Medical Toxicology

Medical Toxicology

Third Edition

Edited by

Richard C. Dart, M.D., Ph.D.

Director
Rocky Mountain Poison and Drug Center
Denver Health
Professor of Surgery (Emergency Medicine)
Medicine and Pharmacy
University of Colorado Health Sciences Center
Denver, Colorado

Authors

E. Martin Caravati, M.D., M.P.H.

Michael A. McGuigan, M.D., C.M., M.B.A.

Ian MacGregor Whyte, M.B.B.S.(Hons), F.R.A.C.P., F.R.C.P.(Edin)

Andrew H. Dawson, M.B.B.S., F.R.C.P., F.R.A.C.P.

Steven A. Seifert, M.D., F.A.C.M.T., F.A.C.E.P.

Seth Schonwald, M.D., F.A.C.E.P., F.A.C.M.T.

Luke Yip, M.D., F.A.C.M.T., F.A.C.E.P., F.A.C.E.M.

Daniel C. Keyes, M.D., M.P.H., A.C.M.T.

Katherine M. Hurlbut, M.D., F.A.C.M.T.

Andrew R. Erdman, M.D.

Richard C. Dart, M.D., Ph.D.

LIPPINCOTT WILLIAMS & WILKINS
A **Wolters Kluwer** Company
Philadelphia • Baltimore • New York • London
Buenos Aires • Hong Kong • Sydney • Tokyo

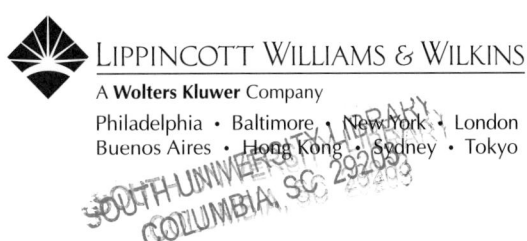

Acquisitions Editor: Anne M. Sydor
Developmental Editor: Raymond E. Reter
Supervising Editor: Mary Ann McLaughlin
Production Editor: Brooke Begin, Silverchair Science + Communications
Manufacturing Manager: Ben Rivera
Cover Designer: Christine Jenny
Compositor: Silverchair Science + Communications
Printer: Quebecor World

530 Walnut Street
Philadelphia, PA 19106 USA
LWW.com

Printed in the USA

Library of Congress Cataloging-in-Publication Data

Medical Toxicology / [edited by] Richard C. Dart.-- 3rd. ed.
p. ; cm.
Rev. ed. of: Ellenhorn's medical toxicology / [edited by] Matthew J. Ellenhorn ... [et al.]. c1997.
Includes bibliographical references and index.
ISBN 0-7817-2845-2
1. Clinical toxicology. 2. Toxicological emergencies. I. Dart, Richard C. II. Ellenhorn's medical toxicology.
[DNLM: 1. Poisoning--diagnosis. 2. Poisoning--therapy. 3. Toxicology--methods. QV 600 M4888 2003]
RA1218.5M43 2003
615.9--dc22

2003060574

---

10 9 8 7 6 5 4 3 2 1

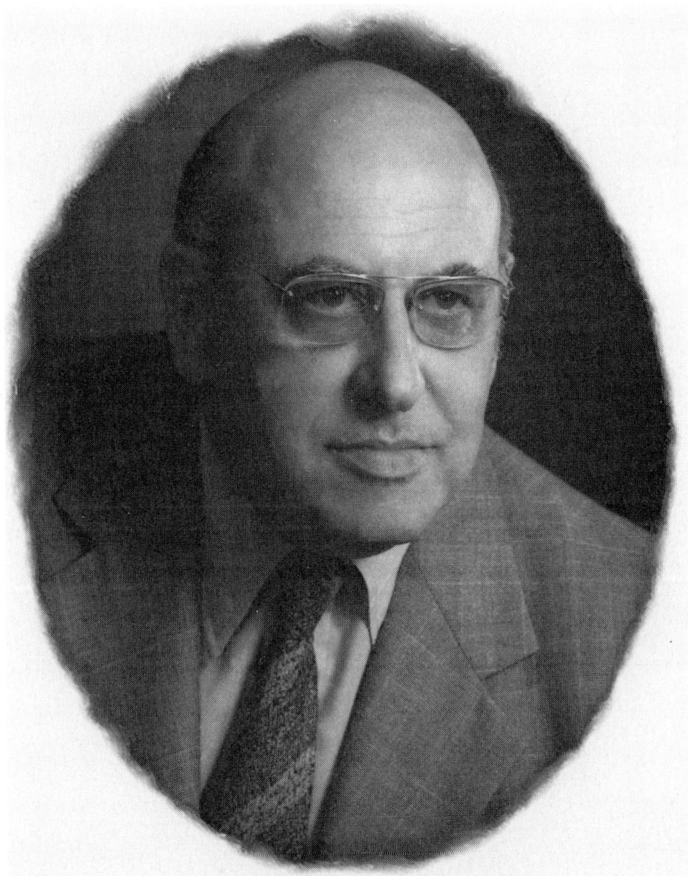

He loved us, supported us, and encouraged us to emulate his lifelong search for excellence.
We proudly pass his legacy to our children.
Leah Ellenhorn Stromberg, M.S.W., L.C.S.W.
Naomi Ellenhorn Davis, M.D., F.A.C.S.
Joshua David Israel Ellenhorn, M.D., F.A.C.S.

Some Thoughts About Dr. Matthew Ellenhorn

Dr. Matthew Ellenhorn was a remarkable clinician and teacher who composed one of the finest and unique textbooks in medical toxicology. Throughout his life he assembled an amazing list of academic credentials. Foremost, he was a very warm and loving man.

Dr. Ellenhorn was a native of Chicago. He was educated at Northwestern University and subsequently at University of Southern California, where he received his medical degree and went on to hold a faculty position in the Department of Chemistry. His postgraduate medical training was at the University of Chicago Clinics and at the University of California Hospitals.

His early interest in toxicology was spawned by a stint at the United States Food and Drug Administration from 1962 to 1965. While there, Dr. Ellenhorn became chief of New Drug Surveillance. He became the U.S. representative for the FDA at several European conferences on pharmacology and on drug toxicity at the World Health Organization in Geneva. He also was instrumental in initiating the International Adverse Drug Reaction Collection System.

During the 1970s and 1980s, Dr. Ellenhorn practiced internal medicine and medical toxicology in Los Angeles. He became Clinical Professor at the Charles R. Drew/University of California, Los Angeles, UCLA School of Medicine, where he gave weekly lectures to emergency medicine residents, paramedics, and students at the Martin Luther King, Jr. General Hospital. These lectures ultimately became the foundation of the first edition of this text, *Medical Toxicology, Diagnosis and Treatment of Human Poisoning*, published by Elsevier with Dr. Donald Barceloux in 1988.

Many other affiliations and services dot the landscape of Dr. Ellenhorn's formidable career. He was author of 50 academic papers on topics ranging from "Allergic Purpura," to phencyclidine to phenytoin toxicity. He gave countless lectures to countless bodies on countless topics and maintained memberships in more than 40 professional and scientific associations. He was diplomate and member of the American Board of Medical Toxicology and American College of Medical Toxicology and was consultant to the regional Poison Center in Los Angeles.

Dr. Ellenhorn was also the devoted husband of Syma Ellenhorn for 41 years. He was the enormously proud father of three children—Leah Ellenhorn Stromberg, Dr. Naomi Ellenhorn Davis, and Dr. Joshua Ellenhorn—and the loving grandfather to four grandchildren—Eliana Rose, Gideon Samuel Stromberg, Amiad Yisrael Davis, and Jacob Abraham Ellenhorn.

Dr. Ellenhorn died on February 2, 1996. The world of Medical Toxicology continues to miss his guidance and insight. We miss his humor and his presence and remain forever indebted for his contributions to our field.

Seth Schonwald, M.D., F.A.C.E.P., F.A.C.M.T.

Dedication: Dr. Patrick McKinney

The third edition of *Medical Toxicology* is dedicated in memory of Dr. Patrick McKinney, one of our finest colleagues. Dr. McKinney recently passed away after a tragic accident. The work he did for the first edition of this text became a springboard for his career in toxicology; therefore, it is with great respect for the doctor that he was and the contributions that he made, that we dedicate this edition to him. His contributions to medical toxicology are numerous and significant, and all demonstrate the unbridled passion that he had for the field and that he brought to his work.

Dr. McKinney started his medical education at the University of Kansas School of Medicine, later entering an Emergency Medicine residency program at Truman Medical Center. He continued his training with a fellowship in Medical Toxicology at the Rocky Mountain Poison and Drug Center in Denver, Colorado. Upon completion of the fellowship, Dr. McKinney joined the faculty of Vanderbilt University School of Medicine in Emergency Medicine and Toxicology. In 1995, he left Tennessee to serve as Medical Director of the New Mexico Poison Center. Against the backdrop of New Mexico's beauty, Dr. McKinney found harmony between his personal aspirations and his professional goals.

Personally, he enjoyed the expanse of New Mexico's outdoors, particularly the hints of toxicology found in nature; he became a mushroom and plant enthusiast. Professionally, in addition to his role at the Poison Center, Dr. McKinney became a tenured faculty member of the Department of Emergency Medicine at the University of New Mexico School of Medicine. He also published extensively on his research, thereby contributing to the growth and development of the field.

Beyond his academic achievements, Dr. McKinney was greatly loved and respected by his peers in the medical toxicology and poison center communities. He was truly a toxicologist's toxicologist—his enthusiasm for the field was contagious. His infectious zeal and captivating lectures continually led him to be one of the residents' favorite faculty members. However, Dr. McKinney's deepest passion was not just for academics but also for using his knowledge to help and enrich the lives of those around him. His loss is deeply felt by those who had the honor to know him, for Dr. McKinney was a great man and a giant in the field of toxicology. His work will continue to enable his colleagues to see farther and expand the breadth of toxicologic knowledge.

Scott D. Phillips, M.D., F.A.C.P., F.A.C.M.T.

Patrick McKinney was a friend and colleague. His accomplishments have been recognized. But, I know that I, along with others, will remember his kindness, his integrity, his inquisitive mind, his half smile, his short staccato laugh, his love of teaching, the fact that he drank warm yogurt from the carton, the fact that he had taught Sam the scientific nomenclature for plants by the age of two, and the fact that he saw a person in each patient. A person lives on in the lives that he has touched. Pat touched all of our lives. We will not forget him.

Donna L. Seger, M.D.

Contents

PART I

General Approach to the Poisoned Patient

SECTION 1: THE PROFESSION OF MEDICAL TOXICOLOGY

SECTION 2: INITIAL MANAGEMENT OF THE POISONED PATIENT

SECTION 3: DIAGNOSIS OF THE POISONED PATIENT: THE TOXICOLOGIST AS SLEUTH

SECTION 4: SUPPORTIVE CARE: GENERAL PRINCIPLES

SECTION 5: ANTIDOTES AND SPECIFIC THERAPIES

SECTION 6: ENHANCEMENT OF ELIMINATION

SECTION 7: PHARMACOKINETICS

SECTION 8: ANALYTICAL AND FORENSIC TOXICOLOGY

PART II

Therapeutic Drugs

PART VI
Mass Incidents

Preface

The specialty of medical toxicology has changed dramatically since the first edition of *Medical Toxicology* (MT1) was introduced in 1988. New poisons and toxins have been discovered. The practice of decontamination has been dramatically altered. New antidotes, such as fomepizole and snake antivenoms, have been introduced. An entire class of poisons, once thought to have ended with World War I, "the war to end all wars," has been resurrected in the form of chemical and biological agents. Sadly, other changes have included the loss of some of our most valued leaders, such as Matthew J. Ellenhorn, M.D., as well as one of the "bright lights" of medical toxicology, Patrick McKinney, M.D.

Some aspects of toxicology have not changed with time. The introduction of MT1 was a success, selling more than 10,000 copies. A distinct achievement for a specialty that did not yet exist officially! In preparation for the 3rd edition (MT3), we spoke with dozens of toxicologists, emergency physicians, pediatricians, and intensivists, as well as other specialist nurses, pharmacists, and physicians regarding their perceptions of *Medical Toxicology*. Their impressions and preferences were remarkably consistent. The most commonly mentioned values of MT1 were consistency, accessibility, and comprehensiveness.

MT1 was a reference text in which one could nearly always find what one was looking for, and readers could count on that information being easy to find in each chapter. Indeed, many of you related that you still go back to MT1 regularly. We chose to follow this proven approach. MT3 strives to be comprehensive. Extensive effort has been made to arrange the material so that the same information is in the same portion of every chapter.

Every classic needs to be updated regularly, and *Medical Toxicology* is not an exception to this rule. In addition to strengthening the consistency and accessibility of the text, new sections have been added. My favorite is the Profession of Medical Toxicology. Although much has been discussed and debated about our specialty, little has been written, collected, and codified. This is not surprising given the relative newness of the specialty. MT3 introduces topics such as The Practice of Medical Toxicology, Specialized Centers for the Treatment of Poisoned Patients, The Medical Toxicology Fellowship, The Medical Toxicologist and Regulatory Agencies, and The Toxicologist in Legal Proceedings. Each of these chapters is written by established toxicologists who have experienced first hand the development of these areas.

Another change in this text is the addition of a section on the diagnosis of the poisoned patient. As any clinician learns quickly, most patients do not present with a sign on their forehead identifying themselves as a "tricyclic antidepressant overdose." It is, therefore, important to provide information on how to evaluate patients who manifest certain clinical syndromes or constellations of findings. Section 3, Diagnosis of the Poisoned Patient: The Toxicologist as Sleuth, includes 25 clinical presentations. The topics range from the more common anticholinergic syndrome through acute liver failure to the more unusual "persistent and progressive pulmonary disease." Many of these chapters provide a new perspective and a unique tool to use in evaluation of the toxicology patient.

It goes without saying that a comprehensive text relies on dedicated and knowledgeable authors to make it a success. Another change in MT3 is the approach to authorship. We were challenged with the task of maintaining the consistency of a textbook authored by just one or two authors. Today, textbooks may include 100 or more authors, which can lead to heterogeneous and fragmented coverage of topics. We enlisted nine coauthors to write most of MT3. In addition, we added distinguished individual authors for selected chapters.

The subspecialty of medical toxicology rests too often on the uncertain foundation of retrospective evidence. Regrettably, toxicology is often a specialty of case reports, case series, and position statements based on insufficient or incomplete information. It is not that we have not tried. Toxicology has come a long way in the centuries since Paracelsus. There have been some very fine studies published, especially since the 1970s. Methods have been refined, more multicenter trials have been performed, and international analysis and exchange have increased. Nevertheless, we remain primarily a specialty of anecdote and retrospective information. The good news is that this leaves wide latitude for personal practice. The bad news is that we often do not know, or at least cannot prove, what is best for the patient.

It is crucial, therefore, that the specialty analyze its scientific content and incorporate important changes quickly. Unfortunately, change tends to proceed slowly in medicine. Medical toxicology is no exception. The ultimate goal of a comprehensive textbook such as MT3 is to summarize concisely and accurately the best evidence available and provide this to a wide audience. Hopefully, MT3 will provoke discussion and provide a reference point for further developments in the practice of medical toxicology.

Richard C. Dart, M.D., Ph.D.

About the Authors

Richard C. Dart, M.D., Ph.D.
Richard C. Dart is the Director of the Rocky Mountain Poison and Drug Center, Denver Health and Hospital Authority, and the Toxicology Consultation Service at Denver Health Medical Center. He is also Professor of Surgery (Emergency Medicine), Medicine, and Pharmacy at the University of Colorado Health Sciences Center. He is active in the American Association of Poison Control Centers (AAPCC), American College of Medical Toxicology (ACMT), American Academy of Clinical Toxicology (AACT), and American College of Emergency Physicians (ACEP). He has served on the governing boards of the AAPCC and ACMT.

Raised in Michigan, Dr. Dart earned his bachelor's degree in biology at Albion College and his medical degree at Wayne State University School of Medicine in Detroit, Michigan. He completed residency training in emergency medicine at the University of Arizona College of Medicine and then completed a fellowship in medical toxicology, as well as a doctorate of Pharmacology and Toxicology at the University of Arizona. After his postgraduate experience, Dr. Dart served as an assistant professor at University of Arizona College of Medicine. In addition, he is board certified by the American Board of Emergency Medicine and the American Board of Medical Toxicology.

Dr. Dart has earned awards for his teaching, research, and leadership endeavors. He was an inaugural member of the Medical Toxicology Subboard of the American Board of Emergency Medicine. In 2002, he was recognized with a special citation from the Commissioner of the U.S. Food and Drug Administration. His research interests include the development of orphan antidotes (antivenoms, metal chelators, and others), the stocking of antidotes, various aspects of analgesic toxicity and their treatments, and adverse drug event reporting.

In 2000, Dr. Dart edited the first edition of *The 5-Minute Toxicology Consult* and is the editor for the 3rd edition of *Medical Toxicology.* He has published more than 125 papers and numerous chapters, reviews, and editorials. He serves on the editorial board of the medical journal *Annals of Emergency Medicine.*

E. Martin Caravati, M.D., M.P.H.
E. Martin Caravati is the Medical Director of the Utah Poison Control Center and the toxicology consult service at the University of Utah Health Sciences Center. He is Professor of Surgery (Emergency Medicine) and Pharmacy Practice at the University of Utah School of Medicine.

Dr. Caravati received a bachelor's degree in chemistry at the University of Virginia and a medical degree from the Medical College of Virginia in 1981. His residency training in emergency medicine was completed at Carolinas Medical Center. He obtained a master's degree in Public Health at the University of Utah. He is board certified in both emergency medicine and medical toxicology. He has served on the Board of Directors for the AAPCC and many other national committees in the area of clinical toxicology. He currently serves on the editorial board of the *Annals of Emergency Medicine.* His research interests include acute poisoning, poisoning epidemiology, and public health. He has more than 60 articles, book chapters, and letters published in the field of clinical toxicology.

Michael A. McGuigan, M.D., C.M., M.B.A.
Michael A. McGuigan is the Medical Director of the Long Island Regional Poison and Drug Information Center at Winthrop-University Hospital in Mineola, New York. He is active in the AAPCC, ACMT, AACT, the Canadian Association of Poison Control Centres (CAPCC), and the European Association of Poisons Centres and Clinical Toxicologists (EAPCCT). He has served on the governing board of the AAPCC and as President of the AACT and the CAPCC.

Raised in Illinois, Dr. McGuigan received his bachelor of arts degree from Miami University (Ohio) and his medical degree from McGill University Faculty of Medicine in Montreal, Quebec, Canada. He completed pediatric training at the University Hospitals in Minneapolis and the Tufts New England Medical Center (Boston Floating Hospital) in Boston. He completed a fellowship in clinical pharmacology at The Children's Hospital (Harvard Medical School) in Boston. After his postgraduate education, Dr. McGuigan moved to Toronto, Ontario to assume the position of medical director of the Ontario Regional Poison Information Centre at The Hospital for Sick Children. He served as an Assistant Professor of Pediatrics and Pharmacology at the University of Toronto Faculty of Medicine before being promoted to Associate Professor. Dr. McGuigan completed his M.B.A. in health services management at McMaster University in Hamilton, Ontario. In addition, he is board certified by the American Board of Pediatrics and the American Board of Medical Toxicology. Dr. McGuigan is a Fellow of the American Academy of Pediatrics, the AACT, and the ACMT. In 2001, Dr. McGuigan moved to Long Island to assume the position of medical director of the Long Island Regional Poison and Drug Information Center. In 2002, Dr. McGuigan was appointed Editor-in-Chief of *Journal of Toxicology—Clinical Toxicology.*

Ian MacGregor Whyte, M.B.B.S.(Hons), F.R.A.C.P., F.R.C.P.(Edin)
Ian MacGregor Whyte is currently employed as Senior Staff Specialist and Director of the Department of Clinical Toxicology and Pharmacology at the Newcastle Mater Misericordiae Hospital in New South Wales, Australia. He is a Professor in the Discipline of Clinical Pharmacology, School of Medical Practice and Population Health, Faculty of Health Sciences, University of Newcastle and is the Director of the Hunter Area Toxicology Service (HATS). He is a clinical toxicologist, clinical pharmacologist, and specialist in internal medicine with Fellowships in the Royal

Australasian College of Physicians and the Royal College of Physicians in Edinburgh.

Professor Whyte is the chair of the Toxicology Editorial Panel of the Australian Medicines Handbook, chair of the Regional Network of the New South Wales Therapeutic Assessment Group, and a member of the editorial boards of POISINDEX and TOXINZ. He is a member of the European Association of Poison Control Centres and Clinical Toxicologists (EAPCCT) and the AACT. He has been an investigator on numerous intervention trials. He is a regular reviewer for numerous international journals. He has published more than 100 papers in peer-reviewed journals and numerous chapters, reviews, editorials, letters, and abstracts.

His current areas of clinical and research interest include deliberate self-poisoning, suicide prevention, and the application of evidenced-based medicine in clinical toxicology. Professor Whyte has a long-term interest in database development for clinical research, particularly in the area of clinical toxicology. He developed and maintains the HATS database. Professor Whyte is one of the authors of *HyperTox*, a computerized educational text designed for emergency ward management of poisoning and undergraduate and postgraduate teaching of clinical toxicology and an essential text for Poisons Information Services in Australia.

Andrew H. Dawson, M.B.B.S., F.R.C.P., F.R.A.C.P.

Andrew H. Dawson is a Senior Staff Specialist in the Department of Clinical Toxicology and Pharmacology and the Hunter Area Toxicology Service (HATS), which is located in Newcastle, Australia. He is also a Professor of Pharmacology in the University of Newcastle.

Dr. Dawson is active in the EAPCCT, the Australasian Society of Clinical and Experimental Pharmacologists and Toxicologists (ASCEPT), and the Asia Pacific Association of Medical Toxicology (APAMT) and the AACT. He has been the convener of the ASCEPT clinical toxicology section and is Vice President of the APAMT.

He completed his undergraduate medical degree at the University of New South Wales, Sydney. He completed postgraduate training in the United Kingdom and Australia training as a physician specializing in clinical pharmacology. His research interests include the integration of clinical care with data collection, the epidemiology of poisoning, and neurotoxicity syndromes. Since 1996, he has been an editor and a principal author of *HyperTox*, a computer-based text. He has published more than 80 papers, in addition to a number of book chapters. He serves on the editorial board of the *Postgraduate Medical Journal*, *Journal of Toxicology—Clinical Toxicology*, and *Toxicology Reviews*.

Steven A. Seifert, M.D., F.A.C.M.T., F.A.C.E.P.

Steven A. Seifert is the Medical Director of the Nebraska Regional Poison Center. He is a Professor of Medical Toxicology in the Department of Surgery, Section of Emergency Medicine at the University of Nebraska Medical Center in Omaha, Nebraska.

Dr. Seifert received a bachelor's degree with honors and with distinction in biology at Cornell University in 1972 and a medical degree from the University of Cincinnati College of Medicine in 1976. He completed a Fellowship in Medical Toxicology at the Rocky Mountain Poison and Drug Center/University of Colorado in 1999. He is certified by the American Board of Emergency Medicine in emergency medicine and medical toxicology. He is a Fellow of the ACEP and the ACMT. He has served on an National Institutes of Health grant review panel, on numerous national committees, and as a national and regional educator and consultant in the area of clinical toxicology. He currently serves on the editorial board of POISINDEX and is a core peer reviewer for the *Journal of Toxicology—Clinical Toxicology* and *Annals of Emergency Medicine*. He is a recipient of the Arizona Governor's Recognition Award and a nominee for a Presidential Service Award for his work in establishing a Sexual Assault Forensic Nurse Examiner program. His research interests include envenomations and medical error. He has more than 100 published medical articles, book chapters, and letters.

Seth Schonwald, M.D., F.A.C.E.P., F.A.C.M.T.

Seth Schonwald is Attending Physician and Director of Medical Toxicology at the East Boston Neighborhood Health Center in East Boston, Massachusetts. He is the author of *Medical Toxicology: A Synopsis and Study Guide* and as a consulting editor on *Medical Toxicology*, 2nd ed.

Dr. Schonwald received a bachelor's degree in biology and English at Brown University in Providence, Rhode Island. His medical degree was completed at the Albert Einstein College of Medicine of Yeshiva University in The Bronx. He completed residency training in Internal Medicine at Harvard Medical School at the Mount Auburn Hospital in Cambridge, Massachusetts, and a second residency in Emergency Medicine at University of California, Los Angeles, UCLA School of Medicine. He also completed a preceptorship in medical toxicology under the guidance of the Massachusetts Poison Control System. He is board certified in internal medicine, emergency medicine, and medical toxicology. He is an avid traveler, United States stamp collector, and world photographer and is actively involved as President of a local investment club.

Luke Yip, M.D., F.A.C.M.T., F.A.C.E.P., F.A.C.E.M.

Luke Yip is a Consultant Toxicologist for the Sydney Poison Information Center and a Consultant Toxicologist and Emergency Physician for Frankston Hospital in Frankston, Victoria (Australia). He is also a faculty member of the Rocky Mountain Poison and Drug Center and an Assistant Professor in the School of Pharmacy of the University of Colorado. Dr. Yip is a section editor on pharmacology, overdoses, and poisonings for the 5th edition of the textbook *Intensive Care Medicine*, is an associate editor for the textbook *The 5-Minute Toxicology Consult*, is on the editorial board of the *Journal of Intensive Care Medicine*, and is a consulting reviewer for *Journal of Toxicology—Clinical Toxicology, Archives of Internal Medicine*, and *Annals of Emergency Medicine*.

Dr. Yip earned a Bachelor of Science degree at the State University of New York at Stony Brook and his medical degree at the Albert Einstein College of Medicine of Yeshiva University in The Bronx. After his residency training in Emergency Medicine at Wayne State University in Detroit, Michigan, he completed preceptorships in Medical Toxicology under the guidance of the Arizona Poison Control System and the Rocky Mountain Poison and Drug Center. Dr. Yip is board certified in medical toxicology and emergency medicine. He is a fellow of the ACMT, the ACEP, and the Australasian College for Emergency Medicine.

Daniel C. Keyes, M.D., M.P.H., A.C.M.T.

Daniel C. Keyes is Chief of the Section of Toxicology and Associate Professor of Surgery in Internal Medicine and Emergency Medicine at the University of Texas Southwestern Medical Center in Dallas and on the faculty of the University of Texas Health Science Center at Houston School of Public Health. Dr. Keyes led the establishment of an emergency medicine residency program in Costa Rica, Central America in 1993 and is also the founder and director of the fully accredited Southwestern Toxicology Training Program. He has also served as Medical Director for the North Texas Poison Center for the past decade. He currently serves on the national consensus panel for the AAPCC.

After graduating from medical school at the University of California, Los Angeles, UCLA School of Medicine, he completed residencies in both Internal Medicine and Emergency Medicine. He also completed Medical Toxicology training while at UCLA and holds a master's degree in public health from Harvard University in Boston, Massachusetts. He is board certified in medical toxicology, internal medicine, and emergency medicine and is a Department of Defense Instructor in domestic preparedness against terrorism. In addition, he has originated several educational programs and grants relating to the medical response to terrorism.

Dr. Keyes has authored numerous publications, including chapters in several major toxicology textbooks. He served as editor of the toxicology section in the textbook entitled, *Emergency Medicine: The Core Curriculum* (Lippincott).

Katherine M. Hurlbut, M.D., F.A.C.M.T.

Katherine M. Hurlbut is Scientific Editor for the POISINDEX Information System and associate editor of *The 5-Minute Toxicology Consult*. She is also a faculty member for the Rocky Mountain Poison and Drug Center; an attending physician in the Department of Emergency Medicine at Denver Health Medical Center, Denver, Colorado; and Clinical Assistant Professor at the University of Colorado Health Sciences Center.

Dr. Hurlbut received a bachelor's degree at the University of Virginia and a medical degree from the East Virginia Medical School of the Medical College of Hampton Roads in 1985. Her residency training in emergency medicine and postgraduate training in clinical toxicology were completed at the University of Arizona. Dr. Hurlbut is board certified in both emergency medicine and medical toxicology and is a Fellow of the ACMT. Dr. Hurlbut's research interests include acute poisonings and heavy metal poisoning. Dr. Hurlbut has published more than 50 articles, book chapters, and letters in the field of clinical toxicology.

Andrew R. Erdman, M.D.

Andrew R. Erdman is currently a Postdoctoral Fellow of Clinical Pharmacology at the University of California, San Francisco and is affiliated with the California Poison Control System. He is actively pursuing research in the areas of pharmacogenetics and biopharmaceuticals under a grant from the National Institutes of Health.

Dr. Erdman received his bachelor's degree in kinesiology from the University of California, Los Angeles in 1992 and his medical degree from the University of California, Davis, School of Medicine in 1996. He completed his residency in emergency medicine at Denver Health Medical Center in 2000 and went on to complete his first postgraduate fellowship in clinical toxicology at the Rocky Mountain Poison and Drug Center in 2002.

Dr. Erdman is a member of the ACMT and of the Alpha Omega Alpha Medical Honor Society. He has recently authored chapters in several major toxicology textbooks and has served as an editorial reviewer for POISINDEX. His areas of interest include pharmacogenetics, toxicogenetics, and chemical/biological warfare agents.

Authors

Richard C. Dart, M.D., Ph.D.
Director
Rocky Mountain Poison and Drug Center
Denver Health
Professor of Surgery (Emergency Medicine)
Medicine and Pharmacy
University of Colorado Health Sciences Center
Denver, Colorado

E. Martin Caravati, M.D., M.P.H.
Professor
Department of Surgery
Division of Emergency Medicine
University of Utah School of Medicine
Medical Director
Utah Poison Control Center
Salt Lake City, Utah

Andrew H. Dawson, M.B.B.S., F.R.C.P., F.R.A.C.P
Associate Professor of Clinical Pharmacology
Department of Clinical Toxicology and Pharmacology
University of Newcastle Faculty of Health Sciences
Waratah, New South Wales, Australia

Andrew R. Erdman, M.D.
Postdoctoral Clinical Pharmacology Fellow
Emergency Physician
Toxicologist
Division of Clinical Pharmacology and Experimental Therapeutics
University of California, San Francisco School of Medicine
San Francisco, California

Katherine M. Hurlbut, M.D., F.A.C.M.T.
Clinical Assistant Professor
Department of Surgery
Division of Emergency Medicine
University of Colorado Health Sciences Center
Physician
Department of Emergency Medicine
Denver Health Medical Center
Denver, Colorado

Daniel C. Keyes, M.D., M.P.H., A.C.M.T.
Associate Professor
Chief
Section of Toxicology
University of Texas
Southwestern Medical Center at Dallas Southwestern Medical School
Dallas, Texas

Michael A. McGuigan, M.D., C.M., M.B.A.
Professor of Emergency Medicine
SUNY at Stony Brook School of Medicine Health Sciences Center
Stony Brook, New York
Medical Director
Long Island Regional Poison and Drug Information Center
Winthrop University Hospital
Mineola, New York

Seth Schonwald, M.D., F.A.C.E.P., F.A.C.M.T.
Director of Toxicology
Department of Urgent Care
East Boston Neighborhood Health Center
Boston Medical Center
Boston, Massachusetts

Steven A. Seifert, M.D., F.A.C.M.T., F.A.C.E.P.
Professor of Medical Toxicology
Department of Surgery
Section of Emergency Medicine
University of Nebraska Medical Center
Medical Director
Nebraska Regional Poison Center
Omaha, Nebraska

Ian MacGregor Whyte, M.B.B.S.(Hons), F.R.A.C.P., F.R.C.P.(Edin)
Professor
Discipline of Clinical Pharmacology
University of Newcastle School of Medicine Practic and Population Health
New Castle, New South Wales, Australia
Director
Department of Clinical Toxicology and Pharmacology
Newcastle Mater Misericordiae Hospital
Waratah, New South Wales, Australia

Luke Yip, M.D., F.A.C.M.T., F.A.C.E.P., F.A.C.E.M.
Sydney Poison Information Center
Consultant Toxicologist and Emergency Physician
Frankston Hospital
Frankston, Victoria, Australia
Assistant Professor
University of Colorado School of Pharmacy
Rocky Mountain Poison and Drug Center
Denver, Colorado

With Contributions From

Cynthia K. Aaron, M.D.
Associate Professor of Emergency Medicine
Director of Clinical Toxicology
Department of Emergency Medicine
Division of Toxicology
University of Massachusetts Medical Center
Worcester, Massachusetts

Timothy E. Albertson, M.D., M.P.H., Ph.D.
Professor of Medicine, Pharmacology/Toxicology, and Anesthesiology
Division of Pulmonary/Critical Care Medicine
University of California, Davis Medical Center
California Poison Control System
VA—Northern California Health Care Systems
Sacramento, California

Ilene B. Anderson, Pharm.D.
Associate Clinical Professor
University of California, San Francisco School of Pharmacy
California Poison Control System, San Francisco Division
San Francisco, California

Thomas C. Arnold, M.D.
Associate Professor and Chairman
Department of Emergency Medicine
Louisiana State University School of Medicine in Shreveport
Medical Director
Louisiana Poison Control Center
Shreveport, Louisiana

Shireen Banerji, Pharm.D., A.B.A.T.
Certified Specialist in Poison Information
Rocky Mountain Poison and Drug Center
Denver Health
Denver, Colorado

William Banner, Jr., M.D., Ph.D.
Clinical Professor of Pediatrics
University of Oklahoma College of Medicine—Tulsa
Medical Director
Children's Hospital at Saint Francis
Tulsa, Oklahoma

Geoffrey L. Bauer, M.D.
Resident Physician
Department of Internal Medicine
Division of Emergency Medicine
Northwestern University Medical School
Chicago, Illinois

Vikhyat S. Bebarta, M.D.
Senior Clinical Instructor
Division of Emergency Medicine
University of Colorado Health Sciences Center
Medical Toxicology Fellow
Rocky Mountain Poison and Drug Center
Denver Health
Denver, Colorado

Yedidia Bentur, M.D.
Lecturer in Toxicology
Director
Israel Poison Information Center
Rambam Medical Center
Haifa, Israel

Jeffrey Bernstein, M.D.
Voluntary Associate Professor
Department of Pediatrics and Medicine
University of Miami School of Medicine
Jackson Memorial Hospital
Medical Director
Florida Poison Information Center—Miami
Miami, Florida

Sheila E. Bloomquist, M.D.
Doctor of Medicine
Family Practice
McGaw Northwestern FP Residency
Glenview, Illinois

John M. Boe, M.D., M.S.
Department of Emergency Medicine
Northwestern University Medical School
Northwestern Memorial Hospital
Evanston Hospital
Chicago, Illinois

G. Randall Bond, M.D., F.A.C.M.T., F.A.A.C.T.
Professor of Clinical Pediatrics and Clinical Emergency Medicine
University of Cincinnati College of Medicine
Medical Director
Drug and Poison Information Center
Cincinnati Children's Hospital Medical Center
Cincinnati, Ohio

Leslie V. Boyer-Hassen, M.D.
Associate Professor of Clinical Pediatrics
University of Arizona College of Medicine
Arizona Poison and Drug Information Center
Tucson, Arizona

George Braitberg, M.B.B.S., F.A.C.E.M.
Associate Professor of Medicine
Department of Emergency Medicine
University of Melbourne Faculty of Medicine
Austin Hospital
Victoria, Australia

Gerald M. Brody, M.D.
Clinical Assistant Professor of Emergency Medicine
SUNY at Stony Brook School of Medicine Health Sciences Center
Stony Brook, New York
Affiliate Professor of Clinical Pharmacy
St. John's University
Jamaica, New York
Chairman
Department of Ambulatory Care
Winthrop University Hospital
Mineola, New York

Alvin C. Bronstein, M.D., F.A.C.E.P.
Assistant Professor of Surgery
Division of Emergency Medicine
University of Colorado Health Sciences Center
Medical Director
Rocky Mountain Poison and Drug Center
Denver Health
Denver, Colorado

D. Eric Brush, M.D.
Instructor of Emergency Medicine
Fellow in Medical Toxicology
Department of Emergency Medicine
Division of Toxicology
University of Massachusetts Medical Center
Worcester, Massachusetts

Nicholas A. Buckley, M.D., F.R.A.C.P.
Associate Professor
Department of Clinical Pharmacology and Toxicology
Australian National University Medical School
Australian Capital Territory, Australia

Jefferey L. Burgess, M.D., M.P.H., F.A.C.M.T.
Associate Professor
Department of Environmental and Community Health
University of Arizona College of Medicine
Tucson, Arizona

Keith K. Burkhart, M.D.
Professor of Emergency Medicine, Medicine, and Pharmacology
Department of Emergency Medicine
Pennsylvania State University College of Medicine
Hershey, Pennsylvania

Thomas R. Caraccio, Pharm.D., D.A.B.A.T.
Associate Professor of Emergency Medicine
SUNY at Stony Brook School of Medicine Health Sciences Center
Stony Brook, New York
Managing Director
Long Island Regional Poison and Drug Information Center
Winthrop University Hospital
Mineola, New York

Gregory L. Carter, M.B., F.R.A.N.Z.C.P.
Doctor
Department of Psychiatry
University of Newcastle Faculty of Health Sciences
Newcastle Misericordiae Mater Hospital
Waratah, New South Wales, Australia

Peter A. Chyka, Pharm.D.
Professor
Department of Pharmacy
University of Tennessee, Memphis College of Medicine
Memphis, Tennessee

Richard F. Clark, M.D.
Professor of Medicine
Division of Medical Toxicology
University of California, San Diego Medical Center
San Diego, California

Barbara Insley Crouch, Pharm.D., M.S.P.H.
Associate Professor (Clinical)
Department of Pharmacy Practice
University of Utah College of Pharmacy
Director
Utah Poison Control Center
Salt Lake City, Utah

Frank F. S. Daly, M.B.B.S., F.A.C.E.M.
Clinical Senior Lecturer
Clinical Toxicologist
Emergency Physician
University of Western Australia
Royal Perth Hospital
Perth, Western Australia, Australia

João H. Delgado, M.D.
Assistant Professor of Emergency Medicine
Department of Traumatology and Emergency Medicine
University of Connecticut School of Medicine
Farmington, Connecticut
Hartford Hospital
Hartford, Connecticut

Christopher R. DeWitt, M.D.
Medical Toxicology Fellow
Rocky Mountain Poison and Drug Center
Denver Health
Denver, Colorado

Jo Ellen Dyer, Pharm.D.
Associate Clinical Professor of Pharmacy
Department of Clinical Pharmacy
University of California, San Francisco School of Pharmacy
California Poison Control System—San Francisco
San Francisco, California

Miguel C. Fernández, M.D.
Associate Professor of Surgery
Division of Emergency Medicine
University of Texas Medical School at San Antonio
South Texas Poison Center
San Antonio, Texas

Robert J. Flanagan, Ph.D., S.R.C.S., C.Chem., F.R.S.C., F.R.C.Path.
Consultant Clinical Scientist
Medical Toxicology Unit
Guy's and St. Thomas' Hospital Trust
London, England, United Kingdom

Lisa M. Forman, M.D.
Assistant Professor of Medicine
Section of Hepatology
University of Colorado Health Sciences Center
Denver, Colorado

Frederick Fung, M.D., M.S.
Clinical Professor of Occupational Medicine
Medical Director of Occupational Medicine
University of California, Irvine College of Medicine
Irvine, California
Sharp Rees-Stealy Medical Group
San Diego, California

Rick A. Gimbel, M.D.
Clinical Instructor
Division of Emergency Medicine
Northwestern University Medical School
Chicago, Illinois
Evanston Northwestern Healthcare
Evanston, Illinois

Barry S. Gold, M.D.
Associate Professor of Medicine
Johns Hopkins University School of Medicine
Baltimore, Maryland

Hernán F. Gómez, M.D., A.C.M.T.
Clinical Associate Professor of Emergency Medicine
University of Michigan Medical School
Ann Arbor, Michigan

Andis Graudins, M.B., Ph.D., B.S.(Hons)
Conjoint Senior Lecturer
Department of Emergency Medicine and Clinical Toxicology
University of New South Wales Faculty of Medicine
Prince of Wales Hospital
Randwick, New South Wales, Australia

Christine A. Haller, M.D., M.S.
Assistant Adjunct Professor of Medicine and Laboratory Medicine
University of California, San Francisco School of Medicine
San Francisco General Hospital
San Francisco, California

Kennon Heard, M.D.
Assistant Professor of Surgery
Section Chief of Medical Toxicology
University of Colorado Health Sciences Center
Rocky Mountain Poison and Drug Center
Denver Health
Denver, Colorado

Judd E. Hollander, M.D.
Professor of Emergency Medicine
University of Pennsylvania School of Medicine
Philadelphia, Pennsylvania

B. Zane Horowitz, M.D., F.A.C.M.T.
Associate Professor of Emergency Medicine
Oregon Health Sciences University School of Medicine
Medical Director
Oregon Poison Center
Portland, Oregon

Geoffrey K. Isbister, M.B., B.Sc., F.A.C.E.M.
Lecturer and Clinical Toxicologist
Clinical Envenoming Research Group
University of Newcastle Faculty of Health Sciences
Newcastle Mater Misericordiae Hospital
Waratah, New South Wales, Australia

Heath A. Jolliff, D.O.
Assistant Clinical Professor
Department of Emergency Medicine
Division of Medical Toxicology
Ohio University College of Osteopathic Medicine—Doctors Hospital
Columbus, Ohio

Alison L. Jones, M.D., B.Sc.(Hons), F.R.C.P.E., F.R.C.P., Fi.B.I.O.L.
Director
Consultant Physician
Clinical Toxicologist
National Poisons Information Service
Guy's and St. Thomas' NHS Trust
London, England, United Kingdom

Mark A. Kostic, M.D.
Fellow in Medical Toxicology
Rocky Mountain Poison and Drug Center
Denver Health
Denver, Colorado

Sunye Kwack, M.D.
Fellow
Division of Pulmonary and Critical Care
Department of Internal Medicine
University of California, Davis Medical Center
Sacramento, California

David C. Lee, M.D.
Clinical Assistant Professor
Department of Emergency Medicine
New York University School of Medicine
New York, New York
Department of Emergency Medicine
North Shore University Hospital
Manhasset, New York

Jana Vander Leest, R.Ph.
Pharmacist
Department of Pharmacy
Rocky Mountain Poison and Drug Center
Denver Health
Denver, Colorado

Jerrold B. Leikin, M.D.
Professor of Medicine and Pharmacology
Rush Medical College of Rush University
Professor of Medicine
Northwestern University Medical School
Chicago, Illinois
Director of Medical Toxicology
Evanston Northwestern Healthcare-OMEGA
Glenbrook Hospital
Glenview, Illinois

Ira M. Leviton, M.D.
Clinical Associate Professor of Medicine
Division of Infectious Diseases
Albert Einstein College of Medicine of Yeshiva University
Montefiore Hospital
Bronx, New York

Erica L. Liebelt, M.D., F.A.C.M.T.
Associate Professor of Pediatrics and Emergency Medicine
University of Alabama School of Medicine
Director
Medical Toxicology Services
University of Alabama Hospitals
Birmingham, Alabama

David E. Lieberman, M.D.
Resident
Department of Emergency Medicine
Cook County Hospital
Chicago, Illinois

Mark Little, M.B.B.S., F.A.C.E.M., M.P.H.&T.M., D.T.M.&H.
Clinical Toxicologist and Consultant Emergency Physician
Department of Emergency Medicine
Sir Charles Gairdner Hospital
Nedlands, Western Australia, Australia

Richard C. Lynton
Attending Physician
Department of Medicine
Veteran's Affairs Medical Center—Sacramento
Mather, California

Scott W. Marshall, Pharm.D.
Clinical Instructor
Specialist in Poison Information
University of Utah College of Pharmacy
Salt Lake City, Utah

Michael Mayersohn, Ph.D.
Professor
Department of Pharmaceutical Sciences
University of Arizona College of Pharmacy
Tucson, Arizona

Christy L. McCowan, M.D.
Research Fellow
Department of Surgery
Division of Emergency Medicine
University of Utah School of Medicine
Salt Lake City, Utah

Robin B. McFee, D.O., M.P.H.
Nova Southeastern University
Center for Bioterrorism Preparedness
Ft. Lauderdale, Florida

Patrick E. McKinney*

Steven A. McLaughlin, M.D.
Assistant Professor
Department of Emergency Medicine
University of New Mexico School of Medicine
Albuquerque, New Mexico

Leslie Ann Mendoza-Temple, M.D.
Academic Fellow
Department of Family Medicine
McGaw Medical Center of Northwestern University
Glenview, Illinois

Matthew N. Meriggioli, M.D.
Assistant Professor of Neurological Sciences
Rush Medical College of Rush University
Chicago, Illinois

*Deceased.

Michael A. Miller, M.D.
Program Director and Medical Toxicologist
Department of Emergency Medicine
Darnall Army Community Hospital
Ft. Hood, Texas

Lindsay M. Murray, M.B.B.S., F.A.C.E.M.
Senior Lecturer
Department of Emergency Medicine
University of Western Australia
Queen Elizabeth II Medical Centre
Nedlands, Western Australia, Australia

Lee S. Newman, M.D., M.A., F.C.C.P.
Professor
Department of Medicine and Preventative Medicine/Biometrics
Division of Environmental and Occupational Health Sciences
University of Colorado Health Sciences Center
National Jewish Medical and Research Center
Denver, Colorado

Dean G. Olsen, D.O.
Toxicology Fellow
Rocky Mountain Poison and Drug Center
Denver Health
Denver, Colorado

Amy L. Olson, M.D.
Clinical Instructor in Medicine
University of Colorado Health Sciences Center
Staff Physician
Denver Veteran's Affairs Medical Center
Denver, Colorado

Kent R. Olson, M.D.
Clinical Professor of Medicine
Department of Pediatrics and Pharmacy
University of California, San Francisco School of Medicine
California Poison Control System—San Francisco
San Francisco, California

Gerald F. O'Malley, D.O.
Director of Toxicology
Department of Emergency Medicine
Albert Einstein Medical Center
Philadelphia, Pennsylvania

Robert B. Palmer, Ph.D., D.A.B.A.T.
Toxicology Section
Department of Surgery
Division of Emergency Medicine
University of Colorado Health Sciences Center
Denver, Colorado
Division of Pharmaceutical Sciences
University of Wyoming School of Pharmacy
Laramie, Wyoming
Department of Chemistry and Biochemistry
University of Northern Colorado
Greeley, Colorado
Toxicology Associates
Rocky Mountain Poison and Drug Center
Denver Health
Denver, Colorado

Scott D. Phillips, M.D., F.A.C.P., F.A.C.M.T.
Associate Clinical Professor of Medicine and Surgery
Division of Clinical Pharmacology and Toxicology
Division of Emergency Medicine
University of Colorado Health Sciences Center
Denver, Colorado

S. Rutherfoord Rose, Pharm.D., F.A.A.C.T.
Associate Professor of Emergency Medicine
Virginia Commonwealth University School of Medicine
Director, Virginia Poison Center
Richmond, Virginia

Stefan P. Rosenbach, M.D.
Associate
Department of Emergency Medicine
Geisinger Medical Center
Danville, Pennsylvania

Barry H. Rumack, M.D.
Clinical Professor of Pediatrics
University of Colorado Health Sciences Center
Director Emeritus
Rocky Mountain Poison and Drug Center
Denver Health
Denver, Colorado

Donna L. Seger, M.D.
Assistant Professor of Medicine and Emergency Medicine
Vanderbilt University Medical Center
Medical Director
Middle Tennessee Poison Center
Nashville, Tennessee

Greene Shepherd, Pharm.D.
Director
North Texas Poison Center
Parkland Health and Hospital System
Dallas, Texas

Marco L. A. Sivilotti, M.D., M.Sc., F.R.C.P.C., F.A.C.E.P.
Assistant Professor
Department of Emergency Medicine and Pharmacology and Toxicology
Queen's University Faculty of Health Sciences
Kingston, Ontario, Canada

Jack W. Snyder, M.D., J.D., Ph.D.
Associate Director
National Library of Medicine
Bethesda, Maryland

Henry A. Spiller, M.S., A.B.A.T.
Director, Kentucky Regional Poison Center
Kosair Children's Hospital
Louisville, Kentucky

Daniel A. Spyker, M.D., Ph.D.
Adjunct Professor
Department of Medicine
Uniformed Services University of the Health Sciences F. Edward Herbert School of Medicine
Bethesda, Maryland
Director of Clinical Pharmacology
Genentech, Inc.
San Francisco, California

Robert L. Stephen, M.D.
Assistant Clinical Professor
Department of Surgery
Division of Emergency Medicine
University of Utah School of Medicine
Salt Lake City, Utah

Jeffrey R. Suchard, M.D.
Associate Clinical Professor of Emergency Medicine
University of California, Irvine Medical Center
Orange, California

Daniel L. Sudakin, M.D., M.P.H.
Assistant Professor
Department of Environmental and Molecular Toxicology
Oregon State University
Corvallis, Oregon

John B. Sullivan, M.D., A.B.M.T.
Associate Professor of Emergency Medicine
University of Arizona College of Medicine
Associate Director
Arizona Poison Center
Tucson, Arizona

Brigham R. Temple, M.D.
Instructor of Clinical Medicine
Division of Emergency Medicine
McGaw Medical Center of Northwestern University
Chicago, Illinois

Steve N. Vogel, M.D.
Associate Professor
Department of Medicine
Division of Emergency Medicine
Northwestern University Medical School
Evanston Hospital
Evanston, Illinois

Javier C. Waksman, M.D.
Assistant Clinical Professor of Medicine
Division of Clinical Pharmacology and Toxicology
University of Colorado Health Sciences Center
Denver, Colorado

Richard Y. Wang, D.O.
Senior Medical Officer
Department of Organic Analytical Toxicology
Division of Laboratory Sciences
National Center for Environmental Health
Centers for Disease Control and Prevention
Atlanta, Georgia

Gary S. Wasserman, D.O., F.A.A.P., F.A.C.M.T., F.A.A.C.T.
Professor of Medicine
Department of Pediatrics
University of Missouri—Kansas City School of Medicine
Chief
Section of Medical Toxicology
Children's Mercy Hospital and Clinic
Kansas City, Missouri

William A. Watson, Pharm.D.
Associate Director, Toxicosurveillance
American Association of Poison Control Centers
Washington, DC

Paul M. Wax, M.D.
Professor of Clinical Emergency Medicine
Department of Medical Toxicology
University of Arizona College of Medicine
Tucson, Arizona
Banner Good Samaritan Medical Center
Phoeniz, Arizona

Lindell K. Weaver, M.D.
Professor
University of Utah School of Medicine
Medical Director, Hyperbaric Medicine
LDS Hospital
Salt Lake City, Utah

Julian White, M.D., M.B., F.A.C.T.M.
Associate Professor
Head of Toxinology
Women's and Children's Hospital
North Adelaide, Australia

Saralyn R. Williams, M.D.
Associate Clinical Professor of Medicine
Division of Medical Toxicology
University of California, San Diego
School of Medicine
La Jolla, California

Alan D. Woolf, M.D., M.P.H.
Associate Professor
Department of Pediatrics
Harvard Medical School
Children's Hospital Boston
Boston, Massachusetts

Robert O. Wright, M.D., M.P.H.
Assistant Professor of Pediatrics
and Environmental Health
Harvard Medical School
Children's Hospital Boston
Boston, Massachusetts

Medical Toxicology

Toxicology Flora and Fauna

FAMILY VIPERIDAE, SUBFAMILY CROTALINAE

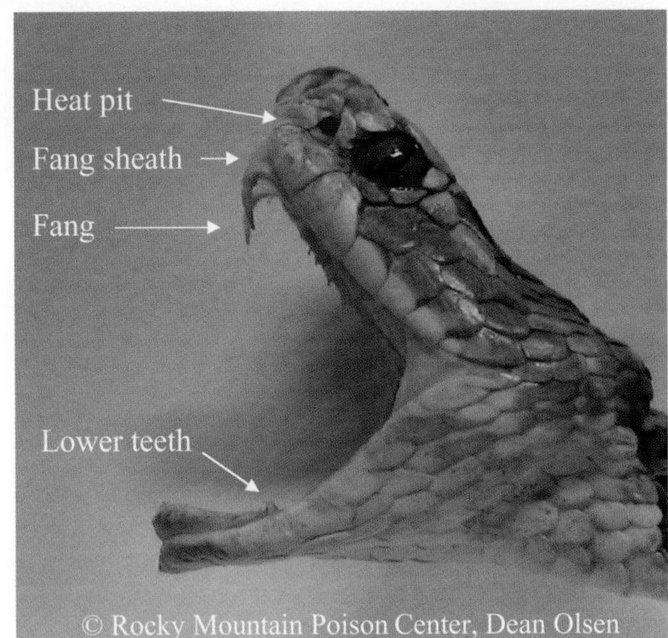

Color Plate 1. Crotaline head (Chapter 245).

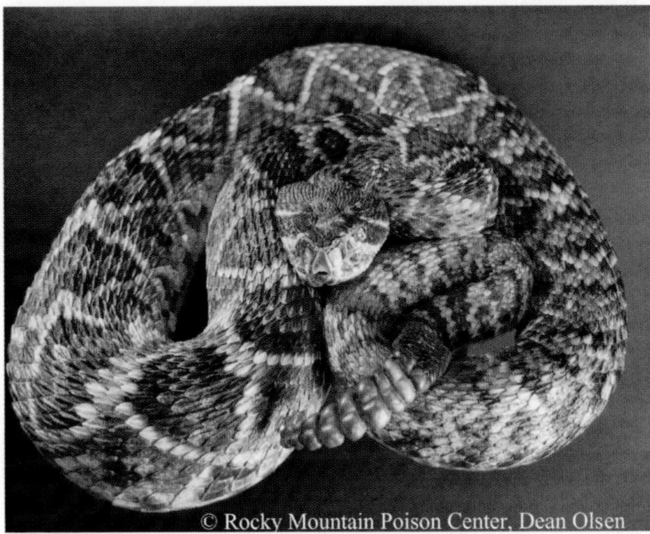

Color Plate 2. Rattlesnake. Example of rattlesnake in defensive pose (Chapter 245).

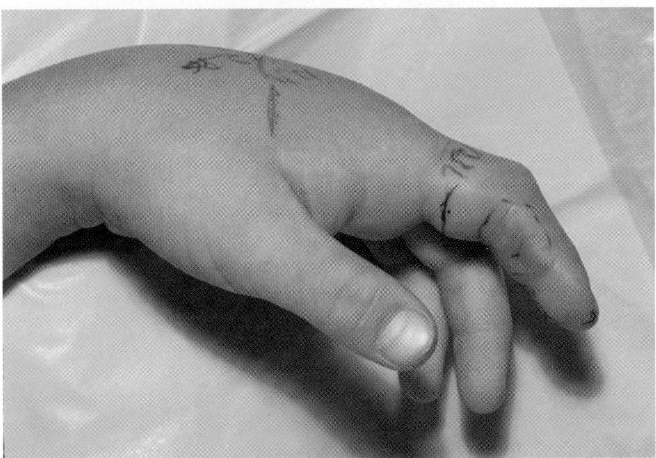

Color Plate 3. Left index hemorrhage after rattlesnake bite (Chapter 245). (Original photograph copyright © 2000 by Dr. Richard C. Dart.)

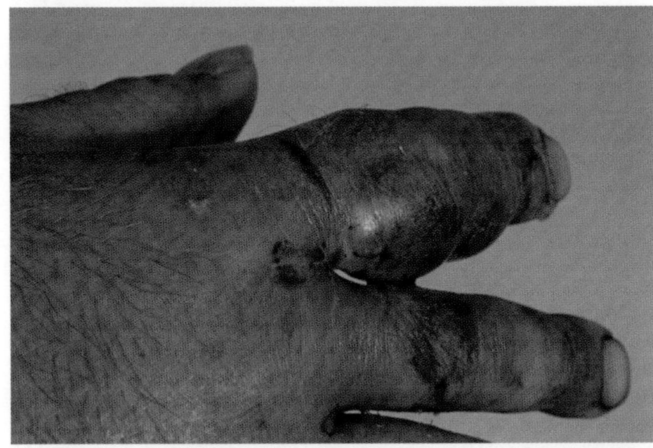

Color Plate 4. Right index bleb. Patient was bitten by Western Diamondback rattlesnake and used belt around base of finger to act as tourniquet. He recovered function after skin graft (Chapter 245).

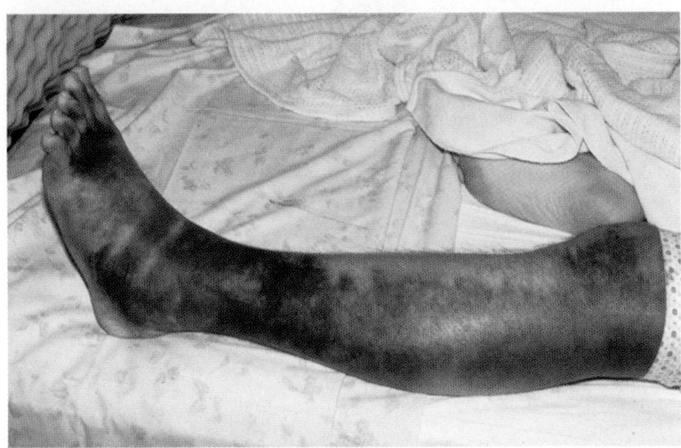

Color Plate 5. Figure 245.2. Left leg hemorrhage. Example of extensive ecchymosis that developed over 24 to 48 hours subsequent to a presumed Western Diamondback rattlesnake bite.

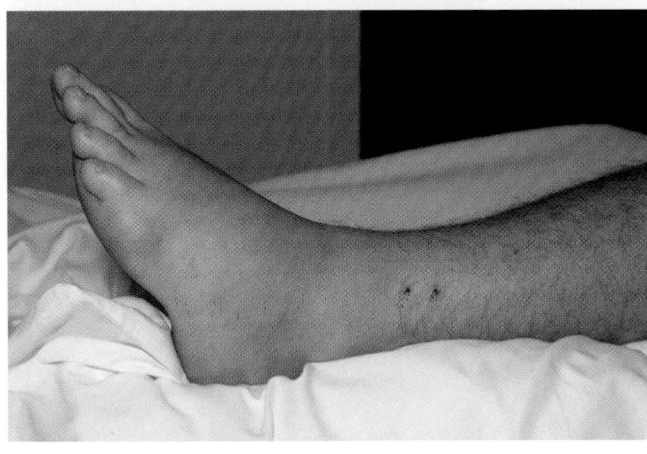

Color Plate 6. Left foot bite. Patient was bitten by unknown snake species. Photograph shows classic bite marks and presence of faint ecchymosis distal to the lateral malleolus (Chapter 245).

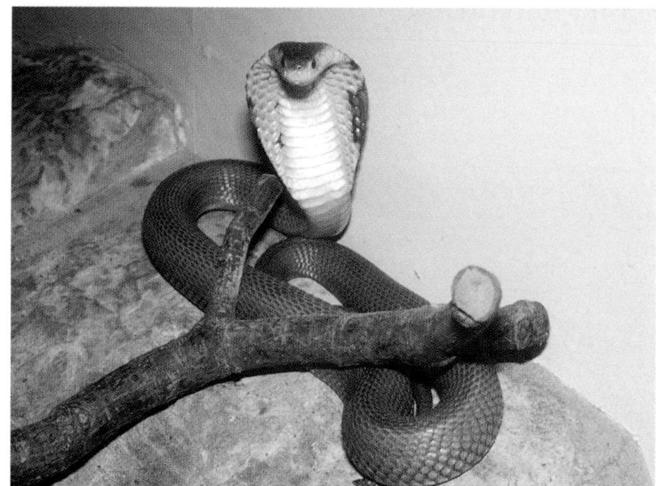

Color Plate 7. Figure 246.1. Indian cobra (*Naja naja*). (Original photograph copyright © by Dr. Julian White.)

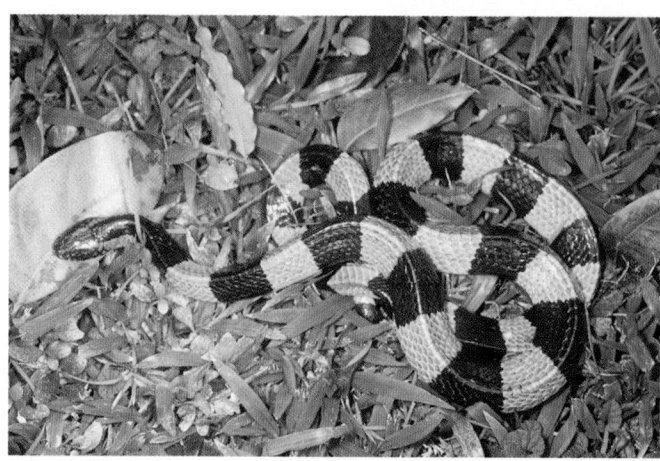

Color Plate 8. Figure 246.10. Banded krait (*Bungarus fasciatus*). (Original photograph copyright © by Dr. Julian White.)

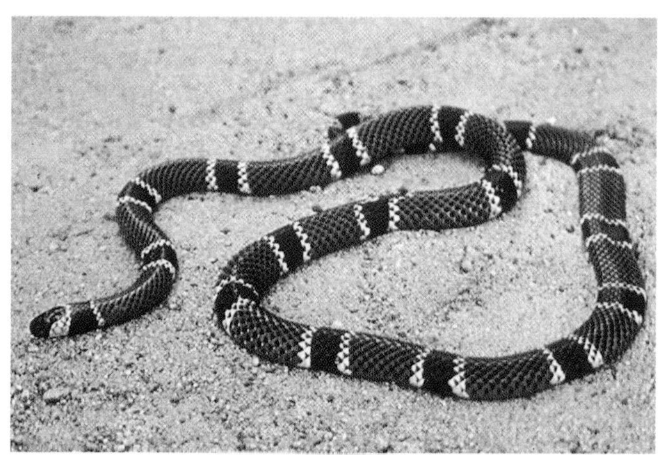

Color Plate 9. Figure 246.13. Painted coral snake (*Micrurus corallinus*). (Original photograph copyright © by Dr. Jurg Meier.)

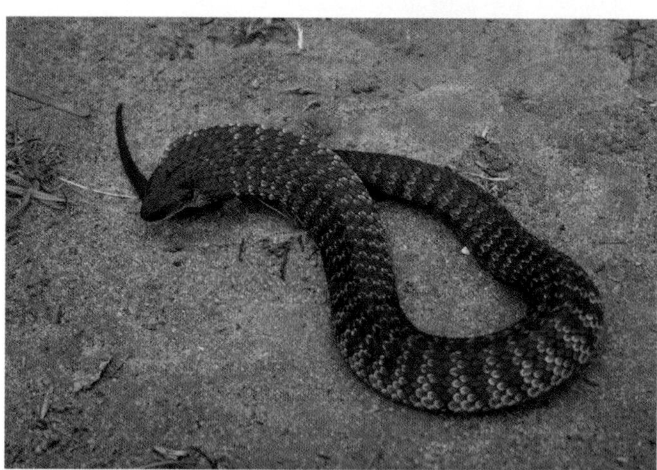

Color Plate 10. Figure 246.21. Common tiger snake (*Notechis scutatus*). (Original photograph copyright © by Dr. Julian White.)

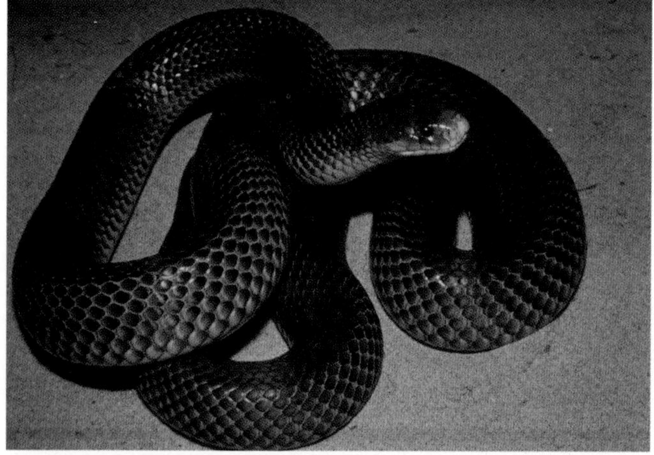

Color Plate 11. Figure 246.25. Mulga snake (*Pseudechis australis*). (Original photograph copyright © by Dr. Julian White.)

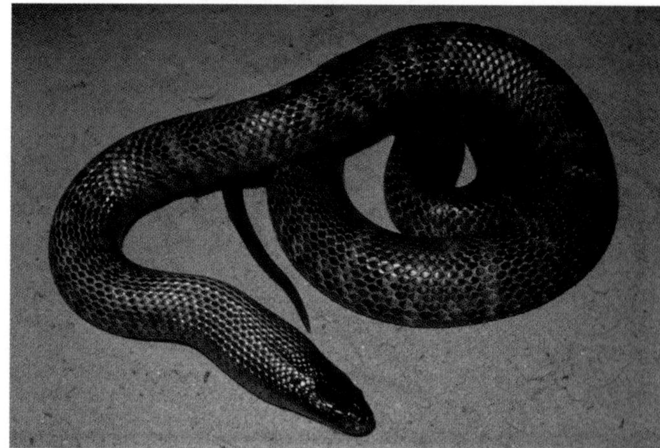

Color Plate 12. Figure 246.26. Collett's snake (*Pseudechis colletti*). (Original photograph copyright © by Dr. Julian White.)

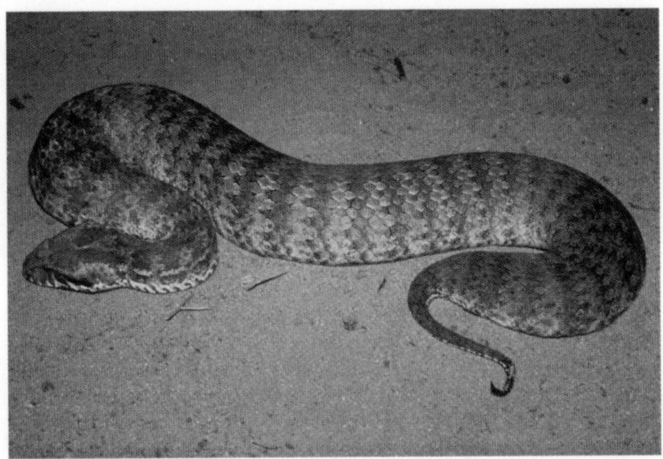

Color Plate 13. Figure 246.30. Common death adder (*Acanthophis antarcticus*). (Original photograph copyright © by Dr. Julian White.)

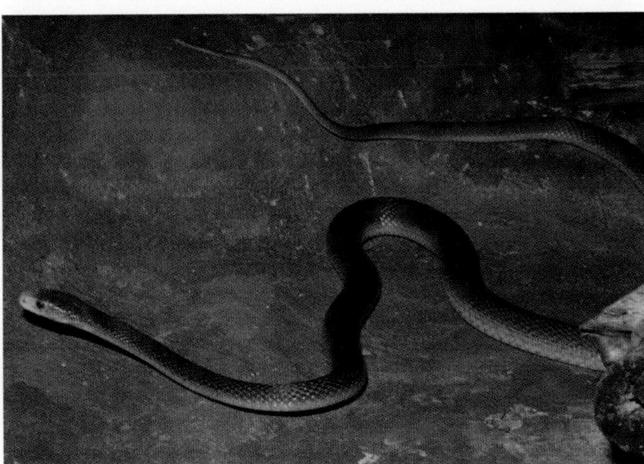

Color Plate 14. Figure 246.32. Common taipan (*Oxyuranus scutellatus*). (Original photograph copyright © by Dr. Julian White.)

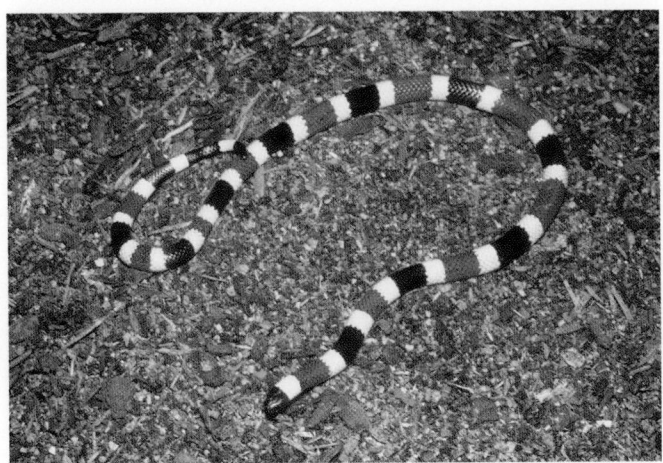

Color Plate 15. Western coral snake (*Micruroides euryxanthus*) (Chapter 246). (Original photograph copyright © by Dr. Julian White.)

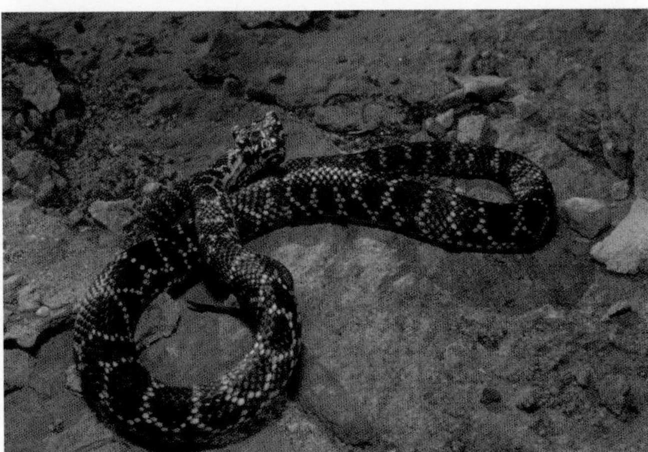

Color Plate 16. Broad-headed snake (*Hoplocephalus bungaroides*) (Chapter 246). (Original photograph copyright © by Dr. Julian White.)

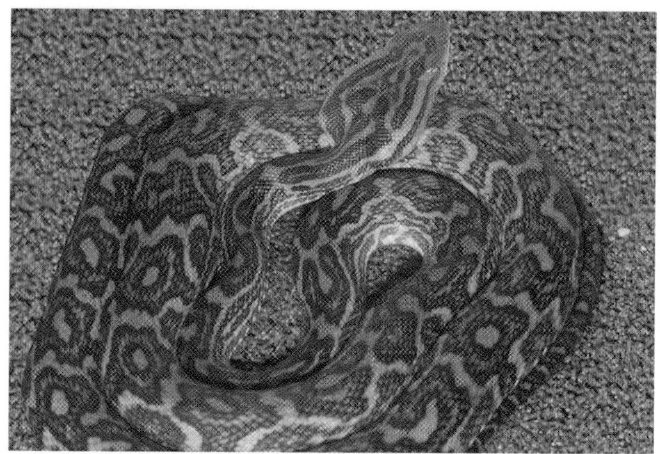

Color Plate 17. Figure 247.29. Habu (*Trimeresurus flavoviridis*). (Original photograph copyright © by Dr. Julian White.)

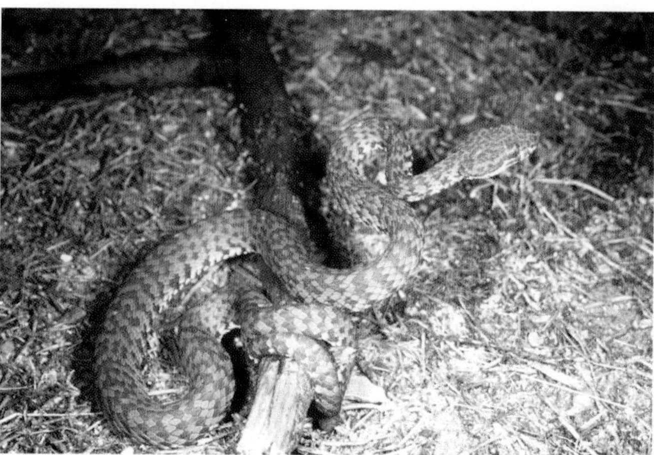

Color Plate 18. Wagler's pit viper (Genus *Tropidolaemus*) (Chapter 247). (Original photograph copyright © by Dr. Julian White.)

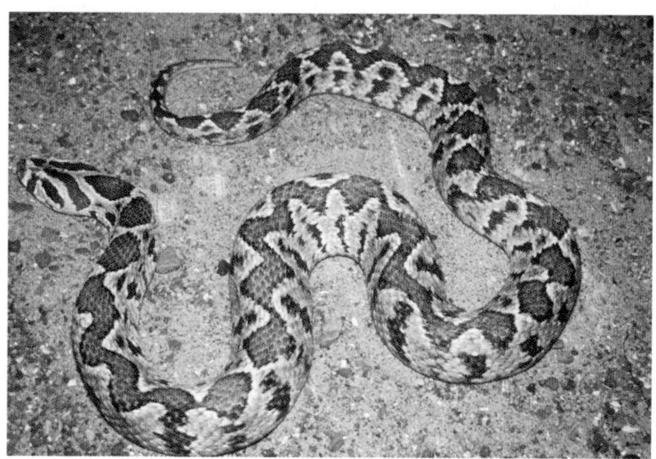

Color Plate 19. Figure 247.3. Palestine viper (*Vipera palestinae*). (Original photograph copyright © by Dr. Julian White.)

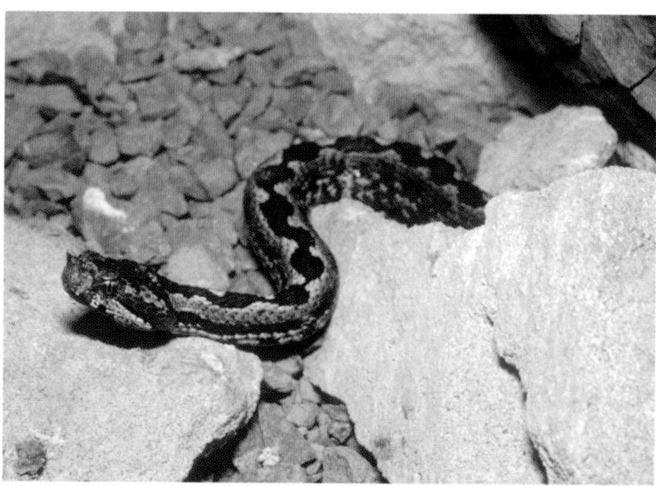

Color Plate 20. Figure 247.4. Balkan viper (Vipera ammodytes). (Original photograph copyright © by Dr. Julian White.)

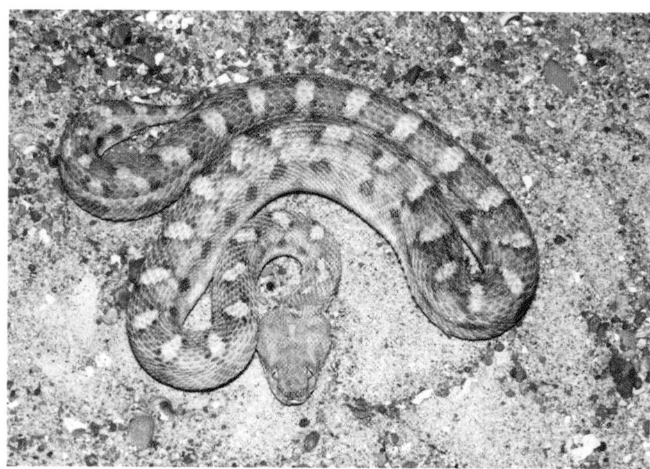

Color Plate 21. Figure 247.6. Burton's carpet viper (*Echis coloratus*). (Original photograph copyright © by Dr. Julian White.)

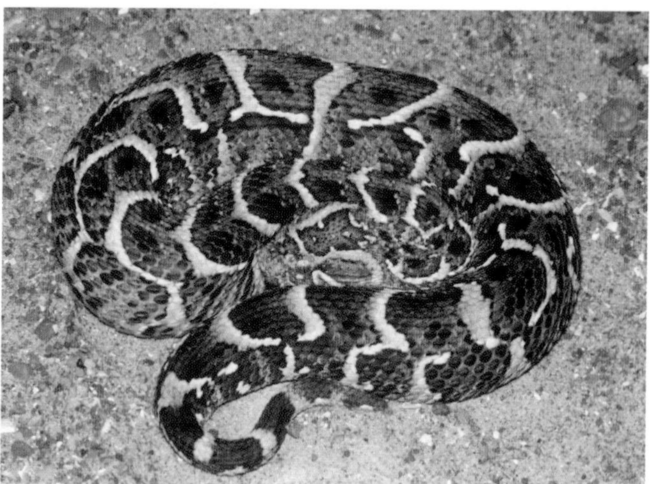

Color Plate 22. Figure 247.10. Puff adder (*Bitis arietans*). (Original photograph copyright © by Dr. Julian White.)

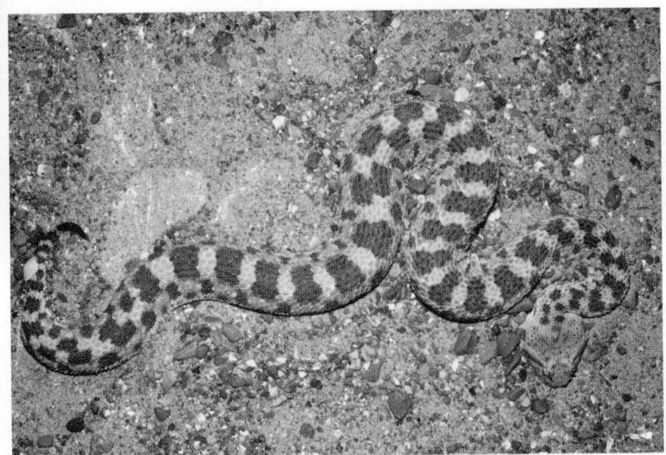

Color Plate 23. Figure 247.12. Horned viper (*Cerastes cerastes*). (Original photograph copyright © by Dr. Julian White.)

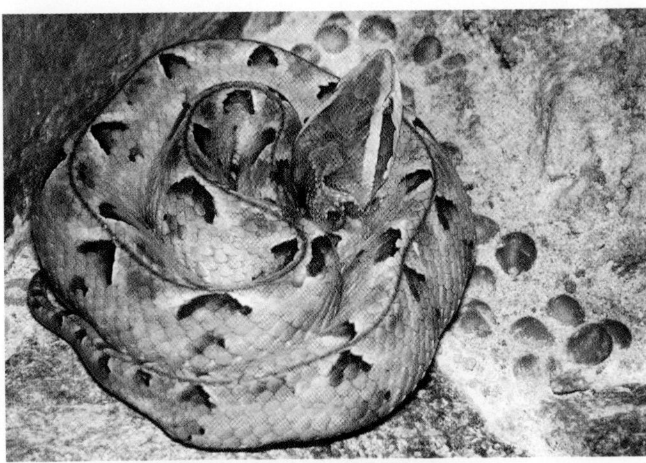

Color Plate 24. Figure 247.19. Malayan pit viper (*Calloselasma rhodostoma*). (Original photograph copyright © by Dr. Julian White.)

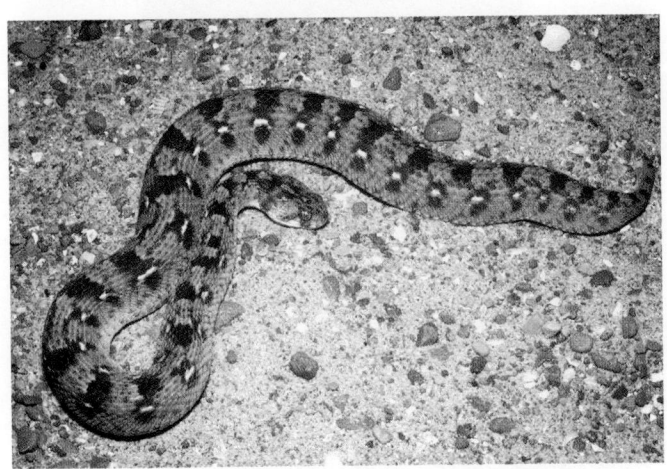

Color Plate 25. West African carpet viper (*Echis ocellatus*) (Chapter 247). (Original photograph copyright © by Dr. Julian White.)

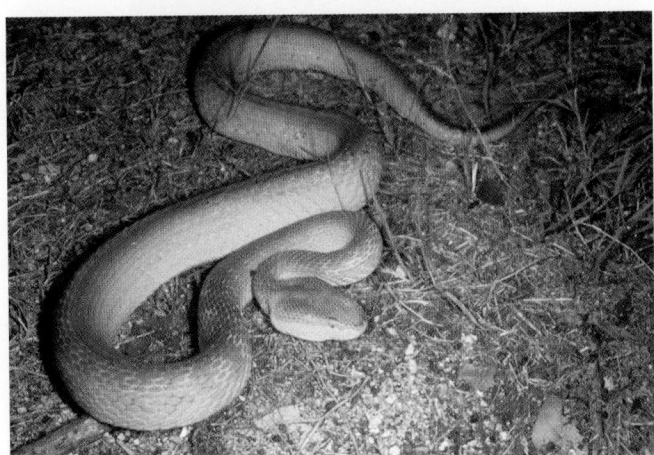

Color Plate 26. Figure 247.28. White-lipped green tree viper (*Trimeresurus albolabris*). (Original photograph copyright © by Dr. Julian White.)

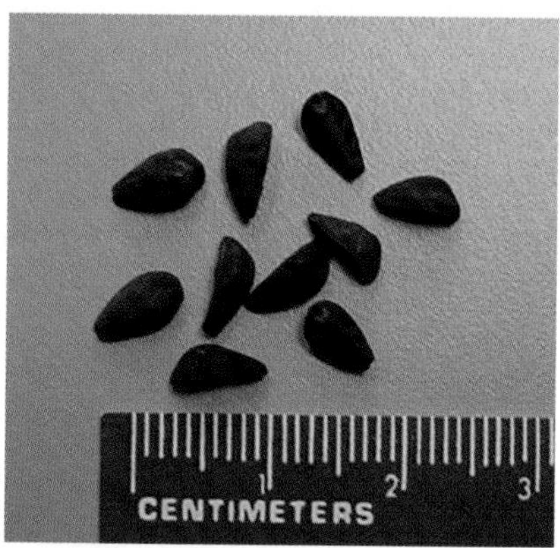

Color Plate 27. Morning Glory seeds (Chapter 255). (Photograph courtesy of Dr. E. M. Caravati.)

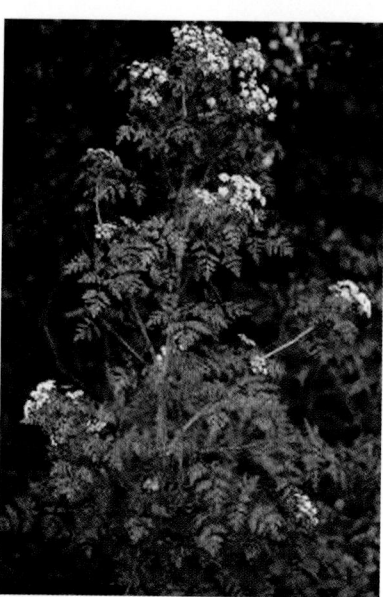

Color Plate 28. Poison Hemlock (*Conium maculatum* L) (Chapter 254). (Photograph courtesy of William and Wilma Follette at USDA-NRCS PLANTS Database/USDA NRCS. 1992. *Western wetland flora: Field office guide to plant species.* West Region, Sacramento, CA.)

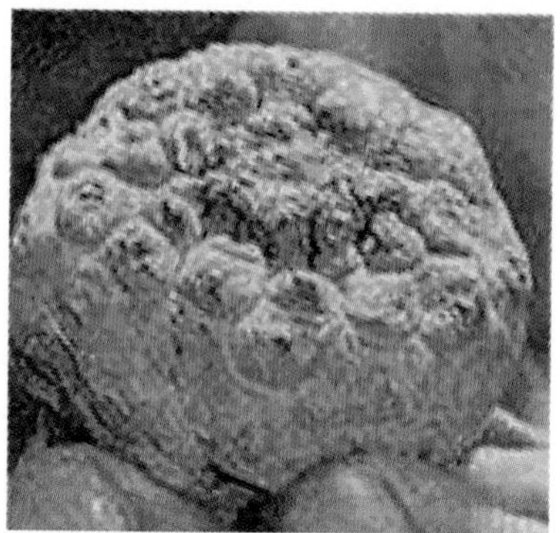

Color Plate 29. Peyote button (Chapter 254). (Photograph courtesy of Drug Enforcement Agency, http://www.dea.gov.)

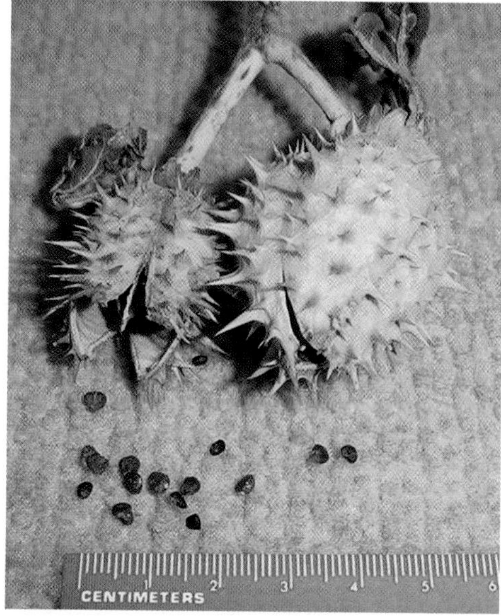

Color Plate 30. Dried jimsonweed pod and seeds (Chapter 255). (Photograph courtesy of Dr. E. M. Caravati.)

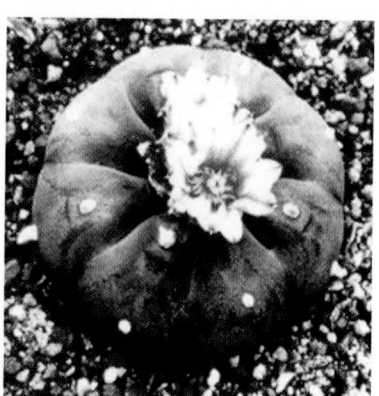

Color Plate 31. Peyote button (Chapter 254). (Photograph courtesy of United Nations Office on Drugs and Crime, http://www.undcp.org.)

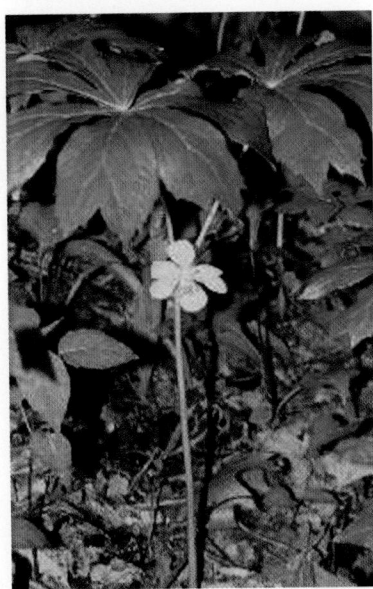

Color Plate 32. Mayapple (Chapter 255). (Photograph courtesy of Jennifer Anderson at USDA-NRCS PLANTS Database.)

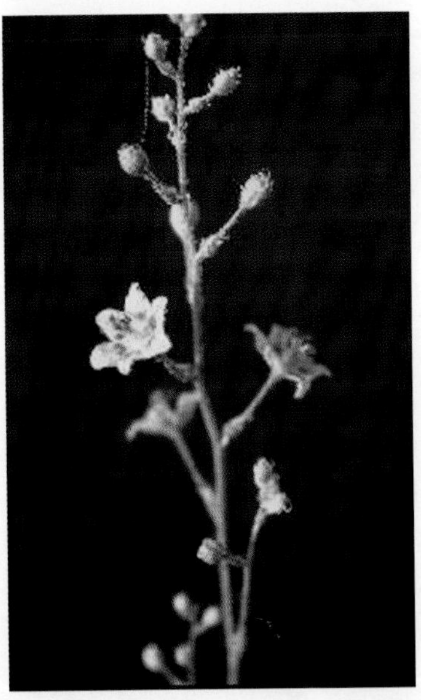

Color Plate 33. Mountain Death camus (Chapter 255). (Photograph courtesy of Lee Casebere at USDA-NRCS PLANTS Database/USDA NRCS. 1995. *Northeast wetland flora: field office guide to plant species.* Northeast National Technical Center, Chester, PA.)

Hazardous Materials

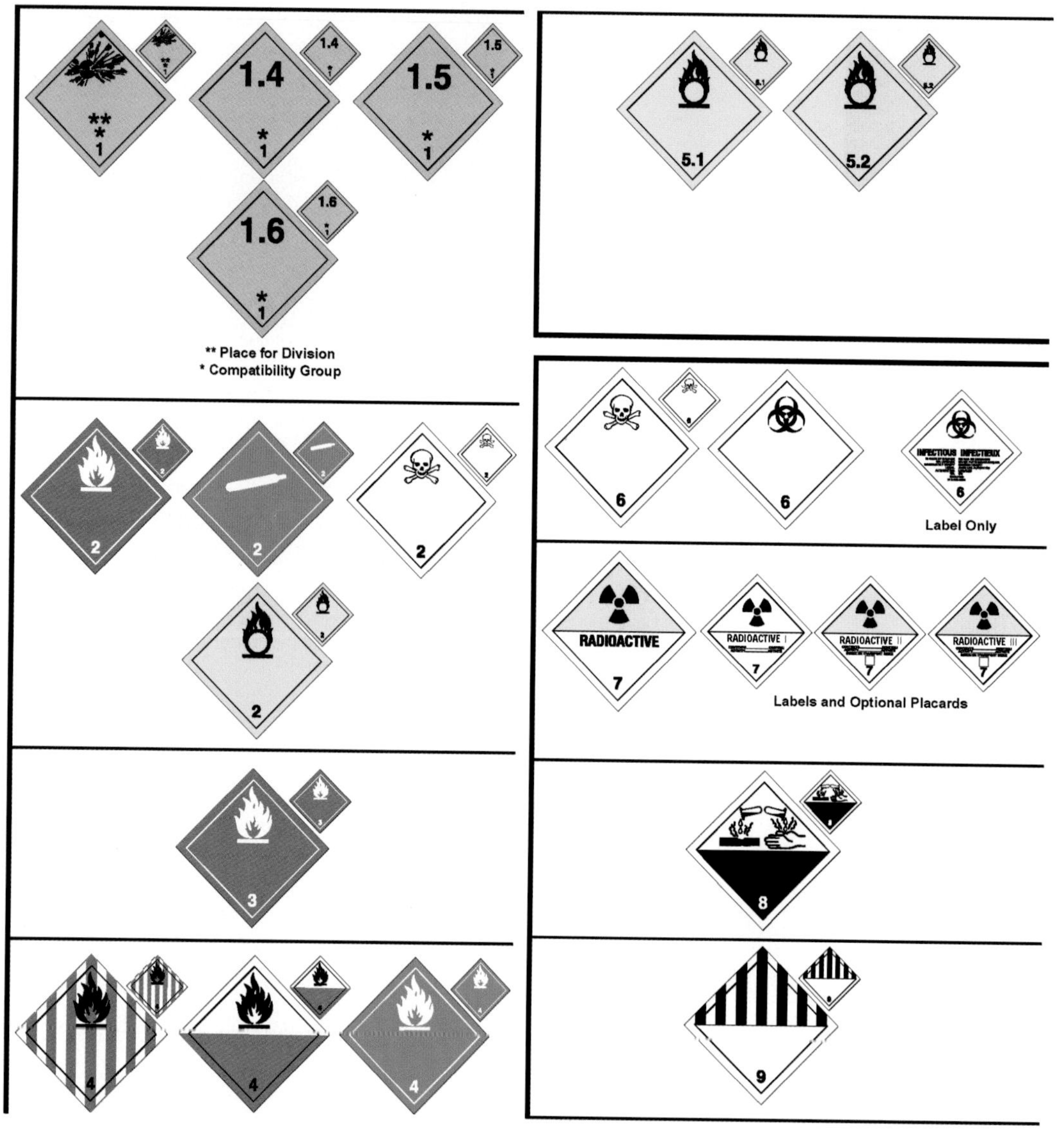

** Place for Division
* Compatibility Group

Label Only

Labels and Optional Placards

Color Plate 34. Figure 259.4. Hazardous materials placards and labels. (See Chapter 259 for complete descriptions.)

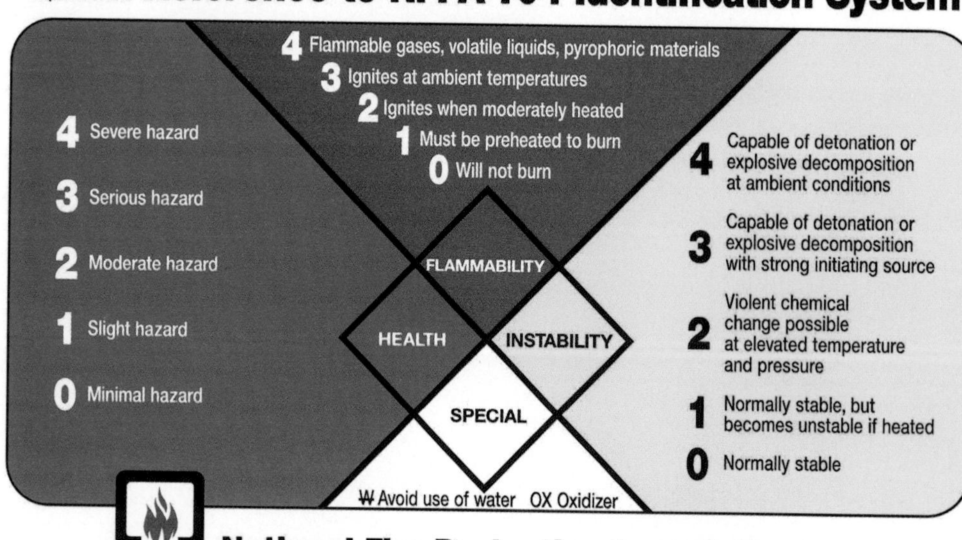

Color Plate 35. Figure 259.5. National Fire Protection Association placard (reproduced with permission).

PART I

General Approach to the Poisoned Patient

SECTION

1

The Profession of Medical Toxicology

Richard C. Dart

Death from poisoning was once the province of naturally occurring poisons, such as venoms, plant toxins, heavy metals, and the like. The industrialization of society has produced innumerable new opportunities for poisoning. Thousands of new industrial chemical entities and pharmaceutical products are introduced annually. Each chemical and drug has a dose that renders it poisonous, creating a public health need to reduce poisoning and its attendant morbidity in the home, the workplace, and the environment.

An important initial response was the creation of poison centers. In the United States, poison centers were first introduced in Chicago. The poison center movement was spearheaded primarily by pediatricians. The need for a public health intervention and similar responses has also emerged in the British Isles, Canada, Australia, France, Germany, and Italy, where poison centers were established as early as the 1960s. Many other countries now have poison centers or are attempting to create them.

Although great strides have been made in the public health aspects of poisoning, it has been persistently apparent that the individual poisoned patient is not optimally managed in many health care systems. Although it varies somewhat by country, the treatment of the individual poisoned patient has not kept pace with the myriad efforts to improve the public health through poison centers, as well as governmental agencies that regulate the safety of the air, water, food, the workplace, as well as medical devices and drugs. A poison center provides crucial advice, but there are many pitfalls in the management of serious poisoning. In many countries, specialized training and related societies have emerged to create facilities to treat the poisoned patient as well as qualified trained health care professionals to work in them. It seems clear that more is needed.

The clinical need created by poisoning has been addressed in the United States by the subspecialty of medical toxicology. The term *clinical toxicology* is often used as well. The practitioners of this clinical science are often physicians, but there are important roles for several disciplines, particularly pharmacy and nursing. There are many facets of medical toxicology, including traditional medical subspecialty clinical activities, public health analysis and intervention, and chemical and pharmaceutical products development, as well as the research needed to create the knowledge base needed for each of these activities.

The chapters of Part I, Section 1, *The Profession of Medical Toxicology*, describe the intellectual development and opportunities available in toxicology. Today, medical toxicology is an exciting, provocative, complex, scientific, political, and progressive aspect of medicine. It is involved in many thorny public health and medical issues affecting civilization today. These range from the population effects of heavy metals, such as lead and arsenic, to determining the role of treatments that could be used on millions of people, such as gastrointestinal decontamination techniques or the use of acetylcysteine.

Currently, the largest employers of medical toxicologists are probably poison centers and emergency departments (often associated with universities), but many other opportunities are available. Toxicology involves the full range of activities in the medical system: hospitals, managed care, occupational injury, public health planning, regulatory activities, and many others (Fig. 1).

The future of the specialty continues to unfold rapidly. A realistic appraisal of labor needs has not yet been developed, but it seems clear that more toxicologists are needed.

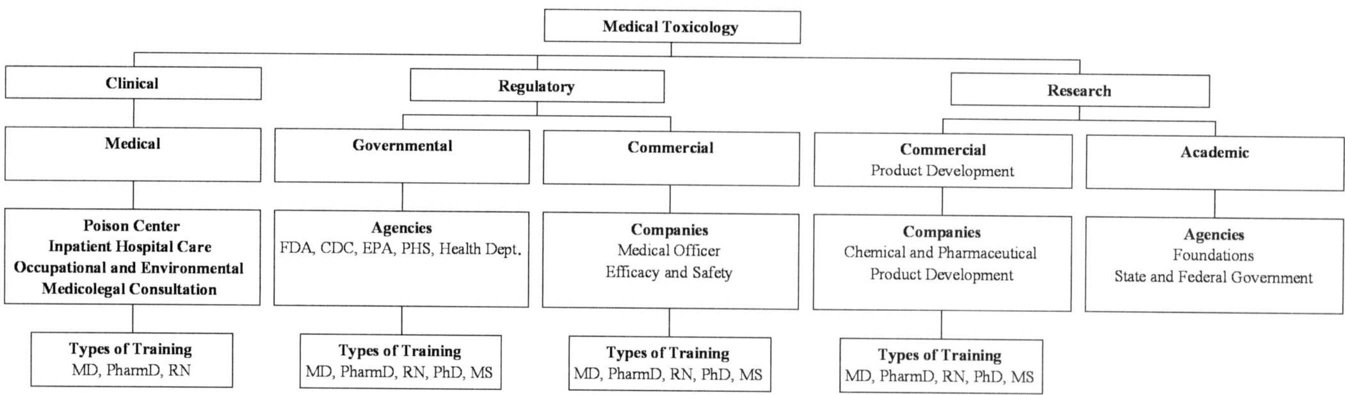

Figure 1. Roles and opportunities in toxicology. CDC, Centers for Disease Control and Prevention; EPA, Environmental Protection Agency; FDA, U.S. Food and Drug Administration; PHS, Public Health Service.

CHAPTER 1

The Practice of Medical Toxicology

Richard F. Clark

Webster's Dictionary defines *toxicology* as "the science which treats of poisons, their effects, antidotes, and recognition . . .," whereas *poison* is listed as "any agent which, when introduced into the animal organism, is capable of producing morbid, noxious, or deadly effect upon it. . . ." The broad implications of these definitions illustrate the difficulty of defining the practice of medical toxicology.

Medical toxicology has grown dramatically over the past 20 years. As recently as 1991, there was no specialty of medical toxicology recognized by the American Board of Medical Specialties. Until that time, independent organizations, such as the American Board of Medical Toxicology, certified practicing physician toxicologists through practice and examination formats. In 1992, the American Board of Medical Specialties reversed its trend against subspecialty recognition and agreed to subspecialty certification in medical toxicology. In 1994, a board examination in medical toxicology was first administered by the primary boards of Emergency Medicine, Pediatrics, and Preventive Medicine. The examination process was followed several years later by accreditation of fellowship programs.

The practice of medical toxicology has evolved during this period. Newer specialties and subspecialties always seek a mechanism of distinguishing themselves. The easiest method in this regard is to develop a technical skill or procedure that is unique, delineating the training and standard by which this skill is learned and practiced. Examples include nephrology and invasive cardiology. More recently, the development of either cost-effective or more lifesaving care than previously practiced has justified medical practice. Today, *hospitalists* manage inpatients on internal medicine services to improve inpatient care, increase billing, and meet regulatory requirements (1). Large medical centers claim significant decreases in hospital length of stay and more efficient use of diagnostic testing when hospitalists are involved in care (2).

Providing "safer" care is a more difficult claim to prove. A good example is trauma care. Large studies suggest that trauma centers save lives and decrease morbidity in certain types of injuries (3,4). Other subspecialties have reported similar cost-effective services (5). However, the cost of maintaining such services is rising rapidly, and many users of these high-cost services are uninsured or underinsured to the degree that these centers may lose millions of dollars annually in providing this care. When these costs are coupled with the rising standards of training and practice of emergency medicine, some urban centers are reevaluating the cost-benefit analysis of trauma centers.

Medical toxicology falls between these models. Similar to subspecialties such as endocrinology, toxicology is a knowledge-based field, thus far lacking both a technical skill to exploit and a large enough patient base to define improved outcomes. For these reasons, the practice of medical toxicology is as diverse as the backgrounds from which its members originate.

CLINICAL PRACTICE

One of the generally accepted goals of medical toxicologists is the establishment of tertiary care consultation and admitting services at the institutions where the presentation and referral of poisonings is frequent (6,7). These centers have been called *regional toxicology treatment centers* (*RTTC*), and it has been proposed that these centers follow certification and designation criteria similar to those for trauma centers (Chapter 2) (6). Although such toxicology services exist now in the United States and internationally, few studies have examined their efficiency or cost effectiveness (8). Whyte et al. published their experience with a centralized toxicology service model for administering care to poisoned patients. They concluded that their model reduced hospital length of stay for poisoned patients but did not affect mortality (9). Lee et al. also reported that their toxicology service decreased the average length of stay for poisoned patients at a teaching hospital in Melbourne, Australia (10). We studied our experience with tricyclic antidepressant poisonings at two urban tertiary care hospitals. Our results suggest that toxicology consultants might improve the efficiency of resource use in these cases, although we were not able to demonstrate significant differences in mortality (11).

There are at least three areas of future research into the feasibility of cost and medical efficacy of the RTTC. The first deals specifically with cost savings of such programs. Financial benefits of RTTC are difficult to assess. Most of the studies that have been published on this subject by other specialties have become outdated owing to the rapid changes that occur in health care economics. The same managed care influences that "carved up" populations into discrete market shares captured by specific hospitals in the 1990s may now be evolving back into a more "economies of scale" approach in which several providers share services. "True" costs of services, medications, and laboratory tests are difficult to calculate owing to agreements between payers and insurers. "Cost-effectiveness analysis" of medical care may not be regarded as favorably in the future.

Another means of examining the effect of an RTTC is resource use. As we found from our study, the outcomes of poisoned or envenomated patients are often unrelated to the number of laboratory tests or decontamination procedures performed. Similar analysis of hospital days spent in the intensive care unit can also be unreliable because one case of unpreventable aspiration can greatly affect endpoints. Resource use is important but unlikely to convince legislators or health care providers of the value of the service.

The most relevant area on which to focus future RTTC research is in outcomes measurement. There may be several methods of this analysis. Morbidity and mortality data are certainly preferable, but the low incidence of severe adverse outcomes and fatalities after poisoning and the great variety of agents that can be involved limit this type of analysis. One method that has been used to study diverse patient populations is to use validated scoring systems. For example, the Glasgow Coma Scale revolutionized the ability to analyze and describe head injuries. Along with the "trauma score," its acceptance has to a large extent enabled trauma centers to define themselves by comparing the outcome of patients with a variety of injuries. Similarly, scoring systems such as the Apache Score have attempted to grade the severity of illness of patients admitted to medical intensive care units. Medical toxicology should strive to develop a widely accepted scoring system to describe the severity of patients. Such a validated approach is necessary if any legitimate comparisons in the outcome of poisoned patients can be undertaken.

Consultation Services

The hospital system in San Diego is carved up into several large health care systems that refer patients to specific affiliated hospitals within their respective organizations. We found ourselves hampered in the creation of an RTTC by practicing in a highly competitive health care market combined with a large proportion of nonpaying patients, such as undocumented immigrants. Physicians and patients in our community would possibly benefit from establishing one source of toxicology referrals. However, the operating costs and revenues of each hospital are so narrow that interfacility transfers are extremely limited. Hospital administrators refuse to bring unfunded cases into their systems, especially when there is not yet a proven upgrade in "level of care" with the transfer of most poisonings.

One solution is to act as a consultant within multiple health care systems. In this model, the medical toxicologist sees inpatients or outpatients at several geographically related facilities. As a consultant, the medical toxicologist must be respected enough to administer care in a similar fashion as the admitting physician and potentially able to order tests or medications and provide recommendations for disposition. In most cases, however, the consultant is not required to maintain as long of a bedside presence as the admitting provider. Currently, the most valuable working relationship as a consultant lies with the emergency department (ED). Similar to the trauma victim, the critical time in the management of poisoned patients is often the first hours after exposure. Most of the "lifesaving" recommendations for care provided by the toxicologist are administered in the ED. It has been vital in our role as consultants to building close relationships with ED physicians and to respond rapidly to calls for assistance. Many of the residency-trained emergency physicians in our community studied toxicology on our service during residency.

Consultants risk having recommendations not followed. We have found that directing our consultation notes toward "educating" the primary provider is effective in generating support and demand for our services. Long notes, including explanations of pathophysiology, pharmacology, and management, are part of the consultation, especially when housestaff are involved in the care of these patients. Over time, the primary providers recognize the importance of the toxicology consultant and the value of their expertise and skills.

Admitting Services

Another viable model for the bedside practice of medical toxicology is to admit patients directly. Admitting the poisoned or overdosed patient adds flexibility for the toxicologist to manage every aspect of care, from initial supportive therapy to disposition. The benefit of this system is the potential to provide the most cost-efficient and therapeutically effective care to these individuals.

Similar to the consulting toxicologist, the referral of patients is critical to success. Effort is required in developing a referral and transfer base that draws cases to one facility, and to be able to receive patients early enough to effect care. Hospital administrators, emergency medical transport services, and ED physicians all need to be involved in the negotiations of providing these services.

The admitting physician must also develop an effective relationship with other specialties, such as psychiatry and social service. Bedside management may require more time as the primary health care provider, but economies of scale can be generated if all of one's patients are located in the same intensive or intermediate care setting. We have developed a blended practice as "consultants who admit patients." Each member of our group has admitting privileges to our primary hospital. Poisonings that we consider unique in clinical presentation and outside the typical practice of other fields of medicine, such as carbon monoxide, mushroom, or snake venom poisoning, are admitted to our service. We also admit the majority of poisonings during times of the year when internal medicine services are crowded. Consultations are exclusively performed on cases seen outside of our host institution. This mix of services has provided us with a balanced practice of providing inpatient care in our community.

Income can be generated by either of these models. In our system, charges are greater when acting as a consultant than as the admitting physician. However, when intensive care time and procedures are factored in, admitting poisoned patients is likely to generate higher gross charges.

Medical toxicology services are becoming more common in the United States and elsewhere. Still, toxicologists are finding that careers in this field often require supplemental income from sources other than inpatient or outpatient management. Many in our specialty still choose to practice part time within their primary field of medicine.

Outpatient Clinics

The consultation and admission service can stimulate referrals in the outpatient setting. It is possible to see new or follow-up cases in a previously arranged clinic, or on an as-needed basis in the ED or urgent care. Once referral patterns are established, outpatient service can draw cases from anywhere within a region. It is, therefore, important for the new toxicologist to meet and advertise their services and expertise throughout the community. Outpatient medical toxicology clinics around the country have focused on a variety of areas. Some medical toxicologists have moved into the area of Multiple Chemical Sensitivity, setting up and running chambers where patients are tested for allergies to environmental and chemical contaminants. Still others work closely with industrial hygienists to test work and home environments for poisons. Outpatient clinic billing tends to be higher than inpatient charges, especially with regard to time investment.

Poison Centers

Medical toxicologists are involved with poison centers either as a referral resource or as an employee. Poison centers can be tremendous referral sources of inpatients and outpatients. Patients frequently call poison centers requesting referral to a physician to evaluate their exposure. Health maintenance organizations often require pre-approval by a primary care provider before seeing a specialist, but most of the internists and family physicians in our area are pleased to refer these cases.

Medical toxicologists can also be found involved with poison centers as a consultant or medical director. The American Association of Poison Control Centers requires involvement of a physician toxicologist in the day-to-day operations of "certified" poison centers. The physicians must participate in the continuing education of specialists and providers and the initiation and maintenance of the medical guidelines that center staff use in the triage and management of exposures. Many centers have several medical toxicologists in rotation for calls when an information specialist requires backup. Some centers use call schedules with experts in certain areas of toxicology, such as envenomation, mushrooms, or hazardous materials, specifically available for these types of cases. Stipends are often available for such involvement.

Occupational Medicine

Occupational physicians are asked increasingly to evaluate patients exposed to toxic agents. Although the vast majority of these exposures are inhalational or topical, the precise source of the toxin is often difficult to determine. Occupational lung diseases are referred to a pulmonary specialist in many institutions. However, the occupational toxicologist is usually able to read and interpret chest radiographs, order and interpret pulmonary function tests, and administer most of the therapy necessary in most inhalational exposures. Management of dermal exposures to toxins is also well within the scope of practice of occupational toxicology, with eczematous reactions being by far the most common disorder encountered.

There are several models for the occupational toxicologist. An occupational medicine provider at the job site (or urgent care contracted by the employer) most often screens patients with potential toxic exposures. Some toxicologists function as primary occupational physicians and are part of this initial screening process. A second type of occupational referral pattern involves the medical toxicologist only as a consultant, when the occupational physician is unsure of the diagnosis or treatment. This is our usual practice, and we have found that these cases are often difficult to definitively diagnose even by a medical toxicologist.

Another role for the occupational toxicologist is to serve as medical review officer. The position of medical review officer is flexible but most often serves to interpret the results of toxicology screening of employees. With many different laboratories using a variety of assays and a range of thresholds for detecting banned substances, toxicologists are often the most knowledgeable specialists to understand and explain the clinical implications of the results.

Pediatric Toxicology

Severe pediatric poisoning cases have fortunately become rare with the rising public awareness of poison prevention, the increasing use of "childproof" containers for medications and household products, and the removal of some products from the market. As pediatric hospital care has centralized in the past decade, many communities rely on a large pediatric referral hospital to handle the most ill children. Toxicologists have become intimately involved with the children's hospital in our city. Because many toxicologists are not trained as pediatricians, acting as consultants in this setting is often the most convenient means of delivering our expertise in these cases.

Pediatric toxicologists most commonly focus outpatient clinical attention to screening for lead and other metal poisonings, because other chronic toxicities are rare in children. In areas in which most housing is relatively new and lead paint is uncommon, such as in San Diego, the opportunity for a consistent source of outpatient toxicology referrals is limited.

MEDICAL-LEGAL CONSULTING

Toxic tort litigation is increasing dramatically in the United States. Attorneys for cases such as environmental exposure, medical malpractice, and product liability are routinely seeking medical toxicologists. Some toxicologists have found that supplementing clinical cases with medical-legal consulting can meet their income needs.

RESEARCH

Creating a research focus for groups of medical toxicologists can assist in substantiating the fund of knowledge of our specialty within our institutions. Many academic and clinical medical centers equate clinical expertise with research experience. Medical toxicology research branches into several broad paths: clinical case-based experience (multicentered), clinical volunteer-based, bench type with animal models, or retrospective reviews of data from registries or case logs. Toxicology research also has great potential with prospective and retrospective designs using poison center databases.

Many academic institutions still recommend a focused style of research interest for career academicians. Notable examples exist of toxicologists with particular interests developing models that can be used to propagate numerous studies and answer several questions. Some of the best recent examples are in the area of venom toxicity and antivenom development. However, product research and development for antidotes or other therapies for the treatment of toxicology-related disorders has not to date drawn significant grant awards from either pharmaceutical companies or the federal government. Often, the potential return on development costs of therapies for toxic exposures is not worth the investment. More recently, the focus on biological and chemical weapons has opened new areas of research for medical toxicologists. The Centers for Disease Control and Prevention, for example, is now becoming more conscious of toxicology-related disorders and has career and research opportunities for toxicologists (Chapter 4).

ADMINISTRATIVE RESPONSIBILITIES

Administrative roles for medical toxicologists exist in many institutions. Perhaps the most obvious responsibility is with medical errors and pharmaceutical use. Medical toxicologists internationally hold many pharmacy and therapeutics committee chair positions. Some medical centers have begun offering stipends to the chair of these committees. In return, hospitals request more time spent on formulary review and management, medication errors, adverse drug reactions, and quality assurance. There are no more qualified individuals for these positions than medical toxicologists.

Another valuable role filled in many institutions by toxicologists is in assisting investigational drug services and investigational review boards. The expertise of the toxicologist in drug toxicity and dosing is a necessity on these committees. In addition, pharmacokinetic knowledge, including drug interactions, can contribute to the committee's assessment of new drug protocols.

TEACHING

The primary role of medical toxicology services in many institutions is teaching. A medical toxicology consultation can provide not only aid in acute management of ill patients but also train housestaff for future care for similar presentations. Our initial consultation notes address all potential classes of drugs involved in the exposure and cover pathophysiology, clinical findings, treatment, and pharmacokinetics. Although housestaff may benefit the most from these reports, attending staff are also often anxious to have us attend work rounds to answer questions and provide more specific didactics.

Within training institutions, rotations in medical toxicology can be offered to housestaff and students. These rotations are very popular among many specialties, and most emergency medicine residencies now require rotations in toxicology. Rotating housestaff on an admitting or consultation service not only provides an audience for teaching, but can also assist in balancing call schedules.

SUMMARY

The specialty of medical toxicology continues to grow nationally and internationally. Admitting and consulting services are becoming viable in many institutions as the number of board-certified and -eligible toxicologists reaches the "critical mass" needed to support call schedules to cover night and daytime admissions and consultations. By combining clinical services with components such as research, teaching, and administrative oversight, medical toxicologists are finding increasing interest in our expertise. Further efforts should be directed toward researching ways to enhance our therapeutic options for critically ill patients and supporting training programs for our fellowships. In these ways, we can improve the international awareness and success of our specialty.

REFERENCES

1. Wachter RM, Goldman L. The hospitalist movement 5 years later. *JAMA* 2002;287:487–494.
2. Reddy JC, Katz PP, Goldman L, et al. A pneumonia practice guideline and a hospitalist-based reorganization lead to equivalent efficiency gains. *Am J Manag Care* 2001;7:1142–1148.
3. Demetriades D, Berne TV, Belzberg H, et al. The impact of a dedicated trauma program on outcome in severely injured patients. *Arch Surg* 1995;130:216–220.
4. Rogers FB, Simons R, Hoyt DB, et al. In-house board-certified surgeons improve outcome for severely injured patients: a comparison of two university centers. *J Trauma* 1993;34:871–877.
5. Pollack MM, Alexander SR, Clarke N, et al. Improved outcomes for a tertiary center pediatric intensive care: a statewide comparison of tertiary and nontertiary care facilities. *Crit Care Med* 1991;19:150–159.
6. Donovan JW, Martin TG. Regional poison systems: roles and titles. *Clin Toxicol* 1993;31:221–222.
7. Banner W, Brent J, Garrettson LK, et al. What's in a name?—Regional toxicology treatment centers. *Clin Toxicol* 1993;31:219–220.
8. Whyte IM, Dawson AH, Buckley A, et al. A model for the management of self-poisoning. *Med J Aust* 1997;167:142–146.
9. Henderson A, Wright M, Pond SM. Experience with 732 acute overdose patients admitted to an intensive care unit over six years. *Med J Aust* 1993;158:28–30.
10. Lee V, Kerr JF, Braitberg G, et al. Impact of a toxicology service on a metropolitan teaching hospital. *Emerg Med* 2001;13:37–42.
11. Clark RF, Williams SR, Nordt SP, et al. Resource-use analysis of a medical toxicology consultation service. *Ann Emerg Med* 1998;31(6):705–709.

CHAPTER 2

Specialized Centers for the Treatment of Poisoned Patients

Frank F. S. Daly, Lindsay M. Murray, Mark Little, and Richard C. Dart

> The American College of Emergency Physicians believes that high-quality toxicology treatment and poison information should be available to all . . . (1).
>
> Proper care of patients with significant or ill-defined poisoning includes a consultation with a medical toxicologist (2).

BACKGROUND AND HISTORY

Deliberate self-poisoning (DSP) and recreational drug abuse are common presentations to the emergency department (ED). These presentations may comprise up to 5% of ED presentations. Studies published since 1965 indicate that between 100 and 400 patients per 100,000 population present to the ED with DSP (3–6).

The development of specialized centers for treatment of the poisoned patient has occurred in parallel with the development of clinical toxicology as a medical discipline. This process started in the nineteenth century when Bonaventure Orfila (1787–1853) was the first to apply rational and scientific principles to the treatment of poisoned patients and recognized that their treatment required skills not found in other areas of clinical medicine and pharmacology. Specialized wards for the treatment of poisoned patients were established in Copenhagen and Budapest in the 1940s (7).

In the United States, recognition of poisoning as a leading cause of pediatric accidents led to the establishment of poison control centers in the 1950s (8). Standards for specialized toxicology treatment units were introduced in 1993 (9).

In 1962, the Atkens report recognized the prevalence of poisoning in the United Kingdom and the need for specialized expertise for poisoned patients (10). The report recommended that all "casualty departments" have poisoning references available, that each district have a designated hospital to treat poisoned patients, and that such centers should be supervised by a clinician experienced in poisoning. The report also recognized that psychosocial morbidity underlies DSP and recommended that the hospitals designated to treat poisoned patients have an on-call psychiatrist.

Over the next 6 years, DSP appeared to increase by 80% in the United Kingdom. In 1968, the Hill report noted that the management of poisoned patients remained fragmented and that few clinicians with specialized expertise were available (11). In addition to the recommendations of the Atkens report, it advocated the establishment of specialized poison treatment units to develop new treatments, facilitate research, and improve training. Again, admission of all DSP patients for psychiatric evaluation was recommended. The Edinburgh poison treatment center published a description of their specialized center in 1969 (3). Over its 90-year history, it had evolved into a self-contained ward of 20 beds adjacent to the ED. All DSP patients were admitted, all received psychiatric evaluation, and a full-time social worker was employed. In 1968, the center admitted 1067 patients and the overall mortality rate was 0.7%. One innovation of the center was prospective collection of medical, laboratory, and psychiatric data for every patient on preformatted punch cards.

Even today, it appears that only a small minority of poisoned patients is treated primarily by clinicians with specialized expertise in toxicology. A recent study of poisoned patients admitted to four large teaching hospitals in the United Kingdom demonstrated heterogeneous and fragmented care (5). Patients were admitted under several different specialties to varied hospital locations. Only 57% of patients were admitted to inpatient services, but those admitted were much more likely to receive a specialist psychosocial assessment. Approximately 53% received specialist psychosocial assessment at the time of attendance. This is probably representative of hospitals around the world.

Throughout North America, the United Kingdom, Europe, and Australasia, telephone consultation with a consultant clinical toxicologist is available, usually through poison information centers. Most poison centers in the United States limit themselves to telephone consultation. The first toxicology fellowship was initiated in the 1970s at Rocky Mountain Poison and Drug Center (Denver). The number of fellowship programs has expanded to more than 20 in 2002. Training fellows typically add technical expertise at their home hospital but do not provide the more comprehensive care characterized by the Edinburgh and other centers. A recent survey of clinical toxicologists in the United States demonstrated that only 54% regard their services to be part of a "center for poison treatment" (12). In addition, only 57% billed for their bedside consultations.

In the late 1980s and early 1990s, widespread discussion of toxicology treatment centers produced a statement regarding the desired characteristics (9). Most important, the guidelines stated the importance of a philosophical and financial commitment to the treatment of poisoned patients (13). Such a commitment should include a multidisciplinary team with integrated psychiatric services; adequate staffing; timely availability of appropriate beds, equipment, and laboratory support; adequate stocking of antidotes; research and education; review and audit; and liaison with poison control or information centers. Thus, the guidelines suggest comprehensive toxicologist coverage and the importance of appropriate facilities. They also include the development of triage and protocols to standardize care in the prehospital and hospital phases of care. Subsequently, the American College of Medical Toxicology revised and endorsed the facility assessment guidelines, renaming them *Centers for Poison Treatment* (14).

PRINCIPLES

It is now recognized that acutely poisoned patients present with an acute, dynamic, and sometimes time-critical medical illness, but many also have complex long-term psychosocial morbidity (15). Toxicology treatment centers attempt to provide an integrated multidisciplinary approach to the treatment of poisoned patients with the aim of improving medical and psychiatric care in a cost-efficient manner.

Benefits of Treatment Centers

MEDICAL

Modern medicine often requires a multidisciplinary approach, and the specialized center offers the opportunity to coordinate and integrate multiple clinical services. An evidence-based approach should form the cornerstone of clinical management, tempered by clinical judgment and experience. Early and informed risk assessment by an experienced clinician allows the recognition of nontoxic exposures, the appropriate and efficient use of gastrointestinal decontamination, early recognition of potentially lethal exposures (thus allowing rapid intervention when required), improved discharge planning, and coordination of aftercare services (4). Daily multidisciplinary rounds may include input from the clinical toxicologist (and fellow), nursing staff, poisons information staff, social worker, drug and alcohol liaison worker, and psychiatrist. This team approach improves work efficiency and job satisfaction, avoids duplication of work, allows multiskilling and cross learning, and facilitates integrated management plans for recurrent patients.

PSYCHIATRIC

DSP is evidence of an underlying chronic psychiatric or social disorder (15). Repeat DSP is relatively common: 4.5% of DSP patients present to hospital again within 28 days, 10% present again within 6 months, and 14% present again within 1 year (16). Furthermore, the long-term mortality of this group is very high. In one study of 940 Danish DSP patients followed for 10 years, 103 had died by suicide and the mortality rate for suicide was 2960 times that of the general population (17).

Current strategies for the deliberate self-harm patient tend to focus on the highest risk patients (18), but this approach may miss the mark. High-risk patients account for only 26% of future suicidal behavior, whereas low-risk patients account for 74% (19). Admission improves access to psychiatric services (4,5), and evidence is emerging that brief admission may improve long-term outcome (20,21). This is despite controversy in the psychiatric literature about the types of interventions that may be most appropriate in this group of patients. However, these recent data reinforce the Atkens report of 40 years ago that recommended admission and psychiatric evaluation for all DSP patients.

ECONOMIC

There are no rigorous data available to assess the economic impact of specialized toxicology treatment centers. There are many promising developments, however. Using a defined team approach that integrates medical and psychiatric care, the Hunter Area Toxicology Service in New South Wales, Australia, has demonstrated that 72% of DSP patients are discharged within 24 hours and 90% of DSP patients are discharged within 48 hours (4). In 1995, the mean length of stay at the Hunter Area Toxicology Service for ages 0 to 17 years was 1.72 days, compared to the national average of 2.25 days for the same discharge codes. For ages 18 to 69 years without complications, the mean length of stay was 1.38 days, compared to 2.6 days for the national average. For ages older than 69 years or in complicated cases (e.g., those requiring intubation and ventilation), the average was 3.78 days, compared to the national average of 4.38 days. Mortality in these groups was unchanged compared to Australian national averages.

The Austin and Repatriation Medical Center Toxicology Service in Victoria, Australia, has reported the effects of establishing an inpatient toxicology admitting service (6). They found the length of stay for uncomplicated poisoning was reduced from 1.97 days to 1.4 days at their hospital. The length of stay for complicated poisoning (e.g., those requiring intubation and ventilation) was reduced from 5.59 days to 1.9 days. These gains were attained without any adverse effect on ED length of stay.

Similar results have been produced in the United States. In San Diego, the impact of a toxicology service was studied in patients presenting with tricyclic antidepressant overdose (22). This retrospective case-controlled chart review indicated fewer admissions to the intensive care unit (ICU), fewer diagnostic procedures, and fewer gastrointestinal decontamination procedures.

MODELS OUTSIDE NORTH AMERICA

The greatest development of specialized centers has occurred outside of North America. Centers in each country bear the mark of the system from which they emerged, and no single model suits all environments. Local requirements are defined by financial, social, political, and geographic factors. For example, centers in the United Kingdom and Australia tend to move the patient to specialized care facilities as found in Edinburgh, Newcastle, or Perth. In the United States, the primacy of the attending physician seems to have overshadowed the role of a facility. The tendency has been to provide advice to the treating physician (who is not a toxicologist) through the regional poison control center. Exceptions to this pattern have emerged where better-integrated systems have developed, such as in Pennsylvania, Arizona, and California, among others.

The Hunter Area Toxicology Service, based in Newcastle, Australia, operates as a 24-hour service for approximately 450,000 people. All toxicology tertiary referral patients requiring admission are diverted to a single hospital. All DSP patients are admitted to inpatient beds under a single multidisciplinary team that includes medical, psychiatric, and drug/alcohol and social services. All DSP patients receive psychiatric evaluation. In 1995, there were 750 admissions to the service (7.5% of all medical admissions to the hospital), and 550 involved DSP. Of these, 16% were admitted to the ICU; overall mortality was 0.2%.

Like Edinburgh in the 1960s, standardized prospective data collection is performed. Since 1990, the systematic prospective collection of clinical data from all toxicology and toxinology presentations to the unit has allowed analysis of important toxicoepidemiologic trends.

The Austin and Repatriation Hospital operates a toxicology treatment service in metropolitan Melbourne with input from emergency medicine, clinical pharmacology, and internal medicine. The hospital is a tertiary referral service for a population of 623,000. Approximately 650 poisoning presentations occur each year (2% of emergency visits). Patients requiring admission for more than 12 hours are admitted to inpatient beds and managed by a multidisciplinary team similar to other centers. There are 200 inpatient hospitalizations each year, of which 30% are admitted to the ICU (6).

In Western Australia, a toxicology service has been established using an appropriately resourced emergency observation unit (EOU). At Sir Charles Gairdner Hospital, a 570-bed tertiary referral center, the service is based in the ED (patient census 38,000 per year). Poisoning or intoxication represents 4.6% of all visits. In 2001, all toxicology patients were admitted to the service (700); 8% required intensive care.

A clinical toxicology team takes overall clinical responsibility for the patient throughout the admission. Strict time-related rules in the EOU have been relaxed to allow a small proportion of patients to stay longer than 24 hours. Toxicologic patients admitted to the ICU are admitted under the clinical toxicologist. Criteria for ICU admission are the requirement for intubation, advanced hemodynamic support, or urgent hemodialysis. As soon as patients no longer fit admission criteria (e.g., they are extubated), they are transferred back to the EOU managed by the multidisciplinary team. Patients are referred to other services if there is end-organ injury that requires specific therapy (e.g., rehabilitation for hypoxic brain injury). Soon after the service was established, the proportion of poisonings managed in the EOU increased from 22% to 70%; however, total bed days used to treat poisoned patients decreased 45% in the same time period (23).

In contrast to specialized units associated with EDs in North America, the United Kingdom, and Australasia, other systems have evolved in Europe. In metropolitan Paris, when severe poisoning is suspected, an intensive care ambulance staffed by a physician and nurse is dispatched to retrieve the patient (24). Advanced resuscitation is commenced at the scene, and the patient is transported directly to a toxicology ICU with specialized expertise in poisoning.

American models for the treatment of poisoned patients are covered in Chapter 3.

SUMMARY

To date, the need for and advantages of specialized treatment centers have not been proven; however, no fatal flaws have been identified. The somewhat idiosyncratic approach in the United States has not yet demonstrated effectiveness. Although further documentation is needed, specialized centers have been successful in the United Kingdom, Europe, and Australia. Evidence has emerged from such centers that treatment centers may result in improved medical, psychiatric, and economic management of all acutely poisoned patients, not just those with unusual or severe poisoning. In addition, such services allow the collection of prospective clinical data, allow toxico-epidemiologic research, and provide a focus for training.

The specific configuration of a treatment center has not been addressed. The relative effectiveness of a wholly self-contained unit (e.g., Edinburgh, Paris), partial unit (e.g., Australian ED observation units), or a specialized service (e.g., San Diego toxicology service) has not been studied. It does seem clear that one key to the success of each of these approaches is close integration of toxicologic, psychiatric, social, and laboratory services.

Other services that might be provided by a center of excellence in toxicology include outpatient services to patients with suspected poisoning; occupational toxicology services; advisory services on adverse drug effects; public health advisory services; and advice to government, regulatory authorities, and international agencies (25).

REFERENCES

1. Poison Information and Treatment Systems. American College of Emergency Medicine Policy Statement. *Ann Emerg Med* 1996;27:686.
2. Martin T. *American College of Medical Toxicology Position Statement: Care of Poisoned Patients.* Available at: http://www.acmt.net/PositionStatements/CareofPoisonedPatient.htm. Accessed February 11, 2003.
3. Matthew H, Proudfoot AT, Brown SS, et al. Acute poisoning: organization and work-load of a treatment centre. *BMJ* 1969;3:489–493.
4. Whyte IM, Dawson AH, Buckley NA, et al. Health care. A model for the management of self-poisoning. *Med J Aust* 1997;167:142–146.
5. Kapur N, House A, Creed F, et al. General hospital services for deliberate self-poisoning: an expensive road to nowhere? *Postgrad Med J* 1999;75:599–602.
6. Lee V, Kerr JF, Braitberg G, et al. Impact of a toxicology service on a metropolitan teaching hospital. *Emerg Med* 2001;13:37–42.
7. Grovaerts M. Poison control in Europe. *Pediatr Clin North Am* 1970;17:729–739.
8. Burda AM, Burda NM. The nation's first poison control center: taking a stand against accidental childhood poisoning in Chicago. *Vet Human Toxicol* 199;39:115–119.
9. American Academy of Clinical Toxicology. Facility assessment guidelines for regional toxicology treatment centers. *J Toxicol Clin Toxicol* 1993;31:2011–217.
10. Anonymous. Emergency treatment of poisoning. *Lancet* 1962;1:470–471.
11. Anonymous. Hospital treatment of acute poisoning. *Lancet* 1968;1:1283–1284.
12. McKay CA. The current practice of bedside medical toxicology in the United States. *Int J Med Toxicol* 2001;5:2.
13. Anonymous. Facility assessment guidelines for regional toxicology treatment centers. American Academy of Clinical Toxicology. *J Toxicol Clin Toxicol* 1993;31(2):211–217.

14. American College of Medical Toxicology. *Center for Poison Treatment Facility Assessment Guidelines*. Available at: http://www.acmt.net. Accessed November 13, 2002.
15. Cameron P, Jelinek G, Kelly A-M, et al. *Textbook of adult emergency medicine*. New York: Churchill Livingstone, 2000.
16. Carter GL, Whyte IM, Ball K, et al. Repetition of deliberate self-poisoning in an Australian hospital-treated population. *Med J Aust* 1999;170:307–311.
17. Nordentoft M, Breum L, Munck LK, et al. High mortality by natural and unnatural causes: a 10 year follow up study of patients admitted to a poisoning treatment centre after suicide attempts. *BMJ* 1993;306:1637–1641.
18. Australasian College for Emergency Medicine and the Royal Australian and New Zealand College of Psychiatrists Guidelines. *Guidelines for the management of deliberate self-harm in young people*. Available at: http://www.acem.org.au. Accessed February 11, 2003.
19. Kreitman N, Foster J. The construction and selection of predictive scales, with special reference to parasuicide. *Br J Psychiatry* 1991;159:185–192.
20. Owens D, Dennis M, Jones S, et al. Self-poisoning patients discharged from accident and emergency: risk factors and outcome. *J R Coll Physicians Lond* 1991;25:218–222.
21. Kapur N, House A, Dodgson K, et al. Effect of general hospital management on repeat episodes of deliberate self poisoning: cohort study. *BMJ* 2002;325:866–867.
22. Clark RF, Williams SR, Nordt SP, et al. Resource-use analysis of a medical toxicology consultation service. *Ann Emerg Med* 1998;31:705–709.
23. Williams AG, Jelinek GA, Rogers IR, et al. The effect on hospital admission profiles of establishing an emergency department observation ward. *Med J Aust* 2000;173:411–414.
24. Riou B, Barriot P, Rimailho A, et al. Treatment of severe chloroquine poisoning. *N Engl J Med* 1988;318:1–6.
25. Vale JA, Meredith TJ. Clinical toxicology in the 1990s: the development of clinical toxicology centers—a personal view. *J Toxicol Clin Toxicol* 1993;31:223–227.

CHAPTER 3
The Medical Toxicology Fellowship

Paul M. Wax

HISTORY OF MEDICAL TOXICOLOGY FELLOWSHIPS

Specialized training in medical toxicology for physicians has been available since the 1970s. Initially, many of these training programs were rather unstructured and consisted of apprenticeships under more seasoned clinical toxicologists. Over the years, formal training programs were initiated and curricula developed. It was not until the year 2000 that formal American Council of Graduate Medical Education (ACGME) recognition of medical toxicology training programs began.

Many of the early training programs in medical toxicology were started at busy poison control centers located in major metropolitan cities. These centers provided the trainees with access to a high volume of poisoning cases and unique clinical experiences that could not be duplicated at a single hospital. Poison centers in Boston, Denver, New York, Phoenix, and San Francisco have trained fellows in medical toxicology since the 1970s. At some of these institutions, the medical toxicology training was under the direct supervision of pediatricians (e.g., Denver, Boston), whereas at other sites the supervision came from emergency physicians (e.g., New York) or occupational medicine physicians (e.g., San Francisco).

Between 1970 and 1997, approximately 147 physicians underwent medical toxicology fellowship training at some 21 medical toxicology fellowship programs across the United States (1). According to a 1997 survey of medical toxicologists, 55% of fellowship-trained toxicologists had competed a residency in emergency medicine, 20% had completed a residency in pediatrics, and 16% had completed a residency in internal medicine. Since 1970, the number of physicians who have chosen to pursue medical toxicology fellowship training has clearly increased. Of the surveyed physicians, 6% completed a fellowship between 1970 and 1979, 35% completed a fellowship between 1980 and 1989, and 59% completed a fellowship between 1990 and 1997.

PHYSICIAN CREDENTIALING IN MEDICAL TOXICOLOGY

The physician credentialing process in medical toxicology has been pivotal to the growth and development of toxicology training programs. Recognizing that a growing number of physicians were spending a major portion of their professional activities engaged in the practice of medical toxicology, the American Academy of Clinical Toxicology established the American Board of Medical Toxicology (ABMT) in 1974. The mandate for ABMT was to develop a certification process for those physicians who possessed special knowledge and skills in the evaluation and treatment of patients exposed to poisons, drugs, and other toxic substances. The initial examination was administered in Kansas City, Missouri, in 1975 under the direction of the first ABMT chairman, Helmut Redetzki (2). Between 1975 and 1992, 209 physicians were certified under the ABMT process. Although this board certification process was independent of the American Board of Medical Specialties (ABMS) credentialing process involving more established medical subspecialties such as cardiology, the ABMT examination was well known for its exceptional rigor and created a high barrier to certification. In addition to standard multiple-choice questions, this examination included an oral examination and a practicum component that tested recognition of visual and odor toxicology clues such as plants.

Entrance criteria to the ABMT examination process evolved over the years. By the late 1980s, candidates were required to have completed specialized training: (a) a 2-year fellowship in medical toxicology, (b) a 3-year supervised preceptorship tutorial in which the candidate had spent at least 150 hours per year involved in toxicologic activities under the supervision of an ABMT diplomate, or (c) a combination of these pathways.

A major change in the credentialing process in medical toxicology occurred in 1992. After much effort, formal ABMS recognition of medical toxicology as a subspecialty occurred. Given the heterogeneous constituency of medical toxicologists, the

American Board of Emergency Medicine, American Board of Pediatrics, and American Board of Preventative Medicine jointly established a Subboard of Medical Toxicology. The American Board of Emergency Medicine was selected to serve as the administrative board for the new subspecialty credentialing process. The eight-person subboard included four appointees from the American Board of Emergency Medicine, two from the American Board of Pediatrics, and two from the American Board of Preventative Medicine.

The first ABMS-recognized examination in medical toxicology was offered in 1994 and is now offered biannually. The examination is based on the *Core Content of Medical Toxicology*, a document that outlines key concepts and toxins in medical toxicology and reflects the considerable breadth of information that specialists in medical toxicology are expected to master. For the first four examination cycles between 1994 and 2000, several different eligibility pathways were available to examination applicants: fellowship training, prior ABMT certification, a practice route, and a combined practice and fellowship-training route. Beginning with the 2002 examination, however, examinees must have completed a 2-year fellowship in medical toxicology within the 5 years preceding the examination date. Unlike the older ABMT examination, the ABMS Medical Toxicology examination is similar in style to other ABMS examinations. It consists solely of single-answer multiple-choice questions, some with visual stimuli. By the end of 2000, a total of 205 physicians had successfully passed the ABMS medical toxicology subboard examination. At present the medical toxicology board certificate is time limited to 10 years. A recertification examination in Medical Toxicology has been created and will be offered for the first time in 2004.

ACCREDITATION OF FELLOWSHIPS

The residency review committee of the sponsoring program conducts the ACGME accreditation process for medical toxicology fellowship programs. At present, fellowship programs in medical toxicology are sponsored by either emergency medicine or preventive medicine [pediatric-based programs are currently sponsored by an EM residency (e.g., Boston Children's)]. In 2002, there were 20 ACGME-approved programs in Medical Toxicology—17 under emergency medicine and three under preventive medicine. A current list of accredited fellowships can be obtained at http://www.acgme.org/adspublic. Each training program must be a minimum of 24 months in duration. Most programs select one to two fellows per year. ACGME requirements for residencies in medical toxicology are found at http://www.acgme.org.

Prerequisite training for fellowship candidates requires completion of an ACGME-accredited residency program, although the exact type of primary training is not specified. Although the majority of candidates for fellowship training have completed a residency in emergency medicine, successful candidates have also come from pediatrics, preventive medicine, internal medicine, and pathology training programs.

Curriculum

Fellowship training in Medical Toxicology provides closely supervised education in all aspects of medical toxicology including direct patient care in inpatient and outpatient sites, poison center consultation, teaching, research, and administration. Whereas some of the fellowship programs are based at pediatric hospitals, most fellowship programs are based at hospitals that admit patients of all ages. Fellowship programs are required to provide clinical experiences from all age groups. The core training teaches prevention, monitoring, evaluation, diagnosis, and treatment of toxic exposures, including intentional, unintentional, occupational, and environmental exposures.

Each toxicology fellowship program requires at least two board-certified medical toxicologists to serve as faculty. Consultants from occupational medicine, pulmonary medicine, disaster and mass casualty incident management, hyperbaric medicine, industrial hygiene, biostatistics, epidemiology, public health, botany, cardiology, dermatology, gastroenterology, nephrology, ophthalmology, pathology, pharmacology, zoology, herpetology, mycology, hazardous materials, weapons of mass destruction, laboratory toxicology, forensic toxicology, and environmental toxicology should also be available.

During the 24-month fellowship period, the fellow must spend at least 12 months actively engaged in clinical care of poisoned patients. The fellow's role may be as the primary physician or consultant physician under the supervision of a toxicology faculty member. The ability to provide direct bedside clinical evaluations is required. Medical toxicology evaluation of critically ill poisoned patients takes place in the intensive care unit as well as the emergency department. In addition to inpatient evaluations, an outpatient experience involving the evaluation of patients with occupational or environmental toxicologic exposures is an essential component of the fellowship program. Optimally, these outpatient evaluations should be performed in a toxicology clinic that serves as a referral center for patients with occupational and environmental toxic exposures. Basic curriculum objectives as outlined by the ACGME are listed in Table 1.

Another important component of the medical toxicology fellowship program is a close association with a regional poison control center. Given the breadth of case material and the large number of toxic exposure cases managed by poison centers, this clinical load offers a unique component that is critical to successful training in medical toxicology. Toxicology fellows-in-training provide 24-hours-per-day, 7-days-per-week medical consulta-

TABLE 1. Sample of toxicology curriculum

The clinical manifestations, differential diagnosis, and management of poisoning
The biochemistry of metabolic processes; the pharmacology; pharmacokinetics; and teratogenesis, toxicity, and interactions of therapeutic drugs
The biochemistry of toxins, kinetics, metabolism, mechanisms of acute and chronic injury, and carcinogenesis
Experimental design and statistical analysis of data as related to laboratory, clinical, and epidemiologic research
Laboratory techniques in toxicology
Occupational toxicology, including acute and chronic workplace exposure to intoxicants and basic concepts of the workplace and industrial hygiene
Prevention of poisoning, including prevention of occupational exposures by intervention methodologies, that take into account the epidemiology, environmental factors, and the role of regulation and legislation in prevention
Environmental toxicology, including identification of hazardous materials and the basic principles of management of large-scale environmental contamination and mass exposures
The function, management, and financing of poison control centers
Oral and written communication skills and teaching techniques
Principles of epidemiology and risk communication, analytical laboratory techniques, and research methodologies in toxicology

From American Council for Graduate Medical Education Web site. Available at: http://www.acgme.org. Accessed September 1, 2002, with permission.

tion to the poison center. The fellow discusses the medical management of the poisoned patient with the referring physician and provides toxicologic expertise as well as information on antidote availability, laboratory capabilities, and tertiary care referral options. A faculty member of the medical toxicology fellowship program supervises each case.

Structured educational conferences and other activities are critical components of successful training. A minimum of 5 hours of conferences per week is required. Conferences generally emphasize basic science, recent medical literature, topic reviews, research methodology, and case reviews. Fellowship training also enables fellows to develop their own teaching skills. On a regular basis, toxicology fellows should deliver lectures to other housestaff, poison center personnel, grand rounds, and other hospitals in the region. Given the heterogeneity of the toxicologic subject matter, interdisciplinary conferences involving toxicologist participation are common at medical centers that support toxicology training. Recent attention to medical errors and biochemical terrorism has increased the role and visibility of toxicologists in the medical center. Presentations at national toxicology meetings such as the North American Congress of Clinical Toxicology annual meeting are encouraged.

Although 2-year medical toxicology fellowships are clinically oriented and are not intended to function as research fellowships, toxicology fellows are required to undertake some sort of research experience—either basic science or clinical—during their fellowship. Typically, during the first year of fellowship, trainees are mentored on how to best prepare for publication an interesting case report, whereas during the second year more time is available to pursue clinical or laboratory investigations. According to fellowship graduates who responded to the 1997 survey, on average, 22% of the fellowship time was devoted to research, whereas 55% was devoted to clinical activities, and 17% was spent on teaching (1).

During the fellowship, the trainees usually have the opportunity to maintain their primary board clinical skills. However, the fellow cannot be required to work more than 12 hours per week on activities not related to medical toxicology.

Career Development

The impact of the medical toxicology fellowship on career development appears to be substantial. Although data are limited, the 1997 survey reported that 91% of fellowship-trained individuals remain at least partly involved in activities relating to medical toxicology (1). Although only 9% of respondents considered themselves "full-time" toxicologists, 47% stated that at least 50% of their professional time was devoted to medical toxicology. Areas of significant impact of the toxicology fellowship on career development include increasing the likelihood of choosing an academic career, developing a toxicology practice, increasing involvement in toxicology training, and decreasing primary practice time.

OTHER TRAINING PATHWAYS

Training programs also exist for nonphysicians desiring specialized training in toxicology. A wide variety of graduate programs with an emphasis on toxicology and the environment are available, including master's programs in Toxicology, Public Health, Industrial Hygiene, and Hazardous Material Management and doctorate programs in Environmental Health and Molecular Toxicology. Those interested in the forensic aspects of toxicology may also pursue doctoral degrees. The American Board of Forensic Toxicology offers a certifying examination to scientists working in the forensic toxicology field. Minimal eligibility requirements include a PhD and at least 3 years of experience in the field.

The American Board of Applied Toxicology offers another pathway for credentialing in toxicology. In 1987, the American Academy of Clinical Toxicology established the American Board of Applied Toxicology to provide an opportunity for nonphysicians to pursue certification in clinical toxicology. A yearly examination is offered. Eligibility, in part, requires either a doctorate degree or at least 5 years working full time in clinical toxicology. Many of these candidates have previously earned a doctorate of pharmacy degree. Completion of at least 12 months of post-doctorate training in a clinical toxicology fellowship is encouraged. Fellowship training in clinical toxicology for nonphysicians is available at certain poison centers across the country.

THE FUTURE

Although some medical toxicology fellowship training programs have now been training future toxicologists for more than 20 years, the recent decision by ACGME to formally accredit toxicology training programs indicates that formal medical toxicology fellowship training is still developing. The field of Medical Toxicology continues to evolve, and workforce needs have not been adequately studied. A major discrepancy exists between the number of medical schools ($N = 122$) and the number of fellowship training programs ($N = 20$) in the United States. Despite the fact that five of six medical schools do not have an affiliated medical toxicology training program, many of the currently accredited programs do not fill their complement of fellow positions on a regular basis. Since many fellowship graduates pursue academic careers, perhaps they may attempt to create toxicology clinical services at academic medical centers that have not previously had a medical toxicology presence. Given the downsizing of some other medical subspecialties (3), a true needs assessment to determine the need for additional toxicology training programs seems warranted.

At present, most toxicology fellowship programs are emergency medicine based. Eighty-five percent of the programs are accredited by the Emergency Medicine Residency Review Committee, and the majority of faculty in these programs have emergency medicine residency training or board certification. The demand for medical toxicology services, however, has metamorphosed significantly beyond caring for acute intoxications. Questions from health care providers, the public, and federal regulatory agencies regarding the recognition, management, treatment, and prevention of low-level environmental or occupational toxic exposures are increasingly directed at medical toxicologists. Expertise regarding the medical aspects of biochemical terrorism also involves the medical toxicologist. In addition, medical toxicologists are frequently consulted on forensic issues including the interpretation of urine drug screens and the results of other biologic monitoring. To stay current with these rapidly changing times, fellowship training programs in the future may need to more heavily emphasize these topics and expend greater effort at integrating preventative and occupational toxicology training into medical toxicology curriculum.

REFERENCES

1. Wax PM, Donovan JW. Fellowship training in medical toxicology, characteristics, perceptions and career impact. *J Toxicol Clin Toxicol* 2000;38:637–642.
2. Comstock EG. Roots and circles in medical toxicology: a personal reminiscence. *J Toxicol Clin Toxicol* 1998;36:401–407.
3. Joiner KA, Powderly WG, Blaser MJ, et al. Fellowship training in infectious diseases: a report from the regional and national meetings of infectious disease division chiefs and program directors. *Clin Infect Dis* 1998;26:1060–1065.

CHAPTER 4

The Medical Toxicologist and Regulatory Agencies

Daniel A. Spyker

This chapter provides a perspective on the role of the medical toxicologist in regulatory medicine—the U.S. Food and Drug Administration (FDA) in particular.

WHAT IS A REGULATORY AGENCY?

It almost suffices to say that a regulatory agency regulates—but gives no flavor of the regulations themselves. One might simply divide regulation into the creation and the enforcement of the rules of commerce.

After legislation is written and approved by Congress, it typically contains little detail of what to do or how to do it. These details are provided in the regulations, often developed by the designated regulatory agency. The regulations developed must undergo public evaluation and comment. Most regulations "become final" through a process of notice and comment wherein the draft regulations are released for public comment [e.g., through the Federal Register (to the public docket)]. The regulatory agency responds to each comment before the regulation becomes final. Such regulations carry the de facto weight of law.

The enforcement of the laws and regulations can be divided into the evaluation of safety and efficacy (termed *review*), and assuring that the rules have been followed (termed *compliance*). The medical review job within a regulatory agency, such as the FDA, involves "due diligence review" of the evidence that a new drug is ready to be evaluated or sold in the United States.

FEDERAL AGENCIES INVOLVED WITH MEDICAL TOXICOLOGY

Agency for Toxic Substances and Disease Registry

The Agency for Toxic Substances and Disease Registry (http://www.atsdr.cdc.gov/about.html), an agency of the U.S. Department of Health and Human Services, serves the public by using the best science, taking responsive public health actions, and providing trusted information to prevent harmful exposures and disease related to toxic substances. The Agency for Toxic Substances and Disease Registry assesses waste sites, consults on specific hazardous substances, maintains health surveillance and registries, responds to emergency hazardous material releases, performs applied research in support of its assessments, develops and disseminates information, and performs education and training about hazardous substances.

Centers for Disease Control and Prevention

The Centers for Disease Control and Prevention (CDC) of the U.S. Department of Health and Human Services (http://www.cdc.gov/aboutcdc.htm) is the lead federal agency for protecting the health and safety of people—at home and abroad—providing credible health information and promoting health through strong partnerships. CDC is the national focus for developing and applying disease prevention and control, environmental health, and health promotion and education activities designed to improve the health of the American population.

Consumer Product Safety Commission

The Consumer Product Safety Commission (http://www.cpsc.gov/about/about.html) is an independent federal agency that reduces the risk of injury or death from consumer products by developing voluntary industry standards, issuing and enforcing mandatory standards or banning consumer products, obtaining the recall or repair of products, conducting research on product hazards, and informing consumers.

Environmental Protection Agency

The Environmental Protection Agency (http://www.epa.gov) protects human health and safeguards the natural environment. The National Environmental Publications Internet site provides access to full images of all original pages and full text, from a collection of more than 9000 documents.

Food and Drug Administration

The FDA (http://www.fda.gov) regulates food, drugs, biologicals, veterinary products, and medical devices. The agency has some responsibility for approximately 25% of goods purchased by U.S. consumers (see following National Center for Toxicology Research section).

National Center for Toxicology Research

The National Center for Toxicology Research (http://www.fda.gov/nctr/) conducts research that supports the regulatory needs of the FDA. This involves peer-reviewed fundamental and applied research designed to define biological mechanisms of action underlying the toxicity of products regulated by the FDA. The goal is the understanding of critical biological events in the expression of toxicity and at developing methods to improve assessment of human exposure, susceptibility, and risk.

National Institute for Occupational Safety and Health

The National Institute for Occupational Safety and Health (http://www.cdc.gov/niosh/about.html) of the CDC conducts research on potentially hazardous working conditions when requested by employers or employees; makes recommendations and disseminates information on preventing workplace disease, injury, and disability; and provides training to occupational safety and health professionals.

National Toxicology Program

The National Toxicology Program (http://ntp-server.niehs.nih.gov/) of the U.S. Department of Health and Human Services coordinates toxicologic testing programs; strengthens the science base in toxicology; develops and validates testing methods; and provides information about potentially toxic chemicals to regulatory and research agencies, scientific and medical communities, and the public. The National Toxicology Program is an interagency program of the National Institutes of Health National Institute of Environmental Health Sciences, CDC/National Institute for Occupational Safety and Health, the FDA National Center for Toxicological Research, and the National Institutes of Health National Cancer Institute.

Occupational Safety and Health Administration

The Occupational Safety and Health Administration (http://www.osha.gov) seeks to protect the health of American workers. The Occupational Safety and Health Administration establishes and enforces protective standards, as well as provides technical assistance and consultation. More than 100 million workers and 6.5 million employers are covered by the Occupational Safety and Health Administration Act of 1970.

STRUCTURE AND FUNCTION OF THE FOOD AND DRUG ADMINISTRATION

The mission of the FDA is to ensure

- Foods, veterinary drugs, biologicals, cosmetics, and radiation emitting and medical devices are safe and effective.
- Regulated products are honestly, accurately, and informatively represented (truth in labeling).
- Products are in compliance with the law and regulations.

The FDA must base regulatory decisions on good science; provide clear standards and advice on meeting them; and collaborate with other agencies, industry, and academia.

What Is a Drug?

Some idea of how a chemical becomes an approved drug is useful in understanding the toxic potential of a drug. The Federal Food, Drug, and Cosmetic Act of 1938 (1) defined a drug as an article

- Recognized in the U.S. Pharmacopoeia, official Homeopathic Pharmacopoeia of the United States, or official National Formulary and
- Intended for use in the diagnosis, cure, mitigation, treatment, or prevention of disease in man or other animals; or
- Other than food intended to affect the structure or function of the body of man or other animals and that is not dependent on being metabolized for the achievement of any of its principal intended purposes.

The act was amended in 1976 to include the definition of a device by "exclusion" as an instrument, apparatus, implement, machine, contrivance, implant, *in vitro* agent, including any component part or accessory, that meets any of the aforementioned criteria for a drug but does not achieve any of its principal intended purposes through chemical action (or on being metabolized) within the body.

Note the use of the word "intended" in these definitions. The intended use or indication must be demonstrated in the clinical trials and can be claimed in the promotion and sale of the product.

Process of Developing a New Drug or Device

Drug development is a complex process that involves multiple stakeholders (Table 1). A manufacturer must demonstrate the safety and efficacy of its drug or device during human use as well as a reliable and safe production process. Data regarding safety and efficacy are gathered during preclinical, clinical (preapproval), and postmarket studies (postapproval). To begin human studies, the manufacturer must receive an investigational new drug or device exemption (Table 2). Table 2 identifies the centers within the FDA and their respective nomenclature for these activities. Further information is available at http://www.fda.gov/cder/handbook/index.htm.

PRECLINICAL DEVELOPMENT—THE INVESTIGATIONAL NEW DRUG

The preclinical development of a drug involves discovery, preclinical evaluation, and development of the chemistry, manufacturing, and controls. A useful and concise discussion of preclinical drug development has been compiled (2). Preclinical (animal) testing refers to *in vivo* animal studies.

CLINICAL STUDIES

The clinical study represents a major "unit of work" in the review of a new drug application (NDA) or medical device application, the premarket approval application. From the regulatory perspective, a clinical study is any form of planned experiment involving patients designed to develop more appropriate treatment of future patients. The special case in which the treatment is assigned by randomization defines the randomized clinical trial.

The clinical development of a drug involves assessment of the toxicology and maximum tolerated dose, pharmacokinetics and pharmacodynamics, as well as assessment of safety and efficacy. Clinical trials are classified in four phases:

Phase I—Feasibility is primarily concerned with treatment safety, usually performed on 20 to 80 human volunteers to determine whether the treatment is tolerated by humans and to generate data permitting studies in patients.

Phase II—Initial Clinical Studies in Patients involve small-scale evaluation of treatment effectiveness and safety, usually involve close monitoring of 100 to 200 patients, and generate data permitting large-scale studies in patients.

Phase III—Full-scale Clinical Evaluation of Treatment addresses large-scale evaluations of treatment effectiveness and safety versus placebo or current standard treatment, usually involves more real-world conditions, must support proposed product label (indications, contraindications), and typically involves 200 to 3000 patients.

Phase IV—Postmarketing Studies address the many unanswered questions remaining after product approval. Long-term studies and large numbers of patient exposures must necessarily await general use. (Promotion exercises designed to bring the product to the attention of a large number of prescribers, sometimes referred to as *market seeding studies*, are not clinical trials.)

TABLE 1. Principal stakeholders in drug and device development

Phase of development	Sponsor	Investigator (clinician)	Regulator (FDA)	Public research (NIH)	Insurance carriers (HCFA)
	Major players/responsibilities				
Preclinical development/ design	Primary	Secondary	Guidance and interaction (review team)	Rare	—
Overall clinical plan	Primary	Secondary	IND or IDE (review team)	Rare	—
Clinical protocol development	Primary	Secondary	IND or IDE (review team)	Rare	Occasional, for HECON
Develop report (valid scientific evidence)	Primary	Secondary	Guidance and interaction (review team)	Rare	—
Validate study results	Secondary (may audit)	Primary (site monitor)	GCP inspection (compliance)	Rare	—
Develop labeling and SSED	Primary (labeling)	? Consultant	Guidance 2o labeling 1o SSED	Rare	—
Demonstrate production capability	Manufacturing site	—	GMP inspection (compliance)	Rare	—
Advertising and promotion	Primary	Occasional	Monitor (DDMAC)	—	—
Reimbursement decisions	Request	Lobby	? Technical consultation	Rare	Primary
Develop new indication	Usually	May initiate	Guidance (review team)	If major public health issue	If major public health issue

DDMAC, Center for Drug Evaluation and Research (CDER) Division of Drug Marketing, Advertising, and Communications; FDA, U.S. Food and Drug Administration; GCP, good clinical practices; GMP, good manufacturing practices; HCFA, Health Care Finance Administration; HECON, health economic; IDE, Investigational Device Exemption; IND, investigational new drug; NIH, National Institutes of Health; SSED, summary of safety and effectiveness data/summary basis of approval.

The Code of Federal Regulations (21 CFR 312 IND application) outlines the elements to safely study a drug in humans (3). This regulation has become the standard of clinical research quality for the world (3). Studies done outside of the United States follow the Declaration of Helsinki (4) or local regulations, whichever provides greater patient protection.

BASIS FOR COMMERCIAL DISTRIBUTION—THE NEW DRUG APPLICATION

When research in the investigational new drug phase has produced acceptable evidence of safety and efficacy, the sponsor must provide this evidence as well as adequate instructions for use [package insert (PI)] to the FDA in the form of an NDA. These fundamental requirements are the same whether the product is a drug, a device, or a biological product. Two adequate and well-controlled (pivotal) studies are needed. Although certainly not a requirement in all cases, a double-blind, concurrent placebo-controlled design with complete access to the raw data (case report forms) is generally considered the "gold standard."

The final NDA package must provide adequate evidence of safety and efficacy and support the PI according to specific guidelines (5). The NDA review and development of the PI is a joint effort of the sponsor and the FDA. The frequent and close interaction of these two teams has been termed *interactive product development*. The review team recommendation of approval or disapproval typically comes 10 or 12 months after submission.

POSTMARKETING ACTIVITIES AND OBLIGATIONS

Approval for a device or drug may have stipulated conditions. Available data at the time of approval must support the safety, effectiveness, and PI, but every approval process generates unanswered questions. The agency review team often recommends follow-up of a subset of patients or additional studies as a condition of approval. Such conditions are generally determined in dis-

TABLE 2. U.S. Food and Drug Administration (FDA) centers and their review activities

CDER Center for Drug Evaluation and Research	**CBER** Center for Biologicals Evaluation and Research	**CDRH** Center for Devices and Radiological Health	**CVM** Center for Veterinary Medicine	**CFSAN** Center for Food Safety and Applied Nutrition
		Approval to begin clinical evaluation		
IND Investigational New Drug	**IND** Investigational New Drug	**IDE** Investigational Device Exemption	**INAD** Investigational New Animal Drug	**FCN** Food Contact Notifications
		Permission to begin commercial marketing		
NDA New Drug Application	**BLA, PMA, NDA** Biologicals License Application	**PMA** Premarket Approval	**NADA** New Animal Drug Application	**FDA 3503 and 3504** Food and Color Additive Applications
ANDA Abbreviated New Drug Application	**510(k)** Premarket Clearance	**510(k)** Premarket Clearance	**ANADA** Abbreviated New Animal Drug Application	**BC** Biotechnology Consultations

cussions with the sponsor, formalized in the Approvable letter, and the sponsor must agree to these conditions in writing before the Approval Order can be issued, which allows the drug to be sold. A more detailed review of these issues is available (6).

ADVERSE EVENTS

In addition to the reporting of adverse events (AE) during the clinical trials, the manufacturer must also report all postmarketing serious AE to the FDA.

Facility Obligations. The Safe Medical Devices Act of 1990 (SMDA 90) requires medical device distributors and user facilities to report serious device-related harm (serious injury, serious illness, or death) to the FDA and to the manufacturer (if known). A user facility is defined as a hospital, ambulatory surgery facility, nursing home, or outpatient diagnostic facility that is not a physician's office. The act provides for civil penalties on user facilities that fail to report.

Practitioner Obligations. Practitioners are encouraged to report serious AE or product problems with a suspected association with a drug or medical device used, prescribed, or dispensed. They should first report to the hospital AE service. If this is not available, a MedWatch report (form 3500) can be filed in several ways: (a) complete form 3500 online at http://www.accessdata.fda.gov/scripts/medwatch/; (b) call 800-FDA-1088 (800-332-1088) to dictate a report; (c) fax a report to 800-332-0178 (download form 3500 from http://www.fda.gov/medwatch/safety/3500.pdf); or (d) mail in the 3500 using the postage-paid form (http://www.fda.gov/medwatch/safety/3500.pdf).

NUTRITIONAL SUPPLEMENTS—A SPECIAL CHALLENGE

The Dietary Supplement Health and Education Act of 1994 inverted the usual drug approval process. Rather than requiring the sponsor to demonstrate safety and efficacy, the sponsor can promote and sell products until the FDA can demonstrate significant harm (http://vm.cfsan.fda.gov/~dms/ds-oview.html). This places greater responsibility on the health care system and individual practitioners to report adverse events to the FDA (see previous Practitioner Obligations section). Of abstracts submitted to the North American Congress of Clinical Toxicology for 1990 to 1995 ($N = 1084$), 21 patient reports were found that could provide useful information on these products to the FDA. None of these reports was present in the MedWatch database (7).

OVERDOSE INFORMATION IN THE PACKAGE INSERT

The *Physicians' Desk Reference* is a common source of drug information. It is a compilation of the official drug product PIs. The 21 CFR part 201.57 stipulates the information required in drug labeling and requires the manufacturer to update information regularly.

An analysis of 20 products in the 1994 *Physicians' Desk Reference* found that 16 (80%) had at least one deficiency, and five (25%) had two or more deficiencies. Thirteen (65%) omitted an indicated specific treatment. Three (15%) entries recommended contraindicated treatments for overdose, and four (20%) advised ineffective treatments with the potential for harm. Only four (20%) had no deficiencies based on the survey criteria (8). Furthermore, Spyker et al. demonstrated that most PIs contained insufficient clinical pharmacology information (9).

Employment Opportunities

The FDA employs thousands of health care professionals, including hundreds of physicians. Physicians are employed primarily as medical officers in the review divisions, which are generally divided along subspecialty lines: cardiology, infectious disease, and so forth. The medical officers serve as managers for the "due diligence" review of the research supporting new medical products. They lead the review teams (including a chemist, pharmacologist, statistician, and pharmacokineticist) in deciding two fundamental questions: Is it safe to begin research with this product in humans? Has the sponsor adequately demonstrated the safety and effectiveness of this product?

A toxicologist may be considered a specialist in the safety side of the assessment since he or she deals primarily with the adverse effects of the drug or chemical. He or she also has experience in making clinical assessments and recommendations based on less-than-complete information. The efficacy assessment, by contrast, tends to be quantitative and statistical in nature. If one's professional goals involve clinical research, especially in drug or medical device development, serving as a medical officer provides the most compressed and varied experience available. In a decade at a Center for Drug Evaluation and Research and Center for Devices and Radiological Health, I was never bored, learned a great deal, and appreciated making decisions based primarily on the public health (http://www.fda.gov/jobs/default.htm).

Information Resources

The Worldwide Web in general and the FDA Web site in particular provide a wealth of information and education opportunities:

- Information. Start with the Center for Drug Evaluation and Research Week list-serve (http://www.fda.gov/cder/cdernew/listserv.html). If you are interested in drug development or seek detail about an approved drug, examine the review package (http://www.fda.gov/cder/da/da.htm).
- Education. Not everyone enjoys a diversion as a clinical fellow, but some do. Programs are available through the University of the Uniformed Health Sciences (http://www.wrair.army.mil/TrainingProgram/ClinicalPharmacology/Fellowship.htm) and the Center for Drug Development Sciences at Georgetown University (http://cdds.georgetown.edu/programs/fellowship.html). For smaller doses, consider participating in the continuing education activities such as MedWatch (http://www.fda.gov/medwatch/articles.htm).
- Observation. To gain insight into the public end of the review and approval process, attend an advisory committee meeting (http://www.fda.gov/cder/meeting/advisorycomyear.htm).
- Participation. The FDA offers a spectrum ranging from submitting MedWatch reports to serving as a member of an advisory committee or other special government employee opportunities.

REFERENCES

1. The Federal Food, Drug, and Cosmetic Act of 1938 [sections 201–903, 52 Stat. 1040 et seq., as amended (21 U.S.C. 301–392)]. U.S. Government Printing Office, ISBN 0-16-041900-X. Available at: http://www.fda.gov/opacom/laws/fdcact/fdctoc.htm.
2. ICH DRAFT guideline on safety pharmacology studies for human pharmaceuticals. International Conference on Harmonization, August 4, 2000. Available at: http://www.fda.gov/cber/gdlns/ichsafety.pdf.
3. 21 CFR 312 Investigational New Drug Application, The Code of Federal Regulations, Title 21, Food and Drugs, Part 312. Available at: http://www.access.gpo.gov/nara/cfr/waisidx_98/21cfr312_98.html.
4. World Medical Association. Declaration of Helsinki—ethical principles for medical research involving human subjects. *JAMA* 2000;284(23):3043–5. Available at: http://www.jama.ama-assn.org/issues/v284n23/

rfull/jco00183.html or available directly from the World Medical Association Web site: http://www.wma.net/e/policy/17-c_e.html.
5. 21 CFR 314 Applications for Food and Drug Administration approval to market a new drug or an antibiotic drug. The Code of Federal Regulations, Title 21, Food and Drugs, Part 314. Available at: http://www.access.gpo.gov/nara/cfr/waisidx_98/21cfr314_98.html.
6. Spyker DA. From concept to operating room: role of the FDA in the development of anesthesia drugs and devices. In: Lake CL, Rice LJ, Sperry RP, eds. *Advances in anesthesia*, vol. 15. New York: Mosby, 1998:375–428.
7. Spyker DA, Love L. Reports of exposure to dietary supplements and traditional remedies to the AAPCC/AACT: the need for cooperation with the FDA. AACT/AAPCC/ABMT Annual Scientific Meeting, 1996.
8. Mullen WH, Anderson IB, Kim SY, et al. Incorrect overdose management advice in the *Physicians' Desk Reference*. *Ann Emerg Med* 1997;29(20):255–261.
9. Spyker DA, Harvey ED, Harvey BE, et al. Assessment and reporting of clinical pharmacology information in drug labeling. *Clin Pharmacol Ther* 2000;67(3):196–200.

CHAPTER 5

The Toxicologist in Legal Proceedings

Jack W. Snyder

Courts, legislatures, and administrative agencies in the United States frequently rely on toxicologists to assist them in legal proceedings. The role of the toxicologist varies with the forum. When agencies develop regulations, for example, toxicologists typically are asked only to review documents and advise regulators on technical issues, either as a matter of personal knowledge or as a matter of expertise. Similarly, the toxicologist's role in court cases is most often limited to reviewing documents and advising litigants. On occasion, in regulatory and in judicial proceedings, the toxicologist contributes further by offering oral or written testimony, or at the request of the agency or tribunal. Rarely, toxicologists may testify before committees of Congress or state legislatures.

Thoughtful toxicologists seeking to make significant contributions to legal process should develop a basic understanding of the law of evidence as it applies to "experts." The rules governing the participation of experts in legal proceedings reflect a compromise between two fundamental principles that determine the competency of scientific or medical evidence. One principle holds that problematic or deficient evidence should never be admitted; the other holds that any problem or deficiency in evidence should influence only the weight, and not the admissibility, accorded that evidence.

RECENT DEVELOPMENTS IN AMERICAN LAW OF EXPERTS

Historically, the law of experts in the United States has focused on two fundamental questions. First, is the subject matter of the expert's opinion appropriate to the matter at hand? Second, is the expert sufficiently qualified to render the opinion? During the last century, three watershed events—a federal court decision in 1923, a federal enactment taking effect in 1975, and a federal court decision in 1993—provided basic answers to these questions.

Since 1923, a decision from the U.S. Court of Appeals for the District of Columbia in *Frye v. United States*, 293 F. 1013, has provided the most recognized standard for admissibility of expert evidence and testimony. Refusing to admit the results of a "lie detector" test, the court wrote, "just when a scientific principle or discovery crosses the line between the experimental and demonstrable stages is difficult to define. Somewhere in this twilight zone the evidential force of the principle must be recognized, and while courts will go a long way in admitting expert testimony deduced from a well-recognized scientific principle or discovery, the thing from which the deduction is made must be sufficiently established to have gained general acceptance in the particular field in which it belongs." By the early 1970s, *Frye* had been approved in the federal courts and in 46 states.

Since 1975, Rules 403 and 701 through 706 of the Federal Rules of Evidence (FRE) have provided an alternative touchstone for determining the admissibility of expert testimony. In 2002, 41 states patterned their evidence codes directly after the Federal Rules. Revised FRE 702 states, "if scientific, technical, or other specialized knowledge will assist the trier of fact to understand the evidence or to determine a fact in issue, a witness qualified as an expert by knowledge, skill, experience, training, or education may testify in the form of an opinion or otherwise, if (1) the testimony is based upon sufficient facts or data, (2) the testimony is the product of reliable principles and methods, and (3) the witness has applied the principles and methods reliably to the facts of the case." By contrast, Revised FRE 701 states, "if the witness is not testifying as an expert, the witness' testimony in the form of opinions or inferences is limited to those opinions or inferences which are (a) rationally based on the perception of the witness and (b) helpful to a clear understanding of the witness' testimony or the determination of a fact in issue, and (c) not based on scientific, technical or other specialized knowledge."

Revised FRE 703 states, "the facts or data in the particular case upon which an expert bases an opinion or inference may be those perceived by or made known to the expert at or before the hearing. If of a type reasonably relied upon by experts in the particular field in forming opinions or inferences upon the subject, the facts or data need not be admissible in evidence in order for the opinion or inference to be admitted. Facts or data that are otherwise inadmissible shall not be disclosed to the jury by the proponent of the opinion or inference unless the court determines that their probative value in assisting the jury to evaluate the expert's opinion substantially outweighs their prejudicial effect."

FRE 704 states, "(a) except as provided in subdivision (b), testimony in the form of an opinion or inference otherwise admissible is not objectionable because it embraces an ultimate issue to be decided by the trier of fact; (b) no expert witness testifying with respect to the mental state or condition of a defendant in a criminal case may state an opinion or inference as to whether the defendant did or did not have the mental state or condition constituting an element of the crime charged or of a defense thereto. Such ultimate issues are matters for the trier of fact alone." (Importantly, FRE 704 does not permit expert witnesses to offer legal conclusions or to directly express opinions about the credibility of other witnesses.)

FRE 705 states, "the expert may testify in terms of an opinion or inference and give reasons therefore without first testifying to the underlying facts or data, unless the court requires otherwise. The expert may in any event be required to disclose the underlying facts or data on cross examination."

FRE 706 states, "the court may on its own motion or on the motion of any party enter an order to show cause why expert witnesses should not be appointed, and may request the parties to submit nominations. The court may appoint any expert witnesses agreed upon by the parties, and may appoint expert witnesses of its own selection. An expert witness shall not be appointed by the court unless the expert witness consents to act. An expert witness so appointed shall be informed of duties by the court in writing or at a conference in which the parties shall have the opportunity to participate. A witness so appointed shall advise the parties of the witness' findings, if any; the witness' deposition may be taken by any party; and the witness may be called to testify by the court or any party. The witness shall be subject to cross-examination by each party, including a party calling the witness."

FRE 403 provides, "although relevant, evidence may be excluded if its probative value is substantially outweighed by the danger of unfair prejudice, confusion of the issues, or misleading the jury, or by considerations of undue delay, waste of time, or needless presentation of cumulative evidence."

In 1993, an opinion from the Supreme Court of the United States in *Daubert v. Merrell Dow Pharmaceuticals, Inc.*, 509 U.S. 579, held that the adoption of the Federal Rules implied the overturn of the *Frye* decision. Importantly, the FRE does not mention the *Frye* test or any need for scientific evidence to be generally accepted. Rather, the FRE replaced the general acceptance test with a validation (reliability) standard derived from the language of FRE 702. According to the *Daubert* court, to be admissible, the expert's testimony must be based on reliable "scientific . . . knowledge." To qualify as *scientific knowledge*, a theory or technique must be validated by the scientific methodology of research and experimentation. However, the approach to scientific knowledge is "flexible," and "its overarching subject is the scientific validity—and thus the evidentiary relevance and reliability—of the principles that underlie a proposed submission." The *Daubert* court also observed that inquiry must be directed to the principles and methodology used by the expert in reaching a conclusion, and not to the conclusion itself.

Factors to be considered in assessing the adequacy (reliability) of the methodology include whether (a) the theory can be falsified by empirical testing, (b) the documentation supporting a theory or technique has been peer reviewed and published, (c) a known or potential rate of error has been determined, and (d) the theory or technique is accepted in the relevant scientific community. Regarding the modern role of the general acceptance test in determining the reliability of evidence, the *Daubert* court stated, "a reliability assessment does not require, although it does permit, explicit identification of a relevant scientific community and an express determination of a particular degree of acceptance within that community." Widespread acceptance can be an important factor in ruling evidence admissible. A technique that attracts only minimal support within the community may properly be viewed with skepticism.

Standards governing the role of the toxicologist as "expert" most likely will continue to evolve from *Frye*, *Daubert*, and the FRE. Currently, federal courts must rely on the FRE and the teachings of *Daubert*, with "general acceptance" providing only one of several factors to be considered in determining admissibility. For example, in *Kumho Tire Co. v. Carmichael*, 526 U.S. 137 (1999), the Supreme Court stated that the factors enunciated in *Daubert* are not exhaustive and do not necessarily apply in every case. The *Kumho* court also said that "whether *Daubert's* specific factors are, or are not, reasonable measures of reliability in a particular case is a matter that the law grants the trial judge broad latitude to determine."

Predictions of the demise of the *Frye* "general acceptance" test have yet to be realized. As of 2002, state courts in at least 17 jurisdictions (Alabama, Arizona, California, Colorado, Florida, Illinois, Kansas, Maryland, Michigan, Minnesota, Mississippi, Missouri, Nevada, New Jersey, New York, Pennsylvania, and Washington) remain committed to *Frye*. Importantly, 75% of these jurisdictions fall within the 25 most populated states, and most fall within the 25 most litigious states. Consequently, most state trials are conducted in *Frye* jurisdictions that may or may not recognize or incorporate *Daubert indicia* (factors) of validity and reliability.

In retaining the "general acceptance" standard, some state supreme courts have refused to follow *Daubert*. Proffered explanations include (a) simple coincidence with random distribution of case outcomes; (b) lack of perceived need, especially in more populous states, to follow the lead of federal courts; (c) satisfaction with the status quo; (d) desire to prevent "inappropriate relaxation" of the standards for introducing scientific testimony; (e) perception that *Frye* "general acceptance" is a more rigorous, cautious, conservative, or higher standard than the more liberal, lenient, or relaxed standard of "validity-reliability" of *Daubert*; and (f) perception that the *Daubert* standard requires judges to make scientific judgments that exceed their competence.

Critics of *Frye*, however, maintain that the scope of application of the "general acceptance" standard is severely limited in many states. These critics argue that *Frye* applies (and often is applied) only to novel theories and techniques of "hard science" and does not permit scrutiny of traditional techniques, "soft science," and nonscientific expertise. By contrast, most *Daubert* courts must examine all types of expert testimony, especially after *Kumho* made it clear that whether the proponent characterizes the proffered expertise as scientific, technical, or specialized, the proponent nevertheless must demonstrate the reliability of the expertise.

Critics of *Frye* also maintain that most trial judges can and do marshall the resources needed to increase their competence and confidence in performing the "gatekeeping" responsibilities mandated by the *Daubert* decision. Judges can appoint experts under FRE 706, use the "special masters" under Rule 53 of the Federal Rules of Civil Procedure, use the Federal Judicial Center's *Reference Manual on Scientific Evidence*, 2nd ed. (2000), and attend forensic science and continuing legal education courses.

Finally, critics of *Frye* point out that determining whether evidence has gained general acceptance in the appropriate field can depend on whether the "field" is defined narrowly or broadly. Although courts have recognized that *Frye* does not require unanimity of view, courts have not provided functional definitions of "general acceptance." Consequently, a clear standard has not emerged for measuring "general acceptance" in the relevant scientific community.

SUBJECT MATTER OF THE EXPERT'S OPINION

Most American courts insist that three basic requirements be met before an individual is permitted to offer testimony as an "expert" witness. First, the testimony must be composed of scientific, technical, or other specialized knowledge. Second, the testimony must assist the fact finder in understanding the evidence or in resolving a factual dispute in the case. Third, the witness must be qualified to render the opinion.

Regarding scientific knowledge, the *Daubert* court explained that "the adjective 'scientific' implies a grounding in the methods and procedures of science. Similarly, the word 'knowledge' connotes more than subjective belief or unsupported speculation. The term applies to any body of known facts or to any body of ideas inferred from such facts or accepted as truths on good grounds. Of course, it would be unreasonable to conclude that the subject of scientific testimony must be 'known' to a certainty; arguably, there are no certainties in science. But, in order to qualify as 'scientific knowledge,' an inference or assertion must be derived by the scientific method. Proposed testimony must be supported by appropriate validation (i.e., 'good grounds') based on what is known. In short, the requirement that an expert's testimony pertain to 'scientific knowledge' establishes a standard of evidentiary reliability."

Regarding assistance to the fact finder, the expert's specialized knowledge must be "helpful." Courts do not agree, however, on the meaning of *helpful*. Some courts believe that "[w]here the subject matter is within the knowledge or experience of laypeople, expert testimony is superfluous," and therefore not helpful. Others hold that there is no requirement that expert testimony be "beyond the jury's sphere of knowledge" before that testimony is deemed helpful.

Regarding qualifications, many courts attempt to characterize the nature of an expert's opinion before deciding on admissibility. Opinions offered by physicians, for example, may address causation, diagnosis, treatment, identity, prognosis, standard of care for diagnosis, and standard of care for treatment. Importantly, American courts are split on the issue of whether nonphysicians may testify against physicians regarding diagnosis, treatment, prognosis, or standards of care. Conversely, American courts also are split on the competency of physicians to testify against nonphysician practitioners. By contrast, nonphysicians and physicians are usually permitted to testify regarding causation and identity.

In malpractice cases, most courts do not require physician experts to practice in, or to be board certified in, precisely the same specialty as the defendant practitioner. Furthermore, in jurisdictions that rely on local or statewide standards of care, it is not necessary that an expert actually live and practice in the locale where alleged malpractice occurred. Some courts allow experts to assert knowledge of local practice through professional contacts, whereas others allow experts to assert that national standards of care apply equally in every location.

FOUNDATION OF THE EXPERT'S OPINION

Before enactment of the FRE in 1975, American courts held that the facts underlying an expert opinion had to be *admitted into evidence* before the expert could state an opinion. In jurisdictions that have adopted FRE 703, however, an expert can base an opinion on personal knowledge, on facts made known or admitted into evidence, and on facts that have not been admitted into evidence and that are themselves inadmissible. FRE 703 "is designed to broaden the basis for expert opinions beyond that current in many jurisdictions and to bring the judicial practice into line with the practice of the experts themselves when not in court. Thus a physician in his own practice bases his diagnosis on information from numerous sources and of considerable variety, including statements by patients and relatives, reports and opinions from nurses, technicians, and other doctors, hospital records, and x-rays. Most of them are admissible in evidence, but only with the expenditure of substantial time in producing and examining various authenticating witnesses. The physician makes life-and-death decisions in reliance upon them. His validation, expertly performed and subject to cross-examination, ought to suffice for judicial purposes."

Regarding the level of scrutiny of facts or data "reasonably relied upon," by experts in a particular discipline, "courts have adopted two judicial approaches to Rule 703: one restrictive, one liberal. The more restrictive view requires the trial court to determine not only whether the data are of a type reasonably relied on by experts in the field, but also whether the underlying data are untrustworthy for hearsay or other reasons. The more liberal view . . . allows the expert to base an opinion on data of the type reasonably relied upon by experts in the field without separately determining the trustworthiness of the particular data involved." *In re "Agent Orange" Product Liab. Litig.*, 611 F. Supp. 1223, 1244 (E.D.N.Y. 1985), *aff'd*, 818 F.2d 187 (2d Cir. 1987), *cert. denied*, 487 U.S. 1234 (1988).

In the Agent Orange cases, the court had to determine the trustworthiness of symptom checklists completed by plaintiffs in preparation for litigation. Are these checklists a type of "datum" reasonably relied on in offering conclusions about diagnosis and causation in the fields of toxicology and epidemiology? The court said, "no," such checklists "are not material that experts in this field would reasonably rely upon and so must be excluded under Rule 703." According to Judge Weinstein, "the court may not abdicate its independent responsibilities to decide if the bases meet minimum standards of reliability as a condition of admissibility. If the underlying data is so lacking in probative force and reliability that no reasonable expert could base an opinion on it, an opinion which rests entirely upon it must be excluded."

Toxicologists should understand that modern courts often analyze expert opinions from two perspectives. Under FRE 702, courts determine whether an opinion is derived from scientific knowledge. Under FRE 703, courts determine whether an opinion has an adequate factual foundation. In courts that follow *Daubert*, the critical focus of inquiry is "reliability." By contrast, in courts that follow *Frye*, the focus remains "general acceptance."

The Supreme Court in *Daubert* did not resolve all of the difficult issues regarding admissibility of expert testimony. One unanswered question is "does the validation (reliability) standard apply only to traditional 'scientific' evidence, or does it also apply to other 'technical,' 'specialized,' or 'social science' evidence?" A second question is "does the validation (reliability) standard apply only to the *methodology* underlying the expert's evidence and opinion, or does it also apply to the *reasoning process* used by the expert in extrapolating or drawing inferences from the underlying scientific evidence to reach his or her conclusion?"

In the *Kumho Tire* decision, 526 U.S. 137 (1999), the Supreme Court held that the "reliability" standard does apply to "less scientific" or "nonscientific" evidence. In *General Electric Co. v. Joiner*, 522 U.S. 136 (1997), the Supreme Court held that both methodology and reasoning should be scrutinized. According to the Court, "[n]othing in either Daubert or the [FRE] requires a district court to admit opinion evidence which is connected to existing data only by the *ipse dixit* of the expert. A court may conclude that there is simply too great an analytical gap between the data and the opinion proffered." In other words, reliability and consequent admissibility require a "good fit" between the expert's methodology and conclusion.

In *Downs v. Perstorp Components, Inc.*, No. 00-5507, 01-04-02, a U.S. Court of Appeals approved a federal district court's scrutiny of a toxicologist's methodology and reasoning. In 1995, defendant purchased a chemical product named Rubiflex SI

30690. Plaintiff, who was contracted to deliver the Rubiflex, found that the packaged product was too large for air transport. Defendant's representative suggested repackaging the Rubiflex in smaller containers. During the repackaging, Rubiflex splashed out of the containers and onto plaintiff's arms and face. Plaintiff was told by the defendant's representative that the chemical was safe. Plaintiff experienced neurologic symptoms, and a physician toxicologist diagnosed chemical encephalopathy caused by exposure to Rubiflex.

The federal magistrate judge excluded the toxicologist's testimony, finding it failed to meet the *Daubert* admissibility standard. Although the expert identified Rubiflex as an epoxy and determined that it contained two toxic substances, he did not identify the components of Rubiflex that were responsible for plaintiff's condition. Furthermore, the expert did not know the amount of Rubiflex to which plaintiff was exposed and did not attempt to independently identify what dose of Rubiflex is necessary to cause the conditions he observed in the plaintiff. Also, the expert could not identify scientific literature showing that Rubiflex caused neurologic problems, and he did not conduct testing to determine the potential human toxicity of Rubiflex. Consequently, the appeals court agreed with the lower court that the expert's opinion should not be admitted because his "methodology primarily involved reasoning backwards from [plaintiff's] condition, and through a process of elimination, concluding that Rubiflex must have caused it."

As the twenty-first century unfolds, the toxicologist expert witness still needs to distinguish *Frye* from *Daubert*. *Frye* jurisdictions remain divided on whether the "general acceptance" test applies to technical, specialized, psychological, or other social science types of evidence. *Frye* courts also disagree on whether "general acceptance" applies not only to an expert's general methodologies but also to his or her conclusions.

The future may bring a melding of analytical principles. Recent state appellate decisions suggest a desire by some courts to adopt a "*Frye* plus reliability" standard for admission of some types of scientific evidence. For example, in *Harris v. Cropmate*, 706 N.E.2d 55 (1999), the Illinois Court of Appeals said, "Illinois utilizes a '*Frye* plus reliability' standard for admission of novel scientific evidence . . . in applying the *Frye* standard the trial court must determine that (1) the scientific test is reliable; and (2) the test's reliability is generally accepted in the particular scientific field to which the test belongs." Furthermore, state trial courts "must not delegate their authority to the scientific community . . . in serving as gatekeepers to keep out scientific evidence that constitutes nothing more than 'junk science' or mere speculation, trial courts should constantly be asking, does the proffered witness have sufficient information, based upon the evidence in this case, to render a *reliable* opinion? Courts should remember that they need not—and should not—accept an expert's opinion on the basis of *ipse dixit*, i.e., such a thing is so because I say it is so."

In *DuPont v. Castillo*, the Florida District Court of Appeals said, "it is the function of the court to not permit cases to be resolved on the basis of evidence for which a predicate of reliability has not been established. Reliability is fundamental to issues involved in the admissibility of evidence. . . . Novel scientific evidence must also be shown to be reliable on some basis other than simply that it is the opinion of the witness who seeks to offer the opinion." Finally, in *Slay v. Keller Industries, Inc.*, No. 1001091, Ala. (2001), the Alabama Supreme Court concluded that "mere assertion of belief, without any supporting research, testing, or experiments, cannot qualify as proper scientific testimony under either the 'general acceptance' standard enunciated in *Frye* or the 'scientifically reliable' standard of *Daubert*."

USE OF LITERATURE AS EVIDENCE

Traditionally, learned treatises and articles could not be admitted as substantive evidence because they were viewed as prohibited forms of hearsay. Such literature could be used, however, during cross-examination to impeach or contradict expert testimony. Modern courts typically require that the treatise or article (a) must have been relied on by the expert in reaching his or her conclusions or (b) must be acknowledged by the witness to be an "authoritative source" or a "recognized authority" in the relevant field. Some courts also permit treatises and articles to be used for impeachment even if the witness does not acknowledge the source as a recognized authority, as long as authoritativeness can be established by judicial notice or through testimony of other witnesses. FRE 803(18), which is best read in conjunction with FRE 703 (see Recent Developments in American Law of Experts section), states, "the following are not excluded by the hearsay rule, even though the declarant is available as a witness: (18) Learned Treatises—To the extent called to the attention of an expert witness upon cross-examination or relied upon by him in direct examination, statements contained in published treatises, periodicals, or pamphlets on a subject of history, medicine, or other science or art, established as a reliable authority by the testimony or admission of the witness or by other expert testimony or by judicial notice. If admitted, the statements may be read into evidence but may not be received as exhibits."

In federal and state forums, the proponents of admissibility of medical and scientific literature argue the following points: (a) the author of an article or treatise has no interest in the outcome of a particular case; (b) the peer review process increases the reliability of published opinions or conclusions; (c) treatises may be more "up-to-date" than the testifying expert; (d) attorneys can attempt to prevent confusion, selective presentation, or presentation out of context; and (e) cross-examination is not necessary when a live expert is available to explain the article or treatise.

By contrast, the opponent of admissibility argues the following points: (a) the author is not available for cross-examination, (b) treatises quickly outdate because medical and scientific knowledge changes rapidly, (c) the trier of fact may be unable to understand complex technical passages that may be presented out of context, and (d) literature is unnecessary as substantive evidence when live expert witnesses are available.

CONCLUSION

Toxicologists can make meaningful and significant contributions to legal proceedings. To function effectively, however, the toxicologist must be willing to do the following: (a) dress appropriately; (b) prepare properly and extensively; (c) leave his or her ego at the door; (d) resist the temptation to elaborate, pontificate, or volunteer information; (e) frequently answer "yes," "no," "I don't know," "I don't recall," and "I don't understand the question"; (f) avoid bringing documents unless specifically asked to do so; (g) expect to be verbally "attacked"; (h) think and react calmly under pressure; (i) recognize the "hypothetical" question; (j) avoid overstatement and use of the words *always* and *never*; (k) avoid hasty answers, so as to enable objections; (l) listen to objections carefully; (m) avoid argument with the examiner; (n) refuse to answer if counsel instructs not to answer; (o) appreciate that, in legal forums, one is an expert only if the tribunal so states; (p) ask to review the entirety of a document before answering questions about parts of it; (q) assert the right to read a transcript of testimony before signing it; and (r) use only those methodologies and state only those conclusions that can be defended before peers in the field of toxicology.

SECTION

2

Initial Management of the Poisoned Patient

Richard C. Dart

It used to be simple to treat the poisoned patient because we had little information on specific poisons. We treated whatever manifestations or complications that the patient developed, using our usual methods. Hypotension was treated with intravenous fluids, bradycardia with atropine, and so on. Nearly all patients received decontamination after an ingestion.

If a 2-year-old child was rushed to the emergency department by her anxious parents after ingesting a whole bottle of ampicillin, for example, we dutifully inserted a nasogastric tube (it only took three of us). We were satisfied with the results when lavage returned a pink fluid. The patient was upset during the procedure, of course, but experienced no long-lasting harm. The parents "knew" that we had done everything possible.

At the time of my training, not *that* long ago, gastric lavage was common. Most patients with an ingestion were treated with lavage. While no harm was done in the case just described, it is inconceivable that the patient benefited from the procedure. The potential benefit was so small that the risk of inserting a nasogastric tube into a struggling patient was unsafe and unwise.

The issue of initial management is not trivial. Today, it is unusual for a patient to die from acute poisoning after reaching medical care. Of those deaths that occur, however, most do so promptly, within hours or a day. A disturbing number of these patients die from unmanaged or mismanaged airway challenges. The resources needed to manage the airway, not to mention intravenous lines; perform decontamination; and perform other activities are substantial. Each procedure is accompanied by the unavoidable possibility of adverse events. In short, all interventions demand a careful risk-benefit analysis.

The challenge is that the study of acute care interventions is very complex, demanding, and rarely leads to definitive answers. These events unfold quickly, involve multiple confounding events, and include disparate patient groups. It is often impossible for one institution to enroll enough patients for a study. Often, a large group of diverse patients is enrolled to create enough statistical power to impress the future journal reviewer. The result is a data set that is less than optimal and often lacks external validity. Nevertheless, the temptation is to extrapolate the results to another group or to subgroups (e.g., applying the decontamination considerations involved in a salicylate overdose to a tricyclic antidepressant overdose). This is unwise. While patients in both groups can and have died from a poorly managed airway, the treatment is very different.

Studies of toxicology interventions typically lack extramural funding: they require "sweat equity." Most toxicologists have committed to such projects at one time or another, revealing the impressive levels of commitment and tenacity that characterize the toxicology community. The problem remains; however, most studies of poisoning lack the resources to enroll large numbers of patients and to focus on a specific problem. There are rarely stakeholders with the financial resources to support large well-designed multicenter trials.

The result has been heroic attempts that provide tantalizing hints but fall short of answering our questions. The story of gastrointestinal decontamination is an excellent example. Several large studies have been performed, typically supported by the home institution and the passion of the research team. Each of the studies made important contributions. However, in their frustrating search for data to help their patients, toxicologists have often extrapolated this information to many different patient groups, willing to overlook the limitations of the studies available. Each of the studies was underpowered in terms of extrapolation attempted. For example, there were too few patients with tricyclic antidepressant or aspirin or cardiac medications enrolled to determine decontamination specific to those groups. Each study also enrolled heterogeneous patient groups. To increase patient numbers at a single site study, wide age groups were used and diverse types of poisons were lumped together. In the assessment of outcome, the old were the same as the young, and the ibuprofen or alcohol ingestion was essentially equivalent to a tricyclic antidepressant. While the methodology of these studies was generally good, evaluation of subgroups was impossible without substantial financial support.

Numerous extrapolations have been performed with the data from these studies, usually by individuals not involved in the study. The primary lesson is that more complete studies that focus on individual agents or at least on individual drug classes are needed. We will not really know how to decontaminate the patient with tricyclic antidepressant, salicylate, or any other potentially lethal intoxication until we have large studies focusing just on the patient with salicylate poisoning. Even then, we would likely need to differentiate certain types of ingestions (acute vs. repeated dose, adult vs. pediatric, mild vs. severe poisoning).

The good news from these studies is that the medical community came to recognize that, for most poisoned patients, decontamination did not have a favorable risk-benefit analysis. Today, we are confident in observing a patient who has ingested a relatively innocuous agent, such as ampicillin (after confirming the history and assuring that no unexpected symptoms or signs are present). This in itself is a significant achievement.

Similar issues bedevil other aspects of early management of the poisoned patient. Are there special considerations in resuscitation of cardiac arrest? Undoubtedly there are, but we do not have the data to know what these will be.

It must be stated plainly: Our efforts at understanding poisoning must be focused and specific to the agent. Whether it be a case report or a multicenter trial, the data produced by our efforts will be limited by the numbers and types of patients that we study. In the world of toxicology, a world limited by insufficient information, a case report with careless documentation of the agent, or a trial extrapolated inappropriately, can change patient management nationwide. To settle for less compromises the care of current patients as well as future patients.

CHAPTER 6

Initial Diagnosis and Treatment of the Poisoned Patient

Daniel C. Keyes and Richard C. Dart

OVERVIEW

Treatment of the acutely poisoned patient requires the integration of multiple aspects of the medical sciences and a broad view of patient care. Perhaps more than other fields, toxicology requires a working knowledge of basic human pharmacology and pathophysiology. It is essential that the clinician apply a thorough approach, including diseases both within and outside of the realm of toxicology.

REGIONAL POISON CENTER

Regional poison centers provide information and advice on the management of a wide variety of poisonings. A network of poison centers exists throughout North America, Northern and Southern Europe, Australia, and New Zealand as well as other regions of the world, providing an important clinical resource. Poison centers in all countries accept calls from health professionals; however, only some countries have the resources to accept calls from patients as well. The typical poison center staff includes nurses or pharmacists trained in providing poison information and advice on toxic exposure. If a patient is referred to a hospital emergency department (ED), the receiving institution receives information about the impending arrival and advice on how to proceed with treatment. Many poison centers also offer the advice of physicians trained in the field of medical toxicology when the complexity of a case merits such consultation. This is a requirement for certified poison centers in the United States. Contact information for poison(s) centers around the world is provided in Appendix V.

DIAGNOSIS

Differential Diagnosis

Many patients have no apparent toxic effects on presentation, even if a toxic agent has been ingested. Others may have findings, but the identity of the toxic agent is unclear. For example, clinical findings may be consistent with infectious, inflammatory, neoplastic, or traumatic origin.

It is often difficult to obtain a reliable history from the poisoned patient. When the patient is coherent, one should interview the patient for the identity and quantity of the drugs ingested, the time of ingestion, and the motive behind the actions. The family or emergency medical services personnel should bring in all medication bottles, paraphernalia, or other containers at the scene. Sending a family member or emergency medical services personnel back to obtain these items at the scene can be extremely useful in selected cases.

A patient who presents with altered mentation is at risk for a variety of life-threatening disorders in addition to poisoning. The proximate cause of death in the intoxicated patient is often trauma. The initial evaluation of the altered patient should therefore include a thorough survey for head injury and other causes of confusion or coma.

A toxidrome is a collection of physical signs that help narrow the diagnosis and identify a type of poison (Table 1). However, toxidromes are often not present, even in patients who truly have been poisoned. The most useful toxidromes are the opioid, the anticholinergic (Chapter 10), the cholinergic (Chapter 13), and the sympathomimetic toxidromes.

Signs and Symptoms

The assessment of the overdose patient requires a systematic evaluation of the vital signs, neurologic function, cardiopulmonary status, abdominal examination, as well as autonomic nervous system signs (dry or moist skin, lacrimation, salivation, and so forth). In an unstable patient, the examination should occur simultaneously with basic supportive interventions: airway, breathing, and circulation.

Vital Signs

The *respiratory rate* is the sign most commonly affected in poisoning. Bradypnea and apnea are usually caused by opioid or sedative-hypnotic medications. Tachypnea and hyperpnea may be difficult to identify clinically. These are most commonly associated with a stimulant drug, underlying hypoxia, or metabolic acidosis. *Hypotension* is caused by myocardial depression,

TABLE 1. Examples of drugs causing toxidromes

Toxidrome	Drugs causing	Manifestations	Chapter
Sympathomimetic	**Direct acting** β-adrenergic agonists (e.g., albuterol, terbutaline) α-adrenergic agonists (e.g., ergot alkaloids, phenylephrine) Predominantly α_1-adrenergic agonists Ephedrine Mephentermine Phenylpropanolamine Pseudoephedrine Inhibitors of norepinephrine uptake Cyclic antidepressants MAO inhibitors Phenelzine Selegiline Tranylcypromine Pargyline Pemoline **Mixed acting** Dopamine Predominantly α_2-adrenergic agonists Yohimbine **Indirect acting** Amphetamines Cocaine Fenfluramine	Increased bowel sounds Moist skin Dilated pupils Tachycardia Hypertension Tachypnea Fever	NA
Anticholinergic	Antidepressants (e.g., tricyclics: amitriptyline, amoxapine, desipramine, doxepin, imipramine, maprotiline, nortriptyline) Antihistamines Antiparkinsonian agents (e.g., carbidopa) Antipsychotics (e.g., phenothiazine) Diphenhydramine Orphenadrine Pemoline Propantheline Trihexyphenidyl Baclofen Benztropine	Decreased bowel sounds Dry skin Dilated pupils Tachycardia Hypertension Tachypnea Fever	10
Cholinergic	Carbamates Organophosphates Pilocarpine	—	13
Opiate	Typical opiates (e.g., morphine, heroin) Atypical opiates Dextromethorphan Pentazocine Propoxyphene	—	NA
Sedative-hypnotic	Opiates Antipsychotics Barbiturates Benzodiazepines Ethanol Meprobamate Methadone Ethchlorvynol Methocarbamol Quinazolines	—	NA
Hallucinogenic/psychedelic	Amphetamines Cannabinoids Indole alkaloids Phencylidine (Mixed effects)	—	19

MAO, monoamine oxidase; NA, not applicable.
Adapted from Rudis MI, Keyes C. Toxic syndromes. In: Aghababian RV, Keyes DC, eds. *Emergency medicine: the core curriculum.* Philadelphia: Lippincott–Raven, 1998.

peripheral vasodilation, or extravascular loss of fluid. Hypertension and hypotension can each be caused by a wide variety of agents (Chapters 36 and 37).

Hyperthermia and *hypothermia* are addressed in Chapter 38. The mechanisms of drug-induced fever and hyperthermic syndromes are varied (Tables 2 and 3) (1,2). In patients experiencing drug-induced fever, temperatures typically range from 39° to 40.6°C. The patient may appear deceptively well. Drug-induced fever can be associated with low-grade eosinophilia and maculopapular rash. Fever usu-

TABLE 2. Drugs that may cause fever, grouped by postulated mechanism[a]

Postulated mechanism	Commonly cause fever	Occasionally cause fever
Hypersensitivity reaction	Methyldopa Penicillins Procainamide	Allopurinol Azathioprine Cephalosporins Hydralazine Iodides Isoniazid Nitrofurantoin Aminosalicylate sodium Rifampin Streptomycin sulfate
Idiosyncratic reaction	Halothane Quinine sulfate Sulfonamides Quinidine Primaquine phosphate	
Administration-related reaction	Amphotericin B Bleomycin sulfate	Streptokinase Vancomycin Cephalosporins Pentazocine Paraldehyde
Pharmacologic action	Antineoplastics Antibiotics[b]	
Altered thermoregulation	Cocaine (abuse) Amphetamines (abuse) Atropine sulfate Antihistamines Levothyroxine sodium	Cimetidine Amphetamines (therapeutic)
Unknown	Phenytoin sodium Salicylates Barbiturates	

[a]Some drugs may cause fever by more than one mechanism.
[b]During treatment of spirochetal disease.
Adapted from Lipsky BA, Hirschmann JV. Drug fever. *JAMA* 1981;245(8):851–854.

ally normalizes within 48 to 72 hours. Dobutamine should be considered as a cause of fever in patients being treated for heart failure (3).

Head, Ears, Eyes, Nose, and Throat

Miosis is usually caused by opiates, cholinesterase inhibitors, or topical miotic agents, or from pontine hemorrhage or infarct. *Papilledema* suggests vitamin A toxicity, severe chronic lead poisoning, methanol toxicity, or a nontoxicologic cause of intracranial hypertension. *Ptosis* may reveal botulism, diphtheria, phenytoin, thallium, neurotoxic snake venom, or Wernicke-Korsakoff syndrome.

Acute and transient *tinnitus* and *hearing loss* are associated with diuretics and antiinflammatory agents (e.g., salicylates). Some antineoplastic agents and aminoglycoside antibiotics are associated with delayed and often irreversible loss of hearing. Drug-associated causes of tinnitus and deafness occurring in the same patient can include erythromycin, aspirin, gentamicin, cisplatin, metronidazole, and naproxen. Deafness without tinnitus is occasionally observed after use of erythromycin, gentamicin, cisplatin, furosemide, metronidazole, and azithromycin. Tinnitus is more common with aspirin, quinine, indomethacin, sulindac, metoprolol, naproxen, and procaine penicillin (4,5).

Skin

Skin *bullae* are rare, usually associated with prolonged coma caused by barbiturates, carbon monoxide, baclofen, or other central nervous system depressants. *Central cyanosis* is classically caused by methemoglobinemia (Chapter 21) but may be observed under a variety of clinical conditions, especially those with cardiovascular depression from a variety of causes. Dermal erythema is caused by anticholinergic agents, niacin, boric acid, vancomycin, and carbon monoxide (postmortem).

Extravasation of some medications can cause severe injury (Chapter 16). Other skin effects include *toxic epidermal necrolysis*, which has been associated with butazones, hydantoins, sulfonamides, barbiturates, antibiotics, and many others (6). Pemphigus may occur secondary to penicillamine, captopril, pyritinol, tiopronin, penicillin, rifampin, pyrazolone compounds, beta-blockers, progesterone, heroin, piroxicam, levodopa, lysine acetyl salicylate, gold, phenobarbital, cephalexin, enalapril, pentachlorophenol, phosphatide, and hydantoin/barbiturate. The incidence of pemphigus with these agents is rare, considering their widespread use (7).

Hair

Hair loss, without other major signs, that develops 2 to 4 months after beginning treatment can be caused by anticoagulants, retinol and its derivatives, interferons, and antihyperlipidemic drugs. Such loss is usually reversible on the interruption of treatment. *Hirsutism* may follow use of testosterone, danazol, corticotropin, metyrapone, anabolic steroids, and glucocorticoids. *Hypertrichosis* is observed after use of cyclosporine, minoxidil, and diazoxide.

Cardiovascular System

Electrocardiogram (ECG) abnormalities are often extremely important findings. A prolonged QRS duration or unexpected ECG right axis deviation is most often caused by blockade of the myocardial fast sodium channel (tricyclic antidepressants, phenothiazines, diphenhydramine, cocaine, others) as well as beta receptor–blocking drugs, anticholinergic drugs, cardiac glycosides, or hypokalemia. A variety of drugs cause cardiac rhythm disturbances (Table 4) (8).

A *prolonged QTc interval* can occur in poisoning from amiodarone, some antihistamines, type 1 antidysrhythmic agents, arsenic, tricyclic antidepressant, fluoride, organophosphates, quinidine, procainamide, propoxyphene, thioridazine and other phenothiazines, hypokalemia, hypomagnesemia, or hypocalcemia. The main risk associated with prolonged QTc is atypical ventricular tachycardia, known as *torsade de pointes*. This rhythm is most commonly caused by the class IA or class III antidysrhythmic drugs, or related drugs. Online registries of drugs that cause prolonged QT interval or torsade de pointes are available (http://www.Torsades.org). The frequency of sudden death from cardiac arrest may be increased by the use of antipsychotic drugs (9). Atrioventricular delay (2° and 3° heart block) may be caused by cardiac glycosides, beta-receptor blockade, and calcium-channel blockers, class I antidysrhythmic agents (procainamide, quinidine), organophosphates, cocaine, clonidine, phenytoin, neuroleptic agents, and cyclic antidepressants (10).

The diagnosis of *hypersensitivity myocarditis* should be considered when new ECG changes, mildly elevated cardiac enzyme levels, cardiomegaly, or unexplained tachycardia is noted in a

TABLE 3. Drug-induced central hyperthermic syndromes

Condition (and mechanism)	Common drug causes	Frequent symptoms	Possible treatment[a]	Clinical course
Hyperthermia (↓ heat dissipation, ↑ heat production)	Atropine Lidocaine Meperidine Nonsteroidal antiinflammatory drug Pheochromocytoma Stimulants Thyrotoxicosis	Hyperthermia, diaphoresis, malaise	Diazepam for agitation or seizure (Chapter 40)	Benign, febrile seizures in children
Malignant hyperthermia (↑ heat production)	Neuromuscular junction blocker (succinylcholine) Halothane (1:50,000)	Hyperthermia Muscle rigidity Dysrhythmias Ischemia[b] Hypotension Rhabdomyolysis Disseminated intravascular coagulation	Dantrolene sodium	Familial 10% mortality if untreated
Tricyclic antidepressant overdose (↑ heat production)	Tricyclic antidepressants	Hyperthermia Confusion Hallucinations Agitation Hyperreflexia Muscle relaxation Anticholinergic effects Dysrhythmias	Sodium bicarbonate (Chapter 75)	Fatalities have occurred if untreated
Autonomic hyperpyrexia (↑ heat production)	Central nervous system stimulants (amphetamines)	Hyperthermia Excitement Hyperreflexia	Lorazepam (Chapter 39)	Reversible High mortality if untreated
Lethal catatonia (↓ heat dissipation)	Lead poisoning	Hyperthermia Intense anxiety Destructive behavior Psychosis		
Neuroleptic malignant syndrome (mixed: hypothalamic, ↑ heat dissipation, ↑ heat production)	Antipsychotics (neuroleptics) Alpha-methyldopamine Reserpine	Hyperthermia Muscle rigidity Diaphoresis Leukocytosis Delirium Rhabdomyolysis Elevated creatine kinase Extrapyramidal symptoms	Bromocriptine Sinemet [carbidopa/levodopa (25/100)] (Chapter 23)	Rapid onset 20% mortality if untreated

[a]Gastric lavage and supportive measures, including cooling, are required in most cases.
[b]Oxygen consumption increases by 7% for every 1°F increase in body temperature.
Adapted from Theoharides TC, Harris RS, Weckstein D. Neuroleptic malignant-like syndrome due to cyclobenzaprine? *J Clin Psychopharmacol* 1995;15(1):79–81.

patient who has an ongoing allergic reaction to a drug, usually with eosinophilia (11).

Respiratory System

The lung can be injured following acute or chronic exposure. *Acute lung injury and persistent progressive lung disease* are addressed in Chapters 27 and 28.

Gastrointestinal Tract and Liver

Medication-induced *esophageal injury* has followed the use of tetracycline, doxycycline, ipratropium bromide, slow-release potassium chloride, acetylsalicylic acid, nonsteroidal antiinflammatory drugs, and quinidine (Table 5). Sudden dysphagia, substernal chest pain, and odynophagia typically occur 4 to 12 hours after ingestion but may be delayed up to several weeks in quinidine-induced cases (12,13).

Drugs can cause *acute pancreatitis*, but, with the exception of ethanol, they rarely cause chronic pancreatitis. Reports of acute pancreatitis are generally anecdotal (Table 6) (14).

The liver is involved in the metabolism and clearance of many drugs. An astonishing array of drugs are capable of causing *acute liver failure*, which is understandable given the importance of the liver in the metabolism and elimination of toxins (Chapter 17).

Kidney and Bladder

Renal injury is induced by a wide variety of agents, including drugs, chemicals, plants, and venoms. Drugs that result in kidney injury when given in excessive dose are summarized in Table 7. Drugs that have been associated with a *hemolytic uremic syndrome* include cyclosporine, anticancer drugs (e.g., mitomycin), ticlopidine, and quinine (15).

Urinary retention is typically caused by anticholinergics, analgesics, and some anesthetics, largely because of decreased

TABLE 4. Rhythm disturbance induced by drugs

Rhythm disturbance	Possible cause
Sinus bradycardia or atrioventricular block	Beta-blockers, calcium antagonists, cyclic antidepressants, digoxin and other cardiac glycosides, organophosphate or carbamate insecticides, phenylpropanolamine, and other α-adrenergic stimulants
Sinus tachycardia	Cocaine, amphetamines, phencyclidine, antihistamines, anticholinergics, cyclic antidepressants, phenothiazines, theophylline, ethanol or sedative-hypnotic withdrawal, carbon monoxide
Prolongation of QRS interval	Cyclic antidepressants, quinidine, procainamide, disopyramide, encainide, flecainide, beta-blockers, calcium antagonists, diphenhydramine (massive dose), phenothiazine (especially thioridazine)
Prolongation of QT interval (including torsade de pointes)	Cyclic antidepressants; quinidine; procainamide; disopyramide; encainide; flecainide; beta-blockers; calcium antagonists; lithium; antihistamines (diphenhydramine, terfenadine, astemizole); phenothiazine; sotalol; dofetilide; pentamidine; cisapride; arsenic; organophosphates
Ventricular tachycardia	Cocaine, amphetamines, chloral hydrate and chlorinated hydrocarbons, theophylline, digoxin and other cardiac glycosides, tricyclic antidepressants

Adapted from Olson KR, Pentel PR, Kelley MT. Physical assessment and differential diagnosis of the poisoned patient. *Med Toxicol* 1987;2(1):52–81.

bladder tone and sphincter contraction. The risk of retention is especially great in men due to prostatic hypertrophy. α-adrenergic blockers may cause decreased sphincter resistance and incontinence (16).

TABLE 5. Drugs that induce esophageal injury

Lower esophageal sphincter tone

- α-adrenergic antagonists
  - Phentolamine
- Anticholinergic agents
  - Atropine, belladonna tincture, dicyclomine, flavoxate, methantheline, oxybutynin, propantheline
- Benzodiazepines
  - Diazepam
- β-adrenergic agonists
  - Caffeine, carbuterol, isoproterenol
- Calcium channel–blocking agents
  - Nifedipine, verapamil
- Dopamine
- Ethanol
- Glucagon
- Narcotic analgesics
  - Meperidine, morphine
- Prostaglandins E_1, E_2, A_2
- Theophylline

Irritate esophageal mucosa

- Captopril
- Chlorazepate
- Clindamycin
- Digoxin
- Ferrous sulfate
- Lincomycin
- Nonsteroidal antiinflammatory drugs
  - Aspirin, ibuprofen, indomethacin, ketoprofen, phenylbutazone, piroxicam
- Penicillin
- Potassium chloride
- Quinidine
- Tetracyclines
  - Doxycycline, tetracycline
- Trimethoprim-sulfamethoxazole
- Vitamin C

From Lee M, Sharfi R. Oxybutynin-induced reflux esophagitis. *DICP Ann Pharmacother* 1990;34:583–585, with permission.

TABLE 6. Drugs associated with acute pancreatitis[a]

Definite association

- Asparaginase
- Azathioprine
- Didanosine
- Estrogens
- Furosemide
- Mercaptopurine
- Pentamidine
- Sulfonamides
- Sulindac
- Tetracyclines
- Thiazides
- Valproic acid

Probable association

- Bumetanide
- Chlorthalidone
- Cimetidine
- Clozapine
- Corticosteroids
- Corticotropin
- Endoscopic retrograde cholangiopancreatography media
- Ethacrynic acid
- Methyldopa
- Metronidazole
- Salicylates
- Sulfasalazine
- Zalcitabine

Questionable association

- Acetaminophen
- Amiodarone
- Ampicillin
- Anticholinesterases
- Carbamazepine
- Cisplatin
- Colchicine
- Cyclosporine
- Cytarabine
- Diazoxide
- Diphenoxylate
- Enalapril
- Ergotamine
- Erythromycin
- Gold compounds
- Interleukin-2
- Isotretinoin
- Ketoprofen
- Lisinopril
- Mefenamic acid
- Metolazone
- Nitrofurantoin
- Octreotide
- Oxyphenbutazone
- Phenformin
- Phenolphthalein
- Piroxicam
- Potassium permanganate
- Procainamide
- Ranitidine
- Roxithromycin
- Tryptophan

[a]Association is considered definite if pancreatitis developed during exposure to the agent, disappeared after withdrawal, and recurred after rechallenge. Association is considered probable if an association is thought to exist, but the three criteria previously mentioned were not all met. Association is considered questionable if published evidence is inadequate or contradictory.
Adapted from Underwood TW, Frye CB. Drug-induced pancreatitis. *Clin Pharm* 1993;12(6):440–448.

Musculoskeletal System

Rhabdomyolysis is addressed in Chapter 29. A *myopathy* can also develop following electrolyte disturbances, muscle compression, ischemia, or autoimmune reactions (17). Repeated injections of antibiotics or drugs of abuse can lead to severe muscle fibrosis and contractures. Clofibrate and ε-aminocaproic acid cause an acute or subacute painful necrotizing myopathy with myoglobinuria and acute renal failure. Other drugs associated with myopathy include lipid-lowering agents, succinylcholine, halothane, corticosteroids, and chloroquine. Drugs that cause a hypokalemic myopathy include the thiazide diuretics, amphotericin, carbenoxolone, emetine, and alcohol. Inflammatory myopathies have followed use of D-penicillamine, procainamide, hydralazine, phenytoin, and penicillin.

Agents associated with *myositis* include foods (adulterated rapeseed oil, L-tryptophan, ciguatera toxin), occupational exposures (silica), and medical devices (collagen implants).

Nervous System

Signs and symptoms relative to individual drugs are described in Table 8. Toxic disorders associated with reversible dementias are listed in Table 9.

TABLE 7. Nephrotoxicity resulting from drugs given in excessive dose

Renal lesion	Drug	Circumstance
Acute interstitial nephritis	Chlorprothixene	Suicide
Acute tubular necrosis	Acetaminophen	Suicide
	Aspirin	Suicide
	Boric acid	Diaper rash
	Bismuth salts	Taken for warts
	Colchicine	Suicide
	Lead	Contaminant of illicit drug
	Nomifensine	Suicide
	Pennyroyal oil	Attempted abortion
	Paraldehyde	Drug overdose
	Triamterene	Suicide
	Uranium	Clinical investigation
Chronic glomerulonephritis	Heroin	Narcotic addiction
	Pentazocine	Narcotic addiction
Chronic interstitial nephritis (analgesic nephropathy)	Nonsteroidal anti-inflammatory drug	Analgesic abuse
Hypercalcemia	Vitamin A	Acne treatment
	Vitamin D	Hypoparathyroidism and metabolic bone disease
Myoglobinuric tubular necrosis	Amoxapine	Suicide
	Amphetamines	Drug overdose
	Barbiturates	Drug overdose
	Cocaine	Drug overdose
	Diazepam	Drug overdose
	Doxepin	Suicide
	Ethanol	Alcoholism
	Glutethimide	Drug overdose
	Heroin	Drug overdose
	Methadone	Drug overdose
	Phencyclidine	Drug overdose
	Phenylpropanolamine	Weight loss, drug overdose
	Strychnine	Mistaken for cocaine
Necrotizing vasculitis	Methamphetamine	Drug overdose
Obstruction (stones)	Magnesium antacid	Antacid abuse
Osmotic nephrosis	Mannitol	Excessive dose
Oxalosis	Intravenous vitamin C	Excessive dose

Adapted from Abuelo JG. Renal failure caused by chemicals, foods, plants, animal venoms, and misuse of drugs. An overview. *Arch Intern Med* 1990;150(3):505–510.

TABLE 8. Drug-induced mental changes

Drug	Clinical state	Physical signs
Amphetamines	Agitation Aggression Paranoia Hallucinations	Pyrexia Hypertension Tachycardia Dysrhythmias Dilated pupils Tremor Convulsions
Barbiturates	Stupor Coma	Hypothermia Hypotension Pupils reactive Oculocephalic reflex absent Apnea Bullous lesions
Benzodiazepines	Stupor, rarely unarousable	Little respiratory depression
Insulin	Stupor Coma	Pallor and sweating Tachycardia Dilated pupils Hyperreflexia and extensor plantar responses
Opiates	Stupor Coma	Hypotension Respiration depression Pulmonary edema Skin cool and moist Pinpoint pupils (but reactive) Fasciculation
Phenothiazines	Drowsiness Coma	Hypotension Dysrhythmias Dystonia
Tricyclic antidepressants	Drowsiness Delirium Coma	Hypotension Dysrhythmias Dilated pupils Warm, dry skin Hyperreflexia and extensor plantar responses Urinary retention Paralytic ileus

Adapted from Morrow JI, Routledge PA. Drug-induced neurological disorders. *Adverse Drug React Acute Poisoning Rev* 1988;7(3):105–133.

The existence of pupillary light reflex, motor response to pain, or spontaneous eye movements is suggestive of a good prognosis from hypoxic-ischemic coma (18), although this has not been verified in overdose. Normally, the eyes follow movement of the head. Loss of cortical influence allows the eyes to move like doll's eyes: opposite the direction of motion. When destruction of the ocular nuclei in the *pons* occurs, the eyes become fixed. Suppression of the medial longitudinal fasciculus produces a dysconjugate ocular response characterized by tonic abduction of the ipsilateral eye and impaired adduction of the contralateral eye. This *internuclear ophthalmoplegia* was present in 10% of one series of toxin-induced coma usually with multiple drug ingestions (19). The drugs most often associated with internuclear ophthalmoplegia are barbiturates, benzodiazepines, phenothiazines, and phenytoin. This sign does not have prognostic value.

The appropriate response to pain is motor activity that localizes to the site of stimulation. The decorticate response is a flexion of elbow and extension of the knee, which occurs in the late diencephalic phase. Midbrain dysfunction produces the decerebrate response: the motor response of extension of both elbow and knee during painful stimulation. Higher flexor responses occur with the arms flexed, whereas initial arm extension and supraorbital stimulation yield more extensor responses (20).

Coma is addressed in Chapter 14. Many clinicians consider the Glasgow Coma Scale, originally developed for trauma patients, as inappropriate for acute poisoning. It does not provide prognostic information, as it does in trauma; however, the Glasgow Coma Scale does offer convenient shorthand for describing the patient's condition, particularly if each of the three components are documented separately (Table 10). Other proposed scales include the Reaction Level Scale (21), Comprehensive Level of Consciousness Scale (22), Clinical Neurological Assessment Tool (23), Coma Recovery Scale (24), Glasgow-Liege Scale (25), Innsbruck Coma Scale (26), and Glasgow Outcome Scale (27). Details of these tests and scoring scales have been summarized, but none have become accepted for the evaluation of coma arising from poisoning (28).

Seizures and *status epilepticus* are often caused by poisoning (Chapter 30). In one survey, the leading causes of seizure associated with poisoning were, in descending order, tricyclic antidepressants, cocaine, isoniazid, theophylline, and amphetamines (29).

TABLE 9. Drugs and chemicals associated with reversible dementias

Drug/chemical	Clinical characteristics	Treatment
Major tranquilizers	Chronic confusional state, parkinsonism	Lower dose or discontinue medication
Antidepressants	Chronic confusional state; tremors, anticholinergic effects	Lower dose or discontinue medication
Sedative-hypnotics	Lethargy, confusional state; withdrawal syndrome	Lower dose or discontinue medication (taper dose)
Narcotics	Pupillary constriction, constipation, respiratory depression, sensitivity to low doses in elderly	Lower dose or discontinue; give naloxone for acute condition
Anticholinergic agents	Memory loss, confusional state, psychosis, dilated pupils, dry skin, tachycardia, wide variety of medications involved	Discontinue medication; give physostigmine in acute state
Antihypertensive agents	Psychomotor slowing, depression; use of methyldopa, reserpine, clonidine, propranolol	Switch to other agents for blood pressure control
Anticonvulsants	Sedation from barbiturates, possibly cerebellar signs with phenytoin use, toxic levels	Switch to another drug
Digoxin	Gastrointestinal and cardiac side effects, confusional state	Adjust dose
Antiparkinsonian agents	Use of levodopa, amantadine, bromocriptine; confusional state; psychosis	Reduce medication dose
Antibiotics	Use of penicillin, chloramphenicol; high doses, often decreased clearance in elderly	Adjust dose
Gastrointestinal agents	Chronic confusional state, cimetidine use, possibly extrapyramidal syndrome with metoclopramide	Adjust or discontinue medication
Antineoplastic agents	Asparaginase, intrathecal administration of methotrexate	Discontinue medication
Lead	Encephalopathy, motor neuropathy, headache, seizures, anemia, lead lines	Institute chelation; eliminate exposure
Arsenic	Somnolence; sensory neuropathy; gastrointestinal symptoms; Mees' lines	Institute chelation; eliminate exposure
Organic solvents	Headache, lethargy, poor concentration, peripheral neuropathy	Eliminate exposure
Insecticides	Irritability, forgetfulness, organophosphates	Avoid exposure

Adapted from Mahler ME, Cummings JL, Benson DF. Treatable dementias. *West J Med* 1987;146(6):705–712.

Benign intracranial hypertension (*pseudotumor cerebri*) is a condition characterized by increased cerebrospinal fluid pressure in the absence of a space-occupying lesion and with cerebral ventricles of normal or even reduced size. Most commonly, the patient is a woman with mild or moderate obesity. There may be diffuse cerebral edema. There are no localizing neurologic signs for this disorder. In most cases, the disorder is of unknown cause, but intracranial thrombosis and drugs are believed to be the most common precipitating factors (30). Drugs most often associated with pseudotumor cerebri include tetracycline, minocycline, nifedipine, nalidixic acid, vitamin A and retinoid analogs, co-trimoxazole, cimetidine, atenolol, and glyceryl trinitrate.

TABLE 10. Glasgow Coma Scale

	Assessment	Score
Eyes		
Open	Spontaneously	4
	To verbal command	3
	To pain	2
	No response	1
Best motor response		
To verbal command	Obeys	6
To painful stimulus	Localizes pain	5
	Flexion—withdrawal	4
	Flexion—abnormal (decorticate rigidity)	3
	Extension (decerebrate rigidity)	2
	No response	1
Best verbal response		
	Oriented and converses	5
	Disoriented and converses	4
	Inappropriate words	3
	Incomprehensible sounds	2
	No response	1
Total		3–15

Adapted from Teasdale G, Jeannett B. Assessment of coma impaired consciousness. *Lancet* 1974;2(7872):81–84.

Drug-induced *movement disorders* may occur during the early phase of neuroleptic (antipsychotic, major tranquilizer) administration (Table 11). *Akathisia* is associated with cyclic antidepressants, monoamine oxidase inhibitors, fluoxetine, lithium, buspirone, and levodopa and prochlorperazine (31–33). Withdrawal from neuroleptic agents is also associated with akathisia (34,35).

Dystonias (oculogyric crises, torticollis, tortipelvis, opisthotonus) are associated principally with phenothiazines, butyrophenones, metoclopramide, and tricyclic antidepressants; with phenytoin, carbamazepine, and propranolol in high doses; and with antiemetics, cocaine, chloroquine, and hydroxychloroquine (36,37). *Chorea* is a movement disorder most commonly associated with the anticonvulsant drugs, especially phenytoin, as well as anabolic steroids, amphetamines, methylphenidate, pemoline, cimetidine, levodopa and dopamine, ethanol, toluene, manganese, and cocaine (38,39).

Tardive dyskinesia is the phenomenon of involuntary athetoid and choreoid movements, which typically occur after prolonged neuroleptic therapy. The disorder typically persists even after the discontinuation of the agent. Phenothiazines are the most common cause. Metoclopramide has also been suspected. The atypical antipsychotics, such as olanzapine, appear less likely to cause this syndrome (40). The risk of tardive dyskinesia increases with age and duration of treatment (41).

A *resting tremor* is a repetitive movement that decreases with activity. This type of tremor is most commonly associated with parkinsonism (Table 12) (42,43). *Postural tremor* is most pronounced with an outstretched hand. This is typical of the sym-

TABLE 11. Agents that induce movement disorders

Compound	Manifestation
Amoxapine	Parkinsonism
Amphetamines	Hyperkinetic movements
Antihistamines	Orofacial dystonia Myoclonic jerking
Black widow spider bite	Rigidity
Butyrophenones	Parkinsonism Orofacial dystonia Opisthotonus, trismus
Caffeine	Myoclonic jerking
Carbamazepine	Orofacial dystonia
Carbon monoxide	Parkinsonism
Chloroquine	Tongue protrusion
Cocaine	Jerking, tremor
Ethylene glycol	Myoclonic jerking
Fluoride	Generalized twitching
Ketamine	Tongue protrusion
Lead (tetraethyl)	Jerking, facial grimacing
Levodopa	Facial grimacing, dystonia Head tossing, flinging extremities
Lithium	Hypertonicity, tongue dystonia, lip smacking, tremor
Metaldehyde	Twitching, hyperreflexia
Methaqualone	Rigidity, hypertonicity
Methylphenidate	Motor and verbal tics
Metoclopramide	Parkinsonism
Monoamine oxidase inhibitors	Rigidity, opisthotonus
1-Methyl-4-phenyl-1,2,3,6-tetrahydropyridine	Parkinsonism
Narcotics (sufentanil)	Chest wall rigidity
Nicotine	Fasciculation progressing to flaccidity
Organophosphates	Fasciculation progressing to flaccidity
Pethidine (meperidine)	Tremor, muscle jerking
Phencyclidine	Generalized rigidity, trismus, orofacial dystonias, twitching, athetosis
Phenothiazines	Orofacial and other dystonias
Phenytoin	Choreoathetosis
Strychnine	Rigidity, opisthotonus, trismus
Toluene (chronic)	Ataxia, jerking eye movements
Tricyclic antidepressants	Twitching, myoclonic jerking

TABLE 12. Agents reported to be associated with parkinsonism

Agent	Source
1-Methyl-4-phenyl-1,2,3,6-tetrahydropyridine	Intravenous drug abuse, occupational
Tranquilizers (flunarizine, cinnarizine, haloperidol, chlorpromazine, etc.)	Psychiatric medication
Antidepressants	Psychiatric medication
Lithium	Psychiatric medication
Phenothiazines	Antiemetic
Reserpine	Antihypertensive, psychiatric
Carbon monoxide	Occupational, environmental
Hydrogen cyanide	Occupational
Postanoxic injury	Environmental
Postencephalitic	Arthropod-borne infection
Carbon disulfide	Occupational (viscose rayon)
Paraquat	Herbicide
Manganese	Occupational (welding)
Mercury	Occupational
Cyanide	Dietary, folk medicine (Asia)
Lathyrus	Dietary (Asia, Africa, World War II)
Rural environment: well water?	Environmental
Suspected protective factors	
Cigarette smoking	Lifestyle
Hydrazine	Lifestyle, occupational
Measles	Environmental

Adapted from Goldsmith JR, Herishanu Y, et al. Clustering of Parkinson's disease points to environmental etiology. *Arch Environ Health* 1990;45(2):88–94.

pathomimetics (beta agonists) such as amphetamines and theophylline, and is also seen in alcohol or benzodiazepine withdrawal (44). It is also described with phenytoin, valproic acid, cyclic antidepressants, monosodium glutamate, lithium, and arsenic. *Cerebellar* (*kinetic*) *tremor* is described as "goal-oriented," being most pronounced with motion. This tremor results from alcoholic cerebellar degeneration, mercury, lithium, and sedative-hypnotic intoxication.

There are many causes of tremor (17). Commonly cited examples include 1-methyl-4-phenyl-1,2,3,6-tetrahydropyridine, a byproduct of designer drug synthesis; clebopride; disulfiram; lithium; organophosphates; metoclopramide; phenylpropanolamine; and antihistamines (42,45). The most frequent causes are the phenothiazine or butyrophenone groups and the major tranquilizers. Tremors are well-described and common manifestations of drug use or withdrawal (46).

Autoimmune (*collagen-vascular*) *disorders* are commonly associated with medications. Up to 10% of cases of systemic lupus erythematosus are drug related (47). While procainamide and hydralazine are most commonly implicated, an association has also been shown for isoniazid, methyldopa, quinidine, and chlorpromazine. Drugs less frequently implicated include many of the anticonvulsants, beta-blockers, sulfasalazine, penicillamine, lithium, and antithyroid drugs. Drug-induced systemic lupus erythematosus usually occurs after long-term (6 to 12 months') high-dose therapy with the suspected drug. Clinical manifestations include arthralgia, arthritis, fever, skin rash, adenopathy, myalgia, pericarditis, pleuritis, pleural effusion, hepatosplenomegaly, and renal and central nervous system involvement. Rapid remission follows discontinuation of the drug. However, the antinuclear antibody test may remain positive for up to 2 years (48).

Scleroderma may follow use of carbidopa, mazindol, 1,5-hydroxytryptophan, diethylpropion, pentazocine, local anesthetics, bromocriptine, phytonadione, cocaine, and appetite suppressants.

The *hypersensitivity syndrome* is a severe multiorgan reaction that manifests with fever, rash, lymphadenopathy, eosinophilia, and hepatitis. It was first described in 1988 but has subsequently been described from exposure to a variety of agents (49,50). Phenytoin, carbamazepine, phenobarbital, and sulfonamides are the most frequent causes of the hypersensitivity syndrome. Other drugs in which it has been described include allopurinol, gold salts, and dapsone. The syndrome typically develops 2 to 6 weeks after a drug is first used—later than most other serious skin reactions. With antiepileptic drugs, fever and rash are the most frequent presenting symptoms. Lymphadenopathy is frequent and usually due to benign lymphoid hyperplasia. Atypical lymphoid hyperplasia and pseudolymphoma occasionally occur. Some of these cases resolve with withdrawal of the drug, but in some cases lymphoma develops. Hepatitis, interstitial nephritis, and hematologic abnormalities (especially eosinophilia and mononucleosis-like atypical lymphocytosis) are also common.

Agents most often associated with vasculitis, serum sickness, and reactions resembling serum sickness are listed in Table 13 (51).

TABLE 13. Agents most often associated with vasculitis, serum sickness, and reactions resembling serum sickness

Vasculitis
Allopurinol
Penicillin
Aminopenicillins
Sulfonamides
Thiazides
Pyrazolones
Hydantoins
Propylthiouracil
Raynaud's disease or digital necrosis
Beta-blockers
Ergot alkaloids
Bleomycin
Serum sickness
Serum preparations (e.g., antivenoms)
Vaccines
Reactions resembling serum sickness
Beta-blockers
Streptokinase
Beta-lactam antibiotics

Adapted from Roujeau JC, Stern RS. Severe adverse cutaneous reactions to drugs. *N Engl J Med* 1994;331(19):1272–1285.

TABLE 14. Basic evaluation of the patient with attempted self-harm

Test	Reason
Essential	
Serum electrolytes, blood urea nitrogen, glucose	To evaluate occult renal, fluid, or electrolyte abnormality; acidosis with increased anion gap indicates certain poisons (Chapter 9)
Serum acetaminophen level	Lethal level is not associated with detectable physical findings
Electrocardiogram	To detect occult and potentially lethal ingestion of sodium-channel blocker, beta-blocker, calcium-channel blocker, or cardiac glycoside
Recommended	
Serum salicylate level	Whereas salicylate does cause symptoms and signs, early signs are easy to overlook clinically
Urine toxicology screen, comprehensive	Typically ordered in patients with altered mental status of unknown etiology or when the patient's manifestations do not agree with the suspected ingestion
Pulse oximetry or arterial blood gas, as appropriate	In patients with respiratory signs; to assess acid-base status
Computerized tomography of the head, lumbar puncture, bacterial cultures	Used to evaluate nontoxicologic causes of altered mental status

DIAGNOSTIC TESTS

Diagnostic tests play an important role in toxicology because the absence of symptoms or signs at presentation does not rule out a potentially serious or fatal ingestion. To evaluate for occult poisoning, a blood sample is typically drawn in all patients in whom a deliberate overdose is likely.

Blood Tests

Screening tests (Table 14) for the patient with deliberate self-poisoning include measurement of serum electrolytes to allow calculation of anion and osmolar gaps (Chapters 9 and 25). *Hyperkalemia* is addressed in Chapter 35. *Hypokalemia* may occur during treatment of hyperkalemia, including increased losses and enhanced intracellular potassium shift (52). Hypokalemia may result from gastrointestinal tract losses; enhanced potassium entry into cells (increased Na-K adenosine triphosphatase activity induced by β_2-agonists, theophylline, insulin); competitive blockade of potassium channels (chloroquine, barium); and with agents causing metabolic alkalosis. The clinical findings associated with hypokalemia include generalized muscle weakness; paralytic ileus; ECG changes (flat or inverted T waves, prominent U waves, ST-segment depression); and cardiac dysrhythmias (atrial tachycardia heart block, atrioventricular dissociation, ventricular tachycardia, ventricular fibrillation) (53).

Hypernatremia follows excessive intake of sodium; salt emetics; enemas; intravenous (IV) saline solutions; excessive water loss; and drugs causing diabetes insipidus, including lithium, phenytoin, and alcohol. Treatment includes cautious replacement of free water and treatment of the underlying cause.

Hyponatremia is best understood in association with serum osmolality or tonicity and is the subject of several reviews (54–57). Drug-induced hyponatremia follows excessive water intake and impaired water excretion by the kidney due to increased activity of antidiuretic hormone resulting from Ecstasy, carbamazepine, chlorpropamide, and nonsteroidal antiinflammatory drug intoxication. Treatment includes water restriction with or without loop diuretics. If the serum sodium level is less than 120 mmol/L and cerebral symptoms are present, sodium should be corrected at no more than 10 mmol/L over 24 hours due to the risk of provoking myelinolysis (58).

Serum *calcium* and *magnesium* are useful in selected cases, primarily in patients who have experienced a seizure, cardiac dysrhythmia, muscle weakness, renal injury, or experienced adverse effects following administration of a cathartic. A calcium level is helpful in ethylene glycol or hydrofluoric acid poisoning.

Liver function tests are useful in selected cases. Acute liver failure is addressed in Chapter 17.

Specific *blood levels* of specific suspected toxicants and therapeutic medications should be obtained when they will affect patient management. Routine urinary toxicology screening is not recommended, but can be helpful when the patient's toxicity cannot be explained by the history of ingestion or the typical diagnostic testing previously described.

An *acetaminophen* level is drawn because it is a potentially lethal overdose and causes no diagnostic effects until treatment is too late to prevent liver injury. A serum *salicylate* level should also be considered. While salicylate does cause signs of intoxication, these may be subtle (e.g., hyperpnea) and easy to overlook by the inexperienced or busy clinician.

Blood cultures, lumbar puncture, and other tests are often needed if there is any doubt about the cause of altered mental status. Lumbar puncture is an often-neglected aspect of evaluation of the poisoned patient. Meningitides, encephalitis, and intracranial bleed have protean presentations. Often, signs with no other immediately apparent cause are ascribed to "poisoning." This premature exclusion of other causes, particularly in the case of altered mental status, is a convenient but dangerous conclusion.

TABLE 15. CHIMPES: a mnemonic for compounds that may be visible on abdominal radiograph

	Agent
C	Calcium carbonate, chloral hydrate
H	Halogenated hydrocarbons (e.g., carbon tetrachloride, chloroform)
I	Iron
M	Metals (arsenic, bismuth, mercury, lead, lithium, zinc)
P	Potassium, phenothiazines, phosphorus
E	Enteric-coated products
S	Salicylate

Electrocardiogram

An ECG is typically ordered for all patients with deliberate self-poisoning to screen for conduction abnormalities and dysrhythmias. A wide variety of agents may affect the ECG by causing either conduction abnormalities (e.g., electrolyte abnormalities, myocardial sodium channel blockade); dysrhythmias (e.g., electrolyte abnormalities); or ischemia (e.g., carbon monoxide, cyanide).

Imaging

Imaging studies are not commonly needed for poisoned patients. Abdominal radiographs may reveal radio-opaque pills or material (Table 15). A chest radiograph is often performed to assess pulmonary complaints (Chapter 27). Other radiographs are appropriate for complaints involving other areas (e.g., computerized tomography of the head for altered mental status).

MANAGEMENT

Initial Stabilization

In the prehospital setting or ED, the ABCs of *a*irway, *b*reathing, and *c*irculation and decontamination always come first (Chapters 7 and 33).

The patient with *altered mental status* should receive certain interventions within the first minutes of care. Essential substrates such as oxygen, glucose, and thiamine are provided without the necessity of laboratory analysis. After determining that the patient has a patent airway, adequate ventilation, and an intact gag reflex, it is appropriate to provide supplemental oxygen by nasal cannula, high-flow nonrebreather mask, or mechanical ventilator. Dextrose must be provided to a hypoglycemic patient within minutes. In light of rapid bedside testing, empiric IV bolus administration of dextrose can often be avoided. After initial management, supportive care is provided until indications for more specific interventions are discovered. Decontamination is addressed in Chapter 7, and specific supportive measures are detailed in Part I, Section 4.

Antidotes

Thiamine may be safely delivered by IV bolus, 100 mg in the adult, to prevent incipient Wernicke's encephalopathy in the at-risk patient, such as an alcoholic (59). Intoxicated patients often have altered mentation, unstable gait, and difficulty cooperating with the extraocular eye examination. This makes it difficult to identify the specific individual at risk of this disorder. Thiamine is not normally administered presumptively to children.

Dextrose is typically administered for three indications: hypoglycemia (blood glucose level below 60 mg/dl or symptoms of hypoglycemia); altered mental status; and hyperkalemia. Diabetic patients who are chronically hyperglycemic may develop hypoglycemic symptoms at "normal glucose" levels. The most commonly encountered cause of hypoglycemia is exogenous insulin. Other causes include sulfonylurea ingestion, salicylate ingestion, alcohol ingestion, and hepatic failure. There are some data suggesting that hyperglycemia worsens outcome in stroke patients (60,61). It is reasonable to withhold dextrose in patients with a history and examination consistent with stroke if glucose levels can be obtained within 5 minutes.

The adult dose of dextrose for hypoglycemia or altered mental status is 50 ml of 50% dextrose solution (25 g) IV push for symptomatic hypoglycemia. The dose for children is 2 to 4 cc/kg of 25% dextrose. The dose for neonates is 2 to 4 cc/kg of 10% dextrose. Profoundly hypoglycemic patients may require multiple doses. Patients with mild hypoglycemia may be treated with oral administration. If repeated doses are needed, it is preferable to use a large-bore IV line or central line. Glucose levels should be checked at least hourly. Octreotide may offer a useful alternative in some patients (Chapter 66).

Hyperkalemia with ECG changes in the adult patient is treated with 50 cc of 50% dextrose (25 g) and 10 units of regular insulin as adjunct therapy for hyperkalemia. Concurrent therapy should also be given (Chapter 35).

Naloxone has traditionally been recommended for all patients with altered mental status on presentation to emergency medical services or the ED (Chapter 65). It is typically administered as 2 mg IV bolus in the adult and as 0.1 mg/kg in the child. More recently, a more thoughtful approach has been advocated, limiting naloxone to patients in whom ventilation is decreased, or starting with very small doses and gradually increasing until the desired effect is achieved (62,63). In the event that the patient's ventilation is suppressed and is not undergoing mechanical ventilation, full dosing of naloxone is appropriate. Patients who are dependent on opiates are often poor candidates for empiric naloxone treatment due to the risk of withdrawal and violent behavior. Opiate withdrawal is almost never life-threatening; however, it causes agitation and may disrupt the ambulance or ED, and put the patient or health care worker at risk of injury.

Flumazenil has also been proposed as an empiric treatment of the patient with altered mental status (Chapter 57). Opposition to this concept has been expressed (64,65). An Israeli paper suggests that its empiric use is safe, if one is careful to administer the drug starting at very low doses and gradually increasing (66). Further, a randomized, prospective trial suggests potential safety and cost savings from using flumazenil (67). A direct comparison of approaches has not been performed.

Acute severe electrolytes abnormalities are treated by providing supplemental dosing (e.g., calcium, magnesium supplementation) and by reducing the underlying cause.

PITFALLS

The most common errors are diagnostic: either overlooking clues to the presence of a toxic etiology or, conversely, inappropriately attributing injury to a toxic etiology when another cause is present (e.g., attributing coma to salicylate intoxication in a patient without acidosis).

REFERENCES

1. Lipsky BA, Hirschmann JV. Drug fever. *JAMA* 1981;245(8):851–854.
2. Theoharides TC, Harris RS, Weckstein D. Neuroleptic malignant-like syndrome due to cyclobenzaprine? *J Clin Psychopharmacol* 1995;15(1):79–81.

3. Chapman SA, Stephan T, Lake KD, et al. Fever induced by dobutamine infusion. *Am J Cardiol* 1994;74(5):517.
4. Palomar Garcia V, Abdulghani Martinez F, Bodet Agusti E, et al. Drug-induced ototoxicity: current status. *Acta Otolaryngol* 2001;121(5):569–572.
5. Griffin JP. Drug-induced ototoxicity. *Br J Aud* 1988;22:195–210.
6. Dolan PA, Flowers FP, Araujo OE, et al. Toxic epidermal necrolysis. *J Emerg Med* 1989;7(1):65–69.
7. Mutasim DF, Pelc NJ, Anhalt GJ. Drug-induced pemphigus. *Dermatol Clin* 1993;11(3):463–471.
8. Olson KR, Pentel PR, Kelley MT. Physical assessment and differential diagnosis of the poisoned patient. *Med Toxicol* 1987;2(1):52–81.
9. Hennessy S, Bilker WB, Knauss JS, et al. Cardiac arrest and ventricular arrhythmia in patients taking antipsychotic drugs: cohort using administrative data. *BMJ* 2002;325:1070–1074.
10. Huff JS, Syverud SA, Tucci MA. Case conference: complete heart block in a young man. *Acad Emerg Med* 1995;2(8):751–756.
11. Taliercio CP, Olney BA, Lie JT. Myocarditis related to drug hypersensitivity. *Mayo Clin Proc* 1985;60(7):463–468.
12. Kikendall JW. Pill esophagitis. *J Clin Gastroenterol* 1999;28:298–305.
13. Klegar KL, Young TL. Pill-induced esophageal injury. *J Tenn Med Assoc* 1992;85(9):417–418.
14. Underwood TW, Frye CB. Drug-induced pancreatitis. *Clin Pharm* 1993;12(6):440–448.
15. Neild GH. Haemolytic-uraemic syndrome in practice. *Lancet* 1994;343(8894):398–401.
16. Drake MJ, Nixon PM, Crew JP. Drug-induced bladder and urinary disorders. Incidence, prevention and management. *Drug Saf* 1998;19(1):45–55.
17. Mastaglia FL. Adverse effects of drugs on muscle. *Drugs* 1982;24(4):304–321.
18. Levy DE, Bates D, Caronna JJ. Prognosis in nontraumatic coma. *Ann Intern Med* 1981;94(3):293–301.
19. Barret LG, Vincent FM, Arsac PL, et al. Internuclear ophthalmoplegia in patients with toxic coma frequency, prognostic value, diagnostic significance. *J Toxicol Clin Toxicol* 1983;20(4):373–379.
20. Barolat-Romana G, Larson SJ. Influence of stimulus location and limb position on motor responses in the comatose patient. *J Neurosurg* 1984;61(4):725–728.
21. Starmark JE, Stalhammar D, Holmgren E. The Reaction Level Scale (RLS85). Manual and guidelines. *Acta Neurochir* 1988;91(1–2):12–20.
22. Stanczak DE, White JG 3rd, Gouview WD, et al. Assessment of level of consciousness following severe neurological insult. A comparison of the psychometric qualities of the Glasgow Coma Scale and the Comprehensive Level of Consciousness Scale. *J Neurosurg* 1984;60(5):955–960.
23. Crosby L, Parsons LC. Clinical neurologic assessment tool: development and testing of an instrument to index neurologic status. *Heart Lung* 1989;18(2):121–129.
24. Giacino JT, Kezmarsky MA, DeLuca J. Monitoring rate of recovery to predict outcome in minimally responsive patients. *Arch Phys Med Rehabil* 1981;72(11):897–901.
25. Born JD. (1988). The Glasgow-Liege Scale. Prognostic value and evolution of motor response and brain stem reflexes after severe head injury. *Acta Neurochir* 1988;91(1–2):1–11.
26. Benzer A, Mitterschiffthaler G, Marosi M, et al. Prediction of non-survival after trauma: Innsbruck Coma Scale. *Lancet* 1991;338(8773):977–978.
27. Jennett B, Bond M. Assessment of outcome after severe brain damage. *Lancet* 1975;1(7905):480–484.
28. Segatore M, Way C. The Glasgow Coma Scale: time for change. *Heart Lung* 1992;21(6):548–557.
29. Olson KR, Kearney TE, Dyer JE, et al. Seizures associated with poisoning and drug overdose. *Am J Emerg Med* 1994;12(3):392–395.
30. Griffin JP. A review of the literature on benign intracranial hypertension associated with medication. *Adverse Drug React Toxicol Rev* 1992;11(1):41–57.
31. Sachdev P. The epidemiology of drug-induced akathisia: Part I. Acute akathisia. *Schizophr Bull* 1995;21(3):431–449.
32. Sachdev P. The epidemiology of drug-induced akathisia: Part II. Chronic, tardive, and withdrawal akathisias. *Schizophr Bull* 1995;21(3):451–461.
33. Drotts DL, Vinson DR. Prochlorperazine induces akathisia in emergency patients. *Ann Emerg Med* 1999;34:469–475.
34. Rosebush PI, Kennedy K, Dalton B, et al. Protracted akathisia after risperidone withdrawal. *Am J Psychiatry* 1997;154(3):437–438.
35. Rosebush PI, Mazurek MF. Complicating factors in the analysis of acute drug-induced akathisia. *Arch Gen Psychiatry* 1995;52(10):878–880.
36. Casey DE. Serotonergic and dopaminergic aspects of neuroleptic-induced extrapyramidal syndromes in nonhuman primates. *Psychopharmacology (Berl)* 1993;112(1):S55–S59.
37. van Harten PN, Hoek HW, Kahn RS. Acute dystonia induced by drug treatment. *BMJ* 1999;319(7210):623–626.
38. Kanazawa Y, Ito H, Ito C, et al. Do blood glucose levels in the elderly have different metabolic significance than in non-elderly subjects? *Japan J Geriat* 1993;30:297–300.
39. Rhee KJ, Albertson TE, Douglas JC. Choreoathetoid disorder associated with amphetamine-like drugs. *Am J Emerg Med* 1988;6(2):131–133.
40. Littrell KH, Johnson CG, Littrell S, et al. Marked reduction of tardive dyskinesia with olanzapine. *Arch Gen Psychiatry* 1998;55(3):279–280.
41. Sweet RA, Pollock BG. Neuroleptics in the elderly: guidelines for monitoring. *Harvard Rev Psych* 1995;2:327–335.
42. Goldsmith JR, Herishanu Y, Abarbanel JM, et al. Clustering of Parkinson's disease points to environmental etiology. *Arch Environ Health* 1990;45(2):88–94.
43. Kordysh EA, Herishanu Y, Goldsmith JR. Chemical exposures and Parkinson's disease in residents of three Negev kibbutzim. *Environ Res* 1997;73(1–2):162–165.
44. Koller W, O'Hara R, Dorus W, et al. Tremor in chronic alcoholism. *Neurology* 1985;35(11):1660–1662.
45. Bachurin SO, Tkachenko SE, Lermontova NN. Pyridine derivatives: structure-activity relationships causing parkinsonism-like symptoms. *Rev Environ Contam Toxicol* 1991;122:1–36.
46. Zesiewicz TA, Hauser RA. Phenomenology and treatment of tremor disorders. *Neurol Clin* 2001;19:651–680.
47. Krop LC. Drug-induced systemic lupus erythematosus. *DICP* 1991;25(2):212–213.
48. Cohen MG, Prowse MV. Drug-induced rheumatic syndromes. Diagnosis, clinical features and management. *Med Toxicol Adverse Drug Exp* 1989;4(3):199–218.
49. Shear NH, Spielberg SP. Anticonvulsant hypersensitivity syndrome. In vitro assessment of risk. *J Clin Invest* 1988;82(6):1826–1832.
50. Carroll MC, Yueng-Yue KA, Esterly NB, et al. Drug-induced hypersensitivity syndrome in pediatric patients. *Pediatrics* 2001;108(2):485–492.
51. Roujeau JC, Stern RS. Severe adverse cutaneous reactions to drugs. *N Engl J Med* 1994;331(19):1272–1285.
52. Gennari FJ. Hypokalemia. *N Engl J Med* 1998;339(7):451–458.
53. Bradberry SM, Vale JA. Disturbances of potassium homeostasis in poisoning. *J Toxicol Clin Toxicol* 1995;33(4):295–310.
54. Adrogue HJ, Madias NE. Hyponatremia. *N Engl J Med* 2000;342(21):1581–1589.
55. Arieff AI. Management of hyponatraemia. *BMJ* 1993;307(6899):305–308.
56. Fraser CL, Arieff AI. Epidemiology, pathophysiology, and management of hyponatremic encephalopathy. *Am J Med* 1997;102(1):67–77.
57. Milionis HJ, Liamis GL, Elisaf MS. The hyponatremic patient: a systematic approach to laboratory diagnosis. *CMAJ* 2002;166(8):1056–1062.
58. Laureno R, Karp BI. Myelinolysis after correction of hyponatremia. *Ann Intern Med* 1997;126(1):57–62.
59. Wrenn KD, Slovis CM. Is intravenous thiamine safe? *Am J Emerg Med* 1992;10(2):165.
60. Capes SE, Hunt D, Malmberg K, et al. Stress hyperglycemia and prognosis of stroke in nondiabetic and diabetic patients: a systematic overview. *Stroke* 2001;32(10):2426–2432.
61. Kagansky N, Levy S, Knobler H. The role of hyperglycemia in acute stroke. *Arch Neurol* 2001;58(8):1209–1212.
62. Hoffman JR, Schriger DL, Luo JS. The empiric use of naloxone in patients with altered mental status: a reappraisal. *Ann Emerg Med* 1991;20(3):246–252.
63. Hoffman RS, Goldfrank LR. The poisoned patient with altered consciousness. Controversies in the use of a "coma cocktail." *JAMA* 1995;274(7):562–569.
64. Barnett R, Grace M, Boothe P, et al. Flumazenil in drug overdose: randomized, placebo-controlled study to assess cost effectiveness. *Crit Care Med* 1999;27:78–81.
65. Gueye PN, Hoffman JR, Taboulet P, et al. Empiric use of flumazenil in comatose patients: limited applicability of criteria to define low risk. *Ann Emerg Med* 1996;27(6):730–735.
66. Weinbroum A, Rudick V, Sorkine P, et al. Use of flumazenil in the treatment of drug overdose: a double-blind and open clinical study in 110 patients. *Crit Care Med* 1996;24(2):199–206.
67. Hojer J, Baehrendtz S, Matell G, et al. Diagnostic utility of flumazenil in coma with suspected poisoning: a double blind, randomised controlled study. *BMJ* 1990;301(6764):1308–1311.

CHAPTER 7

Gastrointestinal Decontamination

Richard C. Dart and G. Randall Bond

OVERVIEW

The *age of gastrointestinal (GI) decontamination* began dramatically in 1831. Presenting to the Academie Française, the physician Tovery survived a self-administered lethal dose of strychnine by concurrently ingesting activated charcoal (AC). Despite the impressive debut, the application of decontamination has produced persistent and contentious debate:

> Gastric lavage (GL) should not be considered unless a patient has ingested a potentially life-threatening amount of a poison and the procedure can be undertaken within 60 minutes of ingestion. Even then, clinical benefit has not been confirmed in controlled studies.—American Academy of Clinical Toxicology/European Association of Poisons Centres and Clinical Toxicologists Position Statement (1)

> Insufficient data are available to guide decisions on a small, but important, subset of patients with life-threatening ingestions. The failure to find supporting evidence in a small subset of data should not be used as a reason to abandon therapies that are logical, safe, rapid, and inexpensive.—Robert S. Hoffman (2)

> The onus is on those who believe a role exists for gastric emptying in these specific subsets to perform a properly conducted, methodologically sound trial to answer the question.—Ian M. Whyte and Nicholas Buckley (3)

The term *gastrointestinal decontamination* refers to any technique that prevents absorption of a drug or chemical. This chapter departs from the traditional approach of addressing GI decontamination by the method of interest (e.g., emesis vs. lavage). Instead, the fundamental decontamination technique is described and then specific patient presentations are addressed:

- The asymptomatic patient with an unknown ingestion.
- Ingestion of a minimally toxic substance in large amounts.
- The patient manifesting signs of toxicity at presentation (e.g., obtundation).
- Early presentation after ingestion of a large or massive ingestion.
- Ingestion of substances that may be absorbed slowly due to their formulation (sustained release compounds) or toxic effects (drugs that impair GI motility).
- The pediatric patient.
- Ingestion of plants.
- Substances that are not bound by AC.
- Body stuffers and packers are addressed in Chapter 12.

DEFINITIONS

There are five types of GI decontamination: induced emesis [syrup of ipecac (SI)]; GL; single dose AC; whole bowel irrigation (WBI); and cathartic administration. GL is the insertion of a large-bore tube into the stomach to irrigate and allow aspiration of gastric contents. In the context of GI decontamination, AC refers to the single administration of activated charcoal. WBI refers to the use of a nonabsorbable electrolyte solution to speed evacuation of drug. Cathartic administration accelerates evacuation of the bowel. Multiple-dose AC is a technique to increase elimination, not to decrease absorption. Sodium polystyrene sulfonate is addressed separately (Chapter 131).

BACKGROUND

Divergent views regarding GI decontamination are not surprising given the paucity of clinically relevant information available. The rationale behind GI decontamination is simple. The fundamental precept of toxicology is that "the dose makes the poison." Toxic effects are usually related to the absorbed dose rather than the ingested dose. For most poisons, GI decontamination decreases the blood concentration, decreases the amount absorbed, and theoretically reduces the severity of poisoning.

Although logical, this hypothesis has not been adequately proven or disproved. It is true that volunteer studies demonstrate that GI decontamination reduces the blood level of an ingested substance. This type of study is not an adequate evaluation of clinical efficacy because efficacy and safety have not been evaluated under "real world" clinical conditions. However, two valid observations can be made from human volunteer trials (Fig. 1). First, each method reduces the blood concentration of the index chemical, if used early. Conversely, none of the methods had an effect if used late. Second, AC reduces absorption under controlled conditions as well as or better than gastric emptying. These data have been cited to support controversial recommendations that GI decontamination must occur within 1 hour to be effective and to assert that AC is as good as other modalities in most clinical settings.

Four often-quoted studies have been used to address the issue of whether GI decontamination affects outcome under clinical conditions. The studies have similar methods and share similar strengths and weaknesses. Kulig et al. studied the efficacy of gastric emptying in 592 acute oral drug overdose patients. All subjects received AC. Before receiving AC, subjects were assigned to receive gastric emptying (SI or GL) or no emptying and followed for 4 hours to record outcome. Early clinical outcome of patients who were awake and alert on presentation to the emergency department (ED) was not affected by SI. GL in obtunded patients led to a better clinical outcome if performed within 1 hour of ingestion. This study opened an important era of investigation and stimulated several subsequent studies (4).

Merigian et al. evaluated cognitive function in 357 symptomatic overdose patients who were assigned on an alternate day basis to receive AC or gastric emptying (5). On emptying days, alert patients received SI, while obtunded patients received GL. AC therapy followed gastric emptying. On nonemptying days, symptomatic patients were treated only with AC. No clinical deterioration occurred in the asymptomatic patients treated without gastric emptying. AC use did not alter outcome measures in asymptomatic patients. Gastric emptying procedures in symptomatic patients did not significantly alter the length of ED

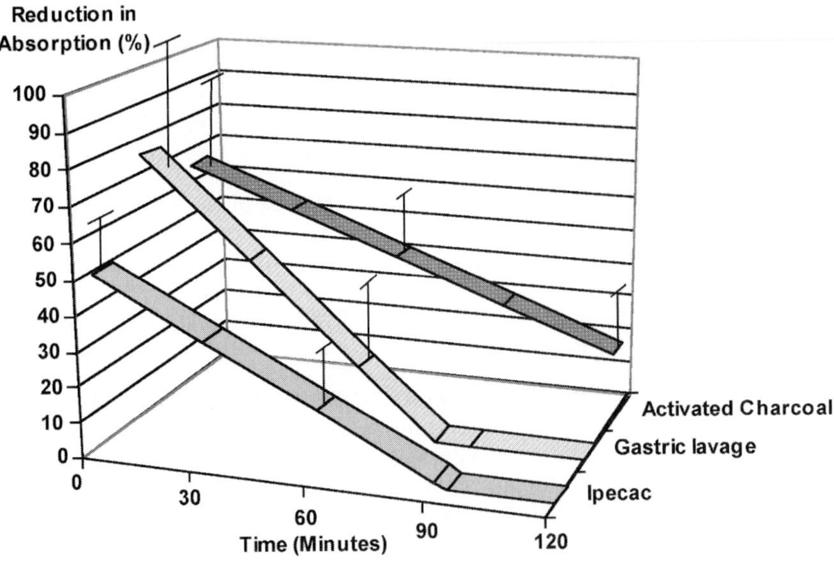

Figure 1. Summary of studies measuring the reduction in blood levels by gastrointestinal decontamination in volunteers. (Adapted from Bond GR. The role of activated charcoal and gastric emptying in gastrointestinal decontamination: a state-of-the-art review. *Ann Emerg Med* 2002;39:273–286.)

stay, mean length of time intubated, or mean length of stay in the intensive care unit. GL was associated with a higher prevalence of intensive care unit admissions and aspiration pneumonia (5).

Albertson et al. compared the clinical effectiveness of SI and AC to that of AC alone in 200 mildly to moderately symptomatic adults with acute ingestion. Patients receiving only AC were discharged from the ED in significantly less time than those receiving both SI and AC. The rate of nonpsychiatric hospitalization was not different between the two groups (11.2% vs. 14.0%). For hospitalized patients, the length of time spent in the intensive care unit or in the hospital was not different between the two groups. A complication rate of 5.4% was found in the SI plus AC group compared with 0.9% in the AC alone group. Three episodes of aspiration pneumonitis occurred after SI plus AC, while none were noted in the AC only group (6).

Pond compared emptying (SI or GL) to nonemptying in 876 consecutive adult overdose patients using alternate day assignment. All patients received AC. There were no significant differences between the emptying and nonemptying groups in outcome when the groups were stratified for severity of the overdose or into subgroups that presented sooner or later than 1 hour after ingestion (7).

These studies address the bulk of patients presenting to the ED with poisoning. Some practitioners have universalized the results of these studies and volunteer studies: "If AC alone is easier to administer and as efficacious as gastric emptying before AC, there is no longer a need to perform gastric emptying." This conclusion is overly broad. Total abandonment of gastric emptying is not advised because the studies all excluded ingestions, like lithium, in which the authors thought gastric emptying important or AC ineffective. Furthermore, extremely cautious interpretation of these studies is needed because their study design compromised their ability to detect a difference. For example, each of the studies included drugs or quantities in which no intervention was likely to change the course. A large ingestion of tricyclic antidepressant had the same weight as an ingestion of ibuprofen tablets. Most of the patients presented hours after ingestion. Patients known to have ingested drugs that delay gastric emptying were not analyzed separately. Few sustained-release products were available at the time of the studies. One study excluded severely symptomatic patients. The primary indicator of severity in the other three studies, central nervous system (CNS) depression, is by itself easy to treat and unlikely to improve in the short period of observation used.

In short, these studies provide general guidance and define issues for further evaluation. However, the overall results cannot be extrapolated to their component parts. If there were few patients who ingested large amounts of cardiotoxic agents, for example, a significant benefit for that subgroup would not be identified by the results of the whole. Few subgroups were assessed. Where subgroups were assessed, it is likely that a conclusion of no significant difference is underpowered (type II error risk). Thus, the studies lacked sufficient subgroup identification and adequate numbers to assess the impact of gastric emptying before AC in all circumstances thought to be high risk. The good news is that these specific circumstances constitute only a fraction of the total number of patients considered for GI decontamination; therefore, the results are reassuring for most of the poisoned patients we treat.

Indeed, there are studies that suggest a true outcome benefit for GI decontamination with specific ingestions. Acetaminophen (APAP) is one of the few poisonings that occurs frequently enough to allow large-scale analysis. Two pediatric studies compared the mean serum APAP level in patients with and without gastric emptying. Bond et al. showed that the APAP level was lower in the children who experienced emesis before 90 minutes as compared with those who did not have emesis (8). Surprisingly, this effect was achieved without controlling for the amount of reported ingestion. In other words, patients were included regardless of the amount of ingestion, and still lower APAP levels were found in the emesis group.

Kirk et al. studied children who received SI within 1 hour of ingestion. The group that received AC within 2 hours of ingestion had lower APAP levels compared to controls without decontamination (9). Another pediatric study compared 7 poison centers, using referral to hospital as an outcome measure (10). The home use of SI reduced the rate of health care facility referral. An Australian study used "need for *N*-acetylcysteine treatment" as an outcome measure of APAP poisoning. *N*-acetylcysteine treatment was used in fewer patients who received AC, thereby sparing some patients the need for hospitalization and treatment (11).

Overall, there is a provocative, incomplete, but growing body of data indicating that GI decontamination may beneficially alter the outcome of selected types of poisonings. The potential benefit of GI decontamination is supported by a reasonable scientific rationale, human volunteer studies, retrospective clinical studies, and a few prospective studies. GI decontamination should be used in circumstances in which there is a potential benefit to the patient and minimal risk. Discerning those circumstances, however, is difficult because of the limited medical literature available.

GASTROINTESTINAL DECONTAMINATION—METHODS AND RISKS

Overview

The most common reported complication of GI decontamination is aspiration. The combination of CNS depression, loss of protective airway reflexes, emesis, and airway manipulation provides an opportunity for aspiration to occur. It is important to realize that prospective data indicate that 5% of patients experienced aspiration *before* decontamination was performed (7). Another 2% of patients in that study experienced aspiration attributed to decontamination. Aspiration occurred in 4% of 93 patients who received emetic decontamination before AC, compared with none of 107 patients in an AC alone group (6). In three of these four cases, aspiration followed the inappropriate use of SI in antidepressant overdose. Aspiration occurred in one of 214 patients (who received ipecac emetic decontamination before AC) compared to no patients of 378 who received either GL plus AC or AC alone (4).

Induced Emesis

The use of SI has produced significant disagreements among toxicologists. A thorough review was unable to clearly condone or condemn its use (12). Like most minor procedures, SI is safe when used appropriately. The rate of aspiration is extremely low (13). Reported adverse events include prolonged emesis (17%), diarrhea (13%), and atypical lethargy (12%) (14). Rare complications of single use include hematemesis resulting from a Mallory-Weiss tear. Furthermore, the wide distribution of SI to homes in the 1960s and 1970s produced few reports of injury.

Ipecac syrup is available over the counter. The U.S. Food and Drug Administration pregnancy classification is C (Appendix I), but it may be relatively contraindicated during late pregnancy due to potential mechanical effects on the uterus.

Although it has fallen out of favor, SI remains a reasonable therapy for a small group of patients (e.g., when the patient has ingested a compound that is expected to produce potentially serious toxicity without early CNS depression and the patient is more than 1 hour from health care). Because the evidence suggests that SI is similar in efficacy to AC, it would also be a reasonable alternative under the same conditions.

SI is not the best approach to GI decontamination in the ED setting. One exception to this rule is potentially serious ingestion in an alert pediatric patient who was too small for effective lavage, had ingested a plant or medication too large to pass through a small-bore tube, or perhaps had ingested a substance not bound by AC.

METHOD

Consultation with a poison center or toxicologist is recommended before home use. The patient must be alert and capable of swallowing voluntarily. For children 6 months to 1 year of age, the SI dose is 15 ml and 30 ml in children 1 to 5 years of age or older than 12 years of age. The same dosage may be repeated in 20 to 30 minutes if vomiting has not occurred. The decision to lavage when SI fails to induce vomiting should be based on the need to remove the toxin, as therapeutic doses of SI are not cardiotoxic. Although the shelf-life of SI is 5 years, evidence suggests potency persists for several years.

ADVANTAGES AND BENEFITS

The primary advantage of SI is its ease of use. It can be administered in the home without the need for special equipment and is more easily accepted by children than AC or GL. When administered early after ingestion, it appears to reduce the amount of toxic substance absorbed to a degree similar to other procedures (Fig. 1).

DISADVANTAGES, RISKS, AND CONTRAINDICATIONS

The primary disadvantage of SI is delay. Emesis occurs after 15 to 30 minutes and persists for an hour or more, thereby delaying subsequent interventions such as AC (15). Relative contraindications include ingestion of a seizure-inducing drug, agents that may quickly depress mentation, hydrocarbons, and corrosives. In addition, SI may cause concern in pregnancy, bleeding diathesis, previous emesis, serious heart disease, or the anticipated use of WBI. Additional relative contraindications include substances that cause bradycardia in the young or old patient. The vomiting caused by ipecac may potentiate bradycardia through vagal effects.

Adverse effects include persistent vomiting (vomiting may persist for hours in rare cases), aspiration of the vomited substance, vagal-induced bradycardia during emesis, esophageal injury (rare Mallory-Weiss tears), stomach herniation into chest, intracranial hemorrhage, and pneumomediastinum.

Because GL would certainly be preferred to SI in the obtunded patient, SI is primarily an agent for use outside of the hospital when the patient has a potentially serious ingestion. In this case, the benefits may outweigh the risks. If both AC and SI are available in the home, they are likely of equal efficacy. The relative safety of SI and single-dose AC is unknown.

Gastric Lavage

Whenever used, the staff undertaking the procedure (whether medical or nursing) should be experienced in its execution. Lavage is not advisable outside of the hospital.

METHOD

Endotracheal or nasotracheal intubation should precede GL in patients who may have a compromised ability to protect their airway. An oral airway should be placed to prevent biting of the endotracheal tube. The patient should be placed in the left lateral head-down position (20-degree tilt on the table) to produce better lavage returns (16). The length of tube to be inserted is estimated and marked before insertion. A wide-bore 36 to 40 French or 30 English gauge tube (external diameter, approximately 12 to 13.3 mm) should be inserted orogastrically in adults, and a 24 to 32 French gauge tube (diameter, 5.3 to 9.3 mm) in children.

Excessive force should not be used to pass the tube. Once the tube is passed, its position should be checked either by air insufflation, while listening over the stomach, or by aspiration with pH testing of the aspirate. Lavage is carried out using small aliquots of liquid. In an adult, 200 to 300 ml of warm (38°C) fluid such as saline or water is used. In a child, 10 to 20 ml/kg body weight of warm fluid should be given. Water should be avoided in young children because of the risk of free-water absorption and hyponatremia. Small volumes are used to minimize the risk of gastric contents entering the duodenum during lavage. Warm fluids avoid the risk of hypothermia in the young and old and those receiving large volumes of lavage fluid. Lavage is continued until the returning lavage solution shows no further particulate matter.

ADVANTAGES AND BENEFITS

The primary advantage is that this procedure allows gastric emptying in patients with altered mental status (after the airway has been secured). It also provides a convenient method to administer AC.

DISADVANTAGES, RISKS, AND CONTRAINDICATIONS

Like other GI decontamination procedures, the most dangerous risk of GL is pulmonary aspiration. The act of GL seems to increase the rate of aspiration. Aspiration was associated with decontamination in 10 of 429 (7.8%) patients who received gastric emptying (either SI or GL) plus AC and 7 of 407 (1.7%) who received AC alone (7).

Complications of GL include epistaxis, laryngospasm, hypoxia, aspiration pneumonia, sinus bradycardia, ST elevation on the electrocardiogram, hyponatremia, hypochloremia, water intoxication, or mechanical injury to the gut (rare). Kulig et al. reported esophageal perforation in 1 of 72 patients who received GL (4). The incidence of perforation was 0 in 216 patients who received lavage in two other prospective studies (5,7). Perforation may allow mediastinal or pleural administration of charcoal (4).

Lavage is absolutely contraindicated in patients with a compromised, unprotected airway, such as obtunded patients and patients at risk of GI hemorrhage or perforation. Relative contraindications include hydrocarbon ingestion, caustic substances, and poisons that have an effective antidote.

An estimation of the risks of GL must include those caused by an unnecessary endotracheal intubation. If paralysis and intubation are performed solely for airway control, the associated adverse events are complications of the lavage. Merigian et al. noted in a prospective study that the rate of endotracheal intubation was four times higher among patients who received GL plus AC instead of just AC (5). If the benefit of GL is unproven, the consequences of intubation are excess costs and morbidity.

Activated Charcoal, Single Dose

Since the 1980s, AC has been chosen increasingly by emergency personnel as the primary means of decontamination based on the perceived lack of adverse effects. It has received endorsement by professional societies (17). AC has theoretical usefulness unless it is known that a drug and coingestants are not bound by charcoal. Substances for which AC administration has not been shown clinically effective include, but are not limited to, mineral acids and bases, ethanol, arsenic, boric acid, bromide, fluoride, iron, iodide, ipecac, lithium, and potassium.

METHOD

The dose of AC is 1 to 2 g/kg. This dose may be too low in children because it is difficult to accurately measure a small amount of AC. It should be administered by drinking (to the alert patient) if possible. The first dose can be administered through a nasogastric (NG) tube while procedures are in progress. Once the patient has been stabilized, lavage with a large-bore orogastric tube can be accomplished, if appropriate.

ADVANTAGES AND BENEFITS

AC appears as effective at reducing drug blood levels as gastric emptying and is likely safer than GL.

DISADVANTAGES, RISKS, AND CONTRAINDICATIONS

The primary adverse effects of single-dose AC are nausea, vomiting, and pulmonary aspiration. Emesis occurs in approximately 15% but is not usually recurrent. Pulmonary injury may result if hydrocarbons have been ingested. Increased esophageal injury may occur when corrosives have been ingested. A rare but potentially serious complication is administration of AC directly into the lung by NG tube.

There were no reported aspiration events in three trials involving a range of patients, including symptomatic patients (5,6,13). The aspiration risk must be minimized because AC may lead to more complications than aspiration of gastric contents alone (18). These observations may be due to a granulomatous reaction, a tissue reaction to coadministered AC suspension agents like sorbitol or povidone iodine, or to increased lung microvascular permeability (19,20).

The major contraindication to AC is lack of airway protection. The need for endoscopic visualization may preclude its use occasionally. It may also adsorb some orally administered antidotes, although no clinically significant complications of this action have been reported.

Although it is often thought that multiple doses increase the probability of AC aspiration, aspiration often occurs during the first administration of AC (21). As with all therapeutic interventions, the risks and benefits of AC should be considered before its use.

Whole Bowel Irrigation

WBI pushes substances through the gut mechanically. Like all decontamination methods, the effect is incomplete (22). Its efficacy is unproven, but WBI is viewed as offering an alternative for selected poisoned patients in whom other decontamination alternatives are not likely to be useful (23).

METHOD

The technique for WBI involves the insertion of an NG tube into the stomach and the instillation of polyethylene glycol electrolyte solution. Alternatively, the solution can be ingested. The use of intravenous metoclopramide (10 mg adults, 0.1 to 0.3 mg/kg body weight) may reduce the incidence of nausea and vomiting. The usual rate of fluid administration is 2 L/hour in adults and 0.5 L/hour (25 to 40 ml/kg body weight) in children younger than 12 years of age. The endpoint occurs when the rectal effluent is similar in appearance to the infusate. The usual infusion lasts 2 to 6 hours. This does not ensure that the toxin or foreign body is eliminated (24).

ADVANTAGES AND BENEFITS

The primary application of WBI is with substances that are not well adsorbed by AC (e.g., lithium, lead, other metals); drugs that are designed for sustained or delayed release; and substances that form concretions (salicylate, enteric-coated preparations, drug packets, etc.).

DISADVANTAGES, RISKS, AND CONTRAINDICATIONS

The primary disadvantage of WBI is delay. It takes a substantial period of time to administer the solution. Large amounts of nursing time may be needed. WBI may reduce the binding of AC with certain compounds. For example, a volunteer study of carbamazepine, theophylline, and verapamil found that WBI added nothing to the effect of AC and increased the absorption of carbamazepine compared to AC alone (25).

Adverse event rates for WBI are largely unknown. Few complications occurred following the use of WBI for preparation of the bowel for radiographic examination or for surgery in either adults or children (26), even in the presence of cardiac, renal, or pulmonary disease (27). Complaints usually are minor and include nausea, vomiting, abdominal distension and cramps, sleep loss, and anal irritation. Polyethylene glycol electrolyte lavage solution may occupy AC binding sites reducing adsorption or displacing toxin from AC, and increasing in toxin bioavailability (28).

Cathartics

The goal of catharsis is to decrease intestinal transit time, thereby expelling the poison before it can be absorbed. Several different cathartics have been tested: magnesium citrate, sodium sulfate, mannitol, and sorbitol. Except for isolated applications, the use of catharsis is discouraged due to lack of efficacy and concerns about safety (29).

One potential application is the combined use of sorbitol with AC. The goal is to speed charcoal through the gut and perhaps to reduce constipation caused by charcoal. In human volunteers, this practice has increased and decreased the amount of drug absorbed (30). There are no prospective clinical trials testing assessing the efficacy of sorbitol (29).

METHOD

Sorbitol is usually provided as a 70% solution. Using the specific gravity, 100 ml of 70% solution equals 90 g of sorbitol. A typical single dose of 70% sorbitol is 1 to 2 ml/kg in adults and 35% sorbitol, 4.3 ml/kg, in children.

DISADVANTAGES, RISKS, AND CONTRAINDICATIONS

Fluid and electrolyte disorders are the primary risks associated with sorbitol. At one time, sorbitol-AC mixtures were administered repeatedly to children for certain poisonings. Although rare, severe hypernatremia and death have resulted (31). Sorbitol should not be used with multiple-dose AC for either adults or children.

SPECIAL ISSUES IN GASTROINTESTINAL DECONTAMINATION

The poisoned patient may present in several ways. First, the drug identity (and therefore the potential risk) may be known or unknown. Second, the patient may be asymptomatic or symptomatic. Finally, the patient may present early or late. While it seems true that a late presentation reduces the effectiveness of GI decontamination, the data are insufficient to precisely define a time. The limit of effectiveness may be 1 hour, 2 hours, or even later. Each of these factors, potential risk, the presence of symptoms, and the time since ingestion affect the decision to use GI decontamination. It is important to remember that symptoms of one drug may mask or delay symptoms of another drug.

In most situations, the research data available do not lead to a clear conclusion; therefore, the individual practitioner and the patient must weigh the risks and benefits in deciding which decontamination method to use or whether decontamination is appropriate at all. In the ED, the choices likely include AC alone, GL, GL plus AC, or WBI. The relative value and safety of these techniques are difficult to investigate, and there is little financial support for research, so better data are unlikely to become available soon.

Ingestion of Substances with Minimal Toxicity

Most patients in this group do not need decontamination because there is little danger and therefore little potential benefit. GI decontamination cannot change the outcome when patients have ingested a nontoxic amount of drug, a large amount of a nontoxic drug, or present so late that the full amount of the drug has already been absorbed. For example, up to 90% of children who ingest a drug are safely managed at home by poison centers (10).

Few ingestions have the potential for major morbidity or mortality. Of 592 patients presenting to a city hospital, only 7% of minimally symptomatic patients and 40% of moderately to severely symptomatic patients were admitted for medical care (4). All of these patients received decontamination; however, the mean time to presentation was more than 3 hours after ingestion, indicating that these patients had absorbed most of the drug before evaluation. Another prospective study found that asymptomatic patients presenting to a large, inner city teaching hospital had the same outcome whether they received AC or no decontamination at all (5). The most likely explanation for these results is that late presenting, asymptomatic patients have identified themselves as having a nontoxic or minimally toxic ingestion. No intervention can alter their course, except to worsen it.

Even the so-called "massive" ingestion is not necessarily a serious ingestion because many ingestants cannot be taken in amounts large enough to cause toxicity (stool softeners, H_2 antagonists, etc.). The issue is not the amount but the net result of the interaction of dose, inherent toxicity of the compound, and the condition of the patient. Guidelines for the nontoxic or minimally toxic ingestion are under development. These guidelines can be used to help create a rational list of substances that do not need decontamination.

In the end, the individual practitioner must assess the potential toxicity of the ingestion and the time since ingestion. If the substance is minimally toxic or enough time has passed that full absorption should have already occurred, GI decontamination is unneeded. Furthermore, it simply exposes the patient to risk without the potential for benefit.

Asymptomatic Patient with an Ingestion of an Unknown Drug

Decontamination of the "unknown overdose" is a particularly challenging clinical problem because neither the drug nor the amount ingested is known. In short, the approach to the asymptomatic patient with an unknown ingestion is to evaluate the patient's condition at a given point in time, observe for a defined period, then discharge if no toxic effects develop. The role of decontamination is less clear. If the provider concludes that a potentially dangerous ingestion has occurred (see Early Presentation after a Potentially Dangerous Ingestion), then GI decontamination is warranted.

Early Presentation after a Potentially Dangerous Ingestion

The "potentially lethal" ingestion is a common clinical challenge. In principle, this group has the greatest potential for benefiting from decontamination because the patient has likely presented before much of the drug has been absorbed. This fact has encouraged physicians to use the potentially dangerous designation to support maximal intervention, including decontamination. Because it is not possible to determine in advance whether the amount of drug is truly dangerous, this common scenario has the potential to greatly expand the numbers of patients who receive GI decontamination.

Truly serious poisonings are infrequent. In the three largest studies available, there were two toxin-related deaths among a total of 2276 patients, and those two outcomes were unlikely to have been influenced by decontamination (4,5,7). This observation suggests one of the following conclusions: (a) serious ingestions are relatively uncommon, (b) many "life-threatening" ingestions were systematically excluded, or (c) serious ingestions are effectively treated by intensive care alone. It is likely that all three factors play a role.

Most overdose deaths are the result of cardiovascular events, respiratory arrest, anoxic brain injury, or hepatic failure (e.g., delayed APAP presentation). Thus, the primary group for consideration of GL in addition to AC in a "life-threatening," acute overdose context is patients who have ingested drugs with severe, difficult-to-treat cardiovascular or respiratory consequences. The most common medications that cause death include calcium-channel blockers, tricyclic antidepressants, aspirin, and APAP. A uniformly effective antidote is available for APAP. Other candidates include the patient with a high lithium level who presents early with minimal toxic effects and perhaps other agents that are not bound by AC. Aggressive intervention can theoretically obviate some of the toxic effects.

There is only a handful of poisonings, therefore, that can potentially benefit from GI decontamination, even if they present before toxicity develops. Bosse et al. reported a prospective, randomized study of patients who ingested tricyclic antidepressants. He compared AC, AC preceded by GL, and AC followed by GL and another dose of AC. Using several outcome measures, no difference between the three groups was found. The size of the groups ($N = 22, 14, 15$, respectively) was small, however, so the ability to detect differences was limited (32).

The need for decontamination in the case of a potentially serious ingestion has not been clarified and is a subjective decision of the medical provider. If the medical provider concludes that a potentially dangerous ingestion has indeed occurred, some risk is justified, and decontamination should be performed. The specific choice of procedures is unclear. A single dose of AC is attractive in its simplicity. However, the asymptomatic patient presenting early with a truly serious ingestion may be the most likely to benefit from aggressive, sequential GI decontamination. The combined use of AC plus GL, followed by an additional dose of AC, likely removes the greatest amount of drug.

Patients with Signs of Toxicity on Presentation

Patients with altered mental status at presentation are of interest because they are easily identified. Two studies have evaluated moderate or severe CNS effects within 1 hour of ingestion (4,7). These data, however, are insufficient to reach a definite conclusion because an insensitive outcome marker was used: the patient's course during the subsequent 4 hours. Furthermore, the studies produced conflicting results. This is not surprising because they were performed in different countries, without control of interventions (except for decontamination procedure) and an insufficient sample size to assess low-frequency events.

Few would debate that GI decontamination would be reasonable in the early presenting patient with altered mental status; however, without specific evidence, the choice of measures is controversial. This is another risk perception issue. If the medical provider concludes that GL is safe, rapid, and inexpensive, it should be used before AC. If the provider believes that it causes unacceptable risk, diverts personnel resources, and delays AC, then AC alone should be used.

In later-presenting symptomatic patients, the benefits of decontamination are even less clear. The likelihood of benefit from decontamination decreases with the time since ingestion (Fig. 1), GI motility, and extended release characteristics of the drug ingested. When drug absorption is likely to be complete, decontamination is not indicated.

Ingestion of Potentially Toxic Substances That May Be Absorbed Slowly

In theory, decreased GI motility should keep toxins in the stomach and available to either gastric emptying or AC. The clinical issue is not whether drug is available in the GI tract; however, the issue is whether performing GL, AC, or both produces a better patient outcome than no intervention at all. A human volunteer ($N = 9$) study of AC efficacy at 1 hour after ingestion found no difference in peak mefenamic acid concentrations with and without the anticholinergic agent hyoscine at the time of ingestion. The time to peak absorption of mefenamic acid was different, but there was no difference in reduction of absorption (36% vs. 42%) (33). Like most studies in GI decontamination, the size and methodology of this study prevent generalizing the conclusions. In summary, little research has addressed this question, and the data are inadequate to reach a conclusion.

Decontamination in the Pediatric Patient

The role of decontamination differs in the pediatric patient. First, the incidence of severe poisoning in pediatric patients is much smaller than in adult patients. Most pediatric poisoning involves tastes and exploration, especially those that are not iatrogenic or induced by a care provider. Poison centers are able to keep more than 90% of these patients at home. Second, children's anatomy is different. It is rare to be able to use a lavage tube with an internal diameter sufficient to remove large pills. Many pills or other poisons cannot be retrieved using lavage. Third, the patient is often unable to cooperate with procedures. Fourth, the substance and timing of ingestion are known with much greater certainty in pediatric than adult ingestions. This allows better determination of the likely benefit of GI decontamination.

If decontamination is desired, AC alone is the preferred method. If a toxic quantity has been ingested but is not bound to AC (e.g., lithium, iron), SI or a large orogastric lavage tube (32F) may be used cautiously. No NG tube and few orogastric tubes pass whole tablets or fragments.

Ingestion of Plants

Few plant ingestions produce clinically significant toxicity. The plant type and quantity are often known or can be determined, and the potential toxicity of most plants is limited to GI irritation. The potential species and toxicity vary by country. In the United States, it typically requires a large ingestion, repeated ingestion (e.g., medicinal herbs), or special processing (e.g., making a tea from oleander leaves) to produce dangerous toxicity in humans.

Medically significant plant ingestions are therefore rare but have occurred with a few plants (foxglove, oleander, a few others) and selected mushrooms. Some of these plants are thought to form a leafy mass in the stomach, but it seems unlikely that such a mass could be retrieved by lavage, even with a large-bore tube. Therefore, some authors have proposed the use of SI for this group of patients. The interaction of SI with plants that increase vagal tone is unlikely early after ingestion when decontamination may be of benefit. Presuming that the usual contraindications to the use of SI are observed (primarily that the patient is not expected to develop an altered level of consciousness), SI seems a reasonable alter-

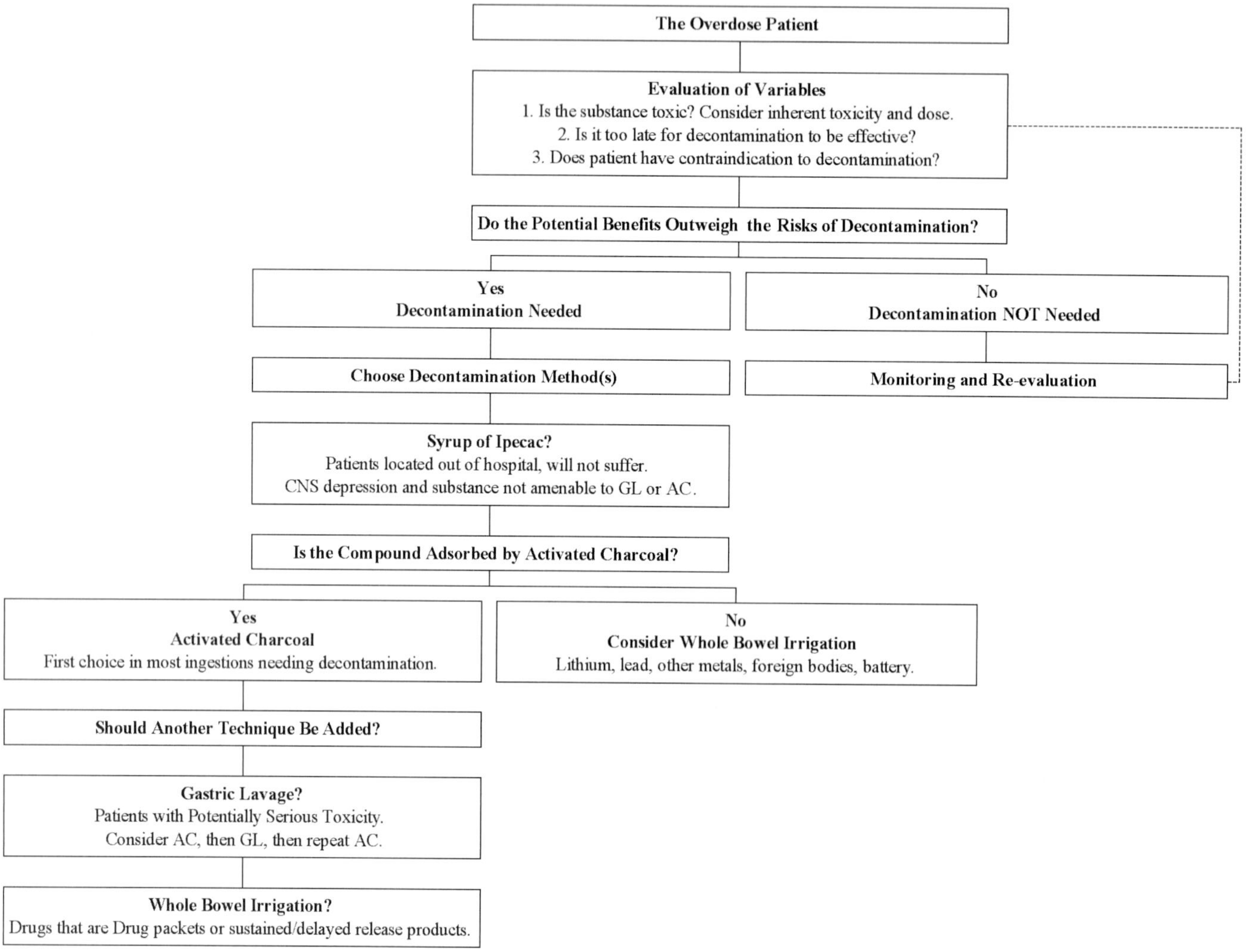

The Overdose Patient

Evaluation of Variables
1. Is the substance toxic? Consider inherent toxicity and dose.
2. Is it too late for decontamination to be effective?
3. Does patient have contraindication to decontamination?

Do the Potential Benefits Outweigh the Risks of Decontamination?

Yes
Decontamination Needed

No
Decontamination NOT Needed

Choose Decontamination Method(s)

Monitoring and Re-evaluation

Syrup of Ipecac?
Patients located out of hospital, will not suffer.
CNS depression and substance not amenable to GL or AC.

Is the Compound Adsorbed by Activated Charcoal?

Yes
Activated Charcoal
First choice in most ingestions needing decontamination.

No
Consider Whole Bowel Irrigation
Lithium, lead, other metals, foreign bodies, battery.

Should Another Technique Be Added?

Gastric Lavage?
Patients with Potentially Serious Toxicity.
Consider AC, then GL, then repeat AC.

Whole Bowel Irrigation?
Drugs that are Drug packets or sustained/delayed release products.

Figure 2. Approach to gastrointestinal decontamination. See text for further explanation of decision points. AC, activated charcoal; CNS, central nervous system; GL, gastric lavage.

native, especially if administered out of hospital or if AC was not available or may be delayed.

RECOMMENDATIONS

Despite the interest and research evolving over decades, controversy and disagreement in the use of GI decontamination persist. Each decision to decontaminate, or not, therefore relies on the risk-benefit assessment of the medical provider in the context of the individual patient. Specific blanket recommendations (e.g., "GI decontamination should only be performed within 1 hour of ingestion") are not justified by the data available and imply simplicity of decision making that is not supported by data nor plausible scientific rationale.

It is recommended that the medical provider use a decision process that focuses on a risk-benefit analysis instead of on blind adherence to an arbitrary protocol (Fig. 2). Some of the variables to be considered, however, are simply unknown. What is the risk of major complication after GL? Has this patient actually ingested a potentially toxic dose? Is it too late to retrieve this drug from the stomach? The decision on whether to use GI decontamination and what technique to use will remain an individual decision far into the future.

REFERENCES

1. Vale JA. Position statement: gastric lavage. American Academy of Clinical Toxicology; European Association of Poisons Centres and Clinical Toxicologists. *J Toxicol Clin Toxicol* 1997;35:711–719.
2. Hoffman R. Importance of gastrointestinal decontamination. *Internet J Med Toxicol* 1999;2:5.
3. Whyte IM, Buckley NA. Progress in clinical toxicology: from case reports to toxicoepidemiology. *Med J Aust* 1995;163:340–341.
4. Kulig K, Bar-Or D, Cantrill SV, et al. Management of acutely poisoned patients without gastric emptying. *Ann Emerg Med* 1985;14:562–567.
5. Merigian KS, Woodard M, Hedges JR, et al. Prospective evaluation of gastric emptying in the self-poisoned patient. *Am J Emerg Med* 1990;8:479–483.
6. Albertson TE, Derlet RW, Foulke GE, et al. Superiority of activated charcoal alone compared with ipecac and activated charcoal in the treatment of acute toxic ingestions. *Ann Emerg Med* 1989;18:56–59.
7. Pond SM, Lewis-Driver DJ, Williams GM, et al. Gastric emptying in acute overdose: a prospective randomized controlled trial. *Med J Aust* 1995;163:345–349.
8. Bond GR, Requa RK, Krenzelok EP, et al. Influence of time until emesis on the efficacy of decontamination using acetaminophen as a marker in a pediatric population. *Ann Emerg Med* 1993;22:1403–1407.
9. Kirk MA, Peterson J, Kulig K, et al. Acetaminophen overdose in children: a comparison of ipecac versus activated charcoal versus no gastrointestinal decontamination. *Ann Emerg Med* 1991;20:472–473(abst).
10. Bond GR. Home use of syrup of ipecac is associated with a reduction in pediatric emergency department visits. *Ann Emerg Med* 1995;25:338–343.
11. Buckley NA, Whyte IM, O'Connell DL, et al. Activated charcoal reduces the need for *N*-acetylcysteine treatment after acetaminophen (paracetamol) overdose. *J Toxicol Clin Toxicol* 1999;37:753–757.
12. Krenzelok EP, McGuigan M, Lheur P. Position statement: ipecac syrup.

American Academy of Clinical Toxicology; European Association of Poisons Centres and Clinical Toxicologists. *J Toxicol Clin Toxicol* 1997;35:699–709.

13. Kornberg AE, Dolgin J. Pediatric ingestions: charcoal alone versus ipecac and charcoal. *Ann Emerg Med* 1991;20:648–651.
14. Czajka PA, Russell SL. Nonemetic effects of ipecac syrup. *Pediatrics* 1985;75:1101–1104.
15. Wrenn K, Rodewald L, Dockstader L. Potential misuse of ipecac. *Ann Emerg Med* 1993;22:1408–1412.
16. Burke M. Gastric lavage and emesis in the treatment of ingested poisons: a review and a clinical study of lavage in ten adults. *Resuscitation* 1972;1:91–105.
17. Chyka PA, Seger D. Position statement: single-dose activated charcoal. American Academy of Clinical Toxicology; European Association of Poisons Centres and Clinical Toxicologists. *J Toxicol Clin Toxicol* 1997;35:721–741.
18. Elliot C, Colby T, Hicks H. Charcoal lung: bronchiolitis obliterans after aspiration of activated charcoal. *Chest* 1989;96:672–674.
19. Menzies D, Busutill A, Prescott L. Fatal pulmonary aspiration of oral activated charcoal. *BMJ* 1988;297:459–460.
20. Arnold TC, Willis BH, Xiao F, et al. Aspiration of activated charcoal elicits an increase in lung microvascular permeability. *J Toxicol Clin Toxicol* 1999;37:9–16.
21. Dorrington C, Johnson D, Brant R, and the MDAC Complication Study Group. Pulmonary aspiration and gastrointestinal obstruction associated with the use of multiple dose activated charcoal. *J Toxicol Clin Toxicol* 2000;38:442A.
22. Scharmann EJ, Lembersky R, Krenzelok EP. Efficiency of whole bowel irrigation with and without metoclopramide. *Vet Human Toxicol* 1992;34:361(abst).
23. Tenenbein M. Position statement: whole bowel irrigation. American Academy of Clinical Toxicology; European Association of Poisons Centres and Clinical Toxicologists. *J Toxicol Clin Toxicol* 1997;35:753–762.
24. Scharman EJ, Lembersky R, Krenzelok EP. Efficiency of whole bowel irrigation with and without metoclopramide pretreatment. *Am J Emerg Med* 1994;12:302–305.
25. Lapatto-Reiniluoto O, Kivisto KT, Neuvonen PJ. Activated charcoal alone and followed by whole-bowel irrigation in preventing the absorption of sustained-release drugs. *Clin Pharmacol Ther* 2001;70:255–260.
26. Sondheimer JM, Sokol RJ, Taylor SF, et al. Safety, efficacy, and tolerance of intestinal lavage in pediatric patients undergoing diagnostic colonoscopy. *J Pediatr* 1991;110:148–152.
27. Goldman J, Reichelderfer M. Evaluation of a rapid colonoscopy preparation using a new gut lavage solution. *Gastrointest Endosc* 1982;28:9–11.
28. Hoffman RS, Chiang WK, Howland MA, et al. Theophylline desorption from activated charcoal caused by whole bowel irrigation. *J Toxicol Clin Toxicol* 1991;29:191–202.
29. American Academy of Clinical Toxicology Position Statement. Available at: http://www.clintox.org/Pos_Statements/Cathartics.html. Accessed March 2003.
30. al-Shareef AH, Buss DC, Allen EM, et al. The effects of charcoal and sorbitol (alone and in combination) on plasma theophylline concentrations after a sustained-release formulation. *Hum Exp Toxicol* 1990;9:179–182.
31. Farley TA. Severe hypernatremic dehydration after use of an activated charcoal-sorbitol suspension. *J Pediatr* 1986;109:719–722.
32. Bosse GM, Barefoot JA, Pfeifer MP, et al. Comparison of three methods of gut decontamination in tricyclic antidepressant overdose. *J Emerg Med* 1995;13:203–209.
33. El-Bahie N, Allen EM, Williams AJ, et al. The effect of activated charcoal and hyoscine butylbromide alone and in combination on the absorption of mefenamic acid. *Br J Clin Pharmacol* 1985;19:836–838.

SECTION

3

Diagnosis of the Poisoned Patient: The Toxicologist as Sleuth

Richard C. Dart

The toxicology patient can present in two ways: the known ingestion and the unknown ingestion. In the case of the known ingestion, the toxicologist is blessed with foreknowledge of the poison involved. Although caution is still warranted, the working diagnosis is apparent. Much more difficult and dangerous is the case of the patient for whom the agent is unknown. The patient attempting self-harm may refuse to provide a history or give false information as a way of continuing his or her act. Other patients may be unable to provide a history due to altered mental status or an occult poisoning. A well-known joke among toxicologists is: "How do you know when the patient is not providing accurate information? Their lips move."

An intensive care unit nurse from a neighboring institution was found unconscious. She had overdosed on several relatively innocuous medications. The evidence was obvious; the pill bottles were found in a wastebasket next to her bed. She had not been seen for at least 24 hours. She received the typical initial evaluations in the emergency department, which were all negative, and was admitted to the intensive care unit. There, she promptly spiraled downward with hypotension refractory to treatment and a regular, but only slightly widened, complex tachycardia. She died days later of multiple organ failure. Later, the empty bottles of desipramine were found stashed away in a remote part of the house. Like an efficient misdirection play in football, the history can mislead as well as inform.

Toxicologists are regularly consulted to answer questions such as, "Could this patient's illness be caused by a poison?" The approach to these patients is always fraught with lack of information and poor timing (often, the question is asked too late to collect useful samples). Nevertheless, there are tools available to make a diagnosis, or at least narrow the diagnosis, in a patient with an unknown or suspect history. The role of the toxicologist becomes sleuth, trying to elucidate the cause of the poisoning from the physical examination and diagnostic tests.

This topic is not typically addressed in textbooks. Most authors find the challenge of describing a disease and its differential diagnosis alone daunting. Without the beginning point of knowing the agent, writing a chapter is even more difficult. The fearless contributors to this book have nevertheless attempted to address some of the thorny presentations that confront the toxicologist. The following section is meant to transfer some of the experience and expertise of an accomplished clinician to the reader. Its focus is on the evaluation of the patient rather than providing specific treatment. Treatment considerations and specific agents are covered in subsequent chapters.

CHAPTER 8

Ascending Paralysis

Robert L. Stephen and E. Martin Caravati

OVERVIEW

Although they occur rarely, there are drugs, chemicals, and venoms that produce ascending paralysis as the primary clinical manifestation. Toxin-induced ascending paralysis is a polyneuropathy. Its manifestations are usually symmetric and generalized. All peripheral fibers are affected, so a combined sensorimotor dysfunction usually dominates over pure motor or sensory loss.

In general, there are no biologic markers for these agents, so the diagnosis relies on a diligent, detailed history of exposure to the etiologic agent. There are also no specific antidotes for these agents. This chapter focuses on the differential diagnosis of toxic exposures that can produce ascending loss of motor function, including agents that produce predominately lower extremity neurologic deficits that may appear as ascending paralysis initially.

PATHOPHYSIOLOGY

Disorders of the peripheral nervous system account for most cases of ascending paralysis. There are four types: (a) myelinopathy, whose hallmark is involvement of the myelin sheath or

Schwann's cell with resultant demyelination of the peripheral nerve; (b) axonopathy, in which the axon itself is initially targeted; (c) neuronopathy, characterized by alterations to the nerve cell body; and (d) transmission neuropathies, distinguished by interference with the release of neurotransmitters or electrical signal propagation. Long and large diameter nerve fibers tend to be more sensitive to toxic injury, explaining why symptoms usually begin distally and progress in an ascending pattern. Neuropathies that involve the progressive dying back of peripheral nerves present with distal weakness that slowly progress to proximal muscles. In contrast, a pattern of descending paralysis is more typical of botulism or diphtheria.

DIAGNOSIS

Patients typically complain of distal lower extremity numbness, gait disturbance, dysesthesia, or progressive weakness. Their symptoms usually progress over days to weeks, and less commonly, months, depending on the toxin. It is important to determine the time course and a detailed temporal relationship of symptoms and the exposure. A detailed history should include diet, work habits, work environment, similar symptoms in coworkers or family members, travel history, hobbies, recreational activities, and any ancillary information that can be obtained from family, friends, and acquaintances. Recent illnesses, other systemic symptoms, and a meticulous drug history are also needed. Particular attention should be given to the possible use of any herbal preparations, vitamins, or supplements.

The physical examination focuses on recording a detailed neurologic examination, including testing of light touch and two-point discrimination in the affected areas. Dermatomal or stocking-glove patterns of sensory deficit should be noted and recorded. Tendon reflexes and motor strength in both upper and lower extremities should be evaluated and graded frequently to detect any deterioration. Any muscle atrophy should be noted. The muscles of flexion and adduction are often affected less severely than those of extension and abduction (1). Motor weakness may rapidly progress to involve the thoracic muscles and affect the patient's ability to breath adequately. The presence of cranial nerve deficits or upper extremity weakness or sensory loss should broaden the differential diagnosis beyond the agents considered in this chapter.

Differential Diagnosis

There are few toxin- or nontoxin-mediated diseases that produce true ascending paralysis (Table 1). Clinically, a distal peripheral neuropathy may suggest, but fail to ultimately manifest, the classic ascending pattern; therefore, these entities are also noted in the following section. Certain neurologic syndromes are known to occur on exposure to specific neurotoxins. When the history and physical findings suggest a novel presentation, an exhaustive search for all causes, toxic and nontoxic, must be pursued by the clinician.

TABLE 1. Causes of ascending paralysis

Toxicologic	Nontoxicologic
Tetrodotoxin	Guillain-Barré syndrome
Sweet pea (*Lathyrus sativa*)	Transverse myelitis
Tick paralysis	Poliomyelitis
Buckthorn (*Karwinskia humboldtiana*)	West Nile virus[a]
N-Hexane	
Intrathecal vincristine	
Clioquinol	

[a]Centers for Disease Control and Prevention. Acute flaccid paralysis syndrome associated with West Nile virus infection—Mississippi and Louisiana, July–August 2002. *MMWR Morb Mortal Wkly Rep* 2002;51:825–828.

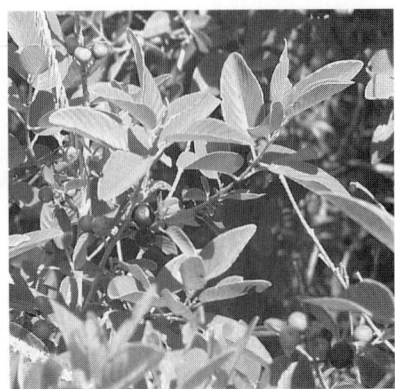

Figure 1. Buckthorn (*Karwinskia humboldtiana*). (Courtesy of Texas A&M Research and Extension Center, Uvalde, Texas.)

Toxins Resulting in Ascending Paralysis

Please see individual chapters for more information on each of these toxins and their treatment.

BUCKTHORN (COYOTILLO, TULLIDORA)

Karwinskia humboldtiana (Fig. 1) is a poisonous shrub found in semi-desert regions of the southern United States, Mexico, Central America, Colombia, and the Caribbean. This is a relatively common cause of ascending paralysis in Mexican children. The plant is often referred to as *buckthorn*, but this name is also associated with other plants found throughout the United States that do not cause neurotoxicity. In Mexico, it may be referred to as *coyotillo* or *tullidora*. A distal, progressive, ascending paralysis devoid of sensory symptoms develops within 1 to 15 days of ingestion. Initial signs are lower extremity weakness or paralysis. Cases with more rapid clinical onset (1 to 2 days) start with diarrhea and vomiting. This is thought to be due to the quantity of fruit ingested, although the exact amount required for toxicity is unclear. It may mimic Guillain-Barré syndrome (GBS), and the diagnosis is difficult without a history of fruit (berry) ingestion. Clinical progression to bulbar paralysis and death can occur. The toxin (T-514 *Karwinskia humboldtiana*) has been detected by thin layer chromatography. Sural nerve biopsy demonstrated segmental demyelination with swelling and phagocytic chambers in Schwann's cells. Recovery is slow but usually complete. Treatment is supportive (2).

N-HEXANE AND METHYL *N*-BUTYL KETONE

Patients may be exposed to *N*-hexane either in an industrial setting by dermal or inhalation routes or from chronic inhalation of glue fumes (Chapter 206). They can develop a progressive quadriparesis resembling GBS. The *N*-hexane and methyl *N*-butyl ketone constituents of the glue are metabolized to the neurotoxin 2,5-hexanedione, which may cause muscle weakness, decreased deep tendon reflexes, and paresthesias similar to GBS. Treatment is the cessation of the industrial exposure or glue sniffing. The effects can be permanent (3).

LATHYRISM (NEUROLATHYRISM)

Lathyrism results from chronic, excessive consumption of *Lathyrus sativus*, the chickling pea and related species. The amino acid, beta-*N*-oxalylamino-*L*-alanine, found in the pea is thought to be responsible. Once widespread, the disease is now found primarily in India, Bangladesh, and Ethiopia. It is a nonprogressive, upper-motor neuron degenerative disease resulting in spastic paraparesis that develops after several weeks to months of eating a daily diet of 400 g/day of the pea. The lower extremities are affected almost exclusively. The effects are permanent, and there is no known treatment (4).

TETRODOTOXIN

Tetraodon poisoning involves the Tetraodontiformes order of fish, all of which contain tetrodotoxin. The most notorious is fugu, a variety of puffer fish eaten as a delicacy in Japan. The toxin interferes with neuromuscular transmission (Chapter 252). Symptoms begin within 5 to 45 minutes of ingestion and are manifested initially by nausea and oral paresthesias. Generalized weakness, dyspnea, diffuse paresthesias, malaise, loss of coordination, fasciculation, dysrhythmias, and ascending paralysis develop over the ensuing 24 hours. The more rapid the onset of symptoms is, the more severe the degree of poisoning that occurs. Buccal bullae can develop, and the cranial nerves can be involved. Mortality approaches 50% in severe cases. Treatment is supportive (5).

TICK PARALYSIS

Tick paralysis is an ascending paralysis with loss of reflexes and intact sensation, mimicking GBS. The neurotoxin is found in the saliva of certain female ticks found in Australia and North America (*Ixodes holocyclus*, *Dermacentor andersoni*, *Dermacentor variabilis*) (Fig. 2). The toxin interferes with acetylcholine release from the presynaptic nerve terminal. Clinical presentation typically begins with nonspecific complaints of irritability, fatigue, restlessness, and muscular pain. Vomiting is uniquely associated with *I. holocyclus*. Ascending paralysis usually occurs 2 to 6 days after exposure. Sensory deficits are uncommon. The diagnosis depends on finding the tick, which may be well hidden in the scalp, neck, or ear. Mortality is due to respiratory muscle paralysis. Treatment is to find and remove the tick, which may require a diligent search. All other care is supportive. Cases involving *I. holocyclus* may continue with progressive muscle weakness for 48 hours after removal of the tick ("coasting" phenomenon). Recovery after removal of *D. andersoni* or *D. variabilis* is usually within 2 or 3 days (6).

VINCRISTINE

Unintentional intrathecal administration of the antineoplastic agent vincristine has resulted in rapidly progressive ascending paralysis and death (Chapter 98). Oral overdose may produce a progressive peripheral neuropathy, particularly in the lower extremities, beginning during the first week after exposure. Muscle weakness and gait disturbance occur 2 to 3 weeks after overdose (7).

CLIOQUINOL

Clioquinol is a halogenated hydroxyquinoline that was indicated for intestinal amoebiasis and for the prophylaxis and treatment of traveler's diarrhea. It was removed from the market because of neurotoxicity that was first reported in Japan in the 1950s. Initial symptoms included abdominal pain and diarrhea, followed by bilateral ascending paresthesia and dysesthesia of the lower extremities. This was occasionally accompanied by loss of visual acuity. The syndrome became known as *subacute myelo-opticoneuropathy*. Green tongue and urine were occasionally found in myelo-opticoneuropathy patients (8).

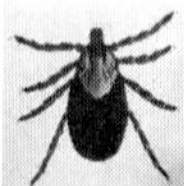

Figure 2. Rocky Mountain wood tick (*Dermacentor andersoni*). (Courtesy of U.S. Centers for Disease Control and Prevention.)

Toxins That May Initially Mimic Ascending Paralysis

Patients may initially present with predominately lower extremity symptoms of motor weakness or sensory symptoms suggestive of an ascending type of neuropathy. These toxins should also be included in the differential diagnosis until causation is definitively established. In most cases, the primary clue to diagnosis is the history of exposure.

ACRYLAMIDE

Subacute acrylamide exposure may cause progressive distal motor neuropathy that may be accompanied by ataxia. The subacute form does not demonstrate the skin manifestations characteristic of chronic acrylamide exposure. Treatment is removal from exposure and supportive care (9).

ETHANOL

Chronic alcoholism may result in a distal sensorimotor polyneuropathy that may primarily affect the lower extremities. It may present as lower extremity weakness, decreased deep tendon reflexes, and dysesthesia.

ETHYLENE OXIDE

Chronic occupational exposures may result in axonal neuropathies of both the upper and lower limbs. This includes numbness of the feet, leg weakness and incoordination, tingling of extremities, absent or decreased reflexes, stocking-and-glove sensory loss, and loss of Achilles tendon reflex (10).

MISONIDAZOLE

Misonidazole, a radiosensitizing drug, was used to treat carcinoma of the pharynx and larynx. It was associated with lower extremity sensory symptoms secondary to an axonal neuropathy that limited its therapeutic use (11).

NITROFURANTOIN

A peripheral neuropathy may occur in patients with renal failure taking nitrofurantoin. Sensory symptoms of burning, painful feet and distal motor weakness may be noted (12).

ORGANIC GOLD

Treatment of rheumatoid arthritis with organic gold has rarely resulted in a peripheral neuropathy resembling GBS. This treatment has largely been replaced with oral methotrexate.

PYRIDOXINE

Large doses of pyridoxine (vitamin B_6) may cause an acute or subacute sensory loss and severe ataxia that may be mistaken for motor weakness (13).

THALLIUM

Thallium toxicity often presents with a painful ascending neuropathy and distal motor weakness that are more pronounced in the lower extremities than upper extremities. Alopecia combined with the painful ascending paresthesias is the hallmark of this disease, but this typically occurs later. Serum or urine levels of thallium may assist in diagnosis (14) (Chapter 231).

TRIORTHOCRESYL PHOSPHATE

Ginger-Jake paralysis occurred in the 1930s due to triorthocresyl phosphate, an organophosphate that contaminated an alcoholic drink distilled from ginger. A polyneuropathy resulted from exposure and was characterized by distal paresthesias, loss of reflexes, and motor weakness that may ascend. Residual paraplegia occurred in some patients (15).

Diagnostic Tests

Laboratory tests in the evaluation of ascending paralysis or lower extremity weakness should include a complete blood count, serum electrolytes, and urinalysis. Other tests to consider are a chest radiograph (paraneoplastic etiologies); sedimentation rate; and a heavy metal screen for thallium, lead, barium, and mercury. Routine comprehensive screening of blood, urine, or hair for neurotoxic chemicals is often unproductive.

Diagnostic procedures include a lumbar puncture for cerebrospinal fluid examination, including immunologic studies, oligoclonal bands, and myelin basic protein determinations. Computerized tomography and magnetic resonance imaging of the brain and spine are indicated to identify structural lesions that may be responsible for the paralysis.

Electromyography and nerve conduction velocity can distinguish axonopathy from myelinopathy and myopathy. However, even a normal test does not absolutely rule out toxicity, as only a small number of normal fibers are needed to give a normal response.

If muscle weakness ascends to the level of the respiratory muscles, serial testing of negative inspiratory force or another measure of respiratory muscle strength should be performed.

MANAGEMENT

In general, the management of this select group of patients is supportive, including the use of intubation and mechanical ventilation in cases of respiratory muscle paralysis. There are no specific antidotes or therapies, although gastrointestinal decontamination with activated charcoal for tetraodon poisoning should be considered for recent ingestion. Metal chelators may be needed if toxic concentrations of lead or thallium are discovered. The source of exposure should be reported to the appropriate agencies, such as the local or state health department, Occupational Safety and Health Administration, or MedWatch.

REFERENCES

1. Wilson JD, Braunwald E, et al. *Harrison's principles of internal medicine*, 12th ed. New York: McGraw-Hill, 1991:2097–2098.
2. Martinez HR, Bermudez MV, Rangel-Guerra RA, et al. Clinical diagnosis in *Karwinskia humboldtiana* polyneuropathy. *J Neurol Sci* 1998;154(1):49–54.
3. Meadows R, Verghese A. Medical complications of glue sniffing. *South Med J* 1996;89:455.
4. Spencer PS, Schaumberg HH. Lathyrism: a neurotoxic disease. *Neurobehav Toxicol Teratol* 1983;5(6):625–629.
5. Sims JK, Ostman DC. Pufferfish poisoning: emergency diagnosis and management of mild human tetrodotoxication. *Ann Emerg Med* 1986;15:1094–1098.
6. Greenstein P. Tick paralysis. *Med Clin N Am* 2002;86:441–446.
7. Manelis J, Freudlich E, Ezekiel E, et al. Accidental intrathecal vincristine administration. Report of a case. *J Neurol* 1982;228:209–213.
8. Tateishi J. Subacute myelo-optico-neuropathy: clioquinol intoxication in humans and animals. *Neuropathology* 2000;20[Suppl]:S20–S24.
9. Igisu H, Goto I, Kawamure Y, et al. Acrylamide encephaloneuropathy due to well water pollution. *J Neurol Neurosurg Psychiatry* 1975;38:581–584.
10. Schroder JM, Hoheneck M, Weis J, et al. Ethylene oxide polyneuropathy: clinical follow-up study with morphometric and electron microscopic findings in a sural nerve biopsy. *J Neurol* 1985;232(2):83–90.
11. Melgaard B, Hansen HS, Kamieniecka Z, et al. Misonidazole neuropathy: a clinical, electrophysiological, and histological study. *Ann Neurol* 1982;12(1):10–17.
12. Cavanagh JB. Peripheral neuropathy caused by chemical agents. *CRC Crit Rev Toxicol* 1973;2:365–417.
13. Schaumburg MD, Kaplan J, Windebank A, et al. Sensory neuropathy from pyridoxine abuse. *N Engl J Med* 1983;309:445–448.
14. Cavanagh JB, Fuller NH, Johnson HR, et al. The effects of thallium salts, with particular reference to the nervous system changes. *QJM* 1974;43:293–319.
15. Aring CD. The systemic nervous affinity of triorthocresyl phosphate (Jamaican ginger palsy). *Brain* 1942;65:34.

CHAPTER 9

Unexplained Acid-Base and Anion Gap Disorders

Steven A. Seifert

ACID-BASE AND ELECTROLYTE HOMEOSTASIS

The poisoned patient may present with a variety of acid-base and electrolyte disturbances. Understanding the normal physiology, the effects of toxins and toxicants on the acid-base system, and the larger differential diagnoses of acid-base disorders allows the toxicologist to help detect substance toxicity, anticipate adverse effects, determine proper therapeutic interventions, and assess the adequacy of supportive and specific care.

The body's buffer and electrolyte system is complex. It contains dependent and independent variables in nonlinear relationships that make precise assessment difficult and create pitfalls for oversimplified analyses. The independent variables of the acid-base system are the partial pressure of arterial carbon dioxide ($PaCO_2$), the strong ion difference (SID), and the total weak acid concentration (the sum of the dissociated and undissociated forms). The dependent variables are the pH, bicarbonate (HCO_3^-) concentration, and hydrogen ion (H^+) concentration. Additionally, information may be obtained from evaluation of blood gases as well as the osmolal gap.

Three broad systems of analysis have been developed (Table 1): (a) *base excess/deficit* (BE/D; determination of the relative amount of buffer base to the normal physiologic state); (b) *SID*

TABLE 1. Definitions/formulas used in acid-base analysis

Normal acid-base status
When the independent variables (Pa_{CO_2}, SID, total weak acid concentration) have normal, empirically established values
BE/D
A condition of BE/D defined relative to pH = 7.4 and Pa_{CO_2} = 40 mm Hg. This does not necessarily indicate completely normal independent variables, although usually HCO_3 is normal. Thus, the BE/D can be 0 while there are still significant acid-base abnormalities
AG
Either the difference between the unmeasured cations and unmeasured anions in plasma *or* the difference between the most common cation(s) (Na with or without K) and commonly measured anions (Cl and HCO_3), which serves as a measure of the unmeasured anion excess; may be corrected for serum Alb
Serum AG = Na – (Cl + CO_2)
nl = 8 – 16 for older methodologies (e.g., flame photometry)
nl = 3 – 9 for newer, ion-selective electrode methodologies (8,37)
Urinary AG = $U_{Na} - (U_{Cl} + U_{CO_2})$
nl = –20 to 0
Alb correction
AG + dAlb × 2.5 = Na – (Cl + CO_2)
Patients with total CO_2 <22 mEq/L, where dAlb is the decrease in Alb from the expected/normal value in g/dl (38)
AG + dAlb × 1.5 = Na – (Cl + CO_2)
Patients with total CO_2 >21 mEq/L, where dAlb is the decrease in Alb from the expected/normal value in g/dl (39)
Delta AG
Delta AG = dAG/dHCO_3 = (AG – 12)/(24 – HCO_3)
Where dAG is the change in the AG from normal in mEq/L, and dHCO_3 is the change of HCO_3 from normal in mEq/L
SID
The difference between completely dissociated cations and completely dissociated anions
SID = 1000 × Kcl × $P_{CO_2}/10^{-pH}$ + 10 × [Alb] × (0.123 × pH – 0.631) + [Pi(tot)] × (0.309 × pH = 0.469)
Where Pi(tot) is total phosphate in mmol/L; Alb is in g/dl; Pa_{CO_2} in mm Hg; and Kcl is 2.46 × 10^{-11} (mEq/L) × 2 mm Hg^{-1} (40) *or*
SID = (Na + K + Ca + Mg) – (Cl + Li)
nl = 40 – 42 mEq/L
Where Pi is phosphate ion, Si is sulfate ion, Ui is urate ion, Li is lactate ion, pK is an averaged pK for proteins with a negative charge (41)
Linear estimation of appropriateness of change in P_{CO_2} for change in HCO_3
Where dHCO_3 is the change in HCO_3, and dPa_{CO_2} is the change in Pa_{CO_2} (see text for discussion) (42)
In metabolic acidosis: dP_{CO_2} = 1.2 × dHCO_3
In metabolic alkalosis: dP_{CO_2} = 0.6 × dHCO_3
In acute respiratory acidosis: dHCO_3 = 0.1 × dP_{CO_2}
In chronic respiratory acidosis: dHCO_3 = 0.35 × dP_{CO_2}
In acute respiratory alkalosis: dHCO_3 = 0.2 × dP_{CO_2}
In chronic respiratory alkalosis: dHCO_3 = 0.5 × dP_{CO_2}
Osmolality
Calculated osmolality = 1.86 × Na (in mEq/L) + glucose (in mg/dl)/18 + blood urea nitrogen (in mg/dl)/2.8
Osmolal gap = measured osmolality – calculated osmolality
ETOH correction factor: ETOH (mg/dl) × 0.217 = contribution to serum osmolality
Isopropanol correction factor: isopropanol (mg/dl) × 0.17 = contribution to serum osmolality
EG correction factor: EG (mg/dl) × 0.2 = contribution to serum osmolality
MeOH correction factor: MeOH (mg/dl) × 0.32 = contribution to serum osmolality

AG, anion gap; Alb, albumin; BE/D, base excess/deficit; EG, ethylene glycol; ETOH, ethanol; HCO_3, bicarbonate; MeOH, methanol; Pa_{CO_2}, partial pressure of arterial carbon dioxide; P_{CO_2}, partial pressure of carbon dioxide; SID, strong ion difference.

[the apparent difference between all of the strong ions (i.e., fully dissociated cations and anions)]; and (c) *anion gap* (AG; an abbreviated determination of SID, with variations). The diagnostic and predictive value of each approach and element to analyzing acid-base and electrolyte status depend on the setting, availability of resources, and knowledge level of the provider.

To evaluate a patient's acid-base balance, some basic principles must be understood. The first is that the body functions optimally in the pH range of 7.35 to 7.45 and has a number of buffer-base systems designed to maintain homeostasis. A physiologic buffer is a weak acid and its salt, which resists changes in H^+ concentration after the addition of an acid or base. The most important physiologic buffer in the body is the carbon dioxide $(CO_2)/HCO_3^-$ system, which accomplishes 80% to 90% of the metabolic acid buffering (1):

$$CO_2 + H_2O \leftrightarrow H_2CO_3 \leftrightarrow H^+ + HCO_3^-$$

Thus, when a patient increases his or her respiratory minute volume to compensate for metabolic acidosis, the CO_2 is reduced. This "pull" decreases the concentration of H_2CO_3, which in turn lowers $H^+ + HCO_3^-$.

A second principle is that plasma is electrically neutral; thus, positively charged ions in the plasma must equal negatively charged ions. It is this relationship that allows us to infer the presence of unmeasured substances in the plasma (metabolic acids or abnormal electrolytes) using changes in the electrolyte pattern. The largest contributors of cations in plasma are sodium (Na^+), potassium (K^+), calcium (Ca^{2+}), magnesium (Mg^{2+}), and, with certain conditions, immunoglobulin G (2). The largest contributors of anions are chloride (Cl^-), HCO_3^-, lactate (La^-), sulfate (SO_4^-), phosphate (PO_4^-), urate, and albumin (Alb).

PATHOPHYSIOLOGY

Many toxic substances disturb acid-base and electrolyte balance. These may be either metabolic or respiratory in nature and may result in a purely metabolic, respiratory, or mixed acid-base disturbance. The terms *acidemia/acidosis* and *alkalemia/alkalosis* are often confused. The suffix *-emia* refers to the pH of the blood. Thus, *acidemia* means that the pH has fallen below 7.35. The suffix *-osis* refers to an electrolyte abnormality. Thus, a metabolic *acidosis* simply means that the serum HCO_3 is below 22 mEq/L. An *-osis* develops before its corresponding *-emia*. For example, the production of La^- drops the serum HCO_3 below 22 mEq/L before the pH falls below 7.35.

Metabolic Acidosis

Organic metabolic acids are constantly generated by metabolism. Under normal circumstances, compensation by buffer consumption and respiratory ventilation (followed by buffer regeneration) keeps the acid-base system in equilibrium. An acidosis may be primarily respiratory (e.g., respiratory depression) or metabolic; both may occur simultaneously. Metabolic acidosis occurs when the rate of acid production or introduction into the body occurs at a rate faster than can be compensated by buffering or increased respiratory ventilation. Because the primary process is one of consumption of buffer base, *metabolic acidosis* is defined as a serum HCO_3^- less than 22 mEq/L. Consumption of HCO_3 generates CO_2. Excess CO_2 is normally removed from the body by increasing respiratory minute ventilation. Severe acidosis in a young person can produce a Pa_{CO_2} as low as 20 mm Hg. Although respiratory compensation begins within minutes of excess acid exposure, full compensation may take longer to develop, and mild acidemia may occur. If the physiologic limits of minute volume (CO_2 excretion) are exceeded, a progressive acidemia will develop.

Normally, pH returns toward normal as a result of respiratory compensation, but even after steady-state compensation is attained, usually does not produce a completely normal pH. The pH will be less than 7.35 and the $PaCO_2$ less than 35 mm Hg unless another process is occurring. Also, as hydrogen ions move intracellularly to be neutralized by other buffer systems, K^+ moves into the extracellular fluid, in part to preserve electrical neutrality. This effect is most pronounced in nonorganic (e.g., exogenous inorganic acids) metabolic acidosis (3,4).

Metabolic Alkalosis

Metabolic alkalosis is defined as a serum HCO_3 greater than 26 mEq/L. The pH is greater than 7.45 and the $PaCO_2$ greater than 45 mm Hg unless another process is occurring. This state is produced by conditions that develop in either a normal or a contracted volume state: excess loss of hydrochloric acid (HCl; gastric fluid from vomiting or nasogastric suction) or loss of Cl^- from villous adenomas, diuretics, or Cl^--deficient diets (e.g., baby formula). Metabolic conditions, such as primary aldosteronism, Cushing's disease, and ectopic production of adrenocorticotropic hormone, occur in a normal volume state and are not responsive to Cl^- replacement. Urinary Cl^- is usually high in these conditions. Respiratory compensation is the opposite of metabolic acidosis by decreasing minute volume (hypoventilation). Hypoxic drive usually prevents complete compensation (pH remains above 7.40), and the $PaCO_2$ rarely exceeds 55 mm Hg (5).

Respiratory Acidosis

Respiratory acidosis is defined as a state in which the $PaCO_2$ is greater than 45 mm Hg. Any agent that can cause central nervous system (CNS) depression can produce respiratory acidosis by depressing ventilation. Many nontoxicologic conditions may also cause a respiratory acidosis, and a wide differential diagnosis should be developed. Respiratory acidosis is caused by hypoventilation and is characterized by an increased $PaCO_2$ and a decreased pH. Compensation is initially accomplished by cellular buffers and later by increased renal absorption of HCO_3 (5). The plasma HCO_3 rises as it shifts extracellularly, but there is no true gain of buffer base. In this case, the body compensates by renal retention of HCO_3. This mechanism requires many hours to develop and may be limited by the rate and degree of renal response. Again, compensation is incomplete, and the resulting pH is less than 7.35 and serum HCO_3 greater than 26 mEq/L unless another process is occurring.

Respiratory Alkalosis

Respiratory alkalosis is defined as a state in which the $PaCO_2$ is less than 35 mm Hg. Initially, the plasma HCO_3 falls as it shifts intracellularly, but there is no true loss of buffer base. Compensation is initially by cellular buffers and later by decreased renal absorption of HCO_3 (5). The renal loss of HCO_3 requires many hours to develop and may be limited by the rate and degree of renal response. The pH is greater than 7.4 and serum HCO_3 less than 22 mEq/L unless another process is occurring.

Common Mixed Disorders

A mixed disorder involves a combined effect of two or more acid-base processes. A primary respiratory alkalosis can result from lactic acidosis, creating a combined metabolic acidosis and increased AG presentation. A related phenomenon occurs with salicylism, which typically begins with respiratory alkalosis caused by stimulation of respiratory centers. The body compensates initially by shifting HCO_3 intracellularly and later by increasing renal excretion of HCO_3. Within hours, a combined picture emerges as metabolic acids are produced and accumulate, causing loss of buffer base. In addition, the kidneys allow loss of HCO_3, resulting in a mixed respiratory alkalosis and metabolic acidosis.

Many CNS depressants cause hypoventilation with a primary respiratory acidosis. At the same time, a metabolic acidosis may develop from either direct properties of the agent or secondarily due to hypoperfusion, hypoxia, rhabdomyolysis, and so forth.

Understanding the Anion Gap

The changes in HCO_3^- as a result of excess acid production provide a method to help diagnose the cause of an acidosis, termed the *AG*. The AG is simply the mathematic difference between commonly measured cations and anions in the plasma:

$$AG = ([Na^+] + [K^+]) - ([Cl^-] + [HCO_3^-])$$

The value for K^+ is often omitted because it contributes little to the total and varies little in living patients. The AG is present even in normal patients. The value for the normal AG depends on the method used to measure electrolyte concentrations and the patient population being studied. In healthy adults, using older technology, the AG is 12 ± 4 mEq/L (6,7). With newer ion-selective laboratory techniques, the normal AG is 10 ± 4 mEq/L (8).

Because the plasma must remain electrically neutral, the "normal" AG is by definition an artifact. It is an artifact caused by the presence of unmeasured anions. In other words, our normal laboratory techniques just happen to measure cations more completely than anions, thus creating an apparent gap. Some of the unmeasured anions undoubtedly arise from Alb, which is not included in the calculation and carries a net negative charge.

Patients with hypoalbuminemic states have a falsely depressed AG because the concentration of Cl^- increases to compensate for the loss of negative ions on Alb. The AG calculation can be enhanced by inclusion of a term to compensate for the serum Alb level. The Alb term is particularly important in patients who are likely to have low serum Alb (e.g., chronic diseases) and can improve the sensitivity of the test (9). The converse condition may also occur. The AG may be falsely depressed with hypergammaglobulinemia because unmeasured cationic charges reduce the apparent gap (2), although others have found a positive correlation between γ-globulin concentrations and AG (10).

Strong Ion Difference

The SID is the difference between completely dissociated cations and completely dissociated anions. Its measurement requires the determination of Ca, Mg, SO_4, uric acid, and lactic acid levels, with those attendant costs and more complex calculations. In one study, the SID detected acid-base abnormalities in cases in which the AG missed an abnormality because of a normal HCO_3^- concentration (9). SID is rarely calculated in clinical practice, and its utility has been questioned (11–13).

Base Excess/Deficit

The condition of BE/D is defined relative to pH = 7.4 and $PaCO_2$ = 40 mm Hg. A BE/D of 0 does not necessarily indicate completely normal independent variables, although HCO_3^- is usually normal. Thus, the BE/D can be 0 while there are still significant acid-base abnormalities. In a comparison of BE/D

TABLE 2. Mnemonic for common causes of increased osmolal gap (MADGAS)

M	Mannitol
A	Alcohols
	Ethanol
	Ethylene glycol
	Isopropanol
	Methanol
	Propylene glycol
D	Diatrizoate
G	Glycerol
A	Acetone
S	Sorbitol

with AG and a physiochemical analysis based on the SID in 152 patients and 9 normal subjects, BE/D did not detect serious acid-base disorders approximately one-sixth of the time, particularly when the plasma concentrations of the non-HCO_3^- buffers (mainly Alb) were abnormal (9).

Osmolal Gap

The osmolal gap (Chapter 25) can be useful in some cases of increased AG acidosis. Osmolality is a measure of the effect of the number of particles dissolved in 1 L of solution and represents the molal concentration of solutes. The *osmolal gap* is the difference between the calculated osmolality and the measured serum osmolality. Many different formulas have been evaluated, but the method of Dorwart is probably the most accurate (14).

Conditions that may increase the measured serum osmolality (and thus the osmolal gap) include renal failure, ketoacidosis, lactic acidosis, and shock, as well as the toxic alcohols (15–18). A mnemonic to remember these causes is *MADGAS* (Table 2).

Evaluating Appropriate Compensation Using the Partial Pressure of Arterial Carbon Dioxide

The relationship between $Paco_2$ and HCO_3^- in blood is logarithmic but can be approximated by a linear formula in the pH range of 7.1 to 7.5: For every 1 mEq/L decrease in plasma HCO_3, the $Paco_2$ should decrease 1.2 mm Hg. If the decrease in $Paco_2$ is less than predicted, a mixed acid-base disturbance may be occurring (e.g., there may be impaired ventilation from CNS depression), the limit of increased minute ventilation has been reached (e.g., the patient cannot increase ventilation further), or an acidosis is developing more rapidly than the respiratory compensation can accommodate.

If the decrease in $Paco_2$ is greater than predicted, a secondary respiratory alkalosis may be occurring (e.g., salicylate intoxication). Similar linear approximations allow a determination of appropriate compensation for other acid-base disorders (see formulas in Table 1).

DIAGNOSIS

The approach to a patient with an acid-base disorder is similar whether the patient presents with a known overdose, an acute illness, or unknown history. History may prove useful but is often lacking or may lag behind treatment imperatives. The physical examination may give clues to the underlying process. Characteristic odors (e.g., acetone or ethanol) and other findings on examination (e.g., calcium oxalate crystals with ethylene glycol or ocular involvement with methanol) may assist in determining an exposure history.

Laboratory evaluation is critical. It is necessary to determine the primary process responsible for the patient's acid-base abnormality. An arterial blood gas provides the most direct and accurate assessment of acid-base status. A venous blood gas (VBG) is not as helpful, obscuring the role of decreased arterial oxygenation and mirroring tissue acidosis, which must then be distinguished from other acidotic processes. An arterialized VBG or even a VBG may be an acceptable alternative in well-perfused children (19). The VBG may also be used in adults when tracking the progress of an already established process.

A stepwise approach to a differential diagnosis can be constructed using the arterial blood gas, electrolytes, renal function, and possibly the serum osmolality. For proper analysis, specimens should be obtained simultaneously. The serum HCO_3^- may be substituted for total CO_2 in calculations if it is directly measured because it accounts for the vast proportion of total CO_2 (20). An acid-base nomogram can assist in determining the primary and secondary processes (Fig. 1).

Differential Diagnosis

NORMAL ANION GAP ACIDOSIS

If an acidosis is due to a gain of both H^+ and Cl^- (e.g., HCl) or a loss of an HCO_3 molecule that is matched by the addition of a Cl^- molecule, there will be no change in the AG because both changes are included in the calculation of AG. The case of a non-AG metabolic acidosis has a specific differential diagnosis (Table 3).

INCREASED ANION GAP ACIDOSIS

In general, a metabolic acidosis that occurs secondary to the presence of any acid increases the AG because unmeasured anions remain in the serum and lower the Cl^- and HCO_3^-. For example, lactic acid composes part of the equilibrium (cations = anions); therefore, the measured anions (Cl^-, HCO_3^-) must go down to accommodate the new (and unmeasured) cation.

The presence of a significantly increased AG is usually indicative of a significant metabolic acidosis (21). There is not necessarily a 1:1 decrease in the HCO_3 for each mEq increase in the AG, however, because excess hydrogen ions are buffered by a variety of buffer systems, the volume of distribution of an anion and HCO_3 may be different, and excretion and metabolism of the anion may not be equal to the regeneration of HCO_3.

Metabolic acidosis may develop in four main ways: (a) generation of lactic acid, (b) generation of ketoacids, (c) drugs that are acids or are metabolized to acids, and (d) uremia. Toxicologic causes of increased AG metabolic acidosis are listed in Table 4.

Some organic anions, such as ketoacids, are normally rapidly excreted in the urine and replaced by Cl^- in the serum. In this instance, there may be a hyperchloremic acidosis also without an AG. Patients with impaired renal function (or decreased glomerular filtration rate secondary to dehydration), however, cannot clear ketoacids as quickly and may develop an AG (21).

Metabolic acidosis has a variety of physiologic effects, some of which are beneficial in terms of compensation and many of which produce immediately detrimental effects. These are summarized in Table 5.

Diagnostic Approach

Identification of the primary acid-base disturbance begins with plotting of the patient's pH and $Paco_2$ and HCO_3 values on a nomogram. When a low plasma HCO_3 is associated with a low

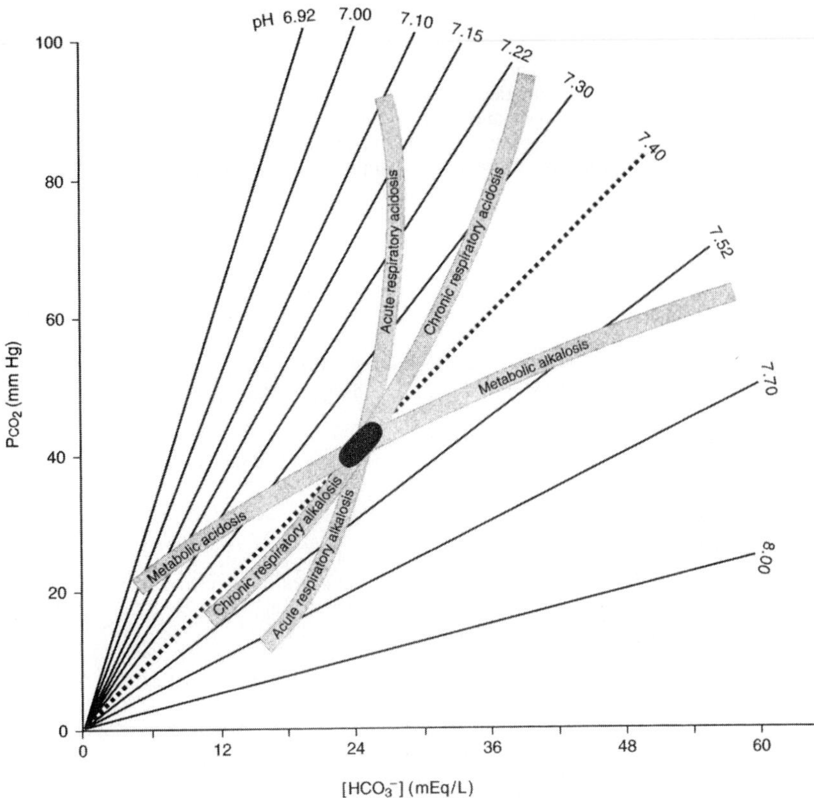

Figure 1. Acid-base map. The region of the map onto which the patient's arterial blood gases fall indicates the primary process and secondary compensatory responses. The center ellipse shows the normal range of values. Shaded areas show the range of values associated with simple acid-base disorders. Two shaded areas are shown for each respiratory disorder: one for acute phase and one for chronic phase. HCO_3^-, bicarbonate; PCO_2, partial pressure of carbon dioxide. (Adapted from Cohen JJ, Kassirer JP. *Acid/base.* Boston: Little, Brown, 1982.)

pH and low $PaCO_2$, a metabolic acidosis is usually the primary process (Fig. 2). Determination of the appropriateness of the decrease in $PaCO_2$ for the decrease in HCO_3 (Table 1) will help to determine whether a second primary (respiratory) process is occurring. The AG is then determined. A normal AG accompanying an acidosis should prompt an evaluation for one of the conditions associated with non-AG acidosis (Table 3). Remember that some mixed acid-base processes can obscure an increased AG and that an acidosis is a dynamic process. A normal AG early in the course may later become an increased AG (e.g., the AG is normal for hours after methanol or ethylene glycol ingestion until enough has been metabolized to reduce the serum HCO_3).

TABLE 3. Differential diagnosis of metabolic acidosis with a normal anion gap

- Drugs
  - Acetazolamide
  - Acids
    - Ammonium chloride
    - Arginine hydrochloride
    - Calcium chloride
    - Hydrochloric acid
    - Lysine hydrochloride
  - Carbonic anhydrase inhibitors
  - Cholestyramine
  - Magnesium chloride
  - Sulfamylon
  - Topiramate (43)
- Gastrointestinal bicarbonate loss
  - Diarrhea
  - Pancreatic fistula
- Miscellaneous
  - Hyperalimentation
  - Posthypocapnia
  - Rapid IV hydration
  - Renal tubular acidosis
  - Ureteroenterostomy

The urine AG (UAG) may also prove useful in assessing acid-base status. Under normal conditions, urine reabsorbs all HCO_3 and the major ions [the cations Na^+, K^+, Ca^{2+}, Mg^{2+}, and ammonium (NH_4^+) and the anions Cl^-, PO_4^-, and SO_4^-]. Because NH_4^+ is the predominant unmeasured cation, the normal UAG is –20 to 0 (Table 1). The normal response to an increased acid load is an increase in renal NH_4^+ excretion, producing an even more negative UAG (–20 to –50 mEq/L). In renal tubular acidosis or other conditions in which normal renal acidification does not occur, however, NH_4^+ excretion is impaired, and the UAG becomes positive (22).

An increased AG is important because it indicates the presence of a metabolic acidosis, even if the process is obscured by a pH that is normal or increased due to compensation by the patient. An AG should be obtained on all patients with a suspected acid-base disorder, and an increased AG should be considered a potential marker of acidosis regardless of the pH. It should be remembered that AGs of 16 to 20 are commonly encountered in the initial evaluation of a drug ingestion and do not necessarily imply the presence of a drug that causes AG acidosis. This may reflect tissue hypoxia; hypoperfusion; seizure; changes in proteins, PO_4^-, or charge equivalents; or other nonspecific effects (20,21,23). With supportive care, these mild elevations usually return to normal within hours.

If the rate of acid production is being adequately compensated by hyperventilation, there may be an *acidosis* (decreased HCO_3^-) but not a significant *acidemia* (pH remains in normal range). Mild or minor acid-base disturbances that seem insignificant on presentation may reflect important processes and

TABLE 4. Toxicologic causes and mechanism of increased anion gap metabolic acidosis

Common causes (mnemonic = MUDPILES)

M	Methanol
U	Uremia
D	Diabetic ketoacidosis
P	Phenformin, paraldehyde, paracetamol (acetaminophen)
I	Iron, isoniazid, inhalants, ibuprofen, inborn errors, idiopathic
L	Lactic acidosis (e.g., carbon monoxide, cyanide, others[a])
E	Ethanol ketoacidosis, ethylene glycol
S	Salicylates, solvents (benzene, toluene), sympathomimetics

Extended list of causes (mechanism) (reference)

Acetaminophen (L) (44)	Nonsteroidal antiinflammatory drugs (L,M)
Aminocaproic acid (M) (45)	Paraldehyde (M)
Benzene (M)	Phenformin (L)
Biguanides (metformin, phenformin) (L)	Polyethylene glycol (low molecular weight) (48)
Carbon monoxide (L)	Propofol (prolonged IV infusion) (U) (49)
Catecholamines (L)	Propylene glycol (L) (50)
Citric acid (M) (46)	Salicylates (L,M)
Cyanide (L)	Streptozotocin (L)
Didanosine (L)	Inorganic sulfur
Diethylene glycol	Sublimed sulfur
Ethanol ketoacidosis (L,K)	Sulfuric acid
Ethylene glycol (M,L)	Sympathomimetics (L)
Fluoride (L)	Amphetamines
Hydrogen sulfide (L)	Cocaine
Hyperphosphatemia (exogenous, pH dependent) (L) (47)	Ephedrine
Iron (L)	Pseudoephedrine
Isoniazid (L)	Theophylline (L)
Lactate (L)	Thiamine deficiency (L)
Metformin (L)	Toluene (M)
Methanol (M,L)	Triethylene glycol (M) (51)
Methionine	Valproic acid (M) (52)
Nalidixic acid (L)	Zidovudine (L)
Niacin (L)	
Nitroprusside (L)	

K, ketoacids; L, lactic acidosis; M, metabolized to organic acids; U, unknown mechanism.
[a]Anything that causes decreased tissue hypoxia may cause lactic acidosis.

TABLE 5. Physiologic effects of metabolic acidosis

Cardiovascular
- Myocardial depression
  - Desensitization of β-adrenergic receptors
  - Antagonism of Ca^{2+} influx and action
- Systemic arterial vascular smooth muscle relaxation
  - Antagonism of Ca^{2+} influx and action
  - Desensitization of alpha-adrenergic receptors
- Systemic venoconstriction and centralization of blood volume
- Pulmonary vasoconstriction
- Enhanced hypoxic pulmonary vasoconstriction
- Sensitization to reentry dysrhythmias and lower threshold for fibrillation

Neuroendocrine
- Sympathetic nervous system stimulation
- Increased cortisol and epinephrine secretion

Cerebral
- Ventilatory stimulation
- Inhibition of metabolism and cell volume regulation
- Increased cerebral blood flow

Respiratory
- Hyperventilation
- Dyspnea and exercise intolerance
- Reduced hemoglobin-oxygen affinity (Bohr effect)
- Improved ventilation-perfusion matching

Metabolic
- Decreased glycolysis
- Increased hepatic and skeletal muscle organic acid uptake
- Decreased insulin sensitivity
- Increased protein degradation

Renal and electrolyte
- Increased HCO_3^- reabsorption and H^+/NH_4^+ excretion
- Hyperkalemia

Others
- Osteoporosis and early epiphyseal closure
- Blunting of cytokine/oxygen radical/nitric oxide formation

From Swenson ER. Metabolic acidosis. *Respir Care* 2001;46:345, with permission.

should not be ignored. An AG that is increasing or failing to resolve despite adequate supportive care or an AG greater than 24 mEq/L usually indicates a significant organic acidosis whose etiology should be sought without delay (20,23).

It should be remembered that many agents require metabolism to produce significant acidosis. There should be periodic clinical and laboratory reevaluation during the first 12 to 24 hours after an ingestion. Regardless, an increased AG should prompt consideration of the differential diagnoses of increased AG metabolic acidosis (Table 4).

A single-agent process produces a delta AG ($dAG{:}dHCO_3$ ratio) within the 0.6 to 1.8 range. An increased AG that falls outside of the 0.6:1.8 ratio to HCO_3 indicates the possibility of a second metabolic process. A low delta AG suggests a non-AG metabolic acidosis. A high delta AG suggests a concomitant metabolic alkalosis (22).

Other laboratory tests may aid in further refining the differential diagnosis. The finding of plasma ketones should indicate the condition of *ketoacidosis*. *Lactic acidosis* is, by definition, an arterial La^- concentration above 5 mmol/L with a pH less than 7.35 (24). An elevated La^- level suggests certain processes. However, lactic acidosis with a toxicologic source is a dynamic process, and rising concentrations should be of concern. Also, because of insensitivity of the AG, with La^- levels between 5.0 and 9.9 mmol/L, 50% of patients have an AG less than 12 mEq/L (25). Finally, both metabolic and respiratory alkaloses may be associated with an increased La^- level, although the AG is usually less than 20 mEq/L. Correction of hypoxia and hypoperfusion should be accomplished and other causes of lactic acidosis considered.

The presence of *renal failure* potentially explains an AG acidosis, but secondary renal failure—from rhabdomyolysis or ethylene glycol, for example—should be considered.

The *osmolal gap* may provide additional incentive to pursue the possibility of toxic alcohols, but this test is limited in the value of either positive or negative results (Chapter 25). An increased osmolal gap may indicate toxic alcohols, but it is also elevated in renal failure, ketoacidosis, lactic acidosis, and other conditions (1). The absence of an osmolal gap cannot exclude the presence of toxic alcohols. Toxic and even potentially fatal doses of some agents that normally increase serum osmolality may not elevate the osmolal gap out of the "normal" range (26). Also, the metabolic products of the parent alcohols may not be as osmotically active, thus further decreasing the diagnostic usefulness of the serum osmolality over time (27). At best, it is an adjunctive test that must be interpreted with caution.

Additional tests that may help to determine the etiology of an AG metabolic acidosis include a serum salicylate level, other specific drug levels as suggested by the patient's history or presentation, urine toxicology, and urinalysis for crystals (e.g., calcium oxalate crystals may indicate the possibility of ethylene glycol ingestion).

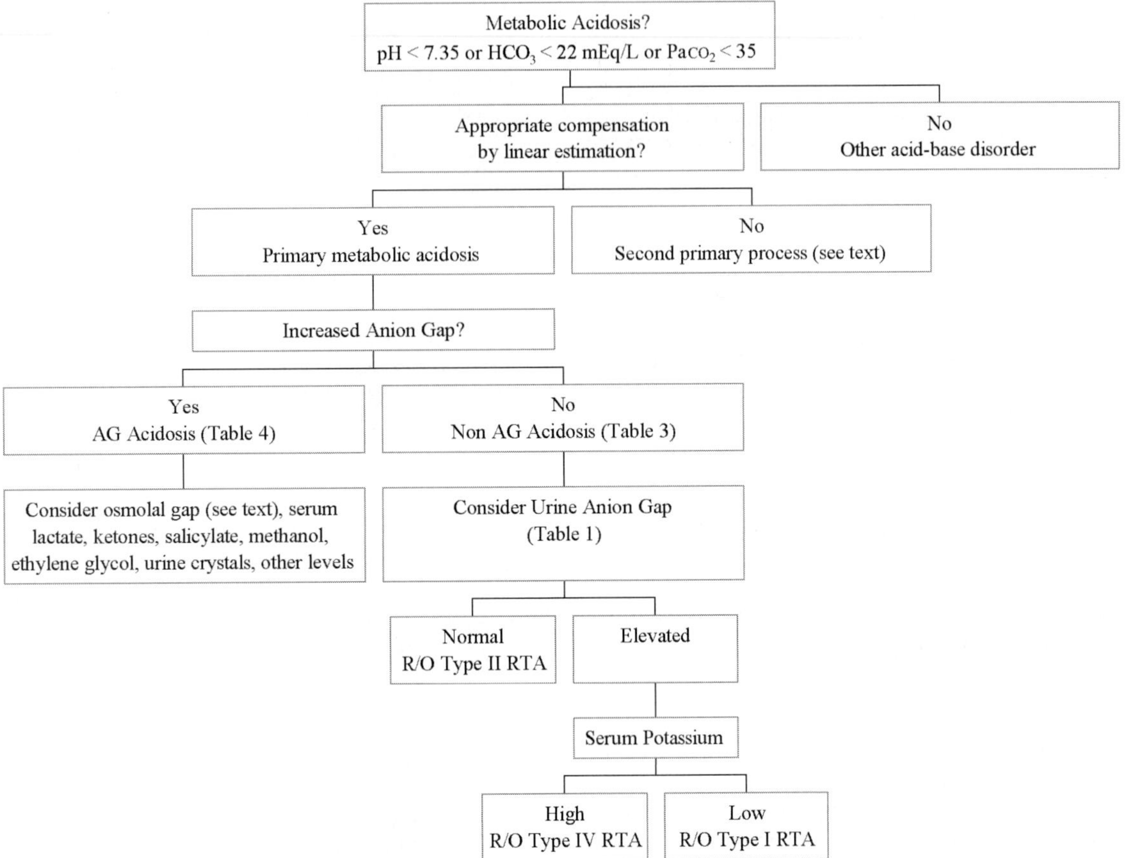

Figure 2. Evaluation of metabolic acidosis. AG, anion gap; HCO_3, bicarbonate; $Paco_2$, partial pressure of arterial carbon dioxide; R/O, rule out; RTA, renal tubular acidosis.

Because of the potential for rapid clinical decline, when an obvious toxicologic cause cannot be confirmed, nontoxicologic etiologies of AG metabolic acidosis should be pursued (Table 6).

Other Acid-Base Abnormalities

A similar stepwise approach to other acid-base abnormalities can help to develop and refine the differential diagnosis.

One condition that requires mention is the finding of a low AG with or without acidosis. This finding suggests either the presence of an unmeasured cation or the loss of an unmeasured anion and may result from limitations in the technology (e.g., bromide being measured as chloride) (Table 7) (28).

MANAGEMENT

The initial treatment of acid-base disorders is symptomatic and supportive, including airway control and volume resuscitation. The initial resuscitation fluid is isotonic normal saline. This is followed by treatment of the underlying conditions and determination of the etiology.

Alcoholic ketoacidosis occurs in the context of volume contraction, thiamine deficiency, and glycogen depletion. Management includes volume replacement, dextrose, and thiamine, with correction of other electrolyte abnormalities, such as hypomagnesemia and hypophosphatemia.

Management of specific toxin-induced acidosis varies. Acidosis secondary to methanol or ethylene glycol requires blockade of alcohol dehydrogenase and consideration of dialysis and

TABLE 6. Nontoxicologic causes of lactic acidosis

Increased oxygen consumption
Chronic hyperventilation
Exercise
Neuroleptic malignant syndrome
Pheochromocytoma
Seizure
Shivering (hypothermic)
Decreased oxygen tissue supply
Decreased cardiac output
Cardiogenic shock
Hypovolemia
Decreased partial pressure of arterial oxygen
Anemia
Hypoxemia
Regional ischemia
Sepsis
Altered metabolic states
Diabetes mellitus (diabetic ketoacidosis)
Decreased lactate clearance
Hepatic failure
Hypoglycemia
Malignancy
Inborn errors of metabolism
Thiamine deficiency
Miscellaneous
Acquired immunodeficiency syndrome
D-Lactic acidosis
Short bowel syndrome/stasis
Renal failure (failure to excrete acids)
Rhabdomyolysis
Starvation ketoacidosis

TABLE 7. Causes of low anion gap

Increased nonmeasured cations
- Not normally present
  - Gammopathies (multiple myeloma, polyclonal gammopathy)
  - Lithium
  - Polymyxin B
- Normally present
  - Hyperkalemia
  - Hypercalcemia
  - Hypermagnesemia

Decreased unmeasured anions
- Hypoalbuminemia (e.g., nutritional deficiency, acquired immunodeficiency syndrome, chronic illness)

Chloride overestimation
- Bromide
- Hypertriglyceridemia (colorimetric assays)
- Iodide

other supportive and adjunctive measures (Chapters 191 and 192). Salicylates typically produce a mixed acid-base picture with an initial respiratory alkalosis followed by a metabolic acidosis (Chapter 127). Treatment is aimed at enhancing elimination by urinary ion trapping and possibly dialysis.

Role of Bicarbonate Therapy

Of note is the controversial aspect of treating acidemia with sodium HCO_3. There is a general consensus that above a pH of 7.1, specific treatment is not required. The need for treatment below a pH of 7.1 is not clear. Cardiac function and numerous enzyme systems are adversely affected by severe acidemia (29). When the HCO_3^- buffering system is compromised by low [HCO_3], the generation of small amounts of H^+ produces significant pH worsening. However, the addition of exogenous HCO_3 in this setting has not been shown to improve outcomes (30). In addition, sodium HCO_3 can cause an increase in the CO_2 production, intracellular acidosis, further depression of cardiac output, a decrease in ionized calcium, a decrease in the partial pressure of arterial oxygen, and an increase in arterial La^- (21). It also decreases oxygen supply to tissues by shifting the oxyhemoglobin dissociation curve to the right (31). Carbicarb, an equimolar mixture of Na^+ carbonate and sodium HCO_3, is $PaCO_2$ neutral and associated with improved hemodynamics (32). It is not available for routine use, however. Insulin inhibits gluconeogenesis and may decrease the amount of precursors for La^- production in metformin and phenformin-induced lactic acidosis (31,33). Dichloroacetate is believed to activate pyruvate dehydrogenase and reduce lactic acid production by that mechanism (31), but no controlled studies have been performed.

PITFALLS

The BE/D and AG methods of acid-base status analysis may miss significant acid-base disorders. One should not rely absolutely on a "normal" AG or BE/D to indicate a normal acid-base status. The AG is sometimes used to make diagnoses beyond its capabilities (34–36).

The absence of an osmolal gap cannot exclude the presence of toxic alcohols.

REFERENCES

1. Swenson ER. Metabolic acidosis. *Respir Care* 2001;46(4):342–353.
2. Schwartz-Goldstein BH, Malik AR, Sarwar A, Brandstetter RD. Lactic acidosis associated with a deceptively normal anion gap. *Heart Lung* 1996;25(1):79–80.
3. Oster JR, Perez GO, Vaamonde CA. Relationship between blood pH, potassium and phosphorus during acute metabolic acidosis. *Am J Physiol* 1978;235:F345–F351.
4. Schwartz SM, Carroll HM, Scharschmidt LA. Sublimed (inorganic) sulfur ingestion: a cause of life-threatening metabolic acidosis with a high anion gap. *Arch Intern Med* 1986;146:1437–1438.
5. Williamson JC. Acid-base disorders: classification and management strategies. *Am Fam Physician* 1995;52(2):584–590.
6. Emmet M, Narins RG. Clinical use of the anion gap. *Medicine* 1977;56:38–54.
7. Witte DL, Rodgers JL, Barret DA. The anion gap: its use in quality control. *Clin Chem* 1976;22:643–646.
8. Winter SD, Pearson R, Gabow PA, et al. The fall of the serum anion gap. *Arch Intern Med* 1990;150:311–313.
9. Fencl V, Jabor A, Kazda A, Figge J. Diagnosis of metabolic acid-base disturbances in critically ill patients. *Am J Respir Crit Care Med* 2000;162:2246–2251.
10. Kirschbaum B. Hyperglobulinemia with an increased anion gap. *Am J Med Sci* 1998;316:393–397.
11. Kowalchuk JM, Scheuermann BW. Acid-base regulation: a comparison of quantitative methods. *Can J Physiol Pharmacol* 1994;72(7):818–826.
12. Piechl RL, Toll PW, Leith DE, et al. Acid-base changes in the running greyhound: contributing variables. *J Appl Physiol* 1992;73(6):2297–2304.
13. Swenson ER. The strong ion difference approach: can a strong case be made for its use in acid-base analysis? Available at: http://www.rcjournal.com/contents/01.99/contents.asp. Accessed 6/02.
14. Dorward WV, Chalmers L. Comparison of methods for calculating serum osmolality from chemical concentrations, and the prognostic value of such calculations. *Clin Chem* 1975;21:190–194.
15. Inaba H, Hirasawa H, Mizuguchi T. Serum osmolality gap in postoperative patients in intensive care. *Lancet* 1987;1:1331–1335.
16. Schelling JR, Howard RL, Winter SK, Linas SL. Increased osmolal gap in alcoholic ketoacidosis and lactic acidosis. *Ann Intern Med* 1990;113:580–582.
17. Sklar AH, Linas SL. The osmolal gap in renal failure. *Ann Intern Med* 1983;98:481–482.
18. Chabali R. Diagnostic use of anion and osmolal gaps in pediatric emergency medicine. *Pediatr Emerg Care* 1997;13(3):204–210.
19. McGillivray D, Ducharme FM, Charron Y, et al. Clinical decision making based on venous versus capillary blood gas values in the well-perfused child. *Ann Emerg Med* 1999;34(1):58–63.
20. Gabow PA. Disorders associated with an altered anion gap. *Kidney Int* 1985;27:472–483.
21. Ishihara K, Szerlip HM. Anion gap acidosis. *Semin Nephrol* 1998;18(1):83–97.
22. Fall PJ. A stepwise approach to acid-base disorders. *Postgrad Med* 2000;107(3):249–263.
23. Gabow PA, Kaehny WD, Fennessey PV, et al. Diagnostic importance of an increased serum anion gap. *N Engl J Med* 1980;303:854–858.
24. Stacpoole PW. Lactic acidosis. *Endocrinol Metab Clin North Am* 1993;22:221–245.
25. Iberti TJ, Leibowitz AB, Papadakos PJ, et al. Low sensitivity of the anion gap as a screen to detect hyperlactatemia in critically ill patients. *Crit Care Med* 1990;18:275–277.
26. Steinhart B. Case report: severe ethylene glycol intoxication with normal osmolal gap—"A chilling thought." *J Emerg Med* 1990;8:583–585.
27. Ammar KA, Heckerling PS. Ethylene glycol poisoning with a normal anion gap caused by concurrent ethanol ingestion: importance of the osmolal gap. *Am J Kidney Dis* 1996;27(1):130–133.
28. Jurado FL, del Rio C, Nassar G, et al. Low anion gap. *South Med J* 1998;91(7):624–629.
29. Orchard CH, Kentish JC. Effects of changes of pH on the contractile function of cardiac muscle. *Am J Physiol* 1990;258:C967–C981.
30. Stacpoole PW, Wright EC, Baumgartner TG, et al. Natural history and course of acquired lactic acidosis in adults. *Am J Med* 1994;97:47–54.
31. Jurovich MR, Wooldridge JD, Force RW. Metformin-associated nonketotic metabolic acidosis. *Ann Pharmacother* 1996;30:53–55.
32. Bersin RM, Arieff AI. Improved hemodynamic function during hypoxia with CarbiCarb®, a new agent for the management of acidosis. *Circulation* 1988;77:227–233.
33. McGuinness ME, Talbert RL. Phenformin-induced lactic acidosis: a forgotten adverse drug reaction. *Ann Pharmacother* 1993;27:1183–1187.
34. Badrick T, Hickman PE. The anion gap: a reappraisal. *Am J Clin Pathol* 1992;98:249–252.
35. DiNubile MJ. The increment in the anion gap: overextension of a concept? *Lancet* 1988;2:951–952.
36. Salem MM, Mujais SK. Gaps in the anion gap. *Arch Intern Med* 1992;152:1625–1629.
37. Sadjadi SA, Fagan T. Lower values and a new range for anion gap in the diagnosis of acid base disorders. *J Am Soc Nephrol* 1993;4:299.
38. Figge J, Jabor A, Kazda A, Fencl V. Anion gap and hypoalbuminemia. *Crit Care Med* 1998;26(11):1807–1810.
39. Carvounis CP, Feinfeld DA. A simple estimate of the effect of the serum albumin level on the anion gap. *Am J Nephrol* 2000;20:369–372.
40. Figge J, Mydosh T, Fencl V. Serum proteins and acid-base equilibria: a follow-up. *J Lab Clin Med* 1992;120(5):713–719.
41. Kellum J. Acid base pHorum. http://www.anes.upmc.edu/mcctp/phorum.html. Accessed June 2002.
42. Narins RG, Emmett M. Simple and mixed acid-base disorders: a practical approach. *Medicine* 1980;59(3):161–187.

43. Wilner A, Raymond K, Pollard R. Topiramate and metabolic acidosis. *Epilepsia* 1999;40(6):792–795.
44. Yale SH, Mazza JJ. Anion gap acidosis associated with acetaminophen. *Ann Intern Med* 2000;133(9):752–753.
45. Budris WA, Roxe DM, Duvel JM. High anion gap metabolic acidosis associated with aminocaproic acid. *Ann Pharmacother* 1999;33:308–311.
46. DeMars CS, Hollister K, Tomassoni A, et al. Citric acid ingestion: a life-threatening cause of metabolic acidosis. *Ann Emerg Med* 2001;38:588–592.
47. Kirschbaum B. The acidosis of exogenous phosphate intoxication. *Arch Intern Med* 1998;158(4):405–408.
48. Erickson TB, Aks SE, Zabaneh R, Reid R. Acute renal toxicity after ingestion of Lava light liquid. *Ann Emerg Med* 1996;27:781–784.
49. Cannon ML, Glazier SS, Bauman LA. Metabolic acidosis, rhabdomyolysis and cardiovascular collapse after prolonged propofol infusion. *J Neurosurg* 2001;95:1053–1056.
50. Glover ML, Reed MD. Propylene glycol: the safe diluent that continues to cause harm. *Pharmacotherapy* 1996;16(4):690–693.
51. Vassiliadis J, Graudins A, Dowsett RP. Triethylene glycol poisoning treated with intravenous ethanol infusion. *J Toxicol Clin Toxicol* 1999;37(6):773–776.
52. Franssen EJF, van Essen GG, Portman AT, et al. Valproic acid toxicokinetics: serial hemodialysis and hemoperfusion. *Ther Drug Monit* 1999;21(3):289–292.

CHAPTER 10

The Anticholinergic Patient

Keith K. Burkhart

OVERVIEW

Historical teaching causes most clinicians, when they hear the term *anticholinergic syndrome,* to think of the classically described mnemonic "Blind as a bat, Hot as Hades, Dry as a bone, Red as a beet, and Mad as a hatter." This mnemonic refers to the anticholinergic consequences of ciliary muscle paralysis (mydriasis); hyperthermia; anhydrosis (dry skin without sweat); vasodilation (flushing); and delirium or psychosis, respectively. A variety of pharmaceuticals and naturally occurring products can produce anticholinergic signs or symptoms. Classes of drugs that can produce the anticholinergic syndrome include antihistamines, antidepressants, antidiarrheals, antiemetics, antiparkinsonian agents, antipsychotics, antispasmodics (including the belladonna alkaloids), bronchodilators, mydriatics, and skeletal muscle relaxants. Some mushrooms and plants (especially jimson weed) produce anticholinergic toxicity. Poisoning from Chinese herbal medicines has also been reported (1).

Many of these drugs have multiple pharmacologic actions. For example, cyclic antidepressants have sympathomimetic and anticholinergic actions that may create overlap of these two syndromes. Likewise, the ingestion of multiple drugs may result in a combination of signs and symptoms differing from each classic syndrome. Anticholinergic toxicity, therefore, has a myriad of presentations for which the expertise of the medical toxicologist will be requested.

Because of the multiple actions of these drugs and polydrug overdoses, the incidence of anticholinergic poisoning is unknown. In addition, the syndrome is often unrecognized and therefore underreported. The elderly who are often subjected to polypharmacy are especially vulnerable (2).

There is potential for serious, life-threatening toxicity and secondary complications from the delirium and coma that may result from anticholinergic syndrome (3,4). Anticholinergic drug-induced coma and respiratory failure often require mechanical ventilation and admission to an intensive care unit (ICU). As with any toxicologic emergency, supportive care is of paramount importance. For anticholinergic poisoning, an effective antidote, physostigmine, is also available. However, controversy surrounds its indications and risks.

PATHOPHYSIOLOGY

By definition, anticholinergic compounds antagonize the effects of the endogenous neurotransmitter acetylcholine (ACh). Receptors for ACh are widely distributed in both the central nervous system and the peripheral nervous system. ACh receptors are divided into muscarinic or nicotinic subtypes. In the peripheral nervous system, muscarinic receptors predominate in the parasympathetic terminals. A detailed review of muscarinic receptor subtypes, including the second messenger systems, is available (5). Nicotinic receptors are found in the autonomic ganglia (sympathetic and parasympathetic) and the motor endplate. Nicotinic receptor stimulation produces tachycardia, hypertension, muscle fasciculation, and receptor fatigue. Paralysis may occur at high doses. Nicotinic antagonists, such as the nondepolarizing muscle relaxants pancuronium and vecuronium, block the action of ACh at the motor endplate and produce paralysis of skeletal muscle. Respiratory failure is the most life-threatening consequence.

The excessive stimulation of muscarinic receptors that may result from poisoning by cholinesterase inhibitors, such as the organophosphate and carbamate insecticides, produces the cholinergic toxidrome (Chapter 13).

Agents that block muscarinic cholinergic receptors may lead to anticholinergic poisoning. Blockade of central nervous system ACh receptors has mind-altering effects that cover a spectrum from agitation to psychosis and delirium to seizures and coma.

Anticholinergic effects may persist for days. Prolonged half-lives, active metabolites, and possibly the persistence of muscarinic receptor binding may explain this phenomenon. For example, many ICU patients awaken from coma in a delirious state. This delirium may represent progressive recovery from anticholinergic coma rather than ICU psychosis. Reversal by physostigmine after the initial phases of poisoning (e.g., cyclic antidepressants) may support this concept (6). Yet another explanation for prolonged symptoms is delayed absorption. Fahy et al. described prolonged coma after a benztropine overdose (7). In this case, serial levels demonstrated falling and then rising levels, suggesting erratic absorption.

TABLE 1. Comparison of anticholinergic, sympathomimetic, and serotonergic syndromes

Symptom/sign	Anticholinergic syndrome	Sympathomimetic syndrome	Serotonergic syndrome
Vital signs			
Fever	++	++	+
Tachycardia	+	++	+
Hypertension	+	++	+
Mental status			
Coma	Common	No	Rare
Agitation	+	+	+
Hallucinations	Common	Some	Some
Motor activity	Myoclonus	Tremor	Myoclonus
Rigidity	–	–	+
Seizures	+	++	+, Delayed
Skin	Dry	Diaphoretic	Diaphoretic
Mydriasis	+	+	+
Ileus	+	–	–
Urinary retention	+	–	–

–, not present; +, ++, indicate strength of manifestation.

DIAGNOSIS

Differential Diagnosis

Other syndromes may overlap with anticholinergic syndrome. For example, sympathomimetic syndrome may also include fever, hypertension, tachycardia, and tremulousness, possibly mistaken for agitation. Differentiating features might include sweating and gastrointestinal symptoms. The serotonin syndrome may include hypertension, tachycardia, fever, agitation, delirium, and myoclonus (Table 1).

History

Historical information often aids or confirms the diagnosis of anticholinergic poisoning. The medical toxicologist searches for evidence that supports access to or exposure to an anticholinergic pharmaceutical or toxin. Attempts should be made to identify all drugs available to the patient and then review their pharmacology for anticholinergic actions. Family and friends may provide historical information on drugs taken or plants ingested. They may provide a description of signs and symptoms that may have preceded delirium or coma.

Signs and Symptoms

The classic mnemonic "Hot as Hades . . ." is used to remember some signs of anticholinergic poisoning. Yet another mnemonic to consider contrasts the cholinergic, "wet syndrome," versus the anticholinergic, "dry syndrome." Whereas *SLUDGE* (*s*alivation, *l*acrimation, *u*rination, *d*efecation, *g*astrointestinal cramping, *e*mesis) describes cholinergic effects, *anti-SLUDGE* describes the lack of or diminished secretions/motility from antimuscarinic actions. The anticholinergic toxidrome can be divided into peripheral and central components (Table 1). Patients may present with primarily peripheral signs and symptoms, primarily central ones, or both. *Central anticholinergic syndrome* refers to symptoms that persist longer than the peripheral manifestations, thereby creating difficulty in diagnosis.

The clinical presentation may also be complicated by other actions of the intoxicant (e.g., tricyclic antidepressants) or the actions of other potentially toxic substances (e.g., salicylates, sympathomimetics). The most serious manifestations include agitated delirium, respiratory failure, hyperthermia, and seizures.

Diagnostic Tests

The tests typically ordered for evaluation of the suicidal patient should be obtained, if appropriate. A general toxicology screen typically adds little to the diagnostic work-up. Many anticholinergic agents are not detected, even on comprehensive screens that take hours to return (8). In addition, routine laboratory tests are not necessary for anticholinergic poisoning except for complications. For example, prolonged agitation should prompt evaluation of altered mental status with a lumbar puncture and perhaps a cranial computed tomography scan. Muscle breakdown can be assessed by measuring the creatine kinase level. Physostigmine administration is a diagnostic test that may also be therapeutic, as explained below (further detail is provided in Chapter 67).

POTENTIAL COMPLICATIONS

Severe agitation and delirium place patients at risk to harm themselves as well as others. For example, deaths have occurred from hyperthermia in the desert environment (3), and jimson weed–poisoned patients have been found outdoors naked in the cold winter environment.

Shortly after exposure, most patients also demonstrate sinus tachycardia and hypertension. These abnormalities are usually mild, however, and rarely require medical intervention. This contrasts with life-threatening hypertension and accompanying tachycardia from sympathomimetic toxicity. Coma and respiratory failure are the most serious derangements from anticholinergic poisoning and may require ICU admission. Monitoring for carbon dioxide retention and respiratory acidosis should be performed. A measurement of the creatine kinase is usually warranted to assess for rhabdomyolysis. Dehydration may also result from agitation, hyperthermia, and poor fluid intake. Urinary retention may also develop.

MANAGEMENT

General supportive care is sufficient in most cases of anticholinergic poisoning. The severity of the agitation and delirium determine the need for pharmacologic intervention. Traditionally, benzodiazepines and occasionally butyrophenones have been used. However, large and heavily sedating doses may be needed such that intubation is required (6). In these cases, physostigmine may be a better alternative.

Antidotes

Physostigmine reversibly binds to acetylcholinesterase and prevents this enzyme from degrading ACh. The neurotransmitter ACh accumulates and competitively reverses muscarinic receptor inhibition at its postsynaptic sites. Unlike the related drugs neostigmine and pyridostigmine, physostigmine is a tertiary rather than a quaternary amine and therefore crosses the blood–brain barrier. As a result, it is effective in reversing central as well as peripheral anticholinergic effects. (See also Chapter 67.) Physostigmine administration can be both a diagnostic and therapeutic aid. Administration in the confused febrile patient may return mental status to normal and reduce fever. These patients may then provide a history that confirms the anticholinergic poisoning, thereby avoiding a lumbar puncture and cranial computed tomography. Some toxicologists have suggested the use of physostigmine for seizures unresponsive to conventional treatment; severe hypertension resulting in acute symptoms or end-organ dysfunction; and supraventricular tachycardias resulting in hemodynamic instability, cardiac ischemia, or other organ dysfunction (9). In practice, however, physostigmine should be used with extreme caution in these patients.

There are contraindications to the use of physostigmine. Enhanced cholinergic neurotransmission might worsen bronchospasm and mechanical obstruction of the intestine or urogenital tract, which are contraindications to physostigmine administration (10). Use physostigmine cautiously in patients with asthma, gangrene, diabetes, or cardiovascular disease and after depolarizing neuromuscular blocking agents (e.g., succinylcholine). Physostigmine should also be avoided in the early (e.g., within the first 6 hours) cyclic antidepressant overdose or any overdose with evidence of cardiac conduction delay (i.e., atrioventricular block or prolonged QRS interval).

In the 1970s, there were a number of reports that purported the benefits of physostigmine for the reversal of altered mental status, including coma, myoclonus, and cardiac complications of cyclic antidepressant and antipsychotic poisoning (11–14). The use of physostigmine in the management of cyclic antidepressant poisoning in later reports, however, allegedly caused cardiac ventricular dysrhythmias (15–17). These case reports and an animal study describe asystole, seizures, and death when physostigmine was used to treat tricyclic antidepressant poisoning. Subsequently, there was a widespread reduction in the use of physostigmine, which remains today.

When administered in excessive amounts or to a patient not in an anticholinergic state, physostigmine often produces signs of cholinergic excess. Any patient receiving physostigmine, therefore, should be observed on a cardiac monitor. The usual starting dose for adults is 0.5 to 2.0 mg. Recommendations for the safe use of physostigmine are centered on its slow intravenous infusion at a rate not to exceed 1 mg/1 to 2 minutes to avoid the complications, seizures, and bradyarrhythmias described above. Slower rates of administration can be used and simply delay the onset of effect. Mental status improvement usually occurs within 10 minutes of administration. If no reversal of anticholinergic effect has occurred after 10 to 20 minutes, an additional 1 to 2 mg may be administered. The recommended dose in pediatric patients is 0.02 mg/kg administered by slow intravenous infusion over 5 to 10 minutes (18).

The duration of action for physostigmine is relatively short compared to many anticholinergic agents. If indications for physostigmine recur, additional doses may be administered. If excessive cholinergic effects are noted, they can be treated with atropine. As the duration of action of physostigmine is relatively brief, atropine would not be needed unless severe cholinergic toxicity developed. In the rare event of a seizure, diazepam is recommended. The half-life of physostigmine is short; therefore, its action after the 2-mg dose typically lasts only 1 hour to as long as 4 hours.

Supportive Care

Gastrointestinal decontamination should be considered for anticholinergically poisoned patients. Induction of emesis is specifically contraindicated in the patient at risk for obtundation or seizures and, therefore, should be avoided in the anticholinergic patient. On the other hand, delayed gastric emptying and slowed gut motility may lead to a benefit several hours after ingestion. Gastric lavage remains an unproved benefit in an already symptomatic anticholinergic patient. Administration of activated charcoal is recommended as the preferred decontamination. Activated charcoal administration or gastric lavage is problematic for the agitated, delirious patient. Physostigmine administration has also been recommended to facilitate gastric decontamination (19,20).

Mildly poisoned patients only require observation or benzodiazepine administration while the anticholinergic agent is cleared. In severely poisoned patients, however, coma may require endotracheal intubation and ICU monitoring. Physostigmine administration may awaken some of these patients, avoiding intubation or facilitating extubation (21). The alternative is to give more and usually high-dose sedation that may keep the patient on a ventilator longer than is necessary. Opportunities may exist to further refine the management of the critically anticholinergically poisoned patients. For example, the use of physostigmine may reduce the use of critical care resources by limiting or shortening intubation and decreasing the length of stay.

REFERENCES

1. Chan TYK. Anticholinergic poisoning due to Chinese herbal medicines. *Vet Hum Toxicol* 1995;37:156.
2. Mintzer J, Burns A. Anticholinergic side-effects of drugs in elderly people. *J R Soc Med* 2000;93:457.
3. Jimson weed poisoning—Texas, New York, and California, 1994. *MMWR Morb Mortal Wkly Rep* 1995;44:41.
4. Rauber-Luthy CH, Giurguis M, Meier-Abt AST, et al. Lethal poisoning after ingestion of a tea prepared from Angels's Trumpet (*Datura suaveolens*). *J Toxicol Clin Toxicol* 1999;37:414 (abst).
5. Goyal RK. Muscarinic receptor subtypes. *N Engl J Med* 1989;321:1022.
6. Burns MJ, Linden CH, Graudins A, et al. A comparison of physostigmine and benzodiazepines for the treatment of anticholinergic poisoning. *Ann Emerg Med* 2000;35:374.
7. Fahy P, Arnold P, Curry SC, et al. Serial serum drug concentrations and prolonged anticholinergic toxicity after benztropine (Cogentin) overdose. *Am J Emerg Med* 1989;7:199.
8. Goldfrank L, Flomenbaum N, Lewin N, et al. Anticholinergic poisoning. *J Toxicol Clin Toxicol* 1982;19:17.
9. Smilkstein MJ. Editorial. *J Emerg Med* 1991;9:275.
10. Product information: Antilirium (physostigmine salicylate). In: *Physicians' desk reference*, 47th ed. Montvale, NJ: Medical Economics, 1993.
11. Burks JS, Walker JE, Rumack BH, et al. Tricyclic antidepressant poisoning: reversal of coma, choreoathetosis, and myoclonus by physostigmine. *JAMA* 1974;230:1405.
12. Manoguerra AS, Ruiz E. Physostigmine treatment of anticholinergic poisoning. *JACEP* 1976;5:125.
13. Tobis J, Das BN. Cardiac complications in amitriptyline poisoning: successful treatment with physostigmine. *JAMA* 1976;235:1474.
14. Weisdorf D, Kramer J, Goldbarg A, Klawans HL. Physostigmine for cardiac and neurologic manifestations of phenothiazine poisoning. *Clin Pharmacol Ther* 1978;24(6):663.
15. Walker WE, Levy RC, Hanenson IB. Physostigmine: its use and abuse. *JACEP* 1976;5:436.
16. Pentel P, Peterson CD. Asystole complicating physostigmine treatment of tricyclic antidepressant overdose. *Ann Emerg Med* 1980;9:588.
17. Vance MA, Ross SM, Millington WR, Blumberg JB. Potentiation of tricyclic antidepressant toxicity by physostigmine in mice. *Clin Toxicol* 1977;11:413.

18. Shannon M. Toxicology reviews: physostigmine. *Pediatr Emerg Care* 1998;14:224.
19. Burkhart KK, Magalski AE, Donovan JW. A retrospective review of the use of activated charcoal and physostigmine in the treatment of jimson weed poisoning. *J Toxicol Clin Toxicol* 1999;37:389(abst).
20. Levy R. Jimson seed poisoning—a new hallucinogen on the horizon. *JACEP* 1977;6:58.
21. Ferraro KK, Burkhart KK, Donovan JW, et al. A retrospective review of physostigmine in olanzapine overdose. *J Toxicol Clin Toxicol* 2001;39:474(abst).

CHAPTER 11

Asthma

João H. Delgado and Lee S. Newman

OVERVIEW

Asthma affects 15 million people in the United States and 5% to 10% of the population worldwide (1). It is the most common occupational pulmonary disease in developed countries (2,3). A National Institutes of Health expert panel defines *asthma* as a "chronic inflammatory disorder of the airways in which many cells and cellular elements play a role. . . . The inflammation also causes an associated increase in the existing bronchial hyperresponsiveness to a variety of stimuli" (1). The toxicologist may be called on to assess asthma that is induced or exacerbated by toxicants.

Clinically, asthma often manifests as dyspnea, wheezing, or coughing. These effects result from airflow obstruction and may reverse spontaneously or after treatment. Asthma exacerbations are typically short-lived, lasting minutes to hours, and interspersed with asymptomatic periods. Chronic asthma, with partial reversibility and persistent airflow obstruction, can occur especially if environmental triggers persist.

Occupational asthma involves asthma that is attributable to a particular working environment and usually not to stimuli encountered outside the workplace (4). It includes both new onset as well as exacerbation of asthma due to workplace exposure. Over 300 substances capable of causing asthma in the workplace have been described (Table 1) (5,6). The proportion of newly diagnosed cases of asthma that can be attributed to occupational exposures is unknown. In the United States, occupational exposure is believed to account for 5% to 17% of adult-onset asthma (7–9).

The reactive airways dysfunction syndrome results from an acute high-dose exposure to an airway irritant (10). Although clinically it may be similar to asthma, it has important differences (Table 2). Most cases of reactive airways dysfunction syndrome follow an accidental occupational exposure. The resulting symptoms are usually self-limited but may persist for months or even years.

TABLE 1. Examples of agents causing occupational asthma and associated occupations

Agent	Occupation
Chemical	
Anhydrides (phthalic, trimellitic, others)	Chemist, epoxy resin worker, paint manufacturer, plastic manufacturer, spray painter, tool setter
Azo dyes	Textile workers
Azodicarbonamide	Plastic and rubber manufacturer
Colophony	Electronics manufacturer, solder flux manufacturer
Cutting oils/machining fluids	Automotive and other machinists
Cyanoacrylate esters	Dentist, nurse
Diisocyanates (hexamethylene, toluene, others)	Auto body worker, chemical worker, plastic manufacturer, polyurethane foam manufacturer
Ethanolamines	Painter, solderer
Ethyleneamines	Rubber manufacturer, photographer, shellac handlers
Fluorine	Pot room worker
Formaldehyde	Laboratory technician, pathologist
Glutaraldehyde	Glove manufacturer, health care worker
Latex	Endoscopy unit worker
Paraphenylenediamine	Chemist, fur dyer
Persulfates (sodium, potassium)	Chemical worker, hairdresser
Plicatic acid (Western Red Cedar)	Cabinetmaker, carpenter, sawmill worker
Polyvinyl chloride	Meat wrapper
Metal	
Aluminum	Aluminum smelter, pot room worker
Chromium	Metal processor, printer, welder
Cobalt	Alloy worker, diamond polisher, metal processor
Nickel	Chemical engineer, metal processor, plater, welder
Platinum	Chemist, platinum refiner
Vanadium	Metal grinder
Pharmaceutical	
Amprolium	Poultry feed mixer
Antibiotics	Pharmaceutical worker/manufacturer
Cimetidine	Pharmaceutical worker/manufacturer
Methyldopa	Pharmaceutical worker/manufacturer
Psyllium	Nurse, pharmaceutical worker/manufacturer
Other	
Animal protein (dander, urine)	Farmer, laboratory worker, meat processor/inspector, veterinarian, veterinary technician
Flour/grains	Baker, brewery worker, farmer, grain elevator worker
Wood	Carpenter, sawmill worker, wood finisher, wood machinist, woodworker

Adapted from Chan-Yeung M, Malo JL. Current concepts: occupational asthma. *N Engl J Med* 1995;333:107–102; and Chan-Yeung M, Malo JL. Aetiological agents in occupational asthma. *Eur Respir J* 1994;7:346–371.

PATHOPHYSIOLOGY

The pathophysiology of asthma is multifactorial and incompletely understood. Airway inflammation plays a central role and can be triggered by many toxins. In response to an inciting stimulus, a variety of inflammatory cells are recruited to the airway: eosinophils, mast cells, macrophages, neutrophils, epithelial cells, and activated T cells. Activation of the resident airway cells and recruited cells results in the release of preformed mediators, such as histamine, bradykinin, leukotrienes, prostaglandins, and platelet-activating factor, and elaboration of newly synthesized mediators. Airway cells, in turn, contribute to this process by releasing a variety of cytokines and chemokines. Regardless of the source, cell-derived mediators can have a profound effect on air-

TABLE 2. Criteria for reactive airways dysfunction syndrome

No history of asthma or asthma-like respiratory disease.
Onset of symptoms after a high-level exposure.
Toxicant is an irritant gas, vapor, fume, aerosol, or dust present in high concentration.
Onset of symptoms is acute, usually developing within minutes to hours, but always within 24 h.
Symptoms simulate asthma (wheezing, dyspnea, persistent cough).
Results of spirometry may be normal or show reversible airflow limitation.

From Draper A. Occupational asthma. *J Asthma* 2002;39:1–10, with permission.

way function: airway edema, inflammatory cell chemotaxis, epithelial disruption, increased number of secretory cells, and airway smooth muscle hypertrophy and hyperplasia.

A characteristic feature of asthma is airway *hyperresponsiveness*, which refers to the exaggerated bronchoconstriction response seen after exposure to certain triggers. This response can be immediate, delayed, or dual. In the immediate phase, bronchoconstriction and a decline in the forced expiratory volume in 1 second (FEV_1) are noted within minutes of exposure. After a several-hour delay, a second decline in FEV_1 may also occur. This late reaction can persist for hours. Less commonly, only the late response occurs. This pattern can pose a diagnostic challenge because the temporal distance between the exposure and the onset of symptoms can obscure the link (11). The variability of peak expiratory flow, the improvement of FEV_1 after bronchodilator administration, and the methacholine challenge test are three frequently used clinical measurements of airway hyperresponsiveness.

Airflow obstruction is a cardinal feature of asthma. The etiology of the obstruction is multifactorial and includes bronchoconstriction, airway edema, mucus plugging, and airway remodeling. The ongoing injury and repair process associated with chronic airway inflammation may lead to subbasement membrane fibrosis. This process is believed to contribute to the persistent airflow abnormalities in some patients (12). Serial spirometry is the most common test used to detect and follow airflow obstruction over time.

Asthma has also been categorized by age of onset. Asthma typically begins during childhood or early adolescence. In such cases, it is usually associated with atopy. Childhood asthma often remits during adolescence or early adulthood. In contrast, atopy is not as commonly seen with adult-onset asthma. The diagnosis of occupational asthma should be entertained whenever an adult is evaluated for new-onset asthma. A significant proportion of adult-onset asthma is work related, and the greatest opportunity for cure comes with early diagnosis and removal from exposure.

DIAGNOSIS

The importance of accurate diagnosis cannot be overemphasized and is the key to developing an appropriate treatment strategy. In the case of occupational asthma, the worker may have to be removed from particular areas or leave the workplace altogether. There may also be implications regarding compensation and disability.

The diagnosis of occupational asthma begins with proving that the worker has asthma. The diagnosis of asthma is established by a compatible history and the presence of three features: (a) episodic symptoms of airflow obstruction, (b) at least partial reversibility of the airflow obstruction, and (c) exclusion of alternative diagnoses (1). When occupational asthma is suspected, the presence of asthma must also be linked to the workplace (Fig. 1).

Differential Diagnosis

The differential diagnosis of asthma is extensive and age dependent (Table 3). If a known or suspected occupational exposure exists, other diseases that can be caused by airway irritants should be considered. These include irritant-induced vocal cord dysfunction, reactive airways dysfunction syndrome, and reactive upper airways dysfunction syndrome (13,14). Alternative diagnoses may be ruled out by historical features, examination findings, or basic diagnostic tests. When the diagnosis remains in doubt, referral to a pulmonologist for additional evaluation is appropriate.

History and Physical Examination

Historical features of asthma include recurrent wheezing, chest tightness, dyspnea, a cough that is worse at night, coughing after exercise, and exacerbation of respiratory symptoms with exposure to certain triggers. A detailed history eliciting symptoms linked to environmental triggers should be performed in all cases. Common environmental and host triggers include airborne pollutants, animal dander, dust mites, exercise, menses, molds, pollen, smoke, upper respiratory infection, cold air, and changes in weather or season.

Symptoms of asthma include wheezing, chest tightness, dyspnea on exertion, and cough. Symptoms tend to be worse at night or in the early morning. Physical examination may reveal wheezing, hyperexpansion of the thorax, and a prolonged expiratory phase. Common ancillary findings include nasal polyps, nasal mucosa hyperemia, and atopic dermatitis. It is important to remember that the signs and symptoms of asthma are episodic; therefore, an unremarkable physical examination does not exclude the presence of asthma.

During an exacerbation, the classic signs are respiratory distress, tachypnea, and polyphonic expiratory wheezing. Lack of wheezing, or a "silent chest," may indicate severe airflow obstruction and impending respiratory failure. Other ominous findings include hypoxia, cyanosis, obtundation, bradypnea, and severe respiratory distress.

For employed patients, a detailed occupational history should be elicited. Occurrence or worsening of symptoms while at work, the presence of similar symptoms in coworkers, progression of symptoms throughout the work week, and improvement during days off are clues to the presence of occupational asthma (15). Because they lack sensitivity, however, the absence of these findings does not rule out the diagnosis. Materials Safety Data Sheets for the substances found in the workplace should be reviewed. A visit to the workplace is frequently helpful in identifying exposure sources and gauging the magnitude of the exposure. A qualified industrial hygienist for workplace testing can also be helpful in these cases.

Diagnostic Tests

The diagnostic approach involves establishing the diagnosis of asthma and then evaluating the potential role of the workplace (Fig. 1). In general, a compelling occupational history in an asthmatic adult is sufficient to make a presumptive diagnosis. For example, if there are known asthma-causing or asthma-aggravating agents in the workplace, and the associated symptoms worsen and remit in parallel with job tasks or work days, the likelihood is high that an occupational etiology is present. On

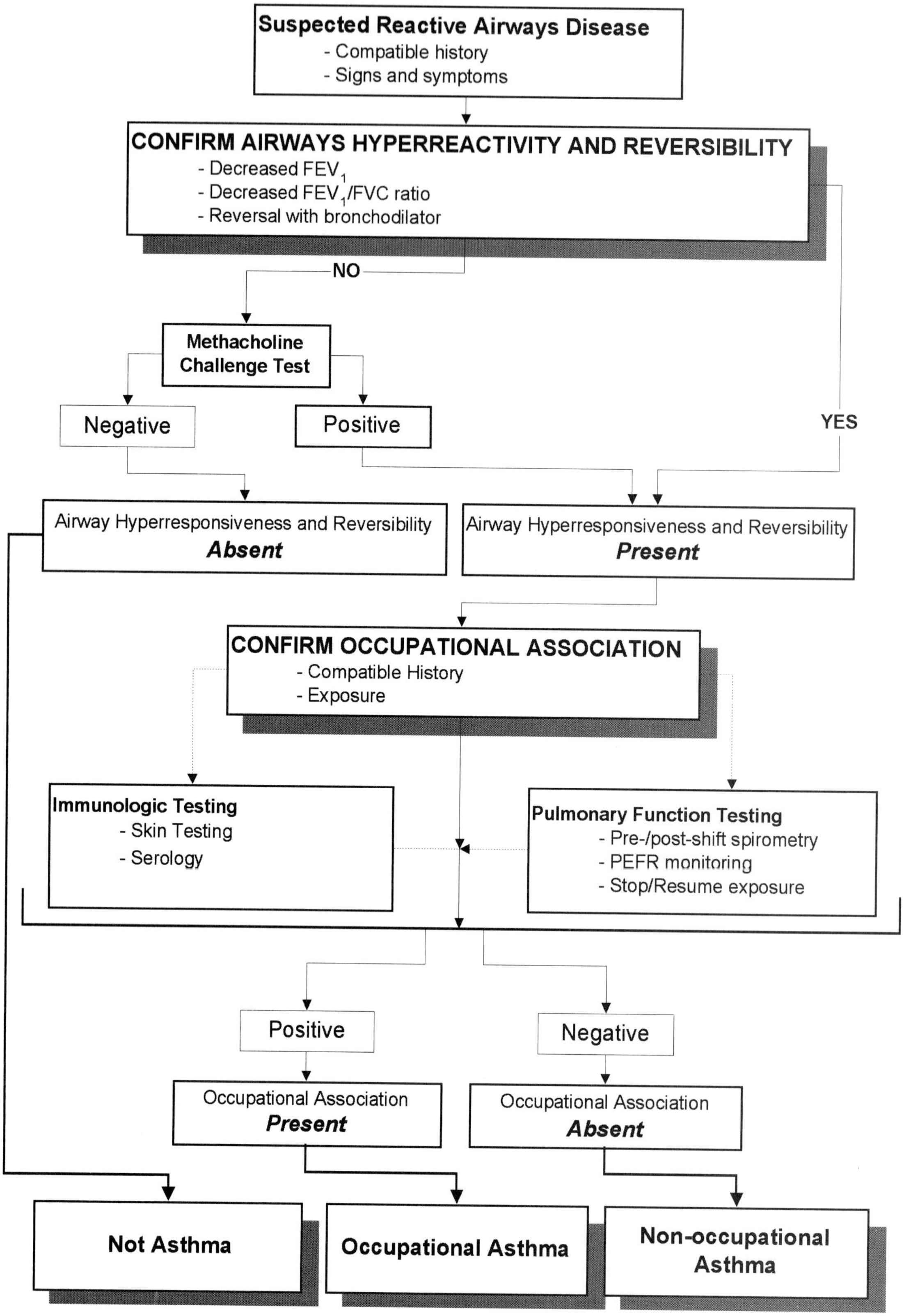

Suspected Reactive Airways Disease
- Compatible history
- Signs and symptoms

CONFIRM AIRWAYS HYPERREACTIVITY AND REVERSIBILITY
- Decreased FEV_1
- Decreased FEV_1/FVC ratio
- Reversal with bronchodilator

NO

Methacholine Challenge Test

Negative

Positive

YES

Airway Hyperresponsiveness and Reversibility ***Absent***

Airway Hyperresponsiveness and Reversibility ***Present***

CONFIRM OCCUPATIONAL ASSOCIATION
- Compatible History
- Exposure

Immunologic Testing
- Skin Testing
- Serology

Pulmonary Function Testing
- Pre-/post-shift spirometry
- PEFR monitoring
- Stop/Resume exposure

Positive

Negative

Occupational Association ***Present***

Occupational Association ***Absent***

Not Asthma

Occupational Asthma

Non-occupational Asthma

Figure 1. Diagnostic approach to occupational asthma. First, the diagnosis of asthma is established. Second, the link to the workplace is evaluated. This approach assumes ongoing or recently discontinued exposure. With more remote exposures, the airway reactivity may have improved or even resolved. FEV_1, forced expiratory volume in 1 second; FVC, forced vital capacity; PEFR, peak expiratory flow rate. (Adapted from Chan-Yeung M, Malo JL. Current concepts: occupational asthma. *N Engl J Med* 1995;333:107–102; and Newman LS. Clinical pulmonary toxicology. In: Sullivan JB Jr, Krieger GR, eds. *Clinical environmental health and toxic exposures*, 2nd ed. Philadelphia: Lippincott Williams & Wilkins, 2001:206–223.)

TABLE 3. Differential diagnosis of asthma

Infants and children	Adults
Allergic rhinitis	Bronchiolitis obliterans
Aspiration of gastric contents (swallowing dysfunction or gastroesophageal reflux)	Chronic aspiration
Bronchial stenosis	Chronic bronchitis
Bronchiolitis	Chronic obstructive pulmonary disease
Bronchopulmonary dysplasia	Drug-induced cough (e.g., angiotensin-converting enzyme inhibitors)
Cystic fibrosis	Hypersensitivity pneumonitis
Congenital heart disease	Laryngeal dysfunction
Foreign body aspiration	Pneumonia
Laryngeal web	Pneumonitis
Laryngotracheomalacia	Pulmonary embolism
Lymphadenopathy (lymphoma)	Sarcoidosis
Tracheal stenosis	Tumors involving airways
Tracheoesophageal fistula	Vocal cord dysfunction
Vascular rings	
Vocal cord dysfunction	

occasion, it is not possible to isolate a specific agent in the workplace either because of insufficient information or because the work environment is complex. In such circumstances, it may still be possible to diagnose work-related asthma, albeit with less confidence. Several common diagnostic aids are listed below, along with their advantages and limitations. A more detailed discussion is available (16).

SPIROMETRY

The clinical suspicion of asthma is typically confirmed with spirometry. Routine spirometry is relatively easy to perform and widely available, although strict attention to procedure and reproducibility are needed to obtain reliable data (17). The parameters most useful for the diagnosis of asthma are the FEV_1 and the FEV_1:forced vital capacity (FVC) ratio before and after the administration of a short-acting β_2-agonist. The results are usually expressed as the percent of the predicted value based on comparison to published standards using age, height, sex, and race (18,19). Confirmatory criteria commonly used for establishing the diagnosis of asthma are a FEV_1:FVC ratio less than or equal to 65% predicted values or significant reversibility as defined by an increase greater than or equal to 12% or greater than or equal to 200 in FEV_1 after inhaling a short-acting β_2-agonist (1).

Asthmatic patients typically demonstrate obstructive airflow impairment (decreased percent predicted FEV_1, decreased FEV_1:FVC ratio) that is at least partially reversible by β_2-agonists. The FEV_1 is the parameter most commonly used to follow patients over time because it varies linearly and inversely with airflow obstruction and is very reproducible (20). The FEV_1:FVC ratio is the most sensitive parameter for determining the presence of mild obstruction and is frequently abnormal even in asymptomatic patients with a normal FEV_1.

As with any diagnostic test, spirometry results must be interpreted within clinical context. For example, many conditions can result in airflow obstruction. This finding alone conclusively establishes the presence of asthma. Conversely, asthmatic patients may not have a demonstrable airflow limitation at the time of testing. In such cases, it is necessary to pursue further confirmatory testing. In workplaces with onsite spirometry, pre- and postshift testing can be useful (21). A decline in FEV_1 of 20% over the workday and a progressive decline in FEV_1 over the workweek are highly suggestive of occupational asthma.

PEAK EXPIRATORY FLOW

Portable peak flow meters can be used by patients to gauge the severity of an attack, measure bronchodilator response, and detect triggers in the environment. Many asthmatics know their baseline peak expiratory flow rate (PEFR) and, thus, are able to compare their values to personal norms and tailor their treatment accordingly. Generally, PEFR values greater than 80% predicted (based on height and gender) are considered to be normal or indicative of mild obstruction. Values between 60% and 80% represent moderate obstruction, whereas values less than 60% represent severe obstruction.

Serial PEFR measurements can be useful in occupational settings if the patient is subject to frequent ongoing exposure (22,23). Four to six PEFR determinations per day for at least 2 weeks are recommended (24). More frequent measurements (every 2 hours) are also used. The monitoring should include periods before, during, and after work, as well as periods away from the exposure, preferably several days. Typical work-related patterns show progressive decrements during a work shift or workweek, with recovery during periods away from work. Such patterns may be obscured by other triggers in the environment, variability in technique, medication usage, and other confounders. Patients should be instructed to maintain a diary and carefully record not only PEFR measurements, but also exposures and medication usage.

An accurate PEFR measurement is effort and technique dependent; therefore, patients should be instructed on the appropriate technique and encouraged throughout the attempt. Children younger than 6 years of age may not have the coordination required to perform this test accurately.

BRONCHOPROVOCATION TESTING

Inhalation of aerosolized methacholine, a muscarinic choline ester, is the most commonly used provocative test for asthma. The test is performed by administering progressively larger doses of methacholine by nebulizer and is halted when the FEV_1 falls by greater than 20% or when five breaths of the highest concentration of methacholine (25 mg/ml) have been administered. The results are usually reported as the PC_{20}, which represents the concentration of methacholine that results in a 20% decline from the baseline FEV_1. The test may also be positive in patients with allergic rhinitis, congestive heart failure, smoking-related flow obstruction, or other chronic pulmonary diseases, although the degree of hyperreactivity is usually mild in these other conditions. Specific bronchoprovocation testing with the suspected causative agent can be performed at specialized centers experienced in the challenge methods and appropriate monitoring. Its routine use is discouraged.

IMMUNOLOGIC TESTING

Referral to an allergist for immunologic testing may also be beneficial when evaluating patients for occupational asthma, in which reactivity may help to link asthma to specific allergens found in the workplace. Examples include skin prick, puddle, or patch testing; radioallergosorbent testing; and enzyme-linked immunosorbent assay. In general, these tests are useful only when the exposure is known, the suspected agent is an allergen, and the test has been well characterized. Although a positive test strengthens the diagnosis, interpretation is problematic because a negative test does not exclude the diagnosis, and a positive test does not conclusively prove causation.

CHEST RADIOGRAPHY

A chest radiograph may help exclude lung disorders that mimic asthma. For example, it can help distinguish bronchiolitis obliterans and pneumonitis from exacerbation of underlying asthma. It is usually not helpful in patients with preexisting asthma who present with a mild to moderate exacerbation. If there is concern for pneumonia causing the exacerbation or if the patient has asymmetric breath sounds, radiography is indicated.

OTHER

Additional tests may help rule out other etiologies: high-resolution computed chest tomography, body plethysmography, and diffusing capacity for carbon monoxide. These tests are usually performed in consultation with a pulmonologist.

COMPLICATIONS

The most serious direct complication of asthma is respiratory failure. Early and aggressive treatment of a severe exacerbation is crucial to mitigate the associated morbidity, including mechanical ventilation, barotrauma, and nosocomial infection. Recent increases in asthma mortality have been documented, although the cause for this remains uncertain. Other less visible complications include lost work time and limitation of activities.

MANAGEMENT

Removal of the exposure is the most critical step for patients with environmental or occupational asthma. For nonspecific irritants, appropriate respiratory protection and workplace remediation may be enough. Many asthmatics can work around irritants if they are appropriately educated and medicated and efforts are made to minimize exposure. If the causative agent is an allergen, however, complete removal of the exposure is usually necessary because even minute exposures can provoke an asthma attack, prolong the illness, and lead to chronic asthma. Significant medical improvement can continue for up to 2 years after exposure to workplace allergens has ceased. Prognosis is related to duration of exposure and degree of impairment at the time of diagnosis. The earlier the patient is removed from the causative agent, the better the prognosis.

The treatment goals for an acute exacerbation are relief of bronchospasm, attenuation of airway inflammation, and ensuring adequate oxygenation. Short-acting β_2-agonists are the mainstay of therapy. Systemically administered corticosteroids are also an integral part of acute management. Attenuation of airway inflammation improves airflow obstruction and prevents early recurrence of symptoms. Supplemental oxygen may be required in more severe cases to maintain oxygenation.

The strategy for the chronic management of all but the mildest cases of asthma focuses on (a) prevention, and (b) control of airway inflammation. Mild asthmatics who have infrequent symptoms can be managed with inhaled β_2-agonists alone. When more frequent symptoms are present, the addition of inhaled corticosteroids and long-acting β_2-agonists is often warranted. Many patients can avoid the use of β_2-agonists altogether by regularly using low-dose, inhaled corticosteroids. Patients whose symptoms and airflow limitation remain uncontrolled should be referred to an asthma specialist.

PITFALLS

The common admonition of "all that wheezes is not asthma" is relevant to the evaluation of new-onset wheezing. Establishing an accurate diagnosis should be a primary concern in all "asthmatic" patients, with particular attention paid to possible workplace and environmental exposures. In patients with previously diagnosed asthma who present with an exacerbation, insufficient treatment may result in progression of symptoms and respiratory failure. Failure to eliminate workplace exposure may result in persistent or worsening symptoms.

REFERENCES

1. Expert panel report II: guidelines for the diagnosis and management of asthma. (NIH publication no. 97-4051.) Bethesda, MD: National Asthma Education and Prevention Program, 1997.
2. Chan-Yeung M, Malo JL. Current concepts: occupational asthma. *N Engl J Med* 1995;333:107–102.
3. Venables KM, Chan-Yeung M. Occupational asthma. *Lancet* 1997;349:1465–1469.
4. Bernstein IL, Chan-Yeung M, Malo JL. Definition and classification of asthma. In: Bernstein IL, Chan-Yeung M, Malo JL, Bernstein DI, eds. *Asthma in the workplace*. New York: Mercel Dekker, 1993:1–4.
5. Draper A. Occupational asthma. *J Asthma* 2002;39:1–10.
6. Chan-Yeung M, Malo JL. Aetiological agents in occupational asthma. *Eur Respir J* 1994;7:346–371.
7. Blanc P. Occupational asthma in a national disability survey. *Chest* 1987;92:613–617.
8. Blanc P, Toren K. Occupational asthma in a community-based survey of adult asthma. *Am J Med* 1999;107:580–587.
9. Reinisch F, Harrison RJ, Cussler S, et al. Physician reports of work-related asthma in California, 1993–1996. *Am J Ind Med* 2001;39:72–83.
10. Brooks SM, Weiss MA, Bernstein IL. Reactive airways dysfunction syndrome (RADS): persistent asthma syndrome after high level irritant exposures. *Chest* 1985;88:376–384.
11. Newman LS. Clinical pulmonary toxicology. In: Sullivan JB Jr, Krieger GR, eds. *Clinical environmental health and toxic exposures*, 2nd ed. Philadelphia: Lippincott Williams & Wilkins, 2001:206–223.
12. Roche WR. Fibroblasts and asthma. *Clin Exp Allergy* 1991;21:545–548.
13. Perkner JJ, Fennelly KP, Balkissoon R, et al. Irritant-associated vocal cord dysfunction. *J Occup Env Med* 1998;40:136–143.
14. Meggs WJ. RADS and RUDS—the toxic induction of asthma and rhinitis. *J Toxicol Clin Toxicol* 1994;32:487–501.
15. Newman LS. Occupational illness. *N Engl J Med* 1995;333:1128–1134.
16. Sood A, Redlich CA. Pulmonary function tests at work. *Clin Chest Med* 2001;22:783–793.
17. American Thoracic Society. Standardization of spirometry: 1994 update. *Am J Respir Crit Care Med* 1995;346:791–795.
18. American Thoracic Society. Lung function testing: selection of reference values and interpretive strategies. *Am Rev Respir Dis* 1991;144:1202–1218.
19. Hankinson JL, Odencrantz JR, Fedan KB. Spirometric reference values from a sample of the general U.S. population. *Am J Respir Crit Care Med* 1999;159:179–187.
20. Enright PL, Lebowitz MD, Cockroft DW. Physiologic measures: pulmonary function tests, asthma outcome. *Am J Resp Crit Care Med* 1994;149:S9–S18.
21. Cote J, Kennedy S, Chan-Yeung MB. Quantitative versus qualitative analysis of peak expiratory flow in occupational asthma. *Thorax* 1993;48:48–51.
22. Moscato G, Godnic-Cvar J, Maestrelli P, et al. Statement on self-monitoring of peak expiratory flow in the investigation of occupational asthma. *Allergy* 1995;50:711–717.
23. Leroyer C, Perfetti L, Trudeau C, et al. Comparison of serial monitoring of peak expiratory flow and FEV1 in the diagnosis of occupational asthma. *Am J Respir Crit Care Med* 1998;158:827–832.
24. Malo JL, Cote J, Cartier A, et al. How many times per day should peak expiratory flow rates be assessed when investigating occupational asthma? *Thorax* 1993;48:1211–1217.

CHAPTER 12

Body Packers and Stuffers

Daniel C. Keyes

OVERVIEW

Each year, more than 1.5 million pounds of cocaine, heroin, marijuana, ecstasy, and other illegal drugs are seized by the U.S. Customs Service (1). The customs agent is faced with the challenge of identifying smugglers. Initial investigation involves questioning and luggage searches. If an individual is determined to be high risk for smuggling, he or she may undergo physical body searches with varying degrees of invasiveness. This must all be undertaken in such a way as not to disrupt the efficient flow of travel for the majority of passengers who are compliant with national and international law.

BODY PACKERS

A commonly reported method used to smuggle drugs is to transport them in the gastrointestinal (GI) tract (Fig. 1). *Body packing* involves the swallowing of drug-filled packets with the intent of smuggling (2). In cases in which suspicion is high or questioning suggests that the traveler might have swallowed packets, radiographic imaging is often necessary to check for the presence of packets. This typically requires the transport of the suspect to a hospital, radiographic evaluation, and then treatment in the emergency department or transportation back to the airport. This process is inconvenient and time consuming, particularly for the occasional law-abiding traveler who comes under suspicion. It is also expensive for law enforcement agencies. In recent years, mobile x-ray services have been used to allow imaging at the site (3). The radiographs are transmitted electronically to radiologists who interpret the films without transporting the suspect.

Mebane and DeVito first described the smuggling of ingested cocaine packets in 1975 (4). This method is also used extensively for other drugs, such as heroin and ecstasy. The person who actually ingests the packets is called a *mule* or *body packer* (2). The packets are swallowed in large numbers just before boarding a flight to the smuggler's destination. An antidiarrheal medication is often taken to delay passage of the ingested packets until checking into a hotel or a "safe house" in the destination city. The most common drug used for this purpose is diphenoxylate hydrochloride with atropine sulfate (Lomotil), which is characterized by opioid and antimuscarinic effects. Some smugglers are apprehended before delivery. If not, the illegal product is sold to drug handlers who repackage and distribute the product to end purchasers.

"Body packets" have evolved over the past 25 years, as the producers of illicit drugs have achieved greater sophistication. In the past, packets were made of drug wrapped in multiple layers of condoms or party balloons and sealed with nonabsorbable suture or other ligature (4). In recent years, the packets are often machine produced, using multiple layers of latex embedded in a wax coating. These newer packets may not be visualized on plain (noncontrast) radiographs of the abdomen.

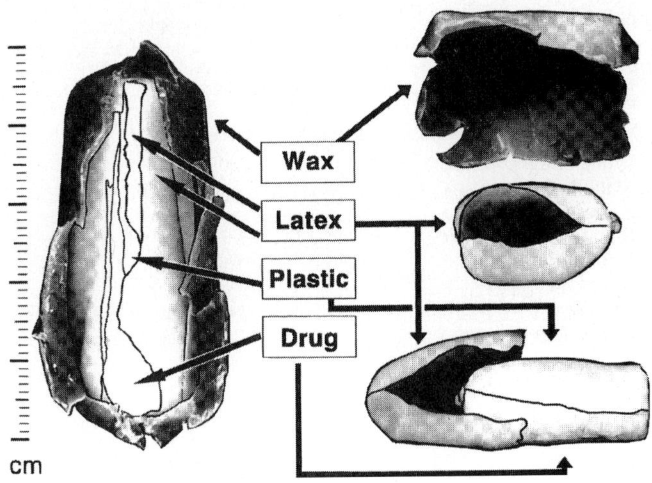

Figure 1. The "anatomy" of a typical internally concealed cocaine package showing several protective layers.

Diagnosis

Custom agents or other law enforcement agencies usually refer the suspect to a hospital. In general, the patient is asymptomatic. The health care practitioner must determine if the patient is indeed body packing, thereby putting the patient at risk of serious intoxication and even death. The history is important in this context, as the clinician must interview the patient regarding packets and their contents, as well as determining the use of a drug to decrease GI motility, such as diphenoxylate-atropine. Patients who initially deny body packing often cooperate with the clinician when spoken to privately and when convinced that the practitioner's intent is to protect their health.

SIGNS AND SYMPTOMS

Irrespective of the patient's history, it is necessary to focus on particular findings when caring for the potential body packer. If an anticholinergic agent has been ingested to retard GI passage of the packets, signs of mydriasis, tachycardia, and dry skin may be present. Bowel sounds are typically decreased. The abdominal examination is usually benign, but occasionally a firm packet may be palpable. If signs of peritonitis are detected, the clinician needs to obtain surgical consultation and prioritize the patient to the highest level of acute care. Rectal examination should be undertaken in all cases, as packets are sometimes directly inserted through the anus or have advanced far enough for detection.

DIAGNOSTIC TESTING

The diagnosis of body packing is enhanced by diagnostic testing, using a combination of urine testing and radiographic imaging. The asymptomatic body packer often admits to ingesting drugs, especially when presented with positive urine testing or other evidence (5). However, the patient may not be accurate regarding the number of packets.

TABLE 1. Urine testing of body packers

Authors (reference)	Year	Number of cases	Method of testing	Comments
Gherardi et al. (7)	1988	60 (ingestion only; additional 58 used rectal insertion)	Urine EMIT	Cocaine and heroin cases also included.
Bogusz et al. (8)	1995	30	Urine EMIT and radiography	Urine testing had lower sensitivity than Gherardi study. Newer technology may defeat attempts at drug testing.
Nihira et al. (22)	1998	16	Urine EMIT and radiography; confirmed with gas chromatography–mass spectrometry	Included five cocaine, two heroin, one opiate, and one marijuana; concluded that urine testing is essential and effective.

EMIT, enzyme-multiplied immunoassay test.

Urine testing is an important tool in cases of suspected body packing (Table 1). The use of drug testing in these patients is highly dependent on the quality and number of cocaine packages present in the GI tract. Cocaine packages have been classified based on the consistency and form of the cocaine and the wrapping materials used (Table 2) (6). Packaging technique influences the risk of leakage and rupture, which may result in rapid death for the courier. Even without rupture, the packets may act as a semipermeable membrane (2). One study tested urine cocaine screening on a large series of patients as an initial detection method (7). The study concluded that urine enzyme-multiplied immunoassay testing for benzoylecgonine, the major urinary metabolite of cocaine, was extremely sensitive for the detection of smugglers. This seemed to confirm the theory of condom semipermeability. However, some years later, Bogusz et al. reexamined the use of initial urine testing and conducted laboratory testing on several cocaine packets to assess their structural integrity. They found that packets may leak occasionally and become detectable on urine testing. Otherwise, the better-wrapped packages used today do not produce positive enzyme-multiplied immunoassay test urine screens, even when very low thresholds for detection are used (8). The evolution of body packet manufacturing suggests that illicit drug producers are aware of the need for quality control and may be aware of the medical literature on the topic.

According to some authors, one can almost always make the diagnosis of body packing with plain abdominal radiographs (9). One specific finding on radiography is known as the "double condom" sign. This consists of two crescents being formed by air trapped between layers of condom wrappings (10). Due to lack of knowledge about the number and characteristics of smugglers who have gone undetected, however, the true sensitivity of a *non*-contrast radiographic detection cannot be evaluated. Contrast studies may be executed using meglumine diatrizoate (Gastrografin) in a dose of 60 ml (0.9 ml/kg) administered on presentation. Radiographs are obtained approximately 5 hours after the contrast is given. Using this method, some investigators have increased the rate of body packet detection (11). The contrast agent may also act as a cathartic.

MEDICAL MANAGEMENT

Several case series involving body packers have been published (Table 3). The largest series describes 215 suspects who were brought to the hospital for evaluation. Approximately 1 in 20 of these individuals suffered intestinal obstruction (9). Two-thirds of body packers used antidiarrheal medicines. Four of five patients were asymptomatic during their medical care. The typical patient was admitted for 3 to 4 days to await passage of the packets. The number of packets ingested ranged from 15 to more than 200, each one containing 3 to 15 g of cocaine. Most couriers originate in South America or the East Indies (9,12). Hence, it is prudent to admit all patients in whom body packing is confirmed to the intensive care unit, due to the potential for rapid deterioration in the event of a packet rupture.

Once the diagnosis of body packing is made, it is important to ensure that complete passage of the packages occurs. Whole

TABLE 2. Classification of cocaine body packets

Characteristics	Classification of bags		
	Type 1	Type 2	Type 3
Color	White	White or light yellow	Yellow
Consistency	Loose powder	Matted power	Rock-hard paste
Covering	None, plastic food wrap, masking tape	None	Aluminum foil
Wrappings	Condoms, toy balloons, finger or latex gloves	Multilayer tubular latex	Multilayer tubular latex
Package ties	Usually prominent	Smooth	Smooth
Radiographic appearance			
Shape	Round or cigar shaped	Oblong	Not seen
Density	Radiopaque or radiolucent	Radiopaque	Radiolucent
Gas	None or irregular	Present and regular "double condom" sign may be seen (see text)	—
Ties	Not apparent or "rosette"	Not apparent	—
Structural integrity	Often break or leach cocaine	No reports of breaking or leaching cocaine	No reports of breaking or leaching cocaine

Modified from McCarron MM, Wood JD. The cocaine "body packer" syndrome. Diagnosis and treatment. *JAMA* 1983;250(11):1417–1420.

TABLE 3. Case series of body packers

Author (reference)	Year of publication	Total cases	Diagnostic methodology	Cases treated surgically	Fatalities
Suarez et al. (15)	1977	3	Plain radiography	3	2
Wetli (2)	1981	11	Plain radiography	1	10
McCarron and Wood (6)	1983	48	Radiography, some with oral barium	1	None
Caruana et al. (16)	1984	50	Plain radiography	9 (6 elective)	None
Gomez Antuñez et al. (9)	1998	215	Radiography	7 (3% of patients)	2 (and 1 brain death)
Bulstrode et al. (12)	2002	180	Radiography	7	None

bowel irrigation with polyethylene glycol electrolyte solution provides rapid, safe removal of packets in the asymptomatic patient (13). Bowel irrigation using polyethylene glycol also enhances the ability to conduct posttreatment GI contrast radiography. Typically, the patient is discharged after the passage of two packet-free stools and negative abdominal radiographs have been obtained.

Potential Complications

The most important complications of the body packer are packet rupture with subsequent overdose from absorbed drug or obstruction of the GI tract. Cocaine is the most commonly smuggled drug by body packers. With rupture, severe toxicity and death are very possible. Cocaine is generally less toxic when ingested than when smoked because it is rapidly hydrolyzed by gastric acid, and it undergoes extensive first-pass metabolism in the liver (14). Bioavailability of cocaine by oral ingestion is approximately 33%. The adult lethal dose for *ingested* cocaine has been estimated as 0.5 to 1.0 g. Individual body packets typically contain 5 to 9 g of cocaine. Hence, the rupture of a single packet is sufficient for severe overdose.

Packets may also cause GI obstruction from inability to pass at narrow points such as the pylorus or terminal ileum. The likelihood of obstruction may be increased by the coingestion of anticholinergic drugs.

In 1977, one author reported three cases of body packing, including two deaths, and advocated the use of surgery in all cases (15). Virtually all other authors advocate a less invasive approach for asymptomatic patients, consisting of observation and decontamination in a monitored hospital setting. Surgical intervention is recommended if bowel obstruction or signs of cocaine toxicity develop, suggesting that packets are leaking or have ruptured. Surgery may also be indicated in patients in whom there is radiologic evidence of packet rupture or if confirmed packets are not passed after several days of observation and catharsis (5,6,16).

BODY STUFFERS

In contrast to the advance preparation of the body packer, the body stuffer ingests an illegal drug urgently, usually to eliminate evidence and avoid prosecution. "Stuffing" is typically precipitated by the presence of law enforcement authorities (17). This "stuffing" is done without time to package the drug carefully, and often the dose ingested is higher than intended for an individual user. Descriptive series of body stuffers are challenged by the difficulty in confirming the actual amount of drug ingested. For example, cocaine can be ingested as "crack," the lipid-soluble free-base form or the water-soluble hydrochloride form, which is likely to be absorbed more rapidly. All illicit drugs can be of variable potency and are often cut with other drugs or fillers.

Diagnosis

Body stuffers are usually brought directly to the emergency department in police custody. The patient may admit to drug ingestion; however, the accuracy of the history is suspect due to the presence of law enforcement officials. The package is often simply a "baggie" or a small piece of foil. Abdominal radiographs are rarely confirmatory, and treatment is usually based on report of the patient or law enforcement or the general suspicion of the clinician. Two case series suggest that only a small percentage of these patients become seriously intoxicated (18,19). Drug testing is often recommended, but it has little impact on the management of the patient. Radiographs of chest or abdomen are rarely useful.

Patients who present after stuffing cocaine or other drugs generally require intravenous access, electrocardiographic monitoring, activated charcoal, and observation. Gastric lavage may not be helpful because of the potential for release of more toxic substances or aspiration of plastic container materials into the trachea. Hoffman and Chiang have suggested a general approach to these patients, which includes early plain radiographic imaging. If these initial images are positive or the patients are symptomatic, then whole bowel irrigation is used (18). Others proceed directly with decontamination, arguing that radiographic imaging has little impact on subsequent management. Whole bowel irrigation may be undertaken simultaneously with activated charcoal, and it may actually enhance the adsorption of cocaine to the activated carbon (20,21).

CONCLUSION

Body packing has become relatively frequent as a method of transporting illegal drugs into developed countries. Illicit drug producers have become increasingly sophisticated in avoiding detection. A high index of suspicion should be exercised in the care of a recent traveler who presents with bowel obstruction or intoxication because death may rapidly ensue if a drug packet ruptures. Most cases may be managed with careful observation, but if cocaine intoxication or bowel obstruction is present, surgical intervention is usually needed. Although cocaine is the drug most commonly associated with body packing, heroin, ecstasy, and hashish have also been transported in this fashion.

Body stuffers present after ingesting cocaine or other drugs that are not well packaged. These patients are generally treated with activated charcoal and emergency department observation. Whole bowel irrigation has also been advocated in this setting, and may be administered concomitantly with activated charcoal.

REFERENCES

1. Winwood C. Hearing on the counterdrug activities of the U.S. Customs Service House Committee on Appropriations Treasury, Postal Service, and General Government Subcommittee: testimony of Acting Commissioner of Customs Charles Winwood. *U S Customs News* 2001;March.

2. Wetli CV, Mittlemann RE. The "body packer syndrome"—toxicity following ingestion of illicit drugs packaged for transportation. *J Forensic Sci* 1981;26(3):492–500.
3. Maston C. Mobile x-ray services provide options for travelers. *U S Customs Today* 2001:April. Available at: http://www.customs.gov/xp/CustomsToday/2001/April/custoday_xray.xml.
4. Mebane C, DeVito JJ. Cocaine intoxication: a unique case. *J Fla Med Assoc* 1975;62(2):19–20.
5. Beck NE, Hale JE. Cocaine "body packers." *Br J Surg* 1993;80(12):1513–1516.
6. McCarron MM, Wood JD. The cocaine "body packer" syndrome. Diagnosis and treatment. *JAMA* 1983;250(11):1417–1420.
7. Gherardi RK, Baud FJ, Leporc P, et al. Detection of drugs in the urine of body-packers. *Lancet* 1988;1(8594):1076–1078.
8. Bogusz MJ, Althoff H, Erkens M, et al. Internally concealed cocaine: analytical and diagnostic aspects. *J Forensic Sci* 1995;40(5): 811–805.
9. Gomez Antuñez M, Cuenca Carvajal C, Farfan Sedano A, et al. [Complications of intestinal transporting of cocaine packets. Study of 215 cases.] *Med Clin (Barc)* 1998;111(9):336–337.
10. Pinsky MF, Ducas J, Ruggere MD. Narcotic smuggling: the double condom sign. *J Can Assoc Radiol* 1978;29(2):79–81.
11. Marc B, Baud FJ, Aelion MJ, et al. The cocaine body-packer syndrome: evaluation of a method of contrast study of the bowel. *J Forensic Sci* 1990;35(2):345–355.
12. Bulstrode N, Banks F, Shrotria S. The outcome of drug smuggling by "body packers"—the British experience. *Ann R Coll Surg Engl* 2002;84(1):35–38.
13. Hoffman RS, Smilkstein MJ, Goldfrank LR. Whole bowel irrigation and the cocaine body-packer: a new approach to a common problem. *Am J Emerg Med* 1990;8(6):523–527.
14. Fattinger K, Benowitz NL, Jones RT, Verotta D. Nasal mucosal versus gastrointestinal absorption of nasally administered cocaine. *Eur J Clin Pharmacol* 2000;56(4):305–310.
15. Suarez CA, Arango A, Lester JL 3rd. Cocaine-condom ingestion. Surgical treatment. *JAMA* 1977;238(13):1391–1392.
16. Caruana DS, Weinbach B, Goerg D, Gardner LB. Cocaine-packet ingestion. Diagnosis, management, and natural history. *Ann Intern Med* 1984;100(1):73–74.
17. Roberts JR, Price D, Goldfrank L, Hartnett L. The bodystuffer syndrome: a clandestine form of drug overdose. *Am J Emerg Med* 1986;4(1):24–27.
18. Hoffman RS, Chiang WK, Weisman RS, Goldfrank LR. Prospective evaluation of "crack-vial" ingestions. *Vet Hum Toxicol* 1990;32(2):164–167.
19. Sporer KA, Firestone J. Clinical course of crack cocaine body stuffers. *Ann Emerg Med* 1997;29(5): 596–601.
20. Makosiej FJ, Hoffman RS, Howland MA, Goldfrank LR. An in vitro evaluation of cocaine hydrochloride adsorption by activated charcoal and desorption upon addition of polyethylene glycol electrolyte lavage solution. *J Toxicol Clin Toxicol* 1993;31(3):381–395.
21. Kirshenbaum LA, Sitar DS, Tenenbein M. Interaction between whole-bowel irrigation solution and activated charcoal: implications for the treatment of toxic ingestions. *Ann Emerg Med* 1990;19(10):1129–1132.
22. Nihira M, Hayashida M, Ohno Y, et al. Urinalysis of body packers in Japan. *J Anal Toxicol* 1998;22(1):61–65.

CHAPTER 13

Cholinergic Syndrome

Thomas C. Arnold

OVERVIEW

The medical toxicologist frequently consults on patients with "cholinergic syndrome." It is likely that the primary care or emergency physician, however, will be confronted first by a patient exhibiting cholinergic effects ranging from subtle to obvious. Cholinergic syndrome involves signs of excess activity of acetylcholine. The classic presentation is a "wet" patient experiencing secretory overdrive manifested by salivation, lacrimation, urination, defecation, vomiting, diarrhea, and increased bronchial secretions. Bronchospasm, bradycardia, altered mental status, muscular fasciculation, weakness, and seizures may also be components.

Cholinergic syndrome is typically the result of exposure to one of the common organophosphate or carbamate insecticides, such as chlorpyrifos or diazinon, but any compound that results in excessive action of the neurotransmitter acetylcholine can produce this syndrome (Table 1). Death from cholinergic syndrome usually arises from respiratory compromise caused by two factors: initial interference of oxygen exchange caused by excessive bronchial secretions obstructing the airways and diminished effort of breathing as a result of muscular paralysis. Therefore, aggressive airway management and support are the keys to the survival of these patients (1).

The most frequent causes of cholinergic poisoning are pesticides, which accounted for 86,880 (4% of total) human exposures reported to American poison control centers in 2000 (2). Both organophosphate and carbamate insecticides produce cholinergic syndrome. In the United States alone, more than 25,000 brands of pesticides are marketed for home and commercial use (3). Additionally, the threat of bioterrorism has served as a

TABLE 1. Products and medications known to cause cholinergic syndrome

Class	Substance
Organophosphate insecticides	Dichlorvos, chlorpyrifos, fenthion, diazinon, dimethoate, malathion, parathion, abate, tetraethylpryophosphate, phorate, mevinphos, demeton, disulfoton, fensulfothion, fonophos, and many others
Chemical warfare nerve agents	Tabun (GA), sarin (GB), soman (GD), VX agents, and others
Carbamate insecticides	Aldicarb, oxamyl, carbofuran, benfuracarb, methomyl, formetanate, aminocarb, dimetilan, dimetan, dioxacarb, methiocarb, propoxur, bendiocarb, primicarb, bufencarb, m-tolyl-N-methyl, 3,4-xylyl-N-methyl carbamate, isoprocarb, carbaryl, and many others
Antimyasthenic agents	Ambenonium, distigmine, edrophonium, neostigmine, pyridostigmine
Direct muscarinic agonists	Acetylcholine, arecholine, bethanechol, carbachol, cevimeline, choline, methacholine, pilocarpine
Ophthalmic preparations (glaucoma)	Demecarium, echothiophate, isoflurophate, physostigmine
Alzheimer's medications	Donepezil, galantamine, rivastigmine, tacrine
Schistosomiasis treatment	Metrifonate (metabolized to dichlorvos)
Mushrooms (group IV)	Inocybe, clitocybe, some *Boletus* species
Nicotine-containing products	Tobacco products (smoke and smokeless), transdermal patches, nicotine gums

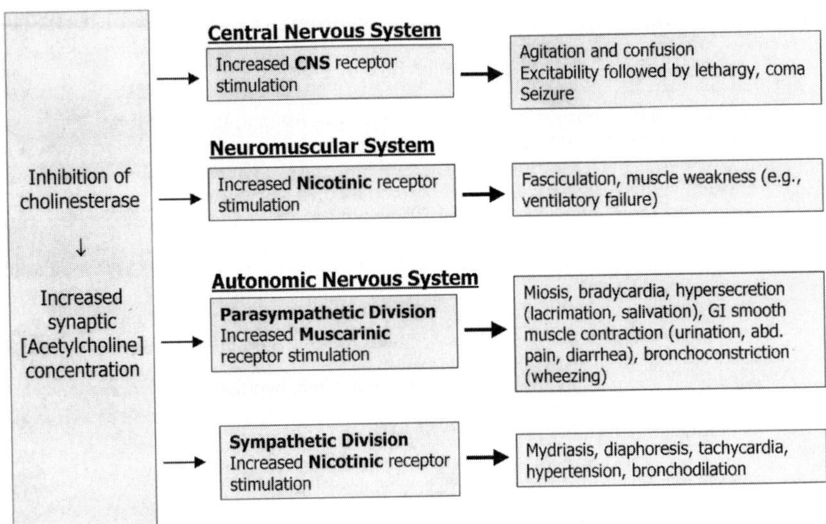

Figure 1. Role of acetylcholine in the human nervous system. abd., abdominal; CNS, central nervous system; GI, gastrointestinal.

reminder that the chemical nerve agents are all extremely potent cholinesterase inhibitors. The chemical warfare agents tabun (GA), sarin (GB), soman (GD), and VX produce cholinergic syndrome rapidly after exposure (Chapter 261) (4). As demonstrated by the Tokyo subway release of sarin in 1995 (6), health care providers must be able to recognize and treat this syndrome and to realize that multiple patients with cholinergic syndrome could be the first sign of a chemical attack.

PATHOPHYSIOLOGY

To understand the complex effects involved in cholinergic syndrome, a basic understanding of the central nervous system, autonomic nervous system, and neuromuscular components is needed (Fig. 1). The *autonomic nervous system* regulates key functions of the body, including activity of the heart, intestinal smooth muscles, and glandular function. It has two divisions: the *sympathetic division* and the *parasympathetic division*. Stimulation of the *sympathetic nervous system* accelerates heart rate, constricts blood vessels, raises blood pressure, and dilates pupils. Stimulation of the *parasympathetic nervous system* slows heart rate, increases intestinal and glandular activity, and relaxes sphincter muscles (Fig. 1).

Acetylcholine is the neurotransmitter of the parasympathetic nervous system—hence the predominance of parasympathetic effects in the cholinergic syndrome. Acetylcholine, epinephrine, and norepinephrine are all represented in the sympathetic nervous system. Epinephrine and norepinephrine produce effects that directly oppose those produced by parasympathetic stimulation. The relative degrees of stimulation of these opposing neurotransmitters account for the variability of some findings such as pupil size, heart rate, and bronchoconstriction in the cholinergic syndrome. Acetylcholine is also the neurotransmitter of neuromuscular transmission. Excess release of acetylcholine at the motor endplate initially results in uncoordinated muscular contraction known as *fasciculation*. Continued excess produces a depolarazing blockade, results in muscular weakness, and culminates in total muscular paralysis (Fig. 1) (7,8).

The increase in synaptic acetylcholine concentration affects both types of acetylcholine receptors. *Muscarinic receptors* are found predominantly in the parasympathetic system in postganglionic nerve endings and control most glandular secretions. In the sympathetic system, muscarinic receptors are found only in postganglionic nerves controlling sweat gland function. Therefore, stimulation of the muscarinic receptors is responsible for the hypersecretory findings associated with cholinergic syndrome. *Nicotinic receptors* are found in the sympathetic and parasympathetic systems, but the predominant symptoms produced by nicotinic receptor activation occur at the neuromuscular junction. Stimulation of nicotinic receptors leads first to muscular fasciculation, followed by motor weakness and paralysis. Hypertension and tachycardia are also a result of nicotinic receptor stimulation (9).

The end result of all cholinergic agents is to increase stimulation of the postsynaptic acetylcholine receptor. Organophosphate and carbamate insecticides do this by binding the acetylcholinesterase enzyme, thereby allowing accumulation of acetylcholine in the synapse (10). Many carbamate compounds are used as insecticides, and some, such as physostigmine, pyridostigmine, and neostigmine, have medical uses (11). There are also several medications for myasthenia gravis that are noncarbamate, reversible cholinesterase inhibitors (e.g., edrophonium). Recently, new products have been developed for use in Alzheimer's disease with the purpose of enhancing central nervous system cholinergic activity (12). Many of these medications cause cholinergic effects during therapeutic use as well as after overdose. Other medications are direct cholinergic agonists: Carbachol, methacholine, and pilocarpine are used as eye drops to produce miosis in patients with glaucoma; bethanechol augments bladder function; and cevimeline is used for xerostomia associated with Sjögren's syndrome (13).

DIAGNOSIS

Differential Diagnosis

Cholinergic syndrome can be confused with many other conditions, depending on whether nicotinic or muscarinic symptoms predominate (Table 2; see also individual chapters for each toxin). The clinician must maintain a high index of suspicion for this diagnosis.

History

A careful history of possible exposure to causative agents should be sought. Insecticide exposures may present with mus-

TABLE 2. Signs, symptoms, and differential diagnosis of cholinergic syndrome

Body system	Cholinergic symptom or sign	Differential diagnosis
General	DUMBELS toxidrome	Ingestion of or exposure to any of the compounds listed in Table 1
Head, ears, eyes, nose, and throat	Diaphoresis, tachycardia, hypertension	Stimulant ingestion (e.g., amphetamines, cocaine, other sympathomimetic amines)
Gastrointestinal	Nausea, vomiting, diarrhea	Gastroenteritis (e.g., viral, bacterial or toxin mediated)
Pulmonary	Hypoxia, respiratory distress, bronchospasm, bronchorrhea	Respiratory compromise (e.g., congestive heart failure, pulmonary edema, acute respiratory distress syndrome, asthma)
Cardiac	Bradycardia, hypotension, and dysrhythmias possible	Cardiotoxic ingestion (e.g., beta-blockers, calcium-channel blockers, digoxin or other cardiac glycosides)
Neurologic	Muscular weakness, fasciculation, and paralysis	Neurologic muscular disorders (e.g., amyotropic lateral sclerosis, multiple sclerosis, myasthenia gravis, Eaton-Lambert syndrome, Guillain-Barré syndrome, polymyositis)
	Seizure	Metabolic derangement or toxin exposure
Genitourinary	Muscular weakness and fatigue	Metabolic abnormality (e.g., anemia, hypocalcemia, hypokalemia, hypomagnesemia, hyponatremia, hypothyroidism)
Dermatologic	Muscular weakness and paralysis	Natural toxins (e.g., botulism; some pit viper, elapid, and scorpion venoms)

DUMBELS, *d*iarrhea, *u*rination, *m*iosis, *b*ronchorrhea and bronchospasm, *e*mesis, *l*acrimation, and *s*alivation.

cular weakness and fatigue several days after the exposure. It is not uncommon for the patient to have initially experienced minimal or no gastrointestinal symptoms shortly after the exposure only to develop significant neurologic symptoms many days later (14,15). Because dermal absorption occurs readily with many of these chemicals, special consideration should be given to the possibility of repetitive small exposures occurring through contact with contaminated clothing, pets, or other materials. The possibility of exposure from multiple sources should be considered. A patient may have contact with flea and tick preparations, plant and garden sprays, and household insecticides simultaneously, especially during the spring and summer months. Commercial agricultural use may occur year round in more temperate climates and is not tightly regulated or monitored in many areas.

A careful medication history should be obtained for Alzheimer's disease, myasthenia gravis, glaucoma, neurogenic bladder, or Sjögren's syndrome. All are treated with cholinergic medications. A history of mushroom ingestion should also be sought, as numerous mushroom species produce cholinergic effects (16).

Physical Examination

The clinical diagnosis of cholinergic syndrome is made by physical examination. The insecticides have a distinct pungent odor, which is usually evident after acute exposure. Signs and symptoms of cholinergic syndrome can be varied depending on the relative degree of muscarinic and nicotinic receptor stimulation (Table 2). Vital sign abnormalities are not specific, as bradycardia with hypotension is seen with predominance of muscarinic signs, and tachycardia with hypertension is seen with nicotinic predominance. The "classic" symptoms responsible for this syndrome are those muscarinic effects represented by the mnemonic *DUMBELS* (*d*iarrhea, *u*rination, *m*iosis, *b*ronchorrhea and bronchospasm, *e*mesis, *l*acrimation, and *s*alivation).

Diagnostic Tests

Diagnostic testing confirms the diagnosis and guides patient management. The diagnosis is confirmed by measuring a depressed cholinesterase level in a patient with appropriate clinical signs. Because the cholinesterase level in the nervous system cannot be measured directly, red blood cell (RBC) and plasma cholinesterase levels are used to estimate the effect on the cholinesterase from an organophosphate or carbamate insecticide (Chapter 236). However, the wide range of normal levels makes interpretation difficult without a baseline value (17). Serial levels drawn over several days may be necessary to demonstrate recovery or continued exposure (18).

In acute poisoning, manifestations of cholinergic syndrome do not generally occur until cholinesterase activity is depressed by 50% of the baseline level (19,20). Workers with potential occupational exposure to these compounds should have baseline reference levels drawn in case a suspected exposure occurs. RBC cholinesterase is more indicative of synaptic inhibition and is preferred for diagnosis (21). However, the RBC cholinesterase must be sent to a reference lab in most hospitals. Plasma cholinesterase is less reliable but is available in most hospitals without the delays associated with the RBC cholinesterase.

Specific testing to guide *patient management* should focus on assessing the adequacy of oxygenation and ventilation. Because most deaths from cholinergic syndrome are a result of respiratory compromise, oxygen saturation, arterial blood gases, and chest radiograph are important parameters to follow. Serum electrolytes, glucose, blood urea nitrogen, creatinine, and urine output should be followed closely to guide fluid replacement decisions. Other testing should include an acetaminophen level if a suicidal gesture is suspected. Cardiac and blood pressure monitoring are warranted because of the potential for dysrhythmias.

POTENTIAL COMPLICATIONS

Potential complications from cholinergic syndrome include permanent hypoxic injury from inadequate ventilation or impaired oxygen exchange. There are several syndromes of delayed or long-term neurologic sequelae associated specifically with organophosphate toxicity (Chapter 236).

MANAGEMENT

The airway is the most important aspect of management in cholinergic syndrome. Bronchorrhea, bronchospasm, and respiratory failure are responsible for early deaths. Administrating oxygen, establishing control of the airway, and providing good pulmonary toilet while simultaneously providing antidotal therapy provide the best opportunity for complete recovery.

Antidotes

Atropine competitively inhibits the action of acetylcholine at the postsynaptic receptor. It is indicated for signs of muscarinic excess, including gastrointestinal distress, salivation, bronchorrhea, bronchospasm, or bradycardia. The initial adult dose is 1 to 4 mg intravenously (IV). Subsequent doses are titrated to response (Chapter 42). The pediatric dose is 0.01 to 0.04 mg/kg IV initially and repeated similarly. The endpoint for treatment is drying of airway secretions, not normalization of pupil size or heart rate. Atropine is also effective intramuscularly and has reportedly been administered by continuous IV infusion, continuous intraosseous infusion, as well as inhalation via nebulization (22–24).

Atropine does not treat the muscular weakness and paralysis seen with cholinergic syndrome (there are no muscarinic receptors in skeletal muscle). *Oximes* such as pralidoxime (2-PAM) or obidoxime (Chapter 69) should always be used in conjunction with atropine if cholinesterase inhibition is suspected. Unlike atropine, an oxime treats muscular weakness and other nicotinic effects. The adult dose of 2-PAM is 1 to 2 g IV over 30 minutes. The dose can be repeated every 2 to 4 hours. A continuous infusion of 500 mg/hour may also be used. The pediatric dose is 20 to 40 mg/kg IV over 15 to 30 minutes and repeated every 2 to 4 hours, or an infusion of 10 mg/kg/hour may be required for severe cases (25,26). Oximes may be used alone in the absence of muscarinic symptoms.

Oximes should be used as early as possible in the course of disease because the organophosphate compound:cholinesterase complex may exhibit aging. Aging is caused by chemical crosslinking that makes the complex resistant to reactivation by 2-PAM or obidoxime (Chapter 69).

Benzodiazepines are the preferred treatment for seizures because their effect is synergistic with oximes for the control of seizures. Many authors recommend prophylaxis of seizures in serious poisoning. Benzodiazepines should be readily available and titrated to effect as for other causes of seizures (Chapter 40).

Supportive Care

Many of the compounds responsible for cholinergic syndrome are readily absorbed through intact skin, necessitating removal of all contaminated clothing and thorough skin decontamination with soap and water (27). Oral activated charcoal may also limit reabsorption by the intestinal lumen and enhance elimination. Ventilatory support may be needed in severe cases if respiratory effort is compromised by muscular weakness. Careful fluid and electrolyte replacement is also imperative for ongoing gastrointestinal losses.

PITFALLS

The most common pitfall in the management of cholinergic syndrome is failure to use adequate amounts of atropine to clear airway secretions. In a significant organophosphate exposure, an entire hospital's supply of atropine could be needed for one patient (28). Another pitfall occurs if 2-PAM is not used soon enough in the course of therapy for organophosphate poisoning. Then, a process called *aging* takes place in which the organophosphate permanently inhibits the cholinesterase to which it is attached. The average person regenerates RBC cholinesterase slowly at a rate of 1% to 2% per day, and recovery is unnecessarily prolonged if the "aging" process is allowed to occur.

Mild cases of cholinergic syndrome may present with relatively few, vague symptoms and are therefore often misdiagnosed as viral gastroenteritis, nonspecific upper respiratory tract illness, or a flu-like illness.

REFERENCES

1. Peter JV, Cherian AM. Organic insecticides. *Anaesth Intensive Care* 2000;28(1):11–21.
2. Litovitz TL, Klein-Schwartz W, White S, et al. 2000 Annual Report of the American Association of Poison Control Centers Toxic Exposure Surveillance System. *Am J Emerg Med* 2001;19(5):337–395.
3. Carlock LL, Chen WL, Gordon EB, et al. Regulating and assessing risks of cholinesterase-inhibiting pesticides: divergent approaches and interpretations. *J Toxicol Environ Health B Crit Rev* 1999;2(2):105–160.
4. Holstege CP, Kirk M, Sidell FR. Chemical warfare. Nerve agent poisoning. *Crit Care Clin* 1997;13(4):923–942.
5. Reference deleted.
6. Suzuki T, Morita H, Ono K, et al. Sarin poisoning in Tokyo subway. *Lancet* 1995;345(8955):980.
7. Besser R, Gutmann L, Weilemann LS. Inactivation of the end-plate acetylcholinesterase during the course of organophosphate intoxications. *Arch Toxicol* 1989;63:412–415.
8. Karalliedde L, Henry JA. Effects of organophosphates on skeletal muscle. *Hum Exp Toxicol* 1993;12:289–296.
9. He F. Neurotoxic effects of insecticides—current and future research: a review. *Neurotoxicology* 2000;21(5):829–835.
10. Gunderson CH, Lehmann CR, Sidell FR, et al. Nerve agents: a review. *Neurology* 1992;42:946–950.
11. Breyer-Pfaff U, Maier U, Brinkmann AM, et al. Pyridostigmine kinetics in healthy subjects and patients with myasthenia gravis. *Clin Pharmacol Ther* 1985;37:495–501.
12. Lamy PP. The role of cholinesterase inhibitors in Alzheimer's disease. *CNS Drugs* 1994;1:146–165.
13. Riley MR, Kastrup EK, Hebel SK, et al., eds. *Drug facts and comparisons*. St. Louis: Facts and Comparisons, 2000.
14. Gadoth N, Fisher A. Late onset of neuromuscular block in organophosphorus poisoning. *Ann Intern Med* 1978;88:654–655.
15. Hierons R, Johnson MK. Clinical and toxicological investigations of a case of delayed neuropathy in man after acute poisoning by an organophosphorus pesticide. *Arch Toxicol* 1978;40:279–284.
16. Koppel C. Clinical symptomatology and management of mushroom poisoning. *Toxicon* 1993;31:1513–1540.
17. Wofsie JH, Winter GD. Statistical analysis of normal human red blood cell and plasma cholinesterase activity values. *Arch Indust Hygiene Occup Med* 1952;6:43–49.
18. Coye MJ, Barnett PG, Midtling JE, et al. Clinical conformation of organophosphate poisoning by serial cholinesterase analysis. *Arch Intern Med* 1987;147:438–442.
19. Hassan RM, Pesce AJ, Sheng P, et al. Correlation of serum pseudocholinesterase and clinical course in two patients poisoned with organophosphate insecticides. *J Toxicol Clin Toxicol* 1981;18:401–406.
20. Midtling JE, Barnett PG, Coye MJ, et al. Clinical management of field worker organophosphate poisoning. *West J Med* 1985;142:514–518.
21. Blaber LC, Creasey NH. The mode of recovery of cholinesterase activity in vivo after organophosphorus poisoning: I. Erythrocyte cholinesterase. *Biochem J* 1960;77:591–596.
22. LeBlanc FN, Benson BE, Gilg AD. A severe organophosphate poisoning requiring the use of an atropine drip. *J Toxicol Clin Toxicol* 1986;24:69–76.
23. Haley KJ, Mortensen ME. Intraosseous infusion of antidote in an organophosphate poisoned child. *Vet Hum Toxicol* 1990;32:370.
24. Shockley LW. The use of inhaled nebulized atropine for the treatment of malathion poisoning. *J Toxicol Clin Toxicol* 1989;27:183–192.
25. Schexnayder S, James LP, Kearns GL. The pharmacokinetics of continuous infusion pralidoxime in children with organophosphate poisoning. *J Toxicol Clin Toxicol* 1998;36(6):549–555.
26. Farrar HC, Wells TG, Kearns GL. Use of continuous infusion of pralidoxime for treatment of organophosphate poisoning in children. *J Pediatr* 1990;116:648–661.
27. Burgess JL, Kirk M, Borron SW, et al. Emergency department hazardous materials protocol for contaminated patients. *Ann Emerg Med* 1999;34(2):205–212.
28. Golsousidis H, Kokkas V. Use of 19,590 mg of atropine during 24 days of treatment after a case of unusually severe parathion poisoning. *Hum Toxicol* 1985;4:339–340.

CHAPTER 14

Coma of Unclear Etiology

Mark A. Kostic and Richard C. Dart

OVERVIEW

The comatose patient with a potential toxicologic source is a common clinical challenge. *Coma* is defined as a state of unconsciousness from which the subject cannot be aroused. Coma is at the far end of a spectrum of alterations in consciousness that can be exhibited by poisoned patients. Generally speaking, etiologies include structural lesions and toxic-metabolic insults.

PATHOPHYSIOLOGY

Alertness is maintained through an intricate and poorly understood interplay of several different neuronal systems. The ascending reticular activating formation, originating in the upper pons and midbrain, is a complex system of neurons that project to the thalamus with relays to both cerebral hemispheres. The roles of acetylcholine, gamma-aminobutyric acid, and glutamate in the function of the ascending reticular activating formation have been elucidated (1–4). Neuronal systems that bypass the thalamus and project directly to the cortex have also been recently described. These use acetylcholine in projections from the basal forebrain to the cortex, serotonin from the brainstem raphe nuclei, norepinephrine from the locus ceruleus, dopamine from the substantia nigra-ventral tegmental area complex, and histamine from the posterior hypothalamus (5,6). Despite this complexity, it is clear that wakefulness is dependent on the integrity of structures in the central gray of the rostral pons and midbrain, the basal forebrain, the hypothalamus, the thalamus, and the cerebral cortex (7). Coma may result from a focal lesion in any of these sites in the brainstem or from diffuse, bilateral cortical dysfunction.

Toxins that produce coma are more often uncharged and lipophilic, allowing them to cross the blood–brain barrier. Mechanisms may vary, yet they all typically result in a global insult to the normal function of both cerebral cortices. Numerous substances are capable of producing coma. Two very general classifications of agents are proposed. First are agents that produce coma through a direct effect on brain cells. Some examples of direct-acting neurotoxins include agents that increase γ-aminobutyric acid effects such as benzodiazepines, alcohols, barbiturates, gamma-hydroxybutyric acid, and propofol. Acetylcholine antagonists, including antihistamines and tricyclic antidepressants as well as acetylcholine agonists such as organophosphates, have a direct, central neuronal effect. Also included are neuroleptics, which are dopamine receptor antagonists, selective serotonin reuptake and monoamine oxidase inhibitors, and presynaptic α_2 receptor agonists such as clonidine and imidazoline compounds. Several anticonvulsants, including phenytoin, carbamazepine, and valproic acid, directly affect neuronal firing by prolonging sodium channel inactivation. Salicylate poisoning may result in coma through cerebral edema. Cyanide and hydrogen sulfide might also be considered in this category due to their direct effect on inhibiting cellular respiration.

The second classification of agents are those in which coma is an indirect result of derangements involving other organ systems. Some examples of indirect agents include those causing hypoxia such as methemoglobin or other agents that decrease oxygen delivery to cells. Agents causing hypotension are included, such as antidysrhythmic drugs and those that block calcium channels and beta receptors. Oral hypoglycemic agents are indirectly implicated in coma, as are those agents that cause severe acid-base, electrolyte, or hepatic disorders.

Carbon monoxide is an example of a substance that likely produces coma via a combination of systemic effects as well as direct cellular toxicity. For a more detailed discussion of individual agents, please see the appropriate chapters.

DIAGNOSIS

History

Once the patient has been stabilized, a thorough history should be sought from all possible sources. Witnesses should be interviewed, and medics, fire, or police personnel should describe the circumstances in which the patient was found and be instructed to retrieve pill bottles or containers from the scene. Family and friends should be questioned as to the patient's medical and psychiatric history, recent state of mind, how the patient was found, when the patient was last seen, how long the patient could have been unconscious, and what drugs or toxins were available to the patient. Medical records should be reviewed.

Physical Examination

The initial examination of the comatose patient helps to identify conditions requiring immediate medical or surgical intervention. After initial stabilization, the physical examination often provides critical clues that narrow the differential diagnosis. Signs of recent head trauma or the presence of lateralizing or asymmetric neurologic findings should prompt an immediate search for a structural lesion. Focal findings on examination greatly reduce the likelihood of a lone toxic or metabolic etiology. Toxidromes, such as those seen in anticholinergic, cholinergic, sympathomimetic, or opiate poisonings, may be helpful if present. These are discussed in more detail in other chapters. Odors can provide useful hints. An odor of acetone may accompany diabetic ketoacidosis, chloral hydrate, or isopropyl alcohol; the scent of bitter almonds with cyanide; and a garlic-like odor with organophosphate toxicity. The presence of track marks is often indicative of intravenous drug use and resultant opiate or sympathomimetic toxicity. Seizure activity, especially if prolonged, is most commonly caused by tricyclic antidepressants, sympathomimetic or anticholinergic agents, and bupropion as well as isoniazid, theophylline, camphor, tramadol, and several others.

Respiratory pattern may be helpful in the comatose patient. Hyperventilation is associated with poisoning with salicylates and any cause of cellular hypoxia (e.g., carbon monoxide, cyanide, others). Most causes of increased hyperventilation ultimately produce respiratory failure if severe or untreated. Hypoventilation or apnea is common with opioid or sedative-hypnotic poisoning. Cheyne-Stokes respiration, defined as alternating hyperpnea and apnea, may represent a structural lesion at the level of the midbrain or be the result of infection, cardiopulmonary disease, or other metabolic disorders. Apneustic breathing, a pattern of breathing punctuated by inspiratory pauses, implies a pontine lesion (7,8).

The size, symmetry, and response of the pupils to light should be determined. Asymmetric dilation implies a structural lesion. In poisoned patients, pupils are typically equal, with an intact but somewhat diminished or delayed light response. Exceptions include opioids, clonidine, imidazoline compounds, organophosphates, and olanzapine, which may produce miotic and fixed pupils. Dilated and fixed pupils are seen with anticholinergic or sympathomimetic poisoning, or with anoxic brain injury. Fixed and midposition pupils occur with barbiturate poisoning. Conjugate eye movement away from the direction of rotation should be noted in poisoned patients while testing for the oculocephalic reflex (doll's eye movements). The oculovestibular reflex, which involves cold-water irrigation of the tympanic membrane, should produce equal bilateral nystagmus with the fast component moving toward the side stimulated.

Papilledema suggests elevated intracranial pressure. Subhyaloid hemorrhages indicate a subarachnoid bleed. Funduscopy can also provide clues to underlying diseases, such as hypertension, diabetes, or endocarditis (7).

The motor examination may reveal focal or asymmetric findings such as decorticate or decerebrate posturing or hemiparesis that should invoke a search for a structural lesion. Clonus is caused by a variety of substances, most commonly sedative-hypnotics and anticonvulsants. Rigidity, clonus, hyperreflexia, and tremor are seen with lithium poisoning. Serotonin syndrome or neuroleptic malignant syndromes typically have a motor component combined with altered mental status and hyperthermia. Compartment syndrome due to prolonged compression of an extremity is a known complication of coma. Therefore, all extremities should be inspected for edema, color change, or vascular deficit.

Diagnostic Tests

A dextrose stick, electrocardiographic monitoring, and pulse oximetry should be immediately obtained on all comatose patients. Cranial computed tomography is generally overused in poisoned patients; however, a scan should be performed if a concern for intracranial injury truly exists. If unrevealing, a lumbar puncture should follow to rule out subarachnoid bleed, meningitis, or encephalitis.

After a structural lesion has been ruled out, further testing is aimed at differentiating metabolic from toxic etiologies. An electrocardiogram should be examined for rate and rhythm disturbance, ST changes indicative of ischemia, AV block, QRS and QT interval prolongation, and right axis deviation. Drugs with myocardial sodium channel–blocking effects often cause electrocardiogram findings of tachycardia, QRS prolongation to greater than 100 ms, and elevated terminal R wave in aVR. On the other hand, cardiac glycosides can present with just about any rhythm disturbance but frequently express a bradycardic rhythm with AV block. This is similar to many calcium channel or beta-blocking agents.

Serum should be sent for electrolytes, ruling out hyponatremia or metabolic acidosis, renal function tests, glucose, and liver function tests. If liver damage is evident, a serum ammonia level may help rule out hepatic encephalopathy (Chapter 17). Coagulation studies can further assess the degree of synthetic liver failure. If an acidosis is present, a serum lactate level as well as a venous pH or arterial blood gas help assess the degree and type of acid-base disorder. The presence of an increased anion gap should be evaluated (Chapter 19). Co-oximetry can rule out poisoning with carbon monoxide or the presence of methemoglobin. The complete blood count, although not typically helpful in the workup of a poisoned patient, is useful if there is a concern for sepsis or severe anemia. Cultures of the blood, urine, and cerebrospinal fluid should also be sent in these cases. A creatine phosphokinase level may be elevated in a comatose patient due to muscle compression. Serum osmolality helps assess for hyperosmolar nonketotic coma. In addition, the osmolal gap may be elevated in cases of poisoning from the toxic alcohols, namely ethylene glycol, methanol, and isopropanol (Chapter 25). Serum thyroid-stimulating hormone screens for myxedema.

A radiograph or computed tomography scan of the chest or abdomen can further evaluate for an infectious source of coma. Urinalysis is part of the workup for an infectious etiology but can also rule out pregnancy and assist in the evaluation of ketosis, hemolysis, and renal injury. A urine screen for benzodiazepines, barbiturates, opiates, cocaine, and amphetamines may occasionally be helpful. The limitations of these "tox screens" vary according to the assay performed (Chapters 80 and 82).

Further laboratory testing can help differentiate between possible toxicologic etiologies. Aspirin and acetaminophen levels should be obtained on all potentially poisoned patients. As stated previously, aspirin causes coma through cerebral edema (typically seen on computed tomography or magnetic resonance imaging). Acetaminophen in massive overdose has also been associated with coma and lactic acidosis in several case reports (9). Many toxins, toxicants, or their resultant effects can be assayed in the serum or urine, have a known correlation with clinical symptoms, and cause coma. Examples include the alcohols; anticonvulsants (phenytoin, carbamazepine, phenobarbital, valproic acid); lithium; carbon monoxide; and methemoglobin. Quantitative levels of tricyclic antidepressants, however, have little correlation with clinical symptoms and are rarely indicated.

MANAGEMENT

General Supportive Care

All comatose patients should be monitored closely, a dextrose stick performed, or glucose administered empirically if the blood sugar is not immediately available. If alcoholic or malnourished, thiamine should be administered due to the concern for Wernicke's encephalopathy.

Oxygen should be administered. Ensuring a secure airway is paramount, and the threshold to intubate is very low. Peripheral intravenous access should be established, and resuscitative fluids provided. In cases of cardiovascular instability, central intravenous access is often necessary. Hypotension is managed with fluids and vasopressor drugs (Chapter 37). Seizure activity is managed initially with benzodiazepines. If seizures are unresponsive, further measures should be pursued because the seizures and acidosis may worsen the underlying poisoning (Chapter 40). Urine output should be maintained due to the concern for rhabdomyolysis (Chapter 29). If compartment syndrome is suspected, intracompartmental pressures should be obtained.

Once the patient has been stabilized, gastrointestinal decontamination should proceed. Activated charcoal is usually indicated and should be given via a nasogastric tube. The use of gastric lavage is questionable, but a benefit has been suggested in patients presenting comatose or obtunded within 1 to 2 hours of ingestion (Chapter 7) (10).

Specific Interventions

Naloxone is a specific opioid antagonist and effectively reverses most opioid toxidromes (see also Chapter 65). If the patient is a known opioid abuser, this agent should preferably be administered only to obviate the need for intubation. Flumazenil is a specific benzodiazepine receptor antagonist and effectively reverses the central nervous system and respiratory depression caused by pure benzodiazepine poisoning. However, the mortality from benzodiazepine poisoning with adequate supportive care is low. Conversely, the potential for provoking an acute benzodiazepine withdrawal state in a chronic user is theoretically high (11). There is also a concern with the indiscriminate administration of this drug to patients in coma. If the causative agent has proconvulsive effects, or if an acute sedative-hypnotic withdrawal state has been elicited, flumazenil may block the effect of benzodiazepine treatment. Thus, the routine use of flumazenil in coma is not recommended (Chapter 57) (11).

Physostigmine inhibits acetylcholinesterase and reverses the antimuscarinic effects of anticholinergic poisoning. The popularity of this agent is once again on the rise, but there are limitations to its use. Cholinergic side effects can occur in patients without anticholinergic poisoning, especially with routine use of this drug as part of a "coma cocktail." Asystole has also been described with the use of physostigmine in patients poisoned with tricyclic antidepressants (12). These issues, along with the fact that supportive care of anticholinergic poisoning is adequate, support the use of physostigmine as a diagnostic rather than a therapeutic tool (Chapter 67).

Ventilation of the comatose patient creates special concerns. A general rule is that the respiratory rate and tidal volume settings should attempt to match the minute ventilation of the patient before intubation. This allows for continued compensation for a metabolic acidosis, if present. Salicylate poisoned patients are a classic example. These patients frequently develop worsening acidemia and deteriorate after being placed on "standard" ventilatory settings.

Hemodialysis is indicated and essential in the treatment of severe ethylene glycol, methanol, and salicylate poisoning. Its efficacy in lithium poisoning has yet to be clearly established.

Repeated-dose activated charcoal is effective at lowering the serum levels of agents with enterohepatic circulation such as carbamazepine, phenobarbital, and theophylline (13). However, clinical benefit has not been adequately demonstrated.

Whole bowel irrigation is another technique aimed at increasing clearance of toxins from the gastrointestinal tract. This should be considered in patients poisoned with compounds that are either not bound well by activated charcoal, are without an effective antidote, or are in a sustained-release preparation. Again, clinical use has not been proven.

COMPLICATIONS

Most comatose poisoned patients do well with aggressive supportive care. Anoxic brain injury can result from prolonged hypoxemia due to apnea, aspiration, or airway obstruction. Rhabdomyolysis and resultant myoglobinuria and acute tubular necrosis can be a direct result of the toxin involved or more commonly from a prolonged period of unresponsiveness, muscle compression, and myoglobin release. Nosocomial infection and iatrogenic injury are also a concern due to the degree of intensive care required by such patients.

PITFALLS

One must always keep in mind that a patient may have more than one cause of coma. For example, the patient with a traumatic subdural hematoma may also be poisoned with salicylates, and the obviously anticholinergic patient may have fallen and struck his head.

Improper or nonaggressive airway management may lead to anoxic brain injury or aspiration. In a patient with elevated creatine phosphokinase levels, inadequate fluid resuscitation and urine output can promote acute tubular necrosis and renal failure.

Failure to repeat drug levels looking for trends, such as with lithium or salicylate, is a common and dangerous error, as many agents have delayed or erratic absorption.

Failure to maintain adequate minute ventilation in patients with metabolic acidosis is a common and potentially fatal error. Finally, it must be remembered that the central nervous system is frequently the first to be affected by drugs or toxins. Therefore, coma is often only the first sign of what may be a multisystem toxic insult.

REFERENCES

1. Steriade M, Glenn L. Neocortical and caudate projections of intralaminar thalamic neurons and their synaptic excitation from midbrain reticular core. *J Neurophysiol* 1982;48:352.
2. Kinomura S, Larsson J, Gulyas B, et al. Activation by attention of the human reticular formation and thalamic intralaminar nuclei. *Science* 1996;271:512.
3. Steriade, M, McCormick D, Sejnowski T. Thalamocortical oscillations in the sleeping and aroused brain. *Science* 1993;262:679.
4. Steriade M. Arousal: revisiting the reticular activating system. *Science* 1996;272:225–226.
5. Foote S, Morrison J. Extrathalamic modulation of cortical function. *Annu Rev Neurosci* 1987;10:67.
6. Kinney H, Samuels M. Neuropathology of the persistent vegetative state. A review. *J Neuropath Exper Neurol* 1994;53:548.
7. Feske S. Coma and confusional states: emergency diagnosis and management. *Neurol Clin* 1998;16:238–243.
8. Schiff H, Sabin T. Alterations in mental state: coma and acute confusional states. In: Noble J, ed. *Textbook of primary care medicine*, 3rd ed. St. Louis: Mosby, 2001:1462–1464.
9. Roth B, Woo O, Blanc P. Early metabolic acidosis and coma after acetaminophen ingestion. *Ann Emerg Med* 1999;33:452–456.
10. Kulig K, Bar-Or D, Cantrill S, et al. Management of acutely poisoned patients without gastric emptying. *Ann Emerg Med* 1985;14:562–567.
11. Gueye P, Hoffman J, Taboulet P, et al. Empiric use of flumazenil in comatose patients: limited applicability of criteria to define low risk. *Ann Emerg Med* 1996;27:733.
12. Pentel P, Peterson C. Asystole complicating physostigmine treatment of tricyclic antidepressant overdose. *Ann Emerg Med* 1980;9:588–590.
13. Position statement: multiple-dose activated charcoal. American Academy of Clinical Toxicology. European Association of Poisons Centres and Clinical Toxicologists. *J Toxicol Clin Toxicol* 1999;37:731–751.

CHAPTER 15

Acute Delirium

Gregory L. Carter and Andrew H. Dawson

OVERVIEW

Delirium is a disorder of impaired cognition and altered level of consciousness. It is a syndromic diagnosis that is estimated to occur in up to 30% of hospital patients. In a hospital population, it is associated with a significant morbidity and mortality, much of which is due to the underlying causes of the delirium. However, prolonged periods of untreated delirium can result in poor outcomes, even for less serious underlying causes (1,2).

Management is based on recognizing the delirium, establishing the causal and contributing etiologies, treating underlying causes, and maintaining patient and staff safety.

TABLE 1. Common diagnostic features of delirium (DSM-IV)

A (Consciousness)	Disturbance of consciousness (i.e., reduced clarity of awareness of the environment) with reduced ability to focus, sustain, or shift attention.
B (Cognition)	A change in cognition (e.g., memory deficit, disorientation, language disturbance) or the development of a perceptual disturbance that is not better accounted for by a preexisting, established, or evolving dementia.
C (Onset)	The disturbance develops over a short period of time (usually hours to days) and tends to fluctuate during the course of the day.
D (Medical)	There is evidence from the history, physical examination, or laboratory findings that the disturbance is caused by the direct physiologic consequences of a general medical condition.
D (Substance intoxication)	There is evidence from the history, physical examination, or laboratory findings of either The symptoms in criteria A and B developed during substance intoxication. Medication use is etiologically related to the disturbance. Note: This diagnosis should be made instead of a diagnosis of substance intoxication only when the cognitive symptoms are in excess of those usually associated with the intoxication syndrome and when the symptoms are sufficiently severe to warrant independent clinical attention.
D (Withdrawal)	There is evidence from the history, physical examination, or laboratory findings that the symptoms in criteria A and B developed during, or shortly after, a withdrawal syndrome. Note: This diagnosis should be made instead of a diagnosis of substance withdrawal only when the cognitive symptoms are in excess of those usually associated with the withdrawal syndrome and when the symptoms are sufficiently severe to warrant independent clinical attention.
D (Multiple etiologies)	There is evidence from the history, physical examination, or laboratory findings that the delirium has more than one etiology (e.g., more than one etiologic general medical condition, a general medical condition plus substance intoxication, or medication side effect).

DSM-IV, *Diagnostic and Statistical Manual of Mental Disorders*, 4th ed.

For purely drug-induced delirium, cessation of the drug(s) often results in resolution of the syndrome. Management also includes reduction of patient distress, reorientation strategies, and maintaining the safety of the patient and staff. Maintaining safety sometimes requires effective sedation and monitoring strategies.

DEFINITION

There are many synonyms for delirium: acute confusional state, exogenous psychosis, reversible toxic psychosis, toxic confusional state, toxic encephalopathy, and toxic psychosis (3).

The *Diagnostic and Statistical Manual of Mental Disorders*, 4th ed., makes the following distinctions: Delirium Due to a General Medical Condition, Substance Intoxication Delirium, Substance Withdrawal Delirium, Delirium Due to Multiple Etiologies, and Delirium NOS (780.09).

PATHOPHYSIOLOGY

Delirium is classified as a mental disorder because of its fluctuating level of consciousness and pervasive impairment in mental, behavioral, and emotional function. However, it is almost always caused by systemic physical disease, organ system failure, central nervous system trauma or illness, or drug effect.

DIAGNOSIS

The *Diagnostic and Statistical Manual of Mental Disorders*, 4th ed., provides general criteria for the diagnosis of delirium (Table 1).

Differential Diagnosis

Multiple potential causes of delirium are possible in any patient (Table 2). Identified risk factors include advanced age, preexisting cognitive impairment, and severe chronic illness.

TABLE 2. Differential diagnosis of delirium

- Delirium: all causes
  - Drugs
    - Intoxication
    - Withdrawal (include toxic ictal delirium)
  - Brain injury
  - Epilepsy postictal, ictal
  - Sepsis
  - Hypoxia
  - Metabolic disturbances
  - Endocrine (thyroid, pituitary, parathyroid)
  - Psychosis (no cognitive impairment)
  - Intoxication
  - Dementia (onset is not acute; fleeting hallucinations and delusions are uncommon)

TABLE 3. Drug classes that commonly produce delirium

Psychiatric and neurologic
- Antidepressant
- Antipsychotic
- Lithium
- Disulfiram
- Antiparkinsonian
- Sedative hypnotic
- Anticonvulsant

Cardiovascular
- Antihypertensive
- Diuretic
- Antidysrhythmic

Antiinfective
- Antibacterial
- Antiviral
- Antimalarial
- Antitubercular agent

Other
- Anticholinergic
- Opioid analgesic
- Nonopioid analgesic
- Corticosteroid
- H_2 receptor antagonist
- Cytotoxic
- Antiemetic

The list of drugs associated with delirium includes drugs from virtually every class (Table 3) (3). In clinical toxicology, drug-induced delirium is commonly due to an anticholinergic drug; a sedative-hypnotic drug; or recreational or habitual use of alcohol, sympathomimetics, opioids, or hallucinogens. Anticholinergic delirium is associated predominantly with specific anticholinergic agents or drugs with mixed pharmacologic activity: neuroleptics, tricyclic antidepressants, and antihistamines. Anticholinergic delirium is often hyperactive with visual or auditory misperceptions or hallucinations.

Sedative-hypnotic drugs including benzodiazepines and anticonvulsants tend to produce a hypoactive type of delirium. Recreational or habitual drug use often involves more than one drug, and mixed forms of delirium are common. Delirium due to drug withdrawal states is often of the hyperactive type, particularly for alcohol, benzodiazepines, and opioids (Table 4).

TABLE 4. Specific syndromes of drug-induced delirium

Syndrome	Physical signs	Specific treatment
Anticholinergic delirium	Agitated delirium with prominent hallucinosis; peripheral stigmata of anticholinergic excess may be present[a]	Physostigmine[b]
Serotonin syndrome	Agitated delirium, hyperreflexia, ankle clonus, ocular clonus, tremor, and diarrhea	Cyproheptadine
Neuroleptic malignant syndrome	Delirium, fever, autonomic dysfunction, extrapyramidal syndrome (history of recent antipsychotic use)	Bromocriptine

[a]Dilated pupils, absent bowel sounds, dry axilla, dry mouth, tachycardia, flushed skin.
[b]Physostigmine is short-acting and may produce bradycardia, asystole, bronchospasm, and seizures. Its clinical usefulness is limited.

History

Toxicologists are often faced with acute presentations of delirious patients at the initial examination. To diagnose delirium and establish the etiology, it is important to get collateral history, especially relating to the pattern and duration of the delirium symptoms and the history of recent prescribed, over-the-counter, and recreational drug use.

The possibly delirious patient usually falls into one of three scenarios. First, there is often a clear history of a drug ingestion strongly associated with delirium. In this case, the diagnosis must be confirmed and appropriate management instituted. Second, there may be no clear history of drug ingestion. In this case, the presence of delirium must be confirmed and non–drug-related causes of delirium investigated. Finally, the onset of delirium may be recognized late in the course, such as after extubation. Although drug-induced delirium is still the most common cause, the patient needs to be assessed for non–drug-related causes of delirium.

Most cases of delirium can be classified as either hyperactive, hypoactive, or mixed in behavioral type. Fluctuations may occur like the other features of delirium (4,5). *Hyperactive delirium* is characterized by a hypervigilant patient with increased psychomotor activity and response to stimuli. *Hypoactive delirium* has reduced psychomotor activity that can resemble complete apathy or withdrawal. Hypoactive delirium is frequently underdiagnosed in the absence of formal cognitive testing. The frequency of each type is approximately 20% hyperactive, 25% hypoactive, and 40% mixed, but with fluctuations (6).

It is important to detect hypoactive delirium as approximately two-thirds of these patients develop a hyperactive phase. There is a large number of diagnostic scoring systems or diagnostic instruments that have been validated in a wide range of clinical settings, which increase detection of delirium (7). Such instruments include the Confusion Assessment Method (8), for use by nonpsychiatric staff, or the Delirium Rating Scale (9), for use by psychiatrically trained staff. The use of such instruments should be considered in any high-risk patient population, because early recognition may be associated with reduced bed stay and resource utilization (10). Once a diagnosis of delirium is made, the patient's progress can be monitored with sequential measurements of instruments including the Delirium Rating Scale or Folstein's Mini-Mental Status Examination.

Signs and Symptoms

The initial physical assessment should be directed at eliciting signs of physical illness and organ failure, particularly fever, evidence of sepsis, head injury, dehydration, or hemodynamic compromise. Fever should prompt investigation for sepsis, even in the presence of anticholinergic drugs. Focal neurologic signs are not a feature of drug-induced delirium. Although seizures can occur with some drugs, alternate causes should be sought. Physical signs of toxidromes may be absent, as the delirium can often persist for longer than the peripheral signs of toxicity. Electrolyte abnormalities such as hypoglycemia, hypoxia, cardiac dysrhythmia, and thyroid dysfunction should be excluded by investigation.

Diagnostic Tests

In many cases of delirium, investigations are only useful to exclude other causes. Repeated clinical observation and assessment of cognition are of more benefit.

Serum chemistry tests are used to detect major electrolyte disturbances or evidence of organ failure. Serum *glucose* excludes hypoglycemia.

An *electrocardiogram* is usually performed as part of the analysis for possible occult overdose. It may show abnormalities that infer tricyclic antidepressant or phenothiazine exposure.

Arterial blood gases effectively establish whether there is hypoxia or any major metabolic disturbance. In the appropriate circumstances, other causes of tissue hypoxia such as carbon monoxide and cyanide should be considered.

A *septic workup* should be performed in any febrile patient. This evaluation typically includes cultures of blood, urine, and cerebrospinal fluid in the acutely delirious febrile patient.

A *urine drug screen* is useful to detect the presence of some recreational drugs but does not in itself establish causation.

In some instances, endocrine disease or intracranial injury (computerized head tomography) should be evaluated.

POTENTIAL COMPLICATIONS

The primary complication of delirium is trauma arising from the patent's inability to perceive his or her environment accurately. Hyperthermic or rhabdomyolysis syndromes may develop from the drug itself or excessive and unusual muscle activity. In addition, the development of renal or liver injury may result from the toxic accumulation of a drug, its metabolites, or other nondrug causes.

MANAGEMENT

Management is based on recognizing the delirium, establishing and treating the causal and contributing etiologies, and maintaining patient and staff safety. It is recognized that delirium in a hospitalized patient "may interfere with his or her management, disrupt ward routine and cause medico-legal complications as a result of patient (or staff) injury" (1).

Delirium is a mental illness, which is also a marker of the presence of systemic, central nervous system, or drug effects, so physician and psychiatrist input is needed. Moreover, clinicians from those countries that share a "common law" legal tradition have a clear *duty of care* to the delirious patient (11). This duty involves an obligation to protect patients from the risk of death or serious physical harm. Hospital systems also owe a *duty of care* for staff and visitor safety, which needs to be considered.

The aims for the management of delirium are fivefold (2):

1. Early detection
2. Identify and reverse (treat) all likely casual factors
3. Supportive medical care
4. Nonpharmacologic management of patient distress, behavior disturbance, and safety
5. Pharmacologic management of patient distress, behavioral disturbance, and safety

Early Detection

The diagnosis is made on clinical grounds; however, the condition is often overlooked; dismissed as transient; or attributed incorrectly to other psychiatric disorders, especially dementia, depression, or psychosis. The duration of delirium may reflect the severity of the underlying causal factors. Longer duration of delirium symptoms, without adequate treatment, increases the recovery time after reversal and increases the chances of central nervous system impairment following resolution of the delirium.

Identify and Reverse (Treat) All Likely Causal Factors

Cases of delirium in general hospital settings are often multifactorial in nature, and drug-induced delirium may involve more than one drug. It is often inadequate to identify and reverse the most recent proximate causal factor once the delirium syndrome has been precipitated. Even after all causes are effectively reversed, it may take some time for resolution of the delirium symptoms.

Supportive Medical Care

Effective management of hydration, electrolytes, nutrition, and pain is important. Thiamine should be administered to patients with a history of alcohol abuse or dependence.

Nonpharmacologic Management

Reassurance, reorientation, maintaining an appropriate level of sensory stimulation, and regular personal contact are essential. This may involve strategies including the use of one-on-one nursing, the bedside presence of family members, appropriate lighting for the time of day, a bedside light, providing familiar objects from home, hearing aids, glasses, radio, television, or a low stimulus environment such as a quiet ward or room.

The patient may require restraint in circumstances in which the patient presents a danger to him- or herself or others. In some situations, brief physical restraint may be indicated while appropriate pharmacologic measures are instituted. There are real dangers in using physical restraint, especially in agitated or elderly patients. Trained staff and approved devices should be used.

Pharmacologic Management

Pharmacologic treatments can be considered as either antidotal or symptomatic. Examples of antidotal treatments include the treatment of anticholinergic delirium with physostigmine; serotonin toxicity with cyproheptadine (Chapter 24); neuroleptic malignant syndrome with bromocriptine (Chapter 23); or alcohol withdrawal with benzodiazepines and barbiturate withdrawal with barbiturates (Table 4). Physostigmine is more effective at reversing anticholinergic delirium than benzodiazepines (Chapter 67) (12). Patients who have ingested anticholinergic agents with a long duration of action may require multiple doses. Neuroleptics may be antidotal for cocaine, amphetamine, and hallucinogens such as lysergic acid diethylamide.

Most pharmacologic treatment is usually symptomatic and "nonspecific," however, aimed at reducing distress, anxiety, cognitive disorganization, psychotic phenomena, or behavior disturbance. These treatments should not be offered as a matter of course but promptly instigated when the clinical indications are evident. This type of "nonspecific" pharmacologic intervention should be reserved for situations in which the risk of harm to self or others is high or when the patient is very distressed.

In clinical practice, rapid control of dangerous behavioral disturbance usually requires intravenous (IV) drug administration. In this situation, the initial dosage needs to be titrated to achieve the necessary clinical effect—physical safety of the patient. Therefore, the patient should be sedated to a reduced level of consciousness but able to maintain an airway and spontaneous ventilation. Reviews of clinical trials of pharmacologic agents in the treatment of delirium report probable benefits for the use of benzodiazepines, neuroleptics, or a combination of both (2). These clinical trials have been predominately carried out in an elderly population and may not be generalized to the acutely delirious toxicology patient.

Benzodiazepines are widely used for acute behavioral control because they are rapidly effective via parenteral administration, have a wide safety margin with no anticholinergic or proconvulsive effects, and are reversible in the event of excessive sedation or respiratory depression. The choices are midazolam (IV or intramuscular), lorazepam (IV or intramuscular), or diazepam (IV only). The dose of these agents is normally titrated against response. If the patient's behavior is not controlled by the acute administration of 60 mg of diazepam (or its equivalent), then supplementary treatment with neuroleptics may be useful.

Adjunctive treatment or alternatives to benzodiazepines are typical neuroleptic medications, particularly haloperidol and droperidol. Both are available in parenteral form. Droperidol is more sedating than haloperidol, but neither produces rapid sedation like the benzodiazepines. Both drugs have the potential to prolong the QT interval, as well as cause extrapyramidal side effects, and should be avoided in patients with preexisting QT prolongation. Droperidol has been withdrawn from the market in some countries.

Patients who require acute chemical restraint require postsedation monitoring of the airway, oxygenation, and hemodynamic status.

When the delirious patient is not exhibiting dangerous behavior disturbance but instead has distress, anxiety, cognitive impairment, or disturbing psychotic phenomena, the clinical goal for pharmacologic management is relief of these symptoms, not sedation.

When distress of the patient is the focus of pharmacologic treatment, a regular oral low-dose approach (using diazepam or haloperidol) for several days may be more useful than single large doses or intermittent dosage, or some combination of those approaches. When psychotic features predominate, haloperidol may be the first drug of choice.

There are some situations when it may be more appropriate to consider sedation and ventilation of the patient. These situations include drug-induced delirium and hyperthermia, respiratory failure, the need for invasive monitoring, or unsuccessful behavior control with pharmacotherapy.

REFERENCES

1. Meagher DJ. Delirium: optimising management. *BMJ* 2001;322(7279):144–149.
2. American Psychiatric Association. Practice guidelines for the treatment of patients with delirium. *Am J Psychiatry* 1999;156:1–20.
3. Carter GL, Dawson AH, Lopert R. Drug-induced delirium. Incidence, management and prevention. *Drug Saf* 1996;15(4):291–301.
4. Camus V, Gonthier R, Dubos G, et al. Etiologic and outcome profiles in hypoactive and hyperactive subtypes of delirium. *J Geriatr Psychiatry Neurol* 2000;13(1):38–42.
5. Camus V, Burtin B, Simeone I, et al. Factor analysis supports the evidence of existing hyperactive and hypoactive subtypes of delirium. *Int J Geriatr Psychiatry* 2000;15(4):313–316.
6. Meagher DJ, O'Hanlon D, O'Mahony E, et al. Relationship between symptoms and motoric subtype of delirium. *J Neuropsychiatry Clin Neurosci* 2000;12(1):51–56.
7. Ely EW, Inouye SK, Bernard GR, et al. Delirium in mechanically ventilated patients: validity and reliability of the confusion assessment method for the intensive care unit (CAM-ICU). *JAMA* 2001;286(21):2703–2710.
8. Inouye SK, van Dyck CH, Alessi CA, et al. Clarifying confusion: the confusion assessment method. A new method for detection of delirium. *Ann Intern Med* 1990;113(12):941–948.
9. Trzepacz PT. The Delirium Rating Scale. Its use in consultation-liaison research. [Review] [35 refs]. *Psychosomatics* 1999;40(3):193–204.
10. Ely EW, Gautam S, Margolin R, et al. The impact of delirium in the intensive care unit on hospital length of stay. *Intensive Care Med* 2001;27(12):1892–1900.
11. Fogel BS, Mills MJ, Landen JE. Legal aspects of the treatment of delirium. *Hosp Community Psychiatry* 1986;37(2):154–158.
12. Burns MJ, Linden CH, Graudins A, et al. A comparison of physostigmine and benzodiazepines for the treatment of anticholinergic poisoning. *Ann Emerg Med* 2000;35(4):374–381.

CHAPTER 16

Extravasation of Drugs

Jana Vander Leest

OVERVIEW

Extravasation is defined as the leakage or direct infiltration of intravenous (IV) drug into the surrounding tissue (1). Others define infiltration and extravasation as the escape of nonvesicant and vesicant substance, respectively, from the vein into subcutaneous tissue (2,3).

The incidence of extravasation ranges from 0.1% to 6.5% of patients receiving IV therapy, and up to 11% in pediatrics (1,4–7). Approximately one-third of all vesicant extravasations progress to ulcer formation requiring surgical intervention (8).

Factors contributing to the risk and severity of extravasation include anatomy (fragile, small, or sclerosed veins; lymphedema; superior vena cava syndrome); physiochemical (amount of infiltrate, duration of tissue exposure); mechanical (poor needle insertion technique, use of metal needles versus plastic cannulas, multiple venipuncture attempts, rapid infusion rate, use of indwelling IV lines, clinician inexperience); and age-related (infants, small children, and unconscious patients are unable to complain of pain at injection site, elderly less likely to complain of discomfort). Additional risk factors include fibrin sheath formation, obesity, tourniquets, prior radiation therapy, vigorous activity, peripheral neuropathy, and use of mental status–altering medication (3,6,8–10).

Irritants

Irritants (mechlorethamine, bisantrene, carmustine, carboplatin, cisplatin, cyclophosphamide, docetaxel, fluorouracil, ifosfamide, paclitaxel, etoposide, thiotepa) produce venous pain caused by local irritation and vessel spasm, impeding blood flow, and fostering phlebitis or sclerosis. Burning, warmth, pain, discomfort, erythema, and tenderness in the area of extravasation may develop, and hyperpigmentation along the vein may follow (1,7,11,12).

Hypersensitizers

Hypersensitizers (doxorubicin, daunorubicin, mechlorethamine) cause urticaria and increased vessel permeability along the course of the vein secondary to histamine release and may leak out despite the absence of a venous break. These reactions usually resolve spontaneously after 30 minutes (7,11,12).

Vesicants

Vesicants (cisplatin, dacarbazine, daunorubicin, doxorubicin, etoposide, teniposide, mechlorethamine, melphalan, mithramycin, mitomycin, vinblastine, vincristine, vindesine) may produce severe tissue damage and necrosis. Pain, erythema, and local swelling may be immediate or delayed for several days to weeks. Within a few days, a painful, indurated lump forms and eventually ulcerates; dry desquamation or blistering may appear. If the extravasated amount is small, symptoms may resolve over several weeks. Necrosis, eschar formation, and ulceration occur with more significant extravasation. These ulcers lack granulation tissue formation, have little epithelial ingrowth, and may gradually expand into surrounding muscles, tendons, vessels, nerves, and bones, resulting in considerable functional and cosmetic damage. Serious sequelae may occur, including nerve compression, permanent joint stiffness, contractures, nerve deficits, and residual sympathetic dystrophy. Vesicants can persist in tissue for months, which may contribute to the chronic and progressive injury (1,6,7,11). Similarly, calcium-containing extravasations may result in skin loss up to 3 weeks after the initial injury (13). Additionally, *recall* can occur as late as 29 weeks after extravasation (8,14). Recall is the reactivation of an apparently healed extravasation injury, associated with further treatment with the same vesicant drug (14,15). It may be precipitated by radiation therapy, alcohol use, and sunlight, which are thought to increase vascular fragility or permeability (16). Recall has been reported to occur with anthracyclines, mitomycin-C, and paclitaxel, and is characterized by severe pain, erythema, induration, hyperpigmentation, and bulla formation (7,16,17).

PATHOPHYSIOLOGY

The literature classifies most drugs as either *irritants* or *vesicants* (18). Irritants chemically injure the venous endothelium, causing phlebitis, flare reactions, and inflammation of the extravascular tissue without necrosis (8,19). *Flare reactions* are characterized by pruritus and redness along the vein or injection site and usually resolve within 30 to 90 minutes (3,8). Unlike extravasation, flares are usually not associated with pain or swelling (3). Although most often seen with irritants such as etoposide and teniposide (8), 3% to 6% of patients receiving doxorubicin also develop flare reactions (20). Vesicants may cause blistering or extravasation-induced tissue necrosis. Vesicants are either nucleic acid–binding agents or nonbinding agents. Agents that bind to deoxyribonucleic acid (DNA) (anthracyclines, mitomycin, mechlorethamine, melphalan) lodge intracellularly and sequentially damage cells, expanding the ulcerated area and prolonging healing rates. Nonbinding agents include hyperosmolar solutions, ischemia-producing drugs, and directly cytotoxic agents. Extravasation of nonbinding agents causes injury similar to a chemical burn, which is usually followed by a normal healing course (19).

Osmolarity

Hyperosmolar solutions cause tissue damage due to an osmotic imbalance across cell membranes. The presence of ions may contribute to inflammatory reactions and prolonged ischemia leading to necrosis. Hypertonic cation-containing solutions such as potassium and calcium chloride, high-concentration dextrose solutions, and hyperalimentation fluid may produce tissue damage due to hyperosmolarity (3,5,21–23). Phenytoin contains 40% propylene glycol, which has extremely high osmolality and can cause connective tissue, muscle, and neuronal necrosis; purple-glove syndrome; and cellulitis that can progress to necrosis requiring amputation, especially in children (24,25).

pH

Highly acidic or alkaline drugs, generally pH below 4.1 or above 9.0 (e.g., phenytoin with a pH of 10.0 to 12.3, acyclovir with a pH of 10.5 to 11.6) may cause precipitation of proteins and vein irritation, potentially causing vasospasm and subsequent leakage of drug (5,10,21–23).

Vasoconstriction

Sympathomimetic drugs (e.g., dopamine, epinephrine, metaraminol, norepinephrine) cause ischemia secondary to vasoconstriction (3,13,22). Irreversible tissue damage likely occurs within 4 to 6 hours of extravasation (26).

Direct Cytotoxicity

Chemotherapeutic agents (e.g., vinca alkaloids) and some antibiotics (e.g., oxacillin, nafcillin) cause direct cytotoxicity (3,9,22,23). Antineoplastic drugs produce cytotoxicity via differing mechanisms. The anthracyclines (e.g., doxorubicin, daunorubicin) intercalate between DNA base pairs, causing steric obstruction of new DNA or ribonucleic acid (RNA) strand formation (19). Doxorubicin and mitomycin-C may cause prolonged tissue damage due to their release from dead cells and subsequent binding to DNA in surrounding tissue (8,16). Doxorubicin can continue to damage live cells for up to 5 months (8). Anthracyclines and mitomycin-C may also form oxygen radicals, altering calcium transport and resulting in irreversible cell membrane damage (16,27,28). Mitomycin is an alkylating agent that is activated intracellularly and cross-links DNA, inhibiting DNA and RNA formation. Mechlorethamine also inhibits DNA and RNA synthesis by forming carbonium ions that cross-link DNA strands. Melphalan (derived from mechlorethamine) alkylates DNA strands after carbonium ion formation. Vinca alkaloids do not bind DNA but rather the microtubular proteins that form the mitotic spindle during cell division; interference with cell division results in cell death (19). Nonchemotherapeutic agents also capable of causing direct cellular toxicity include potassium salts (5). Histologically, extravasation of vesicant chemotherapeutic drugs may cause epidermal and dermal necrosis, including dyskeratotic keratinocytes; vacuolar degeneration of the basal layer; possible inflammatory cell infiltration; collagen necrosis; and calcium deposition, which may continue up to 7 weeks (12).

Mechanical Compression

Large-volume extravasation of any substance can produce mechanical compression and compartment syndromes.

Infection

Infection of the injured site may be a secondary factor responsible for increased tissue damage in an area previously injured by extravasation (3).

MANAGEMENT

Extravasation is a medical emergency. The principles of management are early detection; removal of the extravasated drug, if possible; and early treatment of tissue injury (Tables 1 and 2).

TABLE 1. Extravasation—principles of management

Stop the infusion immediately. The affected extremity should be elevated to decrease capillary hydrostatic pressure and reduce edema but should not compromise arterial inflow or venous drainage.
Do not remove the needle.
Attempt to aspirate any extravasated drug or blood out of the needle and IV tubing. (The amount of drug or solution extravasated should be estimated.)
Use specific antidote if indicated. Do not inject the antidote into the needle; inject it SQ or intradermally.
Do not put pressure on the site.
Remove the needle.
Mark the borders of the affected area.
Put ice pack or warm heat on the affected area, depending on which is recommended.
Elevate the extremity for 48–72 h.
Consider photographing the area for follow-up purposes.

Considerable debate exists regarding application of heat versus cold (2,3,20,29). In animal models, neither heat nor cooling benefited extravasation of alkylating agents (2), whereas dry heat decreased edema after phenytoin extravasation (24) and in healthy volunteers with hyper- and hypotonic saline extravasations (3). Due to the increase in tissue metabolic demand, others advocate topical cooling for all vesicant extravasations except vinca alkaloids (2,3,7,20), to slow cellular metabolic rate and eventually deactivate the extravasated agent (7). Conversely, animal studies show topical cooling intensifies skin toxicity after vinca alkaloid extravasation, whereas mild local warming decreases it (6). Generally, moist towels or soaks should be avoided as skin maceration may occur if underlying tissue is damaged (3,10,29), although case reports indicate warm soaks, elevation, and physical therapy may be of benefit in treating docetaxel extravasation (30).

A surgical consult is recommended if (a) the estimated extravasated volume is greater than 30 ml of ionic or 100 ml of nonionic contrast medium; (b) skin blisters develop; (c) tissue perfusion is altered (decreased capillary refill); (d) pain increases; or (e) if change occurs in sensation at or distal to the site of extravasation (31). A surgical consult is also warranted if conservative measures are ineffective, or if the patient develops ulceration or skin necrosis. Surgical treatment of an extravasation is highly effective (3); suction and saline washout are safe and effective in the treatment of drug and contrast media extravasation injury (32–34).

Antidotes

Antidotes for extravasation injury remain largely anecdotal, due to a lack of randomized clinical trials (15); however, some generally accepted treatment recommendations exist (7,8,14).

HYALURONIDASE

Hyaluronidase is an enzyme that hydrolyzes hyaluronic acid, the tissue cement in connective tissue. The purpose is to decrease interstitial tissue viscosity, increase tissue permeability, and allow increased absorption and distribution of extravasated fluid (26,29,35,36). Onset is immediate, the effects last 24 to 48 hours, and toxicity is minimal (35). Intradermal or subcutaneous injections of hyaluronidase, 15 U/ml in four to five 0.2-ml increments (15 to 300 U have been used clinically) using a 25- or 26-gauge needle have shown benefit in the treatment of injury due to epipodophyllotoxins, vinca alkaloids, carmustine, paclitaxel, aminophylline, calcium, potassium, dextrose, radiocontrast media, nafcillin, parenteral nutrition solution, and phenytoin (3,8,21,29,30,35,36). Ideally, hyaluronidase should be given within 1 hour; however, it has been effective when administered up to 12 hours after extravasation (3,29,35,36). Do not inject hyaluronidase into cancerous areas (29).

The Gault procedure involves making four small punctures around the affected area and injecting the site with hyaluronidase subcutaneously. Saline is then injected into one of the puncture sites using a needle attached to a three-way tap. The saline then flows freely out of the other three puncture sites. Up to 500 ml of saline has been used. Gentle liposuction is then applied to the area (26).

Animal trials indicate hyaluronidase may be used to treat doxorubicin extravasations if drug concentrations are 1 mg/ml or less; if concentrations exceed 10 mg/ml, increased skin necrosis has occurred (37). Hyaluronidase (0.2-ml aliquots of 15 U/ml solution) appeared effective in a toddler patient with phenytoin extravasation (36). Hyaluronidase in conjunction with mild aspiration achieved good results in 10 out of 12 newborn infants with vasoactive and hyperosmolar drug extravasation injuries (26). Chondroitin sulfatase 150 to 200 turbidity-reducing units administered as 6 subcutaneous injections in the affected site may be used interchangeably with hyaluronidase. In addition to hyaluronic acid, chondroitin sulfatase also depolymerizes chondroitin sulfate, another tissue cement component (35,37).

DIMETHYL SULFOXIDE

Dimethyl sulfoxide (DMSO) is a potent free-radical scavenger that may enhance the removal rate of extravasated drug from tissue (38). It also may provide antibacterial, antiinflammatory, analgesic, and vasodilatory effects (3,8). A prospective clinical trial and case reports indicate that a 50% to 99% solution (1 to 2 ml applied topically and allowed to air dry two to six times daily for up to 2 weeks) has successfully treated patients with anthracycline, epirubicin, mitoxantrone, mitomycin, cisplatin, carboplatin, ifosfamide, and fluorouracil extravasation injury (6,7,15,16,18,38). Intermittent local cooling is generally recommended in conjunction with DMSO, unless vinca alkaloids are involved (14,18). DMSO 90% vol/vol in combination with subcutaneous *chondroitin sulfatase* 150 turbidity-reducing units in 3 ml of normal saline (six punctures applied throughout the affected area) effectively treated a patient with dual doxorubicin and vincristine extravasation during a peripheral vein infusion. Necrosis did not develop, and arm movement was virtually normal within 3 weeks (37). DMSO also appears effective in combination with IV dexrazoxane 1000 mg, a strong chelator that prevents anthracycline-induced free radical generation (15).

SODIUM THIOSULFATE

Sodium thiosulfate neutralizes vesicants by creating an alkaline-rich site. Alkylating agents have affinity to the alkaline substrate, binding preferentially to sodium thiosulfate instead of tissue (8). Subcutaneous injection of 5 to 10 ml of a 0.17-mol/L solution into the affected area is recommended for mechlorethamine and dacarbazine extravasation (14); carboplatin (concentrations exceeding 10 mg/ml); cisplatin (more than 20 ml of a 0.5-mg/ml or greater solution); cyclophosphamide; and large carmustine extravasations (18).

PHENTOLAMINE

Phentolamine is an alpha-adrenergic receptor blocker. Although no controlled trials support its efficacy, phentolamine 5 to 10 mg in 10 to 15 ml of normal saline injected with a fine hypodermic needle throughout the affected area decreases tissue injury secondary to vasopressor extravasation (39), especially within 12 hours of the extravasation (26).

TABLE 2. Management of extravasation of antineoplastic agents

Agent	Recommendation	Heat/cold application	Reference(s)
Anthracyclines Daunorubicin Doxorubicin Epirubicin	Topical DMSO: apply 1–2 ml topically two to six times daily for up to 14 d. Consider concurrent treatment with dexrazoxane 1000 mg (typical dose) or 1000 mg/m² (manufacturer's recommended dose) within 5 h of extravasation. Consider GM-CSF, 400 μg SQ once weekly for 3–4 wk. Also consider triamcinolone 70–80 mg IL once weekly for 2 wk.	Cold compress; ice packs may be applied for 15–30 min three to four times daily for 1–3 d or until symptoms resolve.	Albanell et al. (6); Shenaq et al. (7); Bos et al. (15); Drugdex editorial staff (18); Bertelli et al. (38) Whang et al. (12); Shamseddine et al. (42); Ulutin et al. (43)
Mitoxantrone	DMSO 99% topically q8h for 7 d.		Bos et al. (15)
Alkylating agents Carboplatin (≥10 mg/ml) Carmustine Cisplatin (>20 ml of >0.5-mg/ml solution) Cyclophosphamide Dacarbazine	Sodium thiosulfate, 0.17 mol/L; inject 5 ml into affected area.	Cold compress: apply for 1 h every 8 h for 3 d.	Albanell et al. (6); Oostweegel et al. (14); Drugdex editorial staff (18)
Cisplatin Carboplatin Large carmustine extravasations	Consider DMSO 99%. Apply 4 drops/10 cm² of skin surface, covering twice the size of the affected area, q8h for 7 d; allow to air dry without dressings.		Albanell et al. (6); Patel et al. (16); Drugdex editorial staff (18); Bertelli et al. (38)
Ifosfamide	DMSO application only; consider triamcinolone, 70–80 mg IL q1wk for 2 wk.		Whang et al. (12); Drugdex editorial staff (18); Bertelli et al. (38)
Mechlorethamine	Sodium thiosulfate as above.		Drugdex editorial staff (18)
Mitomycin-C	Consider topical collagenase application; may also use triamcinolone cream topically.		Patel et al. (16)
Antimetabolites Fluorouracil (5-FU)	DMSO 99%: apply 4 drops/cm² of skin surface, covering twice the affected area size; air dry without dressings. Consider triamcinolone, 70–80 mg IL qwk for 2 wk; consider topical triamcinolone.	Apply cold pack for 1 h q8h for 3 d.	Whang et al. (12); Patel et al. (16); Bertelli et al. (38)
Plant alkaloids Vinca Vincristine Vindesine Vinorelbine	Hyaluronidase: inject 150–900 IU ID or SQ into affected area. Consider triamcinolone, 70–80 mg IL once weekly for 2 wk.	Apply warm pack for 15–20 min QID for 1–2 d.	Albanell et al. (6); Shenaq et al. (7); Whang et al. (12); Drugdex editorial staff (18)
Etoposide Teniposide	Hyaluronidase per vinca alkaloid protocol.	Apply warm pack for 30–60 min, then alternate on and off every 15 min for 1 d.	Drugdex editorial staff (18)
Paclitaxel Docetaxel	Consider hyaluronidase, 150–300 IU ID or SQ; for mild soft tissue reactions, consider topical cooling only.	Both warm and cold packs used; consider warm soaks for 15–20 min QID for 1–2 d.	Albanell et al. (6); Herrington et al. (17); Drugdex editorial staff (18); Ascherman et al. (30)
Vasoconstrictors Dobutamine Dopamine Epinephrine Norepinephrine	Phentolamine, 5–10 mg, in 10–15 ml NS administered throughout the affected area; consider topical transdermal nitroglycerin 5-mg patch or cream.	Both currently discouraged.	Edwards et al. (24); Casanova et al. (26); Chen et al. (39); Tjon et al. (40)
Antibiotics Penicillins Vancomycin	Hyaluronidase, 15 IU/ml; inject five 0.2-ml increments ID or SQ into affected area (15–300 IU used clinically).	Oxacillin: apply cold pack; alternate 20 min on and off for 3 d.	Fromm et al. (10); Montgomer et al. (29)
Hyperosmolar solutions Calcium Potassium Dextrose (≥10%) Total parenteral nutrition solutions Hypertonic saline	Hyaluronidase, 15 IU/ml: five 0.2-ml injections ID or SQ into affected area (15–300 IU arbitrarily selected in published recommendations).	Recommendations inconsistent; heat may be of benefit.	Hadaway (2); Cohan et al. (3)
Miscellaneous Aminophylline Contrast media (>30 ml of ionic or >100 ml of nonionic)	Hyaluronidase, 15 IU/ml: five 0.2-ml injections ID or SQ into affected area (15–300 IU arbitrarily selected in published recommendations).	Aminophylline and contrast: apply ice pack for 20–60 min TID, PRN	Cohan et al. (3); Drugdex editorial staff (25); Montgomer et al. (29); Sokol et al. (36)
Phenytoin	May also consider applying transdermal nitroglycerin 5-mg patch; some recommend no antidote, only dry warm compresses.	Dry heat may be of benefit.	Edwards et al. (24); Montgomer et al. (29)
Promethazine	Consider hydrocortisone, 100 mg IV.	No specific recommendations available.	Malesker et al. (41)

DMSO, dimethyl sulfoxide; GM-CSF, granulocyte-monocyte colony stimulating factor; ID, intradermally; IL, intralesionally; NS, normal saline.
Table by Jana Vander Leest, RPh; Sarah Largent, PharmD Candidate, University of Colorado, Denver, Colorado.

NITROGLYCERIN

Application of 2% nitroglycerin cream may relieve the ischemia associated with dopamine extravasation (24,40). Both the cream and the patch may relieve vasospasm, aid in reducing edema, and facilitate absorption of the extravasate (24). Case reports suggest that transdermal nitroglycerin 5 mg was beneficial in the treatment of parenteral nutrition (35) and phenytoin extravasation (24). The transdermal patch may be more desirable than the topical cream due to ease of application, predictable release, and absorption of nitroglycerin (40).

STEROIDS

Steroid use is controversial (3,12). Good results have been reported with betamethasone ointment, hydrocortisone injection, and intralesional injection of 7 to 8 ml of triamcinolone 10 mg/ml after various chemotherapeutic agent extravasations (12,16). Hydrocortisone succinate injected once daily was at least partially effective in treating a case of promethazine extravasation (41). Others reject steroid use as histologic studies of chemotherapeutic extravasation ulcers reveal little inflammatory cell response, and steroids may delay healing and increase the risk of local infection (7,8,12,19,38,42).

OTHER AGENTS

The literature contains case reports of treatments that may be of value but require further study. *Granulocyte macrophage-colony stimulating factor* subcutaneously administered weekly for 4 weeks (31.84 to 56.61 μg/cm^2) successfully treated cutaneous ulcers secondary to doxorubicin extravasation in two patients (42); a patient given 400 μg weekly for 3 weeks had complete healing of a 6-month-old doxorubicin extravasation-induced ulcer (43). *Silver sulfadiazine* applied twice daily to blisters at the site of extravasation injury aids in preventing local superinfection and has effectively treated necrosis caused by oxacillin (10). Silver sulfadiazine and ice packs resulted in marked improvement in a patient with blistering secondary to ionic contrast media extravasation (31). *Collagenase ointment* and whirlpool therapy resulted in lesion resolution in a patient with mitomycin-C and fluorouracil extravasation, although residual scarring occurred (16). *Fibrinolysin/deoxyribonuclease ointment* (Elase) has been used to treat calcium, hypertonic, and electrolyte extravasations (29). Fibrinolysin/deoxyribonuclease ointment applied every 8 hours for 3 to 4 weeks successfully treated 15 neonatal intensive care unit patients with full-thickness extravasation injuries (44).

Sodium bicarbonate injection is largely discouraged, as its hyperosmolarity may cause chemical cellulitis, ulceration, and tissue necrosis (6,8,19,20,22).

Additional data are required to determine the role of beta-adrenergics, antioxidants (e.g., butylated hydroxytoluene), and DMSO with vitamin E. Ineffective therapies include antihistamines, *N*-acetylcysteine, lidocaine, procaine, heparin, granulocyte colony-stimulating factor, or locally injected alpha-tocopherol (3,8,43). IV fluorescein may be used to aid in identifying viable tissue (21).

PITFALLS

The diagnosis of extravasation can be difficult, and there is a tendency to underestimate the severity of injury (3). Expected signs and symptoms may not occur immediately, resulting in delayed detection and progressive tissue damage. Extravasation can occur in the presence of good blood return on aspiration, and necrosis and ulceration can ensue despite initial minor and transient irritation (6,18). Available data regarding treatment are often anecdotal or based on animal studies, which may be of limited value in predicting possible human response as skin characteristics may significantly differ (3). Data from human populations do not contain control groups due to ethical considerations, rendering true evidence-based efficacy of antidotal treatment unavailable (3,18).

REFERENCES

1. Susser WS, Whitaker-Worth DL, Grant-Kels JM. Mucocutaneous reactions to chemotherapy. *J Am Acad Dermatol* 1999;40(3):367–398.
2. Hadaway L. Catheter connection . . . treating infiltration and extravasation. *J Vasc Access Device* 2000;5(2):52.
3. Cohan RH, Ellis JH, Garner WL. Extravasation of radiographic contrast material: recognition, prevention, and treatment. *Radiology* 1996;200:593–604.
4. Schulmeister L, Camp-Sorrell D. Chemotherapy extravasation from implanted ports. *Oncol Nurs Forum* 2000;27(3):531–538.
5. Robijns BJ, de Wit WM, Bosma NJ, et al. Localized bullous eruptions caused by extravasation of commonly used intravenous infusion fluids. *Dermatologica* 1991;182:39–42.
6. Albanell J, Baselga J. Systemic therapy emergencies. *Semin Oncol* 2000;27(3):347–361.
7. Shenaq SM, Abbase EA, Friedman JD. Soft-tissue reconstruction following extravasation of chemotherapeutic agents. *Surg Oncol Clin N Am* 1996;5(4):825–845.
8. Kassner E. Evaluation and treatment of chemotherapy extravasation injuries. *J Pediatr Oncol Nurs* 2000;17(3):135–148.
9. Mayo DJ, Pearson DC. Chemotherapy extravasation: a consequence of fibrin sheath formation around venous access devices. *Oncol Nurs Forum* 1995;22(4):675–680.
10. Fromm LA, Graham DL. Oxacillin-induced tissue necrosis. *Ann Pharmacother* 1999;33:1060–1062.
11. Scuderi N, Onesti MG. Antitumor agents: extravasation, management, and surgical treatment. *Ann Plast Surg* 1994;32(1):39–44.
12. Whang SW, Lee SH, Elias PM, et al. Intralesional steroids reduce inflammation from extravasated chemotherapeutic agents [Letter]. *Br J Dermatol* 2001;145:680–682.
13. Kumar RJ, Pegg SP, Kimble RM. Management of extravasation injuries. *ANZ J Surg* 2001;71:285–289.
14. Oostweegel LM, VanWarmerdam LJC, Schot M, et al. Extravasation of topotecan, a report of two cases. *J Oncol Pharm Pract* 1997;3(2):115–116.
15. Bos AM, van der Graaf WT, Willemse PH. A new conservative approach to extravasation of anthracyclines with dimethylsulfoxide and dexrazoxane. *Acta Oncol* 2001;40(4):541–542.
16. Patel JS, Krusa M. Distant and delayed mitomycin C extravasation. *Pharmacotherapy* 1999;19(8):1002–1005.
17. Herrington JD, Figueroa JA. Severe necrosis due to paclitaxel extravasation. *Pharmacotherapy* 1997;17(1):163–165.
18. Drugdex editorial staff. Cytotoxic drug extravasation therapy. In: *Drug consults*. Englewood, CO: Micromedex, Inc., 2001.
19. Mullin S, Beckwith MC, Tyler LS. Prevention and management of antineoplastic extravasation injury. *Hosp Pharm* 2000;35:57–74.
20. How C, Brown J. Extravasation of cytotoxic chemotherapy from peripheral veins. *Eur J Oncol Nurs* 1998;2(1):51–58.
21. MICROMEDEX Healthcare Series. Extravasation injury. In: *POISINDEX managements*. Englewood, CO: Micromedex, Inc., 1998.
22. Tatro DS, Ow-Wing SD. Non-cytotoxic drug extravasation therapy. In: *Drug consults*. Englewood, CO: Micromedex, Inc., 1999.
23. Jones AM, Stanley A. Probe high extravasation rates. *Hosp Pharm Pract* 1997;7:292, 294, 296.
24. Edwards JJ, Bosek V. Extravasation injury of the upper extremity by intravenous phenytoin. *Anesth Analg* 2002;94:672–673.
25. DRUGDEX Editorial Staff. Phenytoin extravasation—treatment. In: *Drug consults*. Englewood, CO: Micromedex, Inc., 1998.
26. Casanova D, Bardot J, Magalon G. Emergency treatment of accidental infusion leakage in the newborn: report of 14 cases. *Br J Plast Surg* 2001;54:396–399.
27. McLoon LK, Wirtschafter J. Local injections of corticotropin releasing factor reduce doxorubicin-induced acute inflammation in the eyelid. *Invest Ophthamol Vis Sci* 1997;38(5):834–841.
28. Cedidi C, Hierner R, Berger A. Plastic surgical management in tissue extravasation of cytotoxic agents in the upper extremity. *Eur J Med Res* 2001;6:309–314.
29. Montgomer LA, Hanrahan K, Kottman K, et al. Guideline for IV infiltrations in pediatric patients. *Pediatr Nurs* 1999;25(2):167–180.
30. Ascherman JA, Knowles SL, Attkiss K. Docetaxel (Taxotere) extravasation: a report of five cases with treatment recommendations. *Ann Plast Surg* 2000;45(4):438–441.
31. Cohan RH, Bullard MA, Ellis JH, et al. Local reactions after injection of iodinated contrast material: detection, management, and outcome. *Acad Radiol* 1997;4(11):711–718.
32. Vandeweyer E, Heymans O, Deraemaecker R. Extravasation injuries and emergency suction as treatment. *Plast Reconstr Surg* 2000;105:109–110.
33. Martin PH, Carver N, Petros AJ. Use of liposuction and saline washout for

the treatment of extensive subcutaneous extravasation of corrosive drugs. *Br J Anaesth* 1994;72:702–704.
34. Vandeweyer E, Deraemaecker R. Early surgical suction and washout for treatment of cytotoxic drug extravasations. *Acta Chir Belg* 2000;100(1):37–38.
35. Gil ME, Mateu J. Treatment of extravasation from parenteral nutrition solution. *Ann Pharmacother* 1998;32:51–55.
36. Sokol DK, Dahlmann A, Dunn DW. Hyaluronidase treatment for intravenous phenytoin extravasation. *J Child Neurol* 1998;13(5):246–247.
37. Comas D, Mateu J. Treatment of extravasation of both doxorubicin and vincristine administration in a Y-site infusion. *Ann Pharmacother* 1996;30:244–246.
38. Bertelli G, Gozza A, Forno GB, et al. Topical dimethylsulfoxide for the prevention of soft tissue injury after extravasation of vesicant cytotoxic drugs: a prospective clinical study. *J Clin Oncol* 1995;13(11):2851–2855.
39. Chen JL, O'Shea M. Extravasation injury associated with low-dose dopamine. *Ann Pharmacother* 1998;32:545–548.
40. Tjon JA, Ansani NT. Transdermal nitroglycerin for the prevention of intravenous infusion failure due to phlebitis and extravasation. *Ann Pharmacother* 2000;34:1189–1192.
41. Malesker MA, Malone PM, Cingle CM, et al. Extravasation of I.V. promethazine. *Am J Health Syst Pharm* 1999;56:1742–1743.
42. Shamseddine AI, Khalil AM, Kibbi AG, et al. Granulocyte macrophage-colony stimulating factor for treatment of chemotherapy extravasation. *Eur J Gynaecol Oncol* 1998;19(5):479–481.
43. Ulutin HC, Guden M, Dede M, et al. Comparison of granulocyte-colony stimulating factor and granulocyte macrophage-colony stimulating factor in the treatment of chemotherapy extravasation ulcers. *Eur J Gynaecol Oncol* 2000;21(6):613–615.
44. Falcone PA, Barrall DT, Jeyarajah DR, et al. Nonoperative management of full-thickness intravenous extravasation injuries in premature neonates using enzymatic debridement. *Ann Plast Surg* 1989;22(2):146–149.

CHAPTER 17

Acute Liver Failure

Richard C. Dart and Lisa M. Forman

OVERVIEW

The medical toxicologist may be asked to evaluate the patient with acute liver injury. In some cases, the clinical issue is the cause of marked serum aminotransferase elevation followed by hepatic failure. In other cases, the etiology of hepatic injury is clear and the clinical concern is the appropriate management of hepatic failure and the optimal time to consider liver transplant.

Acute liver failure (ALF) is defined as the rapid onset of severe hepatic dysfunction, typically over a period of less than 6 months. There are approximately 2000 causes of ALF annually in the United States; many end in death or liver transplantation. The diagnosis is made based on clinical findings and biochemical data. The term *fulminant liver failure* is used to describe ALF with hepatic encephalopathy occurring within 8 weeks of the onset of symptoms in patients without previous history of liver disease. When the onset of encephalopathy occurs more than 8 weeks but less than 6 months after the first symptoms of liver disease, the term *subfulminant* liver failure is used.

A new classification scheme has been proposed based on the time to development of encephalopathy from the onset of jaundice: hyper-ALF, with an onset of encephalopathy of 7 days; ALF, with encephalopathy occurring in less than 28 days; and sub-ALF, with the onset of encephalopathy of less than 3 months (1).

PATHOPHYSIOLOGY

Liver toxins injure the liver through a variety of mechanisms. Direct hepatotoxins themselves injure the hepatocyte by lipid peroxidation, protein arylation, or other mechanisms. Indirect hepatotoxins interfere with metabolic or nutritional pathways that support the liver. Finally, idiosyncratic hepatotoxins (hypersensitivity reactions) cause injury in susceptible individuals.

The fundamental unit of concern in ALF is the hepatocyte. Death of a hepatocyte allows release of cell contents, including the aminotransferase enzymes. When a sufficient portion of the liver is injured, the liver becomes incapable of maintaining normal functions, and the clinical consequences of hepatic failure develop: hypoglycemia, coagulation abnormalities, and jaundice.

The liver parenchyma contains three zones: zone 1 (periportal) has the highest oxygen tension, whereas zone 3 (centrilobular, centrozonal) has the highest concentration of cytochrome P-450 enzymes and the lowest oxygen tension. Zone 2 (midzonal) is intermediate between these zones. Zone 3 is most susceptible to injury from hypoxia and drug metabolites.

DIAGNOSIS

Differential Diagnosis

Worldwide, the most common cause of ALF is viral hepatitis; however, in nations with modern health prevention programs, acetaminophen (paracetamol) is an important cause. The evaluation of aminotransferase enzyme elevation generates a large differential diagnosis (Table 1), particularly in the patient with ALF without known etiology (e.g., no history of an overdose). See individual chapters for more information on specific toxins.

History

The history is a crucial, but problematic, component of determining the cause of acute liver injury. In many cases, a careful history suggests the cause of hepatic injury. Several aspects deserve direct inquiry: over-the-counter medications, illicit drugs, alternative medical treatments, herbal medications, and recent travel should be specifically asked. There are many pitfalls in the history. For example, a past medical history of viral hepatitis, with the possible exception of hepatitis B, is unlikely to explain a more recent and marked elevation of aminotransferase enzymes. A new process should be suspected. Acetaminophen or ibuprofen is used by 23% and 16%, respectively, of American adults in a given week; therefore, a patient with any cause of liver failure may well have a positive acetaminophen level or history of ibuprofen ingestion on presentation. Unless a history of overdose is present, these patients should receive a thorough diagnostic evaluation.

Signs and Symptoms

Hepatic failure results in multiorgan injury. The clinical presentation is dominated in the early course by nonspecific manifestations: malaise, nausea and vomiting, weakness and headache. Right upper quadrant abdominal pain is often present. Tachycardia and hypotension are common due to decreased peripheral resistance. Jaundice is usually present. Encephalopathy may first manifest as confusion or agitation but progresses to generalized depression of the central nervous system. In severe cases, the syndrome is indistinguishable from late septic shock. Seizures or bleeding may complicate the course. Renal failure, hypoglycemia, and acid-base disturbances are common. Ascites and lower extremity edema are usually not present because of the rapid evolution of this condition.

The physical examination may help in determining etiology. A large tender liver suggests hepatic vein thrombosis or malignancy. Kayser-Fleisher rings may be present in Wilson's disease. Spider telangiectasias and gynecomastia suggest chronic liver disease.

Diagnostic Tests

DETERMINING ETIOLOGY

A complete panel of tests for viral hepatitis should be performed: hepatitis A virus, immunoglobulin M, hepatitis B surface antigen, and hepatitis B anticore immunoglobulin M serologies. Hepatitis C virus antibody testing may be negative for several weeks or months after acute infection. Repeat testing may be necessary, but acute hepatitis C virus is a very uncommon cause of fulminant hepatic failure (FHF). If hepatitis C virus is suspected, obtain hepatitis C viral load testing. Other viral studies such as cytomegalovirus, herpes simplex virus, or influenza A may be helpful in the posttransplant setting or when patients are otherwise immunosuppressed. Autoimmune markers such as antinuclear antibody, anti–smooth muscle antibody, and a ceruloplasmin level should be obtained.

By definition, the serum aminotransferases and bilirubin should be increased in ALF. The serum alkaline phosphatase may be increased or normal. An acetaminophen level should be obtained and the results interpreted appropriately, depending on the type of acetaminophen ingestion (Chapter 126). A very high acetaminophen level or a positive level in the presence of known overdose is useful; however, other diagnoses should be considered, especially in patients with minimally elevated acetaminophen levels. Specific drug screening or quantitative levels of known hepatotoxins should be considered (Table 1). Referral clinical laboratories may be able to test for suspected agents.

If the cause of liver failure is not apparent after initial evaluation, ultrasound can establish the patency and flow in the hepatic vein (to exclude Budd-Chiari syndrome), hepatic artery, and the portal vein. Computed tomography or magnetic resonance imaging of the abdomen can define hepatic anatomy and help the clinician exclude other intraabdominal processes. Head computed tomography helps identify cerebral edema and exclude intracranial mass (e.g., hematoma) that may mimic edema from FHF.

Liver biopsy can narrow the diagnosis but may be contraindicated due to coagulopathy. It is rarely of clinical use during the management of ALF. A hepatologist is often helpful in establishing the diagnosis, but up to 20% of all cases of ALF remain unidentified.

TESTS TO GUIDE PATIENT MANAGEMENT

Serum electrolytes and renal function tests are used to detect and guide treatment of complications of liver failure, such as hepatorenal syndrome. Monitoring of the glucose level is important because of glycogen depletion and impaired gluconeogenesis. Serum phosphate may be low and require supplementation. The blood count may show thrombocytopenia, a common complication of ALF. Blood, urine, and other cultures are used to monitor for the common complication of sepsis.

Coagulation studies serve as a marker of liver synthetic function and help to assess prognosis. The prothrombin time or international normalized ratio should be elevated and may become markedly prolonged. Individual coagulation factors become depleted, but this information is not typically used to manage patients. Factor V levels have been proposed as a prognostic indicator (2).

Serial evaluation of acid-base status helps determine prognosis and guides immediate management. In addition, these tests can help estimate the need for liver transplantation (Table 2). The serum lactate is usually elevated due to the combination of inadequate tissue perfusion and decreased clearance by the liver. The serum ammonia level is usually elevated in patients with encephalopathy, but is not reliable and its use is discouraged. An electroencephalogram should be considered to exclude clinically inapparent seizures in comatose patients.

POTENTIAL COMPLICATIONS

The most feared complications of liver failure are hepatic encephalopathy, hepatorenal syndrome, and sepsis. Each greatly reduces prospects for survival. Gastrointestinal bleeding is also common.

MANAGEMENT

General

The principles of management include treatment of the underlying cause and meticulous supportive care. Survival depends on the rapid institution of aggressive medical care. Identification of disease severity is important, and early referral to a transplant center is critical. Endotracheal intubation, hemodialysis, and other invasive procedures are often needed (Table 3). Hypotension is caused by peripheral vasodilation and treated by increasing circulating volume with crystalloid. Some centers use colloid, particularly nonalbumin solutions, but there are no comparative data in ALF and concerns about colloid solutions exist (3,4). If fluid administration is insufficient, norepinephrine may be preferred to dopamine owing to concerns about reduced splanchnic circulation (3).

HEPATOCYTE NECROSIS

Treatment of hepatocyte necrosis depends on the underlying cause. Infectious causes are not addressed in this chapter. Drug causes are often treated with *N*-acetylcysteine, especially in the case of drugs that are metabolized to electrophilic compounds such as acetaminophen (Chapter 64). A randomized trial has demonstrated improved survival in FHF treated with *N*-acetylcysteine. A study of the safety and efficacy of *N*-acetylcysteine in the treatment of ALF not caused by acetaminophen is currently under way.

INCREASED INTRACRANIAL PRESSURE

Increased intracranial pressure due to cerebral edema is a common complication. The use of intracranial pressure monitoring of patients with stage 3 or 4 coma has been recommended but has not been rigorously tested. Determination of cerebral edema can be difficult as computed tomography scans are often nega-

TABLE 1. Selected medications and diseases associated with acutely elevated liver aminotransferases (aspartate aminotransferase or alanine aminotransferase) more than 500 IU/L

Agent	Histopathology remarks	Reference
Infectious hepatitis		
Adenovirus		
Cytomegalovirus	Microvesicular	Duchini et al. (11)
Hepatitis A (acute hepatitis A virus leads to FHF in 0.35%)		
Hepatitis B (approximately 1% of patients go to FHF)		
Hepatitis C		
Hepatitis D (coinfection or superinfection with hepatitis B virus)		
Hemorrhagic fever viruses		
Hepatitis E		
Herpes simplex virus		
Influenza A		Clavell et al. (12)
Paramyxovirus		
Epstein-Barr virus		
Coxsackievirus		
Psittacosis		
Ischemic hepatitis	Zones 2 and 3 necrosis	Seeto et al. (13)
Drugs and chemicals		
Acetaminophen	Zone 3 necrosis, zones 2 and 3 in more severe cases	Smilkstein et al. (14)
Allopurinol	Zone 3 necrosis, zones 2 and 3 in more severe cases	Al-Kawas et al. (15)
Amatoxin (*Amanita phalloides*, other mushrooms)	Zone 3 necrosis	Lampe et al. (16)
Antiretroviral agents		
Inhaled anesthetics (enflurane, halothane, methoxyflurane)		Njoku et al. (17)
Budesonide	Ceroid macrophages	Segir et al. (18)
Bupropion	Zone 1 lymphocytic infiltrate	Hu et al. (19)
Carbamazepine	Zone 3	Hopen et al. (20)
Cetirizine	Zone 3 reticulin collapse, ceroid macrophages	Sanchez-Lombrana et al. (21)
Chlordiazepoxide	Zones 2 and 3	Pickering (22)
Chlortetracycline		Bateman et al. (23)
Clarithromycin	Not reported	Masia et al. (24)
Clindamycin	Zones 2 and 3	Elmore et al. (25)
Chlorazepate (Tranxene)	Zones 2 and 3	Parker (26)
Chlorinated hydrocarbons (e.g., carbon tetrachloride)	Zone 3 necrosis, zones 2 and 3 in more severe cases	Nehoda et al. (27)
Chlorzoxazone		Powers et al. (28)
Clove oil		Hartnoll et al. (29)
Cocaine		Silva et al. (30)
Dacarbazine	Zone 2	Greenstone et al. (31)
Dantrolene	Zones 2 and 3	Utili et al. (32)
Donepezil	Zone 1 eosinophilic infiltrates	Verrico et al. (33)
Ecstasy		Henry et al. (34)
Erythromycin		Gholson et al. (35)
Ethionamide	Zones 2 and 3	Pattyn et al. (36)
Felbamate		Pellock (37)
Fluconazole	Not reported	Crerar-Gilbert et al. (38)
Fluoroquinolone antibiotics (ciprofloxacin, gatifloxacin, trovafloxacin)	Eosinophilic infiltrates	Hennan et al. (39)
Glaphenine	Zone 3 necrosis, massive necrosis, steatosis, cholestasis	Stricker et al. (40)
HMG-CoA reductase inhibitors (atorvastatin, simvastatin)	Zone 1 necrosis and eosinophilic infiltration	Nakad et al. (41)
Indomethacin	Zones 2 and 3	Kelsey et al. (42)
Isoniazid	Zones 2 and 3, submassive or massive	Pessayre et al. (43)
Kava	Zones 2 and 3 with inflammatory infiltrate	Campo et al. (44)
Lamotrigine	Mild eosinophilic portal inflammation	Sauve et al. (45)
LipoKinetix	Not reported	Favreau et al. (46)
Mefloquine	Hepatic steatosis	Gotsman et al. (47)
Metals (salts of arsenic, copper, iron, thallium)		Whitten et al. (48)
Methyldopa	Zones 2 and 3	Rehman et al. (49)
Mercaptopurine	Zones 2 and 3	Popper et al. (50)
Methamphetamine	Zones 2 and 3	Kamijo et al. (51)
Oxacillin	Zone 1	Al-Homaidhi et al. (52)
Nefazodone		Stewart (53)
Nitrofurantoin	"Necrotic hepatic tissue with mononuclear cell infiltrates"	Edoute et al. (54)
Nonsteroidal antiinflammatory agents (aspirin, bromfenac, diclofenac, ibuprofen, sulindac)		Riley et al. (55)
Nonsteroidal antiinflammatory drug–COX 2 inhibitors (celecoxib)	Unknown	Nachimuthu et al. (56)
Paroxetine	Mild zone 3 inflammation	Odeh et al. (57)
Perphenazine	Zones 1, 2, and 3	Popper et al. (50)
Phenprocoumon	Zones 2 and 3	Hinrichsen (58)
Phenobarbital	Zones 2 and 3	Mockli et al. (59)
Phenylbutazone	Zones 1, 2, and 3	Benjamin (60)
Phenytoin	Zones 2 and 3	Brown et al. (61)
Phosphorus, yellow	Zone 1 necrosis	Kelkar et al. (62)
Potassium permanganate		Young et al. (63)
Prochlorperazine	Zones 1, 2, and 3	McFarland (64)
Propylthiouracil	Zones 1, 2, and 3	Mihas et al. (65)
Protease inhibitors		Vergis et al. (66)
Quinidine	Zones 1 and 2	Koch et al. (67)
Ranitidine	Confluent bridging necrosis	Ribeiro et al. (68)
Rifampin	Zones 1 and 2	Pessayre et al. (43)
Sulfadiazine	Zones 1, 2, and 3	Herbut et al. (69)
Sulfamethoxazole	Zones 1, 2, and 3	Ransohoff et al. (70)
Sulfasalazine	Zones 1, 2, and 3	Sotolongo et al. (71)
Terbinafine	Zone 1	Gupta et al. (72)
Thalidomide	Not reported	Fowler et al. (73)
Topiramate	Unknown	Doan et al. (74)
Tricyclic antidepressants (amitriptyline, imipramine)		Danan et al. (75)
Trazodone	Zone 3	Fernandes et al. (76)
Troglitazone		Gitlin et al. (77)
Valproic acid	Zones 1, 2, and 3	Dreifuss et al. (78)
Zafirlukast	Submassive hepatic necrosis with eosinophils	Reinus et al. (79)

FHF, fulminant hepatic failure; HMG-CoA, 3-hydroxy-3-methylglutaryl-coenzyme A.

TABLE 2. Indications for liver transplantation in patients with acute liver failure

King's College criteria [Bernal et al. (3)]	
Acetaminophen induced	**All other causes**
pH <7.3 after fluid resuscitation	INR >7
Or	Or
All of the following	One of the following
INR >7	INR >3.5
Serum creatinine >3.4 mg/dl (300 μmol/L)	Age younger than 10 or older than 40 years
Encephalopathy grade 3 or above	Jaundice to encephalopathy >7 d
	Serum bilirubin >300 μmol/L
	Non–hepatitis A–E; halothane hepatitis, drug reaction

Clichy and Brousse criteria [Bismuth et al. (80)]
Age younger than 30 yr
Factor V <20% and encephalopathy stage 3 or 4
Or
Age older than 30 yr
Factor V <30%

INR, international normalized ratio.

tive. Treatment consists of hyperventilation to decrease intracranial blood volume and mannitol to decrease brain volume. Mannitol at 0.5 to 1.0 g/kg effectively decreases intracranial pressure but is contraindicated in renal failure (5). Other interventions include barbiturates and hypothermia. Hyperthermia and hyperstimulation should be avoided.

RENAL FAILURE

Renal failure occurs in approximately 50% of patients with ALF (6). Hemodialysis is an effective maintenance measure but may significantly lower the arterial pressure and compromise cerebral perfusion. Continuous arteriovenous hemofiltration may be preferable.

INFECTION

Bacterial infection occurs in 80% of patients with ALF; gram-positive organisms predominate, with *Staphylococcus* and *Streptococcus* being the most common (7). Fungemia is also common, occurring in up to 33%, and portends a grim prognosis (8). One should have a low threshold for culturing (urine, sputum, blood) patients and starting empiric antibiotics.

COAGULOPATHY

The treatment of coagulopathy arising from liver failure is controversial. The international normalized ratio is very useful in determining the progression of ALF; therefore, it should not be corrected in the absence of active bleeding or before an invasive procedure.

ELECTROLYTE ABNORMALITIES

Electrolyte abnormalities (hypokalemia, hypomagnesemia, hypophosphatemia) are monitored and replaced as needed. *Nutritional supplementation* may be needed. Large amounts of glucose may be needed. Protein restriction was once used but is no longer recommended.

SPECIALIST CONSULTATION

It is crucial to contact the liver specialty unit or transplantation unit when the patient approaches the transplantation criteria (Tables 2 and 3). Full or partial liver transplantation is the definitive treatment. Transplantation of healthy donor hepatocytes is promising in animal studies but is not yet available for humans.

ARTIFICIAL LIVER SUPPORT

Several types of extracorporeal hepatocyte liver-assist systems have been proposed to provide metabolic assistance to patients with ALF. The devices differ in source of hepatocyte, storage of hepatocyte, membrane type, and therapy duration. They are currently in the initial phase of clinical evaluation. They can improve biochemical indices but have not been shown to improve outcome. A multicenter randomized trial is under way.

Prognosis

Before liver transplantation, the overall prognosis in ALF was grim with a mortality rate as high as 80%. The cause of liver failure can predict survival with a much better survival rate for acute hepatic A and acetaminophen (9). Disease duration is important also; patients with a protracted course are unlikely to spontaneously recover. The overall 1-, 3-, and 5-year patient sur-

TABLE 3. Overview of the management of acute liver failure

Condition	Monitoring	Intervention	Comments
Respiratory depression	Pulse oximetry or arterial blood gas	Endotracheal intubation	—
Electrolyte abnormalities or hypoglycemia	Serum panel monitoring	Supplement as for other causes (e.g., D10W infusion, potassium infusion)	—
Coagulopathy	Factor V levels, INR	—	Do not give FFP unless actively bleeding or before invasive procedures
Encephalopathy	—	Lactulose	Rule out sepsis, gastrointestinal bleed, electrolyte disturbances, and so forth
Cerebral edema	Intracranial pressure monitoring	Elevation of head of bed, hyperventilation, mannitol, fluid restriction, avoid overstimulation	Low threshold for head computed tomography
Sepsis	—	Pancultured Broad spectrum antibiotics Consider empiric antifungal agents	—
Nutritional supplementation	—	Nutritional supplementation	No indication for protein restriction
Renal failure	—	Hemodialysis	Rule out hypovolemia

D10W, dextrose 10% in water; FFP, fresh frozen plasma; INR, international normalized ratio.

vival after liver transplantation is currently estimated at 83.7%, 76.6%, and 66.4%, respectively (10).

PITFALLS

Liver failure is a complex disease with numerous opportunities for misdiagnosis. Do not assume that the first plausible cause uncovered is the true cause of ALF.

REFERENCES

1. O'Grady JG, Shalm SW, Williams R. Acute liver failure: redefining the syndromes. *Lancet* 1993;342:273–275.
2. Izumi S, Langley PG, Wendon J, et al. Coagulation factor V levels as a prognostic indicator in fulminant hepatic failure. *Hepatology* 1996;23:1507–1511.
3. Bernal W, Wendon J. Acute liver failure: clinical features and management. *Gastroenterol Hepatol* 1999;11:977–984.
4. Schierhout G, Roberts I. Fluid resuscitation with colloid or crystalloid solution in critically ill patients: a systematic review of clinical trials. *BMJ* 1998;316:961–964.
5. Canalese J, Gimson A, Davis C, et al. Controlled trial of dexamethasone and mannitol for the cerebral edema of fulminant hepatic failure. *Gut* 1982;23:625–629.
6. Ring-Larsen H, Palazzo U. Renal failure in fulminant hepatic failure and terminal cirrhosis: a comparison between incidence, types, and prognosis. *Gut* 1981;22:585–591.
7. Rolando N, Harvey F, Brahm J, et al. Prospective study of bacterial infection in acute liver failure: an analysis of fifty patients. *Hepatology* 1990;11:49–50.
8. Rolando N, Harvey F, Brahm J, et al. Fungal infection: a common, unrecognized complication of acute liver failure. *J Hepatol* 1991;12:1–9.
9. Williams R. Classification, etiology and considerations of outcome in acute liver failure. *Semin Liver Dis* 1996;16:343–348.
10. *2000 Annual Report of the U.S. Scientific Registry of Transplant Recipients and the Organ Procurement and Transplantation Network: Transplant Data 1989–1998.* Rockville, MD, and Richmond, VA: Health and Human Services/Health Resources and Services Administration/Office of Special Programs/Division of Transplantation and United Network for Organ Sharing, February 16, 2001. Available at: http://www.unos.org/. Accessed October 28, 2002.
11. Duchini A, Viernes E, Nyberg LM, et al. Hepatic decompensation in patients with cirrhosis during infection with influenza A. *Arch Intern Med* 2000;113–115.
12. Clavell M, Barkemeyer B, Martinez B, et al. Severe hepatitis in a newborn with coxsackievirus B5 infection. *Clin Pediatr* 1999;38:739–741.
13. Seeto RK, Fenn B, Rockey DC. Ischemic hepatitis: clinical presentation and pathogenesis. *Am J Med* 2000;109:109–113.
14. Smilkstein MJ, Knapp GL, Kulig KW, et al. Efficacy of oral *N*-acetylcysteine in the treatment of acetaminophen overdose. Analysis of the National Multicenter study (1976 to 1985). *N Engl J Med* 1988;319:1557–1562.
15. Al-Kawas FH, Seeff LB, Berendson RA, et al. Allopurinol hepatotoxicity. Report of two cases and review of the literature. *Ann Intern Med* 1981;95:588–590.
16. Lampe KF, McCann MA. Differential diagnosis of poisoning by North American mushrooms, with particular emphasis on *Amanita phalloides*–like intoxication. *Ann Emerg Med* 1987;16:956–962.
17. Njoku D, Laster MJ, Gong DH, et al. Biotransformation of halothane, enflurane, isoflurane, and desflurane to trifluoroacetylated liver proteins: association between protein acylation and hepatic injury. *Anesth Analg* 1997;84(1):173–178.
18. Segir A, Wettstein M, Oette M, et al. Budesonide-induced acute hepatitis in an HIV-positive patient with ritonavir as a co-medication. *AIDS* 2002;16:1191–1192.
19. Hu K-Q, Tiyyagura L, Kanel G, et al. Acute hepatitis induced by bupropion. *Dig Dis Sci* 2000;45:1872–1873.
20. Hopen G, Nesthus I, Laerum OD. Fatal carbamazepine-associated hepatitis. Report of two cases. *Acta Med Scand* 1981;210:333–335.
21. Sanchez-Lombrana JL, Alvarez RP, Saez LR, et al. Acute hepatitis associated with use of cetirizine intake. *J Clin Gastroenterol* 2002;34:493–495.
22. Pickering P. Hepatic necrosis after chlordiazepoxide therapy. *N Engl J Med* 1966;274:1449.
23. Bateman JC, Barberio Jr, Cromer JK, et al. Investigation of mechanism and type of jaundice produced by large doses of parenterally administered Aureomycin. *Antibiot Chemother* 1953;3:1–15.
24. Masia M, Gutierrez F, Jimeno J, et al. Fulminant hepatitis and fatal toxic epidermal necrolysis (Lyell disease) coincident with clarithromycin administration in an alcoholic patient receiving disulfiram therapy. *Arch Intern Med* 2002;162:474–476.
25. Elmore M, Rissing JP, Rink L, et al. Clindamycin-associated hepatotoxicity. *Am J Med* 1974;57:627–630.
26. Parker JLW. Potassium clorazepate (Tranxene) induced jaundice. *Postgrad Med J* 1979;55:908–910.
27. Nehoda H, Wieser K, Koller J, et al. Recurrent liver failure with severe rhabdomyolysis after liver transplantation for carbon tetrachloride intoxication. *Hepatogastroenterology* 1998;45:191–195.
28. Powers BJ, Cattau EL Jr, Zimmerman HJ. Chlorzoxazone hepatotoxic reactions. *Arch Intern Med* 1986;146:1183–1186.
29. Hartnoll G, Moore D, Douek D. Near fatal ingestion of oil of cloves. *Arch Dis Child* 1993;69:392–393.
30. Silva MO, Roth D, Reddy KR, et al. Hepatic dysfunction accompanying acute cocaine intoxication. *J Hepatol* 1991;12:312–315.
31. Greenstone MA, Dowd PM, Mikhailidis DP, et al. Hepatic vascular lesions associated with dacarbazine treatment. *Br Med J (Clin Res Ed)* 1981;282 (6278):1744–1745.
32. Utili R, Boitnott JK, Zimmerman HJ. Dantrolene-associated hepatic injury. Incidence and character. *Gastroenterology* 1977;72(4 Pt 1):610–616.
33. Verrico MM, Nace DA, Towers AL. Fulminant chemical hepatitis possible associated with donepezil and sertraline therapy. *J Am Geriatr Soc* 2000;48:1659–1663.
34. Henry JA, Jeffreys KJ, Dawling S. Toxicity and deaths from 3,4-methylenedioxymethamphetamine ("ecstasy"). *Lancet* 1992;340:384–387.
35. Gholson CF, Warren GH. Fulminant hepatic failure associated with intravenous erythromycin lactobionate. *Arch Intern Med* 1990;150:215–216.
36. Pattyn SR, Janssens L, Bourland J, et al. Hepatotoxicity of the combination of rifampin-ethionamide in the treatment of multibacillary leprosy. *Intern J Leprosy & Other Mycobacterial Dis* 1984;52:1–6.
37. Pellock JM. Felbamate in epilepsy therapy. Evaluating the risks. *Drug Safety* 1999;21:225–239.
38. Crerar-Gilbert A, Boots R, Fraenkel D, et al. Survival following fulminant hepatic failure from fluconazole induced hepatitis. *Anaesth Intensive Care* 1999;27:650–652.
39. Hennan NE, Zambie MF. Gatifloxacin-associated acute hepatitis. *Pharmacotherapy* 2001;21:1579–1582.
40. Stricker BHC, Blok APR, Bronkhorst FB. Glaphenine-associated hepatic injury. *Liver* 1986;5:63–72.
41. Nakad A, Bataille L, Hamoir V, et al. Atorvastatin-induced acute hepatitis with absence of cross-toxicity with simvastatin. *Lancet* 1999;353:1763–1764.
42. Kelsey W, Scharyj M. Fatal hepatitis probably due to indomethacin. *JAMA* 1967;199:586–587.
43. Pessayre D, Bentata M, Degott C, et al. Isoniazid-rifampin fulminant hepatitis. A possible consequence of the enhancement of isoniazid hepatotoxicity by enzyme induction. *Gastroenterology* 1977;72:284–289.
44. Campo JV, McNabb J, Perel JM, et al. Kava-induced fulminant hepatic failure. *J Am Acad Child Adolesc Psychiatry* 2002;41:631–632.
45. Sauve G, Bresson-Hadni S, Prost P, et al. Acute hepatitis after lamotrigine administration. *Dig Dis Sci* 2000;45:1874–1877.
46. Favreau JT, Ryu ML, Braunstein G, et al. Severe hepatotoxicity associated with the dietary supplement LipoKinetix. *Ann Intern Med* 2002;136:590–595.
47. Gotsman I, Azaz-Livshits T, Fridlender Z, et al. Mefloquine-induced acute hepatitis. *Pharmacotherapy* 2000;20:1517–1519.
48. Whitten CF, Brough AJ. The pathophysiology of acute iron poisoning. *Clin Toxicol* 1971;4:585–595.
49. Rehman OU, Keith TA, Gall EA. Methyldopa-induced submassive hepatic necrosis. *JAMA* 1973;224:1390–1392.
50. Popper H, Rubin E, Gardiol D, et al. Drug-induced liver disease. A penalty for progress. *Arch Intern Med* 1965;115:128–136.
51. Kamijo Y, Soma K, Nishida M, et al. Acute liver failure following intravenous methamphetamine. *Vet Hum Toxicol* 2002;44:216–217.
52. Al-Homaidhi H, Abdel-Haq NM, El-Baba M, et al. Severe hepatitis associated with oxacillin therapy. *South Med J* 2002;95:650–652.
53. Stewart DE. Hepatic adverse reactions associated with nefazodone. *Can J Psychiatry* 2002;47:375–377.
54. Edoute Y, Karmon Y, Roguin A, et al. Fatal liver necrosis associated with the use of nitrofurantoin. *IMAJ* 2001;3:382–383.
55. Riley TR, Smith JP. Ibuprofen-induced hepatotoxicity in patients with chronic hepatitis C: a case series. *Am J Gastroenterol* 1998;93:1563–1565.
56. Nachimuthu S, Volfinzon L, Gopal L. Acute hepatocellular and cholestatic injury in a patient taking celecoxib. *Postgrad Med J* 2001;77:548–550.
57. Odeh M, Misselevech I, Boss JH, et al. Severe hepatotoxicity with jaundice associated with paroxetine. *Am J Gastroenterol* 2001;96:2494–2496.
58. Hinrichsen H, Luttges J, Kloppel G, et al. Idiosyncratic drug allergic phenprocoumon-induced hepatitis with subacute liver failure initially misdiagnosed as autoimmune hepatitis. *Gastroenterology* 2001;36:780–783.
59. Mockli G, Crowley M, Stern R, et al. Massive hepatic necrosis in a child after administration of phenobarbital. *Am J Gastroenterol* 1989;4:820–822.
60. Benjamin SB, Ishak KG, Zimmerman HJ, et al. Phenylbutazone liver injury: a clinical-pathologic survey of 23 cases and review of the literature. *Hepatology* 1981;1:255–263.
61. Brown M, Schubert T. Phenytoin hypersensitivity hepatitis and mononucleosis syndrome. *J Clin Gastroenterol* 1986;8:469–477.
62. Kelkar EJ, Gandhi W. Yellow phosphorus poisoning—an unusual presentation. *J Assoc Phys India* 1995;43:371–372.
63. Young RJ, Critchley JAJH, Young KK, et al. Fatal acute hepatorenal failure following potassium permanganate ingestion. *Hum Exp Toxicol* 1996;15(3):259–261.
64. McFarland RB. Fatal drug reaction associated with prochlorperazine (Compazine). *Am J Clin Pathol* 1963;40:284–290.
65. Mihas AA, Holley P, Koff RS, et al. Fulminant hepatitis and lymphocyte sensitization due to propylthiouracil. *Gastroenterology* 1976;70:770–774.

66. Vergis E, Paterson DL, Singh N. Indinavir-associated hepatitis in patients with advanced HIV infection. *Int J STD AIDS* 1998;9:53.
67. Koch MJ, Seeff LB, Crumley CE, et al. Quinidine hepatotoxicity. A report of a case and review of the literature. *Gastroenterology* 1976;70:1136–1140.
68. Ribeiro JM, Lucas M, Baptista A, et al. Fatal hepatitis associated with ranitidine. *Am J Gastroenterol* 2000;95:559–560.
69. Herbut PA, Scaricaciottolo TM. Diffuse hepatic necrosis caused by sulfadiazine. *Arch Pathol* 1945;40:94–98.
70. Ransohoff DF, Jacobs G. Terminal hepatic failure following a small dose of sulfamethoxazole-trimethoprim. *Gastroenterology* 1981;80:816–819.
71. Sotolongo RP, Neefe LI, Rudzki C, et al. Hypersensitivity reaction to sulfasalazine with severe hepatotoxicity. *Gastroenterology* 1978;75:95–99.
72. Gupta AK, del Rosso JQ, Lynde CW, et al. Hepatitis associated with terbinafine therapy: three case reports and a review of the literature. *Clin Exp Dermatol* 1998;23:64–67.
73. Fowler R, Imrie K. Thalidomide-associated hepatitis: a case report. *Am J Hematol* 2001;66:300–302.
74. Doan RJ, Clendenning M. Topiramate and hepatotoxicity. *Can J Psychiatry* 2000;45:937–938.
75. Danan G, Bernuau J, Moullot X, et al. Amitriptyline-induced fulminant hepatitis. *Digestion* 1984;30:179–184.
76. Fernandes NF, Martin RR, Schenker S. Trazodone-induced hepatotoxicity: a case report. *Am J Gastroenterol* 2000;95:532–535.
77. Gitlin N, Julie NL, Spurr CL, et al. Two cases of severe clinical and histologic hepatotoxicity associated with troglitazone. *Ann Intern Med* 1998;129:36–38.
78. Dreifuss FE, Santilli N, Langer DH, et al. Valproic acid hepatic fatalities: a retrospective review. *Neurology* 1987;37:379–385.
79. Reinus JF, Persky S, Burkiewicz JS, et al. Severe liver injury after treatment with the leukotriene receptor antagonist zafirlukast. *Ann Intern Med* 2000;133:964–968.
80. Bismuth H, Samuel D, Castaing D, et al. Orthotopic liver transplantation in fulminant and subfulminant hepatitis. The Paul Brousse experience. *Ann Surg* 1995;222:109–119.

CHAPTER 18
Gulf War Syndrome

Daniel C. Keyes

OVERVIEW

After the 1990 Iraqi invasion of Kuwait, a coalition of soldiers from several countries was deployed to the Persian Gulf. Approximately 697,000 American soldiers, 45,000 British soldiers, and 4500 Canadian soldiers participated in the campaign (1). After a 39-day air war, ground troops advanced into Iraq over a 4-day period. The number of coalition force casualties was much lower than expected. Iraqi casualties were estimated at more than 85,000 killed and wounded (2–4).

After returning home, veterans from military units of the United States, Great Britain, and Canada reported various combinations of symptoms, including fatigue, insomnia, shortness of breath, headache, skin rashes, chest pain, myalgias, and arthralgias, which have been termed *Gulf War syndrome* (GWS) (5). One British survey found that approximately 17% of Gulf War veterans consider themselves to have GWS (6).

PATHOPHYSIOLOGY

Little agreement exists as to a discrete definition of a "Gulf War syndrome." Various etiologies considered for GWS include depleted uranium shrapnel from "friendly fire," sarin toxicity after the destruction of the Iraqi Kahmisiyah arsenal (7), and pretreatment with pyridostigmine.

Pyridostigmine was used in the Gulf War as a pretreatment to block the nerve agent soman. Soman permanently inactivates the enzyme acetylcholinesterase (AChE). Pyridostigmine is a medicinal carbamate that *reversibly* binds and inhibits AChE. If pyridostigmine is given before soman, it occupies the enzyme active site and prevents soman from binding the active site of AChE. Soman is subsequently cleared from the body, and pyridostigmine leaves AChE, restoring part of its function (8). In short, pyridostigmine "reserves" a portion of the enzyme for use after soman exposure has passed.

Pyridostigmine bromide, 30 mg orally, was self-administered every 8 hours by 41,650 soldiers while under threat of nerve agent attack for 1 to 7 days in January 1991 (9). Approximately one-half of these soldiers noted physiologic changes that were not incapacitating, including increased flatus, abdominal cramps, soft stools, and urinary urgency. Headaches, rhinorrhea, diaphoresis, and tingling of the extremities were occasionally observed. Less than 0.1% of soldiers discontinued the drug. A few experienced acute blood pressure elevation. Pyridostigmine therapy was discontinued for 28 soldiers, including three with exacerbated bronchitis, one asthmatic, two with allergic reactions, two hypertensive patients, and 20 with intolerable nausea and diarrhea (10).

There has been debate regarding the approach to research on GWS. Several groups have performed population surveys and in-person interviews with conflicting results (6,11–14). Some of these surveys have found no definable syndrome, whereas others have concluded that there is in fact an association with certain symptom complexes. Based on the latter, a group of investigators is now advocating for a new phase of clinical research to pursue the findings in surveys (15). Several theories of causation have been proposed, including the large number of inoculations soldiers received before deployment, the psychosocial stressors of the war, post-traumatic stress disorder, organophosphate nerve agent exposure, and pyridostigmine pretreatment strategies (16–18). Several national expert panels have considered the syndrome, including a Presidential Advisory Committee on Gulf War Veterans Illnesses, the Institute of Medicine, the Department of Defense, and the National Institutes of Health (19–21). These panels have not proposed causes of GWS.

Haley et al. used factor analysis and prospective validation techniques to conclude that an organic syndrome involving the nervous system is responsible for the clusters of symptoms experienced by the military personnel involved (5,12,22). They speculated that interactions between pyridostigmine bromide; flea collars (used by some soldiers); low-level chemical nerve agents (such as sarin); and the insect repellant diethyltoluamide may have acted together to cause the syndrome. Three syndromes were identified: "impaired cognition" (syndrome 1), "confusion-ataxia" (syndrome 2), and "central pain" (syndrome 3). The most severely ill subgroup was "confusion-ataxia" or Haley syndrome 2. This

TABLE 1. Differential diagnosis of the Gulf War syndrome

Chronic fatigue syndrome	Occult malignancy
Depression	Systemic lupus erythematosus
Fibromyalgia	Viscerotropic leishmaniasis
Hypokalemia	Irritable bowel syndrome
Hypothyroidism	Post-traumatic stress disorder
Infectious mononucleosis	Undiagnosed chronic infection
Myasthenia gravis	

group had consistently lower levels of paraoxonase-1 type Q arylesterase than others who carried the GWS diagnosis. Paraoxonase-1 type Q is a serum enzyme that hydrolyzes organophosphates such as sarin, soman, and diazinon. These patients did not have distinct pathologic lesions on magnetic resonance imaging. When researchers investigated using the more sensitive technique of magnetic resonance spectroscopy, however, group 2 had evidence of neuronal damage in the basal ganglia and pons (23). This line of research, although promising, has not yet resulted in specific therapeutic modalities for patients with illness related to GWS.

DIAGNOSIS

The diagnosis of GWS is largely undertaken by self-report and interview of Gulf War veterans who experience fatigue, vertigo, memory deficits, and other related problems. Due to the fact that there has not been a single case definition developed or an accepted etiology identified, many of these patients are apprehensive about their health status. Often these individuals exhibit some degree of depression and may have changes in weight or sleep disorders. The differential diagnosis of GWS remains broad (Table 1).

MANAGEMENT

Specific management of GWS is complicated and challenging. Veterans have struggled with a disease that is poorly understood and currently has no specific identity. Although the clinical neurologic research previously described is promising, it does not provide specific management opportunities at this time. Some authors have advocated an approach that centers on

TABLE 2. Recommendations for condition-specific treatments

Condition	Recommendations
Chronic fatigue syndrome	For Gulf War veterans who meet the criteria for diagnosis of chronic fatigue syndrome, the committee recommends Use of cognitive behavioral therapy and exercise therapies because they are likely to be beneficial. Monitoring the results of studies of the efficacy and effectiveness of NADH, dietary supplements, corticosteroids, and antidepressants other than SSRIs. Because immunotherapy and prolonged rest are unlikely to be beneficial, they should not be used as treatments. SSRIs are unlikely to be beneficial and are not recommended unless they are used as treatment for persons with concurrent major depression. Treatments effective for chronic fatigue syndrome should be evaluated in Gulf War veterans who meet the criteria for chronic fatigue syndrome.
Depression	The committee recommends a combination of antidepressant medication and psychotherapy (either cognitive behavioral therapy or interpersonal therapy) as the core therapy for major depression.
Fibromyalgia	The committee recommends that Gulf War veterans who meet criteria for fibromyalgia not receive treatment with opioid analgesics or glucocorticoids. In the absence of therapies of generally proven benefit, results of treatment studies of physical training, tricyclic antidepressants, and acupuncture should be further monitored in Gulf War veterans who meet the criteria for fibromyalgia.
Headache	For Gulf War veterans with chronic headaches not associated with underlying pathology (e.g., tumors, vascular abnormalities), the committee recommends the following treatments: Pharmacologic management of acute episodes, using clinical effectiveness and potential side effects, as listed. Prophylactic pharmacologic management for headaches that occur frequently or are disruptive to the patient's functioning, taking into consideration the clinical effectiveness and potential side effects. Use of behavioral and physical treatments, including relaxation training, thermal biofeedback combined with relaxation training, electromyogram biofeedback and cognitive behavioral therapy, or behavioral therapy combined with preventive drug therapy.
Irritable bowel syndrome	For Gulf War veterans who meet the diagnostic criteria for irritable bowel syndrome, the committee recommends that Cognitive behavioral therapy, tricyclic antidepressants, and smooth-muscle relaxants be considered in appropriate age-specific, carefully selected clinical settings. Results of treatment studies should be monitored to clearly establish therapeutic effectiveness of these agents in the various subgroups of patients diagnosed with irritable bowel syndrome.
Panic disorder	For Gulf War veterans who meet criteria for panic disorder, the committee recommends treatment with antidepressant medication and cognitive behavioral therapy.
Post-traumatic stress disorder	For Gulf War veterans who meet the criteria for post-traumatic stress disorder and with no contraindications, the committee recommends treatment with antidepressant medication and cognitive behavioral therapy.
Medically unexplained symptoms	For Gulf War veterans with unexplained symptoms, the committee recommends that For the purposes of treatment efficacy and effectiveness studies, explicit criteria for medically unexplained physical symptoms (apart from chronic fatigue syndrome, fibromyalgia, and irritable bowel syndrome) be developed and used uniformly in treatment studies. Treatment studies of antidepressant medications, cognitive behavioral therapy, and a stepped intensity-of-care program should be implemented for medically unexplained symptoms.

NADH, the reduced form of nicotinamide adenine dinucleotide; SSRI, selective serotonin reuptake inhibitor.
From Institute of Medicine Committee on Identifying Effective Treatments for Gulf War Veterans' Health Problems. *Gulf War veterans: treating symptoms and syndromes.* Washington, DC: National Academy Press, 2001, with permission.

care of the patient rather than "care of the disease" (20). It is argued that one facet of contemporary society is that a disease is not considered legitimate unless the etiology is clearly identified (24). Under this model, the patient should receive multifaceted treatment of symptoms, and it should be related to the patient that he or she has a legitimate illness.

The U.S. Department of Defense initiated a 3-week-long outpatient "Specialized Care Program" in 1994. Veterans were brought together in groups of three to eight patients with a goal of improving on disabling symptoms experienced by these individuals. The program focused on specific problems including fatigue, headaches, joint pain, skin rash, digestive problems, weight gain or weight loss, and memory problems. The approach taken was to focus on the "establishment of a trusting doctor-patient relationship, negotiations around a common ground of scientific and etiologic beliefs, nonlabeling of the disorder, and work toward recovery in the absence of clear etiologic answers" (25). One common aspect of the GWS is fatigue, and some writers have suggested that cognitive behavioral therapy may be useful; however, this has not been validated by clinical trials in this patient population (25).

If a specific neurochemical etiology is validated through ongoing research, specific therapies may become available in the future. It seems possible that diagnostic tests of specific paraoxonase-1 type Q will aid in the identification and treatment of a subgroup of GWS patients.

General approaches recommended by the Institute of Medicine are listed in Table 2 (26).

REFERENCES

1. Hyams KC, Wignall FS, Roswell R. War syndromes and their evaluation: from the U.S. Civil War to the Persian Gulf War. *Ann Intern Med* 1996;125(5):398–405.
2. Staff. The 1991 Gulf War's toll: quoting the Defense Department, Iraqi government and media reports. *USA Today World* 1996:Sept 3.
3. Defense Science Board. *Report of the Defense Science Board Task Force on Persian Gulf War health effects*. Washington, DC: Office of the Under Secretary of Defense for Acquisition and Technology, 1994.
4. Writer JV, DeFraites RF, Brundage JF. Comparative mortality among US military personnel in the Persian Gulf region and worldwide during Operations Desert Shield and Desert Storm. *JAMA* 1996;275(2):118–121.
5. Haley RW, Kurt TL, Hom J. Is there a Gulf War syndrome? Searching for syndromes by factor analysis of symptoms. *JAMA* 1997;277(3):215–222.
6. Chalder T, Hotopf M, Unwin C, et al. Prevalence of Gulf War veterans who believe they have Gulf War syndrome: questionnaire study. *BMJ* 2001;323(7311):473–476.
7. McCauley L, Lasarev M, Sticker D, et al. Illness experience of Gulf War veterans possibly exposed to chemical warfare agents. *Am J Prev Med* 2002;23(3):200.
8. Lennox WJ, Harris LW, Talbot BG, et al. Relationship between reversible acetylcholinesterase inhibition and efficacy against soman lethality. *Life Sci* 1985;37(9):793–798.
9. Sharabi Y, Danon YL, Berkenstadt H, et al. Survey of symptoms following intake of pyridostigmine during the Persian Gulf War. *Isr J Med Sci* 1991;27(11–12):656–658.
10. Keeler JR, Hurst CG, Dunn MA. Pyridostigmine used as a nerve agent pretreatment under wartime conditions. *JAMA* 1991;266(5):693–695.
11. Doebbeling BN, Clarke WR, Watson D, et al. Is there a Persian Gulf War syndrome? Evidence from a large population-based survey of veterans and nondeployed controls. *Am J Med* 2000;108(9):695–704.
12. Haley RW, Kurt TL. Self-reported exposure to neurotoxic chemical combinations in the Gulf War. A cross-sectional epidemiologic study. *JAMA* 1997;277(3):231–237.
13. Haley RW, Luk GD, Petty F. Use of structural equation modeling to test the construct validity of a case definition of Gulf War syndrome: invariance over developmental and validation samples, service branches and publicity. *Psychiatry Res* 2001;102(2):175–200.
14. Shapiro SE, Lasarev MR, McCauley L. Factor analysis of Gulf War illness: what does it add to our understanding of possible health effects of deployment? *Am J Epidemiol* 2002;156(6):578–585.
15. Haley RW. Will we solve the Gulf War syndrome puzzle by population surveys or clinical research? *Am J Med* 2000;109(9):744–748.
16. Rook GA, Zumla A. Gulf War syndrome: is it due to a systemic shift in cytokine balance towards a Th2 profile? *Lancet* 1997;349(9068):1831–1833.
17. Schumm WR, Reppert EJ, Jurich AP, et al. Pyridostigmine bromide and the long-term subjective health status of a sample of female reserve component Gulf War veterans: a brief report. *Psychol Rep* 2001;88(1):306–308.
18. Shaheen S. Shots in the desert and Gulf War syndrome. Evidence that multiple vaccinations during deployment are to blame is inconclusive. *BMJ* 2000;320(7246):1351–1352.
19. Joellenbeck LM, Hernandez LM. The Institute of Medicine's independent scientific assessment of Gulf War health issues. *Mil Med* 2002;167(3):186–190.
20. Mahoney DB. A normative construction of Gulf War syndrome. *Perspect Biol Med* 2001;44(4):575–583.
21. National Institutes of Health. The Persian Gulf experience and health. NIH Technology Assessment Workshop Panel. *JAMA* 1994;272(5):391–396.
22. Haley RW, Hom J, Roland PS, et al. Evaluation of neurologic function in Gulf War veterans. A blinded case-control study. *JAMA* 1997;277(3):223–230.
23. Haley RW, Marshall WW, McDonald GG, et al. Brain abnormalities in Gulf War syndrome: evaluation with 1H MR spectroscopy. *Radiology* 2000;215(3):807–817.
24. Rosenberg C, Golden J. *Framing disease: studies in cultural history*, 2nd ed. New Brunswick: Rutgers University Press, 1997.
25. Hodgson MJ, Kipen HM. Gulf War illnesses: causation and treatment. *J Occup Environ Med* 1999;41(6):443–452.
26. Committee on Identifying Effective Treatments for Gulf War Veterans' Health Problems. *Gulf War Veterans: treating symptoms and syndromes*. Washington, DC: National Academy Press, 2001.

CHAPTER 19

Hallucinations

Robert L. Stephen and E. Martin Caravati

OVERVIEW

Hallucinations are defined as perceptions that have no basis in external stimulation. In contrast, *illusions* are misperceptions of actual external stimuli and *delusions* are fixed, false beliefs. Hallucinations can occur in either medical (organic) or psychiatric (functional) conditions. Visual, tactile, and gustatory hallucinations are generally indicative of an organic disorder whereas gradual development of auditory hallucinations usually implies a psychiatric etiology. The rapid onset of hallucination over hours to days is more likely to be organic in nature. A toxin-induced delirium is usually associated with visual hallucinations and disorientation whereas a functional psychosis is characterized by the predominance of auditory hallucinations and normal cognition.

Hallucinations are poorly understood. Including all subtypes, the prevalence in the general (noninstitutionalized) population is up to 38.7% (1). Persons with a mental disorder are affected more often. Hypnagogic (occurring at the onset of sleep) and hypnopompic

TABLE 1. Nontoxicologic causes of hallucinations

Infectious
- Meningitis
- Encephalitis
- Sepsis
- Focal infection (e.g., pneumonia)
- Parasitic (malaria)

Metabolic
- Hypoglycemia
- Electrolyte disorder (hyponatremia, hypernatremia, hypoglycemia, hypocalcemia)
- Encephalopathy (hepatic, uremic, Wernicke's encephalopathy)
- Hereditary metabolic disease (e.g., porphyria, mitochondrial cytopathy)
- Endocrine (hypothyroidism, hyperthyroidism, adrenal disease)
- Hypoxia

Environmental
- Hyperthermia
- Hypothermia

Neurologic
- Structural (tumor)
- Temporal lobe epilepsy
- Vascular (intracranial bleed)
- Parkinson's disease

Rheumatologic
- Vasculitis (cerebral)

Psychiatric
- Sleep deprivation
- Schizophrenia
- Acute mania
- Depression
- Factitious

Drug withdrawal
- Ethanol
- Gamma hydroxybutyrate
- Benzodiazepines
- Baclofen [Peng et al. (9)]
- Venlafaxine [Parker et al. (10)]

(occurring on awakening) hallucinations are the most frequent and are generally not associated with any significant pathology. However, those that are persistently frightening are often associated with narcolepsy. Haptic (tactile) and gustatory hallucinations have been associated with the use of hypnotic medications.

Illicit "street drug" usage or withdrawal is a risk factor for all types of hallucinations, particularly tactile and visual. The most common hallucinations in those with psychotic disorders are auditory, haptic, and visual (1). In Parkinson's disease, up to 63% of patients exhibit hallucinations, predominantly visual, sometime during the course of the illness (2). This is thought to be secondary to the chronic pharmacologic therapy used to control symptoms in these patients (2,3).

PATHOPHYSIOLOGY

The pathophysiology of hallucinations is poorly described. Generally, it has been proposed that alterations in various neurotransmitters change the neuronal signal to noise ratio allowing normally extraneous sensory and intrinsic information, which is continuously present and actively processed at a subconscious level, to enter conscious awareness. This aberrant intrusion of unfiltered and unprocessed information into the conscious state results in confusion about reality and is manifested as hallucinations (4).

DIAGNOSIS

The *differential diagnosis* of hallucinations is vast and encompasses non–drug-related medical conditions as well as toxic exposures, drugs of abuse, plants, drug withdrawal syndromes, and idiosyncratic reactions to therapeutic doses of medications (Tables 1–4).

TABLE 2. Drug classes associated with hallucinations

Drug class	Comments	Reference
Sympathomimetic drugs (cocaine, methamphetamine, MDMA)	Overdose or abuse situations	
Anabolic steroids	Usually in abuse situations	
ACE inhibitors	With therapeutic use	
Anticholinergic agents, atropine	More common in elderly and pediatric patients; can occur with scopolamine skin patches and ophthalmic drops	Kortabarria et al. (11); Hamborg-Petersen et al. (12)
Tricyclic antidepressants	Anticholinergic effects can affect elderly; in overdose and acutely manic patients	
Barbiturates	Usually in withdrawal or pediatric and elderly patients	
Benzodiazepines	Either during treatment or withdrawal	
Beta-blockers	With either oral or ophthalmic preparations	Love et al. (13)
Dopamine receptor agonists	During treatment or on withdrawal; especially in elderly or parkinsonian patients	
Fluoroquinolones	With therapeutic use	
H_1 (histamine) blockers (first generation)	In overdose or the elderly	Jones et al. (14)
Inhalants: toluene	Intentional abuse	
Opioids	High doses; abuse; intrathecal morphine; elderly at high risk	
Procaine derivatives (penicillin G, procainamide)	Suspected due to the procaine	Downham et al. (15)
Salicylates	Usually with chronic intoxication more than acute	
Selective serotonin reuptake inhibitors	With therapeutic use or in overdose (serotonin syndrome)	
Sulfonamides	With therapeutic use	Gregor et al. (16)
Hallucinogens (lysergic acid diethylamide, phencyclidine, psilocybin, bufotenine, mescaline, nutmeg, wormwood, peyote, khat, morning glory seeds)	Usually taken intentionally	McCarron et al. (17); Leikin et al. (18)
Phenothiazines	Seen in chronic renal failure	McCallister et al. (19)

ACE, angiotensin-converting enzyme; MDMA, 3,4-methylenedioxymethamphetamine.
Modified from Drugs that may cause psychiatric symptoms. *Med Lett Drugs Ther* 2002;44:59–62.

TABLE 3. Specific drugs associated with hallucinations

Individual drugs	Comments	Reference
Acyclovir	With high doses, especially in renal failure patients	
Amantadine	Elderly; risk increases with duration of therapy	Snoey et al. (20)
Baclofen	Usually with abrupt withdrawal	Peng et al. (9)
Chlorambucil	In high doses	
Chloroquine	More common in children	Garg et al. (21)
Clonidine		
Cyclobenzaprine	Especially in the elderly	
DEET	With excessive or prolonged use	Snyder et al. (22)
Digoxin	Dose dependent, chronic toxicity	
Disopyramide	In the first 24–48 h of treatment	
Efavirenz		
Ergotamine		Gulbranson et al. (23)
Erythropoietin	In dialysis or bone marrow transplant patients	Steinberg et al. (24)
Ifosfamide	Elderly more at risk	
Interleukin-2	At high doses	
Isoniazid		
Ketamine	Emergence phenomena; abuse	
Levodopa	Dose-dependent	
Lidocaine		
Mefloquine	Vivid nightmares and dreams	
Methylphenidate	In pediatric and adult patients	
Methylsergide		
Metronidazole		
Nevirapine		
Pseudoephedrine	In children at usual doses	
Selegiline		
Sildenafil		
Tizanidine	In 3% of patients in clinical trials	
Trazodone		
Vincristine	Possibly dose related	
Zaleplon		
Zolpidem	Higher doses may increase risk; women may be a higher risk; possible interaction with SSRIs	Elko et al. (25)
Clarithromycin	Renal failure patients at high doses	Steinman et al. (26)
Bupropion	In overdose	Tracey et al. (27)

DEET, diethyltoluamide; SSRI, selective serotonin reuptake inhibitor.
Modified from Drugs that may cause psychiatric symptoms. *Med Lett Drugs Ther* 2002;44:59–62.

An accurate history is essential to delineate among the many possible etiologies. The history obtained from an actively hallucinating patient is often unreliable or unobtainable. In this case, additional information from family, friends, coworkers, prehospital personnel, and medical records is invaluable. The information collected should include onset and duration of symptoms, alcohol use or withdrawal, new medications or medication changes, recent ingestions of any type, attendance at functions where substance use is common (e.g., "rave parties," concerts), new diagnoses or illnesses, possible workplace exposures, travel history, and herbal or nontraditional health practices.

Signs and Symptoms

The physical examination may reveal findings that suggest a particular toxicologic or medical syndrome as the cause for the hallucinations. Particular attention should be paid to the patient's vital signs, mental status, pupils, skin, and neurologic examination. Stimulant toxicity, anticholinergic syndrome, thyrotoxicosis, sedative-hypnotic withdrawal, Parkinson's disease, and meningitis all have classic findings that may be detected on physical examination and guide the clinician in the diagnostic evaluation and treatment.

TABLE 4. Nondrug agents associated with hallucinations

Other toxicologic agents	Comments	Reference
Hallucinogenic plants (Table 1)	Intentional abuse	
Molybdenum	Overuse of dietary supplements	Momcilovic (28)
Nutmeg	Abused for hallucinogenic properties	Abernethy et al. (29)
Heavy metals (*Lucor metallicum*)	Arsenic; lead (gasoline sniffing); mercury	Coulehan et al. (30)
Jimson weed	Usually in adolescents and young adults	Klein-Schwartz et al. (31)
Boophane disticha (Buphanine)	South African plant	du Plooy et al. (32)
Angel's trumpet	Usually consumed as a tea; abused for hallucinogenic properties	Gopel et al. (33)

A mental status examination that demonstrates disorientation or confusion suggests an organic etiology rather than a functional psychosis. A depressed affect or well-organized delusion suggests bipolar affective disorder or schizophrenia. Ingestion of lysergic acid diethylamide can produce signs of sympathomimetic activity in a patient who is fully awake, alert, and oriented. Other signs suggestive of the presence of hallucinations include picking at the skin, clothing, or bed covers for nonexistent objects; turning or stopping to answer imaginary questions; or conversing with persons obviously not present.

Diagnostic Tests

Metabolic, infectious, toxic, psychiatric, neurologic, and pharmacologic etiologies, alone or in combination, are possible and common causes of hallucinations. Because the history is often unreliable or initially incomplete, diagnostic testing is an important part of the search for a cause of the hallucinations. When the etiology is unclear, pulse oximetry, complete blood count, serum chemistries, serum electrolytes, urinalysis, as well as blood and urine cultures, among other tests, are all used to evaluate the cause of new-onset hallucinations (Table 1).

Urine screens for drugs of abuse may be helpful. Tests for lysergic acid diethylamide, phencyclidine, tetrahydrocannabinol, stimulant amines, cocaine, metabolites, barbiturates, benzodiazepines, and opiates are often readily available from large diagnostic laboratories and are addressed in their specific chapters.

Other studies (e.g., computerized tomography of the head and lumbar puncture for meningitis) may be advisable. The possibility of an idiosyncratic drug reaction should be kept in mind, especially in the elderly. Because no test is diagnostic of drug reactions, only withdrawal of the offending agent, time, and clinical improvement prove the suspicion correct.

POTENTIAL COMPLICATIONS

The primary complication of xenobiotic-induced hallucination is trauma arising from the poor judgment or altered sensorium caused by the agent. Hyperthermic or rhabdomyolysis syndromes may develop from the drug itself or excessive and unusual muscle activity. In addition, the development of renal or liver injury may result from the toxic accumulation of a drug or its metabolites.

MANAGEMENT

Management of the patient with hallucinations depends on the patient's manifestations as well as the underlying etiology. If the hallucinations are not accompanied by complications such as rhabdomyolysis, the primary goal becomes treatment of the underlying cause. Until the etiology is identified, however, patient safety must be addressed. The presence of family members in the room can be calming for the patient. Antipsychotics and benzodiazepines alone or in combination have been successful when other measures fail (5). In general, the use of observation in a quiet room or pharmacologic therapy is preferable to physical restraints for behavior control of patients actively hallucinating. Physical restraints tend to exacerbate anxiety, agitation, and combative behavior but may be necessary in the initial management for the extremely agitated patient. Restraint of patients in the prone position has resulted in death from asphyxia (6).

Lorazepam and haloperidol have been used successfully for adverse psychotic reactions to lysergic acid diethylamide (7). Acute agitation and psychosis from methamphetamine intoxication have responded to droperidol or lorazepam (8). Withdrawal from central nervous system depressants (e.g., ethanol, benzodiazepine, barbiturate, gamma-hydroxybutyrate) requires sedative administration to control agitation and prevent seizures (Chapter 32). In a suspected anticholinergic syndrome with both central and peripheral signs and symptoms, administration of physostigmine may be diagnostic and curative (Chapter 67). Psychiatric illnesses can be treated with antipsychotics and appropriate referral. Drug reactions are more difficult to diagnose, require prolonged observation, and require repeated examinations to confirm the diagnosis.

Complications are generally treated empirically and do not have substance-specific therapy (i.e., antidote). Hyperthermia, seizures, and rhabdomyolysis are treated supportively (Chapters 29, 38, and 40). All patients should be monitored and observed closely with frequent reassessment of their overall condition and progress.

PITFALLS

Avoid the assumption that hallucinations are the result of a psychiatric illness. Fully consider the other possible causes, many of which are reversible and some of which are potentially fatal without appropriate intervention.

REFERENCES

1. Ohayon MM. Prevalence of hallucinations and their pathological associations in the general population. *Psychiatry Res* 2000;97;153–164.
2. Goetz CG, Leurgans S, Pappert EJ, et al. Prospective longitudinal assessment of hallucinations in Parkinson's disease. *Neurology* 2001;57:2078–2082.
3. Goetz CG, Vogel C, Tanner CM, et al. Early dopaminergic drug-induced hallucinations in Parkinson patients. *Neurology* 1998;51:811–814.
4. Perry EK, Perry RH. Acetylcholine and hallucinations: disease-related compared to drug-induced alterations in human consciousness. *Brain Cogn* 1995;28:240–258.
5. House RM. Delirium and agitation. *Curr Treat Options Neurol* 2000;2(2):141–150.
6. O'Halloran RL, Frank JG. Asphyxial death during prone restraint revisited: a report of 21 cases. *Am J Forensic Med Pathol* 2000;21(1):39–52.
7. Miller PL, Gay GR, Ferris KC, et al. Treatment of acute, adverse psychedelic reactions: "I've tripped and I can't get down." *J Psychoactive Drugs* 1992;24(3):277–279.
8. Richards JR, Derlet RW, Duncan DR. Chemical restraint for the agitated patient in the emergency department: lorazepam versus droperidol. *J Emerg Med* 1998;16(4):567–573.
9. Peng CT, Ger J, Yang CC, et al. Prolonged severe withdrawal symptoms after acute-on-chronic baclofen overdose. *J Toxicol Clin Toxicol* 1998;36(4):359–363.
10. Parker G, Blennerhassett J. Withdrawal reactions associated with venlafaxine. *Aust N Z J Psychiatry* 1998;32(2):291–241.
11. Kortabarria RP, Duran JA, Chacon JR, et al. Toxic psychosis following cycloplegic eyedrops. *DICP* 1990;24(7–8):708–709.
12. Hamborg-Petersen B, Nielsen MM, Thordal C. Toxic effect of scopolamine eye drops in children. *Acta Ophthalmol (Copenh)* 1984;62(3):485–488.
13. Love JN, Handler JA. Toxic psychosis: an unusual presentation of propranolol intoxication. *Am J Emerg Med* 1995;13(5):536–537.
14. Jones J, Dougherty J, Cannon L. Diphenhydramine-induced toxic psychosis. *Am J Emerg Med* 1986;4(4):369–371.
15. Downham TF, Cawley RA, Salley SO, et al. Systemic toxic reactions to procaine penicillin G. *Sex Transm Dis* 1978;5(1):4–9.
16. Gregor JC, Zilli CA, Gotlib IH. Acute psychosis associated with oral trimethoprim-sulfamethoxazole therapy. *Can J Psychiatry* 1993;38(1):56–58.
17. McCarron MM, Schulze BW, Thompson GA, et al. Acute phencyclidine intoxication: clinical patterns, complications, and treatment. *Ann Emerg Med* 1981;10(6):290–297.
18. Leikin JB, Krantz AJ, Zell-Kanter M, et al. Clinical features and management of intoxication due to hallucinogenic drugs. *Med Toxicol Adverse Drug Exp* 1989;4(5):324–350.
19. McCallister CJ, Scowden EB, Stone WJ. Toxic psychosis induced by phenothiazine administration in patients with chronic renal failure. *Clin Nephrol* 1978;10(5):191–195.
20. Snoey ER, Bessen HA. Acute psychosis after amantadine overdose. *Ann Emerg Med* 1990;19(6):668–670.
21. Garg P, Mody P, Lall KB. Toxic psychosis due to chloroquine—not uncommon in children. *Clin Pediatr (Phila)* 1990;29(8):448–450.
22. Snyder JW, Poe RO, Stubbins JF, et al. Acute manic psychosis following the dermal application of N,N-diethyl-m-toluamide (DEET) in an adult. *J Toxicol Clin Toxicol* 1986;24(5):429–439.
23. Gulbranson SH, Mock RE, Wolfrey JD. Possible ergotamine-caffeine-associated delirium. *Pharmacotherapy* 2002;22(1):126–129.
24. Steinberg H, Saravay SM, Wadhwa N, et al. Erythropoietin and visual hallucinations in patients on dialysis. *Psychosomatics* 1996;37(6):556–563.
25. Elko CJ, Burgess JL, Robertson WO. Zolpidem-associated hallucinations and serotonin reuptake inhibition: a possible interaction. *J Toxicol Clin Toxicol* 1998;36(3):195–203.
26. Steinman MA, Steinman TI. Clarithromycin-associated visual hallucinations in a patient with chronic renal failure on continuous ambulatory peritoneal dialysis. *Am J Kidney Dis* 1996;27(1):143–146.
27. Tracey JA, Cassidy N, Casey PB, et al. Bupropion (Zyban) toxicity. *Ir Med J* 2002;95(1):23–24.
28. Momcilovic B. A case report of acute human molybdenum toxicity from a dietary molybdenum supplement—a new member of the "Lucor metallicum" family. *Arh Hig Rada Toksikol* 1999;50(3):289–297.
29. Abernethy MK, Becker LB. Acute nutmeg intoxication. *Am J Emerg Med* 1992;10(5):429–430.
30. Coulehan JL, Hirsch W, Brillman J, et al. Gasoline sniffing and lead toxicity in Navajo adolescents. *Pediatrics* 1983;71(1):113–117.
31. Klein-Schwartz W, Oderda GM. Jimsonweed intoxication in adolescents and young adults. *Am J Dis Child* 1984;138(8):737–739.
32. du Plooy WJ, Swart L, van Huysteen GW. Poisoning with *Boophane disticha*: a forensic case. *Hum Exp Toxicol* 2001;20(5):277–278.
33. Gopel C, Laufer C, Marcus A. Three cases of angel's trumpet tea-induced psychosis in adolescent substance abusers. *Nord J Psychiatry* 2002;56(1):49–52.

CHAPTER 20

Metal Fume Fever

Daniel C. Keyes

OVERVIEW

Metal fume fever (MFF) is a self-limited illness resulting from the inhalation of fumes. It was first reported by Thackrah in 1832, commenting on the effect of zinc oxide fumes on smelter workers: "the brass smelters of Birmingham state their liability also to an intermittent fever, which they term brass-ague" (1). Case reports have also associated MFF with oxides of antimony, aluminum, beryllium, cadmium, copper, magnesium, manganese, tin, and vanadium; however, the causality of these other agents has not been defined conclusively (2). Many names have been used for MFF, including Monday fever, brass chills, zinc ague, welder's ague, spelter shakes, foundry fever, the smothers, and brass founders' ague. Exposure to zinc oxide fumes occurs mainly during welding or the galvanization of steel. It is estimated that as many as one in five welders have experienced MFF by the age of 30 years (2). Other occupations at risk include smelters, shipyard workers, junk metal refiners, electroplaters, metallic pigment makers, metal polishers, and alloy makers.

It has been suggested that MFF be considered part of a spectrum of illnesses known as *inhalation fever* (3–5). These conditions result from exposure to a variety of inhaled agents, including organic dusts, flax, polymers ("polymer fume fever"), and the metal oxides. These exposures share the features of rapid onset of a self-limited illness that includes fever, chills, fatigue, myalgias and dyspnea, and elevated white blood cell count on peripheral smear. Blanc wrote a thoughtful review in 1997 (5).

PATHOPHYSIOLOGY

The lung is the target organ of MFF. Although the clinical syndrome is similar to influenza or a mild bacterial illness, no infectious agent is involved. Exposure to zinc oxide fumes initiates an important pulmonary cellular chemotactic response, which results in the local and systemic findings of this syndrome. Bronchoalveolar lavage performed after symptoms develop in MFF reveals a polymorphonuclear inflammatory infiltrate, which may reach 100 times normal counts (6). Cytokines appear to play an important role, as manifested by an increase in tissue necrosis factor and interleukins (IL-6 and IL-8) after exposure to the fumes (7).

DIAGNOSIS

Differential Diagnosis

Several pulmonary disorders constitute the differential diagnosis of MFF (Table 1). The most common similar complex is caused by influenza. Influenza also runs a rapid, generally benign course in the age range of the industrial worker. It is a diagnosis of exclusion for the inhalational fevers. Influenza may be suspected if the illness is part of an epidemic, particularly if coworkers or family members who are not exposed to fumes have similar symptoms. The diagnosis of MFF is more likely when a geographic and chronologic association exists with known sources of exposure such as welding.

MFF is virtually indistinguishable from other inhalational fevers, except for the occasional report of a metallic taste and the history of welding in association with zinc or galvanized materials. Cadmium exposure from solder and welding fumes may also present with an early fever but may go on to develop a toxic pneumonitis with pulmonary infiltrates and a picture consistent with acute lung injury. Cadmium should be given particular consideration when the worker has been welding through existing solder and steel, because some solders contain cadmium (8–10). Zinc chloride toxicity may also appear like MFF; however, it may cause more severe lung injury. A history of exposure to a police or military smoke bomb is usually obtained (5,11).

Uncomplicated zinc oxide–induced MFF rarely requires admission. Patients experiencing zinc chloride– or cadmium-induced acute lung injury may require admission, or may initially improve, with serous relapse occurring 24 to 48 hours later (12). The important feature of zinc chloride exposure is that it causes a form of acute lung injury, which may be much more serious and even fatal (5).

Exposure to pyrolysis products of fluorine-containing plastics has been associated with a clinical syndrome similar to MFF, called *polymer fume fever*. Acute high concentrations of *ozone* generated during gas metal arc welding of aluminum with argon gas for shielding have been associated with an acute chemical pneumonitis. *Phosgene* and *nitrogen dioxide* in high concentrations are associated with coughing, shortness of breath, and noncardiac pulmonary edema. Exposure to high concentrations of *organic dusts* (contaminated with thermophilic bacteria and fungal spores) has produced symptoms similar to MFF. This has been described mostly in the summer and fall seasons and is associated with shoveling damp wood chips, leaves, or silage. Massive grain dust exposure has also been associated with a febrile reaction similar to the organic dust toxic syndrome. New mill workers' exposure to *cotton dust* is associated with a clinical picture similar to MFF. Tolerance develops with continued exposures.

History

The diagnosis of MFF is usually made when the clinical picture is combined with history of metal fume exposure. A careful

TABLE 1. Differential diagnosis of metal fume fever

Related fume fever syndrome	Presumed etiologic agent (references)
Bronchitis, pneumonia	Virus, bacteria
Cadmium pneumonitis	Cadmium (8–10)
Smoke bomb fever	Hexachloroethane, zinc chloride, aluminum (smoke bombs) (5,11)
Noncardiogenic pulmonary edema	Phosgene, nitrogen oxides
Organic dust toxic syndrome	Organic dusts (15,16)
Mill fever	Cotton dust (17)
Silo filler's disease	Grain dust (18)
Wood trimmer's disease	Wood pulp (19,20)
Polymer fume fever	Polytetrafluoroethylene (21)

TABLE 2. Manifestations of metal fume fever (listed in order of decreasing frequency)

Symptoms	Findings
Headache	Leukocytosis
Sweet metallic taste	Granulocytosis
Myalgias	Fever
Malaise	High erythrocyte sedimentation rate
Cough	Hypoxemia
Thirst	Reduced pulmonary function tests
Chest tightness	Rales
Nausea	High lactate dehydrogenase
Chills	Wheezing
Dyspnea	Tachypnea
Diaphoresis	Tachycardia

Adapted from Blount BW. Two types of metal fume fever: mild vs. serious. *Mil Med* 1990;155(8):372–377.

occupational history should be obtained, with particular attention to fume inhalation. Blount has compared the clinical features of classical MFF (Table 2).

One should determine the chronology of the exposure and the frequency with which the patient has had symptoms related to his or her occupation. The classic history is of symptoms on Monday, symptomatic improvement as the week progresses, with resurgence on returning to work after a weekend off work. Onset of MFF occurs in 4 to 6 hours after exposure begins, typically on the evening after exposure to metal oxide fumes. The symptoms may start when the employee is at home. Fatigue, chills, fever, myalgias, cough, dyspnea, thirst, metallic taste, and salivation are characteristic. The disorder is usually of short duration, lasting no more than 24 to 48 hours. Tachyphylaxis develops in workers but may be lost over the weekend, leading to the term *Monday morning fever* (13). In some cases, it may be useful to contact the employer to clarify the type of exposure experienced by the worker.

Several variations may occur. The patient may describe recurrent flu-like illnesses, which appear to have responded to antibiotics or other intervention (because MFF resolves spontaneously). One should pay particular attention to a history of exposure to cadmium, zinc chloride, or "smoke bombs," as these agents may cause more serious illness requiring specific interventions.

Signs

Physical findings may vary from person to person. Fever, sweating, tachycardia, chills, pleural friction rub, and pulmonary crackles and wheezing have been described. The temperature is commonly elevated to 102° to 104°F, with shaking chills, giving rise to the term *spelter shakes*.

Diagnostic Tests

Laboratory studies include leukocytosis (15,000 to 20,000 cells/mm^3) with excess of polymorphonuclear cells. Zinc levels may be elevated in the serum and urine (14), but the absence of zinc does not rule out exposure of the diagnosis. The chest radiograph may reveal patchy infiltrates but more often is normal.

Pulmonary function study results may be normal or may show acute changes consistent with reduced lung volumes (forced vital capacity and forced expiratory volume in 1 second) and decreased carbon monoxide diffusing capacity. Over time, the pulmonary function abnormalities revert to normal. Bronchoalveolar lavage is not routinely recommended. If bronchoalveolar lavage is performed, lactate dehydrogenase may be elevated with the pulmonary fraction showing the greatest increase.

POTENTIAL COMPLICATIONS

The natural history of MFF is benign, with symptoms resolving over 24 to 36 hours after exposure. There are no known chronic sequelae from repeated exposures; however, it is important to intervene to prevent future episodes through modifications of the site of exposure. Complications may occur from related inhalational or other occupational exposures, and further history may indicate specific testing and follow-up for an individual patient.

MANAGEMENT

The management of MFF is supportive, as no specific intervention, antibiotic, or antidote is known to be of value. Patients may benefit from fluids, rest, and antipyretic therapy. The most important aspect of fever is prevention of future episodes and ensuring that a more dangerous etiology requiring specific therapy is not present. If more serious conditions have been excluded, MFF is most often managed on an outpatient basis, with appropriate clinic follow-up and investigation of the patient's work setting.

Prevention of MFF includes implementation of engineering controls, general room ventilation, local exhaust ventilation, process enclosure, down-draft or cross-draft tables, and use of fume extractors built into welding equipment.

REFERENCES

1. Thackrah C. *The effects of arts, trades, and professions, and of civic states and habits of living on health and longevity*. London: Longman, Ress, Orme, 1832:101–102.
2. Gordon T, Fine JM. Metal fume fever. *Occup Med* 1993;8(3):504–517.
3. Rask-Andersen A, Pratt DS. Inhalation fever: a proposed unifying term for febrile reactions to inhalation of noxious substances. *Br J Ind Med* 1992;49(1):40.
4. Editorial. Inhalation fevers. *Lancet* 1978;1(8058):249–250.
5. Blanc PD. Inhalational fevers. Pulmonary and critical care update, vol. 12 (Lesson 1). 1997. Available at: http://www.chestnet.org/education/online/pccu/vol12/lesson01-02.index.php.
6. Blanc P, Wong H, Bernstein MS, et al. An experimental human model of metal fume fever. *Ann Intern Med* 1991;114(11):930–936.
7. Blanc PD, Boushey HA, Wong H, et al. Cytokines in metal fume fever. *Am Rev Respir Dis* 1993;147(1):134–138.
8. Fuortes L, Leo A, Ellerbeck PG, et al. Acute respiratory fatality associated with exposure to sheet metal and cadmium fumes. *J Toxicol Clin Toxicol* 1991;29(2):279–283.
9. Barnhart S, Rosenstock L. Cadmium chemical pneumonitis. *Chest* 1984;86(5):789–791.
10. National Institute for Occupational Safety and Health. Publication of NIOSH criteria documents on welding, brazing, and thermal cutting and on radon progeny. *MMWR Morb Mortal Wkly Rep* 1988;37(35):545–547.
11. Schenker MB, Speizer FE, Taylor JO. Acute upper respiratory symptoms resulting from exposure to zinc chloride aerosol. *Environ Res* 1981;25(2):317–324.
12. Blount BW. Two types of metal fume fever: mild vs. serious. *Mil Med* 1990;155(8):372–377.
13. Drinker P, Thomson R, Finn J. Metal fume fever: II. Resistance acquired by inhalation of zinc oxide on two successive days. *J Ind Hyg* 1927;9:98–105.
14. Fuortes L, Schenck D. Marked elevation of urinary zinc levels and pleural-friction rub in metal fume fever. *Vet Human Toxicol* 2000;42:164–165.
15. Brinton WT, Vastbinder EE, Greene JW, et al. An outbreak of organic dust toxic syndrome in a college fraternity. *JAMA* 1987;258(9):1210–1212.
16. Rask-Andersen A. Organic dust toxic syndrome among farmers. *Br J Ind Med* 1989;46(4):233–238.
17. Holness DL, Taraschuk IG, Goldstein RS. Acute exposure of cotton dust. A case of mill fever. *JAMA* 1982;247(11):1602–1603.
18. Chan-Yeung M, Ashley MJ, Grzybowski S. Grain dust and the lungs. *CMJ* 1978;118(10):1271–1274.
19. Belin L. Sawmill alveolitis in Sweden. *Int Arch Allergy Appl Immunol* 1987;82(3–4):440–443.
20. Rask-Andersen A, Land CJ, Enlund K, et al. Inhalation fever and respiratory symptoms in the trimming department of Swedish sawmills. *Am J Ind Med* 1994;25(1):65–67.
21. Shusterman DJ. Polymer fume fever and other fluorocarbon pyrolysis-related syndromes. *Occup Med* 1993;8(3):519–531.

CHAPTER 21

Methemoglobinemia

Alan D. Woolf and Robert O. Wright

OVERVIEW

Methemoglobinemia is an uncommon, but not rare, complication of a toxic exposure. Methemoglobin (MetHgb) production refers to the oxidation of ferrous (2+) iron to ferric (3+) iron within the hemoglobin molecule. This reaction impairs hemoglobin's physiologic functions, resulting in tissue ischemia and in severe cases, death. Methemoglobinemia most commonly results from exposure to an oxidizing drug or chemical but may also have genetic, dietary, or idiopathic etiologies.

PATHOPHYSIOLOGY

Red Blood Cell Oxidative Damage

A substance has been oxidized if it loses an electron; when it gains an electron, it has been reduced. Oxidation/reduction reactions (termed *redox* reactions) always occur together; as one substance is reduced, another must be oxidized. Highly reactive, chemically unstable molecules that participate in redox reactions (i.e., *free radicals*) disrupt cell membranes and oxidize cellular enzymes inhibiting their function. Chain reactions can create a cascade of additional radicals capable of progressive cellular and subcellular damage. Some reactions cause the formation of covalent bonds between the arylating oxidant agent and cellular proteins (1). This covalent bond may cause disruption of cellular membrane, interfere with enzyme function, damage deoxyribonucleic acid, and alter gene expression. If unchecked, the process ultimately leads to cell lysis and death (2,3). When these oxidation reactions occur within the heme moiety of hemoglobin, MetHgb is formed.

Whereas some oxidizing agents react only with hemoglobin, most are not specific; thus, methemoglobinemia is often accompanied by some degree of hemolysis. Red blood cells (RBCs) are uniquely susceptible to oxidant stress. They carry oxygen in high concentration and are therefore continuously exposed to oxygen radicals. Unlike other cells, RBCs lack a nucleus and mitochondria. They cannot synthesize new protein and are less efficient at detoxification (4,5). Because the enzymes that detoxify oxygen degrade with time and are not newly synthesized, older RBCs are even more susceptible to oxidation.

Methemoglobin

The iron contained in the porphyrin ring structure in hemoglobin is normally found in the ferrous^{2+} state, but it can be oxidized to the ferric^{3+} state to form MetHgb. Once MetHgb is formed, the hemoglobin unit affected loses its ability to carry molecular oxygen (or CO_2).

Hemoglobin is a tetrameric molecule, and the complete transformation to MetHgb represents a four-electron loss. However, under conditions of oxidative stress, partial oxidation of the individual subunits predominates, and, as such, eight different dimers may exist. Each of the four subunits contains a heme moiety capable of carrying oxygen. During methemoglobinemia, any oxygen that is being carried by a nonoxidized hemoglobin subunit is held onto more tightly and poorly released to tissues. This property is important clinically. For example, a patient with 35% methemoglobinemia has a calculated maximum oxygen-carrying capacity of 65% of his or her hemoglobin. However, the allosteric changes induced by oxidation of one subunit cause oxygen to bind more tightly in the partially oxidized tetrameric hemoglobin molecules, resulting in a left shift in the hemoglobin-oxygen saturation curve. Functional oxygen-carrying capacity is thereby reduced below 35%.

Oxidation also results in a net positive charge to the MetHgb molecule. As such, the molecule has a high affinity for monovalent anions such as cyanide (CN^-), fluoride (F^-), or chloride (Cl^-) as opposed to the uncharged binding ligands (CO_2, CO, and O_2) of normal hemoglobin (6).

Endogenous Methemoglobin Reduction

Even in the absence of exogenous oxidative stress, endogenous oxidation eventually converts enough hemoglobin to MetHgb to impair cellular respiration. Approximately 1% of total hemoglobin is actually in the form of MetHgb at any given time. Several endogenous reduction systems exist to maintain hemoglobin in the ferrous^{2+} state. The cytochrome-b_5 methemoglobin reductase [nicotinamide adenine dinucleotide (NADH) methemoglobin reductase] system accounts for 99% of daily MetHgb reduction. Other endogenous reducing agents include ascorbic acid, glutathione, reduced flavin, tetrahydropterin, cysteamine, and reduced cysteine on protein molecules. The reconversion rate of MetHgb to hemoglobin by endogenous processes in normal individuals (assuming no excessive MetHgb production) is a first-order reaction proceeding at approximately 15% per hour (7). This means that a subject with 40% MetHgb is expected to have a level of 34% 1 hour later (if further MetHgb production does not occur).

Under normal circumstances, only cytochrome-b_5 methemoglobin reductase plays a large role in reduction. However, patients with complete congenital deficiency of the cytochrome-b_5 reductase are able to maintain MetHgb levels below 50%, and sometimes as low as 10%. This suggests that minor pathways (e.g., ascorbic acid, glutathione, and so forth) can compensate and reduce significant amounts of MetHgb when the cytochrome-b_5 reductase pathway is either absent or overwhelmed.

Cytochrome-b_5 Nicotinamide Adenine Dinucleotide (NADH-Dependent)–Methemoglobin Reductase (Diaphorase I)

The predominant pathway by which MetHgb is reduced in the cell is a two-enzyme system known as *diaphorase I*. One of the enzymes is a cytosolic cytochrome, called *cytochrome*-b_5. A second enzyme with a flavin moiety called *cytochrome*-b_5 *reductase* is also necessary to reduce MetHgb. Together, these enzymes are known more commonly as *NADH methemoglobin reductase*. Gly-

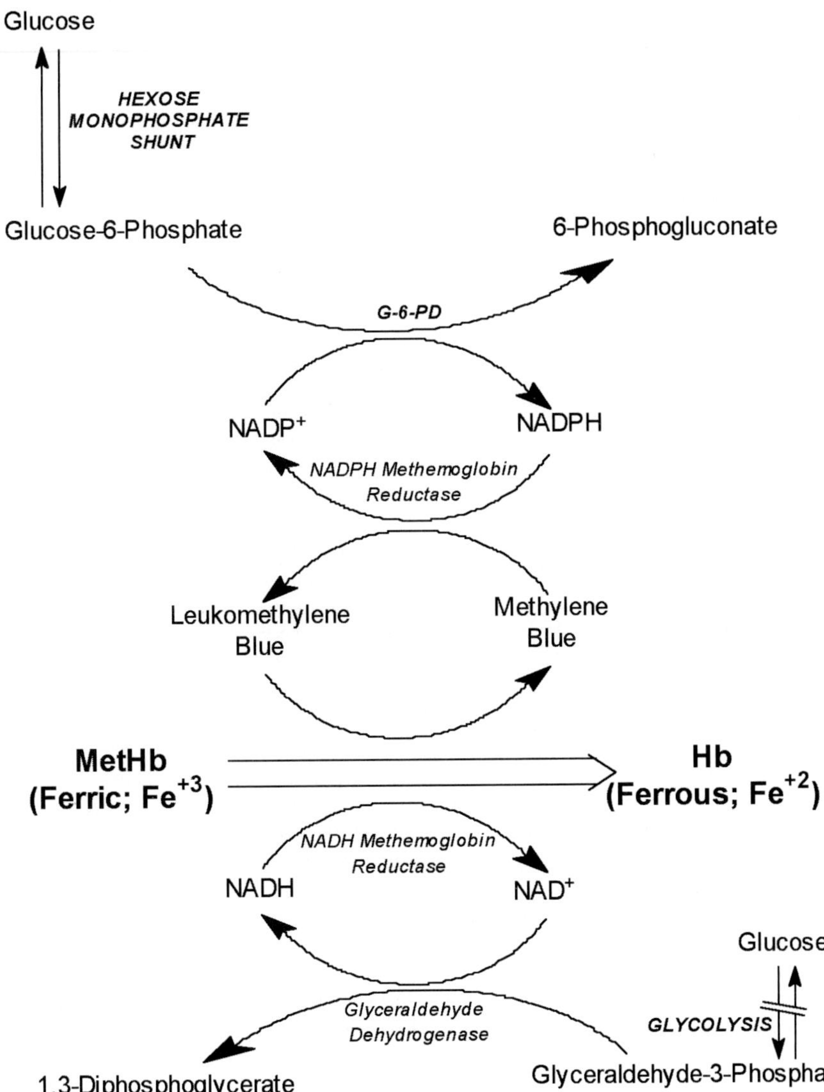

Figure 1. Pathways of methemoglobin metabolism. Nicotinamide adenine dinucleotide (NADH) methemoglobin reductase equals cytochrome-b_5/cytochrome-b_5 reductase equals diaphorase I. G-6-PD, glucose-6-phosphate dehydrogenase; Hb, hemoglobin; MetHb, methemoglobin; NAD+, the oxidized form of nicotinamide adenine dinucleotide; NADP+, the oxidized form of nicotinamide adenine dinucleotide phosphate; NADPH, the reduced form of nicotinamide adenine dinucleotide phosphate.

colytic intermediates, which produce reduced NADH, serve as the original electron donors, and NADH is a necessary cofactor to cytochrome-b_5 reductase. Electrons travel from glycolytic intermediates to NADH to cytochrome-b_5 reductase, to cytochrome-b_5, and finally to MetHgb (Fig. 1).

Nicotinamide Adenine Dinucleotide Phosphate Methemoglobin Reductase (Diaphorase II)

Also known as *nicotinamide adenine dinucleotide phosphate (NADPH)–flavin reductase* and *NADPH methemoglobin-diaphorase II*, this enzyme normally plays a negligible role in reducing MetHgb. It is a generalized reductase with an affinity for dyes, such as methylene blue, Nile blue, and divicine (8–10). In the presence of the cofactor NADPH, this enzyme reduces these dyes (e.g., methylene blue to leukomethylene blue), which in their reduced state subsequently can act to reduce MetHgb (Fig. 1). Present in liver cells as well as RBC, this enzyme is able to reduce riboflavin to hydroriboflavin, which in turn can react with intracellular reactive oxidants. The primary function of NADPH methemoglobin reductase is probably to metabolize oxidant xenobiotics and not MetHgb (11).

Indirect Endogenous Protective Mechanisms

Intracellular sulfation enzymes, ascorbic acid, and glutathione indirectly prevent methemoglobinemia by protecting cells from oxidative stress. Reduced glutathione is quantitatively the most important cellular antioxidant (12), but it is a minor pathway in the reduction of MetHgb. Oxidized glutathione is cytotoxic and diffuses out of cells if it is not reduced back to reduced glutathione, a process requiring the glucose 6 phosphate dehydrogenase (G6PD) cycle (13,14). Hence, oxidative stress in the presence of G6PD deficiency leads to intracellular depletion of total glutathione, rendering the cell vulnerable to further oxidative injury. This explains in part the susceptibility of patients with G6PD deficiency to hemolysis in certain clinical circumstances of oxidative stress.

DIAGNOSIS

Differential Diagnosis of Cyanosis

Cyanosis due to methemoglobinemia must be differentiated from that due to hypoxia (Fig. 2). The differential diagnosis for a small infant with cyanosis is similar to, but much broader than,

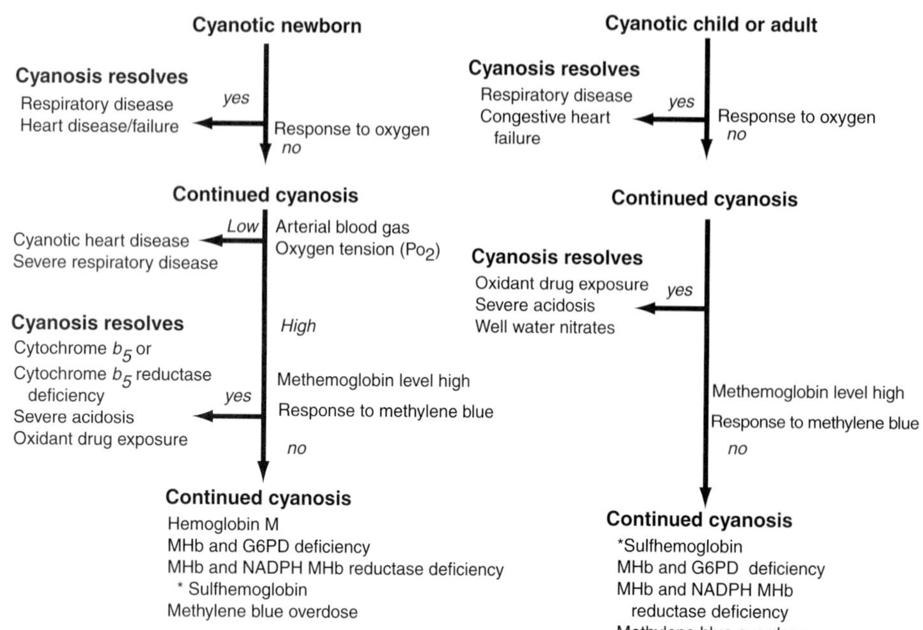

Figure 2. Diagnostic algorithm in cases of cyanosis of unknown origin. *Some co-oximeters may misread sulfhemoglobin as methemoglobin. G6PD, glucose 6 phosphate dehydrogenase; MHb, methemoglobin; NADPH, the reduced form of nicotinamide adenine dinucleotide phosphate. (From Wright RO, Lewander WJ, Woolf AD. Methemoglobinemia: etiology, pharmacology, and clinical management. *Ann Emerg Med* 1999;34:651, with permission.)

that of older children or adults. Pulmonary and cardiac origins for cyanosis include congenital and acquired causes of cardiorespiratory failure, right-to-left shunting, and deoxygenated blood. Sepsis, severe dehydration and acidosis, other poisonings (e.g., carbon monoxide, hydrogen sulfide, or cyanide), or the presence of other dyshemoglobins (e.g., sulfhemoglobinemia) can also cause cyanosis.

Newborns and small infants with congenital methemoglobinemia present like some patients with cyanotic congenital heart disease, having cyanosis that fails to respond to supplemental oxygen, a lack of significant pulmonary findings, and clear chest radiograph. Depending on the degree of cyanosis, there may also be metabolic acidosis. A distinguishing feature of methemoglobinemia is the paradoxical elevation of arterial partial pressure of oxygen (PaO_2) despite clinical cyanosis and normal calculated arterial oxygen saturation. In contrast, children with cyanotic heart disease on supplemental oxygen have a low PaO_2 and low calculated oxygen saturation.

Infants with sepsis may present with symptoms similar to methemoglobinemia but usually respond to supplemental oxygen although the patient with diarrhea, acidosis, and methemoglobinemia may also be septic. Slightly older infants (4 to 6 months of age) may develop methemoglobinemia in the context of severe dehydration, diarrhea, and metabolic acidosis.

Sulfhemoglobin

Sulfhemoglobinemia is much less common than methemoglobinemia but can develop with several drugs: phenacetin, sulfonamides, phenazopyridine, acetanilid, or dapsone. Sulfhemoglobin formation requires that the heme moiety first be oxidized to MetHgb, and then a second reaction occurs in which sulfur is bound to the heme. Most drugs that produce MetHgb can also produce sulfhemoglobin, and sulfhemoglobinemia may be confused with methemoglobinemia (15). Unlike MetHgb, sulfhemoglobin is stable and cannot be reduced to hemoglobin, persisting for the life of the RBC. Symptoms tend to be milder than with methemoglobinemia because the nonsulfated hemoglobin units unload oxygen to tissues more readily (a right-shift hemoglobin dissociation curve), as opposed to methemoglobinemia, which causes a left shift of the hemoglobin dissociation curve (16). Elevated sulfhemoglobin levels in blood confirm the diagnosis (16). Methylene blue is ineffective for sulfhemoglobinemia. Treatment is supportive. In severe cases, exchange transfusion may be needed to improve the patient's functional oxygen-carrying capacity.

Methemoglobinemia

XENOBIOTIC-INDUCED

A variety of chemicals and drugs are associated with MetHgb formation (Table 1). Oxidizing agents can be divided into two groups: Direct oxidizers react with hemoglobin to form MetHgb whereas indirect oxidizers are actually powerful reducing agents that reduce oxygen to the free radical $O_2^{\cdot -}$, or water to H_2O_2, which in turn oxidizes hemoglobin to MetHgb. In children and adults, methemoglobinemia is usually caused by an oxidizing drug such as dapsone (17–24); sulfamethoxazole (25,26); phenazopyridine (27,28); clofazimine (29); nitroglycerin (30); benzocaine (31–35); benzocaine-containing teething gels (36); EMLA anesthetic cream (37); or cocaine adulterated with benzocaine (38), prilocaine (39–41), chloroquine, and primaquine (42); amyl nitrite (43); or liniments or laxatives contaminated with sodium nitrite (44,45). In adolescents and adults, inhalant abuse may lead to methemoglobinemia from volatile nitrites (46). Folk remedies, such as glycerated asafoetida, have also been implicated (47).

Other causes include the nitro-alkanes found in some nail polish removers and other industrial nitrogen-containing compounds. The herbicide paraquat (48) or its vehicle (49) may cause methemoglobinemia. A variety of nitrogen-containing chemicals, dyes, fertilizers, and industrial products can produce occupationally related methemoglobinemia. Aniline is a common precursor for synthetic indigo dyes and also a variety of drugs (e.g., acetanilide, indomethacin, dipyrone, acetaminophen, sulfonamides, sulfones, benzocaine, lidocaine, prilocaine, and phenazopyridine) (50).

Many MetHgb-producing drugs are indirect; they are metabolized to an oxidative free radical. For example, aniline is metabolized to a free radical phenylhydroxylamine, which reacts with

TABLE 1. Drug, chemical, and dietary causes of methemoglobinemia

Drugs and metabolites	Chlorates
Acetanilid	Chlorobenzene
Amyl nitrite	Cobalt preparations
Benzocaine	Dimethylaniline
Cetacaine	Dinitrobenzene
Chloroquine	Dinitrophenol
Chloroquinone	Dinitrotoluene
Clofazimine	Hydroquinone
Dapsone (sulfones)	Inks and shoe polish
Diaminodiphenylsulfone	Isobutyl nitrite
Hydroxylamine	Menthol
Lidocaine	Naphthalene
Menadione	Naphthylamines
Methylene blue	Nitrates/nitrites
Metoclopramide	Nitric oxide
Nitroglycerin	Nitro-alkanes
Nitrosobenzene	Nitrobenzene
Para-aminobenzoic acid	Nitro-chlorobenzene
Para-aminopropiophenone	Nitrofuran
Para-hydroxylaminopropiophenone	Nitrogen oxide
	Nitrogen trifluoride
Phenacetin	Nitroglycerin
Phenazopyridine hydrochloride (Pyridium)	Nitrophenol
	Nitrous gases/nitric oxide
Phenylhydroxylamine	Ozone
Phenytoin	Para-bromoaniline
Potassium permanganate	Paraquat (or monolinuron)
Prilocaine	Para-toluidine
Primaquine	Phenazopyridine
Procaine	Phenetidin
Resorcinol	Phenols
Silver nitrate	Phenylhydrazine
Sodium nitrate	Phenylhydroxylamine
Sodium nitrite	Pyridine
Sodium nitroprusside	Smoke (products of combustion)
Sulfamethoxazole	Sulfones
Sulfanilamide	Toluidine
Sulfapyridine	Trinitrotoluene
Sulfathiazole	Xylidine
Chemicals and other toxic hazards	Foods
Acetanilid	Beets
Alloxan	Cabbage
Ammonium nitrate	Nitrite/nitrate preservatives
Aniline dyes	Nitrogen-rich foods
Antipyrine	Preserved meats
Arsine	Spinach
Benzene derivatives	Well water
Butyl nitrite	

oxygen to form free radicals and then MetHgb. It has been postulated that benzocaine is partly metabolized to aniline, which then is transformed into phenylhydroxylamine and nitrosobenzene, both of which are oxidants.

Because of interindividual variability, not every patient develops methemoglobinemia when exposed to oxidizing agents. Only those who metabolize a significant amount of parent drug to the toxic metabolite are at an increased risk. For example, not every child who ingests benzocaine develops methemoglobinemia. Other factors, such as rate of absorption, enterohepatic recirculation, or ability to reduce MetHgb to Hgb may influence the duration of toxin-induced methemoglobinemia. Nitrites can be absorbed through the skin as well as the gastrointestinal tract, and others, like dapsone, may undergo enterohepatic circulation and produce prolonged MetHgb.

DIARRHEA AND ACIDOSIS

The second most common etiology of MetHgb is idiopathic but related to systemic acidosis. Methemoglobin can be formed in infants younger than 6 months of age who develop severe metabolic acidosis, most commonly due to diarrhea and dehydration (51–55). Several risk factors predispose infants to methemoglobinemia. RBC levels of cytochrome-b_5 reductase are only 50% to 60% of adult levels (56). Fetal hemoglobin is also more easily oxidized than adult hemoglobin, and the higher intestinal pH of infants may promote the growth of organisms that convert nitrates to nitrites, a potent MetHgb inducer. The relative roles of each of these factors are unclear. The syndrome has not been associated with oxidant drugs, and the methemoglobinemia resolves with time, suggesting it is not inherited. An association with certain gram-negative, nitrite-forming bacteria, such as *Escherichia coli* or *Campylobacter jejuni*, has been suggested; however, a consistent pathogen has not been identified (57).

There are also reports of infants with MetHgb and acidosis in the absence of diarrhea, specifically in an infant with renal tubular acidosis and vomiting but no diarrhea (58). It may be that the common endpoint of acidosis is the greatest predisposing factor. Endogenous MetHgb reduction is inhibited by an acidic pH and promoted by an alkaline pH (59,60). In a prospective study of 45 young infants, viral and bacterial pathogens were implicated in MetHgb production, which correlated with both low admission weight percentile and failure to thrive (61). The authors postulated that altered gut flora plays an important role in MetHgb generation and that breast-feeding was protective.

DIETARY SOURCES AND WATER

Nitrogen-containing dietary components have also been shown to cause MetHgb formation (Table 1). Well water contaminated with nitrates deserves special consideration. Because a toxic ingestion is very uncommon in young infants, clinicians may not relate recurrent cyanosis to the water used to make baby formula (62). These very young infants usually live in rural areas where the water source is a shallow well containing high levels of nitrates. Intestinal bacterial flora converts the nitrates to nitrites (63–65). Lactating women on a diet containing high nitrogen levels do not appear to have elevated nitrates in their breast milk (66).

Contaminated water can also produce methemoglobinemia in older patients. An outbreak of methemoglobinemia among school-aged children was traced to soup prepared with water contaminated by a nitrite-containing boiler cleaning solution (67); a second outbreak among six adults was traced to coffee prepared with water contaminated by nitrites (68).

Other dietary sources have been implicated. Six of 17 infants hospitalized with cow's milk or soy protein intolerance had laboratory evidence of MetHgb formation (69). Whether MetHgb is caused by transient dietary protein intolerance itself or the circumstances of infantile diarrhea previously described is unclear. Diets high in nitrogen-containing vegetables such as beets, cabbage, and spinach or meats cured with nitrites have also been associated with methemoglobinemia.

GENETIC

Congenital methemoglobinemia presents at birth or very shortly thereafter. Two different deficiencies may be present: cytochrome-b_5 reductase deficiency or cytochrome-b_5 deficiency (70). Both are transmitted in an autosomal-recessive pattern. These patients have moderately elevated MetHgb levels chronically; their skin may have a slate gray appearance, but they usually tolerate the disorder well.

TABLE 2. Symptoms associated with methemoglobin blood concentrations

Methemoglobin concentration	Total hemoglobin (%)	Symptoms[a]
<1.5 g/dl	<10	None
1.5–3.0 g/dl	10–20	Cyanotic skin discoloration
3.0–4.5 g/dl	20–30	Anxiety, lightheadedness, headache, tachycardia
4.5–7.5 g/dl	30–50	Fatigue, confusion, dizziness, tachypnea, increased tachycardia
7.5–10.5 g/dl	50–70	Coma, seizures, dysrhythmias, acidosis
>10.5 g/dl	>70	Death

Note: Assumes hemoglobin is equal to 15 g/dl. Patients with lower hemoglobin concentrations may experience more severe symptoms for a given percentage methemoglobin level.
[a]Patients with underlying cardiac, pulmonary, or hematologic disease may experience more severe symptoms for a given methemoglobin concentration.

NADPH methemoglobin reductase deficiency has also been described but does not lead to methemoglobinemia. This enzyme is not responsible for endogenous MetHgb reduction and only reduces MetHgb in the presence of an exogenous catalyzing agent such as methylene blue. However, if these patients develop chemically induced methemoglobinemia, they will not respond to methylene blue therapy because methylene blue is dependent on this enzyme to reduce MetHgb (Fig. 1).

M HEMOGLOBINS

Hemoglobin M is a group of diseases of abnormal hemoglobin with autosomal-dominant inheritance. Patients born with one of these genetic variants develop methemoglobinemia because the iron atom, when interacting with the aberrantly formed porphyrin ring, is stabilized in the ferric state.

CLINICAL PRESENTATION

Regardless of etiology, the symptoms of acquired methemoglobinemia are related to the MetHgb level in the blood (Table 2). Levels are conventionally reported as a percentage of total hemoglobin. Approximately 1.5 g/dl of MetHgb (10% to 15% of total Hgb) is necessary to produce visible slate-gray cyanosis, as opposed to 5.0 g/dl of deoxyhemoglobin (30% to 40%) necessary to produce *classic* cyanosis. Higher MetHgb levels provoke respiratory distress, anxiety, confusion, and lethargy. Methemoglobin levels at approximately 70% may cause death.

The patient with life-threatening methemoglobinemia is often cyanotic and comatose. A 50-year-old man presented in coma responsive only to deep pain, with fixed and dilated pupils, and an initial MetHgb level of 81.3%. He responded to methylene blue therapy with complete recovery (71).

Because the MetHgb level is generally reported as a proportion of total hemoglobin, the MetHgb level may not always correspond with symptoms. Other conditions that compromise oxygen delivery may exacerbate the effect of methemoglobinemia. Anemia, acidosis, respiratory compromise, and cardiac disease may make patients more symptomatic than expected for a given MetHgb level. For example, a patient with a MetHgb level of 20% and total hemoglobin of 15 g/dl still has 12 g/dl of functioning hemoglobin, whereas a patient with a MetHgb level of 20% and total hemoglobin of 8 g/dl has only 6.4 g/dl of functioning hemoglobin. Several patient groups are more likely to develop symptoms at lower MetHgb concentrations: newborns, young infants with diarrhea/acidosis, patients with underlying heart disease, fire victims, genetic vulnerability, high-risk occupations, and other illnesses that may compromise the delivery of oxygen to tissues.

HEMOLYSIS AND OTHER TOXICITIES

Oxidant-induced Heinz body hemolysis frequently accompanies methemoglobinemia, although the onset of hemolysis is usually delayed by 12 to 24 hours after drug exposure. Chemicals such as chlorates, chromates, and arsine can cause extreme life-threatening oxidant-induced hemolysis as well as methemoglobinemia.

Other examples of concomitant toxicity include paraquat, which can cause methemoglobinemia and pulmonary fibrosis. Patients overdosing on this herbicide may present with a picture of hypoxia, shortness of breath, and cyanosis, misdiagnosed as an early pulmonary insult unless methemoglobinemia is also considered. Nitrites and nitrates are also potent vasodilators and may lead to significant hypotension, exacerbating the toxicity of the methemoglobinemia. Quinones such as primaquine or chloroquine may produce concurrent cardiotoxicity. A patient who swallowed a fingernail cosmetic presented with symptoms of methemoglobinemia from the toluidine in the product and orogastric burns secondary to its methacrylic acid component (72).

DIAGNOSTIC TESTS

The first step is to confirm the diagnosis of methemoglobinemia. The appearance of cyanosis usually stimulates the performance of pulse oximetry and an arterial blood gas. However, these tests may be normal or near normal in a patient with significant methemoglobinemia and may delay diagnosis.

Arterial Blood Gas Analysis

Arterial blood gas machines are based on electrochemistry. Voltage changes are determined with high impedance electrodes to measure pH and $PaCO_2$; electrical current changes measure PaO_2 (73,74). PaO_2 refers to dissolved gas and not to molecules bound to hemoglobin. Serum bicarbonate is calculated from the pH and $PaCO_2$ using the Henderson-Hasselbalch equation. Similarly, oxygen saturation can be calculated from the pH and PO_2 using the standard oxygen-hemoglobin saturation curve. This conversion assumes the presence of normal hemoglobin. MetHgb, sulfhemoglobin, and carboxyhemoglobin do not carry oxygen but do not affect PaO_2 levels. Subjects with severe methemoglobinemia may have normal PaO_2 levels and falsely elevated arterial blood gas–calculated oxygen saturation.

Pulse Oximetry

The pulse oximeter is a spectrophotometer measuring light absorbance at only two wavelengths: 660 nm and 940 nm. The device measures the pulsatile and background light absorbance to create a pulse-added absorbance at each wavelength, corresponding primarily to arteriolar hemoglobin contributions to absorbance above the tissue and venous background. Both oxy- and deoxyhemoglobin absorb light at 660 and 940 nm; it is the ratio of the absorbance at the two wavelengths that determines oxygen saturation. A ratio of absorbance (660 nm/940 nm) of 0.43 corresponds to 100% oxygen saturation, an absorbance ratio of 1.0 corresponds to an oxygen saturation of 85%, and a ratio of 3.4 corresponds to 0% (75,76).

The machine can output data only as a percent of oxyhemoglobin; it cannot account for changes in light absorption due to dyshemoglobins. MetHgb absorbs light almost equally at both 660 nm and 940 nm; thus, in the theoretical presence of 100% MetHgb, the absorbance ratio of light at 660 nm over 940 nm is approximately 1.0 and the output of the pulse oximeter reading is approximately 85% oxygen saturation. At low levels of MetHgb, oxygen saturation measured by pulse oximetry is slightly lowered, because MetHgb absorbs proportionally more light at 660 nm than does oxyhemoglobin and increases the 660 nm/940 nm ratio above 0.43. However, when MetHgb levels exceed 30%, the light absorbance ratio reaches a plateau, and expressed oxygen saturation values become stable in the 82% to 86% range, independent of actual MetHgb levels. Only the presence of deoxyhemoglobin can lower the pulse oximeter reading below this range. Thus, the pulse oximeter can detect significant levels of MetHgb as mild to moderate oxygen desaturation.

Co-Oximetry

Co-oximetry measures MetHgb accurately. A co-oximeter is also a spectrophotometer, but, unlike a pulse oximeter, it measures light absorbance at four different wavelengths. These wavelengths correspond directly to the absorbance characteristics of deoxyhemoglobin, oxyhemoglobin, carboxyhemoglobin, and MetHgb (630 nm) (77). Sulfhemoglobin has an absorbance peak at 614 nm, which overlaps at 630 nm and may be reported as MetHgb on older machines. Because oxygen saturation values reflect the contributions of all four types of hemoglobin, oxygen saturation measurements are reliable.

Other Measurement Pitfalls

Other errors are possible in MetHgb measurement, even by co-oximetry (78). If analysis is delayed after sample collection, MetHgb can be enzymatically reduced back to hemoglobin, and the measured MetHgb is lower than actual. Because fluoride can interact with MetHgb, producing falsely low levels, it should not be used in collection tubes. MetHgb in blood collected in anticoagulant tubes containing ethylenediaminetetraacetic acid, potassium oxalate, or lithium heparin is stable for up to 2 hours (79). Storage or freeze thawing of blood samples can affect co-oximetry; only fresh blood samples should be analyzed (80). Excessive amounts of fetal hemoglobin in neonatal blood may cause falsely high MetHgb measurements, varying with the specific co-oximetry instrument (81–83). Hyperlipemia may also produce falsely elevated MetHgb levels (84).

Bedside Tests

In the patient with cyanosis, it is important to distinguish whether deoxyhemoglobin or MetHgb is present. Blood containing high concentrations of MetHgb appears chocolate brown as opposed to the dark red or violet of deoxygenated blood (Fig. 3). A simple bedside test is to place a few drops of the patient's blood on white filter paper. The chocolate brown appearance of MetHgb does not change with time; deoxyhemoglobin appears dark red or violet initially but brightens after exposure to atmospheric oxygen. Gently blowing supplemental oxygen onto the filter paper hastens the reaction with deoxyhemoglobin but does not affect MetHgb.

Potassium Cyanide Test

The potassium cyanide test can distinguish between sulfhemoglobin and MetHgb. MetHgb reacts with a few drops of potassium cyanide (Drabkin's reagent) to form cyanomethemoglobin. Cyanomethemoglobin is bright red, as opposed to the chocolate brown color of MetHgb. In contrast, sulfhemoglobin is an inert substance, does not bind cyanide, and remains dark brown when Drabkin's reagent is added (85).

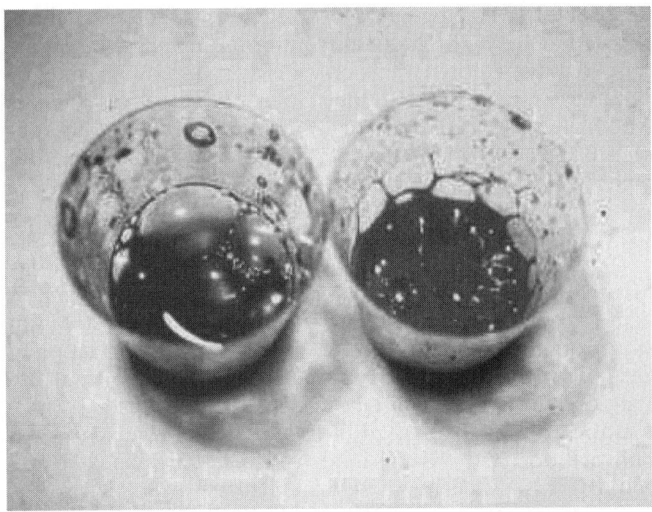

Figure 3. Bedside test for methemoglobinemia. Oxyhemoglobin turns blood bright red after oxygen is bubbled into it; methemoglobin remains dark chocolate brown in appearance.

MANAGEMENT

Initial Care

Once confirmed, life-threatening methemoglobinemia must be treated rapidly. The primary treatment is methylene blue. However, not all patients require the antidotal therapy; many do well with supportive care. Patients with chronic congenital methemoglobinemia can adapt to relatively high levels of MetHgb without overt symptoms except for skin color changes.

The major source of NADH in the RBC is glycolysis. For endogenous reducing enzymes to be effective, glucose must be present. Dextrose is also a key substrate to form NADPH via the hexose monophosphate shunt, which is necessary for methylene blue to be effective. Standard dextrose therapy should be administered to hypoglycemic patients.

Supplemental oxygen should be provided, although the increase in oxygen-carrying capacity is minimal. The role of hyperbaric oxygen in patient management is unclear. Ascorbic acid, a reducing agent, has been used in methemoglobinemia (100 to 500 mg orally or intravenously twice daily), but, because it has a very slow reducing action, it is not considered a clinically important treatment for most patients (86). *N*-Acetylcysteine, a reducing agent, has been shown to reduce MetHgb experimentally but was ineffective in a human volunteer trial (87–89). Cimetidine has been used investigationally to block the formation of the oxidizing metabolites of dapsone (22).

Exchange blood transfusion may rarely be needed in patients with severe, life-threatening methemoglobinemia. Patients who develop severe hemolysis (due to oxidant stress) may require transfusion to correct the lack of functional, oxygen-carrying hemoglobin.

Monitoring

Patients with underlying cardiopulmonary disease or symptoms of ischemia require continuous cardiorespiratory monitoring. Complete blood counts, with reticulocyte determinations, should be obtained serially to monitor for hemolysis and anemia. Hourly determinations of MetHgb concentration may be necessary initially to assess the efficacy of therapy. For patients who have been poisoned with agents causing delayed-onset or recrudescent methemoglobinemia, serial MetHgb measurements may be needed for 3 to 4 days.

Methylene Blue

Methylene blue is addressed in detail in Chapter 63. After an acute exposure, the treatment *action level* is 20% MetHgb in symptomatic patients and 30% in asymptomatic patients. Cyanosis alone does not indicate a need for the antidote; symptoms of hypoxia should also be present. Patients who are symptomatic or have medical problems that compromise oxygen delivery (e.g., heart disease, lung disease, carbon monoxide poisoning, or anemia) should be treated at lower MetHgb levels. Treatment of patients with ischemic heart disease or a prior history of cerebral vascular disease must be individualized. Infants with methemoglobinemia secondary to diarrhea and acidosis may improve with aggressive hydration and bicarbonate to correct the acidosis. However, MetHgb levels greater than 20% should be treated with methylene blue.

Methylene blue comes as a 1% solution (10 mg/ml). The *dose* is 1 to 2 mg/kg (0.1 to 0.2 ml/kg of a 1% solution) or 25 to 50 mg/m^2 intravenously over 3 to 5 minutes. Methylene blue usually alleviates symptoms dramatically and reduces MetHgb levels in less than 1 hour (90). The dose may be repeated at 1 mg/kg if MetHgb does not resolve within 30 minutes but should not exceed a total of 7 mg/kg in any 24-hour period. Interosseous infusion of methylene blue has been used successfully in a 6-week-old infant (91). Methemoglobinemia induced by dapsone has been treated with a continuous infusion (21,24).

FAILURE OF METHYLENE BLUE

Methylene blue therapy may be ineffective in alleviating symptoms. The clinician can use failure to improve with methylene blue infusion as a diagnostic test in considering the differential diagnosis of the patient presenting with evidence of methemoglobinemia (92). In a cyanotic patient with another type of hemoglobin, such as sulfhemoglobinemia, methylene blue does not relieve symptoms.

Other possibilities include either under- or overdosing with methylene blue. Methylene blue is not effective for patients with severe G6PD deficiency. Aniline itself may interfere with the entry of methylene blue into RBC. Recurrence of symptoms despite methylene blue can be explained by inadequate decontamination with activated charcoal or by the toxicokinetics of some agents, such as aniline, benzocaine, or dapsone, which continue to oxidize hemoglobin for hours or even days. These agents are slowly metabolized to reactive metabolites that continue to react with hemoglobin to form MetHgb (93). Continuous infusions of methylene blue, exchange transfusions, and repetitive charcoal have all been used in the management of such patients.

COMPLICATIONS OF METHYLENE BLUE

Paradoxically, methylene blue is actually an oxidant; its metabolite, leukomethylene blue, is the reducing agent. Large doses of the drug (more than 4 mg/kg) may result in proportionately higher levels of the oxidant methylene blue rather than leukomethylene blue (94). The perinatal administration of higher doses of methylene blue given amniotically has been reported to induce hemolysis and methemoglobinemia in non–G6PD-deficient infants (95). Sills and Zinkham reported two neonatal infants given methylene blue who developed Heinz body hemolytic anemia presumably from oxidant stress induced by methylene blue (96).

Patients with G6PD deficiency may develop a Heinz body hemolytic anemia from methylene blue. A second caution is related to the efficacy of the drug in reducing MetHgb in G6PD-deficient patients. The first enzyme in the hexose monophosphate shunt, G6PD is the sole source of NADPH in the RBC. Patients with G6PD deficiency may not produce sufficient NADPH, which is essential to effect the reduction of methylene blue to leukomethylene blue by the enzyme NADPH methemoglobin reductase. This renders methylene blue therapy ineffective for patients with G6PD deficiency who present with methemoglobinemia. Given the increased risk with methylene blue and its potential ineffectiveness, the antidote is relatively contraindicated in those patients with known severe G6PD deficiency, and exchange transfusion should be considered (97).

PITFALLS

The most common error is failure to recognize methemoglobinemia. Co-oximetry should be performed in any cyanotic patient who does not promptly respond to supplemental oxygen. In some hospitals, this test must be specifically requested.

REFERENCES

1. Deleve LD, Kaplowitz N. Glutathione metabolism and its role in hepatotoxicity. *Pharmacol Ther* 1991;52:287–305.
2. Mazor D, Golan E, Philip V, et al. Red blood cell permeability to thiol compounds following oxidative stress. *Eur J Haematol* 1996;57:241–246.
3. Harris JW, Kellermeyer RW. *The red cell.* Cambridge MA: Harvard University Press, 1970.
4. Ogata Y, Goto H, Kimura T, et al. Development of neo red cells (NRC) with the enzymatic reduction system of methemoglobin. *Artif Cells Blood Substit Immobil Biotechnol* 1997;25:417–427.
5. Bernstein SC, Bowman JE, Noche LK. Interaction of sickle cell trait and glucose-6-phosphate dehydrogenase deficiency in Cameroon. *Hum Hered* 1980;30:7–11.
6. Stryer L. *Biochemistry*, 4th ed. New York: WH Freeman & Co., 1995.
7. Finch CA. Treatment of intracellular methemoglobinemia. *Bull N Engl Med Ctr* 1947;6:241–245.
8. Metz EN, Balcerzak SP, Sagon LR. Mechanism of methylene blue stimulation of the hexose monophosphate shunt in the erythrocyte. *J Clin Invest* 1976;58:797–802.
9. Benatti U, Guida L, Grasso M, et al. Hexose monophosphate shunt-stimulated reduction of methemoglobin by divicine. *Arch Biochem Biophys* 1985;242:549–556.
10. Ashmun RA, Hultquist DE, Schultz JS. Kinetic analysis in single, intact cells by microspectrophotometry: evidence for two populations of erythrocytes in an individual heterozygous for glucose-6-phosphate dehydrogenase deficiency. *Am J Hematol* 1986;23:311–316.
11. Hultquist DE, Xu F, Quandt KS, et al. Evidence that NADPH-dependent methemoglobin reductase and administered riboflavin protect tissues from oxidative injury. *Am J Hematol* 1993;42:13–18.
12. Ruffman R, Wendel A. GSH rescue by N-acetylcysteine. *Klin Wochenschr* 1991;69:857–862.
13. Beutler E. Glucose-6-phosphate dehydrogenase deficiency. *N Engl J Med* 1991;324:169–174.
14. Luzatto L, Mehta A. Glucose-6-phosphate dehydrogenase deficiency. In: Stanbury J, Wyngaarden J, Fredrickson D, eds. *Metabolic basis of inherited disease.* New York: McGraw, 1993.
15. Finch CA. Methemoglobin and sulfhemoglobin. *N Engl J Med* 1948:239:470–478.
16. Park CM, Nagel RL. Sulfhemoglobinemia, clinical and molecular aspects. *N Engl J Med* 1984;310:1579–1584.
17. Linakis JG, Shannon M, Woolf A, et al. Recurrent methemoglobinemia after acute dapsone intoxication in a child. *J Emerg Med* 1989;7:477–480.
18. Tingle MD, Mahmud R, Maggs JL, et al. Comparison of the metabolism and toxicity of dapsone in rat, mouse and man. *J Pharmacol Exp Ther* 1997;283:817–823.
19. Tingle MD, Coleman MD, Park BK. An investigation of the role of metabolites, in dapsone-induced methaemoglobinemia using a two compartment in vitro test system. *Br J Clin Pharmacol* 1990;30:829–838.
20. Trillo RA, Aukberg S. Dapsone-induced methemoglobinemia and pulse oximetry. *Anesthesiology* 1992;77:394–398.
21. Berlin G, Brodin B, Hilden JO. Acute dapsone intoxication: a case treated with continuous infusion of methylene blue, forced diuresis, and plasma exchange. *J Toxicol Clin Toxicol* 1985:22:537–540.

22. Coleman MD, Rhodes LE, Scott AK, et al. The use of cimetidine to reduce dapsone dependent methaemoglobinemia in dermatitis herpetiformis. *Br J Clin Pharmacol* 1992:34:244–246.
23. Reigart JR, Trammel HL, Lindsey JM. Repetitive doses of activated charcoal in dapsone poisoning in a child. *J Toxicol Clin Toxicol* 1982–1984;19;1061–1066.
24. Dawson AH, Whyte IM. Management of dapsone poisoning complicated by methaemoglobinemia. *Med Toxicol Adverse Drug Exp* 1989;4:387–392.
25. Reilly TP, Woster PM, Svensson CK. Methemoglobin formation by hydroxylamine metabolites of sulfamethoxazole and dapsone: implications for differences in adverse drug reactions. *J Pharmacol Exp Ther* 1999;288:951–959.
26. Damerois JA, Stoker JM, Aradie JL. Methemoglobinemia after sulfamethoxazole and trimethoprim therapy. *JAMA* 1983;249:590–591.
27. Gavish D, Knobler H, Gottehrer N, et al. Methemoglobinemia, muscle damage, and renal failure complicating phenazopyridine overdose. *Isr J Med Sci* 1986;22:45–47.
28. Avner JR, Henretig FM, McAneney CM. Acquired methemoglobinemia. *Am J Dis Child* 1990;144:1229–1230.
29. De A, Moreira V, De Medeiros BC, et al. Methemoglobinemia secondary to clofazimine treatment for chronic graft-versus-host disease. *Blood* 1998;92:4872–4881.
30. Gibson GR, Hunter JB, Raabe DS, et al. Methemoglobinemia produced by high-dose intravenous nitroglycerin. *Ann Intern Med* 1982;96:615–616.
31. Guertler A, Pearce WA. A prospective evaluation of benzocaine-associated methemoglobinemia in human beings. *Ann Emerg Med* 1994;24:626–630.
32. Collins JF. Methemoglobinemia as a complication of 20% benzocaine spray for endoscopy. *Gastroenterology* 1990;98:211–213.
33. Haggerty RJ. Blue baby due to methemoglobinemia. *N Engl J Med* 1962;267:1303.
34. Dinneen SF, Mohr DN, Fairbanks VF. Methemoglobinemia from topically applied anesthetic spray. *Mayo Clin Proc* 1994;69:886–888.
35. Muchmore EA, Dahl BJ. One blue man with mucositis. *N Engl J Med* 1992;327:133.
36. Gentile DA. Severe methemoglobinemia induced by a topical teething preparation. *Pediatr Emerg Care* 1987;3:176–178.
37. Brisman M, Ljung BML, Otterbom I, et al. Methaemoglobin formation after the use of EMLA cream in term neonates. *Acta Paediatr* 1998;87:1191–1194.
38. McKinney CD, Postiglione KF, Herold DA. Benzocaine-adultered street cocaine in association with methemoglobinemia. *Clin Chem* 1992;38:596–597.
39. Knobeloch L, Goldring J, LeMay W, et al. Prilocaine-induced methemoglobinemia—Wisconsin, 1993. *MMWR Morb Mortal Wkly Rep-CDC* 1994;43:655–657.
40. Duncan PG, Kobrinsky N. Prilocaine-induced methemoglobinemia in a newborn infant. *Anesthesiology* 1983;59:73–76.
41. Nilsson A, Engberg G, Henneberg S, et al. Inverse relationship between age-dependent erythrocyte activity of methemoglobin reductase and prilocaine-induced methemoglobinemia during infancy. *Br J Anesthiol* 1990;64:72–76.
42. Cohen RJ, Sachs JR, Wicker DJ, et al. Methemoglobinemia provoked by malarial chemoprophylaxis in Vietnam. *N Engl J Med* 1968;279:1127–1131.
43. Forsyth RJ, Moulden A. Methemoglobinemia after ingestion of amyl nitrite. *Arch Dis Child* 1991;66:152.
44. Saito T, Takeichi S, Nakajima Y, et al. Experimental studies of methemoglobinemia due to percutaneous absorption of sodium nitrite. *Clin Toxicol* 1997;35:41–48.
45. Ellis M, Hiss Y, Shenkman L. Fatal methemoglobinemia caused by inadvertent contamination of a laxative solution with sodium nitrite. *Isr J Med Sci* 1992;28:289–291.
46. Horne MK, Waterman MR, Simon LM, et al. Methemoglobinemia from sniffing butyl nitrite. *Ann Intern Med* 1979;91:417–418.
47. Kelly KJ, Neu J, Camitta BM, et al. Methemoglobinemia in an infant treated with the folk remedy glycerited asafoetida. *Pediatrics* 1984;73:717–719.
48. Ng LL, Naik RB, Polak A. Paraquat ingestion with methaemoglobinaemia treated with methylene blue. *BMJ* 1982;284:1445–1446.
49. Proudfoot AT. Methaemoglobinaemia due to monolinuron—not paraquat. *BMJ* 1982;285:812.
50. Fairbanks VF. Blue gods, blue oil, and blue people. *Mayo Clin Proc* 1994;69:889–892.
51. Pollack ES, Pollack CV. Incidence of subclinical methemoglobinemia in infants with diarrhea. *Ann Emerg Med* 1994;24:652–656.
52. Yano SS, Danish EH, Hsia YE. Transient methemoglobinemia with acidosis in infants. *J Pediatr* 1982;100:415–418.
53. Lebby T, Roco JJ, Arcinue EL. Infantile methemoglobinemia associated with acute diarrheal illness. *Am J Emerg Med* 1993;11:471–472.
54. Pollack ES, Pollack CV. Incidence of subclinical methemoglobinemia in infants with diarrhea. *Ann Emerg Med* 1994;24:652–656.
55. Gebara BM, Goetting MG. Life-threatening methemoglobinemia in infants with diarrhea and acidosis. *Clin Pediatr* 1994;33(6):370–373.
56. Hjelt K, Lund JT, Scherling B, et al. Methemoglobinaemia among neonates in a neonatal intensive care unit. *Acta Paediatrica* 1995;84:365–370.
57. Smith MA, Shah NR, Lobel JS, et al. Methemoglobinemia and hemolytic anemia associated with *Campylobacter jejuni* enteritis. *Am J Pediatr Hematol Oncol* 1988;10:35–38.
58. Sager S, Grayson GH, Feig SA. Methemoglobin associated with acidosis of probable renal origin. *J Pediatr* 1995;126:59–61.
59. Shugalei IV, L'vov SN, Baev VI, et al. Protective effect of sodium bicarbonate in nitrite ion poisoning. *Ukr Biokhim Zh* 1994;66:109–112(English abst).
60. Klurfeld G, Smith R. Effects of chloride and bicarbonate on methemoglobin reduction in mouse erythrocytes. *Biochem Pharmacol* 1968;17:1067–1077.
61. Hanukoglu A, Danon P. Endogenous methemoglobinemia associated with diarrheal disease in infancy. *J Pediatr Gastroenterol Nutr* 1996;23:1–7.
62. Comly HH. Cyanosis in infants caused by nitrates in well water. *JAMA* 1945;129:112–116.
63. Lukens SN. The legacy of well-water methemoglobinemia. *JAMA* 1987;257:2793–2795.
64. Johnson CJ, Bonrud PA, Dosch TL, et al. Fatal outcome of methemoglobinemia in an infant. *JAMA* 1987;257:2796–2797.
65. Knobeloch L, Krenz K, Anderson H. Methemoglobinemia in an infant—Wisconsin, 1992. *MMWR Morb Mortal Wkly Rep-CDC* 1993;42:217–219.
66. Dusdicker LB, Stumbo PJ, Kross BC, et al. Does increased nitrate ingestion elevate nitrate levels in human milk? *Arch Pediatr Adolesc Med* 1996;150:311–314.
67. Askew GL, Finelli L, Genese CA, et al. Boilerbaisse: an outbreak of methemoglobinemia in New Jersey in 1992. *Pediatrics* 1994;94:381–384.
68. Shih RD, Marcus SM, Genese CA, et al. Methemoglobinemia attributable to nitrate contamination of potable water through boiler fluid additives—New Jersey, 1992 and 1996. *MMWR Morb Mortal Wkly Rep-CDC* 1997;46:202–204.
69. Murray KF, Christie DL. Dietary protein intolerance in infants with transient methemoglobinemia and diarrhea. *J Pediatr* 1993;122:90.
70. Jaffe ER. Enzymopenic hereditary methemoglobinemia: a clinical/biochemical classification. *Blood Cells* 1986;12:81–90.
71. Caudill L, Walbridge J, Kuhn G. Methemoglobinemia as a cause of coma. *Ann Emerg Med* 1990;b19:677–679.
72. Linden CH, Scudder DW, Dowsett RP, et al. Corrosive injury from methacrylic acid in artificial nail primers: another hazard of fingernail products. *Pediatrics* 1998;101:979–984.
73. Blood gas/pH analyzers. *Health Devices* 1995;24:498–501.
74. Else W. Measuring gas in blood. *Nature* 1972;239:47.
75. Ralston AC, Webb RK, Runciman WB. Potential errors in pulse oximetry. III: Effects of interference, dyes, dyshemoglobins and other pigments. *Anaesthesia* 1991;46:291–294.
76. Watcha MF, Connor MT, Hing AV. Pulse oximetry in methemoglobinemia. *Am J Dis Child* 1989;143:845–847.
77. Matthews PJ. Co-oximetry. *Respir Care Clin N Am* 1995;1:47–68.
78. Rausch-Madison S, Mohsenifar Z. Methodologic problems encountered with cooximetry in methemoglobinemia. *Am J Med Sci* 1997;314:203–206.
79. Lim SF, Tan IK. Quantitative determination of methaemoglobin and carboxyhaemoglobin by co-oximetry, and effect of anticoagulants. *Ann Clin Biochem* 1999;36:774–776.
80. Wallace KL, Curry SC. Post collection rise in methemoglobin level in frozen blood specimens. *J Toxicol Clin Toxicol* 2002;40:91–94.
81. de Keijzer MH, Brandts R, Giesendorf BAJ. Comment on the overestimation of methemoglobin concentrations in neonatal samples with the Chiron 800 system co-oximeter module. *Clin Chem* 1999;45:1313–1314.
82. Lynch PLM, Bruns DE, Boyd JC, et al. Chiron 800 system co-oximeter module overestimates methemoglobin concentrations in neonatal samples containing fetal hemoglobin. *Clin Chem* 1998;44:1569–1570.
83. Rausch-Madison S, Mohsenifar Z. Methodologic problems encountered with cooximetry in methemoglobinemia. *Am J Med Sci* 1997;314:203–206.
84. Spurzem JR, Bonekat HW, Shigeoka JW. Factitious methemoglobinemia caused by hyperlipemia. *Chest* 1984;86:84–86.
85. Evelyn KA, Malloy HT. Microdetermination of oxyhemoglobin, methemoglobin and sulfhemoglobin in a single sample of blood. *J Biol Chem* 1938;126:655–662.
86. Dotsch J, Demirakca S, Cryer A, et al. Reduction of NO-induced methemoglobinemia requires extremely high doses of ascorbic acid in vitro. *Intensive Care Med* 1998;24:612–613.
87. Wright RO, Magnani BJ, Shannon MW, et al. N-acetylcysteine reduces methemoglobin in vitro. *Ann Emerg Med* 1996;28:499–503.
88. Wright RO, Woolf AD, Shannon MW, et al. N-acetylcysteine reduces methemoglobin in an in vitro model of glucose-6-phosphate dehydrogenase deficiency. *Acad Emerg Med* 1998;5:225–229.
89. Tanen DA, LoVecchio F, Curry SC. Failure of intravenous N-acetylcysteine to reduce methemoglobin produced by sodium nitrite in human volunteers: a randomized controlled trial. *Ann Emerg Med* 2000;35:369–373.
90. Finch CA. Treatment of intracellular methemoglobinemia. *Bull N Engl Med Ctr* 1947;9:241–245.
91. Herman MI, Chyka PA, Butler AY, et al. Methylene blue by intraosseous infusion for methemoglobinemia. *Ann Emerg Med* 1999;33:111–113.
92. Rosen PJ, Johnson C, McGehee WG, et al. Failure of methylene blue treatment in toxic methemoglobinemia. *Ann Intern Med* 1971;75:83–86.
93. Harvey JW, Keitt AS. Studies of the efficacy and potential hazards of methylene blue therapy in aniline-induced methaemoglobinaemia. *Br J Haem* 1983;54:29–41.
94. Kirsch IR, Cohen HJ. Heinz body hemolytic anemia from the use of methylene blue in neonates. *J Pediatr* 1980;96:276–278.
95. Crooks J. Hemolytic jaundice in a neonate after intra-amniotic injection of methylene blue. *Arch Dis Child* 1982;57:872.
96. Sills MR, Zinkham WH. Methylene blue-induced Heinz body hemolytic anemia. *Arch Pediatr Adolesc Med* 1994;148:306–310.
97. Harrison MR. Toxic methemoglobinemia. A case of acute nitrobenzene and aniline poisoning treated by exchange transfusion. *Anaesthesia* 1977;32:270–272.

CHAPTER 22

Multiple Chemical Sensitivity and Idiopathic Environmental Intolerance

Frederick Fung

OVERVIEW

The medical toxicologist is frequently involved in the evaluation and management of low-level toxic exposure. Most exposures are well below the accepted thresholds and limits for causing potential adverse health effects or long-term impairment.

The human environment is filled with chemicals. Our food, air, water, clothes, books, and countless other things contain chemicals. It is estimated that more than 4 million distinct chemical entities are registered currently, and this number is growing at an average rate of 6000 per week (1). The growing awareness of chemicals has created a wide spectrum of attitudes and understandings toward the impact of chemicals on our physical and mental health. One response is the notion of adverse health effects secondary to low-level chemical exposure leading to a phenomenon termed *multiple chemical sensitivity* (MCS).

The definition and even the existence of MCS are highly controversial. Whenever a new disease is proposed, it is important to use a case definition so that the etiology, differential diagnosis, treatment, and prognosis may be properly defined in research efforts. Randolph proposed several decades ago that patients became ill from exposure to low-level, human-made chemicals, resulting in a new form of chemical sensitivity (2). Over the years, this condition has been called *allergic toxemia, cerebral allergy, chemical sensitivity, ecologic illness, environmental illness, immune system deregulation, total allergy syndrome, twentieth century disease, universal allergy*, and *chemical acquired immunodeficiency syndrome*, among several others.

In the past, clinical ecologists defined *MCS* as a syndrome of toxic effects on the immune system caused by environmental chemicals, which then generated multiple allergies to other chemicals or foods. The American Academy of Environmental Medicine uses the term *environmentally triggered illnesses* instead of *MCS*. Environmentally triggered illnesses have a lengthy and similar description (3). Ever-changing and poorly defined case definitions have hindered the investigation and research of this condition. Cullen proposed a case definition in 1987 that became widely accepted: "An acquired disorder characterized by recurrent symptoms, referable to multiple organ systems, occurring in response to demonstrable exposure to many chemically unrelated compounds at doses far below those established in the general population to cause biologically harmful effects. No single widely accepted test of physiologic function can be shown to correlate with symptoms" (4). Other similar case definitions have been proposed. MCS syndrome has several characteristics: (a) It is acquired after an environmental exposure that may have produced minimal objective evidence of health effects; (b) the symptoms typically wax and wane, include multiorgan and multisystem effects, and may vary in response to other environmental stimuli; (c) the symptoms occur in relationship to low levels of exposure without objective evidence of organ damage or abnormal tests to account for the symptoms; and (d) no known cure exists.

The definition and existence of MCS remain highly contested issues not only in the medical community, but also in insurance, public, media, political, and legal arenas. The prevalence and incidence of MCS are largely unknown. There may be more female patients than male patients who claim to have this condition. A review of eight published studies indicates that 70% to 88% of MCS patients are female (5). However, its significance has not been fully evaluated. Despite our ignorance regarding the natural history, pathophysiology, diagnostic tests, or treatment modalities, MCS has been accepted in numerous states as a compensable illness or injury under workers' compensation laws and as a recognized disability under the Americans with Disabilities Act. As a result, compensation to individuals diagnosed with MCS and accommodation of their home and work environments have been imposed despite the lack of convincing evidence that these measures improve symptoms.

PATHOPHYSIOLOGY

The term *MCS* should more properly be replaced by the term *idiopathic environmental intolerances* (IEI) (6). The use of *IEI* is considered more appropriate because *sensitivity* may be construed inappropriately as an allergic or hypersensitivity pathophysiologic mechanism. Because the scientific basis for an allergic mechanism has not been established, the word *sensitivity* is not appropriate. Additionally, intolerance to electromagnetic fields and foods other than chemicals has been described. The relationship between symptoms and exposure has not been proved. MCS has not been recognized as a clinically defined disease entity with accepted pathophysiologic mechanisms, validated diagnostic criteria, or effective treatment modalities in the position statements by numerous professional societies (6,7–12). Consensus has not emerged as to whether MCS is a new illness, has a biologic basis, diagnostic criteria, therapeutic modalities, or a definable prognosis.

There are multiple hypotheses and proposed mechanisms for IEI (MCS), although none has been widely accepted on the basis of scientific evidence. Proponents typically deemphasize the threshold and dose–response relationship, a common tenet of toxicology. Because science relies on the rejection of the null hypothesis, it is incumbent on the proponents of MCS and IEI to demonstrate a specific disease mechanism or pathophysiology of this condition using the scientific method. A plausible scientific rationale cannot be demonstrated by experimental science and scientific methodology at this time.

Five major theories have been proposed.

1. The *immunologic/allergic theory* is based on the concept of "sensitivity," invoking the rationale that a patient with MCS will experience symptoms on exposure to very low concentrations of chemicals, foods, or drugs. The allergy theory relies on abnormal immune tests among MCS

patients. However, there are interpretation problems and normal variations in the immune test results (13). These tests have also lacked predictability and discrimination between control subjects and alleged MCS patients. Simon et al. showed no significant differences between MCS and control subjects in the prevalence of "positive" immune tests and limited reproducibility during submission of duplicate samples (13).

2. The *toxicologic theory* postulates that MCS patients have experienced a chemical exposure that produced respiratory mucosal irritation, nonspecific inflammation, and results in persistent amplification of the nonspecific immune response to low-level irritants. Such irritant symptoms might be mediated through C fiber neurons and the release of various cell mediators including cytokines. Although this is a plausible explanation for pulmonary complaints, this theory does not account for multisystem complaints. There are no controlled human studies to support that nonspecific inflammation persists after cessation of the chemical exposure.
3. The *neurogenic theory* states that chemical sensitivity may be due to "neuronal-sensitization," suggesting that on exposure to chemicals at low levels, interactions can occur between chemicals and neurons, especially in the limbic and endocrine systems. Because there are multiple neuronal interconnections in the limbic system, exposure to chemicals at low levels may produce multiorgan symptoms in addition to respiratory tract irritation symptoms. It has also been proposed that single high-level or intermittent low-level chemical exposures may produce "limbic kindling." This suggests that electrical or chemical stimuli that do not cause a response initially can eventually induce a response through subsequent repetitive, intermittent stimulation. This phenomenon has been demonstrated in animal studies of seizure disorder; however, these studies used relatively large doses of medications and chemicals rather than low-level exposures. No human-controlled experiments have shown that this phenomenon exists, nor has this theory been borne out by epidemiologic studies.
4. The *behavioral conditioning and stress theory* proposes that MCS is a behavioral-conditioned response to odor. A strong odiferous chemical irritant can cause a direct and unconditioned physiologic response. Subsequently, the odor of irritants at much lower concentrations may cause a conditioned response involving similar symptoms. Although this is not entirely pavlovian conditioning, MCS patients have features similar to conditioning-related phenomena (14). The concept of risk perception is related. If an individual perceives harm associated with an odor, this could exacerbate a psychophysiologic reaction to the smell.

   MCS patients have a high prevalence rate of psychiatric diagnoses, such as depression, anxiety, or somatization, although it is not clear whether psychiatric conditions cause MCS or whether they are simply associated with MCS. MCS patients challenged with triggering substances showed clinical manifestations consistent with anxiety and hyperventilation (15). Binkley used normal saline and sodium lactate to reproduce symptoms in MCS patients, suggesting that MCS may have a neurobiologic component similar to a panic disorder (16). Although there are reports of an increased frequency of symptoms of depression, anxiety, somatization, obsessive-compulsive disorder, other personality disorders, or panic attacks, currently, there is no evidence to suggest that MCS and psychiatric illness are the results of a common neurobiologic mechanism.
5. A final theory proposes that MCS is an *illness of the belief system* (17). Patients labeled with MCS tend to participate in support groups and visit clinicians who believe in MCS as a disease entity. There is a network of clinicians, attorneys, journals, newsletters, and hotlines to support and reinforce a belief in MCS as a disease entity. The medical toxicologist should be aware that the "medical subculture" of MCS does not trust the conventional health care and disability systems. Frequently, these patients view themselves as victims of modern medicine.

DIAGNOSIS

MCS (IEI) is a diagnosis of exclusion. Other traditional medical conditions should be evaluated. The differential diagnosis includes allergic diseases, psychiatric disorders, sick building syndrome, organic solvent syndrome, and specific medical conditions (Table 1).

The symptoms and signs of MCS patients are myriad and diverse. They may present with central nervous system, respiratory, mucous membrane irritation, or gastrointestinal symptoms. Commonly reported symptoms include fatigue, difficulty with concentration, depression, memory loss, general weakness, dizziness, headache, joint pain, muscle pain, constipation, diarrhea, itchy and runny nose, skin rash, and various irritations. Typically, the symptoms start after a known precipitating incident of chemical exposure. Approximately 30% to 40% of MCS patients do not have a known chemical exposure incident, or they developed their symptoms before the exposure occurred. Over time, symptoms may be exacerbated in response to an increasing variety of low-level stimuli, including smell and chemicals that cannot be routinely detected, as well as some foods and drugs. The importance of the history and physical examination in MCS is to diagnose an underlying medical condition that is due to significant toxic exposure or a different disease process.

There are no specific diagnostic tests to establish MCS syndrome. Basic laboratory tests should include complete blood cell count, chemistry panel, and specific endocrine tests whenever indicated to evaluate alternative diagnoses. It is also important to obtain prior medical and treatment records before initiating an extensive laboratory investigation.

Neuropsychiatric testing is not recommended routinely for a toxicology evaluation. If neuropsychiatric testing is to be performed, its limitations should be kept in mind. Neuropsychiatric assessment has low specificity, and there is no biomarker for IEI. Therefore, it is nearly impossible to determine if neurobehavioral findings are related to chemical exposure. Premorbid neuropsychiatric status for IEI patients is usually unknown, making evaluation uncertain as to how much is truly attributed to the exposure. Neuropsychiatric evaluation cannot be used to diagnose IEI, but rather to rule out treatable causes of the symptoms experienced by the patient.

Challenge testing refers to a controlled or uncontrolled environment wherein a patient inhales a low concentration of the offending agent. Such challenge testing is not recommended at this time. There are no controlled studies to demonstrate its sensitivity, specificity, and predictive values. Furthermore, challenge studies with self-identified triggers in IEI patients demonstrate a psychogenic factor in this condition (18). Other tests without proven value that are not recommended for routine toxicologic evaluation of MCS patients include the electroencephalogram, brain electrical activity mapping, brain stem evoked potential, positron emission tomography, as well as serum or blood levels for trace organic chemicals, pesticides,

TABLE 1. Differential diagnosis of multiple chemical sensitivity (MCS)

Differential diagnosis	Pathogenesis	Onset	Symptoms	Diagnostic tests	Management
MCS, idiopathic environmental intolerances	Various hypotheses: immune; toxicologic; neurogenic; behavioral, belief system.	Typically with a history of exposure to an odiferous substance.	Subjective symptoms that wax and wane, neurologic, gastrointestinal, dermal.	No specific diagnostic tests. Immune cytometry, body scans, and so forth are not recommended.	Education and reassurance. Behavioral therapy may help.
Allergic diseases	Type I, immunoglobulin E; type II, cytotoxic; type III, antigen–antibody reaction; type IV, delayed or cell-mediated immune responses.	A sensitization phase is followed by subsequent exposure to the allergen. Symptoms begin within minutes to hours.	Depends on type of allergic reaction; typically respiratory, skin, and gastrointestinal.	Skin prick test, radioallergosorbent test, pulmonary function, nasal smear.	Allergen avoidance, antihistamines, inhaled or nasal corticosteroids, and immunotherapy.
Psychiatric disorders	Serotoninergic, adrenergic, cholinergic, and other neurotransmitter dysfunctions.	Acute or insidious symptom onset depending on the disease.	Depends on the disease.	Psychiatric evaluation.	Pharmachotherapy and behavioral therapy.
Sick building syndrome (see Chapter 31)	Chemical and microbial hypotheses; inadequate fresh air, and so forth.	Insidious.	Nonspecific; typically headache, rash, mucous membrane irritation.	No specific tests. Building-related illness should be ruled out.	Symptoms typically resolve after staying away from the building at issue.
Organic (brain) solvent syndrome	Unclear, lipid-soluble solvents may produce subtle damage to neurons and myelin sheaths.	Insidious. Requires years of exposure to significant levels of organic solvent, such as toluene, xylene, and petrochemicals.	Neurologic fatigue, loss of concentration, memory loss.	Psychological test batteries, electroencephalogram, computed tomography scan of the brain, magnetic resonance imaging.	Supportive. A controversial condition not widely accepted as a true disease entity.

and metals. There is no proven correlation between viral or other immune antibodies and a diagnosis of MCS (13).

POTENTIAL COMPLICATIONS

Patients labeled with MCS (IEI) usually experience unpredictable and episodic symptoms. These symptoms are typically self-limiting with no long-term physical complications. However, it is important to rule out other treatable medical conditions that may produce symptoms of MCS syndrome.

MANAGEMENT

The primary treatment is that of the underlying condition, if one is found. If not, treatment is symptomatic and supportive, with careful attention to the social and psychological aspects of the condition. It is important to remember that MCS patients are usually skeptical of conventional medicine. Therefore, the patient should be treated with respect and empathy. MCS patients should be managed based on a "care rather than cure" approach, as well as a "treat the person and not the environment" approach (19). It is important to acknowledge that the patients experience effects that are real but not fatal. It is paramount to encourage the patient to return to the highest possible level of social and personal function.

There is no known specific *antidote* for MCS syndrome, although a wide spectrum of treatment strategies has been suggested, including rotating diet, antifungal medications, strict avoidance of all exposures to synthetic chemicals, and so forth. These modalities are not supported by controlled clinical trials (6,20). It may be prudent in selected cases to advise a symptomatic patient to avoid known irritant materials and chemicals, even when such exposure is not considered injurious or hazardous. This measure would avoid potential psychological reactions secondary to perceived toxic exposure. The rationale for recommending avoidance must be made clear to the patient, so the patient understands that the physician has not concluded that a toxic reaction has, in fact, occurred.

After rapport has been established, the patient should also be advised to avoid unsubstantiated treatment modalities. It is useful to spend adequate time with the patient periodically, but each encounter should have a focused purpose to avoid off-tangent discussion. For example, the patient could be evaluated and counseled monthly to discuss one or two issues that are most important for the patient. This provides proper education and reassurance about the condition and also provides scientific information concerning MCS from a layperson's perspective. Because isolation from all chemicals is not possible, the patient should be encouraged to expand his or her social contacts to avoid further anxiety and depression. Multivitamins, antioxidants, desensitization shots, heat depuration, and fat purification are unproved and should be avoided.

Most medical toxicologists do not have time to educate or discuss the details of MCS with their patients. Therefore, it may be necessary to manage MCS patients with a primary care provider. However, it is critical to confer with the primary care physician and share the philosophy of management before comanaging MCS patients. Psychiatric evaluation and referral may be necessary when psychiatric disorders are suspected. MCS has been considered a disability under the Americans with Disabilities Act and has been covered by various state workers' compensation laws. At this time, behavioral techniques appear to be the most effective treatment approach for MCS patients.

PITFALLS

There are occasional misdiagnoses among MCS patients. The most common are hypothyroidism, connective tissue disorders and hypocalcemia secondary to other medical conditions, and psychiatric disorders.

REFERENCES

1. Maugh TH. Chemicals: how many are there? *Science* 1978;199:162.
2. Randolph TG. The specific adaptation syndrome. *J Lab Clin Med* 1956;48:934.
3. American Academy of Environmental Medicine. Environmentally triggered illnesses (ETI). http://www.aaem.com. Accessed March 7, 2002.
4. Cullen MR. Workers with multiple chemical sensitivities: an overview. *Occup Med* 1987;2:657–658.
5. Sparks PJ, Daniell W, Black DW, et al. Multiple chemical sensitivity syndrome: a clinical perspective. *J Occup Med* 1994;36:718–730.
6. American Academy of Allergy and Immunology. Position statement on idiopathic environmental intolerances. *J Allergy Clin Immunol* 1999;103:36–40.
7. American Medical Association. AMA Council on Scientific Affairs. Position statement on clinical ecology. *JAMA* 1992;268:3465–3467.
8. American College of Physicians. Position statement on clinical ecology. *Ann Intern Med* 1989;111:168–178.
9. American College of Occupational and Environmental Medicine. Position statement. Multiple chemical sensitivity: idiopathic environmental intolerances. *J Occup Environ Med* 1999;41:940–941.
10. American Academy of Allergy and Immunology. Executive Committee of the American Academy of Allergy and Immunology: clinical ecology. *J Allergy Clin Immunol* 1986;78:269–271.
11. American Lung Association, Environmental Protection Agency, Consumer Product Safety Commission, and American Medical Association. *Indoor air pollution, an introduction for health professionals.* US Government Printing Office Publication No. 1994-525-217-813-22. New York: 1994:20.
12. California Medical Association. Clinical ecology-critical appraisal. *West J Med* 1986;146:145–149.
13. Simon G, Daniell W, Stockbridge H, et al. Immunologic, psychological and neuropsychological factors in multiple chemical sensitivity: a controlled study. *Ann Intern Med* 1993;119:97–103.
14. Giardino ND, Lehrer PM. Behavioral conditioning and idiopathic environmental intolerance. *Occup Med* 2000;15:519–528.
15. Leznoff A. Clinical aspects of allergic disease: provocation challenges in patients with MCS. *J Allergy Clin Immunol* 1997;99:438–442.
16. Binkley KE, Krutcher S. Panic response to sodium lactate infusion in patients with multiple chemical sensitivity syndrome. *J Allergy Clin Immunol* 1997;99:570–574.
17. Staudenmayer H. Idiopathic environmental intolerances (IEI): myth and reality. *Toxicol Lett* 2001;120:333–342.
18. Leznoff A, Binkley KE. Idiopathic environmental intolerance: results of challenge studies. *Occup Med* 2000;15:529–537.
19. Fung F. Multiple chemical sensitivity and environmental toxicology. *Allergy Proc* 1991;12:81–84.
20. Magill MK, Surada A. Multiple chemical sensitivity syndrome. *Am Fam Physician* 1998; 58:721–728.

CHAPTER 23

Neuroleptic Malignant Syndrome

Ian MacGregor Whyte and Gregory L. Carter

OVERVIEW

Neuroleptic malignant syndrome (NMS) is an uncommon syndrome of adverse effects (fever, autonomic dysfunction, and extrapyramidal movement disorder) classically attributed to neuroleptic drugs. NMS has also been reported to occur in relation to other centrally acting dopamine-blocking drugs on withdrawal of dopamine agonist drugs and possibly on exposure to other medications. Knowledge about this syndrome continues to accumulate, although controversies remain. NMS is difficult to diagnose because it is uncommon and because the mild forms of the syndrome or early symptoms may fluctuate as well as mimic many other disorders. There are no laboratory tests or scans that are diagnostic. It remains a clinical diagnosis.

The first description of NMS was French (*syndrom malin*), reported in 1960, and occurred as an adverse effect of haloperidol (1). The first English paper describing NMS was published in 1968 (2). The true initial reports may be earlier. Lethal catatonia existed well before the availability of neuroleptic agents. Its description is nearly identical to that of NMS. Debate continues as to the delineation of NMS from lethal catatonia on clinical and pathophysiologic grounds. There is also debate concerning the delineation of malignant hyperthermia from NMS, although this is now clearer with advances in the understanding of the receptor physiology of malignant hyperthermia (3).

NMS is a drug-induced disorder. Incidence in patients on neuroleptic therapy is estimated as 0.02% to 3.23% (4). NMS occurs predominantly in the setting of drugs that block dopamine receptors in the central nervous system but may also occur after abrupt cessation or reduction of dopamine agonists in patients with idiopathic parkinsonism. It is more likely to occur with exposure to high-potency neuroleptic drugs (e.g., haloperidol) but has been reported in low-potency neuroleptic drugs (e.g., chlorpromazine) and the atypical neuroleptic drugs (e.g., clozapine, risperidone, olanzapine) (5,6). Other drug groups with dopamine-blocking activity, such as antiemetics (e.g., metoclopramide), are also a potential cause. Most cyclic antidepressants [e.g., amitriptyline (7)] and drugs with serotonin reuptake activity [e.g., fluoxetine, venlafaxine (4)] have also had cases reported.

PATHOPHYSIOLOGY

NMS is caused by a relative lack of dopamine at central postsynaptic receptors (4). This may result from dopamine receptor blockade or from inadequate dopamine production. Supporting evidence for this concept includes the occurrence of NMS on exposure to neuroleptic drugs whose prime mechanism of action is dopamine blockade (4). NMS can also occur during therapy with other drugs with dopamine-blocking action [e.g., metoclopramide (8)] and on sudden withdrawal of dopamine therapy in parkinsonian patients (4). When present, NMS usually responds to dopamine agonists (9).

Dopamine-blocking drugs with a high risk of NMS have high binding affinity for dopamine D_2 receptors in the striatum. Atypical antipsychotics (e.g., clozapine) with lower affinities for dopamine D_2 are less likely to cause NMS but may still do so (5,6).

Serotonin can be an inhibitory neurotransmitter on presynaptic dopaminergic neurons, with resultant decrease in dopamine release with increasing serotonin concentrations (10,11). This mechanism may explain observed episodes of NMS during therapy with selective serotonin reuptake inhibitors and some tricyclic antidepressants.

DIAGNOSIS

Several factors are associated with a higher risk of developing NMS (12,13). It is more common in young male patients with greater degrees of psychomotor agitation (particularly with affective disorders), especially if they are dehydrated. Factors related to the use of neuroleptic drugs include a large dose of neuroleptics in the first 24 hours of treatment, a maximum dose in any 24-hour period greater than 600 mg of chlorpromazine (or the equivalent), and depot neuroleptic administration. Patients requiring restraint or seclusion are at greater risk, and there is an association with history of electroconvulsive therapy. Concurrent therapy with lithium and antidepressants increases risk, and it is more common in patients with preexisting brain damage.

NMS may occur from a single dose of a dopamine-blocking drug, but in these cases, there does not seem to be a dose response present, and NMS is extremely rare as a presenting feature of acute neuroleptic drug overdose.

The *Diagnostic and Statistical Manual of Mental Disorders*, 4th ed. (*DSM-IV*) outlines the diagnostic and research criteria for NMS (Table 1) (14). A more useful operational definition requires some essential criteria and then makes the diagnosis based on the presence of major criteria with supporting evidence from some minor features. Delirium is almost always present at some stage and is usually a hypoactive delirium, but delirium is not essential to make the diagnosis. Fever is a major criterion, although cases of normal temperature and hypothermic variants have been reported. The presence of sepsis to account for fever should be considered; however, the presence of sepsis does not exclude NMS, as they can occur simultaneously. For example, an episode of infection may precipitate an episode of NMS. The diagnosis is also supported by a therapeutic response to a dopamine agonist (e.g., bromocriptine).

TABLE 1. Diagnostic and research criteria for neuroleptic malignant syndrome

***DSM-IV* definition of neuroleptic malignant syndrome** (14)

Criterion A. The development of severe muscle rigidity and elevated temperature associated with the use of neuroleptic medication.

Criterion B. Two (or more) of the following
- Diaphoresis
- Dysphagia
- Tremor
- Incontinence
- Changes in level of consciousness ranging from confusion to coma
- Mutism
- Tachycardia
- Elevated or labile BP
- Leukocytosis
- Laboratory evidence of muscle injury (e.g., elevated creatine kinase level)

Criterion C. The symptoms in criteria A and B are not due to another substance (e.g., phencyclidine) or a neurologic or other general medical condition (e.g., viral encephalitis).

Criterion D. The symptoms in criteria A and B are not better accounted for by a mental disorder (e.g., mood disorder with catatonic features).

Alternative diagnostic criteria for neuroleptic malignant syndrome

Essential criteria
- Recent or current therapy with dopamine-blocking drug (a neuroleptic or other drug, such as metoclopramide)

  Or

- Recently stopped treatment with a dopamine agonist (e.g., L-dopa)

Major criteria (all three must be present within a 24-hr period)
- Fever >37.5°C
- Autonomic dysfunction, defined as the presence of two or more of the following:
  - Hypertension or labile BP
    - Systolic BP >30 mm Hg above baseline, *or* diastolic BP >20 mm Hg above baseline, *or* variability of >30 mm Hg systolic BP or >20 mm Hg diastolic BP between readings
  - Tachycardia (pulse >30 beats/min above baseline)
  - Diaphoresis (intense—may be episodic)
  - Incontinence
  - Tachypnea (>25 breaths/min)
- Extrapyramidal features, defined as the presence of two or more of the following:
  - Bradykinesia
  - Lead-pipe or cogwheel rigidity
  - Resting tremor
  - Sialorrhea
  - Dysphagia
  - Dysarthria/mutism
- Additional features (which support but are not required to make the diagnosis) include
  - Increase in creatine kinase
  - Altered sensorium/delirium
  - Leucocytosis >15,000 × 10^9/L
  - Low serum iron (20)

BP, blood pressure; *DSM-IV, Diagnostic and Statistical Manual of Mental Disorders*, 4th ed.

Differential Diagnosis

Perhaps the most common differential diagnostic situation is a neuroleptic-induced extrapyramidal syndrome in a patient with concurrent sepsis (e.g., urinary tract infection exhibiting fever), tachycardia, and other autonomic signs, in addition to leukocytosis and sometimes delirium. Moreover, the presence of a cause for sepsis does not exclude the presence of NMS, having been precipitated by the infection.

The condition may also be confused with serotonin toxicity. NMS and serotonin toxicity have some clinical features in common: fever, autonomic hyperactivity, muscle rigidity, and delirium. In fact, they are two different conditions that have very different etiologies (serotonin excess vs. dopamine blockade) and are usually distinguished by the history of medication exposure, physical examination, and treatment response. Serotonin excess (serotonin toxicity) has a relatively rapid onset after initiating a serotonergic drug or increasing the dose. It responds to serotonin receptor blockade with drugs, such as cyproheptadine and chlorpromazine. Dopamine blockade (NMS) has a relatively slow onset after a neuroleptic drug and responds to dopamine agonists, such as bromocriptine. Clinical features that distinguish between the two conditions are provided in Table 2 of Chapter 24.

The differential diagnosis of NMS also includes numerous causes of fever, leukocytosis, and rigidity. In a patient with fever, stiff neck, and altered mentation (all seen in NMS), meningitis must be ruled out. Other etiologies to consider are primary central nervous system disorders, including infections (viral encephalitis, acquired immunodeficiency syndrome, postinfectious encephalomyelitis), tumors, cerebrovascular accidents, trauma, seizures, and major psychoses (lethal catatonia). Also important to consider are systemic disorders, including infections, metabolic conditions, endocrinopathies (thyroid storm, pheochromocytoma), autoimmune disease (systemic lupus erythematosus), heat stroke, and some toxins (carbon monoxide, tetanus, strychnine).

Diagnostic Tests

Although there is no diagnostic test for the presence of NMS, numerous tests may assist in excluding other conditions. These typically include a complete blood cell count, serum electrolytes, blood urea nitrogen, creatine kinase, cultures of blood, urine and cerebrospinal fluid, and serum iron. In addition, less common tests to evaluate other infectious, malignant, central nervous system, or endocrine disorders may be needed.

MANAGEMENT

High-risk patients should have vital signs and episodes of diaphoresis recorded regularly. On suspecting the diagnosis, all dopamine-blocking drugs must be withdrawn (or previously withdrawn dopaminergic therapy restarted).

Supportive care is important, and the maintenance of adequate hydration is essential. If hyperpyrexia is extreme or ambient temperatures very high, cooling strategies can be used (Chapter 38). Dysphagia may require appropriate feeding techniques. Pulmonary aspiration should be prevented when possible or treated promptly if it occurs. Rhabdomyolysis with secondary renal failure may occur in severe cases, as can cardiac dysrhythmias and intravascular coagulation syndromes. Nonpharmacologic management of delirium should be used for the delirious patient (Chapter 15).

Bromocriptine, a dopamine agonist, is very effective if the patient can take oral therapy (9,15,16). It can be given by nasogastric tube. The dose range is 2.5 mg every 8 hours up to 5 mg every 4 hours. Titration of dosage to clinical response is important for the individual patient. Dosages of 50 mg/day are occasionally needed. Clinical response should be rapid, with resolution of the fever and autonomic instability within 24 hours and clear improvement in the extrapyramidal features within 48 hours. Resolution of the delirium may take several days longer than the resolution of the autonomic and extrapyramidal symptoms. Bromocriptine should be continued for 7 to 10 days after resolution of NMS, with tapering over 1 to 2 weeks more. Even longer therapy may be appropriate when the causal agent is a depot formulation of a neuroleptic.

In the patient with extreme rigidity, very high fever (greater than 40°C), or inability to tolerate oral treatment, dantrolene in a dose of 2 to 3 mg/kg should be used until oral bromocriptine can be started (17). If these pharmacologic measures fail, the diagnosis should be reassessed, and if NMS or lethal catatonia is still likely, electroconvulsive therapy has been used successfully (18,19).

REFERENCES

1. Delay J, Pichot P, Lemperiere T, et al. Un neuroleptique majeur non-phenothiazine et non-reserpine, l'haloperidol, dans la traitment des psychoses. *Ann Med Psychol* 1960;118:145–152.
2. Delay J, Deniker P. Drug-induced pyramidal symptoms. In: Vibken PJ, Bruyn GW, eds. *Handbook of clinical neurology*, 6th ed. New York: Elsevier North Holland Inc., 1968:248–266.
3. Wappler F, Fiege M, Schulte am Esch J. Pathophysiological role of the serotonin system in malignant hyperthermia. *Br J Anaesth* 2001;87(5):794–798.
4. Velamoor VR. Neuroleptic malignant syndrome. Recognition, prevention and management. *Drug Saf* 1998;19(1):73–82.
5. Hasan S, Buckley P. Novel antipsychotics and the neuroleptic malignant syndrome: a review and critique. *Am J Psychiatry* 1998;155(8):1113–1116.
6. Velamoor VR. Atypical antipsychotics and neuroleptic malignant syndrome. *Can J Psychiatry* 2001;46(9):865–866.
7. Baca L, Martinelli L. Neuroleptic malignant syndrome: a unique association with a tricyclic antidepressant. *Neurology* 1990;40(11):1797–1798.
8. Friedman LS, Weinrauch LA, D'Elia JA. Metoclopramide-induced neuroleptic malignant syndrome. *Arch Intern Med* 1987;147(8):1495–1497.
9. Mueller PS, Vester JW, Fermaglich J. Neuroleptic malignant syndrome. Successful treatment with bromocriptine. *JAMA* 1983;249(3):386–388.
10. Millan MJ, Dekeyne A, Gobert A. Serotonin (5-HT)2C receptors tonically inhibit dopamine (DA) and noradrenaline (NA), but not 5-HT, release in the frontal cortex in vivo. *Neuropharmacology* 1998;37(7):953–955.
11. Muramatsu M, Tamaki-Ohashi J, Usuki C, et al. 5-HT2 antagonists and minaprine block the 5-HT-induced inhibition of dopamine release from rat brain striatal slices. *Eur J Pharmacol* 1988;153(1):89–95.
12. Jain KK. *Neuroleptic malignant syndrome. Drug-induced neurological disorders.* Seattle: Hogrefe & Huber Publishers, 1994:347–356.
13. Sachdev P, Mason C, Hadzi-Pavlovic D. Case-control study of neuroleptic malignant syndrome. *Am J Psychiatry* 1997;154(8):1156–1158.
14. American Psychiatric Association. *Diagnostic and statistical manual of mental disorders*, 4th ed. Washington, DC: American Psychiatric Association, 1994.
15. Janati A, Webb RT. Successful treatment of neuroleptic malignant syndrome with bromocriptine. *South Med J* 1986;79(12):1567–1571.
16. Schvehla TJ, Herjanic M. Neuroleptic malignant syndrome, bromocriptine, and anticholinergic drugs [letter]. *J Clin Psychiatry* 1988;49(7):283–284.
17. Ward A, Chaffman MO, Sorkin EM. Dantrolene. A review of its pharmacodynamic and pharmacokinetic properties and therapeutic use in malignant hyperthermia, the neuroleptic malignant syndrome and an update of its use in muscle spasticity. *Drugs* 1986;32(2):130–168.
18. Greenberg RS. Electroconvulsive therapy in treating neuroleptic malignant syndrome. *Convuls Ther* 1986;2(1):61–62.
19. Addonizio G, Susman VL. ECT as a treatment alternative for patients with symptoms of neuroleptic malignant syndrome. *J Clin Psychiatry* 1987;48(3):102–105.

CHAPTER 24

Serotonin Toxicity/Syndrome

Ian MacGregor Whyte

Serotonin toxicity is often known as *serotonin syndrome*. It is not, in fact, a discrete syndrome but represents a spectrum of serotonergic effects, many of which occur at therapeutic doses of a serotonergic agent, whereas some are only seen with toxicity (1–3). For many years, it was believed that serotonin toxicity was mediated through 5-hydroxytryptamine (5-HT_1) receptors (4). It now appears that the predominant receptors involved in toxicity in humans are 5-HT_2 and that 5-HT_1 receptors are responsible for the therapeutic effects of the selective serotonin reuptake inhibitors (SSRIs) (5,6).

Severe serotonin toxicity may be life-threatening with hyperthermia, increased muscle tone that may lead to respiratory failure, and secondary rhabdomyolysis (7). These features should be preventable with sedation, good supportive care, and judicious use of 5-HT_2–blocking agents. Occasionally, more aggressive intervention with muscle paralysis, supported ventilation, and active cooling measures may be required.

Oates first suggested serotonin excess as a medical condition in 1960 (8). His observations involved patients who developed symptoms after receiving tryptophan while on therapy with a monoamine oxidase (MAO) inhibitor. In the 1980s, animal work indicated that the previously documented interaction between meperidine (pethidine) and the irreversible MAO inhibitors was due to excess serotonin. Insel et al. are often quoted as describing the serotonin syndrome (9), although the features had clearly been described previously (8).

PATHOPHYSIOLOGY

Serotonin (5-HT) is a neurotransmitter involved in multiple states, including aggression, pain, sleep, appetite, anxiety, depression, migraine, and emesis. In the human, 5-HT is derived from dietary tryptophan, which is converted to 5-hydroxytryptophan by tryptophan hydroxylase and then to 5-HT by a nonspecific decarboxylase. After transport into cells by a specific transport system, 5-HT is degraded mainly by MAO both within the cell and after release. MAO-A is more significant than MAO-B in this process. The breakdown products are excreted in the urine as 5-hydroxyindoleacetic acid.

The best available evidence supports serotonin toxicity as being mediated primarily by the 5-HT_{2A} receptors (6,10–12) and not by 5-HT_{1A} as originally suggested (4). Early animal models of 5-HT toxicity implicated 5-HT_1 receptors; however, many of the features described were not seen in humans or were not clinically important features. In a more recent rat model, the combined administration of 5-hydroxy-L-tryptophan and clorgyline causes tremulousness with hyperthermia, resembling human serotonin toxicity, and culminates in death (10). This progression is not reversed by dopamine receptor D_2 antagonists such as haloperidol (10) or propranolol (6), a 5-HT_{1A} receptor antagonist. The toxicity is reversed by high doses of nonspecific 5-HT_2 receptor antagonists (e.g., cyproheptadine, chlorpromazine) and by the potent 5-HT_{2A} receptor antagonist ritanserin (6). Risperidone, also a 5-HT_{2A} receptor antagonist (13), has also been shown to reverse the hyperpyrexia and death in this model (10). In humans, there is evidence that cyproheptadine and chlorpromazine (5-HT_2 antagonists) are effective in the treatment of moderate to severe serotonin toxicity (5,11,14).

TABLE 1. Serotonergic drug interactions

Drugs	Mechanism of effect on serotonin
L-Tryptophan, *S*-adenyl-L-methionine, 5-hydroxytryptophan, dopamine	Serotonin precursors
Cocaine	Inhibits serotonin reuptake
Ecstasy (methylenedioxymethamphetamine)	Increases serotonin release and inhibits reuptake
Opioids (dextromethorphan, pentazocine, pethidine)	Inhibit serotonin reuptake
Selective serotonin reuptake inhibitors (escitalopram, citalopram, femoxitene, fluoxetine, fluvoxamine, paroxetine, sertraline), serotonin norepinephrine reuptake inhibitors (clovoxamine, venlafaxine), St. John's wort	Inhibit serotonin reuptake
Tricyclic antidepressants (clomipramine, imipramine)	Inhibit serotonin reuptake
Tramadol	Inhibits serotonin reuptake
Fenfluramine, amphetamines, bromocriptine, dihydroergotamine, gepirone, eltoprazin, quipazine	Serotonin agonists
LSD (lysergic acid diethylamide)	Partial serotonin agonist
MAO inhibitors (clorgyline, isocarboxazid, nialamide, pargyline, phenelzine, tranylcypromine)	Inhibit metabolism of serotonin
Reversible inhibitors of MAO-A (brofaramine, befloxatone, toloxatone, moclobemide)	Inhibit metabolism of serotonin
Lithium	Unknown

MAO, monoamine oxidase.

DIAGNOSIS

Serotonergic excess can be caused by drug interactions, overdose of a serotonergic drug, or as a complication of therapy. Serotonergic drug interactions, particularly when two drugs increase serotonergic transmission through different mechanisms, are common causes of serotonin toxicity (Table 1) (15). Any combination of these drugs may lead to clinical effects of serotonin excess.

Pure SSRI overdose causes clinically significant serotonin toxicity (sufficient to warrant consideration of specific therapy) in approximately 16% of cases (16,17). The combination of an SSRI overdose and a MAO inhibitor or a reversible inhibitor of MAO-A is much more likely to result in serotonin toxicity (55% of cases) and produces the most severe toxicity (29% requiring intubation and neuromuscular paralysis) (18).

Differential Diagnosis

The condition most often confused with serotonin toxicity is neuroleptic malignant syndrome. Although both conditions have autonomic hyperactivity and altered mental status, neuroleptic malignant syndrome has neuromuscular hypoactivity, and they are, in fact, two very different conditions that have very different etiologies (serotonin excess vs. dopamine blockade) and can be distinguished by simple physical examination (Table 2).

Serotonin excess (serotonin toxicity) has a relatively rapid onset after administration of a serotonergic drug and responds to serotonin blockade with drugs such as cyproheptadine and chlorpromazine. Dopamine receptor blockade (neuroleptic malignant syndrome) has a relatively slow onset (days) after administration of a neuroleptic drug and responds to dopamine agonists such as bromocriptine.

Clinical Presentation of Serotonin Excess (Toxicity)

Of the 38 cases summarized by Sternbach (4), the proportion of cases with a particular clinical sign ranged from 42.1% for confusion or hypomania to 13.2% for ataxia or incoordination. The proportion of patients with fever was not recorded. From these cases, diagnostic criteria for the serotonin syndrome were created:

- Coincident with the addition of or increase in a known serotonergic agent to an established medication regimen, at least three of the following clinical features are present: mental status changes (confusion, hypomania), agitation, myoclonus, hyperreflexia, diaphoresis, shivering, tremor, diarrhea, incoordination, fever.
- Other etiologies (e.g., infectious, metabolic, substance abuse or withdrawal) must have been excluded.
- A neuroleptic had not been started or increased in dosage before the onset of the signs and symptoms listed above.

In the context of drug overdose, however, many of these signs may be present without any serotonergic drug being involved. Thus, serotonin toxicity is better characterized (19) as a spectrum of neuroexcitation with a triad of clinical effects:

- Neuromuscular hyperactivity (hyperreflexia, clonus, myoclonus, tremor, and rigidity)
- Autonomic hyperactivity (hyperpyrexia, tachycardia, and diaphoresis)
- Altered mental status (agitation, anxiety, hypomania, and confusion)

Initially, the serotonin-toxic patient is alert, often hypervigilant, with a fine tremor and marked hyperreflexia (especially in the lower limbs). There is ankle clonus, and there may be myoclonus, which can be generalized. Severe myoclonus may be mistaken for seizure activity, which is rare in serotonin toxicity. As toxicity increases, the autonomic features become more evident with hyperpyrexia, sweating, and tachycardia. Rigidity, initially

TABLE 2. Clinical features of serotonin toxicity and neuroleptic malignant syndrome

Feature	Serotonin toxicity	Neuroleptic malignant syndrome
Mental status		
Agitation	++	+
Restlessness	+++	+
Confusion	++	+++
Hypomania	+	–
Motor system		
Inducible clonus	+++	–
Spontaneous clonus	+++	–
Ocular clonus	++	–
Myoclonus	+++	–
Tremor	+++[a]	++[b]
Shivering	++	–
Hyperreflexia	++++	+
Hypertonia/rigidity	++[c]	++++[b]
Bradykinesia	–	+++
Other central nervous system		
Akathisia	–	++
Nystagmus	++	–
Ataxia/incoordination	+	+
Coma	–	+
Oculogyric crisis	–	+
Opisthotonus	–	+
Seizures	–	–
Autonomic system		
Autonomic instability	+	+++
Diaphoresis	++	+++
Tachycardia	+++	++
Flushing	++	+
Mydriasis	++	+
Diarrhea	+	–
Lacrimation	–	–
Other features		
Rhabdomyolysis	+	+++
Fever	++	+++

[a]Action.
[b]Extrapyramidal.
[c]Pyramidal.
From Whyte I. Serotonin syndrome complicating treatment of recurrent depression. *Curr Ther* 1999;40(10):6–7, with permission.

in the lower limbs, is a late sign and indicates greater severity. Characteristically, the neuromuscular signs are predominantly in the lower limbs but become more generalized as the toxicity becomes more severe. As rigidity increases in truncal muscles, respiration becomes impaired; this in conjunction with a rapidly rising temperature heralds life-threatening toxicity.

POTENTIAL COMPLICATIONS

In severe cases, the complications of respiratory insufficiency and rhabdomyolysis may develop. Respiratory failure presumably arises in severe cases from persistent contraction of the trunk and respiratory muscles, leading to decreased ventilation. Rhabdomyolysis occurs in patients with persistent tremors, clonus, and stiffness. It may result in acute renal failure.

MANAGEMENT

Treatment of serotonin toxicity is primarily supportive, with attention to treatment issues indicated by the drug exposure causing the toxicity (see chapters on individual drugs). All serotonergic drugs should be withdrawn until the symptoms have subsided. Maintaining intravenous (IV) access and infusing isotonic fluids are valuable in almost all drug overdose situations. Fever may be treated initially by sedation and acetaminophen.

As many patients with serotonin toxicity are confused or delirious, strategies to manage delirium may be necessary. These include nonpharmacologic management, such as explanation and reorientation strategies by nursing staff, use of family members, and appropriate lighting and other cues to avoid provoking stimuli. Nonspecific pharmacologic management aimed at reducing distress, anxiety, cognitive disorganization, psychotic phenomena, behavioral disturbance, or some combination of these features may be needed. The most common drug group used in these circumstances is the benzodiazepines. This type of nonspecific pharmacologic intervention should be reserved for situations in which the risks of harm to self or others is high or the distress of the patient is unreasonable. These treatments should not be offered as a matter of course but promptly instigated when the clinical indications are evident.

Specific Therapy

Specific treatment using serotonin antagonists has been used successfully (5,11,14). Drugs with 5-HT_2–blocking properties include cyproheptadine and chlorpromazine. Cyproheptadine appears to be well tolerated and safe in overdose (implying safety in high therapeutic doses). It is available only in an oral formulation and, thus, is not helpful in patients unable to tolerate oral therapy or who have recently received activated charcoal. In patients with sufficient neuroexcitation to cause distress either through altered mental status (agitation, confusion), motor activity (marked tremor, myoclonus), or autonomic effects (drenching sweats, temperature up to 38°C), it can often provide relief. The correct dose has not been established, but it appears that larger-than-normal therapeutic doses are required (12). We have found 12 mg orally or by nasogastric tube repeated in 30 minutes, if required, and followed, if necessary, by 4 to 8 mg every 4 to 6 hours to be effective. Response is assessed by clinical observation.

Chlorpromazine has been used in more severe serotonin toxicity [progressive signs, rapidly rising temperature (greater than 38°C), development of rigidity] or when oral therapy is not tolerated (14). The drug is sedating and a potent vasodilator. Because patients with severe toxicity are often febrile and have been unable to consume fluids for hours, fluid resuscitation should precede chlorpromazine administration. The correct dose has not been established. A reasonable starting dose would be 12.5 to 25.0 mg IV initially and then up to 25 mg orally or IV every 6 hours.

Supportive Care

Serotonin toxicity may become life threatening. This usually occurs in the context of combined serotonergic drug overdose (SSRI and MAO inhibitor or reversible inhibitor of MAO-A) or occasionally in single serotonergic drug overdose (e.g., ecstasy). Severe toxicity is heralded by a rapidly rising temperature, which may reach 42° to 43°C, as well as severe tremor, myoclonus, and rigidity. The tremor and myoclonus may be so extensive as to be confused with seizure activity. The rigidity can rapidly progress from the lower limbs to involve the upper limbs and truncal muscles. Impairment of respiration may occur, manifested as a rising partial pressure of arterial carbon dioxide. This is an emergency that requires immediate, aggressive intervention with elective endotracheal intubation, assisted ventilation, and neuromuscular paralysis. Active cooling measures may be necessary to control temperature (Chapter 38), and full barbiturate anesthesia is indicated for the most severe cases.

PITFALLS

A common and potentially life-threatening pitfall is to overlook the early manifestations of increased serotonergic activity. If early signs are detected, simple sedation and discontinuation of the medication lead to complete recovery.

REFERENCES

1. Whyte I. Serotonin syndrome complicating treatment of recurrent depression. *Curr Ther* 1999;40(10):6–7.
2. Gillman PK. Serotonin syndrome: history and risk. *Fundam Clin Pharmacol* 1998;12(5):482–491.
3. Isbister GK, Dawson AH, Whyte IM. Serotonin syndrome and 5-HT2A antagonism. *Ann Pharmacother* 2001;35(9):1143–1144.
4. Sternbach H. The serotonin syndrome. *Am J Psychiatry* 1991;148(6):705–713.
5. Gillman PK. The serotonin syndrome and its treatment. *J Psychopharmacol* 1999;13(1):100–109.
6. Nisijima K, Yoshino T, Yui K, Katoh S. Potent serotonin (5-HT)(2A) receptor antagonists completely prevent the development of hyperthermia in an animal model of the 5-HT syndrome. *Brain Res* 2001;890:23–31.
7. Lane R, Baldwin D. Selective serotonin reuptake inhibitor-induced serotonin syndrome: review. *J Clin Psychopharmacol* 1997;17(3):208–221.
8. Oates J, Sjoerdsma A. Neurologic effects of tryptophan in patients receiving a monoamine oxidase inhibitor. *Neurology* 1960;10:1076–1078.
9. Insel TR, Roy BF, Cohen RM, Murphy DL. Possible development of the serotonin syndrome in man. *Am J Psychiatry* 1982;139(7):954–955.
10. Nisijima K, Yoshino T, Ishiguro T. Risperidone counteracts lethality in an animal model of the serotonin syndrome. *Psychopharmacology (Berl)* 2000;150(1):9–14.
11. Graudins A, Stearman A, Chan B. Treatment of the serotonin syndrome with cyproheptadine. *J Emerg Med* 1998;16(4):615–619.
12. Kapur S, Zipursky RB, Jones C, et al. Cyproheptadine: a potent in vivo serotonin antagonist [letter]. *Am J Psychiatry* 1997;154(6):884.
13. Richelson E, Souder T. Binding of antipsychotic drugs to human brain receptors: focus on newer generation compounds. *Life Sci* 2000;68:29–39.
14. Gillman PK. Successful treatment of serotonin syndrome with chlorpromazine. *Med J Aust* 1996;165(6):345–346.
15. Chan BS, Graudins A, Whyte IM, et al. Serotonin syndrome resulting from drug interactions. *Med J Aust* 1998;169(10):523–525.
16. Whyte IM, Dawson AH. Relative toxicity of venlafaxine and serotonin specific reuptake inhibitors in overdose. *J Toxicol Clin Toxicol* 2001;39(3):255.
17. Whyte IM, Dawson AH. Redefining the serotonin syndrome. *J Toxicol Clin Toxicol* 2002;40(5):668–669.
18. Isbister GK, Hackett LP, Dawson AH, Whyte IM. Moclobemide poisoning, toxicokinetics and occurrence of serotonin syndrome. *Proc Aust Health Med Res Congress* 2002:1165.
19. Isbister GK, Whyte IM. Serotonin toxicity and malignant hyperthermia: role of 5-HT2 receptors. *Br J Anaesth* 2002;88(4):603–604.

CHAPTER 25

Osmolal Gap

Jeffrey R. Suchard

OVERVIEW

The *serum osmolal gap* (OG) is the difference between calculated osmolality (Osm_C) and clinically measured osmolality (Osm_M) and is a value commonly used when evaluating patients potentially poisoned with methanol or ethylene glycol, the so-called toxic alcohols (1–3). The OG can also assist in evaluating exposure to other nonionic low-molecular-weight (MW) toxins including ethanol (ETOH), isopropanol, acetone, and propylene glycol. Calculations based on the OG can estimate serum levels of such toxins. Alternatively, when serum levels are known, their contribution to total osmolality can be compared to the OG to determine if additional osmotically active substances are present. Several nontoxicologic diseases also affect the OG, including diabetic ketoacidosis (DKA) or alcoholic ketoacidosis, lactic acidosis, and renal failure (4–6).

Quantitative determination of toxic alcohol levels is often not available in a clinically relevant time period, and treatment must often precede laboratory confirmation. An elevated OG can support the decision to treat toxic alcohol poisoning empirically. It must be recognized that the OG has several limitations, however, and its use remains more as a screening tool than a diagnostic test.

Osmolality is the number of moles of particles dissolved per kg of solvent. *Serum osmolality* is usually determined by measuring a colligative property [e.g., freezing point depression (FPD)] and then reporting the corresponding osmolality. This value reported is known as the Osm_M. In contrast, the Osm_C is a mathematical construct used in determining the OG, which does not represent any measurable physical attribute. Numerous methods of determining Osm_C have been devised (7–10), which typically include contributions of serum anions and cations, blood urea nitrogen (BUN), and glucose.

The *OG* is the difference between the measured and calculated osmolalities (Eq. 1).

$$OG = Osm_M - Osm_C \qquad \text{[Eq. 1]}$$

The OG represents the contribution to total serum osmolality unaccounted for in the equation used to determine Osm_C.

Osmolarity is easily confused with osmolality. *Osmolarity* is the number of moles of dissolved particles *per L* of solution, whereas *osmolality* is *per kg* of solution. Due to the volume comprised by protein and lipids, the water content of serum is roughly 0.93 kg/L (4,7,11). Dividing serum osmolarity by the serum water content yields serum osmolality (Eq. 2).

$$\frac{\text{serum osmolarity (mOsm/L)}}{\text{serum water content (~0.93 kg/L)}} = \begin{matrix}\text{serum osmolarity}\\ \text{(mOsm/kg)}\end{matrix} \qquad \text{[Eq. 2]}$$

Thus, serum osmolality exceeds the corresponding osmolarity by approximately 7.5% in most patients. Serum water content may vary considerably, depending on hydration status and protein and lipid content. For example, patients with DKA can present with serum water content as low as 0.899 kg/L (4). The lower the serum water content, the larger the apparent OG, even in the absence of exogenous toxins.

The issue of osmolarity versus osmolality is important because laboratory determination of Osm_M is reported in units of mOsm/kg (osmolality) (9,11), whereas the contributors to Osm_C are reported as mEq, mg, or mmol per unit volume (osmolarity). Failing to convert to units of osmolality falsely lowers Osm_C, resulting in a falsely elevated OG. For nonintoxicated patients, this difference is typically minimal; however, among patients with conditions associated with elevated OGs (e.g., ETOH intoxication), the absolute difference becomes greater and may lead the clinician to falsely believe an elevated OG exists.

PATHOPHYSIOLOGY

Calculation of serum osmolality can be accomplished by several methods (7–10). Dissolved electrolytes produce the majority of serum osmolalities. Because serum is electrostatically neutral and sodium comprises most of the cations, most equations for Osm_C reduce the contribution for all electrolytes to twice the measured serum sodium. Glucose and BUN are commonly included, and at normal concentrations, they contribute only a small amount to total osmolality. If all terms were in units of mOsm/kg, the equation for Osm_C is simple:

$$Osm_C = 2[Na^+] + BUN + glucose \quad \text{(molal units)} \qquad \text{[Eq. 3]}$$

In practical use, a number of correction factors affect Equation 3. The use of sodium to represent all ionic solutes is oversimplified. The contribution of ionic solutes is complicated by osmotic activities less than their concentrations (approximately 0.9 times the concentration for univalent ions) and by cations and anions contributing separately (7). For example, the osmotic coefficient of sodium chloride is 1.85[Na^+] (11). In other words, sodium chloride is approximately 93% dissociated in serum water (2). Therefore, the sodium term should be multiplied by 1.86 (0.93 × 2, to include anions and cations) instead of by 2. Because the laboratory reports molar units, the terms are next divided by 0.93 to correct for serum water content. Converting osmolarity to osmolality fortuitously counterbalances the sodium correction factor in the numerator, and the net correction factor for sodium remains 2. The BUN and glucose terms are commonly reported in units of mg/dl, which must be converted into the corresponding amount of mOsm (Eq. 4).

$$\frac{\begin{pmatrix}\text{concentration,}\\ \text{mg/dl}\end{pmatrix} \times \begin{pmatrix}1000\\ \text{mmol/mol}\end{pmatrix} \times \begin{pmatrix}10\\ \text{dl/L}\end{pmatrix}}{(\text{MW, g/mol}) \times (1000\ \text{mg/g})} \qquad \text{[Eq. 4]}$$

$$= \text{concentration, mmol/L}$$

reduces to:

$$\frac{\text{mg/dl}}{\text{MW}/10} = \text{mOsm/L}$$

The laboratory value for any osmotically active substance reported in mg/dl is converted into its corresponding osmolarity by dividing by one-tenth of its MW. The conversion factor for BUN is 2.8 (one-tenth the MW of two nitrogen atoms), and the conversion factor for glucose is 18. Applying these conversion factors yields Equation 5, in which sodium is expressed in mEq/L and BUN and glucose as mg/dl, as commonly reported from the clinical laboratory.

$$Osm_C = \frac{1.86[Na^+] + BUN/2.8 + glucose/18}{0.93} \qquad \text{[Eq. 5]}$$

$$= 2[Na^+] + \frac{BUN/2.8 + glucose/18}{0.93}$$

ETOH is the most common cause of an elevated OG (12,13). The *osmolar* contribution for ETOH is the serum concentration in mg/dl divided by 4.6 (MW of ETOH = 46 g/mol).

$$Osm_C = \frac{1.86[Na^+] + BUN/2.8 + glucose/18 + ETOH/4.6}{0.93}$$

$$= 2[Na^+] + \frac{BUN/2.8 + glucose/18 + ETOH/4.6}{0.93} \qquad \text{[Eq. 6]}$$

$$= 2[Na^+] + \frac{BUN/2.8 + glucose/18}{0.93} + \frac{ETOH}{4.2}$$

Equation 6 shows that when molar units are used, the net correction factor for ETOH becomes approximately 4.2, which has been validated experimentally (7,10).

The OG can be used to calculate alcohol levels (13). The ETOH concentration should be 4.2 times the OG (or 4.6 times the osmolar gap). Studies relating the OG to ETOH levels have shown that the correlation is not ideal. Such calculations overestimate the ETOH concentration because the osmotic coefficient of ETOH is greater than 1, ranging from 1.12 to 1.25 (12,14). Stated otherwise, ETOH exerts more osmotic pressure than expected by its measured serum level.

Investigators have compared different methods of calculating osmolality. A commonly referenced study was performed by Dorwart and Chalmers (7). The most accurate of the 13 equations for Osm_C they compared was

$$Osm_C = 1.86[Na^+] + BUN/2.8 + glucose/18 + 9 \qquad \text{[Eq. 7]}$$

This equation yielded an average OG of zero, with a standard deviation of 6.36 mOsm/kg. Note that this equation uses molar units and is not corrected for serum water content. If the final constant were omitted, the "normal" OG becomes approximately 10 mOsm/kg. This appears to be the origin of the oft-repeated statement that the upper limit of the normal OG is 10 mOsm/kg (11,12,15). The authors of this paper concluded, instead, that "it is rare for noninebriated patients who are not in shock to have measured osmolalities that differ by more than 15 mosmol/kg from calculated osmolalities" (7).

Bhagat et al. empirically derived a formula that fit their data better than Equation 7 and recommended Equation 8 (concentrations are in osm/kg units) (9):

$$Osm_C = 1.86[Na^+] + 1.38[K^+] + 1.03(urea) + 1.08(glucose) + 7.45 \qquad \text{[Eq. 8]}$$

For ease of calculation, the authors suggested a simplified version in which Osm_C = 1.86[Na + K] + urea + glucose + 10.

Hoffman et al. compared three different commonly used methods for calculating osmolality: (a) 2Na + BUN/2.8 + glucose/18 + ETOH/4.6; (b) 1.86Na + BUN/2.8 + glucose/18 + ETOH/4.6; and (c) (2Na + BUN/2.8 + glucose/18 + ETOH/4.6)/0.93, in which all concentrations were in molar units (10). The average baseline OG varied from −2 to 15 mOsm/kg depending on the equation, but the standard deviations of the baseline OG for all equations were grouped in the 5- to 6-mOsm/kg range. This is similar to other reports (7,12,16,17) and probably represents the limits of technical analysis (i.e., laboratory variability in measuring sodium and other osmotic components).

No one equation is likely to be significantly better than another. The most convenient and reliable method should be used. The most attractive option is Osm_C = (1.86[Na^+] + [BUN]/2.8 + [Glucose]/18)/0.93 (3,10), to which should be added an ETOH term to yield Equation 9, in which all concentrations are in molar units, as reported from the clinical laboratory.

$$Osm_C = 2[Na^+] + \frac{BUN/2.8 + glucose/18}{0.93} + \frac{ETOH}{4.2} \qquad \text{[Eq. 9]}$$

Measurement of serum osmolality can be done by the vapor pressure or FPD methods. The FPD method is preferred because most substances in the toxicologic diagnosis of an elevated OG are volatile, and they are not detected by the vapor pressure method (18,19). The vapor pressure method involves heating the sample and allowing volatiles to evaporate; however, they do not recondense with water and, thus, escape detection. Fortunately, up to 100% of teaching hospitals and 89% of nonteaching hospitals measure osmolality by FPD, and most of these use FPD exclusively. Only two-thirds of commercial laboratories, however, use FPD (20).

The use of the OG as a diagnostic test is limited, even after accuracy has been optimized (3,10). First, the normal baseline OG varies considerably. If the standard deviation of the OG is approximately 5 to 6 mOsm/kg, then an "elevated" OG of 10 mOsm/kg still remains within two standard deviations, and using such a criterion for detecting toxic alcohols is nonspecific. The more important thing to know about a patient's OG is how far deviated it is from baseline, and it is doubtful that a patient's baseline OG is available.

Second, it is possible to have clinically significant toxic alcohol poisoning in the absence of an elevated OG. For example, a serum ethylene glycol level of 50 mg/dl corresponds to only 8.7 mOsm/kg, which could easily remain undetected, especially if a patient's baseline OG were somewhat negative.

Furthermore, the OG from methanol or ethylene glycol decreases as they are metabolized. The organic acid metabolites are accounted for in the sodium term for calculating osmolality. These acids dissociate into H^+ and their corresponding anions, producing two dissolved particles; then the H^+ combines with bicarbonate, and two dissolved particles are removed. The net number of dissolved particles (osmolality) decreases as the parent alcohol is metabolized, while the anion gap increases. Thus, late-presenting patients with toxic alcohol poisoning may have a normal OG (21,22). Because isopropanol is metabolized to acetone, which is uncharged and continues to affect the OG, excess osmolality will decrease only by elimination instead of metabolism.

Some authors assert that the OG has "little practical utility in the management of toxic ingestion" (3). It is more accurate to say that "small osmol gaps should not be used to eliminate the possibility of toxic alcohol ingestion" (10). However, a large OG does not prove toxic alcohol ingestion because an OG in the 20 to 25 mOsm/kg range is not uncommon with alcoholic ketoacidosis or DKA (5). An OG greater than 25 mOsm/kg is almost always caused by low-molecular-weight toxins.

If toxic alcohol ingestion is suspected, an elevated OG is presumptive supportive evidence. If such a patient has concurrently elevated anion gaps and OGs, this evidence is probably adequate to initiate empiric therapy. Yet the absence of an elevated OG should not preclude therapy if adequate clinical suspicion exists. In the absence of an elevated anion gap, a normal OG reduces the likelihood, but does not rule out, a significant toxic alcohol ingestion (23).

DIAGNOSIS

The differential diagnosis of an elevated OG includes exogenous substances, nontoxicologic disease states, and sources of artifactual error (Table 1). In theory, high enough levels of any exogenous substance will increase osmolality. However, most drugs or intoxicants cannot be detected using the OG because their serum levels are low or their MWs are high, and they have negligible effects on osmolality (24).

Although lactic acidosis, alcoholic ketoacidosis, and DKA are associated with elevated OGs, it should be noted that lactic acid and the ketoacids themselves do not increase osmolality. As discussed above, even when organic acids accumulate, the conversion of H^+ and bicarbonate into water and carbon dioxide yields a net change of zero in osmolality. The increased osmolality in these disease states comes from other sources, including acetone, glycerol, amino acids, and other unmeasured osmotically active particles, and from decreased serum water content.

The history often elicits the cause of an elevated OG. For unintentional exposures, the history should be straightforward; a typical history involves a child found with an open container of antifreeze or windshield washer fluid. A likely scenario of an elevated OG that could not be easily determined is an alcoholic patient presenting with metabolic acidosis, representing either toxic alcohol ingestion or alcoholic ketoacidosis.

In the poisoned patient, changes in serum osmolality alone do not generally cause clinically evident effects. The clinician should look for signs and symptoms of the disease processes that are associated with changes in the OG.

Measurement of the serum sodium, BUN, glucose, and osmolality by the FPD method are necessary. A serum ETOH level should also be obtained. Arterial blood gas analysis should be considered, because the degree of metabolic acidosis may aid in guiding empiric treatment.

Quantitative determination of all relevant osmotically active substances should be ordered, such as acetone levels in DKA, alcoholic ketoacidosis, and isopropanol ingestion. If available, methanol, ethylene glycol, and isopropanol levels (as appropriate) should be obtained. Routine serum chemistries and osmolality results will return before specific toxic alcohol levels, and calculation of the OG is still a useful tool.

TABLE 1. Differential diagnosis of an elevated osmolal gap

Exogenous causes
- Ethanol
- Methanol
- Ethylene glycol
- Isopropanol
- Acetone
- Propylene glycol
- Paraldehyde
- Isoniazid
- Trichloroethane
- Ethyl ether
- Glycerol
- Dimethyl sulfoxide[a]
- Glycine[a]
- Mannitol[a]
- Osmotic contrast dyes

Disease states
- Alcoholic ketoacidosis
- Diabetic ketoacidosis
- Lactic acidosis
- Chronic renal failure
- Shock/multisystem organ failure
- Very-low-birthweight neonates
- Decreased serum water content
  - Hyperlipidemia
  - Hyperproteinemia

Artifactual
- Lavender top (ethylenediaminetetraacetic acid) tube, 15 mOsm/L
- Gray top (Na F-K-oxalate) tube, 150 mOsm/L
- Blue top (citrate) tube, 10 mOsm/L
- Green top (Li heparin) tube, 6 mOsm/L

[a]When given intravenously.
Adapted from Osterloh JD, Kelly TJ, Khayam-Bashi H, Romeo R. Discrepancies in osmolal gaps and calculated alcohol concentrations. *Am H Clin Pathol* 1973;60:695–699, and with additional material from references 2, 11, 13, and 24.

POTENTIAL COMPLICATIONS

If the OG is interpreted incorrectly and the patient is presumed to have toxic alcohol poisoning when he or she does not, the patient would be subject to unnecessary therapeutic interventions. Conversely, if a "normal" OG is misinterpreted as excluding a toxic alcohol, a patient could experience the effects of untreated methanol or ethylene glycol poisoning.

MANAGEMENT

The major decision-making point in the patient with an elevated OG is to detect a clinically significant toxic alcohol exposure. Any relevant quantitative measurements of osmotically active serum constituents should be obtained and their contribution to the total OG calculated. It is assumed that any excess OG, unaccounted for by the measured substances, could be due to toxic alcohols. In many cases, the only rapidly available toxin level is serum ETOH. Some laboratories are able to measure methanol, isopropyl alcohol, and acetone levels; only a few can provide rapid quantitative measurement of ethylene glycol.

If the apparent OG is accounted for by all of the measured osmotically active constituents, exposure to additional toxic alcohols becomes less likely but not excluded. Other key factors include the time since potential exposure and the remainder of the metabolic evaluation. Patients presenting early after toxic alcohol exposures will have an elevated OG and a normal anion gap. As toxic alcohols are metabolized, the OG decreases, and the anion gap increases. The absence of an OG does not eliminate the possibility of toxic alcohol poisoning in the face of acidosis.

At some point, clinical judgment based on history, physical examination, and laboratory evaluation must come into play. For example, patients with DKA are likely to present with an elevated OG that cannot completely be accounted for by the serum acetone level, yet they will not require toxicologic-directed therapy.

PITFALLS

The biggest pitfall is to use the OG as a true diagnostic test rather than as a screening test. One should not use the OG alone to conclude either that a toxic alcohol is present or absent.

REFERENCES

1. Jacobsen D, Bredesen JE, Eide I, Østborg J. Anion and osmolal gaps in the diagnosis of methanol and ethylene glycol poisoning. *Acta Med Scand* 1982;212:17–20.
2. Gennari FJ. Current concepts: serum osmolality—uses and limitations. *N Engl J Med* 1984;310:102–105.
3. Glaser DS. Utility of the serum osmol gap in the diagnosis of methanol or ethylene glycol ingestion. *Ann Emerg Med* 1996;27:343–346.
4. Davidson DF. Excess osmolal gap in diabetic ketoacidosis explained. *Clin Chem* 1992;38:755–757.
5. Schelling JR, Howard RL, Winter SD, Linas SL. Increased osmolal gap in alcoholic ketoacidosis and lactic acidosis. *Ann Intern Med* 1990;113:580–582.
6. Sklar AH, Linas SL. The osmolal gap in renal failure. *Ann Intern Med* 1983;98:481–482.
7. Dorwart WV, Chalmers L. Comparison of methods for calculating serum osmolality from chemical concentrations, and the prognostic value of such calculations. *Clin Chem* 1975;21:190–194.
8. Weisberg HF. Osmolality—calculated, "delta," and more formulas. *Clin Chem* 1975;21:1182–1185.
9. Bhagat CI, Garcia-Webb P, Fletcher E, Beilby JP. Calculated vs measured plasma osmolalities revisited. *Clin Chem* 1984;30:1703–1705.
10. Hoffman RS, Smilkstein MJ, Howland MA, Goldfrank LR. Osmol gaps revisited: normal values and limitations. *J Toxicol Clin Toxicol* 1993;31:81–93.
11. Smithline N, Gardner KD. Gaps—anionic and osmolal. *JAMA* 1976;236:1594–1597.
12. Pappas AA, Gadsden RH, Taylor EH. Serum osmolality in acute intoxication: a prospective clinical study. *Am J Clin Pathol* 1985;84:74–79.
13. Britten JS, Myers RA, Benner C, et al. Blood ethanol and serum osmolality in the trauma patient. *Am Surg* 1982;48:451–455.
14. Purssell RA, Pudek M, Brubacher J, Abu-Laban RB. Derivation and validation of a formula to calculate the contribution of ethanol to the osmolal gap. *Ann Emerg Med* 2001;38:653–659.
15. Demedts P, Theunis L, Wauters A, et al. Excess serum osmolality gap after ingestion of methanol: a methodology-associated phenomenon? *Clin Chem* 1994;40:1587–1590.
16. Aabakken L, Johansen KS, Rydningen EB, et al. Osmolal and anion gaps in patients admitted to an emergency medical department. *Hum Exp Toxicol* 1994;13:131–134.
17. McQuillen KK, Anderson AC. Osmol gaps in the pediatric population. *Acad Emerg Med* 1999;6:27–30.
18. Lund ME, Banner W, Finley PR, et al. Effect of alcohols and selected solvents on serum osmolality measurements. *J Toxicol Clin Toxicol* 1983;20:115–132.
19. Walker JA, Schwartzbard A, Krauss EA, et al. The missing gap: a pitfall in the diagnosis of alcohol intoxication by osmometry. *Arch Intern Med* 1986;146:1843–1844.
20. Eisen TF, Lacouture PG, Woolf A. Serum osmolality in alcohol ingestions: differences in availability among laboratories of teaching hospital, nonteaching hospital, and commercial facilities. *Am J Emerg Med* 1989;7:256–259.
21. Steinhart B. Case report: severe ethylene glycol intoxication with normal osmolal gap—"a chilling thought." *J Emerg Med* 1990;8:583–585.
22. Darchy B, Abruzzese L, Pitiot D, et al. Delayed admission for ethylene glycol poisoning: lack of elevated serum osmol gap. *Intensive Care Med* 1999;25:859–861.
23. Hoffman R. Reply to letter to the editor: osmolal gap. *J Toxicol Clin Toxicol* 1994;32:97.
24. Glasser L, Sternglanz PD, Combie J, Robinson A. Serum osmolality and its applicability to drug overdose. *Am J Clin Pathol* 1973;60:695–699.

CHAPTER 26

Peripheral Neuropathy

Matthew N. Meriggioli

OVERVIEW

Peripheral neuropathy (PN) is a common manifestation of toxic exposure to environmental, industrial, nutritional, and biologic agents. Hundreds of drugs and chemicals have been associated with PN. For some agents, PN may be the predominant sign of poisoning; in others, the peripheral nervous system may be only one of several target organs. In either case, the signs and symptoms of PN must be recognized before a specific toxin can be implicated. Although treatment options are limited in most instances of toxic neuropathy, early recognition and prompt diagnosis help to reduce cumulative exposure to the offending agent and limit the neurotoxic effects on peripheral nerves.

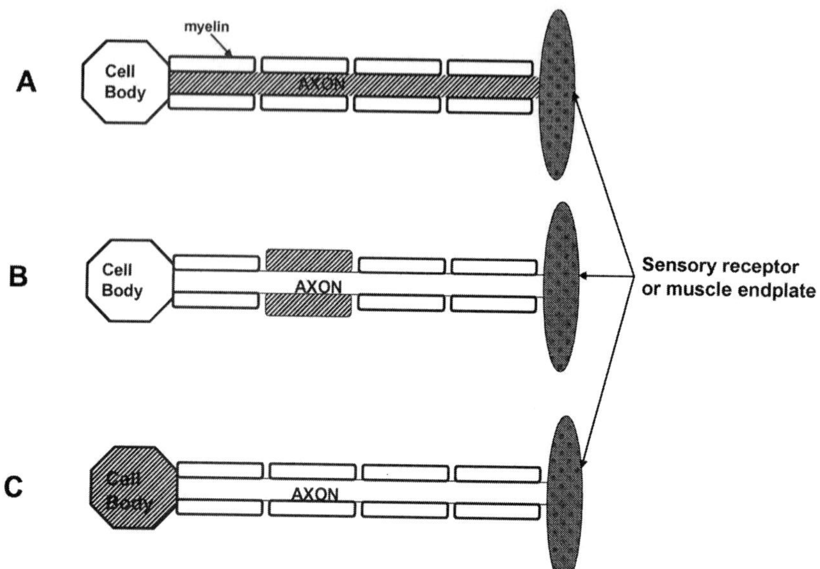

Figure 1. Sites of action of toxic agents on peripheral nerves. **A:** Axonal degeneration (axonopathy). **B:** Segmental demyelination (myelinopathy). **C:** Cell body degeneration (neuronopathy).

PATHOPHYSIOLOGY

The neurons and axons of the peripheral nervous system have a relatively limited repertoire of response to injury (Fig. 1), including (a) axonal degeneration (axonopathy), (b) segmental demyelination (myelinopathy), and (c) nerve cell body degeneration (neuronopathy). Axonal degeneration may occur as a result of focal nerve injury or transection, in which the axon distal to the site of injury degenerates (wallerian degeneration), or may occur due to metabolic or toxic derangements affecting axonal transport mechanisms, resulting in distal axonal breakdown (distal axonopathy). Recovery may occur in these cases if the cause of injury is removed because the peripheral nerve axons are capable of reenervation. The extent of recovery depends on the severity of the original injury. *Segmental demyelination* refers to damage to the myelin sheath with relative sparing of the axon. In this instance, the myelin-forming cells (Schwann's cells) or the myelin sheath itself may be affected, and there is a capacity for recovery by the process of remyelination. In the case of neuronopathies, the primary injury occurs to the neuronal cell body, with secondary axonal degeneration. Recovery is often incomplete in these cases and only occurs if surviving neurons assume the lost function.

Axonopathy is the most common pattern of toxic peripheral nerve injury (1). The most distal part of the axon is usually affected earliest and most severely (distal axonopathy). This is likely due to the metabolic demands of the distal axon. All the proteins and lipids found in the peripheral nerve axon are synthesized in the cell body and must be transported down the axon, in some cases for 1 m or more (2). Toxins causing a distal axonopathy usually interfere with or disrupt this process of axonal transport. Accordingly, the larger the volume of axon cytoplasm (axoplasm), the more challenging the metabolic task of maintaining the axon, and the more vulnerable the axon becomes to the effects of toxins. This is the likely explanation for the fact that most toxins affect larger axons first and most prominently.

On occasion, toxins cause severe injury to the neuronal cell body. In this case, there is secondary axonal degeneration, but this degeneration is not in a "length-dependent" pattern. The entire length of the axon is affected due to inability of the cell body to maintain it. An example is the neuropathy associated with the use of cisplatin in which there is selective injury to the cell bodies in the dorsal root ganglia (3).

Demyelinating neuropathies due to toxic agents are far less common and result from exposure to specific agents such as amiodarone (4). The primary target in these neuropathies may be the myelin sheath or the myelin-producing Schwann's cells. The result is segmental demyelination causing slowing of nerve conduction across the involved segment. It is important to realize that the underlying axon is intact. Once exposure to the toxic agent is removed, remyelination may result in full recovery of nerve function. The situation is frequently not this simple because secondary axonal degeneration may occur with more severe demyelination. In the case of certain toxins, like amiodarone, characteristic lysosomal inclusions visualized on nerve biopsy specimens may aid in confirming a toxic etiology (5).

In addition to having a direct deleterious effect on peripheral nerve axons or myelin, certain agents may precipitate a dysimmune process usually directed toward peripheral nerve myelin. This condition is associated with the use of certain immunomodulating agents, such as tacrolimus (6) and interferon (7). In these cases, patients typically note the subacute onset of sensory and motor symptoms 2 to 10 weeks after beginning therapy. Segmental demyelination, as seen in chronic inflammatory demyelinating polyneuropathy, is demonstrated by electrodiagnostic studies. These patients may respond to plasmapheresis or intravenous immune globulin, suggesting an immune-mediated response. The exact mechanism is not clear, but it is possible that these agents alter the population of T-cell subsets, particularly suppressor T cells, thereby allowing other T lymphocytes to react with autoantigens.

In summary, the most common toxic neuropathy is a distal, symmetric, sensorimotor polyneuropathy. The pathologic finding of distal axonal degeneration is nonspecific in most cases and cannot confirm a toxic etiology. Because most toxic neuropathies are axonal, finding a toxic neuropathy with primary demyelinating pathologic features restricts the list of possible agents to a handful of possibilities, including amiodarone and perhexilene, some of which may have characteristic lysosomal inclusions on nerve biopsy, which may aid in making the diagnosis.

DIAGNOSIS

History

The initial task for the clinician is to establish a diagnosis of PN before confirming a toxic cause. Because most toxic neuropathies are characterized by distal axonal degeneration, the most common presenting symptoms are distal, symmetric sensory and motor dysfunction. Patients typically report paresthesia and sensory loss initially affecting the toes and then gradually progressing proximally. Eventually, a "stocking-glove" distribution of sensory symptoms may become apparent. Patchy, multifocal, or migratory symptoms are unlikely to be due to a toxic neuropathy. Intrinsic foot muscle weakness may be present but is often not noticed by the patient.

There is no specific clinical presentation that definitively distinguishes a toxic PN from one due to other causes. However, particular toxins may have characteristic presentations, accompanying systemic signs, or pathologic findings that may lead to the appropriate diagnosis. Acute toxic exposures, although rare, typically cause fulminant symptoms of neuropathy, usually associated with systemic (nausea, vomiting, stomach cramps) or central nervous system involvement. In these cases, the diagnosis is usually not difficult. However, with chronic exposure, the symptoms may be very similar to PN due to other causes. Furthermore, up to 20% of PN is unexplained even after an exhaustive work-up (8). However, although an "idiopathic PN" is not an unusual occurrence, pursuing a toxic etiology in these cases is rarely rewarding in the absence of a clear history of exposure. In the final analysis, recognition of a toxic neuropathy usually results from a high index of suspicion based on a suggestive history and the systematic elimination of competing causes.

In the rare case of toxic PN resulting in a demyelinating neuropathy, patients are more likely to have proximal symptoms and are usually more functionally disabled. These neuropathies usually evolve more rapidly, progressing over the course of days to weeks.

Finally, with primary involvement of the cell bodies (neuronopathy) in the dorsal root ganglia, the usual symptoms are severe sensory loss and a sensory ataxia. Motor neuron disease due to toxic exposure (i.e., heavy metals) is very rare, but presents with progressive muscle weakness, atrophy, and fasciculations, usually beginning focally.

Physical Examination

A thorough neurologic examination helps to establish the diagnosis. The relative degree of motor and sensory involvement and the anatomic pattern of involvement are important. Most toxic PNs produce sensory signs greater than motor signs with a length-dependent distribution. The extent of muscle stretch reflex loss may help to classify a PN as axonal versus demyelinating. If reflexes are diffusely absent, an underlying demyelinating process is more likely. Absent ankle jerk reflexes, but preserved reflexes more proximally, are the classic finding in axonal sensorimotor PNs. The involvement of motor and autonomic systems varies considerably in different toxic conditions. With certain toxins (e.g., thallium), the presence of cranial nerve abnormalities, particularly optic neuropathy (9), may be an important clue to the etiologic agent.

In the uncommon case of a demyelinating toxic PN, motor impairment is usually much more prominent than in the axonal cases. Muscle stretch reflexes are diffusely hypoactive or absent. Large fiber involvement due to either demyelinating neuropathy or sensory neuronopathy may produce a severe proprioceptive sensory loss and a resultant sensory ataxia. Patients are able to stand with a narrow base with their eyes open but have difficulty maintaining their balance with their eyes closed (positive Romberg's sign).

Concurrent involvement of the central nervous system (pyramidal tracts and cerebellum) may occur with certain toxins (i.e., hexacarbons, organophosphates) and aid in making a specific diagnosis. The presence of systemic signs and symptoms should also be carefully assessed. Weight loss, skin changes, gastrointestinal symptoms, anemia, and alopecia may all be associated with toxic conditions, and the specific systemic sign may be pathognomonic of a particular toxic agent in certain cases (e.g., Mees' lines in arsenic toxicity).

Diagnostic Tests

Electrodiagnostic studies play an important role in the evaluation of toxic neuropathies. These studies can determine the degree of sensory and motor involvement, the distribution and severity of involvement, and the nature of the pathologic process (primarily axonal or demyelinating). Because the pathologic process in toxic PN is usually axonal degeneration, the sensory nerve conduction studies often show low or absent sensory responses in the legs and, to a variable degree, in the arms, depending on the severity and duration of the exposure. The motor responses are most frequently normal or mildly abnormal in chronic, axonal conditions. The reason is that collateral reennervation of denervated muscle fibers by surviving motor axons is sufficient to preserve the response. Obviously, markedly low amplitude or absent motor responses are indicative of a more severe, subacutely evolving, axon-loss process.

Demyelination is characterized on nerve conduction studies as slowing of motor and sensory nerve conduction velocities. It is important to realize that slowed conduction velocities may also be due to degeneration of large diameter axons and may not necessarily indicate a primary demyelinating pathophysiology. Interpretation of the electrodiagnostic findings in light of the clinical presentation is often more crucial to arriving at an appropriate diagnosis than the technical performance of the test itself.

Biochemical diagnosis of a toxic PN is certainly the most direct way of attributing a PN to a specific toxic exposure. Although toxic compounds and metabolites may be identified in serum or urine specimens, the agents of interest must be identified beforehand to guide ordering of the correct test. Screening for the presence of unknown toxins is inefficient and has low diagnostic yield. Other laboratory studies may demonstrate the presence of an anemia or other metabolic disturbance that suggests a toxic etiology.

With a few exceptions, a peripheral nerve biopsy has little to offer in the investigation of a toxic PN. In most cases, a nonspecific axonal degeneration is found. In some cases, certain features of this axonopathy (mitochondrial abnormalities, glycogen accumulation, axonal shrinkage) may point to a toxic cause, but such changes may also occur in nutritional disturbances or after ischemic nerve injury. In the uncommon case of a primary demyelinating toxic PN, nerve biopsy may be helpful by demonstrating characteristic lysosomal inclusions as seen in amiodarone toxicity.

MANAGEMENT

Removal from the toxic exposure is often all that is necessary in the management of toxic PN. Chelation therapy may be indicated with heavy metal exposures. Specific treatments aimed at promoting excretion of the toxic agent may be applicable in certain circumstances (i.e., administration of potassium to increase the rate of thallium excretion). Immune therapy, such as plasmapheresis or intravenous immune globulin, may be effective in demyelinating neuropathy.

Removal from exposure results in improvement in most cases. The extent of recovery is variable, depending on the responsible agent, the magnitude and duration of exposure, and the presence of concomitant systemic or neurologic illness. Clinical worsening for weeks or months after terminating the exposure ("coasting") is typical of hexacarbon intoxication (1) but also occurs in other toxic neuropathies. Painful paresthesias should be treated symptomatically with membrane-stabilizing agents, such as gabapentin. Due to its effects as a sodium-channel blocker, carbamazepine has been reported effective in treating the sensory symptoms of toxicity due to oxaliplatin, which is believed to act on voltage-gated sodium channels, increasing the excitability of sensory neurons (10).

PITFALLS

There are numerous causes of PN. Attributing a particular cause to a toxic etiology requires careful consideration and testing to rule out alternative causes for neuropathy. Appropriate timing of exposure with onset of clinical symptoms is an important part of establishing a cause–effect relationship for a specific toxic agent. Some of the most common toxic PNs are associated with prescription medications, with symptoms sometimes occurring only after years of use. A high index of suspicion and familiarity with the neuropathy associated with the use of prescription medications aids in the recognition of these difficult cases.

Patients with preexisting PN due to other causes, such as diabetes or hereditary neuropathies, may experience acute worsening of neuropathic symptoms after toxic exposure. It is important to recognize this occurrence and remove the exposure rather than attribute the symptoms to progression of the underlying PN.

REFERENCES

1. Jortner BS. Mechanisms of toxic injury in the peripheral nervous system: neuropathologic considerations. *Toxicol Pathol* 2000;28:54–69.
2. Allen RD, Weiss DG, Hayden JH, et al. Gliding movement of and bidirectional transport along single, native microtubules from squid axoplasm: evidence for an active role of microtubules in cytoplasmic transport. *J Cell Biol* 1985;100:1735–1752.
3. Peltier AC, Russell JW. Recent advances in drug-induced neuropathies. *Curr Opin Neurol* 2002;15:633–638.
4. Jacobs JM, Costa-Jussa FR. The pathology of amiodarone toxicity. II. Peripheral neuropathy in man. *Brain* 1985;108:753–769.
5. Hruban Z. Pulmonary and generalized lysosomal storage induced by amphiphilic drugs. *Environ Health Perspect* 1984;55:53–76.
6. Wilson JR, Conwit RA, Eidelman BH, et al. Sensorimotor neuropathy resembling CIDP in patients receiving FK506. *Muscle Nerve* 1994;17:528–532.
7. Meriggioli MN, Rowin J. Chronic inflammatory demyelinating polyneuropathy after treatment with interferon-alpha. *Muscle Nerve* 2000;23:433–435.
8. Lubec D, Mullbacher W, Finsterer J, Mamoli B. Diagnostic work-up in peripheral neuropathy: an analysis of 171 cases. *Postgrad Med J* 1999;75:723–727.
9. Sahenk Z. Toxic neuropathies. *Semin Neurol* 1987;7:9–17.
10. Gamelin E, Gamelin L, Bossi L, Quasthoff S. Clinical aspects and molecular basis of oxaliplatin neurotoxicity: current management and development of preventive measures. *Semin Oncol* 2002;29:21–33.

CHAPTER 27

Pulmonary Disease: Persistent and Progressive

Frederick Fung

OVERVIEW

The evaluation and management of patients with persistent and progressive pulmonary diseases (PPPDs) remain difficult issues for medical toxicologists. The clinical distinction from other nontoxicologic lung diseases is not easy. These diseases are clinically important because patients are frequently severely disabled and require long-term medical treatment, but the underlying disease is often preventable and treatable when recognized early. Despite these difficulties, the toxicologist can apply an organized approach to patients.

Over the last decades, there has been a change in the nature of toxic substances in industry and the environment. Chronic lung diseases, such as pneumoconiosis secondary to asbestos, silica, and coal dust, and beryllium-related lung diseases, are becoming less frequent. On the other hand, PPPDs, such as asthma and hypersensitivity pneumonitis (HP) due to toxic exposures, seem to be more frequent than in the past. New pulmonary syndromes have been associated with biologic toxin and nylon fiber exposures.

PPPD can be defined as a pulmonary disorder involving anatomic or physiologic impairment resulting in progressive, persistent symptoms and frequently disabling lung condition. They can be categorized as interstitial lung disease or bronchoalveolar disorders (see Chapter 11 for asthma and reactive airway disease). Interstitial lung disease includes a diverse group of pulmonary disorders characterized by pathologic changes in the interstitial lung spaces. All of the components of interstitial space may be affected: vasculature, fibroblasts, collagen, and noncollagen proteins. The endpoint of interstitial lung disease is usually pulmonary fibrosis.

PATHOPHYSIOLOGY

In general, the initial insult by a toxic gas, fume, substance, or dust produces a cascade of events, resulting in tissue inflammation and release of cell mediators such as cytokines (1). When the inflammation in the air spaces spreads to adjacent interstitial tissues, chronic and recurrent proliferation of fibroblasts, smooth muscle cells, and collagen will follow. This causes scarring and distortion of the interstitium, interfering with gas exchange and ventilatory function (2).

DIAGNOSIS

Chronic pulmonary disease secondary to toxic exposure is difficult to evaluate and manage (Table 1). The exposure history is fraught with recall bias and long latency time. Furthermore, a typical exposure scenario may only include nonspecific or low-level toxic exposure. PPPD may or may not have an acute phase of illness. The symptoms are usually nonspecific and chronic, and onset is typically insidious. Physical examination is usually normal or nonspecific unless advanced. Pulmonary function and radiographic findings are also nonspecific and may include obstructive and restrictive patterns.

The initial evaluation should include a detailed medical and exposure history. Inquiry into exposure to specific toxins, especially in a detailed chronologic manner, helps to identify the agent and time of exposure and to define the latency period. Because latency may vary from days to more than 20 years, it is important to obtain a chronologic exposure and clinical history simultaneously. Identifying a specific agent is often difficult and may require direct inquiry of current and past employers as well as agencies like the National Institute of Occupational Safety and Health, Occupational Safety and Health Administration, Environmental Protection Agency, Agency for Toxic Substance and Disease Registry, and others.

In contrast to sick building syndrome and multiple chemical sensitivity, the PPPD patient should have objective signs of disease. Although the physical findings vary depending on the severity of the disease, patients with PPPD may appear to be tachypneic or tachycardic at rest or on exertion (Table 2). Chest auscultation may reveal wheezing, rhonchi, basilar end-expiratory rales, or crackles. Clubbing of digits due to cor pulmonale and pulmonary hypertension may be seen on physical examination.

A simple chest radiograph may reveal interstitial lung disease, HP, or simply patchy infiltrates. Specific pneumoconioses have typical findings. For example, silicosis typically demonstrates linear interstitial infiltrates in the middle and upper lung regions. Coal dust pneumoconiosis typically demonstrates infiltrates in the upper lung fields, whereas asbestosis shows interstitial fibrosis and pleural plaques mainly in lower lung fields. High-resolution computed tomography (CT) scanning has become the gold standard in diagnosing early interstitial lung disease.

Pulmonary function testing (PFT) is a useful diagnostic tool, which depends on patient effort. Restrictive lung disease is suggested by a forced vital capacity (FVC) of less than 80% predicted with normal or low-normal forced expiratory volume at 1 second (FEV_1) and FEV_1:FVC ratio greater than 75% predicted. Obstructive disease typically has a FVC greater than 80% predicted, FEV_1 less than 80% predicted, and a ratio of FEV_1:FVC less than 75% predicted. For interstitial lung disease, the diffusion capacity for carbon monoxide (DLCO) is typically less than 75%. There are several formulas for determining the predicted PFT values. In general, individuals are substantially impaired when the FEV_1 falls to 50% or lower of the predicted value.

The methacholine challenge test is a nonspecific airway hyperreactivity test that explores an exaggerated bronchoconstriction response to nonspecific chemical, physical, and pharmacologic stimuli. Despite its nonspecificity, the methacholine challenge test has a good correlation between the degree of bronchial hyperreactivity and the severity of response to the agent at issue.

Special immune testing such as immunoglobulin (Ig)E antibody titer by radioallergosorbent test may be useful in detecting specific IgE antibodies against low-molecular-weight antigens, such as isocyanates and other protein materials, as well as bioaerosols. Serum antibody titer for HP may be useful in confirming a diagnosis of farmer's lung disease. However, serology using IgG and IgM titers should not be used as a screening tool. IgG and IgM antibodies may be present in asymptomatic people; therefore, the presence of the antibody implicates evidence of exposure, not disease. Arterial blood gases and pulse oximetry are useful for hypoxemia evaluation. Pulse oximetry is a useful screening test for detecting hypoxemia; however, the best way to follow PPPD is to assess resting and exercise arterial blood gas over time. Bronchoscopy with bronchoalveolar lavage (BAL) is used when visualization of the bronchial tree, tissue biopsy, and bronchial cytology are indicated.

Finally, exposure assessment is an important factor to establish a causal relationship between lung disease and specific toxic agents. The potential source of toxin, emission factor, uptake, deposition, retention, and degradation of the toxin are important when assessing the exposure. The physical properties such as pH, solubility, concentration, the rate and depth of respiration, and the reactivity of the toxin at tissue level are also important because they determine the deposition and reaction of the toxin in the respiratory tract. Industrial hygiene studies and epidemiologic investigations are often helpful but are beyond the scope of this chapter.

TABLE 1. Clinical and diagnostic tools for evaluating patients with persistent and progressive lung disease

- Initial medical evaluation
  - Medical and exposure history
  - Identification of toxic agent(s)
  - Radiographic studies: chest radiograph
  - Pulmonary function tests: pre- and postbronchodilator, diffusion capacity, lung capacities, oximetry
  - Basic chemistry and blood cell counts
- Specialized testing and review
  - Immune testing and serology on suspected agents
  - High-resolution computed tomography scan
  - Methacholine challenge test
  - Bronchoscopy, bronchoalveolar lavage
  - Material safety data sheets, chemical inventory and environmental reports
- Exposure assessment
  - Industrial hygiene study and environmental assessment
  - Structured epidemiologic investigation

DIFFERENTIAL DIAGNOSIS

There are several substances of toxicologic importance in PPPD (Table 2). (See also Chapters 183, 189, 215, and 256.)

Asbestos

In Greek, *asbestosis* means noncombustible or nondestructible. The term includes a family of naturally occurring fibrous magnesium silicates. The American Thoracic Society defines *asbestosis* as bilateral diffuse interstitial lung fibrosis caused by inhaling asbestos fibers (3).

The pathogenesis of asbestosis involves deposition of asbestos fibers in terminal bronchioles and activation of macrophages leading to release of mediators and inflammation. The result is

TABLE 2. **Persistent and progressive pulmonary diseases of toxicologic importance**

Disease	Toxin	Pathophysiology	Symptoms and signs	Diagnostic testing	Management and comment
Asbestosis	Asbestos (calcium, magnesium silicates with length:diameter ratio >3 μm)	Interstitial fibrosis mainly in the mid- and lower-lung fields	History of exposure >25 yr; dyspnea, dry cough, fatigue; chest pain, weight loss, hemoptysis uncommon	PFT, DLCO, CXR, HRCT	Supportive treatment; threshold of 25 fiber-yr of asbestos exposure
Silicosis	SIO_2	Interstitial fibrosis with eggshell calcification on perihilar lymph nodes; typically involves mid-lung fields	History of exposure >20 yr; exertional dyspnea, chronic cough; may be associated with tuberculosis	PFT, DLCO, CXR, HRCT	Supportive care; threshold of 1.8 mg/m^3 of SIO_2 exposure
Nonspecific interstitial pneumonitis, bronchiolitis	Nylon fiber, coal dust	Various degrees of interstitial inflammation and fibrosis	Cough, dyspnea	PFT, DLCO, CXR, HRCT	Supportive care; exposure avoidance
Bronchiolitis obliterans	Nitrogen dioxide, fly ash, acid vapor	Varying degrees of bronchiole obliteration by connective tissues and fibrosis	Progressive dry cough and dyspnea with interstitial lung infiltrates	PFT, DLCO, CXR, HRCT	Supportive care; exposure avoidance
Reactive airways disease	High-level irritant gases, such as chlorine, ammonia	Varying degrees of bronchoconstriction	Cough, dyspnea, chest pain uncommon	PFT, DLCO, CXR, methacholine challenge test	Supportive care; exposure avoidance
Hypersensitivity pneumonitis	Organic chemicals (isocyanates), biologic agents	Interstitial infiltrates with or without fibrosis	Cough, dyspnea, fever, chest pain uncommon	PFT, CXR, HRCT, BAL, serology panel	Supportive care; exposure avoidance
Pulmonary mycotoxicosis/ organic dust toxic syndrome	Volatile organic chemicals, mycotoxins, glucans, endotoxins(?)	Varying degrees of interstitial inflammation	Latency of a few hours followed by dyspnea, cough, chest pain	BAL showing increase in PMN; rare patchy infiltrates; serology panel normal	Supportive care and respiratory protection; exposure avoidance
Chronic obstructive pulmonary disease/ emphysema	Environmental tobacco smoke, cadmium	Varying degrees of bronchial hypersecretion and destruction of alveoli	Cough, sputum, dyspnea, chest pain	PFT, CXR	Supportive; exposure avoidance
Beryllioisis	Beryllium	Interstitial inflammation with granulomatous changes	History of exposure to beryllium dust; dyspnea, cough, chest pain	BAL, CXR, PFT, DLCO, HRCT	Supportive; exposure avoidance

BAL, bronchoalveolar lavage; CXR, chest radiograph; DLCO, diffusion capacity for carbon monoxide; HRCT, high-resolution computed tomography; PFT, pulmonary function testing; PMN, polymorphonuclear leukocyte; SIO_2, crystalline silica.

fibroblast proliferation, formation of fibrous scar tissue, and loss of pulmonary architecture (4).

A history of asbestos exposure is crucial. In addition to industrial exposures among construction workers, miners, and demolition workers, other environmental and "paraoccupational" exposures involve patients who do not directly handle asbestos (5), such as family members or specialty workers visiting the work site. Disease latency time is an important issue. Pleural thickening and plaques require 10 to 20 years to develop. Unless extensive, they do not produce specific symptoms. Asbestosis typically develops after 20 to 30 years, whereas mesothelioma occurs after 30 to 40 years. Cumulative exposure to asbestos fibers of more than 25 fiber-years may be needed to develop asbestosis. In other words, the dose has to be sufficient and significant in terms of concentration and duration (6).

Symptoms and signs of asbestosis are similar to other interstitial lung diseases. The patient usually presents with shortness of breath first noticed on effort and later at rest. Dry or productive cough becomes more troublesome as the disease progresses. Hemoptysis is rare, as is chest pain. Physical signs include dry basilar rales. Cyanosis and clubbing of the fingers may be present in advanced disease. Complications and mortality are related to intercurrent pneumonia, heart failure, and lung cancer. A typical chest radiograph shows pleural thickening, pleural calcification, and diaphragmatic calcification. The first PFT abnormalities are usually reduction of DLCO and partial pressure of arterial oxygen. A restrictive pattern with reduced lung volumes follows (7).

Diagnosis of asbestosis is based on five criteria: (a) a history of asbestos exposure, (b) radiographic evidence of interstitial fibrosis, (c) PFTs indicating restrictive lung disease, (d) a decrease in DLCO, and (e) clinical evidence of dry rales in lower lung fields. The International Labour Office has provided a system of classifying chest radiographs of pneumoconiosis (8). The chest radiograph is not without false-negatives, however, as 10% to 20% of symptomatic asbestosis patients have a normal radiograph. The high-resolution CT scan is more sensitive for early interstitial changes (9). Lung biopsy is rarely needed (10). Differential diagnosis includes other types of pneumoconiosis and other etiologies of interstitial fibrosis, such as metal, organic dust, drugs, infection, collagen vascular disease, and idiopathic pulmonary fibrosis (Table 2).

Management of asbestosis includes prevention of further exposure and avoidance of cigarette smoking. Other supportive measures (bronchodilators, low-flow oxygen administration, digitalis, and diuretics) may be necessary if right heart failure develops.

Silicosis, coal workers' pneumoconiosis, and metal and other dust-related pneumoconioses are not commonly encountered in

TABLE 3. Exposure-associated hypersensitivity pneumonitis (HP)

Antigen	Source of exposure	Example	Syndrome
Protein	Avian or bird droppings or feathers	Parakeet, pigeon, turkey, and chicken	Pigeon breeder's lung, bird fancier's lung
	Laboratory animals, especially rodents	Rodent urine protein	Lab worker's HP
	Fish meal	Fish protein	Fish meal worker's lung
Bacteria	Moldy hay, grain, and silage	Thermophilic actinomycetes	Farmer's lung
	Moldy sugar cane	Thermophilic actinomycetes	Bagassosis
	Mushroom compost	Thermophilic actinomycetes	Mushroom worker's lung
	Contaminated wood dust in walls	*Bacillus subtilis*	"Familial" HP
	Detergent	*B. subtilis* enzymes	Detergent worker's lung
Fungi	Contaminated water in air conditioning system	*Aureobasidium pullulans*	Air conditioner's lung
	Moldy barley	*Aspergillus fumigatus* or *clavatus*	Malt worker's lung
	Redwood sawdust	*Aureobasidium*	Sequoiosis
	Maple bark	*Cryptostroma corticale*	Maple bark disease
	Oak, cedar, pine dust, or pulp	*Alternaria*	Wood worker's lung
	Moldy cheese	*Penicillium casei*	Cheese worker's lung
	Cork dust	Cork dust mold—*Penicillium*	Suberosis
	Contaminated sauna water	*Aureobasidium*	Sauna taker's lung
	Compost	*Aspergillus*	Compost HP
	Contaminated wood trimmings	*Rhizopus, Mucor*	Wood trimmer's disease
	Dried grasses and leaves	*Saccharomonospora viridis*	Thatched roof disease
	Contaminated fertilizer	*Streptomyces albus*	*Streptomyces* HP
	Contaminated basement/sewage	*Cephalosporium*	Sewage HP
	Mold on tobacco	*Aspergillus*	Tobacco worker's HP
	Mold on grapes	*Botrytis cinerea*	Wine grower's lung
Chemicals	Polyurethane foam, varnish, and foundry casting	Isocyanates (methylene diisocyanate, toluene diisocyanate)	Chemical worker's lung
	Epoxy resin, paints	TMA	TMA pulmonary anemia syndrome

TMA, trimellitic anhydride.

medical toxicology practice. The diagnosis and management of these conditions are similar to asbestosis.

Hypersensitivity Pneumonitis

HP or extrinsic allergic alveolitis is a group of immune-mediated lung diseases secondary to repeated inhalation of finely aerosolized low-molecular-weight chemicals or bioaerosols (Table 3). It is a complex clinical syndrome with different patterns of disease. Chronic low-level exposure to these agents induces a hypersensitivity reaction, resulting in a cascade of inflammatory responses in the bronchioles and alveoli of susceptible patients and the release of cell mediators, leading to tissue damage and granulomatous changes (11). In contrast to bronchiolitis obliterans (BO), reactive airway dysfunction syndrome, and organic dust-toxic syndromes (which typically occur after a single high-dose exposure), HP requires repeated exposure. It has been reported among farmers, pigeon breeders, tobacco workers, chemical workers, and mushroom workers.

The history of exposure is typically repetitive, chronic, and persistent. Symptoms and signs of HP are not uniform. It has acute, subacute, and chronic forms. In the acute form, episodic dyspnea and cough with fever, chills, and malaise occur approximately 4 to 8 hours after exposure and resolve within 24 to 48 hours. The pulmonary volume is decreased with reduced DLCO and hypoxemia. The chronic form is characterized by insidious onset of shortness of breath, eventually leading to symptoms and signs of pulmonary fibrosis. The chronic form may or may not accompany the acute phase. Presence of serum IgG/IgM antibodies implies sufficient exposure to the causative agent to generate an immune response and is simply a marker of exposure, not an indicator of disease. Normal individuals without symptoms may have elevated antibody titers. High-resolution CT scans are considered more sensitive than routine radiographs in detecting early interstitial changes and fibrosis. CT scanning may reveal widespread ground-glass opacity with areas of sparing (12,13).

The diagnosis of HP requires a systematic approach: (a) Identify exposure to a provoking antigen/chemical; (b) demonstrate an immune response to the antigen; (c) establish the relationship of symptoms to antigen exposure; (d) assess the degree of lung impairment, including the extent of radiographic abnormality (Figs. 1–3); (e) consider the need for lung biopsy or BAL; (f) con-

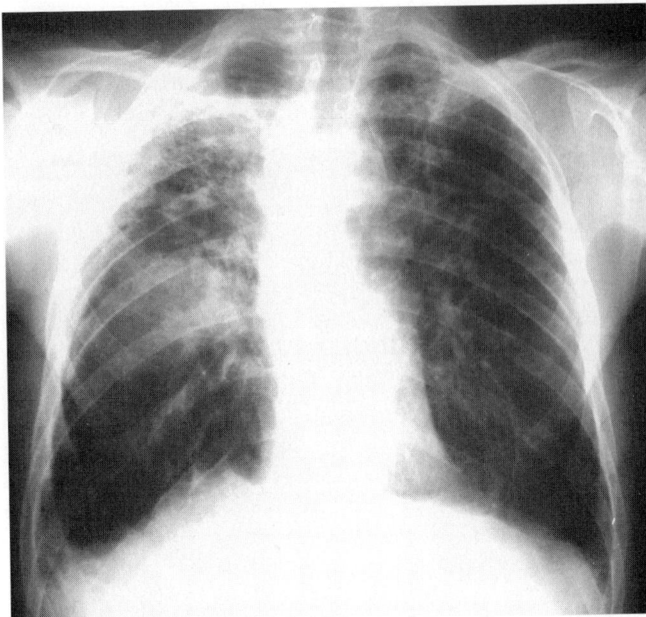

Figure 1. Chest radiograph of a 30-year-old chemical worker with hypersensitivity pneumonitis showing infiltrates most prominent at right mid- and upper-lung zones.

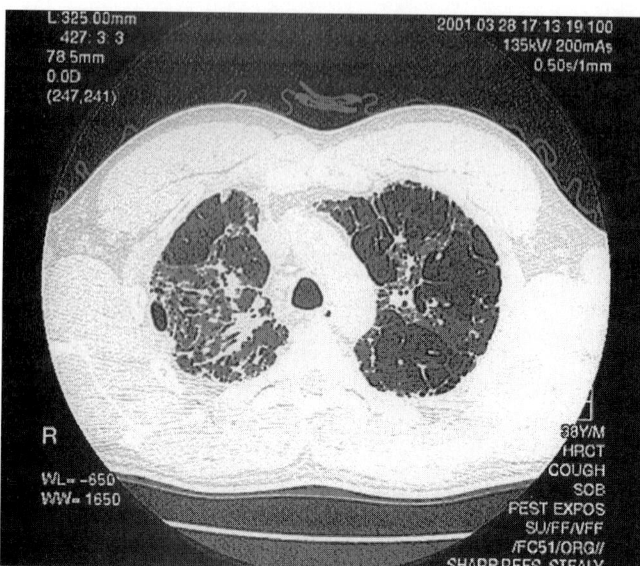

Figure 2. Chest computed tomography of the same chemical worker in Figure 1 showing interstitial fibrosis most prominent in right upper lobe, with honeycombing and scattered interstitial fibrosis in other areas.

sider natural- or laboratory-based challenge study; and (g) exclude alternative diagnoses, such as sarcoidosis and other interstitial lung diseases. It is important to rule out other common chronic lung diseases, such as chronic obstructive pulmonary disease, asthma, reactive airways dysfunction syndrome, and organic dust toxic syndrome.

Treatment is supportive. Antigen avoidance is the key, although discontinuing exposure may not always stop disease progression. A short course of oral steroids has been suggested, but the efficacy has not been documented by controlled studies. Educating individuals at risk in terms of recognizing early symptoms and implementing preventive measures are also important.

Pulmonary Mycotoxicosis

Pulmonary toxicity secondary to mycotoxins or mold metabolism byproduct exposure has been documented in adults (14). This syndrome is also known as *organic dust toxic syndrome*. The issue of whether inhaling mycotoxins can produce pulmonary mycotoxicosis continues to be controversial (15). In agricultural and compost facilities, this condition may occur because the intensity of exposure is typically larger and longer (16). However, the condition has not been well documented in homes and office buildings.

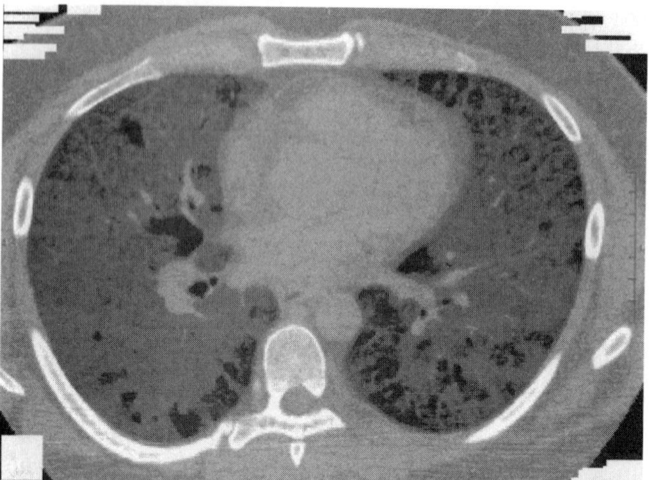

Figure 3. Computed tomography scan (lung window) of a 32-year-old software engineer with fungi-induced hypersensitivity pneumonitis showing extensive ground-glass appearance with some interstitial infiltrates.

Symptoms and signs including dry cough, dyspnea, chills, malaise, myalgia, and headache have been reported in patients exposed to high levels of mold (17,18). The pathogenesis of this syndrome is unrelated to hypersensitivity reactions. More specific pathology has recently been documented in infants exposed to mycotoxins produced by *Stachybotrys atra* (19). There are animal models that demonstrate lung mycotoxicoses induced by certain toxic mold species (20). An extensive review of the human literature on mycotoxin exposure indicates an increase in respiratory symptoms, such as cough, shortness of breath, wheezing, and mucous membrane irritation, when compared to normal, unexposed subjects (21,22). These subjective symptoms may be related to other components of mold (i.e., glucans, volatile organic chemicals, and ergosterols). Despite multiple mycotoxins isolated from various mold species, documented mycotoxin concentrations in literature have been incomplete. Because this condition is not an allergy, immune testing and serology of mold species are not of clinical use.

The diagnosis is based on history of exposure to high mold concentration, industrial hygiene studies, chemical analysis of mycotoxins when available, and symptoms, as well as ruling out HP, infection, and other lung diseases.

Treatment is supportive treatment and avoidance of exposure.

Bronchiolitis Obliterans

BO is an uncommon chronic illness that has been associated with toxic fume exposure (23), such as nitrogen dioxide, sulfur dioxide (24), ammonia, chlorine, phosgene, chloropicrin, hydrogen sulfide, acid vapor, and fly ash (25). Other important causes of BO include infections, connective tissue disorders, bone marrow and major organ transplant, and idiopathic causes. The pathophysiology of BO typically occurs beyond the small bronchioles, resulting in partial or complete obliteration of the bronchiole lumen by organizing connective tissue, fibrosis, and scarring. It is accompanied by interstitial infiltrates with lymphocytes and plasma cells. The key differences with other interstitial lung disease is that the lung architecture is maintained, and there is absence of extensive interstitial fibrosis.

The diagnosis is based on a history of toxic exposure, medical examination, chest radiography, arterial blood gas, PFT, CT scanning, and BAL. Biopsy is rarely indicated. Typically, the patient reports a history of significant toxic fume exposure. Initially, the patient is asymptomatic or only mildly symptomatic; however, cough, dyspnea, and signs of hypoxemia and pulmonary edema develop 24 to 48 hours later. Some patients improve transiently for days to 6 weeks. In the final phase, the patient reports progressive dyspnea, dry cough, chest pain, and hypoxemia. Physical examination is variable and nonspecific. Auscultation may reveal rales, rhonchi, and wheezing. Wheezing is typically unresponsive to bronchodilator and may be accompanied by fever and leukocytosis. The chest radiograph may be normal initially, but then patchy infiltrates or diffused reticulonodular pattern may appear after 24 to 48 hours. A CT scan may show lung hyperinflation, bronchiectasis, or dilatation of the smaller bronchi. PFT typically reveals evidence of low FEV_1 and reduced flow rates. Bronchoscopy is not helpful because the pathology of BO is distal to the visible respiratory tract. BAL may show an increase in lymphocytes; however, this is not a specific finding.

Treatment is symptomatic and supportive. Use of bronchodilators, antibiotics, oxygen, and ventilator may be necessary. Although steroids have been used, their effectiveness is not proved.

Chronic Bronchitis/Emphysema

Chronic bronchitis is characterized by inflammation of the bronchial tree, with persistent cough and sputum production on most days for at least 3 months of the year for 3 successive years (26). Chronic inhalation of irritant dust, fumes, and gases can cause simple chronic bronchitis. Although this can be confounded with smoking, this condition typically occurs among industrial workers who had prolonged exposure to irritants and dust (27). It may develop into permanent respiratory impairment with significant airflow obstruction. Toxic agents capable of producing chronic bronchitis include dust, oil mist, human-made fibers, vanadium, osmium, cotton, cigarette smoke, fire smoke, and engine exhaust. Cadmium oxide fumes are associated with chronic bronchitis and emphysema (28).

The diagnosis is based on a history of exposure with symptoms defined by the American Thoracic Society and PFTs that demonstrate an obstructive ventilatory pattern with no or minimal restrictive effects. Smokers are at high risk of developing respiratory symptoms with exposure to other toxic irritants. Symptoms of mucous membrane irritation may be present. Physical examination may be normal. PFTs show evidence of airway obstruction.

Treatment for chronic bronchitis depends on the etiology. If exposure to a specific toxic agent is discontinued, symptoms typically improve. Bronchodilators, inhaled steroids, and inhaled anticholinergic medications are used with some success.

Synthetic Fibers: Nylon

In general, synthetic fibers and human-made fibers do not produce chronic pulmonary pathology. Recently, synthetic nylon fibers have been associated with "flock workers'" lung secondary to inhaling respirable nylon dust particles. Nylon flocking workers have a higher risk of developing chronic nongranulomatous interstitial lung disease (29). The pathology is nonspecific and may include interstitial pneumonitis, lymphocyte infiltration, and bronchiolitis.

Symptoms include chronic cough, chest tightness, and dyspnea. Physical examination is nonspecific and may include rhonchi, rales, and wheezing. PFT is nonspecific. High-resolution CT typically shows a ground-glass appearance.

Treatment is symptomatic and supportive. Discontinuation of exposure usually alleviates symptoms. Respiratory protection and engineering exposure control are effective in prevention.

REFERENCES

1. O'Shea JJ, Frucht DM, Duckett CS. Cytokines and cytokine receptors. In: Rich RR, Fleisher TA, Shearer WT, et al., eds. *Clinical immunology principles and practice,* 2nd ed. St. Louis: Mosby, 2001.
2. DePaso WJ, Winterbauer RH. *Interstitial lung disease. Disease-a-month.* Littleton, MA: Mosby-Year Book, 1991.
3. American Thoracic Society. Diagnosis of nonmalignant diseases related to asbestos. *Am Rev Respir Dis* 1986;134:363–368.
4. Mossman BT, Churg A. Mechanisms in the pathogenesis of asbestosis and silicosis. *Am J Respir Crit Care Med* 1998;157:1666–1680.
5. Anderson HA, Lilis R, Duam SM, Selikoff IJ. Asbestosis among household contacts of asbestos factory workers. *Ann N Y Acad Sci* 1979;300:386–399.
6. Mossman BT, Gee JBL. Asbestos-related diseases. *N Engl J Med* 1989;320:1721–1730.
7. Miller A. Application of pulmonary function tests to the evaluation of asbestosis. *Ann N Y Acad Sci* 1991;643:145–148.
8. International Labour Office (ILO): guidelines for the use of ILO international classification of radiographs of pneumoconiosis, revised edition. Occupational Safety and Health series No. 22. Geneva, 1980.
9. Aberle DR, Balmes JR. Computed tomography of asbestos-related pulmonary parenchymal and pleural diseases. *Clin Chest Med* 1991;12:115–131.
10. Craighead JE, Abraham JL, Churg A, et al. Report of the Pneumoconiosis Committee of the College of American Pathologists and the National Institute of Occupational Safety and Health. The pathology of asbestos-associated diseases of the lungs and pleural cavities: diagnostic criteria and proposed grading schema. *Arch Pathol Lab Med* 1982;106:544–596.
11. Bourke SJ, Dalphin JC, Boyd G, et al. Hypersensitivity pneumonitis: current concepts. *Eur Respir J* 2001;32:81–92.
12. Richerson HB, Bernstein IL, Fink JN, et al. Report of the Subcommittee on Hypersensitivity Pneumonitis: Guidelines for the Clinical Evaluation of Hypersensitivity Pneumonitis. *J Allergy Clin Immunol* 1989;84:839–843.
13. Jacobs RL, Andrews CP, Coalson J. Organic antigen induced interstitial lung disease: diagnosis and management. *Ann Allergy Asthma Immunol* 2002;88:30–41.
14. Emanuel DA, Wenzel FJ, Lawton BP. Pulmonary mycotoxicosis. *Chest* 1975;67:293–297.
15. Fung F, Clark R, Williams S. *Stachybotrys*: still under investigation. *J Toxicol Clin Toxicol* 1998;36:633–634.
16. Fischer G, Schwalbe R, Ostrowski R, Dott W. Airborne fungi and their secondary metabolites in working places in a compost facility. *Mycoses* 1998;41:383–388.
17. Von Essen S, Robbins RA, Thompson AB, Rennard RI. Organic dust toxic syndrome: an acute febrile reaction to organic dust exposure distinct from hypersensitivity pneumonitis. *J Toxicol Clin Toxicol* 1990;128:389–426.
18. Brinton WT, Vastbinder EE, Greene JW, et al. An outbreak of organic dust toxic syndrome in college fraternity. *JAMA* 1987;258:1210–1212.
19. Pulmonary hemorrhage/hemosiderosis among infants—Cleveland, Ohio, 1993–1996. *MMWR Morb Mortal Wkly Rep* 1997;46:33–35.
20. Nikulin M, Reijula K, Jarvis BB, Hintikka EL. Experimental lung mycotoxicosis in mice induced by *Stachybotrys atra. Intern J Experim Pathol* 1996;77:213–218.
21. Fung F, Clark R, Williams S. *Stachybotrys*, a mycotoxin-producing fungus of increasing toxicologic importance. *J Toxicol Clin Toxicol* 1998;36:79–86.
22. Fung F, Hughson W. Health effects of indoor fungal bioaerosol exposure. *Proc IAQ* 2002;3:46–51.
23. Ezri T, Kunichezky S, Eliraz A, et al. Bronchiolitis obliterans—current concepts. *QJM* 1994,87:1–10.
24. Horvath EP, doPico GA, Barbee RA, Dickie HA. Nitrogen dioxide induced pulmonary disease. *J Occup Med* 1978;20:103–110.
25. Boswell RT, McCunney RJ. Bronchiolitis obliterans exposure to incinerator fly ash. *J Occup Environ Med* 1995;37:850–855.
26. American Thoracic Society. Standards for the diagnosis and care of patients with chronic obstructive pulmonary disease (COPD) and asthma. *Am Rev Respir Dis* 1987;136:225–244.
27. Becklake MR. Chronic airflow limitation: its relationship to work in dusty occupations. *Chest* 1985,88:606–617.
28. Bonnell J, Kazantzis G, King E. A follow-up study of men exposed to cadmium oxide fume. *Br J Ind Med* 1959;16:135–147.
29. Kern DG, Kuhn C 3rd, Ely EW, et al. Flock worker's lung: broadening the spectrum of clinicopathology, narrowing the spectrum of suspected etiologies. *Chest* 2000;117:251–259.

CHAPTER 28

Acute Drug-Induced Respiratory Failure

Sunye Kwack and Timothy E. Albertson

OVERVIEW

The respiratory consequences of an exposure depend on the intrinsic effects of an agent and the extrinsic circumstances of the exposure, as well as host immunity and physiologic reserve. Because drugs that simply depress respiratory drive are common and familiar to practitioners (e.g., opioids, sedative-hypnotics), this chapter addresses acute non–central nervous system causes. Table 1 outlines a method of categorizing acute respiratory failure that is followed throughout this chapter.

PATHOPHYSIOLOGY

Neuromuscular Disease

Diseases of the peripheral nervous system may produce respiratory compromise. These disorders may affect the spinal cord (e.g., poliomyelitis, tetanus), neuromuscular junction (e.g., myasthenia gravis), peripheral nerves (e.g., Guillain-Barré syndrome), or muscles (e.g., muscular dystrophy, steroid myopathy) (1). Some drugs can exacerbate underlying neuromuscular disease and result in respiratory distress (Table 1). For instance, a beta-blocker, an aminoglycoside antibiotic, or phenytoin may precipitate a myasthenic crisis (2,3).

Pleural/Mediastinal Disease

Pleural and mediastinal manifestations commonly involve pneumothoraces and barotrauma. As with iatrogenic barotrauma, attempts to access more central veins (e.g., internal jugular vein during intravenous drug abuse) may result in pneumothorax, with or without pneumomediastinum, tension pneumothorax, hemothorax, empyema, and pyopneumothorax (4,5). Pneumomediastinum and mediastinal hematomas often resolve but can lead to extrinsic obstruction of the trachea or mainstem bronchi (6).

Barotrauma complicates the use of various agents, such as inhalational use of cocaine, amphetamine, and marijuana (Table 1) (5). Intentionally prolonged Valsalva's maneuvers or coughing fits appear to be contributing causative factors. Pneumomediastinum and pneumopericardium have been reported (7). The clinical sequelae are usually mild, although acute respiratory failure from barotrauma has occurred.

Airway Disease

Anaphylactic and anaphylactoid reactions are often indistinguishable (Chapter 34). During anaphylaxis, mast cells and basophils release various preformed inflammatory mediators, triggering a cascade of mediators, such as histamine, leukotrienes, complement activators, and prostaglandins. Collectively, this inflammation causes increased vascular permeability, vasodilatation, stimulation of the autonomic nervous system, and contraction of smooth muscle in the respiratory tract.

A plethora of agents have incited anaphylaxis, with aspirin, beta-lactam antibiotics, nonsteroidal antiinflammatory agents, radiocontrast media, blood products, latex (8), and *Hymenoptera* venom among the more common offenders (9–11). The risk of anaphylaxis increases with increasing exposure intensity (duration, concentration) to an agent, intravenous versus oral administration, prior exposure, and having a history of an anaphylactic reaction. Patients with a history of anaphylaxis to penicillin are at a four- to sixfold increased risk for anaphylaxis with reexposure (12). Although atopic individuals do not appear to experience anaphylaxis reactions more frequently, their fatality rate per episode is slightly increased.

Inhalational injury involves direct physical or chemical effects on the lung. The upper airways and lungs are an interface with the external environment, designed to withstand many types of exposures. Defense mechanisms include the mucociliary assembly, the vocal cords, and the cough and gag reflexes.

The spectrum of inhalational injuries varies from mild tracheobronchitis to acute respiratory distress syndrome (ARDS). Airway inflammation with or without infection may occur with smoking of tobacco, marijuana, or cocaine (13). Aspiration of toxic inhalants, such as isopropyl alcohol, can induce a chemical tracheobronchitis. Bronchorrhea, wheezing, and reversible airway spasm are associated with carbamates and organophosphate insecticides. Fulminant bronchiolitis obliterans with organizing pneumonia (BOOP) involves patchy destruction of the terminal bronchiole and filling of the alveoli with inflammatory cells and loose connective tissue. BOOP has been associated with inhalational or noninhalational exposure to several agents: cocaine, gold, antineoplastic agents, welding fumes, and amiodarone (13–16).

Thermal injuries due to inhalation of smoke or gases are often limited to the supraglottic airways. Airway injury may extend to the lower respiratory tract when steam, other superheated particles, or a closed space exposure are involved. Upper and lower airway burns can also result from caustic materials, such as strong acids or bases. Subsequent edema, necrosis, and sloughing of the airways may obstruct the airway. Laryngospasm occurs but appears to be a less frequent complication of inhalational injuries. Hypoxia and hypoxemia may result as absorption of inhaled oxygen falls or as a systemic toxic effect of the agent ensues. Respiratory insult may also result from direct bronchopulmonary toxicity, as seen with some lower-molecular-weight constituents of smoke via free radical mediators. Additionally, aspiration of foreign material may accompany the inhaled agent (e.g., talc with heroin).

ASTHMA/REACTIVE AIRWAYS DYSFUNCTION SYNDROME

Asthma is a chronic inflammatory disease with airway hyperresponsiveness that is characterized by reversible airway obstruction (Chapter 11) (17–20). The mechanism of drug-induced asthma can be receptor mediated (β-adrenergic receptor antagonists), inflammatory, or allergic/anaphylactoid. Exposure may occur by inhalation, injection, ingestion, dermal, or ophthalmic (18–21). The agent may be difficult to identify and may involve multiple compounds. Exposure to leather protectors (isobutane, isooctane, ethyl acetate, and *n*-heptane mixed with fluoropolymer

TABLE 1. Categories of acute respiratory failure and mechanism of toxicity

Category	Drugs
Neuromuscular failure	Aminoglycoside antibiotics, amiodarone, angiotensin-converting enzyme inhibitors, beta-blockers, calcium-channel antagonists, carbamates, clofibrate, corticosteroids, cyclic antidepressants, D-penicillamine, diuretics (electrolyte imbalance), epsilon-aminocaproic acid, gold, isoniazid, macrolide antibiotics, magnesium sulfate, neuromuscular blockers, nicotine, organophosphates, perhexiline, phenytoin, polymyxin B, procainamide, quinidine, quinine, vaccines, vincristine
Pneumothorax/barotrauma	Amphetamines, bleomycin, BCNU, cocaine, heroin, iron, IV drugs of abuse, marijuana, nitrous oxide
Airways disease	
Inhalational injury	Carbamates, cocaine, heroin, isopropanol, leather protectors, marijuana, organophosphates, smoke, strong acids/bases (e.g., hydrofluoric acid), superheated gases (e.g., cocaine), talc/talc adulterants, tobacco, welding fumes, zinc chloride
Asthma	Adenosine, aminoglycosides, angiotensin-converting enzyme inhibitors, animal danders, antibiotics (e.g., penicillins), aspirin, β-adrenergic receptor antagonists, blood transfusion, cholinergic agents, cotton smoke, diisocyanates, dipyridamole, drugs that increase gastroesophageal reflux (e.g., ethanol), enflurane, indomethacin, inhaled verapamil, interleukin-2, latex, leather protectors (aerosolized), marijuana, methylphenidate, metals (e.g., galvanized steel, nickel, aluminum fluoride), nebulized agents (e.g., pentamidine, beclomethasone), nonsteroidal antiinflammatory drugs, opioids, oral contraceptive drugs, pituitary snuff, plastic/epoxy resins, polymer fumes, polymyxin/colistin, propafenone, propellants and inhaler additives, propofol, protamine, proteolytic enzymes (e.g., subtilisin), radiographic contrast media, suxamethonium, smoked cocaine, sodium metabisulfite preservative, triamterene/hydrochlorothiazide, vaccines/serums, vinblastine/mitomycin-C, vitamin K
Reactive airways dysfunction syndrome	Acetic acid, acids, ammonia fumes, bleaching agents, burned paint fumes, butadiene, calcium oxide, chlorine gas, diphenyl methane diisocyanate, 2-diethylaminoethanol, ether vehicle, ethylene oxide, fire/smoke, floor sealant/cleaner, formaldehyde, fumigating fog, heated acid, hydrazine 35%, hydrochloric acid, hypochlorite sodium, lithium bromide, locomotive exhaust, metal coat remover, metam sodium (sodium *N*-methyldithiocarbamate), methylene chloride (phosgene), perchlorethylene, phosphoric acid, silicon tetrachloride, silo gas, sodium hydroxide, spray paint, sulfur dioxide, sulfuric acid, tear gas, toluene diisocyanate, trochlorosilane, uranium hexafluoride, welding fumes, zinc chloride
Alveolar disease	
Acute respiratory distress syndrome	Acrolein, amiodarone, amphetamines, amphotericin B, bleomycin, blood products, cadmium (high exposure levels), chlorine, cocaine, cyanide, cyclic antidepressants, cyclosporine, cytarabine, dextran-70, epinephrine, ethchlorvynol, ethiodized oil with radioactive iodine, fentanyl (epidural), flurazepam, heparin, hydrochlorothiazide, interleukin-2, leukocyte transfusions, lidocaine, methotrexate (intrathecal and systemic), methyl chloride (inhalation/combustion), mitomycin-C + 5-fluorouracil, mitomycin-C + leukocyte transfusions, moxalactam, nitrofurantoin, nitrogen dioxide, nitroprusside/nitric oxide, opioids/heroin, oxygen (prolonged high exposures), paraquat, D-penicillamine, phenothiazines, phosgene, protamine, pyromellitis dianhydride inhalation, radiation, radiographic contrast material, salicylates, sclerotherapy, smoke inhalation, streptokinase, sulfur dioxide, trichloroethylene (welding-induced inhalation), trimethoprim-sulfamethoxazole, tocolytic agents (e.g., beta agonists, such as terbutaline, ritodrine), tumor necrosis factor/endotoxin, zinc chloride smoke (inhalation)
Cardiogenic pulmonary edema	Antidysrhythmics, beta-blockers, calcium-channel antagonists, colloid and crystalloid, daunorubicin, doxorubicin
Hypersensitivity pneumonitis	Bleomycin, cocaine, cromolyn, dantrolene, hydralazine, isoniazid, L-tryptophan, methotrexate, methylphenidate, nitrofurantoin, penicillin, phenytoin, procarbazine, sulfonamides, thermophilic actinomyces
Interstitial lung disease	
Interstitial pneumonitis	Acrylic resin pneumoconiosis, amiodarone, beryllium, bleomycin, bromine compounds, cemented tungsten carbide, cobalt, cocaine, corneal moisturizer (e.g., Lacri-Lube), flecainide, gold + naproxen, gold salts, hydrogen peroxide (inhalation), IV drug abuse, liquid paraffin, mercury, methotrexate, mexiletine, nitrofurantoin, penicillamine, quinidine, radiation, silica/silicates, sulindac, tocainide, vinblastine + mitomycin-C
Vascular disease	
Pulmonary embolic disease	Cocaine, dextran-40, ethiodized oil/lymphangiography, foreign body additives (e.g., talc), oral contraceptives, therapeutic substance embolization/migration (e.g., Gelfoam, silicone spheres)
Pulmonary hypertension	Amphetamine, aminorex fumarate, cocaine, dexfenfluramine, fat emulsion (intralipid), fenfluramine, paraquat, pyrrolizidine alkaloids (e.g., monocrotaline), sodium morrhuate (e.g., variceal sclerosis)
Pulmonary vascular granulomatosis	Cocaine, cotton fibers, IV use of crushed oral drugs, talc, and cellulose
Pulmonary venoocclusive disease	Bleomycin, BCNU, cyclophosphamide, etoposide, mitomycin-C
Vasculitis	Amphetamines, cocaine, foreign material (i.e., injected during intravenous drug abuse), hydralazine, nitrofurantoin, penicillins, procainamide, sulfonamide
Impaired oxygen delivery	
Reduced cardiac output	Any agent producing bradycardia, antidysrhythmic agents, beta-blockers, cyclic antidepressant overdose, iron
Anemia (hemolytic and nonhemolytic)	Anticonvulsants, azathioprine, chemotherapeutic agents, chloramphenicol, gold salts, hypophosphatemia, methotrexate, methyldopa, nitrous oxide, oxidative drugs (in the setting of glucose 6 phosphate deficiency), penicillin, quinidine, thiouracil, triamterene, trimethoprim
Altered hemoglobin carrying capacity	Acetate, aniline derivatives, benzocaine, carbon monoxide, chlorates, dinitrophenol, ferrocyanide, hydrogen peroxide, mafenide, nitrates, nitrites, nitroglycerin, primaquine, sulfonamides
Impaired cellular use of oxygen	Cyanide, hydrogen sulfide, salicylates, sodium azide

BCNU, carmustine.

resins or carbonyl fluoride) has caused cough, shortness of breath, bronchospasm, and wheezing (22,23). Aspirin and nonsteroidal antiinflammatory drugs have well-established relationships with asthma, as well as angioedema and hives (24). Antileukotriene therapies, such as zileuton, appear to have a particular benefit for the aspirin-intolerant asthmatic (25).

Reactive airways dysfunction syndrome (RADS) develops in a subset of patients with inhalational injury (Table 1). RADS represents a nonimmunologic, asthma-like syndrome induced by irritant inhalation.

UPPER AIRWAY OBSTRUCTION

Upper airway obstruction may be a localized problem or may be associated with more systemic disorders (e.g., asthma or anaphylaxis). For example, nine patients presented with hoarseness or upper airway obstruction after heroin injections into the neck (26), presumably from injury to the recurrent laryngeal nerve. An accompanying cellulitis or abscess may facilitate the diagnosis. Mechanical obstruction with mucous plugs or sloughed epithelium may jeopardize the airway, especially in the setting of an impaired mental status or cough reflex.

Aspiration of foreign bodies has occurred with convulsant agents and central nervous system depressants. Local anesthetics may also lead to aspiration, including a hypodermic needle aspiration by a freebase user of cocaine (27).

Alveolar Disease

ARDS is characterized by noncardiogenic pulmonary edema due to an increase in pulmonary capillary permeability. Sepsis, gastric aspiration, and a variety of drugs and toxins are precipitants of ARDS (Table 1) (13–15,28–33). ARDS generally results in hypoxemic (type I) respiratory failure due to an increase in shunt fraction as alveoli become fluid filled or collapse. Decreased compliance with interstitial inflammation and fluid also adds to the workload of ventilation. The likelihood of ARDS may be modified by the clinical setting. For example, it is more closely associated with amiodarone after cardiopulmonary surgery (1 to 4 days) and pulmonary angiography (1 to 2 hours).

Cardiogenic pulmonary edema is most likely after β-adrenergic receptor antagonist and calcium channel–blocker poisoning. Left ventricular dysfunction may result from negative inotropic or chronotropic effects. Pulmonary hemorrhage can lead to various drug-induced conditions, such as pulmonary vasculitis and ARDS (e.g., dextran 70) (30,34,35).

Interstitial Lung Disease

Interstitial lung disease in its acute form includes an extensive and heterogeneous group: hypersensitivity pneumonitis (HP), eosinophilic pneumonia, and BOOP. *HP*, also known as *extrinsic allergic alveolitis*, is an immunologic reaction of the pulmonary parenchyma to an inhaled antigenic stimulus. Common antigen sources include birds, moldy plant matter, water sources, and synthetic chemicals. Drug-induced interstitial pneumonitis is associated with numerous agents (Table 1).

Vascular Disease

The pulmonary vasculature provides an extensive interface for gas exchange and oxygen delivery. Acute respiratory failure may occur with sudden compromise of the arterial bed and hypoxemia due to ventilation/perfusion mismatching or shunting. Obstruction at the venous level may also be serious but is less prevalent and more likely to be chronic.

Pulmonary embolus (PE) produces shunting and a reduced area for oxygen exchange. The emboli may be the consequence of an induced hypercoagulable state (e.g., oral contraceptives), endogenous material (e.g., fat or amniotic fluid), or exogenous material (e.g., air, talc, cotton fibers) (30,32,36–38). In addition to hypoxemia, acute respiratory failure due to a PE can also reflect a reduction in cardiac output due to an increased afterload on the right ventricle. Right ventricle dysfunction can sometimes be observed by echocardiography in the setting of an extensive PE (39).

Pulmonary hypertension (i.e., pulmonary artery pressure greater than 25 mm Hg at rest or greater than 30 mm Hg with exercise) (40) is associated with several drugs, including amphetamines, cocaine, and paraquat (Table 1) (14,41). There is usually a subacute or chronic disease that appears to result from increased vascular resistance due to proliferation of endothelial smooth muscle (42). Toxins may also produce acute pulmonary hypertension with respiratory failure (hypoxemia) and its typical symptoms. As with PEs, right-sided heart dysfunction or failure (cor pulmonale) can occur in severe cases.

Impaired Oxygen Delivery

The amount of oxygen delivery to the cells depends on both the oxygen content of the blood, as well as cardiac output. The oxygen content of the blood depends on the concentration of oxyhemoglobin and the concentration of dissolved oxygen in blood. In the absence of severe anemia or hyperbaric concentrations, however, dissolved oxygen is a minor contributor to the oxygen content of blood. To maximize oxygen delivery to peripheral tissue, therefore, optimizing hemoglobin levels and cardiac output may often be more effective than augmenting the arterial blood concentration (partial pressure of arterial oxygen) with supplemental oxygen.

Acute respiratory failure may ensue as oxygen delivery fails to meet oxygen demand. Cellular respiration becomes anaerobic, leading to lactic acidosis. The increased work of breathing required to compensate for acidosis may exhaust pulmonary reserves, especially among patients with existing cardiopulmonary dysfunction. Drugs that diminish the ability to increase cardiac output (i.e., negative chronotropic drugs) magnify the ventilatory demands on the pulmonary system.

Other agents disrupt oxygen delivery through noncardiogenic mechanisms (Table 1). Their mechanisms include altering hemoglobin carrying capacity (e.g., carbon monoxide); inducing hemolytic (e.g., oxidative drugs, penicillin) or nonhemolytic (e.g., chemotherapeutic agents) anemia; inducing formation of met- or sulfhemoglobinemia (e.g., nitrites, primaquine, or benzocaine); and uncoupling of cellular oxidative phosphorylation (e.g., cyanide, salicylates, or sodium azide).

DIAGNOSIS

The differential diagnosis of drug-induced respiratory failure is extensive (Table 1). Individual chapters on specific toxins provide additional information. The history can be crucial to establish that an exposure has occurred and to what agent. However, the signs and symptoms are similar among all causes of acute respiratory failure: chest pain, shortness of breath, and cough. In more severe cases, hemoptysis, syncope, and coma may occur. Each of these conditions is characterized by a decreased partial pressure of arterial oxygen and increased partial pressure of arterial carbon dioxide.

Neuromuscular Disease

Neuromuscular diseases are associated with either type II (hypercapnic) respiratory failure or alveolar hypoventilation as the primary defect. Vital capacity may diminish, and tidal volumes smaller than 15 ml/kg are associated with a high risk for ventilatory failure (3). Inability to generate more than 20 cm H_2O of negative inspiratory force is also associated with ventilatory insufficiency. Downward trends in these parameters can lead to impending respiratory difficulties. Although tachypnea may initially compensate for reduced vital capacity, the resulting increase in work of breathing is often difficult to sustain. Respiratory acidosis (increased partial pressure of arterial carbon dioxide) and relatively normal partial pressure of arterial oxygen are common. Depending on the temporal progression of respiratory compromise, the degree of frank acidemia may vary considerably. Hypoxemia may develop in severe cases of type II respiratory failure. It is also important to recognize that the tempo of symptom progression may be affected by an underlying parenchymal lung disease or impaired control of breathing.

Pleural/Mediastinal Disease

Pleural or mediastinal processes typically cause loss of function (e.g., pneumothorax) or physical obstruction (e.g., tension pneumothorax). Chest radiography often reveals barotrauma and pneumothorax.

Airway Disease

Anaphylaxis and anaphylactoid reactions are diagnosed by their acute onset and associated physical signs. Diagnostic tests are of little help in the early course. Anaphylaxis may present with urticaria or angioedema, laryngeal edema, bronchospasm, and hypotension. Shortness of breath, wheezing, nausea, and abdominal cramping may also occur (43). Notably, 5% to 20% of patients have a biphasic response (symptoms recur from 1 to 8 hours postexposure) or protracted response (symptoms persist up to 48 hours despite therapy) (44).

Inhalational injuries can be diagnosed with fiberoptic bronchoscopy. Thermal burns usually manifest early, and maximal effects peak within 48 hours.

Asthma and RADS have reversible obstructive airflow pattern on spirometry, but methacholine challenge testing is generally positive. A key diagnostic criterion of RADS is the absence of preceding respiratory disease in an individual with abrupt onset of persistent asthma-like symptoms within minutes to hours of a documented exposure to excessive concentrations of corrosive or irritating gas, vapor, fumes, or dust (45–47). Although controversial, persistent bronchial hyperresponsiveness and airway obstruction are features of the syndrome. Clinically, cough, wheezing, and dyspnea are common. In contrast to asthma, RADS is not associated with eosinophilia and lymphocytic inflammation within the airway mucosa.

Alveolar Disease

The chest radiograph of ARDS reveals patchy, bilateral infiltrates, which may be mistaken for cardiogenic pulmonary edema. Similarly, computed tomography of the lungs shows patchy airspace disease, with greater alveolar involvement in the gravity-dependent areas.

Clinical findings of cardiogenic pulmonary edema are nonspecific and include respiratory distress, hypoxemia, respiratory acidosis, and increased interstitial markings on chest radiography. Although nonspecific, symptoms of pulmonary hemorrhage may include dyspnea, hemoptysis, cough, and chest pain. Clinical findings of an anemia, coagulopathy, and infiltrates on chest radiography may also suggest the diagnosis. Fiberoptic bronchoscopy can be useful for identifying pulmonary hemorrhage and its sites of involvement.

Interstitial Lung Disease

The clinical symptoms of interstitial pneumonitis may be nonspecific, include progressive dyspnea and a dry cough, and are more often subacute than acute. Acute exacerbation of a more chronic disease process may also occur. The chest radiograph may reveal increased interstitial markings, often with a basilar predominance. Mild hypoxemia can be present as well.

Clinically, the symptoms of HP (e.g., fever, chills, malaise, cough, and dyspnea) often begin within 4 to 6 hours of exposure (48). Delayed symptom onset has been reported (e.g., nitrofurantoin). The symptoms generally last from days to weeks before coming to medical attention. The history often includes exposure to birds (parakeets, pigeons), moldy plant matter (hay, grains, silage, sugar cane, maple bark), and water sources (humidifiers, hot tubs, saunas). Synthetic chemicals have been implicated (Table 1). The physical examination is relatively nonspecific. Tachypnea and diffuse rales may be present. The chest radiograph may reveal interstitial markings in the mid- to lower-lung zones but is often normal. Computed tomography may reveal more extensive interstitial involvement. Bronchoalveolar lavage classically demonstrates lymphocytosis with an increased proportion of CD8 cells. Loosely formed noncaseating granulomas in a peribronchial distribution are the hallmark histopathologic findings of HP. A mononuclear infiltrate and a presence of giant cells can also be prominent.

Vascular Disease

Symptoms of a PE are notoriously nonspecific, including chest pain and shortness of breath. The diagnosis of PE is established by ventilation/perfusion scan, spiral computed tomography, or pulmonary angiography.

POTENTIAL COMPLICATIONS

Complications may be related to respiratory failure or to the underlying cause. Complications of respiratory failure typically arise from hypoxemia (e.g., myocardial infarction, anoxic brain injury). The underlying process may also create complications, such as hyperthermia and rhabdomyolysis after cocaine abuse.

MANAGEMENT

The principles of management are to rapidly intervene when clinically needed (e.g., life-threatening hypoxemia) and then establish the diagnosis. For most of these conditions, immediate airway management is that of advanced life support. Further information is available in chapters on specific agents.

Neuromuscular Disease

In addition to ventilatory support, clinical improvement often depends on identification and removal of the offending drug and improvement of the underlying etiology.

Pleural/Mediastinal Disease

In the absence of acute respiratory failure, conservative measures, such as observation and supplemental oxygen, are effective for most patients with drug-induced barotrauma (7).

Airway Disease

Anaphylaxis and anaphylactoid reactions are addressed in Chapter 34.

Inhalational injury management depends on the nature of the agent and circumstances. Reducing further exposure to the agent is imperative. Antidotes may attenuate ongoing injury, especially if the inhaled compounds are identified quickly. Special consideration should be given to protecting the airway and to anticipating potential complications of airway burns. Judicious use of humidified oxygen and supportive measures addressing bronchospasm, fluid deficits, and other accompanying complications are also especially important in the early stages of management of an inhalational injury. Repeated bronchoscopy to remove casts and mucus may be needed. Treatment of ARDS and BOOP includes removal from further toxic agent exposure, supportive care, and consideration of the use of corticosteroids.

Asthma is treated by removing the patient form further exposure and with the usual therapies for bronchospasm (Chapter 16). RADS is treated by terminating the exposure to the offending agent and administering corticosteroids, either inhaled or systemic. Resolution of RADS is generally observed after 6 weeks to 6 months of therapy.

Upper airway obstruction is managed with bronchoscopic removal of the foreign body. Antibiotics for postobstructive pneumonia and supportive care for other complications may be necessary. Mechanical clearing of debris via fiberoptic bronchoscopy may be required repeatedly to facilitate adequate ventilation.

Alveolar Disease

Treatment of ARDS often requires both positive end-expiratory pressure, oxygen supplementation, and mechanical ventilation. Positive end-expiratory pressure acts by optimizing oxygenation, as well as avoiding end-expiratory decruitment of alveoli. Recently, the benefits of a ventilatory strategy of permissive hypercapnia have been supported by a large, multicenter prospective and randomized trial (49). Using tidal volumes starting at 6 ml/kg while tolerating an arterial pH of 7.3 was effective in decreasing mortality in 861 patients with ARDS. This benefit may be attributable, in part, to the reduced shear injury to alveoli and to a reduced release of injurious inflammatory mediators. Treatment of "chronic" or late-phase ARDS has included corticosteroids.

Overall, mortality with ARDS is estimated at 40% to 50% (50–52). The range of pulmonary sequelae in survivors varies from none to severe impairment at 1 year; only a small minority appears to experience severe pulmonary impairment (53).

Cardiogenic pulmonary edema treatment depends on removal of the offending agent and specific treatment of the cardiogenic failure (oxygen, diuretics, preload and afterload reduction).

Pulmonary hemorrhage is treated by protecting the airway and preserving gas exchange in unaffected areas of the lung. Other supportive measures include supplemental oxygen, fluid resuscitation, and bronchodilators as required. Ultimately, treating an underlying problem is important in preventing progressive injury.

Interstitial Lung Disease

Treatment of HP depends on terminating exposure to the inciting agent; clinical resolution of acute HP usually occurs after 12 hours to a few days. Corticosteroid therapy may accelerate resolution of symptoms but does not appear to alter long-term outcome. Although the risk of recurrence on reexposure to the offending agent is not always clear, ongoing exposure to certain antigens has been associated with progression to more chronic forms of HP (e.g., farmer's lung, bird fancier's lung).

For drug-induced interstitial pneumonitis, withdrawal of the inciting drug is paramount. Corticosteroids may also be an effective adjunct to therapy.

Vascular Disease

PE treatment includes anticoagulants, thrombolytics for severe cases, oxygen, and, in certain circumstances, placement of inferior vena cava filters.

Pulmonary hypertension therapy is directed toward reducing pulmonary pressures (prostacyclin analogs, nitric oxide), treating fluid overload states (diuretics), providing adequate oxygen supplementation, and preventing PEs (anticoagulation).

Alterations in oxygen delivery are treated by restoring oxygen delivery to the cell. Treatment is supportive. Prognosis depends on the underlying etiology.

REFERENCES

1. Epstein SK. An overview of respiratory muscle function. *Clin Chest Med* 1994;15:619–639.
2. Drachman DB. Myasthenia gravis. *N Engl J Med* 1994;330:1797–1810.
3. Ropper AH. Guillain-Barré syndrome. *N Engl J Med* 1992;326:1130–1136.
4. Zorc TG, O'Donnell AE, Holt RW, et al. Bilateral pyopneumothorax secondary to intravenous drug abuse. *Chest* 1988;93:645–647.
5. Hind CRK. Pulmonary complications of intravenous drug misuse: epidemiology and non-infective complications. *Thorax* 1990;45:891–897.
6. Stern WZ, Subbaro K. Pulmonary complications of drug addiction. *Semin Roentgenol* 1983;18:183–197.
7. Seaman ME. Barotrauma related to inhalational drug abuse. *J Emerg Med* 1990;8:141–149.
8. Tanlo SM. Natural rubber latex allergy and asthma. *Curr Opinion Pulm Med* 2001;7:27–31.
9. Kemp SF, Lockey RF, Wolf BL, et al. Anaphylaxis: review of 266 cases. *Arch Intern Med* 1995;155:1749–1754.
10. Yocum MW, Khan DA. Assessment of patients who have experienced anaphylaxis: a 3-year survey. *Mayo Clin Proc* 1994;69:16–23.
11. Ewan PW. Anaphylaxis. *BMJ* 1998;316:1442–1445.
12. Weiss ME, Adkinson NF. Immediate hypersensitivity reactions to penicillins and related antibiotics. *Clin Allergy* 1988;18:515–540.
13. Rosenow EC, Meyers JL, Swensen SF, et al. Drug-induced pulmonary disease: an update. *Chest* 1992;102:239–250.
14. Albertson TE, Walby WF, Derlet RW. Stimulant-induced pulmonary toxicity. *Chest* 1995;108:1140–1149.
15. Cherubin CE, Sapira JD. The medical complications of drug addiction and the medical assessment of the intravenous drug user: 25 years later. *Ann Intern Med* 1993;119:1017–1028.
16. Taskin DP. Pulmonary complications of smoked substance abuse. *West J Med* 1990;152:525–530.
17. National Asthma Education Program Expert Panel. *Guidelines for the diagnosis and management of asthma*, Pub#91-3042. Bethesda, MD: National Institutes of Health, 1991.
18. Hunt LW, Rosenow EC. Asthma-producing drugs. *Ann Allergy* 1992;453–462.
19. Prakash UBS, Rosenow EC. Pulmonary complications from ophthalmic preparations. *Mayo Clin Proc* 1990;65:521–529.
20. Weiss ST. Straightforward diagnosis of occupational lung disease. *Contemp Intern Med* 1991;43–45.
21. Prien T, Traber DC, Richardson JA, et al. Early effects of inhalation injury on lung mechanics and pulmonary perfusion. *Intensive Care Med* 1988;14:25–29.
22. Burkhart KK, Britt A, Petrini G, et al. Pulmonary toxicity following exposure to an aerosolized leather protector. *J Toxicol Clin Toxicol* 1996;34:21–24.
23. Laliberte M, Sanfucon G, Blais R. Acute pulmonary toxicity linked to use of a leather protector. *Ann Emerg Med* 1995;25:841–844.
24. Babu KS, Salvi SS. Aspirin and asthma. *Chest* 2000;118:1470–1476.
25. Dahlen B, Nizankowska E, Szczeklik A, et al. Benefits of adding the 5-lipoxygenase inhibitor zileuton to conventional therapy in aspirin intolerant asthmatics. *Am J Res Crit Care Med* 1998;157:1187–1194.
26. Hillstrom RP, Cohn AM, McCarroll KA. Vocal cord paralysis resulting from neck injections in the intravenous drug use population. *Laryngoscope* 1990;100:503–506.
27. Lacagnina S, Vomero E, Jacobson M, et al. Hypodermic needle aspiration in a freebase cocaine abuser. *Chest* 1990;97:1275–1276.
28. Cooper JAD, White DA, Matthay RA. Drug-induced pulmonary disease: II. Noncytotoxic drugs. *Am Rev Resp Dis* 1966;133:488–505.
29. Heffner JE, Harley RA, Schable SI. Pulmonary reactions from illicit substance abuse. *Clin Chest Med* 1990;11:151–162.
30. Kumar K, Holder WE. Drug-induced pulmonary vascular disease: mechanisms and clinical patterns. *West J Med* 1986;145:343–349.
31. Reed CR, Glauser FL. Drug-induced non-cardiogenic pulmonary edema. *Chest* 1991;100:1120–1124.
32. Rosenow EC. The spectrum of drug-induced pulmonary disease. *Ann Intern Med* 1972;77:977–991.

33. Zitnik RJ. Drug-induced lung disease: antiarrhythmic agents. *J Respir Dis* 1996;17:254–270.
34. Brandt RR, Dunn WF, Ory SJ. Dextran 70 embolization: another cause of pulmonary hemorrhage, coagulopathy and rhabdomyolysis. *Chest* 1993;104:631–633.
35. Kaplan V, Vaur X, Czuppon A, et al. Pulmonary hemorrhage due to inhalation of vapor containing pyromellitic diahydride. *Chest* 1993;104:644–645.
36. Douglas FG, Kafilmont KJ, Patt NL. Foreign particle embolism in drug addicts: respiratory pathophysiology. *Ann Intern Med* 1971;75:865–872.
37. Lewman LV. Fatal pulmonary hypertension from intravenous injection of methyl phenidate (Ritalin) tablets. *Hum Pathol* 1972;3:67–70.
38. Tomashefski JF, Hirsh CS. The pulmonary vascular lesions of intravenous drug abuse. *Hum Pathol* 1980;11:133–145.
39. Benotti JR, Dalen JE. Natural history of pulmonary embolism. *Clin Chest Med* 1984;5:403–410.
40. Pietra GG, Edwards WD, Kay JM, et al. Histopathology of primary pulmonary hypertension: a qualitative and quantitative study of pulmonary blood vessels from 58 patients in the National Heart, Lung and Blood Institute, Primary Pulmonary Hypertension Registry. *Circulation* 1989;80:1198–1206.
41. Rich S, Rubin L, Walker AM, et al. Anorexigens and pulmonary hypertension in the United States: results from the surveillance of North American pulmonary hypertension. *Chest* 2000;117:870–874.
42. Tuder RM, Cool CD, Geraci MW, et al. Prostacyclin synthase expression is decreased in lungs of patients with severe pulmonary hypertension. *Am J Respir Crit Care Med* 1999;159:1925–1932.
43. Bochner BS, Lichtenstein M. Anaphylaxis. *N Engl J Med* 1991;324:1785–1790.
44. Stark BJ, Sullivan TJ. Biphasic and protracted anaphylaxis. *J Allergy Clin Immunol* 1986;78:76–83.
45. Alberts WM, do Pico GA. Reactive airways dysfunction syndrome. *Chest* 1996;109:1618–1626.
46. Brooks SM, Weiss MA, Berstein IL. Reactive airways dysfunction syndrome (RADS) persistent asthma syndrome after high-level irritant exposures. *Chest* 1985;88:376–384.
47. Brooks SM, Hammad Y, Richards I, et al. The spectrum of irritant-induced asthma: sudden and not-so-sudden onset and the role of allergy. *Chest* 1998;113:42–49.
48. Schuyler M, Cormier Y. The diagnosis of hypersensitivity pneumonitis. *Chest* 1997;111:534–536.
49. Ventilation with lower tidal volumes as compared with traditional tidal volumes for acute lung injury and the acute respiratory distress syndrome. The Acute Respiratory Distress Syndrome Network. *N Engl J Med* 2000;342:1301–1308.
50. Zilberberg MD, Epstein SK. Acute lung injury in the medical ICU: comorbid conditions, age, etiology, and hospital outcome. *Am J Respir Crit Care Med* 1998;157:1159–1164.
51. Doyle RL, Szaflarski N, Modin GW, et al. Identification of patients with acute lung injury: predictors of mortality. *Am J Respir Crit Care Med* 1995;152:1818–1824.
52. Sloane PJ, Gee MH, Gottlieb JE, et al. A multicenter registry of patients with acute respiratory distress syndrome: physiology and outcome. *Am Rev Respir Dis* 1992;146:419–426.
53. Hall JB, Schmidt GA,Wood LD, eds. *Principles of critical care*, 2nd ed. San Francisco: McGraw-Hill, 1998:556.

CHAPTER 29
Rhabdomyolysis

Andrew R. Erdman and Richard C. Dart

OVERVIEW

Rhabdomyolysis is defined as the acute destruction of skeletal muscle cells. The release of these cellular contents can lead to end-organ injury and life-threatening sequelae. Its exact incidence is not known, but rhabdomyolysis is a common phenomenon in poisoned patients (1). Most cases (up to 80%) are the result of drugs or alcohol (2,3). Rhabdomyolysis is often not clinically apparent, but a careful history and physical examination generally belie its presence by revealing common predisposing conditions (1,2). The diagnosis can be confirmed by an elevated serum creatine kinase (CK) level or by the presence of significant myoglobinuria.

PATHOPHYSIOLOGY

The toxicologic and nontoxicologic etiologies of rhabdomyolysis can be divided into those that injure muscle cells directly (e.g., myotoxic) or indirectly (e.g., ischemia) (Table 1). The biochemical mechanisms vary depending on the etiology. More than one mechanism may be involved in any given patient. In overdose patients, rhabdomyolysis is most commonly indirect—usually the result of immobilization caused by a variety of drugs or drug combinations leading to prolonged pressure on a muscle group, local ischemia, and cellular necrosis (4,5). Rhabdomyolysis also commonly occurs in patients using cocaine, amphetamines, phencyclidine, or other sympathomimetics (6,7). The resulting motor agitation can deplete the supply of nutrients and rapidly damage myocytes (8).

Energy Imbalance

A common endpoint for many conditions causing rhabdomyolysis is an imbalance in energy utilization and production (1,3). When a myocyte exhausts adenosine triphosphate (ATP), its normal homeostatic, synthetic, and reparative functions deteriorate (9,10). The result is loss of sarcolemmal and cellular membrane integrity and leakage of intracellular contents. Energy imbalance can arise either from inadequate production or increased utilization of ATP. For example, the poisoned patient with central nervous system depression may not respond to ordinary stimuli and shift body position accordingly (11). Prolonged pressure on a muscle group can produce intracompartmental pressures reaching 240 mm Hg, interrupt the normal blood supply, and provide inadequate nutrients for oxidative phosphorylation and diminished ATP production (12). A wide variety of drugs or toxins have caused rhabdomyolysis in this manner (2). In other conditions, such as hypoxemia, methemoglobinemia, or carbon monoxide toxicity, blood flow to muscle may be normal, but oxygen delivery is impaired (13,14), also decreasing ATP production. Cellular asphyxiants (e.g., cyanide or hydrogen sulfide) or uncouplers of oxidative phosphorylation (e.g., salicylates) can also interfere with the production of ATP by the myocytes (15,16).

Alternatively, excessive energy demands on the myocyte can outstrip energy supply and also exhaust ATP stores, leading to

TABLE 1. Common toxicologic and nontoxicologic causes of rhabdomyolysis

- **Primary causes**
  - Toxicologic
    - Ethanol
    - Hydroxymethylglutaryl coenzyme A reductase inhibitors
    - Clofibrate
    - Aminocaproic acid
    - Antimalarials (e.g., quinine)
    - Corticosteroids
    - Amphotericin
    - Pentamidine
    - Heroin
    - Vasopressin
    - Colchicine
    - Retinoids
    - Ethylene glycol
    - Toluene and other solvents
    - Chlorophenoxy herbicides (e.g., 2,4-dichlorophenoxyacetic acid)
    - Animal venoms (e.g., snake, centipede, bee)
  - Nontoxicologic
    - Excessive muscle activity (e.g., exercise, psychiatric agitation/delirium)
    - Seizures
    - Trauma
    - Excessive pressure
    - Hyperthermia
    - Genetic disorders (e.g., muscular dystrophy, McArdle's syndrome)
    - Electrolyte abnormalities (e.g., hypokalemia)
    - Autoimmune (e.g., dermatomyositis)
    - Infections (e.g., viral, bacterial)
    - Electrical current
    - Idiopathic
- **Secondary causes**
  - Seizures
    - Isoniazid
    - Sympathomimetics
    - Tricyclic antidepressants
    - Theophylline
    - Salicylates
    - Tramadol
    - Bupropion
    - Anticholinergics
    - Camphor
    - Mushrooms (e.g., *Gyromitra* sp.)
    - Drug withdrawal
  - Agitation/delirium
    - Sympathomimetics
    - Anticholinergics
    - Phencyclidine
    - Hallucinogens (e.g., lysergic acid diethylamide, psilocybin)
    - Heavy metals
    - Drug withdrawal
  - Sedation
    - Antiepileptics
    - Opioids
    - Benzodiazepines
    - Barbiturates
    - Gamma hydroxybutyrate
    - Ethanol
    - Phenothiazines
    - Carbon monoxide
    - Clonidine
    - Hypoglycemics (e.g., sulfonylureas)
    - Antihistamines
    - Huffing or hydrocarbon inhalation
  - Involuntary muscular contraction
    - Tetanus
    - Dystonia (e.g., neuroleptics)
    - Serotonin syndrome (e.g., serotonin agonists)
    - Neuroleptic malignant syndrome (e.g., neuroleptics)
    - Malignant hyperthermia (e.g., general anesthetics)
    - Succinylcholine
    - Strychnine
    - Lithium
  - Hyperthermia
    - Salicylates
    - Sympathomimetics
    - Anticholinergics
    - Phencyclidine
    - Dinitrophenol
    - Thyroid hormone
    - Monoamine oxidase inhibitors
    - Drug withdrawal
  - Hypokalemia
    - Diuretics
    - Emetics
    - Laxatives
  - Histotoxic hypoxia
    - Carbon monoxide
    - Cyanide
    - Hydrogen sulfide
    - Methemoglobinemia
  - Ischemia
    - Hypotensive agents (e.g., calcium-channel antagonists)
    - Vasospastic agents (e.g., cocaine)

cellular injury. Excessive energy demands may occur during periods of agitation or delirium (psychiatric or drug-induced); struggling against restraints; prolonged or intense exercise; involuntary muscle contraction (e.g., strychnine, serotonin syndrome, extrapyramidal syndromes, neuroleptic malignant syndrome); drug withdrawal states; or convulsions (6,17,18). Similarly, hyperthermia (from any cause) increases metabolic requirements and causes rhabdomyolysis if demand exceeds the available energy supply (19,20). Direct thermal injury to the sarcolemmal membrane may also contribute to the rhabdomyolysis in this case.

Hypokalemia

The mechanism by which hypokalemia leads to myocyte damage is unclear but may be related to the absence of localized potassium-mediated vasodilation in working muscle (21,22). Many drugs and disease states leading to potassium depletion (e.g., diuretics, laxatives, emetics, mineralocorticoids) have been associated with rhabdomyolysis (23,24).

Direct Myocyte Toxicity

Many drugs or toxins appear to cause direct myocyte damage (either in normal or supratherapeutic doses), although the specific mechanisms of sarcolemmal injury have yet to be elucidated. Examples of direct toxins include hydroxymethylglutaryl coenzyme A reductase inhibitors, clofibrate, aminocaproic acid, ethanol, antimalarials, and various animal venoms (25–30).

POTENTIAL COMPLICATIONS

Local complications of rhabdomyolysis are primarily the result of increased muscle compartment pressure caused by muscle edema. Frank compartment syndrome can develop, leading to further muscle damage and ischemia. Permanent nerve or muscle damage may result (31–33).

Systemic complications are common, even from a localized rhabdomyolysis. Injured muscle cells release intracellular enzymes, electrolytes, and other components (myoglobin, CK, myosin, heme proteins, lactic acid, uric acid, potassium) into the blood. Because muscle accounts for more than one-third of total body weight, the amounts released can be massive, leading to end-organ injury or life-threatening complications.

One of these intracellular constituents is myoglobin, which shuttles oxygen from the blood to the mitochondria of the myocytes, where it can be used in aerobic energy production (34). When rhabdomyolysis releases myoglobin into the circulation, it is filtered by the renal glomeruli and tubules where it can cause acute tubular injury and renal failure (35). The mechanisms of injury may include direct nephrotoxicity from myoglobin (the iron-containing moiety is a catalyst in the formation of reactive oxygen species), tubular obstruction from precipitated myoglobin, and afferent arteriolar vasoconstriction from increased distal tubular solute (36–38). Pathologic findings can include acute tubular necrosis, tubular casts and crystals, interstitial edema, inflammatory infiltrates, and sloughing of the tubular epithelial cells (39,40). The renal injury may be compounded by concurrent hypovolemia, uric acid deposition, or tubular damage caused by other precipitated proteins (41,42). The renal failure caused by rhabdomyolysis may be either oliguric or nonoliguric, but it is usually reversible with supportive care and dialysis (2). As many as 8% of acute renal failure cases are the result of rhabdomyolysis (43).

Rhabdomyolysis also releases potassium, and the resultant hyperkalemia can lead to electrocardiogram (ECG) abnormalities and life-threatening dysrhythmias (44). Other systemic complications of rhabdomyolysis include acidosis, other electrolyte abnormalities, and disseminated intravascular coagulation (2).

DIAGNOSIS

Establishing the Diagnosis

Rarely, patients present with symptoms related to rhabdomyolysis. Indeed, only 10% to 50% of patients have any muscular symptoms at all (2). Only 4% of patients have muscular tenderness or swelling (2). Muscle weakness, skin discoloration, or brownish urine is also a rare finding. Dark-colored urine from myoglobinuria or oliguria from renal insufficiency may be the first sign of rhabdomyolysis. More often, patients present for other reasons: drug overdose, trauma, repetitive seizures, or underlying infection.

Health care providers should keep rhabdomyolysis in mind when evaluating a patient with known risk factors, particularly poisoned or overdose patients. Rhabdomyolysis should be suspected in patients with a history of strenuous muscular activity, agitation, prolonged sedation or coma, repetitive or prolonged seizure activity, exposure to drugs or toxins known to be associated with muscular injury, a period of immobilization, significant trauma, a period of hypotension or hypoxemia, or a history of inflammatory muscle disease.

An elevated serum CK is a sensitive marker for rhabdomyolysis. Levels may exceed 100,000 IU/L (2,45,46). Other tests may be more sensitive, particularly for detecting smaller degrees of muscle injury, but the serum CK is sufficient for the purpose of clinical diagnosis. The CK should be fractionated to distinguish myocardial injury from skeletal muscle injury. Higher peak serum CK levels suggest a greater degree of muscle damage, but it has not been demonstrated that patients with higher peak levels have a greater likelihood of complications (45,47). Serial measurements are important for diagnosis and management, because levels may not peak for hours to days after admission (2). A single normal level on presentation does not rule out rhabdomyolysis.

Other laboratory abnormalities that suggest rhabdomyolysis include hyperkalemia, other electrolyte abnormalities, lactic acidosis, hyperuricemia, or a urinalysis positive for hemoglobin but without erythrocytes on microscopic examination (myoglobin cross reacts with hemoglobin on most urine dipstick tests) (2,5,48). Specific testing can distinguish myoglobin in such instances but is rarely necessary unless the diagnosis is not otherwise apparent (43). Other serum enzyme levels such as lactate dehydrogenase and the aminotransferases may also be elevated. An ECG can help estimate the degree of hyperkalemia and guide treatment. If renal injury occurs, it generally is reflected in deteriorating renal function tests within hours to days of the injury.

Determining the Cause of Rhabdomyolysis

No single test exists that can determine the exact etiology in each case, and, in many instances, more than one etiology may contribute. The determination should be based on history, findings at the scene, a review of any medications, physical examination, and laboratory findings. A urine screen for drugs of abuse may indicate recent substance use such as amphetamines or opiates, but it rarely alters patient management. A comprehensive urine screen can detect a wide variety of agents, but its clinical use is limited and often obviated by a good history and review of medications. To evaluate a specific agent, the patient should simply be withdrawn from the suspected agent and monitored. Leukocytosis or elevated sedimentation rate may suggest an infectious or inflammatory cause. Plain radiographs may be helpful in evaluating trauma. Various other rheumatologic or endocrinologic tests may help identify a cause but should be reserved for cases in which more common etiologies have been excluded. Finally, if no other cause for the rhabdomyolysis is readily identified, a muscle biopsy may be indicated.

MANAGEMENT

Management of Underlying Etiology

The goal of management is to terminate ongoing injury and reduce the effects of preceding muscle injury. Agitated patients should not be restrained with physical measures alone. This can exacerbate the undesired behavior and increase muscular activity, thereby worsening rhabdomyolysis and leading to electrolyte or metabolic disorders (49,50). Severe agitation and muscular hyperactivity should be rapidly controlled with sedatives. Parenteral benzodiazepines are the drugs of choice, and large doses may be necessary. Antipsychotics may be added if the patient does not respond to benzodiazepines, but care must be taken, as ECG changes and dysrhythmias may occur. Neuromuscular paralysis and intubation may be necessary in severe cases of rhabdomyolysis or in patients who do not respond to sedation promptly. A nondepolarizing neuromuscular paralytic agent should be used because succinylcholine can induce muscular contractions and worsen rhabdomyolysis. Patients with involuntary muscular hyperactivity, as in neuroleptic malignant syndrome, serotonin syndrome, or strychnine toxicity, should also receive aggressive sedation. Extrapyramidal syndromes usually respond to diphenhydramine or benztropine. If not, sedation should be administered.

Convulsions should be aggressively controlled (Chapter 40). Neuromuscular paralysis should be performed in refractory cases. Anesthetized or sedated patients should be placed on a soft surface to prevent pressure injuries from prolonged immobilization (51,52). Severe hyperthermia should be controlled immediately (Chapter 38). Hypoxemia, hypotension, hypoglycemia, hypokalemia, and other metabolic or electrolyte abnormalities should all be corrected in the usual manner.

Patients with evidence of compartment syndrome require measurement of compartment pressures. If the pressure exceeds 30 mm Hg, surgical consultation is advised. Fasciotomy may be required to relieve the pressure and prevent further damage if patients do not respond to appropriate conservative measures (e.g., mannitol, antivenom) (32,53).

Management of Complications

The management of rhabdomyolysis depends on supportive measures and close monitoring to prevent life-threatening sequelae. Treatment measures should be based on clinical factors such as underlying cause, clinical severity of symptoms, associated comorbid illnesses such as underlying renal insufficiency, degree of hydration, and associated injuries. Serial CK measurements are important for monitoring the progress of muscle injury. A rising level may indicate ongoing injury and the need for further evaluation or more aggressive intervention. It is important to remember that there may be a delay of hours from muscle injury to the time when CK and other intracellular components reach the systemic circulation (2). The absolute level of CK should not be used to dictate treatment decisions. However, CK measurements should be trending downward before supportive measures are discontinued.

Renal injury from myoglobinuria may be ameliorated with hydration; therefore, urine output and fluid status should be monitored closely (54–56). Rapid correction of initial hypovolemia should be followed by continued hydration to maintain a urine output of at least 1 cc/kg/hour. This also prevents decreases in renal blood flow that can contribute to renal injury. Urinary alkalinization by bicarbonate administration has been recommended, but animal and human data on urinary alkalinization are conflicting (56–59). Because urinary alkalinization has adverse effects and its efficacy remains unproven, it should be avoided. Mannitol infusions have also been proposed; however, data in animals are conflicting, and successful human trials are lacking (56,57,60). There is also a potential for hypovolemia with the administration of diuretics. As a result, mannitol and diuretics are not recommended routinely. Renal function should be followed closely for the development of renal insufficiency. If significant renal failure develops, hemodialysis may be necessary until normal function resumes. The indications for hemodialysis are similar to any patient with renal failure.

Frequent evaluation of serum electrolytes and acid-base status is important. If hyperkalemia is present, cardiac monitoring and serial ECGs should be performed to monitor cardiac conduction. Hyperkalemia is treated in the usual manner (Chapter 35). Electrolyte abnormalities such as hypocalcemia and hyperphosphatemia are rarely clinically significant and do not generally require specific treatment. Some have argued that treating asymptomatic hypocalcemia with supplementation may cause calcium deposition in the muscles and exacerbate injury (61). Lactic acidosis usually responds to hydration and other supportive measures. Disseminated intravascular coagulation should be managed in the usual fashion.

The overall prognosis for patients with rhabdomyolysis is good, and most complications, including myoglobinuric renal failure, are reversible with adequate supportive measures (2,62). Rarely, long-term complications occur: neuropathies, muscle contractures or dysfunction, and amputation as a result of irreversible limb damage (5,31,32). Mortality as high as 5% of hospitalized patients has been reported, but this does not include many patients with only minimal rhabdomyolysis. Furthermore, death may be related to the underlying condition rather than to rhabdomyolysis itself.

PITFALLS

The main pitfalls are failures of diagnosis or monitoring that allow rhabdomyolysis to become more severe: (a) missed diagnosis of rhabdomyolysis in patients at risk; (b) failing to rapidly control agitation, seizures, or maintain urinary output; (c) failing to monitor for sequelae such as hyperkalemia, acidosis, or myoglobinuria.

REFERENCES

1. Curry SC, Chang D, Connor D. Drug- and toxin-induced rhabdomyolysis. *Ann Emerg Med* 1989 Oct;18(10):1068–1084.
2. Gabow PA, Kaehny WD, Kelleher SP. The spectrum of rhabdomyolysis. *Medicine* 1982 May;61(3):141–152.
3. Knochel JP. Rhabdomyolysis and myoglobinuria. *Annu Rev Med* 1982;33:435–443.
4. Nicholls K, Niall JF, Moran JE. Rhabdomyolysis and renal failure. Complications of narcotic abuse. *Med J Aust* 1982;2(8):387–389.
5. Penn AS, Rowland LP, Fraser DW. Drugs, coma, and myoglobinuria. *Arch Neurol* 1972;26(4):336–343.
6. Akmal M, Valdin JR, McCarron MM, et al. Rhabdomyolysis with and without acute renal failure in patients with phencyclidine intoxication. *Am J Nephrol* 1981;1(2):91–96.
7. Merigian KS, Roberts JR. Cocaine intoxication: hyperpyrexia, rhabdomyolysis and acute renal failure. *J Toxicol Clin Toxicol* 1987;25(1–2):135–148.
8. Kendrick WC, Hull AR, Knochel JP. Rhabdomyolysis and shock after intravenous amphetamine administration. *Ann Intern Med* 1977;86(4):381–387.
9. McArdle B, Verdi D. Myopathy due to defect in muscle glycogen breakdown. *Clin Sci* 1951;10:13–35.
10. Visweswaran P, Guntupalli J. Rhabdomyolysis. *Crit Care Clin* 1999;15(2):415–428, ix–x.
11. Schreiber S, Liebowitz M, Bernstein L. Limb compression and renal impairment (crush syndrome) following narcotic and sedative overdose. *J Bone Joint Surg (Am)* 1972;54–A:1683–1692.
12. Owen C, Mubarak S, Hargens A, et al. Intramuscular pressures with limb compression. *N Engl J Med* 1979;300:1169–1172.
13. Finley J, Van Beek A, Glover J. Myonecrosis complicating carbon monoxide poisoning. *J Trauma* 1977;17:536–540.
14. Gavish D, Knobler H, Gottehrer N, et al. Methemoglobinemia, muscle damage and renal failure complicating phenazopyridine overdose. *Isr J Med Sci* 1986;22(1):45–47.
15. Skjoto J, Reikvam A. Hyperthermia and rhabdomyolysis in self-poisoning with paracetamol and salicylates. Report of a case. *Acta Med Scand* 1979;205(6):473–476.
16. Vannatta J. Hydrogen sulfide poisoning. Report of four cases and brief review of the literature. *Okla State Med Assoc J* 1982;75:29–32.
17. Cavanaugh JJ, Finlayson RE. Rhabdomyolysis due to acute dystonic reaction to antipsychotic drugs. *J Clin Psychiatry* 1984;45(8):356–357.
18. Mercieca J, Brown EA. Acute renal failure due to rhabdomyolysis associated with use of a straitjacket in lysergide intoxication. *BMJ (Clin Res Ed)* 1984;288(6435):1949–5190.
19. Cohen JD, Jonsson GG, Robins HI. Rhabdomyolysis and temperature. *Lancet* 1990;336(8729):1513–1514.
20. Kitanaka C, Inoh Y, Toyoda T, et al. Malignant brain stem hyperthermia caused by brain stem hemorrhage. *Stroke* 1994;25(2):518–520.
21. Kjellmer I. Potassium ion as a vasodilator during muscular exercise. *Acta Physiol Scand* 1965;63:460–468.
22. Knochel JP, Schlein EM. On the mechanism of rhabdomyolysis in potassium depletion. *J Clin Invest* 1972;51(7):1750–1758.
23. Heitzman E, Patterson J, Stanley M. Myoglobinuria and hypokalemia in regional enteritis. *Arch Intern Med* 1962;110:117–124.
24. Oh S, Douglas J, Brown J. Hypokalemic vascular myopathy associated with chlorthalidone treatment. *JAMA* 1971;216:1858–1859.
25. Brown JA, Wollmann RL, Mullan S. Myopathy induced by epsilon-aminocaproic acid. Case report. *J Neurosurg* 1982;57(1):130–134.
26. Corpier CL, Jones PH, Suki WN, et al. Rhabdomyolysis and renal injury with lovastatin use. Report of two cases in cardiac transplant recipients. *JAMA* 1988;260(2):239–241.
27. Haller RG. Experimental acute alcoholic myopathy—a histochemical study. *Muscle Nerve* 1985;8(3):195–203.
28. Logan JL, Ogden DA. Rhabdomyolysis and acute renal failure following the bite of the giant desert centipede *Scolopendra heros*. *West J Med* 1985;142(4):549–550.
29. Smals AG, Beex LV, Kloppenborg PW. Clofibrate-induced muscle damage with myoglobinuria and cardiomyopathy. *N Engl J Med* 1977;296(16):942.

30. Song S, Rubin E. Ethanol produces muscle damage in human volunteers. *Science* 1972;175:327–328.
31. Howse AJ, Seddon H. Ischaemic contracture of muscle associated with carbon monoxide and barbiturate poisoning. *BMJ* 1966;5481:192–195.
32. Sheridan GW, Matsen FA 3rd. Fasciotomy in the treatment of the acute compartment syndrome. *J Bone Joint Surg (Am)* 1976;58(1):112–115.
33. Thomas MA, Ibels LS. Rhabdomyolysis and acute renal failure. *Aust N Z J Med* 1985;15(5):623–628.
34. Perkoff G, Tyler F. Estimation and physical properties of myoglobin in various species. *Metabolism* 1958;7:751.
35. Koskelo P, Kekki M, Wager O. Kinetic behaviour of 131-I-labelled myoglobin in human beings. *Clin Chim Acta* 1967;17(3):339–347.
36. Heyman SN, Rosen S, Fuchs S, et al. Myoglobinuric acute renal failure in the rat: a role for medullary hypoperfusion, hypoxia, and tubular obstruction. *J Am Soc Nephrol* 1996;7(7):1066–1074.
37. Vetterlein F, Hoffmann F, Pedina J, et al. Disturbances in renal microcirculation induced by myoglobin and hemorrhagic hypotension in anesthetized rat. *Am J Physiol* 1995;268(5 Pt 2):F839–F846.
38. Zager RA, Burkhart K. Myoglobin toxicity in proximal human kidney cells: roles of Fe, Ca^{2+}, H_2O_2, and terminal mitochondrial electron transport. *Kidney Int* 1997;51(3):728–738.
39. Anderson W, Morrison D, Williams E. Pathologic changes following injections of ferrihemate (hematin) in dogs. *Arch Pathol* 1942;3:528–544.
40. Bywaters E, Beall D. Crush injuries with impairment of renal function. *BMJ* 1941;1:427–432.
41. O'Regan S, Fong JS, Drummond KN. Renal injury after muscle extract infusion in rats: absence of toxicity with myoglobin. *Experientia* 1979;35(6):805–806.
42. Stavric B, Johnson WJ, Grice HC. Uric acid nephropathy: an experimental model. *Proc Soc Exp Biol Med* 1969;130(2):512–516.
43. Grossman RA, Hamilton RW, Morse BM, et al. Nontraumatic rhabdomyolysis and acute renal failure. *N Engl J Med* 1974;291(16):807–811.
44. Hendriks F, Kooman JP, van der Sande FM. Massive rhabdomyolysis and life threatening hyperkalaemia in a patient with the combination of cerivastatin and gemfibrozil. *Nephrol Dial Transplant* 2001;16(12):2418–2419.
45. Hess J, Mac Donald R, Frederick R, et al. Serum creatinine phosphokinase activity in disorders of heart and skeletal muscle. *Ann Intern Med* 1964;61:1015.
46. Rosalki SB. Serum enzymes in disease of skeletal muscle. *Clin Lab Med* 1989;9(4):767–781.
47. Ward MM. Factors predictive of acute renal failure in rhabdomyolysis. *Arch Intern Med* 1988;148(7):1553–1557.
48. Akmal M, Bishop JE, Telfer N, et al. Hypocalcemia and hypercalcemia in patients with rhabdomyolysis with and without acute renal failure. *J Clin Endocrinol Metab* 1986;63(1):137–142.
49. Stratton SJ, Rogers C, Brickett K, et al. Factors associated with sudden death of individuals requiring restraint for excited delirium. *Am J Emerg Med* 2001;19(3):187–191.
50. Stratton SJ, Rogers C, Green K. Sudden death in individuals in hobble restraints during paramedic transport. *Ann Emerg Med* 1995;25(5):710–712.
51. Choufane S, Lemogne M, Jacob L. Unexpected rhabdomyolysis with myoglobinuria in a patient in the supine position. *Eur J Anaesthesiol* 1998;15(4):493–496.
52. Targa L, Droghetti L, Caggese G, et al. Rhabdomyolysis and operating position. *Anaesthesia* 1991;46(2):141–143.
53. Vucak MJ. Rhabdomyolysis requiring fasciotomy following heroine abuse. *Aust N Z J Surg* 1991;61(7):533–535.
54. Better OS, Stein JH. Early management of shock and prophylaxis of acute renal failure in traumatic rhabdomyolysis. *N Engl J Med* 1990;322(12):825–829.
55. Bidani AK, Fleischmann LE, Churchill P, et al. Natriuresis-induced protection in acute myohemoglobinuric renal failure without renal cortical renin content depletion in the rat. *Nephron* 1978;22(4–6):529–537.
56. Homsi E, Barreiro MF, Orlando JM, et al. Prophylaxis of acute renal failure in patients with rhabdomyolysis. *Ren Fail* 1997;19(2):283–288.
57. Eneas JF, Schoenfeld PY, Humphreys MH. The effect of infusion of mannitol-sodium bicarbonate on the clinical course of myoglobinuria. *Arch Intern Med* 1979;139(7):801–805.
58. Heyman SN, Greenbaum R, Shina A, et al. Myoglobinuric acute renal failure in the rat: a role for acidosis? *Exp Nephrol* 1997;5(3):210–216.
59. Moore KP, Holt SG, Patel RP, et al. A causative role for redox cycling of myoglobin and its inhibition by alkalinization in the pathogenesis and treatment of rhabdomyolysis-induced renal failure. *J Biol Chem* 1998;273(48):31731–31737.
60. Zager RA, Foerder C, Bredl C. The influence of mannitol on myoglobinuric acute renal failure: functional, biochemical, and morphological assessments. *J Am Soc Nephrol* 1991;2(4):848–855.
61. Davis AM. Hypocalcemia in rhabdomyolysis. *JAMA* 1987;257(5):626.
62. Cadnapaphornchai P, Taher S, McDonald FD. Acute drug-associated rhabdomyolysis: an examination of its diverse renal manifestations and complications. *Am J Med Sci* 1980;280(2):66–72.

CHAPTER 30

Seizures

George Braitberg

OVERVIEW

Seizures are common. Up to 10% of the population has at least one seizure in their lifetime (1). The rate of epilepsy is approximately 15 per 100,000 adults per year. At the age of 50 years, the rate begins to rise, reaching 50 to 75 per 100,000 adults by ages 60 and 75 years, respectively (2). Bleck et al. (3) observed seizures in 61 of 217 patients admitted to an intensive care unit with a primary nonneurologic diagnosis.

The incidence of seizures as a complication of medication therapy is approximately 0.08% (4,5). Most drug-induced seizures are self-limited and without permanent sequelae, but as many as 15% of drug-related seizures develop status epilepticus, especially after overdose (5). The incidence of seizures associated with recreational drug use is not well known. Alldredge et al. (6) reported an incidence of 0.3% of recreational drug-abuse–related medical complications. Recreational drugs were defined as those used unlawfully for psychic effects or addiction. The author acknowledges that this figure may be grossly underestimated.

The presence of epileptic discharges on electroencephalogram (EEG) after a first seizure is a predictor of a subsequent seizure in adults (83% compared with 12% in patients who have a normal EEG) (7).

The terms *seizure* and *convulsion* are often used interchangeably. *Seizure* refers to an episode of abnormal neurologic function caused by an abnormal electrical discharge of neurons. The seizure is the *ictus*, and the postseizure period is the *postictus*. The term *convulsion* refers to an episode of excessive or abnormal motor activity. Convulsions may occur with seizures but also in the absence of central ictal activity (8). These definitions are important because confusion often arises as to whether the observed motor activity is central (neuronal) or peripheral (myonal or myoclonic). The myoclonic jerks caused by strychnine are often treated as seizures. Strychnine acts as a selective, competitive antagonist of glycine at its postsynaptic receptors in the spinal cord and brain stem, causing uncontrollable muscle action, without generally causing seizure (9).

PATHOPHYSIOLOGY

There are primary and secondary mechanisms of seizure. Primary mechanisms refer to the inherent properties of a substance that make it epileptogenic. Primary convulsants affect the central nervous system directly (e.g., stimulants, isoniazid, and so forth). Medication withdrawal causes primary seizures as in alcohol withdrawal seizures (e.g., excessive stimulation of "primed" *N*-methyl-D-aspartate receptors or upregulation of receptors) (10).

Secondary seizures occur as a result of impaired substrate availability or utilization: hypoxia (e.g., opiates); blockade of oxygen utilization (e.g., carbon monoxide, cyanide); reduced oxygen carriage capacity (e.g., methemoglobinemia, anemia); cerebral edema; lack of energy (uncoupling of oxidative phosphorylation-salicylate or dinitrophenol); or disturbances of glucose and electrolyte metabolism (11). Seizures can occur when serum sodium falls below 115 mmol/L (115 mEq/L) or when there is a rapid decrease in sodium concentration. Hypernatremia may also lead to seizures, as can hypomagnesemia (12) and hypocalcemia.

DIAGNOSIS

Differential Diagnosis

A systematic approach is needed in managing the patient with an unknown ingestion who presents with a seizure. A number of risk factors should be considered (Table 1).

One important step is to identify whether the patient has experienced a seizure or a convulsion. The type of motor activity may suggest the drug involved. For example, propofol is an intravenous hypnotic with a modulating action on gamma aminobutyric acid A receptors. There are conflicting reports as to whether propofol causes seizures in susceptible patients or, conversely, is useful in the treatment of seizures (13–15). A recent review (16) found that 30 of 81 patients (43%) were thought to have a generalized tonic clonic seizure on induction, whereas the remaining patients had a variety of twitching or jerking movements. Only 5 of 24 patients had an abnormal EEG after the episode. Sutherland (17) suggests that propofol causes nonepileptic subcortical myoclonus. Regulatory agencies have warned about the use of propofol in patients with epilepsy (18).

In the setting of suspected ingestion, the differentiation of seizure and convulsion may be important. A number of toxidromes cause myoclonic jerking and seizure, such as serotonergic syndrome, sympathomimetic overdose, or tricyclic antidepressant (TCA) poisoning. Myoclonic jerks may be the predominant feature (e.g., anticholinergic syndrome) (19).

TABLE 1. Predisposing risk factors for seizures

Primary factors	Secondary factors
History of seizures	Electroencephalogram abnormalities
Family history of seizures	Brain injury
Intellectual disability	Head trauma
Age-related neurologic conditions (e.g., Alzheimer's disease)	Secondary causes of dementia
Age	Central nervous system vascular or neoplastic disease
Medical illness	Substance abuse or withdrawal
	Polypharmacy

Adapted from Skowron DM, Stimmel GL. Antidepressants and the risk of seizures. *Pharmacotherapy* 1992;12(1):18–22.

In a retrospective study of 190 cases of seizure associated with poisoning, Olsen et al. (20) found that the three most common causes of seizures were TCA, anticholinergic and antihistamine agents, and theophylline. Stimulants and diphenhydramine were more likely to produce brief self-limited seizures, whereas TCA and theophylline were more likely to produce multiple or prolonged seizures and to require intubation.

Drugs That Cause Seizures

An impressive array of drugs are associated with seizure (Table 2).

COCAINE AND OTHER STIMULANTS

Cocaine was reported to cause seizures in 29 of 989 patients (3%) (21). The interval ranged from a few minutes (usually after intravenous use) to 12 hours (21). Alldredge found that cocaine had the shortest time interval between recreational drug use and seizure onset (6).

In humans, amphetamine-induced seizures are also more likely to occur after intravenous use (6). Williams et al. (22) found that 3,4-methylenedioxymethamphetamine (MDMA) was associated with seizures when used with other recreational drugs. Of 48 consecutive MDMA cases, three had seizures (6.3%), and 32 patients reported concurrent use of other illicit drugs or alcohol. None of the 16 patients who used MDMA alone had a seizure.

A review of the literature concluded that acute overdoses of amoxapine, camphor, lindane, cocaine, and strychnine may present suddenly with seizures with minimal or no prior warning (23).

ANTIDEPRESSANTS

Amoxapine was associated with seizure in more than 25% of cases reported to poison centers (24). Overall, the estimated rate of cyclic antidepressant–induced seizure is 3% to 4% (25). Apart from amoxapine, TCA-related seizures are almost always accompanied by widened QRS duration on 12 lead electrocardiogram (20). A QRS duration of 0.10 seconds or longer was moderately predictive of seizures, and an interval of 0.16 seconds or longer was highly predictive of seizures (26). Cyclic antidepressant–overdosed patients are more likely to have multiple or prolonged seizures, which often have abrupt onset, and are more likely to die (20).

Other antidepressants that cause seizures include maprotiline, a tetracyclic antidepressant, which requires higher doses than TCA for seizure (27). Overall, amoxapine, clomipramine, maprotiline, and bupropion are the most likely to produce seizures. Of intermediate potential for seizures are amitriptyline, imipramine, and nortriptyline. Minimal potential are the monoamine oxidase inhibitors such as tranylcypromine (Parnate), which may have anticonvulsant properties (28). Fluoxetine has been reported to cause seizure (29). The selective serotonin reuptake inhibitors and monoamine oxidase inhibitors are more likely to cause seizures in the setting of serotonin syndrome (30). Bupropion causes dose-related seizures at a rate of 2.19% (31).

LITHIUM

Seizure is one of the serious neurologic effects of lithium toxicity (23). The effect of lithium on EEG is characterized by abnormal generalized slowing and paroxysmal diffuse alpha activity. These changes usually occur with supratherapeutic serum levels but occasionally occur at moderate or even low concentrations (28). In acute overdose, there is a good correlation between

TABLE 2. Drug-induced seizures

Antidepressants and lithium salts
  Tricyclic antidepressants (frequent), including classic and "newer" antidepressants (mianserin, maprotiline, amoxapine)
  Monoamine oxidase inhibitors
Antipsychotics
Phenothiazines
Butyrophenones (less frequent)
Antihistamines (H_1-receptor antagonist), more frequent in children
Antiepileptic drugs and their paradoxic proconvulsant activity
Central nervous system stimulants
  Cortical stimulants
  Theophylline
  Cocaine (hyperthermia and cardiac arrhythmias are factors); (body packer's ruptured cocaine-filled condoms)
  Amphetamine (in high-dose "binge" users)
Brain stem stimulants
  Pentetrazol, picrotoxin (rarely used)
  Spinal stimulants: strychnine
  Nonprescription stimulants (caffeine, phenylpropanolamine, ephedrine)
General anesthetics
  Inhalation anesthetics
  Enflurane
  Isoflurane
  IV and nonnarcotic anesthetics
  Ketamine
  Etomidate
  Methohexital
Local anesthetics
  Lidocaine (at high doses)
Antiarrhythmic drugs (including lidocaine)
  Mexiletine
  Tocainide
  Ajmaline
  Disopyramide (severe hypoglycemia)
  Quinidine
Quinine (adulteration of street drugs)
  Propranolol (after high doses)
Opioids and other narcotic analgesics
  Morphine (at high doses in neonates and infants)
  Meperidine (normeperidine)
  Dextropropoxyphene
  Fentanyl and sufentanil
  Parazone
Nonnarcotic analgesics and nonsteroidal antiinflammatory drugs
  Aspirin and salicylates (poisoning depletion of brain glucose?)
  Mefenamic acid (in overdose)
Antimicrobial agents
  β-lactam antibiotics
  Penicillin
  Cephalosporins (rare)
Imipenem/cilastatin
Antitubercular drugs
  Isoniazid (overdose of therapeutic dose)
  Cycloserine
Antifungal agents
  Amphotericin B, miconazole (rare)
Antimalarial drugs
  Chloroquine, pyrimethamine (both in overdoses)
Antineoplastic drugs (infrequent)
  Alkylating agents: chlorambucil, bisulfate, mechlorethamine
Antimetabolites: high-dose methotrexate, cytarabine
  Vinca alkaloids: vincristine
  Others: cisplatin, carmustine, asparaginase (infrequent)
Immunosuppressive drugs
  Cyclosporine (10% neurologic side effects)
Glucocorticoids (occasionally, more often when used with cyclosporine)
Radiologic contrast agents

Data taken from Zaccara G, Muscas GC, Messori A. Clinical features, pathogenesis and management of drug-induced seizures. *Drug Safety* 1990;5(2):109–151.

symptoms and steady-state serum levels (32). Serum levels are less predictive of seizures in chronic lithium toxicity (33).

THEOPHYLLINE

Theophylline-induced seizures may be prolonged, difficult to control, and associated with poor outcome. Eldridge (34) demonstrated the deleterious effect of theophylline as an adenosine antagonist in a cat seizure model. There are two alternating phases of electrical activity in humans and animal models of status epilepticus. High-frequency spikes associated with high cerebral oxygen consumption alternate with interictal periods of isolated spike activity. This spontaneous self-termination is mediated by adenosine (10). Theophylline antagonizes adenosine A_1 and A_2 receptors, preventing cessation of seizures and increasing cerebral metabolism and hypoxia (35).

Seizure incidence in theophylline toxicity varies from 6% to 33% with a 10% mortality rate (23). In acute toxicity, seizures tend to be dose related, with the majority occurring when serum levels exceed 100 μg/ml (36). In chronic theophylline toxicity, seizures occur at lower serum concentrations (23,36).

ANTICHOLINERGIC AGENTS

Olsen et al. (20) identified diphenhydramine and other antihistamines as the third leading cause of drug-induced seizures. These seizures tend to be brief in duration.

ISONIAZID

Isoniazid toxicity causes seizures and severe metabolic acidosis. Through multiple actions, isoniazid and other hydrazines inhibit the gamma aminobutyric acid–mediated inhibitory central nervous system pathways. Seizures may occur without warning, frequently as generalized tonic-clonic or prolonged, and may be resistant to therapy (20,37).

OTHER DRUGS

Some drugs may cause seizures at therapeutic doses in normal patients (Table 3).

SUBSTANCE WITHDRAWAL

Alcohol withdrawal was involved in 41% of seizure presentations to an urban public hospital (38). Alcohol-related seizures typically occur 6 to 48 hours after discontinuation of drinking (11). Rapid benzodiazepine or barbiturate withdrawal may also cause seizures (10). Seizures are most common after sudden withdrawal of short-acting drugs, because drug levels decline rapidly (5). The use of flumazenil can precipitate seizures through this mechanism (39,40).

TABLE 3. Drugs that may cause seizures at therapeutic doses in normal patients

Drug (reference)	Mechanism
Meperidine (40,49)	Normeperidine toxicity
Phenothiazines and butyrophenones (5)	Lower seizure threshold
Beta-lactams (10,40)	$GABA_A$ antagonism
Isoniazid	Inhibition of GABA synthesis
Theophylline	Adenosine antagonism
Anticonvulsants (50)	Nonspecific manifestation of drug intoxication Primary action of drug
Propranolol	Sodium channel blockade

GABA, γ-aminobutyric acid.
Adapted from Garcia PA, Alldredge BK. Drug induced seizures. *Neurol Clin* 1994;12(1):85–89.

TABLE 4. Factors to consider in substance-related seizures

Drug related
- Intrinsic epileptogenicity, including seizure type, drug type
- Factors influencing serum and central nervous system levels (i.e., dosage, drug pharmacokinetics, interaction, compliance issues)

Patient related
- Epilepsy
- Neurologic abnormalities
- Reduced drug elimination capacity
- Breakdown of the blood–brain barrier
- Psychiatric illness

Drug setting
- Recreational, including local drug usage patterns
- Intentional versus accidental ingestion

Adapted from Garcia PA, Alldredge BK. Drug induced seizures. *Neurol Clin* 1994;12(1):85–89.

Other Factors Influencing Seizures

Numerous factors may influence the development of seizures (Table 4).

PATIENT FACTORS

Patients with a preexisting seizure disorder or chronic neurologic condition are at greater risk of seizure after substance ingestion. The elderly are at a higher risk of confusion and medication misuse (41). Antipsychotic-induced seizure activity is more common in the elderly as well as in patients with acute or chronic brain pathology (42). The elderly have reduced excretion and increased sensitivity to epileptiform activity of a wide range of drugs (41). Adolescent adults are ten times more likely to have recreational drug–induced seizures (20).

Medical illness is itself a cause of seizures, although the exact mechanisms are poorly understood. Several factors predispose to seizures in the critically ill, including permeability changes of the blood–brain barrier due to infection, hypoxia, or altered autoregulation of cerebral blood flow, that may allow drugs and toxins to pass across the blood–brain barrier. Conditions such as hypertensive encephalopathy may compromise blood vessel integrity and lead to areas of edema and hemorrhage, which in turn may lead to seizures (11). Seizures in elderly patients are more likely to be associated with other medical complications (20). Seizures are common in cancer, either by direct anatomic central nervous system involvement or cancer-associated vascular disease such as nonthrombotic endocarditis, metabolic derangement, infection, and chemotherapeutic agents (43).

Lithium toxicity may occur at "therapeutic" lithium concentrations, often in the setting of drug interaction or conditions leading to decreased elimination such as low salt diet, dehydration and volume depletion, and cardiac failure and thiazide diuretics (44).

Drug Setting

Substance withdrawal is a common cause of seizures in the elderly. The most commonly encountered withdrawal syndromes are alcohol, benzodiazepines, and barbiturates (45). In the Olsen study (20), there was significant change in the type of drug taken in overdose, compared to 8 years earlier, underscoring the need to consider the clinical setting of the suspected ingestion. For example, the number of stimulant overdoses increased between the two study periods. Since the early 1990s, the prevalence of prescribed selective serotonin reuptake and changing recreational drug usage must be considered.

Alldredge (6) noted that the "prevalence of illicit cocaine usage has continued to rise in recent years" and found that cocaine was the recreational drug most associated with drug-induced seizures in the San Francisco Bay area. The European Monitoring Centre for Drugs and Drug Addiction documented a continued rise in the amount of amphetamine used and the incidence of seizures since 1995 (46). Ecstasy seizures increased until 1996, then stabilized, and increased again in 1999 in all countries except Belgium and Luxembourg. Amounts of ecstasy (methylenedioxymethamphetamine) seized followed the same upward trend since 1985. The highest increases were reported in Finland, Germany, Greece, Portugal, Sweden, and the United Kingdom (46). This trend has been documented in Australia for amphetamine derivative "designer drugs," which have been documented to cause seizures in recreational usage (47). Williams et al. (22) reported that polydrug ingestion was more common than single drug recreational use, and, in the their study of London recreational drug use, amphetamines and cocaine were used more frequently in combination with MDMA. Ling et al. (47) reported two patients with paramethoxyamphetamine "death" ingestion. Seven of 22 urine drug screen–confirmed cases of paramethoxyamphetamine had seizures (32%) compared to only two of 61 (3%) cases of self-reported ecstasy ingestion.

POTENTIAL COMPLICATIONS

Complications may arise from the drug involved, its route of administration, or the act of convulsion. Complications of the act of drug abuse (e.g., pneumothorax) and complications related to specific drugs (e.g., stimulants) are addressed in Part III of this book. Complications of convulsion are essentially the same as other causes of seizure: hypoxia, hypotension, aspiration, hyperthermia, rhabdomyolysis, trauma, and so forth.

MANAGEMENT

The initial approach is the same in any patient presenting with seizure, regardless of suspected etiology (Chapter 40). Management principles involve appropriate resuscitative measures and assessment of neurologic status to determine whether the patient has a focal or nonfocal presentation, indicating the likelihood of a structural lesion. In defiance of the principle of Ockham's razor, a patient occasionally has a drug and structural cause of seizure. A careful history is required to ascertain the setting in which the seizure took place and determine the nature, duration, and number of seizures. A complete physical and neurologic examination is mandatory.

Evidence of head trauma, infection, metabolic insult, and cardiorespiratory injury may all coexist with drug overdose. Of particular importance is evidence of underlying illness, chronic disease, illicit drug use, and complications secondary to the seizure [e.g., shoulder dislocation (48)] or the underlying etiology. After stabilization, appropriate decontamination must be considered if substance ingestion is thought to be likely.

PITFALLS

Seizures should be treated and controlled as soon as possible. This lessens the potential for complications and improves efficacy because seizures are more difficult to control the longer they continue.

REFERENCES

1. Engel J, Starkman S. Overview of seizures. *Emerg Med Clin North Am* 1994;12(4):8895–8923.
2. Hauser WA, Annegers JF, Kurland LT. Incidence of epilepsy and unprovoked seizures in Rochester, Minnesota: 2935–2984. *Epilepsia* 1993;34:453–468.
3. Bleck TP, Smith MC, Pirre-Louis SJ-C, et al. Neurologic complications of critical medical illness. *Crit Care Med* 1993;21:98–103.
4. Porter J, Jick H. Drug induced anaphylaxis, convulsions, deafness and extrapyramidal symptoms. *Lancet* 1977;1:1582–1586.
5. Garcia PA, Alldredge BK. Drug induced seizures. *Neurol Clin* 1994;12(1):85–89.
6. Alldredge BK, Lowenstein DH, Simon RP. Seizures associated with recreational drug abuse. *Neurology* 1989;39:1037–1039.
7. Van Donselaar CA, Schimsheimer RJ, Geerts AT, et al. Value of the electroencephalogram in adult patients with untreated idiopathic first seizures. *Arch Neurol* 1992;49:31–37.
8. Wilkes GR. In: Cameron P, Jelinek G, Kelly AM, et al., eds. *Textbook of emergency medicine*. Churchill Livingstone: Edinburgh, 2000:293–299.
9. Case records of the Massachusetts General Hospital. Weekly clinicopathological exercises. Case 12-2001. A 16-year-old boy with an altered mental status and muscle rigidity. *N Engl J Med* 2001;344(16):1232–1239.
10. Curry SC, Mills KC, Graeme KA. Neurotransmitter. In: Goldfrank L, Flomenbaum N, Lewin NA, et al., eds. *Goldfrank's toxicologic emergencies*, 7th ed. New York: McGraw-Hill, 2002:137–171.
11. Delanty N, Vaughan CJ, French JA. Medical causes of seizures. *Lancet* 1998;352(9125):383–390.
12. Whang R, Hampton EM, Whang DD. Magnesium homeostasis and clinical disorders of magnesium deficiency. *Ann Pharmacother* 1994;28:220–226.
13. Collier C, Kelly K. Propofol and convulsions, the evidence mounts. *Anaesth Intensive Care* 1991;19:573–575.
14. Wood PR, Browne GP, Pugh S. Propofol infusion for the treatment of status epilepticus. *Lancet* 1988;1:480–481.
15. Claassen J, Hirsch LJ, Emerson RJ, et al. Treatment of refractory status epilepticus with pentobarbital, propofol, or midazolam: a systematic review. *Epilepsia* 2002;43(2):146–153.
16. Walder B, Matrin RT, Phil D, et al. Seizure like phenomena and propofol. A systematic review. *Neurology* 2002;58:1327–1332.
17. Sutherland MJ, Burt P. Propofol and seizures. *Anaesth Intensive Care* 1994;22:733–737.
18. Disoprivan 1%. In: Walker G, ed. *ABPI compendium of data sheets and summaries of product characteristics. 1998–9*. London: Datapharm Publications, 1998:1093–1094.
19. Graeme KA, Braitberg G, Kunkel DB, et al. Toxic plant ingestions. In: Auerbach P, ed. *Wilderness medicine*, 4th ed. St. Louis: Mosby–Year Book, 2001:1108.
20. Olsen KR, Kearney TE, Dyer JE, et al. Seizures associated with poisoning and drug overdose. *Am J Emerg Med* 1993;11:565–568.
21. Zaccara G, Muscas GC, Messori A. Clinical features, pathogenesis and management of drug-induced seizures. *Drug Safety* 1990;5(2):109–151.
22. Williams H, Dratcu L, Taylor R, et al. "Saturday night fever": ecstasy related problems in a London accident and emergency department. *J Accid Emerg Med* 1998;15:322–326.
23. Kunisaki TA, Augenstein WL. Drug and toxin induced seizures. *Emerg Med Clin North Am* 1994;12(4):1027–1055.
24. Pimentel L, Trommer L. Cyclic antidepressant overdoses. A review. *Emerg Med Clin North Am* 1994;12(2):533–547.
25. Wedin GP, Odra GM, Klein-Schwartz W, et al. Relative toxicity of cyclic antidepressants. *Ann Emerg Med* 1986;15:797.
26. Boehnert MT, Lovejoy FH. Value of the QRS versus the serum drug level in predicting seizures and ventricular arrhythmias after an acute overdose of tricyclic antidepressants. *N Engl J Med* 1985;313–474.
27. Skowron DM, Stimmel GL. Antidepressants and the risk of seizures. *Pharmacotherapy* 1992;12(1):18–22.
28. Struve FA. Lithium-specific pathological electroencephalographic changes: a successful replication of earlier investigative results. *Clin Electroencephalogr* 1987;18(2):46–53.
29. Braitberg G, Curry SC. Fluoxetine induced seizure after overdose. *Ann Emerg Med* 1995;26:234–237.
30. Mills KC. Serotonin syndrome. A clinical update. *Crit Care Clin* 1997;13(4):763–783.
31. Davidson J. Seizures and bupropion. *J Clin Psychiatry* 1989;50:256–261.
32. Hansen HE, Amdisen A. Lithium intoxication. *Quarterly J Med* 1978;47:123–144.
33. Okusa MD, Jovita LT. Clinical manifestations and management of acute lithium intoxication. *Am J Med* 1994;97(4):383–389.
34. Eldridge FL, Payadrfar D, Scott SC, et al. Role of endogenous adenosine in recurrent generalized seizures. *Exp Neurol* 1989;103:179–185.
35. Dragunow M. Adenosine receptor antagonism accounts for the seizure prolonging effects of aminophylline. *Pharmacol Biochem Behav* 1990;36:751–759.
36. Paloucek FP, Rodvold KA. Evaluation of theophylline overdoses and toxicities. *Ann Emerg Med* 1988;17(2):135–148.
37. Nelson LG. Grand mal seizures following overdose with isoniazid. A report of 4 cases. *Am Rev Resp Dis* 1965;91:600–604.
38. Earnest MP, Yarnell PR. Seizure admission to a city hospital. The role of alcohol. *Epilepsia* 1976;17;387–393.
39. Spivey WH. Flumazenil and seizures. Analysis of 43 cases. *Clin Ther* 1992;14(2):292–305.
40. Thomas RJ. Seizures and epilepsy in the elderly. *Arch Intern Med* 1197;157:605–617.
41. Franson KL, Hay DP, Neppe V, et al. Drug induced seizures in the elderly. Causative agents and optimal management. *Drugs Aging* 1995;7(1):38–48.
42. Logethetis J. Spontaneous epileptic seizures and electroencephalopathic changes in the course of phenothiazine therapy. *Neurology* 1967;17:869–877.
43. Stein DA, Chamberlain MC. Evaluation and management of seizures in the patent with cancer. *Oncology* 1991;5:33–39.
44. Strayhorn JM, Nash JL. Severe neurotoxicity despite "therapeutic" serum lithium levels. *Dis Nerv Syst* 1977;38:107–111.
45. Franson KL, Hay DP, Neppe V, et al. Drug induced seizures in the elderly. Causative agents and optimal management. *Drugs Aging* 1995;7(1):38–48.
46. European Monitoring Centre for Drugs and Drug Addiction Web site. Available at: http://www.emcdda.org/about/index.shtml. Accessed February 27, 2003.
47. Ling LH, Marchant C, Buckley NA, et al. Poisoning with the recreational drug paramethoxyamphetamine ("death"). *Med J Aust* 2001;174(9):453–455.
48. Hartney-Velazco K, Velazco A, Fleming LL. Bilateral anterior dislocation of the shoulder. *South Med J* 1984;77(10):1340–1341.
49. Armstrong PJ, Bersten A. Normeperidine toxicity. *Anaesth Analg* 1986;65:536–538.
50. Perucca E, Gram L, Avanzini G, et al. Antiepileptic drugs as a cause of worsening seizures. *Epilepsia* 1998;39(1):5–17.

CHAPTER 31
Sick Building Syndrome

Frederick Fung

OVERVIEW

Indoor air quality (IAQ) has become an important public health as well as medical issue. The medical toxicologist is often involved in the management and evaluation of IAQ issues. Building-related complaints can be classified as sick building syndrome (SBS) and building-related illnesses (BRIs). SBS has several synonyms, including *tight building* and *abused building syndrome*; however, *SBS* continues to be the most acceptable and recognized term, despite the lack of a clear definition. The World Health Organization presented a classification of symptoms secondary to IAQ complaints (1) but offered no practical solutions to resolve SBS.

From an engineering viewpoint, the American Society for Heating, Refrigerating and Air-Conditioning Engineers (ASHRAE) has published standards on acceptable IAQ since

1970 (2). J. S. Billings was a physician who used carbon dioxide as a measure of impurity emissions from the human body. He calculated that 50 ft^3/minute of ventilating air is needed to keep the carbon dioxide level in a room at 550 parts per million. Billings based his recommendations on the prevention of disease transmission, particularly tuberculosis. On the other hand, engineers were concerned with providing comfort and ensuring the absence of odors in indoor spaces (3). A joint effort of the American Lung Association/Environmental Protection Agency/Consumer Product Safety Committee and American Medical Association defined SBS as ". . . a situation in which reported symptoms among a population of building occupants can be temporally associated with their presence in the building" (4).

Although SBS and BRI are separate illness patterns, outbreaks of BRI encompass specific and nonspecific symptoms. Therefore, SBS may be an early stage of BRI and may progress to BRI.

The prevalence of SBS is unknown. A World Health Organization report (5) estimated that up to 30% of new and remodeled buildings may generate excessive complaints related to IAQ. It has also been reported that 24% of U.S. office workers perceive air quality problems in their work environment, and 20% believe that their work performance has been compromised as the result of poor IAQ (5). Health care costs and lost productivity may amount to $1 billion per year. It has also been estimated that the total cost of operating a building is approximately $350 to $400/$ft^2$ of which only $150/$ft^2$ is attributed to energy costs. Therefore, energy saving is really not a major part of owning and operating a building (6).

PATHOPHYSIOLOGY

Although the specific pathophysiology of SBS is not fully elucidated, three hypotheses are used to explain symptoms experienced by SBS patients. In contrast to multiple chemical sensitivity, there are some epidemiologic and controlled studies to support portions of the SBS hypotheses.

Chemical Hypothesis

The chemical hypothesis proposes that volatile organic chemicals may induce a predictable dose-response relationship involving the irritant receptor, particularly in the eyes and nose (7–9). Respiratory irritants can lead to asthma and rhinitis through interaction with chemical receptors in the airway, resulting in the release of inflammatory mediators (10). Experimental evidence indicates that histamines are released after exposure to a sick building setting (11). More convincing is an exposure chamber study that demonstrates associations between SBS symptoms and exposure to volatile organic compounds (12). However, the relationship between specific symptoms and exposure to levels well below the irritant thresholds of individual chemicals remains to be explained.

Bioaerosol Hypothesis

Cross-sectional studies show that individuals with underlying atopy react to a lower concentration of a volatile organic chemical mixture than do individuals without atopy. Histamine release is induced by allergens as well as by nonimmunologic substances. The reaction can be enhanced by exposure to bacterial endotoxins and mold spores. Mast cell degranulation and the release of inflammatory mediators such as histamine play an important part in bronchoconstriction and inflammatory events of the respiratory tract (13–15).

Host Factors

Individual susceptibility may account for symptoms. As a group, SBS patients have more rapid tear film break-up time and are more likely to experience punctate conjunctivitis (16). These patients also tend to have decreased basal and reflex stimulation leading to dry eye complaints. There is evidence of decreased meibomian gland secretion, allowing rapid evaporation of tear film in the presence of a larger exposed ocular surface during computer screen work (17). Skin complaints appear to be more prevalent among SBS patients, particularly in their description of eczema and irritation, than individuals without such complaints (18). Most patients appear to have psychological components to their discomfort and disease. Work stress and psychosocial factors may explain some variance of symptoms among SBS patients (19).

DIAGNOSIS

Most problem buildings have multiple environmental deficiencies, and the scientific data in most instances are inadequate to establish causal connections between any one factor and the reported health effects (20). Therefore, SBS is a diagnosis of exclusion; however, as soon as a specific cause has been identified, the medical condition under investigation should not be called SBS.

Although it is clinically useful to distinguish between SBS and BRI, patients typically come in with nonspecific complaints that are temporally associated with indoor environments at work or home. Table 1 provides a general overview and guidance of clinically important BRIs. Please see individual chapters for more information on specific diseases and toxins.

History

It is important to recognize potential toxin sources to provide an accurate diagnosis. Toxic pollutants can come from three main sources: outdoors, buildings, and occupant activities (Table 2). The indoor environment can be visualized as the result of constant interactions between outdoor conditions, building systems and materials, furnishings, and the occupants and their activities. A history regarding the general environment, the building or home conditions, and the activities of patients and others in or nearby the building at issue must be obtained to provide sufficient information to make a sound clinical judgment as to whether a patient has experienced potential toxic exposures. Automobile exhaust, bioaerosols (e.g., pollens, mold), and nearby industrial or landfill emissions can find their way indoors. The heating, ventilating, air-conditioning (HVAC) system may be poorly maintained, allowing microbial agents to grow (21). Dust particles, pesticides (22) and combustion products, and emissions from office equipment may not be properly vented, leading to exposure. Leakage of refrigerants, typically Freons, is common in older HVAC systems. Building materials and furnishings such as insulation materials, fiberglass, formaldehyde, volatile organic chemicals, and elevator hydraulic fluid may all contribute to indoor toxic exposure. Occupant activities such as smoking, cooking, housekeeping, janitorial work, exercise, and use of office equipment (photocopying machine) can generate chemicals and dust. Finally, cosmetics and deodorants used by other occupants of the building may also play some part in indoor air pollution.

TABLE 1. **Clinically important building-related syndromes and diseases**

Disease or syndrome	Symptoms/signs	Diagnostic testing	Association factors
Toxic substance			
Toxic gases: carbon monoxide, ozone Chemicals: organic solvents	Headaches, irritability, nausea, visual disturbances.	Carboxyhemoglobin, complete blood count, chemical panel, neuropsychological testing	Exposure to gases/chemicals, solvents, faulty furnace, generator, forklift, etc. Industrial hygiene sampling for specific exposure
Pesticide poisoning	Cholinergic symptoms.	Red blood cell count and serum cholinesterase	History of pesticide/organic phosphorous exposure
Irritation syndromes			
Eye irritation	Eye irritation, burning sensation, excessive tearing, signs of conjunctivitis such as erythema.	Tear film break-up time, slit lamp examination	History of exposure to irritant substances
Nasal irritation	Nasal irritation symptoms, rhinitis, nasal mucosal erythema, and edema.	Rhinometry, nasal lavage, nasal smear	History of exposure to irritants
Contact dermatitis	Itching, dry skin, rash with hives, and eczematous changes.	Patch testing, identification of fiberglass on skin	Exposure to fiberglass, industrial hygiene sampling
Allergy			
Rhinitis/sinusitis	Runny nose, nasal congestion, temporally related to building; symptoms resolve after a few days away. Nasal examination may show pale, erythematous/edematous mucosa.	Skin prick test, radioallergosorbent test, nasal lavage/smear for eosinophils, sinus x-rays, or computed tomography	Positive *in vitro* or *in vivo* immune testing Presence of allergen identified by industrial hygiene sampling
Asthma	Coughing, shortness of breath, chest tightness, wheezing on examination.	Spirometry, peak flow, methacholine challenge test, radioallergosorbent test, skin prick test	Changes on pulmonary function before and after exposure, allergy testing, sampling for sensitizing agents (isocyanates)
Hypersensitivity pneumonitis	Cough, shortness of breath, general fatigue, fever, muscle pain, abnormal lung sounds.	Complete pulmonary function: total lung capacity, diffusion capacity, chest radiography, immunoglobulin G antibody titer, computed tomography scan, open lung biopsy	Exposure to chemical or biologic agents identified by industrial hygiene sampling
Infectious diseases			
Tuberculosis	Cough, fever, night sweating, weight loss for several weeks.	Purified protein derivative (tuberculin), chest x-ray, sputum smear, culture	History of exposure to index case, epidemiologic survey
Legionnaires' disease	Shortness of breath; cough; fever; abnormal lung sounds such as wheezing, rhonchi, and rales.	Chest radiography, sputum culture, blood culture	History of exposure; immune testing; and industrial hygiene survey of the heating, ventilating, air-conditioning system; and response to antibiotics

Signs and Symptoms

Six symptoms are suggestive of SBS: a repeated pattern of nasal, eye, and mucous membrane symptoms, along with lethargy, dry skin, and headaches (23). Please refer to Table 1 for additional information.

Diagnostic Tests

Once a specific source or agent causing SBS is identified, the patient's diagnosis should be changed to the toxin-specific illness. There are no specific diagnostic tests for SBS. However, the following diagnostic procedure should be formulated when

TABLE 2. **Important sources of indoor pollutants and toxins**

Source	Nature	Agent
Outdoors	Biologic	Pollen and mold (*Alternaria, Cladosporium*)
	Chemical	Vehicular exhaust, carbon monoxide, carbon dioxide, smog, and particulate
Building related	Biologic (damp organic materials, standing water)	Bacteria (*Legionella, Thermoactinomyces*), mold, all airborne spores (e.g., *Penicillium, Aspergillus*, etc.), dust mites
	Chemical (from building materials, furniture, janitorial chemicals, pesticides, damp organic materials, carpet)	Formaldehyde, organic solvents, fiberglass, asbestos, pesticides, mycotoxins, glucans
Ventilation system	Improper balance and maintenance of heating, ventilating, air-conditioning system	Relative humidity, temperature, air movement, air distribution, filters, air intake, and fresh make-up air
Occupant activity	Combustion products and chemicals (indoor cooking, machineries, office and janitorial chemicals, office equipment, smoking, personal care products, deodorant, and bioeffluent)	Environmental tobacco smoke (carbon monoxide, nitrogen dioxide), sulfur dioxide, formaldehyde, soot particles, carbonless paper, liquid whiteout (trichloroethene), ozone, butyric acid, and volatile organic chemicals

dealing with patients. First, the presence of a disease should be documented as accurately as possible. For example, if symptoms and signs are consistent with asthma, diagnostic tests should establish that diagnosis. Once a diagnosis is made, treatment may include exposure avoidance and specific treatment of the disease entity, such as a bronchodilator and inhaled corticosteroids for asthma. Second, the source of the toxin should be identified (Table 2). Third, the scope and extent of exposure may need to be assessed by industrial hygiene methods. Fourth, remediation of the exposure should produce symptom resolution or improvement.

POTENTIAL COMPLICATIONS

Because SBS is a nonspecific constellation of symptoms that building occupants experience while in the building, and because their symptoms resolve or improve after they are removed from that building, this condition has no known complications.

MANAGEMENT

The indoor air concentration of toxins is affected by the location or source of a toxin, the air exchange rate, as well as the rate of chemical reaction and deposition. Three approaches are used to manage SBS. The first approach relies on the identification of a specific substance in the building, typically identified through industrial hygiene and environmental assessment. This approach is important for regulatory necessity but is not practical for resolving SBS. Identifying the source or nature of a toxin is important in ensuring that SBS patients do not have a psychological illness, although the situation may be complicated by organizational structure and management-labor relationships. The second approach is based on identifying a disease such as bronchitis, asthma, hypersensitivity pneumonitis, and so forth. Once a disease is identified, then etiologic factors of that disease can be considered. When the diagnosis and treatment of BRI are based on clinical features supplemented with laboratory tests, proper treatment modalities can be instituted and are usually effective. The third approach is based on building design and control. As in any equilibrium, the concentration of indoor toxin is determined by input and elimination: the source of emission and the dilutional ability of the HVAC system. The amount of fresh air that can be brought into the building and the exchange rate of air are both important. Typically, a home without air-conditioning has 0.5 air exchanges per hour. The electronic industry typically has up to 40 air exchanges per hour in sensitive manufacturing areas. In hospital and health care facilities, it has been shown that an inverse relationship exists between transmission of infectious disease and the rate of indoor air exchange (24). A review of the HVAC system, including engineering and architectural designs, may be necessary by nonmedical experts to identify potential factors for SBS. For example, if temperature control or humidity controls are not up to ASHRAE standards (2), occupants of the building may complain of nonspecific symptoms. This approach is useful for the prevention of potential building-related syndromes and diseases.

Table 3 outlines the goals and principles of management. SBS is best managed by prevention. Proper building maintenance and basic knowledge of IAQ standards are important to prevent SBS (Table 4). Because volatile organic chemicals and bioaerosols have been implicated as potential causative factors, industrial hygiene monitoring may be necessary to ensure that toxins

TABLE 3. Goals and principles of sick building syndrome management

Goal	Principle
Recognize sick building syndrome	Establish presence of illness (nonspecific symptoms vs. building-related illness)
Obtain baseline building parameters	Assess building environment; heating, ventilation, and air-conditioning system (i.e., temperature, humidity, and carbon dioxide)
Identify indoor air pollutants	Obtain industrial hygiene study on chemical, biologic agents when scientifically indicated
Establish cause-effect relationship	Demonstrate the presence and adequacy of toxins in environment consistent with disease
Implement control measures	Recommend cost-effective control measures, consider possible psychosocial stress issues, treat specific diseases

TABLE 4. Standards and guidelines on air toxins in the United States

Toxic pollutant	Indoor standards	Outdoor guidelines/standards
Asbestos	Use has been banned by CPSC EPA regulates use in schools	National emissions standard: no visible emissions
Carbon monoxide	None	National ambient air quality standard: 10 mg/m^3 (9 ppm), 8 h. TWA and 40 mg/m^3 (35 ppm), 1 h average
Formaldehyde	Federal standard is 0.4 ppm ambient level	None
Lead	Banned by CPSC in products and paint for consumer use	National ambient air quality: 15 μg/m^3 maximum, quarterly arithmetic mean
Nitrogen dioxide	None	National ambient air quality: 100 μg/m^3 or 0.053 ppm annual arithmetic mean
Ozone	Devices that produce more than 0.05 ppm or 50 ppb prohibited in occupied buildings	National ambient air quality: 235 μg/m^3 of air maximum hourly average or 0.12 ppm
Sulfur dioxide	None	National ambient air quality: 80 μg/m^3 (0.03 ppm) annual arithmetic mean and 365 μg/m^3 (0.14 ppm) 24-h exposure
Biologic toxins	None	None

CPSC, Consumer Product Safety Commission; EPA, Environmental Protection Agency; ppb, parts per billion; ppm, parts per million; TWA, time-weighted average.
Adapted from American Society of Heating, Refrigerating and Air-Conditioning Engineers. *Ventilation for acceptable indoor air quality, 1999.* Atlanta: American Society of Heating, Refrigerating and Air-Conditioning Engineers, 1999; ASHRAE standard 62-1999, with permission.

and agents are kept below the proposed standards. ASHRAE has published standards on temperature, relative humidity, and other levels of chemicals and toxins permitted in indoor environments (2). It has been proposed that total volatile organic chemicals not exceed 3 mg/m^3 of air or approximately 0.9 parts per million of toluene equivalent for a nonindustrial indoor setting to prevent irritant symptoms (25,26).

PITFALLS

The medical toxicologist must be aware that even with a specific agent diagnosis, it may or may not be related to the building involved. A trial of relocating SBS patients to another building or facility may be helpful to alleviate symptoms. However, caution is needed, as patients may take such a measure as "proof" that the building is in fact hazardous to their health, even if it is not.

Because host factors are part of the SBS hypothesis, factors such as organizational structure, risk perception, labor-management issues, and interpersonal relationships may be important in the management of SBS. At a certain point, the building owner, employer, insurance company, and/or other occupants should be informed that such factors play an integral part in resolving SBS (27).

REFERENCES

1. World Health Organization. *Indoor air quality research.* Copenhagen: World Health Organization, 1982; EURO reports and studies 78.
2. American Society of Heating, Refrigerating and Air-Conditioning Engineers. *Ventilation for acceptable indoor air quality, 1999.* Atlanta: American Society of Heating, Refrigerating and Air-Conditioning Engineers, 1999; ASHRAE standard 62-1999.
3. Jansen JE. The history of ventilation and temperature control—the first century of air conditioning. *ASHRAE Journal* 1999;41(9):41–52.
4. American Lung Association, Environmental Protection Agency, Consumer Product Safety Committee, and American Medical Association. Indoor air pollution—an introduction to health professionals. Washington: US Government Printing Office, 1994; publication #1994-523-217/81322.
5. Kreiss K. The sick building syndrome—where is the epidemiologic basis? *Am J Pub Health* 1990;80:1172–1173.
6. Jones W. Sick building syndrome. *App Occup Environ Hyg* 1990;5:74–83.
7. Hempel-Jorgensen A. Sensory eye irritation in humans exposed to mixtures of volatile organic compounds. *Arch Environ Health* 1999;54:416–424.
8. Kjaergaard S. Sensitivity of the eyes to airborne stimuli: influence of individual characteristics. *Arch Environ Health* 1992;47:45–50.
9. Hudnell HK. Exposure of humans to volatile organic mixture II. Sensory. *Arch Environ Health* 1992;47:31–38.
10. Ohm M, Juto JE, Andersson K, et al. Nasal histamine provocation of tenants in a sick building residential area. *Am J Rhinol* 1997;11:167–175.
11. Meggs WJ. RADS and RUDS—the toxic induction of asthma and rhinitis. *J Toxicol Clin Toxicol* 1994;32:487–501.
12. Molhave L. Controlled experiments for studies of the sick building syndrome. In sources of indoor air contaminants—characterizing emissions and health impacts. *Ann N Y Acad Sci* 1992;641:46–55.
13. Norn S. Micro organism-induced for enhanced mediator release: the possible mechanism inorganic dust related diseases. *Am J Indust Med* 1994;25:91–95.
14. Larsen FO, Clementsen P, Hansen M, et al. The indoor micro fungus trichoderma viride potentiates histamine release from human bronchoalveolar cells. *APMIS* 1996;104:673–679.
15. Rylander R. (1-3)-Beta-D-glucan relationship to indoor air-related symptoms, allergy and asthma. *Toxicology* 2000;152:47–52.
16. Franck C, Bach E, Skov P. Prevalence of subjective eye manifestations in people working in office buildings with different prevalences of the sick building syndrome compared with the general population. *Int Arch Occup Environ Health* 1993;65:65–69.
17. Tsubota K, Nakamori K. Dry eyes and video display terminals. *N Engl J Med* 1993;325:584.
18. Eriksson N, Hoog J, Mild KH, et al. The psychosocial work environment and skin symptoms among visual display terminal workers: a case referent study. *Intern J Epidemiol* 1997;26:1250–1257.
19. Eriksson N, Hoog J, Sandstrom M, et al. Facial skin symptoms in office workers. *J Occup Environ Med* 1997;39:108–118.
20. Rosenstock L. NIOSH testimony to the US Department of Labor on IAQ. *Appl Occup Environ Hygiene* 1996;11:1365–1370.
21. Ahearn DG. Fungal colonization of air filters and insulation in a multi-story office building: production of volatile organics. *Current Microbiol* 1997;35:305–308.
22. Hodgson M, Block G, Parkinson D. Organophosphate poisoning in office workers. *J Occup Med* 1986;28:434–437.
23. Finnegan MJ, Pickering CA, Burge PS. The sick building syndrome: prevalence studies. *BMJ* 1984;8:289.
24. Fennelly KP, Nardell EA. The relative efficiency of respirators and room ventilation in preventing occupational tuberculosis. *Infect Control Hosp Epidemiol* 1998;19:754–759.
25. Molhave L. Indoor climate, air pollution and human comfort. *J Expo Anal Environ Epidemiol* 1991;1:63–81.
26. World Health Organization. *Indoor air quality: organic pollutants.* Copenhagen: World Health Organization Regional Office for Europe, 1989; EURO reports and studies 111.
27. Fung F. Indoor air quality in occupational health. *Occup Environ Med Report* 1992;8:60–64.

CHAPTER 32

Withdrawal—Central Nervous System Depressants

Ilene B. Anderson and Jo Ellen Dyer

OVERVIEW

The medical toxicologist is frequently consulted in the management of patients experiencing withdrawal from a central nervous system (CNS) depressant. Despite diverse chemical structures and mechanisms of action, CNS depressants have similar clinical syndromes of neuropsychiatric excitation and autonomic instability during withdrawal. The abstinence syndrome shares features with many other disorders that challenge diagnosis. In addition, the stigma of drug dependence may lead to patient or family denial, further delaying early recognition and appropriate intervention. To combat the difficulties in diagnosing depressant withdrawal, the practitioner should be knowledgeable of the characteristic symptoms of depressant withdrawal, familiar with syndromes that may mimic depressant withdrawal, and able to use the laboratory appropriately to determine a prompt, accurate diagnosis. Once the diagnosis is ascertained, appropriate sedation and supportive care are critical to ensure a satisfactory outcome.

Physiologic dependence is the result of neurologic adaptation from repeated exposure to a substance with evidence of a characteristic syndrome on reduction of drug levels, the *withdrawal syndrome.* Reintroduction of the depressant agent or a closely related substance abates withdrawal symptoms. Sedative-hypnotic drugs including ethanol are a depressant class well known to produce physiologic dependence. *Sedatives* calm activity and depress excitement. Hypnotics cause drowsiness and facilitate sleep (1).

Tolerance usually develops over a period of time and is manifested by the need for escalating doses of a drug to achieve the same effect. *Pharmacodynamic tolerance* occurs due to cellular adaptation and, once attained, can be conferred to other drugs within a class by *cross-tolerance*. *Pharmacokinetic tolerance* occurs as metabolism of a drug is increased. A common example is enhanced drug clearance by induction of hepatic microsomal enzymes (1–3). These biologic phenomena may occur with therapeutic use of a drug and do not require addiction. *Addiction* involves a characteristic behavior pattern of compulsive drug use that persists despite adverse consequences. *Symptom reemergence* may be confused with drug withdrawal; however, it is a reemergence of the original symptoms after cessation of the depressant drug. This phenomenon is common among patients treated for anxiety with benzodiazepines (4). It is less likely to be symptom reemergence if the syndrome waxes and wanes and presents with qualitatively new symptoms (5,6).

CNS depressants are prescribed worldwide for seizure disorders, insomnia, anxiety, chronic pain, preanesthesia, and muscle spasticity of spinal origin. Dependence can result from prolonged administration for the pleasurable reinforcing properties or, more rarely, for therapeutic use. Approximately one-third of patients taking a benzodiazepine for more than 6 weeks experience some withdrawal symptoms if the drug is abruptly discontinued (7). Even a gradual taper may result in some signs of withdrawal, although life-threatening symptoms can be avoided (8). Alcohol has been used for more than 8000 years and still remains the most popular and readily available depressant drug (9). Although delirium tremens was first described in 1787, the development of tolerance, withdrawal, and delirium tremens as a consequence of the dose of ethanol ingested was not definitively demonstrated until 1957 (10). Similar withdrawal syndromes for other depressant drugs have been described: barbiturate dependence in 1950 (11), benzodiazepine withdrawal in 1961 (12), and, most recently, γ hydroxybutyrate (GHB) withdrawal in 2001 (13). In the United States, the annual economic cost of combined alcohol and drug abuse is estimated at more than 246 billion dollars (14).

PATHOPHYSIOLOGY

The depressants share common mechanisms that underlie depressant activity and withdrawal syndromes. One shared pathway is suppression neuronal excitability by activating the γ aminobutyric acid-A (GABA-A) receptor. The resulting increased inward chloride current hyperpolarizes the neuronal membrane and inhibits excitatory impulse propagation. GABA stimulation in combination with benzodiazepines increases the frequency of opening of chloride channels, whereas barbiturates prolong the duration of opening. In high doses, barbiturates also activate the chloride channel directly.

The *N*-methyl-D-aspartate subtype of glutamate receptors is sensitive to ethanol. The presynaptic GABA-B receptor is stimulated by baclofen and hypothesized to be the central site of action for GHB (15). Drugs in the opioid class elicit their acute behavioral effects by binding to specific seven-transmembrane neurotransmitter receptors. Three classes of opioid receptors, mu, sigma, and kappa, have been identified (16).

MECHANISM OF DEPENDENCE

During regular use of a depressant, dependence arises from internal adjustments to maintain homeostasis. Molecular and neuronal pathways are changed to maintain normal function in the presence of inhibiting agents (e.g., receptor down-regulation). The net effect of these is to increase stimulatory activities in the presence of the depressant. If the drug is withdrawn (abstinence), however, the homeostatic adjustments are again off-balance but now in the direction of neuroexcitation. The common symptoms of withdrawal, anxiety, tremor, insomnia, hyperthermia, and seizure, are manifestations of this unchecked CNS excitation that also provokes adrenergic outflow with resulting tachycardia, hypertension, and diaphoresis (17). This persists until the homeostatic processes once again restore normal function.

The severity of the withdrawal syndrome is influenced by dose, duration, history, and drug-specific effects. A study with alcohol indicates that symptom intensity varies directly with the dose and duration of use before abstinence (18). The depressants with shorter half-lives have faster onset, as well as earlier and more intense peak withdrawal effects, compared to longer half-life drugs (6,19,20). The number of prior detoxifications increases the severity of alcohol withdrawal syndrome (21), and the presence of secondary medical complications such as pancreatitis, hepatitis, or infection may worsen the course of withdrawal (22). Finally, patients with codependence on another depressant may experience a more difficult course (23).

DIAGNOSIS

Early diagnosis and intervention are key to the successful management of acute depressant withdrawal. A thorough physical examination, basic laboratories, a "drugs of abuse" screen, an electrocardiogram, a list of the patient's current medications, and interviews with family and friends all aid in the diagnosis. Several illnesses or intoxication may mimic depressant withdrawal (Table 1). Refer to the individual chapters on drug intoxication for additional information.

Signs and Symptoms

The clinical presentation of withdrawal from depressant drugs shares many common features. Selected agents may have distinct clinical features during withdrawal that differ from the majority of depressants (Table 2). In addition, the toxicokinetics may vary depending on the half-life of the drug and the active metabolites (Table 3).

The minimum dose or duration of use required to develop physical dependence is difficult to predict because of wide inter-individual variability. Generally, higher doses and longer duration of use are more likely to result in withdrawal symptoms on abrupt discontinuation. Some patients are at risk of physiologic dependence on benzodiazepines after therapeutic doses for as few as 6 weeks (5).

Depressant agents reported to result in a withdrawal syndrome include benzodiazepines (12,19,20,24); barbiturates (25–27); ethanol (22,28,29); opiates (30,31); carisoprodol (32–34); meprobamate (35,36); GHB (13,37); gamma butyrolactone (38); 1,4-butanediol (39); baclofen (40–46); tramadol (47); chloral hydrate (48); zolpidem (49,50); methaqualone (51); ethchlorvynol (52–56); glutethimide (57–60); and methyprylon (61).

Initially, symptoms may be mild and commonly include anxiety, insomnia, tremor, nausea and vomiting, dizziness, mild tachycardia, and mild hypertension. Without treatment, these

TABLE 1. Selected conditions that mimic sedative-hypnotic withdrawal

Agent	Key differences	Useful diagnostic tests
Amphetamine intoxication	Evidence of chronic IV drug use, formication.	Drug of abuse screen
Anticholinergic syndrome	Absent bowel sounds; dry, flushed skin.	Physostigmine transiently reverses effects
Cocaine intoxication	Short duration of symptoms, evidence of IV drug use, cocaine burns, evidence of chronic smoking/snorting, perforation of nasal septum, pleuritic chest pain.	Drug of abuse screen
Ephedrine, ma huang, or pseudoephedrine intoxication	Resolution of symptoms usually seen within 6 h.	Drug of abuse screen may be positive for amphetamine
Infection, central nervous system	Fever, headache, vomiting, stiff neck, elevated white blood count.	Lumbar puncture, cultures, complete blood count with differential
Levodopa intoxication	History of parkinsonian syndrome.	Monitoring of vital signs and electrocardiogram
MAO inhibitor overdose	Hyperadrenergic state followed by a state of catecholamine depletion (hypotension, bradycardia, etc.).	Monitoring of vital signs
MAO inhibitor interaction with sympathomimetic, tyramine-containing food, or meperidine	May see severe hypertensive crisis, history of MAO inhibitor use, and implicated drug or food.	Monitoring of vital signs
Nicotine poisoning	History of insecticide exposure or presence of strong pesticide odor. A hyperadrenergic state is followed by a state of catecholamine depletion (hypotension, bradycardia, etc.). Muscle weakness, paralysis, miosis may develop.	Monitoring of vital signs
Neuroleptic malignant syndrome	History of antipsychotic use. "Lead-pipe" rigidity.	Monitoring of vital signs
Phencyclidine intoxication	Vertical or rotary nystagmus; behavior oscillating between agitation and lethargy; miosis or mydriasis may be present.	Drug of abuse screen
Pheochromocytoma (110)	Hypertensive crisis. Symptoms may be episodic.	Elevated free plasma and urine normetanephrine and metanephrine
Psychosis (functional)	History of psychiatric disorder; patient is usually oriented; bizarre affect or thought content; vital signs and pupil size are usually normal.	Negative drug of abuse screen (unless patient also concurrently abuses drugs)
Seizure disorder	History of seizure; evidence of urinary or fecal incontinence; tongue biting; gingival hyperplasia (chronic phenytoin use).	Drug levels of common anticonvulsants
Serotonin syndrome	Myoclonic jerking, history of SSRI use or MAO inhibitor use with the addition of a serotonergic agent.	Monitoring of vital signs
Thyroid storm	History of hyperthyroidism; may see hyperbilirubinemia, elevation in prothrombin time, hyperglycemia.	Thyroid function tests
Thyroid hormone intoxication	History of thyroid abnormalities or access to thyroid medications.	Thyroid function tests

MAO, monoamine oxidase; SSRI, selective serotonin reuptake inhibitor.

TABLE 2. Diagnostic clues useful in differentiating depressant withdrawal etiology

Agent	Differentiating clues
Ethanol	History of alcoholism. Tremor, anxiety, brief seizure within 8–12 h of the last drink. Evidence of alcoholic hepatitis or chronic liver disease (hepatic pain or tenderness, hepatomegaly, jaundice, ascites, esophageal varices, elevated transaminases, thrombocytopenia, hypoprothrombinemia, signs of malnutrition), pancreatitis, formication, anemia, various electrolyte and vitamin deficiencies, delirium tremens, Wernicke-Korsakoff syndrome.
Opiates	Piloerection, rhinorrhea, lacrimation, diarrhea, myalgia, muscle cramps, yawning. Rarely develop fever unless infection is present. Patient usually has a clear sensorium without confusion or delirium. Evidence of IV drug use. Patients do not typically develop life-threatening symptoms.
Baclofen	Patients with a history of multiple sclerosis, cerebral palsy, or spinal cord injury. Patients with an intrathecal baclofen pump.
Benzodiazepines	Symptoms may be of longer duration than expected when considering the half-life of the parent compound. Tinnitus may be present in some patients (67).
GHB (13), GBL (38), BD (39)	History of bodybuilding; use of GHB dosing around the clock; anxiety; insomnia. Severe withdrawal symptoms requiring high-dose benzodiazepine treatment. Symptoms tend to occur in an episodic fashion when waning (days 7–14).

BD, butadiene; GBL, gamma butyrolactone; GHB, gamma hydroxybutyrate.

symptoms may abate or may progress to include diaphoresis, weakness, diplopia, mydriasis, nystagmus, hyperreflexia, myoclonic jerking, paranoia, visual, tactile, or auditory hallucinations, and nightmares. More severe symptoms include seizures, combative behavior, confusion, delirium, severe autonomic instability, and psychosis. Alcohol withdrawal may result in the onset of seizures early in the withdrawal syndrome.

Wide patient variability exists regarding the onset, severity, and progression of withdrawal. Medical complications that may occur as a result of severe withdrawal include fluid and electrolyte abnormalities, cardiac arrhythmias, hyperthermia (62), rhabdomyolysis, disseminated intravascular coagulation (41), and death (13,63–65). The duration of withdrawal symptoms is related to the time course of neuroadaptation. After the acute withdrawal syndrome has resolved, milder, subtler symptoms may persist for weeks to months (especially with benzodiazepines) but generally improve with time.

Diagnostic Tests

The onset of withdrawal is largely related to the elimination half-life of the parent drug and active metabolite(s). Withdrawal symptoms usually do not begin until the blood level is low or no longer detectable. The rate of drug elimination may be slower in elderly patients and patients with liver disease. Administration of antagonists (flumazenil and naloxone) usually results in the immediate onset of withdrawal symptoms in dependent patients.

TABLE 3. Toxicokinetics of depressant withdrawal

Agent (references)	Onset	Peak	Duration of acute withdrawal
Baclofen (42–46,81,111,112)	12–72 h	3–5 d	7–9 d or until effectively treated
Barbiturates (12,27,64)	Short-acting: 1 d Long-acting: 2 d	Short-acting: 2–8 d Long-acting: 5–8 d	Short-acting: 3–14 d
Benzodiazepines (4,12,19,24,113)	Short-acting: 1–2 d Long-acting: 2–8 d	Short-acting: 2–5 d Long-acting: 4–7 d	Short-acting: 4–7 d Long-acting: 7–20 d
Ethanol (28)	6–8 h (seizure onset, 8–12 h)	1–2 d; delirium tremens 3–5 d	10–14 d (mild withdrawal resolves within 3 d)
Ethchlorvynol (52,53)	<1–2 d	2–8 d	5–12 d
Gamma hydroxybutyrate (13,37)	1–6 h	24–36 h	5–15 d
Glutethimide (57,59)	<9 h	16–24 h	5–12 d
Meprobamate (35,36,114)	12–36 h	30–96 h	48–96 h
Methaqualone (115)	12–24 h	24–72 h	>72 h
Methyprylon (61)	<1 d	3 d	8–11 d
Opiates	4–6 h; 36–72 h for methadone	36–72 h; 6 d for methadone	5–10 d; 10–14 d for methadone
Tramadol (47)	7 d	9 d	12 d
Zolpidem (49,50)	4–14 h	14 h	4–7 d

Tests to guide patient management before a definitive diagnosis is made include vital signs, physical examination, electrocardiogram, bedside blood glucose test, computed tomography scan of the brain, lumbar puncture, and chest radiograph. Withdrawal is a systemic process that may alter numerous laboratory studies: serum electrolytes, glucose, liver function tests, complete blood count with differential and blood smear, urinalysis, coagulation studies, creatinine phosphokinase, arterial blood gases, drugs of abuse screen, and the comprehensive drug screen. Thyroid function tests should be evaluated if thyroid hormone intoxication or thyroid storm is suspected. Free plasma and urine normetanephrine and metanephrine levels are useful if pheochromocytoma is suspected. Drug levels of common anticonvulsants may be helpful if the patient is suspected of having a seizure disorder.

GHB urine and serum tests are not routinely available but may be useful in diagnosis. However, GHB is usually only detected within 12 hours of the last dose. Ethanol or phenobarbital levels may be useful in diagnosis. Ethanol withdrawal may begin before the level reaches zero in severe dependence.

MANAGEMENT

The primary treatment of withdrawal is supportive care, close monitoring for complications, and the administration of benzodiazepines to control agitation, delirium, hyperthermia, and seizures. More than one drug may be needed in the case of severe withdrawal (e.g., benzodiazepine followed by barbiturate). The combined effect may produce respiratory failure and require emergent airway management.

Benzodiazepines exhibit cross-tolerance with other CNS depressants and are the mainstay of management for withdrawal due to their large therapeutic range, high threshold for respiratory depression, and relative lack of cardiovascular complications. The ability of barbiturates to directly activate the GABA receptor when GABA is diminished or absent provides an alternative or enhancement for withdrawal resistant to benzodiazepine therapy. However, the addition of phenobarbital or pentobarbital in a patient already treated with high doses of benzodiazepines may result in respiratory depression requiring mechanical ventilation. Adjunctive medications may provide further comfort by reducing anxiety, tremor, nausea, insomnia, and depression during withdrawal, but the safety and efficacy of single therapy with these agents have not been demonstrated.

Management of patients with depressant withdrawal in outpatient clinics has been safely accomplished for mild to moderate withdrawal. However, patients expected to undergo severe withdrawal should undergo supervised withdrawal. Severe withdrawal may be predicted by a history of seizures or delirium tremens, use of high doses, use of multiple depressants, prolonged duration of use, or concurrent physical illness (66–68).

Several drug treatment regimens have been used for the treatment of depressant withdrawal. Early recognition of withdrawal allows for *fixed schedule, dose stabilization,* and *gradual taper* with a long half-life benzodiazepine. Other strategies include *tapering of the target drug,* which is more likely to be effective in therapeutic dependence than addiction. The *loading dose technique* has the advantage of establishing the degree of tolerance, as it suppresses the withdrawal symptoms and is effective if combined sedatives have been used or the history is unreliable. More recently, *symptom-triggered therapy* has shown efficacy with lower sedative doses and shorter duration of treatment (69–72). Symptom severity is monitored, using withdrawal scales such as the Clinical Institute Withdrawal Assessment for Alcohol revised (CIWA-Ar) and the CIWA-Benzodiazepines (CIWA-B) proposed for benzodiazepine-like withdrawal (73). Sedatives are administered to suppress withdrawal symptoms based on assessment of severity (74). It is more difficult to manage patients presenting with *severe withdrawal* symptoms, requiring aggressive sedation to control the neuropsychiatric stimulation and autonomic instability (75).

All treatment regimens for CNS depressant withdrawal require frequent patient assessment for efficacy controlling withdrawal symptoms, while avoiding the development of sedative intoxication symptoms: dysarthria, nystagmus, somnolence, ataxia, and Romberg sign. Standardized symptom assessment scales such as CIWA-Ar and CIWA-B may be useful (73,74).

Fixed Schedule—Substitution, Stabilization, and Gradual Taper

Diazepam is substituted for the abused depressant: 40% of equivalent daily dose is divided into four doses given every 6 hours orally. Taper by 10% dose reduction per day thereafter (76).

Phenobarbital substitution dose 30 mg (not the equivalent therapeutic dose) is substituted for each hypnotic dose of depressant. This substitution dose is determined by total daily dose of the target drug, divided by its hypnotic dose, and multiplied by 30 (Table 4). Phenobarbital dose is divided into four doses given every 6 hours. The patient is stabilized 7 days for depressants with a short half-life or 14 days for a long half-life (half-life less than 20 hours), followed by a tapering rate of 30

TABLE 4. Phenobarbital withdrawal substitution[a]

Depressant	Hypnotic dose (mg)	Depressant	Hypnotic dose (mg)
Benzodiazepines		Barbiturates	
Alprazolam	1	Amobarbital	100
Chlordiazepoxide	25	Butabarbital	100
Clonazepam	2	Butalbital	100
Clorazepate	15	Pentobarbital	100
Diazepam	10	Phenobarbital	100
Flurazepam	30	Secobarbital	100
Halazepam	40	Others	
Lorazepam	2	Carisoprodol	350
Oxazepam	30	Chloral hydrate	500
Prazepam	20	Ethanol	1–2 oz 40%
Temazepam	30	Ethchlorvynol	350
Triazolam	0.5	Glutethimide	250
		Meprobamate	200
		Methaqualone	300
		Methyprylon	300

[a]Not phenobarbital equivalent doses.
Data from Smith DE, Wesson DR. Benzodiazepine dependency syndromes. *J Psychoactive Drugs* 1983;15(1–2):85–95; Hayner G, Galloway G, Wiehl WO. Haight Ashbury free clinics' drug detoxification protocols—Part 3: benzodiazepines and other sedative-hypnotics. *J Psychoactive Drugs* 1993;25(4):331–335; and Khantzian EJ, McKenna GJ. Acute toxic and withdrawal reactions associated with drug use and abuse. *Ann Intern Med* 1979;90(3):361–372.

mg per day. Supplemental doses are given for signs of developing withdrawal—anxiety, tremor, or postural hypotension—and the total daily dose is increased by 25% (one dose) (77,78). Symptoms of intoxication are managed by 50% reduction in daily dose (79).

Opiate withdrawal is most commonly managed with methadone. Doses may be administered orally or by injection of 5 to 20 mg after withdrawal onset, repeated every 2 to 6 hours for persistent withdrawal symptoms. A tapering rate of 5 mg daily may begin after a 2-day stabilization period, resolution of the acute medical illness, or completion of the depressant withdrawal. Most patients are controlled with 10 to 40 mg per day (80). The central alpha-adrenergic agonist clonidine can diminish signs and symptoms of withdrawal within 24 hours.

Baclofen withdrawal, a GABA-B–mediated withdrawal syndrome, may be resistant to management with benzodiazepines, although it responds well to reintroduction of baclofen. Improvement is seen within 4 to 72 hours, followed by slow taper by 5 to 10 mg/week (81). Intrathecal baclofen withdrawal is rare and generally results from an unintended mechanical interruption of drug delivery. Intrathecal injection of baclofen has been required to control the withdrawal syndrome (41,82). In some cases, dantrolene in addition to benzodiazepines has been used to control the hyperthermia and rigidity (63,83).

Oral Loading Dose Technique

Diazepam, 20 mg, is administered orally every 2 hours until symptoms of benzodiazepine intoxication are detected (84,85). In an alcohol withdrawal study, 50% of patients responded with three doses and the majority with six doses (86). For alcohol withdrawal, additional doses are rarely given if the loading dose was sufficiently large. One case of alprazolam tolerance required 260 mg diazepam to show signs of intoxication (87).

Phenobarbital, 120 mg, can be administered orally every hour (88) until three of the following signs of intoxication appear: nystagmus, drowsiness, ataxia, dysarthria, or emotional lability. The patient is assessed 1 hour after each dose. The long half-life of phenobarbital provides the tapering effect for short-acting depressants. When withdrawing from a long half-life depressant, additional stabilization time may be required.

Symptom-Triggered Therapy

Administration of sedatives to suppress withdrawal symptoms is guided by assessment of severity with the CIWA-Ar scale (70,71,74). This method has resulted in a lower total benzodiazepine dose and a shorter duration of therapy in uncomplicated withdrawal but requires a trained and motivated nursing staff. Symptom-triggered therapy has also been effective for benzodiazepine withdrawal using a comparative benzodiazepine assessment scale CIWA-B (73).

Diazepam, 10 to 20 mg, or *lorazepam*, 2 to 4 mg, is administered orally followed by assessment after 1 hour. The dose is repeated for an assessment score of 8 to 10.

Sedation for Severe or Resistant Withdrawal

The goal of therapy for the patient admitted with escalating withdrawal symptoms or delirium is rapid sedation to control agitation, fever, and progression of life-threatening symptoms. The dose of sedatives is titrated to control symptoms; occasionally, massive doses are required. For example, a 35-year-old male experiencing GHB withdrawal required intravenous (IV) lorazepam, 1138 mg; fentanyl, 469 μg; and propofol, 155 mg/kg, over the first 4 days of withdrawal (89).

Diazepam, in 5- to 15-mg IV doses, can be administered every 5 to 15 minutes until the patient is calm but awake. The initial calming dose may require 200 mg. The dose over 24 hours may exceed 2000 mg (90). *Lorazepam*, 4 to 8 mg IV every 15 to 20 minutes, is a suitable alternative for patients with encephalopathy or liver dysfunction or lacking IV access (lorazepam can be injected intramuscularly). For rapidly changing symptoms, a lorazepam drip can been titrated to maintain sedation.

Phenobarbital, 260 mg IV with 130 mg every 30 minutes until patient is calm, is an alternative. Mean dose to light sedation in alcohol withdrawal was 598 mg (91). *Pentobarbital* has a faster onset of effect than phenobarbital. Pentobarbital, 1 to 2 mg/kg IV every 30 to 60 minutes, normalized the heart rate and sensorium for 2 to 6 hours in a case of GHB withdrawal (38).

Propofol has been used successfully in resistant alcohol, barbiturate, and 1,4-butanediol withdrawal after intubation (92–95). The initial IV infusion is 5 μg/kg/minute (0.3 mg/kg/hour) for 5 to 10 minutes, repeated until desired sedation is achieved. Sedation is maintained with infusion rates of 5 to 50 μg/kg/minute, titrated to effect (96).

Pancuronium, 0.1 mg/kg IV, is used if skeletal-muscle paralysis is indicated for agitation with rising temperature higher than 104°F. Monitor electroencephalogram for evidence of seizure activity that may be masked by neuromuscular paralysis (97).

Supportive Care

Prolonged poor nutritional intake and withdrawal symptoms of anorexia, vomiting, confusion, diaphoresis, and hyperthermia contribute to *glucose, fluid*, and *electrolyte imbalances*. Evaluate and correct abnormalities in glucose, sodium, potassium, magnesium, calcium, and fluid status, which may contribute to mental status changes.

Vitamins may be administered for nutritional deficits due to selective dieting or poor nutritional intake. Alcoholics may be thiamine deficient, thus at risk to develop Wernicke-Korsakoff syndrome. GHB withdrawal also has presented with global confusion, sixth nerve palsies, and ataxic gait in addition to paranoid delusions and hallucinations (98). GHB is promoted as a treatment for alcohol withdrawal and may be self-administered by patients late in a course of alcoholism. Thiamine administration of 100 mg daily, initial dose by injection; additional vitamins may be given as needed.

Adjunctive Therapy

Clonidine inhibits noradrenergic outflow and hyperexcitability of neurons in the locus ceruleus. This ameliorates adrenergic symptoms in mild to moderate withdrawal; however, it may mask monitoring parameters of progressing withdrawal, leading to premature limitation of benzodiazepine sedation. Low doses have been used as adjunctive therapy for benzodiazepine withdrawal with varied results (99,100). Clonidine at 0.1 mg orally four times a day can be increased to 0.2 to 0.4 mg or 4 to 6 μg/kg/day and divided into three doses given every 8 hours for 2 to 3 days and gradually tapered.

Beta-blockers decrease the severity but not the incidence of symptoms in mild to moderate withdrawal (101). Contraindications to use include hypotension, bronchospastic lung disease, congestive heart failure, and second- or third-degree heart block. A higher incidence of delirium was found in one study (102). Beta-blockers may mask adrenergic symptoms of evolving withdrawal and may not be necessary with adequate sedation.

Carbamazepine has been effective in mild to moderate ethanol withdrawal, although efficacy preventing seizures or delirium has not been demonstrated (103–105). Carbamazepine 600 to 800 mg/day is administered in divided doses over 5 days. For benzodiazepine withdrawal, carbamazepine is administered during the taper of diazepam at 25% per week for 4 weeks and then maintained for an additional 2 to 4 weeks until symptoms of withdrawal are expected to have abated (106). Side effects include vertigo, nausea, vomiting, diplopia, and rash (107).

Neuroleptics (phenothiazines or butyrophenones) reduce some signs and symptoms of withdrawal and may calm agitated patients, but their adverse effect profile is poor: dystonia, aggravation of hypotension, and hyperthermia. Neuroleptics are less effective than benzodiazepines in reducing delirium and seizures and have increased seizures compared to placebo (108).

Antiemetics to limit nausea and vomiting, *antidepressants* for psychiatric diagnoses, and *antihistamines* for sleep are other adjunctive agents that have been helpful ameliorating symptoms of depressant withdrawal.

PITFALLS

Patients may experience withdrawal because an acute illness or complications of dependence have interrupted their usual drug intake. A careful examination for the precipitating event for abstinence may detect an underlying cause. Increased benzodiazepines doses and longer duration of sedation are needed for withdrawing alcoholics with additional illnesses (22).

Multiple drug dependencies easily occur among this population. In addition, benzodiazepines are also used as adjuncts to heroin, either enhancing the euphoria or managing the withdrawal (109). Patients self-treating GHB withdrawal have taken advantage of readily available depressants such as ethanol or opiates (hydrocodone/acetaminophen) when attempting to manage withdrawal symptoms. Combined dependence on CNS depressants and opioids can be managed with methadone maintenance while the patient is stabilized on diazepam or phenobarbital and gradually withdrawn from the CNS depressant. After completion of depressant withdrawal, the methadone can be tapered after 3 to 5 days (78).

Dependence syndromes are chronic medical problems requiring rehabilitation care after detoxification.

REFERENCES

1. Hobbs WRR, Verdoorn TW. Hypnotics and sedatives: ethanol. In: Hardman JG, Limbird LE, eds. *Goodman and Gilman's the pharmacological basis of therapeutics*, 9th ed. New York: MacMillan, 1996:361.
2. Kalant H, LeBlanc AE, Gibbins RJ. Tolerance to, and dependence on, some non-opiate psychotropic drugs. *Pharmacol Rev* 1971;23(3):135–191.
3. American Psychiatric Association. *Diagnostic and statistical manual of mental disorders*, 4th ed. Washington: American Psychiatric Association, 1994.
4. Smith DE, Wesson DR. Benzodiazepine dependency syndromes. *J Psychoactive Drugs* 1983;15(1–2):85–95.
5. Power KG, Jerrom DW, Simpson RJ, et al. Controlled study of withdrawal symptoms and rebound anxiety after six week course of diazepam for generalised anxiety. *BMJ (Clin Res Ed)* 1985;290(6477):1246–1248.
6. Busto U, Sellers EM. Pharmacokinetic determinants of drug abuse and dependence. A conceptual perspective. *Clin Pharmacokinet* 1986;11(2):144–153.
7. Murphy SM, Owen R, Tyrer P. Comparative assessment of efficacy and withdrawal symptoms after 6 and 12 weeks' treatment with diazepam or buspirone. *Br J Psychiatry* 1989;154:529–534.
8. Tyrer P. Dependence as a limiting factor in the clinical use of minor tranquilizers. *Pharmacol Ther* 1988;36(2–3):173–188.
9. Lader M. History of benzodiazepine dependence. *J Subst Abuse Treat* 1991;8(1–2):53–59.
10. Thompson WL. Management of alcohol withdrawal syndromes. *Arch Intern Med* 1978;138(2):278–283.
11. Isbell HA, Kornetsky S, Eisenman CH, et al. Chronic barbiturate intoxication: an experimental study. *Arch Neurol Psychiatry* 1950;64:1–28.
12. Hollister LEM, Motzenbecker FP, Degan RO. Withdrawal reactions from chlordiazepoxide ("librium"). *Psychopharmacologia* 1961;2:63–68.
13. Dyer JE, Roth B, Hyma BA. Gamma-hydroxybutyrate withdrawal syndrome. *Ann Emerg Med* 2001;37(2):147–153.
14. Harwood HJ, Fountain D, Fountain G. Economic cost of alcohol and drug abuse in the United States, 1992. Bethesda, MD: National Institute on Drug Abuse, 1998; National Institutes on Health publication number 98-4327.
15. Carai MAMC, Brunetti G, Melis G, et al. Role of GABA-B receptors in the sedative/hypnotic effect of gamma-hydroxybutyric acid. *Eur J Pharmacology* 2001;428:315–321.
16. Messing RO. Molecular targets of abused drugs. Chapter 386: Biology of addiction. In: Isselbacher KJW, Wilson JD, Martin JB, eds. *Harrison's online*, 15th ed. McGraw-Hill, 2001–2002.
17. Victor M, Adams R. The effects of alcohol on the nervous system. *Res Publ Assoc Res Nerv Ment Dis* 1953;32:526–573.
18. Brown ME, Anton RF, Malcolm R, et al. Alcohol detoxification and withdrawal seizures: clinical support for a kindling hypothesis. *Biol Psychiatry* 1988;23(5):507–514.
19. Rickels K, Schweizer E, Case WG, et al. Long-term therapeutic use of benzodiazepines. I. Effects of abrupt discontinuation. *Arch Gen Psychiatry* 1990;47(10):899–907.
20. Schweizer E, Rickels K, Case WG, et al. Long-term therapeutic use of benzodiazepines. II. Effects of gradual taper. *Arch Gen Psychiatry* 1990;47(10):908–915.
21. Malcolm R, Roberts JS, Wang W, et al. Multiple previous detoxifications are associated with less responsive treatment and heavier drinking during an index outpatient detoxification. *Alcohol* 2000;22(3):159–164.
22. Thompson WL, Johnson AD, Maddrey WL. Diazepam and paraldehyde for treatment of severe delirium tremens. A controlled trial. *Ann Intern Med* 1975;82(2):175–180.
23. Nolop KB, Natow A. Unprecedented sedative requirements during delirium tremens. *Crit Care Med* 1985;13(4):246–247.
24. Busto U, Sellers EM, Naranjo CA, et al. Withdrawal reaction after long-term therapeutic use of benzodiazepines. *N Engl J Med* 1986;315(14):854–859.
25. Fraser H, Isbell H, Eisenmann A, et al. Chronic barbiturate intoxication: further studies. *Arch Intern Med* 1954;94:34–41.
26. Fraser H, Wikler A, Essig C, et al. Degree of dependence induced by secobarbital or pentobarbital. *J Am Med Assoc* 1958;166:126–129.
27. Wikler A. Diagnosis and treatment of drug dependence of the barbiturate type. *Am J Psychiatry* 1968;125(6):758–765.
28. Isbell H, Fraser H, Wikler A, et al. An experimental study of the etiology of "rum fits" and delirium tremens. *Q J Stud Alcohol* 1955;16:1–33.
29. Victor M, Brausch C. The role of abstinence in the genesis of alcoholic epilepsy. *Epilepsia* 1967;8(1):1–20.
30. Petitjean S, Stohler R, Deglon JJ, et al. Double-blind randomized trial of buprenorphine and methadone in opiate dependence. *Drug Alcohol Depend* 2001;62(1):97–104.
31. Avants SK, Margolin A, McKee S. A path analysis of cognitive, affective, and behavioral predictors of treatment response in a methadone maintenance program. *J Subst Abuse* 2000;11(3):215–230.
32. Morse RM, Chua L. Carisoprodol dependence: a case report. *Am J Drug Alcohol Abuse* 1978;5(4):527–530.
33. Luehr JG, Meyerle KA, Larson EW. Mail-order (veterinary) drug dependence. *JAMA* 1990;263(5):657.
34. Sikdar S, Basu D, Malhotra AK, et al. Carisoprodol abuse: a report from India. *Acta Psychiatr Scand* 1993;88(4):302–303.
35. Hazlip TME, Ewing JA. Meprobamate habituation—a controlled clinical study. *N Engl J Med* 1958;258(24):1181–1186.
36. Barkin RL, Stein ZL. Withdrawal symptoms in a postoperative patient. *Hosp Pract (Off Ed)* 1992;27(2):106,108.
37. McDaniel CH, Miotto KA. Gamma hydroxybutyrate (GHB) and gamma

butyrolactone (GBL) withdrawal: five case studies. *J Psychoactive Drugs* 2001;33(2):143–149.
38. Sivilotti ML, Burns MJ, Aaron CK, et al. Pentobarbital for severe gamma-butyrolactone withdrawal. *Ann Emerg Med* 2001;38(6):660–665.
39. Schneir AB, Ly BT, Clark RF. A case of withdrawal from the GHB precursors gamma-butyrolactone and 1,4-butanediol. *J Emerg Med* 2001;21(1):31–33.
40. Kofler M, Arturo Leis A. Prolonged seizure activity after baclofen withdrawal. *Neurology* 1992;42(3 Pt 1):697–698.
41. Reeves RK, Stolp-Smith KA, Christopherson MW. Hyperthermia, rhabdomyolysis, and disseminated intravascular coagulation associated with baclofen pump catheter failure. *Arch Phys Med Rehabil* 1998;79(3):353–356.
42. Kirubakaran V, Mayfield D, Rengachary S. Dyskinesia and psychosis in a patient following baclofen withdrawal. *Am J Psychiatry* 1984;141(5):692–693.
43. Garabedian-Ruffalo SM, Ruffalo RL. Adverse effects secondary to baclofen withdrawal. *Drug Intell Clin Pharm* 1985;19(4):304–306.
44. Stien R. Hallucinations after sudden withdrawal of baclofen. *Lancet* 1977;2(8027):44–45.
45. Terrence CF, Fromm GH. Complications of baclofen withdrawal. *Arch Neurol* 1981;38(9):588–589.
46. Rivas DA, Chancellor MB, Hill K, et al. Neurological manifestations of baclofen withdrawal. *J Urol* 1993;150(6):1903–1905.
47. Freye E, Levy J. Acute abstinence syndrome following abrupt cessation of long-term use of tramadol (Ultram): a case study. *Eur J Pain* 2000;4(3):307–311.
48. Stone CB, Okun R. Chloral hydrate dependence: report of a case. *Clin Toxicol* 1978;12(3):377–380.
49. Aragona M. Abuse, dependence, and epileptic seizures after zolpidem withdrawal: review and case report. *Clin Neuropharmacol* 2000;23(5):281–283.
50. Gericke CA, Ludolph AC. Chronic abuse of zolpidem. *JAMA* 1994;272(22):1721–1722.
51. Inaba DS, Ray GR, Newmeyer JA, et al. Methaqualone abuse. "Luding out." *JAMA* 1973;224(11):1505–1509.
52. Flemenbaum A, Gunby B. Ethchlorvynol (Placidyl) abuse and withdrawal (review of clinical picture and report of 2 cases). *Dis Nerv Syst* 1971;32(3):188–192.
53. Garetz FD. Ethchlorvynol (Placidyl). Addiction hazard. *Minn Med* 1969;52(7):1131–1133.
54. Abuzahra HT, Rossdale M. Ethchlorvynol withdrawal symptoms. *BMJ* 1968;2(602):433–434.
55. Garza-Perez J, Lal S, Lopez E. Addiction to ethchlorvynol. A report of two cases. *Med Serv J Can* 1967;23(5):775–778.
56. Heston LL, Hastings D. Psychosis with withdrawal from ethchlorvynol. *Am J Psychiatry* 1980;137(2):249–250.
57. Vestal RE, Rumack BH. Glutethimide dependence: phenobarbital treatment [Letter]. *Ann Intern Med* 1974;80(5):670.
58. Lucas RE, Montgomery WS. Glutethimide withdrawal syndrome—the ethics of supply and demand. *Aust N Z J Med* 1992;22(6):708.
59. Lingl FA. Irreversible effects of glutethimide addiction. *Am J Psychiatry* 1966;123(3):349–351.
60. Bauer MS, Fus AF, Hanich RF, et al. Glutethimide intoxication and withdrawal. *Am J Psychiatry* 1988;145(4):530–531.
61. Essig CF. Methyprylon. *JAMA* 1966;196:714.
62. Mandac BR, Hurvitz EA, Nelson VS. Hyperthermia associated with baclofen withdrawal and increased spasticity. *Arch Phys Med Rehabil* 1993;74(1):96–97.
63. Green LB, Nelson VS. Death after acute withdrawal of intrathecal baclofen: case report and literature review. *Arch Phys Med Rehabil* 1999;80(12):1600–1604.
64. Fraser H, Shaver M, Maxwell E, et al. Death due to withdrawal of barbiturates: report of a case. *Ann Intern Med* 1953;38:1319–1325.
65. Haque W, Watson DJ, Bryant SG. Death following suspected alprazolam withdrawal seizures: a case report. *Tex Med* 1990;86(1):44–47.
66. Hayner G, Galloway G, Wiehl WO. Haight Ashbury free clinics' drug detoxification protocols—Part 3: benzodiazepines and other sedative-hypnotics. *J Psychoactive Drugs* 1993;25(4):331–335.
67. Marks J. Techniques of benzodiazepine withdrawal in clinical practice. A consensus workshop report. *Med Toxicol Adverse Drug Exp* 1988;3(4):324–333.
68. Hayashida M, Alterman AI, McLellan AT, et al. Comparative effectiveness and costs of inpatient and outpatient detoxification of patients with mild-to-moderate alcohol withdrawal syndrome. *N Engl J Med* 1989;320(6):358–365.
69. Saitz R, O'Malley SS. Pharmacotherapies for alcohol abuse. Withdrawal and treatment. *Med Clin North Am* 1997;81(4):881–907.
70. Saitz R, Mayo-Smith MF, Roberts MS, et al. Individualized treatment for alcohol withdrawal. A randomized double-blind controlled trial. *JAMA* 1994;272(7):519–523.
71. Daeppen JB, Gache P, Landry U, et al. Symptom-triggered vs fixed-schedule doses of benzodiazepine for alcohol withdrawal: a randomized treatment trial. *Arch Intern Med* 2002;162(10):1117–1121.
72. Manikant S, Tripathi BM, Chavan BS. Loading dose diazepam therapy for alcohol withdrawal state. *Indian J Med Res* 1993;98:170–173.
73. Busto UE, Sykora K, Sellers EM. A clinical scale to assess benzodiazepine withdrawal. *J Clin Psychopharmacol* 1989;9(6):412–416.
74. Sullivan JT, Sykora K, Schneiderman J, et al. Assessment of alcohol withdrawal: the revised clinical institute withdrawal assessment for alcohol scale (CIWA-Ar). *Br J Addict* 1989;84(11):1353–1357.
75. Woo E, Greenblatt DJ. Massive benzodiazepine requirements during acute alcohol withdrawal. *Am J Psychiatry* 1979;136(6):821–823.
76. Harrison M, Busto U, Naranjo CA, et al. Diazepam tapering in detoxification for high-dose benzodiazepine abuse. *Clin Pharmacol Ther* 1984;36(4):527–533.
77. Smith DE, Wesson DR. Phenobarbital technique for treatment of barbiturate dependence. *Arch Gen Psychiatry* 1971;24(1):56–60.
78. Smith DE, Wesson DR. A new method for treatment of barbiturate dependence. *JAMA* 1970;213(2):294–295.
79. Khantzian EJ, McKenna GJ. Acute toxic and withdrawal reactions associated with drug use and abuse. *Ann Intern Med* 1979;90(3):361–372.
80. Practice guideline for the treatment of patients with substance use disorders: alcohol, cocaine, opioids. American Psychiatric Association. *Am J Psychiatry* 1995;152[Suppl 11]:1–59.
81. Peng CT, Ger J, Yang CC, et al. Prolonged severe withdrawal symptoms after acute-on-chronic baclofen overdose. *J Toxicol Clin Toxicol* 1998;36(4):359–363.
82. Samson-Fang L, Gooch J, Norlin C. Intrathecal baclofen withdrawal simulating neuroepileptic malignant syndrome in a child with cerebral palsy. *Dev Med Child Neurol* 2000;42(8):561–565.
83. Khorasani A, Peruzzi WT. Dantrolene treatment for abrupt intrathecal baclofen withdrawal. *Anesth Analg* 1995;80(5):1054–1056.
84. Perry PJ, Stambaugh RL, Tsuang MT, et al. Sedative-hypnotic tolerance testing and withdrawal comparing diazepam to barbiturates. *J Clin Psychopharmacol* 1981;1(5):289–296.
85. Sellers EM, Naranjo CA, Harrison M, et al. Diazepam loading: simplified treatment of alcohol withdrawal. *Clin Pharmacol Ther* 1983;34(6):822–826.
86. Koch-Weser J, Sellers EM, Kalant H. Alcohol intoxication and withdrawal. *N Engl J Med* 1976;294(14):757–762.
87. Votolato NA, Batcha KJ, Olson SC. Alprazolam withdrawal. *Drug Intell Clin Pharm* 1987;21(9):754–755.
88. Robinson GM, Sellers EM, Janecek E. Barbiturate and hypnosedative withdrawal by a multiple oral phenobarbital loading dose technique. *Clin Pharmacol Ther* 1981;30(1):71–76.
89. Chin RL. A case of severe withdrawal from gamma-hydroxybutyrate. *Ann Emerg Med* 2001;37(5):551–552.
90. Dill C, Shin S. High-dose intravenous benzodiazepine. *Acad Emerg Med* 2000;7(3):308–310.
91. Young GP, Rores C, Murphy C, et al. Intravenous phenobarbital for alcohol withdrawal and convulsions. *Ann Emerg Med* 1987;16(8):847–850.
92. Coomes TR, Smith SW. Successful use of propofol in refractory delirium tremens. *Ann Emerg Med* 1997;30(6):825–828.
93. Sharma AN, Nelson L, Hoffman RS. Refractory sedative-hypnotic withdrawal treated with propofol. *J Toxicol Clin Toxicol* 2000;38(5):537.
94. Zvosec DL, Smith SW, McCutcheon JR, et al. Adverse events, including death, associated with the use of 1,4-butanediol. *N Engl J Med* 2001;344(2):87–94.
95. McCowan C, Marik P. Refractory delirium tremens treated with propofol: a case series. *Crit Care Med* 2000;28(6):1781–1784.
96. General anesthetics: propofol. In: Wickersham RMN, Burnham TH, Novak KK, et al., eds. *Drug facts and comparisons*. Saint Louis: Wolterskluwer Company, 2001;992.
97. Olson KR. Emergency evaluation and treatment. In: Olson KR, ed. *Poisoning and drug overdose*, 3rd ed. East Norwalk: Appleton & Lang, 1998.
98. Friedman J, Westlake R, Furman M. "Grievous bodily harm": gamma hydroxybutyrate abuse leading to a Wernicke-Korsakoff syndrome. *Neurology* 1996;46(2):469–471.
99. Goodman WK, Charney DS, Price LH, et al. Ineffectiveness of clonidine in the treatment of the benzodiazepine withdrawal syndrome: report of three cases. *Am J Psychiatry* 1986;143(7):900–903.
100. Vinogradov S, Reiss AL, Csernansky JG. Clonidine therapy in withdrawal from high-dose alprazolam treatment. *Am J Psychiatry* 1986;143(9):1188.
101. Tyrer P, Rutherford D, Huggett T. Benzodiazepine withdrawal symptoms and propranolol. *Lancet* 1981;1(8219):520–522.
102. Zilm DH, Jacob MS, MacLeod SM, et al. Propranolol and chlordiazepoxide effects on cardiac arrhythmias during alcohol withdrawal. *Alcohol Clin Exp Res* 1980;4(4):400–405.
103. Klein E, Uhde TW, Post RM. Preliminary evidence for the utility of carbamazepine in alprazolam withdrawal. *Am J Psychiatry* 1986;143(2):235–236.
104. Ries RK, Roy-Byrne PP, Ward NG, et al. Carbamazepine treatment for benzodiazepine withdrawal. *Am J Psychiatry* 1989;146(4):536–537.
105. Malcolm R, Myrick H, Roberts J, et al. The effects of carbamazepine and lorazepam on single versus multiple previous alcohol withdrawals in an outpatient randomized trial. *J Gen Intern Med* 2002;17(5):349–355.
106. Schweizer E, Rickels K, Case WG, et al. Carbamazepine treatment in patients discontinuing long-term benzodiazepine therapy. Effects on withdrawal severity and outcome. *Arch Gen Psychiatry* 1991;48(5):448–452.
107. Hillbom M, Tokola R, Kuusela V, et al. Prevention of alcohol withdrawal seizures with carbamazepine and valproic acid. *Alcohol* 1989;6(3):223–226.
108. Palestine ML, Alatorre E. Control of acute alcoholic withdrawal symptoms: a comparative study of haloperidol and chlordiazepoxide. *Curr Ther Res Clin Exp* 1976;20(3):289–299.
109. Ross J, Darke S. The nature of benzodiazepine dependence among heroin users in Sydney, Australia. *Addiction* 2000;95(12):1785–1793.
110. Lenz T, Gossmann J, Schulte KL, et al. Diagnosis of pheochromocytoma. *Clin Lab* 2002;48(1–2):5–18.
111. Lees AJ, Clarke CR, Harrison MJ. Hallucinations after withdrawal of baclofen. *Lancet* 1977;1(8016):858.
112. O'Rourke F, Steinberg R, Ghosh P, et al. Withdrawal of baclofen may cause acute confusion in elderly patients. *BMJ* 2001;323(7317):870.
113. Owen RT, Tyrer P. Benzodiazepine dependence. A review of the evidence. *Drugs* 1983;25(4):385–398.
114. Greaves DCW, West LJ. Convulsions following withdrawal from meprobamate: report of two cases. *South Med J* 1957;50:1534–1536.
115. Wesson DR, Smith DE, Ling W, et al. Sedative-hypnotics and tricyclics. In: Lowinson JH, Ruiz P, Millman RB, et al., eds. *Substance abuse: a comprehensive textbook*, 3rd ed. Baltimore: Williams & Wilkins, 1997.

SECTION

4

Supportive Care: General Principles

Richard C. Dart

Medical toxicology is an exciting and intellectually stimulating practice that includes both saving lives with timely administration of an antidote and preventing suffering by elucidating the cause of a patient's illness. Although it may appear mundane in some patients, supportive care can also be one of the most satisfying and useful aspects of toxicologic care. Many toxicologists have experienced the "pleasure" of managing a critically ill patient with supportive care only. These patients are alarming, require many more medical resources, and suffer a prolonged illness, but they usually survive. In the practice of toxicology, timely supportive care is more likely to save a life than an astute diagnosis or a dramatic antidote administration.

Supportive care consists of common emergency department and intensive unit care that supports the patient's vital signs and basic functions. The most common interventions are intravenous fluids, pulmonary interventions such as oxygen or endotracheal intubation, and blood pressure support with vasopressors.

As a result of the extraordinary interventions in supportive care, it is now extremely rare in medically developed countries for a poisoned patient to die. In contrast, in less-developed medical systems, 10% or 20% of poisoned patients may expire. Although specific medications such as antidotes undoubtedly account for the survival of many patients, it is likely that supportive care saves the most. For example, in the nineteenth century, the mortality after pit viper envenomation was in the range of 5% to 25% (1–3). By the 1960s, mortality had dropped to less than 1% (1,4). In the 1990s, there were approximately five deaths per year (5). Estimates of the total bites range from 2000 to 8000 annually; the current mortality rate is roughly 0.07% to 0.25%. These estimations are crude, but it appears that a remarkable decrease has occurred.

The question is, "What caused the decrease?" In truth, several developments have improved the prognosis for victims of pit viper poisoning. One was the development of rapid prehospital transport and the proliferation of emergency medical facilities. These services allowed most patients to reach health care facilities and receive immediate supportive care interventions within minutes to hours instead of hours to days. A second was the development of critical care medicine and the construction of intensive care units that provided the ability to support critically ill patients. Finally, the development of a specific antivenom provided an effective method to reduce the venom injury. Because the antivenom for snakebite was not introduced until 1954 and has never been well-stocked in hospital pharmacies, thousands of patients have been treated with supportive care alone over the years.

One secret for the management of crotaline snakebite is early and adequate intravascular volume resuscitation. In some cases, endotracheal intubation and vasopressors are important (6). The same is true of several other conditions. For example, the toxicity of cardiac medications is commonly treated with the nonspecific interventions of oxygen, isotonic fluid resuscitation, vasopressor administration, and hypertonic sodium bicarbonate administration. The lack of immediately available digoxin Fab has forced many patients with hyperkalemia after digoxin ingestion to be treated with sodium bicarbonate and insulin/glucose, but many of them survive.

The following section addresses common aspects of the management of poisoned patients that cross poison categories. The topics included are anaphylaxis, hyperkalemia, hypertension, hypotension, shock, hyperthermia and hypothermia, convulsions, and the psychiatric evaluation of the poisoned patient. These interventions are used for many conditions in addition to poisoning; however, there are specific toxicologic considerations for each.

REFERENCES

1. Russell FE. *Snake venom poisoning*. Great Neck, NY: Scholium International, 1983.
2. Willson P. Snake poisoning in the United States: a study based on analysis of 740 cases. *Arch Int Med* 1908;I:516–570.
3. Barringer PB. The venomous reptiles of the United States, with the treatment of wounds inflicted by them. *South Med Surg Gynec Assoc* 1892;4:283–300.
4. Parrish HM, Goldner JC, Silberg SL. Comparison between snakebites in children and adults. *Pediatrics* 1965;36:251–256.
5. Langley RL, Morrow WE. Deaths resulting from animal attacks in the United States. *Wild Environ Med* 1997;8:8–16.
6. Bush SP, Jansen PW. Severe rattlesnake envenomation with anaphylaxis and rhabdomyolysis. *Ann Emerg Med* 1995;25:845–848.

CHAPTER 33

Airway and Ventilatory Management

Christopher R. DeWitt and Richard C. Dart

OVERVIEW

Advanced airway management is the cornerstone of care for any critically ill patient. Endotracheal intubation allows for airway control, decreases aspiration risk, provides a means for ventilation and oxygenation, and allows for suctioning and drug administration. Because loss of the airway commonly contributes to the death of poisoned patients, effective airway management is crucial. Decontamination and antidote administration do not supersede airway control and maintenance of vital signs. Likewise, appropriate ventilatory management allows time for toxins to be cleared, manipulation of acid-base status, and protection from pulmonary barotrauma and can decrease intracranial hypertension.

GENERAL MANAGEMENT PRINCIPLES

Aside from the technical aspects of intubation, anticipating which patients require intubation is a key management point. Intubation should be considered for the following situations (1):

1. Failure to protect or maintain the airway. In poisoned patients, this occurs from altered mentation and loss of airway reflexes, or from airway obstruction. Airway obstruction arises from copious upper airway secretions; foreign bodies (including vomitus); vocal cord spasm (e.g., airway irritants); or swelling due to caustic injury, thermal insult, or anaphylaxis.
2. Respiratory failure, which is insufficient exchange of oxygen and carbon dioxide between the lungs and blood, or blood and tissues, leading to hypoxia, acidosis, and cell death. Toxicologic causes of respiratory failure are protean, including simple asphyxiants (e.g., methane), toxin-induced pulmonary injury (e.g., irritant gases), hypoventilation from altered mentation or respiratory muscle paralysis (e.g., opioids or botulism), cellular asphyxiants (e.g., cyanide and hydrogen sulfide), inadequate oxygen-carrying capacity or oxygen release to tissues (e.g., carbon monoxide or methemoglobinemia/sulfhemoglobinemia), poison-mediated shock (e.g., calcium-channel blockers or beta-blockers), and acid base disturbances (e.g., salicylates or toxic alcohols).
3. Administration of medicines such as sedatives, or anticipated changes in clinical course such as progressing airway edema from caustic injury, that leads to one of the previous scenarios. Therefore, knowledge of the natural course of a particular poisoning is an important component to airway management.

General management of the ventilated patient involves titration of inspired oxygen, minute ventilation (respiratory rate × tidal volume), and airway pressure to maintain sufficient oxygenation while avoiding hypercarbia, pulmonary injury, and impairment of cardiac output. Most poisoned patients need only basic ventilator settings for respiratory rate (10 to 12 breaths/minute for an adult and age-adjusted in children), tidal volume (10 to 15 ml/kg body weight), and inspired oxygen (initially 100% and weaned to 21% as tolerated).

SPECIFIC MANAGEMENT

Several poisonings require special airway management techniques. Opiate and benzodiazepine drugs have antidotes; however, airway opening maneuvers and assisted ventilation via bag-valve mask should be used while preparing for their use, if indicated. Also, tracheal intubation takes precedence over antidote administration in any unstable patient. Because flumazenil can potentially precipitate seizures and dysrhythmias, it should only be administered when the history of benzodiazepine overdose is supported by physical examination and there is no history of proconvulsant or prodysrhythmic ingestion or of benzodiazepine dependence (2).

Caustics and irritants can produce airway edema that progresses rapidly, altering airway anatomy and making intubation or bag-valve mask ventilation difficult. Thus, patients with airway edema, inability to handle secretions, stridor, or altered mentation require immediate airway management. Muscular tone of the airway may be the only force keeping the airway open; therefore, paralytics should be avoided if possible. Advanced airway techniques such as "awake" nasal intubation, fiberoptic assisted intubation, and surgical cricothyroidotomy may be required. A nonsurgical airway is preferred, if possible, because it may interfere with the surgical esophageal repair (3).

The choice of paralytic used for endotracheal intubation is also important. Nondepolarizing paralytics, rather than succinylcholine, should be used in patients with serotonin syndrome, neuroleptic malignant syndrome, strychnine poisoning, a history of malignant hyperthermia, hyperkalemia, neuropathy or myopathy, and upper motor neuron injury, as well as bradycardia from parasympathetic stimulation (carbamates, organophosphates, and digoxin), who require rapid sequence intubation.

Several poisonings can benefit from specific ventilatory management techniques. Many patients with metabolic acidosis should be hyperventilated. For example, in the setting of salicylate toxicity, hyperventilation produces a respiratory alkalosis that buffers the associated metabolic acidosis. Salicylate poisoned patients who are intubated and are placed on "standard" ventilator settings rapidly become acidemic (Chapter 127). Acidemia allows more salicylate to enter the central nervous system, increasing cerebral edema and elevating intracranial pressure. Therefore, it is imperative that minute ventilation be increased above normal parameters to allow continued ventilatory compensation for the acidosis (4).

Intracranial hemorrhage from sympathomimetic or anticoagulant poisoning can also elevate intracranial pressure. In patients with signs of elevated intracranial pressure (e.g., unilateral mydriasis, posturing), hyperventilation to an arterial car-

TABLE 1. Tests for evaluation of respiratory function

Test	Usefulness
Fiberoptic laryngoscopy/ bronchoscopy	Aid in intubation of the difficult airway, confirmation of endotracheal tube placement, evaluation of airway injury and obstruction.
Pulmonary function testing	Comparison of measured peak expiratory flow rates to expected rates (based on sex, age, and height) can determine the presence of airway obstruction. It should be used to direct therapy and disposition and not the need for intubation. NIF and vital capacity can help guide the need for intubation in poisonings that affect respiratory muscles, such as botulism or organophosphates. A study of patients with respiratory muscle involvement from Guillain-Barré showed a vital capacity <20 ml/kg or NIF <30 cm H_2O is associated with progression to respiratory failure (10).
Peak and plateau airway pressures	To evaluate cause of acute respiratory deterioration in the ventilated patient. Decreased peak inspiratory pressures occur when there is an air leak or hyperventilation. When peak pressures are increased, the plateau pressure must be measured. Elevated plateau pressures occur when compliance is decreased from pulmonary edema, pneumothorax, atelectasis, etc. When the peak pressure increases but the plateau pressure is unchanged, airway or endotracheal tube obstruction is present (11).
Hematocrit	Significant anemia reduces oxygen-carrying capacity.
Serum electrolytes	Hypermagnesemia, hypokalemia, hyponatremia, and hypophosphatemia can cause respiratory muscle weakness.
Pulse oximetry	Evaluates hemoglobin oxygen saturation but is unreliable when dyshemoglobinemias are present (carboxyhemoglobin, methemoglobin, and so forth) (12). Cellular asphyxiants such as cyanide do not change hemoglobin saturation until respiratory failure is present.
Arterial blood gas	Measures oxygenation and ventilation, acid-base status, ventilation-perfusion mismatch, shunting, and detection of impending respiratory failure. Differences between hemoglobin saturation measured by pulse-oximetry and that calculated on the arterial blood gas may provide clues to the presence of dyshemoglobinemia (13). Small differences between arterial and venous oxygen content may indicate presence of a cellular asphyxiant. The presence of a respiratory alkalosis and metabolic acidosis suggest salicylate poisoning.
Co-oximetry	Detection of abnormal hemoglobin (carboxyhemoglobin, methemoglobin; some newer devices can also detect sulfhemoglobin) that interferes with oxygen uptake and delivery.
Chest radiography	Detection of pneumothorax, infiltrates, pulmonary edema, foreign bodies, and endotracheal tube depth. Pulmonary edema with a normal-sized heart, as opposed to cardiomegaly, may suggest ALI/ARDS.
Central venous and Swan-Ganz catheters	Helpful in guiding treatment of patient with renal failure and congestive heart failure when knowledge of volume status and cardiac performance is important. May also be used to differentiate between cardiogenic edema and edema due to ALI/ARDS. Cardiogenic pulmonary edema has elevated central venous and pulmonary capillary wedge pressures with a decreased cardiac output. These parameters should be normal in ALI/ARDS.
Radionucleotide ventriculography and echocardiography	May be needed to differentiate between cardiogenic pulmonary edema and ALI/ARDS.

ALI/ARDS, acute lung injury/acute respiratory distress syndrome; NIF, negative inspiratory force.

bon dioxide partial pressure of 30 to 35 mm Hg can be used as a temporizing measure, until mannitol administration or decompression (5). Respiratory alkalosis via mechanical hyperventilation has also been used to treat cardiotoxicity from tricyclic antidepressant overdose (6). This technique may be used when there is a delay in sodium bicarbonate administration.

Acute lung injury and acute respiratory distress syndrome represent a spectrum of pulmonary injury from various causes that results in increased intraalveolar fluid with a normal cardiac output (7). Opioids, salicylates, irritant gases, hydrocarbons, smoke inhalation, and other toxins are associated with acute lung injury and acute respiratory distress syndrome. Regardless of the cause, treatment is supportive with the use of low tidal volume ventilation (6 to 8 ml/kg) (8). The goal is to allow the lung to heal by avoiding high airway pressures and large pressure fluctuations while maintaining oxygenation. Ideally, a minimal arterial partial oxygen pressure of 55 mm Hg, or oxygen saturation of 88%, is maintained via manipulation of inspired oxygen and positive end expiratory pressure (should be kept under 15 to 20 cm H_2O) (8). This generally allows for acceptable oxygenation while reducing oxygen-mediated lung injury.

USE OF ANCILLARY INFORMATION

Because ventilation and oxygenation are complex processes, multiple ancillary tests may be needed for accurate diagnosis and treatment (Table 1).

PITFALLS

Failure to obtain or recognize the need for intubation commonly leads to the demise of the poisoned patient. Patients with caustic or irritant upper airway injuries require immediate airway attention. Also, succinylcholine should be avoided in patients with hyperkalemia or illness that may potentiate the risk of hyperkalemia, and in patients with increased muscular activity such as neuroleptic malignant syndrome and serotonin syndrome. Finally, inadequate ventilator management can also be a source of morbidity and mortality. Patients with acute lung injury and acute respiratory distress syndrome are at risk for pulmonary barotrauma and require specialized ventilator settings (9). Also, failure to maintain hyperventilation in a patient with an ongoing metabolic acidosis, such as salicylate poisoning, can lead to rapid deterioration.

REFERENCES

1. Walls RM. The decision to intubate. In: Walls RL, Luten RC, Murphy MF, et al., eds. *Manual of emergency airway management*. Philadelphia: Lippincott Williams & Wilkins, 2000:3–7.
2. Hoffman RS, Goldfrank LR. The poisoned patient with altered consciousness. Controversies in the use of the "coma cocktail." *JAMA* 1995;274:562–569.
3. Wu MH, Lai WW. Surgical management of extensive corrosive injuries of the alimentary tract. *Surg Gynecol Obstet* 1993;177:12–16.
4. Yip L, Dart RC, Gabow PA. Concepts and controversies in salicylate toxicity. *Emerg Med Clin North Am* 1994;12:351–363.
5. Chestnut RM. Guidelines for the management of severe head injury: what we know and what we think we know. *J Trauma* 1997;42:S19.

6. Bessen HA, Niemann JT. Improvement of cardiac conduction after hyperventilation in tricyclic antidepressant overdose. *J Toxicol Clin Toxicol* 1986;23:537–546.
7. Bernard GB, Artigas A, Bringham KL. Report of the American-European Consensus conference on acute respiratory distress syndrome: definitions, mechanics, relevant outcomes, and clinical trial coordination. *J Crit Care* 1994;9:72–81.
8. The Acute Respiratory Distress Syndrome Network. Ventilation with lower tidal volumes for acute lung injury and the acute respiratory distress syndrome. *N Engl J Med* 2000;342:1301–1308.
9. Brower RG, Fessler HE. Mechanical ventilation in acute lung injury and acute respiratory distress syndrome. *Clin Chest Med* 2000;21:491–510.
10. Lawn ND, Fletcher DD, Henderson RD, et al. Anticipating mechanical ventilation in Guillain-Barré syndrome. *Arch Neurol* 2001;58:893–898.
11. Marino P. Principles of mechanical ventilation. In: *The ICU book*, 2nd ed. Baltimore: Williams & Wilkins, 1998.
12. Tremper KK, Barker SJ. Using pulse oximetry when dyshemoglobin levels are high. *J Crit Illness* 1988;3:103–107.
13. Hoffman RS. Respiratory principles. In: Goldfrank LR, Flomenbaum NE, Lewin NA, et al., eds. *Goldfrank's toxicologic emergencies*, 7th ed. New York: McGraw-Hill, 2002:303–314.

CHAPTER 34

Anaphylaxis

Richard C. Dart

OVERVIEW

Anaphylaxis is an immediate systemic reaction caused by rapid, immunoglobulin E (IgE)–mediated release of immunohumoral mediators from tissue mast cells and basophils. In toxicology, the common causes include bites and stings as well as the administration of antivenoms. The diagnosis is clinical, based on the temporal relationship to exposure and manifestations of IgE-mediated signs. Most cases involve immediate development of urticaria, tachycardia, hypotension, and wheezing and may result in profound shock and respiratory arrest. Many individual variations of the basic syndrome may occur.

Anaphylactoid reactions are immediate systemic reactions that appear similar to anaphylaxis clinically but are not mediated by IgE. The temporal occurrence of anaphylactic or anaphylactoid reactions is usually immediate but may be delayed depending on the route of exposure.

GENERAL MANAGEMENT PRINCIPLES

The immediate care of anaphylaxis in the prehospital or hospital care is administration of high flow oxygen, establishing large catheter intravenous (IV) access, and providing cardiac monitoring. If exposure to the inciting agent continues, it must be removed (e.g., terminate infusion of antivenom). Airway management may be difficult due to airway edema. In difficult cases, cricothyrotomy or other measures may be necessary to establish an airway. Inhaled beta-agonists should also be administered to patients with wheezing. Initial treatment of hypotension is with aggressive isotonic crystalloid. Infusion of large volumes may be needed in patients refractory to resuscitation.

Treatment is guided by the severity of reaction. Mild reactions with only cutaneous manifestations are treated with a histamine 1 (H_1)–blocker (e.g., diphenhydramine) alone, whereas systemic reactions may require administration of epinephrine, H_1- and histamine 2 (H_2)–blockers, maximum supportive care measures, and corticosteroids. Hypotension is treated initially with prompt infusion of isotonic crystalloid (1 to 2 L in adults or 20 to 30 ml/kg in children initially) and epinephrine, as well as H_1- and H_2-blocking agents. Large volumes of crystalloid may be needed.

Epinephrine

Epinephrine is used parenterally for treatment of angioedema, bronchospasm, or shock as well as subcutaneously (SQ) for isolated urticaria. It is administered SQ, intramuscularly (IM), or IV (or endotracheal tube), depending on the severity of the reaction. The *adult dose* for urticaria or other mild systemic reactions is 0.3 to 0.5 ml of a 1:1000 solution SQ, which may be repeated if needed. If the IM route is used, the thigh is the preferred site of injection (1).

For severe or life-threatening reactions, a solution [1 ml of 1:10,000 concentration is diluted in 10 ml normal saline (NS)] can be administered by slow IV push, repeated as needed. The endotracheal dose is 1.0 ml 1:1000 solution in 10 ml NS. For continuous IV infusion, the dose is 0.1 to 1.0 µg/kg/minute.

Pediatric doses are 0.01 ml/kg SQ or IM of the 1:1000 concentration. The IV dose is 0.01 ml/kg of 1:10,000. The endotracheal dose is 0.01 ml/kg of 1:1000 solution in 1 to 3 ml NS. The IV infusion rate is 0.05 to 1.0 µg/kg/minute (2).

Beta-blockers may cause resistance to epinephrine, and larger than usual doses may be needed. Glucagon has been proposed for these patients. It increases intracellular cyclic adenosine monophosphate levels by a different receptor.

Inhaled Beta$_2$ Receptor Agonists

Beta-agonists are useful for cases of bronchospasm, especially if bronchospasm without serious system effects is present, but they do not replace epinephrine. Numerous inhaled beta-agonists are used for treatment of bronchospasm. Albuterol is a commonly used preparation. The *adult dose* is 0.5 ml of 0.5% solution in 2.5 ml NS nebulized every 15 minutes. However, much larger doses, 5 to 10 mg per dose, have been used with careful cardiovascular monitoring. If large doses are needed in the setting of an acute allergic reaction, it is likely that epinephrine should be administered instead. The *pediatric dose* is 0.03 to 0.05 ml/kg of 0.5% solution in 2.5 ml of saline by nebulizer every 15 minutes (3).

H_1 Receptor Blocking Agents

The *adult dose* of diphenhydramine is 25 to 50 mg IV or IM immediately and then every 4 to 6 hours. Treatment is usually continued orally (50 mg every 4 to 6 hours) for at least 2 days after the initial episode. The *pediatric doses* are 1 to 2 mg/kg IV or IM, or 2 mg/kg orally used in the same manner and intervals as adults (3).

H_2 Receptor Blocking Agents

The effect of H_2-blockers appears additive to H_1 blockade (4–6). Given the safety, ease of administration, and low cost, an H_2 receptor blocker should be administered in most cases of anaphylaxis or anaphylactoid reactions. The *adult dose* of cimetidine is 300 mg by oral, IV, or IM administration initially and then every 6 hours. The *pediatric dose* is 5 to 10 mg/kg by oral, IV, or IM administration.

Corticosteroids

Corticosteroids, like hydrocortisone, are often administered in anaphylaxis, although their effectiveness has not been proved. Typically, the initial doses are administered parenterally and subsequent doses orally. For example, the *adult dose* of methylprednisolone is 50 to 250 mg IV every 6 hours, followed by prednisone, 25 to 100 mg orally per day. The *pediatric dose* is 1 to 4 mg/kg IV every 6 hours, followed by 1 mg/kg orally per day (3).

Other Care

Most patients that experience anaphylaxis after an environmental exposure (i.e., bite or sting) should be prescribed an epinephrine autoinjector. Patients with a severe acute reaction should be referred for evaluation by an allergist to help ascertain the true cause as well as evaluate the potential usefulness of immunotherapy.

SPECIFIC MANAGEMENT

In general, the treatment of anaphylaxis is the same regardless of cause; however, some causes have special considerations.

Insect Bites and Stings

Anaphylaxis after an insect bite or sting is managed as other causes of anaphylaxis. A *large local reaction* is sometimes misdiagnosed as anaphylaxis. A large local reaction involves erythema and swelling that develop over hours. The extent may be large (i.e., an entire limb), but it is not dangerous and resolves with time. Many practitioners prescribe antihistamines only. Epinephrine does not change the course.

Fire ants are a common cause of serious allergic reactions in endemic areas. Documentation of specific IgE sensitivity to imported fire ant is usually performed by skin testing with imported fire ant whole body extract.

Venom immunotherapy is useful in preventing recurrent anaphylaxis and improving quality of life (7).

RADIOGRAPHIC CONTRAST MATERIAL

Although they are not mediated by IgE, radiocontrast-induced anaphylactoid reactions are clinically indistinguishable from IgE-mediated immediate hypersensitivity anaphylactic reactions. Nevertheless, the treatment of anaphylactoid reactions to these agents is the same as other causes. The occurrence of one anaphylactic episode puts the patient at a substantially higher risk of subsequent reactions. Pretreatment regimens for prevention of repeat anaphylactoid reactions include oral glucocorticosteroids, H_1 and H_2 antihistamines, and other medications such as ephedrine.

USE OF ANCILLARY INFORMATION

There are few tests useful during the acute episode. Hypoxia may develop, and pulse oximetry, augmented by arterial blood gases as appropriate, is needed to monitor the patient. An electrocardiogram and cardiac monitoring are needed during the episode because both the process of anaphylaxis and its treatment can produce myocardial ischemia and cardiac dysrhythmias. Radiography is not usually needed, except to assess placement of endotracheal tube after intubation.

It is difficult to identify the cause of the reaction in some cases. Histamine and tryptase levels may be helpful to document the cause. In a randomized trial, histamine levels higher than 1 ng/ml were significantly associated with hypotension, moderate-to-severe rash, and stopped infusion (8). Tryptase is contained in mast cells and is usually increased after IgE-mediated anaphylaxis; however, it may not be elevated in all cases and is not elevated after anaphylactoid reactions (8,9).

PITFALLS

Patients on beta-blocker medications may need higher epinephrine doses or may not respond to epinephrine. In these cases, glucagon may be useful.

REFERENCES

1. Simons FE, Gu X, Simons KJ. Epinephrine absorption in adults: intramuscular versus subcutaneous injection. *J Allergy Clin Immunol* 2001;108:871–873.
2. Carpenter TC, Dobyns EL, Lane J, et al. Critical care. In: Hay WW, et al., eds. *Current pediatric diagnosis and treatment*, 16th ed. New York: Lange Medical Books, 2003:362–399.
3. Boguniewicz M, Leung DYM. Allergic disorders. In: Hay WW, et al., eds. *Current pediatric diagnosis and treatment*, 16th ed. New York: Lange Medical Books, 2003:1051–1098.
4. Lin RY, Curry A, Pesola GR, et al. Improved outcomes in patients with acute allergic syndromes who are treated with combined H_1 and H_2 antagonists. *Ann Emerg Med* 2000;36:462–468.
5. Runge JW, Martinez JC, Caravati EM, et al. Histamine antagonists in the treatment of acute allergic reactions. *Ann Emerg Med* 1992;21:237–242.
6. Schoning B, Lorenz W, Doenicke A. Prophylaxis of anaphylactoid reactions to a polypeptidal plasma substitute by H_1- plus H_2-receptor antagonists: synopsis of three randomized controlled trials. *Klinische Wochenschrift* 1982;60:1048–1055.
7. Oude Elberink JN, De Monchy JG, Van Der Heide S, et al. Venom immunotherapy improves health-related quality of life in patients allergic to yellow jacket venom. *J Allergy Clin Immunol* 2002;110:174–182.
8. Renz CL, Laroche D, Thurn JD, et al. Tryptase levels are not increased during vancomycin-induced anaphylactoid reactions. *Anesthesiology* 1998;89:620–625.
9. Riches KJ, Gillis D, James RA. An autopsy approach to bee sting-related deaths. *Pathology* 2002;34:257–262.

CHAPTER 35
Hyperkalemia

Mark A. Kostic and Richard C. Dart

OVERVIEW

The management of poisoned patients is frequently complicated by *hyperkalemia*, which is defined as a serum potassium (K^+) concentration greater than 5.5 mEq/L.

Potassium homeostasis is normally maintained in two ways. Normally, the kidneys reabsorb potassium efficiently after glomerular filtration. If presented with a potassium load, they are able to increase urinary elimination through decreased reabsorption as well as increased distal tubular secretion. In addition, potassium can also be shifted between intracellular and extracellular fluid compartments. Only 2% of total body potassium is held in the extracellular space. This equilibrium is maintained by several mechanisms, the most important of which is the sodium-potassium adenosine triphosphate–dependent pump [Na^+-K^+ adenosine triphosphatase (ATPase)] (1,2).

ETIOLOGY

Elevated serum potassium may result from increased delivery of potassium to the blood, such as in intravenous or oral overdose during potassium replenishment. It may be a consequence of decreased potassium elimination in acute renal failure or the use of potassium-sparing diuretics, such as spironolactone.

Hyperkalemia may also result from the movement of potassium between compartments. Any condition resulting in acidemia causes the extracellular concentration of potassium to rise. Hemolysis and rhabdomyolysis are examples of other medical conditions that frequently complicate poisonings and may result in hyperkalemia.

A classic example is acute digoxin overdose in which Na^+-K^+ ATPase is poisoned. Other pharmaceutical agents that may cause hyperkalemia include beta-adrenergic antagonists, angiotensin-converting enzyme inhibitors, angiotensin II antagonists, nonsteroidal antiinflammatory drugs, heparin, trimethoprim-sulfamethoxazole, pentamidine, and succinylcholine. Finally, additional causes of hyperkalemia such as aldosterone resistance, hypoaldosteronism, and Addison's disease should be considered. Factitious or pseudohyperkalemia may result from several factors. These include repeated fist clenching (with or without a tourniquet) causing potassium release from skeletal muscle, traumatic venipuncture causing hemolysis, and delayed processing of the blood sample. Other explanations include potassium release from white blood cells in patients with myeloproliferative disorders and from platelets in patients with thrombocytosis, hyperventilation, heparin-coated catheters, and the rare case of familial hyperkalemia (3).

GENERAL MANAGEMENT PRINCIPLES

A general treatment algorithm in the management of hyperkalemia is a useful tool because a specific etiology is often not clinically apparent early in the evaluation (Fig. 1). In a patient with *severe hyperkalemia*, defined as a serum potassium concentration above 7.5 mEq/L, treatment is aimed first at counteracting the effect of potassium on the myocardial cell by administering calcium chloride through a central venous line. If a central line is not available, calcium gluconate may be administered through a peripheral line. Onset of action is 1 to 3 minutes, with a 30- to 60-minute duration of action (4).

The next intervention is aimed at shifting potassium into cells from the extracellular compartment. Sodium bicarbonate is thought to shift potassium into cells due to an increase in serum pH. Onset of effect is 5 to 10 minutes, and the duration of effect is 1 to 2 hours (4). Recently, however, the efficacy of this therapy in patients without acidosis has been questioned (1). Calcium and sodium bicarbonate solutions are incompatible in the same intravenous line.

In severe cases, multiple modalities are usually used simultaneously. Other therapies include insulin and glucose, which is another effective method of shifting potassium into cells. This seems to occur primarily through enhanced activity of Na^+-K^+ ATPase (1). The onset of effect is expected within 30 minutes, lasting approximately 4 to 6 hours (4). Nebulized albuterol is also effective, with an onset of action within 15 minutes and a duration of effect of up to 90 minutes (4). *In vitro* studies have also suggested that epinephrine drives potassium into the cells, although this has yet to be implemented in clinical practice (1).

In some patients, a net loss of potassium from the body is needed. In stable patients with mild to moderate potassium elevation (less than 7.5 mEq/L) and without significant electrocardiographic (ECG) changes (i.e., normal intervals), this may constitute the only necessary treatment. Cation exchange resins, such as sodium polystyrene sulfonate (Kayexalate), slowly lower the potassium concentration over 2 to 6 hours. Diuresis with furosemide increases the urinary excretion of potassium but is limited by the patient's volume and overall clinical status (4).

Hemodialysis efficiently removes potassium from the serum, with or without renal failure. This is often indicated with renal failure as the origin of hyperkalemia. However, this is impractical for emergent treatment of life-threatening hyperkalemia.

SPECIFIC MANAGEMENT PRINCIPLES

Cardiac Glycoside Poisoning

The administration of digoxin Fab is generally indicated in patients acutely poisoned with cardiac glycosides if the potassium concentration exceeds 5.5 mEq/L (Chapter 49). This recommendation does not apply in the case of chronic digoxin poisoning, in which a mildly elevated potassium may be somewhat protective (Chapter 120). Because insulin primarily shifts potassium intracellularly through enhanced activity of Na^+-K^+ ATPase, this modality may theoretically be limited in acute digoxin overdose in which the pump is poisoned. Caution is also warranted with the administration of calcium salts in hyperkalemic patients acutely poisoned with cardiac glycosides. Animal and *in vitro* studies indicate a theoretic concern for cardiac arrest

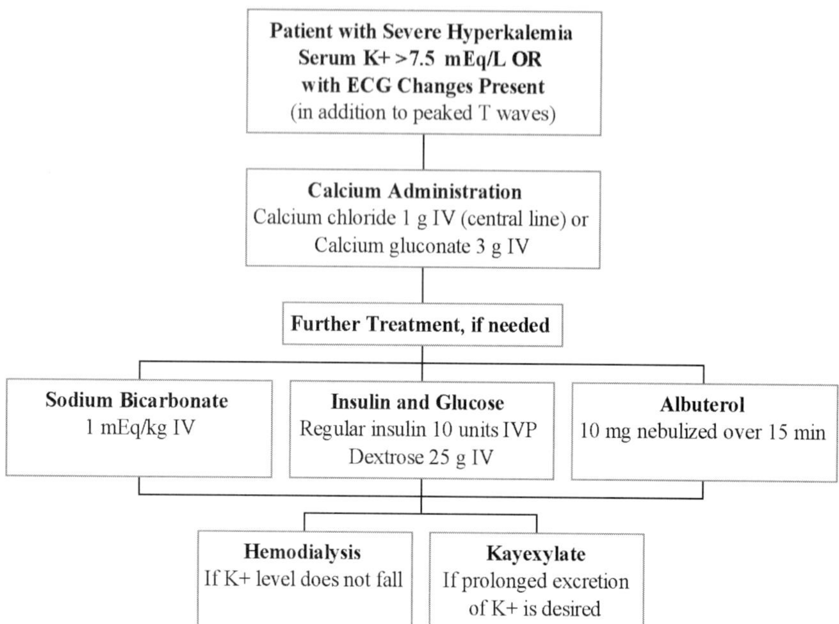

Figure 1. Management of hyperkalemia. Cardiac glycosides are relative contraindication (see text). ECG, electrocardiogram; IVP, intravenous push; K+, serum potassium concentration.

due to exacerbation of the already elevated intracellular levels of calcium in the cardiac myocyte (5–9). In 1936, two case reports suggested a temporal relationship between the administration of calcium salts in digoxin-poisoned patients and cardiac arrest (10). Only one subsequent case was found in the literature (11).

Potassium Overdose

An overdose with potassium can be either parenteral or oral. Acute intravenous overdose is usually iatrogenic, and death, if it occurs, is precipitous. Serious acute oral overdose with potassium is rare. Death was reported in a 26-year-old man who ingested approximately 4 mEq/kg (12) and in a 46-year-old woman who was estimated to have ingested 16 mEq/kg (13). It has been suggested that in a patient with normal renal function, the ability to adequately process an acute overdose of potassium can be overwhelmed with the ingestion of 2.0 to 2.5 mEq/kg (14). If there are no coingestants, oral decontamination with sodium polystyrene sulfonate may be superior to activated charcoal. If pills are visualized, orogastric lavage may remove a large amount. Management of hyperkalemia should proceed as with other causes (Fig. 1). The resulting hyperkalemia may be progressive, however, and preparations for immediate hemodialysis should be made.

Other Medical Conditions

In acute renal failure, serum potassium levels rise due to decreased renal excretion. With acidemia, potassium is excreted from the cell in exchange for hydrogen in an attempt to normalize serum pH. Hemolysis and rhabdomyolysis release excess potassium into the serum through the lysis of red blood cells and muscle cells, respectively. In these situations, the general algorithm (Fig. 1), with special attention to volume status and urine output, is an effective approach to treating the associated hyperkalemia.

USE OF ANCILLARY INFORMATION

The ECG is an important tool because it can guide treatment of hyperkalemia before serum potassium levels are available. "Peaked" T waves, which are tall, tent-shaped T waves with a narrow base, are usually seen best in the precordial leads and appear as the concentration exceeds 5.5 mEq/L. With continued rise, the PR interval prolongs, P-wave amplitude decreases, and the QRS complex widens. As the potassium concentration surpasses 8.0 mEq/L, P waves disappear, intraventricular, fascicular, and bundle branch blocks may arise, and the QRS morphology changes and widens as the axis shifts. Eventually, a "sine-wave" pattern emerges, soon followed by ventricular fibrillation and asystole (15). Repeating the ECG frequently during treatment is crucial because the effect of potassium on cardiac conduction changes rapidly.

The laboratory is useful in the assessment of the etiology of hyperkalemia. The serum potassium concentration may be rapidly acquired through an arterial blood gas. This also provides important information regarding the patient's acid-base status and the ionized calcium level. The latter is helpful in monitoring therapy after calcium has been provided. Serum electrolytes yield information regarding the presence of an acidosis, an anion gap, or hyponatremia (as may occur in adrenal cortical insufficiency). The serum magnesium concentration is important in evaluating patients in renal failure or with an abnormal ECG. Renal function is assessed with blood urea nitrogen and creatinine assays of serum. Urine samples are analyzed for signs of hemolysis and for urine electrolytes. The latter provide information as to the cause of renal failure, if present. The serum potassium concentration should also be repeated frequently to assess the impact of therapy.

Radiographic studies may be useful in the case of an acute overdose of potassium supplements. Visualization of radio-opaque potassium on an abdominal plain film is a clue that the serum levels are likely to rise and may help guide decontamination efforts.

PITFALLS

The most common pitfall is failure to recognize and act on ECG findings consistent with severe hyperkalemia, opting instead to wait for the laboratory results.

The routine withholding of calcium therapy from critically ill patients with hyperkalemia and possible digoxin overdose is also a potential pitfall. Calcium has the fastest onset of action and is the only therapy that directly antagonizes the effect of elevated potassium on the myocyte. If the patient is truly in extremis, it becomes a risk-benefit analysis, and calcium therapy should not be routinely disregarded.

REFERENCES

1. Allon M. Hyperkalemia in end-stage renal disease: mechanisms and management. *J Am Soc Nephrol* 1995;6(4):1134–1142.
2. Hoffman RS. Fluid, electrolyte, and acid-base principles. In: Goldfrank LR, Flomenbaum ME, Lewin NA, et al., eds. *Goldfrank's toxicologic emergencies*, 7th ed. McGraw-Hill, 2002:374–375.
3. Wiederkehr MR, Moe OW. Factitious hyperkalemia. *Am J Kidney Dis* 2000;36(5):1049–1053.
4. American Heart Association. *Handbook of emergency cardiovascular care for healthcare providers*. Dallas: American Heart Association, 2000:73.
5. Khatter JC, et al. Digitalis cardiotoxicity: cellular calcium overload a possible mechanism. *Basic Res Cardiol* 1989;84:553–563.
6. Wagner J, Salzer WW. Calcium-dependent toxic effects of digoxin in isolated myocardial preparations. *Arch Int Pharmacodyn* 1976;223:4–14.
7. Lieberman AL. Studies on calcium VI. Some interrelationships of the cardiac activities of calcium gluconate and scillaren-B. *J Pharmacol Exp Ther* 1933;47:183–192.
8. Smith PK, Winkler AW, Hoff HE. Calcium and digitalis synergism: the toxicity of calcium salts injected intravenously into digitalized animals. *Arch Intern Med* 1936;64:322–328.
9. Gold H, Edwards DJ. The effects of ouabain on heart in the presence of hypercalcemia. *Am Heart J* 1927;3:45–50.
10. Bower JO, Mengle HAK. The additive effect of calcium and digitalis. *JAMA* 1936;106:1151–1153.
11. Kne T, Brokaw M, Wax P. Fatality from calcium chloride in a chronic digoxin toxic patient. *J Toxicol Clin Toxicol* 1997;5:505.
12. Illingworth RN, Proudfoot AT. Rapid poisoning with slow-release potassium. *BMJ* 1980;281:485–486.
13. Saxena K. Death from potassium chloride overdose. *Postgrad Med* 1988;84:97–102.
14. Saxena K. Clinical features and management of poisoning due to potassium chloride. *Med Toxicol Adv Drug Exp* 1989;4:429–443.
15. Mattu A, Brady WJ, Robinson DA. Electrocardiographic manifestations of hyperkalemia. *Am J Emerg Med* 2000;18(6):721–729.

CHAPTER 36
Hypertension

João H. Delgado and Richard C. Dart

OVERVIEW

Hypertension is defined as a persistently elevated systolic or diastolic blood pressure (BP). In adults, it is defined as a systolic BP greater than 140 mm Hg and diastolic BP greater than 90 mm Hg (1). In children, it is defined as a BP greater than the ninetieth percentile for a specific age. Age-specific BPs from birth to 13 years of age are available for boys and girls (2).

Toxicants may cause hypertension by direct mechanisms (receptor stimulation) or indirect mechanisms (agitation). Regardless of cause, acute elevation of BP need not be immediately corrected unless it produces target organ damage (brain, kidney, heart) or unless a concurrent medical illness requires it (e.g., myocardial infarction, aortic dissection). Whenever possible, treatment should be directed toward the underlying cause. This chapter addresses the evaluation and management of the acutely poisoned patient who is hypertensive. Some toxicants that are associated with chronic hypertension are covered in their respective chapters.

GENERAL MANAGEMENT PRINCIPLES

The management of the acutely poisoned hypertensive patient begins with initiation of general supportive care measures. Continuous cardiac monitoring and intravenous (IV) access should be established. Hypertension is frequently caused or exacerbated by agitation. Mild to moderate hypertension in these cases responds to adequate sedation. Pain is also a frequently overlooked etiology that is easily correctable.

The diagnostic evaluation is aimed at detecting evidence of target organ dysfunction and determining the cause of hypertension. In patients with moderate to severe hypertension who are otherwise asymptomatic, an electrocardiogram, serum creatinine, and urinalysis are reasonable screening tests for target organ dysfunction. Additional tests may be indicated by the history and physical examination findings. For example, a head computed tomography is indicated in the hypertensive patient with altered mental status to evaluate for intracranial hemorrhage or other intracranial pathology.

After immediate life threats are addressed, additional specific therapy may be required. The goal of treatment is to reduce the BP gradually to a level that prevents or limits further target organ damage. In patients who have preexisting chronic hypertension or present with stroke symptoms, additional care is needed so that an abrupt decline in BP does not compromise cerebral perfusion. In these cases, initial BP reduction should not exceed 25% of the baseline mean arterial pressure (3).

Some patients remain severely hypertensive despite appropriate supportive care measures. In these patients, parenteral antihypertensive therapy using short-acting titratable agents, such as nitroprusside or esmolol, is appropriate.

SPECIFIC MANAGEMENT

Sympathomimetic Excess

Acute intoxication with a sympathomimetic agent can cause severe hypertension. *Direct* alpha-adrenergic agonists, such as epinephrine, phenylephrine, and ergotamines, bind directly to alpha adrenoceptors resulting in vasoconstriction. *Indirect* agents, such as amphetamines, cocaine, tricyclic antidepressants, and monoamine oxidase inhibitors, act by increasing catecholamine release or decreasing catecholamine reuptake. The hypertension caused by indirect agents may be transient. In fact, hypotension may occur once catecholamine stores are depleted. In general, antihypertensive treatment should be avoided with the following poisons because hypertension is not life threatening and responds to supportive care: clonidine, imidazoline decongestants, bretylium, cocaine, amphetamine, monoamine oxidase inhibitors, tricyclic antidepressants, anticholinergic drugs, beta-receptor agonists, or nicotine.

Benzodiazepines are the first-line agents for sympathomimetic excess from direct or indirect agents. Benzodiazepines reduce central sympathetic outflow and excess circulating catecholamines associated with the use of sympathomimetics (4,5). The choice of the specific benzodiazepine is not critical and should be based on the provider's familiarity with dosing as well as availability. A typical initial adult dose is diazepam, 5 to 10 mg IV, with additional doses titrated to response. For lorazepam, the adult dose is 1 to 2 mg IV, with repeat doses titrated to effect. The initial pediatric doses for diazepam are 0.04 to 0.2 mg/kg IV and for lorazepam, 0.05 mg/kg, both titrated to effect.

The key management point is to titrate whichever agent is chosen such that agitation, heart rate, and BP are well controlled. The clinician should not hesitate to escalate the dose, keeping in mind that very large doses may be required for optimal BP control in severe cases. Endotracheal intubation and neuromuscular blockade may be needed in refractory cases to allow adequate dosing of benzodiazepines and control of motor agitation. These patients should be managed in an emergency department or critical care setting.

Benzodiazepines may be less effective for peripherally active agents. In these cases, the addition of a short-acting titratable agent (e.g., nitroglycerin or nitroprusside) may be useful. The adult and pediatric dose of nitroprusside is 0.5 μg/kg/minute by continuous infusion, which should be titrated upward by 0.25 to 0.5 μg/kg/minute every 5 minutes until the desired BP is reached. An infusion rate above 10 μg/kg/minute is rarely required and may produce cyanide toxicity if prolonged. Nitroprusside should be tapered gradually to avoid rebound hypertension. Intraarterial BP monitoring is recommended for persistent hypertension requiring nitroprusside.

In most cases, adequate sedation is sufficient to control BP. Beta-blockers are generally avoided because of the theoretic concern for unopposed alpha stimulation (see later). In the case of methylxanthines (e.g., caffeine, theophylline), tachycardia is usually more prominent than hypertension. A short-acting beta-blocker like esmolol is useful in treating tachycardia with cardiovascular compromise, despite the theoretic risk of unopposed alpha-receptor stimulation.

Acute coronary syndrome is a controversial challenge in the setting of sympathomimetic toxicity. Beta-blockers decrease myocardial oxygen demand and have been proven to reduce mortality. The phenomenon of paradoxic hypertension after beta-blocker use in the patient with cocaine toxicity has been described. This presumably occurs due to unopposed alpha-adrenergic stimulation (6,7). Because the relative importance of the risks (unopposed alpha stimulation) and benefits (reduction in mortality in the setting of cocaine toxicity) is unknown, it is unclear whether beta-blockers should be used in these situations. Some authors have proposed the use of phentolamine, a selective alpha antagonist, as an alternative in these situations (8).

Withdrawal Syndrome

In general, supportive care and sedation achieve adequate BP control from withdrawal syndromes (Chapter 32). Persistent hypertension may indicate inadequate sedation.

ANCILLARY STUDIES

The electrocardiogram is an essential diagnostic tool. Evidence of left ventricular hypertrophy suggests long-standing hypertension. Evidence of ischemia or infarction should prompt aggressive BP management to decrease myocardial oxygen demand. An elevated creatinine or presence of proteinuria requires prompt and effective BP reduction.

In the patient with altered sensorium, head computed tomography is used to evaluate for intracranial hemorrhage or stroke. Head computed tomography may also reveal evidence of hypertensive encephalopathy in severe cases.

A urine drug screen may provide clues to the etiology of hypertension (e.g., amphetamines, cocaine). Other diagnostic studies may be useful depending on the presenting signs and symptoms.

PITFALLS

Inadequate sedation is the most frequent cause of persistent BP elevation in the poisoned patient. Chronically hypertensive patients who present with a hypertensive emergency, an intracranial hemorrhage, or an ischemic stroke should have their BP decreased cautiously not to compromise cerebral perfusion. The goal is a gradual and modest reduction of the baseline mean arterial pressure. Finally, hypertension may be a clue to the presence of a withdrawal syndrome, which can be effectively treated with sedatives.

REFERENCES

1. 1999 World Health Organization—International Society of Hypertension guidelines for the management of hypertension. Guidelines sub-committee. *Blood Pressure* 1999;1[Suppl]:9–43.
2. Report of the second task force on blood pressure control in children—1987. Task force on blood pressure control in children. National Heart, Lung, and Blood Institute, Bethesda, Maryland. *Pediatrics* 1987;79:1–25.
3. Blumenfeld JD, Laragh JH. Management of hypertensive crises: the scientific basis for treatment decisions. *Am J Hypertension* 2001;14:1154–1167.
4. Guinn MM, Bedford JA, Wilson MC. Antagonism of intravenous cocaine lethality in nonhuman primates. *J Toxicol Clin Toxicol* 1980;16:499–508.
5. Karch SB. Serum catecholamines in cocaine intoxicated patients with cardiac symptoms. *Ann Emerg Med* 1987;16:481.
6. Ramoska E, Sacchetti AD. Propranolol-induced hypertension in treatment of cocaine intoxication. *Ann Emerg Med* 1985;14:1112–1113.
7. Lange RA, Cigarroa RG, Flores ED, et al. Potentiation of cocaine-induced coronary vasoconstriction by beta-adrenergic blockade. *Ann Intern Med* 1990;112:897–903.
8. Hollander JE, Carter WA, Hoffman RS. Use of phentolamine for cocaine-induced myocardial ischemia [Letter]. *New Engl J Med* 1992;327:361.

CHAPTER 37

Hypotension and Shock

Richard C. Dart

OVERVIEW

Hypotension is defined as an abnormally low blood pressure (e.g., a systolic blood pressure less than 90 mm Hg for adults and adolescents, less than 70 mm Hg for ages 5 to 10 years, less than 70 mm Hg for ages 1 to 5 years, and less than 60 mm Hg for newborns younger than 1 year). A definition of shock, however, cannot be based on blood pressure alone because the clinical issue is tissue perfusion. Any condition that provides insufficient oxygen to a tissue can cause injury. The term *shock* is used to describe inadequate perfusion of vital organs leading to tissue injury. Prolonged systemic hypotension is undoubtedly the most common cause of shock. Shock may be caused by inadequate peripheral resistance, decreased cardiac output, loss of effective blood volume, or insufficient substrate delivery to tissue (e.g., hypoxia).

Nearly all poisons have the potential to produce hypotension. For example, acidosis from any cause can manifest as hypotension. Hypotension alone is therefore a poor diagnostic clue for determining the poison involved in a poisoning; however, hypotension may be an important indication for treatment because prolonged hypotension from any cause leads to shock if undertreated.

GENERAL MANAGEMENT PRINCIPLES

The primary treatment of hypotension or shock is reversal of the underlying cause. However, it is usually difficult to reverse the effect quickly unless the poison involved has a specific antidote, such as naloxone for opioid toxicity. In addition to treating the toxin involved, therefore, prompt and aggressive supportive care is needed.

The prehospital treatment of hypotension focuses on prompt transport to a medical facility and the intravenous (IV) administration of isotonic crystalloid fluid. If hypotension in the poisoned patient is unresponsive to initial infusion, the patient should be intubated endotracheally until the cause can be determined. If long transport times are involved, the approach should be similar to that of the emergency department and includes the administration of vasopressor agents.

The aim of emergency department care is to arrest the underlying process by continuing intravascular volume resuscitation as well as increasing peripheral resistance and myocardial contractility. Most patients with hypotension require inpatient treatment.

The airway is an important and too frequently neglected aspect of treatment of hypotension. Hypotension is an indication for endotracheal intubation unless it responds quickly to infusion of IV fluids and the patient has normal mental status. Hypoxia should be immediately treated with supplemental oxygen.

For nearly all poisons, infusion of isotonic crystalloid fluid is the initial treatment of hypotension. The typical initial dose is 20 ml/kg of 0.9% saline IV for either adults or children. If hypotension persists, additional IV fluid administration is guided by the patient's course, the underlying cause (if known), and the use of other supportive measures as described in the following sections. Close monitoring is needed to avoid volume overload, as many agents that cause hypotension are also myocardial depressants (i.e., calcium-channel blockers). If hypotension is initially difficult to reverse or complications arise, invasive hemodynamic monitoring may be needed. Central venous pressure monitoring is usually sufficient. Clinical judgment must be applied during administration of IV fluids to the elderly or patients with likely myocardial dysfunction (i.e., congestive heart failure, poisoning with agent known to impair cardiac contractility).

The endpoint for resuscitation of the poisoned patient has not been established. In general, the goal is to provide adequate oxygenation (oxygen saturation above 70 mm Hg) and tissue perfusion (serum lactate level that is improving) in the presence of reasonable cardiac function (central venous pressure 8 to 15 mm Hg). The goal of resuscitation may well vary by the poison involved, but much more research is needed on resuscitation of the hypotensive poisoned patient.

The presence of a toxin may obscure the clinical findings typically used to guide the treatment of hypotension and shock. For example, drugs that alter myocardial conduction may prevent tachycardia, and an anticholinergic agent could produce a dry patient (although signs of tachycardia should be present).

SPECIFIC MANAGEMENT

Bradycardia

Bradycardia is an abnormal response to hypotension. It may indicate that a poison such as a cardiac glycoside, beta-blocking agent, or calcium-channel blocker has been ingested. Although it is often refractory, bradycardia is usually treated initially with atropine (1). The adult dose is 0.5 to 1.0 mg IV, repeated every 5 minutes if necessary to a maximum dose of 3 mg. For children, the dose is 0.02 mg/kg IV repeated every 5 minutes as needed, up to a total dose of 1 mg in children and 3 mg in adolescents. If bradycardia is refractory, a pacemaker and epinephrine infusion should be considered (1).

Hypotension

There are three approaches to the treatment of hypotension: (a) increase the cardiac output, (b) increase the peripheral resistance, or (c) increase the blood volume. The most common initial approach is to increase cardiac output by administering volume as described previously.

Vasopressors increase cardiac contractility, increase peripheral resistance, or do both. Although authorities agree that vasopressors are an important treatment of hypotension, there is disagreement concerning precisely which pressor to use. In most scenarios, dopamine is the preferred initial agent because it is readily available and health care personnel are familiar with its use. Norepinephrine has been proposed as a preferred pressor for agents that produce alpha receptor blockade, such as tricyclic antidepressant poisoning. However, the data available are mixed (2–4). Clinical studies have used relatively low doses (4). Although it is likely to be as effective as dopamine, its relative unavailability and delays caused by unfamiliarity with its use make it a secondary agent (except in institutions where it is frequently used and readily available).

Dopamine has both alpha and beta receptor agonism and therefore increases cardiac contractility as well as peripheral vascular resistance. A typical starting dose in poisoned patients is 5 to 10 μg/kg/minute by IV infusion, titrated to effect. Doses above 20 μg/kg/minute may be needed in poisoned patients due to the need to overcome receptor blockade. If dopamine does not produce a satisfactory effect, norepinephrine should be added. The dose is 0.1 to 0.2 μg/kg/minute continuous infusion, titrated to effect. In theory, pure alpha receptor agonists may be more effective in reversing hypotension due to alpha receptor blockade. A phenylephrine infusion (0.25 mg/ml in NaCl 0.9%) may be started at 40 μg/minute and titrated to effect. The use of high vasopressor doses is recommended in patients refractory to lower dose therapy (5).

Other agents that may reverse hypotension include calcium chloride for calcium channel–blocker toxicity, glucagon for beta-blocker or calcium channel–blocker toxicity, and sodium bicarbonate for agents that block the sodium channel (see individual chapters for detail). A systematic review noted that naloxone improved blood pressure in hypotensive patients but did not improve survival. This study did not address toxicology patients specifically (6).

Cardiac bypass or the intraaortic balloon pump may be appropriate for selected poisonings refractory to standard therapy. These interventions are theoretically valuable when an improvement in blood pressure for a few hours is likely to allow complete recovery. For example, cardiac bypass can maintain blood pressure (and therefore hepatic perfusion), allowing the elimination of lidocaine (7). Similarly, intraaortic balloon pump may offer transient blood pressure support. For most patients, however, these interventions only prolong their deterioration because recovery is not possible (e.g., anoxic brain damage).

USE OF ANCILLARY INFORMATION

The laboratory may be useful in the assessment of certain causes of hypotension. Serum electrolytes should be determined for hypokalemia or increased anion gap acidosis. An increased serum lactate level confirms one effect of hypotension. Arterial pressure monitoring may be helpful in management of persistent hypotension. Central venous pressure monitoring or Swan-Ganz catheterization may be helpful to assess hemodynamic function and volume status. Radiography is rarely of assistance.

PITFALLS

The most common pitfall is failure to recognize early shock. The result is inadequate treatment that allows the condition to worsen. Clinical and laboratory signs of shock should be monitored frequently and definitive action taken if shock appears to be developing.

A low systolic blood pressure (e.g., 90 mm Hg in an adult woman) may be normal and may not require treatment if evidence of tissue hypoperfusion is not present.

Orthostatic blood pressure determination is unlikely to be helpful. It is often inaccurate even in patients with true hypovolemia and is less likely to be accurate in toxicologic patients in whom the cause of orthostasis is unlikely to be intravascular volume loss.

REFERENCES

1. American Heart Association. *Advanced cardiac life support textbook.* Dallas: American Heart Association, 1997.
2. Follmer CH, Lum BKB. Protective action of diazepam and sympathomimetic amines against amitriptyline-induced toxicity. *J Pharmacol Exp Ther* 1982;222:424.
3. Vernon DD, Banner W Jr, Garrett JS, et al. Efficacy of dopamine and norepinephrine for treatment of hemodynamic compromise in amitriptyline intoxication. *Crit Care Med* 1991;19:544–549.
4. Tran TP, Panacek EA, Rhee KJ, et al. Response to dopamine vs norepinephrine in tricyclic antidepressant-induced hypotension. *Acad Emerg Med* 1997;4:864–868.
5. Albertson TE, Dawson A, de Latorre F, et al. TOX-ACLS: toxicologic-oriented advanced cardiac life support. *Ann Emerg Med* 2001;37:S78–S90.
6. Boeuf B, Gauvin F, Guerguerian AM, et al. Therapy of shock with naloxone: a meta-analysis. *Crit Care Med* 1998;26:1920–1926.
7. Burlington B, Freed CR. Massive overdose and death from prophylactic lidocaine. *JAMA* 1980;243:1036–1037.

CHAPTER 38

Hyperthermia and Hypothermia

Vikhyat S. Bebarta and Richard C. Dart

HYPERTHERMIA

Treatment of the hyperthermic poisoned patient involves not only the management of body temperature but also complications of hyperthermia and the underlying conditions (serotonin syndrome, neuroleptic malignant syndrome, and so forth). It is difficult to define a specific action level for hyperthermia. In most cases, a temperature above 40°C (104°F) should be treated. The goal of treatment is a temperature of 38.3° to 39°C (101.0° to 102.2°F) to avoid hypothermia from temperature overshoot.

GENERAL MANAGEMENT PRINCIPLES

The poisoned hyperthermic patient is often critically ill and at risk for greater mortality. Treatment begins with assuring a secure airway, adequate ventilation and perfusion, and intravenous (IV) access. After the initial assessment is completed and the patient is stabilized, cooling measures should be initiated. Other etiologies such as encephalitis, meningitis, thyroid storm, sepsis, and cerebral hemorrhage must be considered early in the course of management.

In the prehospital setting, hyperthermic patients should be quickly moved to a cool environment. Prehospital providers should obtain as much history as possible and transport promptly to initiate cooling measures in an emergency department rather than staying at the scene. Cooling is initiated en route by removing the patient's clothes and infusing isotonic IV fluids.

Hyperthermic patients are often dehydrated by at least 1000 to 1400 ml, which results in poor perfusion to the skin and impaired heat release (1,2). Therefore, isotonic crystalloidal fluid such as normal saline or lactated Ringer's solution should be administered. If possible, vasopressors should be avoided because they cause vasoconstriction and impair cooling. A urinary catheter should be placed to guide fluid therapy, and a rectal or esophageal thermometer should be used to accurately measure the patient's temperature. Gastric decontamination, if necessary, should be performed after initial stabilization.

Cooling Methods

Evaporation is the most efficient cooling method. Spraying the completely undressed patient with tepid water and placing a fan close to the patient are very effective. Intense cooling of the skin, such as with ice packs placed on the skin, may lead to heat production by shivering and vasoconstriction. Covering the patient with wet sheets is discouraged because it reduces dissipation of heat from the skin. A cooling apparatus used in the Middle East is very effective (3). A modified hammock allows complete patient exposure to tepid water spray and air from a fan. This approach is most effective in a low humidity environment.

Decreasing muscular activity also has an important role in the treatment of hyperthermia. Struggling against restraints can worsen hyperthermia through increased heat production. The combined use of physical and chemical restraints reduces heat generation, whereas evaporative cooling provides increased heat loss. Occasionally, neuromuscular paralysis is needed to sufficiently decrease activity.

Other cooling techniques include immersion in cool water and ice packs. Immersion may be necessary for cases refractory to evaporative cooling. However, it is discouraged due to the need to keep the patient's head out of the water, securing cardiac electrodes and a rectal temperature probe, and the difficulty of performing emergent defibrillation or cardiopulmonary resuscitation if necessary. Ice packs are discouraged because the local intense cooling may cause shivering, which increases heat production.

Iced gastric lavage may be considered in the intubated patient. Peritoneal lavage and bladder irrigation may also be considered. Their relative contribution to the fall in body temperature is unknown, but it is unlikely to be substantial. Finally, cardiopulmonary bypass may be very effective in the patient recalcitrant to other methods of cooling. However, evaporative cooling is effective for the majority of patients.

Complications

Noncardiogenic pulmonary edema may develop during the hyperthermic episode (4). Renal failure may occur either by acute tubular necrosis from dehydration and decreased renal blood flow or by rhabdomyolysis. Centrilobular necrosis in the liver occurs due to direct thermal injury. The liver enzymes are often mildly elevated. The bilirubin is not elevated initially (5). A coagulopathy often develops, perhaps due to thermal injury of the vascular endothelium leading to mild disseminated intravascular coagulation. This results in thrombocytopenia and elevated prothrombin time and partial thromboplastin time. In general, these abnormal values do not require specific therapy.

TABLE 1. Specific management of hyperthermia

Cause	Treatment
Withdrawal from benzodiazepines, barbiturates, or alcohol	Benzodiazepine
Sympathomimetic toxicity	Benzodiazepine
Anticholinergic toxicity	Benzodiazepine
Serotonin syndrome	Benzodiazepine, cyproheptadine
Neuroleptic malignant syndrome	Benzodiazepine, bromocriptine, amantadine
Malignant hyperthermia	Dantrolene
Strychnine	Benzodiazepines, barbiturates, and possibly neuromuscular blockade

Hypokalemia and hypophosphatemia may occur initially, but serum potassium and phosphate may be elevated if the patient has rhabdomyolysis (6,7). Hypocalcemia may also occur with rhabdomyolysis.

Most patients with severe hyperthermia and other systemic symptoms are admitted to the intensive care unit. Those with mild elevation in temperature and resolving symptoms may potentially be observed and discharged from the emergency department if they are stable and appropriate.

SPECIFIC MANAGEMENT

Withdrawal from alcohol, barbiturates, or benzodiazepines is treated with benzodiazepines to decrease heat production from muscular activity (Table 1). Benzodiazepines are effective for most of the sympathomimetic agents (i.e., amphetamines, phencyclidine, cocaine, ephedrine) and anticholinergic agents (including cyclic antidepressants). However, the sympathomimetics also cause hyperthermia by alpha-adrenergic stimulation and decreased vasodilation, which is not addressed by benzodiazepines.

Salicylate, dinitrophenol, pentachlorophenol, and calcium channel– and beta-blocker (Table 1) *toxicity* can cause an increase in body temperature; however, significant hyperthermia with calcium channel– and beta-blocker toxicity is theoretic and has not been reported. There are no specific hyperthermic management principles for these agents other than undressing the patient and using evaporative cooling methods.

Neuroleptic malignant syndrome, serotonin syndrome, monoamine oxidase inhibitor toxicity, and malignant hyperthermia can cause muscular rigidity and hyperthermia (Table 1). Other agents such as strychnine can also generate heat through motor activity. These poisonings are treated by stopping all neuroleptic and serotonergic medications, instituting general cooling measures, and administering benzodiazepines for agitation and muscular activity. Sometimes, intubation and muscular paralysis are necessary to control muscular activity. Anticholinergic medications should be avoided. Neuroleptic malignant syndrome has been treated with amantadine and bromocriptine to decrease rigidity, presumably working as dopamine agonists (Chapter 23) (8,9). Serotonin syndrome has been treated with cyproheptadine, a 5-HT_1 serotoninergic receptor agonist (Chapter 24) (10).

TREATMENT OF COMPLICATIONS

To avoid or minimize renal injury, hyperthermic patients should receive aggressive IV hydration. Mannitol may be considered to increase urinary output as long as the patient is not hypotensive and has been fluid resuscitated. Electrolyte abnormalities should be treated early. Coagulopathies and thrombocytopenia do not need to be treated unless the patient is bleeding.

USE OF ANCILLARY INFORMATION

One of the most concerning complications of hyperthermia is rhabdomyolysis, hyperkalemia, and resultant renal failure. Monitoring the creatine kinase level is helpful in anticipating and treating rhabdomyolysis. The serum phosphate may become elevated if the patient develops rhabdomyolysis and should be monitored closely, along with calcium (which can fall with muscle breakdown) and renal function tests (Chapter 29). An electrocardiogram is helpful to quickly screen for electrolyte abnormalities and to detect dysrhythmias, particularly in the hemodynamically unstable patient. Liver enzymes and function (e.g., international normalized ratio) tests, fibrinogen levels, and a complete blood count should be monitored, especially if the patient is bleeding.

Arterial pressure monitoring may be needed for hypotensive patients. Central venous pressure monitoring or pulmonary artery catheter is helpful if the patient is persistently hypotensive and it is difficult to monitor volume status because of renal insufficiency or pulmonary edema. Radiography is rarely helpful. If the patient is hypoxic, chest radiography may help evaluate for noncardiogenic pulmonary edema. If body packing or stuffing is suspected, an abdominal computed tomogram is helpful in detecting a large source of sympathomimetics in the gastrointestinal tract.

PITFALLS

The most common pitfall is missed diagnosis. Often, the initial temperature is not taken, or hyperthermia develops later in the course of the agitated patient. Standard cooling blankets are often not effective. Antipyretics do not have a role because they simply lower the hypothalamic set point in febrile patients (11). Phenothiazines (e.g., chlorpromazine) and butyrophenones (e.g., haloperidol) can alter hypothalamic function and interfere with cooling and thus are not recommended.

HYPOTHERMIA

Hypothermia is a common complication of overdose. *Mild hypothermia* is defined as a core temperature of 32° to 35°C (89.6° to 95.0°F). Manifestations include tachypnea, tachycardia, ataxia, and dysarthria; shivering generates heat. Moderate hypothermia involves a temperature of 28° to 32°C (82.4° to 89.6°F). Shivering is lost and Osborne J waves (a positive deflection at the end of QRS complex), dysrhythmias, and depressed mentation predominate. *Severe hypothermia* is core temperature below 28°C (82.4°F). At this temperature, loss of reflexes, acidemia, coma, hypotension, ventricular fibrillation, and asystole may occur. Virtually all patients are asystolic at 14° to 20°C. Electronic thermometers may display a falsely high temperature in the severely hypothermic patient.

GENERAL MANAGEMENT PRINCIPLES

In addition to basic life support measures, treatment is directed toward preventing further heat loss; starting warming; and preventing complications, especially cardiac dysrhythmias. Rewarming and specific treatments are initiated while continuing supportive care. Volume resuscitation should be performed with warmed isotonic IV fluid. Mechanical jostling or vigorous movement of the patient may trigger ventricular fibrillation, particularly under 30°C.

Gastrointestinal motility is decreased at low body temperatures. Gastric lavage should likely be avoided in patients with moderate or severe hypothermia to avoid the induction of ventricular dysrhythmias.

Rewarming

Mildly hypothermic patients are rewarmed with external methods along with noninvasive methods such as heated humidified oxygen and warm IV fluids. Moderate hypothermia is treated with warm humidified oxygen, warmed IV fluids, and active external rewarming (e.g., convective blankets or other external heat sources for rewarming). Radiant warmers work only if the patient is fully uncovered. Gastric or peritoneal lavage may be needed if rewarming is proceeding at less than 1°C per hour.

Severe hypothermia mandates active core rewarming. Active core rewarming includes the respiratory system: Nebulizer or ventilator is modified to give 100% humidified air warmed at 40° to 45°C and warm IV fluid (40° to 42°C). Peritoneal lavage and pleural lavage using tube thoracostomy can be useful in patients with severe effects, although cardiac bypass is preferable if available. Gastrointestinal or bladder irrigation may also rewarm central organs but is associated with risks of electrolyte imbalance. If the core temperature is less than 25°C, femoral-femoral bypass should be considered if the facilities are available. For a patient in cardiac arrest, cardiac bypass is the rewarming method of choice. Open pleural lavage for direct cardiac rewarming should be considered if the core temperature remains below 28°C after 1 hour of bypass.

Drug Therapy

Target organs become progressively less responsive to medications as the core temperature falls. Large doses of exogenous insulin or digoxin are ineffective at lower temperatures but can produce a toxic reaction as rewarming progresses. Excessive pharmacologic manipulation of the vasoconstricted and depressed cardiovascular system should be avoided. Infusion of low doses of catecholamine is indicated in patients who have lower blood pressure than is expected for that degree of hypothermia and who are not responding to crystalloid and rewarming.

REFERENCES

1. Al-Harthi SS, Akhtar J, Nouth MS, et al. Evaluation of fluid deficit in pilgrims with heatstroke by hemodynamic monitoring. *Emirates Med J* 1989;7:153.
2. Seraj MA, Channa AB, Al-Harthi SS, et al. Are heatstroke victims fluid-depleted? Importance of monitoring central venous pressure as a simple guideline for fluid therapy. *Resuscitation* 1991;21:33–39.
3. Weiner JS, Khogali M. A physiological body-cooling unit for treatment of heatstroke. *Lancet* 1980;1:507–509.
4. El-Kassimi FA, Al-Mashhadani S, Abdullah AK, et al. Adult respiratory distress syndrome and disseminated intravascular coagulation complicating heatstroke. *Chest* 1986;90:571–574.
5. Kew M, Bersohn I, Seftel H, et al. Liver damage in heatstroke. *Am J Med* 1970;49:192–202.
6. Knochel JP, Caskey JH. The mechanism of hypophosphatemia in acute heat stroke. *JAMA* 1977;238:425–426.
7. Guntupalli KK, Sladen A, Selker RG, et al. Effects of induced total-body hyperthermia on phosphorus metabolism in humans. *Am J Med* 1984;77:250–254.
8. Dhib-Jalbut S, Hesselbrock R, Mouradian MM, et al. Bromocriptine treatment of neuroleptic malignant syndrome. *J Clin Psychiatry* 1987;48:69–73.
9. McCarron MM, Boettger ML, Peck JJ. A case of neuroleptic malignant syndrome successfully treated with amantadine. *J Clin Psychiatry* 1982;43:381–382.
10. Mills KC. Serotonin syndrome: a clinical update. *Crit Care Clin* 1997;13:763–783.
11. Bernheim HA, Block LH, Atkins E. Fever: pathogenesis, pathophysiology, and purpose. *Ann Intern Med* 1979;91:261–270.

CHAPTER 39

Psychiatric Evaluation of the Poisoned Patient

Ian MacGregor Whyte and Gregory L. Carter

OVERVIEW

In the developed world, an episode of deliberate self-harm is the most common presentation of the poisoned patients (1). These patients frequently have significant preexisting psychiatric diagnoses (2). Regardless of the reason for poisoning, many of these patients develop other psychiatric problems, mainly delirium, during their admission (3). Psychiatric assessment of patients presenting with deliberate self-harm is the cornerstone of good treatment with evidence of improved outcomes (4).

BACKGROUND

Deliberate self-poisoning (DSP) is by far the most common form of deliberate self-harm (5). The lifetime suicide attempt rate in the United States is approximately 4.6% (6) and is similar in Canada (3.5%) (7). DSP accounts for 1% to 5% of presentations to the emergency department (8,9) with population-based admission rates varying from 200/100,000/year in Europe (10) and Australia (11) to 400/100,000/year in the United Kingdom (12).

ROLE OF THE PSYCHIATRY SERVICE

When DSP is the reason for presentation, psychiatric assessment and subsequent management are valuable. Integrated multidisciplinary services involving toxicology and psychiatry services have shown significant benefits in terms of shorter lengths of stay and reduced hospital costs (13,14). Although most consensus guidelines recommend that all DSP patients should receive psychiatric assessment, the ability to reach this ideal varies from 50% or less (15) through 78% (16) to nearly 100% (17).

Although the value of psychiatric assessment has been questioned, recent evidence indicates that the very act of psychiatrically assessing these patients reduces the rate of a subsequent self-harm attempt (4). Even without this benefit, the incidence of preexisting psychiatric disorders (2), alcohol- and drug-related disorders (18,19), and personality disorders (20,21) is sufficiently high to warrant intervention. These illnesses are even more marked in patients who make repeated attempts (22–24).

Delirium, potentially from multiple causes, is the most common psychiatric condition to arise in poisoned patients after the overdose (Chapter 15). Another situation in which psychiatric input is helpful is toxic exposures with the potential for long-term neuropsychiatric sequelae such as organophosphates (25,26) and carbon monoxide (27,28).

LEGAL AND ETHICAL ISSUES

The difficulties that arise in managing a poisoned patient who refuses treatment are common and potentially dangerous for the patient and the toxicologist. The potential liability of being found negligent for failing to treat on the one hand or being guilty of assault for treating without consent on the other hand can result in the delay of or even prevent appropriate decision making during the care of these patients. Because legal statutes vary between countries as well as smaller jurisdictions within a country, clear and reliable advice on this issue is hard to find. The use of multidisciplinary management models helps (29), but still some patients refuse treatment.

In the United States, the most common legal action in these circumstances results from failing to prevent patients from harming themselves (30). The duty of care necessary is in proportion to the needs of the patient (30). Informed consent requires that the patient understands the risks and benefits of any intervention and also understands the consequences of any alternative treatments or indeed no treatment (31). Informed consent should be obtained from the patient or his or her appointed guardian for any treatment. When the patient refusing care is legally competent but lacks the capacity to give consent (i.e., an oriented patient with delirium), the situation is much more difficult (31). Some have argued the delirious patient can be treated as having given implied consent (32), whereas in jurisdictions based on English common law, often a common law principle of duty of care exists (33). In a life-threatening emergency, the treating team should treat immediately without fearing legal consequences (31).

Under various acts within the sphere of mental health, most jurisdictions define the circumstances when patients may be detained against their will. In the main, these require that the patients be mentally ill and a danger to themselves or to others. The issue here is the assessment of the degree of dangerousness (34). Once the decision to involuntarily detain is being considered, then ethical issues of being in the patient's best interests and providing the care in the least restrictive setting arise.

REFERENCES

1. Whyte IM, Dawson AH, Buckley NA, et al. Health care. A model for the management of self-poisoning. *Med J Aust* 1997;167(3):142–146.
2. Beaumont G, Hetzel W. Patients at risk of suicide and overdose. *Psychopharmacology (Berl)* 1992;106[Suppl]:S123–S126.
3. Carter GL, Dawson AH, Lopert R. Drug-induced delirium. Incidence, management and prevention. *Drug Saf* 1996;15(4):291–301.
4. Kapur N, House A, Dodgson K, et al. Effect of general hospital management on repeat episodes of deliberate self poisoning: cohort study. *BMJ* 2002;325(7369):866–867.
5. Dennis M, Beach M, Evans PA, et al. An examination of the accident and emergency management of deliberate self harm. *J Accid Emerg Med* 1997;14(5):311–315.
6. Kessler RC, Borges G, Walters EE. Prevalence of and risk factors for lifetime suicide attempts in the National Comorbidity Survey. *Arch Gen Psychiatry* 1999;56(7):617–626.
7. Cote L, Pronovost J, Ross C. [A study of suicidal tendencies in adolescents in the secondary level]. *Sante Ment Que* 1990;15(1):29–45.
8. Thomas SH, Bevan L, Bhattacharyya S, et al. Presentation of poisoned patients to accident and emergency departments in the north of England. *Hum Exp Toxicol* 1996;15(6):466–470.

9. McGrath J. A survey of deliberate self-poisoning. *Med J Aust* 1932;150(6):317–318.
10. Platt S, Bille-Brahe U, Kerkhof A, et al. Parasuicide in Europe: the WHO/EURO multicentre study on parasuicide. I. Introduction and preliminary analysis for 1989. *Acta Psychiatr Scand* 1992;85(2):97–104.
11. Carter GL, Whyte IM, Ball K, et al. Repetition of deliberate self-poisoning in an Australian hospital-treated population. *Med J Aust* 1999;170(7):307–311.
12. House A, Owens D, Storer D. Psycho-social intervention following attempted suicide: is there a case for better services? *Int Rev Psychiatry* 1992;4(1).
13. Hawton K, Gath D, Smith E. Management of attempted suicide in Oxford. *BMJ* 1979;2(6197):1040–1042.
14. Whyte IM, Dawson AH, Buckley NA, et al. Health care. A model for the management of self-poisoning. *Med J Aust* 1997;167(3):142–146.
15. Kapur N, House A, Creed F, et al. General hospital services for deliberate self-poisoning: an expensive road to nowhere? *Postgrad Med J* 1999;75(888):599–602.
16. McFarland AK, Chyka PA. Selection of activated charcoal products for the treatment of poisonings. *Ann Pharmacother* 1993;27(3):358–361.
17. Whyte IM, Dawson AH, Buckley NA, et al. Health care. A model for the management of self-poisoning. *Med J Aust* 1997;167(3):142–146.
18. Hawton K, Fagg J. Deliberate self-poisoning and self-injury in adolescents. A study of characteristics and trends in Oxford, 1976–89. *Br J Psychiatry* 1992;161:816–823.
19. Crumley FE. Substance abuse and adolescent suicidal behavior. *JAMA* 1990;263(22):3051–3056.
20. Casey PR. Personality disorder and suicide intent. *Acta Psychiatr Scand* 1989;79(3):290–295.
21. Crumley FE. The adolescent suicide attempt: a cardinal symptom of a serious psychiatric disorder. *Am J Psychother* 1982;36(2):158–165.
22. Rudd MD, Joiner T, Rajab MH. Relationships among suicide ideators, attempters, and multiple attempters in a young-adult sample. *J Abnorm Psychol* 1996;105(4):541–550.
23. Peterson LG, Bongar B. Repetitive suicidal crises: characteristics of repeating versus nonrepeating suicidal visitors to a psychiatric emergency service. *Psychopathology* 1990;23(3):136–145.
24. Lipowska-Teutsch A, Reder V, Pach J. [Motives and circumstances of repeated suicidal attempts by taking drugs]. *Przegl Lek* 1990;47(6):505–508.
25. Weiner ML, Jortner BS. Organophosphate-induced delayed neurotoxicity of triarylphosphates. *Neurotoxicology* 1999;20(4):653–673.
26. Jamal GA. Long term neurotoxic effects of chemical warfare organophosphate compounds (Sarin) [Editorial]. *Adverse Drug React Toxicol Rev* 1995;14(2):83–84.
27. Chang KH, Han MH, Kim HS, et al. Delayed encephalopathy after acute carbon monoxide intoxication: MR imaging features and distribution of cerebral white matter lesions. *Radiology* 1992;184(1):117–122.
28. Smallwood P, Murray GB. Neuropsychiatric aspects of carbon monoxide poisoning: a review and single case report suggesting a role for amphetamines. *Ann Clin Psychiatry* 1999;11(1):21–27.
29. Whyte IM, Dawson AH, Buckley NA, et al. A model for the management of self-poisoning. *Med J Aust* 1997;167(3):142–146.
30. Bongar B, Maris RW, Berman AL, et al. Inpatient standards of care and the suicidal patient. Part I: general clinical formulations and legal considerations. *Suicide Life Threat Behav* 1993;23(3):245–256.
31. Deaton RJ, Colenda CG, Bursztajn H. Medical-legal issues. In: Stoudemire A, Fogel B, eds. *Psychiatric care of the medical patient*. New York: Oxford University Press, 1993:929–938.
32. Fogel BS, Mills MJ, Landen JE. Legal aspects of the treatment of delirium. *Hosp Community Psychiatry* 1986;37(2):154–158.
33. Plueckhahn VD, Breen KD, Cordner SM. The professional liability of doctors. In: Plueckhahn VD, Breen KD, Cordner SM, eds. *Law and ethics in medicine*. Geelong, Australia: Henry Thacker Print Group, 1994:81–87.
34. Gutheil TG, Bursztajn H, Brodsky A. The multidimensional assessment of dangerousness: competence assessment in patient care and liability prevention. *Bull Am Acad Psychiatry Law* 1986;14(2):123–129.

CHAPTER 40

Treatment of Convulsions

George Braitberg

OVERVIEW

Nearly all seizures related to poisoning are usually treated in the same manner. The standard anticonvulsants used in the acute management of seizures are benzodiazepines and barbiturates. A few drug-induced seizures have specific therapies, and some have contraindications to drug administration (Table 1).

The terms *seizure* and *convulsion* are often used interchangeably. *Seizure* refers to an episode of abnormal neurologic function caused by an abnormal electrical discharge of neurons; the seizure is referred to as the *ictus* and the postseizure period as the *postictus*. The term *convulsion* refers to an episode of excessive or abnormal motor activity. Convulsions may occur with seizures but also in the absence of central ictal activity.

GENERAL MANAGEMENT PRINCIPLES

The treatment of convulsions should be initiated during prehospital care. The approach to care is the same as initial treatment in the emergency department. The immediate goal of treatment is to terminate convulsive activity and then evaluate the cause of seizure or convulsion. There are good data to support the initial use of benzodiazepines intravenously (IV) in patients with seizures and status epilepticus. Lorazepam and diazepam are the most commonly recommended benzodiazepines in the United States (1–3). However, midazolam, given IV, intramuscularly, buccally, or intranasally, is also safe and efficacious. In many parts of the world, clonazepam is the benzodiazepine of choice (4–6). Benzodiazepines increase γ-aminobutyric acid (GABA) neurotransmission by binding to their specific receptors on the GABA-A–chloride ion channel. Benzodiazepines increase the frequency of channel opening, whereas barbiturates increase the duration of channel opening (7).

TABLE 1. Special treatment considerations for drug-induced seizures

Drug	Consideration	Reference
Isoniazid	First-line therapy is pyridoxine. May not respond to gamma-aminobutyric acid-A agonists.	Curry (7); Sullivan (43)
Meperidine	Naloxone may exacerbate seizures.	Knight (44)
Theophylline	Responds poorly to anticonvulsants. Phenytoin may exacerbate.	Eldredge (45); Dragunow (46); Goldberg (47); Blake (48)
Alcohol withdrawal	Responds poorly to phenytoin.	Alldredge (37); Chance (38); Rathlev (39); Young (40)

Adapted from Garcia PA, Alldredge BK. Drug induced seizures. *Neurol Clin* 1994;12(1):85–89.

TABLE 2. Pharmacologic properties of common anticonvulsants

Agent	Special comments	Half-life (h)	Duration of action (h)	IV dose
Diazepam	Rapid redistribution from central nervous system. Can be administered rectally. IM absorption is erratic.	Elimination half-life of 20–48 with active metabolites, hydroxydiazepam, nordiazepam to oxazepam.	0.25–0.50	0.2 mg/kg at 2–5 mg/min. Up to max 20 mg.
Lorazepam	Less lipid soluble than diazepam with slower rise of central nervous system concentrations. Lorazepam is metabolized in the liver mainly to the inactive glucuronide of lorazepam.	Half-life of approximately 2–16.	12–24	0.1 mg/kg at 1–2 mg/min. Up to max 10 mg.
Clonazepam	A correlation between therapeutic effects and side effects with plasma levels of clonazepam and its metabolites has not been established. Can be given as an IV infusion.	Oral doses of 1.5–2.0 mg, 22–54.	6–12	0.008–0.015 mg/kg over 1 min.
Midazolam	Water soluble. Fused imidazole ring provides stability in aqueous solution at low pH and rapid penetration of blood–brain barrier at physiologic pH. Multiple modes of administration.	Short elimination half-life (1.0–2.8) with a large volume of distribution (0.8–1.86 L/kg) and a rapid plasma clearance (0.24–0.73 L/h/kg).	<2	0.1–0.3 mg/kg.

Adapted from Brown AFT, Wilkes GJ. The emergency department management of status epilepticus. *Emerg Med* 1994;6:49–61; pharmacokinetic data from Lowenstein DH, Alldredge BK. Status epilepticus. *N Engl J Med* 1998;338(14):970–976; and benzodiazepine subheadings from Caswell A, ed. MIMS online.version 1.1. Available at: http://www.mims.hcn.net.au. Accessed May 1–July 31, 2002.

Phenytoin is a useful second agent for patients with refractory seizures or patients in status epilepticus (2). Factors such as the need for a rapid infusion, safety, availability, mode of use, and cost guide the physician in selecting between phenytoin and fosphenytoin. Phenobarbital is also a useful second agent and is useful in the treatment of patients who are refractory to the benzodiazepines, as well as in pediatric patients. Propofol can be used to achieve burst suppression in refractory status epilepticus and is an alternative to IV midazolam or clonazepam infusion. However, there is still some controversy about the epileptogenic properties of propofol (8–13).

In pediatric patients with status epilepticus, IV lorazepam is preferred over IV diazepam because of the greater risk of respiratory complications with diazepam use.

Role of Time

Seizures should be treated and controlled promptly (14,15). This not only lessens the potential for complications (e.g., hypoxia, hypotension, aspiration, hyperthermia, trauma, and so forth) but also improves efficacy because seizures are more difficult to control the longer they continue (16–21). Continuing seizure activity itself contributes substantially to neuronal damage despite optimal delivery of glucose and oxygen (4). Drug-induced seizures are more often difficult to control than other causes (22).

Selection of Drug Treatment

BENZODIAZEPINES

Benzodiazepines are safe to use for control of seizures. In a randomized, blinded prehospital trial, benzodiazepines terminated seizures at least twice as frequently as placebo and were without major complications. Patients treated with placebo had more out-of-hospital complications and deaths than the benzodiazepine group (23).

Pharmacologic properties of these agents are summarized in Table 2. Diazepam enters the brain readily and stops seizures quickly. Because it is highly lipid soluble, it redistributes to other fatty tissues causing brain and serum concentrations to fall rapidly; therefore, seizures may recur. A longer acting anticonvulsant is suggested to follow the use of diazepam (1). Diazepam can be effective when given rectally (24). A metaanalysis of anticonvulsants in children concluded that diazepam was not as effective as midazolam, thiopental, or pentobarbital (25).

Lorazepam was recommended as the initial drug of choice in a major review of status epilepticus (17). Alldredge et al. found the odds of seizure termination with lorazepam were more than twice that of diazepam with no difference in complication rate in the prehospital setting (23). In contrast, Leppik et al. found no difference in the efficacy of lorazepam and diazepam (26). Lorazepam was recommended as a first-line agent by Treiman et al. who reviewed 384 patients with a diagnosis of overt generalized convulsive status epilepticus (3). Patients were divided into groups who received diazepam (0.15 mg/kg of body weight) followed by phenytoin (18 mg/kg), lorazepam (0.1 mg/kg), phenobarbital (15 mg/kg), and phenytoin (18 mg/kg). Lorazepam was successful in 64.9% of those assigned to receive it, phenobarbital in 58.2%, diazepam plus phenytoin in 55.8%, and phenytoin alone in 43.6% ($p = .02$ for the overall four-group comparison). Lorazepam was effective significantly more often than phenytoin alone. No difference was found among the treatments in the incidence of hypotension requiring treatment, respiratory depression, or cardiac-rhythm disturbances.

Seizures in children were controlled more quickly with IV diazepam than with intranasal midazolam, although midazolam was as safe and effective as diazepam (6). Buccal midazolam used in 42 students of a residential school (ages 5 to 19 years) was found to be at least as effective as rectal diazepam in the acute treatment of seizures (27). Intranasal midazolam has been shown to be effective in adults and children and is useful when IV access is difficult (28). Some studies have shown midazolam to be more effective than IV diazepam (25).

First used in 1980, clonazepam is not licensed in the United States (29). Clonazepam can be given 0.5 mg IV boluses/minute up to 1 mg (30). There are few data on the comparative efficacy with other benzodiazepines. Its main advantage is the ability to run as an infusion (4).

BARBITURATES

Phenobarbital is effective within 10 to 20 minutes of an IV dose and has a prolonged duration of action (up to 3 days) (4). It was as effective as lorazepam in a blinded, randomized study, with no significant differences in seizure recurrence or adverse events over 30 days. However, it was more difficult to use than lorazepam (3). Apart from central nervous system depression, the primary side effect is hypotension from myocardial depression and decreased venous return, which may necessitate slowing of drug infusion (1).

PHENYTOIN AND FOSPHENYTOIN

Phenytoin is useful for maintaining a prolonged antiseizure effect, especially in combination with diazepam. As a single agent, it was least effective in controlling primary overt generalized convulsive status epilepticus, when compared with the benzodiazepines and barbiturates (3). It is to be avoided in alcohol withdrawal and theophylline-induced seizures. One limitation of use is physician underdosing. The typical 1000-mg loading dose provides inadequate therapy for many adults. Care must be practiced with infusion rates to prevent hypotension and myocardial depression (especially in the elderly) caused by the propylene glycol excipient. This may be avoided by the use of fosphenytoin, a prodrug converted to phenytoin by nonspecific phosphatases (17).

VALPROATE

Rectal valproate has been used in the past (31). IV valproate has limited availability, and human data are insufficient to justify its use at this time, although it was effective in one French study of patients in status epilepticus (32). It may have a limited role in refractory generalized nonconvulsive status epilepticus (33). The theoretical advantage is that it can be continued long-term after the acute episode.

Treatment Algorithm

Lowenstein and Alldredge proposed a treatment algorithm involving a time-based escalation approach, taking the time from last therapy to be deemed a failure before advancing to the next treatment modality in the case of treatment failure (Fig. 1) (17).

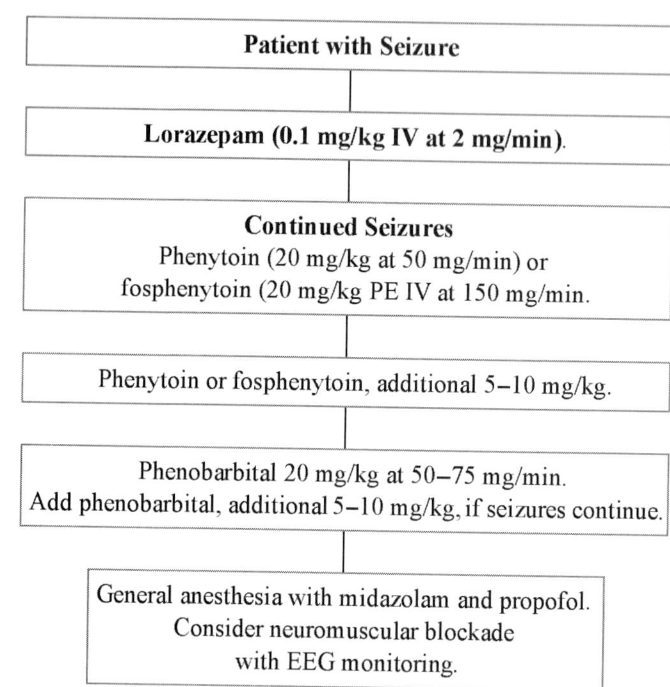

Figure 1. One approach to status epilepticus. EEG, electroencephalogram; PE, phenytoin equivalents. [Modified from Bone RC. Treatment of convulsive status epilepticus. Recommendations of the Epilepsy Foundation of America's Working Group on Status Epilepticus. *JAMA* 1993;270(7):854–859.]

SPECIFIC MANAGEMENT

The type of anticonvulsant drug needed may differ according to the inducing agent. See chapters on individual agents for additional information.

Recreational Drugs

Cocaine-induced seizures were more likely to be controlled by pretreatment with phenobarbitone, whereas methamphetamine-induced seizures were better controlled with diazepam and valproate. In animals, phenytoin had no effect on methamphetamine-induced seizures but profoundly reduced the incidence of cocaine-related clonic seizures (34).

Isoniazid

Isoniazid (INH) and other hydrazines inhibit the formation of pyridoxal phosphate, a necessary cofactor in GABA synthesis. Benzodiazepines and barbiturates bind to receptors on the GABA-A complex to increase the affinity of GABA for its receptor and increase the inhibitory outflow of chloride ions. In the presence of INH poisoning, these anticonvulsants may be ineffectual, as GABA concentrations are low as a result of synthesis inhibition (7). The administration of pyridoxine is effective in terminating INH-induced seizures. The combination of pyridoxine and a benzodiazepine appears to have a synergistic effect (35). If the amount of pyridoxine ingested is unknown, the initial dose is 5 g IV push. The dose may be repeated once in 30 minutes. If the dose of INH is known, the dose of pyridoxine is gram for gram (e.g., 7 g of INH is treated with 7 g of pyridoxine) (36).

Alcohol Withdrawal Seizures

Phenytoin does not prevent alcohol withdrawal seizures. Prospective studies indicate the same rate of seizure in prospective placebo-controlled trials (37,38). A randomized double blind trial comparing IV phenytoin with normal saline placebo after a witnessed alcohol withdrawal seizure found the incidence of seizure to be approximately 20% in both groups (39).

In contrast, a prospective uncontrolled study of 62 patients in acute alcohol withdrawal showed that treatment with phenobarbital allowed 57 patients to be discharged within 4 hours, including those who had presented with seizures, without recurrence of symptoms within the period of observation (40). However, the number of patients enrolled was small, the period of observation limited, and no comparison group was studied.

Theophylline

Pretreatment with a number of anticonvulsants in a rat model of theophylline toxicity demonstrated the lack of effect of phenytoin when compared to clonazepam, diazepam, phenobarbital, and valproic acid. Theophylline brain or serum concentrations at onset of maximal seizures were not statistically different comparing phenytoin (or magnesium) to control. Diazepam and clonazepam, phenobarbital, or valproate significantly raised the concentration required to produce seizure (41).

Tricyclic Antidepressants

The use of phenytoin in a canine experimental model found that there were no differences in multiple variables, including toxicity and the dose required to cause death. Further, the incidence of ventricular dysrhythmias was increased (42). Seizures in tricyclic antidepressants toxicity should be treated in the standard method.

USE OF ANCILLARY INFORMATION

Typically, laboratory tests to assess alternative causes for the seizure are obtained: serum electrolytes, blood urea nitrogen, creatinine, magnesium, and calcium. Rapid glucose testing is needed in all patients. Arterial blood gases are evaluated for acidosis and its course. An electrocardiogram should be performed to assess potential toxin-induced electrocardiogram changes. Serum levels of anticonvulsants are useful in patients with a known preexisting seizure disorder. Other tests may include carboxyhemoglobin, salicylate, theophylline, drugs of abuse or tricyclic antidepressant screen, cholinesterase level, and other tests to establish cause of seizure.

Lumbar puncture and computerized tomography of the head are used to assess presence of structural lesions but may also help evaluate the occasional case of head trauma resulting from a seizure (e.g., fall, automobile accident).

An electroencephalogram should be obtained in patients with seizures refractory to treatment, especially those in whom neuromuscular blockade becomes necessary.

PITFALLS

The empiric use of pyridoxine for the treatment of seizure is often overlooked, even in areas in which tuberculosis is endemic.

REFERENCES

1. Bone RC. Treatment of convulsive status epilepticus. Recommendations of the Epilepsy Foundation of America's Working Group on Status Epilepticus. *JAMA* 1993;270(7):854–859.
2. Lowenstein DH, Alldredge BK. Status epilepticus. *N Engl J Med* 1998;338(14):970–976.
3. Treiman DM, Meyers PD, Walton NY, et al. A comparison of four treatments for generalized convulsive status epilepticus. Veterans Affairs Status Epilepticus Cooperative Study Group. *N Engl J Med* 1998;339(12):792–798.
4. Brown AFT, Wilkes GJ. The emergency department management of status epilepticus. *Emerg Med* 1994;6:49–61.
5. Chamberlain JM, Altieri MA, Futterman C, et al. A prospective, randomized study comparing intramuscular midazolam with intravenous diazepam for the treatment of seizures in children. *Pediatr Emerg Care* 1997;13(2):92–94.
6. Lahat E, Goldman M, Barr J, et al. Comparison of intranasal midazolam with intravenous diazepam for treating febrile seizures in children: prospective randomised study. *BMJ* 2000;321:83–86.
7. Curry SC, Mills KC, Graeme KA. Neurotransmitter. In: Goldfrank L, Flomenbaum N, Lewin N, et al., eds. *Goldfrank's toxicologic emergencies*, 7th ed. New York: McGraw-Hill, 2002:137–171.
8. Disoprivan 1%. In: Walker G, ed. *ABPI compendium of data sheets and summaries of product characteristics. 1998–9.* London: Datapharm Publications, 1998:1093–1094.
9. Claassen J, Hirsch LJ, Emerson RJ, et al. Treatment of refractory status epilepticus with pentobarbital, propofol, or midazolam: a systematic review. *Epilepsia* 2002;43(2):146–153.
10. Collier C, Kelly K. Propofol and convulsions, the evidence mounts. *Anaesth Intensive Care* 1991;19:573–575.
11. Sutherland MJ, Burt P. Propofol and seizures. *Anaesth Intens Care* 1994;22:733–737.
12. Walder B, Matrin RT, Phil D, et al. Seizure like phenomena and propofol. A systematic review. *Neurology* 2002;58:1327–1332.
13. Wood PR, Browne GP, Pugh S. Propofol infusion for the treatment of status epilepticus. *Lancet* 1988;1:480–481.
14. Corsellis JA, Bruton CJ. Neuropathology of status epilepticus in humans. *Adv Neurol* 1983;34:129–139.
15. Sloviter RS. "Epileptic" brain damage in rats induced by sustained electrical stimulation of the perforant path. I. Acute electrophysiological and light microscopic studies. *Brain Res Bull* 1983;10:675–697.
16. DeLorenzo RJ, et al. A prospective, population-based epidemiologic study of status epilepticus in Richmond, Virginia. *Neurology* 1996;46(4):1029–1035.
17. Lowenstein DH, Alldredge BK. Status epilepticus at an urban public hospital in the 1980s. *Neurology* 1993;43:483–488.
18. Meldrum BS, Brierley JB. Prolonged epileptic seizures in primates: ischemic cell change and its relation to ictal physiological events. *Arch Neurol* 1973;28:10–17.
19. Meldrum BS, Vigouroux RA, Brierley JB. Systemic factors and epileptic brain damage: prolonged seizures in paralyzed, artificially ventilated baboons. *Arch Neurol* 1973;29:82–87.
20. Simon RP. Physiologic consequences of status epilepticus. *Epilepsia* 1985;26[Suppl 1]:S58–S66.
21. Walton NY, Treiman DM. Response of status epilepticus induced by lithium and pilocarpine to treatment with diazepam. *Exp Neurol* 1988;101:267–275.
22. Kunisaki TA, Augenstein WL. Drug and toxin induced seizures. *Emerg Med Clin North Am* 1994;12(4):1027–1055.
23. Alldredge BK, Gelb AM, Isaacs SM, et al. A comparison of lorazepam, diazepam and placebo for the treatment of out of hospital status epilepticus. *N Engl J Med* 2001;345:631–637.
24. O'Sullivan C. The use of rectal diazepam for the treatment of prolonged convulsions in children. *Aust Prescr* 1998;21:35–36.
25. Gilbert DL, Gartside PS, Glauser TA, Efficacy and mortality in treatment of refractory generalized convulsive status epilepticus in children: a meta-analysis. *J Child Neurol* 1999;14(9):602–609.
26. Leppik IE, Derivan AT, Homan RW, et al. Double blind study of lorazepam and diazepam in status epilepticus. *JAMA* 1983;249:1452–1454.
27. Scott RC, Besag MC, Neville BGR. Buccal midazolam and rectal diazepam for treatment of prolonged seizures in childhood and adolescence: a randomised trial. *Lancet* 1999;353:623–626.
28. Kendall JL, Reynolds M, Goldberg R. Intranasal midazolam in patients with status epilepticus. *Ann Emerg Med* 1997;29(3):415–417.
29. Gregoriades AD, Frangos. Clinical observations on clonazepam in intractable epilepsy. In: Penry JK, ed. *Epilepsy. The Eighth International Symposium*, 1977:169.
30. McNamara JO. Drugs effective in the therapy of the epilepsies. In: Hardman JG, Limbird LE, Molinoff PB, et al., eds. *Goodman and Gillman's the pharmacological basis of therapeutics.* New York: McGraw-Hill, 1996:478–480.
31. Vajda FJ, Mihaly GW, Miles JL, et al. Rectal administration of sodium valproate in status epilepticus. *Neurology* 1978;28:897–899.
32. Giroud M, Gras D, Escousse A, et al. Use of injectable valproic acid in status epilepticus. *Drug Investigation* 1993;5:154–159.
33. Kaplan PW. Intravenous valproate treatment of generalized nonconvulsive status epilepticus. *Clin Electroencephalogr* 1999;30(1):1–4.
34. Hanson GR, Jensen M, Johnson M, et al. Distinct features of seizures induced by cocaine and amphetamine analogues. *Eur J Pharmacol* 1999;377:167–173.
35. Chin L, Sievers ML, Herrier RN. Potentiation of pyridoxine by depressants and anticonvulsants in the treatment of acute isoniazid intoxication in dogs. *Toxicol Appl Pharmacol* 1981;58:504–509.
36. Wason S, Lacouture PG, Lovely FH. Single high-dose pyridoxine treatment for isoniazid overdose. *JAMA* 1981;246:1102–1104.
37. Alldredge BK, Lowenstein DH, Simon RP. Placebo controlled trial of intravenous diphenylhydantoin for short term treatment of alcohol withdrawal seizures. *Am J Med* 1989;87:645–648.
38. Chance JF. Emergency department treatment of alcohol withdrawal seizures with phenytoin. *Ann Emerg Med* 1991;20:520–522.
39. Rathlev NK, D'Onofrio GD, Fish SS, et al. The lack of efficacy of phenytoin in the prevention of recurrent alcohol related seizures. *Ann Emerg Med* 1994;23(3):513–518.
40. Young GP, Rores C, Murphy CM, et al. Intravenous phenobarbital for alcohol withdrawal and convulsions. *Ann Emerg Med* 1987;16:847–850.
41. Hoffman A, Pinto E, Gihar D. Effect of pretreatment with anticonvulsants on theophylline induced seizures in the rat. *J Crit Care* 1993;8(4):198–202.
42. Callaham M, Schumaker H, Pentel P. Phenytoin prophylaxis of cardiotoxicity in experimental amitriptyline poisoning. *Pharmacol Exp Ther* 1988;245:216–220.
43. Sullivan EA, Geoffroy P, Weisman R, et al. Isoniazid poisonings in New York City. *J Emerg Med* 1998;16:57–59.
44. Knight B, Thomson N, Perry G. Seizures due to norpethidine toxicity. *Aust N Z J Med* 2000;30:513.
45. Eldridge FL, Payadrfar D, Scott SC, et al. Role of endogenous adenosine in recurrent generalized seizures. *Exp Neurol* 1989;103:179–185.
46. Dragunow M. Adenosine receptor antagonism accounts for the seizure prolonging effects of aminophylline. *Pharmacol Biochem Behav* 1990;36:751–759.
47. Goldberg MJ, Spector R, Miller G. Phenobarbital improves survival in theophylline intoxicated rabbits. *Clin Tox J Tox* 1986;24(3):203–211.
48. Blake KV, Massey KL, Hendles L, et al. Relative efficacy of phenytoin for the prevention of theophylline induced seizures in mice. *Ann Emerg Med* 1988;17:1024–1028.

SECTION

5

Antidotes and Specific Therapies

CHAPTER 41

Antidote Stocking

Richard C. Dart

GENERAL

Although the important role of antidotes has been recognized for millennia, recent years have seen a resurgence of interest in antidotes. New antidotes like digoxin immune Fab, fomepizole, and polyvalent crotaline snake antivenom have been introduced. Concerns about chemical warfare and terrorism have expanded the scope of importance for antidotes. Antidotes are now a major concern for hospitals worldwide; however, the data suggest that hospitals do not stock adequate amounts of antidotes, either for single patients or for terrorist events. (Antidotes for warfare and terrorist agents are addressed in Chapter 260.)

Scope of the Problem

More than two million poison exposures are reported by U.S. poison centers each year. Of these, more than 250,000 involve poisons for which an effective antidote is available. In 2001, 44,772 instances of specific antidote use were reported by poison centers, and undoubtedly there were many thousands of instances of other unreported uses by emergency departments and other facilities (1).

Considering the medical need, it seems surprising that hospitals do not routinely monitor and stock antidotes. Numerous articles spanning at least two decades have revealed the international trend in insufficient antidote stocking. In the United States, multiple studies have documented the failure to stock antidotes (2–7). The phenomenon is international in scope, with similar reports arising from Wales and England, Canada, Spain, Taiwan, and Greece (8–13). The potential contribution of drug shortages to inadequate stocking has not been addressed in any study to date (14).

Because the potential number of victims is greater and may involve unusual drugs, stocking of antidotes in preparation for a chemical terrorist attack is even poorer and requires extensive preparation by the medical system (15,16).

Potential Consequences of Inadequate Stocking

The potential consequences of inadequate antidote stocking may seem evident to toxicologists, but research to produce data regarding adverse patient outcomes has not been performed. Most poison centers have encountered inadequate antidote stocking regularly. For example, it is not unusual to be forced to transfer patients or antidotes to obtain the needed antidote. The difficulty is that antidotes like pyridoxine, ethanol, snake antivenom, and several others are often needed immediately. If they are unavailable or their availability is delayed, the patient may die or experience injury that could have been avoided. For example, the use of antivenom has been shown repeatedly to be dependent on time (17). Delay allows tissue injury to progress and leads to prolonged recovery. It seems likely that many patients worldwide die from lack of timely antidote availability. Further, many more patients are likely to have increased injury and prolonged hospital stays due to the lack of antidotes.

SOLUTIONS TO INADEQUATE STOCKING OF ANTIDOTES

It is unlikely that a simple solution exists for this problem. One problem is that the cause of insufficient stocking is not known. Qualitative observations during research have provided some clues, and a review of the medical literature provides some hints as to solutions. For example, some antidotes are commonly stocked in adequate amounts. Naloxone and dextrose are nearly universally stocked. Other relatively well-stocked antidotes include methylene blue and flumazenil. At the other end of the spectrum, several antidotes seem to be routinely understocked, if they are stocked at all: digoxin immune Fab, polyvalent snake antivenom, pyridoxine, ethanol, and fomepizole, among others. It appears that hospitals are capable of consistently stocking some antidotes. The question arises, why aren't other antidotes stocked?

Another potential cause is financial. Antidotes like snake antivenom, digoxin antibody, and fomepizole are expensive. The explanation for this phenomenon is not as simple as expense, however, as many of the cheapest antidotes are not stocked adequately (ethanol, deferoxamine, pyridoxine, and others). Further, the cost of adequate stocking is not prohibitive, ranging from $8000 to perhaps $20,000 depending on the number of antidotes and other factors (4,8). Because antidotes all have a 2- to 3-year expiration date, the cost per year to stock antidotes for one patient amounts to several thousand dollars per year. This is approximately the same cost as one course of antineoplastic chemotherapy or of drotrecogin alfa (Xigris) for sepsis. Because these antidotes prevent major morbidity or death, the investment in antidote stocking does not seem disproportionate. Nevertheless, discussion with hospital pharmacy directors makes it clear that cost is one of the factors limiting antidote stocking (4).

Although many large hospitals also stock antidotes poorly, the size of the hospital has been found to be directly related to antidote stocking. Large hospitals have greater financial and staff resources that may allow them to address the issue of antidote stocking. Bailey and Bussieres documented that the presence of adequate antidote stocking was predicted by the amount of *N*-acetylcysteine consumed in that hospital, the number of annual visits to the emergency department, and the number of hours of pharmacy coverage on weekends (8,18). Juurlink found that higher annual emergency department volume, teaching hospital status, and designation as a trauma center predicted adequate stocking (10). Dart et al. found that lack of adequate antidote stocking was associated with several hospital characteristics: smaller surrounding population, nonteaching institution, smaller bed capacity, and lack of a formal review process for antidote stocking (4). These are all attributes of the smaller hospital.

As a group, these factors can be summarized as indicating the lack of resources to proactively assess and improve the formulary as well as to purchase expensive antidotes. In a small hospital, lack of recent use may create lack of awareness. Further, expensive antidotes consume a larger proportion of the pharmacy budget and create a greater financial strain. Finally, the personnel may not be available to monitor that antidotes are available and stocked in appropriate amounts.

One approach of hospital pharmacies has been to borrow antidotes from neighboring hospitals. This is a common pharmacy practice for rarely used drugs. This is an acceptable approach in many cases. For example, deferoxamine is normally used for chronic iron overload. It is acceptable to delay treatment for hours or a day to obtain the drug. However, this practice can be dangerous when used for emergency antidotes that should be administered within an hour or two. In the case of an acute severe iron overdose, permanent organ injury and death can occur within an hour or two. Although it is often thought by hospital pharmacies that such transfers can be arranged within 1 hour, this is rarely the case. The challenge is the lack of administrative and transportation resources to arrange for transfer and actually move the drug to another hospital. Experience indicates that such transfers typically consume several hours. This time frame is unacceptable for antidotes that are emergently needed (Table 1).

PROCESS OF ANTIDOTE STOCKING

Logically, there are three steps to the adequate stocking of antidotes in most institutions. First, the antidotes and the amount needed for stocking must be determined. Most hospital pharmacies expect the drug prescriber to propose drugs for addition to the formulary. Second, the financial resources to purchase the drugs must be available. Third, the antidote supply in the hospital must be monitored so that consumed or expired antidotes can be restocked.

WHO SPEAKS FOR ANTIDOTES?

Which antidotes should be stocked? In many hospitals, the addition to the hospital formulary is based on a physician's request. In the United States, one consistent observation has been that glucagon is stocked better than expected. Like naloxone, glucagon is a commonly used drug, albeit for endoscopy rather than poisoning. Thus, the gastroenterologist assures that it is on the hospital formulary. Naloxone, atropine, calcium, glucagon, and others are all antidotes that are typically well stocked because they are commonly used or have other uses in the institution. Besides the toxicologist, no physician group seems to be responsible for "orphan" antidotes like the cyanide antidote package, fomepizole, and several others.

No single standard for antidote stocking has been developed. The Joint Commission on Accreditation of Healthcare Organizations regulations state that a hospital must be prepared to treat poisoning, but it does not provide specific requirements. It is also important to consider the hospital's role. The antidotes stocked by hospitals that accept emergency admissions are different than a psychiatric or other hospital without general emergency services. Further, the antidotes and amounts needed are different for hospitals when considering response to chemical terrorism or proximity to industries using hazardous materials.

One approach is to develop consensus recommendations regarding antidotes. The U.S. Health Resource Services Administration supported a national consensus project to develop guidelines for hospitals that accept emergency patients (Table 1) (19). Guidelines have also been developed by the International Programme on Chemical Safety (20). Other local and regional guidelines have been developed. Although telephone contacts from numerous hospital pharmacies indicate some interest in these guidelines, objective data are not encouraging. For example, few changes were found in antidote stocking in the service area of the Rocky Mountain Poison and Drug Center after the publication of consensus guidelines (Table 1) (21). The only antidote that became better stocked was fomepizole. The stocking of all other antidotes on the list remained static. The most likely explanation for the improvement of fomepizole seems to be the manufacturer's marketing program, which was introduced about the same time. Although it is possible that there was a synergistic effect, ineffectiveness of guideline distribution was demonstrated in Greece (13).

Once an antidote and amount have been selected, the monitoring of stocking should be addressed by existing hospital pharmacy systems. At least in the United States, the Joint Commission on Accreditation of Healthcare Organizations requires that all hospital pharmacies have a system in place to monitor the supplies of the drugs they provide. Assuring immediate availability of the antidote may be more difficult. Once a drug has been added to the formulary, it should be available. However, the pharmacy manager often has substantial latitude regarding the purchase of drugs, particularly in small institutions. Simply being on the hospital formulary does not assure that the drug is immediately available. Some pharmacies have to "order out" for drugs that are on the formulary.

The issue of financial resources seems to be a large concern; however, it can easily be argued that this is a false issue. Antidotes constitute a small proportion of pharmacy drug expense. Several authors have tallied the costs of the antidotes included in their research. The cost of stocking the national consensus guidelines was $20,000 in 2000. These prices reflect the average wholesale price; therefore, the total is likely lower for most institutions. This may be another advantage for larger institutions and health care systems.

HOW TO STOCK ANTIDOTES

It is relatively simple for interested people to assure antidotes are stocked in their institution. The critical steps that seem to fail in many hospitals are the designation of an antidote on the hospital formulary and monitoring to assure that the antidote is stocked. The rest of the process is regulated, and the infrastructure should already be present in every hospital.

TABLE 1. U.S. National Consensus Guidelines for stocking of antidotes needed in hospitals accepting emergency patients

Antidote name	Poisoning indication	Stocking recommended? (yes/no)	Number of patients, dose per patient (70 kg patient)	Total stocking amount and cost[a,b] (amount, dollars)	Special comments
Acetylcysteine solution	Acetaminophen	Yes	2 × 19.6 g	39.2 g, 22.32	Because vomiting after acetylcysteine administration is common, the facility should maintain a repeat dose for each patient.
Antivenin (*Crotalidae*) polyvalent	Crotalid snakes	Yes	1 × 10 vials	10 vials, 4504.40	Should be stocked in areas with indigenous crotaline snake species (rattlesnakes, water moccasins, and copperheads). In areas without indigenous crotaline snakes, antivenom should be available due to the practice of collecting nonindigenous snakes. Facilities in areas with snakes that may cause severe envenomation (Eastern diamondback, Western diamondback, Mojave rattlesnake, canebrake rattlesnake) should individually assess their need for antivenom. In many areas, 20 vials and as much as 40 vials can be needed in a severe envenomation.[c]
Antivenin (*Latrodectus mactans*)	Black widow spider	No	1 × 1 vial	1 vial, NA	Although not routinely recommended, antivenin stocking should be considered by hospitals in endemic areas.
Atropine sulfate	Carbamate or organophosphate insecticide	Yes	2 × 75 mg	150 mg, 420.00	Agricultural regions often use organophosphate or carbamate insecticides. Hospitals in these areas should assure that they maintain sufficient stocks of atropine. The amount needed may exceed the standard recommendation.
Calcium gluconate and calcium chloride	Hydrogen fluoride or calcium-channel blocker	Yes	2 × 100 mEq	200 mEq, 67.56	Each institution should assure that both calcium gluconate and calcium chloride forms are available for emergency use. The chloride form is recommended for IV administration. The gluconate form is recommended for dermal application, or intradermal, SQ, intraarterial, or IV injection.
Cyanide kit	Cyanide	Yes	2 × 1 kit	Two kits, 549.12	One kit contains 1 amyl nitrite ampule, 300 mg of sodium nitrite, and 12.5 g of sodium thiosulfate.
Deferoxamine mesylate	Iron	Yes	1 × 8.4 g	8.4 g, 241.35	—
Digoxin immune Fab	Digoxin, digitoxin, or natural product (plants, toads)	Yes	1 × 15 vials	15 vials, 8053.20	—
Dimercaprol	Acute arsenic, inorganic mercury, lead (with encephalopathy)	Yes	1 × 280 mg	280 mg, 74.56	—
Ethylenediaminetetraacetic acid	Lead	No	1 × 1 g	1 g, NA	Although not routinely recommended, hospitals may choose to stock ethylenediaminetetraacetic acid due to endemic lead poisoning.
Ethanol, solution for injection	Methanol or ethylene glycol	Yes	2 × 90.7 ml	181.4 ml absolute alcohol, 798.10	A hospital should stock at least one alcohol dehydrogenase-blocking drug. The panel did not reach consensus regarding which agent is preferred. Either fomepizole or ethanol may be stocked.
Flumazenil	Benzodiazepines	Consensus not achieved	1 × 4 mg	4 mg, NA	If a hospital decides to stock flumazenil due to their patient population, a total of 4 mg is recommended.
Fomepizole (4-methylpyrazole)	Methanol or ethylene glycol	Yes	2 × 1.05 g	2.1 g, 2400.00	A hospital should stock at least one alcohol dehydrogenase-blocking drug. The panel did not reach consensus regarding which agent is preferred. Either fomepizole or ethanol may be stocked.[d]
Glucagon	Beta adrenergic antagonist or calcium-channel blocker	Yes	1 × 50 mg	50 mg, 1922.50	—
Methylene blue	Methemoglobinemia	Yes	2 × 140 mg	280 mg, 133.28	—
Naloxone hydrochloride	Acute opioid poisoning	Yes	2 × 15 mg	30 mg, 411.75	—
Physostigmine salicylate	Anticholinergic agents	Consensus not achieved	2 × 2 mg	4 mg, NA	If a hospital decides to stock physostigmine due to their patient population, a total of 2–4 mg is recommended.
Pralidoxime chloride	Organophosphate insecticide	Yes	2 × 1 g	2 g, 128.26	Agricultural regions often use organophosphate insecticides. Hospitals in these areas should assure that they maintain sufficient stocks of pralidoxime. The amount needed may exceed the standard recommendation.
Pyridoxine	Isoniazid	Yes	1 × 10 g	10 g, 50.00	Hospitals in areas where isoniazid is used frequently (e.g., where tuberculosis is common) should consider stocking 20 g.
Sodium bicarbonate	Tricyclic antidepressant, cocaine, salicylates	Yes	1 × 500 mEq	500 mEq, 32.00	—
Total				**19,808.60**	

NA, not applicable, drug not recommended for all hospitals.
[a]Total stocking amount = [number of patients] × [dose recommended to treat one patient for first 4 hours].
[b]Based on average wholesale price, using generic products when available (22). Please note that the total includes more than one patient for several antidotes.
[c]This antivenom should be stocked by all hospitals in indigenous regions (Florida, Georgia, Alabama, Mississippi, Louisiana, and Texas) but may be stocked by selected hospitals on a regional basis.
[d]Please note that fomepizole is available only in four-vial tray packs. Some institutions have created methods for sharing tray packs.
Modified from Dart RC, Goldfrank LE, Chyka PA. *Ann Emerg Med* 2000;36:126–132.

The initiation process requires the interest of either a physician or pharmacist. This person can request the hospital pharmacy or the Institutional Pharmacy and Therapeutics Committee to address the issue. The monitoring process is likely more problematic. From a regulatory perspective, any hospital in the United States must account for all drugs stocked and dispensed. However, this does not mean that each antidote must be on the shelf and immediately available. An interested clinical can assure that this occurs. The potential approaches are to discuss the issue with the pharmacy director and to periodically inquire about rarely used but life-saving antidotes such as digoxin immune Fab.

REFERENCES

1. American Association of Poison Control Centers. 2001 Annual Report of the American Association of Poison Control Centers Toxic Exposure Surveillance System. Available at: http://www.poison.org. Accessed January 16, 2003.
2. Chyka PA, Conner HG. Availability of antidotes in rural and urban hospitals in Tennessee. *Am J Hosp Pharm* 1994;51:1346–1348.
3. Dart RC, Duncan C, McNally JT. Effect of inadequate antivenin stores on the medical treatment of crotalid envenomation. *Vet Human Toxicol* 1991;33:267–269.
4. Dart RC, Stark Y, Fulton B, et al. Insufficient stocking of poisoning antidotes in hospital emergency departments. *JAMA* 1996;276:1508–1510.
5. Howland MA, Weisman R, Sauter D, et al. Nonavailability of poison antidotes. *N Engl J Med* 1986;314:927–928.
6. Kanatani MS, Kearney TE, Levin RH, et al. Treatment of toxicologic emergencies: an evaluation of Bay Area hospital pharmacies and its impact on emergency planning. *Vet Human Toxicol* 1992;34:319(abst).
7. Woolf AD, Chrisanthus K. On-site availability of selected antidotes: results of a survey of Massachusetts hospitals. *Am J Emerg Med* 1998;15:62–66.
8. Bailey B, Bussieres JF. Antidote availability in Quebec hospital pharmacies: impact of *N*-acetylcysteine and naloxone consumption. *Can J Clin Pharmacol* 2000;7:198–204.
9. Higgins MA, Evans R. Antidotes—inappropriate timely availability. *Human Exp Toxicol* 2000;19:485–488.
10. Juurlink DN, McGuigan MA, Paton TW, et al. Availability of antidotes at acute care hospitals in Ontario. *CMAJ* 2001;165:27–30.
11. Nogue S, Soy D, Munne P, et al. Antidotes: availability, use and cost in hospital and extra-hospital emergency services of Catalonia (Spain). *Arch Toxicol* 1997;19[Suppl]:299–304.
12. Ong HC, Yang CC, Deng JF. Inadequate stocking of antidotes in Taiwan: is it a serious problem? *J Toxicol Clin Toxicol* 2000;38:21–28.
13. Plataki M, Anatoliotakis N, Tzanakis N, et al. Availability of antidotes in hospital pharmacies in Greece. *Vet Human Toxicol* 2001;43:103–105.
14. Tyler LS, Fox ER, Caravati EM. The challenge of drug shortages for emergency medicine. *Ann Emerg Med* 2002;40:598–602.
15. Greenberg MI, Jurgens SM, Gracely EJ. Emergency department preparedness for the evaluation and treatment of victims of biological or chemical terrorist attack. *J Emerg Med* 2002;22:273–278.
16. Sharp TW, Brennan RJ, Keim M, et al. Medical preparedness for a terrorist incident involving chemical and biological agents during the 1996 Atlanta Olympic games. *Ann Emerg Med* 1998;32:214–223.
17. Dart RC, Goldner A, Lindsey D. Efficacy of post envenomation administration of antivenin. *Toxicon* 1988;26:1218–1221.
18. Bussieres JF, Bailey B. Insufficient stocking of antidotes in hospital pharmacies: problem, causes, and solution. *Can J Hosp Pharm* 2000;53:325–337.
19. Dart RC, Goldfrank LF, Chyka PA, et al. Combined evidence-based literature analysis and consensus guidelines for stocking of emergency antidotes in the United States. *Ann Emerg Med* 2000;36:126–132.
20. Pronczuk de Garbino J, Hatines JA, Jacobsen D, et al. Evaluation of antidotes: activities of the International Programme on Chemical Safety. *J Toxicol Clin Toxicol* 1997;35:333–343.
21. Bogdan GM, Hill RE, Dart RC. Effect of poison center recommendations on hospital pharmacy stocking of emergency antidotes. *J Toxicol Clin Toxicol* 1999;37:597(abst).
22. Spoerke DG, Spoerke SE, Rumack BH. International opinion concerning indications, safety and availability of poison centre antidotes and treatment. *Human Toxicol* 1987;6:361–364.

CHAPTER 42

Atropine

Miguel C. Fernández

CH_3 N H O O OH

ATROPINE

Synonyms:	**Atropine sulfate**
Molecular formula and weight:	**$(C_{17}H_{23}NO_3)_2$, H_2SO_4, H_2O, 694.8 g/mol**
SI conversion:	**μg/L × 3.46 = nmol/L**
CAS Registry No.:	**5908-99-6**
Normal or therapeutic levels:	**Not applicable**
Special concerns:	**Overuse of atropine, particularly in a patient without true cholinergic poisoning, can cause anticholinergic syndrome.**

OVERVIEW

Atropine is a white, odorless crystalline powder, occurring in nature only as a racemic mixture of D- and L-hyoscyamine enantiomers, the latter of which is the most biologically active, and is structurally similar to cocaine. Atropos is the name of one of the three fates of ancient Greek cosmology who was responsible for cutting the thread of one's life, thus ending it.

Atropine occurs naturally in plants such as *Atropa belladonna* (deadly nightshade, dwale, poison black cherry, belladonna) and in *Datura* species (jimsonweed, thornapple), sometimes with its related isomer scopolamine (L-hyoscine) (Chapter 255). Although now cultivated throughout the world, *Atropa belladonna* originated in Eurasia where it has been used for centuries as an aphrodisiac and hallucinogen as well as a medicine and poison (1). The name *belladonna*, as in "belladonna alkaloids," is derived from Latin, meaning "beautiful woman" because mydriasis was perceived as more attractive in Roman culture. Atropine sulfate was approved for use in the United States in 1938.

Forms Available

Parenteral atropine sulfate is available in 0.4-mg/ml, 0.4-mg/0.5 ml, 0.5-mg/ml, and 1-mg/ml vials and ampules, and prefilled syringes of 0.05 mg/ml, 0.5 mg/5 ml, and 1 mg/10 ml. It may be purchased in bulk as well (2).

Atropine is also available in an autoinjector as part of the Mark I Nerve Agent Antidote Kit (Meridian Medical Technologies, Columbia, MD) for treatment of nerve agent poisoning. The Mark I Nerve Agent Antidote Kit contains single-unit doses of atropine sulfate and pralidoxime chloride and is designed to be self-injected intramuscularly by individuals when first symptoms occur (3). The autoinjector is a hard plastic tube with a pressure-activated coiled-spring mechanism that, when pressed to the skin surface after removing the safety cap, triggers the 22-gauge needle to inject 2 mg (0.7 ml) of atropine sulfate. The needle is 2 cm in length and can penetrate clothing but not bunker gear. However, the autoinjector is not appropriate for children, although the contents can be discharged and administered intramuscularly to children (4).

A new kit, the Antidote Treatment Nerve Agent autoinjector, is expected to replace the Mark I Nerve Agent Antidote Kit. It is unique in its use of a single prefilled multichambered autoinjector that delivers atropine and pralidoxime in a single injection while maintaining separation of the two drugs in the injector and injection site. A wet/dry multichambered autoinjector that delivers atropine and an H-series oxime is currently in development (5).

Mechanism of Action

Atropine is a competitive antagonist of acetylcholine. It prevents depolarization and thereby nerve conduction by blocking acetylcholine at muscarinic receptors, which are present on the postsynaptic membrane on autonomic synapses in smooth and cardiac muscle, in exocrine glands, and in nerve ganglia. As a parasympatholytic drug, it may act as an anticholinergic neurotoxin in high doses, but it has no significant effect on nicotinic receptors. Atropine crosses the blood–brain barrier and the placenta (6,7).

Its antimuscarinic activity can effectively reverse muscarinic hyperstimulation in organophosphate (OP) poisoning. It therefore antagonizes the OP-induced hypersalivation, bronchorrhea, bronchospasm, bradycardia, hypotension, lacrimation, urinary incontinence, diarrhea, miosis, gastrointestinal cramping, emesis, and central nervous system disturbances.

Sympathomimetic drugs potentiate the anticholinergic properties of atropine and include the catecholamines (dopamine, dobutamine, epinephrine, isoproterenol, norepinephrine); noncatecholamines (amphetamine, ephedrine, methamphetamine, phenylephrine); and selective beta-adrenergic agonists (albuterol, metaproterenol, ritodrine, terbutaline). The anticholinergic effects of atropine can be reversed by the cholinergic actions of bethanechol; methacholine; or, more commonly, physostigmine (8).

INDICATIONS

Bradydysrhythmia

Atropine is used as a first-line medication for symptomatic bradydysrhythmia (e.g., hypotension, lightheadedness, nausea, vomiting, and so forth). It provides positive chronotropic and dromotropic effects. It is often ineffective in poisoning-induced bradycardia, and other interventions may be needed.

Organophosphate and Nerve Agent Poisoning

The clinical indication for atropine administration is bronchospasm or bronchorrhea arising from an excess of acetylcholine. These conditions typically include carbamate or OP insecticides, edrophonium, or other therapeutic cholinesterase inhibitors and nerve agents (Chapters 101 and 260).

Scorpion Envenomation

Atropine can successfully antagonize the cholinergic effects (e.g., hypersalivation) of the *Centruroides* scorpion sting in children (9).

Other Uses

Atropine is used as an antisecretory agent, a bronchodilator, a gastrointestinal antispasmodic, an ophthalmic cycloplegic and mydriatic, and a premedication to anesthesia induction in children.

CAUTIONS AND CONTRAINDICATIONS

Atropine should be used with caution in patients with tachycardia or hypertension because these conditions may be exacerbated. In the case of OP or nerve agent poisoning, catecholamine release may cause tachycardia with or without hypertension and does not contraindicate its careful titration for other effects of cholinergic crisis (10).

Ophthalmic application can produce systemic absorption and toxicity. Ophthalmic preparations are contraindicated in known or suspected acute angle closure glaucoma because of the likelihood of increasing intraocular pressure, especially in the elderly. Prolonged use of atropine in the eye may cause irritation, hyperemia, and edema of the eye (11).

High environmental temperatures may precipitate heat-related illness in patients treated with anticholinergic medications like atropine. Overtreatment with atropine may cause an anticholinergic syndrome.

Atropine sulfate is U.S. Food and Drug Administration pregnancy category C. Atropine passes into breast milk, but clinical toxicity has not been reported.

DOSAGE AND METHOD OF ADMINISTRATION

Bradydysrhythmia

The initial *adult dose* is 0.5 to 1.0 mg intravenously (IV) and the *pediatric dose* is 0.01 mg/kg (0.04 mg/kg). This dose may be repeated every few minutes until heart rate increases. Bradycardia arising from poisoning may be refractory, and other interventions may be needed. Doses less than 0.5 mg for an adult or 0.1 mg for a child should be avoided due to the potential for paradoxical bradycardia. It is generally believed that atropine can be effectively administered endotracheally or intraosseously (12).

Organophosphate and Nerve Agent Poisoning

For the treatment of cholinergic signs (bronchospasm, bronchorrhea) from any OP agent, a full vagolytic *adult dose* is 2 mg IV push and the pediatric dose is 0.05 mg/kg. If possible, the patient should be oxygenated before administration to prevent cardiac dysrhythmia. For known nerve agent poisoning, a larger initial dose (6 mg in adults) should be used. The atropine dose should be repeated every 2 to 5 minutes until drying of airway secretions and improved respiratory status are apparent. Atropine does not treat the muscular weakness and paralysis seen with cholinergic syndrome (there are no muscarinic receptors in skeletal muscle). Concurrent treatment with an OP reactivator may be needed (Chapter 69).

Doses in excess of 1 g have been required over 24 hours for severe OP insecticide poisoning. Nerve agents rarely require massive doses (13).

Atropine is also effective intramuscularly and has reportedly been administered by continuous IV infusion, continuous intraosseous infusion, as well as inhalation via nebulization (12). Because it acts on airway receptors, atropine is expected to be effective by the endotracheal route.

Atropine acts as an effective cycloplegic and mydriatic for as long as 1 to 2 weeks in a dose of 0.6 mg (approximately one drop of a 1% ophthalmic solution).

Scorpion Envenomation

For scorpion envenomation, the pediatric dose for atropine is 0.005 to 0.01 mg/kg IV (9). The precise role in therapy is unclear, but this dose has been used to control copious oral secretions, particularly if secretions may compromise the airway in small children.

Monitoring

Atropine should be administered in an intensive care setting with continuous cardiorespiratory monitoring.

ADVERSE EFFECTS

Atropine causes anticholinergic toxicity (Chapter 10) (e.g., atropism, the typical antimuscarinic symptoms of tachycardia, mental status changes, hyperthermia, visual disturbances, mydriasis, urinary retention, constipation, flushing, and anhydrosis).

PITFALLS

Pitfalls to avoid in using atropine are failure to provide atropine in vagolytic doses during bradydysrhythmic events and failure to provide enough atropine to reverse muscarinic effects of cholinergic poisoning (OP and carbamate insecticides). Significant poisoning by these agents may require the atropine stores of an entire hospital for one patient.

Discontinuation of atropine based on premature development of tachycardia (which may actually be due to sympathomimetic effects from cholinergic stimulation of the adrenal medulla) may not allow control of bronchial secretions.

Lack of miosis should not be used as an indicator to withhold treatment because the nicotinic effects of cholinergic excess may cause mydriasis.

REFERENCES

1. Mann J. *Murder, magic, and medicine*. New York: Oxford University Press, 1992.
2. Geller RJ, Lopez GP, Cutler S, et al. Antidote availability: reformulation of bulk atropine for nerve agent casualties. Presented at Catastrophic Care for the Nation: National Disaster Medical System Conference 1999. Washington; May 11, 1999.
3. Departments of the Army, the Navy, and the Air Force, and Commandant, Marine Corps. Treatment of chemical agent casualties and conventional military chemical injuries. Washington, DC, 1996; FM8-285, Part 1, Chapter 2.
4. Henretig FM, Mechem C, Jew R. Potential use of Autoinjector-packaged antidotes for treatment of pediatric nerve agent toxicity. *Ann Emerg Med* 2002;40:405–408.
5. Meridian Medical Technologies, Inc. Available at: http://www.meridianmeds.com/civdef.html. Accessed September 2002.
6. Van Der Meer MJ. The metabolism of atropine in man. *J Pharm Pharacol* 1986;38:781–784.
7. Kaiser SC, McClain PL. Atropine metabolism in man. *Clin Pharmacol Ther* 1970;11:214–227.
8. Brown JH, Taylor P. Muscarinic receptor agonists and antagonists. In: Gilman A, Goodman LS, Rall TW, et al., eds. *Goodman and Gilman's the pharmacologic basis of therapeutics*, 9th ed. New York: McGraw-Hill, 1996: 149.
9. Suchard JR, Hilder R. Atropine use in *Centruroides* scorpion envenomation. *J Toxicol Clin Toxicol* 2001;39:595–598.
10. Johnson MK, Jacobsen D, Meredith TJ, et al. Evaluation of antidotes for poisoning by organophosphorus pesticides. *Emerg Med* 2000;12:22–37.
11. Lahdes K, Kaila T, Hunponen R, et al. Systemic absorption of topically applied ocular atropine. *Clin Pharmacol Ther* 1988;44:310–314.
12. Prete MR, Hannan CJ Jr, Burkle FM Jr. Plasma atropine concentrations via intravenous, endotracheal, and intraosseous administration. *Am J Emerg Med* 1987;5:101–104.
13. Sidell FR. Nerve agents. In: Sidell FR, Takafuji EJ, Franz DR. *Medical aspects of chemical and biological warfare*. Washington: Borden Institute, Walter Reed Army Medical Center, 1997:129–179.

CHAPTER 43

Benztropine

Alison L. Jones and Robert J. Flanagan

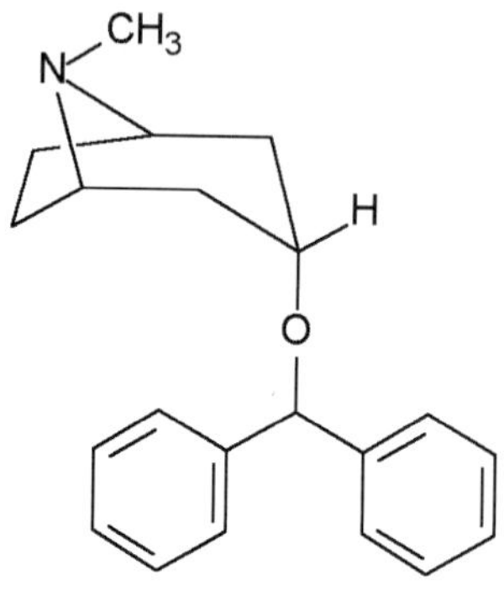

BENZTROPINE

Synonym:	**Benztropine mesylate (Cogentin)**
Molecular formula and weight:	**$C_{21}H_{25}NO$, CH_4O_3S, 403.5 g/mol**
SI conversion:	**mg/L × 3.25 = µmol/L**
CAS Registry No.:	**132-17-2**
Therapeutic level:	**Not recommended or clinically useful**

OVERVIEW

Benztropine is an anticholinergic and antihistaminic medication used in toxicology for dystonias and oculogyric crisis. Its mechanism is competitive inhibition of muscarinic receptors and blockade of dopamine reuptake.

INDICATIONS

Dystonia and Oculogyric Crisis

Benztropine can reverse dystonia associated with neuroleptics, such as haloperidol, phenothiazines, and thioxanthines, and with metoclopramide. It is commonly used to treat the oculogyric crisis that is common in young women given metoclopramide.

Parkinsonism

Benztropine is also effective in drug-induced parkinsonism as well as in true Parkinson's disease.

CAUTIONS AND CONTRAINDICATIONS

Benztropine is U.S. Food and Drug Administration pregnancy category C. It is contraindicated in patients with glaucoma or with prostatic hypertrophy, in whom worsening symptoms would be expected after exposure.

DOSAGE AND ADMINISTRATION

Dystonia and Oculogyric Crisis

For acute dystonia or oculogyric crisis, the *adult dose* is 1 to 4 mg intravenously (IV) or intramuscularly (IM) one to two times daily (1). The *pediatric dose* is 1 to 2 mg IV or IM (2). One dose of benztropine is usually adequate in the case of oculogyric crisis due to metoclopramide. Bioavailability after oral administration is poor and not recommended for acute treatment.

Parkinsonism

The typical dose for Parkinson's disease is 1 to 2 mg/day orally or parenterally.

ADVERSE EFFECTS

Acute adverse effects are anticholinergic (tachycardia, decreased bowel sounds, urinary retention, blurred vision). Most adverse effects occur with chronic administration and involve the central nervous system (memory dysfunction, tardive dyskinesia).

PITFALLS

Patients with dystonias who have been poisoned by long-acting neuroleptics should be given continuation oral therapy for approximately 3 days to prevent relapse (benztropine, 1 to 2 mg twice daily, or diphenhydramine, 25 mg three times daily).

REFERENCES

1. Hasan MY, Schauben JL, Holmes CH. Management of neuroleptic malignant syndrome with anticholinergic medication. *Vet Hum Toxicol* 1999;41:79–81.
2. Dahiya U, Noronha P. Drug-induced acute dystonic reactions in children: alternatives to diphenhydramine therapy. *Postgrad Med* 1984;75:286–290.

CHAPTER 44

Calcium Salts

Alison L. Jones and Robert J. Flanagan

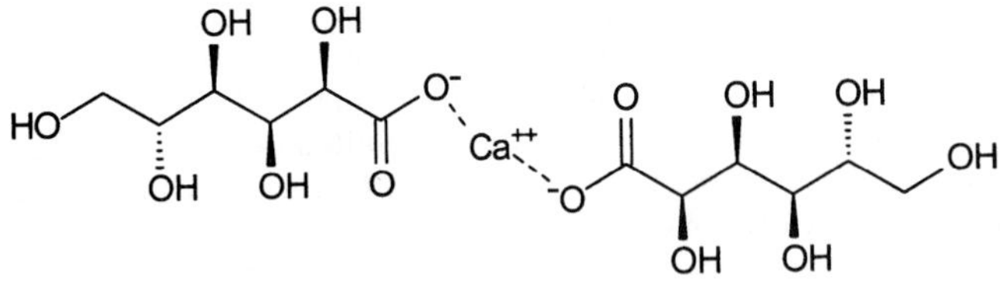

CALCIUM GLUCONATE

Synonyms:	**Calcium chloride, calcium gluconate**
Molecular formula and weight:	**Calcium chloride ($CaCl_2$), 111.0; calcium gluconate ($C_{12}H_{22}CaO_{14}$), 430.4 g/mol**
SI conversion:	**mg/L × 0.025 = mmol/L**
CAS Registry No.:	**10035-04-8 (calcium chloride dihydrate); 18016-24-5 (calcium gluconate monohydrate)**
Normal levels:	**Serum calcium, 8.5–10.5 mg/dl (2.1–2.6 mmol/L); blood ionized calcium, 1.14–1.30 mmol/L**
Special concerns:	**Topical or subcutaneous injection of $CaCl_2$ can cause skin necrosis.**

OVERVIEW

Calcium salts are used to treat hydrofluoric acid (HF) burns or hypocalcemia arising from HF ingestion and calcium channel–blocker toxicity. Calcium chloride is provided as a 10% (100 mg/ml) solution. An ampule contains 10 ml (1 g $CaCl_2$; 13.6 mEq calcium ion). Calcium gluconate is provided as a 10% (100 mg/ml) solution. An ampule contains 10 ml (1 g calcium gluconate; 4.5 mEq calcium ion).

Mechanism of Action

The topical administration of calcium salts allows calcium to bind fluoride ions. Insoluble calcium fluoride is formed, thus preventing further skin penetration of the acid. The administration of calcium salts for HF-induced hypocalcemia maintains an adequate concentration of ionized calcium, thereby preventing cardiac dysrhythmias.

INDICATIONS

Hydrofluoric Acid Skin Exposure

Dermal application of calcium-containing gel is used for mild to moderate pain. More invasive techniques (subcutaneous injection, regional perfusion, or intraarterial infusion) are used for patients with severe and persistent pain (Chapter 207).

Hydrofluoric Acid Ingestion

Ingestion of HF can precipitate cardiovascular collapse quickly. Systemic hypocalcemia, prolonged QTc interval, or other evidence of hypocalcemia are indications for intravenous (IV) calcium treatment. Consider prophylactic use for large or suicidal ingestion (1). Calcium gluconate administration has also been suggested for treating poisoning due to the ingestion of fluoride salts (2).

Calcium Channel–Blocker Overdose

Calcium administration is recommended at the first sign of bradycardia, hypotension, heart block, or any other serious signs of toxicity, although there are doubts about its efficacy (3). Other measures should be instituted if the patient does not improve promptly (Chapter 121).

Other Toxicology Uses

Calcium salts have also been used to antagonize the neuromuscular paralysis associated with hyperkalemia and hypermagnesemia, as well as muscle spasm occurring after *Latrodectus mactans* (black widow spider) envenomation (Chapter 248). Calcium salts have also been used to treat hypocalcemia caused by ethylene glycol toxicity.

CAUTIONS AND CONTRAINDICATIONS

Calcium should not be coadministered with a sodium bicarbonate infusion, as insoluble calcium carbonate will be formed.

Calcium is U.S. Food and Drug Administration pregnancy category C. Calcium preparations are commonly administered to women during pregnancy for a variety of reasons.

DOSAGE AND ADMINISTRATION

Hydrofluoric Acid Burns

Calcium gluconate gel (2.5% weight per weight) is used topically to treat HF burns. Calcium gluconate gel 2.5% can be extemporaneously prepared in the pharmacy using 3.5 g calcium gluconate powder in 150 ml of a water-soluble lubricant, such as K-Y Jelly. The gel should be applied to the affected area for at least 30 minutes, usually longer. If a higher concentration product (e.g., HF concentration greater than 20%) is used or if pain persists, 10% [weight per volume (w/vol)] calcium gluconate can be injected (0.5 ml depots using 30-gauge needle) under the site of the injury to achieve intradermal and subcutaneous penetration. The use of this method is limited because most dermal exposures involve areas, such as the fingers, in which significant volume cannot be injected.

Refractory cases can be treated with regional perfusion of calcium or intraarterial infusion (4). Intraarterial infusion of calcium gluconate [10 ml 10% (w/vol) calcium gluconate diluted with 40 ml 5% (w/vol) dextrose] has also been suggested to treat HF burns in the arms or legs (5–7).

Hydrofluoric Acid Ingestion

Hypocalcemia induced by HF ingestion is often refractory to treatment. Large amounts of calcium are likely to be needed; therefore, calcium chloride is preferred. Calcium chloride 10% is preferred over calcium gluconate. The initial *adult dose* is 1 ampule (10 ml of 10% solution) infused over 5 minutes. The *pediatric dose* is 10 to 25 mg/kg up to 1 ampule per dose. Dose may be repeated every 10 minutes or more frequently as needed using the QTc interval and clinical signs as a guide.

The *adult dose* of calcium gluconate 10% is 10 to 30 ml (i.e., 1 to 3 g) IV over 5 minutes. The *pediatric dose* is 30 to 75 mg/kg over 5 minutes, up to 1 g/dose. This dose may be repeated every 10 minutes as needed.

Calcium Channel–Blocker Overdose

There is 8.9 mg Ca^{2+} in a 10-ml 10% (w/vol) calcium gluconate ampule, whereas there is 27.3 mg Ca^{2+} in 10 ml of 10% (w/vol) calcium chloride; thus, the chloride tends to be preferred in the treatment of calcium channel–blocker overdose (see Chapter 121). The *adult and pediatric dose* is 0.2 to 0.5 ml/kg of a 10% (w/vol) solution of the gluconate or chloride salt (maximum, 10 ml) IV over 5 to 10 minutes. If necessary, the dose may be repeated in 10 to 15 minutes.

Other Toxicology Uses

A similar regimen (0.1 to 0.2 ml gluconate/kg) has been used to reverse hypocalcemia in severe poisoning with ethylene glycol or oxalates. Only symptomatic hypocalcemia should be corrected, however, as excessive administration can lead to increased calcium oxalate deposition in the kidneys and, hence, more serious renal damage.

Monitoring

Monitor serum calcium, preferably ionized calcium, frequently during therapy. In severe calcium channel–blocker overdose, large doses of calcium (producing significant hypercalcemia) may be required.

ADVERSE EFFECTS

Calcium use in the presence of digitalis has been reported to cause cardiac tetany. Transient hypercalcemia may cause cardiac dysrhythmia, hypertension, muscle weakness, and lethargy. Calcium chloride can cause venous thrombosis after IV infusion and skin necrosis if used intradermally, subcutaneously, or topically.

PITFALLS

Large amounts of calcium may be needed to treat hypocalcemia from severe fluoride or calcium channel–blocker poisoning.

Myocardial depression from transient hypercalcemia may occur if calcium is administered IV too rapidly.

REFERENCES

1. Kao WF, Dart RC, Kuffner E, Bogdan G. Ingestion of low concentration hydrofluoric acid: an insidious and potentially fatal poisoning. *Ann Emerg Med* 1999;34:35–41.
2. Lheureux P, Even-Adin D, Askenasi R. Current status of antidotal therapies in acute human intoxications. *Acta Clinica Belgica* 1990;13[Suppl]:29–47.
3. Jaeger A, Le Tacon S, Bosquet C, Sauder P. Effects of poisons on ion channels. *J Toxicol Clin Toxicol* 2000;38:160–161(abst).
4. Graudins A, Burns MJ, Aaron CK. Regional intravenous infusion of calcium gluconate for hydrofluoric acid burns of the upper extremity. *Ann Emerg Med* 1997,30:604–607.
5. Caravati EM. Acute hydrofluoric acid exposure. *Am J Emerg Med* 1988;6:143–150.
6. Vance MV, Curry SC, Kunkel DB, et al. Digital hydrofluoric acid burns: treatment with intraarterial calcium infusion. *Ann Emerg Med* 1986;15:890–896.
7. Velvart J. Arterial perfusion for hydrofluoric acid burns. *Hum Toxicol* 1983;2:233–238.

CHAPTER 45

Calcium Disodium Ethylenediaminetetraacetic Acid ($CaNa_2EDTA$)

Luke Yip

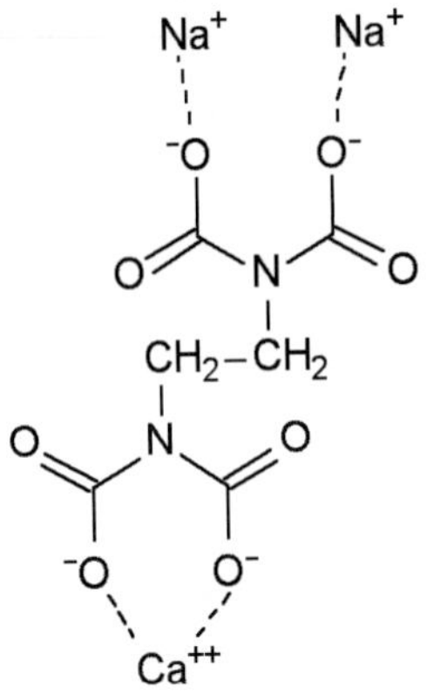

CALCIUM DISODIUM ETHYLENEDIAMINETETRAACETIC ACID

Synonyms:	**Ethylenediaminetetraacetic acid (EDTA), edetate calcium disodium, disodium calcium edetate, calcium disodium versenate, calcium disodium edathamil**
Molecular formula and weight:	**$C_{10}H_{18}N_2Na_2O_{10}$, 372.24 g/mol**
CAS Registry No.:	**36499-65-7**
Normal or therapeutic levels:	**Not applicable**
Special concerns:	**EDTA can potentially worsen lead encephalopathy; it should be first used 4 hours after dimercaprol.**

OVERVIEW

Edetate calcium disodium ($CaNa_2EDTA$) is an intravenous (IV) heavy metal chelating agent. Its primary use, with dimercaprol, is in the treatment of serious lead poisoning and lead encephalopathy.

Mechanism of Action

The calcium component of EDTA can be displaced by divalent and trivalent metals to form a water-soluble complex (chelate) that is readily eliminated by the kidneys. $CaNa_2EDTA$ rapidly and uniformly diffuses throughout the body, but it does not enter red blood cells, and it crosses the blood–brain barrier slowly (1). In animals, $CaNa_2EDTA$ does not effectively reduce total brain lead levels (2). $CaNa_2EDTA$ mobilizes lead from soft tissue stores and, to a lesser extent, increases excretion of endogenous metals, such as zinc, manganese, iron, and copper. Peak urinary lead excretion occurs within the first 24 hours, which represents excretion from soft tissues. Lead is slowly chelated from the skeletal system, as equilibrium is reestablished between bone and soft tissue compartments.

INDICATIONS

Lead

$CaNa_2EDTA$ has been proposed as treatment for lead encephalopathy as well as lesser degrees of lead poisoning. For *lead encephalopathy*, most clinicians advocate the use of British Anti-lewisite (BAL) and $CaNa_2EDTA$. For symptomatic *lead poisoning without lead encephalopathy*, many clinicians advocate the same course of treatment as for those with encephalopathy but with lower doses of BAL and $CaNa_2EDTA$. For *asymptomatic adults or children* with blood lead concentration of 70 to 100 μg/dl and 45 to 70 μg/dl, respectively, chelation therapy with $CaNa_2EDTA$ is recommended as a second-line agent for patients who cannot tolerate or are allergic to succimer (dimercaptosuccinic acid) or who are noncompliant with oral therapy.

Cadmium Poisoning

Treatment with $CaNa_2EDTA$ may be effective when administered immediately after cadmium exposure, as $CaNa_2EDTA$ increases urinary cadmium excretion in rodents (3). The effectiveness of chelation for chronic cadmium poisoning is questionable because of cadmium's long half-life, resulting from high-affinity binding to metallothionein. Because metallothionein is synthesized in large amounts by 24 to 48 hours after exposure, it is unlikely that chelation will be effective.

Cobalt Poisoning

In animal studies, $CaNa_2EDTA$ appears to be protective against cobalt chloride toxicity (4).

Copper Poisoning

$CaNa_2EDTA$ has been used as an adjunct to intramuscular (IM) BAL therapy in treatment of acute severe copper poisoning (5,6). However, the evidence for efficacy is inconclusive.

Uranium Poisoning

Chelation is a potential adjunct therapy that can be considered after a significant acute uranium exposure. Animal data indicate the median lethal dose can be significantly raised by administering polyamine-polycarbonic acid and polyamine-polyalkylphosphonic acids, such as $CaNa_2EDTA$, Na_2Ca_2-diethylenetriamine pentamenthylphosphonic acid, and diethylenetriamine pentaacetic acid (7–11).

Zinc Poisoning

$CaNa_2EDTA$ lowers elevated serum zinc levels (12,13); however, the need to treat acute zinc overdose with chelation therapy has been questioned (14).

CAUTIONS AND CONTRAINDICATIONS

Treatment with $CaNa_2EDTA$ may involve large fluid volumes. Rapid or large-volume IV infusion may exacerbate cerebral edema or the increased intracranial pressure associated with lead encephalopathy. Caution should be exercised with renal failure patients because increased renal lead excretion and renal $CaNa_2EDTA$ accumulation potentially increase the risk of nephrotoxicity.

DOSAGE AND METHOD OF ADMINISTRATION

$CaNa_2EDTA$ can be administered IV or IM, with the former being the preferred and most effective route. The patient's body weight or surface area, the severity of the intoxication, and renal function determine the dose and schedule. Adequate urine output should be established before initiating $CaNa_2EDTA$ therapy. Chelation therapy guidelines are summarized below (15–20). $CaNa_2EDTA$ is incompatible with solutions other than 5.0% dextrose or 0.9% sodium chloride.

Lead Encephalopathy

The priming dose of BAL is 75 mg/m^2 (3 to 5 mg/kg) IM and is administered every 4 hours. The recommended $CaNa_2EDTA$ dose is 1500 mg/m^2/day (30 mg/kg/day) administered as a continuous infusion, starting 4 hours after the initial BAL dose. If evidence of cerebral edema or increased intracranial pressure is present, $CaNa_2EDTA$ (same dosage) should be given by deep IM injection in two to three divided doses every 8 to 12 hours. When the IM route is used, procaine (0.5%) should be given along with $CaNa_2EDTA$ because IM administration is extremely painful. The BAL and $CaNa_2EDTA$ combined regimen is continued for 5 days.

In patients with high body lead burden, cessation of chelation is often followed by a rebound in blood lead level as bone stores equilibrate with soft tissues. A second course of chelation may be considered based on whole blood lead level after 2 days' interruption of chelation treatment and the persistence or recurrence of symptoms. A third course may be required if the whole blood concentration rebounds to 50 µg/dl or greater within 48 hours after the second course of chelation. If a third time is needed, it should begin one week after the last dose of BAL and $CaNa_2EDTA$.

Symptomatic Lead Poisoning without Lead Encephalopathy

The priming dose of BAL is 50 mg/m^2 (2 to 3 mg/kg) IM and is administered every 4 hours. Four hours after the initial BAL dose, a continuous slow IV infusion of $CaNa_2EDTA$ 1000 mg/m^2/day (20 to 30 mg/kg/day) is started. Alternatively, $CaNa_2EDTA$ may be given in two to three divided doses every 8 to 12 hours by deep IM injection. BAL and $CaNa_2EDTA$ may be continued for 5 days with periodic monitoring of whole blood lead levels. BAL may be discontinued any time if the whole blood lead concentration decreases below 50 µg/dl, but $CaNa_2EDTA$ treatment should continue for 5 days. Many practitioners convert the patient to another oral chelating agent during this period, depending on the severity of poisoning and the patient's ability to tolerate oral medications. A second or third course of chelation may be considered based on the same guidelines as discussed in the section Lead Encephalopathy.

Asymptomatic Patients with High Blood Lead Levels

If $CaNa_2EDTA$ is used, the dose is 1000 mg/m^2/day (20 to 30 mg/kg/day) as a continuous slow IV infusion or in two to three divided doses every 8 to 12 hours for 5 days. It is reasonable to allow 10 to 14 days for equilibration of the blood lead level before considering retreatment.

Cadmium Poisoning

The suggested $CaNa_2EDTA$ dose is 75 mg/kg/day in three to six divided doses for 5 days, and the total $CaNa_2EDTA$ dose for the 5 days should not exceed 500 mg/kg (3). A second course of chelation may be considered based on the whole blood cadmium level after 2 days' interruption of therapy.

Cobalt Poisoning

In animal studies, $CaNa_2EDTA$ at 670 mg/kg (1.8 mmol/kg) was completely protective against cobalt chloride toxicity (4). However, no dosing regimens have been studied in humans. If chelation were attempted, a dose of 75 mg/kg/day in three to six divided doses for 5 days, with the total $CaNa_2EDTA$ dose for the 5 days not exceeding 500 mg/kg, may be a reasonable starting point.

Copper Poisoning

Dosing has not been well studied. If chelation were attempted, a reasonable starting point may be the same as for cobalt poisoning.

Uranium Poisoning

In animal studies, $CaNa_2EDTA$ therapy is effective when instituted within 4 hours of exposure but appears most effective within the first hour (9). A suggested dosing schedule is $CaNa_2EDTA$ 4 g daily for several days (9). One patient with nephrotoxicity after ingestion of uranium acetate was treated with IV $CaNa_2EDTA$, 1 g daily for 5 days, followed by a second course of chelation after a 2-week break (21). The clinical efficacy of $CaNa_2EDTA$ remains to be determined.

Zinc Poisoning

$CaNa_2EDTA$ at doses as low as 10 to 15 mg/kg has been found to lower elevated serum zinc levels (12,13). The need to treat acute zinc overdose with chelation therapy has been questioned (14).

Monitoring of Response

Specific details for monitoring metal levels are located in specific metal chapters. In the case of lead poisoning, the $CaNa_2EDTA$ infusion should be stopped for at least 1 hour before obtaining a blood lead level to avoid a falsely elevated value. Lead toxicity causes renal damage independent of chelation. It is important to closely monitor the patient's renal function during $CaNa_2EDTA$ administration and adjust the dose and schedule accordingly (22,23).

ADVERSE EFFECTS

Adverse drug events may occur 4 to 8 hours after the end of the drug infusion and may develop during the night or the following morning (24). The initial systemic symptoms include numbness, tingling, yawning, nasal congestion, and prolonged sneezing and are followed by malaise, fatigue, and excessive thirst. These effects may be followed by acute onset of fever (heralded or followed by chilly sensations or shaking chills), myalgia, frontal headache, anorexia, nausea, vomiting, and urinary frequency and urgency. Periarticular myalgias and joint aches may occur. The fever is usually low grade and persists for 12 to 18 hours. A decrease in white blood cell count without changes in its differential may occur, usually reverting to pretherapy levels within a few days.

$CaNa_2EDTA$ therapy of 2 g or more per day may result in a five- to sixfold increase in urinary zinc excretion (25,26). Histamine-like reactions, such as sneezing episodes, nasal congestion, and occasional lacrimation, may be observed toward the end of a $CaNa_2EDTA$ infusion, commonly at doses of 3 g/day or more (24).

The principal toxic effect of $CaNa_2EDTA$ is on the kidneys, especially with high-dose and prolonged therapy (27,28). It is characterized by hydropic or vacuolated degeneration of renal tubular cells and can result in renal tubular necrosis (28–30). The major sites are the proximal tubule and, to a lesser extent, the distal tubule and glomeruli (27–29,31). With increasing doses and duration of therapy, progressive involvement of the lower nephron down through the loop of Henle to the distal tubule may develop. Urine analysis may show albumin, renal parenchymal cells, granular casts, and red and white cells (24,29). Renal toxicity may be related to the concentration of chelated metal that passes through the renal tubule, release of lead in the kidneys during excretion, and interaction between the chelator and endogenous metals in the proximal tubular cells (28,32). $CaNa_2EDTA$-associated nephrotoxicity appears to be dose related and reversible. Fatal renal failure has been reported in patients treated with either sodium EDTA (90 mg/kg/day for 2 days) or $CaNa_2EDTA$ (125 to 200 mg/kg/day for 2 to 7 days) (27,31).

An acute febrile systemic reaction has been observed after excessively large doses of IV $CaNa_2EDTA$—most commonly greater than 4 g at a single dose administered over 1 to 3 hours (24–26). The fever peaks at 3 to 6 hours after the infusion is initiated and returns to normal within 12 to 24 hours. Syncope has been reported within a few minutes of initiating $CaNa_2EDTA$ 12 g in 500-ml infusion.

$CaNa_2EDTA$ therapy greater than 2 g/day for more than 5 consecutive days may be associated with mucocutaneous lesions (25,26). Sore throat and cheilosis develop, followed by sore mouth and tongue. The tongue may appear magenta in color. Chemosis may be evident. Erythematous, papular, scaly lesions may appear over the face, trunk, and extremities, with oral mucosal bullae and ulcerations of contiguous mucous membranes (e.g., nose, lips, eyes, and rectum). The patient may also develop a persistent fever. In male patients, exfoliative dermatitis of the scrotum followed by a weeping exudate has been reported. The lesions become florid with continued therapy; however, they subside rapidly and heal completely within one week of terminating chelation. Patients who are rechallenged with $CaNa_2EDTA$ develop the same lesions. Pyridoxine, 25 to 75 mg/day, may reduce the incidence and severity of these reactions, whereas vitamin B_{12} and folate provide partial relief (33).

Other adverse drug events include thrombophlebitis, glycosuria, and a decrease in systolic and diastolic pressures (5 to 20 mm Hg) and hemoglobin level (24,26,31).

$CaNa_2EDTA$ may extravasate during IV administration, resulting in local pain, swelling, and erythema, and delayed painful calcinosis may develop at the extravasation site (34). The acute local effects can be managed by warm soaks and splinting, and the calcinosis can be excised.

PITFALLS

$CaNa_2EDTA$ and Na_2EDTA are related compounds; however, Na_2EDTA should not be used as the therapeutic agent because it may produce hypocalcemic tetany at infusion rates greater than 15 mg/minute (24).

Oral $CaNa_2EDTA$ should not be used for lead poisoning. The apparent increase in urinary lead excretion after oral $CaNa_2EDTA$ is due to transfer of lead from the intestine (35,36). Experimental and clinical evidence suggests that lead is absorbed from the gut as the lead chelate, some of the chelate breaks down, and there is an increased lead burden presented to the soft tissues.

Nephrotoxicity may be minimized by limiting the total daily $CaNa_2EDTA$ dose to 50 mg/kg/day (29), and the patient should be well hydrated to maintain good urine output. However, a higher $CaNa_2EDTA$ dose may be needed for patients with lead encephalopathy. If possible, a continuous $CaNa_2EDTA$ infusion should be administered at concentrations of 0.5% or less to minimize the occurrence of thrombophlebitis (24).

$CaNa_2EDTA$ has been advocated as an "alternative" treatment of atherosclerotic heart disease and peripheral atherosclerosis. The rationale for therapy is implausible, however, and controlled trials have not found it effective (37–41).

REFERENCES

1. Foreman H, Trujillo TT. The metabolism of C^{14}-labeled ethylenediaminetetraacetic acid in human beings. *J Lab Clin Med* 1954;43:566–571.
2. Seaton CL, Lasman J, Smith DR. The effects of CaNa(2)EDTA on brain lead mobilization in rodents determined using a stable isotope tracer. *Toxicol Appl Pharmacol* 1999;159:153–160.
3. Cantilena LR, Klaassen CD. Decreased effectiveness of chelation therapy for Cd poisoning with time. *Toxicol Appl Pharmacol* 1982;63:173–180.
4. Llobet JM, Domingo JL, Corbella J. Comparison of the effectiveness of several chelators after single administration on the toxicity, excretion and distribution of cobalt. *Arch Toxicol* 1986;58:278–281.
5. Wahl PK, Lahiri P, Mathur KS, et al. Acute copper sulphate poisoning. *J Assoc Phys Ind* 1963;11:93–103.
6. Walsh FM, Crosson FJ, Bayley M, et al. Acute copper intoxication. *Am J Dis Child* 1977;131:149–151.
7. Catsch A. *Radioactive metal mobilization in medicine*. Springfield, IL: Charles C Thomas, 1964:9, 57, 105–106.
8. Catsch A. Die Wirkung einger Chelatbidner auf die akute Toxicitat von Uranylnitrat. *Klin Wachr* 1959;37:657–666.
9. Dagirmanjian R, Maynard EA, Hodge HC. The effects of calcium disodium ethylenediamine tetraacetate on uranium poisoning in rats. *J Pharmacol Exp Ther* 1956;117:20–28.
10. Ivannikov AT. *On medicative application of complexing agents in the case of uranium intoxication. Central Scientific Institute of Information and Technical Research on Nuclear Science and Technology*. Moscow: TsNIIatominform, 1987:3–15.
11. Lincoln TA, Voelz GL. Management of persons accidentally exposed to uranium compounds. In: Ricks RC, Fry SA, eds. *The medical basis for radiation preparedness II. Clinical experience and follow-up since 1979*. New York: Elsevier, 1990:221–230.
12. Chobanian SJ. Accidental ingestion of liquid zinc chloride: local and systemic effects. *Ann Emerg Med* 1981;10:91–93.
13. Potter JL. Acute zinc chloride ingestion in a young child. *Ann Emerg Med* 1981;10:267–269.
14. Lewis MR, Kokan L. Zinc gluconate: acute ingestion. *J Toxicol Clin Toxicol* 1998;36:99–101.
15. American Academy of Pediatrics Committee on Drugs. Treatment guidelines for lead exposure in children. *Pediatrics* 1995;96:155–160.
16. Centers for Disease Control and Prevention. *Prevention of lead poisoning in young children: a statement by the Centers for Disease Control*. Atlanta: U.S. Department of Health and Human Services, Public Health Service, 1991.
17. Chisolm JJ. The use of chelating agents in the treatment of acute and chronic lead intoxication in childhood. *J Pediatr* 1968;73:1–38.
18. Coffin R, Phillips JL, Staples WI, et al. Treatment of lead encephalopathy in children. *J Pediatr* 1966;69:198–206.
19. Piomelli S, Rosen JF, Chisolm JJ, et al. Management of childhood lead poisoning. *J Pediatr* 1984;105:523–532.

20. Porru S, Alessio L. The use of chelating agents in occupational lead poisoning. *Occup Med* 1996;46:41–48.
21. Pavlakis N, Pollock CA, McLean G, et al. Deliberate overdose of uranium: toxicity and treatment. *Nephron* 1996;72:313–317.
22. Morgan JM. Chelation therapy in lead nephropathy. *South Med J* 1975;68:1001–1006.
23. Osterloh J, Becker CE. Pharmacokinetics of $CaNa_2EDTA$ and chelation of lead in renal failure. *Clin Pharmacol Ther* 1986;40:686–693.
24. Seven MJ. Observations on the toxicity of intravenous chelating agents. In: Seven MJ, Johnson LA, eds. *Metal-binding in medicine proceedings of a symposium sponsored by Hahnemann Medical College and Hospital*. Philadelphia: JB Lippincott, 1960:95–103, 154–159.
25. Perry HM Jr, Schroeder HA. Lesions resembling vitamin B complex deficiency and urinary loss of zinc produced by ethylenediamine tetra acetate. *Am J Med* 1957;22:168–172.
26. Perry HM Jr, Schroeder HA. Depression of cholesterol levels in human plasma following ethylenediamine tetraacetate and hydralazine. *J Chronic Dis* 1955;2:520–533.
27. Dudley HR, Ritchie AC, Schilling A, et al. Pathologic changes associated with the use of sodium ethylene diamine tetra-acetate in the treatment of hypocalcemia: report of two cases with autopsy findings. *N Engl J Med* 1955;252:331.
28. Vogt Von W, Cottier H. Nekrotisierende nephrose nach behandlung einer subakutchronischen bleivergiftung mit versenal in hohen dosen. *Schweiz Med Wochenschr* 1957;87:665–667.
29. Foreman H, Finnegan C, Lushbaugh CC. Nephrotoxic hazards from uncontrolled edathamil calcium disodium therapy. *JAMA* 1956;160:1042–1046.
30. Moel DI, Kumar K. Reversible nephrotoxic reactions to a combined 2,3-dimercapto-1-propanol and calcium disodium ethylenediaminetetraacetic acid regimen in asymptomatic children with elevated blood lead levels. *Pediatrics* 1982;70:259–262.
31. Reuber MD, Bradley JE. Acute versenate nephrosis occurring as the result of treatment for lead intoxication. *JAMA* 1960;174:263.
32. Johnson LA, Seven MJ. Observations on the in vivo stability of metal chelates. In: Seven MJ, Johnson LA, eds. *Metal-binding in medicine proceedings of a symposium sponsored by Hahnemann Medical College and Hospital*. Philadelphia: JB Lippincott, 1960:225–229.
33. Clarke NE, Clarke CN, Mosher RE. The "in vivo" dissolution of metastatic calcium. An approach to atherosclerosis. *Am J Med Sci* 1955;229:142–149.
34. Schumacher HR, Osterman AL, Choi SJ, et al. Calcinosis at the site of leakage from extravasation of calcium disodium edetate intravenous chelator therapy in a child with lead poisoning. *Clin Orthop* 1987;219:221–225.
35. Rieders F. Effects of oral Na_2Ca ethylenediamine tetraacetate on urinary and fecal excretion of lead in rabbits. *Fed Proc* 1954;13:397–398.
36. Rieders F. Effects of oral Na_2Ca ethylenediamine tetraacetate (EDTA) on distribution of Fe, Cu, Zn and Pb in rats. *J Pharmacol Exp Ther* 1955;113:45–46.
37. Guldager B, Faergeman O, Jorgensen SJ, et al. Disodium-ethylene diamine tetraacetic acid (EDTA) has no effect on blood lipids in atherosclerotic patients. A randomized, placebo-controlled study. *Dan Med Bull* 1993;40:625–627.
38. Guldager B, Jelnes R, Jorgensen SJ, et al. EDTA treatment of intermittent claudication—a double-blind, placebo-controlled study. *J Intern Med* 1992;231:261–267.
39. Sloth-Nielsen J, Guldager B, Mouritzen C, et al. Arteriographic findings in EDTA chelation therapy on peripheral arteriosclerosis. *Am J Surg* 1991;162:122–125.
40. Wirebaugh SR, Geraets DR. Apparent failure of edetic acid chelation therapy for the treatment of coronary atherosclerosis. *DICP* 1990;24:22–25.
41. van Rij AM, Solomon C, Packer SG, et al. Chelation therapy for intermittent claudication. A double-blind, randomized, controlled trial. *Circulation* 1994;90:1194–1199.

CHAPTER 46

Cyanide Antidote Package

Andrew R. Erdman

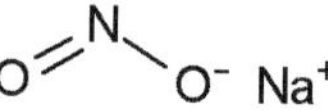

SODIUM NITRITE

Synonyms:	**Lilly Cyanide Antidote Kit**
Molecular formula and weight:	**Amyl nitrite ($C_5H_{11}NO_2$), 117.15 g/mol; sodium nitrite ($NaNO_2$), 69.01 g/mol; sodium thiosulfate ($Na_2S_2O_3$), 158.11 g/mol**
SI conversion:	**mg/L × 0.0217 = mmol/L (nitrite)**
CAS Registry No.:	**463-04-7 (amyl nitrite), 7632-00-0 (sodium nitrite), 7772-98-7 (sodium thiosulfate)**
Normal or therapeutic levels:	**Not clinically applicable**
Special concerns:	**Inappropriate use of sodium nitrite can cause dangerous methemoglobinemia. Hospitals often stock insufficient amounts of cyanide antidote.**

OVERVIEW

The search for an effective cyanide antidote began in the late 1800s when it was reported that both sodium thiosulfate and amyl nitrite individually antagonized cyanide toxicity in animals (1,2). In 1933, Mota successfully treated human cyanide poisoning with sodium nitrite (3). Later that year, Chen et al. discovered that in dogs the combination of sodium nitrite and sodium thiosulfate was more effective than either substance alone (2). Amyl nitrite was also found to act synergistically with sodium thiosulfate (2). In 1934, Viana et al. applied combination therapy to successfully treat human cyanide poisoning (4). Many physicians began using the two drugs routinely. In 1956, Chen reported a series of 48 cyanide victims who were successfully managed using the combination approach (5). The administration of a nitrite followed by sodium thiosulfate has become the standard regimen for cyanide toxicity in the United States.

Forms Available

Each Cyanide Antidote Package (CAP) contains 12 amyl nitrite perles (0.3 ml each) for inhalation; 2 ampules of sodium nitrite 3% solution (10 ml each) for intravenous (IV) injection; and 2 vials of sodium thiosulfate 25% solution (50 ml each) for IV injection. Each component of the kit is also available separately.

Mechanism of Action

Cyanide acts primarily by inhibiting cytochrome-*c* oxidase (complex IV), a key step in the electron transport chain, thereby impairing cellular energy production (6–10). As a result, body tis-

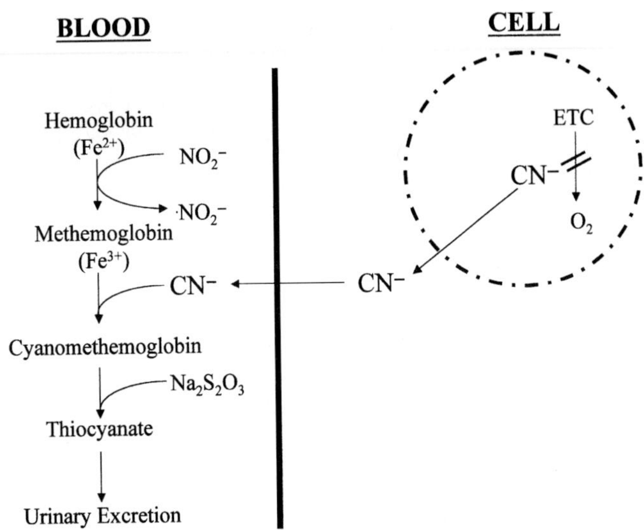

Figure 1. Mechanism for detoxication of cyanide. CN^-, cyanide ion; ETC, electron transport chain; Fe^{2+}, ferrous ion; Fe^{3+}, ferric ion; NO_2^-, nitrite ion; $Na_2S_2O_3$, sodium thiosulfate.

sues must shift from aerobic to anaerobic metabolism, resulting in lactate accumulation and profound acidosis (Chapter 185).

The precise mechanism of action for the agents in the CAP has not been fully elucidated. The nitrites, such as amyl and sodium nitrite, are believed to work by inducing a modest degree of methemoglobinemia in the recipient (3,11). Cyanide has a greater affinity for ferric ions, like those of methemoglobin (MetHgb), than for ferrous ions, like those of cytochrome oxidase (12,13). As a result, MetHgb creates a reservoir or "sink" for ferric ions, diverting cyanide from enzymes in the electron transport chain (Fig. 1) (9). The formation of cyanomethemoglobin cannot only prevent cyanide from inactivating cytochrome oxidase, but it can potentially remove the cyanide ions already bound and, hence, "reactivate" the enzyme (14,15).

Both amyl nitrite and sodium nitrite induce MetHgb formation by oxidation (16–21). Sodium nitrite allows more accurate dosing and more predictable MetHgb formation. Amyl nitrite is inhaled and is more difficult to titrate effectively, and it may not always cause a predictable or even measurable level of MetHgb in practice (22). Amyl nitrite can be administered before IV access is established.

Methemoglobinemia may not be the primary mechanism of nitrite effects. There have been several reports of patients who improved clinically after nitrite administration despite the lack of significant MetHgb formation (23,24). Indeed, most case reports describe clinical improvement after nitrite administration before the development of peak MetHgb levels. Even when pretreated with methylene blue (to prevent MetHgb formation), cyanide-poisoned animals still benefit from nitrite administration (25). Finally, when compared to nonnitrite MetHgb formers, such as 4-dimethylaminophenol or hydroxylamine, the nitrites were more effective despite similar MetHgb levels. One possibility is that the nitrites, as vasodilating agents, might help by improving circulation to critical tissues (26).

Whereas MetHgb can provide a temporary repository for cyanide ions, eventually they must be excreted. Humans have several endogenous mechanisms for the metabolism of cyanide. Probably the most important of these is the reaction of cyanide with thiosulfate to form thiocyanate, a process catalyzed by rhodanese (3,14). Thiocyanate is much less toxic than cyanide and is readily eliminated by the kidney, although it may cause toxicity in patients with renal impairment (27–30). However, endogenous stores of thiosulfate are easily overwhelmed. Evidence suggests a more complex mechanism that may involve other enzyme systems, such as mercaptopyruvate sulfurtransferase, or the formation of sulfane sulfur intermediates (33). Regardless of the exact mechanism, sodium thiosulfate appears to work by donating its sulfur group to cyanide so as to form the more innocuous compound thiocyanate (34).

INDICATIONS

Serious Clinical Effects after Cyanide Exposure

Serious clinical effects after cyanide exposure (hypotension, seizures, altered mental status or coma, respiratory depression, or significant metabolic acidosis) are a clear indication for use of the CAP. Animal studies have found each of the components to be effective. Human efficacy data come primarily from case reports and case series (4,5,23,37–49). In many cases, dramatic improvement of mental status, seizures, cardiorespiratory function, or metabolic acidosis was noted after administration. In other cases, the improvement occurred over hours or even days (50,51), or the patient appeared to show no response (52,53). These reports must be interpreted cautiously because some patients may have improved simply with removal from the exposure.

Known Cyanide Exposure without Clinical Effects

Cyanide toxicity may not be apparent for some time after *ingestion* of cyanide or acetonitrile compounds (or if the substance was not actually cyanide). Because sodium nitrite has significant side effects, it should be reserved for patients with signs of toxicity. However, the thiosulfate component of the kit can be given to asymptomatic patients.

Suspected Cyanide Poisoning

Occult cyanide poisoning may be suspected in conjunction with other toxic exposures (i.e., altered mental status and metabolic acidosis in a smoke inhalation victim). Cyanide toxicity may be uncertain or simply a component of multiple insults (e.g., carbon monoxide and cyanide). In this instance, cyanide detoxification may be desired without consuming more oxygen-carrying capacity with methemoglobinemia. The patient should receive at least the CAP thiosulfate component because there are few risks associated with its use. Whether to give the nitrite components is a decision based on the patient's clinical status, the level of suspicion for cyanide, the nature and severity of the exposure, and any comorbidities that might make administration of nitrites problematic (e.g., preexisting hypotension, hypoxemia, or significant anemia).

The use of nitrites in victims of smoke inhalation has raised the concern that methemoglobinemia may further impair oxygen delivery (54). However, *if the appropriate dose is used*, sodium nitrite produces much smaller MetHgb levels than previously suspected (19,39), and high MetHgb levels are not necessary for clinical benefit (19,23,24). Furthermore, MetHgb levels do not peak until approximately 35 to 70 minutes after administration of sodium nitrite, and carboxyhemoglobin levels are decreasing by this time (19,39).

High-Dose Nitroprusside

High-dose nitroprusside can be treated with the sodium thiosulfate component alone. However, caution should be used in patients with renal failure in whom thiocyanate can accumulate and cause toxicity. To prevent the development of cyanide toxicity, a concomitant infusion of sodium thiosulfate or an admixture of nitroprusside and sodium thiosulfate can be used.

Hydrogen Sulfide Poisoning

Hydrogen sulfide rapidly causes cellular asphyxia (Chapter 186). The data supporting the use of CAP for these patients are limited to animal studies and anecdotal human reports (57–60). Sodium nitrite can be considered for any patient with serious hydrogen sulfide toxicity (e.g., coma, seizures, severe acidosis) that does not respond to initial care, but these effects are usually due to anoxic injury. If used, it should be administered within 15 to 20 minutes of exposure (61).

TABLE 1. Recommended dose of sodium nitrite for children with cyanide poisoning

Hemoglobin (g/100 ml)	Recommended initial dose of sodium nitrite (mg/kg)
7.0	5.8
8.0	6.6
9.0	7.5
10.0	8.3
11.0	9.1
12.0	10.0
13.0	10.8
14.0	11.6

Note: Calculated to produce a methemoglobin level of 26.8% (65).

CAUTIONS AND CONTRAINDICATIONS

Excessive doses of nitrites or their use in susceptible subgroups of patients (e.g., glucose-6-phosphate dehydrogenase deficiency) can lead to life-threatening methemoglobinemia (65). Some patients may not tolerate even a modest degree of methemoglobinemia due to underlying pulmonary or cardiac disease. Nitrites must be used with caution in these patients, with close monitoring of clinical condition and MetHgb levels. The clinical sequelae of excessive MetHgb may include a bluish or brownish discoloration of the skin; increased respiratory rate, decreased blood pressure, or increased heart rate; a deterioration in mental status; evidence of cardiac ischemia; or worsening acidosis.

DOSAGE AND ADMINISTRATION

Serious Clinical Effects after Cyanide Exposure

Recommendations differ little from those of Viana and Chen decades ago (4,5). Amyl nitrite is given only until IV access is established. Sodium nitrite is then infused immediately. Finally, sodium thiosulfate is administered as soon as the nitrite infusion has been completed.

AMYL NITRITE

The perles are crushed and placed in front of the mouth or nose of a breathing patient for 30 seconds of each minute and oxygen administered for the remaining 30 seconds. A new perle should be used every 3 to 5 minutes. The crushed perles can be held in front of the ventilation bag intake valve. Occasionally, patients respond dramatically to amyl nitrite alone (24,42). These are usually patients treated very soon after exposure. In such cases, no further nitrite therapy may be needed. These patients should still receive oxygen, thiosulfate, and close monitoring.

SODIUM NITRITE

The *adult dose* of sodium nitrite is 300 mg IV over 3 to 5 minutes. If hypotension occurs, the rate of infusion can be slowed to 30 minutes. In patients at risk for excessive methemoglobinemia or in those who might not tolerate even modest levels of MetHgb (e.g., significant anemia or hypoxemia), the dose of sodium nitrite may be reduced. However, studies indicate that the normal adult dose rarely results in MetHgb levels above 10% (19,23,24,39).

The *pediatric dose* of sodium nitrite is based on the child's baseline hemoglobin concentration (Table 1). In most clinical situations, treatment needs to precede testing. The initial dose in these cases is 0.33 ml/kg of the 3% solution (approximately 10 mg/kg IV) over a period of several minutes (65). Even this dose may be too high; it is based on calculations to yield a MetHgb level of 26.8%, a level that is higher than needed to produce clinical efficacy.

SODIUM THIOSULFATE

The *adult dose* is 12.5 g IV in adults, and the *pediatric dose* is 400 mg/kg (or approximately 1.65 ml/kg of a 25% solution).

Known Cyanide Exposure without Clinical Effects

A single dose of sodium thiosulfate (12.5 g IV in adults, 400 mg/kg in children) should be given. If the patient develops signs of cyanide toxicity, sodium nitrite should then be administered and the thiosulfate component repeated.

Suspected Cyanide Poisoning

The doses of sodium nitrite and sodium thiosulfate are the same as for a symptomatic patient with known exposure. However, in patients in whom the diagnosis is uncertain, the risks of nitrite administration should be weighed against its potential benefits.

High-Dose Nitroprusside

If toxicity is already present, the sodium thiosulfate component should be given. If high-dose or prolonged nitroprusside treatment is anticipated, an admixture or concurrent infusion with sodium thiosulfate should be considered. The dose is 10 mg for each 1 mg of nitroprusside (e.g., 10 ml of 0.1% nitroprusside solution and 50 ml of 1% sodium thiosulfate).

Hydrogen Sulfide Poisoning

The dose of sodium nitrite is the same as for cyanide poisoning.

Monitoring

All patients should be monitored in an emergency or intensive care setting. Monitoring should include regular assessments of metabolic acidosis using serial arterial blood gases, metabolic panels, or serum lactate determinations. If hypotension develops, the infusion or inhalation of nitrites should be slowed or stopped accordingly, and the patient should be given supplemental fluids or pressors.

If clinical or laboratory signs of cyanide toxicity do not improve within 15 to 30 minutes of CAP administration, the sodium nitrite and sodium thiosulfate portions should be repeated at half the recommended initial dose. They should also be repeated in patients who develop recurrent toxicity after an initial improvement. Recurrent toxicity may also represent ongoing cyanide absorption, so further decontamination should be considered. Patients who do not respond to repeat doses of the CAP should have the diagnosis of cyanide toxicity reconsidered.

A MetHgb level should be checked approximately 30 and 60 minutes after nitrite infusion—earlier if signs of methemoglobinemia develop. The MetHgb level needed for optimal benefit has not been established. Some authors describe a target MetHgb level of 25% to 30%; however, recent evidence suggests that high levels are not necessary for therapeutic benefit (19,23,24). Clinical improvement rather than MetHgb level should be the therapeutic goal.

ADVERSE EFFECTS

If methemoglobinemia compromises the patient's clinical status, methylene blue (1.0 mg/kg IV) should be administered (Chapter 63). Alternatively, at-risk patients may be treated with only the thiosulfate portion of the kit or administered sodium nitrite in smaller doses.

Hypotension is another effect of nitrite administration, particularly with higher doses (23,49,54,67–69). It is due primarily to vasodilation, but large doses also produce myocardial depression in animals (68). Hypotension can usually be avoided by infusing sodium nitrite over a period of 5 minutes or more. There are rare reports of cardiac arrest immediately after nitrite infusion in severely cyanide-poisoned patients (44). It is not clear whether this was an effect of the nitrite or the underlying cyanide toxicity.

Thiosulfate produces few side effects. In patients with renal failure, thiocyanate may accumulate and cause toxicity. The signs of thiocyanate toxicity are generally limited to nausea, vomiting, muscle cramps, and rarely altered mental status or hypotension (27–30,70). In the rare case in which it is necessary to remove the excess thiocyanate, hemodialysis has been used (29). Repeated sodium nitrite dosing combined with sodium thiosulfate has been associated with hypernatremia, although the patient was also receiving IV fluids (49).

PITFALLS

A patient's failure to improve after antidotal therapy may indicate another reason for the original clinical findings (e.g., coexposure, anoxic brain injury, or other diseases).

Hospitals often stock inadequate amounts of the CAP or its components. Treatment is then limited to aggressive supportive care (Chapter 185).

Treatment with the CAP is not innocuous. The "cost" of nitrite therapy is the loss of a certain portion of the body's oxygen-carrying capacity either as MetHgb or as cyanomethemoglobin, neither of which is able to deliver oxygen to the tissues. Excessive methemoglobinemia or nitrite-induced hypotension should be considered in patients who worsen clinically after administration of the CAP.

REFERENCES

1. Pedigo LG. Antagonism between amyl nitrite and prussic acid. *Tr M Soc Virginia* 1888;19:124–131.
2. Chen KK, Rose CL, Clowes GHA. Methylene blue, nitrites, and sodium thiosulphate against cyanide poisoning. *Proc Soc Exp Biol Med* 1933;31:250–253.
3. Chen KK, Rose CL. Nitrite and thiosulfate therapy in cyanide poisoning. *JAMA* 1952;149:113–115.
4. Potter L. The successful treatment of two recent cases of cyanide poisoning. *Br J Industr Med* 1950;7:125–130.
5. Chen KK, Rose CL. Treatment of acute cyanide poisoning. *JAMA* 1956;162:1154–1155.
6. Albaum HG, Tepperman J, Bodansky O. The in vivo inactivation by cyanide of brain cytochrome oxidase and its effect on glycolysis and on the high energy phosphorus compounds in the brain. *J Biol Chem* 1946;64:45–51.
7. Isom GE, Way JL. Effects of oxygen on the antagonism of cyanide intoxication: cytochrome oxidase, in vitro. *Toxicol Appl Pharmacol* 1984;74(1):57–62.
8. Piantadosi CA, Sylvia AL. Cerebral cytochrome a,a3 inhibition by cyanide in bloodless rats. *Toxicology* 1984;33(1):67–79.
9. Piantadosi CA, Sylvia AL, Jobsis FF. Cyanide-induced cytochrome a,a3 oxidation-reduction responses in rat brain in vivo. *J Clin Invest* 1983;72(4):1224–1233.
10. van Buuren KJ, Nicholis P, van Gelder BF. Biochemical and biophysical studies on cytochrome aa 3. VI. Reaction of cyanide with oxidized and reduced enzyme. *Biochim Biophys Acta* 1972;256(2):258–276.
11. Chen KK, Rose CL, Clowes GHA. Amyl nitrite and cyanide poisoning. *JAMA* 1933;100:1920–1922.
12. Ten Eyck RP, Schaerdel AD, Lynett JE, et al. Stroma-free methemoglobin solution as an antidote for cyanide poisoning: a preliminary study. *J Toxicol Clin Toxicol* 1983;21(3):343–358.
13. Ten Eyck RP, Schaerdel AD, Ottinger WE. Stroma-free methemoglobin solution: an effective antidote for acute cyanide poisoning. *Am J Emerg Med* 1985;3(6):519–523.
14. Way JL, Sylvester D, Morgan RL, et al. Recent perspectives on the toxicodynamic basis of cyanide antagonism. *Fundam Appl Toxicol* 1984;4(2 Pt 2):S231–S239.
15. Jandorf BJ, Bodansky O. Therapeutic and prophylactic effect of methemoglobinemia in inhalation poisoning by hydrogen cyanide and cyanogen chloride. *J Indust Hyg Toxicol* 1946;28:125–132.
16. Machabert R, Testud F, Descotes J. Methaemoglobinaemia due to amyl nitrite inhalation: a case report. *Hum Exp Toxicol* 1994;13(5):313–314.
17. Tarburton JP, Metcalf WK. Kinetics of amyl nitrite-induced hemoglobin oxidation in cord and adult blood. *Toxicology* 1985;36(1):15–21.
18. Vick JA, Froehlich H. Treatment of cyanide poisoning. *Mil Med* 1991;156(7):330–339.
19. Kirk MA, Gerace R, Kulig KW. Cyanide and methemoglobin kinetics in smoke inhalation victims treated with the cyanide antidote kit. *Ann Emerg Med* 1993;22(9):1413–1418.
20. Tarburton JP, Metcalf WK. The kinetic differences between sodium nitrite, amyl nitrite and nitroglycerin oxidation of hemoglobin. *Histol Histopathol* 1986;1(3):213–217.
21. Kruszyna R, Kruszyna H, Smith RP. Comparison of hydroxylamine, 4-dimethylaminophenol and nitrite protection against cyanide poisoning in mice. *Arch Toxicol* 1982;49(3–4):191–202.
22. Klimmek R, Krettek C. Effects of amyl nitrite on circulation, respiration and blood homoeostasis in cyanide poisoning. *Arch Toxicol* 1988;62(2–3):161–166.
23. Johnson WS, Hall AH, Rumack BH. Cyanide poisoning successfully treated without "therapeutic methemoglobin levels." *Am J Emerg Med* 1989;7(4):437–440.
24. Vick JA, Froehlich HL. Studies of cyanide poisoning. *Arch Int Pharmacodyn Ther* 1985;273(2):314–322.
25. Holmes RK, Way JL. Mechanism of cyanide antagonism by sodium nitrite. 24. 1982;24:182.
26. Klimmek R, Roddewig C, Fladerer H, et al. Effects of 4-dimethylaminophenol, Co_2EDTA, or $NaNO_2$ on cerebral blood flow and sinus blood homeostasis of dogs in connection with acute cyanide poisoning. *Toxicology* 1983;26(2):143–154.
27. Curry SC, Arnold-Capell P. Toxic effects of drugs used in the ICU. Nitroprusside, nitroglycerin, and angiotensin-converting enzyme inhibitors. *Crit Care Clin* 1991;7(3):555–581.
28. Schulz V. Clinical pharmacokinetics of nitroprusside, cyanide, thiosulphate and thiocyanate. *Clin Pharmacokinet* 1984;9(3):239–251.
29. Pahl MV, Vaziri ND. In-vivo and in-vitro hemodialysis studies of thiocyanate. *J Toxicol Clin Toxicol* 1982;19(9):965–974.
30. Cailleux A, Subra JF, Riberi P, et al. Cyanide and thiocyanate blood levels in patients with renal failure or respiratory disease. *J Med* 1988;19(5–6):345–351.
31. Sylvester DM, Hayton WL, Morgan RL, Way JL. Effects of thiosulfate on cyanide pharmacokinetics in dogs. *Toxicol Appl Pharmacol* 1983;69(2):265–271.
32. Sylvester DM, Sander C, Hayton WL, Way JL. Alteration of the pharmacokinetics of sodium cyanide by sodium thiosulfate. *Proc West Pharmacol Soc* 1981;24:135.
33. Westley J, Adler H, Westley L, Nishida C. The sulfurtransferases. *Fundam Appl Toxicol* 1983;3(5):377–382.
34. Sylvester DM, Hayton WL, Morgan RL, Way JL. Effects of thiosulfate on cyanide pharmacokinetics in dogs. *Toxicol Appl Pharmacol* 1983;69(2):265–271.
35. Burrows GE. Cyanide intoxication in sheep; therapeutics. *Vet Hum Toxicol* 1981;23(1):22–28.
36. Burrows GE, Way JL. Cyanide intoxication in sheep: enhancement of efficacy of sodium nitrite, sodium thiosulfate, and cobaltous chloride. *Am J Vet Res* 1979;40(5):613–617.
37. DiNapoli J, Hall AH, Drake R, Rumack BH. Cyanide and arsenic poisoning by intravenous injection. *Ann Emerg Med* 1989;18(3):308–311.
38. Hall AH, Linden CH, Kulig KW, Rumack BH. Cyanide poisoning from laetrile ingestion: role of nitrite therapy. *Pediatrics* 1986;78(2):269–272.

39. Hall AH, Doutre WH, Ludden T, et al. Nitrite/thiosulfate treated acute cyanide poisoning: estimated kinetics after antidote. *J Toxicol Clin Toxicol* 1987;25(1–2):121–133.
40. Johnson RP, Mellors JW. Arteriolization of venous blood gases: a clue to the diagnosis of cyanide poisoning. *J Emerg Med* 1988;6(5):401–404.
41. van Heijst AN, Douze JM, van Kesteren RG, et al. Therapeutic problems in cyanide poisoning. *J Toxicol Clin Toxicol* 1987;25(5):383–398.
42. Wurzburg H. Treatment of cyanide poisoning in an industrial setting. *Vet Hum Toxicol* 1996;38(1):44–47.
43. Bonsall JL. Survival without sequelae following exposure to 500 mg/m^3 of hydrogen cyanide. *Hum Toxicol* 1984;3(1):57–60.
44. De Busk RF, Seidl LG. Attempted suicide by cyanide. A report of two cases. *Calif Med* 1969;110(5):394–396.
45. Hirsch FG. Cyanide poisoning. *Arch Environ Health* 1964;8:622–624.
46. Litovitz TL, Larkin RF, Myers RA. Cyanide poisoning treated with hyperbaric oxygen. *Am J Emerg Med* 1983;1(1):94–101.
47. Stewart R. Cyanide poisoning. *Clin Toxicol* 1974;7(5):561–564.
48. Yen D, Tsai J, Wang LM, et al. The clinical experience of acute cyanide poisoning. *Am J Emerg Med* 1995;13(5):524–528.
49. Turchen SG, Manoguerra AS, Whitney C. Severe cyanide poisoning from the ingestion of an acetonitrile-containing cosmetic. *Am J Emerg Med* 1991;9(3):264–267.
50. Peters CG, Mundy JV, Rayner PR. Acute cyanide poisoning. The treatment of a suicide attempt. *Anaesthesia* 1982;37(5):582–586.
51. Mueller M, Borland C. Delayed cyanide poisoning following acetonitrile ingestion. *Postgrad Med J* 1997;73(859):299–300.
52. Krieg A, Saxena K. Cyanide poisoning from metal cleaning solutions. *Ann Emerg Med* 1987;16(5):582–584.
53. Carden E. Hyperbaric oxygen in cyanide poisoning. *Anaesthesia* 1970;25(3):442–443.
54. Ma S, Long JP. Central noradrenergic activity and the cardiovascular effects of nitroglycerin and amyl nitrate. *J Cardiovasc Pharmacol* 1992;20(5):826–836.
55. Clark CJ, Campbell D, Reid WH. Blood carboxyhaemoglobin and cyanide levels in fire survivors. *Lancet* 1981;1(8234):1332–1335.
56. Jones J, McMullen MJ, Dougherty J. Toxic smoke inhalation: cyanide poisoning in fire victims. *Am J Emerg Med* 1987;5(4):317–321.
57. Smith RP, Kruszyna R, Kruszyna H. Management of acute sulfide poisoning. Effects of oxygen, thiosulfate, and nitrite. *Arch Environ Health* 1976;31(3):166–169.
58. Hall AH, Rumack BH. Hydrogen sulfide poisoning: an antidotal role for sodium nitrite? *Vet Hum Toxicol* 1997;39(3):152–154.
59. Hoidal CR, Hall AH, Robinson MD, et al. Hydrogen sulfide poisoning from toxic inhalations of roofing asphalt fumes. *Ann Emerg Med* 1986;15(7):826–830.
60. Stine RJ, Slosberg B, Beacham BE. Hydrogen sulfide intoxication. A case report and discussion of treatment. *Ann Intern Med* 1976;85(6):756–758.
61. Beck JF, Bradbury CM, Connors AJ, Donini JC. Nitrite as antidote for acute hydrogen sulfide intoxication? *Am Ind Hyg Assoc J* 1981;42(11):805–809.
62. Stambach T, Haire K, Soni N, Booth J. Saturday night blue—a case of near fatal poisoning from the abuse of amyl nitrite. *J Accid Emerg Med* 1997;14(5):339–340.
63. Mannaioni G, Vannacci A, Marzocca C, et al. Acute cyanide intoxication treated with a combination of hydroxycobalamin, sodium nitrite, and sodium thiosulfate. *J Toxicol Clin Toxicol* 2002;40(2):181–183.
64. Mascarenhas BR, Geller AC, Goodman AI. Cyanide poisoning, medical emergency. *N Y State J Med* 1969;69(12):1782–1784.
65. Berlin CM Jr. The treatment of cyanide poisoning in children. *Pediatrics* 1970;46(5):793–796.
66. Modarai B, Kapadia YK, Kerins M, Terris J. Methylene blue: a treatment for severe methaemoglobinaemia secondary to misuse of amyl nitrite. *Emerg Med J* 2002;19(3):270–271.
67. Moody JM Jr, Bailey SR, Rubal BJ. Subtle features of the hemodynamic response to amyl nitrite inhalation: new aspects of an old tool. *Clin Cardiol* 1993;16(4):331–338.
68. Haley TJ. Review of the physiological effects of amyl, butyl, and isobutyl nitrites. *Clin Toxicol* 1980;16(3):317–329.
69. Hall AH, Kulig KW, Rumack BH. Suspected cyanide poisoning in smoke inhalation: complications of sodium nitrite therapy. *J Toxicol Clin Exp* 1989;9(1):3–9.
70. Barnett HJM, Jackson MV, Spaulding WB. Thiocyanate psychosis. *JAMA* 1951;147:1554–1555.

CHAPTER 47

Dantrolene

E. Martin Caravati

O$_2$N–C$_6$H$_4$–(furan)–CH=N–N(imidazolidinedione)–O$^-$ Na$^+$

DANTROLENE SODIUM

Molecular formula and weight:	**$C_{14}H_9N_4NaO_5$, 399.3 g/mol**
SI conversion:	**mg/L × 3.18 = µmol/L**
CAS Registry No.:	**7261-97-4**
Therapeutic level:	**Not recommended or clinically useful**
Special concerns:	**Hepatotoxicity with repeated use**

OVERVIEW

Dantrolene is reported effective in the treatment of hypermetabolic states, such as malignant hyperthermia, and possibly effective in neuroleptic malignant syndrome (NMS). It may result in rapid resolution of hyperthermia, dysrhythmias, muscle rigidity, tachycardia, hypercapnia, and metabolic acidosis (1). Its efficacy is anecdotal and based on case reports. It has also been used in the treatment of hyperthermia from phenelzine overdose (2,3). Therapeutic efficacy for amphetamine or metheylenedioxy-methamphetamine toxicity is controversial.

Forms Available

The intravenous (IV) form for injection includes 20 mg lyophilized dantrolene powder and 3000 mg mannitol per vial reconstituted with 60 ml sterile water. The IV solution should be protected from light and used within 6 hours of preparation. Orally, dantrolene (Dantrium) is available as 25-, 50-, and 100-mg capsules.

Mechanism of Action

Dantrolene prevents release of skeletal muscle calcium from endoplasmic reticulum into the myoplasm. This results in decreased adenosine triphosphate production and subsequent decrease in energy expenditure, muscle contraction, and heat production. In patients with upper motor neuron disease, it decreases muscle stiffness, clonus, hyperreflexia, and spasticity. It has little or no effect on cardiac or smooth muscle.

When administered orally, absorption is slow and incomplete. Peak concentrations occur approximately 5 hours after oral dosing. It is metabolized primarily by the liver and excreted in the urine. The elimination half-life is approximately 9 hours. Dantrolene is lipid soluble and highly protein bound (97%). It is not dialyzable.

INDICATIONS

Malignant Hyperthermia

Malignant hyperthermia is a rare but potentially fatal syndrome associated with general anesthesia, mainly from halogenated hydrocarbon anesthetics.

Phenelzine Toxicity

The efficacy of dantrolene is demonstrated in case reports only. After external cooling and acetaminophen failed, hyperthermia (41°C), muscle rigidity, trismus, and acidosis improved within 30 minutes after administration of 2.5 mg/kg IV of dantrolene in an adult patient who ingested 2250 mg of phenelzine. Repeated doses of 2.5 mg/kg every 6 hours for 24 hours maintained its reported therapeutic effect (2).

A 44-year-old man developed muscle rigidity, hyperreflexia, tremor, and fever (40.5°C) 3 weeks after beginning phenelzine therapy for depression. He progressed to coma, hypotension, and respiratory failure. His initial serum creatine kinase (CK) was 33,840 IU/L. Dantrolene 2.5 mg/kg/day IV in divided doses was administered in addition to IV fluids, antipyretics, and a cooling blanket. After day 1 of treatment, the hyperthermia, rigidity, tremor, altered mental status, and hyperreflexia resolved. The CK was 13,380 IU/L. Dantrolene was discontinued, and increased muscular rigidity, tremor, and CK level (30,160 IU/L) followed. When dantrolene therapy was resumed, the symptoms again abated, and the CK decreased to 727 IU/L over 4 days (3).

Neuroleptic Malignant Syndrome

Benzodiazepines and nondepolarizing paralytic agents are the drugs primarily indicated in the treatment of NMS. Dantrolene has been associated with improvement in isolated cases of NMS. It does not have U.S. Food and Drug Administration approval for this indication.

An uncontrolled, unblinded study of NMS in 20 patients treated with dantrolene (N = 2), bromocriptine (N = 2), both (N = 4), or supportive care only (N = 12) found that the duration of illness was longer (9.9 vs. 6.8 days) and number of sequelae higher (75% vs. 25%) in the dantrolene/bromocriptine treatment group (4).

A 39-year-old man taking haloperidol and trihexyphenidyl for schizophrenia developed muscle rigidity, tremor, and fever (39.4°C). He was administered 200 mg IV dantrolene over 10 minutes with relief of symptoms within 1 hour. He was maintained on a daily dose of 600 mg/day (6 mg/kg) for 3 days that was tapered over 14 days. He also received 15 mg/day of oral bromocriptine after the initial dose of dantrolene. His plasma dantrolene concentration was 4.4 μg/ml on day 3 and did not change after hemodialysis (5).

Other Toxicology-Related Uses

Dantrolene appears to diminish hyperthermic states and muscle rigidity associated with amphetamine overdose, carbon monoxide poisoning, monoamine oxidase overdose, and organophosphate poisoning (2,6–8). Dantrolene may help control the hypermetabolic state associated with rhabdomyolysis secondary to theophylline poisoning (9). Confirmation of its usefulness for these indications requires further controlled study. Dantrolene was not effective in a controlled study of heatstroke (10,11).

Chronic Spasticity

Dantrolene is used orally in the treatment of spasticity secondary to upper motor neuron disorders, such as cerebral palsy and multiple sclerosis.

CAUTIONS AND CONTRAINDICATIONS

Long-term use of dantrolene has been associated with hepatotoxicity, which may result in death (12,13). Short-term use over a few days has not been associated with apparent hepatotoxicity. The incidence of any hepatic injury was 1.8% of patients in placebo-controlled trials. Approximately half of the patients with hepatotoxicity were asymptomatic when diagnosed. The most common presenting symptoms were jaundice and nausea or vomiting (12). The severity of hepatic injury was related to increasing dose and duration of treatment. The fatalities were associated with doses greater than 200 mg/day. The risk of death increased markedly after 4 months of treatment (12). Histopathology revealed various hepatic lesions, including cirrhosis, chronic active hepatitis, submassive hepatic necrosis, acute hepatitis, and portal inflammation. The etiology of dantrolene-induced hepatitis is unclear but appears to be a subtle, chronic process. It is not a classic hypersensitivity reaction. There are anecdotal reports of patients in the early stages of hepatotoxicity who did not progress to a more severe stage after the drug was withdrawn. Liver function tests should be obtained periodically on all patients treated for more than 1 month, and the drug should be discontinued at the first sign of hepatotoxicity.

Animal studies demonstrate an increase in lethality with a concomitant decrease in seizures when dantrolene is added to theophylline (14).

Complete heart block developed in animals pretreated with verapamil who were then given dantrolene (15).

Each vial of dantrolene contains 3 g of mannitol and should be taken into account if volume overload is a concern.

Chronic therapy with dantrolene is contraindicated if the patient has active liver disease.

DOSAGE AND METHOD OF ADMINISTRATION

Malignant Hyperthermia

In adults and children, the minimum starting dose is 1 mg/kg by rapid IV push, repeated until symptoms resolve or a maximum cumulative dose of 10 mg/kg is reached. An average dose of 2 to 3 mg/kg is usually effective. A 70-kg patient will usually require seven to nine vials of dantrolene (140 to 180 mg) immediately for malignant hyperthermia. Oral dantrolene is not recommended for initial treatment of NMS due to delay in achieving therapeutic levels (16).

After the acute phase of malignant hyperthermia, the dose is 4 to 8 mg/kg/day in four divided doses for 1 to 3 days to prevent recurrence. The stable patient may be converted to oral dantrolene after 48 hours.

The preoperative prophylactic dose is 2.5 mg/kg IV over 1 hour before anesthesia.

Phenelzine Toxicity

In adults, dantrolene 2.5 mg/kg/day IV divided every 6 hours has been recommended as the minimum starting dose (3).

Neuroleptic Malignant Syndrome

Dosage recommendations vary widely (200 to 600 mg/day) (4,5). Begin with 1 mg/kg IV as for malignant hyperthermia.

Chronic Spasticity

The initial adult dose is 25 mg orally per day and increased at weekly intervals as necessary to a maximum dose of 100 mg four times daily. Children begin at 0.5 mg/kg/day to 2 mg/kg three times daily as needed.

Monitoring of Response

Monitor patient's temperature, muscle rigidity, and liver function (aminotransferase levels, total bilirubin, and alkaline phosphatase). Ideal endpoints are normothermia and normal muscle tone. Discontinue treatment if abnormal liver function occurs.

ADVERSE EFFECTS

Acute Effects

After IV administration, dizziness, euphoria, lightheadedness, drowsiness, diarrhea, phlebitis, muscle weakness, respiratory failure, and thrombophlebitis have been reported.

During oral prophylaxis of malignant hyperthermia, nausea, vomiting, dizziness, and diarrhea have been reported.

Chronic Effects

An adult patient who was given daily doses of dantrolene that gradually increased to 250 mg/day developed acute pulmonary edema and severe cardiac insufficiency after 11 days of therapy. Myocardial function returned to normal when drug treatment was stopped (17).

After 1 month of therapy with oral dantrolene, patients (0.1% to 0.2% incidence) may develop hepatotoxicity, which can be fatal. Symptomatic hepatitis may occur in 0.5% of patients treated for more than 30 days (13). Hepatotoxic risk increases with doses of 10 mg/kg/day, female gender, and age older than 35 years. Aplastic anemia, leukopenia, lymphocytic lymphoma, pleural and pericardial effusions, and heart failure have also been reported with long-term therapy.

Drug Interactions

Severe hyperkalemia and cardiovascular collapse have been observed in animals after administration of verapamil and dantrolene (15).

Dantrolene Overdose

Overdoses of dantrolene in three patients (20-month-old child, 25-year-old adult, and 23-year-old second-trimester pregnant woman) were reported after doses of 10 to 12 mg/kg. The child and pregnant woman exhibited no symptoms; only lethargy was noted in the 25-year-old adult. All routine chemistry, hematology, and urinary laboratory tests were normal. The patients were treated supportively and recovered uneventfully. The pregnant patient delivered a healthy child at term (18).

Pregnancy and Lactation

Dantrolene is U.S. Food and Drug Administration pregnancy category C (Appendix I). Dantrolene crosses the placenta. It has been used in a small number of pregnant patients before delivery without adverse effects. It is embryocidal in animals.

PITFALLS

Other supportive measures to decrease the patient's temperature and muscle rigidity should take priority (e.g., cooling techniques, IV fluid administration). The clinical efficacy of dantrolene in conditions other than malignant hyperthermia is anecdotal. It is unlikely to be effective for hyperthermia from causes other than muscular hyperactivity.

REFERENCES

1. Van de Kelft E, de Hert M, Heytens L, et al. Management of lethal catatonia with dantrolene sodium. *Crit Care Med* 1991;19:1449–1451.
2. Kaplan RF, Feinglass NG, Webster W, Mudra S. Phenelzine overdose treated with dantrolene sodium. *JAMA* 1986;255:642–644.
3. Verrilli MR, Virgilio DS, Kozachuk WE, Bennetts M. Phenelzine toxicity responsive to dantrolene. *Neurology* 1987;37:865–867.
4. Rosebush PI, Stewart T, Mazurek MF. The treatment of neuroleptic malignant syndrome: are dantrolene and bromocriptine useful adjuncts to supportive care? *Br J Psychiatry* 1991;159:709–712.
5. Tsujimoto S, Maeda K, Sugiyama T, et al. Efficacy of prolonged large-dose dantrolene for severe neuroleptic malignant syndrome. *Anesth Analag* 1998;86:1143–1144.
6. Barone JA, Peppers MP. Use of dantrolene in the management of amphetamine-induced hyperthermia. *Clin Pharm* 1989;8:324–325.
7. ten Holter JB, Schellens RL. Dantrolene sodium for treatment of carbon monoxide poisoning. *BMJ* 1988;296:1772–1773.
8. Shemesh I, Bourvin A, Gold D, Kutscherowsky M. Chlorpyrifos poisoning treated with ipratropium and dantrolene: a case report. *J Toxicol Clin Toxicol* 1988;26:495–498.
9. Parr MJA, Willatts SM. Fatal theophylline poisoning with rhabdomyolysis: a potential role for dantrolene treatment. *Anaesthesia* 1991;46:557–559.
10. Bouchama A, Cafege A, Devol EB, et al. Ineffectiveness of dantrolene sodium in the treatment of heat stroke. *Crit Care Med* 1991;19:176–180.
11. Channa AB, Seraj MA, Saddique AA, et al. Is dantrolene effective in heat stroke patients? *Crit Care Med* 1990;18:290–293.
12. Chan CH. Dantrolene sodium and hepatic injury. *Neurology* 1990;40:1427–1432.
13. Utili R, Boitnott JK, Zimmerman HJ. Dantrolene-associated hepatic injury. *Gastroenterology* 1977;72:610–616.
14. Tayeb OS. A serious interaction of dantrolene and theophylline. *Vet Hum Toxicol* 1990;32:442–443.
15. Saltzman LS, Kates RA, Corke GC, et al. Hyperkalemia and cardiovascular collapse after verapamil and dantrolene administration in swine. *Anesth Analg* 1984;63:473–478.
16. Wedel DJ, Quinlan JG, Iaizzo PA. Clinical effects of intravenously administered dantrolene. *Mayo Clin Proc* 1995;70:241–246.
17. Robillart A, Bopp P, Vailly B, Dupeyron JP. Cardiac failure due to dantrolene overdose. *Ann Fr Anesth Reanim* 1986;5:617–619.
18. Paloucek FP, Erickson TE, Lundquist S, Ferraro C. Oral dantrolene ingestion: a case series. *Vet Hum Toxicol* 1991;33:362.

CHAPTER 48

Deferoxamine

Steven A. Seifert

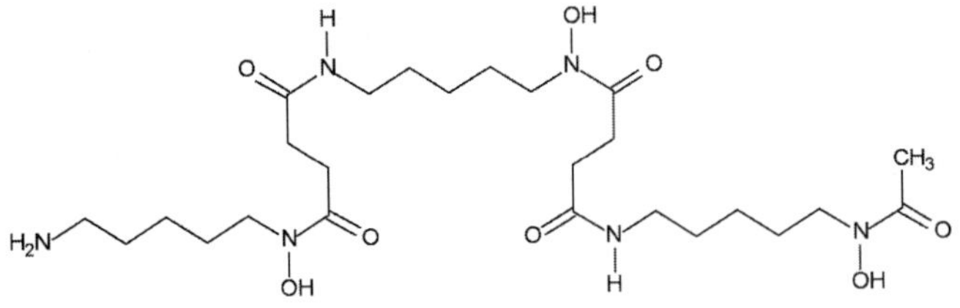

DEFEROXAMINE

Synonyms:	**Deferoxamine mesylate (Desferal, Desferin), desferrioxamine**
Molecular formula and weight:	**$C_{25}H_{48}N_6O_8$, CH_3SO_3H, 656.8 g/mol**
SI conversion:	**mg/L × 1.78 = μmol/L**
CAS Registry No.:	**138-14-7 (desferrioxamine mesylate)**
Normal or therapeutic levels:	**Not clinically applicable**
Special concerns:	**Large doses or rapid infusion may cause hypotension.**

OVERVIEW

Deferoxamine (DFO) is a naturally occurring compound produced by *Streptomyces pilosus*. It is used for the treatment of iron intoxication. DFO is also used for aluminum overload and has been investigated for gastrointestinal (GI) iron decontamination, doxorubicin toxicity (1), paraquat toxicity (2), treatment of sleeping sickness and malaria (3,4), *Pneumocystis carinii* pneumonia (5), aminoglycoside ototoxicity (6), treatment of acetaminophen toxicity (7,8), atherosclerosis (9), and treatment of hyperpigmentation after venous sclerotherapy (10).

Forms Available

DFO is provided as DFO mesylate solution (250 mg/ml) for intravenous (IV), intramuscular (IM), or subcutaneous (SQ) administration. DFO is stable for at least 7 days in normal saline or dextrose 5% in water, at concentrations greater than 180 g/L at 28°C (11).

Mechanism of Action

DFO mesylate strongly complexes the ferric ion of iron to form a hexadentate complex, ferrioxamine. The affinity constant is 10^{30} – 10^{31}, and ferrioxamine, a compound with a small volume of distribution, is readily excreted in the urine (12). DFO is capable of removing iron from transferrin but does not remove iron from cytochromes or hemoglobin, and it does not cause a loss of other trace metals. It is poorly lipophilic. Because of its inability to penetrate into tissues, it chelates iron in the vascular space and, perhaps, the labile pool (13,14). One molecule of DFO chelates one ferric ion so that 1000 mg of DFO can bind 85 mg of ferric iron (15,16).

Only 15% of DFO is absorbed orally. When used for GI decontamination, DFO alone does not appear to reduce the amount of absorbed iron (17,18). Although activated charcoal (AC) poorly adsorbs iron, AC adsorbs iron from solutions that contain DFO, presumably because the DFO-iron chelate is adsorbed in the form of ferrioxamine (19–21). A prospective human volunteer study found that the area under the curve of ferrous sulfate premixed with a DFO-AC slurry (1:3 weight per weight) was lower than when ferrous sulfate was given alone or premixed with only AC (22).

Pretreatment of rats with DFO substantially reduced the peroxidative damage of doxorubicin-treated animals. Protection was not complete and plateaued at a level tenfold that of the doxorubicin dose (1).

PHARMACOKINETICS AND TOXICOKINETICS

After IV administration, the distribution half-life is 5 to 17 minutes, with blood ferrioxamine concentrations peaking at 30 minutes (23,24). The terminal elimination half-life is 3.05 hours, and steady-state concentrations are achieved in 6 to 12 hours during infusion (23). The elimination half-life in renal failure is approximately 26 hours (25). During hemodialysis, the half-life of DFO is approximately 2 hours.

After SQ infusion, plateaus of DFO and ferrioxamine concentrations are reached in 4 to 8 hours, the distribution half-life is 0.56 hours, and the elimination half-life is 9.80 hours (26). The volume of distribution of DFO is 0.60 to 1.33 L/kg (12,23,27) and 0.2 L/kg for the DFO-iron complex (ferrioxamine).

The DFO-aluminum chelate (aluminoxamine) reaches maximum serum levels in 7 to 8 hours (28). The half-life of aluminoxamine is 2 to 4 hours during hemodialysis (29).

DFO is metabolized in the liver by oxidative deamination of the *N* terminus producing multiple metabolites (A–F). The B metabolite is believed responsible for most of the adverse effects (23). The amount and proportion of metabolites are inversely related to the availability of chelatable iron because the DFO-iron complex is not metabolized but rather excreted in the urine (30). A constant infusion of DFO results in significantly decreased amounts of metabolite B compared to higher doses given over shorter infusion periods and results in higher chelation efficiency and lower drug toxicity (26).

INDICATIONS

Acute Iron Poisoning

Specific indications for DFO include clinically significant toxicity (shock, altered mental status, metabolic acidosis), especially if serum iron levels exceed 500 μg/dl, measured on blood drawn 4 to 6 hours after ingestion. A slurry of DFO and AC can be considered to reduce GI absorption of iron when there is evidence of a significant, recent ingestion or ongoing GI absorption (22).

Other common effects of iron intoxication, such as hyperglycemia, leukocytosis, nausea, or radiographic evidence of pill fragments, are not well correlated with toxicity and are not indications for DFO (31–33).

Chronic Iron Poisoning

DFO is also indicated in chronic iron overload, as occurs with multiple blood transfusions, thalassemia, and sickle cell anemia (34).

Aluminum Intoxication

Acute poisoning has been limited to contamination of dialysate solutions in patients with renal failure and in states of acute or chronic aluminum overload in renal failure patients (34–36).

Other Uses in Toxicology

DFO may have a role in treating paraquat toxicity (2).

CAUTIONS AND CONTRAINDICATIONS

DFO is U.S. Food and Drug Administration pregnancy category C. It is unknown whether DFO crosses the placenta; it is charged and larger in size than most drugs that do (37). Animal studies indicate toxicity *in utero* (38,39). There is no human evidence that DFO is teratogenic. There are reports of more than 40 pregnancies in which DFO has been given during several weeks or months of gestation without apparent fetal injury, including two patients treated up to 26 weeks (40).

DFO should not be used alone orally because it may increase the absorption of iron. Because DFO may induce renal failure in patients with decreased intravascular volumes (41), it is recommended that a modest fluid expansion be performed before parenteral administration (42). DFO should be avoided in patients with significant renal impairment unless undergoing hemodialysis because the DFO-metal complex is eliminated renally.

Hypersensitivity reactions to DFO may occur. They are usually dose-rate related. Patients with prior reactions and other toxicity have later received DFO without difficulty, either by another route, by slower administration, or by the use of rapid desensitization dosing schedules (43).

DOSAGE AND METHOD OF ADMINISTRATION

Acute Iron Poisoning

The preferred route of administration is IV. The initial dose for *adults and children* is 15 mg/kg/hour (42,44). This dose chelates only 1.275 mg/kg/hour of iron; however, this dose is often associated with clinical improvement. For severe poisoning, the dose may be titrated upward for signs of iron toxicity, serum iron concentration, and severity of acidosis. Rates of 20 to 25 mg/kg/hour are usually adequate to treat severe poisoning, although rates as high as 40 mg/kg/hour have been used when treating life-threatening iron toxicity. The rate of infusion is tapered as the patient's clinical condition improves and the iron level decreases. Higher dose rates have been safely used, including intermittent dosing at 25 mg/kg/hour (44) and 50 mg/kg/hour as an aluminum challenge test (45). A maximum safe rate of administration has not been established.

Originally, DFO was administered by IM injection, but this route is rarely appropriate today. The *adult* IM dose is 1 g, followed by 500 mg every 4 hours for two doses, with an additional 500 mg every 4 to 12 hours as needed to a maximum total dose of 6 g/day.

The manufacturer recommends a maximum dose of 6 g of DFO per 24 hours, but this amounts to only 6 hours of continuous IV therapy in a 70-kg individual at 15 mg/kg/hour. Because of increased safety of an IV infusion over IM injection, larger iron ingestions, and ongoing symptomatology, this total daily dose is routinely exceeded (46,47), and experience has demonstrated that 15 mg/kg/hour over 24 hours is safe (42).

DFO given to prevent further iron absorption from the GI tract should be given as a slurry combined with AC (1:3 weight per weight) (22).

The appropriate duration of DFO infusion is unclear. Free iron rapidly enters the cell, and free serum iron distribution will be complete within 12 to 24 hours, with serum iron concentrations returning toward "normal" levels. When DFO is given, ferrioxamine may impart a red-orange coloration to the urine, although this does not always occur, and its appearance is not associated with demonstrated clinical benefit. When it is observed in treatment, the return of the urine to a normal coloration generally signals the removal of available free iron. Treatment is traditionally continued until the urine returns to normal (if a color change was noted) *and* clinical indicators, such as hemodynamic stability, metabolic acidosis, the level of consciousness, and liver function, have improved. This usually occurs within 24 hours but may be longer in severe poisoning.

The use of treating with large doses of DFO beyond 24 hours has been questioned, as free iron will have passed intracellularly, where it is relatively inaccessible (13). DFO toxicity is also more likely to occur with prolonged high-dose exposure. Others have proposed intermittent high-dose treatments to chelate free iron redistributing to the central circulation and to minimize DFO and ferrioxamine exposure to the lung, thereby possibly reducing pulmonary toxicity. A schedule of 25 mg/kg/hour for 12 hours, alternating with 12 hours off therapy for 3 days, was successful in treating a 22-month-old boy with an initial serum iron concentration of 16,706 μg/dl (44).

Chronic Iron Poisoning

DFO may be given by SQ bolus, continuous SQ, or IV infusion (35,36). The usual dose of DFO is 1 to 6 g/24 hours, adjusted for serum ferritin (10). For iron overload from multiple blood transfusions, the usual dose is 0.5 to 1.0 g daily. A dose of 2 g IV (15 mg/kg/hour) can be given with each unit of blood transfused (maximum of 6 g/24 hours). Daily doses up to 12 g (15 mg/kg/hour) for 2 years have been well tolerated and effective for patients requiring frequent blood transfusions (48). Because of the potential for serious infections, a lower dosage (5 mg/kg weekly) has been recommended for dialysis patients (49).

Aluminum Poisoning

The usual dose of DFO for chronic aluminum overload is 5 mg/kg/week (49); however, a much lesser dose (0.5 mg/kg, two to three times per week) is efficacious and decreases the possibility of adverse effects (36). The DFO-aluminum chelate is cleared by hemodialysis during treatment with IV or IM DFO (50). Hemodialysis should be performed 6 to 8 hours after DFO administration, corresponding to the maximum blood concentration of aluminoxamine (29,50).

ADVERSE EFFECTS

There are a number of adverse effects of DFO therapy, including hypersensitivity reactions; hypotension; and ocular, otic, encephalopathic, hematologic, and infectious effects (51,52).

Acute Iron Toxicity

Hypotension may occur with IV infusion. It is related to the rate of administration (53) and is believed to be mediated by histamine release (54).

Iron overload itself causes pulmonary injury (55). Prolonged DFO infusions may increase the risk of pulmonary injury. A DFO-related, dose-dependent pulmonary syndrome has been described, consisting of hypoxia, hypocapnia, and bilateral interstitial infiltrates. The pulmonary syndrome followed relatively high-dose IV therapy used to treat acute severe iron overdose (mean daily dose, 166.2 ± 39.6 mg/kg/day for 7.75 ± 2.00 days) in 2 of 17 patients. The syndrome was reversible, with pulmonary functions returning to normal over several months. The syndrome develops after 6 to 10 days of treatment. In one patient, the drug was later reintroduced as an SQ infusion without recurrence (56). Similar findings were reported in four of eight patients with β-thalassemia major receiving doses of 10 to 22 mg/kg/hour for 5 to 9 days (57), and in 8 of 14 patients treated with 15 mg/kg/hour for more than 24 hours (58).

Chronic Use of Deferoxamine

SQ boluses or higher doses given 2 days/week are generally well tolerated (35,59). However, chronic DFO use can produce adverse effects. Bone dysplasia has occurred (60). Sensorimotor neurotoxicity developed in two patients after 5 and 6 months of daily high-dose (120 mg/kg/day) treatment (61). Symptoms resolved with discontinuation of DFO and recurred in one patient on resumption of treatment with DFO.

Ocular toxicity is manifested by decreased visual acuity and disturbance of color vision and is believed to be due to DFO chelation of copper and zinc, as well as interference with iron-dependent enzyme activity in the retina (52,62–64). Electrophysiologic tests of retinal function detect retinal injury earlier than funduscopic examination and may signal the need to discontinue non-lifesaving DFO use (65).

Ototoxicity is manifested by reversible tinnitus (66) and high-frequency sensorineural hearing loss (67,68), which was reversible in some patients. Ototoxicity has been reported in 3.8% to 57.0% of patients undergoing chronic DFO treatment (34,68). Other risk factors for ototoxicity include younger age, higher doses, lower serum ferritin concentrations, peak DFO dose, monthly DFO dose, and increased compliance (34), but not ocular toxicity (69).

The *therapeutic index* is the rate of the mean daily dose divided by the serum ferritin concentration. Ocular toxicity and ototoxicity are increased when the therapeutic index exceeds 0.025 (52,69). A review of 17 patients over 16 years had only one case of retinal toxicity, which occurred when a therapeutic index of 0.025 was briefly exceeded. Reversal of toxicity took place over a period of 9 months (70).

Serious and sometimes fatal infections may accompany the use of DFO, including *Yersinia enterocolitica* (71), mucormycosis (72), and *Aeromonas hydrophila* (73). The DFO-iron complex appears to act as a siderophore, promoting bacterial organism replication in an iron-deficient environment (71,73). Mucormycosis occurred in dialysis patients receiving DFO for aluminum overload (51).

DFO increases the development of Kaposi's sarcoma papules within the drug diffusion area (74), and there is a report of myasthenia gravis after iron chelation for iron overload secondary to sideroblastic anemia (75).

PITFALLS

DFO spuriously lowers the determination of serum iron concentrations by most laboratory methods (13). The total iron-binding capacity is not useful in making decisions regarding treatment and should not be used (31,42). Hospital pharmacies often do not stock DFO in adequate amounts (Chapter 41) (76,77).

REFERENCES

1. Saad SY, Najjar TA, Al-Rikabi AC. The preventive role of deferoxamine against acute doxorubicin-induced cardiac, renal and hepatic toxicity in rats. *Pharmacol Res* 2001;43(3):211–218.
2. Kang SA, Jang YJ, Park H. In vivo dual effects of vitamin C on paraquat-induced lung damage: dependence on release metals from the damaged tissue. *Free Radic Res* 1998;28(1):93–107.
3. Breidbach T, Scory S, Krauth-Siegel RL, Steverding D. Growth inhibition of bloodstream forms of *Trypanosoma brucei* by the iron chelator deferoxamine. *Int J Parasitol* 2002;32(4):473–479.
4. Mabeza GF, Loyevsky M, Gordeuk VR, Weiss G. Iron chelation therapy for malaria. *Pharmacol Ther* 1999;81:53–75.
5. Clarkson AB, Turkel-Parrella D, Williams JH, et al. Action of deferoxamine against *Pneumocystis carinii*. *Antimicrob Agents Chemother* 2001;45(12):3560–3565.
6. Conlon BJ, Perry BP, Smith DW. Attenuation of neomycin ototoxicity by iron chelation. *Laryngoscope* 1998;108:284–287.
7. Sakaida I, Kayano K, Wasaki S, et al. Protection against acetaminophen-induced liver injury in vivo by an iron chelator, deferoxamine. *Scand J Gastroenterol* 1995;30(1):61–67.
8. Schnellmann JG, Pumford NR, Kusewitt DF et al. Deferoxamine delays the development of the hepatotoxicity of acetaminophen in mice. *Toxicol Lett* 1999;106:79–88.
9. Duffy SJ, Biegelsen ES, Holbrook M, et al. Iron chelation improves endothelial function in patients with coronary artery disease. *Circulation* 2001;103(23):2799–2804.
10. Lopez L, Dilley RB, Henriquez JA. Cutaneous hyperpigmentation following venous sclerotherapy treated with deferoxamine mesylate. *Dermatol Surg* 2001;27(9):795–798.
11. Rose C, Cambie C, Forzy G, Mahieu M, et al. Deferoxamine stability in intravenous solution. *Ann N Y Acad Sci* 1998;850:488–489.
12. Keberle H. The biochemistry of desferrioxamine and its relation to iron metabolism. *Ann N Y Acad Sci* 1964;119:758–768.
13. Howland MA. Risks of parenteral deferoxamine for acute iron poisoning. *J Toxicol Clin Toxicol* 1996;34(5):491–497.
14. Ihnat PM, Vennerstrom JL, Robinson DH. Synthesis and solution properties of deferoxamine amides. *J Pharmaceut Sci* 2000;89(12):1525–1536.
15. American Society of Hospital Pharmacists. *AHGS drug information 1990*. Bethesda, MD: American Society of Hospital Pharmacists, 1993:1874–1875.
16. Desferrioxamine (mesylate). In: Sir Colin Dollery, ed. *Therapeutic drugs*. London: Churchill Livingstone, 1991:D28–D32.
17. Dean BS, Oehme FW, Krenzelok EP, et al. Iron complexation with oral deferoxamine in a swine model. *Vet Hum Toxicol* 1996;38(2):96–98.
18. Jackson TW, Long LJ, Washington V. The effect of oral deferoxamine on iron absorption in humans. *J Toxicol Clin Toxicol* 1995;33:325–329.
19. Chang TMS, Barre P. Effect of desferrioxamine on removal of aluminum and iron by coated charcoal haemoperfusion and haemodialysis. *Lancet* 1983;2:1051–1053.
20. Gomez HF, McClafferty H, Horowitz R, et al. Adsorption of iron to a premixed deferoxamine/charcoal slurry. *Vet Hum Toxicol* 1993;35:366 (abst).
21. Yonker J, Banner W, Picchioni A. Absorption characteristics of iron and deferoxamine onto charcoal. *Vet Hum Toxicol* 1980;22[Suppl]:75.
22. Gomez HF, McClafferty HH, Flory D, et al. Prevention of gastrointestinal iron absorption by chelation from an orally administered premixed deferoxamine/charcoal slurry. *Ann Emerg Med* 1997;30(5):587–592.
23. Lee P, Mohammed N, Abeysinghe RD, et al. Intravenous infusion pharmacokinetics of desferrioxamine in thalassaemia patients. *Drugs Metab Disp* 1993;21:640–644.
24. Summers M, Jacobs A, Tudway D, et al. Studies in deferoxamine and ferrioxamine metabolism in normal and iron loaded subjects. *Br J Haematol* 1979;42:547–555.
25. Stivelman J, Schulman G, Fosburg M, et al. Kinetic and efficacy of deferoxamine in iron-overloaded hemodialysis patients. *Kidney Int* 1989;36:1125–1132.
26. Porter JB, Alberti D, Hassan I, et al. Subcutaneous depot desferrioxamine (CGH 749B): relationship of pharmacokinetics to efficacy and drug metabolism. *Blood* 1997;90:265a.
27. Peters G, Keberle K, Schmid K, Brunner H. Distribution and renal excretion of desferrioxamine and ferrioxamine in the dog and rat. *Biochem Pharmacol* 1966;16:93–109.
28. Andriani M, Nordio M, Saporiti E. Estimation of statistical moments for desferrioxamine and its iron and aluminum chelates: contribution to optimisation of therapy in uremic patients. *Nephron* 1996;72:218–224.
29. Verpooten GA, D'Haese PC, Boelaert JR, et al. Pharmacokinetics of aluminoxamine and ferrioxamine and dose finding of desferrioxamine in haemodialysis patients. *Nephrol Dial Transplant* 1992;7:931–938.
30. Porter JB. Deferoxamine pharmacokinetics. *Sem Hematol* 2001;38[1 Suppl 1]:63–68.
31. Chyka PA, Butler AY. Assessment of acute iron poisoning by laboratory and clinical observations. *Am J Emerg Med* 1993;11:99–103.
32. Knasel AL, Collins-Barrow MD. Applicability of early indicators of iron toxicity. *J Natl Med Assoc* 1986;78:1037–1040.

33. Palatnick W, Tenenbein M. Leukocytosis, hyperglycemia, vomiting and positive x-rays are not indicators of severity of iron overdose in adults. *Am J Emerg Med* 1996;14(5):454–455.
34. Kanno H, Yamanobe S, Rybak LP. The ototoxicity of deferoxamine mesylate. *Am J Otolaryngol* 1995;16(3):148–152.
35. Franchini M, Gandini G, de Gironcoli M, et al. Safety and efficacy of subcutaneous bolus injection of deferoxamine in adult patients with iron overload. *Blood* 2000;95(9):2776–2779.
36. Jorge C, Gil C, Possante M, et al. Use of a desferrioxamine "microdose" to chelate aluminum in hemodialysis patients. *Clin Nephrol* 1999;52:335-336.
37. Tenenbein M. Poisoning in pregnancy. In: Koren G, ed. *Maternal-fetal toxicology: a clinician's guide*, 2nd ed. New York: Marcel Dekker, Inc., 1994:223–254.
38. Angeles-Bosque M, Domingo JL, Corbella J. Assessment of the developmental toxicity of deferoxamine in mice. *Arch Toxicol* 1995;69:467–471.
39. Lauro V, Giornelli C, Santilli Giornelli FE, Fanelli A. Effects of iron chelating agent on pregnant rats. Experimental findings. *Arch Obstet Gynecol* 1968;73:269.
40. Singer ST, Vichinsky EP. Deferoxamine treatment during pregnancy: is it harmful? *Am J Hematol* 1999;60:24–26.
41. Koren G, Bentur Y, Strong D, et al. Acute changes in renal function associated with deferoxamine therapy. *Am J Dis Child* 1989;143:1077–1080.
42. Tenenbein M. Benefits of parenteral deferoxamine for acute iron poisoning. *J Toxicol Clin Toxicol* 1996;34(5):485–489.
43. La Rosa M, Romeo MA, Di Gregoria F, Russo G. Desensitization treatment for anaphylactoid reactions to desferrioxamine in a pediatric patient with thalassemia. *J Allergy Clin Immunol* 1996;97(1 Pt 1):127–128.
44. Cheney K, Gumbiner C, Benson B, Tenenbein M. Survival after a severe iron poisoning treated with intermittent infusions of deferoxamine. *J Toxicol Clin Toxicol* 1995;33(1):61–66.
45. Berland Y, Charhon SA, Olmer M, Meunier PJ. Predictive value of desferrioxamine infusion test for bone aluminum deposit in hemodialyzed patients. *Nephron* 1985;40:433–435.
46. Henretig FM, Karl SR, Weintraub WH. Severe iron poisoning treated with enteral and intravenous deferoxamine. *Ann Emerg Med* 1983;12:306–309.
47. Peck MG, Rogers JF, Rivenbark JF. Use of high doses of deferoxamine (Desferal) in an adult patient with acute iron overdosage. *J Toxicol Clin Toxicol* 1982;19:865–869.
48. Cohen AR, Martin M, Schwartz E. Current treatment of Cooley's anemia. Intravenous chelation therapy. *Ann N Y Acad Sci* 1990;612:286–292.
49. De Broe MD, D'Haese PC, Couttenye MM, et al. New insights and strategies in the diagnosis and treatment of aluminium overload in dialysis patients. *Nephrol Dial Transplant* 1993;S1:47–50.
50. Nakamura H, Rose PG, Blumer JL, Reed MD. Acute encephalopathy due to aluminum toxicity successfully treated by combined intravenous deferoxamine and hemodialysis. *J Clin Pharmacol* 2000;40:296–300.
51. Boelaert JR, de Locht M. Side-effects of desferrioxamine in dialysis patients. *Nephrol Dial Transplant* 1993;S1:43–46.
52. Porter JB, Huehns ER. The toxic effects of desferrioxamine. *Clin Haematol* 1989;2:459–474.
53. Leikin S, Vossough P, Mochir-Fatemi F. Chelation therapy in acute iron poisoning. *J Pediatr* 1967;71:425–430.
54. Whitten CF, Givson GW, Good MH, et al. Studies in acute iron poisoning. I. Desferrioxamine in the treatment of iron poisoning: clinical observations, experimental studies, and theoretical considerations. *Pediatrics* 1965;36:322–325.
55. Hoppe J, Marcelli G, Taintenn M. A review of the toxicity of iron compounds. *Am J Med Sci* 1955;558–571.
56. Rego EM, Neto EB, Simoes BP, Zago MA. Dose-dependent pulmonary syndrome in patients with thalassemia major receiving intravenous deferoxamine. *Am J Hematol* 1998;58(4):340–341.
57. Freedman MH, Grisaru D, Olivieri N, et al. Pulmonary syndrome in patients with thalassemia major receiving intravenous deferoxamine infusions. *Am J Dis Child* 1990;144:565.
58. Tenenbein M, Kowalski S, Sienko A, et al. Pulmonary toxic effects of continuous desferrioxamine administration in acute iron poisoning. *Lancet* 1992;339:699.
59. Hagege I, Becker A, Kerdaffrec T, et al. Long-term administration of high-dose deferoxamine 2 days per week in thalassemic patients. *Eur J Haematol* 2001;67:230–231.
60. Chan YL, Chu CW, Chik KW, et al. Deferoxamine-induced dysplasia of the knee: sonographic features and diagnostic performance compared with magnetic resonance imaging. *J Ultrasound Med* 2001;20(7):723–728.
61. Levine JE, Cohen A, MacQueen M, et al. Sensorimotor neurotoxicity associated with high-dose deferoxamine treatment. *J Pedatr Hematol Oncol* 1997;19(2):139–141.
62. Cases A, Kelly J, Sabater F, et al. Ocular and auditory toxicity in hemodialyzed patients receiving desferrioxamine. *Nephron* 1990;56:19–23.
63. Davies SC, Hungerford JL, Arden GB, et al. Ocular toxicity of high dose intravenous deferoxamine. *Lancet* 1983;2:181–184.
64. Pall H, Blake DR, Winyard P, et al. Ocular toxicity of desferrioxamine. An example of copper promoted ayto-oxidative damage? *Br J Ophthalmol* 1989;73:29–31.
65. Haimovici R, D'Amico DJ, Gragoudas ES, Sokol S. The expanded clinical spectrum of deferoxamine renopathy. *Ophthalmology* 2002;109:164–171.
66. Marsh MN, Holbrook IB, Clark C, et al. Tinnitus in a patient with beta-thalassaemia intermedia on long-term treatment with deferoxamine. *Postgrad Med J* 1981;57:582–584.
67. Olivieri NF, Buncic JR, Chew E, et al. Deferal has significant audio-visual neurotoxicity. *Blood* 1984;64[Suppl 1]:40a.
68. Olivieri NF, Buncic JR, Chew E, et al. Visual and auditory neurotoxicity in patients receiving subcutaneous deferoxamine infusions. *N Engl J Med* 1986;314:869–873.
69. Porter JB, Jaswon MS, Huehns ER, et al. Desferrioxamine ototoxicity: evaluation of risk factors in thalassaemic patients and guidelines for safe dosage. *Br J Haematol* 1989;73:403–409.
70. Davis BA, Porter JB. Long-term outcome of continuous 24-hour deferoxamine infusion via indwelling intravenous catheters in high-risk β-thalassemia. *Blood* 2000;95(4):1229–1236.
71. Pallister C, Rotstein OD. *Yersinia enterocolitica* as a cause of intra-abdominal abscess: the role of iron. *Can J Surg* 2001;44(2):135–136.
72. Boelaert JR, de Locht M, Van Cutsem J, et al. Mucormycosis during deferoxamine therapy is a siderophore-mediate infection. In vitro and in vivo animal studies. *J Clin Invest* 1993;91:1979–1986.
73. Lin S-H, Shieh S-D, Lin Y-F, et al. Fatal *Aeromonas hydrophila* bacteremia in a hemodialysis patient treated with deferoxamine. *Am J Kid Dis* 1996;27(5):733–735.
74. Simonart T, Boelaert JR, Van Vooren JP. Enhancement of classic Kaposi's sarcoma growth after intralesional injections of desferrioxamine. *Dermatology* 2002;204(4):290–292.
75. Krishnan K, Trobe JD, Adams PT. Myasthenia gravis following iron chelation therapy with intravenous desferrioxamine. *Eur J Haematol* 1995;55:138–139.
76. Dart RC, Goldfrank LR, Chyka PA, et al. Combined evidence-based literature analysis and consensus guidelines for stocking of emergency antidotes in the United States. *Ann Emerg Med* 2000;36(2):126–132.
77. Sivilotti MLA, Eisen JS, Lee JS, Peterson RG. Can emergency departments not afford to carry essential antidotes? *Can J Emerg Med* 2002;4(1). Available at: http://www.caep.ca/004.cjem-jcmu/004-00.cjem/vol-4.2002/v41-023.htm. Accessed October 23, 2002.

CHAPTER 49

Digoxin Immune Fab

Alison L. Jones and Robert J. Flanagan

Synonyms:	**Anti-Digitale BM, Digibind, DigiFab, Digitalis Antidot**
Molecular weight:	**50,000 daltons**
CAS Registry No.:	**79517-01-4**
Normal or therapeutic levels:	**Not applicable**
Special concerns:	**Many hospital pharmacies do not stock adequate amounts. Recurrence of toxic effects may occur after an initially beneficial response.**

OVERVIEW

Mortality is high in severe digoxin poisoning. Digoxin-specific antibody fragments (DFab) were first used in humans in 1976, and many patients have been treated with them (1–4).

All commercial preparations of DFab contain 40 mg of Fab per vial. Digibind (Glaxo Wellcome) is generally available in North America and in the United Kingdom; DigiFab is available in the United States (Savage Laboratories); and Digitalis Antidot BM (Boeringher Mannheim) is used in Europe (5). All show

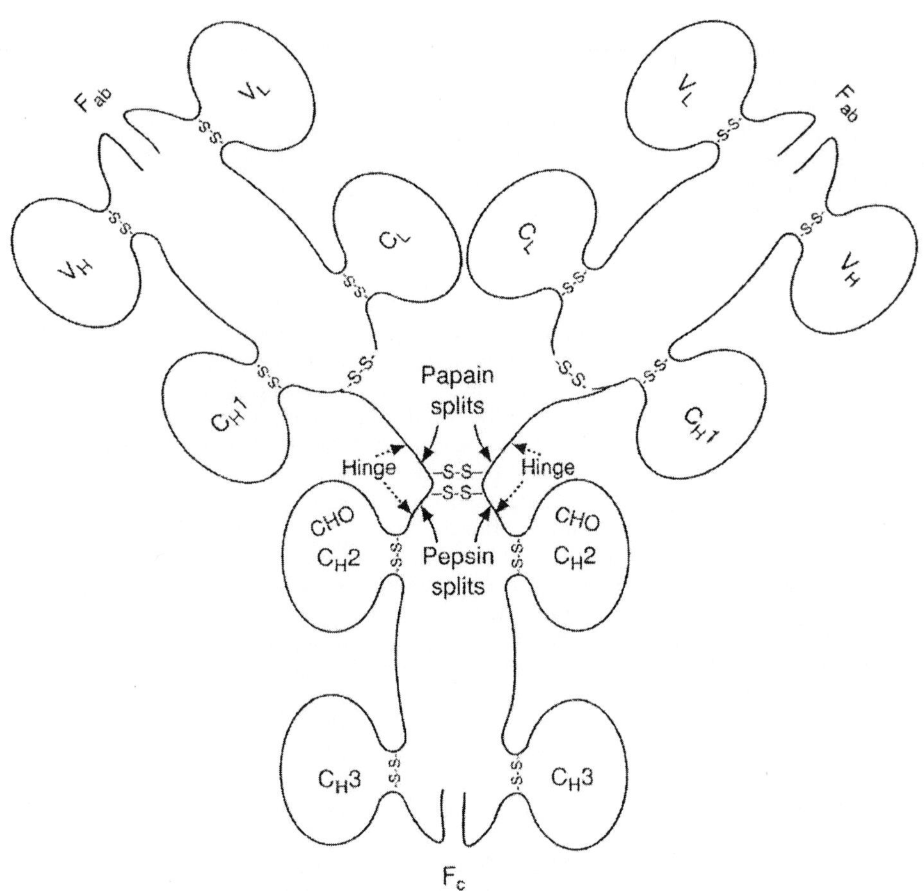

Figure 1. Schematic diagram of the human immunoglobulin G molecule. The molecule is composed of two "heavy" and two "light" polypeptide chains and has two antigen-binding sites (F_{ab}) and a complement fixing site (F_c). V_L and V_H denote light- and heavy-chain variable regions, respectively; C_H1, C_H2, and C_H3 denote "constant" regions on the heavy chain; CL is a constant region of the light chain. (From Kabat, 1982, with permission.)

some cross-reaction with digitoxin (5–8) and lanatoside C (7). Digibind has been shown to reverse β-methyldigoxin– and β-acetyl-digoxin–induced dysrhythmias in guinea pigs (9).

Mechanism of Action

The aim of immunotoxicotherapy is to sequester, extract, or redistribute and eliminate toxins by antigen-antibody binding. For example, the concentration of free digoxin falls immediately to zero after DFab treatment (1). However, the ability to manufacture an antibody with the necessary specificity and affinity, and in large quantities, has limited the application of this approach to poisoning by digoxin, other cardiac glycosides, colchicine, and tricyclic antidepressants (10).

However, whole immunoglobulin G antibodies are themselves immunogenic by virtue of their Fc fragment (Fig. 1), and they are too large to be readily excreted in urine or to be dialyzed (11). Moreover, degradation of the circulating antibody-digoxin complex could theoretically release large quantities of digoxin back into the circulation (12). The use of DFab derived from sheep has overcome these problems (13,14). DFab lack immunogenicity and are small enough (molecular weight, 50,000) to be excreted in the urine.

The use of antibody fragments limits the risk of anaphylaxis but reduces the stability of the toxin-antibody complex. The affinity constant of DFab for digoxin is high (10^{10}) and greater than that of digoxin for its receptor (Na^+K^+-activated adenosine triphosphatase). The affinity constant of the antibody fragment for digitoxin is also high (10^9). DFab bind to circulating glycoside and form relatively stable complexes. The bound digoxin is unable to bind to tissue digitalis receptors. In animals, Fab reverse digoxin effects much more quickly than immunoglobulin G. There is a suggestion that reversal of inotropy lags behind reversal of dysrhythmic effects (15).

Pharmacokinetic/Pharmacodynamic Data

The gastrointestinal tract, kidney, liver, spleen, and lymph nodes are among the potential sites of catabolism of DFab. Circulating DFab are filtered through the glomeruli and rapidly and extensively reabsorbed in the proximal tubules of the kidney. Sixty percent to 70% of Fab total body clearance is nonrenal (10). The elimination half-life of Fab in humans is approximately 12 hours (16). Reported values for the elimination half-life of digoxin after DFab administration are conflicting. Claimed elimination half-lives are 16 to 20 hours (8) and 20 to 30 hours, compared with 160 hours for spontaneous elimination (5). Treatment with DFab increases the renal clearance of digoxin by 20% to 30% (12).

INDICATIONS

Digoxin or Digitoxin Toxicity

Specific indications for administration of DFab have evolved over time and, in clinical practice, vary by practitioner. When Digibind was introduced, the initial recommendations focused on treatment of life-threatening cardiac dysrhythmias. More recent recommendations expand the indication of life-threatening cardiac dysrhythmias to include complete heart block or a serum potassium level above 5.5 mEq/L (17). DFab are also recommended after acute ingestion of more than 4 mg of digoxin in a previously healthy child and 10 mg in a previously healthy adult (18). Finally, administration is recommended if the steady-state serum digoxin level is greater than 10 ng/ml (18). DFab should be used earlier and more freely in elderly patients or those with underlying heart disease (19).

Sixty-three patients with severe digitalis toxicity (life-threatening dysrhythmias or hyperkalemia) were given Digibind over 15 to 30 minutes. They ranged in age from a few days to 85 years, and 28 had taken a massive overdose. Of the 56 patients eligible for the study, 53 recovered completely (8). For Digitalis Antidot BM, 32 of 34 patients were successfully treated (5). Digoxin toxicity resolved in 27 of 29 patients (aged up to 18 years) with severe digoxin poisoning treated with Digibind; 3 patients required additional DFab treatment (20). In no series could death be attributed to failure to reverse digoxin toxicity. Digibind and DigiFab bind digoxin similarly, although the clearance of digoxin in human volunteers was higher for DigiFab (21).

In some cases, the rate of reversal of toxicity has been dramatic: gastrointestinal features of toxicity disappearing almost immediately and hyperkalemia being corrected within 30 to 60 minutes (22). Dysrhythmias were corrected equally as quickly in some patients (22) but more slowly (up to 13.0 hours; mean, 3.2 hours) in others (5). The effects of acute toxicity seem to reverse more quickly than those of chronic toxicity. Even digitoxin-induced thrombocytopenia was improved considerably within hours (6).

Cardiac glycoside toxicity may recur in some patients treated with DFab. Free digoxin levels typically rise again in a mean time of 77 ± 46 hours (23). Recurrence occurs later in patients with renal failure. The clinical implication is that patients require prolonged monitoring for digoxin effects; however, the intensity and type of monitoring needed are unclear.

Other Cardiac Glycosides

Cardiac glycoside toxicity may also arise from plant and animal products. The identity and concentration of cardiac glycosides in these products are unknown. DFab have been useful in several severe cases, although the precise indications for this use are unknown (24,25). A therapeutic trial of DFab is reasonable for signs of cardiac or hemodynamic instability (hypotension, symptomatic bradycardia, or serious cardiac dysrhythmias).

CAUTIONS AND CONTRAINDICATIONS

DFab are U.S. Food and Drug Administration pregnancy category C (Appendix I). DFab should be used in pregnant patients as it is in other patients. DFab should be used very cautiously in patients with a history of allergy to DFab.

DOSAGE AND METHOD OF ADMINISTRATION

Digoxin or Digitoxin Toxicity

The precise dose of DFab after acute digoxin overdose is not well established. Adult patients with severe hemodynamic compromise should be treated with 10 to 20 vials (380 to 760 mg). Stable patients may be treated with dosing based on the ingested amount (if known) or on the steady-state serum level.

If only the amount ingested is known, use Equation 1:

$$\text{Number of DFab vials} = \frac{\text{amount of digoxin}}{\text{ingested (mg)}} \times 0.48 \qquad \text{[Eq. 1]}$$

If the serum digoxin level obtained at least 6 hours after ingestion is known, use Equation 2:

$$\begin{matrix}\text{Number of}\\\text{DFab vials}\end{matrix} = \frac{\begin{matrix}\text{serum digoxin}\\\text{level (ng/ml)}\end{matrix} \times \begin{matrix}\text{ideal body}\\\text{weight (kg)}\end{matrix}}{100} \qquad \text{[Eq. 2]}$$

This calculation should not be used within 6 hours of ingestion because the drug has not had time to distribute; therefore, the level will be misleadingly high.

Patients who develop cardiac toxicity during chronic digoxin therapy usually require much less DFab than those with acute intoxication. Chronic ingestion usually requires less than five vials, whereas toxicity after acute ingestion requires more. When a steady-state serum level is known, Equation 2 may be used to determine the dose of DFab. An alternative for stable patients is to administer two to four vials of DFab and then repeat the dose based on patient response.

Some clinicians have advocated an approach intended to leave some unbound digoxin present in the blood to maintain the desired serum digoxin level. This can be accomplished theoretically using Equation 2 by substituting the term [serum digoxin level (ng/ml) – 1] to maintain a free digoxin level of 1 ng/ml. However, binding varies among patients, and the digoxin level varies depending on the time of serum sampling. Deliberate *partial* reversal of patients (to maintain a therapeutic digoxin level) is likely inaccurate and cannot be recommended.

Other Cardiac Glycoside Toxicity

The appropriate dose for plant and animal sources of cardiac glycosides is unknown. In case reports, the dose has typically been five to ten vials, with additional doses guided by the response to therapy. Large doses have been needed in some cases.

Monitoring Response

The response to therapy is monitored using the patient's vital signs and the electrocardiogram. Toxic effects may recur in some patients, particularly those with renal insufficiency. The time-to-peak rebound of free digoxin levels in five patients with end-stage renal failure and cardiac glycoside toxicity was 127 ± 40 hours—over twice as long as in other patients (23). Although recurrence is often not clinically important, monitoring is recommended, especially if the initial digoxin levels were very high.

ADVERSE EFFECTS

Infusion of DFab is generally well tolerated. Very few immediate or delayed hypersensitivity reactions have been reported (26). However, hypokalemia and exacerbation of congestive heart failure have been reported (5,8,18), and there is concern that renal function could be impaired in some patients. One study found that Fab reduced the glomerular filtration rate in rabbits (27).

PITFALLS

The use of DFab therapy should not delay other therapies. The diagnosis should be reconsidered and other measures instituted to treat hyperkalemia or dysrhythmia as appropriate.

Conventional serum immunoassays of cardiac glycoside concentration are no longer useful when the patient has been treated with DFab (28–31).

All hospitals that accept emergency patients should stock DFab and have it available for immediate use. However, many hospitals currently overlook this responsibility (32).

REFERENCES

1. Antman EM, Wenger TL, Butler VP, et al. Treatment of 150 cases of life-threatening digitalis intoxication with digoxin-specific Fab antibody fragments: final report of a multicenter study. *Circulation* 1990;81:1744–1752.
2. Schaumann W, Kaufmann B, Neubert P, Smolarz A. Kinetics of the Fab fragments of digoxin antibodies and of bound digoxin in patients with severe digoxin intoxication. *Eur J Clin Pharmacol* 1986;30:527–533.
3. Smith TW. New advances in the assessment and treatment of digitalis toxicity. *J Clin Pharmacol* 1985;25:522–528.
4. Sullivan JB. Immunotherapy in the poisoned patient. Overview of present applications and future trends. *Med Toxicol* 1986;1:47–60.
5. Smolarz A, Roesch E, Lenz E, et al. Digoxin specific antibody (Fab) fragments in 34 cases of severe digitalis intoxication. *J Toxicol Clin Toxicol* 1985;23:327–340.
6. Hess T, Riesen W, Scholtysik G, Stucki P. Digitoxin intoxication with severe thrombocytopenia: reversal by digoxin-specific antibodies. *Eur J Clin Invest* 1983;13:159–163.
7. Hess T, Stucki P, Barandun S, et al. Treatment of a case of lanatoside C intoxication with digoxin-specific F(ab')2 antibody fragments. *Am Heart J* 1979;98:767–771.
8. Wenger TL, Butler VP, Haber E, Smith TW. Treatment of 63 severely digitalis-toxic patients with digoxin-specific antibody fragments. *J Am Coll Cardiol* 1985;5(Suppl):118A–123A.
9. GlaxoWellcome, data on file; 1995.
10. Scherrmann JM. Antibody treatment of toxin poisoning—recent advances. *J Toxicol Clin Toxicol* 1994;32:363–375.
11. Berkovitch M, Akilesh MR, Gerace R, et al. Acute digoxin overdose in a newborn with renal failure: use of digoxin immune Fab and peritoneal dialysis. *Ther Drug Monit* 1994;16:531–533.
12. Butler VP, Smith TW, Schmidt DH, Haber E. Immunological reversal of the effects of digoxin. *Fed Proc* 1977;36:2235–2341.
13. Smith TW, Butler VP, Haber E, et al. Treatment of life threatening digitalis intoxication with digoxin-specific Fab antibody fragments. Experience in 26 cases. *N Engl J Med* 1982;307:1357–1362.
14. Smith TW, Haber E, Yeatmen L, Butler VP. Reversal of advanced digoxin intoxication with Fab fragments of digoxin-specific antibodies. *N Engl J Med* 1976;294:797–800.
15. Ochs HR, Vatner SF, Smith TW. Reversal of inotropic effects of digoxin by specific antibodies and their Fab fragments in the conscious dog. *J Pharmacol Exp Ther* 1978;207:64–71.
16. Thanh-Barthet CV, Urtizberea M, Sabouraud AE, et al. Development of a sensitive radioimmunoassay for Fab fragments: application to Fab pharmacokinetics in humans. *Pharm Res* 1993;10:692–696.
17. Bismuth C, Gaultier M, Conso F, Efthymiou ML. Hyperkalemia in acute digitalis poisoning: prognostic significance and therapeutic implications. *J Toxicol Clin Toxicol* 1973;6:153–162.
18. Smith,TW, Willerson JT. Suicidal and accidental digoxin ingestion. Report of five cases with serum digoxin level correlations. *Circulation* 1971;44:29–36.
19. Baud FJ, Lapostolle F, Borron SW, Bismuth C. Acute digitalis poisoning: prognosis and management. EAPPCT International Congress, Amsterdam 2000. *J Toxicol Clin Toxicol* 2000;168–169(abst 10).
20. Woolf AD, Wenger T, Smith TW, Lovejoy FH. The use of digoxin-specific Fab fragments for severe digitalis intoxication in children. *N Engl J Med* 1992;326:1739–1744.
21. Ward SB, Sjostrom L, Ujhelyi MR. Comparison of the pharmacokinetics and in vivo bioaffinity of DigiTAb versus Digibind. *Ther Drug Monit* 2000;22:599–607.
22. Spiegel A, Marchlinski FE. Time course for reversal of digoxin toxicity with digoxin-specific antibody fragments. *Am Heart J* 1985;109:1397–1399.
23. Ujhelyi MR, Robert S, Cummings DM, et al. Influence of digoxin immune Fab therapy and renal dysfunction on the disposition of total and free digoxin. *Ann Intern Med* 1993;119:273–277.
24. Brubacher JR, Lachmanen D, Ravikumar PR, Hoffman RS. Efficacy of digoxin specific Fab fragments (Digibind) in the treatment of toad venom poisoning. *Toxicon* 1999;37:931–942.
25. Shumaik GM, Wu AW, Ping AC. Oleander poisoning: treatment with digoxin-specific Fab antibody fragments. *Ann Emerg Med* 1988;17:732–735.
26. Kirkpatrick CH. Allergic histories and reactions of patients treated with digoxin immune Fab (ovine) antibody. *Am Emerg Med* 1991;9(2 Suppl 1):7–10.
27. Timsina MP, Hewick DS. Digoxin-specific Fab fragments impair renal function in the rabbit. *J Pharm Pharmacol* 1992;44:867–869.
28. Gibb I, Adams PC, Parnham AJ, Jennings K. Plasma digoxin: assay anomalies in Fab-treated patients. *Br J Clin Pharmacol* 1983;16:445–447.
29. Gibb I, Adams PC. Digoxin assay modifications to eliminate interference following immunotherapy for toxicity. *Ann Biol Clin* 1985;43:696(abst).
30. Hursting MJ, Raisys VA, Opheim KE, et al. Determination of free digoxin concentrations in serum for monitoring Fab treatment of digoxin overdose. *Clin Chem* 1987;33:1652–1655.
31. Sinclair AJ, Hewick DS, Johnston PC, et al. Kinetics of digoxin and anti-digoxin antibody fragments during treatment of digoxin toxicity. *Br J Clin Pharmacol* 1989;28:352–356.
32. Dart RC, Goldfrank LR, Chyka PA, et al. Combined evidence-based literature analysis and consensus guidelines for stocking of emergency antidotes in the United States. *Ann Emerg Med* 2000;36:2:126–132.

CHAPTER 50

Dimercaprol

Alison L. Jones and Robert J. Flanagan

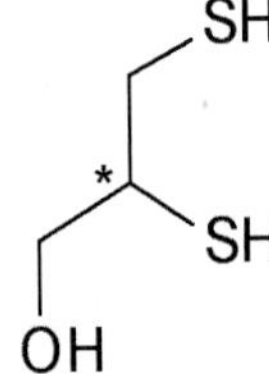

* = chiral center

DIMERCAPROL

Synonyms:	**2,3-dimercaptopropanol, British antilewisite (BAL)**
Molecular formula and weight:	**$C_3H_8OS_2$, 124.2 g/mol**
SI conversion:	**mg/L × 0.0081 = mmol/L**
CAS Registry No.:	**59-52-9**
Normal or therapeutic levels:	**Not clinically applicable**
Special concerns:	**BAL has many dose-dependent adverse effects and is typically used only in lead encephalopathy or when oral chelation is not possible.**

OVERVIEW

Dimercaprol, the first chelating agent to be used clinically, was designed to treat poisoning with the arsenical war gas lewisite (1), hence its original name *British antilewisite.* Dimercaprol is still used to treat arsenic (2), inorganic mercury (3), and gold intoxication and is used as an adjunct to calcium disodium ethylenediaminetetraacetic acid in severe pediatric lead poisoning. Dimercaprol may also be useful in antimony, bismuth, chromium, nickel, tungsten, and zinc poisoning (4,5). It has been used to chelate copper in Wilson's disease and may still play a role in patients allergic to penicillamine. Dimercaprol is widely used in developing countries, possibly because it is cheap and readily available.

Dimercaprol is a 10% solution in a clear, colorless or slightly yellow oily liquid that smells like sulfur (rotten eggs).

Mechanism of Action

Dimercaprol forms relatively stable dimercaptides with metal ions. The optimal effect seems to be obtained if dimercaprol concentrations are sufficient to favor the formation of a 2:1 dimercaprol-metal complex and if it is administered as soon as possible after the exposure (2). The hydroxyl moiety of dimercaprol confers some water solubility and helps excretion of the dimercaprol-metal complex in urine and bile. Dimercaprol-metal chelates are believed to be more stable at higher pH values; thus, maintenance of alkaline urine may protect against toxicity due to liberation of the metal within the kidney. The dimercaprol-mercury complex is removed by dialysis (6).

Dimercaprol is not absorbed orally. It is rapidly absorbed after intramuscular (IM) injection and persists for at least 12 hours (7). Approximately 80% of the dose is absorbed after 1 hour and 90% after 6 hours. Maximal blood concentrations are attained within 1 hour. Hepatic metabolism (by glucuronidation) and excretion are essentially complete within 4 hours. Dimercaprol is the only commonly used chelating agent that readily crosses cellular membranes; as a result, the concentration in certain organs (liver, kidney, small intestine) can be up to five times that in blood.

INDICATIONS

Dimercaprol is used for a variety of heavy metal poisonings, particularly when oral and intravenous administration are unavailable or contraindicated. The list of hazards includes arsenic, lead (encephalopathy), inorganic mercury (3), and gold. It may also be useful in antimony, bismuth, chromium, nickel, tungsten, and zinc poisoning.

CAUTIONS AND CONTRAINDICATIONS

Dimercaprol is said not to cause trace element depletion. As sole therapy, dimercaprol is contraindicated in poisoning with cadmium, iron, selenium, tellurium, and organomercurials, as it may increase tissue uptake of the toxin. Dimercaprol should be avoided, if possible, in patients with hepatic damage, as rats with liver injury showed toxicity with dimercaprol and arsenic (1). Hemolytic anemia may occur in patients with glucose 6 phosphate dehydrogenase deficiency, but many glucose 6 phosphate dehydrogenase deficiencies are partial in nature, so its use is not absolutely contraindicated in this group.

DOSAGE AND ADMINISTRATION

Precise dosages of dimercaprol have not been established for most groups. A typical regimen for all indications is 2.5 to 5.0 mg/kg by deep IM injection every 4 hours for 2 days, then 2.5 mg/kg every 12 hours on day 3, and one to two times daily thereafter for 1 to 2 weeks depending on the response. Many variations on this basic pattern have been used. Hemodialysis or hemodiafiltration may be required to remove the dimercaprol-metal chelate in the presence of renal failure (8,9).

It is believed that dimercaprol may only be effective for up to 9 days after acute poisoning with inorganic arsenic (10). In lead encephalopathy, it is important to administer the dimercaprol first and then the ethylenediaminetetraacetic acid 4 hours later with the second dose of dimercaprol to prevent ethylenediaminetetraacetic acid from increasing the distribution of lead into the brain (Chapter 45).

Monitoring

The level of most metals should be monitored intermittently throughout treatment. Please consult chapters on individual metals for further detail. Monitoring for adverse drug events is usually addressed adequately by typical clinical tests (vital signs, blood cell count, liver enzymes, creatinine).

ADVERSE EFFECTS

Dimercaprol is the most toxic of the currently used chelating agents (median lethal dose, approximately 1 mmol/kg) (11). In clinical use, it causes dose-related increases in both systolic and diastolic blood pressure of up to 50 mm Hg. Its toxicity is dose dependent. The incidence of adverse effects when 4 mg/kg and 5 mg/kg are given rises from 14% to 65%, respectively (2). Adverse effects include nausea; vomiting; abdominal pain; tachycardia; headache; sweating; lacrimation; muscle pain; spasm; a burning sensation in the lips, mouth, throat, and eyes, with rhinorrhea and salivation; and a feeling of constriction in the throat, chest, or hands. These effects peak within 10 to 30 minutes and usually settle spontaneously within 1 hour (2). Febrile reactions sometimes occur, especially in children, and these often persist during therapy. Convulsions and coma have occurred.

PITFALLS

An inadvertent iatrogenic overdose exceeding 4 mg/kg may cause abrupt and severe adverse effects.

REFERENCES

1. Peters RA, Stocken LA, Thompson RHS. British anti-lewisite (BAL). *Nature* 1945;156:616–619.
2. Eagle H, Magnuson HJ. The systemic treatment of 227 cases of arsenic poisoning (encephalitis, dermatitis, blood dyscrasias, jaundice, fever) with 2,3-dimercaptopropanol (BAL). *Am J Syph Gonor Vener Dis* 1946;30:420–441.
3. Longcope WT, Luetscher JA. Clinical uses of 2,3-dimercaptopropanol (BAL). XI. The treatment of acute mercury poisoning by BAL. *J Clin Invest* 1946;25:557–567.
4. Braun HA, Lusky LM, Calvery HO. The efficacy of 2,3-dimercaptopropanol (BAL) in the therapy of poisoning by compounds of antimony, bismuth, chromium, mercury and nickel. *J Pharmacol Exp Ther* 1946;87(Suppl 1):119–125.
5. Petersilge CL. Prolonged anuria following a single injection of a bismuth preparation. Possible response to therapy with BAL. *J Pediatr* 1947;31:580–583.
6. Giunta F, Di Landro D, Chiaranda M, et al. Severe acute poisoning from the ingestion of a permanent wave solution of mercuric chloride. *Hum Toxicol* 1983;2:243–246.
7. Vale JA, Meredith TJ. Antidotal therapy: pharmacokinetic aspects. In: Chambers PL, Gehring P, Sakai F, eds. *New concepts and developments in toxicology*. Amsterdam: Elsevier, 1986:329–338.
8. Mathieu D, Mathieu-Nolf M, Germain-Alonso M, et al. Massive arsenic poisoning—effect of hemodialysis and dimercaprol on arsenic kinetics. *Intensive Care Med* 1992;18:47–50.
9. Vaziri ND, Upham T, Barton CH. Hemodialysis clearance of arsenic. *Clin Toxicol* 1980;17:451–456.
10. Mahieu P, Buchet JP, Roels HA, Lauwerys R. The metabolism of arsenic in humans acutely intoxicated by As_2O_3: its significance for the duration of BAL therapy. *J Toxicol Clin Toxicol* 1981;18:1067–1075.
11. Jones MM. New developments in therapeutic chelating agents as antidotes for metal poisoning. *Crit Rev Toxicol* 1991;21:209–233.

CHAPTER 51

Dimethyl-P-Aminophenol (DMAP)

Alison L. Jones and Robert J. Flanagan

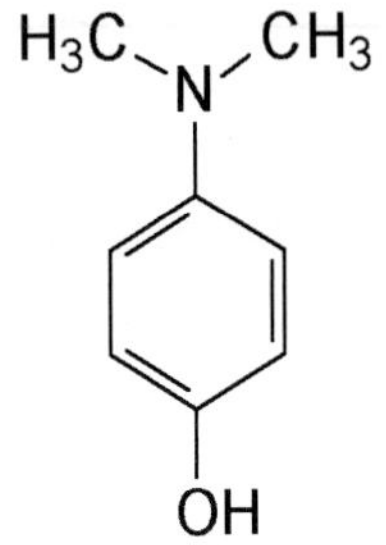

H_3C–N–CH_3 / OH

DIMETHYL-P-AMINOPHENOL

Synonyms:	**4-(*N,N*-dimethylamino)phenol HCl, dimetamfenol, 4-DMAP**
Molecular formula and weight:	**$C_8H_{11}NO$, HCl, 173.6 g/mol**
CAS Registry No.:	**5882-48-4**
Therapeutic level:	**Not recommended or clinically useful**
Special concerns:	**Adverse events are frequent.**

OVERVIEW

4-Dimethylaminophenol hydrochloride (DMAP) is used in the treatment of acute cyanide poisoning as an alternative to sodium nitrite. It is the treatment of choice in Germany for cyanide poisoning in combination with sodium thiosulfate (1). The mechanism by which DMAP catalyzes methemoglobin (MetHgb) formation is complex (2). Although DMAP has not generally found widespread application in treating cyanide poisoning, aminophenones have been investigated for use in prophylaxis, specifically in military situations. 4-Aminopropiophenone is thought to be promising in this regard because of its long half-life (3).

Mechanism of Action

DMAP generates MetHgb more quickly and in larger amounts than either amyl nitrite or sodium nitrite (4). DMAP auto-oxidizes readily at a pH above 7, and this process is accelerated by oxyhemoglobin. The product of auto-oxidation is the 4-(*N,N*-dimethylamino)phenoxyl radical, which in turn rapidly decays to form DMAP and *N,N*-dimethylquinoneimine. The latter product then quickly hydrolyzes to *p*-benzoquinone and dimethylamine, and *p*-benzoquinone reacts with DMAP to form the phenoxyl radical again. This autocatalytic formation of the phenoxyl radical, which is responsible for the oxidation of hemoglobin to MetHgb, is terminated by binding of *N,N*-dimethylquinoneimine to thiol groups of hemoglobin and glutathione in erythrocytes (Fig. 1).

INDICATIONS

The primary indication for DMAP is cyanide poisoning.

CAUTIONS AND CONTRAINDICATIONS

Excessive methemoglobinemia and hemolysis are the two major concerns during therapeutic use. DMAP should be avoided in patients with glucose 6 phosphate dehydrogenase deficiency.

DOSAGE AND METHOD OF ADMINISTRATION

The dose of DMAP recommended in cyanide poisoning is 3 to 5 mg/kg, which oxidizes 30% to 50% of the hemoglobin to MetHgb (2). The reaction is one-half complete within 2 minutes and is complete within 5 to 10 minutes. The preferred route of administration is intravenous because it may cause local pain and swelling with fever when given intramuscularly (e.g., by an autoinjector) (5).

ADVERSE EFFECTS

Many clinicians are cautious about the use of DMAP. There is poor dose-response curve reproducibility, attributed to genetic hemoglobin anomalies, which may produce very high MetHgb levels after even a single dose (2). The need to monitor blood MetHgb after DMAP is often stressed. Children are at particular risk of excessive MetHgb formation because of a comparative lack of MetHgb reductase activity.

Treatment of excess methemoglobinemia during the course of management of cyanide intoxication is controversial. Administration of either methylthionine chloride or tolonium chloride is sometimes recommended, but this merely converts cyanmethemoglobin to hemoglobin with concomitant release of cyanide. Exchange transfusion may, therefore, be the only remaining option. Other complications of DMAP therapy, including hemolysis, may occur, and in animals a Heinz body anemia has been noted (6). DMAP is mutagenic in V79 (Chinese hamster) cells *in vitro* (2).

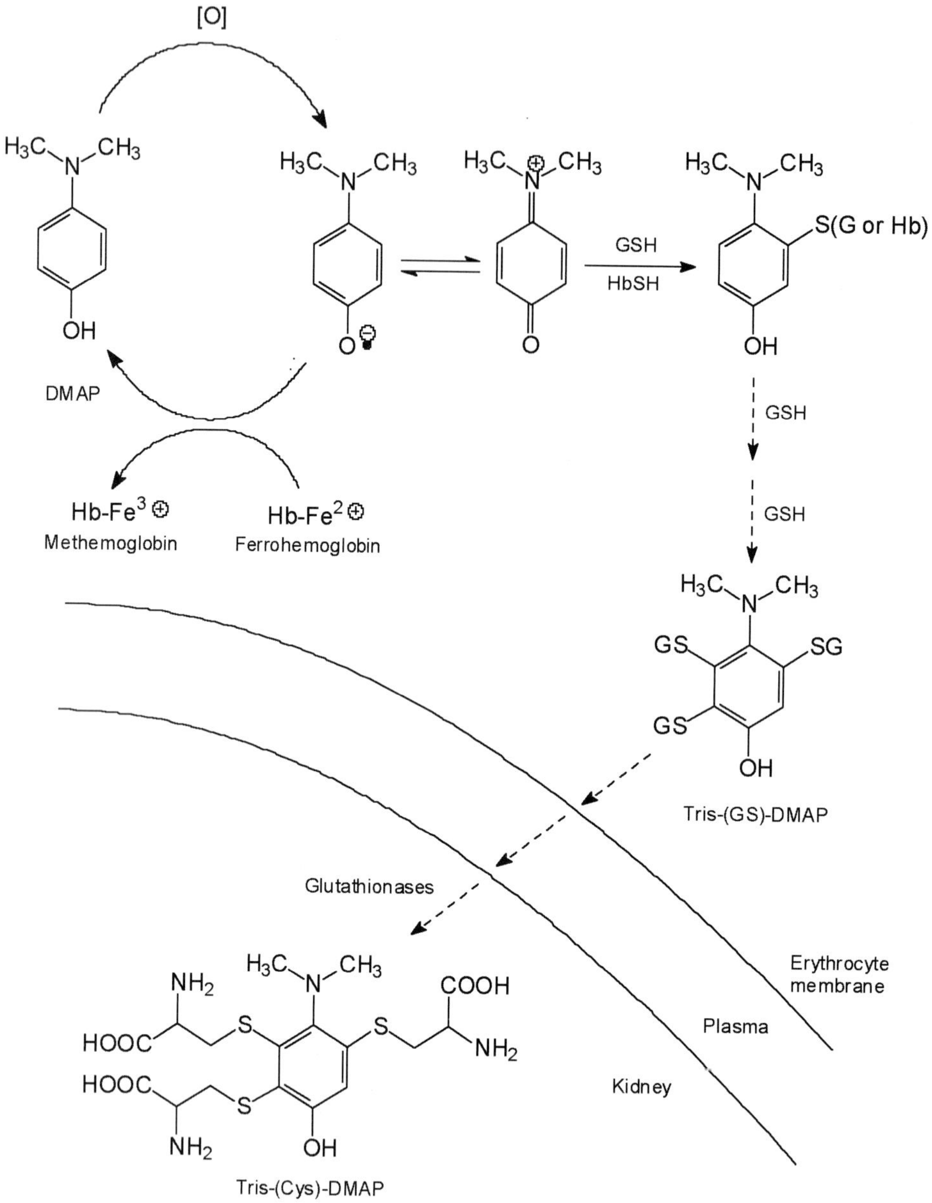

Figure 1. Mechanism of dimethylaminophenol (DMAP). Schematic of the catalytic production of methemoglobin by 4,4'-dimethylaminophenol via formation of the corresponding phenoxyl radical/quinoneimine and the subsequent detoxification of the quinoneimine. GSH, glutathione; Tris-(Cys)-DMAP, S,S,S-(2-dimethylamino-5-hydroxy-1,3,4-phenylene)tris-cysteine; Tris-(GS)-DMAP, S,S,S-(2-dimethylamino-5-hydroxy-1,3,4-phenylene)tris-glutathione.

REFERENCES

1. Jacobs K. [Report on experience with the administration of 4-DMAP in severe prussic acid poisoning. Consequences for medical practice.] *Zentralbl Arbeitsmed* 1984;34:274–277.
2. Meredith TJ, Jacobsen D, Haines JA, et al., eds. *Antidotes for poisoning by cyanide. IPCS/CEC Evaluation of Antidotes Series, Volume 2.* Cambridge, UK: Cambridge University Press, 1993.
3. Bright JE, Marrs TC. Kinetics of methaemoglobin production (2). Kinetics of the cyanide antidote p-aminopropiophenone during oral administration. *Hum Toxicol* 1986;5:303–307.
4. Bhattacharya R. Therapeutic efficacy of sodium nitrite and 4-dimethylamino-phenol or hydroxylamine co-administration against cyanide poisoning in rats. *Hum Exp Toxicol* 1995;14:29–33.
5. Klimmek R, Krettek C, Szinicz L, et al. Effects and biotransformation of 4-dimethylamino-phenol in man and dog. *Arch Toxicol* 1983;53:275–288.
6. Marrs TC, Swanston DW, Scawin J. Heinz-body anaemia produced by 4-DMAP. *Hum Toxicol* 1984;3:332(abstract).

CHAPTER 52
D-Penicillamine

E. Martin Caravati

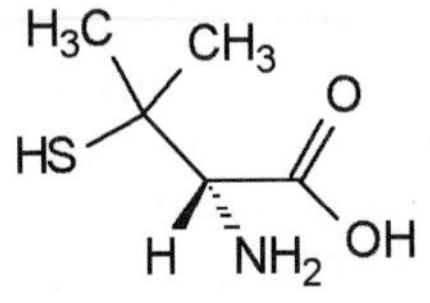

D-PENICILLAMINE

Synonyms:	**Penicillamine, 3-mercapto-D-valine, penicillaminum**
Molecular formula and weight:	**$C_5H_{11}NO_2S$, 149.2 g/mol**
SI conversion:	**mg/L × 0.0067 = mmol/L**
CAS Registry No.:	**52-67-5**
Normal or therapeutic levels:	**Not applicable**
Special concerns:	**Dermatologic, hematologic, and renal toxicity are common during chronic use.**

OVERVIEW

Penicillamine is a monothiol oral chelator that binds copper, iron, mercury, lead, zinc, arsenic, cystine, and possibly other heavy metals. The U.S. Food and Drug Administration has approved D-penicillamine for the treatment of Wilson's disease; cystinuria; and severe, active rheumatoid arthritis. Until the approval of dimercaptosuccinic acid (succimer), it was the only commercially available oral chelating agent. Adverse effects occur in 25% to 63% of patients treated with penicillamine, and deaths have been associated with its use. Succimer has largely replaced penicillamine as an oral chelator, with the possible exception of copper toxicity.

Forms Available

Penicillamine is administered orally. It is available in 125-mg capsules and 250-mg capsules and tablets (Cuprimine capsules, Depen Titratable tablets). The capsules can be opened, and the powder is soluble in water.

Mechanism of Action

Penicillamine is well absorbed orally, with peak concentrations in 1 to 3 hours. It is metabolized by the liver to inactive disulfide compounds and has an initial elimination half-life of 1 to 3 hours. Penicillamine chelates copper, iron, lead, arsenic, zinc, and mercury. One g of penicillamine results in excretion of only approximately 2 mg of copper *in vivo*. It enhances urinary excretion of lead, although not as effectively as other agents. The exact mechanism of chelation is uncertain.

INDICATIONS

Copper Toxicity

Penicillamine is the agent of choice to promote urinary excretion of copper in Wilson's disease (impaired biliary excretion of copper) (1). It has been administered in a case of acute copper sulfate poisoning, but copper excretion was not enhanced appreciably (2).

Lead Poisoning

Penicillamine is not the oral agent of choice for lead poisoning due to adverse effects. It should be considered after succimer and ethylenediaminetetraacetic acid have been tried or are contraindicated. Penicillamine has been used to treat mild lead toxicity or in conjunction with ethylenediaminetetraacetic acid or British antilewisite for moderate to severe toxicity. However, the Centers for Disease Control and Prevention only recommends chelation therapy for blood lead concentrations greater than 45 µg/dl (3). The use of any chelating agent in children is controversial due to lack of data showing that chelation prevents or reverses the effects of lead on cognitive development (4,5). Penicillamine has been used in children with low-level lead poisoning (whole blood lead levels, 25 to 40 µg/dl). The mean blood lead concentration was reduced from 26 to 12 µg/dl in 37 children treated with 15 to 30 mg/kg/day for 11 weeks (4), and the blood lead level decreased by 33% after treatment for 76 days, compared to controls (6).

Arsenic Poisoning

Penicillamine enhances renal excretion of arsenic in children but is not the agent of choice due to adverse effects (7). Its efficacy in humans has been challenged by lack of effectiveness in animal studies (8).

CAUTIONS AND CONTRAINDICATIONS

Lead chelation should not be given on an outpatient basis if exposure to lead is continuing or the physician has doubts about compliance with the therapeutic regimen. Rebound after cessation of therapy may raise the lead level 25% or more above its nadir (4,9). It should be used with caution in patients with renal failure because it is primarily renally excreted. Gastrointestinal absorption of penicillamine is reduced by concurrent use of antacids, ferrous sulfate, and some foods. It can produce a false-positive urine ketone test. It has been associated with autoimmune diseases: systemic lupus erythematosus (mild symptoms to multisystem disease), pemphigus, myasthenia gravis, glomerulonephritis, and autoimmune thyroid disease (see the section Adverse Effects). These effects may be more common during prolonged treatment.

Penicillamine is contraindicated in patients with penicillin allergy, lupus erythematosus, or renal failure. It should not be coadministered with other drugs that have significant hematologic or renal toxicity, such as antimalarials or immunosuppressive agents.

Pregnancy and Lactation

Penicillamine is U.S. Food and Drug Administration pregnancy category D. Penicillamine crosses the placenta. Developmental connective tissue anomalies were noted in 8 out of more than 100 pregnancies in women treated for Wilson's disease, rheumatoid arthritis, and cystinuria. No information is available on its use during lactation or excretion in breast milk (10).

DOSAGE AND METHOD OF ADMINISTRATION

Wilson's Disease

The initial *adult dose* is 1500 to 2000 mg daily in divided doses, then decreased to 750 to 1500 mg/day for maintenance. The dose can be started at 250 mg and titrated up as tolerated. The objective is to increase urinary copper excretion to more than 2 mg/24-hour urine collection and continue for approximately 3 months. The serum-free copper is monitored after the initial urinary copper excretion reaches at least 2 mg/day. The dose needed rarely exceeds 2 g/day. Adequate treatment results in a serum-free copper concentration of less than 10 µg/dl. The *pediatric dose* is 20 mg/kg/day.

Lead Poisoning

The initial *adult dose* is usually 250 mg four times a day. The maximum dose is 2000 mg/day. The *pediatric dose* is 20 to 30 mg/kg/day in three to four divided doses. A lower dose of 15 mg/kg/day may reduce adverse effects without compromising efficacy (11). Side effects can be minimized to an extent by starting with a small dose and increasing it gradually while monitoring for side effects. For example, 25% of the desired dose could be given in week 1, 50% in week 2, and the full dose by week 3 (12).

Arsenic

The dose and schedule for arsenic are the same as for lead poisoning.

ADVERSE EFFECTS

Adverse reactions occurred in 33% of children treated with 25 to 30 mg/kg/day for a mean of 76 days for lead poisoning. Treatment was discontinued in 10% of these patients due to side effects (6). Children with lead poisoning who received a reduced dose of 15 mg/kg/day for 11 weeks had only a 4.5% incidence of rash, a 10% incidence of white blood cell counts below 5000/mm^3, and no renal toxicity (11).

The main side effects of penicillamine are reactions resembling penicillin sensitivity. The incidence and severity of adverse effects increase with duration of therapy and have occurred in up to 62% of patients treated for rheumatoid arthritis (13). Most severe reactions occur during chronic treatment of rheumatoid arthritis, Wilson's disease, or scleroderma. Death has occurred from hematologic adverse effects. Nephrotoxicity, possibly from hypersensitivity reactions, is also reported.

Hypersensitivity effects include urticaria, rash, itching, fever, hematuria, positive antinuclear antibody, proteinuria, eosinophilia, erythema multiforme, and autoimmune bullous syndromes. *Hematologic effects* are leukopenia, thrombocytopenia, hemolytic anemia, agranulocytosis, aplastic anemia, and thrombotic thrombocytopenic purpura. *Liver toxicity* has been seen in a 37-year-old woman who developed cholestatic hepatitis after 10 days of D-penicillamine treatment (14). *Gastrointestinal events* are usually minor (nausea, vomiting, abdominal pain), but pancreatitis has been reported.

Neurologic effects include myasthenia gravis (15) as well as sensory and motor neuropathy. *Endocrine effects* include breast enlargement (gigantism) in both women and men on chronic therapy (16). *Renal toxicity* includes nephrotic syndrome and proteinuria. *Respiratory toxicity* includes Goodpasture's syndrome and obliterative bronchiolitis.

Monitoring

Monitor for symptoms of hypersensitivity reaction, cough, dyspnea, fever, and rash. A complete blood cell count, including platelets and neutrophil count, and a urinalysis should be done every 2 weeks for the first 4 to 6 months and at least monthly thereafter. If the absolute neutrophil count falls below 1500 cells/mm^3, the count should be rechecked immediately, and treatment should be stopped if it falls below 1200 cells/mm^3. Renal function tests should also be checked periodically.

Urine or blood concentrations of the target metal should be obtained periodically to assess the need for continued therapy.

Discontinuation of Treatment

Treatment with penicillamine is terminated immediately if any of the following occurs (17): (a) rise in blood lead level (suggesting ongoing lead exposure); (b) otherwise unexplained generalized urticarial rash; (c) fall in platelet count below 100,000 cells/mm^3; (d) fall in white blood cell count below 4000 cells/mm^3 or neutropenia; and (e) appearance of abnormal urinalysis [proteinuria (greater than 1 on dipstick), hematuria (greater than 10 red blood cells/high-power field), or pyuria (greater than 10 white blood cells/high-power field)].

PITFALLS

Penicillamine is a second- or third-line agent for lead poisoning. When administered, appropriate monitoring for hematologic or nephrotoxic adverse effects is essential.

REFERENCES

1. Loudianos G, Gitlin JD. Wilson's disease. *Semin Liver Dis* 2000;20:353–364.
2. Hantson P, Lievens M, Mahieu P. Accidental ingestion of a zinc and copper sulfate preparation. *J Toxicol Clin Toxicol* 1996;34(6):725–730.
3. Centers for Disease Control and Prevention. *Managing elevated blood lead levels among young children: recommendations from the Advisory Committee on Childhood Lead Poisoning Prevention*. Atlanta: CDC, 2002:49–50.
4. Shannon M, Grace A, Graef JW. Use of penicillamine in children with small lead burdens. *N Engl J Med* 1989;321:979–980.
5. Graziano JH. Use of penicillamine in children with small lead burdens. *N Engl J Med* 1990;322:1887–1889.
6. Shannon M, Graef J, Lovejoy FH. Efficacy and toxicity of D-penicillamine in low-level lead poisoning. *J Pediatr* 1988;12:799–804.
7. Peterson RG, Rumack BH. D-penicillamine therapy of acute arsenic poisoning. *J Pediatr* 1977;9:661–666.
8. Kreppel H, Reichl FX, Forth W, Fichtl B. Lack of effectiveness of D-penicillamine in experimental arsenic poisoning. *Vet Hum Toxicol* 1989;31(1):1–5.
9. Graef J. Lead poisoning management. II. *Clin Toxicol Rev* 1992;14(9):1–2.
10. Briggs GG, Freeman RK, Yaffe SJ. *Drugs in pregnancy and lactation*, 6th ed. Baltimore: Williams and Wilkins, 2002:1076–1077.
11. Shannon MW, Townsend MK. Adverse effects of reduced-dose D-penicillamine in children with mild to moderate lead poisoning. *Ann Pharmacother* 2000;34:15–18.
12. Chisolm JJ Jr, Thomas DJ. Use of 2,3-dimercaptoprane-1-sulfonate in treatment of lead poisoning in children. *J Pharmacol Exp Ther* 1985;235:665–669.
13. Halverson PB, Kozin F, Bernhard GC, et al. Toxicity of penicillamine. A serious limitation to therapy in rheumatoid arthritis. *JAMA* 1978;240:1870–1871.
14. Jacobs JW, van der Weide FR, Druijsen MW. Fatal cholestatic hepatitis caused by D-penicillamine. *Br J Rheumatol* 1994;33(8):770–773.
15. Adelman HM, Winters PR, Mahan CS, Wallach PM. D-penicillamine-induced myasthenia gravis: diagnosis observed by coexisting chronic obstructive pulmonary disease. *Am J Med Sci* 1995;309:191–193.
16. Tchebiner JZ. Breast enlargement induced by D-penicillamine. *Ann Pharmacother* 2002;36:444–445.
17. Liebelt EL, Shannon MW. Oral chelators for childhood lead poisoning. *Pediatr Ann* 1994;23:616–626.

CHAPTER 53

Diethyldithiocarbamate

Luke Yip

$$Na^{+}\ {}^{-}S{-}C({=}S){-}N(CH_2CH_3)_2$$

DITHIOCARB SODIUM

Synonyms:	**DDC, dithiocarb sodium (DTC), sodium diethyldithiocarbamate (DDTC), Imuthiol**
Molecular formula and weight:	**$C_5H_{10}NS_2Na$, 171.25 g/mol**
CAS Registry No.:	**148-18-5**
Therapeutic levels:	**Not applicable**
Special concerns:	**Dithiocarb is usually not immediately available for administration.**

OVERVIEW

Diethyldithiocarbamate (DDC) is a metabolic reduction product of tetraethylthiuram disulfide [disulfiram (Antabuse)] and is a chelator of heavy metals (e.g., nickel, copper, thallium, and cadmium). It is primarily used as treatment for nickel carbonyl poisoning. Neither DDC nor disulfiram appears to be an effective treatment of nickel dermatitis (1–3). DDC has been used in the treatment of human immunodeficiency virus infection (4–6). However, not all of the studies showed the same favorable results (7,8).

DDC is available as Imuthiol capsules from the Merieux Institute (investigational). Each capsule contains 99% DDC.

Mechanism of Action

The therapeutic effect of DDC in acute nickel carbonyl poisoning has been attributed primarily to diminution of the pulmonary nickel burden (9).

INDICATIONS

DDC has been used after exposure to hazardous concentrations of nickel carbonyl and for copper poisoning.

CAUTIONS AND CONTRAINDICATIONS

DDC should be administered with caution to patients who have recently consumed ethanol because of potential disulfiram-like reactions (10). Disulfiram, a close related compound, is U.S. Food and Drug Administration pregnancy category C.

DDC should *not* be used as a chelator in the management of either *nickel* or *thallium* poisoning. The high affinity of the lipophilic nickel- and thallium-DDC complex for lipid-rich tissue results in substantial redistribution of these metals into vital organs (e.g., brain) with potentially devastating consequences. (9,11–16). Similarly, DDC should not be used in cadmium poisoning. Animal studies have shown DDC redistributes cadmium from various organs into the brain (17,18).

DOSAGE AND ADMINISTRATION

Nickel Carbonyl

DDC has not been subjected to controlled clinical studies. The safety and efficacy of DDC for nickel carbonyl poisoning are primarily based on animal studies and clinical experience with patients who did not receive DDC (10,19–21). When DDC use is indicated, it should be administered as soon as possible because a delay in administration may increase nickel carbonyl toxicity.

If the exposure is mild or doubtful (urine nickel concentration less than 10 μg/dl), the *adult dose* of DDC is 250 mg and sodium bicarbonate, 250 mg with water, administered orally every 30 minutes for eight doses. For moderate to severe exposure (urine nickel concentration greater than or equal to 10 μg/dl), the *adult dose* of DDC is 50 mg/kg administered orally over the first 24 hours (e.g., 4000 mg for an 80-kg patient). A suggested dosing schedule for the first day of treatment is 2000 mg (10 × 200-mg capsules) initially, 1000 mg (5 × 200-mg capsules) at 4 hours, 600 mg (3 × 200-mg capsules) at 8 hours, and 400 mg (2 × 200-mg capsules) at 16 hours.

On subsequent days, oral DDC, 400 mg, is administered every 8 hours until the patient is asymptomatic and the urine nickel concentration is in the normal range (less than 5.0 μg/dl). If the patient's condition is critical, DDC may be administered intravenously (IV). The IV solution is prepared by adding 10 ml of a sterile phosphate buffer solution (NaH_2PO_4, 500 mg/dl) to 1000 mg of powdered DDC. The dose is 25 to 100 mg/kg administered over the first 24 hours using the schedule as outlined above.

One molecule of disulfiram is metabolized to two molecules of DDC, and it has been used to treat experimental nickel carbonyl poisoning (22–24). Mortality was reduced when either parenteral disulfiram, 250 mg/kg, or oral disulfiram, 1000 mg/kg, was immediately administered to animals exposed to lethal nickel carbonyl levels. However, clinical experience in this regard is limited, and the efficacy and optimal disulfiram dose remains to be determined. A patient developed a chemical pneumonitis after occupational nickel carbonyl poisoning and was treated with oxygen, continuous positive airway pressure, and oral disulfiram, 0.75 to 2.25 g daily, until DDC (1.2 to 2.8 g daily) was obtained on day 2 (25). Disulfiram was resumed on hospital days 9 to 11 when the DDC supply was exhausted. The patient survived.

Copper Poisoning

Dramatic clinical improvement was reported after a therapeutic trial of IV DDC (600 mg every third day) in a patient with Wilson's disease (10). However, there are conflicting results regarding cupruresis during DDC therapy (10,26).

ADVERSE EFFECTS

Intermittent mental confusion, incoherency, nausea, vomiting, dermatitis, and urticaria were reported during a course of oral DDC (1 g/day) for mercury vapor toxicity (27).

Adverse events have been associated with oral and IV DDC therapy in patients with human immunodeficiency virus infection. Oral DDC 10 mg/kg once a week was associated with unpleasant taste, abdominal discomfort, and nausea (5), whereas IV DDC was associated with gastrointestinal upset, burning at the infusion site, metallic taste, sneezing, confusion, hyperactivity, delusions, and myoclonus. Adverse events appear to be dose related. The maximal tolerated dose varied from 200 mg/m^2 weekly to 800 mg/m^2 twice weekly (28).

PITFALLS

Patients should abstain from consuming any beverage containing alcohol for at least 1 week after DDC or disulfiram therapy because of potentially precipitating a disulfiram reaction.

REFERENCES

1. Kaaber K, Menne T, Veien N, et al. Treatment of nickel dermatitis with Antabuse; a double blind study. *Contact Dermatitis* 1983;9:297–299.
2. van Ketel WG, Bruynzeel DP. The possible chelating effect of sodium diethyldithiocarbamate (DDC) in nickel allergic patients. Patch test procedure with nickel on DDC pretreated skin. *Derm Beruf Umwelt* 1982;30:198–202.
3. Spruit D, Bongaarts PJ, de Jongh GJ. Dithiocarbamate therapy for nickel dermatitis. *Contact Dermatitis* 1978;4:350–358.
4. Hersh EM, Brewton G, Abrams D, et al. Ditiocarb sodium (diethyldithiocarbamate) therapy in patients with symptomatic HIV infection and AIDS. A randomized, double-blind, placebo-controlled, multicenter study. *JAMA* 1991;265:1538–1544.
5. Lang JM, Touraine JL, Trepo C, et al. Randomised, double-blind, placebo-controlled trial of ditiocarb sodium ("Imuthiol") in human immunodeficiency virus infection. *Lancet* 1988;2:702–706.
6. Reisinger EC, Kern P, Ernst M, et al. Inhibition of HIV progression by dithiocarb. German DTC Study Group. *Lancet* 1990;335:679–682.
7. Multicenter, randomized, placebo-controlled study of ditiocarb (Imuthiol) in human immunodeficiency virus-infected asymptomatic and minimally symptomatic patients. The HIV87 Study Group. *AIDS Res Hum Retroviruses* 1993;9:83–89.
8. Shenep JL, Hughes WT, Flynn PM, et al. Decreased counts of blood neutrophils, monocytes, and platelets in human immunodeficiency virus-infected children and young adults treated with diethyldithiocarbamate. *Antimicrob Agents Chemother* 1994;38:1644–1646.
9. Tjalve H, Jasim S, Oskarsson A. Nickel mobilization by sodium diethyldithiocarbamate in nickel-carbonyl-treated mice. *IARC Sci Publ* 1984;53:311–320.
10. Sunderman FW. Nickel and copper mobilization by sodium diethyldithiocarbamate. *J New Drugs* 1964;4:154–161.
11. Belliveau JF, O'Leary GP Jr, Cadwell L, et al. Effect of diethyldithiocarbamate on nickel concentrations in tissues of $NiCl_2$-treated rats. *Ann Clin Lab Sci* 1985;15:349–350.
12. Kamerbeek HH, Rauws AG, ten Ham M, et al. Dangerous redistribution of thallium by treatment with sodium diethyldithiocarbamate. *Acta Med Scand* 1971;189:149–154.
13. Nielsen GD, Andersen O. Effect of tetraethylthiuramdisulphide and diethyl-dithiocarbamate on nickel toxicokinetics in mice. *Pharmacol Toxicol* 1994;75:285–293.
14. Oskarsson A, Tjalve H. Effects of diethyldithiocarbamate and penicillamine on the tissue distribution of $^{63}NiCl_2$ in mice. *Arch Toxicol* 1980;45:45–52.
15. Special communication: thallium poisoning. *Clin Toxicol* 1972;5:89–93.
16. Tjalve H, Borg-Neczak K. Effects of lipophilic complex formation on the disposition of nickel in experimental animals. *Sci Total Environ* 1994;148:217–242.
17. Gale GR, Atkins LM, Walker EM Jr. Effects of diethyldithiocarbamate on organ distribution and excretion of cadmium. *Ann Clin Lab Sci* 1982;12:463–470.
18. Gale GR, Smith AB, Walker EM. Diethyldithiocarbamate in treatment of acute cadmium poisoning. *Ann Clin Lab Sci* 1981;11:476–483.
19. Sunderman FW Sr, Sunderman FW Jr. Nickel poisoning VIII. Dithiocarb: a new therapeutic agent for persons exposed to nickel carbonyl. *Am J Med Sci* 1958;236:26–31.
20. Sunderman FW Sr. The treatment of acute nickel carbonyl poisoning with sodium diethyldithiocarbamate. *Ann Clin Res* 1971;3:182–185.
21. Sunderman FW Sr. Efficacy of sodium diethyldithiocarbamate (dithiocarb) in acute nickel carbonyl poisoning. *Ann Clin Lab Sci* 1979;9:1–10.
22. Baselt RC, Hanson VW. Efficacy of orally-administered chelating agents for nickel carbonyl toxicity in rats. *Res Commun Chem Pathol Pharmacol* 1982;38:113–124.
23. Sunderman FW Sr. Chelation therapy in nickel poisoning. *Ann Clin Lab Sci* 1981;11:1–8.
24. West B, Sunderman FW. Nickel poisoning: VII. The therapeutic effectiveness of alkyl dithiocarbamates in experimental animals exposed to nickel carbonyl. *Am J Med Sci* 1958;236:15–25.
25. Kurta DL, Dean BS, Krenzelok EP. Acute nickel carbonyl poisoning. *Am J Emerg Med* 1993;11:64–66.
26. Hsia YE, Combs JT, Hook L, et al. Hepatolenticular degeneration: the comparative effectiveness of D-penicillamine, potassium sulfide, and diethyldithiocarbamate as decoppering agents. *J Pediatr* 1966;68:921–926.
27. Sunderman FW Sr. Clinical response to therapeutic agents in poisoning from mercury vapor. *Ann Clin Lab Sci* 1978;8:259–269.
28. Kaplan CS, Petersen EA, Yocum D, et al. A randomized, controlled dose response study of intravenous sodium diethyldithiocarbamate in patients with advanced human immunodeficiency virus infection. *Life Sci* 1989;45:iii–ix.

CHAPTER 54

Dimercaptopropanesulfonic Acid (DMPS)

Alison L. Jones and Robert J. Flanagan

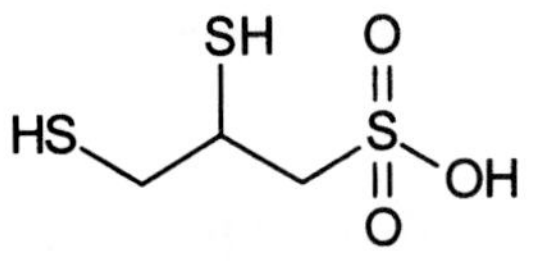

DIMERCAPTOPROPANESULFONIC ACID

Synonyms:	**Sodium D,L-2,3-dimercapto-propanesulfonate (DMPS), unithiol, unitiol, Dimaval**
Molecular formula and weight:	**$C_3H_7NaO_3S_3$, 210.3 g/mol**
SI conversion:	**mg/L × 0.0053 = mmol/L**
CAS Registry No.:	**4076-02-2**
Therapeutic levels:	**Not clinically applicable**
Special concerns:	**DMPS imparts a sulfur odor to bodily secretions.**

OVERVIEW

Sodium D,L-2,3-dimercapto-propanesulfonate (DMPS) is a water-soluble analog of dimercaprol. DMPS was first synthesized as a potential water-soluble chelating agent for arsenic. It has been used to treat Wilson's disease in patients intolerant of other drugs (1). DMPS is less toxic than dimercaprol and more effective when given orally than either dimercaprol or calcium disodium ethylenediaminetetraacetic acid as an antidote for heavy metal poisoning (2–4). However, DMPS is more toxic than 2,3-dimercaptosuccinic acid (DMSA) when administered to laboratory animals (5). Its main use is in treating mercury or arsenic poisoning (2,6). It has also been used to increase excretion of many other metals and compounds (7). DMPS is not approved for use by the U.S. Food and Drug Administration but is allowed to be compounded for individual patients. Animal studies do not indicate embryotoxic or teratogenic effects (7). If chelation must be performed during pregnancy, trace mineral balance should be monitored and supplemented.

Mechanism of Action

The adjacent sulfhydryl groups of DMPS allow it to form stable complexes with heavy metals. DMPS penetrates cell membranes better than succimer but not as well as dimercaprol. This may allow it to chelate metals intracellularly and remove them from biologically important sites, such as the active sites of enzymes.

Oral absorption of DMPS is rapid. Peak levels are reached in 3.4 hours. Protein binding approaches 90%. Elimination is primarily renal with a terminal elimination half-life $(t_{1/2})_{-\alpha}$ of 1.1 hours and $t_{1/2\beta}$ of 27.6 hours.

INDICATIONS

Arsenic Poisoning

DMPS has been found to be effective in arsenic poisoning in humans (2,8). The relative effectiveness or therapeutic indices of these compounds, compared with dimercaprol, have been studied in mice by assessing the protection achieved against a lethal dose of sodium arsenite (9). The relative efficacies found were DMSA:DMPS:dimercaprol in the ratio of 42:14:1. DMPS and DMSA are also more effective than dimercaprol in treating systemic poisoning with lewisite in rabbits (10). Like dimercaprol, DMPS is contraindicated in arsine poisoning.

Mercury Poisoning

Various metal-binding agents were used to treat victims of the 1971 to 1972 methylmercury poisoning disaster in Iraq (11). The mean $t_{1/2}$ obtained were as follows: no treatment, 63 days; and DMPS, 10 days. Clinical improvement was not seen in any group, but it seems reasonable to postulate that reducing the total body burden of methylmercury may limit the progression of central nervous system toxicity. DMPS has also been given in inorganic mercury poisoning after the inhalation of mercury vapor (six patients) and the ingestion of mercuric oxide (one patient) and mercury sublimate (one patient), and it was associated with enhanced urinary mercury excretion (12,13). Fluid replacement and DMPS [250 mg intravenously (IV)], every 4 hours for 60 hours, and then twice daily for 18 days) were used to treat a 53-year-old man who had ingested approximately 50 g mercuric iodide (14). DMPS was commenced approximately 8 hours postingestion, and the patient made an uneventful recovery, with his renal function and other biochemical parameters remaining within normal limits.

In animals, DMSA is more effective than DMPS in removing mercury from the body (2). DMSA appears to remove more organic mercury, whereas DMPS removes more inorganic mercury. A combination of DMSA and DMPS removes mercury from most organs. Although further studies are necessary, DMSA will probably prove to be the treatment of choice for methylmercury poisoning because of its low toxicity and reported efficacy in animal studies. Urinary mercury excretion after DMPS challenge (300 mg orally after an 11-hour fast) appears to be a better diagnostic indicator of low-level mercurialism than unchallenged urinary mercury excretion after exposure to mercury vapor and to mercurous and mercuric salts (3,15,16). Neurologic sequelae, particularly those resulting from exposure to organomercurials, remain a largely irreversible problem despite progress in chelation therapies.

Other Heavy Metals

DMPS has been shown to increase the excretion of arsenic, chromium, cobalt, copper, gold, lead, mercury, polonium, silver, and stibine gas (7). For most of these, the clinical effectiveness of chelation is unknown. DMPS may be a reasonable intervention under selected clinical circumstances or when other treatments have proven ineffective.

The successful treatment with DMPS of 60 men with chronic lead poisoning has been reported from the former Soviet Union (2). They were given 250 mg/day for 20 days, with a resultant gradual reduction in the clinical features of lead toxicity. Treatment with DMPS does not redistribute lead or mercury to the brain of rats (17). However, clinical experience suggests that DMPS is inappropriate for use in lead poisoning in children because succimer had a better efficacy and safety profile (18).

CAUTIONS AND CONTRAINDICATIONS

The U.S. Food and Drug Administration has not classified DMPS. Its safety in pregnancy and lactation has not been studied.

DOSAGE AND ADMINISTRATION

DMPS may be given orally or parenterally. In acute poisoning, 250 mg is given IV every 3 to 4 hours initially, reducing in subsequent days. Hypotension is possible after bolus IV dosage of DMPS; thus, such injections should be given over at least 5 minutes (3). In chronic poisoning, 100 mg is given orally three times per day. The metabolism and pharmacokinetics of DMPS have been studied extensively (3). After DMPS, acyclic and cyclic disulfides of DMPS are found in urine. DMPS does not cross cell membranes extensively (15,19).

ADVERSE EFFECTS

Several adverse effects are shared by all dimercapto-chelating agents (succimer, DMPS, dimercaprol). These include fever, diffuse maculopapular rash, and asymptomatic elevation of aminotransferase levels. Allergic reactions are rare but have occurred. Rare cases of erythema multiforme have been reported during use of DMPS.

PITFALLS

It is often difficult to differentiate the adverse effects of DMPS from the toxicity of the metal under treatment.

REFERENCES

1. Walshe JM. Unithiol in Wilson's disease. *BMJ* 1985;290:673–674.
2. Aposhian HV. DMSA and DMPS—water soluble antidotes for heavy metal poisoning. *Annu Rev Pharmacol Toxicol* 1983;23:193–215.
3. Aposhian HV, Maiorino RM, Gonzalez-Ramirez D, et al. Mobilization of heavy metals by newer, therapeutically useful chelating agents. *Toxicology* 1995;97:23–38.
4. Hruby K, Donner A. 2,3-Dimercapto-1-propanesulphonate in heavy metal poisoning. *Med Toxicol* 1987;2:317–323.
5. Jones MM. New developments in therapeutic chelating agents as antidotes for metal poisoning. *Crit Rev Toxicol* 1991;21:209–233.
6. Campbell JR, Clarkson TW, Omar MD. The therapeutic use of 2,3-dimercaptopropane-1-sulfonate in two cases of inorganic mercury poisoning. *J Am Med Assn* 1986;256:3127–3130.
7. Ruprecht J. *Dimaval (DMPS) scientific monograph*, 6th ed. Houston: Heyltex Corporation, 1997.
8. Moore DF, O'Callaghan CA, Berlyne G, et al. Acute arsenic poisoning: absence of polyneuropathy after treatment with 2,3-dimercaptopropanesulphonate (DMPS). *J Neurol Neurosurg Psychiatr* 1994;57:2233–2235.
9. Aposhian HV, Carter DE, Hoover TD, et al. DMSA, DMPS, and DMPA—as arsenic antidotes. *Fundam Appl Toxicol* 1984;4:S58–S70.
10. Inns RH, Rice P. Efficacy of dimercapto chelating agents for the treatment of poisoning by percutaneously applied dichloro(2-chlorovinyl)arsine in rabbits. *Human Exp Toxicol* 1993;12:241–246.
11. Clarkson TW, Magos L, Cox C, et al. Tests of efficacy of antidotes for removal of methylmercury in human poisoning during the Iraq outbreak. *J Pharmacol Exp Ther* 1981;218:74–83.
12. Dargan PI, Giles L, House IM, et al. A case of severe mercuric sulfate ingestion treated with 2,3-dimercaptopropane-1-sulphonate (DMPS) and hi-flow hemodiafiltration. *J Toxicol Clin Toxicol* 1999;37:622–623(abst).
13. Mant TGK. Clinical studies with dimercaptopropane sulphonate in mercury poisoning. *Hum Toxicol* 1985;4:346(abst).
14. Anderson RA, McAllister WAC, Taylor A. Acute mercuric iodide poisoning. *Ann Clin Biochem* 1996;33:468–470.
15. Aposhian HV, Maiorino RM, Rivera M, et al. Human studies with the chelating agents DMPS and DMSA. *J Toxicol Clin Toxicol* 1992;30:505–528.
16. Maiorino RM, Gonzalez-Ramirez D, Zuniga-Charles M, et al. Sodium 2,3-dimercaptopropane-1-sulphonate challenge test for mercury in humans. III. Urinary mercury after exposure to mercurous chloride. *J Pharmacol Exp Ther* 1996;277:938–944.
17. Aposhian MM, Maiorino RM, Xu Z, Aposhian HV. Sodium 2,3-dimercapto-1-propanesulphonate (DMPS) treatment does not redistribute lead or mercury to the brain of rats. *Toxicology* 1996;109:49–55.
18. Chisolm JJ. BAL, EDTA, DMSA and DMPS in the treatment of lead poisoning in children. *J Toxicol Clin Toxicol* 1992;30:493–504.
19. Gabard B. Distribution and excretion of the mercury chelating agent sodium 2,3-dimercaptopropane-1-sulfonate in the rat. *Arch Toxicol* 1978;39:289–298.

CHAPTER 55

Diethylenetriaminepenta-acetate (DTPA)

Alison L. Jones and Robert J. Flanagan

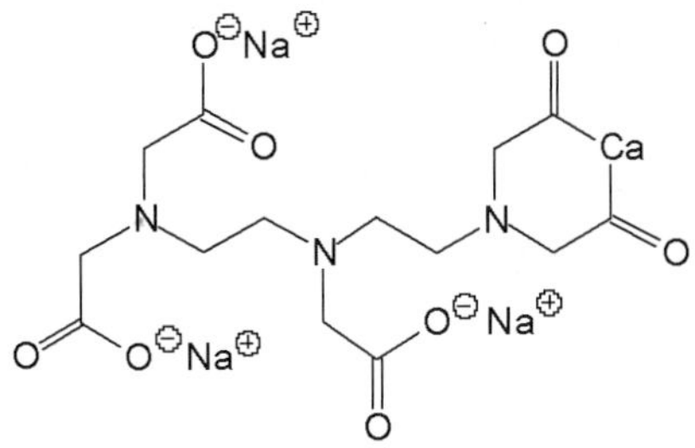

DIETHYLENETRIAMINEPENTAACETATE

Synonyms:	**Calcium trisodium diethylene-triamine pentaacetate, pentetic acid**
Molecular formula and weight:	**$C_{14}H_{18}CaN_3Na_3O_{10}$, 497.4 g/mol**
CAS Registry No.:	**12111-24-9 (calcium trisodium pentetate)**
Therapeutic levels:	**Not clinically applicable**
Special concerns:	**Emergent therapy is performed with Ca-DTPA. Long-term treatment uses Zn-DTPA.**

OVERVIEW

Diethylenetriamine pentaacetic acid (DTPA) is a synthetic polyamino-carboxylic acid similar to ethylenediaminetetraacetic acid (1). As with all chelating agents, DTPA is most effective if administered shortly after exposure. Oral calcium or zinc trisodium DTPA has been used to treat iron-overload patients (2,3). DTPA may be more effective than ethylenediaminetetraacetic acid in treating acute poisoning with cobalt salts (4) but appears to have no advantage over ethylenediaminetetraacetic acid in treating lead poisoning at least in mice (5).

Measures to enhance the excretion of plutonium and other actinides, such as americium, have been studied. The plutonium ion complexes with transferrin in serum. DTPA is the drug of choice because it is administered orally (5). Long-term Zn-DTPA protected against the carcinogenicity of ^{239}Pu in mice (6). DTPA is the most effective at removing plutonium from tissues (5).

DTPA is available as a calcium or zinc salt. The calcium salt chelates more efficiently than the zinc form but is also more toxic. In the United States, Oak Ridge stocks both Ca-DTPA and Zn-DTPA (7). Both drugs are available as 1 g/5 ml diluent. Its plasma half-life is 20 to 60 minutes. Very little is bound to plasma protein. DTPA is rapidly distributed throughout the extracellular fluid; little undergoes metabolism. No accumulation of DTPA in specific organs has been observed. It is promptly cleared by glomerular filtration. Very little radioactively labeled DTPA (less than 3%) is detected in the stool (7).

INDICATIONS

Ca-DTPA and Zn-DTPA effectively chelate several transuranium ions (plutonium, americium, berkelium, curium, and californium). Typical usage has been to treat internal contamination with plutonium and americium. Ca-DTPA should be used initially for large exposures because it is a more effective plutonium chelator. After approximately 24 hours, however, the efficiency of each agent is similar, and Zn-DTPA is preferred because it does not cause zinc or manganese depletion (7). One patient contaminated with more than 1 mCi (converted to becquerel: 1 Ci = 3.7×10^{10} Bq) of americium had 99% of the total body burden removed with prolonged Ca-DTPA/Zn-DTPA therapy over 4 years (7).

CAUTIONS AND CONTRAINDICATIONS

Zn-DTPA should not be used as a chelator for uranium or neptunium. DTPA is U.S. Food and Drug Administration pregnancy category C. The chelates do not significantly cross placental barriers. Studies do not indicate teratogenic effects by Zn-DTPA at doses up to several times the human dose of 28.7 μmol/kg. In these experiments, Zn-DTPA did not show toxicity during pregnancy, but Ca-DTPA did (7).

DOSAGE AND ADMINISTRATION

DTPA is given in a dose range of approximately 1 g/day (approximately 30 μmol/kg) by intravenous (IV) infusion over a few hours. The technique recommended by Oak Ridge Associated Universities is shown in Table 1. It may also be administered intramuscularly (IM), although the use of procaine in the injection is recommended to reduce local pain.

In some cases, treatment has been carried out for 1 or more years intermittently and without adverse effect and with enhanced excretion of small amounts of plutonium and americium. Combined treatment with early inhaled DTPA followed by repeated IV injection is believed likely to be the most effective treatment after inhalation of actinides (8). As zinc depletion may occur during chronic therapy with Ca-DTPA, Zn-DTPA should be used after the first phase of treatment (9).

Inhaled plutonium is difficult to remove with oral DTPA, and bronchioalveolar lavage with the chelating agent enhances removal in such cases. Inhalation of a Zn-DTPA aerosol is more effective than IM or IV injection in mobilizing plutonium from the lung, apparently because distribution to the body from the lung is slower than from muscle (7).

TABLE 1. Oak Ridge guidelines for treatment with Ca-diethylenetriaminepentaacetic acid (DTPA) or Zn-DTPA

The following guidelines are provided to facilitate rapid initiation of treatment.

Is it at all likely that the person has received internal contamination with plutonium, americium, berkelium, curium, or californium?

DTPA is not currently approved for use with uranium or neptunium.

Obtain a history of renal, hematopoietic, bone marrow, cardiac, or respiratory disorders and, if appropriate, the likelihood of pregnancy.

Obtain written informed consent for both Ca-DTPA and Zn-DTPA.

Obtain an initial 24-h urine for radionuclide assay and urinalysis.

If Ca-DTPA contraindicated (e.g., history of or current serious renal disease, bone marrow depression, pregnancy, or age less than 18 yr), use Zn-DTPA.

Administer 1 g of Ca-DTPA or Zn-DTPA by IV push over 3–4 min; IV infusion in 100–250 ml Ringer lactate, dextrose 5% in water, or normal saline; or by inhalation in a nebulizer (1:1 dilution with water or saline). Administration is approved for use by IM injection, but this is not recommended because of pain considerations.

Blood pressure before and after DTPA administration should be routinely monitored.

Follow the remainder of the procedures in the section Therapy Guidelines (http://www.orau.gov/reacts/zinc.htm).

Modified from REAC/TS Resources. Zn-DTPA (trisodium zinc diethylenetriaminepentaacetate). http://www.orau.gov/reacts/zinc.htm. Document dated 2/11/02.

ADVERSE EFFECTS

After chronic Ca- and Zn-DTPA treatment for more than 3 years, trace metal assays showed that zinc was the only metal excreted more rapidly than normal (10). The 132 mg of zinc contained in 1 g of Zn-DTPA compensates for the loss of the 18 mg of zinc that was found to be associated with the injection of 1 g of DTPA salt (7). When given repeatedly, with short intervals for recovery, Zn-DTPA treatment may cause nausea, vomiting, diarrhea, chills, fever, pruritus, and muscle cramps in the first 24 hours.

REFERENCES

1. Hammond PB. The effects of chelating agents on the tissue distribution and excretion of lead. *Toxicol Appl Pharmacol* 1971;18:296–310.
2. Constantoulakis M, Economidou J, Karagiorga M, et al. Combined long-term treatment of hemosiderosis with desferrioxamine and DTPA in homozygous β-thalassemia. *Ann N Y Acad Sci* 1974;232:193–200.
3. Muller-Eberhard U, Erlandson ME, Ginn HE, Smith CH. Effect of trisodium calcium diethylenetriaminepenta-acetate on bivalent cations in thalassemia major. *Blood* 1963;22:209–217.
4. Llobet JM, Domingo JL, Corbella J. Comparison of antidotal efficacy of chelating agents upon acute toxicity of Co(II) in mice. *Res Comm Chem Pathol Pharmacol* 1985;50:305–308.
5. Jones MM. New developments in therapeutic chelating agents as antidotes for metal poisoning. *Crit Rev Toxicol* 1991;21:209–233.
6. Jones CW, Mays CW, Taylor GN, et al. Reducing the cancer risk of ^{239}Pu by chelation therapy. *Radiat Res* 1986;107:296–306.
7. REAC/TS Resources. Zn-DTPA (trisodium zinc diethylenetriaminepentaacetate). http://www.orau.gov/reacts/zinc.htm. Document dated 2/11/02. Accessed 1/16/03.
8. Stather JW, Stradling GN, Gray SA, et al. Use of DTPA for increasing the rate of elimination of plutonium-238 and americium-241 from rodents after their inhalation as the nitrates. *Hum Toxicol* 1985;4:573–582.
9. Taylor DM, Volf V. Oral chelation treatment of injected ^{241}Am or ^{239}Pu in rats. *Health Phys* 1980;38:147–158.
10. Kalkwarf DR, Thomas VW, Nielson KK, Mauch ML. 1976 Hanford americium exposure incident: urinary excretion of trace metals during DTPA treatments. *Health Phys* 1983;45:937–947.

CHAPTER 56

Ethanol

Steven A. Seifert

CH_3CH_2OH

ETHYL ALCOHOL

Synonyms:	**Ethanol, ethyl alcohol**
Molecular formula and weight:	**C_2H_5OH, 46.07 g/mol**
SI conversion:	**g/L × 21.7 = mmol/L**
CAS Registry No.:	**64-17-5**
Therapeutic level:	**100 mg/dl to 130 mg/dl (serum)**
Special concerns:	**Ethanol causes central nervous system and respiratory depression, especially in alcohol-naïve patients.**

OVERVIEW

Ethanol is used therapeutically in the management of poisoning by ethylene glycol, methanol, and other toxic alcohols, such as diethylene glycol, triethylene glycol, propylene glycol, and ethylene glycol butyl ethers. Ethanol is a volatile, mobile, hygroscopic, colorless, flammable liquid. It has a pleasant odor and a burning taste. Intravenous (IV) ethanol is available as 5% or 10% premixed solutions and as a 95% solution for dilution. It is usually diluted in dextrose 5% in water.

Mechanism of Action

Ethanol, methanol, and ethylene glycol are all metabolized by the enzyme alcohol dehydrogenase (ADH), a family of isoenzymes that convert alcohols to their corresponding aldehydes using the oxidized form of nicotinamide adenine dinucleotide as a cofactor (1). The products of methanol and ethylene glycol metabolism are responsible for their toxicity (see Chapters 191 and 192). The affinity of ADH for ethanol is approximately 100-fold greater than its affinity for methanol or ethylene glycol, thus blocking their conversion to aldehydes and acids and allowing elimination of the parent compound by endogenous clearance or by extracorporeal elimination methods.

INDICATIONS

Ethanol has been used for poisoning with ethylene glycol, methanol, propylene glycol, and some glycol ethers. It is more difficult to use than fomepizole but may be the only drug available in some cases.

Ethylene Glycol or Methanol Poisoning

Ethanol therapy should be instituted for an ethylene glycol or methanol level greater than 20 mg/dl or any degree of metabolic acidosis in the setting of possible ethylene glycol ingestion. Some clinicians follow marginal cases of acidosis (e.g., serum bicarbonate of 19 mmol/L); however, clear cases of acidosis or worsening acidosis should be treated promptly. Blocking ADH prevents further production of aldehydes and acids from the parent compound. If levels are not available within 1 to 2 hours, therapy should be instituted for a reliable history of ingestion while further evaluation is performed.

If blood concentrations of ethylene glycol or methanol are not available in a timely manner, ADH blockade must be continued until the time of estimated clearance of the parent compound, and the patient must be followed closely on cessation of therapy for the development of acidosis and other toxicity. In the presence of ethanol, the elimination half-lives of ethylene glycol and methanol are 18 hours and 52 hours, respectively (2,3). Drug elimination is nearly complete after five half-lives, which is approximately 10 days in the case of methanol. Therefore, it is preferable that the patient's blood be transported to a laboratory capable of performing these tests or the patient transferred to a hospital capable of obtaining levels promptly, particularly in cases of likely significant exposure (e.g., known suicidal ingestion).

Other Alcohols and Derivatives

Because of its ability as a competitive inhibitor of ADH, ethanol has been used or proposed for use in the treatment of other toxic "alcohols," such as diethylene glycol, triethylene glycol, propylene glycol, and ethylene glycol butyl ethers.

CAUTIONS AND CONTRAINDICATIONS

Ethanol should be used cautiously in children and novice adult users because they may become comatose at blood ethanol concentrations of 200 mg/dl (4–7). The effects of ethanol are additive or synergistic with a wide range of other central nervous system (CNS) depressants (8,9).

The combination of ethanol with other drugs that are metabolized by ADH (e.g., ethylene glycol, methanol, isopropanol) may result in higher blood concentrations, increased effects, and prolonged half-lives of those agents.

Hypoglycemia develops more readily in patients with small or compromised hepatic glycogen stores, such as children and chronic ethanol users. The hypoglycemic effects of ethanol are not dose dependent (5).

Ethanol should be used cautiously in patients with known cardiovascular dysfunction and in certain ethnic populations. At doses of 1 mg/kg, ethanol produces dysfunction in mitochondrial function, with resultant decreased peripheral oxygen delivery and metabolism, and it may result in hypoxia or shock (10).

Cardiovascular sequelae may develop as a result of sympathomimetic effects involving catecholamine release (positive inotropic and chronotropic responses, vasoconstriction, and hypertension), which may be secondary to the reaction of acetaldehyde with tissue sulfhydryl groups.

Concurrent use of ethanol with disulfiram or other drugs that inhibit aldehyde dehydrogenase (e.g., griseofulvin, trichloroethylene, formamides) can produce an acetaldehyde syndrome (nausea, flushing, and autonomic instability) (8,11,12). Acetaldehyde also acts on the liver to depress mitochondrial function, decrease fatty acid oxidation, enhance glycogenolysis, and decrease gluconeogenesis. These effects may be produced with concentrations of ethanol that are used therapeutically. Other inhibitors of acetaldehyde dehydrogenase include metronidazole; sulfonylurea antidiabetic drugs; the fungicide, thiram; the ink cap mushroom, *Coprinus atramentarius*; and others. Asians often have an inactive aldehyde dehydrogenase variant that causes them to experience high blood acetaldehyde levels when exposed to ethanol, with subsequent development of ethanol intolerance (13).

As a general rule, the fetus is more at risk from the metabolic derangements of the toxic alcohols than from the effects of ethanol itself. However, ethanol passes easily into breast milk, and the fetal level may exceed the maternal level. Breast-feeding should be avoided during ethanol treatment. Ethanol therapy is contraindicated in the rare case of known hypersensitivity (anaphylaxis) to ethanol (14).

DOSAGE AND METHOD OF ADMINISTRATION

Ethylene Glycol or Methanol Poisoning

As an antidote for ethylene glycol or methanol poisoning (or other toxic alcohol), the goal is to maintain a blood alcohol concentration between 100 and 130 mg/dl. A loading dose of ethanol should be given by slow IV infusion or may be given orally if the IV formulation of ethanol is not available. To minimize volume without inducing tissue injury, a 10% ethanol [volume to volume (vol/vol)] solution is recommended. Based on a population average volume of distribution of 0.6 L/kg (15), the loading dose is 750 to 1000 mg/kg (Table 1). This can be infused as 7.5 to 10.0 ml/kg IV of 10% ethanol (vol/vol) in dextrose 5% in water over 30 minutes (16–18). Alternate volumes of different percentage ethanol may be calculated from this formula:

$$X\ (\text{ml}) = Y\ (\text{mg})/[10 \times Z\ (\%)]$$

where X is the volume of ethanol to administer, Y is the desired dose, and Z is the concentration (%) of ethanol to be used.

The maintenance infusion should be started with the loading dose infusion. The initial maintenance dose is 66 mg/kg/hour for nondrinkers (0.66 ml/kg/hour of 10% ethanol) and 154 mg/kg/hour (1.54 ml/kg/hour of 10% ethanol) for chronic drinkers (15–18). When hemodialysis is performed, the maintenance dose of ethanol is increased to 169 mg/kg/hour (1.69 ml/kg/hour of 10% ethanol) for nondrinkers and 257 mg/kg/hour (2.57 ml/kg/hour of 10% ethanol) for chronic drinkers (17).

In the absence of good data, the loading dose and maintenance infusion for children (on a weight basis) should be the same as for adults.

Monitoring of Response

The blood ethanol concentration should be measured at the end of the loading dose and every hour during the initial maintenance dosing. The maintenance dose infusion rate should be adjusted to maintain an ethanol concentration of 100 to 130 mg/dl. Blood glucose and mental status should be monitored frequently during therapy, especially in children because ethanol-induced hypoglycemia and CNS depression are common.

ADVERSE EFFECTS

The primary adverse effect is dose-related CNS depression, ranging from inebriation to coma, respiratory failure, and death.

TABLE 1. Ethanol dosing for ethylene glycol or methanol poisoning

Ethanol dose	Novice drinker	Chronic drinker
Loading dose		
IV, 10% solution		Loading dose is same for novice and chronic drinkers
Amount (mg/kg)	750–1000	
Volume (ml/kg)	7.5–10.0	
Oral, 40% solution (80 proof)		
Volume (ml/kg)	2.5	
Maintenance dose		
IV, 10% solution		
Amount (mg/kg/h)	66	154
Volume (ml/kg/h)	0.66	1.54
Oral, 40% solution (80 proof)		
Volume (ml/kg/h)	0.22	0.51
Maintenance dose during dialysis		
IV, 10% solution		
Amount (mg/kg/h)	169	257
Volume (ml/kg/h)	1.69	2.57
Oral, 40% solution (80 proof)		
Volume (ml/kg/h)	0.56	0.86

Note: The loading dose should be infused over 15 to 20 minutes and the maintenance infusion begun simultaneously. The loading dose is not affected by hemodialysis.

If the patient is starting with an existing blood ethanol level greater than zero, adjust the loading dose by multiplying by the following factor: [100 – blood ethanol (mg/dl)]/100.

Maintenance doses may need to be adjusted up or down, depending on the degree of induction or enhanced clearance by dialysis. If low levels are detected, the patient should receive a repeat bolus of ethanol in addition to increasing the rate. Patients with a blood ethanol level of 0 to 50 mg/dl should receive a bolus of 10 cc/kg (10% solution) and have the infusion rate doubled. Patients with levels of 50 to 80 mg/dl should receive a bolus of 5 cc/kg and have the rate increased 50%. Patients with ethanol levels of 80 to 100 mg/dl should receive a bolus of 2.5 cc/kg and have the rate increased 25%.

In acute ingestion, hypothermia is common (7,19–23). Elevated body temperature has been reported in pediatric cases (5,24). Acutely, alcohol usually causes a modest fall in blood pressure (25), and tachycardia may be present (26). Bradypnea may occur early in the course, and tachypnea may occur in cases of metabolic acidosis.

In acute ingestion, atrial fibrillation (27–29) and atrioventricular block (30) have been reported. Angina may be precipitated (31), and variant angina may occur (32,33). Acute myocardial infarction may occur even in the absence of coronary artery disease (34). Cardiac output may be decreased in persons with or without preexisting cardiac disease (35). Cardiopulmonary arrest occurred in a 2-year-old girl with a blood ethanol concentration of 268 mg/dl after ingesting up to 120 ml of 26.5% ethanol (36).

Respiratory depression and respiratory failure (37,38) may occur with significant ingestions. Because of depressed CNS function and airway reflexes, aspiration pneumonitis may occur (39,40). Cerebral edema may develop as a consequence of prolonged hypoxia secondary to respiratory depression or after aspiration. A 3-year-old with a blood ethanol concentration of 504 mg/dl experienced respiratory arrest and died. A computed tomography scan before death showed impending herniation (36). A 3-year-old boy who ingested up to 500 ml of 40% ethanol had a pulmonary aspiration and died from anoxic encephalopathy (24).

Lethargy and hypotonia are commonly seen in children after acute exposure (41–43). Reflexes are variably affected (44,43). Seizures may occur in children secondary to hypoglycemia (5,6,21,44,45). Various fluid and electrolyte disturbances have been reported. Lactic or ketoacidosis may occur after acute ingestion (21,23,45,46). Hypokalemia has been reported in children (45).

Anaphylaxis after the ingestion of ethanol is rare. Acetaldehyde reactions typically involve facial and trunk flushing and autonomic effects but also may include pulmonary edema, nausea, narcosis, respiratory failure, cardiac dilatation, cardiovascular collapse, congestive heart failure, seizures, and sudden death (47,48).

PITFALLS

Failure to monitor patients properly during ethanol infusion may result in significant ethanol toxicity. Although there is no specific reversal agent for ethanol, flumazenil may improve the mental status of ethanol-intoxicated patients at doses of 2 to 5 mg in adults (49). However, because of the risk of benzodiazepine dependence, coingestants, or the potential need to treat seizures, its use is generally contraindicated.

Due to its effects on mentation and the possibility of hypoglycemia, ethanol treatment usually requires an intensive care setting.

REFERENCES

1. Seitz HK, Oneta CM. Gastrointestinal alcohol dehydrogenase. *Nutr Rev* 1998;56(2 Pt 1):52–60.
2. Peterson CD, Collins AJ, Himes JM, et al. Ethylene glycol poisoning. Pharmacokinetics during therapy with ethanol and hemodialysis. *N Engl J Med* 1981;304:21–23.
3. Palatnick W, Redman LW, Sitar DS, et al. Methanol half-life during ethanol administration: implications for management of methanol poisoning. *Ann Emerg Med* 1995;26:202–207.
4. Litovitz TL, Holm KC, Bailey KM, Schmitz BF. 1991 annual report of the American Association of Poison Control Centers National Data Collection System. *Am J Emerg Med* 1992;10(5):452–505.
5. Hornfeldt CS. A report of acute ethanol poisoning in a child: mouthwash versus cologne, perfume and after-shave. *J Toxicol Clin Toxicol* 1992;30:115–121.
6. Cummins LH. Hypoglycemia and convulsions in children following alcohol ingestion. *J Pediatr* 1961;23–26.
7. Wade T, Gammon A. Ingestion of mouthwash by children (letter). *BMJ* 1999;318:1078.
8. Rall TW. Hypnotics and sedatives; ethanol. In: Gilman AG, Rall RW, Nies AS, et al., eds. *Goodman and Gilman's the pharmacological basis of therapeutics*, 8th ed. New York: Pergamon Press, 1990.
9. VanDierendonk DR, Dire DJ. Baclofen and ethanol ingestion: a case report. *J Emerg Med* 1999;17:989–993.
10. Gutierrez CA, Lambert C, Harrah J, et al. Moderate alcohol intoxication directly reduces peripheral oxygen delivery and utilization (abst). *Acad Emerg Med* 1999;6:391–392.
11. Fett DL, Vukov LF. An unusual case of severe griseofulvin-alcohol interaction. *Am J Emerg Med* 1994;24:95–97.
12. Cox NH, Mustchin CP. Prolonged spontaneous and alcohol-induced flushing due to the solvent dimethylformamide. *Contact Dermatitis* 1991;24:69–70.
13. Harada S, Misawa S, Agarwal DP, Goedde HW. Liver alcohol and aldehyde dehydrogenase in the Japanese: isozyme variation and its possible role in alcohol intoxications. *Am J Hum Genet* 1980;32:8–15.
14. Mallon DF, Katelaris CH. Ethanol-induced anaphylaxis following ingestion of overripe rock melon, *Cucumis melo*. *Ann Allergy Asthma Immunol* 1997;78(3):285–286.
15. Ekins BR, Rollins DE, Duffy DP, et al. Standardized treatment of severe methanol poisoning with ethanol and hemodialysis. *West J Med* 1985;142:337–340.
16. McCoy HG, Cipolle RJ, Ehiers SM, et al. Severe methanol poisoning: application of a pharmacokinetic model for ethanol therapy and hemodialysis. *Am J Med* 1979;67:804–807.
17. Barceloux DG, Krenzelod EP, Olson K, et al. American Academy of Clinical Toxicology Practice Guidelines on the treatment of ethylene glycol poisoning. *J Toxicol Clin Toxicol* 1999;37(5):537–560.
18. Chazal I, Houghton B, Frock J. The "sweet killer": can you recognize the symptoms of ethylene glycol poisoning? *Postgrad Med* 1999;106(4):221–230.
19. Moss MH. Alcohol induced hypoglycemia and coma caused by alcohol sponging. *Pediatrics* 1970;46:445–447.
20. Weyman AE, Greenbaum DM, Grace WJ. Accidental hypothermia in an alcoholic population. *Am J Med* 1974;56:13–21.
21. Selbst SM, De Maio JG, Boenning D. Mouthwash poisoning: report of a fatal case. *Clin Pediatr* 1985;24:162–163.
22. Szpak D, Groszek B, Obara M, et al. Thermoregulatory dysfunction secondary to acute ethanol poisoning. *Przegl Lek* 1995;52:281–283.
23. Lien D, Mader TJ. Survival from profound alcohol-related lactic acidosis. *J Emerg Med* 1999;17:841–846.
24. Vogel C, Caraccio T, Mofenson H, Hart S. Alcohol intoxication in young children. *J Toxicol Clin Toxicol* 1995;33:25–33.

25. Abe H, Kawano Y, Jojima S, et al. Biphasic effects of repeated alcohol intake on 24-hour blood pressure in hypertensive patients. *Circulation* 1994;89:2626–2633.
26. Osborn H. Ethanol. In: Goldfrank LR, Flomenbaum NE, Lewin NA, et al., eds. *Goldfrank's toxicologic emergencies*, 5th ed. Norwalk, CT: Appleton & Lange, 1994:813–824.
27. Ettinger PO, Wu CF, De La Cruz C Jr, et al. Arrhythmias and the "holiday heart": alcohol-associated cardiac rhythm disorders. *Am Heart J* 1978;95:555–562.
28. Thorton JR. Atrial fibrillation in healthy non-alcoholic people after an alcoholic binge. *Lancet* 1984;2:1013–1014.
29. Ridker PM, Gibson CM, Lopez R. Atrial fibrillation induced by breath spray (letter). *N Engl J Med* 1989;320:124.
30. Eilam O, Heyman SN. Wenckebach-type atrioventricular block in severe alcohol intoxication (letter). *Ann Emerg Med* 1991;20:1170.
31. Miwa K, Igawa A, Miyagi Y, et al. Importance of magnesium deficiency in alcohol-induced variant angina. *Am J Cardiol* 1994;73:813–816.
32. Ando H, Abe H, Hisanou R. Ethanol-induced myocardial ischemia: close relation between blood acetaldehyde level and myocardial ischemia. *Clin Cardiol* 1993;16:443–446.
33. Oda H, Suzuki M, Oniki T, et al. Alcohol and coronary spasm. *J Vasc Dis* 1994;45:187–197.
34. Starc R, Brucan A, Bunc M. Acute myocardial infarction induced by alcohol ingestion in an asymptomatic individual. *Europ J Emerg Med* 1999;6:403–406.
35. Sheehy TW. Alcohol and the heart: how it helps, how it harms. *Postgrad Med* 1992;91:271–277.
36. Litovitz TL, Schmitz BF, Holm KC. 1988 annual report of the American Association of Poison Control Centers National Data Collection System. *Am J Emerg Med* 1986;4:427–458.
37. Johnstone RE, Witt RL. Respiratory effects of ethyl alcohol intoxication. *JAMA* 1972;222(4):486.
38. Johnstone RE, Reier CE. Acute respiratory effects of ethanol in man. *Clin Pharmacol Ther* 1973;14:501–508.
39. Dickerman JD, Bishop W, Marks JF. Acute ethanol intoxication in a child. *Pediatrics* 1968;42:837–840.
40. Johnson HRM. At what blood levels does alcohol kill? *Med Sci Law* 1985;25:127–130.
41. Da Dalt L, Dall'Amico R, Laverda AM, et al. Percutaneous ethyl alcohol intoxication in a one-month-old infant. *Pediatr Emerg Care* 1991;7:343–344.
42. Weller-Fahy ER, Berger LR, Troutman WG. Mouthwash: a source of acute ethanol intoxication. *Pediatrics* 1980;66:302–305.
43. Ricci LR, Hoffman SA. Ethanol-induced hypoglycemic coma in a child. *Ann Emerg Med* 1982;11:202–204.
44. Gimenez ER, Vallejo NE, Roy E, et al. Percutaneous alcohol intoxication. *J Toxicol Clin Toxicol* 1968;1:39–48.
45. Leung AKC. Ethyl alcohol ingestion in children: a 15-year review. *Clin Pediatr* 1986;25:617–619.
46. Braden GL, Strayhorn CH, Germain MJ, et al. Increased osmolol gap in alcoholic acidosis. *Arch Intern Med* 1993;153:2377–2380.
47. Brien JF, Loomis CW. Pharmacology of acetaldehyde. *Can J Physiol Pharmacol* 1983;61:1–22.
48. Schootstra R, Bloemhof H, Bouma P, Uges DRA. An unusual case of acetaldehyde intoxication. In: Uges DRA, de Zeeuw RA, eds. *Proceedings of the International Association of Forensic Toxicologists*, 25th Meeting. Groningen, Netherlands: 1988;85–91.
49. Lheureux P, Askenasi R. Efficacy of flumazenil in acute alcohol intoxication: double blind placebo-controlled evaluation. *Human Exp Toxicol* 1991;10:235–239.

CHAPTER 57

Flumazenil

E. Martin Caravati

FLUMAZENIL

Synonyms:	**Anexate, Lanexat, Romazicon**
Molecular formula and weight:	**$C_{15}H_{14}FN_3O_3$, 303.3 g/mol**
SI conversion:	**mg/L × 3.30 = μmol/L**
CAS Registry No.:	**78755-81-4**
Therapeutic levels:	**6 ng/ml (20 to 25 nmol/L)**
Special concerns:	**Flumazenil may induce benzodiazepine withdrawal or unmask the toxic effects of coingestants.**

OVERVIEW

Flumazenil is a 1,4-imidazobenzodiazepine structurally similar to midazolam. It is a specific competitive antagonist at the benzodiazepine receptor site. It improves consciousness, permits return of protective airway reflexes, and lessens the potential for pulmonary aspiration in patients with benzodiazepine toxicity.

The need for gastric lavage, mechanical ventilation, arterial and urinary catheterization, frequent passive position changes, computed tomography of brain, blood culture, lumbar puncture, and electroencephalograms may be lessened in selected patients (1–3). However, a cost analysis of hospitalized patients receiving flumazenil versus placebo for benzodiazepine overdose revealed no economic benefit (4).

Overall, the evidence for using flumazenil as a diagnostic agent in patients with coma of unknown etiology is not compelling. In coma due to multiple-drug overdose, flumazenil reverses the benzodiazepine component of central nervous system (CNS) depression and may help in the diagnosis. Because flumazenil is associated with such risks as seizures, dysrhythmias, and withdrawal symptoms, it cannot be recommended for the patient with coma of unknown origin and a possibly mixed-toxic ingestion. Deaths have followed its use in mixed overdoses (5).

A double-blind, placebo-controlled randomized study of intravenous (IV) flumazenil (1 mg) in patients with coma of uncertain etiology in an intensive care unit demonstrated that invasive procedures, such as urinary catheterization, gastric lavage, endotracheal intubation, artificial ventilation, brain computed tomography, and lumbar puncture, were avoided when compared to the placebo group ($N = 52$). Nine adverse reactions occurred in the flumazenil group ($N = 53$). No seizures or dysrhythmias were noted (3). In another prospective study of 110 consecutive suspected overdose patients, 75% of patients with high benzodiazepine blood concentrations demonstrated improved alertness, but 40% of those relapsed into coma after an average of 18 minutes. Tricyclic antidepressant drugs were ingested by 71% of the cases, and no seizures were noted (6). In a retrospective review, 5 of 35 (14%) consecutive comatose overdose patients who received flumazenil experienced seizures at an average of 28 minutes after the dose (7).

High-performance liquid chromatography and gas-liquid chromatography with nitrogen-phosphorus detection have been used to quantify plasma flumazenil concentrations (8). A gas chromatography–mass spectrometry method is sensitive to 1.0 ng/ml in plasma (9). Flumazenil does not interfere with detection of benzodiazepines by immunologic assay.

Forms Available

Flumazenil is supplied in the United States as a 0.1-mg/ml solution in 5- and 10-ml vials (Romazicon). It is marketed as Anexate in Europe, Australia, and South Africa.

Pharmacokinetics

Flumazenil is 40% to 50% protein bound. The onset of action is usually 1 to 2 minutes after IV injection with peak effect occurring in 5 to 10 minutes. Duration of action after a single IV injection varies from 15 to 140 minutes, depending on the dose (10). Peak levels of flumazenil necessary to achieve reversal of benzodiazepine-induced coma are 20 to 25 nmol/L (6 ng/ml). Maintenance levels of flumazenil are approximately 10 to 20 nmol/L. Therapeutic blood concentrations have been achieved within 1 minute after endotracheal administration of flumazenil (1 mg diluted in 10 ml normal saline) (11). The initial volume of distribution is 0.2 L/kg and 1 L/kg at steady state (12).

After a bolus at the same dose, infusion of 0.5, 1.0, or 3.0 mg/hour produced steady-state plasma concentrations of 6, 13, and 39 μg/L, respectively, at 1.5 hours (13). Plasma concentrations of 10 to 20 μg/L reverse benzodiazepine-induced CNS depression (14). There is an increase in plasma flumazenil concentration in cirrhosis (15).

Flumazenil is rapidly and extensively metabolized in the liver to an inactive metabolite and is excreted predominately in the urine. Less than 0.2% of an IV dose is recovered unchanged in the urine. Metabolism is prolonged with impaired hepatic function. The elimination half-life after IV administration is 40 minutes to 1.3 hours. It is slightly prolonged in patients with cirrhosis and is prolonged two- to fourfold in lung disease (16). Flumazenil and its metabolites are completely eliminated in 48 to 72 hours (17). The pharmacokinetics of flumazenil are not significantly altered in benzodiazepine overdose (17).

Mechanism of Action

The gamma-hydroxybutyrate (GABA)–benzodiazepine receptor complex is a neuronal cell surface protein complex that contains binding sites for benzodiazepines, GABA, barbiturates, steroids, and a chloride (Cl^-) channel (18). The sites are anatomically distinct but closely related functionally (19). Benzodiazepines increase the affinity of GABA for its receptor sites as well as increase the coupling of GABA receptors to the Cl^- channel. When the channel is opened, Cl^- diffuses inside, moves down its concentration gradient, and hyperpolarizes the cell membrane. This hyperpolarized membrane is more resistant to neuronal excitation, resulting in CNS depression (20). Flumazenil antagonizes the actions of benzodiazepines, imidazopyridines (zolpidem), and other compounds that bind to benzodiazepine receptors by competitively inhibiting benzodiazepine activity at the GABA–benzodiazepine receptor complex (21). Flumazenil acts in the CNS but not at peripheral benzodiazepine receptor sites. It does not block the pharmacologic effects of GABA, GABA mimetics, or barbiturates. It has little or no agonist activity. No clinically important hemodynamic changes or increases in levels of plasma catecholamines, glucose, cortisol, vasopressors, or β-endorphins have followed the use of flumazenil (22–24).

Flumazenil, 10 mg IV, produces changes in the electroencephalogram (12,25). Flumazenil (3 mg) induces a reduction in interictal epileptic activity. Flumazenil in high doses may exert an anticonvulsant action (26,27).

INDICATIONS

Benzodiazepine Overdose

ADULT

Flumazenil may be useful in some cases of benzodiazepine overdose. It reverses the sedative effects of benzodiazepines but may not be effective for benzodiazepine-induced respiratory depression. Cardiovascular depression may be reversed with flumazenil. A positive response may obviate the need for invasive procedures and brain computed tomography. On regaining consciousness, the patient can be questioned about the drugs ingested.

PEDIATRIC

Flumazenil reverses recurrent apnea in neonates whose mothers had received benzodiazepines (28,29). The duration of action of flumazenil in children (9 hours) may be longer than in adults (30). Pediatric benzodiazepine toxicity can be managed safely without flumazenil. In a case series of 46 children of mean age 36 months with benzodiazepine ingestion, only two received flumazenil; the rest were treated with activated charcoal and supportive care only. The duration of symptoms was less than 24 hours in 88% of patients (31).

Recovery from Benzodiazepine-Induced Conscious Sedation

ADULT

Flumazenil permits interruption of conscious sedation for diagnostic purposes or to terminate benzodiazepine sedation definitely. Flumazenil reverses sedation and anterograde amnesia associated with midazolam (32–34). Flumazenil reversed the sedation but not the amnesia for gastroscopy induced by benzodiazepines (35). It can be used to reverse adverse effects of midazolam in ophthalmic surgical procedures, such as paradoxic anxiety reaction and upper airway obstruction (36). Despite rapid reversal of sedation with flumazenil, postoperative requirements for narcotic administration are no different than for other postoperative patients (37). Flumazenil may be useful when benzodiazepine sedation has become excessive or suddenly unnecessary (e.g., paradoxic excitement or after day-stay surgery) (38). Resedation may occur in up to 10% of patients during the 3-hour observation period after flumazenil administration.

PEDIATRIC

Flumazenil effectively reversed CNS depression in a case series of children ($N = 107$; average age, 6 years) who underwent conscious sedation with midazolam. Minor adverse events occurred in 35% and consisted of abnormal crying, dizziness, nausea, fever, and headache. Resedation occurred within 50 minutes in 7% of patients (39).

Reversal of General Anesthesia

Flumazenil is effective in reversing sedation associated with midazolam induction and maintenance of general anesthesia (40). Resedation occurs in 10% to 15% of patients. It is not as effective in patients who receive multiple anesthetic agents.

Therapeutic Benzodiazepine Usage

Neurologic deterioration in a patient with chronic obstructive pulmonary disease taking benzodiazepines may be reversed with flumazenil even though serum benzodiazepine levels are not elevated (41). Laryngospasm associated with midazolam for conscious sedation is reversed with flumazenil (42).

Nonbenzodiazepine Antagonism

Flumazenil reverses the sedative effects of imidazopyridine sedative-hypnotics, such as zolpidem and zopiclone (43–45). Flumazenil has been used for ethanol overdose, but reports have been anecdotal and uncontrolled (19). Flumazenil does not improve the CNS depression induced by ethanol intoxication and has no effect on performance after ethanol intoxication (46–48).

Hepatic Encephalopathy

Benzodiazepine-like agonist substances may contribute to hepatic encephalopathy. Flumazenil administration has produced mixed results in clinical studies (49,50). Lack of clinical response may be due to cerebral edema or advanced stages of encephalopathy (51,52). A metaanalysis performed on six double-blind, randomized, controlled trials ($N = 326$, flumazenil treatment, $N = 315$, placebo) found that 27% of patients in the flumazenil group improved compared with 3% of patients in the placebo group (53). The arousal effect of flumazenil in hepatic encephalopathy may be a prognostic factor predicting short-term survival in severe hepatic encephalopathy (54). There are no data on the effect of flumazenil on the morbidity or mortality of acute encephalopathy.

CAUTIONS AND CONTRAINDICATIONS

Flumazenil does not replace the need for adequate respiratory and cardiovascular supportive care. It should be used only if continued observation for recurrence of sedation can be ensured. Flumazenil may unmask the effects of other drugs in a multiple-drug overdose and should be used with caution, especially if tricyclic antidepressants have been ingested (55). An electrocardiogram finding typical of tricyclic antidepressant poisoning is a relative contraindication to flumazenil.

Flumazenil should be avoided in several groups of patients: (a) patients who have ingested a potential convulsive agent (tricyclic antidepressant, isoniazid, cocaine, or propoxyphene) in addition to the benzodiazepine; (b) patients with a history of seizure disorder, head injury, or clinical evidence of impending seizures; and (c) patients treated with benzodiazepines for a prolonged period.

Flumazenil is U.S. Food and Drug Administration pregnancy category C. Reproductive toxicity studies in animals revealed no embryotoxic or teratogenic effects (56). No human data are available.

Allergy to flumazenil, symptomatic tricyclic antidepressant overdose, and administration of a benzodiazepine for a potentially life-threatening condition (e.g., status epilepticus) are contraindications to the administration of flumazenil.

DOSAGE AND ADMINISTRATION

Benzodiazepine Overdose

The *adult dose* of flumazenil is 0.2 mg IV over 30 seconds, followed by 0.3 and 0.5 mg at 1-minute intervals to a maximum dose of 3 mg. To avoid the potential for benzodiazepine withdrawal, slow drug titration using the smallest effective dose is preferable. Pure benzodiazepine overdose often requires a small dose (0.5 to 0.7 mg) to reverse overdose signs. Patients who have only a partial response to a cumulative dose of 3 mg may require additional doses up to a total of 5 mg for a full response. If no response is observed after a cumulative dose of 5 mg, then the sedation is probably not due to a benzodiazepine.

For recurrent sedation, 0.2 to 0.5 mg IV is administered as required every 20 minutes to a total of 1 mg/hour. A continuous infusion of 0.5 to 1.0 mg/hour has been used successfully to prevent resedation in patients with massive benzodiazepine overdose (1,57).

The *pediatric dose* has not been established. A dose of 0.01 to 0.02 mg/kg (0.2 mg maximum) has been used in small children and infants (30,58). A neonate with recurrent apnea from maternal diazepam use responded to a dose of 0.02 mg/kg IV, followed by 0.05 mg/kg/hour for 6 hours (29).

Reversal of Conscious Sedation or General Anesthesia

The *adult dose* involves titration of 0.2-mg doses IV over 15 to 30 seconds at 1-minute intervals until the patient is alert. Most patients respond to a dose of 1 mg. Resedation is treated with repeated 0.2-mg doses. The *pediatric dose* is 0.01 mg/kg (0.2 mg maximum) given over 30 seconds at 1-minute intervals until patient is alert. Maximum cumulative dose is 0.05 mg/kg or 1 mg, whichever is lower.

Hepatic Encephalopathy

Treatment protocols have consisted of 1 to 2 mg IV over 5 to 10 minutes or three sequential boluses of 0.4, 0.8, and 1 mg at 1-minute intervals, followed by infusion rates of 0.25 to 1.00 mg/hour for responders (53).

Monitoring

Flumazenil has a half-life that is often shorter than the drug it is antagonizing. The patient should be closely monitored for recurrence of CNS or respiratory depression for at least 2 to 3 hours (three half-lives) after the last dose of flumazenil. Pulse oximetry and cardiac monitoring with mental status checks every 30 minutes should be performed. Flumazenil does not enhance the elimination of benzodiazepines and does not shorten the period of observation, although it may decrease the need for ventilatory support and intensive monitoring. When the effect of flumazenil declines, patients only return to the level of sedation that would have been present had they not received flumazenil (35).

ADVERSE EFFECTS

Withdrawal Syndrome

Patients who are physiologically dependent on a benzodiazepine may undergo acute withdrawal after flumazenil use. These effects include anxiety, nausea, vomiting, dizziness, headache, agitation, diaphoresis, panic attacks, tachycardia, increased muscle tone, hyperesthesia, and possibly convulsions. Mild reactions are usually short-lived and do not require treatment. Severe symptoms may require large doses of diazepam for control (26,59,60).

Dysrhythmias

Ventricular tachycardia (62–63), bradycardia, complete heart block (64), and death (62) may follow flumazenil use. Flumazenil can precipitate a cardiac dysrhythmia in patients who have overdosed on both a benzodiazepine and a tricyclic antidepressant (63,65). There is one report of bradycardia followed by asystole and death in a patient who ingested a benzodiazepine-antidepressant mixture and received flumazenil (62). Flumazenil, 500 μg, administered to reverse the effects of temazepam, led to a complete heart block within 1 minute; the patient was given atropine and reverted to sinus rhythm. There is one report of nonfatal ventricular tachycardia after administration of flumazenil to a patient who had ingested a benzodiazepine–chloral hydrate mixture (61).

Seizures

Seizures may occur in patients dependent on benzodiazepines or in association with a tricyclic antidepressant overdose. Flumazenil antagonizes the anticonvulsant properties of benzodiazepines and may reveal the epileptogenic activity of a tricyclic antidepressant or any other seizure-inducing drug (65). Refractory seizures resulting in death occurred 2 minutes after administration of flumazenil for a mixed overdose that included a tricyclic antidepressant (5). Seizures may also occur in patients with epilepsy who use benzodiazepine therapy. Barbiturates should be used to treat seizures induced by flumazenil.

Other

Local extravasation during infusion may result in tissue irritation and injury. Postoperative use of flumazenil may exacerbate the sensation of pain with a concomitant increase in consciousness. Flumazenil may increase intracranial pressure in patients with severe head injury (30). Flumazenil has led to a moderate increase in blood pressure and elevation of left ventricular end-diastolic pressure in patients with ischemic heart disease who have received a benzodiazepine. The blood pressure may increase or decrease, and the heart rate may increase (66). Flumazenil for hepatic encephalopathy has resulted in acute psychosis (67).

PITFALLS

Most benzodiazepine toxicity is non–life-threatening. Flumazenil alone is inadequate for treatment of benzodiazepine intoxication. Partial reversal could lead to a fatal delay in instituting rapid tracheal intubation and ventilatory assistance (68). Repeated doses may be required because of the short duration of action of flumazenil compared to most benzodiazepines.

The anticonvulsant and sedative actions of benzodiazepines may be treating more serious toxic effects of another component of a multiple-drug overdose, and the use of flumazenil may result in greater toxic effects from the overdose.

Another etiology should be sought in patients who do not respond to an IV flumazenil dose of 5 mg.

In patients suffering from respiratory depression due to the combined effects of a benzodiazepine and an opioid, flumazenil safely antagonizes the benzodiazepine component. The effect of the opioid may still be present, and respiration is not necessarily restored (18).

Despite rapid reversal of sedation with flumazenil, requirements for narcotic analgesic administration in the postoperative setting are no different than for other postoperative patients (37).

REFERENCES

1. Hojer J, Baehrendtz S, Magnusson A, Gustafsson LL. A placebo-controlled trial of flumazenil given by continuous infusion in severe benzodiazepine overdosage. *Acta Anaesthesiol Scand* 1991;35:584–590.
2. Hojer J, Baehrendtz S. The effect of flumazenil (RO15-1788) in the management of self-induced benzodiazepine poisoning: a double-blind controlled study. *Acta Med Scand* 1988;224:357–365.
3. Hojer J, Baehrendtz S, Matell G, Gustafsson LL. Diagnostic utility of flumazenil in coma with suspected poisoning: a double blind randomised controlled study. *BMJ* 1990;301:1308–1311.
4. Barnett R, Grace M, Boothe P, et al. Flumazenil in drug overdose: randomized, placebo-controlled study to assess cost effectiveness. *Crit Care Med* 1999;27:78–81.
5. Haverkos GP, DiSalvo RP, Imhoff TE. Fatal seizures after flumazenil administration in a patient with mixed overdose. *Ann Pharmacother* 1994;28:1347–1349.
6. Weinbroum A, Rudick V, Sorkine P, et al. Use of flumazenil in the treatment of drug overdose: a double-blind and open clinical study in 110 patients. *Crit Care Med* 1996;24:199–206.
7. Gueye PN, Hoffman JR, Taboulet P, et al. Empiric use of flumazenil in comatose patients: limited applicability of criteria to define low risk. *Ann Emerg Med* 1996;27:730–735.
8. Abernethy DR, Arendt RM, Lauven PM, Greenblatt DJ. Determination of RO15-1788, a benzodiazepine antagonist, in human plasma by gas liquid chromatography with nitrogen–phosphorus detection. *Pharmacology* 1983;26:285–289.
9. Kintz P, Mangin P. Plasma determination of flumazenil, a benzodiazepine antagonist, by immunotoxicology and by capillary gas chromatography/mass spectrometry. *J Anal Toxicol* 1991;15:202–203.
10. Amrein R, Hetzel W. Pharmacology of Dormicum (midazolam) and Anexate (flumazenil). *Acta Anaesthesiol Scand Suppl* 1990;92:6–15.
11. Palmer RB, Mautz DS, Cox K, et al. Endotracheal flumazenil: a new route of administration for benzodiazepine antagonism. *Am J Emerg Med* 1998;16:170–172.
12. Breimer LTM, Hennis PJ, Burm AGL, et al. Pharmacokinetics and EEG effects of flumazenil in volunteers. *Clin Pharmacokinet* 1991;30:491–496.
13. Klotz V, Ziegler G, Reimann N. Pharmacokinetics of the selective benzodiazepine antagonist RO15-1788 in man. *Eur J Clin Pharmacol* 1984;27:115–117.
14. Klotz U, Ziegler G, Ludwig L, et al. Pharmacodynamic interaction between midazolam and a specific benzodiazepine antagonist in humans. *J Clin Pharmacol* 1985;25:400–406.
15. Janssen U, Walker S, Maier K, et al. Flumazenil disposition and elimination in cirrhosis. *Clin Pharmacol Ther* 1989;46:317–323.
16. van der Rijt CC, Drost RH, Schalem SW, Schramel M. Pharmacokinetics of flumazenil in fulminant hepatic failure. *Eur J Clin Pharmacol* 1991;41:501.
17. Rodwell PJL, Maclaren HM, Hughes EW, et al. The pharmacokinetics of flumazenil used as a bolus and an infusion regimen in the treatment of major benzodiazepine self-poisonings. *Ann Emerg Med* 1992;21:471.
18. Amrein R, Hetzel W. Pharmacology of drugs frequently used in ICU's: midazolam and flumazenil. *Intensive Care Med* 1991;17:S1–S10.
19. Votey SR. Flumazenil: a new benzodiazepine antagonist. *Ann Emerg Med* 1991;70:181–188.
20. Kasson BJ. Flumazenil: a specific benzodiazepine antagonist. *J Am Assoc Nurse Anaesth* 1992;60:472–476.
21. Stolarek IH, Ford MJ. Acute dystonia induced by midazolam and abolished by flumazenil. *BMJ* 1990;30:614.
22. Geller E. Flumazenil in clinical medicine: indications and precautions. *Eur J Anaesthesiol* 1988;2:325–329.
23. Geller E, Halpern P, Chernilas J, et al. Cardiorespiratory effects of antagonism of diazepam sedation with flumazenil in patients with cardiac disease. *Anesth Analg* 1991;72:207–211.

24. Geller E, Niv D, Weinbrun A, et al. The use of flumazenil in the treatment of 34 intoxicated patients. *Resuscitation* 1988;16:S57–S62.
25. Hart YM, Meinardi H, Sander JWAS, et al. The effect of intravenous flumazenil on electroencephalographic activity: results of a placebo-controlled study. *J Neurol Neurosurg Psychiatry* 1991;54:305–309.
26. Scollo-Lavizzari G. The clinical anticonvulsant effect of flumazenil, a benzodiazepine antagonist. *Eur J Anaesthesiol* 1988;2:129–138.
27. Scollo-Lavizzari G. The anticonvulsant effects of the benzodiazepine antagonist, RO15-1788: an EEG study in 4 cases. *Eur Neurol* 1984;23:1–6.
28. Dixon JC, Speidel BD, Dixon JJ. Neonatal flumazenil therapy reverses maternal diazepam. *Acta Paediatr* 1998;87:225–226.
29. Richard P, Autret E, Bardol J, et al. The use of flumazenil in a neonate. *J Toxicol Clin Toxicol* 1991;29:137–141.
30. La Fleche RF. Flumazenil. *Clin Toxicol Rev* 1990;12(5):1–2.
31. Wiley CC, Wiley JF 2nd. Pediatric benzodiazepine ingestion resulting in hospitalization. *J Toxicol Clin Toxicol* 1998;36:227–231.
32. Whitman JG. Flumazenil: a benzodiazepine antagonist: many uses possibly including withdrawal from benzodiazepines. *BMJ* 1988;297:999–1000.
33. Whitman JG. The use of midazolam and flumazenil in diagnostic and short surgical procedures. *Acta Anaesthesiol Scand* 1990;34(Suppl 92):16–20.
34. McKay AC, McKinney MS, Clarke RSJ. Effect of flumazenil on midazolam-induced amnesia. *Br J Anaesth* 1990;65:190–196.
35. Pearson RC, McCloy RF, Morns P, Bardhas KD. Midazolam and flumazenil in gastroenterology. *Acta Anaesthesiol Scand* 1990;34(Suppl 92):21–24.
36. Gobeaux D, Sardnal F. Midazolam and flumazenil in ophthalmology. *Acta Anesthesiol Scand* 1990;34(Suppl 92):35–38.
37. Olsen KM, Pablo CS, Ackerman BH. Postoperative analgesic requirements following flumazenil administration. *DICP* 1990;24:1159–1163.
38. Sage DJ. Reversal of sedation with flumazenil in regional anaesthesia: a review. *Eur J Anaesthesiol* 1988;2:201–207.
39. Shannon M, Albers G, Burkhart K, et al. Safety and efficacy of flumazenil in the reversal of benzodiazepine-induced conscious sedation. The Flumazenil Pediatric Study Group. *J Pediatr* 1997;131:582–586.
40. Momose T. A study on the effects of regaining consciousness with flumazenil from anesthesia supplemented with a benzodiazepine and pentazocine. *Clin Pharmacol Ther* 1991;49:185.
41. Appel M, Bron HN, Hooymans PM, Janknegt R. Efficacy of flumazenil in COPD patient with therapeutic diazepam levels. *Lancet* 1989;1:392.
42. Davis DP, Hamilton RS, Webster TH. Reversal of midazolam-induced laryngospasm with flumazenil. *Ann Emerg Med* 1998;32:263–265.
43. Patat A, Naef MM, van Gessel E, et al. Flumazenil antagonizes the central effects of zolpidem, an imidazopyridine hypnotic. *Clin Pharmacol Ther* 1994;56:430–436.
44. Ahmad Z, Herepath M, Ebden P. Diagnostic utility of flumazenil in coma with suspected poisoning. *BMJ* 1991;302:292.
45. Naef MM, Forster A, Nahory A, et al. Flumazenil antagonizes the sedative action of zolpidem, a new iminoazopyridine hypnotic. *Anesthesiology* 1989;4(3A):A297.
46. Flukiger A, Hartmann D, Leishman B, Ziegler WH. Lack of effect of benzodiazepine antagonist flumazenil (RO 15-1788) on the performance of healthy subjects during experimentally induced ethanol intoxication. *Eur J Clin Pharmacol* 1988;34:273–276.
47. Clausen TG, Wolff J, Carl P, Theilgaard A. The effect of the benzodiazepine antagonist, flumazenil, on psychometric performance in acute ethanol intoxication in man. *Eur J Clin Pharmacol* 1990;38:233–236.
48. Lheureux P, Askenasi R. Efficacy of flumazenil in acute alcohol intoxication: double blind placebo-controlled evaluation. *Hum Exp Toxicol* 1991;10:235–239.
49. Grimm G, Ferenci P, Katzenschlager R, et al. Improvement of hepatic encephalopathy treated with flumazenil. *Lancet* 1988;2:1392–1394.
50. Basile AS, Gammal SH. Evidence for the involvement of the benzodiazepine receptor complex in hepatic encephalopathy: implications for treatment with benzodiazepine receptor antagonists. *Clin Neuropharmacol* 1988;11:401–422.
51. Sutherland LR, Minuk GY. Ro 15-1788 and hepatic failure. *Ann Intern Med* 1988;108:158.
52. Klotz U, Walker S. Flumazenil and hepatic encephalopathy. *Lancet* 1989;1:155–156.
53. Goulenok C, Bernard B, Cadranel JF, et al. Flumazenil vs. placebo in hepatic encephalopathy in patients with cirrhosis: a meta-analysis. *Aliment Pharmacol Ther* 2002;16:361–372.
54. Bansky G, Meier PJ, Riederer E, et al. Effects of a benzodiazepine antagonist in hepatic encephalopathy in man. *Hepatology* 1987;7:1103.
55. Hoffman RS, Goldfrank LR. The poisoned patient with altered consciousness: controversies in the use of a "coma cocktail." *JAMA* 1995;274:562–569.
56. Schlappi B, Bonetti EP, Burgin H, Strobel R. Toxicological investigations with the benzodiazepine antagonist flumazenil. *Arzneimittelforschung* 1988;38(2):247–250.
57. Brammer G, Gibly R, Walter FG, et al. Continuous intravenous flumazenil infusion for benzodiazepine poisoning. *Vet Hum Toxicol* 2000;42:280–281.
58. Weinbroum AA, Flaishon R, Sorkine P, et al. A risk-benefit assessment of flumazenil in the management of benzodiazepine overdose. *Drug Saf* 1997;17:181–196.
59. Nutt D, Costello M. Flumazenil and benzodiazepine withdrawal. *Lancet* 1987;2:463.
60. Lopez A, Rebollo J. Benzodiazepine withdrawal syndrome after a benzodiazepine antagonist. *Crit Care Med* 1990;18:1480–1481.
61. Short TG, Maling T, Galletly DC. Ventricular arrhythmias precipitated by flumazenil. *BMJ* 1988;296:1070–1071.
62. Burr W, Sandham P. Death after flumazenil. *BMJ* 1989;298:1713.
63. Marchant B, Wray R, Leach A, Nama M. Flumazenil causing convulsions and ventricular tachycardia. *BMJ* 1989;299:860.
64. Herd B, Clarke F. Complete heart block after flumazenil. *Hum Exp Toxicol* 1991;10:289.
65. Spivey WH. Flumazenil and seizures: analysis of 43 cases. *Clin Ther* 1992;14:292–305.
66. Marty J, Nitenberg A. The use of midazolam and flumazenil in cardiovascular diagnostic and therapeutic procedures. *Acta Anaesthesiol Scand* 1990;34(Suppl 92):33–34.
67. Seebach J, Jost R. Flumazenil-induced psychotic disorder in hepatic encephalopathy. *Lancet* 1992;339:488–489.
68. Lim AG. Death after flumazenil. *BMJ* 1989;299:858–859.

CHAPTER 58

Folic Acid and Leucovorin

Luke Yip

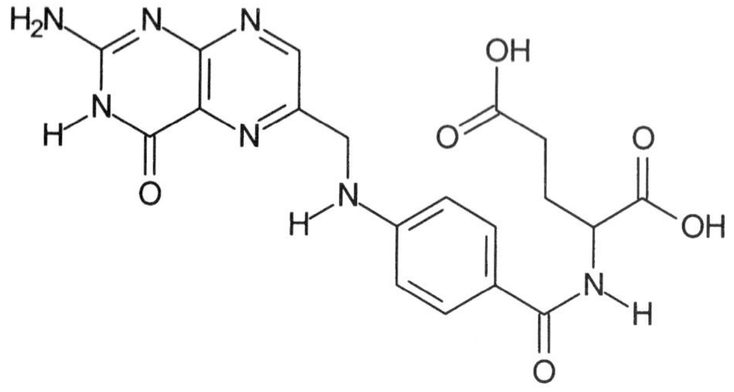

FOLIC ACID

Synonyms:	**Folic acid (folate, pteroylglutamic acid, vitamin BC, vitamin M); leucovorin (5-formyltetrahydrofolic acid, citrovorum factor, folinic acid, 5-FTHFA, tetrahydrofolate)**
Molecular formula and weight:	**Folic acid ($C_{19}H_{19}N_7O_6$), 441.4 g/mol; folinic acid ($C_{20}H_{23}N_7O_7$), 473.4 g/mol**
CAS Registry No.:	**59-30-3 (folic acid); 6484-89-5 (sodium folate); 58-05-9 (folinic acid)**
Therapeutic levels:	**Not clinically applicable**
Special concerns:	**Only leucovorin should be used for methotrexate rescue.**

OVERVIEW

Folic acid is a water-soluble, essential vitamin, and leucovorin is a derivative of tetrahydrofolate, the bioactive form of folic acid. Folic acid in a yellow or yellowish-orange crystalline powder form is suitable for intramuscular or intravenous (IV) administration after reconstitution with sterile water, saline, or dextrose 5% in water (D_5W). It is also available as a tablet for oral administration. Oral preparation is available alone or in combination with other vitamins. Parenteral preparation is available in 5 or 10 mg/ml in 10-ml multidose vials with 1.5% benzyl alcohol. Leucovorin is available as a tablet in 5, 10, 15, and 25 mg. A parenteral preparation is available as calcium leucovorin salt powder in 50-, 100-, and 350-mg vials. It is usually reconstituted to a final concentration of 10 mg/ml.

Mechanism of Action

Folic acid is an essential cofactor in mammalian biosynthetic functions. After active transportation into cells, it is converted to its biologically active form. This process requires folic acid to be reduced to dihydrofolate and then further reduced to tetrahydrofolate. Both reactions are nicotinamide adenine dinucleotide phosphate dependent and catalyzed by dihydrofolate reductase.

Single carbon fragments (e.g., methyl groups) are enzymatically added to tetrahydrofolate in various configurations and may then be transferred during the biosynthesis of other molecules. The transferred carbon groups can exist in a variety of oxidation states and range from highly reduced methyl groups to oxidized formate and methenyl groups. In the transfer process, dihydrofolate is regenerated. In humans, the folate-dependent reactions are syntheses of thymidylate and purines; conversion of serine to glycine, homocysteine to methionine, and histidine to glutamate; and utilization or generation of formate.

Human methanol toxicity is the result of formate accumulation when there is an inadequate folate concentration. This is based on primate studies, which show that formate metabolism is critically dependent on folic acid reserve, and folic acid or leucovorin is highly effective treatment after methanol poisoning (1–3). Pretreatment with folic acid or treatments with leucovorin after methanol administration result in a marked decrease in blood formate levels and absence of metabolic acidosis, without affecting the methanol elimination rate. Leucovorin reverses established methanol toxicity.

In ethylene glycol poisoning, a minor metabolic pathway may produce formic acid, and, theoretically, supplemental folic acid or leucovorin will enhance its elimination. However, the clinical efficacy of folic acid or leucovorin therapy is unknown in this scenario.

Methotrexate is a folic acid analog and is a potent competitive inhibitor of dihydrofolate reductase. When dihydrofolate reductase is inhibited, folic acid cannot be reduced to tetrahydrofolate, and it cannot be regenerated from dihydrofolate. Leucovorin, a tetrahydrofolate derivative, can bypass the inhibited dihydrofolate reductase system and is actively transported into the cell at the same receptor site as folic acid and methotrexate. Administration of leucovorin displaces methotrexate from dihydrofolate reductase, competes with methotrexate intracellular transport, increases methotrexate efflux from the cell, and replenishes intracellular reduced-folate stores (4).

INDICATIONS

It is recommended that leucovorin be administered when there is a high index of suspicion for methanol poisoning.

CAUTIONS AND CONTRAINDICATIONS

The possibility of allergic reactions and seizures should be considered before initiating folic acid or leucovorin therapy. Leucovorin may obscure the diagnosis of pernicious anemia by correcting hematologic manifestations of the disease and allowing neurologic complications to progress. Rare patients have known immunoglobulin E–mediated folic acid or leucovorin allergy.

DOSAGE AND ADMINISTRATION

Leucovorin is preferred to folic acid for all indications. The leucovorin infusion rate should not exceed 160 mg/minute because of the amount of calcium salt present in solution. When leucovorin is reconstituted with bacteriostatic water containing benzyl alcohol, potentially toxic benzyl alcohol doses may be administered during leucovorin infusion at doses greater than 10 mg/m^2. To avoid this potential problem, leucovorin should be reconstituted with sterile water, saline, or D_5W.

Methanol Poisoning

The precise dose of leucovorin is unknown. An *adult and pediatric dose* of leucovorin, 2 mg/kg IV every 4 to 6 hours, appears reasonable based on primate studies and leucovorin pharmacokinetics (2,5). Leucovorin therapy should be continued until methanol (formate) has been eliminated and acidosis has resolved. Folic acid, 50 to 70 mg IV every 4 hours, may be administered if leucovorin is not readily available (6). Folic acid and leucovorin are readily removed during hemodialysis. If hemodialysis is used, a second dose of folic acid or leucovorin should be administered at the completion of dialysis.

Ethylene Glycol Poisoning

Folic acid and leucovorin may be considered as adjunct treatment. The route of administration and dosing are the same as for methanol poisoning.

Methotrexate Overdose

Folic acid is *not* an antidote for methotrexate overdose and should not be substituted for leucovorin in the treatment of methotrexate overdose. Leucovorin should be administered IV as soon as possible, preferably within 1 hour of the overdose. The initial leucovorin dose should be equal to or greater than the estimated ingested methotrexate dose. This dose is repeated every 3 to 6 hours until the methotrexate concentration is less than 10^{-8} mol/L. The methotrexate half-life ranges from 5 to 45 hours depending on the dose and the patient's renal function. The typical duration of leucovorin therapy is 72 hours or longer. If the methotrexate dose is unknown, the recommended initial dose of leucovorin is 10 mg/m^2 IV every 6 hours. Although leucovorin is an antidote, it should be used as adjunct treatment for methotrexate overdose.

Serum creatinine and methotrexate levels should be determined at 24-hour intervals. If the serum creatinine has increased 50% over baseline, if the 24-hour methotrexate level is greater than 5×10^{-6} mol/L, or if the 48-hour level is greater than 9×10^{-7} mol/L, the leucovorin dosage should be increased to 100 mg/m^2 every 6 hours until the methotrexate level is less than 10^{-7} mol/L at 24 hours or 10^{-8} mol/L at any time. If the 24-hour methotrexate level is greater than 5×10^{-5} mol/L or the 48-hour level is greater than 9×10^{-6} mol/L, the leucovorin dose should be increased to 1000 mg/m^2 every 6 hours until the methotrexate level is less than 10^{-7} mol/L at 24 hours or 10^{-8} mol/L at any time.

Leucovorin should be administered IV, *not* intrathecally, after methotrexate overdose. Severe neurotoxicity and death have been reported after intrathecal leucovorin rescue for intrathecal methotrexate overdose (7).

ADVERSE EFFECTS

Folic Acid

Nausea, abdominal distention, discomfort, flatulence, and a constant bad or bitter taste in the mouth have been associated with oral folic acid, 5 mg three times daily (8). Folic acid (400 to 500 μg/kg/day) may interfere with zinc absorption resulting in a decreased serum zinc level (9).

Sleep disturbances, gastrointestinal effects, malaise, overactivity, irritability, and excitability have been reported in healthy volunteers after being on folic acid, 15 mg/day, for 1 month (8). Folic acid therapy may exacerbate psychotic behavior, and behavioral improvement occurred when therapy was discontinued (10). In patients on anticonvulsants for a seizure disorder, oral folic acid supplement has been shown to decrease the seizure threshold and increase seizure frequency (11–17). Oral or intramuscular doses of folic acid have resulted in generalized erythema, pruritus, and urticaria (18). An anaphylactoid reaction has been reported after a single dose of folic acid IV (19). There is a report of a patient who developed an immunoglobulin E–mediated folic acid and leucovorin allergy (20).

Leucovorin

It has been suggested that seizures are associated with high-dose leucovorin and fluorouracil therapy in cancer patients, especially in patients with central nervous system metastases or other predisposing factors (21).

PITFALLS

IV leucovorin administration is preferred, especially if gastrointestinal symptoms are present or if more than 25 mg is to be given, because cellular transport mechanisms for leucovorin become saturated at this amount. The bioavailability of leucovorin decreases from 100% for a 20-mg dose to 78% for a 40-mg dose and 31% for a 200-mg dose (22).

Trimethoprim can interfere with laboratory techniques (e.g., competitive protein binding and enzymatic inhibition) in measuring serum methotrexate levels (23–25). Spectrophotofluorimetric analysis of blood specimens should be avoided during leucovorin rescue therapy because it may be misinterpreted for methotrexate (26).

REFERENCES

1. McMartin KE, Martin-Amat G, Makar AB, et al. Methanol poisoning. V. Role of formate metabolism in the monkey. *J Pharmacol Exp Ther* 1977;201:564–572.
2. Noker PE, Eells JT, Tephly TR. Methanol toxicity: treatment with folic acid and 5-formyl tetrahydrofolic acid. *Alcohol Clin Exp Res* 1980;4:378–383.
3. Johlin FC, Fortman CS, Nghiem DD, et al. Studies on the role of folic acid and folate-dependent enzymes in human methanol poisoning. *Mol Pharmacol* 1987;31:557–561.
4. Jackson RC, Grindey GB. The biochemical basis for methotrexate cytotoxicity. In: Sirotnak FM, ed. *Folate antagonists as therapeutic agents*, Vol. 1. Orlando, FL: Academic Press, 1984:289–315.
5. Straw JA, Newman EM, Doroshow JH. Pharmacokinetics of leucovorin (dl-5 formyltetrahydrofolate) after intravenous injection and constant intravenous infusion. *NCI Monogr* 1987;5:41–45.
6. Osterloh JD, Pond SM, Grady S, et al. Serum formate concentrations in

methanol intoxication as a criterion for hemodialysis. *Ann Intern Med* 1986;104:200–203.
7. Jardine LF, Ingram LC, Bleyer WA. Intrathecal leucovorin after intrathecal methotrexate overdose. *J Pediatr Hematol Oncol* 1996;18:302–304.
8. Hunter R, Barnes J, Oakeley HF, et al. Toxicity of folic acid given in pharmacologic doses to healthy volunteers. *Lancet* 1970;1:61–63.
9. Kakar F, Henderson MM. Potential toxic side effects of folic acid. *J Natl Cancer Inst* 1985;74:263.
10. Prakash R, Petrie WM. Psychiatric changes associated with an excess of folic acid. *Am J Psychiatr* 1982;139:1192–1193.
11. Chanarin I, Laidlaw J, Loughridge LW, et al. Megaloblastic anemia due to phenobarbitone: the convulsant action of therapeutic doses of folic acid. *BMJ* 1960;1:1099–1102.
12. Ch'ien LT, Krumdieck CL, Scott CW Jr, et al. Harmful effect of megadoses of vitamins: electroencephalogram abnormalities and seizures induced by intravenous folate in drug-treated epileptics. *Am J Clin Nutr* 1975;28:51–58.
13. Guidolin L, Vignoli A, Canger R. Worsening in seizure frequency and severity in relation to folic acid administration. *Eur J Neurol* 1998;5:301–303.
14. Houben PF, Hommes OR, Knaven PJ. Anticonvulsant drugs and folic acid in young mentally retarded epileptic patients. A study of serum folate, fit frequency and IQ. *Epilepsia* 1971;12:235–247.
15. Reynolds EH. Mental effects of anticonvulsants, and folic acid metabolism. *Brain* 1968;91:197–214.
16. Reynolds EH. Effects of folic acid on the mental state and fit-frequency of drug-treated epileptic patients. *Lancet* 1967;1:1086–1088.
17. Smith DB, Racusen LC. Folate metabolism and the anticonvulsant efficacy of phenobarbital. *Arch Neurol* 1973;28:18–22.
18. Mathur BP. Sensitivity of folic acid: a case report. *Indian J Med Sci* 1966;20:133–134.
19. Woodliff HJ, Davis RE. Allergy to folic acid. *Med J Aust* 1966;1:351–352.
20. Dyckewicz MS, Orfan NA, Sun W. In vitro demonstration of IgE antibody to folate-albumin in anaphylaxis from folic acid. *J Allergy Clin Immunol* 2000;106:386–389.
21. Meropol NJ, Petrelli NJ, White RM, et al. Seizures associated with leucovorin administration in cancer patients. *J Natl Cancer Inst* 1995;87:56–58.
22. McGuire BW, Sia LL, Haynes JD, et al. Absorption kinetics of orally administered leucovorin calcium. *NCI Monogr* 1987;5:47–56.
23. Bock JL, Pierce R. Trimethoprim interference in methotrexate assays. *Clin Chem* 1980;26:1510–1511.
24. Hande K, Gober J, Fletcher R. Trimethoprim interferes with serum methotrexate assay by the competitive protein binding technique. *Clin Chem* 1980;26:1617–1619.
25. Kitaoka S, Terasawa M, Goto E, et al. Trimethoprim interference in methotrexate assay by an enzyme inhibition assay kit. *Tohoku J Exp Med* 1986;150:481–482.
26. Kinkade JM, Vogler WR, Dayton PG. Plasma levels of methotrexate in cancer patients as studied by an improved spectrophotofluorometric method. *Biochem Med* 1974;10:337–350.

CHAPTER 59

Fomepizole

Steven A. Seifert

H–N—N, ring with CH_3

FOMEPIZOLE

Synonym:	**4-Methylpyrazole**
Molecular formula and weight:	**$C_4H_6N_2$, 82.10 g/mol**
CAS Registry No.:	**7554-65-6**
Normal or therapeutic levels:	**Not applicable**
Special concerns:	**Appropriate use, cost**

OVERVIEW

Fomepizole (Antizol) is an inhibitor of the enzyme alcohol dehydrogenase (ADH) (1). Compared to ethanol, it is a more potent ADH inhibitor in humans; is metabolized and eliminated more slowly; and has more predictable kinetics, simplifying administration and surveillance of treatment (2,3). It is indicated in the management of ethylene glycol (EG) and methanol exposures and may be of value for other glycols, 1,4-butanediol, other precursors of gamma hydroxybutyrate, isopropanol, disulfiram, and disulfiram-like reactions. It is currently the only treatment approved by the U.S. Food and Drug Administration (FDA) (4) and is recommended in the Practice Guidelines of the American Academy of Clinical Toxicology (5).

Forms Available

Fomepizole is produced in 1.5-ml vials containing 1 g/ml (Orphan Medical: Antizol; Antizol-Vet for veterinary use).

Mechanism of Action

Fomepizole is a water-soluble 4-methyl substituted pyrazole (6). It has low protein binding (7) and a small volume of distribution (0.60 to 1.02 L/kg) (6,8,9); thus, it is distributed similarly to EG (10) and methanol (11). Time to peak concentration after ingestion of fomepizole is 0.5 to 2.0 hours (12).

Fomepizole exerts its antidotal effect by preventing the formation of more toxic metabolic products of the parent compounds (EG, methanol, isopropanol, ethanol in disulfiram reactions, and 1,4-butanediol). It blocks ADH metabolism of EG in rats (13), horses (14), dogs (15–18), and monkeys (19). In cats, fomepizole appears to be less effective than ethanol in treating EG toxicity (20). In human adults, prospective, randomized clinical trials and a number of case reports in adults and children support its efficacy and safety in treatment of EG exposure (3,21–24). Fomepizole inhibits human ADH more than ethanol, and the addition of ethanol to fomepizole does not have an additional effect on EG elimination (25).

Similarly, fomepizole effectively blocks ADH metabolism of methanol in rats and monkeys (26–28), and prospective case series and case reports indicate successful treatment of methanol intoxication in humans (2,29–31).

Fomepizole is primarily metabolized by the liver following first-order kinetics, with less than 5% eliminated unchanged in the urine (8,12,32). Recommended doses reliably maintain therapeutic concentrations (3). Maintenance of a therapeutic serum fomepizole concentration effectively blocks ADH metabolism of methanol in animal studies (28,33). Maintenance of the fomepizole concentration above 15 mg/L completely inhibited ADH activity in an adult patient with EG poisoning (21). In a 4-year-old patient with EG poisoning, administration of fomepizole at 15 mg/kg resulted in a 2-hour plasma fomepizole concentration of 18.5 mg/L (22).

Fomepizole is metabolized by and also inhibits cytochrome P-450 isoenzymes, including CYP2E1 (34,35). Fomepizole also induces the activity of several P-450 enzymes, including autoinduction of CYP2E1 (36), and a significant increase in the elimination rate of fomepizole occurs after 30 to 40 hours of use (37).

Fomepizole is known to inhibit retinol dehydrogenase, an isoenzyme of ADH and essential to vision. There is evidence in rats that pyrazole affects dark adaptation (38). Also, patients presenting with retinal injury secondary to methanol metabolism have recovered normal vision after fomepizole therapy (39). Fomepizole inhibition of retinol appears to cause no visual effects or retinal injury.

Fomepizole alters the kinetics of EG and methanol. In 19 patients with EG toxicity treated with fomepizole monotherapy, the half-life of EG was 19.7 ± 1.3 hours, compared with 8.6 ± 1.1 hours when neither fomepizole nor ethanol was used (25). In a mixed methanol and isopropanol ingestion treated with fomepizole, the plasma elimination half-lives of methanol and isopropanol were 47.6 and 27.7 hours, respectively. The effect on the half-life of methanol by the presence of isopropanol (and the reverse) was not able to be determined (40). In four patients with methanol ingestion treated with fomepizole who did not undergo dialysis, the median plasma half-life of methanol was 54 hours. In comparison, methanol has a half-life of between 1.5 and 3.2 hours in subtoxic doses (40).

INDICATIONS

Ethylene Glycol and Methanol

The FDA has approved several indications for the administration of fomepizole:

- The presence of EG or methanol at a serum concentration of 20 mg/dl or greater
- The presence of signs or symptoms of EG or methanol toxicity [e.g., central nervous system (CNS) depression, acidosis, end-organ injury, and osmolal gap greater than 10 mOsm]
- Presumptive exposure sufficient to produce toxicity, while awaiting serum concentrations of EG or methanol
- Prevention of toxicity when unable to determine serum concentrations of EG or methanol

Fomepizole is often preferred over ethanol in the management of EG or methanol exposure for multiple reasons. Compared to ethanol, fomepizole is a better inhibitor of ADH (5,6), has a longer half-life (5,6), and has fewer toxicities and, therefore, has a larger therapeutic index (5,6,41). Furthermore, it is more easily administered because it requires less monitoring (5,6) and does not require a continuous intravenous (IV) infusion or produce CNS depression; thus, it does not require intensive care unit admission in the absence of other toxicity (4). It may obviate the need for dialysis in nonacidotic patients with EG intoxication (3,24,31,42–44).

When fomepizole is given before the development of acidosis or end-organ injury and therapeutic concentrations are maintained, or the parent compound is then removed with hemodialysis, toxicity does not develop. When fomepizole is given to patients with acidosis or end-organ toxicity, further production of metabolic acids from metabolism of EG or methanol is stopped. The acidosis may clear with supportive care or by the institution of hemodialysis. End-organ injury may or may not be reversible (2,29,39).

Other Potential Uses

Fomepizole may be indicated in diethylene glycol and symptomatic polyethylene glycol ingestions. Diethylene glycol is also metabolized by ADH and, like EG, may develop anion gap metabolic acidosis, renal failure, coma, or death. Triethylene glycol is also metabolized by ADH but typically is considered less toxic. A young female patient who ingested a mixture of diethylene glycol and triethylene glycol presented in metabolic acidosis and coma. The metabolic acidosis resolved after administration of fomepizole, and the patient recovered without sequelae (45).

Another potential use of fomepizole is isopropanol ingestion. Some elements of CNS toxicity caused by severe isopropanol toxicity may result from acetone formation, the product of ADH metabolism of isopropanol (46,47). The use of fomepizole prevents acetone formation and slows the clearance of isopropanol but may also prolong CNS obtundation (40). There are no prospective studies to support its use in isopropanol ingestions.

In the event of a disulfiram or disulfiram-like reactions, the use of fomepizole may stop the metabolism of alcohol to acetaldehyde and decrease the progression of symptoms (48). By blocking conversion to gamma hydroxybutyrate, fomepizole may be useful in 1,4-butanediol intoxication (49). Finally, fomepizole decreased hepatotoxicity in a rodent model of acetaminophen toxicity, most likely secondary to CYP2E1 inhibition. It could be of potential use in the unusual circumstance of inability to administer acetylcysteine (50).

CAUTIONS AND CONTRAINDICATIONS

Hypersensitivity to fomepizole or other pyrazoles is a relative contraindication. The manufacturer states that fomepizole should not be given undiluted or by bolus injection. The manufacturer also cautions use in patients with liver disease and renal impairment. Because fomepizole is eliminated primarily by hepatic metabolism, accumulation during long-term use in patients with hepatic failure may occur.

Fomepizole is FDA pregnancy category C (Appendix I). In postnatal rats, treatment with alcohol plus fomepizole resulted in peak blood alcohol concentrations that were at least twice those of pups receiving alcohol alone and demonstrated microencephalopathy as evidence of ethanol toxicity, implicating the importance of functional ADH activity in attenuating alcohol-induced neuroteratogenicity (48).

DOSAGE AND METHOD OF ADMINISTRATION

Ethylene Glycol and Methanol

Fomepizole may be given orally or IV (4,31,51), although the IV route is recommended (4,8). Fomepizole is administered as an IV loading dose of 15 mg/kg, diluted to at least 100 ml of normal saline or 5% dextrose in water, and infused over 30 minutes. The loading dose is followed by maintenance doses of 10 mg/kg IV every 12 hours for four doses. Administration beyond the first five doses should be 15 mg/kg IV every 12 hours.

ETHYLENE GLYCOL

If used as monotherapy, fomepizole administration should be continued until EG concentrations are below 20 mg/dl, and the patient is asymptomatic. In patients with continuing symptoms (acidosis, renal insufficiency) or who presented with end-organ injury, it may be desirable to continue fomepizole until the EG concentrations are undetectable (25).

Without dialysis, the EG half-life is 19.7 ± 1.3 hours when ADH is blocked by fomepizole. All EG half-lives greater than 24 hours occurred in patients with a presenting serum creatinine of 1.5 mg/dl or greater (25). The initial plasma EG level does not predict prolonged elimination or correlate with patient outcome (25). A patient with a serum EG concentration of 103 mg/dl was managed with five doses of fomepizole without dialysis, resulting in estimated savings in intensive care, dialysis, and consultant costs (24). Others have advocated fomepizole as monotherapy with levels greater than 200 mg/dl (25,52). This may be most appropriate when there are other barriers to hemodialysis (e.g., a small child, uncontrolled hypotension, unavailability of dialysis). Some savings will not be realized if patients present in acidosis or otherwise require intensive care. The costs of fomepizole are real expenditures to hospitals, whereas intensive care unit staff, equipment, and perhaps consultant fees may be part of institutional overhead. The risks of dialysis must be weighed against the risks of prolonged hospitalization and perhaps prolonged CNS depression. An optimal management strategy has not been developed.

METHANOL

The use of fomepizole in methanol intoxications raises different issues than in EG. Without dialysis, methanol is cleared with a half-life of 54 hours (29) when ADH is blocked by fomepizole. Therefore, in methanol ingestions with very high plasma concentrations, hemodialysis may be warranted even in the absence of toxicity to prevent prolonged hospitalization (29,30). If used as monotherapy, fomepizole administration should be continued until methanol concentrations are below 20 mg/dl, and the patient is asymptomatic. In patients with continuing symptoms (acidosis, visual symptoms) or who presented with end-organ injury, it may be desirable to continue fomepizole until the methanol concentrations are undetectable (25).

HEMODIALYSIS

Dialysis increases the clearance of fomepizole (9,53); therefore, an increased dose rate is necessary to maintain a therapeutic plasma concentration. The dosing interval should be shortened to every 4 hours (8). If beginning dialysis within 6 hours of a dose of fomepizole, the dose does not have to be repeated. At the end of hemodialysis, the next dose of fomepizole should be administered immediately unless it has been less than 1 hour since the last dose (e.g., during hemodialysis). If it has been between 1 and 3 hours, one-half the dose should be given. If it has been more than 3 hours since the last dose, a full dose of fomepizole should be given at the end of dialysis (8).

ORAL ADMINISTRATION

The oral loading dose of fomepizole is 15 mg/kg. This is followed by 5 mg/kg 12 hours later and then 10 mg/kg every 12 hours until EG plasma levels are undetectable (54).

PEDIATRIC DOSING

Pediatric safety and efficacy have not been established (8). Case reports of successful pediatric use have generally used the same weight-based dosing as for adults (24,30,55).

Monitoring of Response

Monitoring of fomepizole concentrations is not commonly available or required (4). The resolution of metabolic acidosis and possible reversal of end-organ toxicity generally indicate successful ADH blockade.

ADVERSE EFFECTS

Fomepizole is generally well tolerated in therapeutic doses and over an extended period (31). Of 107 dogs treated with fomepizole, one dog developed an observable adverse reaction of tachypnea, gagging, excessive salivation, and trembling after the second dose of fomepizole (16). In a blinded, ascending-dose human study, no side effects were reported at doses up to 20 mg/kg. At 50 mg/kg, slight to moderate nausea, dizziness, and vertigo were reported. At 100 mg/kg, all subjects reported these symptoms (56). In a prospective, multicenter trial of 11 patients treated with fomepizole after presumed methanol exposure, adverse events possibly related to fomepizole were reported in six patients. These were phlebitis, dyspepsia, anxiety, agitation, hiccups, infusion site reaction, transient tachycardia, transient rash, and a "strange" feeling. Slight, transient elevations in serum aminotransferases occur in approximately 40% of patients treated with fomepizole. The elevation is not dose related or apparently mediated through a hypersensitivity reaction (57). Case reports have associated fomepizole with rash (42,58), elevated liver aminotransferases (9,21,58), and eosinophilia (40,42,58). Two patients developed seizures shortly after fomepizole was administered for EG intoxication. The seizures may have been attributable to the underlying intoxication, and the patients received subsequent doses of fomepizole without adverse effect (3).

Drug-Drug Interactions

Fomepizole dosing prolongs the elimination of substances normally metabolized by ADH. Fomepizole prolongs drug-induced sleep times in mice when given in combination with chloral hydrate, pentobarbitone, barbitone, temazepam, and halothane, suggesting a non–ADH-specific effect on the metabolism of these agents (59).

In a double-blind, crossover study of healthy human volunteers, fomepizole caused a 40% reduction in the ethanol elimination rate. Conversely, ethanol inhibited fomepizole metabolism, increasing the duration of therapeutic blood concentrations. Intentional ingestion of EG or methanol may also include ethanol, and the mutual inhibition of fomepizole and ethanol elimination may prolong ADH blockade (32).

PITFALLS

When fomepizole is administered for presumed EG or methanol intoxication without a serum level, an EG or methanol level should be obtained to guide treatment. If concentrations of EG and methanol cannot be obtained, the serum bicarbonate is not useful for monitoring because fomepizole has prevented the metabolism of EG or methanol; therefore, development of acidosis will be delayed until fomepizole is eliminated.

The decision of whether to perform hemodialysis in an EG or methanol exposure is not clear. There were established indications (severe acidosis, end-organ toxicity, renal insufficiency, or clinical deterioration) for hemodialysis when ethanol was the primary antidote. Fomepizole has prompted a reevaluation of what constitutes optimal management. Because of the risks of hemodialysis (i.e., hypotension, iatrogenic error) and the therapeutic benefits of fomepizole relative to ethanol, some cases have been managed with fomepizole alone at plasma levels much higher than have been previously recommended (52). However, the costs and risks associated with prolonged toxicant elimination, prolonged drug administration, and prolonged hospitalization are difficult to assess.

Fomepizole induces a number of P-450 enzymes in the liver and kidney, including CYP2E1, apparently by a posttranscriptional mechanism (36,60). Increases in cytochrome CYP2E1 content and activity result in increased clearance of substances metabolized by this enzyme, including fomepizole (autoinduction) (36,60). As a result, it is recommended to increase the dose of fomepizole after 48 hours to compensate for the increased rate of clearance, although there are no documented cases of injury from reports using dose regimens in which the dose was not increased.

REFERENCES

1. Blomstrand R, Theorell H. Inhibitory effect on ethanol oxidation in man after administration of 4-methylpyrazole. *Life Sci II* 1970;9(11):631–640.
2. Girault C, Tamion F, Moritz F, et al. Fomepizole (4-methylpyrazole) in fatal methanol poisoning with early CT scan cerebral lesions. *J Toxicol Clin Toxicol* 1999;37(6):777–780.
3. Brent J, McMartin K, Phillips S, et al. Fomepizole for the treatment of ethylene glycol poisoning. *N Engl J Med* 1999;340:832–838.
4. Brent J. Current management of ethylene glycol poisoning. *Drugs* 2001;61(7):979–988.
5. Barceloux DG, Krenzelok EP, Olson K, et al. American Academy of Clinical Toxicology practice guidelines on the treatment of ethylene glycol poisoning. *J Toxicol Clin Toxicol* 1999;37:537–560.
6. Jacobsen D, Ostensen J, Bredesen L, et al. 4-Methylpyrazole (4-MP) is effectively removed by haemodialysis in the pig model. *Hum Exp Toxicol* 1996;15(6):494–496.
7. Mayersohn MI, Owens SM, Anaya AL, et al. 4-Methylpyrazole disposition in the dog: evidence for saturable elimination. *J Pharmacol Sci* 1985;74:895–896.
8. Antizol® (fomepizole) injection. Product Information. Minnetonka, MN: Orphan Medical, Inc., 2000.
9. Jobard E, Harry P, Turcant A, et al. 4-Methylpyrazole and hemodialysis in ethylene glycol poisoning. *J Toxicol Clin Toxicol* 1996;34(4):373–377.
10. Jacobsen D, Ostby N, Bredesen JE. Studies on ethylene glycol poisoning. *Acta Med Scand* 1982;212:11–15.
11. Jacobsen D, Jansen H, Wiik-Larsen E, et al. Studies on methanol poisoning. *Acta Med Scand* 1982;212:5–10.
12. Jacobsen D, Barron SK, Sebastian CS, et al. Non-linear kinetics of 4-methylpyrazole in healthy human subjects. *Eur J Clin Pharmacol* 1989;37:599–604.
13. Cornell NE, Hansch C, Kim KH, Henegar K. The inhibition of alcohol dehydrogenase in vitro and in isolated hepatocytes by 4-substituted pyrazoles. *Arch Biochem Biophys* 1983;227:81–90.
14. Dalhbom R, Tolf BR, Akeson A, et al. On the inhibitory power of some further pyrazole derivatives of horse liver alcohol dehydrogenase. *Biochem Biophys Res Commun* 1974;57:549–543.
15. Grauer GF, Thrall MAH, Henre BA, Hjelle JJ. Comparison of the effects of ethanol and 4-methylpyrazole on the pharmacokinetics and toxicity of ethylene glycol in the dog. *Toxicol Lett* 1987;35:307–314.
16. Connally HE, Thrall MA, Forney SD, et al. Safety and efficacy of 4-methylpyrazole for treatment of suspected or confirmed ethylene glycol intoxication in dogs: 107 cases (1983–1995). *J Am Vet Med Assoc* 1996;209:1880–1883.
17. Dial SM, Thrall MA, Hamar DW. 4-Methylpyrazole as treatment for naturally acquired ethylene glycol intoxication in dogs. *J Am Vet Med Assoc* 1989;195(1):73–76.
18. Dial SM, Thrall MA, Hamar DW. Efficacy of 4-methylpyrazole for treatment of ethylene glycol intoxication in dogs. *Am J Vet Res* 1994;55(12):1762–1770.
19. Makar AB, Tephly T. Inhibition of monkey liver alcohol dehydrogenase by 4-methylpyrazole. *Biochem Med* 1975;13:334–342.
20. Dial SM, Thrall MA, Hamar DW. Comparison of ethanol and 4-methylpyrazole as treatments for ethylene glycol intoxication in cats. *Am J Vet Res* 1994;55(12):1771–1782.
21. Harry P, Turcant A, Bouachour G, et al. Efficacy of 4-methylpyrazole in ethylene glycol poisoning: clinical and toxicokinetic aspects. *Hum Exp Toxicol* 1994;13(1):61–64.
22. Harry P, Jobard E, Briand M, et al. Ethylene glycol poisoning in a child treated with 4-methylpyrazole. *Pediatrics* 1998;102(3):E31.
23. Baum CR, Langman CB, Oker E, et al. Fomepizole treatment of ethylene glycol poisoning in an infant. *Pediatrics* 2000;106:1489–1491.
24. Boyer EW, Mejia M, Woolf A, Shannon M. Severe ethylene glycol ingestion treated without hemodialysis. *Pediatrics* 2001;107(1):172–173.
25. Sivilotti ML, Burns MJ, McMartin KE, Brent J. Toxicokinetics of ethylene glycol during fomepizole therapy: implications for management. *Ann Emerg Med* 2000;36(2):114–125.
26. Watkins WD, Goodman JL, Tephly TR. Inhibition of methanol and ethanol oxidation by pyrazole in the rat and monkey *in vivo*. *Mol Pharmacol* 1970;6:567–572.
27. McMartin KE, Makar AB, Martin G, et al. Methanol poisoning. I. The role of formic acid in the development of metabolic acidosis in the monkey and the reversal by 4-methylpyrazole. *Biochem Med* 1975;13:319–333.
28. Blomstrand R, Ostling-Wintzell H, Lof A, et al. Pyrazoles as inhibitors of alcohol oxidation and as important tools in alcohol research: an approach to therapy against methanol poisoning. *Proc Natl Acad Sci U S A* 1979;76:3499–3503.
29. Brent J, McMartin K, Phillips S, et al. Fomepizole for the treatment of methanol poisoning. *N Engl J Med* 2001;344(6):424–429.
30. Brown MJ, Shannon MW, Woolf A, Boyer EW. Childhood methanol ingestion treated with fomepizole and hemodialysis. *Pediatrics* 2001;108(4):E77.
31. Megarbane B, Borron SW, Trout H, et al. Treatment of acute methanol poisoning with fomepizole. *Intensive Care Med* 2001;27(8):1370–1378.
32. Jacobsen D, Sebastian CS, Dies DF, et al. Kinetic interactions between 4-methylpyrazole and ethanol in healthy humans. *Alcohol Clin Exp Res* 1996;20(5):804–809.
33. McMartin KE, Hedstrom KG, Tolf BR, et al. Studies on the metabolic interactions between 4-methylpyrazole and methanol using the monkey as an animal model. *Arch Biochem Biophys* 1980;199:606–614.
34. Feierman DF, Cederbaum AL. Increased sensitivity of the microsomal oxidation of ethanol to inhibition by pyrazole and 4-methylpyrazole after chronic ethanol treatment. *Biochem Pharmacol* 1987;36:3277–3283.
35. Wu DF, Clyan L, Potter B, et al. Rapid decrease of cytochrome P-450 IIE1 in primary hepatocyte culture and its maintenance by added 4-methylpyrazole. *Hepatology* 1990;12:1379–1389.
36. Winters DK, Cederbaum AI. Time course characterization of the induction of cytochrome P-450 2E1 by pyrazole and 4-methylpyrazole. *Biochim Biophys Acta* 1992;1117(1):15–24.
37. Shannon M. Toxicology reviews: fomepizole—a new antidote. *Pediatr Emerg Care* 1998;14:170–172.
38. Raskin NH, Sligar KP, Steinberg RH. Dark adaptation slowed by inhibitors of alcohol dehydrogenase in the albino rat. *Brain Res* 1973;50:496–500.
39. Sivilotti MLA, Burns MJ, Aaron CK, et al. Reversal of severe methanol-induced visual impairment: no evidence of retinal toxicity due to fomepizole. *J Toxicol Clin Toxicol* 2001;39(6):627–631.
40. Bekka R, Borron SW, Astier A, et al. Treatment of methanol and isopropanol poisoning with intravenous fomepizole. *J Toxicol Clin Toxicol* 2001;39(1):59–67.
41. Hantson P, Mahieu P. Pancreatic injury following acute methanol poisoning. *J Toxicol Clin Toxicol* 2000;38(3):297–303.
42. Borron SW, Magarbane B, Baud FJ. Fomepizole in treatment of uncomplicated ethylene glycol poisoning. *Lancet* 1999;354:831.
43. Jacobsen D, McMartin KE. Antidotes for methanol and ethylene glycol poisoning. *J Toxicol Clin Toxicol* 1997;35(2):127–143.
44. Sivilotti MLA, Burns MJ, McMartin KE, et al. A model to predict thylene glycol elimination during fomepizole monotherapy. *J Toxicol Clin Toxicol* 1999;37(5):669–670.
45. Borron SW, Baud FJ, Garnier R. Intravenous 4-methylpyrazole as an antidote for diethylene glycol and triethylene glycol poisoning: a case report. *Vet Hum Toxicol* 1997;39(1):26–28.
46. Daniel DR, McAnalley BH, Garriott JC. Isopropyl alcohol metabolism after acute intoxication in humans. *J Anal Toxicol* 1981;5:110–112.
47. Alexander CB, McBay AJ, Hudson RP. Isopropanol and isopropanol deaths—ten years' experience. *J Forensic Sci* 1982;27:541–548.
48. Chen WJ, McAlhany RE, West JR. 4-Methylpyrazole, an alcohol dehydrogenase inhibitor, exacerbates alcohol-induced microencephaly during the brain growth spurt. *Alcohol* 1995;12(4):351–355.
49. Megarbane B, Fompeydie D, Garnier R, Baud FJ. Treatment of a 1,4-butanediol poisoning with fomepizole. *J Toxicol Clin Toxicol* 2002;40(1):77–80.
50. Brennan RJ, Mankes RF, Lefevre R, et al. 4-Methylpyrazole blocks acetaminophen hepatotoxicity in the rat. *Ann Emerg Med* 1994;23:487–493.
51. Hantson P, Wallemacq P, Brau M, et al. Two cases of acute methanol poisoning partially treated by oral 4-methylpyrazole. *Intensive Care Med* 1999;25(5):528–531.
52. Najafi CC, Hertko LJ, Leikin JB, Korbet SM. Fomepizole in ethylene glycol intoxication. *Ann Emerg Med* 2001;37(3):358–359.
53. Faessel H, Houze P, Baud FJ, Schermann JM. 4-Methylpyrazole monitoring during haemodialysis of ethylene glycol intoxicated patients. *Eur J Clin Pharmacol* 1995;49(3):211–213.
54. Baud FJ, Bismuth C, Garnier R, et al. 4-Methylpyrazole may be an alternative to ethanol therapy for ethylene glycol intoxication in man. *J Toxicol Clin Toxicol* 1987;24:463–483.
55. Brophy PD, Tenenbein M, Gardner J, et al. Childhood diethylene glycol poisoning treated with alcohol dehydrogenase inhibitor fomepizole and hemodialysis. *Am J Kidney Dis* 2000;35(5):958–962.
56. Jacobsen D, Sebastian CS, Blomstrand R, McMartin KE. 4-Methylpyrazole: a controlled study of safety in healthy human subjects after single, ascending doses. *Alcohol Clin Exp Res* 1988;12:516–522.
57. Jacobsen D, Sebastian CS, Barron SK, et al. Effects of 4-methylpyrazole, methanol/ethylene glycol antidote, in healthy humans. *J Emerg Med* 1990;8(4):455–461.
58. Baud FJ, Bismuth C, Garnier R, et al. 4-Methylpyrazole may be an alternative to ethanol therapy for ethylene glycol intoxication in man. *J Toxicol Clin Toxicol* 1986;24:463–483.
59. Taberner PV, Unwin JW. Non-specific prolongation of the effects of general depressants by pyrazole and 4-methylpyrazole. *J Pharm Pharmacol* 1987;39:658–659.
60. Wu D, Cederbaum AI. Characterization of pyrazole and 4-methylpyrazole induction of cytochrome P4502E1 in rat kidney. *J Pharmacol Exp Ther* 1994;270(1):407–413.

CHAPTER 60

Glucagon

Andrew R. Erdman

Synonyms:	**Glucagon hydrochloride, GlucaGen**
Molecular formula and weight:	**$C_{153}H_{225}N_{43}O_{49}S$, 3482.7 g/mol**
CAS Registry No.:	**16941-32-5**
Normal or therapeutic levels:	**Not clinically applicable**
Special concerns:	**Frequently causes vomiting**

OVERVIEW

Glucagon is a polypeptide hormone consisting of 29 amino acids that is produced by the pancreas. Glucagon has been used as an antidote to poisoning by several drugs: insulin, sulfonylureas, beta-receptor blockers, calcium-channel blockers, tricyclic antidepressants, procainamide, and quinidine (1–9).

Glucagon is available in the United States as a lyophilized powder for reconstitution and administration by intravenous (IV), intramuscular (IM), or subcutaneous (SQ) injection. Each vial contains 1 mg of glucagon and a small amount of lactose or hydrochloric acid to adjust the pH (10,11). Older preparations were often packaged with a diluent that contained phenol as a preservative (12), but this has been eliminated. An intranasal form has been used to treat hypoglycemia in clinical trials, and an ocular preparation is also being tested (13–14).

Mechanism of Action

Although glucagon has a wide range of pharmacologic actions, most of these actions appear to share biochemical mechanisms. After binding to specific cell surface receptors, the signal is transduced via a G_S protein system to adenyl cyclase (15,16), which catalyzes the production of cyclic adenosine monophosphate (cAMP) from adenosine triphosphate (17–19). The result is intracellular accumulation of cAMP (20–22). cAMP activates protein kinase A (PKA). Active PKA phosphorylates several intracellular proteins and enzymes, amplifying the original signal and resulting in different pharmacologic actions depending on the target cell (Fig. 1).

GLYCEMIC EFFECTS

The primary action of glucagon is to increase blood glucose by stimulating hepatic glycogenolysis and, later, gluconeogenesis (23–25). It has been used to treat hypoglycemia from insulin or sulfonylureas. The blood glucose rises within 10 minutes of IM or SQ injection, and a maximum hyperglycemic response occurs in 20 to 30 minutes and has a duration of 60 to 90 minutes (10,11,26,27). In the liver, glucagon-induced activation of PKA produces phosphorylation and induction of glycogen phosphorylase (21). Glycogen phosphorylase breaks down glycogen to liberate glucose into the systemic circulation. Glucagon may mobilize glucose in other organs as well. To raise blood glucose appreciably, glucagon depends on the presence of adequate hepatic glycogen stores (28).

INOTROPIC EFFECTS

In the heart, glucagon binds to myocardial receptors that are separate and independent from the beta receptors, although both types appear to work via the same adenyl cyclase system (16,20,29,30). The resulting cAMP-mediated activation of PKA leads to the phosphorylation of at least three major intracellular protein systems. The first, phosphorylation of sarcolemmal calcium channels, increases the amount of calcium that flows intracellularly during excitation (20). Phosphorylation of the enzyme, phospholamban, enhances the sequestration of calcium within the sarcoplasmic reticulum, which subsequently results in the release of more calcium intracellularly during excitation (31). Finally, direct phosphorylation of myofibrillar proteins, myosin binding protein C and troponin I, improves their function (32) (Fig. 1). Although all three mechanisms certainly improve myocardial contractility, glucagon may also act outside of the adenyl cyclase system to enhance cardiac performance. It has been dem-

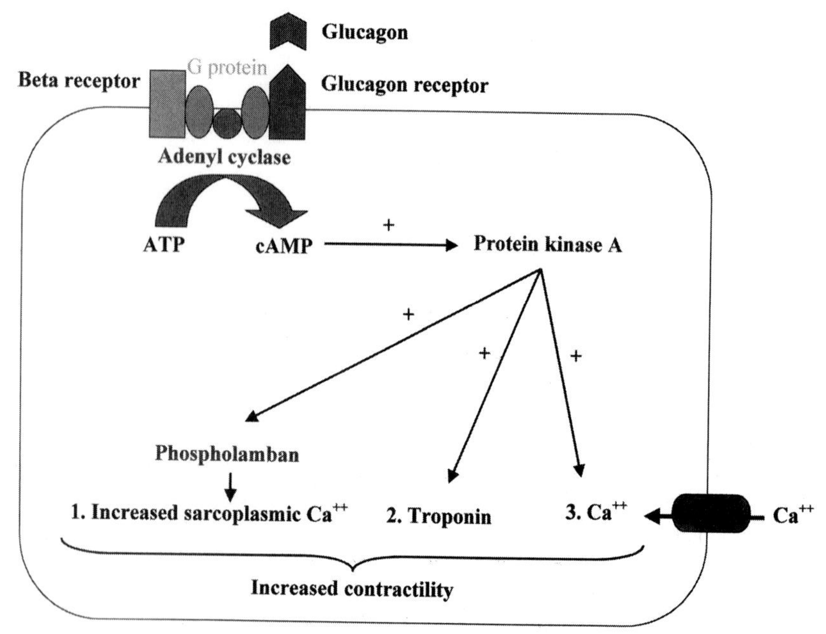

Figure 1. Basic mechanism of action of glucagon in cardiac myocyte. ATP, adenosine triphosphate; cAMP, cyclic adenosine monophosphate.

onstrated to activate phospholipase A_2, resulting in the generation of arachidonic acid which itself has inotropic properties (33). Glucagon also stimulates a modest increase in circulating catecholamines and an increase in cardiac chronotropic activity, but the mechanisms behind both remain unclear (7,20,34).

In the smooth muscle cells of the peripheral vasculature, glucagon-induced increases in cAMP lead to relaxation rather than contraction (35). This may account for a modest vasodilation that is sometimes noted with glucagon administration, as well as the finding that, despite improvements in cardiac output, blood pressure may not return to baseline values in some poisoned patients (27,36). It also suggests, at least in theory, that glucagon might be more effective in some patients if used in conjunction with a pressor that causes vasoconstriction.

The physiologic end result of IV glucagon is improved cardiac performance in both normal subjects and those poisoned with a variety of cardiodepressant drugs, particularly beta-blockers (20,27,37–42). The beneficial effects in patients poisoned with beta-blocker or calcium channel–blocker medications have been demonstrated in human case reports and animal studies, and include dose-dependent increases in heart rate, myocardial contractility, cardiac output, and blood pressure and a decrease in pulmonary capillary wedge pressure (4,5,30,36,43–51). Glucagon may also improve electrical conduction through the myocardium (43,47,52). Higher doses (5 mg or more) are generally required to produce significant improvements. The myocardial effects of a bolus of glucagon occur earlier than its glycemic effects but are more short-lived. Enhanced contractility generally begins within 1 to 3 minutes of IV bolus administration, peaks in 5 to 15 minutes, and lasts up to 10 to 30 minutes (27,43). A few studies have suggested that tachyphylaxis to the cardiac effects may develop after several hours of continuous administration; however, other authors have found no evidence of a desensitization effect (27,37,38,42,53,54).

SMOOTH MUSCLE EFFECTS

Glucagon causes relaxation of the lower esophageal sphincter and upper gastrointestinal smooth muscle (55,56). It has been used for the treatment of esophageal foreign-body or food impactions and as both a diagnostic and therapeutic aid for various gastrointestinal conditions (57).

KINETICS

Maximum plasma concentrations are attained within 1 minute of IV injection, 12 minutes of IM administration, and 20 minutes of SQ administration (10,11,58). Glucagon has a small volume of distribution (0.20 to 0.25 L/kg) (59). The half-life is 6 to 18 minutes after IV administration and reported as 45 minutes after IM administration. It is metabolized extensively in the liver, kidney, and blood. Virtually none of the parent compound is eliminated in the urine.

INDICATIONS

Calcium Channel–Blocker or Beta Receptor–Blocker Toxicity

The first successful use of glucagon to treat cardiovascular collapse in a patient with beta-blocker poisoning was reported in 1971 and in a patient with calcium channel–blocker toxicity in 1991 (4–6). Although there have been no controlled trials in poisoned humans, numerous case reports and several investigations in poisoned animals have documented glucagon's antidotal efficacy (30,44–47,49,60–63). Studies in healthy human volunteers have also demonstrated its inotropic benefits (27,42). High doses are effective at reversing the hypotension, bradycardia, and electrical conduction delays commonly associated with beta-blocker or calcium channel–blocker toxicity and may successfully revive patients otherwise in extremis. Improvements in pulmonary capillary wedge pressure and pulmonary edema are not uncommon, and a patient's obtundation, coma, respiratory depression, and seizures may also respond favorably to glucagon (48–51,64). Its effects generally occur within minutes of IV administration, and large doses are required for optimal benefit (see Dosage and Administration).

Any patient with clinically significant hypotension or bradycardia that is the result of beta-blocker or calcium channel–blocker toxicity should be given a trial of high-dose glucagon therapy. Although a few cases have responded successfully to glucagon alone, it should generally be used in conjunction with judicious fluid resuscitation, pressors, and other supportive measures (64). In most successful reports, glucagon was given in conjunction with a number of other therapeutic measures. Based on these cases, and certainly in theory, glucagon is expected to act synergistically with other pressors such as catecholamines or phosphodiesterase inhibitors. However, limited animal studies have largely failed to find evidence of such a synergistic relationship (21,39,63,65). Notwithstanding, glucagon should be considered a therapeutic adjunct to good supportive care. One potential advantage over other pressors is that glucagon does not appear to increase dysrhythmogenicity or myocardial work (27,38,66–69).

In theory, glucagon should be more effective for beta-blocker poisoning than for calcium channel–blocker poisoning, because it pharmacologically bypasses the blocked receptor of the former, but not the latter. Indeed, a few reports seem to support this contention, suggesting that glucagon is not clinically as successful or as consistent in its benefit for patients with calcium channel–blocker toxicity (20,63,70–72). However, in several of these cases inadequate (<5 mg) doses of glucagon were given. Reports in which higher doses were given showed that patients responded just as well.

Other Drugs Causing Myocardial Depression

The use of glucagon to treat cardiovascular collapse from other myocardial depressant drugs is not well documented, although sporadic cases are encouraging. Glucagon has appeared useful in tricyclic antidepressant poisoning and in patients with procainamide or quinidine toxicity (7–9). Digoxin-induced bradycardia and hypotension have not been shown to respond to glucagon (54,68).

Hypoglycemia

Glucagon has been used to treat hypoglycemia associated with hypoglycemic drugs, ackee fruit, and quinine (1–3). It is not first-line therapy for hypoglycemia. Because its action requires adequate hepatic glycogen stores, there is a delay of several minutes before its peak blood glucose effects occur. Supplemental dextrose is less costly, easier to administer, and more reliable in its effects. Octreotide and diazoxide are also antidotes for sulfonylurea-induced hypoglycemia (Chapter 66) (73,74).

CAUTIONS AND CONTRAINDICATIONS

The most common adverse effect is nausea and vomiting (5,42,43,75). Vomiting is rare with a 1-mg or less dose (27,56). The effects are transient and can usually be controlled with routine antiemetics (60,68). Hypokalemia is relatively common, perhaps as the result of insulin secretion. The potassium level may drop 0.5 to 1.3 mEq/L (26,27,38,64,68). Close monitoring of serum potassium is essential. Other electrolyte abnormalities have not been noted, but both hypo- and hypercalcemia may blunt the myocardial response to glucagon (76).

Hyperglycemia can obviously occur after glucagon, but it is typically mild and rarely requires specific treatment (38,42). On the other hand, glucagon may be ineffective at raising blood glucose in some patients, such as those with hepatic failure, starvation, or other conditions associated with inadequate glycogen stores. Paradoxically, hypoglycemia may also occur after glucagon administration due to its stimulation of insulin release from the pancreas. Patients with inadequate liver glycogen stores and those with insulin hypersecretory states (e.g., insulinomas, sulfonylurea toxicity) may be at particular risk (77–79). Hypoglycemia can also occur in healthy patients; however, in one series, it developed in 1 of 16 patients treated with IV glucagon (38). It can occur immediately after glucagon administration or after the effects of the drug begin to wane.

Glucagon can also induce the release of catecholamines. Therefore, it should be used with caution in patients with pheochromocytomas or other catecholamine hypersecretory conditions (80).

Glucagon, as a polypeptide hormone, may cause hypersensitivity reactions in some patients (81). Severe reactions have not been reported. Patients with a known hypersensitivity to the drug should have other measures attempted before using glucagon. Given the severity and mortality of many beta-blocker and calcium channel–blocker overdoses, however, glucagon might still be considered as a last resort.

DOSAGE AND ADMINISTRATION

Calcium Channel–Blocker or Beta Receptor–Blocker Toxicity

Bolus doses ranging from 1 to 10 mg can improve heart rate, blood pressure, and other indices. The usual *adult dose* is 5 to 10 mg IV as a bolus. The *pediatric* and *neonatal dose* is 50 μg/kg SQ or IV. This dose should be repeated if the hemodynamic response is insufficient (12,82). Smaller doses are often ineffective (19,119). The response is dose dependent (43,47,64). Boluses of up to 17 mg have been used without problems (73). The cardiovascular effects begin within minutes (1,42) and last approximately 15 minutes after a bolus.

Due to its short duration of action, a continuous IV infusion of 1 to 10 mg/hour should be started immediately (54,64,83). The initial infusion rate is typically the same dose per hour as was used in the initial bolus (e.g., 10 mg/hour). Infusions of up to 45 mg over 10 to 15 minutes have been tolerated well (17), except for the occurrence of nausea and vomiting. In one study, patients received as much as 10 mg/hour for 8 days and 16 mg/hour for 3 days without significant side effects (27,38). Although rare, tachyphylaxis to the drug has been described, so patients should be monitored closely and the infusion rate increased if needed (54,84).

The appropriate duration of glucagon infusion has not been determined. Most patients are treated for 24 to 48 hours. The infusion is then tapered slowly as tolerated. Therapy may need to be continued for longer in patients with ongoing drug absorption or those who have ingested sustained-release medications (51).

Hypoglycemia

The *adult dose* for hypoglycemia is 1 mg IV, IM, or SQ. The *pediatric dose* is 0.5 mg IV, IM, or SQ, and the *neonatal dose* is 50 μg/kg SQ or IV. This dose may be repeated or increased to 5 mg as needed (81). Dextrose administration may be needed until the glycemic effect develops. The hyperglycemic effects last only 30 to 60 minutes.

Monitoring

A patient's hemodynamic response to glucagon should be monitored in an intensive care setting. Blood pressure, heart rate, and clinical evidence of adequate perfusion should be checked continually. Invasive hemodynamic monitoring may be necessary.

Because of the potential for both hyper- and hypoglycemia with glucagon use, frequent blood glucose measurements should be performed, particularly during the first hour after initiation or alteration of glucagon therapy and for several hours after the infusion is stopped. Because of the risk of hypokalemia, serum potassium should be measured frequently and regularly and supplemented as necessary.

ADVERSE EFFECTS

Vomiting is a common complication of high-dose glucagon therapy. Antiemetics are generally effective if this complication occurs. Patients with significant sedation or depressed airway reflexes may need endotracheal intubation to prevent aspiration.

Although insulin opposes the effects of glucagon, glucagon stimulates the pancreatic secretion of insulin (32,94,120). Plasma levels of insulin can remain elevated for 30 to 60 minutes after glucagon injection (85,120–122). As a result, glucagon may paradoxically cause hypoglycemia because insulin release may persist and cause hypoglycemia before the onset of hepatic glycogenolysis (i.e., immediately after glucagon administration) (84) or after the hyperglycemic effects of glucagon wear off (32,85). The insulin response may be exaggerated in patients with insulin hypersecretion (e.g., insulinoma or concurrent sulfonylurea ingestion).

PITFALLS

There may be a delay of several minutes before glycemic effects develop. Glucagon may not increase blood glucose in patients with hepatic failure, starvation, or other conditions associated with inadequate glycogen stores.

Hospital pharmacies may not stock enough glucagon to treat a severe poisoning. The gastrointestinal endoscopy suite or other hospitals are likely sources of additional drug.

REFERENCES

1. Elrick H, Witten TA, Arai Y. Glucagon treatment of insulin reactions. *N Engl J Med* 1958;258:476–480.
2. Seltzer HS. Drug-induced hypoglycemia. A review of 1418 cases. *Endocrinol Metab Clin North Am* 1989;18(1):163–183.
3. Harrigan RA, Nathan MS, Beattie P. Oral agents for the treatment of type 2 diabetes mellitus: pharmacology, toxicity, and treatment. *Ann Emerg Med* 2001;38(1):68–78.
4. Kosinski EJ, Stein N, Malindzak GS Jr, Boone E. Glucagon and propranolol (Inderal) toxicity. *N Engl J Med* 1971;285(23):1325.
5. Mullen JT, Walter FG, Ekins BR, Khasigian PA. Amelioration of nifedipine poisoning associated with glucagon therapy. *Ann Emerg Med* 1993;22:1234–1237.
6. Wolf LR, Spadafora MP, Otten EJ. The use of amrinone and glucagon in a case of calcium channel blocker overdose. *Ann Emerg Med* 1993;22:1225–1228.
7. Prasad K, Weckworth P. Glucagon in procainamide-induced cardiac toxicity. *Toxicol Appl Pharmacol* 1978;46(2):517–528.
8. Prasad K. Use of glucagon in the treatment of quinidine toxicity in the heart. *Cardiovasc Res* 1977;11(1):55–63.
9. Sener EK, Gabe S, Henry JA. Response to glucagon in imipramine overdose. *J Toxicol Clin Toxicol* 1995;33(1):51–53.
10. Package insert—GlucaGen. Bedford, OH: Bedford Laboratories, 2001.
11. Package insert—glucagon for injection (rDNA origin). Indianapolis: Eli Lilly and Co., 1998.
12. White CM. A review of potential cardiovascular uses of intravenous glucagon administration. *J Clin Pharmacol* 1999;39(5):442–447.
13. Pontiroli AE, Alberetto M, Pozza G. Metabolic effects of intranasally administered glucagon: comparison with intramuscular and intravenous injection. *Acta Diabetol Lat* 1985;22(2):103–110.
14. Chiou GC, Chuang CY. Treatment of hypoglycemia with glucagon eye drops. *J Ocul Pharmacol* 1988;4(2):179–186.

15. Gilman AG. Nobel Lecture. G proteins and regulation of adenylyl cyclase. *Biosci Rep* 1995;15:65–95.
16. Levey GS, Epstein SE. Activation of adenyl cyclase by glucagon in cat and human heart. *Circ Res* 1969;24(2):151–156.
17. Engelhard VH, Plut DA, Storm DR. Subcellular location of adenylate cyclase in rat cardiac muscle. *Biochim Biophys Acta* 1976;451(1):48–61.
18. Levey GS, Fletcher MA, Klein I, et al. Characterization of 125I-glucagon binding in a solubilized preparation of cat myocardial adenylate cyclase. Further evidence for a dissociable receptor site. *J Biol Chem* 1974;249(9):2665–2673.
19. Rodbell M. The role of hormone receptors and GTP-regulatory proteins in membrane transduction. *Nature* 1980;284(5751):17–22.
20. Chernow B, Reed L, Geelhoed GW, et al. Glucagon: endocrine effects and calcium involvement in cardiovascular actions in dogs. *Circ Shock* 1986;19(4):393–407.
21. Sutherland EW, Robison GA, Botcher RW. Some aspects of the biological role of adenosine 3',5'-monophosphate (cyclic AMP). *Circulation* 1968;37:279–306.
22. Busuttil RW, Paddock RJ, Fisher JW, George WJ. Changes in cyclic nucleotide levels and contractile force in the isolated hypoxic rat heart during perfusion with glucagon. *Circ Res* 1976;38(3):162–167.
23. Exton JH, Park CR. The stimulation of gluconeogenesis from lactate by epinephrine, glucagon, cyclic 3',5'-adenylate in the perfused rat liver. *Pharmacol Rev* 1966;18(1):181–188.
24. Sutherland EW, Cori CF. Influence of insulin preparations on glycogenolysis in liver slices. *J Biol Chem* 1948;172:737–750.
25. Kreisberg RA, Williamson JR. Metabolic effects of glucagon in the perfused rat heart. *Am J Physiol* 1964;207:721–727.
26. Deraney MF. Glucagon? One answer to cardiogenic shock. *Am J Med Sci* 1971;261(3):149–154.
27. Parmley WW, Glick G, Sonnenblick EH. Cardiovascular effects of glucagon in man. *N Engl J Med* 1968;279(1):12–17.
28. Hall-Boyer K, Zaloga GP, Chernow B. Glucagon: hormone or therapeutic agent? *Crit Care Med* 1984;12(7):584–589.
29. Murad F, Vaughan M. Effect of glucagon on rat heart adenyl cyclase. *Biochem Pharmacol* 1969;18(5):1053–1059.
30. Kosinski EJ, Malindzak GS Jr. Glucagon and isoproterenol in reversing propranolol toxicity. *Arch Intern Med* 1973;132(6):840–843.
31. Frank K, Tilgmann C, Shannon TR, et al. Regulatory role of phospholamban in the efficiency of cardiac sarcoplasmic reticulum Ca2+ transport. *Biochemistry* 2000;39(46):14176–14182.
32. Herron TJ, Korte FS, McDonald KS. Power output is increased after phosphorylation of myofibrillar protiens in rat skinned cardiac myocytes. *Circ Res* 2001;89(12):1184–1190.
33. Sauvadet A, Rohn T, Pecker F, Pavoine C. Arachidonic acid drives mini-glucagon action in cardiac cells. *J Biol Chem* 1997;272(19):12437–12445.
34. Whitehouse FW, James TN. Chronotropic action of glucagon on the sinus node. *Proc Soc Exp Biol Med* 1966;122(3):823–826.
35. Okamura T, Miyazaki M, Toda N. Responses of isolated dog blood vessels to glucagon. *Eur J Pharmacol* 1986;125(3):395–401.
36. Glick G, Parmley WW, Wechsler AS, Sonnenblick EH. Glucagon. Its enhancement of cardiac performance in the cat and dog and persistence of its inotropic action despite beta-receptor blockade with propranolol. *Circ Res* 1968;22(6):789–799.
37. Farah A, Tuttle R. Studies on the pharmacology of glucagon. *J Pharm Exp Ther* 1960;129:49–55.
38. Vander Ark CR, Reynolds EW Jr. Clinical evaluation of glucagon by continuous infusion in the treatment of low cardiac output states. *Am Heart J* 1970;79(4):481–487.
39. Lucchesi BR. Cardiac actions of glucagon. *Circ Res* 1968;22(6):777–787.
40. Greenberg BH, Tsakiris AG, Moffitt EA, Frye RL. The hemodynamic and metabolic effects of glucagon in patients with chronic valvular heart disease. *Mayo Clin Proc* 1970;45(2):132–139.
41. Greenberg BH, McCallister BD, Frye RL. Effects of glucagon on resting and exercise haemodynamics in patients with coronary heart disease. *Br Heart J* 1972;34(9):924–929.
42. Smitherman TC, Osborn RC Jr, Atkins JM. Cardiac dose response relationship for intravenously infused glucagon in normal intact dogs and men. *Am Heart J* 1978;96(3):363–371.
43. Love JN, Leasure JA, Mundt DJ, Janz TG. A comparison of amrinone and glucagon therapy for cardiovascular depression associated with propranolol toxicity in a canine model. *J Toxicol Clin Toxicol* 1992;30(3):399–412.
44. Stone CK, May WA, Carroll R. Treatment of verapamil overdose with glucagon in dogs. *Ann Emerg Med* 1995;25(3):369–374.
45. Zaloga GP, Malcolm D, Holaday J, Chernow B. Glucagon reverses the hypotension and bradycardia of verapamil overdose in rats. *Crit Care Med* 1985;13:273.
46. Zaritsky AL, Horowitz M, Chernow B. Glucagon antagonism of calcium channel blocker-induced myocardial dysfunction. *Crit Care Med* 1988;16(3):246–251.
47. Jolly SR, Kipnis JN, Lucchesi BR. Cardiovascular depression by verapamil: reversal by glucagon and interactions with propranolol. *Pharmacology* 1987;35(5):249–255.
48. Smith RC, Wilkinson J, Hull RL. Glucagon for propranolol overdose. *JAMA* 1985;254(17):2412.
49. Ward DE, Jones B. Glucagon and beta-blocker toxicity. *BMJ* 1976;2(6028):151.
50. Jacobsen D, Helgeland A, Koss A. Treatment of beta-blocker poisoning. *Lancet* 1980;1(8176):1031–1032.
51. Doyon S, Roberts JR. The use of glucagon in a case of calcium channel blocker overdose. *Ann Emerg Med* 1993;22(7):1229–1233.
52. Lipski JI, Kaminsky D, Donoso E, Friedberg CK. Electrophysiological effects of glucagon on the normal canine heart. *Am J Physiol* 1972;222(5):1107–1112.
53. Kline JA, Tomaszewski CA, Schroeder JD, Raymond RM. Insulin is a superior antidote for cardiovascular toxicity induced by verapamil in the anesthetized canine. *J Pharmacol Exp Ther* 1993;267(2):744–750.
54. Quezado Z, Lippmann M, Wertheimer J. Severe cardiac, respiratory, and metabolic complications of massive verapamil overdose. *Crit Care Med* 1991;19(3):436–438.
55. Hogan WJ, Dodds WJ, Hoke SE, et al. Effect of glucagon on esophageal motor function. *Gastroenterology* 1975;69(1):160–165.
56. Miller RE, Chernish SM, Greenman GF, et al. Gastrointestinal response to minute doses of glucagon. *Radiology* 1982;143(2):317–320.
57. Marks HW, Lousteau RJ. Glucagon and esophageal meat impaction. *Arch Otolaryngol* 1979;105(6):367–368.
58. Muhlhauser I, Koch J, Berger M. Pharmacokinetics and bioavailability of injected glucagon: differences between intramuscular, subcutaneous, and intravenous administration. *Diabetes Care* 1985;8(1):39–42.
59. Pontiroli AE, Calderara A, Perfetti MG, Bareggi SR. Pharmacokinetics of intranasal, intramuscular and intravenous glucagon in healthy subjects and diabetic patients. *Eur J Clin Pharmacol* 1993;45(6):555–558.
60. Ehgartner GR, Zelinka MA. Hemodynamic instability following intentional nadolol overdose. *Arch Intern Med* 1988;148(4):801–802.
61. Fernandes CM, Daya MR. Sotalol-induced bradycardia reversed by glucagon. *Can Fam Physician* 1995;41:659–660, 663–665.
62. Stone CK, Thomas SH, Koury SI, Low RB. Glucagon and phenylephrine combination vs glucagon alone in experimental verapamil overdose. *Acad Emerg Med* 1996;3(2):120–125.
63. Wolf LR, Spadafora MP, Otten EJ. Use of amrinone and glucagon in a case of calcium channel blocker overdose. *Ann Emerg Med* 1993;22(7):1225–1228.
64. Peterson CD, Leeder JS, Sterner S. Glucagon therapy for beta-blocker overdose. *Drug Intell Clin Pharm* 1984;18(5):394–398.
65. Siegel JH, Levine MJ, McConn R, del Guercio LR. The effect of glucagon infusion on cardiovascular function in the critically ill. *Surg Gynecol Obstet* 1970;131(3):505–515.
66. Parmley WW. The role of glucagon in cardiac therapy. *N Engl J Med* 1971;285(14):801–802.
67. Cohn KE, Agmon J, Gamble OW. The effect of glucagon on arrhythmias due to digitalis toxicity. *Am J Cardiol* 1970;25(6):683–689.
68. Lvoff R, Wilcken DE. Glucagon in heart failure and in cardiogenic shock. Experience in 50 patients. *Circulation* 1972;45(3):534–542.
69. Abel FL. Action of glucagon on canine left ventricular performance and coronary hemodynamics. *Circ Shock* 1983;11(1):45–58.
70. Horowitz BZ, Rhee KJ. Massive verapamil ingestion: a report of two cases and a review of the literature. *Am J Emerg Med* 1989;7(6):624–631.
71. Anthony T, Jastremski M, Elliott W, et al. Charcoal hemoperfusion for the treatment of a combined diltiazem and metoprolol overdose. *Ann Emerg Med* 1986;15(11):1344–1348.
72. Crump BJ, Holt DW, Vale JA. Lack of response to intravenous calcium in severe verapamil poisoning. *Lancet* 1982;2(8304):939–940.
73. Krentz AJ, Boyle PJ, Justice KM, et al. Successful treatment of severe refractory sulfonylurea-induced hypoglycemia with octreotide. *Diabetes Care* 1993;16(1):184–186.
74. Palatnick W, Meatherall RC, Tenenbein M. Clinical spectrum of sulfonylurea overdose and experience with diazoxide therapy. *Arch Intern Med* 1991;151(9):1859–1862.
75. Chernish SM, Maglinte DD. Glucagon: common untoward reactions—review and recommendations. *Radiology* 1990;177(1):145–146.
76. Chernow B, Zaloga GP, Malcolm D, et al. Glucagon's chronotropic action is calcium dependent. *J Pharmacol Exp Ther* 1987;241(3):833–837.
77. Thoma ME, Glauser J, Genuth S. Persistent hypoglycemia and hyperinsulinemia: caution in using glucagon. *Am J Emerg Med* 1996;14(1):99–101.
78. Marri G, Cozzolino G, Palumbo R. Glucagon in sulphonylurea hypoglycaemia? *Lancet* 1968;1(7537):303–304.
79. Oldham J, Campbell RK. Treatment of the hospitalized hypoglycemic patient. *Diabetes Educ* 1987;13(3):310–311.
80. Lawrence AM. Glucagon provocative test for pheochromocytoma. *Ann Intern Med* 1967;66(6):1091–1096.
81. Pollack CV Jr. Utility of glucagon in the emergency department. *J Emerg Med* 1993;11(2):195–205.
82. Robson RH. Glucagon for beta-blocker poisoning. *Lancet* 1980;1(8182):1357–1358.
83. Illingworth RN. Glucagon for beta-blocker poisoning. *Practitioner* 1979;223(1337):683–685.
84. Kline JA, Tomaszewski CA, Schroeder JD, et al. Insulin is a superior antidote for cardiovascular toxicity induced by verapamil in the anesthetized canine. *J Pharmacol Exp Ther* 1993;267(2):744–750.

CHAPTER 61

Hydroxocobalamin

Andrew R. Erdman

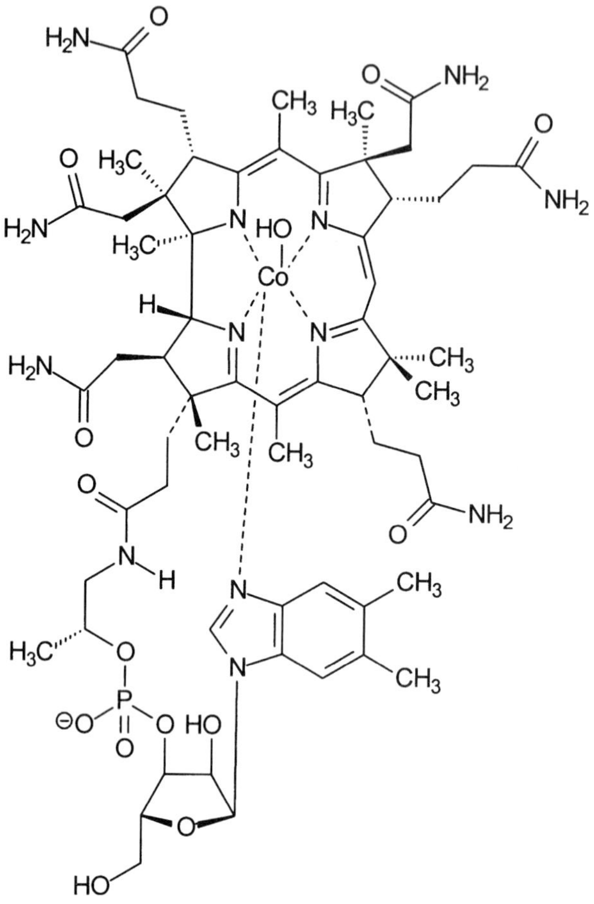

HYDROXOCOBALAMIN

Synonyms:	**Vitamin B_{12a}, Cyanokit**
Molecular formula and weight:	**$C_{62}H_{89}CoN_{13}O_{15}P$, 1346.47 g/mol**
CAS Registry No.:	**13422-51-0**
Therapeutic levels:	**Not clinically applicable**
Special concerns:	**Not generally available in sufficient concentration in most countries to treat cyanide poisoning**

OVERVIEW

Hydroxocobalamin (vitamin B_{12a}) is a vitamin B_{12} (cyanocobalamin) precursor. After *in vitro* studies demonstrated that it binds tightly to cyanide, animal studies revealed that it was an effective antidote for cyanide toxicity (1–3). High doses have since been used to treat poisoned humans, with numerous reports testifying to its efficacy (4,5). Hydroxocobalamin is the preferred antidote for cyanide toxicity in France, where it has been used since the early 1970s (5). It is not generally used in the United States because a concentrated solution is neither readily available nor approved by the U.S. Food and Drug Administration. Hydroxocobalamin has also been used to prevent cyanide toxicity in patients receiving nitroprusside infusion (6).

Forms Available

Hydroxocobalamin is a red crystalline substance that readily forms a dark crimson aqueous solution. It is available in the United States only as a 0.1% injectable solution (1 mg/ml) for the treatment of vitamin B_{12} deficiency. This formulation is too dilute to provide the amount of hydroxocobalamin needed to treat most cases of cyanide poisoning (e.g., 5 g, which would require the administration of 5 L of the 0.1% solution). However, a 5% solution (5 g/100 ml) of hydroxocobalamin is available in France. Hydroxocobalamin has a relatively short shelf-life and must be refrigerated and stored away from light.

Mechanism of Action

Cyanide acts primarily by binding to and inhibiting cytochrome-a_3, a key component in the electron transport chain (7–10). As a result, the tissues must shift to anaerobic metabolism, resulting in lactate accumulation and profound acidosis (Chapter 185).

Hydroxocobalamin has a complex molecular structure, similar to hemoglobin, with a cobalt ion bound to a hydroxy group at its center. Like other cobalt-containing compounds, it has a high affinity for cyanide (11). One cyanide molecule can bind to its central cobalt atom, displacing the hydroxyl group and forming cyanocobalamin (vitamin B_{12}) (1,11,12). Given its molecular weight and molar binding ratio of 1:1, gram quantities are generally required to bind a clinically significant amount of cyanide (3,11).

Cyanocobalamin is relatively harmless even in high doses because its cyanide ion remains tightly complexed (11,13,14). It is readily eliminated by renal excretion (3,15–17). Hydroxocobalamin has a higher affinity for cyanide than cytochrome oxidase does, so it prevents circulating cyanide from entering tissues and inhibiting cellular respiration. It may also reactivate cytochrome oxidase that is already inhibited by removing cyanide from the enzyme.

Some cyanide ions may later dissociate from cyanocobalamin; however, the slow rate of dissociation allows the body's endogenous sulfur donor systems (e.g., thiosulfate) to detoxify them. The end result is a rapid reduction in active cyanide. Indeed, studies in smokers, patients with cyanide toxicity, and those receiving nitroprusside infusions have all confirmed that intravenous (IV) hydroxocobalamin can rapidly lower cyanide levels in the blood and also reduce intracellular cyanide burden (5,6,16,18–20).

Animal studies have consistently demonstrated the efficacy of high-dose hydroxocobalamin therapy for acute cyanide poisoning (3,11,18,21–23). However, very few of these directly compared it to other cyanide antidotes (e.g., components in the Cyanide Antidote Package). One comparative study found that hydroxocobalamin was less effective than sodium nitrite at raising the LD_{50} (lethal dose for 50% of subjects) of cyanide in mice (24). Several others report that it is less effective than sodium thiosulfate under different circumstances (25,26). However, these comparative studies are inconclusive. Their findings may have been the result of inadequate hydroxocobalamin doses, the fact that antidotes were given up to 10 minutes before the induction of cyanide toxicity, or species-related differences in antidotal efficacy. The aggregate clinical experience with hydroxocobalamin in humans suggests that its efficacy is similar to other antidotes (4,5). Additional evidence of its efficacy comes from controlled human trials showing that hydroxocobalamin can lower cyanide levels and prevent toxicity in patients with nitroprusside infusions (6).

In most reports, sodium thiosulfate has been given with hydroxocobalamin; the two drugs appear to work synergistically (11,23). The thiosulfate appears to help accelerate the endogenous detoxification of cyanide to thiocyanate, a process catalyzed by the enzyme rhodanese (Chapter 185). If hydroxocobalamin is given alone, the primary detoxification product is cyanocobalamin (3,4,16). If both hydroxocobalamin and thiosulfate are given, the primary detoxification product becomes thiocyanate, which potentially frees up more hydroxocobalamin to bind additional cyanide (16).

Pharmacokinetics

There are few studies on the pharmacokinetics of high-dose hydroxocobalamin. The elimination half-life ranges from 1.5 to 26.0 hours (12,16,27). Its volume of distribution is low—0.1 to 0.5 L/kg. Hydroxocobalamin appears to be primarily excreted renally (11,12,28). In studies of cyanide-poisoned patients treated with hydroxocobalamin, cyanocobalamin had an elimination half-life of approximately 9 hours (27).

INDICATIONS

Known or Likely Cyanide Poisoning with Serious Clinical Effects

Hydroxocobalamin should be given to patients with evidence of cyanide toxicity (e.g., hypotension, seizures, altered mental status or coma, respiratory depression, or significant metabolic acidosis). It should be followed by the administration of sodium thiosulfate. Improvements in respiratory and hemodynamic parameters as well as mental status are often rapid (within minutes) and dramatic (3–5,22,23). Even patients in extremis or cardiorespiratory arrest may respond favorably. In others, however, recovery is slower (29).

Known Cyanide Exposure but Clinical Effects Have Not Yet Developed

Cyanide toxicity may be delayed in some patients, such as after the ingestion of cyanogenic compounds (e.g., acetonitrile). Because hydroxocobalamin has few significant side effects, it can be safely administered to patients who have not yet developed signs or symptoms of toxicity, preferably in conjunction with sodium thiosulfate (3,18,21,30).

Suspected Cyanide Poisoning

Cyanide poisoning may be suspected in certain critically ill patients (e.g., a patient with altered mental status and metabolic acidosis with access to cyanide or in smoke inhalation). Given its safety compared to other antidotes, hydroxocobalamin should be administered to patients with suspected cyanide toxicity but in whom the diagnosis has not been confirmed. Sodium thiosulfate should also be given.

Hydroxocobalamin has a theoretic advantage over nitrites for smoke inhalation victims, because it does not reduce the oxygen-carrying capacity of blood. It has been used frequently in France for this purpose, and it appears to be safe and effective (12,31).

Prevention of Nitroprusside-Induced Cyanide Toxicity

Both animal and human studies demonstrate that hydroxocobalamin can reduce the accumulation of cyanide and prevent acidosis in subjects on IV nitroprusside (6,18). One animal study has suggested that hydroxocobalamin might be inferior to sodium thiosulfate for this purpose (32).

CAUTIONS AND CONTRAINDICATIONS

Serious allergic reactions, including severe urticaria, bronchospasm, and anaphylactic shock, may occur in patients receiving oral or parenteral hydroxocobalamin (33–35). These reactions are rare and have only been reported in patients who were receiving the drug chronically (i.e., for vitamin deficiency states). Patients with known hypersensitivity to the drug should be treated with a different cyanide antidote.

DOSAGE AND ADMINISTRATION

Known or Likely Cyanide Poisoning with Serious Clinical Effects

The usual initial *adult dose* of hydroxocobalamin is 4 or 5 g, diluted to a volume of at least 200 ml and administered IV over a period of approximately 30 minutes (4,5,16). Based on stoichiometric calculations, a dose of 5 g should bind approximately 100 mg of cyanide. Studies have shown that this dose should be effective for binding blood cyanide levels of up to approximately 40 μmol/L (15). If a patient's cyanide exposure or cyanide level is known to exceed these estimates, a larger initial dose of hydroxocobalamin may be necessary. The *pediatric dose* of hydroxocobalamin has not been determined, but the initial administration of 50 mg/kg is recommended.

Most authors recommend that hydroxocobalamin be followed by a dose of sodium thiosulfate. The usual dose of thiosulfate in these cases is 8 g IV, but 12.5 g can also be used. The two drugs should not be mixed together in the same infusion because thiosulfate may form inactive complexes with hydroxocobalamin (11,23,24).

If patients do not improve clinically within 15 to 30 minutes of the initial treatment or if symptoms of cyanide poisoning recur, the initial doses of hydroxocobalamin and thiosulfate should be repeated. Hydroxocobalamin can safely be used in conjunction with other cyanide antidotes besides sodium thiosulfate. There may in fact be some synergism between therapies (4,29), but the various combinations have not been explored in detail.

Known Cyanide Exposure but Clinical Effects Have Not Yet Developed

The dose is the same as in patients with signs of toxicity.

Suspected Cyanide Poisoning

The dose is the same as in patients with signs of toxicity.

Prevention of Nitroprusside-Induced Cyanide Toxicity

A concurrent IV infusion of hydroxocobalamin should be run at 25 mg/hour during, and for several hours after the cessation of, nitroprusside therapy (6).

Monitoring

All patients suspected of significant cyanide toxicity or cyanide ingestion should be monitored frequently in an intensive care setting. Regular assessments of metabolic acidosis and hyperlactatemia (e.g., arterial blood gases, serum metabolic panels, or serum lactate levels) are needed to assess the response to treatment.

ADVERSE EFFECTS

Human and animal studies indicate that high-dose hydroxocobalamin is generally safe and associated with relatively few significant adverse events (3,11,16,18,21,30). A study of healthy volunteers observed transient hypertension and bradycardia in some subjects, which was believed to be the result of peripheral vasoconstriction (16). There were no adverse clinical sequelae associated with these changes, and no one required specific treatment. The effects resolved within 24 to 48 hours. Animal and *in vitro* studies have demonstrated that hydroxocobalamin has no direct cardiac effects (30,36).

The dose of hydroxocobalamin used in cyanide poisoning frequently causes a benign red or orange discoloration of the patient's skin, urine, plasma, and other bodily fluids (5,12,16, 37). Because of its ultraviolet absorbance, hydroxocobalamin can interfere with lab measurements that employ colorimetric detection. Measurements of liver function, serum electrolytes, serum creatinine, and coagulation are the most frequently affected (16,37,38).

PITFALLS

Failure to improve after adequate doses of hydroxocobalamin should prompt reconsideration of the diagnosis or consideration of the possibility of cointoxicants. A different antidote may be administered if the diagnosis of cyanide poisoning is still suspected.

Recurrent toxicity may represent ongoing cyanide absorption or conversion. Such patients should be reevaluated for the necessity of further decontamination.

REFERENCES

1. Kaczka EA, Wolf DE, Kuehl FA, Folkers K. Vitamin B_{12}: reactions of cyanocobalamin and related compounds. *Science* 1950;112:354–355.
2. Conn JB, Norman SL, Wartman TG. The equilibrium between vitamin B_{12} (cyanocobalamin) and cyanide ion. *Science* 1951;113:658–659.
3. Mushett CW, Kelley KL, Boxer GE, Rickards JC. Antidotal efficacy of vitamin B_{12a} (hydroxo-cobalamin) in experimental cyanide poisoning. *Proc Exp Biol Med* 1952;81:234–237.
4. Hall AH, Rumack BH. Hydroxycobalamin/sodium thiosulfate as a cyanide antidote. *J Emerg Med* 1987;5(2):115–121.
5. Bismuth C, Baud FJ, Djeghout H, et al. Cyanide poisoning from propionitrile exposure. *J Emerg Med* 1987;5(3):191–195.
6. Cottrell JE, Casthely P, Brodie JD, et al. Prevention of nitroprusside-induced cyanide toxicity with hydroxocobalamin. *N Engl J Med* 1978;298(15):809–811.
7. Isom GE, Way JL. Effects of oxygen on the antagonism of cyanide intoxication: cytochrome oxidase, in vitro. *Toxicol Appl Pharmacol* 1984;74(1):57–62.
8. Piantadosi CA, Sylvia AL. Cerebral cytochrome a,a3 inhibition by cyanide in bloodless rats. *Toxicology* 1984;33(1):67–79.
9. Piantadosi CA, Sylvia AL, Jobsis FF. Cyanide-induced cytochrome a,a3 oxidation-reduction responses in rat brain in vivo. *J Clin Invest* 1983,72(4):1224–1233.
10. van Buuren KJ, Nicholis P, van Gelder BF. Biochemical and biophysical studies on cytochrome aa 3. VI. Reaction of cyanide with oxidized and reduced enzyme. *Biochim Biophys Acta* 1972;256(2):258–276.
11. Evans CL. Cobalt compounds as antidotes for hydrocyanic acid. *Br J Pharmacol* 1964;23:455–475.
12. Houeto P, Borron SW, Sandouk P, et al. Pharmacokinetics of hydroxocobalamin in smoke inhalation victims. *J Toxicol Clin Toxicol* 1996;34(4):397–404.
13. Winter CA, Mushett CW. Absence of toxic effects from single injections of crystalline vitamin B12. *J Am Pharm Assoc (Sci Ed)* 1950;39:360–361.
14. Brink NG, Kuehl FA, Folkers K. Vitamin B_{12}: the identification of vitamin B_{12} as a cyano-cobalt coordination complex. *Science* 1950;112:354.
15. Houeto P, Hoffman JR, Imbert M, et al. Relation of blood cyanide to plasma cyanocobalamin concentration after a fixed dose of hydroxocobalamin in cyanide poisoning. *Lancet* 1995;346(8975):605–608.
16. Forsyth JC, Mueller PD, Becker CE, et al. Hydroxocobalamin as a cyanide antidote: safety, efficacy and pharmacokinetics in heavily smoking normal volunteers. *J Toxicol Clin Toxicol* 1993;31(2):277–294.
17. Williams HL, Johnson DJ, McNeil JS, Wright DG. Studies of cobalamin as a vehicle for the renal excretion of cyanide anion. *J Lab Clin Med* 1990;116(1):37–44.
18. Posner MA, Rodkey FL, Tobey RE. Nitroprusside-induced cyanide poisoning: antidotal effect of hydroxocobalamin. *Anesthesiology* 1976;44(4):330–335.
19. Vincent M, Vincent F, Marka C, Faure J. Cyanide and its relationship to nervous suffering. Physiopathological aspects of intoxication. *J Toxicol Clin Toxicol* 1981;18(12):1519–1527.
20. Astier A, Baud FJ. Complexation of intracellular cyanide by hydroxocobalamin using a human cellular model. *Hum Exp Toxicol* 1996;15(1):19–25.
21. Rose CL, Worth RM, Chen KK. Hydroxo-cobalamine and acute cyanide poisoning in dogs. *Life Sci* 1965;4(18):1785–1789.
22. Posner MA, Tobey RE, McElroy H. Hydroxocobalamin therapy of cyanide intoxication in guinea pigs. *Anesthesiology* 1976;44(2):157–160.

23. Friedberg KD, Shukla UR. The efficiency of aquocobalamine as an antidote in cyanide poisoning when given alone or combined with sodium thiosulfate. *Arch Toxicol* 1975;33:103–113.
24. Hatch RC, Laflamme DP, Jain AV. Effects of various known and potential cyanide antagonists and a glutathione depletor on acute toxicity of cyanide in mice. *Vet Hum Toxicol* 1990;32(1):9–16.
25. Mengel K, Kramer W, Isert B, Friedberg KD. Thiosulphate and hydroxocobalamin prophylaxis in progressive cyanide poisoning in guinea-pigs. *Toxicology* 1989;54(3):335–342.
26. Ivankovich AD, Braverman B, Kanuru RP, et al. Cyanide antidotes and methods of their administration in dogs: a comparative study. *Anesthesiology* 1980;52(3):210–216.
27. Astier A, Baud FJ. Simultaneous determination of hydroxocobalamin and its cyanide complex cyanocobalamin in human plasma by high-performance liquid chromatography. Application to pharmacokinetic studies after high-dose hydroxocobalamin as an antidote for severe cyanide poisoning. *J Chromatogr B Biomed Appl* 1995;667(1):129–135.
28. Shearman DJ, Calvert JA, Ala FA, Girdwood RH. Renal excretion of hydroxocobalamin in man. *Lancet* 1965;2(7426):1329–1330.
29. Mannaioni G, Vannacci A, Marzocca C, et al. Acute cyanide intoxication treated with a combination of hydroxycobalamin, sodium nitrite, and sodium thiosulfate. *J Toxicol Clin Toxicol* 2002;40(2):181–183.
30. Riou B, Gerard JL, La Rochelle CD, et al. Hemodynamic effects of hydroxocobalamin in conscious dogs. *Anesthesiology* 1991;74(3):552–558.
31. Baud FJ, Barriot P, Toffis V, et al. Elevated blood cyanide concentrations in victims of smoke inhalation. *N Engl J Med* 1991;325:1761–1766.
32. Hobel M, Engeser P, Nemeth L, Pill J. The antidote effect of thiosulphate and hydroxocobalamin in formation of nitroprusside intoxication of rabbits. *Arch Toxicol* 1980;46(3–4):207–213.
33. Vidal C, Lorenzo A. Anaphylactoid reaction to hydroxycobalamin with tolerance of cyanocobalamin. *Postgrad Med J* 1998;74(877):702.
34. James J, Warin RP. Sensitivity to cyanocobalamin and hydroxocobalamin. *BMJ* 1971;2(756):262.
35. Hovding G. Anaphylactic reaction after injection of vitamin B12. *BMJ* 1968;3(610):102.
36. Riou B, Berdeaux A, Pussard E, Giudicelli JF. Comparison of the hemodynamic effects of hydroxocobalamin and cobalt edetate at equipotent cyanide antidotal doses in conscious dogs. *Intensive Care Med* 1993;19(1):26–32.
37. Curry SC, Connor DA, Raschke RA. Effect of the cyanide antidote hydroxocobalamin on commonly ordered serum chemistry studies. *Ann Emerg Med* 1994;24(1):65–67.
38. Gourlain H, Caliez C, Laforge M, et al. Study of the mechanisms involved in hydroxocobalamin interference with determination of some biochemical parameters. *Ann Biol Clin (Paris)* 1994;52(2):121–124.

CHAPTER 62

Hyperbaric Oxygen

Alison L. Jones and Robert J. Flanagan

Synonym:	**HBO**
Molecular formula and weight:	**O_2, 32 g/mol**
CAS Regsitry No.:	**7782-44-7**
Therapeutic levels:	**HBO at 3 atmosphere absolute can produce arterial partial pressure of oxygen of 1800 mm Hg.**
Special concerns:	**The risks of long-distance emergency medical transport must be balanced over the proposed benefits.**

OVERVIEW

Hyperbaric oxygen (HBO) is the administration of 100% oxygen at pressures above normal atmospheric pressure. It is used to deliver oxygen to tissues when the ability of hemoglobin (Hb) to do so has been seriously compromised [e.g., carbon monoxide (CO), cyanide, or hydrogen sulfide poisoning, or in severe methemoglobinemia]. It is also used to increase solubility of gases and reduce the size of bubbles involved in air embolism. This may have relevance for some poisonings (e.g., hydrogen peroxide).

Equipment

There are single place and multiplace hyperbaric chambers. Both are capable of accommodating critical care devices, such as mechanical ventilators, arterial lines, and Swan-Ganz catheters, although direct current cardioversion is not possible when they are in operation. Only multiplace chambers allow direct patient access by the provider. Monoplace chambers are 8 ft × 3 ft tubular chambers that accommodate one patient. The chamber is pressurized with 100% oxygen, and no mask is worn by the patient. A multiplace chamber can accommodate multiple patients, including benches or gurneys (wheeled stretchers). A nurse or physician can accompany the patient. The chamber interior is pressurized with air (21% oxygen), and each patient wears a facemask that delivers 100% oxygen.

Mechanism of Action

CARBON MONOXIDE POISONING

CO combines with Hb to form carboxyhemoglobin (COHb). Because the affinity of Hb for CO is 200 to 300 times greater than that for oxygen, CO exposure reduces the oxygen-carrying capacity of the blood. COHb also reduces the delivery of oxygen to tissues by shifting the Hb oxygen dissociation curve to the left. In addition, CO inhibits cytochrome-aa_3 and, hence, cellular respiration and reduces cardiac output and tissue perfusion (Chapter 184).

COHb readily dissociates when the partial pressure of CO in the alveolar air falls below that in venous blood. Reducing the partial pressure of inspired CO to zero and increasing the inspired oxygen tension shortens the half-life of CO from 250 minutes when breathing air at normal atmospheric pressure [760 mm Hg; 1 atmosphere absolute (ATA)], but this can be reduced to 50 minutes if 100% oxygen is given at 1 ATA. However, the blood CO half-life can range up to 164 minutes in poisoned patients given 100% oxygen at 1 ATA (1). Administration of HBO (2.5 ATA) reduces the half-life to 22 minutes and also increases the amount of oxygen dissolved in blood from 0.25 to 3.80 ml oxygen per dl blood. This amount is sufficient to allow tissue respiration to proceed in the absence of oxygenated Hb. HBO also dissociates CO from cytochrome-aa_3 and other tissue cytochromes.

MECHANISM OF OXYGEN TREATMENT

Oxygen is an effective treatment for acute CO poisoning, and few acutely poisoned patients, except the elderly or those with preexisting cardiovascular disease, who survive to reach the hospital die. However, neuropsychiatric disturbances (intellectual deterioration; memory impairment; cerebral, cerebellar, and midbrain damage, such as parkinsonism and akinetic mutism; and personality changes, such as irritability, violence, verbal aggressiveness, impulsiveness, and moodiness) may develop some weeks after apparent full recovery (2). At present, there are no reliable prognostic indicators. HBO may reduce the incidence of neuropsychiatric sequelae from 40% to less than 5% (3–5), although this remains controversial (6). It also increases the rate of CO elimination. HBO may also decrease the inflammatory response to hypoxia produced by cellular asphyxiants by decreasing inflammatory cell activity and lipid peroxidation.

INDICATIONS

Widely accepted guidelines for determining which patients should receive HBO have not emerged. A "middle-ground" approach to HBO therapy is recommended.

Carbon Monoxide Poisoning

Because few patients die after arriving at health care facilities, the central issue in HBO treatment is outcome. Do patients who receive HBO have an improved outcome? The primary outcome of clinical interest is neurologic toxicity and has focused specifically on delayed neuropsychiatric sequelae. These sequelae may arise from oxidative damage as oxygen tension rises in a reducing environment (hypoxic/reperfusion injury) (7). Such sequelae develop in approximately 12% of patients, especially elderly patients. At least 80% of these will make a full recovery within one year. However, these sequelae are difficult to quantify precisely.

CHRONIC CARBON MONOXIDE POISONING

Chronic (subacute) CO poisoning may occur as a result of a blocked flue or incomplete combustion of domestic gas in a poorly ventilated room (8). Clinical features of poisoning are vague, and clinicians often miss the diagnosis. The patient usually recovers quickly once the source of exposure is removed. Because the insult is long-standing, HBO is unlikely to be of value in these cases.

ACUTE CARBON MONOXIDE POISONING

Although it is clear that HBO therapy greatly hastens CO elimination and increases oxygen delivery to tissue, debate continues regarding its effect on the outcome of poisoning. There are six controlled trials of HBO for acute CO poisoning. The results reported range from improved to worsened outcome in patients who received HBO. The studies are difficult to compare because the hyperbaric treatment regimens are different, and some studies include patients poisoned in fires and others included patients with simultaneous poisoning by another agent (Table 1). Each study used a unique schedule of HBO treatments. Weaver used a particularly aggressive schedule of HBO treatments with a modest course of normobaric oxygen (9). Scheinkestel used multiple HBO treatments but compared them to oxygen at 1 ATA for 3 days (10). One wonders: Did Scheinkestel show that normobaric oxygen (NBO) was better than expected (and thus HBO was not effective by comparison), or did Weaver show that more intense HBO is better than normobaric oxygen? Another study is needed to find out.

The final decision depends on availability of HBO and the exact clinical scenario. HBO should be considered for the following groups: (a) history of true unconsciousness, especially if prolonged (e.g., more than an hour); (b) conscious patients with neurologic effects (e.g., abnormal neuropsychiatric testing and cerebellar incoordination); (c) patients with markedly elevated COHb concentrations (e.g., greater than 20% to 25%) but without symptoms and signs of CO poisoning; (d) patients with evidence of major end-organ dysfunction (e.g., myocardial ischemia); and (e) pregnant patients with a COHb level above 15%. It is widely believed that the efficacy of HBO declines as the time from exposure increases. Thus, the longer the delay, the more unlikely there will be benefit. This time frame has not been defined but is likely to be in the range of 6 to 24 hours (Table 1).

The patient with transient loss of consciousness poses a serious clinical problem. For example, a patient may experience syncope or have clear signs of confusion after operating a gas-powered tool in a closed space (e.g., basement) for a short period. These patients are nearly always discovered promptly and removed from exposure, which often has not exceeded 30 to 60 minutes. Consciousness returns quickly, and the patient often denies further symptoms and seems to suffer no long-term effects. Until further data are available, HBO therapy is not recommended in these cases unless the patient shows residual signs of cerebellar incoordination (e.g., past pointing, inability to heel-toe walk).

Cyanide Poisoning

HBO may be useful as adjunctive therapy of metabolic acidosis and end-organ dysfunction, which does not respond adequately to antidotal therapy (Chapter 62).

Other Uses in Toxicology

HBO has been used for hydrogen sulfide, carbon tetrachloride, or chloroform poisoning. It has also been used to reduce the size of embolism in severe hydrogen peroxide poisoning and to provide oxygen to the cell when insufficient oxygen-carrying capacity is available (e.g., severe anemia or methemoglobinemia). Further, there are several nontoxicologic uses, such as wound healing.

CAUTIONS AND CONTRAINDICATIONS

Due to the hyperbaric pressure developed, several conditions can be worsened by HBO: (a) recent chest surgery, (b) untreated pneumothorax, (c) hereditary spherocytosis (relative), and (d) patients unable to equalize ear/sinus pressures (relative). HBO should be used cautiously in patients with coma, head injury, extremes of age, history of seizure disorder or ethanol withdrawal, or claustrophobia.

Although concern about the potential teratogenic effect of HBO has been expressed, there is no clinical evidence to support this concern and no biologically plausible explanation for it.

DOSAGE AND ADMINISTRATION

Carbon Monoxide Poisoning

Consultation with a certified and experienced HBO provider is recommended. Chambers are widely distributed throughout

TABLE 1. Comparison of prospective clinical trials of hyperbaric oxygen (HBO) for carbon monoxide (CO) poisoning

Study name (reference)	No. of patients	Design/inclusion criteria	HBO treatment	Outcome	Potential confounders
Raphael (12)	629	Randomized, unblinded comparison of CO patients with or without LOC; included: >14 yr of age; excluded: multiple toxins, pregnancy, contraindication to HBO	One treatment of 2 ATA, 2-h protocol	HBO not improved over NBO.	Not blinded; many patients received HBO >6 h after poisoning.
Ducassé (13)	26	Randomized, noncomatose patients; included: >17 yr of age, duration of CO exposure <12 h, Glasgow Coma Score >12; excluded: pregnancy	One treatment of 2.5 ATA, 2-h protocol	HBO group had better electroencephalogram and single-photon emission computed tomography.	Most patients received treatment started within 1 h of discovery.
Thom (14)	60	Randomized, blinded patients with mild to moderate poisoning; included: acute exposure, increased carboxyhemoglobin; excluded: LOC, cardiac compromise	One treatment of 2.8 ATA × 30 min, 2.0 ATA × 90 min	NBO: 7 of 30 patients developed neuropsychiatric sequelae; HBO: 0 of 30.[a]	Testing was not blinded.
Mathieu (15)	575	Randomized, unblinded; included: noncomatose	One treatment of 2.5 ATA for 90 min	Delayed NP sequelae were lower among noncomatose patients with LOC.	Not blinded.
Scheinkestel (10)	191	Randomized (cluster randomization in some cases), blinded; included: all patients with 24 h of exposure; excluded: pregnancy, children, burn victims	Three or more treatments of 2.8 ATA × 60 min, NBO for 3 d; mean time to treatment, 7.5 h	No improvement with HBO.	Enrollment allowed up to 24 h; only 46% follow-up for NS; many suicide attempters (depression) may have affected NS results; many patients had taken additional poisons.
Weaver (9)	152	Blocked stratified randomization, blinded comparison of acute CO poisoning; included: symptomatic patients >15 yr of age and within 24 hr of exposure, including LOC; excluded: moribund patients, pregnancy	Three treatments: (i) 3 ATA × 75 min, 2 ATA × 75 min; (ii) and (iii) 2 ATA × 120 min	HBO group had lower incidence of selected NP tests.	Average duration of CO exposure much longer in NBO group.

ATA, atmosphere absolute; LOC, loss of consciousness; NBO, normobaric oxygen; NP, neuropsychiatric; NS, neuropsychological sequelae.
[a]Statistically significant difference.

the United States. To locate the nearest chamber, call the Diver Alert Network at Duke University (919-684-8111).

The number of treatments, duration of treatment, and profile of pressure treatment vary substantially by institution. Typically, an initial treatment consists of 30 minutes of 100% oxygen at 3 ATA, then 60 minutes at 2 ATA or until a COHb level less than 10% is achieved. Another common regimen is 2.7 ATA for 30 minutes, then 2.2 ATA for 90 minutes. Often, recovery of consciousness occurs during the treatment. Subsequent treatments depend on local practice and degree of recovery after first treatment.

Another method of administering HBO is with a device known as the *Gamow bag*. This is a folding chamber made of fabric that can be transported. However, it achieves only 1.5 ATA and is usually reserved for out-of-hospital treatment when HBO is unavailable (11).

Cyanide Poisoning

There are no established protocols. In general, patients are treated with a regimen similar to that for CO poisoning. The duration of treatment is varied depending on the clinical conditions. The cyanide-poisoned patient that needs HBO is usually critically ill and refractory to treatment and needs intensive supportive care.

Other Uses in Toxicology

There are no established protocols. In general, patients are treated with a regimen similar to that of CO poisoning. The duration of treatment is varied depending on the clinical conditions.

ADVERSE EFFECTS

Acute oxygen toxicity (seizure) has been reported but only at pressures higher than 2.8 ATA. Other adverse effects are rupture of tympanic membranes and panic reaction due to claustrophobia.

PITFALLS

Complications may be due to associated procedures or underlying disease rather than HBO itself (e.g., seizure can arise from CO poisoning or oxygen toxicity).

Transporting the patient to a hospital is a frequent challenge. Because elapsed time is believed to reduce the efficacy of HBO, assertive attempts to transfer the patient promptly to an HBO facility are needed. However, the dangers of transporting severely ill patients by ambulance are not to be underestimated.

REFERENCES

1. Levasseur L, Galliot-Guilley M, Scherrmann JM, Baud FJ. Effects of mode of inhalation of carbon monoxide and of normobaric oxygen administration on carbon monoxide elimination from the blood. *Hum Exp Toxicol* 1996;15:898–903.
2. Howard RJ, Blake DR, Pall H, et al. Allopurinol/*N*-acetylcysteine for carbon monoxide poisoning. *Lancet* 1987;2:628–629.
3. Mathieu D, Nolf M, Durocher A, et al. Acute carbon monoxide poisoning. Risk of late sequelae and treatment by hyperbaric oxygen. *J Toxicol Clin Toxicol* 1985;23:315–324.
4. Myers RAM, Snyder SK, Emhoff TA. Subacute sequelae of carbon monoxide poisoning. *Ann Emerg Med* 1985;14:1163–1167.
5. Norkool DM, Kirkpatrick JN. Treatment of acute carbon monoxide poisoning with hyperbaric oxygen: a review of 115 cases. *Ann Emerg Med* 1985;14:1168–1171.
6. Tibbles PM, Perrotta PL. Treatment of carbon monoxide poisoning: a critical review of human outcome studies comparing normobaric oxygen with hyperbaric oxygen. *Ann Emerg Med* 1994;24:269–276.
7. Werner B, Persson H, Kulling P. Symposium. Carbon monoxide poisoning: mechanism of damage, late sequelae and therapy. *J Toxicol Clin Toxicol* 1985;23:247–326.
8. Crawford R, Campbell DG, Ross J. Carbon monoxide poisoning in the home: recognition and treatment. *BMJ* 1990;301:977–979.
9. Weaver LK, Hopkins RO, Chan KJ, et al. Hyperbaric oxygen for acute carbon monoxide poisoning. *N Engl J Med* 2002;347:1057–1067.
10. Scheinkestel CD, Bailey M, Myles PS, et al. Hyperbaric or normobaric oxygen for acute carbon monoxide poisoning: a randomised controlled clinical trial. *Med J Aust* 1999;170:203–210.
11. Jay GD, Tetz DJ, Hartigan LF, et al. Portable hyperbaric oxygen therapy in the emergency department with a modified Gamow bag. *Ann Emerg Med* 1995;26:707–711.
12. Raphael JC, Elkharrat D, Jars-Guincestre MC, et al. Trial of normobaric and hyperbaric oxygen for acute carbon monoxide intoxication. *Lancet* 1989;2:414–419.
13. Ducassé JL, Celsis P, Marc-Vergnes JP. Non-comatose patients with acute carbon monoxide poisoning: hyperbaric or normobaric oxygenation? *Undersea Hyperb Med* 1995;22:9–15.
14. Thom SR, Taber RL, Mendiguren II, et al. Delayed neuropsychologic sequelae after carbon monoxide poisoning: prevention by treatment with hyperbaric oxygen. *Ann Emerg Med* 1995;25:474–480.
15. Mathieu D, Wattel F, Mathieu-Nolf M, et al. Randomized prospective study comparing the effect of HBO versus 12 hours NBO in non-comatose CO poisoned patients: results of the interim analysis. *Undersea Hyperb Med* 1996;23[Suppl]:7–8.

CHAPTER 63

Methylene Blue

Greene Shepherd and Daniel C. Keyes

H_3C N CH_3 — N — S ⊕ — Cl⊖ — N CH_3 CH_3

METHYLENE BLUE

Synonym:	**Methylthioninium chloride**
Molecular formula and weight:	**$C_{16}H_{18}ClN_3S$, $3H_2O$, 373.9 g/mol**
CAS Registry No.:	**7220-79-3 (methylene blue trihydrate)**
Therapeutic level:	**Not clinically applicable**
Special concerns:	**Iatrogenic overdose has resulted in serious methemoglobinemia. Treatment of patients with glucose 6 phosphatase deficiency may result in hemolysis.**

OVERVIEW

Methylene blue is a thiazine dye used for several medical purposes, such as a urinary antiseptic. In toxicology, it is used to treat clinically significant methemoglobinemia and ifosfamide-induced encephalopathy. It has dose-dependent oxidation or reduction properties (1). It is available as a dark blue 1% solution (10 mg/ml) for intravenous (IV) injection.

Mechanism of Action

Methemoglobin (MetHgb) results from the oxidation of the iron in hemoglobin from the ferrous (Fe^{2+}) to ferric (Fe^{3+}) states. Under normal oxidative stresses, MetHgb is converted back to normal hemoglobin by a relatively slow reaction catalyzed by nicotinamide adenine dinucleotide–dependent reductase. Increased oxidation of hemoglobin easily overwhelms the capacity of this enzyme, resulting in accumulation of MetHgb. Increasing MetHgb levels can cause tissue hypoxia and central nervous system effects.

At lower doses, methylene blue acts as a reducing agent, whereas at higher doses, it acts as an oxidizing agent. At therapeutic doses, methylene blue is reduced by a nicotinamide adenine dinucleotide phosphate–dependent enzyme system to leukomethylene blue (Fig. 1). This reduced form rapidly converts MetHgb back to hemoglobin. At very high doses, this

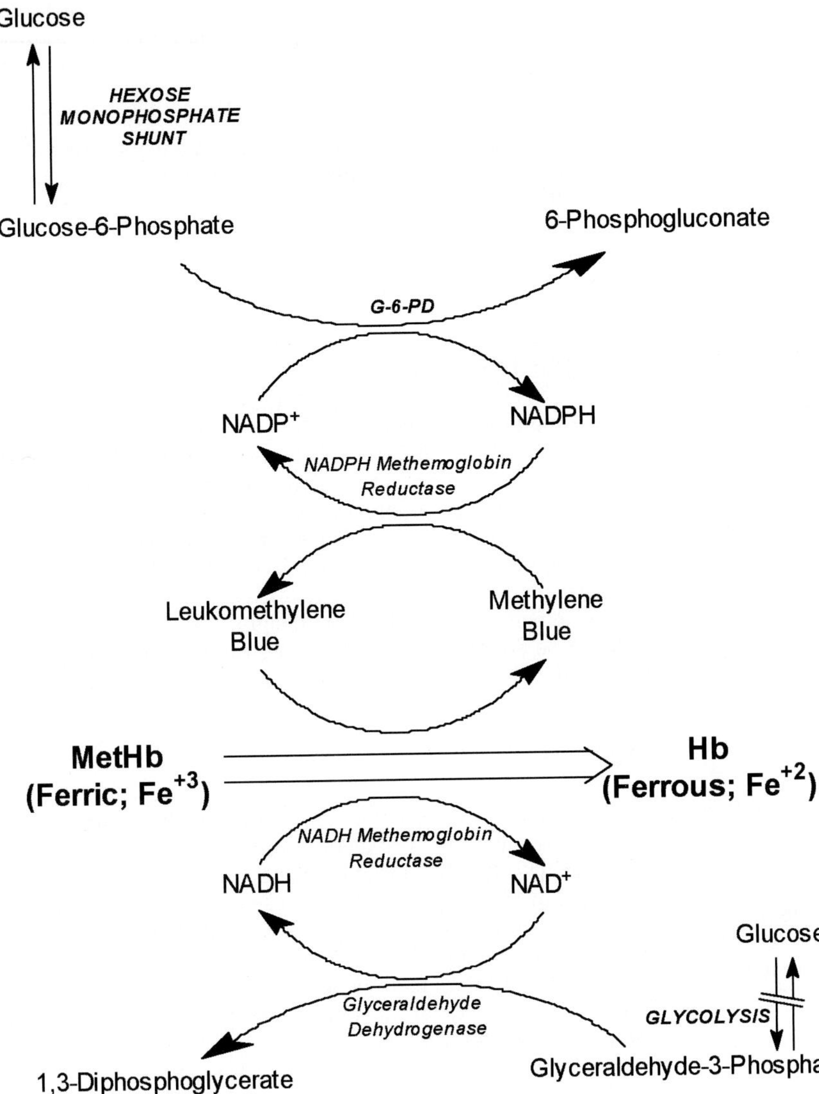

Figure 1. Mechanisms of methemoglobin reduction. G-6-PD, glucose-6-phosphate dehydrogenase; Hb, hemoglobin; MetHb, methemoglobin; NAD^+, the oxidized form of nicotinamide adenine dinucleotide; NADH, the reduced form of nicotinamide adenine dinucleotide; $NADP^+$, the oxidized form of nicotinamide adenine dinucleotide phosphate; NADPH, the reduced form of nicotinamide adenine dinucleotide phosphate.

enzyme is saturated, and the excess methylene blue remains in an oxidized state and may actually produce MetHgb.

INDICATIONS

Methemoglobinemia

Methylene blue is recommended for symptomatic patients with elevated MetHgb levels or asymptomatic patients with MetHgb levels greater than 20% to 30%. Treatment at a lower level may be indicated for patients who cannot tolerate decreased oxygen delivery (e.g., heart disease, lung disease, carbon monoxide poisoning, or severe anemia). Oral doses have been used in the treatment of idiopathic methemoglobinemia, often in conjunction with ascorbic acid or *N*-acetylcysteine.

Other Indications

Methylene blue has been demonstrated to be effective in the treatment and prevention of ifosfamide-induced encephalopathy. Methylene blue may also be used as a genitourinary antiseptic or as a contrast dye.

CAUTIONS AND CONTRAINDICATIONS

Methylene blue should be used cautiously in patients who have glucose 6 phosphate dehydrogenase (G6PD) deficiency (2,3). Patients with G6PD deficiency cannot reduce methylene blue to leukomethylene blue. Therefore, methylene blue is ineffective in these patients, and the high concentration of the methylene blue may cause hemolysis. Exchange transfusion should be seriously considered as an alternative to methylene blue therapy for G6PD patients with methemoglobinemia (Chapter 26).

It may be dangerous to try to reverse the methemoglobinemia caused by the Cyanide Antidote Package (4,5). Because MetHgb combines with cyanide to form cyanomethemoglobin, treatment with methylene blue could theoretically release cyanide and cause clinical deterioration.

Patients with significant renal impairment may require dose adjustments because approximately 75% of the dose is excreted in the urine as unchanged drug or leukomethylene blue.

Relative contraindications for methylene blue include hypersensitivity to methylene blue, significant G6PD deficiency, and severe renal insufficiency. Administration of methylene blue by subcutaneous, intraamniotic, and intrathecal routes is contraindicated (3,6–11). These routes of administration are associated with abscess formation, respiratory depression in neonates, and quadriplegia, respectively.

DOSAGE AND METHOD OF ADMINISTRATION

Methemoglobinemia

The normal *adult* or *pediatric dose* for methylene blue is 1 to 2 mg/kg (0.1 to 0.2 ml/kg of 1% solution) given slowly IV over several minutes. A dose of 25 to 50 mg/m^2 may be used in children. Saline flushes may be used to minimize local infusion pain. Interosseous infusion has been used successfully. The initial response to therapy should be noted within a few minutes, and maximal effect is reached in 30 to 60 minutes. Concurrent administration of dextrose has been recommended because glucose is needed to supply nicotinamide adenine dinucleotide and nicotinamide adenine dinucleotide phosphate (Fig. 1).

The dose may be repeated in 30 minutes and then every 2 to 4 hours as needed. The total dose should not exceed 7 mg/kg as a single dose or 15 mg/kg within 24 hours. The patient should be monitored for clinical resolution of signs and symptoms of excess MetHgb.

If the MetHgb level fails to decrease after methylene blue administration, the cause should be promptly investigated. The patient may have an overwhelming dose of the oxidizing agent or an agent that causes rebound MetHgb levels, an abnormal form of hemoglobin, a genetic enzyme deficiency, or methylene blue toxicity (Table 1).

For asymptomatic cyanosis of patients with hereditary methylene blue reductase insufficiencies, oral methylene blue has been dosed at 300 mg every 4 to 6 hours.

Monitoring involves measurement of oxygen saturation and MetHgb levels by co-oximetry. Repeat hourly until the patient has normalized, then repeat once 4 to 6 hours later to assure that MetHgb levels are not rebounding. Repeated treatment may be needed for compounds with prolonged elimination or those that undergo enterohepatic recirculation (e.g., dapsone).

TABLE 1. Differential diagnosis of failed methylene blue treatment

Diagnosis	Example	Evaluation
Dose of oxidizing toxin that overwhelms dose of methylene blue	Massive dose	Repeat history
Prolonged presence of oxidizing agent in the blood	Dapsone undergoes enterohepatic recirculation	Reevaluate history and doses of methylene blue
Sulfhemoglobinemia	Sulfonamides, phenazopyridine	Co-oximetry
G6PD deficiency	Patient with high penetrance (expression)	Measure G6PD enzyme activity in blood
Nicotinamide adenine dinucleotide phosphate–methemoglobin reductase deficiency	Hereditary condition	Test not readily available; diagnosis of exclusion
Abnormal hemoglobin	Hemoglobin M	Hemoglobin analysis
Iatrogenic overdose of methylene blue	Administration of adult dose to child	Reevaluate dose administered

G6PD, glucose 6 phosphate dehydrogenase.
Note: If the patient does not respond to the initial doses of methylene blue, these conditions should be considered.

Other Indications

Methylene blue has been used for the treatment and prevention of ifosfamide-induced encephalopathy (12–14). Slow IV injection of 50 mg in a 2% aqueous solution up to six times daily may be used for the reversal of this neurotoxicity. Doses of 50 mg every 6 hours, either oral or IV, may be used to prevent further episodes of encephalopathy.

ADVERSE EFFECTS

Common adverse effects of methylene blue include dyspnea, precordial pain, restlessness, and apprehension. Rare effects include tremors, hemolytic anemia, pulmonary edema, and even death. Giving too large a dose saturates the nicotinamide adenine dinucleotide–dependent enzyme system (Fig. 1), resulting in an excess of the oxidant methylene blue. This additional oxidant stress may, paradoxically, increase MetHgb and possibly cause hemolysis. Patients with significant G6PD deficiency will not be able to reduce methylene blue to leukomethylene blue, and it should be avoided (2,15,16).

PITFALLS

Pulse oximeters should not be used, as MetHgb and methylene blue interfere with the wavelengths measured by current pulse oximeters (17–19). The absorption spectra of MetHgb and oxyhemoglobin overlap, causing the pulse oximeter to produce an oxygen saturation value that is inaccurate. For example, the pulse oximeter reads 87% when the true measurement is actually 73%. In addition, methylene blue itself causes the apparent oxygen saturation to rapidly fall artifactually due to wavelength interference. Arterial blood gases with co-oximetry should be used to monitor oxygen saturation and MetHgb levels.

Toxic methemoglobinemia due to substances such as aniline or nitroethane, which have long half-lives and produce metabolites capable of causing MetHgb, can be challenging to manage (20–23). This may require prolonged monitoring and repeated dosing. Animal and *in vitro* models suggest that administering *N*-acetylcysteine, a reducing agent that does not require enzymatic activation, may be a useful adjunct in these situations (24,25). However, it was ineffective in a human volunteer trial of MetHgb produced by sodium nitrite (26).

For therapeutically induced MetHgb, as in the case of cyanide poisoning, administering methylene blue may be counterproductive. However, if the patient is accidentally overdosed with nitrites and develops serious methemoglobinemia, treating with methylene blue is the prudent course of action.

REFERENCES

1. Wright RO, Lewander WJ, Woolf AD. Methemoglobinemia: etiology, pharmacology, and clinical management. *Ann Emerg Med* 1999;34(5):646–656.
2. Rosen PJ, Johnson C, McGehee WG, Beutler E. Failure of methylene blue treatment in toxic methemoglobinemia. Association with glucose-6-phosphate dehydrogenase deficiency. *Ann Intern Med* 1971;75(1):83–86.
3. Harvey JW, Keitt AS. Studies of the efficacy and potential hazards of methylene blue therapy in aniline-induced methaemoglobinaemia. *Br J Haematol* 1983;54(1):29–41.
4. Berlin C. Treatment of cyanide poisoning in children. *Pediatrics* 1970;46:793–796.

5. Douze JM, van Heijst AN. [Recovery of a patient with potassium cyanide poisoning followed by nitrite intoxication.] *Ned Tijdschr Geneeskd* 1973;117(38):1409–1412.
6. Perry PM, Meinhard E. Nectotic subcutaneous abscesses following injections of methylene blue. *Br J Clin Pract* 1974;28(8):289–291.
7. Cowett RM, Hakanson DO, Kocon RW, Oh W. Untoward neonatal effect of intraamniotic administration of methylene blue. *Obstet Gynecol* 1976;48[Suppl 1]:74S–75S.
8. Lee DC, Valente JH. Methylene blue dye-induced knee effusion. *Am J Emerg Med* 1999;17(7):739–740.
9. Crooks J. Haemolytic jaundice in a neonate after intra-amniotic injection of methylene blue. *Arch Dis Child* 1982;57(11):872–873.
10. Nicolini U, Monni G. Intestinal obstruction in babies exposed in utero to methylene blue. *Lancet* 1990;336(8725):1258–1259.
11. Evans JP, Keegan HR. Danger in the intrathecal use of methylene blue. *JAMA* 1960;174:856–859.
12. Pelgrims J, De Vos F, Van den Brande J, et al. Methylene blue in the treatment and prevention of ifosfamide-induced encephalopathy: report of 12 cases and a review of the literature. *Br J Cancer* 2000;82(2):291–294.
13. Kupfer A, Aeschlimann C, Cerny T. Methylene blue and the neurotoxic mechanisms of ifosfamide encephalopathy. *Eur J Clin Pharmacol* 1996;50(4):249–252.
14. Demandt M, Wandt H. [Successful treatment with methylene blue of ifosfamide-induced central nervous system effects.] *Dtsch Med Wochenschr* 1996;121(17):575.
15. Lamont AS, Roberts MS, Holdsworth DG, et al. Relationship between methaemoglobin production and methylene blue plasma concentrations under general anaesthesia. *Anaesth Intensive Care* 1986;14(4):360–364.
16. Goluboff N, Wheaton R. Methylene blue induced cyanosis and acute hemolytic anemia complicating the treatment of methemoglobinemia. *J Pediatr* 1961;58:86–89.
17. Kessler MR, Eide T, Humayun B, Poppers PJ. Spurious pulse oximeter desaturation with methylene blue injection. *Anesthesiology* 1986;65(4):435–436.
18. Barker SJ, Tremper KK. Pulse oximetry: applications and limitations. *Int Anesthesiol Clin* 1987;25(3):155–175.
19. Kirlangitis JJ, Middaugh RE, Zablocki A, Rodriquez F. False indication of arterial oxygen desaturation and methemoglobinemia following injection of methylene blue in urological surgery. *Mil Med* 1990;155(6):260–262.
20. Kearney TE, Manoguerra AS, Dunford JV Jr. Chemically induced methemoglobinemia from aniline poisoning. *West J Med* 1984;140(2):282–286.
21. Christensen CM, Farrar HC, Kearns GL. Protracted methemoglobinemia after phenazopyridine overdose in an infant. *J Clin Pharmacol* 1996;36(2):112–116.
22. Liao YP, Hung DZ, Yang DY. Hemolytic anemia after methylene blue therapy for aniline-induced methemoglobinemia. *Vet Hum Toxicol* 2002;44(1):19–21.
23. Shepherd G, Grover J, Klein-Schwartz W. Prolonged formation of methemoglobin following nitroethane ingestion. *J Toxicol Clin Toxicol* 1998;36(6):613–616.
24. Wright RO, Magnani B, Shannon MW, Woolf AD. *N*-acetylcysteine reduces methemoglobin in vitro. *Ann Emerg Med* 1996;28(5):499–503.
25. Wright RO, Woolf AD, Shannon MW, Magnani B. *N*-acetylcysteine reduces methemoglobin in an in-vitro model of glucose-6-phosphate dehydrogenase deficiency. *Acad Emerg Med* 1998;5(3):225–229.
26. Tanen DA, LoVecchio F, Curry SC. Failure of intravenous *N*-acetylcysteine to reduce methemoglobin produced by sodium nitrite in human volunteers: a randomized controlled trial. *Ann Emerg Med* 2000;35:369–373.

CHAPTER 64

N-*Acetylcysteine*

Richard C. Dart and Alison L. Jones

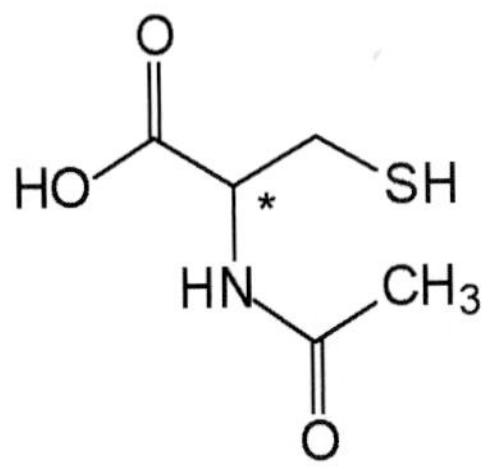

* = Chiral center

N-ACETYLECYSTEINE	
Synonyms:	**NAC, acetylcysteine sodium, *N*-acetyl-L-cysteine, *N*-acetyl-3-mercapto-alanine, mercapturic acid, Mucomyst, Parvolex, Acetadote**
Molecular formula and weight:	**$C_5H_9NO_3S$, 163.2 g/mol**
SI conversion:	**mg/L × 6.1 = µmol/L**
CAS Registry No.:	**616-91-1**
Therapeutic levels:	**Not clinically applicable**
Special concerns:	**NAC should be administered within 8 hours of ingestion of an acetaminophen overdose whenever possible. Attempts to administer NAC orally may delay effective therapy.**

OVERVIEW

Administration of sulfhydryl donors, notably D,L-methionine (racemethionine) or *N*-acetylcysteine (NAC), offers complete protection against acetaminophen (paracetamol) hepatotoxicity and renal toxicity if given within approximately 10 hours of acute ingestion (1,2). Successful use in acetaminophen poisoning was reported for methionine in 1976 (3) and for NAC in 1979 (4). NAC is also routinely used in the management of acetaminophen poisoning, presenting more than 10 hours after ingestion, and in the management of acute liver failure (ALF) due to acetaminophen. Furthermore, its use has been proposed for an array of toxicants that deplete glutathione (GSH), such as pennyroyal, carbon tetrachloride, and chloroform.

NAC is supplied as a 10% or 20% solution for intravenous (IV), oral, or inhalational administration. In the United States, only the oral and inhalation forms are available, although an IV formulation is being developed. In nearly all other countries, NAC is typically given by the IV route. NAC has a strong sulfur odor ("rotten eggs") that discourages its acceptance for oral use.

Mechanism of Action

The cytotoxicity of acetaminophen in early acetaminophen poisoning is mediated by a reactive metabolite, *N*-acetyl-*p*-quinone-imine (NAPQI). NAPQI is an electrophilic oxidant that is normally detoxified by reduced GSH. However, if mitochondrial and cytosolic GSH become depleted to 20% to 30% of normal, covalent binding to cellular macromolecules may lead to liver cell death (Chapter 126).

PREVENTION OF ACETAMINOPHEN TOXICITY

Several mechanisms have been proposed to explain the ability of NAC to prevent acetaminophen toxicity: (a) NAC may increase the amount of GSH available to detoxify NAPQI (5,6); (b) it may directly bind to NAPQI; (c) it may provide inorganic sulfate and promote sulfation; and (d) it may reduce NAPQI back to its parent, acetaminophen. Both L-methionine and NAC require conversion to cysteine by intact hepatocytes before incorporation in GSH—NAC being deacetylated and L-methionine undergoing sequential metabolism by five enzymes.

TREATMENT OF LIVER FAILURE

A prospective trial of acetaminophen-induced ALF found that survival was increased in patients receiving NAC IV (7). The mechanism of action of NAC in patients with liver failure is unclear. The underlying mechanism is a matter of much interest (8). Although once felt to be due to improved tissue microperfusion and, hence, oxygen delivery (9), this view has been challenged using end-tidal carbon dioxide measurements, a more sensitive measure of oxygen kinetics (10). NAC may act by protecting protein thiols against oxidation, by hemodynamic effects on regional blood flow to critical organs (11), by free radical scavenging, or by interfering with production of cytokines (12). It also inhibits neutrophil accumulation (13) and restores some proteolytic enzymes to dispose of arylated protein (14).

Pharmacokinetics

The pharmacokinetics of NAC are complicated because of the variety of forms (free; protein-bound in either reduced or oxidized form; mixed disulfides with other thiols, including protein thiols) in which it occurs. Oral absorption occurs rapidly, but bioavailability is less than 12%, probably due to extensive deacetylation in the intestinal mucosa (15). Plasma half-lives of 2 to 6 hours have been reported after IV administration; 20% to 30% of the dose is excreted unchanged in urine.

In plasma, most of a dose of NAC is present as disulfides. In one study, oral NAC increased free cysteine in plasma, although total cysteine and free and total GSH concentrations remained unchanged (6). Plasma total NAC concentrations soon after the start of an infusion (20 hours' IV regimen on an infusion dose of 150 mg/kg) range from 300 to 900 mg/L, whereas concentrations of only 11 to 90 mg/L are maintained toward the end (20 hours' IV regimen on an infusion dose of 50 mg/kg) (16). These latter plasma concentrations are similar to those attained after oral NAC administration (6).

INDICATIONS

Acute Acetaminophen Poisoning

When administered within 8 to 10 hours of ingestion, NAC usually prevents liver injury (4,17). The decision to administer NAC or methionine is based on the use of a decision tool. In the United States, the Rumack-Matthew nomogram is used, and a similar nomogram is used in the United Kingdom (Fig. 1) (4,18). Treatment is administered if the plasma acetaminophen level falls above a "treatment line" on the respective plots. More detail on the nomogram and its uses is provided in Chapter 126. If a plasma acetaminophen concentration is not available within 8 hours of ingestion, NAC treatment should be commenced and then stopped if the patient's plasma acetaminophen concentration ultimately falls below the treatment line.

A plasma acetaminophen measurement performed within 4 hours of ingestion can be misleading because absorption may be incomplete. New data are emerging; the evidence currently available does not support the reliable use of levels drawn within 4 hours of ingestion.

Several factors complicate the use of the acetaminophen nomogram. The number of patients studied in the original nomogram was small. The time of ingestion may be difficult to determine precisely in a patient who has taken an overdose. The occurrence of coma or vomiting and the risk of adverse reactions should also be considered in the treatment decision. The possibility of higher-risk populations has also been raised, and additional treatment lines have been proposed; however, prospective research has yet to prove the need for additional treatment lines. Although young children seem less susceptible than adults to the hepatorenal toxicity of acetaminophen, those believed to be at risk of hepatorenal damage on the basis of a plasma acetaminophen measurement should be treated in the same way as adults. In a study of 60 pregnant patients who had ingested an overdose of acetaminophen, 24 were believed to be at risk of developing hepatorenal damage on the basis of plasma acetaminophen concentrations and were given oral NAC (19). The incidence of spontaneous abortion or fetal death was increased when treatment was delayed.

Another issue is the time after ingestion beyond which NAC is ineffective. Originally, it appeared that administration of NAC more than 15 hours after ingestion was ineffective (20). However, the clinical practice is to attempt NAC treatment in all patients with liver injury from acetaminophen. This practice is based on the risk-benefit analysis of a relatively safe therapy and a potentially lethal outcome.

Chronic Overdose (Repeated Supratherapeutic Ingestion)

The maximum recommended dose of acetaminophen is 4 g/day. Some patients ingest several acetaminophen doses in succession (i.e., "staggered" overdose). It is unclear if and when these "supratherapeutic"-dose patients should be treated with NAC. The acetaminophen nomogram cannot be used for repeated ingestions.

A *repeated supratherapeutic ingestion* is defined as more than one ingestion of any size occurring over a period exceeding 8 hours that results in a cumulative dose of greater than 4 g of acetaminophen per 24-hour period. A cumulative dose greater than 150 mg acetaminophen per kg of body weight has also been proposed. A method is needed to determine which repeated supratherapeutic ingestion patients should receive NAC. Based on prospectively defined criteria, poison center data indicate that the serum acetaminophen level combined with the serum aspartate aminotransferase or alanine aminotransferase level may be used to determine the need for NAC treatment (21). If the serum acetaminophen level is less than 10 μg/ml, and the serum aspartate aminotransferase and alanine aminotransferase are below 50 IU/L, the patient does not need treatment (21). If either the acetaminophen or hepatic aminotransferase level is increased, the patient is treated with NAC.

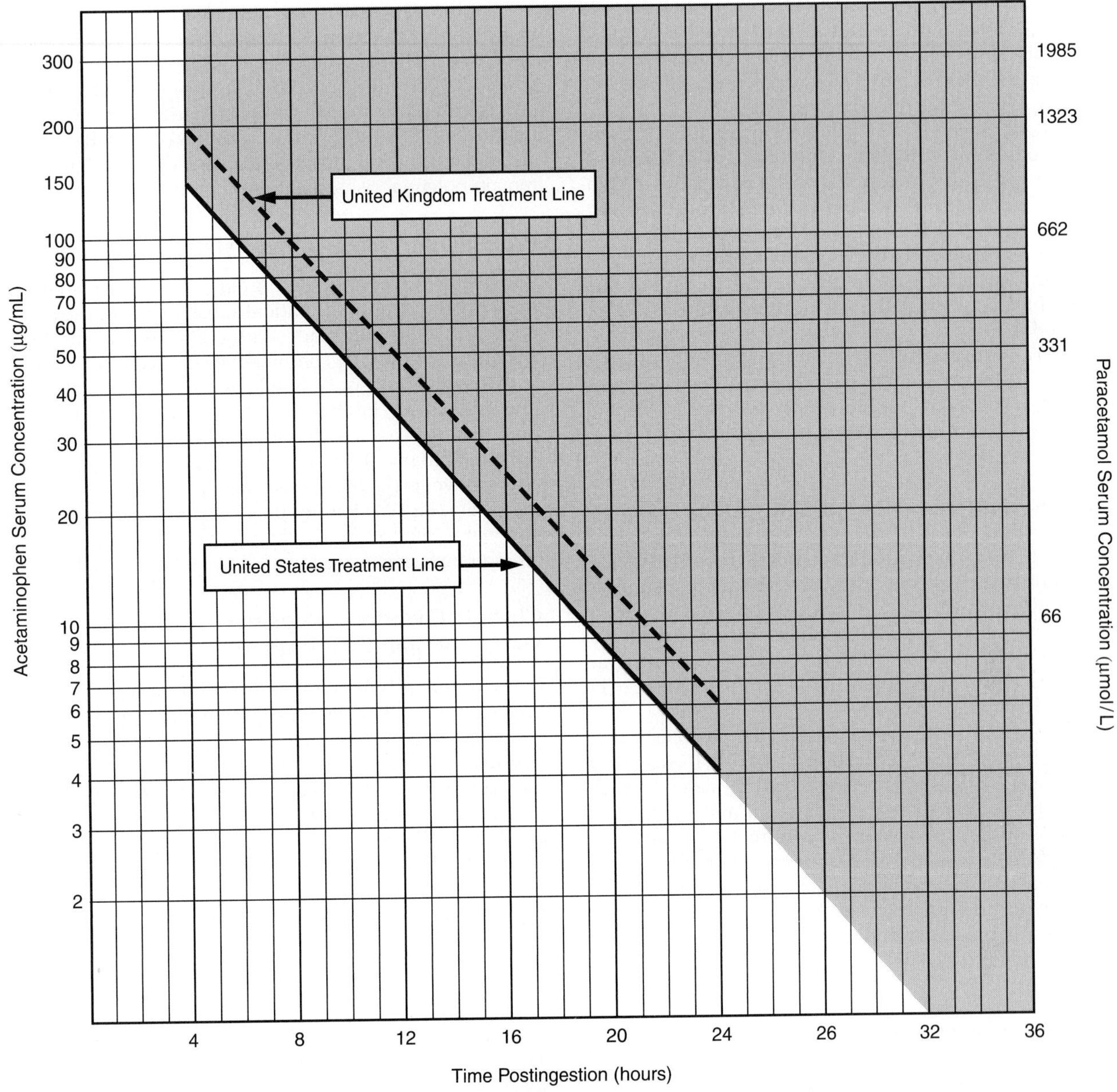

Figure 1. The acetaminophen nomogram. This nomogram incorporates the essential elements of nomograms used in the United Kingdom and the United States. In the case of an acute single ingestion of acetaminophen, the patient's serum concentration of acetaminophen is plotted at the time of sampling postingestion. If the level appears above the line chosen, treatment with acetylcysteine should be commenced. The text addresses potential alterations of the nomogram for selected clinical scenarios.

Drug-Induced Acute Liver Failure

Many other drugs may cause ALF (Chapter 17). Prospective data are available, indicating that NAC improves survival from acetaminophen-induced hepatic failure (7). A U.S. clinical trial of NAC in ALF is currently in progress.

Other Potential Antidotal Uses of *N*-Acetylcysteine

Like many sulfhydryl-containing compounds, NAC also chelates heavy metal ions. Potential advantages over other chelating agents are that NAC is relatively safe and can be given orally in large amounts and that high tissue concentrations are achieved. Clinical studies showing efficacy of NAC as a heavy metal chelating agent are sparse (22), and more effective agents, such as succimer, are now readily available.

In rats, NAC increased chromium VI salt elimination (23). A 25-year-old patient survived after ingesting 16 g of a hexavalent chromium salt when NAC and hemodialysis were used (24). Ascorbate (1 g IV initially every 10 minutes and repeated frequently) and NAC orally or IV in doses equivalent to those used for acetaminophen poisoning should be used together with hemodialysis. NAC has been advocated in acute poisoning with potassium permanganate and with sodium dichromate or chromate (24,25). NAC may also have a protective action against dimethylformamide-induced liver damage (26).

Parenteral dimercaprol and NAC have been used to treat acute poisoning with sodium arsenate (27) and arsenic pentoxide (28). It has been suggested that NAC may enhance gold excretion in patients with sodium aurothiomalate–induced aplastic anemia. However, 1.2 kg NAC over 4 months was associated with the excretion of only 48 mg of gold in a patient given more than 7 g over the previous 5 years (29).

There is a clear theoretic rationale for the use of NAC in the treatment of poisoning with either chloroform or 1,2-dichloropropane. Phosgene ($COCl_2$) is an important metabolite of chloroform. Phosgene depletes GSH to form diglutathionyl dithiocarbonate (GS-CO-SG) and also binds to cell macromolecules and causes tissue necrosis. 1,2-Dichloropropane administration is also associated with hepatic GSH depletion in rats. With carbon tetrachloride, the trichloromethyl free radical (CCl_3) formed initially may bind covalently to macromolecules or react further by several routes. Chloroform is a minor metabolite and may be metabolized to phosgene, but the importance of this is unclear—carbon tetrachloride does not deplete hepatic GSH to the same extent as chloroform in animals (30).

CAUTIONS AND CONTRAINDICATIONS

Animal and human volunteer data indicate that oral NAC is bound by activated charcoal. This raises concern that simultaneous administration will reduce NAC absorption and thereby allow toxicity to develop (31,32). Because of the large dose of NAC administered orally and the lack of data indicating an adverse clinical effect, the potential interaction is not likely to be clinically relevant (33).

NAC is U.S. Food and Drug Administration pregnancy category B. It is commonly used during pregnancy (34). It crosses the placenta and achieves levels in the fetus similar to maternal levels (35). Data are limited, but there are no data indicating teratogenic or other effects during use of NAC for maternal acetaminophen toxicity, and the balance of risk is in favor of its administration to ensure maternal survival and, hence, fetal protection (19).

NAC may be contraindicated in the extremely rare patient with a history of acute anaphylactic response to NAC (most occurring in patients with a history of atopy and asthma).

DOSAGE AND ADMINISTRATION

Acute Acetaminophen (Paracetamol) Poisoning

NAC may be administered either orally or IV. The dosage regimens were derived empirically; therefore, it is difficult to compare the relative efficacy of treatment regimens.

Oral NAC (3% to 5% solution) is used in the United States, although an IV formulation is under development. The *adult* and *pediatric dose* is 140 mg/kg as a loading dose, followed by 70 mg/kg for 17 doses, for a total duration of therapy of 72 hours and a total dose of 1330 mg/kg. If the patient vomits within 1 hour of a dose, the dose should be repeated. Its efficacy is time dependent and decreases if more than 8 to 10 hours elapse between ingestion and NAC administration (17,20). Oral therapy is difficult in patients who refuse it, have a compromised airway, or cannot use their gastrointestinal tract (e.g., caustic coingestion). The inhalation/oral formulation should be used by the IV route in these cases (36). In one case, difficulty in oral administration was associated with an unexpected death after acetaminophen overdose (37).

IV NAC is used extensively around the world to treat acetaminophen poisoning. The initial dose of 150 mg/kg is infused in 200 ml of 5% (weight/volume) dextrose over 15 minutes, followed by 50 mg/kg in 500 ml of 5% dextrose over 4 hours (12.5 mg/kg/hour) and 100 mg/kg in 1 L of 5% dextrose over the next 16 hours (6.25 mg/kg/hour). The total dose is 300 mg/kg NAC over 20 hours. Many clinicians prolong the initial infusion from 15 to 60 minutes to decrease the rate of early adverse effects, extending the total infusion period to 21 hours (38). The quantity of IV fluid used in children should take into account age and weight, but fluid overload and dilutional hyponatremia remain potential risks in patients under 10-kg body weight.

Prolongation of *N*-Acetylcysteine Treatment

With either oral or IV NAC, the clinical practice has been to continue treatment until the patient substantially improves, dies, or undergoes liver transplant. With oral NAC, the most common technique is to simply continue the maintenance doses (70 mg/kg every 4 hours). For IV NAC, the terminal infusion rate is continued (6.25 mg/kg/hour). There are data that indirectly support this approach, but it is primarily based on the severe outcome balanced against a very small incidence of serious adverse events (7). In practice, the NAC infusion is continued at the 50-mg/kg IV rate until the prothrombin time ratio or international normalized ratio shows significant improvement. The aminotransferase levels then follow suit after a delay.

Chronic Overdose (Repeated Supratherapeutic Ingestion)

Many different NAC regimens have been used. One common approach in the United States is to administer the oral loading dose for acute ingestion (140 mg/kg), followed by the typical maintenance dose (70 mg/kg every 4 hours) until the aspartate aminotransferase and alanine aminotransferase improve, the patient dies, or transplant is performed. An alternative is to give the 20-hour IV European regimen until the prothrombin time ratio or international normalized ratio improves.

Drug-Induced Acute Liver Failure

The dose of NAC for ALF unrelated to acetaminophen has not been established. The dose for acetaminophen-induced liver failure is typically used. Either the oral or IV regimen has been used. Because only the IV dose and formulation have been experimentally tested, however, they are likely the best choice for liver failure.

ADVERSE EFFECTS

A systematic review of 93 English-language articles involving the administration of NAC by the IV route to 2219 patients found that minor adverse events are common. Minor events include flushing, rash, urticaria, and wheezing; they nearly always occur during the initial infusion and resolve within 90 minutes (39,40) at the time when the peak plasma concentration of NAC occurs (16). Asthmatics are at special risk—respiratory arrest during the early stages of an infusion in a previously healthy 17-year-old girl with mild asthma has been reported (41,42). Patients who do not need treatment on the basis of the treatment nomogram seem at particular risk. NAC should therefore only be administered for clear clinical indications.

Serious adverse events have been associated with an iatrogenic overdose of NAC rather than a therapeutic dose. Several deaths were caused by iatrogenic NAC overdoses of two- to tenfold. Commonly, bags of IV NAC are made up incorrectly (43). Serious events were typically treated with vasopressor, discontinuation of the infusion, and administration of diphenhydramine (39). If a patient exhibits a severe reaction to NAC but still needs treatment, an antihistamine may be given and the infusion stopped for 30 to 60 minutes before restarting at a lower rate (50 mg/kg). Nearly all patients were continued on IV NAC therapy without further medications despite their initial reactions. No further events developed. Alternatively, oral NAC may be administered if there is no contraindication.

Hepatotoxicity after combined oral and rectal administration of NAC in high doses (106 g in 3 days) to treat meconium ileus equivalent in a 3-year-old boy with cystic fibrosis has also been observed (44).

Donovan et al. reported sudden onset of respiratory distress with resultant fatal cardiac arrest in a patient with preexisting chronic obstructive pulmonary disease who was given NAC IV (20-hour regimen) for acetaminophen overdose (45). Three deaths after accidental NAC IV overdosage have been reported (30).

PITFALLS

Treatment should not await an acetaminophen measurement if the patient presents more than 8 hours after ingesting an acetaminophen dose of more than 150 mg/kg.

Administration of NAC orally creates the potential for overdose. Overdose by the oral route is much less likely due to the large volume needed.

REFERENCES

1. Meredith TJ, Jacobsen D, Haines JA, Berger JC, eds. *Antidotes for poisoning by paracetamol. IPCS/CEC Evaluation of Antidotes Series, Volume 3.* Cambridge, UK: Cambridge University Press, 1995.
2. Vale JA, Proudfoot AT. Paracetamol (acetaminophen) poisoning. *Lancet* 1995;346:547–552.
3. Crome P, Vale JA, Volans GN, et al. Oral methionine in the treatment of severe paracetamol (acetaminophen) overdose. *Lancet* 1976;2:829–830.
4. Prescott LF. The nephrotoxicity and hepatotoxicity of analgesics. *Brit J Clin Pharmacol* 1979;7:453–462.
5. Corcoran GB, Wong BK. Glutathione in prevention of acetaminophen induced hepatotoxicity by N-acetyl-L-cysteine *in vivo*; studies with N-acetyl-D-cysteine in mice. *J Pharmacol Exp Ther* 1986;238:54–61.
6. Burgunder JM, Varriale A, Lauterberg BH. Effect of N-acetylcysteine on plasma cysteine and glutathione following paracetamol administration. *Eur J Clin Pharmacol* 1989;36:127–131.
7. Keays R, Harrison PM, Wendon JA, et al. Intravenous acetylcysteine in paracetamol induced fulminant hepatic failure: a prospective controlled trial. *BMJ* 1991;303:1026–1029.
8. Jones AL. Mechanism of action and value of N-acetylcysteine in the treatment of early and late acetaminophen poisoning: a critical review. *J Toxicol Clin Toxicol* 1998;36:277–285.
9. Harrison PM, Keays R, Bray GP, et al. Improved outcome of paracetamol-induced fulminant hepatic failure by late administration of acetylcysteine. *Lancet* 1990;335:1572–1573.
10. Walsh TS, Hopton P, Philips BJ, et al. The effect of N-acetylcysteine on oxygen transport and uptake in patients with fulminant hepatic failure. *Hepatology* 1998;27:1332–1340.
11. Devlin J, Ellis AE, McPeake J, et al. N-acetylcysteine improves indocyanine green extraction and oxygen transport during hepatic dysfunction. *Crit Care Med* 1997;25:236–242.
12. Jones AL. Recent advances in the management of late paracetamol (acetaminophen) poisoning. *Emerg Med (Aust)* 2000;12:14–21.
13. Mitchell JR. Acetaminophen toxicity. *N Engl J Med* 1988;319:1601–1602.
14. Bruno MK, Cohen SD, Khairallah EA. Antidotal effectiveness of N-acetylcysteine in reversing acetaminophen-induced hepatotoxicity. Enhancement of the proteolysis of arylated proteins. *Biochem Pharmacol* 1988;37:4319–4325.
15. Sjödin K, Nilsson E, Hallberg A, Tunek A. Metabolism of N-acetyl-L-cysteine: some structural requirements for the deacetylation and consequences for the oral bioavailability. *Biochem Pharmacol* 1989;38:3981–3985.
16. Prescott LF, Donovan JW, Jarvie DR, Proudfoot AT. The disposition and kinetics of intravenous N-acetylcysteine in patients with paracetamol overdosage. *Eur J Clin Pharmacol* 1989;37:501–506.
17. Smilkstein MJ, Knapp GL, Kulig KW, Rumack BH. Efficacy of oral N-acetylcysteine in the treatment of acetaminophen overdose. Analysis of the national multicenter study (1976 to 1985). *N Engl J Med* 1988;319:1557–1562.
18. Rumack BH, Peterson RC, Koch GG, Amara IA. Acetaminophen overdose. 662 cases with evaluation of oral acetylcysteine treatment. *Arch Intern Med* 1981;141:380–385.
19. Riggs BS, Bronstein AC, Kulig K, et al. Acute acetaminophen overdose during pregnancy. *Obstet Gynecol* 1989;74:247–253.
20. Prescott LF. Treatment of severe acetaminophen poisoning with intravenous acetylcysteine. *Arch Intern Med* 1981;141:386–389.
21. Daly FFS, Dart RC, Bogdan GM, et al. Repeated supratherapeutic dosing of acetaminophen (APAP): Can serum transaminase levels predict the risk of hepatotoxicity? *J Toxicol Clin Toxicol* 2000;38:580–581(abst).
22. Lund ME, Banner W, Clarkson TW, Berlin M. Treatment of acute methylmercury ingestion by haemodialysis with N-acetylcysteine (Mucomyst) infusion and 2,3-dimercaptopropanesulphonate. *J Toxicol Clin Toxicol* 1984;22:31–49.
23. Banner W, Koch M, Capin DM, et al. Experimental chelation therapy in chromium, lead and boron intoxication with N-acetylcysteine and other compounds. *Toxicol Appl Pharmacol* 1986;83:142–147.
24. Vassallo S, Howland MA. Severe dichromate poisoning: survival after therapy with IV N-acetylcysteine and hemodialysis. *Vet Hum Toxicol* 1988;30:347.
25. Young RJ, Critchley JA, Young KK, et al. Fatal acute hepatorenal failure following potassium permanganate ingestion. *Hum Exp Toxicol* 1996;15:259–261.
26. Buylaert W, Calle P, De Paepe P, et al. Hepatotoxicity of N,N-dimethylformamide (DMF) in acute poisoning with the veterinary euthanasia drug T-61. *Hum Exp Toxicol* 1996;15:607–611.
27. Martin DS, Willis SE, Cline DM. N-Acetylcysteine in the treatment of human arsenic poisoning. *J Am Board Fam Pract* 1990;3:293–296.
28. Gjonovich A, Del Monte D, Petolillo M, et al. Differences in toxicological pattern of acute poisoning from arsenite and arsenate in the light of an extremely rare case of arsenic pentoxide ingestion. *Trace Element Med* 1990;7:63(abst).
29. Hansen RM, Csuka ME, McCarty DJ, Saryan LA. Gold induced aplastic anaemia. Complete response to corticosteroids, plasmapheresis, and N-acetylcysteine infusion. *J Rheumatol* 1985;12:794–797.
30. Flanagan RJ, Meredith TJ. Use of N-acetylcysteine in clinical toxicology. *Am J Med* 1991;91[Suppl 3C]:131S–119S.
31. Renzi FP, Donovan JW, Martin TG, et al. Concomitant use of activated charcoal and N-acetylcysteine. *Ann Emerg Med* 1985;14:568–572.
32. Ekins BR, Ford DC, Thompson MIB, et al. The effect of activated charcoal on N-acetylcysteine absorption in normal subjects. *Am J Emerg Med* 1987;5:483–487.
33. Brent J. Are activated charcoal–N-acetylcysteine interactions of clinical significance? *Ann Emerg Med* 1993;22:1860–1862.
34. Holdiness MR. Clinical pharmacokinetics of N-acetylcysteine. *Clin Pharmacokinet* 1991;20:123–134.
35. Horowitz RS, Dart RC, Jarvie DR, et al. Placental transfer of N-acetylcysteine following human maternal acetaminophen toxicity. *J Toxicol Clin Toxicol* 1997;35:447–452.
36. Yip L, Dart RC, Hurlbut KM. Intravenous administration of oral N-acetylcysteine. *Crit Care Med* 1998;26:40–43.
37. Price LM, Poklis A, Johnson DE. Fatal acetaminophen poisoning with evidence of subendocardial necrosis of the heart. *J Forensic Sci* 1991;36:930–935.
38. Buckley NA, Whyte IM, O'Connell DL, et al. Oral or intravenous N-acetylcysteine: which is the treatment of choice for acetaminophen (paracetamol) poisoning? *J Toxicol Clin Toxicol* 1999;37:759–767.
39. Dart RC, Bogdan GM. Systematic analysis of medical literature regarding safety of intravenous N-acetylcysteine. Rocky Mountain Poison and Drug Center, 2000 (*unpublished*).
40. Dawson AH, Henry DA, McEwen J. Adverse reactions to N-acetylcysteine during treatment for paracetamol poisoning. *Med J Aust* 1989;150:329–331.
41. Reynard K, Riley A, Walker BE. Respiratory arrest after N-acetylcysteine for paracetamol overdose. *Lancet* 1992;340:675.
42. Schmidt LE, Dalhoff K. Risk factors in the development of adverse reaction to N-acetylcysteine in patients with paracetamol poisoning. *Br J Clin Pharmacol* 2001;51:87–91.
43. Ferner RE, Hutchings A, Anton C, et al. The origin of errors in dosage: acetylcysteine as a paradigm. *Br J Clin Pharmacol* 1999;47:581P.
44. Bailey DJ, Andres JM. Liver injury after oral and rectal administration of N-acetylcysteine for meconium ileus equivalent in a patient with cystic fibrosis. *Pediatrics* 1987;79:281–282.
45. Donovan JW, Proudfoot AT, Prescott LF. Adverse effects of intravenous N-acetylcysteine. *Vet Hum Toxicol* 1986;28:487(abst).

CHAPTER 65

Naloxone, Naltrexone, and Nalmefene

Andrew H. Dawson

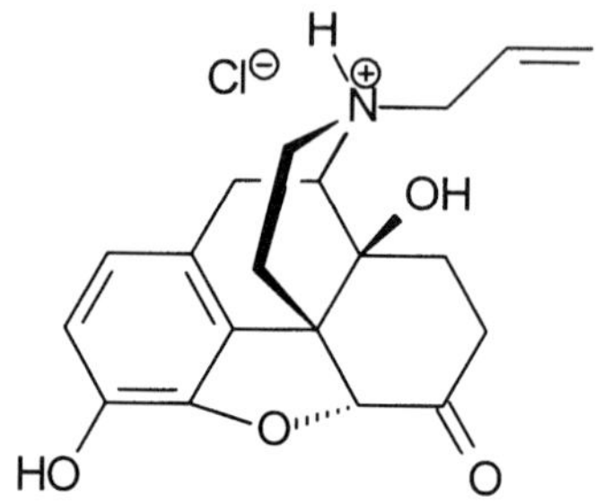

NALOXONE HYDROCHLORIDE

Synonyms:	**Naloxone hydrochloride (Narcan); naltrexone hydrochloride (Nalorex, ReVia, Trexan); nalmefene (Revex)**
Molecular formula and weight:	**Naloxone ($C_{19}H_{21}NO_4$, HCl, $2H_2O$) 399.9 g/mol; naltrexone ($C_{20}H_{23}NO_4$, HCl) 377.9 g/mol; nalmefene ($C_{21}H_{25}NO_3$, HCl) 375.9 g/mol**
CAS Registry No.:	**Naloxone, HCl 51481-60-8; Naltrexone, HCl 16676-29-2; Nalmefene, HCl 58895-64-0**
Therapeutic levels:	**Not clinically applicable**
Special concerns:	**A large dose of an opioid antagonist may precipitate opioid withdrawal.**

OVERVIEW

Naloxone, naltrexone, and nalmefene are synthetic opioid antagonists with high affinity for the μ and κ opioid receptors. The different indications for clinical use are a result of their pharmacokinetic differences.

Naloxone has the longest history of clinical use. Multiple human studies demonstrate that naloxone successfully reverses opioid-induced respiratory depression and has little risk. Most studies were performed in postoperative patients (1–3) or in prehospital and hospital treatment of recreational opioid overdose (4,5).

Naloxone HCl is provided as an aqueous solution (0.02 mg/ml, 0.4 mg/ml, or 1 mg/ml) that is compatible with crystalloidal solutions. Naltrexone is a 50-mg oral tablet primarily used to maintain abstinence in opioid and alcohol dependence. It has no role in the treatment of acute opioid toxicity; however, its inappropriate use in opioid-dependent patients may lead to a severe and protracted withdrawal reaction. Nalmefene is provided as a 0.1-mg/ml or 1-mg/ml aqueous solution. It has an adjunctive role in the treatment of alcohol dependency. It is not first-line therapy but may be of use in acute opioid toxicity when a long duration of antagonist effect is required.

PHARMACOKINETICS AND PHARMACODYNAMICS

All three compounds are absorbed orally but are subject to significant first-pass metabolism. Hepatic metabolism is predominately by glucuronide conjugation. The rapid onset and relatively short duration of clinical effect for naloxone probably reflect more rapid movement into and out of the central nervous system compared to morphine (6).

Nalmefene is metabolized to an inactive glucuronide. Nalmefene and naloxone appear to be equipotent (7). Nalmefene pharmacokinetics are linear; thus, peak concentration increases with increasing dose but no change exists in elimination half-life (8). Both naltrexone and nalmefene may undergo enterohepatic circulation. Naltrexone has an active metabolite, 6-β-naltrexol, which may contribute to its therapeutic effects. Elimination half-life for each drug is provided in Table 1.

INDICATIONS

Acute opioid toxicity is the primary indication for the use of naloxone. Nalmefene is also approved for this indication; however, its pharmacokinetics may make it difficult to titrate an appropriate dose. Kaplan et al. demonstrated similar efficacy between naloxone (2 mg) and nalmefene (1 mg and 2 mg) without an apparent advantage (9). The rate of withdrawal reactions was high in both groups. Naloxone remains the drug of choice for initial treatment. Nalmefene may have a role for opioids with a long duration of action. The major predictor for a response to

TABLE 1. Elimination half-life for opioid receptor antagonists

Compound	Half-life (h)
Naloxone	1
Naltrexone	4
6-β-naltrexol	13
Nalmefene	10

naloxone is a strong clinical history of opioid use and respiratory depression. In the absence of these features, pinpoint pupils alone were less predictive of a response.

Anecdotal reports suggest that naloxone may be effective in septic shock, but randomized trials do not support this use. Naloxone has also been proposed for treatment of a wide variety of intoxications from nonopioid medications, including valproate, alcohol intoxication, clonidine, and angiotensin-converting enzyme inhibitors. There is insufficient evidence to support the routine use of naloxone in nonopioid intoxication.

CAUTIONS AND CONTRAINDICATIONS

Opioid antagonists should be used with caution in patients with hypoxia, hypercapnia, underlying cardiorespiratory disease, or history of opioid dependency. Adverse events (e.g., pulmonary edema, seizure, dysrhythmia) may be more common in these groups.

The elimination of nalmefene is prolonged in renal failure.

Naloxone is U.S. Food and Drug Administration pregnancy category B, naltrexone is category C, and nalmefene is category B (Appendix I).

DOSE AND ADMINISTRATION

In a patient with respiratory depression but measurable blood pressure, there is no difference in response rate between intravenous (IV) or intramuscular administration (5). A randomized trial showed no difference in the time needed to achieve a respiratory rate of 10 breaths/minute when comparing 0.8 mg subcutaneous naloxone and 0.4 mg IV naloxone when IV access had to be established by paramedical staff. Additional naloxone was required in 15% of the subcutaneous group and 35% of the IV group.

Intralingual use is also effective but may be associated with bleeding that is difficult to control and presents a biohazard (10). Endotracheal administration is also effective and has a kinetic profile similar to IV administration (11). Based on the current evidence, the intramuscular route is preferred unless IV access is already available.

The dose of naloxone administered to poisoned patients has been driven largely by clinical protocols. The high incidence of adverse events in these studies (15% to 30%) suggests that overtreatment with antagonists is common (5,9). A prospective study using titrated doses of 0.1 mg reported an estimated incidence of serious adverse events below 3%. The median treatment dose required was 0.2 mg (12). In patients who can be adequately ventilated, the IV dose of naloxone should be titrated at 0.1 mg every 3 minutes. When there are practical difficulties in assisting ventilation, a larger dose of 0.4 mg should be given. For most patients, the goal is to achieve adequate spontaneous respiration without causing opioid withdrawal.

Although doses of naloxone of up to 10 mg have been used to antagonize some synthetic opioids in practice, the need for such doses is rare. If the patient does not respond to 2.0 mg, it is likely that opioids are not the cause or that the patient has a concurrent condition (e.g., sedative drugs or cerebral hypoxia).

Recurrence of opioid toxicity has been reported to occur in one-third of patients, most commonly with long-acting opioids (13). Long-acting opioids include controlled-release preparations (prolonged absorption phase) and those with a long elimination half-life such as methadone. Patients with renal failure may also have a long duration of toxicity due to the accumulation of active glucuronide metabolites of morphine. If prolonged opioid antagonism is clinically appropriate, a continuous infusion of naloxone may be useful. An effective starting regimen is to titrate a bolus of naloxone to achieve an adequate clinical response, then to use two-thirds of that dose each hour as a continuous infusion (14).

MONITORING

Prolonged ongoing careful cardiorespiratory monitoring of the patient is required in all patients treated with an opioid antagonist. Patients who have ingested controlled-release preparations may not reach peak concentrations until 24 hours after ingestion and may need further bolus injections and increased continuous infusion rates.

ADVERSE EVENTS

Similar adverse drugs reactions occur with each of the agents. With the exception of acute narcotic withdrawal, serious events are extremely rare. Adverse events include well-documented reports of sudden death (pulmonary edema, seizures, and asystole) occurring in the postoperative period in which a causal relationship is likely. Such reactions have been more frequently reported in the acutely poisoned patient, but causality has been more difficult to establish because of confounders like medication coingestion and respiratory complications directly related to opioid toxicity. Coingestion of cocaine may be a risk factor for these adverse reactions (15,16).

One putative mechanism for naloxone-related adverse events is excess catecholamine release. Increased catecholamine release is well documented in opioid antagonist-induced narcotic withdrawal. It has also been demonstrated in nonopioid-dependent animal models. The animal models show that catecholamine release is greatly enhanced in the presence of hypercapnea. Maintaining normo- or hypocapnea reduces naloxone-induced catecholamine release and hemodynamic instability in these models (17). Although this technique has not been tested clinically, it would seem prudent to correct hypercapnea and hypoxia before and during opioid reversal whenever possible. This may be of particular importance in high-risk patients such as patients with coexistent cardiac disease, sudden reversal of analgesia, or recreational drug users who also use sympathomimetics such as amphetamine and cocaine.

The most frequently reported adverse reaction is acute behavioral disturbance, which ranges from anger to delirium. These reactions are generally associated with physical signs of acute opioid withdrawal. In prospective studies, the incidence ranges from 15% to 30%. They occur more commonly as the dose of antagonist is increased, suggesting that careful titration of antagonist dose should decrease the incidence (12).

PITFALLS

The duration of the withdrawal syndrome induced by naloxone is less than 1 hour and is not life threatening. However, the associated behavioral disturbance increases the risk of health workers being assaulted.

REFERENCES

1. Drummond GB, Davie IT, Scott DB. Naloxone: dose-dependent antagonism of respiratory depression by fentanyl in anaesthetized patients. *Br J Anaesth* 1977;49(2):151–154.
2. Gerhardt T, Bancalari E, Cohen H, et al. Use of nalotone to reverse narcotic respiratory depression in the newborn infant. *J Pediatr* 1977;90(6):1009–1012.

3. Tigerstedt I. Reversal of fentanyl-induced narcotic depression with naloxone following general anaesthesia. *Acta Anaesthesiol Scand* 1978;22(3):234–240.
4. Wanger K, Brough L, Macmillan I, et al. Intravenous vs subcutaneous naloxone for out-of-hospital management of presumed opioid overdose [see comments]. *Acad Emerg Med* 1998;5(4):293–299.
5. Sporer KA, Firestone J, Isaacs SM. Out-of-hospital treatment of opioid overdoses in an urban setting [see comments]. *Acad Emerg Med* 1996;3(7):660–667.
6. Ngai SH, Berkowitz BA, Yang JC, et al. Pharmacokinetics of naloxone in rats and in man: basis for its potency and short duration of action. *Anesthesiology* 1976;44(5):398–401.
7. Glass PS, Jhaveri RM, Smith LR. Comparison of potency and duration of action of nalmefene and naloxone. *Anesth Analg* 1994;78(3):536–541.
8. Dixon R, Howes J, Gentile J, et al. Nalmefene: intravenous safety and kinetics of a new opioid antagonist. *Clin Pharmacol Ther* 1986;39(1):49–53.
9. Kaplan JL, Marx JA, Calabro JJ, et al. Double-blind, randomized study of nalmefene and naloxone in emergency department patients with suspected narcotic overdose. *Ann Emerg Med* 1999;34(1):42–50.
10. Wasserberger J, Ordog GJ, Kolodny M. Intralingual naloxone injections. *Ann Emerg Med* 1988;17(8):874–875.
11. Tandberg D, Abercrombie D. Treatment of heroin overdose with endotracheal naloxone. *Ann Emerg Med* 1982;11(8):443–445.
12. Osterwalder JJ. Naloxone—for intoxications with intravenous heroin and heroin mixtures—harmless or hazardous? A prospective clinical study [see comments]. *J Toxicol Clin Toxicol* 1996;34(4):409–416.
13. Watson WA, Steele MT, Muelleman RL, et al. Opioid toxicity recurrence after an initial response to naloxone. *J Toxicol Clin Toxicol* 1998;36(1–2):11–17.
14. Goldfrank L, Weisman RS, Errick JK, et al. A dosing nomogram for continuous infusion intravenous naloxone. *Ann Emerg Med* 1986;15(5):566–570.
15. Byck R, Ruskis A, Ungerer J, et al. Naloxone potentiates cocaine effect in man. *Psychopharmacol Bull* 1982;18(4):214–215.
16. Merigian KS. Cocaine-induced ventricular arrhythmias and rapid atrial fibrillation temporally related to naloxone administration. *Am J Emerg Med* 1993;11(1):96–97.
17. Mills CA, Flacke JW, Miller JD, et al. Cardiovascular effects of fentanyl reversal by naloxone at varying arterial carbon dioxide tensions in dogs. *Anesth Analg* 1999;67:730–736.

CHAPTER 66

Octreotide

Steven A. McLaughlin and Patrick E. McKinney

D-Phe-Cys-Phe-D-Trp-Lys-Thr-Cys-NH—CH(CH$_2$OH)—CH(OH)—CH$_3$

OCTREOTIDE

Molecular formula and weight:	**$C_{49}H_{66}N_{10}O_{10}S_2$, x $C_2H_4O_2$; 1019.2 g/mol**
CAS Registry No.:	**79517-01-4**
Normal or therapeutic levels:	**Not applicable**
Special concerns:	**Octreotide should not be used without glucose; it does not produce an immediate increase in blood glucose concentrations.**

OVERVIEW

Severe and recurrent hypoglycemia refractory to glucose therapy may occur during sulfonylurea toxicity (Chapter 158) (1–3). A number of agents have been proposed as *antidotes* for sulfonylurea-induced rebound hypoglycemia, including corticosteroids, glucagon, diazoxide, and octreotide (2,4–6). Corticosteroids do not provide a prompt or reliable hyperglycemic response and are not recommended. Glucagon and diazoxide are difficult to administer and have clinically significant side effects. Glucagon often induces vomiting and may be ineffective if glycogen stores have been depleted. Diazoxide may precipitate hypotension. Only diazoxide and octreotide act by inhibiting the release of insulin from the sulfonylurea-primed pancreatic beta cells, thus directly antagonizing the hypoglycemic action of sulfonylureas. These two antidotes may be useful after the initial hypoglycemia is reversed with dextrose. They may be used to prevent recurrent hypoglycemia, which may decrease or abolish the need for supplemental glucose.

Octreotide is a synthetic analog of the hormone somatostatin. First synthesized in 1980, it is a cyclic octapeptide that mimics many of the effects of somatostatin (7,8). It is normally used for treatment of acromegaly and many other endocrine disorders due to its inhibition of growth hormone, insulin, and glucagon secretion. Octreotide is a more potent and selective inhibitor of insulin, growth hormone, and glucagon secretion than the native hormone and has a half-life of 1.5 hours as compared to 3 minutes for somatostatin (7,9).

Forms Available

Octreotide acetate is available as a solution for subcutaneous injection or intravenous infusion in 50, 100, 200, 500, and 1000 μg glass ampules and multidose vials. A new long-acting suspension is available for depot intramuscular injection (Sandostatin LAR). This long-acting formulation has not been used for treatment of sulfonylurea overdose and is not recommended.

Mechanism of Action

Sulfonylureas produce hypoglycemia by binding to the sulfonylurea receptor (SUR1) on pancreatic beta cells. The SUR1 receptor is associated with an adenosine triphosphate–dependent K^+ channel (10). Sulfonylurea agents inactivate these K^+ channels, which decreases K^+ efflux (11). This is followed by depolarization of the beta cell, opening of voltage-gated Ca^{2+} channels, and subsequent release of preformed insulin (12).

Pancreatic insulin release in response to hyperglycemia is also augmented through this mechanism. This augmented insulin release is responsible for the rebound hypoglycemia seen after glucose therapy in sulfonylurea-poisoned patients.

Octreotide suppresses insulin, growth hormone, and glucagon secretion to basal levels despite stimulation secondary to hyper- or hypoglycemia, respectively (7). Octreotide binds to a second sulfonylurea receptor (SUR2) on pancreatic beta cells, which is coupled to a voltage-gated calcium channel via a G-protein (13,14). Octreotide binding inhibits calcium influx through this channel, thereby reducing the secretion of insulin in response to depolarization.

In glipizide-poisoned volunteers, octreotide was superior to diazoxide in maintaining normal blood glucose concentrations (5). In addition, octreotide effectively suppressed insulin concentrations to baseline levels as compared to the dramatically elevated insulin concentrations measured in the groups treated with diazoxide or glucose. Octreotide has also been used successfully for sulfonylurea-induced hypoglycemia in case reports (1,3–5,15–17). In a retrospective series of nine patients, octreotide greatly reduced the frequency of sulfonylurea-induced hypoglycemia (2). The number of hypoglycemic events recorded per patient before octreotide (mean = 3.2) was greater than the number of hypoglycemic events recorded per patient after octreotide (mean = 0.2), suggesting that octreotide is an effective antidote for recurrent hypoglycemia in this setting (2).

INDICATIONS

Octreotide is indicated for the treatment of sulfonylurea-induced hypoglycemia that recurs after initial glucose therapy. Octreotide appears to be more effective than diazoxide in suppressing insulin secretion and decreasing the need for supplemental glucose in this setting (5). It may also be useful in the treatment of quinine-induced hypoglycemia (18). In the authors' opinion, patients with a history of sulfonylurea exposure but without documented or suspected hypoglycemia can be observed without the need for octreotide administration. Octreotide therapy in patients with a single episode of hypoglycemia that responds to glucose is an option for the conservative clinician. Because of its efficacy and lack of significant side effects during short-term use, octreotide is strongly recommended in patients with even a single episode of recurrent hypoglycemia after initial glucose therapy (2).

Failure of octreotide therapy should suggest inadequate dosing, premature cessation of octreotide therapy, or hypoglycemia due to causes other than sulfonylurea ingestion.

CAUTIONS AND CONTRAINDICATIONS

The only absolute contraindication is hypersensitivity to octreotide. At doses used for the treatment of sulfonylurea overdose, side effects are rare. Octreotide therapy may decrease serum levels and clinical efficacy of cyclosporine. Antidiabetic medications may need to be adjusted in diabetics treated with octreotide.

Octreotide has not been approved by the U.S. Food and Drug Administration for use in children, although there is extensive literature supporting its safety and efficacy in treating pediatric hyperinsulinism (19). Octreotide is U.S. Food and Drug Administration pregnancy category B (Appendix I). Data regarding its use in breast-feeding mothers are lacking.

DOSAGE AND METHOD OF ADMINISTRATION

The optimal dose and duration of octreotide therapy for the treatment of sulfonylurea-induced hypoglycemia have not been clearly defined. Octreotide is most often given as a single subcutaneous injection. In published cases in which a single dose of octreotide was used, doses ranged from 50 to 100 μg in adults and 25 μg in children (3,16,17). Children treated with octreotide for other indications have tolerated doses from 1 to 10 μg/kg without significant side effects (19,20).

Octreotide can also be given as a continuous intravenous infusion in any crystalloid solution. Reported infusion rates in adults range from 100 to 125 μg/hour (1,2). Constant intravenous infusion rates of 30 to 60 ng/kg/minute have been used in adults in research protocols. Mild gastrointestinal symptoms were reported at these higher doses (5,7). Maximal insulin suppression appears to occur at doses of 125 μg/hour or less in adults (7).

The duration of effect of a single subcutaneous dose of 50 to 100 μg of octreotide in sulfonylurea-induced hypoglycemia is not known and likely depends on the severity of the overdose and multiple host factors such as renal and hepatic function (4). The most commonly recommended dosing interval is 12 hours (5,20), and in one case series of nine patients, recurrence of hypoglycemia did not occur within 12 hours of octreotide administration (2). Case reports have described octreotide doses ranging from 50 to 100 μg repeated every 6 to 12 hours over a 24- to 36-hour period (2,4,15).

A reasonable approach for adults is to give 50 to 100 μg of octreotide subcutaneously every 8 to 12 hours and base the duration of treatment on the factors described previously. In most cases of hypoglycemia due to second-generation sulfonylureas, duration of therapy is 24 hours or less. Large overdose or overdoses with extended-release preparations or chlorpropamide may produce hypoglycemia that persists for days or, rarely, weeks (21).

A suggested pediatric starting dose is 25 to 50 μg by subcutaneous injection (3,19,20). A pediatric dose of 1 μg/kg by subcutaneous injection has also been proposed (20). In cases of hypoglycemia refractory to this therapy, a continuous octreotide infusion of 125 μg/hour in adults or 15 ng/kg/minute in children should provide maximal insulin suppression with minimal side effects (1,5,7,20).

Patients treated with octreotide should be serially monitored by clinical observation and glucose testing for hypoglycemia. Most patients should be hospitalized in a monitored setting with close observation. More serious overdoses should be admitted to an appropriate intensive care unit. Existing data do not yet support outpatient management of sulfonylurea-induced hypoglycemia.

ADVERSE EFFECTS

The most frequent side effect of short-term octreotide use is mild steatorrhea, with associated nausea, abdominal cramps, flatulence, and diarrhea (22). These effects start within hours of treatment with octreotide and are dose related (5,7,23). Seven percent of patients have reported mild, transient pain at the site of injection, which resolved within 15 minutes (23).

Long-term use appears to be associated with an increased incidence of gallstone formation (19,23,24). This effect has not been reported with short-term use.

Bradycardia can occur during octreotide administration in up to 21% of patients (25). Reports of bradycardia occur primarily in patients receiving higher doses of octreotide for acromegaly; however, bradycardia has been reported in patients receiving a single 100-μg subcutaneous dose. The mechanism of octreotide-induced bradycardia is unclear but may be related to changes in hepatic blood flow (25). There are no reports of clinically significant side effects from octreotide-induced bradycardia.

Paradoxical hypoglycemia after octreotide administration has been reported in the setting of an insulinoma in a single case (26). Patients with an insulinoma may become dependent on glucagon-stimulated gluconeogenesis for maintenance of euglycemia. Hypoglycemia may theoretically occur after octreotide suppresses glucagon release in these patients (26). Although data are limited, paradoxical hypoglycemia has not been reported with octreotide use in sulfonylurea overdose. If paradoxical hypoglycemia were observed in this setting, glucagon administration may be theoretically useful.

PITFALLS

Potential pitfalls during octreotide use include failure to reverse hypoglycemia with dextrose before or concurrently with octreotide administration. Octreotide itself does not immediately reverse hypoglycemia and must be used in conjunction with supplemental intravenous dextrose.

Octreotide administration does not supplant the need for vigilant monitoring for hypoglycemia.

Octreotide is not effective in reversing hypoglycemia due to exogenous insulin administration.

The sustained-release form of octreotide should not be used for treatment of sulfonylurea toxicity.

REFERENCES

1. Bui L, Alder D, Keller KH. Prolonged octreotide infusion to treat glyburide-induced hypoglycemia. *J Toxicol Clin Toxicol* 2000;38:576(abst).
2. McLaughlin SA, Crandall CS, McKinney PE. Octreotide: an antidote for sulfonylurea-induced hypoglycemia. *Ann Emerg Med* 2000;36:133–138.
3. Mordel A, Sivilotti MLA, Old AC, et al. Octreotide for pediatric sulfonylurea poisoning. *J Toxicol Clin Toxicol* 1998;36:437(abst).
4. Krentz AJ, Boyle PJ, Justice KM, et al. Successful treatment of severe refractory sulfonylurea-induced hypoglycemia with octreotide. *Diabetes Care* 1993;16:184–186.
5. Boyle PJ, Justice K, Krentz AJ, et al. Octreotide reverses hyperinsulinemia and prevents hypoglycemia induced by sulfonylurea overdoses. *J Clin Endocrinol Metab* 1993;76:752–756.
6. Palatnick W, Meatherall RC, Tenenbein M. Clinical spectrum of sulfonylurea overdose and experience with diazoxide therapy. *Arch Intern Med* 1991;151:1859–1862.
7. Krentz AJ, Boyle PJ, Macdonald LM, et al. Octreotide: a long-acting inhibitor of endogenous hormone secretion for human metabolic investigations. *Metabolism* 1994;43:24–31.
8. Pless J, Bauer W, Briner U, et al. Chemistry and pharmacology of SMS 201-995, a long-acting octapeptide analogue of somatostatin. *Scand J Gastroenterol* 1986;21:54–64.
9. Vershoor L, Uitterlinden P, Lamberts SWJ, et al. On the use of a new somatostatin analogue in the treatment of hypoglycaemia in patients with insulinoma. *Clin Endocrinol* 1986;25:555–560.
10. Ashcroft FM, Gribble FM. ATP-sensitive K^+ channels and insulin secretion: their roles in health and disease. *Diabetologia* 1999;42:903–919.
11. Schmidt-Antomarchi H, De Weille J, Fosset M, et al. The receptor for antidiabetic sulfonylureas controls the activity of the ATP-modulated K^+ channel in insulin-secreting cells. *J Biol Chem* 1987;262:15840–15844.
12. Nelson TY, Gaines KL, Rajan AS, et al. Increased cytosolic calcium: a signal for sulfonylurea-stimulated insulin release from beta cells. *J Biol Chem* 1987;262:2608–2612.
13. Hsu WH, Xiang HD, Rajan AS, et al. Somatostatin inhibits insulin secretion by a g-protein-mediated decrease in calcium entry through voltage-dependent calcium channels in the beta cell. *J Biol Chem* 1991;266:837–843.
14. Moldovan S, Atiya A, Adrian TE, et al. Somatostatin inhibits B-cell secretion via a subtype-2 somatostatin receptor in the isolated perfused human pancreas. *J Surg Res* 1995;59:85–90.
15. Graudins A, Linden CH, Ferm RP. Diagnosis and treatment of sulfonylurea-induced hyperinsulinemic hypoglycemia [Letter]. *Am J Emerg Med* 1997;15:95–96.
16. Braatvedt GD. Octreotide for the treatment of sulphonylurea induced hypoglycemia in type 2 diabetes. *N Z Med J* 1997;110:189–190.
17. Hung O, Eng J, Ho J, et al. Octreotide as an antidote for refractory sulfonylurea hypoglycemia. *J Toxicol Clin Toxicol* 1997;35:540–541.
18. Phillips RE, Looareesuwan S, Bloom SR, et al. Effectiveness of SMS 201-995, a synthetic, long-acting somatostatin analogue, in treatment of quinine-induced hyperinsulinaemia. *Lancet* 1986;1:713–716.
19. Barrons RW. Octreotide in hyperinsulinism. *Ann Pharmacother* 1997;31:239–241.
20. Spiller HA. Management of sulfonylurea ingestions. *Pediatr Emerg Care* 1999;15:227–230.
21. Ciechanowski K, Borowiak KS, Potocka BA, et al. Chlorpropamide toxicity with survival despite 27-day hypoglycemia. *J Toxicol Clin Toxicol* 1999;37:869–871.
22. Rosenberg JM. Octreotide: a synthetic analog of somatostatin. *Drug Intell Clin Pharm* 1988;22:748–754.
23. Wass JAH, Popovic V, Chayvialle JA. Proceedings of the discussion, "tolerability and safety of Sandostatin." *Metabolism* 1992;41:80–82.
24. Dowling RH, Hussaini SH, Murphy GM, et al. Gallstones during octreotide therapy. *Metabolism* 1992;41:22–33.
25. Wilinsky MP, Berndt EM. Octreotide acetate (Sandostatin)-induced bradycardia: a case report. *Hosp Pharm* 1997;32:1359–1361.
26. Gama R, Marks V, Wright J, et al. Octreotide exacerbated fasting hypoglycemia in a patient with a proinsulinoma; the glucostatic importance of pancreatic glucagon. *Clin Endocrinol* 1995;43:117–120.

CHAPTER 67

Physostigmine and Pyridostigmine

Steven A. Seifert

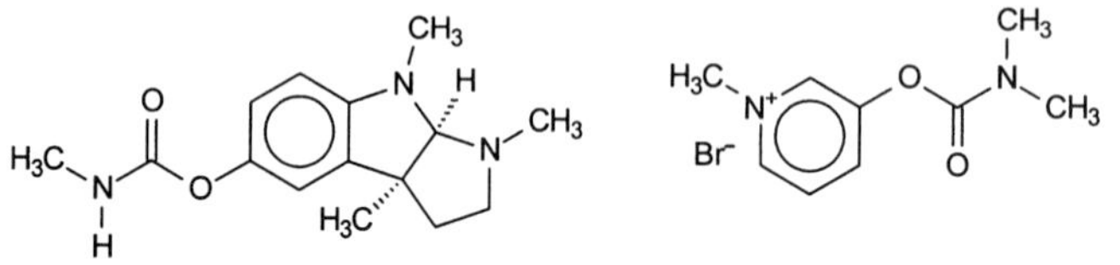

PHYSOSTIGMINE	PYRIDOSTIGMINE
Molecular formula and weight:	**$C_{15}H_{21}N_3O_2$, $C_7H_6O_3$; 413.5 g/mol**
SI conversion:	**mg/L × 2.4 = μmol/L**
CAS Registry No.:	**57-64-7**
Normal or therapeutic levels:	**Not applicable**
Special concerns:	**Administration of high doses may cause cholinergic syndrome. Physostigmine can cause nonspecific arousal and the appearance of partial improvement in patients without anticholinergic toxicity.**

OVERVIEW

There are numerous medications with anticholinergic effects, including anticholinergic agents, antihistamines, phenothiazines, cyclic antidepressants (CA), and antiparkinsonian drugs. Common plant sources include jimsonweed, deadly nightshade, mushrooms, and others. Physostigmine and pyridostigmine are cholinergic agents that act by inhibition of acetylcholinesterase (AChE), decreasing the destruction of acetylcholine at cholinergic synaptic junctions and thereby increasing the transmission of nerve impulses. The degree of cholinesterase inhibition and the location of action determine the effects of these agents.

Physostigmine is a cholinergic agonist, capable of reversible binding to cholinesterase and of reversing anticholinergic effects of drugs. It is a tertiary amine (uncharged) that can cross the blood–brain barrier and is therefore effective centrally and peripherally. It is used routinely in the operating room to reverse the peripheral anticholinergic effects of preoperative anticholinergic agents, to reverse neuromuscular blockade, and as a treatment of closed-angle glaucoma. It is also used antidotally in reversing central anticholinergic syndrome. Because of potentially life-threatening adverse effects, the use of physostigmine to reverse peripheral and central anticholinergic effects of drugs in overdose is controversial.

Pyridostigmine is a monoquaternary amine cholinergic agonist typically active only peripherally (1). Pyridostigmine is used in the treatment of myasthenia gravis and as a pretreatment to protect against possible nerve agent toxicity (2).

Forms Available

Physostigmine for intravenous (IV) injection (Antilirium) is available in 2-ml ampules, 1 mg/ml; vehicle of sodium metabisulfite 0.1%; benzyl alcohol 2.0% as a preservative; in water.

Pyridostigmine bromide is available as a syrup [Mestinon (ICN) 60 mg/5 ml in 5% alcohol]; tablet [Mestinon (ICN) 60 mg]; timespan tablet [Mestinon (ICN) 180 mg]; and for injection [Regonol (Organon) 5 mg/ml in 2- or 5-ml vials].

Mechanism of Action

Physostigmine is a carbamate anticholinesterase derived from the Calabar bean of *Physostigma venenosum*. It is lipophilic, crosses the blood–brain barrier, and is effective centrally and peripherally. It reversibly inhibits AChE at the skeletal neuromuscular junction and at central nervous system (CNS) cholinergic synaptic junctions, allowing acetylcholine to accumulate and competitively reverse muscarinic receptor inhibition. Physostigmine is administered IV and has an onset of action within minutes. The half-life of physostigmine is short, with an effective duration of action of 20 to 60 minutes (1).

Pyridostigmine is a carbamate anticholinesterase. It acts by reversibly inhibiting AChE at the skeletal neuromuscular junction. When used as prophylaxis for war nerve gases, it competes with the nerve agent for binding to AChE (3). Certain types of stresses increase the permeability of the blood–brain barrier to pyridostigmine in some animal models, which may explain reports of CNS symptoms and signs after pyridostigmine use in humans (4–7). Pyridostigmine has a half-life of 3.7 hours after oral administration and is mainly excreted unchanged by the kidney (80% to 90%) (8–10). Lower doses may be needed in patients with renal disease.

INDICATIONS

Physostigmine

Physostigmine is used diagnostically to identify anticholinergic agitated delirium, and therapeutically for anticholinergic effects (Chapter 10). Because of controversy regarding its use, criteria to guide its diagnostic or antidotal use are proposed (Table 1).

TABLE 1. Criteria for using physostigmine (diagnostic/therapeutic)

Diagnostic
- Is this possibly an anticholinergic poisoning or central anticholinergic syndrome?
- Will a positive physostigmine challenge test alter the care of this patient? For example, will clearing of the sensorium avoid a lumbar puncture, head computed tomography, reassure a frantic family, etc.?
- Is this definitely not a cyclic antidepressant poisoning?
- Is physostigmine being given in an appropriate clinical setting (ability to treat seizure or control airway, if necessary)?

Therapeutic
- Is this definitely anticholinergic poisoning? (Have other relatively common etiologies been excluded, such as hallucinogens, etc.?)
- Do the signs and symptoms present really need to be treated? Have they been resistant to standard therapies? Is the benefit to risk ratio in favor of physostigmine?
- Is this definitely not cyclic antidepressant poisoning?
- Is there no bradycardia, and is the QRS duration <100?
- Is physostigmine being given in an appropriate clinical setting (ability to treat seizure or control airway, if necessary)?

DIAGNOSTIC USE

Administration of physostigmine to a patient with anticholinergic syndrome often returns the mental status to normal. An accurate history can then be obtained, confirming the source of symptoms and signs and potentially avoiding a lumbar puncture, head computed tomography, and other diagnostic tests (11).

THERAPEUTIC USE

The duration of action for physostigmine is relatively short compared with anticholinergic toxins. If anticholinergic toxicity recurs, multiple doses or an infusion may be needed to maintain the effect. This is a risk-benefit decision for the individual provider. Repeated use increases the complexity of care and may increase the risk of adverse effects. On the other hand, the agitated patient is subject to complications: sedation, the risk of aspiration, and the need for advanced airway support with alternative therapies (e.g., benzodiazepines) (11).

Physostigmine has been used for toxic agitated delirium of numerous etiologies—belladonna (12), jimsonweed (*Datura stramonium*) (13, phenothiazines (12), ketamine anesthesia (14,15), midazolam (16,17), γ-hydroxybutyrate (GHB) (18–20), heroin (21), and woody nightshade (*Solanum dulcamara*) (22)—and may be useful in reversing propofol anesthesia (23).

Other uses include patients with presumed anticholinergic-induced repetitive or long-lasting seizures, severe sinus or supraventricular tachycardia, or hyperthermia unresponsive to mechanical cooling (24). Physostigmine has been used to reverse the central anticholinergic syndrome that may develop after the use of general anesthetics and other agents (25). Unconsciousness attributed to central anticholinergic syndrome was reversed by physostigmine (40 mg/kg) in an 8-year-old boy after sevoflurane anesthesia, without adverse reactions or recurrence of symptoms (26). Because peripheral anticholinergic manifestations are usually lacking in central anticholinergic syndrome, the diagnosis has been based on the response to physostigmine and the presumption that its cholinergic CNS effects are responsible for the beneficial results.

Pyridostigmine

Pyridostigmine is a component of the Nerve Agent Pre-Treatment System of the United Kingdom (27) and was used as a prophylactic treatment during the Persian Gulf War (2). Pyridostigmine and physostigmine were effective protective treatments against sarin intoxication in a mouse model (28). Pyridostigmine does not reverse the action of nerve agents and is only effective as an adjunct to other antidotal medications

(29). Pyridostigmine has also been used to reverse near vision impairment after transdermal hyoscine use (30).

CAUTIONS AND CONTRAINDICATIONS

Physostigmine

The use of physostigmine for treatment of anticholinergic toxicity is controversial (31,32). The primary concern is its short duration of effects compared to the agent-causing delirium.

TRICYCLIC ANTIDEPRESSANTS

Retrospective reports implicate physostigmine as a potential precipitant of abrupt cardiovascular collapse (seizure and ventricular dysrhythmia) in patients with severe tricyclic antidepressant (TCA) poisoning (24,33–41). The temporal relationship with physostigmine administration suggests at least an additive effect to the seizure risk of the TCA. Between 9% and 12% of patients have been reported to have seizures thought secondary to physostigmine use (35,36). However, it is possible that some fatalities attributed to physostigmine in severe TCA overdosage were the natural progression of TCA toxicity (42).

Animal studies of the TCA-physostigmine interaction have produced some evidence for improvement of TCA-induced electrocardiogram (ECG) changes in dogs (43) but not in cats (44) or rabbits (45). A rat study showed reduced early mortality, but there was no difference by 96 hours (46).

A retrospective study compared physostigmine and benzodiazepines for the treatment of anticholinergic agitation and delirium. Physostigmine was more effective, controlling agitation and reversing delirium in 96% and 87% of patients, respectively. In contrast, benzodiazepines controlled agitation in 24% and were ineffective in controlling delirium. Patients treated initially with physostigmine had significantly fewer complications and shorter recovery times. Side effects and length of stay were not different (11). However, the study design and small enrollment of CA patients leave the issue of safety open.

Various protocols have proposed criteria to reduce potential physostigmine cardiac complications: a 12-lead ECG with right axis deviation, a QTc interval greater than 440 milliseconds, a QRS duration greater than 100 milliseconds (all markers of CA toxicity) (15), other signs of severe CA overdose (11,31), in patients with ingestion of a known CA or similar agents with a higher risk of seizure (amoxapine, maprotiline, pheniramine, dothiepin), in the unknown overdose setting (32) with bradycardia, and in patients with a known underlying seizure disorder or risk factors (31).

It seems prudent to avoid physostigmine if there is ECG evidence of high-dose CA overdose, in the acute phase of a CA or unknown anticholinergic poisoning, with other agents producing significant cardiac conduction abnormalities, and in bradycardic patients. Other situations in which physostigmine should be used with caution in several patient groups: asthma, peripheral vascular disease, intestinal or bladder obstruction, receiving neuromuscular blockers that are metabolized by a cholinesterase, and when the risk of seizure is increased.

γ-HYDROXYBUTYRATE

The use of physostigmine in GHB toxicity lacks a mechanistic basis and is without sufficient supporting data. GHB is not known to affect acetylcholine-mediated nerve transmission (47). Patients who have overdosed on GHB awaken spontaneously after a relatively short period of time, and the temporal relationship between physostigmine administration and awakening may be coincidental.

PREGNANCY

Physostigmine is U.S. Food and Drug Administration pregnancy category C.

CONTRAINDICATIONS

According to the manufacturer, physostigmine is contraindicated when there is documented hypersensitivity to it or in the presence of a history of asthma, gangrene, diabetes, cardiovascular disease, intestinal obstruction, urogenital obstruction, and patients receiving choline esters or depolarizing neuromuscular blockers (48).

Pyridostigmine

Pyridostigmine may cause peripheral symptoms and signs of cholinergic excess (49). In some animals, certain types of stresses can also increase pyridostigmine entry in the CNS (4–7).

PREGNANCY AND LACTATION

Pyridostigmine is U.S. Food and Drug Administration pregnancy category C. It has been used safely in pregnant patients. In rats, it crosses the placenta and can produce growth retardation (50). Its use is considered compatible with breast-feeding. A retrospective study showed no increase in the rate of birth defects in children of Gulf War veterans (51). There is one case report of microcephaly in a patient exposed *in utero* to doses more than four times the recommended dose (52).

CONTRAINDICATIONS

According to the manufacturer, pyridostigmine is contraindicated when there is a documented hypersensitivity to it or in the presence of gastrointestinal or genitourinary obstruction (53).

DOSE AND METHOD OF ADMINISTRATION

Physostigmine (Anticholinergic Delirium)

Physostigmine should be administered in a setting where continuous cardiorespiratory monitoring is available and where potential adverse effects can be managed. A 12-lead ECG should be obtained.

The *adult* dose is 2.0 mg IV at a rate no faster than 1 mg/minute (54). The onset of effect is often delayed for several minutes. A second dose may be repeated if reversal does not occur and if cholinergic effects have not developed (55,56). If the initial doses are effective, repeat doses of physostigmine may be required to further counter anticholinergic symptoms or to prevent recurrence of anticholinergic effects. A maximum dose has not been established. Total physostigmine salicylate doses of 22 mg over 48 hours and 7.5 mg over 3 hours for control of anticholinergic delirium have been reported (57,58). When used to reverse the central effects of ketamine in patients who were otherwise unpremedicated, a dose of 25 μg/kg was used together with 5 μg/kg glycopyrrolate (14).

Physostigmine can be administered transdermally for Parkinson's disease. Bioavailability by this route is 36%, compared with 3% for the oral route as a result of a first-pass effect. There is a lag time of 4 hours to detectable plasma concentrations. After removal of the transdermal patch, the apparent half-life of elimination was 4.9 hours, compared with 0.5 hours for the IV route, suggesting continued drug absorption from a skin depot (59).

The *pediatric* dosage is 0.02 mg/kg IV (not faster than 0.5 mg/minute) (54). The dose can be repeated in 20 minutes or thereafter if reversal has not occurred or if anticholinergic symptoms return (55,56,60). The maximum recommended IV dose in children is 2 mg (61).

Pyridostigmine (Nerve Agent Prophylaxis)

The *adult* dose of pyridostigmine bromide is 30 mg orally every 8 hours (2,27,62). The same dose has been used to reverse near vision impairment from transdermal hyoscine use (30). Safety and effectiveness in the *pediatric* age group has not been established.

Monitoring of Response

Patients treated with physostigmine should be monitored continuously for heart rate, rhythm, and respiratory status. Reversal of central anticholinergic symptoms should occur after a delay of several minutes. The response may be incomplete or unequivocal if other CNS agents are present. Nonspecific arousal should be judged carefully to avoid the incorrect assumption of partial reversal of anticholinergic effect. The patient should be observed closely for the development of cholinergic symptoms.

ADVERSE EFFECTS

Physostigmine

Adverse reactions primarily involve cholinergic excess: abdominal cramping, diarrhea, bronchorrhea, seizures, bradycardia, ventricular dysrhythmias, respiratory arrest, and asystole. Adverse reactions are more likely to be seen if physostigmine is used in a patient who does not have anticholinergic toxicity or if larger doses are used.

Bradycardia caused by physostigmine or pyridostigmine is not related to the degree of cholinesterase inhibition (63). Physostigmine-induced, life-threatening bronchoconstriction, bradycardia, and seizures may respond to atropine sulfate, 0.5 to 1.0 mg IV (24). In addition, standard anticonvulsant therapy should be used (Chapter 30).

Antilirium contains sodium bisulfite and has caused reactive airway exacerbation and type I hypersensitivity reactions, including anaphylaxis. Sulfite sensitivity is seen more frequently in individuals with a prior history of asthma.

Pyridostigmine

A placebo-controlled study of pyridostigmine, 60 mg three times daily, for postpolio syndrome found that 55% of patients in the pyridostigmine group developed diarrhea and 28% had nausea, vomiting, or gastrointestinal upset compared with 19% and 13% of the placebo group, respectively (49). Side effects of pyridostigmine, 30 mg or 60 mg, in volunteers were not correlated with cholinesterase inhibition or plasma levels (2). Nicotinic symptoms of muscle cramps, fasciculation, and weakness can also occur (53). Pyridostigmine bromide has been proposed as a contributor, either singly or in combination with other exposures, in the development of Gulf War illness (Chapter 18).

PITFALLS

Physostigmine

The general analeptic effects of physostigmine may be mistaken for reversal of anticholinergic effect, whereas, in fact, such toxicity does not exist. If nonspecific arousal misleads the practitioner in administering additional doses in the absence of anticholinergic toxicity, potentially severe cholinergic poisoning could occur. Even when anticholinergic effects are present, the presence of coingestants may obscure or limit its effectiveness. In elderly patients on chronic anticholinergic treatment, muscarinic receptor upregulation may increase CNS response to physostigmine (64).

Physostigmine inhibits plasma butyrylcholinesterase and may result in prolonged neuromuscular blockade by agents that are metabolized by plasma cholinesterase (e.g., succinylcholine).

Pyridostigmine

Pyridostigmine inhibits plasma butyrylcholinesterase and may result in prolonged neuromuscular blockade by agents that are metabolized by plasma cholinesterase (e.g., succinylcholine) (27,65). Activity of AChE is reduced 20% to 40% by standard doses. Preliminary studies in military personnel indicate that the degree of prolongation of succinylcholine effect at standard doses is unlikely to be clinically significant (27). The effect of pyridostigmine may be prolonged in elderly men due to decreased clearance of pyridostigmine (66).

REFERENCES

1. Taylor P. Anticholinesterase agents. In: Goodman, Gilman, eds. *The pharmacological basis of therapeutics*. New York: Macmillan, 1996:161–176.
2. Cook MR, Gerkovish MM, Sastre A, et al. Side effects of low-dose pyridostigmine bromide are not related to cholinesterase inhibition. *Aviat Space Environ Med* 2001;72(12):1102–1106.
3. Bardin PG, Moolman JA, Foden AP, et al. Organophosphorus and carbamate poisoning. *Arch Intern Med* 1994;154:1433–1441.
4. Sharabi Y, Danon YL, Berkenstadt H, et al. Survey of symptoms following intake of pyridostigmine during the Persian Gulf War. *Isr J Med Sci* 1991;27(11–12):656–658.
5. Friedman A, Kaufer D, Shemer J, et al. Pyridostigmine brain penetration under stress enhances neuronal excitability and induces early immediate transcriptional response. *Nature Med* 1996;2(12):1382–1385.
6. Hanin I. The Gulf War, stress and a leaky blood-brain barrier. *Nature Med* 1996;2(12):1307–1308.
7. Lallement G, Foquin A, Baubichon D, et al. Heat stress, even extreme, does not induce penetration of pyridostigmine into the brain of guinea pigs. *Neurotoxicology* 1998;19(6):759–766.
8. Breyer-Plti U, Maier U, Brinkmarm AM, et al. Pyridostigmine kinetics in healthy subjects and patients with myasthenia gravis. *Clin Pharmacol Ther* 1985;37:495–501.
9. Cronnelly R, Stanski DR, Miller RD, et al. Pyridostigmine kinetics with and without renal function. *Clin Pharmacol Ther* 1980;28:78–81.
10. Miller RD. Pharmacodynamics and pharmacokinetics of anticholinesterase. In: Ruegheimer E, Zindler M, eds. *Anaesthesiology*. (Hamburg, Germany: Congress, Sept 14–21, 1980:222–223.) (Int Congr. No. 538.) Amsterdam, Netherlands: Excerpta Medica, 1981.
11. Burns MJ, Linden CH, Graudins A, et al. A comparison of physostigmine and benzodiazepines for the treatment of anticholinergic poisoning. *Ann Emerg Med* 2000;35:374–381.
12. Bernards W. Case history number 74: reversal of phenothiazine-induced coma with physostigmine. *Anesth Analg* 1973;52:938–941.
13. Sopchak CA, Stork CM, Cantor RM, et al. Central anticholinergic syndrome due to Jimson weed. Physostigmine: therapy revisited? *J Toxicol Clin Toxicol* 1998;36(1,2):43–45.
14. Hamilton-Davies C, Bailie R, Restall J. Physostigmine in recovery from anaesthesia. *Anaesthesia* 1995;50:456–458.
15. Kuhn M, Caldicott D. Use of physostigmine in the management of gamma-hydroxybutyrate overdose. *Ann Emerg Med* 2001;38(3):347–348.
16. Caldwell CB, Gross JB. Physostigmine reversal of midazolam-induced sedation. *Anesthesiology* 1982;57:125–127.
17. Ebert U, Oertel R, Kirch W. Physostigmine reversal of midazolam-induced electroencephalographic changes in healthy subjects. *Clin Pharmacol Ther* 2000;67(5):538–548.
18. Henderson RS, Holmes CM. Reversal of the anaesthetic action of sodium gamma-hydroxybutyrate. *Anaesth Intensive Care* 1976;4:351–354.
19. Caldicott DGE, Kuhn M. Gamma-hydroxybutyrate overdose and physostigmine: teaching new tricks to an old drug? *Ann Emerg Med* 2001;37:99–102.
20. Yates SW, Viera AJ. Physostigmine in the treatment of gamma-hydroxybutyric acid overdose. *May Clin Proc* 2000;75:401–402.

21. Rupreht J, Dworacek B. Physostigmine versus naloxone in heroin overdose. *J Toxicol Clin Toxicol* 1983;21:387–397.
22. Ceha LJ, Presperin C, Young E, et al. Anticholinergic toxicity from nightshade berry poisoning responsive to physostigmine. *J Emerg Med* 1997;15(1):65–69.
23. Fassoulaki A, Sarantopoulos C, Derveniotis C. Physostigmine increases the dose of propofol required to induce anaesthesia. *Can J Anaesth* 1997;44(11):1148–1151.
24. Reynolds JEF, ed. *Martindale: the extra pharmacopoeia*, 30th ed. London: Pharmaceutical Press, 1993:418.
25. Katsanoulas K, Papaioannou A, Fraidakis O, et al. Undiagnosed central anticholinergic syndrome may lead to dangerous complications. *Eur J Anaesthesiol* 1999;16(11):803–809.
26. Schultz U, Idelberger R, Rossaint R, et al. Central anticholinergic syndrome in a child undergoing circumcision. *Acta Anaesthesiol Scand* 2002;46(2):224–226.
27. Heath KJ, Niemiro LAK, Gosden EA, et al. The effects of nerve agent pretreatment with pyridostigmine on the duration of action of suxamethonium. *Anaesthesia* 1996;51(4):404.
28. Tuovinen K, Kaliste-Korhonen E, Raushel FM, et al. Success of pyridostigmine, physostigmine, eptastigmine and phosphotriesterase treatments in acute sarin intoxication. *Toxicology* 1999;134(2–3):169–178.
29. Medical letter. Prevention and treatment of injury from chemical warfare agents. *Med Lett Drugs Ther* 2002;44(1121):1–4.
30. Alhalel A, Ziv I, Versano D, et al. Ocular effects of hyoscine in double dose transdermal administration and its reversal by low dose pyridostigmine. *Aviat Space Environ Med* 1995;66(11):1037–1040.
31. Burns MJ, Linden CH, Graudins A. Physostigmine versus diazepines for anticholinergic poisoning. *Ann Emerg Med* 2001;37(2):240–241.
32. Oakley P. Physostigmine versus diazepines for anticholinergic poisoning. *Ann Emerg Med* 2001;37(2):239–240.
33. Slovis TL, Ott JE, Teitelbaum DT, et al. Physostigmine therapy in acute tricyclic antidepressant poisoning. *Clin Toxicol* 1971;4:451–459.
34. Tong TG, Benowitz NL, Becker CE. Tricyclic antidepressant overdose. *DICP* 1976;10:712–713.
35. Newton RW. Physostigmine salicylate in the treatment of tricyclic antidepressant overdosage. *JAMA* 1975;231:941–943.
36. Walker WE, Levy RC, Hanenson IB. Physostigmine—its use and abuse. *JACEP* 1976;5:436–439.
37. Pentel P, Peterson CD. Asystole complicating physostigmine treatment of tricyclic antidepressant overdose. *Ann Emerg Med* 1980;9:588–590.
38. Knudsen K, Heath A. Effects of self-poisoning with maprotiline. *BMJ* 1984;228:601–603.
39. Pentel PR, Benowitz NL. Tricyclic antidepressant poisoning—management of arrhythmias. *Med Toxicol* 1986;1:101–121.
40. Frommer DD, Kulig KW, Marx JA, et al. Tricyclic antidepressant overdose—a review. *JAMA* 1987;257:521–526.
41. Shannon M. Toxicology reviews: physostigmine. *Pediatr Emerg Care* 1998;14:224–226.
42. Kulig K, Heath A. Physostigmine and asystole. *Ann Emerg Med* 1981;10:228–230.
43. Brown TCK. Tricyclic antidepressant overdosage: experimental studies on the management of circulatory complications. *Clin Toxicol* 1976;9:255–272.
44. Lum BKB, Follmer CH, Lockwood RH, et al. Experimental studies on the effects of physostigmine and of isoproterenol on toxicity produced by tricyclic antidepressants. *J Toxicol Clin Toxicol* 1982;19:51–65.
45. Goldberger AL, Curtis GP. Immediate effects of physostigmine on amitriptyline-induced ORS prolongation. *J Toxicol Clin Toxicol* 1982;19:445–454.
46. Fleck CH, Braunlich H. Failure of physostigmine in intoxications with tricyclic antidepressants in rats. *Toxicology* 1982;24:335–344.
47. Mullins ME, Dribben W. Physostigmine treatment of gamma-hydroxybutyric acid overdose: appropriate or inappropriate use of a reversal agent? *Mayo Clin Proc* 2000;75:871–872.
48. Antilirium(R), physostigmine [package insert]. St. Louis: Forest Pharmaceuticals, Inc.; 2000.
49. Trojan DA, Collet JP, Shapiro S, et al. A multicenter, randomized, double-blinded trial of pyridostigmine in postpolio syndrome. *Neurology* 1999;53:1225–1233.
50. Levine BS, Parker RM. Reproductive and developmental toxicity studies of pyridostigmine bromide in rats. *Toxicology* 1991;69:291–300.
51. Cowan DN, DeFraites RF, Gray GC, et al. The risk of birth defects among children of Persian Gulf War veterans. *N Engl J Med* 1997;336:1650–1656.
52. Niesen CE, Shah NS. Pyridostigmine-induced microcephaly. *Neurology* 2000;54:1873–1874.
53. Mestinon [package insert]. Costa Mesa, CA: ICN Pharmaceuticals, Inc.; 2002.
54. Physostigmine salicylate injection [package insert]. Elizabeth, NJ: Faulding USA; revised 1995; reviewed Oct 2000.
55. Rumack BH. Anticholinergic poisoning: treatment with physostigmine. *Pediatrics* 1973;52:449.
56. Manoguerra AS, Ruiz E. Physostigmine treatment of anticholinergic poisoning. *J ACEP* 1976;5:125–127.
57. Tobis J, Das BN. Cardiac complications in amitriptyline poisoning. Successful treatment with physostigmine. *JAMA* 1976;235:1474.
58. Beaver KM, Gavin TJ. Treatment of acute anticholinergic poisoning with physostigmine. *Am J Emerg Med* 1998;16:505–507.
59. Walter K, Muller M, Barkworth MF, et al. Pharmacokinetics of physostigmine in man following a single application of a transdermal system. *Br J Clin Pharmacol* 1995;39(1):59–63.
60. Burks JS, Walker JE, Rumack BH, et al. Tricyclic antidepressant poisoning. Reversal of coma, choreoathetosis & myoclonus by physostigmine. *JAMA* 1974;230:1405.
61. Anon. *Guidelines for administration of intravenous medications to pediatric patients*, 2nd ed. Bethesda, MD: American Society of Hospital Pharmacists, 1984.
62. Sidell FR, Borak J Chemical warfare agents: II. Nerve agents. *Ann Emerg Med* 1992;21(7):865–871.
63. Stein RD, Backman SB, Collier B, et al. Bradycardia produced by pyridostigmine and physostigmine. *Can J Anaesth* 1997;44(12):1286–1292.
64. Dukoff R, Wilkinson CW, Lasser R, et al. Physostigmine challenge before and after chronic cholinergic blockade in elderly volunteers. *Biol Psychiatry* 1999;46(2):189–195.
65. Pellegrini JE, Baker AB, Fontenot DJ, et al. The effect of oral pyridostigmine bromide nerve agent prophylaxis on return of twitch height in persons receiving succinylcholine. *Mil Med* 2000;165(4):252–255.
66. Stone JG, Matteo RS, Ornstein E, et al. Aging alters the pharmacokinetics of pyridostigmine. *Anesth Analg* 1995;81:773–776.

CHAPTER 68

Phytonadione (Vitamin K_1)

E. Martin Caravati

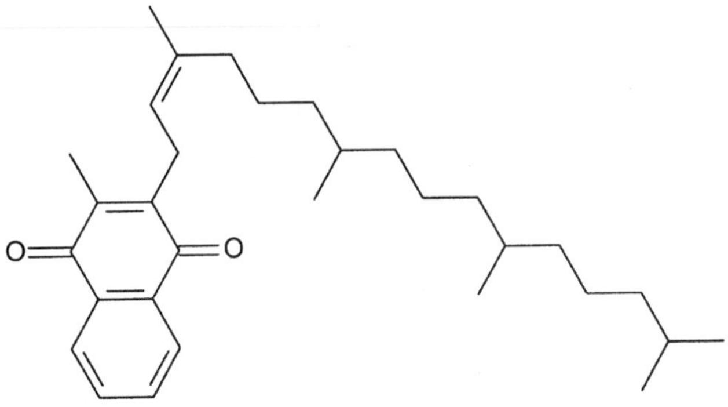

PHYTONADIONE

Synonyms:	Phytomenadione, Mephyton, AquaMEPHYTON
Molecular formula and weight:	$C_{31}H_{46}O_2$, 450.7 g/mol
SI conversion:	ng/L × 2.22 = nmol/L
CAS Registry No.:	84-80-0
Therapeutic levels:	Not clinically applicable
Special concerns:	Large doses or rapid infusion may cause hypotension.

OVERVIEW

Vitamin K_1 is a cofactor in the synthesis of several clotting factors. Phytonadione is a synthetic, fat-soluble naphthoquinone analog of vitamin K_1 and has essentially the same pharmacologic activity as naturally occurring vitamin K_1. It can usually reverse deficiencies in vitamin K–dependent coagulation factors.

Therapeutic use of warfarin may result in excessive anticoagulation. Changing the dose of warfarin eventually corrects the coagulopathy, but this may take several days (1). Administration of vitamin K_1 shortens the time required to achieve the desired level of anticoagulation. Hemorrhage secondary to hypothrombinemia may take several hours to control with phytonadione, and the use of blood products may be needed. Vitamin K_1 does not reverse the anticoagulant effect of heparin.

The daily adequate intake of vitamin K recommended by the National Academy of Sciences for healthy men and women is 120 µg and 90 µg, respectively; 2.0 to 2.5 µg for infants through 6 months of age; and from 30 to 75 µg for ages 1 to 18 years. Foods such as cabbage, spinach, fish, egg yolks, meats, fruits, and dairy products contain natural vitamin K.

Forms Available

Phytonadione is available in most countries. It is supplied as an aqueous solution for injection in 10 mg/ml and 2 mg/ml with benzyl alcohol 0.9% as preservative (AquaMEPHYTON), and as 5-mg tablets (Mephyton). It is compatible with crystalloidal intravenous (IV) infusions. Both formulations are photosensitive and must be shielded from light at all times.

Mechanism of Action

Vitamin K is necessary for the formation of coagulation factors II, VII, IX, and X. The inactive precursors of these factors, as well as proteins S and C, are carboxylated with the assistance of vitamin K. Vitamin K hydroxyquinone (reduced form of vitamin K, KH_2) is converted to inactive vitamin K 2,3-epoxide during the carboxylation process. The epoxide is reduced to vitamin K quinone in the presence of vitamin K 2,3-epoxide reductase, then to active vitamin K hydroxyquinone by vitamin K quinone reductase (Fig. 1).

Warfarin inhibits vitamin K 2,3-epoxide reductase, preventing the formation of active vitamin K, and thus impairs formation of active clotting factors. Administration of exogenous vitamin K overcomes the inhibition of clotting factor synthesis by warfarin and other compounds by providing the substrate necessary for carboxylation of the clotting factor precursors.

Pharmacokinetics/Toxicokinetics

Oral bioavailability varies widely among patients (10% to 63%). Bile salts are needed for absorption in the small intestine. Vitamin K is rapidly metabolized and does not accumulate in tissues. The elimination half-life is approximately 2 hours (2). An increase in blood coagulation factors usually occurs 6 to 12 hours after an oral dose and 3 to 6 hours after IV administration.

INDICATIONS

Warfarin-Induced Excessive Anticoagulation

Management of coagulopathy consists of three options depending on the risk of hemorrhage: (a) decreasing or discontinuing warfarin therapy, (b) administering vitamin K_1, and (c) administering fresh frozen plasma or prothrombin concentrate. Administration of oral vitamin K_1 to excessively anticoagulated patients receiving warfarin reduces the time needed to reach a therapeutic international normalized ratio (INR) (3).

Long-Acting Anticoagulant Rodenticide Poisoning

The long-acting rodenticides include brodifacoum, bromadiolone, difenacoum, and chlorophacinone, among others (Chapter 237). Phytonadione is used to prevent elevation of, or to correct, the prothrombin time (PT) or INR, or to treat the rare case of bleeding.

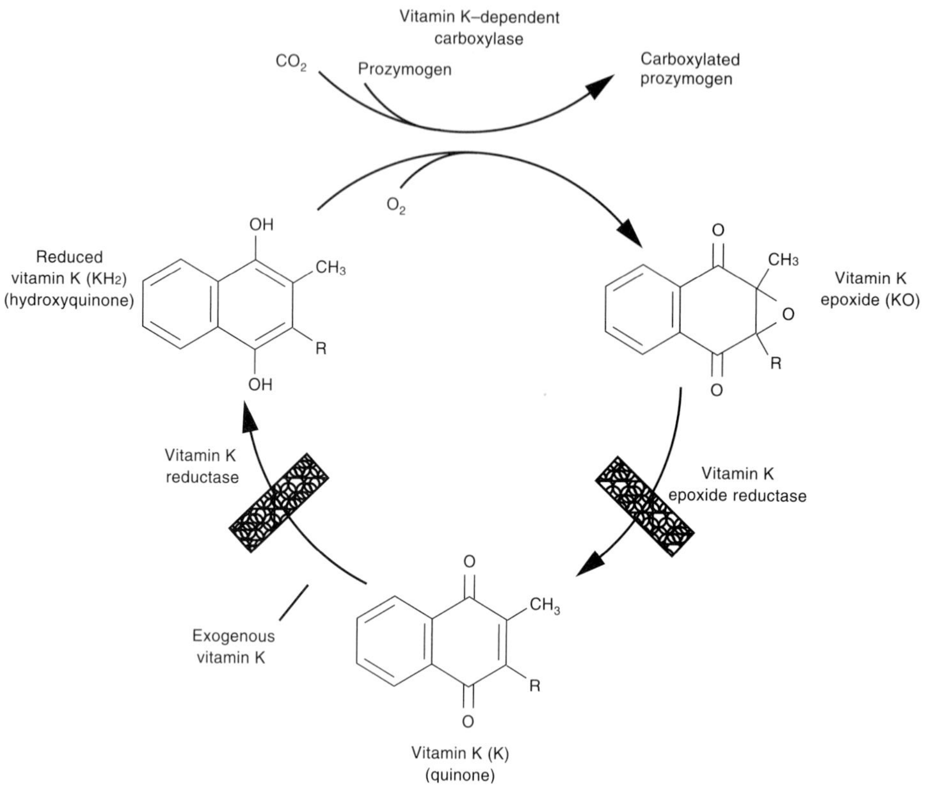

Figure 1. The vitamin K cycle. Hatched areas indicate sites of warfarin inhibition. (From Pineo GF, Hull RD. Adverse effects of coumarin anticoagulants. *Drug Safe* 1993; 9:263–271, with permission.)

Hypoprothrombinemia Secondary to Toxin

Vitamin K_1 may be used in poisoning from salicylates, sulfonamides, quinine, or quinidine when the PT or INR is prolonged.

Hemorrhagic Disease of the Newborn

Phytonadione is used for prevention of hemorrhagic disease of the newborn and treatment of neonates whose mothers received anticonvulsant therapy during pregnancy.

CAUTIONS AND CONTRAINDICATIONS

Allergic reactions to vitamin K have been reported.

Vitamin K is U.S. Food and Drug Administration pregnancy category C. Birth defects have been reported in newborns exposed during the first trimester of pregnancy. The placental transfer of vitamin K_1 is poor. It was nontoxic in doses less than 20 mg/day given to women at term gestation. The use of vitamin K_1 is compatible with breast-feeding. There are no data concerning the treatment of pregnant women with phytonadione for warfarin or long-acting anticoagulant poisoning (4).

Concurrent administration with mineral oil or orlistat may decrease gastrointestinal absorption of vitamin K. The intramuscular route is not recommended due to possible hematoma formation and poor absorption.

DOSAGE AND METHOD OF ADMINISTRATION

The route of administration depends on the severity of the coagulation defect and the risks associated with each route. The risk of bleeding is greater in patients with an INR above 5, in the elderly, or with a history of hypertension.

The oral route is more effective than subcutaneous (SQ) injection (5). Patients with decreased bile secretion require supplemental bile salts with each oral dose of phytonadione (e.g., dehydrocholic acid, 500 mg). An alternative for patients that are unable to absorb phytonadione is to administer it by SQ or IV injection. The SQ route is safest, but absorption by this route is unpredictable and may be delayed (5,6). Due to safety concerns, the IV route is used only when other routes are not feasible. The maximum rate of IV administration is 1 mg/minute. It may be diluted with preservative-free 5% dextrose, normal saline, or 5% dextrose in normal saline.

Warfarin-Induced Anticoagulation

The goal of vitamin K_1 therapy is to lower the INR to a safe level without causing resistance to warfarin when it is restarted. High doses of vitamin K_1 normalize the INR but cause warfarin to be ineffective for up to a week. This places the patient who requires anticoagulation at risk for thromboembolic events. Conservative treatment of nonbleeding patients without the use of vitamin K_1 has been shown to be safe and eliminates many of these concerns (7).

The American College of Chest Physicians has published recommendations for the management of increased INR (Table 1) (8).

Long-Acting Anticoagulant Rodenticide Poisoning

A rodenticide overdose typically requires much higher daily doses of vitamin K_1 than warfarin-induced anticoagulation. Doses ranging from 15 to 600 mg/day divided every 6 to 12 hours have been reported. The starting dose depends on the degree of anticoagulation and risk of bleeding. For a stable patient with an INR greater than 5, a reasonable starting dose is 50 mg orally every 12 hours, titrated to effect over the next 48 hours (9).

TABLE 1. Management of the elevated international normalized ratio (INR)

INR	Significant bleeding present?	Warfarin dose	Vitamin K_1 dose	Other therapy
<5	None	Lower or omit dose until INR therapeutic.	None.	—
5–9	None	Omit next one to two doses.	1.0–2.5 mg PO if bleeding risk. 2–4 mg PO to normalize INR within 24 h. May repeat vitamin K 1–2 mg PO if needed.	Frequent INR monitoring.
>9	None	Omit entirely.	3–5 mg PO should normalize INR in 24–48 h; give more as necessary.	Frequent INR monitoring.
>20	Yes	Omit entirely.	10 mg slow IV infusion; may repeat every 12 h.	Fresh frozen plasma or prothrombin complex concentrate.
—	Life-threatening	Omit entirely.	10 mg slow IV infusion; repeat as necessary.	Prothrombin-complex concentrate; repeat as needed.

Modified from Ansell J, Hirsh J, Dalen J, et al. Managing oral anticoagulant therapy. *Chest* 2001;119:22S–38S.

Due to the long duration of action for rodenticides, weeks or months of treatment may be required. Serum brodifacoum concentrations have been used to predict the duration of vitamin K_1 therapy (10). In one case, a brodifacoum concentration less than 10 ng/ml was not associated with coagulopathy (11). A patient with a PT of 150 seconds due to brodifacoum required 200 mg/day of vitamin K_1 to maintain a normal INR. He tolerated this dose for 5 months without adverse effect (12).

A 52-year-old man developed hypoprothrombinemia and hematuria after ingesting 344 g of D-Con Mouse-Prufe II (0.005% brodifacoum). An empiric dose of 150 mg orally every 6 hours corrected his factor levels after 40 hours. The dose was gradually reduced by 50% over 46 days of outpatient vitamin K_1 treatment while monitoring the PT value. This dose was probably more than required for adequate factor synthesis (10). Parenteral administration would have required a volume of 60 ml/day (10 mg/ml).

Hypoprothrombinemia Secondary to Toxin

For salicylates, sulfonamides, quinine, and quinidine overdose, the *adult dose* of phytonadione is 2 to 25 mg orally or SQ. The dose may be repeated in 8 (parenteral) to 12 hours (oral) depending on the response. Doses more than 25 mg are rarely required, but up to 50 mg may be administered. The *pediatric dose* is 2 mg to infants and 5 to 10 mg to older children, orally or parenterally.

Hemorrhagic Disease of the Newborn

The *neonatal dose* of phytonadione is 0.5 to 1.0 mg intramuscularly after delivery and repeated in 6 to 8 hours if needed. An oral dose of 1 to 2 mg immediately after delivery has also been recommended instead of parenteral dosing. Neonates whose mothers received anticoagulant therapy may require higher doses.

Monitoring of Response

For therapeutic overcoagulation, the PT or INR is typically monitored every 4 to 12 hours during correction with vitamin K_1, depending on patient stability and need for escalating doses of vitamin K_1.

For rodenticide poisoning that has produced coagulopathy, the PT or INR is also monitored frequently during initial vitamin K_1 treatment. Once the PT or INR approaches the therapeutic range, the PT or INR should be monitored on a regular basis every 1 to 2 weeks as an outpatient as a measure of compliance (9). Serial brodifacoum concentrations have been used but often are not needed for management (particularly for pediatric accidental ingestion). In the case of intentional ingestion, they can be obtained every 2 to 3 weeks until less than 10 ng/ml.

Adverse Reactions

INTRAVENOUS USE

Severe reactions, including anaphylaxis, shock, and cardiac arrest, have occurred after or during IV administration (13). Vitamin K_1 should be used IV only when the benefits outweigh the risks of SQ or oral administration. Other symptoms associated with IV use include muscle cramps, chest pain, cyanosis, facial flushing, chest tightness, dyspnea, dizziness, bronchospasm, and decreased level of consciousness (14).

SUBCUTANEOUS

Allergic reactions; pain, swelling, erythema, tenderness at the intramuscular or SQ injection site; hemorrhage or hematoma at the injection site; and skin lesions may progress to indurated, pruritic plaques after repeated injections.

NEWBORNS

Some parenteral products contain benzyl alcohol that may produce toxicity in newborns when given in large amounts (i.e., 100 mg/kg daily). Hyperbilirubinemia and hemolytic anemia has been reported in the newborn after large doses (10 to 20 mg) of vitamin K_1.

PITFALLS

Vitamin K_3 (menadione) is ineffective for the treatment of warfarin and superwarfarin toxicity. It elicits a poor response and should not be used (15,16).

Vitamin K_1 does not reverse the anticoagulant effect of heparin. Vitamin K_1 does not correct hypoprothrombinemia due to hepatocellular injury or disease.

The anticoagulant effect is delayed at least 1 to 2 hours. Fresh frozen plasma or blood should be administered for hemorrhage in addition to vitamin K_1.

Patients who require some degree of anticoagulation due to an underlying thromboembolic risk (e.g., atrial fibrillation) may be at increased risk if anticoagulation is completely reversed.

Administration of vitamin K may interfere with subsequent attempts to achieve oral anticoagulation.

Repeated large doses are not indicated in patients with liver disease who do not respond to initial treatment. Large doses of vitamin K_1 may further depress prothrombin in patients with hepatitis or cirrhosis.

REFERENCES

1. White RH, McKittrick T, Hutchinson R, et al. Temporary discontinuation of warfarin therapy: changes in the international normalized ratio. *Ann Intern Med* 1995;122:40–42.
2. Park BK, Scott AK, Wilson AC, et al. Plasma disposition of vitamin K_1 in relation to anticoagulant poisoning. *Br J Clin Pharmacol* 1984;18:655–662.
3. Doung TM, Plowman BK, Morreale AP, et al. Retrospective and prospective analyses of the treatment of overanticoagulated patients. *Pharmacotherapy* 1998;18:1264–1270.
4. Briggs GG, Freeman RK, Yaffe SJ. *Drugs in pregnancy and lactation*, 6th ed. Baltimore: Williams & Wilkins, 2002:1128–1131.
5. Whitling AM, Bussey HI, Lyons RM. Comparing different routes and doses of phytonadione for reversing excessive anticoagulation. *Arch Intern Med* 1998;158:2136–2140.
6. Raj G, Kumar R, McKinney WP. Time course of reversal of anticoagulant effect of warfarin by intravenous and subcutaneous phytonadione. *Arch Intern Med* 2000;160(7):986.
7. Glover JJ, Morrill GB. Conservative treatment of overanticoagulated patients. *Chest* 1995;108:987–990.
8. Ansell J, Hirsh J, Dalen J, et al. Managing oral anticoagulant therapy. *Chest* 2001;119:22S–38S.
9. Dahl B, Caravati EM. Surreptitious brodifacoum poisoning. *J Toxicol Clin Toxicol* 2001;39:475–476.
10. Bruno GR, Howland MA, McMeeking A, et al. Long-acting anticoagulant overdose: brodifacoum kinetics and optimal vitamin K dosing. *Ann Emerg Med* 2000;36:262–267.
11. Hollinger BR, Pastor TP. Case management and plasma half-life in a case of brodifacoum poisoning. *Arch Intern Med* 1993;153:1925–1928.
12. Sheen SR, Spiller HA, Grossman D. Symptomatic brodifacoum ingestion requiring high-dose phytonadione therapy. *Vet Hum Toxicol* 1994;36:216–217.
13. De la Rubia J, Grau E, Montserrat I, et al. Anaphylactic shock and vitamin K_1. *Ann Intern Med* 1989;110:943.
14. Bjornsson TD, Blaschke TF. Vitamin K_1 disposition and therapy of warfarin overdose. *Lancet* 1978;2:846–847.
15. Kwaan HC, Simon NM, del Greco F. Hemorrhagic diathesis induced by surreptitious ingestion of coumarin drugs. *Med Clin North Am* 1972;56:263–273.
16. Finkel MJ. Vitamin K_1 and vitamin K analogues. *Clin Pharmacol Ther* 1961;2:794–814.

CHAPTER 69

Pralidoxime, Obidoxime, and Other Oximes

Daniel C. Keyes

$Cl^{\ominus}$ $N^{\oplus}$ N OH CH_3

PRALIDOXIME HYDROCHLORIDE

Synonyms:	**Pralidoxime: Hagedorn oximes (2-PAM Cl), Protopam; obidoxime: toxogonin**
Molecular formula and weight:	**Pralidoxime ($C_7H_9ClN_2O$), 172.6 g/mol; obidoxime ($C_{14}H_{16}Cl_2N_4O_3$), 359.2 g/mol**
CAS Registry No.:	**51-15-0 (pralidoxime); 114-90-9 (obidoxime chloride)**
Therapeutic levels:	**Serum concentration of 4 μg/ml**
Special concerns:	**None**

OVERVIEW

Pralidoxime and obidoxime are antidotes for organophosphate (OP) insecticide intoxication. With the recent enhanced interest in responding to terrorism, these and other oximes have taken on renewed importance as treatment for nerve agent exposure (Fig. 1).

Useful reviews of the many clinical studies to evaluate oxime effectiveness have been published in recent years (1,2). Oxime availability varies by region. The oxime routinely available in the United States is pralidoxime chloride (2-PAM Cl), which is the *N*-methyl derivative of 2-pyridinaldoxime. It is available as a parenteral solution and also in autoinjectors developed to provide self-treatment in the battlefield. In the United States, the pralidoxime (2-PAM Cl) autoinjector is packaged with an atropine autoinjector in a package known as the *Mark I kit* (Fig. 2). In the United Kingdom, pralidoxime methanesulfonate (P2S) is the predominant type of oxime available. In Europe, autoinjectors for an alternative oxime, HI-6, are also available. Obidoxime is marketed as an alternative to pralidoxime in Europe and in other parts of the world.

Mechanism of Action

The normal function of the enzyme acetylcholinesterase (AChE) is to catalyze the cleavage of the neurotransmitter acetylcholine (ACh) into acetate and choline. OP insecticides bind AChE, blocking the catalytic site. Cholinergic toxicity results from the accumulation of AChE in the synaptic cleft and myoneural junction, causing an increase in the action potentials transmitted to nerve and muscle.

The toxicity of OP chemicals can be reversed and the bond between AChE, and the OP can be disrupted, allowing normal

Pralidoxime	(pyridinium ring, N^+–Me) CH=NOH
Obidoxime	HON=CH(pyridinium)$\overset{+}{N}CH_2OCH_2\overset{+}{N}$(pyridinium)CH=NOH
HI-6	Cl− Cl− (two pyridinium rings linked by $\overset{+}{N}$–CH_2–O–CH_2–$\overset{+}{N}$; HO–N=CH– and H–C=N–OH substituents)

Figure 1. Structure of common medicinal oximes. Major oximes used for treatment of organophosphate and nerve agent exposure.

AChE activity to return. Initial attempts used choline and hydroxylamine (3,4). Oximes are able to regenerate active AChE through nucleophilic attack on phosphorus (Fig. 3).

Besides activating AChE directly, oximes may neutralize OP molecules directly and possibly exert a direct anticholinergic effect. Oximes are less effective at reversing toxicity at muscarinic sites than at nicotinic sites. Various investigators have demonstrated the direct interaction between certain oximes and OPs (5,6); however, these interactions do not appear to contribute significantly to the therapeutic action of pralidoxime. Similarly, some oximes have shown anticholinergic effects but not to a sufficient degree to have an impact on overall therapy. For example, treatment with atropine and pralidoxime is more efficacious than oxime alone (7).

It has been generally accepted that the minimum serum concentration of oxime required to reverse nerve agent intoxication is 4 µg/ml (8,9). The dose required to produce that level for approximately 1 hour is 10 mg/kg intramuscularly of 2-PAM (10). Required doses have also been measured for HI-6 (250 mg intramuscularly) and toxogonin (11).

After being bound by the toxic OP compound, a limited time is available before the bond ages. The term *aging* refers to the OP-ChE bond becoming covalent and therefore resistant to oxime. Spontaneous reactivation occurs at a small rate that is insufficient for normal function. The time required for aging of the OP-AChE bond varies greatly and is dependent on the type of OP producing the toxicity.

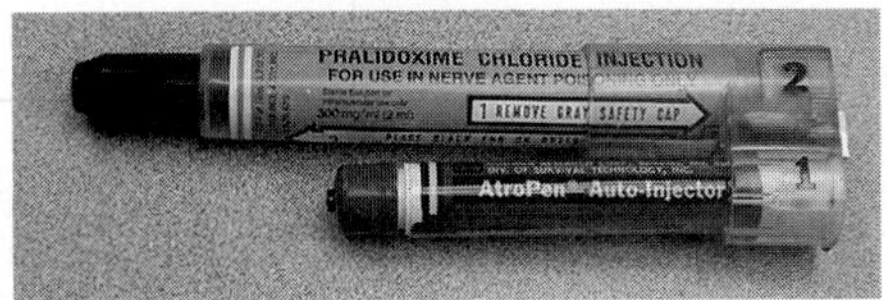

Figure 2. Military autoinjectors, Mark I kit.

The dictum "oxime in time, victim is fine" is true in most, but not all, circumstances. Soman has a short aging time of only 2 to 4 minutes, making it refractory to the use of conventional oximes. One newer oxime, HI-6 (H for Hagedorn), has shown promise as a treatment for soman, even in the context of fully aged OP-AChE complex. A study with rhesus monkeys poisoned by 5 LD_{50} of soman showed survival after treatment with diazepam, atropine, and HI-6. This use of HI-6 was effective in spite of the absence of AChE reactivation (12). Another primate experiment revealed that survival using HI-6 after soman exposure was not associated with reactivation of central nervous system AChE (13). The use of HI-6 as a nerve agent antidote is controversial due to the greater difficulty and expense in manufacture and instability of the aqueous solution (14). Autoinjectors with HI-6 in powder form for mixing immediately before use have been developed and require 5 seconds of mixing before injection (15–17).

INDICATIONS

Organophosphate Insecticides

An oxime should be used in patients with clinically significant OP insecticide poisoning. These typically include nicotinic effects (muscle and diaphragmatic weakness, fasciculation, muscle cramps) and central nervous system effects (coma, seizures). The use of an oxime in carbamate insecticide poisoning is controversial but is recommended, except perhaps in the case of carbaryl. Atropine should also be administered (Chapter 42).

Nerve Warfare Agents

An oxime should be administered in all symptomatic patients that may have experienced exposure to a nerve agent. Atropine should also be administered (Chapter 42).

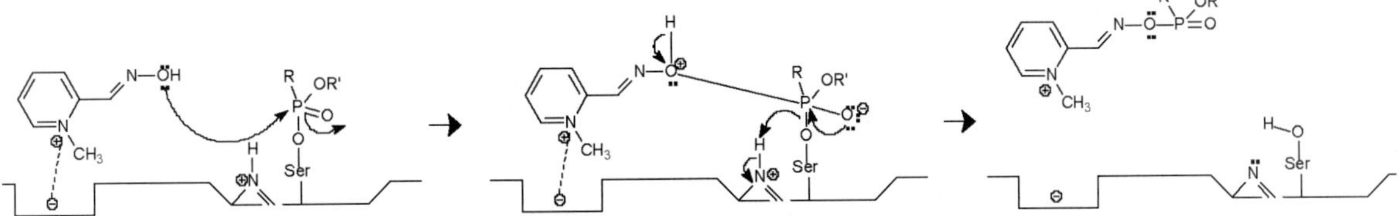

Figure 3. Regeneration of acetylcholinesterase (AChE) by pralidoxime (2-PAM). The organophosphorus (OP) agent is bound to the active site of AChE through a serine (Ser) residue hydroxyl. In regeneration of the enzyme, 2-PAM is held in an appropriate orientation in the active site by a weak electrostatic interaction between the 2-PAM pyridinium nitrogen and an area of the receptor with negative charge character. The nucleophilic oxygen of the oxime moiety of 2-PAM attacks the electrophilic phosphorus of the OP, forcing the electrons of the oxygen-phosphorus double bond onto the oxygen atom. This electron pair then collapses to re-form the double bond and, to maintain the appropriate valence of phosphorus, breaks the bond between the phosphorus and Ser oxygen. The Ser oxygen then acquires a hydrogen atom from a closely adjacent histidine reforming the hydroxyl functionality of the Ser. The OP is now covalently bound to 2-PAM, which falls away from the remaining weak electrostatic attraction to the AChE receptor. In an aged OP-AChE complex, the initially weaker bond between the phosphorus and Ser oxygen becomes strongly covalent, preventing the breaking of that bond when the oxygen-phosphorus double bond reforms.

The use of carbamates before and after intoxication with OP agents has also been investigated (Chapter 67). Attempts were made to use physostigmine and neostigmine to form an unstable bond, which prevents circulating OP from binding to AChE (18,19). Pyridostigmine was used for this purpose in the Gulf War. Carbamates have no use *after* OP poisoning and in fact may worsen the clinical course of the patient (20–22).

CAUTIONS AND CONTRAINDICATIONS

Pralidoxime is largely eliminated by the kidney, and dosing should be adjusted for renal insufficiency. Known previous anaphylactic reaction to pralidoxime is a relative contraindication.

A controversy has developed regarding the use of oximes for the carbamate, carbaryl. Two animal studies reported worsening of clinical outcome with the use of pralidoxime and obidoxime. It was thought that this may be the result of an increased toxicity of the combination of carbamate with carbaryl (23,24). This has not been reported in humans, however, and it is often recommended that antidotal oximes be administered in the event of an unknown toxin, which may be a carbamate as well.

DOSAGE AND ADMINISTRATION

Organophosphate Insecticides

Atropine and an oxime should be administered together in any significant poisoning. The initial *adult dose* of 2-PAM Cl is 1.0 g intravenously. The initial *pediatric dose* is 15 to 25 mg/kg. Pralidoxime may be administered intravenously or by autoinjector. In adults, pralidoxime may also be given as a continuous intravenous infusion of 500 mg/hour, using a 2.5% solution (25). A 5% solution can be used if it is necessary to reduce volume in a patient with pulmonary edema. However, muscle necrosis has been reported if solution is overly concentrated (35% wt/volume) (10). The pediatric dose for continuous infusion is 20 mg/kg/hour. Dosage should be maintained continuously until clinical improvement is established (24 to 48 hours). Because excretion is renal, the dose of pralidoxime should be reduced in patients with renal insufficiency.

Nerve Warfare Agents

Treatment of nerve agent exposure should include the early administration of atropine, pralidoxime, and, if the exposure is severe, diazepam.

The initial dose may be administered as described previously for OP insecticides or by Autoinjector. Military autoinjectors for use after exposure to nerve agents contain 600 mg of pralidoxime (2-PAM Cl) (26). In the United Kingdom, Autoinjectors contain 500 mg of P2S (1). In the United States, atropine and oxime are usually provided in separate autoinjectors (27). They can also be mixed in the same autoinjector solution, as is done in the United Kingdom (1).

ADVERSE EFFECTS

Oximes are generally nonlethal in the doses likely to be prescribed (28) but do cause many mild adverse effects. Mild serum creatine kinase (CK) enzyme elevation may occur. Cardiovascular effects include tachycardia and mild hypertension associated with rapid infusion. Increases in systolic and diastolic blood pressure and inversion of the T wave on electrocardiogram have been described for 2-PAM doses in excess of 30 mg/kg (29). Tachycardia and hypertension, pain at the injection site, and perioral paresthesia and methanol taste were described with toxogonin administration at doses of 2.5 to 10.0 mg/kg (30). Dizziness, headache, drowsiness, and apprehension associated with rapid infusion have been reported. Skin rash may occur. Gastrointestinal effects include nausea and hepatic enzyme elevation. Blurred vision, diplopia, and mydriasis have been reported.

More severe reactions include apnea, hyperventilation, and laryngospasm associated with rapid infusion. High serum pralidoxime concentrations can produce neuromuscular blockade.

PITFALLS

Pralidoxime is not equally effective with all anticholinesterase agents.

The most common error is the inadequate use of atropine early in the treatment regimen before, or simultaneous with, the delivery of oxime therapy. The patient should receive adequate atropinization to relieve respiratory compromise.

Oxime therapy may be required for several days after exposure to highly lipid soluble OPs such as fenthion and chlorfenthion, in which continued OP absorption occurs due to improper decontamination, or when OPs undergo metabolic conversion to other agents (31).

Insufficient stocking of antidotes is prevalent in the United States (32,33). Prudence dictates that health care facilities prepare for the possibility of terrorist chemical attack by maintaining a proper inventory of antidotes.

REFERENCES

1. Dawson RM. Review of oximes available for treatment of nerve agent poisoning. *J Appl Toxicol* 1994;14(5):317–331.
2. van Helden HP, Busker RW, Melchers BP, et al. Pharmacological effects of oximes: how relevant are they? *Arch Toxicol* 1996;70(12):779–786.
3. Wilson IB. Acetylcholinesterase. XI. Reversibility of tetraethyl pyrophosphate inhibition. *J Biol Chem* 1951;199:111–117.
4. Wilson IB. Acetylcholinesterase. XIII. Reactivation of alkyl phosphate-inhibited enzyme. *J Biol Chem* 1952;199:113–120.
5. Wagner-Jauregg T, Hackley BE Jr. Model reactions of phosphorus-containing enzyme inactivators III. Interaction of imidazole, pyridine, and some of their derivatives with dialkyl halogeno-phosphates. *J Am Chem Soc* 1953;75:2125–2130.
6. Lotti M, Becker CE. Treatment of acute organophosphate poisoning: evidence of a direct effect on central nervous system by 2-PAM (pyridine-2-aldoxime methyl chloride). *J Toxicol Clin Toxicol* 1982;19(2):121–127.
7. Lehman RA. Mechanism of the antagonism by pralidoxime and 1,1-trimethylenebis(4-hydroxyiminomethylpyridinium) of the action of echothiophate on the intestine. *Br J Pharmacol Chemother* 1962;18:87–298.
8. Sundwall A. Minimum concentrations of *N*-methylpyridinium-2-aldoxime methanesulphonate (P2S) which reverse neuromuscular block. *Biochem Pharmacol* 1961;8:413–417.
9. Kusic R, Jovanovic D, Randjelovic S, et al. HI-6 in man: efficacy of the oxime in poisoning by organophosphorus insecticides. *Hum Exp Toxicol* 1991;10(2):113–118.
10. Sidell FR, Groff WA. Intramuscular and intravenous administration of small doses of 2-pyridinium aldoxime methochloride to man. *J Pharm Sci* 1971;60(8):1224–1228.
11. Kusic R, Boskovic B, Vojvodic V, et al. HI-6 in man: blood levels, urinary excretion, and tolerance after intramuscular administration of the oxime to healthy volunteers. *Fundam Appl Toxicol* 1985;5(6 Pt 2):S89–S97.
12. Hamilton MG, Lundy PM. HI-6 therapy of soman and tabun poisoning in primates and rodents. *Arch Toxicol* 1989;63(2):144–149.
13. van Helden HP, van der Wiel HJ, de Lange J, et al. Therapeutic efficacy of HI-6 in soman-poisoned marmoset monkeys. *Toxicol Appl Pharmacol* 1992;115(1):50–56.
14. Lundy PM, Hansen AS, Hand BT, et al. Comparison of several oximes against poisoning by soman, tabun and GF. *Toxicology* 1992;72(1):99–105.
15. Eyer P, Hagedorn I, Ladstetter B. Study on the stability of the oxime HI 6 in aqueous solution. *Arch Toxicol* 1988;62(2–3):224–226.
16. Eyer P, Ladstetter B, Schafer W, et al. Studies on the stability and decomposition of the Hagedorn-oxime HLo 7 in aqueous solution. *Arch Toxicol* 1989;63(1):59–67.
17. Schlager JW, Dolzine TW, Stewart JR, et al. Operational evaluation of three

commercial configurations of atropine/HI-6 wet/dry autoinjectors. *Pharm Res* 1991;8(9):1191–1194.
18. Comroe JH Jr, Todd J, et al. The pharmacology of di-isopropyl fluorophosphate (DFP) in man. *J Pharmacol Exp Ther* 1946;87:281–290.
19. Grob D, Lilienthal JL, et al. The administration of di-isopropyl fluorophosphate (DFP) to man. *Bull Johns Hopkins Hosp* 1947;81:217–244.
20. Koster R. Synergisms and antagonisms between physostigmine and di-isopropyl fluorophosphate in cats. *J Pharmacol Exp Ther* 1946;88:39–46.
21. Salerno PR, Coon JM. Drug protection against the lethal action of parathion. *Arch Int Pharmacodyn Ther* 1950;84:227–236.
22. Pelfrene AF. Acute poisonings by carbamate insecticides and oxime therapy. *J Toxicol Clin Exp* 1986;6(5):313–318.
23. Natoff IL, Reiff B. Effect of oximes on the acute toxicity of anticholinesterase carbamates. *Toxicol Appl Pharmacol* 1973;25(4):569–575.
24. Sterri SH, Rognerud B, Fiskum SE, et al. Effect of toxogonin and P2S on the toxicity of carbamates and organophosphorus compounds. *Acta Pharmacol Toxicol (Copenh)* 1979;45(1):9–15.
25. Namba T. Diagnosis and treatment of organophosphate insecticide poisoning. *Med Times* 1972;100(6):100–101(passim).
26. Gunderson CH, Lehmann CR, Sidell FR, et al. Nerve agents: a review. *Neurology* 1992;42(5):946–950.
27. Dunn MA, Sidell FR. Progress in medical defense against nerve agents. *JAMA* 1989;262(5):649–652.
28. Marrs TC. Toxicology of oximes used in treatment of organophosphate poisoning. *Adverse Drug React Toxicol Rev* 1991;10(1):61–73.
29. Calesnick B, Christensen, Richter M. Human toxicity of various oximes. 2-Pyridine aldoxime methyl chloride, its methane sulfonate salt, and 1,1'-trimethylenebis-(4-formylpyridinium chloride). *Arch Environ Health* 1967;15(5):599–608.
30. Sidell FR, Groff WA. Toxogonin: blood levels and side effects after intramuscular administration in man. *J Pharm Sci* 1970;59(6):793–797.
31. Merrill DG, Mihm FG. Prolonged toxicity of organophosphate poisoning. *Crit Care Med* 1982;10(8):550–551.
32. Dart RC, Stark Y, Fulton B, et al. Insufficient stocking of poisoning antidotes in hospital pharmacies. *JAMA* 1996;276(18):1508–1510.
33. Dart RC, Goldfrank LR, Chyka PA, et al. Combined evidence-based literature analysis and consensus guidelines for stocking of emergency antidotes in the United States. *Ann Emerg Med* 2000;36(2):126–132.

CHAPTER 70
Protamine Sulfate

E. Martin Caravati

OVERVIEW

Protamine is derived from fish sperm or roe and consists of the peptides arginine, proline, serine, and valine. Protamine sulfate is used in severe overdose or bleeding caused by heparin, and it partially reverses low-molecular-weight heparins.

Forms Available

Protamine is available as a preservative-free 10-mg/ml intravenous (IV) preparation in 50-mg/5 ml and 250-mg/25 ml vials (protamine sulfate injection).

Mechanism of Action

Protamine combines with heparin, forming an inactive salt that has no anticoagulation activity. This neutralization occurs within 5 minutes of administration. Protamine also neutralizes the antithrombin activity, but only partially the antifactor-Xa effects, of low-molecular-weight heparins. Protamine itself has weak, clinically insignificant anticoagulant activity.

INDICATIONS

The primary indication is bleeding associated with heparin or low-molecular-weight heparin therapy or overdose. Protamine is also used to reverse heparin anticoagulation associated with extracorporal circulation in cardiac surgery or dialysis procedures.

CAUTIONS AND CONTRAINDICATIONS

A history of protamine allergy is the primary contraindication. Fish allergy, vasectomy, infertile males, diabetics who received protamine-containing insulin (isophane), or patients previously treated with protamine may be at increased risk for a hypersensitivity reaction. Fatal anaphylactic reactions have occurred. Resuscitation equipment should be immediately available (1).

Protamine is U.S. Food and Drug Administration pregnancy category C. One case of neonatal central nervous system depression after maternal protamine injection before delivery has been reported (2).

DOSAGE AND ADMINISTRATION

Heparin Neutralization or Overdose

The amount of heparin, route of administration, and time since exposure determine the dose of protamine. Administer protamine by slow IV injection over 10 minutes. The maximum amount administered in any one dose should be 50 mg. If given within minutes of IV heparin injection, 1.0 to 1.5 mg of protamine sulfate is given for each 100 U of heparin administered. If 1 hour has elapsed since the heparin injection, 0.50 to 0.75 mg of protamine can be given for every 100 U of heparin; if more than 2 hours have elapsed, 0.250 to 0.375 mg of protamine can be given for each 100 U of heparin. If heparin was administered by infusion, 25 to 50 mg of protamine is given after stopping the infusion (3).

For heparin administered subcutaneously, give 1.0 to 1.5 mg of protamine per 100 units of heparin. A loading dose of 25 to 50 mg may be given initially by slow IV injection and the rest by continuous infusion over 8 to 16 hours.

Low-Molecular-Weight Heparins

Guidelines for dosing are the same as for heparin, but higher doses may be required due to partial activity against these drugs.

Monitoring of Response

The activated partial thromboplastin time or activated coagulation time can be used to monitor protamine effectiveness 5 to 15 minutes after administration. Repeat monitoring in 2 to 8 hours if there is a concern for heparin rebound.

ADVERSE EFFECTS

Hypersensitivity (anaphylaxis, anaphylactoid) reactions may occur. Acute hypotension, bradycardia, pulmonary hypertension, dyspnea, transient flushing, and a feeling of warmth can occur when protamine is given in doses above 50 mg (10 mg/ml) over 10 minutes or less. Noncardiogenic pulmonary edema has been reported in patients receiving protamine while on cardiopulmonary bypass undergoing cardiac surgery or shortly thereafter (2).

Heparin rebound is the recurrence of anticoagulant activity after adequate neutralization with protamine. It may result in bleeding and is usually associated with cardiopulmonary bypass or dialysis procedures. It occurs 30 minutes to 18 hours after protamine administration despite adequate initial dosing.

Overdose of 600 to 800 mg of IV protamine has resulted in minor, transient anticoagulation.

PITFALLS

Minor bleeding associated with heparin therapy usually resolves within a few hours of discontinuing the heparin, and protamine need not be administered. Major bleeding should also be treated with fresh frozen plasma or blood transfusion.

REFERENCES

1. Holland CL, Singh AK, McMaster PR, et al. Adverse reactions to protamine sulfate following cardiac surgery. *Clin Cardiol* 1984;7:157–162.
2. Wittmaack FM, Greer FR, Fitzsimmons J. Neonatal depression after a protamine sulfate injection. *J Reprod Med* 1994;39:655–656.
3. Protamine, protamine sulfate [package insert]. Indianapolis, IN: Eli Lilly & Co; 1997.

CHAPTER 71

Pyridoxine

Andrew R. Erdman

CH_2OH / HO / CH_2OH / H_3C / N

PYRIDOXINE

Synonyms:	**Vitamin B_6, pyridoxine hydrochloride**
Molecular formula and weight:	**$C_8H_{11}NO_3$, HCl, 205.6 g/mol**
SI conversion:	**1 ng/ml = 4.046 nmol/L**
CAS Registry No.:	**58-56-0**
Normal or therapeutic levels:	**Not applicable**
Special concerns:	**Iatrogenic overdose may cause peripheral neuropathy.**

OVERVIEW

Pyridoxine (vitamin B_6) is a water-soluble vitamin that is an essential cofactor in a variety of enzymatic reactions. It is used for the treatment of pyridoxine deficiency produced by dietary insufficiencies or chronic isoniazid (INH) use. Small doses are given to patients taking chronic INH to prevent the development of neuritis (1,2). In high doses, intravenous (IV) pyridoxine is an effective antidote for the treatment of acute INH or monomethylhydrazine (MMH) poisoning (3–5). Lower doses can be used as adjunctive treatment of acute ethylene glycol poisoning. Pyridoxine has also been used for nausea and vomiting and a variety of other medical conditions (6–8).

Forms Available

Pyridoxine hydrochloride is available as a sterile solution in vials (100 mg/ml) for IV or intramuscular administration. It may be given with any crystalloid fluid. Oral forms of pyridoxine are available for long-term use but are not appropriate for the treatment of acute poisoning.

Mechanism of Action

ISONIAZID TOXICITY

Acute INH toxicity is characterized by obtundation or coma, recurrent seizures, severe metabolic acidosis, and, occasionally, death (5,9–11) (Chapter 91). Seizures probably arise from a reduction in γ-aminobutyric acid (GABA) levels in the brain (12). Normally, GABA suppresses neurotransmission in the central nervous system. Its reduction therefore allows for uncontrolled electrical activity and seizures.

The reduction in GABA is probably the result of several mechanisms. First, INH and its metabolites inhibit the enzyme pyridoxal kinase (13–15). Pyridoxal kinase catalyzes a crucial reaction in the transformation of pyridoxine to its active form, pyridoxal-5-phosphate (PLP) (Fig. 1). PLP is an essential cofactor for the enzyme glutamate decarboxylase, which synthesizes GABA from glutamate (16,17). In addition, INH and its metabolites also appear to inactivate PLP that has already been formed or speed its elimination from the body (13,14). Finally, INH and other hydrazines can combine with pyridoxine, forming hydrazone intermediates that have an even stronger inhibitory effect on GABA synthesis (15,18). The net effect is a decrease in PLP

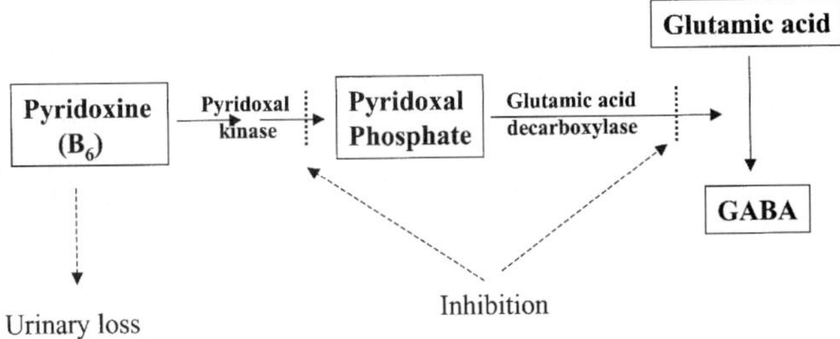

Figure 1. Role of pyridoxine and isoniazid in metabolic activation of glutamic acid. Isoniazid and other hydrazines, hydrazides, or their metabolites may increase urinary loss of pyridoxine and block the enzymes pyridoxal kinase and glutamic acid decarboxylase. GABA, γ-aminobutyric acid.

activity, leading to decreases in central nervous system GABA, with subsequent neuronal disinhibition and seizures (16). Other hydrazine and hydrazide compounds (such as MMH and hydrazine) appear to act in a similar manner (4,15,18–20).

PYRIDOXINE ANTIDOTAL ACTIVITY

Pyridoxine itself is inactive. It is converted in the body to its active form, PLP, in a two-step process involving phosphorylation (catalyzed by pyridoxal kinase) and oxidation (Fig. 1). Treatment with high doses of pyridoxine presumably overcomes inhibition of pyridoxal kinase by hydrazine compounds to replenish PLP and restore GABA synthesis (3,12,16). Both oral and IV doses of pyridoxine result in elevated PLP levels, but PLP production after IV infusion is much greater (perhaps because of a lack of first-pass metabolism in the liver), suggesting that IV pyridoxine is the preferred route in cases of acute toxicity (21).

Little is known about the pharmacokinetics of high-dose pyridoxine. However, it appears that a large proportion of any unused drug gets converted in the liver to pyridoxic acid or other metabolites, which can then be eliminated in the urine (21,22). Pyridoxine has a volume distribution of approximately 0.6 L/kg.

PYRIDOXINE FOR ETHYLENE GLYCOL POISONING

Once in the body, ethylene glycol is converted to glycolate, which contributes to the metabolic acidosis associated with toxicity. Glycolate is subsequently converted to glyoxylate and then oxalate, which is renally excreted. Urinary oxalate excretion causes renal injury. Glyoxylate can also be converted to nontoxic alternatives such as glycine, a reaction that depends on PLP as a cofactor (23,24). It has been proposed that pyridoxine could increase PLP and help facilitate this alternate conversion. There are few data to support this view, although evidence from patients with other forms of hyperoxaluria suggests that pyridoxine can reduce their level of oxalate excretion (25,26).

INDICATIONS

Isoniazid

Pyridoxine is indicated for patients with seizures, altered mental status, or severe metabolic acidosis as the result of acute INH poisoning. The diagnosis may not be known initially, but it should be suspected in any patient with unexplained seizures or severe acidosis, particularly if he or she has a history of tuberculosis or has access to INH. A trial dose of pyridoxine should be considered in any patient with refractory seizures.

High-dose pyridoxine is an effective antidote in animal models of INH poisoning, and successful human case reports attest to its efficacy (3,5,11,16,27–29). There are no controlled human trials, but one case series found that no patient treated with IV pyridoxine developed recurrent seizures or died, compared with historic controls in whom 60% developed recurrent seizures and 7% died (10). Most reports indicate that pyridoxine often results in a dramatic cessation of seizures. In addition, pyridoxine can also improve mental status, coma, and metabolic acidosis associated with severe INH toxicity (10,30,31). A few authors have noted less dramatic results in the reversal of encephalopathy and acidosis, but inadequate doses were used in some of these cases (9,13,32,33). Pyridoxine appears to act synergistically with diazepam for patients with seizures (27).

Monomethylhydrazine

Pyridoxine has not been well studied as an antidote for acute MMH toxicity. In animals, it effectively treats seizures and improves mortality at smaller doses than have been required for INH (4,14,34,35). Patients with significant metabolic or neurologic consequences (e.g., coma, seizures) after MMH exposure should be given a trial of IV pyridoxine.

Hydrazine

The role of pyridoxine in hydrazine toxicity is uncertain. Animal data are conflicting regarding its benefit (18,36,37). Two human case reports in which pyridoxine was used are equivocal (38,39). Given its relative safety and the absence of a better antidote, IV pyridoxine should be considered in patients with severe hydrazine toxicity, particularly in the presence of seizures. Theoretically, pyridoxine may be helpful for poisoning from other hydrazines and hydrazides, or related compounds (e.g., phenelzine) (37,40).

Ethylene Glycol

Intermediate doses of pyridoxine may be used as an adjunctive measure to reduce renal toxicity and acidosis, at least until dialysis can be instituted.

CAUTIONS AND CONTRAINDICATIONS

Pyridoxine should be avoided in patients with known hypersensitivity to the drug or to any of the other ingredients in the injectable solution. The toxic threshold or maximum single dose of pyridoxine has not been well established. Acute doses of up to approximately 20 to 25 g in adults are widely considered to be safe. In general, in the acute setting, cumulative doses should not exceed 1 g/kg (e.g., 70 g in a normal adult).

Pyridoxine is U.S. Food and Drug Administration pregnancy category A. Pyridoxine is often used for the treatment of nausea and vomiting in pregnancy (75 mg/day orally). The use of high doses has not been adequately studied. Excessive chronic oral intake by one mother was reportedly followed by withdrawal seizures in her newborn infant after birth (41).

DOSAGE AND ADMINISTRATION

Isoniazid

The dose of pyridoxine for *adult* or *pediatric* patients with toxicity after INH ingestion is 1 g of pyridoxine IV for each gram of INH ingested (5,10,11,28,42). If the amount of INH is unknown, the adult dose is 5 g IV and the pediatric dose is 70 mg/kg (not to exceed 5 g) (9,10). The dosage is important. Although smaller doses (e.g., 100 to 1000 mg IV) were effective in some cases, most authors have found such doses to be ineffective (29,33,43). One review found that 1:1 dosing was uniformly successful, but 10% to 50% dosing had a seizure recurrence rate of 11%, and patients receiving doses of 10% or less had a seizure recurrence rate of 47% (10).

Benzodiazepines should be given with pyridoxine for convulsions (Chapter 91). In animals, the two drugs appear to act synergistically in reducing seizures and mortality from INH or MMH poisoning (3,4,27). Other anticonvulsants may also be effective (27). Although data are limited, sodium bicarbonate may also be a helpful adjunct in patients with severe metabolic acidosis (29).

Most authors recommend that pyridoxine be infused slowly (5,9,10,30). Based on anecdotal cases, infusion of the initial dose over 5 to 10 minutes appears to be safe and terminates seizures quickly. At least three patients have received 15 to 25 g IV over approximately 30 minutes without apparent problem. If a dose greater than 10 g is needed, it may be wise to infuse the first 5 g as a bolus and run the remaining amount as an infusion, or by repeated injections, over several hours (5,10,22,30,43).

If IV pyridoxine is not available, oral tablets can be crushed and administered enterally as a slurry. The IV route produces higher levels of PLP, however, and there was no apparent protective effect in patients who ingested pyridoxine along with an INH overdose (21,33).

The most important indicator of a positive response to pyridoxine is the cessation or control of seizures. Acid-base status should also be monitored. The initial dose of pyridoxine should be repeated if no clinical response is seen within approximately 5 to 30 minutes.

Monomethylhydrazine

The recommended initial dose of pyridoxine for patients with MMH toxicity is 25 mg/kg IV (4). A repeat dose should be given in 5 to 30 minutes if there is an inadequate clinical response. As with INH, cessation of seizures and acidosis should be monitored.

Hydrazine

No established dose exists for acute hydrazine poisoning. A trial of 5 g (or 70 mg/kg in children) IV may be given for patients with significant toxicity who do not respond to conservative measures. At least one animal study has found that pyridoxine alone is not sufficient to treat hydrazine toxicity; supplemental glucose was also required for full benefit (37).

Ethylene Glycol

The usual dose of pyridoxine for severe ethylene glycol poisoning is 50 mg IV or intramuscularly every 6 hours until toxicity has resolved.

ADVERSE EFFECTS

Large doses of pyridoxine can produce severe peripheral neuropathy, even after a single IV administration (38,44). Neuropathy is more commonly associated with chronic supratherapeutic oral or IV administration (12,45,46). The toxic threshold for neurologic injury is not clear. In one patient, a dose of only 10 g IV was followed by the development of a delayed neuropathy, but this patient had also overdosed on hydrazine, which in itself might have caused or contributed to the injury (38). Massive doses (132 g and 183 g IV) given over 3 days were associated with a severe, debilitating neuropathy (44). Both patients developed long-term deficits including weakness, decreased sensation, paresthesia, ataxia, nystagmus, bowel and bladder dysfunction, and abnormal nerve conduction studies. In most cases, doses of 10 to 25 g (70 to 357 mg/kg) have been given acutely without problems (5,9,10,29,30). A pediatric study found that 30 to 50 mg/kg/day could be administered for several days without problems (8).

In animals, massive doses (more than 1 g/kg) have been associated with peripheral nervous system and central nervous system effects (including seizures, ataxia, paralysis), and doses in excess of 3 to 4 g/kg were often fatal (3,22,47).

The mechanism of neurologic injury is not clear. Most reports describe a sensory axonopathy, but occasionally, motor neurons are also affected (38,48,49). Histopathology generally reveals nuclear changes, neurofilamentous accumulations, and frank necrosis in the dorsal root ganglia and neuronal axons.

Clinically, the patient develops symptoms most consistent with a sensory neuropathy, although motor deficits can occur (12,38,44,50). Symptoms can be severe or debilitating (44). Although histopathologic changes may occur within 24 to 72 hours of administration, clinical symptoms generally do not develop for several days (38,44,49). In most cases, the neuropathy resolves either partially or completely within 3 to 6 months of stopping therapy (12,38,44,50). In some cases, the neuronal injury continues to progress after the cessation of pyridoxine, before finally resolving. In others, neurologic deficits may persist indefinitely (38,44,46).

Chronic therapy with lower doses of pyridoxine also carries the risk of neuropathy (12,45,46). Most of these patients were treated for months or years with daily oral or IV doses before complications developed. The risk appears to be related to the dose and duration of treatment (6,12,46). In general, daily oral doses of less than 500 mg are regarded as safe.

Dermatologic complications, such as a vesicular dermatosis, have been reported after long-term use of high oral doses (2 to 4 g daily) (51).

PITFALLS

Whereas seizures typically respond well to pyridoxine, acidosis and mental status improve more slowly.

Smaller doses than those recommended may be ineffective. At least in the case of INH poisoning, there is a definite dose-response relationship with pyridoxine.

Massive amounts of pyridoxine (especially those exceeding 1 g/kg cumulatively in the acute setting) can lead to significant neurologic injury. Clinicians should follow the dosing recommendations listed previously.

REFERENCES

1. Pellock JM, Howell J, Kendig EL Jr, et al. Pyridoxine deficiency in children treated with isoniazid. *Chest* 1985;87(5):658–661.
2. Snider DE Jr. Pyridoxine supplementation during isoniazid therapy. *Tubercle* 1980;61(4):191–196.
3. Chin L, Sievers ML, Laird HE, et al. Evaluation of diazepam and pyridoxine as antidotes to isoniazid intoxication in rats and dogs. *Toxicol Appl Pharmacol* 1978;45(3):713–722.
4. George ME, Pinkerton MK, Back KC. Therapeutics of monomethylhydrazine intoxication. *Toxicol Appl Pharmacol* 1982;63(2):201–208.
5. Yarbrough BE, Wood JP. Isoniazid overdose treated with high-dose pyridoxine. *Ann Emerg Med* 1983;12(5):303–305.
6. Brush MG, Bennett T, Hansen K. Pyridoxine in the treatment of premenstrual syndrome: a retrospective survey in 630 patients. *Br J Clin Pract* 1988;42(11):448–452.

7. Amadio PC. Pyridoxine as an adjunct in the treatment of carpal tunnel syndrome. *J Hand Surg [Am]* 1985;10(2):237–241.
8. Jiao FY, Gao DY, Takuma Y, et al. Randomized, controlled trial of high-dose intravenous pyridoxine in the treatment of recurrent seizures in children. *Pediatr Neurol* 1997;17(1):54–57.
9. Orlowski JP, Paganini EP, Pippenger CE. Treatment of a potentially lethal dose isoniazid ingestion. *Ann Emerg Med* 1988;17(1):73–76.
10. Wason S, Lacouture PG, Lovejoy FH Jr. Single high-dose pyridoxine treatment for isoniazid overdose. *JAMA* 1981;246(10):1102–1104.
11. Blanchard PD, Yao JD, McAlpine DE, et al. Isoniazid overdose in the Cambodian population of Olmsted County, Minnesota. *JAMA* 1986;256(22):3131–3133.
12. Berger AR, Schaumburg HH, Schroeder C, et al. Dose response, coasting, and differential fiber vulnerability in human toxic neuropathy: a prospective study of pyridoxine neurotoxicity. *Neurology* 1992;42(7):1367–1370.
13. Biehl JP, Vilter RW. Effects of isoniazid on pyridoxine metabolism. *JAMA* 1954;156:1549–1552.
14. Holtz P, Palm D. Pharmacological aspects of vitamin B_6. *Pharmacol Rev* 1964;16:113–178.
15. McCormick DB, Guirard BM, Snell EE. Comparative inhibition of pyridoxal kinase and glutamic acid decarboxylase by carbonyl reagents. *Proc Soc Exp Biol Med* 1960;104:554–557.
16. Wood JD, Peesker SJ. The effect on GABA metabolism in brain of isonicotinic acid hydrazide and pyridoxine as a function of time after administration. *J Neurochem* 1972;19(6):1527–1537.
17. Wood JD, Peesker SJ. A correlation between changes in GABA metabolism and isonicotinic acid hydrazide-induced seizures. *Brain Res* 1972;45:489–498.
18. Medina MA. The in vivo effects of hydrazines and vitamin B6 on the metabolism of gamma-aminobutyric acid. *J Pharm Exp Ther* 1963;140:133–137.
19. Wood JD, Peesker SJ. Development of an expression which relates the excitable state of the brain to the level of GAD activity and GABA content, with particular reference to the action of hydrazine and its derivatives. *J Neurochem* 1974;23(4):703–712.
20. Smith TE. Brain carbohydrate metabolism during hydrazine toxicity. *Biochem Pharmacol* 1965;14(6):979–988.
21. Zempleni J. Pharmacokinetics of vitamin B_6 supplements in humans. *J Am Coll Nutr* 1995;14(6):579–586.
22. Pyridoxine hydrochloride injection [package insert]. Los Angeles: American Pharmaceutical Partners; May 2002.
23. Parry MF, Wallach R. Ethylene glycol poisoning. *Am J Med* 1974;57(1):143–150.
24. Beasley VR, Buck WB. Acute ethylene glycol toxicosis: a review. *Vet Hum Toxicol* 1980;22(4):255–263.
25. Gibbs DA, Watts RW. The action of pyridoxine in primary hyperoxaluria. *Clin Sci* 1970;38(2):277–286.
26. Watts RW, Veall N, Purkiss P, et al. The effect of pyridoxine on oxalate dynamics in three cases of primary hyperoxaluria (with glycolic aciduria). *Clin Sci (Lond)* 1985;69(1):87–90.
27. Chin L, Sievers ML, Herrier RN, et al. Potentiation of pyridoxine by depressants and anticonvulsants in the treatment of acute isoniazid intoxication in dogs. *Toxicol Appl Pharmacol* 1981;58(3):504–509.
28. Katz GA, Jobin GC. Large doses of pyridoxine in the treatment of massive ingestion of isoniazid. *Am Rev Respir Dis* 1970;101(6):991–992.
29. Brown CV. Acute isoniazid poisoning. *Am Rev Respir Dis* 1972;105(2):206–216.
30. Gilhotra R, Malik SK, Singh S, et al. Acute isoniazid toxicity—report of 2 cases and review of literature. *Int J Clin Pharmacol Ther Toxicol* 1987;25(5):259–261.
31. Brent J, Vo N, Kulig K, et al. Reversal of prolonged isoniazid-induced coma by pyridoxine. *Arch Intern Med* 1990;150(8):1751–1753.
32. Miller J, Robinson A, Percy AK. Acute isoniazid poisoning in childhood. *Am J Dis Child* 1980;134(3):290–292.
33. Terman DS, Teitelbaum DT. Isoniazid self-poisoning. *Neurology* 1970;20(3):299–304.
34. Shouse MN. Acute effects of pyridoxine hydrochloride on monomethylhydrazine seizure latency and amygdaloid kindled seizure thresholds in cats. *Exp Neurol* 1982;75(1):79–88.
35. Sterman MB, Kovalesky RA. Anticonvulsant effects of restraint and pyridoxine on hydrazine seizures in the monkey. *Exp Neurol* 1979;65(1):78–86.
36. Cornish HH. The role of vitamin B6 in the toxicity of hydrazines. *Ann N Y Acad Sci* 1969;166(1):136–145.
37. Back KC, Thomas AA. Aerospace problems in pharmacology and toxicology. *Annu Rev Pharmacol* 1970;10:395–412.
38. Harati Y, Niakan E. Hydrazine toxicity, pyridoxine therapy, and peripheral neuropathy. *Ann Intern Med* 1986;104(5):728–729.
39. Nagappan R, Riddell T. Pyridoxine therapy in a patient with severe hydrazine sulfate toxicity. *Crit Care Med* 2000;28(6):2116–2118.
40. Heller CA, Friedman PA. Pyridoxine deficiency and peripheral neuropathy associated with long-term phenelzine therapy. *Am J Med* 1983;75(5):887–888.
41. South M. Neonatal seizures after use of pyridoxine in pregnancy. *Lancet* 1999;353:1940–1941.
42. Sievers ML, Herrier RN. Treatment of acute isoniazid toxicity. *Am J Hosp Pharm* 1975;32(2):202–206.
43. Cameron WM. Isoniazid overdose. *Can Med Assoc J* 1978;118(11):1413–1415.
44. Albin RL, Albers JW, Greeberg HS, et al. Acute sensory neuropathy-neuronopathy from pyridoxine overdose. *Neurology* 1987;37:1729–1732.
45. Schaumburg H, Kaplan J, Windebank A, et al. Sensory neuropathy from pyridoxine abuse. A new megavitamin syndrome. *N Engl J Med* 1983;309:445–448.
46. Parry GJ, Bredesen DE. Sensory neuropathy with low-dose pyridoxine. *Neurology* 1985;35:1466–1468.
47. Unna K. Studies on the toxicity and pharmacology of vitamin B_6 (2-methyl-3-hydroxy-4,5-bis-(hydroxymethyl)-pyridine). *J Pharm Exp Ther* 1940;70:400–407.
48. Sladky JT. Transient ataxia after acute pyridoxine intoxication: electrophysiologic and neuropathologic correlations. *Neurology* 1987;37[Suppl 1]:376.
49. Yue X, Sladky JT, Brown MJ. Proximal to distal axonopathy after acute experimental pyridoxine intoxication. *Neurology* 1987;37[Suppl 1]:310–311.
50. Dalton K, Dalton MJT. Characteristics of pyridoxine overdose neuropathy syndrome. *Acta Neurol Scand* 1987;76:8–11.
51. Friedman MA, Resnick JS, Baer RL. Subepidermal vesicular dermatosis and sensory peripheral neuropathy caused by pyridoxine abuse. *J Am Acad Dermatol* 1986;14:915–917.

CHAPTER 72

Prussian Blue

E. Martin Caravati

OVERVIEW

Prussian blue [also known as *ferric (III) hexacyanoferrate (II), insoluble PB, Berlin blue*] is administered orally and has been shown to decrease absorption and enhance elimination of thallium and cesium-137. It is not absorbed from the gastrointestinal tract and has minimal toxicity.

Forms Available

Prussian blue is not U.S. Food and Drug Administration approved and therefore has limited availability in the United States. It is distributed by Oak Ridge Institute for Science and Education under an investigational protocol (1). Prussian blue (Radiogardase-Cs) is also supplied by the company HEYL GmbH in Germany as a 0.5-g gelatin capsule for oral administration.

Questions regarding the use and availability of Prussian blue may be referred to one of the following co-principal investigators at the Oak Ridge Associated Universities, Post Office Box 117, Oak Ridge, Tennessee 37831-0117: Ronald Goans, PhD, MD (865-576-4049) or Robert Ricks, PhD (865-576-3131). For cesium, contact Robert Townsend, PhD (865-576-3300).

Mechanism of Action

The adsorption of cesium and thallium adsorption by hexacyanoferrates is not fully understood. A chemical ion-exchange mechanism is proposed in which cations of the drug are exchanged with thallium or cesium ions. Thallium is exchanged for potassium in the molecular lattice, and the complex is excreted in the feces. Fecal elimination of thallium and cesium is enhanced.

INDICATIONS

Thallium Poisoning

Prussian blue decreased the half-life of thallium and reduced mortality in an animal model (2).

Cesium-137

Prussian blue is recommended by national and international radiation protection societies for treating internal contamination with radiocesium. One gram of oral Prussian blue decreased cesium absorption from a test meal to 6% of controls (3). Prussian blue caused a cesium dose reduction of approximately 71% in adults exposed to cesium-137 (4). It can reduce the half-life of cesium by approximately 43%.

CAUTIONS AND CONTRAINDICATIONS

The primary contraindication is allergy to Prussian blue. Gastrointestinal motility is needed to eliminate the Prussian blue complexes. There is no U.S. Food and Drug Administration pregnancy category. Prussian blue is not absorbed from the gastrointestinal tract. Teratogenic effects or excretion into breast milk are not expected.

DOSAGE AND ADMINISTRATION

Thallium dosing recommendations vary: (a) 10 g in 100 ml of 15% mannitol twice daily via duodenal tube if the patient is unable to take oral medication or (b) 250 mg/kg/day orally divided into three or four doses and administered with 50 ml of 15% mannitol or 70% sorbitol solution. Initial duration of therapy is usually 2 to 3 weeks.

Cesium dosing should be based on the estimated level of internal contamination. The magnitude of the dose is based on the *annual limit of intake* (ALI). This corresponds to 100 μCi for ingestion and 200 μCi for inhalation. Recommended doses of Prussian blue based on the ALI for cesium-137 are as follows: low (1 to 5 ALI), 3 g daily; intermediate (5 to 10 ALI), 3 to 10 g daily; and high (10 or more ALI), 10 to 20 g daily. All doses should be divided and given three times daily.

Another regimen is 500 mg orally every 2 hours for a total dose of 3 g/day. Duration of therapy is days to weeks depending on the level of fecal contamination with radiocesium.

MONITORING OF RESPONSE

For thallium, Prussian blue is administered until urinary thallium concentration is less than 0.5 to 1.0 mg/24 hours. Monitor serum iron and electrolytes daily. For cesium, whole-body counts, urine, and fecal assays for cesium are monitored. Monitor serum iron and electrolytes daily.

ADVERSE EFFECTS

The reported adverse effects are obstipation and dark (blue) stools.

PITFALLS

Activated charcoal for acute oral thallium overdose should not be delayed awaiting Prussian blue. *In vitro*, the maximum absorptive capacity is 72 mg of thallium per gram of activated charcoal.

REFERENCES

1. Prussian blue [package insert]. Oak Ridge, TN: Oak Ridge Institute for Science and Education; November 8, 1999. Radiation Emergency Assistance Center/Training (REAC/TS): REAC/TS Resources. Available at: http://www.orau.gov/reacts/prussian.htm. Accessed December 28, 2001.
2. Meggs WJ, Hoffman RS, Shih RD, et al. Effects of Prussian blue and N-acetylcysteine on thallium toxicity in mice. *J Toxicol Clin Toxicol* 1997;35:163–166.
3. Dresow B, Nielsen P, Fischer R, et al. In vivo binding of radiocesium by two forms of Prussian blue and by ammonium iron hexacyanoferrate (II). *J Toxicol Clin Toxicol* 1993;31:563–569.
4. Melo DR, Lipsztein JL, de Oliveira CA, et al. 137Cs internal contamination involving a Brazilian accident, and the efficacy of Prussian blue treatment. *Health Phys* 1994;66:245–252.

CHAPTER 73

Scorpion Antivenom

Vikhyat S. Bebarta and Richard C. Dart

OVERVIEW

The only scorpions of medical importance in North America include the genus *Centruroides*. In the United States, the only medically important scorpion is *Centruroides exilicauda* (*Centruroides sculpturatus*), commonly known as the *bark scorpion*. For the past several decades, Arizona State University has produced antivenom for this scorpion from goat serum; however, it does not have U.S. Food and Drug Administration approval, and its production has been terminated. Another scorpion antivenom has achieved orphan drug investigation status but has not yet achieved regulatory approval.

Scorpion envenomation is much more common in other countries, and antivenoms with varying degrees of clinical effectiveness have been developed for most species (Table 1) (1,2).

TABLE 1. Common scorpion antivenoms worldwide

Scorpion	Location of antivenom
Androctonus	Tunisia and Germany
Buthus	Germany
Centruroides	Mexico
Leiurus quinquestriatus	Algeria, Tunisia, and Turkey
Mesobuthus and *Odontobuthus*	Iran
Parabuthus	South Africa
Scorpio	Morocco, Germany, and Iran
Tityus	Brazil

Adapted from Theakston RDG, Warrell DA. Antivenoms: a list of hyperimmune sera currently available for the treatment of envenoming by bites and stings. *Toxicon* 1991;29:1419–1470.

INDICATIONS

Antivenom for scorpion envenomation in the United States is indicated for grade III or IV envenomation, patients with intractable pain or agitation, or patients with possible airway compromise (3). Young patients (younger than 2 years of age) are more likely to present with serious envenomation or airway compromise (4–6). As an alternative to antivenom, supportive care using parenteral analgesics and sedatives (e.g., midazolam) accompanied by aggressive airway management in an intensive care setting may be used (7). The risks and benefits, including monetary costs, must be weighed before choosing a treatment option.

CAUTIONS AND CONTRAINDICATIONS

All antivenoms are capable of producing severe allergic reactions. Acute reactions appear to be more common in patients with a history of asthma or a medication allergy, especially an antibiotic allergy. The only absolute contraindication is an allergy to goat serum.

DOSAGE AND METHOD OF ADMINISTRATION

A skin test, performed by injecting 0.02 ml intradermally, should be conducted before administration. The development of erythema and particularly induration (greater than 10 mm) at 30 minutes, or systemic symptoms, such as bronchospasm, urticaria, or hypotension, are considered positive tests (8). A positive test is not an absolute contraindication to antivenom use.

A therapeutic dose is delivered by diluting 1 antivenom vial into 100 ml of 5% dextrose water or saline and infusing intravenously over 15 to 30 minutes. One dose is usually sufficient, but a second dose may be needed rarely. Because of the risk for anaphylaxis, all antivenoms should be administered in a critical care setting.

ADVERSE EFFECTS

Immediate allergic reactions occur in almost 10% of patients. Slowing the infusion rate and increasing the dilution should lessen the reaction. Serum sickness occurs in up to 60% of cases and correlates with the number of vials given (3,4).

PITFALLS

Due to the high rate of serum sickness and allergic reactions, the antivenom should be given only to those with significant envenomations. Significant allergic reactions to the antivenom skin test and therapeutic dose should be anticipated; failure to do so can lead to airway compromise and increased morbidity.

REFERENCES

1. Abroug F, El Atrous S, Nouira S, et al. Serotherapy in scorpion envenomation: a randomised controlled trial. *Lancet* 1999;354:906–909.
2. Sofer S, Shahak E, Gueron M. Scorpion envenomation and antivenom therapy. *J Pediatr* 1994;124:973–978.
3. Belghith M, Boussarsar M, Haguiga H, et al. Efficacy of serotherapy in scorpion sting: a matched-pair study. *J Toxicol Clin Toxicol* 1999;37:51–57.
4. LoVecchio F, Welch S, Klemens J, et al. Incidence of immediate and delayed hypersensitivity to *Centruroides* antivenom. *Ann Emerg Med* 1999;34:615–619.
5. Curry SC, Vance MV, Ryan PJ, et al. Envenomation by the scorpion *Centruroides sculpturatus*. *J Toxicol Clin Toxicol* 1983–1984;21:417–449.
6. Likes K, Banner W, Chavez M. *Centruroides exilicauda* envenomation in Arizona. *West J Med* 1984;141:634–637.
7. Gibly R, Williams M, Walter FG, et al. Continuous intravenous midazolam infusion for *Centruroides exilicauda* scorpion envenomation. *Ann Emerg Med* 1999;34:620–625.
8. Bond GR. Antivenin administration for *Centruroides* scorpion sting: risks and benefits. *Ann Emerg Med* 1992;21:788–791.

CHAPTER 74

Snake Antivenoms for the United States

Andrew R. Erdman and Richard C. Dart

Synonyms:	**Antivenin (Crotalidae) polyvalent, polyvalent Crotalidae immune Fab (ovine) (FabAV, CroFab), antivenin (*Micrurus fulvius*)**
Molecular weight:	**Fab, 50 to 60 kd; Fab_2, 110 kd; immunoglobulin G (IgG), 150 kd**
Therapeutic levels:	**Not clinically applicable**
Special concerns:	**Delay in antivenom administration may allow tissue injury to progress. All protein products are capable of causing anaphylaxis.**

OVERVIEW

Many treatments have been proposed for snake venom poisoning, ranging from alcohol to strychnine to the application of a split chicken to the site (1). However, nothing has come close in efficacy to the immunotherapies—otherwise known as *antivenoms*. Antivenoms are mixtures of antibodies or antigen-binding antibody fragments, derived from animal serum, that bind and inactivate components of venom. If given in a timely fashion, they can be extremely effective in preventing morbidity and mortality associated with a wide variety of animal envenomations. Snake antivenoms relevant to the United States are addressed in this chapter; other antivenoms are described separately (Chapters 73 and 76).

There is an antivenom available for most species of venomous snakes. A list of available antivenoms worldwide can be accessed online at http://www.toxinology.com. However, local and regional antivenom availability varies widely. Clinicians should be familiar with the venomous snakes in their region and regularly confirm antivenom availability. However, given the fact that zoos, aquariums, and amateur hobbyists are keeping an increasingly global array of snake species in captivity, clinicians need also be familiar with the acquisition of snake antisera for these exotic snake species. In North America, exotic snake antivenoms are generally stocked by a network of legitimate zoos and aquariums. The most complete and up-to-date list of these antivenoms is the *Antivenom Index* (2). The index helps identify which antivenoms can be used for a particular snake species. It also gives information on where to locate the antivenom.

It should be noted that antivenoms are biological agents that differ from other pharmaceuticals in several important aspects: (a) they have no single chemical formula and often have multiple active components; (b) no matter how well they are processed, they are never entirely pure; (c) they may be less stable than typical chemical pharmaceuticals; (d) their activity is difficult to quantify and standardize from batch to batch; and (e) quality control is more difficult to achieve.

The primary advantage of antibodies as therapeutic agents is their specificity. Compared with chemical drugs, which often block the action of many enzymes in addition to the target enzyme, antibodies have a much larger structure, allowing them to conform more closely to the target antigen and imbuing them with remarkable specificity.

History of Antivenoms

Antiserum research began in the late 1800s. The first documented experiment took place in 1887, when pigeons were immunized against snake venom, ameliorating its toxicity (3). The limitations of active immunization became evident quickly—namely, inadequate long-term efficacy and the need to preemptively treat large populations. Passively administered immunotherapies were developed shortly thereafter. These antisera could be given after a bite and only to those who needed it. The first such antisera were reportedly developed in France and Brazil (1,4). Based on simple animal lethality studies (5), these early serum therapies began to be used in humans over the ensuing three decades, with anecdotal success (1,4,6). Mortality from snakebites was reported to drop significantly as a result (1,7).

Antivenoms were not widely available in the United States until Wyeth Laboratories introduced equine hyperimmune serum for rattlesnake bites in 1954 under the name *Antivenin (Crotalidae) Polyvalent* (ACP) (8,9). A variety of other antivenoms began to be commercially produced throughout the world around the same time (10,11). In the United States, ACP proved to be a safe and effective treatment for large numbers of patients with crotaline snake envenomation (12–17). However, some authors continued to argue against its use because of a relatively small but significant risk of allergic reactions, some of which were severe (18). Meanwhile, further refinements in the production of commercial antivenoms occurred—most notably, the development of cleaved antibody fragment–based therapies, such as Fab or Fab_2 antivenoms, and the use of affinity column purification, both of which reduced the risk of adverse reactions associated with the use of antivenom (19–25).

Terms

All current antivenoms are derived from the serum of animals that have been immunized against a target venom or venoms—hence, the interchangeable term *antisera*. Snake antivenoms can be categorized based on preparation and content. *Monovalent antivenom* contains antibodies against the venom of one species. *Polyvalent antivenoms* contain antibodies against more than one species (often a mixture of those species common to a particular geographic region). In general, monovalent antivenoms tend to be more effective and have fewer side effects because their homologous nature allows a lower dose to be administered (26,27). They are, however, impractical in many locales because of multiple endogenous snake species and because choosing the correct antivenom requires identification of the snake, something that is rarely possible. With polyvalent antivenoms, a smaller proportion of their volume is specific for a given snake species, but the mixture of species ensures efficacy for a broad range of snakes.

Some antivenoms contain whole immunoglobulin G (IgG). Others are comprised primarily of immunoglobulin fragments, obtained through enzymatic cleavage of the original IgGs into Fab or Fab_2 fragments (Fig. 1). Antibody fragments are much smaller in size—approximately 50 kd and 110 kd, respectively, for Fab and Fab_2 but still bind to venom. With the Fc portion of the antibody removed, fragmented products may be less immunogenic than their whole immunoglobulin counterparts, reducing the probability of adverse effects (20).

Finally, antivenoms can be classified based on the type of animal from which they are derived. Horses (equine) and sheep (ovine) are the most common animals used in commercial antivenom production. Sheep are preferred by some authors because of a presumed decreased immunogenicity compared to equine serum and because sheep are generally easier to maintain (28,29). Other animals that have been used include dogs, goats, and rabbits (30–32).

Mechanism of Action

Snake venoms are complex mixtures of enzymes, peptides, metalloproteins, and other constituents (33). Their composition varies from species to species and between individual snakes within a species. Despite these differences, there is often a significant degree

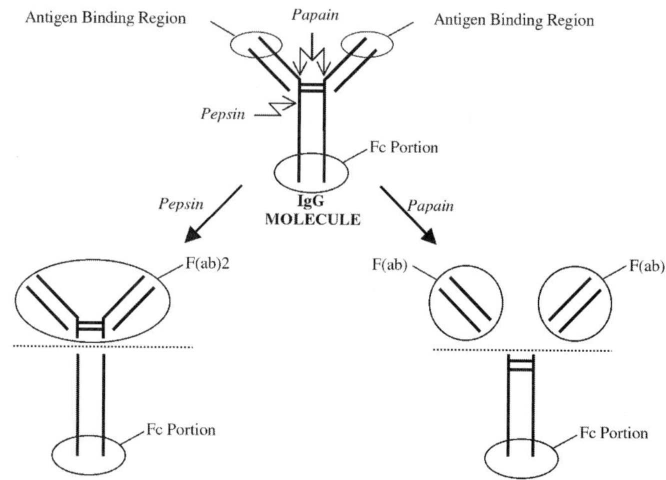

Figure 1. Production of Fab and Fab_2 from whole immunoglobulin G (IgG).

of similarity or cross-reactivity between venoms. Venom components cause local and systemic injury via a number of potential mechanisms including enzymatic degradation (e.g., local tissue injury, fibrinogenolysis); induction of proinflammatory mediators (e.g., local tissue injury); or by binding and sequestering certain constituents within the body (e.g., thrombocytopenia) (34–37). The clinical effects of most snake venoms can be grouped into three general categories: (a) local effects (i.e., swelling, ecchymosis); (b) systemic effects (i.e., hypotension, weakness and paralysis, rhabdomyolysis, altered mental status); and (c) coagulation effects (i.e., thrombocytopenia, hypofibrinogenemia, bleeding).

As complex as the venoms they neutralize, antivenoms are mixtures of different antibodies or antigen-binding antibody fragments. They work through steric hindrance of venom components—by binding or physically interacting with the venom components and thereby blocking their ability to bind to their target tissues. Antivenom binds circulating venom components, but also accumulates at the bite site, inactivating locally deposited venom (38). The inactive antivenom-venom complexes are then removed by the host reticuloendothelial or immune system. In the case of smaller antibody fragments (e.g., Fab), some renal elimination of complexes may occur (20).

Antivenoms often inactivate the venom of snakes that are different than but biologically related to the target species (26,39–43). This phenomenon is termed *cross-reactivity* or *paraspecific activity* and allows the manufacture of one product to have activity against a much wider range of species.

Antivenom Production

The manufacture and processing of antivenoms is a complex, multistep task and varies depending on the product. The general approach, however, is similar. First, animals are immunized against the desired venom(s). This is accomplished by injecting small amounts into the host animal, often in conjunction with an adjuvant to stimulate the animal's immune response. After a period of time, during which antibodies are produced against the venom components, an aliquot of blood is removed and the plasma separated out. The plasma is then fractionated to isolate the IgG portion, but the process leaves a significant amount of other proteins in the product. This "IgG-rich" fraction is often resuspended in solution and further purified. One approach is affinity chromatography (19,21,22,25,44). The chromatography column contains a matrix to which venom components are attached. The antiserum is then run through this column; only those components of the serum that actually bind to venom remain, attached to the column. This fraction is then eluted off to produce a product with enhanced purity and activity. The final concentrated product is sometimes lyophilized (freeze dried by sublimation under a vacuum) to a powder for storage (9,45,46). In other cases, it is packaged and distributed as a concentrated liquid, which may require special storage conditions (19,47).

Antibody fragment–based antivenoms are initially prepared in much the same manner, except that a step involving enzymatic hydrolysis of the whole IgG is added. Depending on the enzyme used, the IgG molecule is cleaved to form a single Fc and two Fab fragments (papain), or a single Fc and one Fab_2 (pepsin) (Fig. 1).

Antivenom Fragments versus Whole Immunoglobulin G

Fragment-based (Fab or Fab_2) antivenoms offer certain potential clinical advantages. Without their Fc portion, antivenom fragments are less immunogenic and less likely to induce a hypersensitivity reaction (20,22,48,49). Because the fragments are also smaller than whole immunoglobulin, they may penetrate tissues more easily (20). Theoretically, this enhances their capacity to neutralize any locally deposited venom; however, an enhanced local effect has not been noted in clinical trials.

Potential disadvantages of Fab and Fab_2 are that their smaller size may make them more easily eliminated from the body or distributed more widely to unwanted tissues (20). Both a shorter elimination half-life and an increased volume of distribution could negatively affect their systemic efficacy. Alternatively, it might lead to a recurrence of venom effects, if the antivenom were removed from circulation at a faster rate than the venom.

Antivenoms in the United States

With the exception of zoos and private collections, the only poisonous snakes found in the United States are the pit vipers (family Viperidae, subfamily Crotalinae), a group that includes rattlesnakes, copperheads, and cottonmouths, and the coral snakes (family Elapidae). Bites by the pit vipers can be managed effectively with Polyvalent Crotalidae immune Fab (ovine). Another antivenom, ACP, has been used since 1954 (13–17) for pit viper envenomations; however, the manufacturer has announced plans for its discontinuation with the advent of polyvalent Crotalidae immune Fab (ovine) Bites by coral snakes can be managed with Antivenin (*M. fulvius*).

Polyvalent Crotalidae immune Fab (FabAV, CroFab) is a Fab-based antivenom that was developed to avoid the severe hypersensitivity reactions associated with ACP (25). FabAV is made by immunizing sheep against the venoms of *Crotalus atrox* (Western diamondback rattlesnake), *Crotalus adamanteus* (Eastern diamondback rattlesnake), *Crotalus scutulatus* (Mojave rattlesnake), and *Agkistrodon piscivorus* (cottonmouth or water moccasin) (46). This breadth of species provides FabAV with a wide paraspecific efficacy, making it effective for virtually all native crotaline species. The product is actually categorized as a mixed monospecific antivenom rather than a polyvalent antivenom, because each animal is immunized against only one species of venom (rather than several venoms at once), and the sera from the four groups of sheep are later pooled. During processing, the IgG fraction is digested with papain and then affinity purified, resulting in a highly specific, pure, and concentrated final product (25). FabAV is effective at ameliorating the local systemic and coagulopathic effects of envenomations by native pit vipers.

Antivenin (*M. fulvius*) was developed to treat envenomation by the Eastern coral snake (*M. fulvius fulvius*). It was introduced in 1967 (before that, U.S. clinicians in the 1950s and 1960s had used a product imported from Brazil) (50). Antivenin (*M. fulvius*) is an equine-based whole IgG, monovalent antivenom (45). Based on several anecdotal reports and case series, it appears effective in ameliorating the neurologic effects of Eastern coral snake envenomation and may prevent the development of paralysis, respiratory failure, and prolonged mechanical ventilation (51).

INDICATIONS

General Indications

In general, antivenom should be given when there is evidence of ongoing, clinically significant venom effects in a victim. A significant effect is one that threatens or has the potential to threaten life or limb. Each patient should be evaluated individually, and, in all cases, the risks of antivenom treatment (i.e., the potential for hypersensitivity reactions) should be weighed against the risks of withholding antivenom (i.e., the likely course of untreated envenomation).

It is also important to remember that snake envenomation is a dynamic process; clinical effects develop and evolve over time. Patients who may not initially meet criteria for antivenom may require treatment later. Such deterioration can occur precipitously or insidiously, so all patients should be monitored closely and for an adequate time period, with adequate stores of antivenom available.

In certain circumstances, it may be appropriate to treat an asymptomatic patient. For example, the neurologic sequelae of Eastern coral snake envenomations may be delayed in appearance, yet they may be irreversible or difficult to manage once present (51). "Prophylactic" antivenom treatment may be indicated in such cases. It has also been proposed for similar reasons for bites by the krait (*Bungarus* spp.) (52).

The indications for treating local effects require some elaboration. Local effects are unlikely to be rapidly reversed by antivenom, in contradistinction to systemic and coagulopathic effects, which often respond quickly (53). The reason is that cellular necrosis, connective tissue injury, loss of vascular integrity, tissue edema, and a local accumulation of inflammatory mediators are essentially irreversible processes that require time for the body's normal healing response to repair them. Antivenom can, however, neutralize any remaining venom components, preventing further damage (17). Essentially, antivenom stops the *progression* of local injury but should not be expected to immediately reverse it.

There are two situations in which antivenom is not needed for snakebite: when no venom has been injected (the so-called dry bite) and when the risks of the antivenom outweigh the benefits of its use. Distinguishing such cases is a difficult clinical decision that creates much of the controversy attending the treatment of venomous snakebite.

Once the decision to treat with antivenom has been made, it should be administered immediately. Earlier treatment may be more effective in certain envenomations (14). It is not known how long after a bite that antivenom is effective, and the time frame depends on the type of snake. With North American crotaline envenomation, for example, it is suggested that antivenom be given within 8 hours of the bite, but it may have some benefit up to 24 to 36 hours later. Circulating venom has even been detected in the victim's blood up to 72 hours after envenomation (13). Regardless of the time since envenomation, if there is clinical or laboratory evidence that effects are continuing to evolve or progress, antivenom should be considered.

Polyvalent Crotalidae Immune Fab (Ovine)

Polyvalent Crotalidae immune Fab (ovine) (FabAV, CroFab) is indicated for progressive local effects, or for clinically significant systemic or coagulation effects, after the bite of a North American crotaline snake. It is used most commonly for treating the progression of local injury: as measured via pain, swelling, or ecchymosis (Chapter 245). Clinically important systemic effects most commonly include remote swelling or tissue injury, hypotension, and, occasionally, neurologic effects (fasciculation, paresthesia, weakness) as well as the rare case of paralysis with bites by the Mojave rattlesnake (*C. scutulatus*). Coagulopathic indications typically include a significant drop in platelet count or fibrinogen level, a significant increase in prothrombin time or international normalized ratio, increased partial thromboplastin time, or frank bleeding.

It has been asserted that copperhead snakebites do not need antivenom treatment because they cause primarily local symptoms. In this scenario, the risks of ACP were believed by many clinicians to outweigh its potential benefit. This view is being reconsidered with the introduction of FabAV. Copperhead venom can cause severe local effects in some cases, leading to significant morbidity, and FabAV has been associated with fewer adverse effects than ACP. Although FabAV was not tested in human trials against copperhead snakebite, it was effective in animal lethality tests, confirming that it binds and neutralizes copperhead venom (41). In light of these arguments, some clinicians have treated copperhead bites like any other crotaline envenomation. The rare systemic or coagulopathic effects ocurring after copperhead bites warrant treatment, as do local effects that are serious and progressive.

The role of antivenom in venom-induced compartment syndrome is controversial. Animal research and anecdotal human experience support its use (Chapter 245), with several large case series suggesting that antivenom can prevent or obviate the need for a fasciotomy in some cases (13,15,54–56). If any sign of compartment syndrome is present, compartment pressures should be measured. If elevated, antivenom should be given, with or without mannitol if indicated, and pressures monitored regularly. In certain instances, conservative treatment using this regimen may prevent an invasive and disfiguring surgical intervention.

Antivenin (*Micrurus fulvius*)

Antivenin (*M. fulvius*) is indicated as soon as a significant bite by an Eastern coral snake is suspected (45,51). This is true even if the patient is asymptomatic. By the time the venom's effects become clinically evident, the antivenom tends to be less effective (51). Features indicating a significant bite include a history of the snake biting, holding on, and chewing; the patient having to shake the snake loose or physically remove it; puncture marks or scratches; and any evidence of local or systemic symptoms.

Administration of the antivenom appears to be effective in most cases at preventing further progression of neurologic effects (51). Rarely, it results in a rapid reversal of systemic effects that are already present. Occasionally, the symptoms of coral snake envenomation continue to progress despite treatment.

Antivenin (*M. fulvius*) also neutralizes the venom of the Texas coral snake (*Micrurus fulvius tener*) (45). It could be considered for use in human envenomations by this species.

CAUTIONS AND CONTRAINDICATIONS

All antivenoms have the potential to cause hypersensitivity reactions in the recipient, regardless of their purity. Early (acute) hypersensitivity reactions are the most serious consequence of antivenom administration. The incidence of acute reactions is difficult to ascertain. Ranges from 0.3% to 76.0% have been reported with different foreign products (11,32,57–59). Severe acute reactions may cause cardiorespiratory failure and death (9,57,59–61). Acute reactions seem to be more common with earlier, less-refined antivenoms and may have been more prevalent when the use of other equine products like tetanus antitoxin was more widespread, because they sensitized large numbers of people to horse serum (11,32). Most antivenom reactions can be managed without significant morbidity or mortality (62).

DOSAGE AND ADMINISTRATION

General

Skin testing before antivenom administration is controversial (11,13,47,51,62,63). Skin testing is a poor predictor of either acute or delayed hypersensitivity reactions. A positive reaction may be helpful in some cases because the patient can then be pretreated with the appropriate medications. In the United States, skin testing is generally recommended before the use of ACP or Antivenin (*M. fulvius*) but not for Polyvalent Crotalidae immune Fab (FabAV).

Many antivenoms are provided as lyophilized powders that must be reconstituted before administration. To do so, the recommended amount of diluent or sterile saline is added to the vial. The vials are then gently swirled or agitated until the powder has dissolved. Reconstitution times vary from several minutes to up to 1 hour, depending on the product. The antivenom solution should then be diluted before administration. Generally, the required number of vials should be mixed in 250 to 500 ml of sterile saline or water (20 ml/kg in children). Immediate hypersensitivity reactions may be more common with concentrated antivenom solutions (11,47).

Although most antivenoms can be given subcutaneously or intramuscularly, the preferred route is intravenously (IV) because it is more effective and easier to control adverse reactions (5,64). However, IV administration may increase the risk of adverse reactions (64).

The antivenom infusion should be started slowly at first to allow for early detection of a reaction. Immediate reactions appear to be more likely with faster infusion rates (11). In general, the infusion should be started at a rate of 10 to 25 ml/hour and then doubled every 5 to 10 minutes as tolerated until the entire volume has been infused. The goal should be to administer the initial dose over a period of 1 hour. The patient should be monitored closely in an emergency department or intensive care unit setting with continuous cardiac, blood pressure, and oximetry measurements. The appropriate medications and tools to manage anaphylaxis should be immediately available.

Polyvalent Crotalidae Immune Fab (FabAV)

The therapeutic goal is to quickly establish control of the crotaline envenomation using an initial dose of antivenom, followed by repeat doses as necessary until initial control is achieved. Smaller "maintenance" doses of antivenom are then given over the ensuing 18 hours to prevent recurrence of effects (Fig. 2).

The initial *adult and pediatric dose* of FabAV is 4 to 6 vials, depending on the severity of envenomation. Patients with severe systemic effects or rapidly progressive local effects should receive 6 vials. Each vial of FabAV is reconstituted with 10 ml of sterile water. Crystalloid fluids, such as normal saline or dextrose 5% in water, have also been used without problem. Reconstitution may take 15 to 45 minutes. The reconstituted vials are then injected into a 250-ml bag of sterile water or saline. A smaller volume can be used in children or patients in whom infusion of large volumes could be detrimental. The initial infusion rate should be slow (e.g., 10 to 25 ml/hour). The rate is then increased every few minutes, as tolerated, until a rate is reached that allows for infusion of the entire dose over a period of 1 hour (e.g., 250 ml/hour). Continuous respiratory and cardiovascular monitoring should be performed.

At the end of the initial infusion, the patient's condition should be reassessed. If significant clinical and laboratory improvement (e.g., cessation of local progression and improvement in systemic and coagulopathic effects) has not occurred, or the patient continues to worsen, the initial dose of antivenom should be repeated. This process is repeated until initial control has been achieved. Occasionally, with severe envenomations, a large number of vials may be required for control. Patients have received as many as 47 vials of CroFab without significant problems (65).

After initial control is established, three maintenance doses of FabAV should be given: 2 vials administered every 6 hours for a total of 6 vials (Fig. 2). In clinical trials, patients receiving scheduled maintenance doses of CroFab had a lower incidence of local recurrence than those assigned to additional doses on an "as needed" basis (66).

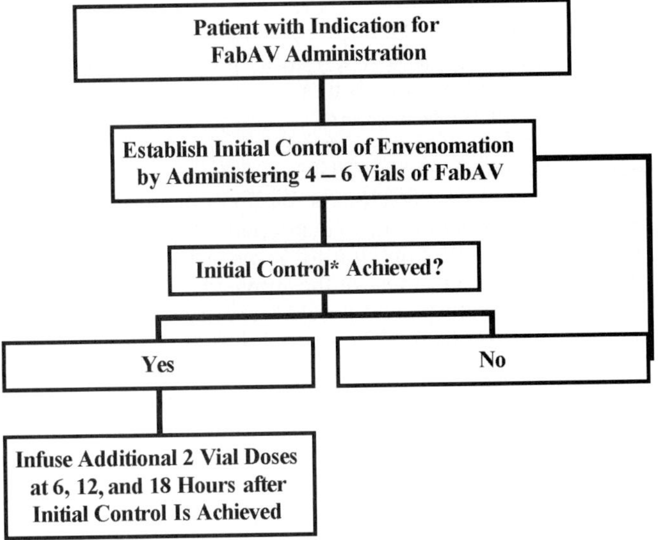

Figure 2. The use of polyvalent Crotalidae immune Fab (ovine). *, initial control is generally defined as arrest of local manifestations and return of coagulation tests and systemic signs to normal.

Recurrence

Recurrence is defined as the return of any venom effect after the abnormality initially resolved (Chapter 245). Recurrences are not peculiar to FabAV; in fact, they probably occur to some degree with most antivenoms (67–70). A *local recurrence* involves return of progressive local swelling after initial control was achieved. *Coagulopathy recurrence* involves the return of thrombocytopenia, prolonged prothrombin time, or elevated fibrin split products.

Local recurrences are uncommon (28,65,66,69,71,72). They usually occur within 12 to 24 hours of treatment, and should be distinguished from simple redistribution of blood/edema, secondary infection, venous thrombosis, and other causes of extremity swelling. Typically, local recurrence is managed with administration of another 2 to 4 vials of FabAV, followed by regular maintenance infusions.

The recurrence of coagulopathy is more common, but usually does not present until after hospital discharge (developing within several days, although it sometimes occurs earlier). Recurrent coagulopathy is often only partially responsive to further antivenom administration. If given early, further FabAV may be effective in correcting the abnormality. However, the benefit may be mild and is often transient (73). For example, a patient 2 days after discharge with a recurrent drop in fibrinogen to 50 mg/dl (normal greater than 150 mg/dl) may only respond to antivenom with an increase in fibrinogen to 125 mg/dl, and the level may simply fall back down to 50 mg/dl again over the next 2 or 3 days. Whether additional antivenom should be administered in such circumstances is controversial (65,67,74). Although coagulation tests are often abnormal, the risk of clinically significant hemorrhage is likely much lower than expected (74). Consequently, current recommendations suggest that recurrent coagulopathy be treated only if it is extreme and involves more than one abnormality, or there is evidence of significant bleeding. Most coagulopathy recurrences can be safely managed expectantly with close serial laboratory monitoring and bleeding precautions. Occasionally, patients may need to be hospitalized until the diathesis is corrected or resolves on its own.

Antivenin (*Micrurus fulvius*)

For bites by the Eastern coral snake or Texas coral snake, a dose of 3 to 5 vials is typically recommended, after skin testing

(45,51). Repeat doses may be given for progressive or recurrent effects. The patient should be monitored for signs of neurologic toxicity (paresthesia, numbness, fasciculation, weakness, hyporeflexia, cranial nerve dysfunction, and confusion) or respiratory insufficiency (rising $PaCO_2$ or falling negative inspiratory force). If neurologic effects develop or worsen after the initial dose, a second dose of 3 to 5 vials is indicated. As many as 20 vials of Antivenin (*M. fulvius*) have been administered without problems (51).

ADVERSE EFFECTS

Hypersensitivity reactions, either acute or delayed, are the primary adverse effects of antivenom treatment (11,32,51,57–59,62,66). They are categorized as either immediate (anaphylactic and anaphylactoid reactions) or delayed (serum sickness). Their incidence varies with the type of antivenom and with various patient factors.

Patient-specific risk factors may include a history of previous antivenom reaction or animal serum reaction, known atopic disease, asthma, and various food or medication allergies. Although pretreatment with antihistamines or epinephrine has been suggested in order to reduce the risk of an allergic reaction, there is little supportive evidence with regard to snake antivenoms (75). One study from Sri Lanka found that epinephrine prevented acute reactions associated with antivenom administration. However, this particular product has a high rate of reactivity, compared to newer U.S. products. The risks of giving epinephrine before U.S. antivenoms may outweigh its potential benefits (76). Another study found that prophylaxis with antihistamines did not prevent early reactions (77). In any event, case reports indicate that pretreatment does not guarantee that a severe reaction is avoidable (78,79). Thus, clinicians must still be prepared to manage such a reaction.

The skin test has been employed as a potential method to predict antivenom reactions. Most studies and case series have indicated that skin testing does not reliably predict either acute or delayed reactions (11,13,47,51,62).

In short, no hypersensitivity reaction can be predicted with certainty; patients without any risk factors can experience a severe reaction, just as patients with several risk factors can develop no problems at all. Moreover, risk factors are not absolute contraindications to antivenom, but should simply serve as cautions. The use of any antivenom is a risk-benefit analysis that must be made for each individual on a case-by-case basis. There may be patients with potentially life- or limb-threatening envenomations in whom the risk of antivenom is outweighed by the risks of untreated envenomation.

For patients with significant risk factors for hypersensitivity, but in whom antivenom is needed, the victim can be pretreated with antihistamines and epinephrine, or the antivenom can be administered with a continuous epinephrine infusion. The rate of epinephrine infusion is adjusted to control the allergic effects.

Early Antivenom Reactions

Early (acute) hypersensitivity reactions range in severity from mild to life-threatening (9,11,51,57,59–62,66,80). Acute reactions can arise from either a type I allergic (anaphylactic) or an anaphylactoid response. Anaphylactic reactions are IgE-mediated responses, caused primarily by the release of histamine and other proinflammatory mediators from mast cells in previously sensitized individuals (25). In contrast, anaphylactoid reactions require no prior exposure or sensitization to the antigen; hence, they cannot be reliably predicted. Anaphylactoid reactions appear to be related to the rate and concentration of antivenom infusion (11,32,64). Studies have suggested they may arise from direct activation of complement (32,47,49). However, other studies have found conflicting results (47,81). Anaphylactoid and anaphylactic reactions, although they differ in underlying mechanism, are clinically similar and should be managed identically.

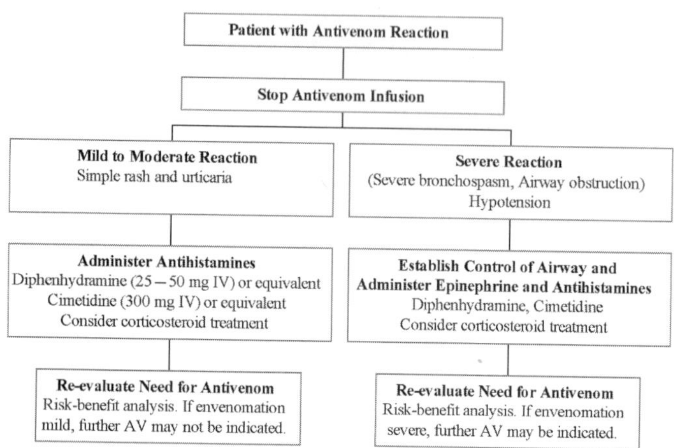

Figure 3. The management of antivenom reactions. AV, antivenom.

Acute reactions present with flushing, pruritus, diaphoresis, and urticaria, to angioedema, bronchospasm, hypotension, anaphylactic shock, and cardiorespiratory arrest. The effects can progress rapidly (32,62,78,80,82), and a few deaths have been reported (9,59,61,83).

If signs of a reaction develop, the infusion should be stopped immediately and the patient treated (Fig. 3). Dermal symptoms can usually be controlled with H_1 and H_2 blockade alone: diphenhydramine, 25 to 50 mg IV, or equivalent, and cimetidine, 300 mg IV, or its equivalent. Occasionally, for severe dermal symptoms, epinephrine may be indicated in otherwise healthy patients without risk of cardiac disease: epinephrine, 0.3 to 0.5 ml of a 1:1000 solution subcutaneously. Bronchospasm can generally be managed with inhaled β_2-receptor agonists (e.g., metered dose inhaler or albuterol, 5 mg by nebulizer). Patients with severe bronchospasm, angioedema, or hypotension are treated as anaphylactic (Chapter 34). Patients on beta-blocking agents who develop anaphylactic shock may respond to IV glucagon if epinephrine is not effective (84). For most acute allergic reactions, corticosteroids (e.g., methylprednisolone, 125 mg IV, or its equivalent) are recommended. They require several hours for full effects; however, some hypersensitivity reactions are biphasic, and steroids may help ameliorate the later phase.

The critical decision then becomes whether to restart the antivenom infusion. If one is available, a different antivenom may be substituted. If the reaction is not limb- or life-threatening, antivenom treatment can be abandoned altogether. However, the antivenom infusion should be restarted if the risks of envenomation exceed those of the antivenom. If the antivenom is to be restarted, the patient should first be treated with antihistamines, epinephrine subcutaneously, and steroids as indicated. The infusion should be restarted at a slower rate and in a more dilute solution. In most cases, this regimen is sufficient to prevent or reduce any further reaction. However, in particularly severe hypersensitivity reactions (e.g., refractory hypotension), an epinephrine infusion can be coadministered, along with the antivenom infusion, and titrated to response (85).

The rate of acute reactions varies with the type of antivenom. Retrospective reports indicate that acute reactions occured with ACP in 3% to 23% of patients (11,13,62,86). Most of these were mild to moderate in severity, but serious reactions and death have been documented (9). The rate of early reactions associated with FabAV has, to date, been lower. Acute reactions developed in approximately 19% of patients in one trial (66). In another, no patient out of 11 developed an acute reaction (28). Postmarketing experience with FabAV has revealed an incidence anywhere from 0% to 13% (65,71,87). No deaths have yet been reported, and the majority of reactions to FabAV have been mild, although in at least two instances, severe reactions have occurred (80,82). Reports of acute reactions to Antivenin (*M. fulvius*) are rare. In one study, one patient out of 17 developed an acute reaction that was classified as severe (51).

Late Antivenom Reactions

Serum sickness is a type III hypersensitivity reaction that is relatively common after antivenom administration (11,32,62,66). It is a flulike illness characterized by symptoms such as fever, chills, myalgia, malaise, arthralgia, rash or flushing, urticaria, nausea, vomiting, lymphadenopathy, and pruritus. It generally develops 5 to 10 days after antivenom treatment. On rare occasions, serum sickness involves complications like bronchospasm, hypotension, glomerulonephritis or proteinuria, or pericarditis (11,32,81,88,89). Serum sickness is believed to be caused by immune complex formation and tissue deposition (81). Administration of foreign serum stimulates an immune response and the production of host antibodies against the foreign immunoglobulins. The host and foreign immunoglobulins combine to form large complexes, which deposit throughout the body. The recipient's immune system is activated by the complexes, resulting in a variety of symptoms and sequelae (49,90). The effects appear to be dose related (11,32,62,91).

Symptoms of serum sickness typically respond to conservative measures such as antipyretics, analgesics/antiinflammatory agents, corticosteroids (e.g., prednisone, 60 mg orally daily for 7 to 14 days), and antihistamines (e.g., diphenhydramine, 25 to 50 mg orally every 6 to 8 hours). Rarely do patients require readmission for severe symptoms (11,62). All patients receiving antivenom should be warned about the occurrence of serum sickness.

The incidence of serum sickness varies markedly between antivenoms. Many studies underestimate the true incidence because follow-up is often problematic, especially in remote areas. A review publication estimated the serum sickness rate for ACP at approximately 75% of recipients (11). FabAV appears to cause far fewer delayed reactions, with postmarketing data suggesting an incidence of approximately 7% (65,66,87).

PITFALLS

The intramuscular and subcutaneous routes of administration should be avoided because of the large volumes required and unpredictable absorption.

Lack of antivenom availability is common. Clinicians should locate and mobilize adequate stores of the appropriate antivenom immediately on learning of a potential snakebite victim.

Insufficient monitoring of venom effects can result in increased morbidity. Venom effects can worsen in a slow, indolent manner. To avoid unnecessary delays in treatment, patients who do not initially meet criteria for antivenom should be monitored every 15 to 30 minutes initially and every 2 to 3 hours thereafter. The effects of envenomation should also be monitored closely after antivenom infusion for improvement. If they continue to progress, more antivenom may be required. Effects may progress slowly or quickly, so patients should be examined regularly by qualified personnel.

Not every bite victim needs antivenom. However, what initially appears to be a mild or dry envenomation can progress over time to become severe, so all patients should be observed for at least 8 hours.

REFERENCES

1. Hutchison RH. On the incidence of snake-bite poisoning in the United States and the results of the newer methods of treatment. *Bull Antivenin Inst Am* 1929;III:43–57.
2. Boyer DM, Index Editor. American Zoo and Aquarium Association antivenom index, 1999 revision ed. San Diego: San Diego Zoo Department of Herpetology, 1999.
3. Sewall H. Experiments on the preventive inoculation of rattlesnake venom. *J Physiol (London)* 1887;8:203–210.
4. Jackson D. Treatment of snake bite. *South Med J* 1929;22:605–608.
5. Martin CJ. Further observations concerning the relation of the toxin and anti-toxin of snake venom. *Proc Roy Soc London* 1898;64:88–94.
6. Crimmins ML. Poisonous snakes and the antivenin treatment. *South Med J* 1929;22:603–604.
7. Do Amaral A. The anti-snake-bite campaign in Texas and in the sub-tropical United States. *Bull Antivenin Inst Am* 1927;1:77–85.
8. Fischer FJ, Ramsey HW, Simon J, et al. Antivenin and antitoxin in the treatment of experimental rattlesnake venom intoxication (*Crotalus adamanteus*). *Am J Trop Med Hyg* 1961;10:75–79.
9. Antivenin (Crotalidae) Polyvalent [package insert]. Marrietta, PA: Wyeth Laboratories, 2001.
10. Taub AM. Antivenins available for the treatment of snake bite. *Toxicon* 1964;2:71–77.
11. Corrigan P, Russell FE, Wainschel J. Clinical reactions to antivenin. *Toxicon* 1978;65[Suppl]:457–465.
12. Offerman SR, Smith TS, Derlet RW. Does the aggressive use of polyvalent antivenin for rattlesnake bites result in serious acute side effects? *West J Med* 2001;175(2):88–91.
13. Wingert WA, Chan L. Rattlesnake bites in southern California and rationale for recommended treatment. *West J Med* 1988;148(1):37–44.
14. Russell FE, Ruzic N, Gonzalez H. Effectiveness of antivenin (Crotalidae) polyvalent following injection of *Crotalus* venom. *Toxicon* 1973;11(6):461–464.
15. Russell FE, Carlson RW, Wainschel J, et al. Snake venom poisoning in the United States. Experiences with 550 cases. *JAMA* 1975;233(4):341–344.
16. Watt CH. Poisonous snakebite treatment in the United States. *JAMA* 1978;240(7):654–656.
17. Grace TG, Omer GE. The management of upper extremity pit viper wounds. *J Hand Surg [Am]* 1980;5(2):168–177.
18. Burch JM, Agarwal R, Mattox KL, et al. The treatment of crotalid envenomation without antivenin. *J Trauma* 1988;28:35–42.
19. Sullivan JB Jr. Past, present, and future immunotherapy of snake venom poisoning. *Ann Emerg Med* 1987;16(9):938–944.
20. Smith TW, Lloyd BL, Spicer N, et al. Immunogenicity and kinetics of distribution and elimination of sheep digoxin-specific IgG and Fab fragments in the rabbit and baboon. *Clin Exp Immunol* 1979;36:384–396.
21. Russell FE, Sullivan JB, Egen NB, et al. Preparation of a new antivenin by affinity chromatography. *Am J Trop Med Hyg* 1985;34(1):141–150.
22. Smith DC, Reddi KR, Laing G, et al. An affinity purified ovine antivenom for the treatment of *Vipera berus* envenoming. *Toxicon* 1992;30:865–871.
23. Consroe P, Egen NB, Russell FE, et al. Comparison of a new ovine antigen binding fragment (Fab) antivenin for United States Crotalidae with the commercial antivenin for protection against venom-induced lethality in mice. *Am J Trop Med Hyg* 1995;53(5):507–510.
24. Chippaux JP, Lang J, Eddine SA, et al. Clinical safety of a polyvalent F(ab')2 equine antivenom in 223 African snake envenomations: a field trial in Cameroon. VAO (Venin Afrique de l'Ouest) Investigators. *Trans R Soc Trop Med Hyg* 1998;92(6):657–662.
25. Sullivan JB, Russell FE. Isolation and purification of antibodies to rattlesnake venom by affinity chromatography. *Proc West Pharmacol Soc* 1982;25:185–192.
26. Mohamed AH, Darwish MA, Hani-Ayobe M. Immunological studies on Egyptian polyvalent antivenins. *Toxicon* 1973;11(6):457–460.
27. Russell FE, Lauritzen L. Antivenins. *Trans R Soc Trop Med Hyg* 1966;60(6):797–810.
28. Dart RC, Seifert SA, Carroll L, et al. Affinity-purified, mixed monospecific crotalid antivenom ovine Fab for the treatment of crotalid venom poisoning. *Ann Emerg Med* 1997;30(1):33–39.
29. Sjostrom L, al-Abdulla IH, Rawat S, et al. A comparison of ovine and equine antivenoms. *Toxicon* 1994;32(4):427–433.
30. Heard K, O'Malley GF, Dart RC. Antivenom therapy in the Americas. *Drugs* 1999;58(1):5–15.
31. Russell FE, Timmerman WF, Meadows PE. Clinical use of antivenin prepared from goat serum. *Toxicon* 1970;8(1):63–65.

32. Sutherland SK, Lovering KE. Antivenoms: use and adverse reactions over a 12-month period in Australia and Papua New Guinea. *Med J Aust* 1979;2(13):671–674.
33. Chippaux JP, Williams V, White J. Snake venom variability: methods of study, results and interpretation. *Toxicon* 1991;29(11):1279–1303.
34. Simon TL, Grace TG. Envenomation coagulopathy in wounds from pit vipers. *N Engl J Med* 1981;305(8):443–447.
35. Thomas RG, Pough FH. The effect of rattlesnake venom on digestion of prey. *Toxicon* 1979;17(3):221–228.
36. Ownby CL, Cameron D, Tu AT. Isolation of myotoxic component from rattlesnake (*Crotalus viridis viridis*) venom. Electron microscopic analysis of muscle damage. *Am J Pathol* 1976;85(1):149–166.
37. Budzynski AZ, Pandya BV, Rubin RN, et al. Fibrinogenolytic afibrinogenemia after envenomation by western diamondback rattlesnake (*Crotalus atrox*). *Blood* 1984;63(1):1–14.
38. McCollough NC, Gennaro JF. Evaluation of venomous snake bite in the southern United States from parallel clinical and laboratory investigations: development of treatment. *J Fla Med Assoc* 1963;49:959–967.
39. Minton SA Jr. Paraspecific protection by elapid and sea snake antivenins. *Toxicon* 1967;5(1):47–55.
40. Minton SA. Polyvalent antivenin in the treatment of experimental snake venom poisoning. *Am J Trop Med Hyg* 1954;3:1077–1082.
41. Consroe P, Egen NB, Russell FE, et al. Comparison of a new ovine antigen binding fragment (Fab) antivenin for United States Crotalidae with the commercial antivenin for protection against venom-induced lethality in mice. *Am J Trop Med Hyg* 1995;53(5):507–510.
42. Cohen P, Dawson JH, Seligmann EB Jr. Cross-neutralization of *Micrurus fulvius fulvius* (coral snake) venom by anti-*Micrurus carinicauda dumerilii* serum. *Am J Trop Med Hyg* 1968;17(2):308–310.
43. Bolanos R, Cerdas L, Abalos JW. Venoms of coral snakes (*Micrurus* spp.): report on a multivalent antivenin for the Americas. *Bull Pan Am Health Organ* 1978;12(1):23–27.
44. Bar-Or D, Sullivan JB Jr, Black E, et al. Neutralization of crotalidae venom induced platelet aggregation by affinity chromatography isolated IgG to *Crotalus viridis helleri* venom. *J Toxicol Clin Toxicol* 1984;22(1):1–9.
45. Antivenin (*Micrurus fulvius*)—North American coral snake antivenin [package insert]. Marietta, PA: Wyeth Laboratories, 2001.
46. CroFab—Crotalidae Polyvalent Immune Fab (Ovine) [package insert]. Melville, NY: Savage Laboratories, 2000.
47. Malasit P, Warrell DA, Chanthavanich P, et al. Prediction, prevention, and mechanism of early (anaphylactic) antivenom reactions in victims of snake bites. *BMJ (Clin Res Ed)* 1986;292(6512):17–20.
48. Hickey AR, Wenger TL, Carpenter VP, et al. Digoxin immune Fab therapy in the management of digitalis intoxication: safety and efficacy results of an observational surveillance study. *J Am Coll Cardiol* 1991;17(3):590–598.
49. Sutherland SK. Serum reactions. An analysis of commercial antivenoms and the possible role of anticomplementary activity in de-novo reactions to antivenoms and antitoxins. *Med J Aust* 1977;1(17):613–615.
50. McCollough NC, Gennaro JF. Coral snake bites in the United States. *J Fla Med Assoc* 1963;49:968–972.
51. Kitchens CS, Van Mierop LH. Envenomation by the Eastern coral snake (*Micrurus fulvius fulvius*). A study of 39 victims. *JAMA* 1987;258(12):1615–1618.
52. Auerbach PS. Wilderness medicine. In: Norris RL, Minton SA. *Non-North American venomous reptile bites*, 4th ed. St. Louis: Mosby, 2001:927–951.
53. Dart RC, Hurlbut KM, Garcia R, et al. Validation of a severity score for the assessment of crotalid snakebite. *Ann Emerg Med* 1996;27(3):321–326.
54. Tanen D, Ruha A, Graeme K, et al. Epidemiology and hospital course of rattlesnake envenomations cared for at a tertiary referral center in Central Arizona. *Acad Emerg Med* 2001;8(2):177–182.
55. Gold BS, Dart RC, Barish RA. Bites of venomous snakes. *N Engl J Med* 2002;347(5):347–356.
56. Stewart RM, Page CP, Schwesinger WH, et al. Antivenin and fasciotomy/débridement in the treatment of the severe rattlesnake bite. *Am J Surg* 1989;158(6):543–547.
57. Christensen PA. Snakebite and the use of antivenom in southern Africa. *S Afr Med J* 1981;59(26):934–938.
58. Moran NF, Newman WJ, Theakston RD, et al. High incidence of early anaphylactoid reaction to SAIMR polyvalent snake antivenom. *Trans R Soc Trop Med Hyg* 1998;92(1):69–70.
59. Trinca GF. The treatment of snakebites. *Med J Aust* 1963;1:275.
60. Clark RF, Wethern-Kestner S, Vance MV, et al. Clinical presentation and treatment of black widow spider envenomation: a review of 163 cases. *Ann Emerg Med* 1992;21(7):782–787.
61. Reid HA. Adder bites in Britain. *BMJ* 1976;2(6028):153–156.
62. Jurkovich GJ, Luterman A, McCullar K, et al. Complications of Crotalidae antivenin therapy. *J Trauma* 1988;28(7):1032–1037.
63. Spaite D, Dart R, Sullivan JB. Skin testing in cases of possible crotalid envenomation. *Ann Emerg Med* 1988;17(1):105–106.
64. Reid HA. Antivenom reactions and efficacy. *Lancet* 1980;1(8176):1024–1025.
65. Ruha AM, Curry SC, Beuhler M, et al. Initial postmarketing experience with crotalidae polyvalent immune Fab for treatment of rattlesnake envenomation. *Ann Emerg Med* 2002;39(6):609–615.
66. Dart RC, Seifert SA, Boyer LV, et al. A randomized multicenter trial of Crotalinae polyvalent immune Fab (ovine) antivenom for the treatment for crotaline snakebite in the United States. *Arch Intern Med* 2001;161(16):2030–2036.
67. Boyer LV, Seifert SA, Cain JS. Recurrence phenomena after immunoglobulin therapy for snake envenomations: part 2. Guidelines for clinical management with crotaline Fab antivenom. *Ann Emerg Med* 2001;37(2):196–201.
68. Seifert SA, Boyer LV. Recurrence phenomena after immunoglobulin therapy for snake envenomations: part 1. Pharmacokinetics and pharmacodynamics of immunoglobulin antivenoms and related antibodies. *Ann Emerg Med* 2001;37(2):189–195.
69. Bogdan GM, Dart RC, Falbo SC, et al. Recurrent coagulopathy after antivenom treatment of crotalid snakebite. *South Med J* 2000;93(6):562–566.
70. Boyer LV, Seifert SA, Clark RF, et al. Recurrent and persistent coagulopathy following pit viper envenomation. *Arch Intern Med* 1999;159(7):706–710.
71. Offerman SR, Bush SP, Moynihan JA, et al. Crotaline Fab antivenom for the treatment of children with rattlesnake envenomation. *Pediatrics* 2002;110(5):968–971.
72. Bush SP, Green SM, Moynihan JA, et al. Crotalidae polyvalent immune Fab (ovine) antivenom is efficacious for envenomations by Southern Pacific rattlesnakes (*Crotalus helleri*). *Ann Emerg Med* 2002;40(6):619–624.
73. Seifert SA, Boyer LV, Dart RC, et al. Relationship of venom effects to venom antigen and antivenom serum concentrations in a patient with *Crotalus atrox* envenomation treated with a Fab antivenom. *Ann Emerg Med* 1997;30(1):49–53.
74. Yip L. Rational use of crotalidae polyvalent immune Fab (ovine) in the management of crotaline bite. *Ann Emerg Med* 2002;39(6):648–650.
75. Lieberman P. The use of antihistamines in the prevention and treatment of anaphylaxis and anaphylactoid reactions. *J Allergy Clin Immunol* 1990;86(4 Pt 2):684–686.
76. Nuchpraryoon I, Garner P. Interventions for preventing reactions to snake antivenom. *Cochrane Database Syst Rev* 2000;(2):CD002153.
77. Fan HW, Marcopito LF, Cardoso JL, et al. Sequential randomised and double blind trial of promethazine prophylaxis against early anaphylactic reactions to antivenom for Bothrops snake bites. *BMJ* 1999;318(7196):1451–1452.
78. Arunanthy S, Hertzberg SR. A life-threatening anaphylactoid reaction to polyvalent snake antivenom despite pretreatment. *Med J Aust* 1998;169(5):257–258.
79. Sutherland SK. A life-threatening anaphylactoid reaction to polyvalent antivenom despite pretreatment. *Med J Aust* 1999;170(2):92–93.
80. Clark RF, McKinney PE, Chase PB, et al. Immediate and delayed allergic reactions to Crotalidae polyvalent immune Fab (ovine) antivenom. *Ann Emerg Med* 2002;39(6):671–676.
81. Nielsen H, Sorensen H, Faber V, et al. Circulating immune complexes, complement activation kinetics and serum sickness following treatment with heterologous anti-snake venom globulin. *Scand J Immunol* 1978;7(1):25–33.
82. Holstege CP, Wu J, Baer AB. Immediate hypersensitivity reaction associated with the rapid infusion of Crotalidae polyvalent immune Fab (ovine). *Ann Emerg Med* 2002;39(6):677–679.
83. Christensen PA. The treatment of snakebite. *S Afr Med J* 1969;43(41):1253–1258.
84. Zaloga GP, DeLacey W, Holmboe E, et al. Glucagon reversal of hypotension in a case of anaphylactoid shock. *Ann Intern Med* 1986;105(1):65–66.
85. Loprinzi CL, Hennessee J, Tamsky L, et al. Snake antivenin administration in a patient allergic to horse serum. *South Med J* 1983;76(4):501–502.
86. Tokish JT, Benjamin J, Walter F. Crotalid envenomation: the southern Arizona experience. *J Orthop Trauma* 2001;15(1):5–9.
87. Bush SP, Green SM, Moynihan JA, et al. Crotalidae polyvalent immune Fab (ovine) antivenom is efficacious for envenomations by Southern Pacific rattlesnakes (*Crotalus helleri*). *Ann Emerg Med* 2002;40(6):619–624.
88. Harkavy J. Cardiac manifestations due to hypersensitivity. *Ann Allergy* 1970;28(6):242–251.
89. Cuzic S, Scukanec-Spoljar M, Bosnic D, et al. Immunohistochemical analysis of human serum sickness glomerulonephritis. *Croat Med J* 2001;42(6):618–623.
90. Birdsey V, Lindorfer J, Gewurz H. Interaction of toxic venoms with the complement system. *Immunology* 1971;21(2):299–310.
91. Campbell CH. Clinical aspects of snake bite in the Pacific area. *Toxicon* 1969;7(1):25–28.

CHAPTER 75

Sodium Bicarbonate

Erica L. Liebelt

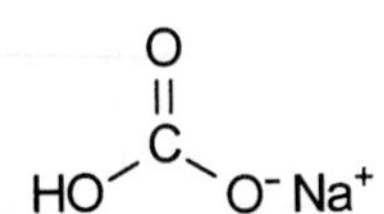

SODIUM BICARBONATE

Synonyms:	**Baking soda, monosodium carbonate**
Molecular formula and weight:	**$NaHCO_3$, 84.01 g/mol**
CAS Registry No.:	**144-55-8**
Normal or therapeutic levels:	**Not applicable**
Special concerns:	**Balancing risk of undertreatment with risk of hypernatremia during therapy.**

OVERVIEW

Sodium bicarbonate ($NaHCO_3$) has a major role in the management of a variety of poisoned patients (Table 1). Sodium bicarbonate is a nonspecific antidotal therapy with several distinct mechanisms and sites of action. Most commonly used for the treatment of tricyclic antidepressant (TCA) and salicylate toxicity, it is also used in the treatment of phenobarbital, chlorpropamide, chlorophenoxy herbicides, and certain antihistamine and antidysrhythmic poisonings. Sodium bicarbonate is also adjunctive therapy for severe metabolic acidosis associated with methanol, ethylene glycol, and isoniazid toxicity as well as cyanide. Finally, it is useful for treatment of hyperkalemia. Most of the literature advocating $NaHCO_3$ therapy comes from isolated case reports and case series. However, its various mechanisms of actions and success have been established in animal models.

Sodium bicarbonate is available in several parenteral formulations. The most commonly used preparations are 8.4% (1 M) and 4.2% solutions (0.5 M). The former contains 1 mEq/ml of $NaHCO_3$ with a calculated osmolarity of 2000 mOsm/L; thus, a 50-ml bottle contains 50 mEq of $NaHCO_3$. The 4.2% solution for neonates is one-half M and contains 25 mEq. The latter formulation is primarily used in neonates. There are also 7.5% and 4.0% solutions.

TABLE 1. Uses of sodium bicarbonate as an antidote

Mechanism	Examples of drugs and chemicals in which therapy may be useful
Altered sodium gradient	Tricyclic antidepressant
Altered interaction between drug and sodium channel	Cocaine
	Encainide
	Flecainide
	Procainamide
	Quinidine
	Quinine
	Diphenhydramine
	Propoxyphene
	Amantadine
	Carbamazepine
Altered drug ionization	Salicylates
	Phenobarbital
	Chlorpropamide
	Chlorophenoxy herbicides
Increased drug solubility to prevent renal tubular precipitation	Methotrexate
Acid neutralization	Chlorine gas
	Cyanide
	Ethylene glycol
	Methanol
Correct metabolic acidosis	Isoniazid

Adapted from Wax PM. Sodium bicarbonate. In: Goldfrank LR, Flomenbaum NE, Lewin NA, et al., eds. *Goldfrank's toxicologic emergencies*, 7th ed. New York: McGraw-Hill, 2002:520.

Mechanism of Action

MYOCARDIAL SODIUM CHANNEL EFFECTS

Numerous drugs produce cardiotoxicity by binding to the myocardial sodium channel and blocking the rapid inward movement of sodium ions through the fast sodium channel. This blockade slows phase 0 depolarization of the action potential in the distal His-Purkinje system as well as the ventricular myocardium. Clinical toxicity is manifested as a wide QRS complex, dysrhythmias, and hypotension. The prototypical drugs exhibiting this toxicity are the TCAs.

In the late 1950s, alkalinization with sodium lactate was proposed as treatment for quinidine toxicity, which also blocks the sodium channel and produces similar cardiotoxic effects (1). Subsequent animal research indicates that hypertonic $NaHCO_3$ reduces QRS prolongation, increases blood pressure, and suppresses ventricular dysrhythmias due to TCA toxicity (2–7). These studies also show that other methods of alkalinization (hyperventilation, and other nonsodium buffer solutions) produce either fewer or equivalent benefits. Cocaine-induced QRS prolongation was reversed by $NaHCO_3$ in a dog model (8,9). The efficacy of $NaHCO_3$ has been demonstrated in animal models for drugs with this mechanism of action: IA antidysrhythmic (e.g., quinidine, procainamide); type IC antidysrhythmic (flecainide, encainide); diphenhydramine; chloroquine; some antihistamines; and phenothiazines (10–14).

Several mechanisms are proposed for the effects of hypertonic $NaHCO_3$. Elevating the blood pH through alkalinization increases the serum protein binding of TCAs, thereby reducing the concentration of the unbound and pharmacologically active drug (15). This mechanism may be least important because of the small fraction of total TCA present in the serum. If free drug is the primary determinant of cardiac toxicity, however, alkalinization could substantially increase TCA bound substantially. Animal studies have produced mixed results. The administration of α_1-acid glycoprotein failed to ameliorate TCA cardiotoxicity (16); however, the use of specific antibody quickly reversed toxicity in an animal model (17).

Because TCAs are weak bases, alkalinization increases the proportion of nonionized drug. This effect may decrease drug-receptor binding, possibly due to a redistribution of the nonionized portion to the periphery (i.e., less "ion trapping"). Increasing the pH accelerates the recovery of sodium channels blocked by TCAs by neutralizing the protonation of the drug-receptor complex, thereby facilitating the egress of the neutral form of the drug from the sodium channel receptor (6,7). Increased bicarbonate concentration lowers the serum potassium levels, which results in membrane hyperpolarization, which, in turn, diminishes the blockade of voltage-dependent sodium channels (5).

Bicarbonate therapy also has pH-independent effects. Animal studies demonstrate improved cardiac conduction after $NaHCO_3$ or NaCl treatment in normal pH and acidemic animals (4,5). Multiple doses of $NaHCO_3$ also appear effective in patients who are already alkalemic (18). These studies suggest not only multiple mechanisms but also another mechanism besides alkalinization for the effects of $NaHCO_3$.

Increasing the extracellular sodium concentration may overcome sodium channel blockade through a gradient effect. This mechanism could explain why animal studies found $NaHCO_3$ more effective in decreasing cardiotoxicity than sodium-free buffers. Hypertonic NaCl loading reversed cardiotoxicity in animal studies (4,19,20). Hypertonic NaCl solution (15 mEq Na/kg) was highly effective in reversing QRS prolongation and hypotension in an animal model, although an adequate direct comparison with $NaHCO_3$ was not available (21). Raising the extracellular sodium concentration also causes dissociation of flecainide from the sodium channel, implying a decrease in the affinity of the channel and drug and allowing the drug to dissociate from the channel (22). However, there are no controlled human studies to determine the relative importance of these mechanisms.

ALTERED DRUG IONIZATION

Sodium bicarbonate increases the ionization of salicylate, phenobarbital, chlorpropamide, and chlorophenoxy herbicides, resulting in enhanced drug elimination and redistribution of drug in the tissues, blood, and urine. These substances are weak acids: salicylates (pK_a, 3.0); chlorpropamide (pK_a, 4.8); 2,4-dichlorophenoxyacetic acid and 2-3-chloro-2-methylphenoxy propionic acid (pK_a of 2.6 and 3.8); and phenobarbital (pK_a, 7.24). When the pH exceeds the pK_a, more of the chemical exists in the ionized form. Ionized molecules do not penetrate membranes (i.e., renal tubular cells, brain cells) as well as nonionized molecules. As a result, these weak acids accumulate and are "trapped" in the alkaline urine or blood where the ionized forms predominate (23,24). *Ion trapping* refers to the filtering of both ionized and nonionized salicylates, while reabsorbing only the nonionized salicylates (25).

Salicylate poisoning is the prototypical example of ion trapping. Without alkalinization, approximately 10% to 20% of salicylate is eliminated unchanged in the urine at a therapeutic blood level. In overdose, saturation kinetics predominate; thus, excretion of free salicylate accounts for 60% to 85% of total elimination in an alkaline urine (26,27).

Some investigators maintain that ion trapping is not the only mechanism of pH-dependent urinary salicylate excretion (28). Indeed, the difference in salicylate ionization at pH 5.0 (99% ionized) compared to pH 8.0 (99.999%) is small, suggesting that decreased tubular reabsorption cannot fully explain the rapid increase in urinary salicylate elimination that occurs above pH 7.0. Increased tubular secretion of nonionized salicylate probably accounts for some of the increase in salicylate elimination caused by an alkaline urine (28). This mechanism can be explained by the persistent concentration gradient formed by the nonionized salicylates in the peritubular fluid and the quickly converted ionized salicylates in the alkaline urine. More nonionized salicylates must pass from the peritubular fluid into the urine in an attempt to reach equilibrium with the small nonionized fraction in the urine.

In addition to the beneficial urinary effects, $NaHCO_3$ may also protect the central nervous system by "trapping" salicylate in the blood and preventing entry into the brain. The acidemia observed in significant salicylate poisoning enhances salicylate transfer into tissues. Raising the blood pH relative to the brain pH through serum alkalinization shifts the equilibrium of the nonionized salicylate from the tissues to the plasma, resulting in decreased salicylate concentration in the brain (29). In an experimental model, lowering the blood pH by inhaling a mixture of 20% carbon dioxide and 80% oxygen, or by infusing ammonium chloride, produced a shift of salicylate into the tissues (30).

INCREASING DRUG SOLUBILITY TO PREVENT TUBULAR PRECIPITATION

Use of high-dose methotrexate treatment may result in renal tubular precipitation of the drug, leading to acute tubular necrosis. Clinical studies indicate that alkalinization with $NaHCO_3$ along with saline diuresis during high-dose methotrexate infusions increases the solubility of methotrexate and increases its elimination (31,32).

ACID NEUTRALIZATION

Inhaled $NaHCO_3$ may neutralize the hydrochloric acid formed when chlorine gas reacts with the water in the airway. In one chlorine-inhalation model, animals treated with 4% nebulized $NaHCO_3$ had a higher PO_2 and lower PCO_2 than did the saline-treated animals, although there was no difference in the mortality or pulmonary histopathology (33). Oral $NaHCO_3$ therapy is not recommended for neutralization of acid ingestion because of the potential problems associated with an exothermic reaction and production of carbon dioxide in the closed gastrointestinal tract.

INDICATIONS

Cardiotoxic Drugs That Affect the Sodium Channel

Sodium bicarbonate therapy plays a major role in the treatment of cardiac toxicity due to TCAs, cocaine, type IA and IC antidysrhythmics, diphenhydramine, and all other drugs affecting the myocardial sodium channels. The mainstay treatment for wide-complex dysrhythmias and hypotension due to TCA toxicity is the combination of serum alkalinization and sodium loading, probably best accomplished with hypertonic $NaHCO_3$. French investigators recommended $NaHCO_3$ for treatment of TCA-induced dysrhythmias in the 1960s (34,35). There are no controlled human studies demonstrating that $NaHCO_3$ is effective; however, numerous reports and extensive clinical experience support its efficacy in treating serious TCA cardiotoxicity (35–39). One large retrospective study noted correction of QRS prolongation and hypotension in the majority of the patients who received $NaHCO_3$ after a TCA overdose (40).

Based on the pathophysiology of cardiotoxicity, indications for $NaHCO_3$ after a TCA overdose include conduction delay (QRS greater than 100 msec, an R wave in lead aVR greater than or equal to 3 mm, or an unexplained or new right bundle branch block), wide-complex tachycardia, or hypotension (41). Many normal electrocardiogram (ECG) tracings have a QRS duration above 100 msec, leading to recommendations of 120 msec or higher as the indication for treatment. Because of the precipitous deterioration associated with TCA toxicity, it is imperative to begin therapy until TCA toxicity can be excluded. It should be administered in patients with acidosis or a normal pH. The value of $NaHCO_3$ therapy for isolated sinus tachycardia and narrow complex supraventricular tachycardia has not been studied. Available evidence does not support prophylactic alkalinization in the absence of cardiovascular toxicity.

Case reports provide most of the evidence regarding the efficacy of $NaHCO_3$ in the treatment of cardiotoxicity from other drugs that impair sodium channel function and cause "quinidine-like effects." Clinical effectiveness has been demonstrated with type IA antidysrhythmic overdoses (procainamide and quinidine) as well as quinine (an optical isomer of quinidine) overdose (13,42,43). Clinical reports have associated improvement of severe cardiotoxicity from flecainide and encainide after $NaHCO_3$ administration (44–46). In addition, $NaHCO_3$ appears effective in narrowing wide-complex dysrhythmias associated with diphenhydramine, other selected antihistamines, and propoxyphene toxicity (47–49). Sodium bicarbonate narrowed the QTc interval but not the QRS interval in one case of amantadine overdose (50). It should be used along with sedation and cooling in treating cardiac toxicity associated with cocaine toxicity (51,52). It is reasonable to consider $NaHCO_3$ treatment for cardiotoxicity induced by drugs like thioridazine, mesoridazine, and carbamazepine, all of which may exhibit type IA–like conduction abnormalities.

Salicylate Poisoning

Treatment with $NaHCO_3$ is indicated for most patients with systemic toxicity. Although validated criteria are not available, some investigators suggest alkalinization for patients with a blood level above 30 mg/dl, even if asymptomatic (53). However, the salicylate concentration needs to be interpreted in the context of the patient's clinical features (mental status changes, hemodynamic instability, hyperpyrexia), degree of metabolic acidosis, age, and etiology of poisoning (acute versus chronic poisoning). Clinical features are more important than the blood level in grading the severity of salicylate poisoning and the need for $NaHCO_3$ therapy or hemodialysis.

Phenobarbital

Sodium bicarbonate may be an adjunctive therapy for phenobarbital toxicity. Although controlled studies of overdose are lacking, one human volunteer study found that urinary alkalinization decreased the elimination half-life of phenobarbital from 148 to 47 hours (54). Serum alkalinization may also enhance the diffusion of phenobarbital out of the brain, thus shortening the duration of central nervous system toxicity. Other barbiturate poisoning is not expected to benefit from $NaHCO_3$ therapy due to its high pK_a and predominant liver elimination.

Chlorpropamide

Sodium bicarbonate should be useful in the treatment of chlorpropamide toxicity because of its long half-life (30 to 50 hours) and increased elimination in an alkaline urine. In one human volunteer study using therapeutic doses, urinary alkalinization to a pH of 8.0 increased renal clearance of chlorpropamide tenfold and reduced the elimination half-life from 50 to 13 hours (55). This therapy has not been studied with other sulfonylurea drugs.

Chlorophenoxy Herbicides

Urinary alkalinization is indicated in the treatment of poisonings with chlorophenoxy compounds such as 2,4-dichlorophenoxyacetic acid and 2-3-chloro-2-methylphenoxy propionic acid, which are commonly found in weed killers. In a case series, alkaline diuresis reduced the half-life of chlorophenoxy compounds through enhanced renal elimination (56). In one patient, resolution of hyperthermia and metabolic acidosis as well as improvement in mental status after alkalinization were associated with transient elevation of the serum concentrations of the chlorophenoxy compounds. These clinical and laboratory observations may reflect the redistribution of chlorophenoxy compounds from the tissues into the more alkalemic blood as seen with salicylates.

Methotrexate

Urinary alkalinization and intensive hydration are indicated as adjunctive therapy along with the specific antidote leucovorin for methotrexate poisoning (31).

Chlorine Gas

Inhalation of $NaHCO_3$ solution with saline may alleviate the respiratory symptoms of chlorine gas exposure (32,57,58). In a review of 86 patients with chlorine gas inhalation, more than 50% showed clinical improvement and were discharged home from the emergency department (59). A trial of nebulized $NaHCO_3$ may be indicated in a patient with significant respiratory symptoms.

CAUTIONS AND CONTRAINDICATIONS

Contraindications to the administration of $NaHCO_3$ include congestive heart failure or pulmonary edema, volume overload, or patients with renal insufficiency in which an osmol load or large quantity of sodium may be detrimental. If $NaHCO_3$ cannot be used, hyperventilation should be used, perhaps with judicious amounts of $NaHCO_3$. Hemodialysis should be initiated promptly in any patient with serious salicylate toxicity and these situations.

DOSAGE AND METHOD OF ADMINISTRATION

Cardiotoxic Drugs Affecting the Sodium Channel

Although not well defined by controlled clinical studies, the typical method is administration of a bolus or rapid infusion over several minutes of hypertonic $NaHCO_3$ (1 mEq/ml) at a dose of 1 to 2 mEq/kg (4,19,35,60). Higher doses have been used successfully, but experience is limited. Additional boluses may be administered until the QRS interval narrows, the amplitude of the R wave in lead aVR decreases, and hypotension improves. To avoid adverse effects, blood pH should be monitored and should not exceed 7.55 (44,60). The use of hypertonic saline solutions (3% to 7% NaCl) or combined $NaHCO_3$ and normal saline solutions (0.9%) for rapid infusion should be effective theoretically; however, these modalities have not been adequately studied, particularly the adverse effects.

The use of continuous $NaHCO_3$ infusions has not been well studied and is unlikely to raise the extracellular concentration of sodium and serum pH to the extent needed for clinical effectiveness in a timely manner. If used, an $NaHCO_3$ infusion can be made by diluting three 50-ml ampules in 1 L of 5% dextrose to run at a fluid rate dependent on blood pH and cardiac hemodynamics. This solution provides 150 mEq of sodium/L. If volume loading with crystalloid is needed, it should be infused through a separate line. Although this technique makes it isotonic and therefore reduces the sodium gradient effect, the beneficial effects of pH elevation may still be present.

Blood pH and resolution of ECG abnormalities and hypotension have been suggested as therapeutic endpoints for $NaHCO_3$ therapy, but optimal duration of therapy has not been established. Careful monitoring to assure the blood pH does not exceed 7.55 is reasonable based on available evidence showing improvements of cardiac toxicity in this range. Some authors advocate continued alkalinization for 12 to 24 hours after the ECG has normalized because of the drug's redistribution from the tissue. However, the time observed for normalization of conduction abnormalities ranges from several hours to days, despite continuous $NaHCO_3$ infusion (61). Alkalinization should be stopped or tapered when the patient has improved clinically as judged by hemodynamic stability, improvement of ECG abnormalities, and resolution of altered mental status.

Salicylates, Phenobarbital, Chlorpropamide, and Chlorophenoxy Herbicides

The $NaHCO_3$ dose in salicylate poisoning depends on the patient's hemodynamics, acid-base status, and the presence of concomitant clinical morbidity (53). In salicylate poisoning, significant acidosis should first be treated with an intravenous bolus of $NaHCO_3$, 1 to 2 mEq/kg (62). Once a blood pH of 7.50 is reached or if the patient already presents alkalemic (secondary to respiratory alkalosis), $NaHCO_3$ should be titrated over the next 4 to 8 hours until the urine pH reaches 7.5 to 8.0 (62,63). Urinary and serum alkalinization can be achieved and maintained with a continuous $NaHCO_3$ infusion of 150 mEq in 1 L of 5% dextrose in water at a rate of 150 to 200 ml/hour or twice the maintenance fluid rate in a child. The goals of therapy are a blood pH of 7.5 and urine pH of 8.0, although the latter may be difficult to reach when the salicylate concentration is high. Frequent monitoring of the acid-base, serum potassium, pulmonary, and hemodynamic status is needed. Blood pH should not exceed 7.55, which may be associated with complications of alkalemia. Fluid rates should also be adjusted to achieve an adequate urine output of 2 to 4 ml/kg/hour. Treatment should be continued until the clinical symptoms resolve and the salicylate concentration falls below 30 mg/dl. Forced diuresis with alkalinization is not recommended. It appears unnecessary and imposes a large fluid load (63–67).

Because the pK_a of phenobarbital is high (7.24), significant urinary elimination occurs when the urinary pH exceeds 7.5 (68). A threefold increase in elimination occurs as the urine pH approaches 8.0. The endpoints for $NaHCO_3$ therapy of phenobarbital, chlorpropamide, or chlorophenoxy herbicide poisoning are not established but typically involve evidence of clinical improvement as well as decreasing phenobarbital or methotrexate levels.

Chlorine Gas Neutralization

Inhaled therapy can be administered by mixing 2 ml of 8.4% $NaHCO_3$ and 2.25 ml of normal saline (3.75% solution) by face mask nebulizer. This therapy may help to relieve the symptoms of chest tightness and burning, throat irritation, cough, and wheezing (31,57,58). The safety of multiple inhalation treatments has not been studied.

ADVERSE EFFECTS

A blood pH exceeding 7.55 may lead to serious sequelae: myocardial depression, hypotension, hypocalcemia with tetany, encephalopathy, and even death (24,26,69,70–72). Hypernatremia along with hyperosmolarity may result in central nervous system sequelae, fluid overload, and pulmonary edema. These effects can be dangerous in infants, the elderly, or any patient with cardiac or renal dysfunction. Excess fluid and osmolarity may be detrimental in salicylate-poisoned patients who are at risk for, or may present with, adult respiratory distress syndrome, acute lung injury, cerebral edema, and renal failure (63,64,66,67).

Urinary and serum alkalinization may cause hypokalemia due to the intracellular shift of potassium. Hypokalemia may make urinary alkalinization difficult because the kidney preferentially reabsorbs potassium in exchange for hydrogen ions in the hypokalemic patient, regardless of total potassium stores (72,73). Chronic potassium depletion increases proximal tubular resorption of bicarbonate, making it difficult to excrete an alkaline urine. However, there are no clinical data specifically addressing the role of potassium supplementation during urinary alkalinization in acute salicylate poisoning. One study found no correlation between serum potassium levels and urinary pH (65). Thus, adequate potassium supplementation by adding 20 to 40 mEq of potassium chloride to each liter of fluid is prudent for hypokalemic and normokalemic patients (74). However, $NaHCO_3$ therapy should not be delayed until normokalemia is achieved.

PITFALLS

Sodium bicarbonate should not be empirically administered to a patient without adequate evidence supporting the diagnosis of a drug or chemical poisoning that would benefit from this therapy. Sodium bicarbonate transiently elevates $PaCO_2$ and intracellular PCO_2 and depresses intracellular pH.

REFERENCES

1. Bellet S, Hamdan G, Somlyo A, et al. The reversal of cardiotoxic effects of quinidine by molar sodium lactate: an experimental study. *Am J Med Sci* 1959;237:165–176.
2. Nattel S, Keable H, Sasyniuk BI. Experimental amitriptyline intoxication: electrophysiologic manifestations and management. *J Cardiovasc Pharmacol* 1984;6:83–89.
3. Nattel S, Mittleman M. Treatment of ventricular tachyarrhythmias resulting from amitriptyline toxicity in dogs. *J Pharmacol Exp Ther* 1984;231:430–435.
4. Pentel P, Benowitz N. Efficacy and mechanism of action of sodium bicarbonate in the treatment of desipramine toxicity in rats. *J Pharmacol Exp Ther* 1984;230:12–19.
5. Sasyniuk BI, Jhamandas V. Mechanism of reversal of toxic effects of amitriptyline on cardiac Purkinje fibers by sodium bicarbonate. *J Pharmacol Exp Ther* 1984;231:387–394.
6. Sasyniuk BI, Jhamandas V. Frequency-dependent effects of amitriptyline on Vmax in canine Purkinje fibers and its alteration by alkalosis. *Proc West Pharmacol Soc* 1986;29:73–75.
7. Sasyniuk BI, Jhamandas V, Valois M. Experimental amitriptyline intoxication: treatment of cardiac toxicity with sodium bicarbonate. *Ann Emerg Med* 1986;15:1052–1059.
8. Beckman KJ, Parker RB, Harmtan RJ, et al. Hemodynamic and electrophysiological actions of cocaine. Effects of sodium bicarbonate as an antidote in dogs. *Circulation* 1991;83;1799–1807.
9. Parker RB, Beckman KJ, Hariman RJI, et al. The electrophysiologic and arrhythmogenic effects of cocaine. *J Pharmacotherapy* 1989;9:176(abst).
10. Keyler DE, Pentel PE. Hypertonic sodium bicarbonate partially reverses QRS prolongation due to flecainide in rats. *Life Sci* 1989;45:1575–1580.
11. Salerno DM, Murakami MM, Johnston RB, et al. Reversal of flecainide-induced ventricular arrhythmia by hypertonic sodium bicarbonate in dogs. *Am J Emerg Med* 1995;13:285–293.
12. Curry SC, Connor DA, Clark RF, et al. The effect of hypertonic sodium bicarbonate on QRS duration and blood pressure in rats poisoned with chloroquine. *J Toxicol Clin Toxicol* 1996;34:73–76.
13. Bou-Abboud E, Nattel S. Relative role of alkalosis and sodium ions in reversal of class I antiarrhythmic drug-induced sodium channel blockade by sodium bicarbonate. *Circulation* 1966;94:1954–1961.
14. Holger JS. Harris CR, Engebretsen KM. Physostigmine, sodium bicarbonate, or hypertonic saline to treat diphenhydramine toxicity. *Vet Hum Toxicol* 2002;44:1–4.
15. Levitt MA, Sullivan JB Jr, Owens SM, et al. Amitriptyline plasma protein building: effect of plasma pH and relevance to clinical overdose. *Am J Emerg Med* 1986;4:121–125.
16. Pentel PR, Keyler DE. Effects of high dose alpha-1-acid glycoprotein on desipramine toxicity in rats. *J Pharmacol Exp Ther* 1988;246:1061–1066.
17. Dart RC, Sidki A, Sulllivan JB, et al. Ovine desipramine antibody fragments reverse desipramine cardiovascular toxicity in the rat. *Ann Emerg Med* 1996;27:309–315.

18. Molloy DW, Penner SB, Rabson J, et al. Use of sodium bicarbonate to treat tricyclic antidepressant-induced arrhythmias in a patient with alkalosis. *Can Med Assoc J* 1984;130:1457–1459.
19. Hoegholm A, Clementson P. Hypertonic sodium chloride in severe antidepressant overdosage. *J Toxicol Clin Toxicol* 1991;29:297–298.
20. McCabe JL, Menegazzi JJ, Cobaugh DJ, et al. Recovery from severe cyclic antidepressant overdose with hypertonic saline/dextran in a swine model. *Acad Emerg Med* 1994;1:111–115.
21. McCabe JL, Cobaugh DJ, Menegazzi JJ, et al. Experimental tricyclic antidepressant toxicity: a randomized, controlled comparison of hypertonic saline solution, sodium bicarbonate, and hyperventilation. *Ann Emerg Med* 1998;32:329–333.
22. Ranger S, Sheldon R, Fermini B, et al. Modulation of flecainide's cardiac sodium channel blocking actions by extracellular sodium: a possible cellular mechanism for the action of sodium salts in flecainide cardiotoxicity. *J Pharmacol Exp Ther* 1993;264:1160–1167.
23. Milne MD, Scribner BR, Crawford MA. Nonionic diffusion and the excretion of weak acids and bases. *Am J Med* 1958;24:709–729.
24. Smith PK, Gleason HL, Soll CC, et al. Studies on the pharmacology of salicylates. *J Pharmacol Exp Ther* 1946;87:237–255.
25. Segar WE. The critically ill child. Salicylate intoxication. *Pediatrics* 1969;44:440–444.
26. Gutman AB, Sirota JH. A study by simultaneous clearance techniques of salicylates excretion in man: effect of alkalinization of the urine by bicarbonate administration; effect of probenecid. *J Clin Invest* 1955;34:711–722.
27. Reimold EW, Worthen HG, Reilly TP. Salicylate poisoning: comparison of acetazolamide administration and alkaline diuresis in the treatment of experimental salicylates intoxication in puppies. *Am J Dis Child* 1983;125:668–674.
28. MacPherson CR, Milne MD, Evans BM. The excretion of salicylates. *Br J Pharmacol* 1955;10:484–489.
29. Hill JB. Experimental salicylates poisoning: observations on the effects of altering blood pH on tissue and plasma salicylates concentrations. *Pediatrics* 1971;47:658–665.
30. Buchanan N, Kundig H, Eyberg C. Experimental salicylates intoxication in young baboons. *J Pediatr* 1975;86:225–232.
31. Christensen ML, Rivera GK, Crom WR, et al. Effect of hydration on methotrexate plasma concentrations in children with acute lymphocystic leukemia. *J Clin Oncol* 1988;6:797–801.
32. Sand TE, Jacobsen S. Effect of urine pH and flow on renal clearance of methotrexate. *Eur J Clin Pharmacol* 1981;19:453–456.
33. Chisholm DV, Singletary EM, Okerberg CV, et al. Inhaled sodium bicarbonate therapy for chlorine inhalation injuries. *Ann Emerg Med* 1989;18:466(abst).
34. Bismuth C, Bodin F, Pebay-Peroula F, et al. Intoxication par l'imipramine avec insuffisance cardiaque aigue. *La Presse Medicale* 1968;76:2277–2278.
35. Prudhommeaux JL, Lechat P, Auclair MC. Etude experimentale de l'influence des ions sodium sur la toxicite cardiaque de l'imipramine. *Therapie (Paris)* 1968;23:675–683.
36. Brown TCK. Sodium bicarbonate treatment for tricyclic antidepressant arrhythmias in children. *Med J Aust* 1976;2:380–382.
37. Brown TCK, Barker GA, Dunlop ME, et al. The use of sodium bicarbonate in the treatment of TCA-induced arrhythmias. *Anaesth Intens Care* 1973;1:203–210.
38. Hoffman JR, McElroy CR. Bicarbonate therapy for dysrhythmias and hypotension in tricyclic antidepressant overdose. *West J Med* 1981;134:60–64.
39. Blackman K, Brown SG, Wilkes GJ. Plasma alkalinization for tricyclic antidepressant toxicity: a systematic review. *Emerg Med* 2001;13:204–210.
40. Hoffman JR, Votey SR, Bayer M, et al. Effect of hypertonic sodium bicarbonate in the treatment of moderate-to-severe cyclic antidepressant overdose. *Am J Emerg Med* 1993;11:336–341.
41. Liebelt EL. Toxicology reviews: targeted management strategies for cardiovascular toxicity from tricyclic antidepressant overdose: the pivotal role for alkalinization and sodium loading. *Ped Emerg Care* 1998;14:293–298.
42. Wasserman F, Brodsky L, Dick MM, et al. Successful treatment of quinidine and procainamide intoxication. *N Engl J Med* 1958;259:797–802.
43. Bodenhamer JE, Smilkstein MJ. Delayed cardiotoxicity following quinine overdose. A case report. *J Emerg Med* 1993;11:279–285.
44. Goldman MJ, Mowry JB, Kirk MA. Sodium bicarbonate to correct widened QRS in a case of flecainide overdose. *J Emerg Med* 1997;15:183–186.
45. Lovechhio F, Berlin R, Brubacher JR, et al. Hypertonic sodium bicarbonate in an acute flecainide overdose. *Am J Emerg Med* 1998;16:534–537.
46. Pentel PR, Goldsmith SR, Salerno DM, et al. Effect of hypertonic sodium bicarbonate on encainide overdose. *Am J Cardiol* 1986;57:878–880.
47. Clark RF, Vance MV. Massive diphenhydramine poisoning resulting in a wide-complex tachycardia: successful treatment with sodium bicarbonate. *Ann Emerg Med* 1992;21:318–321.
48. Stork CM, Redd JT, Fine K, et al. Propoxyphene-induced wide QRS complex dysrhythmia responsive to sodium bicarbonate—a case report. *J Toxicol Clin Toxicol* 1995;33:179–183.
49. Farrell M, Heinrichs M, Tilelli JA. Response of life threatening dimenhydrinate intoxication to sodium bicarbonate administration. *J Toxicol Clin Toxicol* 1991;29:527–535.
50. Farrell S, Lee DC, McNamara RM. Amantadine overdose: considerations for the treatment of cardiac toxicity. *J Toxicol Clin Toxicol* 1995;33:516–517(abst).
51. Kerns W, Garvey L, Owens J. Cocaine-induced wide complex dysrhythmia. *J Emerg Med* 1997;15:321–329.
52. Wang RY. pH-dependent cocaine-induced cardiotoxicity. *Am J Emerg Med* 1999;17:364–369.
53. Whitten CE, Kesaree NM, Goodwin JF. Managing salicylates poisoning in children. *Am J Dis Child* 1961;101:178–194.
54. Frenia ML, Schauben JL, Wears RL, et al. Multiple-dose activated charcoal compared to urinary alkalinization for the enhancement of phenobarbital elimination. *J Toxicol Clin Toxicol* 1996;34:169–175.
55. Neuvonen PJ, Karkkainen S. Effects of charcoal, sodium bicarbonate and ammonium chloride on chlorpropamide kinetics. *Clin Pharmacol Ther* 1983;33:386–393.
56. Flanagan RJ, Meridith TJ, Ruprah M, et al. Alkaline diuresis for acute poisoning with chlorophenoxy herbicides and ioxynil. *Lancet* 1990;335:454–458.
57. Vinsel PJ. Treatment of acute chlorine gas inhalation with nebulized sodium bicarbonate. *J Emerg Med* 1990;8:327–329.
58. Douidar SM. Nebulized sodium bicarbonate in acute chlorine inhalation. *Pediatric Emerg Care* 1997;13:406–407.
59. Bosse GM. Nebulized sodium bicarbonate in the treatment of chlorine gas inhalation. *J Toxicol Clin Toxicol* 1994;32:233–241.
60. Smilkstein MJ. Reviewing cyclic antidepressant cardiotoxicity: wheat and chaff. *J Emerg Med* 1990;8:645–648.
61. Liebelt EL, Ulrich A, Francis PD, et al. Serial electrocardiogram changes in acute tricyclic antidepressant overdoses. *Crit Care Med* 1997;25:1721–1726.
62. Temple AR. Acute and chronic effects of aspirin toxicity and their treatment. *Arch Intern Med* 1981;141:364–369.
63. Snodgrass W, Rumack BH, Peterson RG, et al. Salicylate toxicity following therapeutic doses in children. *J Toxicol Clin Toxicol* 1981;18:247–259.
64. Hormaechea E, Carlson RW, Rogove H, et al. Hypovolemia, pulmonary edema and protein changes in severe salicylates poisoning. *Am J Med* 1979;66:1046–1050.
65. Prescott LF, Balali-Mood M, Critchley A, et al. Diuresis or urinary alkalinization for salicylates poisoning. *BMJ* 1982;285:1383–1386.
66. Temple AR, George DJ, Done AK, et al. Salicylate poisoning complicated by fluid retention. *J Toxicol Clin Toxicol* 1976;9:61–68.
67. Zimmerman GA, Clemmer TP. Acute respiratory failure during therapy for salicylates intoxication. *Ann Emerg Med* 1981;10:104–106.
68. Bloomer HA. A critical evaluation of diuresis in the treatment of barbiturate intoxication. *J Lab Clin Med* 1966;67:898–905.
69. Wrenn K, Smith BA, Slovis CM. Profound alkalemia during treatment of tricyclic antidepressant overdose: a potential hazard of combined hyperventilation and intravenous bicarbonate. *Am J Emerg Med* 1992;10:553–555.
70. Fox GN. Hypocalcemia complicating bicarbonate therapy for salicylates poisoning. *West J Med* 1984;141:108–109.
71. Pentel PR, Benowitz NL. Tricyclic antidepressant poisoning: management of arrhythmias. *Med Toxicol Adverse Drug Exp* 1986;1:101–121.
72. Lawson AAH, Proudfoot At, Brown SS, et al. Forced diuresis in the treatment of acute salicylates poisoning in adults. *Q J Med* 1999;149:31–48.
73. Savege TM, Ward JD, Simpson BR, et al. Treatment of severe salicylates poisoning by forced alkaline diuresis. *BMJ* 1969;1:35–36.
74. Yip L, Dart RC, Gabow PA. Concepts and controversies in salicylates toxicity. *Emerg Med Clin North Am* 1994;12:351–364.

CHAPTER 76

Spider Antivenoms

Steven A. Seifert

Synonyms:	**Antivenin (*Latrodectus mactans*), Antivenom (*Latrodectus hasselti*), funnel web spider antivenom**
Molecular weight:	**Fab_2, 110 kd; IgG, 150 kd**
Therapeutic levels:	**Not clinically applicable**
Special concerns:	**Delay in antivenom administration may allow tissue injury to progress. All protein products are capable of causing anaphylaxis.**

OVERVIEW

There are more than 170,000 species of spiders in the world, but only a limited number are of medical importance. Of those, there are only a handful of antivenoms that have been developed to treat envenomation (Table 1). One of the main applications of antivenom is for widow spiders, which are distributed worldwide (1).

All antivenoms should be administered in a critical care setting capable of managing anaphylaxis (emergency department, intensive care unit, or postanesthesia care unit). Two functioning intravenous (IV) catheters should be in place and continuous cardiac, blood pressure, and oximetry monitoring should be performed during antivenom infusion.

BLACK WIDOW SPIDER ANTIVENOM

Antivenin (*Latrodectus mactans*) is an equine IgG product provided as a lyophilized pellet that must be reconstituted with normal saline. The reconstituted product contains 0.1 mg/ml of mercury in the form of thimerosal.

MECHANISM OF ACTION

The main component responsible for widow spider toxicity, α-latrotoxin, is a mix of proteins with an average molecular weight of 130,000 d. The toxin binds to presynaptic nerves and causes neurotransmitter release from nerve terminals, possibly by increasing permeability of neurons to calcium (2). Clinically, this results in a similar presentation regardless of the specific widow spider and includes muscle spasms, severe pain, and hypertension (3).

Presumably, the venom-specific IgG in the product binds venom components, thereby preventing their action on the neuron. Furthermore, all symptoms can resolve, and the duration of symptoms can be shortened after the use of specific equine-derived *L. mactans* antivenom (4); therefore, the venom components can apparently be removed by the antivenom from their site of action.

INDICATIONS

Indications vary for different widow spider envenomations and antivenoms (5–7). A benefit-risk analysis must be performed before the decision to administer antivenom is made. One difficulty involves spider identification. If the spider was not properly identified, the diagnosis of a spider envenomation may not be correct. There is no pathognomonic symptom, sign, or laboratory test for black widow envenomation. Intractable crying may be the predominant finding in young children (8).

Symptomatic and supportive care is the mainstay of therapy for the black widow spider. Because of the possibility of anaphylaxis, the use of *Latrodectus*-specific antivenom should be restricted to patients with significant neurotoxicity, hemodynamic instability, uncontrolled pain, or prolonged symptomatology. These patients are often refractory to opiates and sedative-hypnotics or are at risk of significant toxicity (e.g., small children, in pregnancy, the elderly) (4). The mortality rate from *Latrodectus* envenomation in the United States since 1965 is far below 1%

TABLE 1. Table of poisonous animals and available antivenins

Producer or distributor	Venoms used in preparation	Trade or common name	Common name of arthropod	Additional venoms neutralized	Comments
Merck, Sharp and Dome, Pennsylvania	*Latrodectus mactans*	Black widow	Black widow (spider)	—	—
Institutio Nacional de Higiene, Lima, Peru	*Loxosceles* sp.	Anti-Loxoscelico	—	—	Ammonium sulfate
Instituto Butantan, Caixa, São Paulo, Brazil	*Phoneutria, Loxosceles, Lycosa*	Antiarachnidico polivalente	—	—	—
Commonwealth Serum Laboratories, Victoria, Australia	*Latrodectus mactans hasselti*	Red back spider antivenom	Red back spider	—	Pepsin digestion and ammonium sulfate precipitation
South African Institute for Medical Research, Johannesburg, South Africa	*Latrodectus*	Black widow	—	—	—

Adapted from Theakston RDG, Warrell DA. Antivenoms: a list of hyperimmune sera currently available for the treatment of envenoming by bites and stings. *Toxicon* 1991;29(12):1419–1470.

(9,10), and the risk to benefit ratio must be determined in each instance. *Latrodectus* antivenom has been used with reported improvement in symptoms as late as 90 hours (11).

A retrospective study found no significant differences in length of hospitalization, ancillary analgesic drug use, or clinical outcome between eight patients given 2.5 ml of *L. mactans* antivenom versus six patients treated with symptomatic care after black widow spider bite (12).

Treatment with antivenom in many circumstances is diagnostic as well as potentially therapeutic. A larger differential diagnosis (trauma, infection, inflammatory conditions, other toxic exposure, and so forth) should always be entertained, and failure to respond to antivenom in the usual doses or timeframe should cast doubt on the diagnosis of spider envenomation.

CAUTIONS AND CONTRAINDICATIONS

L. mactans antivenom is U.S. Food and Drug Administration pregnancy category C. Black widow spider envenomation is associated with abruptio placentae and fetal demise. The antivenom has been used successfully in pregnant women (13).

Contraindications to use include documented hypersensitivity to horse serum or to *L. mactans* antivenom. Previous exposure to horse serum may or may not result in sensitization.

DOSAGE AND ADMINISTRATION

The package insert recommends skin testing for possible allergic reaction to the antivenom. Skin testing is performed by using either horse serum supplied with the antivenom or 0.02 ml of a 1:100 dilution of the antivenom. The test is performed by an intradermal injection and observation for 30 minutes. Induration greater than 10 mm, or systemic symptoms of flushing, bronchospasm, or hypotension, is a positive test. The value of skin testing has been disputed (14). Skin testing with other antivenoms has found poor sensitivity and specificity of this test (15–17).

At best, a positive skin test may suggest the possibility of a reaction and may be used as an indication for pretreatment with antihistamines, which decrease the number of type I hypersensitivity reactions with other agents (18). In addition, antivenom should be diluted in 1000 ml if possible, and the initial infusion rate reduced to 10 to 25 ml/hour (14). A positive skin test should not preclude antivenom use when there are clear indications. A negative test should not be taken as an indication that an adverse reaction will not occur. Skin testing should never be performed unless the physician has already decided to administer antivenom, so as not to risk an unnecessary reaction or to sensitize someone to horse or other serum unnecessarily. Skin testing should not delay administration of antivenom in truly life-threatening situations.

Because the object of antivenom therapy is neutralization of injected venom, dosing is not weight based, and the pediatric dose of antivenom is the same as for adults. To mix the antivenom, dissolve 1 vial in 10 ml of saline with gentle agitation (not shaking; foaming theoretically denatures the protein). The usual *adult and pediatric dose* is 1 to 2 vials. Adverse reactions may be minimized by diluting the antivenom to a total volume of at least 250 ml and administering slowly. Begin the infusion at 1 ml/minute, watching for signs of allergic reaction. If none develop over 15 minutes, increase the rate to complete the infusion over 30 minutes. In children, a total volume of 20 ml/kg, up to 250 ml, may be used. Symptoms usually improve within 1 hour of antivenom administration.

MONITORING

Significant urticaria, airway edema, bronchospasm, or hypotension should result in immediate cessation of the infusion and treatment of anaphylaxis (Chapter 34). It may be possible to restart antivenom after control of an immediate hypersensitivity reaction. Reassessment of the indication for antivenom should be performed. Pre- or concurrent treatment with epinephrine and/or a slower rate of administration may allow successful infusion.

Patients should be followed clinically for at least 2 weeks to detect serum sickness.

ADVERSE EFFECTS

Delayed hypersensitivity to the antivenom or serum sickness occurring after use is infrequently observed. Death has followed antivenom use in a patient with bronchial asthma (5).

The incidence of serum sickness is not well characterized but occurs rarely (5,12). A retrospective study found that one of eight patients receiving *L. mactans* antivenom developed serum sickness. All patients had received antivenom after negative skin testing (12).

PITFALLS

Nearly all patients with true black widow venom toxicity respond to 1 or 2 vials of antivenom. If this dose does not produce improvement, the diagnosis should be reconsidered.

RED BACK SPIDER ANTIVENOM *(LATRODECTUS MACTANS HASSELTI)*

Overview

The red back spider is one of the widow spiders. These spiders share a common toxin, α-latrotoxin; cross-reactivity has been shown among the various antivenoms produced. Between 5000 and 10,000 bites occur per year, with 20% of cases requiring antivenom (19). If untreated, the signs and symptoms may increase in severity for up to 24 hours. In nonfatal cases, symptoms slowly resolve over 1 week. Without specific treatment, symptoms of muscle weakness and spasm may persist for months.

In Australia, red back spider antivenom is available from Commonwealth Serum Laboratories. It is a purified equine-derived IgG-Fab$_2$ produced from the venom of *L. hasselti*. Each vial contains 500 units in a volume of 0.75 ml, including preservative, per ampoule. It is intended for intramuscular use in all except severe envenomations.

Mechanism of Action

The main component responsible for widow spider toxicity is α-latrotoxin, a mix of proteins with an average molecular weight of 130,000 d. The toxin binds to presynaptic nerves and causes neurotransmitter release from nerve terminals, possibly by increasing permeability of neurons to calcium (2). Clinically, this results in a similar presentation regardless of the specific widow spider and includes muscle spasms, severe pain, and hypertension (3).

Indications

The last death in Australia from a red back spider envenomation occurred in 1955. A review of bites in children found antivenom used in 21%, which was comparable to a 21% treatment rate in prior studies with older populations (20,21).

A benefit to risk analysis must be performed before the decision to administer antivenom is made. If the spider was not observed to bite, captured, and properly identified, the diagnosis of a spider envenomation may or may not be correct. Regardless, symptomatic and supportive care is the mainstay of therapy in most spider envenomations.

Significant neurotoxicity, hemodynamic instability, severe muscle spasm, or prolonged symptomatology may require antivenom treatment (22). Pain may be the only symptom, but it may be severe enough or persistent enough to warrant consideration of antivenom. In one series, 76% of patients had local symptoms only (21). Patients at greatest risk, such as children, pregnant patients, the elderly, or those with significant comorbidity or who display severe symptoms (seizures, uncontrolled hypertension, respiratory distress), are the primary candidates for antivenom therapy (5–7).

Treatment with antivenom in many circumstances is diagnostic as well as therapeutic. The antivenom is reported to produce satisfactory results in 94% of cases (19). Multiple vials of antivenom may be required, however (23). There are multiple reports of good response to late treatment with antivenom weeks to months after envenomation (24–27).

Red back spider antivenom prevents toxicity from several *Latrodectus* venoms (*L. hesperus*, *L. mactans*, *L. tredecimguttatus*, *L. lugubrious*, *L. hasselti*) and α-latrotoxin in mice, and would likely be both effective and safer to use in black widow spider envenomation than *L. mactans* antivenom (3,28).

Bites by spiders of the genus *Steatoda*, also known as *false black widow spiders*, may produce similar symptoms to those of *Latrodectus* spiders. The venom neurotoxins are similar, and case reports describe successful treatment with *Latrodectus* antivenom (29,30).

Cautions and Contraindications

The reported incidence of adverse reactions to the Australian *Latrodectus* antivenom is low. Anaphylaxis is reported in 0.5% to 1.0% of cases, and serum sickness may also occur (31).

Dosage and Administration

The usual route of *Latrodectus* antivenom is intramuscularly, although the IV route has been used in severe envenomations (21), and an intravenous regional technique (as for a Bier's block) has been used to treat chronic pain after a red back spider bite (24). Skin testing is not recommended (32). One ampoule is a reasonable initial dose. In retrospective reviews, 76% to 85% of patients required only 1 ampoule, 13% to 18% of patients required 2, and 1.9% to 6.0% required 3 or more ampoules (19,26). Eight vials were required in a patient with chronic lymphedema of the bitten extremity, which presumably reduced penetration of the antivenom at the bite site (23).

Although it is recommended that antivenom be used in the first 24 hours after an envenomation, patients may present up to 1 week after a bite with persistent symptoms and still rapidly respond to antivenom (21), and a favorable response has been reported at 120 hours after envenomation (26). Commonwealth Serum Laboratories recommends pretreatment with a parenteral antihistamine and also recommends consideration of subcutaneous epinephrine with a known allergy to equine protein or in patients who have received antivenom before (32).

Antivenom has been given without adverse effect to patients who had been previously treated. In one case, a patient was given promethazine as a pretreatment. Another was pretreated with promethazine, hydrocortisone, and epinephrine (33). When the antivenom is given IV, the manufacturer recommends diluting the antivenom tenfold in lactated Ringer's (Hartmann's) solution (34). As with other IV antivenoms, starting the infusion slowly (e.g., 1 ml/minute for 15 minutes) and then increasing the rate have minimized the incidence of adverse reactions. In children, a total volume of 20 ml/kg may be used.

Because the object of antivenom therapy is neutralization of injected venom, dosing is not weight based. In one study, unlike adult patients of whom 37% received more than 1 ampoule of antivenom, none of 271 children receiving antivenom received more than 1 ampoule (20,21). It is unclear whether this represented reluctance on the part of clinicians to use the drug in children, lesser toxicity in children than would be expected, or was secondary to other causes.

Monitoring

Significant urticaria, airway edema, bronchospasm, or hypotension should result in immediate cessation of the infusion and treatment of anaphylaxis (Chapter 34). It may be possible to restart antivenom after control of an immediate hypersensitivity reaction. Reassessment of the indication for antivenom should be performed. Pre- or concurrent treatment with epinephrine and/or a slower rate of administration may allow successful infusion.

Patients should be followed clinically for at least 2 weeks to detect serum sickness.

Adverse Effects

The incidence of mild type I hypersensitivity reaction was reported to be 0.54% in 2144 instances of use, and one-half of those cases followed undiluted IV administration (31). There have been no reports of death from this antivenom (19,31,35). Delayed hypersensitivity (serum sickness) occurring after use is infrequent. Serum sickness has been reported in a patient 1 week after receiving antivenom (26).

FUNNEL WEB SPIDER ANTIVENOM

Overview

The funnel web spiders include *Atrax robustus* (the Sydney funnel web spider, which is limited to an area with a radius of approximately 160 km from Sydney); *Hadronyche formidabilis* (Northern or tree-dwelling funnel web spider); *Hadronyche versuta* (Blue Mountains funnel web spider); and *Hadronyche cerebera* (Southern tree-dwelling funnel web spider), all native to Australia. There are 13 recorded deaths from the funnel web spider, but none since the introduction of the antivenom in 1981.

Mechanism of Action

The venom of funnel web spiders has particular mammalian toxicity, especially to humans and monkeys (36). The venom contains numerous low-molecular-weight substances (37) as well as neurotoxins of various molecular weights. The main neurotoxic components of the venom appear to be robustoxin at 4887 d (36) and atraxotoxin, with a molecular weight of 10,000 to 25,000 d (38), which may be a precursor of robustoxin (39,40). The neurotoxins act directly on all nerve membranes, causing spontaneous action potentials with the consequent widespread release of neurotransmitters acetylcholine, epinephrine, and norepinephrine into the synaptic junctions (38,41).

Clinical symptoms include local pain, autonomic instability, and severe neurotoxicity. There is a two-stage clinical syndrome, beginning minutes after envenomation with local piloerection and muscle fasciculation, becoming generalized over 10 to 20 minutes. The second phase occurs 1 to 2 hours after envenomation and includes severe hypertension, tachycardia, hyperthermia, and coma. Death is usually from asphyxia secondary to laryngeal spasm, pulmonary edema, or respiratory muscle paralysis (7,39).

Indications

Use of antivenom should be considered in the event of a symptomatic bite by an *A. robustus*, *H. infensa*, *H. versuta*, or other *Hadronyche* species. Symptoms include muscle fasciculation (in the limb involved or remotely, usually first seen in the tongue or lips); salivation; lacrimation; piloerection; tachycardia; hypertension (late hypotension); dyspnea; disorientation; confusion; or depressed level of consciousness. Because of the rapid onset of severe symptoms, initial symptomatic and supportive care involves the application of firm pressure over the bitten area with a compressive bandage, as with elapid snake envenomation. The compression bandage should not be removed until the patient is in a location where antivenom can be administered, if needed. If symptoms have already occurred or if they develop after the removal of the bandage, it should be reapplied and antivenom administered. If no evidence exists of local muscle fasciculation or systemic envenomations after 4 hours, antivenom is not required and the patient may be discharged.

Although it is raised against male *Atrax robustus* venom, funnel web spider antivenom is safe and effective for both *Atrax* and *Hadronyche* spiders (7,26,42). A benefit-risk analysis must be performed before the decision to administer antivenom is made. If the spider was not properly identified, the diagnosis of a spider envenomation may not be correct.

In an animal model, venom from male *Missulena bradleyi* (Australian Eastern mouse spider) was found to contain a neurotoxic component whose mechanism of action (modifying tetrodotoxin-sensitive sodium channel gating) is similar to that of the γ-atraxotoxins found in the Australian funnel web spider (43).

Cautions and Contraindications

The rate of allergic reactions is unknown, but such reactions should be anticipated, as with all antivenoms.

Dosage and Administration

The initial *adult and pediatric dose* is 1 to 2 ampoules of antivenom IV (100 mg IgG/ampoule) over several minutes, repeated in 15 minutes if there is no improvement. Because the object is neutralization of injected venom, the dose of antivenom is not weight based. Additional antivenom may be required and should be titrated to clinical effect; up to 17 vials have been administered (44). An infant required 6 vials after multiple bites by a male *A. robustus* (45). Skin testing is not recommended; however, pretreatment with antihistamines (H_1 and H_2 receptor antagonists) is suggested.

Monitoring

Significant urticaria, airway edema, bronchospasm, or hypotension should result in immediate cessation of the infusion and treatment of anaphylaxis (Chapter 34). It may be possible to restart antivenom after control of an immediate hypersensitivity reaction. Reassessment of the indication for antivenom should be performed. Pre- or concurrent treatment with epinephrine and/or a slower rate of administration may allow successful infusion.

Patients should be followed clinically for at least 2 weeks to detect serum sickness.

Adverse Effects

No immediate adverse effects have been reported in 50 patients treated with the antivenom (26), although the possibility of a hypersensitivity reaction should be anticipated. A patient treated with 5 vials of antivenom after a confirmed funnel web spider envenomation developed a moderate serum sickness reaction (44).

OTHER SPIDER ANTIVENOMS

The South African Institute for Medical Research produces a *Latrodectus* antivenom raised to *L. mactans* (*indistinctus*) for IV or intramuscular use. Of 27 patients bitten by *L. indistinctus* and treated with South African Institute for Medical Research antivenom, there were 26 with good results and no adverse reactions. Brown widow spiders (*L. geometricus*) may produce typical latrodectism. Four patients with *L. geometricus* envenomation were treated with South African Institute for Medical Research *Latrodectus* antivenom between 6 hours and 5 days postenvenomation, with good results and no adverse effects (6).

Bites by spiders of the genus *Steatoda*, also known as *false black widow spiders*, may produce similar symptoms to that of *Latrodectus* spiders and similarities of the neurotoxins, as well as case reports of successful treatment with *Latrodectus* antivenom (29,30).

In a survey of spider envenomations, 515 patients bitten by wolf spiders (family Lycosidae) developed mild effects, and only three patients received antivenom. Since 1985, Butantan Institute spider antivenom does not include an anti-Lycosid fraction (46,47).

Bites by *Phoneutria* species in South America are typically mild (89.9%), with 8.5% having moderate symptoms and 0.5% severe; 2.3% of cases were treated with intravenous antivenom. No type I hypersensitivity reactions were reported (48).

No commercially produced, U.S. Food and Drug Administration–approved antivenom exists for brown recluse spider (*Loxosceles* spp) envenomation. Several *Loxosceles*-specific antivenoms are available in South America. The efficacy of *Loxosceles* antivenom in treating the dermonecrotic lesion and systemic symptoms is not well documented.

REFERENCES

1. Jelinek GA. Widow spider envenomation (latrodectism): a worldwide problem. *Wilderness Environ Med* 1997;8:226–231.
2. Bittner MA, Krasnoperov VG, Stuenkel EL, et al. A Ca^{2+}-independent receptor for alpha-latrotoxin, CIRL, mediates effects on secretion via multiple mechanisms. *J Neurosci* 1998;18(8):2914–2922.
3. Graudins A, Padula M, Broady K, et al. Red-back spider (*Latrodectus hasselti*) antivenom prevents the toxicity of widow spider venoms. *Ann Emerg Med* 2001;37(2):154–160.
4. Wasserman GS, Anderson PC. Loxoscelism and necrotic arachnidism. *J Toxicol Clin Toxicol* 1983–1984;21:451–472.
5. Clark RF, Wethern-Kestner S, Vance MV, et al. Clinical presentation and treatment of black widow spider envenomation: a review of 163 cases. *Ann Emerg Med* 1992;21:782–787.
6. Muller GJ. Black and brown widow spider bites in South Africa: a series of 45 cases. *S Afr Med J* 1993;83:399–405.
7. Sutherland SK. Treatment of arachnid poisoning in Australia. *Aust Fam Physician* 1990;19:1–10.
8. Byrne GC, Pemberton PJ. Red-back spider (*Latrodectus mactans lasselti*) envenomation in a neonate. *Med J Aust* 1983;2(12):665–666.
9. Maretic Z. Latrodectism: variations in clinical manifestations provoked by Latrodectus species of spiders. *Toxicon* 1983;21(4):457–466.
10. Ennik F. Deaths from bites and stings of venomous animals. *West J Med* 1980;133(6):463–468.
11. O'Malley GF, Dart RC, Kuffner EF. Successful treatment of Latrodectism with Antivenin after 90 hours. *N Engl J Med* 1999;340:657.
12. Moss HS, Binder LS. A retrospective review of black widow spider envenomation. *Ann Emerg Med* 1987;16(2):188–192.

13. Russell FE. Black widow spider envenomation during pregnancy: report of a case. *Toxicon* 1979;17:188–189.
14. Heard K, O'Malley GF, Dart RC. Antivenom therapy in the Americas. *Drugs* 1999;58(1):5–15.
15. Corrigan P, Russell FE, Wainschell J. Clinical reactions to antivenin. In: Rosenberg P, ed. *Toxins: animal, plant and microbial*. Oxford: Pergammon Press, 1978:457–465.
16. Jurkovich GJ, Luterman A, McCullar K, et al. Complications of Crotalidae antivenin therapy. *J Trauma* 1988;28(7):1032–1037.
17. Malasit P, Warrell DA, Chanthavanich P, et al. Prediction, prevention, and mechanism of early (anaphylactic) antivenom reactions in victims of snake bites. *Br Med J (Clin Res Ed)* 1986;292(6512):17–20.
18. Lieberman P. The use of antihistamines in the prevention and treatment of anaphylaxis and anaphylactoid reactions. *J Allergy Clin Immunol* 1990;86(4 Pt 2):684–686.
19. White J. Envenoming and antivenom use in Australia. *Toxicon* 1998;36(1):1483–1492.
20. Mead HJ, Jelinek GA. Red-back spider bites to Perth children, 1979–1988. *J Paediatr Child Health* 1993;29(4):305–308.
21. Jelinek GA, Banham NDG, Dunjey SJ. Red-back spider bites at Freemantle Hospital, 1982–1987. *Med J Aust* 1989;150:693–695.
22. Gala S, Katelaris CH. Rhabdomyolysis due to redback spider envenomation. *Med J Aust* 1992;157:66.
23. Couser GA, Wilkes GJ. A red-back spider bite in a lymphoedematous arm. *Med J Aust* 1997;166(11):587–588.
24. Banham NDG, Jelinek GA, Finsh PM. Late treatment with antivenom in prolonged red-back spider envenomation. *Med J Aust* 1994;161:379.
25. Pincus DR. Response to antivenom 14 days after red-back spider bite. *Med J Aust* 1994;161(3):226.
26. Sutherland SK. Antivenom use in Australia. Premedication, adverse reactions and the use of venom detection kits. *Med J Aust* 1992;157(11–12):734–739.
27. Southcott RV. Red-back spider bite (Latrodectism) with response to antivenene therapy given eighty hours after the injury. *Med J Aust* 1961;1:659–662.
28. Daly FF, Hill RE, Bogdan GM, et al. Neutralization of *Latrodectus mactans* and *L. hesperus* venom by redback spider (*L. hasseltii*) antivenom. *J Toxicol Clin Toxicol* 2001;39(2):119–123.
29. South M, Wirth P, Winkel KD. Redback spider antivenom used to treat envenomation by a juvenile Steatoda spider. *Med J Aust* 1998;169(11–12):642.
30. Graudins A, Gunja N, Broady KW, et al. Clinical and in vitro evidence for the efficacy of Australian red-back spider (*Latrodectus hasselti*) antivenom in the treatment of envenomation by a Cupboard spider (*Steatoda grossa*). *Toxicon* 2002;40(6):767–775.
31. Sutherland SK, Trinca JC. Survey of 2144 cases of red-back spider bites. *Med J Aust* 1978;2(14):620–623.
32. Commonwealth Serum Laboratories. Red back spider antivenom. Victoria, Australia, 1996.
33. Mollison L, Liew D, McDermott R, et al. Red-back spider envenomation in the red centre of Australia. *Med J Aust* 1994;161(11–12):701, 704–705.
34. Brown AFT. Delayed diagnosis of red-back spider envenomation; a timely reminder. *Med J Aust* 1989;151:705–706.
35. White J, Cardoso JL, Fan HW. Clinical toxicology of spider bites. In: Meier J, White J, eds. *Handbook of clinical toxicology of animal venoms and poison*. New York: CRC Press, 1995.
36. Sheumack DD, Claassens R, Whiteley NM, et al. Complete amino acid sequence of a new type of lethal neurotoxin from the venom of the funnel-web spider, *Atrax robustus*. *FEBS Lett* 1985;181:154–156.
37. Duffield PH, Duffield AM, Carroll PR, et al. Analysis of the venom of the Sydney funnel-web spider, *Atrax robustus*, using gas chromatography mass spectrometry. *Biomed Mass Spectrom* 1979;6(3):105–108.
38. Gray MR, Sutherland SK. Venoms of the dipluridae. In: Bettini S, ed., *Arthropod venoms: Handbook of experimental pharmacology*. Berlin: Springer Verlag, 1978.
39. Sutherland SK. The Sydney funnel-web spider (*Atrax robustus*). 3. A review of some clinical records of human envenomation. *Med J Aust* 1972;2:643.
40. Sutherland SK. The Sydney funnel-web spider (*Atrax robustus*). 2. Fractionation of the female venom into five distinct components. *Med J Aust* 1972;2:643.
41. Sutherland SK. Venomous Australian creatures: the action of their toxins and the care of the envenomated patient. *Anaesth Intensive Care* 1974;2(4):316–328.
42. Dieckmann J, Prebble J, McDonogh A, et al. Efficacy of funnel-web spider antivenom in human envenomation by *Hadronyche* species. *Med J Aust* 1989;151(11–12):706–707.
43. Rash LD, Biriny-Strachan LC, Nicholson GM, et al. Neurotoxic activity of venom from the Australian eastern mouse spider (*Missulena bradleyi*) involves modulation of sodium channel gating. *Br J Pharmacol* 2000;130(8):1817–1824.
44. Miller MK, Whyte IM, Dawson AH. Serum sickness from funnelweb spider antivenom. *Med J Aust* 1999;171(1):54.
45. Browne GJ. Near fatal envenomation from the funnel-web spider in an infant. *Pediatr Emerg Care* 1997;13(4):271–173.
46. Lucas S. Spiders in Brazil. *Toxicon* 1988;26(9):759–772.
47. Ribeiro LA, Jorge MT, Presco PV, et al. Wolf spider bites in Sao Paulo, Brazil: a clinical and epidemiological study of 515 cases. *Toxicon* 1990;28:715–717.
48. Bucaretchi F, Deus Reinaldo CR, Hyslop S, et al. A clinico-epidemiological study of bites by spiders of the genus Phoneutria. *Rev Inst Med Trop Sao Paulo* 2000;42(1):17–21.

CHAPTER 77

Succimer

Richard C. Dart

SUCCIMER

Synonyms:	**Meso-2,3-dimercaptosuccinic acid (DMSA), Chemet**
Molecular formula and weight:	**$C_4H_6O_4S_2$, 182.2 g/mol**
CAS Registry No.:	**304-55-2**
Therapeutic level:	**Not applicable**
Special concerns:	**Succimer imparts a sulfur odor to bodily secretions.**

OVERVIEW

Succimer is a heavy metal chelating agent that has been used in the treatment of lead, mercury, and arsenic poisoning. Multiple studies have demonstrated that succimer increases the excretion of these metals; however, improvement of outcome has rarely been tested (1).

Succimer is provided as 100-mg capsules for oral use. The gelatin capsules contain microspheres that may be poured out onto food or drink for small children. The sodium salt has been used parenterally but is not commercially available.

Mechanism of Action

Succimer binds a metal, probably via the sulfhydryl groups, thereby preventing metal effect or possibly removing the metal from binding sites on enzymes or other physiologic proteins. The succimer–heavy metal complex is then excreted renally. Succimer increases urinary excretion of lead, mercury, and arsenic and lowers the blood lead level in humans. Succimer does not result in elimination of clinically significant amounts of trace essential minerals such as zinc, copper, iron, magnesium, and calcium. In animal models, succimer does not appear to redistribute lead from blood into brain.

The pharmacokinetics of succimer and other sulfhydryl-containing drugs are complicated because of the variety of forms (free; protein-bound in either reduced or oxidized form; mixed disulfides with other thiols, including protein thiols) in which it occurs. Succimer is rapidly absorbed orally and undergoes rapid metabolism. It is excreted in the urine with small amounts in the bile and breath. The elimination of total succimer (parent drug plus oxidized metabolites) in three children with lead poisoning, three adults with lead poisoning, and five healthy adult volunteers resulted in half-lives of 3 ± 0.2 hours in the children, 1.9 ± 0.4 hours in the adults with lead poisoning, and 2.0 ± 0.2 hours for volunteers (1).

In a juvenile nonhuman primate model of moderate childhood lead intoxication, succimer reduced the intestinal absorption of lead by 64.9% in controls to 37.0% in treated animals. It also increased the urinary excretion of endogenous lead fourfold and decreased the endogenous fecal lead excretion by approximately 33%. Although succimer reduced the whole-body retention of endogenous lead by approximately 10% compared to vehicle, most (77%) of the lead tracer was retained in the body at 5 days after treatment (2).

INDICATIONS

Lead Poisoning

The labeled indication in the United States is for the treatment of children with blood lead levels above 45 µg/dl. In addition, succimer is often used to treat children with blood lead levels between 20 and 45 µg/dl when removing the child from lead-contaminated environment does not decrease the blood lead level or when significant acute exposure has occurred. Adults with symptoms of lead poisoning or elevated lead levels are also treated with succimer. The exact level at which to chelate is controversial but is usually above 60 µg/dl. Many variations on these basic indications have been used.

The main concern about the use of succimer in lead-poisoned patients is the lack of data demonstrating improved outcome. Rogan et al. performed a large ($N = 780$) trial of succimer in children with blood lead levels of 20 to 44 µg/dl (1.0 to 2.1 µmol/L) in a randomized, placebo-controlled, double-blind trial of up to three 26-day courses of succimer. Follow-up of cognitive, motor, behavioral, and neuropsychological function over 36 months found that the mean blood lead level in the children treated with succimer was 4.5 µg/dl (0.2 µmol/L) lower than the level in the placebo group. The mean IQ score of children in the succimer group was one point lower than the placebo group. The behavior of children given succimer was slightly worse as rated by a parent. However, the children given succimer scored slightly better on the Developmental Neuropsychological Assessment, a battery of tests designed to measure neuropsychological deficits thought to interfere with learning. All these differences were small, and none were statistically significant (3).

Concerns about efficacy are supported by a nonhuman primate trial that found that succimer did not decrease the brain lead level beyond the intervention of simply terminating exposure (4). The cessation of lead exposure alone reduced brain lead 34% compared to pretreatment levels.

It is important to note, however, that these trials did not study subgroups thought to be more responsible to chelation (e.g., children with only recent exposure). Currently, widespread chelation for a blood lead level of less than 45 µg/dl should be used only in selected cases.

Poisoning by Other Heavy Metals

Succimer is often used to increase excretion of antimony, arsenic, bismuth, or mercury in symptomatic adult and pediatric patients (5–10). However, evidence of improved outcome is often unavailable or no effect is found (11). Succimer also increased copper excretion in one study (12).

CAUTIONS AND CONTRAINDICATIONS

Heavy metal chelation is relatively contraindicated in the absence of proof that the exposure has been terminated. Known hypersensitivity to succimer is a contraindication because other chelating agents are usually available.

Succimer is U.S. Food and Drug Administration pregnancy category C. Animal studies have provided conflicting results regarding teratogenesis. Succimer has been used without apparent adverse effect in pregnancy (13).

DOSAGE AND ADMINISTRATION

Lead Poisoning

The *pediatric dose* is 10 mg/kg (or 350 mg/m^2) orally three times a day for 5 days, followed by 10 mg/kg twice a day for 14 days. The use of two courses of 10 mg/kg for 5 days separated by 1 week (i.e., no twice-a-day period) was found to lower blood lead similarly (14). This technique may be useful when compliance is a concern.

Poisoning by Other Heavy Metals

First, a baseline 24-hour urine for the metal of interest is obtained. Succimer is then administered. The proper dose is unknown; therefore, most practitioners use the same dose as lead poisoning. It may be necessary to begin therapy with a parenteral chelator such as dimercaprol or ethylenediaminetetraacetic acid due to vomiting. The patient can often be switched to succimer after a day of parenteral therapy.

The 24-hour urine is repeated during the first day of therapy. This collection should demonstrate a marked increase in metal excretion. If not, succimer is probably not clinically helpful.

Repeated courses of chelation have been used in patients with persistent symptoms of metal toxicity and persistent elevation of urine metal excretion. The exact indications for repeat courses of therapy are not established.

Monitoring

Repeat blood lead level several days after completion of therapy and every 2 to 4 weeks thereafter until level stabilizes. If blood lead level rebounds to above 45 µg/dl, investigate whether repeat exposure could have occurred in interim. If not, repeat course of chelation. If level rebounds to 20 to 45 µg/dl, treatment recommendations are uncertain. Many centers perform at least one more course of chelation.

ADVERSE EFFECTS

A 3-year-old child was given 185 mg/kg of dimercaptosuccinic acid/kg of body weight without apparent adverse effects (15).

Elevations of ALT and aspartate transaminase have occurred during succimer use but have resolved despite continued therapy. Other side effects of oral administration of succimer are rare and mild. They include gastrointestinal discomfort and mild pain, rashes, and eosinophilia, which have not required treatment. One case of hemolysis in a glucose 6 phosphate dehydrogenase–deficient patient has been reported.

PITFALLS

Succimer imparts a sulfur-like odor to the patient's body fluids. This may decrease compliance, especially in adolescents.

Succimer primarily chelates lead in blood and soft tissues. After discontinuation of therapy, blood lead levels often rebound to approximately two-thirds of the original value. This phenomenon is affected by duration of lead poisoning and repeated courses of chelation.

REFERENCES

1. Dart RC, Hurlbut KM, Maiorino RM, et al. Pharmacokinetics of meso-2,3-dimercaptosuccinic acid (DMSA) in lead poisoned patients and normal adults. *J Pediatr* 1994;125:309–316.
2. Cremin JD Jr, Luck ML, Laughlin NK, et al. Oral succimer decreases the gastrointestinal absorption of lead in juvenile monkeys. *Environ Health Perspect* 2001;109:613–619.
3. Rogan WJ, Dietrich KN, Ware JH, et al. The effect of chelation therapy with succimer on neuropsychological development in children exposed to lead. *N Engl J Med* 2001;344:1421–1426.
4. Cremin JR Jr, Luck ML, Laughlin NK, et al. Efficacy of succimer chelation for reducing brain lead in a primate model of human lead exposure. *Toxicol Appl Pharmacol* 1999;161:283–293.
5. Forman J, Moline J, Cernichiari E, et al. A cluster of pediatric metallic mercury exposure cases treated with meso-2,3-dimercaptosuccinic acid (DMSA). *Environ Health Perspect* 2000;108:575–577.
6. Lenz K, Hruby K, Druml W, et al. 2,3-dimercaptosuccinic acid in human arsenic poisoning. *Arch Toxicol* 1981;47:241–243.
7. Ly BT, Williams SR, Clark RF. Mercuric oxide poisoning treated with whole-bowel irrigation and chelation therapy. *Ann Emerg Med* 2002;39:312–315.
8. Reymond JM, Desmeules J. Sodium stibogluconate (Pentosan) overdose in a patient with acquired immunodeficiency syndrome. *Ther Drug Monit* 1998;20:714–716.
9. Shum S, Whitehead J, Vaughn L, et al. Chelation of organoarsenate with dimercaptosuccinic acid. *Vet Human Toxicol* 1995;37:239–242.
10. Slikkerveer A, Noach LA, Tytgat GN, et al. Comparison of enhanced elimination of bismuth in humans after treatment with meso-2,3-dimercaptosuccinic acid and D,L-2,3-dimercaptopropane-1-sulfonic acid. *Analyst* 1998;123:91–92.
11. Guha Mazumder DN, Ghoshal UC, Saha J, et al. Randomized placebo-controlled trial of 2,3-dimercaptosuccinic acid in therapy of chronic arsenicosis due to drinking arsenic-contaminated subsoil water. *J Toxicol Clin Toxicol* 1998;36:683–690.
12. Ren M, Yang R. Clinical curative effects of dimercaptosuccinic acid on hepatolenticular degeneration and the impact of DMSA on biliary trace elements. *Chinese Med J* 1997;110:694–697.
13. Horowitz BZ, Mirkin DB. Lead poisoning and chelation in a mother-neonate pair. *J Toxicol Clin Toxicol* 2001;39:727–731.
14. Farrar HC, McLeane LR, Wallace M, et al. A comparison of two dosing regimens of succimer in children with chronic lead poisoning. *J Clin Pharmacol* 1999;39:180–183.
15. Sigg T, Burda A, Leikin JB, et al. A report of pediatric succimer overdose. *Vet Human Toxicol* 1998;40:90–91.

SECTION 6

Enhancement of Elimination

CHAPTER 78
Elimination Enhancement

Steven A. Seifert

OVERVIEW

Enhancement of elimination of toxic substances encompasses a variety of techniques. To determine that the benefit to risk ratio is in favor of using one of these techniques, a number of questions should be asked. What are the medical benefits of increasing the elimination of the compound? Is the substance of concern causing or likely to cause significant toxicity if it is not removed more rapidly than by endogenous clearance? Is this toxicity likely to cause permanent or significant injury that is not amenable to supportive care? What are the adverse effects and potential complications of these procedures, and what can be done to minimize their occurrence? The answers to these questions inform the decision of whether to apply enhanced elimination measures.

MULTIDOSE ACTIVATED CHARCOAL

Procedure

Activated charcoal (AC) may be repeatedly administered over the course of drug intoxication as a means of interrupting gastrointestinal (GI) recirculation of a drug. This is termed *multiple-dose activated charcoal* (MDAC). The proposed mechanism of action is the binding of a drug that diffuses from the intestinal blood vessels into the GI lumen, a process that has been named *GI dialysis*. It is also possible that drug metabolites excreted in bile are bound before reabsorption.

Numerous dosing schedules have been proposed, but there are no prospective studies to compare efficacies. A typical treatment regimen is 25 to 50 g or 0.5 to 1.0 g/kg orally every 2 to 4 hours.

Possible Applications

The administration of MDAC increases drug elimination significantly in animal and human volunteers (Table 1). It is often used to increase elimination of carbamazepine (CBZ), dapsone, phenobarbital, quinine, or theophylline, because experimental studies confirm enhanced elimination. There are no controlled, prospective studies in poisoned patients that demonstrate a reduction in morbidity or mortality. Other methods of enhanced elimination of these compounds may be appropriate and used concurrently or instead of MDAC. The elimination of other drugs may be increased with MDAC, but data to assess its use with these agents in poisoned patients are lacking (Table 1). The elimination of certain agents is increased by MDAC (Table 1) (1).

Complications

MDAC should be used only when protective airway reflexes are intact or the airway is protected by intubation. Because the latter

TABLE 1. Uses of multiple-dose activated charcoal

Drugs with proven enhanced elimination
Carbamazepine
Dapsone
Phenobarbital
Quinine
Theophylline
Drugs with possible benefit
Amitriptyline
Dextropropoxyphene
Digitoxin
Digoxin
Disopyramide
Nadolol
Phenylbutazone
Phenytoin
Piroxicam
Sotalol
Drugs without enhanced elimination
Astemizole
Chlorpropamide
Doxepin
Imipramine
Meprobamate
Methotrexate
Sodium valproate (valproic acid)
Tobramycin
Vancomycin (may shorten half-life in neonates)

is only partially protective against charcoal aspiration, the potential benefit should outweigh the risks of this therapy. No evidence exists that cathartics are a beneficial adjunct to MDAC in the poisoned patient. In particular, cathartics should be withheld from subsequent doses of AC and in the treatment of children to avoid fluid and electrolyte disturbances.

MDAC also increases the elimination of therapeutic drugs and may reduce therapeutic levels (e.g., use of MDAC for theophylline toxicity could reduce therapeutic phenobarbital levels for a concurrent seizure disorder).

MULTIDOSE SODIUM POLYSTYRENE SULFONATE

Procedure

As with AC, sodium polystyrene sulfonate (SPS) may be given repetitively by a variety of protocols.

Possible Applications

In an animal model of chronic overdosage, multiple-dose SPS lowers lithium levels at 150, 330, and 480 minutes after initiation of treatment, but not at 1440 or 2880 minutes (2). It also lowers lithium levels slightly in human volunteers; however, evidence of clinical efficacy in overdose has not been documented.

Complications

The extent of SPS lowering of serum potassium may limit its use (3).

MULTIDOSE PRUSSIAN BLUE

Procedure

Prussian blue (potassium ferric hexacyanoferrate) is administered via a nasogastric or orogastric tube for thallium poisoning. Various protocols have been advocated, but most commonly, Prussian blue is given as a 3-g bolus followed by multiple doses (every 4 to 12 hours). A dose of 3 g/day is well tolerated; others have advocated up to 250 mg/kg/day. The addition of mannitol as a cathartic has been proposed (50 ml mannitol 15%) (4,5).

Possible Applications

Prussian blue is not absorbed from the GI tract. Potassium ions within the compound's lattice are exchanged for thallium or cesium ions, interfering with enterohepatic circulation and creating a concentration gradient into the intestinal lumen (5,6). Although no controlled studies have been performed, there are numerous case series and reports of its clinical benefit in thallium toxicity (4,7–9). A reduction of cesium body burden and half-life by 43% has been shown in human studies (6).

URINARY ACIDIFICATION

Although urinary acidification enhances the rate of urinary clearance of phencyclidine, quinine, and other weak bases, it is not possible to acidify the urine without decreasing blood pH, which is generally not desirable in the context of most drug toxicities. As a result, urinary acidification is not currently recommended.

URINARY ALKALINIZATION

Procedure

The pH of the urine may be increased as a means of ionizing drugs that have been filtered into the urine, thus preventing their reabsorption back into the renal tubule (*ion trapping*).

Possible Applications

The use of urinary pH manipulation has been questioned by the ability of less care-intensive methods such as repeated-dose charcoal to increase the elimination of many toxins (10). Urinary alkalinization increases renal clearance and reduces the elimination half-life of weak acids such as salicylates, hexachlorophene, phenobarbital, phenoxyacetate herbicides, and chlorpropamide. The use of urinary alkalinization has been called into question by the ability of less care-intensive methods such as MDAC to increase the elimination of many toxins (10).

Complications

Urinary alkalinization increases the elimination of therapeutic drugs with the same characteristics, such as phenobarbital.

EXTRACORPOREAL TECHNIQUES

The efficacy of extracorporeal techniques (dialysis, perfusion, plasma exchange, extracorporeal hemodynamic support) in acute poisoning cannot be easily estimated because of the need to consider concomitant intestinal absorption as well as metabolism and elimination (11). Many reports also involve multiple ingestions, making the contribution of extracorporeal methods to clinical outcome difficult to determine.

The use of extracorporeal techniques in the treatment of poisoning is summarized in Table 2 (C. Koppel, *personal communication*, April 1994) (12). The toxicokinetics of some drugs removed by extracorporeal techniques are summarized in Tables 3 and 4 (12,13). Poisons for which hemoperfusion (HP) and hemodialysis (HD) have been used are listed in Tables 5 and 6 (14). Much of the data on usefulness of these procedures are based on case reports, and the clinical use has evolved since 1983. Extracorporeal techniques are commonly used in severe salicylate, methanol, ethylene glycol, lithium, phenobarbital, and theophylline overdoses and are occasionally used in sedative-hypnotic, industrial, and household poisonings. When the need for extracorporeal measures can be anticipated, access should be available within a short time (15–17).

HEMODIALYSIS

Procedure

HD is an invasive procedure that requires large-lumen vascular access and a trained team. There are a variety of dialysis membranes, dialysates, and flow rates that may affect drug clearance. HD techniques and equipment have improved over the years, which may shorten the duration of dialysis needed to remove a drug.

Possible Applications

If the percentage of free drug in the plasma divided by the apparent volume of distribution (V_d, L/kg) is greater than 80,

TABLE 2. Compounds for which extracorporeal elimination may be the preferred treatment for overdose

Toxic compound	Relative molecular mass	Water soluble	Volume of distribution (L/kg)	Endogenous clearance (ml/min/kg)	Protein binding	Preferred method	Comments
Aminoglycosides	>500	Yes	~0.3	~1.5	<10%	HF	Useful if clearance decreased due to renal failure
Carbamazepine	236	No	~1.4	~1.3	~74%	HP	Clearance increased in patients on long-term treatment
Ethylene glycol	62	Yes	~0.6	~2	0	HD	Clearance decreased as dose increased
Lithium	7	Yes	0.6–1.0	~0.35	0	HD	Useful if clearance decreased due to renal failure
Methanol	32	Yes	~0.7	~0.7	0	HD	—
Phenobarbital	232	No	~0.54	~0.06	24%	HP	—
Procainamide	272	Yes	~1.9	~8	~16%	HD or HP	Clearance decreased in renal failure; active metabolite also removed
Salicylate	138	Yes	~0.17	~0.88	~90%	HD	Clearance and binding decrease with increasing dose
Theophylline	180	Yes	~0.5	~0.65	~56%	HP	—

HD, hemodialysis; HF, hemofiltration; HP, hemoperfusion.
Modified from Pond SM. Extracorporeal techniques in the management of poisoned patients. *Med J Aust* 1991;154:617–622.

HD for 6 hours should remove 20% to 50% of a drug (18). If the percentage of free drug divided by V_d (L/kg) is less than 20, then a small and probably insignificant amount (less than 10%) of the drug is removed during 6 hours of HD. Controlled clinical studies designed to validate these observations have not been performed.

(% Free drug)/V_d (L/kg) >80 = estimated 20% to 50% removed by HD

(% Free drug)/V_d (L/kg) <20 = <10% removed by HD

HD is occasionally combined with HP, either simultaneously (19) or in series.

Complications

Complications of HD include disturbance or dysfunction of hematologic, coagulation, acid-base, fluid and electrolyte, neurologic, and hemodynamic systems as well as complications of vascular access, infections, allergic, and adverse reactions secondary to removal of required medications. The incidence and severity stratification of such complications in the toxicologic setting, when the procedure is often performed emergently, is unknown. Complications of obtaining central venous access are well studied, with an acute complication rate up to 27.2% and a major complication rate of 1% to 5%. Complications of HD are summarized in Table 7.

HEMOPERFUSION

Procedure

HP is the passing of blood through an extracorporeal column or cartridge containing AC. Toxicants in the blood adsorb to AC. Rarely, a synthetic resin may be used instead of AC. The optimal perfusion material may vary based on the toxicant.

Possible Applications

HP may be useful for drugs with a low V_d (less than 1 L/kg) and a low endogenous clearance and that are adsorbed by AC. HP is most commonly used for theophylline, CBZ, phenobarbital, and procainamide (Table 7). In most hospitals, HD can be initiated much more rapidly and may be preferred (even if HP attains higher clearance rates).

Because HP is an invasive procedure, the risk to benefit ratio should be addressed. The poisoning to be treated should be serious and usually involves one or more of these scenarios: (a) disturbance of one or more vital functions with a drug having a small distribution volume and displaying a clear relationship between blood levels and toxic effects; (b) clinical deterioration of an intoxicated patient, despite appropriate conservative treatment; (c) intoxication with a drug known to be metabolized to a more toxic one; (d) intoxication with a drug known to produce delayed toxicity (20); (e) severe intoxication with midbrain dysfunction; (f) development of complications of coma; (g) impairment of normal drug excretory function; or (h) intoxication with an extractable drug that can be removed at a rate greater than that of endogenous elimination (C. Koppel, *personal communication*, April 1994).

The problems that limit the usefulness of HP include late initiation of treatment, presence of compounds with a large V_d or with a rapid distribution, poisonings that are more easily treated with HD, requirement of a trained group, and usefulness of symptomatic therapy during the critical phase (T. Zilker, *personal communication*, April 1994).

Complications

Several complications of HP exist (Table 7). It requires involvement of other specialists to initiate, does not correct acidemia or electrolyte abnormalities, and cannot be performed in severely hypotensive patients.

PERITONEAL DIALYSIS

Procedure

Peritoneal dialysis (PD) requires an abdominal catheter with intermittent or continuous fluid exchange. Acute PD is used principally to treat patients with acute renal failure, especially in

TABLE 3. Pharmacokinetic properties of selected drugs and poisons

Drug name	Apparent volume of distribution, V_d (L/kg)	Plasma clearance (ml/min)	Plasma protein binding (%)	Hemo-dialyzer clearance (ml/min)	Hemo-perfusion clearance (ml/min)	Fractional removal in 4 h (%)		
						Normal patient	With hemodialysis	With hemoperfusion
Central nervous system agents								
Alcohols								
Ethanol	0.6	170–320	0	120–160	—	76	87	—
Isopropanol	0.6	—	0	—	—	—	79	—
Methanol	0.6	44	0	98–176	—	22	56	—
Ethylene glycol	0.8	64	—	—	—	—	—	—
Sedative-hypnotics								
Chloral hydrate	6	600	35–41	120	157–238	29	34	37
Ethchlorvynol	2.8	90	30–50	64	125–300	10	17	23
Glutethimide	2.7	180	45	50	60–250	20	25	32
Meprobamate	0.75	60	0–20	60	85–150	24	42	56
Methaqualone	6	140	80	23	216	8	9	18
Methyprylon	—	—	20–80	5–171	25–171	50	—	—
Pentobarbital	1	36	66	22	50–300	12	18	27
Phenobarbital	0.75	9	25–60	80	80–290	4	33	39
Secobarbital	1.42	5	70	NS	20–119	1	1	16
Analgesics								
Acetaminophen	1	400	10–21[a]	120	125	75	83	83
Aspirin	0.21	45	73–94	20	90	52	65	89
Anticonvulsant drugs								
Carbamazepine	1	59	70–80	NS	80–129	17	17	36
Ethosuximide	0.7	10	0	140	—	5	52	—
Phenytoin	0.57[b]	25	87–93	NS	76–189	14	14	61
Primidone	0.6	40	0	98	98	20	55	55
Sodium valproate	0.15–0.4	10	90–95	23	—	12	33	—
Psychotherapeutic drugs								
Amitriptyline	20	—	96	NS	14–210	—	—	—
Chlordiazepoxide	0.3	25	86–93	NS	—	—	—	—
Chlorpromazine	—	—	90	NS	—	—	—	—
Desipramine	—	—	69–76	NS	—	—	—	—
Diazepam	0.74[c]	35	90	NS	—	15	15	—
Haloperidol	23	1330	90	NS	—	—	—	—
Imipramine	11	1000	86–96	18	—	27	27	—
Lithium carbonate	0.79	20	0	150	—	8	52	—
Nortriptyline	21	740	94	NS	14–210	11	11	12
Cardiovascular agents								
Antiarrhythmic drugs								
Bretylium	7	725	1–6	NS	—	—	—	—
Disopyramide	0.83	93	5–65[d]	123	—	32	40	—
Flecainide	8.7	567	40	NS	—	—	—	—
Lidocaine	1.2	606	66	NS	75–90	82	82	86
Mexiletine	7–10	846	70	NS	—	29	29	—
N-acetylprocainamide[e]	1.5	200	10	41–97	125	37	49	—
Procainamide	2	810	15	65	—	75	78	—
Quinidine	2	270	80–85	11–18	24	37	39	40
Tocainide	3.2	182	10–15	25	—	18	20	—
Antihypertensive drugs								
Acebutolol	1.4	665	11–19	43	—	80	82	—
Atenolol	1.2	176	<5	29–39	—	40	45	—
Diazoxide	0.12	7	94	25	—	18	60	—
Nadolol	2	135	20–30	46–102	—	21	30	—
Cardiotonic agents								
Digitoxin	0.5	3	90	NS	19	2	2	14
Digoxin	7.1	160	20–30	20	80	7	8	11
Spasmolytic agent								
Theophylline	0.45	46	60	70	100–225	30	59	74
Antineoplastic agent								
Methotrexate	0.64[f]	52	50–70	—	54–137	24	—	64
Metals and minerals								
Fluoride	0.5	100	—	100–188	—	—	—	—
Mercury	—	—	99	NS	—	—	—	—
Methylmercury	—	—	99	50–150[g]	—	—	—	—
Herbicides and insecticides								
Demeton-*S*-methylsulfoxide	—	—	—	53	84	—	—	—
Paraquat	2.8	28	—	NS	57–156	—	—	—

NS, not significant.
[a]Data are for the metabolite trichloroethanol.
[b]Concentration dependent.
[c]V_d in uremia is 1.4 L/kg body weight.
[d]V_d in uremia is 2.2 L/kg body weight.
[e]Binding is concentration dependent.
[f]V_d reduced to 0.42 L/kg in end-stage renal disease.
[g]With concurrent L-cysteine infusion.
From Cutler RE, Forland SC, Hammond St JPG, et al. Extracorporeal removal of drugs and poisons by hemodialysis and hemoperfusion. *Annu Rev Pharmacol Toxicol* 1987;27:169–191, with permission.

TABLE 4. Kinetic characteristics of drugs that make them amenable to removal by extracorporeal procedures

Hemodialysis	Hemoperfusion	Hemofiltration
Relative molecular mass <500	Adsorbed by activated charcoal	Relative molecular mass less than the cutoff of the filter fibers, usually <40,000
Water soluble	Small volume of distribution (<1 L/kg)	Small volume of distribution (<1 L/kg)
Small volume of distribution (<1 L/kg)	Poorly bound to plasma proteins	Single-compartment kinetics
Poorly bound to plasma proteins	Single-compartment kinetics	Low endogenous clearance (<4 ml/min/kg)
Single-compartment kinetics	Low endogenous clearance (<4 ml/min/kg)	
Low endogenous clearance (<4 ml/min/kg)		

Adapted from Pond SM. Extracorporeal techniques in the management of poisoned patients. *Med J Aust* 1991;154:617–622.

TABLE 5. Drugs and chemicals removed with dialysis

Barbiturates
Amobarbital
Aprobarbital
Barbital
Butabarbital
Cyclobarbital
Pentobarbital
Phenobarbital
Quinalbital
(Secobarbital)

Nonbarbiturate hypnotics, sedatives, tranquilizers, anticonvulsants
Carbamazepine
Carbromal
Chloral hydrate
(Chlordiazepoxide)
(Diazepam)
(Diphenylhydantoin)
(Diphenylhydramine)
Ethchlorvynol
Ethinamate
Ethosuximide
Galamine
Glutethimide
(Heroin)
Meprobamate
(Methaqualone)
Methsuximide
Methyprylon
Paraldehyde
Primidone
Valproic acid

Antidepressants
(Amitriptyline)
Amphetamines
(Imipramine)
Isocarboxazid
Monoamine oxidase inhibitors
(Pargyline)
(Phenelzine)
Tranylcypromine
(Tricyclics)

Alcohols
Ethanol
Ethylene glycol
Isopropanol
Methanol

Analgesics, antirheumatic agents
Acetaminophen
Acetophenetidin
Acetylsalicylic acid
Colchicine
Methylsalicylate
(D-propoxyphene)
Salicylic acid

Antimicrobial agents/anticancer agents
Amikacin
Dibekacin
Fosfomycin
Gentamicin
Kanamycin
Neomycin
Netilmicin
Sisomicin
Streptomycin
Tobramycin
(Vancomycin)
Bacitracin
Colistin
Ampicillin
Amoxicillin
Azlocillin
Carbenicillin
Clavulanic acid
(Cloxacillin)
(Floxacillin)
Mecillinam
Mezlocillin
(Nafcillin)
Penicillin
Piperacillin
Temocillin
Ticarcillin
(Cefaclor)
Cefadroxil
Cefamandole
Cefazolin
Cefixime
Cefmenoxime
(Cefonicid)
(Cefoperazone)
Ceforanide
(Cefotaxime)
(Cefotetan)
Cefotiam
Cefoxitin
Cefroxadine
Cefsulodin
Ceftazidime
(Ceftriaxone)
Cefuroxime
Cephacetrile
Cephalexin
Cephaloridine
Cephalothin
(Cephapirin)
Cephradine
Aztreonam
Cilastin

Antimicrobial agents/anticancer agents (contd.)
Imipenem
Moxalactam
(Chloramphenicol)
Ciprofloxacin
(Clindamycin)
(Erythromycin)
Metronidazole
Nitrofurantoin
Ornidazole
Sulfonamides
Tetracycline
Tinidazole
Acyclovir
Amantadine
Cycloserine
Ethambutol
5-Fluorocytosine
Isoniazid
(Chloroquine)
Quinine
(Azathioprine)
Bredinin
Cyclophosphamide
5-Fluorouracil
(Methotrexate)

Cardiovascular agents
Acebutolol
N-acetylprocainamide
Atenolol
Bretylium
Captopril
(Diazoxide)
(Digoxin)
(Lidocaine)
Metoprolol
Methyldopa
(Ouabain)
Nadolol
Practolol
Procainamide
Propranolol
(Quinidine)
Sotalol
Tocainide

Metals, inorganics
(Aluminum)*
Arsenic
(Copper)*
(Iron)*
Lead
Lithium
(Magnesium)
(Mercury)*

Metals, inorganics (contd.)
Potassium
Phosphate
Sodium
Strontium
(Tin)
(Zinc)
Bromide
Chloride
Iodide
Fluoride

Miscellaneous drugs
Acipimox
Aminophylline
Aniline
Borates
Boric acid
(Chlorpropamide)
Chromic acid
Cimetidine
Dinitro-*o*-cresol
Folic acid
Mannitol
Methylprednisolone
Potassium dichromate
Sodium citrate
Theophylline
Thiocyanate
Ranitidine

Solvents, gases
Acetone
Camphor
Carbon monoxide
(Carbon tetrachloride)
(Eucalyptus oil)
Thiols
Toluene
Trichloroethylene

Plants, animals, herbicides, insecticides
Alkyl phosphate
Amanitin
Demeton sulfoxide
Dimethoate
Diquat
Methylmercury complex
(Organophosphates)
Paraquat
Snake bite
Sodium chlorate
Potassium chlorate

( ), Not well removed; ( )*, removed with chelating agent.
From Winchester JF. Poisoning: Is the role of nephrologist diminishing? *Am J Kidney Dis* 1989;13:171–183, with permission.

TABLE 6. Drugs and chemicals removed with hemoperfusion

Barbiturates
Amobarbital
Butabarbital
Hexabarbital
Pentobarbital
Phenobarbital
Quinalbital
Secobarbital
Thiopental
Vinbarbital
Nonbarbiturate hypnotics, sedatives, tranquilizers
Carbromal
Chloral hydrate
Chlorpromazine
(Diazepam)
Diphenhydramine
Ethchlorvynol
Glutethimide
Meprobamate
Methaqualone
Methsuximide
Nonbarbiturate hypnotics, sedatives, tranquilizers (contd.)
Methyprylon
Promazine
Promethazine
Analgesics, antirheumatic agents
Acetaminophen
Acetylsalicylic acid
Colchicine
Methylsalicylate
Phenylbutazone
D-propoxyphene
Salicylic acid
Antimicrobial agents/anticancer agents
(Adriamycin)
Ampicillin
Carmustine
Chloramphenicol
Chloroquine
Clindamycin
Dapsone
Doxorubicin
Antimicrobial agents/anticancer agents (contd.)
Gentamicin
Isoniazid
(Methotrexate)
Thiabendazole
Antidepressants
(Amitryptiline)
(Imipramine)
(Tricyclics)
Plants, animals, herbicides, insecticides
Amanitin
Chlordane
Demeton sulfoxide
Dimethoate
Diquat
Methylparathion
Nitrostigmine
Organophosphates
Paraquat
Parathion
Phalloidin
Polychlorinated biphenyls
Cardiovascular agents
N-acetylprocainamide
Digoxin
(Disopyramide)
Procainamide
Quinidine
Metals, inorganics
(Aluminum)*
(Iron)*
Miscellaneous drugs
Aminophylline
Cimetidine
(Fluoroacetamide)
(Phencyclidine)
Phenols
(Podophyllin)
Theophylline
Solvents, gases
Carbon
Tetrachloride
Ethylene oxide
Trichloroethanol

( ), Not well removed; ( )*, removed with chelating agent.
From Winchester JF. Poisoning: Is the role of nephrologist diminishing? *Am J Kidney Dis* 1989;13:171–183, with permission.

TABLE 7. Complications of hemodialysis, hemoperfusion, and hemofiltration

Hypotension
Blood loss
Hematomas
Air embolism
Metabolic disequilibria
Complications specific to hemoperfusion
Thrombocytopenia
Leukopenia
Hypocalcemia
Complications specific to hemodialysis
Hematologic/coagulopathic/thrombotic (90–92)
- Slow flow from clot in line (90)
- Bleeding (90,91), blood loss (12)
- Intracholecystic hemorrhage (93)
- Excessive anticoagulation (heparin) (90), hematomas (12)
- Hemolysis (94,95)
  - With pancreatitis (94,96)
  - From kinked lines (95)
- Anemia (97)
- Leukopenia (98,99)

Acid-base
- Acidosis (100,101)
- Mechanically ventilated patients (101)
- Alkalosis (102)
- Hypoxemia (103,104)

Fluid and electrolyte
- Hypernatremia (105) (from hypertonic dialysate)
- Acute pancreatitis (96) (from hypotonic/hypoosmolality of dialysate); hemolysis (106); hypo- (42) and hypermagnesemia (107); and hypocalcemia (108)

Neurologic/encephalopathic
- Dysequilibrium syndrome (12,100,109)
- Peripheral neuropathy (110)
- Autonomic neuropathy (111)
- Neuritis (112)
- Putaminal hemorrhage
  - With methanol overdoses (113)
- Seizures
  - 12/180 (6.7%) of pediatric cases (114)
- Cerebral edema (associated with leptospiral infection) (115)

Hemodynamic
- Hypotension (12,94,111)
- High efficiency 23/67 (35%) vs. normal dialysis 70/279 (24%) (110)
- Pulmonary edema (105)
- Angina (116)
- Splenic rupture (117)
- Nausea, vomiting (110,116), headache (110,116), leg cramps (110,116, 118) (reported occurring in as high as 96% of chronic dialysis patients)

Complications of vascular access
- Vessel tear (90,119–121)
- Retroperitoneal hemorrhage (120)
- Pneumothorax (121,122)
- Hemothorax (121,123)
- Chylothorax (124)
- Air embolism (12)
- Arterial puncture/cannulation (122,125), pseudoaneurysms (125,126)
- Atrioventricular fistulas (125,126)
- Subclavian stenosis (127)
- Catheter kinking (128)
- Bacteremia (128)
- Subclavian thrombosis (122)
- Vena caval thrombosis (121)

Infections
- Pyrogenic reactions (129)
- Increased prevalence of hepatitis B, C (129)
- Seroconversion, hepatitis C (130–132,139), hepatitis D (133)
- Catheter-related infections (122,134)
- Leptospiral (115)

Allergic
- Hypersensitivity reactions (135)
  - From ethylene oxide (136)
  - With reprocessed hemodialyzers (137)
- Pruritus (117)
- Bronchospasm (117)

Adverse reactions secondary to removal of required medications
- Nitroglycerin, isosorbide dinitrate (138)
- Seizure medications
- Ethanol/fomepizole
- Antiarrhythmics
- Others

TABLE 8. Complications of acute peritoneal dialysis

Pain
Hemorrhage from vascular laceration
Leakage
Inadequate drainage
Perforation of viscus
Superficial subcutaneous infection at catheter insertion site
Bacterial peritonitis
Dysrhythmias
Volume depletion
Volume overload
Pneumonia
Pleural effusion
Hyperglycemia and electrolyte disorders

From Health and Policy Committee, American College of Physicians. Clinical competence in acute hemodialysis. *Ann Intern Med* 1988;108:632–634, with permission.

patients with bleeding disorders or venous access problems or in centers without access to HD. It does not require anticoagulation and uses minimal equipment (21).

Possible Applications

PD is rarely used for poisoning. It is not an acceptable substitute for HD. The mechanism of PD is diffusion of toxins from mesenteric blood vessels across the peritoneal membrane into the dialysate in the peritoneal cavity. The blood-flow rate depends on the mesenteric circulation and cannot be adjusted. The clearance of toxins is consistently much higher with HD than PD. The addition of albumin, lipids, or furosemide to the peritoneal dialysate enhances clearance, but not to the levels achieved with HD. Therefore, the role of PD is limited to the rare patient who is a candidate for HD but for whom the treatment is unavailable or contraindicated (22) and who already has a PD catheter in place.

Complications

Multiple complications have been reported with PD (Table 8) (17).

HEMOFILTRATION

Procedure

During continuous arteriovenous hemofiltration (CAVH), an arteriovenous pressure difference induces a convective transport of solutes through a hollow fiber or flat sheet membrane (Fig. 1). Alternatively, continuous venovenous hemofiltration (CVVH) provides convective mass transport. These techniques permit a substantial flow of plasma water and high permeability to compounds with a molecular weight less than 40,000. Hemofiltration (HF) is similar to HD except that the blood is pumped through a hemofilter. It can be performed intermittently at high ultrafiltrate rates of up to 6 L/hour or continuously at ultrafiltrate flow rates of approximately 100 ml/hour. In the treatment of poisoning, CAVH and CVVH have the advantage of being able to be performed for a long period and reduce the incidence of rebound phenomena.

Possible Applications

The advantage of HF over HD and HP is its ability to remove compounds with a large (<4500 to 40,000) relative molecular weight. Such compounds include the aminoglycoside antibiotics and metal chelate complexes such as aluminum- or iron-

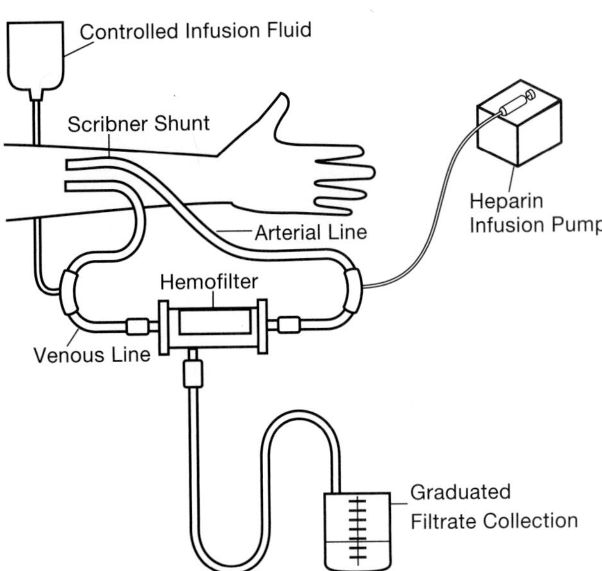

Figure 1. Schematic representation of the continuous arteriovenous hemofiltration system. (From Horton MW, Godley PJ. Continuous arteriovenous hemofiltration: an alternative to hemodialysis. *Am J Hosp Pharm* 1988;45:1361–1368, with permission of the Amicon Division, W.R. Grace & Co., Danvers, MA.)

deferoxamine. CAVH or CVVH may also be useful for eliminating smaller agents like lithium, methanol, metformin, ethanol, ethylene glycol, vancomycin, aminoglycosides, and *N*-acetylprocainamide, but HD is usually more readily available and preferred. CAVH has enhanced the clearance of ethylene glycol when HD was not available (23). Animal studies suggest that CAVH may be a useful technique to remove iron in severe intoxication, particularly in the presence of renal failure (24). CVVH failed to prevent death in a paraquat poisoning (25).

Complications

Complications of HF include clotting of the filter and mild bleeding. Horton et al. have compared CAVH with HD (Table 9) (26).

TABLE 9. Relative advantages and disadvantages of continuous arteriovenous hemofiltration (CAVH) compared with hemodialysis

Advantages
- CAVH maintains consistent homeostasis through slow, gradual shifts in volume status and serum osmolality.
- CAVH avoids hypotensive or dysequilibrium episodes.
- CAVH permits continuous control of fluid balance and reduces the need to restrict fluid administration.
- CAVH requires a lower volume of blood to be circulating outside the body.
- CAVH has no effect on complement or leukocytes.
- CAVH does not require expensive equipment or extensive training of personnel.
- CAVH has greater clearances of mid-molecular-weight solutes.

Disadvantages
- CAVH and hemodialysis require some degree of anticoagulation.
- CAVH and hemodialysis have vascular access complications.
- Staff may be unfamiliar with CAVH.
- CAVH has lower clearance of low-molecular-weight solutes.
- CAVH is not able to maintain nitrogen balance in catabolic patients.

From Horton MW, Godley PJ. Continuous arteriovenous hemofiltration: an alternative to hemodialysis. *Am J Hosp Pharm* 1988;45:1361–1368, with permission.

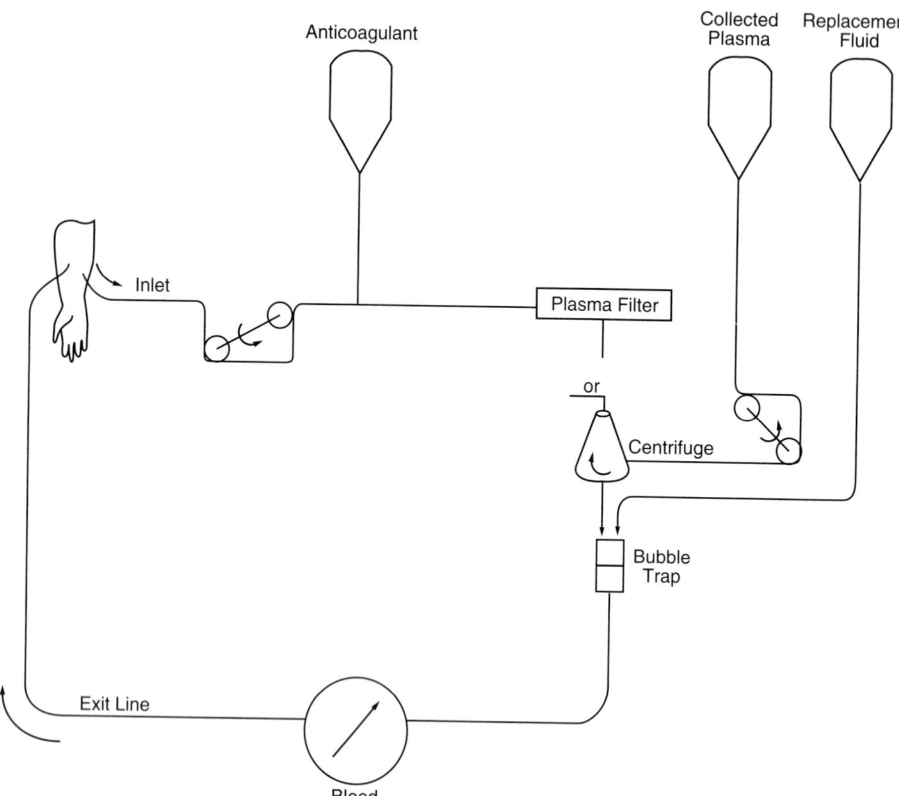

Figure 2. Schematic of plasmapheresis circuit for membrane-based (filter) and centrifugal methods. (From Jones JS, Dougherty J. Current status of plasmapheresis in toxicology. *Ann Emerg Med* 1986;15:474–482, with permission.)

PLASMAPHERESIS/PLASMA EXCHANGE

Procedure

Plasmapheresis separates cellular blood components from plasma. The cells are resuspended in either colloid, albumin, or fresh frozen plasma. The plasma is disposed, removing solutes and drugs. A single plasmapheresis exchange removes a fraction of the plasma, therefore, its efficacy depends on the number of plasma exchanges and the portion of drug in circulation. It eliminates toxic substances but sacrifices part of the patient's plasma proteins (Fig. 2).

Possible Applications

Plasmapheresis is useful in the treatment of heparin-induced thrombocytopenia if started within 4 days of onset (27). When combined with therapies to interrupt absorption, plasmapheresis may be useful in treating amanitin ingestion if started early (28,29). Complexes of mercuric chloride and British antilewisite may have enhanced removal by plasmapheresis in renal failure (30). Plasmapheresis may be an adjunctive therapy in enhancing removal of amiodarone, barbiturates, digoxin antibody complexes, verapamil, CBZ, phenytoin, quinidine, theophylline, trimethoprim-sulfamethoxazole, vancomycin, vincristine, cisplatin, and basiliximab, although other modalities may be more efficacious or more easily performed (29,31–35). Individual case reports on the use of plasmapheresis in overdoses of paxillum, iatrogenic antithymocyte globulin, dapsone, hemlock, orellanine/oreline, oxcarbazepine, phenytoin, propoxyphene, thyroxine, and drug-induced thyrotoxicosis do not suggest a practical role for plasmapheresis with these agents (36–38).

Complications

Complications of plasmapheresis limit its usefulness (Table 10). In addition, plasmapheresis also removes therapeutic drugs, which may then need additional doses.

TABLE 10. Complications of plasmapheresis

Bleeding disorders	Infection
Disseminated intravascular coagulation	Pathogenic
Elevated bleeding times	Opportunistic
Thrombocytopenia	Anaphylaxis
Citrate toxicity	Shock
Paresthesias	Urticaria
Muscle tetany	Angioedema
Nausea	Vascular access
Chills	Vessel perforation
Syncope	Pneumothorax
Cardiac arrhythmias	Air embolism
Dysequilibrium syndrome	Bacteremia
Nausea	Miscellaneous
Vomiting	Seizures
Hypovolemia	Metabolic alkalosis
Fluid overload	Cerebral spasm
Hypertension	Adult respiratory distress syndrome
Congestive heart failure	Cardiac arrhythmias (not associated with calcium)
Hypercoagulation	
Cerebral thrombosis	
Pulmonary embolus	
Myocardial infarction	

From Jones JS, Dougherty J. Current status of plasmapheresis in toxicology. *Ann Emerg Med* 1986;15:479–482, with permission.

HEMODIAFILTRATION

Hemodiafiltration combines continuous HF with HD. It is rarely used for detoxification. Continuous venovenous hemodiafiltration increased clearance of methotrexate. Other methods, such as HD and HP, often show a rebound effect with methotrexate secondary to release from storage tissues, whereas a continuous method, such as continuous venovenous hemodiafiltration, does not (39).

PLASMA PERFUSION

Plasma perfusion is a combination of plasmapheresis and HP that has been used in methylparathion poisoning (40,41). Continuous venovenous hemodiafiltration has been successfully used in a neonate with renal insufficiency and a vancomycin overdose (42).

EXTRACORPOREAL MEMBRANE OXYGENATION AND CARDIOPULMONARY BYPASS

Procedures

Extracorporeal membrane oxygenation (ECMO), cardiopulmonary bypass (CPB), and the intraaortic balloon pump are methods of maintaining oxygenation and circulation when supportive measures have failed. They allow endogenous elimination of a drug from the body by supporting oxygenation and circulation while the substances are cleared by the lungs, kidneys, or liver, and while circulation is mechanically supported.

Possible Applications

A fall in the total serum drug concentration or clinical improvement during or after ECMO or CPB has been reported with aconite, barbiturates, benzodiazepines, cephalosporins, digoxin, diltiazem, etomidate, isoflurane, fentanyl, flecainide, lidocaine, nitroglycerin, propranolol, and quinidine (Table 11) (43–47).

TABLE 11. Drugs for which mechanical support may be useful

Extracorporeal membrane oxygenation/cardiopulmonary bypass
- Aconite
- Barbiturates
- Benzodiazepines
- Calcium-channel blockers
- Cephalosporins
- Digoxin
- Diltiazem
- Etomidate
- Flecainide
- Isoflurane
- Fentanyl
- Flecainide
- Lidocaine
- Nitroglycerin
- Propranolol
- Quinidine

Intraaortic balloon pump
- Verapamil
- Atenolol
- Pyrilamine
- Propranolol
- Toxic mushrooms
- Anaphylaxis secondary to medications or venoms

Severe diltiazem poisoning may be refractory to CPB (T. G. Martin et al., *personal communication*, April 1994) (48). The reported improvement is most plausible for a substance like lidocaine that has a high endogenous clearance rate.

Complications

Each of these procedures is little used in the treatment of poisoning, mostly because of the technical difficulties involved, the need to use a highly invasive intervention before irreversible end-organ damage occurs, and significant morbidity from systemic heparinization and central nervous system vascular compromise (49,50).

SELECTION OF EXTRACORPOREAL TECHNIQUES

None of the extracorporeal techniques (HD, HP, HF, plasmapheresis) have been subjected to controlled clinical trials in poisoned patients. Their clinical benefit and optimal application remain to be established.

Comparison of Hemoperfusion and Hemodialysis

There is little benefit to HP over HD. Clearance of some drugs may be higher with HP, but this is probably not clinically significant. It is likely that HP offers the best opportunity for rapid removal for highly protein-bound poisons (51,52). For dialyzable poisons with a small V_d (e.g., aspirin, theophylline), acute HD appears to be the most reasonable approach. Factors such as more widespread availability as well as the ability to correct acid-base, fluid, or electrolyte imbalance increase the use of HD. In addition, HD appears to have a lower rate of procedural complications (53). Complications of HD, HP, and HF are summarized in Table 7 (12). HD is occasionally combined with HP, either simultaneously (19) or in series (54). For most solutes adsorbed by AC, the order HD-HP gives higher rates of removal. When the characteristics of the agent are of an unfavorable adsorbing solute, the order HP-HD gives higher rates of removal (54).

Hemofiltration, Plasmapheresis, and Other Techniques

If a compound is amenable to removal by HD, its clearance will be greater than that achieved by HF (26,52). Clinical studies suggest that CAVH and CVVH cannot substitute for HD or HP. Both HP and acute HD, however, are short-lived procedures, and the possibility of posttherapy rebound in blood concentration secondary to redistribution of tissue stores exists. If a toxin has a large V_d and is filterable or dialyzable, CAVH, CVVH (either as primary treatments or after HD or HP), or continuous HD may be useful in preventing this rebound phenomenon (52). HF and plasmapheresis generally have higher complication rates compared to HD or HP. Mechanical measures (ECMO, CPB, and intraaortic balloon pump) are reserved for support when oxygenation and circulation cannot be supported by other means.

SPECIFIC AGENTS

Most information regarding extracorporeal elimination relies on case reports and small case series. Because of normal redistribution and endogenous clearance of the toxicant as well as the typical range of interpatient variability, the application of an enhanced elimination technique in a drug toxicity may be followed by a reduction in blood concentrations and/or clinical improvement regardless of efficacy. Caution should be used in attributing a causal relationship between these events.

Acebutolol

ECMO was used to stabilize a patient's clinical condition before commencing HD (55).

Aconite

Two cases of aconitine intoxication with ventricular arrhythmias were treated with charcoal HP with return to normal sinus rhythm soon during and after the procedure (56).

Aluminum

Repetitive chelation with deferoxamine followed by HD over 34 days in a patient with aluminum toxicity and renal insufficiency decreased serum aluminum from 228 µg/L to 17 µg/L with improvement in neurologic function (57).

Amanitin

A review of 14 published investigations concluded that plasmapheresis, combined with interruption of absorption, substantially reduced mortality (28). It is not clear which of these interventions was beneficial. In two adults who received HD and HP (23 hours after ingestion), no enhanced elimination of amanitin was found; however, no amanitin was detectable in the blood preprocedure, leaving open the question of whether plasmapheresis might be effective if the procedure is performed earlier in the course of illness (58). An *in vitro* study showed HP with Amberlite XAD-2 to be more effective than either AC or Amberlite XAD-4 (59).

Baclofen

Nine patients with renal failure and baclofen toxicity who received early HD had shorter recovery times (2.71 days ± 0.42 vs. 9.0 days) (60).

Barium

Three case reports describe correction of serum potassium and increased barium elimination associated with HD (half-life reduced from 18.0 hours to 1.9 hours during dialysis) (61).

Carbamazepine

CBZ is removed by HD or HP (62,63). Charcoal HP reduced CBZ and its 10,11-epoxide metabolite from 54 µg/ml to 23 µg/ml and from 30 µg/ml to 17 µg/ml, respectively, in a 16-month-old with an acute overdose, seizures, coma, and shock (64). MDAC (1 g/kg every 4 hours for 24 hours) shortened the half-life of elimination (9.5 hours vs. 18.0 to 54.0 hours) and increased total body clearance (103.13 ml/minute/kg vs. 75.01 ml/minute/kg) without adverse effects in a series of eight overdose patients (65). Plasmapheresis in a patient with an initial level of 190 µmol/L resulted in a level of 101 µmol/L immediately after the procedure with clinical improvement and without rebound (32).

Chloroquine

The recovery of chloroquine after a severe overdose (10 g) by charcoal HP was only 5.3% of the ingested dose (66).

Cisplatin

A massive cisplatin overdose responded to nine plasma exchanges over 14 days with plasma cisplatin concentrations decreasing from 2470 ng/ml to 216 ng/ml (31).

Diethylene Glycol

Fomepizole and HD in an asymptomatic 17-month-old girl were followed by complete clearance of diethylene glycol (serum level of 1.7 mg/dl) by 12 hours of HD (67).

Diltiazem

Charcoal HP had no apparent effect on the elimination of diltiazem or its desacetyl-metabolite (68).

Doxepin

A patient with a massive doxepin overdose and severe metabolic acidosis was treated with HD and resin HP. The plasma doxepin concentration decreased from 5150 µg/L to 1150 µg/L after HD/HP. This may have represented redistribution of the drug. There was also clinical and electrocardiographic improvement. Despite its large V_d (22 L/kg) and high degree of protein binding (75%), the kinetics/dynamics of massive doxepin overdose may result in prolonged plasma availability and saturation of protein binding sites, allowing clinically significant removal of normally nonperfusable/nondialyzable drugs (69).

Ethylene Glycol

CAVH was used in a patient with multiple organ dysfunction (pH, 6.74) resistant to bicarbonate administration when HD could not be performed. Acidosis corrected within 24 hours, and the ethanol infusion was discontinued after 2 days (23).

Flecainide

CPB was used in a patient who ingested 4 g of flecainide with circulatory failure unresponsive to pacing, inotropes, and sodium bicarbonate. Resolution of cardiac dysfunction occurred over 24 hours, and CPB was stopped at 30 hours. The patient made a full recovery (70). A patient with plasma concentrations 20 times the therapeutic range was successfully resuscitated with 26 hours of ECMO (71).

Ifosfamide

HP combined with HD increased clearance by at least 9% and may have prevented or reversed neuro- and nephrotoxicity (19).

Lithium

A single dose of SPS after a single dose of lithium in a murine model lowered the serum lithium concentration in a dose-related manner, even when given after peak serum levels had been reached (72). Repeated oral doses of SPS effectively lowered plasma lithium concentrations after the administration of lithium to mice in their drinking water (2). High-volume CVVH was successfully used in two cases of acute-on-chronic lithium intoxication, resulting in slow sustained removal of lithium without hemodynamic instability or rebound elevation in lithium concentration (73,74).

Mercury Salts

Standard HD had little to no effect on increasing the clearance of mercury-dimercaptopropane sulfonate complexes. CVVH using a high-flux polysulphone membrane recovered significant amounts of mercury, presumably as mercury-dimercaptopropane sulfonate complexes. Plasma exchanges after CVVH also removed significant amounts of mercury (75).

Methanol

Formate levels are not readily available. Because formate is cleared more rapidly by dialysis than methanol, determination of an endpoint for HD can be accomplished by determining the serum methanol level within 1 hour before dialysis and a second during dialysis (with the interval at least one estimated half-life) and plotting to the desired methanol level with the resulting measured intradialysis half-life (76).

Neuroleptic Malignant Syndrome

Plasmapheresis was used in a patient with neuroleptic malignant syndrome unresponsive to other measures over 6 days. The patient awakened and had stable vital signs after three courses of plasmapheresis but subsequently died from GI bleeding and multiorgan failure. Because most neuroleptics are highly protein bound (92% to 97%) and may have prolonged elimination half-lives, plasmapheresis may contribute to clinical improvement by removal of protein-bound neuroleptics (77). A criticism of this case was that the patient had not received adequate cooling before plasmapheresis, that some or all of the beneficial effect of plasmapheresis may have been due to the use of cooler fluids for volume replacement, and that the subsequently fatal events may have been a complication of this treatment (78).

Pentamidine Isethionate

Charcoal HP was performed for 4 hours after an accidental intravenous overdose (40-fold) of pentamidine. Postfilter blood samples had 141 ng/ml lower concentrations of pentamidine than prefilter samples on average. It was unclear how much the HP contributed to the overall clearance, however. Retrospective analysis indicated that it would have taken several days to achieve complete clearance of the drug by HP (79).

Phenobarbital

A direct comparison between MDAC (six doses AC and two doses sorbitol over 24 hours) and urinary alkalinization demonstrated a clear superiority of MDAC with half-lives of 148 hours, 47 hours, and 19 hours for control, alkalinization, and MDAC, respectively (80). However, a clinical trial failed to document a clinical benefit of MDAC treatment (81). Exchange transfusion (400 ml volume of exchange) reduced the plasma phenobarbital concentration from 112.4 µg/ml to 50.84 µg/ml in a neonate (82).

Phenytoin

Charcoal HP reduced the total and free phenytoin concentrations in a patient with an initial level of 40 µg/ml. Because phenytoin has a low binding constant to serum albumin, the increased clearance was attributed to dissociation of protein-bound phenytoin inside the charcoal column (83).

Quinidine

Eleven days of ECMO allowed cardiovascular stabilization in a 16-month-old with refractory bradydysrhythmias and hypotension after an acute overdose (84).

Valproic Acid

Valproic acid is 90% to 95% protein bound at therapeutic concentrations; however, this process is saturable, and the percentage of free drug may increase in overdose to 75%, making it amenable to HD (85). Charcoal HP reduced plasma valproic acid from 471 to 45 µg/ml, with patient awakening. The half-life was 4.4 hours before HP and 1.8 hours during HP (86).

Vancomycin

High-efficiency dialysis in two patients (plasma concentrations 238 µg/ml and 182 µg/ml) removed 60% of the plasma vancomycin with a half-life of 2 hours, compared with a 40% removal and a half-life of 12.5 hours in a patient treated with charcoal HF (plasma concentration 137 µg/ml) (87). Charcoal HP combined with HD accelerated removal in a 14-month-old after a massive overdose complicated by renal failure and ototoxicity (88). A 17-day-old female with a concentration of 165 µg/ml was treated with MDAC (1 g/kg beginning at 5 hours and every 4 hours for 12 doses). The half-life of vancomycin was 9.4 hours compared with the reported half-life in neonates of 13.4 to 33.7 hours (89).

REFERENCES

1. American Academy of Clinical Toxicology, European Association of Poisons Centres and Clinical Toxicologists. Position statement and practice guidelines on the use of multi-dose activated charcoal in the treatment of acute poisoning. *J Toxicol Clin Toxicol* 1999;37(6):731–751.
2. Linakis JG, Savitt DL, Wu TY, et al. Use of sodium polystyrene sulfonate for reduction of plasma lithium concentrations after chronic lithium dosing in mice. *J Toxicol Clin Toxicol* 1998;36(4):309–313.
3. Scharman EJ. Methods used to decrease lithium absorption or enhance elimination. *J Toxicol Clin Toxicol* 1997;35(6):601–608.
4. Malbrain MLNG, Lambrecht GLV, Zandijk E, et al. Treatment of severe thallium intoxication. *J Toxicol Clin Toxicol* 1997;35(1):97–100.
5. Stevens W, van Peteghem C, Heyndreckx A, et al. Eleven cases of thallium intoxication treated with Prussian blue. *Int J Clin Pharmacol* 1974;10:1–22.
6. Thompson DE, Church CO. Prussian blue for treatment of radiocesium poisoning. *Pharmacother* 2001;21(11):1364–1367.
7. Pau PW. Management of thallium poisoning. *Hong Kong Med J* 2000;6(3):316–318.
8. Van Der Merwe CF. The treatment of thallium poisoning: a report of 2 cases. *S Afr Med J* 1972;46:960–961.
9. Wainwright AP, Kox WJ, House IM, et al. Clinical features of therapy of acute thallium poisoning. *Q J Med* 1988;69:939–944.
10. Garrettson LK, Geller RJ. Acid and alkaline diuresis: when are they of value in the treatment of poisoning? *Drug Saf* 1990;5:220–232.
11. Bismuth C, Muczinski J. *Are extracorporeal techniques of elimination validated in acute poisoning?* Istanbul: Proceedings, European Association of Poison Centres and Clinical Toxicologists; May 1992:69.
12. Pond SM. Extracorporeal techniques in the treatment of poisoned patients [see comments] [Review] [63 refs]. *Med J Aust* 1991;154(9):617–622.
13. Cutler RE, Forland SC, Hammond St JPG, et al. Extracorporeal removal of drugs and poisons by hemodialysis and hemoperfusion. *Annu Rev Pharmacol Toxicol* 1987;27:169–191.
14. Winchester JF. Poisoning: is the role of nephrologist diminishing? *Am J Kid Dis* 1989;13:171–183.
15. Health and Public Policy Committee, American College of Physicians. Clinical competence in continuous arteriovenous hemofiltration. *Ann Intern Med* 1988;108:902–907.
16. Health and Public Policy Committee, American College of Physicians. Clinical competence in acute hemodialysis. *Ann Intern Med* 1988;108:632–634.
17. Health and Public Policy Committee, American College of Physicians. Clinical competence in acute peritoneal dialysis. *Ann Intern Med* 1988;108:763–765.
18. Gwilt PR, Perrier D. Plasma protein binding and distribution characteristics of drugs as indices of their hemodialyzability. *Clin Pharmacol Ther* 1978;24:154–161.

19. Fiedler R, Baumann F, Deschler B, et al. Haemoperfusion combined with haemodialysis in ifosfamide intoxication. *Nephrol Dial Transplant* 2001;16(5):1088–1089.
20. Rommes JH. Haemoperfusion, indications and side effects. *Arch Toxicol* 1992;15[Suppl]:40–49.
21. Shannon M. Extracorporeal drug removal. II. Other methods. *Clin Toxicol Rev* 1990;12(9):1–2.
22. Blye E, Lorch J, Cortrell S. Extracorporeal therapy in the treatment of intoxication. *Am J Kid Dis* 1984;3:321–338.
23. Christiansson LK, Kaspersson KE, Kulling PE, et al. Treatment of severe ethylene glycol intoxication with continuous arteriovenous hemofiltration dialysis. *J Toxicol Clin Toxicol* 1995;33(3):267–270.
24. Banner W, Vernon DD, Ward R, et al. Continuous arteriovenous hemofiltration (CAVH) in experimental iron intoxication. *Vet Hum Toxicol* 1988;30:355.
25. Koo JR, Kim JC, Yoon JW, et al. Failure of continuous venovenous hemofiltration to prevent death in paraquat poisoning. *Am J Kidney Dis* 2002;39(1):55–59.
26. Horton MW, Godley PJ. Continuous arteriovenous hemofiltration: an alternative to hemodialysis. *Am J Hosp Pharm* 1988;45:1361–1368.
27. Robinson JA, Lewis BE. Plasmapheresis in the management of heparin-induced thrombocytopenia. *Semin Hematol* 1999;36[1 Suppl 1]:29–32.
28. Jander S, Bischoff J, Woodcock BG. Plasmapheresis in the treatment of Amanita phalloides poisoning: II. A review and recommendations. *Ther Apher* 2000;4(4):308–312.
29. Kale-Pradhan PB, Woo MH. A review of the effects of plasmapheresis on drug clearance. *Pharmacotherapy* 1997;17(4):684–695.
30. Yoshida M, Satoh H, Igarashi M, et al. Acute mercury poisoning by intentional ingestion of mercuric chloride. *Tohoku J Exp Med* 1997;182(4):347–352.
31. Choi JH, Oh JC, Kim KH, et al. Successful treatment of cisplatin overdose with plasma exchange. *Yonsei Med J (Korea)* 2002;43(1):128–132.
32. Duzova A, Baskin E, Usta Y, et al. Carbamazepine poisoning: treatment with plasma exchange. *Hum Exp Toxicol* 2001;20(4):175–177.
33. Kuhlmann U, Schoenemann H, Muller T, et al. Plasmapheresis in life-threatening verapamil intoxication. *Artif Cells Blood Substit Immobil Biotechnol* 2000;28(5):429–440.
34. Okechukwu CN, Meier-Kriesche HU, Armstrong D, et al. Removal of basiliximab by plasmapheresis. *Am J Kidney Dis* 2001;37(1):E11.
35. Osman BA, Lew SQ. Vancomycin removal by plasmapheresis. *Pharmacol Toxicol* 1997;81(5):245–246.
36. Brophy DF, Mueller BA. Vancomycin removal by plasmapheresis. *Ann Pharmacother* 1996;30(9):1038.
37. Christensen J, Balslev T, Villadsen J, et al. Removal of 10-hydroxycarbazepine by plasmapheresis. *Ther Drug Monit* 2001;23(4):374–379.
38. McClellan SD, Whitaker CH, Friedberg RC. Removal of vancomycin during plasmapheresis. *Ann Pharmacother* 1997;31(10):1132–1136.
39. Jambou P, Levraut J, Favier C, et al. Removal of methotrexate by continuous venovenous hemodiafiltration. *Contrib Nephrol* 1995;116:48–52.
40. Berning T, Krummner T, Glaser T, et al. Plasma perfusion in life-threatening exogenous poisoning. *Schweiz Med Wochenschr* 1987;117:1368–1370.
41. Cnzhnikov EA, Yasoslavsky AA, Molondenkov MV, et al. Plasma perfusion through charcoal in methylparathion poisoning. *Lancet* 1977;1:38–39.
42. Goebel J, Ananth M, Lewy JE. Hemodiafiltration for vancomycin overdose in a neonate with end-stage renal failure. *Pediatr Nephrol* 1999;13(5):423–425.
43. Buylaert WA, Herregots LL, Montier EP, et al. Cardiopulmonary bypass and the pharmacokinetics of drugs: an update. *Clin Pharmacokinet* 1989;17:10–26.
44. Freedman MD, Gal J, Freed CR. Extracorporeal pump assistance: novel treatment of acute lidocaine poisoning. *Eur J Clin Pharmacol* 1982;22:129–135.
45. Holzer M, Sterz F, Schoerkhuber W, et al. Successful resuscitation of a verapamil-intoxicated patient with percutaneous cardiopulmonary bypass. *Crit Care Med* 1999;27(12):2818–2823.
46. Kennedy JH, Barnette J, Flasterstein A, et al. Experimental barbiturate intoxication: treatment by partial cardiopulmonary bypass and hemodialysis. *Cardiovasc Res Center Bull* 1976;14:61–69.
47. Yasui RK, Culclasure TF, Kaufman D, et al. Flecainide overdose: is cardiopulmonary support the treatment? *Ann Emerg Med* 1997;29(5):680–682.
48. Behringer W, Sterz F, Domanovits H, et al. Percutaneous cardiopulmonary bypass for therapy resistant cardiac arrest from digoxin overdose. *Resuscitation* 1998;37(1):47–50.
49. Hendren WG, Schieber RS, Garrettson LP. Extracorporeal bypass for the treatment of verapamil poisoning. *Ann Emerg Med* 1989;18:984–987.
50. Vernon DD, Gleich MC. Poisoning and drug overdose. *Crit Care Clin* 1997;13(3):647–667.
51. Bressolle F, Kinowski J-M, de la Coussaye JE, et al. Clinical pharmacokinetics during continuous haemofiltration. *Clin Pharmacokinet* 1994;26:457–471.
52. Golper TA, Bennett WM. Drug removal by continuous arteriovenous haemofiltration: a review of the evidence in poisoned patients. *Med Toxicol Adverse Drug Exp* 1988;3:341–349.
53. Shannon MW. Comparative efficacy of hemodialysis and hemoperfusion in severe theophylline intoxication. *Acad Emerg Med* 1998;4(7):674–678.
54. Lee CJ, Hsu HW, Chang YL. Performance characteristics of combined haemodialysis/haemoperfusion system for removal of blood toxins. *Med Eng Phys* 1997;19(7):658–667.
55. Rooney M, Massey KL, Jamali F, et al. Acebutolol overdose treated with hemodialysis and extracorporeal membrane oxygenation. *J Clin Pharmacol* 1996;36(8):760–763.
56. Lin CC, Chou HL, Lin JL. Acute aconitine poisoned patients with ventricular arrhythmias successfully reversed by charcoal hemoperfusion. *Am J Emerg Med* 2002;20(1):66–67.
57. Nakamura H, Rose PG, Blumer JL, et al. Acute encephalopathy due to aluminum toxicity successfully treated by combined intravenous deferoxamine and hemodialysis. *J Clin Pharmacol* 2000;40(3):296–300.
58. Mullins ME, Horowitz BZ. The futility of hemoperfusion and hemodialysis in Amanita phalloides poisoning. *Vet Hum Toxicol* 2000;42(2):90–91.
59. Mydlik M, Derzsiova K, Klan J, et al. Hemoperfusion with alpha-amanitin: an in vitro study. *Int J Artif Organs* 1997;20:105–107.
60. Chen KS, Bullard MJ, Chien YY, et al. Baclofen toxicity in patients with severely impaired renal function. *Ann Pharmacother* 1997;31(11):1315–1320.
61. Wells JA, Wood KE. Acute barium poisoning treated with hemodialysis. *Am J Emerg Med* 2001;19(2):175–177.
62. Schuerer DJ, Brophy PD, Maxvold NJ, et al. High-efficiency dialysis for carbamazepine overdose. *J Toxicol Clin Toxicol* 2000;38(3):321–323.
63. Tapolya M, Campbell M, Dailey M, et al. Hemodialysis is as effective as hemoperfusion for drug removal in carbamazepine poisoning. *Nephron* 2002;90(2):213–215.
64. Deshpande G, Meert KL, Valentini RP. Repeat charcoal hemoperfusion treatments in life threatening carbamazepine overdose. *Pediatr Nephrol* 1999;13(9):775–777.
65. Montoya-Cabrera MA, Sauceda-Garcia JM, Escalante-Galindo P, et al. Carbamazepine poisoning in adolescent suicide attempters. Effectiveness of multiple-dose activated charcoal in enhancing carbamazepine elimination. *Arch Med Res* 1996;27(4):485–489.
66. Boereboom FT, Ververs FF, Meulenbelt J, et al. Hemoperfusion is ineffectual in severe chloroquine poisoning. *Crit Care Med* 2000;28(9):3346–3350.
67. Brophy PD, Tenenbein M, Gardner J, et al. Childhood diethylene glycol poisoning treated with alcohol dehydrogenase inhibitor fomepizole and hemodialysis. *Am J Kidney Dis* 2000;35(5):958–962.
68. Luomanmaki K, Tiula E, Kivisto KT, et al. Pharmacokinetics of diltiazem in massive overdose. *Ther Drug Monit* 1997;19(2):240–242.
69. Frank RD, Kierdorf HP. Is there a role for hemoperfusion/hemodialysis as a treatment option in severe tricyclic antidepressant intoxication? *Int J Artif Organs* 2000;23(9):618–623.
70. Corkeron MA, van Heerden PV, Newman SM, et al. Extracorporeal circulatory support in near-fatal flecainide overdose. *Anaesth Intensive Care* 1999;27(4):405–408.
71. Auzinger GM, Scheinkestel CD. Successful extracorporeal life support in a case of severe flecainide intoxication. *Crit Care Med* 2001;29(4):887–890.
72. Linakis JG, Hull KM, Lee CM, et al. Effects of delayed treatment with sodium polystyrene sulfonate on serum lithium concentrations in mice. *Acad Emerg Med* 1995;2(8):681–685.
73. Menghini VV, Albright RC. Treatment of lithium intoxication with continuous venovenous hemodiafiltration. *Am J Kidney Dis* 2000;3(3):E21.
74. van Bommel EF, Kalmeijer MD, Ponssen HH. Treatment of life-threatening lithium toxicity with high-volume continuous venovenous hemofiltration. *Am J Nephrol* 2000;20(5):408–411.
75. Pai P, Thomas S, Hoenich N, et al. Treatment of a case of severe mercuric salt overdose with DMPS (dimercapo-1-propane sulphonate) and continuous haemofiltration. *Nephrol Dial Transplant* 2000;15(11):1889–1890.
76. Burns AB, Bailie GR, Eisele G, et al. Use of pharmacokinetics to determine the duration of dialysis in management of methanol poisoning. *Am J Emerg Med* 1998;16(5):538–540.
77. Gaitini L, Fradis M, Vaida S, et al. Plasmapheresis in neuroleptic malignant syndrome. *Anaesthesia* 1997;52(2)165–168.
78. Priestley GS. Plasmapheresis in neuroleptic malignant syndrome. *Anaesthesia* 1997;52(6):612–613.
79. Watts RG, Conte JE, Zurlinden E, et al. Effect of charcoal hemoperfusion on clearance of pentamidine isethionate after accidental overdose. *J Toxicol Clin Toxicol* 1997;35(1):89–92.
80. Frenia ML, Schauben JL, Wears RL, et al. Multiple-dose activated charcoal compared to urinary alkalinization for the enhancement of phenobarbital elimination. *J Toxicol Clin Toxicol* 1996;34(2):169–175.
81. Pond SM, Olson KR, Osterloh JD, et al. Randomized study of the treatment of phenobarbital overdose with repeated doses of activated charcoal. *JAMA* 1984;251:3104–3108.
82. Sancak R, Kucukoduk S, Tasdemir HA, et al. Exchange transfusion treatment in a newborn with phenobarbital intoxication. *Pediatr Emerg Care* 1999;15(4):268–270.
83. Kawasaki C, Nishi R, Uekihara S, et al. Charcoal hemoperfusion in the treatment of phenytoin overdose. *Am J Kidney Dis* 2000;35(2):323–326.
84. Tecklenburg FW, Thomas NJ, Webb SA, et al. Pediatric ECMO for severe quinidine cardiotoxicity. *Pediatr Emerg Care* 1997;13(2):111–113.
85. Franssen EJ, van Essen GG, Portman AT, et al. Valproic acid toxicokinetics: serial hemodialysis and hemoperfusion. *Ther Drug Monit* 1999;21(3):289–292.
86. Matsumoto J, Ogawa H, Maeyama R, et al. Successful treatment by direct hemoperfusion of coma possibly resulting from mitochondrial dysfunction in acute valproate intoxication. *Epilepsia* 1997;38(8):950–953.
87. Bunchman TE, Valentini RP, Gardner J, et al. Treatment of vancomycin overdose using high-efficiency dialysis membranes. *Pediatr Nephrol* 1999;13(9):773–774.
88. Panzarino VM, Feldstein TJ, Kashtan CE. Charcoal hemoperfusion in a child with vancomycin overdose and chronic renal failure. *Pediatr Nephrol* 1998;12(1):63–64.

89. Kucukguclu S, Tuncok Y, Ozkan H, et al. Multiple-dose activated charcoal in an accidental vancomycin overdose. *J Toxicol Clin Toxicol* 1996;34(1):83–86.
90. Connolly TP, Balsys AJ, King EG. Caval catheter haemodialysis. *Intensive Care Med* 1980;6(2):129–132.
91. Knudsen F, Dyerberg J. Platelets and antithrombin III in uraemia: the acute effect of haemodialysis. *Scand J Clin Lab Invest* 1985;45(4):341–347.
92. Kolb G, Fischer W, Seitz R, et al. Hemodialysis and blood coagulation: the effect of hemodialysis on coagulation factor XIII and thrombin-antithrombin III complex. *Nephron* 1991;58(1):106–108.
93. McFadden DW, Smith GW. Hemodialysis-associated hemorrhagic cholecystitis. *Am J Gastroenterol* 1987;82(10):1081–1083.
94. Daul AE, Schafers RF, Wenzel RR, et al. Acute hemolysis with subsequent life-threatening pancreatitis in hemodialysis. A complication which is not preventable with current dialysis equipment [in German]. *Deutsche Medizinische Wochenschrift* 1994;119(38):1263–1269.
95. Gault MH, Duffett S, Purchase L, et al. Hemodialysis intravascular hemolysis and kinked blood lines. *Nephron* 1992;62(3):267–271.
96. Paus PN, Larsen EW, Sodal G, et al. Pancreatic affection after acute hypotonic hemodialysis. *Acta Medica Scandinavica* 1982;212(1–2):83–84.
97. Barril G, Perez R, Torres T, et al. Acute anemia in a hemodialysis program caused by the appearance of high chloramine levels in the water [in Spanish]. *Medicina Clinica* 1983;80(11):483–486.
98. Craddock PR, Fehr J, Dalmasso AP, et al. Hemodialysis leukopenia. Pulmonary vascular leukostasis resulting from complement activation by dialyzer cellophane membranes. *J Clin Invest* 1977;59(5):879–888.
99. Enia G, Catalano C, Misefari V, et al. Complement activated leucopenia during hemodialysis: effect of pulse methyl-prednisolone. *Int J Artif Organs* 1990;13(2):98–102.
100. Ford DM, Portman RJ, Jurst DL, et al. Unexpected seizures during hemodialysis. Effect of dialysate prescription. *Pediatr Nephrol* 1987;1(4):597–601.
101. Reyes A, Turchetto E, Bernis C, et al. Acid-base derangements during sorbent regenerative hemodialysis in mechanically ventilated patients. *Crit Care Med* 1991;19(4):554–559.
102. Sethi D, Curtis JR, Topham DL, et al. Acute metabolic alkalosis during haemodialysis. *Nephron* 1989;51(1):119–120.
103. Dhakal MP, Kallay MC, Talley TE. Hemodialysis associated hypoxia extends into the post-dialysis period. *Int J Artif Organs* 1997;20(4):204–207.
104. Jones RH, Broadfield JB, Parsons V. Arterial hypoxemia during hemodialysis for acute renal failure in mechanically ventilated patients: observations and mechanisms. *Clin Nephrol* 1980;14(1):18–22.
105. Williams DJ, Jugurnauth J, Harding K, et al. Acute hypernatraemia during bicarbonate-buffered haemodialysis. *Nephrol Dial Transplant* 1994;9(8):1170–1173.
106. Said R, Quintanilla A, Levin N, et al. Acute hemolysis due to profound hypo-osmolality. A complication of hemodialysis. *J Dial* 1977;1(5):447–452.
107. Govan JR, Porter CA, Cook JG, et al. Acute magnesium poisoning as a complication of chronic intermittent haemodialysis. *BMJ* 1968;2(600):278–279.
108. Schulten HK, Sieberth HG, Deck KA, et al. Acute hypercalcaemia as a complication of haemodialysis. *Ger Med Mon* 1968;13(9):429–432.
109. Yoshida S, Tajika T, Yamasaki N, et al. Dialysis dysequilibrium syndrome in neurosurgical patients. *Neurosurgery* 1987;20(5):716–721.
110. Bosl R, Shideman JR, Meyer RM, et al. Effects and complications of high efficiency dialysis. *Nephron* 1975;15(2):151–160.
111. Raine AE. The susceptible patient [Review] [35 refs]. *Nephrol Dial Transplant* 1996;11[Suppl 2]:6–10.
112. Meyrier A, Fardeau M, Richet G. Acute asymmetrical neuritis associated with rapid ultrafiltration dialysis. *BMJ* 1972;2(808):252–254.
113. Giudicissi FM, Holanda CV, Nader NA, et al. Bilateral putaminal hemorrhage related to methanol poisoning: a complication of hemodialysis? Case report. *Arquivos de Neuro-Psiquiatria* 1995;53(3-A):485–487.
114. Glenn CM, Astley SJ, Watkins SL. Dialysis-associated seizures in children and adolescents. *Pediatr Nephrol* 1992;6(2):182–186.
115. Davenport A, Bramley PN, Wyatt JI. Morbidity and mortality due to cerebral edema complicating the treatment of severe leptospiral infection. *Am J Kidney Dis* 1990;16(2):160–165.
116. Collins DM, Lambert MB, Tannenbaum JS, et al. Tolerance of hemodialysis: a randomized prospective trial of high-flux versus conventional high-efficiency hemodialysis. *J Am Soc Nephrol* 1993;4(2):148–154.
117. Zbrog Z, Pawlicki L. Spontaneous rupture of the spleen as a cause of death of a patient with uremia [in Polish]. *Pol Tyg Lek* 1989;44(9):232–233.
118. Sherman RA, Goodling KA, Eisinger RP. Acute therapy of hemodialysis-related muscle cramps. *Am J Kidney Dis* 1982;2(2):287–288.
119. Oropello JM, Leibowitz AB, Manasia A, et al. Dilator-associated complications of central vein catheter insertion: possible mechanisms of injury and suggestions for prevention [see comments]. *J Cardiothorac Vasc Anesth* 1996;10(5):634–637.
120. Pereira BJ, Ramprasad KS, Ravi HR, et al. Retroperitoneal hemorrhage following trauma during femoral vein cannulation for hemodialysis—a therapeutic dilemma. *Ren Fail* 1989–1990;11(4):221–222.
121. Vanholder R, Lameire N, Verbanck J, et al. Complications of subclavian catheter hemodialysis: a 5 year prospective study in 257 consecutive patients. *Int J Artif Organs* 1982;5(5):297–303.
122. Bourquia A, Jabrane AJ, Ramdani B, et al. Complications of the subclavian vascular approach for hemodialysis [Review] [19 refs] [in French]. *Annales de Medecine Interne* 1989;140(2):102–105.
123. Waldman RP, Donner M, Bilsky AC, et al. Delayed onset of hemothorax: an unusual complication of subclavian access for hemodialysis. *Nephron* 1984;37(4):270–272.
124. Hsu LH, Lien TC, Wang JH. Chylothorax: a complication of internal jugular vein catheterization. *Chung Hua i Hsueh Tsa Chih* [Chinese medical journal] 1997;60(1):57–61.
125. Cina G, De Rosa MG, Viola G, et al. Arterial injuries following diagnostic, therapeutic, and accidental arterial cannulation in haemodialysis patients. *Nephrol Dial Transplant* 1997;12(7):1448–1452.
126. Agresti JV, Schwartz AB, Chinitz JL, et al. Delayed traumatic arteriovenous fistula following hemodialysis vascular catheterization. *Nephron* 1987;46(4):350–352.
127. Barrett N, Spencer S, McIvor J, et al. Subclavian stenosis: a major complication of subclavian dialysis catheters. *Nephrol Dial Transplant* 1988;3(4):423–425.
128. Vanholder V, Hoenich N, Ringoir S. Morbidity and mortality of central venous catheter hemodialysis: a review of 10 years' experience. *Nephron* 1987;47(4):274–279.
129. Tokars JI, Alter MJ, Miller E, et al. National surveillance of dialysis associated diseases in the United States—1994. *ASAIO J* 1997;43(1):108–119.
130. Da Porto A, Adami A, Susanna F, et al. Hepatitis C virus in dialysis units: a multicenter study. *Nephron* 1992;61(3):309–310.
131. Oliva JA, Maymo RM, Carrio J, et al. Late seroconversion of C virus markers in hemodialysis patients. *Kidney Int* 1993;41[Suppl]:S153–S156.
132. Simon N. Hepatitis C virus infection in hemodialysis [Review] [33 refs] [in French]. *Pathol Biol (Paris)* 1995;43(8):735–740.
133. Lettau LA, Alfred HJ, Glew RH, et al. Nosocomial transmission of delta hepatitis. *Ann Intern Med* 1986;104(5):631–635.
134. Dahlberg PJ, Agger WA, Singer JR, et al. Subclavian hemodialysis catheter infections: a prospective, randomized trial of an attachable silver-impregnated cuff for prevention of catheter-related infections. *Infect Control Hosp Epidemiol* 1995;16(9):506–511.
135. Lemke HD, Heidland A, Schaefer RM. Hypersensitivity reactions during haemodialysis: role of complement. *Nephrol Dial Transplant* 1990;5(4):264–269.
136. Bommer J, Ritz E. Ethylene oxide (ETO) as a major cause of anaphylactoid reactions in dialysis (a review) [Review] [60 refs]. *Artif Organs* 1987;11(2):111–117.
137. Update: acute allergic reactions associated with reprocessed hemodialyzers—United States, 1989–1990. *MMWR Morb Mortal Wkly Rep* 1991;40(9): 147, 153–154.
138. Imamura T, Tamura K, Taguchi T, et al. Reduction of nitroglycerin and isosorbide dinitrate by hemodialysis in refractory angina pectoris after acute myocardial infarction. *Am J Cardiol* 1988;61(11):954–955.
139. Oliva JA, Ercilla G, Mallafre JM, et al. Markers of hepatitis C infection among hemodialysis patients with acute and chronic infection: implications for infection control strategies in hemodialysis units. *Int J Artif Organs* 1995;18(2):73–77.

SECTION 7

Pharmacokinetics

CHAPTER 79

Principles and Applications of Pharmacokinetics

Michael Mayersohn

This presentation is *not* intended to be a course in mathematics nor, fortunately, does the reader need to be a mathematician to understand and apply the principles of pharmacokinetics. Effort should be expended in understanding the concepts and principles, which, hopefully, is facilitated by the shorthand use of some selected mathematical relationships. The math provides a universal language for developing and discussing the principles. These relationships must make sense (or they are useless), and this occurs if the concepts are understood. That said, it is necessary to use equations to represent the ideas and for calculation purposes. Because one principle or idea draws on those preceding it, try and keep clear "what drives what" (i.e., which is the true *independent* variable and which is the *dependent* variable) and how would a plot of one versus the other appear. Being able to graph one variable against another is important because if one can properly create such a plot, one understands the principle(s) behind the relationship. A graph represents a rapid means of presenting a relationship and often is the starting point for a discussion. By convention, there is only one graphing rule: the dependent variable appears on the y-axis (ordinate) and the independent variable appears on the x-axis (abscissa).

The term *pharmacokinetics* arises from the Greek *pharmacon*, meaning substance (a drug or toxic agent), and *kinetics*, meaning rate process. Pharmacokinetics is the area of study that examines the rates of those processes associated with entry into, disposition through, and exit from the body of a material (i.e., drug or toxin) presented to the body. Further, such study often attempts to relate the pharmacologic response or pharmacodynamic events to the concentration of that substance (or a derivative, such as a metabolite) as a function of time. The latter gives rise to useful pharmacokinetic/pharmacodynamic relationships. By extension, *toxicokinetics* concerns itself with the rate processes associated with a toxic agent (or derivative) entering the body and the consequent concentration and time-related toxicodynamic events. One can contrast pharmacokinetics to pharmacodynamics; the former being what the body does to the drug and the latter representing what the drug does to the body.

The processes that are studied and quantified in pharmacokinetics are often described by the mnemonic *ADME*, *a*bsorption, *d*istribution, *m*etabolism, and *e*xcretion. The three latter processes are associated with *disposition* (i.e., what happens to the drug once in the body, after gaining access to the bloodstream), whereas absorption describes the movement of the drug from the site of application to the bloodstream. In a more general way, these processes may be considered: input (absorption), translocation (distribution), and output (elimination). Critical to our understanding, however, is the ultimate expression of the interaction between the substance and the body, the *biologic outcome*, which is measured as a response or toxic event.

Figure 1 illustrates the important idea of the overlap between the pharmacokinetic events and some corresponding biologic outcome noted as a pharmacodynamic/toxicodynamic event. The driving force for the processes shown is concentration of drug in the blood. For this reason, it is important to understand and characterize the concentration-time profile, as it is critical for all subsequent events (i.e., distribution, elimination, and response). Another important aspect of Figure 1 is that all of the events are occurring at the *same* time, though processes are often sequential. After drug dosing or environmental exposure (on one or multiple occasions), and assuming that the substance is absorbed into the bloodstream, blood concentrations of the substance are achieved. That (driving force) concentration causes movement from the blood to other tissues, including the organs that eliminate the drug (e.g., liver and kidney) as well as the tissues that contain receptors or regions of potential toxicity. Thus, while the drug is being absorbed into the bloodstream, it is simultaneously being distributed to sites of action or toxicity, and it is undergoing elimination. Whereas a response tends to be reversible (increasing or decreasing in some manner related to blood concentration; often directly), elimination processes are almost always irreversible.

A more comprehensive view of the elementary scheme (Fig. 1) is illustrated in Figure 2. The banner cites the basic processes, input-translocation-output, which are further divided into more specific events. Thus, the processes on the left side of the scheme describe the transition steps of disintegration to dissolution to absorption that a solid form of a drug undergoes on ingestion. The dissolution step is often critical because it can rate-limit the overall absorption process, especially for poorly water-soluble

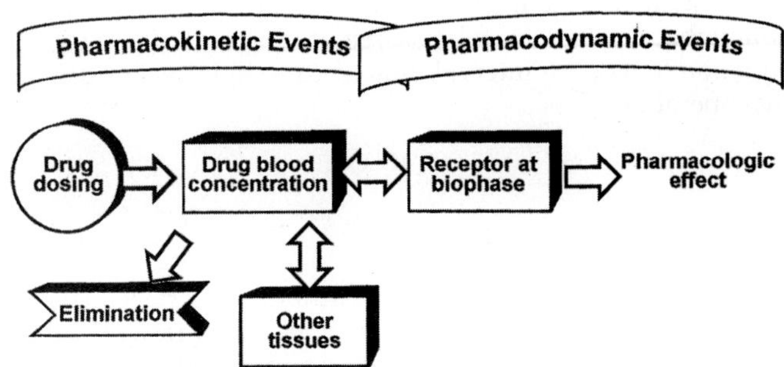

Figure 1. Schematic illustration of the overlap between pharmacokinetic events and biologic outcome noted as pharmacodynamic/toxicodynamic events. Blood concentration is the driving force for all of the events shown. All of the processes are dynamic as they are constantly changing with time. (From M. Mayersohn, *unpublished*, with permission from Saguaro Technical Press, Inc, Tucson, AZ, 2002.)

compounds. Absorption, or the process of passing across one or more biologic membranes into the bloodstream, is a function of the permeability of the molecule (which is related to the oil/water partition coefficient of the chemical). As the molecule moves through the intestinal epithelial cells into the bloodstream, it may undergo metabolism (especially by the CYP-450 oxidative system as well as by conjugation reactions) or encounter efflux transporters (P-glycoprotein), which move the compound from the cell back into the gut lumen. Any absorbed drug then moves via the portal circulation into the liver. Because the latter is the major site of metabolism, the compound could undergo further chemical alteration as it passes through the liver. The *first-pass effect*, also known as *presystemic metabolism*, refers to the movement of compound through the gut wall and liver and its metabolic alteration. The first-pass effect can be quite important in modulating the response to a drug. As noted later, it is the magnitude of metabolic clearance that determines the significance of the first-pass effect (see Nonvascular Input: Absorption and Bioavailability. Once past the liver, the compound (and metabolites) gains access to the bloodstream (the *body*).

Numerous other routes of administration (pulmonary, rectal, subcutaneous, intramuscular, dermal, nasal) may provide alternative and perhaps more efficient modes of administration compared to the oral route (Fig. 2). In each instance, just as with oral dosing, the drug must traverse biologic membranes to gain access to the bloodstream. Each route has its own advantages and disadvantages. The absorption process can be completely bypassed by use of a vascular route, such as intravenous administration. The latter involves either bolus (all at once) dosing or infusion over a specified time. In either approach, the entire absorbed dose enters the body.

Once in the bloodstream, the compound has access to all tissues and organs in the body. During this time the drug distributes to the sites of action or toxicity and it undergoes elimination by the primary eliminating organs, the liver and kidney. Metabolites may form during this time and they in turn distribute to tissues and organs, possibly produce an effect or toxicity, and undergo further elimination from the body. The scheme in Figure 2, although appearing somewhat complex, is a considerable simplification of reality.

Recall that all of the events previously described are occurring at the same time. One needs to understand and relate dose to blood concentration, blood concentration to response, and all of these events with time. This is the challenge and the purpose of pharmacokinetics and toxicokinetics.

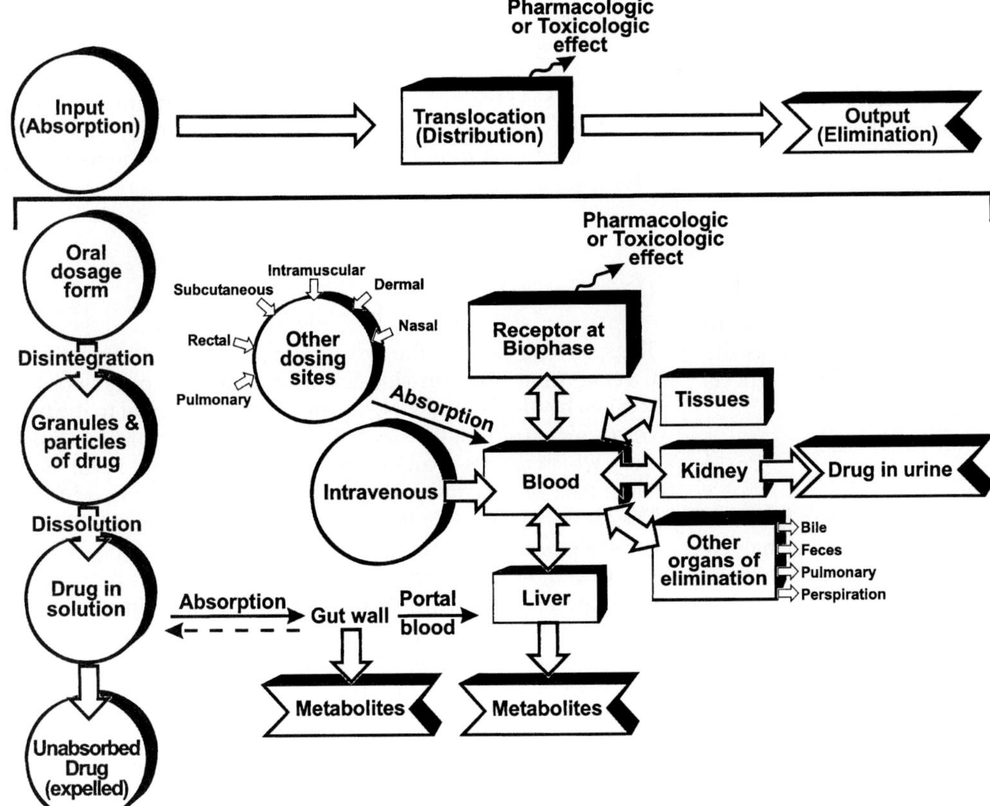

Figure 2. Conceptualized fate of a drug in an animal body after dosing by one or more routes of administration. The left side of the schema represents processes associated with oral absorption (input). The center portion reflects drug movement after gaining access to the body (translocation). The right-hand side of the schema illustrates elimination by various organs (output). (From M. Mayersohn, *unpublished*, with permission from Saguaro Technical Press, Inc, Tucson, AZ, 1998.)

KINETIC PROCESSES

First-Order (Linear) Kinetic Processes

The best place to begin a discussion of pharmacokinetic principles is by first discussing the elimination (or output or loss) process and by making a number of limiting assumptions. To develop a fundamental principle, that of *first-order* or *linear pharmacokinetics*, one first assumes that the drug is given as an intravenous (IV) bolus dose (the entire dose is placed into the bloodstream at one time). Second, one assumes that the drug distributes instantaneously from the blood to the rest of the tissues of the body. That assumption gives rise to the so-called *one-compartment model*. Although the idea of compartments is developed later, for the purpose here, one assumes the simplest possible model (i.e., the one-compartment model).

As long as the body receives doses of the substance that do not exceed the ability of the eliminating processes to handle those doses, one observes a process of elimination referred to as first-order or linear pharmacokinetics. Some important exceptions to this assumption exist (e.g., ethanol), and there are significant pharmacologic and toxicologic implications when they occur. The principle of first-order kinetics, simply stated, is that *the rate of any process is directly related to the concentration or amount of that substance at any given time*. Thus, the driving force for the rate of that process is simply the concentration or amount present at that time. After an IV bolus dose of drug and given the assumptions, the rate of elimination from the body is directly related to the blood concentration or amount present in the body, as shown in equation 1:

$$\text{rate} \propto \text{concentration} \qquad \text{[Eq. 1]}$$

Double the blood concentration (by doubling the dose), and the rate of elimination will double. Halve the concentration (by halving the dose), and the rate will halve. The proportionality sign can be replaced with a constant of proportionality and an equal sign to give

$$\text{rate} = K \cdot \text{concentration} \quad \text{OR} \quad \text{rate} = K \cdot C \qquad \text{[Eq. 2]}$$

in which C is concentration (in blood or plasma or serum), and K is the constant of proportionality. To have a final correct equation, a minus sign needs to be added to one side of the equation to indicate loss or elimination of drug from the body.

$$\text{rate} = -K \cdot C \qquad \text{[Eq. 3]}$$

The sign simply indicates the direction of movement of the substance; in this case, movement out of the body (by elimination) and, therefore, concentrations in the blood are declining with time. The constant of proportionality, K, is referred to as the *apparent overall first-order elimination rate constant*, and it reflects the unchanging relationship between rate and C. Thus,

$$K = \frac{\text{rate}}{C} \qquad \text{[Eq. 4]}$$

Double the concentration, and the rate will double, and K will be unchanged. Halve the concentration, and the rate will be halved and, K will be unchanged. The units of K can be found by substituting the appropriate units for rate and C:

$$K = \frac{\text{rate (concentration/time)}}{\text{C (concentration)}} = \frac{1}{\text{time}} \text{ OR } t^{-1} \qquad \text{[Eq. 5]}$$

The units of a first-order rate constant are always reciprocal time. The meaning of K is described later; however, every compound has a specific average value and range of values for K in a given subject group (or animal species). The problem with the previous rate equations is that they relate concentration and rate rather than what is more useful, concentration and time. To obtain that more useful relationship, it is necessary to integrate equation 3 over the interval, time zero to infinity. Performing that operation gives

$$\int_0^{\infty} \text{rate} = -\int_0^{\infty} K \cdot C \cdot dt \qquad \text{[Eq. 6]}$$

$$C = C^0 \cdot e^{-K \cdot t} \qquad \text{[Eq. 7]}$$

Equation 7 is a classic relationship describing an exponential process, in this case a declining exponential. In contrast, microbiologic growth can be described by an identical but positive exponential equation. Blood concentration, C, at any time after an IV bolus dose is equal to an initial (at time zero) blood concentration, C^0, which is multiplied by some number whose value is declining over time. That number is given by the base, e, raised to a negative exponent, which is formed by the product of the first-order elimination rate constant, K, and time (t), after the IV bolus injection. Because the product of K and t increases as time goes on, the base raised to an increasing negative number results in smaller and smaller values, which, when multiplied by C^0, gives decreasing numerical values for blood concentration. Blood concentration is declining exponentially according to the value of K: The larger the value of K, the more rapidly the compound is lost from the body; the smaller the value of K, the slower it is lost from the body. A plot of blood concentration versus time on a linear (Cartesian coordinate) graphic scale results in a curved line whose concentration values decline exponentially. The initial time zero concentration, C^0, is the result of the IV dose being distributed into some apparent space or volume, generally referred to as the *apparent volume of distribution*, V_d. This somewhat confusing term is discussed in Distribution.

Scientists go through almost any contortion to be able to express data in the form of a straight line (which is easy to analyze). It is not surprising, therefore, that equation 7 is most often presented in one of the two following transformations, which are in the form of straight-line equations.

$$\ln C = \ln C^0 - K \cdot t \qquad \text{[Eq. 8]}$$

Equation 8 is obtained by taking the natural logarithm (ln; base e) of both sides of equation 7. Using the more familiar and common logarithmic form (log; base 10), one obtains the following useful equation:

$$\begin{array}{ccccc} \log C & = & \log C^0 & - & \frac{K}{2.3} \cdot t \\ \Downarrow & & \Downarrow & & \Downarrow \quad \Downarrow \\ Y & = & b & - & m \cdot X \end{array} \qquad \text{[Eq. 9]}$$

Thus, as long as all of the assumptions are correct, a plot of log C versus time results in a log-linear straight line whose slope (m) is given by –K/2.3 and whose y-intercept (b) is equal to the time zero concentration, C^0. In contrast to a graphic plot on linear axes, which results in an exponentially curved line, a plot of the same data on a semilogarithmic scale results in a straight line. The latter has far more useful information compared to the linear scale plot. The data are either transformed to logarithmic values and those plotted on a linear scale or, and the more likely method, semilogarithmic graph paper is used in which the numerical values for concentrations are placed onto the logarithmic y-axis. In fact, what is most often done today is to form a data set in a software program (such as EXCEL), and the data are plotted according to the method of choice. The latter approach often gives the choice of selecting between a linear scale or a logarithmic scale on the y-axis.

Semilogarithmic graph paper has also been called *ratio* paper. Semilogarithmic scales are best suited to the plotting of data that

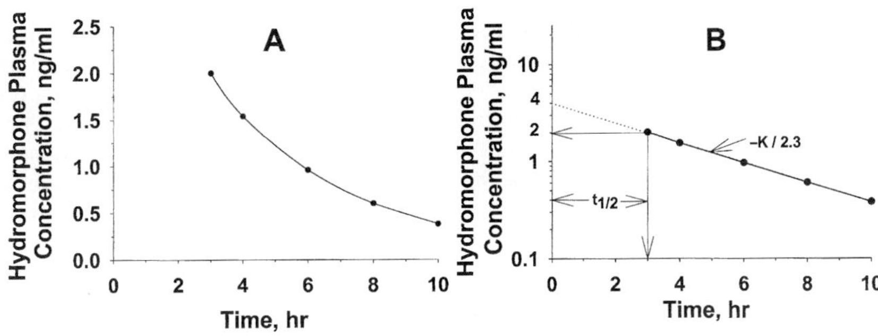

Figure 3. **A:** Plasma concentration-time profile after an intravenous bolus dose of hydromorphone to normal human subjects. The data are plotted on linear (cartesian) scales, and the resulting curvilinearity is an indication of an exponential decline in concentrations with time. **B:** Graph of the same data illustrated in **(A)** but plotted on a semilogarithmic scale. The data are represented by a single log-linear relationship, consistent with an exponential (i.e., first-order) process to describe drug loss from the body. The initial (hypothetical) time zero concentration of this drug, based on extrapolation of the line back to the y-axis, is approximately 4 ng/ml. The slope of the line is given by –K/2.3. The two arrows indicate the time needed for the hypothetical initial concentration (4 ng/ml) to decline by 50% to a value of 2 mg/L. The corresponding intercept on the x-axis (approximately 3 hours) represents the half-life ($t_{1/2}$) of the drug. Any other pair of concentration values in the ratio of 2:1 gives the same value for half-life. Not all of the data have been replotted for this illustration, as discussed later (see Fig. 12). (Data recovered and replotted from Parab PV, Ritschel WA, Coyle DE, et al. Pharmacokinetics of hydromorphone after intravenous, peroral and rectal administration to human subjects. *Biopharm Drug Dispos* 1988;9:187–199. From M. Mayersohn, *unpublished*, with permission from Saguaro Technical Press, Inc, Tucson, AZ, 2002.)

change in an exponential fashion, such as the concentration-time data obtained in pharmacokinetic investigations. The term *ratio* was used to indicate that numbers in the same ratio to each other are the same distance apart on the logarithmic scale. Thus, the following pairs of numbers, which are in the same ratio (of 5:1), are separated by the same distance: 10/2, 100/20, 600/120, and so forth. Similarly, numbers that represent the same percentage increase or decrease are separated by the same distance on the logarithmic scale. The following pairs of numbers, which represent a 10% decrease, are the same distance apart: 100/90, 10/9, and 20/18. Another characteristic of semilog scales is the number of *cycles* that they represent. Each cycle is an order of magnitude (or a factor) of ten. Two-cycle log axis encompasses a 100-fold range (or two orders of magnitude of ten) from, for example, 1 to 10 to 100 or 0.01 to 0.1 to 1.0.

K, the apparent overall first-order elimination rate constant, represents a fractional rate of loss of drug from the body. Thus, for example, if a drug has a value of K of 0.1 hour^{-1} (or 0.1/hour), it is *approximately* correct to say that at the end of any hour *approximately* 10% of drug that was there at the beginning of the hour has now been eliminated. For example, at time zero after giving an IV bolus dose of drug the plasma concentration is 100 mg/L. One hour later, the body has lost *approximately* 10% of 100 mg/L, giving a concentration of 90 mg/L at 1 hour. One hour after that (at 2 hours), another 10% has been lost and the plasma concentration at 2 hours is now *approximately* 81 mg/L. At 3 hours, the concentration is *approximately* 73 mg/L; at 4 hours, *approximately* 67 mg/L; and so forth. If the rate constant had a value of 0.05 year^{-1} (0.05/year), *approximately* 5% of the drug present at the beginning of the year would be lost by the end of that year. There is a more useful and simpler way to express drug loss from the body and it involves the idea of *half-life*, $t_{1/2}$; a term commonly used in many disciplines (i.e., radioactive decay in physics and *in vitro* degradation reactions in chemistry).

Figure 3 illustrates two plasma concentration-time graphs of hydromorphone after IV bolus dosing to a group of normal human subjects (1). For a reason that is explained in Disposition: Models, not all of the data have been replotted in these graphs. The graph on the left (Fig. 3A) is plotted on linear (cartesian) coordinate axes. The data and the corresponding line are curvilinear, consistent with exponential decline in concentration with time. In contrast, the graph on the right (Fig. 3B) is a plot of the same data on semilog axes. This graph, unlike the one using a linear scale, contains useful information and is the starting point for any pharmacokinetic data analysis. It is absolutely essential to plot a data set before beginning any analysis to visualize the behavior of the drug and the system. There are several points that need to be made about Figure 3B. The data are represented by a single, log-linear line, which is expected for any simple (i.e., single) exponential, first-order kinetic process. There is no curvilinearity in the graph for the data plotted, which is consistent with the assumption of instantaneous distribution from the blood to all body tissues (i.e., a one-compartment model). The slope of the line is given by –K/2.3, from which one can estimate the value for the apparent overall first-order elimination rate constant, K. The intercept on the y-axis represents the (hypothetical) time zero plasma concentration, which is never actually measured (it is always estimated by extrapolation of the straight line back to the y-axis).

An important concept illustrated on the semilog graph is the useful and practical idea of a $t_{1/2}$. Unlike a value for K, it is easy to understand the concept of a $t_{1/2}$. By definition, $t_{1/2}$ is the time necessary for any given value of concentration to decline by one-half or by 50%. This is illustrated in Figure 3B by the horizontal arrow indicating where a plasma concentration value of 2 ng/ml is seen on the line and the vertical arrow that indicates the time at which that concentration is achieved. Because the drug level declined 50% (4 to 2 ng/ml) at the 3-hour time point, 3 hours is the value for $t_{1/2}$ for hydromorphone. However, any other pair of concentration values in the ratio of 2:1 could have been used (e.g., 2 to 1 ng/ml) and the same value for $t_{1/2}$ would have been obtained.

Although it does not have meaning at this point, it is good practice to refer to $t_{1/2}$ as the *terminal* $t_{1/2}$. In fact, although a variety of different words are used to qualify the term $t_{1/2}$, including *biologic*, *elimination*, and *disposition*, the one term that is always correct is terminal $t_{1/2}$. *Biologic* $t_{1/2}$ is not a good expression because it can be confused with the decline in pharmacodynamic activity rather than characterization of drug loss from the body. *Elimination* $t_{1/2}$, although commonly used, is only correct when dealing with a one-compartment model, as discussed later. *Disposition* $t_{1/2}$ is often a correct usage; however, it may be incorrect when characterizing plasma concentration-time data after nonvascular dosing (e.g., oral route).

$t_{1/2}$ and K are related. Taking equation 9 and specifying that C is one-half of the starting value, C^0 (which by definition occurs after one $t_{1/2}$) and rearranging,

$$\log C^0 - \log C = \frac{K \cdot t}{2.3}$$

$$\log C^0 - \log[0.5C^0] = \frac{K \cdot t_{1/2}}{2.3}$$

$$\log\left[\frac{C^0}{0.5C^0}\right] = \frac{K \cdot t_{1/2}}{2.3} \quad \text{[Eq. 10]}$$

$$\log[2] = \frac{K \cdot t_{1/2}}{2.3}$$

$$t_{1/2} = \frac{[0.3010] \cdot [2.3]}{K}$$

$$t_{1/2} = \frac{0.693}{K}$$

$t_{1/2}$ and K are inversely related; the greater the K, the smaller the $t_{1/2}$, and the smaller the K, the greater the $t_{1/2}$. Furthermore, notice that $t_{1/2}$ (and K) is *independent* of dose or plasma concentration. This is what is meant by dose-*independent* pharmacokinetics; the parameters describing the disposition of a drug are *not* dependent on dose (this statement also applies to other pharmacokinetic parameters, such as apparent volume of distribution and clearance). In the example cited in Figure 3B, the terminal $t_{1/2}$ value of approximately 3 hours for hydromorphone has a terminal rate constant of 0.693/3 hours, or 0.231 hour^{-1}.

In contrast to the parameters being *independent* of dose, plasma concentration does *depend* on dose; double the dose and plasma concentrations will double, with no change in $t_{1/2}$. These two statements are illustrated in Figure 4. In Figure 4A, three different IV bolus doses have been administered: dose D, dose 2D, and dose 5D. A plot of the concentration-time data on semilog axes gives lines that are parallel to each other, because there is only one value for K or $t_{1/2}$ for that drug. However, the lines intercept the y-axis giving time zero concentrations in the same ratio as the doses: concentration of one unit, concentration of two units, and concentration of five units. As noted above, and as shown in Figure 4B, a plot of $t_{1/2}$ (or K) as a function of dose gives a flat line; there is no dependence of $t_{1/2}$ on dose.

Whereas $t_{1/2}$ is *independent* of dose, the resulting plasma concentrations (as noted in Fig. 4A) are directly *dependent* on dose, as shown in Figure 5A. This is often referred to as dose-proportionality. The idea illustrated in Figure 4A can also be represented by the principle of *superposition*, which states that because doubling the dose results in doubling of plasma concentration, a plot of concentration/dose should give rise to one line that represents the superposition of all concentration and dose pairs. This principle is illustrated in Figure 5B.

One of the most important aspects of first-order or linear kinetics is that everything about the disposition or behavior of a drug is predictable, as can be surmised from the relationships illustrated in Figures 4 and 5. Because parameters remain constant with dose and because concentrations are directly dependent on dose, one is able to predict a concentration-time profile for any given IV dose. In such a linear system, doubling the input results in an exact doubling of the output (e.g., double the dose, double the plasma concentration). When first-order kinetic principles do not apply, all predictability is gone and one faces significant problems in, for example, drug dosing and extrapolating from a subtoxic dose to a toxic dose.

Non–First-Order (Nonlinear) Kinetic Processes

Many physical and biologic processes cannot be simply characterized by first-order kinetic or linear systems behavior. In fact, the world is a nonlinear one in which doubling the input often results in something other than a doubling of the output (less than or more than double the output). The assumption is often made that the system (e.g., the body) behaves in a linear way, or at least that approximation is believed to be correct. In fact, it is true that many of the drugs and toxins that are dealt with behave in a linear manner, at least at medically relevant doses. But, this may not be a reasonable approximation for some doses or levels of exposure, especially at the high end of the range in which the toxicologist becomes involved. All pharmacokinetic processes (absorption, distribution, elimination) may exhibit nonlinear behavior, and there are drug and toxin examples of such behavior for each of those processes.

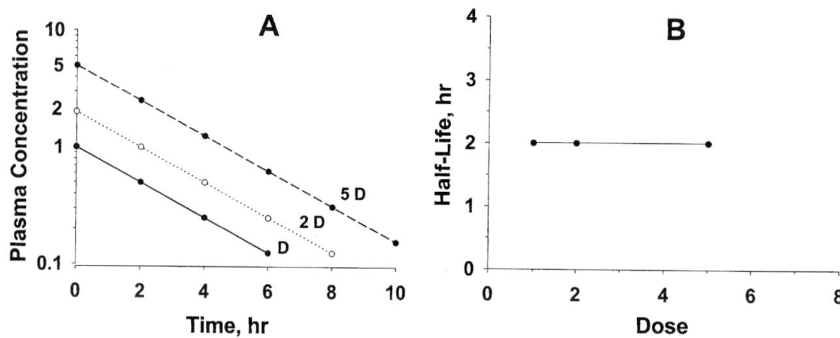

Figure 4. A: Hypothetical semilog plasma concentration-time plots for a drug given at increasing doses of D, 2D, and 5D. Note that the lines are parallel (same slope and, therefore, the same K and half-life), and the intercepts on the y-axis (initial time zero concentrations) are in the same ratio as the doses (1:2:5). These same ratios apply to concentrations resulting from those doses at any given time. **B:** The results of the data in **A** in terms of half-life and its relationship to dose are illustrated in this graph. Note that the half-life is *independent* of dose (or concentration). This behavior is referred to as *dose-independent* pharmacokinetics, which is a characteristic of first-order processes. (From M. Mayersohn, *unpublished*, with permission from Saguaro Technical Press, Inc, Tucson, AZ, 2002.)

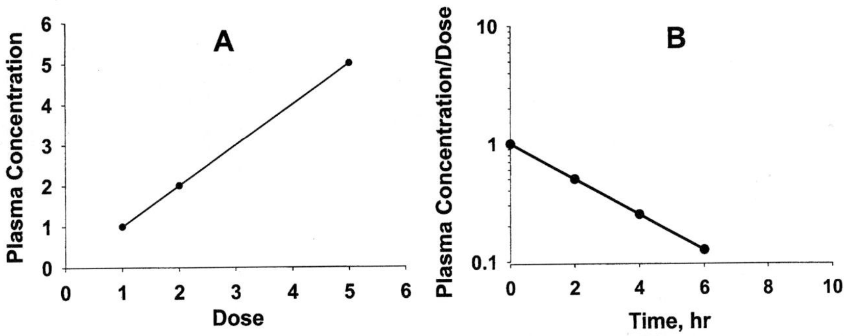

Figure 5. A: The relationship between plasma concentration and dose at any time after an IV bolus dose for the hypothetical drug illustrated in Figure 4A. The points noted are for doses D, 2D, and 5D, and the concentrations are for those seen at time zero. This behavior is often referred to as illustrating *dose-proportionality*. **B:** The concentrations resulting from any given dose are divided by that dose and plotted on semilog axes as a function of dose. This graph illustrates the principle of *superposition* as well as dose-proportionality. (From M. Mayersohn, *unpublished*, with permission from Saguaro Technical Press, Inc, Tucson, AZ, 2002.)

The nonlinear behavior of interest for chemicals and drugs involves the output or elimination process, especially metabolism and urinary excretion. There are some, but few, examples of drugs or toxins that undergo non–first-order or nonlinear elimination. Dosing or exposure to such a compound results in plasma concentrations that exceed the ability of the eliminating organ to efficiently remove that substance. That is, the elimination process is *not able to keep up with* or is *swamped* by the amount of substance that is being presented to it for processing. The latter statement is in contrast with first-order kinetics in which there is a direct relationship between the amount of substance presented and the rate of its being processed (recall: rate $\propto$ concentration).

The most fundamental difference between first-order kinetics and non–first-order (nonlinear) kinetics is illustrated by the relationship between the rate of a given process (e.g., metabolism) and plasma concentration, the driving force for the process. The most useful relationship for the latter process is best expressed in the form of the classical enzyme kinetics equation of Michaelis and Menten. The Michaelis-Menten enzyme kinetic equation expresses the relationship between the rate of enzyme-catalyzed substrate metabolism to the concentration of substrate,

$$\text{rate (or, v)} = \frac{V_{max} \cdot C}{k_{mm} + C} \qquad \text{[Eq. 11]}$$

in which rate (or v for velocity) is a function of a maximal rate (V_{max}), plasma concentration (C), and the Michaelis constant k_{mm}.* The Michaelis constant is equal to the concentration associated with one-half the maximal rate, V_{max} (units of k_{mm} are those of concentration). Equation 11 is in the form of a hyperbola—a relationship commonly noted in biologic systems as a consequence of some nonlinear behavior (e.g., pharmacologic effect versus plasma concentration or receptor or protein binding as a function of concentration). The best way to analyze this relationship is to consider low and high plasma concentrations to simplify the equation by making appropriate approximations.

At low concentrations (i.e., $C << k_{mm}$), C can be ignored in the denominator of equation 11,

$$\text{rate (or, v)} = \frac{V_{max} \cdot C}{k_{mm} + C} \cong \frac{V_{max} \cdot C}{k_{mm}} = \left(\frac{V_{max}}{k_{mm}}\right) \cdot C \qquad \text{[Eq. 12]}$$

*The Michaelis constant is often given the symbol k_m, but it is easily confused with a rate constant, such as a first-order metabolic rate constant. To avoid that confusion, the symbol k_{mm} is used here.

This approximation results in the relationship noted in equation 12, which indicates that at low concentrations, rate is directly proportional to concentration, as would occur for a first-order process. The ratio of the two constants, V_{max} to k_{mm}, is itself a constant, as it is in a first-order process. Thus, at low concentrations, the system behaves according to first-order kinetic principles. The ratio of V_{max} to k_{mm} is a first-order rate constant, and it has also been referred to as *intrinsic clearance*, as is discussed later in the Clearance section. The units of these two terms differ (time^{-1} for a first-order rate constant and volume/time for clearance).

In contrast, at higher concentrations (i.e., $C >> k_{mm}$), k_{mm} is ignored in the denominator of equation 11,

$$\text{rate (or, v)} = \frac{V_{max} \cdot C}{k_{mm} + C} \cong \frac{V_{max} \cdot C}{C} = V_{max} \qquad \text{[Eq. 13]}$$

This approximation results in the relationship shown in equation 13, which indicates that rate becomes a constant, no matter how much concentration increases (or, no matter how the dose increases). At the extreme, this would represent *zero-order kinetics*, but, with few exceptions, true zero-order behavior is rarely actually seen. Instead, *mixed kinetics* is more likely seen—behavior somewhere in between first-order and zero-order kinetics. In a zero-order kinetic process, the rate does not depend on concentration (which is raised to a power of zero, resulting in a constant). Rather, the rate depends on some other factor.

A comparison of this basic behavior (rate vs. concentration) for a linear first-order process and for a nonlinear (Michaelis-Menten) process is illustrated in Figure 6. The graph on the left (Fig. 6A) indicates a direct, linear relationship between rate and concentration for any compound that undergoes first-order elimination. The hypothetical graph shown is for ethanol metabolic rate in humans assuming that ethanol was metabolized according to a first-order process (i.e., using the ratio of V_{max} to k_{mm}, as noted in equation 12). The slope of the line is the first-order rate constant for metabolism or metabolic clearance, depending on units. The graph on the right (Fig. 6B) is a plot of ethanol metabolic rate versus ethanol plasma concentration in humans. This graph is a typical representation of nonlinear elimination, which is characterized by a hyperbolic Michaelis-Menten relationship. Notice that the rate is not directly proportional to concentration, except at low concentrations as shown in the inset graph (i.e., at concentrations much less than the k_{mm} value; in this case, approximately 0.06 g/L). The arrow along the x-axis points to the Michaelis constant (approximately 0.06 g/L), which corresponds to one-half V_{max} (approximately 4.5 g/hour, as shown on the y-axis; V_{max} is approximately 9 g/hour). Aver-

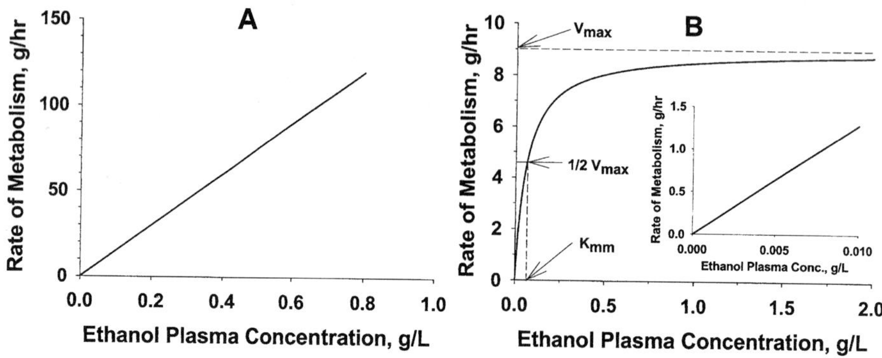

Figure 6. **A:** Hypothetical rate of ethanol metabolism as a function of plasma concentration if ethanol were eliminated by a first-order process. The direct, linear relationship is characteristic of first-order kinetics. The slope of the line is either a first-order rate constant of metabolism or metabolic clearance, depending on units. **B:** Rate of ethanol metabolism as a function of plasma concentration based on the average values of V_{max} (approximately 9 g/hour) and k_{mm} (approximately 0.06 g/L) in humans. The hyperbolic relationship is characteristic of nonlinear or Michaelis-Menten enzyme kinetics. The maximal rate, V_{max}, is the extrapolation on the y-axis of the asymptote of the line (as predicted by equation 13), and k_{mm} is the concentration value on the x-axis corresponding to one-half of V_{max}. Mixed order kinetics is observed over much of the concentration range. The inset graph illustrates the direct, linear relationship between rate and concentration at low concentrations of ethanol (as predicted by equation 12). That line is extended to higher concentrations, assuming first-order kinetics, in **(A)**. (From M. Mayersohn, *unpublished*, with permission from Saguaro Technical Press, Inc, Tucson, AZ, 2002.)

age values in human subjects for V_{max} and k_{mm} have been used in generating the data for these plots.

The consequences of the rate versus concentration relationship for a nonlinear process are extremely important, and there are several significant clinical and toxicologic implications. At low concentrations ($C \ll k_{mm}$), in which first-order kinetics applies, the apparent elimination rate constant is a constant, such that as concentrations increase so do the corresponding rates, as noted on the left side of equation 14. In contrast, as concentrations increase ($C \gg k_{mm}$), rate does not keep up with concentration and the value for K decreases, as noted on the right side of equation 14.

$$C \ll k_{mm}:\ \vec{K} = \frac{rate\uparrow}{C\uparrow} \qquad C \gg k_{mm}:\ K\downarrow = \frac{\overrightarrow{rate}}{C\uparrow} \qquad \text{[Eq. 14]}$$

If the value of K decreases as concentration (or dose) increases, then the $t_{1/2}$ increases. The $t_{1/2}$ is longest at the highest concentrations and then decreases in value as concentrations decrease with time until, finally, a constant terminal $t_{1/2}$ is seen at lower concentrations (i.e., $C \ll k_{mm}$).

The behavior just described is illustrated for ethanol in one human subject in Figure 7 (2) and for the solvent dioxane in rats in Figures 8 and 9 (3). The ethanol blood concentration-time data (2) shown in the large graph is plotted on a linear (y-axis) scale. Most of the data have the appearance of a straight line with curvature at later times when low concentrations are seen. This *hockey-stick* shape occurs when high concentrations exceed k_{mm} and the resulting rate of decline is approximately a constant (i.e., zero-order). This gives rise to a linear concentration-time relationship. At later times (low ethanol concentrations; $C \ll k_{mm}$), the line begins to curve, representing return to an exponential process. In contrast, the semilog plot shown in the inset graph has a line that is continually changing slope until it becomes approximately log-linear at later times (low concentrations; return to first-order kinetics).

The dioxane concentration-time data obtained in rats and shown in Figure 8 are a dramatic example of nonlinear elimination (3). The lowest intravenous dose (3 mg/kg) results in a log-linear decline in concentrations, whereas the two larger doses (100 and 1000 mg/kg) show dramatic curvilinearity, until the terminal log-linear phases are achieved. Notice that the ultimate terminal log-linear lines for all doses are parallel, as they must be for this type of saturable process. The inset graph plots plasma concentration divided by dose as a function of time for the data shown in the large graph. This type of plot illustrates whether the principle of superposition applies. If the lines superimpose at all doses (as noted in Fig. 5B), then first-order, linear kinetics apply. If this does not occur, then there is deviation from linearity and some non–first-order, nonlinear process(es) is being evidenced. The inset graph illustrates that

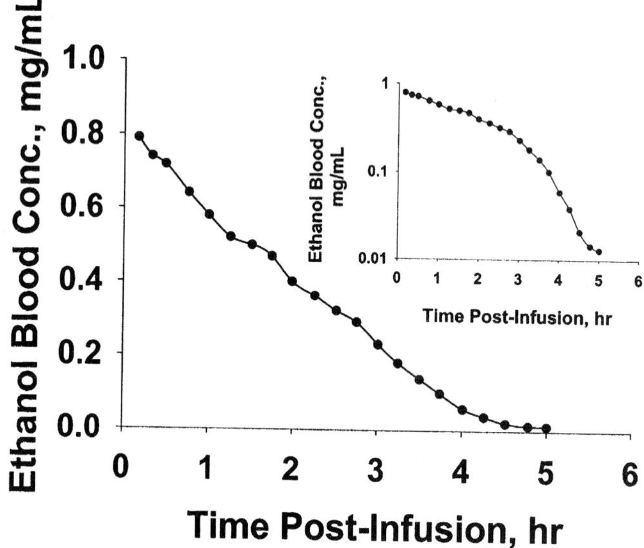

Figure 7. Ethanol blood concentrations as a function of time in one human subject given a 2-hour constant rate intravenous infusion of ethanol (720 ml of 8% v/v ethanol in normal saline). Only the postinfusion data are plotted (i.e., data after the end of the 2-hour infusion; first value deleted). Note that this is a linear scale, and a straight line is obtained until approximately 4 hours after the end of the infusion. The inset graph is a semilogarithmic plot of the same data. Note that a curvilinear line is seen whose slope changes with time until it becomes log-linear only at later times at low concentrations. (Based on data recovered from Wilkinson PK, Sedman AJ, Sakmar E, et al. Blood ethanol concentrations during and following constant-rate intravenous infusion of alcohol. *Clin Pharmacol Ther* 1976;19:213–223. From M. Mayersohn, *unpublished*, with permission from Saguaro Technical Press, Inc, Tucson, AZ, 2002.)

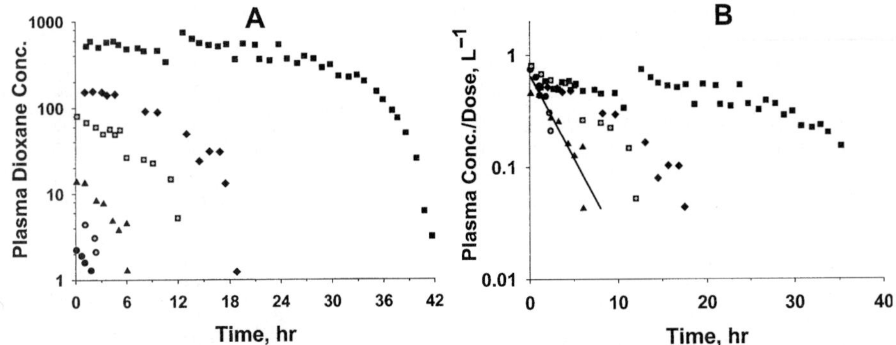

Figure 8. **A:** Semilogarithmic plot of dioxane plasma concentrations as a function of time after the administration of three different intravenous doses to rats. Note that the lowest dose (3 mg/kg) provides a log-linear straight line suggesting first-order kinetics. In contrast, the two higher doses (100 and 1000 mg/kg) result in a typical curvilinear relationship characteristic of a nonlinear saturable process. **B:** Plasma concentrations (for six different doses) divided by dose as a function of time. The principle of superposition (see Fig. 5B) predicts that the resulting data fall onto one line if disposition is described by first-order kinetics. The solid regression line shown represents data from the three smallest doses of dioxane (i.e., 3, 10, and 30 mg/kg). The principle of superposition is violated for all of the larger doses (i.e., 100, 300, and 1000 mg/kg), indicating that some nonlinear, non–first-order process is occurring. Dose key (mg/kg): 3 (●); 10 (○); 30 (▲); 100 (□); 300 (◆); 1000 (■). (Based on data recovered from Young JD, Braun WH, Gehring PJ. The dose-dependent fate of 1,4-dioxane in rats. *J Environ Pathol Toxicol* 1978;2:263–282. From M. Mayersohn, *unpublished*, with permission from Saguaro Technical Press, Inc, Tucson, AZ, 2002.)

linearity applies for the three lowest doses, as expressed by the solid linear regression line. For all other (larger) doses, however, it is clear that dioxane disposition is nonlinear.

The biologic implications of this nonlinear behavior can be appreciated from the graphs illustrated in Figure 9. The general shapes of the relationships shown apply to any first-order (dashed lines) and saturable nonlinear (solid lines) elimination processes; however, the graphs illustrate dioxane behavior in rats. Graph A is a plot of the initial *clearance* of dioxane based on parameter values reported in the literature (3). Because clearance is a measure of the efficiency of elimination (discussed under Clearance Concepts), efficiency decreases with increasing dose, unlike what would be found for a first-order process (dashed line). The apparent $t_{1/2}$ of dioxane is illustrated in graph B and, consistent with the idea of reduced efficiency of removal from the body, the compound stays in the body for a longer and longer time as the dose increases (unlike the behavior of a first-order process; dashed line). Graph C examines what is being referred to as *exposure* as a function of dose. Exposure is related to and often measured by the *area under the plasma concentration-time curve* (AUC), a useful concept that is discussed under Clearance Concepts. For a first-order kinetic process, the greater the dose, the greater the exposure (dashed line); however, exposure increases out of proportion to dose when elimination is saturable. A conse-

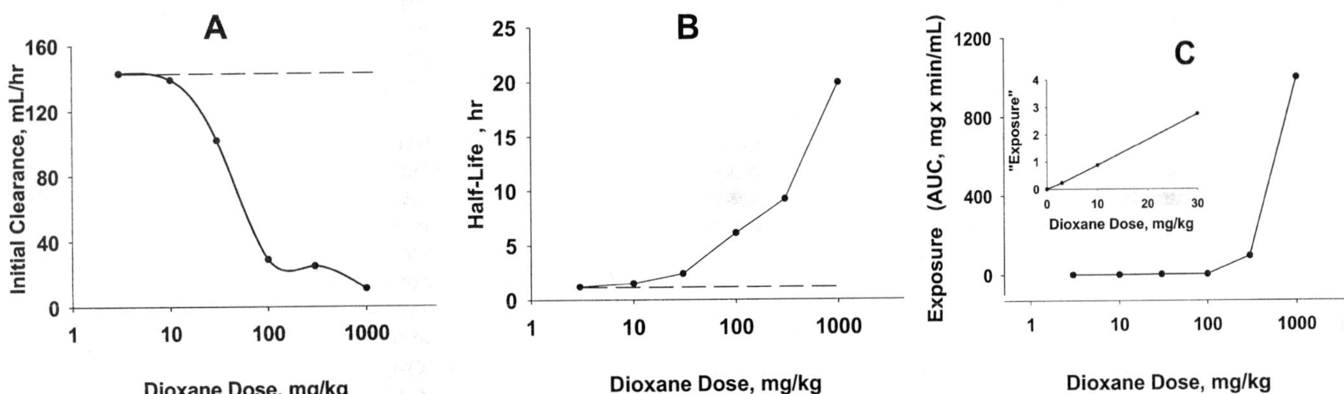

Figure 9. **A:** Initial clearance of dioxane as a function of IV dose given to rats. (The initial clearance was calculated using the parameter values provided in Young JD, Braun WH, Gehring PJ. The dose-dependent fate of 1,4-dioxane in rats. *J Environ Pathol Toxicol* 1978;2:263–282.) Note that clearance, an expression of efficiency of elimination (rate/concentration), decreases as the dose rises. In contrast, clearance is independent of dose for a first-order process (*dashed line*). **B:** Apparent *half-life* of dioxane as a function of IV dose given to rats. The value of *half-life* is based on the initial clearance and apparent volume of distribution. (From Young JD, Braun WH, Gehring PJ. The dose-dependent fate of 1,4-dioxane in rats. *J Environ Pathol Toxicol* 1978;2:263–282, with permission.) Note that *half-life* increases as dose increases. In contrast, half-life is independent of dose for a first-order process (*dashed line*). **C:** *Exposure* to dioxane as a function of IV dose given to rats. *Exposure* is measured as the total area under the dioxane plasma concentration-time curve for each dose. Note that *exposure* increases out of proportion to dose, whereas a linear relationship is expected for a first-order process (*dashed line*). (From M. Mayersohn, *unpublished*, with permission from Saguaro Technical Press, Inc, Tucson, AZ, 2002.)

quence of this behavior is that plasma concentrations on multiple dosing or continued exposure, increase out of proportion to dose (a direct, linear relationship is expected for a first-order process). Furthermore, and of considerable significance, one would expect an abrupt change in the response (or toxicity)-dose relationship at doses above saturation. The graphs illustrated in Figure 9, each representing an important clinical or toxicologic biologic measure, indicate that for a saturable elimination process one does not expect a proportional and predictable relationship with dose. This is in dramatic contrast with a linear, first-order process.

Substrate saturation of enzymatic activity occurs as the result of one of the following conditions: the substrate k_{mm} is small and smaller than plasma concentrations obtained from typical dosing or exposure (e.g., phenytoin); the substrate is ingested in large doses, resulting in plasma concentrations that exceed k_{mm} (e.g., ethanol, salicylates). The latter possibility is especially relevant to the ingestion of a drug overdose or environmental over-exposure and, therefore, is a particularly important consideration in medical toxicology.

There are numerous other mechanisms that may be responsible for nonlinear metabolic behavior, including depletion of metabolic cofactors (e.g., acetaminophen metabolism), reduction in liver blood flow, enzyme induction or inhibition, and substrate-induced hepatic toxicity affecting the previous parameters. Several of these mechanisms suggest that a more inclusive definition of linearity would consider temporal effects. Thus, a *linear system* is one that is both dose and time invariant; the output (or response) is directly related to dose (input) and that relationship remains unchanged at all times. A *nonlinear system* is one that violates either dose or time invariance or both.

Although hepatic metabolism has received the greatest attention with respect to nonlinearity, any route of elimination may undergo nonlinear behavior. For example, the renal excretion of compounds that undergo active tubular secretion (e.g., penicillin) or reabsorption (e.g., nutrients as vitamins, monosaccharides, amino acids) involve transport systems that may be saturated by substrate or inhibited by structurally related compounds. The Michaelis-Menten relationship noted previously applies in an identical fashion to these saturable transport processes, as discussed under Clearance Concepts. Other mechanisms that may result in nonlinear renal excretion include alterations in urine pH (e.g., phencyclidine, methamphetamine) and urine flow (e.g., theophylline) as well as substrate-induced renal toxicity affecting the previous parameters.

DISPOSITION: MODELS

One of the most important functions of any scientific discipline is to make quantitative predictions. This is certainly true in pharmacokinetics, in which one might ask, How does a change in body function or dose affect drug disposition and response? A fairly general approach that is used to make such predictions is through the use of *models*. A model is a hypothetical construct that appears to work in a way similar to that of the system under study—in this case, the human body. A model (any model) only does so, of course, in a limited way. In fact, it is important to bear in mind that "all models are wrong; some models are useful." Useful is often good enough. The human biologic model, which gives rise to a corresponding mathematical model, is usually an abstract notion of how the system is conceived to behave. To create such a model it is necessary to make numerous simplifying assumptions; after all, this is a model and not a duplicate of the system. The correctness of the model predictions is only as good as the quality of the assumptions that have gone into creating the model.

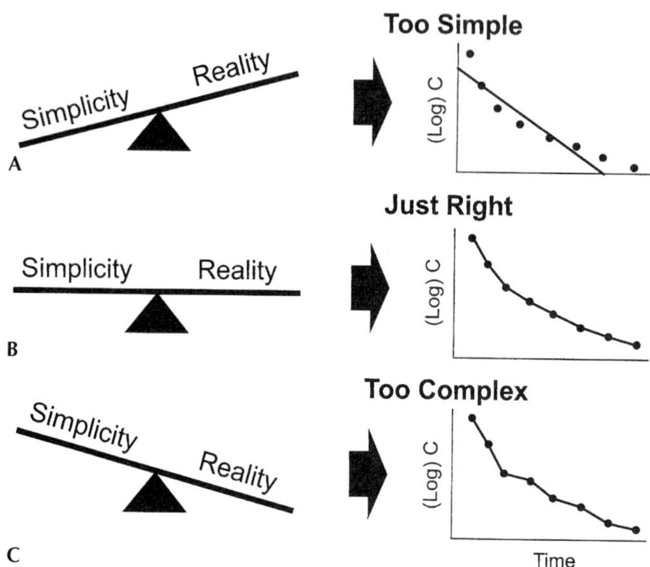

Figure 10. Illustration of the balance needed between simplicity of the model and reality as judged by the plasma concentration-time data. **A:** The model is too simple, as the model-predicted line provides a poor depiction of the actual data. **B:** A reasonable model results in an excellent model-predicted line as it provides a good description of the actual data. A good balance between simplicity and reality is achieved. **C:** The model is unnecessarily complex, resulting in a complicated model equation that exactly connects all of the data points. (From M. Mayersohn, *unpublished*, with permission from Saguaro Technical Press, Inc, Tucson, AZ, 2002.)

All models must balance two opposing needs: simplicity and reality. The model must be simple or it cannot be used in a practical way; we must be able to understand it and write sufficiently simple equations to describe it. The K.I.S.S. principle (*k*eep *i*t *s*imple, *s*tupid) or the rule of parsimony, embodied in the older concept referred to as *Ockham's razor*,* states that the model should be no more complicated than it need be to meet its function, in this case, describing the data. However, if the model is too simple, it does not explain reality (i.e., the data). The simplicity of a model must be balanced by the need of the model to describe the data: If it does not do so, it is useless for predictive purposes. It must also be emphasized, however, that a model can never be any better than the quality of the experimental data that goes into its creation; the experiment and the quality of the data need to be emphasized. In practice, the *best* model is chosen on the basis of statistical comparisons, a discussion of which is beyond the scope of this chapter.

Figure 10 illustrates this idea of balance between simplicity and reality. The model-predicted line in Figure 10A does a poor job in describing the plasma concentration-time data. In this instance the model is too simple, as it does not reflect reality; simplicity is over-weighted. In contrast, the model-predicted line in Figure 10B does a nice job in describing the data. There is a good balance here between simplicity and reality. An unnecessarily complex model and complicated equation results in the predicted line shown in Figure 10C; simplicity is under-weighted.

*Ockham's razor, after William of Ockham (b. 1280 England). "Entia non sunt multiplicanda praeter necessitate"; entities should not be multiplied unnecessarily. Thus, simpler is better. When competing theories lead to the same result, the least complicated is preferred. The simplest most parsimonious explanation for a phenomenon is likely to be the correct one. When seeking to explain a phenomenon, start with the simplest theory. This is opposite a "Rube Goldberg," which uses the most complex methods for completing a task. The *razor* probably represents cutting out the unnecessary details. Einstein takes it one step further: "Everything should be made as simple as possible, but not simpler."

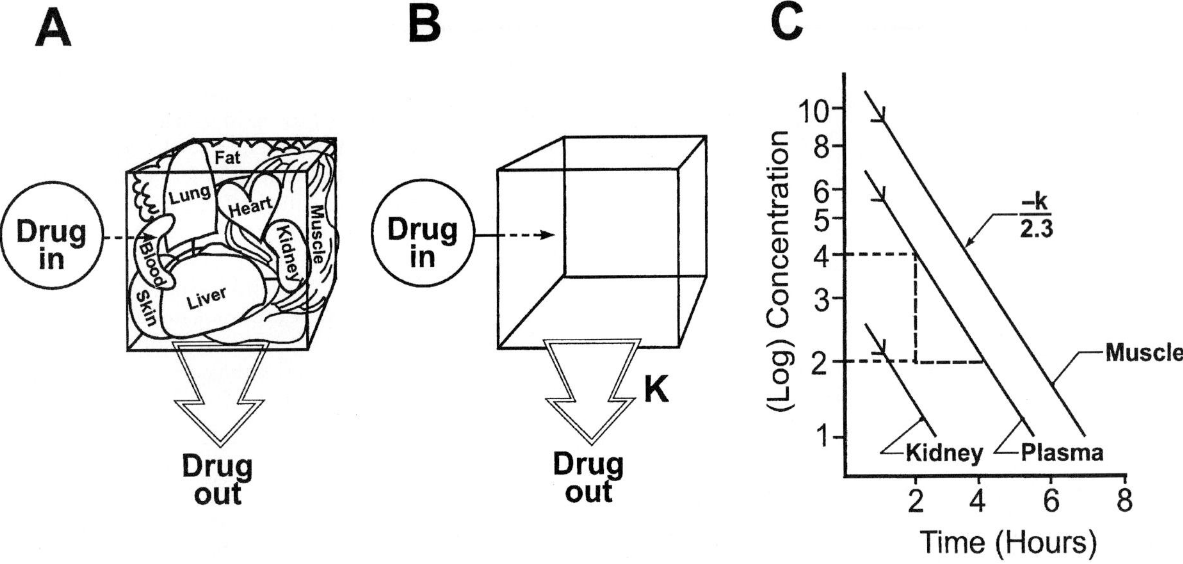

Figure 11. A: A one-compartment open model illustrated from an *anatomic* view. All body tissues and organs are *lumped* together in this single *body* box. Blood connects to all regions. **B:** The one-compartment open model as it is generally presented. K is the apparent overall first-order terminal rate constant. **C:** Semilog concentrations of the drug measured in several tissues after an IV bolus dose. Note that the lines are log-linear at all times after dosing (instantaneous distribution), they are parallel (kinetic homogeneity), but they do not superimpose (lack of concentrational homogeneity). (From Mayersohn M. Toxicokinetics: Measurement of disposition half-life, clearance and residence times. In: Maines M, ed. *Current protocols in toxicology*. New York: John Wiley and Sons, 2000:5.3.3, with permission of Saguaro Technical Press, Inc, 2002, Tucson, AZ.)

Although several approaches are commonly used to analyze data to obtain pharmacokinetic information about a substance, a classic method of data analysis has been referred to as *compartmental modeling*. This approach to modeling visualizes one or more compartments or regions connected together to represent (but are not equivalent to) body tissues. These models are strictly hypothetical and seldom bear any resemblance to physiologic reality, in the sense that real body organs, tissues, or fluids are not actually represented. In contrast, a nonabstract, physiologically meaningful approach exists and is referred to as *physiologically based pharmacokinetic modeling*.

A *compartment* represents body tissues or organs that are lumped together because they behave in the same manner with respect to drug distribution. Thus, body tissues could be lumped together and distinguished from each other as a result of blood flow (well- or poorly perfused) or because they are lean tissues or because they are fatty tissues. The simplest possible model, the *one-compartment open model*, rests on the assumption that all body regions behave the same with regard to drug distribution and this occurs as a result of *instantaneous distribution* to all body regions. Administer an IV bolus dose and the drug instantaneously distributes from the blood to all tissues in the body. Of course, this cannot happen; drug must move at a finite rate from the blood to body tissues, but if this occurs so fast that distribution cannot be accurately measured, then, for practical purposes, distribution is instantaneous. This model and the concentration-time data that it would reflect are illustrated in Figure 11. The data that give rise to this simple model are plotted on semilog axes in Figure 11C. Because the data can be described by a log-linear line, elimination occurs according to first-order kinetics. Because the line is uniformly log-linear at all times (essentially going back to the y-axis), distribution from the blood to all tissues must have occurred rapidly (instantaneously). At least there are no sufficiently early samples taken soon after the IV dose to suggest otherwise. This log-linear line can be described by a single exponential function (i.e., $C = C^0 \cdot e^{-K \cdot t}$) as a result of first-order elimination kinetics and because of instantaneous distribution. Note that the concentration-time lines for different tissues are parallel, indicating that all tissues behave the same kinetically (i.e., *kinetic homogeneity*). The slopes of these lines are identical, and, therefore, values for K and $t_{1/2}$ are the same; there is only one $t_{1/2}$ value for the drug in the body. However, the lines are *not* superimposable. The latter, indicating a lack of concentrational homogeneity, is to be expected as a result of differences in drug binding to different tissues. In the instance shown, muscle tissue, which has higher concentrations than plasma, must bind the drug more than plasma proteins. Plasma concentrations are greater than those in the kidney, suggesting that plasma protein binding must be greater than binding to kidney tissue. This relative ranking of concentrations for the tissues noted is arbitrary and should not be generalized. It is important to recognize that in virtually all experiments it is the *total* concentration of drug that is assayed (i.e., bound and unbound) and plotted. As noted later, the *unbound* concentrations are expected to be identical in all tissues.

The hydromorphone data illustrated in Figure 3B would be interpreted as reflecting first-order kinetics and a one-compartment model, at least for the data plotted. Of course, it is not known what happens before the 3-hour sample. Actually, that is not true; the author of this chapter intentionally deleted the concentration values before 3 hours to illustrate the behavior that was discussed at that point. The complete data set, shown in Figure 12, now indicates a concentration-time curve not consistent with a one-compartment model; the data are behaving in a more complex manner. The display of data, such as that noted in Figure 12, is inconsistent with instantaneous distribution and, therefore, cannot be described by a simple one-compartment model. The initial rapid decline in plasma concentrations that occurs during the first 1 to 2 hours after dosing may be explained by the drug distributing out of the bloodstream and diffusing into other tissues of the body. This movement, unlike the idea of instantaneous distribution, occurs at a measurable rate. This early phase is sometimes referred to as the *distribution phase*, but it is important to keep in mind that elimination also occurs during this phase as

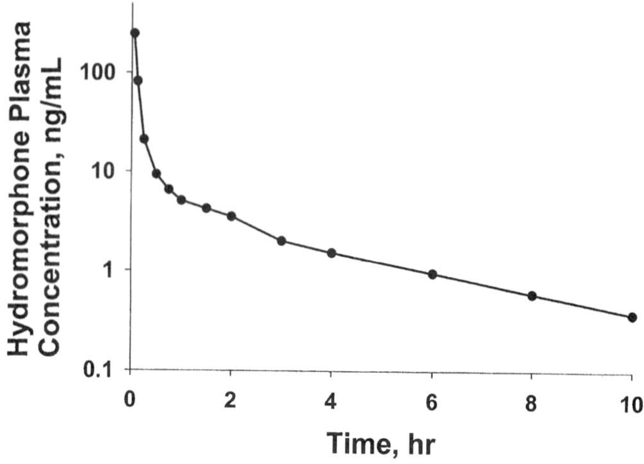

Figure 12. Hydromorphone plasma concentration-time data after an intravenous bolus dose to normal human subjects. The entire data set, which is plotted here, was presented as truncated data shown in Figure 3. The entire data set indicates that drug disposition can be described by a multi-compartment model, rather than by a one-compartment model suggested by the truncated data. Because the terminal data are the same for both plots, the terminal half-life is identical whether all of the data are plotted. (Data recovered and replotted from Parab PV, Ritschel WA, Coyle DE, et al. Pharmacokinetics of hydromorphone after intravenous, peroral and rectal administration to human subjects. *Biopharm Drug Dispos* 1988;9:187–199. From M. Mayersohn, *unpublished*, with permission from Saguaro Technical Press, Inc, Tucson, AZ, 2002.)

well as later times. Once distribution is complete, when there is a type of equilibrium in concentrations between the blood and all other tissues, concentrations in plasma (as well as all other tissues) decline more slowly and these data constitute the *terminal phase*. The latter is sometimes referred to as the elimination phase, but this is not a correct term because the slope of the terminal data depends as much on distribution as it does on elimination. The term noted previously, terminal rate constant or terminal $t_{1/2}$, now has some meaning, as it really does not apply to a one-compartment model (because there is only one phase).

There is need to apply a more complex model, to explain the behavior of the data. Such models require conceiving of the body to be made up of more than one compartment. These *multicompartmental* models require additional compartments consistent with the behavior of the data (e.g., two- or three-compartments). The ultimate selection of the model depends on a statistical comparison of possible choices based on nonlinear regression analysis of the data. Numerous software programs perform the fitting of the data necessary to choose the best model (e.g., WinNonlin, SAAM II, MatLab), but such a discussion is beyond this presentation. A good introduction to nonlinear regression is presented by Motulsky and Ransnas (4).

Reliable parameter values to describe disposition of a drug and the quality of the resulting model depends on experimental design issues, especially analytical parameters (sensitivity, selectivity, reproducibility); frequency; number of samples; and duration of sampling. There is nothing arbitrary about the sampling scheme; it must be designed in accordance with what is known about the disposition of the drug to optimize information about disposition.

The hydromorphone data in Figure 12 suggest that the disposition of the drug can be described by multicompartmental behavior and by, at least, a two-compartment model. A two-compartment (open) model is depicted in Figure 13. Those organs and tissues that receive the drug rapidly are lumped together (*A*, on the left) to form one region or compartment. In this instance those organs include, in addition to blood, the heart, lung, kidney, and liver. In contrast, those regions to which the drug distributes slowly are also lumped together to form another region or compartment (*A*, on the right). The regions depicted are (arbitrarily) the skin, muscle, and fat. As noted in the middle figure, compartment 1 or the *central compartment* is made up of those tissues that receive the drug rapidly. In contrast, the attached compartment 2 or *peripheral compartment* contains tissues that receive drug at a measurable rate. Drug is eliminated from compartment 1 (which contains the major organs of elimination, liver and kidney). Connecting the two compartments are two first-order *micro-rate constants*.

The relationship that is used to describe this profile is in the form of a multiexponential equation: one exponent for each compartment, after IV bolus dosing. The two most commonly used expressions are

$$C = A \cdot e^{-\alpha \cdot t} + B \cdot e^{-\beta \cdot t} \text{ OR } C = A_1 \cdot e^{-\lambda_1 \cdot t} + A_2 \cdot e^{-\lambda_2 \cdot t} \quad \text{[Eq. 15]}$$

The rate constants (α and β or λ_1 and λ_2), which are first-order, have units of reciprocal time. These rate constants are often referred to as *hybrid rate constants*, because they depend on all of the other micro-rate constants in the model, as noted in Figure 13. The terminal $t_{1/2}$ and rate constant, which has a number of symbols (K, β, λ_N, or λ_Z), is as much affected by distribution as elimination of the drug. The coefficients (A and B or A_1 and A_2), which represent intercepts on the y-axis, have units of concentration.

Figure 13C presents a semilog plot of concentrations in plasma and in two other tissues, one in compartment 1 (kidney) and the other in compartment 2 (muscle), as a function of time after an IV bolus dose of drug. The curvilinearity noted in the plasma data is an indication of the need to describe the data according to multicompartmental behavior and, in this instance, by a two-compartment model. The tissues, which are in rapid equilibrium with the blood (and are present in compartment 1), such as the kidney, have a concentration-time curve identical with that of plasma. In contrast, concentrations initially increase in those tissues that receive the drug at a measurable rate (and are present in compartment 2), such as the muscle tissue, and then decline once a type of equilibrium is achieved with plasma concentration. Once the *post–distributive phase* is reached, concentrations in all tissues decline in parallel according to the terminal $t_{1/2}$. However, as noted previously, tissue concentrations do not superimpose due to differences in drug binding to those tissues.

Other, more complex multicompartment models may be necessary to describe the disposition of certain compounds. The necessity to use such models is a consequence of the distribution properties of those compounds. Thus, in addition to its distribution to two other lumped regions, a third compartment may be needed if a tissue, such as adipose, slowly accumulates a lipid-soluble compound. These models are always presented as *mammillary models*, meaning that all compartments feed off or are connected to the central compartment. Furthermore, it has been assumed that all elimination of drug occurs from the central compartment. This may not be the case, for example, if drug is broken down chemically or enzymatically in a tissue that forms part of the peripheral compartment. Such complications have been intentionally avoided here.

Plasma concentration-time data may be analyzed with use of compartmental models, as previously noted. This *parametric* approach requires fitting the data to the best possible model, from which the parameters of the model equation are obtained. Further treatment of those parameters permits the calculation of all disposition characteristics of the drug under study. In contrast, a *noncompartmental* or *nonparametric* approach can also be applied to the same plasma concentration-time data set. In this

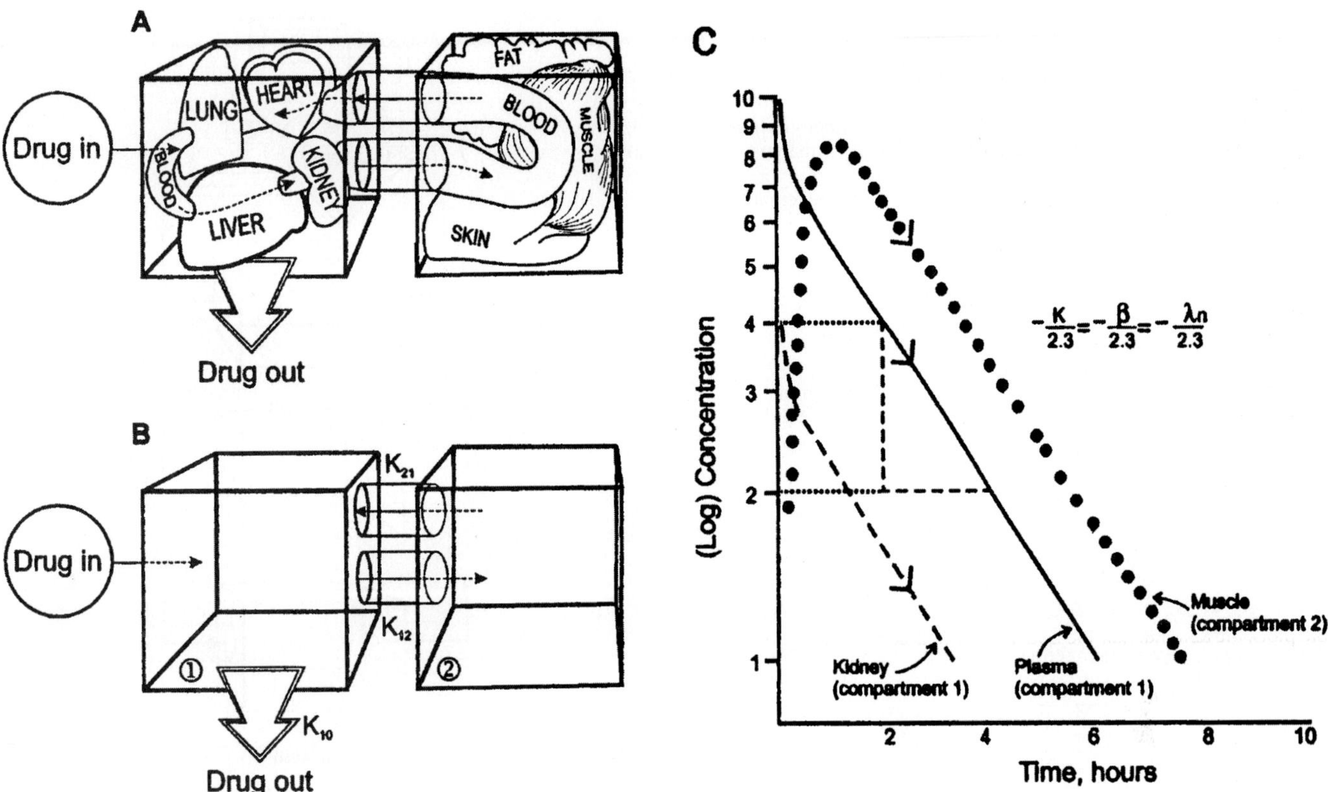

Figure 13. A: An *anatomic* view of a two-compartment open model. Organs and tissues that rapidly receive drug are lumped together in one compartment (*left*), whereas other regions that receive the drug more slowly due to a measurable distribution process are lumped together to form another compartment (*right*). **B:** A conventional scheme used to present a two-compartment open model. Drug enters into the first or central compartment where there is rapid equilibration with blood. Drug is eliminated from this compartment by a first-order rate constant (noted as k_{10} or k_{el}). The second or peripheral compartment into which drug distributes from blood at a measurable rate is connected to the first compartment by first-order micro-rate constants, k_{12} and k_{21}. **C:** The (log) concentration-time, which leads to the necessity for using a multi-compartment model, in this instance, a two-compartment model. Drug has been given as an intravenous bolus. Note that the plasma concentration-time is curvilinear, denoting multi-compartmental behavior. Other tissues associated with the plasma or compartment 1 (e.g., kidney) have lines parallel with the plasma line at all times. Regions contained in compartment 2 (e.g., muscle) have a rising (due to distribution) and then declining concentration-time profile. All of the terminal lines become parallel, giving a single terminal rate constant and half-life, but the concentrations do not superimpose (due to differences in drug binding). The terminal (hybrid) rate constant has a number of symbols, all having the same meaning: K, β, λ_n, or λ_Z. (From Mayersohn M. Toxicokinetics: Measurement of disposition half-life, clearance and residence times. In: Maines M, ed. *Current protocols in toxicology*. New York: John Wiley and Sons, 2000:5.35, with permission of Saguaro Technical Press, Inc, 2002, Tucson, AZ.)

instance, however, it is not necessary to fit the data according to a compartmental model, but rather the useful parameters describing the disposition properties of the drug can be obtained from analysis of the terminal data in conjunction with area analyses. Both approaches provide virtually equivalent parameter values. The disposition parameters of drugs that are of greatest interest are terminal $t_{1/2}$ and rate constant, apparent volume of distribution, and clearance. Other parameters, however, may also be determined such as mean residence time, steady state volume of distribution, and others. These are noted where appropriate. The general type of analysis that may be applied to the curves concerned with here has been given the acronym SHAM, which stands for *s*lope, *h*eight, *a*rea, and *m*oment (5). Consider a plasma concentration-time curve: *slope* gives an estimate of rate constant and $t_{1/2}$; *height* is related to apparent volumes; *area* gives an estimate of exposure from which clearance is calculated; *moments* give rise to residence times. Although many of these calculations are cited later, Table 1 compares the compartmental and noncompartmental approaches for estimation of $t_{1/2}$, apparent volume, and clearance after an IV bolus dose.

Although the previous two methods of analysis are commonly used in characterizing drug disposition, and they are practical methods of data calculation, they are sometimes criticized on the basis of lack of physiologic reality, a charge especially levied against the compartmental approach. In stark contrast to these methods of analysis is an approach referred to as *physiologically based pharmacokinetic models*. As its name implies, it is an attempt to ground the analysis in physiologic reality, and, as all methods of analysis, it has advantages and disadvantages. The prime advantage to this model is that disposition of a drug or chemical is based on real measurements (e.g., concentrations in numerous tissues with time, tissue weights, tissue blood flows, and so forth), as depicted in Figure 14. Each *compartment* is actually a real body organ, tissue, or region that can be removed, weighed, and drug or chemical content determined by assay. Connecting each of these real physiologic areas are real, measurable blood flows (indicated by the arrows), not artificial

TABLE 1. Comparison of compartmental and noncompartmental determination of parameters of disposition

Parameter	Compartmental analysis	Noncompartmental analysis
Half-life, $t_{1/2}$:	From curve fitting: $C = A_1 \cdot e^{-\lambda_1 \cdot t} + A_2 \cdot e^{-\lambda_2 \cdot t}$ λ_2 $t_{1/2} = \frac{0.693}{\lambda_2}$	From the terminal line: λ_2 $t_{1/2} = \frac{0.693}{\lambda_2}$
Apparent volume, V_d:	From curve fitting: $V_d = \frac{\text{IV dose}}{\lambda_2 \cdot \sum_{i=1}^{2} \frac{A_i}{\lambda_i}} = \frac{\text{IV dose}}{\lambda_2 \cdot (AUC)_0^\infty}$	From terminal line and $(AUC)_0^\infty$: $V_d = \frac{\text{IV dose}}{\lambda_2 \cdot (AUC)_0^\infty}$
Clearance, CL_s:	From curve fitting: $CL_s = \frac{\text{IV dose}}{\sum_{i=1}^{2} \frac{A_i}{\lambda_i}} = \frac{\text{IV dose}}{(AUC)_0^\infty}$	From $(AUC)_0^\infty$: $CL_s = \frac{\text{IV dose}}{(AUC)_0^\infty}$

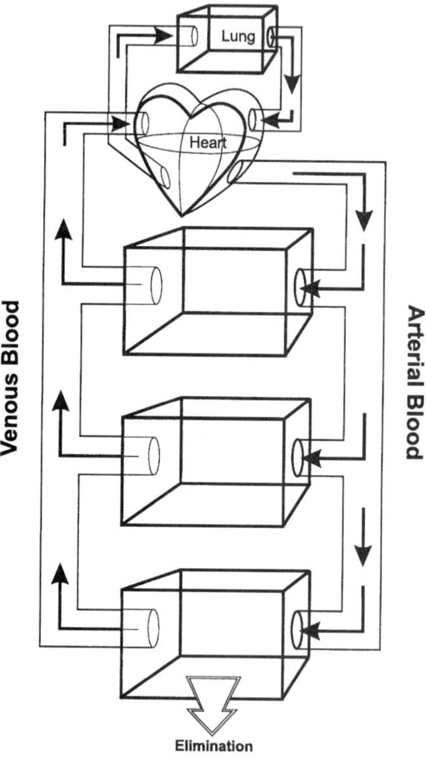

Figure 14. A schematic representation of a simple physiologically based pharmacokinetic model (PB/PK). This model is limited to the heart, lung, and three other organs/tissues, one of which is an eliminating organ (e.g., liver, kidney). The arrows indicate blood flow either entering (arterial) or exiting (venous) the organs (with the exception of the lung, which receives venous flow). The PB/PK model uses real values for blood flows, organ weights, drug partition from blood to tissue, and other potentially important parameters (e.g., binding, V_{max}, k_{mm}, and so forth). The experimental data involve quantitation of the drug (and, perhaps, metabolites) in all tissues/organs of the model as a function of time after dosing or exposure. (From M. Mayersohn, *unpublished*, with permission from Saguaro Technical Press, Inc, Tucson, AZ, 2002.)

intercompartmental transfer rate constants. Furthermore, perhaps the most intriguing and useful aspect of this model is that, although it may be experimentally characterized in the mouse or rat, it has the potential to be scaled up to humans. It is this quality that has most attracted researchers in the area of toxicology and risk-assessment.

The disadvantage to this type of modeling is the large number of experiments and extensive amount of data that must be amassed to thoroughly characterize the drug or chemical in the animal species under study. Scaling up to humans becomes that much more of a challenge. It is well beyond the purpose of this chapter to provide an adequate working presentation of physiologically based pharmacokinetic models, and the reader is referred to several recent publications (6,7).

DISTRIBUTION

Distribution or translocation is the process of a molecule moving from the blood to other areas of the body. The blood acts as the primary communicating system of the body, and this movement of drug or chemical to the receptor(s) at the site of action is essential for production of a desired response or, at higher doses, an exaggerated response that may appear as toxicity. All other processes are irrelevant unless this desired event occurs. The other side to this story, however, is the movement of drug or chemical to other areas of the body not associated with a desired response, but which can give rise to undesired, adverse, or toxic events. The occurrence of these desired and undesired effects is the *ying and yang* of drug therapy, analogous to a two-sided sword, and only in rare cases is this not the prevailing rule.

The distribution process has two components, how fast and how much? The former, how fast, affects the onset of a response and the resulting compartmental model. Thus, rapid-acting IV general anesthetics (e.g., thiopental) distribute quickly from the blood to the brain and result in a fast onset of anesthesia. That rapid movement has a parallel, slower component that describes distribution to other tissues (e.g., adipose tissue) resulting in multicompartmental behavior.

The rate of distribution is a complex function of the physical-chemical properties of the drug molecule, the properties of the tissue and blood flow to that tissue. There are two possible rate-limiting steps to drug distribution from blood to any given organ or tissue: blood flow and permeability. Blood flow is the limiting step for the majority of compounds and for the majority of body regions. The compound needs to have a moderate molecular weight (most drugs are small organic molecules) and a reasonable oil-to-water partition coefficient ($K_{O/W}$), which provides sufficient ability to traverse cell membranes. It has been shown (8) that the $t_{1/2}$ for tissue distribution (or redistribution) is a direct function of the tissue to blood partition coefficient ($K_{Tissue/Blood}$) and inversely related to blood perfusion rate (Q_{Tissue}) per tissue volume (V_{Tissue}), Q_{Tissue}/V_{Tissue}.

$$t_{1/2} \text{ for tissue equilibration} = \frac{0.693 \cdot K_{Tissue/Blood}}{Q_{Tissue}/V_{Tissue}} \quad \text{[Eq. 16]}$$

The tissue to blood partition coefficient ($K_{Tissue/Blood}$) is obtained from the ratio of concentrations of the compound in tissue to that in blood once an equilibrium has been achieved. The greater this number, the greater the *attraction* of the compound for that tissue, which generally means significant binding to tissue proteins. This may seem somewhat counter-intuitive, but having a greater capacity to accumulate a substance translates into taking a longer time to achieve equilibrium. The latter observation is exemplified by the many lipid-soluble environmental poisons (e.g., insecticides, herbicides) that take a long time to achieve equilibrium in adipose tissue, which has a large capacity to accumulate such material. The converse, loss from adipose tissue, also takes a long time. The role of the denominator is to be expected; the poorer the perfusion of the tissue by blood, the longer it takes to achieve equilibrium.

The following comparisons reflect the preceding discussion. For a given compound having the same value of $K_{Tissue/Blood}$ for all tissues, those tissues with the greatest blood perfusion per tissue volume achieve equilibrium the fastest (e.g., brain faster than skin and skin faster than bone). The approach to equilibrium, as judged by increasing $t_{1/2}$, follows the order from the greatest blood perfusion rate to the slowest. In contrast, for different compounds, the $t_{1/2}$ of distribution for a given tissue increases the greater the value of $K_{Tissue/Blood}$.

Blood perfusion may not always be the rate-limiting step to distribution. If the molecule is large or polar and must penetrate a membrane barrier, the rate-limiting step becomes permeability across that barrier. Thus, lipid-solubility and the fraction of the compound that is nonionized at blood pH determine the rate of movement across the blood–brain barrier for a series of, for example, barbiturates. Similar considerations apply to placental and mamillary transfer from the blood.

There are two other issues that substantially complicate a discussion of the distribution process: the apparent volume of distribution and plasma protein binding. The *apparent volume of distribution* (V or V_d) is a hypothetical space into which a substance distributes in the body. It is rarely a real, physiologic space, but it serves several useful functions. First, the value gives some indication of the extent of movement of the substance out of the bloodstream; although, it gives no indication where in the body the substance resides. Thus, the greater the value of V_d, more of the drug is found in tissues outside of the bloodstream. Second, V_d may serve as a useful proportionality constant between the blood concentration and the amount of the substance in the body at any given time. The latter can find use in calculation of residual amounts in the body and in designing dosing regimens. To further complicate this idea is the fact that there are several different apparent volumes of distribution, depending on the compartmental model. In a one-compartment model, there is only one apparent volume of distribution. In a two-compartment model, there is an apparent volume for each of the two compartments (V_1 or $V_{central}$ and V_2 or $V_{peripheral}$). There is also a volume referred to as the *steady state volume of distribution*, and this is noted later.

A useful definition is *the apparent volume of distribution is the imaginary volume that a substance would occupy in the body if it were present throughout the body at the same concentration as in the blood or plasma*. For example, if a substance were present in blood at a concentration of 1 mg/L and the concentration in liver tissue was 100 mg/L, the liver is behaving as if it were equal to approximately 100 L of blood for every liter volume of liver tissue. Obviously, this apparent volume is strictly a hypothetical value. Note that the reference fluid is blood or plasma: the apparent volume is relative to the concentrations of the substance in blood or plasma. This is a reasonable choice of reference fluid because it is readily accessible for sampling and it is the bloodstream that connects to all parts of the body. Another way to look at this volume is to use a different reference tissue. For example, consider the apparent volume of distribution of iodine after an IV dose. Based on the small concentrations that are produced in the blood, iodine appears to have a large apparent volume of distribution; most of that compound resides in tissues outside of the blood. Now, change the reference fluid to be the thyroid tissue, where most of the iodine is located, and one calculates, relative to the thyroid tissue, a small apparent volume of distribution; most of the iodine resides in that reference tissue.

Another way to illustrate this apparent volume is shown in Figure 15. There is a need to determine the exact volume of a tank, which is thought to hold approximately 1000 L of fluid. To do so, 1000 mg of a dye is added to the tank containing water, and the fluid is mixed well. A sample is taken. The resulting concentration of the dye, in the scenario at the top of the figure, is determined to be 1 mg/L. The volume of the tank (amount/concentration) is calculated to be 1000 L—exactly what was expected. The experiment is repeated in another tank (bottom of figure) in an identical fashion, but this time the sample is assayed to contain 0.01 mg/L with a resulting tank volume of 100,000 L. This is not possible: the tank can only hold 1000 L. What happened? As noted in the bottom figure, most of the substance has been adsorbed onto the interior surface of the tank; the molecules have been taken out of the solution. The apparent

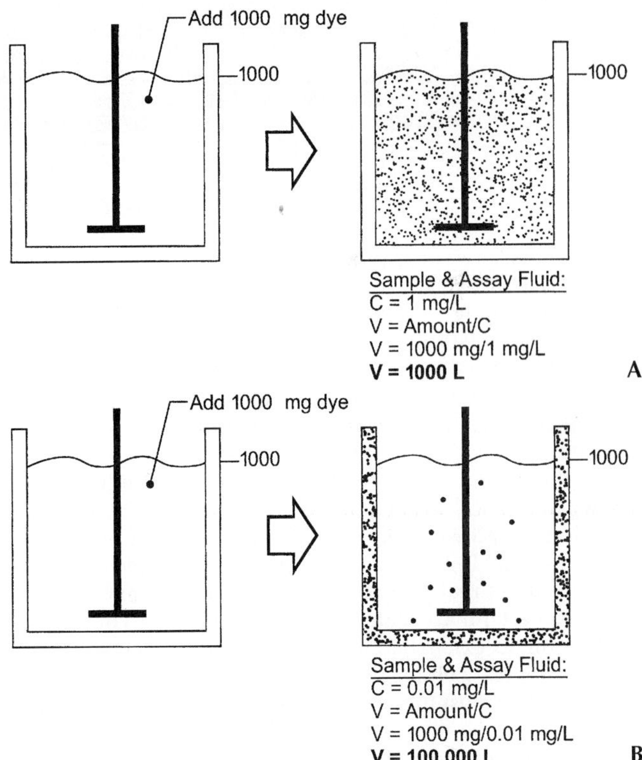

Figure 15. Illustration of the determination and meaning of the apparent volume of distribution. **A:** 1000 mg of a water-soluble dye is added to a tank that holds approximately 1000 L of water. The dye is thoroughly mixed in the fluid of the tank and a sample taken. The sample is assayed to have a concentration of 1 mg/L, and the apparent volume of the tank is determined to be 1000 L, consistent with the actual volume. **B:** The same experiment as noted previously, but this time the assay of the sample gives a concentration of dye of 0.01 mg/L. The resulting (impossible) volume of the tank is calculated to be 100,000 L. Much of the dye has been *distributed* to the surface of the tank (i.e., adsorbed), giving rise to a hypothetically large apparent volume, relative to the reference fluid. (From M. Mayersohn, *unpublished*, with permission from Saguaro Technical Press, Inc, Tucson, AZ, 2002.)

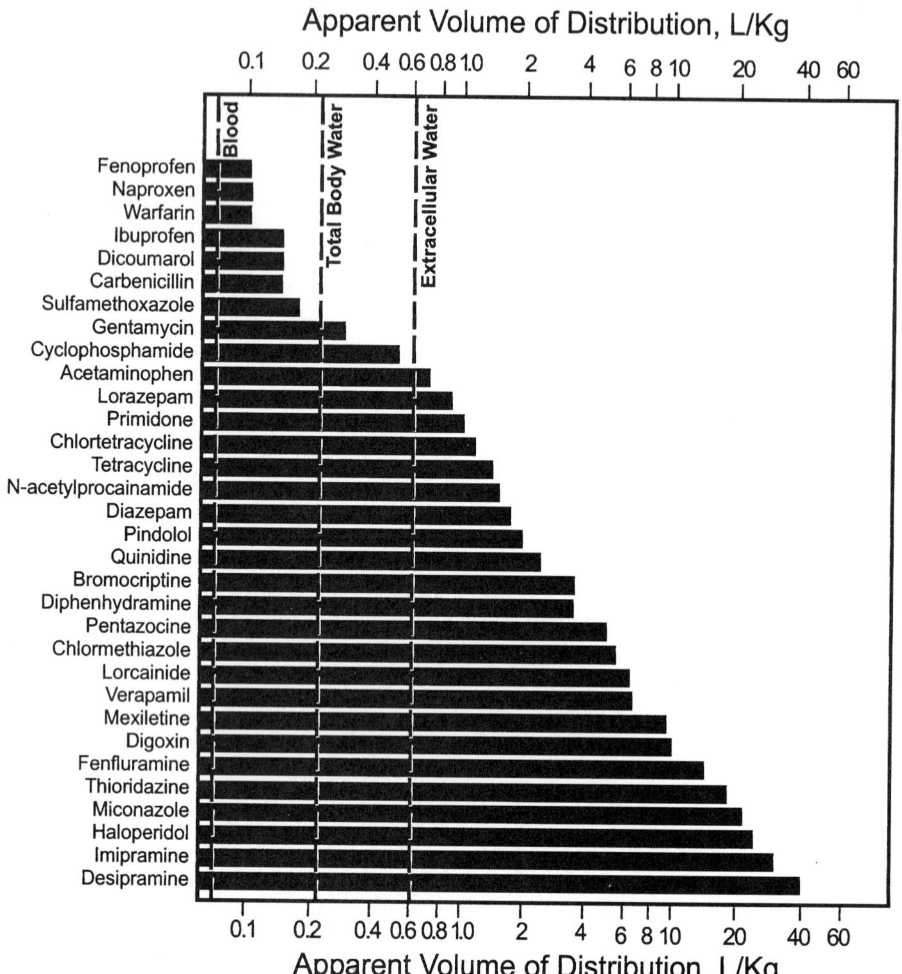

Figure 16. The apparent volumes of distribution of selected drugs (L/kg) illustrating the wide range of values (approximately 0.1 to 40 L/kg). Note that the scale is logarithmic. The three vertical lines that are being used for reference purposes illustrate real physiologic volumes. Those volumes are, from left to right, blood, extracellular water, and total body water. (From M. Mayersohn, *unpublished*, with permission from Saguaro Technical Press, Inc, Tucson, AZ, 2002.)

space that the dye occupies is relative to the remaining concentration of dye in the tank fluid, a small concentration. The resulting volume is huge and not real. This is exactly what happens to compounds after they gain access to the blood; they distribute from the blood to other tissues and they bind there. The compound does not stay in the blood as it did not stay in the tank fluid, the reference fluid.

The wide range of apparent volumes of distribution among selected drugs is illustrated in Figure 16. Note that the scale is logarithmic to accommodate the wide range in values (approximately 0.1 to 40 L/kg). For comparison purposes, vertical lines illustrate three real physiologic spaces (blood, extracellular water, and total body water). The large apparent volumes are attributable to extensive binding to tissue proteins. Clearly, these are not real volumes or physiologic spaces.

Perhaps the most important role that apparent volume plays in drug disposition is as it affects terminal $t_{1/2}$. An important relationship in this regard is the following:

$$t_{1/2} = \frac{0.693 \cdot V_d}{CL_s} \qquad \text{[Eq. 17]}$$

The previous relationship is mathematically and functionally correct. Because this equation is mathematically correct, it can be used to solve for apparent volume or systemic clearance (CL_S). It is important to recognize, however, that the only way to understand the relationship among these parameters is to view them as presented in equation 17; $t_{1/2}$ is *dependent* on apparent volume of distribution and systemic clearance and not the other way around. Compounds that have a large apparent volume, in general, are expected to have a long $t_{1/2}$, unless systemic clearance is high. Again, this reemphasizes the fact that the terminal $t_{1/2}$ depends as much on distribution as it does on elimination (i.e., clearance). Dioxin present in Agent Orange, used as a defoliant during the Vietnam War, has a $t_{1/2}$ in humans of approximately 7 years (9). Compounds with a large apparent volume of distribution have a long $t_{1/2}$ because large quantities reside in areas that are not immediately accessible to the eliminating organs; they must move from the tissue to blood and then through the eliminating organ(s) to be eliminated from the body. Slow movement from such a tissue site to the bloodstream, a process referred to as *redistribution*, essentially rate-limits the elimination process and leads to a prolonged $t_{1/2}$. Recall from a previous discussion, that the rate of redistribution is the reverse of the accumulation process from blood to tissue. The $t_{1/2}$ for both processes is governed by the value, $K_{Tissue/Blood}$; the larger that value, the longer the $t_{1/2}$. Compounds with large values of $K_{Tissue/Blood}$ also have large apparent volumes of distribution.

In an attempt to provide some biologic meaning to the apparent volume of distribution and based on physiologic values in a normal healthy adult man, the following relationship has been developed (10).

$$V_d = 7 + 8 \cdot f_U + V_T\left(\frac{f_U}{f_{U,T}}\right) \qquad \text{[Eq. 18]}$$

The apparent volume of distribution (in liters) is given by a constant (7 L); the unbound or free fraction of drug in the plasma

(f_U); a *tissue* volume (V_T), which represents the space into which the drug distributes minus the extracellular space; and the unbound fraction of drug in the *tissue* ($f_{U,T}$). The unbound fractions (f_U and $f_{U,T}$) are the ratio of unbound drug concentration to total (i.e., bound plus unbound) drug concentration. A drug with a small apparent volume can be approximated by the first two terms, whereas a drug with a large volume is estimated by the last term only.

$$\text{Small volume drug: } V_d \cong 7 + 8 \cdot f_U$$

$$\text{Large volume drug: } V_d \cong V_T\left(\frac{f_U}{f_{U,T}}\right) \quad \text{[Eq. 19]}$$

Thus, the smallest apparent volume of a substance that is totally unbound to plasma (i.e., $f_U \cong 1$) is approximately 15 L, whereas the smallest volume for a substance that is totally bound to plasma proteins (i.e., $f_U \cong 0$) is approximately 7 L. Note that in between these two extremes, a change in plasma protein binding does not lead to a directly proportional change in volume (i.e., as f_U increases, V_d increases in a less than proportional manner).

A compound that has a large apparent volume has a large volume as a result of binding to tissue proteins. That binding is expressed by the value of $f_{U,T}$ in the third term in the general equation 18. Extensive binding to tissue protein results in a small value for $f_{U,T}$, which, in turn, makes the third term large and overwhelmingly larger than the first two terms (which are ignored in the simplification of equation 19). In this instance, any change in the unbound fraction for either plasma or tissue binding results in a directly proportional change in apparent volume. As shown in Figure 16, there are many compounds that have large apparent volumes of distribution. What are considered small and large apparent volumes? There are no definitive rules, but, as an approximation, a volume less than approximate total body water (approximately 0.6 L/kg) might be considered small, whereas a volume greater than approximately 1 L/kg might be considered large. These are arbitrary demarcations, however. Making these approximations becomes useful when attempting to predict how a change in binding might affect the $t_{1/2}$ of a drug, as discussed later under Clearance Concepts.

Plasma protein binding (especially any change in that value) and the disposition and response to a compound is one of the most confusing issues in pharmacokinetics. Many of those ideas are best developed with reference to clearance concepts, which follow this section. Protein binding is generally thought to be a simple, reversible process that may be described by principles of mass action. Binding is determined by an *in vitro* method that requires separation of unbound from total drug. The two most commonly used methods are equilibrium dialysis and ultrafiltration. It is important to keep in mind that all assays used to quantify drug concentrations in blood or plasma (e.g., those reported during therapeutic monitoring or from toxicologic screening) measure *total* concentration and not unbound concentration. This is a consequence of how the samples are handled. Plasma proteins (e.g., albumin) are not able to easily traverse the capillary membrane, and, therefore, it is generally believed that only unbound drug distributes from blood; moves across the capillary membrane; and equilibrates with unbound drug in all tissues, including the receptor at the site of action. As a consequence, it is the unbound drug concentration that drives response and toxicity. It is on this premise that there is great interest in the unbound drug concentration and any changes that may occur to it as a result of, for example, drug-drug interactions or disease states. It can be stated here, although discussed later under Multiple Dosing, that drug displacement interactions are rarely of any clinical importance. Furthermore, although seeming to be illogical and counter intuitive, *the unbound plasma concentration is not determined or affected by plasma protein binding.* This point is discussed later under Multiple Dosing.

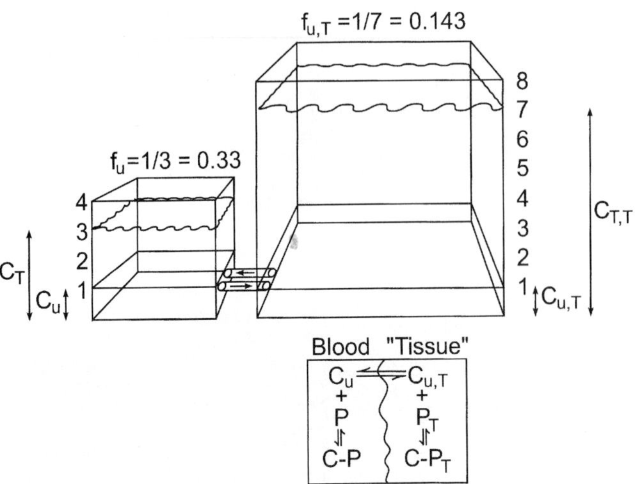

Figure 17. The bottom scheme indicates that three equilibria need to be considered when examining blood and tissue binding. These binding equilibria include: the equilibrium plasma protein binding (*left*), the equilibrium tissue protein binding (*right*), and the equilibrium of unbound drug between blood and tissue. The large graph illustrates these individual equilibrium conditions. The total concentration of drug in the blood (C_T; *left*) is three units, whereas the unbound concentration (C_U) is 1 unit. Thus, the unbound fraction of drug in blood is 0.33. The unbound drug equilibrates between blood and tissue so that the unbound concentration in the tissue ($C_{U,T}$) is the same as in the blood, 1 unit. In contrast, the total concentration of drug in tissue ($C_{T,T}$) is 7 units, giving an unbound fraction in tissue ($f_{U,T}$) of 0.143. Note $f_U \neq f_{U,T}$, but $C_U = C_{U,T}$. (From M. Mayersohn, *unpublished*, with permission from Saguaro Technical Press, Inc, Tucson, AZ, 2002.)

Figure 17 illustrates the equilibrium between blood and some tissue. The bottom part of the figure illustrates the separation by a membrane of blood and some tissue and indicates that three equilibria exist. In the blood, unbound drug (C_U) binds reversibly with protein (P) to form the bound drug complex (C-P). An identical equilibrium exists in the tissue, but now unbound drug in tissue ($C_{U,T}$) binds reversibly with protein in the tissue (P_T) to form a drug-tissue protein complex (C-P_T). There is no reason to believe that those equilibria are the same (i.e., it is not likely that the extent of plasma protein binding is the same as tissue protein binding of drug; $f_U \neq f_{U,T}$). The most important equilibrium is that between blood and tissue and the figure indicates that the unbound concentrations of drug are equal ($C_U = C_{U,T}$; *not* the unbound fractions). The larger graph further illustrates this discussion. The height of the *fluid* in the blood and tissue is analogous to concentrations. The total concentration of drug in blood (left) is 3 units, whereas the unbound concentration is 1 unit (f_U = 0.33). The total concentration of drug in the tissue (on the right) is 7 units—greater than total blood concentration due to greater tissue protein binding. The unbound concentration, 1 unit, is identical to the unbound concentration in blood. Note, however, that the unbound fraction in tissue is 0.143, reflecting the greater tissue protein binding compared to plasma protein binding.

Figure 18 illustrates the wide range of plasma protein binding of drugs in humans, expressed as percent unbound, for selected drugs. Lithium is not bound (f_U = 1; 100% unbound), whereas warfarin is extensively bound to plasma proteins (f_U = 0.01; 1% unbound). For the vast majority of compounds, plasma and tissue protein binding remains constant over a fairly large concentration range, although there are instances of concentration-dependent binding. The latter is most likely to occur for com-

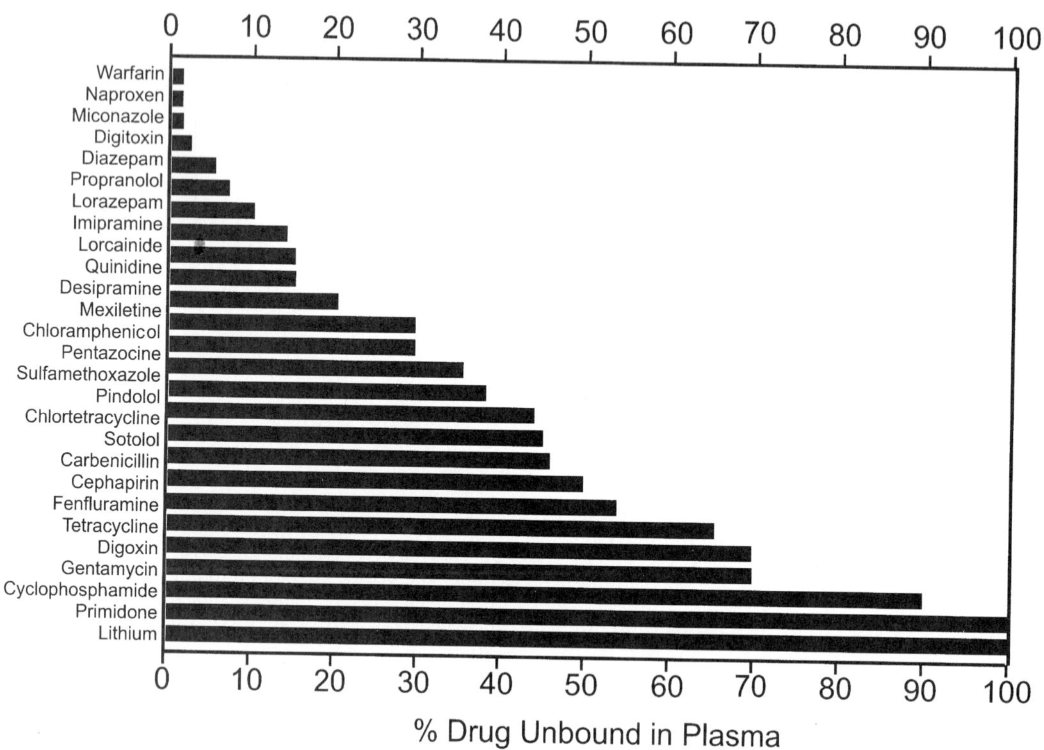

Figure 18. Illustration of the percentage drug unbound to human plasma proteins for a selection of drugs. (From M. Mayersohn, *unpublished*, with permission from Saguaro Technical Press, Inc, Tucson, AZ, 2002.)

pounds present at high concentrations or those compounds that bind to proteins present at low concentrations but that have low binding capacity (e.g., α_1-acid glycoprotein). Plasma protein binding may also be influenced by disease states or age that result in a reduction in plasma protein concentration and, therefore, binding capacity. Displacement interactions can also give rise to a change in plasma protein binding of a drug, but whether these changes in f_U change the unbound plasma concentration is another matter.

Any change in plasma protein binding or tissue protein binding expressed as a change in the unbound fractions, f_U or $f_{U,T}$, results in a change in the apparent volume of distribution, which, in turn, may alter the value for terminal $t_{1/2}$. A change in the apparent volume and the direction and magnitude of change can be judged with reference to the basic volume equation 18 or, more simply, using the approximations noted in equation 19. The relationship between apparent volume and $t_{1/2}$ is illustrated in the following section.

CLEARANCE CONCEPTS

One of the most useful physiologically grounded and predictive concepts in pharmacokinetics is that of *clearance*. Clearance provides a means of understanding the basic, underlying mechanisms associated with organ elimination of a compound and how it may be altered. Clearance also serves as a unifying concept, which permits interrelating other variables and parameters (such as apparent volume, $t_{1/2}$, and plasma protein binding). Finally, clearance is what controls the ultimate plasma concentrations of a substance achieved after multiple dosing or long-term exposure (at steady state). Understanding clearance is essential if one wants to interpret, for example, drug-drug interactions or the effects that a disease state has on drug disposition.

Several measures to characterize drug elimination or loss from the body are available, including rate of elimination, the elimination rate constant, and $t_{1/2}$. The problem with each of these measures is that they cannot stand on their own; they are not *independent* estimates of the efficiency of the removal process. Rate of elimination is a function of concentration, which is usually changing with time after dosing. The rate constant of elimination and $t_{1/2}$ are a function of apparent volume and clearance, as noted in equation 17. Therefore, $t_{1/2}$, although a useful parameter and one easily understood, has little use from the perspective of understanding the physiologic basis of the elimination process or judging the mechanisms responsible for changes in its value. A good illustration of this point is the observation that the $t_{1/2}$ of certain lipid-soluble drugs (primarily eliminated by hepatic metabolism) increase with age in adult humans. This has been noted for the benzodiazepine derivative diazepam (11) and the rapidly acting IV anesthetic thiopental (12). The thiopental example is illustrated in Figure 19, which portrays the relationship between age and the terminal $t_{1/2}$, apparent volume of distribution, and clearance. The relationship between $t_{1/2}$ and age (A), taken by itself, might suggest reduced hepatic elimination efficiency with age. However, as noted in equation 17, $t_{1/2}$ depends on the apparent volume as much as it depends on elimination (given by clearance). In fact, it is the change in apparent volume with age that drives the increase in the terminal $t_{1/2}$ (B). This change in $t_{1/2}$ occurs in the absence of any change in (hepatic) clearance, as noted in the inset figure. The physiologic explanation for this relationship is that adipose tissue represents an increasing percentage of body weight as an individual ages. The consequence of this change in body composition is the expansion of the space that the compound can occupy, which is expressed as an increase in the apparent volume of distribution. This illustration stresses the importance of viewing $t_{1/2}$ in its functional form, as written in equation 17.

Whereas $t_{1/2}$ is governed by distribution and elimination processes and, therefore, reflects what is happening in the entire

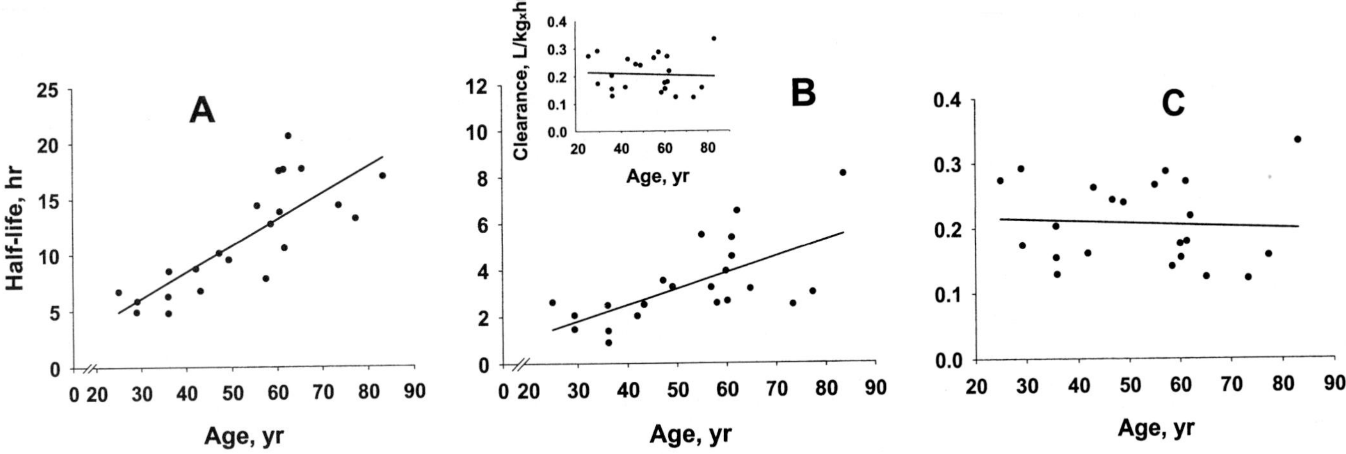

Figure 19. The influence of age (in women undergoing surgery) on the disposition parameters of the lipid-soluble, rapid-acting, intravenous anesthetic agent thiopental. Relationships are shown for terminal half-life **(A)**, apparent volume of distribution (L/kg) **(B)** and systemic clearance (**B**, *inset*). Graph **C** is an enlarged version of the clearance inset in **B**. The lines represent the linear regression equation of the data. (Based on data presented in Jung D, Mayersohn M, Perrier D, et al. Thiopental disposition as a function of age in female patients undergoing surgery. *Anesthesiology* 1982;56:263–268. From M. Mayersohn, *unpublished*, with permission from Saguaro Technical Press, Inc, Tucson, AZ, 2002.)

body, clearance, on the other hand, is a measure of efficiency of elimination or removal by an organ. The basic definition of clearance is essentially a restatement of first-order kinetics.

$$\text{clearance} = \frac{\text{rate of elimination}}{\text{blood or plasma concentration}} = \frac{\text{amount/time}}{\text{amount/volume}} = \frac{\text{volume}}{\text{time}} \quad \text{[Eq. 20]}$$

Notice that the units of clearance are that of a flow, volume/time. The definition of clearance that is often cited is *clearance is the volume of blood that must be acted on and from which all substance is removed per unit of time to account for the rate at which that substance is being eliminated.* Previously, in defining first-order kinetic processes, equation 4 indicated the relationship between rate and concentration, but the proportionality constant was a first-order rate constant and not clearance, as rewritten below:

$$K = \frac{\text{rate of elimination}}{\text{blood or plasma concentration}} = \frac{\text{concentration/time}}{\text{concentration}} = \frac{1}{\text{time}} \quad \text{[Eq. 4]}$$

Clearance and K (or $t_{1/2}$), not surprisingly, are related to each other through the apparent volume of distribution (i.e., $CL = K \cdot V_d$), which is a useful expression, but this does not help in understanding clearance. As for a first-order process, clearance is *independent* of dose or concentration or time after dosing. Every eliminating organ has a corresponding value for clearance; individual organ clearances are additive (as are rate constants) and *independent* of each other. The sum of all clearances for all eliminating processes is referred to as *total body clearance* or *systemic clearance*, CL_S; the latter is the preferred term here.

For any terminal region into which drug is found, such as the urine, bile, or exhaled air, the basic relationship for clearance, equation 20, can be applied experimentally. Thus, renal clearance (CL_R) is assessed by relating the rate of urinary excretion of unchanged drug to plasma concentration at the same time. Similarly, one can experimentally determine biliary clearance (CL_{BILE}) and pulmonary exhalation clearance ($CL_{PULMONARY}$) of unchanged drug. Each of these clearances has one thing in common: a terminal fluid can be collected and assayed for unchanged drug, from which an estimate of rate of drug appearance can be made. How does one go about experimentally determining hepatic clearance (CL_{HEP}) or systemic clearance? The former cannot be done noninvasively, and the latter would require experimentally measuring all possible clearing mechanisms. Some other method must be applied to calculate values for those clearance terms.

The direct answer to this question comes from a common and practical mathematical procedure: convert the rate to an amount through integration. If the rate expression presented in equation 20 is integrated, the following is obtained:

$$\text{systemic clearance} = CL_s = \frac{\text{rate}}{\text{concentration}} = \frac{\int_0^\infty \text{rate} \cdot dt}{\int_0^\infty C \cdot dt} = \frac{\text{IV dose}}{(AUC)_0^\infty} \quad \text{[Eq. 21]}$$

Systemic clearance can be calculated by dividing the IV dose by the corresponding total area under the plasma concentration-time curve (from time zero to infinity) for the unchanged drug. The IV dose is used here because, by definition, the entire IV dose is completely available to the systemic circulation. This is not necessarily true for any other route of administration. Recall that the area may be considered to be an index of exposure to the compound. Systemic clearance can be viewed as affecting the exposure resulting from administration of a given dose. Thus, the greater the clearance, the smaller the exposure from a unit dose of compound. The inverse is also true: a small value of CL_S results in a large exposure to a unit dose of compound. Because clearance is a constant, any increase in dose results in a proportional increase in area under the curve.

Determination of hepatic (or metabolic) clearance requires that the numerator in equation 21 be the rate of metabolite formation, the integral of which is the amount of metabolite formed (not dose). The latter is generally determined after measurement of the fraction of the dose that is converted into metabolite. Another feasible calculation is to subtract all known values for clearance from systemic clearance and assume that the remainder is hepatic or metabolic clearance (e.g., $CL_{HEP} = CL_S - CL_R - CL_{OTHER}$). Also, the ratio of any given organ clearance to systemic clearance gives the fraction of the dose that undergoes

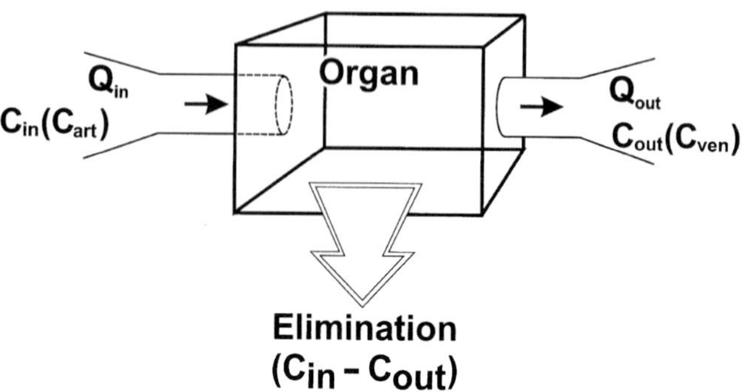

Figure 20. A hypothetical eliminating organ that receives in-flowing (arterial) blood (Q_{in} or C_{art}) and out-flowing (venous) blood (Q_{out} or Q_{ven}). The arterial blood has a concentration of C_{in}, and the venous blood has a concentration of C_{out}. Any difference between C_{out} and C_{in} ($C_{out} < C_{in}$) represents elimination or organ extraction of drug. Extraction ratio, ER, is defined as $C_{in} - C_{out}/C_{in}$. (From M. Mayersohn, *unpublished*, with permission from Saguaro Technical Press, Inc, Tucson, AZ, 2002.)

that pathway. Thus, the ratio of CL_R to CL_S represents the fraction of the dose that is excreted unchanged via the kidney. This is the same fraction that is represented by the ratio of the individual rate constant for urinary excretion (k_U) and the overall elimination rate constant (K).

There are several useful graphical ways to illustrate different aspects of clearance. Figure 20 illustrates a basic term, *extraction ratio* (ER), which provides a measure of efficiency of drug removal by the hypothetical organ illustrated. The organ receives arterial blood flow (Q_{in} or Q_{art}) that contains drug entering the organ at a concentration of C_{in} (or C_{art}). The exiting venous blood flow (Q_{out} or Q_{ven}) contains drug at a concentration of C_{out} (or C_{ven}). If this were a noneliminating organ or tissue, then the concentration exiting the organ would exactly equal the concentration entering ($C_{out} = C_{in}$). In contrast, if some of the drug is eliminated, then the outflowing concentration must be less than the inflowing concentration ($C_{out} < C_{in}$) and the difference, shown by the arrow, is what has been eliminated or extracted by that organ. The efficiency of this process can be expressed by the ER, which is the difference in concentrations normalized by the inflowing concentration.

$$\text{extraction ratio} = \text{ER} = \frac{C_{in} - C_{out}}{C_{in}} \qquad \text{[Eq. 22]}$$

The three possible situations are

I.	$C_{out} = C_{in}$	$= 0$	noneliminating organ
II.	$C_{out} = 0$	$\text{ER} = 1$	extremely efficient eliminating organ
III.	$C_{out} < C_{in}$	$0 < \text{ER} < 1$	varying elimination efficiency

For an eliminating organ, most compounds fall into category III, and every organ has a unique value of ER for a given substance. The ER represents the fractional removal of substance by the organ. Thus, an ER value of 0.2 indicates that 20% of the substance in the blood is removed by the extracting organ as the blood perfuses that organ. The ER value is a measure of efficiency of removal and has no bearing on the extent or completeness of removal by that organ. Thus, two compounds may undergo total hepatic metabolism (i.e., 100% metabolized) yet have different ER values. The former value indicates the primary route of elimination and that ultimately all of the drug is metabolized. The ER value suggests how efficiently the removal process occurs. It seems reasonable that the compound with the greatest ER value is likely to have the shortest $t_{1/2}$, keeping in mind the modulating effect of apparent volume of distribution. It would not be surprising to find that organ clearance is related to ER. This can be easily shown by considering the basic relationship for clearance and with reference to Figure 20. The rate of drug entry into the organ is the product of blood flow in and concentration in, and the rate of drug exit is the product of blood flow out and concentration out:

$$\text{Rate in} = Q_{in} \cdot C_{in} \quad \text{Rate out} = Q_{out} \cdot C_{out} \qquad \text{[Eq. 23]}$$

The rate of elimination or extraction is the difference between the rate in and the rate out:

$$\text{Rate of elimination} = Q_{in} \cdot C_{in} - Q_{out} \cdot C_{out} = Q_{in} \cdot (C_{in} - C_{out}) \qquad \text{[Eq. 24]}$$

Because flow in is equal to flow out, Q_{in} has been factored out and used in the equation. The basic relationship used to define clearance has rate of elimination in the numerator divided by the blood concentration. Substituting equation 24 for the numerator gives

$$\text{clearance} = \frac{\text{rate of elimination}}{\text{blood concentration}} = \frac{Q_{in}(C_{in} - C_{out})}{C_{in}} = Q_{in} \cdot \text{ER} \qquad \text{[Eq. 25]}$$

Clearance by a given organ is the product of the blood flow to that organ multiplied by the organ ER for that compound. Thus, if ER is 0.2, the clearance of that compound is equal to 20% of blood flow; 20% of that compound is removed from the blood as it perfuses the organ. Going back to the three scenarios discussed previously,

I.	$C_{out} = C_{in}$	$\text{ER} = 0$	$\text{CL} = 0$	noneliminating organ
II.	$C_{out} = 0$	$\text{ER} = 1$	$\text{CL} = \text{Q}$	extremely efficient eliminating organ
III.	$C_{out} < C_{in}$	$0 < \text{ER} < 1$	$\text{CL} = \text{ER} \cdot \text{Q}$	varying elimination efficiency

The most interesting aspect of the previous chart is situation II: when ER is the largest possible value, clearance is equal to organ blood flow. This is the statement of a rate-limiting step; *a compound cannot be cleared by an organ any faster than it is delivered (by blood) to that organ.* In fact, there is a clinical application of this principle. Consider diagnostic agents that are used to measure organ blood flow, such as indocyanine green (hepatic blood flow) and para-aminohippurate (PAH) (renal blood flow). These compounds have one pharmacokinetic characteristic in common: they all have a specific organ ER of approximately one. Thus, organ clearance measured *in vivo* after an IV dose cannot exceed organ blood flow. The largest possible value for systemic clearance is total blood flow or cardiac output. Any value of CL_S greater than cardiac output suggests a mechanism of elimination that is independent of blood flow. For example, a compound that is chemically or metabolically altered in the blood *per se* would not be influenced by blood flow, and the resulting clearance could take on any value in excess of cardiac output. The latter appears to be the situation for organic nitrates, such as nitroglycerin, that are metabolized along the surface of blood vessels (13). There are several older but thorough reviews of clearance and blood flow (14,15).

Another way to examine extraction and clearance is illustrated in Figure 21 for three different compounds. The hypothetical organ receives 10 ml of blood per minute and, at time zero, each of the three drugs is present at a concentration of 10 ng/ml. One-

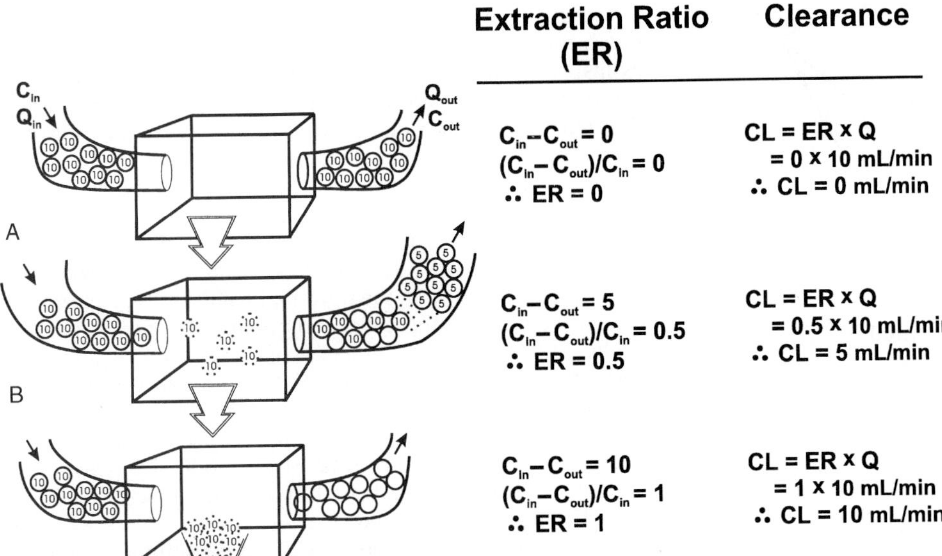

Figure 21. Schematic diagram of the extraction and clearance of three different drugs. The hypothetical organ system receives 10 ml of blood per minute. The compounds have ER, from top to bottom, of 0, 0.5, and 1.0. What is shown is one-minute snapshots of the drug entering and then leaving the organ. At time zero, the concentration in the delivering blood is 10 ng/ml for each compound. **A:** One minute after perfusing the organ, the exiting and incoming concentrations are equal. Thus, this is a noneliminating organ for that drug having an ER and CL of zero. **B:** The exiting concentration of 5 ng/ml is one-half of the entering concentration. The ER value is 0.5, resulting in an organ clearance of 5 ml/minute. Note that what is retained (i.e., eliminated) in the organ is the mass comparable to what was contained in 5 ml of blood. **C:** The exiting concentration of zero gives an ER of 1.0 and a clearance equal to organ blood flow, 10 ml/minute. Again, note that what is eliminated by the organ is the mass comparable to what was contained in the volume cleared. (From M. Mayersohn, *unpublished*, with permission from Saguaro Technical Press, Inc, Tucson, AZ, 2002.)

minute snapshots for each of the three compounds is shown. For the compound at the top of the figure, the exiting concentration equals the incoming concentration, and, therefore, no drug has been extracted or eliminated. The value for ER and CL for this drug is zero; this is a noneliminating organ. The compound in the center has an exiting concentration of 5 ng/ml 1 minute after blood perfuses the organ. The value for ER is the difference between the in and out concentrations divided by the incoming concentration: 10 – 5/10 = 0.5. The resulting value for clearance is ER multiplied by organ blood flow, or 5 ml/minute. The figure illustrates that the organ has retained (or eliminated) the total drug content in 5 ml of blood, or 50 ng. Clearance is the flow equivalent to the mass of compound removed by the organ (what volume of blood contains 50 ng?). The bottom figure indicates

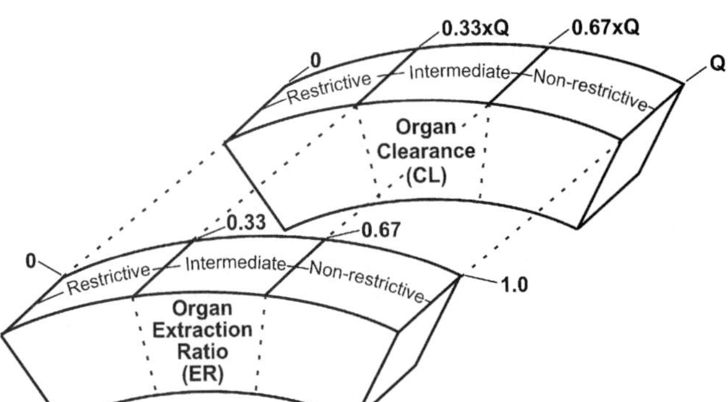

Figure 22. *Rainbows* illustrating the range of organ ERs and CLs. The clearance *rainbow* is connected to the extraction ratio by organ blood flow (CL = ER · Q). Each *rainbow* is divided into thirds. A low ER is less than approximately 0.33, whereas a large ER is greater than approximately 0.67. Intermediate values fall within that range. Drugs with low CL values are less than approximately one-third of organ blood flow, whereas drugs with large CL have a value greater than approximately two-thirds of organ blood flow. Intermediate CL values fall within that range. Note that low clearance drugs are also referred to as being *restrictively* cleared, whereas drugs with high clearance are referred to as being *nonrestrictively* cleared. See text for explanation. (From M. Mayersohn, *unpublished*, with permission from Saguaro Technical Press, Inc, Tucson, AZ, 2002.)

that the exiting concentration is zero, which must indicate total clearance of the compound by the organ (ER = 1 and CL = 10 ml/minute). Extraction can never be more efficient than this; clearance equals organ blood flow.

Figure 22 illustrates *rainbows* for organ ERs and corresponding organ clearances. The ER *rainbow* is in front of the clearance *rainbow* and connected to it by organ blood flow (CL = ER · Q). Values for ER and CL are divided into three parts: low, intermediate, and high. Although the demarcations are arbitrary, a small ER is less than approximately 0.33, whereas a large ER is greater than approximately 0.67. Intermediate vales are in between those ranges. The identical separation is shown for CL, except that the values are multiplied by organ blood flow. Thus, low clearance is any value less than approximately one-third of blood flow, whereas a large clearance is any value greater than approximately two-thirds of blood flow. Intermediate clearances are in between those extremes. Also notice that the term *restrictive* clearance is used to describe those compounds with low clearance and *nonrestrictive* is used to describe those compounds with high clearance. As noted later, the former indicates that clearance is restricted by plasma protein binding, whereas for high clearance compounds, clearance is not restricted by plasma protein binding. Figure 23 illustrates the clearance rainbow with flow values and with drug examples for each division and using the average values for liver blood flow (1500 ml/minute) and renal blood flow (1200 ml/minute) in a normal healthy adult man.

Another way to view clearance is with reference to its basic definition, as illustrated in Figure 24. The panel of three graphs project into the page. The first graph is a linear plot of plasma concentration as a function of time after an IV bolus dose and assuming a one-compartment model. The resulting exponential curve is described by the equation noted to the right. The graph just behind the first is a plot of the rate of elimination versus time, and it is connected by dotted lines to the graph in the front at corresponding times. Because rate of elimination is a function of concentration and a rate constant, K (or clearance, CL), the middle curve declines in parallel with the concentration-time curve, as noted in the equations to the right. Clearance is defined as the relationship between rate of elimination and the driving force concentration. Dividing the middle curve, which describes

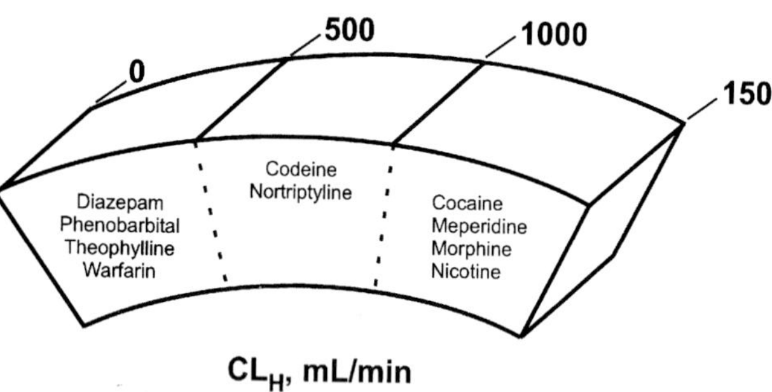

Figure 23. *Rainbows* of extraction ratio and clearance (CL) for drugs that undergo renal CL (CL_R) and hepatic CL (CL_H). The average values for renal (1200 ml/minute) and hepatic (1500 ml /minute) blood flows in a normal 70-kg man have been used and divided into three parts, as noted in Figure 22. Drug examples are provided for each division. (From Mayersohn M. Toxicokinetics: Measurement of disposition half-life, clearance and residence times. In Maines M, ed. *Current protocols in toxicology.* New York: John Wiley and Sons, 2000:5.3.5, with permission of Saguaro Technical Press, Inc, 2002, Tucson, AZ.)

rate of elimination, by the corresponding concentration-time values in the front curve, results in clearance, which is projected onto the back-most graph. Clearance is constant with time, but its magnitude (height) varies from compound to compound. This difference among compounds can be seen in Figure 25. There is a series of three panels, each representing a different drug and each panel is made up of three graphs projecting into the page as described. The compound on the left has the smallest rate of elimination, resulting in a relatively shallow rate versus time curve. The consequence is that clearance, which is a ratio of rate/concentration, is a relatively low value, which can be noted by inspecting the graph in the back of the panel. In contrast, the compound on the right has a rapidly declining concentration-time curve, indicating a large value for the elimination rate constant. The graph just behind indicates a rapid decline in the rate versus time curve. As a consequence, the ratio of rate to concentration or clearance for this compound must be relatively high, as noted in the rear graph. The compound in the center panel is intermediate between the other two compounds. What is it about the compound on the right that results in high clearance? If it is assumed that these three compounds all underwent metabolic clearance by the same enzyme, then there is something about this compound that makes it a better substrate for that enzyme. This difference among compounds can be better understood by expressing a term called *intrinsic clearance* (CL_{int}), which, as noted later, is the ratio of V_{max} to K_{mm}; however, ultimately the explanation lies with how that molecule resides at the active site of the enzyme.

Before discussing the idea of CL_{int}, it is useful to view clearance in yet another way that provides a basis for a comparison between clearance, an expression of organ efficiency, and $t_{1/2}$, which reflects loss of drug from the body. Figure 26 illustrates sequential 1-minute *snapshots* of the extraction of a compound and its movement through the body. The hypothetical compound is given as an IV bolus at a dose of 150,000 ng. The resulting initial plasma concentration is 10 ng/ml. The organ of elimination receives blood flow at the rate of 50 ml/minute and the ER of this compound is 0.3. In the first minute, 50 ml of blood each containing 10 ng of drug perfuses the clearing organ. As the blood traverses the organ, 30% of the compound is removed from the blood during the first minute. This is illustrated by the organ retaining 15 ml of the total of 50 ml of blood, which has perfused the organ. Of course, blood flow is conserved; what is retained by the organ is the total mass of compound contained in 15 ml of blood. Organ clearance is 15 ml/minute (0.3 × 50 ml/minute), and the amount eliminated by the organ is the total content in 15 ml of blood, 150 ng (10 ng/ml × 15 ml). On exit, there are 15 *empty* ml of blood, which reequilibrates with the

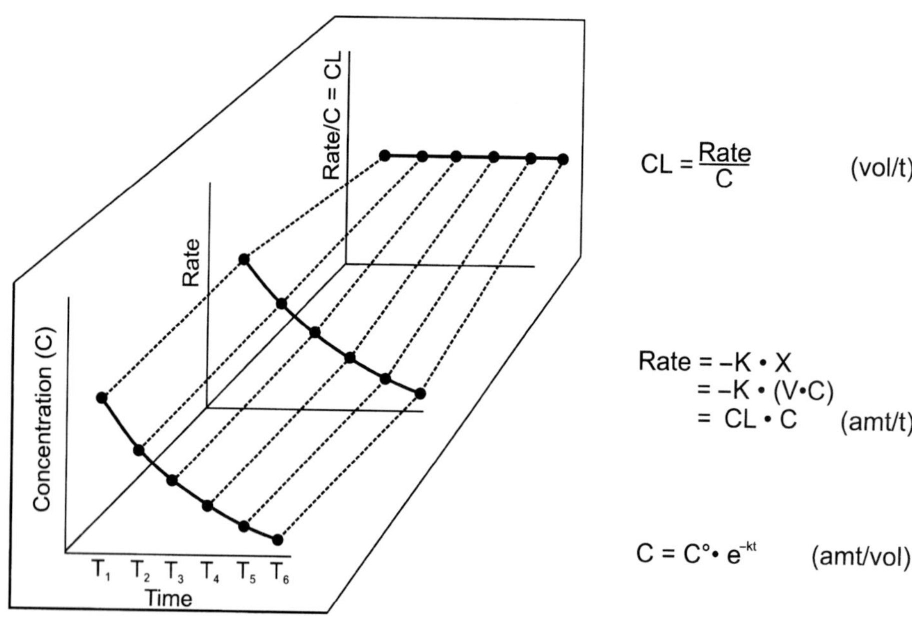

Figure 24. There are three graphs in this panel, which project into the page. The first graph is a linear plot of plasma concentration versus time after an intravenous bolus dose (and assuming a one-compartment model) whose equation is noted to the right. The graph immediately behind is that of rate of elimination versus time. The two graphs are shown connected by dotted lines at the same times. The equations that describe this rate versus time plot are shown to the right. Because the ratio of rate to concentration is defined as clearance (CL), dividing the middle graph by the first graph gives CL, which is noted as the graph in the back. (From M. Mayersohn, *unpublished*, with permission from Saguaro Technical Press, Inc, Tucson, AZ, 2002.)

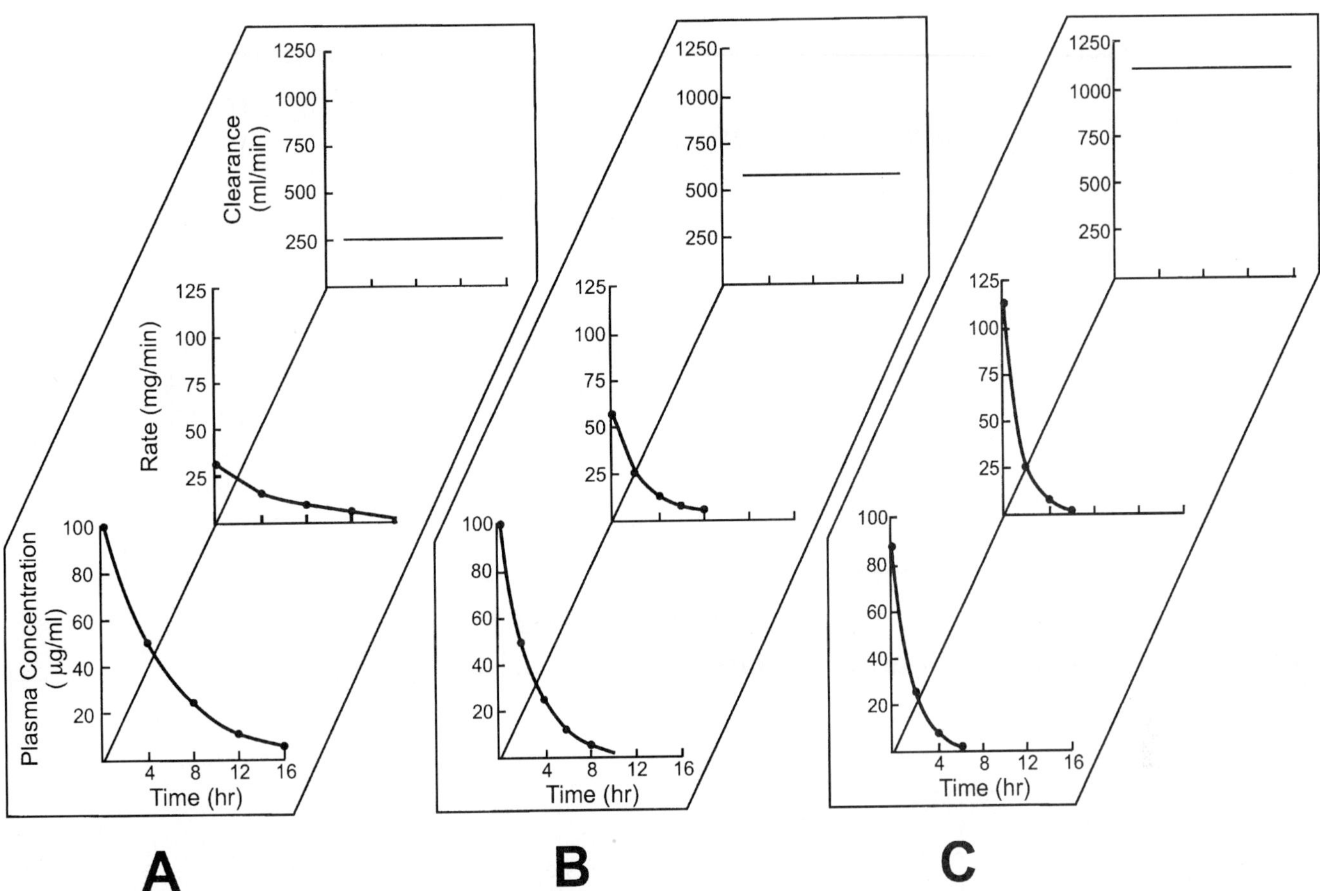

Figure 25. This figure is identical to that described in Figure 24, except three different compounds are being compared. In each of the three panels that project into the page are graphs of, from front to back, plasma concentration versus time, rate of elimination versus time, and rate of elimination/concentration versus time (i.e., clearance vs. time). Each panel represents a different drug with its own rate-concentration (or clearance) relationship. All drugs have the same initial plasma concentration. The terminal rate constant increases (or half-life decreases) when going from **A** to **C**. This is easily seen by comparing the concentration-time curves from **A–C**. Because rate of elimination is lowest for **A**, the ratio of that rate to the corresponding plasma concentration (which is clearance) is low, giving rise to a relatively low clearance. In contrast, **C** has the greatest rate of elimination relative to concentration and, therefore, the ratio of rate to concentration results in a large clearance. **B:** The compound is intermediate between **A** and **C**. (From M. Mayersohn, *unpublished*, with permission from Saguaro Technical Press, Inc, Tucson, AZ, 2002.)

other 35 ml of blood to give a final exiting concentration of 7 ng/ml. Whereas this is a relatively efficient removal of compound from the blood by the organ, does this represent a substantial removal from the *body*? In 1 minute, only 150 ng out of a total dose of 150,000 have been lost from the body. This illustrates the difference between clearance and $t_{1/2}$. In fact, if it were assumed that the ER value was 1.0, the most efficient clearance possible, only 500 ng out of a total of 150,000 ng would be removed in 1 minute. Removal of the compound from the blood results in a trivial change in blood concentration. The $t_{1/2}$ of this compound is approximately 11 hours.

Before the blood perfuses the organ during the second minute, it must mix with the rest of the blood in the body. Because all of the rest of the blood has a concentration of 10 ng/ml, the blood exiting the clearing organ at a concentration of 7 ng/ml results in a trivial dilution of the concentration and the new concentration is 9.99 ng/ml. The process repeats during the second and all subsequent minutes. The ER value and clearance are the same at all times, but the amount extracted by the organ decreases with time as the amount in the body declines. In the second minute, a little less than 150 ng is removed from the blood. The exiting blood concentration has a value of approximately 6.99 ng/ml. When the exiting blood mixes with all of the rest of the blood (at a concentration of 9.99 ng/ml), the resulting concentration is 9.98 ng/ml, which is the new concentration that perfuses the organ during the third minute. This process continues until all of the compound has been eliminated from the body. Of course, this process does not happen in short 1-minute bursts; it is happening all of the time, resulting in a smooth exponential decline in concentration with time.

What is it that drives organ clearance for a specific compound? The ER determines the value for organ clearance. What drives ER? In the model that has been used, which is referred to by several terms (venous equilibrium, blood flow- or perfusion-limited or well-stirred model), the ER is a function of CL_{int}, as noted in the following relationship:

$$\text{extraction ratio} = \frac{CL_{int}}{CL_{int} + Q} \quad \text{[Eq. 26]}$$

Notice that for ER to approach its maximum value of 1.0, CL_{int} must be a large value and larger than organ blood flow (i.e., when $CL_{int} >> Q$; ER $\cong$ 1.0 and CL $\cong$ Q). Such compounds have large values for organ clearance (approximately equal to organ blood flow) and fall into the right side of the organ clearance

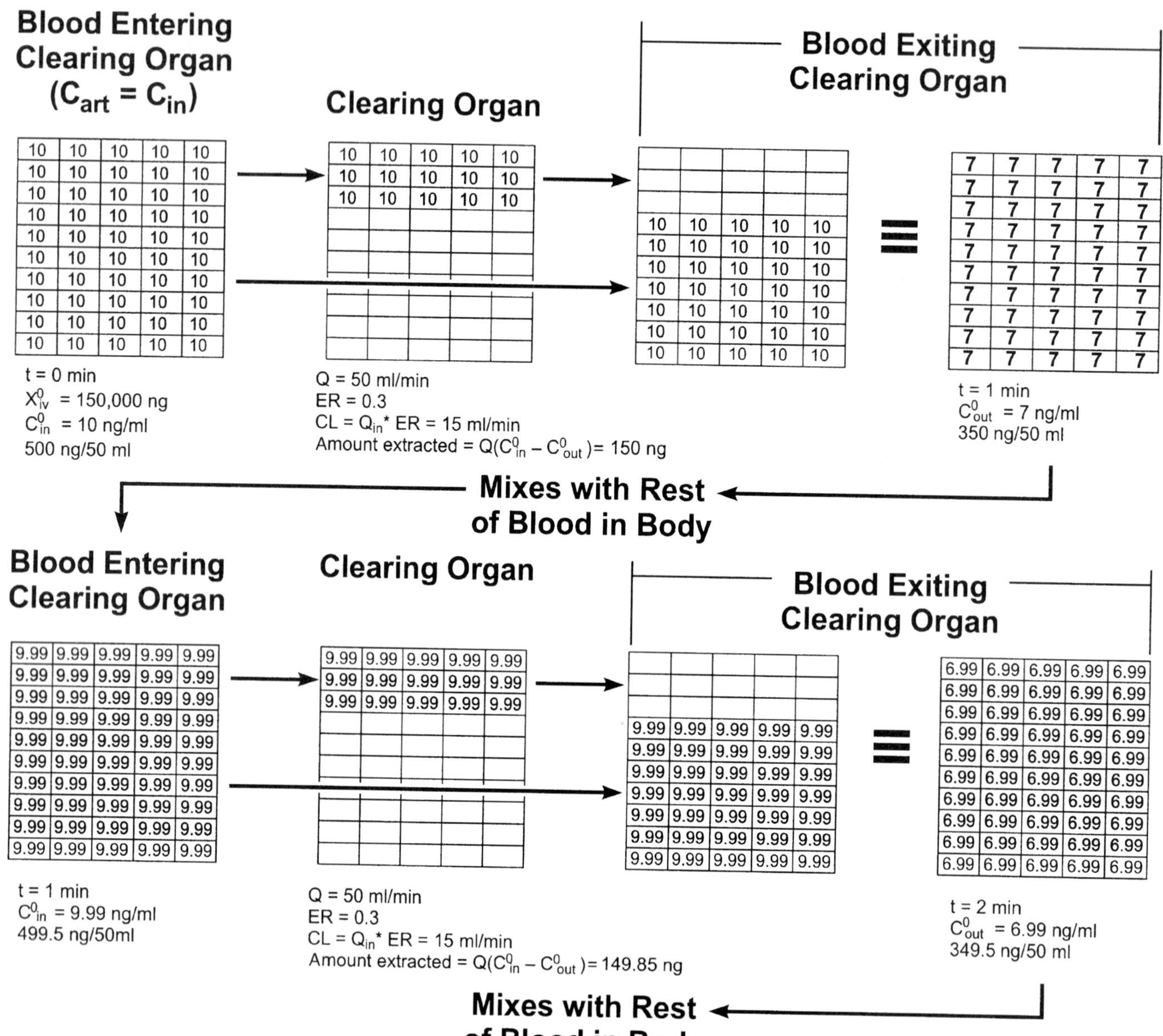

Figure 26. Sequential 1-minute *snapshots* illustrating the extraction of a drug as it traverses the eliminating organ and moves through the body. An intravenous dose is given (150,000 ng), which produces an initial blood concentration of 10 ng/ml. The only organ that eliminates the compound has an extraction ratio (ER) of 0.30, and it receives blood at a rate of 50 ml/minute (Q = 50 ml/minute). At time zero, 50 ml of blood (shown as 50 boxes) at a concentration of 10 ng/ml enters the eliminating organ for the first time. Because the ER is 0.3, 30% of the compound in the blood is removed as blood traverses the organ. This is comparable to saying that the content in 30% of the organ blood volume is removed. This is illustrated with there being 15 boxes or 15 ml of blood (0.3 × 50 ml = 15 ml) devoid of compound. Thus, the clearance (CL) of the compound is 15 ml/minute. As the blood exits the organ, the *empty* boxes now reequilibrate with the rest of the exiting blood to give a homogenous concentration of 7 ng/ml. The organ has removed 30% of the compound that was presented to it in the first minute (i.e., 0.3 × 10 ng/ml × 50 ml/minute = 150 ng removed in the first minute). A physiologic model of this system is shown to indicate that as compound exits the organ, the exiting venous blood concentration is affected by mixing with venous blood perfusing the rest of the body. This mixing results in an increase in the blood concentration before its next entry into the eliminating organ. The exiting venous blood (7 ng/ml) meets up with, mixes, and reequilibrates with the concentration in the rest of the blood (10 ng/ml) to give a concentration of 9.99 ng/ml. This is the new blood concentration that enters the eliminating organ in the second minute. Another 1-minute *snapshot* is shown for the second minute. Fifty milliliters of blood at a concentration of 9.99 ng/ml enters the eliminating organ. Because the ER is the same, 30% of compound once again is removed from the blood (i.e., 0.3 × 9.99 ng/ml × 50 ml/minute = 149.8 ng removed in the second minute). The CL is the same (i.e., 0.3 × 50 ml/minute = 15 ml/minute). On exiting the organ, the concentration of compound reequilibrates to give an exiting concentration of 6.99 ng/ml, which mixes with the rest of the blood (9.99 ng/ml) to give a final venous concentration of 9.98 ng/ml. The latter is now the new concentration entering the organ beginning in minute 3. (From M. Mayersohn, *unpublished*, with permission from Saguaro Technical Press, Inc, Tucson, AZ, 2002.)

rainbow (Fig. 22). In contrast, compounds that have small values for CL_{int}, and that fall into the left side of the organ clearance *rainbow*, have an organ clearance approximately equal to CL_{int} (i.e., when $CL_{int} << Q$; $ER \cong CL_{int}/Q$ and $CL \cong CL_{int}$). The definition of CL_{int} is a *clearance that is not dependent on organ blood flow*. Thus, the rate-limiting step for CL_{int} is not delivery of the compound to the site of clearance (e.g., the hepatic enzymes). In the whole body or for an isolated organ, this cannot apply; blood flow necessarily rate-limits clearance, with the exception of low clearance compounds. Thus, if there were no limit to the ability to pump blood to an organ, at sufficiently large blood flow, CL_{int} would be measurable.

CL_{int} is what is measured in a test tube when a compound is added to some form of enzyme (e.g., pure isozyme, homogenized liver, hepatocytes), and the rate of metabolite formation is determined (or disappearance of parent compound). Adding the compound to the enzyme preparation is instantaneous; there is no measurable delivery rate, as there is in the body via blood flow. The resulting *in vitro* measure of clearance is CL_{int}, because that value is independent of any flow. Numerically, CL_{int} is greater than or approximately equal to organ clearance determined in the body, depending on the magnitude of CL_{int}. The best way to visualize this process is to consider the *in vitro* situation illustrated in Figure 27. Ten molecules of a drug are added to a test tube containing 10 ml of an enzyme solution and rapidly mixed. At time zero, the concentration of drug is 1 mol/ml. One minute later, the enzyme reaction is stopped and the amount of metabolite produced is determined. Four molecules of metabolite have been produced. The rate of metabolite production is 4 mol/minute. The corresponding clearance, which is rate of metabolite formation (4 mol/minute) divided by the starting drug concentration (1 mol/minute), is 4 ml/minute. In 1 minute, 4 ml of starting solution have been completely cleared of drug. This value, 4 ml/minute, is the intrinsic metabolic clearance of that drug. Changing enzyme activity by induction of inhibition alters intrinsic metabolic clearance accordingly.

The equation noted for ER in equation 26 can be substituted for ER in equation 25 to give a more descriptive relationship:

$$CL = \frac{CL_{int} \cdot Q}{CL_{int} + Q} \qquad \text{[Eq. 27]}$$

Low clearance compounds have small values for CL_{int} and because $CL_{int} << Q$, $CL \cong CL_{int}$. An IV bolus dose of such a compound allows determination of the CL_{int} of that compound. In this instance, blood flow does not rate-limit the organ clearance of the compound. Any factor affecting CL_{int} affects clearance. An example is altered enzyme activity by the presence of another compound.

In contrast, high clearance compounds have large values for CL_{int}, and because $CL_{int} >> Q$, $CL \cong Q$. An IV dose of such a compound gives a value of clearance that is actually an estimate of organ blood flow. The clearance of such a compound can only be affected by changes in organ blood flow (e.g., altered cardiac output) and not by changes in CL_{int}.

This analysis has ignored those compounds that fall into an intermediate clearance category. The clearance of such compounds is affected to different degrees by changes in CL_{int} and organ blood flow. Thus, unlike the previous situations, the equation noted in 27 cannot be simplified for intermediate clearance compounds.

There is, finally, one more variable to consider and that is plasma protein binding. Plasma protein binding may affect the clearance of those drugs that have low clearances; these have been referred to as being *restrictively cleared*. The clearance of such compounds is restricted by binding to plasma proteins. This leads to the need to define and illustrate another term, *unbound intrinsic clearance*, $CL_{U,int}$. $CL_{U,int}$ is CL_{int} in the absence of plasma protein binding or adjusted for that binding. This definition is illustrated in Figure 28, which is similar to the scenario noted in Figure 27 and which is for the same compound. In this instance, however, there is binding protein present in the enzyme solution. At time zero, the total concentration of drug is 1 mol/ml. Of that total, 50% is bound to protein, giving an unbound concentration of 0.5 mol/ml. One minute later, two molecules of metabolite are formed giving a rate of formation of 2 mol/minute. The clearance of this compound is 2 mol/minute divided by 1 mol/ml or 2 ml/minute. This value represents the intrinsic metabolic clearance of the drug under the conditions specified. Note that this clearance is one-half the value of CL_{int} when no binding protein was present; the binding has reduced the CL_{int} of the compound (CL_{int}, 4 ml/minute; Fig. 27). If this value of CL_{int} is corrected for only those molecules that are not bound to protein by dividing CL_{int} by the unbound fraction of compound (i.e., 0.5), 4 ml/minute is obtained. The latter value is $CL_{U,int}$ and is identical to the value determined experimentally in the absence of binding protein (Fig. 27). $CL_{U,int}$ is the most fundamental measure of clearance, as it is independent of blood flow and plasma protein bind-

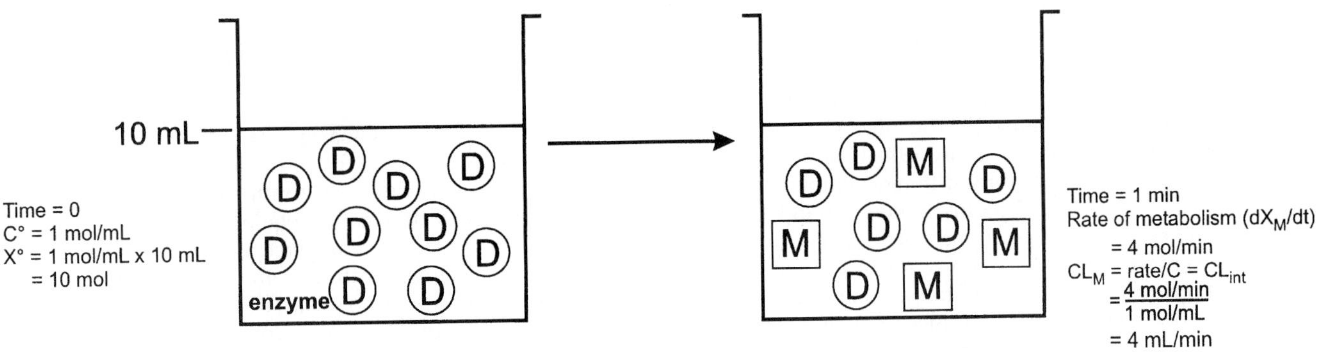

Figure 27. An *in vitro* experiment designed to measure intrinsic metabolic clearance (CL_{int}). At time zero, 10 molecules of drug (D) are added to 10 ml of solution containing enzyme. The initial time zero concentration is 1 mol/ml. One minute later, the reaction is stopped, and the amount of metabolite formed is measured. Four molecules of metabolite (M) are formed in 1 minute; thus, the rate of metabolite formation is 4 mol/min. Because CL is rate (4 mol/minute) divided by concentration (C; 1 mol/ml), the clearance value for this drug is 4 ml/minute. In other words, 4 ml of starting solution have been completely cleared of the drug by having been converted to metabolite. This value of 4 ml/minute is the intrinsic clearance of the drug. (From M. Mayersohn, *unpublished*, with permission from Saguaro Technical Press, Inc, Tucson, AZ, 2002.)

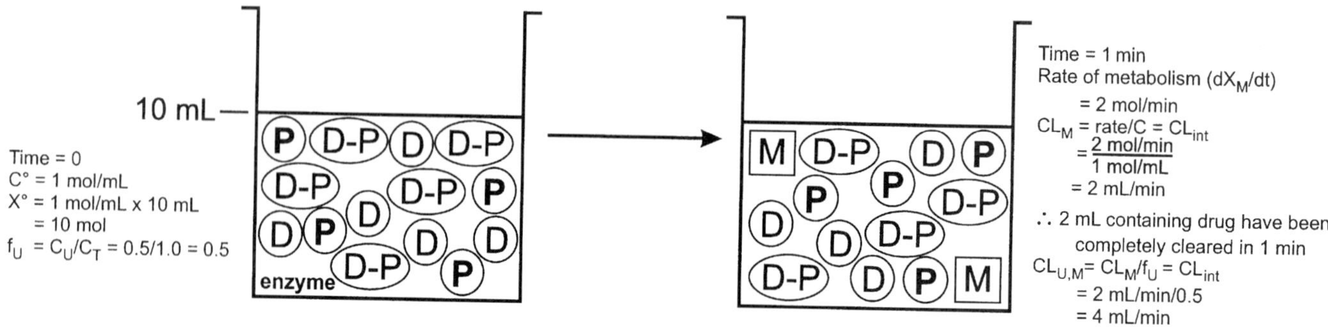

Figure 28. The same scenario as in Figure 27 for the measurement of intrinsic metabolic clearance (CL_{int}). In this instance, however, the enzyme reaction solution contains binding protein. At time zero, ten molecules of drug (D) are added to 10 ml of enzyme solution. One-half of the drug molecules are bound to the protein so that the unbound fraction (f_U) is 0.5. At time zero, the initial total drug concentration is 1 mol/ml, and the unbound concentration is 0.5 mol/ml. One minute later, the reaction is stopped, and the amount of metabolite formed is determined. Two molecules of metabolite (M) are formed in 1 minute; thus, the rate of metabolite formation is 2 mol/minute. Because clearance is rate (2 mol/minute) divided by (total) concentration (1 mol/ml), the clearance value for this drug is 2 ml/minute. In other words, 2 ml of starting solution have been completely cleared of the drug by having been converted to metabolite. This value of 2 ml/minute is the intrinsic clearance of the drug. Note that this is one-half of the value for CL_{int} in the absence of binding protein (4 ml/minute; Fig. 27). The binding protein has protected the drug and reduced its clearance. This leads to the need to estimate unbound intrinsic metabolic clearance, $CL_{U,int}$. The latter is the value of intrinsic clearance corrected for the fraction of drug that is unbound. In this instance, $CL_{U,int}$ is 2 mol/ml divided by 0.5 or 4 ml/minute. The latter value is identical to the one determined in the absence of binding protein in Figure 27. (From M. Mayersohn, *unpublished*, with permission from Saguaro Technical Press, Inc, Tucson, AZ, 2002.)

ing. CL_{int}, is the product of the unbound fraction and $CL_{U,int}$ (i.e., $CL_{int} = f_U \cdot CL_{U,int}$).

Based on the previous development, the final and most useful relationship for defining clearance can be written as follows:

$$CL = \frac{f_U \cdot CL_{U,int} \cdot Q}{f_U \cdot CL_{U,int} + Q} \quad \text{[Eq. 28]}$$

This expression incorporates all factors that can possibly affect the clearance of a compound by an organ, and it is useful in interpreting data and in making predictions. Thus, for a low clearance compound (restrictively cleared), $f_U \cdot CL_{U,int} << Q$ and, therefore, $CL \cong f_U \cdot CL_{U,int}$. The only factors that can affect the clearance of such a compound are those that affect plasma protein binding and/or $CL_{U,int}$. Changes in blood flow should have no effect.

In contrast, for a compound with a large clearance (nonrestrictively cleared), $f_U \cdot CL_{U,int} >> Q$ and, therefore, $CL \cong Q$. Only factors that can affect organ blood flow affect the clearance of this type of drug. Changes in plasma protein binding or in $CL_{U,int}$ are not expected to have an effect. As noted previously, intermediate clearance compounds depend on blood flow, plasma protein binding, and $CL_{U,int}$.

The influence of blood flow and plasma protein binding on clearance is illustrated in Figure 29. The effect of $CL_{U,int}$ is discussed under Multiple Dosing. Figure 29A illustrates the relationship between clearance of three different compounds in the isolated perfused rat liver and perfusate flow through the liver (16). Perfusate flow is a surrogate measure of *blood* flow in the body. The clearance or low clearance (or low CL_{int}) compounds, such as antipyrine, is not expected to be influenced by blood flow. As noted previously, the clearance of such a compound depends only on plasma protein binding and $CL_{U,int}$. This is what is seen in the figure; antipyrine clearance is independent of perfusate flow. In contrast, the clearance of a high clearance (or high CL_{int}) compound, such as lidocaine, is expected to be directly related to blood flow, as is the case shown in the figure. As noted previously, the clearance of such a compound depends only on organ blood flow. The intermediate clearance compound, ethanol, depends on blood flow at low flow rates but then becomes independent of flow at higher flow rates. Knowing the clearance category for a compound allows one to predict the relationship between clearance and organ blood flow.

Figure 29B illustrates the influence of plasma protein binding on the clearance of warfarin in rats (17). The greater the percentage of warfarin unbound in serum, the greater the clearance of the drug. One would conclude that warfarin is a low clearance drug because only for such drugs would one expect plasma binding to affect clearance (i.e., $CL \cong f_U \cdot CL_{U,int}$). Of course, a direct estimation of the clearance category of the drug is to calculate ER by comparing measured clearance with the value of blood flow to the organ responsible for clearance, in this case liver blood flow in the rat. If one knew that warfarin fell into the low clearance category, one would predict the relationship illustrated in Figure 29B.

ER drives clearance and CL_{int} drives ER; what determines CL_{int}? This has been alluded to in a previous discussion of Michaelis-Menten enzyme kinetics. The rate of an enzyme reaction at low concentrations was given by equation 12.

Dividing both sides of the equation by the driving force concentration, C gives the corresponding relationship for enzyme or metabolic clearance:

$$\frac{\text{rate (or, v)}}{C} = \text{Clearance} = \left(\frac{V_{max}}{k_{mm}}\right) \quad \text{[Eq. 29]}$$

Clearance at low *in vitro* concentrations is actually the ratio of the maximal rate of enzymatic metabolism, V_{max}, to the Michaelis constant, k_{mm}. The clearance term noted in the equation is equal to CL_{int}. The magnitude of the CL_{int} of a compound is determined by those factors that affect V_{max} and k_{mm}. $CL_{U,int}$ would be the ratio of V_{max} to k_{mm}, corrected for binding.

What happens to clearance if the system is dose-dependent and becomes nonlinear? Writing the Michaelis-Menten equation expressed as clearance

$$\frac{\text{rate (or, v)}}{C} = \text{Clearance} = \frac{V_{max}}{k_{mm} + C} \quad \text{[Eq. 30]}$$

At low concentrations, as noted previously, $C << k_{mm}$ and clearance is a constant given by V_{max} divided by k_{mm}. At higher concentrations, the denominator becomes larger and larger (i.e., C

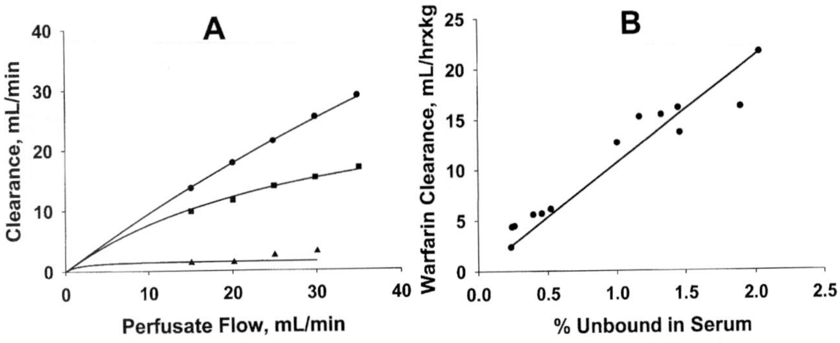

Figure 29. A: Clearance as a function of perfusate (*blood*) flow in the isolated perfused rat liver for three compounds having low, intermediate, and high clearances. The high (lidocaine, ●) and intermediate (ethanol, ■) clearance compounds illustrate a dependence on *blood* flow. The low clearance compound (antipyrine, ▲) has a clearance that does not depend on *blood* flow. (From Sinha V, Brendel K, Mayersohn M. A simplified isolated perfused rat liver apparatus: characterization and measurement of extraction ratios of selected compounds. *Life Sci* 2000;66:1795–1804, used with permission of Saguaro Technical Press.) **B:** Warfarin clearance in rats as a function of the percentage unbound in serum. (Based on data in Levy G. Clinical implications of interindividual differences in plasma protein binding of drugs and endogenous substances. In: Benet LZ, ed. *The effect of disease states on drug pharmacokinetics*. Washington, DC: American Pharmaceutical Association, 1976:137–151.) This relationship indicates that warfarin must fall into a low clearance category because for such compounds, $CL \cong f_U \cdot CL_{U,int}$.

>> k_{mm}), and clearance becomes smaller and smaller and, in theory, approaches zero. Thus, for a saturable or nonlinear system, clearance decreases with concentration, and, as a result, $t_{1/2}$ increases with dose or concentration.

Based on the previous discussions, plasma protein binding or changes in binding affect the apparent volume of distribution (equation 18) and may or may not affect clearance, depending on the category of clearance. It is not at all obvious how such a change in binding affects the $t_{1/2}$ of a drug, because $t_{1/2}$ depends on volume and clearance. In fact, the only rational approach to predicting how a change in plasma protein binding affects $t_{1/2}$ is to consider the fundamental relationship for $t_{1/2}$ as noted in equation 17, and this is illustrated under Nonvascular Input: Absorption and Bioavailability.

ELIMINATION PROCESSES

There are numerous routes of drug elimination, but the most significant are renal excretion and hepatic metabolism. The kidney and liver are anatomically and biochemically well suited for their role in processing drugs and other foreign compounds for their ultimate elimination from the body. Other routes of elimination could become relatively more important, depending on the compound, and these routes include nonhepatic metabolism (e.g., blood, kidney, muscle); biliary excretion; exhalation; perspiration; and so forth. Elimination processes are almost always synonymous with events that occur after a drug has gained access to the body, (i.e., the bloodstream). There are, however, elimination processes that may occur before drug gaining access to the body, and these are best referred to as *presystemic elimination*. The latter events occur at or near the site of drug administration or exposure. An example is chemical breakdown or enzymatic alteration of a compound in muscle tissue after intramuscular dosing. Perhaps the best examined and most significant are the presystemic elimination processes that occur during oral administration and that may substantially affect the dose reaching the systemic circulation. These are discussed in the Absorption and Bioavailability section and include processes such as decomposition or metabolism in gastrointestinal (GI) fluid, metabolism in the GI wall and liver before systemic distribution, and bacterial metabolism in the lower end of the gut.

The elimination process of parent drug from the body is schematically illustrated in Figure 30, which assumes a one-compartment body model that contains the major eliminating organs, the liver and kidney. Each organ is associated with a first-order rate constant for a specific compound, which is represented by k_m for hepatic metabolism and k_u for urinary excretion. The sum of these constants forms the apparent overall elimination rate constant, K. The scheme to the right of the model illustrates the elimination with parallel (or competing) eliminating processes for the kidney and liver. The parent compound in the body, X_B, is excreted via the kidney to form unchanged drug in the urine, X_U, and it is also metabolized by the liver to form metabolite, X_M. The subsequent appearance of metabolite in the urine via the kidney (X_{MU}) is downstream of

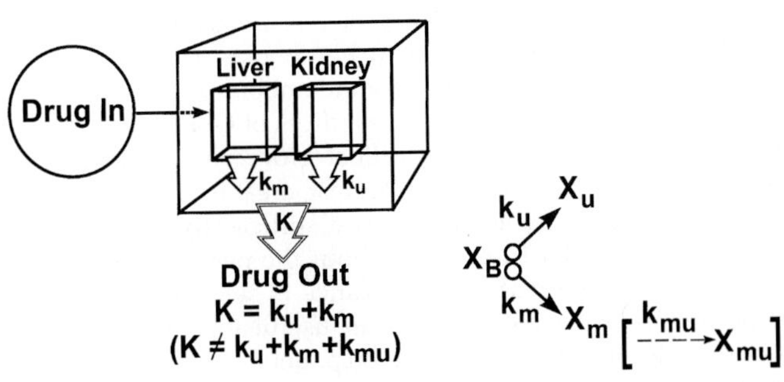

Figure 30. Schematic representation of elimination *via* hepatic metabolism and renal excretion in a one-compartment body model. The apparent overall first-order elimination rate constant, K, is the sum of the individual rate constants associated with loss of parent drug from the body. Thus, K is the sum of the urinary excretion rate constant, k_u, and the hepatic metabolic rate constant, k_m; $K = k_u + k_m$. The scheme used to describe elimination is shown to the right of the model. It is important to note that only those steps responsible for processing the parent drug (indicated as arrows connected to X_B, the amount of parent drug in the body) form part of K. Thus, the down-stream loss of metabolite via urinary excretion by the kidney, k_{mu}, is not part of parent drug elimination. (From Mayersohn M. Toxicokinetics: Measurement of disposition half-life, clearance and residence times. In: Maines M, ed. *Current protocols in toxicology*. New York: John Wiley and Sons, 2000:5.3.5, with permission of Saguaro Technical Press, Inc, 2002, Tucson, AZ.)

parent drug elimination and has no bearing on the value of K. This point is sometimes confused in the literature. Assume that 100% of the compound is metabolized by the liver and that all of that metabolite ultimately appears in the urine. The statement that the *compound is excreted into the urine* is not correct; it is the metabolite that is excreted into the urine and that process is not related to elimination of the parent compound, which is strictly metabolism. In that instance, systemic clearance is equal to hepatic metabolic clearance (renal clearance is zero).

Renal Excretion

The kidney is ideally suited as an organ of elimination on the basis of its specialized anatomy and biochemistry and high blood flow. The functioning unit of the kidney is the nephron, of which there are approximately 1.3 million in each human kidney. The nephron is schematically illustrated in Figure 31. Although not thoroughly illustrated, the nephron consists of the glomerulus, proximal and distal tubules, loop of Henle, and the collecting duct. Approximately 20% of cardiac output (in a normal, lean 70-kg adult man), approximately 1200 ml of blood, perfuses the kidneys each minute. Assuming a hematocrit of approximately 0.5, renal plasma flow is approximately equal to 600 ml/minute. Because only approximately 20% of plasma is filtered by the glomerulus, glomerular filtration rate (GFR) (actually, *filtration clearance*) is approximately 120 ml/minute.* This *filtration fraction* of 0.2 is calculated by the ratio of glomerular filtration clearance (for a compound that only undergoes that process; e.g., inulin, approximately 120 ml/minute) to an estimate of renal plasma flow (as measured by tubular secretion clearance of a compound that exclusively undergoes active tubular secretion; e.g., PAH). Urine production is approximately 1 ml/minute, which represents the difference between what is filtered, approximately 120 ml/minute, and what is reabsorbed, or approximately 119 ml/minute, indicating efficient reabsorption of water.

Arterial blood flows through the glomerulus, which is responsible for the passive filtration of compounds from the blood. The filtered material includes waste products as well as drugs and other foreign chemicals. This passive process is governed by a variety of factors, including glomerular integrity, molecular size of the compound, and binding to plasma proteins. Large molecules, such as proteins, are generally too large to be filtered. Compounds that are highly plasma protein bound are protected from filtration; only the unbound form is filtered. Creatinine and inulin are used as indices of GFR. Although the latter may more accurately reflect glomerular filtration, it requires exogenous dosing. In contrast, creatinine is an endogenous biochemical, which provides a sufficiently accurate estimate of glomerular filtration without the need for exogenous dosing. Because creatinine clearance is seldom determined experimentally in a patient, there are useful approximating relationships for its estimation based on patient gender, age, weight, and serum creatinine concentration.

Because glomerular filtration permits passage of only the unbound form of the material from plasma into the urine, the rate of filtration of the substance is a function of the GFR and the unbound plasma concentration (C_U) of the substance. The latter represents the driving force for filtration,

$$\text{Filtration rate} = GFR \cdot C_U = GFR \cdot f_U \cdot C_{TOTAL} \qquad \text{[Eq. 31]}$$

in which C_{TOTAL} is the total concentration (i.e., bound plus unbound) of the substance in plasma. Therefore, filtration clear-

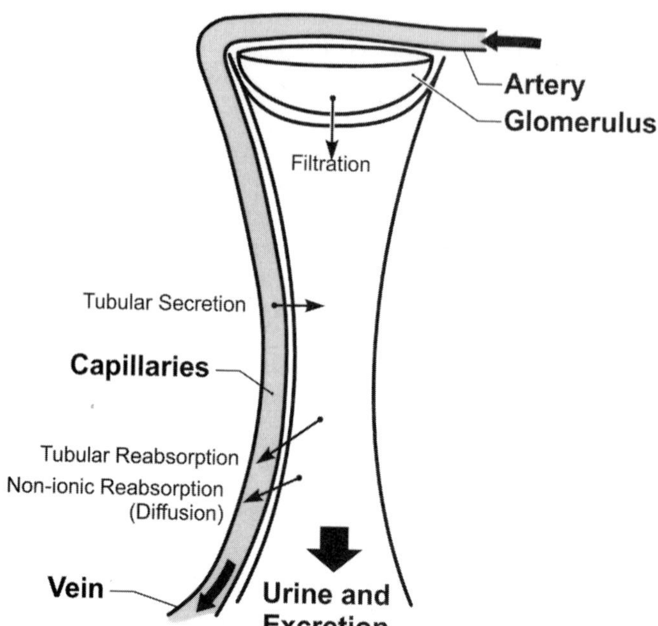

Figure 31. Schematic diagram illustrating the nephron, the functioning unit of the kidney. Arterial blood flow to the glomerulus results in the passive filtration of compound. Tubular secretion is an active, energy-dependent process resulting in movement of a compound against a concentration gradient into the urine. In the distal tubules, compounds present in the urine can undergo active, energy-dependent reabsorption back into the blood. A passive, nonionic diffusion process can also result in reabsorption of certain compounds from the urine back into the blood, depending on their pK_a, oil/water partition coefficient, and urine pH. Filtered and secreted compound is excreted into the formed urine. (From M. Mayersohn, *unpublished*, with permission from Saguaro Technical Press, Inc, Tucson, AZ, 2002.)

ance of a substance is simply the filtration rate divided by the total drug concentration,

$$CL_{FILTR} = \frac{\text{filtration rate}}{C_{TOTAL}} = \frac{GFR \cdot C_{TOTAL} \cdot f_U}{C_{TOTAL}} = GFR \cdot f_U \qquad \text{[Eq. 32]}$$

As a consequence, renal clearance, CL_R, of a substance by glomerular filtration only, should be equal to the GFR of that subject multiplied by the unbound fraction of the substance in plasma. If renal clearance of the compound exceeds the value for CL_{FILTR}, the drug undergoes some tubular secretion. In contrast, if CL_R is less than the value for CL_{FILTR}, the compound undergoes reabsorption. Of course, it is always possible that all of these processes are taking place at the same time. Notice, from equation 32, that CL_{FILTR} is not dependent on plasma concentration of the substance, as long as GFR and plasma protein binding do not change.

In contrast to glomerular filtration, which is a passive process, *tubular secretion* and *tubular reabsorption* are active and saturable, nonlinear processes, much like Michaelis-Menten enzyme kinetics. In fact, the identical relationship can be used to describe those processes, although T_{max}, for transport maximum, sometimes replaces V_{max}. Tubular secretion and tubular reabsorption may be described by the same equation, the only difference is the sign placed in front of the equation, to indicate movement out of or into the body, respectively.

$$\text{Rate of secretion} = \frac{V_{max}^{secr} \cdot C}{k_{mm}^{secr} + C} \qquad \text{Rate of reabsorption} = \frac{V_{max}^{reabs} \cdot C}{k_{mm}^{reabs} + C} \qquad \text{[Eq. 33]}$$

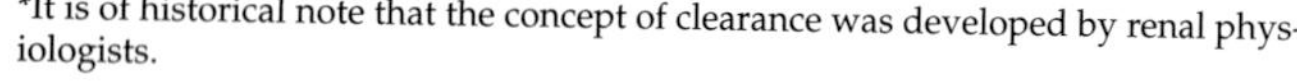

*It is of historical note that the concept of clearance was developed by renal physiologists.

The corresponding relationships for clearance by secretion and reabsorption are

$$CL_{SECR} = \frac{\text{rate of secretion}}{C} = \frac{V_{max}^{secr}}{k_{mm}^{secr} + C} \quad \text{[Eq. 34]}$$

$$CL_{REABS} = \frac{\text{rate of reabsorption}}{C} = \frac{V_{max}^{reabs}}{k_{mm}^{reabs} + C}$$

As plasma concentrations increase as a result of larger doses, secretion clearance and reabsorption clearance decrease; they become less efficient processes, just as one sees with saturable enzyme kinetics. Compounds such as PAH and penicillin undergo active tubular secretion, whereas many endogenous biochemicals (e.g., glucose, amino acids, vitamins, and so forth) undergo tubular reabsorption.

Net urinary excretion rate and renal clearance are a function of all renal mechanisms. Thus, the net urinary excretion rate equals: filtration rate + secretion rate – reabsorption rate – non-ionic reabsorption rate. Dividing each of those rates by plasma concentration gives the corresponding values for clearance.

$$CL_R = CL_{FILTR} + CL_{SECR} - CL_{REABS} - CL_{N.I.REABS} \quad \text{[Eq. 35]}$$

Renal clearance of a compound is determined experimentally by obtaining plasma and urine excretion data and plotting, according to the basic relationship for clearance, rate of urinary excretion versus plasma concentration at the same time or amount excreted versus AUC for corresponding times.

Figure 32A illustrates the rate processes that PAH undergoes as a function of unbound plasma concentration (18). Filtration rate increases directly with concentration, as expected of a passive process. Secretion, in contrast, becomes saturated, and the rate of secretion becomes constant (approaches a V_{max} or a transport maximum, T_{max}). This is exactly what was noted previously for the rate of enzyme metabolism described by Michaelis-Menten kinetics. Because net urinary excretion is the sum of secretion and filtration, that value increases as concentration increases, filtration becoming numerically more important as concentration increases.

The corresponding clearance-concentration relationships are illustrated in Figure 32B. These graphs are obtained by dividing the rates (shown in Figure 32A) by plasma concentrations of PAH. Filtration clearance remains constant, independent of plasma concentration, as expected of a passive, first-order process. Clearance due to secretion decreases as concentrations rise; the process becomes less efficient. Renal clearance, which is the sum of filtration and secretion clearances, decreases as concentrations increase and, ultimately, approaches the value for filtration clearance. The expression for PAH renal clearance is

$$CL_R = CL_{FILTR} + CL_{SECR} = CL_{FILTR} + \frac{V_{max}^{secr}}{k_{mm} + C} \quad \text{[Eq. 36]}$$

As PAH plasma concentrations, C, increase, the term on the right approaches zero and CL_R is approximately equal to CL_{FILTR}.

The comparable graphical relationships for a compound, such as glucose, that undergo tubular reabsorption are illustrated in Figure 33 (19). Rates of the different renal mechanisms as a function of glucose plasma concentration are illustrated in Figure 33A. Filtration increases directly with glucose concentration. Up to a glucose plasma concentration of approximately 2 mg/ml, all of the glucose that has been filtered is reabsorbed back into the body; no glucose appears in the urine. The reabsorption mechanism becomes saturated, as noted for PAH secretion, and rate of secretion becomes constant (a V_{max} or T_{max} is achieved). As a consequence, the net excretion rate is zero until a glucose plasma concentration of approximately 2 mg/ml, beyond which filtration takes over and glucose excretion increases with concentration.

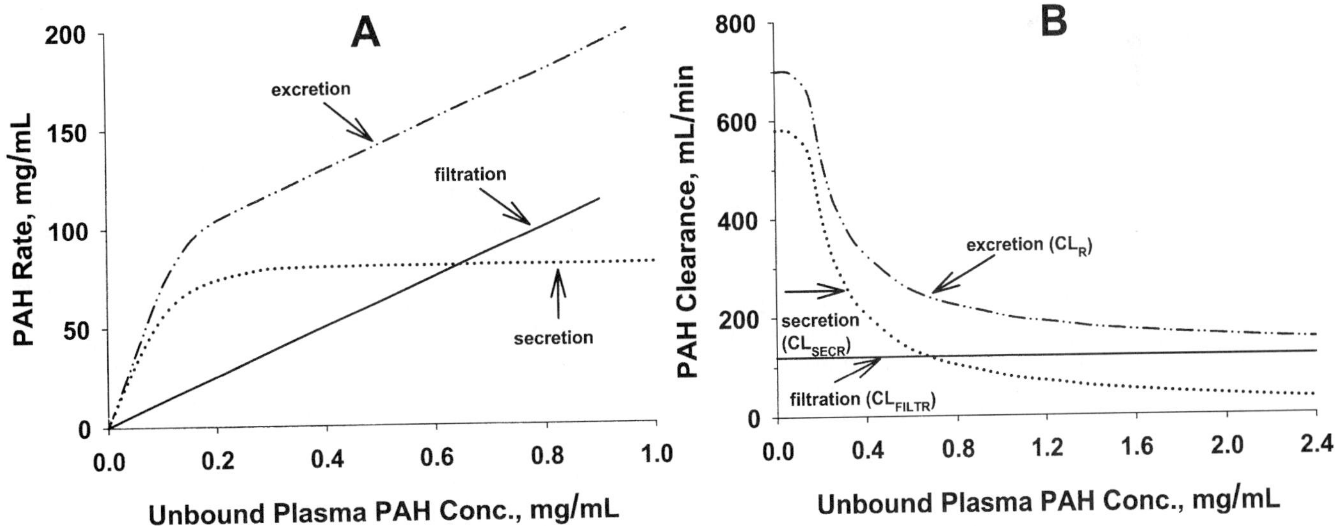

Figure 32. **A:** Rate of para-aminohippurate (PAH) processing by different renal mechanisms as a function of unbound plasma PAH concentrations. Excretion rate is the sum of filtration rate, which remains constant, and secretion rate, which becomes saturated (approximately 80 mg per minute) above a plasma concentration of approximately 0.1 mg/ml. At low plasma concentrations, excretion rate is equal to secretion rate, whereas above saturation concentrations, filtration rate becomes more important. **B:** The rate processes in **A** have been divided by unbound plasma PAH concentrations to give corresponding clearance values plotted as a function of unbound PAH plasma concentrations. Filtration clearance (CL_{FILTR}) remains constant, whereas secretion clearance (CL_{SECR}) decreases with PAH concentration. As a result, net renal clearance (CL_R) of PAH decreases, approaching the value of CL_{FILTR}. (Based on data recovered from Pitts RF. *Physiology of the kidney and body fluids*, 3rd ed. Chicago: Year Book 1974:141–142. From M. Mayersohn, unpublished, with permission from Saguaro Technical Press, Inc, Tucson, AZ, 2002.)

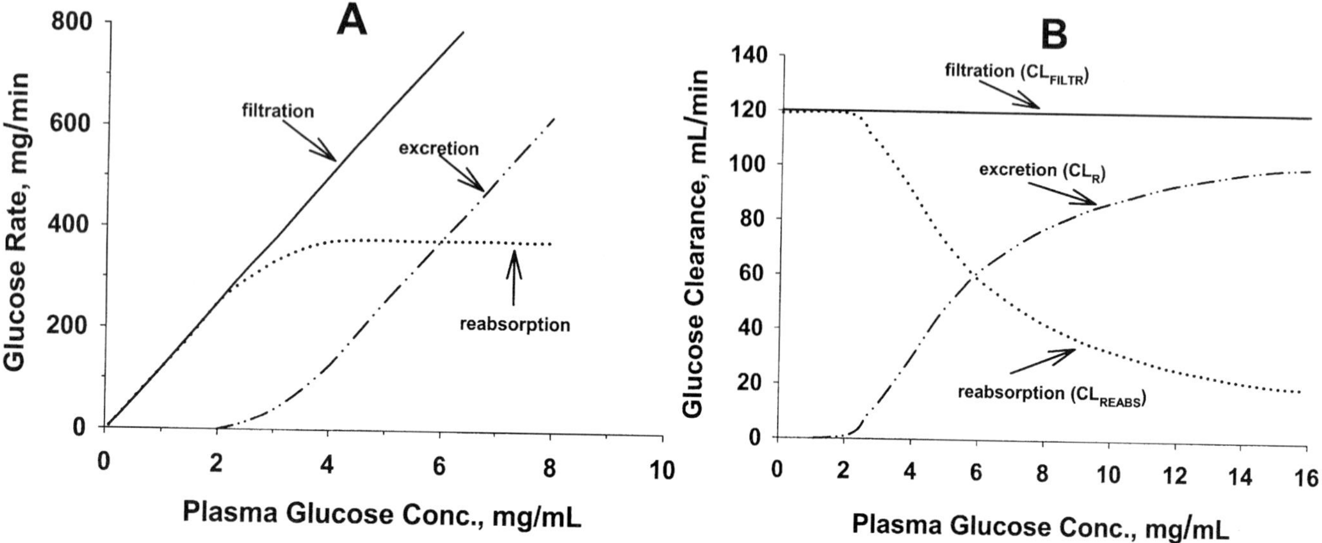

Figure 33. A: Rate of glucose processing by different renal mechanisms as a function of glucose plasma concentrations. Excretion rate is the sum of filtration rate, which remains constant, and reabsorption rate, which becomes saturated (approximately 400 mg/minute) above a plasma concentration of approximately 2 mg/ml. At low plasma concentrations, excretion rate is approximately zero, because what is filtered is reabsorbed. At higher plasma concentrations, filtration exceeds reabsorption, and glucose is excreted into the urine. **B:** The rate processes in **A** have been divided by glucose plasma concentrations to give corresponding clearance values plotted as a function of glucose plasma concentrations. Filtration clearance (CL_{FILTR}) remains constant, whereas reabsorption clearance (CL_{REABS}) decreases with glucose concentration. As a result, net renal clearance (CL_R) of glucose increases, approaching the value of CL_{FILTR}. (Based on data recovered from Pitts RF. *Physiology of the kidney and body fluids*, 3rd ed. Chicago: Year Book 1974:73–74. From M. Mayersohn, *unpublished*, with permission from Saguaro Technical Press, Inc, Tucson, AZ, 2002.)

The corresponding clearance relationships for glucose are illustrated in Figure 33B. Filtration clearance does not change with glucose plasma concentrations. Reabsorption clearance, however, becomes less efficient and decreases with glucose concentration, approaching a value of zero. The net renal clearance increases from zero until it approaches filtration clearance as described by

$$CL_R = CL_{FILTR} - CL_{REABS} = CL_{FILTR} - \frac{V_{max}^{reabs}}{k_{mm} + C} \quad \text{[Eq. 37]}$$

As glucose plasma concentrations, C, increase, the term on the right approaches zero and CL_R is approximately equal to CL_{FILTR}.

The other reabsorption process, which has been referred to as *nonionic reabsorption* or *nonionic diffusion*, is passive, non–energy-requiring transport. To undergo this process, a compound must have sufficient lipophilicity (as measured by oil/water partition coefficient) and an ionization constant (pK_a) such that a reasonable fraction of the compound is unionized at urine pH. The latter are two important factors that affect the movement of any compound across an epithelial membrane. For some compounds, urine flow may also be important. Because the unionized form of a compound has the greatest lipophilicity, and it is that form that most readily penetrates biologic membranes, the urine pH that minimizes ionization is expected to promote reabsorption. Of course, just the opposite is true with regard to renal excretion; the urine pH that increases ionization is expected to decrease reabsorption and promote excretion. The latter observation is the basis for treatment of overdose of certain acidic or basic compounds whose clearance is partially renal. The efficiency of such urine pH manipulation, however, must be viewed cautiously and with consideration of the basic pharmacokinetic properties of the compound. An illustration of the effect of urine pH on the urinary excretion of a basic compound, methamphetamine, is presented in Figure 34 (20). Acidification of urine is expected to ionize the compound in urine and thereby minimize reabsorption and increase renal clearance. In contrast, alkalinization of urine is expected to create the opposite condition: decreased ionization, increased reabsorption, and reduced renal clearance. That is exactly what is seen in Figure 34 for rate of urinary excretion versus time and for the total amount recovered in 16 hours after oral dosing in humans (bar graphs to the right). The rate of urinary excretion is given by excretion rate = $CL_R \cdot C$. Excretion rate increases as a consequence of an increase in renal clearance in the presence of acidified urine. Just the opposite occurs during alkalinization of urine. Under the proper circumstances, alteration of urine pH might prove effective for treatment of overdose for certain weakly acidic or basic compounds.

A good example to illustrate the previous point is urine acidification in an attempt to enhance excretion of the basic drug, phencyclidine (PCP; pK_a = 8.5). Table 2 summarizes the analysis (21). Under uncontrolled urine pH conditions, renal clearance accounts for less than approximately 10% of the elimination of the compound (i.e., $CL_R/CL_S \cong 0.1$), whereas the nonrenal component (CL_{NR}), hepatic metabolism, which represents the major route of elimination, accounts for the remainder, approximately 92%. When the urine is made acidic, the value of nonrenal clearance is not expected to change; it remains approximately 350 ml/minute. It is important to keep in mind that organ clearances are independent of each other, except as a result of some indirect mechanism. In contrast, the renal clearance of PCP increases dramatically from 30 ml/minute to a value approximately four to five times greater, 135 ml/minute. The latter value now represents approximately 28% of systemic clearance (i.e., CL_R/CL_S = 135/485 = 28%). What is the return for this large increase in renal clearance? Systemic clearance, which determines $t_{1/2}$, only increases by 28%, resulting in a decrease in $t_{1/2}$ of a similar magnitude. Thus, a dramatic increase in organ clearance, as noted here for PCP renal clearance,

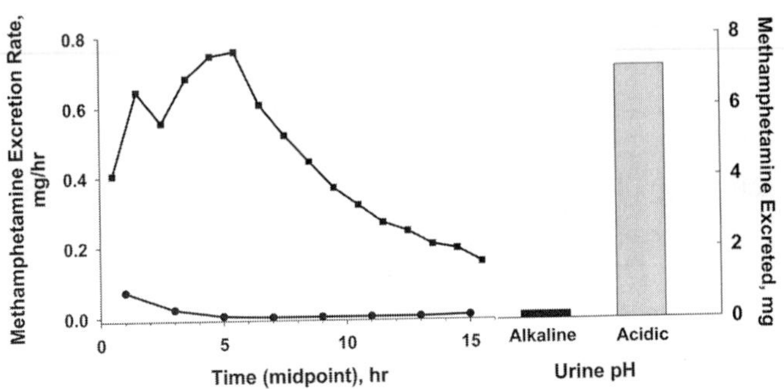

Figure 34. Urinary excretion rate of methamphetamine versus time after the oral administration of 11 mg of the drug to human subjects. The two lines represent different urine pH conditions: acidic pH (■), alkaline pH (●). The total area under the rate curves, which represents the cumulative amount of unchanged methamphetamine excreted into the urine up to 16 hours after dosing, is presented to the right in the form of bar graphs. (Based on data presented in Beckett AH, Rowland M. Urinary excretion kinetics of methylamphetamine in man. *Nature* 1965;206:1260–1261. From M. Mayersohn, *unpublished*, with permission from Saguaro Technical Press, Inc, Tucson, AZ, 2002.)

TABLE 2. Influence of urine acidification on phencyclidine elimination in humans[a]

Parameter	Urine pH: Uncontrolled	Urine pH: Acidic (<5)
Clearance (ml/min)		
Systemic (CL_S)	380	485
Nonrenal (CL_{NR})	350	350
Renal (CL_R)	30	135
CL_R as % CL_S	8	28
Percent increase in Cl_S	—	350
Percent increase in Cl_S	—	28
Elimination $t_{1/2}$(h)	13	10
Percent decrease in $t_{1/2}$	—	23

CL_S, systemic clearance; CL_{NR}, nonrenal clearance; CL_R, renal clearance; $t_{1/2}$, half-life.
[a]Based on data in Mayersohn M. Rational approaches to treatment of drug toxicity: recent considerations and application of pharmacokinetic principles. In: Barnett G, Chiang CN, eds. *Pharmacokinetics and pharmacodynamics of psychoactive drugs.* Foster City, CA: Biomedical Publications, 1985:120–142.

does not necessarily translate into a similar, dramatic change in systemic clearance or $t_{1/2}$. In fact, renal clearance would need to increase by approximately tenfold, for $t_{1/2}$ to decrease by 50%. The success of overdose treatment by manipulating urine pH, in terms of enhancing elimination of a poison and clinical outcome, depends on the contribution of the renal pathway to overall clearance; the greater that fraction, the greater the impact of altered urine pH.

Urine flow is another variable that may affect renal clearance of compounds that undergo reabsorption (22). As noted in Figure 35A, there is a direct relationship between renal clearance of three barbiturates in humans and urine flow. The magnitude of this effect varies among the specific compounds. Figure 35B is a nice illustration of how urine pH alone or with urine flow can affect the renal clearance of a compound, in this case phenobarbital. The renal clearance of the weak acid phenobarbital is increased by urine alkalinization, which promotes ionization, reduces reabsorption, and increases excretion. Increasing urine flow, in conjunction with urine alkalinization, further promotes renal clearance. This observation has led to the idea of *forced alkaline diuresis* for overdose treatment of susceptible organic acids. Compounds that display a pH dependence in renal clearance are also urine flow dependent to an extent that depends on the degree of tubular reabsorption.

Hepatic (Metabolic) Elimination and Metabolite Kinetics

As noted for the kidney, the liver is ideally suited for its role as an eliminating organ by being able to metabolically alter, via

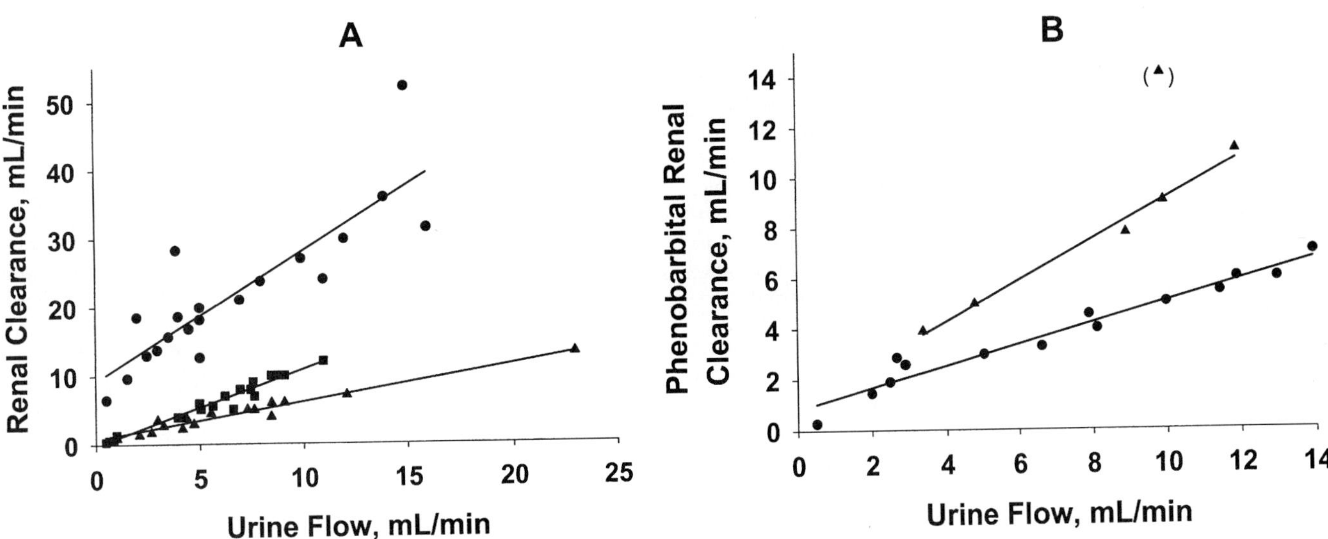

Figure 35. A: Renal clearance of several barbituric acid derivatives in humans as a function of urine flow. Each line represents the linear regression analysis of the data. Amobarbital, ▲; butabarbital, ■; cyclobarbital, ●. **B:** Renal clearance of phenobarbital in humans as a function of urine flow and urine pH. Each line represents the linear regression analysis of the data. One point (in parentheses) has not been used in the regression analysis. Alkalinized urine, pH > 7.6, ▲; uncontrolled urine pH, ●. (Based on the data in Linton AL, Luke RG, Briggs JD. Methods of forced diuresis and its application in barbiturate poisoning. *Lancet* 1967;2:377–380. From M. Mayersohn, *unpublished*, with permission from Saguaro Technical Press, Inc, Tucson, AZ, 2002.)

enzyme action, and endogenous and exogenous compounds. Whereas other tissues (e.g., lung, kidney, muscle) have metabolic enzyme capability, the liver is a virtual storehouse of enzyme activity. The liver, as noted for the kidney, receives a substantial blood flow (approximately 1500 ml per minute). In addition, the liver occupies a unique anatomical position by receiving all absorbed material from the GI tract (for processing) via the portal circulation before systemic distribution. The latter results in the *hepatic first-pass effect*, which is discussed in the Absorption and Bioavailability section. The liver is also capable of extracting compounds from blood and excreting them into bile. The bile then flows to the GI tract where the compound might undergo absorption (*entero-hepatic circulation*), further metabolism (with or without subsequent absorption), or loss via the feces. A discussion of the complex anatomical and biochemical features of the liver is beyond the scope of this chapter.

The process of urinary excretion of a compound (or metabolite) is relatively similar among normal, healthy people, because there are relatively few variables that affect the efficiency of urinary excretion (e.g., urine pH, urine flow). The efficiency of renal function can be gauged rather well with reference to creatinine clearance. The latter measure gives a good *handle* on the functional activity of the kidney, and it serves to relate to and predict the kinetics of drug excretion from the body. There is no comparable measure of liver function that one can use to relate to enzymatic metabolic efficiency; there is not a *handle* on hepatic efficacy as there is with renal function. Furthermore, there are a host of variables that may affect metabolic function, including age, gender, genetics, environmental exposure, nutrition, other drugs, disease states, and so forth. As a consequence, it is not at all surprising to find that the metabolic activity for a given compound varies enormously among even a young, healthy population. This is especially true of $t_{1/2}$ values, which result from the individual variations in both apparent volume of distribution and metabolic clearance.

The metabolite(s) produced by biotransformation reactions are often, but not always, more water-soluble than the parent drug, allowing the metabolite to be excreted into the urine. In general, the metabolite is formed irreversibly, but there are some exceptions in which the metabolite may undergo reversible metabolism to the parent compound. The pharmacologic and toxicologic activity of the parent/metabolite pair allows several possibilities: The metabolite may have less, about the same, or greater activity/toxicity than the parent compound. Understanding which situation applies is obviously of great importance in toxicology and in treatment of overdose. For example, an overdose of methanol or ethylene glycol leads to toxic metabolites. The only appropriate strategy to take in that instance, in addition to maintaining life signs, is to try and reduce the intake, if possible (e.g., reduce absorption), and remove the parent compound from the body while slowing conversion to metabolites. In fact, effective treatment of toxicity created by ingestion of those compounds includes the application of extracorporeal devices (e.g., hemodialysis) to remove the parent compound and administration of ethanol or 4-methylpyrazole to inhibit the metabolism to the toxic metabolites. This specific example is discussed in the next section.

An older but still useful depiction of metabolism of exogenous compounds divides all such events into phase I and phase II processes. This is noted in the following Scheme 1. Phase I processes are those associated with chemical modifications that involve oxidation, hydrolysis, or reduction. The predominant enzymes here are those in the cytochrome P-450 superfamily. Phase II reactions, in contrast, involve addition of chemical groups and are referred to as conjugation reactions. Examples include glucuronidation, glycination, sulfation, acetylation, or methylation. These derivatives are

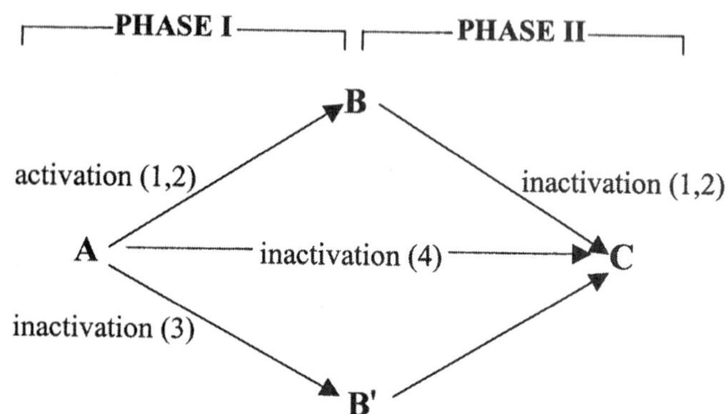

Scheme 1. General scheme depicting drug metabolism reactions falling into phase I and phase II processes.

virtually always more water-soluble than the parent compound and are found excreted into urine or bile. Although conjugates are most often inactive, they can possess pharmacologic activity (e.g., morphine-6-glucuronide) or exert toxicity (e.g., some acyl glucuronides). In the previous scheme, *activation* and *inactivation* may refer to pharmacologic or toxicologic properties. In possibility 1, compound A is inactive and is converted into active compound B, which is then inactivated by conjugation to compound C. Possibility 2 assumes that compound A is active and is converted into compound B, which has similar or different activity from A. In possibility 3, compound A is active and is converted into inactive compound B', which is further metabolized by conjugation into compound C. Finally, compound A is active or inactive and is directly converted into compound C of lesser, equal, or greater activity. The metabolic schemes for a large number of compounds are readily available in the extensive metabolism literature.

As noted in First-Order (Linear) Kinetic Processes, the vast majority of compounds undergoes first-order elimination kinetics. The notable exceptions are those compounds ingested in large doses (perhaps during an overdose) and those relatively rare compounds that have Michaelis constants below the plasma concentrations resulting from ingestion or exposure. The consequences of non–first-order or nonlinear elimination have been discussed in Non–First-Order (Nonlinear) Kinetic Processes. Therefore, the assumption that metabolite formation and subsequent elimination occur by first-order processes can be made here. The relatively simple Scheme 2 considers parallel or competitive elimination of the parent compound and sequential formation and subsequent elimination of the metabolite.

The portion of the scheme that is of interest for this discussion is parent compound to metabolite in body to metabolite in urine (or to another metabolite). This sequential kinetic scheme is sometimes referred to as an *A to B to C* system, and it occurs with some frequency in pharmacokinetics (e.g., it is often used in describing parent drug in the blood after absorption). The plasma concentration of metabolite (C_m) formed as a function of time after IV bolus administration of parent compound is given by the following relationship:

$$C_m = \frac{k_m \cdot X^0}{V_m(k_{mu} - K)} \cdot (e^{-K \cdot t} - e^{-k_{mu} \cdot t}) \equiv A \cdot (e^{-K \cdot t} - e^{-k_{mu} \cdot t}) \quad \text{[Eq. 38]}$$

in which V_m is the apparent volume of distribution of metabolite, X^0 is the IV bolus dose, K is the apparent overall first-order elimination rate constant ($K = k_m + k_u$), and A is a constant equal to the value of the terms shown in the coefficient. An equation containing the difference between two exponential terms rises and declines with time. At time zero, C_m is zero (because e^{-0} is 1 and 1 minus 1 is zero) and at time infinity C_m

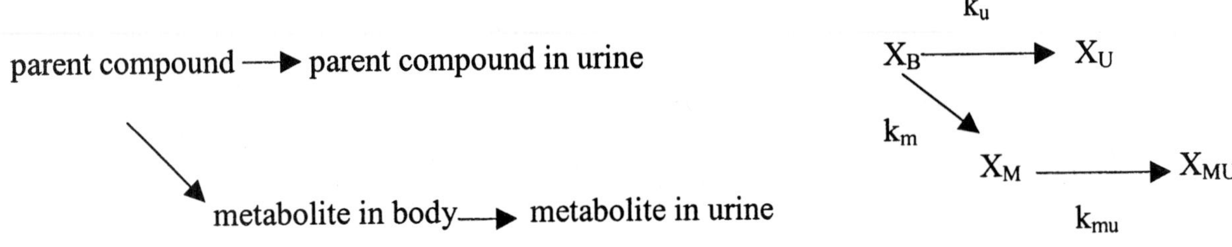

Scheme 2. Simple scheme illustrating parallel (or competitive) elimination of parent compound and consecutive metabolite formation and elimination. The amount of each form (parent or metabolite) is represented by X, and the subscript indicates the form and location.

is zero (because $e^{-\infty}$ is 0). Because one of the two rate constants in the exponential terms must be larger than the other one (i.e., $K > k_{mu}$ or $k_{mu} > K$), the product of that rate constant and time must be greater than the other rate constant and time. The larger product raised as a negative to any base value approaches zero before the other, numerically smaller, exponential term. Thus, at some time, only one exponential term predominates, leading to a log-linear relationship whose slope reflects the smaller of the two rate constants. This is similar to the discussion of multi-compartment models; the terminal slope (e.g., given by β or λ) is always the numerically smallest of all of the rate constants that appear in exponential form (i.e., $\beta < \alpha$ or $\lambda_n < \lambda_{n-1}$). The rule that applies here is that in any sequence of kinetic steps, the slowest step (i.e., smallest rate constant) rate-controls or rate-limits the entire process, and that step (or rate constant) determines the terminal slope of, in this case, plasma metabolite concentration versus time. This idea of a *rate-limiting step* is useful and frequently encountered in pharmacokinetics whenever sequential processes are seen (e.g., as with absorption into the body).

Plasma metabolite concentrations rise after administration of the parent compound as the metabolite is formed, reach a peak, and then decline. When those data are plotted on semilog axes, ultimately there is a log-linear terminal line, indicating that one exponential dominates, and the slope of that line is a function of either K or k_{mu}. If parent compound plasma concentrations are also determined with time, that slope by definition is given by K; then, by comparison, one can ascribe meaning to the slope of the metabolite profile. The slope is the same as the parent compound (i.e., K), in which case, $k_{mu} > K$, or the slope is smaller than that for K, in which case, the slope must be k_{mu} (i.e., $K > k_{mu}$). Consider the two possible cases.

CASE I

If the metabolite is formed slowly but eliminated rapidly, then $k_{mu} > K$. This is referred to as *metabolite formation rate-limited elimination*. Because the rate-limiting step is K, the terminal slope is a function of K. At some time, once the fast exponential term approaches zero, the remaining slower exponential term is given by

$$C_m \cong A \cdot (e^{-K \cdot t}) \qquad \text{[Eq. 39]}$$

This case is quite common. An example is shown in Figure 36 for morphine given as an IV bolus to humans and two formed morphine glucuronide metabolites (23). One of the latter metabolites (morphine-6-glucuronide) has been of considerable interest because of its known analgesic activity; however, a recent study suggests that it contributes relatively little to the overall analgesic activity derived from morphine dosing (24).

Notice that the terminal lines for morphine and each metabolite are parallel, indicating the same value for the terminal slope, which, by definition, must correspond to the terminal $t_{1/2}$ for the parent drug, morphine. This parallelism in lines indicates that the metabolites are formed slowly and then rapidly eliminated.

CASE II

In contrast to the previous situation, the metabolite is formed rapidly but then undergoes slow elimination, slower than the parent compound: $k_{mu} < K$. This is referred to as *excretion rate-limited elimination*. Because the slower and rate-limiting step is k_{mu}, the terminal slope of the metabolite concentration-time data must be governed by that rate constant. In contrast, the terminal slope for the parent compound, by definition, must be given by K. At some time, the exponent containing K approaches zero leaving the other, single (terminal) exponent,

$$C_m \cong A \cdot (e^{-k_{mu} \cdot t}) \qquad \text{[Eq. 40]}$$

A number of parent-metabolite pairs fall into this category. One such example is procainamide and its metabolite, *N*-acetyl-

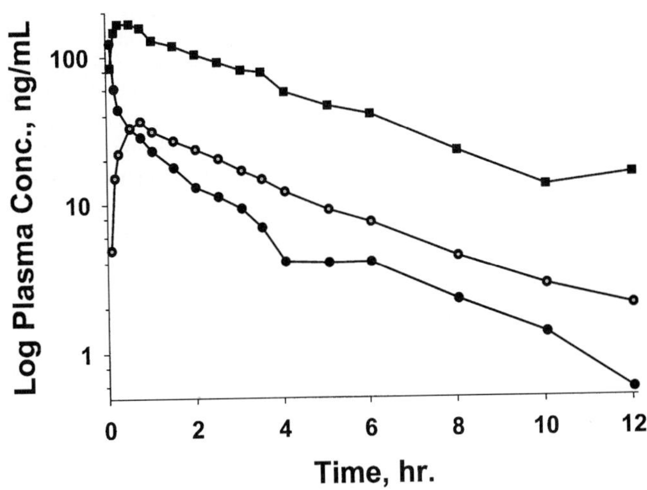

Figure 36. Plasma concentrations of morphine (●) and its formed metabolites, morphine-3-glucuronide (■) and morphine-6-glucuronide (○), after a 5-mg intravenous bolus dose of morphine to ten human subjects. Note that the terminal lines for all compounds are parallel. (Based on the data in Osborne R, Joel S, Trew D, et al. Morphine and metabolite behavior after different routes of morphine administration: demonstration of the importance of the active metabolite morphine-6-glucuronide. *Clin Pharmacol Ther* 1990;47:12–19.)

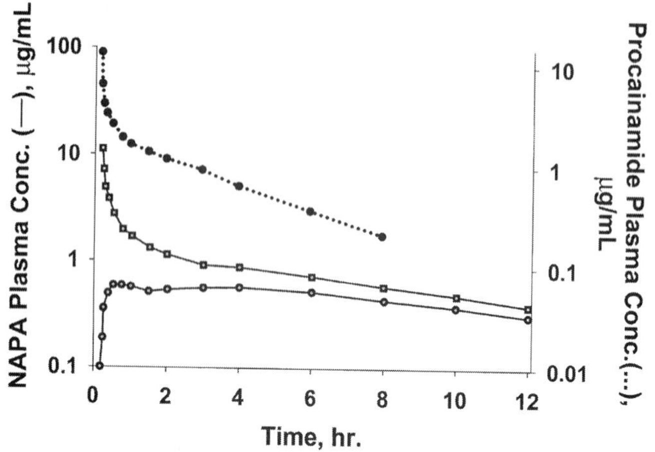

Figure 37. Plasma concentrations of procainamide (●; y-axis on right) and the concentrations of its formed metabolite, *N*-acetylprocainamide, NAPA (○; y-axis on left), after a 436-mg intravenous dose of procainamide in one human subject. Also shown are the concentrations of *N*-acetylprocainamide after a 268-mg intravenous dose of *N*-acetylprocainamide in the same subject (□; y-axis on left). The procainamide plasma concentrations have been plotted on the right-side y-axis using an elevated scale for the two intravenous curves not to coincide. Note that the terminal lines for *N*-acetylprocainamide are parallel to each, but they are not the same as that of procainamide. This is an example of metabolite excretion being slower than its formation. (Based on the data in Dutcher JS, Strong JM, Lucas SV, et al. Procainamide and *N*-acetylprocainamide kinetics investigated simultaneously with stable isotope methodology. *Clin Pharmacol Ther* 1977;22:447–457. From M. Mayersohn, *unpublished*, with permission from Saguaro Technical Press, Inc, Tucson, AZ, 2002.)

procainamide. Figure 37 illustrates the plasma concentrations of procainamide and the formed *N*-acetylprocainamide metabolite after IV dosing of procainamide in a human subject (25). The terminal slopes of those two compounds are not the same; the metabolite concentration-time data results in a shallower slope compared to the parent compound, suggesting rapid metabolite formation and slow subsequent elimination. That conclusion is further supported by the value of the terminal slope of the metabolite data after its IV administration, the slope of which must be given by k_{mu}. The latter line is parallel to the formed *N*-acetylprocainamide line, and neither is equal to the procainamide slope.

Alterations in metabolism may result from increased (induction) or decreased (inhibition) enzymatic activity. The latter are often the result of drug-drug and nutrient-drug interactions. Most of those interactions involve the cytochrome P-450 enzyme family, which is the predominant system responsible for drug metabolism. Among the numerous hepatic isozymes present in the body, only a handful is responsible for the majority of the interactions. One isozyme, CYP 3A4 alone, accounts for approximately 50% of the known interactions (leading to its being referred to as a *promiscuous* enzyme). Approximately 90% of the reported interactions can be accounted for with CYP 3A4 and the following CYP isozymes: 1A2, 2C9/10, 2C19, 2D6, and 2E1. A recent text has provided a thorough review of this area (26).

A simple method to predict the possibility of an interaction resulting from inhibition by a compound can be obtained if certain assumptions are made. Assuming that the inhibition is competitive and that the linear rate versus substrate concentration curve exists, percentage inhibition is approximated by the following relationship:

$$\%\ \text{inhibition} = \frac{100 \cdot (\mathrm{I})}{\mathrm{k_i} + (\mathrm{I})} \qquad \text{[Eq. 41]}$$

Where (I) is the concentration of inhibitor and k_i is an inhibitor constant. The inhibitor constant is the concentration of inhibitor necessary to produce a 50% inhibition in the enzymatic reaction (similar in concept to the Michaelis-Menten constant, k_{MM}). When the inhibitor concentration is low, $(I) < k_i$, inhibition is a function of both (I) and k_i.

$$\%\ \text{inhibition} \cong \frac{100 \cdot (\mathrm{I})}{\mathrm{k_i}} \qquad \text{[Eq. 42]}$$

If, for example, (I) is 10 nM and k_i is 100 nM, an inhibition of approximately 10% is expected. The more serious situation occurs when the inhibitor concentration exceeds the inhibition constant $[(I) > k_i]$. In that case, the relationship approximates 100% inhibition.

There are many recent examples of clinically significant interactions resulting in serious toxicity as a result of inhibition interactions. These include interactions initiated by grapefruit juice and the antifungal agent ketoconazole, both of which inhibit CYP 3A4 metabolism of a variety of drugs. One example involves the first nonsedating antihistamine, terfenadine, which was withdrawn from the marketplace as a result of the inhibition of its metabolism leading to life-threatening cardiotoxicity referred to as torsade de pointes (prolongation of the QT interval). In this instance, it was the parent compound that was responsible for toxicity. The relative importance of these metabolic interactions after oral dosing depends on the value of the hepatic ER of the compound whose metabolism is being inhibited. The greater the hepatic ER, the more dramatic the effect of inhibition on the plasma concentrations and AUCs of the parent compound. Boxenbaum (27) has shown that the ketoconazole-terfenadine interaction results in a greater than 35-fold increase in terfenadine concentration or AUC. Terfenadine has a hepatic ER of approximately 0.95. In contrast, ketoconazole results in an approximate fourfold increase in the AUC of alprazolam whose hepatic ER is 0.065. It is the *first-pass effect*, discussed in the Absorption and Bioavailability section, that accounts for this dramatic dependence on hepatic ER.

In contrast to the previous examples, and one that illustrates the useful side of an interaction, is enzyme inhibition that results in reduced toxicity by minimizing the formation of a toxic metabolite(s). The classic examples are methanol (methyl alcohol; wood alcohol) and ethylene glycol (*antifreeze*). Methanol metabolism via alcohol dehydrogenase leads to the formation of the toxic metabolites formaldehyde and formic acid. Ethylene glycol metabolism via alcohol dehydrogenase results in a series of toxic compounds (glycoaldehyde, glycolic acid, glyoxylic acid, and oxalic acid). In addition to the use of hemodialysis to remove the parent compounds from the body (discussed below), an effective means to reduce the formation of the toxic metabolites is to administer ethanol. Ethanol competitively inhibits the metabolism of methanol and ethylene glycol because it has a greater affinity for the enzyme. Slowing the metabolism of the parent compound prolongs the formation of the toxic metabolites and prevents the metabolites from reaching toxic concentrations. Another compound, 4-methylpyrazole (fomepizole), is also an effective inhibitor or alcohol dehydrogenase, and it offers an alternative to the use of ethanol (28,29).

Extracorporeal Elimination

Increasing the rate of elimination of a compound from the body by enhancing metabolism may present a problem if active/toxic metabolites are produced, as noted for methanol and ethylene glycol. In contrast, efforts at enhancing removal of the parent compound from the body via urinary excretion or other routes/modes of elimination do not offer such a problem. As discussed previously, however, increasing urinary excretion proves efficient only if a substantial portion of the dose can be cleared by renal mechanisms. The latter is not an option for a compound that undergoes primarily hepatic metabolism. One mode that offers an additional route of elimination falls under the category of *extracorporeal* elimination. Such processes offer a new route of elimination from the body that the compound can use. Examples include peritoneal dialysis, hemodialysis, and hemoperfusion.

All dialysis (from the Greek, *to separate*) techniques are based on the same principles. A common laboratory technique referred to as *equilibrium dialysis* uses a semipermeable membrane to separate a protein-bound compound (present on one side of the membrane, for example, in a plasma sample) from unbound material capable of diffusing across the membrane into a solution on the other side of the membrane (generally a buffer). This technique is used to measure plasma protein binding. The unbound form of the compound equilibrates on both sides of the membrane in this, generally, static closed system procedure. By knowing the unbound concentration on one side of the membrane and the total concentration at the beginning of the experiment, the unbound fraction can be calculated. The same idea is applied to the removal of waste materials from the blood of patients with renal failure and, of interest here, for the removal of toxic compounds from the body. In *peritoneal dialysis*, the peritoneal membrane serves as the dialyzing membrane after the peritoneum is filled with dialyzing solution. The exact procedure applied varies and the modes used include intermittent, continuous, continuous ambulatory, and continuous cyclic peritoneal dialysis. Peritoneal dialysis finds its greatest use in the treatment of severe renal impairment. This is generally not an efficient procedure for the rapid removal of a toxic compound from the body after an overdose.

The dialysis method of choice for maintaining renally diseased patients and for treatment of overdose is *hemodialysis*, which has been referred to as the *artificial kidney*. This method is many times more efficient than peritoneal dialysis in removing substances from the blood; however, it is more complex and requires an expensive device. Figure 38 is a diagrammatic sketch of the important aspect of this process: the movement of molecules of the compound present in blood across a semipermeable membrane and into dialyzing fluid. The arterial blood is removed from the body via a pump and placed into a dialyzing machine, which has an extensive network of coils of semipermeable membrane, which are, in turn, filled with dialyzing fluid. The *unbound* form of the compound present in the blood moves down a concentration gradient and diffuses across the membrane into the dialysis fluid. As long as there is a concentration gradient, the compound continues to diffuse across the membrane and is removed from the blood. This is a dynamic process, preventing equilibrium from being achieved, unless the same fluid continues to be recycled through the machine. It is important to note that it is only the *unbound* form that diffuses across the membrane; the protein-bound form does not diffuse. Therefore, it should seem reasonable that highly plasma protein bound compounds are not good candidates for efficient removal by hemodialysis.

As for any other organ of elimination, the efficiency of dialysis removal of a compound from the blood can be judged by a dialysis ER and *dialysis clearance*, CL_D (often referred to in the renal literature as *dialysance*). All of the principles previously developed and discussed for organ clearance apply to hemodialysis clearance. Thus, clearance is from the blood, the fluid containing the compound, and from which extraction occurs. The maximum value for CL_D equals blood flow to the dialysis machine, which is generally approximately 200 ml/minute. Only the unbound form of the compound is dialyzed from the blood. Regardless of the efficiency of dialysis clearance, even

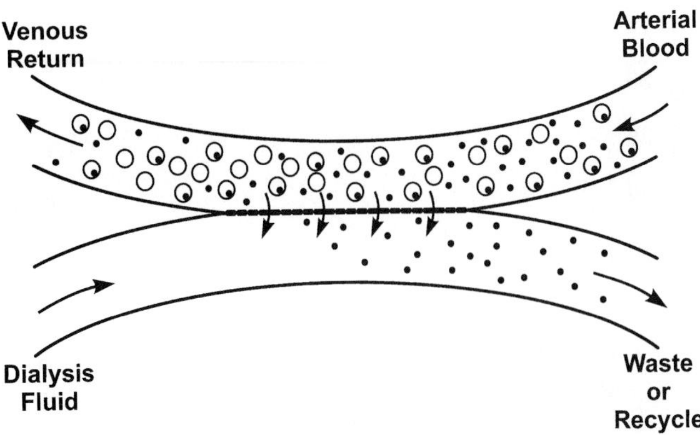

Figure 38. A diagrammatic sketch to illustrate the diffusion of a compound from blood during hemodialysis. Arterial blood is pumped into a hemodialyzer where it is separated from dialyzing fluid by a semipermeable membrane. The unbound form of the compound in the blood (*small solid circles*) moves down a concentration gradient as it diffuses across the membrane into the dialysis fluid, where it is carried away to waste (or is recycled). Note that the protein bound form (*small solid circle within the larger open circle*) is not removed from the blood. This dynamic process continues until the end of the dialysis period. (From M. Mayersohn, *unpublished*, with permission from Saguaro Technical Press, Inc, Tucson, AZ, 2002.)

complete removal of the compound from the bloodstream during a single dialysis period (approximately 4 to 6 hours) does not mean efficient removal from the body (i.e., little change in $t_{1/2}$). This is the identical issue that was discussed previously: efficient removal from the bloodstream versus effective removal from the entire body. Recall that $t_{1/2}$ is a function of clearance and apparent volume of distribution. The larger the apparent volume of distribution, less of the compound is removed from the body during dialysis (i.e., little effect on $t_{1/2}$).

Whether hemodialysis is an effective means for treating an overdose depends on two primary factors: plasma protein binding and the apparent volume of distribution. This has been nicely established by examination of the amount of drug removed from the body during dialysis as a function of those two pharmacokinetic parameters (30). That analysis provides a guideline for predicting the use of hemodialysis in treatment of drug overdose. A somewhat more unified approach is to incorporate both of those parameters into a single parameter, the *unbound apparent volume of distribution*, V_U. The unbound apparent volume of distribution is the apparent volume that the drug would occupy in the body if it were completely unbound to plasma proteins, and it is calculated as the apparent volume divided by the unbound fraction in the plasma (31):

$$V_U = \frac{V}{f_U} \quad \text{[Eq. 43]}$$

The greater the value of V_U, the less efficient is dialysis clearance in removing the compound from the body. This is illustrated in the relationship presented in Figure 39. The y-axis on the left is the reciprocal of the fraction removed from the body; the greater the unbound volume of distribution, the greater that inverse fraction and the smaller the amount removed from the body. The relationship may be seen more directly by referring to the y-axis on the right, which plots the percentage of compound removed from the body and whose values decrease moving up the scale. Thus, the greater the unbound volume of distribution, the smaller the percentage of the compound removed from the body. Efficient hemodialysis removal only occurs for compounds on the left side of the graph, which have small, unbound volumes. Thus, compounds such as digoxin ($V_U \cong 33$ L/kg), methaqualone ($V_U \cong 30$

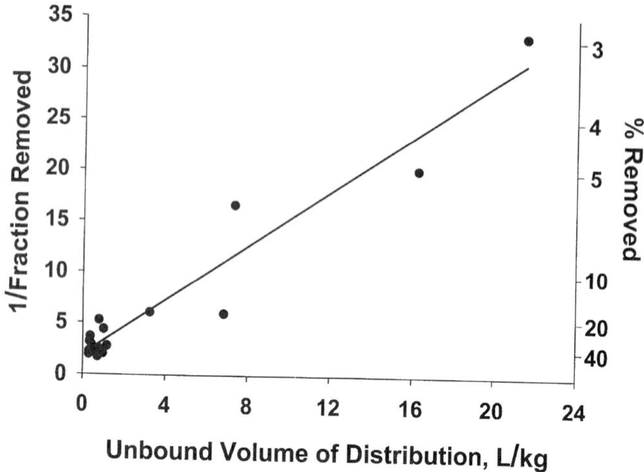

Figure 39. The reciprocal of the fraction of drug removed from the body during a 6-hour hemodialysis period as a function of the unbound apparent volume of distribution (i.e., the apparent volume of distribution divided by the unbound fraction of drug in plasma, V/f_U). The y-axis on the right is the corresponding percentage of the drug removed (note the inverse scale). The equation of the regression line is $Y = 1.33 \cdot X + 2.01$ ($r^2 = 0.930$). (Based on the data reported in Gwilt PR, Perrier D. Plasma protein binding and distribution characteristics of drugs as indices of their hemodialyzability. *Clin Pharmacol Therapeutics* 1978;24:154–161; and from Mayersohn M. Rational approaches to treatment of drug toxicity: recent considerations and application of pharmacokinetic principles. In: Barnett G, Chiang CN, eds. *Pharmacokinetics and pharmacodynamics of psychoactive drugs.* Foster City, CA: Biomedical Publications, 1985:131, with permission.)

L/kg), and flurazepam ($V_U \cong 133$) are poor candidates for hemodialysis removal after an overdose. The basic principle noted here is often overlooked in attempts to apply hemodialysis for the treatment of overdose.

Another issue that is often misinterpreted involves the use of *in vitro* dialysis clearance values as an estimation of the efficiency of hemodialysis for removing a compound from the body. *In vitro* dialysis clearance gives a reasonable estimate of the dialyzer's ability to extract the compound under the experimental conditions, which rarely if ever involves binding of the compound to the *blood* fluid being tested. The latter is most often a simple aqueous solution. The resulting *in vitro* clearance may bear no reasonable relationship to what is observed in the body and, therefore, must be considered an inadequate predictor of *in vivo* dialysis clearance and a poor predictor of the efficiency of removal from the body. This, in fact, has been shown to be the case (30). A group of compounds that might be the exception to this rule are small, polar compounds that do not bind to blood proteins such as methanol, ethanol, ethylene glycol, and so forth. The latter compounds tend to distribute into total body water (approximately 0.6 L/kg), and, therefore, they have a small, unbound volume of distribution: numerically, approximately equal to the apparent volume (because $f_U \cong 1$). In fact, for the compounds just noted, hemodialysis is often used in treatment of overdose, because it is an efficient means of removing those agents from the body. As noted previously, methanol and ethylene glycol overdose treatment often involves both ethanol dosing to reduce the rate of toxic metabolite formation and hemodialysis to remove the parent compound as well as the toxic metabolites that are produced. Figure 40A illustrates the direct dependence of methanol dialysis clearance on blood flow to the dialyzer (32). This relationship suggests a high dialysis ER and that blood flow appears to rate-limit methanol dialysis clearance. The translation of that information into the effect of hemodialysis on methanol (Fig. 40B) and ethylene glycol (Fig. 40C) elimination from the body is also illustrated (33,34). During each dialysis period, methanol and ethylene glycol concentrations decline far more rapidly (decreased $t_{1/2}$) compared to the interdialysis period (longer $t_{1/2}$). Furthermore, several of the toxic metabolites, being small polar molecules, are also effectively removed from the body by dialysis.

It is also important to note that there is no *rebound* effect at the end of a dialysis period. The latter is often seen when blood concentrations drop to low values (i.e., most of the compound is dialyzed from the blood) but then rise again when dialysis stops. This phenomenon (i.e., postdialysis *rebound*) occurs as a result of the tissues reequilibrating with blood, because there is now a concentration gradient from tissue to blood. Compounds that have a large apparent volume of distribution or that reequilibrate slowly with blood

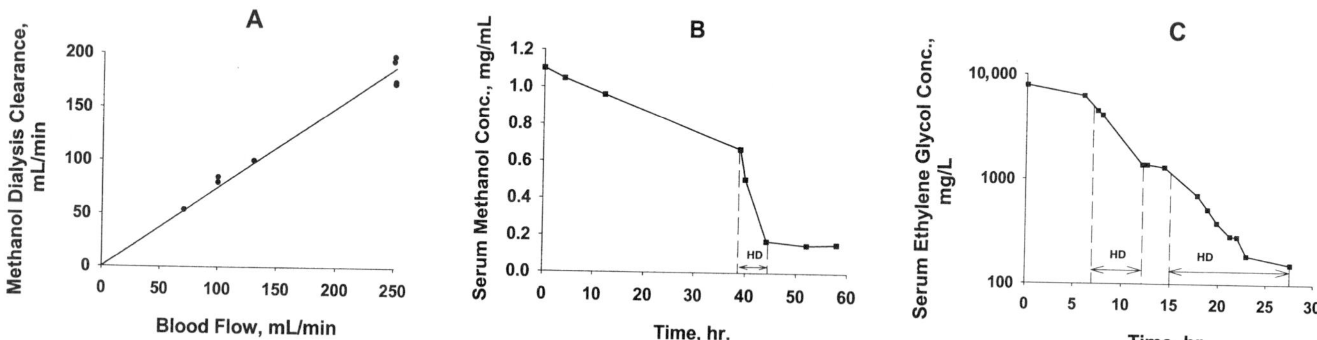

Figure 40. A: Hemodialysis clearance of methanol as a function of blood flow to the dialyzer. This relationship indicates the efficient extraction of methanol from blood by hemodialysis. (Based on the data in Gonda A, Gault H, Churchill D, et al. Hemodialysis for methanol intoxication. *Am J Med* 1978;64:749–758.) **B:** Serum methanol concentrations as a function of time in a 23-year-old male subject who ingested windshield washer fluid. Multiple intravenous doses of ethanol were administered during the time period illustrated. Methanol concentrations dropped dramatically during hemodialysis (HD). (Based on the data in Palatnick W, Redman LW, Sitar DS, et al. Methanol half-life during ethanol administration: implications for management of methanol poisoning. *Ann Emerg Med* 1995;26:202–207.) **C:** Serum ethylene glycol concentrations as a function of time in a 58-year-old male subject who ingested antifreeze. The subject received intravenous ethanol during the time period illustrated. Note the dramatic decline in serum concentrations during each of the two hemodialysis (HD) periods in comparison with the interdialysis periods. (Based on the data in Eder AF, McGrath CM, Dowdy YG, et al. Ethylene glycol poisoning: toxicokinetic and analytical factors affecting laboratory diagnosis. *Clin Chem* 1998;44:168–177. From M. Mayersohn, *unpublished*, with permission from Saguaro Technical Press, Inc, Tucson, AZ, 2002.)

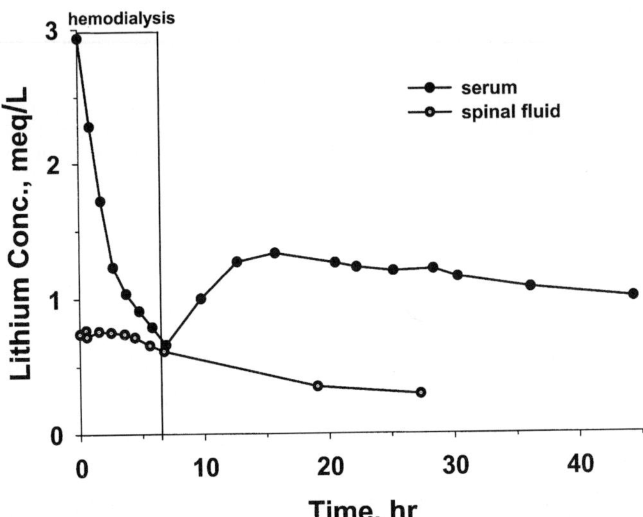

Figure 41. Serum and spinal fluid concentrations of lithium as a function of time during and after a 6.5-hour hemodialysis period. The 48-year-old man subject continued lithium therapy after developing renal failure resulting in toxic lithium concentrations. Note the rapid decline in serum concentrations during hemodialysis, which *rebounds* when dialysis was discontinued as a consequence of tissue redistribution to blood. (Based on the data in Amdisen A, Skjoldborg H. Haemodialysis for lithium poisoning. *Lancet* 1969;2:213.)

display such a profile (e.g., digoxin). An excellent example of this phenomenon is presented in Figure 41 (35). A patient continued lithium therapy after developing renal failure. Because renal excretion is the major route of lithium elimination, lithium accumulated and resulted in toxic concentrations. Serum lithium concentrations declined dramatically during hemodialysis but then rose again when dialysis was discontinued. Spinal fluid concentrations begin to decline only toward the end of and after completion of dialysis as a consequence of the redistribution from tissues to blood.

Another extracorporeal mechanism that holds great promise for treatment of overdose is *hemoperfusion*. Unlike dialysis methods, there is no membrane separating the blood from a dialyzing solution. In hemoperfusion, the blood is pumped out of the body and passed through a solid bed of adsorbing or binding material such as charcoal or ion-exchange resin. Thus, all formed elements of the blood and compounds dissolved in blood mix intimately with the solid phase. This method has the potential to be the most efficient means for removing drug and metabolites from the body. The extraction could be made even more efficient if the solid support contained in a cartridge used material with great affinity for specific drugs or category of drugs. For example, antibodies with a high specificity for the agent to be removed could produce an ER as high as one. Under that circumstance, blood flow through the hemoperfusion material would rate-limit clearance.

In general, the efficiency of dialysis clearance and the amount of compound extracted per unit of time, follows the order hemoperfusion greater than hemodialysis, and hemodialysis greater than peritoneal dialysis. Several publications have reviewed use of extracorporeal methods for treatment of drug overdose (36–38).

NONVASCULAR INPUT: ABSORPTION AND BIOAVAILABILITY

The development of pharmacokinetic principles generally begins with the simplifying assumption of intravenous bolus dosing, as done in the preceding sections. Although the simplicity is useful, it does not reflect the practical, real-world situation. IV bolus drug dosing is relatively uncommon (with the exception of illicit drug use), and when used it is done in a hospital or clinic setting. Drug dosing or exposure in general typically relies on other routes to gain access to the systemic circulation. The primary routes of entry into the body for drugs as well as environmental compounds include oral, buccal (sublingual), dermal, inhalation, subcutaneous, intramuscular, rectal, and vaginal. There are two basic differences between these nonvascular routes and vascular dosing. First, all nonvascular routes require that the substance placed at the site of administration penetrate one or more biologic membrane barriers to gain access to the systemic blood circulation. Second, all nonvascular doses must be formulated into a *dosage form* to permit administration. The dosage form is defined by its physical form (e.g., tablet, liquid, and so forth); by the characteristics of the drug in that form (e.g., crystal form, particle size, salt form, and so forth); and by other formulation factors (e.g., compression forces applied, coatings used, and so forth). The *in vivo* performance of a drug administered as a dosage form may be, and often is, quite different from what is seen from the pure drug or from IV administration. The principles of and some of the factors affecting the concentration-time profile after oral administration are discussed here, but for a more thorough exposition, the readers are referred elsewhere (39).

Gastrointestinal Absorption

The GI tract, which is a major barrier between the body and the environment, has as its primary functions the secretion of specialized fluids, the storage and digestion of ingested food and other materials, and absorption of those processed materials into the bloodstream. The GI tract is lined with epithelial cells specialized for those functions. As with all other membranes of the body, these epithelial cells are best described by the *fluid mosaic* model. The membrane is composed of a lipid bilayer or sandwich that has polar groups reaching into and out of the membrane, separated by two layers of long lipid chains. The latter provide the lipid-like nature of the membrane. Throughout the membrane are transmembrane proteins, and attached to the surface of the membrane are peripheral proteins and carbohydrates. It is this structure that determines the membrane permeability of any drug or chemical. Generally, small polar molecules (e.g., methanol, ethanol, and so forth) are able to traverse such membranes rapidly, whereas larger molecules need to have sufficient ability to partition between an aqueous and a lipid phase. The latter is often measured by the oil to water partition coefficient ($K_{O/W}$).

The vast majority of substances undergo an absorption process that is governed by physical chemical principles, and, therefore, absorption may be described by passive, first-order, or linear kinetics. The most important physical chemical properties of the molecule are its $K_{O/W}$, pK_a, water solubility, and molecular size. The rate of movement across a membrane is given by Fick's first law of diffusion, which may be expressed as

$$\text{Rate of membrane diffusion} = D_M \cdot A_M \cdot P_{M/AQ} \cdot \frac{[C_{gut} - C_{blood}]}{\Delta X_M} \quad \text{[Eq. 44]}$$

In which D_M, A_M, $P_{M/AQ}$, and ΔX_M are the diffusion coefficient through the membrane, the area of the absorbing membrane, the partition coefficient between the membrane, and the aqueous gut solution and the thickness of the membrane, respectively. The driving force for diffusion is the concentration gradient between the substance in the gut fluid (C_{gut}) and that in the compound at absorption site ⟶ compound in body ⟶ compound eliminated

$$X_{ABS} \xrightarrow{k_a} X_B \xrightarrow{K} X_E$$

Scheme 3. Schematic representation of a simple, sequential absorption process. Where X_{ABS}, X_B, and X_E represent the amount of substance at the absorption site, in the body, and eliminated from the body, respectively. The first-order rate constants describe absorption, k_a, and elimination, K.

blood (C_{blood}). This relationship can be simplified by incorporating all of the constant terms into a permeability coefficient, P:

$$\text{Rate of membrane diffusion} = P \cdot [C_{gut} - C_{blood}] \cong P \cdot C_{gut} \quad \text{[Eq. 45]}$$

Because the concentration on the blood side of the membrane is generally small compared to the concentration in the gut fluids (because blood flow carries the absorbed material rapidly away from the site of absorption), the relationship simplifies to a rate equation, which expresses a first-order process. As a consequence, in general, absorption processes for most substances follow first-order kinetic principles (e.g., absorption rate depends on GI fluid concentration or dose; the amount absorbed increases linearly with dose; the fraction of the dose absorbed is constant, independent of dose; and so forth).

As noted in the discussion of metabolite kinetics, the kinetics of absorption may be described by a sequence of steps often referred to as an *A to B to C* system. In which A is the substance in the gut (or any site of absorption), B is that compound in the body (or bloodstream), and C is the substance eliminated from the body (in urine, as metabolite, and so forth). Scheme 3 describes this sequence.

The amount of substance at the absorption site declines exponentially according to the first-order rate constant for absorption, k_a. The amount of drug in the body or plasma concentration is described by a biexponential equation, of a form identical to that used to describe metabolite concentration as a function of time after IV bolus dosing of parent compound (see equation 38). The relationship that describes the plasma concentration of parent compound is given by

$$C = \frac{k_a \cdot F \cdot dose}{V(k_a - K)} \cdot (e^{-K \cdot t} - e^{-k_a \cdot t}) = A \cdot (e^{-K \cdot t} - e^{-k_a \cdot t}) \quad \text{[Eq. 46]}$$

The only new term here that has not been defined is F, the fraction of the dose absorbed intact sometimes referred to as *systemic bioavailability*. The value for F can range from zero to one and it is used, as noted later, to characterize the absorption efficiency of commercial products, and it forms the basis for estimation of *bioequivalence* (i.e., comparability among the same drug products made by different manufacturers). Because all of the terms in the coefficient may be considered to be a constant after a given dose, they may be replaced by a composite constant, A (having units of concentration). A plot of plasma concentration versus time results in a curve that rises and then declines (again, in analogy to the metabolite plasma concentration-time curve after an IV bolus dose of parent compound). As for the metabolite situation or for any sequential process, one of the steps in the sequence must be the slowest and rate-limit the overall process. The terminal slope represents the slowest step. In the absorption scenario, either absorption or elimination is the rate-limiting step. Thus, if absorption is fast, $k_a >> K$, at some time the exponential containing k_a approaches zero before the other exponent, resulting in the terminal slope being given by the overall elimination rate constant, K. This terminal line parallels that seen after IV bolus dosing.

$$C \cong \frac{k_a \cdot F \cdot dose}{V(k_a - K)} \cdot (e^{-K \cdot t}) = A \cdot (e^{-K \cdot t}) \quad \text{[Eq. 47]}$$

In contrast, if absorption is slow, $k_a << K$, the terminal slope is given by the slowest step, the absorption rate constant:

$$C \cong \frac{k_a \cdot F \cdot dose}{V(K - k_a)} \cdot (e^{-k_a \cdot t}) = A \cdot (e^{-k_a \cdot t}) \quad \text{[Eq. 48]}$$

The terminal line in this situation does not parallel the line describing plasma concentrations after IV bolus dosing, but rather it has a smaller slope. The latter situation occurs for drug products designed to release drug slowly (controlled or sustained release dosage forms) to sustain plasma concentrations, for poorly water-soluble compounds in which rate of dissolution rate-limits absorption, or for compounds that have poor membrane permeability.

A comparison of several of these factors is shown in Figure 42. Graph A illustrates the effect of the absorption rate constant on the shape of the curve for the same compound (and same value of K). The smaller the absorption rate constant, the smaller the value of the maximum plasma concentration, C_{max}, and the longer it takes to achieve that concentration, T_{max}. Because the slowest rate constant in all cases is the elimination rate constant, the terminal slope is given by, –K/2.3. Because the same fraction of the dose is absorbed in each case, the total area under the curve must be the same. Graph B illustrates the effect of the fraction of the dose absorbed on the shape of the plasma concentration-time curve. The smaller the value of F, the smaller the value for C_{max}, but there is no change in T_{max}. The most dramatic difference, however, is the total area under the curve: the smaller the value for F, the smaller the AUC. Because the slowest rate constant is the elimination rate constant, the terminal slope is given by, –K/2.3. Graph C illustrates the effect of a change in the rate-limiting step on the plasma concentration-time curve. In one case, the slowest rate constant is the elimination rate constant and the terminal slope is given by –K/2.3. In contrast, for the other case, the slowest rate constant is the absorption rate constant, which now becomes the rate-limiting step. As a consequence, the terminal slope is given by, $-k_a/2.3$. This is sometimes referred to as a *flip-flop model*. For this reason, the $t_{1/2}$ obtained from the log-linear line after nonvascular dosing is always correctly referred to as the terminal $t_{1/2}$. The terminal slope may not reflect the disposition $t_{1/2}$. The value for C_{max} decreases and T_{max} increases when the absorption rate constant gets small (as noted in Fig. 42A); however, the total areas under the curves are the same.

The elimination $t_{1/2}$, although variable among people, remains relatively constant for one individual. Therefore, the major variable affecting the plasma concentration-time curve is the input process: factors relating to the performance of the dosage form and GI absorption. There are four possible factors that may rate-limit the absorption process. The two most significant are dissolution rate and membrane permeability. The other two possible, but generally less important, factors are gastric emptying rate and GI tract blood flow. Two important observations, which have become principles with regard to GI tract absorp-

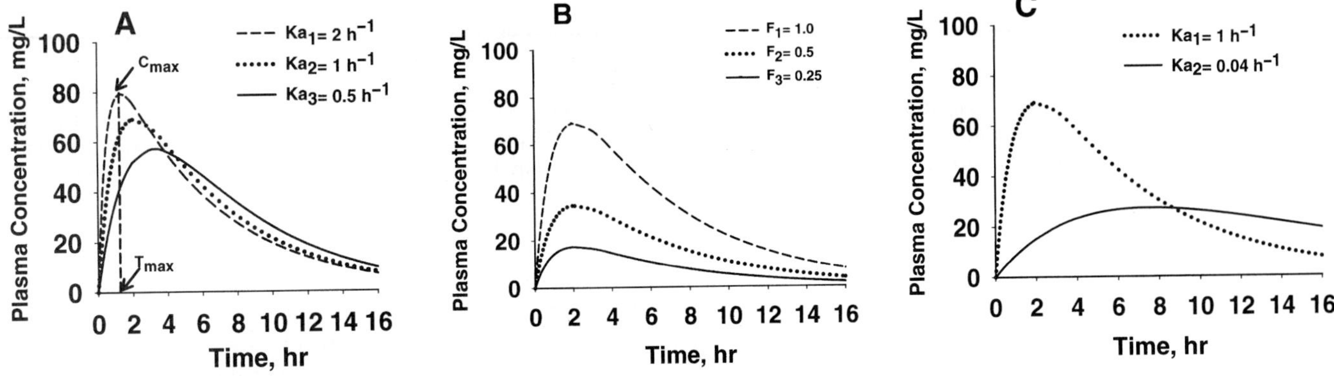

Figure 42. **A:** Hypothetical plasma concentration-time profiles of the same compound administered orally in three different dosage forms. The elimination rate constant is the same for each situation (0.173 hour^{-1}; $t_{1/2}$ = 4 hours); only the absorption rate constants vary. The absorption rate constants are 2.0 hour^{-1}, 1.0 hour^{-1}, and 0.5 hour^{-1}. Note that the smaller the absorption rate constant, the smaller the maximum concentration (C_{max}) and the greater the time of its occurrence (T_{max}). **B:** Hypothetical oral plasma concentration-time profiles for the same compound as shown in **A**, with an elimination rate constant of 0.173 hour^{-1} ($t_{1/2}$ = 4 hour) and absorption rate constant of 1.0 hour^{-1}. The only difference among these curves is the fraction of the dose absorbed (F; bioavailability). The values for F are 1.0, 0.5, and 0.25. **C:** Hypothetical oral plasma concentration-time curves for the same compound as in **A**, with an elimination rate constant of 0.173 hour^{-1} ($t_{1/2}$ = 4 hour). The absorption rate constant is larger than K (k_a = 1.0 hour^{-1}; ···) in one case but smaller than K in the other case (k_a = 0.04 hour^{-1}; —). The terminal slope is given by the smallest rate constant. The situation illustrated for $k_a << K$ is sometimes referred to as a *flip-flop* model. (From M. Mayersohn, *unpublished*, with permission from Saguaro Technical Press, Inc, Tucson, AZ, 2002.)

tion, are the following. For a compound to be absorbed, it must first be in solution in the fluids of the GI tract. The idea of particulate absorption (so-called *persorption*), although it appears to exist, contributes insignificantly to the overall absorption process. This is the reason *dissolution rate* is so important for poorly water-soluble compounds; the faster and the more completely the compound dissolves, the greater the rate and completeness of absorption. Thus, the absorption of poorly water-soluble compounds is frequently dissolution rate-limited. Second, all compounds, whether weak acids or bases, are best absorbed from the small intestine. The idea referred to as the *pH-partition hypothesis*, which suggests that compounds are better absorbed in the environment that favors nonionization, has been misinterpreted. If all other factors along the GI tract were the same, an acidic compound would be best absorbed from the more acidic environment of the stomach, because the nonionized form has a greater oil/water partition coefficient, which would increase the permeability coefficient (see Equation 44) and, thereby, promote absorption. Similarly, basic compounds would be better absorbed from the relatively more alkaline pH of the small intestine. However, the small intestine is uniquely capable of providing the most efficient site for absorption compared to all other regions of the GI tract by virtue of its enormous absorbing surface area (one estimate suggests that the area is similar to that of a tennis court). Thus, all compounds, whether acids or bases, are best absorbed in the small intestine. Another argument against the stomach as being a good site for absorption applies to weak acids that are poorly water-soluble, though such compounds are cited (incorrectly) as undergoing gastric absorption. The rate-limiting step for the absorption of any poorly water-soluble compound, including weak acids, is dissolution rate. In fact, such weak acids dissolve most readily in the relatively more alkaline pH of the small intestine, because ionization favors dissolution.

Restating these two governing principles, a compound must be in solution to be absorbed and all compounds are best absorbed in the small intestine. Therefore, another possible rate-limiting step in absorption is gastric emptying rate. Any delay in the compound moving from the stomach to the small intestine, the primary site of absorption, delays the absorption process. Generally, however, assuming that the compound is stable in the GI tract and is absorbed by passive diffusion, gastric emptying rate is not expected to affect the completeness of absorption. Another possible, but rarely seen, rate-limiting step to absorption is blood flow to the GI tract. Usually that flow is quite high, consistent with one of the primary functions of the GI tract, efficient absorption. If blood flow is slowed sufficiently, then the concentration gradient of the compound between the gut and the blood, the driving force for diffusion, becomes small (see equation 45). This diminution in concentration gradient occurs as a consequence of the compound no longer being carried away rapidly from the site of absorption and the compound accumulating on the blood side of the GI tract membrane. In situations of reduced or relatively static GI tract blood flow, such as might be seen during episodes of fainting or reduced blood volume (e.g., due to blood loss), one may see diminished absorption.

Although the vast majority of compounds move across the absorbing GI tract membrane by passive diffusion, there are many water-soluble nutrients (e.g., monosaccharides, amino acids, vitamins, and so forth) and some drugs (e.g., L-dopa, some aminopenicillins, some aminocephalosporins) whose absorption involves active participation of cell membrane transporters. Such processes are described by specialized (sometimes, active) transport. The absorption kinetics of such compounds are analogous to what has been noted in discussions of renal transport mechanisms (e.g., tubular secretion and reabsorption). Thus, the amount absorbed increases to a maximum value as dose increases and thereafter remains constant (the fraction absorbed decreases with dose). Such specialized processes may be inhibited by other compounds with similar structure.

There is also a family of *efflux transporters*, referred to as *P-glycoproteins*, which are found in epithelial cells of the GI tract (as well as in the liver, kidney, and blood–brain barrier), that are responsible for the movement of substrate out of the absorbing cell back into the gut lumen. These transporters obviously perform a protective role in preventing the systemic absorption of materials that might cause the body harm. These transporters may undergo inhibition or induction in response to certain drugs, which is the basis for a class of drug-drug interactions. Examples of drug substrates that use this transporter include digoxin, quinine, verapamil, and cyclosporin A.

The movement of ingested materials down the GI tract involves esophageal, gastric, intestinal, and colonic transit. Generally, the movement of ingested materials down the esophagus is rapid, especially if a liquid is swallowed alone or with a solid substance. There are instances, however, of solid oral drug dosage forms *attaching* to the esophageal surface and causing erosion of the local tissue. Gastric emptying is a complex process that is influenced by a variety of physiologic factors including the presence and volume of food ingested, the type of food present, and certain drugs. As noted previously, any delay in emptying into the small intestine delays the onset of absorption. Fatty meals are the strongest inhibitor of emptying, and drugs that exert anticholinergic activity, such as narcotic analgesics, slow emptying. Slower gastric emptying rate generally reduces the rate of absorption and results in a lower C_{max} and longer T_{max}. The extent of absorption may be reduced if the compound is unstable in the GI tract fluids or increased if a greater residence time in the GI tract permits more complete dissolution and absorption. Compounds absorbed by a specialized process high in the small intestine (e.g., vitamin C) may evidence more complete absorption in the presence of slow gastric emptying as a result of avoiding saturation of transporters.

Under fasting conditions, the activity of the GI tract is governed by the so-called *migrating motility complex*, or the interdigestive myoelectric complex. This complex cycles approximately every 2 hours. This only occurs, however, during fasting and begins in the proximal stomach and terminates at the ileocecal valve. There are four phases involved in the entire cycle. Phase 1 (45 to 60 minutes) and phase 2 (30 to 45 minutes) are of relatively low activity. It is phase 3, called the *housekeeper wave*, that has intense activity lasting for approximately 5 to 15 minutes, which is responsible for clearing any remaining material from the stomach. This is the only time that relatively large single units (e.g., intact tablets) can be swept into the small intestine. Oral dosing on an empty stomach, relative to the start of the housekeeper wave, determines about how long ingested products remain in the stomach.

Intestinal transit tends to be somewhat more uniform than gastric emptying patterns, and, in general, the average amount of time that it takes a dosage form to transit from the pylorus to the end of the small intestine is approximately 4 hours. This tends to be true regardless of the nature of the substance (solid or liquid) and in the absence or presence of food. Because the small intestine is the major site of absorption, this time *window* for absorption of approximately 4 hours would appear to limit the absorption process. Drug absorption can continue beyond 4 hours after dosing as evidenced by controlled release products and the slow absorption of poorly water-soluble compounds. Compounds can remain in the colon for 24 hours and longer and, therefore, although this is not a particularly efficient site for absorption (due to the small surface area and low fluid volume), the long residence time there may compensate for the lower efficiency.

Efficient oral drug therapy necessitates adequate and, ideally, complete and consistent GI absorption. In contrast, of course, effective treatment of an oral overdose attempts to minimize systemic absorption. This is often the first approach used in treatment along with maintaining life signs but before attempts to removing materials already systemically absorbed (e.g., extracorporeal devices for enhancing elimination). Evacuating and somehow *immobilizing* the orally ingested overdose are the two approaches that may be used. Evacuation may be achieved by inducing vomiting or pumping the stomach or by slow, constant flushing of the gut contents for excretion with fecal material. *Immobilization* is used here to indicate that the overdosed compound is made into a form not available for systemic absorption. The latter may involve the use of specific agents that chemically bind to the toxic compound to prevent further absorption (e.g., chelating agents that form water-insoluble heavy metal chelates to reduce heavy metal poisoning; ion-exchange resins that bind to charged compounds). Alternatively, nonselective materials may be used that are effective for a wide range of toxic compounds, such as activated charcoal and perhaps single or binary phase fluids for lipid-soluble compounds (e.g., nonabsorbable lipids or oil-in-water emulsions). The cardinal rule for the effectiveness of these approaches is the sooner they are applied, the better (for both approaches), and the more used, the better (for *immobilization*). A good example of this idea of *soon and large amount* can be illustrated with charcoal administration. The relative percentage of an acetaminophen dose absorbed after oral administration of a solution of the drug with 5 or 10 g of activated charcoal (given immediately after the acetaminophen solution) was 53% and 39%, respectively. The same 10-g dose of charcoal given 30 minutes after the oral acetaminophen solution resulted in 69% of the dose being absorbed, considerably less efficient compared to immediate administration of charcoal (39%). When administering charcoal in the same ratio to the acetaminophen dose (10:1), less of the drug is absorbed the greater the absolute amount of charcoal (percentage absorbed, g charcoal/g acetaminophen): 42.5%, 5 g/0.5 g; 34.9%, 10 g/1 g; 22.6%, 20 g/2 g; 14.8%, 30 g/3 g (40). An identical observation has been made for the effect of activated charcoal on aspirin absorption (41). In general, the antidotal efficacy of activated charcoal increases with the amount of charcoal administered (42).

Charcoal administration has also been shown to have a dramatic effect on the elimination kinetics of some compounds that are excreted into the bile and that undergo enterohepatic recirculation. An excellent example is phenobarbital whose terminal $t_{1/2}$ was reduced from an average of 110 hours to 45 hours as a result of an increase in CL_S from 4.4 to 12.0 ml/kg per hour (43). Charcoal adsorbs the phenobarbital excreted into the small intestine, interrupting the cycle and, therefore, reduces the $t_{1/2}$ of the compound. In such a circumstance, it is useful to administer charcoal in a multiple dosing fashion to continue to disrupt the cycle (44). Doing so reduced the terminal $t_{1/2}$ of phenobarbital from 110 hours to approximately 20 hours. Other compounds that undergo a similar process include theophylline and carbamazepine. This mode of treatment has been reviewed (45).

A particularly important consideration, especially for GI absorption, is those processes that affect the chemical form of the compound before the parent compound reaching the systemic circulation. In general, these processes are referred to as *presystemic elimination*. The ingested parent compound may be altered, chemically or metabolically, at numerous sites along the GI tract, as illustrated in Figure 43. Perhaps the most significant of the individual sites and processes noted are those that occur in the intestinal wall and liver. The gut wall and liver are virtual storehouses for enzymes. Because the entire absorbed dose must first go through these organs before being systemically distributed, metabolism may represent a significant portion of the dose being altered before systemic absorption. This process has been referred to as the *first-pass effect*, the most important being intestinal wall and hepatic first-pass effects. The importance of any of these first-pass effects depends on the ER or clearance of those individual processes. In addition, it should be appreciated that these effects are sequential, meaning that the net numerical result is multiplicative. Thus, for a compound that undergoes hepatic metabolism, the value of hepatic clearance determines the ER and that, in turn, determines what fraction of the dose survives the first movement through the liver and reaches the systemic circulation. If it is assumed that the orally administered compound is completely absorbed intact

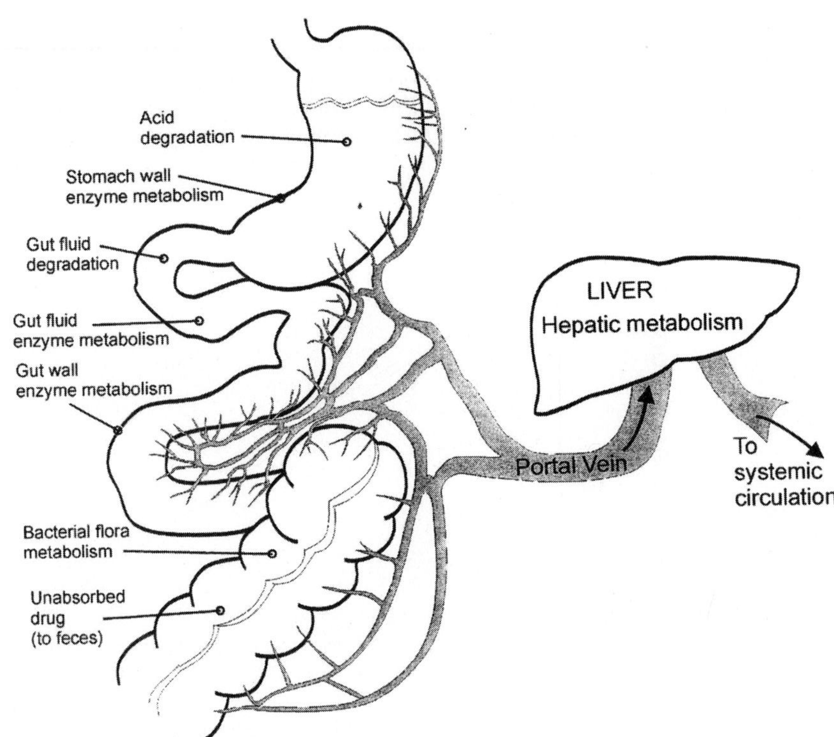

Figure 43. Schematic representation of the numerous sites along the gastrointestinal tract where the orally ingested parent compound may be chemically or metabolically altered. Taken together, these are referred to as *presystemic elimination processes*, and they include intestinal wall and hepatic first-pass effects. (From M. Mayersohn, *unpublished*, with permission from Saguaro Technical Press, Inc, Tucson, AZ, 2002.)

through the intestinal wall and gets into the portal circulation, the fraction of that dose that survives the liver and gets into the systemic circulation intact is given by

$$F = 1 - ER_{HEPATIC} = 1 - \frac{CL_{HEPATIC}}{Q_{HEPATIC}} \quad \text{[Eq. 49]}$$

If all of the possible steps noted in Figure 43 are considered, F is equal to the product of the fractions (f) that survive each sequential step. For example, consider the following sequence of steps: stomach fluid degradation, intestinal wall metabolism, and liver metabolism:

$$F = f_{RELEASED} \cdot f_{GASTRIC\ FLUID} \cdot f_{INTESTINAL\ WALL} \cdot f_{LIVER} \quad \text{[Eq. 50]}$$

The first term represents the fraction of the dose that is released from the form ingested (maximum value is one). All of the other terms represent the fractions that survive each of the individual metabolic steps (i.e., 1-ER). Therefore, if 10% of the dose is chemically altered in gastric fluid (90% survives), and 40% of the dose is extracted by the intestinal wall (60% survives) and 50% of what survives that process is extracted by the liver, the fraction that reaches the systemic circulation is less than approximately 30% of the dose ($0.9 \times 0.6 \times 0.5$). Clearly, this can be an important consideration for those compounds that have high ERs for several of the presystemic elimination steps.

The significance of presystemic elimination needs to be considered with respect to the form of the compound that is pharmacologically and toxicologically active. Assuming, as often happens, that the parent compound is active and toxic, then any of the first-pass effects reduce the magnitude of those responses. Inhibiting such metabolic (or chemical) processes results in enhanced activity. This is especially true for compounds that have a high first-pass effect (i.e., ER >0.9). An interesting example of the latter (discussed previously for terfenadine) is the effect of grapefruit juice and certain drugs (e.g., ketoconazole) on the inhibition of cytochrome P-450 3A4 in the gut wall and liver. Induction of that pathway would have reduced the plasma concentrations of the parent drug, increased the concentration of metabolite (which is active, but not toxic), and minimized the chance of toxicity.

Just the opposite considerations apply for a compound whose metabolite is active or toxic. A classic example is that of the insecticide parathion (46). Parathion is inactive until it is metabolized to paraoxon, which exhibits cholinesterase activity. The infusion of parathion into the portal vein results in greater activity compared to dosing into the vena cava, as a consequence of metabolic activation via the hepatic first-pass effect. In contrast, the active form, paraoxon, is far more active on vena cava administration compared to dosing via the portal vein. In the latter instance, the hepatic route reduces the activity of paraoxon by further metabolism.

It is especially instructive to examine the interactions that are expected to occur for high and low hepatic ER drugs after IV bolus and oral dosing. This comparison is illustrated in Figure 44 assuming inhibition in metabolism. Two compounds that undergo complete hepatic metabolism but with different values for intrinsic hepatic clearance and ER are considered after IV and oral dosing before and after enzyme inhibition. Compound A has a low CL_{int} and ER (150 ml/minute and 0.091) compared to compound B, which has a high CL_{int} and ER (15,000 ml/minute and 0.909). The solid lines in the top panel illustrate the concentration-time profiles after IV dosing (A_{iv}, B_{iv}). In each instance, the values for CL_{int} are cut in half to reflect the inhibition of hepatic clearance. Thus, for A_{iv}, CL_{int} goes from 150 to 75 ml/minute and ER decreases by approximately one-half (0.091 to 0.048) with a similar change in systemic clearance, CL_S (137 to 72 ml/minute). The dotted line indicates the new concentration-time profile after inhibition (top left). $t_{1/2}$ increases by almost twofold (4.0 to 7.6 hours), as does the area under the curve (577 to 1100 ng · hour/ml). All of these changes are not surprising, because, for a low clearance compound, $\downarrow CL_S \cong \downarrow CL_{int} = f_U \cdot \downarrow CL_{U,int}$. Inhibition decreases the value of $CL_{U,int}$ and, in the absence of any change in plasma protein binding, is directly equivalent to the change in CL_{int}. $t_{1/2}$ increases, because in the absence of any change in apparent volume of distribution, $t_{1/2}$ is inversely related to systemic clearance, whose value has decreased: $\uparrow t_{1/2} = (0.693 \cdot V_d)/\downarrow CL_S$

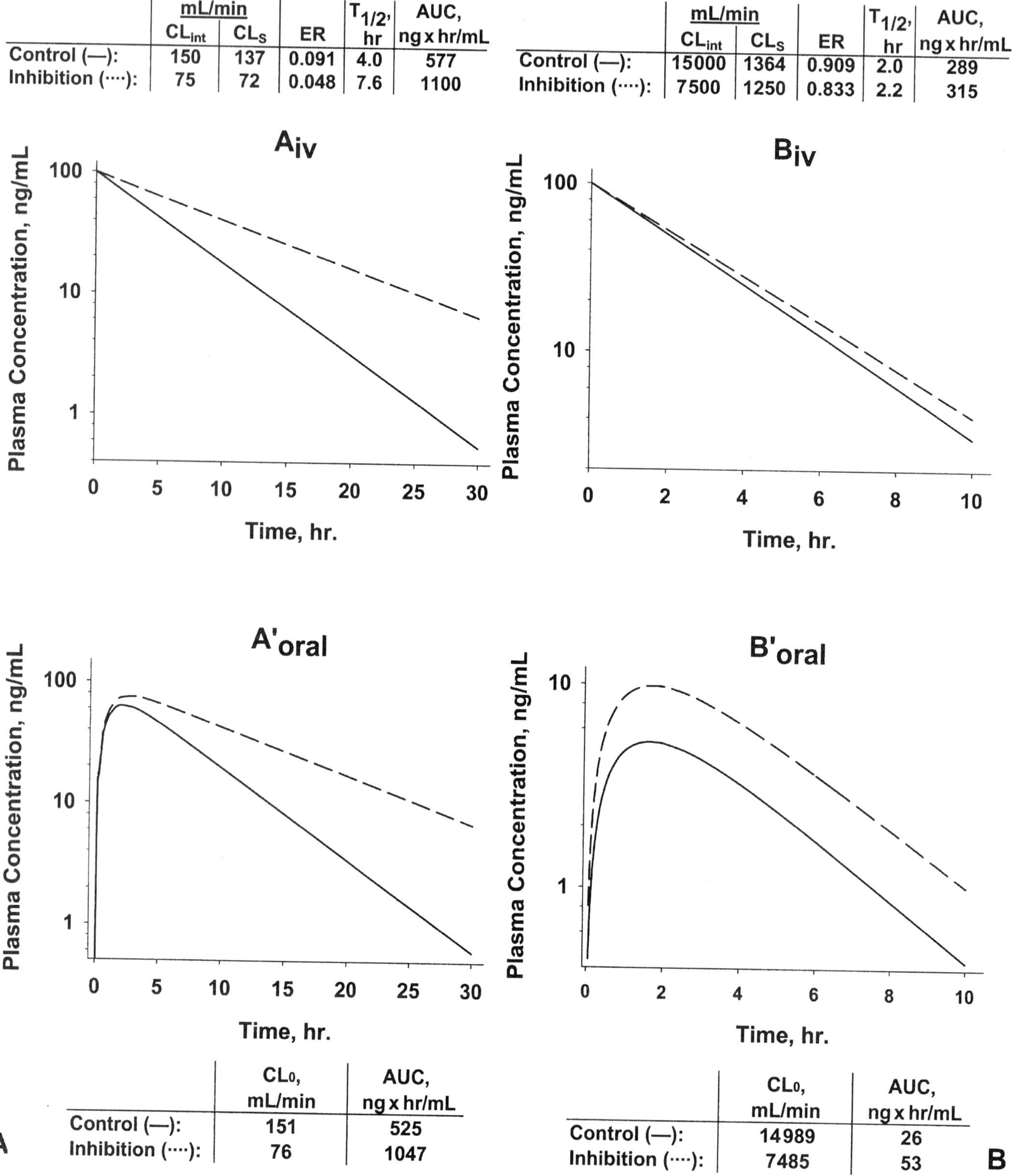

	mL/min		ER	$T_{1/2}$, hr	AUC, ng x hr/mL
	CL_{int}	CL_S			
Control (—):	150	137	0.091	4.0	577
Inhibition (····):	75	72	0.048	7.6	1100

	mL/min		ER	$T_{1/2}$, hr	AUC, ng x hr/mL
	CL_{int}	CL_S			
Control (—):	15000	1364	0.909	2.0	289
Inhibition (····):	7500	1250	0.833	2.2	315

	CL_O, mL/min	AUC, ng x hr/mL
Control (—):	151	525
Inhibition (····):	76	1047

	CL_O, mL/min	AUC, ng x hr/mL
Control (—):	14989	26
Inhibition (····):	7485	53

Figure 44. Hypothetical plasma concentration-time relationships for two drugs (**A** and **B**) given by intravenous bolus (**A'**$_{iv}$, **B'**$_{iv}$) or as oral doses (**A'**$_{oral}$, **B'**$_{oral}$) under control conditions (*solid line*) or after metabolic inhibition (*dashed line*). The control and metabolic inhibition conditions are specified above the graphs. Both compounds are totally metabolized by the liver, whose blood flow is assumed to be 1500 ml/minute. Compound A has a low intrinsic hepatic clearance (150 ml/minute) and extraction ratio (0.091). Compound B has a high intrinsic hepatic clearance (15,000 ml/minute) and extraction ratio (0.909). For both compounds, the intrinsic hepatic clearance is halved under conditions of inhibition. See text for discussion. (From M. Mayersohn, *unpublished*, with permission from Saguaro Technical Press, Inc, Tucson, AZ, 2002.)

The story is different for a high clearance compound given intravenously, as can be seen in B_{iv} (top right). Although the value for CL_{int} is halved, there is a less than a 10% decrease in ER and CL_S. As a consequence, there is little change in $t_{1/2}$ and AUC, as noted by the solid and dotted lines. Given normal experimental variability, the data forming these two lines essentially overlap. Again, this is not surprising because, for a high clearance compound, clearance is approximately equal to organ blood flow ($Q_{hepatic}$ = 1500 ml/minute): $CL_S \cong Q_{hepatic}$. Because there is no change in hepatic blood flow, there is little change in systemic clearance, which leads to little change in area under the curve (289 to 315 ng · hour/ml) and $t_{1/2}$ (2.0 to 2.2 hours). If one were attempting to examine a drug-drug interaction using this protocol, the conclusion of there being no interaction is incorrect. There is, in fact, a substantial change in intrinsic hepatic clearance, but one is unable to view the change experimentally because the IV data do not reflect that change for this compound but, rather, organ blood flow. This would be a failed experiment (actually, the experimenter failed).

The bottom panels of Figure 44 illustrate the identical experiment for the same two compounds but after oral dosing and assuming complete absorption (i.e., 100% of the dose reaches the liver). For the low clearance compound (A'_{oral}), the changes are essentially the same as those seen after IV dosing (A_{iv}) with regard to areas and $t_{1/2}$, because it is intrinsic hepatic clearance that is being measured after oral and IV dosing. Perhaps the most interesting comparison is shown for B'_{oral}, in the lower right-hand graph. The areas under the curve now, unlike the IV data, reflect the 50% decrease in intrinsic hepatic clearance; the interaction can be seen using this oral dosing protocol. The area under the oral dosing curve divided into the oral dose is referred to as *apparent oral clearance* (CL_O or CL_{oral}) and, in this instance, it is equal to intrinsic hepatic clearance, assuming complete absorption. This value is essentially the same measure that is obtained from a test tube experiment in which the compound is incubated with enzyme and which permits determination of CL_{int}. Notice, however, that the terminal line and $t_{1/2}$ have not changed from the control experiment. This is because $t_{1/2}$ still depends on systemic clearance, and, for this compound, that value is approximately equal to hepatic blood flow, which has not changed. Thus, an interaction in metabolism for low or high hepatic clearance compounds can be seen after oral dosing. The only caveat is that there be no interaction in absorption between the test compound and the interactant.

Systemic bioavailability is used to assess the efficiency of absorption by quantitation of the rate and completeness or extent of absorption. Extent of absorption is based on measuring the total area under the plasma concentration-time curve and comparing to some standard. Rate is generally characterized by the values for C_{max} and T_{max}. There are two definitions of bioavailability: absolute and relative. Absolute bioavailability, $F_{absolute}$, compares the total area under the plasma concentration-time curve (AUC_0^∞) obtained after an oral (or any other route) dose to that obtained after an IV dose. Because, by definition, the IV dose is completely absorbed (i.e., F = 1), one determines the absolute amount of the dose absorbed by the nonvascular route. The two appropriate equations and their ratio are

$$(AUC_0^\infty)_{oral} = \frac{F \cdot dose_{oral}}{CL_S} \qquad F = \frac{(AUC_0^\infty)_{oral} \cdot CL_S}{dose_{oral}}$$

$$(AUC_0^\infty)_{iv} = \frac{(1) \cdot dose_{iv}}{CL_S} \qquad 1 = \frac{(AUC_0^\infty)_{iv} \cdot CL_S}{dose_{iv}} \qquad \text{[Eq. 51]}$$

$$F_{absolute} = \frac{F}{1} = \frac{(AUC_0^\infty)_{oral} \cdot CL_S}{(AUC_0^\infty)_{iv} \cdot CL_S} \bullet \frac{dose_{iv}}{dose_{oral}}$$

The study is generally designed so that a crossover protocol is used, and, in that way, it is reasonable to make the assumption that CL_S remains the same in each subject from occasion to occasion. That being true, the basic relationship that is used to calculate bioavailability can be simplified to

$$F_{absolute} = \frac{F}{1} = \frac{(AUC_0^\infty)_{oral}}{(AUC_0^\infty)_{iv}} \bullet \frac{dose_{iv}}{dose_{oral}} \qquad \text{[Eq. 52]}$$

The experimental design should attempt to maximize the correctness of the above assumption by, for example, avoiding any changes from one experiment to the other (e.g., avoid other drugs, alcohol, and so forth). The assumption of constant clearance may not be correct, and it appears to be least correct for those compounds referred to as having highly variable clearance, and, typically, they are compounds with large clearance values.

The other, more practical definition of bioavailability and the one most often used by the U.S. Food and Drug Administration in making decisions about generic drug entry into the marketplace is referred to as *relative bioavailability*, $F_{relative}$. This definition is different from absolute bioavailability in that comparison is not made with reference to an IV dose but rather to some comparable standard product that is already on the market (the innovators product). As a consequence, one only determines how much is absorbed relative to that standard, and the absolute amount absorbed is not determined. Study design and calculations are essentially the same as outlined previously and assuming constant clearance. *Test* refers to the product whose relative bioavailability is being assessed, and *reference* is the innovator's product or some other standard.

$$F_{relative} = \frac{F_{test}}{F_{reference}} = \frac{(AUC_0^\infty)_{test}}{(AUC_0^\infty)_{reference}} \bullet \frac{dose_{reference}}{dose_{test}} \qquad \text{[Eq. 53]}$$

A $F_{relative}$ value of 1.0 gives no information about how completely the dose was absorbed. That value of 1.0 or 100% simply says that the test product is absorbed to the same extent as the reference, which might have an absolute bioavailability of 1% or 100%.

As noted previously, the assumption of constant clearance may not be reasonable for those compounds that have variable clearance, and, if that is the case, one needs to design a study with a large number of subjects to have sufficient statistical power to detect differences between the products. Alternatively, one may use stable or radioactive isotopic forms of the compound. The use of that approach has been reported (47), and it results in a considerable reduction in the number of subjects needed with a gain in statistical power. An example illustrating the effect of changes in the fraction of the dose absorbed on the plasma concentration-time profile was presented in Figure 42B. A good source for information about bioavailability and bioequivalence is the U.S. Food and Drug Administration Web site (http://www.fda.gov).

Intramuscular (IM) and subcutaneous dosing are often thought to result in rapid and complete absorption, comparable to IV dosing and certainly better than oral administration. This may not be the case, however, for several reasons. There are two possible rate-limiting steps to drug absorption after IM dosing. The capillary wall at the site of IM or subcutaneous injection is less of a barrier to absorption than is the GI tract membrane, because the former is more loosely knit. In general, large, polar, and charged molecules have a greater chance of being absorbed by this route than after oral absorption. Thus, this route is commonly used for drugs such as insulin, proteins (e.g., interferons), peptides, and aminoglycosides. This route is also less chemically damaging to those molecules that may be unstable at the low pH of gut fluids. Thus, one possible rate-limiting step in absorption is blood flow to the site of administration, which, in turn, may depend on the specific site used. A good example is that of the water-soluble compound lidocaine, whose absorption is more rapid from the deltoid muscle versus the vastus lateralis. The plasma concentrations rise more rapidly and achieve greater concentrations after deltoid dosing compared to the vastus lateralis, and this results in a greater response from deltoid dosing. The reason for these differences is that there is more rapid blood flow and, therefore, a greater rate of absorption from the deltoid muscle. The buttocks are expected to provide for even a slower rate of absorption and response. There is also, in the latter case, the chance of delivering the drug to deep fat tissue, which further prolongs absorption.

Another possible rate-limiting step that applies to poorly water-soluble drugs after IM dosing is precipitation in the muscle tissue that requires redissolution to be absorbed. The rate-limiting step here, as it is for poorly water-soluble oral drugs, is rate of dissolution. A good example is phenytoin. This drug is poorly water-soluble. It is given in a solution buffered to a pH of approximately 10 or 11, to keep it in solution. On IM administration, the drug meets an aqueous environment of pH 7.4 and it precipitates. The drug then redissolves slowly, and concentrations remain quite constant over a period of several days, essentially performing as a controlled release form. The oral dose is absorbed more rapidly and has a shorter terminal $t_{1/2}$ compared to the IM dose.

Diffusion from the interstitial spaces across the blood capillary wall, as noted previously, allows movement of large, polar, and charged compounds. The upper limit for size, however, is approximately 5000. Compounds of greater molecular weight are not able to diffuse across the capillary wall and these compounds enter the blood primarily via the lymph. Because lymph flow is slow, such compounds are absorbed slowly over a prolonged period of time. Such a process has the appearance of a *flip-flop model*, the terminal phase being quite long and being controlled by lymph flow.

STEADY STATE: INFUSION AND MULTIPLE DOSING

Infusion

It is often desirable, in a clinical setting, to achieve a target plasma concentration associated with a needed response and to then maintain concentrations at or near the target value. In other words, sustain or control the plasma concentrations over a narrow range of values, especially if the drug has a narrow concentration range associated with therapeutic effect. This is the aim of all controlled release products, which may be dosed by several routes (e.g., oral, transdermal, IM, and so forth). Whereas this is most often achieved by multiple dosing, as discussed later, it is instructive to establish the principles using the IV route with continuous dosing.

To maintain precise control over plasma concentrations and desired response, *constant rate intravenous infusion* is used. Mechanically, this may be achieved with use of an infusion pump or with an IV drip. The rate of infusion or input into the body is given by a constant, k_o, with units of amount/time (e.g., mg/minute). The rate of loss of compound from the body is given by the product of clearance and plasma concentration (or the product of the first-order rate constant of elimination, apparent volume of distribution, and plasma concentration): $CL_S \cdot C$ (or, $K \cdot V \cdot C$). The rate of change of the amount of compound in the body is the difference between the rate in and the rate out; rate of change = $k_o - CL_S \cdot C$. When infusion is begun, plasma concentrations rise from a value of zero until the rate of input eventually becomes equal to the rate of loss. When that happens, the rate of change of the concentration of the compound in the body is zero, and the rate in equals the rate out. The latter is said to be a *steady state condition* and it continues for as long as the compound is administered at the same rate. A steady state plasma concentration, C_{SS}, is achieved:

$$\text{rate in} = \text{rate out} \qquad k_o = CL_S \cdot C_{SS} \qquad \text{[Eq. 54]}$$

As a consequence, the steady state plasma concentration, sometimes referred to as the average concentration, depends on the ratio of *rate in* to *rate out*:

$$C_{SS} \equiv C_{average} = \frac{\text{rate in}}{\text{rate out}} = \frac{k_o}{CL_S} \qquad \text{[Eq. 55]}$$

This is an extremely important and useful relationship, which may be expressed in a variety of ways, as illustrated under multiple dosing. There are basically two questions that need to be answered about this relationship: What determines the value of C_{SS}, and how long does it take to get there? For a given value of CL_S, the magnitude of C_{SS} depends directly only on the rate of infusion: the greater the rate of infusion, the greater the plasma concentration (double the k_o, double C_{SS}). This is, as discussed in First-Order (Linear) Kinetic Processes, the simple principle of first-order kinetics or of a linear system: double the input, double the output. Any change in CL_S for a given rate of infusion results in a different C_{SS}. This is shown in Figure 45A for three hypothetical infusion rates. Infusion rates of 10, 20, and 40 mg per hour result in C_{SS} values of 1, 2, and 4 mg/L, respectively. The ratio of any two infusion rates is identical to the ratio of the resulting steady state plasma concentrations.

How long does it take to reach a steady state? Take any of the exponentially increasing plasma concentration-time curves shown in Figure 45A and turn it upside down and a typical exponential decreasing curve just as that seen after an IV bolus dose is seen. The parameter that determines the decline (i.e., slope) of the exponential decreasing curve is the same parameter that determines the rise of an infusion curve, $t_{1/2}$. The time necessary to achieve any fraction of steady state is simply a function of $t_{1/2}$, regardless of rate of infusion. This can be visualized by taking the three curves in Figure 45A, dividing each by infusion rate, and a single superimposed curve is obtained. This is the same idea, superposition, discussed previously for single IV bolus doses, and it is a characteristic of first-order kinetics. Because these infusion rate-normalized curves superimpose, it takes the same amount of time for any of those infusion curves to achieve the same fraction of steady state. It takes one $t_{1/2}$ for an exponential declining curve to reach 50% of the starting concentration; it takes one $t_{1/2}$ for an exponential increasing infusion curve to achieve 50% of its final steady state concentration. After two $t_{1/2}$s, an exponential declining curve has declined by 75% of its starting value; after two $t_{1/2}$s, an infusion curve achieves 75% of its final steady state concentration. After three $t_{1/2}$s, an exponential declining curve has declined to 88% of its starting value; after three $t_{1/2}$s, an infusion curve achieves 88% of its final steady state concentration. This continues for each subsequent $t_{1/2}$. The rise in the infusion curve after a certain number of $t_{1/2}$s (as percentage of the final steady state concentration) is exactly equal to the decline (as percentage of the starting concentration) in an IV bolus plasma concentration-time curve at the same number of $t_{1/2}$s. As a practical general rule, it takes approximately four $t_{1/2}$s to achieve a steady state (actually, 94% of C_{SS}).

The exact equation that describes the concentration-time curve after constant rate IV infusion to steady state, assuming a one-compartment model, is

$$C = \frac{k_0}{CL_S} \cdot (1 - e^{-K \cdot t}) = C_{SS} \cdot (1 - e^{-K \cdot t}) \qquad \text{[Eq. 56]}$$

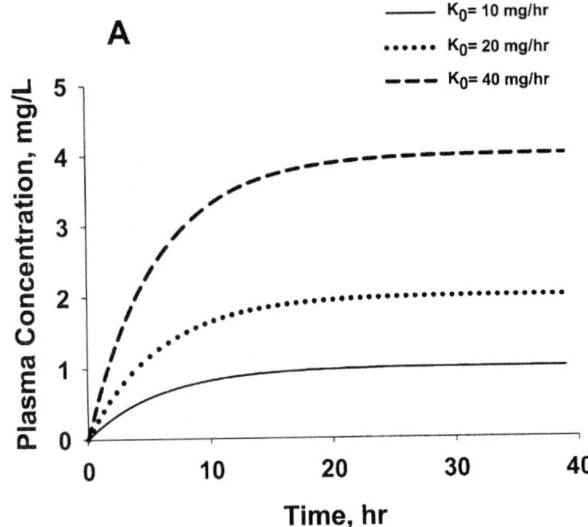

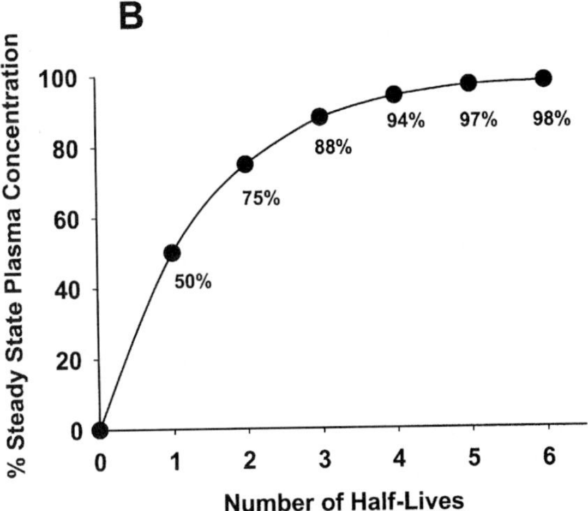

Figure 45. A: Plasma concentration-time profiles for a hypothetical compound given by constant rate intravenous infusion at rates of 10, 20, and 40 mg/hour. The resulting steady state plasma concentrations are directly proportional to the infusion rates: 1, 2, and 4 ng/ml. **B:** The percentage of steady state as a function of the number of half-lives of infusion. The values on the line indicate the percentage steady state achieved at each half-life. (From M. Mayersohn, *unpublished*, with permission from Saguaro Technical Press, Inc, Tucson, AZ, 2002.)

At time zero, the concentration is zero, and, at time infinity, the steady state concentration is reached, and it is equal to k_o/CL_S. This equation describes the curves illustrated in Figure 45A. Once the infusion is stopped, whether a steady state is achieved or not, the concentrations decline in an exponential fashion just as it does after an IV bolus dose. The slope of the line describing the decline is equal to –K/2.3.

The percentage of the steady state plasma concentration that is ultimately achieved after any infusion rate is illustrated in Figure 45B as a function of the number of $t_{1/2}$s of infusion. The values for percentage of steady state achieved are noted on the line for each $t_{1/2}$.

The idea of a steady state plasma concentration applies as much to endogenous biochemicals as it does to exogenously administered compounds. The only difference is that the numerator, rather than being an infusion rate, is a formation or synthesis rate:

$$C_{SS} = \frac{\text{formation rate}}{CL_S} \quad \text{[Eq. 57]}$$

For example, creatinine is formed from muscle metabolism, and the resulting steady state serum creatinine concentrations are a function of its formation rate from muscle and creatinine renal clearance. This idea applies to any biochemical for which there is a source of production, such as serum albumin.

Multiple Dosing

Constant rate IV infusion is useful for establishing the two basic ideas of steady state: What determines the value of the steady state concentration and how long does it take to achieve a steady state. Furthermore, infusion has a place in therapy although its use is limited by the need for a clinical facility and experienced personnel. In some instances, a portable infusion pump can be attached to a patient and thereby permit ambulatory activities to continue. Far and away, however, the most frequent approach to continual therapy and to achieving a steady state is with use of a *multiple dosing regimen*. Although such therapy might involve multiple IV infusions or multiple IV bolus doses (again, in a clinic or hospital setting), other routes, especially oral or subcutaneous administration, are the rule. A multiple dosing regimen requires a maintenance dose (D_M) and, perhaps, a loading dose (D_L), a dosing interval (τ; tau), a route of administration, and a specific drug product. The dosing interval determines the frequency of dosing. Issues of exposure to environmental compounds have identical considerations when it comes to accumulation in the body.

Consider a route of administration that requires absorption into the body, as this results in the most general relationships. The basic relationship, with one alteration, is the same as that developed for constant rate IV infusion. The only difference is that rather than a constant rate infusion, a dose rate is dealt with here. A *dose rate* is the amount of substance that reaches the systemic circulation ($F \cdot D_M$) per dosing interval, τ; dose rate equals $(F \cdot D_M)/\tau$. Therefore, the steady state concentration is given by

$$C_{SS} = C_{average} = \frac{\text{dose rate}}{CL_S} = \frac{F \cdot D_M}{CL_S \cdot \tau} \quad \text{[Eq. 58]}$$

As with the previous relationship, this is an especially useful equation and it can be written in a number of equivalent forms.

$$C_{SS} = C_{average} = \frac{\text{dose rate}}{CL_S} = \frac{F \cdot D_M}{CL_S \cdot \tau} = \frac{F \cdot D_M}{\lambda_n \cdot V \cdot \tau} = \frac{F \cdot D_M \cdot t_{1/2} \cdot (1.44)}{V \cdot \tau} \quad \text{[Eq. 59]}$$

A change in any one variable at a time should lead to a change in C_{SS} that makes sense. Thus, if $t_{1/2}$ were to increase, holding all other variables constant, one would expect the steady state concentration to increase, as the equation predicts. The reason that the term $C_{average}$ is used is because, unlike constant rate IV infusion, multiple dosing actually produces a fluctuating and not a constant steady state, as is illustrated.

Another idea that is different for multiple dosing is that of *accumulation*. As long as one administers a dose of the compound before the prior dose is completely eliminated from the body, the amount of compound in the body continues to accumulate with additional doses until a steady state is reached. What determines the value for C_{SS}? Dose rate and clearance. How long does it take to achieve a steady state? The answer is approximately four $t_{1/2}$s, and it does not matter how often the compound is administered. To illustrate these ideas, consider Figures 46 and 47. A typical multiple dosing plasma concentration-time profile involving absorption is shown in Figure 46A. The compound has a $t_{1/2}$ of 4 hours and it is being dosed every 4 hours. If only the first dose was given, the plasma concentrations continue to decline after reaching a maximum (C_{max}). Also shown is the area under the first dose curve. However, if a sec-

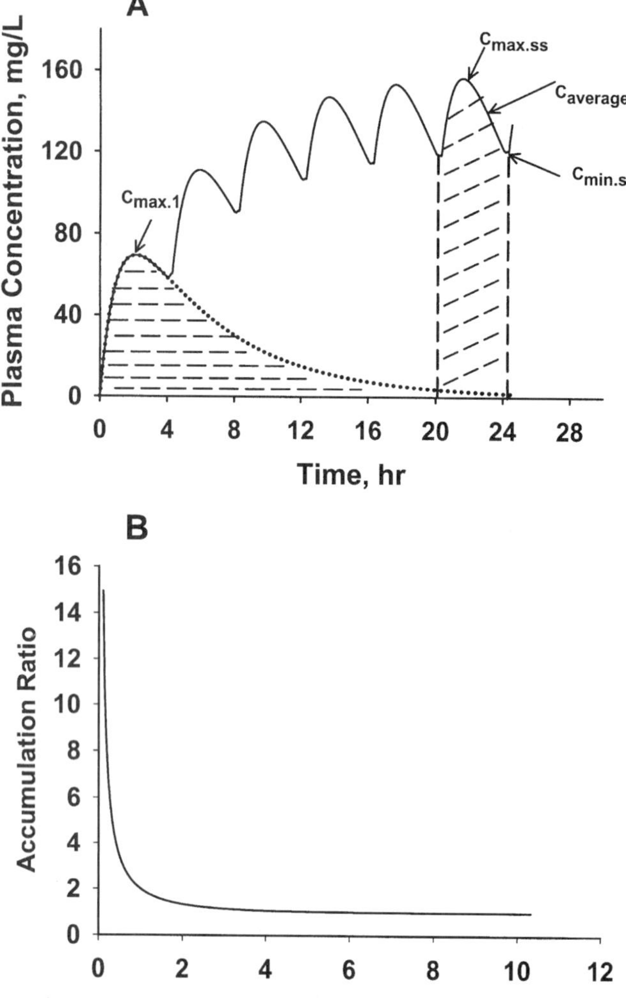

Figure 46. A: Plasma concentration-time profile after the multiple dosing of a compound that undergoes absorption to gain access to the body. The compound has a terminal half-life of 4 hours and is being dosed at a dosing interval (τ) of 4 hours. The concentrations increase with dosing as a result of accumulation, and a steady state concentration is achieved within approximately four half-lives. The first dose is characterized by a maximum plasma concentration ($C_{max\cdot 1}$), and the total area under the curve for the first dose is indicated. At steady state there is a maximum and minimum steady state plasma concentration ($C_{max\cdot ss}$ and $C_{min\cdot ss}$), and an area under the curve during the dosing interval at steady state is indicated. An average steady state concentration ($C_{average}$ or $\bar{C}$) between the maximum and minimum value may also be calculated. **B:** The accumulation ratio as a function of the ratio of dosing interval to half-life, $\tau/t_{1/2}$. The more frequent the dosing (left side of graph), the smaller the value for $\tau/t_{1/2}$ and the greater the compound accumulates. The less frequent the dosing (right side of graph), the greater the value for $\tau/t_{1/2}$ and the smaller the accumulation. Note that when $\tau/t_{1/2} = 1$, the accumulation ratio is 2.0. (From M. Mayersohn, *unpublished*, with permission from Saguaro Technical Press, Inc, Tucson, AZ, 2002.)

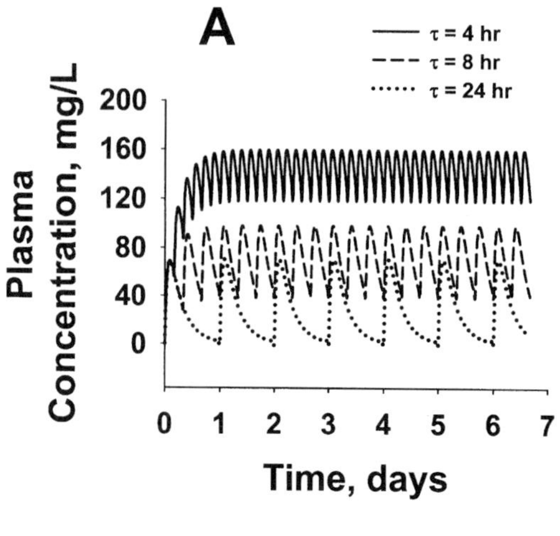

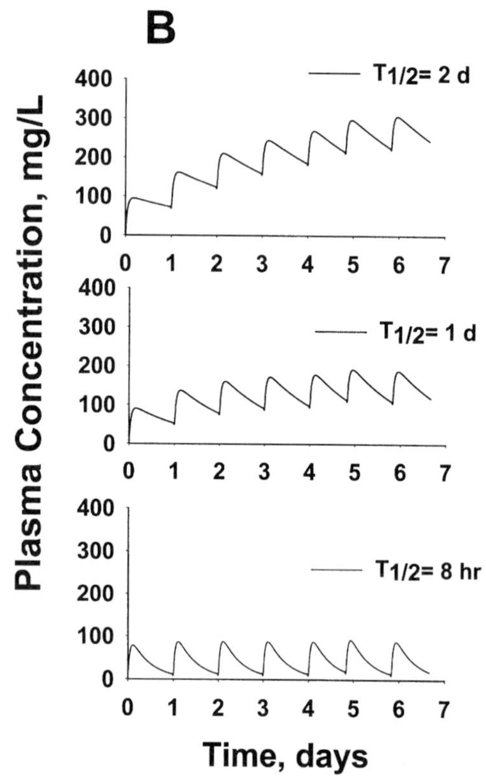

Figure 47. A: Plasma concentration-time profiles for a drug administered in a multiple dosing fashion by a route that requires absorption into the body. The same maintenance dose of the same drug ($t_{1/2}$ = 4 hours), is administered at different dosing intervals (τ = 4, 12, and 24 hours), giving rise to different dose rates and different steady state plasma concentrations. Note that accumulation is greatest for the smallest ratio of $\tau/t_{1/2}$ (i.e., τ = 4 hours). **B:** Plasma concentration-time profiles for different drugs administered in a multiple dosing fashion by a route that requires absorption into the body. Each drug is given at the same dosing interval, τ = 1 day. The half-lives of the drug are 2 days (*top*), 1 day (*middle*), and 8 hours (*bottom*). Note that accumulation is greatest for the smallest ratio of $\tau/t_{1/2}$ (i.e., $t_{1/2}$ = 2 days). (From M. Mayersohn, *unpublished*, with permission from Saguaro Technical Press, Inc, Tucson, AZ, 2002.)

ond and subsequent doses are given every 4 hours, the plasma concentrations rise as a consequence of accumulation. This rise continues until a steady state is achieved and this is seen after approximately four $t_{1/2}$s. All subsequent curves during a dosing interval simply repeat the identical concentration-time pattern (in fact, they are superimposable). Any concentration-time curve during a dosing interval at steady state is characterized by a maximum ($C_{max\cdot ss}$), a minimum ($C_{min\cdot ss}$), and an average ($C_{average}$ or $\bar{C}$; read as *C-bar*) steady state plasma concentration. There are exact equations that may be used to calculate those values. The $C_{average}$ is not the mean of the maximum and minimum concentrations, but rather it is defined as the area under the steady state plasma concentration during a dosing interval divided by the dosing interval, $C_{average} = (AUC_0^{\tau})_{ss}/\tau$. The degree of accumulation is judged by examining the concentration obtained from the first dose and comparing it to the concentration obtained on multiple dosing. For example, the ratio of $C_{max\cdot ss}$ to $C_{max\cdot 1}$ gives an estimate of accumulation. In the example illustrated, the value is approximately 2.0; the drug accumulates to the extent of approximately twofold. The degree of accumulation as judged by the accumulation ratio is illustrated in Figure 46B. Accumulation is a function of the ratio of dosing interval to $t_{1/2}$, $\tau/t_{1/2}$. Thus, the smaller this ratio, the more frequently the dose is given (e.g., τ = 4 hours; $t_{1/2}$ = 24 hours), the greater the accumulation. In contrast, less frequent dosing (e.g., τ = 24 hours; $t_{1/2}$ = 4 hours) gives a large value on the x-axis and little accumulation. A useful index value is an accumulation ratio of 2.0, associated with a $\tau/t_{1/2}$ ratio of 1. That is, dose the drug at a time equal to its $t_{1/2}$ and accumulation is twofold.

The latter ideas are also expressed in Figure 47. Figure 47A illustrates the multiple dosing plasma concentration-time data for a drug that undergoes absorption and that is administered at three different dosing intervals. With a $t_{1/2}$ of 4 hours, this hypothetical drug undergoes greater accumulation when it is given most frequently (i.e., τ = 4 hours) and least accumulation when given infrequently (i.e., τ = 24 hours). Figure 47B illustrates a similar idea except that the dosing interval is held constant (τ = 24 hours) for three different hypothetical drugs with different half-lives (from top to bottom, 2 days, 1 day, and 8 hours). The greater the $t_{1/2}$, the greater the accumulation.

Dosing regimens that use the same dose rate provide identical average steady state plasma concentrations. Thus, the following equivalent dose rates result in identical values for $C_{average}$: 1000 mg/24 hours = 500 mg/12 hours = 250 mg/6 hours. However, the range of maximum to minimum concentrations is different. The least frequent dosing (1000 mg/24 hours) results in a much larger range of concentrations at steady state compared to more frequent dosing (i.e., 250 mg/6 hours). These ranges of concentrations during a dosing interval at steady state for different dosing intervals are illustrated in Figure 48.

One of the most useful applications of clearance concepts is their incorporation into the multiple dosing relationships. Based on the category of clearance of the compound (low or high), one can predict what should happen at steady state as a result of alterations due to, for example, drug-drug interactions or as a result of disease states. In the same way, one can evaluate the results of studies to determine the correct mechanism(s) responsible for the observed changes. This is especially true when trying to understand changes in total and unbound plasma concentrations and $t_{1/2}$ as a result of alterations in plasma protein binding.

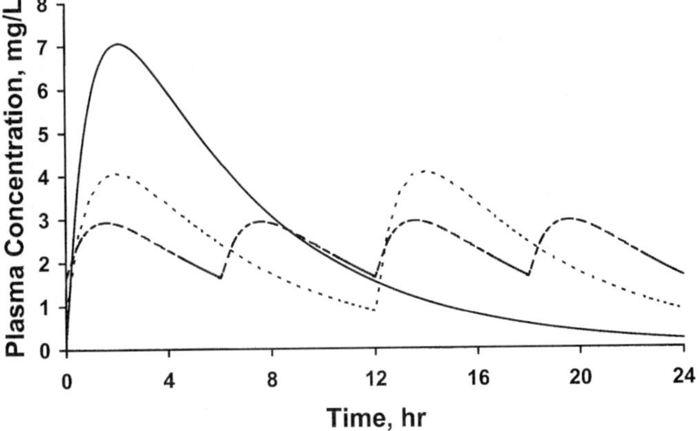

Figure 48. Steady state plasma concentrations of a drug administered in a multiple dosing fashion by a route that requires absorption into the body. The same drug (half-life, 4 hours) was given at different dosing intervals but using equal dose rates. The three dose rates are 1000 mg/24 hours; 500 mg/12 hours; 250 mg/6 hours. Note that the same average steady state plasma concentration is achieved; however, there is a wide range of concentrations when the dosing interval is long. (From M. Mayersohn, *unpublished*, with permission from Saguaro Technical Press, Inc, Tucson, AZ, 2002.)

What effect will a change in plasma protein binding have on total and unbound plasma concentrations? The change in plasma protein binding may be the result of an alteration in plasma protein (e.g., albumin) concentrations or as a consequence of being displaced by another highly bound compound. Total steady state plasma concentration, C_{TOTAL}, is a function of dose rate and clearance, whereas the unbound concentration is that value multiplied by the unbound fraction:

$$C_{TOTAL} = \frac{\text{dose rate}}{CL_S}$$

$$C_{UNBOUND} = f_U \cdot C_{TOTAL} = \frac{f_U \cdot \text{dose rate}}{CL_S} \quad \text{[Eq. 60]}$$

The exact relationship depends on the category of clearance: low or high. For a *low clearance* compound, $CL_S \cong f_U \cdot CL_{U,int}$, and, therefore,

$$C_{TOTAL} \cong \frac{\text{dose rate}}{f_U \cdot CL_{U,int}}$$

$$C_{UNBOUND} = f_U \cdot C_{TOTAL} \cong \frac{f_U \cdot \text{dose rate}}{f_U \cdot CL_{U,int}} = \frac{\text{dose rate}}{CL_{U,int}} \quad \text{[Eq. 61]}$$

Total plasma concentration is affected by changes in plasma protein binding (e.g., an increase in the unbound fraction results in a decrease in total concentration). In sharp contrast, a change in plasma protein binding has *no* effect on unbound plasma concentrations. This important conclusion is sometimes thought to be counter-intuitive, especially when it is stated that *plasma protein binding has no effect on the unbound plasma concentration*. The unbound plasma concentration is influenced only by the $CL_{U,int}$, whereas the total concentration is affected by total clearance. The only way to change the unbound plasma concentration is to alter the $CL_{U,int}$. For example, if the drug is metabolized, any drug-drug interaction causing an increase (induction) or decrease (inhibition) in $CL_{U,int}$ results in a change in the unbound plasma concentration. Because it is the unbound plasma concentration that is in equilibrium with tissues (the likely sites of action), that type of interaction is expected to affect response and/or toxicity. In fact, it is generally correct to state that drug displacement interactions have little if any clinical significance (48).

For a *high clearance* compound, clearance is approximately equal to organ blood flow, $CL_S \cong Q$, and, therefore,

$$C_{TOTAL} \cong \frac{\text{dose rate}}{Q}$$

$$C_{UNBOUND} = f_U \cdot C_{TOTAL} \cong \frac{f_U \cdot \text{dose rate}}{Q} \quad \text{[Eq. 62]}$$

In this instance, total plasma concentrations remain unchanged, but the unbound concentration increases if the unbound fraction increases. This is one of the few categories of drug in which a drug displacement interaction might have clinical relevance (e.g., lidocaine).

An excellent example of the use of these concepts in evaluating literature claims and in examining possible mechanism(s) of interactions is the classical interaction between warfarin and phenylbutazone. It was known that the coadministration of those two compounds resulted in incidents of bleeding. It was also known that both compounds bound extensively to plasma proteins, and displacement from binding sites could be seen in *in vitro* studies. The conclusion reached, which was held for a long time, was that phenylbutazone was displacing warfarin from its plasma protein binding sites. All that is needed to know to assess the correctness of this conclusion is the clearance category of warfarin. Because that compound is totally metabolized by the liver, and its clearance is approximately 100 ml/minute, it is in a low clearance category (ER ≅ 0.067). Equation 61 offers an approximation of total and unbound plasma concentrations for a low clearance compound and it suggests that total concentration should decrease. In fact, total warfarin concentrations were found to decrease in the presence of phenylbutazone in a clinical study. Therefore, that finding is consistent with the suggested mechanism of the interaction being a displacement interaction. However, why would a *decrease* in the concentration of the drug cause an *increased* response (i.e., more bleeding)? Equation 61 also predicts that there should be no change in the unbound plasma concentrations. In fact, in the clinical study, the unbound plasma concentrations were found to *increase* in the presence of phenylbutazone. That increase is consistent with an enhanced response, but how does one explain that change? The only way to explain the findings is to conclude that the $CL_{U,int}$ has decreased, and this is the cause of the increase in the unbound plasma concentrations,

$$\uparrow C_{UNBOUND} \cong \frac{\text{dose rate}}{\downarrow CL_{U,int}} \qquad \text{[Eq. 63]}$$

In other words, there are actually two interactions occurring, but the clinically important one is a result of phenylbutazone inhibiting the metabolism of warfarin, causing a decrease in the $CL_{U,int}$ (49).

These concepts can also be applied in an attempt to predict or interpret the effect of altered plasma protein binding on the terminal $t_{1/2}$. This becomes somewhat more complex because $t_{1/2}$ depends on both apparent volume of distribution and clearance, and both may be affected by plasma protein binding, depending on the clearance category. To conduct this analysis in a practical way, one needs to simplify the volume and the clearance terms: small or large volume, small or large clearance. For example, what effect would an increase in the unbound fraction in plasma have on the terminal $t_{1/2}$ of a small volume and small clearance compound (e.g., warfarin)?

$$t_{1/2} = \frac{0.693 \cdot V_d}{CL_S} \cong \frac{0.693 \cdot (7 + 8 \cdot f_U)}{f_U \cdot CL_{U,int}} \qquad \text{[Eq. 64]}$$

This analysis would conclude that, because the numerator and denominator contain a term for f_U, any change in that value has little if any effect on $t_{1/2}$. Perhaps being a bit more precise (even though this is an approximation only), the numerator goes up in a nonproportional way with an increase in the unbound fraction, whereas the denominator goes up directly, leading to an overall decrease in $t_{1/2}$. This type of simplified analysis is useful and goes a long way in explaining unexpected results and in making reasonable experimental predictions.

REFERENCES

1. Parab PV, Ritschel WA, Coyle DE, et al. Pharmacokinetics of hydromorphone after intravenous, peroral and rectal administration to human subjects. *Biopharm Drug Dispos* 1988;9:187–199.
2. Wilkinson PK, Sedman AJ, Sakmar E, et al. Blood ethanol concentrations during and following constant-rate intravenous infusion of alcohol. *Clin Pharmacol Ther* 1976;19:213–223.
3. Young JD, Braun WH, Gehring PJ. The dose-dependent fate of 1,4-dioxane in rats. *J Environ Pathol Toxicol* 1978;2:263–282.
4. Motulsky HJ, Ransnas LA. Fitting curves to data using nonlinear regression: a practical and nonmathematical review. *FASEB J* 1987;1:365–374.
5. Lassen NA, Perl W. *Tracer kinetic methods in medical physiology*. New York: Raven Press, 1979:102–112.
6. Krishnan K, Andersen ME. Physiologically based pharmacokinetic modeling in toxicology. In: Hayes AW, ed. *Principles and methods of toxicology*, 3rd ed. New York: Raven Press, 1994:149–188.
7. Yang SHR, Andersen MA. Pharmacokinetics. In: Hodgson E, Levi PE, eds. *Biochemical toxicology*, 2nd ed. Norwalk, CT: Appleton & Lange, 1994:49–74.
8. Rowland M, Tozer TN. *Clinical pharmacokinetics—concepts and applications*, 3rd ed. Baltimore: Williams & Wilkins, 1995:137–142.
9. Pirkle JL, Wolfe WH, Patterson LL, et al. Estimates of the half-life of 2,3,7,8-tetrachlorodibenzo-p-dioxin in Vietnam veterans of operation ranch hand. *J Toxicol Environ Health* 1989;27:165–171.
10. Oie S, Tozer TN. Effect of altered plasma protein binding on apparent volume of distribution. *J Pharm Sci* 1979;68:1203–1205.
11. Klotz U, Avant GR, Hoyumpa A, et al. The effects of age and liver disease on the disposition and elimination of diazepam in adult man. *J Clin Invest* 1975;55:347–359.
12. Jung D, Mayersohn M, Perrier D, et al. Thiopental disposition as a function of age in female patients undergoing surgery. *Anesthesiology* 1982;56:263–268.
13. Fung HL, Sutton SC, Kamiya A. Blood vessel uptake and metabolism of organic nitrates in the rat. *J Pharmacol Exp Ther* 1984;228:334–341.
14. Wilkinson GR. Clearance approaches in pharmacology. *Pharmacol Rev* 1987;39:1–47.
15. Wilkinson GR. Pharmacokinetics of drug disposition: hemodynamic considerations. *Annu Rev Pharmacol* 1975;15:11–27.
16. Sinha V, Brendel K, Mayersohn M. A simplified isolated perfused rat liver apparatus: characterization and measurement of extraction ratios of selected compounds. *Life Sci* 2000;66:1795–1804.
17. Levy G. Clinical implications of interindividual differences in plasma protein binding of drugs and endogenous substances. In: Benet LZ, ed. *The effect of disease states on drug pharmacokinetics*. Washington, DC: American Pharmaceutical Association, 1976:137–151.
18. Pitts RF. *Physiology of the kidney and body fluids*, 3rd ed. Chicago: Year Book 1974:141–142.
19. Pitts RF. *Physiology of the kidney and body fluids*, 3rd ed. Chicago: Year Book 1974:73–74.
20. Beckett AH, Rowland M. Urinary excretion kinetics of methylamphetamine in man. *Nature* 1965;206:1260–1261.
21. Mayersohn M. Rational approaches to treatment of drug toxicity: recent considerations and application of pharmacokinetic principles. In: Barnett G, Chiang CN, eds. *Pharmacokinetics and pharmacodynamics of psychoactive drugs*. Foster City, CA: Biomedical Publications, 1985:120–142.
22. Linton AL, Luke RG, Briggs JD. Methods of forced diuresis and its application in barbiturate poisoning. *Lancet* 1967;2:377–380.
23. Osborne R, Joel S, Trew D, et al. Morphine and metabolite behavior after different routes of morphine administration: demonstration of the importance of the active metabolite morphine-6-glucuronide. *Clin Pharmacol Ther* 1990;47:12–19.
24. Skarke C, Darimont J, Schmidt H, et al. Analgesic effects of morphine and morphine-6-glucuronide in a transcutaneous electrical pain model in healthy volunteers. *Clin Pharmacol Ther* 2003;73:107–121.
25. Dutcher JS, Strong JM, Lucas SV, et al. Procainamide and *N*-acetylprocainamide kinetics investigated simultaneously with stable isotope methodology. *Clin Pharmacol Ther* 1977;22:447–457.
26. Levy RH, Thummel KE, Trager WF, et al., eds. *Metabolic drug interactions*. Philadelphia: Lippincott Williams & Wilkins, 2000.
27. Boxenbaum H. Cytochrome P450 3A4 in vivo ketoconazole competitive inhibition: determination of Ki and dangers associated with high clearance drugs in general. *J Pharmaceut Pharmaceut Sci* 1999;2:45–52.
28. Jacobsen D. New treatment for ethylene glycol poisoning. *N Engl J Med* 1999;340:879–881.
29. Brent J, McMartin K, Phillips S, et al. Fomepizole for the treatment of ethylene glycol poisoning. *N Engl J Med* 1999;340:832–838.
30. Gwilt PR, Perrier D. Plasma protein binding and distribution characteristics of drugs as indices of their hemodialyzability. *Clin Pharmacol Ther* 1978;24:154–161.
31. Mayersohn M. Rational approaches to treatment of drug toxicity: recent considerations and application of pharmacokinetic principles. In: Barnett G, Chiang CN, eds. *Pharmacokinetics and pharmacodynamics of psychoactive drugs*. Foster City, CA: Biomedical Publications 1985:131.
32. Gonda A, Gault H, Churchill D, et al. Hemodialysis for methanol intoxication. *Am J Med* 1978;64:749–758.
33. Palatnick W, Redman LW, Sitar DS, et al. Methanol half-life during ethanol administration: implications for management of methanol poisoning. *Ann Emerg Med* 1995;26:202–207.
34. Eder AF, McGrath CM, Dowdy YG, et al. Ethylene glycol poisoning: toxicokinetic and analytical factors affecting laboratory diagnosis. *Clin Chem* 1998;44:168–177.
35. Amdisen A, Skjoldborg H. Haemodialysis for lithium poisoning. *Lancet* 1969;2:213.
36. Tilstone WJ, Winchester JF, Reavey PC. The use of pharmacokinetic principles in determining the effectiveness of removal of toxins from blood. *Clin Pharmacokinet* 1979;4:23–37.
37. Takki S, Gambertoglio JG, Honda DH, et al. Pharmacokinetic evaluation of hemodialysis in acute drug overdose. *J Pharmacokinet Biopharm* 1978;6:427–442.
38. Pond SM. Extracorporeal techniques in the treatment of poisoned patients. *M J Aust* 1991;154:617–622.
39. Mayersohn M. Principles of drug absorption. In: Banker G, Rhodes CT, eds. *Modern pharmaceutics*. New York: Marcel Dekker Inc 2002:23–66.
40. Levy G, Houston JB. Effect of activated charcoal on acetaminophen absorption. *Pediatrics* 1976;58:432–435.

41. Levy G, Tsuchiya T. Effect of activated charcoal on aspirin absorption in man. Part I. *Clin Pharmacol Ther* 1972;13:317–322.
42. Olkkola KT. Effect of charcoal-drug ratio on antidotal efficacy of oral activated charcoal in man. *Br J Clin Pharmacol* 1985;19:767–773.
43. Berg MJ, Berlinger WG, Goldberg MJ, et al. Acceleration of the body clearance of phenobarbital by oral activated charcoal. *N Engl J Med* 1982;307:642–644.
44. Pond SM. Rosl of repeated oral doses of activated charcoal in clinical toxicology. *Med Toxicol* 1986;1:3–11.
45. Holazo AA, Colburn WA. Pharmacokinetics of drugs during various detoxification procedures for overdose and environmental exposure. *Drug Metab Rev* 1982;13:715–743.
46. Davidson AN. The conversion of Schradan (OMPA) and parathion into inhibitors of cholinesterase by mammalian liver. *Biochem J* 1955;61:203–209.
47. Pieniaszek HJ Jr, Mayersohn M, Adams MP, et al. Moricizine bioavailability via simultaneous, dual, stable isotope administration: bioequivalence implications. *J Clin Pharmacol* 1999;39:817–825.
48. Benet LZ, Hoener B-A. Changes in plasma protein binding have little clinical relevance. *Clin Pharmacol Ther* 2002;71:115–121.
49. Schary WL, Lewis RJ, Rowland M. Warfarin-phenylbutazone interaction in man: a long term multiple-dose study. *Res Commun Chem Pathol Pharmacol* 1975;10:633–672.

SUGGESTED READING

Textbooks

Baselt RC. *Disposition of toxic drugs and chemicals in man*, 5th ed. Foster City, CA: Chemical Toxicology Institute, 2000.

Gibaldi M, Perrier D. *Pharmacokinetics*, 2nd ed. New York: Marcel Dekker Inc, 1982.

Gibaldi M. *Biopharmaceutics and clinical pharmacokinetics*, 4th ed. Philadelphia: Lea and Febiger, 1990.

Riggs DS. *The mathematical approach to physiological problems*. Baltimore: Williams and Wilkins, 1963.

Rowland M, Tozer TN. *Clinical pharmacokinetics—concepts and applications*, 3rd ed. Baltimore: Williams & Wilkins, 1995:137–142.

Textbook Chapters

Klassen CD. Principles of toxicology and treatment of disease. In: Hardman JG, Limbird LE, eds. *Goodman and Gilman's the pharmacological basis of therapeutics*, 10th ed. New York: McGraw-Hill, 2001:67–80.

Krishnan K, Andersen ME. Physiologically based pharmacokinetic modeling in toxicology. In: Hayes AW, ed. *Principles and methods of toxicology*, 3rd ed. New York: Raven Press, 1994:149–188.

Renwick AG. Toxicokinetics-pharmacokinetics in toxicology. In: Hayes AW, ed. *Principles and methods of toxicology*, 3rd ed. New York: Raven Press, 1994:101–148.

Wilkinson GR. Pharmacokinetics: the dynamics of drug absorption, distribution, and elimination. In: Hardman JG, Limbird LE, eds. *Goodman and Gilman's the pharmacological basis of therapeutics*, 10th ed. New York: McGraw-Hill, 2001:3–30.

GLOSSARY

A

Absorption: The process of a substance moving from an extravascular (i.e., nonintravenous) site of dosing across one or more biologic membranes (usually down a concentration gradient) and appearing in the systemic (i.e., blood) circulation after administration.

Absorption rate constant: The apparent first-order absorption rate constant describes the relationship between the rate of absorption and the concentration or amount of substance being absorbed from the absorption site; rate of absorption = $k_a \cdot$ amount. Usual symbol is k_A (units, 1/time).

Absolute bioavailability: See *Bioavailability*.

Accumulation: The process of drug amount (and plasma concentration) increasing in the body after multiple dosing. Accumulation occurs when the next dose is given before all drug from the previous dose has been eliminated from the body. Measured by the accumulation ratio.

Accumulation ratio: The extent to which a drug accumulates in the body after a multiple dosing regimen. This value is determined by the ratio of the dosing interval (τ) to elimination half-life ($t_{1/2}$); the smaller that ratio is, the greater the extent of accumulation. Symbol often used is R_C (unitless). For a simple model,

$$R_c = \frac{1}{1-e^{-K \cdot \tau}}$$

Active tubular reabsorption: The active process requiring metabolic energy that is responsible for the movement of a substance from the urine back into the blood. As with all active processes, a specific transport system is required. Such systems are important for homeostasis of required nutrients such as monosaccharides, amino acids, and vitamins. The renal clearance of such substances is approximately zero until the process becomes saturated and at a maximum approaches glomerular filtration. This process is characterized by a V_{max} or T_{max} (transport maximum) and k_m, concentration to achieve one-half T_{max}.

$$CL_{reabs} = \frac{T_{max}}{k_m + C_{urine}} \qquad CL_{reabs} \to 0, \text{ as } C_{urine} \to \infty$$

Active tubular secretion (or transport): When used in the context of the kidney, this refers to the passage of drug directly from the bloodstream (efferent arteriole) into the renal tubule, without going through the glomerulus. The process is *active*, because it requires the input of energy to push the drug from a low concentration in the bloodstream to a high concentration in the renal tubule. Such active processes also have characteristics of site specificity, structural specificity, and may be competitively inhibited. Penicillin is a drug example (inhibited by probenecid; a classic drug-drug interaction). Renal clearance associated with active tubular secretion (approximately 1200 blood/minute or 600 ml plasma/minute) exceeds that of glomerular or passive filtration (approximately 100 to 120 ml plasma/minute). Mathematically, this process can be described by the same relationship as for Michaelis-Menten enzyme kinetics. This process is characterized by a V_{max} or T_{max} (transport maximum) and k_m, concentration to achieve one-half T_{max}. The renal clearance of such substances used to measure renal blood flow (e.g., p-aminohippuric acid) approaches renal blood flow at low plasma concentrations. Clearance approaches zero at high plasma concentrations. At high plasma concentrations, renal clearance approaches glomerular filtration.

$$CL_{secretion} = \frac{T_{max}}{k_m + C_{plasma}} \qquad CL_{secretion} \to 0, \text{ as } C_{plasma} \to \infty$$

ADME: The mnemonic used for *a*bsorption, *d*istribution, *m*etabolism, and *e*xcretion.

p-Aminohippurate (PAH): See *Para-aminohippurate*.

Apparent oral clearance: Determined after an oral dose from $CL_O = \text{dose}/(AUC)_0^\infty$. Sometimes referred to as intrinsic clearance (see *intrinsic clearance*). Apparent oral clearance equals systemic clearance if the fraction of the dose absorbed (F) is equal to 1. Under all other circumstances, oral clearance is greater than systemic clearance (units, volume/time).

Apparent volume of distribution: See *Volume of distribution*. Symbol is V, usually with a subscript to indicate which volume it represents (units, volume).

Area under the curve (AUC): A shorthand term for the area under the plasma concentration-time curve. Unless otherwise specified, AUC_0^∞ is the area from time 0 to infinity. This important measure is directly related to dose (assuming first-order kinetics) and is used to calculate several other important values such as clearance, apparent volume of distribution, and bioavailability. The mathematical equivalent of this graphical area is the integral of the equation that describes the curve (from time 0 to infinity); $AUC_0^\infty = \int_0^\infty C \cdot dt$. The area may be determined by fitting the data (e.g., nonlinear regression analysis), or it may be approximated with any of several techniques (e.g., trapezoidal rule, spline function, and so forth). This area is sometimes referred to as the *zeroth moment*. Conceptually, the AUC_0^∞ may be considered (as it is by pharmacologists and toxicologists) as an index of exposure to the drug. Thus, the greater the area is, the greater the exposure to the drug (units, concentration × time).

B

Bile: A liquid produced by the liver and secreted into the duodenum; it contains water, bile salts, bile pigments, cholesterol, lecithin, and ions. Bile salts make bile a micellar solution. The primary function of bile is to emulsify fats, through micellar solubilization, and it appears to increase the water-solubility and dissolution rate of poorly water-soluble drugs.

Biliary recycling (enterohepatic recirculation): The process whereby a drug or endogenous substance is taken up by the liver, incorporated into bile, secreted into the gut, and reabsorbed back into the systemic circulation. So effective is reabsorption and recycling of bile salts, that greater than 95% of these molecules are reabsorbed from the gut. Biliary recycling of a drug is often observed as a secondary peak in the plasma concentration-time curve, often in association with ingestion of a meal. Disruption of this process increases systemic clearance. The long half-life of phenobarbital (approximately 4 days) appears to be due to enterohepatic recycling. The half-life is reduced dramatically after oral charcoal administration, which disrupts the recycling process.

Bioavailability: A term used to define and quantitate the rate and efficiency of the extravascular absorption process. As a parameter, there are two types of bioavailability: (A) *absolute bioavailability* refers to the fraction of a dose reaching the systemic circulation intact (in reference to an intravenous dose); and (B) *relative bioavailability* is the fraction of a dose of drug reaching the systemic circulation relative to a reference product (*innovator's* product). As an adjective, *bioavailability* refers to the rate and extent of drug absorption (as in a bioavailability study). The symbol F is often used for bioavailability (fraction of the dose absorbed), and the maximum plasma concentration (C_{max}) and the time of occurrence of the maximum concentration (T_{max}) are often used to reflect rate of absorption.

Bioequivalence: The property of two or more dosage forms, which contain the same amount of drug, producing equivalent biologic responses. Regulatory agencies (e.g., U. S. Food and Drug Administration) customarily assume dosage forms are bioequivalent when, from a statistical point of view, they are equally bioavailable. Hence, the term *bioequivalence* is frequently interchanged with bioavailability equivalence. The basis for this determination is often AUC_0^∞ or the amounts of drug excreted into the urine. Numerous statistical approaches are used for this judgment. The Food and Drug Administration has guidances available to define and test bioequivalence.

Biologic half-life: Often used interchangeably with elimination half-life. This term should *not* be used as it is often confused with a response half-life. Symbol $t_{1/2}$ (units, time).

Biopharmaceutics: The study of the influence of physical chemical and formulation factors on the *in vitro* (e.g., dissolution rate) and *in vivo* performance (e.g., absorption) of a drug dosage form. Frequently, however, biopharmaceutics is also used to characterize formulation factors affecting only dissolution.

Biophase: The presumed site of action in which the receptor is located. Drug is thought to bathe this site and be in equilibrium with unbound drug concentration in the blood (see *Effect site*).

Biotransformation: See *Metabolism*.

Bolus: Refers to instantaneous drug input, as an intravenous bolus injection. In veterinary medicine, a bolus refers to a large tablet administered to animals. Symbol often used for an intravenous bolus dose is X_{iv}^{O} (units, mass).

Blood: The fluid that forms the major communication system within the body. Blood is comprised of a fluid (plasma) that is suspended proteins and formed elements (e.g., various cells). Blood is the fluid that delivers and removes drug from tissues that it bathes.

Brush border: See *Microvilli*.

C

Central (or initial) compartment: The compartment or region of a multicompartment model that receives drug and often is the site of elimination of drug. This compartment is *central* to all other compartments in a mammillary model (all others *feed-off* of this compartment) and contains the blood and all other highly blood-perfused tissues. The exact tissues located in this compartment also depend on the drug. Often called the initial compartment.

Clearance: A primary pharmacokinetic parameter characterizing the rate at which drug is removed from plasma. In general, clearances are additive, as, for example, (total) clearance equals metabolic clearance plus renal clearance plus biliary clearance, and so forth. Clearance has units of volume/time. If clearance equals 20 ml/minute, this denotes that total elimination of drug is such that every minute an equivalent amount of drug is irreversibly removed (eliminated) as is contained in 20 ml of plasma (or blood). Clearance may also be viewed as the proportionality constant between plasma concentration and rate of elimination (i.e., plasma concentration × clearance = rate of elimination). When the term *clearance* is used, it refers to total clearance (total body clearance, TBC, or systemic clearance, CL_S), unless specifically denoted otherwise. Clearance is one of if not the most important pharmacokinetic parameters, as it characterizes the functional ability of an eliminating organ and it determines steady-state plasma concentrations resulting from multiple dosing. The fundamental mathematical relationship for clearance is CL = rate of elimination/C_{PLASMA} (units, volume/time).

Compartment: A part of a system, which may be a substance or a space. If a drug and metabolite occupy the same body, there are two compartments, one for the drug and the other for the metabolite. If a drug occurs in two distinct sites in the body, there are two compartments for that drug. The latter, differentiating space or location, is the most frequently used definition. Compartmental models arise from the need to describe measurable rates of drug distribution in the body. Compartmental models are usually arranged in a mammillary format, such that there is a *central* compartment from which all other compartments feed.

Concentration gradient: The difference in concentration of a substance at two different locations. For example, a concentration gradient across a membrane is the driving force for movement across that membrane. When the gradient is zero (i.e., no difference in concentrations on two sides of the membrane), transport ceases. In first-order processes, compounds move down a gradient. Only in active or specialized transport processes is a compound able to go up or against a gradient (e.g., active tubular secretion).

Concentration maximum: See *Maximum plasma concentration*.

Constant of elimination or disposition: See *Disposition rate constant*.

Creatinine (clearance): Creatinine is an endogenous waste product of muscle metabolism. Creatinine is almost completely eliminated by the kidney by glomerular filtration without tubular secretion or reabsorption. Hence, creatinine clearance is a good approximation of glomerular filtration rate. Creatinine clearance is extensively used, because it does not require exogenous drug administration. The value of creatinine clearance may be estimated from a measure of serum creatinine concentration with the aid of one of several equations that incorporate age, body weight, and gender (Cockcroft-Gault equation or Siersback-Nielsen equation).

$$\text{CLCr, ml/min (males)} = \frac{\text{(ideal weight, kg)(144 − age, yr)}}{72 \cdot \text{Scr (mg\%)}}$$

$$\text{CLCr, ml/min (females)} = \frac{0.86\text{(ideal weight, kg)(144 − age, yr)}}{72 \cdot \text{Scr (mg\%)}}$$

in which CLCr is creatinine clearance and Scr is serum creatinine concentration (units, volume/time).
Cytochrome P-450: A large family of enzymes that is responsible for the metabolism of many drugs. Such metabolic processes are described as phase I metabolism. There are numerous isozymes or isoforms, some of which are under genetic control. Also referred to as CYP450.

D

Disintegration: The breaking apart of a dosage form, observed as when an aspirin tablet is placed in water. The tablet initially breaks up into clumps of granules, followed by granules, and then primary particles. This is *not* the same as dissolution, which is a prerequisite step for absorption. Consider a tablet made of granules of cement; the tablet disintegrates but never dissolves.
Distal: Further away from some reference point. For example, the reference point of the gastrointestinal tract is the juncture of the esophagus and stomach. Therefore, the large intestine is more distal than the small intestine.
Disposition: The simultaneous processes of drug distribution and elimination.
Disposition half-life: A term used to describe the terminal log-linear phase of a plot of plasma concentration versus time (or any other plot from which half-life or the rate constant may be determined). This is the preferred term (compared with biologic or elimination half-life) because it implies properly that this half-life is a function of all dispositional processes (i.e., a function of distribution and elimination). The most appropriate relationship for half-life, which shows the dependent and independent variables, is $t_{1/2} = (0.693 \cdot V)/CL$ (units, time).
Disposition rate constant: A constant that acts as a proportionality constant between a rate and the amount or concentration of drug. This rate constant refers to the log-linear terminal phase of a semilog plot of blood concentration versus time. This constant, which has units of reciprocal time, may be viewed as the fractional (or percentage) rate of loss from the body, which involves both processes of distribution and elimination. Symbols often used are K, β, λ_n, or λ_{last}. The disposition half-life is obtained from the value $t_{1/2} = 0.693/K$ (units, 1/time).
Dissolution: The process of dissolving (i.e., changing state from a solid to a liquid). Dissolution rate is often the rate-limiting step in the extravascular absorption process, especially for poorly water-soluble drugs. Dissolution and disintegration are *not* the same processes (see *Disintegration*).
Distribution: Translocation from the plasma to tissues, and *vice versa*.
Distribution equilibrium: This occurs when the ratio of drug concentration in plasma to concentration in tissue remains constant as a function of time. If distribution is instantaneous (which results in a one-compartment model), the plasma/tissue concentration ratios are constant at all times after dosing. If distribution occurs at a measurable rate (leading to a multicompartment model) the plasma/tissue ratios continue to change until an equilibrium is achieved.
Distribution phase: The initial rapid portion of a drug concentration-time profile after an IV bolus dose, which primarily reflects the distribution of drug or movement into other tissues. When this distributive phase occurs, the drug may be described by a multicompartment model. This is often called the *α-phase*.
Dosage form: The physical form in which the drug is dispersed and used for delivery to humans (e.g., tablet, capsule, solution, and so forth).
Dosage regimen: The dosage form, amount, frequency, and route of administration of a multiple dosing scheme (e.g., one 300 mg oral tablet taken every 6 hours).
Dose-dependency: This condition exists whenever drug concentration-time profiles, divided by dose, are not superimposable. A dose-dependent or nonlinear system is one in which there is not a linear relationship between input and output. This process denotes one or more types of nonlinearity. Other terms used are: nonlinearity, capacity-limited, zero-order (but incorrectly), saturable. An example is Michaelis-Menton enzyme kinetics. Dose-dependent generally refers to the relationship between a parameter (e.g., half-life, clearance, volume) and dose. Other forms of nonlinearity are time-dependent.
Dose-response curve: Any linear or (semi)logarithmic plot of drug response (either therapeutic or toxic) as a function of dose. More commonly in pharmacokinetics, concentration-response curves are used.
Dosing interval: Time interval between consecutive doses. Often symbolized by τ (tau) (units, time).
Drug: A substance given for the treatment, cure, or amelioration of disease or physiologic disorders. It may be synthetic, semisynthetic, or derived from natural sources.
Drug metabolism: See *Metabolism*.

E

Effect site: The actual, presumed, or hypothetical site within the body in which receptors generating the pharmacologic effect are located. This site is often called a *biophase* (see *Biophase*).
Elimination: The sum of (bio)chemical and physical removal of drug from the body.
Elimination half-life (or rate constant): A term used to describe the terminal log-linear phase of a plot of plasma concentration versus time (or any other plot from which half-life or the rate constant may be determined). Although this is a commonly used term, it is *not* the preferred term, which is disposition or terminal half-life. See *Disposition half-life*.
Enterohepatic recycling or recirculation: See *Biliary recycling*.
Enzyme: An organic catalyst, frequently a protein.
Enzyme induction: The process whereby exposure to an agent increases the concentration of a drug-metabolizing enzyme, which results in an increase in metabolic clearance. Smoking induces certain forms of cytochrome P-450, which increases the metabolic clearance of certain drugs (e.g., theophylline).
Enzyme inhibition: The reverse of enzyme induction; the process whereby enzyme activity is reduced. This process results in a reduction in metabolic clearance (e.g., cimetidine is a common enzyme inhibitor).
Epithelial cells: These are cells covering internal or external surfaces of the body. Epithelial cells line the villi of the gastrointestinal tract (one layer thick); they are joined and held together by small amounts of a cement-like substance. The junction between any two cells is termed the *tight junction*. Leakage through the tight junction is the major route of drug absorption of dissociated (ionized) molecules. A layer of epithelial cells is termed an *epithelium*.
Ex vivo: Away or removed from life, oftentimes a combination of *in vivo* and *in vitro*. For example, one could study enzyme induction by administering the inducer to rats *in vivo*, then preparing liver homogenates and studying enzymic activity *in vitro*.

Exogenous: Not naturally present in the body. Most drugs are exogenous agents; exceptions are agents like thyroxine, sodium bicarbonate, progesterone, estradiol, and so forth.
Exponential: In pharmacokinetics, referring to any mathematical expression with the number *e* (the base of natural numbers; 2.71828 . . .) or 10 raised to a power. In general, an exponent is the power to which a base is raised (e.g., 10^2; 2 is the exponent of the base 10). Exponential terms most frequently arise in pharmacokinetics as a result of a first-order kinetic process. First-order disposition could be characterized as exponential disposition. Exponential processes occur frequently in nature (e.g., growth of cells). In pharmacokinetics, absorption from an extravascular site is often described by an exponential input of drug into the body; elimination of drug from the body is often described by exponential loss.
Extraction ratio (ER): The fraction of molecules entering an organ or tissue that is irreversibly eliminated from blood as it passes through that organ. For example, a hepatic ER of 0.2 indicates that 20% of all molecules entering the liver are irreversibly eliminated through metabolism, biliary excretion, and so forth. This fraction remains constant with each passage through the eliminating organ assuming first-order kinetics. ER is determined from the following measurement:

$$ER = \frac{C_{in} - C_{out}}{C_{in}}$$

in which C_{in} is the arterial drug concentration entering the eliminating organ and C_{out} is the venous concentration exiting the organ. ER may also be determined from a knowledge of the organ clearance (CL) and with an estimate of organ blood flow (Q): ER = CL/Q.
Extravascular: External to the bloodstream. Any route of administration that does not provide direct entry into the bloodstream. Thus, oral, rectal, pulmonary, transdermal, and so forth are pathways or routes of administration that require passage across one or more biologic membranes before gaining access to the bloodstream.

F

Filtration: See *Glomerular filtration.*
Filtration fraction: The fraction of plasma flow that is filtered through the glomerulus (approximately 20%).
First-order: Denoting direct proportionality between rate and concentration or amount of substance (rate $\propto$ concentration). For example, elimination could be first-order (i.e., directly proportional to plasma drug concentration). The proportionality is represented by a rate constant (rate = K × concentration). This is an important kinetic process that is used to describe the behavior of most drugs. This process is often referred to as linear or dose-independent kinetics. Such pharmacokinetic parameters as half-life, clearance, and volume are dose-independent. See also *Order.*
First-pass effect (presystemic elimination): Drug degradation and/or metabolism after extravascular administration and which occurs before systemic absorption. Oral first-pass effects include lumen degradation/metabolism, gut wall metabolism, and hepatic metabolism before systemic appearance of drug. Oral hepatic first-pass metabolism occurs subsequent to passage into the hepatoportal vein in the *first pass* of drug molecules through the liver, before reaching the heart. The magnitude of the latter is governed by the value of hepatic clearance (or hepatic extraction ratio). This first pass after oral dosing is more significant than after IV dosing because in the latter case the drug is distributed and diluted before its first appearance in the liver (therefore a small mass is cleared). This effect may be avoided by buccal or sublingual administration (e.g., organic nitrates, methyltestosterone). There may also be a pulmonary first-pass effect after IV dosing, dermal first-pass, and so forth. The fraction of the absorbed dose that escapes any of these sequential metabolic processes is given by ($1-ER_i$). See *Hepatic first-pass effect.*
Flip-flop (model): This occurs when rate of drug absorption is slower than disposition, and hence the shape of the plasma concentration-time curve reflects absorption rather than disposition. Penicillin has a disposition half-life of approximately 1 hour; when administered as a depot intramuscular injection, the plasma concentration-time curve decays with a much longer half-life, reflecting the (flip-flop) half-life of absorption. Sustained release products are formulated such that elimination is governed by slow absorption. The slowest step in a sequence of steps (e.g., absorption to blood to elimination) governs the terminal slope of the plasma concentration versus time plot (this is the idea of a *rate-limiting step*).
Fraction unbound: The unbound (or free) fraction of drug in plasma (f_U). See *Unbound fraction.*
Free fraction: Same as fraction unbound. See *Unbound fraction.*

G

Gastric emptying: The process that describes movement out of the stomach and into the small intestine (see *Gastric emptying rate*).
Gastric emptying rate (GER): The rate at which materials (especially food) leave the stomach and enter the small intestine. This rate is different for liquids and solids and is affected by such factors as fat and carbohydrate content, osmotic pressure, position, and so forth. Often measured as a gastric emptying half-time because the process may not be exponential (see *Half-time*). GER may be a limiting factor in controlling rate of absorption because drugs are best absorbed from the small intestine.
Generic: Refers to a product marketed under the pharmaceutical name, as opposed to a proprietary (trade) name.
Genetic polymorphism: A type of genetic variation in which individuals with sharply distinct qualities coexist as normal members of a population. The study of genetic variations in response to drugs falls under the broad heading of *pharmacogenetics*. For example, rapid and slow acetylation of the drug isoniazid represents a pharmacogenetic polymorphism. In such instances a frequency-distribution diagram of clearance or half-life illustrates at least a bimodal shape rather than the usual normal distribution. One CYP-450 isoform that is under genetic control is 2D6.
GI tract: Gastrointestinal tract (or *gut*).
Glomerular filtration: The passive process whereby blood is filtered through the glomerulus of the nephron. All formed elements (e.g., cells) and proteins are not able to penetrate this membrane (this may not be true under disease conditions such as nephritis or nephrosis). As a result, drugs bound to proteins and cellular components are not filtered, and the resulting clearance is less than that for filtration (which is approximately equal to creatinine clearance, approximately 100 to 120 ml/minute). The glomerular filtration clearance of a compound bound to plasma proteins is given by $CL_{FILTRATION} = f_U \cdot CLCr$, in which f_U is the unbound fraction of drug in plasma and CLCr is creatinine clearance (units, volume/time).
Glomerulus: That part of the kidney nephron associated with the passive filtration of unbound substances in plasma (see *Glomerular filtration*).
Gut: Nickname for the gastrointestinal tract.

H

Half-life: An important pharmacokinetic parameter most often used to describe the rate at which a drug is lost from the body.

Although all kinetic processes may be described by a half-life (e.g., absorption half-life, distribution half-life, and so forth), it invariably refers to a first-order process. Half-life describes the time it takes for one-half of the material to be lost from the body (or the site of dosing; absorption half-life) or the time it takes for concentration to decline by one-half. The term strictly applies when there is only one process occurring. Thus, for a drug whose disposition is described by a multicompartment model, after an IV bolus dose half-life refers to the time associated with loss in the terminal or final phase; see *Disposition half-life* and *Terminal half-life* (units, time).

Half-time: Most often used to describe rate of loss by a non–first-order process. Thus, for a saturable elimination process (e.g., ethanol), it is the time it takes for the initial amount or concentration to decline by one-half. Sometimes used to describe gastric emptying rate (gastric emptying half-time) (units, time).

Hematocrit: The volume fraction of blood that is red blood cells. The usual hematocrit (HCT) in humans is approximately 0.45.

Hepatic: Referring to the liver.

Hepatic artery: The major artery supplying blood to the liver.

Hepatic clearance: Clearance of drug by hepatic pathways (also metabolic clearance).

Hepatic first-pass effect: The presystemic elimination or first-pass effect due to hepatic metabolism. After an oral dose the drug moves through the liver via the portal circulation where it undergoes metabolism. The extent of this first-pass effect is directly dependent on the value of hepatic extraction ratio or hepatic clearance, thus, the fraction of the dose escaping this first-pass effect (assuming complete gastrointestinal absorption) is given by

$$1 - ER_{HEPATIC} = 1 - \frac{CL_{HEPATIC}}{Q_{HEPATIC}}$$

See *First-pass effect*.

Hepatoportal: Referring to the blood circulation via the portal vein that enters the liver. Drug absorbed from the gastrointestinal tract first goes to the liver via the portal vein. This movement is what gives rise to the hepatic first-pass effect.

Housekeeper wave: See *Migrating motility complex*.

Hybrid rate constant: A rate constant, usually first-order, that is dependent on other (often micro-) rate constants. For example, the rate constants associated with a two-compartment model (α and β, or λ_1 and λ_2) are hybrid rate constants as they are a function of the micro-rate constants associated with distribution and elimination (units, 1/time).

I

Indocyanine green (ICG): A diagnostic dye used to estimate liver blood flow. Any diagnostic agent used for measurement of organ blood flow must have a high organ extraction ratio or clearance.

In silico: Theoretical experiments or simulations conducted with use of a computer program and computer.

Intramuscular (IM): Route of drug administration whereby the drug is injected into a muscle. The formulation may be a solution, suspension, oil, and so forth.

Inulin: A polysaccharide used to assess glomerular filtration.

In vitro: Literally, *in glass*. It is applied to altered biologic samples studied outside the organism. For example, hepatic enzymes could be purified and studied in a test tube (i.e., *in vitro*).

In vivo: Literally, *in life* or within the living body. Clinical studies in humans are *in vivo* studies.

Intravascular administration: Administration directly into the bloodstream [e.g., intravenous (IV), intra-arterial (IA)].

Intrinsic clearance: The intrinsic or inherent clearance (CL_{int}) of a substance in the absence of any flow (i.e., blood flow delivery to the organ) restrictions. For low clearance drugs, intrinsic clearance is equal to that seen after IV bolus dosing (i.e., systemic clearance). For all drugs that undergo hepatic first-pass metabolism, apparent oral clearance (CL_O) is equal to intrinsic clearance. May be determined experimentally in a test-tube containing enzyme (units, volume/time).

Intrinsic clearance of unbound drug: The maximum hepatic drug metabolism clearance, indicative of access to enzymes and enzymatic activity; theoretically, this occurs when there is no protein binding and hepatic blood flow is nonlimiting (i.e., infinite). Also called *unbound intrinsic clearance* ($CL_{U,INT}$). This clearance is not limited to hepatic enzyme activity, as every clearing process has associated with it an intrinsic unbound clearance (e.g., renal excretion, pulmonary excretion, and so forth). This parameter is simply related to intrinsic clearance and the unbound fraction of drug in plasma: $CL_{int} = f_U \times CL_{u,int}$ or $CL_{u,int} = CL_{int}/f_U$ (units, volume/time).

Isozyme: One of several forms of an enzyme, especially cytochrome P-450. Has the same meaning as *isoform*. See *Cytochrome P-450*.

J

Jejunum: The major portion of the small intestine (following the duodenum) from which most gastrointestinal absorption occurs.

K

Ki: The enzyme inhibition constant that is used to characterize the inhibition of a substrate-enzyme interaction. This value is approximately the concentration needed to reduce the rate of metabolism by 50% (similar in concept to the Michaelis constant) (units, concentration). As an approximation only and assuming competitive inhibition, the percentage inhibition is given by:

$$\%\ \text{inhibition} = \frac{100 \cdot (I)}{(I) + k_i}$$

in which (I) is the inhibitor concentration. Thus, 50% inhibition is seen when the inhibitor is present at a concentration equal to its k_i.

K.I.S.S. principle: Keep it simple, stupid. See *Parsimony, rule of* and *Ockham's razor*.

Km (or Kmm): The Michaelis constant that is used to characterize the substrate-enzyme interaction. This value is the concentration needed to obtain one-half of the maximal rate of metabolism (V_{max}). See *Michaelis-Menten enzyme kinetics* (units, concentration).

L

Lag time: The time delay between the time of administration and the first appearance of drug in the bloodstream (T_{LAG}). This value is associated with disintegration and dissolution processes after an oral dose or the time needed for a compound to reach the small intestine and/or be absorbed into the blood (units, time).

Linearity: In pharmacokinetics, this occurs when drug concentrations, divided by dose, are superimposable. This is another statement of or a characteristic of first-order kinetics. Nonlinearity occurs when the curves are not superimposable. In a linear system, there is a direct relationship between input and output. (See *Dose-dependency* and *First-order kinetics*.)

Loading dose: An initial dose (D_L) given a patient to rapidly achieve a concentration near that to be achieved at steady-state after multiple dosing (units, mass).

M

Maintenance dose: The dose (D_M) that is given repetitively at the dosing interval. This dose (in conjunction with the fraction absorbed and clearance) determines the steady-state plasma concentration (units, mass).
Maximum plasma concentration: The maximum value of the plasma concentration-time curve (C_{MAX}). After an extravascular dose, this value is a function of dose, fraction absorbed, the rate constants of absorption and elimination, and the apparent volume of distribution. The time at which this occurs is referred to as the time of maximum concentration, T_{MAX} (units, concentration).
Metabolic clearance (or metabolite formation clearance): Clearance (CL_M) of drug by enzymatic pathways in the liver (also hepatic clearance). This process represents the formation clearance of the metabolite (units, volume/time).
Metabolism (biotransformation): The biochemical alteration of a drug. Generally metabolism is divided into phase I and phase II processes. Phase I involves some chemical alteration, usually the addition of a group that increases the water-solubility of the parent compound (e.g., hydroxylation, *N*-methylation, and so forth). The resulting compound may be less, equal, or have more activity than the parent compound. Phase II processes are referred to as conjugation reactions because the compound is conjugated with any of several species (e.g., glucuronidation, sulfation). These derivatives are always more water-soluble than the parent compound, and they are usually but not always less active than the parent compound (e.g., morphine glucuronide is more active than morphine).
Metabolite elimination clearance: The clearance of the metabolite (CL_{ME}) by any of several possible pathways (further metabolism, urinary excretion, and so forth). Most directly determined after an IV bolus dose of metabolite. It is more difficult to determine this clearance value after metabolite formation from the parent drug (units, volume/time).
Metabolite induction of metabolism: This occurs rarely when the formed metabolite from the parent drug is able to induce the further metabolism of the parent drug. An example is carbamazepine metabolism in humans.
Metabolite inhibition of metabolism: This occurs rarely when the formed metabolite from the parent drug is able to inhibit further metabolism of the parent drug. An example appears to be phenytoin metabolism in the dog.
Michaelis-Menten elimination (enzyme) kinetics: A kinetic process whose rate may become independent of concentration beyond a certain concentration, unlike first-order kinetics. Such a kinetic process is described by the following relationship (Michaelis-Menten equation):

$$\text{Rate of elimination} = \frac{V_{max} \cdot C}{k_m + C}$$

in which V_{max} is the maximum rate (velocity) of the reaction and k_m is the Michaelis constant (concentration at one-half of V_{max}; note that this is *not* a rate constant but a concentration). The relationship is approximately first-order when $C<<k_m$, and it approaches a constant, V_{max}, when $C>>k_m$. The latter situation is referred to as zero-order kinetics (rate does not depend on concentration). Michaelis-Menten kinetics is also referred to as dose-dependent, saturable, capacity-limited, nonlinear, and zero-order kinetics (the latter is not correct at all concentrations). Note the similarity in form to the equation used to define a pharmacodynamic model.
Microconstant: The first-order rate constant in a multicompartment model used to describe an irreversible movement of drug from one location to another (e.g., K_{12}, K_{21}, K_{10}) (units, 1/time).
Microvilli: Hair-like projections on the outer surface of intestinal epithelial cells. Collectively, microvilli look like the bristles of a brush; consequently, the total microvilli on an epithelial cell are termed the *brush border*.
Migrating motility complex (MMC): A band of regular contractions, migrating slowly (6 to 8 cm per minute) from the proximal stomach to the ileocecal valve. This complex only occurs in the fasting state. Each cycle lasts approximately 100 to 120 minutes and has four phases. Phase III is the most intense and is nicknamed the *housekeeper wave*, sweeping undissolved particles greater than 4 to 10 mm in diameter from the stomach into the duodenum. When an enteric-coated tablet is ingested in a fasting state, it must await the phase III housekeeper to pass into the duodenum. When an enteric-coated tablet is ingested in a fed state, it must await gastric emptying and initiation of phase III of the MMC complex before being passed into the duodenum. An enteric-coated tablet administered after a fatty meal usually takes in excess of 12 hours to pass into the duodenum. The MMC is also called the interdigestive myoelectric complex and the migrating motor complex.
Model: One thing that stands for another. A more formal definition is as follows: If the study of system A leads to an understanding of system B, then system A is a model for system B. Hence, for example, a model could be a pictorial representation of the liver, an equation for clearance or volume of distribution, a hydrodynamic analogy, and so forth. In modeling, one deliberately distorts one aspect of reality to enhance another. For example, one could distort the biophysics of the body (dividing it into two homogeneous compartments, blood and tissues), thereby permitting the easy calculation of the plasma concentration-time on multiple dosing. A model must have two properties: it must be sufficiently simple to explain a system, but, at the same time, it must adequately reflect the behavior of the system (i.e., explain the data). This is a balancing act (simplicity vs. reality). The rule of parsimony suggests that one should always select the simplest model, unless there is sufficient information to the contrary (the KISS principle; keep it simple, stupid). All models are wrong; some models are useful.
Mucosa: The inner surface of the gastrointestinal tract that consists of three layers. From the inside out, they are (a) a single layer of epithelial cells termed the *epithelium*, (b) the lamina propria, and (c) the muscularis mucosae. The epithelial cells are the primary diffusional barrier to drug absorption. The lamina propria consists primarily of connective tissue embedded with blood vessels and lymph nodes. The muscularis mucosae are responsible for gastrointestinal motility.
Multiple dosing: The process whereby a drug is given to a patient as a constant (maintenance) dose every dosing interval.

N

Nephron: The functional unit of the kidney. It consists of a glomerulus (filtering apparatus) and tubule.
Nonlinear kinetics (nonlinearity): See *Dose-dependency*.
Nonrestrictive clearance: Clearance that is not affected by plasma protein binding. Such compounds have a high organ extraction ratio (approximately ER > 0.67) and high organ clearance. Examples include diagnostic agents used to assess organ blood flow (e.g., indocyanine green for liver blood flow and p-aminohippurate for renal blood flow). The latter agents have organ ER values of 1.0. For such compounds, $CL \cong Q$ (units, volume/time).

O

Ockham's razor: After William of Ockham (b. 1280 England). *Entia non sunt multiplicanda praeter necessitate*; entities should not be multiplied unnecessarily. In other words, simpler is better.

When competing theories lead to the same result, the least complicated is preferred. The simplest most parsimonious (see *Parsimony, rule of*) explanation for a phenomenon is likely to be the correct one. When seeking to explain a phenomenon, start with the simplest theory. This is opposite a *Rube Goldberg*, in which the most complex methods are used for completing a task. The *razor* probably represents cutting out the unnecessary details. Einstein's rejoinder, *Everything should be made as simple as possible, but not simpler*.

Oral clearance: See *Apparent oral clearance*.

Order: If rate of change (e.g., metabolism, excretion, and so forth) is proportional to plasma concentration raised to a power, that power is the order. For example, if rate of metabolism is proportional to plasma concentration raised to the power of 1, the system is first-order. If rate of metabolism is proportional to plasma concentration raised to the power of zero, the system is zero order (because anything to the zero power is unity, rate of metabolism in this example is equal to a constant only and is independent of plasma concentration). One frequent goal of formulating a sustained-release product is to achieve zero-order absorption by providing a constant rate of drug release (i.e., a constant absorption rate independent of the amount of drug remaining in the formulation or in the gut).

P

Para-aminohippurate: Diagnostic agent used to assess renal blood flow. As with any such agent, it must have a high organ extraction ratio and high organ clearance.

Parameter: A variable constant (e.g., disposition half-life is a constant, although it varies day-to-day within a subject and also varies between subjects).

Parsimony, rule of: The idea, useful in modeling, that one should always choose the simplest possibility (or model) unless there is information to do otherwise. Also referred to as the K.I.S.S. principle (keep it simple, stupid). See *Ockham's razor*.

Partition coefficient: The concentration ratio of drug between two immiscible or distinct phases or entities. *In vitro*, the most common partition coefficient is the concentration ratio of drug between octanol and water. *In vivo*, the most common partition coefficient is the concentration ratio of drug between tissue and blood. The latter is primarily a reflection of drug binding to the two different tissues.

Per os (po): Latin for *by mouth*.

Percutaneous: Indicates application to the skin. Most percutaneous applications of drugs result in some transdermal absorption.

Perfusion: Usually referring to the flow of blood through a tissue or organ. Tissues are often classified with respect to perfusion: highly perfused lean tissue (e.g., kidney, liver); poorly perfused lean tissue (e.g., muscle, skin); poorly perfused fat tissue (e.g., adipose); negligibly perfused tissue (e.g., nails, hair).

Peripheral: Refers to any body location other than plasma or blood. The *peripheral* compartment in a multicompartment model is a lumping of several different tissues or fluids and does not represent a single real tissue.

Permeability coefficient: Characterization of the rate of movement of a molecule through or across a defined distance and a defined phase (e.g., cell, gut wall, and so forth). The greater the permeability coefficient (P), the more rapidly the compound traverses the membrane. This rate or velocity is often in units of cm/second. Rate of diffusion = P · (ΔC), in which ΔC is the concentration gradient.

pH partition hypothesis: The hypothesis that only undissociated (unionized) molecules can be absorbed from the gastrointestinal tract. Due to pH, weak organic acids are only undissociated (unionized) in the stomach (pH 1 to 4) and are, therefore, presumably only absorbed there. On the other hand, weak organic bases are only undissociated (unionized) at the pH of the intestine (pH 6 to 8) and are only absorbed there. The pH partition hypothesis is a useful concept, but it is incorrect when applied to the gut. However, it is true that undissociated molecules cross the gastrointestinal membrane approximately 1000 to 10,000 times faster than dissociated molecules. This hypothesis was generated in the 1950s and 1960s from scientists at the U.S. National Institutes of Health to help explain drug absorption (e.g., B.B. Brodie). All drugs, acids or bases, are best absorbed from the small intestine regardless of degree of ionization, as a consequence of the large absorbing surface area there. A further critical consideration of this concept is the fact that the pH, which increases ionization, increases dissolution rate, which may be the limiting step for absorption.

Pharmacodynamics: The study of drug responses, frequently as a function of time and/or concentration of drug or metabolite at a presumed active site (but usually in the blood). There is an aphorism that states, *pharmacokinetics is what the body does to the drug, whereas pharmacodynamics is what the drug does to the body*.

Pharmacogenetics: Heredity variations in reactions to drugs and other exogenous compounds. See also *Genetic polymorphism*.

Pharmacokinetics: The kinetics of drug absorption, distribution, metabolism, and excretion of a drug and its metabolites, oftentimes abbreviated ADME, and sometimes KADME. The study of pharmacokinetics often includes examination of the response-time relationship (i.e., pharmacodynamics). The term was coined by the German scientist Gladtke in 1953 in his book *Der Blutspiegel*.

Pharmacokinetic/pharmacodynamic model: A model that attempts to combine the pharmacokinetic (plasma concentration-time data) and pharmacodynamic (response-time data) behaviors of a drug into a single model.

Phase I (metabolism): Those metabolic or biotransformation processes that involve the chemical alteration of a molecule. The resulting molecule is often, but not always, more water-soluble. The metabolite may have less, similar, or greater pharmacologic or toxicologic activity than the parent compound.

Phase II (metabolism): Those metabolic or biotransformation processes that involve the conjugation reactions with a molecule. The resulting molecule is always more water-soluble. The metabolite is usually less active than the parent compound, but there are exceptions (e.g., morphine glucuronide).

Physiologic pharmacokinetic model (PPM) or physiologically based pharmacokinetic model (PB/PK): A pharmacokinetic model that divides the body into real compartments (tissues and organs) that are connected by real blood flows, wherein drug disposition is characterized in terms of blood flow, partitioning, and elimination from each compartment. PPMs are also referred to as physiologically based pharmacokinetic models (PB/PK). This approach has been used by physiologists, anesthesiologists, and chemical engineers. It is attractive to many because it is *real*: There are no artificial compartments that have no physiologic relevance. Furthermore, this approach permits what chemical engineers refer to as *scale-up*, the ability to scale results from a small animal to humans. The latter is attractive in drug development, toxicity, and risk assessment.

Plasma: Fluid in blood in which all material and formed elements are suspended. A plasma sample represents blood devoid of cells but which is anticoagulated so that it contains the coagulation factors. (Compare with serum.)

Plasma protein binding: See *Protein binding*.

Presystemic elimination: The loss of parent drug, usually by chemical breakdown or metabolism, before the parent drug reaching the systemic circulation. Often called the *first-pass effect*. See *First-pass effect*.

Primary pharmacokinetic parameter: Parameters that depend only on protein binding, enzymatic activity, blood flows, and partitioning, and are not dependent on other primary parameters. The most common primary pharmacokinetic parameters are volume of distribution and clearance.
Protein binding: The reversible complexation of drug with plasma proteins. The most common plasma binding proteins are albumin and α_1-acid glycoprotein. Often characterized by the equilibrium association constant (K_{ASSN}) and the unbound fraction (f_U; see *Unbound fraction*).
Proximal: Nearer or closer to some reference point. For example, the reference point of the gastrointestinal tract is the juncture of the esophagus and stomach. Therefore, the small intestine is more proximal than the large intestine. (Also see *Distal*).

R

Rate constant of elimination or disposition: See *Disposition rate constant*.
Rate-limiting step: The slowest step in any sequence of events, which controls/restricts the rate of the overall process. For example, oral absorption may be restricted/controlled (rate-limited) by dissolution, because absorption cannot occur until drug is in solution.
Reabsorption: See *Active tubular reabsorption*.
Receptor: The specific binding site of a drug, which elicits a given response. Receptors are generally believed to be proteins. Drug that binds to a receptor is referred to as substrate.
Relative bioavailability: See *Bioavailability*.
Renal: Refers to the kidney.
Renal clearance: Clearance (CL_R) of a substance from the kidney. This is the sum of clearance as a result of glomerular filtration, active tubular secretion, and active tubular reabsorption (units, volume/time).
Restrictive clearance: Usually applied to hepatic clearance that is directly proportional to unbound fraction in plasma. Protein binding is said to *restrict* clearance. (Unrestricted or nonrestrictive clearance is independent of unbound fraction of drug). Such compounds have a low clearance relative to organ blood flow (or low extraction ratio; usually ER <0.33). In general: $CL \cong f_U \times CL_{U\,INT}$ (units, volume/time).

S

Secondary pharmacokinetic parameter: Parameters that derive from two or more primary pharmacokinetic parameters. The most common secondary parameter is disposition half-life, which is dependent on volume of distribution and clearance:

$$T_{1/2} = \frac{0.693 \cdot V}{CL_S}$$

Secretion: See *Active tubular transport*.
Semilogarithmic plot: Any plot in which one axis is linear and the other is logarithmic. The most common semilog or semilogarithmic plot is log plasma concentration versus time (linear scale). Such graph paper used to be called *ratio* paper, because the distance between any two numbers in the same ratio (e.g., 5/1, 10/2, 100/20) was the same distance apart on the log scale. Also, pairs of numbers that increase or decrease by the same fraction or percentage are the same distance apart (e.g., 100 to 90; 50 to 45; 2 to 1.8; all decrease by 10% and are the same distance apart on the log scale).
Serum (blood serum): Fluid that is obtained from blood after letting the blood coagulate. Thus, this is the same as plasma except that it is devoid of coagulation factors.
S.H.A.M. parameters: The most fundamental parameters used to describe the disposition of a substance. The letters stand for *s*lope, *h*eight, *a*rea, and *m*oment. The latter measures are used to describe a plasma concentration-time profile and from which one can estimate most if not all parameters of disposition.
Steady state: Strictly speaking, steady state exists when rate of input into a system is exactly equal to rate of output from the system; under these conditions, the amount or concentration of drug in the system is constant. In pharmacokinetics, a looser interpretation is applied. Pharmacokinetic steady state exists when a plasma concentration-time pattern repeats itself continuously, as for example when a drug is administered at a constant dose over a constant interval and ceases to accumulate any further. This is actually a fluctuating steady state. Steady state concentration is always expressed as rate in/rate out. In terms of drug dosing, rate in is the dose rate and rate out is clearance. For endogenous compounds, rate in is actually a production rate and rate out is clearance.
Subcutaneous: Underneath the skin (especially, subcutaneous injection, SC).
Sustained-release (SR): Denotes relatively slow release and absorption of a drug from a dosage form relative to a conventional dosage form. Most forms of *extended* release and *controlled* release products are essentially SR products.
Systemic: Referring to a central region; in pharmacokinetics, once a drug molecule has reached the heart, it is systemically available to the body.

T

Terminal rate constant or slope: Along with disposition rate constant or slope, perhaps the best term to apply to the description of the data that appear in the terminal log-linear phase of a semilog plot of plasma concentration versus time. This terminal or last slope from which a rate constant (and half-life) is derived represents the slowest process in a sequence of events. As with the term *disposition*, the word *terminal* does not permit confusion with *elimination* (units, 1/time).
Time invariance: An idea used extensively by engineers to indicate that a given system is invariant or unchanging with time. In completely defining a linear system, the properties of superposition and time invariance should strictly apply. The former is discussed under *Dose-dependency*. Some systems may be nonlinear by virtue of violating the idea of time invariance. For example, a circadian rhythm that changes drug behavior with time; metabolite inhibition of elimination causes a different behavior of parent compound with time and may provide concentration-time profiles that are log-linear or first-order (they are not superimposable, however).
Time of (occurrence) maximum plasma concentration: The time at which the maximum plasma concentration is achieved (see *Maximum plasma concentration*). This value, T_{MAX}, is a function of the rate constants of absorption and elimination and is often used to assess the rate of absorption of a drug in a bioequivalence study (units, time).
Topical: Pertaining to a particular area. In common usage, this almost always refers to a relevant portion of skin.
Total body (or systemic) clearance: Clearance of a substance from the body by all possible routes of elimination ($TBC = CL_S = CL_{RENAL} + CL_{HEPATIC} + CL_{OTHER}$). Calculated as

$$CL_S = \frac{\text{IV dose}}{AUC_0^\infty} \quad \text{or as} \quad CL_S = \frac{F \cdot \text{dose}}{AUC_0^\infty}$$

Toxicokinetics: The application of pharmacokinetics to the understanding and interpretation of toxicity studies.
Transdermal: Through the skin. Percutaneous indicates application to the skin. Most percutaneous applications of drugs result in some transdermal absorption.

Tubular reabsorption: See *Active tubular reabsorption.*
Tubular secretion: See *Active tubular transport.*

U

Unbound fraction: The unbound or free fraction of drug in the plasma (f_U), which is the ratio of unbound or free concentration to the total (i.e., unbound plus bound) concentration. For most drugs, this fraction is constant and independent of plasma drug concentration.
Unbound intrinsic clearance: See *Intrinsic clearance of unbound drug.*
Unbound volume of distribution: The apparent volume of distribution corrected for plasma protein binding, $V_{unbound} = V/f_U$.

V

Volume of distribution (apparent volume of distribution): A primary pharmacokinetic parameter reflecting the reversible uptake of drug by tissues from the blood. The fictitious space or volume that a drug appears to occupy in the body relative to the concentration of drug in the blood. Volume of distribution is the imaginary volume the drug occupies if it is present throughout the body in the same concentration as plasma. Because the reference fluid is always blood, the larger the volume of distribution, the more drug is in tissue relative to plasma. Volume of distribution has units of volume, but is commonly normalized to body weight, as, for example, liters/kg or V/m^2. Volume of distribution multiplied by plasma concentration equals the amount of drug in the body (but with some limitations). This parameter may, therefore, exceed the real volume of the body. There are numerous apparent volumes used in pharmacokinetics, including $V_{extrapolated}$, V_β or V_{AREA}, V_C or V_1, V_P or V_2, V_{SS}. The apparent volume serves two purposes: gives an indication of the magnitude of distribution or movement out of the blood and into tissues (the greater the apparent volume, the less drug is in the blood and more is in tissues); acts as a proportionality constant between the amount of drug in the body and the concentration in the blood.

Z

Zero-order: A rate is zero-order when it is constant, independent of concentration or amount. See *Order.*

CHAPTER 80

Role of the Laboratory in the Diagnosis and Management of Poisoning

Robert J. Flanagan

Analytical toxicology is concerned with the detection, identification, and measurement of drugs and other foreign compounds (xenobiotics) and their metabolites in biologic and related specimens. The analytical toxicologist can play a useful role in the diagnosis and management of poisoning, but to do so, he or she should have a basic knowledge of emergency medicine and intensive care and must be able to communicate effectively with physicians. In addition, a good understanding of clinical chemistry, pharmacology, and toxicology is desirable. The analyst's dealings with a case of suspected poisoning are usually divided into preanalytical, analytical, and post-analytical phases (Table 1).

Many acutely poisoned patients are treated successfully without any contribution from the laboratory other than routine clinical laboratory tests. The analytical toxicologist can only contribute to diagnosis and management if a physician, pathologist, or other person first suspects poisoning. Close collaboration between the analyst and the physician is then important if anything other than the simplest of analyses is to be useful. Many requests for emergency analytical toxicologic investigations are, in fact, requests for advice on the diagnosis or management of poisoning and are best handled by staff of a poisons information service, at least in the first instance.

Toxicologic analyses can play a useful role if the diagnosis of poisoning or the nature of any poison(s) present is in doubt, the administration of antidotes or protective agents is contemplated, or the use of active elimination therapy is being considered. All relevant information about a particular patient should be communicated to the analyst and appropriate specimens must be collected and properly labeled. Information to enable the analyst to assign the appropriate priority to the analysis in such cases is especially vital because, in general, specific therapy is only started when the nature and the amount of the poison(s) involved are known. At the least, a request form should be completed to accompany the specimens to the laboratory.

TABLE 1. Steps in undertaking an analytical toxicologic investigation

Preanalytical	Obtain details of current (suspected) poisoning episode, including any circumstantial evidence of poisoning, and the results of biochemical and hematologic investigations, if any. Also obtain the patient's medical and occupational history, if available, and ensure access to the appropriate samples. Decide the priorities for the analysis.
Analytical	Perform the agreed analysis.
Postanalytical	Interpret the results in discussion with the physician looking after the patient. Perform additional analyses, if indicated, using either the original samples or further samples from the patient. Save any unused or residual samples in case they are required for additional tests.

TABLE 2. Sample requirements for general analytical toxicology

Sample	Notes[a]
Whole blood	10 ml (lithium heparin or EDTA tube—use fluoride/oxalate if ethanol suspected; plastic tube if paraquat suspected; glass or plastic tube with minimal headspace if carbon monoxide or other volatiles suspected).
Plasma/serum	5 ml (send whole blood if volatiles, metals, and some other compounds suspected).
Urine[b]	20–50 ml (plain bottle, no preservative[c]).
Gastric contents[d]	25–50 ml (plain bottle, no preservative).
Scene residues[e]	As appropriate.
Other samples	Vitreous humor, bile, or liver (approximately 5 g) can substitute for urine in postmortem work. Other tissues (brain, liver, kidney, lung, subcutaneous fat—5 g) may also be valuable, especially if organic solvents or other volatile poisons are suspected.

EDTA, ethylenediaminetetraacetic acid.
[a]Smaller volumes may often be acceptable; for example, in the case of children.
[b]All that is normally required for drugs of abuse screening.
[c]Sodium fluoride (1% w/v) should be added if ethanol is suspected and blood is not available.
[d]Includes vomit, gastric lavage (stomach washout) (first sample), and so forth.
[e]Tablet bottles, drinks containers, aerosol canisters, and so forth—pack entirely separately from biologic samples, especially if poisoning with volatiles is a possibility.

TABLE 3. Sample requirements for some metals/trace elements analysis

Element	Sample requirements
Aluminum	10 ml whole blood in plastic (not glass) tube—no anticoagulant/separating beads[a] 20 ml dialysate/supply water in plastic bottle rinsed several times with portions of the intended sample[a]
Antimony	5 ml heparinized whole blood 20 ml urine
Arsenic[b]	5 ml heparinized whole blood 20 ml urine
Bismuth	5 ml heparinized whole blood
Cadmium	2 ml EDTA whole blood[a] 10 ml urine[a]
Chromium	2 ml heparinized whole blood[a,c] 20 ml urine (hard plastic bottle)[a]
Copper	2 ml heparinized or clotted whole blood, or 1 ml plasma/serum 10 ml urine
Iron	5 ml clotted blood or 2 ml serum (no hemolysis) 10 ml urine
Lead	2 ml EDTA whole blood (no clots)
Lithium	5 ml clotted blood or 2 ml serum (*not* lithium heparin tube)
Manganese	1 ml heparinized whole blood or 0.5 ml plasma[a,c]
Mercury	5 ml heparinized whole blood[d] 20 ml urine (hard plastic bottle)[d]
Selenium	2 ml heparinized whole blood or 1 ml plasma/serum
Silver	2 ml heparinized whole blood or 1 ml plasma 10 ml urine
Strontium	2 ml heparinized whole blood or 1 ml plasma
Thallium	5 ml heparinized whole blood 20 ml urine
Zinc	2 ml whole blood (heparinized or clotted but *not* EDTA) or 1 ml plasma/serum

EDTA, ethylenediaminetetraacetic acid.
[a]Send unused sample container from the same batch as used for sample collection to check for possible contamination.
[b]To diagnose chronic poisoning exclude seafood (shell fish and so forth) from diet for 15 days before sample collection.
[c]Use of a plastic cannula to collect blood is advisable.
[d]Send samples promptly to avoid loss of mercury on storage.

SPECIMEN COLLECTION, TRANSPORT, AND STORAGE

Sample requirements for general analytical toxicology are summarized in Table 2. If possible, all biologic specimens should be analyzed immediately or stored at 4°C before analysis. If the amount of sample that can be collected is limited (e.g., a young child is under study), then contact the laboratory beforehand. Special precautions are needed when collecting samples for the analysis of trace elements and toxic metals (Table 3). In such cases, it is prudent to send an empty container from the same batch as that used to collect the sample to test for possible contamination from the container. Contamination with metals can arise from unusual sources. Contamination of blood with chromium and manganese, for example, can occur from an indwelling stainless steel cannula.

Analytical results concerning any specimen submitted for toxicologic investigation may end up under scrutiny in court. It is thus important that all such specimens are clearly labeled with the patient's family or last name and any forenames, the date and time of collection, and the nature of the specimen if this is not self-evident. Hospital and casualty numbers should also be recorded. Attention to these details is especially important if large numbers of patients have been involved in a particular incident, or if a number of specimens have been obtained from one patient. Further problems may arise if one or more blood samples have been centrifuged and the plasma separated in a local laboratory and the original containers discarded.

Sending Samples by Post

In many countries, strict rules govern the transport and storage of biologic specimens. Details should be obtainable from a local hospital laboratory. Specimens should always be stored in labeled biohazard polythene bags. Letters and request forms should be placed in a pouch attached to the bag. Specimens sent by post (first class letter post or Datapost only in the United Kingdom) or courier should be dispatched in post office–approved containers. The polythene bags containing the samples should be sandwiched in the box between absorbent packaging. The lid of the box should be secured with adhesive tape and the package clearly labeled with its destination, its origin, and an indication of its contents (e.g., *pathologic specimen*).

The associated documentation must give full details of any special risk associated with a specimen (hepatitis B, human immunodeficiency virus, and so forth). In the case of human immunodeficiency virus–risk specimens, the specimen container and the request form must all be marked with a *danger of infection* sticker and an indication that the specimen carries an *inoculation risk*. Before dispatch of the specimen, the receiving laboratory must be informed by telephone of the risk, the patient's name, and the investigation required. Records must be kept of all specimens sent by post, taxi, or courier. The minimum information should include type of specimen, destination, and date sent. Additional information to identify specific specimens could be patient's name, laboratory number, name of person packing the sample, request, taxi firm used, and driver's name.

Chain-of-Custody Procedures

If it is clear from the outset that the analyses have medicolegal implications, then strict chain-of-custody procedures should be implemented. The physician or nurse taking the sample should seal the sample with a tamper-proof device and sign and date the seal. A chain-of-custody form should also accompany the specimen. Each person taking possession of the sample should sign and date the form when he or she takes possession. The sample should be secured in a locked container or refrigerator if left unattended before arrival at the laboratory.

After the Analysis

Residues of samples and any unused samples should be saved at 4°C for 4 to 6 weeks in case further analyses are required. In view of the medicolegal implications of some cases, then any specimen remaining should be kept at –20°C or below until investigation of the incident is concluded. This can take several years.

Urine

Urine is useful for *screening* because it is sometimes available in large volumes and usually contains higher concentrations of drugs and some other poisons than blood. The presence of metabolites may sometimes assist identification if chromatographic techniques are used. A 50-ml specimen from an adult, collected into a sealed, sterile container, is sufficient for most purposes. No preservative should be added (e.g., use of Thiomersal (merthiolate) preservative invalidates a urine mercury measurement). The sample should be obtained as soon as possible after admission, ideally before any drug therapy is initiated. Samples taken soon after ingestion, however, may not contain detectable amounts of poison. A further complication is that drugs with anticholinergic activity, such as tricyclic antidepressants, cause urinary retention and, thus, there may be delay in obtaining a specimen, especially if the patient remains conscious or is in shock. Conversely, little poison may remain in specimens taken many hours or days later, though the patient may be ill, as in acute paracetamol (acetaminophen) or paraquat poisoning. If the specimen is obtained by catheterization, there is a possibility of contamination with lignocaine (lidocaine) gel.

Stomach Contents

Stomach contents include vomit, gastric aspirate, and gastric lavage fluid (stomach washings). It is important to obtain the first sample of lavage fluid because later samples may be dilute. At least 20 ml (plain bottle, no preservative) should be collected. This sample can be variable in composition, and additional procedures, such as homogenization followed by filtration and centrifugation, may be required to produce a fluid amenable to analysis. It is the best sample on which to perform certain tests, however, although clearly of little use if the poison has been inhaled or injected. If obtained soon after ingestion, large amounts of poison may be present whereas metabolites, which may complicate some tests, are usually absent. It may be possible to identify tablets or capsules simply by inspection. Emetine from syrup of ipecacuanha may be present, although the use of this mixture is no longer recommended, especially in children.

Scene Residues

It is important that all powders, tablets, bottles, syringes, aerosol, or other containers found with or near the patient (*scene residues*) are retained because they may be related to the poisoning episode. It is usually best to analyze biologic specimens. An exception is one in which topical exposure is suspected because systemic absorption may be undetectable. There is always the possibility that the original contents of containers such as drink bottles have been discarded and replaced either with innocuous material or with more noxious ingredients such as acid, bleach, or pesticides. Care should be taken to assure that containers of volatile materials such as aerosols and organic solvents are packaged entirely separately from biologic specimens to prevent cross-contamination. Indeed, it is best to pack all scene residues entirely separately from biologic samples because the possibility of contamination could be suggested in any future legal proceedings. If police have attended an incident, scene residues may have been removed for forensic analysis.

Blood

Blood plasma or serum is normally used for quantitative assays, but some poisons are best measured in whole blood. A 10-ml sample in a glass or clear hard plastic (polycarbonate) tube containing heparin (or heparinized beads) or sodium ethylenediaminetetraacetic acid (EDTA) should be taken. EDTA is preferred for aminoglycoside antibiotics, carboxyhemoglobin, and for lead and some other metals (Table 3). A fluoride/oxalate tube should be used if ethanol, cocaine, nitrazepam, or clonazepam are suspected. Note that the tubes of this type available commercially contain approximately 0.1% (w/v) fluoride, whereas approximately 1% (w/v) fluoride (40 mg sodium fluoride/2 ml blood) is needed to fully inhibit microbial action in such specimens (1).

The use of disinfectant swabs containing alcohols (ethanol, 2-propanol) before venipuncture should be avoided, as should heparin, which contains phenolic preservatives (chlorbutol, cresol). Use a blood collection site remote from any infusion site. The sample should be dispensed with care: the vigorous discharge of blood through a syringe needle can cause sufficient hemolysis to invalidate a serum iron (or potassium) assay. Do not use a lithium heparin tube if lithium is to be measured. Use plastic tubes if paraquat is to be measured and, ideally, glass if volatiles are suspected.

Use of evacuated blood collection tubes and tubes containing gel separators or soft rubber stoppers are not recommended if a toxicologic analysis is to be performed on the specimen. These tubes may contain phosphate and phthalate plasticizers, which not only interfere in chromatographic methods, but tris(2-butoxyethyl)phosphate can also cause release of many basic drugs from binding sites on α_1-acid glycoprotein. The released drug is then free to diffuse into red blood cells, thereby lowering the plasma concentration (2). Some other compounds present in gel separators dissolve in blood and can thereby affect the solvent extraction characteristics of certain drugs (3). Relatively high concentrations (20 mg/L or more) of ethylbenzene and the xylenes have been detected in blood collected into Sarstedt Monovette serum gel tubes (4).

In general, no significant differences exist in the concentrations of poisons between plasma and serum. However, if a compound is not present to any extent within erythrocytes, then using lysed whole blood results in considerable dilution of the specimen. On the other hand, some poisons such as carbon monoxide, cyanide, and lead are found primarily in erythrocytes and thus whole blood is needed for such measurements. A heparinized or EDTA whole blood sample gives either whole blood or plasma as appropriate. The space above the blood in the tube (*headspace*) should be minimized if carbon monoxide or other volatile poisons are suspected.

Hair

In some circumstances the analysis of hair can provide a record of exposure to a poison and confirm poisoning. However, hair analysis and its interpretation are difficult. For a poison to appear in hair closest to the scalp takes 4 to 7 days. Hair grows at a rate of approximately 1 cm/month. Hair treatment such as bleaching may destroy adsorbed drug, whereas hair-coloring agents may add toxic metals such as lead. A chemical or drug in the air can contaminate hair. Aspects of the collection and analysis of hair specimens from the point of view of testing for drugs of abuse have been reviewed (5).

Breath

Provided absorption is complete, the exhaled air concentration of a volatile compound such as ethanol is related to its blood concentration. Simple electrochemical devices to measure breath ethanol have been available for many years and have proved useful in assessing ethanol intoxication in trauma victims (6). A further simple device is available to measure breath carbon monoxide (hence carboxyhemoglobin) to rapidly diagnose carbon monoxide poisoning and monitor treatment. Ethanol interference can be eliminated by use of a carbon filter (7). Respiratory mass spectrometry has also been developed to assess exposure to other volatiles such as organic solvents but currently is impractical for clinical use.

Other Biologic Specimens

A simple dipstick test for salivary ethanol based on alcohol dehydrogenase has been used but has been largely superseded by breath measuring devices. Apart from this, there has been some interest in measuring salivary concentrations of drugs given in therapy, particularly in children, but in practice such analyses are rare, a major problem being the lack of homogeneity of the sample. Other specimens (sweat, tears, nasal secretions, breast milk, cord blood, meconium, fat biopsy, tissue biopsy, and so forth) may be useful in the context of a particular case.

Postmortem Tissue

Tissue samples may be valuable in the investigation of poisoning fatalities. Vitreous humor is a useful substitute for urine if the bladder is empty and can be used to measure potassium and glucose. Tissue specimens may be especially valuable if death was due to the inhalation of lipophilic compounds, such as many organic solvents, because blood concentrations may be low. Liver, kidney, lung, brain, and subcutaneous fat are the most useful specimens.

PHYSICAL EXAMINATION OF THE SPECIMEN

Physical examination of the specimen may yield valuable diagnostic information. However, appropriate toxicologic investigations are usually needed to confirm such findings.

Urine

High concentrations of some drugs or metabolites can impart characteristic colors to urine (Table 4). Strong-smelling poisons such as camphor, ethchlorvynol, and methyl salicylate (oil of wintergreen) can sometimes be recognized in urine because they are excreted in part unchanged. Acetone may arise from metabolism of 2-propanol (isopropanol), as well as from ingestion/inhalation of acetone or from disordered carbohydrate metabolism. Turbid urine may be due to underlying pathology (blood microorganisms, casts, epithelial cells), or to carbonates, phosphates, or urates in amorphous or microcrystalline forms. Such findings should not be ignored though they may not be related to a poisoning episode. Chronic therapy with sulfonamides may give rise to yellow or green/brown crystals in neutral or alkaline urine. Primidone, sulthiame, and, possibly, phenytoin may form crystals in urine after overdosage, whereas calcium oxalate forms characteristic colorless crystals at neutral pH after ingestion of ethylene glycol (Chapter 192) or of soluble oxalates.

TABLE 4. Some possible causes of colored urine

Color	Possible cause
Yellow/brown	Bilirubin, hemoglobin, myoglobin, porphyrins, urobilin Anthrone derivatives (e.g., from aloin, aloe, cascara, senna, rhubarb, and so forth),[a] bromsulphthalein,[a] carotenes, chloroquine, congo red,[a] cresol, flavins (yellow/green fluorescence), fluorescein, mepacrine, methocarbamol (on standing), methyldopa (on standing), nitrobenzene, nitrofurantoin, pamaquine, phenolphthalein[a], primaquine, quinine, santonin[a]
Red/brown	Bilirubin, hemoglobin, myoglobin, porphyrins, urobilin Aminophenazone, anisindione,[a] anthrone derivatives,[a] bromsulphthalein,[a] cinchophen, congo red,[a] cresol, deferoxamine,[b] ethoxazene, furazolidone, furazolium, levodopa (black on standing), methocarbamol, methyldopa, niridazole, nitrobenzene, nitrofurantoin, phenacetin, phenazopyridine, phenindione,[a] phenolphthalein,[a] phenothiazines, phensuximide, phenytoin, pyrogallol, rifampicin, salazosulphapyridine, santonin,[a] sulphamethoxazole, warfarin
Blue/green	Bile, biliverdin, indican (on standing) Acriflavine (green fluorescence), amitriptyline, azuresin, copper salts, indigo carmine, indomethacin, methylene blue (methylthioinium chloride),[b] nitrofural, phenylsalicylate, resorcinol, toluidine blue,[b] triamterene (blue fluorescence)
Black	Blood (on standing), homogentisic acid, indican (on standing), porphobilin Cascara (on standing), levodopa (on standing), phenols, pyrogallol, resorcinol, thymol

[a]pH dependent.
[b]Usually used to treat poisoning.
From Lentner C, ed. *Geigy scientific tables. Vol. 1. Units of measurement, body fluids, composition of the body, nutrition.* Basle: Ciba-Geigy, 1981:54, with permission.

Stomach Contents and Scene Residues

Characteristic smells may indicate a variety of substances (Table 5). Many other compounds (e.g., ethchlorvynol, methyl salicylate, paraldehyde, phenelzine) also have distinctive smells. Extremes of pH may indicate ingestion of acids or alkali, whereas a green-blue color suggests the presence of iron or copper salts. Examination using a polarizing microscope may reveal tablet or capsule debris. Starch granules used as *filler* in some tablets or capsules may be identified by microscopy using crossed polarizing filters. They appear as bright grains marked with a dark Maltese cross. Undegraded tablets or capsules, and any plant remains or specimens of plants thought to have been ingested, should be examined separately. The local poison center or pharmacy normally has access to publications or other aids for identification.

Blood

Chocolate-brown venous blood suggests methemoglobinemia from exposure to strong oxidizing agents such as nitrites. Cherry-pink blood suggests carbon monoxide poisoning. Pink-brown colored plasma from a carefully collected sample suggests hemol-

TABLE 5. Smells associated with particular poisons[a]

Smell	Possible cause
Almonds	Cyanide
Cloves	Oil of cloves
Fruity	Alcohols (including ethanol), esters
Garlic	Arsenic, phosphine
Mothballs	Camphor
Nail polish remover	Acetone, butanone
Pears	Chloral
Petrol	Petroleum distillates (may be vehicle in pesticide formulation)
Phenolic	Disinfectants, cresols, phenols
Shoe polish	Nitrobenzene
Stale tobacco	Nicotine
Sweet	Chloroform and other halogenated hydrocarbons

[a]CARE, specimens containing cyanides may give off hydrogen cyanide gas (prussic acid), especially if acidified—stomach contents are often acidic. Not everyone can detect hydrogen cyanide by smell. Similarly, phosphides evolve phosphine, and sulfides evolve hydrogen sulfide—the ability to detect hydrogen sulfide (rotten egg smell) is lost at higher concentrations.

ysis and, thus, possible poisoning with compounds such as arsine, chlorates, or dapsone. Orange plasma has been described after ingestion of canthaxanthin as a sun-tanning aid (8,9).

CLINICAL LABORATORY TESTS AND THE POISONED PATIENT

Many routine clinical laboratory tests are helpful in the diagnosis of poisoning and in assessing prognosis. Still more specialized tests may be appropriate depending on the patient's clinical condition, the circumstantial evidence of poisoning and the past medical history, although only larger laboratories may be able to offer all of the tests discussed later on an emergency basis. Tests used in monitoring supportive treatment are not considered here. For further information, see Watson and Proudfoot (10).

Blood Glucose

Marked hypoglycemia often results from overdosage with insulin, sulfonylureas such as tolbutamide, or other antidiabetic drugs. Hypoglycemia may also follow ingestion of salicylates such as aspirin, ethanol (especially in children or fasting adults), and beta-receptor blocking drugs and may also complicate severe poisoning due to a number of hepatotoxic agents, including acetaminophen, chlorinated hydrocarbons such as carbon tetrachloride, isoniazid, phenylbutazone, iron salts, and certain fungi. Hypoglycin is a potent hypoglycemic agent found in unripe akee fruit and is responsible for Jamaican vomiting sickness. Hyperglycemia is a less common complication of poisoning than hypoglycemia but has been reported after poisoning with a variety of compounds (Table 6).

Plasma Electrolytes

Electrolyte disturbances may be simple to monitor and to interpret but are often complex. The correct interpretation of serial measurements requires a detailed knowledge of the therapy administered. Poisons associated with abnormal potassium concentration are shown in Table 7. Hyperkalemia is addressed in Chapter 35. Hypokalemia and metabolic acidosis are features of theophylline and salbutamol overdose. Hypokalemia and metabolic *alkalosis* can be caused by chronic abuse of laxatives

TABLE 6. Poisons reported to cause hyperglycemia

Acetone	Nalidixic acid
Adrenaline	Nifedipine
Aspirin and other salicylates	Phenylbutazone
Cadmium chloride	Phenylpropanolamine
Caffeine	2-Propanol
Clonidine	Salbutamol
Cyanide ion	Sodium azide
Hemlock water dropwort (*Oenanthe crocata*)	Terbutaline
Iron salts	Theophylline
Isoniazid	Verapamil
Methanol	Yew (*Taxus baccata*) leaves
	Zinc chloride

or sodium bicarbonate (12). Hyponatremia can result from many causes, including water intoxication (11), inappropriate loss of sodium, or impaired excretion of water by the kidney. Hypocalcemia can occur after ingestion of ethylene glycol or oxalates, such as oxalic acid, due to sequestration of calcium. Hypocalcemia may also occur as a result of acute poisoning with fluorides.

Plasma Osmolality

Plasma osmolality and the concept of osmolal gap are addressed in Chapter 25. Although the measurement of plasma osmolality and calculation of the osmolal gap (measured osmolality–calculated osmolality) may give useful information, interpretation can be difficult. It is vital, therefore, that toxicologic analyses are performed to confirm any provisional diagnosis. For example, there may be secondary dehydration, as in salicylate poisoning; ethanol may have been taken together with a more toxic, osmotically active substance; or enteral or parenteral therapy may have involved the administration of large amounts of sugar alcohols (mannitol, sorbitol) or formulations containing glycerol or 1,2-propanediol. Note also that a normal plasma osmolality does not exclude severe poisoning with ethylene glycol or methanol.

Plasma Enzyme Activity

Shock, coma, or convulsions are often associated with nonspecific increases in the plasma or serum activities of aspartate aminotransferase and alanine aminotransferase, primarily of hepatic origin, and of lactate dehydrogenase, primarily from heart muscle. Usually the activities increase over a period of a few days and slowly return to normal. Not surprisingly, changes

TABLE 7. Poisons reported to alter plasma potassium concentrations

Hyperkalemia	Hypokalemia	
Atenolol	Barium salts	Oxpentifylline
Cardiac glycosides	Caffeine	Quinine
Disopyramide	Chloroquine	Salbutamol
Fluoride ion	Disopyramide	Sodium bicarbonate
Ibuprofen	Diuretics	Sotalol
Opioids	Insulin	Terbutaline
Oxprenolol	Laxatives	Theophylline
Potassium chloride	Magnesium sulfate	Toluene
Potassium-sparing diuretics	Nalidixic acid	Yew (*Taxus baccata*) leaves
	Nifedipine	

of this nature are of little diagnostic or prognostic value except in the context of poisoning with specific hepato- or myotoxins. Plasma aspartate aminotransferase and alanine aminotransferase activities, for example, may increase rapidly after absorption of toxic doses of hepatotoxins such as paracetamol, carbon tetrachloride, 1,2-dichloropropane (propylene dichloride), and copper salts. It may take several weeks for values to return to normal. Plasma aspartate aminotransferase and alanine aminotransferase activities may also be raised in patients on chronic therapy with drugs such as sodium valproate. Chronic ethanol abuse is usually associated with increased plasma carbohydrate-deficient transferrin and γ-glutamyltransferase activity.

In severe poisoning, especially if a prolonged period of coma, convulsions, hypothermia, or shock has occurred, there is likely to be clinical or subclinical muscle injury associated with rhabdomyolysis and disseminated intravascular coagulation (DIC). Such damage may also occur as a result of chronic parenteral abuse of psychotropic drugs. Frank rhabdomyolysis is characterized by high serum aldolase or creatine phosphokinase activities together with myoglobinuria. This can be detected by test strips, provided there is no hematuria. In serious poisoning, for example with theophylline or with strychnine, or after a prolonged period of convulsions, high serum or plasma potassium, uric acid, and phosphate concentrations may indicate the onset of myoglobinuria and of acute renal failure.

Cholinesterase Activity

Systemic toxicity from carbamate and organophosphorus insecticides is due largely to inhibition of acetylcholinesterase (acetylcholine acetylhydrolase, EC 3.1.1.7) in nerve synapses. Cholinesterase (acylcholine acylhydrolase, EC 3.1.1.8), derived initially from the liver, is also present in plasma, but inhibition of plasma cholinesterase is not thought to be physiologically important. Cholinesterase and acetylcholinesterase are different enzymes: Plasma cholinesterase may be almost completely inhibited, whereas acetylcholinesterase itself may still possess 50% activity. This relative inhibition varies between different compounds and with the route of absorption; with interindividual differences; as well as whether exposure has been acute, chronic, or acute-on-chronic. In addition, individual carbamates and organophosphates differ in the rate at which (acetyl)cholinesterase inhibition is reversed after acute exposure.

In practice, plasma cholinesterase is a useful indicator of exposure to organophosphorus compounds or carbamates, and a normal plasma cholinesterase activity effectively excludes serious poisoning by these compounds. The difficulty lies in deciding whether a low activity is indeed due to poisoning or to some other physiologic, pharmacologic, or genetic cause. The diagnosis can sometimes be assisted by detecting a poison or metabolite in a body fluid. Alternatively, pralidoxime, used as an antidote in poisoning with organophosphorus insecticides, may be added to a second portion of the sample *at an appropriate concentration and the cholinesterase assay repeated*. If the inhibition of cholinesterase activity is reversed by pralidoxime, this obviously suggests the presence of a cholinesterase inhibitor in the sample.

Red blood cell acetylcholinesterase activity can be measured, but this enzyme is membrane-bound, and the apparent activity depends on the methods used in solubilization and separation from residual plasma cholinesterase. Alternatively, quinidine sulfate can be added to inhibit plasma cholinesterase while red blood cell acetylcholinesterase is being measured (13). Red blood cell acetylcholinesterase activity also depends on the rate of erythropoiesis. Newly formed erythrocytes have a high activity, which diminishes with time. Hence, red blood cell acetylcholinesterase activity is a function of the number and age of the cell population. However, if the activities of plasma cholinesterase and red blood cell acetylcholinesterase are low, the likelihood of poisoning due to either organophosphorus compounds or carbamates is strong.

Zinc Protoporphyrin

Lead inhibits ferrochelatase, the enzyme that catalyzes the incorporation of ferrous iron into protoporphyrin IX to form heme. Excessive exposure to lead thus results in an increase in the concentration of protoporphyrin (which is complexed with zinc) in newly formed erythrocytes. Blood zinc protoporphyrin (ZPP) concentrations in unexposed individuals are usually less than 2 μg/g hemoglobin. In the absence of iron-deficiency anemia, which also increases ZPP, blood lead concentrations in the range 350 to 450 μg/L in males (250 to 350 μg/L in females) are associated with increased ZPP concentrations. A blood ZPP concentration of 7 μg/g hemoglobin equates to a blood lead concentration of approximately 500 μg/L if lead exposure is constant. The increase in ZPP is not immediate in newly exposed individuals because it depends on the rate of formation of erythrocytes; the lag period may be up to 2 months in duration. On the other hand, if exposure ceases, blood ZPP may remain elevated for a year or more. This test is used in conjunction with measurement of blood lead concentrations (14).

Ceruloplasmin

Ceruloplasmin is a blue glycoprotein that contains 6 to 8 copper atoms per molecule. Plasma ceruloplasmin normally carries some 95% of the copper in the blood. Normal plasma ceruloplasmin concentrations are 0.2 to 0.4 g/L. In Wilson's disease, plasma ceruloplasmin is less than 0.25 g/L; patients with this disease may have plasma copper concentrations that are 50% of normal, but liver and urine copper concentrations may be greatly elevated.

Blood Clotting

Prolongation of the prothrombin time (normally expressed as a ratio to a control) is a valuable early indicator of hepatic damage in poisoning with compounds such as acetaminophen; chlorinated hydrocarbons (e.g., carbon tetrachloride); isoniazid; iron salts; phenylbutazone and certain fungi, notably *Amanita phalloides*. The prothrombin time and other measures of blood clotting are likely to be abnormal in acute poisoning with rodenticides such as warfarin and related compounds, and after overdosage with heparin or other anticoagulants. Coagulopathies may also occur as a side effect of antibiotic therapy. The occurrence of DIC together with rhabdomyolysis in severe poisoning (prolonged coma, convulsions, shock) has been discussed. DIC occurs commonly after bites from poisonous snakes and has been reported in severe poisoning with monoamine oxidase inhibitors, phencyclidine, and amphetamines and related stimulants.

Carboxyhemoglobin and Methemoglobin

Blood carboxyhemoglobin measurements can be used to assess the severity of acute carbon monoxide poisoning and to monitor exposure to this compound. Blood carboxyhemoglobin measurements are also useful in monitoring methylene chloride exposure because it is metabolized to carbon monoxide (15). However, carboxyhemoglobin is dissociated rapidly once the patient is removed from the contaminated atmosphere, and, thus, the sample should be obtained as soon as possible after admis-

TABLE 8. Blood carboxyhemoglobin saturation and clinical features of toxicity

Carboxyhemoglobin saturation (%)	Clinical features
<1	Endogenous carbon monoxide production
3–8	Cigarette smokers
<15	Heavy (30–50 cigarettes/d) smokers
>20	Headache, weakness, dizziness, impaired vision, syncope, nausea, vomiting, diarrhea (patients with heart disease are at special risk)
>50	Coma, convulsions, bradycardia, hypotension, respiratory depression, death

sion. Even then, blood carboxyhemoglobin correlates poorly with clinical features of toxicity (Table 8).

Methemoglobin (oxidized hemoglobin) may be formed after ingestion of dapsone, phenacetin, and strong oxidizing agents such as chlorates, nitrates, and nitrites [including aliphatic nitrites such as isobutyl and isopentyl (amyl) nitrites (16)]. Methemoglobinemia can also be induced by exposure to aniline and to aromatic nitro-compounds such as nitrobenzene and some of its derivatives. Methemoglobinemia may be indicated by the presence of dark chocolate–colored blood. Blood methemoglobin can be measured but is unstable, and the use of stored samples is thus unreliable.

Hematocrit

Acute or acute-on-chronic poisoning with ethanol, iron salts, indomethacin, salicylates, and other nonsteroidal anti-inflammatory drugs can cause gastrointestinal bleeding leading to anemia. Anemia may also result from chronic exposure to compounds that interfere with heme synthesis, such as lead, or that induce hemolysis either directly (arsine, stibine, mercurials) or indirectly because of glucose 6 phosphate dehydrogenase deficiency (chloroquine, primaquine, chloramphenicol, niridazole, nitrofurantoin). Hemolysis has also been reported in severe poisoning with 1,2-propanediol (17).

Leukocyte Count and Platelet Count

Increases in the leukocyte (white blood cell) count often occur in acute poisoning. This may be in response to metabolic acidosis due to ingestion of, for example, ethylene glycol, methanol, or theophylline, or may be secondary to hypostatic pneumonia after prolonged coma or another source of sepsis such as snakebite. Leukocytopenia and thrombocytopenia may complicate overdosage with colchicine and cytotoxic drugs. Thrombocytopenia may also result from DIC.

ANALYTICAL TOXICOLOGY

A range of powerful chromatographic methods, ligand immunoassays, and other techniques (Tables 9 and 10) are available to the analytical toxicologist. However, it remains impossible to look for all poisons in all samples at the sensitivity required. It is therefore vital that the reason for any analysis is kept clearly in view. Although the underlying principles remain the same in the different branches of analytical toxicology, the nature and amount of specimen available can vary widely, as may the time-scale over which the result is required and the purpose for which the result is to be used. All these factors may in turn influence the choice of methods for a particular analysis. Cases in which toxicologic analyses are requested tend to fall into (a) emergency and general hospital toxicology, including poisons *screening* and (b) more specialized categories, such as forensic toxicology, screening for drugs of abuse, therapeutic drug monitoring (TDM), and occupational/environmental toxicology. There is, however, considerable overlap amongst all of these areas.

TABLE 9. Some methods for the analysis of drugs and other organic poisons in biologic samples

Principle	Technique
Chemical	Color test
Electrochemical	Biosensors
	Differential pulse polarography
Spectrometric	Mass spectrometry, also known as *mass fragmentography*
	Nuclear magnetic resonance
	Spectrophotofluorimetry
	Ultraviolet/visible absorption spectrophotometry
Chromatographic	Gas (liquid) chromatography
	(High-performance) liquid chromatography
	(High-performance) thin-layer chromatography
	Super-critical fluid chromatography
Electrophoretic	Capillary (zone) electrophoresis
Immunoassay	Agglutination inhibition
	Apoenzyme reactivation immunoassay system
	Cloned enzyme donor immunoassay
	Enzyme-linked immunosorbent assay
	Enzyme-multiplied immunoassay technique
	Fluorescence polarization immunoassay
	Hemagglutination inhibition
	Particle concentration fluoroimmunoassay
	Radioimmunoassay
	Substrate-labeled fluoroimmunoassay
Enzyme-based assay	—
Receptor-based assay	—

TABLE 10. Some methods for the analysis of toxic metals in biologic materials

Technique	Mode	Variant
Electrochemical	Potentiometric	Ion selective electrodes
	Coulometric	(Differential pulse) polarography
		Anodic/cathodic stripping voltametry[a]
Spectrophotometric	Atomic emission	Flame photometry[b]
		Flame
		Spark-arc
		Direct current plasma
		Inductively coupled plasma
	Atomic absorption	Flame
		Hydride
		Furnace
		Cold vapor
	X-ray	Fluorescence
	Nuclear	Neutron activation
		Proton activation
Mass spectrometry	—	Spark source (includes isotope dilution)
		Inductively coupled plasma

[a]Also known as *potentiometric stripping analysis*.
[b]Normally refers to the use of filters to select the assay wavelength—used mainly for potassium, lithium, and sodium.

Units of Measurement

In the United Kingdom and in other parts of Europe, some laboratories report analytical toxicology data in *amount concentration* using what purport to be International System of Units (SI) molar units (μmol/L, and so forth), whereas others continue to use mass concentration [so-called "traditional units" (mg/L, and so forth or even mg/dl)], which, in fact, have equal validity as regards SI. The arguments in this debate have been reviewed (18). Reporting the results of analytical toxicology measurements in mass concentration is logical while drugs are still dispensed and pesticides and other chemicals are still quantified for use in mass units. Indeed, mass concentration has to be used in the case of gentamicin and other analytes with no fixed relative molecular mass (*molecular weight*), and mass concentration should also be used if there is uncertainty as to the entity being measured in a particular assay.

Most published analytical toxicology data are presented in SI mass units per milliliter or per liter of the appropriate fluid, or units that are numerically equivalent in the case of aqueous solutions:

$$[\text{parts per million}] = \mu g/g = \mu g/cm^3 = \mu g/ml = mg/L = mg/dm^3 = g/m^3$$

However, although the liter (= dm^3) is a convenient volume for laboratory and domestic use, it is not, in fact, an SI unit, and it can be argued that the cubic meter or submultiples thereof should be used instead. Clinical pharmacologists are, after all, quite accustomed to calculating drug dosage per square meter body surface area, and, thus, expressing drug concentrations per cubic meter of plasma is consistent here. For measurements of concentrations in solid tissues (hair, nails, liver, and so forth), then, SI mass units should be used throughout (e.g., μg/g). Clearly the use of either the solidus or the negative superscript convention to mean *per* or *divided by* in conjunction with symbols in written reports is a matter for local decision taking into account SI guidelines (18). An exception is when preparing written statements for a court of law or other purpose outside the normal reporting channels. In such cases, it is advisable to write out the whole unit of measurement in full (e.g., milligrams per liter) on every occasion.

Conversion from mass concentration (ρ) to amount concentration (c) (*molar units*) and *vice versa* is simple if the molar mass (M) of the compound of interest is known. The following is an example of a compound with a molar mass of 151.2 g/mol:

$$c = \rho/M \text{ [e.g., (1 mol/L) = (151.2 g/L)/(151.2 g/mol)]}$$

$$\rho = c/M \text{ [e.g., (151.2 g/L) = (1 mol/L)} \times \text{(151.2 g/mol)]}$$

However, such conversions always carry a risk of error. Special care is needed in choosing the correct molar mass if the drug is supplied as a salt, hydrate, and so forth. This can cause great discrepancies, especially if the contribution of the accompanying anion or cation is high. Most analytical measurements are expressed in terms of free acid or base and not salt. Relative atomic or molecular masses (atomic or molecular weights) and conversion factors (SI mass and amount concentration) for measurements in blood and other fluids for some compounds of interest are given in Appendices II and III.

GENERAL TOXICOLOGY

Many difficulties may be encountered when performing qualitative and quantitative analyses for poisons, especially if laboratory facilities are limited. The substances that may be present include gases such as carbon monoxide, drugs, solvents, pesticides, metal salts, and naturally occurring toxins. Some poisons may be pure chemicals and others complex mixtures. Plasma concentrations associated with serious toxicity range from μg/L in the case of cardiac glycosides such as digoxin to g/L in the case of ethanol. New drugs, pesticides, and other compounds continually present novel analytical challenges.

Diagnosis of Poisoning

Tests for poisons that a patient is thought to have taken and for which specific therapy is available are often given priority. However, a defined series of tests (a *screen*) is needed in the absence of clinical or other evidence to indicate the poisons involved. If possible, this screen should be tailored to the poisons commonly encountered in a particular country—in Western Europe and North America, for example, drugs have been taken by most poisoned patients admitted to the hospital. However, pesticides are a major problem in many other countries. Screening for pesticides is particularly difficult because such a wide variety of compounds may be encountered. Before starting an analysis, it behoves the analyst to obtain as much information about the patient as possible including medical and social history, especially any history of alcohol or drug abuse; treatment in hospital including drug therapy; and the results of laboratory and/or other investigations. It is also important to be aware of the timing of the sample in relation to the time of the suspected ingestion or exposure because this may influence the interpretation of results.

The specialized nature of analytical toxicologic investigations dictates that facilities are concentrated in centers that are often remote from the patient. The laboratory may undertake a range of analyses in addition to emergency toxicology. Frequently, routine clinical chemical tests are performed at one site, whereas more complex toxicologic analysis is performed by a different department or at a separate site. Despite this, the importance of direct liaison between the physician treating the patient and the analytical toxicologist cannot be overemphasized. Ideally, this liaison should commence before specimens are collected, because some analytes, heavy metals for example, require special precautions in specimen collection (Table 3). At the other extreme, residues of samples held in a clinical chemistry laboratory or by other departments, for example, in the accident and emergency refrigerator, can be invaluable if the possibility of poisoning is only raised in retrospect.

All relevant information about a patient gathered from a clinician, nurse, or poisons information specialist should be recorded in the laboratory using a suitably designed form. A note of a patient's occupation or hobbies can be valuable as this may indicate access to particular poisons. Cyanide poisoning may result from accidents in electroplating establishments, for example, whereas poisoning with sodium barbitone is now encountered most frequently among laboratory workers. Information on the drugs prescribed for the patient, and indeed the patient's relatives, is especially important as this may not only reveal the poisons ingested but also warns that a compound detected may be a drug prescribed for the patient. Chlorpromazine metabolites, for example, may be detected in urine for 18 months after cessation of chronic chlorpromazine therapy as a result of enterohepatic recirculation. Even compounds given inadvertently can cause serious toxicity in exceptional circumstances. Benzyl alcohol used as a preservative in intravenous fluids has caused fatal poisoning in young children. Iodine used intraabdominally after surgery has resulted in death.

The range of analyses that can be offered by specialized laboratories, some on an emergency basis, is shown in Table 11. General toxicologic analyses (poisons *screens*) must use reasonable amounts of commonly available samples (Table 2). If any tests are to influence immediate patient management, the (preliminary) results should be available within 2 to 3 hours of receiving the

TABLE 11. Summary of drugs and other common poisons detected underivatized in blood and in urine by commonly available methods

- Acidic and neutral drugs
  - Barbiturates and anticonvulsants (blood, gas-liquid chromatography)
    - Amylobarbitone
    - Butobarbitone
    - Caffeine
    - Carbamazepine
    - Chlormethiazole
    - Chlorpropamide
    - Ethosuximide
    - Glutethimide
    - Ibuprofen
    - Meprobamate
    - Methaqualone
    - Methocarbamol
    - Methohexitone
    - Methsuximide
    - Methyprylone
    - Metronidazole
    - Paracetamol
    - Pentobarbitone
    - Phenazone
    - Phenobarbitone
    - Phenylbutazone
    - Phenytoin
    - Primidone
    - Propofol
    - Quinalbarbitone
    - Thiopentone
    - Tolbutamide
    - Valproate
  - Barbiturates and anticonvulsants (urine, thin-layer chromatography)
    - Amylobarbitone
    - Butobarbitone
    - Pentobarbitone
    - Phenobarbitone
    - Phenytoin
    - Primidone
    - Quinalbarbitone
    - Thiopentone
    - Theophylline
  - Analgesics (blood/urine, various methods)
    - Acetaminophen (paracetamol)
    - Salicylates[a]
  - Nonsteroidal antiinflammatory drugs (blood, high-performance liquid chromatography)
    - Diflunisal
    - Fenoprofen
    - Ibuprofen
    - Indomethacin
    - Ketoprofen
    - Mefenamic acid
    - Naproxen
    - Piroxicam
  - Antiasthmatics (blood, high-performance liquid chromatography)
    - Caffeine
    - Theophylline
- Basic drugs
  - Detectable in blood after overdose (gas-liquid chromatography)
    - Amisulpride
    - Amitriptyline
    - Amoxapine
    - Amphetamine
    - Atracurium
    - Benzhexol
    - Brompheniramine
    - Cathine
    - Chloroquine
    - Chlorpheniramine
    - Chlorpromazine
    - Citalopram
    - Cocaine
    - Codeine
    - Clomipramine
    - Clozapine
    - Cyclizine
    - Desipramine
    - Dextromoramide
    - Dextropropoxyphene (propoxyphene)[b]
    - Diethylpropion
    - Dihydrocodeine
    - Diltiazem
    - Dipipanone
    - Disopyramide
    - Dothiepin (Prothiden)
    - Doxepin
    - Fenfluramine
    - Fluconazole
    - Fluoxetine
    - Fluvoxamine
    - Haloperidol
    - Hydroxyzine
    - Imipramine
    - Lignocaine (lidocaine)[c]
    - Lofepramine[d]
    - Loxapine
    - Maprotiline
    - Methylenedioxyamphetamine
    - Methylenedioxyethylamphetamine
    - Methylenedioxymethamphetamine
    - Methadone
    - Methylamphetamine
    - Metoclopramide
    - Mianserin
    - Minaprine
    - Mirtazapine
    - Nefopam
    - Nortriptyline
    - Olanzapine
    - Orphenadrine
    - Pethidine (meperidine)
    - Phentermine
    - Phenylpropanolamine
    - Procainamide
    - Procyclidine
    - Propranolol
    - Protriptyline
    - (Pseudo)ephedrine
    - Pyrimethamine
    - Quetipine
    - Quinine/quinidine
    - Remoxipride
    - Risperidone
    - Sertraline
    - Strychnine
    - Sulpiride
    - Terodiline
    - Thioridazine
    - Tranylcypromine
    - Trazodone
    - Trimethoprim
    - Trimipramine
    - Venlafaxine
    - Verapamil
    - Zopiclone
- Drugs/drug groups detectable in urine/gastric contents (gas-liquid chromatography)
  - Most of the drugs previously listed under the heading *Detectable in blood after overdose*, including:
  - β-Adrenoceptor blockers (but not atenolol, sotalol)
  - Amphetamines (includes methylenedioxyamphetamine, methylenedioxyethylamphetamine, and methylenedioxymethamphetamine)
  - Antidysrhythmics (includes disopyramide, flecainide, mexiletine)
  - Antibiotics (includes chloramphenicol, metronidazole, trimethoprim)
  - Anticholinergics (includes dicyclomine, benzhexol, procyclidine)
  - Antihistamines (includes chlorpheniramine, cyclizine, diphenhydramine, terfenadine)
  - Local anesthetics (includes bupivacaine, lidocaine, mepivacaine, prilocaine)
  - Narcotic analgesics (but not heroin/morphine)
  - Pesticides (includes some chlorinated pesticides, and some organophosphorus compounds and carbamates only)
  - Phenothiazines (but not flupentixol and some other low-dose compounds)
  - Tricyclic and related antidepressants (includes amitriptyline, clomipramine, desipramine, dothiepin, imipramine, nortriptyline)
  - Atropine
  - Chlormethiazole
  - Hyoscine (scopolamine)
  - Ketamine
  - Nicotine[e]
  - Propofol
  - Zopiclone
- Drugs detectable in urine/gastric contents (thin-layer chromatography)
  - Those drugs previously listed under the heading *Drugs/drug groups detectable in urine/gastric contents*, β-adrenoceptor blockers, phenothiazines, and also:
  - Cimetidine
  - Heroin
  - Mefenamic acid
  - Morphine
  - Ranitidine
- Hypnotics/anxiolytics
  - Volatile hypnotics (blood, gas-liquid chromatography)
    - Ethchlorvynol
    - Chlormethiazole
    - 2,2,2-Trichloroethanol[f]
  - Benzodiazepines (blood, gas-liquid chromatography–electron capture detection)
    - Alprazolam
    - Bromazepam
    - Chlordiazepoxide
    - Clobazam
    - Clonazepam
    - Diazepam
    - Flunitrazepam
    - Flurazepam
    - Lorazepam
    - Lormetazepam
    - Midazolam
    - Nitrazepam
    - Nordazepam
    - Oxazepam
    - Prazepam
    - Temazepam
    - Triazolam

(continued)

TABLE 11. (*continued*)

- Benzodiazepines (urine, immunoassay)
  - Group identification only
- Solvents and related compounds
  - Volatile substances (blood/urine, gas chromatography) (acetone, ethanol, isopropanol, and methanol commonly measured separately by direct injection gas chromatography; others measured by headspace gas chromatography. More details of the range of compounds that can be encountered are given in Table 20.)
    - Acetone
    - Bromochlorodifluoromethane
    - Butane
    - Butanone
    - Dichloromethane
    - Dimethyl ether
    - Ethanol
    - Halothane
    - Isobutane
    - Isoflurane
    - Isopropanol
    - Methanol
    - Nitrous oxide
    - Paraldehyde
    - Propane
    - Tetrachloroethylene
    - Toluene
    - 1,1,1-Trichloroethane
    - Trichloroethylene
    - Xylene
  - Glycols (blood/urine, gas-liquid chromatography)
    - Ethylene glycol
    - 1,2-Propanediol
  - Essential oils (blood, gas-liquid chromatography)
    - Camphor
    - Cineole
    - Eugenol
- Substance abuse (various methods depending on circumstances; immunoassays often group specific for amphetamines and opiates)
  - Amphetamines (urine)
    - Amphetamine
    - Cathine
    - Diethylpropion
    - Fenfluramine
    - Methylenedioxyamphetamine
    - Methylenedioxyethylamphetamine
    - Methylenedioxymethamphetamine
    - Methylamphetamine
    - Phentermine
    - Phenylpropanolamine
    - (Pseudo)ephedrine
  - Cannabis (urine, as cannabinoids)
  - Cocaine (urine, as benzoylecgonine)
  - Lysergic acid diethylamide (urine)
  - Opiates (urine)
    - Codeine
    - Dihydrocodeine
    - Heroin
    - Morphine
    - Pholcodine
  - Diuretics (urine, thin-layer chromatography)
    - Thiazides
    - Spironolactone
  - Laxatives (urine, thin-layer chromatography)
    - Bisacodyl
    - Danthron
    - Phenolphthalein
    - Rhein (from *Senna*, for example)
- Pesticides
  - Chlorophenoxy and hydroxybenzonitrile herbicides (blood/urine, high-performance liquid chromatography)
    - Bromoxynil
    - 2,4-Dichlorophenoxyacetic acid
    - 2,4-Dichlorophenoxypropionic acid
    - Ioxynil
    - Fenoprop
    - 4-Chloro-2-methylphenoxyacetic acid
    - 4-Chloro-2-methylphenoxypropionic acid
    - 2,4,5-Trichlorophenoxyacetic acid
  - Bipyridilium herbicides (blood/urine, high-performance liquid chromatography)
    - Paraquat
    - Diquat
  - Chlorinated pesticides (blood, gas-liquid chromatography)
    - Chlordane
    - 1,1,1-Trichloro-di-(4-chlorophenyl)ethane
    - Dieldrin
    - Heptachlor
    - Lindane
    - Pentachlorophenol
  - Organophosphorus compounds and carbamate insecticides (blood/urine, gas-liquid chromatography)
    - Carbaryl
    - Dimethoate
    - Malathion
    - Pirimicarb
    - Pirimiphos methyl
- Toxic metals (see also Table 3)
  - Serum
    - Iron
  - Blood
    - Antimony
    - Arsenic
    - Cadmium
    - Lead
    - Mercury
    - Thallium
- Miscellaneous poisons
  - Bromide
  - Carbon monoxide
  - Cyanide
  - Lithium
  - Digoxin

[a]May include aminosalicylate, aspirin, methyl salicylate, and salicylamide if Trinder's test used (see Table 18).
[b]Quantitation by high-performance liquid chromatography recommended.
[c]Common contaminant from catheter lubricant, and so forth.
[d]As desipramine.
[e]Commonly from tobacco smoke.
[f]From chloral hydrate, dichloralphenazone, trichloroethylene, or triclofos (see Table 18).
[g]As carboxyhemoglobin.

specimens (1 hour in the case of acetaminophen and ethanol). In some cases, the presence of more than one poison, for example, may complicate the analysis, and examination of further specimens from the patient may be required. A quantitative analysis carried out on whole blood or plasma is usually needed to confirm poisoning unequivocally, but this may not be possible if laboratory facilities are limited or if the compound is particularly difficult to measure. It is important to discuss the scope and limitations of the tests performed with the clinician concerned and to maintain high standards of laboratory practice, especially when performing tests on an emergency basis. It may be better to offer no result rather than misleading data based on an unreliable test.

Circumstantial evidence of poisoning is often ambiguous, and thus, if an analysis is indicated, it is often advisable to perform a *poisons screen* routinely in all but the simplest cases. Similarly, the analysis should not end after the first positive finding because additional, hitherto unsuspected compounds may be present (19). One exception is provided by sublethal carbon monoxide poisoning, which can be difficult to diagnose even if carboxyhemoglobin measurements are available—circumstantial evidence of poisoning may here prove invaluable. Of course, a *positive* result on a poisons screen does not of itself confirm poisoning, because such a result may arise from incidental or occupational exposure or the use of drugs in treatment.

Selective test ordering based on clinical features (*toxidromes*) has been advocated. This may be acceptable if there is no doubt about the diagnosis and no other clinical indications for performing the tests (20). However, the results of surveys performed to assess the value of general toxicologic analyses are likely to be different if the patient presents either a diagnostic or treatment problem. Indeed, poisoning with certain compounds is not infrequently misdiagnosed, especially if the patient presents in the later stages of an episode. Examples include cardiorespiratory arrest (cyanide), hepatitis (acetaminophen), diabetes (hypoglycemics, including ethanol in young children), paresthesia (thallium), progressive pneumonitis (paraquat), and renal failure (ethylene glycol).

The trend away from indiscriminate prescribing of barbiturates and nonbarbiturate hypnotics such as glutethimide has led to a reduction in the frequency with which such compounds are encountered in acute poisoning in Western Europe and North

TABLE 12. Some compounds not detected by commonly used overdose-screening procedures

Group	Examples
Inorganic ions	Arsenic, barium, bismuth, borate, bromide, cadmium, copper, cyanide, fluoride, iron, lead, lithium, mercury, sulfide, thallium
Organic chemicals	Camphor, carbon disulfide, carbon monoxide, carbon tetrachloride, dichloromethane, ethylene glycol, formates, oxalates, petroleum distillates, phenols, tetrachloroethylene, toluene, 1,1,1-trichloroethane
Drugs	Bretylium, cannabis, clonidine, colchicine, coumarin anticoagulants, dapsone, digoxin, glyceryl trinitrate, lysergic acid diethylamide, metformin, phenformin, salbutamol, tolbutamide
Pesticides	Bromomethane, carbamate insecticides, chloralose, chlorophenoxy herbicides, dinitrophenol pesticides, fluoroacetates, hydroxybenzonitrile herbicides, organochlorine pesticides, organophosphorus insecticides, pentachlorophenol

America. However, these compounds still occur from time to time. Benzodiazepines, tricyclic and related antidepressants, anticonvulsants, narcotic and other analgesics, nonsteroidal antiinflammatory drugs, and, of course, ethanol are all encountered regularly; multiple overdosage is frequent.

Blood is often the easiest specimen to obtain from an unconscious patient and is needed for any quantitative measurements. Urine is also a valuable specimen because drug or metabolite concentrations tend to be higher than in blood, and relatively large volumes are usually available. Some compounds, such as many benzodiazepines, however, are extensively metabolized before excretion, and plasma is then the specimen of choice for detecting the parent compound. Quantitative measurements in urine are generally of little use. All poison screens have limitations (21) (Table 12). Thus, of the drugs commonly used to treat depression, lithium has to be looked for specifically, usually by use of an ion-selective electrode, whereas monoamine oxidase inhibitors have a prolonged action in the body, though plasma concentrations are low even after overdosage. Any unbound drug is rapidly excreted and may be difficult to detect except in a urine specimen obtained soon after the event. Tricyclic antidepressants are lipophilic, and thus urinary concentrations even in fatal poisoning may be below the limit of detection of the method used if death has occurred relatively soon after the ingestion.

Treatment of Poisoning

Treatment of severely poisoned patients may include intravenous administration of anticonvulsants, such as diazepam or chlormethiazole, or of antidysrhythmics, such as lidocaine, all of which may be detected if a toxicologic analysis is subsequently performed. Antidotes such as naloxone and antibiotics such as metronidazole or trimethoprim may also be detected. Lidocaine gel or spray is used as a topical anesthetic and is often an incidental analytical finding after use, for example, during bladder catheterization or endoscopy (22). Acute poisoning with oral or intravenous lidocaine also occurs (23), and thus interpretation of the finding of lidocaine must be undertaken cautiously. Drugs or other compounds may also be given during first aid or investigative procedures such as lumbar puncture or computerized tomographic scans and may be detected on subsequent toxicologic analysis. Iodinated hippuric acids are used as radiographic contrast media. The muscle relaxant atracurium, which gives rise to laudanosine *in vivo*, is frequently given to facilitate mechanical ventilation. Even emetine from syrup of ipecacuanha given to induce vomiting may be detected on subsequent analysis. It is therefore important that details of *all* drugs used in therapy are notified to the laboratory at the time of the initial request.

Antidotes are available for some poisons, and their use is often required before analytical confirmation of the diagnosis can be obtained. Lack of response to a particular antidote, however, must not be used to indicate the absence of particular poisons. Naloxone, for example, rapidly and completely reverses coma due to opioids such as morphine and codeine without risk to the patient, except that an acute withdrawal response may be precipitated in dependent subjects. A lack of response, however, may not mean that no opioids are present because another, non-opioid, drug may be the cause of coma; too little naloxone may have been given; or hypoxic brain damage may have followed a cardiorespiratory arrest. In such cases, a toxicologic analysis is needed to establish the nature of any poisons present.

The measurement of plasma concentrations of some poisons is important because the decision to implement protective treatment, chelation, or active elimination therapy may depend on the result (Table 13). The decision to institute active elimination therapy is not normally determined solely by plasma concentrations but depends also on the clinical picture. The duration of such therapy may again be influenced by plasma concentration measurements. The analytical diagnosis of acetaminophen poisoning is especially important because within the first 24 hours the clinical features of potentially fatal poisoning are often unremarkable. Treatment with *N*-acetylcysteine or methionine, however, must

TABLE 13. Emergency toxicologic analyses that may influence active treatment

Treatment	Poison	Plasma concentration associated with serious toxicity[a]
Protective therapy		
N-Acetylcysteine or methionine	Acetaminophen	200 mg/L at 4 h, 30 mg/L at 16 h
Ethanol	Ethylene glycol	0.5 g/L
	Methanol	0.5 g/L
Antidigoxin Fab antibody fragments	Digoxin	6 μg/L
Chelation therapy		
Desferrioxamine	Aluminium	50–250 μg/L (serum)
	Iron	8 mg/L (serum)
Ethylenediamine tetraacetate/dimercaptosuccinic acid	Lead	600 μg/L (whole blood)
	Antimony	200 μg/L (whole blood)
Dimercaptopropane sulfonate	Arsenic	100 μg/L (whole blood)
	Bismuth	100 μg/L (whole blood)
	Mercury	100 μg/L (whole blood)
Active elimination therapy		
Oral Prussian blue[b]	Thallium	300 μg/L (urine)
Alkaline diuresis	Chlorophenoxy herbicides	0.5 g/L
	Barbitone	300 mg/L
	Phenobarbitone	100 mg/L
	Salicylates	500 mg/L
Hemodialysis/peritoneal dialysis	Barbitone	300 mg/L
	Ethanol	5 g/L
	Ethylene glycol	0.5 g/L
	Lithium	10 mg/L (1.5 mmol/L)
	Methanol	0.5 g/L
	Phenobarbitone	100 mg/L
	2-Propanol	4 g/L
	Salicylates	500 mg/L

[a]Many factors may modify response in a given patient.
[b]Potassium ferrihexacyanoferrate.

TABLE 14. Some factors that may affect interpretation of toxicology results

Acidosis/alkalosis (water-soluble ionizable poisons)	More than one poison present
Age	Nutrition
Burns (state of hydration)	Occupation
Disease	Pregnancy
Drug therapy (long term and recent)	Route of exposure (especially if intravenous or inhalational rather than oral)
Duration of exposure	Shock
Ethanol consumption (short- and long-term)	Site of sampling (especially important if patient undergoing an infusion and in postmortem cases)
Formulation (sustained release, racemate, and so forth)	Surgery
Genetics	Time of sampling relative to exposure and/or death
Hemolysis	Tolerance
Idiosyncrasy	Trauma
Infection	

See also, Flanagan RJ. Interpretation of analytical toxicology results and unit of measurement conversion factors. *Ann Clin Biochem* 1998;35:261–267; and Drummer OH, Gerostamoulos J. Postmortem drug analysis: analytical and toxicological aspects. *Ther Drug Monit* 2002;24:199–209.

be instituted promptly if it is to be effective (Chapter 64). Paracetamol poisoning is so common in the United Kingdom and in the United States that an emergency assay should ideally be performed on samples from all patients aged 10 years or older with suspected intentional overdose (24). The severity of acute poisoning with ethylene glycol and with methanol is best assessed in the early stages by measurement of plasma concentrations.

Interpretation of Results

Patients often respond differently to a given dose of a given compound, especially so far as behavioral effects are concerned. Some of the factors involved, which may include tolerance, age, drug interactions, disease, and the formation of toxic metabolites, are summarized in Tables 14 and 15. In particular, the effects of short- and long-term ethanol consumption on drug and metabolite pharmacokinetics have been reviewed (25). Compilations of data to assist in the interpretation of analytical results are available (26,27). The role of pharmacologically active metabolites has been discussed (28–30).

It is important to bear in mind the time course of the episode when providing interpretation. For example, results obtained from samples taken before absorption or distribution are com-

TABLE 15. Some compounds decomposing *in vivo* or undergoing metabolism to give products of similar or greater toxicity

Compound	Toxic decomposition product/metabolite	Compound	Toxic decomposition product/metabolite
Aldrin	Dieldrin	Hexane (also 2-hexanone)	Hexane-2,5-dione
Alkyl nitriles	Cyanide ion	Hypochlorites	Chlorine
Alkyl nitrites	Nitrite ion	Lofepramine	Desipramine
Aloxiprin	Salicylate	Loxapine	Amoxapine
α-Amanitin	[Reactive intermediates]	Metaldehyde	Acetaldehyde (?)
Amoxapine	7-Hydroxyamoxapine, 8-hydroxyamoxapine	Methanol	Formaldehyde and formate
Aspirin	Salicylate	Methsuximide	*N*-Desmethylmethsuximide
Benorylate	Salicylate and acetaminophen (paracetamol)	Methyl salicylate	Salicylate
Benzene	[Reactive intermediates]	Minoxidil	Minoxidil sulphate
Benzodiazepines[a]	*N*-Demethylated (and/or other) metabolites	Morphine	Morphine-6-glucuronide
Bopindolol	Desbenzoylbopindolol[b]	Nitroprusside	Cyanide ion
Bufuralol	1-Hydroxybufuralol	Paracetamol	[Reactive intermediates]
Bupropion	Hydroxybupropion, *threo*- and *erythro*-hydroxybupropion	Parathion	Paraoxon
Buspirone	1-Pyrimidinylpiperazine	Pethidine	Norpethidine
Camazepam	Temazepam	Phalloidin	[Reactive intermediates]
Carbamazepine	Carbamazepine-10,11-epoxide	Phenacetin	Paracetamol[c]
Carbon tetrachloride	[Reactive intermediates]	Phenothiazines[a]	*N*-Demethylated (and/or other) metabolites
Chloral	2,2,2-Trichloroethanol and trichloracetic acid	Phenylbutazone	Oxyphenbutazone
Chlordane	Oxychlordane, heptachlor epoxide and others	Phenytoin	[Reactive intermediates]
Chloroform	Phosgene	Phosphides	Phosphine
Clorazepate	Nordazepam	Primidone	Phenobarbitone
Clozapine	Norclozapine	Procainamide	*N*-Acetylprocainamide
Cyanogenic glycosides	Cyanide ion	Prontosil	Sulphanilamide
Cyclophosphamide	Acrolein, phosphoramide mustard	Rifampicin	Desacetylrifampicin
Dichloralphenazone	2,2,2-Trichloroethanol and trichloracetic acid	Salicylamide	Salicylate
Dichloromethane	Carbon monoxide	Spironolactone	Canrenone
Dichloropropane	[Reactive intermediates]	Terfenadine	Fexofenadine
3,4-Dihydroxyphenylalanine	3,4-Dihydroxyphenylethylamine (dopamine)	1,1,2,2-Tetrachloroethane	[Reactive intermediates]
Ethylene glycol	Glycolate and oxalate	Theophylline	Caffeine (neonates only)
Fenfluramine	Norfenfluramine	Thiocyanate insecticides	Cyanide ion
Fluoxetine	Norfluoxetine	Trichloroethylene	2,2,2-Trichloroethanol and trichloracetic acid
Flurazepam	Desalkylflurazepam	—	
Halothane	[Reactive intermediates]	Triclofos	2,2,2-Trichloroethanol and trichloracetic acid
Heptachlor	Heptachlor epoxide	—	
Heroin	Morphine and morphine-6-glucuronide	Tricyclic antidepressants	*N*-Demethylated (and/or other) metabolites
Hexamethylmelamine	Pentamethylmelamine, tetramethylmelamine	Trimethadione	Dimethadione

[a]Some compounds only.
[b]*N*-tertiary-Butyl-2-hydroxy-3-(2-methyl-1H-indol-4-yloxy)-1-propylamine.
[c]Hepatorenal toxicity rare possibly because toxic metabolism of paracetamol inhibited by phenacetin.

TABLE 16. Irreversible and delayed toxicity

Compound/group of compounds
Acetaminophen (hepatic, and sometimes renal toxicity)
Acetylcholinesterase inhibitors (organophosphorus insecticides, nerve gases)
Alkyl bromides (e.g., bromomethane)
α-Amanitin (hepatorenal toxicity)
Anticoagulants (e.g., warfarin and other coumarins/indanediones)
Antineoplastic agents (e.g., cyclophosphamide)
Aspirin
Carbon monoxide (neuropsychiatric sequelae)
Carbon tetrachloride (hepatorenal toxicity)
Chloroform (hepatorenal toxicity)
Chloroquine (retinal toxicity)
1,2-Dichloroethane (hepatorenal toxicity)
1,2-Dichloropropane (hepatorenal toxicity)
Ethylene glycol (renal and central nervous system toxicity)
Halothane (hepatic toxicity—rare)
Heavy metals (e.g., cadmium, lead, mercury, thallium)
Hexane and 2-hexanone (peripheral neuropathy)
Iron salts
Methanol (retinal and central nervous system toxicity)
Monoamine oxidase inhibitors
Paraquat (lung toxicity)
Phalloidin (hepatorenal toxicity)
Phenytoin (hepatic toxicity—rare)
Quinine (retinal toxicity)
Sustained-release preparations (e.g., theophylline)

plete may be misleading, as in the case of acetaminophen and with sustained release preparations such as those containing theophylline. Aspects of the pharmacokinetics of drugs in overdose have been reviewed (31). Some compounds giving rise to delayed or irreversible toxicity are listed in Table 16. Plasma concentration measurements are especially valuable in assessing the prognosis in paraquat poisoning (Chapter 239) (32).

There is much current interest in the role of chirality in drug action (33). However, although it has been estimated that some 25% of drugs and pesticides are marketed as racemates, there is in general little need for the enantiomers to be measured separately. Some compounds that are unstable in whole blood or plasma are listed in Table 17; special precautions are obviously needed if these compounds are to be measured. Oxygen rapidly dissociates carboxyhemoglobin and thus a blood sample should be obtained as soon as practicable after carbon monoxide poisoning if measurement of carboxyhemoglobin is to be attempted.

TABLE 17. Some drugs, metabolites, and other poisons unstable in whole blood or plasma

Compound/group of compounds (examples)
Volatile compounds
All (aerosol propellants, anesthetic gases, carbon monoxide, ethanol, mercury, organic solvents, paraldehyde)
Nonvolatile compounds
Acetaminophen (paracetamol)
Alkyl nitrites (glyceryl trinitrate)
Aspirin
Cocaine
Cyanide ion
Cyclosporin[a]
1,4-Dihydropyridines (nifedipine)
Diltiazem
Insulin
N-Glucuronide metabolites (nomifensine)
7-Nitrobenzodiazepines (clonazepam, nitrazepam)
N-Oxide metabolites (alkaline pH)
N-Sulphate metabolites (minoxidil)
Peroxides and other strong oxidizing agents
Phenelzine
Phenothiazines[b]
Physostigmine
Quinol metabolites (4-hydroxypropranolol)
S-Oxide metabolites
Thalidomide
Thiol (sulfydryl-containing) drugs (captopril)
Thiopentone

[a]Redistributes between plasma and red blood cells on standing—use whole blood.
[b]Particularly those without an electron withdrawing substituent at the 2 position.

Reporting the Result

The results of urgent analyses must be communicated verbally or electronically to the appropriate physician without delay, and should be followed by a written report as soon as possible. Most laboratories produce computer-generated reports. Ideally, confirmation from a second, independent method should be obtained before reporting positive findings. However, this may not always be practicable, especially if only simple methods (e.g., colorimetric tests) are available. In such cases, it is vital that the appropriate positive and negative controls have been analyzed together with the specimen.

Although it seems straightforward for the analyst to interpret the results of analyses in which no compounds were detected, such results are sometimes difficult to convey to physicians, especially in writing. This is because it is important to give information as to the poisons *excluded* by the tests performed with all the attendant complications of the scope, limits of sensitivity, and selectivity of the analyses and other factors such as sampling variations. Because of the potential medicolegal and other implications of any toxicologic analysis, it is important to avoid jargon, such as *negative*, or sweeping statements, such as *absent* or *not present*. The phrase *not detected* should convey precisely the laboratory result, especially when accompanied by a statement of the specimen analyzed and the limit of sensitivity of the test (detection limit). However, it can still be difficult to convey the scope of analyses such as that of gas-liquid chromatography (GLC) for acidic and basic drugs as discussed previously. Even with relatively simple tests such as Trinder's test normally performed on plasma or urine to detect aspirin ingestion, a number of other salicylates, including methyl salicylate also react.

One way of giving at least some of this information in a written report is to create a numbered list of the compounds or groups of compounds normally detected by commonly used procedures. If these groups are listed on the back of the report form, for example, then it is a relatively simple matter to refer to the qualitative tests performed by number and, thus, to convey at least some of the information required. Problems may arise if a hospital or other laboratory transcribes a report from a toxicology laboratory onto its own report form that is then forwarded to the physician. The units used for any measurement may be converted (sometimes erroneously) from mass to amount concentration (*molar units*), and any interpretation of the result may be discarded. Information on the drugs looked for but not found may also be lost.

ANALYTICAL METHODS

Drugs and Pesticides

Specialized laboratories use a combination of solvent extraction and thin-layer chromatography (TLC) together with GLC using either flame-ionization or selective (nitrogen/phosphorus, electron capture and/or mass spectrometric) detectors as the basis

TABLE 18. Some commonly used spot tests

Test	Analyte(s)	Fluid	Limit of sensitivity (mg/L)	[Additional] compounds detected
ortho-Cresol/ammonia	Acetaminophen	Urine	1[a]	Aniline[b] Benorylate Nitrobenzene[b] Phenacetin Ethylenediamine[c]
Diphenylamine	Oxidizing agents	Gastric contents[d]	10	Bromates Chlorates Iodates Nitrates Nitrites Peroxides
Dithionite	Paraquat (blue) Diquat (yellow-green)	Urine[e]	1 5	Nil
Ethchlorvynol/diphenylamine	Ethchlorvynol	Urine	1	—
Forrest	Imipramine	Urine	25	Clomipramine Desipramine Trimipramine
FPN[f]	Phenothiazines	Urine	25[g]	—
Fujiwara	Trichloro-compounds	Urine	1[h]	Chloral hydrate Chloroform Dichloralphenazone Trichloroethylene Trichlofos
Trinder's[i]	Salicylates	Plasma Urine Gastric contents[d]	10	Aloxiprin[b] Aminosalicylate Aspirin[b] Benorylate[b] Methyl salicylate[b] Salicylamide[b]

[a]As *para*-aminophenol.
[b]After metabolism or hydrolysis.
[c]From aminophylline, for example.
[d]Includes vomit, stomach wash out, scene residues, and similar samples.
[e]Can be used on plasma in severe cases.
[f]Ferric chloride/perchloric acid/nitric acid.
[g]As chlorpromazine.
[h]As trichloroacetate.
[i]Ketones interfere.
See Flanagan RJ, Braithwaite RA, Brown SS, et al. *Basic analytical toxicology.* Geneva: World Health Organization, 1995, for further details.

for a poisons *screen*. In addition, simple color (*spot*) tests remain useful for some compounds, such as salicylates, acetaminophen, and paraquat (Table 18). Further chromatographic, mass spectrometric, or immunoassay procedures (Table 19) may be used as appropriate.

Color tests are useful in that a minimum of reagents and expertise are required (34). However, sensitivity is limited and the tests are applicable only to urine and other samples likely to contain relatively large amounts of poison, such as stomach contents. False-negatives are rare if a test is used for its intended purpose in appropriate samples. Positive results with poisons such as acetaminophen or paraquat serve to indicate the need for a quantitative measurement in plasma. Other tests, such as the Forrest test for imipramine-type compounds and the ferric chloride, perchloric acid, and nitric acid test for phenothiazines, are less useful and only indicate the need for confirmatory TLC or GLC analysis.

TLC is, in some respects, an extension of the color tests discussed previously because colors formed with various visualization reagents form the basis of compound identifications. However, incorporation of (a) a solvent extraction and concentration step and (b) a chromatographic step enhances sensitivity and selectivity. It is unwise, however, to use TLC without corroboration by another method such as GLC. The resolving power of TLC is limited, and the interpretation of the chromatograms obtained is subjective (35). A commercial TLC *kit* (Toxi-Lab, Varian Inc., Lake Forest, CA) is available and is supplied together with a compendium of color plates and additional information to facilitate interpretation (36). As with TLC in general, problems can arise when attempting to differentiate compounds with similar mobility and color reactions, especially if more than one compound is present. Moreover, the kit is aimed primarily at the U.S. market, and thus, some common United Kingdom drugs are not included. The dangers inherent in the inappropriate use of this kit have been stressed (37).

Spectrophotometry and spectrophotofluorimetry are usually used as detectors for high-performance liquid chromatography (HPLC) or in immunoassays, although in the past these methods were widely used either directly or after sample preparation procedures such as solvent extraction or chromogenic reaction. Spectrophotometric methods are still useful for salicylates and carboxyhemoglobin, amongst other analytes. However, many spectrophotometric and even spectrophotofluorimetric methods experience interference either from metabolites or other drugs. A good example is the use of ultra violet absorption to measure the herbicide 2,4-dichlorophenoxyacetic acid in the presence of the related herbicide ioxynil (38). Methods using derivative spectroscopy or wavelength ratioing techniques can enhance the selectivity of spectrophotometric methods, as in the

TABLE 19. Some immunoassays that have been used in screening for drugs of abuse in urine (consult the manufacturers for current assay availability and sensitivity/selectivity)

Technique	Manufacturer	Drug group	Limit of detection[a] (mg/L)
Agglutination inhibition	Roche Abuscreen Ontrak	Amphetamines	1.0[b]
		Barbiturates	0.2[c]
		Benzodiazepines	0.1[d]
		Cannabinoids[e]	0.05/0.1
		Cocaine	0.3[f]
		Methadone	0.3
		Morphine	0.3
		Phencyclidine	0.025
	Roche Abuscreen Online	Amphetamines	1.0[b]
		Barbiturates	0.2[c]
		Benzodiazepines	0.1[d]
		Cannabinoids[e]	0.1
		Cocaine	0.3[f]
		Methadone	0.3
		Opiates	0.3
		Phencyclidine	0.025
Cloned enzyme Donor Immunoassay	Microgenics	Amphetamines	0.5/1
		Barbiturates	0.2/0.3
		Benzodiazepines	0.2/0.3
		Cannabinoids	0.025/0.05/0.1[e]
		Cocaine	0.15/0.3[f]
		Methadone	0.1
		Opiates	0.3
Enzyme Multiplied Immunoassay Technique	Dade Behring EMIT-ETS/ EMIT II	Amphetamines	0.3/1.0
		Barbiturates	0.2/0.3[c]
		Benzodiazepines	0.2/0.3[g]
		Cannabinoids[e]	0.02/0.05/0.1
		Cocaine	0.15/0.3[f]
		Dextropropoxyphene	0.3
		Methadone	0.3
		Methaqualone	0.3
		Opiates	0.3
		Phencyclidine	0.025
	Dade Behring EMIT-ST	Amphetamines	0.7
		Barbiturates	0.3[c]
		Benzodiazepines	0.3[g]
		Cannabinoids[e]	0.1
	Dade Behring EMIT-ST	Cocaine	0.3[f]
		Dextropropoxyphene	0.3
		Methadone	0.3
		Methaqualone	0.3
		Opiates	0.3
		Phencyclidine	0.075
Fluorescence Polarization Immunoassay (FPIA)	Abbott TDx/ TDxFLx	Amphetamine class	0.5[h]
		Amphetamine/methylamphetamine	0.3[b]
		Barbiturates	0.2[c]
		Benzodiazepines	0.2[d]
		Cannabinoids[e,i]	0.025
		Cocaine	0.3[f]
		Dextropropoxyphene	0.3
		Methadone	0.15
	Abbott TDx/ TDxFLx	Opiates	0.2
		Phencyclidine	0.025
Hemagglutination inhibition	Boehringer Mannheim	Opiates	0.05,[j] 0.5[k]
Radioimmunoassay (^{125}I-label)	Diagnostic Products	Amphetamine	0.5
		Barbiturates	0.05[c]
		Benzodiazepines	0.01[g]
		Buprenorphine	0.0005
		Cannabinoids[e]	0.01
		Cocaine	0.1[f]
		Cotinine	0.1
		Fentanyl	0.00025
		Lysergic acid diethylamide	0.0001
		Methadone	0.005
		Methamphetamine	0.5
		6-Monoacetylmorphin	0.001
		Morphine	0.0025
		Opiates[l]	0.025[k]
		Phencyclidine	0.001

[a] As suggested by the manufacturers but can sometimes be varied.
[b] As dextroamphetamine.
[c] As quinalbarbitone (secobarbitone).
[d] As nordazepam.
[e] 11-Nor-delta-8-tetrahydrocannabinol-9-carboxylic acid.
[f] As benzoylecgonine.
[g] As oxazepam.
[h] As D,L-amphetamine.
[i] 11-Nor-delta-9-tetrahydrocannabinol-9-carboxylic acid calibrators also available.
[j] Free morphine.
[k] Morphine-3-glucuronide.
[l] Veterinary use only.

case of paraquat (39). Wavelength scanning at different pHs can be useful in identifying the constituents of tablets.

Immunoassays, especially those that do not use radioisotopes (so-called nonisotopic immunoassays), have advantages of long shelf life, speed, simplicity of operation, and adaptability to automated equipment (40). The production of monoclonal antibodies has improved selectivity and reproducibility. However, most immunoassay procedures require confirmation using a second method, ideally a chromatographic method, if the results are to withstand scrutiny. This is because few immunoassays are specific for small molecules (such as most drugs). This lack of specificity can be turned to advantage when screening for a number of related compounds, but can cause problems for the unwary. A further factor is that not all compounds that cross-react do so to the same extent at the same concentration. In some cases, cross-reactivity is not confined to compounds of the same chemical class. Some urinary amphetamine immunoassays, for example, also give positive results with tranylcypromine, proguanil, isoxsuprine, labetalol, and phenylethylamine, amongst other compounds, whereas the Dode Behring enzyme-multiplied immunoassay technique antidepressant assay, for example, cross-reacts with phenothiazines after overdosage (41).

Chromatographic techniques, notably GLC and HPLC, have advantages of good selectivity, sensitivity, flexibility, and ability to perform quantitative as well as qualitative measurements, but are expensive. The high resolution of capillary gas chromatography (GC) has made a major impact in analytical toxicology, especially in the analysis of basic drugs, as has the increasing availability of bench-top mass spectrometers, which can give unequivocal identification of many compounds.

Packed column GLC still can be useful in the measurement of basic drugs (42) and in the measurement of ethylene glycol and 1,2-propanediol after formation of the phenylboronate derivatives (43). Note that 2,3-butanediol (44) and 1,2-propanediol (45) have been mistaken for ethylene glycol in other GC assays. HPLC is also often used to analyze specific compounds or groups of compounds, although a screening procedure for the analysis of basic drugs has been developed using silica columns (46). The availability of diode-array detectors and wavelength ratioing techniques has further enhanced the use of HPLC in qualitative analysis. The roles of GLC (47) and of HPLC (48) in analytical toxicology have been reviewed.

Despite major advances in chromatographic and other techniques, there remains a need for simple, reliable methods to detect and identify common poisons for use in smaller hospital laboratories and laboratories in developing countries (34). Although several of the immunoassays available (Table 19) go some way toward this in regards to simplicity in operation and selectivity, there are disadvantages, the least not being the relatively high cost of reagents and potential difficulties in supply. The World Health Organization, the United Nations Environment Programme, and the International Labour Organisation through the International Programme on Chemical Safety are aware of this problem and have sponsored the production of an analytical toxicology manual specifically intended for use in laboratories in developing countries (49).

Ethanol and Other Volatiles

Enzymatic methods for blood ethanol using alcohol dehydrogenase with spectrophotometric measurement of a coenzyme are available in kit form, such as that available for the Abbott TDx/ADx. GC analysis of ethanol by direct injection of blood or urine diluted with internal standard solution, or by static headspace sampling, is also widely used particularly in forensic work. GC is advantageous because methanol, 2-propanol, and acetone may be separated and measured simultaneously. Methanol poisoning from ingestion of synthetic alcoholic drinks is one of the few causes of acute poisoning epidemics, and measurement of blood methanol is important in establishing the diagnosis and in monitoring treatment.

More than 20 additional volatile compounds may be encountered in acute poisoning cases arising, for example, from deliberate inhalation of vapor to become intoxicated [*glue sniffing*, solvent abuse, inhalant abuse, volatile substance abuse (50)]. Some of these substances are listed in Table 20. Static headspace sampling combined with temperature-programmed GC on a capillary column and dual detection (electron capture detector/flame-ionization detector) is the method of choice for these compounds in biologic fluids (51). Some of these volatile compounds have metabolites that may be measured in urine to assess exposure, notably hippuric and methylhippuric (toluric) acids (from toluene and the xylenes, respectively) and trichloroacetic acid (from trichloroethylene). However, most volatiles are excreted unchanged in exhaled air, and thus, whole blood is the best sample in which to detect and identify these compounds.

Many volatiles are relatively stable in blood if simple precautions are taken. The tube should be as full as possible and should only be opened when required for analysis and then only when cold (4°C). An anticoagulant (lithium heparin or EDTA) should be used. If the sample volume is limited, it is advisable to select the container to match the volume of blood so that there is minimal headspace. Specimen storage between –5° and 4°C is recommended (52), and sodium fluoride (1% w/v) should be added to prevent microbial metabolism. In a suspected volatile substance abuse–related fatality, analysis of tissues (especially brain) may prove useful because high concentrations of volatile compounds may be present even if little is detectable in blood.

The value of attempting to measure blood concentrations of substances such as butane, which are gases at room temperature, is questionable, and, in most cases, qualitative identification is all that is needed. In general terms, blood concentrations of less volatile substances such as toluene of 10 to 20 mg/L and above can be associated with serious poisoning. In other words, the pharmacologically effective concentrations of volatile substances such as

TABLE 20. Some volatile substances that may be abused by inhalation

Hydrocarbons
- Aliphatic
  - Acetylene
  - Butane[a]
  - Isobutane (2-Methylpropane)[a]
  - Hexane[b]
  - Propane[a]
- Alicyclic/aromatic
  - Cyclopropane (trimethylene)
  - Toluene (toluol, methylbenzene, phenylmethane)
  - Xylene (xylol, dimethylbenzene)[c]
- Mixed
  - Petrol (gasoline)[d]
  - Petroleum ethers[e]
- Halogenated
  - Bromochlorodifluoromethane (FC 12B1)
  - Carbon tetrachloride (tetrachloromethane)
  - Chlorodifluoromethane (FC 22, Freon 22)
  - Chloroform (trichloromethane)
  - Dichlorodifluoromethane (FC 12, Freon 12)
  - Dichloromethane (methylene chloride)
  - 1,2-Dichloropropane (propylene dichloride)
  - Ethyl chloride (monochloroethane)
  - Halothane (2-bromo-2-chloro-1,1,1-trifluoroethane)
  - Tetrachloroethylene (perchloroethylene)
  - 1,1,1-Trichloroethane (methylchloroform, Genklene)
  - 1,1,2-Trichlorotrifluoroethane (FC 113)
  - Trichloroethylene (*trike*, Trilene)
  - Trichlorofluoromethane (FC 11, Freon 11)

Oxygenated compounds
- Butanone (2-butanone, methyl ethyl ketone)
- Butyl nitrite[f]
- Enflurane (2-chloro-1,1,2-trifluoroethyl difluoromethyl ether)
- Ethyl acetate
- Diethyl ether (ethoxyethane)
- Desflurane [(R,S)-difluromethyl-1,2,2,2-tetrafluoroethyl ether]
- Dimethyl ether (methoxymethane)
- Isobutyl nitrite (*butyl nitrite*)[f]
- Isoflurane (1-chloro-2,2,2-trifluoroethyl difluoromethyl ether)
- Isopentyl nitrite (3-methyl-1-butanol, isoamyl nitrite, *amyl nitrite*)[f,g]
- Methyl acetate
- Methyl isobutyl ketone (isopropyl acetone)
- Methyl *tert*-butyl ether
- Nitrous oxide (dinitrogen monoxide, *laughing gas*)
- Sevoflurane [fluoromethyl 2,2,2-trifluoro-1-(trifluoromethyl)-ethyl ether]

[a]Principal components of liquified petroleum gas.
[b]Commercial *hexane* mixture of hexane and heptane with small amounts of higher aliphatic hydrocarbons.
[c]Mainly *meta*-xylene (1,3-dimethylbenzene).
[d]Mixture of aliphatic and aromatic hydrocarbons with boiling range 40° to 200°C.
[e]Mixtures of pentanes, hexanes, and so forth with specified boiling ranges (e.g., 40° to 60°C).
[f]Abused primarily for its vasodilator properties.
[g]Commercial *amyl nitrite* mainly isopentyl nitrite but other nitrites also present.

many of those listed in Table 20 are similar to those of inhalational anesthetics (27,50) and are thus two or so orders of magnitude lower than those observed in poisoning with relatively water-soluble compounds such as ethanol (Table 13).

The alkyl nitrites, which are abused by inhalation [isobutyl nitrite, isopentyl (*amyl*) nitrite], are a special case. They are extremely unstable and break down rapidly *in vivo* to the corresponding alcohols. Furthermore, they usually contain other isomers (butyl nitrite, pentyl nitrite). Any products submitted for analysis usually contain the corresponding alcohols as well as the nitrites. Propanols and butanols may also arise, for example, by microbial action from normal blood constituents *in vitro* and thus caution is needed in the interpretation of results in cases in which these compounds are detected.

Trace Elements and Toxic Metals

Tests devised in the nineteenth century such as the Reinsch test for arsenic, antimony, bismuth, and mercury are still relevant for the rapid diagnosis of acute poisoning with these compounds. However, to help diagnose chronic poisoning, in which elevations of only a few μg/L of blood or serum can be important, good accuracy and reproducibility are essential (14,53). Sample contamination during collection (e.g., from sample tubes, or even from syringe needles in the case of chromium and manganese) and within the laboratory itself can be serious sources of error. This applies particularly to common elements such as lead and aluminum. Guidelines for sample collection have been given in Table 3. Modern methods for measuring toxic metals in biologic materials (Table 10) vary enormously in terms of complexity, cost, accuracy, and sensitivity. Atomic absorption spectrophotometry with either flame or electrothermal atomization using a graphite furnace is used widely. In the case of serum iron, however, reliable kits based on the formation of a colored complex are available.

Inductively coupled plasma mass spectrometry can detect and measure the various stable isotopes of a metal simultaneously. The relative abundance of the isotopes depends on the source of the metal. Therefore, by measuring the isotope ratios of an element such as lead in a sample from a chronically poisoned patient with those found in material present in the patient's immediate environment, it may be possible to localize the source of exposure (54). Ethnic cosmetics such as surma may contain from 0% to 80% elemental lead, and such products are becoming important causes of acute-on-chronic lead poisoning. So-called "traditional" medicines may also contain toxic doses of salts of lead or other heavy metals (14). Information to assist in the interpretation of results is available (55).

Quality Assurance

Quality assurance (QA) of toxicologic analyses is required not only in regards to results in particular patients, but also to validate data exchange between laboratories. External QA schemes for trace elements (14) and a number of TDM analytes have been operated for some time (56). QA of general toxicology analyses such as poisons screening is complex, but undoubtedly will assume greater importance as analytical standards rise. In analytical toxicology, it is important not only to avoid false-negatives but also to correctly identify any poisons found. Quantitative measurements should also be reliable. QA should begin with properly documented procedures within the laboratory itself, not only in regards to the analyses but also in regards to recording details of telephone calls and so forth.

The organization of QA schemes in analytical toxicology is a difficult area because the choice of appropriate samples and methodology, and correct interpretation of the results, is as important, in some cases perhaps more important, than numerical accuracy. For example, a laboratory using an immunoassay may achieve excellent reproducibility in an external QA scheme providing a synthetic sample containing the drug of interest. A second laboratory may achieve lower reproducibility using HPLC. However, the HPLC method differentiates the drug from a pharmacologically inactive metabolite that is present in real samples at similar concentrations to the parent compound and that cross-reacts in the immunoassay. The obvious answer (adding the metabolite to the QA sample) may not be possible because supplies of the metabolite are not available, whereas use of pooled patient material, if available in sufficient quantity, incurs extra costs because of precautions needed to guard against the risk of transmitting infection. Even then the patient material is likely to contain other compounds, and *spiked* or *weighed-in* values for the analytes (a further valuable parameter) are not available.

The United Kingdom National External Quality Assessment Scheme incorporates serum salicylates, paracetamol, and ethanol. The results of external QA schemes for drug abuse screening have been reported (57), and an attempt has been made to assign a numerical score to reports to facilitate performance assessment (58). There is scope for progress in this area, the nature of analytical toxicology suggesting that combined training/QA programs have the most impact. Ideally, appropriate samples together with a realistic case history should be submitted to test all aspects of laboratory operation (59,60).

Assessing the Role of the Analytical Toxicology Laboratory

In recent years, some authors have attempted detailed consideration of the role of the analytical toxicology laboratory in the diagnosis and management of poisoning (61–66). The symposium edited by Bailey (63) and the review by Dawling and Volans (66) give the most detailed overview of the operation and clinical role of such laboratories. Some other laboratory-based papers emphasize analytical results without reference to outcome (67). Comprehensive assessment of the role of the analytical toxicology laboratory has been undertaken recently, both in the United Kingdom and United States (68,69).

Many clinical papers appear to minimize the value of laboratory work. However, either they include many patients for whom the analytical work requested was unnecessary (70–74), or they lack any insight into the clinical value of the work performed (75). One factor neglected by authors from both sides of the debate, however, is the need for the laboratory to gain and maintain experience in detecting and identifying the drugs commonly and not so commonly encountered in particular types of patients in a particular geographic area, so that the laboratory performs properly when the really important cases come along.

In clinical poisons screening, the main aim is to detect central nervous system depressant drugs and those in which active treatment is indicated (Table 11). Normally, such analyses are performed to help diagnose the cause of serious, often potentially life-threatening conditions such as coma or convulsions (76). It may even be important to establish whether a clinical diagnosis of self-poisoning was correct in the face of denial by the patient. The diagnosis of unauthorized drug administration to children (Munchausen syndrome by proxy) (77) is a particularly specialized area with potentially far-reaching implications (78,79). Excluding the presence of centrally acting drugs such as barbiturates and benzodiazepines has important prognostic implications in suspected brain-stem death (a) if the presenting diagnosis was one of poisoning or poisoning is part of the differential diagnosis and (b) if centrally acting drugs have been given in treatment (80). Toxicologic analyses may also be important in establishing a diagnosis of Münchausen syndrome and in alleviating anxiety in patients who believe they have been poisoned by incidental exposure to, for example, pesticides even though no evidence exists for this belief (81).

SPECIALIZED CATEGORIES

Forensic Toxicology

Toxicologic investigations are often undertaken in murder investigations and in the investigation of other deaths (including deaths in the hospital and in road traffic accidents) in which there is a possibility that drugs or other poisons may have been involved. These include instances in which deliberate (self)-poisoning is a possibility, especially if death has occurred in children or while in police custody or when decomposition has taken place. Nonfatal incidents in which toxicologic investigations may be useful include collapse while in custody, alleged violations of impaired motor vehicle driver laws, allegations of poisoning of relatives or pets, doping in sex offenses, and other cases of assault. It may also be important to analyze samples from a suspect for the presence of drugs such as ethanol, which may have altered perception or behavior during the course of a crime.

The specimens available may range from fresh blood to decomposing tissues recovered from a partial skeleton, whereas the quantity available may range from a kilogram of liver to a dried bloodstain. Breath analysis was introduced in the United Kingdom for the detection of the intoxicated motorist in 1967, initially in the form of indicator tubes using oxidation methods, although now evidential breath ethanol instruments are used. A difficult area is screening for a wide range of compounds that could affect driving performance in, for example, 2 ml of whole blood, while leaving sufficient sample for a quantitative measurement. Here the high sensitivity of radioimmunoassay can often be used to great advantage, and a chromatographic method, frequently involving GC-MS, can be used for any subsequent identification and measurement.

The role of the Coroner in England and Wales and of the Procurator Fiscal in Scotland is primarily to exclude criminal acts as a possible cause of death. Data produced from such courts, however, may be invaluable in monitoring fatal poisoning (82). The importance of adequately documenting all acute poisoning incidents both in the hospital notes and in the laboratory records becomes clear when it is remembered that even an apparently trivial case may, in the end, be reviewed in detail in a coroner's court. Required documentation includes correctly recorded patient details and sample details, including date and time of collection of samples; details of physical examination in the case notes; nature and timing of treatment, particularly drug treatment; results of investigations (including units); and conversations with poisons information services and the laboratory. The laboratory should, of course, fully document all analyses and keep copies of all reports issued. Samples should be kept (–20°C) until the conclusion of the case.

In assessing the evidence of the analytical toxicologist, the courts are concerned especially with the experience of the analyst, the origin and condition of the samples, and the analytical methods used. In all cases, the ability to prove continuous and proper custody of the specimen is important. Normally, at least two unrelated analytical methods should be used before an identification is accepted. The results should be presented together with sufficient information to ensure accurate interpretation of the findings by a coroner, magistrate, judge, and jury. There is always the possibility of an independent examination by a further expert instructed by another party in the case.

Screening for Drugs of Abuse

The value of blood, breath, or urinary measurements in the diagnosis of ethanol abuse and in monitoring abstinence is clear. Screening for drugs of abuse in urine or other appropriate specimen is also valuable in monitoring illicit drug taking in dependent patients and guards against prescribing controlled drugs for patients who are not themselves dependent. These tests may also be valuable in the psychiatric assessment of patients presenting with no overt history of drug abuse. In addition, the diagnosis of maternal drug abuse, either during pregnancy or postpartum, can be important in the management of the neonate. The need for drug abuse screening of personnel in sensitive positions (armed forces, security services, pilots, drivers) or those applying for such positions (*employment* and *pre-employment* screening, respectively) has become accepted in recent years. The detection of illicit drug administration in sport has also assumed importance. In animal sports, the definition of an illicit compound is much easier than in man and can include any substance not normally derived from feedstuffs.

Urine is the specimen of choice in many cases, not only because the concentrations of the compounds of interest tend to be higher than in blood, but also because it is by far the easiest specimen to obtain. Moreover, human urine presents less of a hazard to laboratory staff than blood. The illicit drugs encountered in the United Kingdom include opiates, mainly heroin (diacetylmorphine); barbiturates; benzodiazepines (notably temazepam); cocaine; amphetamines including methylenedioxymethamphetamine (*ecstasy*); and cannabis. In the United States, abuse of cocaine either as the hydrochloride or as the free base (*crack*) is common, and a range of additional compounds may also be encountered, including dextropropoxyphene (propoxyphene), fentanyl, and phencyclidine (*angel dust*).

The purity of street drugs varies widely—heroin may be between 2% and 95% pure, for example. Overdosage either with excessively pure street drug or with drug *cut* with a particularly toxic compound is a further cause of acute poisoning epidemics. Barbiturates may be encountered, either as a result of abuse per se or when mixed with other substances such as heroin. Even compounds such as strychnine, lignocaine, quinine, and chloroquine (83) may be used to cut street drugs. Serious acute poisoning may also occur if tolerance has been reduced through abstinence. Methadone is widely used to treat opioid addiction. Other opioids such as codeine, dihydrocodeine, and pethidine also occur.

The availability of a variety of immunoassay kits (Table 19) has proved invaluable, especially in employment and pre-employment screening, when large numbers of negative results are to be expected and high sensitivity is required. However, TLC is still important because it can resolve controlled drugs—including morphine from opioids such as codeine or pholcodine—which are available without restriction. In addition, TLC is cost-effective and amenable to batch processing of samples. Capillary GC and gc-HS remain valuable in the detection of amphetamines and in the confirmation of TLC results (84).

Ingestion of laxatives and diuretics to produce weight loss is not uncommon and can be difficult to diagnose. Collection of serial urine samples over several days is advisable (85). Detection of the abuse of osmotic laxatives such as lactulose and bulk-formers such as bran is not possible analytically. The covert ingestion of anticoagulants is also well documented and can provide a difficult diagnostic problem (86).

Therapeutic Drug Monitoring

The measurement of plasma concentrations of therapeutic drugs is useful for a small number of compounds for which pharmacologic effect cannot be measured directly and for which the margin between adequate dosage and overdosage is small (Table 21). The

TABLE 21. Some commonly requested plasma/serum therapeutic drug monitoring assays and guidelines for interpretation of results

Group	Drug [metabolite]	Optimal range in an adult (mg/L)
Antiasthmatic	Caffeine	8–50 (neonatal apnea)
	Theophylline	10–20 (6–12 neonatal apnea)
Anticonvulsants	Carbamazepine	8–12 (single drug) 4–8 (multiple therapy)
	[Carbamazepine-10,11-epoxide]	[0.5–5.5][a]
	Clonazepam	0.01–0.07 (may be lower in adults)
	Ethosuximide	40–100
	Lamotrigine	1–4 (upper limit may be 10)
	Phenobarbitone	15–40 (10–25 children)
	Phenytoin	10–20 (lower limit may be 5 or less)
	Primidone	<12 (also measure phenobarbitone)
	Valproate	40–100 (upper limit uncertain)
	Vigabatrin	<45
Antimalarials	Chloroquine	<0.3[b]
	Hydroxychloroquine	<0.5[b]
	Quinine	8–16[b]
Antimicrobial	Chloramphenicol	Trough, <5; peak, 10–25
	Ethambutol	2.5–6.5
	Gentamicin	Trough, <1.5; peak, 4–10
	Kanamycin	Trough, <8; peak, <30
	Tobramycin	Trough, <2; peak, <12–15
	Vancomycin	Trough, 5–10; peak, 20–40
Antineoplastic	Methotrexate	<1.0 (2.2 μmol/L, 24 h post-dose) <0.45 (1 μmol/L, 48 h post-dose)
Cardioactive	Amiodarone	0.5–2.0
	[Desethylamiodarone]	0.5–2.0[a]
	Atenolol	0.2–1.0
	Digoxin	0.0005–0.0020[c]
	Disopyramide	2.0–5.0
	[Desalkyldisopyramide]	[<5.0][a]
	Flecainide	0.2–0.7
	Lidocaine	1.5–5.0
	Perhexiline	0.15–0.6
	Procainamide [+ acecainide[d]]	10–30 (procainamide only 4–8)
	Propafenone	0.1–1
	[5-Hydroxypropafenone]	0.1–1]
	Propranolol	0.01–0.10
	Quinidine	2–5
	Sotalol	0.8–2.0
	Verapamil	0.1–0.2
	[Norverapamil]	[0.1–0.2][a]
Immunosuppressive	Cyclosporin	0.15–0.25 (trough, whole blood)[e]
	Mycophenolic acid	2.5–4.0 (trough)
	Sirolimus	0.005–0.010 (trough, whole blood)
	Tacrolimus	0.01–0.02 (trough, whole blood)
Nonsteroidal antiinflammatory drugs	Salicylates	150–300 (same in children)
Psychoactive	Amitriptyline [+ nortriptyline]	0.08–0.25
	Clomipramine [+ norclomipramine]	<1.0[f]
	Clozapine	>0.35[f]
	Desipramine	0.08–0.16
	Dothiepin [+ nordothiepin]	<0.50[f]
	Doxepin [+ nordoxepin]	0.15–0.25
	Fluoxetine	0.04–0.45
	[Norfluoxetine]	[0.04–0.45]
	Fluvoxamine	0.16–0.22
	Imipramine [+ desipramine]	0.15–0.30
	Lithium	3.5–8.0 (0.5–1.2 mmol/L)
	Mianserin [+ normianserin]	0.03–0.10
	Nortriptyline	0.05–0.15
	Olanzapine	>0.025
	Trazodone	0.8–1.6
	Trimipramine [+ nortrimipramine]	<0.5[f]
	Sulpiride	0.3–0.5

[a]Ratio of metabolite to parent compound guide to duration of therapy and possibly to the likelihood of toxicity.
[b]Possibility of serious toxicity in noninfected subjects.
[c]Assay may be unreliable in some patient groups (e.g., neonates, renal failure, hepatic failure).
[d]N-Acetylprocainamide.
[e]Method dependent.
[f]Adverse effects at higher concentrations limit the dosage that can be tolerated.

availability of a variety of immunoassay and other kits means that many TDM assays can be performed more conveniently by such means than by chromatographic methods. However, chromatographic assays are still important in the case of amiodarone, in which it has proved impossible to produce an antibody that does not cross-react significantly with thyroxine and triiodothyronine, and in general in which active metabolites should be measured as well as the parent compound. Examples here include carbamazepine/carbamazepine-10,11-epoxide, procainamide/*N*-acetylprocainamide, and the tricyclic antidepressants. Aspects of TDM have been reviewed in several publications (87–89).

OCCUPATIONAL AND ENVIRONMENTAL TOXICOLOGY

The monitoring of occupational or environmental exposure to toxins is an important area of analytical toxicology. Metallic elements such as lead and also some organochlorine pesticides such as chlordane and dieldrin have long biologic half-lives, and thus accumulation can occur with prolonged exposure to relatively low concentrations. The manufacture of pharmaceuticals can also present a hazard to those involved via dermal or inhalational absorption (90,91). The abuse of alcohol and controlled drugs is also a subject of much current concern in occupational medicine, especially in regard to screening for drug or substance abuse amongst potential employees and, for example, operators of heavy machinery, pilots, and drivers (see Screening for Drugs of Abuse).

The control of exposure to toxic metals, volatile solvents, and some other poisons is an integral part of industrial hygiene and has been achieved, in part, by monitoring ambient air concentrations of the compound under investigation. However, an individual's work pattern and adherence to safety procedures may greatly influence exposure. *Biologic* monitoring involves blood, urinary, or breath concentrations of a compound or its metabolites to assess an individual worker's exposure. Moreover, skin absorption is obviously best monitored in this way. Some assays that have been found useful in monitoring occupational exposure are given in Table 22. Additional measurements have been considered (92).

The investigation of the accidental release of chemicals into the workplace or environment (so-called *chemical incidents*) is a topic of interest. Recent examples include the Bhopal disaster in India and the Camelford incident in the United Kingdom in which aluminum sulfate was accidentally added to the local drinking water supply (93). Toxicologic analyses can be valuable not only in providing evidence of the nature and magnitude of an exposure but also in demonstrating that no significant exposure has occurred thereby allaying public apprehension. Clearly, the early collection of appropriate biologic samples is essential. In the absence of information to the contrary, it is wise to collect 10 ml whole blood (2 × 5 ml EDTA) and at least 50 ml urine (no preservative) from possibly exposed individuals. Store the samples at 4°C or at –20°C until the appropriate analyses can be arranged. If the incident is investigated in retrospect, then early samples may exist in a local hospital laboratory.

One area that has been neglected somewhat is that of food-derived poisons. Botulinum toxin and other toxins of microbiologic origin are usually considered together with food poisoning. Poisoning from other naturally occurring toxins, which include atropine from *Atropa belladonna*, solanine from potatoes, and cyanide from *Cassava* and from apple pips, also occurs (94). Here, analysis of the foodstuff rather than biologic samples can be more helpful in establishing the diagnosis in individual patients. Acute pesticide poisoning also sometimes occurs after ingestion of contaminated produce, and again analysis of the foodstuff can be helpful (95).

TABLE 22. Biologic measurements valuable in occupational/environmental toxicology

Measurement (fluid)[a]	Indicator of exposure to:
5-Aminolevulinic acid (urine)[b]	Lead
4-Aminophenol (urine)	Aniline
Bromide (serum)	Organobromines[c]
Butoxyacetic acid (urine)	2-Butoxyethanol
Carboxyhemoglobin (whole blood)[b]	Carbon monoxide, dichloromethane
Ceruloplasmin (plasma)[b]	Copper
Cholinesterases (plasma and red cell)[b]	Organophosphorus and carbamate pesticides
2,5-Dichlorophenol (urine)	1,4-Dichlorobenzene
4-(1,1-Dimethylethyl)phenol (urine)	—
Dieldrin (plasma)	Aldrin (also dieldrin itself)
4,6-Dinitro-2-methylphenol	—
Ethoxyacetic acid (urine)	2-Ethoxyethanol, 2-ethoxyethyl acetate
Fluoride (blood and/or urine)	—
Hemoglobin (whole blood)[b]	Lead
Hexachlorobenzene	—
Hippuric acid (urine)	Toluene[d]
Lindane (plasma)	—
Mandelic acid (urine)	Ethylbenzene, styrene[e]
Metals/trace elements (blood and/or urine)[f]	—
N-Methylacetamide (urine)	*N,N*-Dimethylacetamide
4,4'-Methylenebis(2-chloroaniline) (urine)	—
4,4'-Methylenedianiline (urine)	—
N-Methylformamide (urine)	*N,N*-Dimethylformamide
Methylhippuric acids (urine)	Xylenes
2-Methylphenol (urine)	Toluene
4-Nitrophenol (urine)	Parathion
Pentachlorophenol (plasma or urine)	—
Phenol (urine)	—
Polychlorinated biphenyls (blood)	—
Solvents and other volatiles (blood, sometimes urine)[g]	—
2-Thiothiazolidine-4-carboxylic acid (urine)	Carbon disulfide
Trichloroacetic acid (urine)	Trichloroethylene[h]
2,2,2-Trichloroethanol (urine)	Trichloroethylene[h]
Trifluoroacetic acid (urine)	Halothane
Zinc protoporphyrin (blood)[b]	Lead

[a]If specific sample requirements are not known, collect 5 ml ethylenediaminetetraacetic acid blood or 10 ml clotted blood and 25 ml urine.
[b]See Clinical Laboratory Tests and the Poisoned Patient.
[c]Serum bromide concentrations indicative of excessive exposure to organobromines are lower than after use of inorganic bromide as an anticonvulsant.
[d]Not specific indicator of toluene exposure because dietary benzoate [used as a preservative in some drugs and foods (e.g., prawns)] also excreted as hippurate.
[e]Mandelic acid excretion impaired by ingestion of ethanol (96).
[f]See Table 3 for details of sample requirements.
[g]Mainly acetone, benzene, ethylbenzene, tetrachloroethylene, toluene, 1,1,1-trichloroethane, trichloroethylene, and the xylenes.
[h]Ingestion of chloral or triclofos also gives trichloroacetate and 2,2,2-trichloroethanol in urine.

ACKNOWLEDGMENTS

I thank Dr. S. S. Brown, Dr. R. A. Braithwaite, Dr. S. Dawling, Mr. I. House, and Mr. P. Streete for help and advice.

REFERENCES

1. Corry JEL. Possible sources of ethanol ante- and postmortem: its relationship to the biochemistry and microbiology of decomposition. *J Appl Bacteriol* 1978;44:1–56.
2. Borgå O, Piafsky KM, Nilsen OG. Plasma protein binding of basic drugs. I. Selective displacement from α_1-acid glycoprotein by tris(2-butoxyethyl) phosphate. *Clin Pharmacol Ther* 1977;22:539–544.

3. Shang-Qiang J, Evenson MA. Effects of contaminants in blood-collection devices on measurement of therapeutic drugs. *Clin Chem* 1983;29:456–461.
4. Streete PJ, Flanagan RJ. Ethylbenzene and xylene from Sarstedt Monovette serum gel blood collection tubes. *Clin Chem* 1993;39:1344–1345.
5. Wenning R. Potential problems with the interpretation of hair analysis results. *Forensic Sci Int* 2000;107:5–12.
6. Gibb KA, Yee AS, Johnston CC, et al. Accuracy and usefulness of a breath ethanol alcohol analyzer. *Ann Emerg Med* 1984;13:516–520.
7. Kurt TL, Anderson RJ, Reed WG. Rapid estimation of carboxyhaemoglobin by breath sampling in an emergency setting. *Vet Human Toxicol* 1990;32:227–229.
8. Rock GA, Decary F, Cole RS. Orange plasma from tanning capsules. *Lancet* 1981;i:1419–1420.
9. Bareford D, Cumberbatch M, Derrick Tovey L. Plasma discolouration due to sun-tanning aids. *Vox Sang* 1984;46:180–182.
10. Watson I, Proudfoot A. *Poisoning and laboratory medicine*. London: ACB Venture Publications, 2002.
11. Joyce SM, Potter R. Beer potomania: an unusual case of symptomatic hyponatremia. *Ann Emerg Med* 1986;15:745–747.
12. Linford SMJ, James HD. Sodium bicarbonate abuse: a case report. *Br J Psychiatr* 1986;149:502–503.
13. Lewis PJ, Lowing RK, Gompertz D. Automated discrete kinetic method for erythrocyte acetylcholinesterase and plasma cholinesterase. *Clin Chem* 1981;27:926–929.
14. Braithwaite RA, Brown SS. Clinical and sub-clinical lead poisoning: a laboratory perspective. *Human Toxicol* 1988;7:503–513.
15. Peterson JE. Modelling uptake, metabolism and excretion of dichloromethane by man. *Am Ind Hyg Assoc J* 1978;39:41–47.
16. Pierce JM, Nielsen MS. Acute acquired methaemoglobinaemia after amyl nitrite poisoning. *Br Med J* 1989;298:1566.
17. Demey H, Daelemans R, De Broe ME, et al. Propylene glycol intoxication due to intravenous nitroglycerin. *Lancet* 1984;i:1360.
18. Flanagan RJ. SI units: common sense not dogma is needed. *Br J Clin Pharmacol* 1995;39:589–594.
19. Bailey DN. Comprehensive toxicology screening: the frequency of finding other drugs in addition to alcohol. *Clin Toxicol* 1984;22:463–471.
20. Nice A, Leikin JB, Maturen A, et al. Toxidrome recognition to improve the efficiency of emergency urine drug screens. *Ann Emerg Med* 1988;17:676–680.
21. Wiley JF. Difficult diagnoses in toxicology: poisons not detected by the comprehensive drug screen. *Pediatr Clin North Am* 1991;38:725–737.
22. Jameson JS, Kapadia SA, Polson RJ, et al. Is oropharyngeal anaesthesia with topical lignocaine useful in upper gastrointestinal endoscopy? *Aliment Pharmacol Ther* 1992;6:739–744.
23. Dawling S, Flanagan RJ, Widdop B. Fatal lignocaine poisoning: report of two cases and review of the literature. *Human Toxicol* 1989;8:389–392.
24. Ashbourne JF, Olson KR, Khayam-Bashi H. Value of rapid screening for acetaminophen in all patients with intentional drug overdose. *Ann Emerg Med* 1989;18:1035–1038.
25. Lane EA, Guthrie S, Linnoila M. Effects of ethanol on drug and metabolite pharmacokinetics. *Clin Pharmacokinet* 1985;10:228–247.
26. Moffat AC, Osselton D, Widdop B, eds. *Clarke's analysis of drugs and poisons*, 3rd ed. London: Pharmaceutical Press, 2003.
27. Baselt RC. *Disposition of toxic drugs and chemicals in man*, 6th ed. Foster City, CA: Biomedical Publications, 2002.
28. Drayer DE. Pharmacologically active metabolites of drugs and other foreign compounds. Clinical, pharmacological, therapeutic and toxicological considerations. *Drugs* 1982;24:519–542.
29. Garattini S. Active drug metabolites. An overview of their relevance in clinical pharmacokinetics. *Clin Pharmacokinet* 1985;10:216–227.
30. Caccia S, Garattini S. Formation of active metabolites of psychotropic drugs: an updated review of their significance. *Clin Pharmacokinet* 1990;18:434–459.
31. Sue Y-J, Shannon M. Pharmacokinetics of drugs in overdose. *Clin Pharmacokinet* 1992;23:93–105.
32. Proudfoot AT, Stewart MJ, Levitt T, et al. Paraquat poisoning: significance of plasma paraquat concentrations. *Lancet* 1979;ii:330–332.
33. Smith DF. The stereoselectivity of drug action. *Pharmacol Toxicol* 1989;65:321–331.
34. Badock NR. Detection of poisoning by substances other than drugs: a neglected art. *Ann Clin Biochem* 2000;37:146–157.
35. Ojanperä I. Toxicological drug screening by thin-layer chromatography. *Trends Anal Chem* 1992;11:222–230.
36. Michaud JD, Jones DW. Thin-layer chromatography for broad spectrum drug detection. *Amer Lab* 1980;12:104–107.
37. Dawling S, Widdop B. Use and abuse of the Toxi-Lab TLC system. *Ann Clin Biochem* 1988;25:708–709.
38. Flanagan RJ, Ruprah M. HPLC measurement of chlorophenoxy herbicides, bromoxynil and ioxynil in biological specimens to aid the diagnosis of acute poisoning. *Clin Chem* 1989;35:1342–1347.
39. Braithwaite RA. Emergency analysis of paraquat in biological fluids. *Human Toxicol* 1987;6:83–86.
40. Braithwaite RA. Immunoassays—application to analytical toxicology. In: Townshend A, Worsfold P, Macrae R, et al., eds. *Encyclopedia of analytical science*. London: Academic Press, 1995.
41. Schroeder TJ, Tasset JJ, Otten EJ, et al. Evaluation of Syva EMIT toxicological serum tricyclic antidepressant assay. *J Anal Toxicol* 1986;10:221–224.
42. Dawling S, Ward N, Essex EG, et al. Rapid measurement of basic drugs in blood applied to clinical and forensic toxicology. *Ann Clin Biochem* 1990;27:473–477.
43. Flanagan RJ, Dawling S, Buckley BM. Measurement of ethylene glycol (ethane-1,2-diol) in biological specimens using derivatisation and gas-liquid chromatography with flame ionisation detection. *Ann Clin Biochem* 1987;24:80–84.
44. Jones AW, Nilsson L, Gladh Å, et al. 2,3-Butanediol in plasma from an alcoholic mistakenly identified as ethylene glycol by gas-chromatographic analysis. *Clin Chem* 1991;37:1453–1455.
45. Robinson CA, Scott JW, Ketchum C. Propylene glycol interference with ethylene glycol procedures. *Clin Chem* 1983;29:727.
46. Binder SR, Regalia M, Biaggi-McEachern M, et al. Automated liquid chromatographic analysis of drugs in urine by on-line sample cleanup and isocratic multi-column separation. *J Chromatogr* 1989;473:325–341.
47. Flanagan RJ. Gas chromatography in analytical toxicology: principles and practice. In: Baugh PJ, ed. *Gas chromatography—a practical approach*. Oxford: IRL Press, 1993:171–212.
48. Flanagan RJ. High performance liquid chromatography of psychotropic and related drugs. In: Holman RB, Cross AJ, Joseph MH, eds. *High performance liquid chromatography in neuroscience research*. Chichester: Wiley, 1993:321–356.
49. Flanagan RJ, Braithwaite RA, Brown SS, et al. *Basic analytical toxicology*. Geneva: World Health Organization, 1995.
50. Flanagan RJ, Ruprah M, Meredith TJ, et al. An introduction to the clinical toxicology of volatile substances. *Drug Safe* 1990;5:359–383.
51. Streete PJ, Ruprah M, Ramsey JD, et al. Detection and identification of volatile substances by head-space capillary gas chromatography to aid the diagnosis of acute poisoning. *Analyst* 1992;117:1111–1127.
52. Gill R, Hatchett SE, Osselton MD, et al. Sample handling and storage for the quantitative analysis of volatile compounds in blood: the determination of toluene by headspace gas chromatography. *J Analyt Toxicol* 1988;12:141–146.
53. Supraregional Assay Service Trace Element Laboratories. Available at: http://www.sas-centre.org.
54. Delves HT, Campbell MJ. Measurement of total lead concentrations and lead isotope ratios in whole blood by use of inductively coupled plasma source mass spectrometry. *J Anal Atomic Spectrometry* 1988;3:343–348.
55. Friberg F, Nordberg GF, Vouk VB, eds. *Handbook on the toxicology of metals*, 2nd ed. Vol. I, II. Amsterdam: Elsevier, 1986.
56. Wilson JF, Tsanaclis LM, Perrett JE, et al. Performance of techniques for measurement of therapeutic drugs in serum. A comparison based on external quality assessment data. *Ther Drug Monit* 1992;14:98–106.
57. Frings CS, White RW, Battaglia DJ. Status of drug abuse testing in urine: an AACC study. *Clin Chem* 1987;33:1683–1686.
58. Wilson F, Smith BL, Toseland PA, et al. Enteral quality assessment of techniques for the detection of drugs of abuse in urine. *Ann Clin Biochem* 1994;31:335–342.
59. Wilson JF, Toseland PA, Capps NE, et al. External quality assessment of laboratory performance in analysis of toxicological cases. *Forensic Sci Int* 2001;121:27–32.
60. Wilson J. External quality assessment schemes for toxicology. *Forensic Sci Int* 2002;128:98–103.
61. Hepler BR, Sutheimer CA, Sunshine I. The role of the toxicology laboratory in emergency medicine. *Clin Toxicol* 1982;19:353–365.
62. Hepler BR, Sutheimer CA, Sunshine I. Role of the toxicology laboratory in the treatment of acute poisoning. *Med Toxicol* 1986;1:61–75.
63. Bailey DN, ed. Emergency toxicology for the 80's. *J Analyt Toxicol* 1983;7:130–160.
64. Flanagan RJ, Widdop B. Clinical toxicology. In: Curry AS, ed. *Analytical methods in human toxicology*. Part 1. London: Macmillan, 1984;37–66.
65. Ray JE, Reilly DK, Day RO. Drugs involved in self-poisoning: verification by toxicological analysis. *Med J Aust* 1986;144:455–457.
66. Dawling S, Volans GN. Poisons. In: Noe DA, Rock RC, eds. *Laboratory medicine—the selection and interpretation of clinical laboratory studies*. Baltimore: Williams & Wilkins, 1993:580–617.
67. Jammehdiabadi M, Tierney M. Impact of toxicology screens in the diagnosis of a suspected overdose: salicylates, tricyclic antidepressants, and benzodiazepines. *Vet Human Toxicol* 1991;33:40–43.
68. National Poisons Information Service and Association of Clinical Biochemists. Laboratory analyses for poisoned patients: joint position paper. *Ann Clin Biochem* 2002;39:328–339.
69. Wu AH, McKay C, Broussard LA, et al. National academy of clinical biochemistry laboratory medicine practice guidelines: recommendations for the use of laboratory tests to support poisoned patients who present to the emergency department. *Clin Chem* 2003;49:357–379
70. Jacobsen D, Frederichsen PS, Knutsen KM, et al. Clinical course in acute self-poisonings: a prospective study of 1125 consecutive hospitalised adults. *Human Toxicol* 1984;3:107–116.
71. Rygnestad T, Berg KJ. Evaluation of benefits of drug analysis in the routine management of acute self-poisoning. *Clin Toxicol* 1984;22:51–61.
72. Rygnestad T, Aarstad K, Gustaffson K, et al. The clinical value of drug analyses in deliberate self-poisoning. *Human Exptl Toxicol* 1990;9:221–230.
73. Kellermann AL, Fihn SD, LoGerfo JP, et al. Impact of drug screening in suspected overdose. *Ann Emerg Med* 1987;16:1206–1216.

74. Mahoney JD, Gross PL, Stern TA, et al. Quantitative serum toxic screening in the management of suspected drug overdose. *Am J Emerg Med* 1990;8:16–22.
75. Taylor RL, Cohen SL, White JD. Comprehensive toxicology screening in the emergency department: an aid to clinical diagnosis. *Am J Emerg Med* 1985;3:507–511.
76. Helliwell M, Hampel G, Sinclair E, et al. Value of emergency toxicological investigations in differential diagnosis of coma. *BMJ* 1979;2:819–821.
77. Samuels MP, Southall D. Munchausen syndrome by proxy. *Br J Hosp Med* 1992;47:759–762.
78. Rogers D, Tripp J, Bentovim A, et al. Non-accidental poisoning: an extended syndrome of child abuse. *BMJ* 1976;i:793–796.
79. Flanagan RJ, Huggett A, Saynor DA, et al. Value of toxicological investigations in the diagnosis of acute drug poisoning in children. *Lancet* 1981;ii:682–685.
80. Conference of Medical Royal Colleges. Diagnosis of brain death. *BMJ* 1976;2:1187–1188.
81. Hutchesson EA, Volans GN. Unsubstantiated complaints of being poisoned: psychopathology of patients referred to the National Poisons Unit. *Br J Psychiatry* 1989;154:34–40.
82. Flanagan RJ, Rooney C. Recording acute poisoning deaths. *Forensic Sci Int* 2002;128:3–19.
83. O'Gorman P, Patel S, Notcutt S, et al. Adulteration of 'street' heroin with chloroquine. *Lancet* 1987;i:746.
84. Maurer HH. Role of gas chromatography-mass spectrometry with negative ion chemical ionization in clinical and forensic toxicology, doping control, and biomonitoring. *Ther Drug Monit* 2002;24:247–254.
85. de Wolff FA, Edelbroek PM, de Haas EJM, et al. Experience with a screening method for laxative abuse. *Human Toxicol* 1983;2:385–389.
86. O'Reilly RA, Aggeler PM. Covert anticoagulant ingestion: study of 25 patients and review of world literature. *Medicine* 1976;55:389–399.
87. Widdop B, ed. *Therapeutic drug monitoring*. Edinburgh: Churchill Livingstone, 1985.
88. Hallworth M, Capps N. *Therapeutic drug monitoring and clinical biochemistry*. London: ACB Venture Publications, 1993.
89. Gross AS. Best practice in therapeutic drug monitoring. *Br J Clin Pharmacol* 2001;52(Suppl 1):55–105.
90. Baxter PJ, Samuel AM, Aw TC, et al. Exposure to quinalbarbitone sodium in pharmaceutical workers. *Br Med J* 1986;292:660–661.
91. Turci R, Sottani C, Spagnoli G, et al. Biological and environmental monitoring of hospital personnel exposed to antineoplastic agents: a review of analytical methods. *J Chromatogr B* 2003;789:169–209.
92. Mendelsohn HL, Peeters JP, Normandy HJ, eds. *Biomarker and occupational health: progress and perspectives*. Washington, DC: Joseph Henry Press, 1995.
93. Murray V. General medical aspects of chemical incidents. *J Eur Urgences* 1993;6:118–123.
94. de Wolff FA. Nutritional toxicology: the significance of natural toxins. *Human Toxicol* 1988;7:443–447.
95. Stinson JC, O'Gharabhain F, Adebayo G, et al. Pesticide-contaminated cucumber. *Lancet* 1993;341:64.
96. Wilson HK, Robertson SM, Waldron HA, et al. Effect of alcohol on the kinetics of mandelic acid excretion in volunteers exposed to styrene vapour. *Br J Ind Med* 1983;40:75–80.

SECTION

8

Analytical and Forensic Toxicology

CHAPTER 81

Medicinal Chemistry and Toxicology

Robert B. Palmer

BASIC CONCEPTS IN CHEMISTRY

Chemistry is the basis of all life science and is key to the understanding of biology, pharmacology, and toxicology. Many chemical concepts, often not explicitly stated, underlie clinical toxicology. Terms like pK_a, for example, are frequently used without clear understanding. This chapter addresses these concepts for the readers' reference as they read other chapters.

Matter and Its States

All matter is composed of atoms. Matter occurs in three main physical states: solid, liquid, and gas. Interconversion between states is solely a physical change, meaning that the chemical composition of the substance is not altered by the change in physical state. Physical properties describe appearance, whereas chemical properties deal with the composition of a substance. Therefore, a physical change alters appearance only (e.g., solid crack cocaine being heated to become a liquid and then to the vapor that is inhaled), whereas a chemical change involves an alteration of the chemical composition of the material (e.g., the production of hydrogen sulfide when organic matter decays).

The form of matter is determined by the attractive forces between the atoms or molecules that make up the substance. These intermolecular forces include van der Waals forces, ionic forces, dipole-dipole and dipole-ion interactions, and hydrogen bonding. They hold the molecules together in a way that creates the visible appearance. For example, the atoms or molecules of a solid are held in a rigid crystalline lattice, whereas in a liquid, the bonds are less rigid.

Density is simply the mass of a substance per unit volume and is typically reported in units of g/ml. It is constant at any given temperature. It can be determined by weighing a measured volume of the substance. Frequently, clinical laboratories report a related quantity called *specific gravity*. *Specific gravity* is calculated by dividing the density of the substance by the density of a reference standard, typically water. At 20°C, the density of water is 1 g/ml, making the numeric portion of density and specific gravity the same. A key difference, however, is that whereas density has units of mass per volume, specific gravity has no units (i.e., g/L divided by g/L = unitless dimension).

Atomic Structure

An atom can be thought of as containing two general zones, the nucleus and its surrounding electron cloud. Three principal subatomic particles, protons, neutrons, and electrons, are distributed in a specific fashion within these two zones. The nucleus comprises little of the total atomic volume but contains most of the mass of the atom. It is composed of protons (+1 charge) and neutrons (0 charge) and has a net positive charge. In contrast, electrons (–1 charge) have a minimal amount of atomic mass and a net negative charge. Further, the electron cloud comprises most of the total volume of the atom.

The identity of an atom is defined by the number of protons it contains. In its neutral state, the number of protons equals the number of electrons. An alteration in the number of neutrons changes the mass of the atom but not its identity, resulting in isotopes. Protons and neutrons both have a mass of 1.67×10^{-24} g. The mass of an electron (9.11×10^{-28} g) is a small fraction of a proton or neutron.

The *atomic number* provides the identity of a given atom and is defined by the number of protons in the atom. The *mass number* is the sum of the number of protons and neutrons and defines the isotope of the atom. The isotopes of an atom are represented by ${}^{A}_{B}X$ where *A* is the mass number, *B* is the atomic number, and *X* is the atomic symbol. The number of excess or deficient electrons defines ionic charge. Charge is indicated by the oxidation number, which is superscripted after the atomic symbol.

Isotopes exist naturally for atoms. For example, ${}^{12}_{6}C$ (carbon-12) is the primary isotope of carbon and comprises 98.9% of all natural carbon. Two other isotopes, ${}^{13}_{6}C$ (which has one additional neutron) and ${}^{14}_{6}C$ (which has two additional neutrons), also exist in small amounts.

Though it is convenient to think of the overall picture of electrons as being an extranuclear cloud, a closer examination is warranted. Electrons are confined to discrete energy levels called *shells*. Each shell is described by a principal quantum number, N, which is an integer value beginning with 1, the level

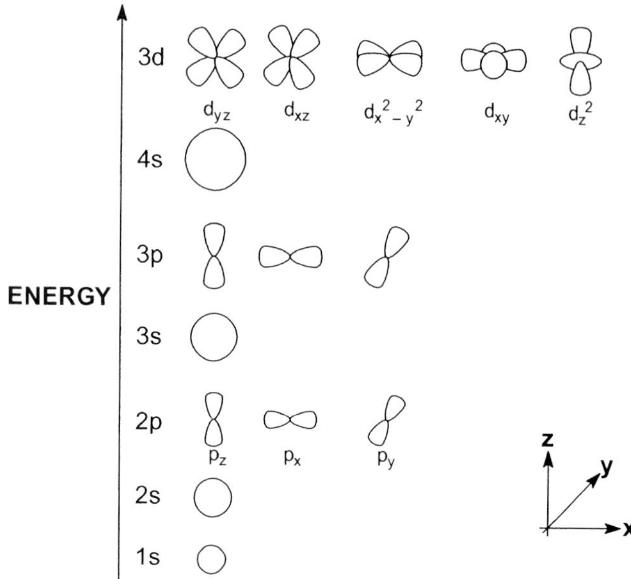

Figure 1. Shapes and relative energies of 1s through 4s atomic orbitals. Note that the 4s orbital is lower in energy than the 3d. The p_x, p_y, and p_z orbitals lie along the axes indicated by the subscript. The lobes of the d_{yz}, d_{xz}, and d_{xy} orbitals lie between the indicated axes, whereas those of the $d_{x^2-y^2}$ lie on the axes. The vertical lobe of the d_{z^2} orbital lies on the z-axis. The shapes of orbitals beyond d are more complicated.

closest to the nucleus. As a general rule, a given shell must be filled with electrons before filling to the next level.

Within each shell exist *subshells*, denoted with lowercase letters *s*, *p*, *d*, and *f* (Fig. 1). Within each subshell are the oribtals in which electrons reside. A given subshell contains a defined number of *orbitals*. An s subshell contains one orbital, a p subshell three orbitals, a d subshell five orbitals, and an f subshell seven orbitals. For convenience, the set of orbitals in a subshell is usually referred to by its *subshell designation*. The s orbital is spherical, and the p orbitals are a set of three dumbbell-shaped lobes.

Orbitals are not physical electron containment vessels; rather, they are mathematic probability maps describing the probable locations of electrons of a given energy. However, it is conceptually useful to think about the orbitals as electron containers. Any given orbital can hold a maximum of two electrons, though a subshell may contain multiple orbitals. In the spherical s orbital, only two electrons can be contained. However, the p subshell can hold six electrons because there are three orbitals, each with a capacity of two electrons.

When constructing an atom, a series of rules for electron addition is followed. Electrons are added to an orbital one at a time (the Aufbau principle), with a single electron being added to each orbital of a given subshell before any orbital has a second electron added (Hund's rule). When a second electron is added to an orbital, it must be of opposite spin (the Pauli exclusion principle). It is worth noting that electron spin is a quantum mechanical property, not a physical difference in polarity or direction of electron travel.

Electron spin plays a strong role in the reactivity of atoms and molecules. Spin is expressed as a quantum number of either plus one-half or minus one-half. The Pauli exclusion principle states that the total magnetic moment of the atom is zero if all electrons are spin-paired. Spin-paired electrons are said to be in a singlet state. If two electrons in an orbital are unpaired (i.e., have the same spin), the molecule is said to be in a triplet state. In a *free radical* (or simply, *radical*), one or more of the electrons is unpaired, resulting in a net magnetic moment and a reactive electron. Free radicals steal an electron from other atoms to resolve their own lack of paired electrons. Although this may satisfy the original radical, removal of an electron from the donor atom creates a new radical at the site of the electron abstraction. This high reactivity is the reason why free radicals are so physiologically damaging.

The outermost atomic shell contains the so-called *valence electrons*. These electrons are those most commonly involved in reactions, because they are farthest from the positively charged nucleus (i.e., they are less tightly held electrostatically) and are on the exterior "surface" of the electron cloud, making them accessible to other reactants.

Ions

Varying the number of electrons alters the atomic charge and creates an *ion*. A negatively charged atom or compound is an *anion*, whereas a positively charged entity is a *cation*. Charged particles do not passively cross membranes because membranes are nonpolar. Ions are active in a variety of biologic processes, however, and may cross membranes through ion channels.

When ions are quantitated in biologic fluids, they are often reported in units of mEq/L. The specific definition of an *equivalent* depends on the reaction taking place in the solution. This is done to account for the magnitude of the charge on each particle as well as its concentration. The current recommendation for reporting concentrations of medically important ions such as sodium, potassium, or chloride is to report them in terms of mmol/L rather than mEq/L because normality is no longer endorsed as an International System of Units unit. Nonetheless, many laboratories still report ion concentrations in terms of milliequivalents. The conversion between the milligram mass of charged particles and the same measurement in terms of milliequivalents must be done in two steps. First, the mass in milligrams is converted to millimoles of ion by multiplying by atomic mass. The number of millimoles is converted to milliequivalents by multiplying by the absolute value of the charge of the ion.

For example, to convert a concentration of 9.0 mg/dl to mEq/L, the following process is followed. First, mg/dl is converted to mg/L:

$$\frac{9.0\text{ mg}}{\text{dl}} \times \frac{10\text{ dl}}{\text{L}} = \frac{90\text{ mg}}{\text{L}}$$

Then, milligrams must be converted to millimoles using the atomic mass of Ca^{2+} (40.08 mg/mmol):

$$\frac{90\text{ mg}}{\text{L}} \times \frac{1\text{ mmol}}{40.08\text{ mg}} = \frac{2.246\text{ mmol}}{\text{L}}$$

Finally, millimoles can be converted to milliequivalents to yield the desired unit set of mEq/L:

$$\frac{2\text{mEq}}{1\text{ mmol}} \times \frac{2.246\text{ mmol}}{\text{L}} = \frac{4.492\text{ mEq}}{\text{L}}$$

Therefore, a calcium concentration of 9.0 mg/dl is equivalent to a calcium concentration of 4.5 mEq/L. Only two digits should be reported to adhere to the rules of significant figures.

Periodic Table

There are three basic classes of elements: metals, nonmetals, and metalloids. These classes are defined by their physical and chemical properties. *Metals* comprise the majority of elements and are located on the left and center of the Periodic Table (Fig. 2). Metals are malleable, ductile, and are efficient heat and electricity con-

Group[a]

Period	1	2	3	4	5	6	7	8	9	10	11	12	13	14	15	16	17	18
	IA	IIA	IIIB	IVB	VB	VIB	VIIB	-------	VIII	----	IB	IIB	IIIA	IVA	VA	VIA	VIIA	vIIIA
	1A	2A	3B	4B	5B	6B	7B		---		1B	2B	3A	4A	5A	6A	7A	8A
1	1 H 1.008																	2 He 4.003
2	3 Li 6.941	4 Be 9.012											5 B 10.81	6 C 12.01	7 N 14.01	8 O 16.00	9 F 19.00	10 Ne 20.18
3	11 Na 22.99	12 Mg 24.31											13 Al 26.98	14 Si 28.09	15 P 30.97	16 S 32.07	17 Cl 35.45	18 Ar 39.95
4	19 K 39.10	20 Ca 40.08	21 Sc 44.96	22 Ti 47.88	23 V 50.94	24 Cr 52.00	25 Mn 54.94	26 Fe 55.85	27 Co 58.47	28 Ni 58.69	29 Cu 63.55	30 Zn 65.39	31 Ga 69.72	32 Ge 72.59	33 As 74.92	34 Se 78.96	35 Br 79.90	36 Kr 83.80
5	37 Rb 85.47	38 Sr 87.62	39 Y 88.91	40 Zr 91.22	41 Nb 92.91	42 Mo 95.94	43 Tc (98)	44 Ru 101.1	45 Rh 102.9	46 Pd 106.4	47 Ag 107.9	48 Cd 112.4	49 In 114.8	50 Sn 118.7	51 Sb 121.8	52 Te 127.6	53 I 126.9	54 Xe 131.3
6	55 Cs 132.9	56 Ba 137.3	57 La* 138.9	72 Hf 178.5	73 Ta 180.9	74 W 183.9	75 Re 186.2	76 Os 190.2	77 Ir 190.2	78 Pt 195.1	79 Au 197.0	80 Hg 200.5	81 Tl 204.4	82 Pb 207.2	83 Bi 209.0	84 Po (210)	85 At (210)	86 Rn (222)
7	87 Fr (223)	88 Ra (226)	89 Ac** (227)	104 Rf (257)	105 Db (260)	106 Sg (263)	107 Bh (262)	108 Hs (265)	109 Mt (266)	110 --- ()	111 --- ()	112 --- ()		114 --- ()		116 --- ()		118 --- ()

* Lanthanide Series	58 Ce 140.1	59 Pr 140.9	60 Nd 144.2	61 Pm (147)	62 Sm 150.4	63 Eu 152.0	64 Gd 157.3	65 Tb 158.9	66 Dy 162.5	67 Ho 164.9	68 Er 167.3	69 Tm 168.9	70 Yb 173.0	71 Lu 175.0
** Actinide Series	90 Th 232.0	91 Pa (231)	92 U (238)	93 Np (237)	94 Pu (242)	95 Am (243)	96 Cm (247)	97 Bk (247)	98 Cf (249)	99 Es (254)	100 Fm (253)	101 Md (256)	102 No (254)	103 Lr (257)

Figure 2. The Periodic Table of the Elements. [a]Groups are noted by three notation conventions. (Courtesy of Los Alamos National Laboratory Chemistry Division.)

ductors. Metals tend to lose electrons, become cations, and are most soluble in an acidic environment. *Nonmetals* reside toward the upper right of the Periodic Table and generally lack the characteristics of metals. Additionally, nonmetals tend to gain electrons and become anions when ionized. *Metalloids* are located in between the metals and nonmetals on the Periodic Table and occur in portions of groups IIIA to VIIA. Metalloids have properties of both metals and nonmetals.

The Periodic Table is divided into columns called *groups* and rows called *periods*. With each addition of an electron into the valence shell plus a proton and neutron to the nucleus, the atomic number is increased by one. This process continues, left to right, across a period until the valence shell is filled and the number of protons equals the number of electrons.

The main divisions of the groups of the Periodic Table are A, B, and O. The A elements are those with a valence shell containing eight electrons. The group B elements (also called *transition elements*) contain d subshells with five degenerate orbitals and can therefore accept an additional ten electrons. The Actinide and Lanthanide series have f subshells that contain seven orbitals with a capacity for 14 additional electrons. The presence of d and f orbitals is largely responsible for the unique trends in reactivity of the group B elements.

Three of the group A families have special names. These are the alkali metals (group IA), alkaline earth metals (group IIA), and the halogens (group VIIA). The group O elements (also sometimes called *group VIIIA*) are called the *Noble Gases*. The alkali and alkaline earth metals (groups IA and IIA) both ionize by losing electrons to form stable monovalent and divalent cations, respectively. Whereas the ions of group IA elements such as Na and K are essential for life functions, in their elemental form, they react violently with water to form their ions. Group VIIA, the halides, gains one electron to form stable monovalent anions. The most stable nonionic form of the halides is as a diatomic molecule. The Noble Gases (group O or group VIIIA) typically exist in a stable monoatomic state.

Polarity—Stability, Polarity, Reactivity

Chemical and physical properties, including lipophilicity and reactivity, are related to electron distribution. It is important to realize that atomic radius increases with progression to the right and down the Periodic Table. As positive charge is contained in the nucleus of the atom, increasing atomic radius results in the negatively charged electrons being further from the positive center and generally held less tightly.

The most stable electron configuration of an atom is that having the outermost electron shell completely filled. For hydrogen and helium, which have only an s orbital, that full complement of electrons is two. The other group A elements follow the *octet rule*, which states that the closer they come to having eight electrons in the outermost (valence) shell, the more stable they are. For an atom such as sodium to achieve its most stable configuration (e.g., eight electrons in the valence shell), it must either gain seven electrons or lose one. Clearly, the path of least resistance is loss of one electron to form a monovalent cation. In contrast, it is far easier for chlorine to gain one electron resulting in a stable monovalent anion than to lose seven electrons. Other atoms, such as carbon, are intermediate and do not form particularly stable anions or cations.

From the principle of ionic stability follows the concept of *electronegativity*. It is simplest to think of electronegativity in an anthropomorphic context—that is, those atoms that "like" electrons versus atoms that do not. In this sense, atoms that tend to accept electrons to attain a more stable configuration are said to be more electronegative. Electronegativity is a crucial concept. In general, electronegativity increases to the right and up in the Periodic Table, making fluorine (electronegativity = 4) the most electronegative atom. Differences in electronegativity between the two atoms involved in any chemical bond dramatically influence the type of bond formed. The type of bond, in turn, affects the reactivity (stability) of the bond.

Chemical bonds are composed of two electrons residing in overlapping orbitals. However, there is not necessarily an equal distribution of these two electrons in a bond. Consider two atoms with dramatically different electronegativities—sodium and chloride. The more electronegative atom, chloride anion (Cl^-, electronegativity = 3.0), donates both electrons required for the chemical bond, whereas the sodium cation (Na^+, electronegativity = 0.9) contributes none. This results in a relatively strong electrostatic attraction called an *ionic bond*. In contrast, two atoms with similar electronegativity, carbon (electronegativity = 2.5) and hydrogen (electronegativity = 2.1), each donate one of the required electrons to the bond and share the two electrons equally. This is the stable *covalent bond*.

When two atoms have moderate differences in electronegativity, such as carbon and chlorine, each atom contributes one electron to the bond, but the electron density on the bond (i.e., the amount of time electrons spend around one atom versus the other) is not equivalent. The electrons have a statistically greater residence time near the more electronegative atom, in this case the chlorine. Those valence electrons not involved in bonding form a cloud about the atoms of the molecule. This electron cloud is distorted such that there is a greater amount of electron density around the more electronegative atom. This unequal distribution of electrons both in the bond and the valence cloud induces partial charges. These partial charges give the bond or molecule a set of electrical poles imparting a property known as *polarity*. The partial positive and partial negative character of these bonds is denoted with the symbols δ^+ and δ^-, respectively. Partial charges are important, affecting important biologic processes such as penetration of the blood–brain barrier, degree of water solubility, and drug-receptor binding. For example, in addition to the ionic full positive charge of the trimethylammonium portion of acetylcholine, this molecule also has a polar bond between the carbonyl carbon (δ^+) and the carbonyl oxygen (δ^-) (Fig. 3). When acetylcholine binds to acetylcholine esterase, the δ^- of the hydroxyl oxygen of the serine-200 residue in the active site is attracted to the carbonyl carbon. At the same time, the ionic attraction between the negatively charged glutamate-237 residue and the acetylcholine ammonium nitrogen holds the neurotransmitter in the active site of the enzyme.

Oxidation-Reduction

The principle of reduction and oxidation (called *redox*) is often misunderstood. The origin of the terms is that an oxidation increases the oxidation number, whereas a reduction decreases (reduces) the oxidation number of an atom. The basis of this type of reaction is, once again, the electron. An *oxidation* is sim-

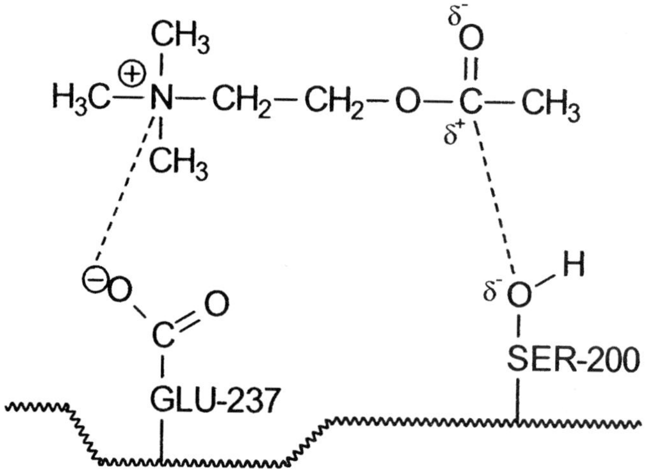

Figure 3. Acetylcholine binding to its receptor site in acetylcholine esterase, showing the ionic attraction between glutamic acid-237 (GLU-237) and the ammonium nitrogen, as well as the dipole-dipole attraction between the hydroxyl of serine-200 (SER-200) and the carbonyl carbon of acetylcholine.

ply a decrease in the number of electrons, whereas a *reduction* is an increase in the number of electrons.

Due to the law of conservation of matter, oxidation and reduction are inextricably linked. If one species is oxidized, another is necessarily reduced, as electrons can be neither created nor destroyed. For example, an increase in the number of oxygen atoms or decrease in the number of hydrogen atoms bonded directly to the atom in question are both oxidations. If a carbon-carbon double or triple bond is converted to a single bond, a reduction has taken place. Likewise, if the oxidized form of nicotinamide adenine dinucleotide is converted to the reduced form of nicotinamide adenine dinucleotide, an electron has been added, meaning a reduction has taken place. Other examples of oxidations are the production of carbon monoxide from incomplete combustion of hydrocarbons, the conversion of ferrous iron to ferric iron in methemoglobinemia, phase I metabolic *N*-dealkylations by P450 enzymes, and the metabolic production of acid metabolites from the toxic alcohols.

Equilibrium/Le Chatelier's Principle

Many chemical reactions proceed until all of the starting materials are consumed and converted to products with no back-conversion to starting materials. These reactions are said to go to *completion*. Not all reactions go to completion. Some attain a state of *equilibrium*, which is the point at which the concentrations of reactants no longer change with time.

Any chemical reaction in a closed system necessarily reaches equilibrium. The position of the equilibrium is often not precisely the midpoint of the reaction. The relative concentrations of reactants and products may be vastly different. The equilibrium may strongly favor the reactants (left side of the equation) or the products (right side of the equation). Anytime the reaction equilibrium is perturbed, the position of the equilibrium adjusts to reestablish equilibrium. The guiding precept for qualitative understanding of equilibrium dynamics is Le Chatelier's principle: If a system at equilibrium is disturbed, the position of the equilibrium shifts in whichever direction reduces that change (reestablish equilibrium).

Equilibrium can also be described quantitatively through calculation of the *equilibrium constant*, K_{eq}. This constant is calculated by dividing the product of the molar concentrations of the products raised to their stoichiometric coefficient powers by the product of the molar concentrations of the reactants raised to their respective stoichiometric coefficient powers.

$$aA + bB \rightleftharpoons yY + zZ$$

$$K_{eq} = \frac{[Y]^y\,[Z]^z}{[A]^a\,[B]^b}$$

The basis for this constant is the *law of mass action*: In a closed system, the ratio of product concentrations to reaction concentrations is constant. This law governs both solution and gas phase equilibria. Regardless of reactant concentrations, there exists a single equilibrium constant for a given reaction at a given temperature.

The use of the equilibrium constant is that it allows prediction of whether a given reaction at equilibrium favors formation of products (K_{eq} >1) or remaining as reactants (K_{eq} <1). Though the position of the equilibrium can be predicted by K_{eq}, the time required for a reaction to achieve equilibrium is unrelated to the magnitude of K_{eq}. That is, K_{eq} demonstrates relative stability between reactants and products, whereas the time required to go from reactants to products is a function of reaction rate. Figure 4 illustrates this by showing that the energy of water is far lower than that of hydrogen peroxide, so the equilibrium lies far to the right, favoring formation of water (i.e., K_{eq} >1). However, the rate of the reaction is dependent on overcoming the energy barrier, E_a, the magnitude of which is not addressed by the equilibrium constant.

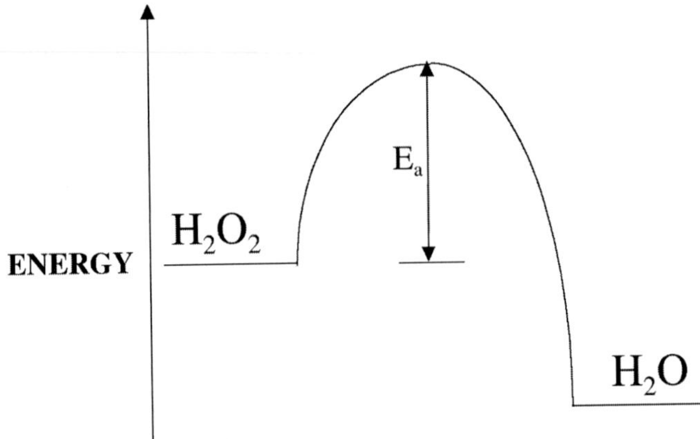

Figure 4. The reaction coordinate diagram for hydrogen peroxide (H_2O_2) becoming water (H_2O). Because water is lower in energy than hydrogen peroxide, K_{eq} >1. This indicates that the reaction equilibrium lies to the right, the extent of which is determined by the difference in energy between the products and reactants. However, the rate at which this reaction occurs is determined by how quickly the activation energy (E_a) can be overcome.

Acid-Base Chemistry

Typically, when one thinks of acids and bases, protons (H^+) are considered the medium of exchange. The greater the concentration of protons, the more acidic the solution. This concept comes from the classic example of an acid (HA) dissociating into a proton (H^+) and its conjugate base (A^-):

$$HA \rightleftharpoons H^+ + A^-$$

An acid-base reaction in which a proton is the medium of exchange is called a *Brønsted-Lowry reaction*. A Brønsted-Lowry acid is an entity capable of donating a proton, whereas a Brønsted-Lowry base is an entity capable of accepting a proton.

There is another theory of acid-base chemistry, named the *Lewis acid-base theory*, which describes acid-base reactions in terms of electrons instead of protons. A Lewis acid is any entity capable of accepting an electron, whereas a Lewis base is any entity capable of donating electrons (Fig. 5). A Lewis acid has an open orbital allowing acceptance of the electron(s) donated by the Lewis base. An example of a Lewis acid-base reaction is chelation of a metal. The metal is the Lewis acid (i.e., has an open orbital), whereas the chelating agent has lone pairs of electrons capable of being donated into the open metal orbital and is therefore the Lewis base. The electrons are shared, but the bond is not fully covalent.

Acidity is measured using the *pH scale*; pH is the negative log of hydrogen ion activity [H^+]. The activity of H^+ is closely approximated by the [H^+]. Because concentration is more easily measured than activity, pH is often described as the negative log of hydrogen ion concentration. The negative log relationship is the reason that the greater the [H^+], the lower the pH. Because the concentrations measured are small, the pH scale uses a logarithmic scale. It is important to remember that the scale is logarithmic, meaning that an increase of one unit in the pH scale represents a tenfold decrease in acidity. Only aqueous solutions can be described using pH. A solution in an organic solvent does not have a pH.

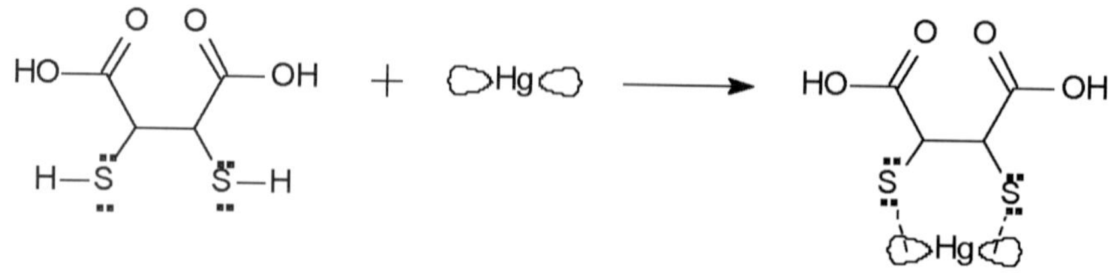

Figure 5. Chemical structures of Lewis base 2,3-dimercaptosuccinic acid (succimer) with Lewis acid Hg^{2+} (shown with vacant orbitals). The chelate is formed by the Lewis acid-base interaction between the two entities.

A great deal of confusion arises from the descriptive terms *strong* and *weak* acids and bases. These adjectives refer only to the extent to which a given acid or base ionizes. The ionization reaction of a strong acid or base goes to completion, whereas that of a weak acid or base does not. The strength of an acid or base has little to do with corrosive or caustic potential.

The extent to which a weak Brønsted-Lowry acid dissociates is described by the equilibrium equation for the reaction. As with any equilibrium equation, there exists a unique constant (K_{eq}) describing the position of the equilibrium, which is calculated as noted previously. In the description of a Brønsted-Lowry acid-base equation, the equilibrium constant is renamed the *acid dissociation constant*, K_a, though it is calculated the same way. Once again, the concentrations of these acids are often small and inconvenient. Therefore, the negative log relationship is also applied to K_a (same as pH), resulting in a new quantity, pK_a, which is useful in describing the ability of a specific proton to dissociate. The negative log relationship once again mandates that a more ionizable proton has a lower pK_a (i.e., is more acidic) than a proton with a larger pK_a. This concept is discussed in greater detail later in this chapter.

Vapor Pressure

There is a key distinction between *vapor* and *gas*. For a substance to be a vapor, it must reside immediately above a liquid pool of the same substance. In contrast, a gas such as nitrogen gas does not exist only above a pool of liquid nitrogen (lest our feet get cold). *Vapor pressure* is the force exerted by a vapor against its containment vessel. The more molecules that are liberated from the liquid into the vapor, the greater the force exerted against the container and, therefore, the greater the vapor pressure. Volatile compounds (e.g., toluene) have a high vapor pressure, whereas nonvolatile compounds have a low vapor pressure.

Vapor is created when the kinetic energy of individual molecules or atoms exceeds the strength of the intermolecular forces holding them together. Vapor is the result of some of the molecules in the liquid phase breaking the intermolecular attractions and being liberated (volatilized) into a gas above the liquid. Molecular kinetic energy is dependent on temperature but not on pressure. Therefore, as long as the temperature is held constant, the vapor pressure of a given substance at sea level is exactly the same as it is at the summit of Mount Everest.

With respect to toxicology, something with a low vapor pressure cannot be smoked. In general, ionic compounds (salts) have low vapor pressures and cannot burn (e.g., NaCl, table salt). Similarly, the salt of cocaine (cocaine HCl) does not melt and volatilize. An exception to this rule is *ice* (methamphetamine HCl). Due to the uniquely high vapor pressure of this salt, it can be smoked.

ORGANIC AND MEDICINAL CHEMISTRY

All life is based on the element carbon, and organic chemistry involves understanding the chemistry of carbon-based compounds. Medicinal chemistry is the study of the organic chemistry of drugs and their actions. Medicinal chemistry is an important aspect of toxicology, as it describes toxic as well as therapeutic effects in carbon-based systems.

Chemistry of Carbon

Carbon is a unique element in its ability to form a nearly infinite array of three-dimensional molecular forms. A carbon can covalently bond four substituents. If this carbon is bonded directly to one other carbon, it is called a *primary carbon*, and if bonded directly to two other carbons, it is *secondary*. Keeping with this theme, a carbon bonded directly to three or four other carbons is classified as *tertiary* or *quaternary*, respectively.

The overall geometry of the molecule depends partly on hybridization of the carbon atom and also on the electronic and spatial requirements of the attached substituents. Hybridization is a method for describing the shape of a carbon atom as well as its reactivity. Recall that electrons reside in orbitals, and carbon has two types of orbitals (s and p) to accommodate its six electrons (Fig. 1). Four of the six electrons are valence electrons. The distribution of the valence electrons is initially expected to be two electrons in the 2s orbital and one each in two of the three 2p orbitals. This would make the electrons in the p orbitals higher in energy than those in the s orbitals. However, it is known that all four valence electrons in carbon are degenerate (i.e., of the same energy). The s and p orbitals of carbon are mathematically "mixed" to form four degenerate "sp^3" *hybrid orbitals*, which adopt a tetrahedral geometry (Fig. 6). By varying the relative ratios of "s" and "p" orbitals in the mathematic mixing, "sp^2" and "sp" hybrids are created, which form double and triple bonds, respectively.

A carbon-carbon single bond whose two electrons come one each from the carbon atoms is a stable (i.e., nonreactive) bond known as a *σ-bond*. Carbon-carbon bonds can also be double or triple bonds. The geometric constraints of orbitals preclude the existence of carbon-carbon quadruple bonds. Multiple bonds contain one σ-bond (end-on overlap of hybrid orbitals) with the rest being two-electron π-bonds (lateral overlap of unhybridized p orbitals). Bond length decreases in going from carbon-carbon single to double to triple bonds; chemical and metabolic reactivity increases due to the π-electrons being less tight than the electrons in the σ-bond.

Functional Groups

The term *functional group* is used to define chemically distinct portions of a molecule on a carbon skeleton. Anything other than an sp^3 hybridized (aliphatic) carbon bearing a hydrogen atom is considered a functional group. Heteroatoms, carbon-carbon multiple bonds, and aromatic rings are all examples of functional groups. From a physiologic or metabolic standpoint, functional groups are the reactive "handles" where metabolic transformations take place. An abbreviated list of functional groups is given in Table 1.

Key to the understanding of functional groups is the classification of groups such as alcohols and amines. Much like carbon atoms, alcohols (an –OH hydroxy functional group) can be primary, secondary, or tertiary. A *primary* alcohol is simply a com-

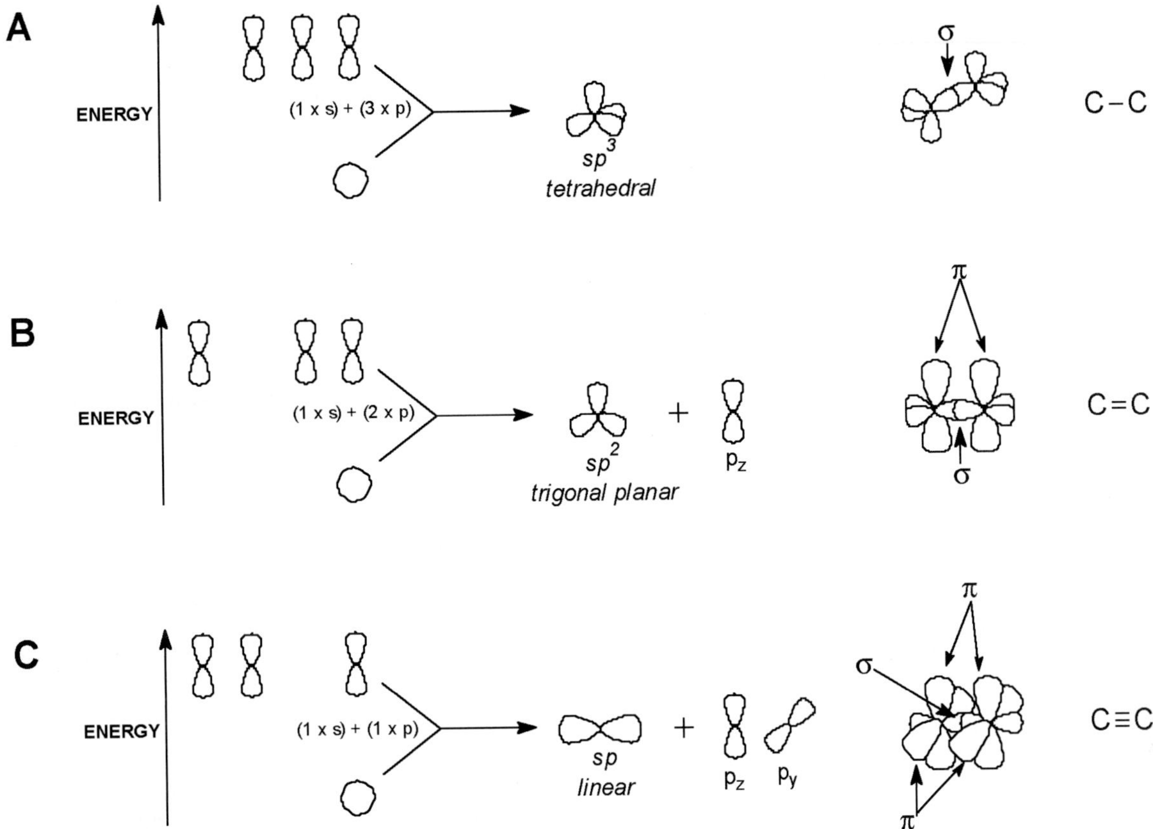

Figure 6. Hybridization of carbon. **A:** Formation of sp^3 hybrid from a single s orbital plus three p orbitals. Carbon-carbon single bonds are formed from sp^3 hybridized carbon atoms. **B:** Formation of sp^2 hybrid from a single s orbital plus two p orbitals. Carbon-carbon double bonds are formed from sp^2 hybridized carbon atoms. **C:** Formation of sp hybrid from a single s orbital plus a single p orbital. Carbon-carbon triple bonds are formed from sp hybridized carbon atoms.

pound in which the carbon bearing the hydroxy group is bonded to only one other carbon. Alcohols in which the carbon bearing the hydroxy group is bonded to two or three other carbons are designated *secondary* and *tertiary*, respectively. A *glycol* is a compound with one hydroxy group on each of two adjacent carbons. The classification of the alcohol determines its ability to be oxidized. For example, a primary alcohol (e.g., ethylene glycol, $HOCH_2CH_2OH$) can be metabolically oxidized from the alcohol through the aldehyde to the carboxylic acid resulting in metabolic acidosis. However, a secondary alcohol such as isopropanol ($H_3CCHOHCH_3$) is oxidized only once to the ketone (acetone), which is not acidic and does not contribute to metabolic acidosis. A tertiary alcohol such as *t*-butanol cannot be oxidized and therefore does not cause acidosis.

Amines can be primary, secondary, tertiary, or quaternary depending on how many substituents are bonded to the nitrogen atom. All but the quaternary form are electrically neutral. A quaternary amine bears a positive charge. This charge can prevent passage of the molecule across a membrane barrier. For example, physostigmine is a tertiary amine (uncharged) and therefore readily crosses the blood–brain barrier, whereas pyridostigmine is a quaternary amine that bears a positive charge and therefore does not (Chapter 10).

Electronic distribution in functional groups is also key to understanding their reactivity. For example, a carbonyl (C=O) is quite polar. The majority of the electron density resides around the oxygen atom, leaving a relative partial positive charge on the carbon (i.e., a so-called *electrophilic carbon*). Therefore, species with a negative charge or substantial negative character (nucleophiles) attack at the carbon atom rather than at the oxygen. Common nucleophiles include the lone pairs on amines, alcohols and thiols, and anions such as hydroxide. The conjugation of reduced glutathione (the nucleophile) with *N*-acetylparabenzoquinoneimine (the electrophile) is an example of a nucleophile attacking an electrophile (Fig. 7) (Chapter 145).

Resonance and Aromaticity

In σ-bonds, the electrons are held tightly in place. However, the electrons in π-bonds are less tightly held and therefore are more available for reaction but also for movement within the molecule itself. If there are p orbitals on adjacent bonded carbons, the orbitals have lateral overlap. Every overlapping p orbital is a place where the π-electrons can travel, meaning the movement of π-electrons may be extensive within the molecule. This free movement of the π-electrons is called *resonance*. The greater the degree of resonance, the more stable the molecule, because the electron charges are not isolated on a single atom but are now spread over a large portion of the molecule. The normally reactive π-electrons are also no longer isolated in a single bond but are now delocalized throughout the area of resonance. The additional stabilization energy imparted on a molecule as a result of resonance is known as *resonance stabilization energy* (Fig. 8).

Another type of molecular stabilization related to resonance is *aromaticity*. Aromaticity refers to a conjugated cyclic system with a greater-than-expected stability. For example, though benzene is often drawn as a cyclic triene with alternating single and double bonds, the compound actually has six carbon-carbon bonds of equal

TABLE 1. Organic functional groups

Functional group name	Structure
Alcohols	
Primary alcohol	R—OH
Secondary alcohol	OH | R—CH—R'
Tertiary alcohol	OH | R—C—R" | R'
Aldehyde	O ‖ R—C—H
Alkane	| | —C—C— | |
Alkene	\ / C=C / \
Alkyne	—C≡C—
Amide	O R' ‖ / R—C—N \ R"
Amines	
Primary amine	R / H—N̈ \ H
Secondary amine	R / H—N̈ \ R'
Tertiary amine	R / R"—N̈ \ R'
Carbamate	R O \ ‖ N—C—O—R" / R'
Carboxylic acid	O ‖ R—C—OH
Ester	O ‖ R—C—O—R'
Ether	R—O—R'
Ketone	O ‖ R—C—R'
Nitrile	R—C≡N
Thioether	R—S—R'

length. These bonds are 1.40 Å in length, midway between the lengths of a carbon-carbon single (1.48 Å) and double (1.32 Å) bonds. The calculated thermodynamic heat of atomization of benzene is less than the equivalent molecule without double bonds (C_6H_6). This additional stability is a result of benzene's aromaticity (Fig. 8).

Di-substituted benzenes have a unique naming convention. Specific relative positions of substituents on a benzene ring can be stated as being *ortho-*, *meta-*, or *para-* to one another. *Ortho-* substituents are attached to adjacent carbons; *meta-* substituents are separated by one carbon; and *para-* substituents are separated by two carbons, directly across from one another (Fig. 8).

Stereochemistry

More than one structure can be constructed from a single molecular formula. Compounds meeting this criterion are called *isomers*. Two principal classes of isomers exist, *constitutional isomers* and *stereoisomers*. Constitutional isomers are based on varying the basic connectivity of the atoms in structures with the same molecular formula. Categories of constitutional isomers include structural and functional group isomers. An example of constitutional isomers is the pair 2-methylpropane and butane, which both correspond to a molecular formula of C_4H_{10}. Functional group isomers are isomers that contain different functional groups such as allyl alcohol and methyl vinyl ether, both of which have the molecular formula C_3H_6O.

Stereoisomers differ from constitutional isomers in that they involve three-dimensional molecular structure at a given sp^3 carbon atom. The four groups covalently σ-bonded to an sp^3 hybridized carbon do not interchange. Rather, they are held rigidly in their respective bonded positions. If the sp^3 hybridized carbon possesses four different groups bonded to that carbon and has no plane of symmetry, that carbon becomes a stereocenter. When a stereocenter is present, a set of nonsuperimposable mirror images called *enantiomers* results. A compound that contains a stereocenter is said to be *chiral*. Of greatest significance with respect to enantiomers in biologic systems, one enantiomer may fit a given receptor, whereas the other does not. In some cases, one enantiomer may be an agonist, whereas the other enantiomer does not even fit the same receptor. This is the case with (–)-levorphanol and its (+)-methoxy derivative, dextromethorphan (Fig. 9). The (–)-levorphanol effectively binds the μ-opioid receptor, whereas (+)-dextromethorphan binds the antitussive receptor but does not bind the opioid receptor.

A chiral compound rotates plane polarized light by a specific amount measured in degrees from the vertical plane. This principle is called *optical isomerism* and explains why enantiomers are also known as *optical isomers* (Fig. 9). The only difference in physical properties between two enantiomers is the direction in which they rotate plane polarized light. All other properties including boiling point, melting point, density, energy, and magnitude (though not direction) of optical rotation are identical for the two enantiomers.

There exist three generally accepted methods for the designation of stereoisomers. These are the optical rotation method, the Cahn-Ingold-Prelog method, and the Fisher method. The optical rotation method is experimentally based and looks only at the direction of rotation of plane polarized light by enantiomers. Enantiomers are designated as either (+) or (–) based on the experimentally observed direction of plane polarized light rotation when this light is passed through an enantiomerically pure solution of the compound. By definition, the (+) isomer rotates plane polarized light to the right, is also called *dextrorotatory*, and is abbreviated *d-*. The other enantiomer, which rotates plane polarized light to the left, is designated *levorotatory* and abbreviated *l-*. Note that these abbreviations are lowercase letters.

Figure 7. Abbreviated scheme of acetaminophen metabolism. Reduced glutathione acts as a nucleophile attacking the electrophilic *N*-acetylparabenzoquinoneimine (NAPQI) to form the nontoxic glutathione conjugate. The glucuronide, sulfate, and mercapturate conjugates are all highly water soluble.

The Cahn-Ingold-Prelog method is empiric and is based on assigning the four substituents on a stereocenter, a priority score based on atomic number. If the priority scores increase when counting to the right (clockwise), the enantiomer is designated *rectus*, abbreviated *R*-. The other enantiomer, in which the priority scores increase going to the left, is designated *sinister*, abbreviated *S*-.

The Fisher method of designating stereoisomers compares a stereocenter to a standard molecule [(+)-glyceraldehyde], which was arbitrarily designated *D*- [and thus by default making the (–)-glyceraldehyde enantiomer *L*-]. The D or L designation for an unknown stereocenter is assigned based on comparison of Fisher projections of the standard with the unknown molecule. Note that the *D* and *L* assigned using the Fisher method are capitalized.

It is imperative to recognize that each of these three methods is independent. It is purely coincidental that R- and S- happen to be equivalent in their assignments of stereochemistry to D and L, respectively. However, there is no such relationship between R/S or D/L and +/– or d/l. The designations R/S and D/L can

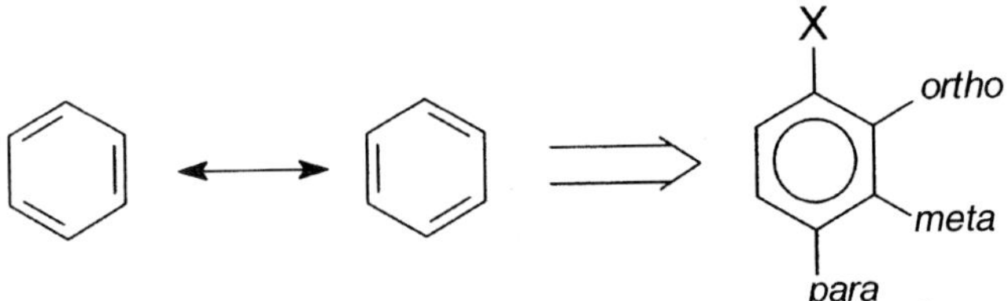

Figure 8. Chemical structures demonstrating the principle of resonance. The nitrogen of an amide is not basic, as the lone pair of electrons is delocalized away from the nitrogen atom owing to resonance **(top)**. The two equivalent resonance structures of benzene are inadequate to represent the fact that all bonds of the ring are of equal length. The most complete representation of benzene has a circle in the middle of the ring, which indicates equal contributions of both resonance forms.

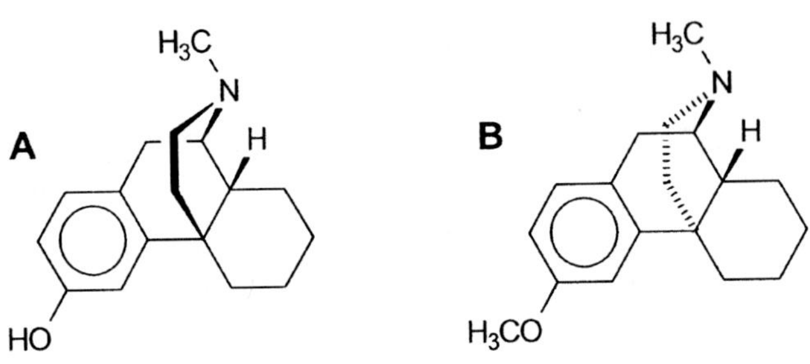

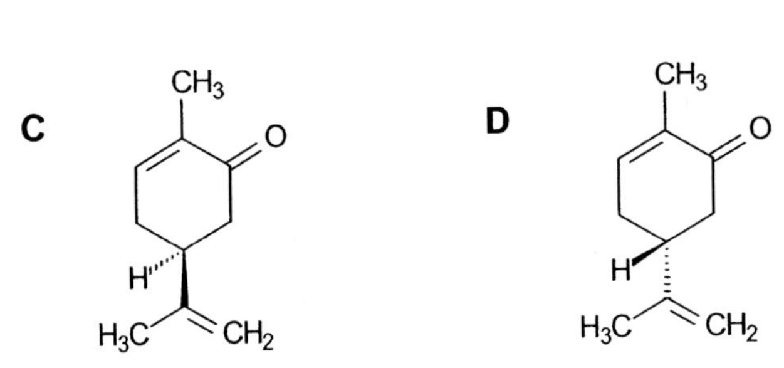

Figure 9. Chemical structures of enantiomeric pairs levorphanol **(A)** and dextromethorphan **(B)** and carvone. The (4S)-(+)-carvone **(C)** is caraway and (4R)-(–)-carvone **(D)** is sweet spearmint.

be used interchangeably; also, d/l and +/– are interchangeable. However, there is no simple relationship between R/S and +/– or between D/L and d/l (i.e., the d and l and D and L definitions are case-sensitive).

If a compound has more than one stereocenter, nonsuperimposable nonmirror images called *diastereomers* can result. Additionally, if a molecule has multiple stereocenters but the molecule contains a plane of symmetry between the stereocenters, the result is a meso compound. Therefore, compounds with multiple stereocenters can exist as enantiomers, diastereomers, and possibly meso compounds.

A compound with multiple stereocenters has 2^n stereoisomers, in which n is the number of stereocenters. So, if a compound has two stereocenters, there are four possible stereoisomers, which are (R,R), (S,S), (R,S), and (S,R). Their relationship to one another is that (R,R) and (S,S) are an enantiomeric pair as are the (S,R) and (R,S). However, if the (R,R) and (R,S) pairs are compared, they are diastereomers, as they are nonsuperimposable and not mirror images of one another. This is also the case in the (S,S)/(S,R) pair.

Both the receptor as well as the ligand can be chiral. For example, differences in tastes and smells of two enantiomers are a result of a specific enantiomer of a compound interacting with a stereospecific receptor. In other words, *smell* and *taste* receptors are chiral. Therefore, only a given enantiomer binds to a given receptor in many cases (Fig. 9). So, the difference in taste/smell is a result of the host's perception, as well as a result of the chemical properties of the compound.

MEDICINAL CHEMISTRY

Drug Solubility, Delivery, and Distribution

A xenobiotic can cause direct effects at the site of entrance (e.g., therapeutic use of β_2-agonists or local tissue damage associated with caustic agents), or it must somehow reach its site of action. For most compounds, initial absorption takes place from the site of primary exposure (lung or intestine) followed by systemic delivery through the bloodstream. Therefore, partitioning across the membranes to enter the bloodstream poses the first challenge, followed by the repartitioning out of the blood and into tissue at the site of action.

Multiple factors determine the extent to which a given compound is absorbed from sites such as the gastrointestinal tract or lungs: molecular size, charge, acidity, lipophilicity, and the availability of active transport mechanisms. Drugs intended for therapeutic use are formulated specifically to deliver the drug to its site of action.

Molecular charge-based solubility is one of the simplest formulations to understand. The human body is an aqueous environment. However, most drugs are organic and therefore have limited water solubility. Indeed, drugs like phenytoin and diazepam are not water soluble and are formulated as lipophilic solutions. Though these formulations are effective in delivering the medication, drugs such as these must be used carefully because the lipophilic diluent can cause adverse effects such as hypotension or tissue necrosis. In an effort to increase the safety with which drugs are delivered, many drugs are converted to a water-soluble form. Typically, the water-soluble form of a compound is an ionic compound called a *salt* (Fig. 10). The reason salts are more soluble is based on the fundamental principle of "like dissolves like." In other words, a polar molecule dissolves in a polar solvent, whereas a nonpolar molecule only dissolves in a nonpolar solvent.

A surprising number of drugs and toxins are plant-derived alkaloids that contain at least one basic nitrogen. This nitrogen is typically in the form of an amine. A basic nitrogen is one that has sufficient localized electron density to accept a proton (i.e., it has no resonance contributors) (Fig. 10). Recall that nitrogen binds three substituents covalently and has a lone pair of electrons left over. This lone pair of electrons is the site that accepts a proton. When a proton combines with the lone pair, the nitrogen atom becomes electron deficient, resulting in a positive charge on the nitrogen atom. The protonation can be reversed with the addition of aqueous base to a solution of ammonium salt. For example, methamphetamine free base is an oil that is only moderately soluble in water, making it inconvenient for illicit distribution. If methamphetamine is converted to its hydrochloride salt, however, it takes on the form of a convenient water-soluble solid that can be easily distributed.

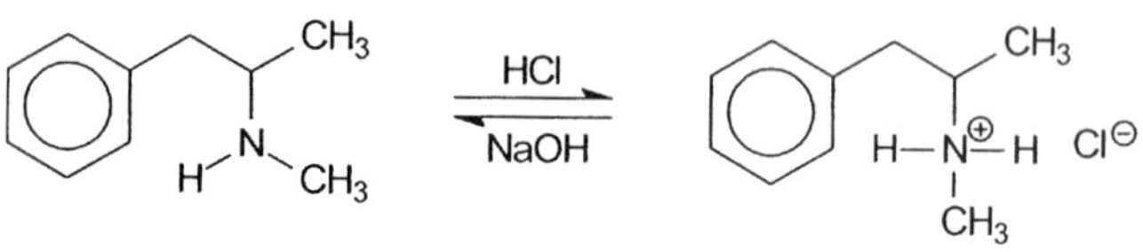

Figure 10. Chemical structures of methamphetamine free base (*left*) and hydrochloride salt (*right*).

Not all nitrogen atoms are basic. For example, though an amine contains a basic nitrogen, the nitrogen atom in an amide is not basic (due to resonance) (Fig. 8). The ability of electrons (in this case, the lone pair on the nitrogen atom) to resonate between different atoms makes them less of a point source of electron density and therefore less available for protonation. Although these examples involve the creation of the acid salt of a basic drug, basic salts of acidic drugs are also made to increase their water solubility. For example, phenobarbital is often formulated as the sodium salt of the drug.

The nitrogen in methamphetamine is an unprotonated secondary amine devoid of resonance forms and is therefore basic (Fig. 10), relatively nonpolar, and soluble in nonpolar solvents (e.g., organic solvents such as ether, methylene chloride, and so forth). This basic nitrogen is free of protonation and still a base. This unprotonated form of the compound is referred to as the *free base*. Note that *free base* is used as a noun. The colloquial verb form of the term refers to isolation of the base for the compound to have sufficient vapor pressure to be smoked. The term *free base* is sometimes used synonymously with the term *alkaloid form*. This is marginally correct, though *free base* is more chemically accurate.

Salts are often impure. They can be purified by a process called *recrystallization*. To do this, a solvent is selected in which the compound is nearly insoluble at low temperature but is soluble at high temperature. For example, acetone is used to purify methamphetamine HCl. The salt is placed in a minimum amount of solvent, and the solvent is heated until all of the salt goes into solution. Then, the solvent is allowed to cool. As it cools, the salt becomes increasingly less soluble and crystallizes out of solution. If cooled quickly, the forming crystals have little time to organize into a well-defined lattice. They tend to be small, resulting in a gritty powder after filtering and drying. However, if the solution is cooled slowly and is not disturbed, large crystals may form with a well-defined crystalline lattice. The slower cooling also improves purity by allowing fewer foreign substances to become trapped in the crystalline lattice. Crystals of methamphetamine HCl are often clear and can be large, creating street names like *glass*, *crystal meth*, or *ice*.

Crack cocaine is the free base of cocaine. The intermolecular forces holding a rock of crack together as a solid are much weaker than those holding a lump of cocaine HCl together. As a result, crack is easily converted to a vapor with heating and can

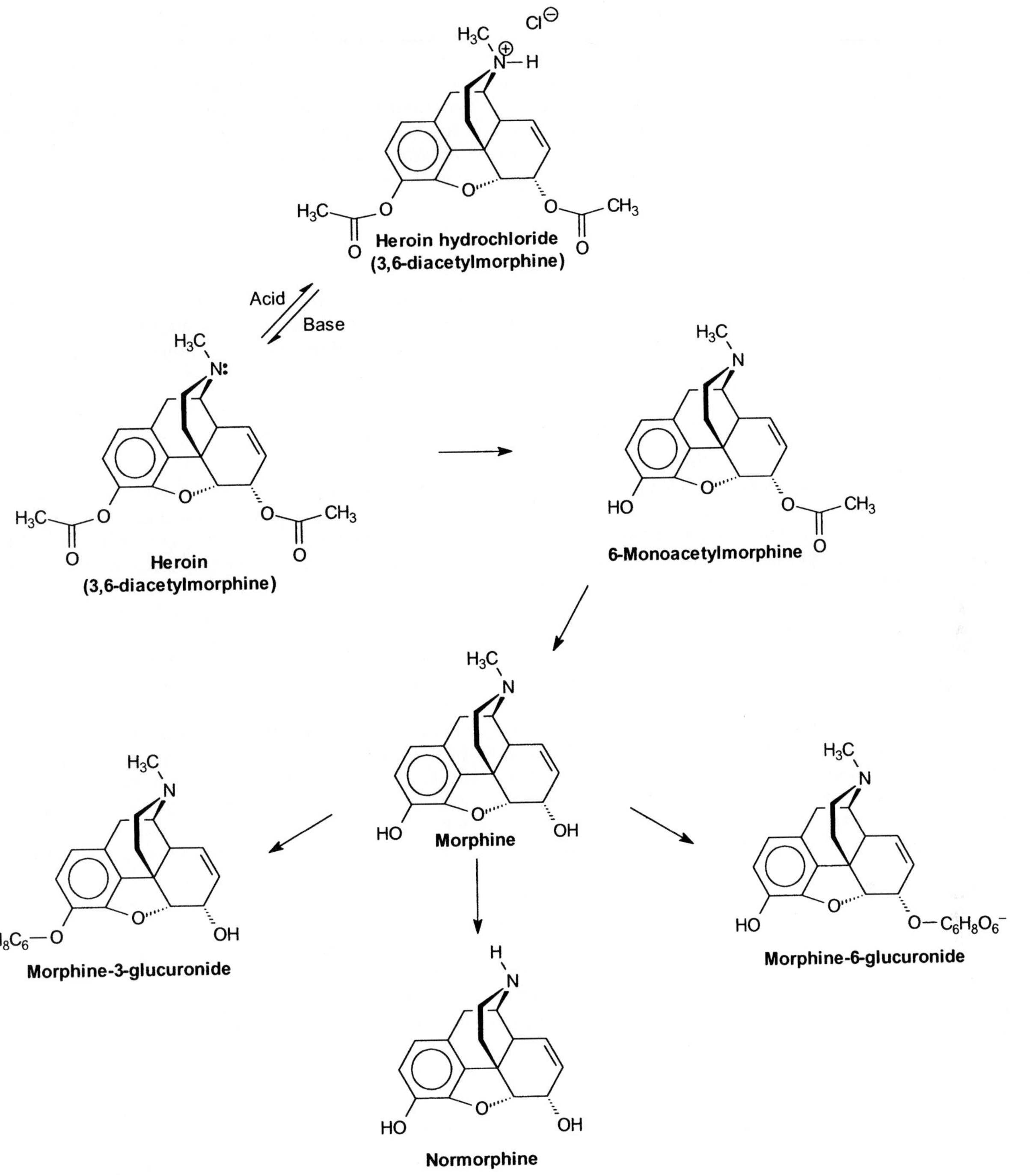

Figure 11. Abbreviated metabolic scheme of heroin.

be smoked. The term *crack* refers to the popping sound it makes when it is heated and gas is liberated.

Additional methods for maximizing drug solubility and delivery include the use of prodrugs such as fosphenytoin or micelle encapsulation of the active drug. Site-specific release matrices and antibody conjugates have been developed for some drugs as well as ion pumps for controlled delivery.

Importance of Strong and Weak Bases

As previously described, pK_a is a measurement of the ease with which a proton can be abstracted (i.e., the acidity of a given proton) from a weak acid. When the pK_a of a given drug is reported, it is a reference to only the proton of lowest pK_a. Removal of this single proton ionizes the compound. However, every proton in an organic compound has an associated pK_a. The pK_a of protons on organic molecules ranges from 0.64 in trichloroacetic acid, to 17 for the hydroxide proton in ethanol, to 47 for the protons of methane.

There is often confusion when attempts are made to relate acid or base strength, pK_a, and pH to the potential for caustic or corrosive injury. The strength of an acid or base speaks only to the extent of ionization in an aqueous solution and not to its corrosive or caustic potential. In aqueous solution, a strong acid or base is fully ionized, whereas a weak acid or base is not. Though the pH of the offending substance is an important feature, so are concentration, thermogenic ability, and physiologic action. For example, both sodium hydroxide (NaOH) drain cleaner and household bleach (NaOCl) have a pH of 12. However, drain cleaner is a profoundly caustic agent, whereas household bleach is only an irritant. Another factor that influences tissue injury is the higher concentration of NaOH in drain cleaner compared to NaOCl in household bleach. With alkaline agents, protein denaturation and tissue and membranous destruction are also significant issues. Further, NaOH also generates a substantial amount of heat when dissolved in water, which may also alter proteins. Finally, some NaOCl is destroyed by endogenous reducing agents, which may also help ameliorate pH-related effects.

Drug Receptor Binding

Most drugs and poisons must bind to a receptor to exert their effect. It is true that some drugs and toxins may not have specific receptors (e.g., caustics) or bind to more than one receptor. In fact, most receptor-specific drugs are actually "dirty"—they bind multiple receptors, particularly at toxic doses.

A number of considerations including complementary polarity, charges, and geometric and stereochemical considerations must be satisfied for a drug to interact with a receptor. After the initial interaction, other intermolecular forces including development of covalent, ionic, and hydrogen bonds, ion-dipole and dipole-dipole attractions, development of charge transfer complexes, and hydrophobic and van der Waals forces may come into play. These forces determine the resident time of the drug binding to that receptor (Fig. 3).

Drug Metabolism

After introduction into the body, xenobiotics are removed. However, the physicochemical properties of many compounds favor retention over elimination. To facilitate removal of xenobiotics from the body, the body performs a series of chemical transformations of the compounds known as *metabolism*. Though the metabolism of compounds may appear complicated, metabolites can be predicted with reasonable accuracy through examination of the structure of the parent compound. In many cases, the metabolism *incidentally* terminates the compound's pharmacologic or toxicologic action.

There are two basic sets of reactions involved in the metabolic transformation of xenobiotics in preparation for their elimination. These steps are known as phase I and phase II transformations. The general purpose of *phase I transformations* is to impart additional polar functionality on the parent compound. The polarity is subsequently used to facilitate conjugation and elimination. Increased polarity can be created through an oxidation, a reduction, or an "unmasking" of a polar heteroatom such as an oxygen or nitrogen by removing carbon-containing substituents from that atom. After phase I, *phase II transformations* conjugate the compound to the larger polar moiety that has been created. The polar prostheses attached during conjugation reactions serve to increase water solubility to facilitate excretion of the metabolites in the urine. For example, the sulfate and glucuronide (phase II) conjugates of acetaminophen are found in the urine (Fig. 7). It is important to realize that parent molecules that possess polar functional groups such as hydroxyls or primary and secondary amines can undergo phase II transformations directly without first undergoing phase I transformation.

SUMMARY

Multiple concepts can be summarized by looking at a single drug (Fig. 11). Heroin has several different organic functional groups, including an aromatic ring, an ether, a double bond, two esters, and an amine. The basic nitrogen of the amine in heroin is commonly converted to the hydrochloride or sulfate salt, making it ionic and, therefore, water soluble. However, the salt has a vapor pressure that is too low for it to be smoked. Therefore, the salt is treated with a base such as NaOH or $NaHCO_3$ to create the *free base* of the drug, which can be volatilized. It is converted metabolically by ester hydrolysis first to 6-monoacetylmorphine (heroin-specific metabolite) and then to morphine by hydrolysis of the second acetate ester. When the heroin base enters the body, it is fairly lipophilic, so a portion of the dose readily crosses the blood–brain barrier into the central nervous system where the hydrolysis of the two esters can take place. Morphine is less lipophilic than heroin and does not cross back across the blood–brain barrier as readily. Morphine readily undergoes the additional phase I metabolic transformation of oxidative *N*-demethylation by CYP2D6. Phase II (conjugation) reactions of morphine include formation of the glucuronide conjugates at the hydroxyl moieties at positions 3 and 6. The glucuronides are then excreted. Note that the aromatic ring stays intact throughout the metabolic transformations, illustrating the stability imparted by aromaticity.

CHAPTER 82

Analytical Toxicology

Robert B. Palmer

OVERVIEW

It seems intuitive to perform laboratory assessments to determine toxin type and concentration in the poisoned patient. However, many hurdles confront the clinician attempting to identify a poison analytically. First, the agent can often be identified clinically from the history, physical examination, and common laboratory tests. It is not necessary to perform a specific analytical determination if that information affects the patient's treatment. Nevertheless, circumstances exist in which treatment may be affected by the results of toxicologic laboratory analysis (Appendix II). However, there are many more cases in which the analysis proves futile. For example, an analytical methodology may not be readily available to determine levels of a given substance. If a level can be determined, it must be emphasized that the presence of a toxicant, or even its concentration, does not directly translate to degree of intoxication or impairment. In those cases in which analytical determinations are available (Appendix II), a fundamental understanding of analytical principles can assist the clinician in assessing the advantages, disadvantages, limitations, and use of an assay and is of significant value in the clinical interpretation of laboratory results.

This chapter provides the clinician with a working understanding of the fundamentals of analytical toxicology. Descriptions of how the various assays and analytical methodologies work are found in many other reference texts and are not presented here in detail, although a brief comparison chart of analytical instrumental techniques is provided (Table 1). This chapter focuses on the information necessary to assess the validity of laboratory results.

This chapter has three sections: Preanalytical Considerations (sample selection, collection, processing, and storage); Analytical Considerations (standards, calibration curves, blanks, controls, and quality control); and Postanalytical Considerations (reporting of results and the use of appropriate significant figures and units).

PREANALYTICAL CONSIDERATIONS

Test Selection: Screening versus Confirmatory Testing

The type of analysis to be performed must be determined before sample collection. The choice of a test dictates the sampling conditions, type of biologic sample to be collected (Appendix II), collection and storage procedures, analytical methodology, and time frame for the analysis. The primary factor influencing this decision is the specificity of the assay. *Specificity* (also called *selectivity*) is the ability to assess an analyte unequivocally in the presence of other components, with a requisite level of accuracy and precision. Additional components include impurities, degradants, metabolites, and the biologic matrix.

Toxicologic analyses fall broadly into two categories: screening and confirmatory. *Screening assays* are rapid and provide qualitative (i.e., presence or absence) or pseudoquantitative (i.e., present or absent above a certain predetermined cutoff concentration) information. Often, this information identifies drug class rather than specific chemical entity (i.e., a positive result indicates the presence of benzodiazepines, but not necessarily diazepam). Common screening methodologies include spot tests and immunoassays. Inherent limitations of spot tests, including a lack of specificity, limit their widespread use, although some standard spot tests are available (Table 2).

A screening *immunoassay* detects a drug by the use of an antibody that binds to a specific portion of the drug. The binding site is a structural component that is common to the drugs of that class. A positive result for an immunoassay is defined as being positive at some concentration greater than a defined "cutoff" concentration. *Cutoff* values are designed to limit the number of false-positives caused by low-level interference from cross-reacting substances. The cutoff value may vary. For example, the cutoff for cocaine metabolite in urine in a laboratory doing work to the standards of the U.S. Department of Health and Human Services (formerly, National Institute of Drug Abuse) is 300 ng/ml, whereas the U.S. Department of Defense cutoff for the same assay is 150 ng/ml. Any value returned by the assay below the designated cutoff is reported as negative. Cutoff values differ from assay limits of detection or quantitation. A cutoff is set far enough above the detection limit of the assay to provide reliable detection of the analyte but low enough that a sufficient time window is available to discern recent drug use. Immunoassay and confirmation cutoff values for common drug classes in urine drug testing programs are listed in Table 3.

Although immunoassays are rapid, they experience numerous analytical limitations and can potentially provide erroneous results. A *false-positive* result is a positive screen when the compound causing the positive reaction is not the analyte of interest. This is often the result of interferences from compounds with structural features similar to the compound of interest. Similarly, a *false-negative* occurs when the compound of interest is actually present but not detected by the assay. This happens when the analyte concentration is too low for detection or when the toxin of interest (parent drug or metabolite) has insufficient reactivity with the antibody, despite belonging to the same drug class for which the antibody was designed. For example, some common benzodiazepine immunoassays detect lorazepam, oxazepam, and temazepam much better if the urine sample is first treated with β-glucuronidase to remove the glucuronide moiety and yield the parent drug. A false-negative or -positive may also result from preanalytical adulteration of the sample, a strategy apparent in the numerous World Wide Web sites providing advice on how to avoid detection of abused substances in urine. Due to the possibility of false-positive results, a positive screening test result should be confirmed using an alternate and more definitive analytical method.

Confirmatory assays identify the specific compound rather than simply the class. These assays are more time and labor intensive and are costly to perform. The gold standard for most drug confirmations is gas chromatography–mass spectrometry. Other toxins such as metals and toxic gases are confirmed using other analytical methodologies. In addition to proving the compound's identity, confirmatory assays are usually quantitative (i.e., provide a specific concentration of the compound in question).

To Test or Not to Test

The first decision to be made is whether a patient's care is enhanced by the use of a drug screen. A drug screen should not be performed on all potentially poisoned patients because a drug screen is able to detect few toxins and because most patients do well with appropriate supportive and intensive care without the exact identity of the drug being known.

A drug screen is appropriate in a few circumstances. The fundamental rule is that the information obtained should alter the patient's care. Altered mental status, tachycardia, or seizures of unclear etiology are common reasons. One overlooked use of a drug screen is to assist in the diagnosis of patients who manifest signs or symptoms that are inconsistent with the reported ingestion (e.g., a small child presenting with agitation in a family setting of opioid abuse). First, the signs are inconsistent with opioid intoxication. A screen could help include another abused drug like cocaine or confirm (exclude) that a paradoxic response to heroin (e.g., hypoxia) was not the cause of transient agitation. This example also demonstrates that the interpretation of drug screen results requires expertise. They must be interpreted carefully in the context of the case. It is necessary for the practitioner to know what drugs and compounds are included in the screen as well as what methodology is used by the laboratory for the screen. This knowledge allows better assessment of possible false results.

Sample Collection, Handling, and Processing

Accurate results of laboratory assays are dependent on the sample collected. The sample itself must be appropriate for the analysis to be conducted, and the collection vessel must preserve the

TABLE 1. Summary of instrumental analytical techniques

	Technique	Relative cost	Relative turnaround time	Advantages	Disadvantages	Applicable analytes	Description
Screening	Thin-layer chromatography	$	🕐🕐	Broad screening capabilities Metabolites can be detected simultaneously with parent drug Many visualization techniques available	Standards required for every analyte Not definitive proof of drug Standards not often available for non-drug toxins Requires experienced technologist Co-eluting spots are possible Not all analytes are amenable	Does work for most drugs Does not work for toxic gases, alcohols, solvents, metals, or proteins	A few microliters of analyte are spotted at the base of thin-layer chromatography plate with analytical standards adjacent. Plate is placed vertically into a tank containing the elution solvent with the spot at the bottom slightly above the level of solvent. Solvent "climbs" the plate through capillary and carries analytes up the plate. Different analytes interact with the stationary phase to different extents and therefore travel varying distances up the plate. Final result is a plate with a series of spots. Each spot corresponds to a chemically different compound. Spots are visualized using light and/or staining reagent. Spots from the sample are compared with the spots from the analytical standards with respect to distance traveled, shape, color, and character using several visualization methods, and a determination of presumptive compound identity is made.
	Immunoassay (radioimmunoassay, enzyme-multiplied immunoassay technique, fluorescence-polarization immunoassay)	$$	🕐	Broad screening capabilities Includes or excludes entire classes of drugs from differential Common technique for pre-employment or abuse monitoring	Screens drug class not specific drug Some drugs of same class cannot be detected due to low concentration Qualitative or semi-quantitative Must have antibody to toxin of interest	Does work for drugs of abuse, acetaminophen, salicylate Does not work for toxic gases, metals	Antibody developed to given molecular epitope of drug or toxin. Antibody is linked to reactive species such as an enzyme. Sample is incubated with enzyme substrate and antibody-enzyme complex. Product of enzyme activity on substrate is measured. If drug or toxin of interest is bound by antibody, enzyme is unable to produce products from substrate, so product concentration drops. Drugs or toxins with similar molecular structures provide varying degrees of cross-reactivity. Often purchased in kit form.
	Gas chromatography	$$$	🕐🕐🕐	Lower limit of detection Can be quantitative Many types of detectors available	Identification based only on retention time Consumes analyte Requires experienced technologist	Does work for most drugs, alcohols, solvents, some toxic gases Does not work for proteins, metals	Analytes volatilized (turned into gases) by intense heating at injector. Gas-phase analytes carried through column by chemically inert gas such as helium. Separation of multiple analytes occurs in column. Column is contained within an oven to prevent condensation of the analytes during passage through column. The analytes then exit the column and pass through a detector. Electronic detector signal is converted to detector response versus time chart.

	High-performance liquid chromatography	$$$	🕒🕒🕒🕒	Many types of detectors available Proteins and enzymes not amenable to gas chromatography can be analyzed Nondestructive technique	Requires experienced technologist Preanalytical sample prep can be extensive	Does work for many drugs, alcohols, proteins, water-soluble compounds Does not work for toxic gases, metals	Analytes are injected into the liquid solvent as a single plug upstream from the column. Pressurized liquid solvent carries analytes through the column where separation takes place. Analytes elute from distal end of the column in solvent and pass through detector. Electronic detector signal is converted to detector response versus time chart.
Confirmatory	Gas chromatography–mass spectrometry	$$$$	🕒🕒🕒🕒	High sensitivity High specificity Some screening capacity	Requires much maintenance Experienced technologist Requires significant sample preparation Destructive technique	Does work for many drugs, alcohols Does not work for proteins, metals	Gas chromatography section identical to that described previously. Mass spectrometry is a specific type of detector. Inside mass spectrometry, sample is struck by high-energy electrons, causing analyte molecules to fragment. Fragments strike detector plate, and this signal is converted to instrument output. The number of fragments striking the detector plate is directly proportional to the amount of compound present. Molecular fragments are characteristic of specific molecules (i.e., molecular identity is confirmed).
	Co-oximetry	$$	🕒🕒	Specific for hemoglobin aberrancies	Interpretation can be complex	Does work for aberrant hemoglobin Does not work for anything else	The basis of this technique is spectrophotometry. Specific light wavelengths are used to quantitate different hemoglobins. This technique provides quantitative results for oxyhemoglobin, desoxyhemoglobin, carboxyhemoglobin, and methemoglobin.
	Atomic absorption	$$$	🕒🕒🕒	Good detection limits Technique of choice for metal analytes	Not useful for nonmetal analytes Destructive technique	Does work for metals Does not work for anything else	Every element has a defined electronic spectrum unique to that atom. Sample is atomized in a high-heat acetylene flame. Atoms then absorb ultraviolet light, which results in electronic transitions to excited states. Excited states relax back to ground states producing a unique emission spectrum.

TABLE 2. "Spot" (noninstrumental) colorimetric tests for poisons

Analyte of interest	Reagent	Color of positive reaction	Other analytes and interferences	Comments
Barbiturates	Cobalt salts (e.g., cobalt nitrate)	Violet-blue	Phenytoin, primidone, glutethimide, chloramine	Reactive species is amine, amide, imide groups. Extraneous biologic species coextracted may also interfere.
Acetaminophen	Orthocresol/ammonia	Blue	Aniline, benorilate, nitrobenzene, phenacetin, ethylenediamine, hyperbilirubinemia	Metabolism or hydrolysis required for positive reaction with aniline, nitrobenzene, and phenacetin.
Salicylates	Trinder's reagent (ferric nitrate, mercuric chloride, hydrogen chloride)	Violet	Aloxiprin, aminosalicylate, aspirin, benorilate, methyl salicylate, salicylamide Diflunisal, labetalol, blue dyes in some medications (e.g., enteric coated Parafon forte), ketones interfere High phenothiazine concentrations	Acid extraction before analysis mitigates phenothiazine interference.
Phenothiazines	Ferric nitrate with sulfuric, perchloric, and nitric acids reagent	Blue to purple/pink	Hyperbilirubinemia Blue dyes in some medications (e.g., enteric coated Parafon forte) High salicylate concentrations	Acid extraction before analysis mitigates salicylate interference.
Trichloro compounds	Fujiwara reagent (10% sodium hydroxide plus redistilled pyridine)	Red	Chloral hydrate, chloroform, dichloralphenazone, trichloroethylene, triclofos, chloramphenicol	Reaction is also called the *Fujiwara reaction.*
Acetone/acetoacetate	Sodium nitroprusside	Purple	Other ketones may cross-react	Acetest tablets contain sodium nitroprusside, glycine, and disodium phosphate. Ketostix are impregnated with buffered mixture of sodium nitroprusside and glycine.
Boric acid	Methanolic turmeric powder	Red to brown (preliminary) Green-black (secondary)	Other boron-containing compounds	Active constituent of turmeric is curcumin. Preliminary test is acidification of sample with dilute HCl and spotting on paper. Secondary test is exposure of preliminarily positive spots to concentrated ammonium hydroxide.
	Carminic acid in sulfuric acid (bright red solution)	Bluish-red or blue		Often used as a quantitative test for boron.
Bromide	Gold chloride	Yellow to bronze	Iodide	A positive test can persist for months after administration of iodinated radiologic contrast agents.
Iron	Thiocyanates, 1,10-phenanthroline, 2,3-bipyridine (some others, too)	Red		Has been used for demonstration of excess iron in gastric aspirates in suspected iron overdose.
Nitrates/nitrites	Diphenylamine in concentrated sulfuric acid	Blue	Bromates, chlorates, iodates, peroxides	
	Sulfanilic acid plus naphthylamine	Red (nitrates)		
Lysergic acid diethylamide	Ethanolic para-dimethylaminobenzaldehyde	Purple	Psilocybin, ergonovine	
Tricyclic antidepressants	Potassium dichromate, sulfuric acid, perchloric acid, nitric acid	Green	Imipramine, clomipramine, desipramine, trimipramine	
Ethchlorvynol	Diphenylamine	Blue	Bromates, chlorates, iodates, nitrates, nitrites, peroxides, other oxidizing agents	
Paraquat/diquat	Dithionite	Blue (paraquat) Yellow-green (diquat)	Benzalkonium, cetylpyridinium chloride	

sample without contaminating it. Preservatives used for one type of analysis may not be suitable for others. A variety of additives are contained within blood collection tubes and are indicated by standardized colors of the stoppers (Table 4). Other preservatives may be added after sample collection, as is commonly done with urine collections.

Physiologic factors can affect the composition of body fluids, thereby influencing the interpretation of laboratory analyses (Appendix II). Such factors include circadian variation, as well as controllable biologic variables such as posture, immobilization, exercise, and physical training. Circadian variations can also be affected by conditions such as blindness and travel.

TABLE 3. Cutoff concentrations for screening and confirmation for common drugs of abuse

	Screening immunoassay (ng/ml)			Confirmation gas chromatography–mass spectrometry (ng/ml)		
Drug class	Target analyte	DHHS/DOT	DoD	Drug	DHHS/DOT	DoD
Amphetamines[a]		1000				
	Amphetamine		500	Amphetamine	500	500
	Methamphetamine		500	Methamphetamine	500[b]	500[b]
Barbiturates	Secobarbital	—	200			
				Amobarbital	—	200
				Butalbital	—	200
				Pentobarbital	—	200
				Secobarbital	—	200
Cannabinoids[a]	Δ^9-THC-COOH	50	50	Δ^9-THC-COOH	15	15
Cocaine[a]	Benzoylecgonine	300	150	Benzoylecgonine	150	100
LSD	LSD	—	0.5	LSD	—	0.2
Opiates[a]	Morphine/codeine	2000	300			
				Morphine	2000	4000
				Codeine	2000	2000
				6-MAM	10	10
PCP[a]	PCP	25	25	PCP	25	25

Δ^9-THC-COOH, 11-nor-Δ^9-tetrahydrocannabinol-9-carboxylic acid; DHHS, Department of Health and Human Services; DoD, Department of Defense; DOT, Department of Transportation; LSD, lysergic acid diethylamide; 6-MAM, 6-monoacetylmorphine (heroin-specific metabolite); PCP, phencyclidine.
[a]A National Institute on Drug Abuse Five analyte included in testing of employees of U.S. federal government and many other testing programs.
[b]Also requires the presence of amphetamine at ≥200 ng/ml.

External factors including time since eating, specific foods ingested, smoking, and alcohol and drug use can also affect the results of laboratory analyses. Medical conditions including fever, shock, trauma, and history of transfusion must also be considered as well as the effects of age, race, gender, menstrual cycle, body habitus, and nutritional status (malnutrition, vegetarianism, starvation/fasting). Most analyses are not affected to a clinically significant degree. The result may not be perfect, but it is good enough for clinical work. Still, the toxicologist must be aware of physiologic factors that affect assays and be able to apply this knowledge to the decisions of whether the analysis is normal or abnormal or whether it simply needs to be repeated or the interpretation adjusted appropriately.

Once the appropriate sample has been collected, correct handling and processing are imperative to ensure that the sample is neither contaminated nor allowed to deteriorate. Sample integrity is affected by storage temperature, elapsed time until cells are separated from plasma or serum, delay between sample acquisition and running, and atmospheric pressure. The storage conditions and length of transport time must be appropriate. In general, cells and clot should be separated from serum or plasma as soon as possible and definitely within 2 hours of collection. Clotting must be complete before centrifugation and removal of serum to prevent formation of residual fibrin clots that can clog instruments. Usually, 20 to 30 minutes at room temperature are sufficient for clotting to be complete. Samples to be held longer than 2 hours before separation should be held at room temperature (cooling to 4°C greatly increases hemolysis). Even with proper storage, there are some analytes of toxicologic importance that are inherently unstable in whole blood or plasma (Appendix II).

Typically, separated samples should be tightly capped to avoid evaporation or loss of volatile components (e.g., ethanol, carbon monoxide) and maintained at 4°C until analysis. Particularly unstable analytes may need to be maintained at –20°C, or even –70°C, depending on the length of storage time and stability of the analyte. However, storage at low temperatures is not always best because some analytes (e.g., isozymes of lactate dehydrogenase) are more stable at room temperature than at 4°C. Boyanton et al. examined the stability of 24 analytes in human serum and plasma, and the study is a reasonable reference regarding short-term stability of common chemistry tests (1).

Chain of Custody

In many laboratories, especially those dealing with forensic specimens, a tracking form called a *chain of custody form* accompanies each sample. Chain of custody refers not only to physical possession of the specimen but to the general procedure that accounts for identification, integrity, and security from the time of collection until final disposition. The chain of custody form tracks handling and storage of the sample at every point from collection through analysis. Each person that takes possession of the sample must complete a line in the form, documenting the person in custody of the sample from the time it is collected. Each person must examine the integrity of seals placed on the specimen at the time of collection for evidence of breakage or tampering and sign, date, and time the chain of custody form, attesting to the integrity of the sample. One must recognize, however, that the chain of custody process is not foolproof. For example, if a sample is substituted or one person within the chain is careless or lacks integrity and does not report a violation of an integrity seal, the validity of the analysis can be questioned. Like any security measure, with enough will and determination, it can be defeated.

Assays take varying amounts of time to perform and may be time intensive for the laboratory technologist. Some tests are run on a when-they-are-received basis (e.g., electrolytes, arterial blood gases), others may be run once or twice per day (e.g., levels of aminoglycosides), whereas still others may be run only once or twice per week (e.g., confirmations of drugs of abuse from urine drug screens). Finally, some tests may be sent to a referral laboratory with results taking days to weeks to be reported. Should the clinician need a result more quickly, the laboratory should be contacted as soon as possible with this request.

However, due to the inherently complicated nature of clinical chemistry, the only way to determine what sample, container, time frame, and storage conditions are required for a given

TABLE 4. Characteristics of commonly used evacuated blood collection tubes[a]

Safety stopper[b] color	Conventional stopper color	Additive	Additive function	General use category	Common analyses	Notes
Gold	Red and black marble	Clot activator and gel separator	Promote clotting and cell separation to provide serum	Chemistry	Serum chemistries	Blood clotting time is approximately 30 min.
Light green	Green and gray marble	Lithium heparin with gel separator	Anticoagulation and cell separation to provide plasma	Chemistry	Plasma chemistries	Not suitable for lithium analysis.
Red	Red	Plastic tube with safety closure: clot activator Glass tube with conventional stopper: no additive	Allow (glass tube) or promote (plastic tube) clotting to provide serum	Chemistry/ serology	Serum chemistries and serologies (plastic or glass) Blood banking (glass)	Glass tubes may be used for blood banking. Plastic tubes containing clot activator are not recommended for blood banking.
Orange	Gray and yellow marble	Thrombin	Promote rapid clotting to provide serum	Chemistry	Immediate chemistries	Complete clotting usually occurs within 5 min.
Royal blue	—	Sodium Heparin Na$_2$EDTA None (serum tube)	Anticoagulation to provide plasma Allow clotting to provide serum	Chemistry	Trace element toxicology and nutritional chemistries	Stopper is specially formulated with low levels of trace elements to prevent sample contamination. Not suitable for chromium, manganese, aluminum, or selenium determinations.
Green	Green	Sodium heparin Lithium heparin	Anticoagulation to provide plasma	Chemistry	Plasma chemistry determinations	Not suitable for lithium analysis.
Gray	Gray	K-oxalate/NaF NaF/Na$_2$EDTA NaF (serum tube)	Oxalate and EDTA: anticoagulation to provide plasma NaF: antiglycolysis Allow clotting to provide serum	Chemistry	Glucose determinations	Commonly used for postmortem samples.
Tan	—	Sodium heparin (glass) K$_2$EDTA (plastic)	Anticoagulation to provide plasma	Chemistry	Lead determination	Tube is certified to contain <0.01 µg/ml (ppm) lead.
Lavender	Lavender	Liquid K$_3$EDTA (glass) Spray dried K$_2$EDTA (plastic)	Anticoagulation for whole blood cell analysis	Hematology	Whole blood hematology determinations	K$_3$EDTA (glass) for whole blood hematology determinations. K$_2$EDTA (plastic) for whole blood hematology determinations and immunohematology testing (ABO grouping, Rhesus typing, antibody screening).
Light blue	Light blue	0.105 M (3.2%) Na-citrate 0.129 M (3.8%) Na-citrate CTAD	Citrate: anticoagulation CTAD: anticoagulation for selected platelet function assays	Coagulation	Citrate: routine coagulation assays (PT/INR, aPTT) CTAD: selected platelet function assays	Some tests require the specimen to be chilled.
Pink	—	Spray dried K$_2$EDTA	Anticoagulation for whole blood cell analysis	Blood banking Hematology	Whole blood hematology studies Immunohematology testing	Has specially designed crossmatch label for AABB-required patient information.
Yellow	Yellow	Acid citrate dextrose *Solution A*: Na$_3$citrate (22.0 g/L), citric acid (8.0 g/L), dextrose (24.5 g/L) *Solution B*: Na$_3$citrate (13.2 g/L), citric acid (4.8 g/L), dextrose (14.7 g/L)	Anticoagulation for blood-banking analysis	Blood banking	Blood bank studies, human leukocyte antigen phenotyping, deoxyribonucleic acid, and paternity testing	*Not* equivalent to yellow-stoppered tubes used for microbiology.
Yellow	Yellow	Sodium polyanethol sulfonate	Anticoagulation for blood culture specimen collection	Microbiology	Blood culture	*Not* equivalent to yellow-stoppered acid citrate dextrose tubes used for blood banking.

aPTT, activated partial thromboplastin time; CTAD, citrate, theophylline, adenosine, dipyridamole; EDTA, ethylenediaminetetraacetic acid; INR, international normalized ratio; ppm, parts per million; PT, prothrombin time.

[a]Portions of information in this table from Becton-Dickenson World Wide Web site at http://www.bd.com/vacutainer.

[b]Safety stopper such as Hemogard (Becton-Dickenson, Franklin Lakes, NJ) closure on Becton-Dickenson blood collection tubes.

assay is to consult the laboratory performing the analysis as well as a reliable reference text.

ANALYTICAL CONSIDERATIONS

Instruments and Reagents

To assure validity of reported results, each instrument must be properly calibrated. A single small malfunction in an instrument may not vary an analytical result by a detectable amount. However, many small malfunctions or worn parts in a given instrument may collectively alter an analytical determination substantially. It is recommended that a qualified technician service all instruments regularly. The manufacturer can be contacted for maintenance guidelines. Records of preventative maintenance should be maintained. Further, all reagents and chemicals must be of an appropriate analytical grade. Records of these calibrations and certificates of analysis should be kept on hand to document use of valid equipment.

Sample Matrices and Extraction

The biologic fluid or tissue (the *matrix*) in which the drug or toxin of interest (the *analyte*) resides often creates important challenges in measurement. Urine can often be used directly in qualitative analyses, such as some immunoassays and thin-layer chromatographic techniques. If quantitation is needed, however, the specimen usually requires some sort of preparation before analysis. Typically, sample preparation involves removal of the analytes from the biologic matrix as well as elimination of as many potential contaminants as possible.

One technique involves manipulation of the sample pH through the addition of acid or base. This can have multiple effects. First, it can precipitate proteins from the solution. More important, it can reduce or increase the ionized fraction of the analyte and allow extraction of the analyte into the organic solvent phase. If the analyte is ionized, as with a basic analyte in an acidic environment, the analyte partitions preferentially into the aqueous phase. When the pH is made basic, the same basic analyte becomes unionized and partitions into the nonpolar organic phase. Serial acid-base extractions are used to remove contaminants and ultimately isolate the analyte of interest in an organic solvent. This can be done with extraction techniques such as liquid-to-liquid organic extraction or through the use of solid-phase columns. Following extraction, the sample may need to be concentrated and chemically derivatized to increase the ability of the instrument to detect them (i.e., increase the analyte concentration in the sample or add a moiety that the instrument can detect).

Liquid matrices (serum, urine, cerebrospinal fluid) are extracted directly, but solid tissues must first be homogenized (typically in a buffer) and centrifuged to remove solid material before extraction. The efficiency of extractions is not 100%. In other words, every molecule of the drug or toxin is not effectively removed in the extraction process. The efficiency of the extraction is measured by recovery. *Recovery* is the amount of the analyte that was successfully extracted. This is measured by spiking the sample with a similar compound before extraction and then quantitating the amount that was actually extracted along with the analyte of interest. Once the recovery is known, analytical results can be corrected for extraction efficiency.

Standards and Calibration Curves

Once the sample is in a liquid, an internal standard is added. A *standard* is a solution with a known composition and concentration. It is typically used to develop an analytical method and act as confirmation that the method is functioning properly. An *external standard* is a standard that is applied to a blank tissue or fluid (i.e., a separate tissue sample that contains none of the analyte of interest). This sample is examined alone, and the only peak on the chromatogram results from the external standard. The area under this peak is compared to subsequently injected patient samples that should contain the analyte of interest. The key point here is the standard is separated from the patient sample (i.e., *external* to the analyte of interest).

An *internal standard* is a compound closely related to the analyte of interest. An internal standard is added directly to the patient's sample, resulting in two chromatogram peaks (one from the internal standard and one from the analyte). The areas under the two peaks in a given chromatogram are compared and a ratio calculated. The key point here is the standard is in the same tube as the patient sample (i.e., *internal* relative to the analyte of interest). An internal standard is a compound that is chemically similar to the analyte but can be analytically distinguished from the analyte. The addition of an internal standard confirms that the extraction worked and that the analytical detection method worked, and it allows for more reliable quantitation.

Calibration standards are used to establish a calibration curve for quantitation. The calibration standards are made in a blank sample matrix (serum, urine, and so forth) that is synthetic or pooled from multiple donors and certified as drug free. The blank matrix is placed in a series of tubes. Into these tubes is added a known amount of analyte covering the concentration range of interest for the assay. Also added to each calibration standard tube is the same amount of internal standard that has been added to each sample tube. The calibration standards are then treated exactly like the patient samples. It is important to include a *zero calibrator* or blank with each assay run. This calibrator does not contain any analyte of interest but does contain internal standard. Therefore, the analyst is able to tell immediately if there is a contaminating interference in the blank matrix, or if sample carryover from the previous sample is a concern. A blank is often run between each set of patient samples to assure no carryover from one patient sample to the next.

A calibration curve can be constructed using either internal or external standards. If using an external standard, the area under the standard peak is plotted against the concentration of the standard. Because the area under the peak is proportional to the concentration, a line can be constructed by using three or more known concentrations of standard. Then, the area of a patient sample can be plugged into the equation of the calibration curve line. When this equation is solved, it yields the concentration of analyte in the patient's sample.

The principle is similar when working with an internal standard. Instead of plotting concentration versus area, however, the plot is made using concentration versus the *ratio* of the internal standard to analyte areas. Solving for an *unknown* concentration is done in the same fashion using the internal standard to analyte ratio in the patient sample.

The calibration curve demonstrates the linearity of the method. *Linearity* of an analytical procedure is its ability to obtain test results that are proportional to the concentration (or amount) of analyte in the sample. Often, only a portion of the calibration curve provides a linear or mathematically predictable response. If this occurs, those values not falling on the linear portion of the graph are said to be beyond the linear range and cannot be reported with any certainty. In this case, the laboratory may report, "exceeds limits of assay." These samples can be diluted until their concentration falls within the assay limits. The lowest concentration calibration standard is called the *limit*

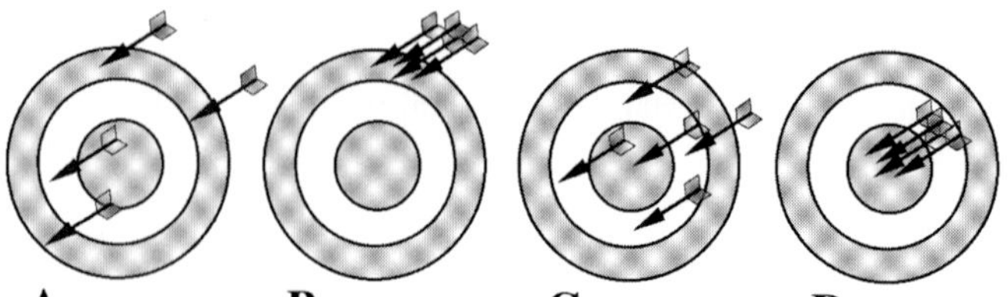

A B C D

Figure 1. Graphic representation of the distinction between precision and accuracy. **Target A:** poor precision, poor accuracy; **Target B:** good precision, poor accuracy; **Target C:** poor precision, good accuracy; **Target D:** good precision, good accuracy.

of quantitation (LOQ). The LOQ is the lowest concentration of the analyte that can be determined with acceptable precision and accuracy under the stated experimental conditions. This is distinctly different from the *limit of detection* for an assay, which is the lowest concentration of analyte in a sample that can be detected (distinguished from baseline with certainty), but not necessarily quantitated, under the assay conditions. The limit of detection can be the same as the LOQ, but it can never be larger than an LOQ.

Controls and Blanks

To discuss the use of controls and standardization of methodologies between laboratories, the terms *accuracy, precision*, and *reproducibility* must be defined (Fig. 1). *Accuracy* is the closeness of agreement between the value found by the method and the value that is accepted either as a conventional true value or a reference value (i.e., a "correct" result). *Precision* refers to the reliability of getting the same result with successive measurements on the same sample in the same laboratory. *Reproducibility* expresses the precision between laboratories and is usually applied to standardization of methodology between multiple laboratories. In other words, if the same sample is analyzed in the same way by multiple laboratories, how well do the results compare? For example, reproducibility of blood lead measurement is assessed by a federal program that sends test samples to laboratories throughout the United States. The concentration measured by a laboratory must be accurate (fall within a predefined range of variation) for the laboratory to be certified.

Different types of standards are used for controls in an analytical procedure. A primary standard is a highly purified compound that can be measured directly producing a substance of exact known concentration. The American Chemical Society purity tolerance for a primary standard is 100 ± 0.02%. A secondary standard is a substance of lower purity whose concentration is determined by comparison with a primary standard. Most biologic specimens are unable to be maintained at these specifications, so primary and secondary standards of physiologic materials analyzed in a clinical laboratory do not exist. As a consequence, the National Institute of Standards and Technology has developed a series of standard reference materials that are certified for use in clinical laboratories. These standard reference materials have been physically and chemically characterized and can be used in place of primary standards in clinical laboratories.

Control samples are composed of matrix containing known amounts of analyte within the concentration range of interest (positive control) or no analyte (negative control or blank). The exact concentration of analyte in the control samples is certified by the selling agency. Concentrations of the controls for pseudoquantitative or quantitative assays usually address three points: 25% below the cutoff value, the cutoff value itself, and 25% above the cutoff value. Controls should be run with each assay batch to assure that the assay is functioning properly. In pseudoquantitative or quantitative assays, the result of analysis of the control must typically be within ± 20% of the certified value for the assay to be considered functioning properly. Controls called *certified reference materials* (CRMs) are available for many clinical laboratory assays. These CRMs can be obtained from private vendors or, in the case of many environmental toxins, the United States National Institute on Standards and Technology.

To prove there is no carryover from one sample to the next, it is necessary to run a blank between each sample analyzed. Any evidence of carryover contamination or aberrance in the absorbance of known standards should prompt immediate investigation of the source of the error and cessation of additional analyses until the source of the error has been located and repaired. This is a common problem in the measurement of ethylene glycol.

Proficiency Testing

Proficiency testing is a process in which the quality of laboratory performance is evaluated through blinded testing of simulated patient samples. In 1967, Congress passed the Clinical Laboratory Improvement Act (CLIA '67) and then the Clinical Laboratory Improvement Amendments (CLIA '88). These laws make proficiency testing a major part of clinical laboratory accreditation to protect patients from poor laboratory quality. Although the major focus of the current accreditation process is the analytical phase of the testing, recommendations have been made to Congress that the "total testing process" must be monitored. The CLIA '88 document serves as the principal guide to clinical laboratory quality in the United States. It requires that studies be performed that include many aspects of laboratory testing (Table 5).

Many of the proficiency testing programs compare results against the group mean of a large group of participating laboratories. A result falling outside the range of 2 SD of the group mean is deemed unacceptable. This method may not detect a laboratory with problems of precision. To best detect poor performance without creating an undue burden, the CLIA '88 guideline for proficiency testing recommends testing five samples three times per year. In this system, a failure is defined as two of five incorrect results on two of three consecutive surveys. Additional proficiency testing at the specialty and subspecialty levels is also performed, although the definitions for a successful or failed survey vary.

Performing blinded comparison of analytical results is essential to document proficiency. Multiple laboratory subscription services exist as part of either formal or informal proficiency testing programs. These programs may be governmental or civilian. Laboratories performing drug testing of federal

TABLE 5. Requirements of the Clinical Laboratory Improvement Amendments '88

Assess the validity, reliability, and accuracy of proficiency testing.
Study the reliability of tests performed.
Study the relationship of internal quality assurance and the accuracy and reliability of tests.
Study the extent and nature of problems in diagnosis and treatment due to inaccurate laboratory test results.
Study the effect of errors in each component of the clinical testing process, including the communications with the attending physician; the selection of tests to be performed; the acquisition, transportation, storage, and analysis of specimens; and the reporting of results.

employees are required to follow the mandatory guidelines or Federal Workplace Drug Testing Programs. Nongovernmental laboratory accreditation programs, such as that administered by the College of American Pathologists, have developed their own guidelines. The College of American Pathologists administers four specific accreditation programs including the Forensic Urine Drug Testing program, which is directed toward workplace drug testing of nonfederal employees.

Subscribers to accreditation programs typically receive samples from the program several times per year. The surveying agency analyzes the results returned from the laboratories tested and releases a compiled report. Enrollment in this program is mandatory in most certified programs. Blinded sample validation and enrollment in a blinded proficiency survey system provide additional credibility to the analytical results obtained by the laboratory. Summaries of the College of American Pathologists interlaboratory comparison results are published regularly in the *Archives of Pathology and Laboratory Medicine*.

Assay Validation

Before reporting any analytical result, the assay used must undergo statistical validation. This process is described in detail in multiple private and government publications (2–5). Statistical validation of an assay involves determination of the limits of detection and quantitation, linearity, sample stability, variability of repeat measurements, and many other assessments. The purpose of validation is to demonstrate that the assay behaves in a reproducible and predictable fashion under the analytical conditions that it will be run. If an assay is properly validated, results returned have an appropriate associated degree of scientific certainty.

POSTANALYTICAL CONSIDERATIONS

Reporting Results

There are two parts to any measurement: the number or value itself, which describes the numeric quantity, and the unit of measurement, which describes the physical dimension of the number. A measurement without units may have qualitative value (i.e., one thing being heavier relative to another) but is quantitatively meaningless. A measurement may initially appear alarming or inconsistent with the observed clinical picture until it is realized that the reported result is being expressed in terms of a set of units unfamiliar to the clinician (e.g., a salicylate level of 250 in an asymptomatic patient is alarming until it is realized that the units are μg/ml, which is equivalent to 25 mg/dl, a result in the therapeutic range).

The concept of significant figures is also important in interpreting laboratory results. The number of significant figures in an analytical result cannot exceed the number of significant figures in the most poorly defined part of the analysis. For example, if the analyte concentration of a calibration standard is known accurately to four significant figures and the analyte concentration of the CRM control is known to five significant figures, no result can be reported to more than four significant figures (the least well-determined value in the materials used). Further, for a given analysis, the number of significant figures cannot change from sample to sample. For example, it is scientifically invalid to report one sample as having a concentration of 1.345 mg/L (four significant figures) and a second sample having an analyte concentration of 16.273 mg/L (five significant figures) despite measurement to the same decimal place. To

TABLE 6. Basic International System of Units

Measurement	Basic unit	Symbol
Mass	Kilogram	kg
Length	Meter	m
Quantity	Mole	mol
Time	Second	s
Temperature	Kelvin	K
Electrical current	Ampere	A
Luminous intensity	Candela	cd
Catalytic amount	Katal	kat

maintain scientific integrity, the second result must be reported as 16.27 mg/L.

Traditionally, scientific disciplines have used various sets of units. In 1960, the International System of Units (SI) was adopted and is the only measurement system used in many countries. The SI units are broadly grouped into three fundamental categories: basic, supplemental, and derived. Only one basic unit is given for any physical quantity. For example, all measurements of length use the meter as the basic unit (Table 6). More complete tables are provided in Appendix II. The basic unit avoids the inherent confusion in using non-SI units systems such as feet, inches, and so forth. Derived units have a mathematic relationship to the base unit. Supplemental units are not categorized as basic or derived and are long-standing, traditionally used units that have such common usage they are simply accepted. Supplemental units include hours, days, angles in degrees, and so forth.

The measurement of temperature deserves specific comment. Although the SI unit for temperature measurement is Kelvin (also known as *absolute* temperature), most clinical laboratories use the Celsius scale. Of note, measurements in Celsius and Fahrenheit scales use increments of the degree. There is no such increment in the Kelvin scale. For example, a temperature is reported as 25 degrees C (25°C), which is equivalent to 298 Kelvin (298 K).

Quality Assurance and Quality Control

In the absence of data from CRM controls, it is not possible to see if there are analytical variations over time that demonstrate trends away from accurate measurements. Multiple methods exist for presenting quality assurance and quality control data. Perhaps the simplest way to address this issue is to use CRM controls and plot the values obtained for these controls on an adaptation of a control chart data sheet. Several types of plots are used, but one of the simplest and most common is the Levey-Jennings control chart (Fig. 2). In this type of plot, the analysis date is on the X-axis, and the measured value for a given CRM control is on the Y-axis. The certified value of the CRM control (i.e., the mean value of its determinations) is in the center of the Y-axis and denoted by a boldface line. Dashed horizontal lines above and below the Y-axis represent plus or minus a specified number of standard deviations from that mean (usually 2 or 3). This variation may also be represented as a percent variation from the certified value. The lot number of the CRM is also recorded, and a new chart is used for each new lot number. To look for trending changes in the observed concentrations of the standards, similar plots should be made for the highest, lowest, and intermediate standards.

By examining these plots over time, it is possible to see if measured values for controls are trending toward a higher or lower value or are randomly getting further from the certified or

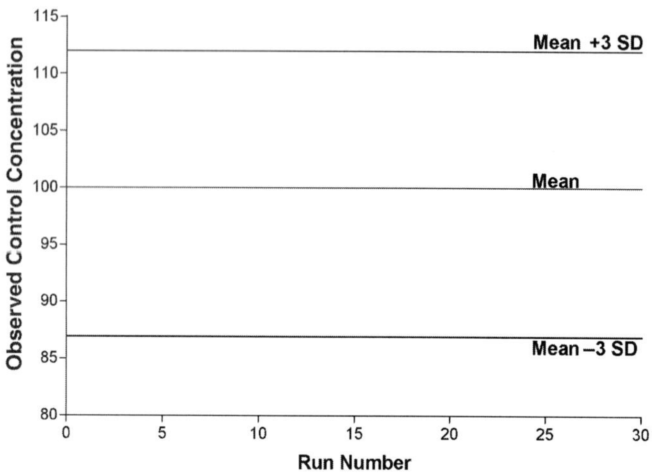

Figure 2. Example of a Levey-Jennings control chart with control limits set at ±3 SD from the mean. Some charts use ±2 SD. With each run, the observed value for the control is plotted versus run number. Control values falling outside control limits must be rejected and explained, and appropriate corrective action must be taken.

TABLE 7. Suggested points for the assessment of analytical validity

Preanalytical
- Sample appropriate for analysis?
- Sample properly collected?
- What were storage conditions, and were they appropriate?
- Transportation of sample was in an appropriate time frame?

Analytical
- Is assay statistically validated?
  - Linearity, limit of detection/limit of quantitation, percentage of relative standard deviation all within acceptable limits?
- Were blanks used between patient runs?
- Were standard reference materials used and within acceptable tolerances?
- Is the laboratory certified/accredited?
- Was the analyst qualified?
- Was the method used specific for the drug, the class of drugs, or only by standard comparison (e.g., retention time, absorbance wavelength, etc.)?

Postanalytical
- Are units reported appropriate?
- Are the significant figures appropriate?
- What quality assurance and quality control programs are in place?

expected value. The real use of this plotting system is that one can detect trends in measurement and initiate corrective intervention long before the CRM controls actually fall out of analytical specification or the control values become unusual. Written procedures should be in place describing how the analyst is to deal with aberrant results in the CRM controls. Such methods are described in many textbooks on laboratory management including *Tietz Fundamentals of Clinical Chemistry*, 5th ed.

Medical Review Officer

A Medical Review Officer (MRO) is a licensed physician with expertise in substance abuse disorders and interpretation of drug test results. The MRO is the individual responsible for receiving the laboratory results and rendering a final decision on whether the sample result is to be reported as positive or negative. In federal drug testing programs, results are sent only to the MRO. The donor provides the MRO with medical records and relevant medical history for review along with the drug testing results. The MRO must allow the donor the opportunity to discuss the result before reporting it to the employer. In the case of a drug screen for employment purposes, if a drug testing result is positive and there exists an alternate medical explanation for the positive result, the MRO reports the results of the drug testing as negative to the employer. Only when there is no reasonable alternate reason for a positive result does the MRO report the result as positive to the employer. As part of the quality control process, the MRO must also review negative results because double blind performance samples may also be sent to the laboratory.

Assessment of Result Validity

The toxicologist is frequently called on to interpret laboratory values in a clinical or forensic setting. In many cases, it is simply assumed that all laboratory assessments performed were done properly and the results valid, even for unusual analytes. Although the process for establishing true analytical validity for a given assay can be quite involved, a brief outline of key points in analytical validity assessment is provided in Table 7.

All phases of the laboratory procedure must be assessed to assure a given result or set of results is valid. Variables that can affect the assay in the preanalytical phase include proper identification of the patient, preparation of the patient for specimen collection, the actual specimen collection, sample transport, sample separation and aliquoting, laboratory logs, turnaround time, and logging and transcribing sample intake information. Variables affecting the analytical phase include appropriate choice of analytical methodology, use of reference and calibrator materials, and maintaining technical competence, among others. Postanalytically, variables such as transcription errors, reporting to the proper patient's chart, legibility of reports, timeliness of reports, and proper interpretation of results must be controlled.

Flanagan Tables

A series of tables summarizing many facets of the laboratory was originally compiled by Flanagan of the Poisons Unit of Guy's and St. Thomas Hospital Trust in London and has been reproduced previously. These useful tables are reprinted in Appendix II.

REFERENCES

1. Boyanton BL, Blick KE. Stability studies of twenty-four analytes in human plasma and serum. *Clin Chem* 2000;48:2242–2247.
2. Jenke DR. Chromatographic method validation: a review of current practices and procedures. I. General concepts and guidelines. *J Liq Chrom Rel Technol* 1996;19:719–736.
3. Jenke DR. Chromatographic method validation: a review of current practices and procedures. II. Guidelines for primary validation parameters. *J Liq Chrom Rel Technol* 1996;19:737–757.
4. Jenke DR. Chromatographic method validation: a review of current practices and procedures. III. Ruggedness, revalidation and system suitability. *J Liq Chrom Rel Technol* 1996;19:1873–1891.
5. U.S. Food and Drug Administration. Reviewer guidance: validation of chromatographic methods. Washington: US Government Printing Office; 1994.

SUGGESTED READING

Bishop ML, Duben-Engelkirk JL, Fody EP, eds. *Clinical chemistry: principles, procedures, correlations*, 4th ed. Philadelphia: Lippincott Williams & Wilkins, 2000.

Burtis CA, Ashwood ER, eds. *Tietz textbook of clinical chemistry*, 3rd ed. Philadelphia: WB Saunders, 1999.

Levine B, ed. *Principles of forensic toxicology*. Washington DC: American Association for Clinical Chemistry Press, 1999.

CHAPTER 83

Interpretation of Analytical Results in Forensic Toxicology

Jerrold B. Leikin and William A. Watson

OVERVIEW

Forensic toxicology includes an understanding of drug use in the immediate antemortem setting, analytical methodologies, and interpretation of the results to determine the role of drug and substance toxicity in causing death. Until the early 1990s, the interpretation of the postmortem blood drug levels was viewed as a relatively simple process. The concentration of drug measured in the postmortem sample was compared to established therapeutic and toxic concentration ranges in the antemortem state (1). Using antemortem concentration ranges for comparison was based on the concept that the drug concentration in the sample does not change after death. This concept has been shown to be incorrect for many substances, and the potential for postmortem changes must be considered for all but a few drugs in which postmortem changes have been demonstrated not to occur (Table 1).

NECROKINETICS

The interpretation of drug concentrations is commonly the most difficult aspect of forensic toxicology. It depends on a number of variables that can result in anatomic site differences of blood levels and changes over time postmortem. The change in drug concentration over time after death was defined as *necrokinetics* in the early 1990s, although the terms *postmortem changes* or *redistribution* are more commonly used and were initially described in the early 1970s (1).

The goal of necrokinetics is to determine whether the drugs measured played a role in the patient's death. This is analogous to clinical toxicology with the exception that the results are not used to determine patient prognosis or treatment requirements. Ideally, the interpretation of postmortem drug concentrations is based on information demonstrating a predictable and consistent relationship between the drug concentration at a specific site (usually venous plasma or serum) at the time of death and the concentration measured in a postmortem sample. Several antemortem factors impact the relationship between the concentration and effect, including the dose administered, the time of administration before death, the route of administration, the development of tolerance to drug effects over time, and whether the drug is at steady-state. The majority of drug concentration–effect relationships are developed in therapeutic situations using trough levels (the concentration immediately before the next dose is administered) at steady-state. In addition, the drug's apparent volume of distribution and pK_a are important determinants of the extent of postmortem changes (1–3).

TABLE 1. Toxins and drugs in which postmortem redistribution does not occur

Alcohols[a]	Nitrazepam
Carbon monoxide	Phenelzine
Carbamazepine	Pheniramine
Chlordiazepoxide	Phenobarbital
Diflunisal	Primidone
Ephedrine	Procyclidine
Hydrocodone	Quinine/Quinidine
Hydroxyzine	Theophylline
Lamotrigine	Xylazine
Lorazepam	Zopiclone
Mirtazapine	

[a]Ethanol level may increase in decomposed bodies due to postmortem fermentation (see Matrix Issues).

Sampling Sites

To understand how these variables impact postmortem drug concentrations, data from both experimental models and human cases are needed. Samples should be collected at various times postmortem and from various sites to determine whether these variables are associated with the changes in drug concentration. To determine whether postmortem redistribution occurs, postmortem samples should be compared to a sample collected immediately before or at the time of death because the rate of redistribution is generally not known. Examples of morphine and barbiturates indicate that redistribution may occur rapidly after death. Significant increases in thiopental and pentobarbital blood concentrations have been demonstrated within 4 hours postmortem (2). When postmortem morphine concentrations are compared to antemortem or perimortem samples, significant increases in concentration are observed in the first few minutes. When the first sample collected is 3 hours or more postmortem, however, no further increase is observed (3–5). Furthermore, collection of samples from multiple sites is important, so that comparisons and standardization of collection sites can be defined. Some sites may have a consistent relation to the blood level at the time of death, whereas others may not.

The assumption that death results in a total cessation of drug movement in the body has obscured the dynamics of drug distribution and transformation that occur in the perimortem and postmortem state (6–15). Because cardiovascular circulation has ended, these dynamics are dependent on the chemical characteristics of the drug and primarily due to several factors: passive concentration-gradient–driven diffusion of the drug as the tissue integrity is lost, fluid shifts, pH, apparent volume of distribution, and the condition of the body. The stomach, liver, bladder, and lungs have all been evaluated as sources of drug for redistribution postmortem. Gravity-dependent blood flow may also play a role in differences among drug concentrations at different sites. For example, diffusion of drug from the stomach primarily accumulates in the left lobe of the liver (14). How-

TABLE 2. Drugs in which postmortem transformation or redistribution may occur

Drug name	Approximate cardiac blood to peripheral blood concentration ratio (C:P ratio)	Drug name	Approximate cardiac blood to peripheral blood concentration ratio (C:P ratio)
Alfentanil	—	Methylenedioxymethamphetamine	2.65
Alprazolam	1.5	Methylfentanyl	—
Amineptine hydrochloride	—	Methyprylon	1.9
Amitriptyline	3.1	Metoprolol	3.8
Amoxapine	1.8	Mexiletine	3.6
Amphetamine	2	Midazolam	4
Benztropine	1.3	Morphine (heroin)	2.2
Brompheniramine	—	*N*-methylbenzodioxazolybutan-amine or MBDB	2.5
Bupropion	1.9	Naproxen	1.5
Chloroquine	3	Nefazodone	—
Chlorpheniramine	3.1	Nicotine	Cotinine-3
Chlorpromazine	4	Nortriptyline	2.4
Clomipramine	1.9	Orphenadrine	1.9
Clonazepam	2	Oxazepam	1.3
Clothiapine	—	Oxycodone	3.1
Clozapine	2.8	Paramethoxyamphetamine	1.6
Cocaine	1.5–2.3	Paroxetine	1.3
Codeine	1.8	Pentazocine	2
Cyanide	1.3	Pethidine or meperidine	2.1
Cyclobenzaprine	2.2	Phencyclidine	1.8
D-Methamphetamine	2.1	Phentermine	1.7
Desipramine	2.4	Phenylbutazone	2.3
Dextromethorphan	2	Phenylpropanolamine	2.4
Diazepam	1.6	Phenytoin	1.4
Diltiazem	2.6	Promethazine	1.6
Diphenhydramine	2.3	Propafenone	2.4
Doxepin or dothiepin	3.0–5.5	Propoxyphene	3.5
Doxylamine	—	Propranolol	2.5
Flunitrazepam	3	Protriptyline	—
Fluoxetine	2.9	Pseudoephedrine	1.5
Flurazepam	3	Quetiapine	—
Fluvoxamine	1.7	Remifentanil	—
Furosemide	1.7	Secobarbital	1.5
Gamma hydroxybutyrate	2	Strychnine	15
Haloperidol	3.6	Sufentanil	—
Hydrochlorothiazide	23	Temazepam	1.6
Ibuprofen	1.8	Tetrahydrocannabinol	—
Imipramine	1.8–2.2	Timolol	2
Indomethacin	1.9	Tranylcypromine	2.2
Ketamine	1.6	Trazodone	1.6
Lidocaine	—	Triazolam	2.8
Maprotiline	3.4	Trichloroethanol	2.0
Meprobamate	1.7	Trimipramine	1.6
Mesoridazine	1.3	Venlafaxine	1.6
Metapramine	—	Verapamil	—
Methamphetamine	2.4	Zolpidem	2.1
Methotrimeprazine	1.3		

ever, if stomach contents reflux from the stomach into the airway, drug may be absorbed into the pulmonary vasculature and result in elevated cardiac and pulmonary vein drug levels (14). The effects of local diffusion are usually not significant when samples are collected from peripheral sites. Ethanol absorption and distribution from the stomach can contaminate pericardial sac blood, a common postmortem sample, when 400 ml of 10% ethanol is present. Ethanol contamination of femoral vein samples under similar conditions is minimal (16).

The cardiac to peripheral blood level ratio of drug concentrations in postmortem blood samples has been evaluated as a measure of the potential for postmortem drug redistribution (Table 2). Drugs that have high ratios are believed to have greater potential for redistribution. In these circumstances, collection of autopsy samples from either a heart chamber or the pericardial sac may result in a drug concentration that is significantly higher than the peripheral concentrations, resulting in inaccurate interpretation of the results.

The position of the body also affects postmortem drug distribution. In general, the supine position is associated with basic drugs in the lungs diffusing into the left heart chambers postmortem (via the pulmonary venous blood movement) (6–15). Additionally, it is known that basic drugs (tricyclic antidepressants, cardiac glycosides, local anesthetics, and opioids) can bind preferentially to the myocardium during life. Diffusion from the myocardium into heart blood may produce increased heart blood concentrations, although this mechanism for anatomic site concentration differences is debated (10–12). Table 2 is a partial list of drugs in which anatomic site differences have been demonstrated (12,13,17–30).

Matrix Issues

A primary difficulty in evaluating postmortem assays is that whole blood is the primary matrix for quantitative autopsy analysis, whereas serum is the usual matrix measured in clinical settings. This can result in a 12% to 18% difference for ethanol values and a factor of 1.6 for cannabinoid samples (to calculate plasma concentrations from whole blood values) (31,32). Further, depending on the time after death that the sample is collected, the consistency of the blood sample changes, with clotting, fluid movement, and cellular components changing. This is potentially important when evaluating postmortem changes for fluoxetine (33).

An analysis of the drugs that have been shown to change in concentration after death can guide the toxicologist to the proper interpretation of postmortem drug levels. It appears that drugs that have a relatively large apparent volume of distribution (greater than 3 L/kg) are candidates for redistribution from tissue into vascular space via passive diffusion from surrounding tissue and extravascular fluid. Postmortem transformation of parent drug to the metabolites is a relatively rare occurrence but has been described with nitrobenzodiazepines (34,35). Ethanol production through fermentation (i.e., when ethanol was not originally present) can occur in substantially decomposed bodies, resulting in blood ethanol levels usually in the range of 0.05 g/dl, although concentrations of up to 0.2 mg% have been reported infrequently (36). Other volatiles such as n-propanol and acetaldehyde can be associated with postmortem ethanol generation through fermentation. Putrefactive ethanol generation usually takes 3 to 10 days to develop. However, cocaethylene, the metabolite resulting from the presence of cocaine and ethanol, cannot be exogenously produced by this mechanism.

Alternative matrices to blood are also usually used to assist in determination of drug-related deaths (Table 3) (37–43). Skeletal muscle (especially the lateral dome of the diaphragm) can serve as a stable matrix for the qualitative determination of drugs (43–44). Bile sequestration of drugs also serves as an excellent site for drug identification for drugs that are found in high concentrations in the bile (Table 4) (13,25,45–47). Drugs identified in adipose tissue are present due to antemortem distribution and not due to postmortem movement (48).

The vitreous humor often serves as the only other matrix from which a quantitative interpretation can be accomplished. The concentration of ethanol in the vitreous is similar to blood, ranging from 0.9 to 1.3 times that of blood concentrations; it also lags well behind blood ethanol concentrations over time (33,49). Vitreous samples can also aid in quantitative analysis of 6-acetylmorphine, benzodiazepines, and electrolytes (30,37,50,51).

TABLE 3. Recommended tissue sampling sites to determine acute fatal poisoning

Drug or chemical	Sampling site
Aconitum alkaloids	Liver, kidneys, ileum, feces
Alimemazine	Brain
Cadmium	Liver or renal cortex
Chloroquine	Liver >150 mg/kg
Colchicine	Bile
Copper	Liver
Digoxin	Kidney >140 μg/kg
Diquat	Kidney >2.4 μg/g
Endrin	Adipose >90 mg/kg
Ethanol	Vitreous
Fentanyl	Liver levels >69 μg/kg associated with overdose
Gold	Renal cortex
Heroin	Brain/cerebellum/vitreous[a]
Insulin	Tissue site injection or femoral blood
Lidocaine	>15 mg/kg in brain, lung, heart, liver, kidney[b]
Platinum	Urine or kidney
Potassium	Vitreous: postmortem interval (h) equals (7.14 times K+) minus 39.1
Silver	Brain/liver
Tricyclic antidepressant	Liver
Xylene	Liver >1 mg/kg
Zopiclone	Right lobe of liver and blood

[a]Cerebellum to blood morphine level ratio is approximately 1 when death occurs within 1 hour and is 3.5 when death occurs within 2 to 48 hours of administration; also, analyzing 6-acetylmorphine in cerebrospinal fluid can detect 46% more heroin-related cases than blood.
[b]Absorption of tracheal lidocaine during intubation (cardiopulmonary resuscitation) results in a kidney to liver lidocaine ratio of less than 1, whereas absorption during intravenous lidocaine treatment results in a ratio of more than 1.

Other Factors Affecting Interpretation of Postmortem Drug Levels

Other selected relevant postmortem blood result interpretations include alcoholic ketoacidosis. The cause of a person's death is ultimately judged unknown in approximately 3% of cases; however, up to 10% of sudden deaths in alcoholic patients may be of unknown cause (52). A blood β-hydroxybutyrate level more than 2500 μmol/L may indicate that the cause of death was alcoholic ketoacidosis (52).

Death due to newer antidepressant or antipsychotic agents can be difficult to identify due to lack of postmortem toxidromes or the presence of coingestants. Some chemicals or drugs produce specific postmortem findings that can help identify the agent responsible for the death. For example, ethylene glycol produces oxalate crystals in the kidney. Some agents have postmortem blood levels that are associated with psychotropic-related fatalities: fluoxetine, 0.63 mg/L; paroxetine, 0.4 mg/L; sertraline, 1.5 mg/L; olanzapine, 0.160 mg/L; and trazodone, 9 mg/L (53–55).

Due to postmortem hemolysis, serum and urinary lactate dehydrogenase, lactic acid, and protein levels may become elevated (56,57). These changes can result in false-positive immunoassays of certain drugs: amphetamines, barbiturates, opiates, cocaine metabolite, propoxyphene, benzodiazepines, ethanol (urine and serum), and low serum phenytoin (high lactate dehydrogenase in blood). C-reactive protein concentrations do not appear to change (58).

Thus, it is clear that the clinical toxicologist must address several issues to properly determine the role of a certain drug in causing death when presented with quantitative results:

1. Were samples collected from multiple sites analyzed for determination of blood drug concentrations? From where were these samples collected?
2. Is the drug either known or suspected to undergo postmortem redistribution (Table 2)?
3. Are there adequate scientific data available to define the concentration-toxicity relationship?
4. Is there adequate clinical information available regarding the drug exposure to insure an accurate interpretation of the results (e.g., tolerance, dosing interval)?
5. Was the drug concentration clinically sufficient to cause, prevent, or be involved directly in the death by affecting the actions of the decedent?
6. Are there characteristic autopsy tissue findings of the overdose (Table 5) (25,48,59,60)?
7. Was the body embalmed (Table 6)? The tricyclic amines and n-ethylamines in the presence of formaldehyde (5% to 20%) are methylated through the Eshweiler-Clark reaction (25,61–68).
8. Does the analyte involved require special sample storage conditions (Table 7) (69–76)?

TABLE 4. Drugs that concentrate in the bile for postmortem analysis

Drug name	Bile to blood ratio in mg/L
Acebutolol	416–22
Acetaminophen	560–248
Amitriptyline	25–2.2
Amoxapine	61–18
Anileridine	2.4–0.9
Antimony	404–4.6
Barium	6.1–1.9
Benzoylecgonine	12–2.4
Bismuth	3.9–0.5
Buprenorphine	25.3–0.004
Chlordiazepoxide	4–2.5
Chlorpromazine	80–1.4
Chlorprothixene	3.9–0.1
Clozapine	454–2.8
Cocaethylene	0.6–0.08
Cocaine	0.7–0.2
Codeine	18–2.8
Colchicine	2.9–0.6
Colchicine	2.9–0.06
Cyproheptadine	8.1–0.5
Desipramine	39–5.6
Diazepam	2.8–0.9
Diltiazem	180–11
Dothiepin	65–3
Doxepin	108–7.4
Ecgonine methyl ester	3.3–1.2
Ethchlorvynol	382–78
Fenfluramine	65–6.5
Fentanyl	0.03–0.01
Flecainide	290–53
Fluoxetine	0.013–0.006
Flurazepam	43–9
Gamma-hydroxybutyrate	57–12
Heroin (morphine)	32–0.43
Hydromorphone	9.2–0.3
Hydroxyzine	122–39
Imipramine	45–3.7
Isoniazid	900–43
Levorphanol	24–2.7
Lidocaine	19–12
Loxapine	16–5
Maprotiline	161–6.2
Methadone	7.5–1.0
Methamphetamine	22–8
Methapyrilene	25–8
Methaqualone	83–8
Methylfentanyl	0.047–0.007
Methylphenidate	5.7–2.8
Metoprolol	254–4.7
Mexiletine	440–38
Mirtazapine	2.5–0.22
Norsertraline	57–0.4
Nortriptyline	11–2
Oxycodone	28–5
Para-methoxyamphetamine	8.0–1.1
Perphenazine	40–4
Phenmetrazine	5–1
Phenylbutazone	475–400
Sertraline	11–0.3
Sodium azide	651–135
Sulindac	2810–130
Thioridazine	9–3
Tramadol	3.5–1.9
Trazodone	45–15
Trichloroethanol	111–79
Trimipramine	2.4–1.3
Venlafaxine	195–45
Zimelidine	1.4–0.7

TABLE 5. Postmortem toxidromes

Drug or chemical	Finding
Dinitro-*o*-cresol	Rapid rigor mortis
Hydrogen sulfide	Discoloration of pennies and dimes (purple/blue)
Carbon monoxide	Cherry red skin appearance (a *classic finding* with <1% prevalence)
Loperamide	Severe abdominal distention in infants younger than 6 mo
Diethyltin	Interstitial edema of brain white matter
Methanol	Putamen/retinal—photoreceptor cell necrosis; optic nerve degeneration
Ethylene glycol	Oxalate nephrosis
Benzene/lead acetate	Bone marrow fibrosis
Anthracycline treatment (chronic)	Hydropic myocardial degeneration
Vitamin D	Ectopic calcification
Fentanyl	Syringe in vein
Arsenic	Necrotic gastroenteritis
Bismuth	Necrotic gastroenteritis
Copper	Necrotic gastroenteritis
Gold	Necrotic gastroenteritis
Iron Salts	Necrotic gastroenteritis
Lead	Necrotic gastroenteritis
Manganese	Necrotic gastroenteritis
Mercury	Necrotic gastroenteritis
Nitrites	Necrotic gastroenteritis
Nickel	Necrotic gastroenteritis
Phosphorus	Necrotic gastroenteritis
Thallium	Necrotic gastroenteritis
Vanadium	Necrotic gastroenteritis
Zinc	Necrotic gastroenteritis

Hair and Nail Analysis

The determination of drug or toxin exposure through postmortem hair or nail testing may have an impact on the medical examiner's findings on the cause and manner of death as well as the circumstances surrounding the event (77). Postmortem hair testing is a useful technique for drug abuse detection, with certain caveats (77–81). The metabolite 6-acetylmorphine is the appropriate biomarker for heroin abuse as compared to acetylcodeine (which is not present in approximately 50% of cases) (79). The biomarker for crack cocaine exposure is anhydro-ecgonine methyl ester, with lidocaine as an appropriate adulterant biomarker in cocaine abusers (82).

Flunitrazepam doses of 1 mg may not result in positive urinary or blood benzodiazepine assays, and their metabolite may be increased in decomposed bodies. However, the metabolite (7-aminoflunitrazepam) may appear in hair in greater concentrations than the parent compound. Flunitrazepam-related deaths

TABLE 6. Drug issues associated with embalming

May introduce artifact, increasing amitriptyline level and decreasing nortriptyline level (conversion rate of 65% in 24 h)
Succinylcholine (postmortem endogenous succinic acid up to 200 mg/kg and 2000 mg/kg may be noted in embalmed brain and liver, respectively)
Slight effect (lowering) on hepatic fentanyl levels
Little effect on strychnine concentrations
May reduce blood ethanol levels
May increase methyl alcohol levels
No apparent effect on morphine analysis
May convert fenfluramine to *N*-methyl fenfluramine
Reduces benzodiazepine levels
Hydrolytic decomposition of phenobarbital to 2-phenylbutyric acid (no apparent effect with pentobarbital or secobarbital)

TABLE 7. Toxins in which specimen storage may be an issue

Cyanide
Acetaldehyde
Chloroform (82% loss when stored for 42 d)
Nicotine (cotinine)
Zopiclone (unstable in alkaline solutions)
Ethchlorvynol (losses up to 90% after 3 mo of storage)
Ethanol
Heroin (6-acetylmorphine is stable at –20°C)
Lysergic acid diethylamide (protect from light or elevated temperature)
Succinylcholine (may disappear from body fluids in 20 d)
Insulin (55% loss in hemolyzed specimen)
Lead
Toluene
Benzene
Trichloroethylene
Zinc (may rise in hemolysis)
Aniline (false-positive when there is concomitant acetaminophen)
Amiodarone
Diltiazem (*in vitro* conversion to desacetyldiltiazem)
γ-hydroxybutyrate (may be artificially elevated in citrate-buffered blood)
Morphine and metabolites (degradation at 4°C, but not –20°C)
Methemoglobin (postcollection rise in frozen-thawed specimens)
Nitrazepam (degrades when exposed to heat, light, or bacteria)
Sarin (store at –20°C/avoid fluoride-containing tubes)
Rifampin (54°C loss within 8 h of storage at room temperature)
Loprazolam (store at –20°C)
Pyridostygmine (store at –20°C)
Ethylbenzene (store at –20°C)
Olanzapine (add ascorbic acid)

have been correlated with maximum flunitrazepam hair levels ranging from 1.8 to 9.5 ng/g (83).

Fingernails are also a useful matrix for several drugs and chemicals (Table 8) (83–86). Hair grows approximately 1 cm per month, fingernails approximately 3 to 5 mm per month, and toenails approximately 1.1 mm per month. Scraping the underside of the nail is essential to remove sweat contamination. Specific drugs/toxin issues in fingernail analysis are detailed in Table 8.

CONCLUSION

Although a drug concentration result may be available from a sample obtained at autopsy, the interpretation and extrapolation of the result to the antemortem state may not always be possible. Although the temptation often exists to interpret the result, the limitations of our knowledge of postmortem necrokinetics can lead to incorrect assumptions (87). Whenever data are available, the drug's postmortem stability and potential for redistribution must be incorporated into the interpretation. The older methods of merely finding pills in gastric contents may be misleading, because these pills may not contain active drug and may be simply a drug-free wax matrix (88). Newer modalities of tissue analysis and hair and nail drug analysis may be helpful in assisting the toxicologist by providing information about the deceased's past use of drugs (89–92). The use of pharmacogenomics (molecular autopsy) can serve as an additional modality in evaluating drug-related death. For example, by genotyping the polymorphic enzyme CYP 2D6 in postmortem blood, an enhanced interpretation of poor and intermediate oxycodone metabolizers and, thus, potential toxicity, can be obtained (94–98). This may be especially useful if a drug interaction is considered as a cause of elevated levels. Newer modalities, such as coupling liquid chromatography with electrospray single quadruple mass-spectrometry (operational in the 100 to 1100 μ mass range in both positive and negative modes) may be useful in drug identification for general unknown screening purposes (99). Forensic entomotoxicology can be useful in qualitative drug analysis in decomposed specimens when insect larvae are involved (100,101). Additional animal research and evaluation of the results obtained at autopsy (especially multiple site analysis and timely antemortem and postmortem assays) are necessary to improve our ability to accurately interpret and report postmortem drug concentrations (102–104).

TABLE 8. Nail analysis

Arsenic (approximately 80% of corresponding hair level)
Amphetamines/methamphetamine
Cocaine/cocaine metabolites/cocaethylene
Cannabis
Morphine/6-monoacetylmorphine/codeine/hydrocodone
Lead (approximately 70% of corresponding hair level)

REFERENCES

1. Winek CL, Wahba WW, Winek CL Jr, et al. Drug and chemical blood-level data 2001. *Forensic Sci Int* 2001;122:107–123.
2. Watson WA, Godley PJ, Garriott JC, et al. Blood pentobarbital concentrations during thiopental therapy. *Drug Intell Clin Pharm* 1986:20;283–287.
3. Koren G, Klein J. Postmortem redistribution of morphine in rats. *Ther Drug Monit* 1992;14:461–463.
4. Logan BK, Smirnow D. Postmortem distribution and redistribution of morphine in man. *J Forensic Sci* 1996;41:37–46.
5. Sawyer WR, Forney RB. Postmortem disposition of morphine in rats. *Forensic Sci Int* 1988;38:259–273.
6. Shepherd MF, Lake KD, Kamps MA. Postmortem changes and pharmacokinetics: a review of the literature and case report. *Ann Pharmacother* 1992;26:510–514.
7. Gomez HF, McKinney PE, Phillips S, et al. Postmortem acetaminophen pharmacokinetics: site and time dependent concentration changes. *J Forensic Sci* 1995;40:980–982.
8. O'Sullivan JJ, McCarth PY, Wren C. Differences in amiodarone, digoxin, flecainide and sotalol concentrations between antemortem serum and femoral postmortem blood. *Hum Exp Toxicol* 1995;14:605–608.
9. Moriya F, Hasimoto Y. Redistribution of basic drugs into cardiac blood from surrounding tissues during early-stages postmortem. *J Forensic Sci* 1999;44(1):10–16.
10. Prouty RW, Anderson WH. The forensic science implications of site and temporal influences on postmortem blood-drug concentrations. *J Forensic Sci* 1990;35:243–270.
11. Bailey DN, Shaw RF. Concentrations of basic drugs in postmortem human myocardium. *J Toxicol Clin Toxicol* 1982;19:197–202.
12. Dalphe-Scott M, Degouffe M, Garbutt D, et al. A comparison of drug concentrations in postmortem cardiac and peripheral blood in 320 cases. *Can Soc For Sci J* 1995;28:113–121.
13. Hilberg T, Rogde S, Marland J. Postmortem drug redistribution—human cases related to results in experimental animals. *J Forensic Sci* 1999;44:3–9.
14. Hilberg T, Ripel A, Slordal L, et al. The extent of postmortem drug redistribution in a rat model. *J Forensic Sci* 1999;44(5):956–962.
15. Baselt RC, ed. *Disposition of toxic drugs and chemicals in man*, 5th ed. Foster City, CA: Chemical Toxicology Institute, 2000.
16. Pounder DJ, Smith DRW. Postmortem diffusion of alcohol from the stomach. *Am J Forensic Med Pathol* 1995;16:89–96.
17. Anderson DT, Fritz KL. Quetiapine (Seroquel) concentrations in seven postmortem cases. *J Anal Toxicol* 2000;24:300–304.
18. Barnhart FE, Fogacci JR, Reed DW. Methamphetamine—a study of postmortem redistribution. *J Anal Toxicol* 1999;23:69–70.
19. Anderson DT, Fritz KL, Muto JJ. Distribution of mirtazapine (Remeron) in thirteen postmortem cases. *J Anal Toxicol* 1999;23:544–548.
20. Logan BK, Smirnow D, Gullberg RG. Lack of predictable site-dependent differences and time-dependent changes in postmortem concentrations of cocaine, benzoylecgonine, and cocaethylene in humans. *J Anal Toxicol* 1997;20:23–31.
21. Kintz P. Interpreting the results of medico-legal analysis in cases of substance abuse. *J Toxicol Clin Toxicol* 2000;38:197–198.
22. Levine B, Wu SC, Smialek JE. Zolpidem distribution in postmortem cases. *J Forensic Sci* 1999;44(2):369–371.
23. Braithwaite RA, Elliott SP, Hale KA. An unusual fatality due to abuse of alfentanil/midazolam mixture. *J Toxicol Clin Toxicol* 2000;38:231.
24. Leikin JB, Paloucek FP. *Poisoning and toxicology handbook*, 3rd ed. Hudson, OH: Lexi-Comp, 2002:1391–1405.
25. Martin TL. Three cases of fatal paramethoxyamphetamine overdose. *J Anal Toxicol* 2001;25:649–651.
26. Levine B, Zhang B, Smialek JE. Citalopram distribution in postmortem cases. *J Anal Toxicol* 2001;25:641–644.
27. Rossum KM, Holt G, Robertson MD. Death by strychnine—a case for postmortem redistribution. *J Anal Toxicol* 2001;25:382.
28. Kemp PM, Sneed GS, George CE, et al. Postmortem distribution of nicotine and cotinine from a case involving the simultaneous administration of multiple nicotine transdermal systems. *J Anal Toxicol* 1997;21(4):310–313.

29. Levine B, Grieshaber A, Pestaner J, et al. Distribution of triazolam and alpha-hydroxytriazolam in fatal intoxication case. *J Anal Toxicol* 2002;26:52–54.
30. DeLetter EA, Clauwaert KM, Lambert WE, et al. Distribution study of 3,4-methylenedioxy-methamphetamine and 3,4-methylenedioxyamphetamine in a fatal overdose. *J Anal Toxicol* 2002;26:113–118.
31. Giroud C, Menetrey A, Augsburger M, et al. Delta (9)-THC, 11-OH-delta(9)-THC and delta(9)-THCCOOH plasma or serum to whole blood concentration distribution ratios in blood samples taken from living and dead people. *Forensic Sci Int* 2001;123(2–3):159–164.
32. Williams RH, Leikin JB. Medicolegal issues and specimen collection for ethanol testing. *Lab Med* 1999;30(8):530–537.
33. Pohland RC, Bernhard NR. Postmortem serum and tissue redistribution of fluoxetine and norfluoxetine in dogs following oral administration of fluoxetine hydrochloride (Prozac). *J Forensic Sci* 1997;42:812–816.
34. Robertson MD, Drummer OH. Postmortem drug metabolism by bacteria. *J Forensic Sci* 1995;40:382–386.
35. Robertson MD, Drummer OH. Postmortem distribution and redistribution of nitrobenzodiazepines in man. *J Forensic Sci* 1998;43(1):9–13.
36. Winek CL. Reliability of 22-hour postmortem blood and gastric alcohol samples. *JAMA* 1975;233:912.
37. Jenkins AJ, Lavins ES. 6-Acetylmorphine detection in postmortem cerebrospinal fluid. *J Anal Toxicol* 1998;22:173–175.
38. Moriya J, Hashimoto Y. Determining the state of the deceased during cardiopulmonary resuscitation from tissue distribution patterns of intubation-related lidocaine. *J Forensic Sci* 2000;45:846–849.
39. Mackey-Bojack S, Kloss J, Apple F. Cocaine, cocaine metabolite and ethanol concentrations in postmortem blood and vitreous humor. *J Anal Toxicol* 2000;24:59–65.
40. Anderson DT, Muto JJ. Duragesic transdermal patch: postmortem tissue distribution of fentanyl in 25 cases. *J Anal Toxicol* 2000;24:627–634.
41. Gorczynski LY, Melbye FJ. Detection of benzodiazepines in different tissues including done, using a quantitative ELISA assay. *J Forensic Sci* 2001;46(4):916–918.
42. Kalasinsky KS, Dixon MM, Schmunk GA, et al. Blood, brain and hair GHB concentrations following fatal ingestion. *J Forensic Sci* 2001;46(3):728–730.
43. Langford AM, Taylor KK, Pounder DJ. Drug concentration in selected skeletal muscles. *J Forensic Sci* 1998;43(1):22–27.
44. Garriott JC. Skeletal muscle as an alternative specimen for alcohol and drug analysis. *J Forensic Sci* 1991;36:60–69.
45. Lemos N, Agarwal A. Significance of bile analysis in drug-induced deaths. *J Anal Toxicol* 1996;20:61–63.
46. Mazzola CD, Miron S, Jenkins AJ. Loxapine intoxication: case report and literature review. *J Anal Toxicol* 2000;24:638–641.
47. Davis G, Park K, Kloss J, et al. Tricyclic antidepressant fatality: postmortem tissue concentrations. *J Toxicol Clin Toxicol* 2001;39(6):649–650.
48. Levisky JA, Bowerman DL, Jenkins WW, et al. Drugs in postmortem adipose tissues: evidence of antemortem disposition. *Forensic Sci Int* 2001;121:157–160.
49. Hardin GG. Postmortem blood and vitreous human ethanol concentrations in a victim of a fatal motor vehicle crash. *J Forensic Sci* 2002;47(2):402–403.
50. Amitai Y. Establishing a cause of death dependent upon time of presentation. *J Toxicol Clin Toxicol* 2001;39(6):651–652.
51. Scott KS, Oliver JS. The use of vitreous humor as an alternative to whole blood for the analysis of benzodiazepines. *J Forensic Sci* 2001;46(3):694–697.
52. Iten PX, Meir M. Beta-hydroxybutyric acid—an indicator for an alcoholic ketoacidosis as cause of death in deceased alcohol abusers. *J Forensic Sci* 2000;45:624–632.
53. Goeringer KE, Raymon L, Christian GD, et al. Postmortem forensic toxicology of selective serotonin reuptake inhibitors: a review of pharmacology and report of 168 cases. *J Forensic Sci* 2000;45:633–648.
54. Robertson MD, McMullin MM. Olanzapine concentrations in clinical serum and postmortem blood specimens—when does therapeutic become toxic? *J Forensic Sci* 2000;45:418–421.
55. Geoeringer KE, Raymon L, Logan BK. Postmortem forensic toxicology of trazodone. *J Forensic Sci* 2000;45:850–856.
56. Coe JJ. Postmortem chemistry update. *Am J Forensic Med Pathol* 1993;14:91–117.
57. Sloop G, Hall M, Simmons GT, et al. False-positive postmortem EMIT drugs of abuse assay due to lactate dehydrogenase and lactate in urine. *J Anal Toxicol* 1995;19:554–556.
58. Uhlin-Hansen U. C-reactive protein (CRP), a comparison of pre- and postmortem blood levels. *Forensic Sci Int* 2001;121:157–160.
59. Simini B. Cherry red discolouration in carbon monoxide poisoning. *Lancet* 1998;352(9134):1154.
60. Graeme KA, Wallace KL, Curry SC, et al. Hydrogen sulfide-induced changes in coin appearance. *J Toxicol Clin Toxicol* 1998;36:469–470.
61. Dettling RJ, Briglia EJ, Dal Cortivo LA, et al. The production of amitriptyline from nortriptyline in formaldehyde containing solutions. *J Anal Toxicol* 1990;14:325–326.
62. Rohrig TP. Comparison of fentanyl concentrations in unembalmed and embalmed liver samples. *J Anal Toxicol* 1998;22:253.
63. Tracy TS, Rybeck BF, James DG, et al. Stability of benzodiazepines in formaldehyde solutions. *J Anal Toxicol* 2001;25:166–173.
64. Skopp G, Potsch L, Klingmann A, et al. Stability of morphine, morphine-3-glucuronide, and morphine-6-glucuranide in fresh blood and plasma and postmortem blood samples. *J Anal Toxicol* 2001;25:2–7.
65. Cingolani M, Froldi R, Mencarelli R, et al. Detection and quantitation of morphine in fixed tissues and formalin solutions. *J Anal Toxicol* 2001;25:31–39.
66. Gannett PM, Hailu S, Daft J, et al. In vitro reaction of formaldehyde with fenfluramine: conversion to N-methyl fenfluramine. *J Anal Toxicol* 2001;25:88–92.
67. Gannett PM, Daft JR, James D, et al. In vitro reaction of barbiturates with formaldehyde. *J Anal Toxicol* 2001;25:443–449.
68. Gransioli MG, Szabo ET, Sunshine I. Detection of methadone as a propoxyphene in stored tissues. *J Anal Toxicol* 1980;4:46–48.
69. Kunsman GW, Presses CL, Rodriguez P. Carbon monoxide stability in stored postmortem blood samples. *J Anal Toxicol* 2000;24:572–578.
70. Koves M, Lawrence K, Mayer JM. Stability of diltiazem in whole blood: forensic implications. *J Forensic Sci* 1998;43(3):587–597.
71. LeBeau MA, Montgomery MA, Jufer RA, et al. Elevated GHB in citrate-buffered blood. *J Anal Toxicol* 2000;24:383–384.
72. Vesey CT, Langford RM. Stabilization of blood cyanide. *J Anal Toxicol* 1998;22:176–178.
73. Darby SM, Miller Ml, Allen RO, et al. A mass spectrometric method for quantitation of intact insulin in blood samples. *J Anal Toxicol* 2001;25:8–14.
74. Moriya F, Hashimoto Y. Potential for error when assessing blood cyanide concentrations in fire victims. *J Forensic Sci* 2001;46(6):1421–1425.
75. Clauwaert KM, Van Bocxlaer JF, De Leenheer AP. Stability study of the designer drugs "MDA, MDMA and MDEA" in water, serum, whole blood and urine under various storage temperatures. *Forensic Science Int* 2001;124:36–42.
76. Wallace KL, Curry SC. Postcollection rise in methemoglobin level in frozen blood specimens. *J Toxicol Clin Toxicol* 2002;40(1):91–94.
77. Selavka C. Drug testing in hair in poisoning and toxicology compendium. In: Leikin JB, Paloucek F, eds. *Poisoning & toxicology handbook.* Hudson, OH: Lexi-Comp, 1997:890–893.
78. Kimura H, Muraids M, Mori A. Detection of stimulants in hair by laser microscopy. *J Anal Toxicol* 1999;23:577–580.
79. Kintz P, Jamey C, Cirimele V, et al. Evaluation of acetylcodeine as a specific marker of illicit heroin in human hair. *J Anal Toxicol* 1998;22:435–429.
80. Cooper GAA, Allen DL, Scott KS, et al. Hair analysis: self-reported use of "speed" and "ecstasy" compared with laboratory findings. *J Forensic Sci* 2000;45(2):400–406.
81. Kintz P. Deaths involving buprenorphine: a compendium of French cases. *Forensic Science Int* 2001;121:65–69.
82. Sporkert F, Pragst F. Determination of lidocaine in hair of drug fatalities by headspace solid-phase microextraction. *J Anal Toxicol* 2000;24:316–322.
83. Negrosz A, Moore C, Deitermann D, et al. Highly sensitive micro-plate enzyme immunoassay screening and NCI-GC-MS confirmation of flunitrazepam and its major metabolite 7-aminoflunitrazepam in hair. *J Anal Toxicol* 1999;23:429–435.
84. Lemos NP, Anderson RA, Valentini R, et al. Analysis of morphine by RIA and HPLC in fingernail clippings obtained from heroin users. *J Forensic Sci* 2000;45(2):407–412.
85. Engelhart DA, Lavins ES, Sutheimer CA. Detection of drugs of abuse in nails. *J Anal Toxicol* 1998;22:314–318.
86. Lemos NP, Anderson RA, Robertson JR. Nail analysis for drugs of abuse: extraction and determination of cannabis in fingernails by RIA and GC-MS. *J Anal Toxicol* 1999;23:147–152.
87. Watson WA, McKinney PE. Necrokinetics: the practical aspects of interpreting postmortem drug concentrations. *J Toxicol Clin Toxicol* 2001;39(3):213–214.
88. Anderson DT, Fritz KL, Muto JJ. OxyContin: the concept of a "ghost pill" and the post mortem tissue distribution of oxycodone in 36 cases. *J Anal Toxicol* 2002:26:448–459.
89. Karch SB. Alternative strategies for postmortem drug testing. *J Anal Toxicol* 2001;25:393–395.
90. Raul J-S, Cirimele V, Ludes B, et al. A single therapeutic treatment with betamethasone is detectable in hair. *J Anal Toxicol* 2002;26:582–583.
91. Kalasinsky KS, Bosy TZ, Schmunk GA, et al. Regional distribution of cocaine in postmortem brain of chronic human cocaine users. *J Forensic Sci* 2000;45(5):1041–1048.
92. Lemos NP, Anderson RA, Valentini R, et al. Analysis of morphine by RIA and HPLC in fingernail clippings obtained from heroin users. *J Forensic Sci* 2000:45(2):407–412.
93. Lester L, Uemura N, Ademola J, et al. Disposition of cocaine in skin, interstitial fluid, sebum and stratum corneum. *J Anal Toxicol* 2002;26:547–553.
94. Jannetto PJ, Wong SH, Gock SB, et al. Pharmacogenomics as molecular autopsy for postmortem forensic toxicology: genotyping cytochrome P450 for oxycodone cases. *J Anal Toxicol* 2002;6:438–447.
95. Jannetto PJ, Wong SH, Gock SB, et al. Pharmacogenomics as molecular autopsy for forensic toxicology: genotyping oxycodone cases for cytochrome: P450 2D6. *J Anal Toxicol* 2003;27:190.
96. Wong SH, Jannetto PJ, Sahin E, et al. DNA electric microarray detection for pharmacogenomics—genotyping CYP-450 mutations as molecular autopsy for certifying drug-related toxicity. *J Anal Toxicol* 2003;27:200.
97. Wong SH, Sahin E, Jannetto PJ, et al. Pharmacogenomics as molecular autopsy genotyping CYP 450 2D6*3/*4/*5/ for certifying antidepressants and selected opioids-related toxicities. *J Anal Toxicol* 2003;27:200–201.
98. Wagner MA, Sakallah S. The potential of a molecular autopsy. Multiplexed CYP 2D6*3,*4,and *6 polymorphism by real time PCR. *J Anal Toxicol* 2003;27:201.
99. Venisse N, Marquet P, Duchoslav E, et al. a general unknown screening procedure for drugs and toxic compounds in serum using liquid chromatography—electrospray—single quadripole mass spectrometry. *J Anal Toxicol* 2003;27:7–114.
100. Peace MR, Poklis A, Byrd JH. Forensic entomotoxicology. A Study of effects of barbituates and amphetamines on the larvae of *Phaenicia sericata*. *J Anal Toxicol* 2003;27:195.
101. Wood M, De Boeck G, Samyn N, et al. Development of a rapid and sensitive method for the quantitation of benzodiazepines in plasma and larvae by LC-MS-MS. *J Anal Toxicol* 2003;27:182–183.
102. Spiller HA, Carlisle RD. Timely antemortem and postmortem concentrations in a fatal carbamazepine overdose. *J Forensic Sci* 2001;46(6):1510–1512.
103. Drummer OH, Gerostamoulos J. Postmortem drug analysis: analytical and toxicological aspects. *Ther Drug Monit* 2002;24(2):199–209.
104. Caplan Y, Yinney JM, Cone EJ. Standardizing terminology for reporting cause of death in cases involving opioid abuse. *J Anal Toxicol* 2003;27:195.

SECTION

9

Pregnancy and Breast-Feeding

CHAPTER 84

Toxic Exposure during Pregnancy and Lactation

Barbara Insley Crouch

OVERVIEW

Toxic exposure during pregnancy and lactation poses several challenges to the clinician. First, the clinician must consider the toxic effects on the mother as well as the fetus, neonate, or infant. In addition, physiologic changes during pregnancy may alter the pharmacokinetics of the toxin. Finally, the clinician must address the immediate and potentially delayed effects, such as teratogenesis in the developing fetus.

An understanding of the potential pharmacokinetic changes can assist the clinician in providing the best care to the mother and unborn child. This chapter focuses on the effect of maternal changes and the role of fetal development on toxic exposures during pregnancy, issues related to toxic exposure during breast-feeding, and specific considerations regarding the treatment of the pregnant overdose patient.

Therapeutic Drug Use

Despite the widespread availability of birth control, some estimate that 50% of pregnancies are unplanned or unwanted. It is common, therefore, that the fetus is unknowingly exposed to drugs and chemicals during the first trimester. *Teratogens* are substances or factors (i.e., maternal disease or chemicals) that affect the development of the fetus and cause structural or functional disability. The thalidomide disaster heightened awareness to the teratogenic potential of drug and environmental exposures during pregnancy. Before thalidomide, it was assumed that the placenta provided a natural barrier and protected the fetus from the effects of drugs and chemicals.

A number of studies have characterized the use of prescription, over-the-counter or illicit drugs, and dietary supplements by women during pregnancy. Women report using a median of 4.7 drugs during pregnancy (1). A more recent study of nonprescription and prescription medications at a university hospital showed that medication use during the first trimester had declined compared to prepregnancy rates but increased during the second and third trimesters. Medication use in the third trimester was greater than prepregnancy rates. The mean number of medications taken during the first trimester was 2.5, compared with 3.3 medications during the second trimester, and 4.1 during the third trimester. Excluding vitamins, acetaminophen was the most common medication taken during pregnancy; its rate of use remained fairly constant (Table 1) (2).

Illicit Drug Use

Drug abuse during pregnancy is not well described. Accurate information is difficult to obtain due to the reliability of the interview. In 100 interviews conducted within 96 hours of delivery at a tertiary care facility in a predominately low-income population, eight women admitted to illicit drug use before pregnancy and four admitted to illicit drug use during the third trimester (2). A study to compare the sensitivity and specificity of maternal interview, hair analysis, and meconium analysis to estimate illicit drug use during pregnancy demonstrated that the interview had a lower sensitivity than maternal hair analysis and meconium analysis. Maternal hair analysis had a relatively

TABLE 1. Medications used during pregnancy—therapeutic use and overdose

Therapeutic use	
First trimester	Second or third trimester
Vitamins	Vitamins
Acetaminophen	Acetaminophen
Iron/calcium	Iron/calcium
Antibiotics	Antacids
Antacids	Antibiotics
Antihistamines	Sympathomimetics
	Antihistamines
Intentional overdose	
Acetaminophen (30%)	Benzodiazepines (7%)
Cough/cold preparations (14%)	Antibiotics (7%)
Vitamins/iron (9%)	

Modified from Splinter MY, Sagraves R, Nightengale B, et al. Prenatal use of medications by women giving birth at a university hospital. *South Med J* 1997;90:498–502; and Perrone J, Hoffman RS. Toxic ingestions in pregnancy: abortifacient use in a case series of pregnant overdose patients. *Acad Emerg Med* 1997;4(3):206–209.

high false-positive result, whereas meconium analysis had the highest sensitivity and specificity and a lower false-positive rate as compared to maternal hair analysis and the maternal interview (3). In 1992, the National Institute on Drug Abuse conducted a nationwide hospital survey to determine the extent of drug abuse among pregnant woman. The survey of 4 million pregnant woman revealed 18.8% consumed ethanol during pregnancy, 20.4% smoked cigarettes, 5.5% used illicit drugs, and 0.3% abused inhalants (4). The most prevalent illicit substances were marijuana and cocaine. Marijuana use was more common in women younger than 25 years of age, and cocaine use was more common in women aged 25 years or older. The survey also evaluated the medical use (prescribed by practitioner) and nonmedical use (not prescribed by practitioner) of selected prescription medications. Analgesics were the most common substances used without a physician's order (1.2%) as well as with a physician's order (7.5%).

Intentional (Self-Harm) Drug Exposures

Suicide rates are generally lower in pregnant women compared to nonpregnant women of childbearing age. However, intentional overdoses are not uncommon. There were 7588 exposures during pregnancy reported to member centers of the American Association of Poison Control Centers in 2001 (5). Of these, 2219 (29%) were intentional self-harm attempts. In two self-harm attempts, fetal death occurred. A 28-year-old woman, 28 weeks pregnant, presented with a refractory metabolic acidosis after an intentional methanol ingestion. The fetus was in severe distress and was delivered by cesarean section. Neither mother nor infant survived. In the second case, a 27-week pregnant woman intentionally ingested acetaminophen. The fetus was in severe distress after delivery by caesarian section and expired shortly thereafter.

Few epidemiologic studies have characterized issues associated with self-poisoning during pregnancy (6–10). The majority of intentional overdoses occur in the first trimester (6,8,10) and result in minimal toxicity to the mother (6,9,10). Intentional overdose early in pregnancy may be associated with fetal loss (6). No significant increase in congenital malformations was identified in two large epidemiologic surveys of infants born to mothers with drug overdoses (7,8). In a study of infants born to mothers who had overdosed, however, infants in the overdose group had lower birth weights compared to those of the control group. Women who overdosed had less education than the control group and were more likely to drink alcohol heavily and smoke as compared to the control group (7). In two studies involving calls to regional poison control centers in the United States, acetaminophen was the most common substance involved in the overdose (Table 1) (9,10).

Abortifacients

For centuries, women have used a variety of pharmacologic agents to induce menses or abortion. Today, the use of substances to induce an abortion is more likely in political entities and cultures that prohibit elective abortions. The use of a toxic substance to induce abortion raises concern regarding toxicity to the woman as well as to the fetus.

The prevalence of the use of abortifacients is not known. In intentional maternal overdose, it is often not known whether the woman intends to harm herself or the fetus. In one study of pregnant women who intentionally overdosed and a regional poison center was contacted, 12% of women ingested a known abortifacient. Abortifacients ingested included misoprostol, quinine, methylergonovine, and oral contraceptives (10). Vaginal bleeding and cramping was described in four of five patients. During the 1- to 3-day follow-up period, fetal demise was not reported.

Abortifacients may be sold on the street or purchased through a dietary supplement outlet. Herbal remedies remain popular choices as abortifacients: pennyroyal oil, black cohosh, blue cohosh, angelica root, and windflower (11). Pennyroyal is a well-known hepatotoxin. Numerous reports of serious toxicity and fatal outcomes have occurred after its use as an abortifacient (12).

CATEGORIZATION OF RISK

Although many women are exposed to many substances unintentionally and intentionally during pregnancy, it is estimated that 2% to 3% of developmental defects are the result of drug or environmental effects (13). The U.S. Food and Drug Administration established a classification system to aid in the interpretation of risk associated with prescription drugs. The system is based on data from humans and animals and includes five categories: A, B, C, D, and X (Appendix I). Category A includes drugs for which there are controlled clinical trials demonstrating no harm to the fetus. Due to legal and ethical concerns, few clinical trials have been performed. Therefore, only three drugs are currently designated category A: thyroid hormone, folic acid, and prenatal vitamins. At the opposite end of the spectrum is category X, which includes drugs in which animal and human studies demonstrate risks to the fetus that outweigh any potential benefit. The majority of drugs fall in category C, which includes drugs that lack sufficient information to clearly identify safety in pregnancy. The current labeling system is inadequate to assist clinicians in evaluating risk. The U.S. Food and Drug Administration is currently evaluating its labeling and improving its system for drugs in pregnancy (14).

MATERNAL CHANGES DURING PREGNANCY

A number of physiologic changes occur during pregnancy that may affect the pharmacokinetics and toxicokinetics of a drug or chemical. Changes are not static during pregnancy and vary throughout the pregnancy (Fig. 1 and Table 2).

The concept of dose-response relationships should also be considered in teratogenesis. The human embryo has remarkable restorative mechanisms. Cell injury and loss during early development can often be replaced by further division and replacement with normal undifferentiated cells. Notable toxicity such as embryo death or major malformation, therefore, has usually been considered a threshold phenomenon. Toxic concentrations below the threshold can cause cell injury and death but are repairable without compromising the developing organism. Toxic exposure exceeding the threshold causes teratogenesis. The concentration achieved is primarily affected by maternal factors such as the dose ingested.

Drug Absorption

The time for gastric emptying is delayed 30% to 50% during pregnancy and may result in delayed absorption and decreased peak serum concentrations (15). Furthermore, gastric acid secretion is decreased, whereas mucous secretion is increased. The net result is an increase in gastric pH that may affect the ionization and absorption of some drugs. Aspirin is more soluble at a higher pH. An increase in the solubility of aspirin increases the dissolution rate, which may lead to an increase in the rate and extent of absorption. Transit time through the small intestine is also prolonged during pregnancy (16). This may lead to more complete

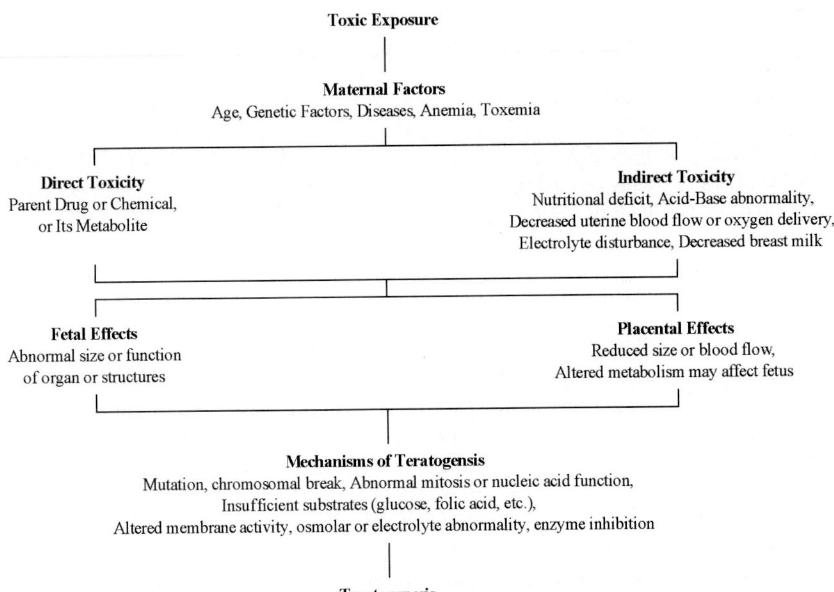

Figure 1. Maternal relationship to fetal toxicity.

absorption of drugs that are absorbed in the small intestine. Nausea and vomiting early in pregnancy may reduce the absorption of drugs after an intentional overdose in pregnancy.

Pulmonary absorption of drugs and chemicals may be enhanced during pregnancy. Pregnant women have larger tidal volumes, hyperventilate chronically (e.g., decreased $PaCO_2$), and have increased pulmonary blood flow during pregnancy. Lower doses of volatile anesthetics may be required (15,17).

Distribution

A woman's blood volume may increase nearly 50% during pregnancy (17). The blood volume starts to increase by the sixth to eighth week of pregnancy, peaks during the second trimester, with a slight increase in the third trimester. The increase in blood volume is due to both an increase in plasma volume and red cell volume. Plasma volume is increased to a greater degree than red cell volume. The hematocrit usually decreases approximately 11% during pregnancy (17). The volume of distribution of drugs that are distributed to total body water increases to a greater extent than those with high tissue distribution. A decrease in peak serum concentration may occur.

Plasma Protein Concentrations

Albumin is the major drug-binding protein in the mother and the fetus. The plasma volume expansion creates a physiologic dilutional hypoalbuminemia. In addition, steroid and placental hormones may occupy protein-binding sites (15). The end result is a decrease in the binding capacity of albumin and a reduced number of binding sites for certain drugs. In therapeutic doses, the increase in free drug concentration is offset by the increase in drug available for metabolism and excretion. In an overdose, the increase in free concentration may be clinically significant. Free concentrations of drugs may more accurately reflect the severity of the exposure. For example, the anticonvulsants phenytoin, carbamazepine, and valproic acid are all highly protein bound. Adjustments in dosing are not usually required during pregnancy because an increase in metabolism and excretion offsets the increase in free concentration of the drug. However, in an acute overdose, it may be useful to monitor free drug concentrations, as total drug concentrations may not reflect the severity of the exposure.

Some basic drugs bind preferentially to $alpha_1$ acid glycoprotein. The concentrations of $alpha_1$ acid glycoprotein are usually unchanged during pregnancy. However, in the fetus, there may be a decrease in the glycoprotein concentration with a resultant increase in free drug concentrations (15).

Metabolism

The proportion of cardiac output that is delivered to the liver is reduced during pregnancy, but the rate of blood flow (e.g., L/minute) does not change (18). Progesterone and estrogen secretion during pregnancy may alter the metabolism of certain drugs. The activity of cytochrome (CYP) 450 enzymes and other enzymes may be changed. Enzymes like CYP1A2, *N*-acetyltransferase, and xanthine oxidase are significantly reduced, whereas the activity of CYP3A4-mediated hydroxylation is increased during pregnancy (19). Women taking drugs metabolized by CYP1A2 may experience increased blood concentrations of the drug. For example, women treated with theophylline during pregnancy should have more frequent therapeutic drug monitoring to determine whether a reduced dose is necessary. Many common drugs are metabolized by CYP1A2 (Table 3).

TABLE 2. Pharmacokinetic changes in pregnant women

Increased gastric pH	Decreased CYP1A2 activity
Increased gastrointestinal transit time	Increased glomerular filtration
Increased volume of distribution	Increased elimination
Decreased protein binding	

TABLE 3. Drugs metabolized by cytochrome P-450–CYP1A2

Caffeine	Haloperidol	Theophylline
Clozapine	Imipramine	R-warfarin
Diazepam	Tacrine	Zileuton
Estradiol		

Due to hormonal enzyme induction, women taking drugs that are metabolized by CYP3A4 may have lower concentrations than expected. Phenytoin and carbamazepine may require an increased dose to achieve the same pharmacologic effect because of increased hydroxylation. A study in pregnant women showed a twofold increase in hydroxylation activity (19). Pregnancy-induced changes in carbamazepine metabolism are more complicated. There may be an increased metabolism of the parent compound to the active metabolite and an increased accumulation of the active metabolite (15). Pregnant women who require anticonvulsant therapy should be monitored closely. The majority of women do not have a change in seizure frequency during pregnancy. In the small numbers who do, multiple factors should be considered. In addition, hepatic clearance; factors such as electrolyte changes, stress, sleep disturbances, and increased respiratory rate; and noncompliance may also contribute to an increased seizure frequency. After overdose, prolonged toxicity may occur with drugs whose primary detoxification is through CYP1A2, xanthine oxidase, or *N*-acetyltransferase. It is not known whether a woman who overdoses on a drug that is metabolized by CYP3A4 would experience less toxicity than a nonpregnant woman.

Elimination

Blood flow to the kidneys, uterus, skin, and mammary glands is increased during pregnancy as a result of increased cardiac output. Increased renal blood flow begins as early as the ninth week of pregnancy and continues to increase through the second trimester and, in total, increases by approximately 45% (17). A slight decrease may occur near term. An increase in the glomerular filtration rate of 50% begins as early as the sixth week of pregnancy and continues to increase into the third trimester. Renal tubular function remains unchanged during pregnancy. Drugs that are primarily excreted via the kidneys have increased elimination during pregnancy and may have lower steady-state serum concentrations. However, the changes may not be significant enough to necessitate dosing changes.

Lithium concentrations may be decreased during pregnancy due to increased elimination. However, patients with significant nausea and vomiting during pregnancy or who have toxemia may be at increased risk for lithium toxicity due to dehydration and sodium restriction. In addition, if the dose of lithium is increased during pregnancy, serum concentrations should be monitored closely and the lithium dose decreased after delivery as renal blood flow and glomerular filtration return to prepregnancy rates.

ROLE OF FETAL DEVELOPMENT

Susceptible Stages of Development

The fetus is not equally susceptible to damage from drugs and environmental factors throughout pregnancy. It is important to remember, however, that the continuum of development for each fetus proceeds at different rates and that many events may overlap.

The *zygote* is formed by the union of egg and sperm. An *embryo* is created by cleavage of the zygote to create a multicelled unit. During the preimplantation period, the embryo moves down the fallopian tube toward the uterus for implantation. The *maternal-placental-fetal* unit begins to develop approximately 2 weeks after conception. Exposures that occur between the time of conception and the development of the maternal-placental-fetal unit generally do not result in congenital malformations. Because the cells are rapidly dividing, a significant insult often results in a catastrophic effect on the embryo and an "all or none" phenomenon. Exposures may be embryocidal and produce significant damage to the embryo to prevent implantation. Pregnancy loss during this time period may go unnoticed. It is also possible that no effect may be seen because the toxin may not achieve critical concentrations in the embryo due to the lack of the maternal-placental-fetal unit.

The three primary germ layers, ectoderm, mesoderm, and endoderm, are formed just after implantation. Insults during this time create eye, brain, and face malformation, indicating damage to the neural plate. This is followed by organization of the rudimentary organs, which is termed *organogenesis*. Organ differentiation is most active during the first trimester; therefore, teratogenic effects are more likely to result from exposures during the first trimester, even in the absence of toxic effects in the mother. The central nervous system continues to grow and differentiate throughout pregnancy and after birth. Therefore, it is possible to see teratogenic effects on the central nervous system throughout pregnancy and in infants who are breast-fed. The peak incidence of teratogenic effects depends on the timing of developmental events in each structure. An insult can be catastrophic in 1 week of gestation and without harm only a week or two later.

In humans, organogenesis ends at approximately 2 months. Subsequent events include tissue differentiation, growth, and maturation. Exposures to drugs and environmental chemicals in the second and third trimester therefore more often affect growth and function, rather than cause teratogenesis.

PLACENTAL TRANSFER

Most drugs cross the placenta. There are a variety of mechanisms that allow nutrients and drugs to cross the placenta into the fetal circulation: (a) simple diffusion, (b) facilitated diffusion, (c) active transport, (d) pinocytosis, and (e) through disruption of cells in the villous tissue. Simple diffusion is the most common process. Factors that affect placental transfer include gestational age, placental blood flow, maternal drug concentration, maternal-fetal blood pH gradient, protein binding, placental metabolism, molecular weight, and certain maternal diseases. Maternal drug concentrations are a major determinant of the amount transferred to the fetus (20). The resultant concentration in the fetus may not be sufficient to achieve a therapeutic or toxic response. Placental transfer of drugs is less early in gestation as compared to term. Fetal-maternal drug concentrations are more likely to approach unity near term.

Throughout gestation, there is a lag time for drugs to reach the fetal circulation. Because of this delay, maternal concentrations may decrease faster than fetal concentrations due to more rapid clearance from the maternal circulation. Diazepam is one drug that can achieve higher concentrations in the fetal circulation as compared to the maternal circulation. It is not known whether the increased fetal concentration is due to an active transport of the drug into the fetus or a more rapid clearance from the maternal circulation. Several other drugs have been studied and noted to have higher concentrations in the fetal compartment as compared to the maternal compartment. These drugs include acyclovir, amoxicillin, ketamine, and valproic acid (21). Most studies of placental transfer are done near term; therefore, it is not known whether the same extent of drug transfer would occur earlier in gestation.

The pH of fetal blood is relatively acidic compared to maternal blood. Acids are more ionized in the maternal circulation and usually have higher concentrations in the maternal circulation as compared to the fetal circulation. Basic drugs tend to have higher concentrations in the fetal circulation.

The blood volume in the fetus varies during gestation. In the first trimester, both total body water and extracellular water are 15% to 20% higher than near term (13). Serum protein concentrations increase, beginning in the fourth week. Near term, the fetus has a higher serum protein concentration than a pregnant woman but a lower concentration compared to a nonpregnant adult. Tightness of protein binding varies during pregnancy.

The fetal liver has phase I (metabolic transformation) and phase II (conjugation) enzymatic processes as early as 7 to 8 weeks of gestation (15). However, the degree of activity of these enzymes is not known, and the majority of elimination of drugs comes from the diffusion back to the maternal circulation.

LACTATION

Most drugs ingested by a lactating woman cross into breast milk to some degree. The risk to the infant depends on a number of factors: (a) concentration of the drug in the serum of the mother, (b) degree of maternal protein binding, (c) molecular weight, (d) degree of ionization at physiologic pH, (e) lipid solubility, and (f) the infant's ability to metabolize and excrete the drug.

Breast milk is relatively acidic compared to blood with a pH of 7.1 (range, 6.7 to 7.4) (22). Basic drugs are relatively less ionized at a physiologic pH and therefore readily cross into breast milk. Because breast milk is relatively acidic, basic drugs can become "trapped" and tend to have higher concentrations in breast milk than the plasma. The ratio of milk:plasma concentrations for weak acids is usually less than 1; for neutral compounds, it is approximately 1, and for weak bases, it is typically greater than 1. The majority of drugs have a milk:plasma ratio less than 1; approximately 25% have a ratio of greater than 1, and approximately 15% have a ratio of greater than 2 (23).

The exposure dose can be estimated if the concentration of the drug in breast milk is known. Infants ingest an average of 150 ml/kg of body weight in breast milk each day. The total daily dose can be calculated and compared to a therapeutic dose in an infant or the adult dose standardized by weight if the therapeutic dose in an infant is not known. Exposure levels less than 10% of the therapeutic dose are generally considered clinically insignificant. If the exposure levels are potentially higher, then the infant may experience some clinical effect. Drugs that have high clearance in infants are unlikely to pose significant problems. Drugs that have low clearance result in higher exposure levels to the infant.

Although not routinely available, evaluation of pharmacokinetic parameters of a drug in breast milk is beneficial in evaluating risk. Parameters such as the maximum quantity in milk, average concentration in milk, percent of adult dose, elimination half-life, time to peak, and the milk:plasma ratio are all useful in evaluating the risk to the infant. Single point estimates have limited usefulness. It is most helpful if pharmacokinetic parameters are averaged over time. In lactating women who overdose, measurement of drug concentrations in breast milk can assist in determining if breast milk is safe for the infant. In the absence of the availability of kinetic information after an intentional overdose, women should express and discard the milk until the drug has been eliminated from the mother. Basic drugs may stay in breast milk slightly longer than acidic drugs.

Information on the safety of drugs when breast-feeding is limited. Often, the data available are from older studies and are estimates based on a single drug concentration. Information about the timing of the sample in relationship to the dose administered is typically not provided. Analytical methods used may not have been as sensitive as methods available today. The majority of the time, it is only possible to determine whether a drug is detected in breast milk and does not provide sufficient information to fully evaluate the risk to the infant. The American Academy of Pediatrics Committee on Drugs periodically publishes a review of drugs and chemicals in human milk (24). This publication is useful to assist health professionals in identifying therapeutic alternatives in women who breast-feed.

CLINICAL MANAGEMENT CONSIDERATIONS

The general approach to the treatment of a pregnant woman after intentional overdose is no different from that of a nonpregnant patient. Emergency stabilization followed by supportive care should be the first line of treatment for any poisoned patient.

Decontamination

Decontamination procedures after an overdose during pregnancy may be effective longer after an overdose as compared to a nonpregnant patient due to pregnancy-induced delays in gastric emptying. However, the clinical significance of delayed emptying is not known. Gastric emptying (ipecac or gastric lavage) is not routinely recommended in the emergency department management of an adult poisoned patient (25,26). Although there are no complete contraindications to either procedure during pregnancy, little benefit is likely to be realized. Activated charcoal should be considered in the treatment of the pregnant overdose victim, especially if the ingestion was recent. Because activated charcoal is not absorbed, no adverse effects to the fetus from activated charcoal are expected. Whole bowel irrigation with a polyethylene glycol solution has been used in the treatment of iron overdose in pregnancy (27,28). Although there is not extensive information about the use of polyethylene glycol solutions in pregnancy, it is considered a nonabsorbed substance. Therefore, adverse effects on the fetus are not expected.

Resuscitation

Rapid maternal stabilization provides the best chance of survival for the mother and the fetus. If the patient requires cardiopulmonary resuscitation, an obstetrician should be part of the resuscitative team as soon as possible. Standard advanced cardiac life support protocols should be followed. If standard doses of medications do not produce the desired results, consider higher doses. The increased blood volume during pregnancy may result in decreased plasma drug concentrations. If the fetus is greater than 24 weeks' gestation, there is evidence that delivery may improve maternal survival. Delivery of the fetus within 5 minutes of maternal arrest markedly increases the chance of survival (29). Alpha-adrenergic agents and combined alpha- and beta-adrenergic agents may produce utero-placental vasoconstriction leading to a decrease in oxygenation and carbon dioxide exchange in the fetus. Whereas standard advanced cardiac life support protocols should be followed during active resuscitation, the least toxic substance should be used after the critical period is over. There are also theoretical concerns about the potential for lidocaine to induce an acidosis in the fetus and beta-blocking agents to cause bradycardia in the fetus.

Benzodiazepines (diazepam or lorazepam) are usually the first line of therapy to treat drug-induced seizures that occur during labor and delivery. Benzodiazepines rapidly cross the placenta and reach equilibrium between the maternal and fetal compartments, placing the fetus at some risk for central nervous system depression. There is controversy as to whether the use of benzodiazepines in pregnancy is associated with the development of major malformations or malformations of the oral cleft. A metaanalysis failed to confirm this association (30). Despite the potential risks to the fetus, benzodiazepines should be considered first-line therapy for the treatment of toxin-induced seizures at any time during pregnancy (31).

Extracorporeal Removal

Hemodialysis is not contraindicated in the pregnant patient. Women with renal disease have been successfully treated with hemodialysis during pregnancy. Chronic hemodialysis during pregnancy is associated with increased complications of pregnancy and intrauterine growth retardation (32). Adjustments made in dialysis frequency, flow rates, and membranes have improved pregnancy outcomes. Hemodialysis should not be withheld in life-threatening situations in a pregnant woman. Hemodialysis has been used successfully in the management of an acute methanol poisoning in late pregnancy (33).

SPECIFIC OVERDOSE MANAGEMENT

The most common substances ingested in an overdose during pregnancy are acetaminophen and iron (9,10). It is also likely that exposures to carbon monoxide are relatively common during pregnancy.

Acetaminophen

Acetaminophen is a common medication used during pregnancy and is one of most common substances involved in intentional overdose during pregnancy (5). In a study conducted by a poison control center, pregnancy outcomes were evaluated in 60 of 113 women who overdosed on acetaminophen and had positive pregnancy tests (34). Acetaminophen overdoses were evenly distributed among the three trimesters. Spontaneous abortions occurred in six women who overdosed in the first trimester, and six women had an elective abortion. All remaining women who overdosed in the first trimester delivered normal term infants. Of women who overdosed in the second trimester, two had a spontaneous abortion, one had an elective abortion, and the remaining women delivered healthy infants. One infant was delivered prematurely. Of women who overdosed in the third trimester, one had a spontaneous abortion, one delivered an infant with a mild deformity of the feet, and the remaining women delivered normal infants. Three infants were delivered prematurely. The administration of *N*-acetylcysteine late and ingestion in the first trimester were significantly associated with fetal death.

The Teratology Information Service in London reported outcomes of 300 women who overdosed on acetaminophen during pregnancy (35). The majority of the exposures occurred in the first trimester (39%). Spontaneous abortions occurred in 16 women, and 54 had an elective abortion. All spontaneous abortions occurred in first trimester exposures, and 63% occurred within 3 weeks of the overdose. The rate of spontaneous abortion was similar to the baseline rate for the United Kingdom. Malformations were noted in 11 infants. None of the malformations occurred in women who had an acetaminophen overdose in the first trimester, and the rate was also similar to the rate of malformations in the general population. Two pregnancies resulted in late fetal death. One occurred at 34 weeks in a woman who had overdosed during week 7. Postmortem examination revealed no clear cause of death. The other death occurred after an exposure in the second trimester. Acetaminophen concentrations were available for 200 women and were less than 100 mg/L at 4 hours in 82%. None of the live-born infants had any signs of hepatic or renal toxicity.

Iron

In a review of 61 patients with iron overdose during pregnancy, there was no relationship between peak serum iron concentration and pregnancy complications, including spontaneous abortion, preterm delivery, malformations, or perinatal death (36). However, there was a significant correlation with the degree of iron toxicity demonstrated and the risk of pregnancy complications. It appears that only transferrin-bound iron crosses the placenta. Therefore, the fetus may be relatively protected from the direct effects of iron but is not protected against the direct effects of maternal toxicity such as shock and metabolic acidosis. In an ovine model, deferoxamine did not cross the placenta (37). Deferoxamine has not been associated with an increased risk of a congenital malformation or fetal demise.

Carbon Monoxide

Carbon monoxide is a leading cause of morbidity and mortality from poisoning. The fetus is particularly sensitive to carbon monoxide exposure due to its dependence on maternal oxygenation as well as the ability of carbon monoxide to diffuse across the placenta. The oxyhemoglobin dissociation curve in the fetus is normally located to the left of the maternal curve. This allows the fetal hemoglobin to pick up oxygen at a lower partial pressure. A small decrease in maternal oxygen tension can significantly decrease fetal oxygen concentration. Before significant carboxyhemoglobin concentrations in the fetus, fetal hypoxia can occur.

In addition, carbon monoxide has a greater affinity for fetal hemoglobin and tends to concentrate in the fetus. Carboxyhemoglobin concentrations in the fetus may be higher than maternal concentrations. In a follow-up study of 40 pregnant women who were exposed to carbon monoxide, no adverse fetal outcomes were noted in women without significant alterations in mental status (38). Adverse fetal outcomes were more common in women who lost consciousness or who had significantly depressed sensorium. Prompt recognition and treatment of carbon monoxide poisoning are critical to treat the mother and the fetus. Pregnant women with carbon monoxide poisoning should be treated more aggressively than other carbon monoxide victims to minimize exposure to the fetus. Hyperbaric oxygen therapy has been used successfully in pregnancy (39).

SOURCES OF INFORMATION

Teratology information services routinely provide information on the safety/risk of drugs, chemicals, radiation, and infections during pregnancy to health professionals and the public. There are more than 24 teratology information services in the United States and Canada. A list of teratology information services in the U.S. and Canada is found on the official World Wide Web site for the Organization of Teratology Information Services at http://www.otispregnancy.org/.

SUMMARY

Toxic exposures during pregnancy and lactation produce unique challenges for the clinician. An understanding of the maternal changes and the role of fetal development can assist the clinician in providing the best possible care for both patients. Likewise, understanding the pharmacokinetics of drugs during lactation can assist the clinician in predicting the risk of toxic exposure to the infant and/or counsel mothers on the appropriate time to discard maternal milk.

REFERENCES

1. Bonati M, Bortolus R, Marchetti F, et al. Drug use in pregnancy: an overview of epidemiological (drug utilization) studies. *Eur J Clin Pharmacol* 1990;38:325–328.
2. Splinter MY, Sagraves R, Nightengale B, et al. Prenatal use of medications by women giving birth at a university hospital. *South Med J* 1997;90:498–502.
3. Ostrea EM, Knapp DK, Tannenbaum L, et al. Estimates of illicit drug use during pregnancy by maternal interview, hair analysis, and meconium analysis. *J Pediatr* 2001;138:344–348.
4. National Institute on Drug Abuse. *National pregnancy and health survey. Drug use among women delivering livebirths: 1992*. Rockville, MD: US Department of Health and Human Services, National Institute on Drug Abuse, 1994.
5. Litovitz TL, Klein-Schwartz W, Rodgers GC, et al. 2001 annual report of the American Association of Poison Control Centers Toxic Exposure Surveillance System. *Am J Emerg Med* 2002;20:391–452.
6. Czeizel AE, Timar L, Susanszky E. Timing of suicide attempts by self-poisoning during pregnancy and pregnancy outcomes. *Int J Gynaecol Obstet* 1999;65:39–45.
7. Czeizel AE, Tomcsik M, Timar L. Teratologic evaluation of 178 infants born to mothers who attempted suicide by drugs during pregnancy. *Obstet Gynecol* 1997;90:195–201.
8. Gunnarskog J, Bengt Kallen AJ. Drug intoxication during pregnancy: a study with central registries. *Reprod Toxicol* 1993;7:117–121.
9. Perrone J, Hoffman RS. Toxic ingestions in pregnancy: abortifacient use in a case series of pregnant overdose patients. *Acad Emerg Med* 1997;4(3):206–209.
10. Rayburn W, Aronow R, DeLancey B, et al. Drug overdose during pregnancy: an overview from a metropolitan poison control center. *Obstet Gynecol* 1984;64:611–614.
11. Netland KE, Martinez J. Abortifacients: toxidromes, ancient to modern—a case series and review of the literature. *Acad Emerg Med* 2000;7:824–829.
12. Anderson IB, Mullen WH, Meeker JE, et al. Pennyroyal toxicity: measurement of toxic metabolite levels in two cases and review of the literature. *Ann Intern Med* 1996;124:726–734.
13. Ward RM. Maternal-placental-fetal unit: unique problems of pharmacologic study. *Clin Pharmacol* 1989;36:1075–1088.
14. Boothby LA, Doering PL. FDA labeling system for drugs in pregnancy. *Ann Pharmacother* 2001;35:1485–1489.
15. Loebstein R, Lalkin A, Koren G. Pharmacokinetic changes during pregnancy and their clinical relevance. *Clin Pharmacokinet* 1997;33:328–343.
16. Parry E, Shields R, Turnbull AC. Transit time in the small intestine in pregnancy. *J Obstet Gynaecol Br Commonw* 1970;77:900–901.
17. Huff RW, Pauerstein CJ, eds. *Human reproduction: physiology and pathophysiology*. New York: John Wiley & Sons, 1979.
18. Frederiksen MC. Physiologic changes in pregnancy and their effect on drug disposition. *Semin Perinatol* 2001;25:120–123.
19. Bologa M, Tang B, Klein J, et al. Pregnancy-induced changes in drug metabolism in epileptic women. *J Pharmacol Exp Ther* 1991;257:735–740.
20. Garland M. Pharmacology of drug transfer across the placenta. *Obstet Gynecol Clin North Am* 1998;25:21–42.
21. Pacifici GM, Nottoli R. Placental transfer of drugs administered to the mother. *Clin Pharmacokinet* 1995;28:235–269.
22. Howard CR, Lawrence RA. Breast-feeding and drug exposure. *Obstet Gynecol Clinics NA* 1998;25:195–217.
23. Ito S. Drug therapy breast-feeding women. *N Engl J Med* 2000;343:118–126.
24. American Academy of Pediatrics, Committee on Drugs. The transfer of drugs and other chemicals into human milk. *Pediatrics* 2001;108:776–789.
25. American Academy of Clinical Toxicology, European Association of Poisons Centres and Clinical Toxicologist. Position statement: ipecac syrup. *J Toxicol Clin Toxicol* 1997;35:699–709.
26. American Academy of Clinical Toxicology, European Association of Poisons Centres and Clinical Toxicologist. Position statement: gastric lavage. *J Toxicol Clin Toxicol* 1997;35:711–719.
27. Van Ameyde KJ, Tennenbein M. Whole bowel irrigation during pregnancy. *Am J Obstet Gynecol* 1989;160:646–647.
28. Turk J, Aks S, Ampuero F, et al. Successful therapy of iron intoxication in pregnancy with intravenous deferoxamine and whole bowel irrigation. *Vet Hum Toxicol* 1993;35(5):441–444.
29. Whitty JE. Maternal cardiac arrest in pregnancy. *Clin Obstet Gynecol* 2002;45:377–392.
30. Dolovich LR, Addis A, Vaillancourt JMR, et al. Benzodiazepine use in pregnancy and major malformations or oral cleft: meta-analysis of cohort and case-control studies. In: Koren G, ed. *Maternal-fetal toxicology*, 3rd ed. New York: Marcel Dekker, 2001:105–114.
31. Jagoda A, Riggio S. Emergency department approach to managing seizures in pregnancy. *Ann Emerg Med* 1991;20:80–85.
32. Chao AS, Huang JY, Lien R, et al. Pregnancy in women who undergo long-term hemodialysis. *Am J Obstet Gynecol* 2002;187:152–156.
33. Hantson P, Lambermont JY, Mahieu P. Methanol poisoning during late pregnancy. *Clin Toxicol* 1997;35:187–191.
34. Riggs BS, Bronstein AC, Kulig K, et al. Acute acetaminophen overdose during pregnancy. *Obstet Gynecol* 1989;74:247–253.
35. McElhatton PR, Sullivan FM, Volans GN. Paracetamol overdose in pregnancy. Analysis of the outcomes of 300 cases referred to the teratology information service. *Reprod Toxicol* 1997;11:85–94.
36. Tran T, Wax JR, Philput C, et al. Intentional iron overdose in pregnancy—management and outcome. *J Emerg Med* 2000;18:225–228.
37. Curry SC, Bond GR, Raschke R, et al. An ovine model of maternal iron poisoning in pregnancy. *Ann Emerg Med* 1990;19:632–638.
38. Bailey B. Carbon monoxide poisoning during pregnancy. In: Koren G, ed. *Maternal-fetal toxicology*, 3rd ed. New York: Marcel Dekker, 2001:257–268.
39. Silverman RK, Montano J. Hyperbaric oxygen treatment during pregnancy in acute carbon monoxide poisoning. A case report. *J Reprod Med* 1997;42:309–311.

PART

II

Therapeutic Drugs

SECTION

1

Antihistamines

CHAPTER 85

Sedating Antihistamines (H_1 Antagonists)

Ian MacGregor Whyte

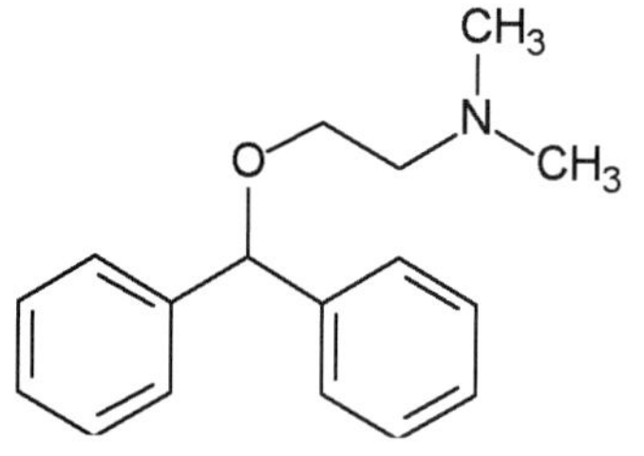

CH_3 — N — CH_3 — O — (diphenylmethyl)

DIPHENHYDRAMINE

Compounds included:	**Antazoline, azatadine, brompheniramine, cinnarizine, clemastine, cyclizine, cyproheptadine, dexchlorpheniramine, dimenhydrinate, diphenhydramine, doxylamine, hydroxyzine, mepyramine (pyrilamine), methdilazine, pheniramine, promethazine, trimeprazine, triprolidine**
Molecular weight:	**See Table 1.**
SI conversion:	**See Table 1.**
Normal levels:	**Triprolidine, 50 µg/L (serum)**
Target organs:	**Central nervous system (acute), heart (acute)**
Antidotes:	**Sodium bicarbonate, physostigmine**

OVERVIEW

Conventional antihistamines (both sedating and nonsedating) antagonize histamine-induced responses at H_1 receptors. The effects of H_1 activation include smooth muscle contraction and dilation of capillaries with an increase in their permeability. Gastric acid secretion is mediated by H_2 receptors. An H_3 receptor, believed to be involved in autoregulation of histamine release, has also been identified.

Sedating antihistamines are used in the management of allergic disorders, motion sickness, vertigo, itch associated with skin disorders, and nausea and for sedation, including premedication. They commonly have anticholinergic and central nervous system adverse effects (sedation due to central H_1 antagonism).

Older H_1 antagonists have sedative (and antimuscarinic) effects and are consequently known as *sedating antihistamines*. The newer H_1 antagonists, which have few or none of these effects, are correspondingly known as *nonsedating antihistamines* and include acrivastine, astemizole, cetirizine, fexofenadine, loratadine, and terfenadine (Chapter 87).

Antihistamine drugs are competitive, reversible inhibitors of the action of histamine at the H_1 receptor. They can prevent, but not reverse, histamine-mediated peripheral effects, such as urticaria, pruritus, and wheal-and-flare responses. Also, the additional pharmacologic effects of the older antihistamines result in effects that can be useful clinically but can also produce adverse effects.

H_1-antagonist overdose is a common poisoning. There are variations among the drugs in their toxicity with the most severe manifestations being seizures and dysrhythmias, although for most, these occur uncommonly. The treatment of minor symptoms, which are mostly due to anticholinergic effects, is best done with sedation and intravenous fluids.

Structure and Classification

There are six structurally distinct groups of antihistamines (Table 1). This structural classification cuts across separation into sedating and nonsedating, as several of the newer agents have very similar structures to the older sedating drugs.

TABLE 1. Structural classification of antihistamines

Structural group	Molecular weight (g/mol)	SI conversion	Comments
Alkylamines			Highly potent, significant sedative action. Acrivastine is a nonsedating alkylamine antihistamine.
Brompheniramine maleate	435.3	μg/L × 3.13 = nmol/L	
Dexchlorpheniramine	390.9	mg/L × 3.64 = μmol/L	
Pheniramine	240.4	mg/L × 4.16 = μmol/L	
Triprolidine	278.4	μg/L × 3.59 = nmol/L	
Acrivastine[a]	—	—	
Monoethanolamines			Pronounced sedative and antimuscarinic action.
Clemastine fumarate	460.0	mg/L × 2.91 = μmol/L	
Dimenhydrinate	470.0	mg/L × 2.13 = μmol/L	
Diphenhydramine	255.4	mg/L × 3.92 = μmol/L	
Doxylamine	270.4	mg/L × 3.70 = μmol/L	
Ethylenediamines			Selective H_1 antagonists, moderate sedation, gastrointestinal upset.
Antazoline HCl	301.8	mg/L × 3.77 = μmol/L	
Mepyramine HCl	321.8	mg/L × 3.39 = μmol/L	
Phenothiazines			Significant sedative effects, pronounced antiemetic and antimuscarinic effects, photosensitivity.
Methdilazine	296.4	mg/L × 3.37 = μmol/L	
Promethazine	284.4	mg/L × 3.52 = μmol/L	
Trimeprazine	298.5	mg/L × 3.35 = μmol/L	
Piperazines			Moderate sedation, significant antiemetic action. Cetirizine causes less sedation.
Cetirizine[a]	—	—	
Cinnarizine	368.5	mg/L × 2.71 = μmol/L	
Cyclizine	266.4	mg/L × 3.75 = μmol/L	
Flunarizine	404.5	mg/L × 2.47 = μmol/L	
Hydroxyzine	374.9	mg/L × 2.67 = μmol/L	
Piperidines			Moderate or low sedation; highly selective for H_1 receptors. Astemizole, loratadine, and terfenadine are nonsedating.
Azatadine[a]	—	—	
Cyproheptadine	287.4	μg/L × 3.48 = nmol/L	
Astemizole[a]	—	—	
Loratadine[a]	—	—	
Terfenadine[a]	—	—	

HCl, hydrochloride.
[a]Low-sedating and nonsedating antihistamines are addressed in Chapter 87.

Toxic Dose

The typical therapeutic dose of a sedating antihistamine may produce adverse effects in a susceptible individual (Table 2). There are no reported overdoses with azatadine, cinnarizine, clemastine, flunarizine, or methdilazine. Very little information on specific toxic doses is available for dexchlorpheniramine, hydroxyzine, or triprolidine. Death after 5 g has been reported for antazoline (1). Brompheniramine is usually part of a combined overdose with sympathomimetic agents (phenylpropanolamine and ephedrine) (2–4).

A cyclizine dose of 5 mg/kg in adults and children is potentially toxic and may produce malaise, tremor, athetoid movement, ataxia, rigidity, and other extrapyramidal signs (5). At 40 mg/kg, approximately 60% of children experience seizures and may have atropine-like effects (hallucination, disorientation, flushed dry skin, mydriasis, and tachycardia) (5). The minimal lethal dose is approximately 80 mg/kg (5).

Cyproheptadine at doses of 0.30 to 6.15 mg/kg has not caused life-threatening effects, although somnolence, excitation, hallucinations, ataxia, tachycardia, and muscle twitching were observed frequently (6). Dimenhydrinate caused status epilepticus and ventricular dysrhythmias in an adult within 1 hour of a 5-g dose (7).

Diphenhydramine can cause delirium during topical or oral therapy (8), particularly with preexisting varicella-zoster skin injury (9). The acute toxicity of oral diphenhydramine is dose dependent. Mild symptoms (somnolence, anticholinergic signs, tachycardia, nausea, vomiting) occurred in 55% to 64% of patients (associated with doses less than 300 mg). Moderate symptoms [isolated and spontaneously resolving agitation, confusion, hallucinations, and electrocardiogram (ECG) disturbances] developed in 22% to 27% of patients (doses of 300 to 1000 mg). Severe symptoms (delirium, psychosis, seizures, coma) occurred in 14% to 18% of patients. For severe symptoms, the critical dose limit was 1 g diphenhydramine (10). It has been suggested that only patients with diphenhydramine ingestions greater than 1 g develop severe symptoms and should be hospitalized (10). Although the frequency of delirium or psychosis remained constant or even decreased, coma and seizures were significantly more frequent in the group that ingested more than 1.5 g, compared with the 1.0- to 1.5-g group (10).

In contrast to diphenhydramine, doxylamine appears to have no correlation between the amount ingested or doxylamine plasma level and the clinical symptomatology (11). In approximately 60% of these cases, 10 to 40 times a single therapeutic dose (25 mg) was ingested.

Pheniramine has resulted in death after ingestion of a minimum of 32 tablets (45.3 mg) of pheniramine (12).

Promethazine produced delirium in two cases of dermal absorption (13). Iatrogenic cardiac arrest occurred in a 2-month-old infant after a tenfold dosing error (14).

TOXICOKINETICS AND TOXICODYNAMICS

The pharmacokinetics and pharmacodynamics of the sedating antihistamines are provided in Table 3 (15). When estimated, most agents have volumes of distribution greater than 4 L/kg

TABLE 2. Typical therapeutic dose of sedating H_1 receptor antagonists

Drug	Adult dose	Pediatric dose
Antazoline	100–200 mg 2–4 times daily	NR
Azatadine	1 mg twice daily	NR
Brompheniramine	4 mg every 4–6 h	0.125 mg/kg every 6 h
Cinnarizine	75 mg once daily	1 mg/kg; maximum, 40 mg once daily
Clemastine	2.68 mg 1–3 times daily	0.5–1.0 mg every 12 h
Cyclizine	50 mg every 4–6 hours	1 mg/kg every 8 h; maximum, 75 mg/day
Cyproheptadine	4 mg 3 times daily	0.2 mg/kg/d; maximum, 16 mg/day
Dexchlorpheniramine	2 mg 4 times daily	0.5–1.0 mg every 4–6 h
Dimenhydrinate	50–100 mg every 4–6 h	1.25 mg/kg every 6 h; maximum, 75 mg/d (younger than 6 yr of age)
Diphenhydramine	25–50 mg 3–4 times daily	1.25 mg/kg every 6 h; maximum, 300 mg/d
Doxylamine	12.5–25.0 mg every 4–6 h	6.25-2.50 mg every 4–6 h (6–12 yr of age)
Flunarizine	20 mg 3 times daily	5–10 mg once daily
Hydroxyzine	25–100 mg 3–4 times daily	0.6 mg/kg
Mepyramine (pyrilamine)	25 mg 3–4 times daily	12.5–25.0 mg every 8 h (older than 6 yr of age)
Methdilazine	8–16 mg twice daily	4 mg 2–4 times daily
Pheniramine	22.65 mg (half a 45.30-mg tablet) 2–3 times daily	3.125 or 3.250 mg every 4–8 h
Promethazine	10–25 mg 2–3 times daily	0.1 mg/kg every 6 h
Trimeprazine	10 mg 3–4 times daily	1.25 mg every 8 h (0.5–3.0 yr of age)
Triprolidine	2.5 mg every 4–6 hours	2 mg every 8 h (1–6 yr of age); 1 mg every 8 h (younger than 1 yr of age)

NR, not reported.

(16). There have been no reported overdoses with azatadine, cinnarizine, clemastine, flunarizine, or methdilazine. Toxic concentrations are unavailable for antazoline, dexchlorpheniramine, dimenhydrinate, pheniramine, promethazine, or triprolidine.

Diphenhydramine levels above 0.1 mg/L have been associated with toxicity (15), whereas 0.5 mg/L has been reported as a lethal blood concentration (17). However, autopsy series suggest that lethal blood diphenhydramine concentrations are usually in the range of 5 to 35 mg/L (18). In approximately 50% of the cases in a large series, between 6 and 40 times a therapeutic dose was ingested, and diphenhydramine plasma levels showed a wide range (0.1 to 4.7 mg/L) with only one death (19).

For doxylamine, no correlation was found between the amount ingested or doxylamine plasma level and the clinical symptomatology (11). Doxylamine plasma concentrations exceeded the maximum plasma level after a therapeutic dose by a ratio of 10:40 in two-thirds of cases (11). No symptoms were observed in 39% of the patients (11).

A plasma hydroxyzine concentration 8.5 hours after an acute ingestion was 102.7 mg/L, with toxicity manifested primarily as generalized seizures and sinus tachycardia (20).

PATHOPHYSIOLOGY

Histamine H_1 receptors are widespread. The competitive inhibition of these receptors provides the desired clinical effects in the management of allergic conditions. Central histamine H_1 inhibition results in sedation, whereas the other receptor effects (antagonism at muscarinic cholinergic, serotonin, or α-

TABLE 3. Pharmacokinetics and pharmacodynamics of sedating antihistamines

Drug	Time to peak (h)	Primary route of excretion	Half-life	Protein binding (%)
Antazoline	NR	NR	NR	NR
Azatadine	1–2	Hepatic	9–12 h	NR
Brompheniramine	3–5	Hepatic	25 h	NR
Cinnarizine	2–4	Hepatic	3–6 h	NR
Clemastine	2–4	Hepatic	21 h	NR
Cyclizine	2	Hepatic to inactive norcyclizine	20 h	NR
Cyproheptadine	NR	Hepatic	NR	NR
Dexchlorpheniramine	2.5–6.0	Hepatic with high first-pass metabolism	2–43 h	70
Dimenhydrinate	NR	NR	NR	NR
Diphenhydramine	1–4	Hepatic with high first-pass metabolism	2.4–9.3 h	85
Doxylamine	2–3	Hepatic	10 h	NR
Flunarizine	2–4	Hepatic	18 d	90
Hydroxyzine	2	Hepatic (increase dose interval in primary biliary cirrhosis)	20 h	NR
Mepyramine (pyrilamine)	NR	NR	NR	NR
Methdilazine	NR	NR	NR	NR
Pheniramine	1.0–2.5	Hepatic	16–19 h	NR
Promethazine	2–3	Hepatic, with high first-pass metabolism	5–14 h	76–93
Trimeprazine	3.5–5.5	Renal	3.6–7.0	>90
Triprolidine	2	Hepatic	3–5 h	90

NR, not reported.

TABLE 4. U.S. Food and Drug Administration (FDA) risk category and breast milk distribution of the sedating antihistamines

Antihistamine	FDA pregnancy risk category[a]	Distribution into breast milk
Antazoline	C	NR
Azatadine	B	NR
Brompheniramine	C	Possible
Cinnarizine	C	NR
Clemastine	B	Yes
Cyclizine	B	NR
Cyproheptadine	B	NR
Dexchlorpheniramine	B	NR
Dimenhydrinate	B	NR
Diphenhydramine	B	Yes
Doxylamine	B	NR
Hydroxyzine	C	NR
Mepyramine (pyrilamine)	NR	NR
Methdilazine	C	NR
Pheniramine	C	NR
Promethazine	C	NR
Trimeprazine	C	NR
Triprolidine	C	Yes

NR, not reported.
[a]Appendix I provides definitions of FDA pregnancy categories.

adrenergic receptors) contribute to the side effects and toxicologic profile (21).

The dose-response relations of H_1 antagonists have been studied by analyzing the inhibition of the wheal-and-flare reaction induced by histamine. All H_1 antagonists inhibit the histamine-induced wheal and flare to some extent. H_1 antagonists decrease the size of the wheal by decreasing vascular permeability and leakage of plasma proteins. They decrease the flare by inhibiting indirect vasodilation caused by stimulation of the histamine-induced axon reflex. The magnitude of the effect, the time to peak effect, and the duration of effect are dose related. Inhibition of this reaction usually begins within 1 hour and is greatest 5 to 7 hours after the dose, several hours after the maximal plasma concentration is reached. There is, therefore, a pharmacodynamic as well as a pharmacologic rationale for giving an H_1 antagonist before an anticipated allergic reaction, whenever possible, to achieve the greatest efficacy (21).

PREGNANCY AND LACTATION

All sedating antihistamines are U.S. Food and Drug Administration pregnancy risk category B or C (Table 4). In most cases, there are no data on distribution into breast milk, but small amounts of drug are expected. It is unclear whether these amounts are clinically significant. Many of these agents block dopamine receptors and could, theoretically, inhibit lactation.

CLINICAL PRESENTATION

Acute Overdose

Many sedating antihistamines are abused recreationally. The incidence and choice of agent vary by country: cyclizine in South Africa (22) and the United States (23), dimenhydrinate in the United States (24) and Canada (25), pheniramine in Australia (26), and promethazine in New Zealand (27).

The effects of overdose differ for the sedating and nonsedating antihistamines. Not surprisingly, sedation is the most common effect of the older antihistamines. Profound coma is uncommon, and patients are usually either drowsy or agitated (usually due to anticholinergic delirium). The anticholinergic effects of these drugs can also lead to nausea, vomiting, delayed gastric emptying, and ileus as well as urinary retention (see Chapter 10). Patients often have dry mouth, absence of sweating, flushing, fever, and dilated pupils.

Seizures have been reported for diphenhydramine and other antihistamines in up to 7% of cases (28) but occur with an unusually high incidence in pheniramine (30% in adults) (26) and cyclizine overdose [60% in children ingesting more than 40 mg/kg (5)], suggesting an additional proconvulsant effect for these drugs.

Sinus tachycardia is common (due to anticholinergic effects), and hypotension (due to peripheral α-adrenergic blockade) may also occur. The dysrhythmias reported have been similar to those reported for tricyclic antidepressant overdose and include ventricular bigeminy, ventricular tachycardia, heart block, and torsades de pointes. QRS and QT prolongation are rare, but, if present, patients should be monitored until these changes resolve.

Rhabdomyolysis has been reported with diphenhydramine overdose (29) and is a potential complication of any sedative drug overdose but seems unusually common with doxylamine poisoning (11,30–32).

Death has been reported after antihistamine overdose and is usually due to cardiac dysrhythmia with or without generalized seizure activity (1,5,7,17,33–35). Nevertheless, most sedating antihistamine overdoses have little major effect and are rarely life-threatening (10,11,19,26,36).

Adverse Reactions

In therapeutic use, the adverse effects are similar for most members of the group. The most common side effect of the sedating antihistamines is central nervous system depression. Effects range from slight drowsiness to deep sleep and include lassitude, dizziness, and incoordination. Paradoxic stimulation may occasionally occur, especially at high doses and in children or the elderly (37). The sedative effects may diminish after a few days of therapeutic use.

Other common adverse reactions include dizziness, tinnitus, blurred vision, euphoria, incoordination, anxiety, insomnia, tremor, nausea, vomiting, constipation, diarrhea, epigastric discomfort, dry mouth, and cough. Infrequently, urinary retention, palpitations, hypotension, headache, hallucination, psychosis, and weight gain (cyproheptadine) may occur. Rarely, leukopenia, agranulocytosis, hemolytic anemia, allergic reactions, dysrhythmias, dyskinesia, seizures, paraesthesia, paralysis, hepatitis, and liver failure (cyproheptadine) are noted (38).

Cinnarizine and flunarizine may cause long-term parkinsonism through their calcium channel–blocking effect or via a direct dopamine blockade in striatal dopaminergic neurons (39,40).

DIAGNOSTIC TESTS

There are no diagnostic tests specific to the sedating antihistamines. Specific drug measurements are not readily available. Plasma concentrations are not indicated for management.

Most testing is directed at assessing other potential causes of central nervous system effects. A complete blood cell count and cultures of blood and cerebrospinal fluid are obtained as needed to rule out other causes of altered mental status. Hepatic and renal function tests are used as indicated. Creatine kinase is measured when rhabdomyolysis is suspected. A urine toxicology screen in patients with persistent tachycardia, QRS widening, prolonged QTc, or altered mental status of unclear etiology may detect tricyclic antidepressants or drugs of abuse.

ECG and cardiac monitoring are used for large ingestions to assess for QRS or QTc prolongation. Measurement of partial pressure of carbon dioxide via expired air or arterial blood gases is the best way to assess respiratory compromise from sedation.

POSTMORTEM CONSIDERATIONS

Postmortem blood brompheniramine concentrations of 0.4 mg/L and greater in children are believed to be indicative of brompheniramine poisoning (3). A postmortem cyclizine blood concentration of 80 μg/ml has been recorded (41). In a fatal case of overdose, the heart blood contained 0.46 mg/L of cyproheptadine (42). A postmortem concentration of doxylamine of 1.2 mg/L in blood with a blood *N*-desmethyldoxylamine of 0.52 mg/L has been reported (43). In a combined overdose death, blood concentrations of doxylamine and pyrilamine were 0.7 and 7.0 mg/L, respectively (44). A fatal blood concentration of trimeprazine (alimemazine) was 6.52 mg/L (45).

TREATMENT

Most patients require only symptomatic and supportive care. Treatment is focused on controlling agitation, maintaining airway, reversing hyperthermia, and supporting hemodynamic function. Gastrointestinal decontamination is not essential, but if not more than 1 hour has elapsed since ingestion of the drug, activated charcoal may be considered. In view of the potential cardiac toxicity in addition to maintenance of the airway, breathing, and circulatory status of the patient, observation for dysrhythmia is warranted. Clinical assessment for signs that may indicate impending seizure activity (hypertonicity, hyperreflexia, or myoclonic jerking) is important. Patients with altered mental status, seizure, abnormal vital signs, or dysrhythmia are typically admitted.

Supportive Care

Agitation and hallucinosis are typically treated with a benzodiazepine or antipsychotic medication (Chapter 10). Physostigmine reverses behavioral effects, but symptoms usually recur within 30 to 60 minutes. Repeated doses of physostigmine are not generally recommended for behavior control.

Cardiac dysrhythmias and hypotension are treated in the manner of tricyclic antidepressants. A 10 to 20 ml/kg bolus of 0.9% sodium chloride followed by a vasopressor should be used (Chapter 133). Limited experience with overdose treatment supports the use of sodium bicarbonate as treatment for the dysrhythmias (46). By analogy with tricyclic antidepressant poisoning, sodium bicarbonate should be considered for the management of seizure activity, especially when accompanied by QRS widening. Changes in the ECG (QRS widening) or ventricular dysrhythmia are treated with sodium bicarbonate, 1 to 2 mEq/kg intravenous bolus repeated as needed for widened QRS. The arterial pH should not exceed 7.55.

Seizures are treated with benzodiazepines and other anticonvulsants (Chapter 40).

Antidotes

The use of physostigmine in anticholinergic poisoning is controversial. Some proponents use it in most patients with serious poisoning, whereas others do not use it at all. Physostigmine may be useful as a diagnostic tool to distinguish altered mental status secondary to anticholinergic toxicity from other causes of agitation and hallucinations (e.g., to avoid extensive testing in a pediatric patient with fever, delirium, and diphenhydramine therapy for chicken pox). Details of administration are provided in Chapter 67. Contraindications include known or suspected tricyclic antidepressant overdose or ECG findings suggestive of TCA overdose (QRS widening, R wave in ECG lead aVR).

Enhancement of Elimination

Hemoperfusion and hemodialysis have been used in diphenhydramine overdose with limited effect (20). These modalities are unlikely to be effective in view of the high volumes of distribution of these agents. The efficacy of forced diuresis has not been established.

Monitoring

Continuous cardiovascular monitoring should be performed until the patient improves. Frequent assessment of mental status is needed, especially when physostigmine is used because the patient often relapses.

REFERENCES

1. Blomquist M, Bostrom K, Fri CG, Ryhage R. Report on a lethal antazoline intoxication. *Z Rechtsmed* 1974;74:313–320.
2. Barone DA, Raniolo J. Facial dyskinesia from overdose of an antihistamine. *N Engl J Med* 1980;303:107.
3. Jumbelic MI, Hanzlick R, Cohle S. Alkylamine antihistamine toxicity and review of Pediatric Toxicology Registry of the National Association of Medical Examiners. Report 4: alkylamines. *Am J Forensic Med Pathol* 1997;18:65–69.
4. Gunn VL, Taha SH, Liebelt EL, Serwint JR. Toxicity of over-the-counter cough and cold medications. *Pediatrics* 2001;108:E52.
5. Resch F, Bachner I, Hruby K, Lenz K. [The intoxication with cyclizin in infancy and adult age (experiences of a contamination-information-central office)]. *Klin Padiatr* 1982;194:42–45.
6. von Muhlendahl KE, Krienke EG. [Toxicity of cyproheptadine. Side effects and accidental overdosage]. *Monatsschr Kinderheilkd* 1978;126:123–126.
7. Winn RE, McDonnell KP. Fatality secondary to massive overdose of dimenhydrinate. *Ann Emerg Med* 1993;22:1481–1484.
8. Bernhardt DT. Topical diphenhydramine toxicity. *Wis Med J* 1991;90:469–471.
9. Chan CY, Wallander KA. Diphenhydramine toxicity in three children with varicella-zoster infection. *DICP* 1991;25:130–132.
10. Radovanovic D, Meier PJ, Guirguis M, et al. Dose-dependent toxicity of diphenhydramine overdose. *Hum Exp Toxicol* 2000;19:489–495.
11. Koppel C, Tenczer J, Ibe K. Poisoning with over-the-counter doxylamine preparations: an evaluation of 109 cases. *Hum Toxicol* 1987;6:355–359.
12. Ogbuihi S, Audick W, Bohn G. [Sudden infant death—fatal poisoning with pheniramine]. *Z Rechtsmed* 1990;103:221–225.
13. Shawn DH, McGuigan MA. Poisoning from dermal absorption of promethazine. *Can Med Assoc J* 1984;130:1460–1461.
14. Brown ET, Corbett SW, Green SM. Iatrogenic cardiopulmonary arrest during pediatric sedation with meperidine, promethazine, and chlorpromazine. *Pediatr Emerg Care* 2001;17:351–353.
15. McGann KP, Pribanich S, Graham JA, Browning DG. Diphenhydramine toxicity in a child with varicella. A case report. *J Fam Pract* 1992;35:210, 213–214.
16. Paton DM, Webster DR. Clinical pharmacokinetics of H1-receptor antagonists (the antihistamines). *Clin Pharmacokinet* 1985;10:477–497.
17. Goetz CM, Lopez G, Dean BS, Krenzelok EP. Accidental childhood death from diphenhydramine overdosage. *Am J Emerg Med* 1990;8:321–322.
18. Karch SB. Diphenhydramine toxicity: comparisons of postmortem findings in diphenhydramine-, cocaine-, and heroin-related deaths. *Am J Forensic Med Pathol* 1998;19:143–147.
19. Koppel C, Ibe K, Tenczer J. Clinical symptomatology of diphenhydramine overdose: an evaluation of 136 cases in 1982 to 1985. *J Toxicol Clin Toxicol* 1987;25:53–70.
20. Magera BE, Betlach CJ, Sweatt AP, Derrick CW Jr. Hydroxyzine intoxication in a 13-month-old child. *Pediatrics* 1981;67:280–283.
21. Simons FE, Simons KJ. The pharmacology and use of H1-receptor-antagonist drugs. *N Engl J Med* 1994;330:1663–1670.
22. Stewart MJ, Moar JJ, Mwesigwa J, Kokot M. Forensic toxicology in urban South Africa. *J Toxicol Clin Toxicol* 2000;38:415–419.
23. Bassett KE, Schunk JE, Crouch BI. Cyclizine abuse by teenagers in Utah. *Am J Emerg Med* 1996;14:472–474.

24. Malcolm R, Miller WC. Dimenhydrinate (Dramamine) abuse: hallucinogenic experiences with a proprietary antihistamine. *Am J Psychiatry* 1972;128:1012–1013.
25. Rowe C, Verjee Z, Koren G. Adolescent dimenhydrinate abuse: resurgence of an old problem. *J Adolesc Health* 1997;21:47–49.
26. Buckley NA, Whyte IM, Dawson AH, Cruickshank DA. Pheniramine—a much abused drug. *Med J Aust* 1994;160:188–192.
27. Bergman J, Wallman P. Promethazine overdose: is it a "Goodnight" after all? *N Z Med J* 1998;111:246–248.
28. Olson KR, Kearney TE, Dyer JE, et al. Seizures associated with poisoning and drug overdose. *Am J Emerg Med* 1993;11:565–568.
29. Emadian SM, Caravati EM, Herr RD. Rhabdomyolysis: a rare adverse effect of diphenhydramine overdose. *Am J Emerg Med* 1996;14:574–576.
30. Lee YD, Lee ST. Acute pancreatitis and acute renal failure complicating doxylamine succinate intoxication. *Vet Hum Toxicol* 2002;44:165–166.
31. Leybishkis B, Fasseas P, Ryan KF. Doxylamine overdose as a potential cause of rhabdomyolysis. *Am J Med Sci* 2001;322:48–49.
32. Mendoza FS, Atiba JO, Krensky AM, Scannell LM. Rhabdomyolysis complicating doxylamine overdose. *Clin Pediatr (Phila)* 1987;26:595–597.
33. Krenzelok EP, Anderson GM, Mirick M. Massive diphenhydramine overdose resulting in death. *Ann Emerg Med* 1982;11:212–213.
34. Bayley M, Walsh FM, Valaske MJ. Fatal overdose from Bendectin. *Clin Pediatr (Phila)* 1975;14:507–509, 514.
35. Bockholdt B, Klug E, Schneider V. Suicide through doxylamine poisoning. *Forensic Sci Int* 2001;119:138–140.
36. Zareba W, Moss AJ, Rosero SZ, et al. Electrocardiographic findings in patients with diphenhydramine overdose. *Am J Cardiol* 1997;80(9):1168–1173.
37. Sweetman S. *Martindale: the complete drug reference*, electronic ed. Greenwood Village, CO: Micromedex, 2003.
38. Allergy and anaphylaxis. In: Rossi S, Vitry A, Hurley E, et al, eds. *Australian medicines handbook*, 3rd ed. Adelaide, Australia: Australian Medicines Handbook Pty Ltd, 2002.
39. Micheli FE, Pardal MM, Giannaula R, et al. Movement disorders and depression due to flunarizine and cinnarizine. *Mov Disord* 1989;4:139–146.
40. Marti-Masso JF, Poza JJ. Cinnarizine-induced parkinsonism: ten years later. *Mov Disord* 1998;13:453–456.
41. Backer RC, McFeeley P, Wohlenberg N. Fatality resulting from cyclizine overdose. *J Anal Toxicol* 1989;13:308–309.
42. Levine B, Green-Johnson D, Hogan S, Smialek JE. A cyproheptadine fatality. *J Anal Toxicol* 1998;22:72–74.
43. Siek TJ, Dunn WA. Documentation of a doxylamine overdose death: quantitation by standard addition and use of three instrumental techniques. *J Forensic Sci* 1993;38:713–720.
44. Wu Chen NB, Schaffer MI, Lin RL, et al. The general toxicology unknown. II. A case report: doxylamine and pyrilamine intoxication. *J Forensic Sci* 1983;28:398–403.
45. Kintz P, Berthault F, Tracqui A, Mangin P. A fatal case of alimemazine poisoning. *J Anal Toxicol* 1995;19:591–594.
46. Clark RF, Vance MV. Massive diphenhydramine poisoning resulting in a wide-complex tachycardia: successful treatment with sodium bicarbonate. *Ann Emerg Med* 1992;21:318–321.

CHAPTER 86

Histamine H_2 Antagonists

Ian MacGregor Whyte

CIMETIDINE

Compounds included:	**Cimetidine (Tagamet), famotidine (Pepcid), nizatidine (Axid), ranitidine (Zantac), roxatidine (Rotane)**
Molecular weight:	**Cimetidine, 252.3; famotidine, 337.4; nizatidine, 331.5; ranitidine, 350.9; roxatidine, 384.9 g/mol**
SI conversion:	**Cimetidine, mg/L × 4.0 = μmol/L; famotidine and nizatidine, mg/L × 3.0 = μmol/L; ranitidine, mg/L × 2.8 = μmol/L; roxatidine, mg/L × 2.6 = μmol/L**
Therapeutic levels:	**Cimetidine, 0.25 to 1.00 μg/ml**
Target organs:	**Heart (acute), central nervous system (acute)**
Antidote:	**None**

OVERVIEW

Conventional antihistamines (both sedating and nonsedating) antagonize histamine-induced responses at the H_1 receptor. Gastric acid secretion is mediated by the H_2 receptor. The concept of a histamine H_2-receptor antagonism began with the discovery of the H_2 receptor in 1972 (1), and the first such drug, cimetidine, was described 3 years later (2). Others in the family include famotidine, nizatidine, ranitidine, and roxatidine. They are now among the largest-selling drugs in the world and are available over the counter in many countries.

Overdoses with H_2 antagonists are usually well tolerated (3), although sinus bradycardia, varying degrees of heart block, and hypotension can occur rarely, and death has been reported (4). These drugs are competitive, reversible inhibitors of the action of histamine at the H_2 receptor. The H_2 antagonists are all structurally dissimilar (Fig. 1). They are used for short-term treatment of duodenal or gastric ulcer, maintenance in recurring ulcers, treat-

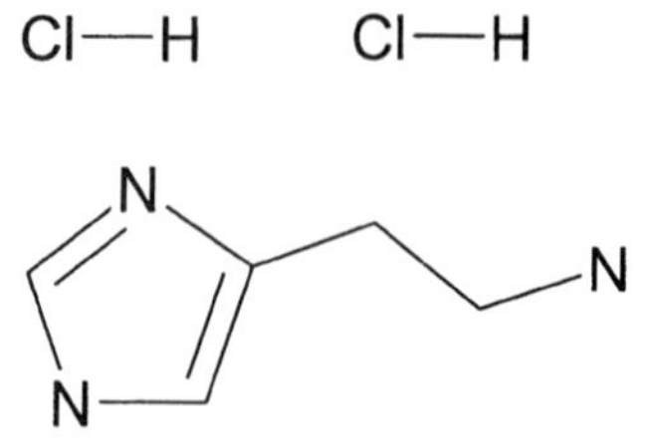

Histamine

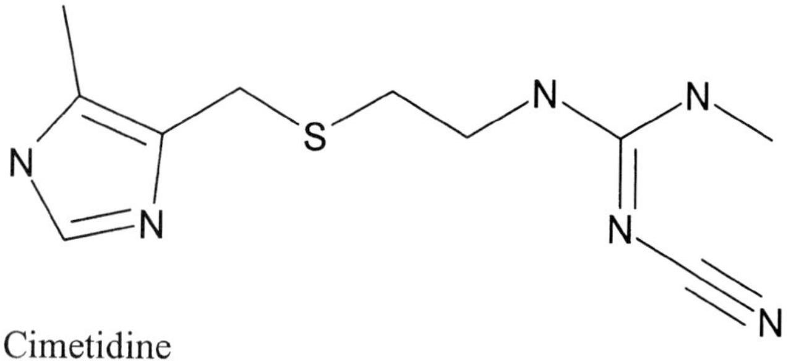

Cimetidine

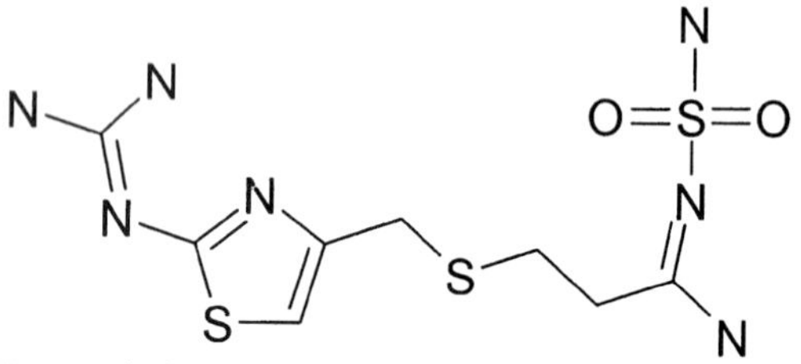

Famotidine

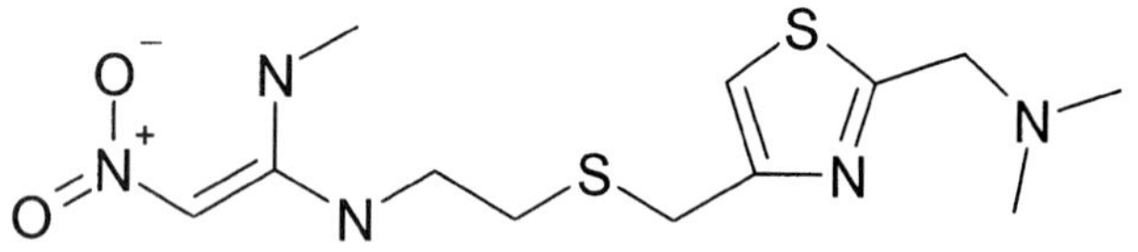

Nizatidine

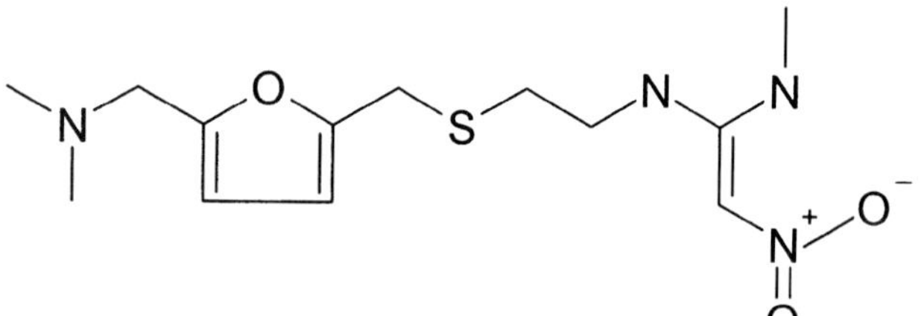

Ranitidine

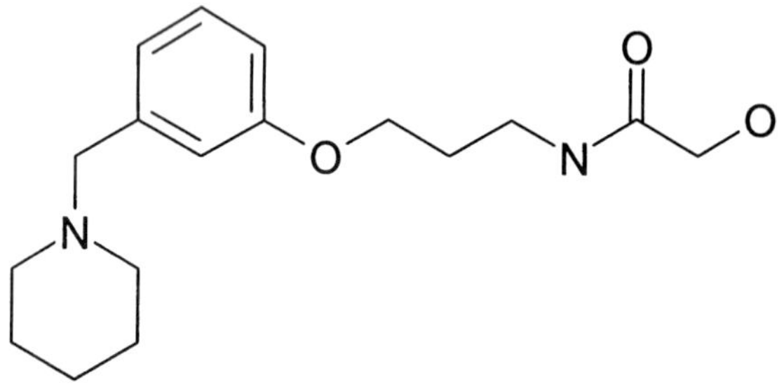

Roxatidine

Figure 1. Structures of histamine H_2 antagonists.

ment of gastroesophageal reflux disease, prophylaxis of stress ulcer in the critically ill patient, and treatment of gastrinoma (Zollinger-Ellison syndrome) and scleroderma esophagus.

TOXIC DOSE

Therapeutic daily doses in adults for each of the H_2 antagonists are shown by indication in Table 1. All are renally excreted and require dosage adjustment in renal failure.

Normal people have ingested massive amounts of cimetidine and developed no neurologic symptoms (5). Three adults remained symptom free after ingestion of 20 g of cimetidine (6). In one case, the blood level was 45.8 µg/ml, 3 hours after the overdose. Therapeutic blood cimetidine concentrations associated with a 50% reduction of stimulated acid secretion range from 0.25 to 1.00 µg/ml (7).

Death has been associated very rarely with administration of an H_2 antagonist, but a causal relationship is often doubtful. A 39-year-old woman ingested 24 g of cimetidine and died (8). No deliberate self-poisonings with famotidine, nizatidine, ranitidine, or roxatidine have been reported, but there are reports of bradycardic cardiac arrests after therapeutic doses of intravenous (IV) famotidine (9) and ranitidine (10).

TOXICOKINETICS AND TOXICODYNAMICS

Pharmacokinetics of the H_2-receptor antagonists are provided in Table 2. Few data regarding toxicokinetics have been reported. A trough concentration of cimetidine greater than 1.25 µg/L has been associated with confusion in critically ill patients (11), whereas concentrations as high as 57 µg/L have been tolerated with little clinical effect in acute overdose (5).

PATHOPHYSIOLOGY

Histamine H_2 receptors are present on the gastric parietal cell. It is the competitive inhibition of these receptors by the H_2 antagonists that prevents stimulation of gastric acid secretion by histamine, pentagastrin, cholinergic agents, caffeine, and food (12). There are chronotropic and inotropic histamine H_2 receptors in cardiac muscle (13), inhibition of which may explain the bradycardic responses occasionally seen after IV H_2 antagonists (9,10). H_2 receptors are also present on T cells, and inhibition of these may alter cell-mediated immune responses (14).

Cimetidine is a potent nonspecific inhibitor of a number of cytochrome P-450 isoenzymes, including CYP3A4, CYP2D6, CYP1A2, CYP2C9, CYP2C11, and CYP2E1 (15). There are many drug interactions that involve cimetidine (Table 3) (15). Famotidine, nizatidine, and roxatidine possess weak cytochrome P-450 inhibitory potential and low drug-drug interaction potential (15). Although ranitidine shows a low inhibitory potential, drug-drug interactions have been reported in some cases (15). The propensity of cimetidine to inhibit hepatic drug metabolism is probably related to the imidazole ring in its structure, similar to other drugs with an imidazole structure that are known to be inhibitors of drug metabolism (ketoconazole, miconazole, itraconazole, metronidazole, omeprazole) (16).

PREGNANCY AND LACTATION

Cimetidine, famotidine, nizatidine, and ranitidine are all U.S. Food and Drug Administration pregnancy category B (Appendix I). Roxatidine is not categorized. Cimetidine is excreted into breast

TABLE 1. Daily dose of H_2 antagonists in adults by indication

Drug name	Daily dose (mg)				
	Acute ulcer	Ulcer maintenance	Gastroesophageal reflux disease	Gastrinoma	Scleroderma esophagus
Cimetidine	800	400	800	1000	1200
Famotidine	40	20	40	80	—
Nizatidine	300	150	300	450	—
Ranitidine	300	150	300	450	—
Roxatidine	150	75	150	—	—

milk in very small quantities (17). Famotidine and nizatidine are excreted into breast milk to a lesser extent than cimetidine or ranitidine and may be the preferred histamine antagonists (18). Negligible amounts of roxatidine are excreted in milk (19).

CLINICAL PRESENTATION

Acute Ingestion

The effects of acute overdose are only known in any detail for cimetidine. An overdose may be associated with dizziness, slurred speech, confusion, dilated pupils, disorientation, and drowsiness, with or without sweating and flushing. Cimetidine use has been associated with bradycardia, hypotension, sinus arrest, and cardiac arrest after overdose (4) as well as after rapid IV infusion. Five patients had cardiac arrests after IV cimetidine (20,21). One recovered with residual cerebral dysfunction, one died after 7 days from respiratory failure (diazepam was also given to this patient), two died immediately, and one died after 14 days from renal failure. No blood levels were reported. Cardiovascular toxicity is very rare.

A review of 881 cases of overdose with up to 15 g of cimetidine revealed that symptoms were absent in 79%. There were no major medical complications and no fatalities in either children or adults. A few patients exhibited vomiting, bradycardia, and drowsiness, all of which were minor and without sequelae (3). In eight cases of cimetidine overdose, blood concentrations ranged from 18.7 to 57.0 µg/ml (5); all recovered. There has been one death involving bradycardia after ingestion of diazepam and cimetidine (4).

Adverse Reactions

Adverse effects are similar for all members of the group. Common adverse reactions to cimetidine, which are rare with other agents, include headache, tiredness, dizziness, confusion (especially in elderly people), diarrhea, constipation, and rash. Infrequent adverse reactions include hypotension and bradydysrhythmias after rapid IV administration. Rarely, thrombocytopenia, agranulocytosis, hepatitis, vasculitis, and reversible involuntary movements (ranitidine) can occur. Cimetidine has been associated with antiandrogenic effects, such as gynecomastia, galactorrhea, impotence, and decreased libido, and is more likely to be involved in drug-drug interactions (Table 3).

Pitfalls

Although a cimetidine overdose is usually well tolerated and lacks serious toxicity, the cardiac effects (hypotension, bradycardia, and potential cardiac arrest) are likely to be dose related and could potentially occur after any H_2-antagonist overdose.

DIAGNOSTIC TESTS

Significant laboratory abnormalities after overdose with cimetidine have not been reported. Specific drug levels are not readily available. Plasma cimetidine values do not appear to correlate well with symptoms. An electrocardiogram for cardiac effects and renal function tests for assessment of clearance are indicated.

TABLE 2. Pharmacokinetics and pharmacodynamics of H_2-receptor antagonists

Parameter	Cimetidine[a]	Famotidine[b]	Nizatidine[c]	Ranitidine[d]	Roxatidine[e]
Onset of effect (min)	45–90	80	30–180	20–70	120–180
Duration of effect (h)	4–8	9–12	9	4–12	12
Volume of distribution (L/kg)	~1.0	1.0–1.3	1.2	1.5	1.7–3.2
Excretion route					
Renal (%)	70	25–70	70	60	95
Hepatic (%)	15	30–35	10	30	—
Elimination half-life (h)	~2.0	2.0–4.0	1.3	1.9	4.0–4.5
Excreted unchanged (%)	40–80	25–70	65–75	50–70	50–60
Active metabolites	None	Unknown	N-2-monodesmethylnizatidine	None	None
Protein binding (%)	20	15–22	27–43	15	6–7

[a]Data from Somogyi A, Gugler R. Clinical pharmacokinetics of cimetidine. *Clin Pharmacokinet* 1983;8:463–495.
[b]Data from Echizen H, Ishizaki T. Clinical pharmacokinetics of famotidine. *Clin Pharmacokinet* 1991;21:178–194.
[c]Data from Callaghan JT, Bergstrom RF, Rubin A, et al. A pharmacokinetic profile of nizatidine in man. *Scand J Gastroenterol Suppl* 1987;136:9–17.
[d]Data from McNeil JJ, Mihaly GW, Anderson A, et al. Pharmacokinetics of the H2-receptor antagonist ranitidine in man. *Br J Clin Pharmacol* 1981;12:411–415.
[e]Data from Collins JD, Pidgen AW. Pharmacokinetics of roxatidine in healthy volunteers. *Drugs* 1988;35[Suppl 3]:41–47.

TABLE 3. Significant drug interactions with cimetidine

Therapeutic class	Drug	Reaction	CYP
Bronchodilator	Theophylline	*N*-demethylation	1A2, 2E1, 3A4
		C^8-hydroxylation	1A2
Central nervous system stimulant	Caffeine	*N*-demethylation	1A2, 2E1
		C^8-hydroxylation	1A2, 2E1, 3A4
Analgesic and anti-inflammatory	Antipyrine	*N*-demethylation	1A2, 2C8, 9, 18, 3A4
		C^3-CH_3-hydroxylation	1A2, 2C9
		C^4-hydroxylation	1A2, 2B6, 3A4
Anesthetic, local	Lidocaine	*N*-deethylation	3A4
Antiarrhythmics	Quinidine	C^3-hydroxylation	3A4
	Verapamil	*N*-dealkylation	1A2, 3A4
Anticoagulants	(*R*)-warfarin	Hydroxylation	1A, 2C19, 3A4
	(*S*)-warfarin	Hydroxylation	1A2, 2C9, 19, 3A4
Antiepileptics	Phenytoin	*p*-Hydroxylation	2C9, 19
	Carbamazepine	10,11-Epoxidation	1A2, 3A4
	Valproic acid	4-ene-Formation (desaturation), C^4- and C^5-hydroxylation	2C9, 19
Antidepressant	Imipramine	*N*-demethylation, C^2-hydroxylation	1A, A2, 2C19, 3A4, 2D6, 2C19
Beta-blockers	Bunitrolol	C^4-hydroxylation	2D6
	Propranolol	C^4-hydroxylation, *N*-dealkylation	1A, 2D6, 2C19
	Metoprolol	O-demethylation	2D6, 2C19
		αC-hydroxylation	2D6
Coronary vasodilator	Nifedipine	Ring oxidation	3A4
Parasympathomimetic	Tacrine	C^1-, C^2-, C^4-, C^7-hydroxylation	1A2
Anxiolytic, sedative, and hypnotic	Diazepam	C^3-hydroxylation	2C19, 3A4
		N-demethylation	2B6, 2C9, 2C19
	Desmethyldiazepam	C^3-hydroxylation	3A4
	Chlordiazepoxide	*N*-demethylation	2C
	Nitrazepam	NO_2-reduction	Reductase

From Rendiæ S. Drug interactions of H_2-receptor antagonists involving cytochrome P450 (CYPs) enzymes: from the laboratory to the clinic. *Croat Med J* 1999;40:357–367, with permission

TREATMENT

Supportive and symptomatic measures form the mainstay of treatment. Limited experience with overdose treatment precludes recommendation for use of specific agents.

Gastrointestinal decontamination is not essential, but if not more than 1 hour has elapsed since ingestion of the drug, activated charcoal may be considered. In view of the occasional report of cardiac problems despite the apparent lack of toxicity of cimetidine, observation for dysrhythmia is warranted. If bradydysrhythmias or other sequelae have not occurred within the first 4 to 6 hours, it is very unlikely they will occur, and the patient is safe to leave acute medical care.

There is no known antidote. Bradydysrhythmias may be treated with atropine. There is no evidence that forced diuresis enhances excretion of cimetidine (6). No studies support the effectiveness of hemoperfusion or hemodialysis.

REFERENCES

1. Black JW, Duncan WA, Durant CJ, et al. Definition and antagonism of histamine H2-receptors. *Nature* 1972;236:385–390.
2. Brimblecombe RW, Duncan WA, Durant GJ, et al. Proceedings: the pharmacology of cimetidine, a new histamine H2-receptor antagonist. *Br J Pharmacol* 1975;53:435–436.
3. Krenzelok EP, Litovitz T, Lippold KP, McNally CF. Cimetidine toxicity: an assessment of 881 cases. *Ann Emerg Med* 1987;16:1217–1221.
4. Hiss J, Hepler BR, Falkowski AJ, Sunshine I. Fatal bradycardia after intentional overdose of cimetidine and diazepam. *Lancet* 1982;2:982.
5. Illingworth RN, Jarvie DR. Absence of toxicity in cimetidine overdosage. *BMJ* 1979;1:453–454.
6. Meredith TJ, Volans GN. Management of cimetidine overdose. *Lancet* 1979;2:1367.
7. Gugler R, Fuchs G, Dieckmann M, Somogyi AA. Cimetidine plasma concentration-response relationships. *Clin Pharmacol Ther* 1981;29:744–748.
8. Litovitz TL, Schmitz BF, Bailey KM. 1989 Annual report of the American Association of Poison Control Centers National Data Collection System. *Am J Emerg Med* 1990;8:394–442.
9. Schoenwald PK, Sprung J, Abdelmalak B, et al. Complete atrioventricular block and cardiac arrest following intravenous famotidine administration. *Anesthesiology* 1999;90:623–626.
10. Hart AM. Cardiac arrest associated with ranitidine. *BMJ* 1989;299:519.
11. Schentag JJ. Cimetidine-associated mental confusion: further studies in 36 severely ill patients. *Ther Drug Monit* 1980;2:133–142.
12. Obrink KJ. Histamine and gastric acid secretion. A review. *Scand J Gastroenterol Suppl* 1991;180:4–8.
13. Kopec P, Korczynska I, Olakowska E. Role of histamine in cardiac muscle function—an attempt at demonstrating the presence of intracellular histaminergic H2-type receptors. *Med Sci Monit* 2001;7:357–362.
14. Kumar A. Cimetidine: an immunomodulator. *DICP* 1990;24:289–295.
15. Rendiæ S. Drug interactions of H2-receptor antagonists involving cytochrome P450 (CYPs) enzymes: from the laboratory to the clinic. *Croat Med J* 1999;40:357–367.
16. Mangini RJ. Clinically important cimetidine drug interactions. *Clin Pharm* 1982;1:433–440.
17. Somogyi A, Gugler R. Cimetidine excretion into breast milk. *Br J Clin Pharmacol* 1979;7:627–629.
18. Hagemann TM. Gastrointestinal medications and breastfeeding. *J Hum Lact* 1998;14:259–262.
19. Bender W, Brockmeier D. Pharmacokinetic characteristics of roxatidine. *J Clin Gastroenterol* 1989;11[Suppl 1]:S6–S19.
20. Shaw RG, Mashford ML, Desmond PV. Cardiac arrest after intravenous injection of cimetidine. *Med J Aust* 1980;2:629–630.
21. Cohen J, Weetman AP, Dargie HJ, Krikler DM. Life-threatening arrhythmias and intravenous cimetidine. *BMJ* 1979;2:768.

CHAPTER 87

Nonsedating Antihistamines

Steven A. Seifert

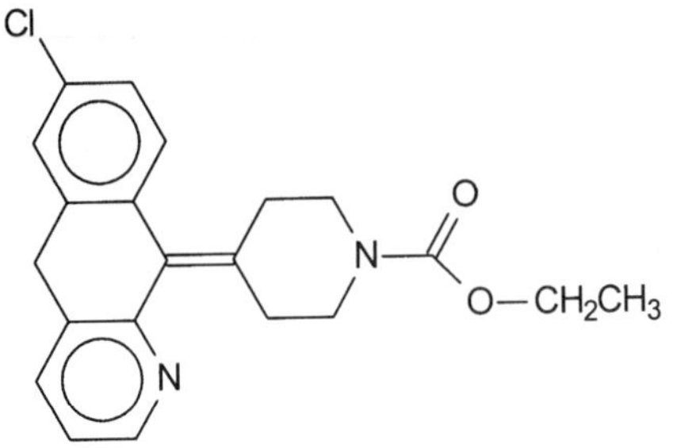

LORATADINE

Compounds included:	**See Table 1.**
Molecular weight:	**Acrivastine, 348.4; astemizole, 458.6; cetirizine hydrochloride, 461.8; desloratadine, 310.8; ebastine, 469.7; fexofenadine hydrochloride, 538.1; ketotifen, 425.5; loratadine, 382.9; mizolastine, 432.5; terfenadine, 471.7 g/mol**
SI conversion:	**See Table 1.**
Normal or therapeutic levels:	**Not applicable**
Special concerns:	**Older, discontinued forms (astemizole, terfenadine) may still be available for use.**
Target organs:	**Cardiac conduction (prolongation of QTc, torsade de pointes); central nervous system (drowsiness, somnolence)**
Antidote:	**None**

OVERVIEW

The second-generation antihistamines are H_1 receptor antagonists that cross the blood–brain barrier to a much smaller extent than first-generation agents. The term *nonsedating antihistamine,* although not completely accurate, is used interchangeably. Agents include acrivastine (Semprex-D), astemizole (withdrawn from the U.S. market), cetirizine hydrochloride (Zyrtec), desloratadine (Clarinex), ebastine (not available in the United States), fexofenadine hydrochloride (Allegra, Allegra-D), ketotifen (investigational in the United States), loratadine (Claritin, Claritin Reditabs, Claritin-D 12 Hour Extended Release Tablets, Claritin-D 24 Hour Extended Release Tablets), mizolastine (not available in the United States), and terfenadine (withdrawn from the U.S. market).

These drugs are used for allergic rhinitis and histamine-related dermatologic disorders and as adjunctive therapy in asthma. Despite their designation as *nonsedating,* some sedation or performance impairment may occur with therapeutic dosing. The most serious adverse reactions in therapeutic use or overdose occur with those agents known to produce a prolonged QTc interval (astemizole and terfenadine). Management is supportive with specific management of prolonged QTc and its sequelae. The diagnostic and therapeutic aspects of these drugs are addressed in the sections Diagnostic Tests and Treatment.

Due to decreased central nervous system penetration, second-generation antihistamines are relatively nonsedating compared to first-generation H_1-blocking agents. Multiple factors produce this effect, including altered lipophilicity, hydrogen- or protein-binding capacity, P-glycoprotein transport, and histamine effects (1). Second-generation antihistamines have differing binding affinities for the H_1 receptor and also other effects in the cell, such as effects on potassium channels and cytosolic calcium levels (2,3).

TABLE 1. Compounds included and SI conversion

Acrivastine (Semprex-D), mg/L × 2.9 = μmol/L	Fexofenadine (Allegra), mg/L × 1.9 = μmol/L
Astemizole (Hismanal), mg/L × 2.2 = μmol/L	Ketotifen (Zaditor), mg/L × 2.4 = μmol/L
Cetirizine hydrochloride (Zyrtec), mg/L × 2.2 = μmol/L	Loratadine (Claritin), mg/L × 2.6 = μmol/L
Desloratadine (Clarinex), mg/L × 3.2 = μmol/L	Mizolastine (Mistamine), mg/L × 2.3 = μmol/L
Ebastine (Kestine), mg/L × 2.1 = μmol/L	Terfenadine, mg/L × 2.1 = μmol/L

ACRIVASTINE

Acrivastine is an alkylamine antihistamine, a structural analog of triprolidine. Acrivastine is indicated in seasonal allergic rhinitis. Semprex-D contains 8 mg of acrivastine and 60 mg of pseudoephedrine. The recommended dose for patients 12 years of age and older is 8 mg every 4 to 6 hours. It is not approved for use in patients younger than 12 years of age. At therapeutic doses, drowsiness was reported 6% more frequently than with placebo (4). Signs and symptoms of pseudoephedrine from combination products may occur.

Overdose experience is limited. A dose of 322 mg was survived uneventfully (4). No fatalities have been reported.

TABLE 2. Selected pharmacokinetic and pharmacodynamic parameters of second-generation antihistamines

Parameter	Acrivastine[a]	Cetirizine hydrochloride[b]	Desloratadine[b]	Loratadine[b]	Fexofenadine hydrochloride[b]
Onset of effect (h)	1.14	1	—	1–3	2–3
Peak plasma concentration (ng/ml)	4 (dose of 5 mg/d)	311 (dose of 10 mg)	4 (dose of 5 mg)	—	142 (dose of 60 mg)
Time of peak concentration (h)	—	1	3	1.3	2–3
Protein binding (%)	50	93	82–87; hydroxydesloratadine, 85–89	97	60–70
Duration of effect (h)	—	24	24	—	12
Volume of distribution (L/kg)	0.82 ± 0.60	—	—	—	—
Metabolism	—	Minimal, hepatic	Hepatic and renal	Hepatic, cytochromes 3A4, 2D6	Minimal, hepatic
Elimination half-life (h)	Parent, 1.9; propionic acid metabolite, 3.5	8.3	28	8.4	14.4

[a]From Product information. Semprex-D. *Physicians' Desk Reference* 2002;56:1172–1174, with permission.
[b]Modified from Kelley C, Good CB. Pharmacy Benefits Management Strategic Healthcare Group Medical Advisory Panel drug class review: non-sedating antihistamines. Available at: http://www.vapbm.org/PBM/reviews.htm. Accessed May 2002.

Toxicokinetics and Toxicodynamics

Only pharmacokinetic and pharmacodynamic data are available (Table 2). Acrivastine is readily absorbed after a therapeutic dose. It is approximately 50% bound to protein, primarily albumin, but also bound to α_1-glycoprotein. Protein-binding displacement is not seen with phenytoin or theophylline. Elimination of acrivastine is 84% in the urine and 13% in feces. Kinetics are linear first order over the therapeutic range. Acrivastine may accumulate in the serum of patients with impaired renal function (4).

Pathophysiology

Acrivastine did not cause significant changes in action potential duration or maximal rate of increase in the action potential in isolated canine Purkinje's fibers at levels ten times higher than plasma levels observed in clinical studies. Acrivastine is considered 60-fold less likely to cause disturbances in cardiac conduction than terfenadine (5).

Pregnancy and Lactation

Acrivastine is U.S. Food and Drug Administration (FDA) pregnancy category B (Appendix I). It is not known whether acrivastine appears in breast milk.

Clinical Presentation

Sedation is possible after an overdose (6). Signs and symptoms of pseudoephedrine from combination products may occur. Acrivastine has an increased incidence of sedation compared to loratadine.

CETIRIZINE HYDROCHLORIDE

Cetirizine hydrochloride is a metabolite of hydroxyzine, a piperazine antihistamine. Cetirizine hydrochloride is indicated in seasonal and perennial allergic rhinitis and chronic idiopathic urticaria. Fatigue and dry mouth were also reported more commonly than with placebo. No clinically significant prolongation of QTc is seen at doses up to six times the maximal daily dose, and no interaction-related increases were found when combined with macrolides or ketoconazole.

The recommended dose in patients 12 years of age and older is 5 or 10 mg once daily; in children 6 to 11 years of age, 5 or 10 mg once daily; and in children 2 to 5 years of age, 2.5 mg once daily. A maximal dose of 5 mg daily is recommended with renal or hepatic impairment.

No specific toxic dose has been established. Cetirizine hydrochloride may cause drowsiness at therapeutic doses and does so reliably in overdose (7,8). At higher therapeutic doses, drowsiness was reported in 13.7% compared with 6.3% of placebo controls. No fatalities have been reported.

Toxicokinetics and Toxicodynamics

Cetirizine hydrochloride is rapidly absorbed (Table 2). Pharmacokinetics are linear for doses up to 60 mg. Food delays the time of peak concentration by 1.7 hours (9). Cetirizine hydrochloride is metabolized by the liver to nonactive metabolites. No clinically significant prolongation of QTc is seen at doses up to six times the maximal daily dose, and no interaction-related increases are seen when combined with macrolides or ketoconazole (9).

Pathophysiology

No prolongation of the action potential was noted in dogs in doses up to 4.5 mg/kg (10).

Pregnancy and Lactation

Cetirizine hydrochloride is FDA pregnancy category B (Appendix I). Cetirizine hydrochloride is excreted in human breast milk, and its use by nursing mothers is not recommended.

Clinical Presentation

Sedation is possible with overdose of cetirizine hydrochloride. Cetirizine hydrochloride has an increased incidence of sedation compared to loratadine (6).

DESLORATADINE

Desloratadine is the major active metabolite of loratadine (the descarboxyethoxyl derivative). It is indicated for the relief of the nasal and nonnasal symptoms of allergic rhinitis and for the symptomatic relief of pruritus and hives in patients with chronic idiopathic urticaria. The recommended dose is 5 mg once daily for patients 12 years of age and older. In patients with liver or renal impairment, an initial dose of one 5-mg tablet every other day is recommended (11).

Human overdose experience is limited. In normal volunteers, single daily doses of 45 mg for 10 days produced an increase in mean heart rate of 9.2 beats/minute and an increase in the QTc interval of 8.1 milliseconds (method of Bazett) and 0.4

milliseconds (method of Fridericia), relative to placebo. No clinical adverse events were reported.

Lethality occurred in rats at oral doses greater than 250 mg/kg. No deaths occurred at oral doses up to 250 mg/kg in monkeys (approximately 810 times the human daily dose on a mg/m^2 basis).

Toxicokinetics and Toxicodynamics

Desloratadine is rapidly absorbed (Table 2). Neither food nor grapefruit juice affects bioavailability. Protein binding of desloratadine and 3-hydroxydesloratadine was unaltered in subjects with impaired renal function (Table 2). Desloratadine is extensively metabolized to 3-hydroxydesloratadine, an active metabolite, which is subsequently glucuronidated. A subset of patients (approximately 7%) are slow metabolizers, with a desloratadine half-life exceeding 50 hours. Slow metabolizers of desloratadine cannot be prospectively identified and may be more susceptible to dose-related adverse events.

Although increased plasma concentrations of desloratadine and 3-hydroxydesloratadine were observed when coadministered with erythromycin, ketoconazole, azithromycin, fluoxetine, and cimetidine, there were no clinically relevant changes in electrocardiographic parameters (including the QTc interval), clinical laboratory tests, vital signs, and adverse events (11).

Pregnancy and Lactation

Desloratadine is FDA pregnancy category C (see Appendix I). There are no adequate human studies. An increase in preimplantation loss and a decreased number of implantations and fetuses were noted in female rats at 24 mg/kg. Desloratadine passes into breast milk (11).

In rats, a higher incidence of hepatocellular tumors was observed in males given 10 mg/kg/day and in males and females given 25 mg/kg/day. The clinical significance of these findings during long-term use of desloratadine is not known. There was no evidence of genotoxic potential in a reverse mutation assay or in two assays for chromosomal aberrations. There was no effect on female fertility in rats at desloratadine doses up to 24 mg/kg/day. Desloratadine had no effect on fertility in rats at an oral dose of 3 mg/kg/day.

Clinical Presentation

At therapeutic doses, the frequency and magnitude of laboratory and electrocardiographic abnormalities were similar in desloratadine- and placebo-treated patients. There were no differences in adverse events for subgroups of patients as defined by gender, age, or race.

Information regarding acute overdosage is limited. In a dose ranging trial, somnolence was reported at doses of 10 mg/day and 20 mg/day. Desloratadine and 3-hydroxydesloratadine are not eliminated by hemodialysis (11).

FEXOFENADINE HYDROCHLORIDE

Fexofenadine hydrochloride is indicated in seasonal allergic rhinitis and chronic idiopathic urticaria. Allegra-D contains fexofenadine hydrochloride, 60 mg, and pseudoephedrine, 120 mg, in an extended-release tablet. Fexofenadine hydrochloride is a metabolite of terfenadine. Unlike terfenadine, there have been no reports of QTc prolongation.

The dose of fexofenadine hydrochloride for patients 12 years of age and older is 60 mg twice a day. For children 6 to 11 years of age, the dosage is 30 mg twice daily.

Although overdose information is limited, single doses up to 800 mg and doses of 690 mg twice a day for 1 month did not produce clinically significant adverse effects and no significant increases in QTc (12).

Toxicokinetics and Toxicodynamics

Pharmacokinetics and pharmacodynamics are provided in Table 2. Approximately 5% of an oral dose is metabolized, and 80% is eliminated unchanged in parent form in the feces and 11% in the urine. Coadministration with erythromycin and ketoconazole increased peak plasma concentration (C_{max}) and the area under the curve (AUC) without QTc prolongation or change in adverse events. There were no effects on the plasma concentrations of erythromycin or ketoconazole.

Pregnancy and Lactation

Fexofenadine hydrochloride is FDA pregnancy category C (Appendix I). There are no adequate human studies. Decreased survival was seen in animal studies (13). It is not known whether fexofenadine hydrochloride is excreted in human milk.

Clinical Presentation

Somnolence should be anticipated. Fexofenadine hydrochloride produced drowsiness more frequently than loratadine (6).

LORATADINE

Loratadine is a piperidine antihistamine. Claritin-D 12 Hour Extended Release Tablets contain loratadine, 5 mg, and pseudoephedrine sulfate, 120 mg. Claritin-D 24 Hour Extended Release Tablets contain loratadine, 10 mg, and pseudoephedrine sulfate, 240 mg. Loratadine has the fewest central nervous system–sedating effects of antihistamines approved for use in the United States (6). Loratadine is indicated for the relief of nasal and nonnasal symptoms of seasonal allergic rhinitis and for the treatment of chronic idiopathic urticaria. Loratadine is also used in treating allergic bronchial asthma. The recommended dose for patients 6 years of age and older is 10 mg once daily, and it is 5 mg once daily for children ages 2 to 5 years. The dose of 24-hour formulation is one tablet daily. The dose of the 12-hour product is one tablet twice daily. Dose adjustment is necessary in patients with liver and renal insufficiency. Patients with a creatinine clearance less than 30 ml/minute should use a starting dose of 10 mg every other day (14). The dose of Claritin-D 12 Hour is one tablet daily, and the dose of Claritin-D 24 Hour is one tablet every other day. In hepatic failure, the dose is 10 mg every other day. The combination product loratadine/pseudoephedrine is not recommended in hepatic insufficiency.

Overdose experience is limited. No QTc prolongation or fatalities have been reported.

Toxicokinetics and Toxicodynamics

Pharmacokinetics and pharmacodynamics are provided in Table 2. The AUC and C_{max} for loratadine rapidly disintegrating tablets (Claritin Reditabs) were 11% and 6% greater than that of loratadine tablets, respectively. Hepatic metabolism is extensive to an active metabolite, descarboethoxyloratadine, followed by renal excretion.

Consuming food before the administration of loratadine (Claritin Reditabs) delays the time of peak concentration of loratadine and descarboethoxyloratadine by 2.4 and 3.7 hours, respectively. With standard loratadine tablets, the time of peak concentration for loratadine and descarboethoxyloratadine was delayed by 1 hour when taken after a meal. C_{max} was not affected (14).

In a study of the extended-release formulation of loratadine/pseudoephedrine, the AUC and the mean C_{max} for loratadine were substantially increased when taken with a fatty breakfast. AUC and C_{max} of descarboethoxyloratadine and pseudoephedrine were unaffected by food (15). When administered with erythromycin, cimetidine, or ketoconazole, plasma concentrations of loratidine were increased by 40%, 103%, and 307%, respectively, without observable clinical effect (14).

In chronic renal failure, both AUC and C_{max} increase for loratadine and its active metabolite (approximately 73% and 120%, respectively). Elimination half-lives in patients with impaired renal function, however, are similar to those with normal renal function (16). Hemodialysis does not affect the pharmacokinetics of loratadine or its active metabolite in subjects with chronic renal impairment (14,16).

The elimination half-lives of loratadine and its active metabolite increase with decreasing hepatic function. In a small sample of 12 elderly patients, the elimination half-life varied widely (14).

Pathophysiology

Therapeutic doses of loratadine have no effect on electroencephalogram-evoked potentials, sleep latency tests, driving performance, and tests of cognitive and psychomotor function (17).

Pregnancy and Lactation

Loratadine is FDA pregnancy category B (see Appendix I). Its active metabolite passes easily into breast milk and achieves concentrations similar to plasma. No effect on the infant is expected from the levels achieved.

Clinical Presentation

In overdose, somnolence, tachycardia, and headache have been reported in adults. In children, extrapyramidal symptoms have been reported.

DIAGNOSTIC TESTS

Serum levels are neither available nor necessary for management of therapeutic use or overdose of second-generation antihistamines. After overdose, an electrocardiograph is used to determine QRS and QTc durations, followed by continuous rhythm monitoring until the acute phase of toxicity has resolved. Second-generation antihistamines known to cause prolonged QTc (astemizole and terfenadine) should be monitored closely for this effect. In sufficient overdose or in combination with other drugs, other agents in this class may demonstrate prolonged QTc and its sequelae (torsades de pointes).

Serum electrolytes, blood urea nitrogen, creatinine, calcium, and magnesium should be determined. Semprex-D and Allegra-D contain pseudoephedrine, and evaluation of sympathomimetic effects maybe needed. Other tests to evaluate the suicidal patient should be considered.

TREATMENT

Treatment is symptomatic and supportive. In overdose, protection of the airway and management of drowsiness and sedation are the main clinical issues.

Decontamination

Gastric emptying is not recommended because of the low probability of serious toxicity and the potential for sedation at high levels. A single dose of activated charcoal without a cathartic may be given within 1 to 2 hours of ingestion, especially if coingestants are possible. Whole bowel irrigation may be considered for very large ingestions presenting past the time when gastric emptying is effective, evidence of a drug bezoar with ongoing significant toxic effects, or when other medications that might require whole bowel irrigation have been taken. Enhanced elimination techniques have not been evaluated.

Antidote

No specific antidote has been developed. Torsades de pointes should be managed in the typical manner with magnesium sulfate, lidocaine, isoproterenol, and overdrive pacing. Administration of agents that can cause QTc prolongation should be avoided.

Disposition

Patients remaining asymptomatic after gastrointestinal decontamination and 6 hours of observation, including a normal QTc, may be discharged after psychiatric evaluation. If QTc prolongation occurs, monitoring should continue until QTc is normal.

PITFALLS

Signs and symptoms of overdose may initially be absent or nonspecific. Cardiac effects with terfenadine have been delayed up to 22 hours (18).

REFERENCES

1. Timmerman H. Why are non-sedating antihistamines non-sedating? *Clin Exp Allergy* 1999;29[Suppl 3]:13–18.
2. Taglialatela M, Castaldo P, Pannaccione A, et al. Cardiac ion channels and antihistamines: possible mechanisms of cardiotoxicity. *Clin Exp Allergy* 1999;29[Suppl 3]:182–189.
3. Letari O, Miozzo A, Folco G, et al. Effects of loratadine on cytosolic Ca2+ levels and leukotriene release: novel mechanisms of action independent of the anti-histamine activity. *Eur J Pharmacol* 1994;266:219–227.
4. Product information. Semprex-D. *Physician's Desk Reference* 2002;56:1172–1174.
5. Lang DG, Wang CM, Wenger TL. Terfenadine alters action potentials in isolated canine Purkinje fibers more than acrivastine. *J Cardiovasc Pharmacol* 1993;22:438–442.
6. Mann RD, Pearce GL, Dunn N, Shakir S. Sedation with "non-sedating" antihistamines: four prescription-event monitoring studies in general practice. *BMJ* 2000;320:1184–1186.
7. Hansen JJ, Feilberg Jorgensen NH. Accidental cetirizine poisoning in a four-year-old boy. *Ugeskr Laeger* 1998;160:5946–5947.
8. Ten Eick AP, Blumer JL, Reed MD. Safety of antihistamines in children. *Drug Saf* 2001;24:119–147.
9. Product information. Zyrtec and Zyrtec-D 12 Hour. *Physician's Desk Reference* 2002;56:2756–2760.
10. Weissenburger J, Noyer M, Cheymol G, Jaillon P. Electrophysiological effects of cetirizine, astemizole and D-sotalol in a canine model of long QT syndrome. *Clin Exp Allergy* 1999;29[Suppl 3]:190–196.
11. Clarinex. Product information. Available at: http://www.clarinex.com/clarinex/productinfo.html. Accessed June 2002.
12. Pratt C, Brown AM, Rampe D, et al. Cardiovascular safety of fexofenadine HCL. *Clin Exp Allergy* 1999;29[Suppl 3]:212–216.
13. Product information. Allegra and Allegra-D. *Physician's Desk Reference* 2002;56:712–716.
14. Product information. Claritin, Claritin-D 12 Hour, and Claritin-D 24 Hour. *Physician's Desk Reference* 2002;56:3100–3106.
15. Nomeir AA, Mojaverian P, Kosoglou T, et al. Influence of food on the oral bioavailability of loratadine and pseudoephedrine from extended release tablets in healthy volunteers. *J Clin Pharmacol* 1996;36:923–930.
16. Matzke GR, Halstenson CE, Opsahl JA, et al. Pharmacokinetics of loratadine in patients with renal insufficiency. *J Clin Pharmacol* 1990;30:364–371.
17. Kay GG, Harris AG. Loratadine: a non-sedating antihistamine. Review of its effects on cognition, psychomotor performance, mood and sedation. *Clin Exp Allergy* 1999;29[Suppl 3]:147–150.
18. Myrenfors PG, Feychting KC. *Serious cardiac effects after terfenadine overdose.* Birmingham, UK: European Association of Poison Centres & Clinical Toxicologists Scientific Meeting; 1993 May 26–28(abst).

SECTION

2

Antiinfective Agents

CHAPTER 88

Sulfonamide and Quinolone Antibiotics

Seth Schonwald and Ira M. Leviton

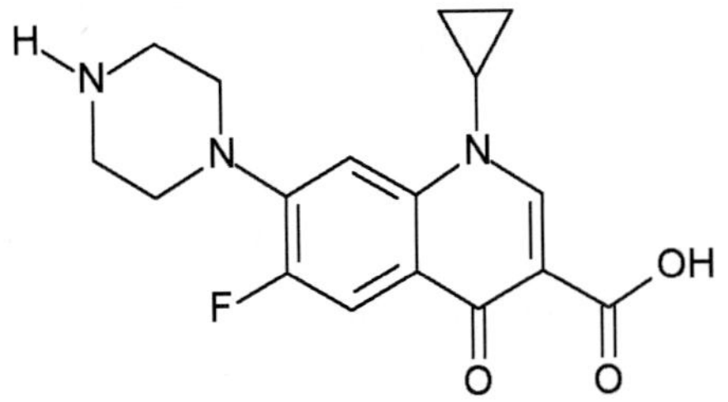

CIPROFLOXACIN

Compounds included:	**See Table 1.**
Molecular weight:	**Trimethoprim, 290.3; ciprofloxacin, 331.4; pefloxacin, 333.15 g/mol**
SI conversion:	**Trimethoprim, mg/L × 3.44 = μmol/L; ciprofloxacin, mg/L × 3.02 = μmol/L; pefloxacin, mg/L × 3.00 = μmol/L**
CAS Registry No.:	**738-70-5 (trimethoprim), 85721-33-1 (ciprofloxacin), 70458-92-3 (pefloxacin)**
Therapeutic levels:	**Trimethoprim, 5 mg/L; ciprofloxacin, 5 mg/L; pefloxacin, 10 mg/L**
Target organs:	**Sulfonamides—allergic reactions, skin rash, methemoglobinemia, bone marrow depression; quinolones—gastrointestinal, cardiac dysrhythmias, psychiatric disturbance**
Antidote:	**None**

SULFONAMIDE ANTIBIOTICS

Sulfonamides were the first modern antimicrobials. Their discovery rapidly resulted in a Nobel Prize for Gerhard Domagk in 1939. They represent a family of antibiotics used to treat a wide range of bacterial infections and are available in oral forms as well as vaginal, ophthalmic, and topical skin preparations.

A poorly absorbable oral preparation of sulfasalazine (Azulfidine) is also used in the treatment of ulcerative colitis and rheumatoid arthritis. This product exerts its effect mainly via the antiinflammatory action of its 5-aminosalicylic acid metabolite, not the antibacterial activity of the sulfapyridine metabolite.

During the past three decades, the combination of trimethoprim and sulfamethoxazole (Bactrim, Cotrim, Septra, and Sulfatrim Pediatric) has occupied a central role in the treatment of several clinical conditions (1), including prophylaxis (2,3), and treatment of urinary tract infections; acute otitis media; exacerbations of chronic bronchitis, spontaneous bacterial peritonitis (4), shigellosis, and bacterial conjunctivitis; and prophylaxis and treatment of *Pneumocystis carinii* infections in acquired immunodeficiency syndrome patients (5,6).

TABLE 1. Compounds included

Sulfonamide antibiotics	Quinolone antibiotics
Silver sulfadiazine (Silvadene, SSD)	Ciprofloxacin (Cipro)
Sodium sulfacetamide (Bleph-10, Sulf-10, Klaron, Vasocidin, Ocusulf-10, Sulamyd)	Enoxacin (Penetrex)
Sulfamethoxazole (Gantanol)	Gatifloxacin (Tequin)
Sulfanilamide (AVC)	Levofloxacin (Levaquin)
Sulfisoxazole (Gantrisin)	Ofloxacin (Floxin)
Triple sulfa (Sultrin)	Moxifloxacin (Avelox)
	Norfloxacin (Noroxin)
	Trovafloxacin (Trovan)

Toxic Dose

Deaths associated with administration of oral sulfonamides have been reported from hypersensitivity reactions, agranulocytosis (7), aplastic anemia, and other blood dyscrasias (8).

Reports of acute toxicity after sulfasalazine ingestion are rare. A case of an acute ingestion of sulfasalazine, 50 g, and paracetamol, 50 g, resulted in severe lactic acidosis, seizures, coagulopathy, hyperglycemia, ketosis, and methemoglobinemia. Despite the ingestion of a large amount of paracetamol with a measured serum paracetamol level of 5486 nmol/L (844 mg/L), significant hepatotoxicity did not occur. The patient recovered fully after administration of *N*-acetylcysteine, methylene blue, sodium bicarbonate, and supportive therapy (9).

A 23-year-old man who ingested 25 g of sulfasalazine in a suicide attempt underwent prompt, supportive treatment and survived with no ill effects (10). A 23-year-old woman who took an overdose of 13 sulfametopyrazine-trimethoprim combination (Kelfiprim) tablets over 5 days developed prolonged fever, agranulocytosis, and anemia. A hypocellular bone marrow with depressed granulopoiesis and hematopoiesis suggested marrow suppression induced by sulfametopyrazine (11).

Toxicokinetics and Toxicodynamics

Sulfonamides are absorbed from the stomach and small intestine and are widely distributed to tissues and bodily fluids, including the central nervous system (12). Approximately 20% of sulfasalazine is absorbed in the small intestine after oral administration. This portion, together with the unabsorbed sulfasalazine, enters the colon where it is split by bacteria into two main metabolites, sulfapyridine and 5-aminosalicylic acid. The peak serum concentration is reached in 3 to 5 hours.

The kidneys excrete sulfonamides and their inactivated metabolites mainly through glomerular filtration after acetylation and glucuronidation (13). Metabolites have no antimicrobial activity. A small percentage of absorbed sulfasalazine is excreted in urine and the rest via bile into the small intestine (enterohepatic circulation). The mean serum half-life of sulfasalazine after a single dose is approximately 6 hours; after repeated doses, it is approximately 8 hours (14).

Pathophysiology

Sulfonamides interfere with the biosynthesis of tetrahydrofolic acid (THF) and folic acid. Sulfonamides are structural analogs of para-aminobenzoic acid, one of the substrates used in the synthesis of THF by the enzyme THF synthetase. This causes a lethal lack of nucleic acids because THF is an essential cofactor in the metabolism of nucleic acids.

Although the sulfonamides rapidly block synthesis of new folate, bacteria can continue to grow for several generations as their preexisting folate pools decline. In contrast to the sulfonamides, trimethoprim rapidly inhibits bacterial growth and is a competitive inhibitor of dihydrofolate reductase, the next enzyme that catalyzes the next step of folic acid synthesis. In the presence of trimethoprim, THF is rapidly depleted and trapped in the unstable dihydrofolate reductase form. Because the reuse of dihydrofolate reductase is prevented, growth inhibition occurs very early.

Pregnancy and Lactation

The sulfonamides are U.S. Food and Drug Administration (FDA) pregnancy category B drugs, whereas trimethoprim and trimethoprim and sulfamethoxazole (Bactrim) are listed as FDA pregnancy category C medications (15). Sulfonamides, including sulfanilamide, readily pass through the placenta and reach fetal circulation. The concentration in the fetus is from 50% to 90% of that in the maternal blood and, if high enough, may cause toxic effects.

Sulfonamides should not be used during the last trimester of pregnancy or during nursing because they can produce jaundice kernicterus in the newborn. The mechanism of this side effect is competition with glucuronyl transferase. Trimethoprim interferes with folate metabolism, and because inadequate folate intake is associated with birth defects in humans, trimethoprim and trimethoprim-sulfamethoxazole probably should be avoided during pregnancy.

Clinical Presentation

ADVERSE EFFECTS

Sulfonamides are among the most common class of drugs that produce allergic reactions. Clinical manifestations range from urticaria and rash to bronchoconstriction, laryngeal edema, hematologic disorders, and other serious reactions (16). Sulfa hypersensitivity reaction is more likely to develop in patients with advanced human immunodeficiency virus infection, and it has been reported that desensitization can restore tolerability to the drug in about two-thirds of those who attempt it (17).

Many drugs induce reactions via altered hepatic metabolism, with production of reactive intermediates that induce a common syndrome of rash and fever plus variable types of other signs. Examples of this reactive metabolite syndrome include the rash and fever in human immunodeficiency virus–infected patients given sulfamethoxazole (18).

DERMATOLOGIC EFFECTS

Sulfonamides may cause Stevens-Johnson syndrome (less than 1% frequency) (19), fixed drug eruption (20), toxic epidermal necrolysis (Lyell's syndrome) (21,22), lichenoid reaction (23), generalized cutaneous depigmentation (24), exfoliative dermatitis, photosensitivity (25), urticaria, and erythema multiforme (26).

HEMATOLOGIC EFFECTS

Hematopoietic disturbances caused by sulfonamides include hemolytic or aplastic anemia (27,28), granulocytopenia, and thrombocytopenia (29).

RENAL EFFECTS

A tubulo-obstructive effect caused by precipitation of sulfonamide crystals (30) was first observed after treatment with sulfonamides in the 1940s. This problem has emerged again because high doses of sulfonamides are given to immunocompromised patients. Acute interstitial nephritis (31) and reversible hyperkalemia (32,33) may follow the use of sulfonamides.

OPHTHALMOLOGIC EFFECTS

Bilateral, anterior uveitis has been precipitated by sulfonamides (34). Myopia has also been reported after sulfonamide use (35,36).

Diagnostic Tests

Rare cases of hyperkalemia dictate that electrolyte determination should be performed in overdose settings. Occasional renal difficulties due to intratubular deposition of sulfonamide crystals suggest that renal function and urine sediment be monitored as well.

Treatment

Fortunately, cases of pure sulfonamide overdose occur rarely. Specific interventions to address these cases have not been described. Decontamination is not typically needed due to the lack of acute toxicity. Supportive care appears sufficient in managing cases in which sulfa drugs have accidentally or intentionally been ingested in excess. There are no specific antidotes.

Hypersensitivity effects are treated according to severity (see Chapter 34). Rash and pruritus may respond to antihistamines, whereas systemic problems, such as bronchospasm, may require inhalers or steroids. Severe dermatologic consequences, such as Stevens-Johnson syndrome, may require corticosteroid therapy as well.

Toxic epidermal necrolysis cases related to sulfonamide use are best managed in specialized burn units. Topical wound care remains an essential factor in the treatment of burn-like syndromes and is a main determining parameter for morbidity and mortality (37).

Toxic nephropathy arising from sulfonamide crystal deposition is managed with hydration, stopping the toxic drug, and close monitoring of renal function.

For the treatment of blood dyscrasias, folinic acid (Leucovorin), 5 to 15 mg per day orally, intramuscularly, or intravenously (IV), may be given. This helps to overcome the inhibition of folic acid synthesis by providing an alternative substrate.

QUINOLONE ANTIBIOTICS

Quinolone antibiotics are particularly effective against gram-negative rods. Older drugs, such as nalidixic acid, cinoxacin, and oxolinic acid, have been supplanted by newer, broad-spectrum fluoroquinolones (also called quinolones). Current products include norfloxacin, ciprofloxacin, enoxacin, ofloxacin, levofloxacin, gatifloxacin, moxifloxacin, and trovafloxacin.

All quinolones are useful for urinary tract infections as well as bacterial prostatitis and bacterial diarrhea, except that caused by *Clostridium difficile*; most are also effective in treatment of gonorrhea, chancroid, pneumonia, skin, soft tissue infections, and osteomyelitis caused by susceptible bacteria. Ofloxacin is approved for treatment of infections caused by *Chlamydia trachomatis* (38).

With the introduction of levofloxacin, gatifloxacin, and moxifloxacin, the traditional gram-negative coverage of quinolones has been expanded to include specific gram-positive organisms and causes of "atypical" pneumonia. Clinical applications beyond genitourinary tract infections include upper and lower respiratory infections, gastrointestinal infections, gynecologic infections, sexually transmitted diseases, and some skin and soft tissue infections (39).

Toxic Dose

No lethal dose of ciprofloxacin or ofloxacin in humans has been reported. A 33-year-old patient ingested 18.75 g of ciprofloxacin and 25 g of pristinamycin. Endoscopy showed gastric ulceration. A renal biopsy disclosed tubular necrosis. The serum creatinine rose on day 4; the serum ciprofloxacin concentration was 3 mg/L. The patient was hemodialyzed and recovered (40). Acute renal failure has also been reported after an overdose with 14 g of ciprofloxacin (41).

A 26-year-old woman inadvertently received 4000 mg of ofloxacin IV instead of 400 mg and survived (42). A 14-year-old patient ingested an unknown amount of ofloxacin and survived (43).

Toxicokinetics and Toxicodynamics

Pharmacokinetic properties of fluoroquinolones are provided in Table 2. Ciprofloxacin, ofloxacin, trovafloxacin, levofloxacin, gatifloxacin, and moxifloxacin are available both IV and orally; the others are available only in oral formulations. Norfloxacin is poorly absorbed orally; the other fluoroquinolones are better absorbed orally, resulting in blood levels adequate for treating systemic infection.

Their bioavailabilities are as follows: ciprofloxacin greater than 70%, enoxacin 90%, norfloxacin 30% to 70%, and ofloxacin 95% to 100%. Food does not impair absorption. Bioavailability is reduced when taken with antacids (aluminum, calcium, or magnesium-containing), laxatives (magnesium-containing, sucralfate, or zinc), ferrous sulfate, or bismuth salicylate.

Nalidixic acid is appropriate for urinary tract treatment but is insufficiently concentrated elsewhere. The fluoroquinolones cross membranes well and are widely distributed to urine, kidney, lung, prostate tissue, stool, bile, bone, and cartilage.

Renal excretion is the primary route of elimination for most quinolones, and doses must be adjusted in renal failure, except for nalidixic acid and pefloxacin.

Pathophysiology

The quinolones are bactericidal and inhibit the activity of DNA gyrase. The older quinolones, nalidixic acid and cinoxacin, are active only against Enterobacteriaceae with no activity against

TABLE 2. Pharmacokinetic properties of some fluoroquinolones

Property	Norfloxacin	Ciprofloxacin	Ofloxacin	Pefloxacin	Enoxacin	Temafloxacin
Oral dose (mg)	400	500	400	400	600	600
Peak levels (μg/ml)	1.5	2.5	5.5	4	4	6
Absorption (%)	35–70	75–85	70–80	80–95	80–90	90
Protein binding (%)	15	20–40	10–20	20–30	30–40	26
Urinary recovery (%)	25	30	90	5	60	65
Half-life (h)	3–4	2–4	5–7	8–12	3–6	7–8
Creatinine clearance (<10 ml/min/1.73 m^2)	8	10	30	12–15	9.4	>10

Modified from Walker RC, Wright AJ. The fluoroquinolones. *Mayo Clin Proc* 1991;66:1249–1259.

gram-positive organisms, *Pseudomonas aeruginosa*, or anaerobes. Furthermore, bacteria tend to become rapidly resistant to these older drugs; older quinolones are used only for urinary tract infections.

The newer quinolones have much greater activity against Enterobacteriaceae and are also active against staphylococci, *P. aeruginosa*, *Mycoplasma* species, *Chlamydia* species, and some streptococci but, with the exception of trovafloxacin and moxifloxacin, are not reliably active against anaerobes.

Ofloxacin, levofloxacin, gatifloxacin, moxifloxacin, and trovafloxacin have the best activity against gram-positive cocci. Resistance has been noted, particularly with *P. aeruginosa* and methicillin-resistant *Staphylococcus aureus*. Resistance to one quinolone generally means resistance to all (44).

Pregnancy and Lactation

The quinolones are FDA pregnancy category C. Ciprofloxacin, ofloxacin, and pefloxacin cross the placenta and produce high concentrations in breast milk (45). Ofloxacin, administered in a dose of 200 mg twice daily for 6 days during the nineteenth week of gestation, led to the normal birth of a full-term infant with no teratogenic abnormalities (46).

Clinical Presentation

GASTROINTESTINAL EFFECTS

Gastrointestinal effects occur in approximately 5% of patients (e.g., nausea, vomiting, and anorexia). These are generally mild and disappear when dosing is stopped. Hepatitis has been observed with ofloxacin use (47). Gatifloxacin-induced fulminant hepatic failure has been reported (48). Trovafloxacin has been associated with hepatic failure (49), leading to death in some cases.

MUSCULOSKELETAL EFFECTS

In testing done before the approval of the newer quinolones, animal experiments indicated that they were chondrotoxic and affected the development of articular cartilage, resulting in irreversible damage in large, weightbearing joints of young animals (50). Therefore, since their introduction, quinolone use in patients younger than 18 years of age has been very limited (51).

A retrospective, observational study was conducted to assess the incidence and relative risk of tendon or joint disorders that occur after use of selected quinolones, compared with azithromycin, a drug with no known effect on cartilage or tendons in humans or animals. The incidence of tendon or joint disorders associated with selected quinolone use in children was less than 1% and was comparable with that of the reference group (52). The newer quinolones have also been associated with a number of cases of spontaneous Achilles' tendon rupture in adults (i.e., in nonexercising and sedentary individuals) (53,54).

RENAL EFFECTS

Renal effects, such as nephrotoxicity, are rare. Allergic nephropathy associated with ciprofloxacin has been described (55). Interstitial nephritis associated with ciprofloxacin use has also been reported (56,57). Acute renal failure secondary to oral ciprofloxacin use has been reviewed (58).

CARDIAC EFFECTS

Animal experiments as well as clinical experience show that the cardiotoxic potentials of sparfloxacin and grepafloxacin are higher than those of the other fluoroquinolones. They cause QT prolongation at rather low doses, thus increasing the risk for severe arrhythmia (torsade de pointes) (59). For this reason, these two quinolones are no longer available, but it should be noted that all quinolones have this effect on the QT interval and may increase the risk for torsade de pointes.

CENTRAL NERVOUS SYSTEM EFFECTS

Central nervous system effects occur in less than 5% of patients and are usually manifested by mild headache, sleep disturbance, dizziness, or mood alteration. All quinolones are γ-aminobutyric acid inhibitors and may cause seizures (60,61). Myasthenia gravis may be exacerbated after ciprofloxacin use (62). Benign intracranial hypertension has been described (63). Reversible visual loss has followed large doses (64).

Psychotoxic effects, including hallucinations (65), agitation, confusion, headaches, vertigo, depression, visual and olfactory disturbances, ataxia, tremor, paresthesia, anxiety, and insomnia, have been reported in approximately 2% to 4% of patients treated with ofloxacin. Seizures occur rarely. Patients with a history of psychiatric disease seem to be at a higher risk of developing psychotoxic effects from ofloxacin (66).

DERMATOLOGIC EFFECTS

Dermatologic effects are primarily photosensitivity rashes, which may be caused by all fluoroquinolones. Lomefloxacin is the most likely to cause this effect.

METABOLIC EFFECTS

Gatifloxacin has been associated with the development of hypoglycemia (67) within the first several days of treatment as well as hyperglycemia after the initial dosing period. This occurs in both diabetics as well as nondiabetics; presumably, patients in the latter group are from the relatively large percentage of undiagnosed diabetics.

Diagnostic Tests

A serum sample obtained 15 minutes after completion of an infusion of 3 g of ofloxacin revealed an ofloxacin level of 39.3 µg/ml. In 7 hours, the level fell to 16.2 µg/ml; in 24 hours, it fell to 2.7 µg/ml (66). After ingestion of an unknown amount of ofloxacin, the plasma levels were 15 µg/ml at 12 hours and 0.2 µg/ml at 24 hours.

Despite the potential for QT prolongation, this side effect is sufficiently rare so that routine electrocardiographic screening or monitoring is not advisable or recommended unless a large overdose has been ingested.

Treatment

DECONTAMINATION

Syrup of ipecac is not advised for treatment of an overdose, as peak blood levels are reached within 1 hour, and there is a danger of seizures. Activated charcoal has not been evaluated but would be expected to bind all quinolones. Gastric lavage may be useful within the first 2 hours of a large ingestion but would not be helpful in smaller ingestions due to the low potential for toxicity.

ENHANCEMENT OF ELIMINATION

The high volume of distribution of ciprofloxacin tends to diminish the effectiveness of hemodialysis or hemoperfusion. Ofloxacin is eliminated, usually 15% to 25%, by hemodialysis during the first 2 hours of dialysis (68), but this procedure is rarely required after an ofloxacin overdose.

SUPPORTIVE CARE

Seizures can be treated with diazepam, phenytoin, and other anticonvulsant drugs. Careful periodic evaluation of renal function (e.g., urinalysis for crystalluria, serum creatinine, and urea nitrogen) is indicated. Adequate hydration (IV fluids) with careful measurement of fluid intake and output should be instituted. Steroid therapy may ameliorate interstitial nephritis as well as arthralgias.

REFERENCES

1. Masters PA, O'Bryan TA, Zurlo J, et al. Trimethoprim-sulfamethoxazole revisited. *Arch Intern Med* 2003;163:402–410.
2. Holland NH, Kazee M, Duff D, et al. Antimicrobial prophylaxis in children with urinary tract infection and vesicoureteral reflux. *Rev Infect Dis* 1982;4:467–474.
3. Sandock DS, Gothe BG, Bodner DR. Trimethoprim-sulfamethoxazole prophylaxis against urinary tract infection in the chronic spinal cord injury patient. *Paraplegia* 1995;33:156–160.
4. Singh N, Gayowski T, Yu VL, et al. Trimethoprim-sulfamethoxazole for the prevention of spontaneous bacterial peritonitis in cirrhosis: a randomized trial. *Ann Intern Med* 1995;122:595–598.
5. Razavi B, Lund B, Allen BL, et al. Failure of trimethoprim/sulfamethoxazole prophylaxis for *Pneumocystis carinii* pneumonia with concurrent leucovorin use. *Infection* 2002;30:41–42.
6. DiRienzo AG, van Der Horst C, Finkelstein DM, et al. Efficacy of trimethoprim-sulfamethoxazole for the prevention of bacterial infections in a randomized prophylaxis trial of patients with advanced HIV infection. *AIDS Res Hum Retroviruses* 2002;18:89–94.
7. Chaimongkol B, Nanthachit N, Navarawong V, et al. Drug-induced agranulocytosis. *J Med Assoc Thai* 1989;72:666–672.
8. Bjorkman A, Phillips-Howard PA. Adverse reactions to sulfa drugs: implications for malaria chemotherapy. *Bull World Health Organ* 1991;69:297–304.
9. Dunn RJ. Massive sulfasalazine and paracetamol ingestion causing acidosis, hyperglycemia, coagulopathy, and methemoglobinemia. *J Toxicol Clin Toxicol* 1998;36:239–242.
10. Minocha A, Dean HA Jr, Mayle JE. Acute sulfasalazine overdose. *J Toxicol Clin Toxicol* 1991;29:543–551.
11. Teo CP, Oh VM, Kueh YK. Agranulocytosis and anaemia induced by sulfametopyrazine in a sulfametopyrazine-trimethoprim combination. *Ann Acad Med Singapore* 1989;18:307–310.
12. Sulfonamides. Available at: http://www.pharmacology2000.com/Chemotherapy/Antibacterial/sulfa1.htm. Accessed April 2003.
13. Chambers HF, Jawetz E. Sulfonamides, trimethoprim, and quinolones. In: Katzung BG, ed. *Basic and clinical pharmacology*. Los Angeles: Appleton-Lange, 1998:761–763.
14. RXmed. Available at: http://www.rxmed.com. Accessed April 2003.
15. Antibiotic use during pregnancy. Available at: http://www.drklein.net/antibioticsandpregnancy.htm. Accessed April 2003.
16. Golembiewski JA. Allergic reactions to drugs: implications for perioperative care. *J Perianesth Nurs* 2002;17:393–398.
17. Ryan C, Madalon M, Wortham DW, et al. Sulfa hypersensitivity in patients with HIV infection: onset, treatment, critical review of the literature. *WMJ* 1998;97:23–27.
18. Shepherd GM. Hypersensitivity reactions to drugs: evaluation and management. *Mt Sinai J Med* 2003;70:113–125.
19. Chan HL, Stern RS, Arndt KA, et al. The incidence of erythema multiforme, Stevens-Johnson syndrome, and toxic epidermal necrolysis. A population-based study with particular reference to reactions caused by drugs among outpatients. *Arch Dermatol* 1990;126:43–47.
20. Ozkaya-Bayazit E, Akar U. Fixed drug eruption induced by trimethoprim-sulfamethoxazole: evidence for a link to HLA-A30 B13 Cw6 haplotype. *J Am Acad Dermatol* 2001;45:712–717.
21. Wagner FF, Flegel WA. Toxic epidermal necrolysis. *N Engl J Med* 1996;334:922.
22. Paquet P, Jacob E, Damas P, et al. Treatment of drug-induced toxic epidermal necrolysis (Lyell's syndrome) with intravenous human immunoglobulins. *Burns* 2001;27:652–655.
23. Bronny AT, Thies RM. Oral mucosal lichenoid reaction to sulfamethoxazole. *Spec Care Dentist* 1990;10:55–57.
24. Martinez-Ruiz E, Ortega C, Calduch L, et al. Generalized cutaneous depigmentation following sulfamide-induced drug eruption. *Dermatology* 2000;201:252–254.
25. Wainwright NJ, Collins P, Ferguson J. Photosensitivity associated with antibacterial agents. *Drug Saf* 1993;9:437–440.
26. Mahboob A, Haroon TS. Drugs causing fixed eruptions: a study of 450 cases. *Int J Dermatol* 1998;37:833–838.
27. Rawson NS, Harding SR, Malcolm E, et al. Hospitalizations for aplastic anemia and agranulocytosis in Saskatchewan: incidence and associations with antecedent prescription drug use. *J Clin Epidemiol* 1998;51:1343–1355.
28. Anti-infective drug use in relation to the risk of agranulocytosis and aplastic anemia. A report from the International Agranulocytosis and Aplastic Anemia Study. *Arch Intern Med* 1989;149:1036–1040.
29. Danielson DA, Douglas SW 3rd, Herzog P, et al. Drug-induced blood disorders. *JAMA* 1984;252:3257–3260.
30. Perazella MA. Crystal-induced acute renal failure. *Am J Med* 1999;106:459–465.
31. Schwarz A, Perez-Canto A. Nephrotoxicity of antiinfective drugs. *Int J Clin Pharmacol Ther* 1998;36:164–167.
32. Marinella MA. Case report: reversible hyperkalemia associated with trimethoprim-sulfamethoxazole. *Am J Med Sci* 1995;310:115–117.
33. Giraud O, Thomas F, Aussavy F, et al. Hyperkalemia and acute renal insufficiency during overdose of trimethoprim-sulfamethoxazole in a patient with AIDS. *Ann Med Interne (Paris)* 1997;148:185–186.
34. Tilden ME, Rosenbaum JT, Fraunfelder FT. Systemic sulfonamides as a cause of bilateral, anterior uveitis. *Arch Ophthalmol* 1991;109:67–69.
35. Drug-induced myopia. *Prescrire Int* 2003;12:22–23.
36. Novack GD. Ocular toxicology. *Curr Opin Ophthalmol* 1994;5:110–114.
37. Atiyeh BS, Dham R, Yassin MF, et al. Treatment of toxic epidermal necrolysis with moisture-retentive ointment: a case report and review of the literature. *Dermatol Surg* 2003;29:185–188.
38. Quinolones. Fluoroquinolones. Available at: http://www.merck.com/pubs/mmanual/section13/chapter153/153g.htm. Accessed April 2003.
39. Oliphant CM, Green GM. Quinolones: a comprehensive review. *Am Fam Physician* 2002;65:455–464.
40. Bouchayer D, Vial T, Mercatello A, et al. Acute renal failure secondary to ciprofloxacin overdose. Proceedings, European Association of Poison Centres. 22 May 1991. Lyon, France.
41. George MJ, Dew RB III, Daly JS. Acute renal failure after an overdose of ciprofloxacin. *Arch Intern Med* 1991;151:620.
42. Kohler PB, Arkins N, Tack NJ. Accidental overdose of intravenous ofloxacin with benign outcome. *Antimicrob Agents Chemother* 1991;35:1239–1240.
43. Koppel C, Hopke T, Menzel J. Central anticholinergic syndrome after ofloxacin overdose and therapeutic doses of diphenhydramine and chlormezanone. *J Toxicol Clin Toxicol* 1990;28:249–253.
44. Quinolones. Fluoroquinolones. Available at: http://www.merck.com/pubs/mmanual/section13/chapter153/153g.htm. Accessed April 2003.
45. Giamarellou H, Kolokythas E, Petrikkos G, et al. Pharmacokinetics of three new quinolones in pregnant and lactating women. *Am J Med* 1989;87(Suppl 5A):49.
46. Peled Y, Friedman S, Hod M, Merlob P. Ofloxacin during the second trimester of pregnancy. *DICP Ann Pharmacother* 1991;25:1181–1182.
47. Glum A. Ofloxacin-induced acute severe hepatitis. *South Med J* 1991;84:1158.
48. Coleman CI, Spencer JV, Chung JO, Reddy P. Possible gatifloxacin-induced fulminant hepatic failure. *Ann Pharmacother* 2002;36:1162–1167.
49. Lazarczyk DA, Goldstein NS, Gordon SC. Trovafloxacin hepatotoxicity. *Dig Dis Sci* 2001;46:925–926.
50. Stahlmann R. Children as a special population at risk—quinolones as an example for xenobiotics exhibiting skeletal toxicity. *Arch Toxicol* 2003;77:7–11.
51. Burstein GR, Berman SM, Blumer JL, et al. Ciprofloxacin for the treatment of uncomplicated gonorrhea infection in adolescents: does the benefit outweigh the risk? *Clin Infect Dis* 2002;35(Suppl 2):S191–S199.
52. Yee CL, Duffy C, Gerbino PG, et al. Tendon or joint disorders in children after treatment with fluoroquinolones or azithromycin. *Pediatr Infect Dis J* 2002;21:525–529.
53. van der Linden PD, Sturkenboom MC, Herings RM, et al. Fluoroquinolones and risk of Achilles tendon disorders: case-control study. *BMJ* 2002;324:1306–1307.
54. Casparian JM, Luchi M, Moffat RE, et al. Quinolones and tendon ruptures. *South Med J* 2000;93:488–491.
55. Rastogi S, Atkinson JL, McCarthy JT. Allergic nephropathy associated with ciprofloxacin. *Mayo Clin Proc* 1990;65:987–989.
56. Murray KM, Wilson MG. Suspected ciprofloxacin-induced interstitial nephritis. *DICP Ann Pharmacother* 1990;24:379–380.
57. Ying LS, Johnson CA. Ciprofloxacin-induced interstitial nephritis. *Clin Pharm* 1989;8:518–521.
58. Hootkins R, Fenves AZ, Stephens MK. Acute renal failure secondary to oral ciprofloxacin therapy: a presentation of three cases and a review of the literature. *Clin Nephrol* 1989;32:75–78.
59. Stahlmann R. Clinical toxicological aspects of fluoroquinolones. *Toxicol Lett* 2002;127:269–277.
60. Semel JD, Allen N. Seizures in patients simultaneously receiving theophylline and imipenem or ciprofloxacin or metronidazole. *South Med J* 1991;84:465–468.
61. Slavich IL, Gleffee RF, Haas EJ. Grand mal epileptic seizures during ciprofloxacin therapy. *JAMA* 1989;261:558–559.
62. Mumford CJ, Ginsberg L. Ciprofloxacin and myasthenia gravis. *BMJ* 1990;301:818.
63. Winrow AP, Supramaniam G. Benign intracranial hypertension after ciprofloxacin administration. *Arch Dis Child* 1990;65:1165–1166.
64. Vriabec TR, Sergott RC, Jaeger EA, et al. Reversible visual loss in a patient receiving high-dose ciprofloxacin hydrochloride (Cipro). *Ophthalmology* 1990;97:707–710.
65. Zaudig M, von Bose M, Weber MM, et al. Psychotic effects of ofloxacin. *Pharmacopsychiatry* 1989;22:11–15.
66. Kohler PB, Arkins N, Tack NJ. Accidental overdose of intravenous ofloxacin with benign outcome. *Antimicrob Agents Chemother* 1991;35:1239–1240.
67. Baker SE, Hangii MC. Possible gatifloxacin-induced hypoglycemia. *Ann Pharmacother* 2002;36:1722–1726.
68. Ciprofloxacin. *Med Lett Drugs Ther* 1988;30:11–13.

CHAPTER 89

Antifungal Drugs

Seth Schonwald and Ira M. Leviton

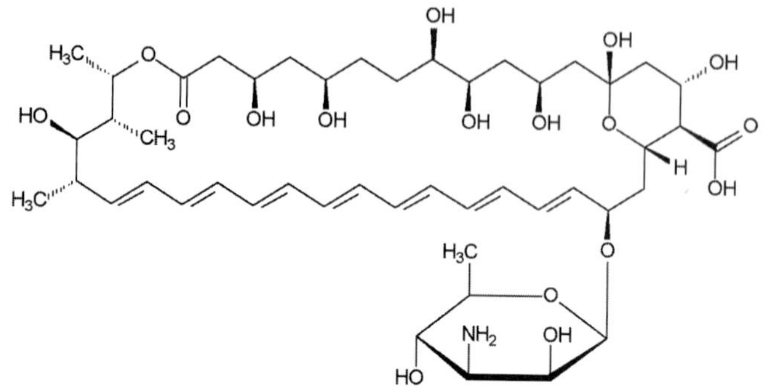

AMPHOTERICIN B

Compounds included:	**Amphotericin (Fungizone, Amphotec, Amphocil, Abelcet, AmBisome); nystatin (Mycostatin, Nilstat); flucytosine (Ancobon); ketoconazole (Nizoral); itraconazole (Sporanox); fluconazole (Diflucan); voriconazole (Vfend); griseofulvin (Grifulvin, Fulvicin); caspofungin (Cancidas); terbinafine (Lamisil); miconazole (Monistat)**
Molecular formula and weight:	**See text.**
SI conversion:	**Amphotericin B, mg/L × 1.1 = μmol/L; flucytosine, mg/L × 7.7 = μmol/L; griseofulvin, mg/L × 2.8 = μmol/L; fluconazole, mg/L × 3.3 = μmol/L; ketoconazole, mg/L × 1.9 = μmol/L; itraconazole, mg/L × 1.4 = μmol/L; miconazole, mg/dL × 2.4 = μmol/L; echinocandins, mg/L × 0.8 = μmol/L**
CAS Registry No.:	**See text.**
Therapeutic levels:	**Not used clinically**
Target organs:	**Heart (acute), kidney (acute and chronic), blood (chronic), allergic (acute), gastrointestinal (acute and chronic), liver (chronic)**
Antidote:	**None**

OVERVIEW

Systemic and mucosal fungal infections are increasing because of immunocompromised patients who are living longer, addiction to intravenous (IV) drugs, and greater use of invasive procedures and broad-spectrum antibiotics. The therapeutic use of systemic antifungal agents will likely continue to increase over the next decade.

The polyene antifungal drug group consists of amphotericin B, natamycin, and nystatin (1). All are used topically for treating superficial candidiasis. Only amphotericin B is used IV; it is an important agent for therapy of systemic fungal infections (2). Overdoses with amphotericin B may be fatal (3–6). The original and relatively toxic deoxycholate salt of amphotericin B (Fungizone) has been used for more than 40 years. Three lipid formulations of amphotericin B with less toxicity are now marketed as well: amphotericin B colloidal dispersion (Amphotec, Amphocil), amphotericin B lipid complex (Abelcet), and liposomal amphotericin B (AmBisome). They have no advantage in efficacy over the original deoxycholate form, and their main difference is less frequent nephrotoxicity.

Nystatin is available in a variety of topical, oral (very poorly absorbed), and vaginal tablet preparations. Natamycin is available only as an ophthalmic suspension.

Flucytosine is a synthetic nucleotide analog used to treat a variety of invasive fungal infections (7). It is the only member of the pyrimidine group of antifungal drugs.

Most of the *imidazoles* are used topically (i.e., clotrimazole, miconazole, econazole, isoconazole, tioconazole). Ketoconazole, itraconazole (8), fluconazole, and voriconazole are active systemically after oral administration. Reports of overdose with miconazole reflect the clinical toxicology of the imidazole group (9,10).

Griseofulvin is used in the treatment of dermatophyte infections as well as a number of nonfungal disease states (e.g., Raynaud's phenomenon, progressive systemic sclerosis, lichen planus, mycosis fungoides, herpes zoster, eosinophilic fasciitis, and molluscum contagiosum) (11).

Caspofungin (Cancidas) represents a new echinocandin type of antifungal agent. It is indicated for invasive aspergillosis and candidiasis in patients who do not respond to alternative treatments. *Ter-*

binafine (12,13) and *naftifine* (14) are allylamines that are active against tinea and dermatophytes; terbinafine is available both topically and as tablets, and naftifine is available only as a topical preparation.

AMPHOTERICIN B

Amphotericin B [Fungizone, Amphotec, Amphocil, Abelcet, AmBisome; $C_{47}H_{73}NO_{17}$; molecular weight (MW), 924.1 g/mol; CAS Registry No., 1397-89-3] is the "gold standard" of antifungal therapy, especially for the systemic mycoses (15–17). Its many drawbacks include its need for IV administration and infusion-related side effects. It also has poor penetration into cerebrospinal fluid (18). Renal dysfunction, hypokalemia, renal tubular acidosis (19), and bone marrow suppression frequently occur with chronic use, and overdosed infants and children have developed life-threatening dysrhythmias and death (2–6). Recently developed lipid-based amphotericin B formulations are less nephrotoxic but still demonstrate a substantial rate of infusion-related side effects.

Toxic Dose

The *adult therapeutic dose* is usually 0.5 to 0.7 mg/kg/day IV and may reach 1.0 mg/kg/day. It is usually given as a slow infusion over 4 to 6 hours. More rapid infusion may cause hypotension, bronchospasm (20), shock, and death.

Up to 14 mg in infants (2) and 200 mg in adults (5) have been ingested with moderate sequelae. Cardiac arrest and death have occurred with doses as low as 5 mg IV.

Toxicokinetics and Toxicodynamics

The pharmacokinetics of antifungal agents (21–25) are summarized in Table 1. The various lipid formulations of amphotericin B have very different pharmacokinetic properties.

Pathophysiology

Amphotericin B binds to ergosterol in fungal cell walls, causing increased membrane permeability and cell death.

Antagonism between amphotericin B and miconazole and ketoconazole has been observed (1). Amphotericin B with gentamicin may induce synergistic nephrotoxicity (26). Similarly, other nephrotoxic drugs may be additive to the nephrotoxic effects of amphotericin B. These drugs include aminoglycosides, capreomycin, colistin, cisplatin, methoxyflurane, polymyxin B, and vancomycin (27).

Because amphotericin B may cause hypokalemia, this effect may be potentiated by corticosteroids. The hypokalemia may potentiate digoxin toxicity (1), may be associated with rhabdomyolysis (28), and may enhance the effect of nondepolarizing (curariform) drugs. The manufacturer warns that amphotericin B should be used with antineoplastic drugs only with great caution (29).

Pregnancy and Lactation

Amphotericin B is U.S. Food and Drug Administration (FDA) pregnancy category B (Appendix I). There are few data on levels of amphotericin B in human milk.

Clinical Presentation

ADVERSE EVENTS

Amphotericin B commonly causes fever, chills, anorexia, rigors, hypotension, and tachypnea, typically beginning 1 to 3 hours after starting an infusion and lasting 1 or more hours.

Cardiac effects include tachycardia and changes in blood pressure, including hypotension if infused too rapidly (30) and hypertension (31). Sinus bradycardia is uncommon. Ventricular fibrillation has also been reported after rapid infusion, especially in patients with renal insufficiency (Table 2).

Renal effects are common after a few days of treatment: measurable decrease in renal function, including a decline in glomerular filtration rate, along with renal tubular acidosis, decreased serum potassium, and diminished renal concentrating ability. This does not alter its pharmacokinetics (32). Some of the decline in renal function is irreversible.

Hematologic effects include normochromic normocytic anemia accompanied by a depression of erythropoietin production that usually occurs in patients on prolonged treatment (33,34).

ACUTE OVERDOSAGE

In infants and very young children, doses of 2.5 to 8.0 mg/kg produced no obvious adverse effects (35,36). In an 8-week-old baby who received 14 mg of amphotericin B, abdominal distention, bloody diarrhea, and thrombocytopenia were observed within 12 hours of overdose; the patient recovered. Hypokalemia and elevated serum levels of γ-glutamyltransferase and aspartate transaminase were observed, but there was no evidence of bone marrow depression or depressed renal function. No permanent renal or bone marrow function abnormalities have been reported after overdose (37).

TABLE 1. Selected pharmacologic properties of systemic antifungal agents

Property	Amphotericin B	Flucytosine	Miconazole	Ketoconazole	Itraconazole	Fluconazole
Oral bioavailability (%)	9	25	75[a]	>70[a]	>80	—
Protein binding (%)	91–95	4	91–93	99	>99	11
Apparent volume of distribution (L/kg)	4.0	0.6–0.7	—[b]	—[c]	—[c]	0.7–0.8
Peak plasma concentration (μg/ml)	1.2–2.0	30.0–45.0	1.2–2.5	1.5–3.1	0.2–0.4	10.2
Dose (mg)	50 IV	2000 PO	400 IV	200 PO	200 PO	200 PO
Time-to-peak plasma concentration (h)	—	2	—	1–4	4–5	2–4
Terminal elimination half-life	15 d	3–6 h	20–24 h	7–10 h[d]	24–42 h[d]	22–31 h
Unchanged drug in urine (%)	3	>75	1	2–4	80	—
Cerebrospinal fluid or plasma concentration (%)	2–4	>75	5–10	>70	—	—

[a]The absolute bioavailability of miconazole and ketoconazole has not been determined because of the absence of a form suitable for intravenous use. The values reported represent the bioavailability of these agents relative to that of an oral solution in normal subjects.
[b]The mean apparent volume of distribution of miconazole in one study of normal subjects was 1474 L/kg of body weight.
[c]The apparent volume of distribution was not assessed in humans because of the absence of a form suitable for intravenous use. In dogs, the apparent volumes of distribution of ketoconazole and itraconazole were 0.87 and 17.00 L/kg, respectively.
[d]Itraconazole and ketoconazole exhibit dose-dependent elimination. Longer terminal elimination half-lives are possible with large daily doses.
From Como JA, Dismukes WE. Oral azole drugs as systemic antifungal therapy. *N Engl J Med* 1994;330:263–272, with permission.

TABLE 2. Adverse events associated with amphotericin B therapy

Gastrointestinal
- Rare diarrhea, nausea, vomiting

Neurologic
- Leukoencephalopathy, hypokalemic paralysis

Renal
- Impairment of renal function in up to 80% of treated patients; increased serum urea nitrogen and creatinine concentrations; decreased glomerular filtration rate and urinary concentrating ability; distal renal tubular acidosis; hypermagnesemia; hyponatruria; hyperkaluria; decreased serum potassium and magnesium levels; rare hematuria, pyuria, proteinuria; recurrent reversible acute renal failure

Skin
- Red man syndrome rash

Heart
- Ventricular fibrillation with hyperkalemia after rapid infusion in anuric patient; transient asystole; premature ventricular contraction in a neonate; malignant hypertensive episodes

Hepatic
- Acute fetal hepatic necrosis

Lungs
- Pulmonary hypertension with liposomal amphotericin B (51), bronchiolitis obliterans

Hematologic
- Normochromic normocytic anemia; thrombophlebitis; pain at injection site; rare thrombocytopenia, leukopenia, agranulocytosis, eosinophilia, and coagulation defects

When given intrathecally
- Headache, nausea and vomiting, urinary retention, pain along lumbar nerves, paresthesia, vision changes, arachnoiditis

Cardiac effects include transient asystole (38), malignant hypertensive episodes (39), ventricular fibrillation (40), and other dysrhythmias (41). Four infants and children developed cardiac arrest and died after ingesting up to 10 to 50 times the recommended dose (Table 3).

Hypersensitivity effects include red man syndrome (42). Allergic reactions to the liposomal component of liposomal amphotericin B are manifested by extensive maculopapular rash and severe itching that resolve with discontinuation of the drug (43). Bronchiolitis obliterans has also been described (44).

Diagnostic Tests

Amphotericin B can be measured by bioassay (45) or high-performance liquid chromatography (46).

Renal function tests (e.g., blood urea nitrogen, serum creatinine, or endogenous creatinine clearance) and liver function tests may become elevated during therapy. Normochromic normocytic anemia, hypokalemia, hypomagnesemia, and elevated liver function tests may also be observed. Clinically significant impairment of liver function is not considered a typical adverse effect of amphotericin B (47).

Treatment

ACUTE OVERDOSAGE

Patients with amphotericin B overdose should be hospitalized for symptomatic and supportive treatment. Cardiac dysrhythmias and central nervous system lesions represent the greatest immediate threats to life. Immediate IV access should be established along with cardiac monitoring for all patients with serious vital sign abnormalities. A chest radiograph and arterial blood gases should be obtained when there is evidence of respiratory depression or distress.

GASTROINTESTINAL DECONTAMINATION

Because amphotericin B is nearly always administered IV, decontamination is only useful if a large amount of ointment, cream, or lozenge is ingested; however, less than 10% of amphotericin B is absorbed orally.

ELIMINATION ENHANCEMENT

Amphotericin B behaves as a colloid in aqueous solution and is poorly dialyzable because of its large molecular size. Its poor dialyzability and high protein binding result in clearance of only negligible amounts by hemodialysis (48).

ANTIDOTE

There is no antidote for amphotericin B toxicity.

SUPPORTIVE MEASURES

Chills and fever are frequent (49). Acetaminophen or ibuprofen can be given 30 minutes before amphotericin B infusion. In addition, hydrocortisone, 25 mg IV, and meperidine, 0.5 mg/kg IV,

TABLE 3. Summary of amphotericin B overdose reports

Age	Weight	Dose of amphotericin B	Adverse effects
21.0 d[a]	0.6 kg	2.5 mg/kg	None
2.0 yr[a]	13.5 kg	3.7 mg/kg	None
Neonate[a]	3.0 kg	8.0 mg/kg	None
8.0 wk[a]	Unknown	14.0 mg	Abdominal distention, bloody diarrhea, thrombocytopenia
5.0 mo	7.0 kg	4.4 mg/kg	None (blood level 4 g/ml)
32.0 d (24.5-wk gestation)	690.0 g at birth	15.0 mg/kg (total dose)	Hypokalemia; elevated γ-glutamyl transpeptidase and aspartate transaminase levels enzymes; half-life, 148.1 d
21.0 yr[a]	—	200.0 mg	No sequelae
5.0 yr[a]	—	3.0 mg/kg	Nausea, vomiting
	—	25.0 mg in 250.0 ml infusion (instead of 5.0 mg in 500.0 ml)	No sequelae
2.0 yr	—	5.0 mg IV	Vomiting, seizure, cardiac arrest; survived
7.0 yr	—	Tenfold overdose	Cardiac arrest, death
4.5 wk	—	25 times higher than intended	Cardiac arrest, death
7.0 wk	—	50 times higher than intended	Cardiac arrest, death

[a]Manufacturer's case reports (Squibb, 1988).
Data from references 37–39.

given approximately 20 minutes before the reaction have been used successfully (50). Patients on chronic amphotericin B treatment may theoretically become addicted when given frequent meperidine treatments (51). Dantrolene does not appear to ameliorate the fever or chills of these patients (52).

Hypokalemia is treated with amiloride, 5 mg twice daily, to reduce the amount of potassium wasting (53). One liter of 0.9% sodium chloride daily should be infused for patients receiving 40 mg of amphotericin B per day or more to help reduce nephrotoxicity (54,55). This intervention is for multiple-day therapy and has no role in treatment of the overdose patient.

MONITORING

The patient must be monitored frequently daily for renal function (serum creatinine, blood urea nitrogen); periodic electrocardiograph (ECG) and other cardiac monitoring and serum electrolyte (sodium, potassium) determinations are also necessary. Hepatic function tests should also be obtained periodically, as should complete blood cell counts, including platelet counts.

FLUCYTOSINE

Flucytosine (Ancobon; $C_4H_4FN_3O$; MW, 129.1 g/mol; CAS Registry No., 2022-85-7), a synthetic, fluorinated pyrimidine analog, is associated with bone marrow suppression, hepatic dysfunction, and diarrhea. Acute or chronic toxicity due to overdose is generally manifested by severe bone marrow suppression or gastrointestinal disorders.

Toxic Dose

The *therapeutic dose* is 150 mg/kg/day in four divided doses. Patients with renal dysfunction require dose reduction (22). A fatal colitis-like condition with multiple intestinal perforations and peritonitis has been observed (56).

Toxicokinetics and Toxicodynamics

The pharmacokinetics of flucytosine are provided in Table 4 (57).

Pathophysiology

Flucytosine is deaminated to 5-fluorouracil and then converted to 5-fluorodeoxyuridylic acid monophosphate, an inhibitor of thymidylate synthetase that interferes with DNA synthesis (22).

Pregnancy and Lactation

Flucytosine is FDA pregnancy category C (Appendix I). Flucytosine is teratogenic to rats.

TABLE 4. Pharmacokinetics of flucytosine and griseofulvin

Property	Flucytosine	Griseofulvin
Peak serum level (μg/ml)	30.0–40.0	0.4–2.0 (in 4.0–8.0 h)
Volume of distribution (L/kg)	0.68	—
Protein binding (%)	2–4	NR
Half-life (h)	2.5–6.0	9.0–24.0
Excreted unchanged in urine (%)	75–90	NR
Oral bioavailability (%)	75–90	25–70

NR, not reported.

Clinical Presentation

Flucytosine toxicity is manifested in rapidly proliferating tissues, particularly the bone marrow, and the lining of the gastrointestinal tract (58). The risk of bone marrow toxicity is increased with prolonged high serum flucytosine concentrations.

Adverse gastrointestinal effects may include nausea, vomiting, anorexia, abdominal bloating, diarrhea, and, rarely, bowel perforation. Elevations of serum hepatic enzyme levels appear to be dose related and reversible.

In the presence of azotemia or concomitant amphotericin B administration, leukopenia, thrombocytopenia, and enterocolitis may occur and may be fatal (22). Such complications are more frequent among patients whose serum flucytosine levels are greater than 100 to 125 μg/ml (59). Anaphylactic reaction has been reported in a patient with acquired immunodeficiency syndrome (60).

Diagnostic Tests

Bioassay (61) and gas chromatographic (62) methods are available. Peak serum levels of 30 to 45 μg/ml are reached within 6 hours after a single 2-g oral dose. Toxicity is associated with prolonged serum concentration greater than 100 to 125 μg/ml. Crystalluria has been observed with doses of 200-mg/kg body weight (63).

Blood studies should include a complete blood cell count, hepatic function tests, and evaluation of renal function. If facilities are available, a serum flucytosine level should be determined and periodically monitored.

Treatment

Airway, breathing, and circulation should be evaluated on examination. All patients should be hospitalized until evidence of bone marrow suppression, serious gastrointestinal disturbance, and hepatic or renal dysfunction has been fully evaluated. Follow-up hematology studies should be scheduled.

GASTROINTESTINAL DECONTAMINATION

Because absorption is slow (2 to 6 hours), gastric emptying or activated charcoal should be considered if the patient is conscious and has a gag reflex and has no obvious internal abdominal pathology after physical examination.

ELIMINATION ENHANCEMENT

Flucytosine may be removed more quickly with the use of extracorporeal methods, such as hemodialysis and peritoneal dialysis, but clinical confirmation is required.

ANTIDOTE

There is no antidote available for flucytosine.

SUPPORTIVE MEASURES

Flucytosine is metabolized to the antimetabolite 5-fluorouracil. Overdose should be treated with all necessary precautions and detailed follow-up, as required in a cytotoxic drug overdose (see Chapter 98).

GRISEOFULVIN

Griseofulvin (Fulvicin, Gris-PEG, Grifulvin; $C_{17}H_{17}ClO_6$; MW, 352.8 g/mol; CAS Registry No., 126-07-8) is an oral fungistatic antibiotic produced by *Penicillium griseofulvin* that is effective in the treatment of dermatophytoses (10). The incidence of adverse reactions with therapeutic doses is very low; there are no overdose reports in the medical literature. The use of griseofulvin has increasingly focused on nonfungal diseases such as Raynaud's phenomenon, progressive systemic sclerosis, lichen planus (64), mycosis fungoides, herpes zoster (65), eosinophilic fasciitis, and molluscum contagiosum (10).

Toxic Dose

The *adult therapeutic dose* of microsize griseofulvin is 500 mg to 1 g daily; ultramicrosize is 330 to 750 mg daily. The *pediatric dose* for the microsize formulation is usually 10 to 11 mg/kg/day; ultramicrosize is 73 mg/kg/day (66). A toxic or lethal dose in humans has not been established.

Toxicokinetics and Toxicodynamics

The pharmacokinetics of griseofulvin are provided in Table 4 (67–69).

Pathophysiology

Although its precise mechanism of action is unknown, griseofulvin is believed to disrupt the fungal mitotic spindle structure and arrest fungal growth in metaphase of cell division.

Pregnancy and Lactation

Griseofulvin formulations have not been rated by the FDA. Griseofulvin may be fetotoxic in the pregnant patient (70).

Clinical Presentation

Therapeutic use can lead to headaches, nausea, vomiting, anorexia, abdominal cramps, flatulence, and diarrhea (71,72). Headaches may occur in up to 15% of patients and may be severe but often remit despite continued treatment. Hypersensitivity reactions to griseofulvin that may be life-threatening include urticaria, erythema multiforme, angioedema, and a reaction resembling serum sickness (71). Erythroid hypoplasia, allergic interstitial nephritis (73), and fatal toxic epidermal necrolysis (71) occur rarely.

Persistent cold urticaria, an acute allergic reaction that often follows a reaction to penicillin, has also been reported with griseofulvin (72). Disabling neurologic phenomena, such as vertigo, blurry vision, mental depression, lethargy, and insomnia, have been observed (74). Rarely, life-threatening hepatotoxicity occurs (74). Griseofulvin may exacerbate attacks of acute porphyria. Renal (75) and hematopoietic toxicity after griseofulvin use is extremely rare (74).

Diagnostic Tests

Serum levels have not been correlated with toxic effects. Liver function tests, renal function tests, and hematopoietic parameters may be abnormal in rare cases.

Treatment

There are no data suggesting specific therapeutic measures for treatment of a griseofulvin overdose. Treatment is symptomatic and supportive. After evaluation of the airway, breathing, and circulatory status, attention must focus on any life-threatening complication, such as a hypersensitivity reaction (angioedema, serum sickness) or a serious hepatotoxic reaction.

GASTRIC DECONTAMINATION

The use of gastric emptying or activated charcoal has not been evaluated.

ANTIDOTES

There is no antidote for griseofulvin.

SUPPORTIVE CARE

Treatment of a hypersensitivity response may require IV fluids, monitoring of central venous pressure or pulmonary wedge pressure in patients with underlying cardiovascular disease, ECG monitoring, epinephrine, diphenhydramine, or either aminophylline or β-adrenergic agonists for bronchospasm (Chapter 34).

Patients with serious renal, hepatotoxic, hematopoietic, or hypersensitivity reactions should be admitted to the hospital and, if required, followed in an intensive care facility with careful respiratory and cardiovascular monitoring. Patients may be discharged after renal, hepatic, and hematopoietic functions have been stabilized, the patient has no neurologic deficit, vital signs are normal, and there is no imminent threat of a recurrent hypersensitivity response.

FLUCONAZOLE

Fluconazole (Diflucan; $C_{13}H_{12}F_2N_6O$; MW, 306.3 g/mol; CAS Registry No., 86386-73-4) differs from other azoles with respect to its toxicokinetic and toxicity profiles. It is used to treat tinea (76), vaginal candidiasis, oropharyngeal and esophageal candidiasis (77), and cryptococcal meningitis (78). There are no published reports of human overdose. Fatal hepatic necrosis, however, has occurred with prolonged use (74,79–81).

Toxic Dose

The *adult therapeutic dose* is 100 to 400 mg/day. The *pediatric dose* is 6 to 12 mg/kg/day. Dosage reduction is necessary for patients with impaired renal function. A minimum lethal dose has not been determined.

Toxicokinetics and Toxicodynamics

Fluconazole may be administered orally or IV, is water soluble, is greater than 90% bioavailable with oral administration, has a long serum half-life and low protein binding, and penetrates well into the cerebrospinal fluid (Table 1) (82).

Fluconazole is eliminated by the kidneys. As the glomerular filtration rate diminishes—even without significant change in the apparent volume of distribution—the half-life (normally approximately 30 hours) becomes prolonged. Dosage must be reduced accordingly.

Pathophysiology

The azole antifungal agents interrupt the conversion of lanosterol to ergosterol, the main sterol of yeast and fungal cell membranes (83). Fluconazole acts by binding to fungal cytochrome P-450, thus inhibiting the demethylase enzyme involved in the synthesis of ergosterol.

Pregnancy and Lactation

Fluconazole is FDA pregnancy category C (Appendix I). Fluconazole attains concentrations in breast milk that may be harmful to a nursing infant (84).

Clinical Presentation

Fluconazole has been associated with abdominal discomfort and nausea and, less commonly, with signs of liver damage. In rare instances, it has been linked to severe skin rashes, such as fixed drug eruption (85), and two cases of fatal hepatic necrosis (86). Dizziness, headache, somnolence, delirium or coma, psychiatric disturbance, malaise, fatigue, and seizures have been reported.

There are rare reports of fever, edema, pleural effusion, oliguria, arthralgia/myalgia, and finger stiffness. Alopecia is commonly associated with higher doses (400 mg/day) of fluconazole given for 2 months or longer. This effect may be severe but is reversed by discontinuing fluconazole therapy or substantially reducing the daily dose (87).

Diagnostic Tests

Fluconazole is analyzed by a high-performance liquid chromatography assay. Mean maximum serum concentrations after fluconazole, 200 mg orally, are 3.43 μg/ml, with a corresponding time-to-peak plasma concentration of 4.0 hours.

Eosinophilia, anemia, leukopenia, neutropenia, thrombocytopenia, hypokalemia (requiring replacement potassium therapy or discontinuance of fluconazole) (88,89), increased serum creatinine and blood urea nitrogen concentrations, and elevated levels of serum bilirubin and transaminases have been observed.

Treatment

Limited information is available on acute toxicity of fluconazole in humans. If acute overdosage occurs, supportive and symptomatic treatment should be initiated.

GASTRIC DECONTAMINATION

Activated charcoal may be of value, but no confirmatory studies are available. There is no evidence to support the use of gastric emptying.

ELIMINATION ENHANCEMENT

Because most of fluconazole is excreted unchanged by the kidneys, consideration should be given to hemodialysis for serious overdoses (90). Hemodialysis reduces the plasma concentrations of fluconazole in severely impaired patients by a mean of 48% during the dialysis period. There are no data to substantiate the use of forced diuresis, peritoneal dialysis, exchange transfusion, charcoal or resin hemoperfusion, plasmapheresis, or whole bowel irrigation after a fluconazole overdose.

ANTIDOTE

There is no antidote for fluconazole toxicity.

SUPPORTIVE MEASURES

Serum potassium levels should be monitored. Blood cell counts should include platelet determination.

KETOCONAZOLE

Ketoconazole (Nizoral; $C_{26}H_{28}Cl_2N_4O4$; MW, 531.4 g/mol; CAS Registry No., 65277-42-1), a synthetic-substituted imidazole derivative structurally related to clotrimazole, miconazole, tioconazole, and econazole, was the first broad-spectrum oral antifungal drug. It has not been associated with acute overdose, although fatalities have been reported in association with hepatotoxic reactions (91).

Toxic Dose

The *adult therapeutic dose* ranges by indication from 300 mg once daily to 800 mg daily for 6 to 12 months (24). Deaths associated with hepatotoxicity have followed treatment with therapeutic doses (92–94). Doses up to 1600 mg have been ingested without apparently serious toxic effects.

Toxicokinetics and Toxicodynamics

Pharmacokinetic parameters for ketoconazole are provided in Table 1 (95,96).

Ketoconazole is poorly absorbed in the absence of gastric acidity (24). H_2 receptor–blocking drugs decrease its absorption. Concurrent use of rifampin markedly decreases serum levels and the effectiveness of ketoconazole because of the induction of ketoconazole metabolism by rifampin via the cytochrome P-450 system. Ketoconazole may increase the effect of oral anticoagulants (97) and the toxicity of cyclosporine, tacrolimus, and corticosteroids (98).

When ketoconazole is used with phenytoin, the serum concentrations of both drugs may be altered. A disulfiram-like reaction can occur with alcohol (24). Transient increases in quinidine concentrations have been observed (99,100). Triazolam concentration is increased by ketoconazole (101).

Pathophysiology

Ketoconazole exerts its antifungal effects by inhibiting the fungal cytochrome P-450 biosynthesis of ergosterol, the main sterol in the membranes of fungi (102). In addition, ketoconazole may inhibit the synthesis of cholesterol in mammalian cells (102). It also interferes with human cytochrome P-450 enzyme systems in several organs (e.g., testes, ovaries, adrenal glands, kidneys, and, especially, the liver).

Pregnancy and Lactation

Ketoconazole is FDA pregnancy category C (Appendix I) (103). Ketoconazole is probably distributed into human milk, suggesting that lactating women receiving the drug should not breastfeed until definitive studies reflect its safety.

Clinical Presentation

Chronic use of ketoconazole may lead to anorexia, nausea or vomiting, pruritus, rash, and dizziness. Anaphylaxis rarely occurs after the first dose. As ketoconazole appears to interfere with gonadal function, it may suppress testosterone production and can lead to gynecomastia, decreased libido, loss of potency in men, and menstrual irregularities in women. High doses may lower plasma cortisol concentrations (99). Adrenal crisis has occurred with its use (104,105). An immunoglobulin G–mediated hemolytic anemia has also occurred (106), and hypoglycemia has been observed (107).

The suppression of testosterone production caused by ketoconazole has been exploited in its use in the treatment of prostatic cancer (108). When high dosages (400 mg orally every 6 to 8 hours) of ketoconazole are used for this purpose, hypertension may be induced secondary to increases in mineralocorticoid levels (109,110). Hallucinations have been infrequently associated with ketoconazole and may reflect its central nervous system penetration (111).

Serious hepatic toxicity occurs in 1 of 15,000 exposed patients (94). Hepatitis associated with ketoconazole is usually reversible when treatment is stopped (112). Fatalities have followed continued use of the drug after the onset of jaundice and other symptoms of hepatitis.

Diagnostic Tests

Serum and plasma levels of ketoconazole have been determined by bioassay (112) and by more sensitive high-performance liquid chromatography methods (113).

In normal subjects given a single oral 200- or 400-mg dose of ketoconazole, peak serum concentrations occur at 2 hours and reach 3 µg/ml. Higher levels are found in patients taking 800 to 1200 mg/day. The drug is undetectable at 24 hours.

Treatment

For most patients with acute ketoconazole overdose, supportive symptomatic therapy, maintenance of life support measures (i.e., airway, respiration, circulation), and administration of sufficient fluids to maintain a urine flow of 3 to 6 ml/kg/hour are adequate.

GASTRIC DECONTAMINATION

Because toxicity occurs during chronic treatment, decontamination is not helpful.

ELIMINATION ENHANCEMENT

Because most of the parent drug ketoconazole is metabolized, and little unchanged drug is found in the urine, extracorporeal methods to enhance elimination do not appear useful.

ANTIDOTES

There is no antidote for ketoconazole toxicity.

SUPPORTIVE MEASURES

If hepatic and renal function tests are normal, and there is no evidence of adrenal or gonadal dysfunction, hypoglycemia, hemolytic anemia, hypertension, or central nervous system abnormalities, the patient can be discharged after being monitored for 24 hours. Although acetaminophen may be a metabolite found in animals, confirmatory studies in humans have not been performed, and there is no clinical evidence to support the use of acetylcysteine.

ITRACONAZOLE

Itraconazole (Sporanox; $C_{35}H_{38}Cl_2N_8O_4$; MW, 705.6 g/mol; CAS Registry No., 84625-61-6) is used for the treatment of onychomycosis, oral candidiasis, candidal esophagitis (114), blastomycosis (115), other endemic fungal diseases, lichen planus (116), and invasive aspergillosis. It can be used both orally (capsule or a solution) and IV (117,118) and undergoes extensive hepatic metabolism via the human cytochrome P-450 system (119). It does not penetrate the brain or cerebrospinal fluid in therapeutic concentrations, has no effect on mammalian steroid biosynthesis, and does not appear to alter pituitary-testicular or adrenal function.

Toxic Dose

The *adult therapeutic dose* is 100 to 400 mg/day in most fungal illnesses (120). The pediatric dose has not been established, but a dose of 5 mg/kg has been used.

Toxicokinetics and Toxicodynamics

Pharmacokinetics for itraconazole are provided in Table 1. Both itraconazole and its major metabolite are inhibitors of CYP3A4. Coadministration of itraconazole and drugs primarily metabolized by CYP3A4 may result in increased plasma concentrations of the drugs. Coadministration of itraconazole with oral midazolam or triazolam has resulted in elevated plasma concentrations of all three drugs. Coadministration of itraconazole and cyclosporine, tacrolimus, or digoxin has led to increased plasma concentrations of the latter three drugs. As with ketoconazole, coadministration of itraconazole and rifampin results in much lower concentrations of itraconazole because of the increased metabolism of itraconazole caused by rifampin.

Pregnancy and Lactation

Itraconazole is FDA pregnancy category C (Appendix I). Excretion into breast milk is unknown.

Clinical Presentation

No fatal reactions have been noted. Gynecomastia and rashes are infrequent occurrences. At doses of 600 mg/day, hypokalemia and hypertension were observed in five of eight patients studied (121). Further studies are required to evaluate the possible relationship of dose to toxicity. Other reactions observed include hypertriglyceridemia, hypokalemia, and hepatic enzyme elevations.

MICONAZOLE

Miconazole (Monistat; $C_{18}H_{14}Cl_4N_2O$; MW, 416.1 g/mol; CAS Registry No., 22916-47-8) has both IV and topical forms. The IV form is no longer in use because of the adverse effects of dysrhythmias, hyponatremia, lethargy, and seizures. Miconazole is a synthetic imidazole-derivative antifungal drug available for topical and vaginal use (122).

Toxic Dose

Two reports of overdose, one in a premature neonate of 31 weeks and one in a 4-month-old infant, have been reported. Both survived (Table 5). A lethal dose has not been reported.

Toxicokinetics and Toxicodynamics

Data available after overdose in a premature infant (8) indicate that the serum level reached 12 µg/ml 6 hours after the last dose. The infant had received 150 mg/kg/day. The level receded to 8.5 µg/ml at 16 hours and 1.4 µg/ml at 40 hours after the last dose.

There appears to be antagonism between miconazole and amphotericin B (123). Miconazole may prolong prothrombin time in patients on warfarin or other coumarin anticoagulants. Severe hypoglycemia has been reported when miconazole has been used

TABLE 5. Summary of miconazole overdose reports

	Patient 1	Patient 2
Age	31 wk[a]	4 mo[b]
Sex	Female	Male
Diagnosis	*Candida* septicemia	? Systemic candidiasis
Dose	50 mg/kg every 8 h IV (instead of 50 mg/kg/d)	500 mg IV
Serum levels	12 µg/ml (6 h)	—
Signs and symptoms	Bradycardia at 72 h; ectopic atrial rhythm; delayed intraventricular conduction; dusky, lethargic, apneic; hyponatremia	Tonic-clonic convulsions
Treatment	Fluid restriction	Diazepam (rectal, IVP)

[a]From Davey PG. New antiviral and antifungal drugs. *BMJ* 1990;300:793–798, with permission.
[b]From Kanarek KS, Williams PR. Toxicity of intravenous miconazole overdosage in a pre-term infant. *Pediatr Infect Dis* 1986;5:486–488, with permission.

with an oral sulfonylurea and diabetic agent. Drug interactions with cyclosporine, phenytoin, and rifampin may occur based on the structural similarity of miconazole to ketoconazole.

Pathophysiology

Miconazole, similar to other imidazoles, exerts its antifungal action by inhibiting ergosterol synthesis and interfering with fungal cytochrome P-450 enzymes.

Pregnancy and Lactation

Miconazole is FDA pregnancy category C (Appendix I). Entry into breast milk is unknown.

Clinical Presentation

ACUTE EXPOSURE

After overdose in an infant, cardiorespiratory depression with bradycardia, delayed intraventricular conduction, seizures, and hyponatremia occurred. There was a concomitant increase in serum miconazole values. These signs responded to supportive and symptomatic therapy.

ADVERSE EVENTS

Adverse events with IV miconazole have included nausea, vomiting, thrombophlebitis, anemia, and hyponatremia. Reactions attributed to the vehicle Cremophor EL (polyoxyethylated castor oil) include hyperlipemia, pruritus, thrombocytosis, and, with too rapid infusion, cardiorespiratory arrest (124). There is one report of three cases of grand mal seizures after miconazole (125,126). Because the commercial miconazole injection contains methylparaben, propylparaben, lactic acid, and polyoxyethylated castor oil, it is not possible to exclude these agents as a cause of seizure activity (9).

Diagnostic Tests

Serum levels of miconazole may reflect evidence of an overdosage. Laboratory examination in an overdose should include complete blood cell count, including platelet count, serum electrolytes, blood lipid profile, chest radiograph, ECG, cardiac monitoring, and appropriate diagnostic neurologic examinations. Cardiac monitoring in an overdose may disclose bradycardia, prolonged intraventricular conduction, and premature atrial beats.

Treatment

The major life-threatening complications of administering IV miconazole either too rapidly (less than 60 minutes) or insufficiently diluted (less than 200 ml of fluid) include cardiac arrest, respiratory arrest, and anaphylaxis (127).

Severely intoxicated patients should receive an IV line, cardiac monitoring, ECG, and oxygen. Mechanical ventilation may be required. If acute shortness of breath, choking, hypotension, cyanosis, or laryngeal edema is observed, immediate treatment with epinephrine, oxygen, and an adequate airway may be indicated.

GASTRIC DECONTAMINATION

Gastric or intestinal decontamination procedures have not been evaluated in imidazole overdoses.

ELIMINATION ENHANCEMENT

Extracorporeal procedures have not been evaluated. Hemodialysis is unlikely to be effective due to the large volume of distribution, high protein binding, extensive metabolism, and minimal renal excretion of unchanged drug.

ANTIDOTES

There is no antidote for miconazole.

SUPPORTIVE MEASURES

Seizures appear to respond best to diazepam (Chapter 40) (9). Hyponatremia may respond to fluid restriction.

VORICONAZOLE

Voriconazole (Vfend; $C_{16}H_{14}N_5F_3O$; MW, 349.3 g/mol; CAS Registry No., 137234-62-9) has features that are similar to those of the previously available triazoles as well as the same mechanism of action (prevention of ergosterol synthesis via inhibition of fungal cytochrome P-450 enzymes) and even broader antifungal activity (128). It is available in tablet and IV formulations, and has numerous potential drug interactions.

Toxic Dose

The *therapeutic dose* for adults and children older than 12 years of age is 4 to 6 mg/kg IV. A minimum toxic or fatal dose has not been established.

Toxicokinetics and Toxicodynamics

Bioavailability is nearly 100% with oral administration. Voriconazole is subject to the same dose adjustments and drug interactions as the other azole drugs.

Pregnancy and Lactation

Voriconazole is FDA pregnancy category D (Appendix I). Entry into breast milk is unknown.

Clinical Presentation

A unique side effect that can appear even with the first dose is visual hyperacuity. Patients report seeing flashes of light, which interfere with normal visual perception. Extensive studies, including funduscopy and visual evoked potentials, have not detected any abnormalities, and this side effect is transient (lasting approximately 30 minutes), although it may recur with additional doses.

ECHINOCANDINS

Caspofungin (Cancidas; $C_{52}H_{88}N_{10}O_{15}$,$2C_2H_4O_2$; MW, 1213.4 g/mol; CAS Registry No., 179463-17-3) represents a new, echinocandin type of antifungal agent (127). It is indicated for invasive aspergillosis (129) and candidiasis (130,131) in patients who do not respond to alternative treatments.

Toxic Dose

The *adult therapeutic dose* is 70 mg/day IV initially, then 50 mg/day thereafter. No pediatric dose has been established.

Toxicokinetics and Toxicodynamics

The protein binding of caspofungin is 97%. The primary mode of drug clearance is distribution rather than biotransformation or excretion. The elimination half-life is 9 to 11 hours. Caspofungin is slowly metabolized via hydrolysis and acetylation. Less than 2% is excreted unchanged in the urine. It is not dialyzable (132).

As caspofungin is not absorbed orally and is a very large molecule, it comes only as an IV form (133).

Pathophysiology

Its mechanism of action is inhibition of 1,3-α-glucan synthetase, an enzyme that is essential for most fungal cell walls (126).

Pregnancy and Lactation

Caspofungin is FDA pregnancy category C (Appendix I). Entry into breast milk has not been determined.

Clinical Presentation

In general, caspofungin appears to be well tolerated. Nausea, vomiting, and anorexia have been reported. Overdoses have not yet been reported. The entire spectrum of toxicity is probably not yet known; it includes local reactions at the injection site, systemic reactions linked to the infusion (especially due to histamine release), and hepatic disorders (134).

ALLYLAMINES

Terbinafine (Lamisil, tablet and topical) and naftifine (Naftin, topical only) represent allylamine antifungal agents. Both are used for tinea, onychomycosis (135), chronic pulmonary aspergillosis (136), and cutaneous candidal infections. Overdoses have not been reported with these agents alone; however, one case of nortriptyline overdose during treatment with terbinafine has been described (137).

REFERENCES

1. McEvoy GK, ed. *AHFS drug information 94.* Bethesda, MD: American Society of Hospital Pharmacists, 1994:94–95, 2288–2289.
2. Daneshmend TK, Warnock DW. Clinical pharmacokinetics of systemic antifungal drugs. *Clin Pharmacokinet* 1983;8:17–42.
3. Brent J, Hunt M, Kulig K, Rumack BH. Amphotericin B overdoses in infants: is there a role for exchange transfusion? *Vet Hum Toxicol* 1990;32:124–125.
4. Koren G, Lau A, Kenyon CF, et al. Clinical course and pharmacokinetics following a massive overdose of amphotericin B in a neonate. *J Toxicol Clin Toxicol* 1990;28:371–378.
5. Spoerke DG. Amphotericin B. In: *Poisindex toxicologic management*. Denver: Micromedex Inc., 1990.
6. Cleary JD, Hayman J, Sherwood J, et al. Amphotericin B overdose in pediatric patients with associated cardiac arrest. *Ann Pharmacother* 1993;27:715–719.
7. Luna B, Drew RH, Perfect JR. Agents for treatment of invasive fungal infections. *Otolaryngol Clin North Am* 2000;33:277–299.
8. Davey PG. New antiviral and antifungal drugs. *Br Med J* 1990;300:793–798.
9. Kanarek KS, Williams PR. Toxicity of intravenous miconazole overdosage in a pre-term infant. *Pediatr Infect Dis* 1986;5:486–488.
10. Coulthard K, Martin J, Matthew N. Convulsions after miconazole overdose. *Med J Aust* 1987;146:57–58.
11. Araujo DE, Flowers FP, King MM. Griseofulvin: a new look at an old drug. *DICP Ann Pharmacother* 1990;24:851–854.
12. Naftifine for fungal skin infections. *Med Lett Drugs Ther* 1988;30:98–99.
13. Lever LR, Thomas R, Dykes PJ, et al. Investigation of the pharmacokinetics of oral and topical terbinafine. *Clin Res* 1989;37:726A; Onychomycosis and terbinafine. *Lancet* 1990;1:636.
14. Stoughton RB, Sefton J, Zeleznick L. In vitro and in vivo cutaneous penetration and antifungal activity of naftifine. *Cutis* 1989;44:333–335.
15. McEvoy GK, ed. *AHFS drug information 94.* Bethesda, MD: American Society of Hospital Pharmacists, 1994:70–74, 2270–2271.
16. Graybill JR, Carven PC. Antifungal agents used in systemic mycoses: activity and therapeutic use. *Drugs* 1983;25:41–62.
17. Douglas KG Jr, Bennett JE. *Anti-infective therapy.* New York: John Wiley & Sons, 1985:307–324.
18. Dismukes WE. Azole antifungal drugs: old and new. *Ann Intern Med* 1988;109:177–179.
19. Sawaya BP, Briggs JP, Schnermann J. Amphotericin B nephrotoxicity: the adverse consequences of altered membrane properties. *J Am Soc Nephrol* 1995;6:154–164.
20. Rolland WA 3rd, Guharoy R, Ramirez L, et al. Respiratory distress secondary to both amphotericin B deoxycholate and lipid complex formulation. *Vet Hum Toxicol* 2000;42:222–223.
21. Atkinson AJ Jr, Bennett JE. Amphotericin B pharmacokinetics in humans. *Antimicrob Agents Chemother* 1978;13:271–276.
22. Starkie JR, Mason EO Jr, Kramer WG, Kaplan SL. Pharmacokinetics of amphotericin B in infants and children. *J Infect Dis* 1987;155:766–774.
23. Drugs for treatment of deep fungal infections. *Med Lett Drugs Ther* 1988;30:30–32.
24. Drugs for treatment of fungal infections. *Med Lett Drugs Ther* 1990;32:58–60.
25. Koren G, Lau A, Klein J, et al. Pharmacokinetics and adverse effects of amphotericin B in infants and children. *J Pediatr* 1988;113:559–563.
26. Baley JE, Meyers C, Kliegman RM, et al. Pharmacokinetics, outcome of treatment and toxic effects of amphotericin B and 5-fluorocytosine in neonates. *J Pediatr* 1990;116:791–797.
27. Antoniskis D, Larsen RA. Acute rapidly progressive renal failure with simultaneous use of amphotericin B and pentamidine. *Antimicrob Agents Chemother* 1990;34:470–472.
28. Drutz DJ, Fan JH, Tai TY, et al. Hypokalemic rhabdomyolysis and myoglobinuria following amphotericin B therapy. *JAMA* 1970;211:824–826.
29. *Physicians' desk reference*, 49th ed. Oradell, NJ: Medical Economics, 1995:523–525.
30. Dele Davies H, King SM, Doyle J, et al. Controlled pilot study of rapid amphotericin B infusions. *Arch Dis Child* 1997;76:165–166.
31. Katz PZ, Cohn RA. Amphotericin B and hypertension. *Pediatr Infect Dis J* 1994;13:839–840.
32. Maddux MS, Barrier SL. A review of complications of amphotericin B therapy: recommendations for prevention and management. *Drug Intell Clin Pharm* 1980;14:177–181.
33. Walker RW, Rosenblum MK. Amphotericin B (AMB)-related leukoencephalopathy. *Neurology* 1991;41[Suppl 1]:199.
34. MacGregor RR, Bennett JE, Erslev AJ. Erythropoietin concentration in amphotericin B-induced anemia. *Antimicrob Agents Chemother* 1978;14:270–273.
35. Hoitsma AJ, Wetzels JFM, Koene RAP. Drug induced nephrotoxicity: aetiology, clinical features and management. *Drug Saf* 1991;6:131–147.
36. Sabra R, Branch RA. Amphotericin B nephrotoxicity. *Drug Saf* 1990;5:94–108.
37. Sacks P, Feliner SK. Recurrent reversible acute renal failure from amphotericin. *Arch Intern Med* 1987;147:593–595.
38. DeMonaco HJ, McGovern B. Transient asystole associated with amphotericin B infusion. *Drug Intell Clin Pharm* 1983;17:547–548.
39. Dukes CS, Perfect JR. Amphotericin B-induced malignant hypertensive episodes. *J Infect Dis* 1990;161:588.
40. Craven PC, Gemillion DH. Risk factors of ventricular fibrillation during rapid amphotericin B infusion. *Antimicrob Agents Chemother* 1985;27:868–871.
41. Googe JH, Walterspiel JN. Arrhythmia caused by amphotericin B in a neonate. *Pediatr Infect Dis* 1988;7:73.
42. Ellio ME, Tharpe W. Red man syndrome associated with amphotericin B. *BMJ* 1990;300:1468.
43. Cesaro S, Calore E, Messina C, et al. Allergic reaction to the liposomal component of liposomal amphotericin B. *Support Care Cancer* 1999;7:284–286.
44. Roncoroni AJ, Corrado C, Besuschio S, et al. Bronchiolitis obliterans possibly associated with amphotericin B. *J Infect Dis* 1990;161:589.
45. Bindschadler DD, Bennett JE. A pharmacologic guide to the clinical use of amphotericin B. *J Infect Dis* 1969;120:427–436.
46. Mayhew JW, Fiore C, Murray T, et al. An internally standardized assay for amphotericin B in tissues and plasma. *J Chromatogr* 1983;274:271–279.
47. Inselmann G, Inselmann U, Heidemann HT. Amphotericin B and liver function. *Eur J Intern Med* 2002;13:288–292.
48. Block ER, Bennett JE, Livoti LG, et al. Flucytosine and amphotericin B: hemodialysis effects on the plasma concentration and clearance. *Ann Intern Med* 1974;80:613–617.
49. Burnett RJ, Reents SB. Premedication for amphotericin B-induced chills. *Clin Pharm* 1989;8:836–837.
50. Oldfield EC III, Burnett RJ, Reents SB. Meperidine for prevention of amphotericin B-induced chills. *Clin Pharm* 1990;9:251–252.
51. Fincannon J. Meperidine addiction associated with amphotericin treatment in leukemia: case study and staff reaction. *Arch Psychiatr Nurs* 1988;2:302–306.
52. DaCamara CC, Lane TW. Dantrolene for amphotericin B-induced rigors. *Arch Intern Med* 1987;147:2220.
53. Smith SR, Galloway MJ, Reilly JT, et al. Amiloride prevents amphotericin B related hypokalemia in neutropenic patients. *J Clin Pathol* 1988;41:494–497.
54. Branch RA. Prevention of amphotericin B-induced renal impairment: a review on the use of sodium supplementation. *Arch Intern Med* 1988;148:2389–2394.
55. Stein RS, Alexander JA. Sodium protects against nephrotoxicity in patients receiving amphotericin B. *Am J Med Sci* 1989;298:299–304.
56. Harder EJ, Hermans PE. Treatment of fungal infections with flucytosine. *Arch Intern Med* 1975;135:231–237.
57. Harper KJ, Sawyer WT. Malabsorption of flucytosine in a pediatric patient with Shwachman syndrome. *DICP Ann Pharmacother* 1989;23:782–783.
58. McEvoy GK, ed. *AHFS drug information 94.* Bethesda, MD: American Society of Hospital Pharmacists, 1994:74–81, 2104–2106.

59. Kauffman C, Frame PT. Bone marrow toxicity associated with 5-fluorocytosine therapy. *Antimicrob Agents Chemother* 1977;11:244–247.
60. Kotani S, Hirose S, Niiya K, et al. Anaphylaxis to flucytosine in a patient with AIDS. *JAMA* 1988;260:3275–3276.
61. Kaspar RL, Drutz DJ. Rapid simple bioassay for 5-fluorocytosine in the presence of amphotericin B. *Antimicrob Agents Chemother* 1975;7:462–465.
62. Harding SA, Johnson GF, Solomon HM. Gas chromatographic determination of 5-fluorocytosine in human serum. *Clin Chem* 1976;22:772–776.
63. Williams KM, Chinwah M, Cobcroft R. Crystalluria during flucytosine therapy. *Med J Aust* 1979;2:617.
64. Eisen D. The therapy of oral lichen planus. *Crit Rev Oral Biol Med* 1993;4:141–158.
65. Castelli M, Zanca A, Giubertoni G, et al. Griseofulvin-methisoprinol combination in the treatment of herpes zoster. *Pharmacol Res Commun* 1986;18:991–996.
66. McEvoy GK, ed. *AHFS drug information 91.* Bethesda, MD: American Society of Hospital Pharmacists, 1991:80–82.
67. Becker LE. Griseofulvin. *Dermatol Clin* 1984;2:115–120.
68. Anderson DW. Griseofulvin: biology and clinical usefulness. *Ann Allergy* 1965;23:103–110.
69. Liu CC, Magat J, Chang R, et al. Absorption, metabolism and excretion of ^{14}C-griseofulvin in man. *J Pharmacol Exp Ther* 1973;187:415–422.
70. Metneki J, Czeizel A. Griseofulvin teratology. *Lancet* 1987;1:1042.
71. Mion G, Verdon R, Le Gulluche Y, et al. Fatal toxic epidermal necrolysis after griseofulvin. *Lancet* 1989;2:1331.
72. Ormerod AD, White MI. Cold urticaria triggered by griseofulvin. *BMJ* 1987;295:612.
73. Haskell LP, Mennemyer RP, Greenman R, Pelezar C. Isolated erythroid hypoplasia and renal insufficiency induced by long-term griseofulvin therapy. *South Med J* 1990;83:1327–1330.
74. Antifungal: fluconazole. In: McEvoy GK, ed. *AHFS drug information 94.* Bethesda, MD: American Society of Hospital Pharmacists, 1994:74–81.
75. Yang DJ, Rankin GO. Nephrotoxicity of antifungal agents. *Adverse Drug React Acute Poisoning Rev* 1985;1:37–49.
76. Farschian M, Yaghoobi R, Samadi K. Fluconazole versus ketoconazole in the treatment of tinea versicolor. *J Dermatol Treat* 2002;13:73–76.
77. Ally R, Schurmann D, Kreisel W, et al. A randomized, double-blind, double-dummy, multicenter trial of voriconazole and fluconazole in the treatment of esophageal candidiasis in immunocompromised patients. *Clin Infect Dis* 2001;33:1447–1454.
78. Yao Z, Liao W, Wen H. Antifungal therapy for treatment of cryptococcal meningitis. *Chin Med J (Engl)* 2000;113:178–180.
79. Fluconazole. *Med Lett Drugs Ther* 1990;32:50–52.
80. Franklin IM, Elias E, Hirsch C. Fluconazole-induced jaundice. *Lancet* 1990;336:565.
81. Fluconazole (systemic). USP DI update, 1990:466–469.
82. Richardson K, Cooper K, Marriott MS, et al. Discovery of fluconazole, a novel antifungal agent. *Rev Infect Dis* 1990;12[Suppl 3]:S267–S271.
83. Force RW. Fluconazole concentrations in breast milk. *Pediatr Infect Dis* 1995;14:235–236.
84. Pasko M, Piscitelli SC, Van Slooton AD. Fluconazole: a new triazole antifungal agent. *DICP Ann Pharmacother* 1990;24:860–867.
85. Heikkila H, Timonen K, Stubb S. Fixed drug eruption due to fluconazole. *J Am Acad Dermatol* 2000;42:883–884.
86. Lazar JD, Wilner XD. Drug interactions with fluconazole. *Rev Infect Dis* 1990;12[Suppl 3]:S327–S333.
87. Pappas PG, Kauffman CA, Perfect J, et al. Alopecia associated with fluconazole therapy. *Ann Intern Med* 1995;123:354–357.
88. German GE. FDA approves the drug fluconazole (alternate treatment for AIDS). *FDA information bulletin.* Washington, DC: U.S. Food and Drug Administration, 1990.
89. Kidd D, Ranaghan EA, Morris TCM. Hypokalaemia in patients with acute myeloid leukaemia after treatment with fluconazole. *Lancet* 1989;1:1017.
90. Toon S, Ross CE, Gokal R, Rowland M. An assessment of the effects of impaired renal function and haemodialysis on the pharmacokinetics of fluconazole. *Br J Clin Pharmacol* 1990;29:221–226.
91. Lake-Bahaar G, Scheuer PJ, Sherlock S. Hepatic reactions associated with ketoconazole in the United Kingdom. *BMJ* 1987;294:419–422.
92. Tabor E. Hepatotoxicity of ketoconazole in men and in patients under 50. *N Engl J Med* 1987;316:1606–1607.
93. Gradnor JD, Sepkowitz DV. Massive hepatic enlargement with fatty change associated with ketoconazole. *DICP Ann Pharmacother* 1990;24:1175–1176.
94. Lyle JH. Ketoconazole. Mechanism of action, spectrum of activity, pharmacokinetics, drug interactions, adverse reactions and therapeutic use. *Pharmacotherapy* 1984;4:343–373.
95. Jacobs PH, Nael N. The action and safety of ketoconazole: a brief literature review. *Cutis* 1988;42:276–282.
96. Daneshmend TK. Diseases and drugs but not food decrease ketoconazole "bioavailability." *Br J Clin Pharmacol* 1990;29:783–784.
97. Wali JP, Aggarwal P, Gupta V, et al. Ketoconazole in treatment of visceral leishmaniasis. *Lancet* 1990;2:810–811.
98. Glynn AM, Slaughter RL, Brass C, et al. Effects of ketoconazole on methylprednisolone pharmacokinetics and cortisol secretions. *Clin Pharmacol Ther* 1986;39:654–659.
99. Van Lyle JH. Ketoconazole. Mechanism of action, spectrum of activity, pharmacokinetics, drug interactions, adverse reactions and therapeutic use. *Pharmacotherapy* 1984;4:343–373.
100. McNulty AM, Lazor JA, Sketch M. Transient increase in plasma quinidine concentrations during ketoconazole-quinidine therapy. *Clin Pharm* 1989;8:222–225.
101. Varhe A, Olkkola T, Neuvonen PJ. Oral triazolam is potentially hazardous to patients receiving systemic antimycotics: ketoconazole as itraconazole. *Clin Pharmacol Ther* 1994;56:601–607.
102. Sonino N. The use of ketoconazole as an inhibitor of steroid production. *N Engl J Med* 1987;317:812–818.
103. McEvoy GK, ed. *AHFS drug information 94.* Bethesda, MD: American Society of Hospital Pharmacists, 1994:87–91, 2282–2284.
104. McCance DR, Ritchie CM, Sheridan B, Atkinson AB. Acute hypoadrenalism and hepatotoxicity after treatment with ketoconazole. *Lancet* 1987;1:573.
105. Khosla S, Wolfson JS, Demerjian Z, Godine JE. Adrenal crises in the setting of high-dose ketoconazole therapy. *Arch Intern Med* 1989;149:802–804.
106. Umstead GS, Babiak LM, Tejwani S. Immune hemolytic anemia associated with ketoconazole therapy. *Clin Pharm* 1987;6:499–500.
107. Lobo BL, Miwa U, Jungnickel PW. Possible ketoconazole-induced hypoglycemia. *Drug Intell Clin Pharm* 1988;22:632.
108. O'Rourke ME. Ketoconazole in the treatment of prostate cancer. *Clin J Oncol Nurs* 2003;7:235–236.
109. Jorgensen JH, Alexander GA, Graybill JR, Drutz DJ. Sensitive bioassay for ketoconazole in serum and cerebrospinal fluid. *Antimicrob Agents Chemother* 1981;20:59–63.
110. Aabo K, De Coster A. Hypertension during high-dose ketoconazole treatment: a probably mineralocorticosteroid effect. *Lancet* 1987;2:637–638.
111. Fisch AZ, Lahad A. Adverse psychiatric reaction to ketoconazole. *Am J Psychiatry* 1989;146:939–940.
112. Bernuau J, Durand F, Pessayre D. Ketoconazole-induced hepatotoxicity. *Hepatology* 1997;26:802.
113. Turner CA, Turner A, Warnock DW. High performance liquid chromatographic determination of ketoconazole in human serum. *J Antimicrob Chemother* 1986;18:757–763.
114. Vazquez JA. Therapeutic options for the management of oropharyngeal and esophageal candidiasis in HIV/AIDS patients. *HIV Clin Trials* 2000;1:47–59.
115. Assaly RA, Hammersley JR, Olson DE, et al. Disseminated blastomycosis. *J Am Acad Dermatol* 2003;48:123–127.
116. Libow LF, Coots NV. Treatment of lichen planus and lichen nitidus with itraconazole: reports of six cases. *Cutis* 1998;62:247–248.
117. Blomley M, Teare EL, de Belder A, et al. Itraconazole and anti-tuberculosis drugs. *Lancet* 1990:336:1255.
118. Sachs MK, Paluzzi RG, Morre JH Jr, et al. Amphotericin-resistant aspergillus osteomyelitis controlled by itraconazole. *Lancet* 1990:335:1475.
119. Frontling RA. Overview of medically important antifungal azole derivatives. *Clin Microbiol Rev* 1988;1:187–217.
120. Denning DW, Tucker RM, Hanson LH. Treatment of invasive aspergillosis with itraconazole. *Am J Med* 1989;86[Suppl 2]:791–800.
121. Tucker AM, Hag Y, Denning DO, Stevens DA. Adverse events associated with itraconazole in 189 patients on chronic therapy. *J Antimicrob Chemother* 1990;26:561–566.
122. Smith AG. Potentiation of anticoagulants by ketoconazole. *BMJ* 1984;288:188–189.
123. McEvoy GK, ed. *AHFS drug information 94.* Bethesda, MD: American Society of Hospital Pharmacists, 1994:91–94, 2284–2286.
124. Fainstein V, Bodey GP. Cardiorespiratory toxicity due to miconazole. *Ann Intern Med* 1980;93:432–433.
125. Jordan WM, Bodey GP, Rodriguez V, et al. Miconazole therapy for treatment of fungal infections in cancer patients. *Antimicrob Agents Chemother* 1979;16:792–797.
126. Letscher-Bru V, Herbrecht R. Caspofungin: the first representative of a new antifungal class. *J Antimicrob Chemother* 2003;51:513–521.
127. Chandrasekar PH, Manavathu EK. Caspofungin. *Drugs Today (Barc)* 2002;38:829–846.
128. Ghannoum MA, Kuhn DM. Voriconazole—better chances for patients with invasive mycoses. *Eur J Med Res* 2002;7:242–256.
129. Chamuleau ME, Deenik W, Zweegman S, et al. Successful treatment of subcutaneously disseminated aspergillosis with caspofungin acetate in an allogeneic peripheral blood stem cell transplantation patient. *Haematologica* 2003;88:ECR10.
130. Vazquez J. Invasive oesophageal candidiasis: current and developing treatment options. *Drugs* 2003;63:971–989.
131. Garbino J, Lew D, Hirschel B, et al. Caspofungin in the treatment of oropharyngeal candidiasis. *Int J Clin Pract* 2003;57:143–144.
132. Index of monographs. Available at: http://home.earthlink.net/~newdrugpb/Monographs/. Accessed 05/06/2003.
133. Cornely OA, Schmitz K, Aisenbrey S. The first echinocandin: caspofungin. *Mycoses* 2002;45[Suppl 3]:56–60.
134. Caspofungin: new preparation. A last resort in invasive aspergillosis. *Prescrire Int* 2002;11:142–143.
135. Darkes MJ, Scott LJ, Goa KL. Terbinafine: a review of its use in onychomycosis in adults. *Am J Clin Dermatol* 2003;4:39–65.
136. Schiraldi GF, Gramegna G, De Rosa C, et al. Chronic pulmonary aspergillosis: current classification and therapy. *Curr Opin Investig Drugs* 2003;4:186–191.
137. Schmutz JL, Barbaud A, Trechot P. Overdose of nortriptyline during treatment with terbinafine (1st reported case). *Ann Dermatol Venereol* 1999;126:647.

CHAPTER 90

Antiparasitics

Steven A. Seifert

$$O_2N\text{-}[\text{imidazole}]\text{-}N\text{-}CH_2CH_2OH,\ CH_3$$

ANTIPARASITIC METRONIDAZOLE

Compounds included:	**Albendazole (Albenza); mebendazole (Vermox); thiabendazole (Mintezol, Eprofil); paromomycin (Humatin); piperazine (Antepar); praziquantel; pyrantel (Antiminth, Ascarel); halogenated hydroxyquinolines: chlorquinaldol (Temetex), clioquinol (Vioform), iodoquinol (Yodoxin)**
Molecular formula and weight:	**See text.**
SI conversion:	**Albendazole, mg/L × 3.8 = µmol/L; mebendazole, mg/L × 3.4 = µmol/L; praziquantel, mg/L × 3.2 = µmol/L; pyrantel, mg/L × 1.7 = µmol/L; piperazine, mg/dl × 1.2 = µmol/L; paromomycin, mg/L × 1.6 = µmol/L; halogenated hydroxyquinolines: chlorquinaldol, mg/L × 4.4 = µmol/L; clioquinol, mg/L × 3.3 = µmol/L; iodoquinol, mg/L × 2.5 = µmol/L**
CAS Registry No.:	**See text.**
Therapeutic levels:	**Not applicable**
Target organs:	**Bone marrow (chronic), central nervous system (chronic), liver (acute or chronic), skin (chronic), many drug interactions**
Antidote:	**None**

OVERVIEW

In 1946, it was estimated that there were 2.3 billion helmintic infections in a human population of 2.2 billion. Since that time, the world's population has doubled, as has the number of helmintic infections (1). It is estimated that helminths infect 25% of the world's population (2).

Toxic effects are most likely to be nonspecific gastrointestinal (GI) upset for oral agents, although liver injury is seen with higher doses and longer treatment regimens. In the treatment of some conditions (e.g., *Cysticercoses*), inflammatory reactions induced by the necrosis of the primary lesions may result in significant toxicity. Toxic effects of topical agents are typically irritation and sensitivity reactions. There are no specific antidotes to any of the antiparasitics. Treatment is primarily symptomatic and supportive.

An overview of the parasitic agents is provided in Table 1. The toxic dose, toxicokinetics, toxic effects, and clinical presentation are provided in Tables 2, 3, and 4.

ALBENDAZOLE

Albendazole [$C_{12}H_{15}N_3O_2S$; molecular weight (MW), 265.3 g/mol; CAS Registry No., 54965-21-8], mebendazole, and thiabendazole are benzimidazole carbamate derivatives and offer the broadest spectrum of action of the anthelmintics. They disrupt tubulin polymerization in a variety of parasites and are effective against trichuris, hookworm, *Strongyloides*, and ascaris (3,4). Adverse effects of high-dose albendazole include blood abnormalities (5) and elevated liver transaminases (6,7).

Toxic Dose

The dose depends on the condition under treatment. The *therapeutic dosage* for adults and children older than 2 years of age ranges from 200 mg twice daily to 400 mg twice daily (3,7,8). For neurocysticercosis, the pediatric dosage is 15 mg/kg for 8 to 30 days, which may be repeated if necessary (7,9).

There is very little experience with overdose of these agents. No toxic dose has been established, and no fatalities have been reported. An oral overdose of at least 16 g taken over 12 hours has been tolerated without symptoms (7).

Toxicokinetics and Toxicodynamics

Albendazole has low bioavailability (less than 5%) (10,11), but its active metabolite, albendazole sulfoxide, reaches therapeutic concentrations in plasma (12). Bioavailability increases four- to five-

TABLE 1. Summary of antimicrobial agents used for treating parasitic infections and their main side effects

Agent	Indications	Contraindications	Primary side effects
Albendazole	Hydatid cyst, intestinal nematodes	Not approved by FDA	Minimal
Allopurinol	Leishmaniasis	Not approved by FDA	Hypersensitivity reactions
Amodiaquine	Malaria	Not available in the United States	Similar to chloroquine
Amphotericin B	Amebic meningoencephalitis, leishmaniasis	Not approved by FDA	Immediate febrile reactions, nephrotoxicity
Azithromycin	Cryptosporidiosis, toxoplasmosis	Not approved by FDA	Unknown
Benzimidazole	American trypanosomiasis	Not approved by FDA	GI upset, dermatitis, neuritis, myelosuppression
Bithionol	*Fasciola hepatica*	Not approved by FDA	Minimal
Chloroquine	Malaria	—	GI upset, pruritus, dermatitis, myelosuppression, hemolysis
Clindamycin	Malaria, babesiosis, toxoplasmosis	Not approved by FDA	Antibiotic-associated diarrhea
Dapsone	*Pneumocystis carinii* pneumonia	Not approved by FDA	GI upset, rash, hemolysis in G6PD deficiency methemoglobinemia
Diethylcarbamazine	Filariasis (not onchocerciasis)	—	Mazzotti reaction (hypersensitivity to dying microfilariae)
Diloxanide furoate	Amebiasis (asymptomatic)	Pregnancy; available from CDC	GI upset, flatulence
Doxycycline	Malaria (prophylaxis)	Pregnancy, children <8 yr of age	GI upset, rash from photosensitivity
Eflornithine (α-difluoromethylornithine)	West African CNS trypanosomiasis	—	Anemia, leukopenia
Emetine	Amebic liver abscess	Pregnancy, children <5 yr of age	GI upset, cardiac toxicity (ECG monitoring needed)
Iodoquinol	Amebiasis (asymptomatic), balantidiasis, *Dientamoeba*	Sensitivity to iodine	GI upset, acne, rash
Ivermectin	Onchocerciasis	Pregnancy, children <5 yr of age	Mazzotti reaction (less than diethylcarbamazine)
Ketoconazole	Leishmaniasis	—	Hepatitis
Mebendazole	Ascariasis, trichuriasis, hookworms, pinworms	Pregnancy	Minimal at usual dose; primarily GI upset
Mefloquine	Malaria	Pregnancy, children <5 yr of age, beta-blocker drugs	GI upset, seizures, acute brain syndrome
Meglumine antimonate	Leishmaniasis	Not approved by FDA	GI upset, rash, pruritus, nephrotoxicity
Melarsoprol (arsenical)	African trypanosomiasis (CNS stage)	—	Encephalopathy, local skin irritation
Metronidazole	Amebiasis, giardiasis	Not approved by FDA for giardiasis	GI upset, disulfiram-like effect
Niclosamide	Tapeworms, especially *Diphyllobothrium latum* and *Taenia solium*	—	GI upset, pruritus
Nifurtimox	American trypanosomiasis	Not approved by FDA; available from CDC	GI upset, polyneuritis, seizures, psychological disturbances
Pentamidine	*P. carinii* pneumonia, leishmaniasis	—	Abscesses at site of IM injection; with IV therapy, fever, hypotension, hypoglycemia, hypocalcemia, nephrotoxicity
Piperazine	Ascariasis	Seizure disorder	Hypersensitivity, neurotoxicity
Praziquantel	Most flukes, tapeworms, and cases of cysticercosis	Ocular cysticercosis	GI upset, dizziness, hypersensitivity to dying cysticerci
Primaquine	Malaria	Pregnancy	Hemolysis in G6PD deficiency, GI upset
Propamidine	*Acanthamoeba* keratitis (topical application)	—	—
Pyrantel pamoate	Alternative for ascariasis, hookworms, pinworms	Pregnancy	GI upset
Pyrimethamine	Malaria, toxoplasmosis (use with clindamycin or sulfadiazine)	—	Mild; sulfa toxicity when combined with sulfadoxine (as Fansidar)
Quinacrine	Giardiasis	Pregnancy, psoriasis	GI upset, yellow staining of skin, psychological disturbances
Quinidine, quinine	Malaria, babesiosis	—	Cinchonism, urticaria, GI upset; with IV therapy, hypotension, heart block
Spiramycin	Cryptosporidiosis, toxoplasmosis	Available from FDA	—
Stibogluconate sodium (antimonial)	Leishmaniasis	Not approved by FDA; available from CDC	GI upset, nephrotoxicity, ECG changes
Sulfonamides: sulfadiazine, sulfadoxine, sulfamethoxazole	Malaria, toxoplasmosis, *P. carinii* pneumonia (treatment and prophylaxis when combined with pyrimethamine or trimethoprim)	Pregnancy, newborns	Allergic reactions, including fever and severe dermatitis, serum sickness, crystalluria, neurotoxicity, and hepatotoxicity
Suramin	African trypanosomiasis (early hemolymphatic stage)	—	GI upset, pruritus, nephrotoxicity (albuminuria), photophobia, paresthesias
Tetracycline	Malaria, balantidiasis	Pregnancy, children <8 yr of age	GI upset, rash from photosensitivity
Thiabendazole	Strongyloidiasis, trichinosis, toxocariasis, trichostrongyliasis, cutaneous larva migrans	Pregnancy	GI upset, rash, pruritus, headache, hypoglycemia, hypotension
Trimethoprim	*P. carinii* pneumonia (treatment and prophylaxis when combined with sulfamethoxazole)	—	See side effects of sulfonamides
Trimetrexate	*P. carinii* pneumonia	Not approved by FDA	Antifolate; must be given with leucovorin to prevent hematotoxicity
Tryparsamide (arsenical)	West African CNS trypanosomiasis (when combined with suramin)	—	Encephalopathy, local skin irritation

CDC, Centers for Disease Control and Prevention; CNS, central nervous system; ECG, electrocardiographic; FDA, U.S. Food and Drug Administration; GI, gastrointestinal; G6PD, glucose 6 phosphate dehydrogenase.
From Rosenblatt JE. Antiparasitic agents. *Mayo Clin Proc* 1992;67:276–287, with permission.

TABLE 2. Therapeutic, toxic, and fatal doses of antiparasitic drugs

Drug	Therapeutic	Toxic	Fatal	Survival
Amodiaquine	200–400 mg[a]	—	—	—
Chloroquine	mg base/kg/24 h (in children)	—	0.75–1.0 g (children), 2–3 g (adults),[b,c] death in 2–3 h	4 g (child)[d]
Halofantrine	8 mg/kg (children)	—	—	—
Hydroxychloroquine	500–800 mg/wk	—	10–12 g[e,f]	—
Ivermectin	0.05–0.20 mg/kg[g]	—	—	—
Mefloquine	1250 ng[h]	900–1000 ng[i]	—	—
Proguanil	100–200 ng/d	Up to 1400 mg[j] (survived)	900 mg and 5 g,[k] 900 mg (children), 1.8–8.0 g (adults)	—

[a]From Reynolds JEF, ed. *Martindale: the extra pharmacopoeia*, 30th ed. London: Pharmaceutical Press, 1993:395–396, with permission.
[b]From Torrey EF. Chloroquine seizures: report of four cases. *JAMA* 1968;204:867–870, with permission.
[c]From Riou B, Barriot P, Rimailho A, Baud FJ. Treatment of severe chloroquine poisoning. *N Engl J Med* 1988;318:1–6, with permission.
[d]From Havena PL, Splaingard ML, Borisonis D, Hofman GM. Survival after chloroquine ingestion in a child. *J Toxicol Clin Toxicol* 1988;26:381–388, with permission.
[e]From Kemmenoe AJ. An infant fatality due to hydroxychloroquine poisoning. *J Anal Toxicol* 1990;14:186–188, with permission.
[f]From Overdose of hydroxychloroquine. *Pharm J* 1963:504, with permission.
[g]From Ette EI, Thomas WOA, Achumba JJ. Ivermectin: a long acting microfilaricidal agent. *DICP Ann Pharmacother* 1990;24:426–433, with permission.
[h]From Lariam. Product literature. Basel, Switzerland: Roche Laboratories, 1990, with permission.
[i]From Patchen LC, Campbell CC, Williams SB. Neurologic reactions after a therapeutic dose of mefloquine. *N Engl J Med* 1989;321:1415–1416, with permission.
[j]From Webster LT Jr. Drugs used in the chemotherapy of protozoal infections. In: Gilman AG, Rall TW, Nies AS, Taylor P, eds. *Goodman and Gilman's the pharmacologic basis of therapeutics*, 8th ed. New York: Pergamon Press, 1991:684–795, with permission.
[k]From Maegrath BG, Tottey MM, Adams ARD, et al. The absorption and excretion of paludrine in the human subject. *Ann Trop Med Parasitol* 1946;40:493–501, with permission.

fold when albendazole is administered with a fatty meal (13). One 400-mg dose of albendazole in healthy adults resulted in a mean maximal drug concentration (C_{max}) of the sulfoxide metabolite of 0.33 μg/ml (range, 0.04 to 1.24 μg/ml) an average of 2.3 hours after administration (12). Albendazole sulfoxide has total protein binding of 75% (12), less than 1% of the total dose cleared in the urine (14). The half-life of the sulfoxide is 8 to 12 hours (5,7,14).

Pathophysiology

Albendazole disrupts the assembly of microtubules and interferes with mitosis. At high doses, albendazole also interferes with microsomal metabolism (15).

Pregnancy and Lactation

Albendazole is U.S. Food and Drug Administration (FDA) pregnancy category C. There is some evidence of fetal toxicity (16). Albendazole sulfoxide inhibits cell proliferation and differentiation in embryonic midbrain and limb bud cultures (17). Albendazole is absorbed to a greater extent than mebendazole; therefore, fetal injury with albendazole may be expected to be higher (18). The excretion of albendazole into breast milk is unknown.

Clinical Presentation

In humans, albendazole produces GI upset at low doses and commonly results in reversible, elevated liver transaminases at higher doses (6). Albendazole had minimal side effects during chronic administration to 1344 children at 400 mg as a single dose (3). Blood abnormalities have been reported in between 1% and 5% of patients: Eosinophilia, pancytopenia, neutropenia, granulocytopenia, agranulocytosis, thrombocytopenia, and amegakaryocytic thrombocytopenic purpura have been described (5,19–21).

Other conditions associated with albendazole include urticarial rashes, headache and increased intracranial pressure, dizziness, headache and vertigo, fever, abdominal pain, and nausea and vomiting as well as jaundice (5%), acute renal failure, and optic neuritis. The incidence of allergic reactions is less than 1% (5,7,22,23).

In the treatment of cysticercosis with albendazole, the manufacturer recommends concomitant treatment with corticosteroids to minimize cerebral hypertension and also recommends consideration of anticonvulsants (7). Steady-state trough concentrations of albendazole sulfoxide are significantly increased (56%) with concomitant dexamethasone administration and may increase adverse effects (7). Concomitant administration of albendazole and praziquantel increases (50%) the mean maximum plasma concentration and area under the plasma concentration–time curve (AUC) of albendazole sulfoxide (24).

Diagnostic Tests

The correlation between blood concentrations and therapeutic effect is not known. Routine qualitative or quantitative blood tests for antiparasitic agents are not required. With albendazole treatment, monitoring of the complete blood cell count (CBC) and liver function tests should be performed at the beginning of treatment and every 2 weeks during therapy (7). The CBC and liver function tests should be monitored in symptomatic patients.

Treatment

Treatment of albendazole toxicity is symptomatic and supportive. Mebendazole (and presumably albendazole) is not significantly removed by hemodialysis (25). There is no specific antidote.

MEBENDAZOLE

Aside from its use as an antiparasitic, mebendazole ($C_{16}H_{13}N_3O_3$; MW, 295.3 g/mol; CAS Registry No., 31431-39-7) is being investigated for the treatment of fibrotic diseases such as pulmonary fibrosis, liver cirrhosis, systemic scleroderma, and others (26). Mebendazole may cause liver transaminase elevations and hepatocellular injury (27–31).

Toxic Dose

The *adult and pediatric dosages* range by indication from a single dose of 100 to 500 mg orally to 100 mg three times a day (32,33). Infants have received a dose of 100 mg twice daily for 3 days (34). Mebendazole dosage should be reduced in patients with hepatic impairment (14).

Overdose experience is limited. No fatalities have been reported. Doses 32 to 62 times the usual therapeutic dose have been well tolerated (35).

TABLE 3. Pharmacokinetics of the major antiparasitic drugs

Parameter	Amodiaquine	Chloro-quine	Halofan-trine	Hydroxy-chloroquine	Iver-mectin	Meflo-quine	Proguanil	Pyrimeth-amine	Quinine
Bioavailability (%)	High	90	—	>90	90	70–80	>90	High	90
Time-to-peak plasma level (h)	0.6–1.3, 3–5 (metabolite)	1.5–3.0	18.0	17	4	7–24	3	2	1–3
Volume of distribution (L/kg)	—	92	100	—	0.5	13–41	—	2.8	1.2–1.7
Protein binding (%)	90	—	—	50	2	98	75	80	70
Elimination half-life	5–8 h, 3–6 h (metabolite)	3–300 h	1–2 d	3 h (30 h after overdose)	—	13–40 d	16–20 h	4–6 d	20 h
Excreted unchanged (%)	—	10–20	—	—	28	—	60	20	<25

From Ette EI, Thomas WOA, Achumba JJ. Ivermerctin: a long acting microfilaricidal agent. *DICP Ann Pharmacother* 1990;24:426–433; Winstanley PA, Edwards G, Orme ML'E, Breckenridge AM. Effect of dose size on amodiaquine pharmacokinetics after oral administration. *Eur J Clin Pharmacol* 1987;33:331–333; Karbwang J, Ward SA, Milton KA, et al. Pharmacokinetics of halofantrine in healthy Thai volunteers. *Br J Clin Pharmacol* 1991;32:639–640; Broom C. The human pharmacokinetics of halofantrine hydrochloride. In: Warhurst DC, Schofield CJ, eds. *Halofantrine in the treatment of multidrug resistant malaria.* Cambridge, UK: Elsevier, 1989:15–20; Bryson HM, Goa KL. Halofantrine: a review of its antimalarial activity, pharmacokinetic properties and therapeutic potential. *Drugs* 1992;43:236–258; Miller DR, Fiechtner JJ, Carpenter JR, et al. Plasma hydroxychloroquine concentrations and efficacy in rheumatoid arthritis. *Arthritis Rheum* 1987;30:567–571; Villalobos D. Plaquenil (hydroxychloroquine) plasmapheresis (PPR) in an overdose. *Vet Hum Toxicol* 1991;33:364; Hall AH, Spoerke DG, Bronsten AC, et al. Human ivermectin exposure. *J Emerg Med* 1985;3:217–219; *Mectizan (ivermectin MSD).* Rahway, NJ: Merck, 1988:35–85; *Ivermectin poison control monograph.* West Point, PA: Merck Sharp & Dohme, Division of Merck, 1985:1–18; Azia MA, Diallo S, Diop IM, et al. Efficacy and tolerance of ivermectin in human onchocerciasis. *Lancet* 1982;2:171–173; Azia MA, Diallo S, Lariviere M, et al. Ivermectin in onchocerciasis. *Lancet* 1982;2:1456–1457; Campbell WC, ed. *Ivermectin and abamectins.* New York: Springer-Verlag, 1989; Edwards G. Pharmacokinetics of antifilarial drugs. *Trop Med Parasitol* 1987;38:64–65; Edwards G, Breckinridge AM. Clinical pharmacokinetics of anthelmintic drugs. *Clin Pharmacokinet* 1988;15:67–93; Edwards G, Dingsdale A, Helsley N, et al. The relative systemic availability of ivermectin after administration as capsule, tablets and oral solution. *Eur J Clin Pharmacol* 1988;35:681–684; Karbwang J, White NJ. Clinical pharmacokinetics of mefloquine. *Clin Pharmacokinet* 1990;19:264–279; Nosten F, Karbwang J, White NJ, et al. Mefloquine antimalarial prophylaxis in pregnancy: dose finding and pharmacokinetic study. *Br J Clin Pharmacol* 1990;30:79–85; Helsby NA, Ward SA, Edwards G, et al. The pharmacokinetics and activations of proguanil in man: consequences of variability in drug metabolism. *Br J Clin Pharmacol* 1990;30:593–598; Maegrath BG, Tottey MM, Adams ARD, et al. The absorption and excretion of paludrine in the human subject. *Ann Trop Med Parasitol* 1946;40:493–501; Wattanagoon Y, Taylor RB, Moody RR, et al. Single dose pharmacokinetics of proguanil and its metabolites in healthy subjects. *Br J Clin Pharmacol* 1987;24:775–780; Taylor RB, Moody RR, Ochekpe NA. Determination of proguanil and its metabolites cycloguanil and 4-chlorphenyl-biguanide in plasma, whole blood and urine by HPLC. *J Chromatog* 1987;416:394–399; Smith CC, Hirig J. Persistent excretion of pyrimethamine following oral administration. *Am J Trop Med Hyg* 1959;8:60–62; Bennett WM, Singer I, Golper T, et al. Guidelines for drug therapy in renal failure. *Ann Intern Med* 1977;86:754–783; Maher JF. Pharmacological aspects of renal failure and dialysis. In: Drukker W, Parsons FM, Maher JF, eds. *Replacement of renal function by dialysis.* Boston: Martinus Nijhoff, 1983:770; La Greca G, Biasioli S, Borin D, et al. Drugs and dialysis. *Int J Artif Organs* 1983;6:135–156; White NJ. Clinical pharmacokinetics of antimalarial drugs. *Clin Pharmacokinet* 1985;10:187–215; Bateman DN, Blain PG, Woodhouse KW, et al. Pharmacokinetics and clinical toxicity of quinine overdosage: lack of efficacy of techniques intended to enhance elimination. *Q J Med N Ser* 1985;54:125–131; Rollo IM. Drugs used in the chemotherapy of malaria. In: Goodman LS, Gilman A, eds. *The pharmacological basis of therapeutics,* 5th ed. New York: MacMillan, 1975:1062–1065; McEvoy GK, ed. *AHFS drug information 86.* Bethesda, MD: American Society of Hospital Pharmacists, 1986:346–349; White NJ, Looareesuwan S, Warrell DA, et al. Quinine pharmacokinetics and toxicity in cerebral and uncomplicated falciparum malaria. *Am J Med* 1982;73:564–572; Brodie BB, Baer JE, Craig LC. Metabolic products of the cinchona alkaloids in human urine. *J Biol Chem* 1951;188:567–581; Bennett WM, Singer I, Golper T, et al. Guidelines for drug therapy in renal failure. *Ann Intern Med* 1977;86:754–783, with permission.

Toxicokinetics and Toxicodynamics

Mebendazole has low bioavailability (14). Different formulations may have variable absorption, with those admixed in oil having increased availability (36). The distribution half-life is 0.2 hours, and the volume of distribution is 1.00 to 2.03 L/kg (14). The time-to-peak plasma concentration (T_{max}) of mebendazole is 2 to 4 hours when given orally (14). Mebendazole is extensively metabolized in the liver (decarboxylated), resulting in several inactive metabolites (14). The elimination half-life of mebendazole is 0.83 to 11.50 hours (14).

Pathophysiology

Mebendazole administration to fibroblast cultures affects protein synthesis and secretion and is reflected in an intracellular accumulation of total proteins and collagen and results in a marked decrease of its deposit in the extracellular matrix (26). The results of these effects in acute or subacute overdosage or in chronic dosing is unknown.

Pregnancy and Lactation

Mebendazole is FDA pregnancy category C. A cross-sectional study in a hookworm endemic area, in which mebendazole was prescribed to 5275 women in the second trimester of pregnancy, showed significantly lower rates of stillbirths, perinatal deaths, and low-birth-weight infants in the mebendazole group compared with controls. Among women who took mebendazole during the first trimester (against advice), an increased incidence of major congenital defects was seen (odds ratio, 1.66; 95% confidence interval, 0.81 to 3.56) (37).

Clinical Presentation

ADVERSE EFFECTS

Mebendazole had minimal side effects during chronic administration to 1344 children at 500 mg as a single dose (3). Children (aged 2 to 16 years) treated with 100 mg of mebendazole twice daily for

TABLE 4. Summary of signs and symptoms of antihelmintic drug overdose

Drug	Age	Toxic dose	Overdose: clinical signs and symptoms
Mebendazole	8 wk	50 mg bid × 3 d	Staring, opisthotonos, respiratory arrest, tachyrhythmias, seizures[a]
Oxamniquine	Adult	6.25 g	Dizziness, convulsions, semicoma, vomiting, diffuse electroencephalograph abnormalities
Pyrantel pamoate	—	>2500 mg	Doses of up to 15,000 mg/d for 10 d taken with no untoward systemic toxicity; diarrhea and nausea may occur with doses >2500 mg
Thiabendazole	Adult	>3 g	May have transient disturbances of vision and psychic alterations; seizures

[a]From Jaeger A, Sauder P, Kopferschmitt J, Flesch F. Clinical features and management of poisoning due to antimalarial drugs. *Med Toxicol* 1987;2:242–273, with permission.

ascaris and *Trichuris* infections developed mild diarrhea as their only adverse reaction (38). Mebendazole, 200 mg three times a day for 5 days, in 50 children (aged 7 to 12 years) produced no reported adverse effects (33). Elevations of liver transaminases occur in 9% to 13% of patients treated with 50 to 100 mg/kg/day (27).

Acute hepatocellular injury has been reported (27–30) after treatment with doses ranging from 600.0 mg/day to 3.5 g/day. Rechallenge has confirmed causality (29,30). Liver biopsy has shown necrosis, inflammatory changes, and eosinophilic infiltration (30). A 53-year-old woman was treated with mebendazole, two times 100 mg/day for 3 days and repeated at 14 days. A febrile illness with elevated liver transaminases (peak alanine aminotransferase, 540 IU/L) began 48 hours after the second treatment course. A liver biopsy revealed granulomas consisting of epithelioid cells, multinucleated giant cells, plasma cells, and lymphocytes (31). A rechallenge was not performed (31).

Other adverse effects reported include leukopenia (35), headache, dizziness, seizures (rarely) (39), and fever [possibly related to necrosis of hydatid cysts (40) or idiosyncratic reactions (41)].

DRUG INTERACTIONS

Drug concentrations of mebendazole are lower with prior or current use of carbamazepine or phenytoin due to increased metabolism, resulting in decreased clinical efficacy of mebendazole (42,43). Increased serum levels may occur in patients concomitantly taking carbamazepine (44). Concurrent cimetidine use may result in increased mebendazole concentrations secondary to decreased metabolism (44).

Diagnostic Tests

The CBC and liver function tests should be monitored in patients receiving prolonged treatment and in symptomatic patients. The relationship of blood levels to toxicity is unknown. Some authors recommend serum levels to substantiate systemic absorption and its effect in symptomatic patients.

Treatment

Treatment is primarily symptomatic and supportive. Mebendazole (and presumably albendazole) is not significantly removed by hemodialysis (25). There is no specific antidote.

THIABENDAZOLE

Thiabendazole ($C_{10}H_7N_3S$; MW, 201.2 g/mol; SI conversion: mg/L × 4.97 = µmol/L; CAS Registry No., 148-79-8) is most commonly used against strongyloidiasis, cutaneous and visceral larva migrans, and trichinosis and as a second-line agent in other parasitic infections.

Toxic Dose

The *therapeutic dosage* is 0.25 g (more than 30 lb body weight) to 1.5 g (more than 150 lb body weight) per day for 1 to 7 days depending on the indication, with a maximum daily dose of 3 g (45).

Overdose experience is limited. There have been no reported fatalities.

Toxicokinetics and Toxicodynamics

The T_{max} of an oral solution of thiabendazole is 1 to 2 hours (45). Thiabendazole is extensively metabolized in the liver to 5-hydroxythiabendazole and excreted in the urine (87% to 90%) as sulfate and glucuronide metabolites (45,46).

Pathophysiology

Cholestasis associated with thiabendazole is believed to be due to a hypersensitivity reaction (47,48).

Pregnancy and Lactation

Thiabendazole is FDA pregnancy category C (45). Excretion in breast milk is unknown.

Clinical Presentation

ADVERSE EFFECTS

Thiabendazole has been associated with reversible leukopenia (45,46). Other reported adverse effects include anorexia, nausea, vomiting and diarrhea, dizziness, headache, rashes (including erythema multiforme and Stevens-Johnson syndrome), cholestatic jaundice, hypersensitivity reactions (including anaphylaxis), and possibly elevated liver transaminases (45,46).

DRUG INTERACTIONS

Thiabendazole can increase the serum levels of theophylline by more than 50% (50,51).

Diagnostic Tests

The CBC and liver function tests should be monitored in patients undergoing prolonged treatment and in symptomatic patients.

Treatment

Treatment is primarily symptomatic and supportive. Other agents in this class are not appreciably removed by dialysis. There is no specific antidote.

PRAZIQUANTEL

Praziquantel ($C_{19}H_{24}N_2O_2$; MW, 312.4 g/mol; CAS Registry No., 55268-74-1) is a trematodicide used to treat schistosome and liver fluke infections.

Toxic Dose

The *therapeutic dosage* of praziquantel ranges from 40 mg/kg/day orally in two divided doses for *Schistosoma haematobium* or *Schistosoma mansoni* to 60 mg/kg/day orally in three divided doses for *Schistosoma japonicum* or *Schistosoma mekongi* to 75 mg/kg/day for 1 day for liver flukes in adults and children older than 4 years of age. Dosage adjustment with liver disease is controversial (14). Hepatic insufficiency should be expected to result in high concentrations of praziquantel, and C_{max} was more than twice as high in patients with moderate liver disease and four times higher in patients with severe liver disease, compared with those with normal liver function. Higher peak plasma concentrations were associated with increased side effects (52). However, other investigators have not found increased concentrations of praziquantel metabolites in patients with liver disease (14). Furthermore, in other studies, the incidence of drug-related adverse effects was not increased in patients with hepatosplenic disease (53). Serum concentrations of praziquantel are increased when the drug is administered with high-carbohydrate food (54).

Overdose experience is limited. There are no reported fatalities.

Toxicokinetics and Toxicodynamics

The bioavailability of praziquantel is 80% (55,56). The bioequivalence of generic manufacturers may not be the same as the original patented preparation (55,57). The T_{max} when administered orally is 1 to 3 hours (54,55,58,59). Protein binding is approximately 80% (14). Cerebrospinal fluid concentrations are 14% to 24% of plasma levels (54,59,60). Metabolism is both by the liver, with the production of inactive metabolites (14,56), and by renal excretion (14,59,61). The elimination half-life of the parent compound is 0.8 to 3.0 hours (52,54,55,59,62) and 4 to 5 hours for the metabolites (59).

Pathophysiology

Treatment of neurocysticercosis may result in a secondary inflammatory reaction and endarteritis caused by destruction of the cysts (63). This may produce cerebral edema, seizures, or infarcts.

Pregnancy and Lactation

Praziquantel is FDA pregnancy category B (55). It is excreted in human breast milk (milk concentration, 25% of plasma) (64). Breastfeeding is not recommended for the 72 hours after a dose (55).

Clinical Presentation

ADVERSE EFFECTS

Adverse effects include fever, dizziness, headache, drowsiness, and malaise (52,65). Headache may occur after even a single low dose of the drug (66). Several cases of a delayed cerebrospinal fluid reaction syndrome have been reported, consisting of nuchal rigidity, papilledema, aphasia, and seizures after treatment for neurocysticercosis (67,68).

Other adverse effects include self-limiting GI toxicity (59), consisting of abdominal pain, nausea, vomiting (65), and diarrhea. Severe abdominal pain followed by bloody diarrhea has been reported (52). Varying degrees of hyperglycemia were seen in one-third of patients treated with 50 mg/kg/day for 15 days (69). A pruritic skin rash lasting several days may occur (70). Hypersensitivity reactions have occurred (71).

DRUG INTERACTIONS

Coadministration of praziquantel and albendazole may increase the mean maximum C_{max} and AUC of the sulfoxide metabolite of albendazole (24). Carbamazepine reduces the AUC of praziquantel by 90% and the C_{max} by 92% (72). Phenytoin also significantly reduces praziquantel's AUC and C_{max}. Cimetidine has been successfully used to counteract the enzyme induction caused by phenytoin and phenobarbital (73). Chloroquine decreases the bioavailability and the C_{max} of praziquantel. Patients with dual infections with malaria and schistosomiasis may require an increased dose of praziquantel when they are also receiving chloroquine (74). Coadministration of praziquantel and dexamethasone results in a 50% reduction of praziquantel serum concentrations (75).

Diagnostic Tests

Monitoring of blood glucose is recommended. With persistent vomiting or diarrhea, the serum electrolytes and fluid balance should be monitored. If significant GI bleeding occurs, the CBC should be followed.

Praziquantel can be quantified in plasma by reversed-phase high-performance liquid chromatography with limits of detection of 15 to 25 ng/ml (76).

Treatment

Treatment is primarily symptomatic and supportive. There is no specific antidote.

Corticosteroids may prevent the delayed cerebrospinal fluid reaction syndrome from occurring (68). However, because of the reduction in praziquantel plasma concentrations from coadministration of corticosteroids, some authors recommend they be avoided as preventative treatment and be reserved for transient therapy of adverse reactions (75). However, authors have stressed the need for early, high-dose, concurrent steroid therapy to treat the anticipated inflammatory response of neurocysticercosis treatment (63).

PYRANTEL

Pyrantel pamoate ($C_{11}H_{14}N_2S{,}C_{23}H_{16}O_6$; MW, 594.7 g/mol; CAS Registry No., 22204-24-6) is an anthelmintic that acts as an agonist of nicotinic receptors of nematodes, depolarizing their muscle membranes and disrupting neuromuscular transmission (77,78).

Toxic Dose

Overdose experience is limited. There are no reported fatalities.

Toxicokinetics and Toxicodynamics

The bioavailability of pyrantel citrate was greater than with the less soluble pyrantel pamoate. The citrate C_{max} was lower, and there was more pyrantel retained in the GI tract with fast transit time diets, although the pamoate was not affected (79). Therapeutically, diets that keep more of the agent in the GI tract are more effective at treating parasitic infections. Systemic toxicity is likely to occur with salts or diets that result in greater bioavailability.

Pathophysiology

Pyrantel is a weak agonist of acetylcholinesterase receptors but has very low efficacy in mammalian systems. It binds to mammalian acetylcholinesterase receptors with an apparent affinity tenfold lower than acetylcholine (78). In rabbits, parenteral administration caused paralysis and death (80).

Pregnancy and Lactation

Pyrantel pamoate is FDA pregnancy category C (81). Exertion in breast milk is unknown.

Clinical Presentation

Common adverse effects include headache, dizziness, drowsiness, insomnia, rashes, anorexia, nausea, vomiting, abdominal pain, and diarrhea. GI distress, including nausea, vomiting, and diarrhea, may occur after therapeutic use of pyrantel pamoate and is transient (82–87).

Transient elevations of serum transaminase levels have been reported (82,87,88). Hyperthermia has been reported after therapeutic dosing of pyrantel pamoate (83,85). Restlessness occurred in two patients, and irritability occurred in one patient after ingesting a single 50-mg/ml dose of a pyrantel pamoate suspension (83).

With concurrent administration of theophylline and pyrantel, serum theophylline concentrations are increased (89). There is an antagonistic interaction between pyrantel and piperazine, and they should not be administered concurrently (86,88,90).

Diagnostic Tests

Pyrantel pamoate can be quantified in plasma by reversed-phase high-performance liquid chromatography with limits of detection of 15 to 25 ng/ml (76). Liver function tests should be monitored in symptomatic patients.

Treatment

Treatment is symptomatic and supportive. There is no specific antidote.

PIPERAZINE

Piperazine ($C_4H_{10}N_2$; MW, 86.14 g/mol; CAS Registry No., 110-85-0) is an antihelmintic agent. It is also used as a corrosion inhibitor, insecticide, and accelerator for curing polychloroprene (91,92). It is no longer produced in the United States.

Toxic Dose

The *adult and pediatric therapeutic dosage* for children and adults is 65 to 75 mg/kg/day (maximum, 3.5 g/day) for 7 days and repeated 1 week later. The precise dose depends on indications. The dosages for piperazine granules, solution, suspension, and tablets are not interchangeable. Furthermore, the dose of piperazine citrate is expressed in terms of the hexahydrate (93). Piperazine citrate tablets are equivalent to 250 mg piperazine hexahydrate, and piperazine citrate syrup is equivalent to 500 mg piperazine hexahydrate per 5 ml. The salts are less hazardous than anhydrous or hexahydrate forms (94). According to the manufacturer, piperazine is contraindicated in renal failure and hepatic dysfunction (95).

Toxicity has been noted at therapeutic doses. Overdose experience is limited. Recovery after ingestion of 11.6 g has been reported.

Toxicokinetics and Toxicodynamics

Approximately 20% to 40% of an oral dose is absorbed. The T_{max} after an oral dose is 1 hour (96). A small amount is metabolized in the liver; 60% to 90% is excreted unchanged in the urine (96).

Pathophysiology

Piperazine paralyzes ascarids by hyperpolarizing the cell membrane. This allows expulsion of the worm by normal peristalsis (46).

Pregnancy and Lactation

Piperazine is FDA pregnancy category B (81). Excretion in breast milk is unknown.

Clinical Presentation

ADVERSE EFFECTS

Seizures may occur at therapeutic doses, including generalized, petit mal, and status epilepticus (93,98,99). The incidence of seizures may be increased when piperazine is combined with other agents that lower seizure threshold (100). Other central nervous system adverse reactions that may occur at therapeutic doses include headache and lethargy (common) (101), cerebellar ataxia (93,98,102–105), coma (101), dementia (99), euphoria, hallucinations, confusional states (106,107), vertigo (106,108), nystagmus (109), blurred vision, and transient visual disturbances may occur (101).

Other adverse effects include nausea, vomiting, myoclonus, tremor, choreiform movements (101,108), muscular weakness (101,106,108), paresthesia (101,106,108), and urticaria (109). Patients with glucose 6 phosphate dehydrogenase may be at risk of developing hemolytic anemia (110).

Piperazine is also a skin and eye irritant. Asthma may occur in workers handling piperazine (111).

DRUG INTERACTIONS

There is an antagonistic interaction between pyrantel and piperazine, and they should not be administered concurrently (86,88,90). Contraindications to piperazine include hypersensitivity to piperazine or its salts or hypersensitivity to ethylenediamine because of reported cross-sensitivity (112–114).

Diagnostic Tests

Plasma piperazine levels are neither available nor clinically useful. In symptomatic patients, electrolytes and renal function tests should be monitored.

Treatment

Because of the potential for central nervous system depression and seizures, induced emesis is contraindicated. Treatment is otherwise symptomatic and supportive. There is no specific antidote for piperazine.

PAROMOMYCIN

Paromomycin (aminosidine; $C_{23}H_{45}N_5O_{14}$, $\times$ H_2SO_4; MW, 615.6 g/mol; CAS Registry No., 7542-37-2 and 59-04-1) is an amebicidal aminoglycoside antibiotic used to treat intestinal amebiasis.

Toxic Dose

The therapeutic dosage varies based on the parasite being treated, ranging from 25 to 60 mg/kg/day for 5 to 10 days (46,115–117). In hepatic coma, the dosage is 4 g a day in divided doses for 5 to 6 days (115,116). Aminosidine has been designated an orphan product for use in the treatment of tuberculosis, *Mycobacterium avium* complex, and visceral leishmaniasis (kala-azar).

Overdose experience is limited. There are no reported fatalities.

Toxicokinetics and Toxicodynamics

Orally administered paromomycin is minimally absorbed (49,81,115).

Pathophysiology

Paromomycin causes malabsorption in volunteers treated with 2 g/day orally for 5 to 7 days (118). Malabsorption may be the result of impaired protein synthesis in the small intestine.

Pregnancy and Lactation

The pregnancy category has not been determined. Because of minimal bioavailability, paromomycin is not expected to be present in significant amounts in breast milk (81,119,120).

Clinical Presentation

Common effects include abdominal pain and cramping, nausea, and diarrhea (49,115,121). Contact dermatitis has been reported when paromomycin was applied topically (122), and vaginal mucosal erosions are common with intravaginal use (123,124). Renal and eighth cranial nerve injury may occur when there is excessive absorption of paromomycin and may occur when it is given with conditions such as ulcerative colitis (116).

Paromomycin is contraindicated in patients with prior hypersensitivity reactions and with intestinal obstruction. Because it is active against normal GI flora, it can enhance overgrowth of nonsusceptible organisms (46).

Diagnostic Tests

Renal function should be monitored when paromomycin is given in conditions that may increase systemic absorption.

Treatment

Treatment is primarily symptomatic and supportive. There is no specific antidote.

HALOGENATED HYDROXYQUINOLINES

The halogenated hydroxyquinolines include chlorquinaldol (Sterosan; $C_{10}H_7Cl_2NO$; MW, 228.1 g/mol; CAS Registry No., 72-80-0), clioquinol (C_9H_5ClINO; MW, 305.5 g/mol; CAS Registry No., 130-26-7), and iodoquinol ($C_9H_5I_2NO$; MW, 397 g/mol; CAS Registry No., 83-73-8). Clioquinol is a chelator that crosses the blood–brain barrier. It has a greater affinity for zinc and copper ions than for calcium and magnesium ions and is under investigation as a treatment for Alzheimer's disease (125). The toxicity of topical preparations is primarily local irritation and sensitivity reactions (126–128).

Toxic Dose

Chlorquinaldol is used as a 1% to 3% ointment or cream and usually combined with a topical corticosteroid for dermatomycoses. Overdose experience is limited. There are no reports of fatalities.

Clioquinol has an *adult therapeutic dose* for Alzheimer's disease of 20 to 80 mg/day (125). For the treatment of acrodermatitis enteropathica and other conditions, doses of 500.00 mg to 2.25 g per day of clioquinol have been used (129). Clioquinol overdose experience is limited. There have been cases of neurologic toxicity in which the total dosage was less than 100 g (130). The risk of adverse neurologic effects is generally dose dependent. Patients have taken up to 500 to 700 mg/day of clioquinol for more than 1 year without experiencing toxicity (131), and doses of 750 mg/day for 4 weeks or less caused little or no risk of serious adverse reactions. The incidence of neurotoxicity is 1% at a dose of 750 to 1500 mg/day for less than 2 weeks. The risk increases to 35% at doses of 750 to 1500 mg/day more than 2 weeks. With higher doses, toxicity may start within 24 hours of initiation of treatment (132).

Iodoquinol has an *adult therapeutic dosage* of 630 to 650 mg three times a day for 20 days (133). The pediatric dose is 40 mg/kg daily in three divided doses for 20 days (maximum of 650 mg/dose or 1950 mg/day) (133). Overdose experience is limited. No fatalities have been reported.

Toxicokinetics and Toxicodynamics

Hydroxyquinolines are irregularly absorbed from the GI tract (5). The half-life of chlorquinaldol is 7 hours, with a steady-state plasma concentration of 0.8 to 1.0 mg/dl (129). Systemic absorption from its topical preparations varies from 4.2% to 40.0%. The bulk of chlorquinaldol (98%) is excreted as a glucuronide, 1.3% as a sulfate, and 0.8% unchanged. Approximately 70% of the dose is excreted within 24 hours (134).

Iodoquinol has a bioavailability of 8% (116). Absorption is reduced if taken with food (129,135).

Pathophysiology

For clioquinol, degenerative changes in the visual pathways, the lateral corticospinal tracts of the lower spinal cord, and the rostral portions of the gracile fasciculi seem to be responsible for the adverse visual effects (136,137). A subacute myelo-opticoneuropathy appears to be from retrobulbar optic nerve damage and degenerative changes in the spinal cord long tracts (138).

Pregnancy and Lactation

Iodoquinol is FDA pregnancy category C (81). The other halogenated hydroxyquinolines are not rated by the FDA. Entry into breast milk is unknown.

Clinical Presentation

Topical chlorquinaldol may cause skin irritation and sensitivity in approximately 1% of patients (126,127). Overall adverse effects were reported in 4.7% of patients treated with a 1% cream combined with a steroid for dermatomycoses (128). When hydroxyquinolines have been used to treat leg ulcers secondary to chronic venous insufficiency, 6% of patients develop contact sensitivity reactions (139).

There is some degree of cross-reactivity of hydroxyquinolines. A retrospective review of 698 patients patch tested for hydroxyquinoline sensitivity found 1.4% positive to clioquinol. Of those, five had been tested to chlorquinaldol, and two were positive (140). A study of 16 patients sensitive to clioquinol found that eight were sensitive to chlorquinaldol (140), and a patient previously diagnosed with contact allergy to clioquinol developed a reaction to chlorquinaldol (141). It is important to note that a negative patch test to one agent does not guarantee that a patient will not be sensitive to others in the class (140). Also, it is possible that oral or mucosal application of hydroxyquinolines in topically sensitized patients may cause a generalized dermatitis (141) or systemic allergic reaction. Sensitization may be secondary to other substances in topical preparations, notably parabens. A patient with a bullous dermatitis after chlorquinaldol use was found to have a positive patch test to methyl- and propylparaben, used as preservatives in the ointment (142).

Clioquinol produced no adverse events in a uncontrolled study of 20 Alzheimer's patients treated with low doses for 21 days (125), but serious ocular and neurologic adverse reactions have been reported at the higher doses used to treat acrodermatitis enteropathica (129).

High-dose systemic administration of hydroxyquinolines causes more serious adverse reactions. The first reaction is optic atrophy (143,144), optic neuritis (5), and neurologic effects, consisting of confusion, ataxia, and polyneuropathy (5,129,131). Seizure developed in one case of iodoquinol, 420 mg for 12 days (145). Such reactions have been seen with clioquinol, iodoquinol, diodoquin, and broxyquinoline at doses ranging from 500.0 mg to 3.6 g/day. Although the neurologic effects generally improved after withdrawal of the drug, visual impairment persisted (129). The second type of adverse neurologic effect is subacute myelo-opticoneuropathy, reported in up to 10,000 patients in Japanese studies (146). Symptoms and signs are of subacute onset of myelopathy, optic neuropathy, and peripheral neuropathy (87,132,147).

Iodoquinol is contraindicated in patients with impaired kidney or liver function (5,116), hypersensitivity to halogenated hydroxyquinolines or iodine (5), and chronic diarrhea (association with optic atrophy and vision loss) (116,148). Caution should also be used when there is thyroid disease (interference with iodine measurement) (5,116), neurologic disorders (5), topical application in infants and children (because of up to 40% systemic absorption) (149), and high-dose or long-term use.

Diagnostic Tests

Chlorquinaldol can be detected by extractive alkylation in combination with gas-liquid chromatography (150). A highly accurate and precise method of reversed-phase high-performance liquid chromatography has been developed for the analysis of clioquinol and iodoquinol (151).

Treatment

Treatment is symptomatic and supportive. There is no specific antidote.

REFERENCES

1. Krishnaiah YSR, Raju PV, Kumar BD, et al. Development of colon targeted drug delivery systems for mebendazole. *J Control Release* 2001;77:87–95.
2. Grover JK, Vats V, Uppal G, Yadav S. Anthelmintics: a review. *Trop Gastroenterol* 2001;22:180–189.
3. Anonymous. Intestinal helminths. Anthelmintic drug trial. *Wkly Epidemiol Rec* 1995;70:25–28.
4. Winstanley P. Albendazole for mass treatment of asymptomatic trichuris infections. *Lancet* 1998;352:1080–1081.
5. Reynolds JEF, ed. *Martindale: the extra pharmacopoeia* (electronic version). Denver: Micromedex, Inc., 1990.
6. Horton RJ. Chemotherapy of echinococcus infection in man. *Trans R Soc Trop Med Hyg* 1989;83:97–102.
7. Albenza, albendazole. Product information. Philadelphia: SmithKline Beecham Pharmaceuticals, 2000.
8. Caumes E. Treatment of cutaneous larva migrans. *Clin Infect Dis* 2000;30:811–814.
9. USPDI. *Drug information for the health care professional*, 20th ed. Englewood, CO: Micromedex, Inc., 2000
10. Zentel. Technical information. 1990.
11. Dominguez L, Fagiolino P, Gordon S, et al. Bioavailability comparison between albendazole and albendazole sulphoxide in rats and man. 1995;50:697–702.
12. Marriner SE, Morris DL, Dickon B, Bogan JA. Pharmacokinetics of albendazole in man. *Eur J Clin Pharmacol* 1986;30:705–708.
13. Lange H, Eggers R, Bircher J. Increased systemic availability of albendazole when taken with a fatty meal. *Eur J Clin Pharmacol* 1988;34:315–317.
14. Edwards G, Breckenridge AM. Clinical pharmacokinetics of anthelmintic drugs. *Clin Pharmacokinet* 1988;15:67–93.
15. Steiger U, Cotting J, Reichen J. Albendazole treatment of echinococcosis in humans: effects on microsomal metabolism and drug tolerance. *Clin Pharmacol Ther* 1990;47:347–353.
16. Gottscall DW, Theodorides VJ, Waang R. The metabolism of benzimidazole anhelmintics. *Parasitol Today* 1990;6:115–124.
17. Whittaker SG, Faustman EM. Effects of albendazole and albendazole sulfoxide on cultures of differentiating rodent embryonic cells. *Toxicol Appl Pharmacol* 1991;109:73–84.
18. Auer H, Kollaritsch J, Juptner J, et al. Albendazole and pregnancy. *Appl Parasitol* 1994;35:146–147.
19. Fernandez FJ, Rodriguez-Vidigal FF, Ledesma L, et al. Aplastic anemia during treatment with albendazole [Letter]. *Am J Hematol* 1996;53:53–54.
20. Eskazole, albendazole. Technical information. Bristol, TN: SmithKline Beecham Pharmaceuticals, 1990.
21. Yildiz BO, Haznedaroglu IC, Coplu L. Albendazole-induced amegakaryocytic thrombocytopenic purpura [Letter]. *Ann Pharmacother* 1998;32:842.
22. El-Mufti M, Kamag A, Ibrahim H, et al. Albendazole therapy of hydatid disease: 2-year follow-up of 40 cases. *Ann Trop Med Parasitol* 1993;87:241–246.
23. Tandon R, Sihota R, Dada T, el al. Optic neuritis following albendazole therapy for orbital cysticercosis. *Aust N Z J Ophthalmol* 1998;26:339–341.
24. Albenza. Product information. Philadelphia: SmithKline Beecham Pharmaceuticals, 1996.
25. Allgayer H, Zahringer J, Bach P, et al. Lack of effect of haemodialysis on mebendazole kinetics: studies in a patient with echinococcosis and renal failure. *Eur J Clin Pharmacol* 1984;27:243–245.
26. Soto H, Masso F, Cano S, de Leon LD. Effects of mebendazole on protein biosynthesis and secretion in human-derived fibroblast cultures. *Biochem Pharmacol* 1996;52:289–299.
27. Stricker BHCH. *Drug-induced hepatic injury*, 2nd ed. Amsterdam, Netherlands: Elsevier, 1992.
28. Bekhti A, Pirotte J. Hepatotoxicity of mebendazole. Relationship with serum concentrations of the drug. *Gastroenterol Clin Biol* 1987;11:701–703.
29. Seitz R, Schwerk W, Arnold R. Hepatocellular drug reactions caused by mebendazole therapy in cystic echinococcosis. *Z Gastroenterol* 1983;21:324–329.
30. Junge U, Mohr W. Mebendazole-hepatitis. *Z Gastroenterol* 1983;21:736–738.
31. Colle I, Naegels S, Hoorens A, et al. Granulomatous hepatitis due to mebendazole. *J Clin Gastroenterol* 1999;28:44–48.
32. Bulut BU, Gülnar SB, Aysev D. Alternative treatment protocols in Giardiasis: a pilot study. *Scand J Infect Dis* 1996;28:493–495.
33. Sadjjadi SM, Alborzi AW, Mostovfi H. Comparative clinical trial of mebendazole and metronidazole in giardiasis of children. *J Trop Pediatr* 2001;47:176–178.
34. Scragg JN, Proctor EM. Mebendazole in the treatment of severe symptomatic trichuriasis in children. *Am J Trop Med Hyg* 1977;26:198–203.
35. Miskovitz PF, Javitt NB. Leukopenia associated with mebendazole therapy of hydatid disease. *Am J Trop Med Hyg* 1980;29:1356–1358.
36. Dawson M, Watson TR. The effect of dose form on the bioavailability of mebendazole in man. *Br J Clin Pharmacol* 1985;19:87–90.
37. De Silva NR, Sirisena JLGJ, Gunasekera DPS, et al. Effect of mebendazole therapy during pregnancy on birth outcome. *Lancet* 1999;353:1145–1149.
38. Rafi S, Memon A, Billo AG. Efficacy and safety of mebendazole in children with worm infestation. *J Pak Med Assoc* 1997;47:140–141.
39. Vermox, mebendazole chewable tablets. Product information. *Physician's desk reference* (electronic version). Englewood, CO: MICROMEDEX, Inc., 1998.
40. Murray-Lyon IM, Reynolds KW. Complications of mebendazole treatment for hydatid disease. *Br Med J* 1979;2:1111–1112.
41. Harris A. Pyrexia and mebendazole. *Br Med J* 1979;2:1365.
42. Luder PJ, Siffert B, Witassek F, et al. Treatment of hydatid disease with high oral doses of mebendazole. Long-term follow-up of plasma mebendazole levels and drug interactions. *Eur J Clin Pharmacol* 1986;31:443–448.
43. Bekhti A, Pirotte J, Woestenborghs R. A correlation between serum mebendazole concentrations and the aminopyrine breath test. Implications in the treatment of hydatid disease. *Br J Clin Pharmacol* 1986;21:223–226.
44. Bekhti A, Pirotte J. Cimetidine increases serum mebendazole concentrations. Implications for treatment of hepatic hydatid cysts. *Br J Clin Pharmacol* 1987;24:390–392.
45. Mintezol, thiabendazole tablets and suspension. Product Information. West Point, PA: Merck & Company, Inc., 1998.
46. Gilman AG, Rall TW, Nies AS, et al., eds. *Goodman and Gilman's the pharmacological basis of therapeutics*, 8th ed. New York: Macmillan Publishing Co, 1990.
47. Jalota R, Freston JW. Severe intrahepatic cholestasis due to thiabendazole. *Am J Trop Med* 1974;23:676.
48. Feregrino Goyos M, Lifshitz Guinzberg A, Hernandez Berumen A, et al. Intrahepatic cholestasis due to thiabendazole, treated with phenobarbital. *Prensa Med Mex* 1976;41:167–171.
49. Reference deleted.
50. Sugar AM, Kearns PJ, Haulk AA, et al. Possible thiabendazole-induced theophylline toxicity. *Am Rev Respir Dis* 1980;122:501–503.
51. Lew G, Murray WE, Lane JR, et al. Theophylline-thiabendazole drug interaction. *Clin Pharm* 1989;8:225–227.
52. Watt G, White NJ, Padre L, et al. Praziquantel pharmacokinetics and side effects in *Schistosoma japonicum*-infected patients with liver disease. *J Infect Dis* 1988;157:530–535.
53. Wegner DH. The profile of the trematodicidal compound praziquantel. *Arzneimittelforschung* 1984;34:1132–1136.
54. Sotelo J, Jung H. Pharmacokinetic optimisation of the treatment of neurocysticercosis. *Clin Pharmacokinet* 1998;34:503–515.
55. Biltricide, praziquantel tablets. Product information. West Haven, CT: Bayer Corporation, 2000.
56. *Drug facts and comparisons*. St. Louis: Wolters Kluwer Health, 2003:1479.
57. Kaojarern S, Nathakarnkikool S, Suvanakoot U. Comparative bioavailability of praziquantel tablets. *Drug Intell Clin Pharm* 1989;23:29–32.
58. Pehrson PO, Bengtsson E, Diekmann HW, et al. Treatment with praziquantel in a patient with schistosomiasis and chronic renal failure. *Trans R Soc Trop Med Hyg* 1983;77:687–688.
59. Pearson RL, Guerrant RL. Praziquantel: a major advance in anthelmintic therapy. *Ann Intern Med* 1983;99:195–198.
60. Jung H, Hurtado M, Sanchez M, et al. Plasma and CSF levels of albendazole and praziquantel in patients with neurocysticercosis. *Clin Neuropharmacol* 1990;13:559–564.
61. Katz M. Praziquantel. *Pediatr Infect Dis* 1983;2:144–145.
62. Ofori-Adjei D, Adjepon-Yamoah K, Lindstrom B. Oral praziquantel kinetics in normal and *Schistosoma haematobium*-infected subjects. *Ther Drug Monit* 1988;10:45–49.
63. Bang OY, Heo JH, Choi SA, et al. Large cerebral infarction during praziquantel therapy in neurocysticercosis. *Stroke* 1997;28:211–213.
64. Leopold G, Ungenthum W, Groll E, et al. Clinical pharmacology in normal volunteers of praziquantel, a new drug against schistosomes & cestodes. *Eur J Clin Pharmacol* 1978;14:281–291.
65. El-Alamy MA, Habib MA, McNeeley DF, et al. Preliminary results of chemotherapy using praziquantel on a large scale in Qalyub Bilharziasis

Project where simultaneous infection with *S. mansoni* and *S. haematobium* exists. *Arzneimittelforschung* 1981;31:612–615.
66. Flisser A, Madrazo I, Plancarte A, et al. Neurological symptoms in occult neurocysticercosis after single taeniacidal dose of praziquantel [Letter]. *Lancet* 1993;342:748.
67. Ciferri F. Delayed CSF reaction to praziquantel. *Lancet* 1988;1:642–643.
68. Fong GCY, Cheung RTF. Caution with praziquantel in neurocysticercosis [Letter]. *Stroke* 1997;28:1648–1649.
69. Webbe G. Human cysticercosis: parasitology, pathology, clinical manifestations and available treatment. *Pharmacol Ther* 1994;64:175–200.
70. Jong EC, Wasserheit JN, Johnson RJ, et al. Praziquantel for the treatment of *Clonorchis/Opisthorchis* infections: report of a double-blind, placebo-controlled trial. *J Infect Dis* 1985;152:637–640.
71. Huang SW. A clinical approach to a patient with praziquantel hypersensitivity. *J Allergy Clin Immunol* 1992;90:867–868.
72. Bittencourt PR, Gracia CM, Martins R, et al. Phenytoin and carbamazepine decrease oral bioavailability of praziquantel. *Neurology* 1992;42:492–496.
73. Dachman WD, Adubofour KO, Bikin DS, et al. Cimetidine-induced rise in praziquantel levels in a patient with neurocysticercosis being treated with anticonvulsants. *J Infect Dis* 1994;169:689–691.
74. Masimirembwa CM, Naik YS, Hasler JA. The effect of chloroquine on the pharmacokinetics and metabolism of praziquantel in rats and in humans. *Biopharm Drug Dispos* 1994;15:33–43.
75. Vazquez ML, Jung H, Sotelo J. Plasma levels of praziquantel decrease when dexamethasone is given simultaneously. *Neurology* 1987;37:1561–1562.
76. Morovjan G, Csokan P, Makranszki L, et al. Determination of fenbendazole, praziquantel and pyrantel pamoate in dog plasma by high-performance liquid chromatography. *J Chromatog* 1998;797:237–244.
77. Forrester JE, Bailar JC, Esrey SA, et al. Randomised trial of albendazole and pyrantel in symptomless trichuriasis in children. *Lancet* 1998;352:1103–1108.
78. Rayes D, De Rosa MJ, Spitzmaul G, Bouzat C. The anthelmintic pyrantel acts as a low efficacious agonist and an open-channel blocker of mammalian acetylcholine receptors. *Neuropharmacology* 2001;41:238–245.
79. Hennessy DR, Praslicka J, Bjorn H. The disposition of pyrantel in the gastrointestinal tract and effect of digesta flow rate on the kinetic behaviour of pyrantel in the pig. *Vet Parasitol* 2000;92:277–285.
80. Bescansa E, Nicolas M, Aguado C, et al. Myasthenia gravis aggravated by pyrantel pamoate. *J Neurol Neurosurg Psychiatry* 1991;54:563.
81. Briggs GG, Freeman RK, Yaffe SJ. *Drugs in pregnancy and lactation: a reference guide to fetal and neonatal risk*, 5th ed. Baltimore: Williams & Wilkins, 1998.
82. Antiminth. Product information, 1974.
83. Cervoni WA, Oliver-Gonzalez J. Clinical evaluation of pyrantel pamoate in helminthiasis. *Am J Trop Med Hyg* 1971;20:589–591.
84. Drugs for parasitic infections. *Med Lett Drugs Ther* 1995;37:99–107.
85. Anonymous. Drugs for parasitic infections. *Med Lett Drugs Ther* 1990;32:23–32.
86. Lenoir G. Antiparasitic medications in children, neonates, and the fetus: pharmacokinetics, tolerance, toxicity. *Arch Fr Pediatr* 1985;42:965–969.
87. Sweetman S, ed. *Martindale: the complete drug reference*. London: Pharmaceutical Press (electronic version); Greenwood Village, CO: Micromedex, 2002.
88. McEvoy GK, ed. *American hospital formulary service 97*. Bethesda, MD: American Society of Health-System Pharmacists, Inc., 1997.
89. Hecht L, Murray WE. Theophylline-pyrantel pamoate interaction [Letter]. *DICP* 1989;23:258.
90. Hardman JG, Limbird LE, Molinoff PB, et al., eds. *Goodman and Gilman's the pharmacological basis of therapeutics*, 9th ed. New York: McGraw-Hill, 1996.
91. Budavari S, ed. *The Merck index*, 11th ed. Rahway, NJ: Merck & Co, Inc., 1989:1185.
92. Sax NI, Lewis RJ. *Hawley's condensed chemical dictionary*, 11th ed. New York: Van Nostrand Reinhold Company, 1987:921.
93. USPDI. *Drug information for the health care professional*, 15th ed. US Rockville, MD: Pharmaceutical Convention, 1995.
94. Clayton GD, Clayton FE, eds. *Patty's industrial hygiene and toxicology, Vol. 2A. Toxicology*, 3rd ed. New York: John Wiley & Sons, 1981:2690–2693.
95. Antepar, piperazine citrate. Product information. Research Triangle Park, NC: Burroughs Wellcome, 1986.
96. Chasseaud LF, Hawkins DR, Moore DH, et al. The confirmation in man of the metabolic data for ethyl-4 (3,4,5-trimethoxycinnamoyl) piperazinyl acetate in animals. *Arzneimittelforschung* 1972;22:2003–2005.
97. Reference deleted.
98. Conners GP. Piperazine neurotoxicity: worm wobble revisited. *J Emerg Med* 1995;13:341–343.
99. Graf W, Haldimann B, Flury W. Piperazine intoxication in long-term hemodialysis. *Schweiz Med Wochensch* 1978;108:177–181.
100. Boulos BM, Davis LE. Hazard of simultaneous administration of phenothiazine and piperazine. *N Engl J Med* 1969;280(22):1245–1246.
101. Miller CG, Carpenter R. Neurotoxic side effects of piperazine. *Lancet* 1967;1:895–896.
102. Gupta SR. Piperazine neurotoxicity and psychological reaction. *J Indian Med Assoc* 1976;66:33.
103. Bomb BS, Bedi HK. Neurotoxic side-effects of piperazine. *Trans R Soc Trop Med Hyg* 1976;70:358.
104. Neff L. Another severe psychological reaction to side effects of medication in an adolescent. *JAMA* 1966;197:218.
105. Nickey LN. Possible precipitation of petit mal seizures with piperazine citrate. *JAMA* 1966;195:1069.
106. Combes B, Damon A, Gottfried E. Piperazine (Antepar) neurotoxicity. *N Engl J Med* 1956;254:223–224.
107. Schuch P, Stephan U, Jacobi G. Neurotoxic side-effects of piperazines [Letter]. *Lancet* 1966;1:1218.
108. Parsons AC. Piperazine neurotoxicity: "worm wobble." *BMJ* 1971;4:792.
109. Reynolds JEF, ed. *Martindale: the extra pharmacopeia* (CD-ROM version). Micromedex, Inc., 1989.
110. Buchanan N, Cassel R, Jenkins T. G-6-PD deficiency and piperazine. *BMJ* 1971;2:110.
111. Hagmar L, Bellander T, Ranstam J, et al. Piperazine-induced airway symptoms: exposure-response relationships and selection in an occupational setting. *Am J Ind Med* 1984;6:347–357.
112. Wright S, Harman RRM. Ethylenediamine and piperazine sensitivity. *BMJ* 1983;287:463.
113. Burry JN. Ethylenediamine sensitivity with a systemic reaction to piperazine citrate. *Contact Dermatitis* 1978;4:380.
114. Calnan CD. Occupational piperazine dermatitis. *Contact Dermatitis* 1975;1:126.
115. Humatin, paromomycin sulfate capsules. Product information. Morris Plains, NJ: Parke-Davis, Division of Warner-Lambert Company, 1999.
116. Olin BR, ed. *Drug facts and comparisons*. St. Louis: Facts and Comparisons, 1990.
117. Humatin, paromomycin. Product information. Morris Plains, NJ: Parke-Davis, 1990.
118. Keusch GT, Troncale FJ, Buchanan RD, et al. Malabsorption due to paromomycin. *Arch Intern Med* 1970;125:273–276.
119. Hill DR. Giardiasis: issues in diagnosis and management. *Infect Dis Clin North Am* 1993;7:503–525.
120. Ziv G, Sulman FG. Distribution of aminoglycoside antibiotics in blood and milk. *Res Vet Sci* 1974;17:68–74.
121. Daikos GK, Kontomichalou P, Bilalis D, et al. Intestinal flora ecology after oral use of antibiotics. *Chemotherapy* 1968;13:146–160.
122. Ozgoztasi O, Baydar I. A randomized clinical trial of topical paromomycin versus oral ketoconazole for treating cutaneous leishmaniasis in Turkey. *Int J Dermatol* 1997;36:61–63.
123. Poppe WAJ. Nitroimidazole-resistant vaginal trichomoniasis treated with paromomycin. *Eur J Obstet Gyn Reprod Biol* 2001;96:119–120.
124. Nyirjesy P, Sobel JD, Weitz MV, et al. Difficult-to-treat trichomoniasis: results with paromomycin cream. *Clin Infect Dis* 1998;26:986–988.
125. Regland B, Lehmann W, Abedini I, et al. Treatment of Alzheimer's disease with clioquinol. *Dement Geriatr Cogn Disord* 2001;12:408–414.
126. Murphy JC. Chlorquinaldol (Sterosan) in dermatologic therapy. *Rocky Mtn Med J* 1959;55:53.
127. Fox HH. Topical therapy with chlorquinaldol and hydrocortisone. *Antibiot Med* 1959;6:85.
128. Maeder E, Schindlery C, Macarol V, Schoenenberger PM. A comparative multicentre trial of halometasone/Triclosan cream and diflucortolone valerate/chlorquinaldol cream in the treatment of acute dermatomycoses. *J Int Med Res* 1983;11[Supp 1]:48–52.
129. Hagermark O, Wahlberg JE, Germanis M. Determination of oxyquinoline concentrations in plasma in a patient treated for Acrodermatitis enteropathica—an aid in therapeutic control. *Dermatologica* 1974;149:29–38.
130. Rose FC, Gawel M. Clioquinol neurotoxicity: an overview. *Acta Neurol Scand* 1984;70:137–145.
131. Selby G. Subacute myelo-optic neuropathy in Australia. *Lancet* 1972;1:123–125.
132. Ellenhorn MJ, Barceloux DG. *Medical toxicology: diagnosis and treatment of human poisoning*. New York: Elsevier, 1988.
133. Yodoxin, iodoquinol tablets. Product information. *Physicians' desk reference* (electronic version), Englewood, CO: Micromedex, Inc., 1999.
134. Degen PH, Moppert J, Schmid K, Weirich EG. Percutaneous absorption of chlorquinaldol (Sterosan). *Dermatologica* 1979;159:239–244.
135. Hagermark O, Hoglund S. Iron metabolism in tetracycline-treated acne patients. *Acta Derm Venerol* 1974;54:45–48.
136. Tateishi J, Kuroda S, Saito A, et al. Experimental myelo-optic neuropathy induced by clioquinol. *Acta Neuropathol* 1973;24:304–320.
137. Schaumburg HH, Spencer PS, Krinke G, et al. The CNS distal axonopathy in dogs intoxicated with clioquinol. *J Neuropathol Exp Neurol* 1978;37:686a.
138. Hanakago R, Uono M. Clioquinol intoxication occurring in the treatment of acrodermatitis enteropathica with reference to SMON outside of Japan. *J Toxicol Clin Toxicol* 1981;18:1427–1434.
139. Le Coz DJ, Scrivener Y, Santinelli F, Heid E. Contact sensitization in leg ulcers. *Ann Dermatol Venereol* 1998;125:694–699.
140. Myatt AE, Beck MH. Contact sensitivity to chlorquinaldol. *Contact Derm* 1983;9:523.
141. Rodriguez A, Cabrerizo S, Barranco R, et al. Contact cross-sensitization among quinolines. *Allergy* 2001;56:795.
142. Schamberg IL. Allergic contact dermatitis to methyl and propyl paraben. *Arch Derm* 1967;95:626–628.
143. Berggren L, Hansson O. Treating acrodermatitis enteropathica. *Lancet* 1966;1:52.
144. Berggren L, Hansson O. Absorption of intestinal antiseptics derived from 8-hydroxyquinolines. *Clin Pharmacol Ther* 1968;9:67–70.
145. Fisher A, Walter FG, Szabo S. Iodoquinol associated seizures and radiopacity. *Vet Hum Toxicol* 1991;33:392.
146. Tsubaki T, Honma Y, Hoshi M. Subacute myelo-optic neuropathy following abdominal symptoms: a clinical and pathological study. *Jpn J Med* 1965;4:181.

147. Wadia NH. SMON as seen from Bombay. *Acta Neurol Scand* 1984;70:159–164.
148. Yaffe SJ, Bierman CW, Cann HW, et al. Blindness and neuropathy from diiodohydroxyquin-like drugs. *Pediatrics* 1974;54:378–379.
149. Kauffman RE, Banner W, Blumer JL, et al. Clioquinol (iodochlorhydroxyquin, Vioform) and iodoquinol (diiodohydroxyquin): blindness and neuropathy. *Pediatrics* 1990;86:797–798.
150. Degen PH, Schweizer A. Quantitative determination of drugs in biological materials by means of extractive alkylation and gas-liquid chromatography. *J Chromatog* 1977;142:549–557.
151. Rizk M, Belal F, Ibrahim F, et al. LC of pharmaceutically important halogenated 8-hydroxyquinolines after precolumn derivatization with Pd (II). *J Pharm Biomed Anal* 2002;27:813–820.

CHAPTER 91

Antituberculosis Drugs

Michael A. McGuigan

H
N
O
NH_2
N

ISONIAZID

Compounds included:	**Aminosalicylic acid (Paser); capreomycin (Capastat, Ogostal); cycloserine (Seromycin); ethambutol (Myambutol); ethionamide (Trecator); isoniazid (Nydrazid); pyrazinamide (Rifater); the rifamycin derivatives: rifabutin (Mycobutin), rifampin (Rifadin, Rimactane), rifapentine (Priftin)**
Molecular formula and weight:	**See text.**
SI conversion:	**Aminosalicylic acid, mg/L × 6.5 = µmol/L; capreomycin, mg/L × 1.5 = µmol/L; cycloserine, mg/L × 9.8 = µmol/L; ethambutol, mg/L × 3.6 = µmol/L; isoniazid, mg/L × 7.3 = µmol/L; pyrazinamide, mg/L × 8.1 = µmol/L; rifamycin, mg/L × 1.2 = µmol/L**
CAS Registry No.:	**See text.**
Therapeutic levels:	**Serum cycloserine 5 to 20 µg/ml; serum isoniazid 20 mg/L**
Target organs:	**Central nervous system (acute); gastrointestinal (acute or chronic); hematologic (chronic); kidney (chronic); ear (chronic); eye (acute or chronic); liver (acute or chronic); muscle (acute); peripheral nervous system (acute or chronic); skin (acute or chronic)**
Antidotes:	**Pyridoxine, benzodiazepines**

OVERVIEW

Antituberculosis drugs can be divided into first-line drugs [ethambutol, isoniazid (INH), pyrazinamide, rifampin, streptomycin], second-line drugs (amikacin, aminosalicylic acid, capreomycin, ciprofloxacin, cycloserine, ethionamide, kanamycin, ofloxacin), and drugs used primarily for the treatment of *Mycobacterium avium* disease complex (azithromycin, clarithromycin, fluoroquinolones, rifabutin, rifapentine). The drugs addressed in this chapter are aminosalicylic acid, capreomycin, cycloserine, ethambutol, ethionamide, INH, pyrazinamide, and the rifamycin derivatives (rifabutin, rifampin, rifapentine).

Due to the diverse drugs included in this group, a wide variety of adverse events and toxicity may occur. Antitubercular drugs are frequently used in combination, so there is always a potential for drug-drug interactions and additive or synergistic effects. Treatment of clinical toxicity is primarily symptomatic and supportive care.

AMINOSALICYLIC ACID

Aminosalicylic acid [Paser; 4-aminosalicylic acid, para-aminobenzoic acid; $C_7H_7NO_3$; molecular weight (MW), 153.1 g/mol; CAS Registry No., 65-49-6] is a bacteriostatic agent. Adverse effects are primarily limited to topical gastrointestinal (GI) effects and hypersensitivity reactions. Therapeutic preparations are most commonly available as coated granules.

Toxic Dose

The *adult therapeutic dose* is 12 g/day in three divided doses. The *pediatric dose* is 150 mg/kg/day in three or four divided doses up to 12 g/day. Doses exceeding 12 g/day are poorly tolerated due to GI effects.

No fatalities due to aminosalicylic acid have been reported in either adults or children.

Toxicokinetics and Toxicodynamics

The coated granular form of aminosalicylic acid has an oral bioavailability of 60% to 65%. The time-to-peak plasma concentration (T_{max}) after a therapeutic dose is 6 hours (range, 1.5 to 24.0 hours). Protein binding is 50% to 60% at therapeutic levels. The apparent volume of distribution (V_d) is 24% of body weight with low concentrations in the cerebrospinal fluid (1). If aminosalicylic acid is administered unprotected by coating, approximately 10% is decarboxylated in simulated gastric acid to *m*-aminophenol, a known hepatotoxin.

More than 50% of the drug is acetylated in the liver. Approximately 84% of an ingested dose is excreted in the urine within 24 hours (21% as the parent compound, 63% as the acetylated metabolite). After an oral dose of the granules, the elimination half-life is 1.1 to 1.6 hours; the half-life after the ingestion of an immediate-release formulation is 45 to 60 minutes.

Pathophysiology

Pathophysiology is related to local (topical) GI effects (10% to 20% of patients), hypersensitivity reactions (5% to 10% of patients), or thrombocytopenia.

Pregnancy and Lactation

Aminosalicylic acid is U.S. Food and Drug Administration (FDA) pregnancy category C (Appendix I). No documented effects on the fetus were found in limited data (2). Small amounts enter breast milk. When the maternal plasma level is 70 µg/ml at 2 hours, the breast milk concentration at 3 hours is 1 µg/ml.

Clinical Presentation

ACUTE OVERDOSAGE

No cases of acute overdose have been reported.

ADVERSE REACTIONS

Anorexia, nausea, epigastric pain, and diarrhea are common. High fever, malaise, arthralgia, sore throat, or skin eruptions may occur. Hematologic abnormalities may include leukopenia, agranulocytosis, lymphocytosis, or thrombocytopenia; acute hemolytic anemia has been reported (3).

Diagnostic Tests

A complete blood cell count (CBC) may be needed to begin assessment of hematologic effects and hypersensitivity reactions. Abdominal distress due to aminosalicylic acid needs to be distinguished from peptic ulcer disease.

Treatment

Treatment is symptomatic and supportive. Induced emesis is not recommended. A single dose of activated charcoal may bind aminosalicylic acid after an acute overdose. The use of a cathartic or whole bowel irrigation is not recommended.

ENHANCEMENT OF ELIMINATION

Aminosalicylic acid and its acetyl metabolite are removed by hemodialysis (4). The clinical indications for dialysis have not been established. Multiple-dose activated charcoal is not recommended.

ANTIDOTES

There is no antidote to aminosalicylic acid.

PITFALLS

Aminosalicylic acid is 4-aminosalicylic acid and does not produce salicylate toxicity. It should not be confused with mesalamine (5-aminosalicylic acid), which may cause clinical effects similar to acetylsalicylic acid.

CAPREOMYCIN

Capreomycin [Capastat, Ogostal; $C_{25}H_{44}N_{14}O_8$; MW, 668.7 g/mol; CAS Registry No., 1405-37-4 (capreomycin sulfate)] is a cyclic polypeptide antimycobacterial drug with adverse effects of ototoxicity, nephrotoxicity, ocular toxicity, eosinophilia, and pain at the intramuscular (IM) injection site. Capreomycin is used only in conjunction with other drugs for the treatment of "resistant" tuberculosis.

Toxic Dose

The *adult therapeutic dose* is 1 g/day IM (not to exceed 20 mg/kg/day). Although the *pediatric dose* has not been established, doses of 15 to 30 mg/kg/day IM have been used.

The lethal or minimum toxic dose has not been established for either adults or children. The subcutaneous lethal dose in mice is 514 mg/kg (5).

Toxicokinetics and Toxicodynamics

Capreomycin is poorly absorbed after oral administration. The V_d is approximately 0.4 L/kg (6). The T_{max} is 2 hours after an IM injection. Capreomycin is almost entirely excreted unchanged through the kidneys. The elimination half-life has been reported as 2 to 5 hours with normal renal function and increases depending on the creatine clearance (7,8). The intrinsic clearance rate is 0.61 ml/minute/kg.

Pathophysiology

The mechanisms of capreomycin toxicity have not been established. Its therapeutic mechanism of action is not established, but mycobacterial species that have become resistant to other agents are typically susceptible to capreomycin.

Pregnancy and Lactation

Capreomycin is FDA pregnancy category C (Appendix I). Excretion of capreomycin in breast milk has not been studied.

Clinical Presentation

ACUTE OVERDOSAGE

Cases of acute or subacute overdose have not been reported.

ADVERSE EVENTS

During chronic use, nephrotoxicity, ototoxicity, or ocular toxicity may develop. Nephrotoxicity consists of elevations in urea and creatinine along with changes in electrolytes (9). As many as 66% of patients experience mild proteinuria (10). Severe renal tubular dysfunction and tubular necrosis have been reported. Ototoxicity occurs in 11% of patients and consists of vertigo, tinnitus, and hearing loss. Possibly as many as 5% of patients experience decreases in visual acuity.

Diagnostic Tests

ACUTE OVERDOSAGE

No acute or subacute overdoses have been reported.

ADVERSE EVENTS

Patients receiving capreomycin should be screened for nephrotoxicity (urea, creatinine, electrolytes, urinalysis), ototoxicity (audiometry), and ocular toxicity (funduscopic examination and visual acuity tests). CBCs with differentials should help to identify rare hematologic adverse events (e.g., eosinophilia).

In symptomatic patients, the diagnostic tests chosen to evaluate capreomycin toxicity depend on the presenting symptoms and signs.

Treatment

Treatment is primarily symptomatic and supportive.

GASTROINTESTINAL DECONTAMINATION

GI decontamination is unnecessary after an acute ingestion because capreomycin is so poorly absorbed.

ENHANCEMENT OF ELIMINATION

Capreomycin has a hemodialysis clearance reported as high as 2.7 L/hour (6) and may be used after large parenteral overdoses with renal compromise.

ANTIDOTES

There is no antidote for capreomycin.

MONITORING

Physical examination should include a careful evaluation of the ocular fundi. Laboratory tests should include renal function tests, serum electrolytes, and blood gases. Serial audiometric and visual acuity tests are recommended for patients who are symptomatic.

CYCLOSERINE

Cycloserine (Seromycin; $C_3H_6N_2O_2$; MW, 102.1 g/mol; CAS Registry No., 68-41-7) is most commonly used as a second-line therapy in the treatment of tuberculosis or other mycobacterial infections that are resistant to other antibiotics. The most commonly reported adverse effects from cycloserine use involve the central nervous system.

Toxic Dose

The *adult therapeutic dose* is 500 to 1000 mg/day in divided doses. The *pediatric dose* is 10 to 15 mg/kg/day in two divided doses.

No acute overdoses have been reported, and the lethal or minimum toxic doses have not been established.

Toxicokinetics and Toxicodynamics

Although cycloserine is rapidly destroyed in an acidic medium, it is well absorbed from the GI tract. The T_{max} is 2 to 3 hours of an oral dose. The V_d is 0.10 to 0.25 L/kg. Cerebrospinal fluid levels approximate plasma levels.

A small amount of cycloserine is metabolized in the liver; 50% of a parenteral dose of cycloserine is excreted unchanged in the urine. The renal clearance with normal renal function is 0.110 to 0.013 L/hour/kg (11), The elimination half-life is 10 to 25 hours and is affected by renal function.

Pathophysiology

Cycloserine interferes with cell wall synthesis. The mechanism by which it produces neurotoxicity is unclear but may be related to pyridoxine deficiency. Cycloserine is believed to be a partial agonist at the glycine recognition site on the *N*-methyl-D-aspartate receptor (12,13).

Pregnancy and Lactation

Cycloserine is FDA pregnancy category C (Appendix I). Approximately 0.6% of the adult dose of cycloserine is excreted in breast milk (14), with the breast milk concentration being 72% of the concomitant serum concentration (15). However, breast-feeding is not contraindicated while being treated with cycloserine (16).

Clinical Presentation

ACUTE OVERDOSAGE

No cases of acute or subacute overdose have been reported.

ADVERSE EVENTS

Adverse reactions to cycloserine tend to appear within 2 weeks of beginning therapy and resolve when the drug is discontinued (17,18). The toxicity of cycloserine is closely related to excessive blood levels caused by high dosage or inadequate renal clearance. Milder clinical manifestations include somnolence, headache, tremor, dysarthria, vertigo, confusion, nervousness, or irritability. More severe psychiatric reactions include psychosis with suicidal tendencies, paranoia, catatonia, or depression. Generalized paresis and tonic-clonic convulsions have occurred. A history of psychological problems is believed to be a contributing factor. Chronic or excessive concurrent use of ethanol is claimed to increase the possibility of convulsions; and the risk of cycloserine-induced convulsions appears to be increased in alcoholics.

Diagnostic Tests

ACUTE OVERDOSAGE

No acute or subacute overdoses have been reported.

ADVERSE EVENTS

Patients taking cycloserine should have their hematologic, renal, and liver function tests and cycloserine blood levels monitored. Adverse effects of cycloserine are more common when serum levels exceed 30 μg/ml (19).

Treatment

Treatment of an acute overdose or chronic toxicity should be treated with drug withdrawal and symptomatic supportive care. Hemodialysis may be used to enhance the removal of cycloserine.

GASTROINTESTINAL DECONTAMINATION

The induction of emesis is not indicated because the patient may develop convulsions. The administration of activated charcoal within 2 hours of ingestion is expected to reduce cycloserine absorption. The administration of a cathartic or whole bowel irrigation is not indicated.

ENHANCEMENT OF ELIMINATION

Multiple-dose activated charcoal is not indicated. Hemodialysis may be useful in removing cycloserine in patients with a large overdose or in those with renal compromise. More than 50% of a 500-mg dose was recovered during hemodialysis (20).

ANTIDOTES

No antidote has been recommended, but pyridoxine may be useful in treating convulsions (Chapter 71).

MONITORING

A careful neurologic and psychiatric examination is appropriate for symptomatic patients. Patients taking cycloserine should have their hematologic, renal, and liver function tests and cycloserine blood levels monitored (should not exceed 30 µg/ml).

SUPPORTIVE CARE

Typical supportive care should include seizure and suicide precautions.

ETHAMBUTOL

Ethambutol (Myambutol; $C_{10}H_{24}N_2O_2$,2HCl; MW, 277.2 g/mol; CAS Registry No., 1070-11-7) is a synthetic drug used primarily for the treatment of infections with *Mycobacterium tuberculosis*, *Mycobacterium kansasii*, or *M. avium* complex. Adverse effects have affected the central and peripheral nervous systems, GI tract, hematologic system, liver, and joints. Acute overdose may produce nausea, abdominal pain, fever, mental confusion, visual hallucinations, and optic neuropathy.

Toxic Dose

The *adult therapeutic dose* is 15 mg/kg/dose as a single daily dose. Alternative treatment regimens use larger doses three times weekly or twice weekly. Patients with renal insufficiency require dosage adjustment. The *pediatric dose* is 15 to 25 mg/kg/dose daily or 50 mg/kg/dose twice weekly up to a maximum of 2.5 g/dose (21). Ethambutol is not recommended in children who may be too young (younger than 6 to 8 years of age) or otherwise unable to undergo reliable visual acuity testing (22).

No definitive acute lethal dose or minimum toxic dose has been established for either adults or children. The prevalence of visual disturbances appears to be dose related: 1.6% of patients taking more than 15 mg/kg/day, 2.8% of patients taking 25 mg/kg/day (23), and 15.0% of patients taking 35 mg/kg/day or more (24). An acute overdose of INH, rifampin, and ethambutol, 10 g, was associated with optic neuritis (25).

Toxicokinetics and Toxicodynamics

Approximately 80% of ethambutol is absorbed after ingestion, with a maximal drug concentration of 2 to 4 hours. Total protein binding is 10% to 30%. Cerebrospinal fluid concentrations are 20% to 80% of serum concentrations. The apparent V_d is 1.6 to 3.9 L/kg. Approximately 50% of an oral dose is excreted unchanged in the urine, and 20% is excreted unchanged in the feces; up to 20% undergoes hepatic metabolism to inactive aldehyde metabolites. Renal clearance is 6.0 to 8.5 ml/minute/kg and is prolonged in renal failure (26). The elimination half-life is 2.5 to 3.6 hours at therapeutic levels.

Pathophysiology

Two types of retrobulbar neuritis have been identified. In the first, involvement of the central fibers of the optic nerve produces blurred vision, diminished visual acuity, a central scotoma, and difficulty with color vision. In the second, involvement of the peripheral fibers of the optic nerve results in a constriction of peripheral visual fields but no loss of visual acuity or change in color vision (27). The mechanism of the optic neuritis is unclear. It has been hypothesized that because ethambutol chelates the zinc, the optic neuritis may be related to an abnormality in zinc metabolism (28). Factors which may increase the potential for ethambutol ocular toxicity include elderly age (29), impaired renal function, and optic neuritis due to other causes (e.g., tobacco, ethanol, diabetes mellitus).

Pregnancy and Lactation

Ethambutol is FDA pregnancy category B (Appendix I) (30). Ethambutol is compatible with breast-feeding (31).

Clinical Presentation

ACUTE OVERDOSAGE

Reported overdoses often involve other antituberculosis agents such as INH or rifampin. Acute overdose of ethambutol may produce nausea, abdominal pain, fever, mental confusion, visual hallucinations, and optic neuropathy. Acute overdose involving both ethambutol and INH may result in synergistic nervous system toxicity.

ADVERSE EVENTS

Optic neuritis is the principal side effect of ethambutol (32). It is usually dose related and often reversible (27). However, after chronic ethambutol therapy, the optic neuritis is not always reversible, particularly in the elderly (33). Permanent visual disability may result. In four cases of optic neuritis, symptoms developed 2.5, 7.5, 8.0, and 12.0 months after therapy. Three cases had irreversible neuritis, with one patient developing permanent visual impairment (32). In ten consecutive patients with severe ethambutol ocular toxicity, five patients had improvement in visual acuity over 1 to 3 years, and the other five patients recovered visual acuity 4 to 11 months after withdrawal of ethambutol (33).

Anorexia, nausea, vomiting, and abdominal pain may occur. Rare adverse effects include confusion, disorientation, hallucinations; peripheral neuropathy; neutropenia, thrombocytopenia; cholestatic jaundice; and gouty arthritis secondary to hyperuricemia.

Diagnostic Tests

ACUTE OVERDOSAGE

CBC and smear, renal function tests, and liver function tests are recommended. Ocular funduscopic examination, color vision, and visual acuity tests are recommended in overdoses exceeding 10 g.

ADVERSE EVENTS

Renal function tests are needed to determine the correct dose of ethambutol and should be followed at regular intervals. CBCs and uric acid levels should be measured routinely. Periodic visual acuity tests and funduscopic examination should be performed; visual evoked potentials may identify subclinical optic nerve damage.

Treatment

GASTROINTESTINAL DECONTAMINATION

Ethambutol is likely bound by activated charcoal and should be given up to 2 hours after ingestion. There are no data supporting the use of a cathartic or whole bowel irrigation.

ENHANCEMENT OF ELIMINATION

Based on chemistry and pharmacokinetics, ethambutol is likely to be removed by hemodialysis.

ANTIDOTES

Parenteral doses of prednisolone or vitamin B_{12} have been tried in the treatment of optic neuritis with unclear results (34,35).

PITFALLS

An overdose of ethambutol should be taken seriously; the potential for optic nerve damage after large overdose is real.

Most overdoses of antitubercular drugs involve more than one antimycobacterial drug. Drug interactions must be considered in the management of these patients.

ETHIONAMIDE

Ethionamide (Trecator; $C_8H_{10}N_2S$; MW, 166.2 g/mol; CAS Registry No., 536-33-4) is active against a number of atypical mycobacteria. Common adverse effects are GI, neurologic, and dermatologic. No dose-related toxicity has been reported. Ethionamide is a second-line therapy used only in combination with other agents when first-line agents have failed. Concomitant administration of pyridoxine is usually recommended.

Toxic Dose

The *adult therapeutic dose* is 0.5 to 1.0 g/day. The *pediatric dose* is 15 to 20 mg/kg/day in divided doses (maximum of 750 mg/dose or 1 g/day).

No lethal or minimum toxic dose has been reported for adults or children. An adult tolerates 90 mg/kg once per week (36). The oral lethal dose in mice is 1000 mg/kg (37).

Toxicokinetics and Toxicodynamics

Ethionamide is nearly completely absorbed from the GI tract and does not undergo substantial first-pass metabolism. The maximal drug concentration is 90 to 180 minutes after ingestion of a therapeutic dose. It is rapidly distributed to tissues, and total protein binding is 30%. The apparent V_d is approximately 1.2 L/kg. Hepatic metabolism accounts for nearly all of an administered dose. The primary metabolite is the sulfoxide conjugate. Only 1% of a therapeutic dose is excreted unchanged in the urine.

Pathophysiology

The mechanism of encephalopathy is unclear. It is clinically similar to the encephalopathy of pellagra, and nicotinamide blood levels have been decreased during the concomitant administration of INH and ethionamide (38).

Pregnancy and Lactation

Ethionamide is FDA pregnancy category B (Appendix I). There are no data specifically for ethionamide in breast milk, but it has been estimated that with most antituberculosis drugs, a nursing infant receives no more than 20% of a usual therapeutic dose (39).

Clinical Presentation

ACUTE OVERDOSAGE

No cases of acute or subacute overdosage have been reported.

ADVERSE EVENTS

Adverse effects at therapeutic doses have included nausea, vomiting, diarrhea, headache, encephalopathy, psychosis, alopecia, rashes, and hypoglycemia in diabetics. Hepatotoxicity and hypothyroidism may occur.

A reversible encephalopathy in two patients taking ethionamide began with depression and personality changes and progressed to dementia and an inability to walk with plantar extensor responses and painful flexor spasms. Other patients have experienced confusion, irritability, incontinence, difficulty standing and walking, ataxia, slowed mentation, and abnormal reflexes (38). A mild sensory neuropathy has been described as a complication of prolonged ethionamide therapy (40,41).

Hepatotoxicity consists of elevations in serum transaminases, bilirubin, and alkaline phosphatase. In a series of 32 patients treated with ethionamide for tuberculosis or leprosy, nine (28%) patients developed hepatotoxicity (42).

Diabetic patients appear to be more susceptible to the development of hypoglycemia; management is more difficult, and hepatotoxicity may occur more often in this group.

Diagnostic Tests

ACUTE OVERDOSAGE

No cases of acute or subacute overdosage have been reported.

ADVERSE EVENTS

Hepatic and thyroid function tests should be performed regularly. Blood glucose levels, especially in diabetic patients, should be monitored regularly during therapy. Patients with symptoms and signs of peripheral neuropathy should be evaluated by a neurologist.

Treatment

Encephalopathy and neuropathy resolve once ethionamide is discontinued. Adverse reactions or chronic toxicity should be treated with discontinuation of the ethionamide.

GASTROINTESTINAL DECONTAMINATION

A single dose of activated charcoal is recommended within 2 hours of an oral overdose. The use of a cathartic or whole bowel irrigation is not indicated.

ENHANCEMENT OF ELIMINATION

Ethionamide is not dialyzable; only 2.1% of a 500-mg dose was recovered in dialysate (43).

ANTIDOTES

Nicotinamide (100 to 150 mg/day orally) and pyridoxine (100 to 150 mg/day orally) and other B vitamins may be useful in treating toxic encephalopathy. Prophylactic use of vitamins has not been beneficial.

ISONIAZID

Isonazid [Nydrazid; isonicotinic acid hydrazide (INH); $C_6H_7N_3O$; MW, 137.1 g/mol; SI conversion, mg/L × 7.29 = μmol/L; CAS Registry No., 54-85-3] is a first-line antimycobacterial agent that is structurally similar to nicotinic acid. The most common adverse effects are peripheral neuropathy and hepatotoxicity. Acute overdose results in convulsions and metabolic acidosis.

Toxic Dose

The *adult therapeutic dose* of INH is 5 mg/kg/day (up to 300 mg) orally given as a single dose. The *pediatric dose* for preventive therapy is 10 mg/kg/day (up to 300 mg) given orally as a single dose.

Acute ingestion of 10 to 15 g (80 to 150 mg/kg), if untreated, is frequently fatal (44). Acute ingestion of 2 to 3 g (35 to 40 mg/kg) may produce convulsions. Chronic doses of 3 to 5 mg/kg/day are associated with 2% or less toxicity, whereas 10% to 20% of patients have toxic symptoms when the total dose is 10 mg/kg/day (45).

Toxicokinetics and Toxicodynamics

INH is rapidly and completely absorbed orally. The T_{max} is 1 to 2 hours. INH is 10% to 15% protein bound. Cerebrospinal fluid levels are essentially equal to plasma levels 3 to 6 hours after an oral dose (46). The apparent V_d is 0.7 L/kg.

INH is metabolized by the liver at a rate determined by acetylator phenotype. Approximately 50% to 65% of whites, blacks, South Asian Indians, and Mexicans are slow acetylators, whereas 80% to 90% of Inuit, Japanese, and Chinese populations are rapid acetylators (47,48). Fast acetylators excrete approximately 94% of an INH dose as acetyl INH and its metabolites and 6% as free INH and hydrazone conjugates. Slow acetylators excrete approximately 63% of an INH dose as acetyl isoniazid and its metabolites and 37% as free INH and hydrazone conjugates (49). After therapeutic doses, the elimination half-life of INH is 0.7 to 2.0 hours for rapid acetylators and 2.3 to 3.5 hours for slow acetylators (48).

Pathophysiology

INH inhibits a number of enzymes, binds pyridoxal phosphate, and acts as an inactive replacement for nicotinic acid.

INH overdose causes convulsions as a result of a series of events (50). Normally, pyridoxine is converted in the liver to pyridoxal, which, in turn, is converted by pyridoxal kinase to pyridoxal phosphate. Pyridoxal phosphate is a cofactor for the decarboxylation process that converts glutamate to γ-aminobutyric acid, an inhibitory neurotransmitter. In overdose, INH binds with pyridoxine and pyridoxal to form hydrazone complexes, which inhibit pyridoxal kinase and, perhaps, the decarboxylase enzyme. Inhibition of pyridoxal kinase reduces the formation of pyridoxal phosphate. Reduced levels of pyridoxal phosphate (which has an elimination half-life of 2.5 hours) and inhibition of decarboxylation combine to result in reduced levels of γ-aminobutyric acid. Also, reduced conversion of glutamate to γ-aminobutyric acid may result in relatively higher levels of glutamate. Decreased γ-aminobutyric acid reduces inhibition, and increased glutamate increases excitation, resulting in convulsions.

The excessive muscular activity in a generalized tonic-clonic convulsion results in anaerobic metabolism, which produces lactic acid. INH inhibits the conversion of lactate to pyruvate, thus favoring the development of a profound and long-lasting metabolic acidosis.

The cause of INH-induced hepatotoxicity is unknown but may be due to the intracellular accumulation of acetylhydrazine, a metabolite of INH (50). The cause of INH-induced peripheral neuritis is unclear but may be related to pyridoxine deficiency.

Pregnancy and Lactation

INH is FDA pregnancy category C (Appendix I) (51). INH crosses the placenta, and the fetal blood level is similar to the maternal level. After maternal ingestion of INH, 0.75% to 2.30% of the dose is excreted into breast milk in 24 hours. The amount ingested by nursing infants ranged from 0.64 to 2.00 mg/kg. The risk of adverse effects to infants of nursing mothers receiving INH is very low (52).

Clinical Presentation

ACUTE OVERDOSAGE

The hallmark of an acute INH overdose is the rapid development of generalized convulsions and metabolic acidosis. Convulsions often begin within 2 hours and tend to be recurrent as well as resistant to treatment. As a result of the convulsions, a severe metabolic (lactic) acidosis develops, and coma may ensue. Secondary effects may include hypotension, hyperglycemia, elevated hepatic transaminases, rhabdomyolysis, and renal failure.

ADVERSE EVENTS

Peripheral neuritis occurs in 2% to 20% of patients unless pyridoxine is taken concurrently. Factors predisposing to the development of peripheral neuritis include higher doses of INH (more than 5 mg/kg/day), absence of pyridoxine supplements, slow acetylator status, diabetes mellitus, poor nutrition, or anemia. Clinical findings include stocking-glove paresthesias, which may progress proximally and, less common, myalgia and weakness (53,54).

INH-induced hepatotoxicity is more likely with increasing age, slow acetylator status, and initiation of INH therapy within 2 months. Clinical effects include anorexia, nausea, malaise, fatigue, and jaundice; abnormalities in laboratory tests include elevated transaminases and bilirubin (50).

Diagnostic Tests

ACUTE OVERDOSAGE

Blood gas determinations assess metabolic acidosis after convulsions. A CBC, electrolytes, and blood glucose level are recommended. Severe toxicity correlates with serum INH levels above 30 mg/L, although INH blood levels are rarely useful. If the origin of seizures is uncertain, other tests to evaluate their cause should be obtained (Chapter 30).

ADVERSE EVENTS

The diagnosis of hepatotoxicity is based on changes in liver function tests. Serum transaminase levels five times above normal are an indication to discontinue the drug. Peripheral neuropathy may need to be evaluated (Chapter 26).

POSTMORTEM CONSIDERATIONS

Postmortem INH blood levels of 65 to 168 mg/L were found in three patients who died within a few hours of ingestion (55).

INH-induced hepatotoxicity is characterized as bridging and multilobular hepatonecrosis (50).

Treatment

Treatment of the acute overdose should focus primarily on the treatment of convulsions and secondarily on the treatment of metabolic acidosis.

GASTROINTESTINAL DECONTAMINATION

Induced emesis is contraindicated because of the risk of convulsion. A single dose of activated charcoal may be considered within 1 hour of ingestion. The risk of convulsions may preclude its use. Control of the airway should be assured. The use of a cathartic or whole bowel irrigation is not indicated.

ENHANCEMENT OF ELIMINATION

Multiple-dose activated charcoal is not useful. Average removal of the total dose by hemodialysis within 5 hours is 73% (56). The hemodialysis clearance rate of INH is 24 to 49 ml/minute.

ANTIDOTES

Pyridoxine and a benzodiazepine (e.g., diazepam) are always used together for the treatment of INH-induced convulsions (Chapter 71). Although early pyridoxine administration may be associated with fewer complications (57), suggestions that pyridoxine could be used prophylactically in asymptomatic patients with a history of a large INH overdose may be premature. In severely symptomatic patients with seizures, acidosis, and coma, pyridoxine should be given intravenous push (in addition to a benzodiazepine) until seizures are controlled and coma resolves (44,58,59). The amount of pyridoxine should equal the amount of INH ingested. When the INH amount is uncertain, the initial dose of pyridoxine should be 5 g. However, it must be remembered that pyridoxine is not an anticonvulsant.

Diazepam is the anticonvulsant of choice because it acts synergistically with pyridoxine, has strong γ-aminobutyric acid A agonist activity, and has a relatively long duration of action. The initial adult dose of diazepam is 5 to 10 mg IV initially, repeated every 5 to 10 minutes as needed. The pediatric dose is 0.2 to 0.5 mg/kg IV, repeated every 5 minutes as needed.

Midazolam and lorazepam have been suggested as anticonvulsants because of the rapidity of their anticonvulsant effects and because, like diazepam, they have inherent γ-aminobutyric acid A agonist activity. The relatively short duration of action of midazolam may require repeated dosing if prolonged anticonvulsant activity is required. Documented efficacy of midazolam or lorazepam in treating INH-induced convulsions is lacking. Phenobarbital also has γ-aminobutyric acid A agonist activity but is a potent central nervous system depressant. Phenytoin is not recommended in the treatment of INH-induced convulsions.

MONITORING

Observe for symptoms and signs of peripheral neuritis (numbness, tingling, burning or pain in hands or feet, blurred vision, or loss of vision) and liver toxicity in patients receiving INH chronically. Liver function tests should be monitored in patients receiving INH chronically.

MANAGEMENT PITFALLS

The primary pitfalls in the management of an acute INH overdose are inadequate doses of pyridoxine and use of an anticonvulsant other than a benzodiazepine.

PYRAZINAMIDE

Pyrazinamide (Rifater; $C_5H_5N_3O$; MW, 123.1 g/mol; CAS Registry No., 98-96-4) is a synthetic pyrazine analog of nicotinamide used as a first-line agent in the therapy of tuberculosis and has been effective in the treatment of atypical mycobacterial infections. The primary adverse effects are hepatotoxicity and hyperuricemia. No acute toxicity has been reported.

Toxic Dose

The *adult and pediatric dose* for the treatment of tuberculosis is 15 to 30 mg/kg/day up to a maximum of 2 g/day. Larger doses have been used to treat tuberculosis in patients with acquired immunodeficiency syndrome. Alternative treatment regimens use larger doses two or three times weekly.

No fatalities due to pyrazinamide have been reported in adults or children. Daily doses of 40 to 50 mg/kg result in hepatotoxicity in 15% of patients.

Toxicokinetics and Toxicodynamics

Pyrazinamide is very well absorbed from the GI tract; T_{max} is 2 hours after a therapeutic dose. The drug is 10% protein bound, and the apparent V_d is 0.7 L/kg. Pyrazinamide is metabolized to two primary metabolites (pyrazinoic acid and 5-hydroxypyrazinoic acid); less than 4% of the drug is excreted in the urine as unchanged drug. Renal clearance is by glomerular filtration. The elimination half-life is 9 to 10 hours. Dosage reduction is recommended in patients with end-stage renal disease.

Pathophysiology

Pyrazinoic acid, the major metabolite of pyrazinamide, inhibits the renal tubular secretion of uric acid, causing serum uric acid concentrations to rise.

Pregnancy and Lactation

Small amounts of pyrazinamide enter the breast milk (1.5 mg/L after a maternal dose of 1 g). Pyrazinamide should be used with caution in nursing mothers (60).

Clinical Presentation

ACUTE OVERDOSAGE

No cases of acute or subacute overdosage have been reported.

ADVERSE EVENTS

The primary adverse effect of pyrazinamide is liver toxicity. Daily doses of 40 to 50 mg/kg/day result in hepatotoxicity (elevated transaminase levels are the earliest sign) in 15% of patients. Pyrazinamide elevates serum uric acid levels. Uric acid levels above 12 mg/dl occurred in 3.3% of patients receiving a daily regimen of pyrazinamide and rifampin (61). Elevations of serum uric acid concentrations are much more marked during daily rather than intermittent treatment with pyrazinamide (62). The mean uric acid level increased from 3.7 to 5.7 mg/dl in 92% of children receiving pyrazinamide, 20 to 25 mg/kg daily. After cessation of the drug, serum uric acid normalized in all subjects (63).

Other adverse effects associated with pyrazinamide include arthralgia, pellagra, acne, photosensitivity, and, rarely, reversible sideroblastic anemia. Pyrazinamide may make blood glucose control difficult in patients with diabetes mellitus (64).

Diagnostic Tests

ACUTE OVERDOSAGE

No cases of acute or subacute overdosage have been reported.

ADVERSE REACTIONS

Investigations should include a serum uric acid, liver function tests, CBC with differential and smear, and blood glucose levels in diabetic patients.

Treatment

GASTROINTESTINAL DECONTAMINATION

Activated charcoal may prevent absorption of pyrazinamide if given within 1 hour of ingestion. The use of a cathartic or whole bowel irrigation is not indicated.

ENHANCEMENT OF ELIMINATION

Hemodialysis beginning 2 hours after a pyrazinamide dose of 1000 mg results in a median dialysate recovery of 45%. Pyrazinoic acid concentrations are not determined (65).

ANTIDOTES

There are no antidotes for pyrazinamide.

MONITORING

Patients should be monitored for arthralgias developing within the first 1 or 2 months of therapy (66).

RIFAMYCIN DERIVATIVES

The rifamycin derivatives include rifabutin (Mycobutin), rifapentine (Priftin), and rifampin (rifampicin, Rifadin, Rimactane, Rifater; $C_{43}H_{58}N_4O_{12}$; MW, 822.9 g/mol; SI conversion, mg/L × 1.22 = μmol/L; CAS Registry No., 13292-46-1). Common adverse effects include rash, GI intolerance, and neutropenia for rifabutin; hyperuricemia, neutropenia, and lymphopenia for rifapentine; and hepatitis for rifampin.

Rifampin is a first-line agent in the treatment of pulmonary and extrapulmonary tuberculosis. Rifapentine is also used for treatment of pulmonary tuberculosis and has a longer duration of action and potentially greater antimycobacterial efficacy than rifampin. Rifabutin is used for the prevention of *M. avium* disease complex in patients with advanced human immunodeficiency virus infection.

Toxic Dose

The *adult therapeutic doses* of rifamycin derivatives are: rifabutin, 300 mg/day (range, 150 to 600 mg/day) orally; rifampin, 600 mg/day (dosage adjustments should be considered in patients with liver disease); and rifapentine, 600 mg twice weekly in the intensive phase, less frequently in the subsequent continuation phase.

The *pediatric therapeutic doses* of rifamycin derivatives are: rifabutin, 5 mg/kg daily; and rifampin, 10 to 20 mg/kg/day up to a maximum of 600 mg/day (dosage adjustments should be considered in patients with liver disease). The safety and efficacy of rifapentine in children younger than 12 years of age have not been established. The pharmacokinetics in children weighing less than 45 kg who received 450 mg were similar to adults and adolescents receiving 600 mg.

The minimal lethal or toxic doses are not well established. Rifampin doses of 14 and 60 g have been fatal in adults (67,68). No fatalities have been reported due to rifabutin or rifapentine. Children aged 1 to 4 years given rifampin, 100 mg/kg, developed acute toxicity (69). Minimum toxic doses of rifabutin or rifapentine have not been established.

A single 10-g rifampin dose in adults usually produces brownish-red to orange discoloration of the skin, saliva, tears, sweat, urine, and feces. A rifampin dose of 12 g resulted in vomiting and mild liver impairment (70). Healthy volunteers who received single, oral rifapentine doses of 1.2 g experienced no serious adverse events. In clinical trials, patients who received rifapentine, 600 mg daily for up to 20 days, had no evidence of serious adverse effects (71).

Toxicokinetics and Toxicodynamics

Rifabutin (72) has an oral bioavailability of 50%, protein binding of 85%, and an apparent V_d of 9.3 L/kg. The T_{max} is 2 to 4 hours after an oral therapeutic dose. The drug is metabolized in the liver, with an elimination half-life of 45 hours. Approximately 50% is renally excreted.

Rifampin has an oral bioavailability of 90%, protein binding of 90%, and an apparent V_d of 0.9 to 1.6 L/kg. The T_{max} is 2 to 4 hours after an oral therapeutic dose. Rifampin is deacetylated in the liver and eliminated in the bile (70%) and urine (20%). Unchanged rifampin undergoes enterohepatic circulation. Rifampin is a potent inducer of the hepatic microsomal enzyme system. The elimination half-life is 2.1 hours but may be as long as 5 hours in overdose (73).

Rifapentine has a 70% oral bioavailability, protein binding of 98%, and an apparent V_d of 70.2 L/kg. The T_{max} is 3 to 9 hours after an oral therapeutic dose. Rifapentine is metabolized by esterase enzymes to produce a 25-desacetyl–active metabolite. Rifapentine is a potent inducer of hepatic mixed-function oxidase activity. The elimination half-life is 14 to 17 hours (74). Less than 20% is excreted in the urine.

Pathophysiology

The mechanism of toxicity from rifamycin derivatives is unknown.

Pregnancy and Lactation

All three rifamycin derivatives are FDA pregnancy category C (Appendix I).

Rifampin crosses the placenta to produce clinically significant levels in the fetus (75). After maternal ingestion of rifampin, 600 mg, 0.05% of the dose is excreted into breast milk. The amount of rifampin ingested by nursing infants is estimated to be 0.085 mg/kg or 0.57% of the usual pediatric dose (76). Rifapentine is teratogenic in animals at doses similar to those used in humans (on basis of body surface area).

Clinical Presentation

ACUTE OVERDOSAGE

Acute overdose of rifampin typically presents with nausea, vomiting, mental status changes, and a reversible brown-red-orange discoloration of skin, saliva, tears, sweat, urine, and feces ("red man syndrome") (73,77). The average time of onset of the pigmentation is 2.2 hours (range, 0.5 to 24.0 hours) (78). Periorbital or facial edema, red-orange skin discoloration, head pruritus, vomiting, headache, and diarrhea were seen in 19 children, aged 1 to 4 years, inadvertently given rifampin, 100 mg/kg; symptoms began 30 to 240 minutes after ingestion and lasted up to 72 hours (69). Overdoses may result in transiently elevated liver transaminases and can rarely result in seizures, dysrhythmias, pulmonary edema, and death.

ADVERSE EVENTS

Hepatitis secondary to rifampin alone or in combination with INH has been reported frequently. Hepatitis and jaundice may be noted after chronic therapeutic administration of rifamycin derivatives and are most common among patients with chronic liver disease, alcoholism, and old age. Elevated transaminases may occur with therapeutic doses (77).

High and intermittent doses of rifampin have resulted in acute renal failure, acute pancreatitis, thrombocytopenia, hemolysis, and bronchospasm. Rifabutin use has been associated with uveitis (79) and arthralgia. Rifapentine use has been associated with hyperuricemia, neutropenia, and lymphopenia. Rifabutin may cause rash, GI intolerance, neutropenia, or uveitis.

Diagnostic Tests

ACUTE OVERDOSAGE

Liver function tests should be performed on all overdose patients. A chest radiograph should be performed because overdose with these drugs can rarely result in pulmonary edema. An electrocardiogram is needed to evaluate cardiac conduction abnormalities.

ADVERSE EVENTS

All patients should be monitored closely for signs and symptoms of liver, kidney, and hematologic toxicity.

POSTMORTEM CONSIDERATIONS

Death was attributed to pulmonary edema in one case (68). Nonspecific interstitial shadowing on chest radiograph in a fatal rifampin overdose has been reported (67).

Treatment

Treatment is symptomatic and supportive. The red man syndrome resolves spontaneously.

GASTROINTESTINAL DECONTAMINATION

The rifamycin derivatives should be bound by activated charcoal. Administration within 2 hours is recommended. The use of a cathartic or whole bowel irrigation is not indicated.

ENHANCEMENT OF ELIMINATION

Extracorporeal removal techniques are unlikely to result in significant clearance of these drugs.

ANTIDOTES

There are no specific antidotes to the rifamycin derivatives.

MONITORING

Elevated hepatic transaminases should be followed until they return to normal. Monitoring for thrombocytopenia and neutropenia is appropriate.

REFERENCES

1. Peloquin CA, Henshaw TL, Huitt GA, et al. Pharmacokinetic evaluation of para-aminosalicylic acid granules. *Pharmacotherapy* 1994;14:40–46.
2. Briggs GG, Freeman RK, Yaffee SJ. *Drugs in pregnancy and lactation: a reference guide to fetal and neonatal risk,* 5th ed. Baltimore, MD: Williams & Wilkins, 1998.
3. Nariman S. Adverse reactions to drugs used in the treatment of tuberculosis. *Adverse Drug React Acute Poisoning Rev* 1988;4:207–227.
4. Malone RS, Fish DN, Spiegel DM, et al. The effect of hemodialysis on cycloserine, ethionamide, para-aminosalicylate, and clofazimine. *Chest* 1999;116:984–990.
5. Registry of Toxic Effects of Chemical Substances. National Institute for Occupational Safety and Health, Cincinnati (Internet version). Englewood, CO: Micromedex, Inc, 2000.
6. Lehmann CR, Garrett LE, Winn RE, et al. Capreomycin kinetics in renal impairment and clearance by hemodialysis. *Am Rev Respir Dis* 1988;138:1312–1313.
7. Bennett WM, Aronoff GR, Golper TA. Drug prescribing. In: *Renal failure,* 3rd ed. Philadelphia: American College of Physicians, 1994.
8. Hardman JE, Limbird LE. *Goodman & Gilman's the pharmacological basis of therapeutics,* 9th ed. New York: McGraw-Hill, 1996:1712–1792.
9. Mandell GL, Petri WA Jr. Antimicrobial agents (continued). In: Hardman JE, Limbird LE, eds. *Goodman & Gilman's the pharmacological basis of therapeutics,* 9th ed. New York: McGraw-Hill, 1996:1155–1174.
10. Kropp R, Jungbluth H, Radenbach KL. Influence of capreomycin on renal function (preliminary results). *Antibiot Chemother* 1970;16:59–68.
11. Zhu M, Nix DE, Adam RD, et al. Pharmacokinetics of cycloserine under fasting conditions and with high-fat meal, orange juice, and antacids. *Pharmacotherapy* 2001;21:891–897.
12. Goff DC, Tsai G, Manoach DS, et al. D-Cycloserine added to clozapine for patients with schizophrenia. *Am J Psychiatry* 1996;153:1628–1630.
13. Tsai GE, Falk WE, Gunther J, Coyle JT. Improved cognition in Alzheimer's disease with short-term D-cycloserine treatment. *Am J Psychiatry* 1999;156:467–469.
14. Snider D, Powell KE. Should women taking antituberculosis drugs breastfeed? *Arch Int Med* 1984;144:589–590.
15. Mandell GL, Bennett JE, Dolin R. *Principles and practice of infectious diseases,* 4th ed. New York: Wiley Medical Publication, 1995.
16. American Academy of Pediatrics Committee on Drugs. The transfer of drugs and other chemicals into human milk. *Pediatrics* 1994;93:137–150.
17. Mandell GL, Petri WA Jr. Antimicrobial agents (continued). In: Hardman JE, Limbird LE, eds. *Goodman & Gilman's the pharmacological basis of therapeutics,* 9th ed. New York: McGraw-Hill, 1996:1155–1174.
18. Helmy B. Side effects of cycloserine. *Scand Respir Dis Suppl* 1970;71:220–225.
19. Seromycin, cycloserine. Product information. Indianapolis: Eli Lilly and Company, 1995.
20. Malone RS, Fish DN, Spiegel DM, et al. The effect of hemodialysis on cycloserine, ethionamide, para-aminosalicylate, and clofazimine. *Chest* 1999;116:984–990.
21. Benitz WE, Tatro DS. *The pediatric drug handbook,* 3rd ed. St. Louis: Mosby-Year Book, Inc., 1995.
22. Anonymous. Treatment of tuberculosis and tuberculosis infection in adults and children. *Am J Respir Crit Care Med* 1994;149:1359–1374.
23. Roberts SM. A review of the papers on the ocular toxicity of ethambutol hydrochloride, (Myambutol), an anti-tuberculous drug. *Am J Optom Physiol Opt* 1974;51:987–992.
24. Citron KM, Thomas GO. Ocular toxicity from ethambutol. *Thorax* 1986;41:737–739.
25. Ducobu J, Dupont P, Laurent M, Bruart J. Acute isoniazid/ethambutol/rifampin overdose [Letter]. *Lancet* 1982;1:632.
26. Aronoff GR, Berns JS, Brier ME, et al., eds. *Drug prescribing in renal failure,* 4th ed. Philadelphia: American College of Physicians, 1999:56.
27. Schild HS, Fox BC. Rapid-onset reversible ocular toxicity from ethambutol therapy. *Am J Med* 1991;90:404–406.
28. Lessell S. Histopathology of experimental intoxication. *Invest Ophthalmol Vis Sci* 1976;15:765–769.
29. Fledelius HC, Petrera JE, Skjodt K, Trojborg W. Ocular ethambutol toxicity. A case report with electrophysiological considerations and a review of Danish cases 1972-81. *Acta Ophthalmol (Copenh)* 1987;65:251–255.
30. Briggs GG, Freeman RK, Yaffe SJ. *Drugs in pregnancy and lactation,* 5th ed. Baltimore: Williams & Wilkins, 1998.
31. American Academy of Pediatrics Committee on Drugs. The transfer of drugs and other chemicals into human milk. *Pediatrics* 1994;93:137–150.
32. Sivakumaran P, Harrison AC, Marschner J, Martin P. Ocular toxicity from ethambutol: a review of four cases and recommended precautions. *N Z Med J* 1998;111:428–430.
33. Tsai RK, Lee YH. Reversibility of ethambutol optic neuropathy. *J Ocul Pharmacol Ther* 1997;13:473–477.
34. Chatterjee VK, Buchanan DR, Friedmann AI, Green M. Ocular toxicity following ethambutol in standard dosage. *Br J Dis Chest* 1986;80:288–291.
35. Guerra R, Casu L. Hydroxycobalamine for ethambutol-induced optic neuropathy. *Lancet* 1981;2:1176.
36. Anonymous. A controlled trial of daily and intermittent rifampicin plus ethambutol in the retreatment of patients with pulmonary tuberculosis: results up to 30 months. *Tubercle* 1975;56:179–189.
37. Registry of Toxic Effects of Chemical Substances. National Institute for Occupational Safety and Health, Cincinnati (Internet version). Englewood, CO: Micromedex, Inc., 2001.
38. Swash M, Roberts AH, Murnaghan DJ. Reversible pellagra-like encephalopathy with ethionamide and cycloserine. *Tubercle* 1972;53:132–136.
39. Holdiness MR. Clinical pharmacokinetics of the antituberculosis drugs. *Clin Pharmacokinet* 1984;9:511–544.

40. Girling DJ. Adverse effects of antituberculosis drugs. *Drugs* 1982;23:56–74.
41. Hudgson P. Adverse drug reactions in the neuromuscular apparatus. *Adverse Drug React Acute Poisoning Rev* 1982;1:35–64.
42. de Carsalade GY, Wallach D, Spindler E, et al. Daily multidrug therapy for leprosy; results of a fourteen-year experience. *Int J Lepr Other Mycobact Dis* 1997;65:37–44.
43. Malone RS, Fish DN, Spiegel DM, et al. The effect of hemodialysis on cycloserine, ethionamide, para-aminosalicylate, and clofazimine. *Chest* 1999;116:984–990.
44. Sievers ML, Herrier RN, Chin L, Picchioni AL. Treatment of isoniazid overdose. *J Am Med Assoc* 1982;247:583–584.
45. Kastrup ED. *Facts and comparisons*. St. Louis: JB Lippincott Co., 1986:384.
46. Donald PR, Gent WL, Seifart HI, et al. Cerebrospinal fluid isoniazid concentrations in children with tuberculous meningitis: the influence of dosage and acetylation status. *Pediatrics* 1992;89:247–250.
47. Iselius L, Evans DA. Formal genetics of isoniazid metabolism in man. *Clin Pharmacokinet* 1983;8:541–544.
48. Ellard GA. The potential clinical significance of the isoniazid acetylator phenotype in the treatment of pulmonary tuberculosis. *Tubercle* 1984;65:211–227.
49. Holdiness MR. Clinical pharmacokinetics of the antituberculosis drugs. *Clin Pharmacokinet* 1984;9:511–544.
50. Mandell GL, Petri WA Jr. Antimicrobial agents (continued). In: Hardman JE, Limbird LE, eds. *Goodman & Gilman's the pharmacological basis of therapeutics*, 9th ed. New York: McGraw-Hill, 1996:1155–1174.
51. Briggs GG, Freeman RK, Yaffe SJ. *Drugs in pregnancy and lactation*, 5th ed. Baltimore: Williams & Wilkins, 1998.
52. Snider DE, Powell KE. Should women taking anti-tuberculosis drugs breastfeed? *Arch Intern Med* 1984;144:589–590.
53. Holdiness MR. Neurological manifestations and toxicities of the antituberculosis drugs—a review. *Med Toxicol* 1987;2:33–51.
54. Siskind MS, Thienemann D, Kirlin L. Isoniazid-induced neurotoxicity in chronic dialysis patients: report of three cases and a review of the literature. *Nephron* 1993;64:303–306.
55. Baselt RC. *Disposition of toxic drugs and chemicals in man*, 5th ed. Foster City, CA: Chemical Toxicology Institute, 2000:446–449.
56. Gold CH, Buchanan N, Tringham V, et al. Isoniazid pharmacokinetics in patients with chronic renal failure. *Clin Nephrol* 1976;6:355–359.
57. Cash JM, Zawada ET. Isoniazid overdose; successful treatment with pyridoxine and hemodialysis. *West J Med* 1991;155:644–646.
58. Yarbrough BE, Wood JP. Isoniazid overdose treated with high-dose pyridoxine. *Ann Emerg Med* 1983;12:303–305.
59. Brent J, Vo N, Kulig K, Rumack BH. Reversal of prolonged isoniazid-induced coma by pyridoxine. *Arch Intern Med* 1990;150:1751–1753.
60. Holdiness MR. Antituberculosis drugs and breast-feeding [Letter]. *Arch Int Med* 1984;144:1888.
61. Gordin F, Chaisson RE, Matts JP, et al. Rifampin and pyrazinamide vs isoniazid for prevention of tuberculosis in HIV-infected persons. An international randomized trial. *J Am Med Assoc* 2000;283:1445–1450.
62. Ellard GA, Haslam RM. Observations on the reduction of the renal elimination of urate in man. *Tubercle* 1976;57:97–103.
63. Sanchez-Albisua I, Vidal ML, Joya-Verde G, et al. Tolerance of pyrazinamide in short course chemotherapy for pulmonary tuberculosis in children. *Pediatr Infect Dis J* 1997;16:760–763.
64. Nariman S. Adverse reactions to drugs used in the treatment of tuberculosis. *Adverse Drug React Acute Poisoning Rev* 1988;4:207–227.
65. Malone RS, Fish DN, Spiegel DM, et al. The effect of hemodialysis on cycloserine, ethionamide, para-aminosalicylate, and clofazimine. *Chest* 1999;116:984–990.
66. Horsfall PA, Plummer J, Allan WG, et al. Double blind controlled comparison of aspirin, allopurinol and placebo in the management of arthralgia during pyrazinamide administration. *Tubercle* 1979;60:13–24.
67. Broadwell RO, Broadwell SD, Comer PB. Suicide by rifampin overdose. *J Am Med Assoc* 1978;240:2283–2284.
68. Plomp TA, Battista HJ, Unterdorfer H, et al. A case of fatal poisoning by rifampicin. *Arch Toxicol* 1981;48:245–252.
69. Bolan G, Laurie RE, Broome CV. Red man syndrome: inadvertent administration of an excessive dose of rifampin to children in a day-care center. *Pediatrics* 1986;77:633–635.
70. Product information. Rifampin. Strasbourg, Germany: Hoechst Marion Roussel, 1996.
71. Product information. Rifapentine. Strasbourg, Germany: Hoechst Marion Roussel, 1998.
72. Skinner MH, Hsieh M, Torseth J, et al. Pharmacokinetics of rifabutin. *Antimicrob Agents Chemother* 1989;33:1237–1241.
73. Wong P, Bottorff MB, Heritage RW, et al. Acute rifampin overdose: a pharmacokinetic study and review of the literature. *J Pediatr* 1984;104:781–783.
74. Vital Durand D, Hampden C, Boobis AR, et al. Induction of mixed function oxidase activity in man by rifapentine (MDL 473), a long-acting rifamycin derivative. *Br J Clin Pharmacol* 1986;21:1–7.
75. Ginsburg CM, McCracken GH. Comparison of salivary concentrations of rifampin and cefaclor: a rationale for chemoprophylaxis of *Haemophilus influenzae* type b disease. *Clin Pediatr* 1982;21:397–399.
76. Snider DE, Powell KE. Should women taking anti-tuberculosis drugs breastfeed? *Arch Int Med* 1984;144:589–590.
77. Villarino ME, Ridzon R, Weismuller PC, et al. Rifampin preventive therapy for tuberculosis infection. Experience with 157 adolescents. *Am J Respir Crit Care Med* 1997;155:1735–1738.
78. Holdiness MR. A review of the red man syndrome and rifampicin overdosage. *Med Toxicol Adverse Drug Exper* 1989;4:444–451.
79. Vaudaux JD, Guex-Crosier Y. Rifabutin-induced cystoid macular edema. *J Antimicrob Chemother* 2002;49:421–422.

CHAPTER 92

Antiviral Drugs

Katherine M. Hurlbut

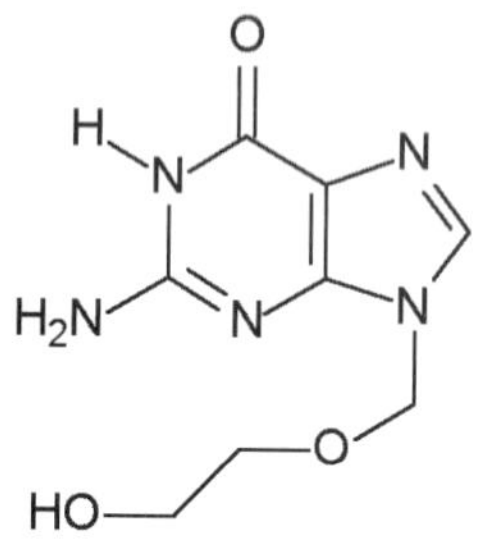

O
H N N
H₂N N N
O
HO

ACYCLOVIR

Compounds included:	**See Table 1.**
Molecular formula and weight:	**See text.**
SI conversion:	**See Table 1.**
CAS Registry No.:	**See text.**
Therapeutic levels:	**Not used clinically**
Target organs:	**Kidney (acute or chronic), liver (chronic), bone marrow (chronic), heart (acute or chronic), central nervous system (acute or chronic), electrolyte disturbances (acute or chronic)**
Antidote:	**None**

ACYCLOVIR

Acyclovir [Zovirax; $C_8H_{11}N_5O_3$; molecular weight (MW), 225.2 g/mol; CAS Registry No., 69657-51-8] is used in various varicella and herpes infections. It is supplied as capsules of 100 mg, 400 mg, or 800 mg as well as suspensions and as an ointment.

Toxic Dose

The usual *adult therapeutic dose* is 5 to 20 mg/kg intravenously (IV). Oral regimens range from 200 mg five times daily to 800 mg five times daily, depending on the type of infection being treated (1). The usual *pediatric dosage* is 5 to 20 mg/kg every 8 hours IV. The oral dose for varicella is 20 mg/kg four times daily (1). The dose is reduced in patients with renal insufficiency.

Two neonates who received 60 mg/kg and 100 mg/kg acyclovir IV, respectively, did not develop evidence of neurologic or renal toxicity (2). Overdoses of up to 20 g in adults have resulted in lethargy, agitation, coma, seizures, and acute renal failure. A lethal dose has not been established.

Toxicokinetics and Toxicodynamics

Pharmacokinetic parameters of acyclovir are provided in Table 2. The half-life is prolonged in patients with impaired renal function.

Pathophysiology

Acyclovir triphosphate (formed intracellularly) binds viral DNA polymerase in competition with guanosine and is incorporated into viral DNA, preventing further elongation of the chain (3).

Pregnancy and Lactation

Acyclovir is U.S. Food and Drug Administration (FDA) category B (Appendix I). Acyclovir is concentrated in breast milk, and the milk to serum ratio is 0.6:4.1 (4,5). Because the amount ingested by the nursing infant is small, it is considered compatible with breast-feeding (6).

Clinical Presentation

ACUTE OR REPEATED OVERDOSAGE

The manufacturer reports overdoses of up to 20 g in adults. Overdoses reported to the manufacturer have resulted in acute renal failure, agitation, coma, seizures, and lethargy (1).

A neonate received 100 mg/kg three times a day for 4 days and developed transient renal insufficiency. Peak creatinine was 211 µmol/L on the fifth day (7). Another neonate received acyclovir, 750 mg IV (220 mg/kg/dose), after having received five dos-

TABLE 1. Compounds included and SI conversion

Compound	SI conversion
Acyclovir (Vistide, Zovirax)	mg/L × 4.4 = µmol/L
Adefovir (Hepsera)	mg/L × 3.6 = µmol/L
Alpha interferons (Roferon-A, Intron A, Alferon N, Infergen)	—
Amantadine hydrochloride (Symmetrel, Protexin)	mg/L × 5.3 = µmol/L
Cidofovir (Vistide)	mg/L × 3.6 = µmol/L
Famciclovir (Famvir)	mg/L × 3.1 = µmol/L
Foscarnet (Foscavir, Virudin)	mg/L × 3.3 = µmol/L
Ganciclovir (Cytovene, Vitrasert)	mg/L × 3.6 = µmol/L
Oseltamivir (Tamiflu)	mg/L × 2.4 = µmol/L
Palivizumab (Synagis)	—
Peginterferon alphas (Pegasys, PEG-Intron)	—
Ribavirin (Rebetol, Virazole)	mg/L × 4.1 = µmol/L
Rimantadine (Flumadine)	—
Valacyclovir (Valtrex)	mg/L × 2.8 = µmol/L
Valganciclovir (Valcyte)	mg/L × 2.5 = µmol/L
Zanamivir (Relenza)	mg/L × 3.0 = µmol/L

ages at 10 mg/kg/dose every 8 hours. A clinically insignificant transient rise in serum creatinine from 0.5 to 0.7 mg/dl, which returned to baseline within 66 hours, was the only manifestation of toxicity noted (8). A 2-year-old child developed increasing agitation and confusion over several hours after being given acyclovir, 800 mg IV. Serum creatinine levels increased but gradually returned to normal over the next 2 days (9).

ADVERSE EVENTS

A 68-year-old man with chronic renal failure developed progressive somnolence progressing to coma after receiving acyclovir, 600 mg orally four times daily for 1 week. Neurologic and renal function improved after 3 days of intermittent hemodialysis (10). A 77-year-old woman developed delayed neurotoxicity 24 to 48 hours after receiving 6 g IV over 2 days (11).

Neurotoxicity develops in approximately 1% of patients receiving IV acyclovir. It is more common after IV administration rather than after oral administration and occurs more frequently with high-dose therapy and in patients with renal insufficiency. Common manifestations of neurotoxicity include confusion, lethargy, hallucinations, fasciculations, and myoclonic jerks; agitation and coma occur in severe cases (12). Headache, nausea, and vomiting are also common with therapeutic doses. Increases in serum blood urea nitrogen and creatinine are common and may develop in up to 10% of patients receiving IV bolus therapy or high oral doses (13,14). Renal insufficiency is usually reversible. Acute renal failure has also been reported. Precipitation of acyclovir crystals may be noted in the urine (15).

Diagnostic Tests

Monitor renal function, urinalysis, and urine output in all overdose patients. Acyclovir crystals (fine, elongated, rectangular crystals) are sometimes identified on microscopic examination of the urine (16).

Acyclovir concentration can be determined in plasma by radioimmunoassay or high-performance liquid chromatography (11,17). Acyclovir concentrations are useful to confirm overdose but do not guide patient management or predict outcome. An oral 400-mg dose in pregnant women (36 to 38 weeks) produced a maximum acyclovir concentration of 0.7 μg/ml (18).

Treatment

GASTROINTESTINAL DECONTAMINATION

Oral activated charcoal is sufficient decontamination after overdose ingestion.

ENHANCEMENT OF ELIMINATION

Acyclovir can be removed by hemodialysis (1). Although use of hemodialysis has not yet been reported in the management of overdose, it might be warranted in a patient with preexisting renal insufficiency and severe overdose.

ANTIDOTES

There is no antidote for acyclovir overdosage.

SUPPORTIVE CARE

Administer sufficient IV fluids to maintain brisk urine output in an attempt to minimize the precipitation of acyclovir crystals in renal tubules. Monitor intravascular volume carefully. Alterations in mental status generally resolve over several days with discontinuation of the drug. Seizures are usually not protracted and respond to benzodiazepines.

ADEFOVIR

Adefovir dipivoxil (Hepsera; $C_{20}H_{32}N_5O_8P$; MW, 273.2 g/mol; CAS Registry No., 142340-99-6) is used primarily for human immunodeficiency virus and hepatitis B infections. It is available as a 10-mg tablet.

Toxic Dose

The usual *adult dose* for hepatitis B is 10 mg/day orally. No overdose data are available.

Toxicokinetics and Toxicodynamics

Pharmacokinetic parameters of adefovir are provided in Table 2. Oral form (adefovir dipivoxil) is converted to active adefovir by enzymes in intestinal epithelium. Forty-five percent of an oral dose and 98% of an IV dose are excreted unchanged in urine.

Pathophysiology

Adefovir is phosphorylated intracellularly to its active form (adefovir diphosphate), which inhibits reverse transcriptase/DNA polymerase by competing with deoxyadenosine triphosphate and causing DNA chain termination after incorporation into viral DNA (19,20).

Pregnancy and Lactation

Adefovir is FDA pregnancy category C (Appendix I). Excretion into breast milk is unknown.

Clinical Presentation

ACUTE OVERDOSAGE

No overdose data are available.

ADVERSE EVENTS

Headache, fatigue, nausea, vomiting, and diarrhea are common adverse effects with therapeutic use. Long-term therapy is associated with a relatively high incidence of nephrotoxicity. Nephrotoxicity is more common in patients with underlying renal insufficiency. In one study, 35% of patients treated for 48 weeks developed an increase in serum creatinine of 0.5 mg/dl or more, and 50% of patients developed a creatinine increase of that magnitude after 72 weeks of therapy (21).

Elevated serum transaminases are common, and hepatic failure has been reported (20). In a study of patients receiving adefovir, 20% developed an increase in serum aspartate aminotransferase, whereas 28% developed increased serum alanine aminotransferase concentrations (21).

Diagnostic Tests

Monitor renal function tests and hepatic enzyme concentrations after overdose and during therapeutic use.

Treatment

Medical care is primarily symptomatic and supportive.

GASTROINTESTINAL DECONTAMINATION

Activated charcoal is sufficient gastrointestinal decontamination.

ENHANCEMENT OF ELIMINATION

Based on pharmacokinetic parameters, it is likely that adefovir could be removed by hemodialysis.

TABLE 2. Selected pharmacokinetic/pharmacodynamic parameters of antiviral drugs

Parameter	Acyclovir[a]	Adefovir[b]	Amantadine[c]	Cidofovir[d]	Famciclovir[e]	Foscarnet[f]	Ganciclovir[g]	Oseltamivir[h]	Palivizumab[i]
Time to maximum serum concentration (h)	1.5–2.4	1.75	1.5–8.0	NR	0.7–0.9	NR	NR	1–4 (animals)	48
Bioavailability (%)	10–20	59	86–94	NR	75–77	Poor	5	75	Good
Protein binding (%)	9–33	4	59–67	0.5	<20	14–17	1–2	42	NR
Apparent volume of distribution	0.8 L/kg	0.4 L/kg	4.5–4.8 L/kg	0.5 L/kg	1.08 L/kg	0.30–0.74 L/kg	0.74 ± 0.15 L/kg	23–26 L	NR
Metabolism	NR	Negligible, hepatic	Little	Minimal	Extensive hepatic to active form penciclovir	NR	NR	Hepatic (extensive); also blood and peripheral tissue esterases	NR
Renal excretion (%)	62–91	45, PO; 98, IV	Primarily unchanged	84–98	73 (negligible unchanged)	73–94	81–100	99	NR
Terminal half-life	2.5 h	7.5 h	10–14 h	2.5 h	2.0–2.3 h	3–6 h	2–5 h	1–3 h; 6–10 h oseltamivir carboxylate (active)	13–27 d

NR, not reported.
[a]From Kimberlin DE, Weller S, Whitley RJ, et al. Pharmacokinetics of oral valacyclovir and acyclovir in late pregnancy. *Am J Obstet Gynecol* 1998;179:486–491; Zovirax, acyclovir. Product information. Research Triangle Park, NC: Glaxo Wellcome Inc., 2002; and de Miranda P, Good SS, Laskin OL, et al. Disposition of intravenous radioactive acyclovir. *Clin Pharmacol Ther* 1981;30:662–672, with permission.
[b]From references 19 and 20.
[c]From Aoki FY, Sitar DS. Clinical pharmacokinetics of amantadine hydrochloride. *Clin Pharmacokinet* 1988;14:35–51; Wu MJ, Ing TS, Soung LS, et al. Amantadine hydrochloride pharmacokinetics in patients with impaired renal function. *Clin Nephrol* 1982;17:19–23; and Symmetrel, amantadine. Product information. Wilmington, DE: DuPont Pharmaceuticals, 2001, with permission.
[d]From Cundy KC, Petty BG, Flaherty J, et al. Clinical pharmacokinetics of cidofovir in human immunodeficiency virus-infected patients. *Antimicrob Agents Chemother* 1995;39:1247–1252, with permission.
[e]From reference 47.
[f]From reference 49.
[g]From Cytovene, ganciclovir injection and capsules. Product information. Nutley, NJ: Roche Laboratories, Inc., 2002; Jung D, Griffy K, Wong R, et al. Absolute bioavailability and dose proportionality of oral ganciclovir after ascending multiple doses in human immunodeficiency virus (HIV)-positive patients. *J Clin Pharmacol* 1998;38:1122–1128; and Laskin OL, Cederberg DM, Mills J, et al. Ganciclovir for the treatment and suppression of serious infections caused by cytomegalovirus. *Am J Med* 1987;83:201–207, with permission.
[h]From references 76 and 77.
[i]From Subramanian KNS, Weisman LE, Rhodes T, et al. Safety, tolerance and pharmacokinetics of a humanized monoclonal antibody to respiratory syncytial virus in premature infants and infants with bronchopulmonary dysplasia. *Pediatr Infect Dis J* 1998;17:110–115; and Product information. Synagis, Palivizumab. Gaithersburg, MD: Medimmune Inc., 2003, with permission.

ANTIDOTES

There is no antidote.

SUPPORTIVE CARE

Maintain adequate urine output. Admit patients with elevated renal function tests or hepatic enzyme levels after overdose.

AMANTADINE

Amantadine hydrochloride (Symmetrel, Protexin, many others; $C_{10}H_{17}N,HCl$; MW, 187.7 g/mol; CAS Registry No., 665-66-7) is used in the treatment of influenza and for Parkinson's disease. It is available as a 100-mg capsule and a 10-mg/ml syrup. It has been reported to cause anticholinergic and cardiac toxicity.

Toxic Dose

The usual *adult therapeutic dosage* is 200 mg/day. The usual *pediatric dosage* for children younger than 10 years of age (or less than 40 kg regardless of age) is 5 mg/kg/day. The dosage should not exceed 150 mg/day in children younger than 10 years of age.

Fatalities in adults have been reported after ingestion of as little as 2 g (22). Ingestion of 2.8 g by an adult and 600 mg by a 2-year-old child caused agitated delirium, but both patients survived (23,24).

Toxicokinetics and Toxicodynamics

Pharmacokinetic parameters of amantadine are provided in Table 2. Amantadine is primarily excreted unchanged in urine, with 0.6% fecal elimination.

Parameter	Ribavirin[j]	Rimantadine[k]	Valacyclovir[l]	Valganciclovir[m]	Zanamivir[n]	Interferon-alpha-2a[o]	Interferon-alpha-2b[p]	Interferon-alpha-n3[q]	Interferon-alphacon-1[r]
Time to maximum serum concentration (h)	1.0–1.6	2–6	1–3	0.50–0.75	0.75–2.0, PO; 1–2, nasal	4, IM; 7, SQ	3–12	6, IM; 8.5, SQ	6, IM; 4–6, SC
Bioavailability (%)	20–64	~100	55	60	2, PO; 10, nasal	80, IM; 90, SQ	NR	NR	80% (animals)
Protein binding (%)	None	40	13–18	NR	NR	NR	NR	NR	NR
Apparent volume of distribution	802 L	720–986 L	NR	NR	16 L	0.22–0.75 L/kg	NR	NR	NR
Metabolism	NR	Extensive hepatic	Extensive hepatic to active form acyclovir	Hydrolyzed in plasma to active ganciclovir	Minimal	Minimal, hepatic	Minimal	Minimal	NR
Renal excretion (%)	40	92 (<1 unchanged)	42 (<1 unchanged)	NR	87, IV	Completely	Completely	Completely	NR
Terminal half-life	24–36 h, single dose; 151 h, prolonged therapy	20–37 h	<30 min	0.4–0.6 h	1.6–5.1 h	3.7–8.5 h	2–3 h	4.4–6.8 h	0.5–7.0 h

[j]From references 94 and 95.
[k]From Wintermeyer SM, Nahata MC. Rimantadine: a clinical perspective. *Ann Pharmacother* 1995;29:299–310; and Hayden FG, Minocha A, Spyker DA, et al. Comparative single-dose pharmacokinetics of amantadine hydrochloride and rimantadine hydrochloride in young and elderly adults. *Antimicrob Agents Chemother* 1985;28:216–221, with permission.
[l]From Weller S, Blum MR, Doucette M, et al. Pharmacokinetics of the acyclovir pro-drug valaciclovir after escalating single- and multiple-dose administration to normal volunteers. *Clin Pharmacol Ther* 1993;54:595–605; and Acosta EP, Fletcher CV. Valacyclovir. *Ann Pharmacother* 1997;31:185–191, with permission.
[m]From references 112 and 113.
[n]Cass LMR, Efthymiopoulos C, Bye A. Pharmacokinetics of zanamivir after intravenous, oral, inhaled or intranasal administration to healthy volunteers. *Clin Pharmacokinet* 1999;36[Suppl 1]:1–11, with permission.
[o]From Roferon-A, interferon alfa-2a recombinant. Product information. Nutley, NJ: Roche Laboratories, 2001; and Wills RJ, Dennis S, Spiegel HE, et al. Interferon kinetics and adverse reactions after intravenous, intramuscular, and subcutaneous injection. *Clin Pharmacol Ther* 1984;35:722–727, with permission.
[p]From reference 65, with permission.
[q]From Sturgill MG, Rashidbaigi A, Liao MJ, et al. Extravascular administration of interferon alpha-N3 increases serum exposure and 2-5(A) synthetase activity. *J Clin Pharmacol* 2000;40:606–615, with permission.
[r]From Neidhart JA, Schmidt S, Rosenblum M, et al. Phase I study of recombinant methionyl human consensus interferon (r-metHuIFN-Con1). *J Biol Resp Modifiers* 1988;7:240–248, with permission.

Pathophysiology

The antiviral mechanism has not been completely elucidated. Amantadine blocks penetration of virus into host cells and blocks uncoating of virus and release of nucleic acids once viral penetration has occurred (25). Amantadine also increases dopaminergic activity in the peripheral nervous system and central nervous system (CNS) by augmenting the release and inhibiting reuptake of dopamine (26).

Pregnancy and Lactation

Amantadine is FDA pregnancy category C (Appendix I). Amantadine does enter breast milk, and breast-feeding is contraindicated.

Clinical Presentation

ACUTE OVERDOSAGE

Anticholinergic effects, such as tachycardia, mydriasis, urinary retention, and dry mouth, are fairly common after amantadine overdose (27–29). Severe hyperthermia (up to 42°C) has been reported after overdose and may persist for several days (28,30).

Severe overdose can cause prolonged QTc and QRS widening (28). These patients may progress to torsade de pointes, ventricular tachycardia, or ventricular fibrillation (30,31). Acute respiratory distress syndrome may develop in patients with severe manifestations of overdose, most often in those with significant cardiac toxicity (28,30,31).

Agitated delirium with hallucinations, disorientation, aggression, and confusion can develop after significant overdose (22–24,27,32). Seizures develop in a minority of these patients (23,27,28). Ataxia, lethargy, CNS depression, and severe cases of coma have also been reported (30,33). Rhabdomyolysis has been reported in patients with agitated delirium (27,28).

ADVERSE EVENTS

CNS adverse effects are common with amantadine therapy. Confusion, disorientation, mood and memory disturbance, delusions, paranoia, nightmares, and insomnia are among the more common CNS effects reported (29,34,35). Neuroleptic malignant syndrome has rarely been reported after withdrawal or dose reduction of amantadine (36,37).

Diagnostic Tests

Monitor serum electrolytes and electrocardiogram (ECG), with special attention to QTc interval. Monitor creatine kinase in patients with prolonged agitation or severe hyperthermia.

Treatment

GASTROINTESTINAL DECONTAMINATION

Gastric lavage should be considered after a large, recent ingestion, as overdose can cause fatal ventricular dysrhythmias. Administer activated charcoal. Meticulous monitoring for ECG changes and dysrhythmias and evaluation of mental status are crucial.

ENHANCED ELIMINATION

Hemodialysis is not effective for amantadine.

ANTIDOTES

QRS widening may respond to sodium bicarbonate. Administer an initial dose of 1 to 2 mEq/kg IV bolus and repeat as needed. Monitor serial ECG and arterial blood gases. The arterial pH should not exceed 7.55 (Chapter 75). In one case report, QTc prolongation improved after administration of IV sodium bicarbonate (28).

Torsade de pointes is treated with magnesium (2 g IV infusion over 5 minutes, repeated if recurrent dysrhythmias develop). Monitor ECG, neurologic examination, and serum magnesium levels. Overdrive pacing or isoproterenol infusion are alternatives in patients who are not responsive to magnesium.

Agitation is usually responsive to sedation with benzodiazepines. Physostigmine has been used successfully to treat anticholinergic delirium from amantadine poisoning (29,38). Because amantadine overdose can cause dysrhythmias and seizures, benzodiazepines are generally preferred.

CIDOFOVIR

Cidofovir (Vistide; $C_8H_{14}N_3O_6P$; MW, 279.2 g/mol; CAS Registry No., 149394-66-1) is associated primarily with ocular, hematologic, and renal toxicity.

Toxic Dose

The usual *therapeutic dosage* for cytomegalovirus (CMV) retinitis is 5 mg/kg once weekly for 2 weeks then 5 mg/kg every other week (39). Intravitreal doses of 20 µg have been used (40). In adults, single doses of up to 17.4 mg/kg have been tolerated without significant clinical toxicity or renal insufficiency.

Toxicokinetics and Toxicodynamics

Pharmacokinetic parameters of cidofovir are provided in Table 2. Cidofovir has minimal systemic metabolism and extensive intracellular phosphorylation.

Pathophysiology

Cidofovir diphosphate (formed intracellularly) interferes with viral DNA polymerase (41).

Pregnancy and Lactation

Cidofovir is FDA pregnancy category C (Appendix I). Excretion into breast milk has not been reported.

Clinical Presentation

ACUTE OVERDOSAGE

Only two cases of overdose have been reported. Two adults received single injections of 16.3 mg/kg and 17.4 mg/kg, respectively. Both were also receiving probenecid and IV hydration. Each patient was hospitalized and treated with oral probenecid (1 g three times daily) and vigorous IV hydration with normal saline for 3 to 5 days. Neither developed significant changes in renal function, and other toxicity was not reported (39).

ADVERSE EVENTS

Anterior uveitis is common after intravitreal administration (up to 44% of patients) and has also occurred after IV administration (42). Iritis and decreases in intraocular pressure appear less common. Headache, fatigue, nausea, vomiting, and diarrhea are common with therapeutic use.

Nephrotoxicity is the dose-limiting effect, developing in 59% of patients in one clinical trial of patients receiving 5 mg/kg every other week (39). Nephrotoxic manifestations may include proteinuria, glycosuria, decreases in serum phosphate and uric acid, renal tubular acidosis, and nephrogenic diabetes insipidus as well as increased serum creatinine and decreased creatinine clearance (43–45). Acute renal failure may develop after one or two doses in high-risk patients (taking other nephrotoxic agents, preexisting renal disease) (46).

Neutropenia is another common adverse effect, occurring in up to 24% of patients in clinical trials (39).

Diagnostic Tests

Diagnostic testing includes a complete blood cell count (CBC) and monitoring of renal function, urinalysis, and urine output.

Treatment

GASTROINTESTINAL DECONTAMINATION

Decontamination is not needed because cidofovir is administered parenterally.

ENHANCEMENT OF ELIMINATION

Cidofovir can be removed from circulation by hemodialysis, but this has not been attempted after overdose.

ANTIDOTES

Probenecid blocks uptake of cidofovir by the cells of the proximal renal tubule and may prevent nephrotoxicity. Initiate aggressive IV hydration and probenecid (1 g three times daily) to prevent nephrotoxicity after overdose.

FAMCICLOVIR

Famciclovir (Famvir; $C_{14}H_{19}N_5O_4$; MW. 321.3 g/mol; CAS Registry No., 104227-87-4) is used primarily for herpes simplex and zoster infections. Headache, nausea, vomiting, and diarrhea are the most common adverse effects reported.

Toxic Dose

The *adult therapeutic dosage* ranges from 125 mg twice daily to 500 mg every 8 hours, depending on the indication (47). A toxic dose has not been reported.

Toxicokinetics and Toxicodynamics

Pharmacokinetic parameters of famciclovir are provided in Table 2. It has negligible excretion of unchanged drug. Fecal elimination is 27%.

Pathophysiology

Penciclovir, the active metabolite, is phosphorylated intracellularly to penciclovir triphosphate, which is a competitive inhibitor of DNA polymerases. Viral replication is prevented by inhibition of viral DNA synthesis (47,48).

Pregnancy and Lactation

Famciclovir is FDA pregnancy category B (Appendix I). It is excreted in breast milk in experimental animals (47).

Clinical Presentation

No data on clinical presentation after overdose are available.

Diagnostic Tests

Monitor serum electrolytes in patients with significant vomiting or diarrhea.

Treatment

Treatment is symptomatic and supportive. Enhancement of elimination is unlikely to be clinically effective.

FOSCARNET

Foscarnet sodium (Foscavir, Virudin; $CNa_3O_5P{,}6H_2O$; MW, 300 g/mol; CAS Registry No., 34156-56-4) is used for herpes and CMV infections and as a pyrophosphate analog. It is supplied as a 24-mg/ml solution for IV administration.

Toxic Dose

The usual *adult therapeutic dosage* for CMV retinitis is an induction dose of 90 mg/kg infused over 1.5 to 2.0 hours every 12 hours for 2 to 3 weeks, followed by a maintenance dose of 90 to 120 mg/kg/day infused over 2 hours (49). Concurrent hydration is important to reduce the risk of nephrotoxicity.

Overdoses up to eight times the recommended dose have resulted in seizures, coma, renal insufficiency, paresthesia, and electrolyte abnormalities. One patient died after receiving 12.5 g/day for 3 days.

Toxicokinetics and Toxicodynamics

Pharmacokinetic parameters of foscarnet are provided in Table 2. Foscarnet is poorly absorbed after ingestion.

Pathophysiology

Foscarnet acts as a noncompetitive inhibitor of many viral RNA and DNA polymerases as well as human immunodeficiency virus reverse transcriptase.

Pregnancy and Lactation

Foscarnet is FDA pregnancy category C (Appendix I). It is unknown if it is excreted in breast milk.

Clinical Presentation

ACUTE OVERDOSAGE

The manufacturer reports ten patients who inadvertently received overdoses of foscarnet during clinical trials, with one fatality (49). One patient received 12.5 g/day for 3 days (intended dose, 10.9 g). He had a grand mal seizure, then became comatose, and died 3 days later. The other nine patients received 1.14 to 8.0 times the intended dose (average, four times the intended dose). Three patients developed seizures, three developed renal insufficiency, five had paresthesias (limb or perioral), and five had electrolyte disturbances (primarily hyperphosphatemia and hypocalcemia).

ADVERSE EVENTS

Nephrotoxicity is the dose-limiting toxicity. In clinical trials, 33% of patients developed a serum creatinine level of 2 mg/dl or greater (49). In another study, the serum creatinine increased at least 25% above baseline in 37 of 56 (66%) courses of foscarnet (50). Anemia has occurred in 33% to 50% of patients and granulocytopenia in 17% of patients receiving foscarnet therapy, although it is rarely severe enough to require discontinuation of therapy (51,52).

Electrolyte disturbances are common with foscarnet therapy. Hyperphosphatemia develops in approximately 6% of patients, and the incidence may be higher in patients with acquired immunodeficiency syndrome (AIDS) (53). It is generally not associated with clinical symptoms. Parathyroid levels generally rise during long-term therapy, and hyperphosphatemia resolves (54). Transient decreases in ionized calcium levels are common during infusion (15% to 30% of patients) and are believed to be secondary to calcium chelation by foscarnet. Hypercalcemia has been reported less frequently during long-term therapy (53). Hypokalemia occurs in 16% to 48% of patients, generally within 2 weeks of beginning therapy. It may be resistant to correction with oral potassium supplements (55).

Fever is also common, developing in up to 65% of patients in clinical trials (49). Seizures have been reported after overdose and in approximately 10% of patients in clinical trials (49). Other common, but less serious, adverse effects include nausea, vomiting, diarrhea, headache, and fatigue.

Diagnostic Tests

Monitor serum electrolytes (including phosphorus and calcium), renal function, CBC with differential, urinalysis, and urine output.

Treatment

ACUTE OVERDOSAGE

Management is symptomatic and supportive. Decontamination may not be needed because it is poorly absorbed orally. Convulsions are treated in the usual manner (Chapter 40).

ADVERSE EVENTS

Administer sufficient IV fluids to maintain brisk urine output. Correct hypocalcemia or other electrolyte abnormalities. Seizures are usually responsive to benzodiazepines. Clinical signs of hypocalcemia can be reduced by slowing the rate of infusion (49).

ENHANCEMENT OF ELIMINATION

Foscarnet can be removed from serum by hemodialysis, but this has not yet been performed in the overdose setting.

ANTIDOTES

There is no antidote for foscarnet toxicity.

GANCICLOVIR

Ganciclovir (Cytovene, Vitrasert; $C_9H_{12}N_5NaO_4$; MW, 277.2 g/mol; CAS Registry No., 107910-75-8) is used primarily for CMV infection in immunocompromised patients. It is available as a 250-mg tablet (ganciclovir sodium), a 4.5-mg vitreous implant, and a 500-mg vial for IV administration.

Toxic Dose

The usual *adult therapeutic dosage* for CMV retinitis, esophagitis, and colitis is induction of 5 mg/kg IV over 1 hour every 12 hours for 14 to 21 days, followed by maintenance dosing of 5 mg/kg IV daily or 1000 mg orally three times per day (56). The *pediatric dosage* has not been established, but dosages of 30 to 50 mg/kg/dose orally three times daily have been used for prevention of CMV disease in a small number of patients (57). Overdose of oral ganciclovir has not yet been reported.

Toxicokinetics and Toxicodynamics

Pharmacokinetic parameters of ganciclovir are provided in Table 2.

Pathophysiology

Ganciclovir is converted to ganciclovir triphosphate by intracellular enzymes. Ganciclovir triphosphate competitively inhibits the binding of deoxyguanosine triphosphate to DNA polymerase, inhibiting DNA synthesis and terminating DNA elongation (58).

Pregnancy and Lactation

Ganciclovir is FDA pregnancy category C (Appendix I). Its excretion into breast milk is unknown.

Clinical Presentation

ACUTE OVERDOSAGE

IV overdoses have resulted in granulocytopenia, pancytopenia, hepatitis, acute renal failure, and seizures. Temporary visual loss and retinal artery occlusion secondary to increased intraocular pressure developed in one patient after intravitreal overdose.

An adult male cardiac transplant recipient received a dose of 50 mg/kg every 12 hours for three doses (total dose of 8.25 g, a tenfold overdose). No adverse sequelae were noted over 12 months of follow-up (59). The manufacturer reports 17 cases of overdose with IV ganciclovir (13 adults and 4 children younger than 2 years of age) (56). Five of these patients had no adverse sequelae: an adult who received seven doses of 11 mg/kg over 3 days; an adult who received one dose of 3500 mg; a 4-month-old child who received a single dose of 500 mg (72.5 mg/kg) followed by 48 hours of peritoneal dialysis; an 18-month-old child who received a single dose of approximately 60 mg/kg followed by exchange transfusion; and a 21-month-old child who received two doses of 500 mg instead of 31 mg.

A man with AIDS and CMV colitis developed pancytopenia after receiving 3000 mg/day ganciclovir IV for 2 consecutive days. He developed acute renal failure requiring short-term dialysis. The patient's pancytopenia persisted for several months until his death from a malignancy (56). Another adult developed persistent neutropenia and thrombocytopenia after a single dose of 6000 mg IV. Four adults developed reversible neutropenia or granulocytopenia after inadvertent administration of overdoses ranging from 8 mg/kg daily for 4 days to a single dose of 25 mg/kg.

Hepatitis developed in one adult (10 mg/kg daily) and an infant (single 40-mg dose). An adult developed acute renal failure (creatinine, 5.2 mg/dl) after a single dose of between 5000 and 7000 mg. Another adult developed transient worsening of hematuria after a single 500-mg dose. An adult with a known seizure disorder had a seizure after treatment with 9 mg/kg/day for 3 days.

An adult who received 0.4 ml (instead of 0.1 ml) of intravitreal ganciclovir developed temporary loss of vision and central retinal artery occlusion secondary to increased intraocular pressure related to the injected fluid volume (56).

ADVERSE EVENTS

Approximately 25% of patients treated with ganciclovir develop bone marrow toxicity (60). Neutropenia is the most common manifestation; anemia occurs often as well. Thrombocytopenia occurs much less frequently. Bone marrow toxicity is more common in patients receiving IV ganciclovir and in patients with AIDS (56).

Elevation of hepatic enzyme concentrations has been reported after ganciclovir therapy (58,61,62), although this was not a common adverse effect in early clinical trials. Ventricular tachycardia has been reported in two patients receiving ganciclovir; in one patient, ventricular tachycardia recurred on rechallenge (63).

Diagnostic Tests

Patients with acute overdose and chronic exposure should undergo monitoring of CBC with differential and platelet counts, electrolytes, renal function tests and serum transaminase concentrations, urinalysis, and urine output after overdose.

Treatment

Treatment is symptomatic and supportive. Administer IV fluids and maintain adequate urine output. Pancytopenia and hepatitis generally improve without specific therapy.

GASTROINTESTINAL DECONTAMINATION

Activated charcoal should be administered after oral overdose.

ENHANCEMENT OF ELIMINATION

Ganciclovir can be cleared by hemodialysis, but its effect on outcome is unclear.

ANTIDOTES

There are no antidotes for ganciclovir toxicity.

INTERFERON-ALPHA

The alpha interferons [alpha-2a (Roferon-A), alpha-2b (Intron A), alpha-n3 (Alferon N), alfacon-1 (interferon consensus, Infergen)] are a group of immunomodulators that are used in the treatment of chronic hepatitis B and C, various malignancies, and condyloma acuminatum (alpha-n3). They are available as injectable solutions for IV, intramuscular, subcutaneous, or intralesional administration, depending on the product and the indication for treatment. The dosing is not standardized among these products, increasing the potential for medication errors.

Toxic Dose

INTERFERON-ALPHA-2A

The usual *adult therapeutic dosage* ranges from 3 million IU intramuscularly (IM) or subcutaneously (SQ) three times a week for 12 months for chronic hepatitis C to 36 million U IM or SQ daily for 10 to 12 weeks for AIDS-related Kaposi's sarcoma (64). The *pediatric dosage* is 2.5 to 5.0 million IU/m^2 IM daily (64).

INTERFERON-ALPHA-2B

The usual *adult dosage* ranges from 3 million IU IM or SQ three times a week for up to 24 months for hepatitis C to 30 million IU/m^2 IM or SQ three times per week for up to 6 months for AIDS-related Kaposi's sarcoma (65). The *pediatric dosage* is initially 3 million IU/m^2 SQ three times a week for 1 week followed by 6 million IU/m^2 three times a week for 16 to 24 weeks, with a maximum of 10 million IU three times per week (65).

INTERFERON-ALPHA-N3

The usual *adult dosage* for CMV prophylaxis after renal transplant is 3 million IU three times a week for 6 weeks followed by the same dose twice weekly for 8 weeks (66).

INTERFERON-ALFACON-1

The usual *adult dosage* for chronic hepatitis C infection is 9 μg SQ three times weekly for 24 weeks (67).

Toxicokinetics and Toxicodynamics

Pharmacokinetic parameters of alpha interferons are provided in Table 2. Alpha interferons undergo complete glomerular filtration and rapid proteolytic degradation during tubular reabsorption (68). Interferon alpha-2b undergoes proteolytic degradation in the kidneys (68).

Pathophysiology

Interferons inhibit viral replication in infected cells, suppress cell proliferation, enhance the phagocytic activity of macrophages, augment cytotoxicity of natural killer cells, and increase antibody-dependent cellular cytotoxicity of polymorphonuclear leukocytes (64,65,69).

Pregnancy and Lactation

All the alpha interferons are FDA pregnancy category C (see Appendix I). Alpha interferons are excreted in breast milk in animals; no human data are available.

Clinical Presentation

ACUTE OVERDOSAGE

There are few reports of overdose with alpha interferons in humans. Their effects have been extensions of their reported adverse events. One patient, who was inadvertently given interferon alpha-2a IV rather than interferon alpha-2b, developed severe hypotension that resolved once the infusion was stopped (70).

ADVERSE EVENTS

An acute "flu-like" syndrome is common after administration of interferons; the most common effects are fever, chills, tachycardia, myalgia, arthralgia, headache, fatigue, dizziness, diaphoresis, and malaise (71). Onset is generally within 2 hours of administration, and duration is approximately 24 hours (72,73). Patients may develop tolerance to these effects over time.

A decrease in white blood cell count (approximately 50% of baseline) usually occurs within a few hours of administration (73). Thrombocytopenia is also common. Neutropenia and thrombocytopenia become more clinically significant at higher doses (10 million U daily); recovery is usually rapid after drug discontinuation. Anemia may also occur, generally in fewer than 30% of patients (72,73).

Elevation in serum transaminase levels, often with simultaneous elevation of bilirubin, lactic dehydrogenase, and alkaline phosphatase, is also common with alpha interferons, more frequently with higher doses and IV regimens (73). Rarely, hepatic failure has developed (74).

Nausea, vomiting, diarrhea, and abdominal pain are also common with alpha-interferon therapy (73,75).

Diagnostic Tests

Patients with acute overdose and chronic exposure should undergo monitoring of CBC with differential and platelet count and serum transaminase concentrations.

Treatment

Treatment is primarily symptomatic and supportive. Myelosuppression and hepatic injury generally reverse without specific therapy. Acetaminophen or nonsteroidal antiinflammatory agents may provide relief of flu-like symptoms.

GASTROINTESTINAL DECONTAMINATION

Decontamination is not needed because of parenteral administration. If ingested, alpha interferons would likely be degraded before absorption.

ENHANCEMENT OF ELIMINATION

The interferons have large MWs and are not amenable to hemodialysis.

OSELTAMIVIR

Oseltamivir phosphate (Tamiflu; $C_{16}H_{28}N_2O_4,H_3PO_4$; MW, 410.4 g/mol; CAS Registry No., 204255-11-8) is used for the prophylaxis and treatment of influenza. It is available as a 75-mg capsule and as a solution of 12 mg/ml.

Toxic Dose

The usual *adult therapeutic dosage* is 75 mg twice daily for 5 days. The *pediatric dosage* for children ranges from 30 mg twice daily for patients weighing less than 15 kg to 75 mg for patients more than 40 kg (76). Overdose information is very limited. Doses of up to 1000 mg have caused only nausea and vomiting.

Toxicokinetics and Toxicodynamics

Pharmacokinetic parameters of oseltamivir are provided in Table 2. It undergoes hepatic metabolism as well as metabolism in blood and peripheral tissue by esterases to the active form oseltamivir carboxylate (77). Oseltamivir carboxylate is eliminated almost entirely (99%) by renal excretion.

Pathophysiology

Oseltamivir is metabolized to oseltamivir carboxylate, a selective inhibitor of influenza A and B neuraminidase (77). Neuraminidase is an enzyme expressed on the viral surface that hydrolyzes terminal sialic acid residues from glycoproteins, oligosaccharides, and glycolipids and is required for infectivity of influenza virus (77,78).

Pregnancy and Lactation

Oseltamivir is FDA pregnancy category C (Appendix I). It is excreted in breast milk in rats; no human data are available.

Clinical Presentation

ACUTE OVERDOSAGE

Single doses up to 1000 mg have been associated with only nausea and vomiting; no other overdose information is available (76).

ADVERSE EVENTS

Nausea and vomiting are also the primary effects noted with therapeutic administration, occurring in approximately 11% of patients (79). Dizziness, headache, fatigue, and elevated liver enzyme levels have been reported less frequently (76).

Diagnostic Tests

Serum electrolytes should be monitored in patients with severe vomiting.

Treatment

Treatment is symptomatic and supportive. Administer IV fluids and antiemetics as indicated for vomiting. Recovery is expected with supportive care.

PALIVIZUMAB

Palivizumab (Synagis) is a monoclonal antibody used in the prevention of respiratory syncytial virus (RSV) infection. It is available as 100-mg vial for intramuscular injection only.

Toxic Dose

For prevention of RSV in high-risk infants, the usual dosage of palivizumab is 15 mg/kg monthly (80). No overdose data are available.

Toxicokinetics and Toxicodynamics

Pharmacokinetic parameters of palivizumab are provided in Table 2.

Pathophysiology

Palivizumab is a human monoclonal antibody directed against the fusion protein of RSV.

Pregnancy and Lactation

Palivizumab is FDA pregnancy category C (Appendix I). Entry into breast milk is unknown.

Clinical Presentation

No overdose information is available. Diarrhea, vomiting, increases in serum transaminase levels, rash, localized irritation at the site of injection, and rare cases of anaphylaxis have been reported after therapeutic administration (81,82).

Diagnostic Tests

Monitor serum electrolytes and transaminase levels after overdose.

Treatment

Treatment is symptomatic and supportive. Administer IV fluids and antiemetics as indicated in patients with vomiting and diarrhea.

PEGINTERFERON ALPHA

Peginterferon alpha [peginterferon alpha-2a (Pegasys), peginterferon alpha-2b (PEG-Intron)] is used in the treatment of hepatitis C and other infections.

Toxic Dose

The usual *adult therapeutic dosage* of peginterferon alpha-2a is 180 µg SQ once a week (83). The adult dosage of peginterferon alpha-2b administered SQ weekly ranges from 40 µg for patients weighing 37 to 45 kg to 150 µg for patients more than 137 kg (84). The toxic dose has not been reported.

Toxicokinetics and Toxicodynamics

Pharmacokinetic parameters of peginterferon alpha-2a are as follows: time to maximum serum concentration, 45 to 80 hours; bioavailability, at least 60%; volume of distribution, 8 to 12 L; half-life, 60 to 90 hours (85). Pharmacokinetic parameters of peginterferon alpha-2b are as follows: time to maximum serum concentration, 15 to 44 hours; volume of distribution 1 L/kg; elimination half-life, 22 to 60 hours (86,87).

Pathophysiology

Peginterferons are covalent conjugates of straight-chain polyethylene glycol and recombinant interferon alpha-2a or alpha-2b in a 1:1 ratio. Linkage with polyethylene glycol (pegylation) reduces clearance and may enhance the efficacy of alpha interferon due to more prolonged exposure (86,88).

Pregnancy and Lactation

Both products are FDA pregnancy category C (Appendix I). Entry into breast milk is unknown.

Clinical Presentation

No overdose data are available. In three large studies, the most common adverse effects reported with subcutaneous peginterferons were headache, fatigue, rigors, myalgia, fever, nausea, abdominal pain, dizziness, insomnia, and depression; inflammation at the site of injection was also reported in many patients (87,89–91). Alopecia is common with peginterferon alpha-2b therapy (86). A flu-like syndrome (fever, headache, myalgias, rigors, fatigue) is common within 24 hours of administration (86,87). Severity is dose related and tends to diminish with subsequent doses.

Patients with cirrhosis secondary to chronic hepatitis C have developed exacerbation of neutropenia and thrombocytopenia, usually within 2 weeks of starting therapy (89). Anemia has also been reported.

Diagnostic Tests

Monitor the CBC with differential and platelet count and serum transaminase concentrations after overdose.

Treatment

Treatment is symptomatic and supportive. Myelosuppression and hepatic injury generally reverse without specific therapy. Acetaminophen or nonsteroidal antiinflammatory agents may provide relief of flu-like symptoms.

RIBAVIRIN

Ribavirin (Rebetol, Virazole; $C_8H_{12}N_4O_5$; MW, 244.2 g/mol; CAS Registry No., 36791-04-5) is used in the treatment of hepatitis C and RSV in infants. It is available as a 200-mg capsule or a 6-g/dl solution for aerosolization.

Toxic Dose

The *adult therapeutic dosage* for hepatitis C is 400 mg in the morning and 600 mg at night for patients weighing less than 75 kg and 600 mg twice daily for patients more than 75 kg (92). For aerosolized ribavirin to treat RSV in infants, 20 mg/ml ribavirin (Virazole) is added as the starting solution in the drug reservoir of the small particle aerosol generator–2 unit, with continuous aerosol administration for 12 to 18 hours per day for 3 to 7 days (93).

An *overdose* of 10 g ribavirin was not associated with any clinical toxicity.

Toxicokinetics and Toxicodynamics

Pharmacokinetic parameters of ribavirin are provided in Table 2. The elimination half-life is 24 to 36 hours after a single dose, longer (151 hours) after several weeks of dosing (94,95).

Pathophysiology

Ribavirin is phosphorylated intracellularly to active mono and triphosphate forms, which interfere with viral nucleic acid synthesis.

Pregnancy and Lactation

Ribavirin is FDA pregnancy category X (Appendix I). Pregnant health care workers should preferably not administer ribavirin. If pregnant workers cannot avoid close patient contact, ribavirin should be administered in a negative pressure room with adequate ventilation (at least six air exchanges per hour). The aerosol should be administered with scavenging devices; turn off the small particle aerosol generator–2 for 5 to 10 minutes before prolonged patient contact; and wear an appropriate respiratory filter mask. Surgical masks do not adequately filter ribavirin particles (93,96).

Clinical Presentation

ACUTE OVERDOSAGE

Data regarding overdose is limited. The manufacturer reports that the maximum overdose reported during clinical trials was a dose of 39 million U of interferon alpha-2b (13 subcutaneous injections of 3 million IU each) taken with 10 g of ribavirin (fifty 200-mg capsules). The patient was observed for 2 days, and no adverse effects were noted (92).

ADVERSE EVENTS

Hemolytic anemia is common during therapeutic use. It develops in approximately 10% of treated patients, with onset 1 to 2 weeks after beginning therapy and resolution 4 to 8 weeks after therapy. Anemia is generally more severe in patients taking higher doses (97,98). Increases in serum bilirubin and uric acid levels are common during therapy. Conjunctivitis is common with aerosolized ribavirin and usually resolves within several hours (99). Decreases in pulmonary function may occur with aerosolized ribavirin, particularly in patients with underlying asthma or chronic obstructive pulmonary disease (93).

Health care workers exposed to aerosolized ribavirin commonly develop headache, conjunctivitis, rhinitis, nausea, rash, dizziness, lacrimation, or pharyngitis (93).

Diagnostic Tests

Monitor the CBC and serum bilirubin. In patients with evidence of hemolysis, monitor renal function, urinalysis, and urine output.

Treatment

Treatment is symptomatic and supportive. After ingestion, administer activated charcoal. Maintain adequate hydration and brisk urine output (2 to 3 ml/kg/hour) in patients with hemolysis to minimize nephrotoxicity.

RIMANTADINE

Rimantadine (Flumadine) is used in the treatment of influenza A. It is available as a 100-mg capsule and a 10-mg/ml syrup.

Toxic Dose

The *adult therapeutic dosage* is 100 mg orally twice per day. The *pediatric dose* is 5 mg/kg for children younger than 10 years of age. No overdose data are available.

Toxicokinetics and Toxicodynamics

Pharmacokinetic parameters of rimantadine are provided in Table 2.

Pathophysiology

Rimantadine interferes with replication of influenza A virus by interfering with viral uncoating (100).

Pregnancy and Lactation

Rimantadine is FDA pregnancy category C (Appendix I). Rimantadine should not be used while breast-feeding. In rats, concentrations in milk were twice those in serum, and adverse effects developed in nursing pups (101).

Clinical Presentation

No overdose data are available. Adverse effects are less common and less severe than with amantadine. Headache, fatigue, dizziness, insomnia, nausea, vomiting, anorexia, and dry mouth are the most common adverse effects. Seizures have been reported occasionally (102). Patients taking higher than recommended doses have developed diaphoresis, fever, and lacrimation (101). Anticholinergic effects developed in 1.5% of patients in one study (103).

VALACYCLOVIR

Valacyclovir hydrochloride (Valtrex; $C_{13}H_{20}N_6O_4$,HCl; 360.8 g/mol; CAS Registry No., 124832-27-5) is used for herpes zoster and genital herpes. It is available as 500-mg or 1-g capsules.

Toxic Dose

The usual *adult therapeutic dosage* ranges from 1 g/day for suppression of recurrent genital herpes to 1 g three times daily for herpes zoster. Dosages of 2000 mg four times daily are associated with diarrhea and nausea (104). The pediatric dose has not been established. There is no information available concerning overdosage.

Toxicokinetics and Toxicodynamics

Pharmacokinetic parameters of valacyclovir are provided in Table 2.

Pathophysiology

Valacyclovir is metabolized to acyclovir, which is phosphorylated intracellularly to acyclovir triphosphate. Acyclovir triphosphate binds viral DNA polymerase in competition with guanosine and is incorporated into viral DNA, preventing further elongation of the chain (3).

Pregnancy and Lactation

Valacyclovir is FDA pregnancy category B (Appendix I). Breast-feeding is contraindicated.

Clinical Presentation

ACUTE OVERDOSAGE

No overdose data are available. As valacyclovir is metabolized to acyclovir, similar toxicity is expected in significant overdose.

ADVERSE EVENTS

Anemia, neutropenia, and thrombotic thrombocytopenic purpura with hemolytic uremic syndrome have been reported in immunosuppressed patients receiving valacyclovir therapy; these effects have not been reported in immunocompetent patients (105,106). Headache, nausea, and vomiting are common adverse effects. Isolated cases of aseptic meningitis, encephalopathy, and choreiform movements have been reported in association with valacyclovir therapy (107–109). Elevation in serum transaminase levels occurs with therapeutic use, and abnormal aspartate aminotransferase levels developed in 1% to 4% of patients in clinical trials (110).

Diagnostic Tests

As for acyclovir, monitor renal function, urinalysis, and urine output in all overdose patients. Acyclovir crystals (fine, elongated rectangular crystals) may be identified on microscopic examination of the urine. Acyclovir concentration can be determined in plasma by radioimmunoassay or high-performance liquid chromatography (11,17). Acyclovir concentrations are useful to confirm overdose but do not guide patient management or predict outcome.

Treatment

Treatment is symptomatic and supportive. Oral activated charcoal is generally sufficient decontamination after overdose ingestion.

ENHANCEMENT OF ELIMINATION

Acyclovir can be removed by hemodialysis (1). Although use of hemodialysis has not yet been reported in the management of overdose, it might be warranted in a patient with preexisting renal insufficiency and severe overdose.

ANTIDOTE

There is no antidote for valacyclovir.

SUPPORTIVE CARE

Any patient with alteration of mental status, seizures, or an increase in serum creatinine after overdose should be admitted. Administer sufficient IV fluids to maintain brisk urine output in an attempt to minimize the precipitation of acyclovir crystals in renal tubules. Alterations in mental status generally resolve over several days with discontinuation of the drug. Seizures are usually not protracted and respond to benzodiazepines.

VALGANCICLOVIR

Valganciclovir hydrochloride (Valcyte; $C_{14}H_{22}N_6O_5$,HCl; MW, 390.8 g/mol; CAS Registry No., 175865-59-5) is used to treat CMV retinitis. It is available as a 450-mg tablet.

Toxic Dose

The usual *adult therapeutic dosage* is 900 mg twice a day induction for 21 days followed by 900 mg/day administered with food (111). A tenfold *overdosage* for several days resulted in death from bone marrow aplasia.

Toxicokinetics and Toxicodynamics

Pharmacokinetic parameters of valganciclovir are provided in Table 2.

Pathophysiology

Valganciclovir is rapidly hydrolyzed in plasma to ganciclovir, which is converted to ganciclovir triphosphate by intracellular enzymes. Ganciclovir triphosphate competitively inhibits the binding of deoxyguanosine triphosphate to DNA polymerase, inhibiting DNA synthesis and terminating DNA elongation.

Pregnancy and Lactation

Valganciclovir is FDA pregnancy category C (Appendix I). Excretion into breast milk is unknown.

Clinical Presentation

Fatal bone marrow aplasia developed in a male patient who was treated for several days with a dose that was at least tenfold greater than appropriate for his degree of renal impairment (111). Because valganciclovir is metabolized to ganciclovir, similar toxicity might develop.

Anemia and neutropenia develop in approximately 25% of treated patients; thrombocytopenia is less common (111). Nausea, vomiting, diarrhea, abdominal pain, headache, and insomnia are also quite common with therapeutic use (112,113). Paresthesia and peripheral neuropathy develop in approximately 9% of treated patients (112,113).

Diagnostic Tests

Monitor the CBC with differential and platelet count, renal function, serum transaminase levels, urinalysis, and urine output after overdose. Nerve conduction studies may be useful in patients with evidence of neuropathy.

Treatment

Treatment is symptomatic and supportive. Administer activated charcoal after acute ingestion. Administer IV fluids and maintain adequate urine output. Pancytopenia and hepatitis generally improve without specific therapy. Ganciclovir can be cleared by hemodialysis, but there are no reports of its use in the management of overdose. Consider granulocyte colony-stimulating factor in patients with severe persistent granulocytopenia.

ZANAMIVIR

Zanamivir (Relenza; $C_{12}H_{20}N_4O_7$; MW, 332.3 g/mol; CAS Registry No., 139110-80-8) is used in the treatment of influenza. It is available as an inhaler.

Toxic Dose

The *therapeutic dosage* in adults and children 7 years of age and older is 10 mg by inhalation twice daily (114). IV doses up to 1200 mg/day and intranasal doses up to 96 mg/day caused minor adverse effects in volunteers.

Toxicokinetics and Toxicodynamics

Pharmacokinetic parameters of zanamivir are provided in Table 2.

Pathophysiology

Zanamivir inhibits neuroaminidase in influenza A and B viruses. This inhibits the release of newly formed viruses from the surface of infected cells, preventing viral spread (115).

Pregnancy and Lactation

Zanamivir is FDA pregnancy category C (Appendix I). Entry into breast milk is unknown.

Clinical Presentation

In volunteer studies, doses of 600 mg IV did not cause adverse effects, whereas dosages of 1200 mg/day IV for 5 days caused adverse effects similar to those seen at therapeutic doses. Intranasal doses up to 96 mg/day and inhaled doses up to 64 mg/day are well tolerated (114). Bronchospasm and declines in pulmonary function have been reported with therapeutic use, primarily in patients with underlying asthma or chronic obstructive pulmonary disease (114,116).

Treatment

Symptomatic and supportive care is sufficient. Bronchospasm is treated in the usual manner.

REFERENCES

1. Zovirax, acyclovir. Product information. Research Triangle Park, NC: Glaxo Wellcome Inc., 2002.
2. McDonald LK, Tartaglione TA, Mendelman PM, et al. Lack of toxicity in two cases of neonatal acyclovir overdose. *Pediatr Infect Dis J* 1989;8:529–532.
3. King DH. History, pharmacokinetics, and pharmacology of acyclovir. *J Am Acad Dermatol* 1988;18:176–179.
4. Lau RJ, Emery MG, Galinsky RE. Unexpected accumulation of acyclovir in breast milk with estimation of infant exposure. *Obstet Gynecol* 1987;69:468–471.
5. Briggs GG, Freeman RK, Yaffe SJ. *Drugs in pregnancy and lactation*, 5th ed. Baltimore: Williams & Wilkins, 1998.
6. Anonymous. Committee on Drugs, American Academy of Pediatrics: the transfer of drugs and other chemicals into human milk. *Pediatrics* 2001;108:776–789.
7. Rauber-Luthy CH, Lanzicher L, Guirguis M, et al. Acyclovir overdose in a newborn with consecutive renal impairment. *J Toxicol Clin Toxicol* 2001;39:506–507(abst).
8. Baker KL, Baker SD, Morgan DL. High dose acyclovir given to an eleven day old child. *J Toxicol Clin Toxicol* 2002;40:638(abst).
9. Sigg T, Burda AM, Dimanno J, et al. Inadvertent IV administration of acyclovir 800 mg to a child. *J Toxicol Clin Toxicol* 2001;39:505–506(abst).
10. Bradley J, Forero N, Pho H, et al. Progressive somnolence leading to coma in a 68-year-old man. *Chest* 1997;112:538–540.
11. Haefeli WE, Schoenenberger RAZ, Weiss P, et al. Acyclovir-induced neurotoxicity: concentration-side effect relationship in acyclovir overdose. *Am J Med* 1993;94:212–215.
12. Adair JC, Gold M, Bond RE. Acyclovir neurotoxicity: clinical experience and review of the literature. *South Med J* 1994;87:1227–1231.
13. Johnson GL, Limon L, Trikha G, et al. Acute renal failure and neurotoxicity following oral acyclovir. *Ann Pharmacother* 1994;28:460–463.
14. Brigden D, Whiteman P. The mechanism of action, pharmacokinetics and toxicity of acyclovir—a review. *J Infect* 1983;6[Suppl 1]:3–9.
15. Krieble BF, Rudy DW, Glick MR, et al. Case report: acyclovir neurotoxicity and nephrotoxicity—the role for hemodialysis. *Am J Med Sci* 1993;305:36–39.
16. Peterslund NA, Larsen ML, Mygind H. Acyclovir crystalluria. *Scand J Inf Dis* 1988;20:225–228.
17. Boulieu R, Gallant C, Silberstein N. Determination of acyclovir in human plasma by high performance liquid chromatography. *J Chromatogr B Biomed Sci Appl* 1997;693:233–236..
18. Kimberlin DE, Weller S, Whitley RJ, et al. Pharmacokinetics of oral valacyclovir and acyclovir in late pregnancy. *Am J Obstet Gynecol* 1998;179:486–491.
19. Cundy KC, Barditch-Crovo P, Walker RE, et al. Clinical pharmacokinetics of adefovir in human immunodeficiency virus type 1-infected patients. *Antimicrob Agents Chemother* 1995;39:2401–2405.
20. Hepsera, adefovir dipivoxil tablets. Product information. Foster City, CA: Gilead Sciences, Inc., 2002.
21. Kahn J, Lagakos S, Wulfsohn M, et al. Efficacy and safety of adefovir dipivoxil with antiretroviral therapy. *JAMA* 1999;282:2305–2312.
22. Simpson DM, Ramos F, Ramirez LF. Death of a psychiatric patient from amantadine poisoning [Letter]. *Am J Psychiatry* 1988;145:267–268.
23. Fahn S, Craddock G, Kumin G. Acute toxic psychosis from suicidal overdose of amantadine. *Arch Neurol* 1971;25:45–48.
24. Berkowitz CD. Treatment of acute amantadine toxicity with physostigmine. *J Pediatr* 1979;95:144–145.
25. Hirsch MS, Swartz MN. Antiviral agents. *N Engl J Med* 1980;302:903–904.
26. Shannon KM, Goetz CG, Carroll VS, et al. Amantadine and motor fluctuations in chronic Parkinson's disease. *Clin Neuropharmacol* 1987;10:522–526.

27. Yang CC, Deng JF. Anticholinergic syndrome with severe rhabdomyolysis—an unusual feature of amantadine toxicity. *Intensive Care Med* 1997;23:355–356.
28. Farrell S, Lee DC, McNamara B. Amantadine overdose: considerations for the treatment of cardiac toxicity. *J Toxicol Clin Toxicol* 1995;33:516–517(abst).
29. Halpern JS. Amantadine: antiviral agent for influenza A. *J Emerg Nurs* 1985;11:158–160.
30. Brown CR, Hernandez S, Kelly MT. Hyperthermia and death from amantadine overdose. *Vet Hum Toxicol* 1987;29:463(abst).
31. Sartori M, Pratt CM, Young JB. Torsade de pointe malignant cardiac arrhythmia induced by amantadine poisoning. *Am J Med* 1984;77:388–391.
32. Snoey ER, Bessen HA. Acute psychosis after amantadine overdose. *Ann Emerg Med* 1990;19:668–670.
33. Macchio GJ, Ito V, Sahgal V. Amantadine-induced coma. *Arch Phys Med Rehabil* 1993;74:1119–1120.
34. Keyser LA, Karl M, Nafziger AN, et al. Comparison of central nervous system adverse effects of amantadine and rimantadine used as sequential prophylaxis of influenza A in elderly nursing home patients. *Arch Intern Med* 2000;160:1485–1488.
35. Rego MD, Giller EL Jr. Mania secondary to amantadine treatment of neuroleptic-induced hyperprolactinemia. *J Clin Psychiatry* 1989;50:143–144.
36. Weller M, Kornhuber J. Amantadine withdrawal and neuroleptic malignant syndrome [Letter]. *Neurology* 1993;43:2155.
37. Hamburg P, Weilburg JB, Cassem NH, et al. Relapse of neuroleptic malignant syndrome with early discontinuation of amantadine therapy. *Compr Psychiatry* 1986;27:272–275.
38. Casey DE. Amantadine intoxication reversed by physostigmine. *N Engl J Med* 1978;298:516.
39. Vistide Injection, cidofovir. Product information. Foster City, CA: Gilead Sciences, Inc., 1999.
40. Kirsch LS, Arevalo JF, Chavez-de la Paz EC, et al. Intravitreal cidofovir (HPMPC) treatment of cytomegalovirus retinitis in patients with acquired immune deficiency syndrome. *Ophthalmology* 1995;102:533–543.
41. Neyts J, De Clercq E. Mechanism of action of acyclic nucleoside phosphonates against herpes virus replication. *Biochem Pharmacol* 1994;47:39–41.
42. Akler ME, Johnson DW, Burman WJ, et al. Anterior uveitis and hypotony after intravenous cidofovir for the treatment of cytomegalovirus retinitis. *Ophthalmology* 1998;105:651–657.
43. Higgins G. Unique agent under development for CMV infection. *Inpharma* 1994; 967:9–10.
44. Kay TD, Hogan PG, McLeod SE, et al. Severe irreversible proximal renal tubular acidosis and azotemia secondary to cidofovir [Letter]. *Nephron* 2000;86:348–349.
45. Schliefer K, Rockstroh JK, Spengler U, et al. Nephrogenic diabetes insipidus in a patient taking cidofovir. *Lancet* 1997;350:413–414.
46. Skiest DJ, Duong M, Park S, et al. Complications of therapy with intravenous cidofovir: severe nephrotoxicity and anterior uveitis. *Infect Dis Clin Pract* 1999;8:155–157.
47. Famvir, famciclovir tablets. Product information. Philadelphia: SmithKline Beecham Pharmaceuticals, 2001.
48. Vere Hodge RA, Cheng YC. The mode of action of penciclovir. *Antivir Chem Chemother* 1993;4[Suppl 1]:13–24.
49. Foscavir, foscarnet sodium. Product information. Wilmington, DE: AstraZeneca LP, 2002.
50. Deray G, Martinez F, Katlama C, et al. Foscarnet nephrotoxicity: mechanism, incidence, and prevention. *Am J Nephrol* 1989;9:316–321.
51. Wagstaff AJ, Bryson HM. Foscarnet: a reappraisal of its antiviral activity, pharmacokinetic properties and therapeutic use in immunocompromised patients with viral infections. *Drugs* 1994;48:199–226.
52. Fanning MM, Read SE, Benson M, et al. Foscarnet therapy of cytomegalovirus retinitis in AIDS. *J AIDS* 1990;3:472–479.
53. Jacobson MA, O'Donnell JJ, Mills J. Foscarnet treatment of cytomegalovirus retinitis in patients with the acquired immunodeficiency syndrome. *Antimicrob Agents Chemother* 1989;33:736–741.
54. DeTorres O. Focus on foscarnet: a pyrophosphate analog for use in CMV retinitis and other viral infections. *Hosp Formul* 1991;26:929–947.
55. Gearhart MO, Sorg TB. Foscarnet-induced severe hypomagnesemia and other electrolyte disorders. *Ann Pharmacother* 1993;27:285–289.
56. Cytovene, ganciclovir injection and capsules. Product information. Nutley, NJ: Roche Laboratories, Inc., 2002.
57. Frenkel LM, Capparelli EV, Dankner WM, et al. Oral ganciclovir in children: pharmacokinetics. Safety, tolerance, and antiviral effects. *J Infect Dis* 2000;182:1616–1624.
58. Anonymous. Collaborative DHPG Treatment Study Group: treatment of serious cytomegalovirus infections with 9-(1,3-dihydroxy-2-propoxymethyl)guanine in patients with AIDS and other immunodeficiencies. *N Engl J Med* 1986;314:801–805.
59. Kostis EB, Nanas JN, Moulopoulos SD. Absence of toxicity after overdose of ganciclovir in a cardiac transplant recipient [Letter]. *Eur J Cardiothorac Surg* 1999;15:876.
60. Drucker JL, King DH. Management of viral infections in AIDS patients. *Infection* 1987;15:S32–S33.
61. Figge HL, Bailie GR, Briceland LL, et al. Possible ganciclovir-induced hepatotoxicity in patients with AIDS. *Clin Pharmacokinet* 1992;11:432–434.
62. Shea BF, Hoffman S, Sesin GP, et al. Ganciclovir hepatotoxicity. *Pharmacotherapy* 1987;7:223–226.
63. Cohen AJ, Weiser B, Afzal Q, et al. Ventricular tachycardia in two patients with AIDS receiving ganciclovir (DHPG). *AIDS* 1990;4:807–809.
64. Roferon-A, interferon alfa-2a recombinant. Product information. Nutley, NJ: Roche Laboratories, 2001.
65. Intron A, interferon alfa-2b, recombinant. Product information. Kenilworth, NJ: Schering Corporation, 2001.
66. Hirsch MS, Schooley RT, Cosimi AB, et al. Effects of interferon-alpha on cytomegalovirus reactivation syndromes in renal-transplant recipients. *N Engl J Med* 1983;308:1489–1493.
67. Infergen, interferon alfacon-1. Product information. Thousand Oaks, CA: Amgen, 1997.
68. Wills RJ. Clinical pharmacokinetics of interferons. *Clin Pharmacokinet* 1990;19:390–399.
69. Alferon N, interferon alfa-n3. Product information. Norwalk, CT: Purdue Frederick, 1998.
70. Hanson DS, Leggette CT. Severe hypotension following inadvertent intravenous administration of interferon alfa-2a [Letter]. *Ann Pharmacother* 1997;31:371–372.
71. Jones GJ, Itri LM. Safety and tolerance of recombinant interferon alfa-2a (Roferon-A) in cancer patients. *Cancer* 1986;57[Suppl]:1709–1715.
72. Balmer CM. The new alpha interferons. *Drug Intell Clin Pharm* 1985;19:887–893.
73. Quesada JR, Talpaz M, Rios A, et al. Clinical toxicity of interferons in cancer patients: a review. *J Clin Oncol* 1986;4:234–243.
74. Lock G, Reng CM, Graeb C, et al. Interferon-induced hepatic failure in a patient with hepatitis C [Letter]. *Am J Gastroenterol* 1999;94:2570–2571.
75. Sriskandan K, Garner P, Watkinson J, et al. A toxicity study of recombinant interferon-gamma given by intravenous infusion to patients with advanced cancer. *Cancer Chemother Pharmacol* 1986;18:63–68.
76. Tamiflu, oseltamivir phosphate. Product information. Nutley, NJ: Roche Laboratories Inc., 2002.
77. Li W, Escarpe PA, Eisenberg EJ, et al. Identification of GS 4104 as an orally bioavailable prodrug of the influenza virus neuraminidase inhibitor GS 4071. *Antimicrob Agents Chemother* 1998;42:647–653.
78. Mendel DB, Tai CY, Escarpe PA, et al. Oral administration of a prodrug of the influenza virus neuraminidase inhibitor GS 4071 protects mice and ferrets against influenza infection. *Antimicrob Agents Chemother* 1998;42:640–646.
79. Hayden FG, Atmar RL, Schilling M, et al. Use of the selective oral neuraminidase inhibitor oseltamivir to prevent influenza. *N Engl J Med* 1999;341:1336–1343.
80. Synagis, palivizumab. Product information. Gaithersburg, MD: MedImmune, Inc.
81. Subramanian KNS, Weisman LE, Rhodes T, et al. Safety, tolerance and pharmacokinetics of a humanized monoclonal antibody to respiratory syncytial virus in premature infants and infants with bronchopulmonary dysplasia. *Pediatr Infect Dis J* 1998;17:110–115.
82. Anonymous. Palivizumab, a humanized respiratory syncytial virus monoclonal antibody, reduces hospitalization from respiratory synctial virus infection in high-risk infants. *Pediatrics* 1998;102:531–537.
83. Pegasys, peginterferon alfa-2a. Product information. Nutley, NJ: Hoffmann-LaRoche.
84. PEG-Intron Powder for Injection, peginterferon alfa-2b. Product information. Kenilworth, NJ: Schering Corporation.
85. Perry CM, Jarvis B. Peginterferon-alpha-2a (40 kD): a review of its use in the management of chronic hepatitis C. *Drugs* 2001;61:2263–2288.
86. Glue P, Rouzier-Panis R, Raffanel C, et al. A dose-ranging study of pegylated interferon alfa-2b and ribavirin in chronic hepatitis C. *Hepatology* 2000;32:647–653.
87. Glue P, Fang JWS, Rouzier-Panis R, et al. Pegylated interferon-alfa2b: pharmacokinetics, pharmacodynamics, safety, and preliminary efficacy data. *Clin Pharmacol Ther* 2000;68:556–567.
88. Gordon D. Pegylated interferon for treatment of hepatitis C. *Gastroenterology* 2001;120:4.
89. Heathcote EJ, Shiffman ML, Cooksley WG, et al. Peginterferon alfa-2a in patients with chronic hepatitis C and cirrhosis. *N Engl J Med* 2000;343:1673–1680.
90. Zeuzem S, Feinman SV, Rasenack J, et al. Peginterferon alfa-2a in patients with chronic hepatitis C. *N Engl J Med* 2000;343:1666–1672.
91. Reddy KR, Wright TL, Pockros PJ, et al. Efficacy and safety of pegylated (40-kd) interferon alpha-2a compared with interferon alpha-2a in noncirrhotic patients with chronic hepatitis C. *Hepatology* 2001;33:433–438.
92. Rebetol, ribavirin capsules. Product information. Kenilworth, NJ: Schering Corp., 2002.
93. Virazole, ribavirin. Product information. Costa Mesa, CA: ICN Pharmaceuticals, 2002.
94. Laskin OL, Longstreth JA, Hart CC, et al. Ribavirin disposition in high-risk patients for acquired immunodeficiency syndrome. *Clin Pharmacol Ther* 1987;41:546–555.
95. Lertora JJL, Rege AB, Lacour JT, et al. Pharmacokinetics and long-term tolerance to ribavirin in asymptomatic patients infected with human immunodeficiency virus. *Clin Pharmacol Ther* 1991;50:442–449.
96. Shults RA, Baron S, Decker J, et al. Health care worker exposure to aerosolized ribavirin: biological and air monitoring. *J Occup Environ Med* 1996;38:257–263.
97. Cosgriff TM, Hodgson LA, Canonico PG, et al. Morphological alterations in blood and bone marrow of ribavirin-treated monkeys. *Acta Haematol* 1984;72:195–200.
98. Hall CB, Douglas RG Jr, Schnabel KC, et al. Infectivity of respiratory syncytial virus by various routes of inoculation. *Infect Immun* 1981;33:779–783.
99. Hall CB, McBride JT, Gala CL, et al. Ribavirin treatment of respiratory syncytial viral infection in infants with underlying cardiopulmonary disease. *JAMA* 1985;254:3047–3051.
100. Hoffman CE. Structure, activity and mode of action of amantadine HCl and related compounds. *Antibiotics Chemother* 1980;27:233–250.

101. Flumadine, rimantadine. Product information. St. Louis: Forest Pharmaceuticals, Inc.
102. Wintermeyer SM, Nahata MC. Rimantadine: a clinical perspective. *Ann Pharmacother* 1995;29:299–310.
103. Hayden FG, Gwaltney JM, Van de Castle RL, et al. Comparative toxicity of amantadine hydrochloride and rimantadine hydrochloride in healthy adults. *Antimicrob Agents Chemother* 1981;19:226–233.
104. Weller S, Blum MR, Doucette M, et al. Pharmacokinetics of the acyclovir pro-drug valaciclovir after escalating single- and multiple-dose administration to normal volunteers. *Clin Pharmacol Ther* 1993;54:595–605.
105. Jacobson MA, Gallant J, Wang LH, et al. Phase I trial of valaciclovir, the L-valyl ester of acyclovir, in patients with advanced human immunodeficiency virus disease. *Antimicrob Agents Chemother* 1994;38:1534–1540.
106. Rivaud E, Massiani MA, Vincent F, et al. Valacyclovir hydrochloride therapy and thrombotic thrombocytopenic purpura in a HIV-infected patient. *Arch Intern Med* 2000;160:1705–1706.
107. Fobelo MJ, Corzo Delgado JE, Alonso AR, et al. Aseptic meningitis related to valacyclovir [Letter]. *Ann Pharmacother* 2001;35:128–129.
108. Maru MC, Fialkow RZ, Haria DM. Choreiform movements in dialysis patient taking valacyclovir and famciclovir. *South Med J* 2001;94:655.
109. Linssen-Schuurmans CD, van Kan EJM, Feith GW, et al. Neurotoxicity caused by valacyclovir in a patient on hemodialysis. *Ther Drug Monit* 1998;20:385–386.
110. Valtrex, valacyclovir hydrochloride caplets. Product information. Research Triangle Park, NC: GlaxoWellcome Inc.
111. Valcyte. Product information. 2001.
112. Brown F, Banken L, Saywell K, et al. Phamacokinetics of valganciclovir and ganciclovir following multiple oral dosages of valganciclovir in HIV- and CMV-seropositive volunteers. *Clin Pharmacokinet* 1999;37:167–176.
113. Jung D, Dorr A. Single-dose phamacokinetics of valganciclovir in HIV- and CMV-seropositive subjects. *J Clin Pharmacol* 1999;8:800–804.
114. Relenza, zanamivir for inhalation. Product information. Research Triangle Park, NC: Glaxo Wellcome.
115. Waghorn SL, Goa KL. Zanamivir. *Drugs* 1998;55:721–725.
116. Williamson JC, Pegram PS. Respiratory distress associated with zanamivir. *N Engl J Med* 2000;342:661–662.

CHAPTER 93

Antiretroviral Drugs

Katherine M. Hurlbut

N OH H OH N N N H_3C H_3C C N O O H_3C H

INDINAVIR

Compounds included:	**See Table 1.**
Molecular formula and weight:	**See text.**
SI conversion:	**See Table 1.**
CAS Registry No.:	**See text.**
Therapeutic levels:	**Not used clinically**
Target organs:	**Gastrointestinal (acute), liver (chronic), skin (chronic), peripheral nervous system (chronic), metabolic acidosis (chronic), central nervous system (chronic)**
Antidote:	**None**

OVERVIEW

The antiretroviral agents are all used in the treatment of infection by human immunodeficiency virus (HIV) and acquired immunodeficiency syndrome. Because of their similarities and the limited information available concerning overdosage, the *diagnostic tests and treatment for these agents are addressed as a group* at the end of this chapter.

The antiretroviral agents are divided into four categories: (a) *fusion inhibitors*: pentafuside; (b) *nucleosides*: pyrimidine nucleoside analogs (didanosine, lamivudine, zalcitabine), thymidine nucleoside analogs (fialuridine, stavudine, zidovudine), carboxylic nucleoside analog (abacavir), acyclic nucleoside phosphonates (adefovir; tenofovir), thiacytidine nucleoside analog (emtricitabine); (c) *nonnucleosides*: atevirdine, delavirdine, efavirenz, emivirine, nevirapine; (d) *protease inhibitors*: amprenavir, indinavir, lopinavir, ritonavir, nelfinavir, and saquinavir mesylate.

There is little information about overdose with these agents. Zidovudine overdose has caused lethargy, bone marrow suppression, and seizures. Chronic therapy with nucleoside analogs

TABLE 1. Compounds included and SI conversion

Compound	SI conversion
Abacavir (Ziagen)	mg/L × 1.5 = μmol/L
Amprenavir (Agenerase)	mg/L × 2.0 = μmol/L
Atevirdine	mg/L × 2.6 = μmol/L
Delavirdine mesylate (Rescriptor)	mg/L × 1.8 = μmol/L
Didanosine (Videx)	mg/L × 4.2 = μmol/L
Efavirenz (Sustiva, Stocrin)	mg/L × 3.2 = μmol/L
Emivirine (Coactinon)	mg/L × 3.3 = μmol/L
Enfuvirtide (pentafuside)	mg/dl × 2.2 = μmol/L
Indinavir sulfate (Crixivan)	mg/L × 1.4 = μmol/L
Lamivudine (3TC, Epivir, Heptovir)	mg/L × 4.4 = μmol/L
Lopinavir (Kaletra)	mg/L × 1.6 = μmol/L
Nelfinavir mesylate (Viracept)	mg/L × 1.5 = μmol/L
Nevirapine (Viramune)	mg/L × 3.8 = μmol/L
Ritonavir (Norvir)	mg/L × 1.4 = μmol/L
Saquinavir mesylate (Invirase)	mg/L × 1.3 = μmol/L
Stavudine (Zerit)	mg/L × 4.5 = μmol/L
Zalcitabine (Hivid)	mg/L × 4.7 = μmol/L
Zidovudine (Retrovir)	mg/L × 3.7 = μmol/L

TABLE 2. Selected pharmacokinetic parameters of nonnucleoside reverse transcriptase inhibitors

Parameter	Atevirdine[a]	Delavirdine mesylate	Efavirenz	Emivirine[b]	Nevirapine[c]
Time to maximum serum concentration (h)	0.5–1.0	1	3–5	1	2–4
Apparent volume of distribution (L/kg)	Unknown	Unknown	Unknown	NR	1.4
Route of excretion (%)	Hepatic metabolism	51 renal	14–34 renal, most as unchanged drug	—	<5 renal
Elimination half-life (h)	18–46	2–11	52–76 after single dose; 40–55 after multiple doses	6–8	40 after single dose; 25–30 after multiple doses
Excreted unchanged (%)	NR	<5	NR	NR	<5
Active metabolites	NR	NR	NR	NR	NR
Protein binding (%)	98	98–99	99	78–96	50–60

NR, not reported.
[a]From Rosser LM, O'Donnell AM, Lee KM, et al. In vitro protein-binding characteristics of atevirdine and its N-dealkylated metabolite. *Antiviral Res* 1994;25:193–200; and Been-Tiktak AMM, Vrehen HM, Schneider MME, et al. Safety, tolerance, and pharmacokinetics of atevirdine mesylate (U-87201E) in asymptomatic immunodeficiency virus-infected patients. *Antimicrob Agents Chemother* 1995;39:602–607, with permission.
[b]From Furman PA, Moxham C. MKC-442: non-nucleoside reverse transcriptase inhibitor. *Drugs Future* 1998;23:718–724, with permission.
[c]From Cheeseman SH, Hattox SE, McLaughlin MM, et al. Pharmacokinetics of nevirapine: initial single-rising-dose study in humans. *Antimicrob Agents Chemother* 1993;37:178–182; Nevirapine. Product information. Ridgefield, CT: Boehringer Ingelheim, 2002; and Hoetelmans RMW. Pharmacology of antiretroviral drugs. *Antiviral Ther* 1999;4[Suppl 3]:29–41, with permission.

has caused lactic acidosis, often associated with hepatic microsteatosis, pancreatitis, myopathy, and neuropathy. This syndrome may progress to fatal multiorgan system failure. It is associated with female gender, obesity, and prolonged courses of therapy.

FUSION INHIBITORS: ENFUVIRTIDE

Enfuvirtide [pentafuside; $C_{204}H_{301}N_{51}O_{64}$; molecular weight (MW), 4491.9 g/mol; CAS Registry No., 159519-65-0] is available in injectable form only.

Toxic Dose

The *adult therapeutic dose* is 100 mg subcutaneously twice daily. Overdose has not been reported.

Toxicokinetics and Toxicodynamics

The bioavailability of enfuvirtide is 75%; the half-life is 2 to 3 hours in animals (1).

Pathophysiology

Pentafuside is a synthetic peptide that prevents viral fusion and entry into cells by binding to one of two peptide domains within gp41 of the HIV virus, blocking the peptide ability to form a natural coil structure (2–5). The tip of the gp41 protein does not effectively penetrate the host cell membrane, and the virus cannot infect the host cell with its RNA.

NONNUCLEOSIDES

Atevirdine

Atevirdine (U-87201E; $C_{21}H_{25}N_5O_2$; MW, 379.5 g/mol; CAS Registry No., 138540-32-6) is provided in an injectable form only.

TOXIC DOSE

The *adult therapeutic dosage* is 600 mg three times daily (6). No overdose data are available.

TOXICOKINETICS AND TOXICODYNAMICS

The pharmacokinetics of atevirdine are provided in Table 2.

PATHOPHYSIOLOGY

Atevirdine inhibits the RNA- and DNA-directed DNA polymerases of HIV-1 reverse transcriptase (7).

PREGNANCY AND LACTATION

The U.S. Food and Drug Administration (FDA) category of atevirdine has not been established.

CLINICAL PRESENTATION

No overdose data are available. Rash, elevated serum triglyceride levels, and elevated transaminase levels have been reported during therapeutic use.

Delavirdine Mesylate

Delavirdine mesylate (Rescriptor; $C_{22}H_{28}N_6O_3S,CH_4O_3S$; MW, 552.7 g/mol; CAS Registry No., 147221-93-0) is available as 100- and 200-mg capsules.

TOXIC DOSE

The *adult therapeutic dose* is 400 mg three times daily. No overdose data are available.

TOXICOKINETICS AND TOXICODYNAMICS

The pharmacokinetics of delavirdine mesylate are provided in Table 2. It has nonlinear elimination at steady-state due to inhibition of P-450 3A metabolism.

PATHOPHYSIOLOGY

Delavirdine mesylate inhibits HIV reverse transcriptase, preventing viral replication. It also inhibits CYP3A and 2C9.

PREGNANCY AND LACTATION

Delavirdine mesylate is FDA pregnancy category C (Appendix I); it is unknown if excreted in breast milk.

CLINICAL PRESENTATION

The are no overdose data available. Adverse events during therapeutic use include headache, fatigue, nausea, vomiting and abdominal pain, and rashes. Elevation of serum transaminase levels, proteinuria, and myalgias are also described.

Efavirenz

Efavirenz (Sustiva, Stocrin; $C_{14}H_9ClF_3NO_2$; MW, 315.7 g/mol; CAS Registry No., 154598-52-4) is supplied as 50-, 100-, and 200-mg capsules and a 600-mg caplet.

TOXIC DOSE

The *adult therapeutic dosage* is 600 mg/day. The *pediatric dosage* ranges from 200 mg/day for patients weighing 10- to 15-kg body weight to 600 mg/day for patients weighing more than 40-kg body weight (8).

TOXICOKINETICS AND TOXICODYNAMICS

The pharmacokinetics of efavirenz are provided in Table 2. Efavirenz induces its own metabolism (CYP3A4 and CYP2B6); the half-life is 52 to 76 hours after a single dose, 40 to 55 hours after multiple doses.

PATHOPHYSIOLOGY

Efavirenz inhibits HIV reverse transcriptase, preventing viral replication.

PREGNANCY AND LACTATION

Efavirenz is FDA pregnancy category C (Appendix I). It is unsafe for breast-feeding.

CLINICAL PRESENTATION

An adult developed a manic syndrome with agitation, irritability, disinhibition, and aggressiveness after ingesting 90 efavirenz tablets (9). Increased central nervous system adverse effects and involuntary muscle contractions have been reported in patients who inadvertently took twice the normal daily dose (8).

ADVERSE EVENTS

Adverse central nervous system effects are common, including dizziness, insomnia, impaired concentration, somnolence, abnormal dreams, and occasionally hallucinations. Nausea, vomiting, and diarrhea are common. Rashes are quite common (26% of adults and 45% of children); rarely, Stevens-Johnson syndrome or toxic epidermal necrolysis may develop.

Emivirine

Emivirine (Coactinon; $C_{17}H_{22}N_2O_3$; MW, 302.4 g/mol; CAS Registry No., 149950-60-7) is usually used in combination with other drugs.

TOXIC DOSE

The *adult therapeutic dosage* is 750 mg twice daily (10). No toxic dose has been reported.

TOXICOKINETICS AND TOXICODYNAMICS

The pharmacokinetics of emivirine are provided in Table 2.

PATHOPHYSIOLOGY

Emivirine inhibits reverse transcriptase of HIV-1.

PREGNANCY AND LACTATION

Emivirine appears to be safe in pregnancy. No FDA pregnancy category has been established.

CLINICAL PRESENTATION

No overdose data are available. Headache, dizziness, nausea, vomiting, diarrhea, and increased γ-glutamyltransferase are common with therapeutic doses.

Nevirapine

Nevirapine (Viramune; $C_{15}H_{14}N_4O$; 266.3 g/mol; CAS Registry No., 129618-40-2) is provided as a 200-mg tablet and as a10-mg/ml suspension.

TOXIC DOSE

The *adult therapeutic dosage* is 200 mg/day initially, increased to twice daily after 2 weeks. The *pediatric dosage* for children 2 months to 8 years of age is initial dose, 4 mg/kg/day, increased to twice a day after 2 weeks (11).

TOXICOKINETICS AND TOXICODYNAMICS

The pharmacokinetics of nevirapine are provided in Table 2. The bioavailability is 90% (11,12). It has extensive hepatic metabolism, less than 5% renal excretion. The elimination half-life of 40 hours decreases to 25 to 30 hours after multiple doses because it induces its own metabolism (13).

PATHOPHYSIOLOGY

Nevirapine inhibits reverse transcriptase activity and replication of HIV-1.

PREGNANCY AND LACTATION

Nevirapine is FDA pregnancy category C (Appendix I). It is excreted into breast milk (concentration is 60% of serum) (14).

CLINICAL PRESENTATION

No overdose data are available. Relatively common adverse events include nausea, diarrhea, headache, somnolence, fatigue, fever, and rashes. Severe hepatotoxicity has been reported, and fatal hepatic failure has occasionally been reported. Stevens-Johnson syndrome and toxic epidermal necrolysis occur rarely. Nevirapine increases the metabolism of methadone and may induce withdrawal in patients on methadone maintenance (15).

NUCLEOSIDES

Abacavir

Abacavir (Ziagen; $C_{14}H_{18}N_6O_2, H_2SO_4$; MW, 670.7 g/mol; CAS Registry No., 188062-50-2) is available as a 300-mg tablet and as a 20-mg/ml solution.

TOXIC DOSE

The *adult therapeutic dosage* is 300 mg twice daily. The *pediatric dosage* is 8 mg/kg (maximum, 300 mg) twice daily.

TOXICOKINETICS AND TOXICODYNAMICS

The pharmacokinetics of abacavir are provided in Table 3. Bioavailability is approximately 83%. It undergoes extensive

TABLE 3. Selected pharmacokinetic parameters of nucleoside reverse transcriptase inhibitors

Paramater	Abacavir[a]	Didanosine[b]	Lamivudine[c]	Stavudine[d]	Zalcitabine[e]	Zidovudine[f]
Time to maximum serum concentration (h)	2	0.15–1.50	1.0–1.5	1	1–2	0.5–1.5
Apparent volume of distribution	0.85 L/kg	0.8–1.0 L/kg	0.9–1.7 L/kg	58 L	0.54–0.64 L/kg	1.6 L/kg
Route of excretion (%)	NR	18 renal	Renal	NR	62 renal, 10 fecal	18 renal
Elimination half-life (h)	1.0	1.3–1.5	3–7	0.9–1.6	1–3	0.5–3.0
Excreted unchanged (%)	<1	NR	70	40	NR	NR
Active metabolites	Abacavir monophosphate	Dideoxyadenosine triphosphate	Lamivudine triphosphate	Stavudine triphosphate	Zalcitabine triphosphate	Zidovudine triphosphate
Protein binding (%)	50	<5	<36	Negligible	<5	<38

NR, not reported.

[a]From Chittick GE, Gillotin C, McDowell JA, et al. Abacavir: absolute bioavailability, bioequivalence of three oral formulations, and effect of food. *Pharmacotherapy* 1999;19:932–942, with permission.

[b]From Lambert JS, Siedlin M, Reichman RC, et al. 2',3'-Dideoxyinosine (ddI) in patients with the acquired immunodeficiency syndrome or AIDS-related complex: a phase I trial. *N Engl J Med* 1990;322:1333–1340; and Videx, didanosine. Product information. Princeton, NJ: Bristol-Myers Squibb Company, 2002, with permission.

[c]From van Leeuwen R, Lange JM, Hussey EK, et al. The safety and pharmacokinetics of a reverse transcriptase inhibitor, 3TC, in patients with HIV infection: a phase I study. *AIDS* 1992;6:1471–1475, with permission.

[d]From Zerit, stavudine. Product information. Princeton, NJ: Bristol-Myers Squibb, 2002; and Browne MJ, Mayer KH, Chafee SBD, et al. 2',3'-Didehydro-3'-deoxythymidine (d4T) in patients with AIDS or AIDS-related complex: a phase I trial. *J Infect Dis* 1993;167:21–29, with permission.

[e]From Gustavson LE, Fukuda EK, Rubio FA, et al. A pilot study of the bioavailability and pharmacokinetics of 2',3'-dideoxycytidine in patients with AIDS or AIDS-related complex. *J AIDS* 1990;3:28–31; Klecker RW, Collins JM, Yarchoan RC, et al. Pharmacokinetics of 2',3'-dideoxycytidine in patients with AIDS and related disorders. *J Clin Pharmacol* 1988;28:837–842; and Adkins JC, Peters DH, Faulds D. Zalcitabine. An update of its pharmacodynamic and pharmacokinetic properties and clinical efficacy in the management of HIV infection. *Drugs* 1997;53:1054–1080, with permission.

[f]From Yarchoan R, Weinhold KJ, Lyerly HK, et al. Administration of 3'-azido-3'-deoxythymidine, an inhibitor of HTLV-III/LAV replication, to patients with AIDS or AIDS-related complex. *Lancet* 1986;1:575–580; Retrovir tablets, capsules, and syrup, zidovudine. Product information. Research Triangle Park, NC: GlaxoSmithKline, 2001; and Spear JB, Kessler HA, Lehrman SN, et al. Zidovudine overdosage. *Ann Intern Med* 1988;109:76–77, with permission.

hepatic metabolism, primarily by alcohol dehydrogenase and glucuronyl transferase; less than 1% is excreted unchanged in urine (16).

PATHOPHYSIOLOGY

Abacavir is a competitive inhibitor of HIV-RNA/DNA reverse transcriptase. Lactic acidosis has been postulated to be secondary to interference with mitochondrial DNA replication.

PREGNANCY AND LACTATION

Abacavir is FDA pregnancy category C (Appendix I). Excretion into breast milk is unknown.

CLINICAL PRESENTATION

Little overdose information is available. Adverse neurologic effects common during therapy include headache, sleep disturbance, dizziness, and fatigue (17). Fever and rash are the most common manifestations. Nausea, vomiting, diarrhea, and anorexia are also common. Nausea, vomiting, diarrhea, anorexia, headache, and fatigue are common at therapeutic doses. A hypersensitivity reaction may develop in 2% to 5% of patients and can be fatal (18,19).

Respiratory effects, such as dyspnea and cough, as well as pharyngitis may also be a component. Other nonspecific effects may include malaise, lethargy, myalgia, arthralgias, headache, and paresthesia. Physical findings may include lymphadenopathy, conjunctivitis, and oral ulcerations. In severe cases, anaphylaxis, liver or renal failure, hypotension, and death may ensue. Onset can be within hours after rechallenge with abacavir, even in patients without previous history of hypersensitivity (19).

A syndrome of lactic acidosis, with or without hepatomegaly, hepatic steatosis, and elevated serum transaminase levels has been reported in patients treated with abacavir and other nucleoside reverse transcriptase inhibitors. Pancreatitis, neuropathy, and myopathy may also develop. It is most common after prolonged therapy (more than 6 months) and may progress to fatal multiple-organ system failure.

Didanosine

Didanosine (Videx; $C_{10}H_{12}N_4O_3$; MW, 236.23 g/mol) is available as chewable tablets of 25, 50, 100, and 150 mg; single-dose packets of 100, 167, and 250 mg; and a pediatric powder for oral solution of 2 and 4 g.

TOXIC DOSE

The *adult therapeutic dosage* is 125 mg twice a day for patients weighing less than 60 kg and 200 mg twice a day for patients weighing more than 60 kg. The *pediatric dosage* (children 8 months of age or older) is 120 mg/m^2 twice a day (20).

Limited overdose data are available. When administered at ten times the recommended dose, pancreatitis, peripheral neuropathy, diarrhea, hyperuricemia, and hepatic injury have been reported (20).

TOXICOKINETICS AND TOXICODYNAMICS

The pharmacokinetics of didanosine are provided in Table 3. Its oral bioavailability is 21% to 43%.

PATHOPHYSIOLOGY

Didanosine inhibits HIV replication in T cells and monocytes. It is converted to an active metabolite that inhibits HIV reverse transcriptase and blocks DNA synthesis (21). The adverse effect of lactic acidosis has been postulated to be secondary to interference with mitochondrial DNA replication.

PREGNANCY AND LACTATION

Didanosine is FDA pregnancy category B (Appendix I). It is excreted into the breast milk of rats; no human data are available (20).

CLINICAL PRESENTATION

No information is available about single acute overdose. Chronic administration of doses ten times the therapeutic dose caused pancreatitis, peripheral neuropathy, diarrhea, hyperuricemia, and hepatic injury.

Painful, symmetrical distal neuropathy is a dose-limiting toxicity associated with therapeutic use. It is more common at higher doses and in patients at more advanced stages of HIV disease (22). Pancreatitis is another major toxicity associated with didanosine therapy, developing in 1% to 13% of treated patients. It is often associated with severe lactic acidosis and may be fatal. It appears to be more common at higher doses (20).

A syndrome of lactic acidosis with hepatomegaly, steatosis, pancreatitis, and elevated serum transaminase levels reported with other nucleoside reverse transcriptase inhibitors has also been reported with didanosine (23). This syndrome appears to be more common in pregnant women taking didanosine and stavudine in combination with other antiretroviral drugs (24).

Other adverse effects reported with therapeutic use include seizures, hypokalemia, hyperuricemia, thrombocytopenia, dysrhythmias, heart failure, and rashes. Optic neuritis and retinal depigmentation have been reported primarily in children. Concurrent use with zalcitabine may increase the risk of peripheral neuropathy. Concurrent use with ganciclovir increases didanosine concentrations (increases bioavailability) and may result in didanosine toxicity (20).

Lamivudine

Lamivudine (3TC, Epivir, Heptovir; $C_8H_{11}N_3O_3S$; MW, 229.3 g/mol; CAS Registry No., 131086-21-0, 134678-17-4) is available as 100- or 150-mg tablets and 5- or 10-mg/ml solutions.

TOXIC DOSE

The usual *adult therapeutic dosage* is 300 mg/day for HIV and 100 mg/day for hepatitis B infection. The *pediatric dosage* for children ages 3 months to 16 years is 4 mg/kg twice daily (25).

TOXICOKINETICS AND TOXICODYNAMICS

The pharmacokinetics of lamivudine are provided in Table 3.

PATHOPHYSIOLOGY

Lamivudine is converted to an active metabolite that inhibits HIV reverse transcriptase and blocks DNA synthesis. Lactic acidosis has been postulated to arise from interference with mitochondrial DNA replication.

PREGNANCY AND LACTATION

Lamivudine is FDA pregnancy category C (Appendix I). Small amounts are excreted into breast milk, with a mean concentration of 1.22 µg/ml (26).

CLINICAL PRESENTATION

Acute Overdosage. Ingestion of 6 g by an adult caused no symptoms and no laboratory or hematologic toxicity. Two children, one ingesting a single dose of 7 mg/kg and the other treated with 5 mg/kg twice daily for 30 days, did not develop evidence of toxicity (25).

Adverse Events. Bone marrow suppression, peripheral neuropathy, nausea, vomiting, and diarrhea are the most common adverse effects at therapeutic doses.

Stavudine

Stavudine (Zerit; $C_{10}H_{12}N_2O_4$; MW, 224.2 g/mol; CAS Registry No., 3056-17-5) is available as 15-, 20-, 30-, and 40-mg tablets and as a 1-mg/ml solution.

TOXIC DOSE

The usual *adult therapeutic dosage* is 40 mg every 12 hours for patients weighing more than 60 kg and 30 mg every 12 hours for patients weighing less than 60 kg. It should not be administered with zidovudine. The *pediatric dose* ranges from 0.8 mg/kg/dose for infants from birth to 13 days of age to the adult dose for children weighing 30 kg or more (27).

TOXICOKINETICS AND TOXICODYNAMICS

The pharmacokinetics of stavudine are provided in Table 3. Stavudine undergoes hepatic metabolism, with 40% of a dose excreted unchanged in urine (28).

PATHOPHYSIOLOGY

Stavudine is phosphorylated to an active metabolite (stavudine triphosphate) that inhibits HIV reverse transcriptase and blocks DNA synthesis. Lactic acidosis has been postulated to be secondary to interference with mitochondrial DNA replication.

PREGNANCY AND LACTATION

Stavudine is FDA pregnancy category C (Appendix I). It is excreted into breast milk in rats; no human data are available (27). Pregnant women should generally avoid the combination of stavudine and didanosine because of the risk of fatal lactic acidosis.

CLINICAL PRESENTATION

No clinical effects were noted in patients treated with 12 to 24 times the recommended daily dose (27).

Headache, nervousness, rashes, nausea, vomiting, and diarrhea are common adverse effects. Peripheral neuropathy may also occur. Lactic acidosis with hepatomegaly, steatosis, and marked elevation in transaminase levels has occurred with stavudine monotherapy or in combination with other antiretrovirals. A Guillain-Barré–like syndrome has also occurred in this setting.

Zalcitabine

Zalcitabine (Hivid; $C_9H_{13}N_3O_3$; MW, 211.2 g/mol; CAS Registry No., 7481-89-2) is supplied as 0.375- and 0.75-mg tablets.

TOXIC DOSE

The *adult therapeutic dosage* is 0.75 mg orally every 8 hours: Intravenous dosages of 0.03 to 0.09 mg/kg every 4 hours have been used (29). The *pediatric dosage* is 0.015 to 0.040 mg/kg every 6 hours (30).

TOXICOKINETICS AND TOXICODYNAMICS

The pharmacokinetics of zalcitabine are provided in Table 3.

PATHOPHYSIOLOGY

Zalcitabine is phosphorylated to a metabolite that inhibits HIV reverse transcriptase and blocks DNA synthesis. Lactic acidosis has been postulated to be secondary to interference with mitochondrial DNA replication.

PREGNANCY AND LACTATION

Zalcitabine is FDA pregnancy category C (Appendix I). Entry into breast milk is unknown.

CLINICAL PRESENTATION

Acute Overdosage. In children, inadvertent overdose of 1.5 mg/kg produced no clinical evidence of toxicity. Mixed overdoses in adults (up to 18.75 mg zalcitabine) have resulted in drowsiness, vomiting, increased creatine kinase, and γ-glutamyltransferase (31).

Adverse Events. Peripheral neuropathy is common at therapeutic doses, occurring in 22% to 35% of patients (32). The neuropathy is in a stocking-glove distribution (primarily lower extremities) and is initially painful but may progress to numbness (32). It is more common in patients with advanced HIV. In early studies, all patients receiving six times the current total recommended daily dose developed peripheral neuropathy by the tenth week; 8% of patients receiving two times the currently recommended daily dose developed peripheral neuropathy by the twelfth week (31).

A syndrome of rash with fever, lymphadenopathy, and aphthous ulcers is fairly common, usually developing within 4 to 6 weeks (33). Neutropenia, thrombocytopenia, and, less often, anemia may occur with therapeutic doses. Pancreatitis and hepatic failure with metabolic acidosis, hepatic steatosis, and hepatomegaly are rare but life-threatening adverse effects with zalcitabine (31).

Drug Interactions. Concurrent use with didanosine may increase risk of peripheral neuropathy (31). Cimetidine and probenecid decrease renal excretion of zalcitabine and may cause toxicity (31).

Zidovudine

Zidovudine (Retrovir; $C_{10}H_{13}N_5O_4$; MW, 267.2 g/mol; CAS Registry No., 30516-87-1) is available as a 100-mg capsule, 300-mg tablet, 10-mg/ml solution, and 10-mg/ml syrup.

TOXIC DOSE

The *adult therapeutic dosage* is 600 mg/day divided in two or three doses. The *pediatric dosage* for children 6 weeks to 12 years of age is 160 mg/m^2 every 8 hours (maximum, 200 mg every 8 hours) (34).

TOXICOKINETICS AND TOXICODYNAMICS

The pharmacokinetics of zidovudine are provided in Table 3. It undergoes extensive hepatic metabolism with significant first-pass effect; renal clearance is 18% (34). Elimination half-life is 0.5 to 3.0 hours after therapeutic dosing, 1 hour after overdose (35).

PATHOPHYSIOLOGY

Zidovudine is phosphorylated to a metabolite that inhibits HIV reverse transcriptase and blocks DNA synthesis. Lactic acidosis has been postulated to be secondary to interference with mitochondrial DNA replication.

PREGNANCY AND LACTATION

Zidovudine is FDA pregnancy category C (Appendix I). It is excreted into human breast milk at a concentration similar to that in serum (34).

CLINICAL PRESENTATION

Acute Overdosage. Clinical toxicity after acute overdose is limited. An adult who ingested 3.6 g remained asymptomatic, whereas another developed only lethargy after ingesting 3 g (36,37). A 20-g ingestion was associated with lethargy and mild myelosuppression (38). An adult developed a single tonic-clonic seizure 3 hours after ingesting 36 g (39). In adults ingesting overdoses of up to 50 g, most developed nausea and vomiting; mild myelosuppression was common, and transient neurologic effects, such as lethargy, headache, dizziness, and confusion, developed in some patients (34). A 27-month-old child was asymptomatic after ingesting 130 mg (40).

Adverse Events. Myelosuppression, seizures, nausea, vomiting and anorexia, and fingernail discoloration are adverse effects that are fairly common after therapeutic use. A syndrome of lactic acidosis with hepatic steatosis, hepatic injury, and hepatomegaly has been reported with zidovudine use.

Drug Interactions. Concurrent administration with other drugs that cause myelosuppression (e.g., dapsone, doxorubicin, flucytosine, ganciclovir, interferon-alpha, vinblastine, vincristine) may increase the risk of myelosuppression (34). Interferon-beta-1A, methadone, probenecid, valproic acid, and sulfacytine reduce zidovudine clearance and may cause toxicity (41–44).

PROTEASE INHIBITORS

Amprenavir

Amprenavir (Agenerase; $C_{25}H_{35}N_3O_6S$; MW, 505.6 g/mol; CAS Registry No., 161814-49-9) is supplied as 50- and 150-mg capsules and 15-mg/ml solution.

TOXIC DOSE

The *adult therapeutic dosage* is 1200 mg twice daily. The *pediatric dosage* is 20 mg/kg twice daily for children weighing less than 50 kg, with a maximum daily dose of 2400 mg. Amprenavir solution is contraindicated in infants and children younger than 4 years of age.

TOXICOKINETICS AND TOXICODYNAMICS

The pharmacokinetics of amprenavir are provided in Table 4. It undergoes extensive hepatic metabolism by cytochrome CYP3A4; less than 3% is excreted unchanged in urine (45).

PATHOPHYSIOLOGY

Amprenavir binds to the active site of HIV protease, preventing the binding of viral protein precursors, resulting in the formation of immature, noninfectious viral particles.

PREGNANCY AND LACTATION

Amprenavir is FDA pregnancy category C (Appendix I). The solution is contraindicated in pregnancy because of propylene glycol excipient.

CLINICAL PRESENTATION

No overdose information is available. Headache, nausea, vomiting, diarrhea, rashes, and peripheral neuropathy manifesting as perioral peripheral paresthesias are the most common adverse effects associated with chronic therapy (45,46). Hyperglycemia and new-onset diabetes mellitus have also been reported. Amprenavir solution contains propylene glycol as an excipient, which may cause seizures, central nervous system depression, tachycardia, lactic acidosis, and nephrotoxicity in large doses, especially in susceptible populations (infants and young children, pregnancy, hepatic and renal failure).

Indinavir Sulfate

Indinavir sulfate (Crixivan; $C_{36}H_{47}N_5O_4{,}H_2SO_4$; MW, 711.9 g/mol; CAS Registry No., 157810-81-6) is available as 100-, 200-, 333-, and 400-mg capsules.

TABLE 4. Selected pharmacokinetic parameters of protease inhibitors

Parameter	Amprenavir[a]	Indinavir[b]	Lopinavir[c]	Ritonavir[d]	Nelfinavir[e]	Saquinavir[f]
Time to maximum serum concentration (h)	1–2	0.8	5	2–4	2–4	3
Volume of distribution	430 L	195 L	NR	0.41 L/kg	2–7 L/kg	700 L
Elimination (%)	—	—	—	11 renal, 86 fecal	1–2 renal, 87 fecal	1–3 renal, 81–88 fecal
Elimination half-life (h)	7–10	1.5–2.0	5–6	3.0–3.5	3.5–5.0	13
Excreted unchanged (%)	<3	Little	Little	3.5	Little	Little
Active metabolites	—	—	—	NR	NR	NR
Protein binding (%)	90	60	98–99	98–99	99	98

NR, not reported.
[a]From Adkins JC, Faulds D. Amprenavir. *Drugs* 1998;55:837–842; and Agenerase, amprenavir. Product information. Research Triangle Park, NC: Glaxo Wellcome Inc., 2002, with permission.
[b]From Hoetelmans RMW. Pharmacology of antiretroviral drugs. *Antiviral Ther* 1999;4[Suppl 3]:29–41; Crixivan, indinavir sulfate. Product information. Whitehouse Station, NJ: Merck & Co., Inc., 2002; and Letendre SL, Capparelli EV, Ellis RJ, et al. Indinavir population pharmacokinetics in plasma and cerebrospinal fluid. *Antimicrob Agents Chemother* 2000;44:2173–2175, with permission.
[c]From Bertz R, Lam W, Brun S, et al. Multiple-dose pharmacokinetics (PK) of ABT-378/ritonavir (ABT-378/r) in HIV+ subjects (abstract 327). Abstract of the 39th Interscience Conference on Antimicrobial Agents and Chemotherapy. September 26–29 1999:15; and Kaletra. Product information. North Chicago, IL: Abbott Laboratories, 2002, with permission.
[d]From Norvir. Product information. North Chicago, IL: Abbott Laboratories, 2002; and Kempf DJ, Marsh KC, Denissen JF, et al. ABT-538 is a potent inhibitor of human immunodeficiency virus protease and has high oral bioavailability in humans. *Proc Natl Acad Sci U S A* 1995;92:2484–2488, with permission.
[e]From Viracept, nelfinavir. Product information. La Jolla, CA: Agouron Pharmaceuticals, Inc., 2002, with permission.
[f]From Williams PEO, Muirhead GJ, Madigan MJ, et al. Disposition and bioavailability of the HIV-proteinase inhibitor, Ro 31-8959, after single oral doses in healthy volunteers. Proceedings of the BPS, 1992 April 8–10:155P–156P; and Invirase, saquinavir mesylate. Product information. Nutley, NJ: Roche Laboratories Inc., 2002, with permission.

TOXIC DOSE
The *adult therapeutic dosage* is 800 mg orally every 8 hours. The *pediatric dose* is not approved, but dosages of 350 to 500 mg/m^2 orally every 8 hours have been reported.

TOXICOKINETICS AND TOXICODYNAMICS
The pharmacokinetics of indinavir sulfate are provided in Table 4. It undergoes extensive hepatic metabolism by CYP3A4 (47).

PATHOPHYSIOLOGY
Indinavir interferes with HIV protease, preventing processing of viral protein precursors, resulting in the formation of immature, noninfectious viral particles.

PREGNANCY AND LACTATION
Indinavir is FDA pregnancy category C (Appendix I). It is excreted into breast milk in rats; no human data are available.

CLINICAL PRESENTATION
Acute Overdosage. Ingestion of 8 g resulted in nausea, dizziness, and extremity paresthesia, which resolved within 4 hours (48). In more than 60 cases of acute or chronic overdose of up to 23 times the maximum daily dose, flank pain, hematuria, nephrolithiasis, nausea, vomiting, and diarrhea were the most common effects (47).

Adverse Events. Nephrolithiasis develops in 4% to 12% of treated patients, related to crystallization of drug in the urine (49,50). Other common adverse effects include hepatotoxicity (usually reversible), nausea, vomiting, and diarrhea. Hypertension and new-onset diabetes mellitus are less common adverse effects (47,51).

Lopinavir

Lopinavir (Kaletra; $C_{37}H_{48}N_4O_5$; MW, 628.8 g/mol; CAS Registry No., 192725-17-0) is available as a capsule containing lopinavir/ritonavir (133.3 mg/33.3 mg) or a solution (80 mg/20 mg/ml).

TOXIC DOSE
The *adult therapeutic dosage* is 400 mg (with 100 mg ritonavir) twice daily. The *pediatric dosage* for children 6 months to 12 years of age who weigh 7 to 15 kg is 12 mg/kg lopinavir and 3 mg/kg ritonavir twice daily (52).

TOXICOKINETICS AND TOXICODYNAMICS
The pharmacokinetics of lopinavir are provided in Table 4. Bioavailability in humans is unknown, but it is low in animals (53). Bioavailability increases when administered with ritonavir secondary to decreased first-pass metabolism (53). It undergoes extensive hepatic metabolism, primarily by CYP3A4.

PATHOPHYSIOLOGY
Lopinavir interferes with HIV protease, preventing processing of viral protein precursors, resulting in the formation of immature, noninfectious viral particles.

PREGNANCY AND LACTATION
Lopinavir is FDA pregnancy category C (Appendix I). Breast-feeding is considered unsafe.

CLINICAL PRESENTATION
No overdose data are available. Nausea, vomiting, diarrhea, and abdominal pain are common. Mild elevations in serum transaminase concentrations are seen less often. Pancreatitis is rare, but fatal cases have been reported (52).

Ritonavir

Ritonavir (Norvir; $C_{37}H_{48}N_6O_5S_2$; MW, 720.9 g/mol; CAS Registry No., 155213-67-5) is available as a 100-mg tablet or solution (80 mg/ml).

TOXIC DOSE
The *adult therapeutic dosage* is 600 mg orally twice daily. The *pediatric dosage* is 400 mg/m^2 twice daily (54).

TOXICOKINETICS AND TOXICODYNAMICS
The pharmacokinetics of ritonavir are provided in Table 4. It is well absorbed; bioavailability is 80% in animals (55). It undergoes extensive hepatic metabolism by CYP3A4.

PATHOPHYSIOLOGY
Ritonavir interferes with HIV protease, preventing processing of viral protein precursors, resulting in the formation of immature, noninfectious viral particles.

PREGNANCY AND LACTATION

Ritonavir is FDA pregnancy category C (Appendix I). Entry into breast milk is unknown.

CLINICAL PRESENTATION

Paresthesias have been reported after overdose. Ingestion of 1500 mg/day for 2 days resulted in paresthesias that resolved after dose reduction. Renal failure with eosinophilia has also been reported after overdose of an unknown quantity (54).

Nausea, vomiting, diarrhea, and increased serum cholesterol and triglyceride levels are common adverse effects with therapeutic use (54,56). Circumoral and peripheral paresthesias are common, occurring in up to 15% and up to 7%, respectively, in treated patients (56). Hepatotoxicity is common, developing in 30% of patients in two studies (56,57). Although elevations in serum transaminase levels are usually mild, severe hepatotoxicity and fatal liver failure have been reported (58). Renal insufficiency is common, developing in 14% of patients in one study (59). Acute renal failure is uncommon (60). Pancreatitis is a rare adverse effect, but fatal cases have occurred (54,61).

Nelfinavir Mesylate

Nelfinavir mesylate (Viracept; $C_{32}H_{45}N_3O_4S,CH_4O_3S$; MW, 663.9 g/mol; CAS Registry No., 159989-65-8) is available as 250-mg tablets and 50-mg/g powder.

TOXIC DOSE

The *adult therapeutic dosage* is 750 mg three times daily or 1250 mg twice daily. The *pediatric dosage* for children ages 2 to 13 years is 20 to 30 mg/kg/dose three times daily (62).

TOXICOKINETICS AND TOXICODYNAMICS

The pharmacokinetics of nelfinavir mesylate are provided in Table 4. It undergoes extensive hepatic metabolism; urinary excretion is 1% to 2%; fecal elimination is 87% (78% as oxidative metabolites, 22% as unchanged drug) (62).

PATHOPHYSIOLOGY

Nelfinavir mesylate interferes with HIV protease, preventing processing of viral protein precursors, resulting in the formation of immature, noninfectious viral particles.

PREGNANCY AND LACTATION

Nelfinavir mesylate is FDA pregnancy category C (Appendix I). It is excreted into breast milk in rats.

CLINICAL PRESENTATION

No information on clinical effects in overdose is available. Headache, fatigue, nausea, and diarrhea are common adverse effects. Mild anemia and neutropenia have been reported in children (63). Urticaria has developed in less than 2% of treated patients and recurs with rechallenge (64). Symptomatic junctional bradycardia was reported in a 45-year-old man on nelfinavir mesylate. It resolved when the drug was withdrawn and recurred with rechallenge on three separate occasions (65).

Saquinavir Mesylate

Saquinavir mesylate (Invirase; $C_{38}H_{50}N_6O_5,CH_4O_3S$; MW, 766.9 g/mol; CAS Registry No., 149845-06-7) is available as a 200-mg capsule.

TOXIC DOSE

The *adult therapeutic dosage* is 600 mg orally three times a day. The pediatric dose has not been reported.

TOXICOKINETICS AND TOXICODYNAMICS

The pharmacokinetics of saquinavir mesylate are provided in Table 4. Bioavailability of the hard gelatin capsule is 4%; the soft gelatin capsule is believed to have a bioavailability 331% higher (66). It undergoes hepatic metabolism, primarily by CYP3A4 with extensive first-pass effect (66).

PATHOPHYSIOLOGY

Saquinavir mesylate interferes with HIV protease, preventing processing of viral protein precursors, resulting in the formation of immature, noninfectious viral particles.

PREGNANCY AND LACTATION

Saquinavir mesylate is FDA pregnancy category B (Appendix I). It is unknown if it is excreted into breast milk.

CLINICAL PRESENTATION

Acute Overdosage. A patient who ingested 8 g remained asymptomatic. Another patient who ingested 2.4 g saquinavir mesylate and 600 mg ritonavir developed throat pain that resolved after 6 hours. Chronic administration of 7200 mg/day for 25 weeks did not result in serious toxicity (67).

Adverse Events. Nausea, diarrhea, dyspepsia, abdominal pain, and asthenia are common. Paresthesia and peripheral neuropathy have been reported in 4% to 5% of patients. Mild neutropenia and anemia have been reported as well as rare cases of hemolytic anemia (67,68).

DIAGNOSTIC TESTS

The antiretroviral drugs rarely require diagnostic tests to establish the diagnosis. Most diagnostic testing is directed at adverse events.

Acute and Subacute Overdosage

Monitor serum electrolytes and glucose, renal function tests, and serum transaminase concentrations in symptomatic patients after overdose.

Adverse Events

Multiple organ systems are often involved. The complete blood cell count with differential is monitored to detect bone marrow suppression. Monitor bilirubin and international normalized ratio in patients with elevated transaminase levels. For the nucleoside agents, measure the serum lipase concentration if clinical presentation suggests pancreatitis. Monitor urinalysis and evaluate for clinical evidence of nephrolithiasis after indinavir overdose.

Nerve conduction velocities may be useful in evaluating patients with paresthesias or dysesthesias. Computerized tomography of the kidneys, ureters, and bladder or intravenous pyelogram may be used to confirm nephrolithiasis in patients with suggestive symptoms after indinavir sulfate overdose.

TREATMENT

With few exceptions, the retroviral drugs are treated primarily with symptomatic and supportive care.

Gastrointestinal Decontamination

Life-threatening toxicity is unusual after acute overdose with these agents. A single dose of activated charcoal is adequate in most patients.

Enhancement of Elimination

There are no reports of the use of any enhanced elimination technique in the treatment of overdose. Didanosine and stavudine are known to be cleared by hemodialysis.

Antidotes

There are no antidotes for any of the antiretroviral agents. Riboflavin may be useful as described in the section Supportive Care.

Supportive Care

Life-threatening toxicity is not yet reported after acute overdose with these agents. Intravenous hydration with normal saline to maintain a urine output of 2 to 3 ml/kg/hour is recommended after indinavir sulfate overdose, as urinary calculi may form secondary to crystallization of the drug in urine.

Patients who present with lactic acidosis and hepatic injury with or without pancreatitis may progress to life-threatening toxicity, hypotension, and multiorgan system failure. They should be admitted to an intensive care setting, with careful monitoring of mental status, vital signs, renal and hepatic function, acid-base balance, and serum lactate. Hypotension should be treated with intravenous normal saline. Central venous pressure monitoring may be useful in guiding fluid therapy in patients with persistent hypotension. Vasopressors, such as dopamine or norepinephrine, may be needed.

Case reports suggest that riboflavin (50 mg/day) may help reverse lactic acidosis in the setting of nucleoside reverse transcriptase toxicity (69,70). Data are limited to a handful of cases, and there are no controlled trials or animal models evaluating this therapy.

Management Pitfalls

Most patients taking antiretrovirals are on complex drug regimens. The potential for drug interactions is great, and it is important to gain accurate information about all the medications to which a patient has access that may be responsible for an overdose or toxic effect.

REFERENCES

1. Johnson MR, Lambert DM, Hopkins S, et al. T-20: a peptide-based membrane fusion inhibitor directed against HIV-1 gp41 (abstract 335). Third conference on retroviruses and opportunistic infections; 1996 Jan 28:115.
2. Lambert DM, Barney S, Lambert AL, et al. Peptides from conserved regions of paramyxovirus fusion (F) proteins are potent inhibitors of viral fusion. *Proc Natl Acad Sci U S A* 1996;93:2186–2191.
3. Reference deleted.
4. Wild CT, Shugars DC, Greenwell TK, et al. Peptides corresponding to a predictive alpha-helical domain of human immunodeficiency virus type 1 gp41 are potent inhibitors of virus infection. *Proc Natl Acad Sci U S A* 1994;91:9770–9774.
5. Johnson MR, Lambert DM, Hopkins S, et al. Pentafuside (T-20): an amphipathic helical peptide-based membrane fusion inhibitor directed against HIV-1 gp41 (abstract 252). 211th American Chemical Society National Meeting; 1996 March 24.
6. Brew BJ, Dunbar N, Druett JA, et al. Pilot study of the efficacy of atevirdine in the treatment of AIDS dementia complex. *AIDS* 1996;10:1357–1360.
7. Althaus IW, Chou JJ, Gonzales AJ, et al. Steady-state kinetic studies with the non-nucleoside HIV-1 reverse transcriptase inhibitor U-87201E. *J Biol Chem* 1993;268:6119–6124.
8. Sustiva, efavirenz. Product information. Princeton, NJ: Bristol-Myers Squibb Company, 2002.
9. Blanch J, Corbella B, Garcia F, et al. Manic syndrome associated with efavirenz overdose [Letter]. *Clin Infect Dis* 2001;33:270–271.
10. Johnson D, Sanne I, Baraldi E, et al. A phase II, open-label study to evaluate the antiviral activity, safety, and tolerability of emivirine (EMV, MKC-442) with stavudine (d4T) + didanosine (ddI) (abstract 502). Abstract from the 39th ICAAC, San Francisco; 1999 Sept 26–29:470.
11. Viramune, nevirapine. Product information. Columbus, OH: Roxane Laboratories, Inc., 2002.
12. Cheeseman SH, Hattox SE, McLaughlin MM, et al. Pharmacokinetics of nevirapine: initial single-rising-dose study in humans. *Antimicrob Agents Chemother* 1993;37:178–182.
13. Hoetelmans RMW. Pharmacology of antiretroviral drugs. *Antiviral Ther* 1999;4[Suppl 3]:29–41.
14. Musoke P, Guay LA, Bagenda D, et al. A phase I/II study of the safety and pharmacokinetics of nevirapine in HIV-1-infected pregnant Ugandan women and their neonates (HIVNET 006). *AIDS* 1999;13:479–486.
15. Altice FL, Friedland GH, Cooney EL. Nevirapine induced opiate withdrawal among injection drug users with HIV infection receiving methadone. *AIDS* 1999;13:957–962.
16. Chittick GE, Gillotin C, McDowell JA, et al. Abacavir: absolute bioavailability, bioequivalence of three oral formulations, and effect of food. *Pharmacotherapy* 1999;19:932–942.
17. Staszewski S, Katlama C, Harrer T, et al. A dose-ranging study to evaluate the safety and efficacy of abacavir alone or in combination with zidovudine and lamivudine in antiretroviral treatment-naive subjects. *AIDS* 1998;12:F197–F202.
18. Saag MS, Sonnerborg A, Torres RA, et al. Antiretroviral effect and safety of abacavir alone and in combination with zidovudine in HIV-infected adults. *AIDS* 1998;12:F203–F209.
19. Ziagen, abacavir. Product information. Research Triangle Park, NC: Glaxo Wellcome Inc., 2002.
20. Videx, didanosine. Product information. Princeton, NJ: Bristol-Myers Squibb Company, 2002.
21. Lambert JS, Siedlin M, Reichman RC, et al. 2',3'-Dideoxyinosine (ddI) in patients with the acquired immunodeficiency syndrome or AIDS-related complex: a phase I trial. *N Engl J Med* 1990;322:1333–1340.
22. Moore RD, Wong WME, Keruly JC, et al. Incidence of neuropathy in HIV-infected patients on monotherapy versus those on combination therapy with didanosine, stavudine, and hydroxyurea. *AIDS* 2000;14:273–278.
23. Coghlan ME, Sommadossi JP, Jhala NC, et al. Symptomatic lactic acidosis in hospitalized antiretroviral-treated patients with human immunodeficiency virus infection: a report of 12 cases. *Clin Infect Dis* 2001;33:1914–1921.
24. Anonymous. FDA Talk Paper: FDA/Bristol Myers Squibb issues caution for HIV combination therapy with Zerit and Videx in pregnant women. January 5, 2001. Available at: http://www.fda.gov/bbs/topics/ANSWERS/ANS01063.html.
25. Epivir, lamivudine. Product information. Research Triangle Park, NC: GlaxoSmithKline, 2002.
26. Moodley J, Moddley D, Pillay K, et al. Pharmacokinetics and antiretroviral activity of lamivudine alone or when coadministered with zidovudine in human immunodeficiency virus type 1-infected pregnant women and their offspring. *J Infect Dis* 1998;178:1327–1333.
27. Zerit, stavudine. Product information. Princeton, NJ: Bristol-Myers Squibb, 2002.
28. Browne MJ, Mayer KH, Chafee SBD, et al. 2',3'-Didehydro-3'-deoxythymidine (d4T) in patients with AIDS or AIDS-related complex: a phase I trial. *J Infect Dis* 1993;167:21–29.
29. Yarchoan R, Thomas RV, Allain JP, et al. Phase I studies of 2',3'-dideoxycytidine in severe human immunodeficiency virus infection as a single agent and alternating with zidovudine (AZT). *Lancet* 1988;1:76–81.
30. Pizzo PA, Butler K, Balis F, et al. Dideoxycytidine alone and in an alternating schedule with zidovudine in children with symptomatic human immunodeficiency virus infection. *J Pediatr* 1990;117:799–808.
31. HIVID, zalcitabine. Product information. Nutley, NJ: Roche Laboratories, 2002.
32. Blum AS, Dal Pan GJ, Feinberg J, et al. Low-dose zalcitabine-related toxic neuropathy: frequency, natural history, and risk factors. *Neurology* 1996;46:999–1003.
33. Broder S. Pharmacodynamics of 2',3'-dideoxycytidine: an inhibitor of human immunodeficiency virus. *Am J Med* 1990;88[Suppl 5B]:2S–7S.
34. Retrovir tablets, capsules, and syrup, zidovudine. Product information. Research Triangle Park, NC: GlaxoSmithKline, 2001.
35. Spear JB, Kessler HA, Lehrman SN, et al. Zidovudine overdosage. *Ann Intern Med* 1988;109:76–77.
36. Heard JM, Slovis CM. Zidovudine (AZT) (Retrovir) overdose. *Vet Hum Toxicol* 1988;30:365–366(abst).
37. Stern RA, van der Horst CM, Hooper SR, et al. Zidovudine overdose in an asymptomatic HIV seropositive patient with hemophilia. *Psychosomatics* 1992;33:454–457.
38. Pickus OB. Overdose of zidovudine [Letter]. *N Engl J Med* 1988;318:1206.
39. Routy JP, Prajs E, Blanc AP, et al. Seizure after zidovudine overdose [Letter]. *Lancet* 1989;1:384–385.
40. Moore EC, Cohen F, Kauffman RE, et al. Zidovudine overdose in a child (letter). *N Engl J Med* 1990;322:408–409.
41. Ruedy J, Schechter M, Montaner JS. Zidovudine for early human immunodeficiency virus (HIV) infection: who, when, and how? *Ann Intern Med* 1990;112:721–723.
42. McCance-Katz EF, Rainey PM, Jatlow P, et al. Methadone effects on zidovudine disposition (AIDS clinical trials group 262). *J Acquir Immune Defic Syndr Hum Retrovirol* 1998;18:435–443.
43. Kornhauser DM, Petty BG, Hendrix CW, et al. Probenecid and zidovudine metabolism. *Lancet* 1989;2:473–475.
44. Lertora JJ, Rege AB, Greenspan DL, et al. Pharmacokinetic interaction between zidovudine and valproic acid in patients infected with human immunodeficiency virus. *Clin Pharmacol Ther* 1994;56:272–278.
45. Adkins JC, Faulds D. Amprenavir. *Drugs* 1998;55:837–842.
46. Agenerase, amprenavir. Product information. Research Triangle Park, NC: Glaxo Wellcome Inc., 2002.

47. Crixivan, indinavir sulfate. Product information. Whitehouse Station, NJ: Merck & Co., Inc., 2002.
48. Burkhart KK, Kemerer K, Donovan JW. Indinavir overdose [Letter]. *J Toxicol Clin Toxicol* 1998;36:747.
49. Reiter WJ, Schon-Pernerstorfer H, Dorfinger K, et al. Frequency of urolithiasis in individuals seropositive for human immunodeficiency virus treated with indinavir is higher than previously assumed. *J Urol* 1999;161:1082–1084.
50. Daudon M, Estepa L, Viard JP, et al. Urinary stones in HIV-1-positive patients treated with indinavir. *Lancet* 1997;349:1294–1295.
51. Hewitt R, Hernandez F, Shelton M. Systemic hypertension associated with indinavir (abstract). Presented at the 39th Interscience Conference on Antimicrobial Agents and Chemotherapy; September 26, 1999; San Francisco.
52. Kaletra. Product information. North Chicago, IL: Abbott Laboratories, 2002.
53. Sham HL, Kempf DJ, Molla A, et al. ABT-378, a highly potent inhibitor of the human immunodeficiency virus protease. *Antimicrob Agents Chemother* 1998;42(12):3218–3224.
54. Norvir. Product information. North Chicago, IL: Abbott Laboratories, 2002.
55. Kempf DJ, Marsh KC, Denissen JF, et al. ABT-538 is a potent inhibitor of human immunodeficiency virus protease and has high oral bioavailability in humans. *Proc Natl Acad Sci U S A* 1995;92:2484–2488.
56. Markowitz M, Saag M, Powderly WG, et al. A preliminary study of ritonavir, an inhibitor of HIV-1 protease, to treat HIV-1 infection. *N Engl J Med* 1995;333:1534–1539.
57. Sulkowski MS, Thomas DL, Chaisson RE, et al. Hepatotoxicity associated with antiretroviral therapy in adults infected with human immunodeficiency virus and the role of hepatitis C or B virus infection. *JAMA* 2000;283:74–80.
58. Arribase JR, Ibanez C, Ruiz-Antoran B, et al. Acute hepatitis in HIV-infected patients during ritonavir treatment. *AIDS* 1998;12:1722–1724.
59. Bochet MV, Jacquiaud C, Valantin MA, et al. Renal insufficiency induced by ritonavir in HIV-infected patients [Letter]. *Am J Med* 1998;105:457.
60. Deray G. Ritonavir-induced acute renal failure [Letter]. *Clin Drug Invest* 1998;16:175.
61. Perry RC, Cushing HE, Deeg MA, et al. Ritonavir, triglycerides, and pancreatitis. *Clin Infect Dis* 1999;28:161–162.
62. Viracept, nelfinavir. Product information. La Jolla, CA: Agouron Pharmaceuticals, Inc., 2002.
63. Krogstad P, Wiznia A, Luzuriaga K, et al. Treatment of human immunodeficiency virus 1-infected infants and children with the protease inhibitor nelfinavir mesylate. *Clin Infect Dis* 1999;28:1109–1118.
64. Demoly P, Messaad D, Trylesinski A, et al. Nelfinavir-induced urticaria and successful desensitization. *J Allergy Clin Immunol* 1998;102:875–876.
65. Landovitz RJ, Sax PE. Symptomatic junctional bradycardia after treatment with nelfinavir. *Clin Infect Dis* 1999;29:449–450.
66. Fortavase, saquinavir soft gelatin capsule. Product information. Nutley, NJ: Roche Laboratories Inc., 2002.
67. Invirase, saquinavir mesylate. Product information. Nutley, NJ: Roche Laboratories Inc., 2002.
68. Kitchen VS, Skinner C, Ariyoshi K, et al. Safety and activity of saquinavir in HIV infection. *Lancet* 1995;345:952–955.
69. Fouty B, Frerman F, Reves R. Riboflavin to treat nucleoside analogue-induced lactic acidosis. *Lancet* 1998;352:291–292.
70. Luzzati R, Bravo PD, Perri GD, et al. Riboflavine and severe lactic acidosis (letter). *Lancet* 1999.

CHAPTER 94

Antimalarial Agents

Ian MacGregor Whyte

CH_2CH_3 N CH_2CH_3 H N CH_3 N Cl

CHLOROQUINE

Compounds included:	**See Table 1.**
Molecular formula and weight:	**See Table 3.**
SI conversion:	**Chloroquine, mg/L × 3.13 = μmol/L; hydroxychloroquine, mg/L × 2.98 = μmol/L; quinine, mg/L × 3.08 = μmol/L**
CAS Registry No.:	**See Table 3.**
Therapeutic levels:	**Chloroquine, 0.3 mg/L; quinine, 1 to 3 mg/L**
Target organs:	**Eyes (acute), heart (acute), central nervous system (acute), blood (acute)**
Antidotes:	**Folinic acid, methylene blue, benzodiazepines, beta-receptor agonists**

OVERVIEW

The toxicity of antimalarial drugs varies greatly because the drugs come from several different chemical classes with very different structures. Antimalarial drugs can be classified by their structure and by the stage of the parasitic life cycle they affect (Tables 1 and 2). Most of the current drugs are quinoline-related compounds, which include the highly toxic quinine, chloroquine, and hydroxychloroquine. Several antimalarials have other indications that serve to increase the availability of these drugs in populations not prone to malaria. Examples include chloroquine and hydroxychloroquine for rheumatic diseases, quinine for leg cramps, and pyrimethamine and primaquine in human immunodeficiency virus infection.

Several drugs used in the treatment of malaria are covered in other sections of this book: the 4-methanolquinoline, quinidine (optical isomer of quinine); the sulfone, dapsone; the tetracyclines, doxycycline and tetracycline; the sulfonamides, sulfadoxine and sulfametopyrazine; and the lincosamide antimicrobial, clindamycin.

TABLE 1. Structural classification of antimalarial agents

Group	Structural subgroup	Examples
Quinoline-related compounds	4-Methanolquinolines	Quinine, mefloquine
	4-Aminoquinolines	Amodiaquine, amopyroquine, chloroquine, hydroxychloroquine
	8-Aminoquinolines	Primaquine
	4-Piperazinoquinolines	Piperaquine, hydroxypiperaquine
Antifolates	Biguanides	Chlorproguanil, proguanil (cycloguanil)
	Diaminopyrimidines	Pyrimethamine
Antimicrobials	Hydroxynaphthoquinones	Atovaquone
Artemisinin derivatives	Sesquiterpene lactones	Artemether, artemisinin, artesunate
Others	9-Phenanthrenemethanols	Halofantrine
	Dichlorobenzylidenes	Lumefantrine

Adapted from Sweetman S. *Martindale: the complete drug reference.* London: Pharmaceutical Press, electronic ed. Greenwood Village, CO: Micromedex, 2003.

TOXIC DOSE

The *therapeutic dose* of most antimalarials (Table 3) can produce adverse effects in a susceptible individual. There are no acute poisonings recorded for amopyroquine, artemether, artemisinin, artesunate, chlorproguanil, hydroxypiperaquine, lumefantrine, piperaquine, or primaquine.

Amodiaquine may produce involuntary movements at high therapeutic doses (1), and a potentially fatal toxic hepatitis may occur during therapy (2–4). In four reported cases of overdose, there were no symptoms recorded (5). *Atovaquone* produced no effects after an ingestion of 9 g (6). Overdoses up to 31.5 g of atovaquone have been reported without significant adverse effects (7). *Artesunate* has produced severe allergic reactions at therapeutic doses (8).

TABLE 2. Functional classification of antimalarial agents

Primary mode of action	Examples	Notes
Blood schizonticides	Amodiaquine, artemisinin, atovaquone, chloroquine, halofantrine, hydroxychloroquine, mefloquine, quinine	Act on the erythrocytic stages of the parasite; cannot produce a radical cure of ovale or vivax malaria
	Chlorproguanil, proguanil, pyrimethamine	Slow acting
Tissue schizonticides	Chlorproguanil, primaquine, proguanil, pyrimethamine	Act on the exoerythrocytic stages of the parasite; can produce radical cures of vivax and ovale malaria
Gametocytocides	Amodiaquine, atovaquone, chloroquine, hydroxychloroquine, primaquine, quinine	Destroy the sexual forms of the parasite; interrupt transmission of the infection to the mosquito vector
Sporontocides	Chlorproguanil, primaquine, proguanil, pyrimethamine	Prevent sporogony in the mosquito

Adapted from Sweetman S. *Martindale: the complete drug reference.* London: Pharmaceutical Press, electronic ed. Greenwood Village, CO: Micromedex, 2003.

Chloroquine causes retinopathy, which is more likely if a daily dose of 3.5 to 4.0 mg/kg ideal body weight is exceeded (9). A 26-year-old man developed toxicity after taking 1.0 g chloroquine daily instead of weekly (10). Chloroquine in doses of 1000 mg daily for 3 or 5 days can result in dysrhythmia (torsade de pointes) (11). More than 2 g of chloroquine has been regarded as a clinically significant poisoning (12), whereas moderately severe intoxication has been defined as an ingested dose of 2 g or more but less than 4 g (13). Nevertheless, a 13-year-old boy developed ventricular fibrillation after the ingestion of only 750 mg of chloroquine base (14). A 16-year-old girl who ingested 1.95 g developed apnea with subsequent survival (15). A 39-year-old patient was found unconscious after having taken 2.5 g of chloroquine (16). A dose of 3.75 g of chloroquine resulted in deep coma (17).

Ingestion of more than 5 g of chloroquine is said to be an accurate predictor of a fatal outcome in the absence of specific treatment (18). A 17-year-old boy ingested 8 g of chloroquine, and cardiac arrest occurred within 1 hour (19). Cardiac and respiratory arrest followed by death occurred after 7.5 g of chloroquine base was ingested by a 14-year-old girl (20). A 20-year-old woman who ingested 9 g developed ventricular tachycardia and subsequently died (21). In children, two to three times the adult therapeutic dose (620 to 930 mg of chloroquine base) may be rapidly fatal (22), and death has been reported from ingestion of as little as one tablet (300 mg) (23,24).

Halofantrine consistently causes QT prolongation in therapeutic doses (25) as well as sudden death in both children and adults (26,27) and ventricular fibrillation without preceding QTc prolongation (28). Ingestion of 16.5 g over 11 days resulted in minor clinical symptoms and recovery within 48 hours (29).

Hydroxychloroquine is more likely to produce retinopathy if a daily dose of 6.0 to 6.5 mg/kg ideal body weight is exceeded (9). A 4-g dose in an adult can produce life-threatening toxicity (30). A 16-year-old girl ingested a handful of hydroxychloroquine 200-mg tablets and developed severe toxicity within 30 minutes (31). A 24-year-old man ingested 12 g and developed hypotension with sinus tachycardia, a QRS of 160 milliseconds and respiratory depression with ultimate survival (32). An 18-year-old woman survived ingestion of 20 g of hydroxychloroquine, although life-threatening toxicity occurred (33). Ingestion of 14 g resulted in deep coma and cardiac arrest within minutes and death at 22 hours (30). A 2.5-year-old boy died after an estimated ingestion of as many as sixty 200-mg tablets (12 g) (34).

Mefloquine has caused serious central nervous system (CNS) events during standard therapy in 1:1200 Asians and 1:200 whites or Africans. Risk factors include dosage, concomitant drug use or interactions, previous history of a CNS event, and disease severity. Re-treatment (within a month) increases the risk in Asians by sevenfold (35). A 39-year-old man received 3500 mg mefloquine over 3 days in addition to 3250 mg chloroquine and 175/3500 mg sulfadoxine/pyrimethamine. He developed severe neuropsychiatric symptoms (36).

Primaquine produces methemoglobinemia in high therapeutic doses (37) as well as hemolysis, particularly in patients with glucose 6 phosphate dehydrogenase deficiency (38). *Proguanil* causes megaloblastic anemia and pancytopenia when renal failure (39) and hemodialysis (40) cause accumulation of proguanil and its metabolites. A 14.5 g overdose is reported with no clinical sequelae (41).

Pyrimethamine, 350 mg, resulted in seizures in an adult (42). A 7-week-old infant survived sustained overdose (ten times the usual dose for 10 days) (43). Another tenfold dosing error in an 8-month-old infant resulted in a seizure on the second day of treat-

TABLE 3. Usual adult oral dose of antimalarial agents

Drug	Molecular formula	Molecular weight (g/mol)	CAS Registry No.	Prophylactic dose	Therapeutic dose
Amodiaquine (Camoquin, Flavoquine)	$C_{20}H_{22}ClN_3O$	355.9	86-42-0	NA	35 mg of amodiaquine base per kg given over 3 d
Artemether (Paluther)	$C_{16}H_{26}O_5$	298.4	71963-77-4	NA	80 mg; then 80 mg at 8, 24, 36, 48, and 60 h (total dose, 480 mg)
Artemisinin	$C_{15}H_{22}O_5$	282.3	63968-64-9	NA	25 mg/kg on d 1; 12.5 mg/kg on d 2 and 3
Artesunate (Plasmotrim)	$C_{19}H_{27}O_8Na$	406.4	88495-63-0	NA	5 mg/kg on d 1; 2.5 mg/kg on d 2 and 3
Atovaquone (Mepron, Wellvone)	$C_{22}H_{19}O_3Cl$	366.8	95233-18-4	250 mg daily	1000 mg daily for 4 d
Chloroquine (Aralen)	$C_{18}H_{26}ClN_3$	319.9	54-05-7	310 mg of chloroquine base once a wk	620 mg of chloroquine base followed by 310 mg 6 h later; then 310 mg on d 2 and 3 (total dose of 25 mg/kg body weight)
Chlorproguanil	$C_{11}H_{15}Cl_2N_5,HCl$	324.6	15537-76-5	20 mg twice weekly	2 mg/kg once daily for 3 d
Halofantrine (Halfan)	$C_{26}H_{30}Cl_2F_3NO,HCl$	536.9	36167-63-2	NA	500 mg; then 500 mg at 6 and 12 h (total dose, 1500 mg); repeat in 1 wk
Hydroxychloroquine (Plaquenil)	$C_{18}H_{26}ClN_3O,H_2SO_4$	434.0	747-36-4	400 mg once a wk	800 mg followed by 400 mg 6 to 8 h later; then 400 mg on d 2 and 3
Lumefantrine	$C_{30}H_{32}Cl_3NO$	528.9	82186-77-4	NA	480 mg; then 480 mg at 8, 24, 36, 48, and 60 h (total dose, 2.88 g)
Mefloquine (Lariam)	$C_{17}H_{16}F_6N_2O,HCl$	414.8	51773-92-3	250 mg of mefloquine base once a wk	750 mg of mefloquine base followed by 500 mg after 6–8 h
Primaquine (Primacin)	$C_{15}H_{21}N_3O,2H_3PO_4$	455.3	63-45-6	30 mg of primaquine base daily	15 mg of primaquine base daily for 14 d after primary treatment with chloroquine
Proguanil (Malarone)	$C_{11}H_{16}ClN_5,HCl$	290.2	637-32-1	100–200 mg daily	400 mg daily for 4 d
Pyrimethamine (Daraprim)	$C_{12}H_{13}ClN_4$	248.7	58-14-0	12.5 mg once a wk	75 mg as a single dose
Quinine (Legatrin, Quinamm)	$C_{20}H_{24}N_2O_2$	782.9	6119-70-6	NA	600 mg of quinine sulfate every 8 h for 7 d

NA, not applicable.
Note: Many of these drugs are given only in combination. Doses given are for the individual components of combination therapy. For detailed information on treatment or prophylaxis of malaria, consult an appropriate reference source.

ment (44). Accidental ingestion of 450 mg by a 14-month-old child resulted in initial vomiting, coma, seizures, and hyperpyrexia followed by blindness and deafness (45). Pyrimethamine, 1625 mg, caused death in a 16-month-old child, whereas 625 mg caused nonfatal seizures in a 2.5-year-old child (46).

Quinine causes cinchonism at therapeutic doses. High-tone hearing loss occurs, but irreversible auditory or ocular effects are very rare (35). One study showed that 100 mg of quinine in tonic water is sufficient to produce positional abnormalities on electronystagmography (47). A 25-year-old woman had no light perception 14.5 hours after ingesting 3.7 to 4.7 g of quinine (48). Two patients had no light perception vision and dilated, nonreactive pupils within hours of ingesting 13 to 15 g in addition to other drugs (49). Death occurred in a 24-year-old man who ingested 8 g of quinine sulfate (50). Quinine and chloroquine are among the very few drugs that are potentially fatal for a 10-kg toddler on ingestion of one commercially available dose unit (24).

TOXICOKINETICS AND TOXICODYNAMICS

Pharmacokinetic parameters for the antimalarial drugs are provided in Table 4. Little or no information is available on the toxicokinetics or toxicodynamics of amodiaquine, artemether, artemisinin, artesunate, chlorproguanil, halofantrine, lumefantrine, mefloquine, or primaquine.

Atovaquone has a therapeutic plasma concentration of 20 mg/L (51). Ingestion of 9 g produced a level of 9.50 mg/L at 9 hours postingestion (6).

Chloroquine kinetics fit a two-compartment model with a distribution phase that is much more rapid than the terminal elimination phase (Table 4) (52). It is likely that this distribution phase is more relevant to toxicity than is the prolonged elimination phase. Whole blood concentrations are five to ten times greater than plasma concentrations (53). Therapeutic plasma concentrations for treatment of malaria are 1.9 mg/L or less (54). Even within that range, there is a relationship between plasma concentration and adverse effects, with no effects observed at concentrations less than 0.38 mg/L. In contrast, 80% of patients with concentrations greater than 0.8 mg/L had side effects (55).

The terminal elimination half-life of chloroquine correlates well with the peak plasma concentration (41), suggesting dose-dependent kinetics in overdose as has been observed in therapeutic dosing (55). In a severe 10-g chloroquine poisoning in a 52-year-old woman, the apparent volume of the central compartment was 181 L, whereas the apparent volume of distribution was 1137 L. The half-life in the distribution phase was 6.4 hours; half-life in the elimination phase was 392.8 hours; and total body clearance was 2.01 L/hour (56).

Hydroxychloroquine plasma concentration was 29.87 mg/L 2 hours after ingestion of 20 g, and the elimination half-life was 22 hours (33), although this is more likely to be a distribution

TABLE 4. Pharmacokinetics of the antimalarial agents

Drug	Time to peak (h)	Primary route of excretion	Volume of distribution (L/kg)	Terminal elimination half-life	Protein binding (%)
Amodiaquine	4	Hepatic (by CYP2C8) to active metabolite (desethylamodiaquine)	17–34	1–3 wk	90
Artemether	4	Hepatic to active metabolite (dihydroartemisinin)	NA	1.9 h	95.4 (33% to α_1-acid glycoprotein)
Artemisinin	2	Hepatic (induces CYP2C19 and its own metabolism)	3–4	30–40 min	77
Artesunate	0.5–1.0 (dihydroartemisinin)	Plasma cholinesterases (prodrug of dihydroartemisinin)	0.77–1.01 (dihydroartemisinin)	40–64 min (dihydroartemisinin)	NA
Atovaquone	2–4	Excreted unchanged in bile	3	77 h	99.9
Chloroquine	1.5–3.0	70% unchanged in urine	200	6–50 d (distribution half-life, 6 h)	50–65
Chlorproguanil	NA	Hepatic (CYP2C19) to chlorcycloguanil	NA	12.6 h	NA
Halofantrine	3.4–6.0	Hepatic (CYP3A4)	100–570	1.3–6.6 d	NA
Hydroxychloroquine	2.0–4.5	16% to 25% unchanged in urine	78–630	40 d	37–64
Lumefantrine	8–10	Hepatic (CYP3A4)	3.8	3–5 d	NA
Mefloquine	1–6	Hepatic (CYP3A4, mainly fecal elimination)	13.5–19.1	13.6–33.0 d	98
Primaquine	1–3	Hepatic (CYP3A4)	2.9	5.4–7.1 h	—
Proguanil	2–4	60% unchanged in urine and 30% as cycloguanil (via CYP2C19)	—	15–20 h	75
Pyrimethamine	2–6	Hepatic	2.9	80–95 h	87
Quinine	1–3	Hepatic (CYP3A4, 20% unchanged in urine)	1.8	9–15 h	70–89

NA, not available.
Data from reference 41; Krishna S, White NJ. Pharmacokinetics of quinine, chloroquine and amodiaquine. Clinical implications. *Clin Pharmacokinet* 1996;30:263–299; Rolan PE, Mercer AJ, Tate E, et al. Disposition of atovaquone in humans. *Antimicrob Agents Chemother* 1997;41:1319–1321; Winstanley P, Watkins W, Muhia D, et al. Chlorproguanil/dapsone for uncomplicated *Plasmodium falciparum* malaria in young children: pharmacokinetics and therapeutic range. *Trans R Soc Trop Med Hyg* 1997;91:322–327; Colussi D, Parisot C, Legay F, Lefevre G. Binding of artemether and lumefantrine to plasma proteins and erythrocytes. *Eur J Pharm Sci* 1999;9:9–16; and Davis TM, Phuong HL, Ilett KF, et al. Pharmacokinetics and pharmacodynamics of intravenous artesunate in severe falciparum malaria. *Antimicrob Agents Chemother* 2001;45:181–186.

half-life. Hydroxychloroquine kinetics are similar to those of chloroquine (57).

Proguanil, 10 mg orally, produces a therapeutic concentration of 0.1 mg/L (41). Serum proguanil may reach 1.03 mg/L in renal failure with bone marrow toxicity (39).

Pyrimethamine, 1 mg/kg intravenously (IV), produced a mean peak plasma concentration of 2.1 mg/L. The mean elimination half-life was 140 hours (58). Initial plasma concentration of pyrimethamine was 6.22 mg/L after ten times the usual dose for 10 days in a 7-week-old infant (43).

Quinine has a therapeutic concentration of 1 to 3 mg/L. Plasma quinine concentrations (within the first 20 hours) greater than 10 mg/L are associated with increased risks of permanent visual damage; concentrations greater than 15 mg/L are associated with cardiac dysrhythmias (59). Initial quinine concentrations greater than 20 mg/L were associated with blindness in 87% of patients. For concentrations between 10 and 15 mg/L, it was 37%; for less than 10 mg/L, it was 16.5% (60). Plasma quinine concentration related to time from ingestion was found to be a useful predictor of visual toxicity (61).

A 19-year-old patient became blind with a serum quinine concentration of 10.5 mg/L, measured 13 hours after ingestion (62). Two cases of acute blindness presented with quinine concentrations of 13.6 mg/L and 18.6 mg/L, respectively. In addition, tinnitus, decreased hearing, vomiting, abdominal pain, and confusion were noted in one patient, and the other experienced decreased hearing, headache, confusion, tachycardia, later bradycardia, and first-degree atrioventricular block (63). In five symptomatic patients with acute quinine poisoning, the mean admission plasma concentration was 11.1 mg/L (64). Two cases of acute bilateral blindness from quinine presented with cinchonism, including nausea, vomiting, and tinnitus and serum quinine concentrations of 5.3 mg/L and 13.0 mg/L (65).

The elimination half-life of quinine is longer after overdose (mean, 25 to 26 hours) than after therapeutic doses (9 to 15 hours) (59). Activated charcoal halves the quinine elimination half-life after therapeutic doses (66) and in overdose (64).

PATHOPHYSIOLOGY

The mechanism and degree of toxicity of the antimalarials varies markedly between the structural groups and even within groups. Within the quinoline-related compounds, *chloroquine* and *hydroxychloroquine* have the most severe toxicity, which appears to be mediated by similar mechanisms. These drugs may have a direct toxic effect on the CNS via effects on voltage-dependent Na^+ channels (67), or their CNS manifestations may be secondary to cerebral hypoperfusion from the cardiac effects. The cardiac effects are related to blocking of several inward and outward membrane currents (68). The order of potency is as follows: inward rectifying potassium current [I(K1)] greater than rapid delayed rectifying potassium current [I(Kr)] greater than sodium current [I(Na)] greater than L-type calcium current [I(Ca-L)]. Chloroquine blocks the rapid component of the delayed rectifying outward current, I(Kr), but not the slow component, I(Ks). This provides the cellular mechanism for the prolonged QT interval, impaired ventricular conduction, and increased automaticity that are responsible for its prodysrhythmic effects (68). Hypotension and cardiogenic shock are due to a direct cardiodepressant effect rather than peripheral vasodilation (69). The prominent hypokalemia is believed to be due to a transport-dependent mechanism (54).

Quinine also causes hypokalemia, but the mechanism is unclear (70,71). It induces both hearing loss and tinnitus via blocking neuronal potassium currents (IK) in a voltage-dependent manner. At higher concentrations, quinine also reduces the size of neuronal sodium currents (INa) in a use-dependent manner, while leaving calcium currents (ICa) relatively unaffected (72). The ocular toxicity occurs via a direct effect on retinal cells by an unclear mechanism (48,73–77). In spite of recent reports of interventions aimed at reversing vasospasm (78) or hypoxia (49), there is little or no support for these mechanisms being involved (61,79). Quinine produces myocardial sodium-channel blockade that is similar to but less potent than quinidine, its optical isomer.

Amodiaquine, mefloquine, amopyroquine, piperaquine, and *hydroxypiperaquine*, although structurally related, have substantially less toxicity than the other quinolines.

Primaquine toxicity in the red cell (methemoglobinemia and hemolysis) is due to 5-hydroxylated metabolites rather than the parent drug. There is a dual mechanism for the oxidative effects, involving auto-oxidation of the 5-hydroxy-8-aminoquinolines and their coupled oxidation with oxyhemoglobin. The initial products of these processes are drug metabolite free radicals, superoxide radical anions, hydrogen peroxide, and methemoglobin. Further free radical reactions lead to oxidation of glutathione, hemoglobin, and probably other cellular constituents. In the glucose 6 phosphate dehydrogenase–deficient erythrocyte, the oxidation of hemoglobin and glutathione leads to Heinz-body formation and eventually to hemolysis, the mechanisms of which are yet unclear (80).

Pyrimethamine, chlorproguanil (and its active metabolite chlorcycloguanil), and *proguanil* (and its active metabolite cycloguanil) have differing structures but have similar mechanisms of hematologic toxicity via competitive inhibition of dihydrofolate reductase. The mechanism of the neurologic toxicity is unknown.

Atovaquone stops synthesis of pyrimidines, which results in protozoan cell death with little toxicity in human cells, which can reuse existing pyrimidines (81).

The *artemisinin derivatives*, which act mainly through dihydroartemisinin, have little evident toxicity but have been reported to cause neurotoxicity with a discrete distribution in the brain stems of rats and dogs after multiple doses, although the neuronal target is unknown (82).

Halofantrine causes dose-dependent QT prolongation with repolarization changes that indicate a class III antidysrhythmic effect (83). Lumefantrine does not share this effect (84).

PREGNANCY AND LACTATION

Pregnancy categorization and lactation information is provided in Table 5.

TABLE 5. Pregnancy and lactation information for antimalarial drugs

Drug	U.S. Food and Drug Administration pregnancy risk category	Distribution into breast milk
Amodiaquine	NA	NA
Artemether	NA (ADEC category B3)	NA
Artemisinin	NA	NA
Artesunate	NA	NA
Atovaquone	C (ADEC category B2)	NA
Chloroquine	C (prophylaxis: ADEC category A; treatment: ADEC category D)	Milk to plasma ratio, 1.96:4.26[a]
Chlorproguanil	NA	NA
Halofantrine	C	NA
Hydroxychloroquine	C (ADEC category D)	Detectable in milk[b]
Lumefantrine	NA	NA
Mefloquine	C (ADEC category B3)	Milk to plasma ratio, 0.13:0.16[c]
Primaquine	C (ADEC category B3)	NA
Proguanil	NA (ADEC category B2)	Small amounts insufficient for protection against malaria
Pyrimethamine	C (ADEC category B3)	Milk to plasma ratio, 0.46:0.66[a]
Quinine	X (ADEC category D)	Milk to plasma ratio, 0.11:0.53[d]

ADEC, Australian Drug Evaluation Committee; NA, not available.
[a]Edstein MD, Veenendaal JR, Newman K, Hyslop R. Excretion of chloroquine, dapsone and pyrimethamine in human milk. *Br J Clin Pharmacol* 1986;22:733–735.
[b]Ostensen M, Brown ND, Chiang PK, Aarbakke J. Hydroxychloroquine in human breast milk. *Eur J Clin Pharmacol* 1985;28:357.
[c]Edstein MD, Veenendaal JR, Hyslop R. Excretion of mefloquine in human breast milk. *Chemotherapy* 1988;34:165–169.
[d]Phillips RE, Looareesuwan S, White NJ, et al. Quinine pharmacokinetics and toxicity in pregnant and lactating women with falciparum malaria. *Br J Clin Pharmacol* 1986;21:677–683.

CLINICAL PRESENTATION

Acute Overdose

There are no acute poisonings recorded for amopyroquine, artemether, artemisinin, artesunate, chlorproguanil, hydroxypiperaquine, lumefantrine, piperaquine, or primaquine.

Chloroquine is said to be one of the most frequently used drugs for committing suicide in the Orient and Far East (85) and is the most common cause of pharmaceutic poisoning admission in Zimbabwe, with a mortality rate of 5.7% (86). It is the most severe and frequent cause of intoxications with antimalarial drugs (41). From the limited information available, hydroxychloroquine has a similar toxicity profile (30).

Chloroquine and *hydroxychloroquine* toxicity is rapid in onset (within minutes to 3 hours of ingestion) and potentially life-threatening. Possible predictors for death from chloroquine poisoning include systolic blood pressure less than 85 mm Hg, dose ingested greater than 5 g, QRS duration of 0.12 second or more, and blood chloroquine concentration greater than 8 mg/L (87). Initial drowsiness after rapid onset of CNS depression is common (41). Coma can occur but is usually in the context of cardiovascular collapse. Other CNS manifestations include blurred vision with occasional, transient, completely reversible blindness (5); dizziness; vomiting; and headache (41). Seizures can occur but appear mainly related to primary cardiac toxicity with hypotension and cardiac arrest.

Cardiac toxicity may be the initial presentation or may rapidly follow the initial CNS effects. It occurs in 50% to 60% of presentations (5,41) and is the usual mode of death. Hypotension occurs early and is often severe, progressing rapidly to cardiogenic shock. Electrocardiogram (ECG) changes due to cardiac-channel blockade are evident with QT prolongation, appearance of U waves, ST segment depression, and QRS widening. Cardiac dysrhythmias may ensue with ventricular tachycardia and ventricular fibrillation early (first few hours) and ventricular extrasystoles and torsade de pointes late (after 8 hours) (41). Hypokalemia is almost always present in severe chloroquine poisoning and may itself be severe (less than 3 mmol/L). It appears within the first 3 hours of ingestion and is inversely correlated with severity of poisoning (54,88). If the first few hours are survived, allowing time for redistribution of drug, then survival is more likely, provided no life-threatening injury has been sustained during the period of critical illness.

Quinine toxicity causes quinine amblyopia and cinchonism (41). In overdose, the clinical features include visual disturbance, CNS effects, and cardiac effects (dysrhythmias and myocardial depression). Cinchonism is common in quinine poisoning and includes nausea, vomiting, tinnitus, deafness, headache, vasodilation, and slightly disturbed vision (41). The mean time of onset after ingestion was 3.5 hours in one study (61). CNS depression is not uncommon, although usually mild. However, coma and convulsions have been reported, particularly in children with severe poisoning and myocardial depression (60).

Quinine blindness (amblyopia) is a common and often dramatic effect of poisoning. It appears in 20% to 40% of acute overdoses (60,61), with a mean time of onset of 9 hours after ingestion (61). Thus, the eye changes may appear the next day or after the patient awakens. Patients complain of seeing badly in a bright light and of "misty" vision. Partial or complete blindness is often sudden. It may pass after 14 to 24 hours; however, such changes may last up to 10 weeks or more. Of those developing blindness, one-third achieve full recovery within 1 to 3 weeks (79). In two-thirds, central vision recovers without treatment, with varying degrees of residual peripheral field constriction (61). Occasionally, patients may remain blind permanently (3%) (79).

The typical ophthalmoscopic findings of pallor of the optic disks, extreme contraction of the arteries and veins of the retina, cherry spot at the macula, and retinal edema appear after the onset of blindness. Most authors believe them to be secondary changes rather than causal (48,73–75,79,89,90). This is supported by animal work (76,77). The electroretinogram may be almost normal during the initial marked loss of vision; it becomes abnormal during the phase of visual improvement and parallels the changes in visual acuity on the second or third day (48). Visual evoked potential, dark adaptation, and color testing measurements are often abnormal.

Quinine cardiac effects are less severe than with quinidine, chloroquine, or hydroxychloroquine, although conduction abnormalities and dysrhythmias can occur (41). Sinus tachycardias with ST-T wave changes and increased QT interval are the most common cardiac findings (91). In more severe poisoning, these may progress to increased PR interval, widening of the QRS, and the appearance of bundle branch blocks (60,61). Ventricular tachycardia and cardiogenic shock may supervene, rarely (41). Hypokalemia can occur (70).

Amodiaquine poisoning is very rare and produced no symptoms in four reported cases (5). There may be the possibility of neurologic effects with the dose-dependent production of involuntary movements (1).

Mefloquine overdose has not been reported, but severe neuropsychiatric symptoms have been reported after ingestion of 3500 mg of mefloquine over 3 days (in combination with chloroquine and sulfadoxine/pyrimethamine) (36).

Atovaquone seems very well tolerated in overdose, with no significant adverse effects in doses ranging from 9.0 g (6) to 31.5 g (8).

Proguanil appears well tolerated in overdose, with an overdose of 14.5 g producing no adverse effects (41). If overdose does occur, features of folate antagonism are possible in the presence of renal failure (39).

Pyrimethamine poisoning produces gastrointestinal (GI) symptoms with vomiting followed by CNS manifestations (restlessness, tremor, ataxia, coma, and prominent seizures) (44,45,92,93). Later, features of megaloblastic anemia or pancytopenia may appear (94), and residual blindness and deafness have been reported (45). Death has been reported in children (46).

Halofantrine has no reported acute overdoses, but severe cardiotoxicity could potentially occur with QT prolongation and ventricular fibrillation (25,28). A chronic overdose of halofantrine involving 16.5 g ingested over 11 days resulted in minor clinical symptoms with full recovery within 48 hours (29).

Adverse Reactions

Chloroquine causes fewer adverse effects at the dosage for malaria than when it is used in higher dosages for rheumatoid arthritis. Common effects are nausea, diarrhea, anorexia, abdominal cramps, rash, itch, and alopecia. Infrequently noted are vomiting, muscle weakness, vertigo, tinnitus, nerve deafness, headache, nervousness, psychotic episodes, anxiety, personality changes, visual disturbances (large doses), reversible corneal opacities, and irreversible retinopathy (occurs with cumulative doses exceeding 100 g). Rarely, agranulocytosis, aplastic anemia, thrombocytopenia, bleaching of hair, seizures, erythema multiforme, Stevens-Johnson syndrome, cardiomyopathy, hepatitis, photosensitivity, blue-black pigmentation of mucous membranes and skin, reversible myopathy, elevation of thyroid-stimulating hormone, and seizures occur (95).

Hydroxychloroquine causes effects similar to those of chloroquine (95).

Quinine effects usually occur only with higher dosages (greater than 1.8 g daily). They commonly include GI disturbances, CNS disturbances, cinchonism (tinnitus, headache, nausea, vertigo, and visual disturbances), fever, rash, thrombocytopenia, hypoglycemia, and ECG changes. Rarely, angioedema, intravascular hemolysis, and acute renal failure can occur (95).

Amodiaquine also causes effects similar to chloroquine, except that it was associated with hepatitis and a much higher incidence of agranulocytosis when used for malaria prophylaxis (96).

Amopyroquine has little information available but is expected to be similar to its analog amodiaquine. *Piperaquine* and *hydroxypiperaquine* have little information available.

The adverse effects of *mefloquine* are dose related and commonly include nausea, diarrhea, abdominal pain, headache, dizziness, and difficulty in performing skilled tasks. Infrequently, rash, myalgia, paresthesia, visual disturbances, elevated liver enzymes, asymptomatic bradycardia, and neuropsychiatric effects (e.g., delirium, stupor) that can be severe and prolonged may occur. Rarely, hyperpyrexia, blood dyscrasias, and erythema multiforme may ensue (95).

Primaquine usually causes minimal effects, but abdominal pain and gastric distress are more common. Larger doses may cause nausea and vomiting. Methemoglobinemia may occur occasionally. Hemolytic anemia can occur in people with glucose 6 phosphate dehydrogenase deficiency. Other uncommon effects include mild anemia and leukocytosis. Hypertension and cardiac dysrhythmias occur rarely. Primaquine produces leukopenia or agranulocytosis rarely (96).

Proguanil produces few effects, apart from mild GI intolerance, and some reports of aphthous ulceration (96). Infrequently, vertigo, reversible alopecia, and scaling of skin have been reported; whereas rarely, megaloblastic anemia and pancytopenia [more likely with renal impairment (39)], disseminated intravascular coagulation, hepatitis, allergic reactions, convulsions, and psychosis may occur (95). There is little information on tolerability of chlorproguanil.

Pyrimethamine commonly causes a reversible photosensitive rash. Larger doses, used for toxoplasmosis, may cause GI symptoms, anemia, leukopenia, CNS effects (including headache, ataxia, seizures), and pulmonary eosinophilia (95).

Atovaquone causes rash, nausea, vomiting, diarrhea, headache, fever, insomnia, abdominal pain, and anemia as well as hyponatremia and increased amylase, alkaline phosphatase, and transaminases (may need to stop drug if more than three to five times the upper limit of normal). Rarely, erythema multiforme, dementia, increase in serum bilirubin, increase in blood urea, and increase in serum creatinine occur that may require cessation of atovaquone (95).

Artemisinin derivatives appear to be well tolerated. There have been reports of mild GI disturbance, dizziness, tinnitus, neutropenia, elevated liver enzyme values, and ECG abnormalities, including prolongation of the QT interval. Bradycardia and acute cerebellar dysfunction have also been reported (96).

Halofantrine causes diarrhea, abdominal pain, nausea, vomiting, pruritus, and skin rash. Transient elevation of serum transaminases, intravascular hemolysis, and hypersensitivity reactions have been reported. Halofantrine can also cause QT interval prolongation. Serious ventricular dysrhythmias have been reported, and fatalities have occurred (1).

Lumefantrine is marketed in combination with artemether. Adverse effects of the combination commonly include headache, dizziness, sleep disturbance, palpitations, GI disturbances, anorexia, pruritus, rash, cough, arthralgia, myalgia, and fatigue (96).

DIAGNOSTIC TESTING

Specific drug measurements are not readily available for most antimalarial agents. Nevertheless, plasma concentrations of quinine and chloroquine correlate well with outcome and would be useful if available acutely. High plasma concentrations of chloroquine are associated with cardiotoxicity and have been associated with death when they exceed 3.0 mg/ml (88,97), although a plasma concentration of chloroquine of only 1.3 mg/L was recorded in a 13-year-old boy who developed ventricular fibrillation (14). In poisonings resulting in shock or cardiac arrest, plasma concentrations are usually higher than 5 mg/L (41). Death was reported in a 12-month-old child with a plasma concentration of 4.4 mg/L (23). In one review, no patient with a plasma concentration of more than 8 mg/L survived (18). The blood concentration in a chloroquine-related death was 16.71 mg/L (98). In a review of 191 consecutive cases, the mean plasma chloroquine level was 8.4 mg/L. Plasma potassium varied directly with the systolic blood pressure and inversely with the QRS and QT and plasma chloroquine. The degree of hypokalemia predicted the seriousness of the poisoning (54,99).

Many of these drugs have significant cardiac effects, so an ECG and cardiac monitoring are mandatory. Hepatic and renal function tests are indicated. Serum potassium is of prognostic value in chloroquine, hydroxychloroquine, and possibly quinine poisoning. For primaquine, a full blood count and possibly measurement of methemoglobinemia and hemolysis are indicated. For the folate antagonists, full blood count and estimates of serum folate (and vitamin B_{12}) may be of value.

Assessment of vision in quinine poisoning is important and may be of value in poisoning by chloroquine, hydroxychloroquine, or pyrimethamine as well. This involves ophthalmoscopy and may also require formal visual field testing, electroretinography, color testing, and visual evoked responses. Measurement of partial pressure of carbon dioxide in expired air or arterial blood gases is the best way to assess respiratory compromise from sedation.

POSTMORTEM CONSIDERATIONS

Postmortem femoral blood to antemortem drug concentration ratios may be very high for chloroquine probably due to its extremely high volume of distribution and the high blood to plasma concentration ratio. It is doubtful that the femoral drug concentration at autopsy represents the antemortem level (100). A liver concentration of 150 mg/kg is a useful discriminator between overdose and nonoverdose cases at autopsy (101).

TREATMENT

Supportive and symptomatic measures form the mainstay of treatment for all of the antimalarial drugs. In drugs with potential cardiac toxicity, in addition to maintenance of the airway, breathing, and circulatory status of the patient, observation for dysrhythmia is warranted. Clinical monitoring for signs that may indicate impending seizure activity (hypertonicity, hyperreflexia, or myoclonic jerking) is important.

Gastrointestinal Decontamination

In view of the life-threatening nature of chloroquine, hydroxychloroquine, quinine, or pyrimethamine poisoning, GI decontamination with activated charcoal should be instituted if the patient presents within an hour of ingestion (102). For quinine, there is evidence that repeated doses of activated charcoal significantly shorten quinine elimination half-life. It seems a reasonable therapeutic maneuver, although it is unclear whether this improves outcome (64,103).

Enhanced Elimination

Hemodialysis and hemoperfusion are not useful in chloroquine poisoning due to the high volume of distribution.

Charcoal hemoperfusion, hemodialysis, plasma exchange, peritoneal dialysis, exchange transfusion, and forced diuresis have been shown to be ineffective in increasing quinine elimination (59,62). The only effective method of shortening quinine elimination half-life is repeated doses of activated charcoal (64).

Antidotes

Apart from supportive care, folinic acid has been suggested for pyrimethamine toxicity to prevent or ameliorate megaloblastic anemia and pancytopenia (94). There is no information on whether this is helpful in other folate antagonist overdoses (proguanil, chlorproguanil).

If symptomatic methemoglobinemia occurs in a pyrimethamine overdose, methylene blue is the mainstay of treatment (see Chapter 63). For less severe poisonings, one or two doses of 1 to 2 mg/kg of a 1% solution may be given IV over a period of several minutes. The repeat dose may be given after 1 hour if required. If more than two doses are required, a methylene blue infusion should be used as in dapsone poisoning (104), as pyrimethamine has an even longer half-life.

Specific treatment for chloroquine poisoning is controversial. Based on animal work in rats (105) and pigs (106), a benefit of high-dose IV diazepam was postulated. Because the cardiac-depressant effects of chloroquine were not reversed by diazepam in rat cardiac papillary muscle *in vitro* (107), the use of separate inotrope therapy was required. In a nonrandomized clinical trial, combined treatment of elective intubation using thiopentone induction followed by gastric lavage and activated charcoal, high-dose diazepam (2 to 3 mg/kg), and epinephrine appeared to dramatically improve the outcome compared with historical controls (18). However, the historical controls were selected on the basis of their poor outcome. Further, a study of the effect of diazepam using unselected controls demonstrated no significant improvement in outcome with the routine use of diazepam (12). Subsequently, a randomized, controlled trial of diazepam in poisonings of moderate severity failed to demonstrate a significant benefit (13).

The effect of diazepam was originally believed to be on peripheral benzodiazepine receptors (which are less sensitive to diazepam and thus require very large doses for effect) (105). However, even in animal models, the effect is small and appears more likely to be an effect on CNS γ-aminobutyric acid receptors, as IV clonazepam and intracerebral diazepam are more effective than IV diazepam (108,109). Diazepam and clonazepam have no beneficial effects in a rat model of chloroquine poisoning in which the rats were anesthetized with barbiturates (110). However, this may have been due to an adverse effect of barbiturates, as a case series suggests that barbiturates themselves may be harmful (88). Epinephrine, as well as increasing blood pressure, may act as a pharmacologic overdrive pacer and thus suppress early afterdepolarizations and triggered dysrhythmias. In a rat model of chloroquine poisoning, isoproterenol provided more protection against the cardiovascular effects of chloroquine than epinephrine, and pure alpha-agonist activity appeared to be harmful (110).

These data have led to a recommended treatment for severe chloroquine poisoning of high-dose clonazepam (0.1 mg/kg IV push), elective intubation without barbiturate anesthesia (maintaining sedation with benzodiazepines), and epinephrine or isoproterenol (titrated to maintain blood pressure and heart rate) (111). Given the very similar toxicity profile (30) and closely related structure of hydroxychloroquine, a similar management strategy is appropriate for severe hydroxychloroquine poisoning (32).

Supportive Care

Treatment of specific complications of chloroquine poisoning requires some changes from conventional practice. Seizures should be treated with benzodiazepines as usual, but clonazepam should be considered early as an alternative if diazepam is unsuccessful. Barbiturates should not be used (88).

The treatment of dysrhythmia is also somewhat different. Magnesium is normally the drug of choice for treating torsade de pointes, but its calcium channel–blocking activity may aggravate the hypotension and heart block that can complicate chloroquine poisoning. Isoproterenol or overdrive pacing (heart rate, 120 to 140 beats/minute) are indicated for torsade de pointes and should be considered for all tachydysrhythmias. Any acidosis should be corrected, and there is some suggestion that hypertonic sodium bicarbonate may be beneficial (112). Beta-blockers (including sotalol) are contraindicated (113) as are class 1A antidysrhythmic drugs.

The blindness of quinine poisoning has been the focus of many postulated interventions. Most proposals have revolved around means to improve blood flow and oxygenation to the retina (49,78,114,115). However, as quinine-induced blindness is due to direct retinal toxicity and the vascular changes are secondary, there is no anticipated benefit in these procedures. In particular, stellate ganglion block is not effective and is a procedure with significant risk (41,60,74,79,90,116). High-dose diazepam, in a manner analogous to the treatment of chloroquine poisoning, has been tried in quinine poisoning with apparent effect (117), but there are no controlled trials of its use.

REFERENCES

1. Akindele MO, Odejide AO. Amodiaquine-induced involuntary movements. *Br Med J* 1976;2:214–215.
2. Larrey D, Castot A, Pessayre D, et al. Amodiaquine-induced hepatitis. A report of seven cases. *Ann Intern Med* 1986;104:801–803.
3. Bernuau J, Larrey D, Campillo B, et al. Amodiaquine-induced fulminant hepatitis. *J Hepatol* 1988;6:109–112.
4. Raymond JM, Dumas F, Baldit C, et al. Fatal acute hepatitis due to amodiaquine. *J Clin Gastroenterol* 1989;11:602–603.
5. Vitris M, Aubert M. [Chloroquine poisoning: our experience apropos of 80 cases]. *Dakar Med* 1983;28:593–602.
6. Cheung TW. Overdose of atovaquone in a patient with AIDS. *AIDS* 1999;13:1984–1985.
7. Product information. Mepron suspension. Atovaquone. Research Triangle Park, NC: Glaxo Wellcome Inc., 2001.
8. Leonardi E, Gilvary G, White NJ, Nosten F. Severe allergic reactions to oral artesunate: a report of two cases. *Trans R Soc Trop Med Hyg* 2001;95:182–183.
9. Ochsendorf FR, Runne U. [Chloroquine and hydroxychloroquine: side effect profile of important therapeutic drugs]. *Hautarzt* 1991;42:140–146.
10. Ochsendorf FR, Runne U. [Subacute chloroquine overdosage]. *Dtsch Med Wochenschr* 1991;116:1513–1516.
11. Demaziere J, Fourcade JM, Busseuil CT, et al. The hazards of chloroquine self prescription in west Africa. *J Toxicol Clin Toxicol* 1995;33:369–370.
12. Demaziere J, Saissy JM, Vitris M, et al. [Effects of diazepam on mortality from acute chloroquine poisoning]. *Ann Fr Anesth Reanim* 1992;11:164–167.
13. Clemessy JL, Angel G, Borron SW, et al. Therapeutic trial of diazepam versus placebo in acute chloroquine intoxications of moderate gravity. *Intensive Care Med* 1996;22:1400–1405.
14. Collee GG, Samra GS, Hanson GC. Chloroquine poisoning: ventricular fibrillation following "trivial" overdose in a child. *Intensive Care Med* 1992;18:170–171.
15. Semb SO, Jacobsen D. [Chloroquine poisoning]. *Tidsskr Nor Laegeforen* 1996;116:478–480.
16. Rajah A. The use of diazepam in chloroquine poisoning. *Anaesthesia* 1990;45:955–957.
17. Altrock G, Lange A, Munster P. [Acute chloroquine poisoning]. *Dtsch Med Wochenschr* 1997;122:225–228.
18. Riou B, Barriot P, Rimailho A, Baud FJ. Treatment of severe chloroquine poisoning. *N Engl J Med* 1988;318:1–6.
19. Hantson P, Ronveau JL, De Coninck B, et al. Amrinone for refractory cardiogenic shock following chloroquine poisoning. *Intensive Care Med* 1991;17:430–431.
20. Muhm M, Stimpfl T, Malzer R, et al. Suicidal chloroquine poisoning: clinical course, autopsy findings, and chemical analysis. *J Forensic Sci* 1996;41:1077–1079.
21. Henderson A, Adamson M, Pond SM. Death from inadvertent chloroquine overdose. *Med J Aust* 1994;160:231.
22. Cann HM, Verhulst HL. Fatal acute chloroquine poisoning in children. *Pediatrics* 1961;27:95–102.
23. Kelly JC, Wasserman GS, Bernard WD, et al. Chloroquine poisoning in a child. *Ann Emerg Med* 1990;19:47–50.
24. Koren G. Medications which can kill a toddler with one tablet or teaspoonful. *J Toxicol Clin Toxicol* 1993;31:407–413.
25. Nosten F, ter Kuile FO, Luxemburger C, et al. Cardiac effects of antimalarial treatment with halofantrine. *Lancet* 1993;341:1054–1056.
26. Akhtar T, Imran M. Sudden deaths while on halofantrine treatments—a report of two cases from Peshawar. *J Pak Med Assoc* 1994;44:120–121.
27. Malvy D, Receveur MC, Ozon P, et al. Fatal cardiac incident after use of halofantrine. *J Travel Med* 2000;7:215–216.
28. Gundersen SG, Rostrup M, von der LE, et al. Halofantrine-associated ventricular fibrillation in a young woman with no predisposing QTc prolongation. *Scand J Infect Dis* 1997;29:207–208.
29. Vincent MP, Becquart JP, Receveur MC, et al. [Halofantrine overdosage]. *Presse Med* 1992;21:131.
30. Isbister GK, Dawson A, Whyte IM. Hydroxychloroquine overdose: a prospective case series. *Am J Emerg Med* 2002;20:377–378.
31. Marquardt K, Albertson TE. Treatment of hydroxychloroquine overdose. *Am J Emerg Med* 2001;19:420–424.
32. Pruchnicki SA, Good TF, Watson PD. Severe hydroxychloroquine poisoning reversed with diazepam. *J Toxicol Clin Toxicol* 1996;33:582.
33. Jordan P, Brookes JG, Nikolic G, Le Couteur DG. Hydroxychloroquine overdose: toxicokinetics and management. *J Toxicol Clin Toxicol* 1999;37:861–864.
34. Kemmenoe AV. An infant fatality due to hydroxychloroquine poisoning. *J Anal Toxicol* 1990;14:186–188.
35. Phillips-Howard PA, ter Kuile FO. CNS adverse events associated with antimalarial agents. Fact or fiction? *Drug Saf* 1995;12:370–383.
36. Burgmann H, Winkler S, Uhl F, et al. [Mefloquine and sulfadoxine/pyrimethamine overdose in malaria tropica]. *Wien Klin Wochenschr* 1993;105:61–63.
37. Sin DD, Shafran SD. Dapsone- and primaquine-induced methemoglobinemia in HIV-infected individuals. *J Acquir Immune Defic Syndr Hum Retrovirol* 1996;12:477–481.
38. Motulsky AG. Hemolysis in glucose-6-phosphate dehydrogenase deficiency. *Fed Proc* 1972;31:1286–1292.
39. Boots M, Phillips M, Curtis JR. Megaloblastic anemia and pancytopenia due to proguanil in patients with chronic renal failure. *Clin Nephrol* 1982;18:106–108.
40. Tattersall JE, Greenwood RN, Baker LR, Cattel WR. Proguanil poisoning in a hemodialysis patient. *Clin Nephrol* 1987;28:104.
41. Jaeger A, Sauder P, Kopferschmitt J, Flesch F. Clinical features and management of poisoning due to antimalarial drugs. *Med Toxicol Adverse Drug Exp* 1987;2:242–273.
42. Grisham RS. Central nervous system toxicity of pyrimethamine (Daraprim) in man. *Am J Ophthalmol* 1962;54:1119–1121.

43. Tracqui A, Mikail I, Kintz P, Mangin P. Nonfatal prolonged overdosage of pyrimethamine in an infant: measurement of plasma and urine levels using HPLC with diode-array detection. *J Anal Toxicol* 1993;17:248–250.
44. Cheron G, Saint-Raymond A, Castot A. [Congenital toxoplasmosis, convulsions and overdose of pyrimethamine]. *Arch Fr Pediatr* 1987;44:824.
45. Akinyanju O, Goddell JC, Ahmed I. Pyrimethamine poisoning. *BMJ* 1973;4:147–148.
46. Davies CS. Two cases of Daraprim (pyrimethamine) poisoning. *Cent Afr J Med* 1956;2:364.
47. Balfour AJ. The bite of Jesuits' bark. *Aviat Space Environ Med* 1989;60:A4–A5.
48. Brinton GS, Norton EW, Zahn JR, Knighton RW. Ocular quinine toxicity. *Am J Ophthalmol* 1980;90:403–410.
49. Wolff RS, Wirtschafter D, Adkinson C. Ocular quinine toxicity treated with hyperbaric oxygen. *Undersea Hyperb Med* 1997;24:131–134.
50. Goldenberg AM, Wexler LF. Quinine overdose: review of toxicity and treatment. *Clin Cardiol* 1988;11:716–718.
51. Hughes W, Leoung G, Kramer F, et al. Comparison of atovaquone (566C80) with trimethoprim-sulfamethoxazole to treat *Pneumocystis carinii* pneumonia in patients with AIDS. *N Engl J Med* 1993;328:1521–1527.
52. Aderounmu AF, Salako LA, Lindstrom B, et al. Comparison of the pharmacokinetics of chloroquine after single intravenous and intramuscular administration in healthy Africans. *Br J Clin Pharmacol* 1986;22:559–564.
53. Ducharme J, Farinotti R. Clinical pharmacokinetics and metabolism of chloroquine. Focus on recent advancements. *Clin Pharmacokinet* 1996;31:257–274.
54. Clemessy JL, Favier C, Borron SW, et al. Hypokalaemia related to acute chloroquine ingestion. *Lancet* 1995;346:877–880.
55. Frisk-Holmberg M, Bergkvist Y, Domeij-Nyberg B, et al. Chloroquine serum concentration and side effects: evidence for dose-dependent kinetics. *Clin Pharmacol Ther* 1979;25:345–350.
56. Boereboom FT, Ververs FF, Meulenbelt J, Van Dijk A. Hemoperfusion is ineffectual in severe chloroquine poisoning. *Crit Care Med* 2000;28:3346–3350.
57. Tett SE, Cutler DJ, Day RO, Brown KF. A dose-ranging study of the pharmacokinetics of hydroxy-chloroquine following intravenous administration to healthy volunteers. *Br J Clin Pharmacol* 1988;26:303–313.
58. Almond DS, Szwandt IS, Edwards G, et al. Disposition of intravenous pyrimethamine in healthy volunteers. *Antimicrob Agents Chemother* 2000;44:1691–1693.
59. Bateman DN, Blain PG, Woodhouse KW, et al. Pharmacokinetics and clinical toxicity of quinine overdosage: lack of efficacy of techniques intended to enhance elimination. *QJM* 1985;54:125–131.
60. Boland ME, Roper SM, Henry JA. Complications of quinine poisoning. *Lancet* 1985;1:384–385.
61. Dyson EH, Proudfoot AT, Prescott LF, Heyworth R. Death and blindness due to overdose of quinine. *Br Med J (Clin Res Ed)* 1985;291:31–33.
62. Sabto JK, Pierce RM, West RH, Gurr FW. Hemodialysis, peritoneal dialysis, plasmapheresis and forced diuresis for the treatment of quinine overdose. *Clin Nephrol* 1981;16:264–268.
63. Smilkstein MJ, Kulig KW, Rumack BH. Acute toxic blindness: unrecognized quinine poisoning. *Ann Emerg Med* 1987;16:98–101.
64. Prescott LF, Hamilton AR, Heyworth R. Treatment of quinine overdosage with repeated oral charcoal. *Br J Clin Pharmacol* 1989;27:95–97.
65. Wolf LR, Otten EJ, Spadafora MP. Cinchonism: two case reports and review of acute quinine toxicity and treatment. *J Emerg Med* 1992;10:295–301.
66. Lockey D, Bateman DN. Effect of oral activated charcoal on quinine elimination. *Br J Clin Pharmacol* 1989;27:92–94.
67. Dargent B, Jullien F, Couraud F. Internalization of voltage-dependent sodium channels in fetal rat brain neurons: a study of the regulation of endocytosis. *J Neurochem* 1995;65:407–413.
68. Sanchez-Chapula JA, Salinas-Stefanon E, Torres-Jacome J, et al. Blockade of currents by the antimalarial drug chloroquine in feline ventricular myocytes. *J Pharmacol Exp Ther* 2001;297:437–445.
69. Britton WJ, Kevau IH. Intentional chloroquine overdosage. *Med J Aust* 1978;2:407–410.
70. Reimold WV, Larbig D, Kochsiek K. [Hypopotassemia and heart rhythm disorders due to quinine poisoning]. *Dtsch Med Wochenschr* 1970;95:517–521.
71. Padmaja UK, Adhikari P, Periera P. Experience with quinine in falciparum malaria. *Indian J Med Sci* 1999;53:153–157.
72. Lin X, Chen S, Tee D. Effects of quinine on the excitability and voltage-dependent currents of isolated spiral ganglion neurons in culture. *J Neurophysiol* 1998;79:2503–2512.
73. Zahn JR, Brinton GF, Norton E. Ocular quinine toxicity followed by electroretinogram, electro-oculogram, and pattern visually evoked potential. *Am J Optom Physiol Opt* 1981;58:492–498.
74. Bacon P, Spalton DJ, Smith SE. Blindness from quinine toxicity. *Br J Ophthalmol* 1988;72:219–224.
75. Canning CR, Hague S. Ocular quinine toxicity. *Br J Ophthalmol* 1988;72:23–26.
76. Cibis GW, Kolder H. [Fluoresceinangiography in experimental quinine poisoning (author's transl)]. *Klin Monatsbl Augenheilkd* 1974;164:789–794.
77. Cibis GW, Burian HM, Blodi FC. Electroretinogram changes in acute quinine poisoning. *Arch Ophthalmol* 1973;90:307–309.
78. Barrett NA, Solano T. Quinine ocular toxicity: treatment of blindness using therapy for vasospasm. *Anaesth Intensive Care* 2002;30:234–235.
79. Dyson EH, Proudfoot AT, Bateman DN. Quinine amblyopia: is current management appropriate? *J Toxicol Clin Toxicol* 1985;23:571–578.
80. Fletcher KA, Barton PF, Kelly JA. Studies on the mechanisms of oxidation in the erythrocyte by metabolites of primaquine. *Biochem Pharmacol* 1988;37:2683–2690.
81. Artymowicz RJ, James VE. Atovaquone: a new antipneumocystis agent. *Clin Pharm* 1993;12:563–570.
82. Wesche DL, DeCoster MA, Tortella FC, Brewer TG. Neurotoxicity of artemisinin analogs in vitro. *Antimicrob Agents Chemother* 1994;38:1813–1819.
83. Touze JE, Heno P, Fourcade L, et al. The effects of antimalarial drugs on ventricular repolarization. *Am J Trop Med Hyg* 2002;67:54–60.
84. Bindschedler M, Lefevre G, Degen P, Sioufi A. Comparison of the cardiac effects of the antimalarials co-artemether and halofantrine in healthy participants. *Am J Trop Med Hyg* 2002;66:293–298.
85. Maier RD, Benkert B. [Toxicological aspects of fatal chloroquine poisoning over a period of several days]. *Z Rechtsmed* 1984;92:27–33.
86. Ball DE, Tagwireyi D, Nhachi CF. Chloroquine poisoning in Zimbabwe: a toxicoepidemiological study. *J Appl Toxicol* 2002;22:311–315.
87. Wilkinson R, Mahatane J, Wade P, Pasvol G. Chloroquine poisoning. *BMJ* 1993;307:504.
88. Clemessy JL, Taboulet P, Hoffman JR, et al. Treatment of acute chloroquine poisoning: a 5-year experience. *Crit Care Med* 1996;24:1189–1195.
89. Francois J, De Rouck A, Cambie E. Retinal and optic evaluation in quinine poisoning. *Ann Ophthalmol* 1972;4:177–185.
90. Guly U, Driscoll P. The management of quinine-induced blindness. *Arch Emerg Med* 1992;9:317–322.
91. Bateman DN, Dyson EH. Quinine toxicity. *Adverse Drug React Acute Poisoning Rev* 1986;5:215–233.
92. Duveau E, Chomienne F, Seguin G. [Convulsions associated with pyrimethamine overdose]. *Arch Pediatr* 1996;3:286–287.
93. Todt H, Gmyrek D. [Seizure within the scope of poisoning with pyrimethamine (Tindurin)]. *Z Arztl Fortbild (Jena)* 1988;82:1089–1090.
94. Aguemon AR, Atchade D, Houngbe F, Fayomi B. [A case of acute pyrimethamine poisoning]. *Bull Soc Pathol Exot* 1997;90:117–119.
95. Antimalarials. In: *Australian medicines handbook*, 3rd ed. Adelaide, Australia: Australian Medicines Handbook Pty. Ltd, 2002.
96. Sweetman S. *Martindale: the complete drug reference*. London: Pharmaceutical Press, Electronic ed. Greenwood Village, CO: Micromedex, 2003.
97. Croes K, Augustijns P, Sabbe M, et al. Diminished sedation during diazepam treatment for chloroquine intoxication. *Pharm World Sci* 1993;15:83–85.
98. Kintz P, Ritter-Lohner S, Lamant JM, et al. Fatal chloroquine self-poisoning. *Hum Toxicol* 1988;7:541–543.
99. Clemessy JL, Lapostolle F, Borron SW, Baud FJ. [Acute chloroquine poisoning]. *Presse Med* 1996;25:1435–1439.
100. Hilberg T, Rogde S, Morland J. Postmortem drug redistribution—human cases related to results in experimental animals. *J Forensic Sci* 1999;44:3–9.
101. Kuhlman JJ Jr, Mayes RW, Levine B, et al. Chloroquine distribution in postmortem cases. *J Forensic Sci* 1991;36:1572–1579.
102. Chyka PA, Seger D. Position statement: single-dose activated charcoal. American Academy of Clinical Toxicology; European Association of Poisons Centres and Clinical Toxicologists. *J Toxicol Clin Toxicol* 1997;35:721–741.
103. Position statement and practice guidelines on the use of multi-dose activated charcoal in the treatment of acute poisoning. American Academy of Clinical Toxicology; European Association of Poisons Centres and Clinical Toxicologists. *J Toxicol Clin Toxicol* 1999;37:731–751.
104. Dawson AH, Whyte IM. Management of dapsone poisoning complicated by methaemoglobinaemia. *Med Toxicol Adverse Drug Exp* 1989;4:387–392.
105. Crouzette J, Vicaut E, Palombo S, et al. Experimental assessment of the protective activity of diazepam on the acute toxicity of chloroquine. *J Toxicol Clin Toxicol* 1983;20:271–279.
106. Riou B, Rimailho A, Galliot M, et al. Protective cardiovascular effects of diazepam in experimental acute chloroquine poisoning. *Intensive Care Med* 1988;14:610–616.
107. Riou B, Lecarpentier Y, Barriot P, Viars P. Diazepam does not improve the mechanical performance of rat cardiac papillary muscle exposed to chloroquine in vitro. *Intensive Care Med* 1989;15:390–395.
108. Gnassounou JP, Advenier C. Les effets antagonistes du diazepam et du RO5-4864 dans l'intoxication aigue par la chloroquine chez le rat et chez le cobaye sont-ils de nature cantrale ou peripherique? *Rean Soins Intens Med Urg* 1988;4:61–62.
109. Gnassounou JP, Dabire H, Advenier C. Le clonazepam est plus actif que le diazepam comme antagoniste de la chloroquine. *Rean Soins Intens Med Urg* 1988;4:467.
110. Buckley NA, Smith AJ, Dosen P, O'Connell DL. Effects of catecholamines and diazepam in chloroquine poisoning in barbiturate anaesthetised rats. *Hum Exp Toxicol* 1996;15:909–914.
111. Buckley NA, Dawson AH, Whyte IM. Chloroquine. In: *HyperTox: assessment and treatment of poisoning*, Vol. 1229. Newcastle, Australia: MediTox Pty. Ltd, 2002.
112. Curry SC, Connor DA, Clark RF, et al. The effect of hypertonic sodium bicarbonate on QRS duration in rats poisoned with chloroquine. *J Toxicol Clin Toxicol* 1996;34:73–76.
113. Sofola OA. The effects of chloroquine on the electrocardiogram and heart rate in anaesthetized dogs. *Clin Physiol* 1983;3:75–82.
114. Bricknell PP, Middleton HG, Hollingsworth A, Evans EM. Stellate ganglion block in treatment of total blindness due to quinine. *BMJ* 1967;4:400–401.
115. Browne GF, Coppel DL. Management of quinine overdose. *Hum Toxicol* 1984;3:399–402.
116. Bateman DW, Loydon CR, Ryan DW, Dyson EH. Stellate ganglion block and quinine overdose. *Anaesthesia* 1984;39:71–72.
117. Hachfi-Soussi F, Coudert V, Biron R, Barois A. [Acute quinine poisoning treated with high dose of diazepam]. *Arch Fr Pediatr* 1993;50:485–488.

CHAPTER 95

Dapsone

Ian MacGregor Whyte

DAPSONE

Molecular formula and weight:	**$C_{12}H_{12}N_2O_2S$, 248.31 g/mol**
SI conversion:	**mg/L × 4.03 = µmol/L**
CAS Registry No.:	**80-08-0**
Therapeutic level:	**Serum, 0.5 to 5.0 mg/L**
Special concerns:	**Methemoglobinemia, sulfhemoglobinemia, hemolysis, and anemia**
Antidotes:	**Repeated doses of activated charcoal increase clearance; methylene blue reduces methemoglobinemia**

OVERVIEW

Dapsone is the main drug used in the management of leprosy (1). It has been used in the treatment of malaria (2,3) and, more recently, as prophylaxis for *Pneumocystis carinii* pneumonia in patients infected with human immunodeficiency virus (4). It has been used extensively in a variety of skin conditions for its anti-inflammatory and immunosuppressive effects (5,6). The main limitation in its clinical use is its hematologic effects (7).

Dapsone (4,4'-diaminodiphenylsulfone) is a sulfone. In the late 1930s, sulfones were found to be capable of killing a variety of pathogenic bacteria (8). Although there were problems with toxicity, dapsone was established in the treatment of leprosy by the early 1940s (8) and remains the mainstay of current combination treatment (1). Dapsone was tried with serendipitous success in dermatitis herpetiformis (6). Dapsone was tried with success in the treatment of malaria (2,3) and has been used for prophylaxis for *Pneumocystis* pneumonia (4) and toxoplasmosis (9). It is used for the treatment of actinomycotic mycetoma (10).

The introduction of alternative antibiotics has altered the medical use of dapsone. Its main applications are now in the treatment of noninfectious inflammatory, autoimmune, and bullous diseases: acne, Behçet's disease, bullous and cicatricial pemphigoid, epidermolysis bullosa acquisita, erythema elevatum diutinum, Kaposi's sarcoma, linear immunoglobulin A bullous dermatosis, cutaneous discoid lupus erythematosus, lobular panniculitis associated with α_1-antitrypsin deficiency, pemphigus, pemphigus herpetiformis and immunoglobulin A pemphigus, pyoderma gangrenosum, relapsing polychondritis, subcorneal pustular dermatosis (Sneddon-Wilkinson disease), urticarial vasculitis syndrome, and leukocytoclastic vasculitis (6). It has also been recommended for the treatment of necrotic reactions to spider bite (Chapter 249).

TOXIC DOSE

The *adult therapeutic dose* varies by indication, ranging from 50 mg daily to 100 mg twice daily (11). The *pediatric dose* is 1 to 2 mg/kg, up to a maximum dose of 100 mg.

In the largest series of cases (274 patients, aged 1 month to 50 years), severe methemoglobinemia (median methemoglobin of 38%) occurred at doses greater than 750 mg (12). Adult ingestion of 1.4 to 6.0 g (13), 1 to 10 g (14), 3 g (15), 4 g (16), 7.5 g (17), 8 to 9 g (18), 10 g (19), and 14 g (20) has caused marked methemoglobinemia, some sulfhemoglobinemia, and varying degrees of hemolysis with ultimate survival. Survival of the initial phase followed by death at 10 days from sepsis-induced multiorgan failure occurred after an ingestion of 5 g (21). Death occurred in three cases of dapsone overdose in adults in which methylene blue was not available (22) and in another case in which treatment details were unclear (23).

An ingestion of 37.5 mg/kg in a child was survived after methemoglobinemia (24). A 23-month-old child died after ingesting 5 g of dapsone. Methylene blue was not used, as methemoglobin was not detected (25).

In the largest series of cases, the median dapsone concentration of 29 mg/L was achieved at doses greater than 2 g (12). A concentration of 80 mg/L was reached after an overdose of 15 g (20). A concentration of 3.9 mg/L occurred 24 hours after ingestion of an unknown amount in a 3.5-year-old child (26). Both patients survived. Three adults reported as ingesting 10 g achieved concentrations of 120 mg/L (19), 30 mg/L (14), and 120 mg/L (27). All three survived.

A hypersensitivity reaction to dapsone in therapeutic doses has resulted in death (28).

TOXICOKINETICS AND TOXICODYNAMICS

The pharmacokinetic parameters of dapsone are provided in Table 1. Dapsone is metabolized by two routes: *N*-acetylation [via *N*-acetyltransferase to monoacetyl dapsone (MADDS)] and *N*-hydroxylation (29). The hematologic toxicity of dapsone, in particular, methemoglobin formation and hemolytic anemia, is due to the hydroxylamine metabolites of dapsone and MADDS produced by *N*-hydroxylation (30). These metabolites are mainly produced by CYP2E1 (31), although CYP3A4 (32), CYP2C6, CYP2C11, and CYP3A1 have all been implicated (33). There are fast and slow acetylators of dapsone as well as fast and slow *N*-hydroxylators of dapsone and MADDS (29). Hematologic toxicity is greater in slow acetylators (more dapsone is available for *N*-hydroxylation), fast *N*-hydroxylators, and, especially, in combination.

There is a linear relationship between hydroxylamine-dependent methemoglobin formation and conversion of dapsone hydroxylamine to dapsone in red cells (34). There may be a cycle between the hepatic *N*-hydroxylation of dapsone to its hydroxylamine form and reduction to amine within the red cell (35).

In overdose, methemoglobinemia correlates well with the dapsone concentration, resolving as the level declines to the therapeutic range (12,19,36). The apparent half-life of both dapsone [88 hours (19) and 40 to 100 hours (14)] and MADDS [67 hours (19)] may be prolonged in overdose. This is likely due to continuing absorption and enterohepatic recirculation as the

TABLE 1. Pharmacokinetics of oral dapsone

Time-to-peak serum concentration	4 h
Absorption half-life	1.1 h
Bioavailability	70–80%
Volume of distribution	1.5 L/kg
Route of excretion	Hepatic with enterohepatic circulation
Elimination half-life	30 h
Metabolites	Main metabolite is MADDS (half-life, 20 h; 100% protein bound; nontoxic); hydroxylamine metabolites of both dapsone and MADDS cause the hemolysis[a]
Protein binding	70–90%

MADDS, monoacetyl dapsone.
[a]Data from reference 30.
Adapted from Zuidema J, Hilbers-Modderman ES, Merkus FW. Clinical pharmacokinetics of dapsone. *Clin Pharmacokinet* 1986;11:299–315.

ratio of MADDS to dapsone remains constant (suggesting the elimination is not saturable) (36). This observation is supported by the marked reductions in apparent half-life of dapsone after repeated doses of activated charcoal (14,19,37).

The acetylation ratio (MADDS:dapsone) shows a genetically determined bimodal distribution, indicating that there are "slow" and "rapid" acetylators (38).

PATHOPHYSIOLOGY

Dapsone acts against bacteria and protozoa by inhibition of dihydrofolic acid synthesis through competition with para-aminobenzoate for the active site of dihydropteroate synthetase (6). The antiinflammatory action of the drug is unrelated to its antibacterial action and is still not fully understood. An inflammatory disease that responds to dapsone is almost invariably associated with marked polymorphonuclear leukocyte infiltration (39). It appears that neutrophils and neutrophil products are the major targets for the antiinflammatory action of dapsone (6).

The methemoglobin formation and hemolytic anemia of dapsone are due to the hydroxylamine metabolites of dapsone and MADDS (30). The conversion of dapsone hydroxylamine to dapsone in red cells is directly related to methemoglobin formation (34). Subsequent *N*-hydroxylation of dapsone to its hydroxylamine form provides more toxic metabolites for reduction to amine within the red cell (35).

PREGNANCY AND LACTATION

Dapsone is U.S. Food and Drug Administration pregnancy category C (Appendix I). Dapsone distributes into milk in significant quantities and can cause hemolytic anemia in the breast-feeding infant (40).

CLINICAL PRESENTATION

Acute Overdosage

Early gastrointestinal features (nausea and vomiting) in dapsone poisoning are nonspecific. Within a few minutes (in massive overdose) to as much as 24 hours (for minor overdose), cyanosis develops due to methemoglobinemia. In a series of 274 patients, cyanosis occurred in 65.7% of the patients and in all children younger than 5 years of age (12).

Sulfhemoglobinemia has been reported infrequently (7,15), but it is also not clinically evaluated in most patients. When measured, its onset has been later than that of methemoglobinemia (7,15). Signs of hypoxia ensue if the amount of altered hemoglobin (methemoglobin plus sulfhemoglobin) is sufficient (usually greater than 20% in nonanemic patients). As the severity of the hypoxia increases, signs include headache, lethargy, dizziness, fatigue, syncope, dyspnea, and increasing central nervous system depression followed by coma, seizures, dysrhythmias, shock, and death. Concomitant tachycardia and hypertension or hypotension are expected, as is the potential for end-organ injury (hepatic, renal, central nervous system, myocardial) if the hypoxia is severe or prolonged.

Because of the prolonged absorption and enterohepatic recirculation of dapsone, methemoglobinemia may persist for several days (7,15,19–21,26,41), by which time hemolytic anemia may complicate the clinical picture (16,17,19,20). This is particularly likely in patients with preexisting glucose 6 phosphate dehydrogenase (G6PD) deficiency or abnormal hemoglobin (42–44). Hemolysis may complicate therapy with methylene blue (45). This would be more likely if methemoglobinemia was not present (see Pitfalls).

Macular injury, possibly an unusual complication of hemolysis and hypoxia, may occur (17,46–48). Peripheral neuropathy is a rare dose-dependent complication of chronic therapy [usually either an inappropriately high chronic dose (49,50) or in slow acetylators (29)] that may also occur after acute overdose (46).

Adverse Events

Adverse effects may be dose related or idiosyncratic. The common dose-related effects are asymptomatic anemia and methemoglobinemia, anorexia, nausea, vomiting, headache, and rash (in 30% to 40% of human immunodeficiency virus patients). Infrequent effects are fever, hepatitis, albuminuria, psychosis, and motor neuropathy (increased risk if used with zalcitabine). Rarely, agranulocytosis, neutropenia, and severe cutaneous reactions (e.g., exfoliative dermatitis) may occur (11).

An idiosyncratic hypersensitivity syndrome may occur in the first 6 weeks of therapy and includes rash, which is always present, fever, jaundice, and eosinophilia. It usually resolves rapidly after discontinuation; corticosteroid therapy may help (11).

Pitfalls

The onset of the methemoglobinemia, sulfhemoglobinemia, and hemolysis may be significantly delayed. Patients may need observation and repeated hematologic investigation for several days to a week or more. Sulfhemoglobinemia is clinically indistinguishable from methemoglobinemia but is unresponsive to methylene blue.

DIAGNOSTIC TESTING

Acute Overdosage

Specific drug concentrations are not readily available. In overdose, serial measurement of methemoglobin using a cooximeter, sulfhemoglobin (if possible), hemoglobin, and hematocrit helps assess severity and guides treatment in the early phase. Assessment of hemolysis by haptoglobin, free hemoglobin, reticulocyte counts, and urinary hemoglobin may be required. Arterial blood gas measurement is useful to assess acid-base balance. Assessments of liver and renal function tests help assess end-organ damage from hypoxia.

TREATMENT

Management of toxicity focuses on increasing the elimination of dapsone and its metabolite as well as treating methemoglobinemia.

Gastrointestinal Decontamination

Decontamination with activated charcoal should be instituted for all patients who have ingested an overdose within 1 hour of ingestion.

Enhancement of Elimination

For an ingestion with clinical evidence of methemoglobinemia, repeated doses of activated charcoal should be administered (Chapter 7). An activated charcoal dose of 20 g four times a day has significantly shortened half-lives of both dapsone and MADDS after overdose (19) and increased clearance in volunteers and overdose patients (37). The increase in clearance is equivalent to that achieved with hemodialysis (14). Repeat-dose charcoal (1 g/kg three to six times/day) is also well tolerated in children with dapsone poisoning (51). Although 12 of 18 children had a methemoglobin level above 30% and required methylene blue, only one dose was required with no continuing methemoglobinemia, suggesting some benefit from the elimination of dapsone and its metabolites (51). Charcoal hemoperfusion markedly shortens the elimination half-life of dapsone (to 1.5 hours) and has been used in one case (16). Plasma exchange is not helpful (20). In most cases, exchange transfusion provides little clinical benefit and is a difficult procedure (22,27). In a 2-year-old child, exchange transfusion reduced methemoglobin with clinical improvement (52).

Antidotes

Methylene blue is the mainstay of treatment for methemoglobinemia (Chapters 21 and 63). For less severe poisonings, one or two doses of 1 to 2 mg/kg intravenously of a 1% solution may be given over several minutes. A repeat dose may be given after 1 hour if required. If more than two doses are required, or in more severe poisonings, sulfhemoglobin should be measured, as it produces the same clinical symptoms but does not respond to methylene blue. If sulfhemoglobin is not a problem, then the methemoglobinemia is likely to be prolonged, and a methylene blue infusion should be used (7,20,50). Initial dose should be 0.2 mg/kg/hour titrated to effect. Methylene blue in large doses, by intermittent injection or by infusion can result in methemoglobinemia and hemolysis (45) (particularly in G6PD-deficient individuals), so repeated measurement of methemoglobin and assessment for hemolysis are needed during treatment.

Supportive Care

Hemolysis may require transfusion, particularly in G6PD-deficient patients in whom the hemolysis is more severe (53). If hemolysis is severe, assessment of vision and macular function is warranted (17,46–48). Clinical assessment for late onset of a peripheral neuropathy is appropriate after very high-dose poisonings (46).

Monitoring

The presence of G6PD deficiency should be excluded before using dapsone. The complete blood cell count and liver function should be tested before starting treatment and the blood cell count monitored weekly during the first month of therapy and then monthly during treatment. If the patient is receiving concomitant folate antagonists, monitor more frequently. Methemoglobinemia is common at treatment dosing levels.

REFERENCES

1. Ramos-e-Silva, Rebello PF. Leprosy. Recognition and treatment. *Am J Clin Dermatol* 2001;2:203–211.
2. DeGowin RL, Eppes RB, Carson PE, Powell RD. The effects of diaphenylsulfone (DDS) against chloroquine-resistant *Plasmodium falciparum*. *Bull World Health Organ* 1966;34:671–681.
3. Sheehy TW, Reba RC, Neff TA, et al. Supplemental sulfone (dapsone) therapy. Use in treatment of chloroquine-resistant falciparum malaria. *Arch Intern Med* 1967;119:561–566.
4. Cruciani M, Bertazzoni ME, Mirandola M, et al. Twice-weekly dapsone for primary prophylaxis against *Pneumocystis carinii* pneumonia in HIV-1 infection: efficacy, safety and pharmacokinetic data. *Clin Microbiol Infect* 1996;2:30–35.
5. Zhu YI, Stiller MJ. Dapsone and sulfones in dermatology: overview and update. *J Am Acad Dermatol* 2001;45:420–434.
6. Wolf R, Matz H, Orion E, et al. Dapsone. *Dermatol Online J* 2002;8:2.
7. Dawson AH, Whyte IM. Management of dapsone poisoning complicated by methaemoglobinaemia. *Med Toxicol Adverse Drug Exp* 1989;4:387–392.
8. Doull J. Sulfone therapy of leprosy. Background, early history and present status. *Int J Lepr Other Mycobact Dis* 1963;31:143–160.
9. Payen MC, De Wit S, Sommereijns B, Clumeck N. A controlled trial of dapsone versus pyrimethamine-sulfadoxine for primary prophylaxis of *Pneumocystis carinii* pneumonia and toxoplasmosis in patients with AIDS. *Biomed Pharmacother* 1997;51:439–445.
10. Poncio MR, Negroni R, Bonifaz A, Pappagianis D. New aspects of some endemic mycoses. *Med Mycol* 2000;38[Suppl 1]:237–241.
11. Anti-infectives. In: *Australian medicines handbook*, 3rd ed. Adelaide, Australia: Australian Medicines Handbook Pty. Ltd, 2002.
12. Carrazza MZ, Carrazza FR, Oga S. Clinical and laboratory parameters in dapsone acute intoxication. *Rev Saude Publica* 2000;34:396–401.
13. Casey PB, Tracey JA. Methemoglobinemia following dapsone overdose. EAPCCT XIX International Congress abstract. *J Toxicol Clin Toxicol* 1999;37:411–412.
14. Neuvonen PJ, Elonen E, Haapanen EJ. Acute dapsone intoxication: clinical findings and effect of oral charcoal and haemodialysis on dapsone elimination. *Acta Med Scand* 1983;214:215–220.
15. Lambert M, Sonnet J, Mahieu P, Hassoun A. Delayed sulfhemoglobinemia after acute dapsone intoxication. *J Toxicol Clin Toxicol* 1982;19:45–50.
16. Endre ZH, Charlesworth JA, Macdonald GJ, Woodbridge L. Successful treatment of acute dapsone intoxication using charcoal hemoperfusion. *Aust N Z J Med* 1983;13:509–512.
17. Kenner DJ, Holt K, Agnello R, Chester GH. Permanent retinal damage following massive dapsone overdose. *Br J Ophthalmol* 1980;64:741–744.
18. Ferguson AJ, Lavery GG. Deliberate self-poisoning with dapsone. A case report and summary of relevant pharmacology and treatment. *Anaesthesia* 1997;52:359–363.
19. Elonen E, Neuvonen PJ, Halmekoski J, Mattila MJ. Acute dapsone intoxication: a case with prolonged symptoms. *J Toxicol Clin Toxicol* 1979;14:79–85.
20. Berlin G, Brodin B, Hilden JO, Martensson J. Acute dapsone intoxication: a case treated with continuous infusion of methylene blue, forced diuresis and plasma exchange. *J Toxicol Clin Toxicol* 1984;22:537–548.
21. Wagner A, Marosi C, Binder M, et al. Fatal poisoning due to dapsone in a patient with grossly elevated methaemoglobin levels. *Br J Dermatol* 1995;133:816–817.
22. Sahoo SK, Tripathy N, Debi BP. Acute fatal DDS poisoning. (Report of 4 cases). *Lepr India* 1979;51:244–248.
23. Singhal SK. Suicide with dapsone. *Indian J Lepr* 1988;60:87–89.
24. MacDonald RD, McGuigan MA. Acute dapsone intoxication: a pediatric case report. *Pediatr Emerg Care* 1997;13:127–129.
25. Davies R. Fatal poisoning with Udolac (Diaminodiphenylsulphone). *Lancet* 1950;905–906.
26. Linakis JG, Shannon M, Woolf A, Sax C. Recurrent methemoglobinemia after acute dapsone intoxication in a child. *J Emerg Med* 1989;7:477–480.
27. Szajewski JM, Dorywalski T, Tomecka Z, Sabiniewicz M. [Case of severe poisoning with diamino-diphenylsulfone (DDS)—an antileprotic drug]. *Pol Arch Med Wewn* 1972;49:181–186.
28. Frey HM, Gershon AA, Borkowsky W, Bullock WE. Fatal reaction to dapsone during treatment of leprosy. *Ann Intern Med* 1981;94:777–779.
29. Bluhm RE, Adedoyin A, McCarver DG, Branch RA. Development of dapsone toxicity in patients with inflammatory dermatoses: activity of acetylation and hydroxylation of dapsone as risk factors. *Clin Pharmacol Ther* 1999;65:598–605.
30. Grossman SJ, Jollow DJ. Role of dapsone hydroxylamine in dapsone-induced hemolytic anemia. *J Pharmacol Exp Ther* 1988;244:118–125.
31. Mitra AK, Thummel KE, Kalhorn TF, et al. Metabolism of dapsone to its hydroxylamine by CYP2E1 in vitro and in vivo. *Clin Pharmacol Ther* 1995;58:556–566.
32. Fleming CM, Branch RA, Wilkinson GR, Guengerich FP. Human liver microsomal N-hydroxylation of dapsone by cytochrome P-4503A4. *Mol Pharmacol* 1992;41:975–980.
33. Vage C, Svensson CK. Evidence that the biotransformation of dapsone and monoacetyldapsone to their respective hydroxylamine metabolites in rat liver microsomes is mediated by cytochrome P450 2C6/2C11 and 3A1. *Drug Metab Dispos* 1994;22:572–577.
34. Coleman MD, Jacobus DP. Reduction of dapsone hydroxylamine to dapsone during methaemoglobin formation in human erythrocytes in vitro. *Biochem Pharmacol* 1993;45:1027–1033.
35. Coleman MD, Jacobus DP. Reduction of dapsone hydroxylamine to dap-

sone during methaemoglobin formation in human erythrocytes in vitro—II. Movement of dapsone across a semipermeable membrane into erythrocytes and plasma. *Biochem Pharmacol* 1993;46:1363–1368.
36. Woodhouse KW, Henderson DB, Charlton B, et al. Acute dapsone poisoning: clinical features and pharmacokinetic studies. *Hum Toxicol* 1983;2:507–510.
37. Neuvonen PJ, Elonen E, Mattila MJ. Oral activated charcoal and dapsone elimination. *Clin Pharmacol Ther* 1980;27:823–827.
38. Zuidema J, Hilbers-Modderman ES, Merkus FW. Clinical pharmacokinetics of dapsone. *Clin Pharmacokinet* 1986;11:299–315.
39. Lang PG Jr. Sulfones and sulfonamides in dermatology today. *J Am Acad Dermatol* 1979;1:479–492.
40. Sanders SW, Zone JJ, Foltz RL, et al. Hemolytic anemia induced by dapsone transmitted through breast milk. *Ann Intern Med* 1982;96:465–466.
41. Reigart JR, Trammel HLJ, Lindsey JM. Repetitive doses of activated charcoal in dapsone poisoning in a child. *J Toxicol Clin Toxicol* 1982;19:1061–1066.
42. Scott GL, Rasbridge MR. The in vitro action of dapsone and its derivatives on normal and G6PD-deficient red cells. *Br J Haematol* 1973;24:307–317.
43. Manfredi G, De Panfilis G, Zampetti M, Allegra F. Studies on dapsone induced haemolytic anaemia. I. Methaemoglobin production and G-6-PD activity in correlation with dapsone dosage. *Br J Dermatol* 1979;100:427–432.
44. Lachant NA, Tanaka KR. Dapsone-associated Heinz body hemolytic anemia in a Cambodian woman with hemoglobin E trait. *Am J Med Sci* 1987;294:364–368.
45. Goldstein BD. Exacerbation of dapsone-induced Heinz body hemolytic anemia following treatment with methylene blue. *Am J Med Sci* 1974;267:291–297.
46. Abhayambika K, Chacko A, Mahadevan K, Najeeb OM. Peripheral neuropathy and haemolytic anaemia with cherry red spot on macula in dapsone poisoning. *J Assoc Physicians India* 1990;38:564–565.
47. Seo MS, Yoon KC, Park YG. Dapsone maculopathy. *Korean J Ophthalmol* 1997;11:70–73.
48. Chakrabarti M, Suresh PN, Namperumalsamy P. Bilateral macular infarction due to diaminodiphenyl sulfone (4,4' DDS) toxicity. *Retina* 1999;19:83–84.
49. Sirsat AM, Lalitha VS, Pandya SS. Dapsone neuropathy—report of three cases and pathologic features of a motor nerve. *Int J Lepr Other Mycobact Dis* 1987;55:23–29.
50. Southgate HJ, Masterson R. Lessons to be learned: a case study approach: prolonged methaemoglobinaemia due to inadvertent dapsone poisoning; treatment with methylene blue and exchange transfusion. *J R Soc Health* 1999;119:52–55.
51. Bucaretchi F, Miglioli M, Pereira FT, et al. Acute dapsone exposure and methemoglobinemia: a pediatric case series. EAPCCT XIX International Congress abstract. *J Toxicol Clin Toxicol* 1999;37:412.
52. Kumar A, Antony TJ, Kurein KM, et al. Exchange transfusion for dapsone poisoning. *Indian Pediatr* 1988;25:798–800.
53. Hansen DG, Challoner KR, Smith DE. Dapsone intoxication: two case reports. *J Emerg Med* 1994;12:347–351.

CHAPTER 96

Urinary Antiinfective Drugs

Steven A. Seifert

NH_2 N H_2N N=N

PHENAZOPYRIDINE

Compounds included:	**Fosfomycin (Monurol), methenamine (Hiprex, Mandelamine), nitrofurantoin (Furadantin, Macrodantin, Macrobid), phenazopyridine (Pyridium, Uristat), trimethoprim (Bactrim, Septra)**
Molecular formula and weight:	**See text.**
SI conversion:	**Fosfomycin, mg/L × 7.2 = µmol/L; methenamine hippurate, mg/L × 3.1 = µmol/L; methenamine mandelate, mg/L × 3.4 = µmol/L; nitrofurantoin, mg/L × 4.2 = µmol/L; phenazopyridine, mg/L × 4.0 = µmol/L; trimethoprim, mg/L × 3.4 = µmol/L**
CAS Registry No.:	**See text.**
Therapeutic levels:	**Serum levels are not clinically useful.**
Target organs:	**Gastrointestinal (acute), liver (chronic), skin (acute), lungs (chronic), electrolyte abnormalities (chronic), central nervous system (chronic)**
Antidote:	**Methylene blue (phenazopyridine)**

OVERVIEW

The drugs used to treat urinary tract infections are a mixed group, with different structures, modes of action, effectiveness against particular pathogens, and toxicities. Management of toxicity is generally symptomatic and supportive, with recognition of the causative nature of symptoms and signs and cessation of the responsible agent.

FOSFOMYCIN

Fosfomycin [Monurol; $C_3H_7O_4P$; molecular weight (MW), 138.1 g/mol; CAS Registry No., 78964-85-9] is a phosphonic acid with activity against most urinary tract pathogens. It is available as fosfomycin tromethamine, fosmidomycin, and as a calcium salt. Fosfomycin is also known to protect against cisplatin-induced ototoxicity, without inhibiting its tumoricidal efficacy (1–3).

Toxic Dose

The *adult therapeutic dose* is a single 3-g oral dose. It may also be given as 3 g daily for up to 3 days for more serious or resistant infections. The *pediatric dose* is 2 g orally.

There is no reported minimum toxic dose or lethal dose.

Toxicokinetics and Toxicodynamics

Oral fosfomycin tromethamine has a bioavailability of 34% to 41% (4–6), with a large volume of distribution (V_d) of 140 L (7) and a peak serum level of 2.0 to 2.5 hours (8). Fosfomycin is excreted unchanged in the urine (99.5%) by glomerular filtration (9), with a mean elimination half-life of 5.7 hours (10). Elimination is prolonged when combined with food or metoclopramide (8) or in patients with renal impairment (11). The peak serum concentration of the tromethamine salt is approximately two times higher, and the half-life is two to four times longer than the other formulations (12).

Pregnancy and Lactation

Fosfomycin is U.S. Food and Drug Administration (FDA) pregnancy category B (Appendix I) (10). Fosfomycin crosses the placenta, but fetotoxicity has not been reported (13,14). Concentrations in human milk are 10% of simultaneous serum concentrations (15).

Clinical Presentation

ADVERSE EVENTS

Adverse events are usually mild, last only 1 to 2 days, and usually resolve without treatment (16,17). The overall incidence is 6% with oral therapeutic dosing (18) and 17% with parenteral administration (19). Gastrointestinal (GI) complaints, primarily diarrhea, are most frequent. Other effects include dizziness, headache, and vaginitis. Adverse events are lower when the drug is given as a single dose. Less common events are angioedema, aplastic anemia, asthma exacerbation, cholestatic jaundice, hepatic injury, toxic megacolon, pseudomembranous colitis, and possibly optic neuritis (10,20). Recurrent fosfomycin-induced hepatic toxicity was reported with drug rechallenge in a woman with cystic fibrosis (21).

DRUG INTERACTIONS

Concomitant administration of metoclopramide lowers serum and urinary concentrations of fosfomycin tromethamine (22).

Diagnostic Tests

Fosfomycin serum concentrations are not clinically useful. Liver transaminases and function tests should be followed during long-term or high-dose use or in symptomatic patients. A complete blood cell count (CBC) or renal function tests should be obtained as clinically indicated.

Treatment

The drug should be withdrawn if significant adverse effects occur. Management of toxicity is primarily symptomatic and supportive. Enhanced elimination with dialysis is possible in patients with renal impairment but rarely should be required. There is no specific antidote.

METHENAMINE

Methenamine hippurate (Hiprex; $C_6H_{12}N_4$,$C_9H_9NO_3$; MW, 319.4 g/mol; CAS Registry No., 5714-73-8) and methenamine mandelate (Mandelamine; $C_6H_{12}N_4$,$C_8H_8O_3$; MW, 292.3 g/mol; CAS Registry No., 587-23-5) are used for long-term prophylactic suppression of urinary infection. Methenamine decomposes to generate low concentrations of formaldehyde in the urine. Because the production of formaldehyde is enhanced in an acidic environment, ascorbic acid or cranberry juice is often given with methenamine. Significant levels of formaldehyde are not found in the GI tract or tissues (23). The hippurate salt is less well tolerated than trimethoprim (24). Side effects are primarily GI with indigestion and nausea.

Toxic Dose

The *adult therapeutic dose* of methenamine hippurate is 1 g/day orally (25), and methenamine mandelate is 1 g four times a day orally (26). The *pediatric dosage* (children ages 6 to 12 years) is 25 to 50 mg/kg/day divided every 12 hours as the hippurate salt or 50 to 75 mg/kg/day divided every 6 hours as the mandelate salt.

There is no reported minimum toxic dose or lethal dose.

Toxicokinetics and Toxicodynamics

Methenamine mandelate is relatively unique among antibacterial salts in that its biologic activity derives from both ions (27). Approximately 90% of the drug is converted to urinary formaldehyde within 3 hours. Hypersensitivity reactions may occur, particularly in patients who are also sensitive to tartrazine and salicylates.

Pregnancy and Lactation

Methenamine is FDA pregnancy category C (Appendix I) (28). It is present in breast milk in approximately the same concentration as in serum. No adverse effects on breast-feeding infants have been reported.

Clinical Presentation

Methenamine hippurate may produce a photosensitivity reaction (29). Overdose experience is limited. An 8-g overdose in a 2.5-year-old child resulted in hemorrhagic cystitis, mild metabolic acidosis, elevated blood urea nitrogen, and lower urinary tract irritation (30). Vulvovaginal rash or irritation may occur (24).

Diagnostic Tests

Plasma methenamine levels are not clinically useful. In symptomatic patients, a baseline CBC, renal and hepatic function tests, and urinalysis should be obtained and followed as indicated. Methenamine mandelate may be detected by cerimetric titration. Methenamine in therapeutic doses or overdose may produce a spurious elevation of urinary catecholamine, 17-hydroxycorticosteroid, and vanillylmandelic acid and a decrease in urinary hydroxyindoleacetic acid (28,31).

Treatment

The drug should be withdrawn if significant adverse effects occur. Management is primarily symptomatic and supportive. Interruption of absorption by gastric emptying or activated charcoal should be used for large ingestions presenting within 1 to 2 hours after exposure. There is no specific antidote.

NITROFURANTOIN

Nitrofurantoin (Furadantin, Macrodantin, Macrobid; $C_8H_6N_4O_5$; SI conversion, mg/L × 4.20 = μmol/L; CAS Registry No., 17140-

81-7; MW, 238.16 g/mol) is rapidly absorbed and concentrated in the urine (32). Few reports of nitrofurantoin overdose are available despite its extensive use. In the elderly, the dose is often reduced to 50 mg four times daily (32).

Toxic Dose

The *adult therapeutic dose* is 50 to 100 mg four times daily. The *pediatric dose* is 5 to 7 mg/kg/24 hours in four divided doses. There is no reported minimum toxic dose or lethal dose.

Toxicokinetics and Toxicodynamics

The oral bioavailability of nitrofurantoin is 90%. The peak serum level is 2 hours with a V_d of 0.6 L/kg. It is 90% bound to plasma proteins, with 33% of the drug converted to active metabolites (32–34). The elimination half-life in individuals with normal renal function is 0.3 to 1.0 hour but may be prolonged in those with impaired creatinine clearance.

Pathophysiology

Nitrofurantoin undergoes cyclic oxidation and reduction. However, the association between this process and its toxicity is not clear (35). Nitrofurantoin also depletes cellular glutathione and protein thiols, which may be a cause or effect of oxidative stress (36). The acute phase of pulmonary toxicity is believed to be a hypersensitivity reaction, whereas chronic pulmonary injury is believed to be direct oxygen radical injury to the lung by oxygen radicals (37,38). Hepatic toxicity may be mediated by the induction of cytotoxic T-cell activation against hepatocytes (39), and antibody-mediated pulmonary, hepatic (40), and ocular injury (41) may also occur.

Pregnancy and Lactation

Nitrofurantoin is FDA pregnancy category B (Appendix I) (28). It is actively transported into human milk, with concentrations exceeding serum (42).

Clinical Presentation

The most frequent adverse reactions are anorexia, nausea, and vomiting, occurring more often when the dose exceeds 7 mg/kg/day (32). Excessive doses induce nausea and vomiting.

Pulmonary toxicity has both acute and chronic manifestations. Acute toxicity occurs within 1 month of initiating therapy, whereas the chronic form develops after 2 months to 5 years of continuous therapy (38,43). Acute pulmonary reactions are more common in the elderly and rare in children (44). Chronic pulmonary toxicity has an incidence of 0.0009% (45). Interstitial edema and pulmonary fibrosis occur with chronic toxicity (37,38), resulting in bronchiolitis obliterans organizing pneumonia and other conditions (46,47). Its incidence is 0.0002% (45). The incidence of hepatotoxicity is 0.0003% (39,45).

There are rare reports of acute interstitial nephritis (48). Ocular myasthenia has been reported (41). Hematologic reactions may be seen in patients who have glucose 6 phosphate dehydrogenase deficiency. Hematologic adverse effects occur with an incidence of 0.0004% (45). Peripheral neuropathy can begin within 2 to 8 weeks of starting treatment, and the severity is not related to dose or renal function (49). Total or partial recovery is common, but irreversible injury has been reported (49,50). The incidence is 0.0007% (45).

Hypersensitivity reactions occur in 1% to 5% of patients and may rapidly subside after cessation of therapy. There are a number of reports of severe recurrent toxicity in patients who were rechallenged with nitrofurantoin after a previous reaction (49).

Diagnostic Tests

Nitrofurantoin serum concentrations are not clinically useful. A CBC and renal and liver function tests should be obtained in symptomatic patients.

A chest radiograph should be obtained if there are pulmonary symptoms. A reticular pattern on high-resolution computed tomography scan correlates with the fibrosis of chronic pulmonary toxicity. Fibrosis may improve after discontinuation of the drug (38). Lung biopsy may occasionally be needed, but it is usually not performed when drug-induced lung disease is likely, based on exposure history and improvement after drug withdrawal.

Treatment

Treatment is largely symptomatic and supportive. Interruption of absorption by gastric emptying or activated charcoal should be used for a large ingestion presenting within 1 to 2 hours of ingestion. A high fluid intake should be provided to promote urinary excretion of the drug. Enhanced elimination with hemodialysis is possible in severe overdose or in patients with impaired renal function. There is no specific antidote.

With chronic pulmonary toxicity, withdrawal of the drug and use of oral corticosteroids have been advocated (46,47).

PHENAZOPYRIDINE

Phenazopyridine hydrochloride (Pyridium, Uristat; $C_{11}H_{11}N_5$,HCl; MW, 249.7 g/mol; CAS Registry No., 136-40-3) is used primarily as a urinary tract analgesic and anesthetic. As with other azo compounds, it may cause hemolytic anemia in patients with or without glucose 6 phosphate dehydrogenase deficiency (51,52).

Toxic Dose

The *adult therapeutic dose* is 200 mg three times orally per day, with therapy not to continue beyond 2 days when used in combination with a urinary antiinfective. The *pediatric dose* is 12 mg/kg/day orally divided thrice daily for 2 days.

There is no reported minimum toxic dose or lethal dose.

Toxicokinetics and Toxicodynamics

Phenazopyridine is metabolized by cleavage of the azo bond. After a therapeutic dose, 90% is excreted in the urine in the first 24 hours, with 8% of the dose eliminated as aniline (53).

Pathophysiology

Azo compounds produce oxidative stress within the red blood cell. This may be an effect of the 2,3,6-triaminopyridine metabolite, which has been shown to generate superoxide radicals and hydrogen peroxide (54). Sulfhemoglobinemia also occurs (55). Phenazopyridine can cause hemolytic anemia in patients with or without glucose 6 phosphate dehydrogenase deficiency. Methemoglobinemia can occur during therapeutic dosing in patients with normal renal function (56), but it occurs more commonly in individuals with decreased renal function (57). It is more common after overdose, perhaps as a result of the production of aniline (51–53,58).

Acute renal injury in the absence of methemoglobinemia or hemolytic anemia has been reported and may be due to direct tubular injury (59). Phenazopyridine hydrochloride may crystallize and increase the size of urinary calculi (60). Hepatic injury occurs rarely in humans and may be either from direct injury or by a hypersensitivity reaction (61). Phenazopyridine also results in red blood cell abnormalities and methemoglobinemia when given to cats (62).

Pregnancy and Lactation

Phenazopyridine is FDA pregnancy category B (Appendix I). Entry into breast milk is unknown.

Clinical Presentation

ACUTE OVERDOSAGE

Life-threatening effects can occur (63). Phenazopyridine can cause hemolytic anemia in patients. Methemoglobinemia after phenazopyridine use or overdose may be protracted and require multiple doses of methylene blue (58).

ADVERSE EVENTS

Acute renal failure may occur during therapeutic use (59). Aseptic meningitis, confirmed by rechallenge, has also been reported (64). When given to patients with a preexisting urinary tract calculus, it may serve as a nidus for deposition of phenazopyridine crystals, thus causing a rapid enlargement of the calculus (60). Yellow skin and nail discoloration may occur (65). Chronic, surreptitious use of phenazopyridine has been reported, and it may be a cause of a chronic anemia (66).

Diagnostic Tests

Phenazopyridine concentrations are not clinically useful. After overdose, the patient should be observed for the development of hemolysis or methemoglobinemia. A baseline CBC should be obtained and followed as clinically indicated.

Phenazopyridine may be determined by column chromatography, spectrophotometry, and high-performance liquid chromatography (67). Phenazopyridine may interfere with the visual interpretation of protein, nitrite, and leukocyte esterase test strips (68).

Treatment

Treatment is largely symptomatic and supportive. The drug should be withdrawn for adverse events. Interruption of absorption by gastric emptying or activated charcoal should be used for large ingestions presenting within 1 to 2 hours after exposure. Methemoglobinemia is treated with methylene blue (Chapter 63). In overdose, multiple doses of methylene blue may be required (58). Hemolytic anemia may require red blood cell transfusion and severe methemoglobinemia or sulfhemoglobinemia may require exchange transfusions (63).

TRIMETHOPRIM

Trimethoprim [Polytrim, 2,4=diamino-5-(3,4,5-trimethoxybenzyl) pyrimidine $C_{14}H_{18}N_4O_3$; MW, 290.3 g/mol; SI conversion, mg/L × 3.44 = μmol/L; CAS Registry No., 738-70] is a dihydrofolate reductase inhibitor. Trimethoprim is used alone and in combination with sulfamethoxazole [trimethoprim-sulfamethoxazole (TMP-SMX)] for synergistic action as an antibacterial agent. The commercial product contains a 5:1 ratio of sulfamethoxazole to trimethoprim.

Toxic Dose

The *adult therapeutic dose* is 100 mg orally every 12 hours. TMP-SMX is administered in doses of two tablets every 12 hours (equivalent to trimethoprim, 160 mg every 12 hours). The *pediatric dose* is 6 mg/kg/day in two divided doses.

Trimethoprim has been ingested in an overdose of 8000 mg. The patient survived (69). Twenty tablets of TMP-SMX was accidentally administered at one time. The patient was hospitalized and discharged in 2 days. There have been no fatalities from trimethoprim alone or in combination products.

Toxicokinetics and Toxicodynamics

Trimethoprim is readily and almost completely absorbed from the GI tract (70). The peak serum concentration is approximately 1 μg/ml, and the peak serum level is 1 to 4 hours after an oral dose. Trimethoprim is 40% to 70% bound to plasma proteins. Steady-state serum concentrations of 1.2 to 3.2 μg/ml follow trimethoprim, 160 mg every 12 hours.

Oral TMP-SMX is rapidly and well absorbed. A single dose of trimethoprim, 160 mg, and sulfamethoxazole, 800 mg, produces a peak serum concentration of 1 to 2 μg/ml trimethoprim and 36 to 40 μg/ml sulfamethoxazole in 1 to 4 hours. Sulfamethoxazole is 66% bound to plasma proteins.

The apparent V_d for trimethoprim is approximately 1.4 L/kg, and the apparent V_d of sulfamethoxazole is 0.14 L/kg (70a). Ten percent to 30% of trimethoprim is metabolized in the liver to oxide and hydroxylated metabolites. Sulfamethoxazole is also metabolized in the liver, where it is acetylated and conjugated with glucuronic acid. Approximately 40% to 60% of trimethoprim and 20% of sulfamethoxazole are excreted as unchanged drug. The elimination half-life of trimethoprim is 8 to 11 hours, 10 to 13 hours for sulfamethoxazole. The total clearance of trimethoprim is 0.12 L/hour/kg (71,72).

Pathophysiology

Trimethoprim is a dihydrofolate reductase inhibitor and thus impairs folate-dependent processes, including DNA synthesis (73,74). Trimethoprim also induces interleukin-6 production in peripheral white blood cells in trimethoprim-sensitive individuals and is likely the trigger for the observed clinical reactions such as aseptic meningitis (75). Trimethoprim exerts a potassium-sparing effect approximately tenfold less than amiloride or triamterene (76). Trimethoprim also augments urinary uric acid excretion and thus reduces serum uric acid levels.

Pregnancy and Lactation

Trimethoprim and sulfamethoxazole are FDA pregnancy category C (Appendix I). Both cross the placenta and are found in breast milk (69,71).

Clinical Presentation

ACUTE OVERDOSAGE

Trimethoprim poisoning causes nausea, vomiting, headache, swollen face, epigastric pain, and weakness (69). TMP-SMX may produce nausea, vomiting, diarrhea, confusion, facial swelling, headache, bone marrow depression, and a slight increase in levels of serum transaminases (77).

ADVERSE EVENTS

Hyponatremia (115 mmol/L) (78), hyperkalemia, and hypouricemia (79) have been reported during therapeutic dosing. Aseptic meningitis and a systemic inflammatory response syndrome, characterized by headache, fever, chills, and general malaise are well-recognized adverse events (75,80). High-dose trimethoprim treatment may cause hyperkalemia, hyponatremia, renal salt wasting, prerenal azotemia, and metabolic acidosis (76,81). Hypersensitivity reactions to trimethoprim, including anaphylaxis, have been reported (82).

Deaths after TMP-SMX ingestion have been due to drug-induced hemolytic anemia and toxic epidermal necrolysis (83,84). Trimethoprim alone or with sulfamethoxazole can cause renal insufficiency and renal failure (85).

DRUG INTERACTIONS

Trimethoprim inhibits CYP2C8 activity. Drugs metabolized by this enzyme may exhibit higher blood concentrations and effects (e.g., phenytoin, tolbutamide, and warfarin) (86–89). It also decreases the renal clearance of procainamide (90). TMP-SMX should be used with caution with methotrexate, as sulfonamides can displace methotrexate from plasma protein-binding sites.

Diagnostic Tests

Trimethoprim may be quantitated in the serum by a high-performance liquid chromatographic method; the limit of detection is 0.2 μg/ml (90a). Simultaneous measurement of trimethoprim and sulfamethoxazole is available with the use of high-performance liquid chromatography with sensitivity limits of 0.02 and 0.20 μg/ml, respectively (91).

Serum levels are not clinically useful. The serum trimethoprim concentration after ingestion of 8000 mg was 19.6 μg/ml. This is approximately 20 times more than that observed after a single dose of 200 mg (69).

Hemolytic anemia may occur. Serum transaminase levels may be elevated after overdose with trimethoprim. After overdose or in symptomatic patients, baseline CBC and renal and liver function tests should be obtained and followed as clinically indicated. Hematologic evaluation may include a bone marrow study according to clinical judgment.

Postmortem Considerations

A suicide patient after trimethoprim overdose had a blood level of 133 μg/ml postmortem (92). It is unclear what dose of trimethoprim was ingested.

Treatment

Treatment is usually symptomatic and supportive. For toxicity during therapeutic dosing, discontinuation of the medication has resulted in correction of electrolyte disturbances (81). Acidification of the urine may enhance the elimination of trimethoprim but is generally not recommended. Hemodialysis may remove only moderate amounts of trimethoprim in view of its protein binding and large V_d (72). There is no specific antidote. Folinic acid (leucovorin) has not been studied. Seizures can be treated with diazepam (Chapter 40).

Monitoring

Electrolytes should be determined and replaced together with adequate fluid replacement. Patients should be followed for any evidence of hematologic depression, both in hospital and as outpatients in the following weeks. If patients are asymptomatic and able to eat without difficulty, they can be discharged to be followed as outpatients.

REFERENCES

1. Schweitzer VG. Cisplatin-induced ototoxicity: the effect of pigmentation and inhibitory agents. *Laryngoscope* 1993;103:1–52.
2. Hayashi M, Numaguchi M, Watabe H, et al. Cisplatin-induced nephrotoxicity and the protective effect of fosfomycin on it as demonstrated by using a crossover study of urinary metabolite levels. *Acta Obstet Gynecol Scand* 1997;76:590–595.
3. Jordan JA, Schwade ND, Truelson JM. Fosfomycin does not inhibit the tumoricidal efficacy of cisplatinum. *Laryngoscope* 1999;109:1259–1262.
4. Bergan T, Thorsteinsson SB, Albini E. Pharmacokinetic profile of fosfomycin trometamol. *Chemotherapy* 1993;39:297–301.
5. Bergan T. Degree of absorption, pharmacokinetics of fosfomycin trometamol and duration of urinary antibacterial activity. *Infection* 1990;18[Suppl 2]:65–69.
6. Wilson P, Williams JD, Folandi E. Comparative pharmacokinetics of fosfomycin tormetamol, sodium fosfomycin and calcium fosfomycin in humans. In: Neu H, Williams JD, eds. *New trends in urinary tract infections*. Basel, Switzerland: Karger, 1988:136–142.
7. Reeves DS. Fosfomycin trometamol. *J Antimicrob Chemother* 1994;34:853–858.
8. Bergan T, Mastropaolo G, Di Mario F. Pharmacokinetics of fosfomycin and influence of cimetidine and metoclopramide on the bioavailability of fosfomycin trometamol. In: Neu HC, Williams JD, eds. *New trends in urinary tract infections*. Basel, Switzerland: Karger, 1988:157–166.
9. Bergan T. Pharmacokinetics of fosfomycin. *Rev Contemp Pharmacother* 1995;6:55–62.
10. Monurol. Package insert. New York: Forest Laboratories Inc., 1996.
11. Janknegt R, Hooymans PM, Fabius GT, et al. Urinary concentrations of fosfomycin after a single 3g dose of fosfomycin to elderly nursing-home patients. *Pharm World Sci* 1994;16:149–153.
12. Bergan T. Pharmacokinetic comparison between fosfomycin and other phosphonic acid derivatives. *Chemotherapy* 1990;36[Suppl 1]:10–18.
13. Ragni N, Pivetta C, Paccagnella F, et al. Urinary tract infections in pregnancy. In: Neu HC, Williams JD, eds. *New trends in urinary tract infections*. Basel, Switzerland: Karger, 1988:197–206.
14. Reeves DS. Clinical efficacy and safety of fosfomycin trometamol in the prevention and treatment of urinary tract infections. *Rev Contemp Phamacother* 1995;6:71–83.
15. Ferreres L, Paz M, Martin G, Governado M. New studies on placental transfer of fosfomycin. *Chemotherapy* 1977;23[Suppl 1]:175–179.
16. De-Jong Z, Pontonnier F, Plante P. Single-dose fosfomycin trometamol (Monuril) versus multiple-dose norfloxacine: results of a multicenter study in females with uncomplicated lower urinary tract infections. *Urol Int* 1991;46:344–348.
17. Jardin A. A general practitioner multicenter study: fosfomycin trometamol single dose versus pipemidic acid multiple dose. *Infection* 1990;18[Suppl 2]:89–93.
18. Naber KG. Fosfomycin trometamol in treatment of uncomplicated lower urinary tract infections in adult women—an overview. *Infection* 1992;20:S310–S311.
19. Fujii R. Fosfomycin in the treatment of bacterial infections: summary of clinical trials in Japan. *Chemotherapy* 1977;23[Suppl 1]:234–246.
20. Mayama T, Yokota M, Shimatani I, Ohyagi H. Analysis of oral fosfomycin calcium (Fosmicin) side-effects after marketing. *Int J Clin Pharmacol Ther Toxicol* 1993;31:77–82.
21. Durupt S, Josserand RN, Sibille M, Durieu I. Acute, recurrent fosfomycin-induced liver toxicity in an adult patient with cystic fibrosis. *Scand J Infect Dis* 2001;33:391–392.
22. Patel SS, Balfour JA, Bryson HM. Fosfomycin tromethamine: a review of its antibacterial activity, pharmacokinetic properties and therapeutic efficacy as a single-dose oral treatment for acute uncomplicated lower urinary tract infections. *Drugs* 1997;53:637–656.
23. Musher DM, Griffith DP. Generation of formaldehyde from methenamine: effect of pH and concentration, and antibacterial effect. *Antimicrob Agents Chemother* 1974;6:708–711.
24. Brumfitt W, Hamilton-Miller JM, Gargan RA, et al. Long-term prophylaxis of urinary infections in women: comparative trial of trimethoprim, methenamine hippurate and topical povidone-iodine. *J Urol* 1983;130:1110–1114.
25. Hiprex, methenamine hippurate. Product information. Cincinnati: Merrell-National Laboratories, 1994.
26. Mandelamine, methenamine mandelate. Product information. Morris Plains, NJ: Parke-Davis, 1996.
27. Chafetz L, Gaglia CA. Assay of methenamine mandelate and its pharmaceutical dosage forms by direct cerimetric titration. *J Pharm Sci* 1966;55:854–856.

28. Hebel SK, Kastrup EK, eds. *Drug facts and comparisons*. St. Louis: Facts and Comparisons, 2002.
29. Selvaag E, Thune P. Photosensitivity reaction to methenamine hippurate. A case report. *Photodermatol Photoimmunol Photomed* 1994;10:259–260.
30. Ross RR, Conway GF. Hemorrhagic cystitis following accidental overdose of methenamine mandelate. *Am J Dis Child* 1970;119:86–87.
31. Gleckman R, Alvarez S, Joubert DW, et al. Drug therapy review: methenamine mandelate and methenamine hippurate. *Am J Hosp Pharm* 1979;36:1509–1512.
32. Shah RR, Wade G. Reappraisal of the risk/benefit of nitrofurantoin: review of toxicity and efficacy. *Adverse Drug React Acute Poisoning Rev* 1989;8:183–201.
33. Mannisto PT, Lamminsiu V. Nitrofurantoin is highly bound to plasma protein. *J Antimicrob Chemother* 1982;9:327–328.
34. Cunha BA. Nitorfurantoin: current concepts. *Urology* 1988;32:67–71.
35. Adam A, Smith LL, Cohen GM. An assessment of the role of redox cycling in mediating the toxicity of paraquat and nitrofurantoin. *Environ Health Perspect* 1990;85:113–117.
36. Hoener B, Noach A, Andrup M, Yen TS. Nitrofurantoin produces oxidative stress and loss of glutathione and protein thiols in the isolated perfused rat liver. *Pharmacology* 1989;38:363–373.
37. Martin WJ. Nitrofurantoin: evidence for the oxidant injury of lung parenchymal cells. *Am Rev Respir Dis* 1983;127:482–486.
38. Sheehan RE, Wells AU, Milne DG, Hansell DM. Nitrofurantoin-induced lung disease: two cases demonstrating resolution of apparently irreversible CT abnormalities. *J Comput Assist Tomogr* 2000;24:259–261.
39. Kelly BD, Heneghan MA, Bennani F, et al. Nitrofurantoin-induced hepatotoxicity mediated by CD8+ T cells. *Am J Gastroenterol* 1998;93:819–821.
40. Schattner A, Von der Walde J, Kozak N, Sokolovskaya N. Nitrofurantoin-induced immune-mediated lung and liver disease. *Am J Med Sci* 1999;317:336–340.
41. Wasserman BN, Chronister TE, Stark BI, Saran BR. Ocular myasthenia and nitrofurantoin. *Am J Ophthalmol* 2000;130:531–533.
42. Gerk PM, Kuhn RJ, Desai NS, McNamara PJ. Active transport of nitrofurantoin into human milk. *Pharmacotherapy* 2001;21:669–675.
43. Hailey FJ, Glascock HWJ, Hewitt WF. Pleuropneumonic reactions to nitrofurantoin. *N Engl J Med* 1969;281:1087–1090.
44. Chudnofsky DR, Otten EJ. Acute pulmonary toxicity to nitrofurantoin. *J Emerg Med* 1989;7:15–19.
45. D'Arcy PF. Nitrofurantoin. *Drug Intell Clin Pharm* 1985;19:540–547.
46. Cameron RJ, Kolbe J, Wilsher ML, Lambie N. Bronchiolitis obliterans organising pneumonia associated with the use of nitrofurantoin. *Thorax* 2000;55:249–251.
47. Fawcett IW, Ibrahim NB. BOOP associated with nitrofurantoin. *Thorax* 2001;56:161.
48. Kahn SR. Acute interstitial nephritis associated with nitrofurantoin. *Lancet* 1996;348:1177–1178.
49. Bialas MC, Shetty HGM, Houghton J, et al. Nitrofurantoin rechallenge and recurrent toxicity. *Postgrad Med J* 1997;73:519–520.
50. Spring PJ, Sharpe DM, Hayes MW. Nitrofurantoin and peripheral neuropathy: a forgotten problem? *Med J Aust* 2001;174:153–154.
51. Greenberg MS, Wong H. Methemoglobinemia and Heinz body hemolytic anemia due to phenazopyridine hydrochloride. *N Engl J Med* 1964;271:431–435.
52. Galun E, Oren R, Glikson M, et al. Phenazopyridine-induced hemolytic anemia in G-6-PD deficiency. *Drug Intell Clin Pharm* 1987;21:921–922.
53. Jeffery WH, Zelicoff AP, Hardy WR. Acquired methemoglobinemia and hemolytic anemia after usual doses of phenazopyridine. *Drug Intell Clin Pharm* 1982;16:157–159.
54. Munday R, Fowke EA. Generation of superoxide radical and hydrogen peroxide by 2,3,6-triaminopyridine, a metabolite of the urinary tract analgesic, phenazopyridine. *Free Radic Res* 1994;21:67–73.
55. Halvorsen SM, Dull WL. Phenazopyridine-induced sulfhemoglobinemia: inadvertent rechallenge. *Am J Med* 1991;91:315–317.
56. Landman J, Kavaler E, Waterhouse RL. Acquired methemoglobinemia possibly related to phenazopyridine in a woman with normal renal function. *J Urol* 1997;158:1520–1521.
57. Nathan DM, Siegel AJ, Bunn HF. Acute methemoglobinemia and hemolytic anemia with phenazopyridine: possible relation to acute renal failure. *Arch Intern Med* 1977;137:1636–1638.
58. Christensen CM, Farrar HC, Kearns GL. Protracted methemoglobinemia after phenazopyridine overdose in an infant. *J Clin Pharmacol* 1996;36:112–116.
59. Rule KA, Biggs AW. Transient renal failure following phenazopyridine overdose. *Urology* 1984;24:178–179.
60. Crawford ED, Mulvaney WP. Rapid increase in calculous size: a possible hazard of phenazopyridine hydrochloride therapy in the presence of already formed stones. *J Urol* 1978;119:280–281.
61. Badley BW. Phenazopyridine-induced hepatitis. *BMJ* 1976;2:850.
62. Harvey JW, Kornick HP. Phenazopyridine toxicosis in the cat. *J Am Vet Med Assoc* 1976;169:327–331.
63. Truman TL, Dallessio JJ, Weibley RE. Life-threatening Pyridium plus intoxication: a case report. *Pediatr Emerg Care* 1995;11:103–106.
64. Herlihy TE. Phenazopyridine and aseptic meningitis. *Ann Intern Med* 1987;106:172–173.
65. Amit G, Halkin A. Lemon-yellow nails and long-term phenazopyridine use. *Ann Intern Med* 1997;127:1137.
66. Thomas RJ, Doddabele S, Karnad AB. Chronic severe hemolytic anemia related to surreptitious phenazopyridine abuse. *Ann Intern Med* 1994;121:308.
67. Du Preez JL, Botha SA, Lotter AP. High-performance liquid chromatographic determination of phenazopyridine hydrochloride, tetracycline hydrochloride and sulphamethizole in combination. *J Chromatogr* 1985;333:249–252.
68. Kerr JE, Magee-Nolan C, Schuster BL. Interference by phenazopyridine with the leukocyte esterase dipstick. *JAMA* 1986;256:38–39.
69. Hoppu K, Partanen S, Koskela E. Trimethoprim poisoning. *Lancet* 1980;1:778.
70. Cockerill FR III, Edson RS. Trimethoprim sulfamethoxazole. *Mayo Clin Proc* 1987;62:921–929.
70a. McEvoy GK, ed. *AHFS drug information 91*. Bethesda, MD: American Hospital Formulary Service, 1991:461–464, 468–474.
71. Hutabarat RM, Unadkat JP, Sahajwalla C, et al. Disposition of drugs in cystic fibrosis. 1. Sulfamethoxazole and trimethoprim. *Clin Pharmacol Ther* 1991;49:402–409.
72. Wathen GG, Winnehy RJ. High dose co-trimoxazole for patients receiving hemodialysis. *BMJ* 1987;295:333.
73. Abou-Eisha A, Creus A, Marcos R. Genotoxic evaluation of the antimicrobial drug, trimethoprim, in cultured human lymphocytes. *Mutat Res* 1999;440:157–162.
74. Steinberg SE, Campbell CL, Rabinovitch PS, Hillman RS. The effect of trimethoprim-sulfamethoxazole on friend erytholeukemia cells. *Blood* 1980;55:501–504.
75. Antonen J, Saha H, Hulkkonen J, et al. Increased in vitro production of interleukin 6 in response to trimethoprim among persons with trimethoprim induced systemic adverse reactions. *J Rheumatol* 1999;26:2585–2590.
76. Gabriels G, Stockem E, Greven J. Potassium-sparing renal effects of trimethoprim and structural analogues. *Nephron* 2000;86:70–78.
77. Goff O. Renal failure induced by co-trimoxazole. *Hosp Ther* 1989;14:61–67.
78. Dreiher J, Porath A. Severe hyponatremia induced by theophylline and trimethoprim. *Arch Intern Med* 2001;161:291–292.
79. Don BR. The effect of trimethoprim on potassium and uric acid metabolism in normal human subjects. *Clin Nephrol* 2001;55:45–52.
80. Redman RC, Miller JB, Hood M, De Maio J. Trimethoprim-induced aseptic meningitis in an adolescent male. *Pediatrics* 2002;110:e26.
81. Kaufman AM, Hellman G, Abramson RG. Renal salt wasting and metabolic acidosis with trimethoprim-sulfamethoxazole therapy. *Mt Sinai J Med* 1983;50:238–239.
82. Alfaya T, Pulido Z, Gonzalez-Mancebo E, et al. Anaphylaxis to trimethoprim. *Allergy* 1999;54:766–767.
83. Taraszewski R, Harvey R, Rosman P. Death from drug induced hemolytic anemia. *Postgrad Med* 1989;85:79–81.
84. Carmichael AJ, Tan CY. Fatal toxic epidermal necrolysis associated with co-trimoxazole. *Lancet* 1989;2:808–809.
85. Smith GW, Cohen SB. Hyperkalemia and non-oliguric renal failure associated with trimethoprim. *BMJ* 1994;308:454.
86. Hansen JM, Kampmann JP, Siersbaek-Nielsen K, et al. The effect of different sulfonamides on phenytoin metabolism in man. *Acta Med Scand Suppl* 1979;624:106–110.
87. Wing LM, Miners JO. Cotrimoxazole as an inhibitor of oxidative drug metabolism: effects of trimethoprim and sulphamethoxazole separately and combined on tolbutamide disposition. *Br J Clin Pharmacol* 1985;20:482–485.
88. O'Reilly RA. Stereoselective interaction of trimethoprim-sulfamethoxazole with the separated enantiomorphs of racemic warfarin in man. *N Engl J Med* 1980;302:33–35.
89. Wen X, Wang J-S, Backman JT, et al. Trimethoprim and sulfamethoxazole are selective inhibitors of CYP2C8 and CYP2C9, respectively. *Drug Metab Dispos* 2002;30:631–635.
90. Kosoglou T, Rocci ML, Blasses PH. Trimethoprim alters the disposition of procainamide and N-acetylprocainamide. *Clin Pharmacol Ther* 1988;44:467–477.
90a. Metherall R. High performance liquid chromatographic determination of trimethoprim in serum. *Ther Drug Monit* 1989;11:79–83.
91. De Angelis DV, Woolley JL, Sigel CW. High performance liquid chromatographic assay for the simultaneous measurement of trimethoprim and sulfamethoxazole in plasma or urine. *Ther Drug Monit* 1990;12:382–392.
92. Dawling S, Widdop B. A fatal case involving trimethoprim. *Bull Int Assoc Forensic Toxicol* 1986;19:34–35.

CHAPTER 97

Miscellaneous Antiinfective Agents

Steven A. Seifert

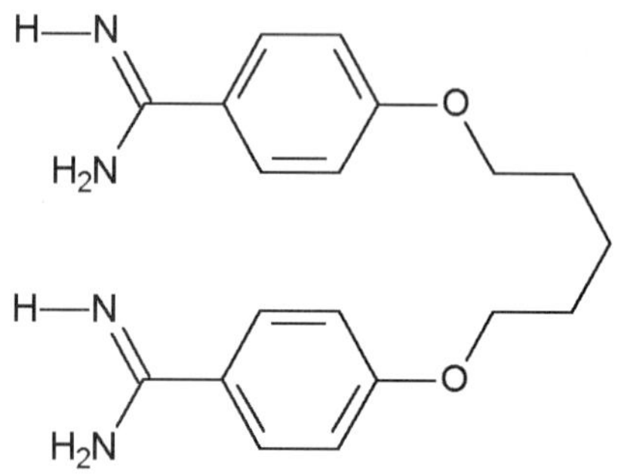

PENTAMIDINE

Compounds included:	**Clofazimine (Lamprene); co-trimoxazole (many others); furazolidone (Furoxone); linezolid (Zyvox); metronidazole (Flagyl); pentamidine isethionate (Pentam); trimetrexate (Neutrexin)**
Molecular formula and weight:	**See text.**
SI conversion:	**Clofazimine, mg/L × 2.1 = μmol/L; co-trimoxazole, mg/L × 1.8 = μmol/L; furazolidone, mg/L × 4.4 = μmol/L; linezolid, mg/L × 3.0 = μmol/L; metronidazole, mg/L × 5.8 = μmol/L; pentamidine, mg/L × 1.7 = μmol/L; trimetrexate, mg/L × 1.8 = μmol/L**
CAS Registry No.:	**See text.**
Target organs:	**Gastrointestinal tract (acute and chronic), heart (acute), skin (chronic), cornea (chronic), hematologic (chronic), kidney (chronic), liver (chronic), endocrine (chronic), central nervous system (chronic)**
Antidotes:	**Magnesium, glucose, vasopressors**

OVERVIEW

The drugs in this section are used to treat a variety of bacterial and other infections. They are a mixed group, with different structures, modes of action, effectiveness against particular pathogens, and toxicities. Management of toxicity is generally symptomatic and supportive, with recognition of the causative nature of symptoms and signs and cessation of the responsible agent.

CLOFAZIMINE

Clofazimine [Lamprene; $C_{27}H_{22}Cl_2N_4$; molecular weight (MW), 473.4 g/mol; CAS Registry No., 2030-63-9] is an antileprosy agent with antimycobacterial and antiinflammatory activity. It is also used to treat mycobacterium avian complex and pyoderma gangrenosum.

Toxic Dose

The usual *adult therapeutic dose* for treating leprosy is 100 to 200 mg/day with meals and usually in combination with other antileprosy agents (1). Dose adjustments should be considered in patients with severe hepatic insufficiency. Acute overdose experience is limited.

Toxicokinetics and Toxicodynamics

The oral bioavailability is 45% to 70% (1,2). Absorption is increased when taken with food (3). It is highly lipophilic and deposits primarily in fatty tissue (1). Clofazimine is primarily metabolized in the liver (4) and has a half-life of elimination of the parent compound of 70 days (1,5). A significant amount is also excreted in the feces with an average of 11% to 59% of a single dose over 3 days (5).

Pregnancy and Lactation

Clofazimine is U.S. Food and Drug Administration (FDA) pregnancy category C (Appendix I). Three neonatal deaths occurred in 15 pregnancies during which clofazimine was being taken (6).

Clofazimine produces a red tint to breast milk (1,6,7). The ratio of milk to plasma drug concentration ranges from 1.0:1.7, corresponding to an infant dose of 22.1% of the maternal dose (8).

Clinical Presentation

ADVERSE EVENTS

The most common complaints are gastrointestinal (GI), including abdominal pain, nausea, vomiting, and diarrhea in as many as 40% to 50% of patients and usually of mild severity. Constipation, eosinophilic enteritis, and bowel obstruction occur infrequently but may be fatal (1,9). Hepatitis is reported, with elevated transaminases and bilirubin (1).

Skin pigmentation, varying from pink to red/brownish-black, occurs in 75% to 100% of patients, appears to be dose-dependent, and usually occurs within a few weeks of initiation of therapy. Deposition of clofazimine crystals in tissues and a drug-induced ceroid lipofuscinosis (caused by the accumulation of a ceroid lipofuscin within lipid-laden macrophages) are responsible for the discoloration (10,11). Reversibility of pigmentary changes occurs slowly after discontinuation of the drug and may take months to years (1). Depression secondary to skin pigmentary changes may be severe. Other dermatologic conditions include ichthyosis and pruritus, phototoxicity, and other rashes, including exfoliative dermatitis (1,12).

Hyperglycemia may be seen, and reddish discoloration of secretions is reported (1). Conjunctival and corneal pigmentation have occurred and are secondary to deposition of clofazimine crystals (1). Corneal changes have been partially or completely reversible with discontinuation of clofazimine (13). Bull's eye maculopathy and generalized retinal degeneration in a patient with acquired immunodeficiency syndrome (AIDS) have been reported (14). There have been reports of leukopenia during therapeutic dosing, although a cause and effect relationship was not established (15). Also reported are anemia, eosinophilia, elevated erythrocyte sedimentation rates, and thromboembolism (1). Metabolic acidosis, which resolved after discontinuation of the drug, was reported in four patients with AIDS who were treated with clofazimine for at least 6 weeks (16).

DRUG INTERACTIONS

Concurrent use of clofazimine and phenytoin or fosphenytoin may result in reduced serum concentrations and reduced efficacy of phenytoin (17).

Diagnostic Tests

Plasma concentrations of clofazimine are not clinically relevant. In symptomatic patients, it is prudent to monitor the complete blood cell count (CBC) and renal and liver function. Patients with significant vomiting or diarrhea should have their fluid and electrolyte status followed.

Clofazimine can be detected by a variety of techniques, with limits of detection of high-performance liquid chromatography (HPLC) at 10 μg/L and of thin-layer chromatography at 5 μg/L (3).

Treatment

Management of toxic effects is primarily symptomatic and supportive. Toxicity during therapeutic dosing generally responds to this and withdrawal of the medication. The decision regarding medication withdrawal must be made with regard to the need for the antimicrobial effects of the drug as well as available alternative agents.

In acute overdose, the decision regarding interruption of absorption by gastric lavage or activated charcoal must be made on an individual basis and may often be made with regard to possible coingestants. Because of the high lipophilicity and tissue deposition, hemodialysis and hemoperfusion are unlikely to be of benefit. There is no specific antidote to clofazimine.

CO-TRIMOXAZOLE

Co-trimoxazole (MW, 543.60 g/mol; CAS Registry No., 8064-90-2) is a compound drug that is a mixture of five parts sulfamethoxazole and one part trimethoprim. The adverse effects are those of its components (Chapter 88) and include serious adverse effects during therapeutic dosing.

Toxic Dose

The *adult therapeutic dosage* of co-trimoxazole is 160 mg/800 mg twice daily for 5 to 14 days. Dosages up to 10 to 20 mg/kg/day (of the trimethoprim component) for 14 to 21 days are used in the treatment of *Pneumocystis carinii* pneumonia (PCP), for which the drug may be given intravenously (IV). Co-trimoxazole is contraindicated when the creatinine clearance is less than 15 ml/minute (18).

The usual *pediatric dose* of co-trimoxazole in children is: 6 weeks to 5 months of age, 60 mg twice daily; up to 240 mg twice daily for ages 6 to 12 years. Co-trimoxazole is generally not used in infants younger than 6 weeks of age because of the risk of kernicterus, although it has been used in infants from 4 weeks of age for the treatment or prophylaxis of PCP.

For patients with a documented hypersensitivity reaction and for whom treatment is imperative, there are graded desensitization protocols available (19,20).

Toxicokinetics and Toxicodynamics

Absorption after ingestion is 90% to 100%. Protein binding of trimethoprim is 40% to 60% and of sulfamethoxazole is 60% to 70%. The volume of distribution (V_d) for sulfamethoxazole and trimethoprim is 360 ml/kg and 2 L/kg, respectively. They cross the blood–brain barrier and achieve therapeutic concentrations in the cerebrospinal fluid (CSF). At therapeutic dosing, the half-life of sulfamethoxazole is 8 to 11 hours and 6 to 17 hours for trimethoprim. The drugs are extensively metabolized in the liver. The half-lives of both drugs are prolonged in renal failure (20 to 30 hours or more) and may be prolonged in overdose.

Plasma concentrations of trimethoprim to sulfamethoxazole may vary from 1:2:1:3 or more. The ratio is usually lower in tissues (1:2:1:5) because trimethoprim is more lipophilic and penetrates better than sulfamethoxazole. In urine, the ratio varies from 1:1:1:5 and is pH dependent.

Pregnancy and Lactation

Trimethoprim is FDA pregnancy category C (Appendix I) (21). Sulfamethoxazole is FDA pregnancy category C (see Appendix I) (21). There is a report of two cases of severe spinal malformations in the fetuses of women treated with combination antiretroviral therapy and co-trimoxazole (22).

Both trimethoprim and sulfamethoxazole are excreted into breast milk but in low concentrations. Except in premature infants or infants with hyperbilirubinemia or glucose 6 phosphate dehydrogenase deficiency, breast-feeding is not contraindicated (23).

Clinical Presentation

ADVERSE EVENTS

Adverse events include hypersensitivity reactions, blood dyscrasias, a variety of skin rashes, diarrhea, pancreatitis, nephrotoxicity, urolithiasis, and hepatotoxicity.

Deaths associated with the use of co-trimoxazole are primarily related to blood dyscrasias and skin reactions. Serious skin reactions include toxic epidermal necrosis and Stevens-Johnson syndrome. Blood effects include agranulocytosis, aplastic anemia, hemolytic or megaloblastic anemia, hypoprothrombinemia, leukopenia, methemoglobinemia, neutropenia, pancytopenia, and thrombocytopenia (18,24). The overall incidence of serious blood and skin reactions is 5.6 and 2.8/100,000 population, respectively (25).

There is a marked increase of serious adverse events with increasing age. In patients younger than 40 years of age, there were 0.25 reported deaths per million prescriptions. In a 1985 study, the incidence was more than 15-fold higher for patients older than 65 years of age (26). A follow-up study in 1995 found a similar pattern of serious adverse reactions, with most fatalities caused by blood dyscrasias and generalized skin disorders, occurring mainly in the elderly (27).

Patients with AIDS, and perhaps others with compromised immune systems, appear to be at increased risk of adverse reactions during therapeutic dosing. Rashes and leukopenia develop in 30%, compared with less than 5% for each complication in patients without AIDS (28). A syndrome of fever, malaise, nausea, and headache is commonly reported. The overall incidence of adverse effects may be greater than 80% in such patients (29–31).

DRUG INTERACTIONS

Sulfamethoxazole displaces bilirubin and sulfonylureas from their protein-binding sites (1,32), potentially resulting in kernicterus when given to premature infants and inducing hypoglycemic reactions in patients on sulfonylureas.

Sulfamethoxazole impairs hepatic metabolism of warfarins, increasing their therapeutic effect (33). Trimethoprim causes decreased renal tubular secretion of digoxin and may increase digoxin serum concentrations by 30% to 50% (34).

Concurrent use of angiotensin converting–enzyme inhibitors and trimethoprim has resulted in severe hyperkalemia, presumably from the combined effects of potassium secretion inhibition and aldosterone reduction (35,36).

Trimethoprim may result in decreased phenytoin clearance and possibly phenytoin toxicity (37,38). Similarly, decreased renal clearance of procainamide and its metabolite *N*-acetylprocainamide may also result in increased procainamide toxicity (39,40).

Concurrent administration of co-trimoxazole with a number of antiretroviral drugs (zidovudine, lamivudine) may cause increased serum levels and increased adverse effects of these medications (41). Trimethoprim causes inhibition of dihydrofolate reductase, and sulfamethoxazole may displace methotrexate from plasma proteins and decrease its renal clearance (42,43). Combination of trimethoprim with other agents that are folic acid antagonists (e.g., pyrimethamine) may result in increased hematologic toxicity.

Disulfiram-like reactions may occur when IV co-trimoxazole is combined with metronidazole (secondary to the 10% ethanol base of the co-trimoxazole) (44) and when co-trimoxazole is combined with ethanol and was presumably due to inhibition of aldehyde dehydrogenase (45).

Diagnostic Tests

Co-trimoxazole may cause a reduction in serum-thyroxine and triiodothyronine concentrations, although it does not produce clinical hypothyroidism (46,47). Co-trimoxazole may interfere with the laboratory determination of methotrexate, theophylline, and serum creatinine, depending on the methodology used (48). Hematologic evaluation may include a bone marrow study according to clinical judgment.

Treatment

For most patients with co-trimoxazole overdose, treatment is symptomatic and supportive. For toxicity during therapeutic dosing, discontinuation of the medication has resulted in correction of electrolyte disturbances (49). Patients should be hospitalized if cardiac monitoring, IV fluids, or oxygen is required. Seizures can be treated with diazepam (see Chapter 40). Electrolytes should be determined and replaced together with adequate fluid replacement. Patients should be followed for any evidence of hematologic depression both in hospital and as outpatients in the following weeks. If patients are asymptomatic and able to eat without difficulty, they can be discharged to be followed as outpatients.

ANTIDOTES

There is no specific antidote. Folinic acid (Leucovorin) has not been studied.

ENHANCEMENT OF ELIMINATION

Acidification of the urine may enhance the elimination of trimethoprim but is generally not recommended. Approximately 50% of the dose of trimethoprim and sulfamethoxazole is removed with a 4-hour hemodialysis session (18,50).

FURAZOLIDONE

Furazolidone (Furoxone; $C_8H_7N_3O_5$; MW, 225.2 g/mol; CAS Registry No., 67-45-8) is an antiinfective agent primarily used in the treatment of giardiasis and other bacterial GI infections. Toxicity during therapeutic use is primarily GI, with important adverse effects related to monoamine oxidase (MAO) inhibition, hemolytic anemia in glucose 6 phosphate dehydrogenase deficiency states, and disulfiram-like reactions. Furazolidone is available as a 100-mg tablet and a 50 mg/15 ml liquid (51).

Toxic Dose

The *adult therapeutic dosage* for giardiasis is 100 mg four times a day for 7 to 10 days (51). The *pediatric dosage* is based on weight: 1.25 to 2.00 mg/kg/dose four times a day. Use in infants younger than 1 month of age is not recommended (51).

No specific toxic dose has been identified. The maximum recommended oral dose for children is 8.8 mg/kg/day (51).

Toxicokinetics and Toxicodynamics

Furazolidone is well-absorbed orally (52,53). It is extensively metabolized in the intestine (54). Renal excretion is variable. Between 5% and 65% is excreted in the urine as parent drug and metabolites (53).

Pathophysiology

The main toxic effects of furazolidone are GI; a cumulative, irreversible MAO inhibition secondary to metabolites; and aldehyde dehydrogenase blockade, potentially producing a disulfiram-like reaction.

Pregnancy and Lactation

Furazolidone is FDA pregnancy category C (Appendix I). Furazolidone crosses into breast milk. Because of the risk of hemolytic anemia, breast-feeding is not recommended for infants younger than 1 month of age (53).

Clinical Presentation

ADVERSE EVENTS

One study (55) evaluated 10,433 patients on furazolidone therapy. During therapeutic dosing, nausea, vomiting, abdominal pain, and diarrhea occur in approximately 8% of patients (55).

Hemolytic anemia may also be induced in children younger than 1 month of age and in patients with glucose 6 phosphate dehydrogenase deficiency (53). Other hematologic effects include agranulocytosis, anemia, eosinophilia, leukopenia, leukocytosis, and purpura. Hematologic effects occur in approximately 0.36% of patients (55).

Neurologic events occur in approximately 1.34% of patients and include headache and vertigo (51,55). Other effects were reported regarding neurologic, hepatic, respiratory, dermatologic, endocrine (hypoglycemia), and immunologic (hypersensitivity reactions) systems (51,55).

DRUG INTERACTIONS

Because of its MAO inhibitor (MAOI) effect, MAOI drugs, tyramine-containing foods, and directly acting sympathomimetic amines (i.e., phenylephrine, ephedrine, amphetamine) should generally be avoided (51). No such reactions have been reported. An adverse reaction, consisting of an acute, toxic psychosis, occurred in a patient concurrently receiving amitriptyline (56).

In addition to the MAO inhibition, furazolidone may also alter catecholamine uptake and metabolism, resulting in potential drug-drug interactions with tricyclic antidepressants, sympathomimetics, selective serotonin reuptake inhibitors, meperidine, and other drugs and foods.

Diagnostic Tests

Measurement of furazolidone levels is not clinically useful. Concentrations in the serum may be determined by ultraviolet spectrometry, HPLC with ultraviolet spectrometry, or high-performance thin-layer chromatography with spectrometric determination (57–60).

In overdose or toxicity during therapeutic dosing, CBC, electrolytes, and renal and hepatic function tests should be obtained. Monitor pulse oximetry or arterial blood gas, chest radiograph, and pulmonary function tests in patients with pulmonary symptoms.

A false-positive result for urinary glucose may occur with cupric sulfate reagent tests (e.g., Clinitest) (54). Furazolidone use may discolor the urine a rust-yellow to brown color (53,61).

Treatment

Treatment is generally symptomatic and supportive. If adverse reactions occur (disulfiram-like reaction, hemolytic anemia, MAOI interactions), furazolidone therapy should be discontinued and specific monitoring and specific management of these conditions commenced. In acute overdose, the decision regarding interruption of absorption by gastric lavage or activated charcoal must be made on an individual basis and may often be made with regard to possible coingestants.

ENHANCEMENT OF ELIMINATION

There have been no studies regarding enhanced elimination of furazolidone.

ANTIDOTES

There is no specific antidote to furazolidone.

SUPPORTIVE CARE

Patients with diffuse pulmonary infiltrates and pulmonary eosinophilia may respond to corticosteroid therapy.

LINEZOLID

Linezolid (Zyvox, Zyvoxam; $C_{16}H_{20}FN_3O_4$; MW, 337.3 g/mol; CAS Registry No., 165800-03-3) is an oxazolidinone antibiotic with activity against antibiotic-resistant gram-positive cocci. It is commonly used in the treatment of vancomycin-resistant enterococcal infections, nosocomial or community-acquired pneumonia, and skin infections. Human overdose information is limited. The adverse effects that may commonly occur after therapeutic administration include nausea, diarrhea, headache, tongue discoloration, rash, and thrombocytopenia. Elevated liver transaminases are reported infrequently.

Toxic Dose

The *adult therapeutic dosage* is 600 mg IV or orally every 12 hours for 10 to 28 days, depending on the indication (62). No dosage adjustment is needed in patients with renal or mild to moderate hepatic insufficiency (62).

Studies of safety and efficacy in children have not been performed. The half-life of linezolid is shorter in children, which may affect efficacy (62). There are case reports of use in patients of at least 28 days of age with multiresistant gram-positive infections (63).

Toxicokinetics and Toxicodynamics

The bioavailability approaches 100% orally, with a time-to-peak plasma concentration (T_{max}) of 2 hours (62). Protein binding is 31% (62,64). The V_d in adults is 40 to 60 L (62,64,65) and 0.66 L/kg in children (66). It distributes into the CSF (67), the pleural space (68), and pancreatic fluid (69). Linezolid is metabolized 50% to 75% in the liver (70), with saturable metabolism at higher doses (65). Linezolid is not metabolized by, nor is it an inducer of, P-450 liver enzymes (62). Approximately 30% of the dose is excreted unchanged by the kidneys, and renal excretion of parent and metabolites constitutes 80% to 85% of dose (62,70,71); 7% to 12% is excreted in the feces (70). The elimination half-life is approximately 5 hours in adults (62,64) and 2.7 hours in children (3 months to 16 years of age) (66).

Pathophysiology

Reversible myelosuppression, similar to that seen with chloramphenicol, is reported. Linezolid exhibits weak, reversible MAOI activity (72), potentiates the hypertensive effect of sympathomimetics, and may induce a serotonin syndrome when combined with selective serotonin reuptake inhibitors.

Pregnancy and Lactation

Linezolid is FDA pregnancy category C (Appendix I) (62). Excretion in breast milk is unknown.

Clinical Presentation

Reversible myelosuppression, including anemia, neutropenia, and thrombocytopenia, during therapeutic dosing is reported. Reversal has occurred after discontinuation (68,73,74).

Other adverse reactions reported include headache (up to 11.3%), GI complaints (up to 18%), rare rashes and hepatic transaminase elevations (62), and vaginal yeast superinfections (up to 36%) (75). Linezolid potentiates the hypertensive response to pseudoephedrine and phenylpropanolamine (76) and may rarely precipitate a serotonin syndrome when concomitantly administered to patients on selective serotonin reuptake inhibitors (77) and a MAOI reaction when combined with meperidine (78).

Diagnostic Tests

In overdose or toxicity during therapeutic dosing, CBC, electrolytes, and renal and hepatic function tests should be obtained. Measurement of linezolid serum concentrations are not clinically useful. Linezolid and its metabolites are detectable by HPLC (71).

Treatment

Treatment is generally symptomatic and supportive. If adverse reactions occur (myelosuppression, severe headache, clinically significant GI disturbances, or drug-drug/drug-food interactions), linezolid therapy should be discontinued and specific monitoring and specific management of these conditions commenced.

GASTROINTESTINAL DECONTAMINATION

In acute overdose, the decision regarding interruption of absorption by gastric lavage or activated charcoal must be made on an individual basis and may often be made with regard to possible coingestants.

ENHANCED ELIMINATION

There is no information on enhanced elimination. Linezolid and its major metabolites are removable by hemodialysis (62).

ANTIDOTES

There is no specific antidote to linezolid.

METRONIDAZOLE

Metronidazole (Flagyl; $C_6H_9N_3O_3$; MW, 171.2 g/mol; CAS Registry No., 443-48-1) is used to treat anaerobic bacterial infections, bacterial vaginosis, giardia, *Helicobacter pylori*, pseudomembranous colitis, amebic liver abscesses, and other infections. Metronidazole has orphan drug status in the treatment of rosacea and perioral dermatitis.

Toxic Dose

The *adult therapeutic dosage* varies by indication from 15 mg/kg IV followed by 7.5 mg/kg IV or by mouth every 6 hours for 7 to 10 days to 750 mg three times a day for 5 to 10 days. Higher doses and treatment courses for up to several weeks are used for more serious infections. For vaginal trichomoniasis, a single 2-g oral dose is usually given. Extemporaneous preparations may not have equal concentrations throughout the liquid unless shaken well and are generally stable for 30 days if refrigerated. A maximum dose of 4 g per 24 hours IV should not be exceeded (79,80). Because patients with severe hepatic disease metabolize metronidazole more slowly, lower doses should be given (79–81).

The *pediatric dose* also varies by indication, ranging from 35 to 50 mg/kg/day to 80 mg/kg/day. IV, oral, and topical routes have been used in children.

Acute ingestion up to 15 g has been tolerated with minimal effects.

Toxicokinetics and Toxicodynamics

The T_{max} of metronidazole is 1 to 2 hours after an oral dose (79,82), with a bioavailability of 100% (83). With vaginal use, systemic bioavailability is 19% (82). Total protein binding is less than 20% (79). The V_d is 0.25 to 0.85 L/kg (84). The elimination half-life is 6 to 14 hours (79,84) and 34 hours in patients with total renal failure (85). The drug is metabolized in the liver to an active metabolite. Approximately 20% of a dose is excreted unchanged in the urine. Metronidazole and its active metabolites are dialyzable (84).

Pregnancy and Lactation

Metronidazole is FDA pregnancy category B (Appendix I) (79). Metronidazole crosses the placenta and can be detected in the fetal circulation (86). It is contraindicated in the first trimester (79). Metronidazole is excreted in breast milk in concentrations close to those in serum (87,88).

Clinical Presentation

ACUTE OVERDOSAGE

After acute overdose, severe toxicity is uncommon. Acute ingestion up to 15 g has been tolerated with minimal effects. There is a report of green/black discoloration of the urine in a 15-year-old girl after an overdose.

ADVERSE EVENTS

Adverse effects include leukopenia, seizures, and peripheral neuropathy. These effects are usually seen during prolonged use. Pseudomembranous colitis has been reported. A disulfiram-like reaction with ethanol is well described (89) and may also occur after intravaginal use (90). Hypersensitivity reactions may occur (91,92). Metronidazole has demonstrated cross-sensitivity with tinidazole (93).

DRUG INTERACTIONS

Metronidazole inhibits aldehyde dehydrogenase, resulting in a disulfiram-like reaction when combined with ethanol. Metronidazole is a substrate and inhibitor of CYP3A4 hepatic enzymes and may affect the metabolism of other drugs metabolized by this pathway. Metronidazole inhibits warfarin metabolism, resulting in an enhanced anticoagulant effect (79). Metronidazole inhibits the metabolism of carbamazepine, resulting in significantly increased carbamazepine concentrations (94). Drugs that induce hepatic enzymes, such as phenytoin, may result in increased metabolism and lower serum concentrations of metronidazole, but there is no apparent way to predict which drugs will be influenced by metronidazole administration (95). Increased serum lithium levels have been reported with the concurrent use of metronidazole and lithium (79,96).

Diagnostic Tests

Metronidazole and its metabolites are detectable by HPLC (97).

Treatment

Treatment of acute overdose is generally symptomatic and supportive. If adverse reactions occur during therapeutic use, (neuropathy, drug-drug interactions, disulfiram-like reaction), metronidazole therapy should be discontinued and specific monitoring and specific management of these conditions commenced.

GASTROINTESTINAL DECONTAMINATION

In acute overdose, the decision regarding interruption of absorption by gastric lavage or activated charcoal must be made on an individual basis and may often be made with regard to possible coingestants.

ENHANCED ELIMINATION

Metronidazole and metabolites are rapidly removed by dialysis, and no dosing adjustment is required in patients undergoing dialysis (79,80,98).

ANTIDOTES

There is no specific antidote for metronidazole.

PENTAMIDINE

Pentamidine isethionate (Pentam, NebuPent, Pneumopent; $C_{19}H_{24}N_4O_2.2C_2H_6O_4S$; MW, 592.7 g/mol; CAS Registry No.,

140-64-7) is an antiprotozoal agent used in the treatment of PCP, leishmaniasis, and trypanosomiasis.

Toxic Dose

The *adult* and *pediatric therapeutic dosage* of pentamidine is 2 to 4 mg/kg/day intramuscularly or IV for 12 to 14 days (99,100). Aerosolized pentamidine, 300 mg every 4 weeks, is used for the prevention of PCP (101). Renal clearance is only 2.1%, and no dosage adjustment is necessary in renal impairment or during dialysis (102,103).

Toxicokinetics and Toxicodynamics

Pentamidine is poorly absorbed from the GI tract. The T_{max} is reached within 60 minutes (104). The V_d is 821 L IV and 2725 L intramuscularly (104). Tissue binding is extensive, resulting in detectable levels in plasma for 6 to 8 weeks postdosing (105). The elimination half-life is 6.4 to 9.0 hours (104).

Pathophysiology

The mechanism by which pentamidine causes dysrhythmias has not been clearly established, but the similarity of its structure to procainamide may contribute to its prodysrhythmic effects (106).

Pregnancy and Lactation

Pentamidine is FDA pregnancy category C (Appendix I) (99).

Clinical Presentation

Overdose experience is limited.

ADVERSE EVENTS

Fatalities have resulted from severe hypotension, hypoglycemia, and ventricular dysrhythmias after treatment with pentamidine.

Cardiac effects with pentamidine therapy include hypotension, torsade de pointes, other dysrhythmias, and cardiac arrest. Hypotension occurs in approximately 5% of patients receiving intramuscular or IV pentamidine (99,107,108). In one study, 10 of 32 patients had QT interval prolongation (109). Torsade de pointes and other dysrhythmias may recur repeatedly for up to 2 weeks after discontinuing therapy (106). Ventricular fibrillation secondary to pentamidine-induced nephrotoxicity with hyperkalemia was reported in a 28-year-old man with AIDS (110). Other cardiovascular effects that have been reported with an incidence of less than 1% include cerebrovascular accidents, hypertension, palpitations, phlebitis, syncope, vasculitis, and vasodilation (99,101).

Neurologic effects are common. Dizziness is reported in up to 47% of patients receiving nebulized pentamidine. Headache is less common but reported in up to 5% of patients during inhalation therapy. Other effects include ataxia, confusion, insomnia, neuropathies and neuralgias, seizures, and vertigo (99,101). In addition, anxiety, depression, hallucinoses, and paranoid ideation are reported (99,101).

Hematologic effects during therapeutic dosing include anemia, leukopenia, and thrombocytopenia (99,111). During aerosol treatments, adverse hematologic effects occur with an incidence of approximately 1% (101). Megaloblastic anemia is rarely reported, and decreased serum folic acid levels have been reported (112,113), although coadministration of folic acid with pentamidine therapy is not recommended (114,115).

Nephrotoxicity during therapy is common, occurring in 25% of patients treated with parenteral drug (99,116). Elevated serum creatinine may progress to acute renal failure.

Hepatic toxicity may also occur during therapy. Abnormal transaminases may occur in up to 10% of patients receiving parenteral drug (99,117).

GI effects include decreased appetite and a metallic taste in up to 72% of patients (99). Nausea, vomiting, diarrhea, and abdominal pain occur, and there are individual reports of gingival effects, gastric ulcer, alterations of salivation, GI bleeding, esophagitis, pancreatitis, and colitis (99).

Metabolic disturbances are seen with therapeutic pentamidine use, including hypoglycemia, hyperglycemia, hypocalcemia, hypomagnesemia, and hyperkalemia. Hypoglycemia is common, occurring in up to 40% of patients receiving intramuscular or IV therapy and is believed to be secondary to inappropriate insulin secretion (111). Inhalational therapy rarely causes this effect (118). Risk factors for development of hypoglycemia include prolonged duration of therapy, previous pentamidine exposure, and azotemia during treatment. (119). Hyperglycemia is also reported, often in association with the development of pancreatitis, diabetes mellitus (111,120), and ketoacidosis (118). Hypocalcemia, hypomagnesemia, or hypokalemia occurs rarely and is believed to result from pentamidine-induced renal injury (111).

Other effects seen during therapeutic use include ocular (conjunctivitis and blurred vision), respiratory (cough and bronchospasm), and dermatologic (pruritus, desquamation, urticaria, and Stevens-Johnson syndrome) effects. Stevens-Johnson syndrome is reported in 0.2% of patients receiving pentamidine parenterally (99). Cellulitis and local tissue injury with necrosis secondary to extravasation at the infusion site are reported (99). Fatal hypersensitivity reactions have also occurred.

DRUG INTERACTIONS

Combination of pentamidine with nephrotoxic drugs, such as cidofovir and foscarnet, results in increased incidence of renal toxicity (121). Combination of pentamidine with other drugs known to increase the QT interval, such as the fluoroquinolones, resulted in increased QT intervals and the risk of torsade de pointes, and pentamidine should be used cautiously in this setting (122,123).

Diagnostic Tests

Symptomatic patients should have a CBC, serum glucose and electrolytes and renal and liver function determined and followed. Measurement of pentamidine levels is not clinically useful. A 12 lead electrocardiogram should be obtained before administration and periodically assessed for QT interval prolongation. Low serum magnesium and calcium should be corrected if abnormal. In acute overdose, the QT interval should be monitored until normalizing.

Treatment

Overdose experience is limited. Management focuses on the detection of adverse events such as QT prolongation. Treatment is symptomatic and supportive. Type I hypersensitivity reactions should be treated in the usual manner (see Chapter 34).

GASTROINTESTINAL DECONTAMINATION

The risks of attempts to interrupt absorption must be weighed against potential benefits, and such decisions may be driven by considerations of timing and coingestants.

ENHANCED ELIMINATION

Because of extensive tissue binding, hemodialysis is unlikely to result in significantly enhanced elimination. A 17-month-old child developed severe hypotension after a 40-fold overdose. Blood pressure stabilized during a standard 4-hour course of hemoperfusion (124).

ANTIDOTES

Torsade de pointes should be managed with IV magnesium, isoproterenol (2 to 10 μg/minute), antidysrhythmics not known to cause QT interval prolongation (with the possible exception of amiodarone), and overdrive pacing, if necessary. Avoid class Ia (quinidine, disopyramide, procainamide) and most class III antidysrhythmic agents (e.g., sotalol).

Significant hypoglycemia may require parenteral glucose. Oral diazoxide (100 mg q6h for 3 days) was found to be effective in treating ongoing, pentamidine-induced hypoglycemia (125).

SUPPORTIVE CARE

Because of the risk of hypotension, patients should be supine when the drug is administered parenterally and blood pressure closely monitored. Correction of hypotension should be accomplished by proper positioning, fluid expansion, and pressors as needed (see Chapter 37). Patients with significant toxicity should have their serum glucose, electrolytes, CBC, and liver and renal functions followed. Low serum potassium, calcium, or magnesium may contribute to prolonged QT intervals (126).

MONITORING

Serial electrocardiography should be undertaken before pentamidine therapy as well as continuous cardiac monitoring after significant overdose or with evidence of toxicity during therapeutic dosing. Patients with complications related to QT interval prolongation or a QTc interval greater than 500 milliseconds should be monitored closely until the QT interval normalizes. Resolution of the QT interval may take up to 7 days after discontinuation of therapy (127).

TRIMETREXATE

Trimetrexate glucuronate (Neutrexin; $C_{19}H_{23}N_5O_3,C_6H_{10}O_7$; MW, 563.6 g/mol; CAS Registry No., 82952-64-5) is a dihydrofolate reductase inhibitor similar to methotrexate. Trimetrexate, with concurrent folinic acid administration, is used as an alternate therapy for PCP in immunocompromised patients. Trimetrexate is also being investigated as an antineoplastic agent. The major dose-limiting toxicity of trimetrexate is myelosuppression. Nonhematologic adverse effects include hepatic and renal toxicity, stomatitis, nausea and vomiting, diarrhea, and rash. Myelosuppression associated with trimetrexate, stomatitis, and GI toxicity can usually be ameliorated with concurrent folinic acid administration.

Toxic Dose

The *adult therapeutic dosage* for PCP is 45 mg/m^2 once a day IV over 60 to 90 minutes for 21 days with concurrent folinic acid for 24 days. Folinic acid should be administered for 72 hours after the last dose of trimetrexate. The dose may require adjustment in patients with renal insufficiency. The pediatric dose has not been established, but trimetrexate was used in two children (9 months and 15 months of age) without serious or unexpected adverse effects at the same body surface area dose as adults (128).

Toxicokinetics and Toxicodynamics

Oral absorption is rapid, with a bioavailability of 44% (range, 19% to 67%) and a T_{max} of 2 hours (129). The V_d is 0.62 L/kg in adults (130) and 0.46 L/kg in children (131). Trimetrexate is cleared renally, with 10% to 30% of the drug excreted unchanged in the urine (128,132). Trimetrexate also undergoes extensive hepatic metabolism (133), and up to 8% is excreted in the feces (130). At therapeutic concentrations, protein binding is extensive (95% to 98%) (133). At higher concentrations, a greater percentage of unbound drug is present (128). The elimination half-life is 15 to 17 hours (130) but decreases to 7 to 15 hours when coadministered with folinic acid (128).

Pathophysiology

Trimetrexate is a dihydrofolate reductase inhibitor similar to methotrexate. This limits the cell production of tetrahydrofolate, which in turn limits the conversion of deoxyuridylate to thymidylate, the limiting nucleotide in the synthesis of DNA.

Pregnancy and Lactation

Trimetrexate is FDA pregnancy category D (Appendix I) (128).

Clinical Presentation

ACUTE OVERDOSAGE

Overdose experience is limited, but significant exacerbation of adverse effects seen during therapeutic dosing can be expected.

ADVERSE EVENTS

Toxicity with therapeutic dosing often occurs during the first treatment cycle (134). The primary toxicity of trimetrexate is myelosuppression with granulocytopenia and thrombocytopenia (135,136). Nausea and vomiting are reported in up to 31% of patients (135) and diarrhea in 22% (137). A diarrhea-related fatality has been reported (134). Stomatitis is also common, occurring in 24% of patients (135). Reversible elevations in serum creatinine (130,133), liver transaminases, and bilirubin (130) are reported. Hypoalbuminemia and hypoproteinemia are at increased risk of experiencing severe toxic effects (138). Generalized erythematous skin rashes and postinflammatory hyperpigmentation are reported (139). Because trimetrexate inhibits histamine metabolism, anaphylactoid (non–immunoglobulin E–mediated) hypersensitivity reactions may occur when the drug is given as a bolus (128).

DRUG INTERACTIONS

Trimetrexate concentrations and adverse effects may increase when it is coadministered with drugs that inhibit CYP3A4 P-450 enzymes (cimetidine, clotrimazole, erythromycin, fluconazole, itraconazole, ketoconazole, and miconazole) (128). Drugs that induce CYP3A4 (rifabutin and rifampin) may cause increased hepatic metabolism, lower plasma concentrations, and decreased trimetrexate efficacy (128). Concurrent administration of trimetrexate and zidovudine should be avoided because of additive myelosuppressive effects (140). Because cell-mediated immunity may be compromised during therapeutic dosing, live virus immunizations should be avoided (141).

Diagnostic Tests

Measurement of trimetrexate levels is not routinely performed.

Treatment

Acute overdose experience is limited. After acute overdose, because of the potential for serious toxicity, interruption of absorption by lavage or the administration of activated charcoal should be considered. Such measures are most effective if initiated within 1 hour of ingestion (Chapter 7).

ENHANCEMENT OF ELIMINATION

Because of the high degree of protein binding, hemodialysis is generally ineffective in removing trimetrexate at therapeutic concentrations. In patients with renal failure, however, high flux hemodialysis has been shown to remove significant amounts of methotrexate (142). Hemodialysis may also be useful in overdose, in which there is a greater free fraction of the drug. Charcoal hemoperfusion alone and in sequence with hemodialysis has been used to increase removal of methotrexate (143–146). Hemofiltration has also been shown to effectively remove methotrexate when excessive concentrations were present (147–149).

ANTIDOTES

Folinic acid is a specific antidote for trimetrexate. It supplies the cofactor for tetrahydrofolate, the synthesis of which is blocked by trimetrexate. Because folic acid must be converted to folinic acid by dihydrofolate reductase, which is blocked by trimetrexate, folic acid is not an effective antidote. Folinic acid is most effective if given within the first hour and may not provide antidotal efficacy if given beyond 4 hours postoverdose. The optimal dose has not been determined. In overdose or with signs of toxicity, it is generally recommended that doses of folinic acid equal to or greater than the ingested dose of trimetrexate be given. Lower doses are used during therapy in an attempt to protect normal body cells from injury. A high-dose loperamide regimen has been used for control of severe diarrhea (134).

With methotrexate, precipitation in the kidney can be prevented by alkalinization of the urine. It is not known whether this is the case with trimetrexate, but maintenance of adequate urine flow and possibly alkalinization of the urine should be considered in significant overdose.

Thymidine rescues cells from the cytotoxic effects of methotrexate. It is unknown whether this provides protection from the effects of trimetrexate. In methotrexate toxicity, it is dosed as 8 g/m^2/day as a continuous IV infusion for a minimum of 48 hours. In addition, carboxypeptidase has been used to increase the metabolism of methotrexate. The dose for methotrexate toxicity is 50 U/kg IV over 5 minutes. It is given every 4 hours for three doses. It is unknown whether carboxypeptidase is of benefit with trimetrexate toxicity.

INTRATHECAL ADMINISTRATION

Although trimetrexate is not normally given intrathecally, methotrexate is, and accidental intrathecal trimetrexate may be given inadvertently. When excessive doses of methotrexate are injected intrathecally, drainage of 20 ml of CSF can remove 95% of the injected dose if performed within 15 minutes of the exposure. Ventriculolumbar perfusion (150) and CSF exchange (151) have also been used in this setting. Steroids are commonly given to prevent arachnoiditis. Intrathecal leucovorin is not recommended because it can cause severe neurotoxicity (152).

SUPPORTIVE CARE

Trimetrexate treatment should be stopped if liver transaminases increase by more than five times the upper limit of normal, if serum creatinine is greater than 2.5 mg/dl, for mucosal toxicity interfering with intake or if uncontrolled fever greater than 105°F (128).

REFERENCES

1. Lamprene, clofazimine. Product information. East Hanover, NJ: Novartis Pharmaceuticals Corporation, 1999.
2. Vischer WA. The experimental properties of G 30 320 (B 663)—a new antileprotic agent. *Lepr Rev* 1969;40:107–110.
3. Holdiness MR. Clinical pharmacokinetics of clofazimine. A review. *Clin Pharmacokinet* 1989;16:74–85.
4. Feng PC, Fenselau CC, Jacobson RR. Metabolism of clofazimine in leprosy patients. *Drug Metab Disp* 1981;9:521–524.
5. Levy L. Pharmacologic studies of clofazimine. *Am J Trop Med* 1974;23:1097–1109.
6. Farb H, West DP, Pedvis-Leftick A. Clofazimine in pregnancy complicated by leprosy. *Obstet Gynecol* 1982;59:122–123.
7. Freerksen E, Seydel JK. Critical comments on the treatment of leprosy and other mycobacterial infections with clofazimine. *Arzneimittelforschung* 1992;42:1243–1245.
8. Venkatesan K, Mathur A, Girdhar A, Girdhar BK. Excretion of clofazimine in human milk in leprosy patients. *Lepr Rev* 1997;68:242–246.
9. Venencie PY, Cortez A, Orieux G, et al. Clofazimine enteropathy. *J Am Acad Dermatol* 1986;15:290–291.
10. Job CK, Yoder L, Jacobson RR, Hastings RC. Skin pigmentation from clofazimine therapy in leprosy patients: a reappraisal. *J Am Acad Dermatol* 1990;23:236–241.
11. Fitzpatrick JE. New histopathologic findings in drug eruptions. *Dermatol Clin* 1992;10:19–36.
12. Pavithran K. Exfoliative dermatitis after clofazimine [Letter]. *Int J Lepr* 1985;53:645–646.
13. Ohman L, Wahlberg L. Ocular side-effects of clofazimine. *Lancet* 1975;2:933–934.
14. Cunningham CA, Friedberg DN, Carr RE. Clofazamine-induced generalized retinal degeneration. *Retina* 1990;10:131–134.
15. Karat AB, Jeevaratnam A, Karat S, et al. Double-blind controlled clinical trial of clofazimine in reactive phases of lepromatous leprosy. *BMJ* 1970;1:198–200.
16. Soriano V, Moreno V, Alba A, et al. Kussmaul respiration and abdominal pain secondary to metabolic acidosis in AIDS patients with disseminated *Mycobacterium avium* complex infection receiving clofazimine. *AIDS* 1993;7:894–895.
17. Cone LA, Woodard DR, Simmons JC, et al. Drug interactions in patients with AIDS [Letter]. *Clin Infect Dis* 1992;15:1066–1068.
18. Septra, trimethoprim and sulfamethoxazole. Product information. Research Triangle Park, NC: Burroughs Wellcome, 2000.
19. Demoly P, Messaad D, Sahla H, et al. Six-hour trimethoprim-sulfamethoxazole-graded challenge in HIV-infected patients. *J Allergy Clin Immunol* 1998;102:1033–1036.
20. Caumes E, Guermonprez G, Lecomte C, et al. Efficacy and safety of desensitization with sulfamethoxazole and trimethoprim in 48 previously hypersensitive patients infected with human immunodeficiency virus. *Arch Dermatol* 1997;133:465–469.
21. Hebel SK, ed. *Drug facts and comparisons*. St. Louis: Wolters Kluwer, 2002.
22. Richardson MP, Osrin D, Donaghy S, et al. Spinal malformations in the fetuses of HIV infected women receiving combination antiretroviral therapy and co-trimoxazole. *Eur J Obstet Gynecol Reprod Biol* 2000;93:215–217.
23. Briggs GG, Freeman RK, Yaffe SJ. *Drugs in pregnancy and lactation: a reference guide to fetal and neonatal risk*, 4th ed. Baltimore: Williams & Wilkins, 1994.
24. Tapp H, Savarirayan R. Megaloblastic anaemia and pancytopenia secondary to prophylactic cotrimoxazole therapy. *J Paediatr Child Health* 1997;33:166–167.
25. Myers MW, Jick H. Hospitalization for serious blood and skin disorders following co-trimoxazole. *Br J Clin Pharmacol* 1997;43:649–651.
26. Committee on Safety of Medicines. Deaths associated with co-trimoxazole, ampicillin and trimethoprim. *Curr Probl* 1985;15.
27. Committee on Safety of Medicines. Revised indications for co-trimoxazole (Septrin, Bactrim, various generic preparations). *Curr Probl* 1995;21:6.
28. Masur H. Treatment of infections and immune defects. In: Fauci AS, moderator. Acquired immunodeficiency syndrome: epidemiologic, clinical, immunologic, and therapeutic considerations. *Ann Intern Med* 1984;100:92–106.
29. Gordin FM, Simon GL, Wofsy CB, Mills J. Adverse reactions to trimethoprim-sulfamethoxazole in patients with the acquired immunodeficiency syndrome. *Ann Intern Med* 1984;100:495–499.
30. Jaffe HS, Abrams DI, Ammann AJ, et al. Complications of co-trimoxazole in treatment of AIDS-associated Pneumocystis carinii pneumonia in homosexual men. *Lancet* 1983;2:1109–1111.
31. Mitsuyasu R, Groopman J, Volberding P. Cutaneous reaction to trimethoprim-sulfamethoxazole in patients with AIDS and Kaposi's sarcoma. *N Engl J Med* 1983;308:1535–1536.
32. Diabinese, chlorpropamide. Product information. New York: Pfizer Inc., 1995.
33. Kaufman JM, Fauver HE Jr. Potentiation of warfarin by trimethoprim-sulfamethoxazole. *Urology* 1980;16:601–603.
34. Petersen P, Kastrup J, Bartram R, et al. Digoxin-trimethoprim interaction. *Acta Med Scand* 1985;217:423–427.
35. Thomas RJ. Severe hyperkalemia with trimethoprim-quinapril. *Ann Pharmacother* 1996;30:413–414.
36. Bugge JF. Severe hyperkalaemia induced by trimethoprim in combination with an angiotensin-converting enzyme inhibitor in a patient with transplanted lungs. *J Intern Med* 1996;240:249–251.
37. Gillman MA, Sandyk R. Phenytoin toxicity and co-trimoxazole [Letter]. *Ann Intern Med* 1985;102:559.

38. Hansen JM, Kampmann JP, Siersbaek-Nielsen K, et al. The effect of different sulfonamides on phenytoin metabolism in man. *Acta Med Scand Suppl* 1979;624:106–110.
39. Vlasses PH, Kosoglou T, Chase SL, et al. Trimethoprim inhibition of the renal clearance of procainamide and N-acetylprocainamide. *Arch Intern Med* 1989;149:1350–1353.
40. Kosoglou T, Rocci ML Jr, Vlasses PH. Trimethoprim alters the disposition of procainamide and N-acetylprocainamide. *Clin Pharmacol Ther* 1988;44:467–477.
41. Trizivir, abacavir sulfate, lamivudine, and zidovudine. Product information. Research Triangle Park, NC: GlaxoSmithKline, 2002.
42. Ferrazzini G, Klein J, Sulh H, et al. Interaction between trimethoprim-sulfamethoxazole and methotrexate in children with leukemia. *J Pediatr* 1990;117:823–826.
43. Methotrexate sodium. Product information. Philadelphia: ESI Lederle Inc., 1999.
44. Edwards DL, Fink PC, Van Dyke PO. Disulfiram-like reaction associated with intravenous trimethoprim-sulfamethoxazole and metronidazole. *Clin Pharm* 1986;5:999–1000.
45. Heelon MW, White M. Disulfiram-cotrimoxazole reaction. *Pharmacotherapy* 1998;18:869–870.
46. Cohen HN, Beastall GH, Ratcliffe WA, et al. Effects on human thyroid function of sulphonamide and trimethoprim combination drugs. *BMJ* 1980;281:646–647.
47. Cohen HN, Pearson DW, Thomson JA, et al. Trimethoprim and thyroid function. *Lancet* 1981;1:676–677.
48. Gantanol, sulfamethoxazole. Product information. Nutley, NJ: Roche Laboratories Inc., 1998.
49. Kaufman AM, Hellman G, Abramson RG. Renal salt wasting and metabolic acidosis with trimethoprim-sulfamethoxazole therapy. *Mt Sinai J Med* 1983;50:238–239.
50. Nissenson AR, Wilson C, Holazo A. Pharmacokinetics of intravenous trimethoprim-sulfamethoxazole during hemodialysis. *Am J Nephrol* 1987;7:270–274.
51. Furazolidone, Furoxone. Product information. Norwich, NY: Norwich Eaton Pharmaceuticals, 1996.
52. White AH. Absorption, distribution, metabolism, and excretion of furazolidone. A review of the literature. *Scand J Gastroenterol Suppl* 1989;169:4–10.
53. USPDI. Drug information for the health care professional (Internet version). Greenwood Village, CO: Micromedex, 2001.
54. AHFS. American Hospital Formulary Service Drug Information 88. American Society of Hospital Pharmacists. Bethesda, MD: 1988:452–453.
55. Altamirano A, Bondani A. Adverse reactions to furazolidone and other drugs. A comparative review. *Scand J Gastroenterol* 1989;24[Suppl 169]:70–80.
56. Aderhold RM, Muniz CE. Acute psychosis with amitriptyline and furazolidone. *JAMA* 1970;213:2080.
57. Elsayed L, Hassan SM, Kelani KM, et al. Simultaneous spectrophotometric determination of nifuroxime and furazolidone in pharmaceutical preparations. *J Assoc Off Anal Chem* 1980;63:992–995.
58. Smallidge RL, Rowe NW, Wadgaonkar ND, et al. High performance liquid chromatographic determination of furazolidone in feed and feed premixes. *J Assoc Off Anal Chem* 1981;64:1100–1104.
59. Cieri UR. Quantitative thin layer chromatographic determination of furazolidone and nitrofurazone in animal feeds. *J Assoc Off Anal Chem* 1978;61:92–95.
60. Rauter H. Determination of furazolidone in feeds with high-performance thin-layer chromatography (Ger). *Landwirtsch Forsch* 1979;32:232–236.
61. Knoben JE, Anderson PO, eds. *Handbook of clinical drug data*, 6th ed. Hamilton, IL: Drug Intelligence Publications, Inc., 1988.
62. Zyvox, linezolid. Product information. Kalamazoo, MI: Pharmacia & Upjohn Co, 2001.
63. Birmingham MC, Zimmer GS, Hafkin B, et al. Initial results of linezolid in patients with multi drug resistant gram positive infections. Presented at the 38th Interscience Conference on Antimicrobial Agents and Chemotherapy, Sept. 24–27, 1998; San Diego.
64. Pawsey SD, Daley-Yates PT, Wajszczuk CP, et al. U-100766 safety, toleration and pharmacokinetics after oral and intravenous administration. First European Congress of Chemotherapy: May 14, 1996; F151. Presented at the 38th Interscience Conference on Antimicrobial Agents and Chemotherapy, Sept. 24–27, 1996; San Diego (abst).
65. Turnak MR, Forrest A, Hyatt JM, et al. Multiple-dose pharmacokinetics of linezolid-200, 400, and 600 mg PO Q12 h. Presented at the 38th Interscience Conference on Antimicrobial Agents and Chemotherapy, Sept. 24–27, 1998; San Diego.
66. Kearns GL, Abdel-Rahman SM, Blumer JL, et al. Single dose pharmacokinetics of linezolid in infants and children. *Pediatr Infect Dis J* 2000;19:1178–1184.
67. Shaikh ZHA, Peloquin CA, Ericsson CD. Successful treatment of vancomycin-resistant *Enterococcus faecium* meningitis with linezolid: case report and literature review. *Scand J Infect Dis* 2001;33:375–379.
68. Kaplan SL, Patterson L, Edwards KM, et al. Linezolid for the treatment of community-acquired pneumonia in hospitalized children. *Pediatr Infect Dis J* 2001;20:488–494.
69. Rao GG, Steger A, Tobin CM. Linezolid levels in pancreatic secretions. *J Antimicrob Chemother* 2001;48:931–932.
70. Feenstra KL, Slatter JG, Stalker DJ, et al. Metabolism and excretion of the oxazolidinone antibiotic linezolid (PNU-100766) following oral administration of (C)PNU-100766 to healthy volunteers. Presented at the 38th Interscience Conference on Antimicrobial Agents and Chemotherapy, Sept. 24–27, 1998; San Diego.
71. Slatter JG, Stalker DJ, Feenstra KL, et al. Pharmacokinetics, metabolism, and excretion of linezolid following an oral dose of [(14)C]linezolid to healthy human subjects. *Drug Metab Dispos* 2001;29:1136–1145.
72. Norrby R. Linezolid—a review of the first oxazolidinone. *Expert Opin Pharmacother* 2001;2:293–302.
73. Green SL, Maddox JC, Huttenbach ED. Linezolid and reversible myelosuppression. *JAMA* 2001;285:1291.
74. Waldrep TW, Skiest DJ. Linezolid-induced anemia and thrombocytopenia. *Pharmacotherapy* 2002;22:109–112.
75. Turnak MR, Forrest A, Hyatt JM, et al. Multiple-dose pharmacokinetics of linezolid-200, 400, and 600 mg PO Q12h. Presented at the 38th Interscience Conference on Antimicrobial Agents and Chemotherapy. September 24–27, 1998; San Diego, CA.
76. Hendershot PE, Antal EJ, Welshman IR, et al. Linezolid: pharmacokinetic and pharmacodynamic evaluation of coadministration with pseudoephedrine HCl, phenylpropanolamine HCl, and dextromethorphan HBr. *J Clin Pharmacol* 2001;41:563–572.
77. Wigan CL, Goetz MB. Serotonin syndrome and linezolid. *CID* 2002;34:1651–1652.
78. Hammerness P, Parada H, Abrams A. Linezolid: MAOI activity and potential drug interactions. *Psychosomatics* 2002;43:248–249.
79. Flagyl, metronidazole. Product information. Chicago: Searle Labs, 1999.
80. Flagyl IV/RTU, metronidazole. Product information. Chicago: Searle Labs, 1999.
81. Plaisance KJ, Quintiliani R, Nightingale CH. The pharmacokinetics of metronidazole and its metabolites in critically ill patients. *J Antimicrob Chemother* 1988;21:195–200.
82. Fredricsson B, Hagstrom B, Nord CE, et al. Systemic concentrations of metronidazole and its main metabolites after intravenous oral and vaginal administration. *Gynecol Obstet Invest* 1987;24:200–207.
83. Ralph ED. Clinical pharmacokinetics of metronidazole. *Clin Pharm* 1983;8:43–62.
84. Bennett WM, Aronoff GR, Golper TA, et al. *Drug prescribing in renal failure: dosing guidelines for adults*, 3rd ed. Philadelphia: American College of Physicians, 1994.
85. Houghton GW, Dennis MJ, Gabriel R. Pharmacokinetics of metronidazole in patients with varying degrees of renal failure. *Br J Clin Pharmacol* 1985;19:203–209.
86. Noritate, metronidazole. Product information. Collegeville, PA: Dermik Laboratories, 1999.
87. Anonymous. American Academy of Pediatrics: the transfer of drugs and other chemicals into human milk. *Pediatrics* 2001;108:776–789.
88. Passmore CM, McElnay JC, Rainey EA, et al. Metronidazole excretion in human milk and its effect on the suckling neonate. *Br J Clin Pharmacol* 1988;26:45–51.
89. Giannini AJ, DeFrance DT. Metronidazole and alcohol—potential for combinative abuse. *J Toxicol Clin Toxicol* 1984;20:509–515.
90. Plosker GL. Possible interaction between ethanol and vaginally administered metronidazole. *Clin Pharm* 1987;6:192–193.
91. Pearlman MD, Yashar C, Ernst S, et al. An incremental dosing protocol for women with severe vaginal trichomoniasis and adverse reactions to metronidazole. *Am J Obstet Gynecol* 1996;174:934–936.
92. Kurohara ML, Kwong FK, Lebherz TB, et al. Metronidazole hypersensitivity and oral desensitization. *J Allergy Clin Immunol* 1991;88:279–280.
93. Thami GP, Kanwar AJ. Fixed drug eruption due to metronidazole and tinidazole without cross-sensitivity to secnidazole. *Dermatology* 1998;196:368–370.
94. Patterson BD. Possible interaction between metronidazole and carbamazepine [Letter]. *Ann Pharmacother* 1994;28:1303–1304.
95. Blyden GT, Scavone JM, Greenblatt DJ. Metronidazole impairs clearance of phenytoin but not alprazolam or lorazepam. *J Clin Pharmacol* 1988;28:240–245.
96. Teicher MH, Altesman RI, Cole JO, et al. Possible nephrotoxic interaction of lithium and metronidazole [Letter]. *JAMA* 1987;257:3365–3366.
97. Jensen JC, Gugler R. Single- and multiple-dose metronidazole kinetics. *Clin Pharmacol Ther* 1983;34:481–487.
98. Roux AF, Moirot E, Delhotal B, et al. Metronidazole kinetics in patients with acute renal failure on dialysis: a cumulative study. *Clin Pharmacol Ther* 1984;36:363–368.
99. Pentam 300, pentamidine. Product information. Deerfield, IL: Fujisawa Pharmaceutical, 1997.
100. Centers for Disease Control and Prevention. Guidelines for preventing opportunistic infections among HIV-infected persons—2002 recommendations of the U.S. Public Health Service and the Infectious Diseases Society of America. *MMWR Morb Mortal Wkly Rep* 2002;51:1–48.
101. NebuPent, pentamidine. Product information. Rosemont, IL: Lyphomed, Inc., 1997.
102. Conte JE, Upton RA, Lin ET. Pentamidine pharmacokinetics in patients with AIDS with impaired renal function. *J Infect Dis* 1987;156:885–890.
103. Conte JE Jr. Pharmacokinetics of intravenous pentamidine in patients with normal renal function or receiving hemodialysis. *J Infect Dis* 1991;163:169–175.
104. Conte JE, Upton RA, Phelps RT, et al. Use of a specific and sensitive assay to determine pentamidine pharmacokinetics in patients with AIDS. *J Infect Dis* 1986;154:923–929.

105. Avery GS, ed. *Drug treatment*, 2nd ed. New York: ADIS Press, 1980.
106. Cortese LM, Gasser RA, Bjornson DC, et al. Prolonged recurrence of pentamidine-induced torsades de pointes. *Ann Pharmacother* 1992;26:1365–1369.
107. Helmick CG, Green JK. Pentamidine-associated hypotension and route of administration. *Ann Intern Med* 1985;103:480.
108. Navin TR, Fontaine RE. Intravenous versus intramuscular administration of pentamidine. *N Engl J Med* 1984;311:1701–1702.
109. Stein KM, Fenton C, Lehany AM, et al. Incidence of QT interval prolongation during pentamidine therapy of *Pneumocystis carinii* pneumonia. *Am J Cardiol* 1991;68:1091–1094.
110. Balslev U, Berild D, Nielsen TL. Cardiac arrest during treatment of *Pneumocystis carinii* pneumonia with intravenous pentamidine isethionate. *Scand J Infect Dis* 1992;24:111–112.
111. O'Brien JG, Dong BJ, Coleman RL, et al. A 5-year retrospective review of adverse drug reactions and their risk factors in human immunodeficiency virus-infected patients who were receiving intravenous pentamidine therapy for *Pneumocystis carinii* pneumonia. *Clin Infect Dis* 1997;24:854–859.
112. Lillehei JP, Funke JL, Drage CW, et al. *Pneumocystis carinii* pneumonia. Needle-biopsy diagnosis and successful treatment. *JAMA* 1968;206:596–600.
113. Western KA, Penera DR, Schultz MD. Pentamidine isethionate in the treatment of *Pneumocystis carinii* pneumonia. *Ann Intern Med* 1970;73:695–702.
114. Kovacs JA, Heimenz JW, Macher AM, et al. *Pneumocystis carinii* pneumonia: a comparison between patients with the acquired immunodeficiency syndrome and patients with other immunodeficiencies. *Ann Intern Med* 1984;100:495–499.
115. Kovacs JA, Hiemenz JW, Macher AM, et al. *Pneumocystis carinii* pneumonia: a comparison between patients with the acquired immunodeficiency syndrome and patients with other immunodeficiencies. *Ann Intern Med* 1984;100:663–671.
116. Wispelwey B, Pearson R. Pentamidine. A risk-benefit analysis. *Drug Saf* 1990;5:212–219.
117. Walzer PD, Perl DP, Krogstad DJ, et al. *Pneumocystis carinii* pneumonia in the United States. Epidemiologic, diagnostic, and clinical features. *Ann Intern Med* 1974;80:83–93.
118. Herchline TE, Plouffe JF, Para MF. Diabetes mellitus presenting with ketoacidosis following pentamidine therapy in patients with acquired immunodeficiency syndrome. *J Infect* 1991;22:41–44.
119. Waskin H, Stehr-Green JK, Helmick CG, et al. Risk factors for hypoglycemia associated with pentamidine therapy for pneumocystis pneumonia. *JAMA* 1988;260:345–347.
120. Villamil A, Hammer RA, Rodriguez FH. Edematous pancreatitis associated with intravenous pentamidine. *South Med J* 1991;84:796–798.
121. Foscavir, foscarnet sodium. Product information. Westborough, MA: Astra USA, Inc., 1994.
122. Vistide, cidofovir injection. Product information. Foster City, CA: Gilead Sciences, Inc., 1996.
123. Raxar, grepafloxacin hydrochloride. Product information. Research Triangle Park, NC: Glaxo Wellcome Inc., 1999.
124. Watts RG, Conte JE, Zurlinden E, et al. Effect of charcoal hemoperfusion on clearance of pentamidine isethionate after accidental overdose. *J Toxicol Clin Toxicol* 1997;35:89–92.
125. Fitzgerald DB, Young IS. Reversal of pentamidine-induced hypoglycaemia with oral diazoxide. *J Trop Med Hyg* 1984;87:15–19.
126. Wharton JM, Demopulos PA, Goldschlager N. Torsade de pointes during administration of pentamidine isethionate. *Am J Med* 1987;83:571–576.
127. Gonzalez A, Sager PT, Akil B, et al. Pentamidine-induced torsade de pointes. *Am Heart J* 1991;122:1489–1492.
128. Neutrexin, trimetrexate glucuronate for injection. Product information. Gaithersburg, MD: MedImmune Oncology, Inc., 2002.
129. Rogers P, Allegra CJ, Murphy RF, et al. Bioavailability of oral trimetrexate in patients with acquired immunodeficiency syndrome. *Antimicrob Agents Chemother* 1988;32:324–326.
130. Lin JT, Cashmore AR, Baker M, et al. Phase I studies with trimetrexate: clinical pharmacology, analytical methodology, and pharmacokinetics. *Cancer Res* 1987;47:609–616.
131. Balis FM, Patel R, Luks E, et al. Pediatric phase I trial and pharmacokinetic study of trimetrexate. *Cancer Res* 1987;47:4973–4976.
132. Amsden GW, Kowalsky SF, Morse GD. Trimetrexate for *Pneumocystic carinii* pneumonia in patients with AIDS. *Ann Pharmacother* 1992;26:218–226.
133. Fanucchi MP, Walsh TD, Fleisher M, et al. Phase I and clinical pharmacology study of trimetrexate administered weekly for three weeks. *Cancer Res* 1987;47:3303–3308.
134. Blanke CK, Messenger M, Taplin SC. Trimetrexate: review and current clinical experience in advanced colorectal cancer. *Semin Oncol* 1997;24[Suppl 18]:S18–57, S18–S63.
135. Stewart JA. Safety and tolerance of trimetrexate: results of a phase II multicenter study in patients with metastatic cancer refractory to conventional therapy or for which no conventional therapy exists. *Semin Oncol* 1988;15[Suppl 2]:10–16.
136. Allegra CJ, Chabner BA, Tuazon CU, et al. Trimetrexate for the treatment of *Pneumocystis carinii* pneumonia in patients with the acquired immunodeficiency syndrome. *N Engl J Med* 1987;317:978–985.
137. Szelenyi H, Hohenberger P, Lochs H, et al. Sequential trimetrexate, 5-fluorouracil and folinic acid are effective and well tolerated in metastatic colorectal carcinoma. *Oncology* 2000;58:273–279.
138. Grem JL, Ellenberg SS, King SA, Shoemaker DD. Correlates of severe of life-threatening toxic effects of trimetrexate. *J Natl Cancer Inst* 1988;80:1313–1318.
139. Weiss RB, James WD, Major WB, et al. Skin reactions induced by trimetrexate, an analog of methotrexate. *Invest New Drugs* 1986;4:159–163.
140. Young FE, Nightingale SL. FDA's newly designated treatment INDs. *JAMA* 1988;260:224–225.
141. General recommendations on immunization. *MMWR Morb Mortal Wkly Rep* 1989;38:205–214, 219–227.
142. Wall SM, Johansen MJ, Molony DA, et al. Effective clearance of methotrexate using high-flux hemodialysis membranes. *Am J Kid Dis* 1996;28:846–854(abst).
143. Bouffet E, Frappaz D, Laville M, et al. Charcoal haemoperfusion and methotrexate toxicity [Letter]. *Lancet* 1986;1:1497.
144. Molina R, Fabian C, Cowley B. Use of charcoal hemoperfusion with sequential hemodialysis to reduce serum methotrexate levels in a patient with acute renal failure. *Am J Med* 1987;82:350–352.
145. McIvor A. Charcoal hemoperfusion and methotrexate toxicity. *Nephron* 1991;58:378.
146. Grimes DJ, Bowles MR, Buttsworth JA, et al. Survival after unexpected high serum methotrexate concentrations in a patient with osteogenic sarcoma. *Drug Saf* 1990;5:447–454.
147. Montagne N, Milano G, Caldani C, et al. Removal of methotrexate by hemodiafiltration. *Cancer Chemother Pharmacol* 1989;24:400–401.
148. Goto E, Tomojiri S, Okamoto I, et al. Methotrexate poisoning with acute hepatorenal dysfunction. *J Toxicol Clin Toxicol* 2001;39:101–104.
149. Jambou P, Levraut J, Favier C, et al. Removal of methotrexate by continuous venovenous hemodiafiltration. In: *Continuous extracorporeal treatment in multiple organ dysfunction syndrome*. New York: Basel, 1995;116:48–52.
150. Spiegel RJ, Cooper PR, Blum RH, et al. Treatment of massive intrathecal methotrexate overdose by ventriculolumbar perfusion. *N Engl J Med* 1984;311:386–388.
151. Jakobson AM, Kreuger A, Mortimer A, et al. Cerebrospinal fluid exchange after intrathecal methotrexate overdose. A report of two cases. *Acta Pediatr* 1992;81:359–361.
152. Jardine LF, Ingram LC, Bleyer WA. Intrathecal leucovorin after intrathecal methotrexate overdose. *J Pediatr Hematol Oncol* 1996;18:302–304.

SECTION 3

Antineoplastic Drugs

CHAPTER 98

Antineoplastic Drugs

Seth Schonwald

OVERVIEW

Antineoplastic drugs are characterized as alkylating agents, antimetabolites, natural products, hormone inhibitors, or other miscellaneous products (Table 1). Within each group of drugs, the toxic effects exhibited by one member of the class are not easily translated to others within the same group.

Cytotoxic drugs administered in overdose by the oral route, inadvertently or self-induced, seldom result in an immediate life-threatening emergency. When these agents are administered in overdose or by the wrong route [e.g., intrathecally instead of intravenously (IV)], however, predictable (e.g., bone marrow suppression) and unpredictable (e.g., brain damage after inadvertent intrathecal use) toxic reactions may follow.

Treatment of most antineoplastic overdoses is symptomatic and supportive and managed without antidotes. Treatment of antineoplastic agents is addressed for all agents at the end of this chapter. Extravasation is covered separately.

ACTINOMYCIN D

Actinomycin D (dactinomycin) is used to treat Ewing's sarcoma, rhabdomyosarcoma, Wilms' tumor, gestational trophoblastic disease, Kaposi's sarcoma, melanoma, optic nerve glioma, osteogenic sarcoma, testicular cancer, and endometrial cancer.

Typical adult IV dosing is 1.25 mg/m^2 every other week or 1 to 2 mg/m^2 (25 to 50 µg/kg) every 3 to 4 weeks. A typical dose in children is 45 µg/kg every 3 weeks IV and 15 µg/kg/day IV for 5 days every 5 to 8 weeks. The maximum single dose is 500 µg.

Actinomycin D overdose has rarely been reported (1). A large dactinomycin overdose in an 18-month-old child resulted in multisystem failure and prolonged hypotension (2).

Toxicokinetics and Toxicodynamics

Actinomycin D is poorly absorbed orally. It crosses the placenta but not the blood–brain barrier. Plasma protein binding is 5% (3). The terminal elimination half-life of actinomycin D is 36 to 48 hours. Although 15% is eliminated hepatically, there are no active metabolites. Parent drug is excreted in the stool (15%) and in the urine (15%) over the first week.

Pathophysiology

At low concentrations, dactinomycin inhibits DNA-primed RNA synthesis by intercalating with guanine residues. At higher concentrations, it also inhibits DNA synthesis. Interstrand and DNA-protein cross-links may occur. Dactinomycin is cell cycle phase nonspecific (4–6).

Pregnancy and Lactation

Actinomycin D is U.S. Food and Drug Administration (FDA) pregnancy risk category D (Appendix I). Breast-feeding is not recommended.

Clinical Presentation

Overdose may result in seizures, hyponatremia, hypovolemia, hypocalcemia, hypomagnesemia, thrombocytopenia, oral mucositis, diarrhea, and fever.

Immediate effects of a therapeutic dose include anaphylaxis; vein irritation; nausea and vomiting (onset, 1 to 6 hours, duration, 4 to 20 hours); loss of appetite; allergic reactions; flushing; rare hypocalcemia; and radiation recall reaction. Early effects include myelosuppression (nadir, 14 to 21 days; recovery, 21 to 25 days); stomatitis; mild to moderate alopecia; diarrhea; folliculitis; and liver problems. Delayed effects may include cancer (rare) (3).

Actinomycin D is a rare cause of hepatotoxicity and veno-occlusive disease (7). Toxicity may manifest as increased aminotransferase and bilirubin levels, ascites, and liver enlargement. In some cases, thrombocytopenia may accompany hepatotoxicity. Severe hepatotoxicity is associated with concurrent use of other hepatotoxic agents, using single-dose dactinomycin as opposed to a 5-day regimen, doses of dactinomycin of 60 µg/kg or greater, and radiation.

Dactinomycin may enhance radiation injury to tissues before, concurrent with, or even after its administration. Recur-

TABLE 1. Cancer chemotherapeutic agents

Alkylating agents	Exemestane
Busulfan	Flutamide
Busulfan injection	Goserelin
Carboplatin	Letrozole
Carmustine	Leuprolide
Cisplatin	Megestrol
Cyclophosphamide	Mitotane
Dacarbazine	Nilutamide
Ifosfamide	Tamoxifen
Lomustine	Toremifene
Streptozocin	Monoclonal antibodies
Temozolomide	Alemtuzumab
Antibiotics	Gemtuzumab ozogamicin
Bleomycin	Imatinib mesylate
Dactinomycin	Rituximab
Daunorubicin	Trastuzumab
Doxorubicin	Nitrogen mustard derivatives
Epirubicin	Chlorambucil
Idarubicin	Estramustine
Mitomycin-C	Mechlorethamine
Plicamycin	Melphalan
Valrubicin	Thiotepa
Antimetabolites	Plant alkaloids
Capecitabine	Docetaxel
Cladribine	Etoposide
Cytarabine	Irinotecan
Floxuridine	Paclitaxel
Fludarabine	Teniposide
5-Fluorouracil	Topotecan
Gemcitabine	Vinblastine
Hydroxyurea	Vincristine
Mercaptopurine	Vinorelbine
Methotrexate	Others
Pentostatin	Alitretinoin
Thioguanine	Altretamine
Biologicals	Arsenic trioxide
Aldesleukin	Asparaginase
Denileukin diftitox	*Escherichia coli* strain
Interferon alpha-2a (recombinant)	BCG live (intravesical)
Interferon alpha-2b (recombinant)	Bexarotene
Hormonal agents	Mitoxantrone
Aminoglutethimide	Pegaspargase
Anastrozole	Procarbazine
Bicalutamide	Tretinoin

Adapted from Adams VR. Guide for the administration and use of cancer chemotherapeutic drugs. *Pharm Pract News* 2001;4:21.

rent injury may occur weeks to months after radiation (3). Dactinomycin may also potentiate radiation pneumonitis (8).

Tissue necrosis with extravasation may occur days to weeks after treatment.

Diagnostic Tests

Diagnostic testing is aimed at assessing end organ effects (e.g., myelosuppression). Renal and bone marrow function should be assessed frequently. Complete blood counts (CBCs) and liver function tests (LFTs) should be checked with each treatment. Dactinomycin levels are not used to guide therapy.

Treatment

See Antineoplastic Treatment Guidelines Hemodialysis is probably ineffective in treating actinomycin overdose (9). There is no specific antidote.

ALDESLEUKIN

Aldesleukin, a synthetic version of interleukin-2 (IL-2), is used to treat metastatic renal cell cancer and metastatic melanoma. It is being investigated in acute myelogenous leukemia (AML), non-Hodgkin's lymphoma, human immunodeficiency virus (HIV) infection, nasopharyngeal carcinoma, Kaposi's sarcoma, and leprosy.

The dose of aldesleukin is 600,000 IU/kg administered every 8 hours IV over 15 minutes for 5 days for a maximum of 14 doses (cycle 1). Following a rest period of 6 to 10 days, a second 5-day cycle is administered. IL-2 has rarely been administered in overdose (10).

Pathophysiology

IL-2 is a lymphokine produced by normal T lymphocytes. It is central to both cellular and humoral arms of the immune system and regulates lymphocyte proliferation and differentiation (3). The use of aldesleukin in the treatment of acquired immune deficiency syndrome patients is not FDA approved; however, aldesleukin increases the CD4 T-cell count in HIV-infected individuals without an associated increase in viral load (11).

Pregnancy and Lactation

Aldesleukin is FDA pregnancy risk category C (Appendix I).

Clinical Presentation

Neurologic and psychiatric disturbances with moderate or severe mental status changes, including paranoia and hallucinations, are common and sometimes treatment limiting. These are less common if used subcutaneously (SQ). Drowsiness, sleep disturbances, headache, fatigue, weakness, malaise, loss of appetite, visual changes, and alterations or loss of taste may occur (12).

Hypothyroidism is a major endocrine complication, and antithyroid antibodies have been detected in approximately 50% of patients (12). Anemia occurs in 75% of patients and may necessitate blood transfusion. A low platelet count occurs in two-thirds of patients, and low white blood cell count occurs in one-third (3). Autoimmune hemolytic anemia has been described in a patient with chronic lymphocytic leukemia (CLL) and renal cell carcinoma after treatment with high-dose IV bolus IL-2 (13).

Cardiovascular effects include myocarditis (14), angina pectoris, and myocardial infarction, occurring in the first days of treatment. Supraventricular dysrhythmias are the most common rhythm disorder. Decreases in myocardial contractility and cardiomyopathy may occur (15).

Capillary leak syndrome following aldesleukin therapy can cause renal dysfunction (16). Increased platelet adherence induced by IL-2 caused by effects on the endothelium could result in microvascular thrombus formation and contribute to organ dysfunction (17).

Itching occurs in one-half of all patients, and rash occurs in one-fourth. Occasionally, fixed drug eruptions can be severe (18). A burning itchy erythema occurs in many patients (19). Nausea or vomiting occurs in most patients, and diarrhea occurs in three of every four patients. Abdominal pain or constipation is unusual. Liver tests become abnormal in most patients, and jaundice may result from reversible cholestasis (20). Pancreatitis has been associated with IL-2 use as well (21).

Diagnostic Tests

Diagnostic testing is aimed at assessing end organ effects (e.g., myelosuppression, thyroid, cardiac, hepatic, and renal). Renal and bone marrow function should be assessed frequently. CBC and LFTs should be checked with each treatment. Aldesleukin levels are not used to guide therapy.

Treatment

See Antineoplastic Treatment Guidelines at the end of this chapter. Aggressive and proactive management of aldesleukin toxicity can help facilitate completion of therapy (11). There is no specific antidote.

ANASTROZOLE

Aromatization of androgen precursors in peripheral tissues is the major source of estrogens in postmenopausal women. Inhibition of the aromatase enzyme offers an effective means of inducing regression of estrogen-responsive breast cancer (22).

A new generation of aromatase inhibitors offers effective and convenient aromatase inhibition (23). Anastrozole and letrozole are used in the treatment of advanced postmenopausal breast cancer after failure of tamoxifen (24).

Maximal estrogen suppression is produced by a 1-mg dose (25). A single dose of anastrozole that results in major toxicity has not been established. Single doses up to 60 mg in healthy men volunteers and 10 mg daily given to postmenopausal women with advanced breast cancer were well tolerated (26).

Toxicokinetics and Toxicodynamics

Anastrozole is rapidly and almost completely absorbed orally. Food reduces absorption (27). Metabolism is primarily in the liver, resulting in *N*-dealkylation, hydroxylation, and glucuronidation. Postmenopausal women excrete approximately 10% of the dose as unchanged drug in urine within 72 hours and approximately 60% of the dose as metabolites (26).

Pathophysiology

The goal of hormone therapy in breast cancer is to deprive tumor cells of estrogens, which are implicated in the development or progression of tumors (28). Anastrozole is a reversible aromatase inhibitor. Aromatase catalyzes the final and rate-limiting step in the conversion of androgens to estrogens in peripheral tissues. This occurs mainly in adipose tissue as well as normal and malignant breast tissues and provides the main source of estrogen in postmenopausal women.

Pregnancy and Lactation

Anastrozole is FDA pregnancy risk category D (Appendix I) (29). Breast-feeding is not recommended (30).

Clinical Presentation

Toxicity from anastrozole is generally mild or moderate and transient (31). The most common adverse events are gastrointestinal (GI) disturbances (incidence 29% to 33%). Other reported adverse events include headache (18%), asthenia (16%), pain (15%), hot flushes and bone pain (12%), back pain and dyspnea (11%), and peripheral edema (9%) (32).

Nonspecific symptoms such as fatigue and weight gain have been reported with anastrozole (33). Thromboembolic events and vaginal bleeding were reported in fewer patients treated with anastrozole than with tamoxifen in postmenopausal women with breast cancer (34).

Diagnostic Tests

Diagnostic testing is rarely needed for drug effects. Specific levels of aldesleukin are not available or clinically useful.

Treatment

See Antineoplastic Treatment Guidelines at the end of this chapter. Anastrozole is probably dialyzable, but this intervention has not been needed. There is no specific antidote.

ASPARAGINASE

Asparaginase (or L-Asparaginase) is an immune modulator used to treat acute lymphoblastic leukemia (ALL), AML, acute nonlymphoid leukemia, acute myelomonocytic leukemia, CLL, Hodgkin's disease, melanosarcoma, and non-Hodgkin's lymphoma.

It is estimated that 3% to 10% of children with ALL experience acute, transient neurotoxicity during induction chemotherapy. One report describes two children who died from unexpected, acute fatal neurologic toxicity during induction chemotherapy for ALL (35).

Toxicokinetics and Toxicodynamics

Bioavailability after intramuscular (IM) injection is markedly decreased. It has a prolonged elimination half-life up to 50 hours.

Pathophysiology

Asparaginase acts by deaminating extracellular L-asparagine, an amino acid that appears essential for protein synthesis by some tumor cells lacking adequate levels of asparagine synthetase. Asparaginase from *Erwinia carotovora* is serologically and biochemically distinct from asparaginase from *Escherichia coli*, although its antineoplastic activity and toxicity are similar (4).

Pregnancy and Lactation

Asparaginase is FDA pregnancy risk category C (Appendix I).

Clinical Presentation

Asparaginase may produce hypersensitivity reactions with a 1% mortality rate from anaphylaxis. Patients with a history of atopy or allergy, previous drug exposure, intermittent IV as opposed to intermittent IM administration, and use of drug alone have a higher risk. Hypersensitivity reactions are rare when asparaginase is given IV on a daily basis (36,37). Asparaginase has also been associated with toxic epidermal necrolysis (38).

Hepatotoxicity is frequent (39). Biochemical changes include decreased serum albumin, elevation of aminotransferases, bilirubin, and alkaline phosphatase. Hepatic dysfunction may produce decreased levels of factors II, VII, IX, X, and fibrinogen and, possibly, contribute to coagulation disorders. Liver abnormalities typically resolve a few days to weeks after therapy (40).

Pancreatitis also occurs and can be fatal (41). Hemorrhagic and thrombotic events as well as thrombus formation in the extremities occur in 1% to 2% of patients receiving asparaginase (42). Most children receiving asparaginase have deficiencies in hemostatic proteins, but it is difficult to predict which child will develop these complications. Headache, obtundation, hemiparesis, and seizure (43) may result from intracranial thrombi, whereas extremity thrombi can manifest as local pain, swelling, and discoloration (43). The outcome of these events is usually good; however, some authors recommend prophylactic pretreatment with fresh frozen plasma in patients who have manifested coagulopathy problems.

Cerebral dysfunction occurs in 21% to 60% of patients and is manifested by lethargy, drowsiness, depression, confusion, and personality changes. In children with ALL, acute arterial or sagittal sinus thrombosis secondary to L-asparaginase has been reported (44). A delayed form of organic brain syndrome can occur a week after asparaginase administration and can last several weeks. There appears to be no clinically significant difference in the neurotoxic potential of *E. coli* or *Erwinia* asparaginase (45).

L-Asparaginase can cause hypoparathyroidism, which can yield hypocalcemia, hypophosphatemia, and hyperphosphaturia (46). Hyperglycemia occurs in approximately 10% of leukemic children treated with asparaginase and prednisone. Transient diabetes mellitus may develop in these settings (47) but is usually reversible when the drug is discontinued. Risk factors in children for the development of hyperglycemia include age older than 10 years, obesity, family history of diabetes mellitus, and Down syndrome.

Diagnostic Tests

Diagnostic testing is aimed at assessing end organ effects (e.g., pancreas). Renal and bone marrow function should be assessed frequently. CBC and LFTs should be checked with each treatment. Serum amylase levels should be obtained before each cycle of therapy. An elevated amylase level suggests pancreatitis, but pancreatitis may develop despite normal amylase concentrations. Specific levels of asparaginase are not used to guide therapy.

Treatment

See Antineoplastic Treatment Guidelines at the end of this chapter. Asparaginase therapy should be discontinued if pancreatitis is diagnosed (48). Insulin may be needed to treat hyperglycemia. No specific antidote is available.

BICALUTAMIDE

Bicalutamide is approved to treat prostate cancer (49). It may be useful for hirsutism and priapism. The oral daily dose for prostate cancer is 50 mg (range, 50 to 150 mg) (50). No adjustment is required for renal or hepatic disease. The dose for hirsutism is 25 mg daily.

Toxicokinetics and Toxicodynamics

Bicalutamide is extensively absorbed and unaffected by food (51). Absolute bioavailability is not known (52). Time-to-peak plasma concentration is up to 48 hours (53). Plasma protein binding is 96%. Hepatic metabolism produces an inactive metabolite (54).

Pathophysiology

Bicalutamide is a nonsteroidal antiandrogen without other endocrine activity that competes for androgen receptors. Prostate cancer is mostly androgen dependent. Antiandrogen monotherapy is consistently equivalent to castration (55) but is considered for patients who want to maintain sexual potency (56). Bicalutamide does not suppress androgen production and may increase serum androgen concentrations (57).

Pregnancy and Lactation

Bicalutamide is FDA pregnancy risk category X (Appendix I). Breast-feeding is not recommended.

Clinical Presentation

Breast tenderness, gynecomastia (58), and hot flashes may occur with bicalutamide use (58). Interstitial pneumonitis (59) and eosinophilic lung disease (60) have also been reported.

Diagnostic Tests

Dyspnea during treatment should be evaluated with chest radiography and arterial blood gas analysis if severe. Bicalutamide concentrations are not used to manage therapy.

Treatment

See Antineoplastic Treatment Guidelines at the end of this chapter. Dialysis is not likely to remove significant amounts due to protein binding (54). No specific antidote is available.

BLEOMYCIN

Bleomycin is used in combination chemotherapy for patients with germ cell tumors; Hodgkin's disease; non-Hodgkin's lymphoma; squamous cell cancer of the vulva, cervix, penis, or skin; head and neck cancer; osteogenic sarcoma; and testicular cancer. Still other uses are malignant pleural effusion, renal cell cancer, soft tissue sarcoma, and leukoplakia.

The fatality rate of bleomycin pulmonary toxicity (BPT) is 1% to 2% and is dose related. The reported incidence of nonfatal BPT appears to be 5% to 10%, and fatal BPT has been reported in approximately 2% of treated cases (61,62). The incidence of pulmonary toxicity is low but increases significantly at doses above 500 U.

Toxicokinetics and Toxicodynamics

Bleomycin is not absorbed orally. High concentrations are found in skin, lung, kidney, peritoneum, and lymphatics. Bleomycin crosses the placenta but not the blood–brain barrier. The V_d is 0.27 L/kg and plasma protein binding is less than 10% (63). Enzymes in many tissues, including the liver, inactivate bleomycin. Bleomycin is excreted in urine. The alpha half-life of bleomycin is 10 to 20 minutes, and the beta half-life is 2 to 4 hours (3).

Pathophysiology

Bleomycin causes single- and double-strand DNA breaks through formation of an intermediate iron complex. DNA synthesis and, to a lesser degree, RNA and protein synthesis are inhibited. Bleomycin is cell cycle phase specific (4,64).

Pregnancy and Lactation

Bleomycin is FDA pregnancy risk category D (Appendix I). Unknown if excreted in breast milk.

Clinical Presentation

Immediate effects include anaphylaxis (pretreatment is recommended), fever, chills, nausea and vomiting, phlebitis, and rare radiation recall reactions. Early effects may include rash, reversible hyperpigmentation, nail changes, stomatitis, alopecia, rare disseminated intravascular coagulation, and rare Raynaud's syndrome. Delayed effects may include lung problems (10% interstitial pneumonitis, 1% chronic fibrosis) and reversible hyperpigmentation (3).

A dry, hacking cough; dyspnea; tachypnea; fever; and cyanosis characterize BPT. Early and late pulmonary toxicity have distinct pathologic and radiographic features. BPT may occur in the form of acute pneumonitis, chronic pulmonary fibrosis, or acute respiratory distress syndrome (most common postoperatively) (65). Symptoms may develop as long as 3 months after treatment. Risk factors include age older than 40 years; cumulative dose above 450 units; renal failure; concomitant administration of cisplatin, cyclophosphamide, methotrexate (MTX), and doxorubicin; chest irradiation; and positive fluid balance during prolonged surgical procedures (66). Other risks include smoking, previous exposure to bleomycin within 6 months, and bolus dosing. Animal studies have demonstrated that supplemental oxygen may be an additional risk factor for lung toxicity (67), but human data are less clear. Multivariate analyses in two large retrospective reviews have not identified high flow oxygen as a risk factor (68).

Skin changes occur in approximately 50% of patients. Bleomycin can cause unusual pigmentation consisting of linear streaks with crisscross patterns on the trunk (69,70).

Fever and chills occur in approximately 50% of patients and may occur after every injection, starting 4 to 10 hours after treatment and lasting up to 48 hours.

Bleomycin may enhance radiation injury to tissues (71). Although often called *radiation recall reactions*, the timing of the radiation may be before, concurrent, or even weeks after bleomycin administration.

Hemolytic uremic syndrome has rarely been reported in association with cisplatin, bleomycin, or vincristine therapy and is frequently fatal in patients older than 50 years with squamous cell cancers (72).

Diagnostic Tests

Laboratory monitoring during each treatment should include CBC, kidney function, and liver function. Lung function should be monitored periodically.

Treatment

See Antineoplastic Treatment Guidelines at the end of this chapter. Specific modalities to treat bleomycin in overdose have rarely been described in the literature (73). There is no specific antidote.

Topical steroids may be useful. Skin ulceration and peeling on fingertips may be painful and can require discontinuation of bleomycin.

Numerous recommendations have been proposed to manage BPT. Caution regarding oxygen therapy should be observed. If supplemental oxygen is required, the lowest FIO_2 that maintains adequate tissue oxygenation should be provided (3).

Pneumonitis is treated with corticosteroids to prevent progression to fibrosis (74,75). Steroids are of questionable benefit once interstitial fibrosis has occurred. Bleomycin should be withheld if pulmonary diffusing capacity of lung for carbon monoxide falls to 40% of initial value, if forced vital capacity falls to less than 25% of initial value, or if there are any clinical or radiographic features indicating pulmonary toxicity.

Recreational use of high flow oxygen (e.g., scuba diving) should be discouraged. Depending on severity, hypersensitivity reactions to bleomycin use can be successfully managed by interrupting the infusion and administering steroids, antihistamines, benzodiazepines, nebulized β-agonists, and/or pressors (76).

BUSULFAN

Busulfan is used to treat chronic myeloid leukemia (CML) and other leukemias, multiple myeloma, myeloproliferative disorders, non-Hodgkin's lymphoma, and polycythemia rubra vera.

The IV induction dose in adults is 0.06 mg/kg/day or 1.8 mg/m^2/day (range, 1 to 12 mg daily). The maintenance dose is 2 mg weekly to 4 mg daily. In children, the IV induction dose is 0.06 mg/kg/day or 4 mg/m^2/day. A 4.6-kg infant received an overdose of busulfan. Hemodialysis was immediately performed and resulted in accelerated clearance of busulfan (77).

The total dose for pulmonary toxicity has ranged between 500 and 5700 mg, with a mean of 3000 mg. Pulmonary toxicity has not been reported under 500 mg.

Toxicokinetics and Toxicodynamics

Oral absorption is variable and subject to first pass metabolism. Busulfan is rapidly eliminated from plasma, crosses the placenta, and crosses the blood–brain barrier. The V_d in adults is 0.6 to 1.0 L/kg and in children is 1.4 to 1.6 L/kg. Plasma protein binding is 7% to 55% (3).

There is extensive hepatic metabolism, 25% to 35% as methanesulfonic acid, an inactive substance. Excretion is primarily as metabolites in urine. The half-life in adults is 2.3 to 2.6 hours, in older children is 2.7 hours, and in younger children is 1.7 to 2.8 hours (78).

Pathophysiology

Busulfan is a bifunctional alkylating agent. Carbonium ions are rapidly formed after absorption, leading to DNA alkylation. This results in DNA breaks and cross-linking, thus interfering with DNA replication and transcription of RNA (4,5).

Pregnancy and Lactation

Busulfan is FDA pregnancy risk category D (Appendix I). Impotence or irreversible loss of fertility can occur. Fetal death or congenital malformations may occur during the first trimester of pregnancy. Intrauterine growth may be retarded or fetal gonads damaged during the second and third trimesters. Breast-feeding is not recommended (3).

Clinical Presentation

Immediate effects include rare anaphylaxis; hyperuricemia; allergic reactions (rash, fever, facial swelling, joint pain); nausea; vomiting; diarrhea; and seizure. Early effects may include myelosuppression and pancytopenia (nadir, 11 to 30 days; recovery, 24 to 54 days), hyperpigmentation, alopecia, and veno-occlusive disease.

Delayed effects may include heart problems (endocardiac fibrosis, rare), leukemia, lung problems, cholestatic hepatitis, infertility, delayed pubertal development, decreased gonadal function, gynecomastia, ovarian suppression, amenorrhea, menopausal symptoms, and cataracts (rare; only with long-term use) (3).

Pancytopenia (79) develops if treatment is maintained despite falling counts. Counts may continue to fall for a month or more after discontinuation of busulfan. Although pancytopenia can last from 1 month to 2 or more years, it is generally reversible.

High-dose busulfan (16 mg/kg) used as part of preparative regimens for bone marrow transplantation can cause seizures (80). Phenytoin or clobazam (81) for seizure prophylaxis in this setting has been recommended.

Busulfan causes hyperpigmentation, which may become persistent with prolonged therapy (82). The symptoms mimic Addison's disease and usually resolve when busulfan is stopped.

Dyspnea, dry cough, fever, and rales characterize pulmonary toxicity. It has distinct pathologic and radiographic features and is related to prolonged treatment (83). The incidence of clinical symptoms is 3%. Risk factors include thoracic irradiation.

The course is rapid in some instances and slow in others, with progression to pulmonary insufficiency and death in many patients. Treatment with prednisone and discontinuation of busulfan may be of some benefit.

Pubertal development and gonadal function may be adversely influenced by high-dose busulfan therapy in children and adolescents.

Diagnostic Tests

Laboratory monitoring during induction should include a CBC weekly. During maintenance, a CBC biweekly is recommended. Periodic monitoring of uric acid and LFTs should also occur.

Treatment

See Antineoplastic Treatment Guidelines at the end of this chapter. There is no specific antidote. Patients may require supplementation with appropriate gonadal hormones.

CARBOPLATIN

Carboplatin is an analog of cisplatin used to treat a wide variety of tumors.

Toxicokinetics and Toxicodynamics

Carboplatin is poorly absorbed orally. Whereas cisplatin is highly protein bound, carboplatin is less reactive, and only a minimal amount of intrinsic platinum becomes protein bound. Platinum is widely distributed to SQ fat, kidney, bone, pancreas, liver, and hair (84). Erythrocytes represent an important deep compartment for oxaliplatin and a little less for cisplatin. Carboplatin is quickly extruded from erythrocytes and is largely excreted unchanged in urine. The half-life of total platinum is approximately 6 days (3).

Pathophysiology

Like cisplatin, carboplatin contains a platinum atom but is more stable and less nephrotoxic, neurotoxic, ototoxic, and emetogenic (3). The mechanism of action is not known. Carboplatin undergoes intracellular activation to form reactive platinum complexes that are believed to inhibit DNA synthesis by forming interstrand and intrastrand cross-linking. Carboplatin is a radiation-sensitizing agent (3).

Pregnancy and Lactation

Carboplatin is FDA pregnancy risk category D (Appendix I) (85).

Clinical Presentation

Nausea and vomiting usually begin 6 to 12 hours after treatment and may persist 24 hours or longer. Acute vomiting is most common in patients with prior or concurrent emetogenic cytotoxic therapy. The incidence of nausea and vomiting may be lower when carboplatin is given as a 24-hour continuous infusion or in divided doses over 5 consecutive days (86).

At conventional doses, carboplatin causes only minor transient elevations in urinary enzymes. Nephrotoxicity is less common or severe than with cisplatin, and concomitant IV hydration and diuresis are generally not needed with carboplatin (87). The risk and severity of nephrotoxicity are increased with high-dose regimens, especially with concurrent nephrotoxic chemotherapy (88).

Carboplatin rarely causes peripheral neurotoxicity (89); however, some patients may demonstrate sensory loss and paresthesia with cumulative doses exceeding 400 mg/m^2. Neurotoxicity such as peripheral sensory neuropathy (e.g., paresthesias) is less frequent or severe than with cisplatin. Ototoxicity is rare with conventional doses (90). Peripheral neuropathy is more common in patients older than 65 years of age, receiving prolonged treatment, or with prior cisplatin therapy. Patients with preexisting cisplatin-induced peripheral neurotoxicity generally do not worsen during carboplatin therapy.

Myelosuppression is the dose-limiting toxicity, usually manifested as thrombocytopenia and less commonly as leukopenia, neutropenia, and anemia. Risk factors include prior cytotoxic therapy (especially cisplatin), old age, impaired renal function, and concurrent myelosuppressive therapy (91). Myelosuppression is dose dependent and closely related to the renal clearance of carboplatin. Anemia is more common with increased carboplatin exposure, and blood transfusions may be needed during prolonged carboplatin therapy.

Hypersensitivity is reported in 2% of patients receiving carboplatin alone and in 9% to 12% of patients receiving carboplatin with other cytotoxic drugs (92). Reactions are similar to those seen with other platinum agents: pruritus, rash, palmar erythema, fever, chills, rigors, swelling (face, tongue, and at the infusion site), GI upset, dyspnea, wheezing, tachycardia, hypertension, or hypotension (93). Reactions can develop hours to days after administration.

Diagnostic Tests

Laboratory monitoring with each treatment should include CBC, electrolytes, and kidney function. Periodically, uric acid, hearing function, and neurologic function should be tested.

Treatment

See Antineoplastic Treatment Guidelines at the end of this chapter. There is no specific antidote.

CARMUSTINE

Carmustine is used to treat brain tumors, GI cancers, Hodgkin's disease, malignant melanoma, multiple myeloma, breast cancer, non-Hodgkin's lymphoma, and pancreatic cancer.

Typical adult regimens include 150 to 200 mg/m^2 IV every 5 to 8 weeks or 75 to 100 $mg/m^2/day \times 2$ days every 6 to 8 weeks. Up to 600 mg/m^2 is used for bone marrow transplants. Topical dosing is 10 to 20 mg/day for 4 to 8 weeks as a solution or ointment. In children, the dose is 60 mg/m^2 or 2 mg/kg IV, then 30 to 45 mg/m^2 or 1.0 to 1.5 mg/kg IV every 6 weeks.

One multivariate regression analysis of glioma patients, which corrected for survival time bias, suggested increased risk of pulmonary toxicity when total dose exceeded 1400 mg/m^2 (94).

Toxicokinetics and Toxicodynamics

Carmustine is readily and completely absorbed. It is highly lipid soluble, with the highest concentrations found in spleen, liver, and ovaries. It may be found in breast milk and crosses the blood–brain barrier [cerebrospinal fluid (CSF) equilibrates within 1 hour to 30% to 97% of plasma levels]. The V_d is 2.6 to 3.3 L/kg, and plasma protein binding *in vitro* is 80% (3). There is rapid and extensive metabolism by the hepatic microsomal enzyme oxidation system to active and inactive metabolites. Excretion is predominantly urinary (30% within 24 hours), although 6% to 10% is eliminated by respiratory excretion and 1% in feces. The alpha half-life is 1.4 minutes, and the beta half-life is 0.3 to 1.5 hours (3).

Pathophysiology

Carmustine is a highly lipophilic nitrosourea compound that undergoes hydrolysis *in vivo* to form reactive metabolites. These metabolites cause alkylation and cross-linking of DNA. Other biologic effects include inhibition of DNA repair and some cell cycle phase specificity. Nitrosoureas generally lack cross-resistance with other alkylating agents (3).

Pregnancy and Lactation

Carmustine is FDA pregnancy risk category D (Appendix I). Breast-feeding is not recommended.

Clinical Presentation

Immediate effects may include phlebitis, flushing, nausea and vomiting, and myocardial ischemia with high doses. Early effects include mucositis, esophagitis, diarrhea, skin discoloration along veins, elevated LFTs, glomerular and renal tubular lesions, and central nervous system (CNS) problems (e.g., acute encephalopathy with intracarotid administration, dizziness, loss of balance, and ataxia). Delayed effects include myelosuppression (nadir, 25 to 60 days; recovery, 35 to 85 days); reversible, elevated LFTs; pulmonary fibrosis; azotemia; infertility; and leukemia (3). Effects on bone marrow are dose related and cumulative.

Local burning occurs at the injection site. Rapid IV infusion may produce facial flushing. These effects are thought to be secondary to the alcohol diluent. Extravasation tissue necrosis may occur weeks to months after treatment. Patients must be observed for delayed reactions, and prior injection sites must be carefully inspected.

The pulmonary toxicity of high-dose carmustine may manifest as severe interstitial pneumonitis, most frequently in patients with recent (months) mediastinal radiation. Pulmonary fibrosis can develop. Risk factors include preexisting lung disease, smoking, cyclophosphamide therapy, and recent thoracic radiation. Clinical signs include dyspnea, tachypnea, and a dry hacking cough. Incidence of pulmonary fibrosis is 20% to 30%, and mortality is 24% to 80% (95).

Nausea and vomiting may be severe, beginning soon after administration and lasting 4 to 6 hours. When used in high doses, toxicity can include severe nausea and vomiting, encephalopathy, hepatotoxicity, and pulmonary toxicity. Infusion-related hypotension during infusion of high-dose carmustine can hasten renal dysfunction (16).

Damage to the corneal and conjunctival epithelium has followed high doses (96).

Diagnostic Tests

Monitoring during each treatment includes CBC and electrolytes. Blood counts should be monitored for at least 6 weeks after dose (3). Uric acid, liver function, kidney function, and lung function should be ascertained periodically.

Treatment

See Antineoplastic Treatment Guidelines at the end of this chapter. Steroids and cyclosporine have been used with varying degrees of success to treat carmustine-induced pulmonary toxicity (97).

CHLORAMBUCIL

Chlorambucil is the slowest acting and least toxic of the nitrogen mustard–alkylating agents. It is used to treat CLL, non-Hodgkin's lymphomas, Hodgkin's disease, multiple myeloma, amyloidosis, mycosis fungoides, uveitis, Behçet's syndrome, necrobiotic xanthogranuloma, nephrotic syndrome, pyoderma gangrenosum, dermatomyositis, sarcoidosis, primary biliary cirrhosis, Waldenström's macroglobulinemia, and Sézary syndrome.

Therapeutic doses in adults and children range from 0.1 to 0.2 mg/kg/day IV. At total doses of 4 to 6 mg/kg in adults, myoclonus and seizures may occur. Dosages of 1.5 to 6.8 mg/kg have been associated with lethargy, irritability, myoclonus, vomiting, abdominal pain, ataxia, seizures, transient electroencephalogram changes, and coma.

A 22-month-old, 10-kg child ingested 32 mg of chlorambucil and developed irritability, myoclonic-like muscle jerks, an exaggerated startle reflex, vomiting, and electroencephalogram changes within a few hours. The neurologic symptoms improved overnight, and the patient was discharged at approximately 28 hours post-ingestion. During the 3 weeks of follow-up, mild bone marrow suppression occurred and resolved (98).

Toxicokinetics and Toxicodynamics

Chlorambucil is orally absorbed with a bioavailability of 70% to 80% (10% to 20% with food). The half-life of chlorambucil is 2 hours. Tissue distribution is homogeneous, crosses the placenta, and is found in ascitic fluid. The V_d is 0.14 to 0.24 L/kg, and plasma protein binding is 99% (3). Metabolism is mostly by the hepatic microsomal enzyme oxidation system. Phenylacetic acid mustard is an active metabolite. Chlorambucil and metabolites are probably not dialyzable.

Pathophysiology

Chlorambucil is a derivative of mechlorethamine and is closely related in structure to melphalan. Alkylation of DNA results in breaks in the DNA molecule as well as cross-linking, thus interfering with DNA replication and RNA transcription. Like other alkylators, it is cell cycle phase nonspecific (4,5).

Pregnancy and Lactation

Chlorambucil is FDA pregnancy risk category D (Appendix I). It has been used in late pregnancy if the mother has a life-threatening condition (99,100).

Clinical Presentation

Immediate toxicity includes rare anaphylaxis, increased uric acid levels, nausea, and vomiting. Myelosuppression may occur (nadir, 7 to 14 days; recovery, 14 to 21 days). Myelosuppression is more severe with continuous administration than intermittent high-dose chlorambucil. Prolonged therapy or excessive doses may result in pancytopenia or irreversible bone marrow damage. Intermediate symptoms may include rash, rare mucositis, double vision, liver necrosis, and seizures with high dosing. Late toxicity includes cancer (e.g., leukemia, solid tumors), keratitis, chronic pulmonary fibrosis, and infertility (3).

Pulmonary toxicity similar to bleomycin can occur. Pulmonary toxicity is usually associated with prolonged therapy (6 to 24 months) and a total dose greater than 2 g. Partial recovery can occur several weeks after discontinuing therapy. In other patients, pulmonary complications can progress, and death has occurred (101).

Anecdotal reports of chlorambucil-induced seizures have appeared (102). Most cases involved patients on high-dose therapy and children with nephrotic syndrome (103). In adults without a seizure history, seizures have occurred only in patients treated with high-dose chlorambucil or in overdose (104). Myoclonus may occur in adults receiving therapeutic dosages of chlorambucil (105).

Acute cholestatic hepatitis due to chlorambucil has been reported (106).

Diagnostic Tests

Laboratory monitoring during induction should include a CBC weekly. CBC biweekly should be checked during maintenance, and uric acid and liver function should be checked periodically.

Treatment

See Antineoplastic Treatment Guidelines at the end of this chapter. There is no specific antidote.

CISPLATIN

Cisplatin is used to treat a wide range of cancers: bladder, small cell lung, ovarian, testicular, non–small cell lung, adrenocortical, brain, breast, cervical, vulvar, endometrial, GI, germ cell tumors, esophageal, head and neck, and thyroid, as well as gynecologic sarcoma, hepatocellular carcinoma (HCC), malignant melanoma, neuroblastoma, non-Hodgkin's lymphoma, osteosarcoma, and mesothelioma.

The dose range in adults is 25 to 120 mg/m^2 IV every 1 to 4 weeks or 20 to 60 mg/m^2/day for 2 to 5 days every 2 to 4 weeks. The intraperitoneal dose is 120 mg every week with escalations, 60 to 90 mg/m^2 every 3 weeks, and 270 mg/m^2 every 3 weeks with sodium thiosulfate. The intraarterial dose is 75 to 150 mg/m^2 every 2 to 5 weeks. The dose in children is 60 to 120 mg/m^2 IV every 3 weeks or 3 mg/kg IV every 3 weeks (for children less than 10 kg) or 20 mg/m^2/day times 4 days continuous IV every 7 weeks.

A 59-year-old man received a massive cisplatin dose of 300 mg/m^2. Toxic effects included severe emesis, myelosuppression, renal failure, mental deterioration with hallucinations, dim vision, and hepatotoxicity. Plasmapheresis was effective in lowering the platinum concentration from 2979 ng/ml to 185 ng/ml and appeared to be of clinical benefit (107). A 68-year-old woman received a massive cisplatin dose without IV hydration due to the substitution of cisplatin for carboplatin. She developed emesis, myelosuppression, renal failure, and deafness. Plasmapheresis lowered the platinum concentration from above 2900 ng/ml to 200 ng/ml and appeared to be of clinical benefit. Even after the onset of renal failure, hydration increased urinary excretion of platinum (108).

Toxicokinetics and Toxicodynamics

Cisplatin is not orally absorbed. Protein binding is 80% to 85%. The platinum is widely distributed to SQ fat, kidney, bone, pancreas, liver, intestines, and hair (84). Erythrocytes represent an important deep compartment for oxaliplatin and a little less for cisplatin. Cisplatin is found in breast milk, distributes into ascites and pleural fluid, and may cross the placenta. The V_d is 0.17 to 1.47 L/kg. Cisplatin and metabolites react with small proteins containing sulfhydryl groups, such as glutathione, cysteine, and methionine, and then with high-molecular-weight proteins, such as albumin and gamma-globulins. The alpha half-life is 6 to 13 minutes, beta half-life is 25 to 49 minutes, and gamma half-life is 2 to 96 hours (3).

Cisplatin renal excretion is complex, combining reabsorption and secretion processes. Of the current platinum agents, only carboplatin can be adjusted based on creatinine clearance measurement thanks to its simple renal excretion.

Pathophysiology

Cisplatin is an inorganic complex formed by an atom of platinum surrounded by chlorine and ammonia atoms in the *cis* position. Intracellularly, water displaces the chloride to form highly reactive charged platinum complexes. These complexes inhibit DNA through covalent binding DNA cross-linking. Experimental and clinical data suggest that cisplatin enhances radiation therapy effects. Cisplatin has complex and variable effects on the cell cycle (5,109).

Pregnancy and Lactation

Cisplatin is FDA pregnancy risk category D (Appendix I). Cisplatin excretion into breast milk has been documented (110,111). The outcome of infants exposed to cisplatin through milk is not known.

Clinical Presentation

Immediate effects may include anaphylaxis. Moderate to severe nausea and vomiting occurs in most patients. Onset occurs in 1 to 4 hours and may persist for 1 to 7 days. Early effects include myelosuppression in 25% to 30% of patients (nadir, 18 to 23 days; recovery may take 39 days). Other early effects include toxic nephropathy, hypomagnesemia, electrolyte disturbances, rare electrocardiographic (ECG) changes, elevated liver tests, hemolytic anemia, and encephalopathy. Delayed effects may include peripheral neuropathy, encephalopathy, retinopathy, optic neuropathy, ototoxicity, infertility, and Raynaud's disease (3).

Cumulative nephrotoxicity develops in 28% to 36% of patients and is manifested by acute tubular necrosis. Cisplatin reduces glomerular filtration (112) and may require saline hydration and mannitol diuresis to eliminate potentially lethal renal damage. Furosemide diuresis may be hazardous due to potentially additive ototoxicity. Renal tubular abnormality such as acidosis, hypomagnesemia, or hypokalemia may be present with normal glomerular function. Hypomagnesemia may become severe enough to cause tetany and may persist after treatment.

Peripheral neurotoxicity is a dose-limiting complication (89). Neuropathies are sensory in nature but can also include motor difficulties, reduced deep-tendon reflexes, and leg weakness. Loss of vibration sense, paresthesia, and sensory ataxia may develop after several treatment cycles. Symptoms usually occur after prolonged therapy (4 to 7 months) and may be irreversible. Seizures, altered taste, slurred speech, and memory loss have each occurred rarely.

Ototoxicity is cumulative, dose related, and generally irreversible. Clinical hearing loss occurs in 6% and tinnitus in 9%. Audiogram abnormalities develop in 24% of patients, usually involving the high frequency range (113), but may affect the normal hearing range. Hearing loss may be more severe in children. Cranial irradiation may lower the cumulative dose at which cisplatin causes hearing loss. Vestibular ototoxicity is rare (114). Cisplatin has also caused vocal cord paralysis (115) and optic neuritis (116).

Cisplatin can cause mild hematologic toxicity (117). Leukopenia and thrombocytopenia (onset, 6 to 26 days) may occur. Erythropoietin-responsive anemia can occur with prolonged therapy.

Hemolytic uremic syndrome is a rare complication of cisplatin, bleomycin, or vincristine therapy and is frequently fatal in patients older than 50 years of age with squamous cell cancers (72).

Diagnostic Tests

Laboratory monitoring with each treatment should include CBC, electrolytes, and kidney function. Uric acid, hearing function, and neurologic function should be tested periodically. Pure-tone threshold audiometry (or auditory brainstem response in young children) should be done before the first dose of cisplatin, after the first dose, and at regular intervals thereafter, especially after reaching a cumulative dose of 360 mg/m^2.

Treatment

See Antineoplastic Treatment Guidelines at the end of this chapter. Hemodialysis used to clear platinum after renal insufficiency due to an accidental cisplatin dosage of 205 mg/m^2 instead of 100 mg/m^2 was of "limited usefulness" (118). A 48-year-old man received a massive cisplatin toxic overdose (400 mg/m^2 of cisplatin over 4 days) without IV hydration. From day 5 to 19, he underwent nine cycles of plasma exchange, which reduced his plasma cisplatin concentration from 2470 ng/ml to 216 ng/ml. He recovered without sequelae. There are no previous reports of survival without complication after a high cisplatin dosage without hydration (119).

No proven antidotes have been established. An accidental overdose in a child resulting in acute renal failure was managed successfully with sodium thiosulfate (120). Cisplatin-induced renal toxicity was possibly reversed by *N*-acetylcysteine treatment in another (121). A combination of ondansetron, dexamethasone, and lorazepam provided better emetic control with fewer adverse reactions than metoclopramide, dexamethasone, and lorazepam in the acute nausea and vomiting phase after receiving cisplatin (122). After ondansetron failure, another 5FT(3)-receptor antagonist, granisetron, may be used instead (123).

CLADRIBINE

Cladribine (2-chlorodeoxyadenosine) is used to treat hairy cell leukemia, AML, CLL, CML, cutaneous T-cell lymphoma, Sézary syndrome, non-Hodgkin's lymphoma, and Waldenström's macroglobulinemia.

Typical adult dosing regimens range from 0.09 to 0.1 mg/kg/day IV for 7 days or 4.0 to 8.9 mg/m^2/day for 5 to 7 days every 4 to 5 weeks. In children, dosing is 6.2 to 8.9 mg/m^2/day for 5 days by continuous infusion.

Toxicokinetics and Toxicodynamics

Oral absorption is minimal as the drug is acid labile. Bioavailability is 34% to 48%. The drug crosses the blood–brain barrier to 25% of plasma levels. The V_d is 9.2 L/kg, and plasma protein binding is 20% (3). Metabolism of prodrug, activated by intracellular phosphorylation, produces the active metabolite 2-chloro-2'-deoxy-β-D-adenosine triphosphate (CdATP). From 10% to 30% is excreted in urine. The alpha half-life is 3 to 35 minutes, and the beta half-life is 5.4 to 14.2 hours.

Pathophysiology

Cladribine is structurally related to fludarabine. It is phosphorylated to its corresponding nucleotide, CdATP, which accumulates and is incorporated into the DNA of cells such as lymphocytes. CdATP leads to DNA strand breaks, inhibition of DNA synthesis, and cell death. Unlike other antimetabolite drugs, cladribine has cytotoxic effects on resting as well as proliferating lymphocytes (124).

Pregnancy and Lactation

Cladribine is FDA pregnancy risk category D (Appendix I). Breast-feeding is not recommended (125).

Clinical Presentation

Immediate effects may include increased uric acid levels. Early effects include myelosuppression (nadir, 7 to 14 days; recovery, 28 to 56 days), fever, fatigue, mild nausea, rash, headache, injection site reactions, immunosuppression, and renal impairment. Delayed effects may include fatigue, rash, headache, immunosuppression, and nerve problems (paraparesis, quadriparesis, 35% with bone marrow transplant doses) (3).

Cumulative myelotoxicity and prolonged thrombocytopenia can occur after multiple cycles. Pancytopenia occurs in 20% of patients with mycosis fungoides. Cladribine can cause a reduction in CD4 (helper) and CD8 (suppressor) T lymphocytes, which can last for years. Fever is common in hairy cell leukemia patients but appears to correspond to the time of maximal cell lysis rather than a direct reaction. Fever does not usually occur when cladribine is used for other malignancies.

High-dose cladribine, in conjunction with cyclophosphamide and total body radiation in preparation for bone marrow transplantation, has been associated with severe, irreversible neurologic toxicity (paraparesis, quadriparesis) and acute renal impairment (some patients required dialysis).

Diagnostic Tests

Diagnostic testing is aimed at assessing end organ effects (e.g., bone marrow). Laboratory monitoring with each treatment should include CBC, electrolytes, kidney function, and uric acid (repeat during infusion). Specific levels of cladribine are not used to guide clinical management.

Treatment

See Antineoplastic Treatment Guidelines at the end of this chapter. Infections are common (lungs and venous access sites), and septicemia has been reported. Hairy cell leukemia patients with pancytopenia and especially lymphopenia appear to be at increased risk.

CYCLOPHOSPHAMIDE

Cyclophosphamide is a nitrogen mustard–alkylating agent used to treat ALL, AML, breast cancer, CLL, CML, Ewing's sarcoma, Hodgkin's disease, small cell lung cancer, multiple myeloma, mycosis fungoides, neuroblastoma, non-Hodgkin's lymphoma, rhabdomyosarcoma, osteogenic sarcoma, retinoblastoma, and soft tissue sarcoma. Other uses include pediatric brain tumors, ovarian cancer, testicular cancer, endometrial cancer, gestational trophoblastic tumors, and non–small cell lung cancer.

Adult oral dosing is typically 1 to 5 mg/kg/day or 60 to 120 $mg/m^2/day$ continuously, 40 to 50 mg/kg every 2 to 4 weeks (may be over 2 to 5 days), or 200 $mg/m^2/day$ for 4 days every 4 weeks. The IV dose ranges from 3 to 5 mg/kg twice weekly to 40 to 50 mg/kg every 2 to 4 weeks (may be over 2 to 5 days). Pediatric oral dosing is 150 $mg/m^2/day$ for 7 days every 3 weeks. An IV single dose is up to 2 g/m^2 and 600 to 1000 mg/m^2 every 2 to 8 weeks.

Toxicokinetics and Toxicodynamics

The oral bioavailability of cyclophosphamide is 75% to 100%. Distribution occurs to most tissues. It crosses the placenta and the blood–brain barrier and is present in breast milk and ascites. The V_d is 0.34 to 1.2 L/kg, and the plasma protein binding of parent drug is 12% to 14% (3).

Cyclophosphamide is mainly activated by the hepatic microsomal enzymes, and there is some activation peripherally as well. It is transformed to the active alkylating metabolites of acrolein and phosphoramide mustard. The kidney excretes drug and metabolites where some tubular reabsorption occurs. Its half-life is 4 to 10 hours in adults and 1.0 to 6.5 hours in children.

Pathophysiology

Cyclophosphamide is a cyclic phosphoramide ester of mechlorethamine. Cyclophosphamide causes prevention of cell division primarily by cross-linking DNA strands. It is cell cycle phase nonspecific (126,127).

Pregnancy and Lactation

Cyclophosphamide is FDA pregnancy risk category D (Appendix I). Cyclophosphamide is contraindicated in pregnancy due to a high risk of congenital malformations. A 29-year-old woman with ALL maintained remission with daily cyclophosphamide and intermittent prednisone treatment. She delivered a male twin with multiple congenital abnormalities who subsequently developed papillary thyroid cancer and stage III neuroblastoma (128). Adverse events, including neutropenia (129) and leukopenia (130), occurred in two infants exposed during breast-feeding. Breast-feeding should be terminated before use.

Clinical Presentation

Immediate effects include rare anaphylaxis, facial burning, nausea and vomiting, phlebitis, hyperuricemia, hemorrhagic cystitis, syndrome of inappropriate antidiuretic hormone secretions (SIADH), hyponatremia, and rare radiation recall reactions. Early effects may include myelosuppression (nadir, 8 to 15 days; recovery, 17 to 28 days), reversible alopecia, anorexia, rare stomatitis, skin problems (radiation recall reaction, rare; hyperpigmentation of skin or fingernails), interstitial pneumonitis, and rare cardiac necrosis. Delayed effects include hemorrhagic cystitis, interstitial pneumonitis, pulmonary fibrosis, and fertility problems (e.g., amenorrhea, azoospermia). Secondary malignancies including bladder cancer, nonlymphocytic leukemia, and non-Hodgkin's lymphoma have developed (3).

Dose-related hemorrhagic cystitis occurs due to direct contact with bladder mucosa of active and toxic metabolites that accumulate in concentrated urine (131). This occurs in 10% of patients receiving chronic low-dose or intermittent high-dose cyclophosphamide and may occur during treatment or several months after treatment. Hemorrhagic cystitis occurs in more than 40% of patients receiving high-dose cyclophosphamide for bone marrow transplantation (3).

Unless contraindicated, hydration and diuresis to maintain high urine flow should be provided prophylactically. Mesna is used to treat this complication (132). Concurrent or previous pelvic radiation therapy may increase the risk of this complication. Grade II–IV graft-versus-host disease, use of busulfan, and younger age at transplant were related to an increased risk of hemorrhagic cystitis after bone marrow transplantation (133). Children appear to be at higher risk of hemorrhagic cystitis, but this may be due to the relatively high doses given to children.

Interstitial pneumonitis (134) and pulmonary fibrosis occur occasionally. Discontinuation of cyclophosphamide and treatment with corticosteroids are followed by clinical recovery in approximately 50% of patients and, in some cases, reversal of the lung injury (135). Pulmonary fibrosis may be fatal. Lung biopsy is the only sure method of diagnosis.

Administration of cyclophosphamide in doses higher than 30 to 40 mg/kg has been associated with water retention and dilutional hyponatremia (136). Children may be especially susceptible. Decreased urine flow, decreased serum osmolarity, and increased urine osmolarity occur 4 to 12 hours after cyclophosphamide and resolve within 24 hours.

Cardiac toxicity (e.g., hemorrhagic necrosis) can occur (137,138), especially with high doses used in preparing patients for marrow transplantation (greater than 120 mg/kg). Concomitant doxorubicin or daunorubicin therapy and radiation to cardiac vessels or heart are risk factors. Clinical signs include dyspnea, tachypnea, fluid retention, increased systemic venous pressure, and shock.

Cyclophosphamide may enhance radiation injury to tissues. Although termed *radiation recall reactions*, the timing of the radiation may be before, concurrent with, or even after cyclophosphamide administration. Recurrent injury to a previously radiated site may occur weeks to months following the radiation.

Testicular atrophy and sterility may occur in males (139). Amenorrhea and ovarian failure may occur in women. Gonadal dysfunction may reverse with time, but future reproductive capacity is uncertain.

Diagnostic Tests

Testing is aimed at assessing the end organ effects (e.g., bone marrow, cardiac, lung, gonadal). Laboratory monitoring with each treatment should include CBC, electrolytes, and kidney function. Specific levels of cyclophosphamide are not used to guide management.

Treatment

See Antineoplastic Treatment Guidelines at the end of this chapter. Prophylactic measures to reduce hemorrhagic cystitis include catheter bladder drainage, bladder irrigation, hyperhydration, forced diuresis, and the administration of mesna. Cyclophosphamide should be given early in the day to decrease the amount of drug remaining in the bladder overnight. The drug should not be used in patients developing this complication.

Several methods to treat hematuria are currently advocated, depending on the severity (140). Mild cases are treated with saline or water bladder irrigation. Intravesical instillation of astringents [e.g., alum (141,142) or silver nitrate (143)] or systemic administration of antifibrinolytics may be effective. For moderate bladder hemorrhage, cystoscopy is used to evacuate bladder clots and continuous bladder irrigation instituted to prevent recurrent clot formation.

Following cystoscopy for severe hematuria, treatment may require intravesical formalin (144), phenol (145), or intravesical prostaglandin (146) and may proceed to surgical intervention. Electrocautery (147), hyperbaric oxygen (148,149), yttrium-aluminum-garnet laser (150), cryosurgery, vasopressin (151), diversion of urine flow (152,153), hypogastric artery ligation, and cystectomy (154) have all been advocated.

Hyperuricemia during periods of active cell lysis can be minimized with allopurinol and hydration. In hospitalized patients, the urine may be alkalinized if tumor lysis is expected (3).

CYTARABINE

Cytarabine (cytosine arabinoside, Ara C) is used to treat AML, meningeal leukemia, ALL, CML, erythroleukemia, Burkitt's lymphoma, and non-Hodgkin's lymphoma.

The usual IV induction dose range in adults is 100 to 200 mg/m^2/day for 5 to 10 days every 2 to 4 weeks or 2 to 6 mg/kg/day for 5 to 10 days every 2 to 4 weeks. Maintenance dose is 1.0 to 1.5 mg/kg IM/SQ every 1 to 4 weeks. High-dose applications may use 2000 to 3000 mg/m^2 every 12 hours for 4 to 12 doses every 2 to 3 weeks. Cytarabine is also administered intrathecally. In children, IV schedules include 75 to 150 mg/m^2/day for 5 days every 4 weeks. The SQ dose is 150 mg/m^2/day IV/SQ infusion for 5 days, and high dose is 1 to 3 g/m^2/dose every 12 hours for 4 to 12 doses.

Accidental administration of 200-mg cytarabine intrathecally to a 4-year-old boy caused dilated pupils during the first hour. CSF exchange with isotonic saline was started 1 hour after overdose, and approximately 27% of the administered dose was recovered (155). One month later, an unsteady gait and mild intention tremor in his hands were noted.

Adverse effects from high-dose cytarabine (2 to 3 g/m^2) are qualitatively similar but quantitatively different from usual doses of cytarabine. Severe and occasionally fatal CNS, GI, or pulmonary toxicity may occur.

Toxicokinetics and Toxicodynamics

Cytarabine is poorly absorbed orally. Bioavailability is less than 20%. Cytarabine is rapidly and widely distributed and crosses the placenta and the blood–brain barrier. The V_d is 31.9 L/kg, and plasma protein binding is 13% (3). Cytarabine is rapidly and extensively metabolized by cytidine deaminases in the liver and kidneys; 70% to 80% is cleared in the urine within 24 hours (7% to 8% as intact drug) after IV use (3).

Pathophysiology

Cytarabine is metabolized intracellularly into its active form, cytosine arabinoside triphosphate. This metabolite damages DNA by multiple mechanisms, including the inhibition of alpha-DNA polymerase, inhibition of DNA repair through an effect on beta-DNA polymerase, and incorporation into DNA. The latter mechanism is probably the most important (4,5).

Pregnancy and Lactation

Cytarabine is FDA pregnancy risk category D (Appendix I). There are many case reports of normal babies after first-trimester exposure (156); however, at least two malformations have been reported (157). Breast-feeding is not recommended (158).

Clinical Presentation

Immediate effects include rare anaphylaxis, hyperuricemia, cerebellar toxicity, cerebral dysfunction, and seizures. CNS toxicity after intrathecal treatment may include arachnoiditis, seizures, and paraplegia. Other effects include nausea and vomiting, a flu-like syndrome, and injection site pain and thrombophlebitis. Early effects may include myelosuppression (first nadir, 7 to 9 days; second nadir, 15 to 24 days; recovery, 25 to 34 days), pulmonary edema, conjunctivitis, stomatitis, alopecia, hematemesis, diarrhea, abdominal pain, hepatotoxicity, rare peripheral neuropathy, rash, freckling, and megaloblastosis. Infertility may be a late sequela (3).

Cerebellar toxicity (dysarthria, dysdiadochokinesia, dysmetria, and ataxia) (159,160) occurs in approximately 10% of patients treated with high doses of cytarabine. Cerebral dysfunction (somnolence, confusion, memory loss, psychosis, or seizures) often occurs concurrently. Seizures are usually self-limited and do not recur once therapy is stopped (161). In most patients, neurologic dysfunction resolves in 5 to 10 days, but may be irreversible or fatal. There is a high incidence of recurrent cerebellar toxicity in patients with a previous episode. Intrathecal cytarabine may cause arachnoiditis (162) and myelopathic syndromes. Adverse effects associated with intrathecal use include nausea and vomiting, headache, fever, paresthesias, and seizures (163).

Conjunctivitis may occur with high doses (3 g/m^2) and can be minimized by prophylactic use of ophthalmic corticosteroids (164). Although even low doses can increase LFTs, high-dose regimens can cause hepatotoxicity (165). Significant liver injury may require discontinuation.

Noncardiogenic pulmonary edema has been reported (166). Pulmonary insufficiency from high-dose Ara-C varies in severity and may be fatal (167).

Diagnostic Tests

Testing is aimed at assessing end organ effects (e.g., bone marrow, liver, lung, brain, gonadal). Laboratory monitoring during treatment should include CBC, electrolytes, and kidney function. Periodically, uric acid and liver function should be followed. Specific levels of cytarabine are not used to guide management.

Treatment

See Antineoplastic Treatment Guidelines at the end of this chapter. High-dose steroids have been used to treat cytarabine-induced pulmonary edema (168).

DACARBAZINE

Dacarbazine is used to treat Hodgkin's disease, malignant melanoma, neuroblastoma, and soft tissue sarcomas. The usual dose in adults is 375 mg/m^2 IV every 15 days, 850 mg/m^2 every 3 to 4 weeks, 2.0 to 4.5 mg/kg/day for 10 days every 3 weeks. In children, typical IV dose regimens are 375 mg/m^2 every 2 weeks and 750 mg/m^2 every 6 to 8 weeks.

Toxicokinetics and Toxicodynamics

Oral absorption is erratic, slow, and incomplete. Less than 15% crosses the blood–brain barrier. The V_d is 0.63 L/kg, and plasma protein binding is less than 5%. Dacarbazine is oxidized by hepatic enzymes into active metabolites. The major inactive metabolite is amino imidazole carboxamide. Excretion is subject to renal tubular secretion (30% to 45% in urine within 6 hours, 50% as amino imidazole carboxamide). Alpha half-life is 3 minutes, and beta half-life is 0.58 to 0.68 hours (3).

Pathophysiology

Dacarbazine is an imidazole carboxamide derivative with structural similarity to certain purines. Its primary mode of action appears to be alkylation of nucleic acids. Dacarbazine is cell cycle phase nonspecific (4,5).

Pregnancy and Lactation

Dacarbazine is FDA pregnancy risk category C (Appendix I). Healthy babies have been born to mothers treated during pregnancy (169). Its safe use in pregnancy and its effects on fertility have not been established. Breast-feeding is not recommended (170,171).

Clinical Presentation

Immediate effects may include rare anaphylaxis, phlebitis, frequent nausea and vomiting, occasional diarrhea, facial flushing, facial paresthesia, and photosensitivity. Early effects may include myelosuppression (nadir, 16 to 28 days; recovery, 21 to 35 days); flu-like symptoms; liver problems (e.g., rare, elevated LFTs, veno-occlusive disease, allergic vasculitis); kidney problems (e.g., increased blood urea nitrogen and rare renal impairment); and reversible alopecia (3).

Nausea and vomiting occur in most patients and are most severe on the first day. Hepatic veno-occlusive disease and Budd-Chiari syndrome have been fatal complications (172,173). A flu-like syndrome (fever, myalgia, and malaise) occurs in less than 10% of patients, starting 2 to 7 days after treatment and lasting 7 to 21 days, especially after large doses.

A 44-year-old woman patient developed recall dermatitis due to dacarbazine in a site previously irradiated for the treatment of malignant melanoma (174).

Diagnostic Tests

Testing is aimed at assessing the end organ effects (e.g., bone marrow, liver, kidney). Laboratory monitoring during treatment should include CBC, electrolytes, and kidney function. Specific levels of cytarabine are not used for management.

Treatment

See Antineoplastic Treatment Guidelines at the end of this chapter. The use of prophylactic and continuing antiemetic medication is generally necessary.

DAUNORUBICIN

Daunorubicin is an antitumor, anthracycline antibiotic used to treat ALL, acute non-lymphocytic leukemia, CML, Ewing's sarcoma, Hodgkin's disease, non-Hodgkin's lymphoma, Wilms' tumor, and rhabdomyosarcoma.

Typical adult regimens include 1 to 2 mg/kg/day IV for 3 to 12 days and 30 to 60 mg/m^2/day for 3 to 12 days. In children, schedules include 60 mg/m^2/day IV for 2 days and 20 mg/m^2/day for 4 days every 10 days for 2 courses, then every 3 weeks.

A 3.5-year-old girl with ALL was inadvertently given a 17-mg intrathecal injection of daunorubicin. She died despite CSF exchange, drainage, and supportive care (175).

Risk factors for daunorubicin-induced congestive heart failure (CHF) are high cumulative dose, thoracic radiation, preexisting heart disease, and prior anthracycline therapy (176). Clinical cardiotoxicity in children increases rapidly at a cumulative dose of 450 mg/m^2, but individual patients may have a lower threshold and develop toxicity at a significantly lower dose.

Toxicokinetics and Toxicodynamics

Daunorubicin is not orally absorbed. Distribution after IV infusion is rapid with highest levels appearing in liver, kidneys, lungs, spleen, heart, and small intestine. V_d is 20 to 39 L/kg, and plasma protein binding is 50% to 60%.

Metabolism in liver and other tissues produces active metabolites, including daunorubicinol, as well as inactive metabolites. Hepatobiliary secretion in feces is the predominant route of elimination (40%) with 14% to 23% excreted in urine within 3 days. The alpha half-life is 45 to 180 minutes, and the beta half-life is 20 to 30 hours (3).

Pathophysiology

Daunorubicin damages DNA by intercalation of the anthracycline portion, metal ion chelation, or by generation of free radicals. Daunorubicin also inhibits DNA polymerases and affects regulation of gene expression. Cytotoxic activity is cell cycle phase nonspecific (126,177).

Pregnancy and Lactation

Daunorubicin is FDA pregnancy risk category D (Appendix I). A normal baby was born to a woman with acute promyelocytic leukemia treated with daunorubicin from the ninth week of gestation (178). Breast-feeding is not recommended (3).

Clinical Presentation

Immediate effects may include anaphylaxis (rare), pain during injection, facial flushing, flare reaction due to histamine release, frequent nausea and vomiting, reddish urine discoloration (lasts 1 to 2 days), rare radiation recall reaction, skin rash and fever, irregular heartbeat, and hyperuricemia. Early effects may include myelosuppression (nadir, 6 to 13 days; recovery, 21 to 24 days), stomatitis, alopecia, diarrhea, hyperpigmentation, and nail changes.

Cardiomyopathy and CHF may occur in weeks to months following use (3). Cardiac toxicity is cumulative across the anthracycline (doxorubicin, epirubicin, idarubicin, daunorubicin) and anthracenedione (mitoxantrone) families. Toxicity is divided into early, non–dose-related ECG abnormalities in 1% of patients and cumulative dose-dependent cardiomyopathy. Early ECG changes are reversible and do not indicate impending cardiomyopathy. Diminished QRS voltage may be dose-related. The mortality associated with CHF can reach 79%.

Tissue necrosis from extravasation may occur days to weeks after treatment.

Daunorubicin has the potential to enhance radiation injury. Radiation recall reactions may occur before, concurrently, or even weeks to months after daunorubicin treatment.

Diagnostic Tests

Testing is aimed at assessing end organ effects (e.g., bone marrow). Laboratory monitoring during treatment should include CBC, electrolytes, and kidney function. Specific levels of daunorubicin are not used to guide management.

An echocardiogram (ECHO) should be done at 3, 6, and 12 months following therapy, with radionucleotide angiocardiography as a confirmatory test, if possible, at 12 months following therapy. For children receiving anthracyclines, it is recommended that monitoring include ECHO or radionucleotide angiocardiography as baseline (179). ECHO should be repeated before each course of anthracycline when the cumulative dose is less than 300 mg/m^2. ECHO (or radionucleotide angiocardiography) should be done before each course of anthracycline when the total cumulative dose is less than 300 mg/m^2, and mediastinal radiation is greater than 1000 rads. ECHO and radionucleotide angiocardiography should be done before each course of anthracycline when the total course is 400 mg/m^2.

Treatment

See Antineoplastic Treatment Guidelines at the end of this chapter. Daunorubicin-induced CHF is managed by discontinuation of drug and standard CHF treatment. Pediatric patients with daunorubicin-induced CHF are very sensitive to digitalis. The total digitalizing dose required is 0.01 to 0.02 mg/kg of digoxin with a maintenance less than one-fourth of the original dose.

Cardiomyopathy has been successfully treated with angiotensin converting enzyme inhibitors (180). Experimental work on cardiac prophylaxis includes possible protection by razoxane (ICRF-159), dexrazoxane (ICRF-187) (181), adenosine, dextran conjugation (182), and pretreatment with cardiac glycoside.

DOXORUBICIN

Doxorubicin (Adriamycin) is an anthracycline antineoplastic used to treat ALL, AML, acute non-lymphocytic leukemia, breast cancer, Ewing's sarcoma, Hodgkin's disease, small cell lung cancer, non-Hodgkin's lymphoma, osteogenic sarcoma, ovarian cancer, rhabdomyosarcoma, and soft tissue sarcomas. It has been used on many other malignancies as well.

Typical adult IV regimens are 60 to 90 mg/m^2 every 3 to 4 weeks and 20 to 30 mg/m^2 every week. Intraarterial dosing is 25 mg/m^2/day for 3 days every 3 to 4 weeks. Intravesical dosing is 40 to 80 mg every 3 to 4 weeks. In children, IV dosing is 45 to 75 mg/m^2 every 3 to 8 weeks, and intraarterial dosing is 20 to 30 mg/m^2/day for 3 days.

The risk of cardiotoxicity with doxorubicin increases with total dose. Cardiomyopathy may be fatal (183). The incidence of CHF is 0.1% to 1.2% with a cumulative dose of less than 550 mg/m^2 in contrast to 30% with a cumulative dose above 550 mg/m^2. Continuous infusion may be safer than bolus doses (184). Patients who have reached 450 mg/m^2 with their tumors responding should have careful cardiac assessment before continuing treatment. Children younger than 15 years of age appear more likely to develop CHF from cumulative doses above 550 mg/m^2.

Patients who have received prior mediastinal radiotherapy (specifically to the heart) should not receive a total cumulative dose greater than 300 mg/m^2. Enhancement of radiation injury to the esophagus and GI tract is most severe when the drug and radiation are given concomitantly.

Toxicokinetics and Toxicodynamics

Doxorubicin is not absorbed orally. Highest concentrations are found in liver, spleen, kidney, heart, small intestines, and lung. It crosses the placenta and is found in breast milk. The V_d is 25 L/kg, and plasma protein binding is 79% to 85% (3).

The liver is the major site of doxorubicin metabolism. Active metabolites include doxorubicinol. Elimination is primarily via the biliary system with 40% to 50% appearing in feces within 7 days; 4% to 5% appears in urine over 5 days. The alpha half-life is 12 minutes, beta half-life is 3.3 hours, and gamma half-life is 29.6 hours (3).

Pathophysiology

Daunorubicin and its 14-hydroxy derivative, doxorubicin, are anthracycline antibiotics. Doxorubicin damages DNA by intercalation of the anthracycline portion, metal ion chelation, or generation of free radicals. Doxorubicin inhibits DNA cleavage and inhibits DNA and RNA synthesis by intercalating between DNA base pairs. Doxorubicin has also been shown to inhibit DNA topoisomerase II, which is critical to DNA function (3).

Pregnancy and Lactation

Doxorubicin is FDA pregnancy risk category D (Appendix I). Doxorubicin has been shown to have mutagenic and carcinogenic properties in experimental models. Its safe use in pregnancy and its effects on fertility have not been established. In one report, low levels of doxorubicin were found in breast milk although infant outcome was not known (111). Breast-feeding is not recommended (185).

Clinical Presentation

Immediate effects include anaphylaxis (rare), pain during injection, phlebitis, facial flushing, flare reaction due to histamine release, nausea, vomiting, diarrhea, reddish urine discoloration (lasts 1 to 2 days), rare radiation recall reaction, irregular heartbeat, and hyperuricemia. Acute encephalopathy, dysuria, gait disturbances, coma, seizures, mydriasis, myelotoxicity, mucositis, and elevated CSF protein levels have been observed with its use. Early effects include myelosuppression (nadir, 6 to 13 days; recovery, 21 to 24 days), stomatitis, conjunctivitis, alopecia, diarrhea, rash, fever, and chills. Delayed effects include cardiomyopathy, CHF, hyperpigmentation, nail changes, and infertility (3).

Cardiac toxicity is cumulative across the anthracycline (doxorubicin, epirubicin, daunorubicin, idarubicin) and anthracenedione (mitoxantrone) families. Cumulative doses required to produce cardiac toxicity are lower in patients who have received radiation to the mediastinal area or therapy with other cardiotoxic agents such as cyclophosphamide (186).

Cardiotoxicity can be divided into an acute effect with transient ECG abnormalities and a later cumulative, dose-dependent cardiomyopathy. Acute ECG changes are usually reversible, unrelated to total dose, return to baseline readings within a few days to two months, and not an indication to discontinue the doxorubicin. The mortality rate for cardiomyopathy (0.4% to 9.0% of all patients) is as high as 61%. Risk factors include total dose, schedule, increased age, preexisting cardiac disease, mediastinal radiotherapy, and antineoplastic drugs. The onset of cardiomyopathy may be delayed 6 months or more after therapy (3).

Doxorubicin flare reactions (red streaking along the vein) generally resolve within 45 minutes (187). The injection may be continued, more slowly in the same site, or may be changed to another site. Tissue necrosis following extravasation may happen days to weeks after treatment.

Doxorubicin has the potential to enhance radiation injury to tissues (188). *Radiation recall reactions* may occur before, concurrent with, or even after doxorubicin (189). The skin is most commonly affected, resulting in erythema followed by dry desquamation. Skin reactions generally occur only if the drug is given within 7 days of the radiation.

Diagnostic Tests

Testing is aimed at end organ effects (e.g., bone marrow, heart, heart). Laboratory monitoring during treatment should include CBC, electrolytes, and kidney function. Specific levels of doxorubicin are not used to guide management. Cardiac monitoring should be performed as described in the Daunorubicin section. Early decline in left ventricular ejection fraction predicts cardiotoxicity in lymphoma patients (190).

Treatment

See Antineoplastic Treatment Guidelines at the end of this chapter. Diphenhydramine 25 mg (1 mg/kg/dose in children), or hydrocortisone 100 mg (1 mg/kg/dose in children), by slow IV push may hasten clearing of the *daunorubicin flare* reaction.

Management of CHF is discontinuation of drug and standard CHF treatment. Pediatric patients with CHF are sensitive to digitalis. The total digitalizing dose required is 0.01 to 0.02 mg/kg of digoxin with maintenance less than one-fourth of the original dose.

Cardiomyopathy has been successfully treated with angiotensin converting enzyme inhibitors (180). Experimental work on cardiac prophylaxis includes possible protection by razoxane (ICRF-159), dexrazoxane (ICRF-187) (181), dextran conjugation (182), adenosine, probucol (191), and pretreatment with cardiac glycosides.

ETOPOSIDE

Etoposide (VP-16) is a semisynthetic podophyllotoxin used to treat ALL, AML, germ cell tumors, Hodgkin's disease, small cell or non–small cell lung cancer, non-Hodgkin's lymphoma, gestational trophoblastic tumors, retinoblastoma, testicular cancer, brain tumors, Ewing's sarcoma, histiocytosis X, Kaposi's sarcoma, neuroblastoma, ovarian cancer, gestational trophoblastic disease, vasculitis, and rhabdomyosarcoma.

Typical oral adult regimens include 120 to 200 mg/m^2/day for 5 days every 3 to 4 weeks and 50 to 100 mg daily for 1 to 2 months. The IV regimens include 35 to 150 mg/m^2/day for 3 to 5 days every 2 to 5 weeks. The bone marrow transplantation dose is 1200 to 2400 mg/m^2. In children, the IV dose is 100 to 150 mg/m^2/day for 3 to 5 days every 3 to 4 weeks.

Overdose may lead to decreased leukocyte counts, T lymphocytes, and blast transformation. Delayed toxicity may manifest as rash, alopecia, peripheral neuropathy, mucositis, and leukemia.

Toxicokinetics and Toxicodynamics

Oral absorption is approximately 50%. Bioavailability is variable. Bioavailability of low oral doses of 100 mg may be better than higher doses. Drug is widely distributed to saliva, liver, spleen, kidneys, cardiac tissue, and brain tumor tissue. The V_d is 0.36 L/kg, and plasma protein binding is 94% (3).

Metabolism to active and inactive metabolites occurs in the liver. The primary route of elimination is renal (42% to 88% within 48 hours, 67% as unchanged drug), and 0% to 16% is recovered in the feces. Alpha half-life after IV use is 1.5 hours and 0.44 hours after oral use. Beta half-life after IV use is 4 to 11 hours and 6.8 hours after oral use (3).

Pathophysiology

Etoposide causes single-strand DNA breaks. Etoposide also causes DNA damage through inhibition of topoisomerase II and activation of oxidation-reduction reactions to produce derivatives that bind to DNA (4,5).

Pregnancy and Lactation

Etoposide is FDA pregnancy risk category D (Appendix I). Breast-feeding is not recommended (192).

Clinical Presentation

Immediate effects include anaphylaxis, phlebitis, nausea and vomiting, hypotension with rapid IV infusion, rash (193), and palmar erythema (194) with high dose. Early effects include myelosuppression (nadir, 7 to 14 days; recovery, 20 to 28 days), reversible alopecia, stomatitis, anorexia, rare peripheral neuropathy, elevated LFTs, and acidosis with high doses. Leukemia is a recognized late effect (3).

Anaphylactoid reactions occur in 0.7% to 2.0% of patients. Signs include chest discomfort, dyspnea, bronchospasm, and hypotension (195). Fewer hypersensitivity reactions may occur if the infusion rate is slow (i.e., over at least 30 minutes). Rare cases of hypersensitivity reactions occurring months after use have been recorded (196).

Stomatitis and mucositis (197) are likely to occur in patients treated with radiation to the head and neck region and have been the dose-limiting toxicity on high-dose etoposide protocols. Adverse GI effects are more common following oral use. Hepatitis has been reported following standard-dose treatments of etoposide (198).

The development of Lhermitte's sign accompanied by cervical motor neuropathy, dorsal column myelopathy, and sensory neuropathy has been reported in a patient treated with cisplatin and etoposide for small cell lung cancer (199).

The use of etoposide has been associated with secondary AML and myelodysplastic syndrome (200,201). Once weekly or twice weekly dosing schedules show a higher risk than less frequent dosing.

Ultraviolet recall or sunburn reactivation is an infrequently reported phenomenon. It is an erythematous eruption in the distribution of previous ultraviolet-induced sunburn. The case of a young man who developed ultraviolet recall after treatment with etoposide (VP-16) and cyclophosphamide has been reported (202).

Diagnostic Tests

Testing is aimed at end organ effects (e.g., bone marrow, heart). Laboratory monitoring during treatment should include CBC, electrolytes, and kidney function. Specific levels of etoposide are not used to guide management.

Treatment

See Antineoplastic Treatment Guidelines at the end of this chapter. If a hypersensitivity reaction occurs, etoposide should be discontinued and vasopressor, corticosteroids, antihistamines, or plasma volume expanders administered. Patients can be rechallenged.

FLOXURIDINE

Floxuridine, an antineoplastic antimetabolite, is effective in the palliative management of GI adenocarcinoma metastatic to the liver when given by continuous regional intraarterial infusion in carefully selected patients who are considered incurable by other means (203,204).

The dosage schedule of floxuridine by continuous arterial infusion is 0.1 to 0.6 mg/kg/day. The higher dosage ranges are usually used for hepatic artery infusion because the liver metabolizes the drug, thus reducing the potential for systemic toxicity. Safety and effectiveness in pediatric patients have not been established.

Toxicokinetics and Toxicodynamics

When floxuridine is given by rapid intraarterial injection, it is rapidly catabolized to 5-fluorouracil (5-FU) (205). Rapid injection of floxuridine produces the same toxic and antimetabolic effects as 5-FU. Floxuridine is metabolized in the liver.

Pathophysiology

Floxuridine and its metabolite, 5-FU, act by three main mechanisms. Principally, the intermediate metabolite fluorodeoxyuridine monophosphate inhibits an important enzyme in pyrimidine biosynthesis, namely thymidylate synthase. 5-FU is also metabolized to ribo- and deoxy-ribonucleotides, which act as false bases for incorporation into RNA and DNA (206).

Pregnancy and Lactation

Floxuridine is FDA pregnancy risk category D (Appendix I). It is not known whether floxuridine is excreted in human milk (207). Breast-feeding is not recommended.

Clinical Presentation

Adverse reactions to floxuridine are generally related to the procedural complications of regional arterial infusion. The more common adverse reactions to the drug are nausea, vomiting, diarrhea, enteritis, stomatitis, and localized erythema. GI effects may include vomiting, diarrhea, enteritis, stomatitis (208), duodenal ulcer, duodenitis, gastritis, bleeding, gastroenteritis, glossitis, pharyngitis, anorexia, cramps, abdominal pain, and possible intra- and extrahepatic biliary sclerosis (209), as well as acalculous cholecystitis.

Dermatologic effects may include alopecia, dermatitis, nonspecific skin toxicity, and rash. Other effects include myocardial ischemia, fever, lethargy, malaise, and weakness.

Diagnostic Tests

More common laboratory abnormalities are anemia, leukopenia, thrombocytopenia, and elevations of alkaline phosphatase, serum transaminase, serum bilirubin, and lactic dehydrogenase. Patients who have been exposed to an overdosage of floxuridine should be monitored hematologically for at least 4 weeks.

Treatment

See Antineoplastic Treatment Guidelines at the end of this chapter.

FLUDARABINE

Fludarabine is used as a second-line agent for advanced CLL, hairy cell leukemia, non-Hodgkin's lymphomas, mycosis fungoides, and Waldenström's macroglobulinemia.

Typical adult IV regimens include 18 to 30 mg/m^2/day for 5 days every 4 weeks and 20 mg/m^2 bolus followed by 30 mg/m^2/day for 2 days as continuous infusion every 4 weeks. In children, the IV loading dose is 8 mg/m^2, then 23.5 mg/m^2/day for 5 days as continuous infusion.

Toxicokinetics and Toxicodynamics

Oral bioavailability is 70%. The V_d is 44 to 96 L/m^2 in adults and 10.8 L/m^2 in children (3).

Fludarabine is rapidly dephosphorylated to the active metabolite F-Ara-ATP, which is necessary for cellular uptake. The peak concentration of F-Ara-ATP in leukemia cells is achieved 4 hours after start of fludarabine infusion (210). Most excretion is via the kidneys (41% to 60%). The half-life is 0.6 to 1.64 hours. In children, the alpha half-life is 1.6 hours.

Pathophysiology

Fludarabine is metabolized to F-Ara-ATP, which inhibits DNA polymerases and prevents elongation of DNA strands through direct incorporation into DNA (211).

Pregnancy and Lactation

Fludarabine is FDA pregnancy risk category D (Appendix I). Breast-feeding is not recommended.

Clinical Presentation

Immediate effects may include nausea and vomiting, fever in most patients, chills, fatigue, rash, and hyperuricemia. Early effects include myelosuppression (nadir, 13 to 16 days; recovery, 37 to 45 days), diarrhea, stomatitis, and increased LFTs. Rare peripheral neuropathy can be late sequelae as can interstitial pneumonitis (3).

The major causes of morbidity associated with fludarabine in CLL are infections and febrile episodes (212). These occur more frequently in previously treated patients and those with advanced disease. Cryptococcal meningitis has been reported after fludarabine therapy (213–215).

Myelosuppression is dose limiting, and a small proportion of CLL patients develop moderate to severe and, sometimes, protracted myelosuppression (216).

Progressive multifocal leukoencephalitis has been reported with standard doses in three CLL patients (217,218). Severe irreversible CNS effects, including blindness, coma, and death, may occur in patients receiving more than the recommended dose for CLL.

Fludarabine use in CLL patients has been associated with paraneoplastic pemphigus (219).

Diagnostic Tests

Testing is aimed at end organ effects (e.g., bone marrow, brain). Laboratory monitoring during treatment should include CBC, electrolytes, and kidney function. Neurologic assessment and LFTs are recommended periodically. Specific levels of fludarabine are not used to guide management.

Treatment

See Antineoplastic Treatment Guidelines at the end of this chapter.

FLUOROURACIL

5-FU is an antimetabolite agent used to treat colorectal, esophageal, gastric, hepatic, and breast cancers. Other uses include basal cell carcinoma, choriocarcinoma, bladder, cervical, endometrial, head and neck, non–small cell lung, pancreatic, prostate and ovarian cancers, as well as actinic keratosis and glaucoma (220).

An overdose of 5-FU may cause nausea, vomiting, diarrhea, GI ulceration, bleeding, and bone marrow depression. Life-threatening cardiotoxicity is manifested by atrial and ventricular dysrhythmias, CHF, myocardial ischemia, and sudden death.

Toxicokinetics and Toxicodynamics

Oral absorption is 28% to 100%. 5-FU distributes into body water, crosses the placenta, and is found in malignant effusions. Its V_d is 0.25 L/kg, and plasma protein binding is approximately 10% (3).

Approximately 80% of a dose is eliminated by the liver, 60% to 80% is excreted as carbon dioxide by the respiratory route, and 2% to 3% is excreted by the biliary system. The 5-FU half-life is 10 to 20 minutes (3).

Pathophysiology

5-FU is a fluorinated pyrimidine that is metabolized intracellularly to its active form, fluorodeoxyuridine monophosphate. Leucovorin is used to enhance the activity of 5-FU by stabilizing the bond of its active metabolite (5-fluorodeoxyuridine monophosphate) to the enzyme thymidylate synthetase. The active form inhibits DNA synthesis by inhibiting the normal production of thymidine (3).

Pregnancy and Lactation

5-FU is FDA pregnancy risk category D (Appendix I). Normal infants have been born after the use of 5-FU during pregnancy (221). Breast-feeding is not recommended (222).

Clinical Presentation

Immediate effects include rare anaphylaxis, phlebitis, nausea and vomiting, lacrimation, conjunctivitis, rare angina pectoris and ECG changes, rare radiation recall reaction, and erythema with topical use. Early effects include myelosuppression (nadir, 7 to 14 days; recovery, 22 to 24 days); stomatitis; diarrhea; alopecia; hyperpigmentation; photosensitivity; rash; nail changes; hand-foot syndrome; lacrimation; megaloblastosis; acute cerebellar syndrome; acute encephalopathy; and red, blistering skin with topical use. Delayed effects also include rare radiation recall reaction, tear duct fibrosis, and CNS problems (3).

Although cardiotoxicity associated with 5-FU administration is infrequent, there are reports of acute coronary syndromes. Acute myocardial infarction, ischemic ECG changes, and coronary vasospasm have been reported (137,223).

Excessive lacrimation occurs frequently. Transient blurred vision, eye irritation, and nasal discharge have also been reported (224). Eye symptoms may occur at any time during treatment. 5-FU has been demonstrated in tear fluid causing acute and chronic conjunctivitis that can lead to tear duct fibrosis. Ectropion secondary to bolus injection of 5-FU has been reported (225).

5-FU can cause acute and delayed neurotoxicity (encephalopathy or as cerebellar syndrome). Seizures are rare. Acute neurotoxicity due to 5-FU is dose related and self-limiting. A 44-year-old man developed 5-FU neurotoxicity with organic brain syndrome and progression to multifocal leukoencephalopathy (226). Acute cerebellar syndrome involves ataxia of the trunk or extremities, disturbance of gait and speech (227), coarse nystagmus, and dizziness. Ataxia syndrome is related to peak plasma 5-FU levels rather than cumulative dose (228).

Palmar-plantar erythrodysesthesia or hand-foot syndrome (229) has been noted with protracted and high-dose continuous 5-FU infusion. The syndrome begins with dysesthesia of the palms and soles that progresses to pain and tenderness associated with symmetric swelling and erythema (230). The syndrome resolves with cessation of drug infusion.

5-FU is associated with radiation recall reactions before, concurrent with, or even after 5-FU administration (3). When 5-FU is applied to a lesion, erythema is usually followed by vesiculation, erosion, ulceration, necrosis, and epithelization (231,232). The cream is preferably applied with a nonmetal applicator or glove. Allergic contact dermatitis has been reported (233,234).

Diagnostic Tests

Testing is aimed at end organ effects (e.g., bone marrow, heart, brain). Laboratory monitoring during treatment should include CBC, electrolytes, and kidney function. Neurologic assessment and LFTs are recommended periodically. Specific levels of 5-FU are not used to guide management.

Treatment

See Antineoplastic Treatment Guidelines at the end of this chapter. Treatment with 50 or 150 mg of pyridoxine daily is used to reverse the palmar-plantar erythrodysesthesia syndrome. If 5-FU is applied with the fingertips, the hands should be washed immediately. Frequent local reactions include pruritus, hyperpigmentation, and pain at the application site (235).

FLUTAMIDE

Flutamide is used to treat prostate cancer, acne, hirsutism, congenital adrenal hyperplasia, and polycystic ovary syndrome. The typical adult oral dose is 250 mg orally three times daily. Low-dose flutamide (125 mg/day) has been used to treat hirsutism. There are no pediatric indications. Doses up to 1500 mg/day for periods up to 36 weeks have produced gynecomastia, breast tenderness, and elevated aminotransferases. A dose of flutamide associated with symptoms of overdose or considered life-threatening has not been established.

Toxicokinetics and Toxicodynamics

Flutamide is well absorbed orally. Plasma protein binding is 94% to 96%. Flutamide is metabolized in the plasma, urine, and feces. Active metabolites include 2-hydroxyflutamide. Approximately 4% is excreted in feces within 72 hours, and 28% is excreted in urine in 24 hours. Its alpha half-life is 5 to 6 hours, and its beta half-life is approximately 10 hours.

Pathophysiology

Flutamide is a nonsteroidal antiandrogen that inhibits androgen uptake and nuclear binding of androgen in target tissues. As monotherapy, it increases plasma testosterone by blocking feedback inhibition of the hypothalamus and pituitary by testosterone. The increase does not occur when flutamide is used in combination with a luteinizing hormone releasing hormone (LHRH) agonist, nor in a previously orchiectomized patient (3).

Pregnancy and Lactation

Flutamide is FDA pregnancy risk category D (Appendix I).

Clinical Presentation

Immediate effects may include nausea and vomiting. Early effects may include breast swelling or soreness, galactorrhea, appetite or bowel changes, and fatigue. Late effects may include edema, thromboembolism, rare myocardial infarction, depression, elevated LFTs, rare blurred vision, and reduced sperm counts (3).

The most common adverse effect is gynecomastia (236), sometimes with galactorrhea. Flutamide apparently does not affect libido or potency. Toxic hepatitis has rarely been associated with flutamide (237–239). Diarrhea has been associated with flutamide as well (240). A photosensitive drug eruption was reported in a 68-year-old man treated with flutamide (241).

Diagnostic Tests

Testing is aimed at end organ effects (e.g., heart, liver). Laboratory monitoring during treatment should include CBC, electrolytes, and kidney function. LFTs are recommended periodically. Specific levels of flutamide are not used to guide management.

Treatment

See Antineoplastic Treatment Guidelines at the end of this chapter. Low-dose tamoxifen may be useful in treating painful gynecomastia for patients on flutamide/finasteride combination therapy (242).

GEMCITABINE

Gemcitabine, a pyrimidine analog, is an antimetabolite used to treat non–small cell lung, pancreatic, and bladder cancers. Other uses include breast, cervical, head and neck, small cell lung, and ovarian cancers, as well as cutaneous T-cell lymphoma, Hodgkin's lymphoma, and mesothelioma.

A typical adult dose is 1000 mg/m^2 on days 1, 8, and 15 of each 28-day cycle. Fatal pulmonary toxicity has been reported in patients receiving gemcitabine (243).

Toxicokinetics and Toxicodynamics

Gemcitabine is widely distributed and may be found in ascitic fluid. Its V_d within 70 minutes of infusion is 50 L/m^2 and 370 L/m^2 in 70 to 285 minutes. Plasma protein binding is less than 10% (3).

Gemcitabine is metabolized intracellularly by nucleoside kinases to the active metabolites gemcitabine diphosphate and gemcitabine triphosphate. It is also metabolized intracellularly and extracellularly by cytidine deaminase to the inactive metabolite difluorodeoxyuridine. Excretion after a single dose is mainly renal (92% to 98% in urine over 1 week; 89% as difluorodeoxyuridine, less than 10% as gemcitabine). The half-life is 0.7 to 1.6 hours (3).

Pathophysiology

Gemcitabine is metabolized to two active metabolites, gemcitabine diphosphate and gemcitabine triphosphate. The cytotoxic effects of gemcitabine are exerted through incorporation of gemcitabine triphosphate into DNA with the assistance of gemcitabine diphosphate, resulting in inhibition of DNA synthesis and induction of apoptosis. Gemcitabine is a radiation-sensitizing agent (3).

Pregnancy and Lactation

Gemcitabine is FDA pregnancy risk category D (Appendix I). Breast-feeding is not recommended (244).

Clinical Presentation

Hemolytic uremic syndrome occurs rarely after gemcitabine use (245,246). The syndrome can present either acutely with severe hemolysis, thrombocytopenia, and rapidly progressive renal failure or insidiously with mild or no thrombocytopenia and slowly progressive renal failure.

Gemcitabine causes transient and reversible elevations of liver function enzymes in approximately two-thirds of patients (247). Gemcitabine is frequently associated with flu-like symptoms (248) such as fever, headache, chills, cough, rhinitis, myalgia, fatigue, sweating, and insomnia. These symptoms are usually mild and transient and rarely dose limiting.

Acute dyspnea may sometimes occur but is usually self-limiting. Severe pulmonary toxicities such as pulmonary edema, interstitial pneumonitis (249), and adult respiratory distress syndrome (166) are rare.

Gemcitabine can cause a macular or maculopapular pruritic eruption on the trunk and extremities. It is not dose limiting and usually responds to antihistamines and topical corticosteroids. Erysipeloid skin reactions confined to areas of impaired lymphatic drainage after application of gemcitabine have been reported (250).

Radiation recall from gemcitabine chemotherapy is rare but can potentially arise in any site that has been previously irradiated (251).

Diagnostic Tests

Testing is aimed at the end organ effects (e.g., bone marrow, kidney, liver). Laboratory monitoring during treatment should include CBC, electrolytes, and kidney function. LFTs are recommended periodically. Specific levels of gemcitabine are not used to guide management.

Treatment

See Antineoplastic Treatment Guidelines at the end of this chapter. Pulmonary toxicity is treated by discontinuation of gemcitabine and early supportive care with bronchodilators, corticosteroids, diuretics, and oxygen. Although pulmonary toxicity may be reversible, fatal recurrence of severe pulmonary symptoms has been reported in one patient after rechallenge with gemcitabine.

HYDROXYUREA

Hydroxyurea is used to treat CML, AML, chronic myelomonocytic leukemia, and certain brain tumors. Other uses include squamous cell, ovarian, and gastric cancers, as well as malignant melanoma, psoriasis, sickle cell anemia, and polycythemia vera.

Toxicokinetics and Toxicodynamics

Hydroxyurea is readily absorbed orally. It is widely distributed, crosses the placenta and blood–brain barrier, and is found in ascitic fluid. Its V_d is 0.5 L/kg (3). Approximately 50% of hydroxyurea is metabolized in the liver, and 50% is recovered in the urine within 12 hours, mainly as intact drug. The rest is exhaled as carbon dioxide. Its half-life is 2 to 4 hours.

Pathophysiology

Hydroxyurea acts primarily as an inhibitor of ribonucleotide reductase that depletes essential DNA precursors. Another proposed mechanism involves direct chemical damage to DNA by hydroxyurea or a metabolite. Repair of DNA damaged by chemotherapy or radiation is inhibited, offering potential synergy between hydroxyurea and radiation or alkylating agents (3). It has been suggested that hydroxyurea acts against the episomes responsible for drug resistance.

Pregnancy and Lactation

Hydroxyurea is FDA pregnancy risk category D (Appendix I). Hydroxyurea is teratogenic in animals and has the potential to be mutagenic. Its safe use in pregnancy and its effects on fertility have not been established, although it has been used to treat chronic myeloid leukemia during pregnancy (252). Breast-feeding is not recommended.

Clinical Presentation

Immediate effects include allergic reactions manifested by fever or serum sickness, nausea and vomiting, diarrhea, anorexia, hyperuricemia, and rare radiation recall reaction. Early effects include myelosuppression (nadir, 7 days; recovery, 14 to 21 days), anemia (megaloblastosis), stomatitis, alopecia, nail changes, facial erythema, drowsiness, renal insufficiency, and hyperuricemia. Hyperpigmentation and rash may be delayed or late effects (3).

Hepatitis has been associated with hydroxyurea use (253,254). Nail and skin pigmentation have been reported in patients treated with hydroxyurea (255). Other less common findings include xerosis, diffuse alopecia, edema of the legs, dermatomyositis (256), oral ulcers (257), and actinic psoriasis (258). Leg ulcers have also been reported (259,260).

Hydroxyurea may cause radiation recall reactions before, concurrent with, or even after its administration. Recurrent injury to a previously radiated site may occur weeks to months after radiation (3).

Diagnostic Tests

Testing is aimed at end organ effects (e.g., bone marrow, liver). Laboratory monitoring during treatment should include CBC, electrolytes, and kidney function. LFTs are recommended periodically. Specific levels of hydroxyurea are not used to guide management.

Treatment

See Antineoplastic Treatment Guidelines at the end of this chapter.

IFOSFAMIDE

Ifosfamide is a nitrogen mustard agent used to treat cervical, breast, small cell and non–small cell lung, ovarian, pancreatic, and bladder cancers as well as soft tissue sarcoma, pediatric brain tumors, Ewing's sarcoma, Burkitt's lymphoma, Hodgkin's disease, leukemias, neuroblastoma, non-Hodgkin's lymphoma, osteogenic sarcoma, hepatoblastoma, malignant schwannoma, Wilms' tumor, and rhabdomyosarcoma.

Therapeutic doses of ifosfamide range from 1.2 to 2.5 g/m^2/day IV. The maximum tolerated dose reported has been 17 g/m^2 by continuous IV infusion over 120 hours with mesna uroprotection. Dose-limiting renal toxicity has been observed at 18 g/m^2. High total dose was the only risk factor identified regarding ifosfamide nephrotoxicity in children. Cumulative doses more than 100 g/m^2 should be avoided in children with cancer (261).

Nausea and vomiting are minimal at 10 mg/kg (400 mg/m^2) and mild at 20 mg/kg, whereas 95% of patients experience severe nausea and vomiting at 150 mg/kg (6000 mg/m^2).

Toxicokinetics and Toxicodynamics

Oral bioavailability is 100%. Distribution is limited to body water. Ifosfamide may be found in breast milk and ascites. Its V_d is 0.34 to 0.85 L/kg, and there is minimal plasma protein binding (3). Ifosfamide is activated by the hepatic microsomal oxidation. Chloroacetaldehyde is one of the main products of hepatic ifosfamide metabolism and may be responsible for its nephrotoxicity (262). The half-life of ifosfamide is 4.1 to 15.2 hours (3); 60% to 80% is excreted in the urine in 72 hours (50% to 60% as unchanged drug).

Pathophysiology

Ifosfamide is a structural analog of cyclophosphamide. Its mechanism of action is presumed to be identical. Ifosfamide is cell cycle phase nonspecific. CNS toxicity and nephrotoxicity may be related to the metabolite chloracetaldehyde, which is structurally similar to chloral hydrate. The sedative effects of narcotics, antihistamines, and some antiemetics may add to these CNS effects and should be used with caution.

Pregnancy and Lactation

Ifosfamide is FDA pregnancy risk category D (Appendix I). Two women had successful pregnancies after high-dose cyclophosphamide and ifosfamide treatment (263). Breast-feeding is not recommended.

Clinical Presentation

Immediate effects include rare anaphylaxis, dose-related nausea and vomiting, hematuria, dysuria, frequency, hemorrhagic cystitis, and phlebitis. Early effects include myelosuppression (nadir, 8 to 10 days; recovery, 14 to 21 days), reversible alopecia, persistent hematuria, dysuria, frequency, and hemorrhagic cystitis. Other early effects include kidney injury (e.g., proximal tubular damage, metabolic acidosis, SIADH), rare dysrhythmias at high doses, and encephalopathy. Delayed effects include proximal renal tubular damage, interstitial pneumonitis, gonadal damage, and sterility (3).

Urologic toxicity can affect 40% of patients. Cumulative dose of ifosfamide and concomitant cisplatin administration may influence not only the incidence but also the severity of renal toxicity. Preliminary studies suggest young age as a risk factor for nephrotoxicity (264). Irreversible severe renal failure, which appears due to nephrotoxic damage of renal tubular epithelium and the renal microvasculature, may develop. Neither large cumulative doses of ifosfamide nor prior cisplatin treatment are necessary for this toxicity to occur (265). Proximal tubular damage may present as Fanconi's syndrome (266) (characterized by hypophosphatemia or growth failure), renal tubular acidosis, or diabetes insipidus (267). Mesna does not appear to be protective against the proximal tubular abnormalities induced by ifosfamide.

In children, CNS toxicity may manifest as mental status changes (e.g., somnolence, disorientation, and lethargy), cerebellar dysfunction, transient weakness, cranial nerve dysfunction, or seizure activity. This toxicity may be transient and reversible; however, progressive cerebellar and then temporal and frontocortical degeneration leading to death has occurred

(268). Mutism and a confusional state were reported in two patients (269). Peripheral neuropathy is a less well-known side effect that may limit its use (270).

High-dose ifosfamide may be associated with severe but usually reversible myocardial depression and malignant dysrhythmias (271). Dysrhythmias appeared to be reversible on discontinuation of the drug (272).

Diagnostic Tests

Laboratory manifestations of ifosfamide-induced nephrotoxicity include low serum phosphate, low serum bicarbonate, glucosuria, aminoaciduria, and hypochloremic metabolic acidosis.

Treatment

See Antineoplastic Treatment Guidelines at the end of this chapter. There are no antidotes. Dialysis may be useful in view of the favorable toxicokinetics (i.e., low apparent V_d).

Patients receiving ifosfamide with mesna uroprotection can tolerate considerable dose escalation over usual prescribed doses before nonhematologic toxicity becomes dose limiting (273). In one patient, neurotoxicity was reportedly reversed with methylene blue (274).

Methods to treat mild hematuria include saline or water bladder irrigation. Intravesical instillation of astringents [e.g., alum (141,142) or silver nitrate (143)] or systemic administration of antifibrinolytics may be effective. For moderate bladder hemorrhage, cystoscopy is used to evacuate the bladder of clots and continuous irrigation instituted to prevent recurrent clot formation. Following cystoscopy for severe hematuria, treatment may require intravesical formalin (144), phenol (145), or prostaglandin (146) and may proceed to surgical intervention. Electrocautery (147); hyperbaric oxygen (148,149); yttrium-aluminum-garnet laser (150); cryosurgery; IV vasopressin (151); diversion of urine flow (152,153); hypogastric artery ligation; and cystectomy (154) have all been advocated in certain cases.

INTERFERON

Interferon (interferon-alpha) is used to treat CML, hairy cell leukemia, hemangiomas of childhood, Kaposi's sarcoma, mycosis fungoides, essential thrombocythemia, non-Hodgkin's lymphoma, renal cell carcinoma, basal cell carcinoma, immune thrombocytopenic purpura, condyloma acuminata, bladder cancer, melanoma, multiple myeloma, hepatitis C, and hepatitis B.

Interferon-alpha doses of 1 to 9 million units (MU) are generally well tolerated, but doses of 18 to 36 MU yield moderate to severe toxicity. Doses greater than 36 MU can induce significant toxicity (3). At doses greater than 10 MU, daily reduction in hemoglobin levels and in neutrophil and platelet counts occurs. Myelosuppression seldom requires dose reduction. Psychiatric problems have occurred in patients receiving more than 20 MU. Doses greater than 100 MU produce marked lethargy, confusion, dysphagia, and overall mental and motor slowing occurs. Rarely, seizures have occurred at high doses.

Toxicokinetics and Toxicodynamics

Interferon is not used orally, as it is degraded in the stomach. Its V_d is 0.4 L/kg. It is catabolized in renal tubular cells during reabsorption. There are only inactive metabolites. There is an initial distributive half-life of 7 minutes and a beta half-life of 2 to 5 hours.

Pathophysiology

Interferons are a group of naturally occurring proteins that are antiviral, antiproliferative, cytostatic, immunomodulatory, differentiating, and inhibitory of cellular genes, including oncogenes. Interferons can act on tumor cells as well as effector cells such as natural killer cells, T cells, and macrophages.

Pregnancy and Lactation

Interferons are FDA pregnancy risk category C (Appendix I).

Clinical Presentation

Immediate effects include rare allergic reactions, dysrhythmias, hypotension, common flu-like symptoms (e.g., fever, fatigue, chills), nausea, vomiting, injection site problems, and paresthesia. Early effects include diarrhea, myelosuppression (nadir, 17 to 22 days), anorexia, nausea and vomiting, elevated LFTs, reversible alopecia, rash, confusion, depression, headache, rare seizures, rare visual problems, and pulmonary effects (3).

The most common adverse effect is a flu-like syndrome consisting of fever, chills, fatigue, myalgia, anorexia, and headache (275). These effects are transient, dose-related, and reversible within 72 hours. Tolerance to the flu syndrome develops over several months. Symptoms may be reduced if the interferon is given as a continuous infusion over 12 to 18 hours.

Elevation in LFTs occurs frequently (276), especially at doses more than 10 MU daily, but generally decreases despite continued treatment and return to preexisting levels within 2 weeks after cessation of treatment.

CNS toxicity (confusion, depression, headache, and rare visual problems) is dose related and generally reversible, but resolution may take up to 3 weeks. Psychiatric problems may occur (277,278). At high doses, marked lethargy, anxiety (279), confusion, akathisia (280), dysphagia, and overall mental and motor slowing occurs. Seizures have occurred at high doses (281,282).

Cardiovascular effects, especially dysrhythmias, are correlated with preexisting cardiac dysfunction and prior cardiotoxic therapy. Hypotension may occur during, or up to 2 days after, interferon therapy. Bradycardia (283) and giant negative T waves (284) have been reported. Cardiogenic shock has been attributed to interferon as well (285).

Adverse reactions to the intralesional administration of interferon are common but mild to moderate in severity and usually resolve within 24 hours. Minor reactions include erythema, eczema, and depilation. Necrosis and vasculitis can require interruption of treatment (286). Interferon-induced cutaneous sarcoidosis is well documented (287).

Nephrotic syndrome occurs rarely, but it can occur anytime after the start of therapy. Physicians treating hepatitis C must be aware of this idiosyncratic adverse event (288).

Diagnostic Tests

The CBC should be monitored throughout treatment. CNS toxicity may require computed tomography scanning and chemistry profile to rule out other possible causes.

Treatment

See Antineoplastic Treatment Guidelines at the end of this chapter. Paroxetine has been suggested for interferon-induced depression (289). Seizures from interferon may require anticonvulsant therapy but have stopped spontaneously with cessation of therapy (290).

IRINOTECAN

Irinotecan is used to treat colorectal cancer as well as cervical, esophageal, gastric, small cell lung, and pancreatic cancers and glioma and mesothelioma.

Toxicokinetics and Toxicodynamics

Time-to-peak plasma concentration is 1 to 2 hours. Drug is detected in pleural fluid (291), sweat, and saliva (292). The V_d of a 125-mg/m^2 dose is 110 L/m^2 and of 340 mg/m^2 is 234 L/m^2. Plasma protein binding of parent drug is 30% to 68% and of SN-38 is 95% (3).

Metabolism is primarily hepatic. It is rapidly converted to its active metabolite, SN-38, by hepatic carboxylesterase enzymes. Excretion is biliary, urinary, and fecal. The half-life of a 340-mg/m^2 dose is 11.7 hours for irinotecan and 21 hours for SN-38 (3).

Pathophysiology

Irinotecan and SN-38 inhibit the action of topoisomerase I, an enzyme that produces reversible single-strand breaks in DNA during DNA replication. These single-strand breaks relieve torsional strain and allow DNA replication to proceed (293).

Pregnancy and Lactation

Irinotecan is FDA pregnancy risk category D (Appendix I). Breast-feeding is not recommended.

Clinical Presentation

Irinotecan is relatively well tolerated. Dose-limiting toxicities are diarrhea, nausea and vomiting, leukopenia, and neutropenia (294). In addition to myelosuppression and febrile neutropenia (295), irinotecan-induced immune thrombocytopenia has been described (296).

Irinotecan can cause both early and late onset diarrhea. Early onset diarrhea is usually transient, infrequently severe, and thought to be mediated by increased cholinergic activity caused by the parent compound. Other cholinergic symptoms include rhinitis, hypersalivation, miosis, flushing, lacrimation, diaphoresis, and abdominal pain. Cholinergic effects are more likely at higher doses and are associated with peak irinotecan levels (297). Late onset diarrhea occurs more than 24 hours after infusion and can be prolonged, leading to potentially life-threatening dehydration and electrolyte imbalance. This form is thought to be related to increased secretion of water and electrolytes by the intestinal mucosa (298).

Severe liver enzyme abnormalities, observed in less than 10% of patients, are typically seen in patients with known hepatic metastases. The use of irinotecan in patients with significant hepatic dysfunction has not been established. Individuals with Gilbert syndrome have deficient uridine diphosphate glucuronosyltransferase activity, which is involved in the active metabolite of irinotecan. Hence, Gilbert syndrome may increase the risk of irinotecan-induced toxicity (299). Screening for Gilbert syndrome using direct and indirect bilirubin is suggested (300).

Dizziness may represent symptomatic orthostatic hypotension due to dehydration. Dysarthria has been associated with irinotecan use (301).

A potentially life-threatening syndrome consisting of dyspnea, fever, and reticulonodular pattern on chest radiograph occurred in some patients with preexisting lung tumors or nonmalignant pulmonary diseases in early clinical trials. Irinotecan-associated interstitial pneumonitis has been described (302).

Some evidence exists linking therapy with topoisomerase I inhibitors, such as irinotecan, to the development of acute leukemias associated with specific chromosomal translocations.

Diagnostic Tests

The CBC should be regularly followed throughout treatment. Electrolyte determination is indicated in cases of severe diarrhea. Stool cultures should be sent to rule out pathogens.

Treatment

See Antineoplastic Treatment Guidelines at the end of this chapter. The cholinergic syndrome that occurs within the first 24 hours is easily controlled with atropine (303), 0.25 to 1.0 mg IV or SQ, repeated as needed (303). Prophylactic atropine may be required for subsequent treatments (304).

Late onset diarrhea is treated with loperamide. Octreotide is effective for loperamide-refractory diarrhea resulting from irinotecan-based chemotherapy (305). Thalidomide may reduce the dose-limiting GI effects (306). Oral neomycin may also be useful in modulating diarrhea (307).

LETROZOLE

Anastrozole and letrozole are second-line endocrine treatments of advanced postmenopausal breast cancer after failure of tamoxifen (24). Letrozole is also used to treat endometrial stromal sarcoma.

Maximal estrogen suppression is produced by a 0.1-mg dose, although a higher dose (i.e., 2.5 mg/day) was associated with increased clinical responses (308).

Toxicokinetics and Toxicodynamics

Letrozole is rapidly and completely absorbed orally (309). Food decreases its absorption. It is rapidly distributed into tissues. Its V_d is 1.9 L/kg, and plasma protein binding is 60% (310).

Letrozole is metabolized by hepatic cytochrome P-450 (3A4 and 2A6). Excretion is mainly renal; 6% is excreted in urine as unchanged drug and 84% as metabolites (311). The half-life of letrozole is 48 hours.

Pathophysiology

The goal of hormone therapy in breast cancer is to deprive tumor cells of estrogens, which are implicated in the development or progression of tumors (28,312). Maximal estrogen suppression occurs 48 to 78 hours after a single dose of letrozole (313). Letrozole is a reversible (type II), nonsteroidal aromatase inhibitor. Aromatase catalyzes the final and rate-limiting step in the conversion of androgens to estrogens in peripheral tissues. This occurs mainly in adipose tissue, but also in normal and malignant breast tissue, and provides the main source of estrogen in postmenopausal women.

Pregnancy and Lactation

Letrozole is FDA pregnancy risk category D (Appendix I). If exposed to letrozole during pregnancy, the patient should be apprised of the potential fetal hazard and risk for loss of the pregnancy. It is not known if letrozole is excreted in human milk (314).

Clinical Presentation

In general, letrozole is well tolerated. Weight gain (315), headache, hair thinning, and diarrhea have been reported (316). Other common effects include fatigue, increased appetite, musculoskeletal pain, and nausea (317). One patient with advanced breast cancer involving the pleural space, unresponsive to chemotherapy, experienced tumor lysis syndrome after initiation of letrozole (318).

Diagnostic Tests

Rare cases of tumor lysis syndrome require electrolyte determination. Fatigue may require search for other clinical entities, and headache, if severe, may require computed tomography scanning.

Treatment

No overdoses have been reported, and there is no specific antidote.

LEUPROLIDE

Leuprolide is used to treat prostate, breast, and ovarian cancers as well as central precocious puberty.

Toxicokinetics and Toxicodynamics

Plasma protein binding is 7% to 15%. Metabolism to amino acids is extensive at unknown sites. Excretion of leuprolide is urinary. Its half-life is 3 hours.

Pathophysiology

Leuprolide is a synthetic analog of gonadotropin releasing hormone that antagonizes LHRH. It inhibits LHRH without initial stimulation of the LHRH receptor (319). Continuous treatment produces initial stimulation then suppression of hormones to castrate or produce postmenopausal levels. In males, it reduced testosterone to castration levels within 2 to 4 weeks. In women, both ovarian estrogen and androgen synthesis are inhibited (320).

Pregnancy and Lactation

Leuprolide is FDA pregnancy risk category X (Appendix I). Leuprolide may impair male and female fertility. Breast-feeding is not recommended.

Clinical Presentation

Immediate effects include nausea and vomiting, disease flare, and irritation at the injection site. Early effects include swelling of the hands, feet, or lower legs; flushing; hot flashes (321); impotence; decreased sex drive (322); vaginal bleeding; gynecomastia; testicular atrophy; amenorrhea; constipation; blurred vision; anorexia; dizziness; depression; headache; irritability; insomnia; paresthesia; increased blood urea nitrogen; and increased creatinine. Delayed effects include persistent breast swelling or tenderness, decrease in testicle size, and blurred vision (3).

The initial pituitary stimulation produces an acute increase in plasma testosterone. This can produce a disease flare in 5% to 10% of patients and transient prostate enlargement in 30% to 50% (323). Increased bone pain and, less frequently, symptoms of urinary tract obstruction (e.g., dysuria, hematuria) or spinal cord compression (e.g., weakness of lower extremities) can occur during this flare in patients with prostate cancer. Prostate-specific antigen can also flare with leuprolide therapy (324).

Leuprolide is generally well tolerated. Toxicity is mostly confined to hot flashes that occur in most patients receiving the drug (325). Severe ovarian hyperstimulation syndrome occurred after the administration of leuprolide to suppress multicystic ovaries in one case (326).

Diagnostic Tests

Laboratory monitoring periodically should include tumor markers and serum testosterone (optional).

Treatment

See Antineoplastic Treatment Guidelines at the end of this chapter. To completely avert prostate-specific antigen flare in prostate cancer patients, treatment with flutamide for 2 weeks before leuprolide administration is effective (327).

LOMUSTINE

Lomustine is a nitrosourea-alkylating agent used to treat brain tumors such as medulloblastoma. Other uses include breast, lung, ovarian, and pancreatic cancers; Hodgkin's disease; malignant melanoma; multiple myeloma; non-Hodgkin's lymphoma; and renal cell carcinoma.

Lomustine is usually administered in doses of 100 to 130 mg/m^2 orally every 4 to 6 weeks. A 28-year-old woman with anaplastic astrocytoma took lomustine 1400 mg over 1 week, her regular dose being 200 mg on day 1 of the regimen. Pancytopenia developed within a week after the last dose. Approximately 3 weeks later, the patient developed multiorgan dysfunction and died (328).

Toxicokinetics and Toxicodynamics

Oral lomustine is completely absorbed in 30 to 60 minutes. There is rapid and extensive tissue distribution. The CSF achieves more than 50% of plasma levels. Lomustine is oxidized by the hepatic microsomal system into active metabolites. Approximately 50% is excreted in urine within 24 hours as metabolites. The half-life is 4 to 5 hours for metabolites and 15 minutes for parent.

Pathophysiology

Lomustine is a highly lipophilic nitrosourea compound that undergoes hydrolysis to form reactive metabolites. These metabolites cause alkylation and cross-linking of DNA. Lomustine also inhibits DNA synthesis and has some cell cycle phase specificity. Nitrosoureas generally lack cross-resistance with other alkylating agents (4,5).

Pregnancy and Lactation

Lomustine is FDA pregnancy risk category D (Appendix I). Breast-feeding is not recommended (329).

Clinical Presentation

Immediate effects include nausea and vomiting. Early effects include stomatitis and transient elevation of LFTs. Nausea and vomiting occur in approximately one-half of patients. Vomiting may occur 45 minutes to 6 hours after an oral dose and usually abates within 24 hours.

Delayed effects include myelosuppression (nadir, 24 to 60 days; recovery, 38 to 65 days), lung problems (rare, infiltrates, or fibrosis), kidney problems, transient elevation of LFTs, stomatitis, alopecia, CNS problems (rare), infertility, and leukemia (3).

Myelosuppression is cumulative. After repeated courses of treatment, recovery of blood cell count is slower, and bone marrow hypoplasia may persist. Pulmonary fibrosis (330) has been reported at cumulative doses above 1100 mg/m^2. There is one report of pulmonary toxicity at a cumulative dose of 600 mg (331). The onset of toxicity has varied from 6 months to 15 years.

Diagnostic Tests

Testing is aimed at end organ effects (e.g., bone marrow). Laboratory testing during treatment should include CBC, electrolytes, and kidney function. LFTs are recommended periodically. Specific levels of lomustine are not used to guide management.

Treatment

See Antineoplastic Treatment Guidelines at the end of this chapter.

MECHLORETHAMINE

Mechlorethamine is used to treat Hodgkin's disease, mycosis fungoides, CLL, CML, small cell lung cancer, malignant effusions, medulloblastoma, and non-Hodgkin's lymphoma.

The usual adult dose is 0.4 mg/kg IV every 3 to 6 weeks. Topical dosing is 10 mg daily, and intracavitary dosing is 0.2 to 0.4 mg/kg. In children, the dose is 6 mg/m^2 IV every 4 weeks.

Toxicokinetics and Toxicodynamics

Oral absorption occurs but is irritating to the GI tract. The drug is highly reactive and cleared from blood within minutes. Mechlorethamine ionizes in solution to an active form and combines with reactive compounds. Its half-life is 15 minutes, and 50% is excreted in urine as metabolites within 24 hours (3).

Pathophysiology

Mechlorethamine is a polyfunctional-alkylating agent that interferes with DNA replication and RNA transcription through alkylation. Alkylation produces breaks in the DNA molecule as well as cross-linking of its twin strands. Mechlorethamine is cell cycle phase nonspecific (127).

Pregnancy and Lactation

Mechlorethamine is FDA pregnancy risk category D (Appendix I). Nicholson reviewed 11 pregnancies with nitrogen mustard use, six during the first trimester. One pregnancy was terminated, and three ended as spontaneous abortion. Of the seven live births, none had a malformation (332). Numerous healthy children have been born to pregnant mothers treated with a regimen of mechlorethamine, Oncovin (vincristine), procarbazine, and prednisone for Hodgkin's disease (333).

Clinical Presentation

Immediate effects include rare anaphylaxis, phlebitis, nausea and vomiting in most patients, a metallic taste, drowsiness, tinnitus, and hearing loss. Early effects include myelosuppression (nadir, 7 to 14 days; recovery, 28 days), vein irritation and sclerosis, rare stomatitis, anorexia, diarrhea, rash, contact dermatitis with topical use, hyperuricemia, and alopecia. Delayed effects include infertility, contact dermatitis, and cancer (e.g., leukemia, lymphoma, and skin cancer) (3).

Extravasation into SQ tissue is painful and can result in induration and sloughing (334). Phlebitis and pain at the injection site during or after injection may occur (335).

Confusion, disorientation, hallucinations, tremor, lethargy, and seizures have been reported after mechlorethamine use for bone marrow transplantation (336). Reproductive effects include delayed menstruation, oligomenorrhea, and temporary or permanent amenorrhea. In males, mechlorethamine can impair spermatogenesis (337). Patients can develop an allergic contact or bullous (338) dermatitis to topical mechlorethamine.

Diagnostic Tests

Testing is aimed at end organ effects (e.g., bone marrow). Testing during treatment should include CBC, electrolytes, and kidney function. Specific levels of mechlorethamine are not used to guide management.

Treatment

See Antineoplastic Treatment Guidelines at the end of this chapter. A 55-year-old man was accidentally given 30 mg of mechlorethamine IM. Approximately 5 hours later, one-sixth M sodium thiosulfate was infused around the site. Although systemic responses to the mechlorethamine developed, expected muscular and adjacent skin destruction did not occur (339).

Mechlorethamine-induced dermatitis is treated with discontinuation of the drug and either systemic prednisone or topical glucocorticoids until the reaction has subsided. Systemic toxicity associated with topical mechlorethamine is minimal.

MEGESTROL

Megestrol is a synthetic progestin used to treat breast cancer. Other uses include endometrial and prostate cancers and cancer cachexia to stimulate appetite in patients with growth hormone deficiency, chronic obstructive pulmonary disease, HIV, and end-stage renal disease, and as a hormone replacement in menopausal women who cannot tolerate estrogens.

The usual dose range in adults is 120 to 160 mg/day orally. The dose for cancer cachexia is 480 to 800 mg/day. There are no pediatric indications.

Toxicokinetics and Toxicodynamics

Oral absorption is rapid and extensive. Megestrol is distributed to breast milk. Metabolism of megestrol is mainly in the liver to free steroids and glucuronide conjugates. There are no active metabolites. The half-life of megestrol is 15 to 38 hours (3). Excretion is primarily renal.

Pathophysiology

Megestrol probably acts locally to inhibit growth of hormone sensitive cells. It is not cell cycle phase specific but may be maximal in the G1 phase of dividing cells (3).

Pregnancy and Lactation

Megestrol is FDA pregnancy risk category X (Appendix I).

Clinical Presentation

Immediate effects include mild nausea. Early (days to weeks) effects include fluid retention, carpal tunnel syndrome, hot flushes, hypercalcemia, improved appetite, and weight gain. Delayed effects include rare deep vein thrombosis, alopecia, and vaginal bleeding (3). Spotting may occur during megestrol treatment. Vaginal bleeding (340) is common following withdrawal of megestrol. Cushing syndrome was induced by high-dose megestrol in a patient with renal insufficiency (341) and in three patients treated for breast cancer (342).

Diagnostic Tests

Laboratory monitoring should periodically include liver function and blood glucose determinations.

Treatment

See Antineoplastic Treatment Guidelines at the end of this chapter.

MELPHALAN

Melphalan is a nitrogen mustard–alkylating agent used to treat multiple myeloma, breast cancer, Ewing's sarcoma, malignant melanoma, neuroblastoma and medulloblastoma, ovarian cancer, amyloidosis, myelofibrosis, and myeloid metaplasia.

After a dose of more than 125 mg/m² IV, GI side effects such as hemorrhagic diarrhea or even bowel perforation may be observed. One patient died 6 days after 290 mg/m² of melphalan, probably due to cardiac dysrhythmia before onset of marrow failure (343). SIADH and electrolyte disturbances may cause death before infectious or bleeding complications.

Rare cases of melphalan overdose have been reported (73,344). A 52-year-old woman with acute oliguric renal failure was erroneously treated with high-dose IV melphalan (60 mg/m²). Treatment with granulocyte colony-stimulating factor was initiated. Pronounced leukopenia developed, and the patient was treated with hemodialysis. Within 10 days, the patient no longer required hemodialysis (345). Two other cases of IV melphalan overdose (less than 100 mg/m²) recovered from marrow aplasia within 3 weeks without major complication.

Toxicokinetics and Toxicodynamics

Oral absorption ranges from 25% to 89% (346). The V_d is 0.5 to 0.6 L/kg, and 90% to 95% is plasma protein bound. Melphalan is not metabolized, but it spontaneously degrades to mono- and dihydroxy products. Fecal excretion is 20% to 50% within 6 days, and urinary excretion is 10% to 15% as intact drug within 24 hours. The alpha half-life of melphalan has been estimated at 8 minutes after IV dosing, and the beta half-life at 1.8 hours (347).

Pathophysiology

Melphalan is a phenylalanine derivative of mechlorethamine. Alkylation of DNA results in breaks in the DNA molecules as well as cross-linking of the twin strands, thus interfering with DNA replication and RNA transcription. Melphalan is cell cycle phase nonspecific (4,5).

Pregnancy and Lactation

Melphalan is FDA pregnancy risk category D (Appendix I).

Clinical Presentation

Bronchopulmonary dysplasia and pulmonary interstitial fibrosis have been reported with melphalan use (348). Clinical effects include dry cough, dyspnea, tachypnea, fever, and cyanosis. There are no identifiable risk factors for melphalan pulmonary toxicity, including dose or duration of therapy. Patients may recover with complete resolution or die from progressive pulmonary disease. Cardiotoxicity occurs rarely. Acute left ventricular heart failure has occurred with melphalan and fludarabine combination chemotherapy before allogeneic stem cell transplantation (349).

Diagnostic Tests

Testing is aimed at the end organ effects (e.g., bone marrow, lung). CBC, electrolytes, and kidney function should be followed during treatment. Specific levels of melphalan are not used to guide management.

Treatment

See Antineoplastic Treatment Guidelines at the end of this chapter. There are no antidotes. In view of its toxicokinetic properties, hemodialysis or hemoperfusion would likely not be effective. Colony-stimulating factors such as granulocyte-macrophage colony-stimulating factor and granulocyte colony-stimulating factor may improve the prognosis of moderate-to-severe overdose (343).

MERCAPTOPURINE

Mercaptopurine [6-mercaptopurine (6-MP)] is used to treat ALL, AML, and CML as well as histiocytosis X. Hepatotoxic reactions are most common when daily doses exceed 2.5 mg/kg. These effects are usually reversible on discontinuation of the drug.

Toxicokinetics and Toxicodynamics

Oral absorption is incomplete and variable. Bioavailability is 5% to 37% largely due to first-pass hepatic metabolism (350). 6-MP is widely distributed and is found in breast milk. The V_d is 0.56 to 0.9 L/kg, and protein binding is 19% (3).

Rapid intracellular activation of 6-MP yields active metabolites. At conventional doses, clearance is primarily hepatic. Renal clearance may become important at high doses with 50% of an oral dose excreted in urine in 24 hours. Its half-life is 0.3 to 1.0 hour after infusion (3).

Pathophysiology

6-MP is a 6-thiopurine analog of the naturally occurring purine bases hypoxanthine and guanine. Intracellular activation results in *de novo* inhibition of purine synthesis and incorporation into DNA. Cytotoxicity is cell cycle phase specific (S phase) (3).

Pregnancy and Lactation

6-MP is FDA pregnancy risk category D (Appendix I).

Clinical Presentation

In overdose, dizziness, headache, abdominal pain, and a rise in serum bilirubin may be seen. Characteristic hepatotoxic features are cholestasis and parenchymal cell necrosis. Elevation of serum bilirubin may forewarn of cholestasis, which may prove fatal (351).

Pancreatitis has also resulted from 6-MP use (352). Serum sickness with acute lobular panniculitis and vasculitis developed in a patient with Crohn's disease treated with 6-MP (353). Myelosuppression is the main hematotoxic effect of 6-MP. Immune hemolytic anemia was reported in a 67-year-old man with chronic myelomonocytic leukemia (354).

Diagnostic Tests

Testing is aimed at end organ effects (e.g., liver). Specific levels of 6-MP are not used to guide management.

Treatment

See Antineoplastic Treatment Guidelines at the end of this chapter. The dose should be reduced to 25% of the usual dose if allopurinol is given (355,356).

MESNA

Mesna is a uroprotectant used to prevent hemorrhagic cystitis caused by cyclophosphamide or ifosfamide (357). Although some adverse effects (e.g., hemorrhagic cystitis) of ifosfamide can be overcome by the coadministration of mesna, others, such as nephrotoxicity, cannot (264).

The usual dose is expressed as a percentage of the ifosfamide or cyclophosphamide dose. Oral dose is 40% orally for three doses (0, 4, and 8 hours). The IV dose is 20% for three doses (0, 4, and 8 hours), and continuous IV dose is 20% prechemotherapy, 50% to 100% with chemotherapy, then 25% to 50% for 12 hours (358). In children, the dose is 60% to 160% of oxazaphosphorine doses.

Toxicokinetics and Toxicodynamics

Oral absorption is 50%. The V_d of mesna is 0.65 L/kg, and plasma protein binding is 10% (359). The half-life is 0.3 to 4.0 hours.

Pathophysiology

Mesna reacts with acrolein and other urotoxic metabolites of cyclophosphamide or ifosfamide to form stable, nontoxic compounds. Mesna does not have any antitumor activity, nor does it appear to interfere with the antitumor activity of antineoplastic drugs (5).

Pregnancy and Lactation

Mesna is FDA pregnancy risk category B (Appendix I). Breast-feeding is not recommended (5).

Clinical Presentation

Fatal hypokalemia (360), encephalopathy (361,362), and seizures (363) have been associated with ifosfamide/mesna chemotherapy. Drug eruptions attributed to mesna have been reported after cyclophosphamide treatment of patients with systemic lupus erythematosus and dermatomyositis (364). Mesna has been reported to induce urticaria as well (365).

METHOTREXATE

MTX is used to treat ALL, breast, bladder, head and neck, and lung cancers, as well as graft-versus-host disease (prophylaxis), non-Hodgkin's lymphoma, osteogenic sarcoma, adult soft tissue sarcoma, choriocarcinoma, primary biliary cirrhosis, rheumatoid arthritis, ectopic pregnancy, primary sclerosing cholangitis, psoriasis, and mycosis fungoides.

Steroid therapy, in combination with other antileukemic drugs or in cyclic combinations with MTX, has appeared to produce ALL remission. When used for induction, doses of 3.3 mg/m^2 in combination with 60 mg/m^2 of prednisone produced remissions in 50% of patients, usually within a period of 4 to 6 weeks (366).

A 52-year-old woman took 112.5 mg MTX over 5 days. Extensive erosions with necrotic changes were noted in her mouth, groin, and vulvar mucous membranes. The patient died on the twenty-second day from pneumonia and extensive mycosis (367).

A 9-year-old boy with non-Hodgkin's lymphoma who received 650 mg intrathecally died. He sustained immediate necrotizing leukoencephalopathy despite early CSF exchange, IV leucovorin, and dexamethasone. Although CSF exchange removed 78% of the administered dose, the CSF and serum MTX levels were 50- to 100-fold higher than normal (368).

A 24-month-old girl received 170 mg/m^2 intrathecally but developed only mild headaches with IV leucovorin and oral dexamethasone (369). An 80-year-old woman took her weekly MTX dose on 4 consecutive days. She developed pancytopenia and mucositis and was treated with antibiotics and folinic acid with complete recovery (370).

Stomatitis is rare with weekly doses of 30 mg/m^2, whereas doses of 20 mg/m^2 on 5 consecutive days produce stomatitis in most patients.

Toxicokinetics and Toxicodynamics

MTX is well absorbed orally. Highest levels are found in kidney, gallbladder, spleen, liver, and skin. Drug crosses the placenta and may be found in breast milk and malignant effusions. The V_d is 16.4 L/m^2, and plasma protein binding is 50% (3).

MTX is metabolized in the liver to polyglutamate products. Excretion is principally renal (80%). Biliary excretion is less than 10%. The alpha half-life of MTX is 1.5 to 3.5 hours, and beta half-life is 8 to 15 hours (3).

Pathophysiology

MTX and its active metabolites compete for the folate-binding site of the enzyme dihydrofolate reductase. Folic acid must be reduced to tetrahydrofolic acid by this enzyme for DNA synthesis and cellular replication to occur. Competitive inhibition of the enzyme leads to blockage of tetrahydrofolate synthesis; depletion of nucleotide precursors; and inhibition of DNA, RNA, and protein synthesis (127).

Pregnancy and Lactation

MTX is FDA pregnancy risk category D (Appendix I). Successful pregnancies have followed the use of MTX before conception (371). When administered to a pregnant woman, abortion may occur. MTX is excreted into breast milk in minimal amounts (372), and single weekly doses are unlikely to pose substantial risk. Breast-feeding is not recommended.

Clinical Presentation

Immediate effects include rare anaphylaxis, dose-related nausea and vomiting, fever and chills, radiation recall reaction, chemical meningitis with intrathecal use, pulmonary edema, and pleuritic chest pain. Early effects include myelosuppression (nadir, 7 to 14 days; recovery, 14 to 21 days), dose-related stomatitis, diarrhea, bleeding, perforation, elevated LFTs, pigmentation changes, photosensitivity, rash, anorexia, alopecia, interstitial pneumonitis, conjunctivitis, acute encephalopathy, megaloblastosis, and kidney problems.

MTX can cause hepatic fibrosis (373) or cirrhosis (374). Acute elevation of hepatic enzymes occurs more frequently in patients receiving high-dose therapy and is reversible. Chronic hepatic fibrosis is more common in patients receiving long-term, low-dose therapy (375). In most patients, MTX-induced liver cirrhosis is not aggressive. The continued use of liver biopsies in the surveillance of MTX-treated psoriasis and other conditions has been advocated (376) but is controversial.

Renal toxicity may be related to precipitation of MTX in the renal tubules and collecting ducts. The risk of renal failure due to high-dose MTX (greater than 1 g/m^2) can be minimized by brisk diuresis and alkalinization of the urine. Acute renal failure has been treated successfully with leucovorin and thymidine (377).

The incidence and severity of stomatitis vary with dose and schedule (378). Risk factors for stomatitis include renal dysfunction, irradiation to the head and neck area, and prolonged infusion. Administration of leucovorin and oral folate decreases the risk of stomatitis.

Myelosuppression may develop with any dosage schedule but is more severe with high doses, with daily administration of lower doses, in malnourished patients, in patients with decreased renal function, and in patients with effusions, ascites, or significant edema. Low-dose MTX is uncommonly associated with hematologic toxicity (379).

MTX has the ability to enhance radiation injury to tissues (380) before, concurrent with, or even after treatment. Recurrent injury to a previously radiated site may occur weeks to months following radiation.

MTX-induced neurotoxicity is a frequent complication of therapy for patients with malignant and inflammatory diseases. Neurotoxicity can occur after intrathecal MTX or after low-, intermediate-, or high-dose systemic administration. Symptoms can present in the acute, subacute, or late setting and can range from affective disorders, malaise, and headaches to somnolence, focal neurologic deficits, and seizures (381). Other CNS toxicities can include an acute encephalopathy consisting of aphasia or hemiparesis. Progressive leukoencephalopathy, occurring months to years after MTX, can be severe or fatal (382). This rare complication is usually associated with some combination of cranial irradiation and systemic and intrathecal MTX.

The most common toxic effect of intrathecal MTX is chemical arachnoiditis (383), which is generally mild and occurs soon after injection and resolves within several days. Spinal cord and nerve damage can result in reversible or ascending paraplegia (384) and may result in death. Patients can also develop encephalopathy, dementia, seizures, coma, and death. The toxicity of intrathecal MTX may partially be related to preservatives such as benzyl alcohol.

Chemical meningitis may occur with intrathecal MTX (385), beginning 2 to 4 hours after injection and lasting for 12 to 72 hours. Symptoms include stiff neck, headache, nausea and vomiting, fever, and lethargy. The syndrome may be subacute or chronic, transient or permanent. Progression to spasticity, quadriplegia (transient or permanent), visual disturbances, leukoencephalopathy (386), seizures, and slurred speech can occur (387).

Pulmonary toxicity can be immediate (chest pain, pulmonary edema) or delayed (fibrosis). MTX also causes acute hypersensitivity pneumonitis (388). Pulmonary toxicity appears to be schedule-dependent, because daily or weekly dosing is more toxic than every 2 to 4 week dosing. Pulmonary toxicity occurs in 0.5% to 14.0% of patients receiving low-dose MTX (389). Leucovorin does not appear to protect against pulmonary toxicity. Corticosteroids may hasten recovery.

Diagnostic Tests

Testing is aimed at end organ effects (e.g., bone marrow, lung, brain, liver, kidney). CBC, electrolytes, and kidney function should be followed during treatment. MTX levels are usually obtained in conjunction with high-dose MTX and leucovorin rescue (Chapter 58). Post–high-dose MTX levels are used to adjust leucovorin doses (i.e., prolong the duration and/or increase the dose). Occasionally, levels are used to characterize MTX kinetics in individual patients with subsequent adjustment in dose (390).

Treatment

See Antineoplastic Treatment Guidelines at the end of this chapter. In overdose, prompt leucovorin rescue (Chapter 58) with charcoal hemoperfusion to reduce plasma MTX concentration appears effective if used early. Venovenous hemodiafiltration has been used to successfully remove MTX (391). Exchange transfusion was not effective in treating MTX toxicity in a 19-year-old patient (392). Dextromethorphan effectively treated subacute neurotoxicity in one report (381).

Excessive intrathecal administration is treated with immediate lumbar puncture and CSF drainage. Drainage of 30 ml of CSF within the first 15 minutes removes up to 95% of the dose. A delay of 2 hours removes less than 20% of the dose. CSF drainage alone is insufficient for a massive MTX overdose, because toxic amounts remain. With doses more than 100 mg, CSF drainage must be accompanied by ventriculolumbar perfusion. Thymidine rescue is used 24 hours after intrathecal MTX overdose. The dose is 8 g/m^2/day by continuous infusion.

Fluid balance should be carefully maintained to avoid cerebral edema. Cerebral edema may be ameliorated with mannitol, and phenytoin has been used to prevent seizures. Steroids are not recommended. Urinary alkalinization has been proposed to promote urinary excretion of MTX; however, there are no controlled studies to support this procedure.

MITHRAMYCIN

Mithramycin (plicamycin) is used to treat hypercalcemia of malignancy (393) as well as CML and testicular cancer. The dose for adult testicular cancer is 25 to 30 μg/kg/day IV for 8 to 10 days. The dose for hypercalcemia is 25 μg/kg/day, with repeat doses of 1 mg/m^2 for 2 to 3 doses every 2 days. In children, the IV dose is 25 μg/kg every 3 to 4 days as needed.

Toxicokinetics and Toxicodynamics

Oral absorption is nil. Mithramycin is cleared from plasma in 2 hours and crosses the blood–brain barrier. It is not protein bound. The major route of elimination is urinary (40% within 15 hours). Its half-life is 2 to 24 hours.

Pathophysiology

Mithramycin lowers serum calcium levels by blocking parathyroid hormone action on osteoclasts.

Pregnancy and Lactation

Mithramycin is FDA pregnancy risk category D (Appendix I). Breast-feeding is not recommended.

Clinical Presentation

Immediate effects may include vein irritation, nausea and vomiting in the majority of patients, hypocalcemia, and fever. Early effects may include elevated LFTs, hepatic necrosis, coagulopathy, and mild myelosuppression (nadir, 5 to 10 days; recovery, 10 to 18 days). Late effects may include acute hepatic necrosis and acute tubular necrosis of the kidney (3).

Mithramycin lowers serum calcium at doses much lower than are needed to treat sensitive cancers. Serum calcium falls within hours of injection, and peak effectiveness is reached within 72 hours. Weekly doses have been successful in managing hypercalcemia of malignancy.

Tissue necrosis from extravasation (394) may occur days to weeks after mithramycin use. Bleeding is rare with doses used to treat hypercalcemia and with alternate day dosing. Nausea and vomiting persisting for several hours occur in the majority of patients receiving a 25- to 50-μg/kg infusion.

Azotemia occurs in 40% of patients at doses of 25 to 50 μg/kg for 5 consecutive days. Declining renal function is related to cumulative doses (395). Mithramycin given as a single dose for the treatment of hypercalcemia has reportedly caused nephrotoxicity (396).

Diagnostic Tests

Testing is aimed at end organ effects (e.g., bone marrow, liver, kidney). CBC, electrolytes, and kidney function should be followed during treatment. Specific levels of mithramycin are not used to guide management.

Treatment

See Antineoplastic Treatment Guidelines at the end of this chapter.

MITOMYCIN

Mitomycin is a purple antineoplastic agent used to treat bladder, gastric, colorectal, breast, cervical, head and neck, non–small cell lung, ovarian, pancreatic, and *primary unknown* cancers, as well as osteogenic sarcoma. The usual adult dose is 10 to 20 mg/m^2 IV every 4 to 8 weeks or 2 mg/m^2/day for 5 days weekly for 2 weeks every 6 to 8 weeks.

Toxicokinetics and Toxicodynamics

Oral absorption is erratic. The V_d of mitomycin is 16 to 56 L/m^2. Prodrug is activated *in vivo*. Primary means of elimination is by hepatic metabolism. Mitomycin is excreted in urine (4% to 27%) and detected in bile and feces. Its half-life is 8 minutes (3).

Pathophysiology

Mitomycin is activated *in vivo* to a bifunctional and trifunctional alkylating agent. Binding to DNA leads to cross-linking and inhibition of DNA synthesis and function (397).

Pregnancy and Lactation

Mitomycin is FDA pregnancy risk category C (Appendix I). Breast-feeding is not recommended.

Clinical Presentation

Immediate side effects may include fever, phlebitis, cystitis with bladder instillation, nausea, and vomiting. Early effects may include myelosuppression (nadir, 24 to 28 days; recovery, 42 to 56 days). Interstitial pneumonitis, stomatitis, elevated LFTs, hair loss, rash, blue bands in nails, encephalopathy, blurred vision, and amenorrhea may occur within weeks. Tissue necrosis with extravasation may happen days to weeks after treatment. Late effects can include pulmonary fibrosis, renal failure, and microangiopathic hemolytic anemia (3).

Pulmonary toxicity presenting with dyspnea, nonproductive cough for weeks to months, and basilar rales have been reported; approximately 40% of these patients die of progressive fibrosis (398). Steroids may be of some benefit.

The incidence of cardiotoxicity may be increased in patients receiving mitomycin in combination with doxorubicin or in patients who have had prior exposure to anthracycline antineoplastics (399).

Mitomycin has the potential to enhance radiation injury to tissues before, concurrent with, or after its administration. Recurrent injury to a previously radiated site may occur weeks to months after radiation (3).

Diagnostic Tests

Testing is aimed at the end organ effects (e.g., bone marrow, lung, liver). CBC, electrolytes, and kidney function should be followed during treatment. Liver function should be monitored periodically. Specific levels of mitomycin are not available or used to guide management.

Treatment

See Antineoplastic Treatment Guidelines at the end of this chapter.

MITOTANE

Mitotane causes direct necrosis and atrophy of the adrenal cortex and is used to treat adrenocortical cancer (400), a rare, aggressive tumor that is often detected in an advanced stage (401).

The usual adult dose initially is 500 mg orally, four times/day, escalated by 1000 mg/day every 1 to 2 weeks to a maximum tolerated dose. In children, the dose is 0.5 to 1.0 g daily, escalated to 1 to 4 g/day.

Toxicokinetics and Toxicodynamics

Oral absorption is approximately 40%. Mitotane is distributed to all tissues, primarily to fat (402). The liver and kidney metabolize small amounts of mitotane: 60% is excreted unchanged in feces, and 10% to 25% as metabolites in urine. The half-life of mitotane is approximately 8 minutes (403).

Pathophysiology

Mitotane acts mainly as an inhibitor of intramitochondrial pregnenolone and cortisol synthesis (404). Mitotane is probably metabolized to reactive intermediates (405).

Pregnancy and Lactation

Mitotane is FDA pregnancy risk category C (Appendix I).

Clinical Presentation

Mitotane causes adrenocortical suppression and can cause adrenal crisis (406). Supplementation with exogenous steroids is necessary. GI toxicity occurs in 80% of patients. An erythematous eruption of the palms and soles may develop (407).

Adverse CNS effects occur in 40% of patients: lethargy, somnolence, dizziness, depression, irritability, confusion, and tremors. Rare CNS side effects include speech difficulty, memory loss, ataxia, and hallucinations (408). Retinopathy has been reported (409). Long-term use can cause permanent CNS damage. Behavior and neurologic assessments should be performed periodically when continuous use exceeds 2 years (410,411).

Diagnostic Tests

Periodic monitoring includes mitotane levels, electrolytes, dehydroepiandrosterone, liver function, kidney function, blood pressure, and neurologic assessment. The therapeutic mitotane level is 14 to 20 μg/ml (412).

Treatment

See Antineoplastic Treatment Guidelines at the end of this chapter. Patients may require fludrocortisone 0.1 mg daily for mineralocorticoid deficiency causing orthostatic hypotension (413). If shock or infection occurs, mitotane should be temporarily discontinued and steroids given immediately. When mitotane is discontinued, the steroid should be tapered slowly but may need to be continued indefinitely.

MITOXANTRONE

Mitoxantrone is used to treat AML, acute non-lymphocytic leukemia, non-Hodgkin's lymphoma, multiple myeloma, multiple sclerosis, ALL, and CML, as well as gastric, liver, ovarian, multiple, and prostate cancers. A 9-year-old girl inadvertently received a bolus IV injection of 100 mg/m^2. Severe but transient myelotoxicity was induced. Sequential ECHOs demonstrated a reversible decrease of the shortening fraction of the left ventricle (414).

The main side effects in three patients who received 100 mg/m^2 to 183 mg/m^2 were moderate nausea and vomiting, shaking chills, and profound but reversible neutro- and thrombocytopenia. There was no immediate cardiac toxicity (415). Overdoses of 140 to 180 mg/m^2 have resulted in severe leukopenia, thrombocytopenia, infection, and death.

Toxicokinetics and Toxicodynamics

Oral absorption is poor. The V_d of mitoxantrone is 1875 to 2248 L/m^2, and plasma protein binding is 78% (3). The liver metabolizes mitoxantrone; excretion is mainly biliary, with a small amount in urine. The alpha half-life of mitoxantrone is 0.14 hours, and the beta half-life is 3.1 hours (3).

Pathophysiology

The exact mechanism of action is unknown but includes intercalation with DNA to cause inter- and intrastrand cross-linking. It also causes DNA strand breaks through binding with the phosphate backbone of DNA (3).

Pregnancy and Lactation

Mitoxantrone is FDA pregnancy risk category D (Appendix I). Mitoxantrone causes chromosomal aberrations in animals. Breast-feeding is not recommended (416).

Clinical Presentation

Immediate effects include rare anaphylaxis, nausea and vomiting, blue-green urine discoloration, and occasional phlebitis. Early effects include myelosuppression (nadir, 10 days; recovery, 21 days), stomatitis, alopecia, diarrhea, anorexia, elevated LFTs, transient dysrhythmias, CHF, and cardiomyopathy. Delayed effects include transient dysrhythmias, CHF, cardiomyopathy, and renal damage (3).

Cardiotoxicity is cumulative across members of the anthracycline (e.g., daunorubicin, doxorubicin, epirubicin, idarubicin) and anthracenedione (e.g., mitoxantrone) class of drugs. The cumulative dose for cardiotoxicity is lower in patients who have received mediastinal radiation or therapy with other cardiotoxic agents. Mitoxantrone-induced acute left heart failure has been reported after intrapleural administration (417).

Mitoxantrone can cause discoloration of the nails (418), as well as skin hyperpigmentation (419).

Diagnostic Tests

Testing is aimed at end organ effects (e.g., bone marrow, heart, liver). CBC, electrolytes, and kidney function should be followed during treatment. Liver function should be monitored periodically. Specific levels of mitoxantrone are not used to guide management.

Treatment

See Antineoplastic Treatment Guidelines at the end of this chapter. Hemoperfusion was inefficient in increasing clearance of mitoxantrone in a 9-year-old who received an accidental overdose (414).

Cardiac monitoring (e.g., ECHO with ejection fraction) is advisable every two to three cycles, and before every cycle in patients who have received a cumulative dose of 140 mg/m^2 (approximately ten courses). The cumulative dose required to produce cardiotoxicity is reportedly lower in children and in patients who have received radiation to the mediastinal area or concomitant therapy with other cardiotoxic agents.

NILUTAMIDE

Nilutamide is used to treat prostate cancer and HCC. The dose is 100 mg every 8 hours. Nilutamide poisoning is rare. A 79-year-old man ingested 13 g of nilutamide (170 mg/kg) following 300 mg/day for 2 weeks. On admission, he underwent gastric lavage, followed by AC, and received an IV infusion of glucose in balanced salt solution. During the first 12 hours, he developed vomiting and diarrhea. No adverse effects previously described with daily nilutamide were noted (420).

Toxicokinetics and Toxicodynamics

Nilutamide is well absorbed orally. Plasma protein binding is 84%. Nilutamide metabolism involves the hepatic microsomal oxidation system. Excretion is 49% to 78% in the urine as metabolites. Fecal excretion is 1.4% to 7.0%. The half-life is 56 hours (421).

Pathophysiology

Nilutamide is a pure antiandrogen with affinity for androgen receptors (but not for progestogen, estrogen, or glucocorticoid receptors). Nilutamide blocks the action of androgens of adrenal and testicular origin that stimulates the growth of normal and malignant prostate tissue (422).

Pregnancy and Lactation

Nilutamide is FDA pregnancy risk category X (Appendix I).

Clinical Presentation

Nilutamide can cause neutropenia (423). Acute hepatitis (424) and fatal fulminant hepatitis have been induced by nilutamide (425). Nilutamide can delay adaptation to darkness after exposure to bright light. This often improves with maintenance doses and resolves when discontinued (426).

Nilutamide can cause a disulfiram-like reaction with alcohol. Hot flushes are common in patients who have been surgically castrated and may be the result of the surgery rather than nilutamide (3). Depression has been reported with nilutamide use (427). Interstitial pneumonitis was associated with neoadjuvant leuprolide and nilutamide for prostate cancer (428).

Diagnostic Tests

Testing is aimed at end organ effects (e.g., bone marrow, heart, liver). CBC and electrolytes should be followed during treatment. Liver function should be monitored periodically. Specific levels of nilutamide are not used to guide management.

Treatment

See Antineoplastic Treatment Guidelines at the end of this chapter.

PACLITAXEL

Paclitaxel (Taxol) is used to treat breast, ovarian, head and neck, non–small cell lung, and gastric cancers as well as germ cell tumors, astrocytomas, and Kaposi's sarcoma. The usual adult dose is 135 to 200 mg/m^2 IV every 3 weeks. In children the dose is 350 mg/m^2 IV every 3 weeks.

Toxicokinetics and Toxicodynamics

Paclitaxel is not absorbed orally. Its V_d is 55 to 182 L/m^2. It does not cross the blood–brain barrier. Plasma protein binding is 89% to 97% (3). Paclitaxel is metabolized in the liver. Urinary excretion of unchanged drug is 2% to 13%. The alpha half-life of paclitaxel is 16 to 29 minutes, and beta half-life is 6.4 to 12.7 hours (3).

Pathophysiology

Unlike other agents (e.g., vincristine, colchicine) that inhibit mitotic spindle formation, paclitaxel promotes assembly of microtubules, stabilizes them against depolymerization, and inhibits cell replication.

Pregnancy and Lactation

Paclitaxel is FDA pregnancy risk category D (Appendix I). A woman was treated with paclitaxel during pregnancy and gave birth to a normal child (429). Breast-feeding is not recommended.

Clinical Presentation

Immediate effects include anaphylaxis and allergic reactions. Other immediate effects include nausea and vomiting, diarrhea, bradycardia, hypotension during infusion, vein irritation, and rare radiation recall reactions. Early effects may include myelosuppression (nadir, 8 to 11 days; recovery, 15 to 21 days), alopecia, peripheral neuropathy, muscle and joint pain, mucositis, ECG changes, and elevated LFTs (3).

Peripheral neuropathy may be dose limiting. Paclitaxel-induced neuropathy is mostly sensory and begins after the first or second dose (430). Common symptoms include numbness, tingling, and burning pain in a glove-and-stocking distribution. The symptoms are generally tolerable but may be disabling in patients treated with 250 mg/m^2 or more, in treatment combined with cisplatin, and in those at high risk of developing neurotoxicity (e.g., prior exposure to neurotoxic agents such as cisplatin and the vinca alkaloids, diabetes mellitus, or chronic alcoholism). Bilateral facial nerve palsy after a single cycle of high-dose paclitaxel therapy (825 mg/m^2) has been described (431).

Myelosuppression does not appear to be cumulative but is increased in heavily pretreated patients who received myelosuppressive or radiation therapy. Anemia and thrombocytopenia are rarely significant with paclitaxel.

Hypersensitivity reactions typically occur within 10 minutes of starting the infusion (432). Reactions are neither dose-related nor dependent on prior exposure to paclitaxel and may be caused by histamine release mediated by the Cremophor EL diluent (433). Paclitaxel has the potential to enhance radiation injury to tissues (434).

Diagnostic Tests

Testing is aimed at end organ effects (e.g., bone marrow, peripheral nerves). CBC and electrolytes should be followed during treatment. Liver function should be monitored periodically. Specific levels of paclitaxel are not used to guide management.

Treatment

See Antineoplastic Treatment Guidelines at the end of this chapter. Glutamate is a neuroprotectant against paclitaxel neuropathy in a rat model (435). Coadministration of paclitaxel with prosaptides prevented paclitaxel-induced thermal hypoalgesia in a rat study (436).

PEGASPARGASE

Pegaspargase (polyethylene glycol-L-asparaginase) is a *pegylated* version of L-asparaginase. It is used to treat patients with ALL (437) who have developed hypersensitivity to native L-asparaginase (438).

The recommended dose for adults and children with a body surface area greater than 0.6 m^2 is 2500 IU/m^2 every 14 days IV or IM (IM is the preferred route because of the lower incidence of hepatotoxicity, coagulopathy, and GI and renal disorders). The dose for children with a body surface area less than 0.6 m^2 is 82.5 IU/kg administered every 14 days.

Three patients received 10,000 IU/m^2 of pegaspargase IV. One patient experienced a slight increase in liver enzymes. A second patient developed a rash that was treated by slowing the rate and an antihistamine. A third patient did not experience any reaction (439).

Toxicokinetics and Toxicodynamics

Plasma half-life does not appear to be influenced by dose levels or correlated with age, sex, surface area, renal or hepatic function, diagnosis, or extent of disease. The V_d is 2093 ml/m^2, similar to L-asparaginase, indicating that pegaspargase is mainly localized in the plasma (440).

Pathophysiology

Polyethylene glycol modified L-asparaginase reduces the immune response and extends half-life. Leukemic cells lack asparagine synthetase and are dependent on an exogenous source of asparagine for survival. Rapid depletion of asparagine by L-asparaginase kills the leukemic cells. Normal cells are less affected due to their ability to synthesize asparagine (441).

Pregnancy and Lactation

Pegaspargase is FDA pregnancy risk category C (Appendix I).

Clinical Presentation

The most frequent adverse effects are allergic reactions, aminotransferase increase, nausea and vomiting, fever, and malaise. Less common effects are anaphylactic reactions, dyspnea, injection site hypersensitivity, lip and peripheral edema, rash, urticaria, abdominal pain, chills, pain in the extremities, hypotension, tachycardia, thrombosis, anorexia, diarrhea, jaundice, abnormal LFTs, decreased anticoagulant effect, diffuse intravascular coagulation, decreased fibrinogen, hemolytic anemia, leukopenia, pancytopenia, thrombocytopenia, injection site pain, hyperbilirubinemia, hyperglycemia, hyperuricemia, hypoglycemia, hypoproteinemia, arthralgia, myalgia, convulsion, headache, night sweats, and paresthesia (439).

The use of pegaspargase is sometimes limited by hypersensitivity reactions (442). Pancreatitis has been reported in children with ALL treated with pegaspargase (443). L-asparaginase–induced disturbances of clotting homeostasis may result in thrombosis or hemorrhage. Thrombotic occlusion of cerebral veins has been reported in patients with ALL.

A 16-year-old boy with non-Hodgkin's lymphoma developed a focal motor seizure 15 minutes after receiving pegaspargase. Brain imaging demonstrated multiple cortical and subcortical lesions that likely represented focal brain edema due to thrombotic venous occlusion. The patient improved within 3 days and completely resolved within 3 weeks without specific intervention (444).

Diagnostic Tests

Testing is aimed at end organ effects (e.g., bone marrow, liver). CBC and electrolytes should be followed during treatment. Liver function should be monitored periodically. Specific levels of pegaspargase are not used to guide management.

Treatment

See Antineoplastic Treatment Guidelines at the end of this chapter.

PENTOSTATIN

Pentostatin is used to treat hairy cell leukemia, CLL, mycosis fungoides, non-Hodgkin's lymphoma, melanoma, graft-versus-host disease, and T-cell lymphoma. The usual adult dose is 4 mg/m^2 IV every 2 weeks. There are no pediatric indications. Neurotoxicity is rarely dose limiting at less than 5 mg/m^2. Severe renal, hepatic, pulmonary, and CNS toxicity, leading in some cases to death, occurred in phase I studies that used 20 to 50 mg/m^2 per course. Lower doses (e.g., 4 mg/m^2) are better tolerated.

Toxicokinetics and Toxicodynamics

Pentostatin is not absorbed orally. The V_d is 20 L/m^2, it penetrates the blood–brain barrier, and plasma protein binding is 4% (3). A small amount is metabolized to active metabolites. It is mainly excreted unchanged by the kidneys. The alpha half-life is 9 to 85 minutes, and beta half-life is 6 hours (3).

Pathophysiology

Pentostatin, a structural analog of deoxyadenosine, is a potent inhibitor of adenosine deaminase. Adenosine deaminase, an important enzyme in purine metabolism, is found in high concentrations in lymphatic tissue. This inhibition results in the arrest of cells in the G1 or S phase of the cell cycle and subsequent cell dysfunction or death (445).

Pregnancy and Lactation

Pentostatin is FDA pregnancy risk category D (Appendix I). Breast-feeding is not recommended.

Clinical Presentation

Immediate effects include nausea and vomiting, which last up to 48 hours (446). Early effects include myelosuppression (recovery, 11 to 18 days), rash, lethargy, fatigue, seizures, and rare coma. Other effects include transiently elevated LFTs, anorexia, diarrhea, myalgia, elevated creatinine, acute renal failure, and painful keratoconjunctivitis.

Pentostatin produces immunosuppression, often manifested by herpes simplex and herpes zoster outbreaks, skin infections, and other opportunistic infections (447). Patients with severe preexisting infections should not receive this agent (448). The recovery of dose-related immunosuppression (e.g., reduction of CD4 cells) occurs slowly over several months.

Skin rash may occur early in therapy without recurrence during continued treatment. A fatal erythroderma has been reported (449). Acute renal failure, generally mild and reversible, has been reported (16). Keratitis with corneal ulceration and severe pain has been reported (450).

Diagnostic Tests

Testing is aimed at end organ effects (e.g., bone marrow, liver). CBC and electrolytes should be followed during treatment. Liver function should be monitored periodically. Specific levels of pentostatin are not used to guide management.

Treatment

See Antineoplastic Treatment Guidelines at the end of this chapter. Patients with CNS toxicity should not be treated until these have resolved (451). Subsequent treatment with pentostatin should use lower doses. Vigorous hydration should be maintained if possible. Other known nephrotoxic agents (e.g., aminoglycosides) should be avoided.

PROCARBAZINE

Procarbazine is part of the regimen of mechlorethamine, Oncovin (vincristine), procarbazine, and prednisone used to treat Hodgkin's disease. Other uses include non-Hodgkin's lymphoma and certain brain tumors.

Toxicokinetics and Toxicodynamics

Oral absorption is rapid and complete. Procarbazine rapidly crosses the blood–brain barrier (3). Metabolism of procarbazine occurs in the liver via the microsomal oxidation system. Excretion is predominantly in urine as *N*-isopropyl-terpthalamic acid (25% to 42% within 24 hours). The alpha half-life of procarbazine is 7 to 10 minutes, and the beta half-life is 1 hour (3).

Pathophysiology

Procarbazine has multiple sites of action. It inhibits incorporation of small DNA precursors, as well as RNA and protein synthesis. Procarbazine can also directly damage DNA by alkylation.

Pregnancy and Lactation

Procarbazine is FDA pregnancy risk category D (Appendix I). No congenital anomalies were found in six children of mothers treated during pregnancy with regimens that included procarbazine. Only one of these women was treated during the first trimester (452). Breast-feeding is not recommended.

Clinical Presentation

Immediate effects include anaphylaxis (453), radiation recall reaction, serum sickness, fever, a flu-like syndrome, nausea, and vomiting. Early effects include myelosuppression (nadir, 14 to 21 days; recovery, 28 days), lung injury (acute infiltrates, edema, cough), diplopia, stomatitis, alopecia, anorexia, rash, urticaria, hyperpigmentation, hemolytic anemia, amenorrhea, azoospermia, and CNS depression. Late effects may include leukemia, peripheral neuropathy, persistent hyperpigmentation, and infertility with amenorrhea, or azoospermia (3).

Hypersensitivity pneumonitis can occur within hours. Patients usually recover following discontinuation of procarbazine; however, the pneumonitis can be severe and irreversible (454). Procarbazine is a weak monoamine oxidase inhibitor (455). Neurotoxicity may involve altered consciousness, peripheral neuropathy, ataxia, or effects of monoamine oxidase inhibition. Peripheral neuropathy consists of paresthesias, decreased deep tendon reflexes, and myalgia (456).

In addition to myelosuppression with normal use, prolonged thrombocytopenia has been described (457). Hypersensitivity to procarbazine characterized by a nonpigmented fixed drug eruption has been reported (458). Maculopapular rash and urticaria have also been reported (459,460). Procarbazine can cause azoospermia (461), which is often irreversible, and amenorrhea in women.

Procarbazine can enhance radiation injury before, concurrent with, or even after its administration. Recurrent injury to a previously radiated site may occur weeks to months following radiation (3).

Diagnostic Tests

Testing is aimed at end organ effects (e.g., bone marrow, lung, liver, neuropathy). CBC and electrolytes should be followed during treatment. Liver function should be monitored periodically. Specific levels of procarbazine are not used to guide management.

Treatment

See Antineoplastic Treatment Guidelines at the end of this chapter.

RITUXIMAB

Rituximab is a chimeric murine/human monoclonal antibody directed against the CD20 antigen found on normal and malignant B lymphocytes (462). It is used to treat B-cell non-Hodgkin's lymphoma, transplant-related lymphoma, cold agglutinin disease, autoimmune hemolytic anemia, and B-cell purging in autologous bone marrow transplant. A typical adult dose is 375 mg/m^2 IV weekly for 4 weeks. Doses have not been established in children.

Toxicokinetics and Toxicodynamics

The half-life of rituximab was 3.2 days following a single infusion but increases with dose and repeated dosing.

Pathophysiology

Rituximab binds specifically to the CD20 antigen located on pre-B, mature B lymphocytes, and more than 90% of B-cell non-Hodgkin's lymphomas. The CD20 antigen regulates the activation process for cell cycle initiation and differentiation.

Pregnancy and Lactation

Rituximab is FDA pregnancy risk category C (Appendix I). Because IgG crosses the placenta, women of childbearing age should use birth control during and up to 12 months after rituximab therapy. Breast-feeding is not recommended.

Clinical Presentation

Severe pulmonary events such as bronchospasm, dyspnea, hypoxia, pulmonary infiltrates, and acute respiratory failure may occur with rituximab therapy (463). Patients with preexisting pulmonary insufficiency or tumor infiltration are at higher risks. Infusion-related adverse effects include allergic reactions and other symptoms (e.g., flushing, hypotension, rhinitis, nausea, asthenia, and headache) (464). Symptoms usually occur 30 minutes to 2 hours after starting the infusion and may be related to the release of cytokines and other mediators. There are no apparent risk factors for infusion-related syndrome (465). Cytokine release syndrome may occur within 24 hours of the first infusion and can be fatal (466). Symptoms begin 1 to 2 hours after starting the infusion and can include severe dyspnea, bronchospasm, hypoxia, pulmonary infiltrates, acute respiratory failure, fever, chills, rigors, urticaria, angioedema, and tumor lysis syndrome (467,468). Tumor lysis syndrome consists of hyperuricemia, hyperkalemia, hypocalcemia, acute renal failure, elevated lactate dehydrogenase, and high fevers. It usually occurs within 1 to 2 hours but may be delayed until 12 to 24 hours after the first infusion. It is more common in patients with high numbers of circulating malignant lymphocytes and probably due to rapid lysis of B lymphocytes (469).

Rare severe mucocutaneous reactions similar to Stevens-Johnson syndrome have been noted. The onset varies from days to months after therapy. Rituximab should be discontinued (470).

Diagnostic Tests

Testing is aimed at end organ effects (e.g., lung, tumor lysis). CBC and electrolytes should be followed during treatment. Specific levels of rituximab are not used to guide management.

Treatment

See Antineoplastic Treatment Guidelines at the end of this chapter. During infusion, vital signs should be monitored frequently. If a reaction occurs, the infusion should be stopped immediately. Because initial improvement may be followed by deterioration, patients should be closely monitored until tumor lysis syndrome and pulmonary infiltration have been ruled out. Mild infusion reactions are treated with diphenhydramine, acetaminophen, β-agonist nebulizers, or IV saline. Severe reactions are treated with epinephrine, antihistamines, and steroids. Most patients with mild reactions can complete the full therapy.

STREPTOZOCIN

Streptozocin is used to treat pancreatic islet cell, colon, hepatic, pancreatic, and prostatic cancers as well as carcinoid tumor, Hodgkin's disease, and insulinomas. The adult dose is 1 g/m^2 IV weekly for 2 weeks and then increased according to patient response. A maximal single dose is 1.5 g/m^2 or 500 mg/m^2/day for 5 days every 6 weeks. In children, the dose is 500 mg/m^2/day IV every 4 weeks for 5 days.

Toxicokinetics and Toxicodynamics

Streptozocin is poorly absorbed orally. It is distributed to the liver, kidney, and pancreas. The V_d is 0.5 L/kg. Metabolism is by liver and kidney. It also spontaneously degrades to methylcarbonium ion. Active metabolites include a methylated metabolite and methylcarbonium ion. Excretion is renal (60% to 72% in 24 hours; 10% to 20% as unchanged drug). The alpha half-life is 5 to 15 minutes, and the beta half-life is 35 to 40 minutes (3).

Pathophysiology

Streptozocin inhibits DNA synthesis (471), interferes with nicotinamide adenine dinucleotide and the reduced form of nicotinamide adenine dinucleotide, and inhibits some gluconeogenic enzymes. It is cell cycle phase nonspecific and non–cross-resistant with other nitrosoureas (4).

Pregnancy and Lactation

Streptozocin is FDA pregnancy risk category C (Appendix I). Breast-feeding is not recommended (472).

Clinical Presentation

Immediate effects include severe nausea and vomiting, fever, chills, hypoglycemia, and burning or pain on injection. Early effects include myelosuppression (nadir, 7 to 14 days; recovery, 21 days), nephrotoxicity in 65% of patients, loss of diabetic control, diarrhea, anorexia, elevated LFTs, and nail changes. Late effects may include persistent nephrotoxicity, leukemia, and renal neoplasms (3). Tissue necrosis may occur.

Nephrotoxicity is the dose-limiting toxicity, occurs in 65% of patients, and may be fatal. Signs of nephrotoxicity include hypophosphatemia, hypokalemia, hypouricemia, renal tubular acidosis, glucosuria, acetonuria, and aminoaciduria (16). Transient, reversible proteinuria and Fanconi syndrome have also been documented.

In some patients, insulin may be released suddenly, resulting in hypoglycemia within 24 hours of treatment. Glycosuria has been observed.

Diagnostic Tests

Testing is aimed at end organ effects (e.g., bone marrow, kidney, liver). CBC, electrolytes, liver enzymes, and fasting insulin levels should be followed with each treatment. Periodic blood glucose and uric acid determinations are recommended. Specific levels of streptozocin are not used to guide management.

Treatment

See Antineoplastic Treatment Guidelines at the end of this chapter. Monitor for the proteinuria or a decline in creatinine clearance. The role of hydration in decreasing nephrotoxicity has not been clearly defined. Forced diuresis was used to reduce nephrotoxicity in metastatic insulinoma (473).

TAMOXIFEN

Tamoxifen is used to treat breast cancer, brain tumors, endometrial cancer, malignant melanoma, pancreatic cancer in postmenopausal women, and prostate cancer. Adult dose regimens include 20 mg orally/day, 20 mg/m^2 orally/day, up to 40 mg orally four times a day for 7 days (for malignant melanoma).

Toxicokinetics and Toxicodynamics

Tamoxifen is well absorbed orally and distributed primarily to uterus, endometrium, breast, prostate, and ovary. Hepatic microsomal oxidation produces active metabolites such as *N*-desmethyltamoxifen and inactive metabolites (474). Excretion is primarily biliary. Tamoxifen undergoes enterohepatic circulation and is slowly excreted in feces and less than 1% in urine. The alpha half-life is 7 to 14 hours after a single dose and 7 days at steady-state.

Pathophysiology

Tamoxifen is thought to competitively block estrogen receptors and suppress the breast cancer cell genome. Other effects include interaction with protein kinase C and stimulation of human natural killer cells. Approximately 25% of malignant melanomas have estrogen receptors, and occasional responses to tamoxifen have been reported. Similar observations have been made in normal and malignant pancreas.

Pregnancy and Lactation

Tamoxifen is FDA pregnancy risk category D (Appendix I).

Clinical Presentation

Tamoxifen is usually well tolerated, and serious side effects are rare. Immediate effects include nausea and vomiting. Early effects include hot flushes, headache, transient increase in bone or tumor pain, hypercalcemia, menstrual irregularities, edema, rare vaginal discharge or bleeding, vulvar itching, and dizziness (3). Other effects include transient myelosuppression, rash, dermatomyositis, and elevated LFTs. Delayed effects include infrequent pulmonary emboli or thromboses, depression, retinopathy, corneal opacities, and rare endometrial cancer (3).

The most serious effect is hypercalcemia, which develops in 4% to 5% of metastatic breast cancers (475). A transient increase in bone pain, local disease flare (swelling and redness), and hypercalcemia may occur at initiation in patients with metastatic disease (476,477).

Greatly thickened endometria are often observed in vaginal sonography in patients taking tamoxifen (478,479). Endometrial polyps have been attributed to tamoxifen use (480,481). Tamoxifen therapy increases the relative risk of endometrial cancer slightly (482,483). The incidence of other tumors is not increased by tamoxifen treatment.

Tamoxifen may precipitate nonalcoholic steatohepatitis in predisposed persons by exacerbating insulin resistance, central obesity, diabetes, and hypertriglyceridemia (484,485). Submassive hepatic necrosis (486), pancreatitis (487,488), and the development of HCC (489) have also been attributed to tamoxifen.

Ocular problems [e.g., retinopathy (490,491), corneal opacities, and keratopathy] have been reported in patients who received a high dose or standard doses (492). Hot flashes are the most prominent side effect of tamoxifen (493). Severe dermatomyositis has occurred with tamoxifen use (494). Total alopecia has also been reported (495).

Diagnostic Tests

Testing is aimed at end organ effects (e.g., bone marrow, liver, hypercalcemia). CBC and electrolytes should be followed during treatment. Serum calcium should be monitored 3 to 7 days after starting treatment in patients with extensive bony metastatic disease. Specific levels of tamoxifen are not used to guide management.

Treatment

See Antineoplastic Treatment Guidelines at the end of this chapter. Hot flushes, nausea, and vomiting occur in up to 25% of patients but are rarely severe enough to discontinue treatment. These may be controlled by a decreased or divided dose. Night sweats may be treated by taking tamoxifen in the morning. Clonidine, 0.05 mg bid (496), or belladonna-ergotamine-phenobarbital tablets have been used to alleviate severe hot flushes, but with limited success.

TENIPOSIDE

Teniposide is a semisynthetic podophyllotoxin (497) used to treat ALL, non-Hodgkin's lymphoma, Hodgkin's disease, small cell lung cancer, brain metastases, multiple myeloma, and retinoblastoma. The adult dose is up to 250 mg/m^2 IV (with vincristine) weekly for 4 to 8 weeks. The pediatric dose is up to 250 mg/m^2 IV (with vincristine) weekly for 4 to 8 weeks.

Toxicokinetics and Toxicodynamics

Distribution of teniposide is highest in liver, kidneys, small intestine, and adrenals. Teniposide may be found in ascitic fluid and crosses the blood–brain barrier. Its V_d is approximately 30% of body weight, and plasma protein binding is 99.4% (3). Teniposide is metabolized to active and inactive metabolites. Fecal excretion is 0% to 10% within 3 days, and 44.5% is excreted in urine within 72 hours, 21.3% as unchanged drug. Alpha half-life is 45 minutes, and beta half-life is 2.8 to 4.0 hours (3).

Pathophysiology

Teniposide causes single-strand DNA breaks and also causes DNA damage through inhibition of the enzyme topoisomerase II and activation of oxidation-reduction reactions to produce derivatives that bind directly to DNA (498).

Pregnancy and Lactation

Teniposide is FDA pregnancy risk category D (Appendix I).

Clinical Presentation

Immediate effects include allergic reactions, hemolytic anemia, anaphylaxis (499), phlebitis, nausea and vomiting, and hypotension after rapid administration. Early effects include myelosuppression (nadir, 7 to 14 days; recovery, 22 to 28 days), alopecia, diarrhea, stomatitis, anorexia, nephrotoxicity, elevated LFTs, and rare peripheral neuropathy. AML has been reported as a potential late effect (3,500).

Teniposide appears to cause more reactions than etoposide, possibly due to the presence of the surfactant Cremophor EL in the teniposide preparation (501). Type 1 hypersensitivity reactions account for the majority of effects (e.g., urticaria, angioedema, flushing, or rashes) (502). More severe reactions may produce bronchospasm, cyanosis, chest pain, and/or hypotension. No fatalities have been reported (503).

The use of teniposide in children has been associated with the development of secondary AML (504) and acute promyelocytic leukemia (505).

Diagnostic Tests

Testing is aimed at end organ effects (e.g., bone marrow). The CBC should be followed during treatment. Specific levels of teniposide are not used to guide management.

Treatment

See Antineoplastic Treatment Guidelines at the end of this chapter. Discontinuing the infusion and administering an antihistamine can relieve most allergic symptoms.

TESTOLACTONE

Testolactone is adjunctive therapy in the palliative treatment of advanced or disseminated breast cancer in postmenopausal women. It is also used to treat precocious puberty, congenital adrenal hyperplasia, gynecomastia, desmoid tumors, and male infertility. The adult dose is 250 mg four times a day orally. Safety and effectiveness in children have not been established. There are no reports of acute overdosage.

Toxicokinetics and Toxicodynamics

Testolactone is well absorbed. It is metabolized hepatically and undergoes urinary excretion.

Pathophysiology

Its principal action is reported to be inhibition of steroid aromatase activity (506) and consequent reduction in estrone synthesis from adrenal androstenedione, the major source of estrogen in postmenopausal women. Despite its similarity to testosterone, testolactone has no androgenic effect (507).

Pregnancy and Lactation

Testolactone is FDA pregnancy risk category C (Appendix I). It is not known whether this drug is excreted in human milk.

Clinical Presentation

Toxic effects include maculopapular erythema, increase in blood pressure, paresthesia, malaise, aches and edema of the extremities, glossitis, anorexia, and nausea and vomiting. Alopecia alone and with associated nail growth disturbance has been reported rarely; these side effects subsided without interruption of treatment (507).

Diagnostic Tests

Testing is aimed at end organ and metabolic effects (e.g., hypocalcemia). Specific levels of testolactone are not used to guide management.

Treatment

See Antineoplastic Treatment Guidelines at the end of this chapter.

THIOGUANINE

6-Thioguanine (6-TG) is used to treat childhood ALL, AML, CML, and psoriasis. The adult dose for induction is 75 to 200 mg/m^2/day orally for 5 to 7 days/course or 2 to 3 mg/kg/day orally. The maintenance dose is 2 mg/kg/day orally. In children, the induction dose is 2 to 3 mg/kg/day orally and 75 to 200 mg/m^2/day orally for 5 to 7 days. Maintenance dose is 2 mg/kg/day orally.

Toxicokinetics and Toxicodynamics

Oral bioavailability is 14% to 46%. 6-TG crosses the placenta. Metabolism is mainly hepatic. 2-Amino-6-methylmercaptopurine is an active metabolite. Excretion is mainly urinary (24% to 46% within 24 hours); however, hemodialysis is unlikely to decrease toxicity. The alpha half-life of thioguanine is 15 minutes, and the beta half-life is 11 hours (3).

Pathophysiology

Intracellular activation of thioguanine results in incorporation into DNA as a false purine base (508). It is also incorporated into RNA. Thioguanine is cross resistant with 6-MP.

Pregnancy and Lactation

6-TG is FDA pregnancy risk category D (Appendix I). 6-TG has been followed by the birth of a normal child (509); however, fetal death (510) and chromosomal abnormalities have also occurred.

Clinical Presentation

Immediate effects include nausea, vomiting, and hyperuricemia. Early effects include myelosuppression (nadir, 7 to 14 days; recovery, 14 to 21 days), stomatitis, diarrhea, anorexia, rash, and liver problems (e.g., elevated LFTs, veno-occlusive disease, and jaundice). Delayed effects may include birth defects, loss of vibration sensitivity, and unsteady gait. "Painful red hands" have been described in patients receiving cytosine arabinoside, 6-TG, and adriamycin for leukemia (3,511).

Diagnostic Tests

Laboratory monitoring for each treatment should include a CBC. Periodic monitoring should include serum uric acid, kidney function, and liver function. Specific levels of 6-TG are not available or used to guide management.

Treatment

See Antineoplastic Treatment Guidelines at the end of this chapter. Unlike 6-MP, 6-TG metabolism is not inhibited by allopurinol (3).

THIOTEPA

Thiotepa is used to treat transitional cell, breast, and ovarian cancers, as well as pediatric brain tumors, Hodgkin's disease, non-Hodgkin's lymphoma, and osteogenic sarcoma. Intrathecal thiotepa has been used for leptomeningeal metastases.

Toxicokinetics and Toxicodynamics

Oral absorption is incomplete. Distribution of thiotepa is rapid. The V_d of thiotepa is 47 to 72 ml/m^2, and plasma protein binding is 10% to 40% (3). It enters the brain but is rapidly cleared. Thiotepa is metabolized in the liver to the active metabolite triethylenephosphoramide. Excretion is urinary (60% within 72 hours). Alpha half-life is 6 to 24 minutes, and beta half-life is 1.3 to 2.2 hours.

Pathophysiology

Thiotepa is a polyfunctional-alkylating agent that produces DNA breaks as well as cross-linking. Thiotepa is cell cycle phase nonspecific (4).

Pregnancy and Lactation

Thiotepa is FDA pregnancy risk category D (Appendix I). Thiotepa is teratogenic. Breast-feeding is not recommended.

Clinical Presentation

Immediate effects include rare anaphylaxis, allergic reactions, nausea and vomiting, cystitis with bladder instillation, and CNS problems (e.g., somnolence, and seizures with bone marrow transplant doses). Elevated bilirubin may follow bone marrow transplant doses and paresthesias may be associated with the intrathecal route. Early effects include myelosuppression (nadir, 10 to 21 days; recovery, 18 to 40 days) and alopecia. Bone marrow transplant doses may yield stomatitis, diarrhea, and hyperpigmentation. Delayed effects may include infertility, amenorrhea, impaired spermatogenesis, and leukemia (3,200). GI effects may include stomatitis (512), esophagitis, nausea, vomiting, and diarrhea.

Intrathecal administration can cause lower extremity weakness, discomfort, transient paresthesia, myelopathy (513), and rare spinal cord demyelination. Eosinophilic cystitis has developed after intravesical instillation of thiotepa (514). Myelosuppression may follow the intravesical instillation (515,516). Skin toxicity from high-dose therapy typically presents as a sunburn-like redness that becomes hyperpigmented (517) and peels off after several weeks.

Diagnostic Tests

Testing is aimed at end organ effects (e.g., bone marrow, liver). Specific levels of thiotepa are not used to guide management.

Treatment

See Antineoplastic Treatment Guidelines at the end of this chapter.

TOPOTECAN

Topotecan is used to treat relapsed ovarian, small cell lung, non–small cell lung, and pancreatic cancers, as well as gliomas, AML, chronic myelomonocytic leukemia, multiple myeloma, myelodysplastic syndrome, neuroblastoma, retinoblastoma, HCC, non-Hodgkin's lymphoma, rhabdomyosarcoma, and Ewing's sarcoma. The dose is 1.5 mg/m^2 by IV infusion over 30 minutes daily for 5 days. A minimum of four courses is recommended. Pediatric use has not been established.

Toxicokinetics and Toxicodynamics

Oral absorption is 30% to 40%, and time-to-peak plasma concentration is 1 to 2 hours (518). Drug is evenly distributed between blood cells and plasma (519). V_d is 130 L, and plasma protein binding is 35% (520). Topotecan undergoes reversible, pH-dependent hydrolysis of the active lactone moiety to the inactive hydroxyacid (carboxylate) form. A relatively small amount is metabolized by hepatic enzymes to an active metabolite, *N*-desmethyltopotecan (521). Extent of biliary excretion is not determined, and 20% to 60% of dose is excreted in the urine (522). The half-life is 2 to 3 hours.

Pathophysiology

Topotecan is a semisynthetic, water-soluble derivative of camptothecin. Topotecan inhibits the action of topoisomerase I. Topotecan binds to the topoisomerase I–DNA complex and prevents relegation of the DNA strand, resulting in double-strand DNA breakage and cell death (3).

Pregnancy and Lactation

Topotecan is in FDA pregnancy risk category D (Appendix I). Topotecan may cause fetal harm *in utero* (523). Breast-feeding is not recommended.

Clinical Presentation

Hematologic toxicity is the predominant side effect. Noncumulative myelosuppression has limited its use (524). High-risk patients include those with more than six cycles of chemotherapy containing an alkylating agent, with radiation to more than 25% of marrow-bearing bones, and with a history of myelosuppression or renal impairment. By reducing the topotecan dose, myelosuppressive effects, as evidenced by neutropenia (525) and thrombocytopenia, may be lessened or prevented without reducing the antitumor response (526).

Topotecan has been associated with a scleroderma-like illness (527). Neutrophilic eccrine hidradenitis, a self-restricted inflammatory condition, is also associated with topotecan use (528).

Diagnostic Tests

Testing is aimed at end organ effects (e.g., bone marrow, liver). Specific levels of topotecan are not used to guide management.

Treatment

See Antineoplastic Treatment Guidelines at the end of this chapter. Hemodialysis may effectively clear topotecan and can be considered in selected situations (e.g., overdose, severe renal dysfunction) (529). The mean duration of neutropenia from topotecan was reduced by granulocyte-macrophage colony-stimulating factor priming in one study (530).

TOREMIFENE

Toremifene is used as a substitute for tamoxifen in breast cancer patients (531). The dosage is 40 or 60 mg, once daily, orally (532). Treatment is generally continued until disease progression is observed. There is no pediatric indication. Toremifene is well tolerated over a wide range of doses (10 to 680 mg/day). The major side effects are hot flashes, nausea, and vomiting (533). In postmenopausal breast cancer patients, toremifene 400 $mg/m^2/day$ caused dose-limiting nausea and dizziness, as well as hallucinations and ataxia in one patient (534).

Toxicokinetics and Toxicodynamics

Toremifene is well absorbed orally. C_{max} is reached within 4 hours (535). The apparent V_d is 580 L, and drug binds extensively to serum proteins, mainly albumin. Toremifene is extensively metabolized by P-450 enzymes (536). Toremifene is eliminated as metabolites in the feces and slightly (10%) in the urine during a 1-week period. Elimination of toremifene is slow, in part because of enterohepatic circulation. The half-life is approximately 5 days, and steady-state is reached in 6 weeks depending on the dose.

Pathophysiology

Toremifene binds to estrogen receptors and may exert estrogenic or antiestrogenic (or both) activities. The antitumor effect is mainly due to its antiestrogenic effects.

Pregnancy and Lactation

Toremifene is FDA pregnancy risk category D (Appendix I). Toremifene is embryotoxic and fetotoxic in animals. Breast-feeding is not recommended.

Clinical Presentation

Common adverse effects include vasomotor symptoms such as hot flashes and vaginal discharge (537). Toremifene may induce fatty liver and nonalcoholic steatohepatitis in breast cancer patients (538).

After a total cumulative exposure to toremifene of 140,000 patient-years, only nine cases of endometrial carcinoma have been reported. The annual hazard rate (per 1000 patient-years) of developing endometrial carcinoma in breast cancer patients on adjuvant toremifene is 1.14 (vs. tamoxifen, 2.0, and placebo, 0.4). Although toremifene (being a partial agonist) may unmask preexisting endometrial tumors, there are no clinical data implying that it causes endometrial carcinoma (539).

Diagnostic Tests

Testing is aimed at end organ effects (e.g., bone marrow, liver). Periodic CBC, calcium levels, and LFTs should be obtained. Specific levels of toremifene are not used to guide management.

Treatment

See Antineoplastic Treatment Guidelines at the end of this chapter. There is no specific antidote.

VALRUBICIN

Valrubicin is used as intravesical therapy of Bacille Calmette-Guérin (BCG)–refractory carcinoma *in situ* of the urinary bladder in patients for whom surgery is inappropriate (540). The intravesicular dose in adults is 800 mg once weekly for 6 weeks (541).

Toxicokinetics and Toxicodynamics

Action is primarily local, and systemic absorption is negligible. Drug is excreted by voiding of instillate.

Pathophysiology

Valrubicin is an anthracycline (542) that inhibits the incorporation of nucleosides into nucleic acids, causes extensive chromosomal damage, and arrests the cell cycle in G2. Valrubicin metabolites interfere with the normal DNA breaking-resealing action of DNA topoisomerase II.

Pregnancy and Lactation

Valrubicin is FDA pregnancy risk category C (Appendix I).

Clinical Presentation

Early effects include dizziness, headache, malaise, weakness, and pneumonia. Other effects include chest pain, vasodilation, abdominal pain, diarrhea, flatulence, nausea, and vomiting.

Effects after intravesical instillation include bladder spasm, cystitis, dysuria (543), hematuria, red urine, urinary incontinence, urinary tract infection, urinary urgency, local burning, nocturia, urethral pain, and urinary retention. Other reported effects include rash, peripheral edema, anemia, hyperglycemia, and back pain (3). Dose-limiting toxicities are leukopenia and neutropenia, beginning within 1 week of dose administration, with nadirs by the second week and recovery generally by the third week.

Diagnostic Tests

Testing is aimed at end organ effects (e.g., bone marrow, liver). Periodic CBC, calcium levels, and LFTs should be obtained. Specific levels of valrubicin are not used to guide management.

Treatment

See Antineoplastic Treatment Guidelines at the end of this chapter.

VINBLASTINE

Vinblastine is used to treat breast, testicular, bladder, cervical, non–small cell lung, and renal cell cancers, as well as Hodgkin's disease, Kaposi's sarcoma, choriocarcinoma, germ cell neoplasms, histiocytosis X, mycosis fungoides, and non-Hodgkin's lymphoma.

The usual IV dose in adults is 3.0 to 18.5 mg/m^2 every 1 to 4 weeks. In children, the usual IV dose range is 6.0 to 6.5 mg/m^2 IV every 1 to 2 weeks. Overdose has resulted in SIADH (544). A pediatric vinblastine overdose resulted in neurologic toxicity (e.g., seizures, coma) and marrow aplasia, which improved and gradually resolved. The child was given salvage therapy with steroids and citrovorum factor and survived (545).

Toxicokinetics and Toxicodynamics

Oral absorption is erratic. Vinblastine is extensively bound to tissues and to peripheral blood elements. Its V_d is 27.3 L/kg, and plasma protein binding is 43% to 99% (3). The liver produces the active metabolite desacetylvinblastine as well as inactive metabolites. Vinblastine is slowly excreted in urine and feces. The half-life is 19 to 25 hours.

Pathophysiology

Vinblastine binds to the microtubular proteins of the mitotic spindle, leading to crystallization of the microtubule and mitotic arrest or cell death. Vinblastine has some immunosuppressant effects. The vinca alkaloids are cell cycle phase specific.

Pregnancy and Lactation

Vinblastine is FDA pregnancy risk category D (Appendix I). No congenital anomalies were found in ten children born to women treated during pregnancy with vinblastine. Four of these women were treated during the first trimester. Their growth, intellectual development, and cytogenetic analysis were normal in ages ranging from 3 to 19 years at the time of the follow-up (546). Breast-feeding is not recommended (547).

Clinical Presentation

Immediate effects include rare anaphylaxis, pain on injection, vasoconstriction, parotid gland pain, muscle and tumor pain, and vomiting. Early effects may include alopecia, myelosuppression (nadir, 4 to 9 days; recovery, 7 to 21 days), neuropathy, constipation, urinary retention, autonomic neuropathy, stomatitis, SIADH, hyperuricemia, and photosensitivity. Delayed effects may include infertility (3). Vinblastine may be lethal if injected intrathecally.

Neurotoxicity may manifest as numbness, paresthesia, mental depression, loss of deep tendon reflexes, headache, malaise, dizziness, seizures, or psychosis. Cranial neuropathy may lead to vocal cord paresis or paralysis (548,549), oculomotor nerve dysfunction, and bilateral facial nerve palsies. Cranial nerve toxicity tends to be bilateral and reversible when vinblastine is stopped. Autonomic neuropathy is manifested as constipation, abdominal pain, ileus, and urinary retention (550). GI symptoms are seen with high doses (e.g., more than 20 mg). Tissue necrosis may develop after extravasation (334).

Diagnostic Tests

Testing is aimed at end organ effects (e.g., bone marrow, electrolytes, liver). Periodic CBC, serum electrolytes, and LFTs should be obtained. Specific levels of vinblastine are not used to guide management.

Treatment

See Antineoplastic Treatment Guidelines at the end of this chapter. Fluid restriction may be required for SIADH. Please see Methotrexate section for information regarding toxicity following intrathecal use.

VINCRISTINE

Vincristine (Oncovin) is used to treat ALL, Ewing's sarcoma, Hodgkin's disease [Oncovin is the "O" in the MOPP regimen (mechlorethamine, Oncovin [vincristine], procarbazine, and prednisone), non-Hodgkin's lymphoma, Wilms' tumor, rhabdomyosarcoma, brain tumors, CLL, CML, Burkitt's lymphoma, hepatoblastoma, Kaposi's sarcoma, melanoma, multiple myeloma, neuroblastoma, osteogenic and soft tissue sarcomas, gestational trophoblastic tumors, hemangiomas, and thrombotic thrombocytopenic purpura, as well as small cell lung, breast, cervical, colorectal, and testicular cancers.

A 53-year-old patient received 14 mg (4 mg/m^2/day for 2 days) of vincristine instead of vinblastine. Life-threatening effects included "paresthesias, bone marrow depression, severe oral mucositis, paralytic ileus, bladder atony, myalgia, muscle weakness, high fever, derangement of various organs (liver, heart), hypertension, and insomnia" (551). Other than extremity paresthesias, the patient recovered completely with intensive symptomatic and supportive care (551).

An esophageal cancer patient with bilateral lung and neck lymph node metastases received 24 mg of vincristine instead of vinblastine. Central and peripheral neuropathy with muscle atrophy, GI symptoms, bone marrow suppression, and mucocutaneous involvement occurred (552).

Vincristine can be lethal if given intrathecally (553). There are no successful antidotes.

Following overdose, fever, nausea, and vomiting usually begin in the first day and resolve within 1 week. Peripheral neuropathy may progress during the first week, associated with diminished reflexes, particularly in the lower extremities; paresthesias in 10 days; and muscle weakness and disturbed gait in 2 to 3 weeks. Slow recovery may occur over 30 to 45 days (3).

Neurotoxicity is dose related such that drug therapy has to be stopped after a cumulative dose of 30 to 50 mg. Neurotoxicity is usually reversible on interruption, but the recovery is slow and takes several months (554).

Vincristine overdoses (7.5 mg/m^2) were accidentally administered to three children. Treatment included double-volume exchange transfusion, phenobarbital prophylaxis, and folinic acid rescue, 18 mg every 3 hours for 16 doses. Two patients developed peripheral neuropathy on day 4, bone marrow toxicity on day 5, GI toxicity on day 6, and hypertension on days 7, and survived. The third patient died of liver and marrow toxicity on day 9 (555).

Toxicokinetics and Toxicodynamics

Vincristine is not absorbed orally. The V_d is 8.4 L/kg, and plasma protein binding is 44%. Metabolism is hepatic. Drug and metabolites are excreted into bile and feces (67% within 72 hours, 40% to 50% as metabolites), and urine (12% within 72 hours, 50% as metabolites). The half-life is 85 hours (3).

Pathophysiology

Vincristine crystallizes microtubules of the mitotic spindle, causing mitotic arrest or cell death. The vinca alkaloids are considered cell cycle phase specific (127,556).

Pregnancy and Lactation

Vincristine is FDA pregnancy risk category D (Appendix I). Normal babies have been delivered after first-, second-, or third-trimester exposures (156,557,558); however, vincristine was associated with early fetal loss in 124 nurses preparing chemotherapy (559). Breast-feeding is not recommended.

Clinical Presentation

Neurotoxicity with the vinca alkaloids is qualitatively similar but quantitatively different. Regarding toxicity, vincristine is greater than vindesine, and vindesine is greater than vinblastine. Predisposition for chemotherapy-induced neuropathy has been observed in nerves previously damaged by diabetes mellitus, alcohol, or inherited neuropathy (89).

The most frequent manifestation is peripheral neuropathy, the earliest indication of which is depression of the Achilles reflex (560). After three or more weekly doses, loss of other deep tendon reflexes occurs and is accompanied by peripheral paresthesias, pain, and tingling. If therapy is prolonged or high doses are administered, wrist and foot drop, ataxia, a slapping gait, and difficulty in walking may occur. Young children may refuse to walk due to extremity pain. Peripheral neuropathy may be more common in HIV-infected individuals (561). Loss of deep tendon reflexes does not necessarily require dosage reduction. For severe motor neuropathy, vincristine should be omitted.

Cranial neuropathy may lead to vocal cord paresis (547) or paralysis (562) (hoarseness, weak voice); ocular motor nerve dysfunction [ptosis (563), strabismus]; bilateral facial nerve palsies; or jaw pain. Severe jaw pain can occur within a few hours of the first dose (564). Jaw pain is not an indication to stop or modify dose and is treated with analgesics. Ptosis or hoarseness is an indication to hold doses until recovery from this symptom. Cranial nerve toxicity is usually reversible when vincristine is discontinued.

Autonomic neuropathy is manifested as constipation (565), abdominal pain, urinary retention, paralytic ileus, and abnormal variation in blood pressure on standing (566). These symptoms resolve with time. If bladder atony occurs, vincristine should be held until symptoms resolve. Other signs of central neurotoxicity include headache, malaise, dizziness, seizures (567,568), mental depression, hallucinations (569), and psychosis. Sensory disturbances may begin during the first week, progress to lethargy and disorientation by the second week, and resolve over 2 to 4 weeks. Intrathecal administration may cause ascending paralysis and death in weeks.

Infants are more susceptible to neurotoxicity. Symptoms of neurotoxicity in infants include a characteristic aphonic cry, irritability, poor feeding, and peripheral motor weakness. Infants are also more susceptible to ileus, SIADH, and hematologic toxicity from vincristine.

Bone marrow depression is characterized by leukopenia (nadir, 10 days; recovery, within 3 weeks). Tissue necrosis may occur after extravasation. Hemolytic uremic syndrome occurs rarely (72). SIADH may begin in 3 to 7 days and may be associated with seizures that do not appear directly related to hyponatremia. At least 76 cases of SIADH have been identified (570).

Diagnostic Tests

Testing is aimed at end organ effects (e.g., bone marrow, electrolytes, liver). Periodic CBC, serum electrolytes, and LFTs should be obtained. Specific concentrations of vincristine are not used to guide management.

Treatment

See Antineoplastic Treatment Guidelines at the end of this chapter. Fluid restriction may be required for SIADH. Please see Methotrexate section for information regarding toxicity following intrathecal use.

Vincristine is highly protein bound and cannot be dialyzed. Plasmapheresis was used to treat a tenfold vincristine overdose in an 18-year-old patient (571). Leucovorin does not appear to significantly alter toxicity (572).

VINDESINE

Vindesine is a vinca alkaloid used to treat ALL, CML, as well as breast, colorectal, non–small cell lung, and renal cell cancers. Typical dosing is 2 to 4 mg/m^2 IV every 1 to 2 weeks or 1.5 $mg/m^2/day$ for 5 to 7 days every 3 to 4 weeks as a continuous infusion. Typical pediatric IV dosing is 4 mg/m^2 every week.

Toxicokinetics and Toxicodynamics

Vindesine is not absorbed orally. It is rapidly distributed but does not cross the blood–brain barrier. The V_d of vindesine is 8.11 L/kg. Vindesine is metabolized in the liver and excreted via the biliary system (19%) and urine within 84 hours. The half-life is 20 to 24 hours (3).

Pathophysiology

Vindesine is a synthetic derivative of vinblastine (573). It crystallizes microtubular proteins, causing mitotic arrest or cell death. It is cell cycle phase specific (127).

Pregnancy and Lactation

Vindesine is FDA pregnancy risk category D (Appendix I). One normal baby in a mother treated with vindesine and other agents has been reported (574). Breast-feeding is not recommended (3).

Clinical Presentation

Vindesine overdose has been associated with generalized muscle pain, tinnitus, diarrhea, sleeplessness, a burning sensation in the mouth, and hiccups (575). Patients usually respond to supportive treatment.

Immediate adverse effects include rare anaphylaxis, nausea and vomiting, severe jaw pain, and cranial neuropathy. Early effects include alopecia; myelosuppression (nadir, 3 to 6 days; recovery, 7 to 10 days); increased platelet count; peripheral, cranial nerve, and autonomic neuropathy; abdominal cramping; constipation; paralytic ileus; phlebitis; stomatitis; and rash (3).

Neurotoxicity with the vinca alkaloids is qualitatively similar but quantitatively different. Regarding toxicity, vincristine is greater than vindesine, and vindesine is greater than vinblastine. Peripheral paresthesias are similar to vincristine neurotoxicity. Abdominal cramping is common with infrequent constipation (576). Paralytic ileus is rarely dose limiting. Urinary retention and postural hypotension have been noted rarely.

Hoarseness and, sometimes, severe transient jaw pain are infrequent. Cortical blindness has been described with vindesine use (577,578). Tissue necrosis may follow extravasation.

Diagnostic Tests

Testing is aimed at end organ effects (e.g., bone marrow, electrolytes, liver). Periodic CBC, serum electrolytes, and LFTs should be obtained. Specific levels of vindesine are not used to guide management.

Treatment

See Antineoplastic Treatment Guidelines at the end of this chapter. Fluid restriction may be required for SIADH. Please see Methotrexate section for information regarding toxicity after intrathecal use.

VINORELBINE

Vinorelbine is used to treat breast, cervical, non–small cell lung, small cell lung, and ovarian cancers. Numerous dosing schedules exist. One dosing regimen is 25 mg/m^2 in combination with cisplatin given weekly every 4 weeks. Vinorelbine is currently being studied in children.

Toxicokinetics and Toxicodynamics

There is large interpatient variability when given IV (579). The V_d is 25.4 to 40.1 L/kg, and plasma protein binding is 80% to 91% (3). Metabolism of vinorelbine is by hepatic P-450 enzymes (580). Active metabolites include desacetylvinorelbine. Vinorelbine and its metabolites are excreted in the bile, urine, and feces (46%). The half-life in adults is 28 to 44 hours and approximately 15 hours in children (3).

Pathophysiology

Vinorelbine inhibits cell growth by binding to the tubulin of the mitotic microtubules (3).

Pregnancy and Lactation

Vinorelbine is FDA pregnancy risk category D (Appendix I). In one report, no adverse effects were noted in a baby delivered to a mother treated with vinorelbine (581). Breast-feeding is not recommended.

Clinical Presentation

Mild to moderate peripheral neuropathy is the most frequently reported neurologic toxicity of vinorelbine and is usually reversible on discontinuation of the drug (582). Prior treatment with paclitaxel may result in cumulative neurotoxicity (583).

Extravasation can produce extravasation injury (584). Dyspnea (585,586) and severe bronchospasm occur infrequently. Subacute pulmonary reactions occur within 1 hour and may be characterized by cough, dyspnea, hypoxemia, and interstitial infiltration.

An acute pain syndrome at the tumor site can occur within 30 minutes of the first dose (587). The pain usually lasts for 1 hour or less. The theory is that prior surgery and radiation cause a nerve lesion and that subsequent vinorelbine causes neuralgic pain.

Diagnostic Tests

Testing is aimed at end organ effects (e.g., bone marrow, electrolytes, liver). Periodic CBC, serum electrolytes, and LFTs should be obtained. Specific levels of vinorelbine are not used to guide management.

Treatment

See Antineoplastic Treatment Guidelines at the end of this chapter. Fluid restriction may be required for SIADH. Please see Methotrexate section for information regarding toxicity following intrathecal use. Pulmonary reactions may respond to corticosteroid therapy. Oxygen may provide symptomatic relief (588). Tumor pain can be managed with nonsteroidal antiinflammatory drugs or corticosteroids (589) and may sometimes require narcotic analgesics.

ANTINEOPLASTIC TREATMENT GUIDELINES

Breast-feeding

Anticancer chemotherapeutic drugs are generally incompatible with breast-feeding because even low levels of exposure can prove toxic. If breast-feeding is continued, drug levels in milk and infant plasma, and infant hematologic parameters, should be monitored.

Conjunctivitis

Ocular exposures to antineoplastic agents are treated with normal saline irrigation and ophthalmologic consultation as needed. Conjunctivitis is often treated with antibiotic drops or ointments. Conjunctivitis may occur with high doses of cytarabine, MTX, 5-FU, and pentostatin and is minimized with prophylactic ophthalmic corticosteroids.

Electrolyte Abnormalities

Hyponatremia, hypokalemia, hypocalcemia, and hypomagnesemia are treated with supplementation and volume restriction, as appropriate. Certain electrolyte abnormalities may be seen with tumor lysis syndrome. Significant ECG abnormalities indicate aggressive management of electrolyte abnormalities in a monitored setting.

Encephalopathy

Electrolyte and glucose determination is performed as in all cases of mental status change. Computerized tomography, electroencephalogram, lumbar punctures for CSF analysis, and nuclear magnetic resonance studies may be required to rule out other causes of altered mental status.

Fever

Fever is evaluated with blood, urine, sputum, and other culture sources. Broad-spectrum antibiotics, addressing *Pseudomonas* and other gram-negative organisms, as well as gram-positive coverage, are vital when treating febrile leukopenic patients. Reverse isolation procedures may be indicated.

Hematologic Effects

Thrombocytopenia may be treated with platelet transfusions in severe cases, and significant anemia is treated with red blood cell transfusions. The decision to administer platelet transfusions should incorporate individual clinical characteristics of the patients and not simply be a reflexive reaction to the platelet count (590). Frequent physical examinations addressing sources of occult bleeding, such as stool guaiac checks, are indicated in all anemic patients.

The availability and efficacy of hematopoietic growth factors such as granulocyte colony-stimulating factor or granulocyte-macrophage colony-stimulating factor and erythropoietin have had a considerable impact on supportive care in cancer patients. Several randomized trials have shown a reduction of neutropenia and the frequency of severe infections in elderly patients treated with granulocyte colony-stimulating factor following myelotoxic chemotherapy (591).

Hypersensitivity Reactions

Hypersensitivity reactions are treated in the usual manner (Chapter 34). The infusion should be stopped immediately. Mild reactions are treated with diphenhydramine. Anaphylactic reactions require IV access, fluids, close monitoring, epinephrine, and steroids. β-agonists may relieve bronchospasm.

Intrathecal Antineoplastic Overdose

Currently, four therapeutic agents are available for intrathecal treatment: MTX, ara-C, sustained-release ara-C, and thiotepa (592). Prompt *cerebral washout* or CSF drainage is required as soon as possible after intrathecal injection of MTX or other agents. See Methotrexate section for additional details.

Mucositis and Oral Complications

Mucositis, xerostomia, osteoradionecrosis, and local infections are the most common oral complications. From the standpoint of dose limitation, treatment breaks, quality of life, and health economic outcomes, mucositis is the most significant acute oral toxicity (593). Currently, no intervention is completely successful at preventing or treating oral mucositis (594).

Weak evidence exists that allopurinol mouthwash and vitamin E improve mucositis (595,596). Fluconazole oral suspension and amphotericin B oral suspension have successfully been used (597). Filgrastim (recombinant human granulocyte colony-stimulating factor) has also been used to treat mucositis (598). Laser therapy significantly reduced the incidence and the severity of mucositis in chemotherapy patients in one study (599). Parenteral sources of nutrition may be necessary when oral intake is severely limited. Antibiotics are used to treat superinfected oral lesions.

Nausea and Vomiting

Serotonin receptors appear to be principal mediators of the emetic reflex. Numerous *antiemetic cocktails* have been proposed. Several studies have confirmed the efficacy of high-dose metoclopramide and, more recently, serotonin antagonists, with and without dexamethasone, in the prophylaxis of cisplatin (600) and other chemotherapeutic-induced nausea and vomiting. Others agents include phenothiazines (e.g., prochlorperazine), butyrophenones (e.g., droperidol), benzodiazepines (e.g., lorazepam), and 5-HT_3 receptor antagonists (e.g., ondansetron and granisetron). Vomiting from intrathecal chemotherapy can be greatly reduced by IV ondansetron before the procedure, and severe vomiting can be virtually eliminated (601).

Dehydration after significant antineoplastic-induced emesis is treated with IV fluids, with careful attention to urine output and central venous pressure as indicated. Dronabinol (i.e., delta-9-tetrahydrocannabinol, Marinol) may be effective for patients in whom conventional antiemetics fail (602).

Seizures

Seizures are managed as those from other toxicologic causes (Chapter 30).

Skin Exposures

Skin exposures to antineoplastic splashes are generally treated with soap and water. Vesicant exposures should be flooded with saline.

Syndrome of Inappropriate Antidiuretic Hormone

SIADH has followed the use of certain antineoplastics [e.g., ifosfamide, melphalan (343), vinblastine (543), and cyclophosphamide]. The syndrome is treated with fluid restriction, diuretics to promote water excretion, sodium replacement, and careful attention to fluid and electrolyte balance (603). Declomycin, a drug used to promote nephrogenic diabetes insipidus, has been used to treat certain cases of SIADH (604). Antidiuretic hormone assay may be helpful.

Tumor Lysis Syndrome

The tumor lysis syndrome results from the abrupt release of intracellular ions into the blood stream due to rapid tumor cell death. It occurs more frequently in hematologic malignancies and lymphomas. Hyperuricemia during periods of active cell lysis can be minimized with allopurinol (in doses up to 500 mg/m^2) and hydration. Despite prophylactic therapy with allopurinol and volume repletion, patients may still develop acute renal failure with tumor lysis syndrome (605). In hospitalized patients, the urine may be alkalinized by addition of sodium bicarbonate to IV fluids if tumor lysis syndrome is expected.

Serum electrolytes, creatinine, blood urea nitrogen, uric acid, calcium, phosphorus, and lactic acid dehydrogenase should be monitored until stable and then every few days. Hemodialysis may be considered in severe cases. Suggested criteria include serum of potassium 6 mEq/L or more, serum uric acid 10 mg/dl or more, and serum phosphorus 10 mg/dl or more.

REFERENCES

Actinomycin

1. Choonara IA, Kendall-Smith S, Bailey CC. Accidental actinomycin D overdosage in man, a case report. *Cancer Chemother Pharmacol* 1988;21(2):173–174.
2. Brogan TV, Mellema JD, Jardine DS. Severe dactinomycin overdose in an 18-month-old child. *Med Pediatr Oncol* 1999;33(5):506–507.
3. de Lemos ML, ed. *B.C. Cancer Agency cancer drug manual*, 3rd ed. Vancouver, British Columbia: B.C. Cancer Agency, 2001. Available at: http://www.bccancer.bc.ca.

4. Haskell CM, ed. *Cancer treatment*, 3rd ed. Philadelphia: WB Saunders, 1990.
5. Chabner BA, Myers CE. Clinical pharmacology of cancer chemotherapy. In: DeVita VT, Hellman S, Rosenberg SA, eds. *Cancer: principles and practice of oncology*, 3rd ed. Philadelphia: JB Lippincott Co, 1989.
6. Riggs CE. Antitumor antibiotics and related compounds. In: Perry MC, ed. *The chemotherapy source book.* Baltimore: Williams & Wilkins, 1992:330–332.
7. D'Antiga L, Baker A, Pritchard J, et al. Veno-occlusive disease with multi-organ involvement following actinomycin-D. *Eur J Cancer* 2001;37(9):1141–1148.
8. Cohen IJ, Loven D, Schoenfeld T, et al. Dactinomycin potentiation of radiation pneumonitis: a forgotten interaction. *Pediatr Hematol Oncol* 1991;8(2):187–192.
9. Sauer H, Fuger K, Blumenstein M. Modulation of cytotoxicity of cytostatic drugs by hemodialysis in vitro and in vivo. *Cancer Treat Rev* 1990;17(2–3):293–300.

Aldesleukin

10. Chen CS, Seidel K, Armitage JO, et al. Safeguarding the administration of high-dose chemotherapy: a national practice survey by the American Society for Blood and Marrow Transplantation. *Biol Blood Marrow Transplant* 1997;3(6):331–340.
11. Sundin DJ, Wolin MJ. Toxicity management in patients receiving low-dose aldesleukin therapy. *Ann Pharmacother* 1998;32(12):1344–1352.
12. Vial T, Descotes J. Clinical toxicity of interleukin-2. *Drug Saf* 1992;7(6):417–433.
13. Schlegel PJ, Samlowski WE, Ward JH. Autoimmune hemolytic anemia in a patient with chronic lymphocytic leukemia and renal cell carcinoma after treatment with high-dose intravenous bolus interleukin-2. *J Immunother* 2000;23(4):507–508.
14. Matsumori A, Yamada T, Suzuki H, et al. Increased circulating cytokines in patients with myocarditis and cardiomyopathy. *Br Heart J* 1994;72(6):561–566.
15. Goel M, Flaherty L, Lavine S, et al. Reversible cardiomyopathy after high-dose interleukin-2 therapy. *J Immunother* 1992;11(3):225–9.
16. Kintzel PE. Anticancer drug-induced kidney disorders. *Drug Saf* 2001;24(1):19–38.
17. Lentsch AB, Edwards MJ, Miller FN. Interleukin-2 induces increased platelet-endothelium interactions: a potential mechanism of toxicity. *J Lab Clin Med* 1996;128(1):75–82.
18. Bernand S, Scheidegger EP, Dummer R, et al. Multifocal fixed drug eruption to paracetamol, tropisetron and ondansetron induced by interleukin 2. *Dermatology* 2000;201(2):148–150.
19. Wolkenstein P, Chosidow O, Wechsler J, et al. Cutaneous side effects associated with interleukin 2 administration for metastatic melanoma. *J Am Acad Dermatol* 1993;28(1):66–70.
20. Fisher B, Keenan AM, Garra BS, et al. Interleukin-2 induces profound reversible cholestasis: a detailed analysis in treated cancer patients. *J Clin Oncol* 1989;7(12):1852–1862.
21. Kusske AM, Rongione AJ, Reber HA. Cytokines and acute pancreatitis. *Gastroenterology* 1996;110(2):639–642.

Anastrozole

22. Manni A. Clinical use of aromatase inhibitors in the treatment of breast cancers. *J Cell Biochem Suppl* 1993;17G:242–246.
23. Dowsett M, Lonning PE. Anastrozole—a new generation in aromatase inhibition: clinical pharmacology. *Oncology* 1997;54[Suppl 2]:11–14.
24. de Jong PC, Blijham GH. New aromatase inhibitors for the treatment of advanced breast cancer in postmenopausal women. *Neth J Med* 1999;55(2):50–58.
25. Geisler J, King N, Dowsett M, et al. Influence of anastrozole (Arimidex), a selective, non-steroidal aromatase inhibitor, on in vivo aromatisation and plasma oestrogen levels in postmenopausal women with breast cancer. *Br J Cancer* 1996;74(8):1286–1291.
26. Anastrozole overdose. Rx List Web site. Available at: http://www.rxlist.com/cgi/generic2/anastr_od.htm. Accessed March 2003.
27. Plourde PV, Dyroff M, Dukes M. Arimidex: a potent and selective fourth-generation aromatase inhibitor. *Breast Cancer Res Treat* 1994;30:103–111.
28. Santen RJ, Harvey HA. Use of aromatase inhibitors in breast carcinoma. *Endocr Relat Cancer* 1999;6(1):75–92.
29. Anastrozole. USP DI. Vol. 1. *Drug information for the health care professional*, 20th ed. Englewood, Colorado: Micromedex, Inc., 2000.
30. Arimidex [package insert]. Mississauga, Ontario: AstraZeneca Pharmacy; 2000.
31. Castiglione-Gertsch M. New aromatase inhibitors: more selectivity, less toxicity, unfortunately, the same activity. *Eur J Cancer* 1996;32A(3):393–395.
32. Wiseman LR, Adkins JC. Anastrozole. A review of its use in the management of postmenopausal women with advanced breast cancer. *Drugs Aging* 1998;13(4):321–332.
33. Lavrenkov K, Man S, Geffen DB, et al. Experience of hormonal therapy with anastrozole for previously treated metastatic breast cancer. *Isr Med Assoc J* 2002;4(3):176–177.
34. Bonneterre J, Thurlimann B, Robertson JF, et al. Anastrozole versus tamoxifen as first-line therapy for advanced breast cancer in 668 postmenopausal women: results of the tamoxifen or Arimidex randomized group efficacy and tolerability study. *J Clin Oncol* 2000;18(22):3748–3757.

Asparaginase

35. Ray M, Marwaha RK, Trehan A. Chemotherapy related fatal neurotoxicity during induction in acute lymphoblastic leukemia. *Indian J Pediatr* 2002;69(2):185–187.
36. Billett AL, Carls A, Gelber RD, et al. Allergic reactions to Erwinia asparaginase in children with acute lymphoblastic leukemia who had previous allergic reactions to Escherichia coli asparaginase. *Cancer* 1992;70:201–206.
37. Weiss RB, Bruno S. Hypersensitivity reactions to cancer chemotherapeutic agents. *Ann Intern Med* 1981;94:66–72.
38. Rodriguez AR. L-asparaginase and toxic epidermal necrolysis. *J Med Assoc Ga* 1980;69(5):355, 357.
39. Jenkins R, Perlin E. Severe hepatotoxicity from Escherichia coli L-asparaginase. *J Natl Med Assoc* 1987;79(7):775, 779.
40. McEvoy GK, ed. American hospital formulary service: drug information 1993. Bethesda: American Society of Hospital Pharmacists, 1993:524–526.
41. Sahu S, Saika S, Pai SK, et al. L-asparaginase (Leunase) induced pancreatitis in childhood acute lymphoblastic leukemia. *Pediatr Hematol Oncol* 1998;15(6):533–538.
42. Priest JR, Ramsay NK, Steinherz PG, et al. A syndrome of thrombosis and hemorrhage complicating L-asparaginase therapy for childhood lymphoblastic leukemia. *J Pediatr* 1982;100:984–989.
43. Foreman NK, Mahmoud HH, Rivera GK, et al. Recurrent cerebrovascular accident with L-asparaginase rechallenge. *Med Pediatr Oncol* 1992;20(6):532–534.
44. Packer RJ, Rorke LB, Lange BJ, et al. Cerebrovascular accidents in children with cancer. *Pediatrics* 1985;76(2):194–201.
45. Feinberg WM, Swenson MR. Cerebrovascular complications of L-asparaginase therapy. *Neurology* 1988;38:127–133.
46. O'Regan S, Carson S, Chesney RW, et al. Electrolyte and acid-base disturbances in the management of leukemia. *Blood* 1977;49(3):345–353.
47. Uysal K, Uguz A, Olgun N, et al. Hyperglycemia and acute parotitis related to L-asparaginase therapy. *J Pediatr Endocrinol Metab* 1996;9(6):627–629.
48. Sadoff J, Hwang S, Rosenfeld D, et al. Surgical pancreatic complications induced by L-asparaginase. *J Pediatr Surg* 1997;32(6):860–863.

Bicalutamide

49. Schellhammer PF, Sharifi R, Block NL, et al. Clinical benefits of bicalutamide compared with flutamide in combined androgen blockade for patients with advanced prostatic carcinoma: final report of a double-blind, randomized, multicenter trial. Casodex Combination Study Group [see comments]. *Urology* 1997;50(3):330–336.
50. Iversen P, Tyrrell CJ, Kaisary AV, et al. Bicalutamide monotherapy compared with castration in patients with nonmetastatic locally advanced prostate cancer: 6.3 years of followup. *J Urol* 2000;164(5):1579–1582.
51. Casodex [package insert]. Mississauga, Ontario: AstraZeneca Pharmacy; 1995.
52. Goa KL, Spencer CM. Bicalutamide in advanced prostate cancer. A review [published erratum in: *Drugs Aging* 1998;13(1):41]. *Drugs Aging* 1998;12(5):401–422.
53. Cockshott ID, Cooper KJ, Sweetmore DS, et al. The pharmacokinetics of Casodex in prostate cancer patients after single and during multiple dosing. *Eur Urol* 1990;18[Suppl 3]:10–17.
54. Bicalutamide. USP DI. Vol. 1. *Drug information for the health care professional*, 20th ed. Englewood, Colorado: Micromedex, Inc., 2000.
55. Blackledge G, Kolvenbag G, Nash A. Bicalutamide: a new antiandrogen for use in combination with castration for patients with advanced prostate cancer. *Anticancer Drugs* 1996;7(1):27–34.
56. Joyce R, Fenton MA, Rode P, et al. High dose bicalutamide for androgen independent prostate cancer: effect of prior hormonal therapy. *J Urol* 1998;159(1):149–153.
57. Kolvenbag GJ, Blackledge GR. Worldwide activity and safety of bicalutamide: a summary review. *Urology* 1996;47[1A Suppl]:70–9; discussion 80–84.
58. See WA, Wirth MP, McLeod DG, et al. Bicalutamide as immediate therapy either alone or as adjuvant to standard care of patients with localized or locally advanced prostate cancer: first analysis of the early prostate cancer program. *J Urol* 2002;168(2):429–435.
59. McCaffrey JA, Scher HI. Interstitial pneumonitis following bicalutamide treatment for prostate cancer. *J Urol* 1998;160(1):131.
60. Wong PW, Macris N, DiFabrizio L, et al. Eosinophilic lung disease induced by bicalutamide: a case report and review of the medical literature. *Chest* 1998;113(2):548–550.

Bleomycin

61. Jules-Elysee K, White DA. Bleomycin-induced pulmonary toxicity. *Clin Chest Med* 1990;11(1):1–20.
62. Comis RL. Bleomycin pulmonary toxicity: current status and future directions. *Semin Oncol* 1992;19[2 Suppl 5]:64–70.

63. Alberts DS, Chen HS, Woolfenden JM, et al. Pharmacokinetics of bleomycin in man. III. Bleomycin 57Co Vs bleomycin. *Cancer Chemother Pharmacol* 1979;3(1):33–40.
64. Dorr RT, Fritz WL, eds. *Cancer chemotherapy handbook*. New York: Elsevier Science, 1980:274–283.
65. Goldiner PL, Carlon GC, Cvitkovic E, et al. Factors influencing postoperative morbidity and mortality in patients treated with bleomycin. *BMJ* 1978;1(6128):1664–1667.
66. Sutherland J. Bleomycin associated lung toxicity. A guideline for oxygen therapy for patients who have received bleomycin systemic therapy. [British Columbia Cancer Agency Web site]. Available at: http://www.bccancer.bc.ca/. Accessed July 2000.
67. Hay JG, Haslam PL, Dewar A, et al. Development of acute lung injury after the combination of intravenous bleomycin and exposure to hyperoxia in rats. *Thorax* 1987;42(5):374–382.
68. Donat SM, Levy DA. Bleomycin associated pulmonary toxicity: is perioperative oxygen restriction necessary? *J Urol* 1998;160(4):1347–1352.
69. Von Hilsheimer GE, Norton SA. Delayed bleomycin-induced hyperpigmentation and pressure on the skin. *J Am Acad Dermatol* 2002;46(4):642–643.
70. Nigro MG, Hsu S. Bleomycin-induced flagellate pigmentation. *Cutis* 2001;68(4):285–286.
71. Stelzer KJ, Griffin TW, Koh WJ. Radiation recall skin toxicity with bleomycin in a patient with Kaposi sarcoma related to acquired immune deficiency syndrome. *Cancer* 1993;71(4):1322–1325.
72. Gardner G, Mesler D, Gitelman HJ. Hemolytic uremic syndrome following cisplatin, bleomycin, and vincristine chemotherapy: a report of a case and a review of the literature. *Ren Fail* 1989;11(2–3):133–137.
73. Thomas LL, Mertens MJ, von dem Borne AE, et al. Clinical management of cytotoxic drug overdose. *Med Toxicol Adverse Drug Exp* 1988;3(4):253–263.
74. Maher J, Daly PA. Severe bleomycin lung toxicity: reversal with high dose corticosteroids. *Thorax* 1993;48(1):92–94.
75. Hartmann LC, Frytak S, Richardson RL, et al. Life-threatening bleomycin pulmonary toxicity with ultimate reversibility. *Chest* 1990;98(2):497–499.
76. Robinson JB, Singh D, Bodurka-Bevers DC, et al. Hypersensitivity reactions and the utility of oral and intravenous desensitization in patients with gynecologic malignancies. *Gynecol Oncol* 2001;82(3):550–558.

Busulfan

77. Stein J, Davidovitz M, Yaniv I, et al. Accidental busulfan overdose: enhanced drug clearance with hemodialysis in a child with Wiskott-Aldrich syndrome. *Bone Marrow Transplant* 2001;27(5):551–553.
78. Cremers S, Schoemaker R, Bredius R, et al. Pharmacokinetics of intravenous busulfan in children prior to stem cell transplantation. *Br J Clin Pharmacol* 2002;53(4):386–389.
79. Fernandez LA, Zayed E. Busulfan-induced sideroblastic anemia. *Am J Hematol* 1988;28(3):199–200.
80. Kami M, Hamaki T, Maruta Y, et al. Limitations of oral busulfan in preparative regimen before hematopoietic stem-cell transplantation. *Haematologica* 2002;87(2):ELT10.
81. Schwarer AP, Opat SS, Watson AL, et al. Clobazam for seizure prophylaxis during busulfan chemotherapy. *Lancet* 1995;346(8984):1238.
82. Simonart T, Decaux G, Gourdin JM, et al. Hyperpigmentation induced by busulfan: a case with ultrastructure examination. *Ann Dermatol Venereol* 1999;126(5):439–440.
83. Morgan M, Dodds A, Atkinson K, et al. The toxicity of busulphan and cyclophosphamide as the preparative regimen for bone marrow transplantation. *Br J Haematol* 1991;77(4):529–534.

Carboplatin

84. Vandiver F, Duffield FV, Yoakum A, et al. Determination of human body burden baseline data of platinum through autopsy tissue analysis. *Environ Health Perspect* 1976;15:131–134.
85. Carboplatin. USP DI. Vol. 1. *Drug information for the health care professional* [update monographs]. Englewood, Colorado: Micromedex, Inc., 2000.
86. McEvoy GK, ed. *AHFS 2000 drug information*. Bethesda, Maryland: American Society of Health-System Pharmacists, Inc.; 2000.
87. Go RS, Adjei AA. Review of the comparative pharmacology and clinical activity of cisplatin and carboplatin. *J Clin Oncol* 1999;17(1):409–422.
88. Beyer J, Rick O, Weinknecht S, et al. Nephrotoxicity after high-dose carboplatin, etoposide and ifosfamide in germ-cell tumors: incidence and implications for hematologic recovery and clinical outcome. *Bone Marrow Transplant* 1997;20(10):813–819.
89. Quasthoff S, Hartung HP. Chemotherapy-induced peripheral neuropathy. *J Neurol* 2002;249(1):9–17.
90. Ding DL, Wang J, Salvi R, et al. Selective loss of inner hair cells and type-I ganglion neurons in carboplatin-treated chinchillas. Mechanisms of damage and protection. *Ann N Y Acad Sci* 1999;884:152–170.
91. Paraplatin-aq [package insert]. Montreal, Quebec: Bristol-Myers Squibb; 1994.
92. Markman M, Kennedy A, Webster K, et al. Clinical features of hypersensitivity reactions to carboplatin. *J Clin Oncol* 1999;17(4):1141–1145.
93. Weidmann B, Mulleneisen N, Bojko P, et al. Hypersensitivity reactions to carboplatin. Report of two patients, review of the literature, and discussion of diagnostic procedures and management. *Cancer* 1994;73(8):2218–2222.

Carmustine

94. Weinstein AS, Diener-West M, Nelson DF, et al. Pulmonary toxicity of carmustine in patients treated for malignant glioma. *Cancer Treat Rep* 1986;70(8):943–946.
95. Patterson DL, Wiemann MC, Lee TH, et al. Carmustine toxicity presenting as a lobar infiltrate. *Chest* 1993;104(1):315–317.
96. Cruciani F, Tamanti N, Abdolrahimzadeh S, et al. Ocular toxicity of systemic chemotherapy with megadoses of carmustine and mitomycin. *Ann Ophthalmol* 1994;26(3):97–100.
97. Zappasodi P, Vitulo P, Volpini E, et al. Successful therapy with high-dose steroids and cyclosporine for the treatment of carmustine-mediated lung injury. *Ann Hematol* 2002;81(6):347–349.

Chlorambucil

98. Vandenberg SA, Kulig K, Spoerke DG, et al. Chlorambucil overdose: accidental ingestion of an antineoplastic drug. *J Emerg Med* 1988;6(6):495–498.
99. Ostensen M, Ramsey-Goldman R. Treatment of inflammatory rheumatic disorders in pregnancy: What are the safest treatment options? *Drug Saf* 1998;19(5):389–410.
100. Ostensen M. Treatment with immunosuppressive and disease modifying drugs during pregnancy and lactation. *Am J Reprod Immunol* 1992;28(3–4):148–152.
101. Giles FJ, Smith MP, Goldstone AH. Chlorambucil lung toxicity. *Acta Haematol* 1990;83(3):156–158.
102. Jourdan E, Topart D, Pinzani V, et al. Chlorambucil/prednisone-induced seizures in a patient with non-Hodgkin's lymphoma. *Am J Hematol* 2001;67(2):147.
103. Salloum E, Khan KK, Cooper DL. Chlorambucil-induced seizures. *Cancer* 1997;79(5):1009–1013.
104. Byrne TN Jr, Moseley TA 3rd, Finer MA. Myoclonic seizures following chlorambucil overdose. *Ann Neurol* 1981;9(2):191–194.
105. Wyllie AR, Bayliff CD, Kovacs MJ. Myoclonus due to chlorambucil in two adults with lymphoma. *Ann Pharmacother* 1997;31(2):171–174.
106. Pichon N, Debette-Gratien M, Cessot F, et al. Acute cholestatic hepatitis due to chlorambucil [in French]. *Gastroenterol Clin Biol* 2001;25(2):202–203.

Cisplatin

107. Jung HK, Lee J, Lee SN. A case of massive cisplatin overdose managed by plasmapheresis. *Korean J Intern Med* 1995;10(2):150–154.
108. Chu G, Mantin R, Shen YM, et al. Massive cisplatin overdose by accidental substitution for carboplatin. Toxicity and management. *Cancer* 1993;72(12):3707–3714.
109. Raefsky EL, Wasserman TH. Combined modality therapy. In: Perry MC, ed. *The chemotherapy source book*. Baltimore: Williams & Wilkins, 1992:114–116.
110. De Vries EG, van der Zee AG, Uges DR, et al. Excretion of platinum into breast milk [Letter] [published erratum in: *Lancet* 1989;1(8641):798]. *Lancet* 1989;1(8636):497.
111. Egan PC, Costanza ME, Dodion P, et al. Doxorubicin and cisplatin excretion into human milk. *Cancer Treat Rep* 1985;69(12):1387–1389.
112. Ward JM, Young DM, Fauvie KA, et al. Comparative nephrotoxicity of platinum cancer chemotherapeutic agents. *Cancer Treat Rep* 1976;60(11):1675–1678.
113. Nagy JL, Adelstein DJ, Newman CW, et al. Cisplatin ototoxicity: the importance of baseline audiometry. *Am J Clin Oncol* 1999;22(3):305–308.
114. Black FO, Gianna-Poulin C, Pesznecker SC. Recovery from vestibular ototoxicity. *Otol Neurotol* 2001;22(5):662–671.
115. Taha H, Irfan S, Krishnamurthy M. Cisplatin induced reversible bilateral vocal cord paralysis: an undescribed complication of cisplatin. *Head Neck* 1999;21(1):78–79.
116. Mansfield SH, Castillo M. MR of cis-platinum-induced optic neuritis. *AJNR Am J Neuroradiol* 1994;15(6):1178–1180.
117. McKeage MJ. Comparative adverse effect profiles of platinum drugs. *Drug Saf Clin Toxicol* 1991;29:467–472.
118. Lagrange JL, Cassuto-Viguier E, Barbe V, et al. Cytotoxic effects of long-term circulating ultrafiltrable platinum species and limited efficacy of hemodialysis in clearing them. *Eur J Cancer* 1994;30A(14):2057–2060.
119. Choi JH, Oh JC, Kim KH, et al. Successful treatment of cisplatin overdose with plasma exchange. *Yonsei Med J* 2002;43(1):128–132.
120. Erdlenbruch B, Pekrun A, Schiffmann H, et al. Topical topic: accidental cisplatin overdose in a child: reversal of acute renal failure with sodium thiosulfate. *Med Pediatr Oncol* 2002;38(5):349–352.
121. Sheikh-Hamad D, Timmins K, Jalali Z. Cisplatin-induced renal toxicity: possible reversal by N-acetylcysteine treatment. *J Am Soc Nephrol* 1997;8(10):1640–1644.
122. Manusirivithaya S, Chareoniam V, Isariyodom P, et al. Comparison of ondansetron-dexamethasone-lorazepam versus metoclopramide-dexamethasone-lorazepam in the control of cisplatin induced emesis. *J Med Assoc Thai* 2001;84(7):966–972.

123. de Wit R, de Boer AC, Linden GH, et al. Effective cross-over to granisetron after failure to ondansetron, a randomized double blind study in patients failing ondansetron plus dexamethasone during the first 24 hours following highly emetogenic chemotherapy. *Br J Cancer* 2001;85(8):1099–1101.

Cladribine

124. Beutler E. Cladribine (2-chlorodeoxyadenosine). *Lancet* 1992;340:952–956.
125. Piro LD. 2-Chlorodeoxyadenosine treatment of lymphoid malignancies. *Blood* 1992;79(4):843–845.

Cyclophosphamide

126. Perry MC, ed. *The chemotherapy source book.* Baltimore: Williams & Wilkins, 1992.
127. Dorr RT, Fritz WL, eds. *Cancer chemotherapy handbook.* New York: Elsevier Science, 1980.
128. Zemlickis D, Lishner M, Erlich R, et al. Teratogenicity and carcinogenicity in a twin exposed in utero to cyclophosphamide. *Teratog Carcinog Mutagen* 1993;13:139–143.
129. Amato D, Niblett JS. Neutropenia from cyclophosphamide in breast milk [Letter]. *Med J Aust* 1977;1(11):383–384.
130. Durodola JI. Administration of cyclophosphamide during late pregnancy and early lactation: a case report. *J Natl Med Assoc* 1979;71(2):165–166.
131. Walker RD. Cyclophosphamide induced hemorrhagic cystitis. *J Urol* 1999;161(6):1747.
132. Haselberger MB, Schwinghammer TL. Efficacy of mesna for prevention of hemorrhagic cystitis after high-dose cyclophosphamide therapy. *Ann Pharmacother* 1995;29(9):918–921.
133. Seber A, Shu XO, Defor T, et al. Risk factors for severe hemorrhagic cystitis following BMT. *Bone Marrow Transplant* 1999;23(1):35–40.
134. Ozsahin M, Belkacemi Y, Pene F, et al. Interstitial pneumonitis following autologous bone-marrow transplantation conditioned with cyclophosphamide and total-body irradiation. *Int J Radiat Oncol Biol Phys* 1996;34(1):71–77.
135. Segura A, Yuste A, Cercos A, et al. Pulmonary fibrosis induced by cyclophosphamide. *Ann Pharmacother* 2001;35(7–8):894–897.
136. Moses AM, Miller M. Drug-induced dilutional hyponatremia. *N Engl J Med* 1974;291(23):1234–1239.
137. Gharib MI, Burnett AK. Chemotherapy-induced cardiotoxicity: current practice and prospects of prophylaxis. *Eur J Heart Fail* 2002;4(3):235–242.
138. Buja LM, Ferrans VJ. Myocardial injury produced by antineoplastic drugs. *Recent Adv Stud Cardiac Struct Metab* 1975;6:487–497.
139. Charak BS, Gupta R, Mandrekar P, et al. Testicular dysfunction after cyclophosphamide-vincristine-procarbazine-prednisolone chemotherapy for advanced Hodgkin's disease. A long-term follow-up study. *Cancer* 1990;65(9):1903–1906.
140. West NJ. Prevention and treatment of hemorrhagic cystitis. *Pharmacotherapy* 1997;17(4):696–706.
141. Murphy CP, Cox RL, Harden EA, et al. Encephalopathy and seizures induced by intravesical alum irrigations. *Bone Marrow Transplant* 1992;10(4):383–385.
142. Seear MD, Dimmick JE, Rogers PC. Acute aluminum toxicity after continuous intravesical alum irrigation for hemorrhagic cystitis. *Urology* 1990;36(4):353–354.
143. Jerkins GR, Noe HN, Hill DE. An unusual complication of silver nitrate treatment of hemorrhagic cystitis: case report. *J Urol* 1986;136(2):456–458.
144. Redman JF, Kletzel M. Cutaneous vesicostomy with direct intravesical application of formalin: management of severe vesical hemorrhage resulting from high dose cyclophosphamide in boys. *J Urol* 1994;151(4):1048–1050.
145. Duckett JW Jr, Peters PC, Donaldson MH. Severe cyclophosphamide hemorrhagic cystitis controlled with phenol. *J Pediatr Surg* 1973;8(1):55–57.
146. Levine LA, Jarrard DF. Treatment of cyclophosphamide-induced hemorrhagic cystitis with intravesical carboprost tromethamine. *J Urol* 1993;149(4):719–723.
147. Ohhara M, Okumura S, Tsuboi N, et al. Severe cyclophosphamide hemorrhagic cystitis controlled with transurethral electrocoagulation: a case report. *Hinyokika Kiyo* 1985;31(6):1045–1048.
148. Cho PA, George JL. Treatment of cyclophosphamide induced hemorrhagic cystitis with hyperbaric oxygen: a case report. *Can J Urol* 1998;5(5):652–653.
149. Etlik O, Tomur A, Deveci S, et al. Comparison of the uroprotective efficacy of mesna and HBO treatments in cyclophosphamide-induced hemorrhagic cystitis. *J Urol* 1997;158(6):2296–2299.
150. Gweon P, Shanberg A. Treatment of cyclophosphamide induced hemorrhagic cystitis with neodymium:YAG laser in pediatric patients. *J Urol* 1997;157(6):2301–2302.
151. Pyeritz RE, Droller MJ, Bender WL, et al. An approach to the control of massive hemorrhage in cyclophosphamide-induced cystitis by intravenous vasopressin: a case report. *J Urol* 1978;120(2):253–254.
152. Sneiders A, Pryor JL. Percutaneous nephrostomy drainage in the treatment of severe hemorrhagic cystitis. *J Urol* 1993;150(3):966–967.
153. Zagoria RJ, Hodge RG, Dyer RB, et al. Percutaneous nephrostomy for treatment of intractable hemorrhagic cystitis. *J Urol* 1993;149(6):1449–1451.
154. Koc S, Hagglund H, Ireton RC, et al. Successful treatment of severe hemorrhagic cystitis with cystectomy following matched donor allogeneic hematopoietic cell transplantation. *Bone Marrow Transplant* 2000;26(8):899–901.

Cytarabine

155. Lafolie P, Liliemark J, Bjork O, et al. Exchange of cerebrospinal fluid in accidental intrathecal overdose of cytarabine. *Med Toxicol Adverse Drug Exp* 1988;3(3):248–252.
156. Schardein JL. *Chemically induced birth defects.* New York and Basel: Marcel Dekker Inc, 1993:480.
157. Wagner VM, Hill JS, Weaver D, et al. Congenital anomalies in a baby born to cytarabine treated mother. *Lancet* 1980;2:98–100.
158. Krogh CME, ed. *Compendium of pharmaceuticals and specialties,* 27th ed. Ottawa: Canadian Pharmaceutical Association, 1992:268–269.
159. Zawacki T, Friedman JH, Grace J, et al. Cerebellar toxicity of cytosine arabinoside: clinical and neuropsychological signs. *Neurology* 2000;55(8):1234.
160. Hwang TL, Yung WK, Estey EH, et al. Central nervous system toxicity with high-dose Ara-C. *Neurology* 1985;35(10):1475–1479.
161. Baker WJ, Royer GL Jr, Weiss RB. Cytarabine and neurologic toxicity. *J Clin Oncol* 1991;9(4):679–693.
162. Jaeckle KA, Phuphanich S, Bent MJ, et al. Intrathecal treatment of neoplastic meningitis due to breast cancer with a slow-release formulation of cytarabine. *Br J Cancer* 2001;84(2):157–163.
163. Resar LM, Phillips PC, Kastan MB, et al. Acute neurotoxicity after intrathecal cytosine arabinoside in two adolescents with acute lymphoblastic leukemia of B-cell type. *Cancer* 1993;71(1):117–123.
164. Barletta JP, Fanous MM, Margo CE. Corneal and conjunctival toxicity with low-dose cytosine arabinoside. *Am J Ophthalmol* 1992;113(5):587–588.
165. Ganesan TS, Barnett MJ, Amos RJ, et al. Cytosine arabinoside in the management of recurrent leukaemia. *Hematol Oncol* 1987;5(1):65–69.
166. Briasoulis E, Pavlidis N. Noncardiogenic pulmonary edema: an unusual and serious complication of anticancer therapy. *Oncologist* 2001;6(2):153–161.
167. Shearer P, Katz J, Bozeman P, et al. Pulmonary insufficiency complicating therapy with high dose cytosine arabinoside in five pediatric patients with relapsed acute myelogenous leukemia. *Cancer* 1994;74(7):1953–1958.
168. Larouche G, Denault A, Prenovault J. Corticosteroids and serious cytarabine-induced pulmonary edema. *Pharmacotherapy* 2000;20(11):1396–1399.

Dacarbazine

169. Dipaola RS, Goodin S, Ratzell M, et al. Chemotherapy for metastatic melanoma during pregnancy. *Gynecol Oncol* 1997;66(3):526–530.
170. Krogh CME, ed. *Compendium of pharmaceuticals and specialties,* 28th ed. Ottawa: Canadian Pharmaceutical Association, 1993:386.
171. USP DI. *Drug information for the health care professional,* 12th ed. Rockville: United States Pharmacopeial Convention Inc., 1992:1115–1118.
172. Paschke R, Heine M. Pathophysiological aspects of dacarbazine-induced human liver damage. *Hepatogastroenterology* 1985;32(6):273–275.
173. Asbury RF, Rosenthal SN, Descalzi ME, et al. Hepatic veno-occlusive disease due to DTIC. *Cancer* 1980;45(10):2670–2674.
174. Kennedy RD, McAleer JJ. Radiation recall dermatitis in a patient treated with dacarbazine. *Clin Oncol (R Coll Radiol)* 2001;13(6):470–472.

Daunorubicin

175. Mortensen ME, Cecalupo AJ, Lo WD, et al. Inadvertent intrathecal injection of daunorubicin with fatal outcome. *Med Pediatr Oncol* 1992;20(3):249–253.
176. Von Hoff DD, Layard M. Risk factors for development of daunorubicin cardiotoxicity. *Cancer Treat Rep* 1981;65[Suppl 4]:19–23.
177. Dorr RT, Fritz WL, eds. *Cancer chemotherapy handbook.* New York: Elsevier Science, 1980:373–379.
178. Alegre A, Chunchurreta R, Rodriguez-Alarcon J, et al. Successful pregnancy in acute promyelocytic leukemia. *Cancer* 1982;49(1):152–153.
179. Steinherz LJ, Graham T, Hurwitz R, et al. Guidelines for cardiac monitoring of children during and after anthracycline therapy: report of the Cardiology Committee of the Childrens Cancer Study Group. *Pediatrics* 1992;89(5 Pt 1):942–949.
180. Hauser M, Wilson N. Anthracycline induced cardiomyopathy: successful treatment with angiotensin converting enzyme inhibitors. *Eur J Pediatr* 2000;159(5):389.
181. Lemez P, Maresova J. Efficacy of dexrazoxane as a cardioprotective agent in patients receiving mitoxantrone- and daunorubicin-based chemotherapy. *Semin Oncol* 1998;25[4 Suppl 10]:61–65.
182. Shinozawa S, Gomita Y, Araki Y. Protective effects of various drugs on adriamycin (doxorubicin)-induced toxicity and microsomal lipid peroxidation in mice and rats. *Biol Pharm Bull* 1993;16(11):1114–1117.

Doxorubicin

183. Singal PK, Iliskovic N. Doxorubicin-induced cardiomyopathy. *N Engl J Med* 1998;339(13):900–905.
184. Lipshultz SE, Giantris AL, Lipsitz SR, et al. Doxorubicin administration by

continuous infusion is not cardioprotective: the Dana-Farber 91–01 acute lymphoblastic leukemia protocol. *J Clin Oncol* 2002;20(6):1677–1682.
185. Karp GI, von Oeyen P, Valone F, et al. Doxorubicin in pregnancy: possible transplacental passage. *Cancer Treat Rep* 1983;67:773–777.
186. Dunn J. Doxorubicin-induced cardiomyopathy. *J Pediatr Oncol Nurs* 1994;11(4):152–160.
187. Curran CF, Luce JK, Page JA. Doxorubicin-associated flare reactions. *Oncol Nurs Forum* 1990;17(3):387–389.
188. Vegesna V, Withers HR, McBride WH, et al. Adriamycin-induced recall of radiation pneumonitis and epilation in lung and hair follicles of mouse. *Int J Radiat Oncol Biol Phys* 1992;23(5):977–981.
189. Cassady JR, Richter MP, Piro AJ, et al. Radiation-adriamycin interactions: preliminary clinical observations. *Cancer* 1975;36(3):946–949.
190. Nousiainen T, Jantunen E, Vanninen E, et al. Early decline in left ventricular ejection fraction predicts doxorubicin cardiotoxicity in lymphoma patients. *Br J Cancer* 2002;86(11):1697–1700.
191. Siveski-Iliskovic N, Kaul N, Singal PK. Probucol promotes endogenous antioxidants and provides protection against adriamycin-induced cardiomyopathy in rats. *Circulation* 1994;89(6):2829–2835.

Etoposide

192. Krogh CME, ed. *Compendium of pharmaceuticals and specialties*, 28th ed. Ottawa: Canadian Pharmaceutical Association, 1993:1307–1308.
193. Yokel BK, Friedman KJ, Farmer ER, et al. Cutaneous pathology following etoposide therapy. *J Cutan Pathol* 1987;14(6):326–330.
194. Fitzpatrick JE. New histopathologic findings in drug eruptions. A review. *Dermatol Clin* 1992;10(1):19–36.
195. Siderov J, Prasad P, De Boer R, et al. Safe administration of etoposide phosphate after hypersensitivity reaction to intravenous etoposide. *Br J Cancer* 2002;86(1):12–13.
196. Hoetelmans RM, Schornagel JH, ten Bokkel Huinink WW, et al. Hypersensitivity reactions to etoposide. *Ann Pharmacother* 1996;30(4):367–371.
197. Raber-Durlacher JE, Weijl NI, Abu Saris M, et al. Oral mucositis in patients treated with chemotherapy for solid tumors: a retrospective analysis of 150 cases. *Support Care Cancer* 2000;8(5):366–371.
198. Tran A, Housset C, Boboc B, et al. Etoposide (VP 16-213) induced hepatitis. Report of three cases following standard-dose treatments. *J Hepatol* 1991;12(1):36–39.
199. List AF, Kummet TD. Spinal cord toxicity complicating treatment with cisplatin and etoposide. *Am J Clin Oncol* 1990;13(3):256–258.
200. Hosing C, Munsell M, Yazji S, et al. Risk of therapy-related myelodysplastic syndrome/acute leukemia following high-dose therapy and autologous bone marrow transplantation for non-Hodgkin's lymphoma. *Ann Oncol* 2002;13(3):450–9.
201. Ng A, Taylor GM, Eden OB. Secondary leukemia in a child with neuroblastoma while on oral etoposide: What is the cause? *Pediatr Hematol Oncol* 2000;17(3):273–279.
202. Williams BJ, Roth DJ, Callen JP. Ultraviolet recall associated with etoposide and cyclophosphamide therapy. *Clin Exp Dermatol* 1993;18(5):452–453.

Floxuridine

203. Kemeny M. Hepatic artery infusion of chemotherapy as a treatment for hepatic metastases from colorectal cancer. *Cancer J* 2002;8[Suppl 1]:S82–S88.
204. Carroll NM, Alexander HR Jr. Isolation perfusion of the liver. *Cancer J* 2002;8(2):181–193.
205. Ensminger WD. Intrahepatic arterial infusion of chemotherapy: pharmacologic principles. *Semin Oncol* 2002;29(2):119–125.
206. Thomas DM, Zalcberg JR. 5-Fluorouracil: a pharmacological paradigm in the use of cytotoxics. *Clin Exp Pharmacol Physiol* 1998;25(11):887–895.
207. Floxuridine warnings. RxList Web site. Available at: http://www.rxlist.com/cgi/generic2/floxuridine_wcp.htm. Accessed March 2000.
208. Lorenz M, Staib-Sebler E, Koch B, et al. The value of postoperative hepatic arterial infusion following curative liver resection. *Anticancer Res* 1997;17(5B):3825–3833.
209. Hohn DC, Rayner AA, Economou JS, et al. Toxicities and complications of implanted pump hepatic arterial and intravenous floxuridine infusion. *Cancer* 1986;57(3):465–470.

Fludarabine

210. Gandhi V, Plunkett W. Cellular and clinical pharmacology of fludarabine. *Clin Pharmacokinet* 2002;41(2):93–103.
211. Ross SR, McTavish D, Faulds D. Fludarabine: a review of its pharmacological properties and therapeutic potential in malignancy. *Drugs* 1993;45(5):737–759.
212. Schmitt B, Wendtner CM, Bergmann M, et al. Fludarabine combination therapy for the treatment of chronic lymphocytic leukemia. *Clin Lymphoma* 2002;3(1):26–35.
213. Leenders A, Sonneveld P, de Marie S. Cryptococcal meningitis following fludarabine treatment for chronic lymphocytic leukemia. *Eur J Clin Microbiol Infect Dis* 1995;14(9):826–828.
214. Chim CS, Liang R, Wong SS, et al. Cryptococcal infection associated with fludarabine therapy. *Am J Med* 2000;108(6):523–524.
215. Costa P, Luzzati R, Nicolato A, et al. Cryptococcal meningitis and intracranial tuberculoma in a patient with Waldenström's macroglobulinemia treated with fludarabine. *Leuk Lymphoma* 1998;28(5–6):617–620.
216. Keating MJ, Estey E, O'Brien S, et al. Clinical experience with fludarabine in leukaemia. *Drugs* 1994;47[Suppl 6]:39–49.
217. Gonzalez H, Bolgert F, Camporo P, et al. Progressive multifocal leukoencephalitis (PML) in three patients treated with standard-dose fludarabine (FAMP). *Hematol Cell Ther* 1999;41(4):183–186.
218. Vidarsson B, Mosher DF, Salamat MS, et al. Progressive multifocal leukoencephalopathy after fludarabine therapy for low-grade lymphoproliferative disease. *Am J Hematol* 2002;70(1):51–54.
219. Gooptu C, Littlewood TJ, Frith P, et al. Paraneoplastic pemphigus: an association with fludarabine? *Br J Dermatol* 2001;144(6):1255–1261.

Fluorouracil

220. Recchia F, Sica G, De Filippis S, et al. Phase II study of epirubicin, mitomycin C, and 5-fluorouracil in hormone-refractory prostatic carcinoma. *Am J Clin Oncol* 2001;24(3):232–236.
221. Dreicer R, Love RR. High total dose 5-fluorouracil treatment during pregnancy. *Wis Med J* 1991;90(10):582–583.
222. Krogh CME, ed. *Compendium of pharmaceuticals and specialties*, 28th ed. Ottawa: Canadian Pharmaceutical Association, 1993:29–30,403–404,465–468.
223. Tsavaris N, Kosmas C, Vadiaka M, et al. Cardiotoxicity following different doses and schedules of 5-fluorouracil administration for malignancy—a survey of 427 patients. *Med Sci Monit* 2002;8(6):PI51–PI57.
224. Loprinzi CL, Love RR, Garrity JA, et al. Cyclophosphamide, methotrexate, and 5-fluorouracil (CMF)-induced ocular toxicity. *Cancer Invest* 1990;8(5):459–465.
225. Reeder RE, Mika RO. Ectropion secondary to bolus injection of 5-fluorouracil. *Optometry* 2001;72(2):112–116.
226. Ki SS, Jeong JM, Kim SH, et al. A case of neurotoxicity following 5-fluorouracil-based chemotherapy. *Korean J Intern Med* 2002;17(1):73–77.
227. Serrano-Castro PJ, Aguilar-Castillo MJ. Comment: fluorouracil-induced aphasia: neurotoxicity versus cerebral ischemia. *Ann Pharmacother* 2001;35(6):785–786.
228. Koenig H, Patel A. The acute cerebellar syndrome in 5-fluorouracil chemotherapy: a manifestation of fluoroacetate intoxication. *Neurology* 1970;20(4):416.
229. Chiara S, Nobile MT, Barzacchi C, et al. Hand-foot syndrome induced by high-dose, short-term, continuous 5-fluorouracil infusion. *Eur J Cancer* 1997;33(6):967–969.
230. Nagore E, Insa A, Sanmartin O. Antineoplastic therapy-induced palmar plantar erythrodysesthesia ("hand-foot") syndrome. Incidence, recognition and management. *Am J Clin Dermatol* 2000;1(4):225–234.
231. Pearlman DL. Weekly pulse dosing: effective and comfortable topical 5-fluorouracil treatment of multiple facial actinic keratoses. *J Am Acad Dermatol* 1991;25(4):665–667.
232. Zesch A. Adverse reactions of externally applied drugs and inert substances. *Derm Beruf Umwelt* 1988;36(4):128–133.
233. Sanchez-Perez J, Bartolome B, del Rio MJ, et al. Allergic contact dermatitis from 5-fluorouracil with positive intradermal test and doubtful patch test reactions. *Contact Dermatitis* 1999;41(2):106–107.
234. Nadal C, Pujol RM, Randazzo L, et al. Systemic contact dermatitis from 5-fluorouracil. *Contact Dermatitis* 1996;35(2):124–125.
235. Umstead GS, Fryer NL, Decker DA. Local tissue reaction to intravenous fluorouracil and leucovorin. *DICP* 1991;25(3):249–250.

Flutamide

236. McLeod DG. Tolerability of nonsteroidal antiandrogens in the treatment of advanced prostate cancer. *Oncologist* 1997;2(1):18–27.
237. Kraus I, Vitezic D, Oguic R. Flutamide-induced acute hepatitis in advanced prostate cancer patients. *Int J Clin Pharmacol Ther* 2001;39(9):395–399.
238. Pontiroli L, Sartori M, Pittau S, et al. Flutamide-induced acute hepatitis: investigation on the role of immunoallergic mechanisms. *Ital J Gastroenterol Hepatol* 1998;30(3):310–314.
239. Wallace C, Lalor EA, Chik CL. Hepatotoxicity complicating flutamide treatment of hirsutism. *Ann Intern Med* 1993;119(11):1150.
240. Delaere KP, Van Thillo EL. Flutamide monotherapy as primary treatment in advanced prostatic carcinoma. *Semin Oncol* 1991;18[5 Suppl 6]:13–18.
241. Yokote R, Tokura Y, Igarashi N, et al. Photosensitive drug eruption induced by flutamide. *Eur J Dermatol* 1998;8(6):427–429.
242. Staiman VR, Lowe FC. Tamoxifen for flutamide/finasteride-induced gynecomastia. *Urology* 1997;50(6):929–933.

Gemcitabine

243. Pavlakis N, Bell DR, Millward MJ, et al. Fatal pulmonary toxicity resulting from treatment with gemcitabine. *Cancer* 1997;80(2):286–291.

244. Gemcitabine. USP DI. Vol. 1. *Drug information for the health care professional* [update monographs]. Englewood, Colorado: Micromedex, Inc., 1999.
245. Fung MC, Storniolo AM, Nguyen B, et al. A review of hemolytic uremic syndrome in patients treated with gemcitabine therapy. *Cancer* 1999;85(9):2023–2032.
246. Gross M, Hiesse C, Kriaa F, et al. Severe hemolytic uremic syndrome in an advanced ovarian cancer patient treated with carboplatin and gemcitabine. *Anticancer Drugs* 1999;10(6):533–536.
247. Martin C, Pollera CF. Gemcitabine: safety profile unaffected by starting dose. *Int J Clin Pharmacol Res* 1996;16(1):9–18.
248. Aapro MS, Martin C, Hatty S. Gemcitabine—a safety review. *Anticancer Drugs* 1998;9(3):191–201.
249. Attar EC, Ervin T, Janicek M, et al. Side effects of chemotherapy. Case 3. Acute interstitial pneumonitis related to gemcitabine. *J Clin Oncol* 2000;18(3):697–698.
250. Brandes A, Reichmann U, Plasswilm L, et al. Time- and dose-limiting erysipeloid rash confined to areas of lymphedema following treatment with gemcitabine—a report of three cases. *Anticancer Drugs* 2000;11(1):15–17.
251. Jeter MD, Janne PA, Brooks S, et al. Gemcitabine-induced radiation recall. *Int J Radiat Oncol Biol Phys* 2002;53(2):394–400.

Hydroxyurea

252. Fadilah SA, Ahmad-Zailani H, Soon-Keng C, et al. Successful treatment of chronic myeloid leukemia during pregnancy with hydroxyurea. *Leukemia* 2002;16(6):1202–1203.
253. Weissman SB, Sinclair GI, Green CL, et al. Hydroxyurea-induced hepatitis in human immunodeficiency virus-positive patients. *Clin Infect Dis* 1999;29(1):223–224.
254. Heddle R, Calvert AF. Hydroxyurea induced hepatitis. *Med J Aust* 1980;1(3):121.
255. Aste N, Fumo G, Contu F, et al. Nail pigmentation caused by hydroxyurea: report of 9 cases. *J Am Acad Dermatol* 2002;47(1):146–147.
256. Varma S, Lanigan SW. Dermatomyositis-like eruption and leg ulceration caused by hydroxyurea in a patient with psoriasis. *Clin Exp Dermatol* 1999;24(3):164–166.
257. Paleri V, Lindsey L. Oral ulcers caused by hydroxyurea. *J Laryngol Otol* 2000;114(12):976–977.
258. Kumar B, Saraswat A, Kaur I. Mucocutaneous adverse effects of hydroxyurea: a prospective study of 30 psoriasis patients. *Clin Exp Dermatol* 2002;27(1):8–13.
259. Sirieix ME, Debure C, Baudot N, et al. Leg ulcers and hydroxyurea: forty-one cases. *Arch Dermatol* 1999;135(7):818–820.
260. Weinlich G, Fritsch P. Leg ulcers in patients treated with hydroxyurea for myeloproliferative disorders: What is the trigger? *Br J Dermatol* 1999;141(1):171–172.

Ifosfamide

261. Skinner R, Pearson AD, English MW, et al. Risk factors for ifosfamide nephrotoxicity in children. *Lancet* 1996;348(9027):578–580.
262. Dubourg L, Taniere P, Cochat P, et al. Toxicity of chloroacetaldehyde is similar in adult and pediatric kidney tubules. *Pediatr Nephrol* 2002;17(2):97–103.
263. Sharon N, Neumann Y, Kenet G, et al. Successful pregnancy after high-dose cyclophosphamide and ifosfamide treatment in two postpubertal women. *Pediatr Hematol Oncol* 2001;18(4):247–252.
264. Aleksa K, Woodland C, Koren G. Young age and the risk for ifosfamide-induced nephrotoxicity: a critical review of two opposing studies. *Pediatr Nephrol* 2001;16(12):1153–1158.
265. Berns JS, Haghighat A, Staddon A, et al. Severe, irreversible renal failure after ifosfamide treatment. A clinicopathologic report of two patients. *Cancer* 1995;76(3):497–500.
266. Garcia AA. Ifosfamide-induced Fanconi syndrome. *Ann Pharmacother* 1995;29(6):590–591.
267. Negro A, Regolisti G, Perazzoli F, et al. Ifosfamide-induced renal Fanconi syndrome with associated nephrogenic diabetes insipidus in an adult patient. *Nephrol Dial Transplant* 1998;13(6):1547–1549.
268. Shuper A, Stein J, Goshen J, et al. Subacute central nervous system degeneration in a child: an unusual manifestation of ifosfamide intoxication. *J Child Neurol* 2000;15(7):481–483.
269. Primavera A, Audenino D, Cocito L. Ifosfamide encephalopathy and nonconvulsive status epilepticus. *Can J Neurol Sci* 2002;29(2):180–183.
270. Frisk P, Stalberg E, Stromberg B, et al. Painful peripheral neuropathy after treatment with high-dose ifosfamide. *Med Pediatr Oncol* 2001;37(4):379–382.
271. Quezado ZM, Wilson WH, Cunnion RE, et al. High-dose ifosfamide is associated with severe, reversible cardiac dysfunction. *Ann Intern Med* 1993;118(1):31–36.
272. Kandylis K, Vassilomanolakis M, Tsoussis S, et al. Ifosfamide cardiotoxicity in humans. *Cancer Chemother Pharmacol* 1989;24(6):395–396.
273. Antman KH, Elias A, Ryan L. Ifosfamide and mesna: response and toxicity at standard- and high-dose schedules. *Semin Oncol* 1990;17[2 Suppl 4]:68–73.
274. Kupfer A, Aeschlimann C, Wermuth B, et al. Prophylaxis and reversal of ifosfamide encephalopathy with methylene-blue. *Lancet* 1994;343(8900):763–764.

Interferon

275. Kirkwood J. Cancer immunotherapy: the interferon-alpha experience. *Semin Oncol* 2002;29[3 Suppl 7]:18–26.
276. Barone AA, de Paula Cavalheiro N, Suematsu S. Response in patients with chronic HCV hepatitis to treatment with interferon-alpha. *Braz J Infect Dis* 1999;3(3):118–128.
277. Capuron L, Gumnick JF, Musselman DL, et al. Neurobehavioral effects of interferon-alpha in cancer patients: phenomenology and paroxetine responsiveness of symptom dimensions. *Neuropsychopharmacology* 2002;26(5):643–652.
278. Adams F, Quesada JR, Gutterman JU. Neuropsychiatric manifestations of human leukocyte interferon therapy in patients with cancer. *JAMA* 1984;252(7):938–941.
279. Caraceni A, Gangeri L, Martini C, et al. Neurotoxicity of interferon-alpha in melanoma therapy: results from a randomized controlled trial. *Cancer* 1998;83(3):482–489.
280. Horikawa N, Yamazaki T, Sagawa M, et al. A case of akathisia during interferon-alpha therapy for chronic hepatitis type C. *Gen Hosp Psychiatry* 1999;21(2):134–135.
281. Valentini P, Mariotti P, Ngalikpima CJ, et al. Seizures in an interferon-treated child. *Dig Liver Dis* 2001;33(4):363–365.
282. Ameen M, Russell-Jones R. Seizures associated with interferon-alpha treatment of cutaneous malignancies. *Br J Dermatol* 1999;141(2):386–387.
283. Sasaki M, Sata M, Suzuki H, et al. A case of chronic hepatitis C with sinus bradycardia during IFN therapy. *Kurume Med J* 1998;45(1):161–163.
284. Fujiwara T, Kiura K, Ochi K, et al. Giant negative T waves during interferon therapy in a patient with chronic hepatitis C. *Intern Med* 2001;40(2):105–109.
285. Teragawa H, Hondo T, Amano H, et al. Cardiogenic shock following recombinant alpha-2b interferon therapy for chronic hepatitis C. A case report. *Jpn Heart J* 1996;37(1):137–142.
286. Charron A, Bessis D, Dereure O, et al. Local cutaneous side effects of interferons [in French]. *Presse Med* 2001;30(31 Pt 1):1555–1560.
287. Cogrel O, Doutre MS, Marliere V, et al. Cutaneous sarcoidosis during interferon alfa and ribavirin treatment of hepatitis C virus infection: two cases. *Br J Dermatol* 2002;146(2):320–324.
288. Willson RA. Nephrotoxicity of interferon alfa-ribavirin therapy for chronic hepatitis C. *J Clin Gastroenterol* 2002;35(1):89–92.
289. Kraus MR, Schafer A, Faller H, et al. Paroxetine for the treatment of interferon-alpha-induced depression in chronic hepatitis C. *Aliment Pharmacol Ther* 2002;16(6):1091–1099.
290. Shakil AO, Di Bisceglie AM, Hoofnagle JH. Seizures during alpha interferon therapy. *J Hepatol* 1996;24(1):48–51.

Irinotecan

291. Friedman HS, Petros WP, Friedman AH, et al. Irinotecan therapy in adults with recurrent or progressive malignant glioma. *J Clin Oncol* 1999;17(5):1516–1525.
292. Abigerges D, Chabot GG, Armand JP, et al. Phase I and pharmacologic studies of the camptothecin analog irinotecan administered every 3 weeks in cancer patients. *J Clin Oncol* 1995;13(1):210–221.
293. Irinotecan. USP DI. Vol. 1. *Drug information for the health care professional*, 20th ed. Englewood, Colorado: Micromedex, Inc., 2000.
294. Gershenson DM. Irinotecan in epithelial ovarian cancer. *Oncology (Huntingt)* 2002;16[5 Suppl 5]:29–31.
295. Bleiberg H, Cvitkovic E. Characterisation and clinical management of CPT-11 (irinotecan)-induced adverse events: the European perspective. *Eur J Cancer* 1996;32A[Suppl 3]:S18–S23.
296. Bozec L, Bierling P, Fromont P, et al. Irinotecan-induced immune thrombocytopenia. *Ann Oncol* 1998;9(4):453–455.
297. Camptosar [package insert]. Mississauga, Ontario: Pharmacia and Upjohn; 1999.
298. Saliba F, Hagipantelli R, Misset JL, et al. Pathophysiology and therapy of irinotecan-induced delayed-onset diarrhea in patients with advanced colorectal cancer: a prospective assessment. *J Clin Oncol* 1998;16(8):2745–2751.
299. Wasserman E, Myara A, Lokiec F, et al. Severe CPT-11 toxicity in patients with Gilbert's syndrome: two case reports. *Ann Oncol* 1997;8(10):1049–1051.
300. B.C. Cancer Agency Gastrointestinal Tumor Group. *BCCA protocol summary for second-line palliative treatment for fluorouracil-refractory metastatic colorectal cancer using irinotecan (GIIR)*. Vancouver, British Columbia: BC Cancer Agency, 2000.
301. Baz DV, Bofill JS, Nogueira JA. Irinotecan-induced dysarthria. *J Natl Cancer Inst* 2001;93(18):1419–1420.
302. Madarnas Y, Webster P, Shorter AM, et al. Irinotecan-associated pulmonary toxicity. *Anticancer Drugs* 2000;11(9):709–713.
303. Hecht JR. Gastrointestinal toxicity of irinotecan. *Oncology (Huntingt)* 1998;12[8 Suppl 6]:72–78.
304. Cersosimo RJ. Irinotecan: a new antineoplastic agent for the management of colorectal cancer. *Ann Pharmacother* 1998;32(12):1324–1333.
305. Barbounis V, Koumakis G, Vassilomanolakis M, et al. Control of irinotecan-

induced diarrhea by octreotide after loperamide failure. *Support Care Cancer* 2001;9(4):258–260.
306. Govindarajan R, Heaton KM, Broadwater R, et al. Effect of thalidomide on gastrointestinal toxic effects of irinotecan. *Lancet* 2000;356(9229):566–567.
307. Kehrer DF, Sparreboom A, Verweij J, et al. Modulation of irinotecan-induced diarrhea by cotreatment with neomycin in cancer patients. *Clin Cancer Res* 2001;7(5):1136–1141.

Letrozole

308. Lipton A, Demers LM, Harvey HA, et al. Letrozole (CGS 20267). A phase I study of a new potent oral aromatase inhibitor of breast cancer. *Cancer* 1995;75(8):2132–2138.
309. Sioufi A, Gauducheau N, Pineau V, et al. Absolute bioavailability of letrozole in healthy postmenopausal women. *Biopharm Drug Dispos* 1997;18(9):779–789.
310. Sioufi A, Sandrenan N, Godbillon J, et al. Comparative bioavailability of letrozole under fed and fasting conditions in 12 healthy subjects after a 2.5 mg single oral administration. *Biopharm Drug Dispos* 1997;18(6):489–497.
311. Lamb HM, Adkins JC. Letrozole. A review of its use in postmenopausal women with advanced breast cancer. *Drugs* 1998;56(6):1125–1140.
312. Njar VC, Brodie AM. Comprehensive pharmacology and clinical efficacy of aromatase inhibitors. *Drugs* 1999;58(2):233–255.
313. Femara [product insert]. Dorval, Quebec: Novartis Pharmaceuticals Canada Inc.; 2000.
314. Letrozole warnings. RxList Web site. Available at: http://www.rxlist.com/cgi/generic2/letroz_wcp.htm. Accessed March 2003.
315. Hamilton A, Piccart M. The third-generation non-steroidal aromatase inhibitors: a review of their clinical benefits in the second-line hormonal treatment of advanced breast cancer. *Ann Oncol* 1999;10(4):377–384.
316. Buzdar A, Douma J, Davidson N, et al. Phase III, multicenter, double-blind, randomized study of letrozole, an aromatase inhibitor, for advanced breast cancer versus megestrol acetate. *J Clin Oncol* 2001;19(14):3357–3366.
317. Dombernowsky P, Smith I, Falkson G, et al. Letrozole, a new oral aromatase inhibitor for advanced breast cancer: double-blind randomized trial showing a dose effect and improved efficacy and tolerability compared with megestrol acetate. *J Clin Oncol* 1998;16(2):453–461.
318. Zigrossi P, Brustia M, Bobbio F, et al. Flare and tumor lysis syndrome with atypical features after letrozole therapy in advanced breast cancer. A case report. *Ann Ital Med Int* 2001;16(2):112–117.

Leuprolide

319. Stricker HJ. Luteinizing hormone-releasing hormone antagonists in prostate cancer. *Urology* 2001;58[2 Suppl 1]:24–27.
320. Krogh CME, ed. *Compendium of pharmaceuticals and specialties*, 27th ed. Ottawa: Canadian Pharmaceutical Association, 1992:635–636.
321. Dowsett M, Jacobs S, Aherne J, et al. Clinical and endocrine effects of leuprorelin acetate in pre- and postmenopausal patients with advanced breast cancer. *Clin Ther* 1992;14[Suppl A]:97–103.
322. Chrisp P, Sorkin EM. Leuprorelin. A review of its pharmacology and therapeutic use in prostatic disorders. *Drugs Aging* 1991;1(6):487–509.
323. Cersosimo RJ, Carr D. Prostate cancer: current and evolving strategies. *Am J Health Syst Pharm* 1996;53(4):381–96;quiz,446–448.
324. Tsushima T, Nasu Y, Saika T, et al. Optimal starting time for flutamide to prevent disease flare in prostate cancer patients treated with a gonadotropin-releasing hormone agonist. *Urol Int* 2001;66(3):135–139.
325. Dowsett M, Mehta A, Mansi J, et al. A dose-comparative endocrine-clinical study of leuprorelin in premenopausal breast cancer patients. *Br J Cancer* 1990;62(5):834–837.
326. Droesch K, Barbieri RL. Ovarian hyperstimulation syndrome associated with the use of the gonadotropin-releasing hormone agonist leuprolide acetate. *Fertil Steril* 1994;62(1):189–190.
327. Noguchi K, Uemura H, Harada M, et al. Inhibition of PSA flare in prostate cancer patients by administration of flutamide for 2 weeks before initiation of treatment with slow-releasing LH-RH agonist. *Int J Clin Oncol* 2001;6(1):29–33.

Lomustine

328. Trent KC, Myers L, Moreb J. Multiorgan failure associated with lomustine overdose. *Ann Pharmacother* 1995;29(4):384–386.
329. Krogh CME, ed. *Compendium of pharmaceuticals and specialties*, 28th ed. Ottawa: Canadian Pharmaceutical Association, 1993:210–211.
330. Block M, Lachowiez RM, Rios C, et al. Pulmonary fibrosis associated with low-dose adjuvant methyl-CCNU. *Med Pediatr Oncol* 1990;18(3):256–260.
331. Stone MD, Richardson MG. Pulmonary toxicity of lomustine. *Cancer Treat Rep* 1987;71(7–8):786–787.

Mechlorethamine

332. Nicholson HO. Cytotoxic drugs in pregnancy: review of reported cases. *J Obstet Gynaecol Br Commonw* 1968;75:307–312.
333. Aviles A, Neri N. Hematological malignancies and pregnancy: a final report of 84 children who received chemotherapy in utero. *Clin Lymphoma* 2001;2(3):173–177.
334. Kassner E. Evaluation and treatment of chemotherapy extravasation injuries. *J Pediatr Oncol Nurs* 2000;17(3):135–148.
335. Kaufman S, Robinson E. Chemical phlebitis after nitrogen mustard injection. *Clin Oncol* 1976;2(4):405–406.
336. Sullivan KM, Storb R, Shulman HM, et al. Immediate and delayed neurotoxicity after mechlorethamine preparation for bone marrow transplantation. *Ann Intern Med* 1982;97(2):182–189.
337. Marmor D, Duyck F. Male reproductive potential after MOPP therapy for Hodgkin's disease: a long-term survey. *Andrologia* 1995;27(2):99–106.
338. Goday JJ, Aguirre A, Raton JA, et al. Local bullous reaction to topical mechlorethamine (mustine). *Contact Dermatitis* 1990;22(5):306–307.
339. Owen OE, Dellatorre DL, Van Scott EJ, et al. Accidental intramuscular injection of mechlorethamine. *Cancer* 1980;45(8):2225–2226.

Megestrol

340. Logmans A, Mous HV, Bontenbal M, et al. Results of curettage for postmenopausal vaginal bleeding in women treated with tamoxifen and megestrol acetate for progressive metastatic breast carcinoma. *Eur J Obstet Gynecol Reprod Biol* 1994;56(3):173–176.
341. Caparros GC, Zambrana JL, Delgado-Fernandez M, et al. Megestrol-induced Cushing syndrome. *Ann Pharmacother* 2001;35(10):1208–1210.
342. Harte C, Henry MT, Murphy KD, et al. Progestogens and Cushing's syndrome. *Ir J Med Sci* 1995;164(4):274–275.

Melphalan

343. Jost LM. Overdose with melphalan (Alkeran): symptoms and treatment. A review. *Onkologie* 1990;13(2):96–101.
344. Coates TD. Survival from melphalan overdose. *Lancet* 1984;2(8410):1048.
345. Pecherstorfer M, Zimmer-Roth I, Weidinger S, et al. High-dose intravenous melphalan in a patient with multiple myeloma and oliguric renal failure. *Clin Investig* 1994;72(7):522–525.
346. Alberts DS, Chang SY, Chen H-SG, et al. Oral melphalan kinetics. *Clin Pharmacol Ther* 1979;26:737–745.
347. Alberts DS, Chang SY, Chen H-SG, et al. Kinetics of intravenous melphalan. *Clin Pharmacol Ther* 1979;26:73–80.
348. Akasheh MS, Freytes CO, Vesole DH. Melphalan-associated pulmonary toxicity following high-dose therapy with autologous hematopoietic stem cell transplantation. *Bone Marrow Transplant* 2000;26(10):1107–1109.
349. Ritchie DS, Seymour JF, Roberts AW, et al. Acute left ventricular failure following melphalan and fludarabine conditioning. *Bone Marrow Transplant* 2001;28(1):101–103.

Mercaptopurine

350. Zimm S, Collins JM, Riccardi R, et al. Variable bioavailability of oral mercaptopurine. *N Engl J Med* 1983;308:1005–1009.
351. Laidlaw ST, Reilly JT, Suvarna SK. Fatal hepatotoxicity associated with 6-mercaptopurine therapy. *Postgrad Med J* 1995;71(840):639.
352. Underwood TW, Frye CB. Drug induced pancreatitis. *Clin Pharm* 1993;12:440–448.
353. Andersen JM, Tiede JJ. Serum sickness associated with 6-mercaptopurine in a patient with Crohn's disease. *Pharmacotherapy* 1997;17(1):173–176.
354. Pujol M, Fernandez F, Sancho JM, et al. Immune hemolytic anemia induced by 6-mercaptopurine. *Transfusion* 2000;40(1):75–76.
355. Krogh CME, ed. *Compendium of pharmaceuticals and specialties*, 27th ed. Ottawa: Canadian Pharmaceutical Association, 1992:947–948.
356. Pinkel D. IV 6-mercaptopurine. Life begins at 40. *J Clin Oncol* 1993;11:1826–1831.

Mesna

357. deVries CR, Freiha FS. Hemorrhagic cystitis: a review. *J Urol* 1990;143(1):1–9.
358. Dorr RT. *Mesnex (mesna) injection. Dosing and administration guide.* Evansville: Bristol Laboratories, 1989.
359. James CA, et al. Pharmacokinetics of intravenous and oral sodium 2-mercaptoethane sulfonate (mesna) in normal subjects. *Br J Clin Pharmacol* 1987;23:561–568.
360. Husband DJ, Watkin SW. Fatal hypokalaemia associated with ifosfamide/mesna chemotherapy. *Lancet* 1988;1(8594):1116.
361. Verdeguer A, Castel V, Esquembre C, et al. Fatal encephalopathy with ifosfamide/mesna. *Pediatr Hematol Oncol* 1989;6(4):383–385.
362. Cantwell BM, Harris AL. Ifosfamide/mesna and encephalopathy. *Lancet* 1985;1(8431):752.
363. Somma-Mauvais H, Farisse P, Viallat JR. Epileptic seizures and treatment with ifosfamide-mesna [in French]. *Rev Neurol (Paris)* 1994;150(4):307–308.
364. Zonzits E, Aberer W, Tappeiner G. Drug eruptions from mesna. After cyclo-

phosphamide treatment of patients with systemic lupus erythematosus and dermatomyositis. *Arch Dermatol* 1992;128(1):80–82.
365. Pratt CB, Sandlund JT, Meyer WH, et al. Mesna-induced urticaria. *Drug Intell Clin Pharm* 1988;22(11):913–914.

Methotrexate

366. Methotrexate indications. RxList Web site. Available at: http://www.rxlist.com/cgi/generic/mtx_ids.htm. Accessed March 2003.
367. Porawska W. Overdose of methotrexate with a fatal outcome in a patient with rheumatoid arthritis. *Pol Arch Med Wewn* 1995;93(4):346–350.
368. Ettinger LJ. Pharmacokinetics and biochemical effects of a fatal intrathecal methotrexate overdose. *Cancer* 1982;50(3):444–450.
369. Ettinger LJ, Freeman AI, Creaven PJ. Intrathecal methotrexate overdose without neurotoxicity: case report and literature review. *Cancer* 1978;41(4):1270–1273.
370. Brown MA, Corrigan AB. Pancytopenia after accidental overdose of methotrexate. A complication of low-dose therapy for rheumatoid arthritis. *Med J Aust* 1991;155(7):493–494.
371. Green DM, Zevon MA, Lowrie G, et al. Congenital anomalies in children of patients who received chemotherapy for cancer in childhood and adolescence. *New Engl J Med* 1991;325:141–146.
372. Johns DG, Rutherford LD, Leighton PC, et al. Secretion of methotrexate into human milk. *Am J Obstet Gynecol* 1972;112(7):978–980.
373. Brass EP. Hepatic toxicity of antirheumatic drugs. *Cleve Clin J Med* 1993;60(6):466–472.
374. ter Borg EJ, Seldenrijk CA, Timmer R. Liver cirrhosis due to methotrexate in a patient with rheumatoid arthritis. *Neth J Med* 1996;49(6):244–246.
375. Langman G, Hall PM, Todd G. Role of non-alcoholic steatohepatitis in methotrexate-induced liver injury. *J Gastroenterol Hepatol* 2001;16(12):1395–1401.
376. Zachariae H, Sogaard H, Heickendorff L. Methotrexate-induced liver cirrhosis. Clinical, histological and serological studies—a further 10-year follow-up. *Dermatology* 1996;192(4):343–346.
377. van den Bongard HJ, Mathjt RA, Boogerd W, et al. Successful rescue with leucovorin and thymidine in a patient with high-dose methotrexate induced acute renal failure. *Cancer Chemother Pharmacol* 2001;47(6):537–540.
378. Jones KW, Patel SR. A family physician's guide to monitoring methotrexate. *Am Fam Physician* 2000;62(7):1607–12, 1614.
379. Calvo-Romero JM. Severe pancytopenia associated with low-dose methotrexate therapy for rheumatoid arthritis. *Ann Pharmacother* 2001;35(12):1575–1577.
380. Camidge DR. Methotrexate-induced radiation recall. *Am J Clin Oncol* 2001;24(2):211–213.
381. Drachtman RA, Cole PD, Golden CB, et al. Dextromethorphan is effective in the treatment of subacute methotrexate neurotoxicity. *Pediatr Hematol Oncol* 2002;19(5):319–327.
382. Antunes NL, Souweidane MM, Lis E, et al. Methotrexate leukoencephalopathy presenting as Klüver-Bucy syndrome and uncinate seizures. *Pediatr Neurol* 2002;26(4):305–308.
383. Brain E, Alexandre J, Minozzi C, et al. High-dose methotrexate and cerebral neurotoxicity. Apropos of a case of arachnoiditis [in French]. *Presse Med* 1997;26(6):265–268.
384. Werner RA. Paraplegia and quadriplegia after intrathecal chemotherapy. *Arch Phys Med Rehabil* 1988;69(12):1054–1056.
385. Chaudhry VP, Marwa RK. Intrathecal methotrexate induced meningitis. *Indian Pediatr* 1979;16(1):87–89.
386. Shore T, Barnett MJ, Phillips GL. Sudden neurologic death after intrathecal methotrexate. *Med Pediatr Oncol* 1990;18(2):159–161.
387. Maytal J, Grossman R, Yusuf FH, et al. Prognosis and treatment of seizures in children with acute lymphoblastic leukemia. *Epilepsia* 1995;36(8):831–836.
388. Dawson JK, Graham DR, Desmond J, et al. Investigation of the chronic pulmonary effects of low-dose oral methotrexate in patients with rheumatoid arthritis: a prospective study incorporating HRCT scanning and pulmonary function tests. *Rheumatology (Oxford)* 2002;41(3):262–267.
389. Zisman DA, McCune WJ, Tino G, et al. Drug-induced pneumonitis: the role of methotrexate. *Sarcoidosis Vasc Diffuse Lung Dis* 2001;18(3):243–252.
390. Bressler L. Antineoplastic drugs—general principles of use. University of Illinois at Chicago Web site: pharmacy practice. Available at: http://www.uic.edu/classes/pmpr/pmpr652/Final/bressler/antineo.html.
391. Jambou P, Levraut J, Favier C, et al. Removal of methotrexate by continuous venovenous hemodiafiltration. *Contrib Nephrol* 1995;116:48–52.
392. Benezet S, Chatelut E, Bagheri H, et al. Inefficacy of exchange-transfusion in case of a methotrexate poisoning. *Bull Cancer* 1997;84(8):788–790.

Mithramycin

393. Schaiff RAB. Medical treatment of hypercalcemia. *Clin Pharm* 1989;8:108–121.
394. Soble MJ, Dorr RT, Plezia P, et al. Dose-dependent skin ulcers in mice treated with DNA binding antitumor antibiotics. *Cancer Chemother Pharmacol* 1987;20(1):33–36.
395. Vogelzang NJ. Nephrotoxicity from chemotherapy: prevention and management. *Oncology (Huntingt)* 1991;5(10):97–102, 105, discussion 105, 109–111.
396. Benedetti RG, Heilman KJ 3rd, Gabow PA. Nephrotoxicity following single dose mithramycin therapy. *Am J Nephrol* 1983;3(5):277–278.

Mitomycin

397. Dorr RT, Fritz WL, eds. *Cancer chemotherapy handbook*. New York: Elsevier Science, 1980:548–555.
398. Okuno SH, Frytak S. Mitomycin lung toxicity. Acute and chronic phases. *Am J Clin Oncol* 1997;20(3):282–284.
399. Villani F, Comazzi R, Lacaita G, et al. Possible enhancement of the cardiotoxicity of doxorubicin when combined with mitomycin C. *Med Oncol Tumor Pharmacother* 1985;2(2):93–97.

Mitotane

400. Vassilopoulou-Sellin R, Schultz PN. Adrenocortical carcinoma. Clinical outcome at the end of the 20th century. *Cancer* 2001;92(5):1113–1121.
401. Kopf D, Goretzki PE, Lehnert H. Clinical management of malignant adrenal tumors. *J Cancer Res Clin Oncol* 2001;127(3):143–155.
402. McEvoy GK, ed. *American hospital formulary service: drug information 1993*. Bethesda: American Society of Hospital Pharmacists, 1994:672.
403. Dorr RT, Von Hoff DD, eds. *Cancer chemotherapy handbook*, 2nd ed. Norwalk: Appleton & Lange, 1994:726–729.
404. Kasperlik-Zaluska AA. Clinical results of the use of mitotane for adrenocortical carcinoma. *Braz J Med Biol Res* 2000;33(10):1191–1196.
405. Andersen A, Kasperlik-Zaluska AA, Warren DJ. Determination of mitotane (o,p-DDD) and its metabolites o,p-DDA and o,p-DDE in plasma by high-performance liquid chromatography. *Ther Drug Monit* 1999;21(3):355–359.
406. Pardo C, Boix E, Lopez A, et al. Adrenal crisis due to mitotane therapy. *Med Clin (Barc)* 2002;118(7):278.
407. Zuehlke RL. Erythematous eruption of the palms and soles associated with mitotane therapy. *Dermatologica* 1974;148(2):90–92.
408. du Rostu H, Krempf M, Mussini JM, et al. Neurotoxicity of mitotane therapy of adrenocortical carcinoma (5 cases) and Cushing's syndrome (7 cases). *Presse Med* 1987;16(19):951–954.
409. Fraunfelder FT, Meyer SM. Ocular toxicity of antineoplastic agents. *Ophthalmology* 1983;90(1):1–3.
410. Gutierrez ML, Crooke ST. Mitotane (o,p'-DDD). *Cancer Treat Rev* 1980;7:49–55.
411. Boven E, Vermorken JB, Van Slooten H, et al. Complete response of metastasized adrenal cortical carcinoma with o,p'-DDD: case report and literature review. *Cancer* 1984;53:26–29.
412. Terzolo M, Pia A, Berruti A, et al. Low-dose monitored mitotane treatment achieves the therapeutic range with manageable side effects in patients with adrenocortical cancer. *J Clin Endocrinol Metab* 2000;85(6):2234–2238.
413. Samaan NA, Hickey CR. Adrenal cortical carcinoma. *Semin Oncol* 1987;14:292–296.

Mitoxantrone

414. Hachimi-Idrissi S, Schots R, DeWolf D, et al. Reversible cardiopathy after accidental overdose of mitoxantrone. *Pediatr Hematol Oncol* 1993;10(1):35–40.
415. Siegert W, Hiddemann W, Koppensteiner R, et al. Accidental overdose of mitoxantrone in three patients. Med Oncol Tumor Pharmacother. 1989;6(4):275–278.
416. Krogh CME, ed. Compendium of pharmaceuticals and specialties, 28th ed. Ottawa: Canadian Pharmaceutical Association, 1993:832–833.
417. Kahles H, Bastian HJ, Schiffmann O, et al. Mitoxantrone-induced acute left heart failure after intrapleural administration [in German]. *Herz* 1997;22(4):217–220.
418. Scheithauer W, Ludwig H, Kotz R, et al. Mitoxantrone-induced discoloration of the nails. *Eur J Cancer Clin Oncol* 1989;25(4):763–765.
419. Kumar L, Kochipillai V. Mitoxantrone induced hyperpigmentation. *N Z Med J* 1990;103(883):55.

Nilutamide

420. Rouger-Barbier D, Delefosse D, Pamphile R, et al. Absence of clinical and biological manifestations after massive absorption of nilutamide. *J Toxicol Clin Exp* 1989;9(2):77–82.
421. Budman DR. Investigational drugs. In: Perry MC, ed. *The chemotherapy source book*. Baltimore: Williams & Wilkins, 1992:473.
422. Harris MG, Coleman SG, Faulds D, et el. Nilutamide—a review of its pharmacodynamic and pharmacokinetic properties and therapeutic efficacy in prostate cancer. *Drugs and Aging* 1993;3:9–25.
423. Eaton VS, Blackmore TK. Nilutamide-induced neutropenia. *BJU Int* 2001;88(7):801–802.
424. Hammel P, Ducreux M, Bismuth E, et al. Nilutamide-induced acute hepatitis. *Gastroenterol Clin Biol* 1991;15(6–7):557.
425. Pescatore P, Hammel P, Durand F, et al. Fatal fulminant hepatitis induced by nilutamide (Anandron). *Gastroenterol Clin Biol* 1993;17(6–7):499–501.

426. Dijkman GA, Klotz LH, Diokno AC, et al. Comment: clinical experiences of visual disturbances with nilutamide. *Ann Pharmacother* 1997;31(12):1550–1552.
427. Maroy B, Pitrou P. Acute depressive syndrome possibly due to nilutamide (Anandron) treatment. *Therapie* 1997;52(1):79–81.
428. Wieder JA, Soloway MS. Interstitial pneumonitis associated with neoadjuvant leuprolide and nilutamide for prostate cancer. *J Urol* 1998;159(6):2099.

Paclitaxel

429. Sood AK, Shahin MS, Sorosky JI. Paclitaxel and platinum chemotherapy for ovarian carcinoma during pregnancy. *Gynecol Oncol* 2001;83(3):599–600.
430. Forsyth PA, Balmaceda C, Peterson K, et al. Prospective study of paclitaxel-induced peripheral neuropathy with quantitative sensory testing. *J Neurooncol* 1997;35(1):47–53.
431. Lee RT, Oster MW, Balmaceda C, et al. Bilateral facial nerve palsy secondary to the administration of high-dose paclitaxel. *Ann Oncol* 1999;10(10):1245–7.
432. Weiss RB, Donehower RH, Wiernik PH, et al. Hypersensitivity reactions from taxol. *J Clin Oncol* 1990;8:1263–1268.
433. Price KS, Castells MC. Taxol reactions. *Allergy Asthma Proc* 2002;23(3):205–8.
434. Bokemeyer C, Lampe C, Heneka M, et al. Paclitaxel-induced radiation recall dermatitis. *Ann Oncol* 1996;7(7):755–756.
435. Boyle FM, Wheeler HR, Shenfield GM. Amelioration of experimental cisplatin and paclitaxel neuropathy with glutamate. *J Neurooncol* 1999;41(2):107–116.
436. Campana WM, Eskeland N, Calcutt NA, et al. Prosaptide prevents paclitaxel neurotoxicity. *Neurotoxicology* 1998;19(2):237–244.

Pegaspargase

437. Kurre HA, Ettinger AG, Veenstra DL, et al. A pharmacoeconomic analysis of pegaspargase versus native Escherichia coli L-asparaginase for the treatment of children with standard-risk, acute lymphoblastic leukemia: the Children's Cancer Group study (CCG-1962). *J Pediatr Hematol Oncol* 2002;24(3):175–181.
438. Clavell LA, Gelber RD, Cohen HJ, et al. Four-agent induction and intensive asparaginase therapy for treatment of childhood acute lymphoblastic leukemia. *N Engl J Med* 1986;315(11):657–663.
439. L-asparaginase description. RxList Web site. Available at: http://www.rxlist.com/cgi/generic2/pegaspargase.htm. Accessed March 2003.
440. Ho DH, Brown NS, Yen A, et al. Clinical pharmacology of polyethylene glycol-L-asparaginase. *Drug Metab Dispos* 1986;14(3):349–352.
441. Capizzi RL, Holcenberg JS. Asparaginase. In: Holland JF, Frei E 3rd, eds. *Cancer medicine*, 3rd ed. Philadelphia: Lea & Febiger, 1993.
442. Alfieri DR. Pegaspargase. *Pediatr Nurs* 1995;21(5):471–474, 490.
443. Alvarez OA, Zimmerman G. Pegaspargase-induced pancreatitis. *Med Pediatr Oncol* 2000;34(3):200–205.
444. Bushara KO, Rust RS. Reversible MRI lesions due to pegaspargase treatment of non-Hodgkin's lymphoma. *Pediatr Neurol* 1997;17(2):185–187.

Pentostatin

445. Kane BJ, Kuhn JG, Roush MK. Pentostatin: an adenosine deaminase inhibitor for the treatment of hairy cell leukemia. *Ann Pharmacother* 1992;26:939–947.
446. Lindley CM, Bernard SA, Robertson JD. Vomiting associated with pentostatin and pentostatin plus alpha-interferon: unique pattern and potential mechanisms. *J Pain Symptom Manage* 1990;5(4):262–264.
447. Samonis G, Kontoyiannis DP. Infectious complications of purine analog therapy. *Curr Opin Infect Dis* 2001;14(4):409–413.
448. Dorr RT, Von Hoff DD, eds. *Cancer chemotherapy handbook*, 2nd ed. Norwalk: Appleton & Lange, 1994:774–779.
449. Ghura HS, Carmichael AJ, Bairstow D, et al. Fatal erythroderma associated with pentostatin. *BMJ* 1999;319(7209):549.
450. Spiers AS, Ruckdeschel JC, Horton J. Effectiveness of pentostatin (2'-deoxycoformycin) in refractory lymphoid neoplasms. *Scand J Haematol* 1984;32(2):130–134.

Procarbazine

451. Cheson BD, Vena DA, Foss FM, et al. Neurotoxicity of purine analogs: a review. *J Clin Oncol* 1994;12(10):2216–2228.
452. Aviles A, Diaz-Maqueo JC, Talavera A, et al. Growth and development of children of mothers treated with chemotherapy during pregnancy. Current status of 43 children. *Am J Hematol* 1991;36:243–248.
453. Lokich JJ, Moloney WC. Allergic reaction to procarbazine. *Clin Pharmacol Ther* 1972;13(4):573–574.
454. Mahmood T, Mudad R. Pulmonary toxicity secondary to procarbazine. *Am J Clin Oncol* 2002;25(2):187–188.
455. Pfefferbaum B, Pack R, van Eys J. Monoamine oxidase inhibitor toxicity. *J Am Acad Child Adolesc Psychiatry* 1989;28(6):954–955.
456. Macdonald DR. Neurologic complications of chemotherapy. *Neurol Clin* 1991;9(4):955–967.
457. Hadjiyanni M, Valianatou K, Tsilianos M, et al. Prolonged thrombocytopenia after procarbazine "overdose." *Eur J Cancer* 1992;28A(6–7):1299.
458. Giguere JK, Douglas DM, Lupton GP, et al. Procarbazine hypersensitivity manifested as a fixed drug eruption. *Med Pediatr Oncol* 1988;16(6):378–380.
459. Coyle T, Bushunow P, Winfield J, et al. Hypersensitivity reactions to procarbazine with mechlorethamine, vincristine, and procarbazine chemotherapy in the treatment of glioma. *Cancer* 1992;69(10):2532–2540.
460. Andersen E, Videbaek A. Procarbazine-induced skin reactions in Hodgkin's disease and other malignant lymphomas. *Scand J Haematol* 1980;24(2):149–151.
461. Howell SJ, Shalet SM. Testicular function following chemotherapy. *Hum Reprod Update* 2001;7(4):363–369.

Rituximab

462. Kosits C, Callaghan M. Rituximab: a new monoclonal antibody therapy for non-Hodgkin's lymphoma. *Oncol Nurs Forum* 2000;27(1):51–59.
463. Kanelli S, Ansell SM, Habermann TM, et al. Rituximab toxicity in patients with peripheral blood malignant B-cell lymphocytosis. *Leuk Lymphoma* 2001;42(6):1329–1337.
464. McLaughlin P, Hagemeister FB, Grillo-Lopez AJ. Rituximab in indolent lymphoma: the single-agent pivotal trial. *Semin Oncol* 1999;26[5 Suppl 14]:79–87.
465. Davis TA, White CA, Grillo-Lopez AJ, et al. Single-agent monoclonal antibody efficacy in bulky non-Hodgkin's lymphoma: results of a phase II trial of rituximab. *J Clin Oncol* 1999;17(6):1851–1857.
466. Dillman RO. Infusion reactions associated with the therapeutic use of monoclonal antibodies in the treatment of malignancy. *Cancer Metastasis Rev* 1999;18(4):465–471.
467. Winkler U, Jensen M, Manzke O, et al. Cytokine-release syndrome in patients with B-cell chronic lymphocytic leukemia and high lymphocyte counts after treatment with an anti-CD20 monoclonal antibody (rituximab, IDEC-C2B8). *Blood* 1999;94(7):2217–2224.
468. Byrd JC, Waselenko JK, Maneatis TJ, et al. Rituximab therapy in hematologic malignancy patients with circulating blood tumor cells: association with increased infusion-related side effects and rapid blood tumor clearance. *J Clin Oncol* 1999;17(3):791–795.
469. Yang H, Rosove MH, Figlin RA. Tumor lysis syndrome occurring after the administration of rituximab in lymphoproliferative disorders: high-grade non-Hodgkin's lymphoma and chronic lymphocytic leukemia. *Am J Hematol* 1999;62(4):247–250.
470. Rituxan [package insert]. Mississauga, Ontario: Hoffmann-LaRoche; 2001.

Streptozocin

471. Uchigata Y, Yamamoto H, Kawamura A, et al. Protection by superoxide dismutase, catalase, and poly(ADP-ribose) synthetase inhibitors against alloxan- and streptozotocin-induced islet DNA strand breaks and against the inhibition of proinsulin synthesis. *J Biol Chem* 1982;257(11):6084–6088.
472. Krogh CME, ed. *Compendium of pharmaceuticals and specialties*, 27th ed. Ottawa: Canadian Pharmaceutical Association, 1992:1318–1319.
473. Tobin MV, Warenius HM, Morris AI. Forced diuresis to reduce nephrotoxicity of streptozotocin in the treatment of advanced metastatic insulinoma. *Br Med J (Clin Res Ed)* 1987;294(6580):1128.

Tamoxifen

474. Sridar C, Kent UM, Notley LM, et al. Effect of tamoxifen on the enzymatic activity of human cytochrome CYP2B6. *J Pharmacol Exp Ther* 2002;301(3):945–952.
475. Nikolic-Tomasevic Z, Jelic S, Popov I, et al. Tumor 'flare' hypercalcemia—an additional indication for bisphosphonates? *Oncology* 2001;60(2):123–126.
476. Harvey HA. Issues concerning the role of chemotherapy and hormonal therapy of bone metastases from breast carcinoma. *Cancer* 1997;80[8 Suppl]:1646–1651.
477. Reddel RR, Sutherland RL. Tamoxifen stimulation of human breast cancer cell proliferation in vitro: a possible model for tamoxifen tumour flare. *Eur J Cancer Clin Oncol* 1984;20(11):1419–1424.
478. Neis KJ, Brandner P, Schlenker M. Tamoxifen-induced hyperplasia of the endometrium. *Contrib Gynecol Obstet* 2000;20:60–68.
479. Juneja M, Jose R, Kekre AN, et al. Tamoxifen-induced endometrial changes in postmenopausal women with breast carcinoma. *Int J Gynaecol Obstet* 2002;76(3):279–284.
480. Nomikos IN, Elemenoglou J, Papatheophanis J. Tamoxifen-induced endometrial polyp. A case report and review of the literature. *Eur J Gynaecol Oncol* 1998;19(5):476–478.
481. Neven P, De Muylder X, Van Belle Y. Tamoxifen-induced endometrial polyp. *N Engl J Med* 1997;336(19):1389;discussion,1389–1390.
482. Pukkala E, Kyyronen P, Sankila R, et al. Tamoxifen and toremifene treatment of breast cancer and risk of subsequent endometrial cancer: a population-based case-control study. *Int J Cancer* 2002;100(3):337–341.
483. White IN. The tamoxifen dilemma. *Carcinogenesis* 1999;20(7):1153–1160.
484. Farrell GC. Drugs and steatohepatitis. *Semin Liver Dis* 2002;22(2):185–194.

485. Nemoto Y, Saibara T, Ogawa Y, et al. Tamoxifen-induced nonalcoholic steatohepatitis in breast cancer patients treated with adjuvant tamoxifen. *Intern Med* 2002;41(5):345–350.
486. Storen EC, Hay JE, Kaur J, et al. Tamoxifen-induced submassive hepatic necrosis. *Cancer J* 2000;6(2):58–60.
487. Elisaf MS, Nakou K, Liamis G, et al. Tamoxifen-induced severe hypertriglyceridemia and pancreatitis. *Ann Oncol* 2000;11(8):1067–1069.
488. Artac M, Sari R, Altunbas H, et al. Asymptomatic acute pancreatitis due to tamoxifen-induced severe hypertriglyceridemia in a patient with diabetes mellitus and breast cancer. *J Chemother* 2002;14(3):309–311.
489. Law CH, Tandan VR. The association between tamoxifen and the development of hepatocellular carcinoma: case report and literature review. *Can J Surg* 1999;42(3):211–214.
490. Yanyali AC, Freund KB, Sorenson JA, et al. Tamoxifen retinopathy in a male patient. *Am J Ophthalmol* 2001;131(3):386–387.
491. Lee AG. Tamoxifen retinopathy. *J Neuroophthalmol* 1998;18(4):276.
492. Noureddin BN, Seoud M, Bashshur Z, et al. Ocular toxicity in low-dose tamoxifen: a prospective study. *Eye* 1999;13(Pt 6):729–733.
493. Loprinzi CL, Zahasky KM, Sloan JA, et al. Tamoxifen-induced hot flashes. *Clin Breast Cancer* 2000;1(1):52–56.
494. Harris AL, Smith IE, Snaith M. Tamoxifen-induced tumour regression associated with dermatomyositis. *Br Med J (Clin Res Ed)* 1982;284(6330):1674–1675.
495. Puglisi F, Aprile G, Sobrero A. Tamoxifen-induced total alopecia. *Ann Intern Med* 2001;134(12):1154–1155.
496. Pandya KJ, Raubertas RF, Flynn PJ, et al. Oral clonidine in postmenopausal patients with breast cancer experiencing tamoxifen-induced hot flashes: a University of Rochester Cancer Center Community Clinical Oncology Program study. *Ann Intern Med* 2000;132(10):788–793.

Teniposide

497. Damayanthi Y, Lown JW. Podophyllotoxins: current status and recent developments. *Curr Med Chem* 1998;5(3):205–252.
498. Gordaliza M, Castro MA, del Corral JM, et al. Antitumor properties of podophyllotoxin and related compounds. *Curr Pharm Des* 2000;6(18):1811–1839.
499. O'Dwyer PJ, King SA, Fortner CL, et al. Hypersensitivity reactions to teniposide (VM-26): an analysis. *J Clin Oncol* 1986;4:1262–1269.
500. Murphy SB. Secondary acute myeloid leukemia following treatment with epipodophyllotoxins (editorial). *J Clin Oncol* 1993;11:199–201.
501. Eschalier A, Lavarenne J, Burtin C, et al. Study of histamine release induced by acute administration of antitumor agents in dogs. *Cancer Chemother Pharmacol* 1988;21(3):246–250.
502. Kellie SJ, Crist WM, Pui CH, et al. Hypersensitivity reactions to epipodophyllotoxins in children with acute lymphoblastic leukemia. *Cancer* 1991;67(4):1070–1075.
503. Siddall SJ, Martin J, Nunn AJ. Anaphylactic reactions to teniposide. *Lancet* 1989;1(8634):394.
504. Womer RB. Epipodophyllotoxins and secondary leukemia. *Pediatr Hematol Oncol* 1993;10(2):xi–xiii.
505. Lopez-Andrew JA, Ferris J, Verdeguer A, et al. Secondary acute promyelocytic leukemia in a child treated with epipodophyllotoxins. *Am J Pediatr Hematol Oncol* 1994;16(4):384–386.

Testolactone

506. Cocconi G. First generation aromatase inhibitors—aminoglutethimide and testolactone. *Breast Cancer Res Treat* 1994;30(1):57–80.
507. Testolactone indications and uses. RxList Web site. Available at: http://www.rxlist.com/cgi/generic2/testolactone_ids.htm. Accessed March 2003.

Thioguanine

508. Karran P. Mechanisms of tolerance to DNA damaging therapeutic drugs. *Carcinogenesis* 2001;22(12):1931–1937.
509. Taylor G, Blom J. Acute leukemia during pregnancy. *South Med J* 1980;73(10):1314–1315.
510. Volkenandt M, Buchner T, Hiddemann W, et al. Acute leukemia during pregnancy. *Lancet* 1987;2:1521–1522.
511. Shall L, Lucas GS, Whittaker JA, et al. Painful red hands: a side-effect of leukaemia therapy. *Br J Dermatol* 1988;119(2):249–253.

Thiotepa

512. Eder JP, Antman K, Elias A, et al. Cyclophosphamide and thiotepa with autologous bone marrow transplantation in patients with solid tumors. *J Natl Cancer Inst* 1988;80(15):1221–1226.
513. Watterson J, Toogood I, Nieder M, et al. Excessive spinal cord toxicity from intensive central nervous system-directed therapies. *Cancer* 1994;74(11):3034–3041.
514. Choe JM, Kirkemo AK, Sirls LT. Intravesical thiotepa-induced eosinophilic cystitis. *Urology* 1995;46(5):729–731.
515. Soloway MS, Ford KS. Thiotepa-induced myelosuppression: review of 670 bladder instillations. *J Urol* 1983;130(5):889–891.
516. Heney NM. First-line chemotherapy of superficial bladder cancer: mitomycin vs thiotepa. *Urology* 1985;26[4 Suppl]:27–29.
517. Horn TD, Beveridge RA, Egorin MJ, et al. Observations and proposed mechanism of N,N′,N″-triethylenethiophosphoramide (thiotepa)-induced hyperpigmentation. *Arch Dermatol* 1989;125(4):524–527.

Topotecan

518. Kollmannsberger C, Mross K, Jakob A, et al. Topotecan—a novel topoisomerase I inhibitor: pharmacology and clinical experience. *Oncology* 1999;56(1):1–12.
519. Cersosimo RJ. Topotecan: a new topoisomerase I inhibiting antineoplastic agent. *Ann Pharmacother* 1998;32(12):1334–1343.
520. Hycamtin [package insert]. Oakville, Ontario: SmithKline Beecham; 1999.
521. Topotecan. USP DI. Vol. 1. *Drug information for the health care professional* [update monographs]. Englewood, Colorado: Micromedex, Inc., 2000.
522. O'Reilly S, Rowinsky E, Slichenmyer W, et al. Phase I and pharmacologic studies of topotecan in patients with impaired hepatic function. *J Natl Cancer Inst* 1996;88(12):817–824.
523. Topotecan warnings. RxList Web site. Available at: http://www.rxlist.com/cgi/generic2/topotec_wcp.htm. Accessed March 2003.
524. Rodriguez M, Rose PG. Improved therapeutic index of lower dose topotecan chemotherapy in recurrent ovarian cancer. *Gynecol Oncol* 2001;83(2):257–262.
525. Zamboni WC, D'Argenio DZ, Stewart CF, et al. Pharmacodynamic model of topotecan-induced time course of neutropenia. *Clin Cancer Res* 2001;7(8):2301–2308.
526. Anastasia PJ. Nursing considerations for managing topotecan-related hematologic side effects. *Clin J Oncol Nurs* 2001;5(1):9–13.
527. Ene-Stroescu D, Ellman MH, Peterson CE. Topotecan and the development of scleroderma or a scleroderma-like illness. *Arthritis Rheum* 2002;46(3):844–845.
528. Marini M, Wright D, Ropolo M, et al. Neutrophilic eccrine hidradenitis secondary to topotecan. *J Dermatolog Treat* 2002;13(1):35–37.
529. Herrington JD, Figueroa JA, Kirstein MN, et al. Effect of hemodialysis on topotecan disposition in a patient with severe renal dysfunction. *Cancer Chemother Pharmacol* 2001;47(1):89–93.
530. Janik JE, Miller LL, Korn EL, et al. A prospective randomized phase II trial of GM-CSF priming to prevent topotecan-induced neutropenia in chemotherapy-naive patients with malignant melanoma or renal cell carcinoma. *Blood* 2001;97(7):1942–1946.

Toremifene

531. Bertelli G, Queirolo P, Vecchio S, et al. Toremifene as a substitute for adjuvant tamoxifen in breast cancer patients. *Anticancer Res* 2000;20(5C):3659–3661.
532. Ellmen J, Werner D, Hakulinen P, et al. Dose-dependent hormonal effects of toremifene in postmenopausal breast cancer patients. *Cancer Chemother Pharmacol* 2000;45(5):402–408.
533. Hamm JT. Phase I and II studies of toremifene. *Oncology (Huntingt)* 1997;11[5 Suppl 4]:19–22.
534. Bishop J, Murray R, Webster L, et al. Phase I clinical and pharmacokinetics study of high-dose toremifene in postmenopausal patients with advanced breast cancer. *Cancer Chemother Pharmacol* 1992;30(3):174–178.
535. Anttila M, Valavaara R, Kivinen S, et al. Pharmacokinetics of toremifene. *J Steroid Biochem* 1990;36(3):249–252.
536. Berthou F, Dreano Y, Belloc C, et al. Involvement of cytochrome P450 3A enzyme family in the major metabolic pathways of toremifene in human liver microsomes. *Biochem Pharmacol* 1994;47(10):1883–1895.
537. Taras TL, Wurz GT, Linares GR, et al. Clinical pharmacokinetics of toremifene. *Clin Pharmacokinet* 2000;39(5):327–334.
538. Hamada N, Ogawa Y, Saibara T, et al. Toremifene-induced fatty liver and NASH in breast cancer patients with breast-conservation treatment. *Int J Oncol* 2000;17(6):1119–1123.
539. Maenpaa J, Holli K, Pasanen T. Toremifene. Where do we stand? *Eur J Cancer* 2000;36[Suppl 4]:S61–S62.

Valrubicin

540. Randall S. Valrubicin: an alternative to radical cystectomy for carcinoma in situ of the bladder. *Urol Nurs* 2001;21(1):30–31, 34–36.
541. Steinberg G, Bahnson R, Brosman S, et al. Efficacy and safety of valrubicin for the treatment of Bacillus Calmette-Guerin refractory carcinoma in situ of the bladder. The Valrubicin Study Group. *J Urol* 2000;163(3):761–767.
542. Sweatman TW, Parker RF, Israel M. Pharmacologic rationale for intravesical N-trifluoroacetyladriamycin-14-valerate (AD 32): a preclinical study. *Cancer Chemother Pharmacol* 1991;28(1):1–6.
543. Patterson AL, Greenberg RE, Weems L, et al. Pilot study of the tolerability and toxicity of intravesical valrubicin immediately after transurethral resection of superficial bladder cancer. *Urology* 2000;56(2):232–235.

Vinblastine

544. Winter SC, Arbus GS. Syndrome of inappropriate secretion of antidiuretic hormone secondary to vinblastine overdose. *Can Med Assoc J* 1977;117(10):1134.
545. Conter V, Rabbone ML, Jankovic M, et al. Overdose of vinblastine in a child with Langerhans' cell histiocytosis: toxicity and salvage therapy. *Pediatr Hematol Oncol* 1991;8(2):165–169.
546. Aviles A, Diaz-Maqueo JC, Talavera A, et al. Growth and development of children of mothers treated with chemotherapy during pregnancy: current status of 43 children. *Am J Hematol* 1991;36:243–248.
547. Krogh CME, ed. *Compendium of pharmaceuticals and specialties*, 28th ed. Ottawa: Canadian Pharmaceutical Association, 1993.
548. Burns BV, Shotton JC. Vocal fold palsy following vinca alkaloid treatment. *J Laryngol Otol* 1998;112(5):485–487.
549. Brook J, Schreiber W. Vocal cord paralysis: a toxic reaction to vinblastine (NSC-49842) therapy. *Cancer Chemother Rep* 1971;55(5):591–593.
550. Hansen SW. Autonomic neuropathy after treatment with cisplatin, vinblastine, and bleomycin for germ cell cancer. *BMJ* 1990;300(6723):511–512.

Vincristine

551. Chae L, Moon HS, Kim SC. Overdose of vincristine: experience with a patient. *J Korean Med Sci* 1998;13(3):334–338.
552. Maeda K, Ueda M, Ohtaka H, et al. A massive dose of vincristine. *Jpn J Clin Oncol* 1987;17(3):247–253.
553. Dettmeyer R, Driever F, Becker A, et al. Fatal myeloencephalopathy due to accidental intrathecal vincristin administration: a report of two cases. *Forensic Sci Int* 2001;122(1):60–64.
554. Legha SS. Vincristine neurotoxicity. Pathophysiology and management. *Med Toxicol* 1986;1(6):421–427.
555. Kosmidis HV, Bouhoutsou DO, Varvoutsi MC, et al. Vincristine overdose: experience with 3 patients. *Pediatr Hematol Oncol* 1991;8(2):171–178.
556. Krogh CME, ed. *Compendium of pharmaceuticals and specialties*, 28th ed. Ottawa: Canadian Pharmaceutical Association, 1993:865–7,1318–1319.
557. Caligiuri MA, Mayer RJ. Pregnancy and leukemia. *Semin Oncol* 1989;16(5):388–396.
558. Doll DC, Ringenberg QS, Yarbro JW. Antineoplastic agents and pregnancy. *Semin Oncol* 1989;16(5):337–346.
559. Selevan SG, Lindbohn ML, Hornung RW, et al. A study of occupational exposure to antineoplastic drugs and fetal loss in nurses. *N Engl J Med* 1985;313(19):1173–1178.
560. Pal PK. Clinical and electrophysiological studies in vincristine induced neuropathy. *Electromyogr Clin Neurophysiol* 1999;39(6):323–330.
561. Othieno-Abinya NA, Nyabola LO. Experience with vincristine-associated neurotoxicity. *East Afr Med J* 2001;78(7):376–378.
562. Ryan SP, DelPrete SA, Weinstein PW, et al. Low-dose vincristine-associated bilateral vocal cord paralysis. *Conn Med* 1999;63(10):583–584.
563. Albert DM, Wong VG, Henderson ES. Ocular complications of vincristine therapy. *Arch Ophthalmol* 1967;78(6):709–713.
564. Ridgway D, Renholds DC, Neerhout RC, et al. Vincristine in the etiology of toxicity of high-dose methotrexate therapy. *Cancer* 1980;46(12):2571–2572.
565. Hancock BW, Naysmith A. Vincristine-induced autonomic neuropathy. *BMJ* 1975;3(5977):207.
566. Roca E, Bruera E, Politi PM, et al. Vinca alkaloid-induced cardiovascular autonomic neuropathy. *Cancer Treat Rep* 1985;69(2):149–151.
567. Hurwitz RL, Mahoney DH Jr., Armstrong DL, et al. Reversible encephalopathy and seizures as a result of conventional vincristine administration. *Med Pediatr Oncol* 1988;16(3):216–219.
568. Dallera F, Gamoletti R, Costa P. Unilateral seizures following vincristine intravenous injection. *Tumori* 1984;70(3):243–244.
569. Ghosh K, Sivakumaran M, Murphy P, et al. Visual hallucinations following treatment with vincristine. *Clin Lab Haematol* 1994;16(4):355–357.
570. Hammond IW, Ferguson JA, Kwong K, et al. Hyponatremia and syndrome of inappropriate anti-diuretic hormone reported with the use of Vincristine: an over-representation of Asians? *Pharmacoepidemiol Drug Saf* 2002;11(3):229–234.
571. Pierga JY, Beuzeboc P, Dorval T, et al. Favourable outcome after plasmapheresis for vincristine overdose. *Lancet* 1992;340(8812):185.
572. Thomas LL, Braat PC, Somers R, et al. Massive vincristine overdose: failure of leucovorin to reduce toxicity. *Cancer Treat Rep* 1982;66(11):1967–1969.

Vindesine

573. Cersosimo RJ, Bromer R, Licciardello JT, et al. Pharmacology, clinical efficacy and adverse effects of vindesine sulfate, a new vinca alkaloid. *Pharmacotherapy* 1983;3(5):259–274.
574. Fassas A, Kartalis G, Klearchou N, et al. Chemotherapy for acute leukemia during pregnancy. Five case reports. *Nouv Rev Fr Hematol* 1984;26(1):19–24.
575. Fiorentino MV, Salvagno L, Chiarion Sileni V, et al. Vindesine overdose. *Cancer Treat Rep* 1982;66(5):1247–1248.
576. Turpin F, Tubiana-Hulin M, Meeus L, et al. Complications of antitumor and antileukemic chemotherapy. *Sem Hop* 1982;58(36):2047–2057.
577. Rowinsky EK, Donehower RC. Vinca alkaloids and epipodophyllotoxins. In: Perry MC, ed. *The chemotherapy source book*. Baltimore: Williams & Wilkins, 1992:366–368.
578. Heran F, Defer G, Brugieres P, et al. Cortical blindness during chemotherapy: clinical, CT, and MR correlations. *J Comput Assist Tomogr* 1990;14(2):262–266.

Vinorelbine

579. Rowinsky EK, Noe DA, Trump DL, et al. Pharmacokinetic, bioavailability, and feasibility study of oral vinorelbine in patients with solid tumors. *J Clin Oncol* 1994;12(9):1754–1763.
580. Gregory RK, Smith IE. Vinorelbine—a clinical review. *Br J Cancer* 2000;82(12):1907–1913.
581. Janne PA, Rodriguez-Thompson D, Metcalf DR, et al. Chemotherapy for a patient with advanced non-small-cell lung cancer during pregnancy: a case report and a review of chemotherapy treatment during pregnancy. *Oncology* 2001;61(3):175–183.
582. Navelbine [package insert]. Mississauga, Ontario: Glaxo Wellcome; 1998.
583. Vinorelbine. USP DI. Vol. 1. *Drug information for the health care professional* [update monographs]. Englewood, Colorado: Micromedex, Inc., 2000.
584. Cicchetti S, Jemec B, Gault DT. Two case reports of vinorelbine extravasation: management and review of the literature. *Tumori* 2000;86(4):289–292.
585. Kouroukis C, Hings I. Respiratory failure following vinorelbine tartrate infusion in a patient with non-small cell lung cancer. *Chest* 1997;112(3):846–848.
586. Tassinari D, Sartori S, Gianni L, et al. Is acute dyspnoea a rare side effect of vinorelbine? *Ann Oncol* 1997;8(5):503–504.
587. Gebbia V, Testa A, Valenza R, et al. Acute pain syndrome at tumour site in neoplastic patients treated with vinorelbine: report of unusual toxicity [Letter]. *Eur J Cancer* 1994;30A(6):889.
588. Hohneker JA. A summary of vinorelbine (Navelbine) safety data from North American clinical trials. *Semin Oncol* 1994;21[5 Suppl 10]:42–46;discussion,6–7.
589. Kornek GV, Kornfehl H, Hejna M, et al. Acute tumor pain in patients with head and neck cancer treated with vinorelbine [Letter]. *J Natl Cancer Inst* 1996;88(21):1593.

Antineoplastic Treatment Guidelines

590. Wandt H, Ehninger G, Gallmeier WM. New strategies for prophylactic platelet transfusion in patients with hematologic diseases. *Oncologist* 2001;6(5):446–450.
591. Bokemeyer C, Honecker F, Wedding U, et al. Use of hematopoietic growth factors in elderly patients receiving cytotoxic chemotherapy. *Onkologie* 2002;25(1):32–39.
592. Kim L, Glantz MJ. Neoplastic meningitis. *Curr Treat Options Oncol* 2001;2(6):517–527.
593. Sonis ST, Fey EG. Oral complications of cancer therapy. *Oncology (Huntingt)* 2002;16(5):680–6; discussion 686,691–692,695.
594. Demarosi F, Bez C, Carrassi A. Prevention and treatment of chemo- and radiotherapy-induced oral mucositis. *Minerva Stomatol* 2002;51(5):173–186.
595. Worthington HV, Clarkson JE, Eden OB. Interventions for treating oral mucositis for patients with cancer receiving treatment. *Cochrane Database Syst Rev* 2002;(1):CD001973.
596. Wadleigh RG, Redman RS, Graham ML, et al. Vitamin E in the treatment of chemotherapy-induced mucositis. *Am J Med* 1992;92(5):481–484.
597. Lefebvre JL, Domenge C. A comparative study of the efficacy and safety of fluconazole oral suspension and amphotericin B oral suspension in cancer patients with mucositis. *Oral Oncol* 2002;38(4):337–342.
598. Crawford J, Tomita DK, Mazanet R, et al. Reduction of oral mucositis by filgrastim (r-metHuG-CSF) in patients receiving chemotherapy. *Cytokines Cell Mol Ther* 1999;5(4):187–193.
599. Wong SF, Wilder-Smith P. Pilot study of laser effects on oral mucositis in patients receiving chemotherapy. *Cancer J* 2002;8(3):247–254.
600. Malik I, Moid I, Khan Z, et al. Prospective randomized comparison of tropisetron with and without dexamethasone against high-dose metoclopramide in prophylaxis of acute and delayed cisplatin-induced nausea and vomiting. *Am J Clin Oncol* 1999;22(2):126–130.
601. Parker RI, Prakash D, Mahan RA, et al. Randomized, double-blind, crossover, placebo-controlled trial of intravenous ondansetron for the prevention of intrathecal chemotherapy-induced vomiting in children. *J Pediatr Hematol Oncol* 2001;23(9):578–581.
602. Tramer MR, Carroll D, Campbell FA, et al. Cannabinoids for control of chemotherapy induced nausea and vomiting: quantitative systematic review. *BMJ* 2001;323(7303):16–21.
603. Kinzie BJ. Management of the syndrome of inappropriate secretion of antidiuretic hormone. *Clin Pharm* 1987;6(8):625–633.
604. Miyagawa CI. The pharmacologic management of the syndrome of inappropriate secretion of antidiuretic hormone. *Drug Intell Clin Pharm* 1986;20(7–8):527–531.
605. Jeha S. Tumor lysis syndrome. *Semin Hematol* 2001;38[4 Suppl 10]:4–8.

SECTION

4

Autonomic Drugs

CHAPTER 99

Adrenergic Agents

David E. Lieberman

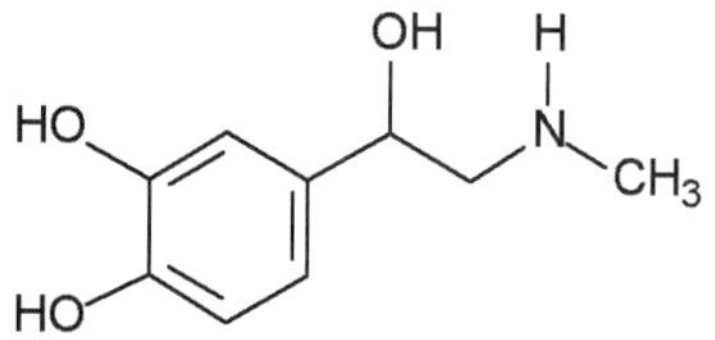

EPINEPHRINE

Compounds included:	**Dobutamine (Dobutrex), dopamine (Intropin), epinephrine (Adrenalin), isoproterenol (Isuprel), mephentermine (Wyamine), metaraminol (Aramine), methoxamine (Vasoxyl), norepinephrine (Levophed), phenylephrine (Neo-Synephrine)**
Molecular formula and weight:	**See Table 1.**
SI conversion:	**See Table 1.**
CAS Registry No.:	**See Table 1.**
Therapeutic levels:	**Not applicable**
Target organs:	**Cardiovascular system**
Antidotes:	**β-receptor agonists, glucagon, insulin, and glucose**

OVERVIEW

The adrenergic agents include a wide array of agents whose mechanism of action involves the α, β, or combined adrenergic receptor stimulation (Table 2). Many of the adrenergic receptor actions can be understood in terms of the known physiologic effects of catecholamines. Most of the available agonists are structural analogs of epinephrine and norepinephrine as these are the endogenous catecholamines. The synthetic adrenergic agents have some advantages in therapy including better oral bioavailability, specificity for particular receptor subtype, duration of action, and side effect profile. Many direct acting sympathomimetic agents influence both types of adrenergic receptors, but the ratio of activity at each receptor subtype varies in a spectrum from predominantly α activity (phenylephrine) to purely β activity (isoproterenol). Each class of agent, α or β, is addressed as a class in the following.

Each agent is addressed individually in this chapter. The diagnosis and treatment of all adrenergic agents is similar and is addressed in a combined section at the end of this chapter.

DOBUTAMINE

Dobutamine hydrochloride (Dobutrex) is a cardioselective, synthetic sympathomimetic amine that was developed to reduce the deleterious effects associated with previous inotropic agents. Dobutamine is a β_1-adrenergic agonist and acts primarily as an inotropic agent with modest peripheral vasodilating properties (1). Although dobutamine was thought to be a relatively selective β_1-adrenergic agonist, its pharmacologic effects include a modest α_1 adrenoceptor–mediated vasoconstriction and β_2 adrenoceptor–mediated vasodilation (2–4).

The primary difference between dobutamine and dopamine is related to the greater activity of dopamine as an agonist of α-1 receptors, which is partially mediated through dopamine-induced release of norepinephrine from nerve endings (2,5–8). Unlike dopamine, dobutamine does not cause endogenous release of norepinephrine (5,9,10) and does not stimulate renal dopaminergic receptors (2,9,11). The predominant mechanism of action of dobutamine is augmentation of myocardial contractility via β_1 stimulation.

Dobutamine is used when parenteral therapy is necessary for inotropic support in the short-term treatment of cardiac decompensation due to depressed contractility resulting either from

TABLE 1. Physical characteristics and therapeutic dose for adrenergic agents

Name	Molecular formula, molecular weight (g/mol), CAS Registry No.	SI conversion	Therapeutic dose: Adult (mg)	Therapeutic dose: Children (mg/kg)
Dobutamine hydrochloride	$C_{18}H_{23}NO_3$,HCL; 301.39; 49745-95-1	μg/L × 0.0033 = μmol/L	2.5–15 μg/kg/min IV up to 40 μg/kg/min, titrate to desired response	2.5–15 μg/kg/min IV, titrate to desired response
Dopamine hydrochloride	$C_8H_{11}NO_2$,HCL; 153.18; 51-61-6, 62-31-7	μg/L × 0.0065 = μmol/L	1–5 μg/kg/min IV up to 50 μg/kg/min, titrate to desired response	1–20 μg/kg/min IV, up to 50 μg/kg/min, titrate to desired response
Epinephrine hydrochloride	$C_9H_{13}NO_3$,HCl; 183.20; 51-43-4	μg/L × 0.0054 = μmol/L	0.2–0.5 mg SQ every 2 h as required; 0.3 mg IM (0.3 ml of a 1:1000 solution); 1 mg IV initially, may be repeated as necessary every 3–5 min; 0.1 mg/kg ET (0.1 ml/kg of a 1:1000 solution)	0.01 ml/kg/dose SQ; up to 0.4–0.5 ml; 0.01 mg/kg IM; 0.01 mg/kg IV (0.1 ml/kg of a 1:10,000 solution), may be repeated every 3–5 min as needed; 0.1 mg/kg ET (0.1 ml/kg of a 1:1000 solution)
Isoproterenol	$C_{11}H_{17}NO_3$,HCL; 211.24; 7683-59-2, 51-30-9, 299-95-6, 6700-39-6	μg/L × 0.0047 = μmol/L	10–20 mg SL; 0.5–5.0 μg/min IV up to 2–20 μg/min, titrate to desired response	5–10 mg SL; 0.5–5 μg/min IV up to 2–20 μg/min, titrate to desired response
Mephentermine	$C_{12}H_{19}N$; 163.25; 83915-83-7	μg/L × 0.0061 = μmol/L	0.5 mg/kg IM; 30–45 mg IV	NR
Metaraminol	$C_9H_{13}NO_2$ $C_4H_6O_6$; 167.20; 33402-03-8	μg/L × 0.0060 = μmol/L	2–10 IM or SQ; 0.5–5.0 IV	NR
Methoxamine	$C_{11}H_{17}NO_3$,HCl; 247.7; 390-28-3, 61-16-5	μg/L × 0.0034 = μmol/L	10 to 20 mg IM; 3 to 10 mg IV	NR
Norepinephrine	$C_8H_{11}NO_3$; 169.18; 51-41-2, 51-40-1, 6981-49-5	μg/L × 0.0059 = μmol/L	Begin 4 μg/min IV up to 8–12 μg/min, titrate to desired effect	0.05–0.1 μg/kg/min IV, titrate to desired effect
Phenylephrine	$C_9H_{13}NO_2$,HCl; 203.67; 59-42-7, 61-76-7	μg/L × 0.0060 = μmol/L	2–5 mg IM or SQ; bolus 0.1–0.5 mg/dose, IV infusion begin 100–180 μg/min	0.1 mg/kg IM or SQ; bolus 5–20 μg/kg IV, infusion 0.1–0.5 μg/kg/min

ET, endotracheal; NR, not reported.

organic heart disease or from cardiac surgical procedures (12,13). In doses that produce similar increases in cardiac output, dobutamine as compared to isoproterenol may produce a smaller increase in heart rate, a smaller decrease in peripheral resistance, and a smaller decrease in diastolic blood pressure (14,15). At low doses (2 to 15 μg/kg/minute) dobutamine increases cardiac output, reduces systemic vascular resistance, lowers central venous and pulmonary wedge pressures, improves renal blood flow, and relieves the signs and symptoms of congestive heart failure. Urine output increases with dobutamine due to increased renal perfusion. In addition, a non–U.S. Food and Drug Administration (FDA) labeled indication for dobutamine is in its use for pharmacologic stress testing, an acceptable alternative in patients unable to perform exercise stress testing.

Toxic Dose

Adult and pediatric therapeutic doses are provided in Table 1. Few patients with overdose have been reported (1–5). Toxic symptoms and signs are usually related to excessive cardiac beta-receptor stimulation. There have been no reported fatalities due to an overdose. A patient with an acute myocardial infarction received 40 μg/kg/minute and survived (16). Dobutamine, 50 mg, was administered as a bolus injection to a 36-year-old patient in cardiogenic shock. There were no significant immediate sequelae (17). One 56-year-old patient accidentally received 70-μg/kg/minute dobutamine and survived but died 10 days later of an arterial embolus (18). A 47-year-old patient inadvertently received 130 μg/kg/minute for 30 minutes; there were no sequelae (19). A 2-hour infusion of 30 μg/kg/minute in one patient and a 5-minute infusion of 80 μg/kg/minute did not produce any life-threatening reactions (20).

Toxicokinetics and Toxicodynamics

The pharmacokinetic data for dobutamine are provided in Table 3. Dobutamine is inactive after oral administration because of first-pass effect (21). Infusion of 2 μg/kg/minute produces a

TABLE 2. Sympathomimetic amine–induced responses of effector organs subserved by α, β_1, and β_2 adrenoceptors

Subserved by the α adrenoceptor: Effector organ	Response	Subserved by the β_1 adrenoceptor: Effector organ	Response	Subserved by the β_2 adrenoceptor: Effector organ	Response
Vascular smooth muscle	Vasoconstriction	Heart	Augmented pacemaker; augmented contractility	Vascular smooth muscle	Vasodilatation
Liver	Glycogenolysis	Vascular smooth muscle; coronary; intestine	Relaxation	Tracheal and bronchial smooth muscle	Relaxation
Intestinal smooth muscle	Relaxation	Adipose tissue (white)	Lipolysis Lipogenesis	Skeletal muscle	Contraction Glycogenolysis
				Potassium uptake	Hypokalemia

Adapted from Paradis NA, Koscove EM. Epinephrine in cardiac arrest: a critical review. *Ann Emerg Med* 1990;19(11):1288–1301.

TABLE 3. Pharmacokinetics of angiotensin-converting enzyme inhibitors

Parameter	Dobutamine	Dopamine	Epinephrine	Isoproterenol	Mephentermine	Metaraminol	Methoxamine	Norepinephrine	Phenylephrine
Bioavailability (%)	—	—	Oral: none; SQ: 100%	Readily absorbed	—	—	—	Poor	Oral: 38%
Onset of action	IV: 1–2 min	5 min	SQ: less than 1 h	Inhalation: within 1 min	IM: 5–15 min; IV: immediate	IM: 10 min; IV: 1–2 min	IM: 15–20 min; IV: 0.5–2 min	1–2 min	IM: 10–15 min
Volume of distribution	0.2 L/kg	1.81 to 2.45 L/kg	—	0.5 L/kg	—	—	—	—	5 L/kg
Elimination half-life (h)	2.4 ± 0.7 min	2 min	1 min	Biphasic: first phase 2.5–5.0 min; second phase 3–7 h	17 to 18 h	—	—	1 min	2.5 h
Protein binding (%)	—	—	—	65	—	—	—	—	—
Metabolism	L	L, R, P	L	L	L	L	L	L, R, P	L
Metabolites	Glucuronide conjugate; 3-0-methylated dobutamine	Homovanillic acid; norepinephrine (active); 3-methoxytyramine	Metadrenaline; derivatives of mandelic acid	3-O-methylisoproterenol	Normephentermine, P-hydroxynormephentermine	—	—	Normetanephrine, vanilmandelic acid	Phenolic conjugates
Urine excretion (unchanged) (%)	66	80	—	50–80	NR	—	NR	4–16	80–86
Pregnancy category	B	C	C	C	C	C	C	C	C
Placental transfer	—	NR	Y	—	—	—	—	Y	NR
Breast milk	NR	NR	NR	NR	NR	NR	NR	NR	NR
Removed by hemodialysis	NR	—	—	—	—	—	—	—	—

L, liver; N, no; NR, not reported; P, plasma; R, renal; Y, yes.

serum dobutamine level of approximately 20 ng/ml in approximately 10 minutes (22,23) Onset of action is 1 to 2 minutes intravenously (IV), and the duration of action is less than 10 minutes (24) However, one study demonstrated in 17 of 25 patients a continued beneficial effect from dobutamine for at least 1 week after the infusion had been discontinued (23). In children, infusions of dobutamine ranging from 2 to 15 mg/kg/minute result in plasma levels of 6.4 to 347 ng/ml (24a). Dobutamine toxicokinetics in children follow a first-order kinetic model (24b). The threshold plasma level for increasing cardiac output in children is approximately 8 ng/ml, and that for an increase in systolic blood pressure is approximately 34 ng/ml (25).

The dobutamine apparent volume of distribution (V_d) is 0.20 to 0.08 L/kg in patients with low-output cardiac failure (23,24) and 3.2 L/kg in children after open-heart surgery (26). The plasma half-life of dobutamine is approximately 2 minutes (26a). Dobutamine is metabolized by catechol-*O*-methyltransferase in the liver and other tissues to an inactive compound, 3-*O*-methyldobutamine, and by conjugation with glucuronic acid. Conjugates of dobutamine and 3-*O*-methyldobutamine are excreted mainly in the urine (27). Total body clearance values in children vary from 32 to 625 ml/kg/minute (24a). Plasma clearance in children averages approximately 15 ml/kg/minute (25,28).

Pathophysiology

Dobutamine exerts its cardiovascular action through its β_1-adrenergic agonist activity. It also induces α_1-adrenoceptor–mediated vasoconstriction and β_2-adrenoceptor–mediated vasodilation. The (*d*) enantiomer acts on β_1 adrenoceptors to increase cardiac contractility, on β_2 receptors to cause vasodilation (29), and as an α-adrenergic antagonist to decrease vascular resistance. The (*l*) enantiomer acts on α_1 adrenoceptors to increase vascular resistance (30,31). Because dobutamine is available as a racemic mixture, the α-adrenergic properties of the two enantiomers offset each other (and the mixture's net effect is to increase cardiac contractility through β_1 stimulation) and cause vasodilation (through β_2 stimulation) with little change in heart rate (30,32,33). Dobutamine has no action on dopamine receptors and unlike dopamine, dobutamine does not cause release of endogenous norepinephrine.

Pregnancy and Lactation

Dobutamine is FDA pregnancy category B (see Appendix I). Excretion in breast milk is unknown (28). Animal studies have revealed no teratogenic effects or evidence of impaired fertility (28).

Clinical Presentation

ACUTE OVERDOSAGE

Dobutamine excess induces a decrease in systemic vascular resistance with hypotension and oliguria; supraventricular tachycardia; stuffy nose, hoarseness, red warm skin (18); feelings of anxiousness, jitteriness, tachypnea; palpitations, anginal, or chest pain; paresthesias of the upper extremities; enuresis; and urinary incontinence (19). Signs and symptoms usually clear within 2 hours (17). Sinus tachycardia is common after epinephrine overdose and was observed with dobutamine overdose (19).

Positive inotropic and chronotropic effects of dobutamine on the myocardium may cause hypertension, tachydysrhythmias, myocardial ischemia, and ventricular fibrillation (VF) (13,31,34). A 47-year-old woman with urosepsis presented with hypertension, tachycardia, tachypnea, jitteriness, palpitations, chest pains, paresthesia, vomiting, and urinary incontinence when she was inadvertently given dobutamine at a rate more than 130 μg/kg/minute for 30 minutes. Her symptoms resolved after 2 hours (19).

CHRONIC OVERDOSE/WITHDRAWAL

Many patients with severe decompensated ventricular failure who have been hemodynamically stabilized with dobutamine develop an intolerance to dobutamine withdrawal with a worsening of symptoms of dyspnea, systemic hypertension, or a deterioration of renal function. Hemodynamic intolerance to dobutamine withdrawal is defined as (a) a decrease in cardiac index to less than 2.2 L/minute/m^2 or, if the baseline measure was less than this, a 10% decrease in cardiac index; (b) an increase in pulmonary wedge pressure to 20 mm Hg or an increase of 10% over the baseline value; and (c) a decrease in systolic blood pressure to less than 70 mm Hg (35). Use of continuous or intermittent infusions in patients with severe heart failure is considered controversial because tolerance can develop and does not improve survival (36–39). Continuous infusions have been associated with an increase in mortality, clinical event rates (e.g., myocardial infarction, worsening heart failure), and do not appear to improve quality of life in patients with severe heart failure (40).

ADVERSE EVENTS

Contraindications to the use of dobutamine include hypersensitivity to dobutamine and idiopathic hypertrophic subaortic stenosis. The more common adverse effects are chest pain, hypertension, palpitations, tachycardia, dyspnea, headache, hypokalemia, and nausea. The more serious effects include dysrhythmias, eosinophilic myocarditis, and thrombocytopenia (rare).

The commercial dobutamine solution contains sodium bisulfite, which can induce allergic-type reactions including anaphylaxis or a life-threatening clinical state. Sulfite sensitivity is frequently seen in asthmatics. Hypersensitivity-type local erythema and pruritus develop 4 to 12 days after dobutamine use at the site of IV administration (33).

Adverse effects related to the use of dobutamine include hypertension, tachycardia, dysrhythmias, and alterations in coronary blood flow. Dobutamine can increase systolic pressure. In clinical studies, approximately 7.5% of patients developed systolic pressure increases of 50 mm Hg or greater, which can be minimized by decreasing the dose (28). Two hypertensive patients developed marked systolic hypertension (blood pressure greater than 190 mm Hg) during dobutamine infusion (41).

Major cardiac dysrhythmias are not a common problem with dobutamine, however the following have occurred: nodal escape beats, unifocal and multifocal ventricular ectopic beats, and ventricular bigeminy (2,42,43). Torsade de pointes and QT prolongation have been reported; hypokalemia may have contributed to the event (44). Dobutamine can precipitate or exacerbate ventricular ectopic activity; approximately 5% of patients treated have had increased premature ventricular contractions (PVCs) during infusion, which are dose-related (28). Sustained ventricular tachycardia (VT) or VF are rare but have been reported at higher doses (45).

The results of one study indicate that dobutamine stress echocardiography does not significantly increase dysrhythmias during the following 24 hours. In this study, adverse effects during administration of dobutamine were primarily ventricular (*N* = 14) and atrial (*N* = 4) premature contractions; however, three patients exhibited nonsustained ventricular contractions. There were no sustained episodes of supraventricular tachycardia or VT (46). Dobutamine can provoke coronary spasm in some patients with coronary spastic angina. When dobutamine stress echocardiography is performed to evaluate coronary artery disease, not only fixed coronary stenosis but also coronary spasm should be considered as a genesis of asynergy (47).

Other reports have described deleterious effects of dobutamine in patients with coronary artery disease (43,48,49). Angina, palpitations, and nonspecific chest pain have been reported in 1% to 3% of patients who receive dobutamine therapy (28,41). Angina may be more likely to occur in elderly patients (49a). Low-dose dobutamine can result in myocardial ischemia in patients with significant coronary obstruction who are not in heart failure. One study evaluated the effect of low-dose dobutamine in patients with coronary artery disease and near normal or normal left ventricular function at rest and during atrial pacing (49). Dobutamine was given in doses of 3.8 µg/kg/minute. Three of 14 patients at rest developed chest pain, ST segment depression increases, and decreases in myocardial lactate extraction, associated with increases in heart rate, coronary sinus flow, and myocardial oxygen consumption. Acute myocardial infarction as a complication of dobutamine stress echocardiography is described in two patients during or shortly after undergoing the procedure. Both clinical events resulted in characteristic elevations in cardiac enzymes and the development of new electrocardiographic Q waves in the inferior leads (50).

Syncope caused by cardiac asystole during dobutamine stress echocardiography occurred in a 60-year-old woman presenting with chest pain and a nondiagnostic exercise test. Cardiac asystole was not associated with myocardial ischemia and was attributed to a powerful cardioinhibitory vagal reflex elicited by the stimulation by the drug of cardiac and aortic mechanoreceptors. Cardiac asystole was promptly reversed by the administration of atropine with no significant sequelae (51).

Other events that occurred during dobutamine stress echocardiography include generalized tetany that developed in a 49-year-old woman who was coadministered dobutamine and atropine (52). The incidence of eosinophilic myocarditis may be as high as 7% and results from the sulfite stabilizer found in the infusions (53).

Necrosis of the skin has been reported secondary to a constant infusion of dobutamine at 2.5 µg/kg/minute (54). It is speculated that dobutamine-induced pruritus is secondary to receptor stimulation in the papillary layer of the dermis (55). Local dermal hypersensitivity reactions characterized by erythema, pruritus, and phlebitis with or without bullae formation have been described, at the site of injection, after IV dobutamine infusions (56).

In contrast to other catecholamines, which generally produce platelet-aggregating properties, dobutamine has been demonstrated *in vivo* and *in vitro* to inhibit platelet function (57). A significant decrease in plasma potassium (4.6 to 4.2 mEq/L) has been reported in 13 patients with congestive heart failure after an IV infusion of dobutamine (10 µg/kg/minute). After discontinuing the infusion, the decrease in potassium persisted for at least 45 minutes (58). An association between the decrease in potassium and the development or worsening of dysrhythmias, in three of the patients, was suggested, though not clearly established.

Several patients experienced urinary urgency during a high dose, 10-minute dobutamine infusion. Urgency ceased when the infusion was discontinued (59). Also, dobutamine-induced hyperthermia has been reported (60).

DOPAMINE

Dopamine (Intropin) is a catecholamine and the immediate precursor of norepinephrine. The effects that dopamine produces in the body are directly related to its actions on α, β, and dopaminergic receptor sites (Table 4) (61,62). When these receptors are stimulated cyclic adenosine monophosphate levels increase, increasing calcium transport into the cell (63–68). The amount of dopamine determines which receptors are predominantly stimulated. At infusion rates more than 5 to 10 µg/kg/minute, alpha-receptor stimulation predominates, resulting in peripheral vasoconstriction, with a rise in blood pressure. At infusion rates greater than 20 µg/kg/minute, the vasoconstrictive effect can be greater than the β_1 effect (69).

TABLE 4. Peripheral actions of dopamine

Receptor	Location	Response
α	Blood vessels	Vasoconstriction
β	Heart	Cardiac stimulation; increased rate and force
	Blood vessels	Vasodilation (minor)
DA_2 (prejunctional)	Sympathetic ganglia and prejunctional sympathetic nervous system nerve terminal	Inhibition of norepinephrine release; decreased rate; passive vasodilation
DA_1 (postjunctional)	Blood vessels, renal tubules	Vasodilation; increased renal flow; diuresis; natriuresis

DA_1, dopamine agonist receptor type 1; DA_2, dopamine agonist receptor type 2.
From Rosenkranz RP, McClelland DL. An historical perspective of dopamine and its analogs. *Proc West Pharmacol Soc* 1990;33:15–19, with permission.

Dopamine is a commonly used pressor agent used for the shock syndrome due to myocardial infarctions, trauma, endotoxic septicemia, open heart surgery, renal failure, and chronic cardiac decompensation as in congestive failure. It stimulates α-adrenergic receptor sites to induce peripheral vasoconstriction, which may become so severe that it compromises the peripheral arterial circulation and can lead to gangrene. Few cases of accidental overdose and fatalities have been reported, but tissue extravasation can cause tissue necrosis.

Toxic Dose

Adult and pediatric therapeutic doses are provided in Table 1. The maximum recommended IV dose for dopamine in pediatric patients is 50 µg/kg/minute (70). IV dopamine in dosages greater than 10 µg/kg/minute may induce sufficient α-adrenergic stimulation to cause excessive peripheral vasoconstriction and gangrene. A 30-year-old woman died after receiving daily doses of dopamine ranging from 14 to 115 µg/kg/minute and doses of dobutamine from 9 to 54 µg/kg/minute (71). A 1-day-old, 29-week premature infant received an overdose of 125 µg/kg per minute during a 1-hour period and died within 1 hour (72).

Toxicokinetics and Toxicodynamics

The pharmacokinetic data for dopamine are provided in Table 3. Dopamine is inactivated after oral administration and therefore is administered only by the IV route. Dopamine administered in dosages of 1, 3, 6, 9, and 14 µg/kg/minute leads to plasma levels that correlate with the infusion rate, increasing from 0.04 µg/L to 208 µg/L during the highest infusion rates. The so-called renal dose of dopamine (3 µg/kg/minute) corresponds to a plasma level of 57 µg/L. This is higher than the plasma level, which affects most metabolic (glucose, nonesterified fatty acids) and cardiovascular (systolic, diastolic, blood pressure, heart rate) variables (73–75). As a normal constituent of plasma, most dopamine (99%) is conjugated to sulfate (75).

The V_d is 0.89 L/kg in adults and 1.81 L/kg in newborns (76). Steady-state plasma concentrations are achieved in 5 to 10 minutes. In infants such steady-state concentrations ranged from 0.013 to 0.3 μg/ml (77). Clearance may be more rapid in infants. Dopamine does not cross the blood–brain barrier and therefore does not affect D_1 and D_2 receptors in the central nervous system (CNS). Unlike adults, dopamine crosses the blood–brain barrier in preterm infants (78).

Dopamine is eliminated from plasma with a half-life of approximately 9 minutes. The pharmacologic half-life of an IV bolus dose is approximately 2 minutes, and the duration of action is approximately 10 minutes. Total body clearance of dopamine is approximately 73 ml/kg/minute (3) and averages 115 ml/kg/minute in newborns (76). Dopamine is extensively metabolized in the liver. Less than 10% of a dose is recovered unchanged in the urine (79). Hepatic metabolism results in inactive metabolites (75% of the dose) and norepinephrine (active, 25% of the dose) in the adrenergic nerve terminals (80,81). The principal means of elimination appear to be *O*-methylation by catechol-*O*-methyltransferase to form 3-methoxytyramine, followed either by sulfoconjugation (by phenosulfotransferase) or by deamination [by monoamine oxidase (MAO)] to homovanillic acid. Approximately 80% of the drug is excreted in the urine as homovanillic acid, homovanillic acid metabolites, and norepinephrine metabolites within 24 hours. A small portion is excreted unchanged (80,81). Approximately 20% of dopamine is also cleared by the lungs, especially when plasma dopamine levels are elevated (82).

Pathophysiology

The effects of dopamine are directly related to its actions on α, β, and dopaminergic receptor sites (83,84). When these receptors are stimulated cyclic adenosine monophosphate levels increase, permitting an increase in calcium transport into the cell (63–68). At low dosages (0.5 to 2.0 μg/kg/minute), D_1 and D_2 receptors are activated. D_1 receptors are located on vascular smooth muscle and participate in renal, mesenteric, cerebral, and coronary vascular dilation (84).

The D_2 receptor is located on postganglionic sympathetic neuron endings and autonomic ganglia. D_2 receptor activation inhibits norepinephrine release from sympathetic nerve endings. Blood pressure remains stable or may decrease (85). Renal plasma flow, glomerular filtration rate, and sodium excretion usually increase (86–88). At higher dosages (2 to 5 μg/kg/minute), β adrenoceptors are activated leading to increased cardiac contractility, heart rate, and atrioventricular conduction. Dopamine acts on β_1 receptors to release norepinephrine from myocardial storage sites; cardiac output and systolic blood pressure increase. After an increase in dosage (more than 5 μg/kg/minute), α_1 and α_2 receptors are activated (89). These are located on vascular effector cells and, when activated by dopamine, cause vasoconstriction. Activation of α_2 adrenoceptors on the prejunctional sympathetic nerve terminals leads to inhibition of noradrenalin release. Systolic and diastolic pressures increase.

Pregnancy and Lactation

Dopamine is FDA pregnancy category C (Appendix I). Dopamine is unlikely to be excreted in breast milk. Any that is excreted is probably inactivated by the neonate before reaching the systemic circulation. Animal studies indicate that dopamine interferes with vitamin B_1 metabolism (83). A dopamine infusion at a rate of 1 to 5 mg/kg/minute has been effective in treating preeclamptic women with oliguria (90). Use of the drug in animals indicated that offspring treated with dopamine had a greater incidence of abnormalities than a nontreated group (91).

Clinical Presentation

ACUTE OVERDOSAGE

Patients with prior vascular disease may be subject to excess ischemic effects from the α-adrenergic–stimulated vasoconstriction induced by dopamine (92–96). Such ischemic effects often begin after 24 hours of dopamine use and may progress to gangrene of an extremity (often requiring amputation); they are more likely to occur at dopamine infusion levels of 10 μg/kg/minute or more. One patient developed bilateral retinal infarctions after dopamine infusion at a rate of 14 to 115 μg/kg/minute (71). A newborn died within 1 hour of receiving an overdose of 125 μg/kg/minute (72). Extravasation and infiltration of dopamine may lead to ischemia, gangrene, and amputation of an extremity (72,97).

ADVERSE EVENTS

Skin ischemia, necrosis, and gangrene are uncommon but known complications of dopamine extravasation. In most cases, these complications are associated with the use of high-dosage dopamine infusion. A neonate received a dopamine infusion after birth. He developed cyanosis of his extremity immediately after dopamine was started via peripheral line, which improved spontaneously after dopamine was stopped. This happened repeatedly at various sites and at lower concentrations of dopamine. Subsequently, dopamine was replaced by dobutamine and the patient did well (98). IV dopamine was infused peripherally (in the antecubital fossa) to two patients in the cardiac intensive care unit in an attempt to enhance renal blood perfusion and urine output. Dopamine extravasation occurred in both patients while the low dose (less than 3 μg/kg/minute) was infused. Significant local tissue injury was observed in both patients (99).

Ventricular dysrhythmias may occur during dopamine infusion. A report describes an infant with circulatory failure who experienced an episode of paroxysmal supraventricular tachycardia while receiving dopamine (100). In 15 patients that developed hypotension (unresponsive to other inotropic agents), dopamine in doses of 6 to 33 μg/kg/minute increased heart rates of 120 to 180 with dosage ranges from 3 to 25 μg/kg/minute (101). One other patient developed VT associated with a convulsive seizure after doses of dopamine (6 μg/kg/minute) in addition to isoproterenol (1 μg/minute). Another study (102) evaluated the effect of dopamine infusion on ventricular hemodynamics in normal subjects. Dopamine was infused in 15 patients at a rate of 400 μg/minute over a period of 20 minutes. Variable changes in heart rate were noted (± 20 beats/minute). One patient developed supraventricular tachycardia within 1 minute of infusion, which necessitated discontinuation of dopamine. Two patients developed extrasystoles (102). Paroxysmal supraventricular tachycardia occurred in an infant receiving dopamine to treat circulatory failure. Dopamine 10 μg/kg/minute was initiated and then gradually increased to 17 μg/kg/minute (103). Dopamine has exacerbated atrial fibrillation/flutter. Dopamine 3 μg/kg/minute was administered to a 55-year-old man with controlled atrial fibrillation/flutter. Atrioventricular conduction was enhanced by the low dose of dopamine, inducing the return of atrial fibrillation/flutter (104).

Anginal pain, tachycardia, ventricular premature beats, and palpitations have been reported (105,106).

Delusions, hallucinations, and periods of confusion have been reported after intraventricular infusion of dopamine (4 to 15 mg/day) in the treatment of Parkinson's disease (107,108).

Dysuria and urgency were reported in a 71-year-old man treated with a dopamine infusion at a rate of 4.3 µg/kg/minute. The symptoms cleared completely after drug withdrawal. A similar course of events took place on retrial and subsequent discontinuation of dopamine (109).

Reversible dopamine-induced diabetes insipidus that was resistant to vasopressin developed in an 18-year-old woman being treated for hypotension. Polyuria and urine hypo-osmolarity occurred after IV administration of dopamine (12 µg/kg/minute). Urine output decreased within an hour after discontinuation of dopamine. Re-challenge with dopamine 2 days later resulted in hypotonic polyuria (110). Polyuria was described in a 75-year-old black man during dopamine infusion for hypotension (111). During infusion of 9 to 19 µg/kg/minute, the patient voided between 100 to 1000 ml/hour, and an output of greater than 5 L was observed over an 8-hour period. Withdrawal of dopamine and substitution with norepinephrine resulted in a drop in urine volume (less than 100 ml/hour).

Bilateral retinal infarction occurred in a 30-year-old IV drug abuser with fulminant non-A-non-B hepatitis treated with a dopamine dose ranging from 14 to 115 µg/kg/minute (71). Dopamine has been implicated with pulmonary hypertension. A 40-year-old woman being treated for toxic goiter and malignant exophthalmus with large doses of dexamethasone developed pulmonary hypertension at a dopamine dose of 5.6 µg/kg/minute. It resolved when dopamine was discontinued (112).

Infiltration of dopamine into the tissues after extravasation has occurred after 5.9 and 7 µg/kg/minute (113). In both patients, amputation was required. Pedal gangrene, symmetric peripheral gangrene, and necrosis have been reported to occur at the injection site and other nonadjacent limbs (114–116a). Doses as low as 1 to 1.5 µg/kg/minute have caused gangrene (115,117). One group (114) reported four cases of gangrene after the use of dopamine infusion. Phentolamine was used successfully in one patient when given directly into the skin of the involved area. Dramatic improvement in color occurred after approximately 90 minutes.

In mechanically ventilated critically ill patients, low-dose (4 µg/kg/minute) dopamine may adversely affect gastroduodenal motility during fasting and nasogastric feeding (118). It has been suggested that administration of dopamine may have an inhibitory effect on sodium-potassium adenosine triphosphatase pump activity in low-birth-weight preterm neonates leading to hyperkalemia in this patient population (119,120).

EPINEPHRINE

Epinephrine is a direct-acting sympathomimetic agent with pronounced effects on α- and β-adrenergic receptors. Epinephrine has been used for anaphylaxis, status asthmaticus, and as a myocardial stimulant in cardiopulmonary resuscitation. The toxic effects include anxiety, tachycardia, dyspnea, weakness, tremor and headache. More serious reactions include dysrhythmias, pulmonary edema, and hypertensive crisis.

Toxic Dose

Adult and pediatric therapeutic doses are provided in Table 1. Cardiac Arrest Advanced Cardiac Life Support standards recommend 7.5 to 15.0 µg/kg of epinephrine (0.5 to 1.0 mg in an adult) in cardiac arrest (121). The Adrenergic Agonist Panel concluded that the standard IV bolus dosage of epinephrine should be simplified to 1.0 mg every 3 to 5 minutes. Higher doses of epinephrine (over 0.2 mg/kg), 1 to 15 mg (bolus doses), may improve initial resuscitation rates in children but has been disappointing in adults (122,123). An IV bolus dose of 50 µg/kg or more is considered a high-dose epinephrine therapy (124). The endotracheal dosing of epinephrine should be at least 2.0 to 2.5 times larger than the peripheral IV dosage (125).

The minimum lethal human dose by subcutaneous (SQ) injection is estimated as 4 mg (126). One patient died immediately after receiving 3 mg IV (126). A 37-year-old man experienced myocardial ischemia, VF, and refractory hypotension resulting in death 26 days later after self-injection of 82.5 mg of epinephrine from Primatene Mist (127). Two patients with histories of IV drug abuse have been reported who self-injected 1.1 and 20 mg IV and survived (128,129).

A 23-year-old man self-injected 20 mg IV and gradually became comatose, with widely dilated pupils that were nonreactive to light (129).

Toxicokinetics and Toxicodynamics

The pharmacokinetic data for epinephrine are provided in Table 3. Circulating epinephrine is metabolized in the liver and is taken up into adrenergic neurons and metabolized by MAO and catechol-*O*-methyltransferase to metadrenaline, sulfate conjugates, and hydroxy derivatives of mandelic acid (130,131). Its onset of action is within 1 minute IV and within 3 to 5 minutes by inhalation. Mean maximum plasma epinephrine levels are achieved significantly faster after intramuscular (IM) compared to SQ administration. Mean peak plasma epinephrine concentrations are significantly higher after IM injection into the thigh than after IM or SQ injection into the upper arm (132,133). Elimination half-life is 1 minute.

Pathophysiology

Epinephrine is a direct-acting sympathomimetic agent with pronounced effects on α- and β-adrenergic receptors. Its use results in dramatic increases in blood pressure, with greater increases in systolic pressure than diastolic, resulting in an increase in pulse pressure. The chief vascular effects of the drug are exerted on the small arterioles and precapillary sphincters, resulting in a reduction in cutaneous blood flow after injection; blood flow to skeletal muscles and coronaries is increased by therapeutic epinephrine doses (134). Epinephrine is a direct cardiac stimulant, acting directly on β_1 receptors of myocardium as well as cells of the pacemaker in conducting tissues, resulting in increased cardiac output and increased oxygen consumption. Epinephrine results in decreases in the amplitude of T-waves in the electrocardiogram (ECG).

The effects of epinephrine on smooth muscles include relaxation of gastrointestinal smooth muscle, relaxation of the detrusor muscle of the bladder, and contraction of the splenic capsule. Epinephrine is a potent bronchodilator and is effective in the setting of bronchial asthma. The drug increases respiratory rate and tidal volume, resulting in a reduction in alveolar carbon dioxide content in normal subjects (134,135).

Metabolic effects of epinephrine are diverse, including elevations in blood glucose and lactate and inhibition of insulin secretion via alpha-receptors and enhancement by activation of beta-receptors, with the predominant effect on insulin being inhibition. The concentration of free fatty acids in blood is elevated after epinephrine use, and the drug has a significant calorigenic action, reflected by an increase of 20% to 30% in oxygen consumption after conventional doses (134).

Pregnancy and Lactation

Epinephrine is FDA pregnancy category C (Appendix I). Excretion in breast milk is unknown. In a prospective study, one group (136) reported that the use of inhaled beta-agonist bronchodilators for the therapy of asthma during pregnancy was not associated with an increased frequency of adverse maternal or infant perinatal outcomes, including congenital defects. No differences were observed between the asthmatic patients who used inhaled bronchodilators and the patients who did not use bronchodilators with regard to perinatal mortality, congenital malformations, preterm births, numbers of low-birth-weight infants, mean birth weight, numbers of infants who were small-for-gestational-age or had low Apgar scores, labor and delivery complications, or postpartum bleeding.

Clinical Presentation

ACUTE OVERDOSAGE

Symptoms of pallor, cyanosis, headache, diaphoresis, hypertension, tachycardia, ECG evidence of myocardial ischemia, PVCs, bigeminal rhythm, precordial chest discomfort, palpitations, numbness and paresthesias of the hands and feet, and abdominal pain commonly develop within seconds to minutes after injection of excessive amounts of epinephrine, depending on the route (137). Metabolic acidosis, hypotension, and pulmonary edema have a delayed onset (138,139).

A 37-year-old man experienced diaphoresis, chest pain, vomiting, and collapsed after an intentional injection of Primatene Mist (82.5 mg epinephrine). He was found to be in VF, have myocardial damage (initial isoenzyme of creatine kinase with muscle and brain subunits of 40.3 ng/ml), acidemia, and rhabdomyolysis with peak CK of 9646 IU/L. Marked hypotension requiring continuous pressor infusions were required, but the patient died 26 days after exposure (127).

Accidental intraarterial injection of 3 mg of epinephrine led to unconsciousness, hypotension, and VT with marked pallor of the arm. Phentolamine 5 mg injected through the same arterial catheter led to rapid return of perfusion to the arm (140,141). IV epinephrine in doses of 1333 μg/minute (80 mg/hour) was used to restore blood pressure after an overdose of 5600 to 7000 mg of labetalol (142).

Acute myocardial infarction resulted in a 29-year-old woman after self-injection of a solution extracted from Primatene Mist inhaler. An estimated 82.5 to 124 mg of epinephrine was injected, approximately 25 times a normal dose. The woman experienced atrial fibrillation, acidemia, and significant hypotension within an hour of the injection, and developed anterior myocardial infarction by the next day (143).

A 5-year-old boy received 1.75 mg epinephrine SQ and developed junctional bigeminy, PVC, and two brief nonsustained runs of VT. One to three mm ST segment depression in leads V_1–V_6 were reported on an ECG (144).

Pulmonary edema with rales, rhonchi, dyspnea, frothy or bloody sputum, and an atypical chest x-ray picture may occur after an epinephrine overdose (126,137,139,145,146). Pulmonary edema usually develops within 20 minutes (147). It is unclear whether this pulmonary edema is cardiogenic or acute lung injury (128). In one case of an unintentional tenfold dose increase in an epinephrine-soaked gauze placed over a large area of wound débridement, a delayed-onset (more than 1 hour after dose) pulmonary edema occurred (147).

ADVERSE EVENTS

Unintentional digit injections of epinephrine, often from autoinjector devices, have resulted in intense vasoconstriction leading to tissue ischemia, sometimes irreversible. Rapid onset of local symptoms, including pallor, loss of sensation and function, pain, and swelling, can develop (148). Significant vasoconstriction resulting in numbness and paleness of the left index finger after epinephrine autoinjection of the digit has been reported (149). A 45-year-old man unintentionally given epinephrine into the right brachial artery during resuscitation efforts developed marked pallor of the distal right arm. Phentolamine was given through the catheter and rapid return of perfusion was noted.

Serious cardiac complications have occurred with the use of epinephrine. VT, progressing to VF, occurred during anesthesia in a 12-year-old girl after the instillation of 6 ml of 1:1000 epinephrine (240 μg/kg) in two divided doses into the external auditory canal (150).

Myocardial infarction has been reported in a pediatric patient after multiple doses of nebulized racemic epinephrine for croup and severe respiratory distress (150a). Myocardial ischemia was reported in a 23-year-old woman after IV injection of 0.3 mg epinephrine for anaphylactic shock. After injection, the patient developed severe retrosternal chest pain, diaphoresis, and dizziness (151). Other cardiovascular effects that have been described include profound bradycardia with cyanosis in a racemic-epinephrine–overdosed infant (137) and sinus tachycardia after epinephrine overdose (128,152,153).

Acute renal failure, accompanied by myocardial infarction, atrial fibrillation, and metabolic acidosis developed in a 29-year-old woman after self-injection of Primatene Mist inhalant (82.5 to 124.0 mg epinephrine). Peak serum creatinine and blood urea nitrogen were reported to be 14.2 mg/dl and 105 mg/dl, respectively, and decreased to 7.5 mg/dl and 85 mg/dl, respectively, within 24 hours without dialysis (143). Inadvertent intraaortic administration of epinephrine was reported to result in renal failure, hypertension, acidemia, and tachycardia in a premature neonate. Anuria persisted for approximately 20 hours followed by a 12-hour oliguric phase and then a brisk diuresis (153a).

Epinephrine is capable of constricting the mesenteric vasculature and has the potential to produce constriction, ischemia, and bowel necrosis in patients whose intestinal blood flow is already compromised (154).

Hypokalemia has been reported with epinephrine overdose (128). The proposed mechanism is intracellular redistribution of potassium mediated by an increase in intracellular 3,5-cyclic adenosine monophosphate concentrations (155).

Syncope has been reported in pediatric patients after administration of 0.05 to 0.2 ml of epinephrine in the treatment of asthma attacks. Syncope is often accompanied with pallor, unconsciousness, weakness, tachycardia, and hypotension (156).

Ocular administration of epinephrine in 1% and 2% concentration by the topical route in the treatment of glaucoma has been reported to result in ocular pigmentation, which can result in deterioration of vision, conjunctival pigmentation, and pigmentation of the cornea (157–160).

Gas gangrene after IM administration of epinephrine has been reported. Three cases of gas gangrene after IM injection of epinephrine have occurred subsequent to administration of the drug into either the buttock or thigh. Two cases have resulted in death and only one case had appropriate treatment with gas gangrene antiserum, steroids, and antibiotics that resulted in survival of the patient (161–163). It appears that clostridium organisms become deposited into muscle tissue during penetration of the skin and that the vasoconstrictor properties of adrenaline enhance the effects of the infection.

ISOPROTERENOL

Isoproterenol (Isuprel) is a synthetic sympathomimetic drug with potent, nonselective β-adrenergic agonist activity and low affinity for α-adrenergic receptors. Isoproterenol has strong inotropic and chronotropic properties, which result in increased cardiac output. However, a reduction in mean blood pressure occurs due to peripheral vasodilation.

Isoproterenol is used to stimulate heart rate in patients with bradycardia or heart block, particularly in anticipation of inserting an artificial cardiac pacemaker or in patients with torsade de pointes. FDA-labeled indications include use in Adams-Stokes attack, bronchospasm, cardiac arrest, hypoperfusion, and as adjunctive therapy in shock or sepsis. In addition, isoproterenol is effective in some cases of pulmonary hypertension.

Toxic Dose

Adult and pediatric therapeutic doses are provided in Table 1. The maximum recommended dose for isoproterenol in pediatric patients (17 years and younger) is 1 μg/kg/minute IV (164). There are few reported cases in which isoproterenol resulted in toxicity and several reported fatalities. The doses given in most of these case reports were either unknown or within therapeutic parameters.

A 46-year-old woman inhaled an unknown amount of isoproterenol aerosol for an acute asthmatic attack, developed asystole, and died in the hospital (165). Necropsy revealed no underlying pathologic conditions. It is unclear whether asystole was secondary to isoproterenol or the propellant gas in the inhalant.

Toxicokinetics and Toxicodynamics

The pharmacokinetic data for isoproterenol are provided in Table 3. Isoproterenol is metabolized primarily in the liver and other tissues to 3-*O*-methyl-isoproterenol by catechol-*O*-methyltransferase (166,167). After IV administration of isoproterenol, 25% to 35% is metabolized by catechol-*O*-methyltransferase to the 3-*O*-methyl metabolite (167). The 3-*O*-methyl metabolite is either excreted unchanged in the urine or as the sulfate conjugate. It possesses weak beta-blocker activities but has a short half-life (167,168).

Oral isoproterenol is irregularly absorbed and rapidly metabolized in the gastrointestinal tract. After an IV dose of isoproterenol, approximately 50% is excreted unchanged in the urine (167). After an aerosol dose of isoproterenol, 80% is excreted in the urine as the sulfate conjugate (167). The duration of action of isoproterenol is 8 minutes with low doses and up to 50 minutes with large doses (169). After IV administration of radioactive-labeled isoproterenol in children, serum radioactivity was shown to decrease in a biphasic manner, with a half-life (rapid phase) of 2.5 to 5.0 minutes. The half-life of the slower second phase was 3 to 7 hours (170).

Pathophysiology

Isoproterenol is a β_1- and β_2-adrenergic receptor agonist. When given systemically, the drug stimulates beta receptors in the heart, which produces positive inotropic and chronotropic effects and results in increased cardiac output. Isoproterenol also increases myocardial oxygen requirements that may precipitate myocardial ischemia. Systemic isoproterenol also lowers peripheral vascular resistance, especially in skeletal muscle, and lowers mean arterial blood pressure (171). Stimulation of receptors in the smooth muscle of the bronchi produces bronchodilation. In asthma patients, besides bronchodilation, isoproterenol may be beneficial by inhibiting antigen-induced histamine release (171).

Pregnancy and Lactation

Isoproterenol is FDA pregnancy category C (Appendix I). Excretion in breast milk is unknown. The use of inhaled β-agonist bronchodilators for asthma during pregnancy was not associated with an increased frequency of adverse maternal or infant perinatal outcomes, including congenital malformations (172).

In a randomized, double blind study, the hemodynamic variables in 60 nonlaboring women at term were studied 5 minutes before and for 10 minutes after an IV injection of either 5 μg isoproterenol or saline. Maternal heart rate did not change after saline but increased significantly after injection of isoproterenol. Uterine blood flow also increased significantly after isoproterenol during the same time interval. Umbilical blood flow did not change. Other hemodynamic variables did not change (173).

Clinical Presentation

ACUTE OVERDOSAGE

A 45-year-old man was given 2.5 mg isoproterenol instead of diazepam via IV bolus. Within 30 seconds, his heart rate increased to 190 beats/minute, and a blood pressure was unobtainable. The patient complained of palpitations, faintness, and angina. A supraventricular tachydysrhythmia was diagnosed, and cardioversion was attempted but was unsuccessful. Reevaluation showed the dysrhythmia to be sinus tachycardia.

Tachycardia was reported in healthy subjects after isoproterenol inhalations (0.44 to 22.0 mg daily) were reported (174). Average increase in heart rate (with 0.44 mg inhalation) was 28 beats/minute. Average increase after 3 inhalations was 44 beats/minute. Average duration of tachycardia was 30 minutes. On discontinuation of inhalation, tachycardia was abolished in all patients.

A 17-year-old man with anorexia nervosa developed atypical prolongation of his corrected QT interval when placed on isoproterenol for profound sinus bradycardia. His corrected QT interval normalized after the infusion was discontinued. Autonomic imbalance may explain the observed corrected QT interval lengthening.

There are several reports of IV isoproterenol-induced myocardial ischemia that occurred during active treatment of status asthmaticus. A 14-year-old boy developed ECG findings consistent with myocardial ischemia during an IV isoproterenol infusion of 0.11 μg/kg/minute (175). The patient admitted to the use of metaproterenol by hand nebulizer as often as every hour for the previous 24 hours before admission. A 17-year-old girl developed chest pain, hypotension, cardiomegaly, pulmonary edema, and ECG changes consistent with myocardial ischemia during IV isoproterenol therapy for status asthmaticus (176). The patient had received an isoproterenol dose of 3000 μg/kg over 30 hours when the drug was discontinued. An ECG taken several hours later while she was experiencing chest pain, dizziness, and tachycardia revealed marked ST-T elevation consistent with myocardial ischemia.

A case of fatal myocardial toxicity occurred during an isoproterenol infusion in an 18-year-old woman with an acute asthma attack (177). The patient was also receiving aminophylline, hydrocortisone, aerosolized isoethane, and oxygen. The cardiac arrest occurred after 36 hours of therapy during the isoproterenol taper. The isoproterenol infusion during this time reached a maximum of 0.32 μg/kg/minute. Autopsy revealed multiple small areas of myocardial necrosis.

Excessive use of isoproterenol aerosol has been associated with myocardial necrosis. A 39-year-old woman received a total of 675 mg isoproterenol by inhalation over a period of less than 3 days for acute asthmatic attacks. The patient developed acute respiratory distress with marked diaphoresis, heart rate of 120/minute, blood pressure 230/160 mm Hg, respiratory rate of 40 per minute.

ADVERSE EVENTS

Adverse events related to isoproterenol predominantly involve the cardiovascular system. VT has been reported (178,179), as well as ventricular ectopic beats (180). Atrioventricular junctional tachycardia is a complication of IV isoproterenol therapy (180a).

Cardiomyopathy has been reported secondary to isoproterenol (181,182). On retrospective analysis, 15 of 19 cases in which isoproterenol was used to treat severe childhood asthmatics showed an increase in CPK-MB (myocardial band enzymes of creatine phosphokinase) (mean value 204 IU/L) and MB band (mean, 6.05%). A significant number also had abnormal ECGs (183).

Contact allergic laryngitis occurred in a 48-year-old man after inhalation of larger than recommended doses of isoproterenol for a period of 2 years (184). Skin testing revealed positivity to isoproterenol that remained for 6 months. Several cases of asthma induced by isoproterenol aerosol have been reported (185,186). Severe, refractory wheezing occurred in patients receiving large amounts of isoproterenol aerosol (5 to 60 times normal dose) (187).

Dizziness, faintness, headache, nervousness, tremor, urinary hesitancy, blurred vision, dry mouth, and weakness have occurred during isoproterenol therapy (188,189). Sublingual administration of isoproterenol has been shown to increase gastric secretions and concentration (190). Ulcerations have occurred after the use of sublingual isoproterenol tablets (188,191).

MEPHENTERMINE

Mephentermine (Wyamine) is an indirect-acting sympathomimetic drug that shares similar properties as other paraphenylethylamines. It acts to release norepinephrine. This agent may also stimulate β-adrenergic receptors (192,193), and the change in heart rate is variable, depending on vagal tone (192).

Mephentermine is used in the treatment of hypotension secondary to the use of ganglionic blockers or spinal anesthesia (194). Although mephentermine is not recommended as corrective therapy for shock of hypotension due to hemorrhage, this agent may be used as an emergency measure to maintain blood pressure until blood or blood substitutes can be administered (194). Mephentermine (5 mg IV) has been beneficial for the treatment of cardiogenic shock. Because mephentermine has no chronotropic or inotropic effects but induces peripheral vasoconstriction, this agent is effective for controlling persistent hypotension (195). Some studies indicate that mephentermine may increase survival rate of patients experiencing cardiogenic shock (196).

Toxic Dose

Adult and pediatric therapeutic doses are provided in Table 1. The toxic effects of mephentermine are similar to those of other paraphenylethylamines including dysrhythmias and hypertension especially in patients with heart disease (194,197).

Toxicokinetics and Toxicodynamics

The pharmacokinetic data for mephentermine are poorly established. Mephentermine undergoes hepatic metabolism to inactive metabolites and undergoes renal excretion (198). Excretion is more rapid with acidic urine, but essentially unaffected by urine flow (194). Elimination half-life is around 17 to 18 hours.

Pathophysiology

Mephentermine is a sympathomimetic drug that indirectly releases norepinephrine. This agent may also stimulate β-adrenergic receptors (192,193) and the change in heart rate is variable, depending on vagal tone (192). The elevation in blood pressure is probably related to an increase in cardiac output predominantly from enhanced cardiac contraction and also an increase in peripheral resistance from peripheral vasoconstriction (192,194).

Pregnancy and Lactation

Mephentermine is FDA pregnancy category C (Appendix I). Excretion in breast milk is unknown. An IV infusion of mephentermine increases the intensity and frequency of uterine contractions as well as resting uterine tone (199).

Clinical Presentation

ACUTE OVERDOSAGE

There are reports of inadvertent intraarterial injection of mephentermine causing vasoconstriction leading to ischemia and possibly necrosis of distal extremities (200,201). Mephentermine may produce CNS stimulation, especially with overdoses; anxiety, drowsiness, incoherence, and convulsions have been reported (198).

ADVERSE EVENTS

Reports of psychosis with disturbed behavior and vivid visual, auditory, and olfactory hallucinations have developed after the abuse of inhalers that at one time contained mephentermine (202). Dependence on mephentermine associated with chronic psychosis has been reported (203).

METARAMINOL

Metaraminol (Aramine) is a sympathomimetic amine that acts directly and indirectly at alpha-receptor and beta-receptor sites to cause a vasopressor effect. It is an effective agent for the treatment of acute hypotensive states. The advantage of metaraminol is the IM dosing. Metaraminol provides reliable and predictable blood pressure control during spinal or subarachnoid anesthesia. It is an effective adjunctive therapy for hypotension caused by hemorrhage, surgical complications, brain injury, or drug reactions (204). In addition, metaraminol is used to produce cardiac stimulation and increased blood pressure in patients with shock, which persists after adequate fluid volume replacement. It has also been used to relieve attacks of paroxysmal atrial tachycardia, especially with coexisting hypotension, and as an alternative to phenylephrine in the treatment of low flow priapism in a limited number of patients (205–209).

Toxic Dose

Adult and pediatric therapeutic doses are provided in Table 1. Although no fatalities have been reported with use of metaraminol, toxicity can arise from their overuse. The blood pressure was elevated to 200 mm Hg after an intracavernous dose of 5 mg in a 6-year-old boy (206).

Toxicokinetics and Toxicodynamics

The pharmacokinetic data for metaraminol are poorly established. Metaraminol undergoes hepatic metabolism and is excreted renally and in the bile mostly as metabolites. It is not known whether these metabolites are active.

Pathophysiology

Metaraminol has both a direct effect on α-adrenergic receptors and an indirect effect on sympathetic nerve endings releasing norepinephrine. The action of metaraminol is not solely dependent on the release of norepinephrine, but prolonged use may deplete norepinephrine from nerve endings. Repeated use may result in tachyphylaxis. The α-adrenergic effects may be beneficial in many shock patients because blood is preferentially directed to vital organs (210). However, it may be detrimental in patients in which vasoconstriction is a significant factor in shock. The peripheral blood flow to vital organs may be decreased secondary to vasoconstriction (211–214).

In low doses, metaraminol stimulates β-adrenergic receptors in the heart, which increases cardiac contractile force and cardiac output. At larger doses it stimulates α-adrenergic receptors, leading to constriction of blood vessels in the skin, kidneys, and gastrointestinal tract.

Metaraminol increases the oxygen requirement of the left ventricle by increasing cardiac workload and it causes vasoconstriction and possible organ ischemia. Vasoconstriction is especially detrimental in cardiogenic shock because it usually occurs as part of the clinical presentation of the condition (215).

Pregnancy and Lactation

Metaraminol is FDA pregnancy category C (Appendix I). Excretion in breast milk is unknown. Metaraminol should be avoided during pregnancy. Contraction of uterine blood vessels decreases uterine blood flow, which may adversely affect the fetus.

Clinical Presentation

ACUTE OVERDOSAGE

The blood pressure was elevated to 200 mm Hg after an intracavernous dose of 5 mg was administered to a 6-year-old boy. In this case, the penis was strangulated after administration of metaraminol in addition to the systemic effects (206).

ADVERSE EVENTS

Tachyphylaxis may develop during prolonged administration of metaraminol (216–218). Existing factors such as tissue hypoxia, acidosis, reduced cardiac output, severity of myocardial injury, or the previous use of catecholamine-depleting drugs may alter the expected vasopressor response from metaraminol (213). When metaraminol is discontinued the patient should be monitored closely for hypotension (214).

The more common adverse effects include chest pain, palpitations, and hypertension. Serious adverse effects include acute pulmonary edema, dysrhythmias, cerebral hemorrhage, or cardiac arrest (can be precipitated by excessive pressor response), acute tubular necrosis, malaria relapse, and metabolic acidosis (prolonged administration). Major adverse effects include tachydysrhythmias, hypertension, dysrhythmias, rebound hypotension, metabolic acidosis, acute tubular necrosis, pulmonary edema, and tissue necrosis with SQ administration. Absolute contraindications include concomitant anesthesia with cyclopropane or halothane and hypersensitivity to metaraminol or its sulfites.

A leukemoid reaction has been reported after intermittent use of metaraminol in a 68-year-old white man treated for shock due to possible myocardial infarction and gram-negative bacteremia. The patient developed a white blood cell count of 73,750/mm (3), in the absence of other conditions (219).

Cardiac dysrhythmias have been reported, especially in patients with myocardial infarctions or during rapid induction of a hypertensive response (214). Rebound hypotension after abrupt cessation of metaraminol has been reported (214). Acute hypertension has been reported after metaraminol use for paroxysmal supraventricular tachycardia (220). Pulmonary edema has been reported after an IV infusion of metaraminol for paroxysmal supraventricular tachycardia (220).

SQ administration may cause skin necrosis (213,220). In patients who have contracted malaria in the past, metaraminol may cause a relapse (214). Oral metaraminol has caused a syndrome resembling pheochromocytoma (221).

METHOXAMINE

Methoxamine (Vasoxyl) is a sympathomimetic with mainly α-adrenergic activity; β-adrenergic activity is not demonstrable and β-adrenoceptor blockade has been postulated. Methoxamine causes prolonged peripheral vasoconstriction and consequently a rise in arterial blood pressure. Despite the lack of clinical trials, methoxamine is used almost solely to prevent or treat hypotension occurring during anesthesia, particularly spinal anesthesia. It has also been used to terminate paroxysmal supraventricular tachycardia and priapism. The principal toxic effects include a marked pilomotor effect but does not stimulate the CNS or cause bronchodilation. It may also induce a desire to micturate and markedly reduces renal blood flow.

Toxic Dose

Adult and pediatric therapeutic doses are provided in Table 1. Methoxamine can produce extreme increases in blood pressure resulting in headache and vomiting (222,223).

Toxicokinetics and Toxicodynamics

Methoxamine undergoes hepatic metabolism, but information on its excretion is not reported. In addition, it is not known whether it is metabolized to an active metabolite. Onset of action is 0.5 to 2.0 minutes IV and 15 to 20 minutes IM. Duration of action of these two routes is approximately 10 to 15 minutes and approximately 1.5 hours, respectively. Methoxamine produces a predictable rise in systolic and diastolic pressures for 60 to 90 minutes after IV or IM administration.

Pathophysiology

Methoxamine is a potent, relatively pure parenteral α-adrenergic receptor agonist similar to phenylephrine. Methoxamine lacks beta-receptor effects in smooth muscle. It produces rapid and prolonged increase in peripheral vasoconstriction, resulting in increased blood pressure, with virtually no stimulant effects on the heart. Unlike epinephrine, methoxamine prolongs the ventricular action potentials and refractory period and slows atrioventricular conduction (224).

Tachyphylaxis has not been reported (222,225,226). Although a reflex bradycardia may occasionally occur secondary to a carotid sinus reflex mediated via the vagus nerve, it has little effect on the heart, and cardiac output remains unchanged or may decrease (222,227).

Pregnancy and Lactation

Methoxamine is FDA pregnancy category C (Appendix I). Excretion in breast milk is unknown. No epidemiologic studies of congenital anomalies among infants born to women treated with methoxamine during pregnancy have been reported. Increased uterine contraction was observed in women treated with methoxamine late in pregnancy (228). Increased hypoxia, hypercarbia, and metabolic acidosis occurred in the fetuses of near-term pregnant ewes after treatment with methoxamine in doses sufficient to correct maternal hypotension produced by spinal anesthesia (229). There is one reported case of fetal death associated with methoxamine use. However, multiple drug exposures were involved (223).

Clinical Presentation

ACUTE OVERDOSAGE

Piloerection, hypertension, bradycardia, headache, and cold extremities are the primary manifestation of methoxamine use. Nausea and vomiting has also been reported to occur in the acute setting (222,223). Less common effects include premature ventricular ectopic beats, fetal bradycardia, extravasation injury, sinus bradycardia, sinus tachycardia, dysrhythmias (ventricular), and vasoconstriction. Other effects include mania, urinary urgency, and nystagmus (223).

ADVERSE EVENTS

In a placebo-controlled, double blind crossover study in women with stress incontinence, methoxamine evoked nonsignificant increases in maximum urethral pressure and diastolic blood pressure but caused a significant rise in systolic blood pressure and significant fall in heart rate at maximum dosage. The predominant systemic side effects in this study included piloerection, headache, and cold extremities, which were experienced in all subjects (230).

Tingling and coldness of the extremities were reported after IV injection, primarily with high doses (222,231). Inhalation of methoxamine has been reported to decrease airway conductance slightly in normal volunteers. This effect was abolished with concomitant phentolamine administration (232).

NOREPINEPHRINE

Norepinephrine (Levophed) is a direct-acting sympathomimetic that stimulates both α- and β_1-receptors, leading to increased atrial and ventricular contractility; increased heart rate; enhancement of conduction through the ventricles; and arteriole constriction in skin, gut, and kidney (233). It is used as a cardiac stimulant and to raise blood pressure in patients with shock. It is indicated for the adjunctive treatment of cardiac arrest and profound hypotension and contraindicated in hypotension due to hypovolemia. In the treatment of shock, norepinephrine should be limited to final attempts to maintain blood pressure in patients with severe shock and should not be used if severe peripheral vasoconstriction exists because it may be ineffective and cause further reductions in blood flow to vital organs.

Toxic Dose

Adult and pediatric therapeutic doses are provided in Table 1. Norepinephrine produces a wide range of adverse effects, and these may occur at therapeutic doses. Cardiovascular adverse effects include stimulation of α-adrenergic receptors producing gangrene, hypertension, cerebral hemorrhage, reflex bradycardia, dysrhythmias, anginal pain, palpitations, cardiac arrest, and sudden death (234). A case is described of sudden death occurring after the use of a local anesthetic in a preparation containing 1:25,000 noradrenaline. Autopsy revealed a massive subarachnoid hemorrhage after a ruptured cerebral aneurysm (235).

Toxicokinetics and Toxicodynamics

The pharmacokinetic data for norepinephrine are provided in Table 3. Norepinephrine is metabolized by catechol-*O*-methyltransferase and MAO to the inactive metabolites normetanephrine and vanilmandelic acid. Four percent to 16% of an administered dose of norepinephrine is excreted unchanged in the urine (236). Onset of action is 1 to 2 minutes and duration is 1 to 2 minutes. Norepinephrine given by the SQ route has poor bioavailability (236). Elimination half-life is 1 minute.

Pathophysiology

Norepinephrine constitutes 10% to 20% of the catecholamine content of the adrenal medulla. It is a potent agonist at a receptor and has relatively little action on β_2 receptors. Systolic, diastolic pressures, and pulse pressure are usually increased. Cardiac output is unchanged or decreased, and total peripheral resistance is unchanged. A compensatory vagal reflex slows the heart, and stroke volume is increased. Norepinephrine constricts mesenteric vessels and reduces splanchnic, hepatic, and renal blood flow. Coronary flow is usually increased.

Pregnancy and Lactation

Norepinephrine is FDA pregnancy category C (Appendix I). Excretion in breast milk is unknown. Because it is poorly absorbed orally, absorption by the infant is minimal and is thus considered safe for breast-feeding. Norepinephrine may stimulate uterine contractions (237).

Clinical Presentation

ACUTE OVERDOSAGE

Severe peripheral and visceral vasoconstriction, decreased renal perfusion and urine output, poor systemic blood flow despite normal blood pressure, tissue hypoxia, and lactate acidosis may occur if norepinephrine is administered in the presence of blood volume deficit (238).

Central effects of norepinephrine include fear, anxiety, restlessness, tremor, insomnia, confusion, irritability, weakness, and psychosis (234). In addition, norepinephrine may cause nausea, vomiting, altered glucose metabolism, difficulty in micturition, and urinary retention (234).

Creatinine clearance was decreased 13.1 ml/minute and insulin clearance 17.3 ml/minute in seven healthy subjects given norepinephrine in dosage sufficient to increase blood pressure 40 mm Hg (239).

Numerous reports of local skin necrosis secondary to extravasation of norepinephrine into local tissue around IV injection site have been reported (240,241). A 55-year-old man receiving norepinephrine every 2 days to maintain blood pressure postoperatively developed gangrene of the lower limb below the site of infusion (242). Ischemia of the hand secondary to norepinephrine extravasation has been described in two patients (243). No benefit was derived from surgical decompression or phentolamine local injection. Both patients subsequently died.

PHENYLEPHRINE

Phenylephrine (Neo-Synephrine), like methoxamine, is a powerful alpha receptor stimulant with little effect on cardiac beta receptors. Phenylephrine causes peripheral vasoconstriction and consequently a rise in systolic and diastolic blood pressure due to constriction of most vascular beds. Marked reflex bradycardia occurs, which was formerly used clinically to terminate episodes of paroxysmal atrial tachycardia (244). Phenylephrine is the drug of choice topically to produce mydriasis in ophthalmology. Parenterally, phenylephrine is used to treat hypotension during spinal anesthesia, shock, drug-induced hypotension, and hypersensitivity reactions. It is used orally and topically as a decongestant and is also used in the treatment of priapism. Additional FDA indications include use in paroxysmal supraventricular tachycardia.

Toxic Dose

Adult and pediatric therapeutic doses are provided in Table 1. There have been a few reported cases in which phenylephrine resulted in toxicity and one reported fatality. These cases involved fatal hypertension after topical administration of phenylephrine. Some of these cases were complicated by bradycardia or depressed myocardial contractility in patients administered either α-blockers (due to unopposed α-adrenoreceptor activity) or calcium antagonists to treat this emerging hypertension (245). Both nonfatal and fatal cases of severe myocardial ischemia have occurred after topical use of phenylephrine (both ophthalmic and nasal) (245,246).

A 4-year-old boy became hypertensive to 180/110 mm Hg and tachycardia to 160 beats/minute rapidly after nasal application of 3 drops of 0.5% phenylephrine to each nostril for local hemostasis. Labetalol were given which was associated with further deterioration. The child died despite aggressive resuscitative efforts. Labetalol use was deemed responsible for worsening of cardiac output and contributing to development of pulmonary edema (245).

Seven cases of cardiac arrest resulted after instillation of 10% phenylephrine ophthalmic solution for pupillary dilatation for fluorescein angiography (247). Phenylephrine was implicated due to the lack of reported cardiovascular toxicity of fluorescein. All patients were elderly and had serious cardiovascular disease.

Toxicokinetics and Toxicodynamics

The pharmacokinetic data for phenylephrine are provided in Table 3. Phenylephrine undergoes hepatic and intestinal metabolism by MAO to hydroxymandelic acid and inactive phenolic conjugates. Metabolism to phenolic conjugates occurs primarily after oral administration and to a lesser extent after IV administration (248). Elimination in the urine approaches 90%. Onset of action is 0.5 to 2.0 minutes IV and 15 to 20 minutes IM. Duration of action of these two routes is approximately 10 to 15 minutes and approximately 1.5 hours, respectively. Half-life of the drug is 2 to 3 hours (248).

Pathophysiology

Phenylephrine is a sympathomimetic agent, differing from epinephrine by lacking a hydroxyl (OH) group in the 4 position on the benzene ring. The drug is a potent, relatively pure parenteral α-adrenergic receptor agonist similar to methoxamine and lacks beta-receptor effects on the heart. It causes vasoconstriction of the arterioles of the nasal mucosa and conjunctiva producing rapid and prolonged increases in systolic and diastolic blood pressure. The drug also causes pupillary constriction. Sympathomimetics with indirect/mixed activity such as phenylephrine cause the release of norepinephrine, and the use of MAO inhibitors results in more norepinephrine being made available at nerve receptor sites through inhibition of catecholamine degradation; concurrent use leads to greater amounts of norepinephrine, which increases sympathetic activity (249).

Pregnancy and Lactation

Phenylephrine is FDA pregnancy category C (Appendix I). Excretion in breast milk is unknown. Because phenylephrine is poorly absorbed orally, absorption by the infant is minimal and is thus considered safe for breast-feeding (250,251).

Clinical Presentation

ACUTE OVERDOSAGE

A 1-year-old boy received topical 2.5% phenylephrine (6 to 7 mg) for bleeding that occurred during a procedure. Within seconds his systolic pressure increased to 200 mm Hg. Though the dosage used was extremely large, care should be taken with administration of 2.5% phenylephrine topically in small, anesthetized children (252).

Self-administered phenylephrine nasal solution to five to ten times the normal dose several times daily resulted in palpitations, dizziness, and dyspnea, as well as an acute leukocytosis to 38,200 cells/mm^3 (253).

ADVERSE EVENTS

Although rare, sympathomimetic psychosis may occur with the prolonged use of intranasal phenylephrine preparations. Chronic hallucinosis occurred in a 61-year-old man using phenylephrine intranasally for a chronic sinus condition (254). A 26-year-old woman with a 13-year history of self-prescribed phenylephrine use sprayed into both nostrils every 15 minutes during waking hours presented with a self-described feeling of panic associated with difficult breathing just before using the drops. At the time of presentation, she exhibited symptoms of visual and tactile hallucinations, visual illusions, and paranoid delusions consistent with a toxic psychosis (255).

Hypertension is one of the more common cardiovascular effects of phenylephrine. Premature neonates, the elderly, and those with idiopathic orthostatic hypotension are at a greater risk for hypertension especially after use of the 10% ophthalmic solution (256–260). Severe hypertension and PVCs developed in a 57-year-old man (260/120 mm Hg) minutes after 4 drops of 10% phenylephrine were inadvertently instilled into his eye. Three hours later, he complained of chest pain and developed a non–Q-wave myocardial infarction (261). Coadministration of indirect-acting sympathomimetics and an MAO inhibitor has resulted in serious hypertension (262–264).

Hypertensive crisis may occur due to the synephrine content found in oral bitter orange preparations. Oral bitter orange preparations are often standardized to 6% synephrine, a sympathomimetic similar to phenylephrine. These products contain 15 mg to 72 mg of synephrine per dose (265,266). Sympathomimetics with indirect/mixed activity (phenylephrine, synephrine, and pseudoephedrine) cause the release of norepinephrine, which may lead to adverse cardiac effects. The risk of adverse cardiac events may increase when these agents are used concomitantly (249).

Hypertension, left ventricular failure, and pulmonary edema followed within 15 minutes after subconjunctival administration of approximately 5 mg phenylephrine (0.2 ml, 2.5% solution) in a 2-month-old, 5-kg infant with congenital cataracts (267). Adverse systemic reactions to topical ocular application of phenylephrine 10% in pledget form have also occurred. All cases occurred after a single exposure; most patients noted systemic effects within minutes of phenylephrine application; and the adverse systemic reactions included severe hypertension, pulmonary edema, cardiac dysrhythmia, cardiac arrest, and subarachnoid hemorrhage (268).

Patients who received phenylephrine had a 275% greater chance of experiencing myocardial ischemia than those in whom the same mean blood pressure and stump pressure were maintained without phenylephrine in 60 patients undergoing carotid endarterectomy (269).

Nasal use of phenylephrine may cause local irritation and swelling of the nasal mucosa (270,271). Burning, stinging, sneezing, or increased nasal discharge may occur at higher than recommended doses (272). Contact dermatitis has been described after topical application of an ophthalmic solution (273,274). A 66-year-old man developed a conjunctivitis-like reaction after administration of a phenylephrine-containing solution during ophthalmic examinations. Additional cases of contact dermatitis resulting from use of a hemorrhoidal ointment containing phenylephrine are reported (275).

DIAGNOSTIC TESTS FOR ADRENERGIC AGENTS

Serum Drug Concentrations

Therapeutic drug monitoring is not used clinically for the adrenergic agents. In general, levels are not readily available nor are they very useful because of the short duration of action for these agents.

Other Tests

Other diagnostic tests are directed at assessing the organ effects of noradrenergic drug toxicity. An ECG, serum electrolytes, blood glucose, and blood pressure should be monitored. Also, chest radiography and arterial blood gases should be obtained if pulmonary edema, severe respiratory, or CNS depression occurs.

TREATMENT OF ADRENERGIC AGENTS

The principle of treatment is to terminate the exposure and then administer drugs that antagonize the toxic effect. The rate of drug infusion should be reduced or temporarily discontinued until the patient's condition stabilizes.

Decontamination

Gastrointestinal decontamination is not needed for these agents because they are poorly absorbed and are degraded in the stomach.

Enhancement of Elimination

Due to the short half-lives of these agents, extracorporeal elimination is not expected to be clinically useful.

Antidotes

Most toxic effects of the adrenergic agents are mediated through the α-adrenergic receptor. These include local vasospasm causing tissue necrosis and malignant hypertension. Both are effectively antagonized using phentolamine (Regitine). Beta-Receptor blockade is usually avoided because it may allow unopposed alpha-receptor stimulation.

Epinephrine intradigital injections may be treated with warm soaks, compresses and massage, phentolamine and lidocaine standard digital block, terbutaline digital injection, or application of nitroglycerin paste (276). Local SQ injection of epinephrine is treated with topical nitroglycerin or digital block with lidocaine. If these are not effective, phentolamine 1.5 mg (0.3 ml Regitine) locally infiltrated may produce hyperemia, a warm digit, and normal capillary refill within 5 minutes (277). Others have found the local injection of a mixture of 0.5 mg phentolamine (in 1-ml solution) with 1 ml 2% lidocaine to be effective in restoring circulation (140,278). Accidental injections of epinephrine into main arteries (brachial) can be treated with phentolamine to counteract arterial vasospasm.

Extravasation of norepinephrine or dopamine can cause tissue necrosis. If extravasation occurs, the area should be infiltrated as soon as possible with 10 to 15 ml of saline solution containing 5 to 10 mg phentolamine in an attempt to prevent tissue necrosis and sloughing (Chapter 16) (238). A syringe with a fine hypodermic needle should be used and the solution infiltrated liberally throughout the area of extravasation (easily identified as having a cold, hard, pallid appearance). Sympathetic blockade with phentolamine causes immediate and conspicuous local hyperemic changes if the area is infiltrated within 12 hours. Therefore, phentolamine should be given as soon as possible after the extravasation is noted (80,99,Inotropin, 1991). Blood pressure should be monitored. The half-life of phentolamine is approximately 20 minutes.

If extravasation of metaraminol occurs, the area should be liberally infiltrated as soon as possible with 10 to 15 ml of 0.9% sodium chloride injection containing 5 to 10 mg of phentolamine using a fine hypodermic needle (197).

Hypertension should be first treated with benzodiazepine administration. This reduces adrenergic tone and also effectively treats agitation. Severe and prolonged hypertension can be effectively treated with nitroprusside or with an α-blocking agent such as phentolamine. Atropine may be given if reflex bradycardia occurs. Adrenergic blocking agents and vasodilators should be used with caution because of the frequent biphasic hypertensive-hypotensive nature of adrenergic drug overdose. Fluids should be given with caution and with careful monitoring because of the possible late development of pulmonary edema.

Dobutamine withdrawal symptoms and signs may be ameliorated by hydralazine 25 mg immediately before the first reduction in the dobutamine infusion, and every 4 hours thereafter to a maximal dose of 150 mg (35).

Short-term use of risperidone (mean dosage, 1.1 mg per day) improves the psychopathology of patients with Parkinson's disease who have dopamine-induced psychosis without adversely affecting the symptoms of Parkinson's disease (279).

For isoproterenol, the combined use of a beta-blocking agent and a nitrate completely reverses the abnormal ECG findings induced by isoproterenol (181,182).

Monitoring

All patients should be monitored for cardiovascular effects. Blood pressure and heart monitoring are indicated, and an ECG should be obtained. Monitor pulse, ECG, serum potassium, blood sugar, and cardiac enzymes. Monitor the chest radiograph and arterial blood gases if pulmonary edema occurs.

REFERENCES

1. Wood M. Drugs and the sympathetic nervous system. In: Wood M, Wood AJJ, eds. *Drugs and anesthesia: pharmacology for anesthesiologists*. Baltimore: Williams & Wilkins, 1990:395.
2. Leier CV, Unverferth DV. Diagnosis and treatment: drugs five years later: dobutamine. *Ann Intern Med* 1983;99:490–496.
3. Henakin TP. An in vitro quantitative analysis of the alpha adrenoceptor partial agonist activity of dobutamine and its relevance to inotropic selectivity. *J Pharmacol Exp Ther* 1981;216:210–219.
4. Williams RS, Bishop T. Selectivity of dobutamine for adrenergic receptor subtypes: in vitro analysis by radioligand binding. *J Clin Invest* 1981;67:1703–1711.
5. Tuttle RR, Mills J. Dobutamine: development of a new catecholamine to selectively increase cardiac contractility. *Circ Res* 1975;36:185–196.
6. Nash CW, Wolff SA, Ferguson BA. Release of tritiated noradrenaline from perfused rat hearts by sympathomimetic amines. *Can J Physiol Pharmacol* 1968;46:35–39.

7. Berkowitz C, McKeever L, Croke RP, et al. Comparative responses to dobutamine and nitroprusside in patients with chronic low output cardiac failure. *Circulation* 1977;56:917–924.
8. Goldberg L, Hsich Y, Resnekov L. Newer catecholamines for treatment of heart failure and shock: an update on dopamine and a first look at dobutamine. *Prog Cardiovasc Dis* 1977;19:327–340.
9. Robie NW, Nutter DO, Moody C, et al. In vivo analysis of adrenergic receptor activity of dobutamine. *Circ Res* 1974;34:663–671.
10. Lumley P, Broadley KJ, Levy GP. Analysis of the inotropic: chronotropic selectivity of dobutamine and dopamine in anaesthetized dogs and guinea pig isolated atria. *Cardiovasc Res* 1977;11:17–25.
11. Vatner SF, McRitchie RJ, Brunwald E. Effects of dobutamine on left ventricular performance, coronary dynamics and distribution of cardiac output in conscious dogs. *J Clin Invest* 1974;53:1265–1273.
12. Mueller HS. Inotropic agents in the treatment of cardiogenic shock. *World J Surg* 1985;9:3–10.
13. *Physicians' desk reference*. 46th ed. Montvale, NJ: Medical Economics, 1992:1259–1260.
14. McEvoy GK, ed. *AHFS drug information 92*. Bethesda, MD: American Society of Hospital Pharmacists, 1992:669–670.
15. Parmley WW, Chatterjee K, Francis GS, et al. Congestive heart failure: new frontiers. *West J Med* 1991;154:427–441.
16. Gillespie TA, Ambos HD, Sobel BE, et al. Effects of dobutamine in patients with acute myocardial infarction. *Am J Cardiol* 1977;39:588–593.
17. Gabry AL, Pourriat J-L, Hoang The Dan Ph, et al. Choc cardiogenique au cours d'une intoxication neuroleptique: reversibilite par bolus de dobutamine. *Presse* 1982;11:2225–2226.
18. Goethals M, Demey H. Massive dobutamine overdose in a cardiovascular compromised patient. *Acta Cardiol* 1984;39:373–378.
19. Paulman PM, Cantral K, Meade JG, et al. Dobutamine overdose. *JAMA* 1990;264:2386–2387.
20. Gillespie TA, Ambos HD, Sobel BE, et al. Effects of dobutamine in patients with acute myocardial infarction. *Am J Cardiol* 1977;39:588–593.
21. Dollery C, ed. *Therapeutic drugs*. Edinburgh: Churchill Livingstone, 1991:D196–D201.
22. McEvoy GK, ed. *AHFS drug information 92*. Bethesda, MD: American Society of Hospital Pharmacists, 1992:669–670.
23. Leiser CV, Unverferth DV, Kates RE. The relationship between plasma dobutamine concentrations and cardiovascular responses in cardiac failure. *Am J Med* 1979;66:238–242.
24. Kates RE, Leier CV. Dobutamine pharmacokinetics in severe heart failure. *Clin Pharmacol Ther* 1978;24:537–541.
24a. Banner W, Vernon DD, Minton SD, et al. Nonlinear dobutamine pharmacokinetics in a pediatric population. *Crit Care Med* 1991;19:871–873.
24b. Habil DM, Padbury JF, Anas NG, et al. Dobutamine pharmacokinetics and pharmacodynamics in pediatric intensive care patients. *Crit Care Med* 1992;20:601–608.
25. Padbury JF, Perkin RM, Anas NG, et al. Dobutamine pharmacokinetics in pediatric intensive care patients. *Clin Res* 1989;37:176A.
26. Blumer JL, Ruggerie DP, Witte WK, et al. Polymorphic clearance (I) of dopamine (DA) and dobutamine (DB) in children (K). *Clin Pharmacol Ther* 1989;45:140.
26a. Thomas RL, Watson D, Marshall LE, et al. Review of intermittent dobutamine infusions for congestive cardiomyopathy. *Pharmacotherapy* 1987;7:47–53.
27. Murphy PJ, Williams TL, Kare DLK. Disposition of dobutamine in the dog. *J Pharmacol Exp Ther* 1976;199:423–431.
28. Product information: Dobutrex, dobutamine. Indianapolis: Eli Lilly & Co, (PI revised 9/97) reviewed 1/2000.
29. Broadley KJ. Cardiac adrenoceptors. *J Auton Pharmacol* 1982;2:119.
30. Ruffalo RR Jr, Spradlin TA, Pollock GD, et al. Alpha- and beta-adrenergic effects of the stereoisomers of dobutamine. *J Pharmacol Exp Ther* 1981;219:447–452.
31. Wu C-C, Chen W-J, Cheng J-J, et al. Local dermal hypersensitivity from dobutamine hydrochloride (Dobutrex solution) injection. *Chest* 1991;99:1547–1548.
32. Tuttle RR, Mills J. Dobutamine: development of a new catecholamine to selectively increase cardiac contractility. *Circ Res* 1975;36:185–196.
33. Ruffalo RR Jr, Yaden EL. Vascular effects of the stereoisomers of dobutamine. *J Pharmacol Exp Ther* 1983;224:46–50.
34. Majerus TC, Dasta JS, Bauman JL, et al. Dobutamine: ten years later. *Pharmacotherapy* 1989;9:245–259.
35. Binkley PF, Starling RC, Hammer DF, et al. Usefulness of hydralazine to withdraw from dobutamine in severe congestive heart failure. *Am J Cardiol* 1991;68:1103–1106.
36. Leier CV, Binkley PF. Parenteral inotropic support for advanced congestive heart failure. *Prog Cardiovasc Dis* 1998;41(3):207–224.
37. Roberts R. The role of diuretics and inotropic therapy in failure associated with myocardial infarction. *Arch Int Physiol Biochim* 1984;92:S33–S48.
38. Leier CV, Huss P, Lewis RP, et al. Drug-induced conditioning in congestive heart failure. *Circulation* 1982;65:1382–1387.
39. Unverferth DV, Magorian RD, Lewis RP, et al. Long-term benefit of dobutamine in patients with congestive cardiomyopathy. *Am Heart J* 1980;100:622–630.
40. O'Connor CM, Gattis WA, Uretsky BF, et al. Continuous intravenous dobutamine is associated with an increased risk of death in patients with advanced heart failure: insights from the Flolan International Randomized Survival Trial (FIRST). *Am Heart J* 1999;138(1):78–86.
41. Dukes MNG. *Meyler's side effects of drugs*, vol. 9. New York: Excerpta Medica, 1980.
42. Dukes MNG. *Meyler's side effects of drugs*, ann. 3. New York: Excerpta Medica, 1979.
43. Rabinovitch MA, Kalff V, Chan W, et al. The effect of dobutamine on exercise performance in patients with symptomatic ischemic heart disease. *Am Heart J* 1984;107:81–85.
44. La Vecchia L, Ometto R, Finocchi G, et al. Torsade de pointes ventricular tachycardia during low dose intermittent dobutamine treatment in a patient with dilated cardiomyopathy and congestive heart failure. *PACE* 1999;22:397–399.
45. Poldermans D, Fiorette PM, Boersma E, et al. Safety of dobutamine-atropine stress echocardiology in patients with suspected or proven coronary artery disease. *Am J Cardiol* 1994;73:456–459.
46. Chauvel C, Cohen A, Khireddine M. Safety of dobutamine stress echocardiography: a 24 h Holter monitoring study. *Eur Heart J* 1996;17:1898–1901.
47. Kawano H, Fujii H, Motoyama T, et al. Myocardial ischemia due to coronary artery spasm during dobutamine stress echocardiography. *Am J Cardiol* 2000;85(1):26–30.
48. Kupper W, Waller D, Hanrath P, et al. Hemodynamic and cardiac metabolic effects of inotropic stimulation with dobutamine in patients with coronary artery disease. *Eur Heart J* 1982;3:29–34.
49. Pacold I, Kleinman B, Gunnar R, et al. Effects of low dose dobutamine on coronary hemodynamics, myocardial metabolism, and anginal threshold in patients with coronary artery disease. *Circulation* 1983;68:1044–1050.
49a. Renard M, Bernard R, Melot C, et al. Hemodynamic effects of dobutamine in patients below and over 65 years, with left heart failure secondary to an acute myocardial infarction. *Gerentology* 1984;30:408–413.
50. Lewis WR, Arena FJ, Galloway *MT*, et al. Acute myocardial infarction associated with dobutamine stress echocardiography. *J Am Soc Echocardiogr* 1997;10(5):576–578.
51. Lanzarini L, Previtali M, Diotallevi P. Syncope caused by cardiac asystole during dobutamine stress echocardiography. *Heart* 1996;75(3):320–321.
52. Abbas AE, Loftis R, Lester SJ, et al. Generalized tetany: an unusual complication during dobutamine stress echocardiography. *J Am Soc Echocardiogr* 2002;15(11):1414–1416.
53. Levine TB, Levine AB, Elliott WG, et al. Dobutamine as bridge to angiotensin-converting enzyme inhibitor-nitrate therapy in endstage heart failure. *Clin Cardiol* 2001;24:231–236.
54. Hoff JV, Peatty PA, Wade JL. Dermal necrosis from dobutamine. *N Engl J Med* 1979;300:1280.
55. McCauley CS, Blumenthal MS. Dobutamine and pruritus of the scalp. *Ann Intern Med* 1986;105:966.
56. Wu C-C, Chen W-J, Cheng J-J, et al. Local dermal hypersensitivity from dobutamine hydrochloride (Dobutrex solution) injection. *Chest* 1991;99:1547–1548.
57. Smith RE, Briggs B, Unverferth DV, et al. Dobutamine-induced inhibition of platelet function. *Int J Clin Pharm Res* 1982;2:89–97.
58. Goldenberg IF, Olivari MT, Levine TB, et al. Effect of dobutamine on plasma potassium in congestive heart failure secondary to idiopathic or ischemic cardiomyopathy. *Am J Cardiol* 1989;63:843–846.
59. Dukes MNG. *Meyler's side effects of drugs*, vol. 9. New York: Excerpta Medica, 1980.
60. Robison-Strane SR, Bubik JS. Dobutamine-induced fever. *DICP* 1992;26:1523–1524.
61. Haeusler G, Lues I, Minck K-O, et al. Pharmacological basis for antihypertensive therapy with a novel dopamine agonist. *Eur Heart J* 1992;13[Suppl. D]:129–135.
62. Budny J, Anderson-Drews K. IV inotropic agents: dopamine, dobutamine and amrinone. *Crit Care Nurse* 1991;10:54–62.
63. Creese I, Sibley DR, Leff S, et al. Dopamine receptors: subtypes, localization and regulation. *Fed Proc* 1981;40:147–152.
64. Waddington JL, O'Boyle KM. Dogs acting on brain dopamine receptors: a conceptual re-evaluation five years after the first selective D_1 antagonist. *Pharmacol Ther* 1989;43:1–52.
65. Strange PG. D_1/D_2 dopamine receptor interaction at the biochemical level. *Trends Pharmacol Sci* 1991;12:48–49.
66. Strange PG. Aspects of the structure of the D_2 dopamine receptor. *Trends Neurol Sci* 1990;13:373–378.
67. Sokoloff P, Girus B, Martres M-P, et al. Molecular cloning and characterization of a novel dopamine receptor (D_3) as a target for neuroleptics. *Nature* 1990;347:146–151.
68. Mercuri NB, Calabresi P, Bernardi G. Physiology and pharmacology of dopamine D_2 receptors: their implications in dopamine-substitute therapy for Parkinson's disease. *Neurology* 1989;39:1106–1108.
69. Whipple JK, Medicus-Bringa MA, Schimel BA, et al. Selected vasoactive drugs: a readily available chart reference. *Crit Care Nurs* 1992;12:23–29.
70. Anonymous. *Guidelines for administration of intravenous medications to pediatric patients*, 2nd ed. Bethesda: American Society of Hospital Pharmacists, 1984.
71. Opremcak EM, Davidorf FH. Bilateral retinal infarction associated with high dose dopamine. *Ann Ophthalmol* 1985;17:141–144.
72. Curel HE. Personal communication. DuPont Pharmaceuticals, January 30, 1992.

73. Ensinger H, Schulich S, Grunert A, et al. Dopamine: cardiovascular and metabolic effects in relation to plasma levels. *Crit Care Med* 1990;18:S179.
74. Padbury JF, Agata Y, Baylen BG, et al. Pharmacokinetics of dopamine in critically ill newborn infants. *J Pediatr* 1990;17:472–476.
75. Eldrup E, Hagen C, Christensen NJ, et al. Plasma free and sulfoconjugated dopamine in man: relationship to sympathetic activity, adrenal function and meals. *Dan Med Bull* 1988;35:291–294.
76. Bhatt-Mehta V, Nahata MC, McClead RE, et al. Dopamine pharmacokinetics in critically ill newborn infants. *Eur J Clin Pharmacol* 1991;40:593–597.
77. Eldadah MK, Schwartz PH, Harrison R, et al. Pharmacokinetics of dopamine in infants and children. *Crit Care Med* 1991;19:1008–1011.
78. Seri I, Tulassay T, Kiszel J, et al. Effect of low-dose dopamine therapy on catecholamine values in cerebrospinal fluid in preterm neonates. *J Pediatrics* 1984;105:489–491.
79. Notterman DA, Greenwald BM, Moran F, et al. Dopamine clearance in critically ill infants and children: effect of age and organ system dysfunction. *Clin Pharmacol Ther* 1990;48:138–147.
80. Product information: dopamine hydrochloride injection, USP. North Chicago: Abbott Laboratories, (PI revised 3/1997) reviewed 06/2002.
81. Goodall McC, Alton H. Dopamine (3-hydroxy-tyramine) replacement in metabolism in sympathetic nerve and adrenal medullary depletions after prolonged thermal injury. *J Clin Invest* 1969;48:1761.
82. Sumikawa K, Hayashi Y, Yamatodani A, et al. Contribution of the lungs to the clearance of exogenous dopamine in humans. *Anesth Analg* 1991;72:622–626.
83. Weir MR, Keniston RC, Enriquez JI Sr, et al. Depression of vitamin B_6 levels due to dopamine. *Vet Hum Toxicol* 1991;33:118–121.
84. Frederickson ED, Bradley TJ, Goldberg LI. Block of the renal effects of dopamine in the dog by the DA_1 antagonist, SCH 23390. *Am J Physiol* 1985;249:F236–F240.
85. Levinson PD, Goldstein PS, Mundson PJ, et al. Endocrine, renal and hemodynamic responses to graded dopamine infusions in normal men. *J Clin Endocrinol Metab* 1985;60:821–826.
86. McDonald RH, Goldberg LI, McNay JL. Effects of dopamine in man: augmentation of sodium excretion, glomerular filtration rate and renal plasma flow. *J Clin Invest* 1964;43:1116–1124.
87. Goldberg LI. Cardiovascular and renal actions of dopamine: potential clinical applications. *Pharmacol Rev* 1972;24:1–29.
88. Parker S, Carlon GC, Isaacs M, et al. Dopamine administration in oliguria and oliguric renal failure. *Crit Care Med* 1981;9:630–632.
89. Greenlaw CW, Null LW II. Dopamine-induced ischemia. *Lancet* 1977;2:555.
90. Mantel GD, Makin JD. Low dose dopamine in postpartum pre-eclamptic women with oliguria: a double-blind, placebo controlled, randomised trial. *Br J Obstet Gynaecol* 1997;104:1180–1183.
91. Samojlek E, Khing OJ, Chang MC. Effects of dopamine on reproductive processes and fetal development in rats. *Am J Obstet Gynecol* 1969;104:578.
92. Greenlaw CW, Null LW II. Dopamine-induced ischemia. *Lancet* 1977;2:555.
93. Alexander CS, Sako Y, Mikulic E. Pedal gangrene associated with the use of dopamine. *N Engl J Med* 1975;293:591.
94. Valdes ME. Post-dopamine ischemia treated with chlorpromazine. *N Engl J Med* 1976;295:1081–1082.
95. Goldbranson FL, Lurie L, Vance RM, et al. Multiple extremity amputations in hypotensive patients treated with dopamine. *JAMA* 1980;243:1145–1146.
96. Maggi JC, Angelats J, Scott JP. Gangrene in a neonate following dopamine therapy. *J Pediatr* 1982;100:323–325.
97. Ebels TJ, Homan van der Heide JN. Dopamine-induced ischaemia. *Lancet* 1977;2:762.
98. Goenka S, Mehta AV, Powers PJ. An unusual peripheral vascular response to dopamine in a neonate. *Tennessee Medicine* 1999;92(10):375–376.
99. Chen JL, O'Shea M. Extravasation injury associated with low-dose dopamine. *Annals of Pharmacotherapy* 1998;32(5):545–548.
100. Shahar E, Lotan D, Barzilay Z. Dopamine-induced paroxysmal supraventricular tachycardia in an infant. *Clinical Pediatrics* 1981;20(8):541–543.
101. Rosenblum R, Frieden J. Intravenous dopamine and the treatment of myocardial dysfunction after open heart surgery. *Am Heart J* 1972;83:743.
102. Bucher HW, Kroiss G, Stucki P. On the effect of dopamine on left and right ventricular hemodynamics. *Schweiz Med Wochenschr* 1972;102:414.
103. Shahar E, Lotan D, Barzilay Z. Dopamine-induced paroxysmal supraventricular tachycardia in an infant. *Clin Pediatr* 1981;20:541–543.
104. Gelfman DM, Ornato JP, Gonzalez ER. Dopamine-induced increase in atrioventricular conduction in atrial fibrillation-flutter. *Clin Cardiol* 1987;10:671–673.
105. Rosenblum R, Tai AR, Lawson D. Dopamine in man: cardiorenal hemodynamics in normotensive patients with heart disease. *J Pharm Exp Ther* 1972;183:256.
106. Anonymous. Dopamine for treatment of shock. *Med Lett Drug Ther* 1975;17:13.
107. Kulkarni J, Horne M, Butler E, et al. Psychotic symptoms resulting from intraventricular infusion of dopamine in Parkinson's disease. *Biol Psychiatry* 1992;31:1225–1227.
108. Venna N, Sabin TD, Ordia JI, et al. Treatment of severe Parkinson's disease by intraventricular injection of dopamine. *Appl Neurophysiol* 1984;47:62–64.
109. Oneglia C, Maestri M. Dysuria as a side effect of dopamine therapy. *Cardiovasc Drugs Ther* 1994;8:515.
110. Oppenheim A, Pizov R, Elhallel-Darnitzki M, et al. Intravenous dopamine associated with nephrogenic diabetes insipidus-like syndrome. *Clin Drug Invest* 1999;17(2):167–169.
111. Polansky D, Eberhard N, McGrath R. Dopamine and polyuria. *Ann Intern Med* 1987;107:941.
112. Klausen NO, Qvist J, Brynjolf I, et al. Pulmonary hypertension in a patient with ARDS—a possible side-effect of dopamine treatment. *Intensive Care Med* 1982;8:155–158.
113. Boltax RS, Dineen JP, Scarpa FJ. Gangrene resulting from infiltrated dopamine solution. *N Engl J Med* 1977;296:823.
114. Alexander CS, Sako Y, Mikulic E. Pedal gangrene associated with the use of dopamine. *N Engl J Med* 1975;293:591.
115. Greene SI, Smith JW. Dopamine gangrene. *N Engl J Med* 1976;294:114.
116. Golbranson FL, Lurie L, Vance RM, et al. Multiple extremity amputations in hypotensive patients treated with dopamine. *JAMA* 1980;243:1145–1146.
116a. Park JY, Kanzler M, Swetter SM. Dopamine-associated symmetric peripheral gangrene. *Arch Dermatol* 1997;133:247–249.
117. Julka WK, Nova JR. Gangrene aggravation after use of dopamine. *JAMA* 1976;235:2812.
118. Dive A, Foret F, Jamart J, et al. Effect of dopamine on gastrointestinal motility during critical illness. *Intensive Care Med* 2000;26:901–907.
119. Vasarhelyi B, Nobilis A, Machay T, et al. Inhibitory effect of dopamine treatment on Na+/K+-ATPase activity in preterm infants. *Eur J Pediatr* 1997;156:79–80.
120. Matsuo Y, Hasegawa K, Doi Y, et al. Erythrocyte sodium-potassium transport in hyperkalaemic and normokalaemic infants. *Eur J Pediatr* 1995;7:571–576.
121. Callaham M. High-dose epinephrine in cardiac arrest. *West J Med* 1991;155:289–292.
122. Barton C, Callaham M. High-dose epinephrine improves the return of spontaneous circulation rates in human victims of cardiac arrest. *Ann Emerg Med* 1991;20:722–725.
123. Martin D, Werman HA, Brown CG. Four case studies: high dose epinephrine in cardiac arrest. *Ann Emerg Med* 1990;19:232–236.
124. Callaham M, Barton CW, Kayser S. Potential complications of high-dose epinephrine therapy in patients resuscitating from cardiac arrest. *JAMA* 1991;265:1117–1122.
125. Ornato JP. Members of the Use of Adrenergic Agonists During CPR Panel. Use of adrenergic agonists during CPR in adults. *Ann Emerg Med* 1993;22:411–416
126. Freedman BJ. Accidental adrenaline overdosage and its treatment with piperoxan. *Lancet* 1955;2:575–578.
127. Scalzo A, Keith G, Thompson M. Fatal outcome after massive epinephrine overdose by intravenous injection of an OTC asthma inhaler. *J Toxicol Clin Toxicol* 1995;33:501–502(abst).
128. Hall AH, Kulig KW, Rumack BH. Intravenous epinephrine abuse. *Am J Emerg Med* 1987;5:64–65.
129. Kolendorf K, Moller BB. Lactic acidosis in epinephrine poisoning. *Acta Med Scand* 1974;196:465–466.
130. Alton H, Goodall M. Metabolic products of adrenaline (epinephrine) during long-term constant rate intravenous infusion in the human. *Biochem Pharmacol* 1968;17:2163.
131. Gilman AG, Goodman LS, Rall TW, et al., eds. *Goodman and Gilman's the pharmacological basis of therapeutics*, 7th ed. New York: Macmillan Publishing Co, 1985.
132. Simons FER, Gu X, Simons KJ. Epinephrine absorption in adults: intramuscular versus subcutaneous injection. *J Allergy Clin Immunol* 2001;108:871–873.
133. Simons FER, Roberts JR, Gu X, et al. Epinephrine absorption in children with a history of anaphylaxis. *J Allergy Clin Immunol* 1998;101:33–37.
134. Gilman AG, Goodman LS, Gilman LG. *Goodman and Gilman's the pharmacological basis of therapeutics*, 6th ed. New York: Macmillan Publishing Co, 1980.
135. Reynolds JEF, ed. *Martindale: the extra pharmacopeia*, 28th ed. London: Pharmaceutical Press, 1982.
136. Schatz M, Zeiger RS, Harden KM, et al. The safety of inhaled beta-agonist bronchodilators during pregnancy. *J Allergy Clin Immunol* 1988;82:686–695.
137. Kurachek SS, Rochoff MA. Inadvertent intravenous administration of racemic epinephrine. *JAMA* 1985:253:1441–1442.
138. Egoz N, Firestone SC. Adrenaline-induced pulmonary edema and its treatment. A report of two cases. *Br J Anaesth* 1971;43:709–712.
139. Novey HS, Meleyco IN. Alarming reaction after intravenous administration of 30 mL of epinephrine. *JAMA* 1969;209:2435–2441.
140. Deshmukh N, Tollard JT. Treatment of accidental epinephrine injection in a finger. *J Emerg Med* 1989;7:408.
141. Roberts JR, Krisanda TJ. Accidental intra-arterial injection of epinephrine treated with phentolamine. *Ann Emerg Med* 1989;18:424–453.
142. Hicks PR, Rankin APN. Massive adrenaline doses in labetalol overdose. *Anaesth Intensive Care* 1991;19:447–450.
143. Woodard ML, Brent LD. Acute renal failure, anterior myocardial infarction, and atrial fibrillation complicating epinephrine abuse. *Pharmacotherapy* 1998;18:656–658.
144. Davis C, Wax PM. Prehospital epinephrine overdose in a child resulting in ventricular dysrhythmias and myocardial ischemia. *Pediatr Emerg Care* 1999;15:116–118.
145. Carter BT, Westfall VK, Heironimus TW, et al. Severe reaction to accidental subcutaneous administration of large doses of epinephrine. *Anesth Analg* 1971;50:175–178.

146. McCarroll KA, Roszler MH. Lung disorders due to drug abuse. *J Thorac Imaging* 1991;6:30–35.
147. Liu HP, Wu KC, Lu PP, et al. Delayed-onset epinephrine-induced pulmonary edema. *Anesthesiology* 1999;91:1169–1170.
148. Barkhordarian AR, Wakelin SH, Paes TRF. Accidental digital injection of adrenaline from an autoinjector device [Letter]. *Br J Dermatol* 2000;143:1359.
149. Mol CJ, Gaver J. Case reviews: a 39-year-old nurse with accidental discharge of an epinephrine autoinjector into the left index finger. *J Emerg Nurs* 1992;18:306–307.
150. Bennie RE, Miyamoto RT. Epinephrine-induced ventricular fibrillation during anesthesia for myringotomy and tube insertion. *Otolaryngology Head Neck Surg* 1994;111:824–826.
150a. Butte MJ, Nguyen BX, Hutchison TJ, et al. Pediatric myocardial infarction after racemic epinephrine administration (abstract). *Pediatrics* 1999;104(1):103–104.
151. Horak A, Raine R, Opie LH, et al. Severe myocardial ischaemia induced by intravenous adrenaline. *Br Med J (Clin Res)* 1983;286:519.
152. Paulman PM, Cantral K, Meade JG, et al. Dobutamine overdose [Letter]. *JAMA* 1990;264:2386.
153. Lapostolle F, Agostinucci JM, Borron SW. Abuse of epinephrine as a stimulant [Letter]. *Ann Intern Med* 2002;136:174–175.
153a. Levine DH, Levkoff AH, Pappu LD, et al. Renal failure and other serious sequelae of epinephrine toxicity in neonates. *South Med J* 1985;78:874–877.
154. Stemmer E, Connolly J. Mesenteric vascular insufficiency. *Calif Med* 1973; 118:18.
155. Heath A, Hulten BA. Terbutaline concentrations in self-poisoning: a case report. *Hum Toxicol* 1987;6:525–526.
156. Speer F, Tapay NJ. Syncope in children following epinephrine. *Ann Allergy* 1970;28:50.
157. Kolker AE, Becker B. Epinephrine maculopathy. *Arch Ophthalmol* 1968;79:552.
158. Mooney D. Pigmentation after long-term topical use of adrenaline compounds. *Br J Ophthalmol* 1970;54:823.
159. Madge GE, Geeraets WJ, Guerry D III. Black cornea secondary to topical epinephrine. *Am J Ophthalmol* 1971;71[Suppl]:402–405.
160. Spaeth GL. Nasolacrimal duct obstruction caused by topical epinephrine. *Arch Ophthalmol* 1967;77:355.
161. Maguire WB, Langley NR. Gas gangrene following an adrenaline-in-oil injection into the left thigh with survival. *Med J Aust* 1967;1:973.
162. Harvey PW, Purnell GV. Fatal case of gas gangrene associated with intramuscular injections. *BMJ* 1968;1:744.
163. Van Hook R, Vandevelde AG. Gas gangrene after intramuscular injection of epinephrine: report of a fatal case [Letter]. *Ann Intern Med* 1975;83:669.
164. Anonymous. *Guidelines for administration of intravenous medications to pediatric patients*, 2nd ed. Bethesda: American Society of Hospital Pharmacists, 1984.
165. Dodds WN, Soler NG, Thompson H. Death in asthma. *BMJ* 1975;4:345.
166. Product information: Isuprel, Mistometer, isoproterenol. *Physicians' desk reference* (electronic version). Englewood, CO: Micromedex, Inc, 1997.
167. Blackwell EW, Briant RH, Conolly ME, et al. Metabolism of isoprenaline after aerosol and direct intrabronchial administration in man and dog. *Br J Pharmacol* 1974;50:587.
168. Wade A, ed. *Martindale: the extra pharmacopoenia*, 27th ed. London: The Pharmaceutical Press, 1977:1925.
169. Conolly ME, Davies DS, Dollery CT, et al. Metabolism of isoprenaline in dog and man. *Br J Pharmacol* 1972;46:458.
170. Kadar D, Tang HY, Conn AW. Isoproterenol metabolism in children after intravenous administration. *Clin Pharmacol Ther* 1974;16:789.
171. Gilman AG, Goodman LS, Nies AS, et al., eds. *Goodman and Gilman's the pharmacological basis of therapeutics*, 8th ed. New York: Macmillan Publishing Co, 1990.
172. Schatz M, Zeiger RS, Harden KM, et al. The safety of inhaled beta-agonist bronchodilators during pregnancy. *J Allergy Clin Immunol* 1988;82:686–695.
173. Marcus MA, Vertommen JD, Van Aken H, et al. Hemodynamic effects of intravenous isoproterenol versus saline in the parturient. *Anesth Analg* 1997;84(5):1113–1116.
174. Paterson JW, Conolly ME, Davis DS, et al. Isoprenaline resistance and the use of pressurized aerosols in asthma. *Lancet* 1968;2:426.
175. Matson JR, Loughlin GM, Strunk RC. Myocardial ischemia complicating the use of isoproterenol in asthmatic children. *J Pediatr* 1978;92:776–778.
176. Page R, Gay W, Friday G, et al. Isoproterenol-associated myocardial dysfunction during status asthmaticus. *Ann Allergy* 1986;57:402–404, 429–430.
177. Kurland G, Williams J, Lewiston NJ. Fatal myocardial toxicity during continuous infusion intravenous isoproterenol therapy of asthma. *J Allergy Clin Immunol* 1979;63:407–411.
178. Wood DW, Downes JJ. Intravenous isoproterenol in the treatment of respiratory failure in childhood status asthmaticus. *Ann Allergy* 1973;31:607.
179. Wood DW, Downes JJ, Scheinkof H, et al. Intravenous isoproterenol in the management of respiratory failure in childhood status asthmaticus. *J Allergy* 1972;50:75.
180. Wosornu JL, Easmon CO. Intravenous isoprenaline in treatment of septic shock in man. *Br Med J* 1970;1:723.
180a. Fisch C. AV dissociation: the use of isoproterenol. *J IN Med Assoc* 1969;62:48.
181. Mills BF, Winsor T. Isoproterenol myocardiopathy. *Am Soc Pharmacol Ther* 1970;71:37.
182. Winsor T, Wright RW, Berger HJ. Isoproterenol toxicity. *Am Heart J* 1975;89:814.
183. Maguire JF, Geha RS, Umetsu DT. Myocardial specific creatine phosphokinase isoenzyme elevation in children with asthma treated with intravenous isoproterenol. *J Allergy Clin Immunol* 1986;78:631–636.
184. Warth J, Rappaport A. Atypical reaction to isoproterenol. *JAMA* 1969;209:417.
185. Reisman RE. Asthma induced by adrenergic aerosols. *J Allergy* 1970;46:162–177.
186. Reisman RE. Asthma induced by adrenergic aerosols. *Chest* 1973;63 [Suppl]:16S.
187. Van Metre TE. Adverse effects of inhalation of excessive amounts of nebulized isoproterenol in status asthmaticus. *J Allergy* 1969;43:101.
188. Dukes MN, ed. *Meyler's side effects of drugs*, vol. VIII. Amsterdam: Excerpta Medica, 1975.
189. Klock LE, Miller TD, Morris AH, et al. A comparative study of atropine sulfate and isoproterenol hydrochloride in chronic bronchitis. *Am Rev Respir Dis* 1975;112:371.
190. Anshelevich IuV, Okun KV. The effect of adrenergic drugs on gastric acid and alkaline secretion. *Ter Arkh* 1972;44(10):47–49.
191. Brown RD, Bolas G. Isoprenaline ulceration of the tongue. *Br Dent J* 1973;134:336.
192. Gilman AG, Rall TW, Nies AS, et al., eds. *Goodman and Gilman's the pharmacological basis of therapeutics*, 8th ed. New York: Pergamon Press, 1990.
193. Smith NT: Acute haemodynamic effects of mephentermine in man. *Br J Anaesth* 1972;44:452–459.
194. Sifton DW. *PDR generics*, 3rd ed. Montvale, NJ: Medical Economics, 1997.
195. Zoll PM. Rational use of drugs for cardiac arrest and after cardiac resuscitation. *Am J Cardiol* 1971;27:645–649.
196. Mills LC, Moyer JH. Indications for adrenergic stimulators in shock. *Intern Zeitschrift fur Klinische Pharm, Therapy, Toxicol* 1991;4:385–395.
197. Olin B, ed. *Facts and comparisons*. St Louis: JB Lippincott, 1990.
198. Reynolds JEF, ed. *Martindale: the extra pharmacopoeia* (electronic version). Denver: Micromedex, Inc, 1997.
199. Levinson G, Shnider SM. Pharmacology of adjuvant drugs. *Clin Anesth* 1973;10:78–109.
200. Nahrwold ML, Phelps M Jr. Inadvertent intra-arterial injection of mephenteramine. *Rocky Mountain Med J* 1973;70:38–39.
201. Hawkins LG, Lischer CG, Sweeney M. The main line accidental intra-arterial drug injection. *Clin Ortho Related Res* 1973;94:268–274.
202. Angrist BM, Schweitzer JW, Gershon S, et al. Mephentermine psychosis: misuse of the Wyamine inhaler. *Am J Psychiatry* 1970;126:149–151.
203. Joshi UG, Bhat SM. Mephentermine dependence with psychosis: a case report. *Br J Psychiatry* 1988;152:129–131.
204. Chiles BW III, Cooper PR. Acute spinal injury. *N Engl J Med* 1996;334:514–520.
205. Koga S, Shiraishi K, Saito Y. Post-traumatic priapism treated with metaraminol bitartrate: case report. *J Trauma* 1990;30:1591–1593.
206. Mizutani M, Nakano H, Sagami K, et al. Treatment of post-traumatic priapism by intracavernous injection of alpha-stimulant. *Urol Int* 1986;41:312–314.
207. Branger B, Ramperez P, Oules R, et al. Metaraminol for haemodialysis associated priapism (letter). *Lancet* 1985;641.
208. Stanners A, Colin-Jones D. Metaraminol for priapism. *Lancet* 1984;2:978.
209. Lindoro J, Castro JC, Cruz F, et al. Treatment of priapism [Letter]. *Lancet* 1984;2:1348–1349.
210. Rice V. Shock management part II: pharmacologic intervention. *Crit Care Nurse* 1985;5:42–57.
211. Olin B, ed. *Facts and comparisons*. St Louis: JB Lippincott Co, 1990.
212. Gilman AG, Goodman LS, Rall TW, et al., eds. *Goodman and Gilman's the pharmacological basis of therapeutics*, 7th ed. New York: Macmillan Publishing Co, 1985.
213. Reynolds JEF, ed. *Martindale: the extra pharmacopoeia* (electronic version). Denver: Micromedex, Inc, 1990.
214. Product information: Aramine(R), metaraminol bitartrate injection. *Physicians' desk reference* (electronic version). Englewood, CO: MICROMEDEX, Inc, (PI revised 9/1996) reviewed 9/2000.
215. Bourdarias JP, Dubourg O, Gueret P, et al. Inotropic agents in the treatment of cardiogenic shock. *Pharm Ther* 1983;22:53–79.
216. Perlroth MG, Harrison DC. Cardiogenic shock: a review. *Clin Pharmacol Ther* 1969;10:449–467.
217. Brown RS, Carey JS, Woodward NW, et al. Hemodynamic effects of sympathomimetic amines in clinical shock. *Surg Gynecol Obstet* 1966;122:303–307.
218. Binder MJ. Effect of vasopressor drugs on circulatory dynamics in shock following myocardial infarction. *Am J Cardiol* 1965;16:834–840.
219. Watts FB. Myocardial infarction, gram-negative bacteremia, prolonged shock, and leukemoid reaction. *Am Heart J* 1965;69:253.
220. Dukes MNG. *Meyler's side effects of drugs*, vol 9. New York: Excerpta Medica, 1980.
221. Portioli I, Valcavi R: Factitious phaeochromocytoma: a case for Sherlock Holmes. *BMJ* 1981;283:1660–1661.
222. Gilman AG, Goodman LS, Rall TW, et al., eds. *Goodman & Gilman's the pharmacological basis of therapeutics*, 7th ed. New York: Macmillan Publishing Co, 1985.
223. Product information: Vasoxyl, methoxamine hydrochloride injection. *Physicians' desk reference* (electronic version). Englewood, CO: MICROMEDEX, Inc, (PI revised 12/97) reviewed 2/2000.

224. Gilbert JL, Lange G, Polevoy I, et al. Effects of vasoconstrictor agents on cardiac irritability. *J Pharmacol Exp Ther* 1958;123:9–15.
225. Aviado DM. Cardiovascular effects of some commonly used pressor amines. *Anesthesiology* 1959;20:71.
226. Eckstein JW, Abbaud FM. Circulatory effects of sympathomimetic amines. *Am Heart J* 1962;63:119–135.
227. Smith NT, Whitcher C. Acute hemodynamic effects of methoxamine in man. *Anesthesiology* 1967;28:735–748.
228. Senties L, Arellano G, Casellas A, et al. Effects of some vasopressor drugs upon uterine contractility in pregnant women. *Am J Obstet Gynecol* 1970;107(6):892–897.
229. Shnider SM, deLorimier AA, Asling JH, et al. Vasopressors in obstetrics. II. Fetal hazards of methoxamine administration during obstetric spinal anesthesia. *Am J Obstet Gynecol* 1970;106(5):680–686.
230. Radley SC, Chapple CR, Bryan NP, et al. Effect of methoxamine on maximum urethral pressure in women with genuine stress incontinence: a placebo-controlled, double-blind crossover study. *Neurourol Urodyn* 2001;20(1):43–52.
231. AMA Department on Drugs. *AMA drug evaluations*, 4th ed. Littleton, MA: PSG Publishing Co, 1986.
232. Anthracite RF, Vachon L, Knapp PH. Alpha-adrenergic receptors in the human lung. *Psychosomatic Med* 1971;33:481–489.
233. Koch-Weser J: Dobutamine: a new synthetic cardioactive sympathetic amine. New Engl J Med 1979; 300:17-22.
234. Reynolds JEF, ed. *Martindale, the extra pharmacopoeia*, 29th ed. London: The Pharmaceutical Press, 1989.
235. Okada Y, Suzuki H, Ishiyama I. Fatal subarachnoid haemorrhage associated with dental local anaesthesia. *Australian Dental Journal* 1989;34(4):323–325.
236. Goodman LS, Gilman A. *The pharmacological basis of therapeutics*, 5th ed. New York: Macmillan Publishing Co, 1975.
237. Amy JJ, Karum SM. Intrauterine administration of l-noradrenaline and propranolol during the second trimester of pregnancy. *J Obstet Gynaecol Br Comm* 1974;81:75–83.
238. Product information: Norepinephrine bitartrate injection, USP. North Chicago: Abbott Laboratories, (PI revised 10/1992) reviewed 06/2002.
239. Renner E, Edel HH, Gurland HJ. Vergleichende untersuchungen uber die wirkung von ahtyladrianol und nor-adrenalin auf die neiren hamodynamik des grsunden. *Med Klin* 1965;60:546–548.
240. Fritz H, Hagstam K, Lindqvist B. Focal skin necrosis after intravenous infusion of norepinephrine, and the concept of endotoxinaemia. *Acta Med Scand* 1965;178:403–416.
241. Oglesby JE, Baugh JH. Tissue necrosis due to norepinephrine. *Am J Surg* 1968;115:408–412.
242. Jaconelli J. Massive gangrene of the lower limb following use of continuous noradenaline intravenous infusion. *Med J Aust* 1965;52:79–80.
243. Weeks PM. Ischemia of the hand secondary to levarterenol bitartrate extravasation. Methods of management. *JAMA* 1966;196:288–290.
244. Eckstein JW, Abboud FM. Circulatory effects of sympathomimetic amines. *Am Heart J* 1962;63:119–135.
245. Jones J, Greenberg L, Groudine S, et al. Phenylephrine advisory panel report. *Int J Pediatr Otorhinolaryngol* 1998;45:97–99.
246. Diamond JP. Systemic adverse effects of topical ophthalmic agents: implications for older patients. *Drugs Aging* 1997;11(5):352–360.
247. Wesley RE. Phenylephrine eyedrops and cardiovascular accidents after fluorescein angiography. *J Ocular Ther Surg* 1983;Jul–Aug:212–214.
248. Hengstmann JH, Goronzy J. Pharmacokinetics of 3H-phenylephrine in man. *Eur J Clin Pharmacol* 1982;21:335–341.
249. Gilman AG, Rall TW, Nies AS, et al., eds. *Goodman and Gilman's the pharmacological basis of therapeutics*, 8th ed. New York: Macmillan Publishing Co, 1990.
250. White GJ, White MK. Breastfeeding and drugs in human milk. *Vet Human Toxicol* 1980;22:1–43.
251. Wilson JT, Brown RD, Cherek DR, et al. Drug excretion in human breast milk: principle pharmacokinetics and projected consequences. *Clin Pharmacokinet* 1980;5:1–66.
252. Wellwood M, Goresky GV. Systemic hypertension associated with topical administration of 2.5% phenylephrine. *Am J Ophthalmol* 1982;93:369–370.
253. Huycke MM, Muttiana DS, Morrison A, et al. A leukemoid reaction caused by a nasal sympathomimetic. *Clin Infect Dis* 1992;15:885–886.
254. Escobar JI, Karno M. Chronic hallucinosis from nasal drops. *JAMA* 1982;247:1859–1860.
255. Snow SS, Logan TP, Hollender MH. Nasal spray 'addiction' and psychosis: a case report. *Br J Psychiatry* 1980;136:297–299.
256. Diamond JP. Systemic adverse effects of topical ophthalmic agents: implications for older patients. *Drugs Aging* 1997;11(5):352–360.
257. Duffin RM, Pettit TH, Straatsma BR. 2.5% v 10% phenylephrine in maintaining mydriasis during cataract surgery. *Arch Ophthalmol* 1983;101:1903–1906.
258. Lees BJ, Cabal LA. Increased blood pressure following pupillary dilation with 2.5% phenylephrine hydrochloride in preterm infants. *Pediatrics* 1981;68:231–234.
259. Rosales T, Isenberg S, Leake R, et al. Systemic effects of mydriatics in low weight infants. *J Pediatr Ophthalmol Strabismus* 1981;18:42–44.
260. Robertson D. Contraindication to the use of ocular phenylephrine in idiopathic orthostatic hypotension. *Am J Ophthalmol* 1979;87:819–822.
261. Lai YK. Adverse effect of intraoperative phenylephrine 10%: case report. *Br J Ophthalmol* 1989;73:468–469.
262. Smookler S, Bermudez AJ. Hypertensive crisis resulting from an MAO inhibitor and an over-the-counter appetite suppressant. *Ann Emerg Med* 1982;11:482–484.
263. Cuthbert MF, Greenberg MP, Morley SW. Cough and cold remedies: a potential danger to patients on monoamine oxidase inhibitors. *BMJ* 1969;1:404–406.
264. Terry R, Kaye AH, McDonald M. Sinutab [Letter]. *Med J Aust* 1975;1:763.
265. Anonymous. Vitacost, 2002. Available at: http://www.vitacost.com/store/products/ProductSearch.cfm. Accessed November 7, 2002.
266. Anonymous. Bitter orange extract. Natures Way, 1999. Available at: http://www.naturesway.com. Accessed October 31, 2002.
267. Greher M, Hartmann T, Winkler M, et al. Hypertension and pulmonary edema associated with subconjunctival phenylephrine in a 2-month-old child during cataract extraction. *Anesthesiology* 1998;88:1394–1396.
268. Fraunfelder FW, Fraunfelder FT, Jensvold B. Adverse systemic effects from pledgets of topical ocular phenylephrine 10%. *Am J Ophthalmol* 2002;134(4):624–625.
269. Smith JS, Roizen MF, Cahalan MK, et al. Does anesthetic technique make a difference? Augmentation of systolic blood pressure during carotid endarterectomy: effects of phenylephrine versus light anesthesia and of isoflurane versus halothane on the incidence of myocardial ischemia. *Anesthesiology* 1988;69:846–853.
270. AMA Department of Drugs. *AMA drug evaluations*, 4th ed. Chicago: American Medical Association, 1980.
271. Dukes MN. *Meyler's side effects of drugs*, vol. 9. New York: Excerpta Medica, 1980.
272. Product information: Neo-Synephrine(R) Nasal, phenylephrine. Bayer Corporation, 1997.
273. Wigger-Alberti W, Elsner P, Wuthrich B. Allergic contact dermatitis to phenylephrine. *Allergy* 1998;53:217–218.
274. Tosti A, Bardazzi F, Tosti G, et al. Contact dermatitis to phenylephrine. *Contact Dermatitis* 1987;17:110–111.
275. Wilkinson SM, Kingston TP, Beck MH. Allergic contact dermatitis from phenylephrine in a rectal ointment. *Contact Dermatitis* 1993;29:100–101.
276. Mrvos R, Anderson BD, Krenzelok EP. Accidental injection of epinephrine from an autoinjector: invasive treatment not always required. *South Med J* 2002;95:318–320.
277. McCauley WA, Gerace RV, Scilley C. Treatment of accidental injection of epinephrine with an auto-injector. *Vet Hum Toxicol* 1990;33:375.
278. Maguire WA, Reisdorff EJ, Smith D, et al. Epinephrine-induced vasospasm reversed by phentolamine digital block. *Am J Emerg Med* 1990;8:46–47.
279. Inotropin product literature (dopamine HCl injection, USP): 6227-1/Rev. Du Pont Pharmaceuticals, January 1991.

CHAPTER 100

Antimuscarinic Drugs

Andrew H. Dawson

See Figure 1.

Compounds included:	**Atropine, benztropine (Cogentin, BETE), dicyclomine (Bentyl, Spasmoban), homatropine (Hycodan), ipratropium (Atrovent, Itrop), orphenadrine (Myotrol, Norflex), oxybutynin (Ditropan), pirenzepine (Gastrozepin), procyclidine (Kemadrin), scopolamine (Transderm Scop, Donnagel, many others), tirolidine (Tirolaxo), trihexyphenidyl (Artane)**
Molecular formula and weight:	**See Table 1.**
SI conversion:	**See Table 1.**
CAS Registry No.:	**See Table 1.**
Therapeutic levels:	**Not used clinically**
Target organs:	**Central nervous system (acute)**
Antidote:	**Physostigmine**

OVERVIEW

Antimuscarinic drugs competitively inhibit the muscarinic effects of acetylcholine. They are also known as *parasympatholytic, atropinic, atropine-like,* or *anticholinergic agents.* Atropine is the prototypic antimuscarinic agent. The major clinical problem associated with the toxicity of the antimuscarinic drugs is central nervous system (CNS) toxicity. This toxicity is typically manifested as delirium (central anticholinergic syndrome) in combination with peripheral antimuscarinic effects. Control of the delirium is the most common clinical problem. Severe toxicity includes hyperpyrexia and seizures. Clinically significant toxicity can last for days, reflecting a combination of prolonged absorption and long half-life. Toxicity can result from an exaggerated response to therapeutic dose (1), an overdose, recreational abuse (2,3), or inadvertent use with adulterated street drugs (4,5), as well as from some foods or herbal preparations (6–9). Although most anticholinergic poisonings require only supportive care, some antimuscarinic drugs have direct cardiotoxicity that requires specific management. Within the antimuscarinic class, orphenadrine appears to have the greatest risk of death as a result of ventricular dysrhythmias, respiratory depression, seizures, and hypoglycemia.

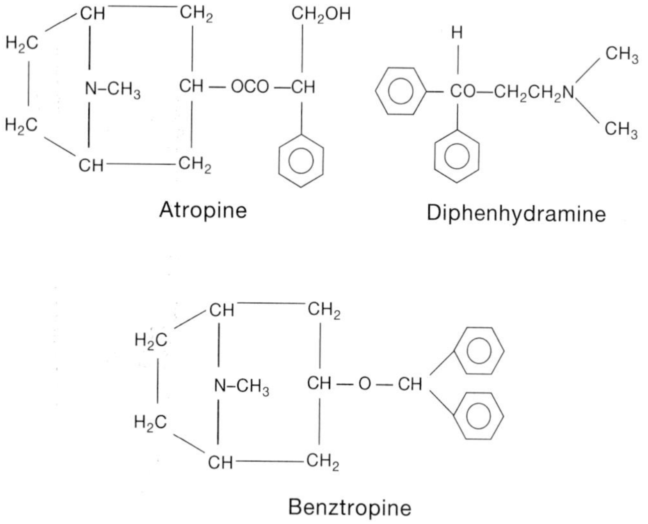

Figure 1. Structures of atropine, diphenhydramine, and benztropine. (From Howrie DL, Rowley AH, Krenzelok EP. Benztropine-induced acute dystonic reaction. *Ann Emerg Med* 1986;15:594-596, with permission.)

Classification and Uses

Antimuscarinic agents can be classified on the basis of their source (natural, semisynthetic, or synthetic) and their cationic structure (tertiary amine or quaternary ammonium compounds). Atropine, hyoscyamine, and scopolamine are naturally occurring tertiary amines (Table 2) produced by the roots, leaves, and beans of plants of the Solanaceae family, of which the deadly nightshade *(Atropa belladonna)* is the best known. These alkaloids can be synthesized, but plant extraction is less expensive. *Duboisia myoporoides* is now the main source, in addition to *Atropa belladonna* and *Datura stramonium* (jimsonweed).

Antimuscarinic agents are used for a wide range of medical conditions spanning all age groups. Atropine is used as an antidote in organophosphate and other cholinergic drug poisonings to treat bradycardia and muscarinic symptoms (Chapter 42). It has been used in cardiac glycoside poisoning and in situations in which enhanced vagal tone due to nausea, intubation, or oropharyngeal stimulation contributes to bradycardia from beta-blockers or calcium-channel blockers. It is also used in sinus node dysfunction tests and in assessment of coronary artery disease (10). Nebulized atropine had been used as a bronchodilator, but unacceptable systemic side effects occurred.

Orphenadrine, which is a congener of diphenhydramine without sharing its soporific effect, is an antimuscarinic tertiary amine with actions and uses similar to those of benzhexol (trihexyphenidyl). It also has weak antihistaminic and local anesthetic properties.

Terodiline has actions similar to those of atropine. It is also reported to possess calcium channel–blocking activity. It was used for the relief of urinary incontinence. In 1991, it was withdrawn from the market in all countries because of its association with cardiac dysrhythmias.

Atropine, scopolamine, and glycopyrrolate have all been used as preoperative medication to inhibit salivation, diminish excessive

TABLE 1. Formulation, dose, and indication for antimuscarinic agents

Drug, molecular formula, molecular weight (g/mol), CAS Registry No.	SI conversion	Formulation	Common adult dosage	Indication
Atropine sulfate; $(C_{17}H_{23}NO_3)_2,H_2SO_4,H_2O$; 694.8; 5908-99-6	ng/ml × 3.46 = nmol/L	0.6-mg tablets; 0.1, 0.6, 1.2 mg/ml solution[a]	0.3–1.2 mg, 2 mg every 5 min or continuous infusion	Preoperative, cardiac; cholinesterase inhibitor toxicity
		0.5%, 1% drops	1–2 drops, 2–4 times/d	Mydriasis and cycloplegia for refraction; inflammatory eye disorders
Benzhexol hydrochloride (trihexyphenidyl); $C_{20}H_{31}NO,HCl$; 337.9; 52-49-3	ng/ml × 3.32 = nmol/L	2 mg, 5 mg (extended release)	1–5 mg, 3 times/d	Parkinson's syndrome and antipsychotic extrapyramidal drug effects
Benztropine mesylate; $C_{21}H_{25}NO,CH_4O_3S$; 403.5; 132-17-2	ng/ml × 3.25 = nmol/L	0.5-, 1.0-, 2.0-mg tablets	1–2 mg/d	Parkinson's syndrome and antipsychotic extrapyramidal drug effects
		2 mg in 2-ml ampule	1–2 mg	Acute dystonic reactions
Biperiden hydrochloride; $C_{21}H_{29}NO,HCl$; 347.9; 1235-82-1	ng/ml × 3.21 = nmol/L	2 mg	1–4 mg, 3 times/d	Parkinson's syndrome and antipsychotic extrapyramidal drug effects
Cyclopentolate hydrochloride; $C_{17}H_{25}NO_3,HCl$; 327.8; 5870-29-1	µg/L × 3.43 = nmol/L	0.50%, 1%	1–2 drops, 4 times/d	Mydriasis and cycloplegia for refraction; higher strength for pigmented eyes
Dicyclomine hydrochloride; $C_{19}H_{35}NO_2,HCl$; 345.9; 67-92-5	µg/ml × 3.23 = µmol/L	10-, 20-mg capsules; 1 mg/ml syrup[b]	20–40 mg, 4 times/d	Gastrointestinal spasm
		10 mg/5 ml	20 mg, 4 times/d	
Glycopyrrolate bromide; $C_{19}H_{28}BrNO_3$; 398.3; 596-51-0	ng/ml × 3.14 = nmol/L	0.2 mg/ml	—	Preoperative
Homatropine hydrobromide; $C_{16}H_{21}NO_3,CH_3Br$; 370.3; 80-49-9	ng/ml × 3.63 = nmol/L	0.5%, 2.0%, 5.0%	1–2 drops, every 4 h	Mydriasis and cycloplegia for refraction, inflammatory eye disorders
Hyoscine butylbromide, $C_{21}H_{30}BrNO_4$, 440.4, 149-64-4	pg/ml × 0.0033 = nmol/L	10 mg	20 mg, 4 times/d	Gastrointestinal spasm
		20 mg/ml	20–40 mg IMI or IVI	Biliary or renal colic
Ipratropium bromide; $C_{20}H_{30}BrNO_3,H_2O$; 430.4; 66985-17-9	ng/ml × 3.0 = nmol/L	21, 44 mg/metered dose	44–88 mg, 3 times/d	Allergic rhinitis
		20, 40 mg per metered dose	40–80 mg, 4 times/d	Bronchospasm
		0.25 mg/ml, 0.5 mg/ml	0.25–0.5 mg, 3 times/d	Bronchospasm
Orphenadrine citrate; $C_{18}H_{23}NO,C_6H_8O_7$; 461.5; 4682-36-4	ng/ml × 3.71 = nmol/L	100 mg extended release[b]	100 mg, 2 times/d	Musculoskeletal pain, Parkinson's syndrome, antipsychotic extrapyramidal drug effects
Oxybutynin hydrochloride; $C_{22}H_{31}NO_3,HCl$; 393.9; 1508-65-2	ng/ml × 2.8 = nmol/L	5-mg tablets, 5 mg/5 ml syrup	5 mg, 3 times/d	Urinary incontinence
Pirenzepine hydrochloride; $C_{19}H_{21}N_5O_2$, 2HCl,H_2O; 442.3; 29868-97-1	µg/ml × 2.85 = µmol/L	50 mg	50 mg, 3 times/d	Gastric ulcer
Procyclidine hydrochloride; $C_{19}H_{29}NO,HCl$; 323.9; 1508-76-5	µg/ml × 3.48 = µmol/L	5-mg tabs, 2.5, 5.0 mg in 5 ml	5–10 mg, 3 times/d	Parkinson's syndrome and antipsychotic extrapyramidal drug effects
		10 mg in 2 ml	5–10 mg IMI or IV	
Scopolamine transdermal (see also Hyoscine)		1.5 mg	Released over 3 d	Released over 3 d
Terodiline	µg/ml × 3.15 = µmol/L	Withdrawn from market	—	QT prolongation
Tiotropium bromide, $C_{19}H_{22}BrNO_4S_2$, 472.4, 139404-48-1	ng/ml × 2.55 = nmol/L	Capsule for use in inhaler	18 mg once daily	
Trihexyphenidyl		See Benzhexol	—	—
Tropicamide, $C_{17}H_{20}N_2O_2$, 284.4, 1508-75-4	ng/ml × 3.52 = nmol/L	0.50%, 1%	1–2 drops, 4 times/d	Mydriasis and cycloplegia for refraction; higher strength for pigmented eyes

IMI, intramuscular injection; IVI, intravenous injection.
[a]Extemporous preparations of higher strength are available.
[b]May be found as a component of multiingredient preparations.
From HyperTox, 2003. Available at: http://members.ozemail.com.au/~ouad/index.html. Accessed July 2003, with permission.

secretions, and reduce postoperative nausea. Scopolamine is used in palliative care to dry secretions and reduce "death rattle" (11). Transdermal scopolamine is used to prevent motion sickness.

Oxybutynin, propantheline, and dicyclomine are used in the treatment of urinary incontinence predominately by modifying detrusor and bladder outlet tone. Dicyclomine has been used in irritable bowel syndrome and for infantile colic. Benztropine, orphenadrine, benzhexol, and trihexyphenidyl are used as adjunctive treatment in Parkinson's disease and for drug-induced extrapyramidal reactions.

Atropine, homatropine hydrobromide, and cyclopentolate are available as topical ophthalmic preparations to induce mydriasis and cycloplegia for examination of the retina and optic disk and for measurement of refractive error. They are also used to maintain a dilated pupil and prevent posterior synechiae following glaucoma surgery (trabeculectomy with peripheral iridectomy) or acute inflammatory conditions in the uveal tract.

Pirenzepine is a selective M(1) tertiary amine antimuscarinic, which therefore does not readily cross the blood-brain barrier. It acts on the gastric mucosa, reducing secretion of gastric acid.

Toxic Dose

The adult and pediatric therapeutic doses are detailed in Table 1. Although clinical toxicity has been associated with a wide dose range, there is in general a dose-response relationship. Death

TABLE 2. Classification of antimuscarinic agents

Tertiary	Quaternary	Selective
Atropine	Atropine	Pirenze-
Atropine sulfate	Methobromide	pine
Benzhexol hydrochloride	Atropine methonitrate	hydro-
Benztropine mesylate	Clidinium bromide	chloride
Biperiden hydrochloride	Diphemanil	Telenzepine
Biperiden lactate	Methylsulfate	
Cyclopentolate hydrochloride	Emepronium bromide	
Dicyclomine hydrochloride	Glycopyrronium	
Homatropine	Bromide homatropine	
Homatropine hydrobromide	Methobromide	
Hyosceine	Hyoscine	
Hyosceine hydrobromide	Butylbromide	
Hyosceyamine	Hyoscine methonitrate	
Methixene hydrochloride	Ipratropium bromide	
Oxybutynin hydrochloride	Isopropamide iodide	
Oxyphencyclimine hydrochloride	Mepenzolate bromide	
Procyclidine hydrochloride	Octatropine	
Tropicamide	Methylbromide	
	Otilonium bromide	
	Oxitropium bromide	
	Pipenzolate bromide	
	Prifinium bromide	
	Poldine	
	Methylsulfate	
	Propantheline	
	Bromide tiemonium	
	Iodide tiemonium	
	Methylsulfate	
	Timepidium bromide	
	Valethamate bromide	

From Reynolds JEF, ed. *Martindale: the extra pharmacopoeia*, 30th ed. London: Pharmaceutical Press, 1993:418, with permission.

has been reported with most antimuscarinic agents but is relatively rare. In addition to the risk from direct pharmacologic effects, patients with anticholinergic delirium are at increased risk of physical harm through misadventure.

Atropine has been associated with death with doses as low as 1.6 mg (12) and as high as 100 mg in children (13). An adult survived ingestion of 1 g (14). Seizures occurred after the therapeutic use of atropine eye drops in a child (15). An oral dose of 30 mg/mg/kg produced a peak serum level of 6.7 nmol/L at 2 hours (16). Ketchum et al. (17) observed that 175 mg/mg/kg intramuscularly produced initial peripheral autonomic effects such as tachycardia and dryness of mouth. Concomitant with these effects were central disturbances: somnolence, restlessness, ataxia, incoordination, hyperreflexia, hyperthermia and hypertension, disruption of awareness, and incoherent speech or inability to carry out instructions lasting 10 to 12 hours. Atropine sulfate, 0.5 mg via nebulizer every 4 hours, led to central anticholinergic intoxication; the patient recovered (18).

Homatropine eye drops have caused antimuscarinic CNS toxicity in children (19) and adults (20,21). After ingestion of 0.5 mg per breast-feed for 1 week, a 2-month-old boy presented with coma, mydriasis, and a temperature of 107.4°F (41.9°C), tachypnea, and tachycardia. He responded to cooling measures (22).

Atropine methonitrate caused CNS signs (dilated pupils, irritability, and restlessness) in eight infants aged 1 to 27 weeks who received doses of 0.39 to 3.55 mg/kg. Toxicity lasted 24 to 60 hours. All recovered with supportive treatment (23). Accidental administration of 32 mg by inhalation to a 65-year-old man produced only a transient headache. Quaternary ammonium congeners of atropine may have a wider therapeutic margin than atropine sulfate when inhaled (24).

A benztropine dose of 4 to 120 mg produced anticholinergic delirium and peripheral signs of toxicity in 12 patients (25). All patients received tacrine to treat the delirium and recovered. The duration of symptoms ranged from 4 to 58 hours. Clinical toxicity may last for up to 9 days (26,27). At least three fatalities have been reported (28–30); complications of hyperthermia appear to be the likely mechanism.

A dicyclomine ingestion of 300 mg by a 15-month-old boy was survived (31). A 1-year, 8-month-old child ingested 200 mg, experienced a toxic delirium, and was discharged in 1 day (32). A 3-year-old boy ingested an unknown quantity of doxyl-amine succinate (Debenox, Bendectin), and anticholinergic delirium and peripheral effects developed. He responded to treatment and was discharged in 1 day (33). Administration of 10 mg dicyclomine to two infants aged 5 and 6 weeks resulted in apnea and cyanosis in one case and rigidity and apnea in the second; both patients recovered (34). Other infants have experienced similar symptoms (35), including, in one case, respiratory arrest (35). Two fatalities have been attributed to dicyclomine alone (36); the rest have occurred with combination preparations commonly containing doxylamine succinate. An 18-month-old ate a bottle full of extended-release doxyl-amine succinate tablets; signs of anticholinergic toxicity and respiratory and cardiac arrest developed, and he died (31). A 3-year-old ingested 100 bendectin tablets; developed restlessness, disorientation, ataxia, and tonic-clonic seizures; and later died in cardiorespiratory arrest (37).

Ipratropium and tiotropium in escalating oral, subcutaneous, intravenous, and inhaled doses of ipratropium produce anticholinergic toxicity in animals (38). Direct contact with the eye in patients with poor puffer technique can cause mydriasis and precipitate glaucoma (39–41).

A 100-mg dose of oxybutynin caused anticholinergic effects, including stupor, followed by delirium, dilated pupils, dry skin, and retention of urine in an adult. The patient also had ventricular ectopic beats and bigeminy for 30 hours (42). Anticholinergic delirium has been reported in children (43). Therapeutic doses have been implicated as a cause of severe hyperpyrexia (44).

No deaths from pirenzepine have been reported. The risk of CNS effects is low because it does not cross the blood–brain barrier. Procyclidine has caused anticholinergic delirium lasting 42 hours after ingestion of an unknown quantity (45). It is also a recreational drug of abuse (46) and has caused delirium in other cases (47,48).

Scopolamine toxicity usually arises from adulterated products or ingestion of scopolamine-containing plants, producing classic anticholinergic syndrome (8,49–52). Adults as well as children have developed central anticholinergic syndrome with hallucinations and incontinence after being treated with a single transdermal patch (53–55).

Terodiline was withdrawn from the worldwide market in 1991 after it was found to be associated with torsade de pointes (56-58). CYP2C19 deficiency appears to increase the risk of toxicity (59). A trihexyphenidyl (benzhexol) ingestion of 300 mg caused anticholinergic toxicity, with recovery after 1 week (60). An adult ingested 150 mg, which led to lip-smacking, disorientation, delirium, and visual hallucinations; the patient recovered in 3 to 4 days (61). Deaths have occurred (62).

A 35 mg/kg orphenadrine ingestion in a child produced delirium and ataxia within 1 hour followed by seizures and ventricular tachycardia, which responded to lignocaine (63). In a 3-year-old boy, central anticholinergic toxicity developed after ingestion of up to 12.5 mg/kg (64). Confusion, generalized tonic-clonic seizures, and sustained ventricular tachycardia developed in a 3-year-old boy after ingestion of an unknown quantity, which was reversed by administration of physostigmine (65). Orphenadrine is over-represented in deaths when compared with other antimuscarinics or antipsychotics (66,67). The adult lethal dose ranges from 2 to 3 g (68,69). Death has been suggested to be associated with ingestion of greater than 22 mg/kg in adults and 72 mg/kg in children (68–70).

TOXICOKINETICS AND TOXICODYNAMICS

Pharmacokinetics

Pharmacokinetic information is largely restricted to studies involving young healthy volunteers given single doses. In general, this class of drugs is rapidly absorbed after ingestion. Oral bioavailability is variable between the different drugs, ranging from 30% to more than 70%. All drugs appear to have a large volume of distribution and rapid distribution to tissues. All have relatively low hepatic clearance and appear to be extensively metabolized, primarily to N-dealkylated and hydroxylated metabolites. Excretion of parent drug and metabolite is via the urine and bile (71). In healthy volunteers there is no clear relationship between concentration and peripheral anticholinergic effects, indicating significant pharmacodynamic variation (72). The elderly and patients with Down syndrome are more prone to side effects.

Atropine eye drops have a bioavailability of 63% (73). The time to peak serum concentration (T_{max}) is 1 to 2 hours after ingestion of atropine, 0.03 mg/kg, with a peak concentration (C_{max}) of 6.7 nmol/L. The corresponding result after intramuscular administration was a peak level of 5.7 nmol/L at 0.5 hour (16). The terminal half-life is 2 to 4 hours.

Ipratropium bromide bioavailability is 3.3%, with a half-life of 98 minutes (74). Dicyclomine ingestion of one 40-mg sustained-release tablet resulted in a C_{max} of 80 ng/ml and T_{max} of 2 hours. Within the next 2 hours the level dropped to approximately 25 ng/ml (75).

Oxybutynin at therapeutic doses has a T_{max} of 1 to 2 hours after ingestion, with a mean C_{max} of 8.0 to 12.0 ng/ml after a 5-mg dose and a half-life of 2 hours (76,77). Similar concentrations are reported after administration in the bladder (78).

Procyclidine ingestion of 10 mg produces a mean C_{max} of 116 ng/ml and mean bioavailability of 75%. The volume of distribution is 1 L/kg, and the half-life is 12 hours. Peripheral effects are maximal at about 1 to 2 hours after oral dosing (79).

Benzhexol ingestion of 4 mg produces a C_{max} of 7.15 ng/ml and T_{max} of 1.32 hours, with an elimination half-life of 32.7 ± 6.35 hours (80). Orphenadrine ingestion of 100 mg produces an elimination half-life ranging from 13.2 to 20.0 hours but becomes longer with repeated dosing (81).

Toxicokinetics and Toxicodynamics

As absorption is rapid, clinical toxicity is normally evident within 2 hours of ingestion. Anticholinergic effects may cause delayed gastric emptying, resulting in late peak levels or cyclic absorption (27). The duration is often prolonged either due to a long half-life or to a delayed absorption phase.

Atropine tablets caused death after ingestion. The atropine blood level was 200 ng/ml, and a urine level was 1.5 mg/ml. A healthy adult ingested 1 g atropine, and an anticholinergic syndrome developed. The blood atropine level several hours later was 129 ng/ml (82). Inadvertent injection of 2 mg atropine into children led to relatively mild symptoms of atropinization. Serum atropine levels ranged from 7.5 to 69 ng/ml (83).

Benztropine toxicokinetics have not been systematically studied. Patients who received 4 mg per day exhibited plasma levels of 19 to 125 ng/ml (84). An adult with acute anticholinergic poisoning syndrome (agitation, active hallucinations, and combativeness) had a serum benztropine level of 100 ng/ml. It decreased in an erratic course until it reached 9 ng/ml, at which time there was no further evidence of anticholinergic toxicity (27). Urine levels of 5.3 to 123 ng/ml were observed after 4 mg/day was ingested by four patients (84).

A dicyclomine blood concentration of 505 ng/ml in a 2-year-old caused unresponsiveness. Another 2-month-old child became apneic and died with a blood dicyclomine concentration of 221 ng/ml. These concentrations represent ten and four times the adult therapeutic concentration, respectively (36).

Procyclidine blood concentrations in overdose have averaged 2.7 mg/ml (85). An orphenadrine ingestion of 35 mg/kg in a child produced an initial peak level of 3.55 mg/ml and a calculated elimination half-life of 10.2 hours (86).

PATHOPHYSIOLOGY

Antimuscarinic drugs competitively inhibit the effects of acetylcholine at muscarinic receptors. They do not diminish the production of acetylcholine. The muscarinic receptor has at least five subtypes. Although there is a considerable overlap of regions, the different receptor subtypes display different tissue distributions within the body. For example, M1 receptors are located primarily in the CNS, whereas M2 receptors are located in the brain and heart; M3 receptors are located in salivary glands, and M4 receptors are present in the brain and lungs (87). Benztropine and trihexyphenidyl have a higher affinity for the M1 receptor than do other antimuscarinics (88).

In the periphery, the antimuscarinic agents block autonomic effectors innervated by postganglionic cholinergic nerves or on smooth muscles that do not contain cholinergic innervation. CNS effects of atropine and related drugs result from their central antimuscarinic actions. In usual doses, they produce mild vagal stimulation and decrease of heart rate.

The cardiac toxicity of antimuscarinic agents is most probably due to sodium channel blockade (89). Orphenadrine is a diphenhydramine derivative that has effects on noradrenaline reuptake (90), serotonin (91), and *N*-methyl-D-aspartate receptors. In animal models, the unventilated animal dies from respiratory arrest, whereas in ventilated animals the mode of death is cardiac arrest preceded by sinus node dysfunction and heart block (92).

PREGNANCY AND LACTATION

Pregnancy and lactation information for the antimuscarinic drugs is provided in Table 3.

TABLE 3. Pregnancy category and breast milk penetrance for antimuscarinic agents

Drug	FDA pregnancy risk category	Australian pregnancy risk category	Use during breast-feeding
Atropine	C	A	Safe to use
Benztropine	B	B2	Unknown
Biperiden	C	B2	Unknown
Dicyclomine	B	NR	Unknown
Glycopyrrolate	B	NR	NR
Ipratropium	B	B1	Safe to use
Orphenadrine	C	B2	Unknown
Oxybutynin	B	B1	Unknown
Pirenzepine	NR	NR	Unknown
Procyclidine	C	NR	Unknown
Scopolamine	C	B2	Safe to use
Terodiline	NR	NR	Withdrawn
Trihexyphenidyl	NR	B1	Unknown

NR, not recorded; FDA, U.S. Food and Drug Administration.

CLINICAL PRESENTATION

Acute Overdosage

The major toxicity common to all the antimuscarinic drugs is an anticholinergic syndrome secondary to muscarinic receptor blockade. This can be divided into central and peripheral anticholinergic effects. Some agents also have additional toxicity, which is not mediated by muscarinic receptor blockade. Antimuscarinic drugs are also components of multidrug preparations that have separate or synergistic toxicity.

Central anticholinergic syndrome is most commonly manifested as a hyperactive (agitated) delirium, often with pressured and incoherent speech and visual and auditory hallucinations. Patients may have visual perceptual abnormalities and be seen to be picking at objects on their bed sheets. This can be determined by asking patients to pick up small pieces of white tissue; they are either unable to distinguish the tissue or continue to pick at nonexistent tissue. Hypoactive and mixed delirium syndromes also occur, although it is usual for most patients to have a period of hyperactive delirium. The delirium can persist after many of the peripheral signs resolve; this is thought to reflect the higher affinity of M1 receptors for some agents. Seizures and coma are reported in severe cases. Dystonia and movement disorders have been reported after overdose.

Peripheral anticholinergic syndrome is composed of (in descending order of frequency) thirst, dry mouth, dilated pupils, tachycardia, flushed face, slowed gastric emptying and decreased bowel sounds, dry skin, hyperthermia, and urinary retention. Patients often complain of a dry mouth and difficulty in swallowing. Vision may be blurred. Pupils are dilated and respond poorly to light. Some coingestions may reduce pupil size, but the pupillary reactions remain sluggish. The axilla or groin may be dry. Bowel sounds may be absent, and patients may present with pseudo-obstruction. Sinus tachycardia is common; blood pressure may be either low secondary to peripheral vasodilation or elevated (often as a response to an agitated delirium).

The absence of tachycardia in a symptomatic anticholinergic ingestion should prompt an examination for a concurrent cardiotoxic drug ingestion. Fever is a marker of severity. Peripherally, the cause of fever is a combination of decreased heat loss and increased heat production. Centrally mediated temperature dysregulation may also be present.

Orphenadrine poisoning is associated with rapid onset of anticholinergic syndrome, seizures, and cardiac effects. Seizures occurred within 2 hours and ventricular tachycardia at 4 hours; delirium persisted for 84 hours (93). Death has occurred within 2.5 hours of ingestion (94). A prolonged absorptive phase is possible (95). The electrocardiogram (ECG) may show QRS or QT changes.

Adverse Events

Exaggerated antimuscarinic responses to therapeutic doses are similar to those seen after overdose. Signs and symptoms may follow use by any route (eye, oral, intramuscular, intravenous, or inhalation). The most common symptoms are dry mouth and blurred vision. Patients older than 60 are more likely to experience cognitive impairment at therapeutic doses (96,97).

Unilateral and bilateral mydriasis has occurred with scopolamine patches and inadvertent exposure of the eye to ipratropium. Diagnosis contamination can be confirmed by prompt and extensive constriction of the pupil on instillation of 0.5% to 1.0% pilocarpine hydrochloride in the affected eye (98). Acute angle-closure glaucoma has occurred with all antimuscarinic agents including ipratropium (41,99).

Orphenadrine decreases CYP2D6 activity by 80% to 90% and decreases the metabolism of drugs that use that enzyme (100). Intravenous atropine has caused immunoglobulin E–mediated anaphylactic shock (101). Allergic contact dermatitis is reported with scopolamine patches (102). Paradoxic bronchospasm has occurred with ipratropium (103) and may be due to preservatives in some preparations (104). Patients with Down syndrome have increased sensitivity to atropine, which may result from the genetic imbalance imposed by the extra chromosome 21 in this syndrome (105).

Withdrawal

An antimuscarinic withdrawal syndrome has been described (106). Nausea, vomiting, and perspiration developed 1 day after cessation of long-term use of atropine eye drops for the management of amblyopia. All symptoms resolved within 24 hours (107). The author has observed a similar syndrome in recreational users of benztropine. When transdermal scopolamine has been used for longer than 3 days, withdrawal of its use has occasionally been followed by dizziness, nausea, vomiting, headache, and disturbance of equilibrium (108,109).

DIAGNOSTIC TESTS

Plasma levels are not readily available and do not guide management, which must be based on clinical evaluation. An ECG is most likely to show sinus tachycardia. With the exception of orphenadrine, QRS and QT prolongation should suggest other drug ingestion or preexisting cardiac disease. Full biochemistry and blood gases should be taken. In patients with no complications, the serum electrolytes, renal and hepatic tests, creatine kinase, and acid-base status should be normal. In some cases, multiple tests are needed to evaluate altered mental status. These may include urine drug screening as well as lumbar puncture and culture and computed tomography of the head.

Postmortem Considerations

A benzhexol ingestion (unknown dose) that resulted in death showed blood and liver concentrations to be 120 ng/ml and 0.5 mg/kg, respectively (62). Postmortem blood concentrations of benztropine revealed that 183 ng/ml was reported after ingestion of an unknown amount of benztropine (110). A 19-year-old male who was found dead 2.5 hours after last being seen alive was found to have orphenadrine blood concentration of 18.1 mg/ml and 1452 mg in the stomach (94). In a series of ten autopsy cases, concentrations ranged from 5.5 to 37.0 mg/ml (111).

TREATMENT

Patients should be admitted for observation. Symptomatic patients normally require close observation best delivered in a specialist unit, high dependency care, or intensive care. Patients with ECG abnormalities or those who have taken cardiotoxic drugs require prolonged monitoring. All patients require assessment of the adequacy of airway, ventilation, and circulation.

Decontamination

If present, transdermal patches should be removed. After ingestion of any anticholinergic drug, gastric emptying may be delayed, and oral activated charcoal should be considered for patients who present within 4 hours of ingestion. Patients who have ingested orphenadrine, who are unconscious, or who have ECG abnormalities should have elective intubation, consideration of gastric lavage, and activated charcoal.

Enhancement of Elimination

Extracorporeal elimination methods such as hemodialysis or hemoperfusion are not indicated or likely to be effective.

Antidotes

Physostigmine and other anticholinesterases act by reversibly inhibiting the enzyme acetylcholinesterase, thereby increasing the concentration of acetylcholine at the muscarinic receptor and overcoming the competitive receptor blockade. To be effective in the treatment of central anticholinergic toxicity, the drug needs to cross the blood–brain barrier. Physostigmine (112,113), tacrine (25,114), and galanthamine (115) have all been reported to have efficacy in reversing delirium and peripheral anticholinergic toxicity.

The greatest experience has been with physostigmine. It has been used most commonly in patients with extensive delirium or agitation; other possible indications are repetitive or long-lasting seizures, severe sinus tachycardia or supraventricular tachycardia, or extensive hyperthermia that is unresponsive to mechanical cooling. Physostigmine does not protect against any of the more serious complications that are due to the membrane-blocking, cardiac (116), or antihistamine effects of some of these drugs (i.e., seizures and dysrhythmias).

Physostigmine appears to be relatively safe in the treatment of pure anticholinergic toxicity. Patients should be monitored during administration. Because physostigmine can cause bronchospasm, a history of asthma is a relative contraindication to its use, and all patients should be observed for evidence of bronchial constriction during administration. The initial dose should be 1 to 2 mg intravenously, given slowly (Chapter 67). Delirium normally resolves within minutes, and the duration of effect varies between 30 and 90 minutes. The usual pediatric intravenous dose of physostigmine salicylate recommended by the manufacturer is 0.02 mg/kg.

Repeated doses of physostigmine may be required; 20 doses were given over 8 days to treat benztropine toxicity (26). Tacrine appears to give a longer duration of response, but it is difficult to obtain the intravenous form. Excessive doses of cholinesterase inhibitors may produce cholinergic toxicity (e.g., bradycardia, increased salivation, diarrhea, seizures, or respiratory arrest). Physostigmine-induced life-threatening bronchoconstriction, bradycardia, and seizures may respond to intravenous administration of 0.5 to 1.0 mg atropine sulfate. Neostigmine, a quaternary ammonium cholinesterase inhibitor that does not cross the blood–brain barrier, has been used successfully to reverse anticholinergic induced pseudo-bowel obstruction (117).

Supportive Care

Seizures are treated with benzodiazepines, phenobarbital, and then more aggressive interventions if needed (Chapter 40). Fever is treated with hydration, antipyretics, and cooling in the usual manner (Chapter 38). Urinary retention often requires bladder catheterization.

Delirium is treated by placing the patient in a quiet and supportive environment and providing reorientation. If these measures do not control the delirium, pharmacologic treatment as described for physostigmine in the section Antidotes may be indicated. Phenothiazines and other drugs with anticholinergic effects should not be used. In practice, parenterally administered benzodiazepines may make the patient more manageable but do not appear to diminish the delirium and also increase the likelihood that the patient may need mechanical ventilation (112). Cholinergic agents such as physostigmine provide better control of the delirium and probably reduce the need for other drug therapy.

Dysrhythmias are difficult to treat because the mechanism is generally unknown, and no animal or human studies have been done. Potassium and magnesium deficiency should be corrected. The pKa of orphenadrine is 8.4, which indicates that alkalinization may alter ion channel binding. It would be reasonable to try any of the following treatments, which have been used in other drugs with antidysrhythmic drug effects: sodium bicarbonate (Chapter 75) (89), lidocaine (93), magnesium, or overdrive pacing.

REFERENCES

1. German E, Siddiqui N. Atropine toxicity from eyedrops. *N Engl J Med* 1970;282(12):689.
2. Al Nsour TS, Hadidi KA. Investigating the presence of a common drug of abuse (benzhexol) in hair; the Jordanian experience. *J Clin Forensic Med* 2002;9(3):119–125.
3. Carlini EA. Preliminary note: dangerous use of anticholinergic drugs in Brazil. *Drug Alcohol Depend* 1993;32(1):1–7.
4. From the Centers for Disease Control and Prevention. Scopolamine poisoning among heroin users—New York City, Newark, Philadelphia, and Baltimore, 1995 and 1996. *JAMA* 1996;276(2):92–93.
5. Hamilton RJ, Perrone J, Hoffman R, et al. A descriptive study of an epidemic of poisoning caused by heroin adulterated with scopolamine. *J Toxicol Clin Toxicol* 2000;38(6):597–608.
6. Bjorndal N, Frewald B. [Pronounced addiction to procyclidine (Kemadrin). Case report.] [Danish] *Ugeskr Laeger* 1977;139(42):2512–2513.
7. Boyd R, Rintoul R, Nichol N, et al. Atropine poisoning after drinking Indian tonic water. *Eur J Emerg Med* 1997;4(3):172–173.
8. Chan TYK. Anticholinergic poisoning due to Chinese herbal medicines. *Vet Hum Toxicol* 1995;37(2):156–157.
9. Ramirez M, Rivera E, Ereu C. Fifteen cases of atropine poisoning after honey ingestion. *Vet Hum Toxicol* 1999;41(1):19–20.
10. Mathias W Jr, Arruda A, Santos FC, et al. Safety of dobutamine-atropine stress echocardiography: a prospective experience of 4,033 consecutive studies. *J Am Soc Echocardiogr* 1999;12(10):785–791.
11. Bennett M, Lucas V, Brennan M, et al. Using anti-muscarinic drugs in the management of death rattle: evidence-based guidelines for palliative care. *Palliative Med* 2002;16(5):369–374.
12. Heath WE. Death from atropine poisoning. *BMJ* 1950;2:608.
13. Legroux P. A propos d'un cas d'intoxication mortelle par un collyre a l'atropine. *Ann Ocul* 1962;195:48–52.
14. Alexander E Jr, Eslick RL, Morris DP. Atropine poisoning: report of a case with recovery after ingestion of one gram. *N Engl J Med* 1946;234:258.
15. Wright BD. Exacerbation of akinetic seizures by atropine eye drops. *Br J Ophthalmol* 1992;76(3):179–180.
16. Saarnivaara L, Kautto UM, Iisalo E, et al. Comparison of pharmacokinetic and pharmacodynamic parameters following oral or intramuscular atropine in children. Atropine overdose in two small children. *Acta Anaesthesiol Scand* 1985;29(5):529–536.
17. Ketchum JS, Sidell FR, Crowell EB Jr, et al. Atropine, scopolamine, and ditran: comparative pharmacology and antagonists in man. *Psychopharmacologia* 1973;28(2):121–145.
18. Herschman ZJ, Silverstein J, Blumberg G, et al. Central nervous system toxicity from nebulized atropine sulfate. *J Toxicol Clin Toxicol* 1991;29(2):273–277.
19. Hoefnagel D. Toxic effects of atropine and homatropine eyedrops in children. *N Engl J Med* 1961;264:168–171.
20. Tune LE, Bylsma FW, Hilt DC. Anticholinergic delirium caused by topical homatropine ophthalmologic solution: confirmation by anticholinergic radioreceptor assay in two cases. *J Neuropsychiatry Clin Neurosci* 1992;4(2):195–197.
21. Reid D, Fulton JD. Tachycardia precipitated by topical homatropine. *BMJ* 1989;299(6702):795–796.
22. Purcell MJ. Atropine poisoning in infancy. *BMJ* 1966;5489:738.
23. Meerstadt PW. Atropine poisoning in early infancy due to Eumydrin drops. *BMJ* 1982;285(6336):196–197.
24. Gross NJ, Skorodin MS. Massive overdose of atropine methonitrate with only slight untoward effects. *Lancet* 1985;2(8451):386.
25. Dawson A, Oakley P, Isbister G, et al. Tacrine in the treatment of anticholinergic delirium. *J Toxicol Clin Toxicol* 2003;41:412–413.
26. Arnold P, Beaird D, Curry S. Serial plasma benzotropine concentrations after overdose. *Vet Hum Toxicol* 1987;29:482.
27. Fahy P, Arnold P, Curry SC, et al. Serial serum drug concentrations and prolonged anticholinergic toxicity after benztropine (Cogentin) overdose. *Am J Emerg Med* 1989;7(2):199–202.
28. Lynch MJ, Kotsos A. Fatal benztropine toxicity. *Med Sci Law* 2001;41(2):155–158.
29. Catterson ML, Martin RL. Anticholinergic toxicity masquerading as neuroleptic malignant syndrome: a case report and review. *Ann Clin Psychiatry* 1994;6(4):267–269.

30. Forester D. Fatal drug-induced heat stroke. *JACEP* 1978;7(6):243–244.
31. Meadow SR, Leeson GA. Poisoning with delayed-release tablets. Treatment of debendox poisoning with purgation and dialysis. *Arch Dis Child* 1974;49(4):310–312.
32. Greenblatt DJ, Allen MD, Koch-Weser J, et al. Accidental poisoning with psychotropic drugs in children. *Am J Dis Child* 1976;130(5):507–511.
33. Clarkson SG, Glanvill AP. Debendox overdosage in children. *BMJ* 1977;2(6084):459–460.
34. Williams J, Watkins-Jones R. Dicyclomine: worrying symptoms associated with its use in some small babies. *BMJ* 1984;288(6421):901.
35. Dicyclomine in babies. *BMJ* 1984;288(6425):1230–1231.
36. Garriott JC, Rodriquez R, Norton LE. Two cases of death involving dicyclomine in infants. Measurement of therapeutic and toxic concentrations in blood. *J Toxicol Clin Toxicol* 1984;22(5):455–462
37. Bayley M, Walsh FM, Valaske MJ. Fatal overdose from bendectin. *Clin Pediatr* 1975;14(5):507–509.
38. Sarafana L, Clark GC, Stotzer H. [Toxicological studies on ipratropium bromide (author's translation).] [German] *Arzneimittelforsch* 1976;26(5a):985–989.
39. Bond DW, Vyas H, Venning HE. Mydriasis due to self-administered inhaled ipratropium bromide. *Eur J Pediatr* 2002;161(3):178.
40. Calderin Morales MP, Gallego M, Aguilar HE, et al. Pupillary asymmetry secondary to local administration of ipratropium bromide. [Spanish] *Acta Pediatrica Española* 2001;59(4):219–221.
41. Lellouche N, Guglielminotti J, Saint-Jean M, et al. Acute glaucoma induced by ipratropium and salbutamol aerosol treatment [1]. [French] *Presse Med* 1999;28(19):1017.
42. Banerjee S, Routledge PA, Pugh S, et al. Poisoning with oxybutynin. *Hum Exp Toxicol* 1991;10(3):225–226.
43. Choulot JJ, Mensire A, Saint MJ. [Overdose of anticholinergic agents and confusional syndrome.] [French] *Ann Pediatr (Paris)* 1989;36(10):714.
44. Adubofour KO, Kajiwara GT, Goldberg CM, et al. Oxybutynin-induced heatstroke in an elderly patient. *Ann Pharmacother* 1996;30(2):144–147.
45. Teoh R, Page AV, Hardern R. Physostigmine as treatment for severe CNS anticholinergic toxicity. *Emerg Med J* 2001;18(5):412.
46. McGucken RB, Caldwell J, Anthon B. Teenage procyclidine abuse. *Lancet* 1985;1(8444):1514.
47. Caston JC, Randels PM, Keeler MA. Intoxication with procyclidine (Kemadrin): report of three cases. *J SC Med Assoc* 1973;69(2):37–39.
48. Coid J, Strang J. Mania secondary to procyclidine ("Kemadrin") abuse. *Br J Psychiatry* 1982;141:81–84.
49. Balikova M. Collective poisoning with hallucinogenous herbal tea. *Forensic Sci Int* 2002;128(1-2):50–52.
50. Goldfrank L, Flomenbaum N, Lewin N, et al. Anticholinergic poisoning. *J Toxicol Clin Toxicol* 1982;19(1):17–25.
51. Nogue S, Sanz P, Munne P, et al. Acute scopolamine poisoning after sniffing adulterated cocaine. *Drug Alcohol Depend* 1991;27(2):115–116.
52. Urich RW, Bowerman DL, Levisky JA, et al. *Datura stramonium*: a fatal poisoning. *J Forensic Sci* 1982;27(4):948–954.
53. Holland MS. Central anticholinergic syndrome in a pediatric patient following transdermal scopolamine patch placement. *Nurse Anesthes* 1992;3(3):121–124.
54. Minagar A, Shulman LM, Weiner WJ. Transderm-induced psychosis in Parkinson's disease [Comment]. *Neurology* 1999;53(2):433–434.
55. Mego DM, Omori JM, Hanley JF. Transdermal scopolamine as a cause of transient psychosis in two elderly patients. *South Med J* 1988;81(3):394–395.
56. Connolly MJ, Astridge PS, White EG, et al. Torsades de pointes ventricular tachycardia and terodiline [Comment]. *Lancet* 1991;338(8763):344–345.
57. Thomas SH, Higham PD, Hartigan-Go K, et al. Concentration dependent cardiotoxicity of terodiline in patients treated for urinary incontinence. *Br Heart J* 1995;74(1):53–56.
58. Hartigan-Go K, Bateman DN, Daly AK, et al. Stereoselective cardiotoxic effects of terodiline. *Clin Pharmacol Ther* 1996;60(1):89–98.
59. Ford GA, Wood SM, Daly AK. CYP2D6 and CYP2C19 genotypes of patients with terodiline cardiotoxicity identified through the yellow card system. *Br J Clin Pharmacol* 2000;50(1):77–80.
60. Ananth JV. Toxic psychosis induced by benzhexol hydrochloride. *Can Med Assoc J* 1970;103(7):771.
61. Stephens DA. Psychotoxic effects of benzhexol hydrochloride (Artane). *Br J Psychiatry* 1967;113(495):213-218.
62. Gall JAM, Drummer OH, Landgren AJ. Death due to benzhexol toxicity. *Forensic Sci Int* 1995;71(1):9-14.
63. Van H, Mertens K, Maes V, et al. Orphenadrine poisoning in a child: clinical and analytical data. *Intensive Care Med* 1999;25(10):1134-1136.
64. Garza MB, Osterhoudt KC, Rutstein R. Central anticholinergic syndrome from orphenadrine in a 3 year old. *Pediatr Emerg Care* 2000;16(2):97–98.
65. Danze LK, Langdorf MI. Reversal of orphenadrine-induced ventricular tachycardia with physostigmine. *J Emerg Med* 1991;9(6):453–457.
66. Buckley N, McManus P. Fatal toxicity of drugs used in the treatment of psychotic illnesses [Comment]. *Br J Psychiatry* 1998;172:461–464.
67. Gjerden P, Engelstad KS, Pettersen G, et al. [Fatalities caused by anticholinergic antiparkinsonian drugs. Analysis of findings in an 11-year national material] [Comment]. [Norwegian] *Tidsskr Nor Laegeforen* 1998;118(1):42–44.
68. Sangster B, Van Heijst AN, Zimmerman AN, et al. Intoxication by orphenadrine HCl; mechanism and therapy. *Acta Pharmacol Toxicol* 1977;41[Suppl 2]:129–136.
69. Sangster B, Van Heijst AN, Zimmerman AN. Treatment of orphenadrine overdose. *N Engl J Med* 1977;296(17):1006.
70. Bozza-Marrubini M, Frigerio A, Ghezzi R, et al. Two cases of severe orphenadrine poisoning with atypical features. *Acta Pharmacol Toxicol* 1977;41[Suppl 2]:137–152.
71. Brocks DR. Anticholinergic drugs used in Parkinson's disease: an overlooked class of drugs from a pharmacokinetic perspective [Review]. *J Pharm Sci* 1999;2(2):39–46.
72. Guthrie SK, Manzey L, Scott D, et al. Comparison of central and peripheral pharmacologic effects of biperiden and trihexyphenidyl in human volunteers. *J Clin Psychopharmacol* 2000;20(1):77–83.
73. Kaila T, Korte JM, Saari KM. Systemic bioavailability of ocularly applied 1% atropine eyedrops. *Acta Ophthalmol Scand* 1999;77(2):193–196.
74. Ensing K, de Zeeuw RA, Nossent GD, et al. Pharmacokinetics of ipratropium bromide after single dose inhalation and oral and intravenous administration. *Eur J Clin Pharmacol* 1989;36(2):189–194.
75. Meffin PJ, Moore G, Thomas J. Determination of dicyclomine in plasma by gas chromatography. *Anal Chem* 1973;45(11):1964–1966.
76. Gupta SK, Sathyan G. Pharmacokinetics of an oral once-a-day controlled-release oxybutynin formulation compared with immediate-release oxybutynin. *J Clin Pharmacol* 1999;39(3):289–296.
77. Douchamps J, Derenne F, Stockis A, et al. The pharmacokinetics of oxybutynin in man. *Eur J Clin Pharmacol* 1988;35(5):515–520.
78. Lehtoranta K, Tainio H, Lukkari-Lax E, et al. Pharmacokinetics, efficacy, and safety of intravesical formulation of oxybutynin in patients with detrusor overactivity. *Scand J Urol Nephrol* 2002;36(1):18–24.
79. Whiteman PD, Fowle AS, Hamilton MJ, et al. Pharmacokinetics and pharmacodynamics of procyclidine in man. *Eur J Clin Pharmacol* 1985;28(1):73–78.
80. He H, McKay G, Wirshing B, et al. Development and application of a specific and sensitive radioimmunoassay for trihexyphenidyl to a pharmacokinetic study in humans. *J Pharm Sci* 1995;84(5):561–567.
81. Labout JJ, Thijssen C, Keijser GG, et al. Difference between single and multiple dose pharmacokinetics of orphenadrine hydrochloride in man. *Eur J Clin Pharmacol* 1982;21(4):343–350.
82. Michelson EA, Schneider SM, Martin TG. Adult inadvertent massive oral atropine overdose. *Vet Hum Toxicol* 1991;(33):360.
83. Amitai Y, Singer R, Almog S, et al. Atropine poisoning in children from automatic injectors during the Gulf crisis. *Vet Hum Toxicol* 1991;(33).
84. Jindal SP, Lutz T, Hallstrom C, et al. A stable isotope dilution assay for the antiparkinsonian drug benztropine in biological fluids. *Clin Chim Acta* 1981;112(3):267–273.
85. Baselt RC, Cravey RH. *Disposition of toxic drugs and chemicals in man*, 3rd ed. Chicago: Year Book, 1989:720–721.
86. Van H, I, Mertens K, Maes V, et al. Orphenadrine poisoning in a child: clinical and analytical data. *Intensive Care Med* 1999;25(10):1134–1136.
87. Brann MR, Jorgensen HB, Burstein ES, et al. Studies of the pharmacology, localization, and structure of muscarinic acetylcholine receptors [Review]. *Ann N Y Acad Sci* 1993;707:225–236.
88. Bolden C, Cusack B, Richelson E. Antagonism by antimuscarinic and neuroleptic compounds at the five cloned human muscarinic cholinergic receptors expressed in Chinese hamster ovary cells. *J Pharmacol Exp Ther* 1992;260(2):576–580.
89. Clark RF. Orphenadrine poisoning and review of physostigmine. *J Emerg Med* 1993;11(1):97.
90. Pubill D, Canudas AM, Pallas M, et al. Assessment of the adrenergic effects of orphenadrine in rat vas deferens. *J Pharm Pharmacol* 1999;51(3):307–312.
91. Hunskaar S, Rosland JH, Hole K. Mechanisms of orphenadrine-induced antinociception in mice: a role for serotonergic pathways. *Eur J Pharmacol* 1989;160(1):83–91.
92. Sangster B, Nieuwland G, Zimmerman AN, et al. The influence of orphenadrine HCl in overdose alone and in combination with droperidol on respiration and circulation in the rat. *Toxicol Eur Res* 1979;2(2):93–97.
93. Van H, Mertens K, Maes V, et al. Orphenadrine poisoning in a child: clinical and analytical data. *Intensive Care Med* 1999;25(10):1134–1136.
94. Wilkinson LF, Thomson BM, Pannel LK. A report on the analysis of orphenadrine in post mortem specimens. *J Anal Toxicol* 1983;7:72–75.
95. How J, Strachan RW. Acute dilatation of stomach as late complication of drug overdose. *BMJ* 1976;1(6009):563–564.
96. Flicker C, Ferris SH, Serby M. Hypersensitivity to scopolamine in the elderly. *Psychopharmacologia* 1992;107(2–3):437–441.
97. Nakra BR, Margolis RB, Gfeller JD, et al. The effect of a single low dose of trihexyphenidyl on memory functioning in the healthy elderly. *Int Psychogeriatr* 1992;4(2):207–214.
98. Price BH. Anisocoria from scopolamine patches. *JAMA* 1985;253(11):1561.
99. Hamill MB, Suelflow JA, Smith JA. Transdermal scopolamine delivery system (TRANSDERM-V) and acute angle-closure glaucoma. *Ann Ophthalmol* 1983;15(11):1011–1012.
100. Guo Z, Raeissi S, White RB, et al. Orphenadrine and methimazole inhibit multiple cytochrome P450 enzymes in human liver microsomes. *Drug Metab Dispos* 1997;25(3):390–393.
101. Aguilera L, Martinez-Bourio R, Cid C, et al. Anaphylactic reaction after atropine. *Anaesthesia* 1988;43(11):955–957.
102. Gordon CR, Shupak A, Doweck I, et al. Allergic contact dermatitis caused by transdermal hyoscine. *BMJ* 1989;298(6682):1220–1221.
103. Facchini G, Antonicelli L, Cinti B, et al. Paradoxical bronchospasm and cutaneous rash after metered-dose inhaled bronchodilators. *Monaldi Arch Chest Dis* 1996;51(3):201–203.

104. Beasley CR, Rafferty P, Holgate ST. Bronchoconstrictor properties of preservatives in ipratropium bromide (Atrovent) nebuliser solution. *Br Med J Clin Res Ed* 1987;294(6581):1197–1198.
105. Harris WS, Goodman RM. Hyper-reactivity to atropine in Down's syndrome. *N Engl J Med* 1968;279(8):407–410.
106. Kajimura N, Mizuki Y, Kai S, et al. Memory and cognitive impairments in a case of long-term trihexyphenidyl abuse. *Pharmacopsychiatry* 1993;26(2):59–62.
107. Schafer WD, Sauerland HJ. [Observations on long term medication with atropine eye-drops (author's translation).] [German] *Klin Monatsbl Augenheilkd* 1976;168(3):421–423.
108. Kjeldaas L. [Scopoderm depot plasters—confusions and hallucinations.] [Norwegian] *Tidsskr Nor Laegeforen* 1986;106(5):436–437.
109. Saxena K, Saxena S. Scopolamine withdrawal syndrome. *Postgrad Med* 1990;87(1):63–66.
110. Rosano TG, Meola JM, Wolf BC, et al. Benztropine identification and quantitation in a suicidal overdose. *J Anal Toxicol* 1994;18(6):348–353.
111. Robinson AE, Holder AT, McDowall RD, et al. Forensic toxicology of some orphenadrine-related deaths. *Forensic Sci* 1977;9(1):53–62.
112. Burns MJ, Linden CH, Graudins A, et al. A comparison of physostigmine and benzodiazepines for the treatment of anticholinergic poisoning [Comment]. *Ann Emerg Med* 2000;35(4):374–381.
113. Beaver KM, Gavin TJ. Treatment of acute anticholinergic poisoning with physostigmine. *Am J Emerg Med* 1998;16(5):505–507.
114. Mendelson G. Central anticholinergic syndrome reversed by tetrahydroaminacrine (tha). *Med J Aust* 1975;2(24):906–909.
115. Cozanitis DA. Galanthamine hydrobromide, a longer acting anticholinesterase drug, in the treatment of the central effects of scopolamine (Hyoscine). *Anaesthesist* 1977;26(12):649–650.
116. Zandberg P, Sangster B. The influence of physostigmine on respiratory and circulatory changes caused by overdoses of orphenadrine or imipramine in the rat. *Acta Pharmacol Toxicol* 1982;50(3):185–195.
117. Isbister GK, Oakley P, Whyte I, et al. Treatment of anticholinergic-induced ileus with neostigmine. *Ann Emerg Med* 2001;38(6):689–693.

CHAPTER 101

Cholinergic Drugs

Andrew H. Dawson

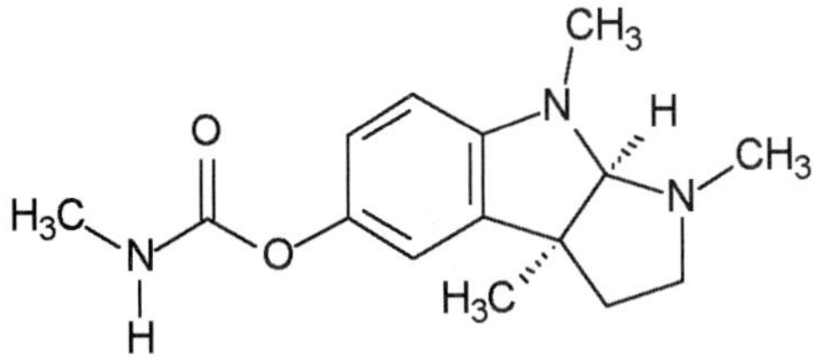

PHYSOSTIGMINE

Compounds included:	**Ambenonium, bethanechol (Duvoid, Urecholine), donepezil (Aricept), edrophonium (Enlon, Tensilon), galantamine (Reminyl), neostigmine (Prostigmin), physostigmine (Antilirium), pyridostigmine (Mestinon, Rogonon), rivastigmine (Exelon), tacrine (Cognex)**
Molecular formula and weight:	**See Table 1.**
SI conversion:	**See Table 1.**
CAS Registry No.:	**See Table 1.**
Target organs:	**Peripheral and central cholinergic system**
Antidote:	**Atropine**

OVERVIEW

The therapeutic and toxic effects of cholinergic drugs are mediated by reversible inhibition of cholinesterase enzymes, thereby increasing the acetylcholine (ACh) concentration and increasing cholinergic nerve transmission. As the understanding of the role of cholinergic transmission increases, their use has found wider clinical indications.

Physostigmine was isolated from the Calabar bean (Physostigma venenosum) in 1864. It was used in the "ordeal by poison" in the Calabar Province of Nigeria. In this ritual, an accused person drinks a solution of poisonous beans, dying if guilty and surviving if innocent (1). Physostigmine was subsequently noted to antagonize the effects of atropine and curare. The observation of curare antagonism led Mary Walker to use physostigmine in myasthenia gravis (2). Efficacy in this disorder led to the development of an understanding of the mechanism of that disease and new therapeutic compounds. Subsequent use was mainly restricted to this disease and reversal of anesthesia.

Evidence of efficacy in Alzheimer's dementia led to the registration of tacrine in 1993. A number of other centrally acting cholinesterase inhibitors with less toxic side effect profiles were subsequently developed. Current research is exploring the efficacy of these agents in other neurologic and psychiatric diseases (3–6), and it is therefore likely that the indications and extent of use of these compounds will expand. The clinical pattern of cholinergic toxicity is determined by the extent to which each drug inhibits acetylcholinesterase and butylcholinesterase and to whether it crosses the blood–brain barrier.

Structure, Classification, and Uses

Physostigmine is predominantly used for the treatment of anticholinergic delirium (Chapter 67) as it crosses the blood–brain barrier. Neostigmine is predominantly used for the reversal of neuromuscular blockade induced by nondepolarizing neuromuscular blocking agents. As it is a quaternary ammonium compound, it does not cross the blood–brain barrier. It can be used in treating myasthenia gravis when a parenteral medica-

TABLE 1. Physical characteristics and dosage of cholinergic medications

Drug (reference), CAS Registry No.	Molecular formula, molecular weight, (g/mol), SI conversion	Formulation	Dose (oral route, unless specified)
Ambenonium chloride, 52022-31-8	$C_{28}H_{42}Cl_4N_4O_2$, 608.5, NR	No longer available	5–75 mg, 3 or 4 times daily
Bethanechol chloride, 590-63-6	$C_7H_{17}ClN_2O_2$, 196.7, NR	5 mg/ml solution; 5-, 10-, 25-, 50-mg tablets	10–30 mg 4 times daily
Donepezil chloride (12), 120011-70-3	$C_{24}H_{29}NO_3$,HCl, 416.0, NR	5-, 10-mg tablets	5–10 mg daily
Edrophonium chloride (13), 116-38-1	$C_{10}H_{16}ClNO$, 201.7, NR	10-mg/ml solution	2–10 mg IV
Galantamine hydrobromide (12), 1953-04-4	$C_{17}H_{21}NO_3$,HBr, 368.3, NR	4-mg/ml solution; 4-, 8-, 12-mg tablets	4–12 mg 2 times daily
Neostigmine bromide (13), 114-80-7	$C_{12}H_{19}BrN_2O_2$, 303.2, mg/L × 4.48 = nmol/L	0.5, 1.0, 2.5 mg/ml solution; 15-mg tablet	Myasthenia gravis: adult, SQ/IM 1.0–2.5 mg; child, SQ/IM 200–500 µg. Reversal of neuromuscular blockade: adult, IV 50–70 µg/kg, up to 5 mg; child, IV 50-µg/kg/dose, up to 2.5 mg
Physostigmine salicylate (13), 57-64-7	$C_{15}H_{21}N_3O_2$,$C_7H_6O_3$, 413.5, µg/L × 3.63 = nmol/L	0.5, 1.0 mg/ml solution; 0.25, 0.5% ophthalmic solution	0.5–2.0 mg IV
Pyridostigmine bromide (13), 101-26-8	$C_9H_{13}BrN_2O_2$, 261.1, mg/L × 5.52 = µmol	10-, 100-mg tablets; 180-mg controlled release	300–720 mg daily in divided doses
Rivastigmine tartrate (12), 129101-54-8	$C_{14}H_{22}N_2O_2.C_4H_6O_6$, 400.4, NR	1.5-, 3-, 4.5-, 6-mg capsules, 2 mg/ml liquid	1.5–6.0 mg 2 times daily
Tacrine hydrochloride, 1684-40-8	$C_{13}H_{14}N_2$,HCl, 234.7, NR	10-, 20-, 30-, 40-mg capsules	10–40 mg 4 times daily

NR, not reported.

tion is required. It has been shown to have efficacy in colonic pseudo-obstruction from all causes (7) and following benztropine poisoning (8). Ambenonium was used for similar indications but is no longer available.

Pyridostigmine is a quaternary cholinesterase inhibitor that is the first-line treatment for oral maintenance therapy of myasthenia gravis. It is available as an oral formulation and has a slower onset and longer duration of action than neostigmine.

Edrophonium is a quaternary cholinesterase inhibitor that is used primarily in the diagnosis of myasthenia gravis. It is extremely short acting. Patients are given 2 mg and re-examined; if there is no effect, they can be given up to a further 6 mg. Small doses can be used to distinguish between a myasthenic crisis (which should improve) and cholinergic toxicity (which is exacerbated). *Bethanechol* is used to increase bladder contraction by parasympathomimetic stimulation.

Donepezil, galantamine, rivastigmine, and *tacrine* have all been shown to have efficacy in Alzheimer's disease. Their primary mechanism of action is to improve central cholinergic transmission. The drugs also increase amyloid precursor protein metabolism and may be disease modifying (9). Their use has been investigated in the treatment of other neurologic disorders (3–5), and they have been reported to be used in the treatment of anticholinergic (10,10a) and nonanticholinergic delirium (11). Tacrine's side effect profile has led it to be the least preferred treatment option for drugs in this class. Controlled-release preparations of physostigmine are also effective but are not released commercially.

Toxic Doses

The *adult and pediatric therapeutic doses* for cholinergic agents are provided in Table 1. The toxic dose of physostigmine varies considerably. Doses of 1 mg have been associated with seizures in the setting of tricyclic toxicity, whereas patients with clear anticholinergic toxicity tolerate high and repeated doses. Powdered physostigmine salicylate, 1 g, produced paradoxically dilated pupils and central and peripheral cholinergic symptoms, including seizures. Symptoms started 10 minutes after ingestion. Cholinesterase activity was depressed and returned to the lower limit of normal 26 hours after ingestion. Atropine (1.05 mg) was associated with development of multifocal ventricular ectopic beats and tachycardia; 1 g aldoxime was given without any evidence or cholinesterase reactivation (14).

Neostigmine in a dose of 45 mg produced severe toxicity in a volunteer (15). An intravenous dose of 2 mg for acute colonic pseudo-obstruction in 18 patients produced transient abdominal pain in 13, increased salivation in 8, and symptomatic bradycardia that required atropine in 2 patients (7). Edrophonium chloride, 10 mg intravenously, caused an atropine-responsive sinus bradycardia and asystole in a 66-year-old woman who had been admitted 17 days previously for myocardial infarction (16).

Nine cases of pyridostigmine self-poisoning with doses of 390 to 900 mg resulted in mild to moderate cholinergic symptoms, such as abdominal cramps, diarrhea, emesis, nausea, hypersalivation, urinary incontinence, fasciculations, muscle weakness, and blurred vision. No central nervous system (CNS) manifestations were evident. The symptoms were associated with cholinesterase depression ranging from 25% to 79%, which was thought to correspond with severity. The symptoms developed within several minutes and lasted up to 24 hours. Atropine (1 to 8 mg) was required in only three patients (17). Pyridostigmine bromide administered in doses of either 120 mg orally four times a day or as a sustained-release dose of 180 mg is sufficient to produce bromide intoxication (18).

A donepezil ingestion by a 74-year-old resulted in drowsiness for 4 to 5 hours; her subsequent recovery was uneventful (19). A 79-year-old received 50 mg donepezil instead of her usual 5-mg dose. She experienced nausea, vomiting, and persistent bradycardia. She required intermittent doses of 0.2 mg atropine to treat bradycardia; a total of 3.0 mg was administered over 18 hours. Each bolus kept her pulse rate above 60 beats/minute for 0.5 to 2.0 hours. Her pulse rate returned to baseline by day 2 (20).

TABLE 2. Pharmacokinetics of cholinergic agents

Name	Bioavailability (%)	T_{max} (h)	Half-life (h)	Protein binding (%)	Metabolism
Tacrine	17–33	1–2	1.3–2.0	75	CYP1A2, CYP2D6
Donepezil	100	3–5	70–80	96	CYP2D6, CYP3A4
Rivastigmine	40	0.5–2.0	2	40	Nonhepatic
Physostigmine	3–22	0.75	0.3	50	Hepatic cholinesterase
Galantamine	85–100	0.5–1.0	5–7	18	CYP2D6, CYP3A4

Adapted from Cummings JL. Cholinesterase inhibitors: a new class of psychotropic compounds. *Am J Psychiatry* 2000;157(1):4–15, and Jann MW, Shirley KL, Small GW. Clinical pharmacokinetics and pharmacodynamics of cholinesterase inhibitors. *Clin Pharmacokinet* 2002;41(10):719–739.

TOXICOKINETICS AND TOXICODYNAMICS

The pharmacokinetics of the reversible quaternary cholinesterase inhibitors neostigmine, pyridostigmine, and edrophonium are relatively similar. Oral bioavailability is low: 10% for pyridostigmine and even lower for neostigmine. One to 2 hours after oral administration of 60 mg pyridostigmine, peak plasma concentrations of 40 to 60 μg/L are observed, whereas the plasma concentrations of neostigmine after a 30-mg oral dose are only 1 to 5 μg/L. Plasma clearance ranges from 0.5 to 1.0 L/kg per hour, and their apparent volumes of distribution range from 0.5 to 1.7 L/kg. Elimination half-lives are short, on the order of 30 to 90 minutes, but are longer in the presence of severe renal failure (4).

After intravenous administration, physostigmine had very rapid plasma elimination, with a plasma clearance ranging from 47 L/hour to 163 L per hour (mean, 92.5 L/hour). The volume of distribution was 46.5 L, and distribution and plasma elimination half-lives were 2.3 and 22.0 minutes, respectively (21). Oral bioavailability was 25.3 minutes (22).

The kinetics and pharmacodynamics of tacrine, rivastigmine, galantamine, and donepezil have been studied more intensively than those of the other agents (Table 2). The measure of "efficacy" used in these studies is the degree of cholinesterase inhibition. At the upper end of the therapeutic dose range, inhibition of cholinesterase activity ranges from 60% to 80%. The therapeutic range is considered to be 40% to 70% inhibition; however, inhibition of peripheral cholinesterase correlates poorly with central cholinesterase inhibition (23,24).

PATHOPHYSIOLOGY

Cholinesterase inhibitors inhibit the enzymes acetylcholinesterase and butylcholinesterase, thereby reducing synaptic degradation of ACh. The resultant increase in synaptic ACh concentration produces stimulation of muscarinic and nicotinic cholinergic receptors in the CNS and in the peripheral nervous system. Normally, ACh binds to an esteratic and an anionic site in a "gorge" within the enzyme. Further esteratic and anionic sites are located peripherally, figuratively at the entrance to the gorge region of the enzyme. Cholinesterase inhibitors bind to at least one gorge site inhibiting ACh breakdown, and in addition some cholinesterase inhibitors may bind to a peripheral site, inhibiting entry of ACh into the gorge (Table 3). The nature of the binding determines the duration of action of each cholinesterase agent. In addition, some cholinesterase inhibitors (galantamine, physostigmine) bind to the nicotinic ACh receptor (25), which may increase ACh release. Tacrine may have some direct effects on the muscarinic receptor (26).

PREGNANCY AND LACTATION

Each of these agents is U.S. Food and Drug Administration pregnancy category C (Appendix I). Donepezil is Australian pregnancy category B3, galantamine is category B1, neostigmine is category B2, and pyridostigmine is category C (12). Information on breast-feeding is not available for the cholinergic agents, except for neostigmine and pyridostigmine, which are considered safe for use by breast-feeding mothers (28).

CLINICAL PRESENTATION

Acute Exposure

Onset of symptoms is usually rapid following ingestion. The clinical syndrome may be thought of as a varying combination of peripheral and central cholinergic signs. The variability in the clinical picture relates to the relative selectiveness for the enzymes that degrade the cholinergic agents (acetylcholinesterase and butylcholinesterase) combined with the physiochemical properties that determine whether the drug crosses the blood–brain barrier.

Central symptoms include CNS excitation, delirium, seizures, and respiratory depression. Peripheral symptoms and signs of ACh excess include abdominal cramps, diarrhea, emesis, nausea, hypersalivation, urinary incontinence, fasciculation, muscle weakness, miosis, blurred vision, bronchospasm, bronchorrhea, and bradycardia. The combination of muscle weakness, bronchospasm, and bronchorrhea can lead to respiratory failure.

TABLE 3. Sites of action and esterase preference for the cholinergic drugs

Name	Class	Selectivity	Enzymatic site of action
Tacrine	Acridine	BChE > AChE (4-fold) (27)	Anionic[g]
Donepezil	Piperidine	AChE >> BChE (188-fold) (27)	Anionic[gp]
Rivastigmine	Carbamate	AChE = BChE	Anionic[g] and esteratic[g]
Physostigmine	Carbamate	BChE > AChE (2-fold) (27)	Esteratic
Galantamine[a]	Phenanthrene alkaloid	AChE > BChE (9-fold) (27)	Esteratic[gp]

[a], active O-demethyl metabolite; AChE, acetylcholinesterase; BChE, butylcholinesterase; [g], gorge site; [gp], gorge and peripheral.
Adapted from Cummings JL. Cholinesterase inhibitors: a new class of psychotropic compounds. *Am J Psychiatry* 2000;157(1):4–15, and Jann MW, Shirley KL, Small GW. Clinical pharmacokinetics and pharmacodynamics of cholinesterase inhibitors. *Clin Pharmacokinet* 2002;41(10):719–739.

Physostigmine may produce paradoxic pupil dilation at high doses (14,29). The risk of toxicity may be increased when physostigmine is administered with lithium (30).

Pyridostigmine overdose may lead to a cholinergic crisis with increased cholinergic effects (e.g., excessive sweating, involuntary defecation and urination, miosis, nystagmus, bradycardia, hypotension, increased muscle weakness leading to fasciculation and paralysis), CNS effects (e.g., ataxia, convulsions, agitation, and coma), and death due to respiratory failure or cardiac arrest. Distinction between a cholinergic crisis (overtreatment) and a myasthenic crisis (undertreatment) may be difficult and may require an edrophonium test. Normally, a cholinergic crisis occurs within an hour of ingestion, whereas a myasthenic crisis occurs later when drug concentrations fall.

Adverse Events

Physostigmine eye drops may cause local conjunctival hyperemia, discomfort from ciliary muscle contraction, and contact allergic blepharoconjunctivitis (29). Dose-dependent side effects were common in clinical trials of various cholinergic agonists in patients with Alzheimer's disease. These trials generally used fixed escalating dose regimens that may not reflect individual clinical management. At the upper end of the normal, the suggested therapeutic dose range nausea occurred in 11% to 50% of patients, vomiting in 11% to 35%, and diarrhea in 10% to 17% (24). Other common dose-related side effects included abdominal pain, dyspepsia, headache, insomnia, fatigue, dizziness, tremor, weight loss, muscle cramps, urinary incontinence, and increased sweating. Infrequent or rare side effects included syncope, bradycardia, heart block, seizure, agitation, hallucination, confusion, gastrointestinal hemorrhage, and hypertension.

Tacrine causes elevation of the serum transaminase in approximately 40% of patients, requiring strict monitoring; it should not be used in new patients. Risk appears to be associated with deficiencies of two glutathione S-transferase isoenzymes and is not clearly dose related (31). Tacrine in high doses caused myocyte damage in rats, possibly from increased nicotinic stimulation (32).

Given the known effects of cholinergic stimulation, the use of cholinergic drugs is relatively contraindicated in patients with a history of ulcer disease, sick sinus syndrome, seizures, bradydysrhythmia, asthma, or obstructive pulmonary disease.

DIAGNOSTIC TESTS

Measurement of the cholinergic agents in the blood is not clinically useful. However, measurement of the serum cholinesterase activity was found to be a reliable and sensitive diagnostic tool in pyridostigmine poisoning. Red cell and serum cholinesterase are depressed by therapy with all the cholinesterase inhibitors in clinical use (24); cholinesterase measurement should be a sensitive marker of exposure. No clear correlation was found between the extent of cholinesterase inhibition and the incidence or severity of the cholinergic signs (17).

Pyridostigmine bromide may cause bromide toxicity and spuriously elevate the serum chloride values (33). Other testing may be needed to evaluate the toxic effects of altered mental status, seizure, or cardiac dysrhythmia.

TREATMENT

Patients should have cardiac monitoring and frequent assessment of the adequacy of respiration and neuromuscular function. Cholinergic symptoms should be treated with atropine, and seizures are treated with benzodiazepines as described below.

Decontamination

Activated charcoal should be offered to patients who present within 1 hour. Repeated doses of activated charcoal or whole bowel irrigation should be considered following ingestion of controlled-release medications.

Enhancement of Elimination

Hemoperfusion and hemodialysis are not indicated and are in any case unlikely to be effective in view of the kinetics of these agents.

Antidotes

In clinical practice the first line of treatment is repeated doses of atropine titrated against clinical response (Chapter 42). Animal modes of physostigmine toxicity have confirmed that muscarinics such as atropine and benztropine that penetrate the CNS improve survival compared with agents that do not cross the blood–brain barrier (34). The combination of atropine and diazepam improved survival from physostigmine poisoning in a mouse model, whereas atropine and pralidoxime did not show any benefit over atropine alone (35).

Following a symptomatic physostigmine ingestion of 1 g, atropine (1.05 mg) was associated with development of multifocal ventricular ectopics and tachycardia; 1 g aldoxime was given without any evidence of cholinesterase reactivation (14). Atropine-associated tachycardia reported in a physostigmine-toxic patient was controlled with intravenous propranolol (36). In situations in which bronchospasm is prominent, patients could receive adjunctive treatment with ipratropium; this has been effective in exacerbation of chronic obstructive pulmonary disease by cholinesterase inhibitors (37,38).

Three of nine cases of pyridostigmine self-poisoning required atropine (1 to 8 mg) to relieve symptoms (17). An elderly woman required a total of 3.0 mg atropine in an 18-hour period to treat bradycardia (20).

Pretreatment of animals with clonidine reduced mortality in rats poisoned with physostigmine, but not those poisoned by neostigmine. This suggested that central cholinergic neurons involved in the regulation of respiration and fine motor control may be inhibited by clonidine acting on alpha receptors (39).

Supportive Care

Patients should have intravenous access, cardiorespiratory monitoring, supplemental oxygen, and seizure precautions provided. Hypotension is managed with isotonic crystalloidal intravenous fluids followed by vasopressor support, if necessary (Chapter 37). After stabilization of the airway, seizures should be with benzodiazepines followed by more aggressive interventions if needed (Chapter 40).

REFERENCES

1. Rygnestad T. [Development of physostigmine from a poisonous plant to an antidote. One of the most important drugs in the development of modern medicine?] [Norwegian]. *Tidsskrift for Den Norske Laegeforening* 1992;112(10):1300–1303.
2. Keesey JCM. Contemporary opinions about Mary Walker: a shy pioneer of therapeutic neurology. *Neurology* November 1998;51(5):1433–1439.
3. Fabbrini G, Barbanti P, Bonifati V, et al. Donepezil in the treatment of progressive supranuclear palsy. *Acta Neurol Scand* 2001;103(2):123–125.

4. Aquilonius SM, Hartvig P. Clinical pharmacokinetics of cholinesterase inhibitors. *Clin Pharmacokinet* 1986;11(3):236–249.
5. Nicolodi MM, Galeotti NP, Ghelardini CP, et al. Central cholinergic challenging of migraine by testing second-generation anticholinesterase drugs. *Headache* 2002;42(7):596–602.
6. Cummings JL. Cholinesterase inhibitors: a new class of psychotropic compounds. *Am J Psychiatry* 2000;157(1):4–15.
7. Ponec RJ, Saunders MD, Kimmey MB. Neostigmine for the treatment of acute colonic pseudo-obstruction. *N Engl J Med* 1999;341(3):137–141.
8. Isbister GK, Oakley P, Whyte I, et al. Treatment of anticholinergic-induced ileus with neostigmine. *Ann Emerg Med* 2001;38(6):689–693.
9. Giacobini E. Long-term stabilizing effect of cholinesterase inhibitors in the therapy of Alzheimer's disease. *J Neural Transm Suppl* 2002;(62):181–187.
10. Cozanitis DA. Galanthamine hydrobromide, a longer acting anticholinesterase drug, in the treatment of the central effects of scopolamine (Hyoscine). *Anaesthetist* 1977;26(12):649–650.
10a. Dawson A, Oakley P, Isbister G, et al. Tacrine in the treatment of anticholinergic delirium. *J Toxicol Clin Toxicol* 2003;41:412–413.
11. Fischer P. Successful treatment of nonanticholinergic delirium with a cholinesterase inhibitor. *J Clin Psychopharmacol* 2001;21(1):118.
12. Anticholinesterases. In: Rossi S, ed. *Australian medicines handbook*. Adelaide: Australian Medicines Handbook Pty Ltd, 2002.
13. Acetylcholinesterase inhibitors. In: Rossi S, ed. *Australian medicines handbook*. Adelaide: Australian Medicines Handbook Pty Ltd, 2002.
14. Cumming G, Harding LK, Prowse K. Treatment and recovery after massive overdose of physostigmine. *Lancet* 1968;2(7560):147–149.
15. Goodman LS, Bruckner WJ. The therapeutics of prostigmin. A warning concerning its oral use based on a personal experience. *JAMA* 1937;108:965–968.
16. Rossen RM, Krikorian J, Hancock EW. Ventricular asystole after edrophonium chloride administration. *JAMA* 1976;235(10):1041–1042.
17. Almog S, Winkler E, Amitai Y, et al. Acute pyridostigmine overdose: a report of nine cases. *Isr J Med Sci* 1991;27(11–12):659–663.
18. Schumm WR, Reppert EJ, Jurich AP, et al. Pyridostigmine bromide and the long-term subjective health status of a sample of female reserve component Gulf War veterans: a brief report. *Psychol Rep* 2001;88(1):306–308.
19. Greene YM, Noviasky J, Tariot PN. Donepezil overdose. *J Clin Psychiatry* 1999;60(1):56–57.
20. Shepherd G, Klein-Schwartz W, Edwards R. Donepezil overdose: a tenfold dosing error. *Ann Pharmacother* 1999;33(7–8):812–815.
21. Hartvig P, Wiklund L, Lindstrom B. Pharmacokinetics of physostigmine after intravenous, intramuscular and subcutaneous administration in surgical patients. *Acta Anaesthesiol Scand* 1986;30(2):177–182.
22. Hartvig P, Lindstrom B, Pettersson E, Wiklund L. Reversal of postoperative somnolence using a two-rate infusion of physostigmine. *Acta Anaesthesiol Scand* 1989;33(8):681–685.
23. Sramek JJ, Cutler NR. RBC cholinesterase inhibition: a useful surrogate marker for cholinesterase inhibitor activity in Alzheimer disease therapy? *Alzheimer Dis Assoc Disord* 2000;14(4):216–227.
24. Jann MW, Shirley KL, Small GW. Clinical pharmacokinetics and pharmacodynamics of cholinesterase inhibitors. *Clin Pharmacokinet* 2002;41(10):719–739.
25. Lilienfeld S, Parys W. Galantamine: additional benefits to patients with Alzheimer's disease. *Dement Geriatr Cogn Disord* 2000;11[Suppl 1]:19–27.
26. Becerra MA, Herrera MD, Marhuenda E. Action of tacrine on muscarinic receptors in rat intestinal smooth muscle. *J Auton Pharmacol* 2001;21(2):113–119.
27. Greig NH, De Micheli E, Holloway HW, et al. The experimental Alzheimer drug phenserine: preclinical pharmacokinetics and pharmacodynamics. *Acta Neurol Scand Suppl* 2000;102[Suppl 84].
28. Briggs GG, Freeman RK, Yaffe SJ. *Drugs in pregnancy and lactation*, 6th ed. Philadelphia: Lippincott Williams & Wilkins, 2002.
29. Grant WM, Schuman JS. *Toxicology of the eye*, 4th ed. Springfield, IL: Charles C Thomas Publisher, 1993.
30. Davis WM, Hatoum NS. Synergism of the toxicity of physostigmine and neostigmine by lithium or by a reserpine-like agent (Ro4-1284). *Toxicology* 1980;17(1):1–7.
31. Simon T, Becquemont L, Mary-Krause M, et al. Combined glutathione-S-transferase M1 and T1 genetic polymorphism and tacrine hepatotoxicity. *Clin Pharmacol Ther* 2000;67(4):432–437.
32. Jeyarasasingam G, Yeluashvili M, Quik M. Tacrine, a reversible acetylcholinesterase inhibitor, induces myopathy. *Neuroreport* 2000;11(6):1173–1176.
33. Ruff RL. Spuriously elevated serum chloride values caused by pyridostigmine bromide. *Arch Neurol* 1981;38(5):321.
34. Niemegeers CJ, Awouters F, Lenaerts FM, et al. Prevention of physostigmine-induced lethality in rats. A pharmacological analysis. *Arch Int Pharmacodyn Ther* 1982;259(1):153–165.
35. Klemm WR. Efficacy and toxicity of drug combinations in treatment of physostigmine toxicosis. *Toxicology* 1983;27(1):41–53.
36. Valero A. Treatment of severe physostigmine poisoning. *Lancet* 1968; 2(7565):459-460.
37. Robinet G, Leroyer C, Andre J, et al. [Value of ipratropium (Atrovent) in the treatment of chronic obstructive lung diseases in myasthenic patients treated with anticholinesterase agents. Apropos of a case.] [French]. *Rev Pneumol Clin* 1989;45(4):161–163.
38. Liggett SB, Daughaday CC, Senior RM. Ipratropium in patients with COPD receiving cholinesterase inhibitors. *Chest* 1988;94(1):210–212.
39. Buccafusco JJ. Mechanism of the clonidine-induced protection against acetylcholinesterase inhibitor toxicity. *J Pharmacol Exp Ther* 1982;222(3):595–599.

CHAPTER 102

Ergotamines

Saralyn R. Williams

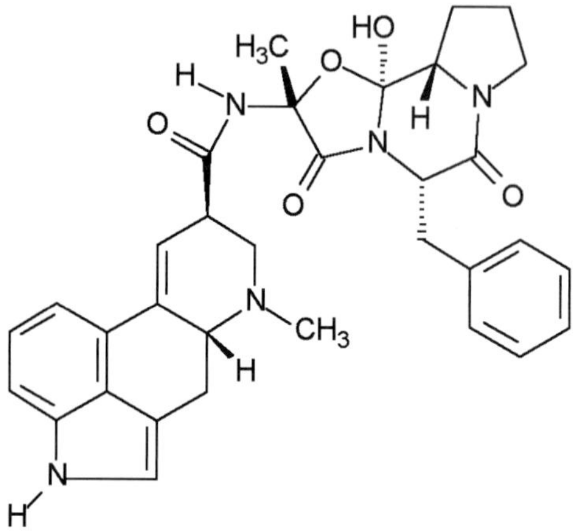

ERGOTAMINE

Compounds included:	**Dihydroergotamine (D.H.E. 45, Migranal), ergotamine (Ergomar, many others), ergonovine (ergometrine, Ergotrate), bromocriptine (Parlodel), methylergonovine (Methergine), methysergide (Desiril, Sansert), pergolide (Permax)**
Molecular formula and weight:	**See Table 1.**
SI conversion:	**Dihydroergotamine, μg/L × 1.71 = nmol/L; bromocriptine, μg/L × 1.55 = nmol/L; ergonovine, μg/L × 3.07 = nmol/L**
CAS Registry No.:	**See Table 1.**
Therapeutic levels:	**Dihydroergotamine, 10 μg/L; bromocriptine, 1 μg/L; ergonovine, 1 μg/L**
Special concerns:	**Extreme vasoconstriction can cause organ ischemia.**
Antidotes:	**Nitroglycerin, nitroprusside, other vasodilators**

OVERVIEW

The ergots are a diverse group of alkaloids that are nonselective agonists of adrenergic, dopaminergic, and serotonergic receptors. Ergot may be contained in natural products or pharmaceutical products (bromocriptine, ergotamine derivatives, methylergonovine, methysergide).

ERGOT ALKALOIDS

Naturally occurring ergots are the product of a fungus, *Claviceps purpurea*, that contaminates rye and other grains. Ingestion of the contaminated grain results in epidemics of ergotism. *C. purpurea* is parasitic to the grain and grows particularly well in wet seasons. Initial descriptions of the fungus were found in Assyrian tablets describing a "noxious pustule in the ear of grain" in 600 B.C. In one of the books of Parsees (400 to 300 B.C.), there is reference to "noxious grasses that cause pregnant women to drop the womb and die in childbed" (1).

Written descriptions during the Middle Ages allude to the severe vasospasm that occurred in affected people. Burning pain so severe in nature that the limbs were said to be consumed by the Holy Fire was described. Significant gangrene of extremities was reported, and occasionally the tissue would separate without bleeding. *St. Anthony's fire* was another name used for the disease. St. Anthony was the saint whose shrine offered relief from the agony. It is speculated that the pilgrims who sought the shrine actually did experience relief, as they were not exposed to the contaminated grains during the pilgrimage. Abortions were another complication from ergotism, although later ergot was known as an obstetric herb and used by midwives before recognition by the medical profession (1).

Large outbreaks of ergot poisoning have occurred in Russia in 1926, Ireland in 1929, and France in 1953. They were associated with improper storage and processing of grain (2). In modern times, government inspections of grain fields prevent sale of grain that is more than 0.3% contaminated with ergot, thereby eliminating the condition (1).

Classification and Uses

Ergot alkaloid drugs are derivatives of the tetracyclic 6-methylergoline. Ergotamine was first derived in 1920, and ergonovine

TABLE 1. Physical characteristics and dose of ergot alkaloid pharmaceuticals

Drug	Molecular formula, molecular weight (g/mol), CAS Registry No.	Formulation	Dose	
			Adult	Pediatric
Dihydroergotamine mesylate	$C_{33}H_{37}N_5O_5$, CH_4O_3S; 679.8; 6190-39-2	1 mg/ml solution; 1, 4 mg/ml sprays	1 mg IV, IM, or SQ	Not recommended
Ergonovine maleate	$C_{19}H_{23}N_3O_2$,$C_4H_4O_4$; 441.5; 129-51-1	0.2 mg/ml solution, 0.2-mg tablet	0.2 mg IM/IV q2–4h, 0.2–0.4 mg PO	Not recommended
Ergotamine tartrate	$(C_{33}H_{35}N_5O_5)_2$,$C_4H_6O_6$; 1313.4; 379-79-3	2-mg tablet, 1-mg tablet with 100 mg caffeine	1–2 mg	Not recommended
Methylergonovine maleate	$C_{20}H_{25}N_3O_2$,$C_4H_4O_4$; 455.5; 57432-61-8	0.2 mg/ml solution, 0.2-mg tablet	0.2 mg q6–8h	Not recommended
Bromocriptine mesylate	$C_{32}H_{40}BrN_5O_5$, CH_4O_3S; 750.7; 22260-51-1	2.5-mg tablet, 5-, 10-mg capsules	2.5 mg, 2–3 times daily	Not recommended
Methysergide maleate	$C_{21}H_{27}N_3O_2$,$C_4H_4O_4$; 469.5; 129-49-7	2-mg tablets	4–8 mg PO/day in divided doses	Not recommended

was isolated in 1932. Classification of the ergots includes the amine alkaloids, amino acid alkaloids, and hydrogenated alkaloids (Table 2). The amine alkaloids include ergonovine, methylergonovine, methysergide, and D-lysergic acid diethylamide. The ergonovine types lack a peptide side chain and have less adrenergic activity (3) The amino acid derivatives include ergotamine and bromocriptine. Dihydrogenation of the lysergic acid nucleus increases α-adrenergic blocking activity (3). A variety of adverse reactions are associated with ergotamines and vary according to the activity of the specific drug (Table 3).

Ergot alkaloids have been used for treatment of migraines since the 1920s. Their oxytocic effects have been known for centuries. Because the gravid uterus is quite sensitive to the ergots, few systemic effects may be seen at low doses. Use is primarily to maintain uterine contraction to reduce bleeding, primarily in the postpartum period (3). Suppositories usually include 2 mg ergotamine tartrate and 100 mg caffeine.

Toxic Dose

The therapeutic dose of ergot pharmaceutical agents is provided in Table 1. Oral ergotamine can be combined with 100 mg caffeine. The dose required to cause signs and symptoms of ergotism is quite variable, as even therapeutic dosing has been associated with vasospasm. In adults, ergotism has occurred in patients who have taken one dose of the medication. Ergotism has also occurred in patients who have been maintained on a stable regimen.

One 14-month-old child ingested 12 Cafergot tablets (1 mg ergotamine tartrate and 100 mg caffeine per tablet) and died with cerebral edema and hemorrhagic gastritis. Another 13-month-old child took Bellergal tablets that contained ergotamine in addition to phenobarbitone and belladonna. The child was comatose and hypotensive with peripheral cyanosis but recovered (4). A 2977-g neonate was accidentally given 0.1 mg methylergonovine via intramuscular injection instead of phytonadione. Doppler evaluation of the major vessels demonstrated reduced flow through the superior mesenteric artery during diastole. The infant remained asymptomatic, and the flow profiles were normal within 72 hours (5).

TABLE 2. Classification of the ergot alkaloids

Amine alkaloids	Amino acid alkaloids	Hydrogenated alkaloids
Ergonovine	Bromocriptine	Dihydroergotamine
Methylergonovine	Ergotamine	Dihydroergocristine
Methysergide	Ergocristine	Dihydroergosine
Lergotrile	Ergosine	Dihydroergocornine
D-Lysergic diethylamide (LSD)	Ergocornine	
	Ergocryptine	

Toxicokinetics and Toxicodynamics

Most ergots are absorbed within 30 minutes of ingestion with a peak plasma concentration (T_{max}) of approximately 2 hours (6). Interindividual variation occurs. In some patients, plasma concentrations are undetectable after ingestion of ergotamine (7). Bioavailability is poor after oral dosing due to the large first-pass effect. Rectal administration also results in interindividual variation of plasma concentrations (8). The T_{max} after intramuscular injection was 30 minutes. Bioavailability is variable. Theories for this variability include self-limited absorption due to vasoconstriction (9).

Concurrent use of caffeine may increase the rate of oral absorption (10). However, peak concentrations were not different between human volunteers who ingested ergotamine/caffeine compared with those who were given plain ergotamine (7,8). The volume of distribution (V_d) for most ergotamines is approximately 2 L/kg. The V_d for methylergonovine is 0.5 L/kg (11).

Ergotamines are metabolized in the liver, and this is followed by biliary excretion (6,9). The pathways for metabolism are unclear, although ergots may have some effect on the P450 mixed oxidase system. After intravenous administration, 80% to 90% of the drug is excreted in the feces as metabolites (6). Although the plasma half-life is 2 to 6 hours, the pharmacodynamic effects may be more prolonged. The prolonged pharma-

TABLE 3. Clinical effects of the ergot alkaloids

Ergot	Emesis	Psychosis	Myometrial stimulation	Vasoconstriction	Fibrosis
Methylergonovine	+	None	+++	++	None
Methysergide	+	+	+	+	+++
Ergotamine	+++	+	+++	+++	+
Bromocriptine	++	+++	None	++	+

+, low association; ++, moderate association; +++, high association.

codynamic effects could be related to active metabolites or high potency of the ergotamines (9).

Pathophysiology

Ergots have complex pharmacologic properties. They were initially described as potent adrenergic receptor antagonists; however, partial agonist activity may also be seen. The activity of the ergot varies depending on the vascular bed. They have partial agonist and antagonist properties at a variety of other receptors including dopaminergic and serotonergic (5-HT_1, 5-HT_2). Dihydroergotamine has activity at 5-HT_1, 5-HT_{2A}, 5-HT_{2B}, D_2, α_1, and α_2 receptors (3).

Pregnancy and Lactation

Most ergotamines are oxytocic, and methylergonovine has been used for this purpose. Ergotamines produce prolonged uterine tone, resulting in fetal hypoxia. Ergotamines for treatment of headache in pregnant patients are considered contraindicated and are classified as U.S. Food and Drug Administration (FDA) pregnancy category X (Appendix I). Methylergonovine is class C; however, it is considered contraindicated for use during pregnancy because of the potential to cause sustained tetanic uterine contractions. Teratogenic potential is low with small, infrequent doses; however, larger doses may result in maternal or fetal vascular disruption.

An intentional ingestion of ten ergotamine tablets by a 17-year-old woman resulted in fetal demise approximately 13.5 hours after the ingestion (12). Accidental administration of methylergonovine to a patient during the first stage of labor resulted in uterine hypertonus and bradycardia, followed by acidosis and tachycardia, as the hypertonus did not respond to treatment. The infant was delivered by cesarean section (13).

The American Academy of Pediatrics considers ergotamines to be contraindicated in the breast-feeding mother (14). Ergotamines are excreted into breast milk, and signs of ergotism may develop in nursing infants. Ergotamines may also inhibit lactation (15). No adverse effects in infants exposed to methylergonovine have been reported. Although structurally related, its effects on inhibition of prolactin are markedly less than bromocriptine (15).

Clinical Presentation

ACUTE OVERDOSAGE

Ergotamines cause vasoconstriction in a variety of blood vessels. Presentation may include cold, cyanotic, and painful extremities. Poor perfusion with delayed capillary refill is usually present. Pulses are generally diminished or absent (16–22). Claudication may also be an initial complaint (21,23). Abdominal pain, nausea, and vomiting are complaints associated with ergot-induced mesenteric ischemia (24,25). Carotid involvement may present as neurologic signs (26,27). Chest pain in a patient who has been taking ergotamines should be evaluated for myocardial ischemia.

ADVERSE EFFECTS

The most commonly reported complication from ergots is the vasospasm, usually in the lower or upper extremity (16–22,28). One patient had recurrence of vasospasm after she restarted her ergotamine/caffeine suppositories. She was challenged with a therapeutic dose of ergotamine/caffeine on her third visit, and her symptoms and signs returned (29). Vasoconstriction of the right internal carotid artery occurred in a patient who was taking ergotamine and methysergide and presented with ptosis of the left eye and a mild left facial droop (26). Another patient had bilateral paralysis of the upper and lower facial muscles with anisocoria, ptosis, and external strabismus of the right side. Angiography revealed filling defects of the external carotid arteries (27). Vasospasm of the circle of Willis was reported in a woman who presented with expressive aphasia and right-sided sensorimotor weakness (30).

Myocardial ischemia related to the use of ergotamine may occur. Cluster headaches developed in a 31-year-old man who had used methysergide for treatment of developed chest pressure, and he had abnormalities on the electrocardiogram that were different than a previous electrocardiogram. His enzymes did not increase, and a subsequent stress test was normal (31). A 29-year-old man sustained a myocardial infarction after taking 120 mg ergotamine (32). Other cases of infarction and ischemia have been reported (33,34). Mesenteric vessel vasospasm has also been associated with ergotamine tartrate (24). Concomitant vasoconstriction of vessels to the lower extremities and the superior mesenteric artery were demonstrated in a woman with lower extremity pain and claudication (25).

Complications from the use of ergotamine have included development of fibrotic cardiac valves. They have been reported with the mitral and the aortic valves (35,36), and one patient required replacement of the mitral, aortic, and tricuspid valves (37).

DRUG INTERACTIONS

Vasospasm may be precipitated by the concurrent use of macrolide antibiotics. An initial case was reported in 1969 with the use of triacetyloleandomycin and ergotamine tartrate (38). Several cases have been associated with erythromycin. One case involved a patient who was taking erythromycin and developed ergotism after taking a total dose of 6 mg ergotamine for a migraine headache (39). Another patient took erythromycin for 3 weeks and the following week developed ergotism after taking his usual dose of ergotamine tartrate/caffeine (40). In a similar case a patient presented with severe bilateral upper extremity ischemia after the use of erythromycin while taking ergotamine tartrate (41). An acute case of lingual ischemia was reported with the use of ergotamine tartrate and clarithromycin (42). Bilateral lower extremity ergotism was reported after routine use of caffeine-ergotamine tartrate and 7 days of clarithromycin (43).

Although the mechanism is not clear, a study in rhesus monkeys demonstrated that troleandomycin could increase the blood concentrations of dihydroergotamine (44). It was proposed that macrolide antibiotics may complex with P450 mixed oxidase enzymes and interfere with the metabolism of ergotamines. A similar interaction has been described with protease inhibitors, including ritonavir (16,28,30,45), indinavir (23), and nelfinavir (46).

Diagnostic Tests

Detection of ergotamines in plasma or serum may be difficult due to the low bioavailability. High-performance liquid chromatography has been used for a variety of ergot alkaloids (47). Gas chromatography–mass spectrometry techniques have also been developed (48). In 12 cases of nonfatal poisoning, plasma concentrations of 9 to 0.003 µg/ml were reported 1.7 to 5.0 hours after ingestion (11). Levels do not necessarily correlate with toxicity or clinical effects.

Diagnosis of vasospasm is usually made by angiography of the affected limb(s) or vessels (18,20,21). Duplex sonography may also demonstrate vessel narrowing. Magnetic resonance angiography has been used as well, particularly for intracranial vessels (30).

Treatment

Initial treatment includes cessation of the medication involved. Alternative therapies should be used to treat headache syndromes.

DECONTAMINATION

For a large oral ingestion, activated charcoal can be given if the ingestion is recent. Because absorption is rapid with the ergotamines, delayed presentation may negate the need for decontamination.

ENHANCEMENT OF ELIMINATION

Administration of multiple-dose activated charcoal has not been studied in this clinical setting even though the majority of ergotamines are excreted via the biliary system.

ANTIDOTES

No specific antidote is available for ergots. A variety of vasodilating agents have been used in clinical practice to reverse vasoconstriction. Vasodilators have been used when ischemic changes occur in the extremities or the myocardium. The vasodilator dose is titrated upward until organ perfusion is improved. Nitroglycerin infusion would be first choice for myocardial ischemia. Nitroglycerin has also been used for treatment of extremity ergotism with improved peripheral pulses. During the treatment of one case, the nitroglycerin infusion was stopped and the peripheral pulses disappeared, only to return on restarting the infusion (49). An *in vitro* model using temporal artery segments exposed the vessel segments to ergotamine. Ergotamine increased the isometric tension. The addition of nitroglycerin to the solution returned the tension back to baseline (49). Complications from nitroglycerin infusion were described in a patient with ergotism involving the circle of Willis. Hypotension and worsening neurologic symptoms developed with the infusion of nitroglycerin (30).

Nitroprusside has also been used as a vasodilator with reported improvement of symptoms (19,50,51). After an epidural block failed, the infusion of nitroprusside was associated with clinical improvement. When the infusion was interrupted, the signs of vasoconstriction returned (51). Direct intraarterial infusion of nitroprusside after systemic infusion did not result in immediate improvement (52). Intra-arterial infusion may circumvent the hypotension that may occur with systemic administration of nitroprusside.

Nifedipine has been used due to its peripheral vasodilation (53). Intravenous or intraarterial phentolamine has been recommended because it is a nonselective alpha-receptor antagonist. Other dilators, such as prazosin and prostaglandin E_1 infusion, have also been tried (54,55). In addition, sympathectomy has been described in anecdotal reports, but improvement is delayed and may be due to spontaneous resolution (19,51,56).

SUPPORTIVE CARE

Initial therapy for peripheral vasoconstriction with ischemic signs would include isotonic fluid administration and analgesia. Fluid administration is recommended to improve perfusion to the affected organs. Heparin in therapeutic doses should be considered early in the presentation, as the differential of ischemic changes includes arterial thrombus. Heparin also has been recommended in the setting of ergot-related vasospasm to reduce the possible risk of thrombus formation. Low-molecular-weight fractionated heparin can be considered, although there is a paucity of data with its use. Antiplatelet medications have also been recommended, with aspirin being most commonly used. Neither the glycoprotein IIb/IIIa inhibitors nor thrombolytics have been studied.

BROMOCRIPTINE

Bromocriptine is a semisynthetic ergot alkaloid that was approved for clinical use in 1978. It is a brominated ergopeptide that is classified as an amino acid ergot alkaloid. As an ergot alkaloid, it has pronounced activity at dopaminergic receptors. Pergolide is another ergot derivative similar to bromocriptine that has similar activity at dopamine 2 (D_2) receptors (57).

Current uses for bromocriptine include treatment for Parkinson's disease, lactation suppression, and acromegaly. Other uses include treatment of amenorrhea, galactorrhea, and female infertility due to hyperprolactinemia (58). Bromocriptine has been used for prolactinomas. In addition to suppressing prolactin levels, reduction of tumor size of macroadenomas has been reported (58). It has also been used for treatment of patients with clinical syndromes suggestive of neuroleptic malignant syndrome (59,60).

Toxic Dose

The adult and pediatric therapeutic doses are provided in Table 1. Higher doses are used in patients whose galactorrhea is due to neuroleptic medications or associated with markedly elevated hyperprolactinemia. Acromegaly is usually treated with 5 to 20 mg three times a day. Parkinson's disease can be treated with a range of dosages depending on the sensitivity of the receptor. Monotherapy or combination therapy with other antiparkinsonian medications has been used. The range includes 1.25 to 40.0 mg, but up to 300 mg per day has been used (58,61,62).

Ingestion of 50 mg and 75 mg bromocriptine in two adults resulted in vomiting. One of these patients had mild hypotension (63). A case report described mild to moderate effects after ingestion by a 160-kg adult of approximately 225 mg bromocriptine, 2.25 g cortisone, 30 Actifed tablets, and 30 mg cyclobenzaprine. Dry mucous membranes and a brief period of hallucinations developed (64).

A pediatric ingestion of 25 mg in a 2-year-old boy resulted in lethargy, combativeness, and mydriasis. Vomiting and lethargy occurred in a 2.5-year-old boy who ingested 7.5 mg bromocriptine. No weights were provided (65). Lethargy developed in an 18-month-old child who ingested an unknown number of tablets. The recovery was uneventful (66).

Toxicokinetics and Toxicodynamics

Absorption of bromocriptine after ingestion is nearly complete and rapid, within 30 minutes (67). Because an extensive first-pass effect occurs, the oral bioavailability is only 3% to 6% (57). The V_d is 2 to 3 L/kg (57). Protein binding is approximately 90% (68). The liver metabolizes bromocriptine. Elimination occurs in two distinct phases. The α phase is approximately 5 hours, with a β phase of 45 hours (67). The majority of the dose is in the bile (68). A minimal amount of bromocriptine is excreted in the urine. The metabolites are inactive (69).

Pathophysiology

Five dopamine receptors have been identified, but due to lack of selective agonists for each receptor type, the classification system is divided into those that are similar to D_1 and those that are similar to D_2. D_1-like receptors include D_1 and D_5. These receptors are linked to adenylate cyclase. D_2-like receptors may inhibit adenylate cyclase and include D_2, D_3, and D_4 receptors (69). Postsynaptic D_2 receptor stimulation is used for treatment of Parkinson's disease. Bromocriptine has strong agonist effects at the D_2 receptor and partial antagonist effects at D_1. It also has less affinity as an antagonist for α_1 and α_2 receptors than dihydroergotamines (57). Bromocriptine is a weak antagonist of serotonin receptors (57,69). The effects of bromocriptine on hyperprolactinemia and acromegaly are due to stimulation of D_2 receptors in the pituitary that inhibits the release of prolactin. Bromocriptine also inhibits the prolactin release from the effect of thyrotropin-releasing hormone (57,62).

Pregnancy and Lactation

Bromocriptine is FDA pregnancy category C (Appendix I). Because it has been used for infertility treatment from hyperprolactinemia, many pregnancies have had exposure in the embryonic stage. No pattern of anomalies has been detected (70). Bromocriptine is used therapeutically to suppress lactation, and it is considered contraindicated for use by breast-feeding mothers (71).

Clinical Presentation

ACUTE OVERDOSAGE

Bromocriptine overdosage may result in nausea, vomiting, and mild hypotension. Psychosis and hallucinations may occur as well. In the patient on high-dose bromocriptine for Parkinson's disease, psychosis may occur. Although rare, cardiovascular effects such as myocardial ischemia have been associated with bromocriptine.

ADVERSE EVENTS

Adverse effects from dosages used for treatment of Parkinson's disease include nausea, vomiting, and orthostatic hypotension (58,69). Choreic and dystonic movements similar to those seen with levodopa have also been observed (62).

Postpartum psychosis has been associated with low-dose bromocriptine for suppression of lactation (72,73). The diagnosis is difficult because the clinical features of postpartum psychosis in the absence of bromocriptine and bromocriptine-induced psychosis are similar (74). One review suggests that bromocriptine may increase the incidence of these problems, but the current evidence is anecdotal (74).

Bromocriptine-associated psychosis has also occurred during the treatment of amenorrhea, hyperprolactinemia, and acromegaly (75–78). In one patient psychosis developed after she took low-dose bromocriptine for amenorrhea. Her condition improved after discontinuation of the bromocriptine. A follow-up letter by the same authors revealed that this patient had recurrence of her hallucinations, requiring the use of haloperidol. The authors suggest that their case points toward a predisposition to bromocriptine psychosis (75,79). This is similar to a patient who had stable schizophrenia that worsened after administration of low-dose bromocriptine for hyperprolactinemia (76). Of the patients in whom bromocriptine-associated psychosis developed, the greatest number are reported in parkinsonian patients who receive a higher dose of bromocriptine (74). There appears to be a correlation between the dose, length of time on the drug, and severity of symptoms (74).

The use of bromocriptine in psychiatric patients is not necessarily associated with worsening psychosis. A randomized placebo-controlled double-blinded trial of 16 psychiatric patients placed on daily bromocriptine for 10 weeks revealed no differences in the mean neuroleptic dose of the two groups (80). One theory proposed is that thresholds of tolerance of dopamine agonist activity exist even in those patients with a predisposition to psychosis (74).

Bromocriptine has been implicated as the possible cause of myocardial infarction in postpartum women (81–85). Some of the cases have co-morbidities such as concomitant use of ergonovine (81), previous cocaine use, and pregnancy-induced hypertension (83). An inferior transmural infarction from total occlusion of the right coronary artery occurred in a 32-year-old woman who used bromocriptine to suppress lactation. A month after her angioplasty, acute narrowing of the right coronary artery was documented after a single dose of bromocriptine. The vasoconstriction resolved with intracoronary nitroglycerin administration (84). An anterolateral infarction with 90% narrowing of the first diagonal branch was diagnosed in a 34-year-old woman using bromocriptine. Repeat catheterization 2 months later revealed no identifiable lesion in the diagonal artery (85).

Acute cerebral thrombosis and death occurred in a 30-year-old woman who had been taking bromocriptine for approximately 3 weeks after her delivery (86). Postpartum use of bromocriptine has also been associated with onset of severe headaches, with one case progressing to loss of vision and convulsions when a patient was concurrently treated with phenylpropanolamine and guaifenesin. This patient had angiography that demonstrated spasm of the left vertebral, left basilar, and posterior cerebral arteries (87). Postpartum cerebral angiopathy was also reported in a patient who took 5 days of low-dose bromocriptine (88).

Retroperitoneal fibrosis has rarely been reported in patients being treated for Parkinson's disease (89). Cases of pleuropulmonary fibrosis have been associated with use of bromocriptine in the therapy of Parkinson's disease (90). Pergolide has also been associated with pericardial, pleural, and retroperitoneal fibrosis (91,92).

Skin manifestations include erythromelalgia-like syndrome, reported in nine patients with Parkinson's disease. Clinical manifestations include erythema, edema, and tenderness of the lower extremities up the knee bilaterally. Withdrawal of bromocriptine was associated with disappearance of the rash in one patient (93). One case of cutaneous pseudolymphoma has been reported with bromocriptine therapy for macroprolactinoma. The nodular skin lesions resolved 8 weeks after cessation of bromocriptine (94).

Bromocriptine-associated hepatitis has been described in a patient with Parkinson's disease. The patient was started on a 5-mg twice-a-day dose, and transaminitis developed after 4 days of therapy. Serologic work-up was negative, and all medications were discontinued. The transaminitis improved but recurred on rechallenge (95).

Diagnostic Tests

No tests are available to establish the diagnosis of bromocriptine toxicity. Serum concentrations can be measured in reference laboratories but do not affect clinical management.

Treatment

DECONTAMINATION

For the intentional ingestion, decontamination with use of single-dose activated charcoal may be beneficial if given soon after the ingestion. Cathartic or whole bowel irrigation has little role considering the rapid and complete absorption of bromocriptine.

ENHANCEMENT OF ELIMINATION

Extracorporeal elimination has no role.

ANTIDOTES

No specific antidotes are available for bromocriptine toxicity.

SUPPORTIVE CARE

Treatment for the poisoned patient is primarily supportive. He or she should be monitored for alteration in mental status, and airway management may be required. Antiemetics can be used for persistent vomiting. Hypotension is usually transient and responds to intravenous fluids. A direct α-agonist can be used for recalcitrant, persistent hypotension. For the adverse effect of psychosis in the setting of therapeutic dosing, most symptoms improve with cessation of the bromocriptine. Clozapine has been used for treatment in one case report (96).

METHYSERGIDE

Methysergide is a semisynthetic ergot alkaloid that is a congener of methylergonovine. Methysergide has an active metabolite, methylergometrine, that may have more activity than the parent compound (97). Its primary use is for the prophylaxis of migraines, and it is not beneficial for treatment of an acute migraine attack. It has been used in patients with carcinoid tumor to reduce the diarrhea (97).

Toxic Dose

The adult and pediatric therapeutic doses are provided in Table 1. The onset of the protective effect to reduce the risk of headache appears delayed after onset of dosing. Drug withdrawal every 6 months is recommended to reduce the risk of the adverse effects. Few data regarding the toxic dose in the overdose are available.

Pathophysiology

Methysergide has antagonist activity at 5-HT_{2A} and 5-HT_{2C}. It may have some partial agonist effects, as it has been noted to be nonselective at serotonin receptors. It has weak vasoconstrictor effect and weak oxytocic effects.

Pregnancy and Lactation

Methysergide is FDA pregnancy category D (Appendix I). Few data regarding the use of methysergide in pregnant or lactating women are available.

Clinical Presentation

Toxicity from acute overdosage has not been reported. Adverse events include primarily retroperitoneal fibrosis. Two cases were initially reported in 1964 in a case series discussing the use of methysergide for headache in 500 patients (98). A series of 27 patients with retroperitoneal fibrosis was reported in 1966. Presentations were variable, including abdominal pain, leg edema, and pain in the lower back. Intravenous pyelography revealed hydronephrosis that was usually bilateral. Fourteen of the 27 patients were treated with surgical lysis (99). Mesenteric ischemia and gangrenous bowel from severe mesenteric adventitial fibrosis have been described (100). Iliocaval manifestations occurred in a 25-year-old woman who was on methysergide for 18 months (101). Cessation of methysergide is usually associated with partial or complete improvement of the retroperitoneal fibrosis.

Development of cardiac murmurs has also been associated with methysergide. In the 1966 case series by Graham (102), significant cardiac murmurs also developed in 7 of the original 27 patients with retroperitoneal fibrosis. Graham described an additional 29 patients who developed cardiac murmurs while taking methysergide. Fibrosis of the aortic root and the aortic valve leaflets developed in one patient. Another patient received aortic and mitral valves (102). After cessation of methysergide, the cardiac manifestations did not improve as dramatically as the retroperitoneal fibrosis (99,102).

Pleuropulmonary fibrosis has also been related to the use of methysergide. The presentation includes chest pain, shortness of breath, and fevers. Pleural friction rubs and effusions were noted in these patients. Symptoms and signs improved after cessation of the drug. One patient had a relapse when he restarted his methysergide. A pulmonary biopsy of one patient revealed fibrosis around the vessels and terminal bronchioles. Pleural biopsy demonstrated acute fibrinous exudates and fibrosis (102).

Akathisia has been reported in a 35-year-old man in whom restlessness and persistent compulsion to move developed after a trial of methysergide. A similar reaction occurred when the patient restarted the drug (103). One case of methysergide-associated psychosis has been reported, which resolved with drug discontinuation (104).

Vasospasm of the lower extremity resulting in gangrene and amputation of the foot occurred after methysergide use for 2 to 3 years (105). Another case occurred in a 48-year-old woman who had been taking methysergide for 2 years. Angiography demonstrated narrowing of the superficial femoral and popliteal arteries. The pulses returned within 48 hours after cessation of the methysergide (106).

Diagnostic Tests

Serum levels have not been studied in correlation of the adverse effects with methysergide.

Treatment

The primary treatment for the adverse effects of methysergide is cessation of the medication. In one series of retroperitoneal fibrosis, symptoms improved markedly after the medication was discontinued, although approximately half of the patients required lysis of adhesions and ureterolysis (99). Removal of gangrenous bowel was required for the case of severe mesenteric adventitial fibrosis (100). The associated cardiac effects may have more long-term complications, including congestive heart failure and the need for valve replacement (102). The pleuropulmonary complications typically improve after cessation of methysergide, although one patient required decortication (102).

REFERENCES

1. Hardman JG, Limbird LE, eds. *Goodman and Gilman's the pharmacological basis of therapeutics*, 9th ed. New York: McGraw-Hill, 1996.
2. MacGuire AM, Cassidy JT. Modern ergotism. *Am Fam Physician* 1984;30:179–183.
3. Hardman JG, Limbird LE, eds. *Goodman and Gilman's the pharmacological basis of therapeutics*, 10th ed. New York: McGraw-Hill, 2001.
4. Jones EM, Williams B. Two cases of ergotamine poisoning in infants. *BMJ* 1966;5485:466.
5. Baum CR, Hilpert PL, Bhutani VK. Accidental administration of an ergot alkaloid to a neonate. *Pediatrics* 1996;98:457–458.
6. Aellig WH, Nüesch E. Comparative pharmacokinetic investigations with tritium-labeled ergot alkaloids after oral and intravenous administration in man. *Int J Clin Pharmacol* 1977;15:106–112.
7. Ala-Hurula V, Myllylä VV, Arvela P, et al. Systemic availability of ergotamine tartrate after three successive doses and during continuous medication. *Eur J Clin Pharmacol* 1979;16:355–360.
8. Ala-Hurula V, Myllylä VV, Arvela P, et al. Systemic availability of ergotamine tartrate after oral, rectal and intramuscular administration. *Eur J Clin Pharmacol* 1979;15:51–55.
9. Perrin VL. Clinical pharmacokinetics of ergotamine in migraine and cluster headaches. *Clin Pharmacokinet* 1985;10:334–352.
10. Schmidt R, Fanchamps A. Effect of caffeine on intestinal absorption of ergotamine in man. *Eur J Clin Pharmacol* 1974;7:213–216.
11. Moffat AC, Jackson JV, Moss MS, Widdop B, eds. *Clarke's isolation and identification of drugs*, 2nd ed. London: Pharmaceutical Press, 1986.
12. Au KL, Woo JSK, Wong VCW. Intrauterine death from ergotamine overdosage. *Eur J Obstet Gynecol Reprod Biol* 1985;19:313–315.
13. Moise KJ Jr, Carpenter RJ Jr. Methylergonovine-induced hypertonus in term pregnancy. A case report. *J Reprod Med* 1988;33:771–773.
14. American Academy of Pediatrics Committee on Drugs. The transfer of drugs and other chemicals into human milk. *Pediatrics* 1994;93:137–150.
15. Briggs GG, Freeman RK, Yaffe SJ, eds. *Drugs in pregnancy and lactation*, 6th ed. Philadelphia: Lippincott Williams & Wilkins, 2002.
16. Caballero-Granado FJ, Viciana P, Cordero E, et al. Ergotism related to concurrent administration of ergotamine tartrate and ritonavir in an AIDS patient. *Antimicrob Agents Chemother* 1997;41:1207.
17. Yao ST, Goodwin DP, Kenyon JR. Case of ergot poisoning. *BMJ* 1970;3:86–87.
18. Imrie CW. Arterial spasm associated with oral ergotamine therapy. *Br J Clin Pract* 1973;27:457–460.
19. Bongard O, Bounameaux H. Severe iatrogenic ergotism: incidence and clinical importance. *Vasa* 1991;20:153–156.
20. Voyvodic F, Hayward M. Case report: upper extremity ischaemia secondary to ergotamine poisoning. *Clin Radiol* 1996;51:589–591.
21. Garcia GD, Goff JM Jr, Hadro NC, et al. Chronic ergot toxicity: a rare cause of lower extremity ischemia. *J Vasc Surg* 2000;31:1245–1247.
22. Vila A, Mykietiuk A, Bonvehì, et al. Clinical ergotism induced by ritonavir. *Scand J Infect Dis* 2001;33:788–789.
23. Rosenthal E, Sala F, Chichmanian RM, et al. Ergotism related to concurrent administration of ergotamine tartrate and indinavir. *JAMA* 1999;281:987.
24. Christopoulos S, Szilagyi A, Kahn SR. Saint-Anthony's fire. *Lancet* 2001;358:1694.

25. Greene FL, Ariyan S, Stansel HC Jr. Mesenteric and peripheral vascular ischemia secondary to ergotism. *Surgery* 1977;81:176–179.
26. Richter AM, Banker VP. Carotid ergotism. A complication of migraine therapy. *Radiology* 1973;106:339–340.
27. Lazarides MK, Karageorgiou C, Tsiara S, et al. Severe facial ischaemia caused by ergotism. *J Cardiovasc Surg* 1992;33:383–385.
28. Liaudet L, Buclin T, Jaccard C, et al. Drug points: severe ergotism associated with interaction between ritonavir and ergotamine. *BMJ* 1999;318(7186):771.
29. Curry RW Jr, Yalamanchili RR. Recurrent ergotism: a case report. *J Fam Pract* 1978;6:769–773.
30. Spiegel M, Schmidauer C, Kampfl A, et al. Cerebral ergotism under treatment with ergotamine and ritonavir. *Neurology* 2001;57:743–744.
31. Galer BS, Lipton RB, Solomon S, et al. Myocardial ischemia related to ergot alkaloids: a case report and literature review. *Headache* 1991;31:446–450.
32. Carr P. Self-induced myocardial infarction. *Postgrad Med J* 1981;57:654–655.
33. Klein LS, Simpson RJ Jr, Stern R, et al. Myocardial infarction following administration of sublingual ergotamine. *Chest* 1982;82:375–376.
34. Snell NJ, Russell-Smith C, Coysh HL. Myocardial ischaemia in migraine sufferers taking ergotamine. *Postgrad Med J* 1978;54:37–39.
35. Hauck AJ, Edwards WD, Danielson GK, et al. Mitral and aortic valve disease associated with ergotamine therapy for migraine. *Arch Pathol Lab Med* 1990;114:62–64.
36. Austin SM, El-Hayek A, Comianos M, et al. Mitral valve disease associated with long-term ergotamine use. *South Med J* 1993;86(10):1179–1181.
37. Wilke A, Hesse H, Hufnagel G, et al. Mitral, aortic, tricuspid valvular heart disease associated with ergotamine therapy for migraine. *Eur Heart J* 1997;18:701.
38. Hayton AC. Precipitation of acute ergotism by triacetyloleandomycin. *N Z Med J* 1969;69:42.
39. Ghali R, De Léan J, Douville Y, et al. Erythromycin-associated ergotamine intoxication: arteriographic and electrophysiologic analysis of a rare cause of severe ischemia of the lower extremities and associated ischemic neuropathy. *Ann Vasc Surg* 1993;7:291–296.
40. Karam B, Farah E, Ashoush R, et al. Ergotism precipitated by erythromycin: a rare cause of vasospasm. *Eur J Vasc Endovasc Surg* 2000;19:96–98.
41. Bird PA, Sturgess AD. Clinical ergotism with severe bilateral upper limb ischaemia precipitated by an erythromycin-ergotamine drug interaction. *Aust N Z J Med* 2000;30:635–636.
42. Horowitz RS, Dart RC, Gomez HF. Clinical ergotism with lingual ischemia induced by clarithromycin-ergotamine interaction. *Arch Intern Med* 1996;156:456–458.
43. Ausband SC, Goodman PE. An unusual case of clarithromycin associated ergotism. *J Emerg Med* 2001;21:411–413.
44. Azria M, Kiechel JR, Lavenne D. Contribution à l'étude de l'interaction de la triacelyloléandomycine avec l'ergotamine ou la dihydroergotamine. *J Pharmacologie* 1979;10:431–438.
45. Blanche P, Rigolet A, Gombert B, et al. Ergotism related to a single dose of ergotamine tartrate in an AIDS patient treated with ritonavir. *Postgrad Med J* 1999;75(887):546–547.
46. Mortier E, Pouchot J, Vinceneux P, et al. Ergotism related to interaction between nelfinavir and ergotamine. *Am J Med* 2001;110:594.
47. Gill R, Key JA. High-performance liquid chromatography system for the separation of ergot alkaloids with applicability to the analysis of illicit lysergide (LSD). *J Chromatogr* 1985;346:423–427.
48. Feng N, Minder EI, Grampp T, et al. Identification and quantification of ergotamine in human plasma by gas chromatography–mass spectrometry. *J Chromatogr* 1992;575:289–294.
49. Tfelt-Hansen P, Østergaard JR, Gøthgen I, et al. Nitroglycerin for ergotism. Experimental studies in vitro and in migraine patients and treatment of an overt case. *Eur J Clin Pharmacol* 1982;22:105–109.
50. Carliner N, Denune DP, Finch CS Jr, et al. Sodium nitroprusside treatment of ergotamine-induced peripheral ischemia. *JAMA* 1974;227:308–309.
51. Andersen PK, Christensen KN, Hole P, et al. Sodium nitroprusside and epidural blockade in the treatment of ergotism. *N Engl J Med* 1977;296:1271–1273.
52. Dierckx RA, Peters O, Ebinger G, et al. Intraarterial sodium nitroprusside infusion in the treatment of severe ergotism. *Clin Neuropharmacol* 1986;9:542–548.
53. Dagher FJ, Pais SO, Richards W, et al. Severe unilateral ischemia of the lower extremity caused by ergotamine: treatment with nifedipine. *Surgery* 1985;97:369–373.
54. Cobaugh DS. Prazosin treatment of ergotamine induced peripheral ischemia. *JAMA* 1980;244:1360.
55. Edwards RJ, Fulde GWO, McGrath MA. Successful limb salvage with prostaglandin infusion: a review of ergotamine toxicity. *Med J Aust* 1991;155:825–827.
56. Atwell D, Pois A, Morledge J, et al. Severe unilateral ischemia secondary to ergot intoxication. *Wis Med J* 1976;75:S33–S34.
57. Hardman JG, Limbird LE, eds. *Goodman and Gilman's the pharmacological basis of therapeutics*, 10th ed. New York: McGraw-Hill, 2001.
58. Vance ML, Evans WS, Thorner MLO. Drugs five years later: bromocriptine. *Ann Intern Med* 1984;100:78–91.
59. Rosenberg MR, Green M. Neuroleptic malignant syndrome. *Arch Intern Med* 1989;149:1927–1931.
60. Sakkas P, Davis JM, Hua J, Wang Z. Pharmacotherapy of neuroleptic malignant syndrome. *Psych Ann* 1991;21:157–164.
61. Hardman JG, Limbird LE, eds. *Goodman and Gilman's the pharmacological basis of therapeutics*, 9th ed. New York: McGraw-Hill, 1996.
62. Parkes D. Bromocriptine. *N Engl J Med* 1979;301:873–878.
63. Descotes J, Frantz P, Bourrat C. Intoxication aigue par ingestion volontare de bromocriptine: a propos de 2 observations personnelles. *Bull Med Leg Toxicol* 1979;22:487–490.
64. Warren DE, Nakfoor E. Acute overdose of bromocriptine. *Drug Intell Clin Pharm* 1983;17:374.
65. Vermund SH, Goldstein RG, Romano AA, Atwood SJ. Accidental bromocriptine ingestion in childhood. *J Pediatr* 1984;105(5):838–840.
66. Mack RB. Mairzy doats and dozy doats and a kiddle eat almost anything. Bromocriptine (Parlodel) overdose. *N C Med J* 1988;49:17–18.
67. Aellig WH, Nüesch E. Comparative pharmacokinetic investigations with tritium-labeled ergot alkaloids after oral and intravenous administration in man. *Int J Clin Pharmacol* 1977;15:106–112.
68. Moffat AC, Jackson JV, Moss MS, Widdop B, eds. *Clarke's isolation and identification of drugs*, 2nd ed. London: Pharmaceutical Press, 1986.
69. Deleu D, Northway MG, Hanssens Y. Clinical pharmacokinetic and pharmacodynamic properties of drugs used in the treatment of Parkinson's disease. *Clin Pharmacokinet* 2002;41(4);261–309.
70. Turkalj I, Braun P, Krupp P. Surveillance of bromocriptine in pregnancy. *JAMA* 1982;247:1589–1591.
71. American Academy of Pediatrics Committee on Drugs. The transfer of drugs and other chemicals into human milk. *Pediatrics* 1994;93:137–150.
72. Canterbury RJ, Haskins B, Kahn N, et al. Postpartum psychosis induced by bromocriptine. *South Med J* 1987;80:1463–1464.
73. Reeves RR, Pinkofsky HB. Postpartum psychosis induced by bromocriptine and pseudoephedrine. *J Fam Pract* 1997;44:164–166.
74. Boyd A. Bromocriptine and psychosis: a literature review. *Psychiatr Q* 1995;66:87–95.
75. Einarson TR, Turchet EN. Psychotic reaction to low-dose bromocriptine. *Clin Pharm* 1983;2:273–274.
76. Procter AW, Littlewood R, Fry AH. Bromocriptine induced psychosis in acromegaly. *BMJ* 1983;286(6358):50–51.
77. Shukla S, Turner WJ, Newman G. Bromocriptine-related psychosis and treatment. *Biol Psychiatry* 1985;20:326–328.
78. Le Feuvre CM, Isaacs AJ, Frank OS. Bromocriptine-induced psychosis in acromegaly. *BMJ* 1982;285:1315.
79. Einarson TR, Turchet EN. Follow-up on bromocriptine-induced psychosis. *Clin Pharm* 1983;2:512.
80. Perovich RM, Lieberman JA, Fleischhacker WW, et al. The behavioral toxicity of bromocriptine in patients with psychiatric illness. *J Clin Psychopharmacol* 1989;9:417–422.
81. Iffy L, TenHove W. Frisoli G. Acute myocardial infarction in the puerperium in patients receiving bromocriptine. *Am J Obstet Gynecol* 1986;155:371–372.
82. Ruch A, Duhring JL. Postpartum myocardial infarction in a patient receiving bromocriptine. *Obstet Gynecol* 1989;74:448–451.
83. Bakht, FR, Kirshon B, Baker T, et al. Postpartum cardiovascular complications after bromocriptine and cocaine use. *Am J Obstet Gynecol* 1990;162:1065–1066.
84. Larrazet F, Spaulding C, Lobreau HJ, et al. Possible bromocriptine-induced myocardial infarction. *Ann Intern Med* 1993;118:199–200.
85. Hopp L, Weisse AB, Iffy L. Acute myocardial infarction in a healthy mother using bromocriptine for milk suppression. *Can J Cardiol* 1996;12(4):415–418.
86. Maurel C, Abhay K, Schaeffer A, et al. Acute thrombotic accident in the postpartum period in a patient receiving bromocriptine. *Crit Care Med* 1990;18(10):1180–1181.
87. Kulig K, Moore LL, Kirk M, et al. Bromocriptine-associated headache: possible life-threatening sympathomimetic interaction. *Obstet Gynecol* 1991;78:941–943.
88. Comabella M, Alvarez-Sabin J, Rovira A, et al. Bromocriptine and postpartum cerebral angiopathy: a causal relationship? *Neurology* 1996;46:1754–1756.
89. Kains JP, Hardy JC, Chevalier C, et al. Retroperitoneal fibrosis in two patients with Parkinson's disease treated with bromocriptine. *Acta Clin Belg* 1990;45:306–310.
90. McElvaney NG, Wilcox PG, Churg A, et al. Pleuropulmonary disease during bromocriptine treatment of Parkinson's disease. *Arch Intern Med* 1988;148:2231–2236.
91. Shaunak S, Wilkins A, Pilling JB, et al. Pericardial, retroperitoneal, and pleural fibrosis induced by pergolide. *J Neurol Neurosurg Psychiatry* 1999;66:79–81.
92. Balachandran KP, Stewart D, Berg GA, et al. Chronic pericardial constriction linked to the antiparkinsonian dopamine agonist pergolide. *Postgrad Med J* 2002;78:49–50.
93. Eisler T, Hall RP, Kalavar KA, et al. Erythromelalgia-like eruptions in parkinsonian patients treated with bromocriptine. *Neurology* 1981;31:1368–1370.
94. Wiesli P, Joos L, Galeazzi RL, et al. Cutaneous pseudolymphoma associated with bromocriptine therapy. *Clin Endocrinol* 2000;53:656–657.
95. Liberato NL, Poli M, Bollati P, et al. Bromocriptine-induced acute hepatitis. *Lancet* 1992:340:969–970.
96. Al-Semaan YM, Clay HA, Meltzer HY. Clozapine in treatment of bromocriptine-induced psychosis. *J Clin Psychopharmacol* 1997;17:126–128.
97. Hardman JG, Limbird LE, eds. *Goodman & Gilman's the pharmacological basis of therapeutics*, 10th ed. New York: McGraw-Hill, 2001.
98. Graham JR. Methysergide for the prevention of headache; experience in five hundred patients over three years. *N Engl J Med* 1964;270:67–72.
99. Graham JR, Suby HI, LeCompte PR, et al. Fibrotic disorders associated with methysergide therapy for headache. *N Engl J Med* 1966;274(7):359–368.
100. Regan JF, Poletti BJ. Vascular adventitial fibrosis in a patient taking methysergide maleate. *JAMA* 1968;203:1069–1071.
101. Bucci JA, Manoharan A. Methysergide-induced retroperitoneal fibrosis: successful outcome and two new laboratory features. *Mayo Clin Proc* 1997;72:1148–1150.
102. Graham JR. Cardiac and pulmonary fibrosis during methysergide therapy for headache. *Am J Med Sci* 1967;254:1–12.
103. Bernick C. Methysergide-induced akathisia. *Clin Neuropharmacol* 1988;11(1):87–89.
104. Skorzewska A, Lal S. Methysergide-induced psychosis: case report with long-term follow-up. *Neuropsychobiology* 1989;22:125–127.
105. Bagby RJ, Cooper RD. Angiography in ergotism. Report of two cases and review of the literature. *AJR Am J Roentgenol* 1972;116:179–186.
106. Tanner JR. St. Anthony's fire, then and now: a case report and historical review. *Can J Surg* 1987;30:291–293.

SECTION

5

Skeletal Muscle Relaxants

CHAPTER 103

Paralytic Agents

B. Zane Horowitz

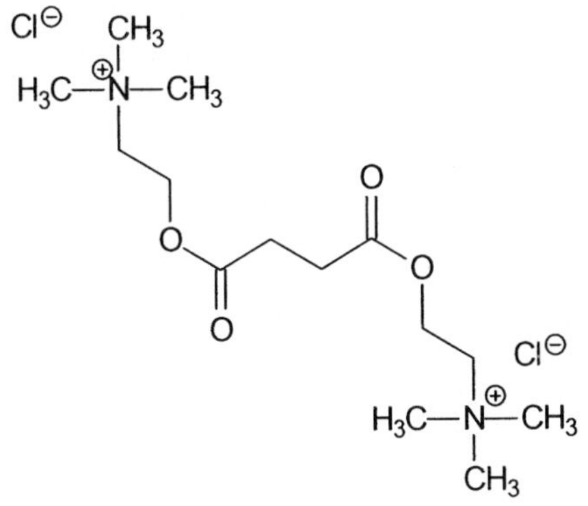

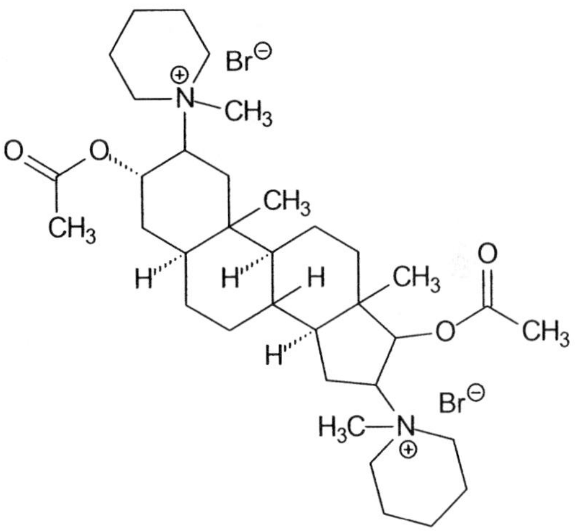

SUCCINYLCHOLINE CHLORIDE

Depolarizing neuromuscular-blocking agents

Compounds included:	**Suxamethonium, succinylcholine, diacetylcholine**
Molecular formula and weight:	**$C_{14}H_{30}Cl_2N_2O_4$, $2H_2O$, 397.3 g/mol**
SI conversion:	**mg/L × 2.5 = μmol/L**
CAS Registry No.:	**306-40-1**
Normal levels:	**Not applicable**
Therapeutic levels:	**Not applicable**
Special concerns:	**May produce bradycardia in children; causes hyperkalemia with some conditions (burns, muscle injury, paraplegia, multiple sclerosis, upper motor neuron injury or extensive denervation of skeletal muscle, muscular dystrophy); also causes malignant hyperthermia**
Target organs:	**Muscle, neuromuscular junction**
Antidote:	**None**

PANCURONIUM BROMIDE

Nondepolarizing neuromuscular-blocking agents

Synonym:	**Pancuronium**
Molecular formula and weight:	**$C_{35}H_{60}Br_2N_2O_4$, 732.7 g/mol**
SI conversion:	**mg/L × 1.4 = μmol/L**
CAS Registry No.:	**15500-66-0**
Normal levels:	**Not applicable**
Therapeutic levels:	**Not applicable**
Special concerns:	**Numerous drug-drug and drug-disease interactions**
Target organs:	**Muscle, neuromuscular junction**
Antidotes:	**Neostigmine, pyridostigmine, atropine, glycopyrrolate**

OVERVIEW

Curare has been used for centuries as an arrow poison by tribes of the Amazon basin. Derived from the plants of the *Strychnos* species, curare was used to coat the tips of arrows that were blown through a reed into their prey (1). The prey was immobilized and could easily be killed. The chemist Claude Bernard experimented with curare in 1856 (2), but clinical uses did not occur until 1932, when it was tried in the treatment of tetanus (3). Curare was first suggested for use in electroconvulsive therapy in 1940 (4) and for neuromuscular blockade in general anesthesia in 1942 (5). Succinylcholine was discovered in 1906 but was not used until 1952 (6).

The toxiferines compounds, which cause neuromuscular paralysis, are derived from the plants *Chododendron tomentosum*, *Strychnos toxifera*, and *Malouetia bequaertiana* (1). The first semisynthetic neuromuscular blocker, alcuronium chloride, was derived from *S. toxifera* (1).

CLASSIFICATION AND CHARACTERISTICS OF THE DRUG CLASS

The neuromuscular-blocking drugs can be classified by mechanism: (a) the *competitive nondepolarizing inhibitors* of acetylcholine (ACh) at the neuromuscular junction (peripheral nicotinic receptor site N_M), of which succinylcholine (Anectine, Quelicin) is the only agent available, and (b) the *noncompetitive agents*, which cause myocyte depolarization and act similarly to ACh. There are two broad chemical classifications in the nondepolarizing neuromuscular-blocking agents: aminosteroid and benzylisoquinolinium compounds (7). The benzylisoquinolinium compounds include D-tubocurarine (curare), metocurine (Metubine), atracurium (Tracrium), *cis*-atracurium (Nimbex), doxacurium (Nuromax), and mivacurium (Mivacron). These agents classically were more likely to release histamine; however, the two newest agents, doxacurium and *cis*-atracurium, do not. The aminosteroidal compounds include pancuronium (Pavulon), vecuronium (Norcuron), pipecuronium (Arduan), rocuronium (Zemuron), and rapacuronium (Raplon). These agents were historically free of histamine release; however, the newest agent, rapacuronium, does release histamine and causes bronchospasm (8). Therefore, the old rule relating histamine to chemical structure is obsolete.

Succinylcholine is the only depolarizing agent available for clinical use. In contrast to nondepolarizing agents, depolarizing agents produce fasciculation before the onset of paralysis (9). Succinylcholine is essentially a dimer of the neurotransmitter ACh linked by an acetate methyl group (1). It is noncompetitive in that increasing the availability of ACh at the neuromuscular junction does not reverse the blockade.

The nondepolarizing agents are competitive with ACh for the nicotinic receptors at the neuromuscular junction; by increasing the amount of ACh available with reversal agents that inhibit the breakdown of ACh, nondepolarizing agents competitively reverse the degree of blockade (7). Conversely, an agent that depletes cholinesterase prolongs the duration of action.

Succinylcholine is used chiefly to facilitate tracheal intubation. The nondepolarizing agents are indicated for induction of neuromuscular paralysis for intubation, during surgery, and in the intensive care unit (ICU) to facilitate mechanical ventilation, control severe muscle activity (e.g., tetanus), and decrease intracranial pressure.

Intubation of a patient's trachea optimally requires complete relaxation of all muscles. The agents capable of rapid onset are succinylcholine (9) and rapacuronium (8,10), both capable of complete paralysis in approximately 60 seconds. The advantage to using succinylcholine, which cannot be reversed but has a short duration of action, is its rapid onset of action that creates intubating conditions in the shortest period of time of all agents. Rapacuronium has almost identical onset of complete paralysis as succinylcholine; however, it was withdrawn from the market in the United States due to bronchospasm (8).

The agents atracurium (11–17) and rocuronium (18,19) are capable of inducing complete paralysis in less than 3 minutes. Mivacurium and atracurium both release histamine, making them less acceptable as agents for rapid induction of complete paralysis (11–17).

Succinylcholine has the shortest duration of action, with its effects wearing off in 8 minutes in most patients, compared with 10 to 180 minutes for other agents (Table 1). Succinylcholine stimulates muscarinic receptors (20) and causes vagal stimulation, which, in susceptible populations, such as children, causes bradycardia and junctional escape rhythms (9,21).

Many of the older agents suffered from some degree of vagolytic (antimuscarinic) effects. The agent with the most potency as an antimuscarinic agent is gallamine. However, alcuronium and pancuronium also have vagolytic effects (7,22).

Some of these agents cause histamine release and produce vasodilatation, bronchospasm, hypotension, and facial flushing. The older agents all cause histamine release (7,20): D-tubocurarine, gallamine, metocurine, and alcuronium (7,20,23,24). Pancuronium causes less histamine release than these older agents (25). Succinylcholine may cause some histamine release and is associated with the largest number of allergic reactions (9). Atracurium and mivacurium produce histamine release, especially when administered by rapid boluses (11,13). *Cis*-atracurium, a stereoisomer of atracurium, does not release histamine (26).

The older agents, D-tubocurarine, metocurine, and alcuronium, have ganglionic blockade effects via nicotinic (N_N) stimulation of the sympathetic ganglia. These effects can cause hypertension and tachycardia (20).

The general use and impact on clinical practice of the neuromuscular-blocking agents involve neuromuscular relaxation (27). None of these agents provides sedation or amnesia, and all should be used with a drug that first—or, at the least, simultaneously—produces unconsciousness. The faster-onset agents (succinylcholine, rocuronium, and vecuronium) may be used for rapid sequence intubation (RSI) (9,26).

Intermediate-duration agents are used for short surgical procedures and in the ICU to maintain paralysis to facilitate mechanical ventilation (27). The longer-duration agents are used for longer surgical procedures (7,28). These agents may be adjuncts in the treatment of tetanus, strychnine poisoning, and refractory seizure disorders when used in conjunction with either a benzodiazepine or propofol for conscious sedation and seizure control (1,27).

PATHOPHYSIOLOGY OF THE CLASS

ACh is the neurotransmitter at the neuromuscular junction (29). It is synthesized in the motor neuron from choline and acetyl coenzyme A—a reaction catalyzed by the enzyme choline *O*-acetyltransferase—in the cytoplasm. ACh is then stored in synaptic vessels near the nerve terminus. These synaptosomes are arranged in rows adjacent to the neuron cell membrane, awaiting the chemical signal that initiates docking and fusion of the synaptosome with the cell membrane. When an action potential of the presynaptic motor neuron occurs, a voltage-gated calcium channel is opened, increasing the intracellular calcium level and triggering exocytosis; the synaptosome vesicle docks and fuses with the nerve terminal cellular membrane, creating a fusion pore with the cell membrane. Each depolarization causes the exocytosis of 50 to 100 synaptosomes. One of the most potent paralytic toxins, botulinum toxin, inhibits the exocytosis of the synaptosome and produces paralysis by preventing ACh release. The neuromuscular-blocking agents, however, all act at the postsynaptic receptor.

The synaptic cleft spans only 20 nm. ACh diffuses across the synapse and binds to nicotinic ACh receptors (N_M). In adults,

TABLE 1. Neuromuscular-blocking agents by classification

Class and drug	Initial dose (mg/kg)	Onset (min)	Duration of action (min)	Maintenance dose
Depolarizing agents				
Succinylcholine (Anectine, Quelicin)	0.6–1.0	IV: 0.5–1.0	6–10	—
		IM: 4	15–30	
Nondepolarizing agents				
Aminosteroidal compounds				
Pancuronium (Pavulon)	0.06–0.12	2–3	60–120	0.010–0.015 mg/kg intermittent bolus
Vecuronium (Norcuron)	Normal: 0.08–0.1	4–5	30–40	0.8–2.0 μg/kg/min
	High: 0.28	1.5–2.0	174	
Pipecuronium (Arduan)	0.085–0.1	2–3	80–120	0.005–0.010 mg/kg intermittent bolus
Rocuronium (Zemuron)	IV: 0.6–1.0	1–3	30–75	8–12 μg/kg/min
	0.45	1.5		
	0.6	1.0		
	Adult IM: 1.8	3–8		
	IM children <1 yr: 1.0	4		
	IM children >1 yr: 1.8	4		
Rapacuronium (Raplon)	1.5 –2.5	1	8–16	9 μg/kg/min
Benzylisoquinolinium compounds				
D-Tubocurarine (Curare)	0.1–0.2	3	60–100	0.10–0.15 mg/kg
Metocurine (Metubine)	0.4–0.5	0.2–0.4	—	0.05 –0.10 mg/kg
Atracurium (Tracrium)	0.4–0.6	IV: 2–3	60–70	4–12 μg/kg/min
		IM: 10		
Cis-atracurium (Nimbex)	Adult: 0.15–0.2	1.5 –3.0	40–75	1–2 μg/kg/min
	Pediatric: 0.1			
Doxacurium (Nuromax)	0.05–0.08	4–5	55–160[a]	0.005–0.010 mg/kg intermittent bolus
Mivacurium (Mivacron)	0.15–0.25	IV: 2–3	15–20	3–15 μg/kg/min
		IM: >10		
Miscellaneous agents				
Gallamine (Flaxedil)	1.0–3.0	2	90–120	0.3–0.5 mg/kg
Alcuronium	0.2–0.3	3	60–120	0.05–0.10 mg/kg

[a]Prolonged in the elderly.

the nicotinic receptor is a pentamer of four distinct subunits: two alpha, one beta, one epsilon, and one delta. In the fetus and denervated adult muscle, the epsilon subunit is replaced with a gamma subunit, rendering it insensitive to ACh stimulation. In the adult, ACh binding sites are at the alpha-epsilon and the alpha-delta interfaces. When two ACh molecules bind at these sites, they stimulate a conformational change in the ligand-gated receptor, which opens the ion channel in the center of the pentameric receptor. This channel allows sodium and calcium to enter the motor cell and potassium to exit and thereby depolarizes the postsynaptic cell, resulting in muscle contraction.

Succinylcholine also binds to the ACh receptor and initiates depolarization and is, therefore, a depolarizing-neuromuscular blocker. The other neuromuscular-blocking agents are all non-depolarizing-competitive inhibitors. These agents do not open the postsynaptic ion channel.

There are other nicotinic receptors at the sympathetic and parasympathetic autonomic ganglia, at the adrenal medulla, and in the central nervous system (CNS). These N_N receptors may be cross-stimulated by some of the agents that cause neuromuscular blockade, resulting in undesirable side effects with the use of these agents. Muscarinic receptors on secretory glands, on bronchial smooth muscle, and in the cardiac conduction tissue may also be antagonized by some of the nondepolarizing agents.

ACh is normally degraded in the synapse by the enzyme acetylcholinesterase (AChE), which hydrolyzes ACh to choline and acetic acid. Choline is then pumped back into the nerve terminus to be used in the synthesis of more ACh. Small amounts of ACh also stimulate presynaptic receptors, which act by assisting in the mobilizing of more ACh for subsequent packaging into synaptosomes. AChE is the enzyme responsible for the normal hydrolysis of ACh in neural transmission. AChE also exists in red blood cells, and this is the source of the "true" or red blood cell cholinesterase that is measured by the laboratory.

ACh is broken down quickly by AChE, but succinylcholine is not affected by it. There is another cholinesterase called *pseudocholinesterase*, which is synthesized in the liver and circulates in the plasma. Pseudocholinesterase is referred to as *plasma cholinesterase* or *butyrylcholinesterase*. Pseudocholinesterase does not reside in the synaptic cleft and does not contribute to normal ACh degradation, but it is the enzyme responsible for degradation of the neuromuscular-blocking agents succinylcholine and mivacurium. These agents must diffuse back out of the synaptic cleft to be metabolized by the plasma cholinesterase. Once the concentration of succinylcholine or mivacurium falls in the synapse, normal neuromotor function is restored and paralysis resolves.

Some patients have an inherited or drug-induced deficiency of pseudocholinesterase; these patients have a prolonged action of succinylcholine and mivacurium (30,31). All forms of cholinesterase can be inhibited by carbamate and organophosphate compounds (32). Carbamate compounds can be used therapeutically to hasten the reversal of neuromuscular blockade after the use of nondepolarizing agents. These drugs include physostigmine, neostigmine, and pyridostigmine, which inhibit the enzyme AChE and the breakdown of ACh (33) by allowing more ACh to compete for the N_M receptor, competitively reversing the action of the nondepolarizing neuromuscular-blocking agents.

DEPOLARIZING AGENTS: SUCCINYLCHOLINE

Succinylcholine is the only depolarizing agent in clinical use. It causes depolarization and, therefore, fasciculation of the muscle followed by flaccid paralysis. It may cause histamine release, inducing hypotension, bronchospasm, flushing, or rash (9). Succinylcholine can stimulate the vagus nerve at the muscarinic receptor sites. This results in bradycardia and bradydysrhythmias. Succinylcholine can stimulate the sympathetic ganglia, releasing catecholamines, which may cause tachycardia (9). It transiently elevates intraocular pressure and should be avoided in patients with an open eye injury (34).

The advantage to using succinylcholine, which has an ultrashort duration of action, is its rapid onset of action. It produces intubating conditions in the shortest period of time. Another advantage is that it can be stored at room temperature for up to 4 weeks. Once reconstituted from its lyophilized powder, however, it should be used or discarded within 24 hours (35).

Succinylcholine is used to facilitate intubation in emergency conditions when immediate airway control is critical (36). It does not cross the blood–brain barrier and has no sedative effects. It should always be used with a rapid onset sedative hypnotic agent that can produce unconsciousness and amnesia. Although use for maintenance of neuromuscular paralysis during surgery has been described, infusions of succinylcholine convert from causing a phase I block to a phase II block similar to the nondepolarizing agents (20). Some tachyphylaxis occurs due to its effect during continuous infusions, and higher doses may be needed to produce the same degree of phase II block. Inhalation anesthetic gases potentiate the phase II block. Due to these factors, it is safer to provide ongoing neuromuscular paralysis with a nondepolarizing agent. Succinylcholine is often the agent of choice for short procedures, such as reduction of a dislocated joint, brief endoscopy, and electroconvulsive therapy.

A test dose of 0.1 mg/kg may be given 1 to 2 minutes before the doses described below (37). This dose diminishes the degree of fasciculation, potassium release, and muscle pain experienced by the patient. In addition, it may provide a useful warning because there should be negligible muscle relaxation with this dose. If the patient has a pseudocholinesterase deficiency, these patients often develop paralysis or respiratory depression from the test dose, thereby indicating a depressed serum pseudocholinesterase. If prolonged paralysis occurs, then the patient should be evaluated for a genetic deficiency of pseudocholinesterase.

The standard *adult dose* for RSI is 0.6 to 1.0 mg/kg intravenously (IV) (Table 1). If IV access is not possible and airway management is critical, an intramuscular (IM) dose of 2.5 mg/kg of succinylcholine may be used (do not exceed 150 mg total) (38). Continuous IV infusion of 0.5 to 10.0 mg/minute has been used for short procedures. An intermittent bolus method of 0.04 to 0.07 mg/kg to maintain relaxation has also been described. In general, a nondepolarizing agent should be used to maintain paralysis instead of succinylcholine.

The *pediatric dose* for RSI is 1.0 to 2.0 mg/kg IV (39,40). In children younger than 5 years of age, atropine, 0.02 mg/kg IV (minimum dose, 0.1 mg; maximum dose, 1.0 mg), or glycopyrrolate, 4.4 to 8.8 μg/kg IM, should be used. Succinylcholine should be used only when the need for an emergency airway exceeds the risks of using succinylcholine (36,41,42). If the airway cannot be obtained with a single dose, one must weigh the risk that in children subsequent doses of succinylcholine may produce bradycardia or asystole (42,43). An alternative agent should be used if there is a continued need for an emergent airway. Continuous infusions and intermittent bolusing should never be used in children.

Toxic Pediatric Dose

Due to several reports of asystole and hyperkalemic cardiac arrest occurring within minutes after administration of succinylcholine, it should not be used for routine airway management (43,44). It may only be indicated for emergency intubation. The highest risk group is children younger than 8 years of age, and boys may be more susceptible than girls. Some instances may be due to subclinical cases of Duchenne's or Becker's muscular dystrophy (42,45). Cases of severe hyperkalemia, rhabdomyolysis, and malignant hyperthermia (MH) have occurred in otherwise apparently healthy children and adolescents (46,47).

Children have an exaggerated physiologic response to laryngoscopy with bradycardia (41,42). Hypoxia and vagal stimulation enhance this effect. Profound bradycardia, brady-escape dysrhythmias, and asystole have occurred in children given succinylcholine.

Pharmacokinetics and Pharmacodynamics

ABSORPTION AND DISTRIBUTION

Succinylcholine is not absorbed orally. Total muscle paralysis is complete within 30 to 60 seconds (Table 1) (48,49). The duration of action is 6 to 10 minutes. IM absorption is less predictable. After an IM injection, the time of onset is 2 to 3 minutes, and duration of action ranges from 15 to 30 minutes (49). Succinylcholine does not cross the blood–brain barrier.

ELIMINATION

Succinylcholine is eliminated primarily by rapid metabolism by pseudocholinesterase in the plasma (90%); 10% is excreted unchanged in the urine (Table 2). The metabolite is succinylmonocholine, which has a ratio of 1:20 the activity of succinylcholine (28,49). After IV injection, most of the drug is metabolized by plasma cholinesterase before it binds to the nicotinic receptor. Recovery from succinylcholine neuromuscular blockade involves the diffusion of succinylcholine off the ACh nicotinic receptor back into plasma where it is metabolized.

Succinylmonocholine may cause a nondepolarizing, rather than a depolarizing, neuromuscular block. Succinylmonocholine is slowly hydrolyzed to succinate and choline, neither of which are active. The portion of succinylmonocholine that is not hydrolyzed is excreted renally; it can accumulate in patients with renal failure or patients treated with repeated doses or constant infusions and can produce prolonged neuromuscular blockade. The phenomenon is referred to as *phase II blockade*, and recovery from it is slower, similar to the nondepolarizing-neuromuscular agents (20).

Pseudocholinesterase, correctly called *butyrylcholinesterase*, is produced by the liver. Its half-life is 11 days (50). A variety of disease states and medications can alter its metabolism (Table 3). When pseudocholinesterase levels are depressed, the duration of action of succinylcholine is also prolonged (31). Other agents may prolong the action of succinylcholine without depressing the level of pseudocholinesterase (Table 4).

Pseudocholinesterase levels are dependent on having both alleles of the E1 gene that synthesizes pseudocholinesterase. Patients with an enzymatic deficiency of one or both alleles of E1 have a prolonged response to succinylcholine. The incidence of the heterozygous deficiency is approximately 1:480 (51). The patient with a heterozygote that lacks a single normal allele may experience doubling of the duration of effect after receiving succinylcholine. The rare patient with a homozygous deficiency (approximately 1:3200 people) may experience paralysis of 4 to 8 hours after succinylcholine (51–54).

A patient who requires more than 10 to 15 minutes to recover muscular function after a single intubating dose of succinylcholine should be evaluated for pseudocholinesterase deficiency (31). There are two methods. The first technique is by measuring the absolute amount of pseudocholinesterase in the blood. The second is by using the

TABLE 2. Pharmacokinetics and pharmacodynamics of neuromuscular-blocking agents

Class and drug	Protein binding (%)	Metabolism	Clearance	Half-life
Depolarizing agents				
Succinylcholine (Anectine, Quelicin)	None	Pseudocholinesterase in plasma, 90% of dose	Renal, 10% of dose	<1 min
Nondepolarizing agents				
Aminosteroidal compounds				
Pancuronium (Pavulon)	7–11	20% liver deacetylation	Renal	Normal: 90–140 min; renal failure: 257 min; cirrhosis: 208 min
Vecuronium (Norcuron)	30	30% liver, active metabolite with 80% potency of parent	Renal	71 min
Pipecuronium (Arduan)	32	<5% liver	Renal	137–161 min
Rocuronium (Zemuron)	30	Minimal hepatic	Biliary	84–131 min; liver disease: 142 min
Rapacuronium (Raplon)	50–88	Liver deacetylation; active metabolite with twice the potency	Renal	72–175 min
Benzylisoquinolinium compounds				
D-Tubocurarine (Curare)	—	Hepatic	Renal	—
Metocurine (Metubine)	—	Hepatic	Renal	—
Atracurium (Tracrium)	82	—	Hoffmann elimination; hypothermia below 34°C reduces clearance	16–20 min
Cis-atracurium (Nimbex)	Unknown	—	Hoffmann elimination	22–31 min
Doxacurium (Nuromax)	30	—	Renal, unchanged; bile, small amount	Normal: 72–96 min; chronic renal failure: 221 min; liver disease: 115 min
Mivacurium (Mivacron)	Unknown	Plasma cholinesterase; duration lengthened threefold in anhepatic subjects; duration 3–4 h longer in cholinesterase deficiency	Duration lengthened 10–15 min in renal failure	1.8–2.0 min

dibucaine number, which gives a percentage of inhibition of the patient's pseudocholinesterase with dibucaine, a known inhibitor of pseudocholinesterase. A dibucaine number greater than 85% is normal, whereas a dibucaine number less than 63% suggests homozygous deficiency (31). Genetic testing of leukocytes can characterize whether a deficiency exists (31). At least 12 additional human pseudocholinesterase variants have been discovered (55,56).

TABLE 3. Disease states and drugs that inhibit or lower pseudocholinesterase levels

Disease states	Drugs
Pregnancy	Organophosphate pesticides and nerve agents
Malignancy	Anticholinesterase-reversal agents (neostigmine, edrophonium)
Liver disease	Anticholinesterase agents for Alzheimer's disease (tacrine, donepezil, rivastigmine, galantamine)
Malnutrition	Anticholinesterase eyedrops (echothiophate, isoflurophate)
Severe anemia	Anticholinesterases used for myasthenia gravis [pyridostigmine bromide (Mestinon)]
Burns	Physostigmine salicylate (Antilirium)
Myxedema	Cocaine
Severe dehydration	Oral contraceptives
Uremia	Metoclopramide
	Phenothiazines
	Monoamine oxidase inhibitors (especially phenelzine)
	Corticosteroids
	Cyclophosphamide
	Bambuterol (prodrug of terbutaline)
	Propanolol
	Aprotinin
	Thiotepa

Pregnancy and Lactation

Succinylcholine is classified as U.S. Food and Drug Administration (FDA) pregnancy category C (Appendix I). Nevertheless, succinylcholine should be avoided in pregnancy if possible because serum pseudocholinesterase levels may be depressed up to 24%, prolonging its duration of action (57). Succinylcholine crosses the placenta in quantities too small to have effects on the fetus (57). Succinylcholine has been used for induction for emergent cesarean section. It is not believed to affect the uterine muscles. No studies on lactation or excretion in breast milk have been done.

Clinical Presentation

HYPERKALEMIA

Succinylcholine may raise the serum potassium by 0.5 to 1.0 mEq/L transiently in normal patients (58,59). Patients with

TABLE 4. Drugs that may potentiate the neuromuscular blockade with succinylcholine via mechanisms other than depletion of pseudocholinesterase

Sodium channel–blocking agents	
Quinine	Procainamide
Quinidine	Lidocaine
Chloroquine	Promazine
Miscellaneous effects on the neuromuscular junction	
Lithium	Polymyxin
Magnesium	Clindamycin
Furosemide at low doses <1 mg/kg	Cyclosporin
	Tetracycline
Calcium-channel blockers	Metoclopramide
Terbutaline	Inhalation anesthetics
Aminoglycosides	Oxytocin

TABLE 5. Clinical features of the neuromuscular-blocking agents

Class and drug	Histamine release	Cardiovascular effects
Depolarizing agents		
Succinylcholine (Anectine, Quelicin)	Yes	Stimulates vagus nerve (bradycardia) and sympathetic ganglia (tachycardia)
Nondepolarizing agents		
Aminosteroidal compounds		
Pancuronium (Pavulon)	Minimal	Moderate vagolytic; no ganglionic blockade
Vecuronium (Norcuron)	None	Weakly vagolytic; no ganglionic blockade
Pipecuronium (Arduan)	None	Weakly vagolytic; no ganglionic stimulation
Rocuronium (Zemuron)	None	Minimal
Rapacuronium (Raplon)	Yes	Vasodilatation via calcium-channel blockade
Benzylisoquinolinium compounds		
D-Tubocurarine (Curare)	Yes	No vagolytic effect
Metocurine (Metubine)	Yes	No vagolytic effect
Atracurium (Tracrium)	Yes, especially doses >0.5 mg/kg	No vagolytic or ganglionic blockade
Cis-atracurium (Nimbex)	None	No vagolytic or ganglionic blockade
Doxacurium (Nuromax)	None	No vagolytic or ganglionic blockade; rare cases of hypotension
Mivacurium (Mivacron)	Yes, especially rapid bolus	No vagolytic or ganglionic blockade
Miscellaneous agents		
Gallamine (Flaxedil)	None	Strong vagolytic
Alcuronium	Little	Slight vagolytic

underlying muscle disease (60), burns (61), and spinal cord injury (62-64) may experience excess potassium release from myocytes from succinylcholine. Although the use of succinylcholine in patients with renal disease has been a concern, it may be used safely if there is no preexisting hyperkalemia (65-67). The risk is greatest in patients with untreated renal failure and potassium overload who may experience an increase in their potassium and are unable to excrete it (66). Patients with digitalis toxicity (68) or diabetic ketoacidosis or a hemodialysis patient who has missed several treatments is also at great risk of having preexisting hyperkalemia. Hyperkalemia has also occurred in patients with intraabdominal infections who have been given succinylcholine (69) and patients placed on a prolonged infusion of succinylcholine (70).

FASCICULATION

Succinylcholine causes fasciculation when administered at full dose (71,72). A "priming" dose (10% of the full dose) can be given 1 to 2 minutes before the full dose to blunt fasciculation. Administering a pre-fasciculation dose of a nondepolarizing neuromuscular-blocking agent before succinylcholine also diminishes fasciculation (73,74). Severe fasciculation may cause transient myoglobinuria (72,75,76) or elevated creatine kinase (77) or induce hyperkalemia (58,59,78). Masseter spasm has been described rarely in children (79). Muscle pain may result and may not be proportional to the degree of fasciculation (73,74,79,80). Pretreatment with nondepolarizing-neuromuscular blockers (73,74,80), dantrolene (78), or benzodiazepines (71) may reduce muscle pain.

CARDIAC DYSRHYTHMIAS

Succinylcholine stimulates nicotinic receptors on both parasympathetic and sympathetic ganglia (Table 5) as well as muscarinic receptors in the heart (82). At standard doses, bradycardia and junctional escape rhythms may occur due to excess muscarinic stimulation (83). Young children and patients receiving a second dose of succinylcholine are more susceptible to this effect (84). Prior administration of atropine may blunt the bradydysrhythmias (83,85). Premedicating with a pre-fasciculation dose of a nondepolarizing neuromuscular-blocking agent may blunt fasciculation and potassium release (20,42).

Ventricular dysrhythmias may occur due to the release of catecholamines from the sympathetic ganglia (86). Hypoxia, hypercarbia, and electrolyte disturbances may produce an additive effect (87). Cardiac sensitizing drugs, including some inhalational anesthetics, digitalis, monoamine oxidase inhibitors, and tricyclic antidepressants, may also predispose to ventricular dysrhythmias (20).

INTRAOCULAR PRESSURE

Intraocular pressure increases within 1 minute of IV injection, peaks in 2 to 4 minutes, and resolves by 6 minutes (34,87–90). The pathophysiology involves contraction of the iris myofibrils and transient dilation of choroidal blood flow (20,91). Pretreatment with a nondepolarizing agent diminishes this effect (92). In the patient with a possible penetrating eye injury, RSI should be induced using a nondepolarizing agent alone or as a priming dose for succinylcholine (93).

INTRAGASTRIC PRESSURE

As a result of abdominal muscle fasciculation, succinylcholine may increase intragastric pressure and facilitate regurgitation (94). This effect may be proportional to body size and is less common in infants (95). Administering a pre-fasciculation dose of a nondepolarizing-neuromuscular blocker may diminish the effect (96).

INTRACRANIAL PRESSURE

Succinylcholine may increase intracranial pressure (97). Pretreatment with a pre-fasciculation dose of a nondepolarizing agent may diminish this effect (98). Some studies in intensive care patients with intracranial monitoring catheters in place who were given succinylcholine did not show an appreciable change in intracranial pressure (99,100).

Diagnostic Tests

Succinylcholine levels are not clinically useful but may be of value in suspected suicide or homicide. Ion-paired, thin-layer chromatography detects succinylcholine and its derivatives (101). Patients with more than 10 to 15 minutes of motor paralysis after a single dose of succinylcholine should have pseudocholinesterase levels checked (31). Patients with masseter spasm or a family history of MH should have a muscle biopsy for a caffeine stimulation test (102,103). Patients who develop

MH need numerous critical care tests to assess complications and guide therapy.

Treatment

Treatment strategies focus on maintaining adequate ventilation until the neuromuscular blockade resolves. Initial assistance with a bag-valve-mask device or even mouth-to-mouth resuscitation is required for maintenance of respiration. If prolonged paralysis is anticipated, then endotracheal intubation should be established. Rare side effects, such as bradycardia, bronchospasm, hypotension, dysrhythmias, heat production, and hyperkalemia, require immediate recognition and supportive care.

BRADYCARDIA

The treatment of bradycardia begins by terminating the intubation attempt and ensuring appropriate ventilation. Atropine is administered if bradycardia does not respond.

CARDIAC ARREST

If cardiac arrest occurs within minutes of administering succinylcholine, hyperkalemia must be suspected (42,46,47). Immediate treatment with IV calcium chloride, sodium bicarbonate, insulin, and glucose should be commenced (Chapter 44) (42).

MALIGNANT HYPERTHERMIA

MH is a rare autosomal-dominant inherited trait affecting skeletal muscle (104,105). It occurs in 1 in 50,000 to 100,000 individuals (106,107), but its incidence in children undergoing general anesthesia may be as high as 1 in 15,000 (107). Mutations occur on chromosome 19 in the gene for the ryanodine-1 receptor on skeletal muscle, which is responsible for the activation of the calcium-releasing channel (108). Many different amino acid substitutions are associated with variants of the ryanodine-1 receptor (109). This may account for variability in expressivity of the hyperthermia syndrome. Studies in countries with high incidence likely overestimate the incidence of the gene in an unselected population (110). Defects of the ryanodine-2 receptor in cardiac muscle have been associated with polymorphous ventricular dysrhythmias and sudden death (111).

In MH, the myocyte sarcoplasmic reticulum releases excess calcium, causing sustained contraction and heat production (104,112). Much of the pathophysiology is derived from studies of porcine MH, a similar disorder (113). Animal research has shown that the myocyte's intracellular calcium levels are three times normal (114), and when triggered by succinylcholine, excess calcium release may elevate intracellular ionized calcium levels 17-fold (115). This hypercalcemia inhibits troponin and allows sustained contraction of actin and myosin (112). It also breaks down adenosine triphosphate (ATP). At the same time, it activates phosphorylase kinase, regenerating ATP via glycolysis (116). This cycle of ATP creation and destruction creates a hypermetabolic state consuming glycogen, ATP, and oxygen as well as increasing heat production, pyruvate to lactic conversion, and anaerobic metabolism (116). Rhabdomyolysis occurs, and myocyte damage leads to entry of potassium, creatinine, creatinine kinase, phosphate, and myoglobin into the blood (104,112,116). Excessive myoglobin is precipitated in the renal tubules in hypovolemia and acidosis, leading to acute tubular necrosis (117,118). Dantrolene blocks the release of calcium from the sarcoplasmic reticulum, disrupting the initiating event in MH (119).

Clinically, MH is characterized by sudden chest wall rigidity and difficulty ventilating the patient (104,112,116,120). Shunting of oxygenated blood to the hypermetabolic muscles causes venous desaturation and a sudden rise in end-tidal carbon dioxide (CO_2), which is pathognomonic of this disorder (104,116). Elevated end-tidal CO_2 may occur before perceptible changes in vital signs or muscle rigidity (121). With the onset of muscle rigidity, hyperthermia, hyperkalemia, and rhabdomyolysis usually occur (122). Hyperkalemia may cause dysrhythmias and cardiac arrest. When children sustain a cardiac arrest immediately after being intubated using succinylcholine, it may be due to excess potassium release from undiagnosed myotonic dystrophy rather than MH (44–46).

Treatment of MH can be difficult.* It involves immediate cessation of anesthesia, hyperventilation with 100% oxygen in an effort to blow off CO_2, and rapid cooling with iced saline gastric lavage (104,116,123). A venous blood sample may help to confirm the diagnosis if it shows diminished oxygen and high CO_2. Dantrolene is the cornerstone of treatment (Chapter 62) (104,116). Dantrolene blocks the release of calcium from the sarcoplasmic reticulum and may antagonize the interaction of actin, myosin, troponin, and tropomyosin (119,124). Clinical improvement of muscle tone and heat production should be evident within 20 minutes (116). Dantrolene should be administered as a 2.5- to 3.0-mg/kg IV bolus every 10 minutes for three doses (116). Each vial of dantrolene, 20 mg, contains 3 g of mannitol to increase diuresis. In rare circumstances, patients refractory to the initial three boluses (a total of 7.5 to 9.0 mg/kg) require a dose of 10 mg/kg IV (116).

After the acute phase of hyperthermia, the patient must be carefully monitored for metabolic acidosis, rhabdomyolysis, myoglobinuria, volume depletion, hyperkalemia, ventricular dysrhythmias, and acute pulmonary edema (104). Hemolysis and disseminated intravascular coagulopathy may develop in severe cases (104). Additional doses of dantrolene, 1 mg/kg every 6 to 8 hours, should be given for most cases (116). Adjuncts to management include IV sodium bicarbonate to correct the serum pH and fluid boluses to maintain a urine output of 2 ml/kg/hour (116). Both these interventions may help prevent the effects of myoglobin-induced renal injury (116–118). Patients should be observed in an ICU for 24 to 48 hours, with careful monitoring for signs of volume overload and acute pulmonary edema as well as compartment syndrome due to fluid uptake by the muscle (104,116). If the patient experiences tachydysrhythmias or hypertension, calcium-channel blockers are contraindicated, as they interact with dantrolene to further elevate serum potassium (116,125).

MASSETER SPASM

Masseter spasm occurs in up to 1% of children given succinylcholine (126,127). There is debate as to whether isolated masseter spasm in children represents a variant form of MH or only a more severe form of "masseter tetany" that is ultimately associated with MH (116,128). If a patient experiences masseter spasm after induction with succinylcholine, he or she should be carefully observed for 15 minutes. If the spasm persists after paralysis resolves, or if end-tidal CO_2 begins to rise, then treatment with dantrolene should be instituted (116). If the patient remains asymptomatic, some sources advocate ICU monitoring for at least 24 hours.

*Resources for treatment of malignant hyperthermia: Cases of malignant hyperthermia are difficult to treat, and the technical assistance of anesthesiologists experienced in its management can be accessed at the Malignant Hyperthermia Hotline: 1-800-MH-HYPER. If calling from outside of the United States, the international phone number is 001-315-464-7079. Posters outlining MH treatment are also available from the Malignant Hyperthermia Association of the United States (MHAUS; 1-800-98-MHAUS) for display in areas where succinylcholine or volatile anesthetics are used. The MHAUS Web site (http://www.mhaus.org) also contains up-to-date information on the location of muscle biopsy testing sites.

Patients with masseter spasm or MH and their family members should be referred for muscle biopsy testing (102). The Malignant Hyperthermia Association of the United States (http://www.mhaus.org) has information on laboratories that perform this procedure. One caveat in obtaining the muscle biopsy is to avoid premedication with either dantrolene or droperidol, both of which may falsely normalize the caffeine stimulation test (129). The North American caffeine/halothane stimulation test has a sensitivity of 97% and a specificity of 78% for MH (103). The European *in vitro* contracture test has a sensitivity of 99% and a specificity of 94% (130).

Treatment involves supportive care and treatment of complications as described above. There are no methods to enhance elimination, although neostigmine has been used to reverse phase II blockade from prolonged succinylcholine infusion (131). Succinylcholine usually has a short duration of action; however, patients with pseudocholinesterase deficiency may exhibit prolonged effects. Prolonged respiratory support is indicated for this group of patients, although theoretically, an infusion of fresh frozen plasma could restore plasma cholinesterase levels to normal and reverse the neuromuscular blockade. There is no role for the use of oral activated charcoal, diuresis, hemodialysis, or hemoperfusion. Experimentally, the germine derivatives can reverse blockade (132).

NONDEPOLARIZING AGENTS

The *nondepolarizing agents* are a group of similar agents used to produce neuromuscular relaxation. The faster-onset agents can be used as a substitute for succinylcholine for RSI. Intermediate-duration agents are used for short surgical procedures and in the ICU to maintain paralysis and facilitate mechanical ventilation. The longer-duration agents are used for longer surgical procedures (27). These agents may be adjuncts in the treatment of tetanus, strychnine poisoning, and refractory seizure disorders (27). Each agent is discussed individually, but due to their similarities, their diagnosis and treatment are presented as a group at the end of this section.

Pathophysiology

The nondepolarizing agents are competitive inhibitors of ACh at the neuromuscular junction. By blocking receptor binding of ACh, flaccid paralysis is produced. Because ACh is competitive with the nondepolarizing agents, increasing the amount of ACh available at the neuromuscular junction competitively antagonizes the effects of the nondepolarizing agents. This is the rationale behind using anticholinesterase agents for reversal (7,132).

Pancuronium

Pancuronium (Pavulon) is a long-acting agent. It is not commonly used for intubation. The weak vagolytic and histamine-releasing effects of this agent cause slight increase in heart rate and blood pressure; therefore, it should be avoided in patients who cannot tolerate these effects, such as the patient with coronary disease (25,133,134).

TOXICOKINETICS AND TOXICODYNAMICS

Pharmacokinetics and pharmacodynamics are provided in Table 2.

VULNERABLE POPULATIONS

Pancuronium is FDA pregnancy category C (Appendix I). It should be used with caution in patients who may not tolerate tachycardia. Cardiovascular side effects include tachycardia and no ganglionic blockade. The duration of action is increased 20% in renal failure and 65% in liver disease.

CLINICAL PRESENTATION

Table 1 provides typical doses, onset, and duration of action. Table 5 addresses histamine release and cardiovascular effects.

Vecuronium

Vecuronium (Norcuron) is the 2-desmethyl analog of pancuronium. It has a short duration of action and, unlike pancuronium, does not cause an increase in heart rate or blood pressure (135). However, it is deacetylated in the liver to an active metabolite, which is then further metabolized and renally excreted. It should be used with caution in patients with renal or hepatic disease.

TOXICOKINETICS AND TOXICODYNAMICS

Pharmacokinetics and pharmacodynamics are provided in Table 2.

VULNERABLE POPULATIONS

Vecuronium is FDA pregnancy category C (Appendix I). Use with caution in liver and renal disease, obesity, the elderly, and children younger than the age of 1 year.

CLINICAL PRESENTATION

Table 1 provides typical doses, onset, and duration of action. Table 5 addresses histamine release and cardiovascular effects.

Rocuronium

Rocuronium (Zemuron) has fast onset of action, making it an acceptable substitute for RSI (18,136). However, it must be stored under refrigeration at 2° to 8°C and, once it is warmed to room temperature, should be used within 30 days.

VULNERABLE POPULATIONS

Rocuronium is FDA pregnancy category B (Appendix I). It is not recommended for RSI in cesarean sections. Use with caution in patients with liver disease; the duration of action is increased by 40%. The elderly may also have prolonged duration of action.

CLINICAL PRESENTATION

Table 1 provides typical doses, onset, and duration of action. Table 5 addresses histamine release and cardiovascular effects.

Pipecuronium

Pipecuronium (Arduan) is a derivative of pancuronium that possesses 20% to 30% more potency and long duration of action (20). It is ideally used in surgical procedures lasting longer than 90 minutes.

VULNERABLE POPULATIONS

Pipecuronium is FDA pregnancy category C (Appendix I). Use with caution in renal disease.

CLINICAL PRESENTATION

Table 1 provides typical doses, onset, and duration of action. Table 5 addresses histamine release and cardiovascular effects.

Atracurium

Atracurium (Tracrium) is a mixture of ten stereoisomers, which are eliminated in the plasma by Hoffmann elimination, an enzymatic process (137). Because there is no hepatic metabolism or renal clearance, it can be used in patients with liver and renal disease (12). High doses or rapid infusion cause histamine release, which may be significant (23). Pretreatment with an H_2-blocker may blunt the effect of histamine (24). Like rocuronium, it must be refrigerated. It should be used within 14 days of rewarming. It should not be used IM due to tissue irritation. Hypothermia below 34°C reduces clearance.

VULNERABLE POPULATIONS

Atracurium is FDA pregnancy category C (Appendix I). Avoid prolonged infusions in the ICU with seizure patients due to the accumulation of laudanosine. Avoid in patients with a history of anaphylaxis or multiple drug allergies. Use cautiously in patients with coronary heart disease because of histamine release.

CLINICAL PRESENTATION

Table 1 provides typical doses, onset, and duration of action. Table 5 addresses histamine release and cardiovascular effects.

Cis-Atracurium

Cis-*atracurium* (Nimbex) is a single *cis-cis* isomer of atracurium and is also cleared by Hoffmann elimination (138). This potent isomer from atracurium increases potency, and onset of action is reduced. It also does not cause histamine release in normal doses (139). Therefore, it is an excellent agent for cardiovascular surgery, use in renal or hepatic disease, and in children.

VULNERABLE POPULATIONS

Local anesthetic agents may prolong duration. *Cis*-atracurium is FDA pregnancy category B (Appendix I).

CLINICAL PRESENTATION

Table 1 provides typical doses, onset, and duration of action. Table 5 addresses histamine release and cardiovascular effects.

Mivacurium

Mivacurium (Mivacron) is a mixture of three stereoisomers, which are metabolized by plasma cholinesterase, similar to succinylcholine (12). It is a short-acting agent with a duration of approximately three times that of succinylcholine. Histamine release occurs with rapid IV bolus; the effects are usually transient and may be blunted by the use of H_2-blockers (16,17). It is ideally used for nonemergent intubation for short surgical procedures.

VULNERABLE POPULATIONS

Use with caution in homozygous cholinesterase deficiency states and coronary artery disease. Mivacurium is FDA pregnancy category C (Appendix I). It has been used in emergency cesarean sections.

CLINICAL PRESENTATION

Table 1 provides typical doses, onset, and duration of action. Table 5 addresses histamine release and cardiovascular effects.

Doxacurium

Doxacurium (Nuromax) is a long-acting neuromuscular blocker that is relatively free of cardiac side effects and is used primarily for long surgical procedures (7,20).

VULNERABLE POPULATIONS

Use with caution in renal failure. Doxacurium is FDA pregnancy category C (Appendix II).

CLINICAL PRESENTATION

Table 1 provides typical doses, onset, and duration of action. Table 5 addresses histamine release and cardiovascular effects.

Rapacuronium

Rapacuronium (Raplon) is an analog of vecuronium (10). It has a fast onset of action and a short duration, making it attractive as an agent for RSI. Postmarketing surveillance indicated a 5% incidence of bronchospasm (8). It has been withdrawn from use.

VULNERABLE POPULATIONS

Use with caution in reactive airway disease and coronary disease. Rapacuronium is FDA pregnancy category C (Appendix I).

CLINICAL PRESENTATION

Table 1 provides typical doses, onset, and duration of action. Table 5 addresses histamine release and cardiovascular effects.

Pharmacokinetics and Pharmacodynamics

ABSORPTION, PROTEIN BINDING, AND DISTRIBUTION

Nondepolarizing agents are not well absorbed orally. Rapid onset with initial muscle weakness within 1 minute and complete muscle paralysis within 3 minutes are common to all agents after IV injection (Table 1). After IM injection, there is a variable onset of action. Only rocuronium has an acceptable onset of action after IM use (Table 1) (140).

The neuromuscular-blocking agents are distributed to plasma and tissue compartments. The clinical manifestations are dependent on the concentration at the neuromuscular junction. As the plasma level declines, a slower equilibration with neuromuscular junction levels occurs, and the blockade is slowly reversed (29). Patients with burns may have altered sensitivity to these agents and experience severe hyperkalemia (141). These drugs remain mostly in the extracellular compartment, with little penetration of the blood–brain barrier. These agents can cross the placenta during the first trimester of pregnancy.

METABOLISM

Vecuronium, pipecuronium, pancuronium, and rapacuronium are deacetylated in the liver and excreted in the urine (Table 2) (20). Vecuronium and pancuronium have active metabolites. Pancuronium is deactivated to 3-desacetyl pancuronium, which has two-thirds the activity of pancuronium but accounts for only a small percent of the metabolic degradation (142,143). Vecuronium is deactivated to 3-desacetyl vecuronium, which has 80% of the activity of vecuronium and accounts for approximately 12% of metabolites (143,144). The metabolite 3-desacetyl rapacuronium (ORG 9488) is two to three times more potent than rapacuronium (ORG 9487) and has a longer half-life (145,146). These metabolites are excreted in bile, cleared renally, and may accumulate in renal failure.

Rocuronium is metabolized in the liver and excreted renally (147). The onset and duration of action of rocuronium are prolonged in liver disease (148). Pipecuronium has only a small amount of metabolites (149).

The older agents, D-tubocurarine and metocurine, undergo biliary excretion after hepatic metabolism (20).

HOFFMANN ELIMINATION

Atracurium and *cis*-atracurium are metabolized by *Hoffmann elimination*, which is plasma enzymatic hydrolysis at normal body temperature and pH (12,150,151). Acidosis slows the enzymatic degradation reaction, as does decreased body temperature (20). In hypothermia, atracurium may have a marked prolongation of action. These agents can be used safely in liver failure or renal impairment, although due to limited renal elimination of *cis*-atracurium, its half-life may be prolonged in chronic renal failure (151). *Atracurium* is a mixture of ten optical isomers, and cis-*atracurium* is a single *cis-cis* isomer and can be used at lower doses than atracurium (151). One of atracurium's metabolites, laudanosine, can cause CNS excitation and seizures in very high doses in animal models (152,153). However, it does not accumulate to a clinically important level in doses used in human studies (153,154). Laudanosine is eliminated by hepatic metabolism and renal excretion and theoretically may accumulate in high doses or prolonged infusions in these patients (155,156).

PLASMA CHOLINESTERASE METABOLISM

Mivacurium is metabolized by plasma cholinesterases (14). It actually consists of three stereoisomers: *cis-trans*, *cis-cis*, and *trans-trans*. The *cis-trans* and *trans-trans* isomers, which make up 95% of the pharmaceutical preparation, are rapidly hydrolyzed with a half-life of 2 to 3 minutes (157). The remaining 5% is the *cis-cis* isomer, which has a half-life of 55 minutes but only a ratio of 1:10 the activity of the other isomers (157,158). The net result is that mivacurium has a short duration of action, which is not significantly affected by the longer half-life of the *cis-cis* isomer (15). However, mivacurium is still longer in duration than succinylcholine, which is also metabolized by plasma cholinesterases (13). When using mivacurium in patients who have an enzymatic deficiency of the plasma cholinesterase, the duration of action is prolonged (159). Liver disease (lower pseudocholinesterase levels) also prolongs its duration of action (160).

RENAL ELIMINATION

Only gallamine is excreted unchanged in the urine (20). Doxacurium does not undergo any hepatic metabolism, but up to 50% may be excreted unchanged in the urine (161,162).

Drug and Disease Interactions

Multiple drugs potentiate or antagonize the effects of the nondepolarizing agents (Tables 6 and 7). Inhalation anesthetics enhance the effect of nondepolarizing-neuromuscular blockers (163). Isoflurane, sevoflurane, desflurane, and enflurane have greater effects than halothane. To maintain the same level of neuromuscular blockade, infusion rates of a nondepolarizing agent may be reduced when used with inhalational anesthesia. Monitoring with twitch response can help gauge the depth of blockade during surgical anesthesia (164). Isoflurane and sevoflurane have been reported to prolong the recovery time from vecuronium (163-166).

The aminoglycosides potentiate nondepolarizing agents. In high doses, they may induce neuromuscular blockade (167). Even oral neomycin may cause the reversal agents to be less effective after induction with rocuronium (168).

Patients with myasthenia gravis may be more sensitive to the nondepolarizing agents (7,169,170). These patients may be taking AChE inhibitors for treatment (e.g., pyridostigmine), which increase the availability of ACh. These same agents are used as reversal agents for nondepolarizing agents and cause resistance to their effect (170).

Duchenne's muscular dystrophy is an X-linked recessive genetic disorder characterized by muscle weakness, usually presenting in the preschool age with leg weakness (171). *Myotonic dystrophy* is an autosomal dominant disease that is characterized by a blockade of calcium reuptake at the sarcoplasmic reticulum (172). Although succinylcholine is contraindicated in these disorders, the nondepolarizing agents can be safely administered but at reduced doses (171,172).

All the nondepolarizing agents may be used in patients with MH except for the older agents, gallamine and D-tubocurarine (103,116). However, inhalation anesthetics must be avoided.

Mivacurium should be avoided in patients with homozygous cholinesterase deficiency (14,159). Patients with heterozygous cholinesterase deficiency may have a prolongation of effect of mivacurium by only 10 minutes.

Patients with burns may be resistant to nondepolarizing agents, and larger doses may be needed (173). Resistance is greatest with burns covering more than 25% body surface area, begins 7 days after injury, peaks at 14 to 40 days, and then gradually decreases but may persist for 18 months (173–175).

TABLE 6. Drugs that potentiate the nondepolarizing neuromuscular-blocking agents

Inhalational anesthetics	Cardiovascular agents
Isoflurane	Verapamil
Sevoflurane	Propanolol
Desflurane	Lidocaine
Enflurane	Quinidine
Anesthetic adjuncts	Quinine
Local anesthetics (e.g., prilocaine)	Procainamide
Ketamine	Nitroglycerin infusion
Midazolam	Immunosuppressive agents
Dantrolene	Corticosteroids
Antibiotics	Cyclosporine
Aminoglycosides	Azathioprine
Polymyxin	Miscellaneous agents
Clindamycin	Amphotericin B
Tetracyclines	Ketorolac
Electrolytes	
Magnesium	
Lithium	

Diagnostic Tests

TRAIN-OF-FOUR STIMULATION

The easiest and most used mechanism to monitor for adequate paralysis is the train-of-four (TOF) stimulus technique (176–179). With TOF stimulus, four sequential stimuli of 2 Hz each are applied for 2 seconds each at 0.5-second intervals (176). The ratio of the fourth to the first response indicates the degree of blockade and is expressed as a fraction or a percent. A TOF ratio greater than 0.7 indicates recovery from neuromuscular blockade (177). The TOF stimulus is usually applied to the ulnar nerve with measurement of the contraction of the adductor pollicis muscle of the thumb (176). A portable nerve stimulator is available for use in non–operating-room situations, such as the emergency department, ICU, or during helicopter transport.

TABLE 7. Drugs that antagonize nondepolarizing neuromuscular-blocking agents

Carbamates	Oxcarbazepine
Phenytoin	Theophylline
Fosphenytoin	Ranitidine
Carbamazepine	

There is good correlation between the visual assessment of relaxation of the adductor pollicis or the orbicularis oculi muscles and intubating conditions (180,181). To compare the potency of neuromuscular-blocking agents, the ratios used are the dose required to produce a 50% reduction in muscle twitch height [median effective dose (ED_{50})], or the dose required to produce a 95% reduction (ED_{95}) (176). Neuromuscular-blocking agents produce large muscle weakness first and diaphragmatic paralysis and vocal cord relaxation last. Vocal cord relaxation, the key element for optimal intubating conditions, usually requires almost twice as much neuromuscular relaxant than that required for suppression of the adductor pollicis. A dose twice the ED_{95}, or four times the ED_{50}, is usually considered adequate for optimal tracheal intubation (20).

When a TOF of 0.7 occurs during recovery from neuromuscular blockade, spontaneous tidal volume should have returned to normal, and negative inspiratory force is usually 20 to 25 cm H_2O (176,177). This degree of recovery correlates clinically with the ability of the patient to lift his or her head on command and sustain it elevated for 5 seconds or the ability to contract the masseter muscle or grip the examiner's hand. It is at this level of recovery that reversal agents may be safely used (177).

The TOF technique is used for nondepolarizing neuromuscular-blocking agents. With succinylcholine, all four twitches are suppressed simultaneously (176). However, a pattern of response with a TOF ratio of less than 0.3 after a constant infusion of succinylcholine indicates a phase II block, which may be reversed with anticholinesterase agents (176).

SINGLE TWITCH RESPONSE

A single twitch response to a 0.1- to 1.0-Hz stimulus has also been used to assess degree of block (176,182,183). Twitch depression is expressed as percent of baseline. Observed depression of the single twitch response correlates with 70% blockade (183).

TETANIC CONTRACTION

A sustained, painful muscle contraction can be induced by high-frequency stimulation. A tetanic contraction to a 50-Hz stimulus applied for 5 seconds indicates normal neuromuscular function, which indicates normal ACh stores (176,177). The ability to suppress this completely indicates deep neuromuscular blockade. There is a fade in the tetanic contraction once 70% receptor occupancy occurs with a neuromuscular-blocking agent, correlating with a TOF ratio of 0.7. Because it is painful, an awake baseline measurement is rarely used, but the tetanic stimulus may be used in the technique of posttetanic potentiation that is used under deep neuromuscular blockade (184).

POSTTETANIC POTENTIATION

Normal individuals not undergoing neuromuscular blockade respond to a single twitch after tetanic stimulation with increased muscle contraction. This is due to stimulation of synthesis and mobilization of ACh, which lasts for 30 minutes after a tetanic burst (176). With nondepolarizing-neuromuscular blockade, this posttetanic potentiation phenomenon is exaggerated. This monitoring technique uses a 50-Hz tetanic for 5 seconds followed by a single twitch stimulus of 1 Hz (184,185). The number of posttetanic contractions (PTC) after the single twitch stimuli are then counted. PTC occur before recovery of twitches with a TOF stimulus. A PTC of two to three indicates that pancuronium-induced block will be measurable by TOF in 20 to 30 minutes, and vecuronium induced-block will be measurable by TOF in 7 to 8 minutes (47). This technique can be used to monitor when to redose a patient with neuromuscular-blocking agent to maintain the deep neuromuscular block required for abdominal surgery; it also can be used as an indicator of early recovery and to anticipate the need as to when reversal may be used (185). Once a PTC of six to seven occurs, the first twitch from a TOF stimulus can be seen, correlating with a 70% blockade (47). PTC may also be used to distinguish the phase I from phase II block, which could occur with succinylcholine. PTC are absent after the use of succinylcholine but occur with phase II block (47).

DOUBLE BURST

Two sequential bursts of three stimuli each at a frequency of 50 Hz are applied at 750 milliseconds (176). This produces two visible muscle contractions. The ratio of the second contraction to the first contraction correlates with the degree of neuromuscular block. The ability to estimate a TOF of less than 0.3, which occurs with succinylcholine phase II block, is difficult, and double burst may be preferred (176).

Treatment

ANTIDOTES

The nondepolarizing neuromuscular-blocking agents can be antagonized by increased concentrations of ACh (1). Drugs that antagonize the enzyme AChE may be used to reverse nondepolarizing agents once significant recovery from neuromuscular blockade occurs (186). As described in the section Nondepolarizing Agents: Diagnostic Tests, 70% recovery is regarded as the minimum recovery necessary before a reversal agent can be used (187). The AChE inhibitors commonly used are neostigmine, pyridostigmine, and edrophonium, which do not cross the blood–brain barrier (186). The *neostigmine adult dose* is 0.04 to 0.08 mg/kg (2.5 to 5.0 mg). The *neostigmine pediatric dose* is 0.02 mg/kg. The *pyridostigmine dose* is 0.2 to 0.4 mg/kg. The *edrophonium dose* is 0.5 to 1.0 mg/kg.

Because the ACh generated by these agents acts at both the nicotinic and muscarinic receptors, the reversal agents are given with an antimuscarinic agent to reduce the side effects of muscarinic stimulation (186). Either atropine or glycopyrrolate is used in combination with the AChE inhibitors for this reason. When edrophonium, a fast-onset agent, is used, atropine is preferred over glycopyrrolate. The speed of onset is rarely an important issue if airway control is maintained. The combination usually used to reverse the effects of the longer-acting neuromuscular-blocking agents is neostigmine with glycopyrrolate (188). There is no reason to use the AChE inhibitors for the short-acting neuromuscular-blocking agents, and they should not be given when a bolus of succinylcholine has been used in the last 10 minutes (189). Because succinylcholine and mivacurium are metabolized by AChE, the AChE agents may prolong their duration of action (20,190,191). However, when constant infusions of succinylcholine have been used, a phase II block may occur; in this instance, reversal agents have been tried (131).

Glycopyrrolate and *atropine* are used as secondary antidotes (antimuscarinic agents). The *adult dose* of *glycopyrrolate* (Robinul) is 0.01 to 0.02 mg/kg or, when used as an adjunct for reversal of neuromuscular blockade, 0.2 mg IV for each 1 mg of neostigmine, or each 5 mg pyridostigmine, administered simultaneously. Glycopyrrolate in doses of 0.010 to 0.015 mg/kg is effective in protecting against neostigmine-induced cardiac and secretory effects when given simultaneously with doses of 0.05 mg/kg neostigmine (192,193). Glycopyrrolate is generally not used in conjunction with edrophonium because the onset of glycopyrrolate is slower than that of edrophonium (194).

The *adult dose* of *atropine* is 0.02 to 0.03 mg/kg. The *pediatric dose* is a minimum of 0.1 mg and a maximum of 1.0 mg. The usual IV dose of atropine sulfate for adult patients is 0.6 to 1.2 mg for each 0.5 to 2.5 mg of neostigmine or for each 10 to 20 mg of pyridostigmine. Atropine is the preferred antimuscarinic with edrophonium because both have a fast onset (194). In the presence of bradycardia, atropine sulfate should be administered IV before the anticholinesterase to increase the pulse to approximately 80 beats/minute. *Infants* may receive a 0.02-mg/kg dose of atropine with a 0.02- to 0.04-mg/kg dose of neostigmine; however, for atropine, the pediatric dose should never be below 0.1 mg, as paradoxic bradycardia may develop (193). Some reports suggest that children with Down syndrome may be more susceptible to atropine, and they also are more likely to have narrow angle glaucoma, a contraindication to using atropine (195–197).

Scopolamine is usually not used as an antimuscarinic for reversal because it has 5 to 15 times the CNS potency of atropine and, hence, more sedating effects. However, it is an excellent antisialagogue that decreases secretions and may be used preoperatively for this reason (1,47).

MISCELLANEOUS REVERSAL AGENTS

4-Aminopyridine (Pymidin) is available in parts of Europe as an alternative agent for reversal of nondepolarizing agents (198). The dose is 0.3 mg/kg IV, which has an onset of action within 10 minutes and a reported full recovery of motor function within 30 minutes. Perioral paresthesias may develop. It is sometimes used with lower doses of neostigmine to take advantage of the synergistic effects and to avoid the atropine side effects (199). 4-Aminopyridine increases the release of ACh presynaptically through blockade of potassium channels (198). It is postulated to enhance calcium influx and has been investigated as an antidote to calcium channel–blocking agents (200,201). However, it enters the brain and has side effects of nonspecific stimulatory and analeptic activity. Its diamino derivatives, 3,4-diaminopyridine and 2,4-diaminopyridine, are more potent and have less CNS penetrance (202,203). Overdoses and therapeutic errors involving 4-aminopyridine cause jitteriness, diaphoresis, hypersalivation, and seizures (203). It is available in the United States as an orphan drug for Eaton-Lambert syndrome (204).

4-Aminopyridine is also available to licensed exterminators as an avicide (Avitrol, Queletox, Starlicide). It repels birds by causing hyperactivity and disorganized flight, which causes other birds to avoid the feeding grounds where the sick bird has eaten (205).

OLDER PARALYZING AGENTS NO LONGER IN WIDE USAGE

D-Tubocurarine

D-Tubocurarine [dTc (Curare)] was the first muscular relaxant. Its major limitation was histamine causing a decrease in blood pressure. Histamine release levels after a rapid bolus increase tenfold, but this effect may be decreased by a slow infusion (24).

Metocurine

Metocurine (Metubine) was synthesized from dTc in 1935 but was not introduced in anesthesia practice until 1948. It has twice the potency of dTc but only 50% of its histamine-releasing properties (24). Its advantage over dTc was fewer cardiovascular effects.

MISCELLANEOUS AGENTS

Gallamine

Gallamine triethiodide (Flaxedil) was the first synthetic neuromuscular-blocking agent but is no longer in clinical use. Allergies can be triggered in iodine-sensitive persons (20).

Alcuronium

Alcuronium was a semisynthetic, long-acting agent introduced in 1964. Anaphylactic reactions have limited its use (20,206). It is excreted unchanged in the urine and, to a small extent, in the bile. It is unavailable in the United States but is available in Australia, Europe, and Asia.

REFERENCES

1. Hardman JG, Limbird LE, eds. *Goodman & Gilman's the pharmacological basis of therapeutics*, 9th ed. New York: McGraw-Hill Publishers, 1996.
2. Bernard C. Analyse physiologique des proprietes des systemes musculaires et nerveux au moyen du curare. *C R Acad Sci (Paris)* 1856;43:825–829.
3. West R. Curare in man. *Proc R Soc Med* 1932;25:1107–1116.
4. Bennett AE. Preventing traumatic complications in convulsive shock therapy by curare. *JAMA* 1940;114:322–324.
5. Griffith HR, Johnson GE. The use of curare in general anesthesia. *Anesthesiology* 1942;3:418–420.
6. Foldes FF, McNall PG, Borrego-Hinojosa JM. Succinylcholine, a new approach to muscular relaxation in anaesthesiology. *N Engl J Med* 1952;247–596.
7. Hunter JM. New neuromuscular blocking drugs. *N Engl J Med* 1995;332:1691–1699.
8. Onrust SV, Foster RH. Rapacuronium bromide: a review of its use in anaesthetic practice. *Drugs* 1999;58:887–918.
9. Orebaugh SL. Succinylcholine: adverse effects and alternatives in emergency medicine. *Am J Emerg Med* 1999;17:715–721.
10. Goulden MR, Hunter JM. Rapacuronium (ORG 9487): do we have a replacement for succinylcholine? *Br J Anaesth* 1999;82:489–492.
11. Lennon RL, Olson RA, Gronert GA. Atracurium or vecuronium for rapid sequence endotracheal intubation. *Anesthesiology* 1986;64:510–513.
12. Miller RD, Rupp SM, Fisher DM, et al. Clinical pharmacology of vecuronium and atracurium. *Anesthesiology* 1984;61:444–453.
13. Goldberg ME, Larijani GE, Azad SS, et al. Comparison of tracheal intubating conditions and neuromuscular blocking profiles after intubating doses of mivacurium chloride or succinylcholine in surgical outpatients. *Anesth Analg* 1989;69:93–99.
14. Cook DR, Stiller RL, Weakly JN, et al. In vitro metabolism of mivacurium chloride (BW B1090U) and succinylcholine. *Anesth Analg* 1989;68:452–456.
15. Diefenbach C, Mellinghoff H, Lynch J, et al. Mivacurium: dose-response relationship and administration by repeated injection or infusion. *Anesth Analg* 1992;74:420–423.
16. Shanks CA, Fragen RJ, Pemberton D, et al. Mivacurium-induced neuromuscular blockade following single bolus doses and with continuous infusion during either balanced or enflurane anesthesia. *Anesthesiology* 1989;71:362–366.
17. Goudsouzian NG, Alifimoff JK, Eberly C. Neuromuscular and cardiovascular effects of mivacurium in children. *Anesthesiology* 1989;70:237–242.
18. Cooper R, Mirakhur RK, Clarke RSJ, et al. Comparison of intubating conditions after administration of ORG 9426 (Rocuronium) and suxamethonium. *Br J Anaesth* 1992;69:269–273.
19. Tang J, Joshi GP, White PF. Comparison of rocuronium and mivacurium to succinylcholine during outpatient laparoscopic surgery. *Anesth Analg* 1996;82:994–998.
20. Savarese JJ, Caldwell JE, Lien CA, Miller RD. Pharmacology of muscle relaxants and their antagonists. In: Miller RD, ed. *Anesthesia*, 5th ed. New York: Churchill Livingstone, 2000.
21. Sorensen M, Engbaek J, Viby-Mogensen J, et al. Bradycardia and cardiac asystole following a single injection of suxamethonium. *Acta Anaesthesiol Scand* 1984;28:232–235.
22. Stoelting RK. The hemodynamic effects of pancuronium and D-turbocurarine in anesthetized patients. *Anesthesiology* 1972;36:612–615.
23. Basta SJ, Savarese JJ, Ali HH, et al. Histamine releasing properties of atracurium, dimethyl turbocurarine, and turbocurarine. *Br J Anaesth* 1983;55:105S–106S.
24. Basta SJ. Modulation of histamine release by neuromuscular blocking drugs. *Curr Opin Anaesth* 1992;5:572–577.
25. Brauer FS, Ananthanarayan CR. Histamine release by pancuronium. *Anesthesiology* 1978;49:434–435.
26. Meakin GH. Recent advances in myorelaxant therapy. *Paediatr Anaesth* 2001;11:523–531.
27. Murray MJ (chair), Task Force of the American College of Critical Care Medicine. Clinical practice guidelines for sustained neuromuscular blockade in the adult critically ill patient. *Am J Health Syst Pharm* 2002;59:179–195.
28. Degarma BH, Dronen S. Pharmacology and clinical use of neuromuscular blocking agents. *Ann Emerg Med* 1983;12:48–55.
29. Prior C, Marshall IG. Neuromuscular junction physiology. In: Hemmings HC, Hopkins PM, eds. *Foundations of anesthesia basic and clinical sciences.* London: Mosby, 2000.
30. Ostergaard D, Rasmussen SN, Viby-Mogensen, et al. The influence of drug-induced low plasma cholinesterase activity on the pharmacokinetics and pharmacodynamics of mivacurium. *Anesthesiology* 2000;92:1581–1587.
31. Cerf C, Mesguish M, Gabriel I. Screening patients with prolonged neuro-

muscular blockade after succinylcholine and mivacurium. *Anesth Analg* 2002;94:461–466.
32. Karalliedde L. Organophosphate poisoning and anesthesia. *Anaesthesia* 1999;54:1073–1088.
33. Lien CA, Savarese JJ. Neuromuscular junction pharmacology. In: Hemmings HC, Hopkins PM, eds. *Foundations of anesthesia basic and clinical sciences*. London: Mosby, 2000.
34. Cook JH. The effect of suxamethonium on intraocular pressure. *Anaesthesia* 1981;36:359–365.
35. Boehm J, Dutton DM, Poust RI. Shelf life of unrefrigerated succinylcholine chloride injection. *Am J Hosp Pharm* 1984;41:300–302.
36. Thompson JD, Fish S, Ruiz E. Succinylcholine for endotracheal intubation. *Ann Emerg Med* 1982;11:526–529.
37. Cass NM, Doolan LA, Gutteridge GA. Repeated administration of suxamethonium in a patient with atypical plasma cholinesterase. *Anaesth Intensive Care* 1982;10:25–28.
38. Liu LM, DeCook TH, Goudsouzian NG, et al. Dose response to intramuscular succinylcholine in children. *Anesthesiology* 1981;55:599–602.
39. Cook DR, Fisher CG. Neuromuscular blocking effects of succinylcholine in infants and children. *Anesthesiology* 1975;27:124–130.
40. Meakin G, McKiernan EP, Morris P, et al. Dose-response curves for suxamethonium in neonates, infants, and children. *Br J Anaesth* 1989;62:655–658.
41. Gerardi MJ, Sacchetti AD, Cantor RM. Rapid sequence intubation of the pediatric patient. *Ann Emerg Med* 1996;28:55–74.
42. Goudsouzian NG. Muscle relaxants in children. In: Cote CJ, Todres ID, Ryan JF, Goudsouzian NG, eds. *A practice of anesthesia for infants and children*, 3rd ed. Philadelphia: WB Saunders, 2001.
43. Morell RC, Berman JM, Royster RI, et al. Revised label regarding use of succinylcholine in children and adolescents. *Anesthesiology* 1994;80:242–245.
44. Salem MR, Bennett EJ, Schweiss JF, et al. Cardiac arrest related to anesthesia: contributing factors in infants and children. *JAMA* 1975;233:238–241.
45. Henderson WA. Succinylcholine induced cardiac arrest in unsuspected Duchenne muscular dystrophy. *Can Anaesth Soc J* 1984;31:444–446.
46. Larach MG, Rosenberg H, Gronert GA, et al. Hyperkalemic cardiac arrest during anesthesia in infants and children with occult myopathies. *Clin Pediatr* 1997;36:9–16.
47. Keneally JP, Bush GH. Changes in serum potassium after suxamethonium in children. *Anaesth Intensive Care* 1974;2:147–150.
48. Duvaldestin P. Pharmacokinetics in intravenous anaesthetic practice. *Clin Pharmacokinet* 1981;6:61–82.
49. Bevan DR. Succinylcholine. *Can J Anaesth* 1994;41:465–468.
50. Ostergaard D, Viby-Morgensen J, Hanel H, et al. Half-life of plasma cholinesterase. *Acta Anaesthesiol Scand* 1988;32:266–269.
51. Jokanovic M, Maksimovic M. Abnormal cholinesterase activity: understanding and interpretation. *Eur J Clin Chem Biochem* 1997;35:11–16.
52. Ostergaard D, Jensen FS, Viby-Mogensen J. Pseudocholinesterase deficiency and anticholinesterase toxicity. In: Ballantyne B, Marrs TC, eds. *Clinical and experimental toxicology of organophosphates and carbamates*. London: Butterworth–Heinemann, 1992.
53. Pantuck E. Plasma cholinesterase: gene and variations. *Anesth Analg* 1993;77:380–386.
54. Whittaker M. *Cholinesterase*. New York: Karger, 1986.
55. Lockridge O, Masson P. Pesticides and susceptible populations: people with butyrylcholinesterase genetic variants may be at risk. *Neurotoxicology* 2000;21:113–126.
56. Primo-Parmo SL, Bartels CF, Wiersema B, et al. Characterization of 12 silent alleles of the human butyrylcholinesterase gene. *Am J Hum Genet* 1996;58:52–64.
57. James FM. Pharmacology of anesthetics. *Clin Ob Gyn* 1981;24:561–573.
58. Birch AA, Mitchell GD, Playford GA, et al. Changes in serum potassium response to succinylcholine following trauma. *JAMA* 1969;210:490–495.
59. Gronert GA, Theye RA. Pathophysiology of hyperkalemia induced by succinylcholine. *Anesthesiology* 1975;43:89–99.
60. Cooperman LH. Succinylcholine induced hyperkalemia in neuromuscular disease. *JAMA* 1970;213:1867–1871.
61. Schamer PJ, Brown RL, Kirsey THD, et al. Succinylcholine induced hyperkalemia in burned patients. *Anesth Analg* 1969;48:764–770.
62. Cooperman LH, Strobel GE, Kennel EM. Massive hyperkalemia after administration of succinylcholine to the traumatized patient. *Anesthesiology* 1969;32:161–164.
63. Mazze RI, Escue HM, Houston JB. Hyperkalemia and cardiovascular collapse following administration of succinylcholine to the traumatized patient. *Anesthesiology* 1969;31:540–547.
64. Cooperman LH, Strobel GE, Kennel EM. Massive hyperkalemia after administration of succinylcholine. *Anesthesiology* 1970;32:161–164.
65. Powell JN, Golby M. The pattern of potassium liberation following a single dose of suxamethonium in normal and uremic rats. *Br J Anesth* 1971;43:662–668.
66. Miller RD, Way WL, Hamilton WK, et al. Succinylcholine induced hyperkalemia in patients with renal failure, *Anesthesiology* 1972;36:138–141.
67. Kohlschutter B, Baur H, Roth F. Suxamethonium induced hyperkalemia in patients with severe intra-abdominal infections. *Br J Anaesth* 1976;48:557–562.
68. Bismuth C, Gaultier M, Conso F, et al. Hyperkalemia in acute digitalis poisoning: prognostic significance and therapeutic implications. *J Toxicol Clin Toxicol* 1973;6:153–162.
69. Lee G, Antogninin JF, Gronert GA. Complete recovery after prolonged resuscitation and cardiopulmonary bypass for hyperkalemia cardiac arrest. *Anesth Analg* 1994;79:172–174.
70. Markewitz BA, Elstad MR. Succinylcholine induced hyperkalemia following prolonged pharmacologic neuromuscular blockade. *Chest* 1997;111:248–250.
71. Choi WW, Gergis SD, Sokoll MD. Controversies in muscle relaxants. *Semin Anesth* 1985;4:73–80.
72. Blanc VF, Vaillancourt G, Brisson G. Succinylcholine, fasciculations and myoglobinaemia. *Can Anaesth Soc J* 1986;33:178–184.
73. Brodksy JB, Brock-Utne JG, Samuels SI. Pancuronium pretreatment and post-succinylcholine myalgias. *Anesthesiology* 1979;51:259–261.
74. Bennetts FE, Khalil KI. Reduction of post-suxamethonium pain by pretreatment with four non-depolarizing agents. *Br J Anaesth* 1981;53:531–536.
75. Ryan JF, Kagen LJ, Hyman AI. Myoglobinemia after a single dose of succinylcholine. *N Engl J Med* 1971;285:824–827.
76. Laurence AS. Serum myoglobin release following suxamethonium administration to children. *Eur J Anaesthesiol* 1988;5:31–38.
77. Miller ED, Saunders DB, Rowlingson JC, et al. Anesthesia induced rhabdomyolysis in a patient with Duchenne's muscular dystrophy. *Anesthesiology* 1978;48:146–148.
78. Laurence AS, McKean JF. Dantrolene and suxamethonium: myalgia, biochemical changes and serum dantrolene levels following oral dantrolene pre-treatment in laparoscopy patients. *Eur J Anaesthesiol* 1990;7:493–500.
79. Habre W, Sims C. Masseter spasm and elevated creatinine kinase after intravenous induction in a child. *Anaesth Intensive Care* 1996;24:496–499.
80. McLaughlin C, Elliot P, McCarthy G, et al. Muscle pains and biochemical changes following suxamethonium administration after six pretreatment regimens. *Anaesthesia* 1992;47:202–206.
81. Oxorn DC, Whatley GS, Knox WD, et al. The importance of activity and pretreatment in the prevention of suxamethonium myalgias. *Br J Anaesth* 1992;69:200–201.
82. Galindo AHF, Davis TB. Succinylcholine and cardiac excitability. *Anesthesiology* 1962;23:32–38.
83. Stoelting RK, Peterson C. Heart-rate slowing and junctional rhythm following intravenous succinylcholine with and without intramuscular atropine preanesthetic medication. *Anesth Analg* 1975:54:705–709.
84. Rosenberg H, Gronert GA. Intractable cardiac arrest in children given succinylcholine. *Anesthesiology* 1992;77:1054.
85. Lerman J. The heart rate response to succinylcholine in children: a comparison of atropine and glycopyrrolate. *Can Anaesth Soc J* 1984;31:382–394.
86. Nigrovic V, McCullough LS, Wajskol A, et al. Succinylcholine induced increases in plasma catecholamine levels in humans. *Anesth Analg* 1983;62:627–632.
87. Leiman BC, Katz J, Butler BD. Mechanisms of succinylcholine induced arrhythmias in hypoxic or hypercarbic dogs. *Anesth Analg* 1987;66:1292–1297.
88. Metz HS, Venkatesh B. Succinylcholine and intraocular pressure. *J Pediatr Ophthalmol Strabismus* 1981;18:12–14.
89. Craythorne NWB, Rottenstein HS, Dripps RD. The effect of succinylcholine on intraocular pressure in the adults, infants, and children during general anesthesia. *Anesthesiology* 1960;21:59–63.
90. Pandey K, Badola RP, Kumar S. Time course of intraocular hypertension produced by suxamethonium. *Br J Anaesth* 1972;44:191–196.
91. Kelley RE, Dinner M, Turner LS, et al. Succinylcholine increases intraocular pressure in the human eye with the extraocular muscles detached. *Anesthesiology* 1993;9:948–952.
92. Miller RD, Way WL, Hickey R. Inhibition of succinylcholine induced increased intraocular pressure by non-depolarizing muscle relaxants. *Anesthesiology* 1968;29:123–126.
93. Libonati MM, Leahy JJ, Ellison N. The use of succinylcholine in open eye surgery. *Anesthesiology* 1985;62:637–640.
94. Smith G, Dalling R, Williams TR. Gastroesophageal pressure gradient changes produced by induction of anesthesia and suxamethonium. *Br J Anaesth* 1978;50:1137–1140.
95. Salem MR, Wong AY, Lin YH. The effect of suxamethonium on the intragastric pressure in infants and children. *Br J Anaesth* 1972;44:166–170.
96. Miller RD, Way WL. Inhibition of succinylcholine induced increased intragastric pressure by nondepolarizing muscle relaxants and lidocaine. *Anesthesiology* 1971;34:185–188.
97. Cottrell JE, Hartung J, Griffin JP, et al. Intracranial and hemodynamic changes after succinylcholine in cats. *Anesth Analg* 1983;62:1006–1009.
98. Minton MD, Grosslight K, Stirt JA, et al. Increases in intracranial pressure from succinylcholine: prevention by prior nondepolarizing blockade. *Anesthesiology* 1986;65:165–169.
99. Kovarick WD, Mayberg TS, Lam AM, et al. Succinylcholine does not change intracranial pressure, cerebral blood flow velocity or the electroencephalogram in patients with neurologic injury. *Anesth Analg* 1994;78:469–473.
100. Brown MM, Parr MJ, Manara AR. The effect of suxamethonium on the intracranial pressure and the cerebral perfusion pressure in patients with severe head injury following blunt trauma. *Eur J Anaesth* 1996;13:474–477.
101. Stevens HM, Moffat AC. A rapid screening procedure for quaternary ammonium compounds in fluids and tissues with special reference to suxamethonium. *J Forensic Sci Soc* 1974;14:141–148.
102. Rosenberg H, Antognini JF, Muldoon S. Testing for malignant hyperthermia. *Anesthesiology* 2002,96:232–237.

103. Allen GC, Larach MG, Kunselman AR, et al. The sensitivity and specificity of the caffeine-halothane contracture test: a report from the North American malignant hyperthermia registry. *Anesthesiology* 1998;88:579–588.
104. Denborough M, Lovell R. Anesthetic deaths in a family. *Lancet* 1960;2:45–46.
105. Tomarken JL, Britt BA. Malignant hyperthermia. *Ann Emerg Med* 1987;16:1253–1265.
106. Britt BA, Kalow W. Malignant hyperthermia: statistical review. *Can Anaesth Soc J* 1970;17:293–315.
107. Relton JE, Britt BA, Steward DJ. Malignant hyperpyrexia. *Br J Anaesth* 1973;45:269–275.
108. McCarthy TV, Healy JM, Heffron JJ, et al. Localization of the malignant hyperthermia susceptibility locus to human chromosome 19q12-13.2. *Nature* 1990;343:562–564.
109. Manning BM, Quane KA, Lynch PJ, et al. Identification of novel mutations at amino acid position 614 in the ryanodine receptor in malignant hyperthermia. *Br J Anaesth* 1997;79:332–337.
110. Fagerlund TH, Islander G, Twetman ER, et al. A search for three known RYR1 gene mutations in 41 Swedish families with predisposition to malignant hyperthermia. *Clin Genet* 1995;48:12–16.
111. Marks AR, Priori S, Memmi M, et al. Involvement of the cardiac ryanodine receptor/calcium release channel in catecholaminergic polymorphic ventricular tachycardia. *J Cell Physiol* 2002;190:1–6.
112. Loke J, MacLennan DH. Malignant hyperthermia and central core disease: disorders of calcium release channels. *Am J Med* 1998;104:470–486.
113. Hall GM, Lucke JN, Lister D. Malignant hyperthermia—pearls out of swine? *Br J Anaesth* 1980;52:165–171.
114. Lopez JR, Allen PD, Alamo L, et al. Myoplasmic free calcium during a malignant hyperthermia episode in swine. *Muscle Nerve* 1988;11:82–88.
115. Kim DH, Sreter FA, Ohnishi ST, et al. Kinetic studies of calcium release from sarcoplasmic reticulum of normal and malignant hyperthermia susceptible pig muscles. *Biochem Biophys Acta* 1984;775:320–327.
116. Bissonnette B, Ryan JF. Temperature regulation: normal and abnormal (malignant hyperthermia). In: Cote CJ, Todres ID, Ryan JF, Goudsouzian NG, eds. *A practice of anesthesia for infants and children*, 3rd ed. Philadelphia: WB Saunders, 2001.
117. Holt S, Moore K. Pathogenesis of renal failure in rhabdomyolysis: the role of myoglobin. *Exp Nephrol* 2000;8:72–76.
118. Zager RA. Rhabdomyolysis and myohemoglobinuric acute renal failure. *Kidney Int* 1996;49:314–326.
119. Nelson TE, Flewellen EH. Rationale for dantrolene vs. procainamide for treatment of malignant hyperthermia. *Anesthesiology* 1979;50:118–122.
120. Hopkins PM. Malignant hyperthermia: advances in clinical management and diagnosis. *Br J Anaesth* 2000;85:118–128.
121. Triner L, Sherman J. Potential value of expiratory carbon dioxide measurement in patients considered susceptible to malignant hyperthermia. *Anesthesiology* 1981;55:482.
122. Nelson TE. Heat production during anesthetic induced malignant hyperthermia. *Biosci Rep* 2001;21:169–179.
123. Bertorini TE. Myoglobinuria, malignant hyperthermia, neuroleptic malignant syndrome and serotonin syndrome. *Neurol Clin* 1997,15:649–671.
124. Fruen BR, Mickelson JR, Louis CF. Dantrolene inhibition of sarcoplasmic reticulum calcium release by direct and specific action at skeletal muscle ryanodine receptors. *J Biol Chem* 1997;272:26965–26971.
125. Saltzman LS, Kates RA, Corke BC, et al. Hyperkalemia and cardiovascular collapse after verapamil and dantrolene administration in swine. *Anesth Analg* 1984;63:473–478.
126. Schwarz L, Rockoff MA, Koka BV. Masseter spasm with anesthesia: incidence and implications. *Anesthesiology* 1984;61:772–775.
127. Littleford JA, Patel LR, Bose D, et al. Masseter muscle spasm in children. *Anesth Analg* 1991;72:151–160.
128. Larach MG, Allen GC, Kunselman AR, et al. Do patients who experience masseter muscle rigidity as part of a malignant hyperthermia episode differ from patients with isolated masseter muscle rigidity? *Anesthesiology* 1996;85:A1057.
129. Isaacs H, Badenhorst M. False-negative results with muscle caffeine halothane contracture testing for malignant hyperthermia. *Anesthesiology* 1993;79:5–9.
130. Islander G, Twetman ER. Comparison between the European and North American protocols for diagnosis of malignant hyperthermia susceptibility in humans. *Anesth Analg* 1999;88:1155–1160.
131. Ramsey FM, Lebowitz PW, Savarese JJ, et al. Clinical characteristics of long term succinylcholine neuromuscular blockade during balanced anesthesia. *Anesth Analg* 1980;59:110–116.
132. Miller RD. Antagonism of neuromuscular blockade. *Anesthesiology* 1976;44:318–329.
133. Orkin FK, Pegg JRP. Cardiac effects of pancuronium bromide. *JAMA* 1973;224:630.
134. Stoelting RK. The hemodynamic effects of pancuronium and d-turbocurarine in anesthetized patients. *Anesthesiology* 1972;36:612–615.
135. Fahey MR, Morris RB, Miler RD, et al. Clinical pharmacology of ORG NC 45 (Norcuron): a new nondepolarizing muscle relaxant. *Anesthesiology* 1981;55:6–11.
136. Mendez DR, Goto CS, Abramo TJ, et al. Safety and efficacy of rocuronium for controlled intubation with paralytics in the pediatric emergency department. *Pediatr Emerg Care* 2001;17:233–236.
137. Basta SJ, Ali HH, Savarese JJ, et al. Clinical pharmacology of atracurium besylate (BW33A): a new non-depolarizing muscle relaxant. *Anesth Analg* 1982;61:723–729.
138. Lepage JY, Malinovsky JM, Maalinge M, et al. Pharmacodynamic dose-response and safety study of cisatracurium (51W89) in adult surgical patients during N2O-O2 opioid anesthesia. *Anesth Analg* 1996;83:823–829.
139. Doenicke A, Soukup J, Hoernecke R, et al. The lack of histamine release with cisatracurium: a double-blind comparison with vecuronium. *Anesth Analg* 1997;84:623–628.
140. Reynolds LM, Lau M, Brown R, et al. Intramuscular rocuronium in infants and children: dose ranging and tracheal intubating conditions. *Anesthesiology* 1996;85:231–239.
141. Martyn JA, Goldhill DR, Goudsouzian NG, et al. Clinical pharmacology of muscle relaxants in patients with burns. *J Clin Pharmacol* 1986;26:680–685.
142. Miller RD, Agoston S, Booij LH, et al. The comparative potency and pharmacokinetics of pancuronium and its metabolites in anesthetized man. *J Pharmacol Exp Ther* 1978;207:539–543.
143. Larijani GE, Gratz I, Silverberg M, et al. Clinical pharmacology of the neuromuscular blocking agents. *Ann Pharmacother* 1991;25:54–64.
144. Caldwell JE, Szenohradszky J, Segredo V, et al. The pharmacodynamics and pharmacokinetics of the metabolite 3-desacetylvecuronium (ORG 7268) and its parent compound, vecuronium, in human volunteers. *J Pharmacol Exp Ther* 1994;270:1216–1222.
145. Schiere S, Proost JH, Schuringa M, et al. Pharmacokinetics and pharmacokinetics-dynamic relationship between rapacuronium (ORG 9487) and its 3-desacetylmetabolite (ORG 9488). *Anesth Analg* 1999;88:640–647.
146. Larijani GE, Zafeiridis A, Goldberg ME. Clinical pharmacology of rapacuronium bromide, a new short acting neuromuscular blocking agent. *Pharmacology* 1999;19:1118–1122.
147. Szenohradszky J, Fisher DM, Segredo V, et al. Pharmacokinetics of rocuronium bromide (ORG 9426) in patients with normal renal function or patients undergoing cadaver renal transplants. *Anesthesiology* 1992;77:899–904.
148. van Miert MM, Eastwood NB, Boyd AH, et al. The pharmacokinetics and pharmacodynamics of rocuronium in patients with hepatic cirrhosis. *Br J Clin Pharmacol* 1997;44:139–144.
149. Wierda JM, Szenohradszky J, De Wit AP, et al. The pharmacokinetics, urinary and biliary excretion of pipecuronium bromide. *Eur J Anaesthesiol* 1991;8:451–457.
150. Basta SJ, Ali HH, Savarese JJ, et al. Clinical pharmacology of atracurium besylate (BW33A): a new non-depolarizing muscle relaxant. *Anesth Analg* 1982;61:723–729.
151. Boyd AH, Eastwood NB, Parker CJ, et al. Pharmacodynamics of 1R cis-1'R cis isomer of atracurium (51W89) in health and chronic renal failure. *Br J Anaesthesia* 1995;74:400–404.
152. Tateishi A, Zornow MH, Scheller MS, et al. Electroencephalographic effects of laudanosine in an animal model of epilepsy. *Br J Anaesth* 1989;62:548–552.
153. Manthous CA, Chatila W. Atracurium and status epilepticus? *Crit Care Med* 1995;23:1440–1442.
154. Farenc C, Lefrant JY, Audran M, et al. Pharmacokinetics of atracurium and laudanosine in intensive care patients with acute respiratory distress syndrome undergoing mechanical ventilation. *Clin Drug Invest* 2000;19:143–150.
155. Ward S, Boheimer N, Weatherley BC, et al. Pharmacokinetics of atracurium and its metabolites in patients with normal renal function and in patients with renal failure. *Br J Anaesth* 1987;59:697–706.
156. Ward S, Neill EA. Pharmacokinetics of atracurium in acute hepatic failure (with acute renal failure). *Br J Anaesth* 1983;55:1169–1172.
157. Savarese JJ, Ali HH, Basta SJ, et al. The clinical neuromuscular pharmacology of mivacurium chloride (BW B1090U): a short-acting nondepolarizing ester neuromuscular blocking drug. *Anesthesiology* 1988;68:723–732.
158. Savarese JJ, Lien CA, Belmont MR, et al. The clinical and basic pharmacology of mivacurium: a short-acting nondepolarizing benzylisoquinolinium diester neuromuscular blocking drug. *Acta Anaesth Scand* 1995;106:18–22.
159. Goudsouzian NG, D'Hollander AA, Viby-Mogensen J. Prolonged neuromuscular block from mivacurium in two patients with cholinesterase deficiency. *Anesth Analg* 1993;77:183–185.
160. Cook DR, Freeman JA, Lai AA, et al. Pharmacokinetics of mivacurium in normal patients and in those with hepatic or renal failure. *Br J Anaesth* 1992;69:580–585.
161. Cashman JN, Luke JJ, Jones RM. Neuromuscular block with doxacurium (BW A938U) in patients with normal or absent renal function. *Br J Anaesth* 1990;64:186–192.
162. Martlew RA, Harper NJ. The clinical pharmacology of doxacurium in young adults and in elderly patients. *Anaesthesia* 1995;50:779–782.
163. Swen J, Rashkovsky OM, Ket JM, et al. Interaction between nondepolarizing neuromuscular blocking agents and inhalational anesthetics. *Anesth Analg* 1989;69:752–755.
164. Morita T, Kurosaki D, Tsukagoshi H, et al. Sevoflurane and isoflurane impair edrophonium reversal of vecuronium induced neuromuscular block. *Can J Anaesth* 1996;43:799–805.
165. Pittet J, Melis A, Rouge J, et al. Effect of volatile anesthetics on vecuronium induced neuromuscular blockade in children. *Anesth Analg* 1990;70:248–252.
166. Ahmed AA, Kumagai M, Otake T, et al. Sevoflurane exposure time and neuromuscular blocking effect of vecuronium. *Can J Anaesth* 1999;46:429–432.
167. Dupuis JY, Martin R, Tetrault JP. Atracurium and vecuronium interaction with gentamicin and tobramycin. *Can J Anaesth* 1989;36:407–411.

168. Hasfurther DL, Bailey PL. Failure of neuromuscular blockade reversal after rocuronium in a patient who received oral neomycin. *Can J Anaesth* 1996;43:617–620.
169. Buzello W, Noeldge G, Krieg N, et al. Vecuronium for muscle relaxation in patients with myasthenia gravis. *Anesthesiology* 1986;64:507–509.
170. Chan KH, Yang MW, Huang HH. A comparison between vecuronium and atracurium in myasthenia gravis. *Acta Anaesth Scand* 1993;37:679–682.
171. Morris P. Duchenne muscular dystrophy: a challenge for the anaesthetist. *Pediatr Anaesth* 1997;7:1–4.
172. Mitchell MM, Ali HH, Savarese JJ. Myotonia and neuromuscular blocking agents. *Anesthesiology* 1978;49:44–48.
173. Martyn J, Goldhill DR, Goudsouzian NG. Clinical pharmacology of muscle relaxants in patients with burns. *J Clin Pharmacol* 1986;26:680–685.
174. Ward JM, Martyn J. Alterations in neuromuscular function following thermal injury. *Biochem Soc Trans* 1991;19:191S.
175. Marathe PH, Dwersteg JF, Pavlin EG, et al. Effect of thermal injury on the pharmacokinetics and pharmacodynamics of atracurium in humans. *Anesthesiology* 1989;70:752–755.
176. Crowley MP, Ali HH. Monitoring neuromuscular function. In: Blitt CD, Hines RL, eds. *Monitoring in anesthesia and critical care medicine*, 3rd ed. New York: Churchill Livingstone, 1995.
177. Ali HH, Savarese JJ, Lebowitz PW, et al. Twitch, tetanus, and train-of-four as indices of recovery from non-depolarizing neuromuscular blockade. *Anesthesiology* 1981;54:294–297.
178. Stoelting RK, Miller RD. Neuromuscular blocking drugs. In: Stoelting RK, Miller RD, eds. *Basics of anesthesia*, 4th ed. New York: Churchill Livingstone, 2000.
179. McCoy EP, Connolly FM, Mirakhur RK, et al. Nondepolarizing neuromuscular blocking drugs and train-of-four fade. *Can J Anaesth* 1995;42:213–216.
180. Riamaniol JM, Dhonneur G, Sperry L, et al. A comparison of the neuromuscular blocking effects of atracurium, mivacurium, and vecuronium on the adductor pollicis and the orbicularis oculi muscle in humans. *Anesth Analg* 1996;83:808–813.
181. Le Corre F, Plaud B, Benhamou E, et al. Visual estimation of onset time at the orbicularis oculi after five muscle relaxants: application to clinical monitoring of tracheal intubation. *Anesth Analg* 1999;89:1305–1310.
182. Curran MJ, Donati F, Bevan DR. Onset and recovery of atracurium and suxamethonium induced neuromuscular blockade with simultaneous train-of-four and single twitch stimulation. *Br J Anaesth* 1987;59:989–994.
183. Kopman AF, Klewicka MM, Neuman GC. The relationship between acceleromyographic train-of-four and single twitch depression. *Anesthesiology* 2002;96:583–587.
184. Gibson FM, Mirakhur RK. Tetanic fade following administration of nondepolarizing neuromuscular blocking drugs. *Anesth Analg* 1989;68:759–762.
185. Saitoh Y, Fujii Y, Toyooka H, et al. Post-tetanic burst count: a stimulating pattern for profound neuromuscular blockade. *Can J Anaesth* 1995;42:1096–1100.
186. Mirakhur RK. Basic pharmacology of reversal agents. *Anesth Clin North Am* 1993;11:237–246.
187. Baurain MJ, Hoton F, D'Hollander AA. Is recovery of neuromuscular transmission complete after the use of neostigmine to antagonize block produced by rocuronium, vecuronium, atracurium, and pancuronium? *Br J Anaesth* 1996;77:496–499.
188. McCoy EP, Mirakhur RK. Comparison of the effects of neostigmine and edrophonium on the duration of action of suxamethonium. *Acta Anaesth Scand* 1995;39:744–747.
189. Joshi G, Garg SA, Hailey A, et al. The effects of antagonizing residual neuromuscular blockade by neostigmine and glycopyrrolate on nausea and vomiting after ambulatory surgery. *Anesth Analg* 1999;89:628–631.
190. Hart PS, Wright PM, Brown R, et al. Edrophonium increases mivacurium concentrations during constant mivacurium infusions, and large doses minimally antagonize paralysis. *Anesthesiology* 1995;82:912–918.
191. Szenohradszky J, Fogarty D, Kirkegaard-Nielsen H, et al. Effect of edrophonium and neostigmine on the pharmacokinetics and neuromuscular effects of mivacurium. *Anesthesiology* 2000;92:708–714.
192. Mirakhur RK. Antagonism of the muscarinic effects of edrophonium with atropine or glycopyrrolate: a comparative study. *Br J Anaesth* 1985;57:1213–1216.
193. Mirakhur RK, Jones CJ. Atropine and glycopyrrolate: changes in cardiac rate and rhythm in conscious and anaesthetized children. *Anaesth Intensive Care* 1982;10:328–332.
194. Mirakhur RK, Dundee JW, Clarke RS. Glycopyrrolate-neostigmine mixture for antagonism of neuromuscular block: comparison with atropine-neostigmine mixture. *Br J Anaesth* 1977;49:825–829.
195. Harris WS, Goodman RM. Hyper-reactivity to atropine in Down's syndrome. *N Engl J Med* 1968;279:407–410.
196. Kobel M, Creighton RE, Steward DJ. Anaesthetic considerations in Down's syndrome: experience with 100 patients and a review of the literature. *Can Anaesth Soc J* 1982;29:593–599.
197. Caputo AR, Wagner RS, Reynolds DR, et al. Down syndrome: clinical review of ocular features. *Clin Pediatr* 1989;28:355–358.
198. Soni N, Kam P. 4-Aminopyridine: a review. *Anaesth Intensive Care* 1982;10:120–126.
199. Miller RD, Booij LHDJ, Agoston S, et al. 4-Aminopyridine potentiates neostigmine and pyridostigmine in man. *Anesthesiology* 1976;50:416–420.
200. Biessels PTM, Agoston S, Horn AS. Comparison of the pharmacological actions of some new 4-aminopyridine derivatives. *Eur J Pharmocol* 1985;106:319–325.
201. ter Wee PM, Hovinga TKK, Uges DRA, et al. 4-Aminopyridine and haemodialysis in the treatment of verapamil intoxication. *Hum Toxicol* 1985;4:327–329.
202. Plewa MC, Martin TG, Menegazzi JJ, et al. Hemodynamic effects of 3,4-diaminopyridine in a swine model of verapamil toxicity. *Ann Emerg Med* 1994;23:499–507.
203. Stork CM, Hoffman RS. Characterization of 4-aminopyridine in overdose. *J Toxicol Clin Toxicol* 1994;32:583–587.
204. McEvoy KM, Windebank AJ, Daube JR, et al. 3,4-Diaminopyridine in the treatment of Eaton-Lambert myasthenic syndrome. *N Engl J Med* 1989;321:1567–1571.
205. Schafer EW, Bruton RB, Cunningham DJ. A summary of the acute toxicity of 4-aminopyridine to birds and mammals. *Toxicol Appl Pharmacol* 1973;26:532–538.
206. Chan CS, Yeung ML. Anaphylactic reaction to alcuronium. *Br J Anaesth* 1972;44:103–105.

CHAPTER 104

General Muscle Relaxants

Katherine M. Hurlbut

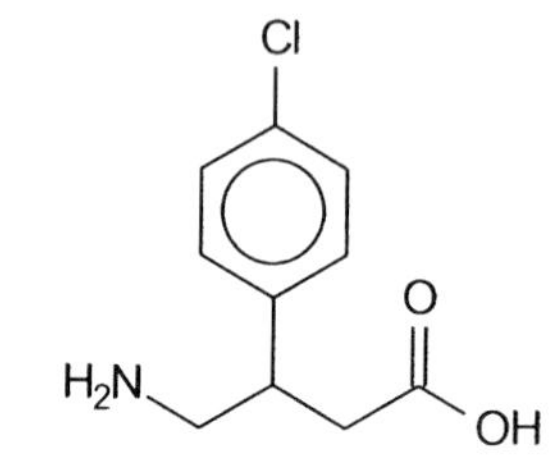

BACLOFEN

Compounds included:	**See Table 1.**
Molecular weight:	**Baclofen, 213.7; carisoprodol, 260.3; chlorphenesin, 245.7; chlorzoxazone, 169.6; cyclobenzaprine, 311.8; metaxalone, 221.3; methocarbamol, 241.2; orphenadrine, 461.5; tizanidine, 290.2 g/mol**
SI conversion:	**See Table 1.**
Therapeutic levels:	**Therapeutic drug levels are not used clinically.**
Special concerns:	**Baclofen can produce profound coma that is prolonged for several days.**
Antidote:	**Flumazenil has been proposed but is rarely needed.**

OVERVIEW

Skeletal muscle relaxants are used to relieve spasticity and muscle spasm. Baclofen (Lioresal, Baclospas), chlormezanone, chlorphenesin carbamate (Maolate), chlorzoxazone (Paraflex, Parafon), metaxalone (Skelaxin), methocarbamol (Delaxin, Robaxin, Robomol, Marbaxin, Lumirelax, Miowas), carisoprodol, cyclobenzaprine (Flexeril), orphenadrine (Norflex), and tizanidine are addressed in this chapter. The diagnostic and therapeutic aspects of treatment are similar for these drugs and are addressed in the sections Diagnostic Tests and Treatment. Other chapters address benzodiazepines (Chapter 132) and dantrolene (Chapter 47).

Effects of overdose with these agents are usually an exaggeration of therapeutically desired effects, diminished consciousness or coma, profound muscle hypotonia, absent limb reflexes, and respiratory depression. Laboratory studies are usually normal. Patients given good supportive care usually survive (1). Management is supportive with specific management of prolonged QTc and its sequelae.

BACLOFEN

Baclofen is the β-*p*-chlorophenol derivative of the inhibitory neurotransmitter γ-aminobutyric acid (2). As γ-aminobutyric acid is a strongly polar and hydrophilic substance and cannot penetrate the blood–brain barrier, a lipophilic substance is added to the molecule (3).

TABLE 1. Compounds included and SI conversions

Compound	SI conversion
Baclofen	mg/L × 4.7 = μmol/L
Carisoprodol (Soma)	mg/L × 3.8 = μmol/L
Chlorphenesin (Germazide)	mg/L × 4.1 = μmol/L
Chlorzoxazone (Paraflex)	mg/L × 5.9 = μmol/L
Cyclobenzaprine (Flexeril)	mg/L × 3.2 = μmol/L
Metaxalone (Skelaxin)	mg/L × 4.5 = μmol/L
Methocarbamol (Robaxin)	mg/L × 4.2 = μmol/L
Orphenadrine (Norflex)	mg/L × 2.2 = μmol/L
Tizanidine (Zanaflex)	mg/L × 3.5 = μmol/L

Baclofen is used to alleviate spasticity, clonus, spinal automatic movements, flexor spasms, and associated pain in patients with multiple sclerosis and spinal disorders (4,5). Intrathecal baclofen is available in the United States for amelioration of spasticity caused by multiple sclerosis or for spinal cord injury in patients unresponsive to oral baclofen. Respiratory depression, somnolence, and coma have been observed with this route of administration (6). Baclofen is often the preferred antispasticity drug because it is usually effective at doses that are free of undesired side effects. Baclofen has been effective in relieving intractable hiccups.

The *adult dose* of baclofen is 40 to 80 mg/day orally. Baclofen has been administered as a continuous intrathecal infusion for severe spasticity. The usual intrathecal dose is 300 to 800 μg/day. Adult patients have ingested up to 2 g of baclofen and survived (7). Serious poisoning has occurred with doses of 150 and 300 mg in adults. Intrathecal administration of 1.5 to 10.0 mg in adults and adolescents has caused central nervous system (CNS) and respiratory depression with recovery. Ingestion of 1250 to 2500 mg by one patient led to fatality (8). A 30-year-old man who probably ingested between 1000 and 1800 mg of baclofen, became comatose and died in 5 days (9).

The *pediatric dose* is 10 to 15 mg/day divided 8 hourly up to 40 mg/day. A 22-month-old patient had a respiratory arrest after ingesting 120 mg (10).

Baclofen has been used recreationally as a drug of abuse by adolescents. Hypothermia, bradycardia, mild hypertension, seizures, and respiratory and CNS depression have all been described after recreational abuse (11). Intensive supportive care and ventilatory assistance may be required in these patients.

Toxicokinetics and Toxicodynamics

Pharmacokinetic and pharmacodynamic data are provided in Table 2. Baclofen is almost completely absorbed orally (2). Its bioavailability is 70% to 80% (12). A single oral dose of 40 mg begins to

TABLE 2. Selected pharmacokinetic and pharmacodynamic parameters of the skeletal muscle relaxants

Parameters	Baclofen (reference)	Cyclobenzaprine (reference)	Chlormezanone (reference)	Chlorphenesin (reference)	Chlorzoxazone (reference)	Carisoprodol (reference)	Methocarbamol (reference)	Metaxalone (reference)	Orphenadrine (reference)	Tizanidine (71)
Onset of effect	30–45 min (13)	Unknown; T_{max}, 4 h (56)	15–30 min (83)	Unknown; T_{max}, 1.9 h (84)	1 h (63)	30 min (63)	30 min (63)	1 h (63)	Unknown; T_{max}, 2–4 h (87)	Unknown; T_{max}, 1.5 h, 5.7 h after sustained release formulation
Duration of effect	4–8 h	Unknown	6 h (83)	Unknown	Unknown	4–6 h (63)	24 h (85)	4–6 h (63)	Unknown	Unknown
Volume of distribution	0.8 L/kg (12); 2.4 L/kg in overdose (14)	Unknown	Unknown	1.27 L/kg (84)	Unknown	Unknown	Unknown	Unknown	Unknown	2.4 L/kg
Route of excretion	Renal, 85–90% (2)	Renal, 51% (57)	Renal, 40% (49)	Renal (63)	Renal, 74%[a]	Renal	Renal, 65%; fecal, small amount (86)	Renal	Renal, 60% (88)	Renal, 60%; fecal, 20%
Elimination half-life	3.6 h (12); 34.6 h in overdose (16)	18 h (56)	19–24 h; prolonged in elderly (54 h) and overdose (29 h)	3–4 h (84)	1.1 h (63)	8 h (63)	0.9–2.0 h (86)	2–3 h (63)	13–20 h (87)	2.5 h
Excreted unchanged	85% (2)	1% (57)	None	None	Little	Little	10–15% (86)	Little	Unknown	Not reported
Active metabolites	Not reported	Not reported	Unknown	Not reported	Not reported	Not reported	Not reported	Not reported	Not reported	No
Protein binding	30% (2)	93% (57)	48% (49)	Unknown	Unknown	Unknown	Unknown	Unknown	Unknown	30%

T_{max}, time of maximal concentration.
[a]Paraflex. Product information. Raritan, NJ: Ortho-McNeil Pharmaceutical, 1991.

act in 30 to 45 minutes (13). Plasma levels for the unchanged drug peak within 2 hours (0.3 to 0.6 µg/ml). A metabolite formed by deamination and oxidation (β-*p*-chlorophenol–γ-hydroxybutyric acid) peaks at 4 hours (peak less than 0.2 µg/ml). The activity of the metabolite has not been evaluated. Total peak drug levels (drug and metabolites) for a 10-mg oral dose average approximately 0.3 µg/ml; for 20 mg, 0.4 µg/ml; and for 40 mg, 0.6 µg/ml (2).

Baclofen has a distribution time of 1.29 ± 0.70 hours (alpha half-life, 0.54 hour) (12). The apparent volume of distribution is approximately 0.8 L/kg (12). The apparent volume of distribution increases to 2.4 L/kg after overdose (14). Animal studies indicate wide tissue distribution (liver, kidneys) with slow release from brain and nervous tissue (2,4). Approximately 30% of baclofen is protein bound in humans (2).

Approximately 85% to 90% of an oral dose is excreted unchanged in the urine; 10% is excreted in the feces (2,4). Before excretion, perhaps 15% is deaminated in the liver, where it also undergoes oxidation and enters the Krebs cycle (15). The elimination half-life averages approximately 3.6 hours and ranges from 2 to 6 hours (2,12). Baclofen half-life in overdose may increase to 34.6 hours or longer (16). The intrathecal baclofen elimination half-life ranges from 0.9 to 5.0 hours, and the clearance ranges from 8 to 13 ml/hour, suggesting that baclofen persists in the cerebrospinal fluid longer than in the plasma (17).

Pathophysiology

Baclofen acts mainly as a mimetic of γ-aminobutyric acid in the spinal cord, blocking the excitatory effects of the sensory input from limb muscles. It inhibits both monosynaptic (H reflex) and polysynaptic flexor transmissions but has no effect on neuromuscular transmission (4). Baclofen is not a γ-aminobutyric acid receptor agonist, but it appears to act at a novel site on the nerve terminal (18). However, it is as active as γ-aminobutyric acid in reducing evoked transmitter output (18). Baclofen is also believed to inhibit substance P, which normally acts to stimulate monoaminergic neurons in the brainstem (19). In animals, baclofen produces a diminution of norepinephrine and epinephrine content in heart muscle (20). In humans, baclofen produces deep coma and respiratory depression. The mechanisms of action for these effects have not been elucidated (20).

Pregnancy and Lactation

Baclofen is U.S. Food and Drug Administration (FDA) pregnancy category C (Appendix I). At 7 days of age, an infant of a mother treated with baclofen, 80 mg/day, as well as oxybutynin and trimethoprim developed generalized seizures that were resistant to treatment. Baclofen 1 mg/kg/day in four divided doses stopped the seizures with the first dose (21).

Clinical Presentation

TOXICITY AFTER ACUTE OVERDOSE

The clinical features of baclofen overdose in both adults and children include coma, muscle flaccidity, hyporeflexia, and respiratory depression (22). Within 3 to 5 hours, patients may become flaccid; lose limb reflexes; develop deep coma; become unresponsive to painful stimuli; have no spontaneous respirations; and exhibit absence of the ciliospinal reflex, doll's eyes response, and ice-water caloric response (20,23,24). Involuntary movements may be observed initially, with grand mal seizures developing 6 hours after ingestion (11,16,20).

Muscle twitching and jerking are often present throughout toxicity. Behavior disturbances and delirium have been observed (8). Akinetic mutism followed a single 10-mg dose of baclofen in an adult with end-stage renal failure (24a).

Inadvertent intrathecal injection of 10 mg of baclofen into a brain-injured patient produced somnolence, flaccidity, nystagmus, and respiratory depression. Treatment with physostigmine produced no response. Status epilepticus improved after the removal of 30 ml of cerebrospinal fluid (25). In another study, seven events of intrathecal baclofen overdose occurred in five patients. The doses resulting in coma ranged from 50 µg administered as a bolus to 1500 µg/24 hours infused continuously. Physostigmine was not always effective in reversing these symptoms. Lumbar puncture drainage (e.g., 30 ml) was useful in cases involving intrathecal toxicity. Lumbar puncture combined with symptomatic treatment (cardiac respiratory monitoring, airway patency, oxygenation, and ventilation) in an intensive care environment probably offers a safer alternative than physostigmine used alone as an antidote (26).

Mild bradycardia is common after baclofen overdose (11,27). Hypotension and hypertension have been observed after baclofen overdose (8,24,78). First-degree atrioventricular block, premature ventricular contractions, premature atrial contractions, and supraventricular tachydysrhythmia occur rarely (11,28–30).

Hypothermia may develop (11,31,32). Mydriasis is common (22,33). Consciousness and muscle and neurologic function may not return for several days, perhaps due to the slow elimination rate of baclofen from nerve tissue (2) or the use of diazepam to control convulsions (16). Evidence of cerebral edema has been found at autopsy (8). A 10-mg bolus of baclofen was inadvertently delivered intrathecally. Within 80 minutes, the patient developed nystagmus, flaccidity, absence of tendon jerks, and coma; recovery occurred after 6 days of symptomatic therapy (34).

ADVERSE REACTIONS

Fatigue, lassitude, giddiness, mental confusion, depression, headaches, euphoria, and muscle weakness may develop (4). Nausea, vomiting, and diarrhea have been observed. In two patients with epilepsy, electroencephalographic deterioration developed (4). Patients with unrecognized renal insufficiency may develop baclofen toxicity after therapeutic doses (35–37).

Abrupt cessation of baclofen after many months of use may lead to grand mal seizures, auditory and visual hallucinations, paranoid ideas, insomnia, confusion, buccolingual dyskinesias, sleeplessness, agitation, belligerence, hyperactivity, and grandiose ideas within 12 to 96 hours (13,23,29). In severe cases, hyperthermia, hypotension, severe spasticity, and disseminated intravascular coagulation may develop and may last up to 8 days (29). These effects are similar to those produced by withdrawal from benzodiazepines, chlormezanone, and many sedative-hypnotic drugs (19,23,29,38). Restoring baclofen in normal dosage with gradual tapering may be an effective approach to management (38). An acute withdrawal syndrome was particularly severe after cessation of intrathecal baclofen in a patient with spasticity (39–42). Case reports suggest that patients with preexisting brain dysfunction or a family history of seizures may be at increased risk of baclofen withdrawal seizures, even after short-term administration (34).

DRUG INTERACTIONS

As baclofen is a neuronal depressant in the CNS, it may potentiate the effects of other sedative drugs, such as diazepam and alcohol (20). Ibuprofen-induced renal insufficiency led to baclofen toxicity in one 64-year-old man under treatment for spinal cord injury (43).

CARISOPRODOL

Carisoprodol is used to treat painful muscle spasm, and its mechanism of action is unclear but may be related to general sedative effects. Information on overdose is limited. The usual *adult dose* and the dose for *children 12 years of age or older* are 350 mg four times daily.

Toxicokinetics and Toxicodynamics

Pharmacokinetic and pharmacodynamic data are provided in Table 2. Onset of effects is 30 minutes with a duration of 4 to 6 hours. Carisoprodol undergoes hepatic metabolism, and very little drug is excreted unchanged in urine. Elimination half-life is 8 hours.

Pregnancy and Lactation

Carisoprodol is FDA pregnancy category C (Appendix I).

Clinical Presentation

CNS depression is the primary effect expected. Agitation and delirium may be more common than appreciated (44).

CHLORMEZANONE

Chlormezanone is mainly a tranquilizer that may have some muscle relaxant qualities (45). The major manufacturer has withdrawn this drug from the market due to cases of toxic epidermal necrolysis.

The *adult dose* is 150 to 225 mg/day. Ingestion of 4 g and 1500 mg of diclofenac sodium caused transient confusion and hypotonia, followed by complete recovery (46). Ingestion of 7 to 11 g in adults has produced CNS depression, hypotension, and anticholinergic effects (47,48). The *pediatric dose* is 50 to 100 mg three or four times daily for children 5 to 12 years of age.

Toxicokinetics and Toxicodynamics

Pharmacokinetic and pharmacodynamic data are provided in Table 1. Chlormezanone peaks in 1 to 2 hours and is 48% protein bound (49). Chlormezanone is hepatically metabolized followed by urinary elimination as metabolites (40%). It has a half-life of 19 to 24 hours, prolonged in elderly patients (54 hours) and slightly prolonged (29 hours) in overdose (47,49).

Pregnancy and Lactation

Insufficient data are available regarding chlormezanone.

Clinical Presentation

Mild tachycardia and hypotension and CNS depression have been reported after overdose (46,47). Therapeutic dosages may be associated with a hypersensitivity type of hepatitis with onset 1 to 2 months after initiation of therapy. Overdose (12 g) has been followed by an abrupt elevation of liver enzymes (50).

CHLORPHENESIN

The usual *adult dose* of chlorphenesin is 800 mg three times daily until pain is controlled, then reduced to 400 mg four times daily.

Toxicokinetics and Toxicodynamics

Pharmacokinetic and pharmacodynamic data are provided in Table 1. Peak chlorphenesin blood levels are reached 2 hours after therapeutic dosing. The volume of distribution is 1.3 L/kg. Chlorphenesin is primarily excreted in the urine as metabolites, with an elimination half-life of 3 to 4 hours.

Pathophysiology

The mechanism of action is unknown. Its muscle relaxant properties are probably related to sedative effects.

Pregnancy and Lactation

Insufficient data are available regarding chlormezanone.

Clinical Presentation

Overdose data are extremely limited; CNS depression is the most likely manifestation.

CHLORZOXAZONE

Chlorzoxazone is used for symptomatic relief of muscle spasm. The usual *adult dose* is 250 to 750 mg three or four times per day. The *pediatric dose* is 20 mg/kg/day in three or four doses.

Toxicokinetics and Toxicodynamics

Pharmacokinetic and pharmacodynamic data are provided in Table 1. Chlorzoxazone is 100% bioavailable orally, with peak serum levels 1 to 2 hours after a therapeutic dose. It is metabolized by cytochrome P-450 2E1 and may inhibit metabolism of other substances metabolized by this enzyme (51). The elimination half-life is 1.1 hours, and volume of distribution is 13.7 L (52).

Pregnancy and Lactation

Chlorzoxazone is FDA pregnancy category C (Appendix I).

Clinical Presentation

Overdose data are limited, but CNS and respiratory depression requiring intubation have been reported (53).

CYCLOBENZAPRINE

Cyclobenzaprine is a tricyclic amine, structurally similar to amitriptyline, which is used in acute, painful skeletal muscle conditions. The usual *adult dose* of cyclobenzaprine is 10 mg three times daily. Adults have survived ingestion of 260 to 900 mg of cyclobenzaprine; ingestion of 100 mg by an adult generally does not result in toxicity (54,55).

Toxicokinetics and Toxicodynamics

Pharmacokinetic and pharmacodynamic data are provided in Table 1. Bioavailability of cyclobenzaprine is 55% due to extensive first-pass metabolism. The peak concentration is reached in blood 3.8 to 4.0 hours after a therapeutic dose (56). It is 93% bound to plasma proteins, extensively metabolized in the liver, and eliminated as glucuronide conjugates (57).

Pathophysiology

Cyclobenzaprine has anticholinergic, antihistaminic, and sedative properties. It is a weak inhibitor of presynaptic norepinephrine and serotonin reuptake. Its skeletal muscle relaxant activity is primarily due to brain stem–mediated inhibition of γ- and α-motor neurons (58).

Pregnancy and Lactation

Cyclobenzaprine is FDA pregnancy category C (Appendix I).

Clinical Presentation

Anticholinergic effects and lethargy are common. Hypotension, coma, and respiratory depression requiring endotracheal intubation may occur with severe overdose (55). Sinus tachycardia is common after overdose (55). Mild hypertension and hypotension have been reported occasionally (55,59). Ventricular dysrhythmias and conduction delays are of theoretic concern because of structural similarity to amitriptyline but have not been reported with pure cyclobenzaprine overdose.

Anticholinergic effects, such as mydriasis, dry skin and mucous membranes, and decreased bowel sounds, may develop (54). Rhabdomyolysis complicated by renal insufficiency has been reported but is rare (60). Hallucinations have been reported in the elderly (61).

Surreptitious cyclobenzaprine toxicity may be diagnosed by a false-positive tricyclic antidepressant screen (62).

METAXALONE

With use of metaxalone, muscle relaxant effects are likely secondary to CNS depression. It has also been proposed to treat diabetic peripheral neuropathy. The usual *adult dose* is 800 mg three to four times daily.

Toxicokinetics and Toxicodynamics

Pharmacokinetic and pharmacodynamic data are provided in Table 2. Onset of effects occurs in 1 hour, and duration of effects lasts 4 to 6 hours (63). It is excreted in urine as metabolites and has a half-life of 2 to 3 hours (63). Metaxalone peaks in 2 hours (63).

Pathophysiology

Metaxalone does not directly affect skeletal muscle. Most of its therapeutic effects come from actions on the CNS.

Pregnancy and Lactation

Very little information is available, but description indicates that it is equivalent to FDA category C (Appendix I).

Clinical Presentation

Extremely little information is available. Sedation and CNS depression are the primary expected effects.

METHOCARBAMOL

The *adult dose* of methocarbamol is 6 to 8 g/day in divided doses for acute conditions. The *pediatric dose* for the treatment of tetanus is 15 mg/kg/day; however, the solution is hypertonic and may cause extravasation injury.

Toxicokinetics and Toxicodynamics

Pharmacokinetic and pharmacodynamic data are provided in Table 2. Methocarbamol, 1.5 g orally, induces a peak blood level of approximately 23 μg/ml in 1.1 hours. Protein binding ranges between 46% and 50% (64). Therapeutic blood levels are reported to range from 16 to 41 μg/ml (65). Methocarbamol exhibits a half-life of 1.14 hours in normal control subjects (64).

Pregnancy and Lactation

Methocarbamol is FDA pregnancy category C (Appendix I).

Clinical Presentation

Drowsiness and dizziness are common at the therapeutic dose. Overdose data are limited; CNS depression is the most likely manifestation.

ORPHENADRINE

The normal *adult dose* is 100 mg orally twice a day. Although not well documented, death does not occur until several grams have been ingested. Even then, a dose several times the daily dose typically causes only mild anticholinergic effects.

Toxicokinetics and Toxicodynamics

Pharmacokinetic and pharmacodynamic data are provided in Table 1.

Pregnancy and Lactation

Orphenadrine is FDA pregnancy category C (Appendix I).

Clinical Presentation

Patients with mild overdoses may develop typical anticholinergic effects, such as mydriasis, tachycardia, agitation, confusion, hallucinations, urinary retention, and decreased gastrointestinal motility (66). Cardiac dysrhythmia, including nonsustained ventricular tachycardia, has been reported (67,68).

TIZANIDINE

Tizanidine is an imidazole derivative with α_2-adrenergic agonist effects (69). Tizanidine is used to treat spasticity associated with multiple sclerosis or spinal cord injury. The usual *adult dose* is 4 to 8 mg three times daily, maximum 36 mg/day.

An adult survived ingestion of 120 mg tizanidine (70).

Toxicokinetics and Toxicodynamics

Pharmacokinetic and pharmacodynamic data are provided in Table 2. Bioavailability is only 40% due to extensive first-pass metabolism (71). Protein binding is 30%, and volume of distribution is 2.4 L/kg (71). Tizanidine undergoes hepatic metabolism (95%), followed by renal (60%) and fecal (20%) elimination. It has a half-life of 2.5 hours (71).

Pathophysiology

Tizanidine has α_2-adrenergic agonist effects; at therapeutic doses, it has minimal antihypertensive effects compared to clonidine.

Pregnancy and Lactation

Tizanidine is FDA pregnancy category C (Appendix I).

Clinical Presentation

Hypotension, bradycardia, first-degree atrioventricular block, and Wenckebach type II atrioventricular block have been reported after tizanidine overdose (70,72).

ACUTE AND SUBACUTE OVERDOSE OF CENTRALLY ACTING MUSCLE RELAXANTS

Diagnostic Tests

LABORATORY TESTS

Quantitative blood levels of these agents are available only from referral laboratories. Blood levels are not typically used for clinical management but may be helpful occasionally in confirming exposure and source of toxic effects. Other typical laboratory tests are usually normal or reflect tissue injury from other effects (e.g., muscle injury from prolonged coma). The creatine kinase should be monitored in patients with prolonged seizures or coma (28). Occasional transient elevations of lactic dehydrogenase and aspartate transaminase levels have been observed (20).

Accurate plasma levels of baclofen are available with the use of a gas-liquid chromatography method (73). A reverse-phase high-performance liquid chromatography (HPLC) method can detect quantities of baclofen in plasma and urine to 5 ng (9,74). HPLC with ultraviolet detection can rapidly quantitate baclofen and its γ-hydroxy metabolite in urine (75). A secondary blood level peak is observed after recovery of consciousness (16,32) and may reflect either a release of the lipophilic drug from lipid stores or evidence of enterohepatic recycling of baclofen. Toxic blood levels have been reported from 1100 to 3500 ng/ml (therapeutic plasma trough concentrations after baclofen, 15 to 90 mg, range from 100 to 400 ng/ml) (9). Blood levels after a baclofen ingestion of probably between 1000 and 1800 mg averaged 17 μg/ml (17,000 ng/ml). The urine baclofen concentration was 760 μg/ml (9). Ingestions of baclofen, 1.0 to 1.8 g, led to coma and death in 5 days with serum and urine baclofen concentrations of 17 and 760 μg/ml, respectively (9).

Plasma methocarbamol concentrations are fluorometrically determined by HPLC with a sensitivity to 200 ng/ml (64).

Cyclobenzaprine can be detected in biologic fluids by gas-liquid chromatography (76). Distinguishing cyclobenzaprine from tricyclic antidepressants can be difficult using thin-layer chromatography, immunoassays, or HPLC (77). Surreptitious cyclobenzaprine toxicity may be diagnosed by a false-positive tricyclic antidepressant screen (62).

ANCILLARY TESTS

The electrocardiogram and chest radiograph are usually normal. If abnormal, they typically reflect injury induced by other drug effects (e.g., hypotension, pulmonary aspiration). Computed tomography of the head and lumbar puncture may be needed to evaluate other causes of CNS depression, such as trauma, meningitis, and encephalitis (Chapters 14 and 19).

Treatment

OVERVIEW

The patient may be conscious on admission but quickly lapse into a deep coma with profound respiratory and generalized flaccidity. Close monitoring for respiratory compromise and prompt endotracheal intubation may be needed. Airway support may be needed for several days. After intrathecal baclofen overdose, withdraw 30 to 50 ml of cerebrospinal fluid as soon as possible (78,79).

GASTROINTESTINAL DECONTAMINATION

Syrup of ipecac is contraindicated because skeletal muscle relaxants cause mental status depression. The need for endotracheal intubation for airway protection should be assessed early. Administer activated charcoal as soon as possible after overdose ingestion. Gastric lavage with endotracheal intubation may be considered in patients who present 1 to 2 hours after large overdose.

SUPPORTIVE CARE

The airway should be maintained by endotracheal intubation if respiratory depression or obstruction occurs. Assisted ventilation is frequently required early after an overdose because of the severe respiratory depression that quickly supervenes (10,15).

Supportive management is the mainstay of care for overdose with antispasticity drugs. Coma with baclofen may continue for several days after an overdose despite its therapeutic half-life of 3 to 4 hours. An intensive care unit is usually needed.

SEIZURES

Seizures after baclofen overdose are managed similar to other toxin-induced seizures (Chapter 30). The initial drug is intravenous (IV) diazepam. If there is an inadequate response to diazepam, then IV phenobarbital or phenytoin may be required.

CARDIOVASCULAR TOXICITY

Hypotension can be managed by placing the patient in Trendelenburg position, starting an infusion of IV fluid, and administering pressor amines (dopamine or norepinephrine). IV atropine, 600 μg, was temporarily effective in elevating depressed body temperature, increasing respiratory tidal volume, and restoring depressed heart rate and blood pressure (31). Sinus tachycardia generally does not require treatment.

NEUROLOGIC TOXICITY

Baclofen withdrawal hallucinations can be managed by reintroducing the drug and tapering it gradually. Withdrawal reactions occur after use of baclofen for many months and have not been reported after acute poisonings (85). See also Chapter 32.

ANTIDOTES

No specific antidote is available for the treatment of overdose with baclofen, chlormezanone, or methocarbamol. There are anecdotal reports suggesting that both flumazenil and physostigmine may be effective in reversing respiratory and CNS depression after intrathecal baclofen overdose as well as after chlorzoxazone or carisoprodol overdose (5,53,80,81). Other case reports suggest that these agents are not always effective (25,30,78). In addition, flumazenil administration in this setting carries the risk of seizures as baclofen has a proconvulsant effect, and many baclofen-treated patients also take benzodiazepines chronically (82). Use of flumazenil for baclofen overdose has been associated with the development of cardiac arrest (6,26). Given the short half-life of flumazenil and the fact that patients recover uneventfully with intensive supportive care, use of flumazenil and physostigmine is generally not warranted.

ENHANCEMENT OF ELIMINATION

Forced diuresis may theoretically be useful in view of the excretion of baclofen (largely unchanged) in the urine (4,8,10). However, there is no evidence that this improves outcome or shortens length of stay after overdose, and nearly all patients recover with intensive supportive care. Enhancement of elimination of baclofen by extracorporeal means (peritoneal dialysis, hemodialysis, hemoperfusion) has not been evaluated; however, the low degree of protein binding and the excretion of almost all baclofen as unchanged drug suggest that these modalities may speed drug elimination after overdose. As the majority of patients do well with intensive supportive care, extracorporeal elimination techniques should only be considered in patients with severe toxicity not responding to conventional care.

MONITORING

Continuous monitoring of electrocardiogram, pulse (bradycardia), respiration, and temperature (hypothermia frequent in overdose) and periodic evaluation of renal and hepatic function are useful during coma and after return of consciousness.

Monitoring of vital signs and CNS and respiratory function provides guidelines for determination of time of discharge from the intensive care unit.

REFERENCES

1. Lebby TI, Dugger K, Lipscomb JW, et al. Skeletal muscle relaxant ingestion. *Vet Hum Toxicol* 1990;32:133–135.
2. Faigle JW, Keberle H. The chemistry and kinetics of Lioresal. *Postgrad Med J* 1972;48:9–13.
3. Katogi Y, Tamaki N, Adachi M, et al. Simultaneous determination of dantrolene and its metabolite, 5-hydroxydantrolene, in human plasma by high-performance liquid chromatography. *J Chromatogr* 1982;228:404–408.
4. Brogden RN, Speight TM, Avery GS. Baclofen: a preliminary report of its pharmacological properties and therapeutic efficacy in spasticity. *Drugs* 1974;8:1–14.
5. Muller-Schwefe G, Penn RD. Physostigmine in the treatment of intrathecal baclofen overdose. *J Neurosurg* 1989;71:273–275.
6. Penn RD, Kroin JS. Failure of physostigmine in treatment of acute severe intrathecal baclofen intoxication. *N Engl J Med* 1990;322:1533–1534(letter).
7. Gerkin R, Curry SC, Vance MV, et al. First-order elimination kinetics following baclofen overdose. *Ann Emerg Med* 1986;15:843–846.
8. Haubenstock A, Aruby K, Jager U, et al. Baclofen (Lioresal[R]) intoxication: report of 4 cases and review of the literature. *J Toxicol Clin Toxicol* 1983;20(1):59–68.
9. Fraser AD, MacNeil W, Isner AF. Toxicological analysis of a fatal baclofen (Lioresal[R]) ingestion. *J Forens Sci* 1991;36:1596–1602.
10. Blankenship JMK, Moses ES. Baclofen overdose in a child resulting in respiratory arrest. *Vet Hum Toxicol* 1983;25[Suppl 1]:45–46.
11. Perry HE, Wright RO, Shannon MW, et al. Baclofen overdose: drug experimentation in a group of adolescents. *Pediatrics* 1998;101:1045–1048.
12. Kochak GM, Rakhit A, Wagner WE, et al. The pharmacokinetics of baclofen derived from intestinal infusion. *Clin Pharmacol Ther* 1985;38:251–257.
13. Garabedian-Ruffalo SM, Ruffalo RL. Adverse effects secondary to baclofen withdrawal. *Drug Intell Clin Pharm* 1985;19:304–306.
14. Anderson P, Noher H, Swahn CG. Pharmacokinetics in baclofen overdose. *J Toxicol Clin Toxicol* 1984;22:11–20.
15. May CR. Baclofen overdose. *Ann Emerg Med* 1983;12:171–173.
16. Ghose K, Holmes KM, Matthewson K. Complications of baclofen overdosage. *Postgrad Med J* 1980;56:865–867.
17. Parr MJ, Willatts SM. Fatal theophylline poisoning with rhabdomyolysis: a potential role for dantrolene treatment. *Anaesthesia* 1991;46:557–559.
18. Morison DH. Placental transfer of dantrolene. *Anesthesiology* 1983;59:265.
19. Bowery NG, Hill DR, Hudson AL, et al. Baclofen decreases neurotransmitter release in the mammalian CNS by an action at a novel GABA receptor. *Nature* 1980;283:92–94.
20. Paulson GW. Overdose of Lioresal. *Neurology* 1976;26:1105–1106.
21. Ratnayaka BD, Dhaliwal H, Watkin S. Neonatal convulsions after withdrawal of baclofen. *BMJ* 2001;323:85.
22. Cooke DEM, Glasstone MA. Baclofen poisoning in children. *Vet Human Toxicol* 1994;36:448–450.
23. Arnold ES, Rudd SM, Kirshner H. Manic psychosis following rapid withdrawal from baclofen. *Am J Psychiatry* 1980;137:1466–1467.
24. Ostermann ME, Young B, Sibbald WJ, et al. Coma mimicking brain death following baclofen overdose. *Intensive Care Med* 2000;26:1144–1146.

24a. Parmar MS. Akinetic mutism after baclofen. *Ann Intern Med* 1991;115:499–500.

25. Salturari L, Baumgartner H, Kofler M, et al. Failure of physostigmine in treatment of acute severe intrathecal baclofen intoxication [letter]. *N Engl J Med* 1990;322:1533–1534.
26. Delhaas EM, Brouwers JR. Intrathecal baclofen overdose: report of 7 events in 5 patients and review of the literature. *Int J Clin Pharmacol Ther Toxicol* 1991;29:274–280.
27. Peng CT, Ger J, Yang CC, et al. Prolonged severe withdrawal symptoms after acute-on-chronic baclofen overdose. *J Toxicol Clin Toxicol* 1998;36:359–363.
28. Lee TH, Chen SS, Su SL, et al. Baclofen intoxication: report of four cases and review of literature. *Clin Neuropharmacol* 1992;15:56–62.
29. Nugent S, Katz MD, Little TE. Baclofen overdose with cardiac conduction abnormalities: case report and review of the literature. *J Toxicol Clin Toxicol* 1986;24:321–328.
30. Roberge RJ, Martin TG, Hodgman M, et al. Supraventricular tachyarrhythmia associated with baclofen overdose. *J Toxicol Clin Toxicol* 1994;32:291–297.
31. Ferner RE. Atropine treatment for baclofen overdose. *Postgrad Med J* 1981;57:580–581.
32. Lipscomb DJ, Meredith TJ. Baclofen overdose. *Postgrad Med J* 1980;56:108–109.
33. Chapple D, Johnson D, Connors R. Baclofen overdose in two siblings. *Ped Emerg Care* 2001;17:110–112.
34. Kofler M, Saltuari L, Schumatzhard E, et al. Electrophysiological findings in a case of severe intrathecal baclofen overdose. *Electroencephalogr Clin Neurophysiol* 1992;83:83–86.
35. Bassilios N, Launay-Vacher V, Mercadal L, et al. Baclofen neurotoxicity in a chronic haemodialysis patient. *Nephrol Dial Transplant* 2000;15:715–716.
36. Chen KS, Bullard MJ, Chien YY, et al. Baclofen toxicity in patients with severely impaired renal function. *Ann Pharmacother* 1997;31:1315–1320.
37. Choo YM, Kim GB, Choi JY, et al. Severe respiratory depression by low-dose baclofen in the treatment of chronic hiccups in a patient undergoing CAPD. *Nephron* 2000;86:546–547.
38. Lees AJ, Clarke CR, Harrison MJ. Hallucinations after withdrawal of baclofen. *Lancet* 1977;1:858.
39. Green LB, Nelson VS. Death after acute withdrawal of intrathecal baclofen: case report and literature review. *Arch Phys Med Rehabil* 1999;80:1600–1604.
40. Sampathkumar P, Scanlon PD, Plevak DJ. Baclofen withdrawal presenting as multiorgan system failure. *Anesth Analg* 1998;87:562–563.
41. Samson-Fang L, Gooch J, Norlin C. Intrathecal baclofen withdrawal simulating neuroleptic malignant syndrome in a child with cerebral palsy. *Dev Med Child Neurol* 2000;42:561–565.
42. Siegfried RN, Jacobson L, Chabal C. Development of an acute withdrawal syndrome following the cessation of intrathecal baclofen in a patient with spasticity. *Anesthesiology* 1992;77:1048–1050.
43. McChesney EW, Banks WF Jr, Portmann GA, et al. Metabolism of chlormezanone in man and laboratory animals. *Biochem Pharmacol* 1967;16:813–826.
44. Roth BA, Vinson DR, Kim S. Carisoprodol-induced myoclonic encephalopathy. *J Toxicol Clin Toxicol* 1998;36:609–612.
45. Baldessarini RJ. Drugs and the treatment of psychiatric disorders. In: Gilman AG, Goodman LS, Rall TW, et al., eds. *The pharmacological basis of therapeutics*, 7th ed. New York: Macmillan, 1985:437.
46. Netter P, Lambert H, Larcan A, et al. Diclofenac sodium-chromezanone poisoning. *Eur J Clin Pharmacol* 1984;26:535–536.
47. Armstrong D, Braithwaite RA, Vale JA. Chlormezanone poisoning. *BMJ* 1983;286:845–846.
48. Kirkham BW, Edelman JB. Overdose of chlormezanone: a new clinical picture. *BMJ* 1986;292:732.
49. Koppel C, Tenczer J, Wagemann A. Metabolism of chlormezanone in man. *Arzneimittelforschung* 1986;36:1116–1118.
50. Sheu BS, Lin CY, Chen KW, et al. Severe hepatocellular damage induced by chlormezanone overdose. *Am J Gastroenterol* 1995;90:833–835.
51. Ernstgard L, Gullstrand E, Johanson G. Toxicokinetic interactions between orally ingested chlorzoxazone and inhaled acetone or toluene in male volunteers. *Toxicol Sci* 1999;48:189–196.
52. Desiraju RK, Renzi NL, Nayak RK, et al. Pharmacokinetics of chlorzoxazone in humans. *J Pharm Sci* 1983;72:991–994.
53. Roberge RJ, Atchley B, Ryan K, et al. Two chlorzoxazone (Parafon Forte) overdoses and coma in one patient: reversal with flumazenil. *Am J Emerg Med* 1998;16:393–395.
54. Linden CH, Mitchiner JC, Lindzon RD, et al. Cyclobenzaprine overdosage. *J Toxicol Clin Toxicol* 1983;20:281–288.
55. Spiller HA, Winter ML, Mann KV, et al. Five year multicenter retrospective review of cyclobenazprine toxicity. *Vet Hum Toxicol* 1994;36:370.
56. Winchell GA, King JD, Chavez-Eng CM, et al. Cyclobenzaprine pharmacokinetics, including the effects of age, gender, and hepatic insufficiency. *J Clin Pharmacol* 2002;42:61–69.
57. Share NN. Pharmacological properties of cyclobenzaprine, in clinical evaluation of Flexeril (cyclobenzaprine HCL/MSD). *Postgrad Med Comm* 1978;14–18.
58. Share NN, McFarlane CS. Cyclobenzaprine: a novel centrally acting skeletal muscle relaxant. *Neuropharmacology* 1975;12:675–684.
59. Levine B, Jones R, Smith ML, et al. A multiple drug intoxication involving cyclobenzaprine and ibuprofen. *Am J Forensic Med Pathol* 1993;14:246–248.
60. O'Riordan W, Gillette P, Calderon J, et al. Overdose of cyclobenzaprine, the tricyclic muscle relaxant. *Ann Emerg Med* 1986;15:592–593.
61. Douglass MA, Levine DP. Hallucinations in an elderly patient taking recommended doses of cyclobenzaprine. *Arch Intern Med* 2000;160:1373.
62. Matos ME, Burns MM, Shannon MW. False-positive tricyclic antidepressant drug screen results leading to the diagnosis of carbamazepine intoxication. *Pediatrics* 2000;105:E66.
63. Elenbaas JK. Centrally acting oral skeletal muscle relaxants. *Am J Hosp Pharm* 1980;37:1313–1323.
64. Sica DA, Comstock TJ, Davis J, et al. Pharmacokinetics and protein binding of methocarbamol in renal insufficiency and normals. *Eur J Clin Pharmacol* 1990;39:193–194.
65. Ferslew KE, Hagardorn AN, McCormick WF. A fatal interaction of methocarbamol and ethanol in an accidental poisoning. *J Forens Sci* 1990;35:477–482.

66. Garza MB, Osterhoudt KC, Rutstein R. Central anticholinergic syndrome from orphenadrine in a 3 year old. *Pediatr Emerg Care* 2000;16:97–98.
67. Dilaveris P, Pantazis A, Vlasseros J, et al. Non-sustained ventricular tachycardia due to low-dose orphenadrine. *Am J Med* 2001;111:418–419.
68. Van Herreweghe I, Mertens K, Maes V, et al. Orphenadrine poisoning in a child: clinical and analytical data. *Intensive Care Med* 1999;25:1134–1136.
69. Eyssette M, Rohmer F, Serratrice G, et al. Multi-centre, double-blind trial of a novel antispastic agent, tizanidine, in spasticity associated with multiple sclerosis. *Curr Med Res Opin* 1988;10:699–708.
70. Luciani A, Brugioni L, Serra L, et al. Sino-atrial and atrio-ventricular node dysfunction in a case of tizanidine overdose. *Vet Hum Toxicol* 1995;37:556–557.
71. Zanaflex, tizanidine hydrochloride. Product information. San Francisco: Athena Neurosciences, 1998.
72. Chu J, Nelson LS, Hoffman RS. Hypotension in an unintentional overdose with tizanidine. *J Toxicol Clin Toxicol* 2001;39:283.
73. Terrence CF, Fromm GH. Complications of baclofen withdrawal. *Arch Neurol* 1981;38:588-589.
74. Wuis EW, Dirks RJ, Vree TB, et al. High performance liquid chromatographic analysis of baclofen in plasma and urine of man after precolumn extraction and derivitization with ophthaldialdehyde. *J Chromatogr Biomed Appl* 1985;337:341–350.
75. Wuis EW, Van Beijsterveldt LE, Dirks RJ, et al. Rapid simultaneous determination of baclofen and its gamma-hydroxy metabolite in urine by high-performance liquid chromatography with ultraviolet detection. *J Chromatogr* 1987;420:212–216.
76. Constanzer ML, Vincek WC, Bayne WF. Determination of cyclobenzaprine in plasma and urine using capillary gas chromatography with nitrogen-selective detection. *J Chromatogr* 1985;339:414–418.
77. Poklis A, Edinboro LE. REMEDI drug profiling system readily distinguishes between cyclobenzaprine and amitriptyline in emergency toxicology urine specimens [letter]. *Clin Chem* 1992;38:2349–2350.
78. Fakhoury T, Abou-Khali B, Blumenkopf B. EEG changes in intrathecal baclofen overdose: a case report and review of the literature. *Electroencephalogr Clin Neurophysiol* 1998;107:339–342.
79. Merchant J, Hollis G. Intrathecal baclofen overdose. *J Emerg Med* 1997;9:221–225.
80. Roberge RJ, Lin E, Krenzelok EP. Flumazenil reversal of carisoprodol (Soma) intoxication. *J Emerg Med* 2000;18:61–64.
81. Saissy JM, Vitris M, Demaziere J, et al. Flumazenil counteracts intrathecal baclofen-induced central nervous system depression in tetanus. *Anesthesiology* 1992;76:1051–1053.
82. Chern TL, Kwan A. Flumazenil-induced seizure accompanying benzodiazepine and baclofen intoxication. *Am J Emerg Med* 1996;14:231–232.
83. Trancopral, chlormezanone. Product information. New York: Winthrop Pharmaceuticals, 1996.
84. Forist AA, Judy RW. Comparative pharmacokinetics of chlorphenesin carbamate and methocarbamol in man. *J Pharm Sci* 1971;60:1686-1688.
85. Levine IM, Jossmann PB, Rudd J, et al. The quantitative evaluation of intravenous methocarbamol in the relief of spasticity. *Neurology* 1968;18:69–74.
86. Esplin DW. Centrally acting muscle relaxants; drugs for Parkinson's disease. In: Goodman LS, Gilman A, eds. *The pharmacological basis of therapeutics*, 4th ed. London: Macmillan Co., 1970:226–236.
87. Labout JM, Thijssen CT, Keijser GG, et al. Difference between single and multiple dose pharmacokinetics of orphenadrine hydrochloride in man. *Eur J Clin Pharmacol* 1982;21:343–350.
88. Cedarbaum JM. Clinical pharmacokinetics of anti-parkinsonian drugs. *Drugs* 1987;13:141-178.

CHAPTER 105

Nicotine

Michael A. McGuigan

N

H_3C—N

NICOTINE

Molecular formula and weight:	**$C_{10}H_{14}N_2$, 162.23 g/mol**
CAS Registry No.:	**54-11-5**
SI conversion:	**mg/L × 6.2 = μmol/L**
Normal or therapeutic levels:	**Not applicable**
Special concerns:	**Mild toxicity is common. Severe toxicity is rare and develops early in course.**
Antidote:	**None**

OVERVIEW

Nicotine was first isolated from the tobacco plant in 1828. Nicotine has been used as an insecticide, in medicines, and in tanning, but its primary use is as a recreational drug in tobacco products. This chapter addresses the medical toxicology of nicotine; it does not include the chronic health effects of smoking tobacco or of the *Nicotiana* plant.

Nicotine commonly produces adverse effects: dermal exposure may cause skin irritation; oral exposure may cause mucous membrane irritation and gastrointestinal (GI) effects; inhalation can cause upper airway irritation; neurologic effects include headaches, paresthesias, nervousness, dizziness, lightheadedness, sleep disturbances and depression; and cardiovascular effects include chest pain, hypertension, and tachycardia. Acute nicotine toxicity involves the GI tract and central nervous system and cardiovascular system stimulation followed by organ system depression.

Nicotine is available in a free state or as a dihydrochloride, salicylate, sulfate, or bitartrate salt. Nicotine has a pK_a of 8.5 and, as a 0.05 mol/L solution, a pH of 10.2 (1). Natural exposure results from contact with the plants *N. tabacum* and *N. rustica*.

Sources of exposure include occupational exposure—occurring during the harvesting, processing, and extracting of tobacco—or during the mixing, storage, and application of nicotine-containing insecticides. Other sources of exposure include the chewing or ingestion of any tobacco-containing consumer product and nicotine transdermal patches, sprays, or chewing gums. Rarely, exposure may be from the administration of tobacco enemas to treat intestinal parasites.

Standards

Commercial nicotine is entirely a byproduct of the tobacco industry. The permissible exposure limit:time-weighted average is 0.5 mg/m^3 (skin); threshold limit value:time-weighted average is 0.5 mg/m^3 (skin); threshold limit value is 0.2 mg/m^3 of nicotine sulfate mist; and the immediately dangerous to life or health limit value is 35 mg/m^3. No standards for short-term exposure limit or ceiling limit have been developed.

Toxic Dose

Toxicity and fatalities can occur from nicotine in liquid forms, tobacco, gum, spray, and transdermal patches absorbed through GI, dermal, or rectal routes. Extrapolation of nicotine dose from the amount of tobacco in any product is unreliable and problematic.

The *adult toxic dose* of nicotine is not well documented. Ingestion of 1.0 and 4.5 mg of liquid nicotine produced systemic toxicity (2). A dose of 2 to 5 mg may produce nausea and vomiting. In dogs, nicotine, 10 mg/kg buccally, is potentially fatal (3). Other animal data suggest an oral median lethal dose range of 3.3 to 200.0 mg/kg, depending on the nicotine formulation, route of administration, and animal species (4,5). The commonly accepted potentially lethal oral dose for adults is 40 to 60 mg, but data supporting the statement "the acutely fatal dose of nicotine for an adult is probably in the neighborhood of 60 mg" (6) are not available.

The *pediatric toxic dose* has not been established. A dose of 1 mg or more may cause symptoms in a small child. The lethal dose is estimated as 1 mg/kg. Oral exposure of children to cigarettes or cigarette butts has caused significant systemic toxicity. It is not possible to establish a "toxic dose" based on nicotine content, and it is difficult to do so using the number of cigarettes or butts reported. No data are available correlating cigarette exposure and clinical effects with serum nicotine levels.

Four retrospective or poison center studies have attempted to establish a toxic dose, but each lacks confirmation of the ingestion history. A retrospective study reported that all six children who "ingested" half a cigarette were asymptomatic, whereas all four children who ingested two cigarettes developed serious toxicity (7). A poison center study reported that 47% of 17 children who ingested fewer than one cigarette developed mild self-limited symptoms, whereas all eight children who ingested one to one and one-half cigarettes developed more serious effects (8). A prospective poison center study found that 18.8% of 656 children who ingested fewer than two cigarettes or six butts and 45.5% of 44 children who ingested more than 2 cigarettes or 6 butts developed mild self-limited symptoms; all other children were asymptomatic (9). In 1996, a retrospective review of cigarette exposures in children up to 6 years of age found that 18.8% of 209 children who ingested one or fewer cigarettes or butts and 50% of the 14 children who ingested more than one cigarette or butt developed mild self-limited symptoms; all other children were asymptomatic (10).

Unintentional exposures of children to transdermal nicotine patches have caused mild self-limited clinical toxicity when the nicotine doses were at least 0.01 mg/kg (11).

TOXICOKINETICS AND TOXICODYNAMICS

Absorption occurs rapidly from buccal mucosa, intestine (12), respiratory tract, and skin (13,14). The bioavailability of nicotine depends on its chemical formulation, the pH of the environment, and the site of absorption. The free base is more readily absorbed than a salt. Nicotine is absorbed better in an alkaline medium: Only 3% of an ingested nicotine solution was absorbed over a 15-minute period at pH 1; absorption increased to 8.3% at pH 7.4 and to 18.6% at pH 9.8 (15). Buccal absorption is also pH dependent.

The amount of nicotine absorbed from nicotine gum also depends on the amount of nicotine and the rate and vigor of chewing (16,17). Rapid and vigorous chewing produces higher peak levels and is associated with more adverse effects. After 30 minutes of chewing, 72% to 96% of the nicotine is absorbed (16,18). Swallowing the gum without chewing results in 15% bioavailability in dogs (19). Nicotine is a base, so absorption from the stomach is limited (15). Nicotine undergoes significant first-pass hepatic clearance (16) and may undergo significant enterohepatic or enteroenteric recirculation (20).

Protein binding ranges from 5% (21) to 20% (22). The apparent volume of distribution is 2.6 L/kg and ranges from 1.0 L/kg to 3.1 L/kg (23,24). Nicotine passes through the placenta and is found in both amniotic fluid (1.5 to 23.0 ng/ml) and umbilical cord blood (0.5 to 25.0 ng/ml) (25).

Nicotine has an elimination half-life of approximately 2 hours (26). Up to 90% of absorbed nicotine is metabolized primarily in the liver but also in the kidney and lung (27). Cotinine is the major metabolite; nicotine-1'-*N*-oxide, 3-hydroxycotinine, and conjugated metabolites are produced in lesser quantities. Both nicotine (10% to 20% of an absorbed dose) and its metabolites are excreted in the urine, with the extent of nicotine excretion being pH dependent: 23% is excreted unchanged with a urine pH less than 5, whereas 2% is excreted unchanged with a urine pH greater than 7 (23).

PATHOPHYSIOLOGY

Nicotine affects a variety of sites and can stimulate or inhibit both sympathetic and parasympathetic receptors (27). The response of any given organ is a result of both the initial stimulatory and subsequent inhibitory effects of nicotine.

Central nervous system effects are the result of stimulation and then depression of central motor and respiratory activities. Nicotine also stimulates the emetic center of the medulla oblongata and the release of antidiuretic hormone. Small doses of nicotine stimulate the autonomic ganglia cells of the peripheral nervous system. After larger doses, transient stimulation is followed by more persistent blockade of transmission at sympathetic and parasympathetic ganglia. The effects on the adrenal gland are similar—small doses cause release of catecholamines, and larger doses prevent their release. The stimulation phase at the neuromuscular junction is obscured by a rapidly developing paralysis due in part to receptor desensitization. Nicotine initially stimulates salivary and bronchial secretions, which are followed by inhibition.

Cardiovascular stimulation is the result of nicotine's effects at the sympathetic and parasympathetic ganglia, the adrenal medulla, and the chemoreceptors of the carotid and aortic bodies. GI effects are the result of parasympathetic stimulation and activation of cholinergic nerve endings, which increase muscle tone and motor activity.

VULNERABLE POPULATIONS

Nicotine is a possible human teratogen. Developmental abnormalities in the cardiovascular system were observed in the offspring of a woman who ingested nicotine. Teratogenic effects have been reported in monkeys, mice, and chickens but not in several other species (28). Nicotine is excreted in breast milk in small quantities (2 to 62 ng/ml), and infant serum concentrations range from less than 0.2 to 1.6 ng/ml (25).

Migrant populations working in tobacco fields are at risk for developing *green tobacco sickness*, a mild form of nicotine poisoning caused by uncured tobacco leaves (29,30).

CLINICAL PRESENTATION

Acute and Subacute Exposure

Clinical effects often begin within 30 minutes of exposure and last 1 to 2 hours after mild exposure or up to 18 to 24 hours in more severe intoxication. Stimulatory effects characterize a mild poisoning as well as the early phase of severe intoxication; the late phase of severe poisonings is characterized by depressed organ function. Symptoms and signs that begin within 30 minutes of an oral exposure are most likely due to the buccal absorption of nicotine during chewing.

GI effects include a burning sensation in the mouth, throat, esophagus, and stomach. Other effects include increased salivation, nausea, vomiting, abdominal pain, cramps, and diarrhea.

Central nervous system effects include headache, dizziness, confusion, agitation or restlessness, and tremor followed by lethargy, convulsions, and coma. Peripheral nervous system signs consist of weakness, fasciculation, hypotonia, and decreased deep tendon reflexes, progressing to paralysis. Ocular findings include lacrimation and miosis followed by mydriasis. Nicotine-induced nystagmus is relatively common and can be produced by smoking a cigarette or chewing nicotine gum (31). Skin pallor and excessive sweating may be noted.

Cardiovascular findings include hypertension and tachycardia. Constriction of the coronary arteries may occur. Delayed effects include hypotension and bradycardia. Cardiac arrest is rare. Respiratory signs include tachypnea and bronchorrhea; dyspnea and bradypnea may develop later. Death is due to respiratory failure with apnea and may occur as early as 1 hour postingestion (32).

Chronic Exposure

Green tobacco sickness is characterized by nausea and vomiting several hours after working with wet, uncured tobacco leaves (33). Chronic exposure to nicotine may be associated with dermatoses and hypercholesterolemia.

DIAGNOSTIC TESTS

The vital signs and electrocardiogram should be monitored closely in symptomatic patients. Urine cotinine levels can be used to monitor occupational exposures. Plasma nicotine levels are neither clinically useful nor readily available. Serum electrolytes, urea, creatinine, creatine phosphokinase, urinalysis, and urine myoglobin should be measured, and respiratory function should be monitored in severe cases.

Postmortem blood nicotine levels range from 11 to 63 mg/L in people who ingest 10 to 25 g of nicotine sulfate (34).

TREATMENT

The exact product and route or routes of exposure need to be identified. In suicide, other drugs should be considered because nicotine is an unusual choice. Adults who deliberately placed multiple transdermal nicotine patches on themselves were likely to have ingested other substances in suicide attempts (35).

Gastric emptying is not indicated because the patient is often vomiting already and because of the risk of rapid-onset convulsions or coma. Activated charcoal may bind nicotine, but persistent nicotine-induced emesis may preclude its use. Neither emesis nor activated charcoal is recommended for unintentional ingestion of tobacco. The role of GI decontamination for ingestion of nicotine gum or the transdermal patch is unclear.

Nicotine is lipid soluble and rapidly penetrates the skin (36,37). As soon as possible, remove contaminated clothing and wash affected areas thoroughly with mild soap and copious amounts of cold running water to reduce dermal absorption (38).

Enhancement of Elimination

Because nicotine accumulates in acidic fluids, multiple-dose activated charcoal could enhance its elimination, but there are no data to confirm this hypothesis, and its routine use is not recommended (15). The use of hemodialysis or other extracorporeal clearance techniques for the treatment of nicotine poisoning has not been reported. Urinary acidification enhances the renal clearance of nicotine (23), but there are no data assessing its effectiveness or clinical benefit.

Antidotes

The use of atropine sulfate to reduce cholinergic effects (lacrimation, bronchorrhea, diarrhea, sweating) has a sound pharmacologic basis. Despite the fact that there are no data demonstrating improved patient outcome, its use should be considered when cholinergic effects have reached clinically significant levels. The use of an antacid, H_2-blocking agent, or proton pump inhibitor is contraindicated because nicotine is better absorbed in an alkaline medium (15).

Monitoring

Monitoring should include fluid balance, cardiorespiratory function, and neuromuscular paralysis. Ongoing laboratory monitoring should include arterial blood gases, blood glucose levels, renal function tests, urinalysis, and myoglobinuria.

Supportive Care

Cardiovascular and respiratory support are crucial. Appropriate fluid balance must be maintained despite significant insensible fluid losses. Benzodiazepines should be used to treat extreme agitation, restlessness, or convulsions.

Pitfalls

A patient on lithium and nicotine transdermal patches developed nausea, diaphoresis, and tremor after smoking cigarettes and was misdiagnosed with lithium toxicity (39). Most patients exposed to nicotine have minor self-limited toxicity. Those who have more serious exposures deteriorate very quickly.

REFERENCES

1. Oil and hazardous materials technical assistance data system. U.S. Environmental Protection Agency, Washington, DC (CD-ROM version). Englewood, CO: Micromedex, Inc, 1997.
2. McGuigan HA. Pharmacology of ganglia. In: *Applied pharmacology*. St. Louis: Mosby, 1940:587–594.
3. Franke FE. *Proceedings of the society for experimental biology*. 1932;29:1177–1179.
4. Registry of Toxic Effects of Chemical Substances. National Institute for Occupational Safety and Health, Cincinnati (CD-ROM version). Denver: Micromedex, Inc, 2000.
5. Larson PS, Haag HB, Silvette H. Toxicology. In: *Tobacco. Experimental and clinical studies*. Baltimore: Williams & Wilkins, 1961:428–514.
6. Goodman LS, Gilman A. Autonomic blocking agents (continued) III. Drugs inhibiting skeletal muscles and autonomic ganglia. In: *Goodman & Gilman's the pharmacological basis of therapeutics*, 2nd ed. New York: Macmillan, 1955:596–643.
7. Malizia E, Andreucci G, Alfani F, et al. Acute intoxication with nicotine alkaloids and cannabinoids in children from ingestion of cigarettes. *Hum Toxicol* 1983;2:315–316.
8. Smolinske SC, Spoerke DG, Spiller SK, et al. Cigarette and nicotine chewing gum toxicity in children. *Hum Toxicol* 1988;7:27–31.
9. McGee D, Brabson T, McCarthy J, et al. Four-year review of cigarette ingestions in children. *Pediatr Emerg Care* 1995;11:13–16.
10. Sisselman SG, Mofenson HC, Caraccio TR. Cigarette and nicotine chewing gum toxicity in children [Letter]. *Lancet* 1996;347:200–201.
11. Woolf A, Burkhart K, Caraccio T, et al. Childhood poisoning involving transdermal nicotine patches. *Pediatrics* 1997;99:E4.

12. Busto U, Bendayan R, Sellers EM. Clinical pharmacokinetics of non-opiate abused drugs. *Clin Pharmacokinet* 1989;16:1–26.
13. Svensson CK. Clinical pharmacokinetics of nicotine. *Clin Pharmacokinet* 1987;12:30–40.
14. Lavoie FW, Harris TM. Fatal nicotine ingestion. *J Emerg Med* 1991;9:133–136.
15. Ivey KJ, Trigg EJ. Absorption of nicotine by the human stomach and its effect on gastric ion fluxes and potential difference. *Am J Dig Dis* 1978;23:809–814.
16. Benowitz NL, Jacob P 3rd, Savanapridi C. Determinants of nicotine intake while chewing nicotine polacrilex gum. *Clin Pharmacol Ther* 1987;41:467–473.
17. Nemeth-Coslett R. Physiologic effects of nicotine polacrilex. *Biomed Pharmacother* 1989;43:5–10.
18. Nyberg G, Panfilov V, Sivertsson R, et al. Cardiovascular effects of nicotine chewing gum in healthy non-smokers. *Eur J Clin Pharmacol* 1982;23:303–307.
19. Ferno O. A substitute for tobacco-smoking. *Psychopharmacologia* 1973;31:201–204.
20. Andersson G, Hansson E, Schmiterlow CG. Gastric secretion of C14-nicotine. *Experientia* 1965;15:211–213.
21. Benowitz NL, Jacob P 3rd, Jones RT, et al. Interindividual variability in the metabolism and cardiovascular effects of nicotine in man. *J Pharmacol Exper Ther* 1982;221:368–372.
22. Schievelbein H. Nicotine, resorption and fate. *Pharmacol Ther* 1982;18:233–248.
23. Rosenberg J, Benowitz NL, Jacob P 3rd, et al. Disposition kinetics and effects of intravenous nicotine. *Clin Pharmacol Ther* 1980;28:517–522.
24. Perez-Stable EJ, Herrera B, Jacob P 3rd, et al. Nicotine metabolism and intake in black and white smokers. *JAMA* 1998;280:152–156.
25. Luck W, Nau H. Exposure to the fetus, neonate, and nursed infant to nicotine and cotinine from maternal smoking [Letter]. *N Engl J Med* 1984;311:672.
26. Benowitz NL, Jacob P 3rd. Nicotine and cotinine elimination pharmacokinetics in smokers and nonsmokers. *Clin Pharmacol Ther* 1993;53:316–323.
27. Taylor P. Agents acting at the neuromuscular junction and autonomic ganglia. In: Hardman JE, Limbird LE, eds. *Goodman & Gilman's the pharmacological basis of therapeutics,* 9th ed. New York: McGraw-Hill, 1996:177–197.
28. Registry of Toxic Effects of Chemical Substances. National Institute for Occupational Safety and Health, Cincinnati, OH (CD-ROM version). Englewood, CO: Micromedex, Inc, 1997.
29. McKnight RH, Kryscio RJ, Mays JR, et al. Spatial and temporal clustering of an occupational poisoning: the example of green tobacco sickness. *Stat Med* 1996;15:747–757.
30. Arcury TA, Quandt SA, Preisser JS, et al. The incidence of green tobacco sickness among Latino farmworkers. *J Occup Environ Med* 2001;43:601–609.
31. Pereira CB, Strupp M, Eggert T, et al. Nicotine-induced nystagmus: three-dimensional analysis and dependence on head position. *Neurology* 2000;55:1563–1565.
32. Singer J, Janz T. Apnea and seizures caused by nicotine ingestion. *Pediatr Emerg Care* 1990;6:135–137.
33. McKnight RH, Levine EJ, Rodgers GC. Detection of green tobacco sickness by a regional poison center. *Vet Hum Toxicol* 1994;36:505–510.
34. Baselt RC. *Disposition of toxic drugs and chemicals in man,* 5th ed. Foster City, CA: Chemical Toxicology Institute, 2000.
35. Woolf A, Burkhart K, Caraccio T, et al. Self-poisoning among adults using multiple transdermal nicotine patches. *J Toxicol Clin Toxicol* 1996;34:691–698.
36. Benowitz NL, Lake T, Keller KH, et al. Prolonged absorption with development of tolerance to toxic effects after cutaneous exposure to nicotine. *Clin Pharmacol Ther* 1987;42:119–120.
37. Zorin S, Kuylenstierna F, Thulin H. In vitro test of nicotine's permeability through human skin. Risk evaluation and safety aspects. *Ann Occup Hyg* 1999;43:405–413.
38. Hipke ME. Green tobacco sickness. *South Med J* 1993;86:989–992.
39. Weiss RD. Nicotine toxicity misdiagnosed as lithium toxicity. *Am J Psychiatry* 1996;153:132.

SECTION

6

Products Affecting Blood Formation

CHAPTER 106

Hematopoietic Agents

Peter A. Chyka and William Banner, Jr.

Fe^{2+} ferrous sulfate structure

FERROUS SULFATE

Iron compounds:	**Iron fumarate, gluconate, sulfate, carbonyl iron (Feosol), iron-polysaccharide (Niferex), iron dextran (INFeD), iron sucrose (Venofer), sodium ferric gluconate (Ferrlecit)**
Erythroid-stimulating drugs:	**Epoetin alfa (rHuEPO, Epogen, Procrit); darbepoetin alfa (Aranesp)**
Myeloid-stimulating drugs:	**Filgrastim (Neupogen); pegfilgrastim (Neulasta); sargramostim (Leukine)**
Molecular formula and weight:	**See Table 1.**
SI conversion:	**Iron, mg/L × 17.92 = μmol/L**
CAS Registry No.:	**See Table 1.**
Normal or therapeutic levels:	**Iron, 75 to 150 μg/dl (serum)**
Target organs:	**For oral iron, gastrointestinal tract (acute), cardiovascular system (acute), liver (acute or chronic)**
Antidote:	**Deferoxamine (for iron)**

OVERVIEW

Several different drug categories with unique actions are used to treat hematopoietic insufficiency states. Iron compounds provide an exogenous source of iron when the body's demand for iron is high or the dietary intake is insufficient. Erythroid-stimulating agents, such as recombinant darbepoetin alfa and epoetin alfa, increase the production of erythrocytes when it is insufficient due to disease or drug therapy. Myeloid-stimulating agents, such as Filgrastim, pegfilgrastim, and sargramostim, increase the production of neutrophils, granulocytes, and macrophages, depending on the drug, when it is insufficient due to disease or drug therapy.

ORAL IRON PHARMACEUTICALS

Oral iron pharmaceuticals cause life-threatening poisoning after unintentional ingestion, as in preschool-aged children, and intentional overdose, as in a suicide attempt (1–3). There are numerous products available. Multivitamins have lower amounts of elemental iron. The different chemical forms of iron contain specific amounts of elemental iron. The elemental iron content of a drug is the basis for estimations of toxicity (Table 1).

Toxic Dose

The typical adult therapeutic dose for iron is 20 to 30 mg of elemental iron, which for most products is one tablet daily. The pediatric dose varies with age but is approximately 1 mg/kg of elemental daily as one or two doses.

Toxic doses of iron on acute ingestion are primarily derived from poison center–based triage guidelines (2–5). Some degree of gastrointestinal (GI) distress, such as nausea, vomiting, and diarrhea, will develop when a dose of 5 to 20 mg/kg of elemental iron is ingested. An ingestion of 60 mg/kg or more of elemental iron often causes systemic symptoms and may be life-threatening. Ingestion of iron-polysaccharide forms may be less likely to produce iron toxicity compared to other oral iron compounds (6).

TABLE 1. Physical characteristics of iron-containing pharmaceuticals

Drug	Molecular formula, molecular weight, CAS Registry No.	Content of elemental iron (%)
Oral iron formulations		
Ferrous fumarate	$C_4H_2FeO_4$, 169.9 g/mol, 141-01-5	33
Ferrous gluconate	$C_{12}H_{22}FeO_{14}$,H_2O, 12389-15-0	12
Ferrous sulfate	$FeSO_4$,$7H_2O$, 278.0 g/mol, 7782-63-0	20 (65 mg elemental iron in 325-mg tablet)
Carbonyl iron	$C_9Fe_2O_9$, 363.8 g/mol, '7439-89-6, 15321-51-4	50 mg/tablet[a]
Iron-polysaccharide	NR	50 mg/tablet, 150 mg/capsule[a]
Parenteral iron products		
Iron dextran	NR, 165 kd, 9004-66-4	50 mg/ml[a]
Iron sucrose	NR, 34–60 kd, 8047-67-4	20 mg/ml[a]
Sodium ferric gluconate	$C_{12}H_{22}FeO_{14}$,H_2O, 289–440 kd, 12389-15-0	12.5 mg/ml[a]

[a]Reflects iron content of drug products available in 2003. Verify values for current products.

Toxicokinetics and Toxicodynamics

The toxicokinetics of iron are based on pharmacokinetic studies in human volunteers and case reports of overdosage (7,8). The bioavailability of iron in therapeutic doses varies from 5% to 30%, depending on the body's need for iron. The extent to which this regulation of iron absorption is maintained with acute overdosage is unknown, but it is speculated to be overwhelmed, allowing massive absorption of iron (2,3). Iron is distributed throughout the body and is bound in the blood to several different proteins that act as transient carriers of iron (transferrin) or as storage forms of iron (hemosiderin, ferritin). The effect of protein binding on overdosage is not well characterized. Once absorbed, iron exhibits essentially a closed pharmacokinetic elimination model, with elimination occurring only through small daily losses in sweat, stool, urine, and epithelial desquamation (1 mg/day) and through blood loss (1 mg/ml). With therapeutic doses, iron undergoes redistribution into tissues, such as bone marrow, liver, and the reticuloendothelial system (RES) (9), and presumably does the same with acute overdose. A distributive serum half-life of approximately 6 hours has been observed with acute overdoses (7,8,10).

In evaluating acute overdose, there has been considerable interest in the time to achieve a peak serum iron concentration (T_{max}). As there are few case reports with serial iron determinations, information is primarily based on studies in human volunteers. The T_{max} after ingestion of a single therapeutic dose of ferrous sulfate occurs at 2 to 5 hours (11), but T_{max} for prenatal iron preparation was not reached for 5 to 6 hours (12,13). The T_{max} for crushed ferrous fumarate tablets was not reached within 6 hours, but was only 4 hours for chewed multiple vitamins with iron (in the same subjects) (14). In overdose, determination of T_{max} is further complicated by a potential delay in the absorption of iron tablets, which can sometimes be retrieved from the GI tract 8 to 16 hours after ingestion.

Pathophysiology

Iron is toxic to multiple organs and is commonly presented as having five stages of acute toxicity (2,3,5). When ingested in sufficient amounts, iron has a direct effect on mucous membranes. There is often ulceration and erosion of the stomach lining (15,16). Tablets may in fact become embedded in the wall of the stomach. Bleeding may occur into the gut lumen, and diffuse inflammation may lead to dramatic fluid losses, especially as this process continues into the small bowel. The bowel may acutely decompensate and undergo necrosis with air in the bowel wall (17–19).

After the first phase , or GI phase, a quiescent period (phase 2) may ensue during which GI symptoms abate, but iron absorption continues. Phase 3 of acute iron toxicity occurs 2 to 12 hours after ingestion and is characterized by shock and metabolic acidosis (Fig. 1). As iron is absorbed into the circulation its conversion from the 3^+ form (ferric iron) to the 2^+ form (ferrous iron) contributes a hydrogen ion to the circulation, leading to a metabolic acidosis. Studies have also pointed to the direct effects of iron on the circulation by both fluid loss (20) and direct depres-

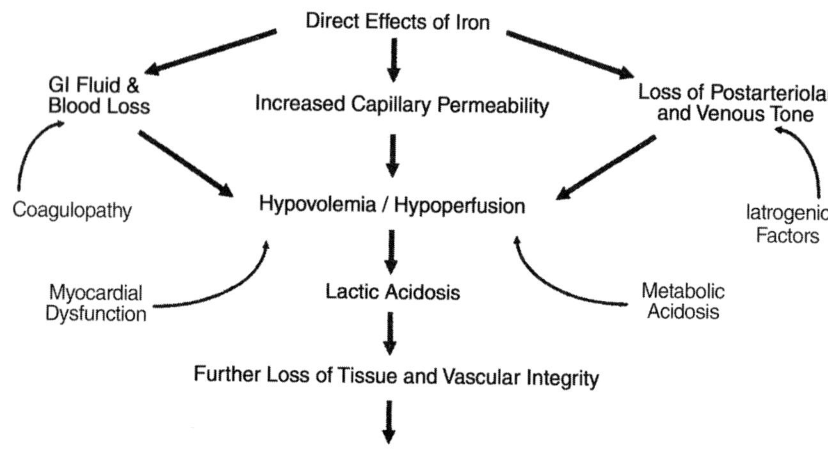

Figure 1. Pathophysiology of shock in acute iron poisoning. (From Banner W Jr, Tong TG. Iron poisoning. *Pediatr Clin North Am* 1986;33:393–409, with permission.)

sion of myocardial contractility (21). Cardiac output has been shown to deteriorate despite maintenance of adequate preload and without compensation by means of increasing heart rate (22). When taken together, all of these factors contribute to the rapid evolution of shock (Fig. 1), the systemic inflammatory response, and coagulopathy that may be the terminal event within several hours of ingestion (23,24).

Phase 4 develops on days 2 to 4. Hepatic injury may be related to the uptake of iron by the RES and in particular the Kupffer cells of the liver. The intracellular concentration of iron may reach a point of toxicity, and so the liver can become a target of iron poisoning (25,26). Apart from this isolated organ involvement, the majority of other organ toxicity seems to be related to the effects of shock rather than direct effects of iron itself.

Phase 5 follows the acute phases of iron toxicity. There may be residual scarring of the stomach causing contraction and scarring and leading to outflow tract obstruction (27). This may require surgical correction. Aggressive overgrowth of *Yersinia enterocolitica* from "feeding" with the deferoxamine/iron complex, which acts as a nutrient siderophore, may cause septicemia (28,29).

Pregnancy and Lactation

Iron is U.S. Food and Drug Administration (FDA) pregnancy category C (see Appendix I). It is clearly indicated during pregnancy and lactation for nutritional support and is routinely prescribed. Acute iron overdose during pregnancy increases the risk of stillborn births and spontaneous abortions (30). Peripartum availability and physiologic alterations may also contribute to the frequency of this overdose during pregnancy (30,31). It is this high availability during times when older siblings may be present that can permit exposure.

Clinical Presentation

In the past 50 years, most iron toxicity arose from acute ingestion. Increasing use of blood products for hematologic disorders has established chronic iron overload syndromes as a more common presentation. Recent implementation of packaging requirements has reduced the potential for iron ingestion by toddlers.

ACUTE OVERDOSAGE

The acute toxicity of iron is commonly presented as having five stages of acute toxicity (2,3,5). The first, or GI, phase involves the stomach and GI tract. There is often ulceration and erosion of the stomach lining (15,16). Tablets may become imbedded in the wall of the stomach. Many patients who ingest a toxic amount of iron vomit spontaneously, and the vomitus may contain tablet fragments, thereby limiting the dose. The clinical manifestations are initially vomiting with abdominal distention followed by bloody diarrhea that may produce immediate hypotension due to volume loss. Abdominal pain with diarrhea and bleeding suggest the severity of the ingestion and may serve as a warning of things to come. The abdomen may evolve from cramping abdominal pain to the findings of a perforated viscus requiring emergent surgical intervention. A decrease in level of consciousness is not necessarily from iron but rather from circulatory insufficiency, leading to central nervous system depression.

The second phase, or quiescent period, may ensue during which GI symptoms abate but iron absorption continues. This period is short or nonexistent in severe poisoning. This may simply be a time when the symptoms that presage overt shock are not being closely observed (2).

Phase 3 occurs 2 to 12 hours after ingestion and is characterized by shock and metabolic acidosis. Cardiac output decreases despite supportive care. Together, these factors contribute to the rapid evolution of shock, the systemic inflammatory response, and coagulopathy that may be fatal within several hours of ingestion (23,24).

Phase 4 involves the liver and develops on days 2 to 4. The clinical manifestations of liver injury are variable in onset and include the appearance of hyperbilirubinemia and biochemical markers of liver injury. In rare cases, a fatal outcome has been described with this, and transplantation has been used to manage this problem (32).

Phase 5 follows the acute phases of iron toxicity. Some patients develop strictures that create signs of obstruction such as feeding and projectile vomiting.

As is generally true in the pediatric patient, the onset of shock may not be heralded by hypotension but rather by indicators of circulatory insufficiency such as tachycardia, poor peripheral pulses, perfusion, and mild changes in mental status. Hypotension may thereby develop precipitously.

CHRONIC OVERDOSAGE

Chronic toxicity from oral ingestion is rare. Hemochromatosis developed in a 10-year-old girl who ingested 300 mg of elemental iron daily for 5 years. She exhibited elevated liver function tests, a serum iron concentration of 215 mg/dl, and an elevated serum ferritin concentration of 1190 ng/ml; she also had three-plus siderosis of hepatic parenchymal cells. Treatment included ten isovolemic phlebotomies during 4 months, with an estimated 4.5 g of iron removed. She has been in good health for the subsequent 10 years (33).

Chronic iron overload primarily occurs in the setting of hypertransfusion or hemochromatosis. In these cases, there is a primary disorder responsible for abnormalities in heme handling or excessive turnover of red blood cells causing a total body excess of iron. Chelation therapy has been used in these settings to offset iron overload using a variety of agents.

ADVERSE EVENTS

Adverse reactions during intended use of iron products are generally mild. GI discomfort is one of the most commonly reported side effects and may be avoided by timing and dilution of the iron product.

Diagnostic Tests

Serum iron concentration is an important diagnostic tool, but the relation between the serum iron concentration and clinical effects have not been established. Normal serum iron is 75 to 150 μg/dl. The existing data are affected by inconsistent or unknown sampling times and potential colorimetric assay interference with deferoxamine. In one series, serum iron concentrations obtained from 2 to 9 hours after ingestion ranged from 205 to 1500 μg/dl and were associated with cardiovascular instability in six pediatric patients, whereas the serum iron of 12 asymptomatic children ranged from 17 to 513 μg/dl. Subsets of 44 patients with only GI symptoms had concentrations in the range of 155 to 500 μg/dl, and 30 patients with central nervous system changes (with or without GI distress) were in the range of 159 to 523 μg/dl. Two of the children died and exhibited serum iron concentrations in excess of 1000 μg/dl (34). Patients with serum iron concentrations of 300 to 500 μg/dl after acute ingestion may exhibit some symptoms, and a few may exhibit serious toxicity. Patients with serum iron concentrations in excess of 500 µg/dl are likely to experience systemic toxicity, but generally recover with appropriate therapy. Generally, concentrations in excess of 1000 µg/dl are associated with life-threatening symptoms and death (2,3,35,36).

In the minimally symptomatic child, only the serum iron concentration is usually needed. In patients with a high serum iron level or signs of toxicity, testing should include complete cell blood count, serum electrolyte panel, renal function, liver enzymes, and coagulation tests.

An abdominal radiograph can demonstrate multiple densities either in the stomach or distributed throughout the GI tract (37). Typically, only full-strength iron compounds, with undissolved, hard tablet coating (e.g., ferrous sulfate) is detected in this manner. Radiography can be repeated after GI decontamination to document resolution of the densities. Endoscopy and upper GI radiographic studies may be needed in patients with signs of esophageal or gastric strictures.

Treatment

Generally, ingestion of more than 20 mg/kg of iron or the presence of symptoms (e.g., repeated vomiting) should lead to medical evaluation. At lower doses and in the absence of symptoms, close observation for at least 6 hours after ingestion is warranted.

DECONTAMINATION

Routine induction of emesis with ipecac syrup may obscure an important symptom of iron poisoning; namely, vomiting. There are no scientific data to support or refute the use of ipecac syrup, but there may be little benefit in its use for the patient who has already vomited spontaneously. The value of gastric lavage is also questionable, particularly when the small lumen size used in children limits the ability to retrieve whole tablets or tablet fragments. Activated charcoal has been shown to have variable results in adsorbing iron or reducing its absorption, but it is not routinely used due to a lack of demonstration of its value and because subsequent emesis from its use may obscure assessing the degree of toxicity. A systematic literature review of lavage and activated charcoal for iron poisoning (38,39) found few articles that provided data for evaluation, except that one report suggested a potential role for activated charcoal combined with deferoxamine (40).

Whole-bowel irrigation has been used to flush the intestine of iron tablets and thereby reduce the potential load of iron (Chapter 7) (41). These patients typically had tablets identified on abdominal radiographs before whole-bowel irrigation, and iron tablets were detected in the intestinal outflow during this therapy. Many patients also received supportive and deferoxamine therapy, which complicates the evaluation of whole-bowel irrigation. Generally, whole-bowel irrigation for the treatment of poisoning is not associated with serious adverse effects, and it may prove to be a routine therapy when iron tablets are suspected to be present in the GI tract.

ENHANCEMENT OF ELIMINATION

Multiple doses of activated charcoal appears to have a fairly limited role in elimination of iron. It does adsorb a small amount of iron, but it does not appear to significantly impact the overall amount in the stomach. In addition, the binding of deferoxamine to charcoal with subsequent binding to iron does not appear to increase the overall amounts that can be bound. Although it may be theoretically possible for activated charcoal in repeated doses to alter the kinetics of the deferoxamine/iron complex, this has not been demonstrated in either animals or patients.

Hemodialysis, exchange transfusion (42), charcoal hemoperfusion, and continuous venovenous hemoperfusion (43) have been reported experimentally and in acute iron intoxication. The iron molecule does not appear to transit membranes very effectively. It can be removed by continuous venovenous hemofiltration, however, when bound to deferoxamine. The iron-deferoxamine complex (ferrioxamine) can be removed by peritoneal dialysis, but this does not appear to offer any advantage in clearance over renal excretion, except in the patient with renal failure. The acute effects of iron on the GI tract preclude the use of this technique.

ANTIDOTE

The primary antidote for iron is deferoxamine (35,44–46). Details of the administration and adverse effects of deferoxamine are provided in Chapter 48. Although the absolute threshold for chelation is controversial, children with iron concentrations of less than 500 µg/dl should receive chelation only in the presence of other clinical manifestations of iron intoxication (34). A blood specimen should be obtained approximately 4 to 6 hours postingestion to avoid values that do not contribute to management.

Deferoxamine has significant side effects and should not be used casually (47,48). Rapid infusion of deferoxamine can produce severe hypotension and death. Early use by rapid infusion led to a restricted dose that was administered intramuscularly (IM). Subsequently, an intravenous (IV) protocol that delivers a larger total dose but at a lower rate (15 mg/kg/hour) has proven safe and reliable. At this rate, the amount of iron that is actually being bound is relatively small compared to the amount that is ingested. It is presumed, however, that the amount actually in the circulation is a relatively small fraction of the amount ingested, and thus deferoxamine is effective in improving outcome (49).

In the past, when iron overdosage was more common and the cases more severe, the appearance of "vin rose" urine was used as an indicator of iron toxicity and the efficacy of deferoxamine. The binding of iron by deferoxamine forms ferrioxamine. Ferrioxamine creates a reddish vin rose color in urine. This sign is useful only when positive. The lack of vin rose urine does not indicate that iron toxicity has not occurred. Although deferoxamine can be administered IM, this seems imprudent in a patient in shock from severe iron toxicity. Higher infusion rates may be tolerated but need to be titrated on a case-by-case basis (50,51). Iron may be bound to other compounds, some of which have been studied in acute ingestions (52). These are also useful in the setting of chronic iron overload associated with some chronic hematologic disorders (53).

SUPPORTIVE CARE

The seriously ill patient requires cardiovascular support and chelation therapy to avoid significant residual effects of iron. The most demanding situation involves iron concentrations in excess of 1000 µg/dl when more heroic efforts may be considered. There are no prospective data on which to compare exchange transfusion, acute dialysis, and continuous venovenous hemofiltration, but all modalities have been suggested for improving the clearance of iron, especially when renal insufficiency is evolving. Whether these actually alter outcome is not clear. There exist case reports of survival with iron concentrations of more than 5000 µg/dl, but deaths have occurred with much lower concentrations (3,34). Obviously, there is a poor correlation between serum iron measurements and the total body manifestations of iron intoxication.

Hypotension should be treated with an IV bolus of isotonic crystalloid (10 to 20 ml/kg normal saline) and correction of acidosis and electrolyte abnormalities (Chapter 37). Large volumes of crystalloid may be needed. An animal model study demonstrated that despite adequate hydration, loss of cardiac output still contributes to circulatory insufficiency, suggesting that vasopressor catecholamines are warranted early to induce an increase in resistance and preserve perfusion (22).

MONITORING

In suspected intoxication, efforts at monitoring the patient during the supposed period of stability should include adequacy of hydration, including urine output, capillary refill, mental status, and serial assessment of acid-base balance to assess the onset of metabolic acidosis. Current pediatric practice recognizes the evolution of shock well before overt hypotension has occurred. Tachycardia, increased capillary refill time, depressed level of consciousness, and tachypnea may all precede the more terminal manifestations of shock and should be closely monitored. Hyperglycemia, leukocytosis, and acidosis were once thought to be prognostic indicators of clinically significant iron poisoning. These indicators have fallen from use as more recent studies have questioned their validity (34,54,55).

The serum iron concentration would be the most appropriate laboratory value to follow in conjunction with therapy. The total iron binding capacity has been demonstrated to be erroneously elevated in the presence of toxic amounts of iron (56).

The most typical scenario of iron intoxication is that of a young child taking a multivitamin with iron or with prenatal vitamin ingestion. Over time, an extremely conservative approach has been taken to these patients using a general guideline of 20 mg/kg of elemental iron acutely ingested as the lower threshold dose of concern to initiate treatment. The reality is that the vast majority of patients ingesting less than 60 mg/kg of elemental iron have no discernible symptoms (2). This wide range of potential toxicity may result in some patients being overtreated. The majority of these patients require observation for the onset of more severe symptoms after basic decontamination has been undertaken.

MANAGEMENT PITFALLS

The literature on iron intoxication is full of innovative therapies that have proven to be more deadly than iron intoxication itself. The use of phosphate solutions for lavage is one such example (57). The failure to recognize the severity of an iron intoxication is probably the single most significant contributor to poor outcome. In particular, the period of relative stability that actually reflects the onset of shock may go unrecognized.

PARENTERAL IRON PHARMACEUTICALS

Iron dextran (DexFerrum, INFeD) is indicated for the treatment of iron deficiency anemia when oral iron therapy is unsatisfactory or impossible; whereas, iron sucrose (Venofer) and sodium ferric gluconate (Ferrlecit) are primarily indicated for the treatment of iron deficiency anemia in patients undergoing hemodialysis and receiving erythropoietin (57a,58). In the United States, iron dextran has been available since 1974, and the other products were approved in the late 1990s; however, these latter products have been used for several years in other countries. All products are administered by IV infusion, with the INFeD brand of iron dextran also administered by deep IM injection.

Iron dextran is a complex of ferric hydroxide and partially hydrolyzed low-molecular-weight dextran with a molecular weight (MW) of 165 kd. Iron sucrose is a complex of polynuclear ferric hydroxide and sucrose with an MW of approximately 34 to 64 kd. Sodium ferric gluconate contains ferric oxide hydrate that is bound to sucrose and chelated with gluconate with an MW of 350 kd. Iron content of these parenteral iron products varies (Table 1).

Toxic Dose

The adult therapeutic dose for parenteral iron is 100 to 125 mg of elemental iron at intervals of one to three times weekly, depending on the specific product. Evidence-based guidelines for the treatment of anemia of chronic renal failure address usage and dosage of these agents (58). The manufacturer's recommended maximum rates of IV administration to avoid hypotension for these agents is 1 ml/minute for iron dextran injection, 1 ml/minute for injection or 100 mg in 100 ml over 15 minutes as an infusion for iron sucrose, and 125 mg in 100 ml over 1 hour as an infusion of sodium ferric gluconate. Severe reactions with iron dextran are typically associated with single doses in excess of 500 mg of elemental iron.

A 9-year-old child developed no signs of toxicity after receiving 1300 mg of IV elemental iron over 48 hours. The problem was detected 8 hours after the infusion, and the serum iron was 1830 µg/dl. The serum iron concentration declined to normal values in 3 days (59). A 4-year-old girl received IV iron dextran, 2000 mg. Despite aggressive treatment, she died of sepsis after 9 days.

Toxicokinetics and Toxicodynamics

The kinetic characteristics of parenteral iron products are complex. The iron complex is distributed in the vascular space, it is taken up by the RES, iron is dissociated, then it is transported by transferrin in the bloodstream, and finally undergoes similar kinetic patterns of oral iron preparations (57a,60). After injection of iron dextran IM, 60% of the dose is absorbed within 3 days, and 90% is absorbed in 1 to 3 weeks. Once absorbed, iron dextran appears to be taken up by the RES at a rate of 10 to 20 mg/hour. After IV injection, the serum half-life of distribution has been reported as 6 hours and up to 87 hours. The kinetic variables for the other two agents are less developed, but the general sequence would also apply.

Pathophysiology

All three drugs are taken up by the RES, where iron is dissociated and released into the systemic circulation via transferrin (57a). IM injection of INFeD (iron dextran) is absorbed by the lymphatic system in a biphasic manner that may take several weeks for full absorption and to be taken up by the RES. Toxicity due to parenteral iron overdose is rare and may be related to the absence of direct GI contact and subsequent injury, or to the much slower rate of iron introduction into the systemic circulation (60).

Pregnancy and Lactation

Iron dextran is FDA pregnancy category C (Appendix I) due to teratogenic and embryocidal effects noted in animals. It can cross the placenta. Iron sucrose and sodium ferric gluconate are pregnancy category B. For all three drugs, human data are inadequate; use is generally not recommended during the first trimester of pregnancy. Iron dextran appears in breast milk, but problems have not been reported in humans (57).

Clinical Presentation

ACUTE OVERDOSAGE

Only case reports and abstracts form the basis of experience with acute overdosage of parenteral iron products. A 4-year-old girl with biliary atresia was given IV iron dextran, 2000 mg.

After a 12- to 24-hour delay, she developed arthralgias, vomiting, metabolic acidosis, bradycardia, and depressed level of consciousness. The serum iron concentration was 54,500 μg/dl, which represented all iron present in the serum, including the iron dextran. She was treated with deferoxamine, hemodialysis, and plasmapheresis, which led to improvement, but she died 9 days later due to sepsis. Objective measures of the effectiveness of the therapies were not reported (61).

The case of a 39-year-old woman with a learning disability who had received an appropriate dose of iron dextran demonstrates the problem in assessment. She complained of nausea, vomiting, headache, lethargy, lightheadedness, and abdominal cramps, which she attributed to receiving "too much iron." Approximately 6 hours after dosing, deferoxamine was given, and the serum iron concentration was 1404 μg/dl. Therapy was stopped when it was recognized shortly thereafter that she had received an appropriate therapeutic dose and was experiencing typical adverse effects. The authors proposed that iron dextran falsely elevates serum iron concentrations and can thereby lead to more aggressive therapy than is warranted (62).

ADVERSE EVENTS

Adverse effects during the therapeutic use of parenteral iron drugs occurs in one-third of patients (57a,60,63–66). Anaphylactic reactions (e.g., shock, coma, dyspnea, and seizures) are more frequently associated with iron dextran (0.7% of patients) and may reflect greater usage or sensitivity to dextran, but hypersensitivity reactions can also occur with the other products (66). A test dose is strongly recommended for all products before use, except that it is an option for iron sucrose. There is little evidence for cross reactivity among the products if a hypersensitivity reaction occurs with one agent (57a).

Other reactions also occur. Hypotension is a common adverse effect that may be related to the rate of infusion or total dose of iron (63). Other symptoms include myalgia, headache, nausea, vomiting, metallic taste, and abdominal pain (60). Iron dextran has been associated with a delayed reaction of fever, arthralgia, myalgia, headache, and lymphadenopathy that starts 4 to 48 hours after administration and may last for 3 to 7 days (67). Local reactions vary among the three drugs, but discomfort at the injection site and phlebitis are possible. Because patients have serious underlying illness and usually receive multiple medications, it is difficult to distinguish adverse effects that result from use of these drugs exclusively.

Treatment

Experience with the treatment of overdosage of parenteral iron drugs is limited.

DECONTAMINATION

GI decontamination should not be appropriate, because all reported cases involved iatrogenic overdose of parenteral iron products by injection. It is unknown whether iron is absorbed from the GI tract in the unusual event that these agents are ingested.

ENHANCEMENT OF ELIMINATION

Iron dextran is not appreciably removed by hemodialysis. There is less evidence for the effect of dialysis on iron sucrose and sodium ferric gluconate, but the large MW of these drugs would tend to make hemodialysis unsuccessful.

ANTIDOTES

It is not clear whether deferoxamine chelates iron, which is still bound to the dextran, sucrose, or gluconate, or whether chelation occurs as iron is released from the RES. In the absence of clear guidelines, deferoxamine should be considered when symptoms of serious iron poisoning (e.g., acidosis, shock, and coma) become evident several hours after injection, and the symptoms are not those related to the more immediate anaphylactic reaction (Chapter 48).

SUPPORTIVE CARE

Anaphylactic reactions are treated in the usual manner (Chapter 34). Hypotension should be treated with an IV bolus of isotonic crystalloid (10 to 20 ml/kg normal saline) and correction of acidosis and electrolyte abnormalities (Chapter 37). Other symptoms, such as myalgia and headache, typically respond to simple analgesics.

MONITORING

It would seem prudent to monitor patients with overdoses of parenteral iron products in a manner similar to that for overdosage of oral iron pharmaceuticals. The signs and symptoms of toxicity are the sole reliable means to assess toxicity. The administration of these agents may cause serum iron concentrations to rise to levels typically associated with life-threatening symptoms after the ingestion of iron, but few, if any, serious symptoms of acute iron poisoning may develop with the parenteral administration of iron (67). This phenomenon requires further study.

ERYTHROID-STIMULATING DRUGS

Biosynthetic forms of erythropoietin mimic the endogenous glycoprotein hormone to stimulate the production of erythrocytes. Two recombinant forms are currently available as epoetin alfa [EPO, rHuEPO, Epogen, Procrit; MW, 30 kd; CAS number, 113427-24-0) and darbepoetin alfa (Aranesp; MW, 30 to 37 kd). Darbepoetin alfa is similar to epoetin alfa except for the addition of two oligosaccharide chains that impart a longer half-life and biologic activity. None of these agents have an appreciable effect on levels of other formed blood elements. In general, these drugs are used to reduce allogeneic blood transfusion requirements or for autologous blood donation in patients before undergoing elective surgery and to treat anemia associated with chronic renal failure, acquired immunodeficiency syndrome (AIDS), cancer, and other chronic diseases.

Virtually all patients receiving erythroid-stimulating drugs also require supplemental iron therapy, typically parenteral iron, due to increased demand for iron incorporation into hemoglobin when red blood cell production is increased (68,69). These drugs have also been misused to enhance athletic performance, particularly for participants in high-aerobic demand, endurance-type events such as bicycling, marathon running, and cross-country skiing (70,71). Because of increased erythrocyte count and resultant oxygen-carrying capacity of the blood after misuse of these drugs, the ergogenic effects are expected to be similar to erythrocyte transfusion or "blood doping." Due to an illicit demand and the high cost of these drugs, there is an underground market of stolen, or counterfeit erythropoietin products.

Toxic Dose

The adult therapeutic dose of erythroid-stimulating drugs can be guided by evidence-based guidelines for the treatment of anemia of chronic renal failure (58). A typical dose of epoetin alfa is 50 to 300 U/kg three times a week by the IV or subcutaneous (SC) routes. The initial dose of darbepoetin alfa is 0.45–

2.25 μg/kg IV or SC, depending on the underlying cause of the anemia, followed by smaller weekly doses. Doses are modified at monthly intervals to maintain an acceptable hemoglobin level without exceeding a hemoglobin of 12 g/dl or an increase in hemoglobin of greater than 1 g/dl in 2 weeks.

The maximum dosage of these agents has not been determined. In patients with end-stage renal disease, no direct toxicity was detected with doses of 1500 U/kg three times weekly for 3 to 4 weeks (68,69). Doses of up to 8 μg/kg weekly and 15 μg/kg every 3 weeks have been administered to cancer patients for up to 12 to 16 weeks.

Toxicokinetics and Toxicodynamics

A dose-dependent increase in hemoglobin is typically observed within 2 to 6 weeks of administration of erythroid-stimulating drugs. Doses of 500 μg/kg epoetin alfa increased the hematocrit from 18% to 31% within 4 weeks of therapy (72). The response varies with underlying illness, iron stores, and dose.

The T_{max} occurs 8 to 24 hours after SC administration of epoetin alfa and darbepoetin. The drugs are rapidly distributed throughout the plasma compartment. The half-life of epoetin alfa ranges from 4 to 16 hours and that of darbepoetin is typically 21 to 89 hours. The majority of both drugs undergo hepatic metabolism, with less than 10% of the drugs excreted unchanged in the urine (68,73).

Pathophysiology

The pathophysiology of toxicity from epoetin alfa and darbepoetin alfa is primarily based on the relatively abrupt and supraphysiologic increase in the level of erythrocytes (71,73). As the hematocrit exceeds the normal range, the relative oxygen transport capacity of the blood decreases due to increasing blood viscosity. The target hemoglobin concentration for therapeutic indications should not exceed 12 g/dl. In clinical trials, an increase in hemoglobin greater than approximately 1 g/dl in 2 weeks was associated with a higher frequency of cardiac arrest, seizures, strokes, exacerbations of hypertension, chronic heart failure, acute myocardial infarction, and fluid overload and edema (69,71,74).

Pregnancy and Lactation

Epoetin alfa and darbepoetin alfa are both FDA pregnancy category C (Appendix I). Entry into breast milk is unknown (68).

Clinical Presentation

CHRONIC OVERDOSAGE

No overdose effects are expected from a single overdose, because the effects of erythroid-stimulating drugs require multiple injections over time. In contrast, repeated overdosage can lead to serious effects, which are typically an extension of the therapeutic action. Two case reports form the basis for evaluation. A 62-year-old man self-administered unknown amounts of epoetin alfa with daily injections for several weeks. He exhibited markedly labored breathing, cyanosis, diaphoresis, rales and rhonchi, hypotension, tachycardia, and acidosis. The patient was intubated and placed on a ventilator and given antibiotics and vasopressors. On admission, his hemoglobin was 23.4 g/dl, his hematocrit was 70.4%, and his leukocytes were 12,000 cells/mm^3. He was treated with serial phlebotomy and IV hydration to achieve a hematocrit of 48%. His hospitalization was complicated by several episodes of angina, hypertension, and barotrauma-related pneumothorax (75).

The other case report involved a 42-year-old with AIDS and Kaposi's sarcoma with abdominal pain and pain and swelling of his feet. Due to confusion, he had self-administered epoetin alfa 10,000 U/day for several weeks instead of 20,000 U/week. His physical examination was normal except for confusion and blackened skin at the tips of his toes bilaterally with decreased pulses and pitting edema. His hemoglobin was 22.3 g/dl, and the hematocrit was 77.1%. A repeat hemoglobin was 21.3 g/dl, and hematocrit was 72.3%. He was treated with IV fluid and emergent erythropheresis through a peripheral 18-gauge catheter that reduced his hematocrit to 50%. During hospitalization, he received phlebotomy and erythropheresis to maintain his hemoglobin below 55%. He recovered without complications (76).

ADVERSE EVENTS

It is difficult to identify the adverse effects of erythroid-stimulating drugs because patients typically have serious underlying chronic illness and receive multiple medications. Adverse effects have included bone pain, myalgia, and fever. Other mild adverse effects include headache, conjunctivitis, nausea, vomiting, and diarrhea (68). Hypertension is observed in 3% to 30% of patients (77). It is typically observed in patients with end-stage renal disease and is associated with a rapid rise in hematocrit that is quicker and larger than expected (58,71). Thrombotic events have included renal and temporal vein thrombosis, and cardiovascular effects have included transient ischemic attacks, stroke, and myocardial infarction (58). The cardiovascular and thrombotic effects have been observed primarily in patients with end-stage renal disease. Seizures, visual disturbances, headache, and hypertensive encephalopathy have been associated with epoetin alfa administration (68). Local reactions, such as redness and pain at the injection site, can occur after SC administration of either drug.

Diagnostic Tests

The complete blood cell count should be measured serially for several weeks after exposure to erythroid-stimulating drugs. The risk of cardiovascular adverse effects is greater when the hemoglobin increases beyond 12 g/dl, and several studies suggest that levels should be maintained below 14 g/dl (58,74). Others suggest that the goal of treating overdoses of epoetin alfa is to reduce the hematocrit to below 45% (76).

Exogenous forms of erythropoietin cannot be readily differentiated from the endogenous hormone, making the detection of abuse difficult through analytic means. The International Olympic Committee for the 2002 Winter Games adopted an integrated approach of measuring recombinant epoetin concentrations in the serum and urine via isoelectric patterning and correlating the results with markers of enhanced erythropoiesis such as hematocrit, serum epoetin, macrocytic erythrocytes, and serum transferrin (70).

Treatment

Supportive care and monitoring for the clinical effects of increased blood viscosity and clotting form the basis of management of overexposure to erythroid-stimulating drugs.

DECONTAMINATION

Because erythroid-stimulating drugs are not appreciably active when ingested, gastric decontamination would not be warranted for the patient who ingests these drugs.

ENHANCEMENT OF ELIMINATION

Neither of the erythroid-stimulating drugs is amenable to removal by hemodialysis, owing in part to their large MWs.

ANTIDOTE

There is no antidote for erythropoietin toxicity.

SUPPORTIVE CARE

Adequate hydration and urine output should be assured in overexposure to erythroid-stimulating drugs. Phlebotomy and electropheresis (76) have been used for symptomatic overdoses for epoetin alfa and would appear appropriate for darbepoetin alfa.

MYELOID-STIMULATING DRUGS

Endogenous colony-stimulating growth factors on hematopoietic cells are recombinant forms of endogenous hormone-like glycoproteins (cytokines) that act on specific cell surface receptors to stimulate and differentiate myeloid progenitor cells and end-cell functional activation (78). Filgrastim [granulocyte colony-stimulating factor (CSF), recombinant granulocyte CSF (Neupogen); MW, 18.8 kd] and pegfilgrastim [recombinant granulocyte CSF covalently conjugated with monomethoxypolyethylene glycol (Neulasta); MW, 19 kd] share the same mechanism of action, which is primarily to increase neutrophil granulocytes. Sargramostim [granulocyte-macrophage CSF, recombinant granulocyte-macrophage CSF (Leukine); MW, 15.5, 16.8, and 19.5 kd; CAS Registry No., 123774-72-1] acts on less mature progenitor cells and promotes formation of granulocyte and macrophage colonies to increase concentrations of neutrophils, eosinophils, and monocytes. None of these agents have an appreciable effect on levels of erythrocytes or platelets. In general, these agents are used to treat severe neutropenia associated with fever due to cancer chemotherapy, acceleration of myeloid recovery after autologous or allogeneic bone marrow or stem cell transplantation, and neutropenia associated with AIDS complications and antiretroviral therapy. The limited availability and high cost of myeloid-stimulating drugs has led to thefts of filgrastim from pharmacies (79).

Toxic Dose

The adult and pediatric therapeutic doses of myeloid-stimulating drugs are available as evidence-based guidelines (80). A typical dose of filgrastim is 5 to 10 μg/kg/day IV or SC. The dose of pegfilgrastim is 6 mg SC once per chemotherapy cycle for patients who weigh more than 45 kg. The dose of sargramostim is 250 $\mu g/m^2$ IV over 2 hours.

Filgrastim has been administered up to 115 to 138 μg/kg daily without serious toxic effects. Pegfilgrastim in single doses of 300 μg/kg has produced leukocytosis, with a mean maximum white blood cell count of $67 \times 10^9/L$ and a peak value of $120 \times 10^9/L$ without serious adverse effects. Sargramostim has been given at dosages 16 times the recommended dose for 7 to 18 days without serious toxic effects (79,81).

Toxicokinetics and Toxicodynamics

Within an hour of administration of myeloid-stimulating drugs, circulating neutrophils, monocytes, and eosinophils decrease and rebound to baseline or beyond baseline within 2 to 4 hours. The initial peak effect of filgrastim is 24 hours, and sargramostim achieves an initial plateau in leukocyte count after 3 to 7 days. The peak effect varies with underlying illness and dose (78).

After SC administration, the agents are detected in the serum within 5 minutes, and T_{max} is 2 to 8 hours. The clearance of these agents is dependent on the number of neutrophils; with low counts, the clearance is increased. The elimination half-life of filgrastim is approximately 3.5 hours and that of pegfilgrastim is 15 to 80 hours. The half-life of sargramostim ranges from 1 to 3 hours (82,83).

Pathophysiology

Myeloid-stimulating drugs stimulate the normal production and developmental process for myeloid cells. In addition to regulating proliferation and release of cells, they also modulate the activities of mature cells. Filgrastim specifically promotes proliferation and maturation of neutrophil granulocytes. In contrast, pegfilgrastim stimulates all granulocytes, affecting neutrophil granulocytes, eosinophilic granulocytes, macrophages, and megakaryocytes. Pegfilgrastim also stimulates the proliferation and activation of monocyte-macrophages and induces these cells to produce cytokines, including tumor necrosis factor and interleukin-1. Filgrastim does not have this effect. Another action of filgrastim is to act with interleukin-3 to support other cell lines, such as megakaryocytes and platelets.

Pregnancy and Lactation

All myeloid-stimulating drugs are FDA pregnancy category C (Appendix I). It is not known whether these agents appear in breast milk; problems have not been reported in humans.

Clinical Presentation

There is little information on the toxic effects of myeloid-stimulating drugs on single or multiple overdose. A single dose of pegfilgrastim has produced leukocytosis, with a mean maximum white blood cell count of $67 \times 10^9/L$ and the highest value of $120 \times 10^9/L$ without serious adverse effects. The leukocytosis lasted for 6 to 13 days.

It is difficult to identify the adverse effects of these drugs because patients typically have serious underlying illness and receive multiple medications. Adverse effects from all three agents have included bone pain, myalgia, fever, skin rashes, pruritus, and redness and pain at the injection site. Rarely, sargramostim may produce a first-dose reaction characterized by flushing, hypotension, syncope, and weakness. High daily doses of sargramostim (32 μg/kg) has also been rarely associated with a capillary leak syndrome of fluid retention, peripheral edema, and pleural or pericardial effusions (78).

Diagnostic Tests

Transient elevations of alkaline phosphatase, lactic dehydrogenase, and uric acid typically occur as a physiologic response to the rise in neutrophil count.

Treatment

Because serious toxicity after overdosage of myeloid-stimulating drugs has yet to be reported, therapy for unintentional, suicidal, or iatrogenic overdose includes supportive and symptomatic care, with monitoring of the patient's condition and white blood cell count for 1 to 2 weeks. Gastric decontamination would not be warranted in the rare instance of ingestion.

Adequate hydration and urine output should be assured. These agents are not amenable to removal by hemodialysis owing in part to their large MWs. The manufacturer lists leukapheresis as a treatment option for symptomatic overdoses of filgrastim and pegfilgrastim, but the use of such therapy has not been reported to date in the literature (81).

REFERENCES

1. Morris CC. Pediatric iron poisonings in the United States. *South Med J* 2000;93:352–358.
2. Banner W, Tong TG. Iron poisoning. *Pediatr Clin North Am* 1986;33:393–409.
3. Fine JS. Iron poisoning. *Curr Probl Pediatr* 2000;30(3):71–90.
4. Klein-Schwartz W, Oderda GM, Gorman RL, et al. Assessment of management guidelines: acute iron ingestion. *Clin Pediatr* 1990;29:316–321.
5. Mills KC, Curry SC. Acute iron poisoning. *Emerg Med Clin North Am* 1994;12:397–413.
6. Klein-Schwartz W. Toxicity of polysaccharide—iron complex exposures reported to poison control centers. *Ann Pharmacother* 2000;34:165–169.
7. Barr DGD, Fraser DKB. Acute iron poisoning in children: role of chelating agents. *BMJ* 1968;1:737–741.
8. Chyka PA, Butler AY. Assessment of acute iron poisoning by laboratory and clinical observations. *Am J Emerg Med* 1993;11:99–103.
9. Ricketts C, Cavill I. Ferrokinetics: methods and interpretation. *Clin Nuclear Med* 1978;3:159–164.
10. Leikin S, Vossough MD, Mochir-Fatemi F. Chelation therapy in acute iron poisoning. *J Pediatr* 1967;71:425–430.
11. Dietzfelbinger H. Bioavailability of bi- and trivalent oral iron preparations. Investigations of iron absorption by postabsorption serum iron concentration curves. *Arnzneimettel-Forshung* 1987;37:107–112.
12. Biswas MK, Pernoll MJ, Mabie WC. A placebo-controlled comparative trial of various prenatal vitamin preparations in pregnant women. *Clin Ther* 1984;6:763–769.
13. Babior BM, Peters WA, Briden PM, Cetrulo CL. Pregnant women's absorption of iron from prenatal supplements. *J Reproductive Med* 1985;30:355–357.
14. Linakis JG, Lacouture PG, Woolf A. Iron absorption from chewable vitamins with iron versus iron tablets: implications for toxicity. *Pediatr Emerg Care* 1992;8:321–324.
15. Foxford R, Goldfrank L. Gastrotomy—a surgical approach to iron overdose. *Ann Emerg Med* 1985;14:1223–1126.
16. Pestaner JP, Ishak KG, Mullick FG, Centeno JA. Ferrous sulfate toxicity: a review of autopsy findings. *Biolog Trace Element Res* 1999;69:191–198.
17. Hosking CS. The small intestine in experimental acute iron poisoning. *Br J Exp Pathol* 1971;52:7–13.
18. Nayfield SG, Kent TH, Rodman NF. Gastrointestinal effects of acute ferrous sulfate poisoning in rats. *Arch Pathol Lab Med* 1976;100:325–328.
19. Smith WL, Franken EA, Grosfeld JL, et al. Pneumatosis of the bowel secondary to acute iron poisoning. Radiological quiz. *Radiology* 1977;122:192, 246.
20. Whitten CF, Chen YC, Gibson GW. Studies in acute iron poisoning. 3. The hemodynamic alterations in acute experimental iron poisoning. *Pediatr Res* 1968;2:479–485.
21. Artman M, Olson RD, Boucek RJ, et al. Acute effects of iron on contractile function in isolated rabbit myocardium. *Dev Pharmacol Ther* 1984;7:50–60.
22. Vernon DD, Banner W, Dean JM. Hemodynamic effects of experimental iron poisoning. *Ann Emerg Med* 1989;18:863–866.
23. Whitten CF, Brough AJ. The pathophysiology of acute iron poisoning. *Clin Toxicol* 1971;4:585–595.
24. Tenenbein M, Israels SJ. Early coagulopathy in severe iron poisoning. *J Pediatr* 1988;113:695–697.
25. Tenenbein M. Hepatotoxicity in acute iron poisoning. *J Toxicol Clin Toxicol* 2001;39:721–726.
26. de Castro FJ, Jaeger R, Gleason WA. Liver damage and hypoglycemia in acute iron poisoning. *Clin Toxicol* 1977;10:287–289.
27. Tenenbein M, Littman C, Stimpson RE. Gastrointestinal pathology in adult iron overdoses. *J Toxicol Clin Toxicol* 1990;28:311–320.
28. Hadjiminas JM. Yersiniosis in acutely iron-loaded children treated with desferrioxamine. *J Antimicrob Chemother* 1988;21:680–681.
29. Mofenson HC, Caraccio TR, Sharieff N. Iron sepsis: *Yersinia enterocolitica* septicemia possibly caused by an overdose of iron. *N Engl J Med* 1987;316:1092–1093.
30. Tran T, Wax JR, Philput C, et al. Intentional iron overdose in pregnancy—management and outcome. *J Emerg Med* 2000;18:225–228.
31. Lacoste H, Goyert GL, Goldman LS, Wright DJ, Schwartz DB. Acute iron intoxication in pregnancy: case report and review of the literature. *Obstet Gynecol* 1992;80(3 Pt 2):500–501.
32. Kozaki K, Egawa H, Garcia-Kennedy R, et al. Hepatic failure due to massive iron ingestion successfully treated with liver transplantation. *Clin Transplant* 1995;9:85–87.
33. Pearson HA, Ehrenkranz RA, Rinder HM, Riely CA. Hemosiderosis in a normal child secondary to oral iron medication. *Pediatrics* 2000;105:429–431.
34. Chyka PA, Butler AY, Holley JE. Serum iron concentrations and symptoms of acute iron poisoning in children. *Pharmacotherapy* 1996;16:1053–1058.
35. Westlin WF. Deferoxamine in the treatment of acute iron poisoning: clinical experience with 172 children. *Clin Pediatr* 1966;5:531–535.
36. McEnery JT. Hospital management of acute iron ingestion. *Clin Toxicol* 1971;4:603–613.
37. Everson GW, Oukjhane K, Young LW, et al. Effectiveness of abdominal radiographs in visualizing chewable iron supplements following overdose. *Am J Emerg Med* 1989;7:459–463.
38. Jones S. Activated charcoal and gastric absorption in iron compounds. *Emerg Med J* 2002;19:49.
39. Teece S. Gastric lavage and iron overdose. *Emerg Med J* 2002;19:251–252.
40. Gomez HF, McClafferty HH, Flory D, et al. Prevention of gastrointestinal iron absorption by chelation from an orally administered premixed deferoxamine/charcoal slurry. *Ann Emerg Med* 1997;30:587–592.
41. Tenenbein M. Whole bowel irrigation in iron poisoning. *J Pediatr* 1987;111:142–145.
42. Movassaghi N, Purugganan GG, Leikin S. Comparison of exchange transfusion and deferoxamine in the treatment of acute iron poisoning. *J Pediatr* 1969;75:604–608.
43. Banner W Jr, Vernon DD, Ward RM, Sweeley JC, Dean JM. Continuous arteriovenous hemofiltration in experimental iron intoxication. *Crit Care Med* 1989;17:1187–1190.
44. Whitten CF, Gibson GW, Good MH, et al. Studies in acute iron poisoning. I. Desferrioxamine in the treatment of acute iron poisoning: clinical observations, experimental studies, and theoretical considerations. *Pediatrics* 1965;36:322–335.
45. Whitten CF, Chen YC, Gibson GW. Studies in acute iron poisoning. II. Further observations on desferrioxamine in the treatment of acute experimental iron poisoning. *Pediatrics* 1966;38:102–110.
46. Tenenbein M. Benefits of parenteral deferoxamine for acute iron poisoning. *J Toxicol Clin Toxicol* 1996;34:485–489.
47. Howland MA. Risks of parenteral deferoxamine for acute iron poisoning. *J Toxicol Clin Toxicol* 1996;34:491–497.
48. Koren G, Bentur Y, Strong D, et al. Acute changes in renal function associated with deferoxamine therapy. *Am J Dis Child* 1989;143:1077–1080.
49. Cheney K, Gumbiner C, Benson B, et al. Survival after a severe iron poisoning treated with intermittent infusions of deferoxamine. *J Toxicol Clin Toxicol* 1995;33:61–66.
50. Peck M, Rogers J, Riverbach J. Use of high doses of deferoxamine (Desferal) in an adult patient with acute iron overdosage. *J Toxicol Clin Toxicol* 1982;19:865–869.
51. Shannon M. Desferrioxamine in acute iron poisoning (letter). *Lancet* 1992;339:1601.
52. Berkovitch M, Livne A, Lushkov G, et al. The efficacy of oral deferiprone in acute iron poisoning. *Am J Emerg Med* 2000;18:36–40.
53. Bergeron RJ, Wiegand J, Brittenham GM. HBED ligand: preclinical studies of a potential alternative to deferoxamine for treatment of chronic iron overload and acute iron poisoning. *Blood* 2002;99:3019–3026.
54. James JA. Acute iron poisoning: assessment of severity and prognosis. *J Pediatr* 1970;77:117–119.
55. Palatnick W, Tenenbein M. Leukocytosis, hyperglycemia, vomiting, and positive x-rays are not indicators of severity of iron overdose in adults. *Am J Emerg Med* 1996;14:454–455.
56. Tenenbein M, Yatscoff RW. The total iron-binding capacity in iron poisoning: is it useful? *Am J Dis Child* 1991;145:437–439.
57. Geffner ME, Opas LM. Phosphate poisoning complicating treatment for iron ingestion. *Am J Dis Child* 1980;134:509–510.

57a. McEvoy GK. Iron preparations. In: McEvoy GK, ed. *AHFS drug information*. Bethesda, MD: American Society of Health-System Pharmacists, 2002:1394–1410.

58. National Kidney Foundation. K/DOQI clinical practice guidelines for anemia of chronic kidney disease, 2000. *Am J Kidney Dis* 2001;37[Suppl 1]:S182–S238. Available at: http://www.kidney.org/professionals/doqi/guidelines/an (accessed April 21, 2003).
59. Rodgers G, Matyunas N, Ross M. Lack of toxicity following a large inadvertent overdose of iron-dextran: a case report (abstract). *J Toxicol Clin Toxicol* 1995;33:515–516.
60. Besarab A, Frinak S, Yee J. An indistinct balance: the safety and efficacy of parenteral iron therapy. *J Am Soc Nephrol* 1999;10:2029–2043.
61. Douidar SM, Snodgrass WR. Fatal iron-dextran poisoning: a combined iron toxicity and dextran-induced immune block (abstract). *Vet Hum Toxicol* 1989;31:342.
62. Harchelroad F, Rice S. Iron dextran: treatment or overdose? (abstract). *Vet Hum Toxicol* 1992;34:329.
63. Fletes R, Lazarus JM, Gage J, et al. Suspected iron dextran-related adverse drug events in hemodialysis patients. *Am J Kidney Dis* 2001;37:743–749.
64. Charytan C, Levin N, Al-Saloum M, et al. Efficacy and safety of iron sucrose for iron deficiency in patients with dialysis-associated anemia: North American clinical trial. *Am J Kidney Dis* 2001;37(2):300–307.
65. Van Wyck DB, Cavallo G, Spinowitz BS, et al. Safety and efficacy of iron sucrose in patients sensitive to iron dextran: North American clinical trial. *Am J Kidney Dis* 2000;36(1):88–97.
66. Burns DL, Pomposelli JJ. Toxicity of parenteral iron dextran therapy. *Kidney Int* 1999;55[Suppl 69]:S:119–124.
67. Choulis NH, Dukes MNG. Metals. In: Dukes MNG, Aronson JK, eds. *Meyler's side effects of drugs*, 14th ed. Amsterdam: Elsevier, 2000:683–713.
68. McEvoy GK. Hematopoietic agents. In: McEvoy GK, ed. *AHFS drug information*. Bethesda, MD: American Society of Health-System Pharmacists, 2002:1488–1520.
69. Markham A, Bryson HM. Epoetin alfa: a review of its pharmacodynamic and pharmacokinetic properties and therapeutic use in nonrenal applications. *Drugs* 1995;49:232–254.
70. Wilber RL. Detection of DNA-recombinant human epoetin-alfa as a pharmacological ergogenic aid. *Sports Med* 2002;32:125–142.
71. Overbay DK, Manley HJ. Darbepoetin-α: a review of the literature. *Pharmacotherapy* 2002;22:889–897.
72. Eschbach JW, Egrie JC, Downing MR, et al. Correction of the anemia of end-

stage renal disease with recombinant human erythropoietin: results of a combined phase I and II clinical trial. *N Engl J Med* 1987;316:73–78.
73. Spivak JL. Erythropoietin use and abuse: when physiology and pharmacology collide. *Adv Exp Med Biol* 2001;502:207–224.
74. Anon. Product information: Aranesp (darbepoetin alfa), annotated complete prescribing information. Thousand Oaks, CA: Amgen, July 19, 2002.
75. Brown KR, Carter W Jr, Lombardi GE. Recombinant erythropoietin overdose. *Am J Emerg Med* 1993;11(6):619–621.
76. Hoffman RS, Cobrin G, Nelson LS, Howland MA. Erythropoietin overdose treated with emergency erythropheresis. *Vet Hum Toxicol* 2002;44:157–159.
77. Novak BL, Force RW, Mumford BT, Solbrig RM. Erythropoietin-induced hypertensive urgency in a patient with chronic renal insufficiency: case report and review of the literature. *Pharmacotherapy* 2003;23(2):265–269.
78. Anon. Colony stimulating factors. In: USPDI: drug information for the health care professional. Greenwood Village, CO: Micromedex, 2001.
79. Klausner MA. Counterfeiting of Procrit (epoetin alfa). Ortho Biotech Products. Available at http://www.procrit.com/counterfeit/letter.html. Accessed June 2003.
80. Ozer H, Armitage JO, Bennett CL, et al. 2000 Update of recommendations for the use of hematopoietic colony-stimulating factors: evidence-based, clinical practice guidelines. *J Clin Oncol* 2000;18:3558–3585.
81. Anon. Product information: Neulasta (pegfilgrastim), complete prescribing information. Thousand Oaks, CA: Amgen, January 31, 2002.
82. Anon. Pegfilgrastim. In: USPDI: drug information for the health care professional, internet version. Greenwood Village, CO: Micromedex, 2002.
83. Anon. Pegfilgrastim (Neulasta) for prevention of febrile neutropenia. *Med Lett* 2002;44:44–45.

CHAPTER 107

Dicoumarol Anticoagulants

Henry A. Spiller

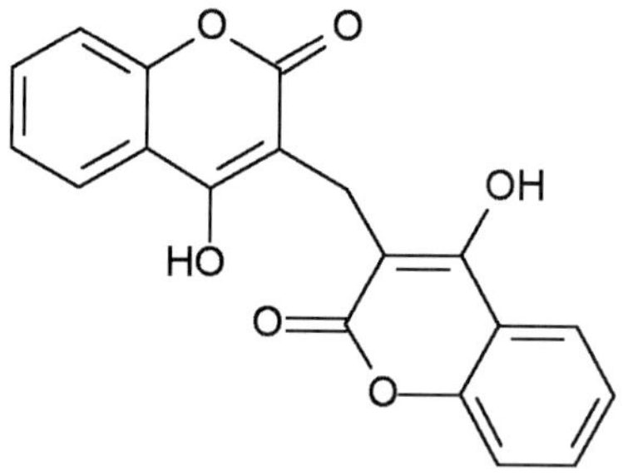

DICOUMAROL

Compounds included:	**Anisindione (Miradon); dicoumarol, dicumerol, dicoumarin, bishydroxycoumarin; warfarin (Coumadin)**
Molecular formula and weight:	**Anisindione ($C_{16}H_{12}O_3$), 252.3; dicoumarol ($C_{19}H_{12}O_6$), 336.3; warfarin ($C_{19}H_{16}O_4$), 308.35 g/mol. Structures are provided in Figure 1.**
SI conversion:	**Anisindione, mg/L × 3.9 = µmol/L; dicoumarol, mg/L × 2.9 = µmol/L; warfarin, mg/L × 3.2 = µmol/L**
CAS Registry No.:	**117-37-3 (anisindione); 66-76-2 (dicoumarol); 81-81-2 (warfarin)**
Therapeutic levels:	**Two- to threefold prolongation of prothrombin time or international normalized ratio**
Special concerns:	**Spontaneous bleeding, skin necrosis, purple toe syndrome**
Target organs:	**Coagulation system**
Antidote:	**None**

OVERVIEW

The oral anticoagulants, which include the coumarins (dicumarol and warfarin [Coumadin]) and the indandione derivatives (anisindione [Miradon]), function by interfering with the hepatic synthesis of the vitamin K–dependent clotting factors. They are used in the treatment and prophylaxis of venous thrombosis, atrial fibrillation with embolism, and pulmonary embolism and as an adjunct treatment of coronary occlusion. Warfarin may be used as an adjunct treatment of small cell carcinoma of the lung. In overdose, their main toxic effect is coagulopathy and bleeding due to lack of clotting factors. Long-acting anticoagulants are used as rodenticides (Chapter 237).

TOXIC DOSE

The adult therapeutic dose of warfarin is usually initiated at 2 to 5 mg/day. Maintenance doses of 2 to 10 mg/day are then titrated to an international normalized ratio (INR) of 2.0:3.0. The adult dose of dicoumarol is 25 to 200 mg/day titrated to prothrombin time (PT) response. The adult dose of anisindione is 300 mg on the first day, 200 mg on the second day, and 100 mg on the third day, with a maintenance dose of 25 to 250 mg titrated to the PT.

Warfarin is most toxic when ingested daily over a period of 5 to 7 days. In humans, drug interactions that reduce hepatic clearance or altered protein binding are the most common cause of toxicity (1). The acute lethal dose is not known. Acute inges-

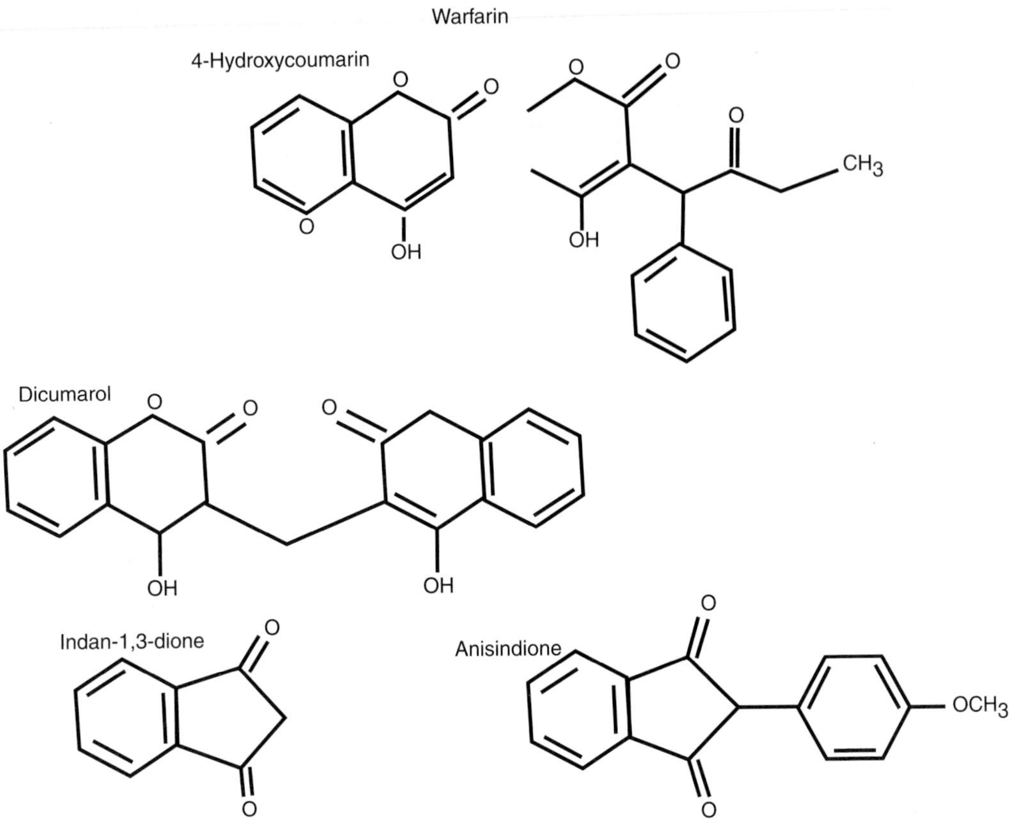

Warfarin

4-Hydroxycoumarin

Dicumarol

Indan-1,3-dione

Anisindione

Figure 1. Structures of the dicoumarol anticoagulants.

tion of 250 and 280 mg of warfarin in adults has resulted in elevated PT and INR (2,3). Ingestion of warfarin, 567 mg over 6 days, by a man produced bleeding and a PT greater than 4 minutes (4). Acute ingestion of more than 2.0 mg/kg is expected to increase the INR and the risk of bleeding (5). Ingestion of 4.4 mg/kg by a 20-month-old child produced an elevated PT but no evidence of bleeding (6).

TOXICOKINETICS AND TOXICODYNAMICS

Pharmacokinetic parameters are provided in Table 1. Oral anticoagulants are rapidly and completely absorbed via oral, inhalational, and parenteral routes (7,8). Slow but significant dermal absorption also occurs (9). The oral anticoagulants are highly protein bound (97% to 99%), primarily to albumin (7). Any

TABLE 1. Pharmacokinetic parameters of oral anticoagulants

	Warfarin	Dicoumarol	Anisindione
Time-to-peak prothrombin time changes (d)	0.5–4.0	1.0–3.0	1.0–3.0
Duration of effect, therapeutic (d)	2–5	2–10	1–6
Duration of effect, overdose (d)	5–10	NR	NR
Volume of distribution (L/kg)	0.11–0.20	NR	NR
Elimination half-life (d)	0.5–3.0	1.0–2.0	3.0–5.0
Elimination half-life in overdose (d)	0.9–2.2	NR	NR
Protein binding (%)	97–99	>97	>97

NR, not reported.

drugs affecting the protein binding may significantly increase the risk of an adverse bleeding event.

Warfarin is metabolized via cytochrome P-450 oxidation and reduction to stereoisomeric alcohols. The *S*- and *R*-isomers of warfarin are metabolized by distinct pathways. Genetic variation in the activity of the cytochrome P-450 family may account for variation in dose response and effect (10). *S*-warfarin exhibits approximately two to five times the anticoagulant activity of *R*-enantiomer. In general, oral anticoagulants are excreted in the bile as inactive metabolites, resorbed, and then excreted in the urine.

PATHOPHYSIOLOGY

γ-Carboxylation of the precursor proteins of the clotting factors II (prothrombin), VII (proconvertin), IX (Christmas factor or plasma thromboplastin component), and X (Stuart-Prower factor) is the final stage in activation for these clotting factors (Chapter 68). Carboxylation requires the presence of the reduced vitamin K species hydroxyquinone (vitamin KH_2), oxygen, and carbon dioxide. The oral anticoagulants bind to and inhibit vitamin K–epoxide reductase and, to a lesser extent, vitamin K reductase, eliminating the pathway for cyclical regeneration of the reduced vitamin K species hydroxyquinone. The result is synthesis of dysfunctional clotting factors. As the circulating functional clotting factors are depleted, the ability to form clots is compromised. The rate of depletion of functional vitamin K–dependent clotting factors depends on their individual rate of degradation: II (60 hours), VII (4 to 6 hours), IX (20 to 24 hours), and X (48 to 72 hours). Administration of exogenous vitamin K can circumvent this depletion by providing a substrate for vitamin K reductase, the second reductase in the vitamin K cycle, which is less sensitive to oral anticoagulant inhibition.

PREGNANCY AND LACTATION

Coumarin and anisindione are U.S. Food and Drug Administration pregnancy category D (Appendix I). All of these compounds cross the placenta. The American Academy of Pediatrics considers warfarin and dicoumarol compatible with breastfeeding. In a large study of postpartum women treated with dicoumarol, no adverse events or changes in PT were noted in any of the infants (11). Indandione derivatives (anisindione) should be avoided by lactating women.

CLINICAL PRESENTATION

Acute and Subacute Overdosage

The effects from overdose are primarily an extension of the therapeutic effect. Onset of prolonged PT/INR from acute overdose is expected to be delayed from 18 to 48 hours (6,12). Onset is more rapid in patients with preexisting anticoagulation from therapeutic use (3,13). Patients may exhibit epistaxis, lower back and flank pain, hematuria, petechial rash, bruising, gingival bleeding, ecchymosis, retinal hemorrhage, headache, and cerebral hemorrhage (2,4,13).

Chronic Use

Bleeding is the most serious complication from chronic use of oral anticoagulants. In one prospective study, bleeding complications were found in 153 of 2745 consecutive patients at 34 anticoagulation clinics (14). Over a 30-month period, 84 patients presented to one emergency department with an INR greater than 6.0. Of these patients, major bleeding occurred in 16.7%, and minor bleeding occurred in 17.8% (15). A prospective study of ambulatory patients over a 1-year period found 114 patients who developed an INR greater than 6.0: Ten (8.8%) patients experienced abnormal bleeding, and five (4.4%) experienced a major hemorrhage (16). Other reported effects secondary to over-coagulation are cardiac tamponade, pulmonary hemorrhage, hemothorax, intracranial hemorrhage, gastrointestinal bleeding with hemoculture-positive stools, lower back/flank pain, hematuria, and retinal hemorrhage.

There are several risk factors in oral anticoagulant–induced bleeding: (a) age older than 60 years (1.6-fold increased risk), (b) female gender (1.3-fold increased risk), and (c) presence of malignancy (2.2-fold increased risk) (17).

TABLE 2. Warfarin-induced adverse drug events

Drugs that may cause an increased response to the oral anticoagulants secondary to inhibition of hepatic metabolism
Amiodarone
Amitriptyline (dicumarol)
Cimetidine
Chloramphenicol
Erythromycin
Fluconazole
Ifosfamide
Ketoconazole
Lovastatin
Metronidazole
Miconazole
Nortriptyline (dicumarol)
Omeprazole
Phenylbutazone
Propafenone
Propoxyphene
Quinidine
Sulfamethoxazole and trimethoprim
Sulfinpyrazone
Drugs that may increase response by displacing oral anticoagulants from protein-binding sites
Chloral hydrate
Loop diuretics
Nalidixic acid
Drugs that may increase response of oral anticoagulants by effects on platelets
Cephalosporins
Diflusinal
Penicillins
Salicylates
Drugs that may increase response of anticoagulants by other or unknown mechanisms
Acetaminophen
Androgens
Clofibrate
Thyroid hormones (increase catabolism of clotting factors)
Gemfibrozil
Glucagon
Phenytoin (may initially increase effects, then decrease effects with chronic therapy)
Influenza virus vaccine
Isoniazid
Moricizine
Tamoxifen
Urokinase

Adverse Reactions

Many drugs interact to produce increased anticoagulation (Table 2). Oral anticoagulant–induced necrosis or gangrene of the skin is a rare complication with a prevalence of 0.01% to 0.10% (18). It usually occurs early after initiation of anticoagulant therapy (1 to 10 days) and may occur after the first dose (19,20). It usually occurs in females and in areas of high-fat content: breast, abdomen, legs, and buttocks (18). The necrosis usually begins as painful erythematous patches that progress to dark hemorrhagic areas. It is believed that the sudden decrease in protein C activity is the precipitant (18). Hereditary protein C deficiency is considered a major risk factor but is not the sole risk factor. Protein C generally inhibits coagulation by inactivating factors V and VII and facilitating fibrinolysis. A rapid decline in protein C, before full decline of other vitamin K–dependent clotting factors, results in a short-term hypercoagulable state. This leads to thrombotic occlusion of the microvasculature with resulting necrosis. Skin necrosis usually occurs when the hypercoagulable state is maximal.

The purple toe syndrome has been attributed to cholesterol crystal emboli released as a result of warfarin-induced bleeding into atherosclerotic plaques (21,22). Purple toe syndrome usually occurs 3 to 10 weeks after initiation of therapy. The syndrome is typically characterized by purple discoloration of the plantar surface of the toes and feet and may include pain and tenderness to touch. It may be bilateral (22).

DIAGNOSTIC TESTS

Acute Overdose

Patients should have the PT and INR monitored periodically. Changes in INR may not develop for 24 to 48 hours postingestion. If needed, levels of the individual factors can be measured. The levels of vitamin K–dependent clotting factors (II, VII, IX, X) should be decreased. Warfarin concentration testing is available from reference laboratories. In a case of massive ingestion, peak warfarin concentration was 111 mg/L and remained above 2.0 mg/L for 7 days (13). A number of methods for assaying warfarin and its metabolites have been developed.

Chronic Use

Therapy is guided by PT and INR. The INR is maintained at 2.0:3.0, except for prophylaxis after artificial heart valve replacement when it may be 2.0:3.5. An INR greater than 6.0 presents an increased risk of hemorrhage (16). Serum levels of warfarin are not usually measured. Prothrombin complex synthesis is inhibited 50% when the warfarin concentration is 1.5 mg/L.

TREATMENT

A distinction should be made between (a) a single acute ingestion, and (b) a chronic ingestion or (c) an acute ingestion in an already anticoagulated patient. The onset of anticoagulation is delayed after an acute ingestion. In the case of chronic toxicity, the effects may be more severe or already evident on patient presentation. Priority should be given to assessment of coagulation status and control of bleeding. Hemorrhage is treated as from any cause, with local pressure, fluid resuscitation, and pressors, if refractory to treatment.

Unintentional ingestion less than 2.0 mg/kg in a child is unlikely to produce significant risk of bleeding. In accidentally over-anticoagulated patients, therapy is guided by the INR and the presence or absence of active bleeding. Three therapies are applied depending on the risk present: temporary discontinuation of warfarin therapy, administration of vitamin K, and transfusion of fresh frozen plasma.

Decontamination

Emesis is contraindicated in any already coagulated patient due to the risk of a Valsalva's maneuver increasing intracranial pressure and causing intracranial hemorrhage. Activated charcoal may be warranted in the event the ingestion is large and recent. However, these drugs do not cause immediate effects; therefore, the patient may not present in a time period appropriate for decontamination.

Enhanced Elimination

Enhanced elimination via multiple-dose activated charcoal or extracorporeal removal has no role in oral anticoagulant management. Oral cholestyramine has been suggested to increase elimination of warfarin, but data are limited on its value, and it cannot be routinely recommended (12,23,24).

Antidote

Vitamin K reverses the effects of the oral anticoagulants. However, it may take 1 to 10 days to correct the INR in severely anticoagulated patients (2,25). The approach to individual patients is based largely on clinical judgment. In the presence of bleeding, fresh frozen plasma or prothrombin complex concentrate rapidly corrects the coagulopathy. Details of the use and administration of vitamin K are provided in Chapter 68. The recommendations of the American College of Chest Physicians are shown in Table 3.

Management Pitfalls

Too rapid reversal of anticoagulation in the setting of a patient requiring anticoagulation therapy, such as patients with prosthetic heart valves, may result in prolonged oral anticoagulant resistance and the possibility of thrombosis or thromboemboli (26).

TABLE 3. Guidelines for the reversal of anticoagulation therapy

Indication	International normalized ratio (INR) range	Recommendation
In absence of clinically significant bleeding	<5.0	Hold next warfarin dose and resume therapy at lower dose when INR is therapeutic.
	5.0–9.0	Hold 1–2 doses and resume warfarin at lower dose when INR is therapeutic; *OR* hold 1 dose of warfarin and give vitamin K, 1.0–2.5 mg PO.
	>9.0	Hold warfarin and give vitamin K, 3.0–5.0 mg PO.
Rapid reversal indicated	5.0–9.0 and surgery planned	Hold warfarin and give vitamin K, 2–4 mg PO, approximately 24 h before procedure; an additional dose of vitamin K, 1–2 mg PO, may be given.
	>20.0 or serious bleed	Give vitamin K, 10 mg by slow IV infusion. Fresh frozen plasma or prothrombin complex concentrate may also be indicated depending on urgency of situation. May repeat vitamin K every 12 h as needed.

From Hirsh J, Dalen JE, Anderson DR, et al. Oral anticoagulants: mechanism of action, clinical effectiveness, and optimal therapeutic range. *Chest* 1998;114:445S–469S, with permission.

REFERENCES

1. Beyth RJ, Landerfeld CS. Anticoagulants in older patients. A safety perspective. *Drugs Aging* 1995;6:45–54.
2. Bates D, Mintz M. Phytonadione therapy in the multiple-drug overdose involving warfarin. *Pharmacotherapy* 2000;20:1208–1215.
3. Bjornsson TD, Blaschke TF. Vitamin K disposition and therapy of warfarin overdose. *Lancet* 1978;2:846–847.
4. Holmes RW, Love J. Suicide attempt with warfarin. *JAMA* 1952;148:935–937.
5. O'Reilly RA, Aggeler PM. Studies on coumarin anticoagulant drugs. Initiation of warfarin therapy without a loading dose. *Circulation* 1968;38:169–177.
6. Montanio CD, Wruk KM, Kulig KW, et al. *Am J Disease Child* 1993;147:609–610.
7. Holford NH. Clinical pharmacokinetics and pharmacodynamics of warfarin. *Clin Pharmacokinet* 1986;11:483–504.
8. Breckenridge AM, Orme M. Kinetics of warfarin absorption in man. *Clin Pharmcol Ther* 1973;14:955–961.
9. Abell TL, Merigian KS, Lee JM, et al. Cutaneous exposure to warfarin-like anticoagulant causing an intracerebral hemorrhage: a case report. *J Toxicol Clin Toxicol* 1994;32:69–73.
10. Takahashi H, Echizen H. Pharmacogenetics of warfarin elimination and its clinical implications. *Clin Pharmacokinet* 2001;40:587–603.
11. Brambel CE, Hunter RE. Effect of dicumarol on the nursing infant. *Am J Obstet Gynecol* 1950;59:1153–1159.
12. Renowden S, Westmoreland D, White JP, Routledge PA. Oral cholestyramine increases elimination of warfarin after overdose. *BMJ* 1985;291:513–514.
13. Hackett LP, Llett KF, Chester A. Plasma warfarin concentrations after massive overdose. *Med J Aust* 1985;142:642–643.
14. Palareti G, Leali N, Coccheri S, et al. Bleeding complications of oral anticoagulant treatment: an inception-cohort prospective collaborative study. *Lancet* 1996;248:423–428.
15. Cruickshank J, Ragg M, Eddy D. Warfarin toxicity in the emergency department: recommendation for management. *Emerg Med (Fremantle)* 2001;13:91–97.
16. Hylek EM, Chang Y, Skates SJ, et al. Prospective study of the outcome of ambulatory patients with excessive warfarin anticoagulation. *Arch Intern Med* 2000;160:1612–1617.
17. Ebell MH. Determining the risk of bleeding in warfarin therapy. *J Fam Pract* 1999;48:413.
18. Chen YC, Valenti D, Mansfield AO, Stansby G. Warfarin induced necrosis. *Br J Surg* 2000;87:266–272.

19. Slutzki S, Bogokowsky H, Gliboa Y, Halpern Z. Coumadin-induced skin necrosis. *Int J Dermatol* 1984;23:117–119.
20. Haynes CD, Mathews JW, Gwaltney N, Lazenby WD. Breast necrosis complicating anticoagulation therapy. *South Med J* 1983;76:1091–1093.
21. Sallah S, Thomas DP, Roberts HR. Warfarin and heparin-induced skin necrosis and the purple toe syndrome: infrequent complications of anticoagulant treatment. *Thromb Haemost* 1997;78:785–790.
22. Raj K, Collins B, Rangarajan S. Purple toe syndrome following anticoagulant therapy. *Br J Haematol* 2001;114:740.
23. Roberge RJ, Rao P, Miske GR, Riley TJ. Diarrhea associated over anticoagulation in a patient taking warfarin: therapeutic role of cholestyramine. *Vet Hum Toxicol* 2000;42:351–353.
24. Isbister GK, Whyte IM. Management of anticoagulant poisoning. *Vet Hum Toxicol* 2001;43:117–118.
25. Hung A, Singh S, Tait RC. A prospective randomized study to determine the optimal dose of intravenous vitamin K in reversal of over-warfarinization. *Br J Haematol* 2000;109:537–539.
26. Baglin T. Management of warfarin overdose. *Blood Rev* 1998;12:91–98.

CHAPTER 108

Heparin and Low-Molecular-Weight Heparins

Henry A. Spiller

Compounds included:	**Heparin; enoxaparin (Lovenox, Clexane, Plausina); tinzaparin (Innohep, Logiparin); dalteparin (Boxol, Fragmin); danaparoid (Orgaran)**
SI conversion:	**Not applicable.**
CAS Registry No.:	**9041-08-1 (heparin sodium); 9041-08-1 (enoxaparin); 9041-08-1 (tinzaparin); 9041-08-1 (dalteparin); 83513-48-8 (danaparoid sodium)**
Therapeutic levels:	**Heparin target activated partial thromboplastin time of 50 to 70 seconds; low-molecular-weight heparins 0.5–1.2 antifactor Xa IU/ml**
Special concerns:	**Spontaneous bleeding, heparin-induced thrombocytopenia**
Target organs:	**Coagulation system**
Antidote:	**None**

OVERVIEW

The heparin anticoagulants include unfractionated heparin (heparin sodium), the low-molecular-weight heparins (LMWH; enoxaparin, tinzaparin and dalteparin), and low-molecular-weight heparinoids (danaparoid). They are used in the prophylaxis and treatment of venous thrombosis, pulmonary embolism, and peripheral arterial embolism; in the diagnosis and treatment of consumptive coagulopathies (disseminated intravascular coagulation); and in the prevention of clotting in arterial and heart surgery, extracorporeal circulation, and dialysis procedures. Bleeding is the main toxic effect of these agents.

Heparin is a glycosaminoglycan found in the secretory granules of mast cells. It is commonly extracted from porcine intestinal mucosa or bovine lung. LMWH are isolated from unfractionated heparin by gel-filtration chromatography or depolymerization of unfractionated porcine heparin; they differ from heparin in both their pharmacologic properties and mechanisms of action. Heparin interacts with antithrombin III to produce a substance that immediately neutralizes thrombin (factor IIa) by forming a heparin-antithrombin-thrombin complex. Heparin increases the thrombin-antithrombin reaction 100- to 1000-fold. In contrast, LMWH produce their anticoagulant effect mainly through inhibition of factor Xa because they lack the molecular length to bind thrombin and antithrombin simultaneously (1). Danaparoid is made of three closely related glycosaminoglycans derived from porcine intestinal mucosa, consisting of heparin sulfate (84%), dermatan sulfate (12%), and chondroitin sulfate (4%), with actions and uses similar to those of LMWH (2–4).

TOXIC DOSE

The *adult therapeutic dose* of heparin is 4000 U by intravenous (IV) bolus, followed by 20,000 to 40,000 U/day as a continuous IV infusion. The adult therapeutic dose of enoxaparin is 30 mg every 12 hours subcutaneously (SQ) for 7 to 10 days. Do not administer intramuscularly. Tinzaparin is dosed as 175 IU/kg SQ once daily for 6 days until adequately anticoagulated by warfarin. The dose of dalteparin is 120 IU/kg SQ every 12 hours for 5 to 8 days. The dose of danaparoid is 750 anti-Xa U SQ twice daily.

A typical *pediatric therapeutic dose* of heparin is 50 U/kg IV bolus, followed by 20,000 U/m^2/24 hours as a continuous infusion. The enoxaparin dose for children older than 2 months is 0.62 to 1.00 mg/kg every 12 hours. Pediatric dosing has not been established for other agents.

The acute toxic dose is not clear because there are limited case reports of acute overdose (5,6). An infusion of heparin, 550,000 U over 24 hours, resulted in death (5). A bolus infusion of more than 100 to 150 U/kg is expected to double the activated partial thromboplastin time (aPTT), although there is some variance in response to heparin dosage.

TOXICOKINETICS AND TOXICODYNAMICS

Information after overdose is not available. The pharmacokinetic parameters for these agents are presented in Table 1. Heparins are not absorbed via the oral or dermal route and must be administered parenterally. The LMWH should be administered SQ only. Animal studies of new methods for oral delivery of

TABLE 1. Pharmacokinetic parameters of heparin and low-molecular-weight heparins

Drug	Bioavailability (%)	Time to maximum serum concentration (h)	Volume of distribution	Elimination half-life (h)
Heparin, IV	100	Rapid/immediate	0.06 L/kg	0.5–1.5, dose dependent
Heparin, SQ	Not reported	2–4	0.06 L/kg	0.5–1.5, dose dependent
Enoxaparin	92	3–5	6 L	4.5
Tinzaparin	86.7	3.7	3.1–5.0 L	3–4
Dalteparin	87	4	2.8–4.2 L	3–5
Danaparoid	100	2–5	8–9 L	24

heparin and LMWH are promising (7,8). Phase II human trials were successful, and clinical trials are planned (9,10).

PATHOPHYSIOLOGY

Heparin binds with and produces a conformational change in antithrombin III. This complex is approximately 100 to 1000 times more active than antithrombin III alone in neutralization of the activated clotting factors XIIa, XIa, IXa, Xa, and thrombin (IIa) (Fig. 1) (11). The major effect appears to be against factor Xa, as this halts any further conversion of prothrombin (II) to thrombin (IIa) in both the intrinsic and extrinsic pathways. In addition, heparin has high affinity for vascular endothelium and von Willebrand's factor, thereby inhibiting platelet aggregation.

Heparin-induced thrombocytopenia (HIT) is mediated by immunoglobulin. The pathogenic antibody, usually immunoglobulin G, recognizes a multimolecular complex of heparin and platelet factor 4, resulting in platelet activation. In addition to platelet activation, there is a concomitant activation of coagulation, marked by increased thrombin generation (12).

Heparin suppresses aldosterone synthesis by inhibition of the renin-angiotensin system as well as other poorly defined mechanisms (13). The most important—but probably not the only—mechanism appears to involve reduction in both number and affinity of the angiotensin II receptors in the zona glomerulosa. Aldosterone suppression results in hyponatremia, hyperkalemia, and, rarely, hyperchloremic metabolic acidosis (Fig. 2) (13).

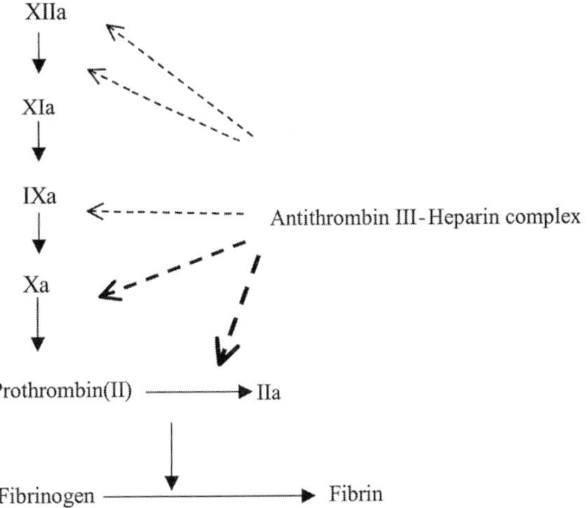

Figure 1. Inhibitory effect of the antithrombin III-heparin complex on clotting pathway. Thrombin (IIa) and Xa are the most sensitive to the effects of antithrombin III heparin.

PREGNANCY AND LACTATION

Heparin is in U.S. Food and Drug Administration (FDA) pregnancy category C (Appendix I). Heparin appears to have major advantages over the oral anticoagulants because its high molecular weight prevents placental transfer and entry into breast milk (14,15). Dalteparin, enoxaparin, and tinzaparin are FDA pregnancy category B. Excretion in breast milk has not been determined for danaparoid, enoxaparin, and tinzaparin.

A once-daily dose of dalteparin, 2500 IU SQ, produced anti-Xa activities in breast milk, ranging from less than 0.005 to 0.037 IU/L of breast milk. This is equivalent to a milk:plasma ratio of less than 0.025:0.224 and indicates no clinically relevant effect on the nursing infant (16).

CLINICAL PRESENTATION

Acute Overdosage

Overdose of heparin results in rapid prolongation of coagulation time and may cause active bleeding. Hematuria, epistaxis, or tarry stools may be the first signs of bleeding. Easy bruising and petechial formation may progress to frank bleeding. Heparin overdose should be considered in the neonate with bleeding, prolonged prothrombin time and aPTT, and normal platelets (17,18). Additionally, unintended overdosage may occur from "heparin flush syndrome" caused by multiple IV flushes containing heparin (19–21). Further, heparin ampules of significantly different strengths may appear identical (20).

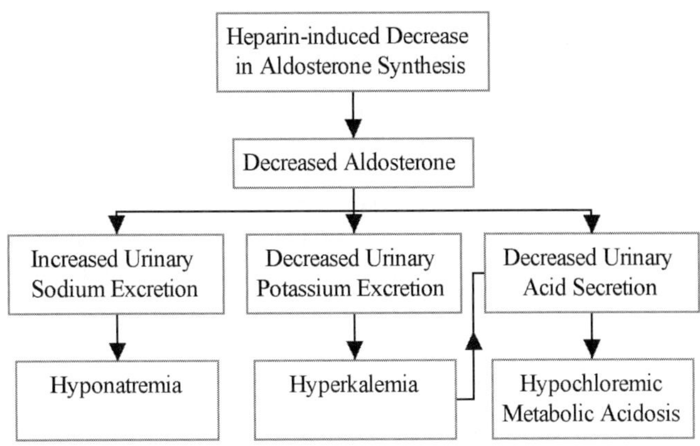

Figure 2. The effect of heparin on aldosterone activity. Heparin-induced aldosterone suppression results in hyponatremia, hyperkalemia, and, rarely, hyperchloremic metabolic acidosis.

TABLE 2. Heparin drug interactions

Drugs that may increase risk of bleeding when administered with heparin
Cephalosporins
Penicillins
Platelet inhibitors
Ibuprofen
Aspirin
Indomethacin
Dipyridamole
Hydroxychloroquine
Nonsteroidal antiinflammatory drugs
Ticlopidine
Phenylbutazone
Dextran
Drugs that may decrease the pharmacologic effect of heparin
Nitroglycerin
Digitalis
Tetracycline
Nicotine
Antihistamines

Adverse Reactions

Drug interactions for heparin are provided in Table 2.

HEPARIN-INDUCED THROMBOCYTOPENIA

HIT is diagnosed on both clinical and serologic features (1). HIT antibody formation causes an unexpected decrease in platelet count (more than 50%) or skin lesions (erythematous plaques or necrosis) at injection site. Complications of HIT are venous thrombotic events (deep venous thrombosis, venous limb gangrene, pulmonary embolism, cerebral sinus thrombosis, adrenal hemorrhagic infarction), arterial thrombosis, graft occlusion, and myocardial infarction (12,22). HIT typically occurs 5 to 8 days after starting heparin therapy and affects approximately 3% of patients (12). However, it may be delayed up to 19 days after stopping heparin therapy (22). There is a 50% risk of thrombosis during the subsequent 30 days (12). HIT is more common in patients receiving unfractionated heparin than patients treated with LMWH (23).

HEPARIN-INDUCED ALDOSTERONE SUPPRESSION AND HYPERKALEMIA

Heparin is a predictable and potent inhibitor of aldosterone production (13). Aldosterone suppression results in natriuresis, hyponatremia, and, less predictably, hyperkalemia and hyperchloremic acidosis (Fig. 2) (13). Decreases in aldosterone levels may occur with heparin doses as low as 5000 U twice per day. Hyperkalemia occurs in approximately 7% of patients receiving heparin, often occurring within 8 to 14 days of initiating therapy. Increased risk factors are renal insufficiency, diabetes mellitus, and the use of potassium salts or angiotensin-converting enzyme inhibitors (13).

HEPARIN-INDUCED OSTEOPOROSIS

During pregnancy, heparin or LMWH are preferred over the oral anticoagulants for long-term therapy (women with mechanical heart valves or venous thromboembolism and prevention of fetal loss in women with antiphospholipid antibodies) (1). Significant reductions in bone density and fractures have been reported in approximately 30% of patients receiving heparin for 1 month or more (1,24,25). LMWH carry a lower risk of osteoporosis than unfractionated heparin (1,26). Heparin-induced osteoporosis is not rapidly reversible after discontinuation of heparin therapy, possibly because of sequestration of heparin in bone (27).

DIAGNOSTIC TESTS

Acute Overdose

Under normal conditions, circulating endogenous heparin levels cannot be detected in the blood. An aPTT and activated clotting time may be used to monitor the effects of heparin overdose. Anti-Xa activity may be monitored. Complete blood cell count and platelet counts should be obtained.

Chronic Therapy

The serum potassium level should be measured every 3 to 4 days. Patients on chronic therapy or those who have received heparin in the previous 100 days may be at risk for HIT. Platelets should be monitored. Enzyme-linked immunosorbent assays for the diagnosis of HIT immunoglobulin are commercially available (12).

Heparin drug monitoring involves assays that measure the inhibition of added factor Xa or IIa by the antithrombin-III/heparin complex. Heparin assays may underestimate drug levels in neonates due to neonatal antithrombin III deficiency and may lead to over heparinization, placing them at a higher risk of bleeding (28,29).

TREATMENT

Decontamination of these drugs is not feasible because of parenteral administration.

Acute Overdose or Adverse Events

Heparin therapy should be withdrawn in the event of adverse effects. Hemorrhage is treated as from any cause, with local pressure, fluid resuscitation, vasopressors, and blood products, if refractory to treatment. If bleeding is minimal, no treatment may be necessary due to the short half-life of heparin. If bleeding is severe or a substantial heparin dose has been administered, consider administration of protamine sulfate.

Antidote

Protamine sulfate is a strongly basic protein that forms a stable salt with heparin, resulting in the loss of anticoagulant activity. Its use is described in more detail in Chapter 70. The neutralization of heparin occurs within 30 to 60 seconds after injection. One mg of protamine sulfate neutralizes 90 U of heparin derived from lung tissue and 115 U derived from intestinal mucosa. If given immediately after the heparin overdose, administer 1 mg protamine sulfate for every 100 U of heparin. It should be given IV slowly over 10 minutes to reduce risk of anaphylaxis or anaphylactoid reaction. For each hour postoverdose, the dose of protamine should be reduced by one-half—at 1 hour postoverdose, administer 0.5 mg of protamine sulfate for each 100 U of heparin; at 2 hours, 0.25 mg of protamine for each 100 U of heparin. The aPTT should be obtained 5 to 15 minutes after protamine administration to help guide therapy. In a substantial overdose, continue to monitor aPTT for potential heparin rebound.

Protamine is also used for LMWH, although it is less effective in treating the LMWH than unfractionated heparin. The dose is 1 mg protamine sulfate for each 100 U of anti-Xa activity for dalteparin and tinzaparin and 1 mg of protamine for each 1 mg of enoxaparin. Protamine may not be effective on the heparinoids (danaparoid).

Because of the potential for acute allergic reactions, resuscitation equipment and epinephrine should be immediately available during administration of protamine. The half-life of protamine is shorter than heparin; therefore, there may be a rebound effect from the heparin.

Heparin-Induced Thrombocytopenia

The treatment of HIT includes discontinuation of heparin and substitution of an alternate anticoagulant to avoid thrombosis. Initial therapy with lepirudin, a recombinant hirudin, or danaparoid sodium is recommended (12,30,31). LMWH have a high rate of *in vitro* cross-reactivity with HIT immunoglobulin G antibodies and are not recommended. Because the oral anticoagulants require 2 to 3 days to produce effective anticoagulation and there is a potential risk of venous limb gangrene, warfarin therapy should not be instituted until the platelet count has fully recovered (12). Protamine sulfate has no role in HIT because the cause of the process is not the anticoagulant effects of the heparin but rather due to the antigenic properties.

REFERENCES

1. Hirsh J, Warkentin TE, Shaughnessy SG, et al. Heparin and low-molecular-weight-heparin: mechanism of action, pharmacokinetics, dosing, monitoring, efficacy and safety. *Chest* 2001;119:64S–94S.
2. Meuleman DG. Orgaran (Org 10172): its pharmacologic profile in experimental models. *Haemostasis* 1992;22:58–65.
3. Danhof M, de Boer A, Magnani HN, Stiekema JC. Pharmacokinetic considerations on orgaran (Org 10172) therapy. *Haemostasis* 1992;22:73–84.
4. Bradbrook ID, Magnani HN, Moelker HC, et al. ORG 10172: a low molecular weight heparinoid anticoagulant with a long half-life in man. *Br J Clin Pharmacol* 1987;23:667–675.
5. Missliwetz J, Korninger C, Denk W. [A fatality caused by heparin overdose.] *Z Rechtsmed* 1989;103:147–153.
6. Hackett LP, Iiett KF, Chester A. Plasma warfarin concentrations after a massive overdose. *Med J Aust* 1985;142:642–643.
7. Jiao Y, Marchand-Arvier M, Vigneron C, et al. In vitro and in vivo evaluation of oral heparin-loaded polymeric nonoparticles in rabbits. *Circulation* 2002;105:230–235.
8. Welt FG, Woods TC, Edelman ER. Oral heparin prevents neointimal hyperplasia after arterial injury: inhibitory potential depends on type of vascular injury. *Circulation* 2001;104:3121–3124.
9. Pineo GF, Hull RD, Marder VJ. Orally active heparin and low-molecular-weight heparin. *Curr Opin Pulm Med* 2001;7:344–348.
10. Lee Y, Nam JH, Shin HC, Byun Y. Conjugation of low molecular weight heparin and deoxycholic acid for the development of a new oral anticoagulant agent. *Circulation* 2001;104:3116–3120.
11. Harrington R, Ansell J. Risk-benefit assessment of anticoagulant therapy. *Drug Saf* 1991;6:54–69.
12. Warkentin TE. Heparin-induced thrombocytopenia. *Drug Saf* 1997;17:235–340.
13. Oster JR, Singer I, Fishman LM. Heparin-induced aldosterone suppression and hypokalemia. *Am J Med* 1995;98:575–586.
14. Chaplin S, Sanders GL, Smith JM. Drug excretion in human breast milk. *Adverse Drug React Acute Poison Rev* 1982;1:255–287.
15. Heparin. In: Briggs GG, Freeman RK, Yaffe SJ, eds. *Drugs in pregnancy and lactation*, 6th ed. Philadelphia: Lippincott, Williams & Wilkins, 2002:644–647.
16. Richter C, Sitzmann J, Lang P, et al. Excretion of low molecular weight heparin in human milk. *Br J Clin Pharmacol* 2001;52:708–710.
17. Moncino MD, Kutzberg J. Accidental heparinization in the newborn: a case report and brief review of the literature. *J Perinatol* 1990;10:399–402.
18. Galant SP. Accidental heparinization of a newborn infant. *Am J Dis Child* 1967;114:313–319.
19. Passannante A, Macik BG. The heparin flush syndrome: a cause of iatrogenic hemorrhage. *Am J Med Sci* 1988;96:71–73.
20. Williams PE, Dawes J, Dearden NM, et al. Coagulation disorder due to apparent inadvertent heparin administration. *Clin Lab Haematol* 1989;11:101–104.
21. Morgan SK, Grush OC, Jernigan D. Unexplained bleeding associated with central venous catheter care. *Am J Pediatr Hematol Oncol* 1989;11:447–449.
22. Warkentin TE, Kelton JG. Delayed-onset heparin-induced thrombocytopenia and thrombosis. *Ann Intern Med* 2001;135:502–506.
23. Warkentin TE, Levine MN, Hirsh J, et al. Heparin-induced thrombocytopenia in patients treated with low-molecular-weight heparin or unfractionated heparin. *N Engl J Med* 1995;332:1330–1335.
24. Dahlman TC, Sjoberg HE, Ringertz H. Bone mineral density during long-term prophylaxis with heparin in pregnancy. *Am J Obstet Gynecol* 1994;170:1315–1320.
25. Dahlman TC. Osteoporotic fractures and the recurrence of thromboembolism during pregnancy and the puerperium in 184 women undergoing thromboprophylaxis with heparin. *Am J Obstet Gynecol* 1993;168:1265–1270.
26. Muir JM, Hirsh J, Weitz JI, et al. A histomorphometric comparison of the effects of heparin and low-molecular-weight heparin on cancellous bone in rats. *Blood* 1997;89:3236–3242.
27. Shaughnessy SG, Hirsh J, Bhandari M, et al. A histomorphometric evaluation of heparin-induced bone loss after discontinuation of heparin treatment in rats. *Blood* 1999;93:1231–1236.
28. Schmidt B, Mitchell L, Ofosu F. Standard assays underestimate the concentration of heparin in neonatal plasma. *J Lab Clin Med* 1988;112:641–643.
29. Schmidt B, Wais U, Pringsheim W, Kunzer W. Plasma elimination of antithrombin III (heparin cofactor activity) is accelerated in term newborn infants. *Eur J Pediatr* 1984;141:225–227.
30. Deitcher SR, Carman TL. Heparin induced thrombocytopenia: natural history, diagnosis and management. *Vasc Med* 2001;6:113–119.
31. Deitcher SR, Toppulos AP, Bartholomew JR, Kichuk-Chrisant MR. Lepirudin anticoagulation for heparin-induced thrombocytopenia. *J Pediatr* 2002;140:264–266.

CHAPTER 109

Lepirudin

Henry A. Spiller

Molecular formula and weight:	**$C_{287}H_{440}N_{80}O_{111}S_6$, 6980 g/mol**
SI conversion:	**mg/dl × 1.4 = μg/L**
CAS Registry No.:	**138068-37-8**
Therapeutic level:	**Variable, 0.5 to 1.5 mg/L**
Special concerns:	**Renal impairment or renal failure causes significant prolongation of half-life and potential for coagulopathy.**
Antidote:	**None**

OVERVIEW

Lepirudin (Refludan) and desirudin (Revasc) are recombinant hirudins that directly inhibit both free and clot-bound thrombin. Lepirudin is an anticoagulant used in the treatment of heparin-induced thrombocytopenia. It has been investigated for use in the treatment of acute coronary syndromes, prevention of venous thrombosis, and cardiac pulmonary bypass surgery (1,2). In overdose, the primary toxic effect is coagulopathy and bleeding due to inhibition of thrombin.

Lepirudin is a recombinant hirudin that directly inhibits the active site pocket and the fibrinogen-binding site of free and clot-bound thrombin (1). Desirudin differs from lepirudin in the first two *N*-amino acids. Antithrombin activity is 18,000 U/mg for lepirudin and 16,000 U/mg for desirudin. Lepirudin may be more effective than the low-molecular-weight heparins in the treatment of heparin-induced thrombocytopenia.

TABLE 1. Manufacturer-recommended dosing adjustments for lepirudin in patients with renal failure

Creatinine clearance (ml/min)	Serum creatinine (mg/dl)	Bolus dose (mg/kg)	Infusion rate
>60	<1.6	0.4	0.1500 mg/kg/h
45–50	1.6–2.0	0.2	0.0750 mg/kg/h
30–44	2.1–3.0	0.2	0.0450 mg/kg/h
15–29	3.1–6.0	0.2	0.0225 mg/kg/h
<15	> 6	0.2	0.1000 mg/kg bolus every other day if activated partial thromboplastin time <1.5 times baseline

TOXIC DOSE

The *therapeutic dose* of lepirudin is 0.4 mg/kg intravenous bolus followed by an infusion rate of 0.15 mg/kg/hour. The rate is adjusted for impaired renal function (Table 1). Although few data are available, the same dose has been used in children. Antihirudin antibodies may significantly enhance the anticoagulant effect of lepirudin, probably by decreased renal clearance of the lepirudin-immunoglobulin complex (1,3). Dosing may have to be adjusted in patients treated with lepirudin for more than 5 days (3). Lepirudin is not recommended for long-term therapy; however, treatment for 8 months with subcutaneous lepirudin has been reported without complication (4).

Limited information is available on toxic dose. An inadvertent 30-fold increase in dose in a patient with renal failure produced a blood concentration greater than 5 mg/L (5). The patient was rapidly treated with hemodiafiltration, and no bleeding complications occurred.

TOXICOKINETICS AND TOXICODYNAMICS

Pharmacokinetic data are provided in Table 2. Data regarding toxicokinetics and toxicodynamics have not been reported.

PATHOPHYSIOLOGY

Thrombin is responsible for activation of platelets and factor V and VIII. It also stabilizes and enlarges existing thrombi by cleavage of fibrinogen to fibrin and activation of factor XIII. Fibrin-bound thrombin mediates platelet recruitment into existing thrombi. Lepirudin and desirudin directly inhibit the active site pocket and the fibrinogen-binding site of free and clot-bound thrombin, causing it to lose its effect on coagulation and platelets (1). The significant differences between the recombinant hirudins and heparin are: (a) The recombinant hirudins are direct inhibitors of thrombin, whereas the heparins require the cofactor antithrombin III; (b) the recombinant hirudins are able to inactivate clot-bound thrombin as well as circulating thrombin, whereas the heparins only inactivate circulating thrombin; and (c) lack of effect on platelet factor 4.

TABLE 2. Pharmacokinetic parameters for lepirudin

Bioavailability is 100%.
T_{max} (intravenous) is 5–18 min.
T_{max} (subcutaneous) is 3–4 h.
Volume of distribution is 0.2 L/kg.
Protein binding is <10%.
Terminal elimination half-life is dependent on renal function. In healthy volunteers, half-life is 0.8–1.7 h, which may lengthen to 150 h in renal failure.
Route of excretion is 90% renal.
Excreted unchanged is 38–65%.
Active catabolic metabolite is 30%.

T_{max}, time-to-peak plasma concentration.

PREGNANCY AND LACTATION

There are no data on use of lepirudin in pregnancy or breast-feeding. At this time, it cannot be recommended.

CLINICAL PRESENTATION

Acute Overdose

The major effects expected are prolongation of bleeding time and hemorrhage. In trials of lepirudin treatment of heparin-induced thrombocytopenia, minor bleeding was more frequent in the lepirudin treatment group than in historical controls, 39% versus 27%, respectively. However, there was no significant difference in bleedings requiring transfusions (1). Major bleeding is expected to be more common in overdose. In the single reported overdose, an inadvertent 30-fold increase in dose in a patient with renal failure produced a blood concentration greater than 5 mg/L (5). The patient was rapidly treated with hemodiafiltration, and no bleeding complications occurred.

Adverse Reactions

Renal impairment and antilepirudin immunoglobulins (often produced after more than 5 days of therapy) both reduce lepirudin elimination and may require a reduction adjustment of dosage. Combined use of lepirudin with aspirin or glycoprotein IIb/IIIa inhibitors could increase the risk of bleeding.

DIAGNOSTIC TESTS

Assays for specific drug concentrations are not widely available and therefore are of limited clinical value for routine monitoring. The therapeutic range is 0.5 to 1.5 mg/L. Lepirudin is best monitored by the ecarin clotting time, but limited availability of the ecarin clotting time may reduce its use (6). The activated partial thromboplastin time is routinely used to monitor therapy; in overdose, serial measurement of the complete blood cell count and activated partial thromboplastin time should be made (1).

TREATMENT

Decontamination is not feasible because lepirudin and desirudin are administered parenterally. The drugs should be discontinued. Hemorrhage is treated, as from any cause, with local pressure, fluid resuscitation, and pressors, if necessary. If bleeding is minimal and the patient has adequate renal function, no treatment may be necessary due to the short half-life of the drug.

Enhanced Elimination

Extracorporeal elimination of lepirudin is highly variable. Hemodialysis has no effect on clearance (6–8). Hemofiltration and modified ultrafiltration commonly used during cardiopulmonary bypass surgery and hemodiafiltration using high-flux capillary dialyzer polysulfone can significantly increase the elimination of lepirudin (5,9). The filtering capability is determined more by the electrostatic charge of the membrane material than by pore size (9). Plasmapheresis filters are more effective hemofilters but have the disadvantage of potentially removing large amounts of plasma proteins, including the circulating clotting factors (9). The hemofilter systems removed between 15% and 42% of circulation lepirudin. The plasmapheresis filter systems removed 63% to 65% of circulating lepirudin (9).

Antidote

There is no specific antidote for lepirudin or desirudin available (1). Small trials of desmopressin show a reversing effect (10,11), but more information is needed before it can be recommended.

REFERENCES

1. Greinacher A, Lubenow N. Recombinant hirudin in clinical practice: focus on lepirudin. *Circulation* 2001;103:1479–1483.
2. Eriksson BI, Ekman S, Kalebo P, et al. Prevention of deep-venous thrombosis after total hip replacement: direct thrombin inhibition with recombinant hirudin, CGP 39393. *Lancet* 1996;347:635–639.
3. Eichler P, Friesen HJ, Lubenow N, et al. Antihirudin antibodies in patients with heparin-induced thrombocytopenia treated with lepirudin: incidence, effects on aPTT and clinical relevance. *Blood* 2000;96:2373–2378.
4. Andreescu AC, Cushman M, Hammond JM, Wood ME. Trousseau's syndrome treated with long-term subcutaneous lepirudin. *J Thromb Thrombolysis* 2001;11:33–37.
5. Bauersachs RM, Lindhoff-Last E, Ehrly AM, et al. Treatment of hirudin overdosage in a patient with chronic renal failure. *Thromb Haemost* 1999;81:323–324.
6. Wittkowsky AK, Kondo M. Lepirudin dosing in dialysis-dependent renal failure. *Pharmacotherapy* 2000;20:1123–1128.
7. VanHolder R, Camez A, Veys N. Pharmacokinetics of recombinant hirudin in haemodialyzed end-stage renal failure patients. *Thromb Haemost* 1997;77:650–655.
8. Van Wyk V, Badenhorst PH, Luus HG, Kotze HF. A comparison between the use of recombinant hirudin and heparin during hemodialysis. *Kidney Int* 1999;56[Suppl 72]:46S–50S.
9. Koster A, Merkle F, Hansen R, et al. Elimination of recombinant hirudin by modified ultrafiltration during simulated cardiopulmonary bypass: assessment of different filter systems. *Anesth Analg* 2000;91:265–269.
10. Ibbotson SH, Grant PJ, Kerry R, et al. The influence of infusions of 1-desamino-8-D-arginine vasopressin (DDAVP) in vivo on the anticoagulant effect of recombinant hirudin (CGP39393) in vitro. *Thromb Haemost* 1991;65:64–66.
11. Amin DM, Mant TG, Walker SM, et al. Effect of a 15-minute infusion of DDAVP on the pharmacokinetics and pharmacodynamics of REVASC during a four-hour intravenous infusion in healthy male volunteers. *Thromb Haemost* 1997;77:127–132.

CHAPTER 110

Coagulants

Andrew R. Erdman

H_2N … OH, O

AMINOCAPROIC ACID

Compounds included:	**Aminocaproic acid (Amicar); aprotinin (Trasylol, Antagosan); factor VIII (antihemophilic factor) (Alphanate, Hemofil M, Humate-P, Koāte-DVI, Monarc-M, Monoclate-P, Hyate:C, Bioclate, Helixate, Helixate FS, Kogenate, Kogenate FS, Recombinate); thrombin (factor IIa, Thrombin-JMI, Thrombogen, Topostasin)**
Molecular formula and weight:	**See Table 1.**
SI conversion:	**See Table 1.**
CAS Registry No.:	**60-32-2 (aminocaproic acid); 9087-70-1 (aprotinin); 9002-04-4 (thrombin)**
Therapeutic levels:	**Not clinically applicable**
Special concerns:	**Hypersensitivity reactions, hypercoagulability and systemic thrombosis (theoretic)**
Antidote:	**None**

AMINOCAPROIC ACID

Aminocaproic acid (ACA; ε-ACA or 6-aminohexanoic acid) is a synthetic antifibrinolytic agent used for the management of patients with bleeding that involves excessive fibrinolysis. Fibrinolysis is the process that results, ultimately, in the dissolution of blood clots within the body. The crucial component of fibrinolysis is the activation of the circulating protein and plasminogen by various activators to form plasmin. Plasmin in turn catalyzes the cleavage of fibrin (as well as its precursor fibrinogen), one of the essential components of all blood clots. Excessive fibrinolysis can lead to a bleeding diathesis. Conditions often associated with fibrinolysis include the postsurgical period (particularly after cardiac bypass), cirrhosis, placental abruption, cancer, and various hematologic disorders (1).

ACA antagonizes fibrinolysis by competitively inhibiting various plasminogen activators (Fig. 1) (2–6). It does so probably because of its structural similarity to lysine and arginine, the amino acids in plasminogen to which various plasminogen activators bind. In addition, ACA may bind directly to both plas-

TABLE 1. Molecular formula and weight for coagulants

Drug	Molecular formula	Molecular weight (g/mol)	SI conversion
Aminocaproic acid	$C_6H_{13}NO_2$	131.17	mg/L × 7.62 = µmol/L
Aprotinin	$C_{284}H_{432}N_{84}O_{79}S_7$	6512	NA
Factor VIII			NA
Human light chain	—	Approximately 80,000	NA
Human heavy chain	—	Approximately 90,000–210,000	NA
Thrombin	—	Approximately 37,000	NA

minogen and active plasmin to form complexes with an altered conformation and decreased functionality (7). The end clinical result is an inhibition of fibrinolysis and a shift in the balance away from clot breakdown (8).

ACA is indicated for the management of patients with ongoing bleeding due, at least in part, to excessive fibrinolysis. The drug has also been used in patients with a variety of other bleeding disorders and prophylactically for certain high-risk individuals, with variable success; also it has been used in the management of patients with angioneurotic edema (9–19). It is typically not recommended for patients with disseminated intravascular coagulation, a type of secondary fibrinolysis, because it may predispose such patients to intravascular thrombosis, which in turn can exacerbate both disseminated intravascular coagulation and any fibrinolysis (19).

ACA is available as a 500-mg tablet, a syrup of 1250 mg/5 ml, and a 250-mg/ml intravenous (IV) solution.

Toxic Dose

The usual *adult therapeutic dose* is 5 g IV over 1 hour followed by a continuous infusion of 1 g/hour for 8 hours or until excessive bleeding has stopped. Up to 48 g/day has been used in certain patients (1,16). The oral dose is the same as the IV dose, but other regimens have been proposed (20). The toxic dose of ACA is not known. One report of renal failure occurred after a dose of 12 g, but others have tolerated doses of 100 g without significant problems (1).

Toxicokinetics and Toxicodynamics

An oral therapeutic dose of ACA is rapidly absorbed with a peak plasma drug level of 1 to 2 hours or 30 minutes after IV infusion (1). Peak clinical effects occur 15 to 60 minutes after infusion (1,8,21). Its volume of distribution (V_d) is 0.4 L/kg (1,8). ACA is primarily eliminated by renal excretion of the unchanged drug (60% to 95% of an ingested dose) and of its primary metabolite, adipic acid (8,22,23). The terminal elimination

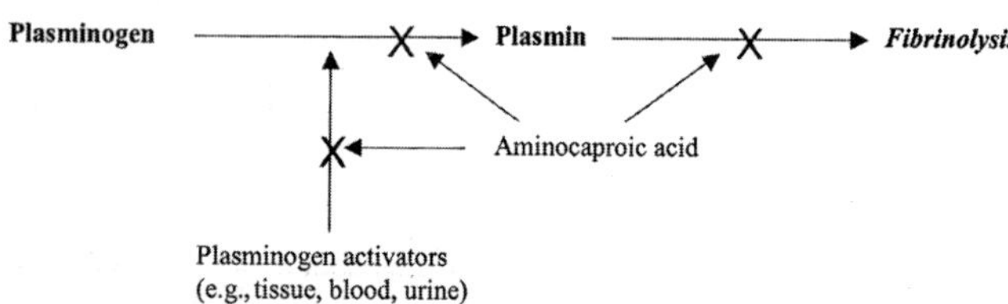

Figure 1. Diagram of fibrinolytic system and its primary and secondary mechanisms of inhibition by aminocaproic acid.

half-life of ACA is 2 hours, and the duration of effect is approximately 3 hours (1,19,21,23). These values may differ after overdose. In patients with renal failure, ACA or its metabolites can accumulate and lead to toxicity (24,25). A reduction in dosing may be necessary in patients with renal insufficiency.

Pathophysiology

Little is known about ACA overdose. Reported effects range from no toxicity to transient hypotension to acute renal failure (1,26). One death has occurred in a patient who developed renal failure. At lower doses, the hypotension is generally mild and transient; however, it may be more severe or sustained with larger doses or rapid infusions (1,14,17,27,28). The reason for hypotension is unclear. Tachy- or bradydysrhythmias may also occur with rapid or high-dose infusions, as may seizures and delirium (1,19,29–31). Their pathophysiology is uncertain.

Renal insufficiency may develop with ACA use (26). It may be secondary to hypotension, rhabdomyolysis, or genitourinary tract obstruction by blood clots in patients with significant hematuria. Cases of rhabdomyolysis and severe myopathy have been reported (32–34). The pathophysiology is unknown but appears to be a direct effect.

Because ACA inhibits fibrin breakdown and disrupts the normal equilibrium between clot formation and breakdown, its use has been associated with the development of intravascular thrombosis, in some cases, with life-threatening complications (25,35–38). The exact incidence of thrombosis associated with ACA use is not clear, and some studies have found no increased risk at all (27,39,40). Conversely, other authors have found high doses (greater than 24 g/day) to be associated with prolonged bleeding times and a paradoxic bleeding diathesis, probably as the result of platelet dysfunction (41).

Blood clots formed in the presence of ACA may fail to undergo spontaneous lysis and resolution if they occur in the pleural or pericardial spaces or in other body cavities. Similarly, patients with hematuria who are treated with ACA may develop urinary tract clots that can obstruct the normal flow of urine, leading to renal insufficiency.

Hypersensitivity reactions have been reported. They may be localized or systemic (e.g., anaphylactic or anaphylactoid shock, nasal congestion, conjunctival irritation, or pruritus) (39,42). ACA may also cause dose-dependent nausea, metabolic acidosis, hyperkalemia, and various dermatologic manifestations such as dermatitis and bullae formation (1,24,39,43,44).

Pregnancy and Lactation

ACA is U.S. Food and Drug Administration (FDA) pregnancy category C (Appendix I). It is teratogenic in rats (45). Excretion into human breast milk is not known.

Clinical Presentation

OVERDOSAGE

There are few reports of ACA overdose. Effects have ranged from no demonstrable sequelae to transient hypotension to acute renal failure (1,26). One death occurred in a patient who developed renal failure. The adverse effects associated with therapeutic use may theoretically occur after overdoses.

ADVERSE EVENTS

Patients may develop signs and symptoms of hypotension with IV use (e.g., weakness, dizziness, syncope). At normal doses, the decrease in blood pressure is generally mild and transient; however, with larger doses or rapid infusions, hypotension may be more severe or sustained (1,14,17,27,28). Tachy- or bradydysrhythmias may also occur with rapid or high-dose infusions, as may seizures and delirium (1,19,29–31).

Renal insufficiency is heralded by the onset of oliguria or rising serum creatinine levels (26). Rhabdomyolysis and myopathy may present with muscle pain or weakness, myoglobinuria, elevated serum creatine phosphokinase levels or, in some cases, renal insufficiency (32–34).

Signs and symptoms of spontaneous arterial or venous thrombosis depend on their location, size, and degree of obstruction. Obstructive clots in the genitourinary system generally present with decreased urine output, flank pain, and sudden cessation of hematuria.

Hypersensitivity reactions may be mild to severe, with symptoms ranging from pruritus, urticaria, or a dermal rash, to nausea, vomiting, fever, dyspnea, chest tightness, wheezing, angioedema, stridor, tachycardia, hypotension, and cardiovascular collapse. ACA may also cause dose-dependent nausea, metabolic acidosis, hyperkalemia, and various dermatologic manifestations such as dermatitis and bullae formation (1,24,39,43,44).

Diagnostic Tests

There are no readily available tests to diagnose poisoning. Plasma ACA levels can be performed but are not readily available and are not commonly used. They could be helpful in corroborating the diagnosis retrospectively. Levels of 130 μg/ml have been associated with clinically significant inhibition of fibrinolysis and improvement in hemostasis and are generally considered therapeutic (23,24).

A complete blood cell count, serum electrolytes, renal function tests and urinalysis, coagulation tests, creatine kinase, and other tests may be needed in symptomatic patients to assess adverse effects. Patients with evidence of intravascular thrombosis generally require radiographic or angiographic studies to confirm the diagnosis, depending on the location and symptoms.

Treatment

The management of overdose or toxicity is supportive and symptomatic. Given its duration of action (approximately 3 hours), most of the clinical effects are likely to be short-lived unless underlying renal insufficiency or ongoing absorption is present.

DECONTAMINATION

Decontamination measures have not been evaluated. Patients should receive activated charcoal if the patient presents early. Gastric lavage and other decontamination measures are unlikely to be necessary unless life-threatening coingestants are suspected.

ENHANCED ELIMINATION

ACA appears to be removed by hemodialysis (46).

ANTIDOTE

There is no specific antidote for ACA toxicity.

SUPPORTIVE CARE

Hypotension, dysrhythmias, hypersensitivity reactions, and seizures are treated in the usual manner (Chapters 37, 34, and 40, respectively). Mild hypersensitivity reactions generally resolve spontaneously after cessation of the ACA infusion (8). Patients with renal failure may require hemodialysis, using the usual indications. The use of dialysis specifically to remove ACA or reduce any signs of toxicity has not been evaluated.

Patients with blood clots after ACA therapy are treated like any other patient with intravascular thrombosis, except that such patients may be more resistant to thrombolytic drugs.

APROTININ

Aprotinin is a naturally occurring serine protease inhibitor derived from bovine lung tissue. It inhibits a wide range of proteins. The precise mechanism underlying its hemostatic action is unclear, but it involves several major pathways (47). For one, it antagonizes fibrinolysis by competitively inhibiting plasmin (48). It further reduces fibrinolysis by inhibiting plasma kallikrein and tissue kallikrein, which normally help to convert plasminogen to plasmin (49,50). During cardiac bypass surgery, aprotinin prevents the extracorporeal decrease in platelet aggregability, probably by preserving various platelet glycoproteins (51–53). Aprotinin also inhibits the activation of the intrinsic clotting cascade, a process that normally initiates both coagulation and subsequent fibrinolysis (54). In doing so, it prevents inappropriate activation of coagulation during cardiac bypass. Finally, aprotinin at higher doses may inhibit proinflammatory cytokine release and prevent an extracorporeal-induced inflammatory response (55–60).

Aprotinin is indicated for prophylactic use to minimize perioperative blood loss in patients undergoing cardiac bypass surgery (61–66). It has also been used prophylactically for other surgeries in which significant blood loss is common, such as orthopedic and transplantation procedures; in patients on extracorporeal life support; in patients with active postsurgical hemorrhage; and for patients with pancreatitis (67–71). Aprotinin is available as a colorless, isotonic solution for IV administration, which contains 10,000 kallikrein-inhibiting unit (KIU)/ml (1.4 mg/ml) and is packaged in vials of 100 or 200 ml. Occasionally, it is also found in topical fibrin sealant preparations (72,73).

Toxic Dose

The recommended *adult therapeutic dose* for prophylactic use of aprotinin in patients undergoing cardiac bypass surgery is an IV load (through a central line) of 2 million KIU (280 mg) given over 20 to 30 minutes before cannulation, followed by a constant infusion of 500,000 KIU/hour (70 mg/hour) until the surgery is finished, and given along with a "pump prime" dose of 2 million KIU added to the recirculating priming fluid of the cardiac bypass circuit before bypass (61). A test dose to screen for hypersensitivity reactions is recommended by the manufacturer, but false-negative reactions may occur (61).

No cases of overdose have been reported. One patient received more than 15 million KIU over 24 hours and later died with postoperative hepatic and renal failure; however, the relationship to aprotinin is not clear (61). Doses up to 17.5 million KIU have been administered to other subjects over 24 hours without significant adverse effects (61).

Toxicokinetics and Toxicodynamics

Aprotinin levels peak almost instantaneously, then fall as the drug is rapidly distributed to the extracellular space. The terminal elimination half-life is approximately 7 to 10 hours (61,74–76). Drug elimination is primarily via renal metabolism (20,61). Aprotinin is filtered by the glomerulus and then actively reabsorbed by the proximal tubules, where it is stored in the phagolysosomes and metabolized to smaller peptides and amino acids (77). Less than 10% is excreted unchanged in the urine. One study suggests that clearance of the drug decreases, and its elimination half-life increases in patients with impaired creatinine clearance (76). Its pharmacokinetics in patients with underlying hepatic insufficiency are not known.

Pathophysiology

When used therapeutically, the drug is extremely safe (78,79). Its primary adverse effects are hypersensitivity reactions, ranging from mild (e.g., dermal rash, pruritus) to severe and life-threatening (e.g., bronchospasm, shock) (61,72,80). The incidence of hypersensitivity reactions ranges from 2.7% to 5.0% in those who have had prior exposure to the drug (especially within the previous 6 months) and from 0.1% to 0.6% in patients without prior exposure (61,78).

In some studies, aprotinin has been associated with early vein graft occlusion after coronary bypass surgery (78,81–83). However, other significant thrombotic sequelae have not been reported in humans, and studies have not found an increase in the overall risk of thrombotic events when compared with placebo (61,67,78,84). The use of aprotinin is associated with minimal transient increases in postoperative serum creatinine, but clinically significant renal insufficiency was not found in controlled trials (64,85).

Pregnancy and Lactation

Aprotinin is FDA pregnancy category B (Appendix I). Animal studies have not shown evidence of fetotoxicity or teratogenicity (61). Entry into human breast milk is unknown.

Clinical Presentation

ACUTE OVERDOSAGE

There are no reports of acute or chronic aprotinin overdose in the literature. One poorly documented case noted the death of a patient with postoperative hepatic and renal failure after receiving more than 15 million KIU over 24 hours; however, the relationship of these effects to aprotinin is not clear (61).

ADVERSE REACTIONS

Hypersensitivity reactions may be mild to severe, with symptoms ranging from pruritus, urticaria, or a dermal rash, to nausea, vomiting, fever, dyspnea, chest tightness, wheezing, angioedema, stridor, tachycardia, hypotension, and cardiovascular collapse (61,72,80). Signs and symptoms typically begin within minutes of starting or increasing the drug infusion.

Patients with premature venous graft occlusion may be asymptomatic or present with signs and symptoms of myocardial infarction.

Diagnostic Tests

Plasma aprotinin levels are not readily available. Aprotinin may prolong partial thromboplastin time (PTT) and activated clotting time to varying degrees, depending on how each test is performed (86–88). However, it is not clear if these tests can serve as a reliable surrogate marker for aprotinin concentrations. Moreover, the clinical significance of such findings is unclear because aprotinin has not been associated with significant bleeding complications.

Treatment

Treatment is primarily symptomatic and supportive. The short half-life and duration of action indicate that toxicity is likely to be short-lived after the infusion is stopped.

DECONTAMINATION

If aprotinin toxicity or hypersensitivity is suspected, the infusion should be stopped immediately. Aprotinin, as a protein, is broken down in the stomach and is therefore unlikely to be toxic after ingestion.

ENHANCEMENT OF ELIMINATION

Given its size and molecular weight, aprotinin is unlikely to cross dialysis membranes.

ANTIDOTES

There is no specific antidote for aprotinin.

SUPPORTIVE CARE

The treatment of hypersensitivity reactions depends on their severity (Chapter 34). Patients with postsurgical venous graft occlusion should be managed in the usual fashion. Patients on aprotinin may be resistant to treatment with thrombolytic agents.

MONITORING

Patients with suspected or confirmed aprotinin overdose should be monitored clinically for the development of hypersensitivity reactions. Measurements of renal function (e.g., serum creatinine) and coagulation should be performed (e.g., activated clotting time, PTT) and followed serially if abnormal. Patients suspected of aprotinin toxicity should be monitored for a period of several hours or until clinical effects resolve.

FACTOR VIII (ANTIHEMOPHILIC FACTOR)

Endogenous factor VIII (antihemophilic factor) is an essential cofactor in the intrinsic blood coagulation cascade. In the process of hemostasis, factor VIII is activated and then serves as a cofactor for activated factor IX, which converts factor X to activated factor X. Endogenous factor VIII is bound to von Willebrand's factor, which helps stabilize the association between its two chains. Certain patients, such as those with hemophilia A or von Willebrand's disease, have deficient or dysfunctional factor VIII. In such patients, the administration of exogenous factor VIII can prevent and control bleeding (89–91). There are three types of commercially available exogenous factor VIII: human, porcine, or recombinant DNA. The recombinant form is currently considered the preparation of choice for most patients with hemophilia.

Human-derived factor VIII (antihemophilic factor, human) is a lyophilized powder prepared from pooled human plasma. It is indicated for the management and prevention of hemorrhage in patients with hemophilia A or acquired factor VIII deficiency. A variety of preparations are available (92,93). The potency of each preparation is expressed in antihemophilic factor units (AFU) or international units. As defined by the World Health Organization, 1 AFU equals 1 IU, which equals, approximately, the quantity of factor VIII contained in 1 ml of normal pooled human plasma.

Porcine-derived factor VIII (antihemophilic factor, porcine) is a lyophilized powder prepared from porcine plasma. It is structurally similar to endogenous human factor VIII and has nearly identical biologic effects. Its potency is expressed in porcine units of antihemophilic factor activity. The preparation available in the United States also contains porcine von Willebrand's factor (94).

Antihemophilic factor (recombinant) is a lyophilized powder prepared using recombinant DNA techniques (95,96). Recombinant factor VIII is structurally and functionally similar to the endogenous form. Some preparations also contain human albumin. Like antihemophilic factor (human), the potency of the recombinant product is expressed in IU or AFU.

All three antihemophilic factor preparations must be reconstituted with saline and are meant to be administered via IV infusion.

Toxic Dose

The *therapeutic dose* of exogenous antihemophilic factor depends on the patient's endogenous factor level, the clinical significance of any bleeding, the particular product being used, and the patient's inhibitor status (91). No cases of overdose with antihemophilic factors have been reported.

Toxicokinetics and Toxicodynamics

The initial instantaneous increase in coagulant activity is followed by a rapid initial decline in activity, representing equilibration of the drug with the extravascular space, and then later by a slower, steady decline, representing drug metabolism, use, or degradation (97). The half-life of recombinant antihemophilic factor is 12.7 to 15.8 hours (95,96,98). The half-life of antihemophilic factor (human) is similar, ranging from 16.1 to 17.9 hours (92,93,97,99). The half-life of the porcine product is slightly shorter, averaging approximately 10 to 11 hours (94,100). The volume of distribution of antihemophilic factor at steady-state ranges from 0.04 to 0.06 L/kg. The half-life values may decrease significantly in patients with hemophilia or circulating antihemophilic factor inhibitors or in the postsurgical period.

Pathophysiology

In one abstract, the authors indicate that massive doses of antihemophilic factor (human) can lead to hemolytic anemia, increased bleeding tendency, and hyperfibrinogenemia (101,102). The underlying pathophysiology of these effects and whether they are dose related is unclear.

The primary adverse effects of antihemophilic factors are hypersensitivity reactions and factor inhibitor formation. Infrequently, transmission of certain infectious diseases, blood-group incompatibility reactions, and thrombocytopenia may occur. These adverse effects may theoretically occur after overdoses as well as therapeutic use. Cases of thrombosis due to antihemophilic factor have not been reported.

Both anaphylactic and anaphylactoid reactions may occur. Their incidence ranges from 0.7% to 15.0%, but their overall frequency has declined in recent years due to the advent of purer, more refined formulations (92–96,103–108). Significant hypersensitivity reactions have not been reported with the current recombinant products (95,96).

Treatment with antihemophilic factor may induce or exacerbate the formation of factor VIII–inhibiting immunoglobulin G antibodies (antihemophilic inhibitors), which can neutralize, and hence reduce, the efficacy of future antihemophilic factor infusions (92–96,109–113). The inhibiting antibodies formed against human antihemophilic factor may also react to varying degrees with porcine antihemophilic factor and vice versa.

As a pooled human blood product, antihemophilic factor (human) carries the risk of disease transmission (e.g., hepatitis, parvovirus, Creutzfeldt-Jakob disease) (114). Hepatitis A seroconversion after treatment with U.S. antihemophilic factor (human) has occurred (92,93,115,116), but no cases of human immunodeficiency virus, hepatitis B or C, or other major infectious disease have been noted. There have been no reports of disease transmission to humans from the porcine product (94).

In addition, antihemophilic factor (human) contains trace amounts of blood groups A and B isohemagglutinins; therefore, large amounts given to individuals of the opposite blood type may rarely cause hemolysis and anemia (117–119). The porcine product has been associated with mild, transient thrombocytopenia, which generally does not affect hemostasis (120,121). The mechanism appears to be platelet aggregation caused by small amounts of porcine von Willebrand's factor in the preparation.

Pregnancy and Lactation

Factor VIII is FDA pregnancy category C (Appendix I). Entry into breast milk is unknown.

Clinical Presentation

ACUTE OR CHRONIC OVERDOSAGE

There are no reports of acute or chronic antihemophilic factor overdose in the literature. One author has reported that massive doses of antihemophilic factor (human) can lead to hemolytic anemia, increased bleeding tendency, and hyperfibrinogenemia (101,102).

ADVERSE REACTIONS

Hypersensitivity reactions may vary in severity, from mild to life-threatening, with symptoms ranging from burning, pruritus, urticaria, or a dermal rash, to nausea, vomiting, fever, dyspnea, chest tightness, wheezing, angioedema, stridor, tachycardia, hypotension, and cardiovascular collapse. Signs and symptoms typically begin within minutes of beginning or increasing the factor infusion (92–96,103–108).

Hemolysis after the use of human antihemophilic factor may be heralded by fever, chills, jaundice, anemia, evidence of hemolysis on peripheral blood smear, hemoglobinuria, and elevated serum lactate dehydrogenase levels or decreases in serum haptoglobin levels (117–119).

Inhibiting antibodies may become evident to clinicians when patients are noted to have a reduced clinical response to further factor infusions or when their presence is specifically measured in the laboratory.

Diagnostic Tests

Circulating factor VIII levels are often used to monitor antihemophilic factor therapy. Given that the assay is time consuming and that toxic levels have not been established, the test is unlikely to be useful in acute overdose.

A complete blood cell count should be checked because of the association between some antihemophilic factor products and hematologic abnormalities such as hemolytic anemia and thrombocytopenia. If hemolysis is suspected, serum haptoglobin and lactate dehydrogenase levels or tests for urinary hemoglobin may be helpful.

Therapeutic use of antihemophilic factor may be associated with normalization in PTTs, but it is unclear how overdoses of the drug would affect this assay. Various diagnostic tests can be performed to look for seroconversion, if a transfusion-associated infectious disease transmission is suspected.

Treatment

DECONTAMINATION

If toxicity or hypersensitivity are suspected, the drug infusion should be stopped. Because it is a protein, antihemophilic factor is broken down in the stomach and therefore unlikely to cause toxicity after ingestion.

ENHANCED ELIMINATION

There is no role for dialysis or other enhanced elimination techniques in the treatment of antihemophilic factor toxicity.

ANTIDOTES

There is no antidote for antihemophilic factor.

MONITORING

Patients should be monitored clinically for hypersensitivity reactions. Platelet and red blood cell counts should be monitored for hemolytic anemia (with human antihemophilic factor) or thrombocytopenia (with porcine antihemophilic factor). Patients should be monitored for clinical signs of bleeding and, if evident, coagulation tests should be performed.

SUPPORTIVE CARE

The treatment of hypersensitivity reactions depends on their severity (Chapter 34). Thrombocytopenia associated with the use of the porcine product does not typically require more than cessation of therapy. If needed, the patient may be switched to an alternative antihemophilic product. Severe thrombocytopenia or thrombocytopenia associated with bleeding complications may require platelet transfusions. Hemolytic anemia associated with the use of the human product should be managed by cessation of therapy and supportive measures (e.g., serial blood cell counts, hydration, and transfusions if required). If further factor replacement is necessary, the recombinant or porcine preparations should be considered.

THROMBIN

Endogenous thrombin (factor IIa) is a glycoprotein serine protease. Thrombin is formed *in vivo* from its precursor protein, prothrombin (factor II), a process catalyzed by activated factor X (factor Xa). Once formed, thrombin catalyzes the cleavage of fibrinogen to fibrin, which plays a critical role in normal hemostasis. Thrombin also activates factor XIII, which further strengthens the fibrin clot by cross-linking its monomeric subunits. Furthermore, thrombin enhances platelet aggregation and degranulation and affects the coagulation and inflammatory pathways in a variety of other complex ways.

Exogenous thrombin (factor IIa, Thrombin-JMI, Thrombogen, Topostasin) is a safe and effective topical hemostatic agent used in surgery for minor venous or capillary bleeding (122–125). It can be used with absorbable gelatin sponges for surgical hemostasis (126). It is sometimes used in conjunction with fibrinogen—this combination is typically referred to as *fibrin glue* (127).

The only commercially available product in the United States is bovine prothrombin that has been treated with calcium and thromboplastin in order to activate it (128). Thrombin is available as a lyophilized powder, in vials of varying strengths (1000 U, 5000 U, 10,000 U, 20,000 U, and 50,000 U).

Toxic Dose

The *therapeutic dose* of thrombin depends on the indication but generally solutions of 100 to 2000 U/ml are applied topically (128). No cases of overdose have been reported.

Toxicokinetics and Toxicodynamics

Little has been reported about the systemic pharmacokinetics of bovine thrombin preparations. Significant systemic absorption after topical administration has not been reported.

Pathophysiology

IV administration of bovine thrombin has not been reported but could lead to systemic intravascular coagulation and thrombosis. Excessive topical application has not been reported but could theoretically lead to systemic absorption and hypercoagulability. Therapeutic use of topical bovine thrombin has been associated with bleeding and significant coagulation abnormalities such as prolongation of prothrombin time and PTT (129–132). This is due to the formation of antibodies against the bovine prothrombin or factor V contained in the product, which then cross-react with and inhibit the function of the patient's endogenous coagulation factors.

Hypersensitivity reactions to topical thrombin have been reported in rare instances (128,133).

Pregnancy and Lactation

Bovine thrombin is FDA pregnancy category C (Appendix I). Excretion into breast milk is not known.

Clinical Presentation

IV administration or significant parenteral absorption through excessive topical application onto large open vessels could theoretically lead to intravascular clotting and thrombotic complications (e.g., stroke, myocardial infarction, pulmonary embolism).

Hypersensitivity reactions have occurred after topical use of bovine thrombin (128,133). Hypersensitivity reactions may be mild to severe, with symptoms ranging from burning, pruritus, urticaria, or a dermal rash, to nausea, vomiting, fever, dyspnea, chest tightness, wheezing, angioedema, stridor, tachycardia, hypotension, and cardiovascular collapse.

Coagulation abnormalities due to inhibitor formation and cross-reaction with endogenous clotting factors may present with signs of excessive bleeding or prolongation of prothrombin time or PTT.

Diagnostic Tests

Circulating thrombin levels can be measured. However, their use in cases of suspected overdose or toxicity has not been assessed. The patient's prothrombin time and PTT should be measured after overdoses or suspected toxicity. The work-up for suspected intravascular thrombosis could necessitate various laboratory studies, radiography, or angiography, depending on the suspected location and the patient's associated symptoms.

Treatment

Treatment of suspected overdoses or toxicity is generally supportive and symptomatic.

DECONTAMINATION

Application of the drug should be stopped and the site irrigated thoroughly. As a protein, thrombin is broken down in the stomach, and ingestion is not expected to result in clinical toxicity. Therefore, gastrointestinal decontamination is unnecessary unless significant coingestants are suspected.

ENHANCEMENT OF ELIMINATION

There is no role for dialysis or other enhanced elimination techniques in the elimination of bovine thrombin.

ANTIDOTE

There is no antidote for thrombin, although heparin may help antagonize its effects through the enhancement of antithrombin III activity.

SUPPORTIVE CARE

Patients with hypersensitivity reactions should be treated in the usual fashion, depending on the severity of symptoms

(Chapter 34). Patients with intravascular thrombosis may require treatment with heparinization or thrombolytics, if necessary, until clot resolution. However, patients with significant systemic absorption of thrombin may be resistant to the effects of these medications, and physicians should adjust the doses accordingly.

There is no specific treatment for patients who develop bleeding or coagulopathy associated with factor inhibitor formation. Further treatment with topical bovine thrombin should be avoided. Ongoing bleeding, depending on its location and severity, may necessitate blood product transfusions. One author has reported apparent temporal improvement with the use of IV immunoglobulins and steroids (129).

REFERENCES

1. Mikart I. Prescribing Information—aminocaproic acid. 2001.
2. Burchiel KJ, Hoffman JM, Bakay RA. Quantitative determination of plasma fibrinolytic activity in patients with ruptured intracranial aneurysms who are receiving epsilon-aminocaproic acid: relationship of possible complications of therapy to the degree of fibrinolytic inhibition. *Neurosurgery* 1984;14:57–63.
3. Ambrus CM, Ambrus JL, Lassman HB, Mink IB. Studies on the mechanism of action of inhibitors of the fibrinolysin system. *Ann N Y Acad Sci* 1968;146:430–447.
4. Ablondi FB, et al. Inhibition of plasmin and trypsin in the streptokinase activated fibrinolytic system by epsilon-aminocaproic acid. *Arch Biochem* 1959;82:153.
5. Alkjaersig N, Fletcher AP, Sherry S. Epsilon-aminocaproic acid: an inhibitor of plasminogen activation. *J Biol Chem* 1959;234:832.
6. Nilsson IM, Sjoerdsma A, Waldenstrom J. Antifibrinolytic activity and metabolism of epsilon-aminocaproic acid in man. *Lancet* 1960;1:1322.
7. Violand BN, Sodetz JM, Castellino FJ. The effect of epsilon-aminocaproic acid on the gross conformation of plasminogen and plasmin. *Arch Biochem Biophys* 1975;170:300–305.
8. Frederiksen MC, Bowsher DJ, Ruo TI, et al. Kinetics of epsilon-aminocaproic acid distribution, elimination, and antifibrinolytic effects in normal subjects. *Clin Pharmacol Ther* 1984;35:387–393.
9. Epsilon aminocaproic acid. *BMJ* 1967;4:725–726.
10. Landymore RW, Murphy JT, Lummis H, Carter C. The use of low-dose aprotinin, epsilon-aminocaproic acid or tranexamic acid for prevention of mediastinal bleeding in patients receiving aspirin before coronary artery bypass operations. *Eur J Cardiothorac Surg* 1997;11:798–800.
11. Jordan D, Delphin E, Rose E. Prophylactic epsilon-aminocaproic acid (EACA) administration minimizes blood replacement therapy during cardiac surgery. *Anesth Analg* 1995;80:827–829.
12. Henry DA, Moxey AJ, Carless PA, et al. Anti-fibrinolytic use for minimising perioperative allogeneic blood transfusion. *Cochrane Database Syst Rev* 2001:CD001886.
13. Kutner B, Fourman S, Brein K, et al. Aminocaproic acid reduces the risk of secondary hemorrhage in patients with traumatic hyphema. *Arch Ophthalmol* 1987;105:206–208.
14. Palmer DJ, Goldberg MF, Frenkel M, et al. A comparison of two dose regimens of epsilon aminocaproic acid in the prevention and management of secondary traumatic hyphemas. *Ophthalmology* 1986;93:102–108.
15. Garewal HS, Durie BG. Anti-fibrinolytic therapy with aminocaproic acid for the control of bleeding in thrombocytopenic patients. *Scand J Haematol* 1985;35:497–500.
16. Adams HP Jr, Nibbelink DW, Torner JC, Sahs AL. Antifibrinolytic therapy in patients with aneurysmal subarachnoid hemorrhage. A report of the cooperative aneurysm study. *Arch Neurol* 1981;38:25–29.
17. Gardner FH, Helmer RE 3rd. Aminocaproic acid. Use in control of hemorrhage in patients with amegakaryocytic thrombocytopenia. *JAMA* 1980;243:35–37.
18. Frank M, Gelfand JA, Alling DW, Sherins RJ. Epsilon aminocaproic acid for hereditary angioedema. *N Engl J Med* 1977;296:1235–1236.
19. Griffin JD, Ellman L. Epsilon-aminocaproic acid (EACA). *Semin Thromb Hemost* 1978;5:27–40.
20. Verstraete M. Clinical application of inhibitors of fibrinolysis. *Drugs* 1985;29:236–261.
21. Bergin JJ. The complications of therapy with epsilon-aminocaproic acid. *Med Clin North Am* 1966;50:1669–1678.
22. Dvorchik BH, Katlic KL, Hayes AH Jr, Eyster ME. Effect of probenecid on the kinetics of epsilon-aminocaproic acid. *Clin Pharmacol Ther* 1980;28:223–228.
23. McNicol GP, Fletcher AP, Alkjaersig N, Sherry S. The absorption, distribution, and excretion of epsilon-aminocaproic acid following oral or intravenous administration to man. *J Lab Clin Med* 1962;59:15–24.
24. Budris WA, Roxe DM, Duvel JM. High anion gap metabolic acidosis associated with aminocaproic acid. *Ann Pharmacother* 1999;33:308–311.
25. Naeye RL. Thrombotic state after hemorrhagic diathesis, a possible complication of therapy with epsilon-aminocaproic. *Blood* 1962;19:694.
26. Manjunath G, Fozailoff A, Mitcheson D, Sarnak MJ. Epsilon-aminocaproic acid and renal complications: case report and review of the literature. *Clin Nephrol* 2002;58:63–67.
27. Nilsson IM, Andersson L, Bjorkman SE. Epsilon-aminocaproic acid (E-ACA) as a therapeutic agent based on 5 year's clinical experience. *Acta Med Scand Suppl* 1966;448:1–46.
28. Swartz C, Onesti G, Ramirez O, et al. Cardiac and renal hemodynamic effects of the antifibrinolytic agent, epsilon aminocaproic acid. *Curr Ther Res Clin Exp* 1966;8:336–342.
29. Rabinovici R, Heyman A, Kluger Y, Shinar E. Convulsions induced by aminocaproic acid infusion. *DICP* 1989;23:780–781.
30. Wysenbeek AJ, Sella A, Blum I, Yeshurun D. Acute delirious state after epsilon-amino caproic acid administration. *J Toxicol Clin Toxicol* 1979;14:93–95.
31. Feffer SE, Parray HR, Westring DW. Seizure after infusion of aminocaproic acid. *JAMA* 1978;240:2468.
32. Seymour BD, Rubinger M. Rhabdomyolysis induced by epsilon-aminocaproic acid. *Ann Pharmacother* 1997;31:56–58.
33. Winter SS, Chaffee S, Kahler SG, Graham ML. ε-Aminocaproic acid-associated myopathy in a child. *J Pediatr Hematol Oncol* 1995;17:53–55.
34. Kane MJ, Silverman LR, Rand JH, et al. Myonecrosis as a complication of the use of epsilon amino-caproic acid: a case report and review of the literature. *Am J Med* 1988;85:861–863.
35. Fanashawe MP, Shore-Lesserson L, Reich DL. Two cases of fatal thrombosis after aminocaproic acid therapy and deep hypothermic circulatory arrest. *Anesthesiology* 2001;95:1525–1527.
36. Haddy SM, Shely WW, Rice N. Intravascular thrombosis after exsanguination in a patient treated with epsilon-aminocaproic acid. *J Cardiothorac Vasc Anesth* 1996;10:510–512.
37. Hocker JR, Saving KL. Fatal aortic thrombosis in a neonate during infusion of epsilon-aminocaproic acid. *J Pediatr Surg* 1995;30:1490–1492.
38. Hoffman EP, Koo AH. Cerebral thrombosis associated with Amicar therapy. *Radiology* 1979;131:687–689.
39. Vinnicombe J, Shuttleworth KE. Aminocaproic acid in the control of haemorrhage after prostatectomy. Safety of aminocaproic acid—a controlled trial. *Lancet* 1966;1:232–234.
40. Black WD, Hatch FE, Acchiardo S. Aminocaproic acid in prolonged hematuria of patients with sicklemia. *Arch Intern Med* 1976;136:678–681.
41. Glick R, Green D, Ts'ao C, et al. High dose epsilon-aminocaproic acid prolongs the bleeding time and increases rebleeding and intraoperative hemorrhage in patients with subarachnoid hemorrhage. *Neurosurgery* 1981;9:398–401.
42. Yien HW, Hseu SS, Chan KH, Lee TY. Suspected anaphylactoid shock to aminocaproic acid (plaslloid) during operation. *Zhonghua Yi Xue Za Zhi (Taipei)* 1992;50:415–419.
43. Perazella MA, Biswas P. Acute hyperkalemia associated with intravenous epsilon-aminocaproic acid therapy. *Am J Kidney Dis* 1999;33:782–785.
44. Brooke CP, Spiers EM, Omura EF. Noninflammatory bullae associated with epsilon-aminocaproic acid infusion. *J Am Acad Dermatol* 1992;27:880–882.
45. Dubin NH, Cummings DB, Blake DA, King TM. Effect of epsilon amino caproic acid, a fibrinolytic inhibitor, on implantation and fetal viability in the rat. *Biol Reprod* 1980;23:553–557.
46. Haug MT 3rd, Mauro VF, Davis HH. Effect of renal failure and hemodialysis on aminocaproic acid plasma concentrations. *DICP* 1989;23:922–923.
47. Royston D. The serine antiprotease aprotinin (Trasylol): a novel approach to reducing postoperative bleeding. *Blood Coagul Fibrinolysis* 1990;1:55–69.
48. Longstaff C. Studies on the mechanisms of action of aprotinin and tranexamic acid as plasmin inhibitors and antifibrinolytic agents. *Blood Coagul Fibrinolysis* 1994;5:537–542.
49. Campbell DJ, Dixon B, Kladis A, et al. Activation of the kallikrein-kinin system by cardiopulmonary bypass in humans. *Am J Physiol Regul Integr Comp Physiol* 2001;281:R1059–R1070.
50. Hoffmann H, Siebeck M, Thetter O, et al. Aprotinin concentrations effective for the inhibition of tissue kallikrein and plasma kallikrein in vitro and in vivo. *Adv Exp Med Biol* 1989;247B:35–42.
51. Tabuchi N, De Haan J, Boonstra PW, et al. Aprotinin effect on platelet function and clotting during cardiopulmonary bypass. *Eur J Cardiothorac Surg* 1994;8:87–90.
52. van Oeveren W, Harder MP, Roozendaal KJ, et al. Aprotinin protects platelets against the initial effect of cardiopulmonary bypass. *J Thorac Cardiovasc Surg* 1990;99:788–796; discussion 796–797.
53. Wendel HP, Schulze HJ, Heller W, Hoffmeister HM. Platelet protection in coronary artery surgery: benefits of heparin-coated circuits and high-dose aprotinin therapy. *J Cardiothorac Vasc Anesth* 1999;13:388–392.
54. de Smet AA, Joen MC, van Oeveren W, et al. Increased anticoagulation during cardiopulmonary bypass by aprotinin. *J Thorac Cardiovasc Surg* 1990;100:520–527.
55. Coeugniet E. Lymphokines and thrombosis. Thrombocyte and coagulation activation by culture supernatants of concanavalin-A-stimulated human lymphocytes. Some physicochemical properties and inhibition by chemical compounds. *Scand J Haematol Suppl* 1979;34:90–102.
56. Hill GE, Taylor JA, Robbins RA. Differing effects of aprotinin and epsilon-aminocaproic acid on cytokine-induced inducible nitric oxide synthase expression. *Ann Thorac Surg* 1997;63:74–77.
57. Gilliland HE, Armstrong MA, Uprichard S, et al. The effect of aprotinin on interleukin-8 concentration and leukocyte adhesion molecule expression in an isolated cardiopulmonary bypass system. *Anaesthesia* 1999;54:427–433.

58. Greilich PE, Okada K, Latham P, et al. Aprotinin but not epsilon-aminocaproic acid decreases interleukin-10 after cardiac surgery with extracorporeal circulation: randomized, double-blind, placebo-controlled study in patients receiving aprotinin and epsilon-aminocaproic acid. *Circulation* 2001;104[12 Suppl 1]:I265–I269.
59. Asimakopoulos G, Lidington EA, Mason J, et al. Effect of aprotinin on endothelial cell activation. *J Thorac Cardiovasc Surg* 2001;122:123–128.
60. Wachtfogel YT, Kucich U, Hack CE, et al. Aprotinin inhibits the contact, neutrophil, and platelet activation systems during simulated extracorporeal perfusion. *J Thorac Cardiovasc Surg* 1993;106:1–9; discussion 9–10.
61. Trasylol (aprotinin injection). Prescribing information. West Haven, CT: Bayer Corporation, 2001.
62. Wildevuur CR, Eijsman L, Roozendaal KJ, et al. Platelet preservation during cardiopulmonary bypass with aprotinin. *Eur J Cardiothorac Surg* 1989;3:533–537; discussion 537–538.
63. Fremes SE, Wong BI, Lee E, et al. Metaanalysis of prophylactic drug treatment in the prevention of postoperative bleeding. *Ann Thorac Surg* 1994;58:1580–1588.
64. Ehrlich M, Grabenwoger M, Cartes-Zumelzu F, et al. Operations on the thoracic aorta and hypothermic circulatory arrest: is aprotinin safe? *J Thorac Cardiovasc Surg* 1998;115:220–225.
65. Harder MP, Eijsman L, Roozendaal KJ, et al. Aprotinin reduces intraoperative and postoperative blood loss in membrane oxygenator cardiopulmonary bypass. *Ann Thorac Surg* 1991;51:936–941.
66. Levy JH, Pifarre R, Schaff HV, et al. A multicenter, double-blind, placebo-controlled trial of aprotinin for reducing blood loss and the requirement for donor-blood transfusion in patients undergoing repeat coronary artery bypass grafting. *Circulation* 1995;92:2236–2244.
67. Samama CM, Langeron O, Rosencher N, et al. Aprotinin versus placebo in major orthopedic surgery: a randomized, double-blinded, dose-ranging study. *Anesth Analg* 2002;95:287–293.
68. Molenaar IQ, Begliomini B, Grazi GL, et al. The effect of aprotinin on renal function in orthotopic liver transplantation. *Transplantation* 2001;71:247–252.
69. Porte RJ, Molenaar IQ, Begliomini B, et al. Aprotinin and transfusion requirements in orthotopic liver transplantation: a multicentre randomised double-blind study. EMSALT Study Group. *Lancet* 2000;355:1303–1309.
70. Biswas AK, Lewis L, Sommerauer JF. Aprotinin in the management of life-threatening bleeding during extracorporeal life support. *Perfusion* 2000;15:211–216.
71. Trapnell JE, Rigby CC, Talbot CH, Duncan EH. A controlled trial of Trasylol in the treatment of acute pancreatitis. *Br J Surg* 1974;61:177–182.
72. Scheule AM, Beierlein W, Wendel HP, et al. Fibrin sealant, aprotinin, and immune response in children undergoing operations for congenital heart disease. *J Thorac Cardiovasc Surg* 1998;115:883–889.
73. Sirieix D, Chemla E, Castier Y, et al. Comparative study of different biological glues in an experimental model of surgical bleeding in anesthetized rats: platelet-rich and -poor plasma-based glue with and without aprotinin versus commercial fibrinogen-based glue. *Ann Vasc Surg* 1998;12:311–316.
74. Kaller H, Patzschke K, Wegner LA, Horster FA. Pharmacokinetic observations following intravenous administration of radioactive labeled aprotinin in volunteers. *Eur J Drug Metab Pharmacokinet* 1978;3:79–85.
75. Naito S, Hirano M, Yoshihara H, Ohta M. Pharmacokinetics on blood concentration of aprotinin (Trasylol) in humans. *Basic Pharmacol Ther* 1980;8:3613–3627.
76. O'Connor CJ, Brown DV, Avramov M, et al. The impact of renal dysfunction on aprotinin pharmacokinetics during cardiopulmonary bypass. *Anesth Analg* 1999;89:1101–1107.
77. Just M, Habermann E. The renal handling of biologically active peptides. *Contrib Nephrol* 1975;1:62–68.
78. Peters DC, Noble S. Aprotinin: an update of its pharmacology and therapeutic use in open heart surgery and coronary artery bypass surgery. *Drugs* 1999;57:233–260.
79. Rich JB. The efficacy and safety of aprotinin use in cardiac surgery. *Ann Thorac Surg* 1998;66[5 Suppl]:S6–S11; discussion S25–S28.
80. Cohen DM, Norberto J, Cartabuke R, Ryu G. Severe anaphylactic reaction after primary exposure to aprotinin. *Ann Thorac Surg* 1999;67:837–838.
81. Alderman EL, Levy JH, Rich JB, et al. Analyses of coronary graft patency after aprotinin use: results from the International Multicenter Aprotinin Graft Patency Experience (IMAGE) trial. *J Thorac Cardiovasc Surg* 1998;116:716–730.
82. Kalangos A, Tayyareci G, Pretre R, et al. Influence of aprotinin on early graft thrombosis in patients undergoing myocardial revascularization. *Eur J Cardiothorac Surg* 1994;8:651–656.
83. Cosgrove DM 3rd, Heric B, Lytle BW, et al. Aprotinin therapy for reoperative myocardial revascularization: a placebo-controlled study. *Ann Thorac Surg* 1992;54:1031–1036; discussion 1036–1038.
84. Murkin JM, Haig GM, Beer KJ, et al. Aprotinin decreases exposure to allogeneic blood during primary unilateral total hip replacement. *J Bone Joint Surg Am* 2000;82:675–684.
85. Lemmer JH Jr, Stanford W, Bonney SL, et al. Aprotinin for coronary artery bypass grafting: effect on postoperative renal function. *Ann Thorac Surg* 1995;59:132–136.
86. Wang JS, Lin CY, Hung WT, et al. In vitro effects of aprotinin on activated clotting time measured with different activators. *J Thorac Cardiovasc Surg* 1992;104:1135–1140.
87. Hunt BJ, Segal H, Yacoub M. Aprotinin and heparin monitoring during cardiopulmonary bypass. *Circulation* 1992;86[5 Suppl]:II410–II412.
88. Hendrice C, Schmartz D, Pradier O, et al. Effects of aprotinin on blood loss, heparin monitoring tests, and heparin doses in patients undergoing coronary artery bypass surgery. *J Cardiothorac Vasc Anesth* 1995;9:245–249.
89. Mannucci PM, Chediak J, Hanna W, et al. Treatment of von Willebrand disease with a high-purity factor VIII/von Willebrand factor concentrate: a prospective, multicenter study. *Blood* 2002;99:450–456.
90. Powell JS, Bush M, Harrison J, et al. Safety and efficacy of solvent/detergent-treated antihaemophilic factor with an added 80 degrees C terminal dry heat treatment in patients with haemophilia A. *Haemophilia* 2000;6:140–149.
91. Abildgaard CF, Simone JV, Corrigan JJ, et al. Treatment of hemophilia with glycine-precipitated factor 8. *N Engl J Med* 1966;275:471–475.
92. Alphanate [antihemophilic factor (human)]. Prescribing information. Los Angeles: Alpha Therapeutic Corporation, 2000.
93. Koate-DVI [antihemophilic factor (human)]. Prescribing information. West Haven, CT: Bayer Corporation, 2000.
94. Hyate:C [antihemophilic factor (porcine)]. Prescribing information. Berkshire, UK: Ipsen Biopharm Ltd, 2000.
95. Kogenate [antihemophilic factor (recombinant)]. Prescribing information. West Haven, CT: Bayer Corporation, 1998.
96. Helixate FS [antihemophilic factor (recombinant)]. Prescribing information. King of Prussia, PA: Aventis Behring Ltd, 2002.
97. Rousell RH, Kasper CK, Schwartz RS. The pharmacology of a new pasteurized antihemophilic factor concentrate derived from human blood plasma. *Transfusion* 1989;29:208–212.
98. Lee C. The use of recombinant factor VIII products in previously treated patients with hemophilia A: pharmacokinetics, efficacy, safety, and inhibitor development. *Semin Thromb Hemost* 2002;28:241–246.
99. Dobrkovska A, Krzensk U, Chediak JR. Pharmacokinetics, efficacy and safety of Humate-P in von Willebrand disease. *Haemophilia* 1998;4[Suppl 3]:33–39.
100. Hermans C, Owens D, Longo G, et al. Single-dose pharmacokinetics of porcine factor VIII (Hyate C). *Thromb Haemost* 2002;87:352–353.
101. Hathaway WE, Mahasandana C, Clarke S, Humbert JR. Paradoxical bleeding in intensively transfused hemophilics: alteration of platelet function. *Transfusion* 1973;13:6–12.
102. Hathaway WE, Mahasandana C, Clarke S. Alteration of platelet function after transfusion in hemophilia. *Proc 14th Ann Mtg, Am Soc Hematol* 1971; abstract 58:88(abst).
103. Eyster ME, Bowman HS, Haverstick JN. Adverse reactions to factor VIII infusions. *Ann Intern Med* 1977;87:248.
104. Prager D, Djerassi I, Eyster ME, et al. Pennsylvania state-wide hemophilia program: summary of immediate reactions with the use of factor VIII and factor IX concentrate. *Blood* 1979;53:1012–1013.
105. Brettler DB, Forsberg AD, Levine PH, et al. The use of porcine factor VIII concentrate (Hyate:C) in the treatment of patients with inhibitor antibodies to factor VIII. A multicenter US experience. *Arch Intern Med* 1989;149:1381–1385.
106. Bove JR, McIntosh S. Anaphylactic reaction to purified anti-hemophilic factor concentrate. *Transfusion* 1988;28:603.
107. Erskine JG, Davidson JF. Anaphylactic reaction to low-molecular-weight porcine factor VIII concentrates. *Br Med J (Clin Res Ed)* 1981;282:2011–2012.
108. Helmer RE 3rd, Alperin JB, Yunginger JW, Grant JA. Anaphylactic reactions following infusion of factor VIII in a patient with classic hemophilia. *Am J Med* 1980;69:953–957.
109. Brackmann HH, Schwaab R, Effenberger W, et al. Antibodies to factor VIII in hemophilia A patients. *Vox Sang* 2000;78[Suppl 2]:187–190.
110. de Biasi R, Rocino A, Papa ML, et al. Incidence of factor VIII inhibitor development in hemophilia A patients treated with less pure plasma derived concentrates. *Thromb Haemost* 1994;71:544–547.
111. Hay CR, Ludlam CA, Colvin BT, et al. Factor VIII inhibitors in mild and moderate-severity haemophilia A. UK Haemophilia Centre Directors Organisation. *Thromb Haemost* 1998;79:762–766.
112. Hoyer LW. Factor VIII inhibitors. *Curr Opin Hematol* 1995;2:365–371.
113. Kreuz W, Ettingshausen CE, Zyschka A, et al. Inhibitor development in previously untreated patients with hemophilia A: a prospective long-term follow-up comparing plasma-derived and recombinant products. *Semin Thromb Hemost* 2002;28:285–290.
114. Berntorp E. Viral safety issues: plasma-derived factor VIII. *Ann Hematol* 1994;68[Suppl 3]:S35–S36.
115. From the Centers for Disease Control and Prevention. Hepatitis A among persons with hemophilia who received clotting factor concentrate—United States, September–December 1995. *JAMA* 1996;275:427–428.
116. Soucie JM, Robertson BH, Bell BP, et al. Hepatitis A virus infections associated with clotting factor concentrate in the United States. *Transfusion* 1998;38:573–579.
117. Egberg N, Blomback M. High frequency of low plasma haptoglobin values found in hemophilia A patients on prophylactic treatment with factor VIII concentrates—a sign of hemolysis? *Thromb Haemost* 1981;46:554–557.
118. Hach-Wunderle V, Teixidor D, Zumpe P, et al. Anti-A in factor VIII concentrate: a cause of severe hemolysis in a patient with acquired factor VIII:C antibodies. *Infusionstherapie* 1989;16:100–101.
119. Orringer EP, Koury MJ, Blatt PM, Roberts HR. Hemolysis caused by factor VIII concentrates. *Arch Intern Med* 1976;136:1018–1020.

120. Kernoff PB, Thomas ND, Lilley PA, et al. Clinical experience with polyelectrolyte-fractionated porcine factor VIII concentrate in the treatment of hemophiliacs with antibodies to factor VIII. *Blood* 1984;63:31–41.
121. Gatti L, Mannucci PM. Use of porcine factor VIII in the management of seventeen patients with factor VIII antibodies. *Thromb Haemost* 1984;51:379–384.
122. Lupinetti FM, Stoney WS, Alford WC Jr, et al. Cryoprecipitate-topical thrombin glue. Initial experience in patients undergoing cardiac operations. *J Thorac Cardiovasc Surg* 1985;90:502–505.
123. Ofodile FA, Sadana MK. The role of topical thrombin in skin grafting. *J Natl Med Assoc* 1991;83:416–418.
124. Jasani B, Baxter-Smith DC, Donaldson LJ, et al. Topical thrombin and control of wound haematoma. *Lancet* 1977;2:332–333.
125. Hashemi K, Donaldson LJ, Freeman JW, et al. The use of topical thrombin to reduce wound haematoma in patients receiving low-dose heparin. *Curr Med Res Opin* 1981;7:458–462.
126. Krill D, Savord EG. Topical thrombin and powdered gelfoam: an efficient hemostatic treatment for surgery. *J Tenn Dent Assoc* 1986;66:26–27.
127. Thompson DF, Letassy NA, Thompson GD. Fibrin glue: a review of its preparation, efficacy, and adverse effects as a topical hemostat. *Drug Intell Clin Pharm* 1988;22:946–952.
128. Thrombin-JMI [thrombin, topical U.S.P (bovine origin)]. Prescribing information. Middleton, WI: GenTrac Incorporated, 2000.
129. Adams JD, Jones S, Brost BC. Development of antibodies to topical bovine thrombin after abdominal hysterectomy. A case report. *J Reprod Med* 2001;46:909–912.
130. Dorion RP, Hamati HF, Landis B, et al. Risk and clinical significance of developing antibodies induced by topical thrombin preparations. *Arch Pathol Lab Med* 1998;122:887–894.
131. Christie RJ, Carrington L, Alving B. Postoperative bleeding induced by topical bovine thrombin: report of two cases. *Surgery* 1997;121:708–710.
132. Ortel TL, Charles LA, Keller FG, et al. Topical thrombin and acquired coagulation factor inhibitors: clinical spectrum and laboratory diagnosis. *Am J Hematol* 1994;45:128–135.
133. Rothenberg DM, Moy JN. Anaphylactic reaction to topical bovine thrombin. *Anesthesiology* 1993;78:779–782.

CHAPTER 111

Hemorrheologic Agents

Andrew R. Erdman

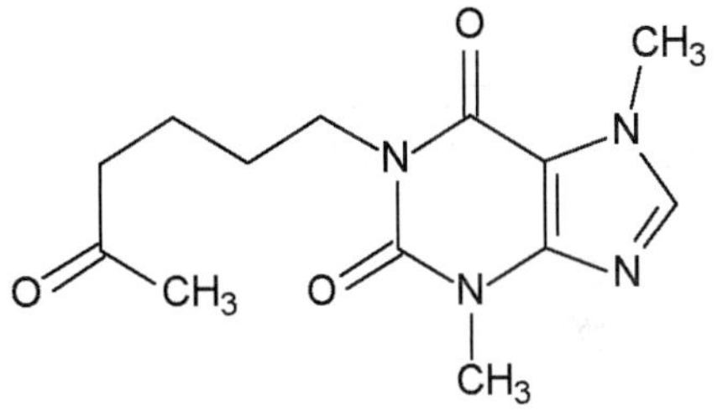

PENTOXIFYLLINE

Compound included:	**Trental**
Molecular formula and weight:	**$C_{13}H_{18}N_4O_3$, 278.31 g/mol**
SI conversion:	**mg/L × 3.59 = µmol/L**
CAS Registry No.:	**6493-05-6**
Therapeutic levels:	**Serum 5 mg/L; not routinely available**
Special concerns:	**Potential drug interaction with theophylline**
Target organs:	**Heart (acute), central nervous system (acute), electrolytes (acute and chronic), gastrointestinal (acute and chronic)**
Antidote:	**None**

OVERVIEW

Hemorrheologic agents improve the viscosity and enhance the flow characteristics of blood. In so doing, they can improve microcirculation and the delivery of oxygen to peripheral tissues. They are used in the management of patients with occlusive peripheral arterial disease. Pentoxifylline (Trental) is currently the only hemorrheologic agent available in the United States. In patients with occlusive peripheral arterial disease, randomized trials indicate that it ameliorates claudication and improves overall functional capacity (1,2). Pentoxifylline is a dimethylxanthine, similar in structure to theophylline but with different pharmacologic effects. Pentoxifylline is available as a 400-mg extended-release tablet.

Pentoxifylline also has a wide variety of immunomodulatory and cardiovascular actions. For these reasons, its use has been investigated for other medical conditions, including sepsis, chemical-induced hepatic or pulmonary fibrosis, drug- (e.g., cyclosporine, interleukin, amphotericin) or radiation-related organ damage, various inflammatory disorders, venous leg ulcers, and as an adjunctive agent in patients with human immunodeficiency virus (3–12).

TOXIC DOSE

The recommended therapeutic *adult dosage* for patients with claudication is 1200 mg/day in three divided doses (1,13). A *pediatric dose* has not been established, but doses of to 10 to 20 mg/kg/day have been used safely in children with sickle cell anemia or Kawasaki disease (14,15).

The toxic dose of pentoxifylline has not been established. In one study, patients receiving oral doses of 7.2 g/day tolerated the drug well, with little more than gastrointestinal effects (6). Overdoses have only rarely been reported. In a poison center series from France, patients taking up to 80 mg/kg developed symptoms of moderate to severe toxicity (16). In a separate abstract, the authors report an infant who ingested 80 mg/kg of pentoxifylline along with 6 mg/kg of clobazam and several hours later developed life-threatening effects, which resolved with supportive care (17).

TOXICOKINETICS AND TOXICODYNAMICS

Pentoxifylline is well absorbed after ingestion (19–21). The time-to-peak serum concentration is 30 to 60 minutes, 2 to 4 hours for the extended-release form (21). Pentoxifylline undergoes extensive hepatic first-pass metabolism, producing major metabolites of 5-hydroxyhexyl (metabolite I) and 3-carboxypropyl (metabolite V) (13). These metabolites begin to appear in the blood almost immediately after ingestion, and their concentrations generally run parallel to and exceed those of the parent compound (19,22). Both of the metabolites are pharmacologically active (22,23). A small amount of reductive metabolism of pentoxifylline by erythrocytes may also occur, but its significance is unclear (22).

Elimination of pentoxifylline is hepatic (mainly oxidation and demethylation), followed by renal excretion of the metabolites (13). The elimination half-life of the parent compound is 30 to 60 minutes and 1 to 2 hours for its metabolites (19). These values may increase significantly after overdoses if hepatic metabolism or renal excretion become saturated. However, no data on the metabolism and elimination of pentoxifylline after overdose are available. In patients with renal insufficiency or renal failure, both the parent compound and its major active metabolites can accumulate as their elimination half-lives become prolonged (24,25). The same is true for patients with cirrhosis (26). Drugs, such as cimetidine, may impair pentoxifylline metabolism (27).

PATHOPHYSIOLOGY

Pentoxifylline inhibits the function of phosphodiesterase (PDE) in certain cells, leading to an increase in intracellular cyclic adenosine monophosphate (28). The role of cyclic adenosine monophosphate in the drug's diverse clinical effects is uncertain; however, PDE inhibition does not appear to be the mechanism underlying its rheologic benefits (22,29). Pentoxifylline's ability to inhibit PDE does not appear to be as strong as the other methylxanthine derivatives (30).

Clinically, pentoxifylline causes a reduction in blood viscosity, mediated through a combination of improved erythrocyte flexibility, enhanced leukocyte deformability, and reduced platelet aggregation and plasma fibrinogen levels (13,22,31–39). Blood flow through the microcirculatory system and past arterial stenoses is improved along with overall oxygen delivery to peripheral tissues (31,40–42). Both the parent compound and its major metabolites contribute to its rheologic activity (23). The mechanism for these rheologic effects is unknown. PDE inhibition does not appear to be the etiology because other PDE-inhibiting drugs lack similar rheologic properties and because therapeutic doses of pentoxifylline do not produce other clinical effects of PDE inhibition (22,29).

In animal studies and after intravenous administration to humans, pentoxifylline causes peripheral vasodilation (31,43–46). At doses typically used to treat claudication, however, it does not appear to have significant vascular effects (47). Its vasodilatory action is consistent with PDE inhibition, but the release of vascular endothelially derived relaxing factors and prostacyclin and increases in vascular cell nitric oxide levels may all play a role (45,48–51).

In addition to its effects on the blood and vasculature, pentoxifylline also has immunomodulatory properties, including reducing tumor necrosis factor and interleukin-8 secretion, reducing fibroblast proliferation, and inhibiting leukocyte polarization and extravasation (52–55). The pharmacologic mechanisms underlying these actions are not known.

The effects of pentoxifylline on the heart are not as prominent as with other methylxanthine drugs, but therapeutic doses do improve cardiac contractility in patients with cardiomyopathy. These inotropic effects are probably the result of PDE inhibition, but in patients with cardiomyopathy, decreases in tumor necrosis factor may also play a role (56–58).

Information on acute overdose is limited, and in the few cases that have been reported in the literature to date, no distinct or predictable pattern of clinical effects has emerged. However, significant PDE inhibition may result in vasodilation, hypotension, and reflex tachycardia (Chapter 123). Indeed, hypotension and shock have been reported in the literature (16,18). Other cases of hypotension due to pentoxifylline use have been recorded by the manufacturer (13).

Pentoxifylline appears to have a different and unique spectrum of pharmacologic effects at therapeutic oral doses than other methylxanthines (e.g., theophylline), but overdoses could theoretically result in signs and symptoms similar to methylxanthine toxicity.

PREGNANCY AND LACTATION

Pentoxifylline is U.S. Food and Drug Administration pregnancy category C. The limited animal data available do not indicate teratogenicity. No human data on teratogenicity, fetotoxicity, or breast-feeding are available. Both pentoxifylline and its major metabolites are excreted in breast milk (13,59).

CLINICAL PRESENTATION

Acute Overdosage

In the few cases that have been reported to date, no distinct or predictable pattern of clinical effects has emerged (13,16–18,60). Toxic effects have included flushing, fever, hypothermia, agitation, myoclonus, somnolence, loss of consciousness, coma, seizures, and hypotension. Bradycardia, atrioventricular block, and asystole have been reported (17,60). Hypokalemia has also been noted (60). Hypotension seems to be common among the few reported cases. Death has occurred after massive ingestion as a result of irreversible shock (18). Gastrointestinal side effects, such as nausea and vomiting, have been noted with large therapeutic oral doses and are expected after overdose (6,61).

Theophylline-like toxicity has not been reported despite the chemical similarities of the drugs, but it might theoretically occur after overdoses. Clinical toxicity related to the rheologic and immunologic actions of pentoxifylline has not been reported.

Symptoms generally develop within 1 to 2 hours but may not manifest for 4 to 5 hours after ingestion of the extended-release preparation (13,16,17,60). Clinical effects of toxicity typically resolve within 12 to 24 hours but could theoretically last much longer after massive overdoses, particularly those involving the extended-release product or with the coingestion of agents that impair gut motility.

There are no reports of significant toxicity associated with chronic, excessive pentoxifylline use. Gastrointestinal effects, such as nausea and vomiting, are common (13,61). Based on its pharmacologic actions, hypotension and reflex tachycardia might be expected.

Adverse Events

Occasional reports of angina, dysrhythmias, and hypotension have occurred during therapeutic use, but their relation to pentoxifylline is unclear (13). Gastrointestinal effects are also a common side effect with oral therapy, particularly at higher doses (61). One patient taking pentoxifylline therapeutically developed hepatotoxicity (62).

Drug Interactions

The concomitant use of pentoxifylline and theophylline may lead to elevated theophylline levels and symptoms of theophylline toxicity (63). This appears to be the result of interference with theophylline's metabolism due to the similarity in chemical structure between the two agents.

Because pentoxifylline reduces blood viscosity and affects platelet aggregation and fibrinogen levels, it might be expected to exacerbate any ongoing bleeding. However, there have been no reports of significant hemorrhage associated with either overdose or therapeutic use. Therapeutic doses do not appear to significantly affect any of the coagulation parameters, even in patients on concomitant warfarin therapy, although the manufacture recommends close monitoring in patients taking both medications (13,64).

DIAGNOSTIC TESTS

The diagnosis of pentoxifylline toxicity is made on clinical grounds. Pentoxifylline levels in the blood and urine can be obtained by spectrophotometry or chromatography, but these tests are not readily available (65,66). Quantitative levels may help to confirm a suspected overdose retrospectively.

If overdose is suspected, an electrocardiogram should be performed to check for conduction delays, and serum electrolytes should be drawn to look for hypokalemia (60). Measurements of coagulation may be considered, although the drug has not been directly linked to either coagulopathy or bleeding. Liver function tests should be performed. Patients taking theophylline should have levels confirmed because pentoxifylline can interfere with its metabolism; however, pentoxifylline and its metabolites do not appear to interfere with laboratory assays for theophylline (63,67,68).

TREATMENT

Management of pentoxifylline overdose consists of supportive and symptomatic care.

Decontamination

Decontamination measures to reduce the absorption of pentoxifylline have not been evaluated. Oral administration of activated charcoal should be considered for patients with significant recent acute ingestion of pentoxifylline or if other coingestants are suspected. If a recent, potentially life-threatening ingestion is suspected, gastric lavage should be considered. Because the drug is available as an extended-release tablet, decontamination measures might be more effective later in the course.

Enhanced Elimination

Enhanced elimination measures for pentoxifylline have not been studied. Patients with evidence of a large gastrointestinal burden of the extended-release tablets and ongoing toxicity might benefit from the use of repeated-dose charcoal or whole bowel irrigation.

Antidotes

There is no specific antidote for pentoxifylline.

Monitoring

Patients suspected of significant pentoxifylline ingestion should be observed for at least 8 hours, particularly with extended-release tablets. Continuous cardiac, blood pressure, and oximetry monitoring for hypotension, tachycardia, cardiac conduction delays, decreased respirations, or coma should be performed. Serial measurements of electrolytes and measurements of coagulation should be considered. Evaluation for concurrent theophylline toxicity must be considered in patients on both medications (Chapter 123).

Supportive Care

Because hypotension due to pentoxifylline is likely to be the result of vasodilation rather than direct cardiac toxicity, α-adrenergic pressors should be considered. Clinically significant bradycardia generally responds well to atropine (60). Seizures should be managed with the usual anticonvulsants. Electrolyte deficiencies should be replaced as necessary. Gastrointestinal effects generally respond well to the usual antiemetics.

REFERENCES

1. Porter JM, Cutler BS, Lee BY, et al. Pentoxifylline efficacy in the treatment of intermittent claudication: multicenter controlled double-blind trial with objective assessment of chronic occlusive arterial disease patients. *Am Heart J* 1982;104:66–72.
2. Strano A, Davi G, Avellone G, et al. Double-blind, crossover study of the clinical efficacy and the hemorrheological effects of pentoxifylline in patients with occlusive arterial disease of the lower limbs. *Angiology* 1984;35:459–466.
3. Jull A, Waters J, Arroll B. Pentoxifylline for treatment of venous leg ulcers: a systematic review. *Lancet* 2002;359:1550–1554.
4. Ohsaki Y, Ishida S, Fujikane T, Kikuchi K. Pentoxifylline potentiates the antitumor effect of cisplatin and etoposide on human lung cancer cell lines. *Oncology* 1996;53:327–333.
5. Peterson TC, Neumeister M. Effect of pentoxifylline in rat and swine models of hepatic fibrosis: role of fibroproliferation in its mechanism. *Immunopharmacology* 1996;31:183–193.
6. Dezube BJ, Lederman MM, Spritzler JG, et al. High-dose pentoxifylline in patients with AIDS: inhibition of tumor necrosis factor production. National Institute of Allergy and Infectious Diseases AIDS Clinical Trials Group. *J Infect Dis* 1995;171:1628–1632.
7. Desmouliere A, Xu G, Costa AM, et al. Effect of pentoxifylline on early proliferation and phenotypic modulation of fibrogenic cells in two rat models of liver fibrosis and on cultured hepatic stellate cells. *J Hepatol* 1999;30:621–631.
8. Albornoz LE, Sanchez SB, Bandi JC, et al. Pentoxifylline reduces nephrotoxicity associated with cyclosporine in the rat by its rheological properties. *Transplantation* 1997;64:1404–1407.
9. Kudoh I, Ohtake M, Nishizawa H, et al. The effect of pentoxifylline on acid-induced alveolar epithelial injury. *Anesthesiology* 1995;82:531–541.
10. Koo DJ, Yoo P, Cioffi WG, et al. Mechanism of the beneficial effects of pentoxifylline during sepsis: maintenance of adrenomedullin responsiveness and downregulation of proinflammatory cytokines. *J Surg Res* 2000;91:70–76.
11. Bacher A, Mayer N, Klimscha W, et al. Effects of pentoxifylline on hemodynamics and oxygenation in septic and nonseptic patients. *Crit Care Med* 1997;25:795–800.
12. Staubach KH, Schroder J, Stuber F, et al. Effect of pentoxifylline in severe sepsis: results of a randomized, double-blind, placebo-controlled study. *Arch Surg* 1998;133:94–100.

13. Trental. Prescribing information. Strasbourg, France: Aventis Pharmaceuticals Inc., 2002.
14. Aronoff SC, Quinn FJ Jr, Carpenter LS, Novick WJ Jr. Effects of pentoxifylline on sputum neutrophil elastase and pulmonary function in patients with cystic fibrosis: preliminary observations. *J Pediatr* 1994;125:992–997.
15. Furukawa S, Matsubara T, Umezawa Y, et al. Pentoxifylline and intravenous gamma globulin combination therapy for acute Kawasaki disease. *Eur J Pediatr* 1994;153:663–667.
16. Fournier PE. Bilan de Sept annees d'observation du torental (pentoxifylline) par le Centre Antipoisons de Paris, 17.
17. Garnier R, Riboulet-Delmas G, Chatenet T, Efthymiou ML. [Acute pentoxifylline poisoning in children]. *Ann Pediatr (Paris)* 1986;33:62–63.
18. Suarez-Penaranda JM, Rico-Boquete R, Lopez-Rivadulla M, et al. A fatal case of suicidal pentoxifylline intoxication. *Int J Legal Med* 1998;111(3):151–153.
19. Smith RV, Waller ES, Doluisio JT, et al. Pharmacokinetics of orally administered pentoxifylline in humans. *J Pharm Sci* 1986;75:47–52.
20. Bryce TA, Chamberlain J, Hillbeck D, Macdonald CM. Metabolism and pharmacokinetics of 14C-pentoxifylline in healthy volunteers. *Arzneimittelforschung* 1989;39:512–517.
21. Hinze HJ, Grigoleit HG, Rethy B. Bioavailability and pharmacokinetics of pentoxifylline from "Trental 400" in man. *Pharmatherapeutica* 1976;1:160–171.
22. Aviado DM, Porter JM. Pentoxifylline: a new drug for the treatment of intermittent claudication. Mechanism of action, pharmacokinetics, clinical efficacy and adverse effects. *Pharmacotherapy* 1984;4:297–307.
23. Ambrus JL, Stadler S, Kulaylat M. Hemorrheologic effects of metabolites of pentoxifylline (Trental). *J Med* 1995;26:65–75.
24. Paap CM, Simpson KS, Horton MW, et al. Multiple-dose pharmacokinetics of pentoxifylline and its metabolites during renal insufficiency. *Ann Pharmacother* 1996;30:724–729.
25. Silver MR, Kroboth PD. Pentoxifylline in end-stage renal disease. *Drug Intell Clin Pharm* 1987;21:976–978.
26. Rames A, Poirier JM, LeCoz F, et al. Pharmacokinetics of intravenous and oral pentoxifylline in healthy volunteers and in cirrhotic patients. *Clin Pharmacol Ther* 1990;47:354–359.
27. Mauro VF, Mauro LS, Hageman JH. Alteration of pentoxifylline pharmacokinetics by cimetidine. *J Clin Pharmacol* 1988;28:649–654.
28. Nandi JS, Nair KG, Deo S. Inhibition cAMP-phosphodiesterase in the rat heart by pentoxifylline—a new xanthine derivative. *Adv Myocardiol* 1980;1:359–365.
29. Sato Y, Miura T, Suzuki Y. Interaction of pentoxifylline with human erythrocytes. III. Comparison of fluidity change of erythrocyte membrane caused by S-adenosyl-L-methionine with that by pentoxifylline. *Chem Pharm Bull (Tokyo)* 1991;39:468–473.
30. Grossmann M, Braune J, Ebert U, Kirch W. Dilatory effects of phosphodiesterase inhibitors on human hand veins in vivo. *Eur J Clin Pharmacol* 1998;54:35–39.
31. Di Perri T, Carandente O, Vittoria A, et al. Studies of the clinical pharmacology and therapeutic efficacy of pentoxifylline in peripheral obstructive arterial disease. *Angiology* 1984;35:427–435.
32. Ehrly AM. The effect of pentoxifylline on the deformability of erythrocytes and on the muscular oxygen pressure in patients with chronic arterial disease. *J Med* 1979;10:331–338.
33. Schneider R. Results of hemorheologically active treatment with pentoxifylline in patients with cerebrovascular disease. *Angiology* 1989;40:987–993.
34. Ambrus JL, Anain JM, Anain SM, et al. Dose-response effects of pentoxifylline on erythrocyte filterability: clinical and animal model studies. *Clin Pharmacol Ther* 1990;48:50–56.
35. Weithmann KU. Reduced platelet aggregation by effects of pentoxifylline on vascular prostacyclin isomerase and platelet cyclic AMP. *Gen Pharmacol* 1983;14:161–162.
36. Muller R. Hemorheology and peripheral vascular diseases: a new therapeutic approach. *J Med* 1981;12:209–235.
37. Yamac K, Kaptan KM, Beyan C, et al. Comparison of the hematological effects of a sustained release chitosan formulation of pentoxifylline with a commercial formulation. *Arzneimittelforschung* 2000;50:827–831.
38. Schroer RH. Antithrombotic potential of pentoxifylline. A hemorheologically active drug. *Angiology* 1985;36:387–398.
39. Ferrari E, Fioravanti M, Patti AL, et al. Effects of long-term treatment (4 years) with pentoxifylline on haemorheological changes and vascular complications in diabetic patients. *Pharmatherapeutica* 1987;5:26–39.
40. Ehrly AM. The effect of pentoxifylline on the flow properties of human blood. *Curr Med Res Opin* 1978;5:608–613.
41. Ehrly AM, Saeger-Lorenz K. Influence of pentoxifylline on muscle tissue oxygen tension (pO2) of patients with intermittent claudication before and after pedal ergometer exercise. *Angiology* 1987;38:93–100.
42. Accetto B. Beneficial hemorheologic therapy of chronic peripheral arterial disorders with pentoxifylline: results of double-blind study versus vasodilator-nylidrin. *Am Heart J* 1982;103:864–869.
43. Krysztopik RJ, Bentley FR, Wilson MA, et al. Vasomotor response to pentoxifylline mediates improved renal blood flow to bacteremia. *J Surg Res* 1996;63:17–22.
44. Sonkin PL, Chen LE, Seaber AV, Hatchell DL. Vasodilator action of pentoxifylline on microcirculation of rat cremaster muscle. *Angiology* 1992;43:462–469.
45. Kaye AD, Ibrahim IN, Kadowitz PJ, Nossaman BD. Analysis of responses to pentoxifylline in the pulmonary vascular bed of the cat. *Crit Care Med* 1996;24:263–267.
46. Kamphuis J, Smits P, Thien T. Vascular effects of pentoxifylline in humans. *J Cardiovasc Pharmacol* 1994;24:648–654.
47. Kruuse C, Jacobsen TB, Thomsen LL, et al. Effects of the non-selective phosphodiesterase inhibitor pentoxifylline on regional cerebral blood flow and large arteries in healthy subjects. *Eur J Neurol* 2000;7:629–638.
48. Berkenboom G, Fang ZY, Unger P, et al. Endothelium-dependent effects of pentoxifylline in rat aorta. *Eur J Pharmacol* 1991;193:81–86.
49. Kim NY, Pae HO, Kim YC, et al. Pentoxifylline potentiates nitric oxide production in interleukin-1beta-stimulated vascular smooth muscle cells through cyclic AMP-dependent protein kinase A pathway. *Gen Pharmacol* 2000;35:205–211.
50. Sinzinger H. Pentoxifylline enhances formation of prostacyclin from rat vascular and renal tissue. *Prostaglandins Leukot Med* 1983;12:217–226.
51. Kaputlu I, Sadan G. Pentoxifylline-induced vasodilatation is not endothelium-dependent in rabbit aorta. *J Basic Clin Physiol Pharmacol* 1994;5:295–304.
52. Zabel P, Schonharting MM, Schade UF, Schlaak M. Effects of pentoxifylline in endotoxinemia in human volunteers. *Prog Clin Biol Res* 1991;367:207–213.
53. Krakauer T. Pentoxifylline inhibits ICAM-1 expression and chemokine production induced by proinflammatory cytokines in human pulmonary epithelial cells. *Immunopharmacology* 2000;46:253–261.
54. Dominguez-Jimenez C, Sancho D, Nieto M, et al. Effect of pentoxifylline on polarization and migration of human leukocytes. *J Leukoc Biol* 2002;71:588–596.
55. Entzian P, Zahringer U, Schlaak M, et al. Comparative study on effects of pentoxifylline, prednisolone and colchicine in experimental alveolitis. *Int J Immunopharmacol* 1998;20:723–735.
56. Robinson DA, Wang P, Chaudry IH. Pentoxifylline restores the depressed cardiac performance after trauma-hemorrhage and resuscitation. *J Surg Res* 1996;66:51–56.
57. Skudicky D, Bergemann A, Sliwa K, et al. Beneficial effects of pentoxifylline in patients with idiopathic dilated cardiomyopathy treated with angiotensin-converting enzyme inhibitors and carvedilol: results of a randomized study. *Circulation* 2001;103:1083–1088.
58. Sliwa K, Skudicky D, Candy G, et al. Randomised investigation of effects of pentoxifylline on left-ventricular performance in idiopathic dilated cardiomyopathy. *Lancet* 1998;351:1091–1093.
59. Witter FR, Smith RV. The excretion of pentoxifylline and its metabolites into human breast milk. *Am J Obstet Gynecol* 1985;151:1094–1097.
60. Sznajder I, Bentur Y, Taitelman U. First and second degree atrioventricular block in oxpentifylline overdose. *Br Med J (Clin Res Ed)* 1984;288:26.
61. Dezube BJ, Fridovich-Keil JL, Bouvard I, et al. Pentoxifylline and wellbeing in patients with cancer. *Lancet* 1990;335:662.
62. Saez-Royuela F, Lopez-Vazquez A, Lopez-Morante A, et al. Pentoxifylline-induced acute hepatitis. *J Hepatol* 1995;23:482–484.
63. Ellison MJ, Horner RD, Willis SE, Cummings DM. Influence of pentoxifylline on steady-state theophylline serum concentrations from sustained-release formulations. *Pharmacotherapy* 1990;10:383–386.
64. Ingerslev J, Mouritzen C, Stenbjerg S. Pentoxifylline does not interfere with stable coumarin anticoagulant therapy: a clinical study. *Pharmatherapeutica* 1986;4:595–600.
65. Rieck W, Platt D. Determination of 3,7-dimethyl-1-(5-oxohexyl)-xanthine (pentoxifylline) and its 3,7-dimethyl-1-(5-hydroxyhexyl)-xanthine metabolite in the plasma of patients with multiple diseases using high-performance liquid chromatography. *J Chromatogr* 1984;305:419–427.
66. Mancinelli A, Pace S, Marzo A, et al. Determination of pentoxifylline and its metabolites in human plasma by high-performance liquid chromatography with solid-phase extraction. *J Chromatogr* 1992;575:101–107.
67. Morton MR, Parish RC, Spruill WJ. Lack of theophylline assay interference from pentoxifylline and its metabolites. *Ther Drug Monit* 1989;11:347–348.
68. Cohen IA, Johnson CE, Wesolowicz L, Converse-Swastek K. Effect of pentoxifylline and its metabolites on three theophylline assays. *Clin Pharm* 1988;7:457–461.

CHAPTER 112

Platelet Aggregation Inhibitors

Richard C. Dart

Molecular formula and weight:	**Abciximab, 47,615; eptifibatide ($C_{35}H_{49}N_{11}O_9S_2$), 831.96; tirofiban ($C_{22}H_{36}N_2O_5S$), 495.08; clopidogrel bisulfate ($C_{16}H_{16}Cl,NO_2SO_4$), 419.9 g/mol**
SI conversion:	**Abciximab, µg/L × 0.021 = µmol/L; eptifibatide, µg/L × 0.0012 = µmol/L; tirofibon, µg/L × 0.0020 = µmol/L; clopidogrel bisulfate, µg/L × 0.0024 = µmol/L**
CAS Registry No.:	**148031-34-9 (eptifibatide), 150915-40-5 (tirofiban), 120202-66-6 (clopidogrel)**
Normal or therapeutic levels:	**Not applicable**
Target organs:	**Platelets**
Antidote:	**None**
Note:	**The structure is not applicable to this chapter—too many structures, minor clinical relevance to the medical toxicologist.**

OVERVIEW

The antiplatelet agents include inhibitors of the platelet glycoprotein (GP) IIb/IIIa receptor [abciximab (ReoPro), eptifibatide (Integrilin), lamifiban, sibrafiban, tirofiban (Aggrastat)] or the adenosine diphosphate (ADP) receptor [ticlopidine hydrochloride (Ticlid, Tiklid, Ticlodone), clopidogrel bisulfate (Plavix)]. These drugs are used for the treatment of atherosclerotic disease. In overdose, their main toxic effect is coagulopathy and bleeding due to lack of platelet activity. Aspirin is covered in Chapter 127.

INHIBITORS OF GLYCOPROTEIN IIB/IIIA RECEPTOR

Abciximab is a mouse and human chimeric monoclonal Fab that binds to the GP IIb/IIIa receptor and the $\alpha_v\beta_3$ (vitronectin) receptor, whereas eptifibatide, lamifiban, sibrafiban, and tirofiban are synthetic nonpeptide compounds that bind to the GP IIb/IIIa receptor. Each agent has been shown in randomized trials to improve the outcome from ischemic complications of atherosclerotic heart disease.

The *therapeutic dose* for abciximab is typically 0.25 mg/kg by intravenous (IV) bolus 10 to 60 minutes before the percutaneous coronary intervention, followed by an infusion of 0.125 µg/kg/minute (to a maximum of 10 µg/minute) for 12 hours. Tirofiban is administered IV at an initial rate of 0.4 µg/kg/minute for 30 minutes and then continued at 0.1 µg/kg/minute. The rate is halved in patients with severe renal insufficiency. Eptifibatide dosage for acute coronary syndrome is an IV bolus of 180 µg/kg, followed by an infusion of 2 µg/kg/minute until hospital discharge or initiation of surgery for up to 72 hours. For percutaneous coronary intervention without an acute coronary syndrome, a bolus of 135 µg/kg is administered before the procedure, followed by an infusion of 0.5 µg/kg/minute for 20 to 24 hours.

Intentional *overdosage* has not been reported; however, each of these drugs increases the rate of major bleeding events during therapeutic use (1). Iatrogenic overdosage up to ten times the usual dose has occurred during use of eptifibatide and tirofiban. The most frequently reported effect was bleeding, primarily minor mucocutaneous bleeding events and minor bleeding at sites of catheterization.

Toxicokinetics and Toxicodynamics

Only pharmacokinetic and pharmacodynamic data are available (Table 1).

Pathophysiology

Expression of GP IIb/IIIa is the final common pathway of platelet aggregation. Inhibitors of the GP IIb/IIIa receptor reduce platelet aggregation by blocking that route of activation. Abciximab is a protein and may produce immune responses. One case of anaphylaxis has been reported (2). A second administration of abciximab could theoretically include allergic reactions, thrombocytopenia, and neutralization of injected abciximab by antibodies formed during its first administration. However, abciximab has been success-

TABLE 1. Selected pharmacokinetic and pharmacodynamic parameters of glycoprotein IIb/IIIa receptor inhibitors

Parameters	Abciximab[a]	Eptifibatide[b]	Tirofiban[c]
Onset of effect	Within 2 h	Within 1 h	5 min
Duration of effect (h)	12	2–4	3–8
Volume of distribution	Not reported	185 ml/kg	22–42 L
Route of excretion	Not reported	Renal, 71%	Renal, 65%; fecal, 25%
Elimination half-life	Not reported	1.1–2.5 h	90–180 min
Excreted unchanged	Not reported	36%	—
Active metabolites	Not reported	No	No
Protein binding	Not reported	25%	Low

[a]From Abciximab. Product literature, healthcare series, vol. 112. Greenwood Village, CO: MICROMEDEX, 2002, with permission.
[b]From Alton KB, Kosoglou T, Baker S, et al. Disposition of C(14)-eptifibatide after intravenous administration to healthy men. *Clin Ther* 1998;20:307–323, with permission.
[c]From Tirofiban. Product literature, healthcare series, vol. 112. Greenwood Village, CO: MICROMEDEX, 2002, with permission.

fully readministered to 500 patients without an allergic reaction or any apparent change in efficacy (3).

Pregnancy and Lactation

Abciximab is U.S. Food and Drug Administration (FDA) pregnancy category C. Eptifibatide and tirofiban are category B. (See Appendix I for pregnancy categories.) Tirofiban is likely excreted into breast milk in significant quantities. Information regarding other agents is unknown.

Clinical Presentation

The effect of overdosage is primarily an extension of the therapeutic effect. Major bleeding is the primary adverse effect and is expected to be more common in overdose.

The most common adverse reaction is bleeding. These drugs are used in conjunction with heparin, and bleeding is common; however, the rate of major bleeding events appears to be reduced without loss of efficacy by using a low-dose heparin treatment. A metaanalysis found that the rate of major bleeding during use for percutaneous coronary intervention was 5.8% for abciximab and 3.8% for eptifibatide or tirofiban (4). In addition to inhibition of platelet aggregation, severe absolute thrombocytopenia has occurred in 1% to 2% of patients treated with abciximab, eptifibatide, or tirofiban. Thrombocytopenia may occur within hours or after a delay of several days and returns to normal if therapy is discontinued (5). Diffuse alveolar hemorrhage and hemoptysis (without severe thrombocytopenia) have occurred during appropriate use of abciximab and tirofiban and may be fatal (6).

Specific diagnostic tests and drug levels are not readily available. In overdose, serial measurement of the complete blood cell count and bleeding time may assess severity. The bleeding time is often markedly prolonged, but the clinical use of this information is not clear.

Treatment

After overdosage or an adverse event, the drug should be discontinued. Decontamination is not feasible because these drugs are administered IV. Hemorrhage is treated with local pressure, fluid resuscitation, and pressors if needed. Profound thrombocytopenia has been corrected with platelet transfusion, but the precise indications and dose are unknown (7). The effects of abciximab have been successfully reversed by platelet transfusion. Eptifibatide and tirofiban are expected to be effectively cleared from plasma by hemodialysis; however, the efficacy of this technique has not been assessed. Platelet transfusions have not been as effective with these drugs (8). Diffuse alveolar hemorrhage is treated supportively with discontinuation of antiplatelet and anticoagulant medications, blood transfusion using the usual indicators, and respiratory support guided by the severity of illness.

ADENOSINE DIPHOSPHATE RECEPTOR INHIBITORS

Ticlopidine hydrochloride (Ticlid, Tiklid, Ticlodone) and clopidogrel bisulfate (Plavix) are thienopyridine structure drugs that inhibit platelet aggregation. Ticlopidine hydrochloride is indicated for prevention of stroke and perhaps other thromboembolic states. It has also been used to maintain vascular graft patency, to prevent platelet loss during extracorporeal circulatory procedures, and in the treatment of vaso-occlusive complications of sickle cell crisis. Clopidogrel bisulfate is used for reduction of ischemic events, such as myocardial infarction or stroke, in patients with atherosclerotic disease.

The *therapeutic dosage* of ticlopidine hydrochloride is 500 mg/day in two divided doses. Clopidogrel bisulfate dosage is 75 mg/day. There is no need for dosage adjustment for age, gender, or renal disease. No pediatric dose is available for either drug. *Toxic dosages* for ticlopidine hydrochloride and clopidogrel bisulfate have not been established. One report of acute ingestion of ticlopidine hydrochloride, 10 g, resulted in major toxicity in an adult (9). The pediatric toxic dose is unknown.

Toxicokinetics and Toxicodynamics

Only pharmacokinetic and pharmacodynamic data are available (Table 2).

Pathophysiology

Both agents competitively interfere with one route of platelet activation—binding of ADP to the ADP receptor (10). Ticlopidine hydrochloride inhibits platelet aggregation induced by ADP, collagen, arachidonic acid, thrombi, and platelet aggregation factor. It also reduces plasma fibrinogen (blood viscosity) and increases red cell deformability. These effects are associated with a dose-dependent prolongation of bleeding time, which peaks in 3 days and persists for up to 10 days. Unlike aspirin, ticlopidine hydrochloride does not interfere with the prostacyclin-thromboxane pathway (11).

Pregnancy and Lactation

Both agents are FDA pregnancy category B (Appendix I). Excretion in breast milk has not been evaluated.

Clinical Presentation

Little information is available for toxicity from acute overdose. Ticlopidine hydrochloride increases the bleeding time and may increase alanine aminotransferase concentration. After a 10-g ingestion of ticlopidine hydrochloride, a 69-year-old man developed agitation, confusion, and tachycardia. Three hours after admission, he became lethargic and developed hypotension, hypoxia, and metabolic acidosis. During hospitalization, he developed ecchymosis, hematuria, epistaxis, and guaiac-positive stools. Bleeding time was greater than 15 minutes for several days (9).

Adverse effects for either clopidogrel bisulfate or ticlopidine hydrochloride have included abdominal pain, diarrhea (12), rash, prolongation of bleeding time (13), decreased platelet func-

TABLE 2. Selected pharmacokinetic and pharmacodynamic parameters of the adenosine diphosphate receptor inhibitors

Parameters	Ticlopidine hydrochloride[a]	Clopidogrel bisulfate[b]
Bioavailability	90%	>50%
Peak plasma level	0.3–2.0 μg/ml	0.1–3.0 ng/ml
Time-to-peak plasma level (h)	1–3	<1
Elimination half-life (h)	24–36; 96 with repeated dosing	8
Excreted unchanged	<1%	Not reported
Active metabolites	2-Keto derivative	Not reported
Protein binding	98%	98%

[a]From Balsano F, Cocchei S, Libretti A, et al. Ticlopidine in the treatment of intermittent claudication: a 21 month double-blind trial. *J Lab Clin Med* 1989;114:84–91, with permission.
[b]From Van Hecken, Depre M, Wynants K, et al. Effect of clopidogrel on naproxen-induced gastrointestinal blood loss in healthy volunteers. *Drug Metab Drug Interact* 1998;14:193–205, with permission.

tion, and hepatic dysfunction. Gastrointestinal symptoms often subside spontaneously. Naproxen-induced fecal blood loss is increased by clopidogrel bisulfate (14). Ticlopidine hydrochloride inhibits CYP2C19 and appears to inhibit the clearance of phenytoin (15). Clopidogrel bisulfate does not appear to affect hepatic drug metabolism (16). Clopidogrel bisulfate has been associated with acute arthritis (17).

The adverse effects of ticlopidine hydrochloride include neutropenia or thrombocytopenia, which occurs in 2% to 3% of patients; aplastic anemia has also been reported (18,19). Blood cell counts usually return to normal within 3 weeks of discontinuation (12). Cholestasis has occurred infrequently (20). Because it shares structural similarities to ticlopidine hydrochloride, neutropenia is also a concern with clopidogrel bisulfate, although this effect has not been reported. Diffuse skin reactions have been associated with ticlopidine hydrochloride use, occurring 2 to 20 days after initiation. The most common forms are pruritus and an urticarial eruption or maculopapular rash that subsides even if the drug is not discontinued (21).

Thrombotic thrombocytopenic purpura has been associated with the use of ticlopidine hydrochloride. The incidence is approximately 0.009% to 0.040%, has occurred within 2 weeks of initiating therapy, and is associated with 20% mortality in a retrospective study (21). Thrombotic thrombocytopenic purpura is also associated with clopidogrel bisulfate and may occur within the first 2 weeks of therapy (22).

Diagnostic Tests

Plasma levels are available from reference laboratories. In overdose, serial measurement of the complete blood cell count and perhaps bleeding time may be used to assess severity. The bleeding time is often markedly prolonged. Thrombocytopenia may develop. The use of these laboratory studies in clinical management has not been described.

For adverse events, bleeding time, other measures of coagulopathy, and serial evaluation of liver enzymes is recommended. Patients treated with ticlopidine hydrochloride should be evaluated serially for blood, skin, and liver toxicity during the first 3 months.

Treatment

No agent-specific information is available for gastrointestinal decontamination after acute overdosage. These drugs lack immediate effects, and the patient is unlikely to seek care in time for decontamination. If a patient presents very early, gastrointestinal decontamination may be plausible to reduce absorption and ultimate drug effect.

No agent-specific information is available regarding enhancement of elimination. There are no data concerning enterohepatic recirculation. Hemodialysis would not be expected to be helpful for either ticlopidine hydrochloride or clopidogrel bisulfate due to extensive protein binding (10).

There is no antidote available for either agent. In most cases, the drug should be discontinued. Treatment is primarily symptomatic and supportive care. Profound thrombocytopenia has been treated with platelet transfusion, but the precise indications and dose are unknown (1). Corticosteroids and granulocyte colony-stimulating factor have been reported in related clinical situations; however, the precise indications and use are unknown (23).

REFERENCES

1. The EPIC investigators. Use of a monoclonal antibody directed against the platelet glycoprotein IIb/IIIa receptor in high-risk coronary angioplasty. *N Engl J Med* 1994;330:956–961.
2. Guzzo JA, Nichols TC. Possible anaphylactic reaction to abciximab. *Catheter Cardiovasc Interv* 1999;48:71–73.
3. Tcheng JE, Kereiakes DJ, Braden GA, et al. Safety of abciximab retreatment: final clinical report of the ReoPro readministration registry. *Circulation* 1998;19:1–17(abst).
4. Brown DL, Fann CS, Chan CJ. Meta-analysis of effectiveness and safety of abciximab versus eptifibatide or tirofiban in percutaneous coronary intervention. *Am J Cardiol* 2001;87:537–541.
5. Blankenship JC. Bleeding complications of glycoprotein IIb-IIIa receptor inhibitors. *Am Heart J* 1999;138:S287–S296.
6. Ali A, Patil S, Grady KJ, Schreiber TL. Diffuse alveolar hemorrhage following administration of tirofiban or abciximab: a nemesis of plate glycoprotein IIb/IIIa inhibitors. *Catheter Cardiovasc Interv* 2000;49:181–184.
7. Berkowitz SD, Harrington RA, Rund MM, et al. Acute profound thrombocytopenia following c7E3 Fab (abciximab) therapy. *Circulation* 1997;95:809–813.
8. Ferguson JJ, Lao TK. Safety of the use of IIb/IIIa receptor blockers with or without the use of other anticoagulants. *Semin Interv Cardiol* 1999;4:97–102.
9. Horowitz RS, Dart RC. Cardiopulmonary instability, mental status changes and hemorrhage associated with overdose of ticlopidine. *Vet Hum Toxicol* 1993;35:344(abst).
10. Ito MK, Smith AR, Lee ML. Ticlopidine: a new platelet aggregation inhibitor. *Clin Pharm* 1992;11:603–617.
11. Coller BS. Platelets and thrombolytic therapy. *N Engl J Med* 1990;322:33–42.
12. Guedon C, Bruna T, Ducrotte P, et al. Altered small bowel motility in severe chronic diarrhea with ticlopidine. *Gastroenterol Clin Biol* 1989;13:934–937.
13. Balsano F, Cocchei S, Libretti A, et al. Ticlopidine in the treatment of intermittent claudication: a 21 month double-blind trial. *J Lab Clin Med* 1989;114:84–91.
14. van Hecken, Depre M, Wynants K, et al. Effect of clopidogrel on naproxen-induced gastrointestinal blood loss in healthy volunteers. *Drug Metab Drug Interact* 1998;14:193–205.
15. Donahue S, Flockhart DA, Abernethy DR. Ticlopidine inhibits phenytoin clearance. *Clin Pharmacol Ther* 1999;66:563–568.
16. Pierce CH, Houle JM, Dickinson JP, et al. *Semin Thromb Hemost* 1999;25[Suppl 2]:35–39.
17. Garg A, Radvan J, Hopkinson N. Clopidogrel associated with acute arthritis. *BMJ* 2000;320:483.
18. Bousser MG, Roberts RS, Gent M. Ticlopidine and clopidogrel in secondary stroke prevention. *Cerebrovasc Dis* 1997;7:17–23.
19. Steinhubl SR, Tan WA, Foody JM, Topol EG. Incidence and clinical course of thrombotic thrombocytopenic purpura due to ticlopidine following coronary stenting. *JAMA* 1999;281:806–810.
20. Iqbal M, Goenka P, Young M, et al. Ticlopidine-induced cholestatic hepatitis. *Dig Dis Sci* 1998;43:2223–2226.
21. Yosipovitch G, Rechavia E, Feinmesser M, David M. Adverse cutaneous reactions to ticlopidine in patients with coronary stents. *J Am Acad Dermatol* 1999;41:473–476.
22. Bennett CL, Connors JM, Carwile JM, et al. Thrombotic thrombocytopenic purpura associated with clopidogrel. *N Engl J Med* 2000;342:1773–1777.
23. Mataix R, Ojeda E, Perez MDC, Jimenez S. Ticlopidine and severe aplastic anemia. *Br J Haematol* 1992;80:125–132.

CHAPTER 113

Thrombolytic Agents

Katherine M. Hurlbut

Compounds included:	**Alteplase, reteplase, streptokinase (SK), tenecteplase (TNK)**
Molecular formula and weight:	**Alteplase (rt-PA; $C_{2569}H_{3894}N_{746}O_{781}S_{40}$), 59011.291; reteplase (r-PA; $C_{1736}H_{2653}N_{499}O_{522}S_{22}$), 39571.1; tenecteplase (TNK; $C_{2558}H_{3872}N_{738}O_{781}S_{40}$), 58750.08; urokinase mixture of low and high molecular mass forms, 33,000 and 54,000 g/mol**
SI conversion:	**Not applicable**
CAS Registry No.:	**105857-23-6 (alteplase); 133652-38-7 (reteplase); 191588-94-0 (tenecteplase); 9039-53-6 (urokinase)**
Therapeutic levels:	**Not applicable**
Special concerns:	**Adverse effects are common at therapeutic doses.**
Target organs:	**Coagulation system (plasminogen activator)**
Antidotes:	**Aminocaproic acid, aprotinin**

OVERVIEW

The thrombolytic agents are used for the treatment of acute myocardial infarction, pulmonary embolism, and thromboembolic stroke and to restore patency to occluded central venous catheters. Streptokinase (SK) was the original thrombolytic agent introduced. Urokinase is used primarily for catheter patency and for selected procedures in interventional radiology. *Alteplase* (rt-PA) is tissue plasminogen activator created using recombinant DNA technology. *Anistreplase* is a complex of bacterially derived SK and human Lys-plasminogen in equimolar amounts. It is used primarily in the treatment of acute myocardial infarction. *Reteplase* is a nonglycosylated deletion mutant of recombinant tissue plasminogen activator and tenecteplase. All of these products are administered parenterally.

Overdose with thrombolytic agents can be associated with severe hemorrhage, which may be fatal. Bleeding may occur, especially at puncture sites. Treatment involves the use of antifibrinolytics, cryoprecipitates, fresh frozen plasma, packed red blood cells, and platelets.

TOXIC DOSE

The toxic dose is difficult to define because the therapeutic dose is intended to produce anticoagulation.

Alteplase

The adult therapeutic dose for myocardial infarction in patients weighing more than 67 kg is 15 mg by intravenous (IV) bolus followed by 50 mg infused over 30 minutes, then 35 mg infused over 60 minutes. The dose for patients weighing less than 67 kg is 15 mg followed by 0.75 mg/kg infused over 30 minutes, then 0.50 mg/kg infused over 60 minutes. The dose for pulmonary embolism is 100 mg IV over 2 hours (1).

Anistreplase

The adult therapeutic dose is a 30-U IV bolus over 2 to 5 minutes.

Reteplase

The adult therapeutic dose is a 10-U IV bolus over 2 minutes followed by a second 10-U bolus given 30 minutes after the first.

Tenecteplase

The adult therapeutic dose is 30 to 50 mg as a single dose.

Streptokinase

The adult therapeutic dose for myocardial infarction is 1,500,000 IU of SK given as a continuous infusion over up to 60 minutes (2). For pulmonary embolism, loading dose is 250,000 IU infused over 30 minutes followed by 100,000 IU of SK per hour for 24 hours (2).

TOXICOKINETICS AND TOXICODYNAMICS

Pharmacokinetic and pharmacodynamic parameters for thrombolytic agents are in Table 1.

PATHOPHYSIOLOGY

All of the tissue plasminogen activators act by increasing the amount of plasmin. Plasmin degrades fibrin. Some agents also affect other coagulation factors, particularly at higher doses.

PREGNANCY AND LACTATION

rt-PA, anistreplase, reteplase, and SK are all U.S. Food and Drug Administration pregnancy category C. Excretion into human breast milk has not been reported.

TABLE 1. Selected pharmacokinetic and pharmacodynamic parameters of thrombolytic agents

Parameter	Alteplase	Anistreplase	Reteplase[a]	Streptokinase	Tenecteplase[b]
Peak plasma level (ng/ml)	1000–4000	NR	4000	NR	>1000
Volume of distribution	0.07 L/kg	NR	NR	5.68 L[c]	6–15 L
Route of excretion	Hepatic	NR	Hepatic and renal	Renal	Hepatic
Elimination half-life (min)					
Alpha phase	5–10	70–120[d]	13–16	18	11–20
Beta phase	72	—	98–135	83	41–138
Active metabolites	None	None	None	Unknown	None

NR, not reported.
[a]Retavase (reteplase, recombinant). Product information. Gaithersburg, MD: Boehringer Mannheim Corporation, Therapeutics Division, 1997.
[b]Retevase (reteplase). Package insert. Gaithersburg, MD: Boehringher Mannheim Corporation, 1996.
[c]Gemmille JD, Hogg KJ, Burns JMA, et al. A comparison of the pharmacokinetic properties of streptokinase and anistreplase in acute myocardial infarction. *Br J Clin Pharmacol* 1991;31:143–147.
[d]Bennett WM, Aronoff GR, Golper TA, et al. *Drug prescribing in renal failure*, 3rd ed. Philadelphia: American College of Physicians, 1994.

CLINICAL PRESENTATION

Adverse events are common, with hemorrhage being the most common adverse event of thrombolytic therapy (3–7) (Table 2). The risk of bleeding is high in patients in whom invasive procedures are performed or who are given heparin concurrently or subsequently. Strokes and intracerebral bleeding have occurred and are more common in elderly patients (8). Major bleeds require transfusion. Minor bleeds include gross hematuria, hematemesis, hematomas, and oozing from vascular access (9). Fatal hemorrhages range from 0% to 4%. A fall in fibrinogen levels to less than 100 mg/ml during or after thrombolytic therapy has been associated with an increased risk of bleeding (10).

Cholesterol embolization can occur after use of thrombolytic therapy for treatment of occlusive arterial thrombi (11–18). Effects can include peripheral gangrene, hypertension, acute renal failure, pancreatitis, cerebral or spinal cord infarction, retinal artery occlusion, bowel infarction, and rhabdomyolysis.

Hypersensitivity responses follow SK use and anistreplase infusion in 1% to 8% of patients (3,19) and occur rarely after use of other thrombolytic agents. Hypotension follows use of all thrombolytic agents in 10% to 20% of patients after either rapid infusion or high-dose infusion. Other effects include serum sickness, headaches, backaches, renal dysfunction, reversible hepatic dysfunction, nausea, vomiting, and fever. SK has been associated with Guillain-Barré syndrome and, rarely, with hemolysis (8,20,21).

Drug interactions include other anticoagulant drugs and the nitrates. Any drug that impairs the coagulation system (aspirin, heparin, low-molecular-weight heparin, glycoprotein inhibitors, warfarin) should be used with extreme caution. All of these increase the chance of bleeding but may be indicated in selected circumstances. Nitrates may increase clearance of rt-PA, reducing the likelihood of reperfusion and increasing the risk of reocclusion (22). One group found that tenecteplase was not affected by concomitant nitrate therapy (23).

DIAGNOSTIC TESTS

During treatment, monitor the complete blood cell count, platelets, serum electrolytes and renal function tests, international normalized ratio, activated partial thromboplastin time, fibrinogen, and liver enzymes.

rt-PA has been assayed in human plasma using spectrophotometry, enzyme-linked immunosorbent assay, antibody radioimmunoassay, and an enzyme immunoassay (24).

TREATMENT

The treatment of thrombolytic agents focuses on the detection and immediate treatment of bleeding complications followed by the replacement of coagulation factors in severe cases. Vital signs and clinical evidence of bleeding or allergic reaction should be evaluated frequently. Minor bleeding generally does not require therapy. Serious bleeding may require transfusion (packed red blood cells, fresh frozen plasma, cryoprecipitate). Aminocaproic acid and aprotinin have been used in reversing bleeding associated with SK therapy, but experience is limited.

TABLE 2. Risk factors for bleeding with thrombolytic agents

Risk category	Peripheral or systemic bleeding	Intracranial bleeding
Major (thrombolytic therapy contraindicated)	Major surgery or organ biopsy within 6 wk; major trauma within 6 wk; gastrointestinal or genitourinary bleeding within 6 mo; history of a bleeding diathesis; known or suspected aortic dissection; known or suspected pericarditis	Known intracranial tumor; previous neurosurgery; stroke within 6 mo; head trauma within 1 mo
Important (a relative contraindication to thrombolysis)	Puncture of a noncompressible vessel or cardiopulmonary resuscitation for >10 min	Acute severe hypertension; remote thrombotic stroke; recent transient ischemic attacks; older age; female sex; small body size; history of hypertension
Minor (increased risk of bleeding, but no definite contraindication to thrombolysis)	Diabetic retinopathy; cardiopulmonary resuscitation for <10 min; older age; small body size; female sex	Acute severe hypertension; remote thrombotic stroke; recent transient ischemic attacks; older age; female sex; small body size; history of hypertension

Modified from Anderson HV, Willerson JT. Thrombolysis in acute myocardial infarction. *N Engl J Med* 1993;329:703–709.

Hypotension is treated by discontinuing the infusion and restarting at a lower rate.

Bleeding

Management of bleeding involves applying direct pressure to bleeding sites, if possible, and discontinuing the lytic agent as well as other anticoagulants such as heparin. If bleeding occurs within 4 hours of heparin administration, consider the use of protamine sulfate (Chapter 70). Intravascular volume is replaced with isotonic IV fluids as required. Pressure is applied to bleeding sites for 15 to 30 minutes. If bleeding continues, blood product transfusion may be needed. Cryoprecipitate, 10 U, may be given. Fibrinogen levels guide further doses. Transfusion is usually not required if the level of fibrinogen is 100 mg/dl or more.

If the patient continues to bleed or has fibrinogen levels below 100 mg/dl, 2 to 6 U of fresh frozen plasma may be necessary. If bleeding continues after cryoprecipitate and fresh frozen plasma are administered, obtain a bleeding time to assess platelet function. If the bleeding time is more than 7 minutes, 10 U of platelets and antifibrinolytic drugs is recommended. If the bleeding time is less than 9 minutes, only antifibrinolytic agents are required.

Antidotes

Aminocaproic acid, aprotonin, and tranexamic acid are available antifibrinolytic agents, but experience in their use to reverse thrombolytic agents is limited. The dose of aminocaproic acid for treatment of acute bleeding due to elevated fibrinolytic activity is 16 to 20 ml (4 to 5 g) in 250-ml diluent administered as an IV infusion over 1 hour, followed by a continuous infusion at a rate of 4 ml (1 g) in 50-ml diluent per hour for 8 hours or until bleeding is controlled (25). Aprotonin has been used to control bleeding in patients requiring surgery after receiving SK. The dose (administered 1 to 5 hours after SK infusion) was 2 million KIU before bypass, with an additional 1 to 2 million KIU added to the pump prime and a continuous infusion of 0.5 million KIU/hour during surgery (26).

REFERENCES

1. Activase (alteplase), recombinant. Product information. San Francisco: Genentech, Inc., 1996.
2. Streptase (streptokinase). Product information. *Physicians' desk reference* (electronic version). Englewood, CO: Micromedex, Inc., 1998.
3. Nazar J, Davison R, Kaplan K, Fintel D. Adverse reactions to thrombolytic agents: implications for coronary reperfusion following myocardial infarction. *Med Toxicol Adverse Drug Exp* 1987;2:274–286.
4. Guidry JR, Raschke RA, Mortunas AE. Anticoagulants and thrombolytics. *Crit Care Clin* 1991;7:533–554.
5. Sane DC, Califf RM, Topol EJ, et al. Bleeding during thrombolytic therapy for acute myocardial infarction: mechanisms and management. *Ann Intern Med* 1989;111:1010–1022.
6. Verstraete M. The pharmacokinetics of anisoylated plasminogen streptokinase activation complex, tissue-type plasminogen activator, and simple-chain urokinase-type plasminogen activator. In: Julian DG, Kubler W, Norris RM, et al., eds. *Thrombolysis in cardiovascular disease.* New York: Marcel Dekker, 1989:69–86.
7. Verstraete M, Vaughan DE. Latest update in thrombolysis. In: Julian DG, Kubler W, Norris RM, et al., eds. *Thrombolysis in cardiovascular disease.* New York: Marcel Dekker, 1989:409–431.
8. Califf RM, Topol EJ, George BS, et al. Hemorrhagic complications associated with use of intravenous tissue plasminogen activator in treatment of acute myocardial infarction. *Am J Med* 1988;85:353–359.
9. Cairns JA, Collins R, Fuster V. Coronary thrombolysis. *Chest* 1989;95:235.
10. Fletcher AP, Alkjaersig NR. The hematologic consequences of thrombolytic therapy. *Proc Hematol* 1986;14:183–200.
11. Baldwin SH, Musa J. Cholesterol emboli syndrome occurring after administration of tissue plasminogen activator. *J Miss State Med Assoc* 2002;43:108.
12. Bhardwaj M, Goldweit R, Erlebacher J, et al. Tissue plasminogen activator and cholesterol crystal embolization [Letter]. *Ann Intern Med* 1989;111:687–688.
13. Adorati M, Pizzlitto S, Franzon R, et al. Cholesterol embolization and acute interstitial nephritis: two adverse effects of streptokinase thrombolytic therapy in the same patient. *Nephrol Dialysis Transplant* 1998;13:1262–1264.
14. Wright DA, Forni LG, Carr P, et al. Cholesterol embolization after systemic streptokinase. *Br J Hosp Med* 1997;57:51–52.
15. Schwartz MV, McDonald GB. Cholesterol embolization syndrome. Occurrence after intravenous streptokinase therapy for myocardial infarction. *JAMA* 1987;258:1934–1935.
16. Ridker PM, Michel T. Streptokinase therapy and cholesterol embolization. *Am J Med* 1989;87:357–358.
17. Pirson Y, Honhon B, Cosyns JP, van Ypersele C. Cholesterol embolism in a renal graft after treatment with streptokinase. *BMJ* 1988;6619:394–395.
18. Queen M, Biem HJ, Moe GW, Sugar L. Development of cholesterol embolization syndrome after intravenous streptokinase for acute myocardial infarction. *Am J Cardiol* 1990;65:1042–1043.
19. Tisdale JE, Stringer KA, Antalek M, Matthews GE. Streptokinase-induced anaphylaxis. *DICP* 1989;23:984–987.
20. Kalra PA, Coady AM, Iqbal A, et al. Acute tubular neurosis induced by coronary thrombolytic therapy. *Postgrad Med* 1991;67:212.
21. Mathiesen O, Grunner N. Haemolysis after intravenous streptokinase. *Lancet* 1989;1:1016–1017.
22. Romeo F, Rosano GM, Martuscelli E, et al. Concurrent nitroglycerin administration reduces the efficacy of recombinant tissue-type plasminogen activator in patients with acute anterior wall myocardial infarction. *Am Heart J* 1995;130:692–697.
23. Modi N, Eppler S, Breed J, et al. Pharmacokinetics of a slower clearing tissue plasminogen activator variant, TNK-tPA, in patients with acute myocardial infarction. *Thromb Haemost* 1998;79:134–139.
24. Ziller FP, Spinler SA. Alteplase: a tissue plasminogen activator for acute myocardial infarction. *Drug Intell Clin Pharm* 1988;22:6–14.
25. Amicar (aminocaproic acid). Product information. Florence, KY: Xanodyne Parmacol, Inc., 2002.
26. Akhtar TM, Goodchild CS, Boylan MKG. Reversal of streptokinase-induced bleeding with aprotonin for emergency cardiac surgery. *Anaesthesia* 1992;47:226–228.

SECTION

7

Cardiovascular Drugs

CHAPTER 114

Antihyperlipidemia Drugs

Sheila E. Bloomquist and Richard C. Dart

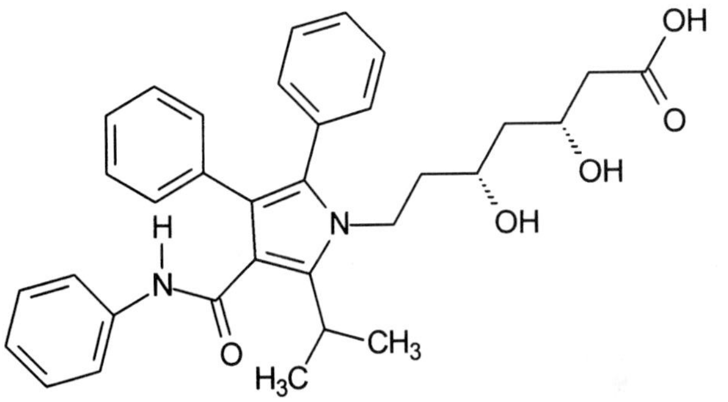

ATORVASTATIN

Compounds included:	**See Table 1.**
Molecular formula and weight:	**See Table 1.**
SI conversion:	**See Table 1.**
CAS Registry No.:	**See Table 1.**
Therapeutic levels:	**Not used clinically**
Special concerns:	**Life-threatening rhabdomyolysis may occur, primarily with statins. Hepatic necrosis may occur during chronic therapy.**
Antidote:	**None**

BILE ACID SEQUESTRANTS

Cholestyramine

Cholestyramine (Questran) is used in the treatment of hypercholesterolemia, pruritus, and pseudomembranous colitis. It is relatively contraindicated in hypersensitivity, biliary obstruction, and constipation.

TOXIC DOSE

Adult and pediatric therapeutic doses are provided in Table 1. Chronic dosing 15% above the normal dosage can cause deficiency of vitamins A, D, E, and K and folic acid as a result of decreased absorption.

TOXICOKINETICS AND TOXICODYNAMICS

Cholestyramine is not absorbed systemically. It binds bile acid and is then excreted in the feces (1).

PATHOPHYSIOLOGY

Cholestyramine is an anion-exchange resin. It inhibits reabsorption of cholesterol by binding bile acids in the intestine and increasing their excretion in the feces. The loss of bile acids activates the enzyme cholesterol 7-α-hydroxylase to make more bile acids. As these acids are produced, they consume intrahepatic cholesterol stores, which in turn increase the number of low-density lipoprotein (LDL) receptors in the liver and enhance the clearance of LDL-cholesterol from the circulation (2,3).

PREGNANCY AND LACTATION

Cholestyramine is U.S. Food and Drug Administration (FDA) pregnancy category C (Appendix I). Although cholestyramine resin is not absorbed, it should be used cautiously in nursing women due to decreased absorption of fat-soluble vitamins.

CLINICAL PRESENTATION

Acute overdosage has not been reported. Adverse events include fecal impaction. More common events are constipation, flatulence, nausea, dyspepsia, abdominal pain, anorexia, sour taste in the mouth, headache, urticaria, rash, hematuria, fatigue, weight loss, and bleeding gums. Cholestyramine can also cause hypochloremic acidosis arising from increased chloride supply from the resin.

TABLE 1. Physical characteristics and dose of the antihyperlipidemia drugs

Compounds included	Molecular formula, molecular weight (g/mol), CAS Registry No.	SI conversion	Formulation	Therapeutic dose (oral)	
				Adults	Children
Bile acid binders					
Cholestyramine (Questran)	NR, >1 million, 11041-12-6	NA	4 g/bar; chewable bar, 4 g oral powder	4–24 g in divided doses	80 mg/kg 3 times daily
Colesevelam (Welchol)	NR, very high, 182815-44-7	NA	625-mg tablet	1875–4275 mg/d	Not approved for use
Colestipol (Colestid)	NR, very high, 37296-80-3	NA	1-g tablet, 5 g/dose oral suspension	2–16 g/d	Not approved for use
Lipolysis inhibitors					
Clofibrate (Atromid)	$C_{12}H_{15}ClO_3$, 242.7, 637-07-0	mg/L × 4.1 = µmol/L	—	1–2 g/d in divided doses	Not approved for use
Fenofibrate (Tricor, Lipidil)	$C_{20}H_{21}ClO_4$, 360.8, 49562-28-9	mg/L × 2.8 = µmol/L	54-, 160-mg tabs	67–201 mg/d	Not approved for use
Gemfibrozil (Lopid)	$C_{15}H_{22}O_3$, 250.3, 25812-30-0	mg/L × 4.0 = µmol/L	300-mg capsule, 600-mg tablet	600 mg twice daily	Not approved for use
HMG-CoA reductase inhibitors					
Atorvastatin (Lipitor)	$C_{66}H_{68}CaF_2N_4O_{10}3H_2O$, 1209.4, 134523-03-8	mg/L × 0.8 = µmol/L	10-, 20-, 40-, 80-mg tablets	10–80 mg/d	10–20 mg/d
Cerivastatin (Baycol)	$C_{26}H_{33}FNNaO_5$, 481.5, 143201-11-0	mg/L × 2.1 = µmol/L	NR	0.2–0.8 mg/d	Not approved for use
Fluvastatin (Lescol)	$C_{24}H_{25}FNNaO_9$, 433.4, 93957-55-2	mg/L × 2.3 = µmol/L	—	—	—
Lovastatin (Mevacor)	$C_{24}H_{36}O_5$, 404.5, 75330-75-5	mg/L × 2.5 = µmol/L	10-, 20-, 40-mg tablets	10–80 mg/d	10–40 mg/d
Pravastatin (Pravachol)	$C_{23}H_{35}O_7Na$, 446.5, 81131-70-6	mg/L × 2.2 = µmol/L	10-, 20-, 40-, 80-mg tablets	40–80 mg/d	20–40 mg/d
Simvastatin (Zocor)	$C_{25}H_{38}O_5$, 418.6, 79902-63-9	mg/L × 2.4 = µmol/L	5-, 20-, 40-, 80-mg tablets	5–80 mg/d	Not approved for use
Other					
Ezetimibe (Zetia)	—	—	10-mg tab	10 mg/d orally	Not approved for use
Niacin (Niaspan, many others)	$C_6H_5NO_2$, 123.1, 59-67-6	mg/L × 8.1 = µmol/L	50 mg/5 ml elixir; 375-, 500-, 750-, 1000-mg sustained-release tablet or capsule; 50-, 100-, 250-, 500-, 750-mg tablets	100 mg–2 g orally 3 times daily	100–250 mg/d in 3 divided doses with meals; up to 10 mg/kg/d

HMG-CoA, hydroxymethylglutaryl coenzyme A; NA, not applicable; NR, not reported.

Drug interactions include decreased efficacy of thiazides, amiodarone, statins, and thyroid hormone. Cholestyramine should be avoided in patients with phenylketonuria or similar disorders.

DIAGNOSTIC TESTS

Serum electrolytes may be needed to evaluate hyperchloremia in symptomatic volume-depleted patients. Coagulation and liver function tests may be needed in symptomatic patients.

TREATMENT

No experience with overdosage has been reported. Treatment of adverse events involves discontinuation of therapy, followed by symptomatic and supportive care. Gastrointestinal (GI) decontamination has not been reported or evaluated. No information is available regarding enhancement of elimination or antidotes.

Colesevelam

Colesevelam (Welchol) is a nonabsorbed polymer that binds bile acids (4). It must be taken with meals. In higher doses, the bile acid binders can cause deficiencies of vitamins A, D, E, and K. Supplementation with a multivitamin is recommended.

The drug is contraindicated in patients with a history of allergic reaction to colesevelam, GI obstruction, triglyceride levels above 300 mg/dl, GI motility disorders, dysphagia, and a history of major GI surgery.

TOXIC DOSE

Adult and pediatric therapeutic doses are provided in Table 1. At doses above 4.5 g/day, vitamin K deficiency can develop.

PATHOPHYSIOLOGY

Colesevelam tightly binds bile acids, acts in the intestinal lumen, and is excreted in the feces. Oral absorption is minimal.

PREGNANCY AND LACTATION

Colesevelam is FDA pregnancy category B (Appendix I). It is considered safe in breast-feeding.

CLINICAL PRESENTATION

Acute overdosage has not been reported. Adverse events include vitamin K deficiency at doses above 4.5 g/day, which can cause hemorrhage. Other adverse effects include constipation, dyspepsia, and flatulence.

Drug interactions involve decreased absorption of verapamil by colesevelam.

DIAGNOSTIC TESTS

Coagulation tests may be needed in symptomatic patients.

TREATMENT

No experience with overdosage has been reported. Treatment of adverse events involves discontinuation of therapy, followed by symptomatic and supportive care. No information is available regarding GI decontamination, enhancement of elimination, or antidotes.

Colestipol

Colestipol (Colestid) is an insoluble, high-molecular-weight basic anion-exchange resin that is used in the treatment of hypercholesterolemia (5). Its use is relatively contraindicated in patients with chronic constipation.

TOXIC DOSE

Adult and pediatric therapeutic doses are provided in Table 1. The toxic dose has not been established.

PATHOPHYSIOLOGY

Colestipol is an insoluble resin that is not absorbed. It acts by binding bile acids in the intestine and is then excreted in the feces.

PREGNANCY AND LACTATION

Colestipol is FDA pregnancy category C (Appendix I). It is considered safe during breast-feeding.

CLINICAL PRESENTATION

Acute overdosage has been followed by hepatotoxicity in one report. Adverse events include fecal impaction, rarely complicated by GI obstruction. Difficulty swallowing and transient esophageal obstruction have occurred rarely. Other reported events include GI bleeding. More common occurrences are constipation, abdominal pain, bloating, flatulence, dyspepsia, liver dysfunction (6), musculoskeletal pain, chest pain, and anorexia. The fasting blood glucose and serum insulin concentration may be increased during treatment (7).

Drug interactions involve interference with vitamin absorption (vitamins A, D, E, K; folic acid; multivitamins). It can decrease the efficacy of thiazides, statins, amiodarone, and digoxin. Colestipol decreases absorption of tetracycline, furosemide, penicillin G, hydrochlorothiazide, and gemfibrozil.

DIAGNOSTIC TESTS

In symptomatic patients, liver function tests, creatine kinase (CK), and coagulation tests should be evaluated. GI obstruction is assessed in the usual manner with contrast radiographic studies and endoscopy.

TREATMENT

No experience with overdosage has been reported. Treatment of adverse events involves discontinuation of therapy, followed by symptomatic and supportive care. No information is available regarding GI decontamination, enhancement of elimination, or antidotes.

LIPOLYSIS INHIBITORS

Gemfibrozil

Gemfibrozil (Lopid) is used in the treatment of hypertriglyceridemia and hypercholesterolemia. It is relatively contraindicated in hypersensitivity, gallbladder disease, concomitant use of cerivastatin, hepatic dysfunction, severe renal disease, or impaired renal function. It should be used with caution with other statins.

TOXIC DOSE

Adult and pediatric therapeutic doses are provided in Table 1. A dose of 9 g or less was associated with clinical effects and spontaneous recovery in a 7-year-old child.

TOXICOKINETICS AND TOXICODYNAMICS

Gemfibrozil is well absorbed orally and is 99% bound to serum proteins (8). It is extensively oxidized in the liver, and renal excretion is 70%. It is excreted as the glucuronide conjugate. The elimination half-life is 1.5 hours (8).

PATHOPHYSIOLOGY

Gemfibrozil is thought to reduce hepatic triglyceride production by inhibiting peripheral lipolysis and decreasing the hepatic extraction of plasma free fatty acids. The drug may also inhibit synthesis of very-low-density lipoprotein carrier apoproteins (9).

PREGNANCY AND LACTATION

Gemfibrozil is FDA pregnancy category C (Appendix I). It is considered unsafe for use during breast-feeding.

CLINICAL PRESENTATION

Acute Overdosage. Abdominal cramps, abnormal liver function tests, diarrhea, increased serum CK, joint and muscle pain, nausea, and vomiting developed in a 7-year-old child after he ingested up to 9 g gemfibrozil. He recovered without complication (8).

Adverse Events. Common events include an increase in liver function tests, abdominal pain, dyspepsia, diarrhea, fatigue, nausea and vomiting, and elevated CK. Serious events are rare and include thrombocytopenia, anemia, leukopenia, myositis, myopathy, rhabdomyolysis, cholelithiasis, cholestatic jaundice, hypersensitivity, exfoliative dermatitis, acute appendicitis, and atrial fibrillation.

Some animal evidence of liver nodules and cancer has been found. Gemfibrozil may cause peroxisome proliferation and possible carcinogenicity in rats.

Drug Interactions. Gemfibrozil may increase the risk of rhabdomyolysis if used with statin-type drugs. It may increase the serum triglyceride level with beta-receptor blockers or thiazide diuretics. Gemfibrozil increases the risk of gallbladder disease and increases the triglyceride level with oral contraceptive pills. It also increases the effect of warfarin (Coumadin).

DIAGNOSTIC TESTS

Although little information has been reported, diagnostic testing should be directed at the anticipated effects of liver injury and coagulopathy (liver function tests, prothrombin time or international normalized ratio, complete blood count).

TREATMENT

Treatment of acute overdosage is symptomatic and supportive. GI decontamination has not been reported or evaluated. Enhancement of elimination is not expected to be successful because of the high degree of protein binding. No antidote is available for gemfibrozil poisoning.

Clofibrate and Fenofibrate

Clofibrate (Atromid) and fenofibrate (Tricor) are used for hypertriglyceridemia, hypercholesterolemia, and mixed dyslipidemia. Contraindications to the use of fenofibrate include hypersensitivity, severe renal disease, hepatic dysfunction, unexplained increase in liver function tests, gallbladder disease, and primary biliary cirrhosis. These drugs should be used with caution in patients with impaired renal function. The risk of pancreatitis is increased (increased triglycerides or gallbladder sludge).

TOXIC DOSE

Adult and pediatric therapeutic doses are provided in Table 1. The toxic dose has not been established.

TOXICOKINETICS AND TOXICODYNAMICS

Fenofibrate is metabolized via conjugation with glucuronic acid and excreted in the urine. A small amount is reduced to benzhydrol and excreted 25% in feces, with the rest in urine. Its half-life is 20 hours.

PATHOPHYSIOLOGY

The mechanism of action is unknown. Fibrates inhibit synthesis of triglycerides and stimulate catabolism of triglyceride-rich lipoproteins.

PREGNANCY AND LACTATION

Clofibrate and fenofibrate are FDA pregnancy category C (Appendix I). Neither should be used during breast-feeding.

CLINICAL PRESENTATION

Acute Overdosage. No data are available for acute overdosage.

Adverse Events. Common events include an increase in liver function tests, respiratory distress, abdominal pain, back pain, headache, increased CK, nausea, constipation, and rhinitis. Serious events include hepatitis, cirrhosis (rare), cholelithiasis, pancreatitis, myositis, rhabdomyolysis (rare), hypersensitivity, Stevens-Johnson syndrome (rare), toxic epidermal necrolysis (rare), thrombocytopenia (rare), and agranulocytosis (rare).

The myopathy associated with fibrates usually starts after a few days of medication but may develop after prolonged use. The patient notes muscle weakness and pain, and the serum CK is markedly increased. Renal failure may develop, and death may occur (10).

Alkaline phosphatase, γ-glutamyl transferase, and bilirubin levels are often decreased without apparent undesirable effect. Studies indicate increased lithogenicity; however, there has been no evidence of a significant rise in the incidence of cholelithiasis in the clinical trials (11,12).

Clofibrate has been associated with cholangiocarcinoma and dermatitis. Some evidence exists of carcinogenesis in animal studies: hepatotoxicity, peroxisome and pancreatic acinar adenomas, and adenocarcinomas.

Drug Interactions. The fibrates have multiple drug interactions. Use with thiazides, oral contraceptives, and beta-blockers increases triglyceride levels and decreases their efficacy. The risk of rhabdomyolysis is increased with statins and niacin. Interaction with ezetimibe increases hepatobiliary side effects. Fibrates increase the effect of warfarin.

DIAGNOSTIC TESTS

Although little information has been reported, diagnostic testing should be directed at the anticipated effects of liver injury and coagulopathy (liver function tests, prothrombin time or international normalized ratio, complete blood count).

TREATMENT

Treatment of acute overdosage is symptomatic and supportive. GI decontamination has not been reported or evaluated. Enhancement of elimination is not expected to be successful because of the high degree of protein binding. No antidote is available for gemfibrozil poisoning.

HYDROXYMETHYLGLUTARYL COENZYME A REDUCTASE INHIBITORS

The hydroxymethylglutaryl coenzyme A (HMG-CoA) reductase inhibitors include atorvastatin (Lipitor), cerivastatin (Baycol, Lipobay), fluvastatin (Lescol), lovastatin (Mevacor), pravastatin (Pravachol), and simvastatin (Zocor). Also known as the *statins*, the HMG-CoA reductase inhibitors block the rate-limiting step in the conversion of mevalonic acid to cholesterol. Cerivastatin was approved in 1999 and withdrawn from the U.S. market in 2001 because of the risk of rhabdomyolysis.

The HMG-CoA reductase inhibitors are indicated for the treatment of hypercholesterolemia, hypertriglyceridemia, and dysbetalipidemia. They reduce LDL and very-low-density lipoproteins, increase high-density lipoproteins, and are used in primary and secondary prevention in cardiovascular events.

General contraindications to the HMG-CoA reductase inhibitors are a history of hypersensitivity to the agent, active liver disease, an unexplained increase in liver function tests, pregnancy, and lactation. These drugs should be used cautiously in patients with a history of liver disease, ethanol abuse, or severe renal disease or when used concomitantly with fibrates, cyclosporine, niacin, amiodarone, or verapamil.

Toxic Dose

Adult and pediatric therapeutic doses are provided in Table 1. The few cases of overdosage reported have involved doses of less than 10 g and have produced no specific toxic effects.

Toxicokinetics and Toxicodynamics

The metabolism of atorvastatin, lovastatin, and simvastatin is primarily by CYP3A4 (13). Pravastatin has minimal CYP3A4 metabolism and is cleared renally. Fluvastatin is metabolized by CYP2C9, and cerivastatin is metabolized by CYP3A4 and CYP2C8 (13). Medications that inhibit CYP3A4 increase serum concentrations of selected statins and the risk of rhabdomyolysis. It is important to note that individual variation in CYP3A4 activity can vary tenfold (14).

Pathophysiology

Several theories exist regarding the cause of statin-associated rhabdomyolysis. The most common theory is that a synthetic pathway blocked by statin results in depletion of cholesterol in skeletal muscle cell membranes. Data regarding this theory are mixed (15). Other theories are that the levels of isoprenoids (i.e., ubiquinone) or regulatory proteins are reduced, leading to muscle injury, or that a small guanosine triphosphate binding protein is involved in the myotoxicity of statins (15).

Pregnancy and Lactation

All of the HMG-CoA reductase inhibitors are FDA pregnancy category X (Appendix I). All should be avoided by breast-feeding mothers.

Individual cases have implicated lovastatin with VATER (*v*ertebral anomalies, *a*nal atresia, *t*racheoesophageal fistula with *e*sophageal atresia, *r*enal and radial dysplasias) (16). Many statins are teratogenic in animals.

Clinical Presentation

ACUTE OVERDOSAGE

Several episodes of overdosage have been reported, without the development of specific toxic effects (17).

ADVERSE EVENTS

The first generation of statins in particular have many interactions, which are listed in the section Drug Interactions. Common adverse events include dyspepsia, constipation, flatulence, abdominal pain, diarrhea, nausea, rash, asthenia, myalgia, muscle weakness, increased CK, increased liver function tests, and eczema/ichthyosis/psoriasis.

The most serious events are rhabdomyolysis (rare) and hepatotoxicity (rare). The incidence of rhabdomyolysis (per 1 million

TABLE 2. Drugs that increase the risk of statin-associated rhabdomyolysis

Advicor	Fluconazole
Amiodarone	Fluvoxamine
Azole antifungals	Griseofulvin
Cimetidine	H_2 receptor blockers
Clarithromycin	Imatinib
Clopidogrel	Macrolide antibiotics
Cyclosporine	Nefazadone
Dalfopristin	Niacin
Danazol	Protease inhibitors
Delavirdine	Proton pump inhibitors
Diltiazem	Quinupristin-dalfopristin
Erythromycin	Verapamil
Fibric acid derivatives (gemfibrozil, clofibrate, fenofibrate)	Voriconazole
	Warfarin

prescriptions) is estimated for the statins: lovastatin, 0.19; pravastatin, 0.04; simvastatin, 0.12; fluvastatin, 0; atorvastatin, 0.04; and cerivastatin, 3.16 (18).

The relation between the complaint of myalgia and the development of rhabdomyolysis is unclear. Although a patient with rhabdomyolysis nearly always has myalgia, asymptomatic rhabdomyolysis has been reported (19). It is interesting that myalgia is a common complaint of patients with familial hypercholesterolemia, but the rate of myalgia in these patients is not different when they are treated with a statin or placebo (20).

The risk of rhabdomyolysis is dose related. In addition, factors that reduce the volume of distribution (e.g., body size and gender) and factors that reduce metabolism (renal or hepatic dysfunction, age, hypothyroidism, debilitation, and diabetes) increase the risk of rhabdomyolysis (15).

All HMG-CoA reductase inhibitors have the potential to cause adrenal and gonadal dysfunction if prolonged or high doses are used (through blunting of the cholesterol synthesis pathways). Pancreatitis has occurred rarely in patients treated with HMG-CoA reductase inhibitors.

DRUG INTERACTIONS

Many drugs cause an increase in serum statin levels and thereby increase the risk of adverse events such as rhabdomyolysis. Numerous drugs increase the risk of rhabdomyolysis when used with a statin (15) (Table 2).

Warfarin interactions occur with fluvastatin and simvastatin. Simvastatin decreases the therapeutic dose of diltiazem and cisapride. It increases the effect of warfarin. It decreases the efficacy of rifampin, bile acid binders, bosentan, efavirenz, and griseofulvin. It increases liver function tests with ezetimibe (Zetia) and causes hypoglycemia with repaglinide. Pravastatin results in decreased efficacy with bile acid resin and rifampin and an increase in liver function tests with ezetimibe.

Diagnostic Tests

Although various regimens have been proposed, the most common is to determine baseline liver function tests and CK levels before therapy and then to monitor every 3 to 6 months. Some experienced authors do not recommend regular monitoring of asymptomatic patients (15). These tests should also be ordered if patients' complaints are consistent with myopathy or hepatitis.

Treatment

Because acute overdose does not cause severe toxicity, supportive care is appropriate. Acute GI decontamination is not needed unless toxic coingestants are present. Enhancement of elimination has not been proposed or studied for statin toxicity. No antidotes are available.

Supportive Care

The treatment of all adverse effects involves prompt discontinuation of therapy and intensive supportive care. Statins have been restarted in some patients who have recovered from rhabdomyolysis, but this should be avoided if possible (13).

Patients with myalgia should be evaluated. If the CK is not elevated, they can continue therapy if their symptoms are tolerable. Alternatively, they can be switched to another statin (15). In many cases their symptoms persist, and they should be changed to another form of lipid-lowering therapy.

OTHER AGENTS

Niacin

Niacin is one of the water-soluble vitamins. It is an effective antihyperlipidemia agent but has suffered from adverse events at doses sufficient to lower lipid levels. Extended-release forms (Niaspan) or a combination of lower doses of niacin with other antihyperlipidemic agents offer a better adverse event profile. Nicotinamide is a metabolite of niacin that does not reduce lipid levels.

Niacin is relatively contraindicated in patients with unstable angina or a history of coronary artery disease, atrial fibrillation or other dysrhythmias, orthostatic hypotension, allergies to yellow dye No. 5, known peptic ulcer disease, active liver disease, or asthma (may increase thromboxane and leukotriene synthesis).

TOXIC DOSE

Adult and pediatric therapeutic doses are provided in Table 1. A single dose of 500 mg can cause flushing and other effects in the niacin-naïve individual.

TOXICOKINETICS AND TOXICODYNAMICS

The oral bioavailability of immediate or extended release is 60% to 76% (21,22). The plasma elimination half-life is approximately 45 minutes (21).

PATHOPHYSIOLOGY

The mode of action is not well defined. Niacin may inhibit hepatic synthesis of lipoproteins (23), promote lipoprotein lipase activity (24), and reduce free fatty acid release from adipose tissue.

PREGNANCY AND LACTATION

Niacin is FDA pregnancy category A (Appendix I). It enters breast milk but is considered safe for use during breast-feeding.

CLINICAL PRESENTATION

Acute Overdosage. Acute overdosage may produce flushing, abdominal distress, and a feeling of warmth. Death from acute overdosage has not been reported.

Adverse Events. The most common reactions involve flushing, warmth, and pruritus. The response is dose and formulation dependent. Doses above 1 g/day of the immediate-release form cause many reactions, and 40% of patients have withdrawn from trials. In contrast, although approximately 65% of patients who receive higher doses of the extended-release form report flushing, many fewer discontinue therapy (25).

Chronic use has been associated with hyperpigmentation/acanthosis nigricans, orthostatic hypotension, dyspepsia, vomiting, diarrhea, peptic ulceration, jaundice, abnormal liver function tests, dry skin, decreased glucose tolerance, hyperuricemia, gout, toxic amblyopia, headache, and macular edema. Doses of 1 g/day do not affect glycemic control, but higher doses may need adjustment of the antidiabetic therapy (25). The most serious events have involved atrial fibrillation, ventricular dysrhythmias, hepatotoxicity, and fulminant hepatic necrosis.

Drug Interactions. The most serious interaction is to increase the risk of rhabdomyolysis when used with a statin. Niacin also increases the risk of hyperglycemia with insulin, metformin, thiazolidinediones, and sulfonylureas. It may increase uric acid levels and decrease the efficacy of uricosurics. It decreases the efficacy of bile acid binders and increases the risk of hepatotoxicity with ethanol.

DIAGNOSTIC TESTS

Laboratory tests should be directed toward the known adverse effects: serum CK for patients with myalgia or similar complaints, liver function tests in evidence of liver injury, and serum electrolytes and glucose for diabetics. In a 71-year-old man with nicotinic acid–induced retinopathy, optical coherence tomography demonstrated cystoid spaces in the outer plexiform layer and inner nuclear layer (26).

TREATMENT

Treatment of adverse events involves discontinuation of therapy followed by symptomatic and supportive care. Immediate flushing reactions resolve spontaneously. GI decontamination has not been reported or evaluated. No information is available regarding enhancement of elimination or antidotes.

Ezetimibe

Ezetimibe is indicated for familial homozygous-type hypercholesterolemia and familial sitosterolemia. It is a novel inhibitor of cholesterol absorption that does so without affecting the absorption of triglycerides or fat-soluble vitamins. Ezetimibe inhibits intestinal cholesterol absorption, whereas statins inhibit cholesterol production.

TOXIC DOSE

Adult and pediatric therapeutic doses are provided in Table 1. The toxic dose has not been established.

TOXICOKINETICS AND TOXICODYNAMICS

The maximum serum concentration was 3.4 to 5.5 ng/ml at 4 to 12 hours after a single 10-mg dose in fasted adults (27). Ezetimibe and its active metabolite, ezetimibe glucuronide, are highly protein bound (more than 90%) (27). Ezetimibe does not appear to interact with cytochrome P-450 enzymes (28). The elimination half-life is 22 to 24 hours (28).

PATHOPHYSIOLOGY

Ezetimibe inhibits cholesterol absorption in the gut, decreases LDL by 80%, and increases high-density lipoproteins by 2%. It does not affect absorption of triglycerides or fat-soluble vitamins.

PREGNANCY AND LACTATION

Ezetimibe is FDA pregnancy category C (Appendix I). Entry into breast milk is unknown.

CLINICAL PRESENTATION

Acute overdosage. Acute overdosage has not been reported.

Adverse Events. Adverse events include diarrhea, abdominal pain, arthralgia, back pain, and fatigue.

Drug Interactions. Ezetimibe can be used with statins or in patients who have experienced statin-associated rhabdomyolysis (29). It may rarely cause an increase in liver function tests or toxicity when used with bile acid binders, cyclosporine, fibric acid derivatives, and statins.

DIAGNOSTIC TESTS

Serum liver function tests, CK levels, and electrolytes are often monitored.

TREATMENT

No experience with acute overdosage has been reported. Treatment of adverse events involves discontinuation of therapy followed by symptomatic and supportive care. No information is available regarding enhancement of elimination or antidotes.

REFERENCES

1. Questran, cholestyramine product information. Princeton, NJ: Bristol-Myers Squibb, 1997.
2. LaRosa J. Review of clinical studies of bile acid sequestrants for lowering plasma lipid levels. *Cardiology* 1989;76[Suppl 1]:55–64.
3. Shepherd J. Mechanism of action of bile acid sequestrants and other lipid lowering drugs. *Cardiology* 1989;76[Suppl 1]:65–74.
4. Davidson MH, Dillon MA, Gordon B, et al. Colesevelam hydrochloride (Cholestagel): a new potent bile acid sequestrant associated with a low incidence of gastrointestinal side effects. *Arch Intern Med* 1999;159:1893–1900.
5. Heel RC, Brogden RN, Pakes GE, et al. Colestipol: a review of its pharmacological properties and therapeutic efficacy in patients with hypercholesterolemia. *Drugs* 1980;19:161–180.
6. Sirmans SM, Beck JK, Banh HL, et al. Colestipol-induced hepatotoxicity. *Pharmacotherapy* 2001;21:513–516.
7. Lithell H, Vessby B, Boberg J, et al. The effects of colestipol when combined with clofibrate in the treatment of severe hyperlipidemia. Short-term and long-term studies. *Atherosclerosis* 1980;37:175–186.
8. Lopid, gemfibrozil product information. Morris Plains, NJ: Parke-Davis Co, 1998.
9. Kaukola S, Manninen V, Malkonen M, et al. Gemfibrozil in the treatment of dyslipidaemias in middle-aged male survivors of myocardial infarction. *Acta Med Scand* 1981;209:69–73.
10. Hodel C. Myopathy and rhabdomyolysis with lipid-lowering drugs. *Toxicol Lett* 2002;128:159–168.
11. Blane GF. Comparative toxicity and safety profile of fenofibrate and other fibric acid derivatives. *Am J Med* 1987;83(5B):26–36.
12. Roberts WC. Safety of fenofibrate—US and worldwide experience. *Cardiology* 1989;76:169–179.
13. Omar MA, Wilson JP, Cox TS. Rhabdomyolysis and HMG-CoA reductase inhibitors. *Ann Pharmacother* 2001;35:1096–1107.
14. Bottorff M, Hansten P. Long-term safety of hepatic hydroxymethyl glutaryl coenzyme A reductase inhibitors: the role of metabolism—monograph for physicians. *Arch Intern Med* 2000;160:2273–2280.
15. Thompson PD, Clarkson P, Karas RH. Statin-associated myopathy. *JAMA* 2003;289:1681–1690.
16. Ghidini A, Sicherer S, Willner J. Congenital abnormalities (VATER) in baby born to mother using lovastatin. *Lancet* 1992;339:1416–1417.
17. Mevacor, lovastatin. Product information. West Point, PA: Merck & Co, Inc, 1999.
18. Staffa JA, Chang J, Green L. Cerivastatin and reports of fatal rhabdomyolysis. *N Engl J Med* 2002;346:539–540.
19. Phillips PS, Haas RH, Bannykh S, et al. Statin-associated myopathy with normal creatine kinase levels. *Ann Intern Med* 2002;137:581–585.
20. Medical Research Council/British Heart Foundation. Heart protection study of cholesterol lowering with simvastatin in 20,536 high-risk individuals: a randomized placebo-controlled trial. *Lancet* 2002;360:7–22.
21. Hebel SK, Burnham TH, eds. *Drug facts and comparisons*. St. Louis: Facts and Comparisons, Inc, 2002.
22. Niaspan, niacin extended-release tablets, product information. Miami: Kos Pharmaceuticals, Inc, 1997.
23. Grundy SM. Drug therapy in dyslipidemia. *Scand J Clin Lab Invest* 1990a;50[Suppl 199]:63–72.
24. Odetti P, Cheli V, Carta G, et al. Effect of nicotinic acid associated with retinol and tocopherols on plasma lipids in hyperlipoproteinaemic patients. *Pharmatherapeutica* 1984;4:21–24.

25. Grundy Scott M, Vega GL, et al. Efficacy, safety, and tolerability of once-daily niacin for the treatment of dyslipidemia associated with type 2 diabetes: results of the assessment of diabetes control and evaluation of the efficacy of Niaspan trial. *Arch Intern Med* 2002;162:1568–1576.
26. Spirn MJ, Warren FA, Guyer DR, et al. Optical coherence tomography findings in nicotinic acid maculopathy. *Am J Ophthalmol* 2003;135:913–914.
27. Zetia, ezetimibe, product information. Kenilworth, NJ: Schering Corp.
28. Bays HE, Moore PB, Drehobl MA, et al. Effectiveness and tolerability of ezetimibe in patients with primary hypercholesterolemia: pooled analysis of two phase II studies. *Clin Ther* 2001;23:1209–1230.
29. Ballantyne CM, Houri J, Notarbartolo A, et al. Effect of ezetimibe coadministered with atorvastatin in 628 patients with primary hypercholesterolemia: a prospective, randomized, double-blind trial. *Circulation* 2003;2409–2415.

CHAPTER 115

Angiotensin-Converting Enzyme Inhibitors

Shireen Banerji

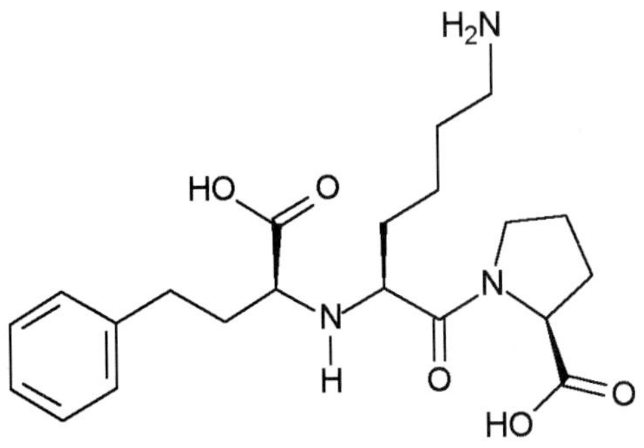

LISINOPRIL

Compounds included:	**Benazepril (Lotensin), captopril (Capoten), enalapril (Vasotec), fosinopril (Monopril), lisinopril (Prinivil, Zestril), moexipril (Univasc, Perdix), perindopril (Aceon), quinapril (Accupril), ramipril (Altace), trandolapril (Mavik), enalaprilat (Vasotec IV)**
Molecular formula and weight:	**See Table 1.**
SI Conversion:	**See Table 1.**
CAS Registry No.:	**See Table 1.**
Therapeutic level:	**Not recommended or clinically useful**
Target organs:	**Angiotensin II, bradykinin (renin-angiotensin system); may cause hypotension**
Antidote:	**None**

OVERVIEW

Angiotensin-converting enzyme (ACE) inhibitors encompass a widely prescribed group of antihypertensive drugs (Table 1). Worldwide, there are approximately 16 different ACE inhibitors available. ACE inhibitors are also used in the treatment of congestive heart failure (CHF), diabetic nephropathy, and post-myocardial infarction. Many ACE inhibitors are available in combination products containing a thiazide diuretic or a calcium channel blocker. The principal toxic effect of ACE inhibitor overdose is hypotension, although hyperkalemia and renal failure may occur. Angiotensin receptor blockers are addressed in Chapter 116.

ACE inhibitors can be divided into three subgroups: sulfhydryl-containing (captopril), carboxyl- or dicarboxyl-containing ACE inhibitors (lisinopril, benazepril, enalapril, ramipril, quinapril, moexipril, trandolapril, perindopril), and the phosphorus- or phosphinyl-containing ACE inhibitor (fosinopril). They all share the same mechanism of action on the renin-angiotensin system: binding to the zinc site of ACE, thus preventing conversion of angiotensin I to angiotensin II (1).

TOXIC DOSE

Adult and pediatric therapeutic doses are provided in Table 1. Although not commonly used in the pediatric population, ACE inhibitors may be used in children with CHF, hypertension, and nephropathy. Among ACE inhibitor overdosage reported in the literature, the majority of cases involved coingestants and thus toxicity as a result of the added drugs (2,3). Fatalities from an isolated ACE inhibitor overdose are rare. A 75-year-old male ingested 90 2.5-mg captopril tablets, and the postmortem plasma concentration of captopril was 60.4 mg/L (4).

Accidental pediatric ingestion of adult doses of ACE inhibitors is not expected to produce toxicity. A prospective poison center study of captopril, enalapril, and lisinopril overdose in children suggests home management of patients younger than 6 years of age who ingest less than 4 mg/kg captopril, less than 1 mg/kg enalapril, or less than 1 mg/kg lisinopril (5). Alternatively, a retrospective review of 48 children younger than 6 years of age found that an estimated ingestion of 12.5 to 300 mg captopril or 5 to 30 mg enalapril produced no symptoms. Children ingesting more than 100 mg captopril were decontaminated with syrup of ipecac (6).

TABLE 1. Physical characteristics and therapeutic dose for angiotensin-converting enzyme inhibitors

Name	Molecular formula, molecular weight (g/mol), and CAS Registry No.	SI conversion	Therapeutic dose	
			Adult (mg)	Children (mg/kg)
Benazepril	$C_{24}H_{28}N_2O_5$,HCl, 424.50, 86541-74-4	mg/L × 2.4 = μmol/L	5–80 daily single or divided dosage	NR
Captopril	$C_9H_{15}NO_3S$, 217.3, 62571-86-2	mg/L × 4.6 = μmol/L	6.25–150 two to three times daily	0.05–0.5 three times a day
Enalapril	$C_{20}H_{28}N_2O_5$,$C_4H_4O_4$, 376.45, 76095-16-4	mg/L × 2.7 = μmol/L	2.5–40 single or divided dosage	0.1–0.5 once daily
Fosinopril	$C_{30}H_{45}NNaO_7P$, 563.67, 88889-14-9	mg/L × 1.8 = μmol/L	10–80 single or divided dosage	NR
Lisinopril	$C_{21}H_{31}N_3O_5$,$2H_2O$, 441.5, 83915-83-7	mg/L × 2.3 = μmol/L	5–40 single or divided dosage	NR
Moexipril	$C_{27}H_{34}N_2O_7$,HCl, 535.0, 82586-52-5	mg/L × 1.9 = μmol/L	7.5–30 single or divided dosage	NR
Perindopril	$C_{19}H_{32}N_2O_5$,$C_4H_{11}N$, 368.47, 107133-36-8	mg/L × 2.7 = μmol/L	4–16 single or divided dosage	NR
Quinapril	$C_{25}H_{30}N_2O_5$,HCl, 438.52, 82586-55-8	mg/L × 2.3 = μmol/L	5–80 single or divided dosage	NR
Ramipril	$C_{23}H_{32}N_2O_5$, 416.5, 87333-19-5	mg/L × 2.4 = μmol/L	1.25–20 single or divided dosage	NR
Trandolapril	$C_{24}H_{34}N_2O_5$, 430.5, 87679-37-6	mg/L × 2.3 = μmol/L	1–4 daily	NR

NR, not reported.

TOXICOKINETICS AND TOXICODYNAMICS

Only pharmacokinetic data are available (Table 2). ACE inhibitors differ amongst each other with regard to two properties: potency and pharmacokinetics (7). Most ACE inhibitors (fosinopril is the exception) are cleared by the renal route. For this reason, the dosages of ACE inhibitors should be reduced in patients with impaired renal function. Besides pharmacokinetic differences, some ACE inhibitors rely on conversion from a prodrug to an active metabolite. Consequently, conversion from the prodrug to the active metabolite may be delayed or incomplete in patients with hepatic dysfunction.

PATHOPHYSIOLOGY

On a molar basis, angiotensin II is approximately 40 times more potent than norepinephrine (8). ACE is an enzyme found in lung and vascular endothelium. In addition to angiotensin II, it also catalyzes the breakdown of bradykinin, a potent vasodilator, to inactive substances. The principal pharmacologic and clinical benefits of ACE inhibitors seem to arise from the suppression of angiotensin II and consequently aldosterone secretion. This results in decreased blood pressure due to vasodilatation and reduced sodium and water retention; decreased peripheral vascular resistance; increased cardiac output; as well as increased coronary, renal, and cerebral flow. ACE inhibitors increase bradykinin levels, which stimulate prostaglandin synthesis. The bradykinin–nitric oxide generation is an important action of ACE inhibitors and this may further add to the vasodilatory effect. Another system that may mediate the hemodynamic effects of ACE inhibitors is the endogenous opioid system. The use of naloxone in treatment of ACE inhibitor overdose is addressed later in Antidotes.

PREGNANCY AND LACTATION

The U.S. Food and Drug Administration pregnancy category for all ACE inhibitors is C during the first trimester and category D during the second and third trimesters (Appendix I). ACE inhibitors are potential teratogens and their use during the second and third trimesters of pregnancy is contraindicated. Defects in skull ossification, pulmonary hypoplasia, oligohydramnios, neonatal hypertension, renal failure, anuria, and fetal death have been reported after fetal exposure to ACE inhibitors during the second and third trimesters (9). Fatal acute enterocolitis occurred in a neonate with *in utero* exposure to captopril throughout pregnancy (10). Congenital renal dysgenesis may have resulted from the ingestion of captopril throughout pregnancy (11).

Transfer of captopril to breast milk is minimal. The American Academy of Pediatrics considers captopril to be compatible with breast-feeding (12). Excretion of these agents into breast milk varies by agent (Table 2). Benazepril appears to be safe to administer to lactating mothers because less than 0.1% of the maternal dose of benazepril and benazeprilat would be ingested by a breast-feeding infant. Fosinopril used by nursing mothers is not recommended. Neither ramipril nor its metabolites were detectable in breast milk after a single 10-mg dose. Data from multiple dosing are not available; breast-feeding during ramipril use is not recommended. Breast-feeding is not recommended while taking trandolapril.

CLINICAL PRESENTATION

Acute Overdosage

Mild hypotension is the primary manifestation. Although hyperkalemia, bradycardia, and renal failure may occur, these effects are uncommon.

Adverse Events

ACE inhibitors are well tolerated. Hypotension may be expected after the first dose of an ACE inhibitor, especially in patients who are volume-depleted or with elevated plasma renin activity. Treatment with an ACE inhibitor should be initiated using small doses in patients that are salt-depleted, experience CHF, or are treated with multiple antihypertensive medications.

A nonproductive, dry, hacking cough is the most common adverse reaction reported. It is not dose-related, occurs in 5% to 20% of patients, occurs more frequently in women than in men, and usually develops between 1 week and 6 months after starting therapy (8). The cough usually disappears within 1 to 4 days after drug withdrawal but can rarely take as long as 4 weeks to subside (13). The presumed explanation for the ACE inhibitor–induced cough is due to the accumulation of bradykinin, substance P, and prostaglandins in the lung tissues (8). A genetic polymorphism has also been suggested (14). ACE inhibitor–induced cough does not affect standard pulmonary function tests. Patients with a primary airway disease such as asthma and chronic obstructive pulmonary disease are apparently not at increased risk of developing ACE inhibitor–induced cough (13,15).

TABLE 2. Pharmacokinetics of angiotensin-converting enzyme inhibitors

	Captopril	Benazepril	Enalapril	Lisinopril	Quinapril	Ramipril	Fosinopril	Perindopril	Trandolapril	Moexipril
Bioavailability (%)	70–75	37	60	25	50	60	30–36	75, 20–30 (M)	10, 40–60 (M)	13–22
Time to peak (h)	0.5–1.5	0.5–1.0, 1–4 (M)	1, 4–6 (M)	6–8	0.5–2.0	0.7–2.0, 2–4 (M)	3–4	1, 3–7 (M)	0.5–2.0, 4–10 (M)	1.5
Volume of distribution	0.7 L/kg	8.7 L	NR	1.6 L/kg	NR	NR	10 L	0.22 L/kg, 0.16 L/kg (M)	18 L	183 L
Elimination half-life (h)	1.9	0.6, 22 (M)	1.3, 11 (M)	12	0.8, 2 (M)	1–5, 13–17 (M)	<1, 11.5–12 (M)	0.8–1.0, 3–10 (M)	0.6–1.6, 16–24 (M)	1, 2–10 (M)
Protein binding (%)	25–30	97, 89–95 (M)	50–60	Minimal	97	73	89–99	10–20, 60 (M)	80, 94 (M)	50–70
Renal clearance	0.4 L/kg/h	1.36 L/h	9.48 L/h	6.3 L/h	3.96 L/h	0.64 L/h	16–20 ml/kg/h	1.5 L/h	1–4 L/h	NR
Metabolism	L	L	L	Minimal	L	L	L	L	L	L
Active metabolite	N	Benazeprilat	Enalaprilat	N	Quinaprilat	Ramiprilat	Fosinoprilat	Perindoprilat	Trandolaprilat	Moexiprilat
Urine excreted unchanged (%)	40–50	20 (M)	18, 43 (M)	29	NR	<2	NR	2.6	0.5, 14 (M)	1, 7 (M)
Placental transfer	NR	Y	NR	NR	NR	NR	NR	NR	NR	NR
Breast milk	Minimal	Minimal	Minimal	NR	Y	NR	Y	NR	Y	NR
Removed by hemodialysis	Y	N	Y	Y	N	Y	N	Y	NR	NR

L, liver; M, metabolite; N, no; NR, not reported; R, renal; Y, yes.

Hyperkalemia has been reported with therapeutic use, especially in patients with renal insufficiency and those taking nonsteroidal antiinflammatory drugs. A clinically significant increase in serum potassium is rare in nondiabetic patients with normal renal function and who are not taking concomitant potassium-retaining medications.

ACE inhibitors can induce acute renal insufficiency in patients with bilateral renal artery stenosis or with stenosis of the artery to a single remaining kidney (8). This results when angiotensin II is blocked from constricting the efferent arteriole, resulting in inadequate renal perfusion and insufficient glomerular filtration. Abrupt deterioration in renal function while on ACE inhibitor therapy has also been seen in patients with severe renal damage, marked volume depletion, and severe cardiac decompensation (13).

A maculopapular rash with or without pruritus has been described in patients prescribed captopril as well as other ACE inhibitors. The sulfhydryl component of captopril was initially attributed as the cause; however, because it occurs with other ACE inhibitors, the cause is not clearly elucidated.

Angioneurotic edema or angioedema is a rare but serious effect that occurs in 0.1% to 0.2% of patients (8,14,16–18). This condition is characterized by a rapid swelling in the upper respiratory tract, which can result in life-threatening respiratory distress, airway obstruction, and death. In rare cases, angioedema may manifest as isolated dysphagia or edema of the gastrointestinal tract. The increase in capillary blood flow and permeability leading to an increase in interstitial fluid may occur as a result of antigen-antibody interactions, bradykinin, or components of the complement system (14,16,18). Whereas ACE inhibitor–induced angioedema typically occurs within hours of the first dose or through the first week of therapy, this serious reaction may occur any time during therapy. It reverses with drug withdrawal. Many cases of mild angioedema are missed, leading to significant morbidity. Patients with prior history of idiopathic angioedema may be at increased risk for ACE inhibitor–induced angioedema.

Neutropenia is a rare side effect of ACE inhibitors. It occurs predominantly in hypertensive patients with collagen-vascular or renal parenchymal disease (8).

Patients treated with ACE inhibitors are often on concurrent aspirin therapy. The interaction between ACE inhibitors and aspirin in patients with CHF has been the subject of increasing interest. Cyclooxygenase blockers such as aspirin may interfere with ACE inhibitor via opposing effects on prostaglandin production. A study evaluating 26 patients with New York Heart Association class II or III dilated cardiomyopathy showed that aspirin in conjunction with ACE inhibitor therapy worsened exercise performance and pulmonary gas exchange as compared to the group who did not receive an ACE inhibitor (19,20).

DIAGNOSTIC TESTS

ACE inhibitor levels are neither useful nor readily available. Serum electrolytes and renal function tests should be assessed, particularly in patients with underlying renal disease or on concurrent diuretic therapy. An electrocardiogram may be needed to help assess hyperkalemia (Chapter 35).

TREATMENT

Decontamination

Because acute toxicity is not severe, gastric emptying should be avoided. Administration of activated charcoal within 1 to 2 hours of ingestion is recommended.

Enhancement of Elimination

ACE inhibitors are dialyzable but are not usually needed because supportive care is highly effective.

Antidotes

An infusion of angiotensin II would be an ideal antidote for treating ACE inhibitor–induced hypotension; however, availability is limited and the response to intravenous fluids and vasopressors is excellent so it is not used. Angiotensin amide is identical to naturally occurring angiotensin II and was approved by the U.S. Food and Drug Administration in June 1962. A case of hypotension refractory to traditional therapy in a patient with dilated cardiomyopathy responded to an infusion of angiotensin II to elevate the blood pressure (21).

Naloxone may also have a role in treatment of ACE inhibitor–induced hypotension as ACE inhibitors may inhibit the metabolism of enkephalins, potentiate endogenous opioids, and thereby lower blood pressure. A case of intentional captopril overdose with marked hypotension was treated with naloxone with prompt resolution in hypotension (22). The use of naloxone in ACE inhibitor overdose remains unclear.

Supportive Care

Hypotension should initially be treated with isotonic crystalloid fluid resuscitation followed by inotropic support if needed (Chapter 37). Intravascular volume expansion alone has been successful in restoring and maintaining blood pressure.

The cough acquired from ACE inhibitor therapy does not mandate cessation of therapy unless the patient finds it intolerable. Because cough involves a weighty differential diagnosis, a 4-day trial of withdrawal of the ACE inhibitor or substitution of a different type of antihypertensive agent is suggested in one review, to determine if the ACE inhibitor is the cause of the chronic cough (14). The ACE inhibitor cough generally does not respond well to classic antitussive agents. One controlled study suggests that sodium cromoglycate is effective (23).

The treatment of angioedema depends on its severity (16). Nasopharyngeal airway may suffice, depending on the site of obstruction. If the situation dictates, more invasive procedures may be needed (Chapter 33). Most cases are effectively controlled by standard anti-allergic drug therapy (subcutaneous epinephrine, intravenous antihistamines, and corticosteroids). The patient should be given an outpatient regimen consisting of oral antihistamines and a short course of corticosteroids. However, ACE inhibitor–induced angioedema is not associated with an increase in IgE, thus these interventions may be ineffective. The physician should be alert to a possible rebound phenomenon and closely observe the patient. Patients should be counseled to avoid ACE inhibitors and consult their primary physician for alternative medications. The use of angiotensin II receptor blockers in this patient population is cautioned against.

REFERENCES

1. Gavras H, Gavras I. Angiotensin-converting enzyme inhibitors. Properties and side effects. *Hypertension* 1988;11[Suppl II]:37–41.
2. Dawson AH, Harvey D, Smith AJ, et al. Lisinopril overdose. *Lancet* 1990;335:487–488.
3. Augenstein WL, Kulig KW, Rumack BH. Captopril overdose resulting in hypotension. *JAMA* 1988;259:3302–3305.
4. Park H, Purnell GV, Mirchandani HG. Suicide by captopril overdose. *J Toxicol Clin Toxicol* 1990;28:379–382.
5. Hogue-Murray K, Horowitz R, Dart RC. Outcome of ACE inhibitor ingestion in children under the age of six years [abstract]. *J Toxicol Clin Toxicol* 1995;33:509.

6. Spiller HA, Udicious TM, Muir S. Angiotensin-converting enzyme inhibitor ingestion in children. *J Toxicol Clin Toxicol* 1989;27:345–353.
7. Furberg CD. Class effects and evidence-based medicine. *Clin Cardiol* 2000;23[Suppl. IV]:IV 15–IV 19.
8. Jackson EK, Garrison JC. Renin and angiotensin. In: Hardman JG, Limbird LE, Molinoff PB, et al., eds. *Goodman & Gilman's the pharmacological basis of therapeutics*, 9th ed. New York: McGraw-Hill, 1996:733–758.
9. Brent RL, Beckman DA. Angiotensin-converting enzyme inhibitors: an embryopathic class of drugs with unique properties: information for clinical teratology counselors. *Teratology* 1991;43:543–546.
10. De Carolis MP, Muzii U, Romagnoli C, et al. Neonatal necrotizing enterocolitis (NEC) and maternal treatment with captopril. *Clin Exp Hypertension* 1991:Pt B10:264.
11. Knott PD, Thorpe SS, Lamont CAR. Congenital renal dysgenesis possibly due to captopril. *Lancet* 1989;1:451.
12. Capoten [package insert]. MICROMEDEX Healthcare Series Vol. 113; expires Sept. 2002.
13. Israili ZH, Hall WD. Cough and angioneurotic edema associated with angiotensin-converting enzyme inhibitor therapy. *Ann Intern Med* 1992;117:234–242.
14. Ram CV, Fenves A. Clinical pharmacology of antihypertensive drugs. *Cardiol Clin* 2002;20:265–280.
15. Packard KA, Wurdeman RL, Arouni AJ. ACE inhibitor-induced bronchial reactivity in patients with respiratory dysfunction. *Ann Pharmacother* 2002;36:1058–1067.
16. Finley CJ, Silverman MA, Nunez AE. Angiotensin-converting enzyme inhibitor-induced angioedema: still unrecognized. *Am J Emerg Med* 1992;10:550–552.
17. Slater EE, Merril DD, Guess HA, et al. Clinical profile of angioedema associated with angiotensin-converting enzyme inhibition. *JAMA* 1988;260:967–970.
18. Rees RS, Bergman J, Ramirez-Alexander R. Angioedema associated with lisinopril. *Am J Emerg Med* 1992;10:321–322.
19. Guazzi M, Pontone G, Agostoni P. Aspirin worsens exercise performance and pulmonary gas exchange in patients with heart failure who are taking angiotensin-converting enzyme inhibitors. *Am Heart J* 1999;138:254–260.
20. Teerlink JR, Massie BM. The interaction of ACE inhibitors and aspirin in heart failure: torn between two lovers. *Am Heart J* 1999;138:193–197.
21. Trilli LE, Johnson KA. Lisinopril overdose and management with intravenous angiotensin II. *Ann Pharmacother* 1994;28:1165–1168.
22. Varon J, Duncan SR. Naloxone reversal of hypotension due to captopril overdose. *Ann Emerg Med* 1991;20:1125–1127.
23. Hargreaves HR, Berson MK. Inhaled cromoglycate in angiotensin-converting enzyme inhibitor cough. *Lancet* 1995;345:13–16.

CHAPTER 116

Angiotensin Receptor Blockers

Shireen Banerji

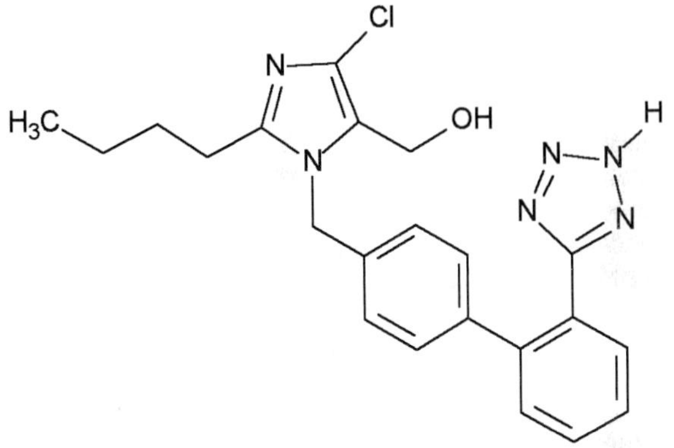

Cl N H_3C N OH N N H N N

LOSARTAN

Compounds included:	**Losartan (Cozaar), valsartan (Diovan), irbesartan (Avapro), candesartan (Atacand), telmisartan (Micardis), eprosartan (Teveten)**
Molecular formula and weight:	**See Table 1.**
SI conversion:	**See Table 1.**
CAS Registry No.:	**See Table 1.**
Therapeutic levels:	**Not clinically useful**
Target organs:	**Angiotensin II (renin-angiotensin system)**
Antidote:	**None**

OVERVIEW

Angiotensin receptor blockers (ARBs) represent an important therapeutic advance in the blockade of the renin-angiotensin pathways. Losartan was approved by the U.S. Food and Drug Administration in 1995. There are currently six ARBs marketed in the United States for treatment of hypertension: losartan, valsartan, irbesartan, candesartan, telmisartan, and eprosartan. Like angiotensin-converting enzyme (ACE) inhibitors, ARBs cause regression of left ventricular hypertrophy.

Early evidence suggests that ARBs improve hemodynamic parameters in patients with heart failure and may reduce mortality, but multiple large-scale trials are lacking (1). There is increasing interest in the field of cardiology in using an ACE inhibitor and an ARB together as combination therapy based on their different mechanisms of action (2,3).

TOXIC DOSE

The *adult and pediatric therapeutic doses* for ARBs are provided in Table 1 (4). Overdosage information is limited. A 45-year-old woman recovered without sequelae after intentional ingestion of candesartan cilexetil 160 mg along with other drugs (5).

TABLE 1. Physical characteristics and therapeutic dosage of angiotensin receptor blocking agents

Name	Molecular formula, molecular weight (g/mol), CAS Registry No.	SI conversion	Maximum single dose	
			Adult (mg)	Children
Candesartan	$C_{33}H_{34}N_6O_6$, 610.7, 145040-37-5	mg/L × 1.6 = μmol/L	8–32 once daily or divided doses	NR
Eprosartan	$C_{23}H_{24}N_2O_4S{,}CH_4O_3S$, 520.6, 144143-96-4	mg/L × 1.9 = μmol/L	400–800 once daily or divided doses	NR
Irbesartan	$C_{25}H_{28}N_6O$, 428.5, 138402-11-6	mg/L × 2.3 = μmol/L	150–300 once daily	75–150 once daily
Losartan	$C_{22}H_{22}ClKN_6O$, 461.0, 124750-99-8	mg/L × 2.2 = μmol/L	25–100 once daily or divided doses	NR
Telmisartan	$C_{33}H_{30}N_4O_2$, 514.6, 144701-48-4	mg/L × 1.9 = μmol/L	40–80 once daily	NR
Valsartan	$C_{24}H_{29}N_5O_3$, 435.5, 137862-53-4	mg/L × 2.3 = μmol/L	80–320 once daily or divided doses	NR

NR, not reported.

TOXICOKINETICS AND TOXICODYNAMICS

Only pharmacokinetic data are available (Table 2). Unlike ACE inhibitors, most ARBs do not have active metabolites. ARBs are eliminated either unchanged in the feces or through a variable proportion of urinary and biliary excretion.

PATHOPHYSIOLOGY

ACE inhibitors indirectly suppress the formation of angiotensin II by blocking conversion from angiotensin I to angiotensin II. However, angiotensin II can be formed by enzymes other than ACE, such as chymase. After long-term therapy with ACE inhibitors, angiotensin II levels tend to return to normal (1). ARBs block the receptor for angiotensin II on the blood vessel, heart, adrenal cortex, and possibly other tissues; this leads to reversal of vasoconstriction, myocardial and vascular hypertrophy, and inhibition of aldosterone (4). The current angiotensin II analogs lack agonist activity, and all clinically significant effects are attributed to the direct antagonism on the AT_1 receptor.

The six ARBs on the market differ only by their kinetic profiles. Their blood pressure–lowering properties are comparable to ACE inhibitors, but their side effect profiles are more favorable (6). Unlike ACE inhibitors, ARBs do not potentiate the effects of bradykinin and this may explain the reduced rate of cough reported among patients being treated with ARBs. However, this attenuation of bradykinins effect may remove the advantageous vasodilatory effect on cardiac and renal vasculature.

PREGNANCY AND LACTATION

The ARB drugs are all U.S. Food and Drug Administration category C (Appendix I) for women in their first trimester and category D for women in their second and third trimesters. Entry into breast milk is unknown (Table 2).

CLINICAL PRESENTATION

Acute Overdosage

The most likely manifestations of overdosage are hypotension and tachycardia; bradycardia could occur from parasympathetic (vagal) stimulation. Hyperkalemia may also occur in patients with renal disease or in patients taking potassium-sparing medications.

Adverse Events

Side effects from therapeutic doses of ARBs include headache, dizziness, and gastrointestinal complaints. The incidence of cough is 5% to 20% for patients treated with ACE inhibitors but is considerably less with ARBs.

Despite the promise of eliminating the potential for angioneurotic edema or angioedema by switching from an ACE inhibitor to an ARB, this complication was reported occasionally in patients treated with an ARB (6–8). A review of the literature identified 19 patients who experienced angioedema;

TABLE 2. Pharmacokinetics of the angiotensin receptor blocking drugs

	Losartan	Valsartan	Irbesartan	Candesartan	Telmisartan	Eprosartan
Absorption (%)	25	25	60–80	15	42	13
T_{max} (h)	1–1.5	2–4	1.5–2	3–4	0.5–1.0	4
V_d	34 L	17 L	53–93 L	0.13 L/kg	500 L	308 L
Elimination half-life (h)	1.5–2.0	6–9	11–15	NR	24	6
Protein binding (%)	98.7	94–95	90	>99	99.5	98
Renal clearance	2.6–4.5 L/h	0.62 L/h	0.18–0.20 L/h	0.01 L/kg/h	NR	2.3–2.7 L/h
Metabolism	Liver	Liver	Liver	Intestinal wall	Liver	Liver
Active metabolites	E-3174	No	No	Candesartan (Candesartan cilexetil is a prodrug)	No	No
Urine excreted unchanged (%)	3–5, 6–8 (M)	13	31–56	26	NR	80
Placental transfer	NR	NR	NR	Yes	NR	NR
Breast milk	NR	NR	NR	NR	NR	NR
Removed by hemodialysis	No	No	No	No	No	NR

M, metabolite; NR, not reported; T_{max}, time to maximum serum concentration; V_d, apparent volume of distribution.

six of the patients had a history of ACE inhibitor–induced angioedema (7).

DIAGNOSTIC TESTS

Specific diagnostic tests and drug levels are not readily available.

TREATMENT

After overdosage or angioedema, the drug should be discontinued. Early gastrointestinal decontamination with activated charcoal is indicated after overdosage. Treatment is supportive; the use of intravenous isotonic crystalloid therapy followed by vasopressors should be administered for significant hypotension. Close monitoring of vital signs and chemistries should be included in the management of ARB overdose.

REFERENCES

1. Califf RM, Cohn JN. Cardiac protection: the evolving role of ARBs. *Am Heart J* 2000;139:S15–S22.
2. Carson PE. Rationale for the use of combination angiotensin-converting enzyme inhibitor/angiotensin II receptor blocker therapy in heart failure. *Am Heart J* 2000;140:361–366.
3. Houghton AR, Harrison M, Cowley AJ, et al. Combined treatment with losartan and an ACE inhibitor in mild to moderate heart failure: results of a double-blind, randomized, placebo-controlled trial. *Am Heart J* 2000;140:e25.
4. Ram CV, Fenves A. Clinical pharmacology of antihypertensive drugs. *Cardiol Clin* 2002;20:265–280.
5. Atacand(R), candesartan cilexetil tablets [package insert]. Wilmington, DE: AstraZeneca; revised Sept 2001.
6. Ferdinand KC. Update in pharmacologic treatment of hypertension. *Cardiol Clin* 2001;19:279–294.
7. Warner KK, Visconti JA, Tschampel MM. Angiotensin II receptor blockers in patients with ACE inhibitor-induced angioedema. *Ann Pharmacother* 2000;34:526–528.
8. Chiu AG, Krowiak EJ, Deeb ZE. Angioedema associated with angiotensin II receptor antagonists: challenging our knowledge of angioedema and its etiology. *Laryngoscope* 2001;111:1729–1731.

CHAPTER 117

Clonidine

Richard C. Dart and Donna L. Seger

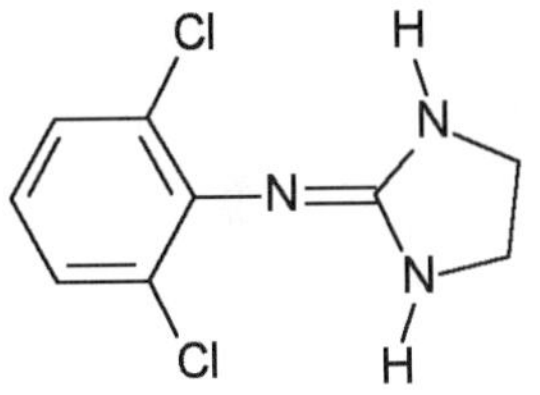

CLONIDINE

Compounds:	**Clonidine (Catapres, Catapres TTX, Duraclon), apraclonidine (Lopidine)**
Molecular formula and weight:	**Clonidine ($C_9H_9Cl_2N_3$,HCl), 266.6 g/mol; apraclonidine ($C_9H_{10}Cl_2N_4$,HCl), 281.6 g/mol**
SI conversion:	**μg/L × 4.35 = nmol/L**
CAS Registry No.:	**4205-91-8 (clonidine); 73218-79-8 (apraclonidine)**
Therapeutic level:	**2 μg/L (serum)**
Target organs:	**Clonidine causes respiratory depression and apnea, and transient hypertension followed by hypotension.**
Antidote:	**Naloxone**

OVERVIEW

Clonidine is an α_2-receptor agonist and antihypertensive agent. It is also used for many other conditions: attention deficit disorder; conduct and oppositional disorder; Tourette's syndrome; narcotic, nicotine, or alcohol withdrawal; preanesthesia; menopausal symptoms; and postural hypotension in patients with autonomic failure. It is available as a 100-μg/ml solution; 0.1-, 0.2-, and 0.3-mg tablets; and as 2.5-, 5-, and 7.5-mg patches.

Apraclonidine is used in the treatment of glaucoma. Like clonidine, it is an α_2-receptor agonist but also binds some α_1-receptors. Apraclonidine is more polar than is clonidine, which reduces its penetration through the blood–brain barrier and suggests that it causes more peripheral rather than central effects. It is available as 0.1% and 0.5% solutions.

TOXIC DOSE

The *adult therapeutic dose* of clonidine is 0.1 mg orally twice daily, which is titrated upward to a maximum dose of 2.4 mg/day. The *pediatric dose* for hypertension is 5 to 10 μg/kg/day in divided doses, up to 0.9 mg/day. A typical dose of apraclonidine is 1 drop in each eye three times a day.

Significant symptoms have followed ingestion of 0.2 mg clonidine by small children (1,2). A 5-year-old child who weighed 17.5 kg received 50 mg of clonidine (1000-fold overdosage), producing a serum concentration of 64 ng/ml at 17 hours postingestion (3). To subdue potential victims, thieves have added up to 8 mg of clonidine solution to alcoholic beverages. One victim developed hypotension, bradycardia, hypothermia, cyanosis, and impaired consciousness, and recovered with supportive care (4).

TOXICOKINETICS AND TOXICODYNAMICS

Clonidine is well absorbed; bioavailability is 100%. The plasma concentration and its hypotensive effect peak at 1 to 3 hours. The elimination half-life is 6 to 24 hours; approximately 50% of a dose is excreted unchanged in the urine (5). Binding to plasma proteins is 20% to 40% (6). The apparent volume of distribution is 1 to 2 L/kg (7).

PATHOPHYSIOLOGY

Clonidine causes hypotension through several actions. It decreases the sympathetic outflow from the central nervous system (7). It stimulates the α_2-adrenergic receptor and the imidazoline receptor. There are three subtypes of the α_2-receptor: α_{2a}, α_{2b}, and α_{2c}. Stimulation of α_{2a} by clonidine decreases norepinephrine release and inhibits sympathetic outflow in the central nervous system, but it also stimulates the α_{2b} peripherally and causes vasoconstriction. Stimulation of imidazoline receptors also decreases sympathetic outflow, by an unknown mechanism. Clonidine probably stimulates γ-aminobutyric acid, opioid or serotonin neurons (8), which produces additional sources for hypotension. Interaction of the imidazoline receptor and the α_2-receptor appear to be needed for the hypotensive action of clonidine (9,10). Finally, clonidine also increases the production of nitric oxide in a dose-dependent manner. Overall, clonidine has some effects that increase blood pressure (peripheral α agonism) and others that decrease blood pressure (central α_2 agonism, imidazoline agonism, γ-hydroxybutyrate agonist, and increased nitric oxide release).

PREGNANCY AND LACTATION

Clonidine is U.S. Food and Drug Administration pregnancy category C (Appendix I). Entry into breast milk has not been reported.

CLINICAL PRESENTATION

Acute Overdosage

The initial effect is usually mental status depression, which occurs within an hour of ingestion. Life-threatening signs of clonidine poisoning include apnea, coma, bradycardia, and hypotension. It also causes miosis and hypothermia. Cardiovascular effects usually follow central nervous system effects.

Hypotension is usually mild but may be more severe after large ingestion. The more direct and dangerous effect is hypoventilation and apnea from central respiratory failure. Coma and apnea are common effects after a large overdose. The mental status change is curious in that tactile stimulation has been noted to awaken the patient. For example, testing for a Babinski reflex may transiently awaken a formerly unresponsive patient.

Hypertension may be caused by clonidine toxicity, although it is not addressed frequently in the medical literature. Hypertension usually occurs early in the course and may be followed by a more prolonged period of hypotension. A review of multiple small case series reports indicates that the incidence of hypertension in children ranged from 18% to 48% (11). After ingestion of 1.95 mg, a 9-month-old child became comatose. Her blood pressure peaked at 140/90 mm Hg at 6 hours. Her lowest heart rate was 60 beats/minute at 5 hours. Heart rate and blood pressure normalized by 10 hours postingestion (12). Hypertension has also been reported in adults with preexisting hypertension. A 60-year-old woman ingested 20 mg of clonidine. Her initial blood pressure was 100/70 mm Hg, but she became hypertensive within 30 minutes and was treated with nitroprusside.

Adverse Events

Rare but serious effects that occur during therapeutic use include atrioventricular block, other minor dysrhythmias, Raynaud's phenomenon, and congestive heart failure. Other effects include confusion, hallucination, dry mouth, hypotension, nausea, vomiting, constipation, pruritus, contact dermatitis, tinnitus, and sedation.

Drug Interactions

The addition of mirtazapine (an α_2-agonist) caused a hypertensive urgency in a patient with essential hypertension controlled by clonidine (13). Similar effects have been noted with multiple drugs that are α-receptor agonists.

DIAGNOSTIC TESTS

Quantitation of the serum clonidine concentration is not clinically useful. In clinical research, toxicity was associated with a plasma clonidine level of 25 to 50 ng/ml, compared to a concentration of 1 to 2 ng/ml produced by a therapeutic dose (6). Testing is dictated by the clinical effects of overdosage, including evaluation of coma and the detection of hypotension and its sequelae. Typically, the complete blood count, serum electrolytes, and renal function are measured. Evaluation of respiratory function with pulse oximetry and arterial blood gases in more severe poisoning is important. An electrocardiogram is performed, especially if bradycardia is present. Computerized tomography of the head may be needed to evaluate coma.

TREATMENT

Supportive care with appropriate airway management is the mainstay of treatment. Endotracheal intubation for several hours or a day is usually sufficient to allow spontaneous recovery.

Decontamination

Induced emesis should be avoided because of potential for altered mental status. The risk of gastric lavage is justified only in a recent and large ingestion (Chapter 7). A dose of oral activated charcoal within 1 to 2 hours of ingestion is reasonable in patients with a protected airway. Whole bowel irrigation is theoretically useful in the case of a transdermal patch ingestion.

Enhancement of Elimination

Hemodialysis, multiple dose activated charcoal, and urinary alkalinization have not been demonstrated effective. Clonidine is likely marginally amenable to dialysis, but its use in case reports has not been followed by clinical improvement.

Antidotes

There is no proven antidote for clonidine poisoning. Naloxone has often been proposed as an antidote, although justified only by small case series (14,15). Furthermore, personal experience indicates that in some cases the response may be to the stimulation of inserting an intravenous line for insertion. However, there is a plausible scientific rationale for response in some patients (11). Thus, a therapeutic trial is warranted, especially in severe cases in which complications of the airway, bradycardia, or hypotension prove difficult to manage (Chapter 65). Theoretically, patients may respond to high dose naloxone (10 mg), even if they have not responded to lower doses. These are likely the patients with increased sympathetic tone (11).

Supportive Care

Symptomatic bradycardia typically fails to respond to atropine. Hypotension should initially be treated with isotonic crystalloid fluid resuscitation followed by inotropic support if needed (Chapter 37). Naloxone has been reported to reverse coma and hypotension.

Hypertension may occur and be followed by hypotension. Treatment of hypertension should be avoided, if possible. However, in the rare case that end organ damage develops, a titratable and reversible antihypertensive such as nitroprusside should be used.

Monitoring

Admit small children with history of ingestion and adults who develop toxic effects.

REFERENCES

1. Olsson JM, Pruitt AW. Management of clonidine ingestion in children. *J Pediatr* 1983;103:646–650.
2. Fiser DH, Moss MM, Walker W. Critical care for clonidine poisoning in toddlers. *Crit Care Med* 1990;18:1124–1128.
3. Romano MJ, Dinh A. A 1000-fold overdose of clonidine caused by a compounding error in a 5-year-old child with attention-deficit/hyperactivity disorder. *Pediatrics* 2001;108:471–472.
4. Lusthof KJ, Lameijer W, Zweipfenning PGM. Use of clonidine for chemical submission. *J Toxicol Clin Toxicol* 2000;38:329–332.
5. Oats JA. Antihypertensive agents and the drug therapy of hypertension. In: Harman JG, Limbird LE, Molinoff PB, eds. *Goodman and Gilman's the pharmacological basis of therapeutics*, 9th ed. New York: McGraw-Hill, 1996:780–806.
6. Dollery CT, Davies DS, Draffan GH, et al. Clinical pharmacology and pharmacokinetics of clonidine. *Clin Pharmacol Ther* 1976;19:11–17.
7. Nishina K, Miawa K, Shiga M, et al. Clonidine in paediatric anaesthesia. *Paediatr Anaesth* 1999;9:187–202.
8. Moulderings GJ. Imidazoline receptors: basic knowledge, recent advances and future prospects for therapy and diagnosis. *Drugs Future* 1997;22:757–772.
9. Head GA, Chan CKS, Burke SL. Relationship between imidazoline and α_2-adrenoceptors involved in the sympatho-inhibitory actions of centrally acting antihypertensive agents. *J Auton Nerv Syst* 1998;72:163–169.
10. Bousquet P, Brauban V, Schann S, et al. Participation of imidazoline receptor and alpha$_2$-adrenoceptors in the central hypotensive effects of imidazoline-like drugs. *Ann N Y Acad Sci* 1999;881:272–278.
11. Seger DL. Clonidine toxicity revisited. *J Toxicol Clin Toxicol* 2002;40:145–155.
12. Yagupsky PY, Gorodischer R. Massive clonidine overdose in a 9-month-old infant. *Pediatrics* 1983;72:500–502.
13. Abo-Zena RA, Bobek MB, Dweik RA. Hypertensive urgency induced by an interaction of mirtazapine and clonidine. *Pharmacotherapy* 2000;20:476–478.
14. Bamshad MJ, Wasserman GS. Pediatric clonidine intoxications. *Vet Hum Toxicol* 1990;32:220–223.
15. Banner W, Lund ME, Clawson L. Failure of naloxone to reverse clonidine toxic effect. *Am J Dis Child* 1983;137:1170–1171.

CHAPTER 118

Type I Antidysrhythmic Agents

E. Martin Caravati

See Figures 1 through 3.

Compounds included:	**Type IA: disopyramide (Norpace, Dirythmin), procainamide (Procan, Pronestyl), quinidine (Cardioquin, Kinidin, Quinaglute); type IB: lidocaine, tocainide (Tonocard), mexiletine (Mexitil), and phenytoin (Chapter 130); type IC: ajmaline (Aritmina), cibenzoline (Cibed Timecelles), encainide (Enkaid), flecainide (Tambocor), prajmaline (Neorhythmin), propafenone (Rythmol, Rytmonorm), and moricizine (Ethmozine)**
Molecular formula and weight:	**See Table 1.**
SI conversion:	**See Table 1.**
Therapeutic levels:	**See Table 1.**
Special concerns:	**Anticholinergic properties, ventricular dysrhythmias, and conduction blocks; QT prolongation (acute, chronic), torsade de pointes (acute, chronic), cinchonism, seizures, agranulocytosis (chronic), pulmonary fibrosis (chronic)**
Antidotes:	**Sodium bicarbonate, magnesium**

OVERVIEW

Type I antidysrhythmic agents are fast sodium channel blockers in the myocardium. They are primarily indicated for life-threatening ventricular dysrhythmias and are divided into three subtypes (A through C). Type IA and IC also block potassium channels and prolong refractoriness in addition to decreasing conduction velocity in normal cardiac tissue. Type IB has only mild to moderate sodium channel blockade, primarily in ischemic tissue, and enhances repolarization. All type I agents

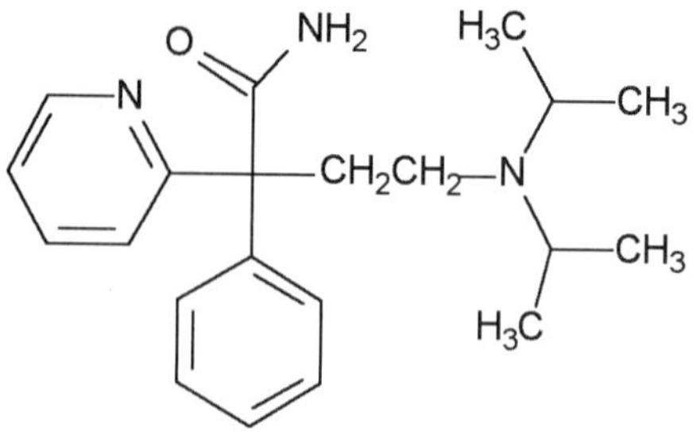

Figure 1. Disopyramide.

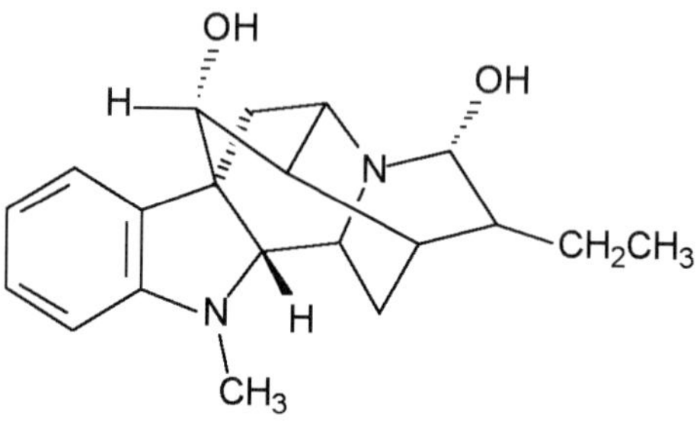

Figure 3. Ajmaline.

can depress conduction, automaticity, and contractility in toxic doses. These agents have a narrow therapeutic index. Each type I agent is metabolized by the cytochrome P-450 system except procainamide and are prone to drug-drug interactions (1).

Prodysrhythmia and Class I Drugs

Aggravation or provocation of dysrhythmias is known as *prodysrhythmia* (2). All types of bradydysrhythmia and tachydysrhythmia, whether supraventricular or ventricular, can be worsened or provoked by antidysrhythmic drugs. Torsade de pointes is the prototype of ventricular tachydysrhythmia provoked by antidysrhythmic drugs. Incessant monomorphic ventricular tachycardia (VT) is another common manifestation. This dysrhythmia is often caused by class IC antidysrhythmic agents and usually has a QRS complex with a long duration so that it appears *sinusoidal* in contour.

During therapy with class IA drugs, the risk of developing prodysrhythmia is increased by the presence of bradycardia, hypokalemia, or hypomagnesemia. Atrial fibrillation also seems to increase the risk of prodysrhythmia. Other risk factors for prodysrhythmia include toxic blood concentration due to old age, renal disease, hepatic disease, heart disease, severe ventricular dysfunction (i.e., an ejection fraction less than 35%), serious presenting dysrhythmia (i.e., sustained VT or VF), concomitant digitalis therapy, hypokalemia or hypomagnesemia, bradycardia or intermittent long RR intervals on background electrocardiogram (ECG), and certain drug combinations (e.g., type IA plus type III, and type IA plus a tricyclic antidepressant drug) (3).

Treatment Strategies

Overdose of these agents is potentially life threatening so aggressive gut decontamination with activated charcoal shortly after ingestion, cardiac monitoring and intravenous (IV) access are reasonable. Sodium bicarbonate has been associated with reversing cardiac toxicity from quinidine, procainamide, and flecainide overdose in case reports. Based on pharmacology it may also be helpful in sodium channel blockade toxicity from other type I agents (4). Phenytoin has type IB effects on cardiac conduction and should be avoided in the treatment of seizures associated with type IB agents. Hemodialysis may be of benefit in disopyramide (DP), procainamide, and tocainide toxicity. Treatment is discussed for each agent individually.

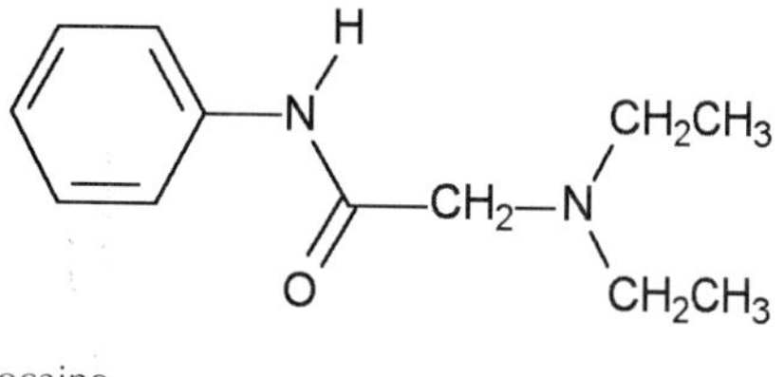

Figure 2. Lidocaine.

TYPE IA AGENTS

Disopyramide

DP (Norpace, Dirythmin) is a membrane-stabilizing agent with actions similar to quinidine and procainamide. It decreases myocardial excitability and conduction velocity and may depress contractility. It possesses anticholinergic properties. DP is used to suppress and prevent the recurrence of life-threatening ventricular dysrhythmias. It is contraindicated with complete heart block, cardiogenic shock, and angle-closure glaucoma. It must be used with caution in patients with heart failure, conduction defects, hypokalemia, history of urinary retention, family history of glaucoma, and myasthenia gravis.

TOXIC DOSE

The *adult therapeutic dose* is 200 to 300 mg as an oral loading dose for rapid control of ventricular dysrhythmias, followed by 150 mg every 6 hours of the regular-release capsules or 300 mg orally every 12 hours as extended-release capsules. The total daily dose is 400 to 800 mg. Dosage adjustments are required for renal, hepatic, or cardiac failure. The *pediatric dose* ranges from 6 to 30 mg/kg daily divided every 6 hours.

The mean lethal dose in a series of 106 adult overdoses was 2.8 g (5). A 19-year-old girl ingested 3.75 mg and developed hypotension, apnea, and seizures within 1 hour. Five hours post ingestion she developed ventricular fibrillation (VF) and died (6). A 16-year-old girl ingested 2000 mg, experienced a cardiac arrest and survived (7). One case series of 106 adult overdoses estimates 1.5 g as toxic in healthy adults (5). A 2-year-old child ingested 600 mg and died 12 hours later (8). One capsule (100 mg) could be toxic.

PHARMACOKINETICS AND PHARMACODYNAMICS

DP is rapidly absorbed. The time to peak serum concentration (T_{max}) is 2 to 3 hours. Protein binding varies inversely with plasma concentration and is 50% to 65% at therapeutic concentrations. The volume of distribution (V_d) is 0.6 to 1.3 L/kg. DP is partially metabolized via the cytochrome P-450 system of the liver to the major metabolite, mono-*N*-dealkylated DP (nordisopyramide), which has approximately 50% of the activity of the parent compound. The major route of elimination is renal; 50% unchanged drug, 20% *N*-dealkylated metabolite, and 10% other metabolites. The elimination half-life is 4 to 10 hours and increases in renal, hepatic, and cardiac failure.

PATHOPHYSIOLOGY

DP binds to fast sodium channels and inhibits recovery after repolarization. It suppresses automaticity in the His-Purkinje system, decreases automaticity of ectopic pacemakers, and decreases conduction velocity in the atria and ventricles. In therapeutic doses it has little effect on the atrioventricular (AV) node. Negative inotropic effects result in a decrease of cardiac

TABLE 1. Molecular formula, weight, therapeutic levels, and conversions for the type I antidysrhythmic drugs

Class/drug name	Molecular formula, molecular weight (g/mol)	Therapeutic blood level (μg/ml)	SI conversion
Type 1A			
Disopyramide	$C_{21}H_{29}N_{30}$, 339.5	2–7	mg/L × 3.36 = μmol/L
Procainamide	$C_{13}H_{21}N_{30}$,HCl, 271.8	3–10	mg/L × 4.25 = μmol/l
Quinidine	$C_{20}H_{24}N_2O_2$, 324.4	2–5	mg/L × 3.08 = μmol/L
Type 1B			
Lidocaine	$C_{14}H_{22}N_{20}$, 234.3	1.5–5.0	mg/L × 4.27 = μmol/L
Mexiletine	$C_{11}H_{17}NO$,HCl, 215.7	0.5–2	mg/L × 5.58 = μmol/L
Tocainide	$C_{11}H_{16}N_{20}$, HCl, 228.7	4–10	mg/L × 5.20 = μmol/L
Type IC			
Ajmaline	$C_{20}H_{26}N_2O_2$, 326.4	0.01–0.03	mg/L × 3.06 = μmol/L
Cibenzoline	$C_{18}H_{18}N_2$, 262.3	0.20–0.60 (trough)	mg/L × 3.81 = μmol/L
Encainide	$C_{22}H_{28}N_2O_2$,HCl, 388.9	0.015–0.100	mg/L × 2.84 = μmol/L
Flecainide	$C_{17}H_{20}F_6N_2O_3$,$C_2H_4O_2$, 474.4	0.2–1.0	mg/L × 2.41 = μmol/L
Prajmaline	$C_{23}H_{33}N_2O_2$,$C_4H_5O_6$, 518.6	0.17–0.44	mg/L × 2.71 = μmol/L
Propafenone	$C_{21}H_{27}NO_3$,HCl, 377.9	0.5–2.0	mg/L × 2.93 = μmol/L
Moricizine	$C_{22}H_{25}N_3O_4S$,HCl, 464.0	NR	mg/L × 2.34 = μmol/L

NR, not reported.

output of approximately 10% to 15%. It also possesses anticholinergic properties.

PREGNANCY AND LACTATION

DP is U.S. Food and Drug Administration (FDA) pregnancy category C (Appendix I). It has demonstrated oxytocic effects and produced uterine contractions and abdominal pain. No adverse effects have been reported in nursing infants, and it is considered compatible with breast-feeding (9). It crosses the placenta and is distributed into breast milk. DP and its metabolite *N*-monodesalkyl DP (NMD) have been found in breast milk in concentrations 1.06 and 6.24 times the serum levels of DP and NMD, respectively. Cord blood contained 26% (DP) and 43% (NMD) of the maternal concentrations (10).

CLINICAL PRESENTATION

Acute Overdosage. Clinical effects typically appear within 1 or 2 hours of overdose and are dose related. Minor anticholinergic side effects occur, including urinary retention, blurred vision, and dry mouth. A variety of ventricular dysrhythmias and conduction blocks may result. In a case series of 106 adult overdoses, 60 developed significant symptoms of cardiogenic shock (24 patients), cardiac arrest (17 cases), AV block (21 cases), intraventricular block (24 cases), and ventricular dysrhythmias (12 cases) (5). Several case reports were characterized by an initial resuscitation after cardiac arrest, followed by progressive deterioration over 6 to 12 hours leading to death (11). Cardiovascular collapse and apnea usually appear within several hours after a serious overdose, but the anticholinergic properties of DP may theoretically delay symptoms.

A 16-year-old girl ingested 2000 mg DP. Within 2 hours she was comatose, apneic, and pulseless with fixed and dilated pupils. Asystole was treated with epinephrine (1 mg), isoproterenol (0.9 μg/kg/minute), and calcium chloride (3.0 g total) over 75 minutes. The heart rhythm changed to atrial fibrillation with blood pressure of 70/50 mm Hg. Ten hours after admission she was conscious and extubated. Her serum DP concentration 4 hours after exposure was 11.0 μg/ml. The plasma half-life was 11.9 hours (7).

Adverse Events. Rapid IV injection (not FDA approved) may cause diaphoresis and hypotension.

Most common effects with therapeutic use are antimuscarinic (dry mouth, blurred vision, urinary hesitancy) and are dose-related. The following affects may be seen with therapeutic use: mydriasis, blurred vision, acute glaucoma; nausea and abdominal pain; heart failure, prolonged QT interval, ventricular dysrhythmias, and torsade de pointes (12); cholestatic jaundice, disseminated intravascular coagulation; granulocytopenia (13); agitation, paranoia, auditory, and visual hallucinations; peripheral neuropathy; urinary retention.

Drug Interactions. DP is a CYP3A3/4 enzyme substrate. Toxicity and cardiac effects may be additive when administered with other class I antidysrhythmic agents, propranolol, phenytoin, or verapamil. Erythromycin, azithromycin (14), or clarithromycin added to a regimen of DP may induce QT_c prolongation, polymorphic ventricular tachycardias, and elevation of DP serum concentrations. Erythromycin interferes with the hepatic dealkylation of DP, thus increasing DP and decreasing metabolite serum levels (15).

Rifampin decreases serum levels of DP when administered concurrently (16). A fatal torsade de pointes type of ventricular dysrhythmia may follow DP use in patients with acute hepatocellular dysfunction. DP should be discontinued when jaundice or acute hepatocellular dysfunction occurs (12).

DIAGNOSTIC TESTS

Acute and Subacute Overdose. Serum concentrations of 2 to 4 μg/ml are required to suppress ventricular dysrhythmias, and up to 7 μg/ml are required for refractory VT. Toxicity is associated with plasma concentrations greater than 9 μg/ml. A 16-year-old girl ingested 2000 mg and had a 4-hour post-ingestion concentration of 11.0 μg/ml (7).

In therapeutic doses, DP has little effect on the PR or QRS intervals, but the QT_c may be prolonged. Toxic concentrations produce sinus tachycardia, prolonged QRS and QT intervals, bundle branch block, and ventricular dysrhythmias.

Postmortem Considerations. A 41-year-old person ingested an unknown dose of DP, developed cardiac arrest, and died. Concentrations of postmortem blood disclosed a DP concentration of 49 μg/ml and a mono-*N*-dealkylated metabolite concentration of 9 μg/ml (17). A 40-year-old man died after reportedly ingesting 3600 mg of DP. His blood concentration of DP was 63 μg/ml at autopsy (18).

A postmortem DP concentration of 41.3 μg/ml was found in a child (19). The following postmortem tissue levels were found in a 44-year-old woman with an unknown ingestion: blood 27 mg/L, liver 36 mg/L, bile 349 mg/kg, and kidney 147 mg/kg (20).

TREATMENT

Gastrointestinal Decontamination. Induction of emesis is contraindicated because of its rapid onset of action. Gastric lavage may be indicated within 1 to 2 hours after a large overdose. Activated charcoal shortly after ingestion has been shown to decrease absorption in humans (21).

Enhancement of Elimination. In a human volunteer study, activated charcoal at 4, 6, 8, and 12 hours after ingestion reduced the mean serum level of the parent drug and main metabolite (mono-*N*-dealkyldisopyramide) by 40% and the serum half-life by 67% (22).

Hemodialysis has been effective in reducing the serum half-life of DP in chronic hemodialysis patients and may be useful in cases in which supportive care is not effective (23). Gosselin suggests that clearance is greater with hemoperfusion than with hemodialysis, but their data were limited to dogs and one patient (11). Jaeger reported that hemoperfusion increased clearance by only 5% in two patients (5).

Antidotes. There are no specific antidotes for DP.

Supportive Care. All persons who overdose with DP should be admitted to an intensive care unit (ICU). Continuous cardiac monitoring should be instituted on admission. Discontinue DP therapy and avoid other type I antidysrhythmic agents if possible. Hypotension should initially be treated with isotonic crystalloid fluid resuscitation (Chapter 37) followed by inotropic support if needed. Ventricular dysrhythmias should be treated with standard doses of lidocaine. Consider dialysis early if the clinical condition deteriorates with supportive care.

High doses of calcium chloride (0.5 g every 5 minutes up to a total dose of 3.0 g), in combination with conventional therapy and cardiopulmonary resuscitation, appeared to reverse the electromechanical dissociation (EMD) following a 2000-mg DP overdose (7).

Prolonged cardiopulmonary resuscitation may be required. A 16-year-old girl who presented in asystole was resuscitated after 75 minutes of cardiopulmonary resuscitation and survived with complete neurologic recovery (7). A 28-year-old man developed hypotension and ventricular flutter after ingesting 8400 mg of DP. He was maintained on percutaneous cardiopulmonary support for 36 hours until his cardiac function became normal (24).

Monitoring. Patients with evidence of hypotension, dysrhythmias, or significant conduction delay should have continuous monitoring of blood pressure and cardiac rhythm in an intensive care setting. Frequent ECGs should be obtained to assess the QT and QRS intervals and the effectiveness of therapy. Serial serum DP concentrations may be helpful in assessing the effectiveness of any elimination enhancement techniques used during treatment. Based on the tricyclic antidepressant toxicity experience, a minimum of 6 hours of observation and monitoring is recommended.

Procainamide

Procainamide (Procan, Pronestyl) is a type IA antidysrhythmic with properties similar to quinidine. It is indicated for treatment of ventricular dysrhythmias and may be used to maintain sinus rhythm after cardioversion of atrial fibrillation. It is contraindicated for patients with systemic lupus erythematosus, heart block, or known hypersensitivity to it or procaine. It should be used with caution in patients with heart failure, renal failure, hypotension, or myasthenia gravis.

TOXIC DOSE

The *adult therapeutic dose* for ventricular dysrhythmias ranges up to 50 mg/kg/day orally of the immediate release capsules divided every 3 to 6 hours for adults with normal renal function. The IV dose is 100 mg every 5 minutes given at a maximum rate of 50 mg/minute until dysrhythmia is corrected, adverse effects occur, or a maximum of 500 mg is given. More than 500 to 600 mg is not usually required. The maintenance rate is 2 to 6 mg/minute. The *pediatric dose* is 15 to 60 mg/kg daily dose divided every 3 to 6 hours, maximum 4 g/day.

A 2 to 3 g dose is potentially dangerous, especially in patients who are slow acetylators or have decreased renal function or heart disease. A 67-year-old woman ingested 7000 mg of procainamide and developed hypotension, renal failure, and life-threatening cardiac toxicity (25).

TOXICOKINETICS AND TOXICODYNAMICS

Procainamide is almost completely absorbed with a T_{max} of 90 minutes. Plasma protein binding is 14% to 23% and it is widely distributed (V_d 2 L/kg). A significant portion of the parent compound is metabolized by the liver to the active metabolite *N*-acetylprocainamide (NAPA). *Slow acetylators* metabolize 16% to 21% and *fast acetylators* metabolize 24% to 33% of procainamide to NAPA. Both compounds are excreted primarily in the urine. Accumulation of the parent drug and metabolite may occur with renal insufficiency (26). The mean elimination half-life is 1.7 hours in children and 5.3 hours in neonates. The half-life in adults with normal renal function is 3 to 4 hours for procainamide and 7 hours for NAPA. Renal insufficiency and advanced age prolongs the elimination half-life.

PATHOPHYSIOLOGY

Procainamide binds with fast sodium channels and is a myocardial depressant. It decreases cardiac excitability and conduction velocity and increases the effective refractory period of the atria, His-Purkinje system, and ventricles. Toxic concentrations may prolong AV conduction or induce AV block. It has weak vagal blocking action, no α-adrenergic blockade, and less myocardial depression than quinidine. It also has anticholinergic properties. It has local anesthetic effects similar to procaine. The major metabolite, NAPA, possesses type III antidysrhythmic activity.

PREGNANCY AND LACTATION

Procainamide is FDA pregnancy category C (Appendix I). It crosses the placenta, but has not been associated with congenital defects. Fetal to mother blood concentration ratios of 0.28 to 1.1 have been demonstrated. The parent compound and NAPA accumulate in breast milk in 4:1 milk to maternal serum concentration ratio. Procainamide is considered compatible with breast-feeding (27).

CLINICAL PRESENTATION

Acute Overdosage. Acute toxicity primarily affects the central nervous system (CNS) and cardiovascular system. CNS effects include confusion, agitation, seizures, and drowsiness. Cardiovascular effects are hypotension, ventricular dysrhythmias such as VT, VF, torsade de pointes, and conduction delays. Anticholinergic symptoms such as dry mouth, mydriasis, tachycardia, and decreased bowel motility may also be observed. Acute weakness associated with myasthenia gravis has been reported (28).

A 14-year-old boy (weight, 74 kg) ingested a large amount of procainamide and developed abdominal pain, weakness, and dizziness. Two hours after ingestion, his vital signs were normal, pupils dilated (10 mm), and mouth dry. Within 30 minutes, he vomited and had a brief tonic-clonic seizure. Anticholinergic symptoms resolved within 8 hours. The ECG showed sinus rhythm with a PR interval 123 milliseconds, QRS interval 76 milliseconds, and QTc interval of 371 milliseconds. His serum procainamide was 63 mg/L (normal range, 4 to 8 mg/L) and serum NAPA was 80.4 mg/L (normal range, 2 to 8 mg/L). Cardiac toxicity did not develop and hemodialysis was not required (29).

Adverse Events. Cerebellar ataxia has been reported in a patient with supratherapeutic serum procainamide concentrations that resolved within 3 days of discontinuing therapy (30). Respiratory arrest and myasthenic crisis developed after administration of procainamide to a myasthenia gravis patient (28). Pure red cell aplasia has followed prolonged use of sustained-release procainamide (31).

Cardiovascular effects including hypotension with rapid IV infusion may result in hypotension, VF, and asystole. Prolongation of QRS and QT intervals is observed with therapeutic dosing and toxicity. Procainamide administered to control recurrent ventricular dysrhythmias may delay removal of ventilatory support because it produces muscle weakness and associated respiratory insufficiency (32).

CNS effects include dizziness and generalized skeletal muscle weakness. Gastrointestinal (GI) effects include anorexia, nausea, vomiting, bitter taste, and diarrhea at high oral doses. Hepatomegaly and elevated transaminases have been reported.

A 45-year-old woman developed acute psychosis within 72 hours of initiating therapy. Her symptoms resolved within 24 hours of discontinuing the drug. Serum procainamide and NAPA concentrations were therapeutic (33).

A systemic lupus erythematosus-like syndrome is reported as high as 30% in chronic administration. Symptoms include arthralgias, arthritis, myalgias, pleural effusion, pericarditis, and fever. Antinuclear antibodies are present. Angioedema, skin rashes, pruritus, urticaria, flushing, and hypergammaglobulinemia may also occur. This usually responds to withdrawal of the drug, but corticosteroids may be necessary.

Hematologic effects with a reported 0.5% incidence include neutropenia, agranulocytosis (20% to 25% mortality), thrombocytopenia, hemolytic anemia, and pancytopenia. Most events begin during the first 12 weeks of therapy and resolve within 1 month of discontinuing the drug but may be life threatening.

Drug Interactions. Amiodarone can produce an increased serum procainamide level and development of clinical signs of toxicity (34). Respiratory failure due to neuromuscular weakness was produced by procainamide intoxication in a patient with preexisting neuropathy caused by amiodarone (35). Cimetidine appeared to increase the average steady-state blood concentrations of procainamide and NAPA (36). Famotidine does not appear to interact.

Trimethoprim is associated with decreased renal clearance of procainamide and NAPA (37). Concomitant use of propranolol, histamine H_2 antagonists, and quinidine with procainamide may increase serum procainamide levels. Procainamide may potentiate the effects of succinylcholine, pancuronium, and tubocurarine. Alcohol consumption may enhance acetylation to NAPA and reduce the half-life of procainamide.

DIAGNOSTIC TESTS

Acute and Subacute Overdose. Plasma procainamide concentrations of 3 to 10 µg/ml are generally required to suppress ventricular dysrhythmias. Mild toxicity may occur in the range 12 to 16 µg/ml, and serious toxicity occurs when procainamide levels exceed 16 µg/ml (38). Interpretation of the plasma level is complicated by active metabolites. Procainamide and NAPA concentrations are needed to assess therapeutic concentrations. Total procainamide and NAPA therapeutic levels range from 5 to 30 µg/ml. True *in vivo* plasma procainamide levels may differ from measured levels when freshly drawn and separated blood samples are not used for analysis. In storage, procainamide continues to diffuse into red blood cells and undergoes metabolism to both active (NAPA) and inactive metabolites. A 35% decrease in procainamide and 24% increase in NAPA concentration have been noted when whole blood is stored at room temperature (39). Plasma NAPA concentrations of 33 to 52 µg/ml have been associated with VT (40). In an overdose case, junctional tachycardia and conduction defects appeared at total procainamide and NAPA levels exceeding 42 µg/ml, and severe hypotension and lethargy, at levels above 60 µg/ml (25).

Adverse Events. Therapeutic concentrations may produce sinus tachycardia, widened QRS interval, and prolonged QT and PR intervals. Torsade de pointes is infrequent but may develop with renal insufficiency. Prolongation of the QT_c may be associated with elevated NAPA values (41). If the QRS interval increases more than 25% or marked prolongation of the QT interval occurs during therapy, then potential toxicity should be considered. Reduction in dosage is recommended if the QRS increases by 50%.

Periodically obtaining a complete blood count, serum creatinine, and ECG are useful to detect possible hematologic effects, risk of decreased drug clearance, and cardiac toxicity. An increasing ANA titer may precede the onset of symptomatic lupoid syndrome. IgG antibodies to histone complex H2A–H2B appear to be sensitive and specific markers of procainamide-induced lupus (42).

Postmortem Considerations. The postmortem procainamide serum concentration in four fatal overdose cases averaged 145 mg/L (range, 80 to 260 mg/L) (43).

TREATMENT

Gastrointestinal Decontamination. Induced emesis is contraindicated. Given the serious potential toxicity, decontamination is an appropriate intervention. Gastric lavage within 1 to 2 hours after a large ingestion and activated charcoal may be useful but have not been systematically studied.

Enhancement of Elimination. There are no data evaluating multiple dose activated charcoal. Hemodialysis increases procainamide and NAPA clearance at rates of 47 to 88 ml/minute and 22 to 104 ml/minute, respectively. Hemoperfusion clearance of procainamide and NAPA are reported to be 47 to 103 ml/minute and 47 to 151 ml/minute, respectively (25,29,44).

Nguyen reported that using a high-clearance dialyzer for 4 hours decreased the serum NAPA concentration from 43 to 20 µg/ml with resolution of torsade de pointes in one patient (40). Kar reported increased clearance of NAPA by combining high-efficiency hemodialysis and charcoal hemoperfusion. The overall clearance of NAPA was 153 ml/minute. The hemodialysis clearance averaged 102 ml/minute and the hemoperfusion averaged 88 ml/minute, a 50% increase in clearance over high-efficiency hemodialysis alone (45).

Redistribution of NAPA after hemodialysis may occur in 12 to 24 hours and result in rebound serum concentrations. Continuous hemofiltration or more frequent intermittent hemodialysis treatments based on serum concentration continue to remove NAPA as it is redistributed to the vascular compartment.

Antidotes. Because procainamide binds with fast sodium channels, conduction delays and ventricular dysrhythmias may respond to IV sodium bicarbonate (Chapter 75). A reasonable starting dose is 1 to 2 mEq/kg as an IV bolus, repeated as needed to maintain an arterial pH of 7.45 to 7.55.

Supportive Care. All patients with potential toxicity should have IV access and continuous cardiac monitoring. Other type IA agents should be avoided. Lidocaine and phenytoin are antidysrhythmic agents of choice for persistent dysrhythmias. Torsade de pointes may respond to magnesium, 2 g IV bolus, isoproterenol infusion, or overdrive cardiac pacing. Hypotension should initially be treated with isotonic fluid resuscitation and inotropic support if needed (Chapter 37). Seizures are treated with benzodiazepines, followed by phenytoin and more invasive procedures in patients with refractory seizures (Chapter 40).

Pacemaker insertion should be considered early with signs of increasing AV block or polymorphic VT.

Monitoring. Frequent monitoring of the ECG and vital signs is needed to detect toxicity during procainamide loading orally or IV. Overdose patients should be monitored for at least 6 hours for mental status changes, conduction delays, dysrhythmia, or hypotension. Procainamide and NAPA concentrations can help guide elimination enhancement during toxicity.

Quinidine

Quinidine (Cardioquin, Kinidin, Quinaglute) is an alkaloid derived from *Cinchona* or *Remijia pedunculata*. It is the dextrorotatory isomer of quinine. It is a type IA agent used to maintain sinus rhythm after conversion of atrial fibrillation and suppression of symptomatic atrial and ventricular dysrhythmias. Oral products include the sulfate, gluconate, and polygalacturonate salts. IV quinidine is available as the gluconate but its clinical usefulness is limited by hypotension.

TOXIC DOSE

The *adult therapeutic dose* of quinidine sulfate is 200 to 400 mg orally three or four times per day. Maximum dose is 4 g/day. The IV dose is 800 mg in 50 ml dextrose 5% in water at 1 ml/minute. The *pediatric dose* for cardiac dysrhythmias in children is 30 mg/kg or 900 mg/m^2 daily in 5 divided doses.

An adult who ingests more than 1 g is expected to exhibit toxicity. A 4-g ingestion by a 57-year-old woman who had no previous history of cardiovascular disease produced conduction delays, hypotension, coma, and convulsions (46). An adult ingestion of 8 g led to severe hypotension and dysrhythmias, which required overdrive pacing and an intraaortic balloon pump (47). A patient who reportedly ingested 20 g survived with supportive care, despite hypotension and anuria (48). Quinine sulfate may display similar toxicity with an average toxic dose of 4 g. A 2-year-old child ingested 5 g of a sustained release preparation and died in 28 hours (49).

TOXICOKINETICS AND TOXICODYNAMICS

Quinidine is well absorbed and undergoes some first-pass metabolism. The bioavailability is 70% to 80% after oral use. The T_{max} of the sulfate salt is 60 to 120 minutes. The V_d averages 2 L/kg in healthy adults. Congestive heart failure (CHF) reduces the V_d by one-third, and chronic liver disease increases it by 30%. Quinidine is highly bound to albumin: 80% to 90% in adults and 60% to 70% in neonates. Cirrhosis increases the portion of unbound drug due to hypoalbuminemia.

Procainamide is metabolized by the liver to several metabolites that are excreted in the urine: 3-hydroxyquinidine *N*-oxide, 2'-oxoquinidinone, desmethylquinidine, and quinidine *N*-oxide. The usual plasma half-life is 6 to 8 hours and increases with chronic liver disease (50). Hepatic failure increased the half-life from 66 to 99 hours in a 57-year-old man and resulted in a serum concentration of 3.1 μg/ml and torsade de pointes (51). CHF reduces clearance by one-half. Urinary excretion is dependent on urinary pH and increases with acidic urine (pH less than 6). Alkaline urine promotes formation of nonionized drug and tubular reabsorption that can lead to increase serum concentrations. Approximately 10% to 50% of a dose is excreted unchanged in 24 hours.

PATHOPHYSIOLOGY

Quinidine affects the fast sodium channels, which causes decreased myocardial excitability, conduction velocity, and contractility. It is a myocardial depressant and suppresses automaticity in the His-Purkinje system similar to lidocaine, but its anticholinergic properties may antagonize this effect at high concentrations. It also possesses α-blocking activity.

Quinidine produces toxic effects similar to those of procainamide. There is a dose-related decrease in conduction velocity that is reflected by increases in the PR, QRS, and QT intervals (52). High plasma quinidine levels cause high-grade AV block, bundle-branch block, and asystole resembling that of hyperkalemia. In contrast to procainamide, QT prolongation with quinidine occurs at therapeutic levels. In therapeutic doses, quinidine may decrease automaticity depending on the anticholinergic effect, and in high doses it may increase automaticity.

Hypotension and reflex tachycardia may result at high concentrations. IV quinidine depresses contractility and decreases systemic vascular resistance primarily by α-adrenergic receptor blockade. High blood levels of quinidine increase left ventricular end-diastolic pressure through its negative inotropic effect.

PREGNANCY AND LACTATION

Quinidine is FDA risk category C (Appendix I). There are no reports of congenital defects associated with quinidine. Neonatal thrombocytopenia has been reported after maternal use. It crosses the placenta; fetal levels approximate the mother's. High quinidine doses have resulted in abortion secondary to its oxytocic properties. Quinidine is secreted into breast milk and is considered compatible with breast-feeding (53). A patient at 33 weeks of gestation was administered quinidine for treatment of a fetal supraventricular tachycardia. The patient had evidence of quinidine toxicity at low to mid-therapeutic serum levels of quinidine, but markedly elevated levels of 3-hydroxyquinidine. Elevated levels of 3-hydroxyquinidine may be associated with quinidine toxicity even in the presence of a nontoxic serum quinidine level (54).

Clinical Presentation

ACUTE OVERDOSAGE

Acute poisoning may result in cardiovascular, respiratory, GI, and neurologic signs and symptoms. Cardiovascular effects result from delayed conduction, myocardial depression, and α-adrenergic blockade. This produces heart block; widening of the PR, QT, and QRS intervals; ventricular dysrhythmia; asystole; syncope; and hypotension (55). Conduction defects are always present in overdose although QT prolongation may be present at therapeutic levels.

CNS effects include irritability, lethargy, ataxia, delirium, hallucinations, generalized seizures, and coma. Neurologic symptoms may appear without cardiovascular depression (56). Respiratory depression or apnea has been observed. Pulmonary edema developed after an 8-g quinidine ingestion despite normal pulmonary capillary wedge pressures (47). Pulmonary edema may result from depressed myocardial contractility in patients with underlying cardiovascular disease.

A 16-year-old girl ingested 8 g of quinidine and developed coma, seizures, dysrhythmias, and hypotension. She had a serum quinidine concentration of 21 mg/L 10 hours post-ingestion (47).

ADVERSE EVENTS

Approximately 2% to 8% of patients on chronic therapy develop QT interval prolongation and torsade de pointes. This generally occurs at therapeutic concentrations. *Quinidine syncope* is a loss of consciousness due to paroxysmal VT or torsade de pointes that occurs with therapeutic doses.

Cinchonism is a toxic syndrome after therapeutic use of *Cinchona* alkaloids (quinidine, quinine). It is usually associated with increased serum concentrations of quinidine. Symptoms may mimic salicylate toxicity. Clinical manifestations include headache, fever, mydriasis, visual field and visual acuity abnormalities, tinnitus, hearing loss, nausea, vomiting, abdominal pain, rash, and an organic brain syndrome that varies from memory impairment to delirium. Chronic organic brain syndrome may be the only symptom of cinchonism (56). Coma, convulsions, and cardiorespiratory arrest may occur in patients with severe cinchonism. Mild cases can be managed with a reduction on quinidine dose.

Quinine amblyopia is a vision loss that may be complete and sudden. This phenomenon is addressed in Chapter 94.

Quinidine therapy is commonly associated with nausea and diarrhea. Diarrhea-associated hypokalemia may predispose to ventricular dysrhythmias (torsade de pointes).

Many adverse events are not related to plasma concentration. Manifestations include drug fever, cholestatic hepatitis, systemic lupus erythematosus (57), asthma, anaphylaxis, thrombocytopenia, hemolytic anemia (especially in glucose 6 phosphate dehydrogenase deficiency), hypoprothrombinemia, uveitis, and polyarthritis. Thrombocytopenia is the most common reaction and usually resolves with withdrawal of the drug. Skin changes include maculopapular eruptions, thrombocytopenic purpura, cutaneous vasculitis (58), photosensitivity, and bullous lesions. IV quinidine for malaria treatment has been associated with hypoglycemia (59).

DRUG INTERACTIONS

Quinidine may potentiate the effect of depolarizing and nondepolarizing neuromuscular blocking agents such as succinylcholine and pancuronium bromide. The anticholinergic effects may be additive with those of other anticholinergic drugs.

Administering verapamil in the presence of quinidine may result in hypotension. Amiodarone, ketoconazole, itraconazole, carbonic anhydrase inhibitors, and cimetidine may increase the serum quinidine concentration. Drugs that alkalinize the urine may increase quinidine concentrations via reduced clearance (e.g., acetazolamide, sodium bicarbonate, and thiazide diuretics).

Phenytoin and phenobarbital may increase the metabolism of quinidine. Nifedipine is reported to decrease serum concentrations of quinidine. Quinidine increases the serum concentration of digoxin two- to threefold.

DIAGNOSTIC TESTS

Plasma concentrations are difficult to use in overdose due to different sensitivities between laboratory methods and individual patient variation in protein binding. Therapeutic quinidine concentrations may vary depending on the type, severity, and duration of the cardiac dysrhythmia. When using nonspecific assay methods of analysis, the therapeutic concentration ranges from 2 to 7 µg/ml. Levels greater than 5 µg/ml may be associated with toxic symptoms. Concentrations greater than 14 µg/ml have been associated with cardiac toxicity in a majority of patients. If more specific assay methods for the parent compound are used, then the therapeutic range may be lower.

On the ECG, QT and QRS prolongation are excellent markers of significant ingestion if obtained after peak plasma concentrations are achieved. Widening of QT and QRS intervals usually begins to occur when plasma concentrations exceed 2 µg/ml and definitely occur at plasma levels greater than 8 µg/ml (59). A 50% increase in the QT interval or QRS complex indicates a toxic quinidine concentration. Patients with quinidine-induced torsade de pointes usually have QT intervals exceeding 550 milliseconds. Patients at risk are patients with preexisting QT prolongation, bradycardia not corrected by a pacemaker, hypokalemia or hypomagnesemia, a history of torsade de pointes with other type I agents, and genetic abnormalities in drug metabolism.

Serum levels of electrolytes (sodium, potassium, calcium, phosphorus, and magnesium) should be checked in all cases of serious poisoning.

Postmortem Considerations. A 2-year-old child ingested approximately 5 g and died 28 hours after ingestion. The blood concentration was 45 mg/L (49).

TREATMENT

Acute overdose of quinidine may be life threatening. GI decontamination should be undertaken and the patient continuously monitored for hypotension, dysrhythmias, and signs of conduction delay for at least 6 hours. Treatment is primarily supportive.

Gastrointestinal Decontamination. Induced emesis is contraindicated. Given the serious potential toxicity, decontamination is an appropriate intervention. Gastric lavage within 1 to 2 hours after a large ingestion and activated charcoal may be useful but have not been systematically studied. Activated charcoal adsorbs quinidine *in vitro*. If a sustained-release product has been ingested, a repeat dose of activated charcoal may be warranted to prevent further delayed absorption.

Enhancement of Elimination. Although oral charcoal reduced the serum concentration of quinidine in rabbits (60), the large volume of distribution and high protein binding of quinidine indicate that methods to enhance elimination are unlikely to be effective.

An acidic urine increases the renal excretion of unmetabolized quinidine, but this technique has not been clinically evaluated (61). Attempts to acidify the urine may cause systemic metabolic acidosis and electrolyte abnormalities that complicate treatment. Forced diuresis has not been studied. The adverse effects of acid or forced diuresis outweigh any possible increase in quinidine elimination that theoretically may occur.

Dialysis does not remove a clinically significant amount of quinidine and should be used only in the presence of renal failure. Hemoperfusion for 6 hours was associated with a mean quinidine clearance of 24 ml/minute and a reduction in the serum quinidine concentration of 36%. The patient improved during the procedure (62).

Antidotes. Hypertonic sodium bicarbonate is theoretically promising, but there are no systematic human studies to support its efficacy. A reasonable starting dose is 1 to 2 mEq/kg IV push and repeated as needed to maintain an arterial pH of 7.45 to 7.55 (Chapter 75). This therapy may alkalinize the urine and potentially decrease drug clearance.

Glucagon had a positive inotropic effect and corrected conduction delays in quinidine poisoned dogs, but its clinical efficacy has not been evaluated in humans (63). *Bretylium* antagonizes quinidine-induced toxic effects on ventricular fibers, but it may enhance quinidine-induced reduction in AV conduction (64).

Supportive Care. All patients with potential toxicity should have IV access and continuous cardiac monitoring. Quinidine therapy should be discontinued and other type IA agents avoided. Drugs that alkalinize the urine (acetazolamide, thiazide diuretics) should be avoided.

When atypical VT presents, the goal is to reduce the QT interval. Infusion of isoproterenol at 2 to 8 μg/minute may be effective, but usually overdrive pacing (120 to 140/minute) is necessary. Torsade de pointes may also respond to magnesium, 2 g IV bolus. Lidocaine and procainamide are not effective and may be deleterious. Be sure to correct electrolyte imbalances, especially hypokalemia.

Hypotension should initially be treated with isotonic crystalloid fluid resuscitation followed by inotropic support if needed (Chapter 37). Isoproterenol and norepinephrine have been used successfully. Refractory hypotension has responded to the placement of an intraaortic balloon pump (47). Seizures are treated with benzodiazepines, followed by phenytoin and more invasive procedures in patients with refractory seizures (Chapter 40).

Extracorporeal membrane oxygenation (ECMO) was successfully used to maintain cardiovascular stability in a 16-month-old child that developed bradydysrhythmias and hypotension after an acute overdose (65).

Monitoring. Patients with evidence of hypotension, dysrhythmias, or significant conduction delay should have continuous monitoring of blood pressure and cardiac rhythm in an intensive care setting. Frequent ECGs should be obtained to assess the QT and QRS intervals and the effectiveness of therapy.

Chronic diarrhea may cause hypokalemia and predispose to dysrhythmia. Patients should have potassium concentrations monitored if experiencing diarrhea-associated quinidine use.

TYPE IB AGENTS

Lidocaine

Lidocaine (lignocaine) is an amide-type local anesthetic used topically and by injection. It is used as a type IB antidysrhythmic agent. It has been used off-label for the treatment of status epilepticus. Contraindications include hypersensitivity to amide-type local anesthetics, severe heart block, or Adams-Stokes syndrome. Caution should be used for patients with CHF, liver failure, and Wolff-Parkinson-White syndrome.

TOXIC DOSE

The *adult therapeutic dose* is 3 mg/kg/dose topically every 2 hours. The IV dose is 1.0- to 1.5-mg/kg bolus over several minutes. Repeated smaller doses may be administered, up to a maximum of 3 mg/kg. The continuous infusion rate is 1 to 4 mg/minute.

Unintentional IV doses of 250 to 2000 mg in six adult patients resulted in death (66). A 1-month-old child experienced a respiratory arrest, seizures, and coma after receiving a 50 mg (12 mg/kg) IV bolus (67).

TOXICOKINETICS AND TOXICODYNAMICS

Lidocaine is well absorbed from mucous membranes and the GI tract. It has significant first-pass metabolism. Oral administration does not produce adequate serum concentrations. The onset of action after a single bolus is 45 to 90 seconds with duration of 10 to 20 minutes. It crosses the blood–brain barrier and has a V_d of 1 to 2 L/kg. The V_d is decreased in CHF and liver failure. Protein binding is 60% to 80% to α_1 acid glycoprotein.

It is 90% metabolized by the liver to the active metabolites monoethylglycinexylidide and glycinexylidide. The initial half-life is 7 to 30 minutes (distribution phase) and the terminal half-life is 1 to 2 hours in adults (hepatic metabolism). The half-life is prolonged to 3 hours in neonates and infants. It increases with liver disease, CHF, shock, and renal failure. Approximately 3% to 14% of the drug is excreted unchanged in the urine in 24 hours. The elimination half-lives of plasma and unbound lidocaine were 3.8 and 2.7 hours, respectively, after a 2-g overdose (68).

PATHOPHYSIOLOGY

Lidocaine blocks myocardial sodium channels with greater effect on slowing conduction in ischemic tissue. It decreases automaticity by decreasing the slope of phase 4 of the action potential. There is no effect on the PR or QRS intervals but the QT may be slightly shortened. It has little or no myocardial depressant effect. The action potential duration is unaffected or slightly shortened. The net effect is to reduce the frequency and duration of ventricular dysrhythmias.

It is a CNS depressant with sedative, analgesic, and anticonvulsant properties. Seizures result from high concentrations that depress the inhibitory motor pathways in the brain. Motor nerve paralysis may cause respiratory arrest. It also suppresses the cough and gag reflexes.

PREGNANCY AND LACTATION

Lidocaine is FDA pregnancy category C (Appendix I). There are no reports of congenital defects associated with lidocaine. Neonatal thrombocytopenia has been reported after maternal use. It rapidly crosses the placenta and fetal concentration ranges between 50% to 70% of the mother's serum concentration after IV and epidural anesthesia. Lidocaine may produce CNS depression in newborns with high serum concentrations. Lidocaine is secreted into breast milk but is compatible with breast-feeding (69).

CLINICAL PRESENTATION

Acute Overdosage. Toxicity may result from many routes of exposure including unintentional intravascular administration during regional anesthesia, rapid injection of therapeutic doses, excessive subcutaneous administration, urethral and rectal instillation, and from swallowed or topical application of viscous or topical preparations.

Neurologic toxicity appears in some patients near the upper limit of therapeutic plasma lidocaine concentration. Early effects are lightheadedness, dizziness, drowsiness, confusion, dysarthria, tremor, nystagmus, ataxia, hearing loss, and euphoria. Visual disturbances, agitation, and muscle fasciculation indicate more toxic concentrations and often precede convulsions and coma. Seizures may present with plasma levels greater than 8 μg/ml (67). Apnea and hypotonia occur in massive overdose.

Cardiovascular toxicity occurs primarily in massive overdose due to depressed myocardial contractility and delay bundle-branch conduction. Large IV doses in adults (1 to 2 g) have resulted in immediate asystole, apnea, and multiple seizures (70,71). Toxicity may persist for hours or days after the levels of lidocaine have become subtherapeutic. This is probably due to persistent metabolites (67).

An IV bolus of 50 mg of lidocaine (12 mg/kg) administered to a 6-month-old child produced cardiovascular collapse, respiratory arrest, seizures, and coma. The patient was treated with phenobarbital. Consciousness returned within 18 hours but tremors persisted for 48 hours. Recovery was complete. Plasma lidocaine concentrations were 3.8 and 1.5 μg/ml at 1.2 and 3.5 hours after administration, respectively (67).

A 2-year-old child ingested viscous lidocaine that was followed by coughing and choking. Seizures began within 10 to 15 seconds. Two intraosseous phenobarbital doses plus lorazepam 20 mg/kg were needed for complete control of seizures. Suctioning of the airway revealed viscous material. The patient developed bilateral infiltrates, adult respiratory distress syndrome, syndrome of inappropriate antidiuretic hormone, and bilateral pneumothoraces. The patient required 14 days of ECMO before recovery. A lidocaine concentration at 4 hours post-ingestion was 0.5 μg/ml (72).

Adverse Events. CNS events include tremor, dizziness, tinnitus, blurred vision, anxiety, euphoria, paresthesias, and psychosis. Rapid infusion of a large dose may result in a generalized seizure. Cardiovascular events include bradycardia, hypotension, and heart block. Administration to patients with atrial fibrillation may result in increased ventricular rate. Respiratory events include dyspnea, bronchospasm, and adult respiratory distress syndrome (73).

Other events include rash, pruritus, nausea, vomiting, altered taste, thrombophlebitis, allergic reactions, edema, and urticaria. Case reports associate the therapeutic use of lidocaine with the onset of adult respiratory distress syndrome (Howard) and the development of acute methemoglobinemia in a patient with a normal hemoglobin electrophoresis and methemoglobin reductase level (74).

Drug Interactions. Lidocaine is a CYP1A2 enzyme inhibitor and a CYP1A2, 2B6, and 3A3/4 substrate. Inhibitors of CYP3A/4 may increase its serum concentration. St. John's Wort may decrease lidocaine concentration. Neuromuscular blocking effect of succinylcholine may be enhanced by lidocaine.

DIAGNOSTIC TESTS

Acute Overdosage. The therapeutic concentration is 1.5 to 5.0 μg/ml, with concentrations greater than 6 μg/ml being potentially toxic. Plasma and unbound concentrations of 17.7 and 12.0 μg/ml, respectively, resulted from 2 g of IV lidocaine. Hypotension, decreased heart rate, tremors, and unresponsiveness to stimuli were observed. The patient moved his extremities when suctioned at a total plasma level of 8.9 μg/ml and an unbound concentration of 4.98 μg/ml. The patient became alert and recovered spontaneous respiration when the total and unbound concentrations were 6.8 and 3.7 μg/ml, respectively. The CNS effects induced by lidocaine required support when the total plasma lidocaine concentration was more than 7 μg/ml. Complete recovery was observed at a total plasma level less than 5 μg/ml (68).

Fatal outcome has been associated with plasma levels of 40 and 53 μg/ml in adults (75). An estimated 1.2 g IV over 1 hour in a 20 kg man produced hypotension and asystole; the serum lidocaine level was 19.2 μg/ml 1 hour postarrest (76). A 13-month-old child died after an oral lidocaine overdose. The serum lidocaine concentration was 19.5 μg/ml, and that of the metabolite (monoethylglycylxylidide), 6.5 μg/ml (77).

Lidocaine concentrations may be lowered by 25% after contact with the stoppers of Vacutainer tubes (78).

Postmortem Considerations. Postmortem lidocaine levels after overdose have ranged from 6 to 33 μg/ml. In most cases, the blood lidocaine level exceeds 15 μg/ml (79). Tracheal topical lidocaine used during cardiac resuscitation has been found in left ventricular blood postmortem (80).

TREATMENT

Gastrointestinal Decontamination. Induced emesis is contraindicated. Given the serious potential toxicity, decontamination is an appropriate intervention. Gastric lavage within 1 to 2 hours after a large ingestion and activated charcoal may be useful but have not been systematically studied.

Enhancement of Elimination. Due to its large volume of distribution and high protein binding, methods to enhance elimination are unlikely to be effective. Lidocaine is not dialyzable. Due to its high hepatic clearance, augmented circulation (cardiac bypass, intraaortic balloon pump) may provide sufficient temporary support for the liver to reduce lidocaine levels quickly (81).

Antidotes. There are no specific antidotes. Hypertonic sodium bicarbonate infusion theoretically may have some benefit in treating conduction delay, but there are no clinical studies to support its efficacy.

Supportive Care. All patients with potential toxicity should have supplemental oxygen, IV access, and continuous cardiac monitoring. Discontinue lidocaine therapy and avoid other type IB agents. Supportive care should suffice for most overdoses in view of the short half-life of lidocaine. Adequate ventilation and acid-base balance must be ensured because hypoxia and hypercapnia may increase cerebral penetration of lidocaine (82). Metabolic acidosis may be corrected with fluids and sodium bicarbonate. Dopamine, intubation, epinephrine, atropine, and cardiac pacing may be necessary for massive doses.

Seizures are treated with benzodiazepines, followed by phenytoin and more invasive procedures in patients with refractory seizures (Chapter 40). Transvenous cardiac pacing may be useful for heart block or cardiac arrest (83).

Monitoring. Most patients should have continuous monitoring of blood pressure and cardiac rhythm in an intensive care setting. Frequent ECGs should be obtained to assess the QT and QRS intervals and the effectiveness of therapy.

Mexiletine

Mexiletine (Mextil) is considered an oral analog of lidocaine and has similar properties. It blocks the rapid inward sodium current and has minimal effect on sinus node function and AV node and His-Purkinje system conduction. It has less negative inotropic effect than procainamide. It has a narrow therapeutic index. Acute overdose may result in bradycardia, complete heart block, torsade de pointes, asystole, hypotension, and seizures. Treatment is primarily supportive.

TOXIC DOSE

The *adult therapeutic dose* is 150 to 400 mg orally every 6 to 8 hours, maximum 1.2 g/day. Ingestion of twice the daily therapeutic dose may be life threatening. A 41-year-old woman ingested 18 g, developed seizures, and survived (84). Death has been reported with doses of 4 to 8 g (85).

TOXICOKINETICS AND TOXICODYNAMICS

Mexiletine is rapidly absorbed with bioavailability of 80% to 90%. The T_{max} is 1 to 3 hours. It is metabolized by the liver. The elimination half-life is 10 to 14 hours and increases with heart or liver failure. Protein binding is 50% to 70%, and the V_d is 5 to 7 L/kg. Approximately 10% to 15% is excreted in the urine. Urinary alkalization decreases excretion.

PATHOPHYSIOLOGY

Mexiletine inhibits the inward sodium current, similar to lidocaine and tocainide, which reduces the rate of rise of the action potential. In therapeutic doses it does not prolong the PR, QRS, or QT intervals. Decreased cardiac output, increased systemic vascular resistance, and depressed myocardial function have been observed.

PREGNANCY AND LACTATION

Mexiletine is FDA pregnancy category C (Appendix I). There are no reports of congenital defects associated with mexiletine in animals or humans. It crosses the placenta and is secreted into breast milk in concentrations greater than maternal serum, but it is considered compatible with breast-feeding (86).

CLINICAL PRESENTATION

Acute Overdosage. Overdose has resulted in drowsiness, confusion, bradycardia, complete heart block, torsade de pointes, hypotension, seizures, status epilepticus, respiratory failure, and asystole. Ingestion of 4400 mg resulted in paresthesias of the tongue, nausea, seizures, asystole, and death in 2 hours (87). After ingestion of 2400 mg by two adults and 1000 mg by another, dizziness, drowsiness, and mild disorientation persisted for approximately 6 hours; two experienced bradycardia (88). Sudden cardiac arrest and hypokalemia after ingestion of 8000 mg of mexiletine responded to treatment with gastric lavage, atropine, and cardiopulmonary resuscitation (89,90). Status epilepticus has been observed without cardiovascular toxicity (84).

Adverse Events. Adverse reactions to mexiletine are primarily GI (up to 40%) and neurologic (10%). Symptoms include nausea, vomiting, heartburn, esophageal spasm, tremor, dizziness, extremity paresthesias, blurred vision, seizures, ataxia, and dyskinesia (91). Prodysrhythmic effects occur in 10% and heart block in 1% of patients taking therapeutic doses. Thrombocytopenia, hypereosinophilia, liver dysfunction, and skin rashes may occur during therapeutic use (92,93).

Drug Interactions. Mexiletine is a CYP2D6 enzyme substrate and CYP1A2 inhibitor. Quinidine, fluvoxamine, and urinary alkalization may increase serum concentrations of mexiletine, but cimetidine had no effect on the pharmacokinetics of mexiletine. Mexiletine is a potent inhibitor of theophylline metabolism. Prodysrhythmic effects may be enhanced in patients receiving mexiletine and theophylline concurrently (94). Concurrent administration of phenytoin or lidocaine, both type 1B antidysrhythmics, may increase the risk of neurotoxicity of mexiletine.

DIAGNOSTIC TESTS

Acute Overdosage. The therapeutic serum level of mexiletine is 0.5 to 2 μg/ml; levels greater than 2 μg/ml are associated with toxicity. A serum concentration of 4 μg/ml was associated with agitation, confusion, and tremors in a 62-year-old man (95). A serum concentration of 20 μg/ml was associated with status epilepticus in a 41-year-old woman (84).

Postmortem Considerations. Mexiletine may demonstrate postmortem redistribution. Heart to peripheral blood concentration ratios averaged 3.6 in two fatalities (85). The following tissue distribution of mexiletine was found in a fatal overdose: heart blood, 44.8 μg/ml; femoral blood, 10.0 μg/ml; vitreous, 8.6 μg/ml; liver, 171.6 μg/g; brain, 84.0 μg/g; and gastric contents, 1464 mg (96).

TREATMENT

Gastrointestinal Decontamination. Induced emesis is contraindicated. Given the serious potential toxicity, decontamination is an appropriate intervention. Gastric lavage within 1 to 2 hours after a large ingestion and activated charcoal may be useful, but have not been studied. In an *in vitro* study using a polyethylene glycol solution medium, 328 mg of mexiletine was adsorbed per gram of charcoal.

Enhancement of Elimination. Mexiletine has a large volume of distribution and high protein binding, indicating that it is unlikely to be amenable to enhancement of elimination.

Antidotes. There is no specific antidote for mexiletine toxicity. Hypertonic sodium bicarbonate infusion theoretically may have some benefit in treating conduction delay but there are no clinical studies to support its efficacy (Chapter 75).

Supportive Care. All patients with potential toxicity should have supplemental oxygen, IV access, and continuous cardiac monitoring. Discontinue mexiletine therapy and avoid other type IB agents such as lidocaine and phenytoin. Hypotension should initially be treated with isotonic crystalloid fluids followed by inotropic support if needed (Chapter 37).

Seizures have responded to benzodiazepines and pentobarbital (84). Benzodiazepines are the first line agent for seizure treatment. Phenytoin should be used with caution, if at all, because of its type 1B antidysrhythmic properties.

Monitoring. Patients with evidence of hypotension, dysrhythmias, or significant conduction delay should have continuous monitoring of blood pressure and cardiac rhythm in an intensive care setting. Frequent ECGs should be obtained to assess the QT and QRS intervals and the effectiveness of therapy.

Tocainide

Tocainide (Tonocard) is a structural oral analog of lidocaine with similar pharmacology and toxicity. It is indicated for life-threatening ventricular dysrhythmias.

TOXIC DOSE

The *adult therapeutic dose* is 400 to 600 mg orally every 6 to 8 hours; maximum, 2400 mg/day. It is contraindicated for patients allergic to amide type local anesthetics, or in second or third degree heart block. Ingestion of twice the therapeutic dose is potentially life threatening. A 70-year-old man ingested 16 g and developed seizures, complete heart block, hypotension, and asystole unresponsive to cardiac pacing (97).

TOXICOKINETICS AND TOXICODYNAMICS

Tocainide is well absorbed; T_{max} is 30 to 160 minutes. Tocainide avoids first pass metabolism and has high oral bioavailability. Metabolism is 60% hepatic and 40% renal (unchanged drug). Renal insufficiency decreases clearance and may lead to toxicity. Protein binding is 10% to 50% and the V_d is 3 L/kg. It has a half-life 11 to 14 hours. Renal failure prolongs the half-life to 27 hours and heart failure to 37 hours.

PATHOPHYSIOLOGY

The pharmacologic properties and physiologic effects are similar to lidocaine. It decreases myocardial cell excitability and increases the effective refractory period through dose-dependent decreases in sodium and potassium conductance. It does not prolong the PR, QRS, or QT intervals in therapeutic doses.

PREGNANCY AND LACTATION

Tocainide is FDA classification C (Appendix I). It appears to be concentrated in breast milk. In one case, it was administered at 6 months' gestation. The patient delivered a normal baby 1-month prematurely (98).

CLINICAL PRESENTATION

Acute Overdosage. The clinical presentation is similar to mexiletine and lidocaine. Vomiting, diarrhea, headache, tremor, confusion, coma, seizures, complete heart block, hypotension, and asystole occur in overdose. The QRS and QT are usually normal but may be prolonged in severe toxicity.

Adverse Events. Prodysrhythmic effects occur in 1% to 8% of patients taking therapeutic doses (99). Bradycardia and hypotension have been reported after IV administration. Pulmonary fibrosis and interstitial pneumonitis may occur (100). GI effects include nausea (15%), vomiting, and diarrhea. CNS effects include headache (5%), tremor (dose-related), dizziness (8% to 15%), paresthesias (4% to 9%), ataxia (dose-related), blurred vision, confusion, paranoia, and visual hallucinations. Blood dyscrasias (0.18% of patients) usually occur within the first 3 months of therapy and include neutropenia, agranulocytosis (25% mortality), thrombocytopenia, and aplastic anemia. Dermatologic events include rash (1% to 8%), Stevens-Johnson syndrome, erythema multiforme, exfoliative dermatitis (101).

Drug Interactions. Tocainide may increase serum levels of theophylline. Therapeutic levels of tocainide lowered the seizure threshold to lidocaine in dogs. Lidocaine should be used with caution and in lower doses in patients on tocainide (102).

DIAGNOSTIC TESTS

Therapeutic plasma concentrations are 4 to 10 μg/ml (103). A rapid high performance liquid chromatography assay can determine free and total plasma tocainide levels (104). Monitor the complete blood count to evaluate for hematologic toxicity. Perform chest radiograph for pulmonary symptoms to detect pulmonary fibrosis, interstitial pneumonitis, alveolitis, pulmonary edema, and pneumonia.

Postmortem Considerations. A postmortem serum level of 68 mg/L was found in a 26-year-old woman who experienced ventricular dysrhythmias and coma after overdose. The vitreous humor tocainide concentration was 9.3 mg/L and bile 11 mg/L (105).

TREATMENT

Gastrointestinal Decontamination. Induced emesis is contraindicated. Given the serious potential toxicity, decontamination is an appropriate intervention. Gastric lavage within 1 to 2 hours after a large ingestion and activated charcoal may be useful but have not been systematically studied.

Enhancement of Elimination. There are no data available indicating that multiple dose activated charcoal is effective. One patient ingested 400 mg of tocainide and developed a blood level of 34 μg/ml. Hemodialysis for 4 hours appeared to be useful in enhancing clinical recovery and reducing the blood concentration (103).

Antidote. Because tocainide causes sodium channel blockade, hypertonic sodium bicarbonate infusion theoretically may have some benefit.

Supportive Care. All patients with potential toxicity should have supplemental oxygen, IV access, and continuous cardiac monitoring. Discontinue tocainide therapy and avoid other type IB agents. Hypotension should initially be treated with isotonic crystalloid fluid resuscitation followed by inotropic support if needed (Chapter 37).

IV benzodiazepines are the first line agent for seizure treatment. Phenytoin should be used with caution, if at all, because of its type IB antidysrhythmic properties.

TYPE IC AGENTS

Type IC drugs have a narrow therapeutic index. Severe intoxication with type IC antidysrhythmics is associated with an average mortality rate of 23% (106). Specific antidotes are not available. Sodium bicarbonate infusion has been administered with inconsistent results (106,107). The Cardiac Arrhythmic Suppression Trial was the first long-term, multicenter, multidrug, placebo-controlled trial of the safety and efficacy of antidysrhythmic drug therapy in reducing sudden death. Results indicated that the use of encainide and flecainide induced lethal ventricular dysrhythmias and substantially increased the rate of sudden death and total mortality (108,109). Encainide has been voluntarily removed from the market. Physicians should use these drugs only for life-threatening dysrhythmias. Atrial life-threatening prodysrhythmic effects also may follow use of class IC antidysrhythmic drugs (110).

Ajmaline

Ajmaline (Aritmina) was first discovered among the rauwolfia alkaloids in 1931. Ajmaline has class IC and IA antidysrhythmic effects and is associated with high mortality in overdose. In Paris, ajmaline was responsible for 38 cases of poisoning resulting in nine deaths (111). In the German series, overdose with ajmaline led to deaths in 4 of 12 cases. It is available in Austria, Italy, Germany, Belgium, and Spain.

TOXIC DOSE

The *adult therapeutic dose* is 100 to 300 mg/day orally. The IV dose is 1 mg/kg at a maximum rate of 10 mg/minute. The intramuscular dose is 50 to 150 mg daily. Ingestion of twice the therapeutic dose is potentially life threatening.

Three patients survived doses of 1050 mg, 2240 mg, and 750 mg (112,113). A dose of 18 mg/kg resulted in VT for 10 hours and the patient recovered (114). No correlation between ingested overdose and outcome was found in a case series of 12 patients (115). Fatal intoxication has been observed with doses of 500 mg and 2500 mg (115,116). Ataxia, clonic-tonic seizures, loss of consciousness, and apnea were observed in a 17-month-old person after ingestion of 250 mg (117). A 4-year-old infant died 3 hours after ingesting approximately 850 mg of ajmaline (118).

TOXICOKINETICS AND TOXICODYNAMICS

Ajmaline is 5% bioavailable orally. The distribution half-life is 6 minutes; the elimination half-life is 95 minutes. The V_d is 2 to 3 L/kg; protein binding is 75% (115,119). Ajmaline undergoes hepatic metabolism, and approximately 5% of an ajmaline dose is excreted unchanged in the urine. The main metabolite is hydroxyajmaline (119,120). The toxicity of oral ajmaline may be due to saturation of a metabolic enzyme with resultant rise in plasma concentrations (115). Impairment of liver function or cardiogenic shock leads to a reduced clearance. After phenobarbital enzyme induction, the total plasma clearance of ajmaline is increased fivefold (119).

PATHOPHYSIOLOGY

Ajmaline diminishes cardiac excitability, slows the heart rate, and slows AV conduction. In high doses, ajmaline appears to have a negative inotropic effect. AV and intraventricular blocks are common. Similar to quinidine, it has led to asystole and VF after rapid injection. The drug may affect the CNS, resulting in respiratory depression, and convulsions (117). It does not appear to have the sedative qualities of other rauwolfia alkaloids.

PREGNANCY AND LACTATION

There have been no controlled studies demonstrating clinical evidence of safety of either the mother or the fetus when ajmaline is administered during pregnancy.

CLINICAL PRESENTATION

Onset of symptoms is rapid. Overdose may also be characterized by GI symptoms of nausea and vomiting. Cardiac toxicity may include bradycardia, AV block, intraventricular block, VT, prolongation of the QT interval, and cardiac arrest (121). In a case series of 59 patients, cardiac arrest occurred only in patients with a QRS of 200 milliseconds or more. The duration of the cardiac effects was less than 12 hours (122). Cardiac arrest has been observed after IV use in elderly patients (123). Cardiac arrest was observed in 9 of 38 overdoses (111).

A 4-year-old child developed grade 1 AV block with QT prolongation. He was treated with supportive measures and recovered (124). Ataxia, clonic-tonic seizures, loss of consciousness, and apnea followed by supraventricular tachycardia, left bundle-branch block, and a prolonged QT interval were observed in a 17-month-old child after ingestion of 250 mg (117). A 4-year-old infant died 3 hours after ingesting approximately 850 mg of ajmaline (118).

Adverse Reactions. Acute hepatitis and prolonged cholestasis were reported in three patients who received the drug for 8 to 16 days. Fever, eosinophilia, and portal inflammatory infiltration suggested an autoimmune etiology (125). Agranulocytosis, eye twitching, seizures, torsade de pointes (126) and respiratory depression have also been reported.

Drug Interactions. Hepatic microsomal enzyme inducers such as phenobarbital accelerate metabolism of ajmaline and increase its excretion (119). Patients under halothane or Fluothane anesthesia appear to be more sensitive to ajmaline. Increased plasma concentrations of ajmaline are seen when administered concurrently with quinidine (127).

DIAGNOSTIC TESTS

Blood levels of ajmaline measured after IV administration indicate that the desirable therapeutic level ranges from 0.01 to 0.03 μg/ml and that 0.15 μg/ml is toxic (128,129). Overdose patients with ventricular dysrhythmias and cardiac arrest have had serum ajmaline concentrations from 0.8 to 6 mg/L (121). A blood ajmaline concentration of 5.5 μg/ml was measured in a 4-year-old girl who died 3 hours after ingesting 850 mg (118). A blood level of 10 μg/ml was measured in a woman aged 56 years who died 2 hours after ingesting 2500 mg (130). Within 150 minutes of ingesting 1000 mg, a 57-year-old man had a blood level of 3 μg/ml and a urine level of 12.6 μg/ml. On day two, the blood level was zero and the urine level was 6.09 μg/ml (131).

An ECG should be obtained on all patients who overdose or manifest signs of toxicity. Bradycardia, AV block, intraventricular block, VT, and QT prolongation may be observed.

TREATMENT

Gastrointestinal Decontamination. Induced emesis is contraindicated. Given the serious potential toxicity, decontamination is an appropriate intervention. Gastric lavage within 1 to 2 hours after a large ingestion and activated charcoal may be useful but have not been systematically studied. Vagal stimulation induced by gastric lavage tube placement may precipitate or worsen bradycardia.

Enhancement of Elimination. Due to its large volume of distribution and high protein binding, methods to enhance elimination are unlikely to be effective.

Antidotes. There are no known antidotes.

Supportive Care. All patients with potential toxicity should have supplemental oxygen, IV access, and continuous cardiac monitoring. Cardiopulmonary bypass may be required in certain cases (132). Discontinue ajmaline therapy and avoid other type IC agents. Hypotension should be treated with isotonic crystalloid fluid followed by inotropic support if needed (Chapter 37). Pacemaker insertion should be considered early with signs of increasing bradycardia, AV block, or ventricular dysrhythmias.

Monitoring. All persons who overdose with ajmaline should be admitted to an ICU. Patients with evidence of hypotension, dysrhythmias, or significant conduction delay should have continuous monitoring of blood pressure and cardiac rhythm. Frequent ECGs should be obtained to assess the QT and QRS intervals and the effectiveness of therapy.

Prajmaline

Prajmaline (prajmalium bitartrate, Neorhythmin) has type IA and IC properties similar to those of ajmaline and quinidine. It is the *N*-propyl derivative of ajmaline. Overdose reports (132–134) indicate a high fatality rate. It is available in Germany, Italy, Spain, Switzerland, and Austria.

TOXIC DOSE

The adult therapeutic dose is 40 to 80 mg/day orally in 3 to 4 divided doses. The maintenance dose is 20 to 100 mg orally in divided daily doses. Ingestion of twice the therapeutic dose is potentially life threatening. Overdoses with less than 20 of the 20-mg tablets have been fatal (133).

TOXICOKINETICS AND TOXICODYNAMICS

Prajmaline has an oral bioavailability of 80% to 100%, T_{max} of 1 to 2 hours, V_d of 2 to 3 L/kg, and elimination half-life of 4 to 7 hours. It is 60% plasma protein bound. There are two main metabolites, 21-carboxyprajmaline and hydroxyprajmaline. Slow metabolizers may have a half-life of 26 hours. Approximately 30% is eliminated in the urine as unchanged drug (132).

PATHOPHYSIOLOGY

Prajmaline is a sodium and calcium channel antagonist. It depresses phase 0 and prolongs the action potential duration and effective refractory period. It also has quinidine-like effects and delays depolarization and repolarization. It prolongs the HV intervals in the bundle of His. It also inhibits platelet aggregation *in vitro*.

PREGNANCY AND LACTATION

Prajmaline crosses the placenta. Doses of 5 mg/kg/day were embryotoxic in rabbits. There are no controlled studies demonstrating its safety for either the mother or the fetus.

CLINICAL PRESENTATION

Clinical symptoms after overdose are similar to those of ajmaline. Koppel reported on 47 cases of prajmaline overdose and symptoms included vomiting, bradycardia, tachycardia, and hypotension. Prajmaline had the highest fatality rate (36%) of the type IC drugs studied (132).

Adverse Events. Cholestatic jaundice (incidence, 1:12,000–15,000), intrahepatic cholestasis with eosinophilia, and anicteric hepatitis may occur. Hematologic effects include leukopenia and thrombocytopenia. Cardiovascular events include bradycardia, heart block, conduction disturbances, and VF.

Drug Interactions. Avoid coadministering drugs that prolong the QT interval such as dofetilide, gatifloxacin, levofloxacin, sotalol, and other type I antiarrhythmic agents.

DIAGNOSTIC TESTS

Blood levels do not correlate well with outcome. Patients may have adverse effects in the therapeutic range of 154 to 991 ng/ml (135). A single dose of 40 mg resulted in an average maximal plasma concentration of 228 ng/ml.

A 12-lead ECG should be obtained on all patients who overdose or manifest signs of toxicity. Bradycardia, AV block, intraventricular block, VT, and prolongation of the QT interval may be observed.

TREATMENT

Gastrointestinal Decontamination. Induced emesis is contraindicated. Given the serious potential toxicity, decontamination is an appropriate intervention. Gastric lavage within 1 to 2 hours after a large ingestion and activated charcoal may be useful but have not been systematically studied.

Enhancement of Elimination. Due to its large volume of distribution and high protein binding, methods to enhance elimination are unlikely to be effective. Resin hemoperfusion appeared to assist in survival in one case (133) but did not prevent fatality in two others (132).

Antidotes. There are no specific antidotes.

Supportive Care. All patients with potential toxicity should have supplemental oxygen, IV access, and continuous cardiac monitoring. Continuous cardiac monitoring should be instituted on admission. Discontinue prajmaline therapy and avoid other type IA and IC agents. Hypotension should initially be treated with isotonic crystalloid fluid followed by inotropic support if needed (Chapter 37). Pacemaker insertion should be considered early with signs of increasing bradycardia, AV block, or ventricular dysrhythmias. Cardiopulmonary bypass may be required in certain cases (132).

Monitoring. All persons who overdose with prajmaline should be admitted to an ICU. Patients with evidence of hypotension, dysrhythmias, or significant conduction delay should have continuous monitoring of blood pressure and cardiac rhythm. The ECG should be monitored frequently to assess the QT and QRS intervals and the effectiveness of therapy.

Cibenzoline

Cibenzoline (cifenline, Cipralan, Cibed Timecelles) is chemically unrelated to other antidysrhythmic drugs. Its electrophysiologic properties are similar to those of quinidine (136–138). It possesses type IA, IC, III, and IV activity.

TOXIC DOSE

The *adult therapeutic dose* is 130 mg initially, then 4 to 6 mg/kg or 260 to 390 mg daily. The dose should be reduced with renal insufficiency. Ingestion of twice the therapeutic dose is potentially life threatening. An adult ingested 3250 mg of cibenzoline and survived with supportive care. Ingestion of 3900 mg and 5200 mg has been associated with rapidly fatal circulatory failure.

TOXICOKINETICS AND TOXICODYNAMICS

Cibenzoline is 90% bioavailable. The T_{max} is 1 hour. It is 50% bound to plasma protein. Plasma concentrations correlate with its therapeutic effect; levels of 215 to 405 ng/ml result in a 90% reduction of premature ventricular complex frequency (138). Its V_d is 4 to 6 L/kg. Approximately 60% of a dose is excreted unchanged in the urine. Elimination half-life is 6 to 15 hours and is independent of dose. In renal failure, its half-life increases to 22 hours (136). Total clearance is approximately 9 ml/minute/kg (139). Renal clearance declines with age.

PATHOPHYSIOLOGY

It possesses type I, III, and IV antidysrhythmic activity. Cibenzoline lengthens AH and HV intervals and ventricular myocardial effective refractory periods (140). ECG findings reflect a dose-related prolongation of the PR and QRS intervals with slight QT_c prolongation (140,141).

PREGNANCY AND LACTATION

There have been no controlled studies demonstrating clinical evidence of safety for either the mother or the fetus.

CLINICAL PRESENTATION

Overdose with cibenzoline resulted in hypotension, loss of consciousness, nausea, vomiting, and intraventricular block in a 60-year-old man. Toxic effects were refractive to potassium loading; sodium lactate, 500 ml IV; and calcium chloride, 2 g IV. The cardiogenic shock was refractory to dobutamine, 10 mg/kg/minute; glucagon, 3 mg; and additional sodium lactate. The patient died in 12 hours with a serum level of 2550 ng/ml. Sodium lactate, reported elsewhere as being effective with other type I agents (142), was ineffective in this patient (143).

A myastheniform syndrome with acute respiratory failure occurred after overdose in a patient with renal failure. Muscle strength recovered as the serum cibenzoline concentration fell. Neuromuscular blockade was demonstrated by repetitive nerve stimulation (144). Hypoglycemia has been reported after cibenzoline use (145,146).

Adverse Events. An 80-year-old woman was taking 300-mg cibenzoline daily for 1 month and presented in cardiogenic shock and CHF. The ECG showed a QRS, 0.20 sec, and QTc, 0.64 sec, and *pacing failure*. She had evidence of renal insufficiency. The admission plasma cibenzoline concentration was 2580 ng/ml. She recovered with vasopressor support, ventricular pacing, and charcoal hemoperfusion (147).

Adverse Reactions. Adverse effects with cibenzoline are infrequent: nausea, vomiting, and diarrhea; headache, visual disturbances, tremor, and vertigo; dry mouth, urinary retention; asymptomatic liver transaminase elevation; and hypoglycemia. There appears to be an eightfold risk of hypoglycemia in patients taking cibenzoline therapeutically (146).

Drug Interactions. Cimetidine increases the blood concentration and half-life of cibenzoline (148).

DIAGNOSTIC TESTS

All potentially toxic patients should have a metabolic panel obtained to evaluate acid-base status, serum glucose, and renal and hepatic function. An ECG should be obtained to evaluate conduction delays and dysrhythmias and repeated frequently until toxicity is resolved.

Serum cibenzoline concentrations are available but usually do not guide treatment. Patients with elevated concentrations and significant symptoms of toxicity may be candidates for enhanced elimination by charcoal hemoperfusion.

TREATMENT

Gastrointestinal Decontamination. Induced emesis is contraindicated. Given the serious potential toxicity, decontamination is an appropriate intervention. Gastric lavage within 1 to 2 hours after a large ingestion and activated charcoal may be useful but have not been systematically studied. Vagal stimulation induced by gastric lavage tube placement may precipitate or worsen bradycardia.

Elimination Enhancement. Due to its large volume of distribution and high protein binding, methods to enhance elimination are unlikely to be effective. There are no data available indicating that multiple dose activated charcoal is effective. In a study of subtherapeutic dosing in healthy volunteers and renal failure patients, hemodialysis accounted for only 13% of drug clearance (136).

Charcoal hemoperfusion increased the clearance of cibenzoline in an 80-year-old woman with chronic toxicity. Charcoal hemoperfusion was performed for 5 hours with a DHP-1 containing 100 g activated charcoal coated with poly-HEMA at a flow rate of 150 ml/minute. The plasma cibenzoline concentration decreased from 1450 ng/ml to 930 ng/ml during hemoperfusion. The elimination half-life during hemoperfusion was 9.8 hours compared to 92 hours before hemoperfusion. The mean hemoperfusion clearance was 117.6 ml/minute, whereas hemodialysis clearance is reported to be only 30 ml/minute (147).

Antidote. There is no specific antidote.

Supportive Care. All patients with potential toxicity should have supplemental oxygen, IV access, and continuous cardiac monitoring. Discontinue cibenzoline therapy and avoid other type I antiarrhythmic agents. Hypotension should initially be treated with isotonic crystalloid fluid resuscitation followed by inotropic support if needed (Chapter 37). Pacemaker insertion should be considered early with signs of increasing bradycardia, AV block, or ventricular dysrhythmias. Cardiopulmonary bypass may be required in certain cases.

Molar sodium lactate (500 ml IV over 30 minutes) with potassium chloride resulted in an improvement in clinical status with narrowing of the QRS in four patients (142), although one report indicated it was of no value (143). Hypoglycemia may occur and should be treated with supplemental IV glucose administration as needed.

Monitoring. All persons who overdose with cibenzoline should be admitted to an ICU. Patients with evidence of hypotension, dysrhythmias, or significant conduction delay should have continuous monitoring of blood pressure and cardiac rhythm. Frequent ECGs should be obtained to assess the QT and QRS intervals and the effectiveness of therapy.

Encainide

Encainide (Enkaid) is a class IC antidysrhythmic that was withdrawn in the United States in December 1991 because of increased mortality rates in the Cardiac Dysrhythmia Suppression Trial (149). It may be still available to patients through their physicians via the Continuing Patient Access Program.

TOXIC DOSE

The *adult therapeutic dose* is 25 mg orally every 8 hours. The maximum single dose is 75 mg and maximum total daily dose is 200 mg/day. Unintentional ingestion of extra single doses of encainide has caused ventricular dysrhythmias in patients with cardiac disease. A 3 to 4 g overdose of encainide in an adult produced obtundation, seizures, QT prolongation, bradycardia, and hypotension (150). A 6-month-old infant reportedly ingested a single 25-mg encainide tablet and within 40 minutes developed VT and VF (151).

TOXICOKINETICS AND TOXICODYNAMICS

Encainide is rapidly absorbed with a bioavailability of 25% to 90%. The T_{max} is 1 to 3 hours after ingestion. Encainide is metabolized by the liver to two major active metabolites, *O*-demethyl encainide (ODE) and 3-methoxy-*O*-demethyl encainide (MODE). The metabolites have longer half-lives and equal or greater potency than the parent compound (152). Encainide has two distinct phenotypes for metabolism, extensive (90% of white population) and slow (10%). Extensive metabolizers have an encainide half-life of approximately 2 hours, producing the two active metabolites ODE and MODE, with 50% of the drug excreted unchanged in the urine. Slow metabolizers have an encainide half-life of 9.8 hours, producing the inactive metabolite *N*-demethyl encainide. Effective plasma levels of ODE for suppression of dysrhythmia are 100 to 300 ng/ml, whereas plasma levels of MODE are 60 to 280 ng/ml during long-term therapy in extensive metabolizers. Slow metabolizers require concentrations of encainide greater than 265 ng/ml for therapeutic effects. Plasma levels of encainide are 250 to 1000 ng/ml in slow metabolizers, 20 times higher than those in extensive metabolizers, due to the greater oral bioavailability and longer half-life of elimination. Toxicity with ODE is seen at concentrations above 300 ng/ml. Protein binding is 70% and 78% for extensive and slow metabolizers, respectively. The V_d is 172 to 375 L.

PATHOPHYSIOLOGY

Encainide is a sodium channel antagonist that is much more potent than procainamide. Electrophysiologic effects are related to the route of administration of the drug. Acute IV administration causes slowing of phase 0 depolarization. This results in a prolonged QRS duration with little increase in the QT interval. Chronic therapy (more than 3 days) causes decreased conduction in the AV node and His-Purkinje system, increased refractoriness in the atrium and ventricle, and increased QRS and QT intervals. The metabolites account for most of the electrophysiologic effects during chronic therapy. It also possesses local anesthetic properties similar to lidocaine. Encainide differs from quinidine and tricyclic antidepressants in its lack of anticholinergic, α-adrenergic antagonist, and vasodilator properties.

PREGNANCY AND LACTATION

Encainide is FDA pregnancy category B (Appendix I). Encainide and its active metabolites cross the placenta and are excreted into human breast milk. Encainide has been used successfully to treat fetal cardiac dysrhythmias *in utero* (153).

CLINICAL PRESENTATION

Acute Overdosage. The onset of symptoms is rapid, usually within an hour of ingestion, and consists of CNS depression, seizures, hypotension, bradycardia, ventricular dysrhythmias, and cardiovascular collapse (150). Metabolic acidosis may occur in association with generalized seizure activity.

A 6-month-old boy ingested one 25-mg encainide tablet. He developed a wide-complex tachycardia (QRS, 0.16 sec) followed by pulseless VT within 40 minutes. He was resuscitated using chest compressions and cardioversion with 1 J/kg and had a normal ECG 72 hours later (151).

Adverse Reactions. The most common adverse effects are sudden death in post-myocardial infarction patients (7.7%), dysrhythmias, dizziness, visual changes, headache, tremors, ataxia, hyperglycemia, fatigue, memory or speech impairment, nausea, vomiting (6%), and metallic taste. Withdrawal of chronic encainide therapy led to a fatal episode of VT and VF (154).

Drug Interactions. Coadministration of encainide and cimetidine may increase encainide plasma concentrations and its major metabolites by 30% to 40% (155). However, no clinically significant adverse effects were seen in a retrospective evaluation of 33 patients who received both drugs (156).

DIAGNOSTIC TESTS

Acute Overdosage. The therapeutic concentration of encainide is reported to be 15 to 100 ng/ml. The therapeutic concentrations of its major metabolites are ODE 180 to 220 ng/ml and MODE 140 to 185 ng/ml. A 6-month-old child reportedly ingested 25 mg of encainide and 1 hour later had an encainide concentration of 180 ng/ml (15 to 100 ng/ml), ODE concentration 464 ng/ml (100 to 300 ng/ml), and MODE concentration 126 (60 to 300 ng/ml) (151).

Prolongation of QRS interval, ventricular dysrhythmias, and bradycardia may occur.

Metabolic acidosis secondary to tissue hypoperfusion or seizure activity may be observed.

Adverse Events. Encainide exacerbates hyperglycemia in some patients. Serum glucose levels should be monitored when encainide therapy is begun in patients with type II diabetes mellitus and when encainide is discontinued in patients receiving insulin therapy (157).

TREATMENT

Ingestion of a single tablet could be lethal in infants or children and immediate transport to the nearest hospital for evaluation is warranted, even if the patient is asymptomatic (151).

Gastrointestinal Decontamination. Induced emesis is contraindicated. Given the serious potential toxicity, decontamination is an appropriate intervention. Gastric lavage within 1 to 2 hours after a large ingestion and activated charcoal may be useful but have not been systematically studied. Vagal stimulation induced by gastric lavage tube placement may precipitate or worsen bradycardia.

Elimination Enhancement. Due to its large volume of distribution and high protein binding, methods to enhance elimination are unlikely to be effective. There is no data available indicating that multiple dose activated charcoal is effective.

Antidotes. Hypertonic sodium bicarbonate or sodium chloride may be beneficial in reversing cardiotoxic effects of encainide overdose, but data is limited. The usual loading dose is 1 to 2 mEq/kg IV bolus to achieve a target blood pH of 7.50 to 7.55 (Chapter 75). Infusion of 100 mEq sodium bicarbonate was followed promptly by resolution of bradycardia and hypotension in a patient who had ingested 3000 to 3500 mg of encainide. The patient's QRS duration decreased from 200 milliseconds on presentation to 130 milliseconds 6 hours post-ingestion (150). However, sodium bicarbonate infusion had no significant effect on the duration of the QRS, PR, or QT interval in a controlled study of patients taking therapeutic doses of flecainide or encainide (156).

Supportive Care. Hospital admission should be considered for selected patients in whom encainide therapy is to be discontinued (154). All patients with potential toxicity should have supplemental oxygen, IV access, and continuous cardiac monitoring in an ICU. Discontinue encainide therapy and avoid other type I antidysrhythmic agents. Hypotension should initially be treated with isotonic crystalloid fluid resuscitation followed by inotropic support if needed (Chapter 37). Pacemaker insertion should be considered early with signs of increasing bradycardia, AV block, or ventricular dysrhythmias. Cardiopulmonary bypass may be required in certain cases.

Seizures are treated with benzodiazepines, followed by phenytoin and more invasive procedures in patients with refractory seizures (Chapter 40).

Monitoring. Patients with evidence of hypotension, dysrhythmias, or significant conduction delay should have continuous monitoring of blood pressure and cardiac rhythm in an intensive care setting. Frequent ECGs should be obtained to assess the QT and QRS intervals and the effectiveness of therapy.

Flecainide

Flecainide (Tambocor) is available in 50-, 100-, and 150-mg tablets. Its prodysrhythmias substantially limit its therapeutic use (158). Severe bradycardia, ventricular tachydysrhythmias, and seizures occur in overdose.

TOXIC DOSE

The *adult therapeutic dose* is 50 to 100 mg orally every 12 hours up to a maximum of 400 mg/day. Daily doses of 200 to 400 mg are associated with an 11% to 27% widening of the QRS interval, 3% to 11% increase in the PR interval, and a 3% to 11% prolongation of the QT interval (159). The *pediatric dose* is 3 to 6 mg/kg/day in three divided doses; maximum dose is 11 mg/kg/day.

Flecainide has a narrow therapeutic range. Ingestion of twice the therapeutic dose in an adult or a single tablet in a child should be considered potentially life threatening. A 38-year-old woman ingested 1000 mg and developed hypotension, conduction delay (QRS 220 milliseconds), and recovered (160). A 45-year-old woman ingested 2000 mg and developed VF and cardiac arrest (161). An 18-year-old person ingested an estimated 1200 mg and died within 90 minutes (162). Ingestion of 900 mg of flecainide daily by an adult led to symptoms of blurred vision, headache, photophobia, paresthesias, and generalized weakness (163).

TOXICOKINETICS AND TOXICODYNAMICS

GI absorption is rapid and complete (90% bioavailable). The T_{max} is 2 to 3 hours. The liver metabolizes approximately 50% of a dose; the kidney excretes approximately 25% to 30% unchanged. Protein binding is 40% and the V_d is 5 to 12 L/kg. The elimination half-life is 7 to 23 hours in adults, 11 to 12 hours in infants, and 8 hours in children. It is prolonged with CHF. End-stage renal disease may prolong the half-life to 51 to 58 hours. The elimination curve of a patient who ingested approximately 9 g is illustrated in Figure 4 (164).

PATHOPHYSIOLOGY

Flecainide slows cardiac conduction by inhibition of sodium channels. This results in prolonged PR, QRS, and QT intervals.

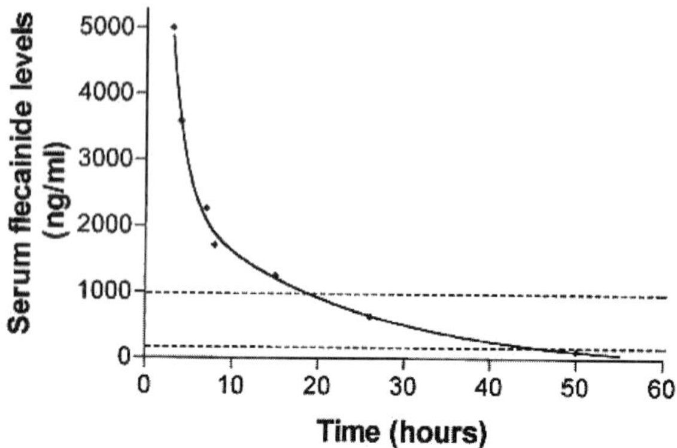

Figure 4. The elimination curve from a patient who ingested approximately 9 g of flecainide. (From Hanley NA, Bourke JP, Gascoigne AD. Survival in a case of life-threatening flecainide overdose. *Int Care Med* 1998;24:740–742, with permission.)

It increases the electrical stimulation threshold of the ventricle and His-Purkinje system. It also has local anesthetic and negative inotropic effects that may result in seizures and hypotension.

PREGNANCY AND LACTATION

Flecainide is FDA pregnancy category C (Appendix I). Flecainide crosses the placenta and concentrates in the breast milk. It has been used to treat fetal tachycardias (165). A patient who received 200 mg of flecainide and 160 mg of sotalol daily delivered a normal baby by cesarean section 3 weeks before term. The maternal milk to maternal plasma ratio was 1.57:1 to 2.18:1, indicating excretion of flecainide in breast milk (166). The expected average steady-state plasma concentration in a newborn consuming all its mother's milk (700 ml/day) would not be expected to exceed approximately 62 ng/ml. Few toxic effects have occurred at plasma levels of 100 to 900 ng/ml (167).

CLINICAL PRESENTATION

Acute Overdosage. Symptoms usually begin within 30 minutes of ingestion. Toxic effects include blurred vision, dry mouth, dizziness, nausea, vomiting, dizziness, lethargy, coma, seizures, hypotension, and conduction delays (160,168). Severe bradycardia and ventricular tachydysrhythmias may occur. Polymorphic VT, VF, variable AV block, and asystole have been reported. In 25 patients (average age 21 years) with flecainide overdose, a dose 200 to 3600 mg caused nausea and vomiting in 50%; bradycardia, hypotension in 10%; and two died. Nausea typically occurred within 30 minutes and cardiac effects were observed at 30 to 120 minutes after ingestion. Vomiting early in the course seemed to indicate better outcome (168).

A 30-year-old man ingested 6000 mg and was unconscious, cyanotic, and had a wide-complex bradycardia with a heart rate of 26 beats/minute within 1 hour of ingestion. He had three generalized seizures en route to the hospital. His plasma flecainide concentration was 20.5 μg/ml. Transvenous and transcutaneous cardiac pacing attempts failed. Idioventricular rhythm, nonsustained VT, atrial fibrillation, junctional rhythm, and sinus rhythm with first-degree AV block occurred. He was supported with ECMO and recovered (169).

A 37-year-old woman intentionally overdosed on an unknown amount of flecainide and alcohol. She presented unconscious with fixed and dilated pupils. The peak flecainide concentration 3 to 10 hours post-ingestion was 6160 ng/ml (six times therapeutic). She developed VF that was successfully defibrillated. An idioventricular rhythm with marked QRS widening and QT prolongation was observed. Torsade de pointes

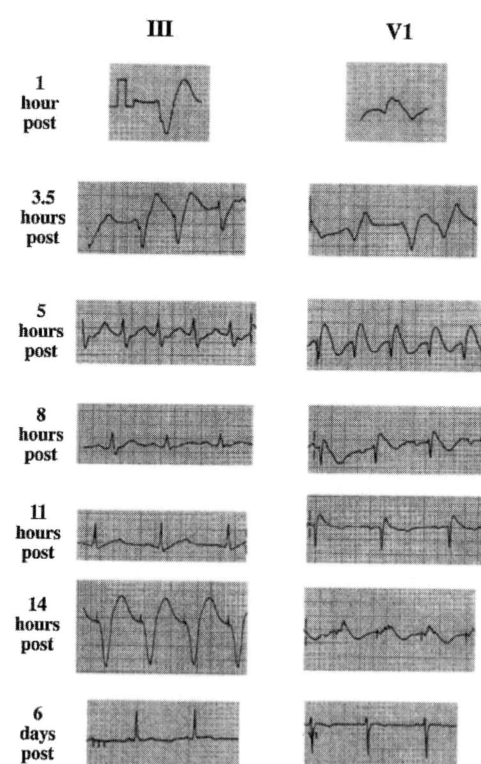

Figure 5. Electrocardiographic changes associated with flecainide overdose. (From Hanley NA, Bourke JP, Gascoigne AD. Survival in a case of life-threatening flecainide overdose. *Intensive Care Med* 1998;24:741, with permission.)

was treated with high doses of lidocaine (4 g daily) and repeat defibrillation. She recovered and was discharged 37 days after admission with no permanent sequelae (170).

Generalized tonic-clonic seizures followed ingestion of 1500 mg of flecainide in a 12-year-old girl (171). The initial flecainide level was greater than 4 μg/ml and the QRS was markedly prolonged. She recovered in 48 hours with supportive care.

A 15-year-old girl ingested 9000 mg of flecainide. She presented in coma with fixed dilated pupils, bradycardia, and unobtainable blood pressure. She received gastric lavage, activated charcoal, and was resuscitated with IV fluids and endotracheal intubation. Three hours after overdose she was comatose with a wide complex irregular bradycardia (Fig. 5). IV adrenaline infusion (0.25 μg/kg/minute) was started. Five hours post-ingestion she developed episodes of VT that was converted with 100 mg of lidocaine after direct current cardioversion failed. Additional episodes of VT responded to lidocaine infusion. A prophylactic transvenous ventricular pacing wire was inserted. At 36 hours she was hemodynamically stable and extubated (164).

Adverse Events. An increase in the QRS duration of 50%, the PR interval of 30%, or QTc interval of 15% over baseline values suggests flecainide toxicity and corresponds to high concentrations of drug. However, patients may develop acute toxicity due to chronic drug accumulation without warning (159). Sudden withdrawal of flecainide may be associated with exacerbation of underlying life-threatening ventricular dysrhythmias (172).

In one series of patients with a prior history of serious ventricular dysrhythmias, the flecainide dose of 200 mg twice daily was associated with the development of VT demonstrating an unusual sinusoidal QRS complex (173). CNS effects are most common and consist mainly of dizziness and visual disturbances (30% of patients). Nausea, vomiting, headache, tremor, peripheral neuropathy, ataxia, and paresthesia may also occur and respond to decreased dosing. Corneal deposits, pulmonary fibrosis, and pneumonitis have occurred during treatment.

Drug Interactions. Flecainide is a CYP2D6 enzyme substrate, and concentrations may be increased by concurrent administration of amiodarone, cimetidine, digoxin, propranolol, quinidine, and ritonavir. Additive negative inotropic effects may be seen with beta-blockers. Drugs that alkalinize the urine (bicarbonate, carbonic anhydrase inhibitors) may decrease renal clearance and increase serum concentration.

DIAGNOSTIC TESTS

The therapeutic serum range of flecainide is 0.2 to 1.0 μg/ml. Plasma levels exceeding 1 μg/ml are probably toxic (174). Serum concentrations of 2 to 3 μg/ml have been associated with AV nodal block with escape rhythm and QRS interval prolongation (175), dysarthria and hallucinations (176), and hypotension and conduction delay (160). An acute overdose of 2000 mg in a 45-year-old woman who survived resulted in a 5-hour post-ingestion concentration of 850 μg/ml.

The ECG usually demonstrates conduction delay within the first 2 hours of overdose. The PR, QRS, and QT intervals may be markedly prolonged. AV block and wide complex dysrhythmias such as idioventricular rhythms and VT also occur (Fig. 5) (164,168–171,177).

Ingestion of 900 mg of flecainide daily by an adult resulted in broadening of P waves, prolongation of the PR interval, and widening of the QRS with a plasma level of 2.5 g/ml. The QT interval lengthened at concentrations of 1.86 to 1.1 μg/ml. At 0.49 μg/ml, the QT interval normalized and giant T waves appeared (163). Ingestion of 1800 mg of flecainide resulted in absent P waves, a wide QRS complex, and an increased QT interval (178). A patient ingested 3800 mg of flecainide with 50 mg of diazepam, 20 mg of loperamide, and 100 g of ethanol. In 2 hours the flecainide serum level was 3.7 μg/ml. The ECG showed a prolonged QT, QRS, and PR intervals with a VT that deteriorated to polymorphous VT. Sinus rhythm was restored after infusion of dopamine, sodium bicarbonate, and physostigmine. Normalization of the ECG was correlated with diminishing serum levels of flecainide (159).

Postmortem Considerations. Postmortem blood levels of 16 μg/ml (162) and 13 μg/ml have been reported (179). Flecainide was detected by gas chromatography/electron capture detector in the following tissue distribution: femoral blood 7.7 mg/kg, bile 0.26 mg/kg, liver 18 mg/kg, cerebrospinal fluid 0.22 mg/kg, and urine 28.9 mg/kg, total gastric contents 43 mg (180). Postmortem levels in an 18-year-old male with Marfan's syndrome who died within 90 minutes of ingestion were as follows: blood (16.3 mg/L), liver (111 mg/kg), and stomach contents (4.26 g/L) (162). The postmortem distribution of flecainide in a patient with a blood concentration of 13 mg/L was bile, 160 mg/L; urine, 54 mg/L; vitreous humor, 7.4 mg/L; liver, 180 mg/L; kidney, 74 mg/L; and stomach contents, 120 mg (179). Two fatalities from suicidal ingestion of flecainide, ages 33 and 15 years, were found to have postmortem blood concentrations of 93.7 and 100 μg/ml (181).

TREATMENT

Gastrointestinal Decontamination. Induced emesis is contraindicated. Given the serious potential toxicity, decontamination is an appropriate intervention. Gastric lavage within 1 to 2 hours after a large ingestion and activated charcoal may be useful but have not been systematically studied. A single dose of activated charcoal (30 g) has been shown to prevent absorption shortly after ingestion of 200 mg of flecainide in human volunteers (182).

Enhancement of Elimination. Due to its large volume of distribution and high protein binding, methods to enhance elimination are unlikely to be effective. Hemodialysis did not prevent death in a patient with a flecainide plasma concentration of 6500 ng/ml. Hemoperfusion was associated with "substantial stabilization of cardiac function" in one overdose case and was not helpful in another (168). Hemoperfusion was ineffective in significantly enhancing the plasma clearance of flecainide in other cases (183,184). Clinical improvement followed combined hemodialysis and charcoal hemoperfusion in one case. A 34-year-old woman ingested 3000 mg of flecainide that resulted in seizures, AV and intraventricular block, and asystole. The maximum flecainide plasma concentration was 4.9 μg/ml. The plasma half-life during hemodialysis/hemoperfusion was 4.5 to 8.5 hours and her conduction delays improved (185).

Antidotes. Sodium ions compete with the binding of flecainide to receptors in the cardiac sodium channel, reversing the action of flecainide on phase 0 of the action potential. Alkalization of the serum may also decrease the active-ionized fraction of flecainide required for sodium channel blockade (186). Hypertonic sodium bicarbonate (100 mEq over 5 minutes) was well tolerated by patients taking therapeutic doses of flecainide or encainide. These patients had baseline prolonged QRS (mean, 119 milliseconds) and PR (mean, 213 milliseconds) intervals, and sodium bicarbonate infusion had no significant effect on the duration of the QRS, PR, or QT interval (187). Hypotension and QRS prolongation (220 milliseconds) responded to two boluses of 100 mEq sodium bicarbonate (8.4%) followed by continuous infusion to maintain a serum pH of 7.5 to 7.55 (160).

A 16-year-old patient with wide complex tachycardia and hypotension within 1 hour of ingestion cardioverted to a normal sinus rhythm after 100 mEq sodium bicarbonate and 50 mg of lidocaine IV. Two subsequent episodes of QRS widening responded rapidly to infusions of 150 mEq and 50 mEq of sodium bicarbonate (177).

Supportive Care. All patients with potential toxicity should have supplemental oxygen, IV access, and continuous cardiac ICU monitoring. Discontinue flecainide therapy and avoid other type I agents if possible. Hypotension should initially be treated with isotonic crystalloid fluid resuscitation followed by inotropic support if needed (Chapter 37). Pacemaker insertion should be considered early with signs of increasing bradycardia, AV block, or ventricular dysrhythmias.

Seizures are treated with benzodiazepines, followed by phenytoin and more invasive procedures in patients with refractory seizures (Chapter 40).

Cardiopulmonary Bypass Support. Hemodynamic support has been provided by cardiopulmonary bypass support (CBS) to allow the liver to metabolize flecainide to nontoxic concentrations. A 20-year-old woman developed hypotension and bradycardia after ingesting flecainide. She remained unstable after hypertonic saline infusion and cardiac pacing, and 2 hours after arrival was placed on CBS at a rate of 4 L/minute. The patient became anuric but improved hemodynamically over the next 2 hours. CBS was discontinued after 10 hours due to hemorrhage. During CBS, the flecainide half-life was approximately 6 hours (Fig. 6). The patient died 87 hours after exposure of kidney failure (188).

A 20-year-old woman ingested 4 g of flecainide and developed cardiogenic shock unresponsive to an inotrope, bicarbon-

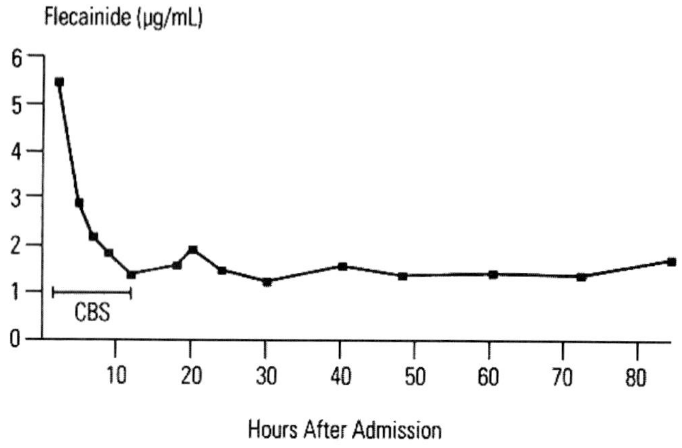

Figure 6. Plasma flecainide concentration during cardiopulmonary bypass support (CBS). (From Yasui RK, Culclasure TF, Kaufman D, et al. Flecainide overdose: is cardiopulmonary support the treatment? *Ann Emerg Med* 1997;29:680–682, with permission.)

ate infusion, and cardiac pacing. She was placed on CBS for 30 hours during which her cardiac failure recovered. She made a full recovery despite developing coma and unresponsive, dilated pupils (189).

Extracorporeal Membrane Oxygenation. ECMO can also provide hemodynamic support to allow the metabolism and clearance of flecainide. A 30-year-old man with EMD and cardiovascular collapse after a flecainide overdose was supported successfully with ECMO for 26 hours and made a full recovery (169).

Treatment of Cardiac Dysrhythmias. Cardioversion has not been evaluated in many patients with flecainide toxicity. It failed to convert VT in one case (164). Prophylactic insertion of a transvenous pacing wire should be considered in symptomatic patients (164,190). Transcutaneous pacing is an option until the patient is more stable. Ventricular capture has not always been successful (169).

Lidocaine infusion (100-mg bolus) was followed by conversion of VT to sinus rhythm after DC cardioversion failed in one case report (164). An idioventricular rhythm with marked QRS widening and QT prolongation was observed in another case. Torsade de pointes subsequently developed, which was treated with high doses of lidocaine (4 g daily) and repeat defibrillation. The patient recovered and was discharged 37 days after admission with no permanent sequelae (170).

The proarrhythmic effects of flecainide may be suppressed by high-dose amiodarone (191). A 45-year-old woman ingested 2000 mg, developed VF, and was converted to a spontaneous rhythm after IV amiodarone. A continuous amiodarone infusion was maintained for 72 hours and the patient recovered (192). Caution is advised as the administration of amiodarone has increased serum flecainide concentrations (193).

Monitoring. Hospital admission should be considered for selected patients with a history of ventricular dysrhythmias in whom flecainide therapy is to be discontinued. Acute overdose patients who appear initially asymptomatic should be monitored for a minimum of 4 to 6 hours. All patients with evidence of hypotension, dysrhythmias, or conduction delay should have continuous monitoring of blood pressure and cardiac rhythm in an intensive care setting. Frequent ECGs should be obtained to assess the QT and QRS intervals and the effectiveness of therapy.

Propafenone

Propafenone (Rythmol, Rytmonorm) is available in Europe and the United States. It has been marketed in the United States for oral treatment of life-threatening ventricular dysrhythmias. It may have a role in treating supraventricular tachydysrhythmias (194). The structure of propafenone is similar to many beta-blockers. Propafenone appears as a racemic of D and L isomers (195). It is supplied as 150, 225, and 300 mg tablets.

TOXIC DOSE

The *adult therapeutic dose* of propafenone is 150 to 300 mg orally every 8 hours. Due to nonlinear kinetics, a threefold increase in dosage may lead to a tenfold elevation in plasma concentration (196). Propafenone has a narrow therapeutic range. Ingestion of twice the therapeutic dose in an adult or a single tablet in a child should be considered life threatening.

A 57-year-old patient ingested 1350 mg of propafenone and survived (197). Intentional ingestion of 2.4 g and 2.7 g of propafenone resulted in third-degree heart block and generalized tonic-clonic seizures in two young adults (198,199). A 53-year-old female developed coma, seizures, hypotension, metabolic acidosis, and ECG changes after ingesting 3.6 g (200). A 28-year-old male experienced generalized seizures, coma, mild hypotension, a QRS interval of 289 milliseconds, and survived after ingesting 8.1 g (201). Doses of 4800 mg (202) and 9000 mg (203) were fatal. A 2-year-old child ingested 1800 mg (133 mg/kg), developed seizures, hypotension, right bundle branch block, EMD, and recovered (204).

TOXICOKINETICS AND TOXICODYNAMICS

Propafenone is well absorbed (95%) with a bioavailability of 12%. Its V_d is 1.1 to 3.6 L/kg, and it is 95% protein bound. It exhibits extensive first-pass hepatic metabolism to two active metabolites: 5-hydroxy propafenone (5-HP) and *N*-depropylpropafenone. Both metabolites have activity comparable to that of propafenone. Formation of the 5-HP metabolite is a saturable process mediated by the CYP2D6 isozyme. Small increases in dose can lead to large increases in plasma concentration. Propafenone half-life ranges from 2 to 32 hours due to polymorphic metabolism. Extensive metabolizers have half-lives of 2 to 10 hours (mean, 5 hours), poor metabolizers, 10 to 32 hours (mean, 17 hours). In the 10% of patients who are poor metabolizers, 5-HP is absent or largely diminished (205,206). Renal clearance of propafenone is 12 ml/minute/kg. The terminal half-life of 5-HP is 8 to 16 hours. Less than 1% of the dose is eliminated unchanged in the urine.

The C_{max} after a single dose of 300 mg is approximately 400 ng/ml for the parent compound and 180 ng/ml for 5-HP (207). After 150 mg three times a day, the steady-state plasma propafenone level is approximately 400 ng/ml, the 5-HP level is approximately 240 ng/ml, and *N*-depropylpropafenone level is approximately 90 ng/ml (208). The T_{max} of the drug and its metabolite is 1 to 4 hours. After 1 month of treatment, blood levels of the drug and its 5-HP metabolite rise. There is poor correlation between plasma propafenone concentration and suppression of dysrhythmias (208).

PATHOPHYSIOLOGY

Propafenone is a sodium channel blocker that may also block potassium channels similar to flecainide. The S-(+) enantiomer has weak β-adrenergic blocking properties. It prolongs the PR and QRS intervals. It suppresses nonsustained ventricular dysrhythmias. Propafenone slows intraatrial and AV nodal conduction by prolonging atrial refractoriness (209). It also prolongs, to a lesser extent, the ventricular effective refractory period. Dysrhythmia suppression occurs at the same dose level in extensive and poor metabolizers (205,206). Increases (15% to 25%) in PR, QRS, QT_c, AH, and HV intervals follow its use (208).

Propafenone possesses approximately 5% of the beta-blocking activity of propranolol. The degree of beta blockade is increased in the 7% to 10% of the population with a genetic deficiency in the ability to metabolize the parent drug to its metabolite, 5-HP (210).

PREGNANCY AND LACTATION

Propafenone is FDA pregnancy category C (Appendix I). There are few data available to assess its safety. It was embryotoxic in doses of 10 and 40 times the maximum recommended dose (211). Propafenone and 5-HP are detectable in newborn plasma and in maternal milk at concentrations lower than those in maternal plasma (212).

CLINICAL PRESENTATION

Acute Overdosage. The onset of toxicity may occur within 30 minutes, but cardiac toxicity may be delayed up to 120 minutes. Nausea, vomiting, hypotension, CNS depression, bradycardia, recurrent generalized seizures, acidosis, heart block, ventricular dysrhythmias, and cardiac arrest may occur (197,201–204,213,214). Koppel evaluated 34 propafenone overdose patients (213). The mean age was 14 years with doses ranging from 300 to 3000 mg. One-half of the patients had no symptoms. The following symptoms were found: nausea and vomiting (50%), bradycardia (75%), and hypotension (18%). Fatalities occurred in 8% of cases. Vomiting early in the course seemed to increase the chance of survival.

A 53-year-old female was unresponsive with seizure activity after ingesting 3600 mg of propafenone. Her blood pressure was 60/30 mm Hg and heart rate 45 beats/minute. The ECG demonstrated right bundle branch block (RBBB) and left posterior hemiblock. She responded to normal saline, 100 mEq sodium bicarbonate, dopamine, and epinephrine infusions. She was extubated 16 hours after admission and recovered (200).

A 28-year-old man ingested 8.1 g and was unconscious with a blood pressure of 90 mm Hg approximately 1 hour post-ingestion. He developed EMD, widened QRS interval (up to 400 milliseconds), bradycardia, and recurrent seizure activity. The seizures responded to diazepam and his blood pressure was supported with an epinephrine infusion. A transcutaneous pacemaker failed to capture, but a transvenous pacemaker was successful after epinephrine therapy. Sodium bicarbonate infusion (6 doses of 1 to 2 mEq/kg) did not narrow the QRS complex. Serum propafenone concentration 10 hours post-ingestion was 3200 ng/ml. The patient became alert 16 hours after ingestion (201).

A 2-year-old boy ingested 1800 mg (133 mg/kg) and experienced a generalized seizure 50 minutes post-ingestion. The QRS interval was 200 milliseconds with a RBBB pattern and hypotension. After a second seizure, he was treated with phenytoin (135 mg over several minutes), which was followed in 30 minutes by progressive widening of the QRS and QT intervals, bradycardia, and EMD. This was treated with atropine, sodium bicarbonate, and dopamine resulting in return of the ECG to normal over several hours (204).

Adverse Events. Approximately 20% of patients experience some mild side GI effects: constipation; nausea; vomiting; and, rarely, diarrhea. A bitter taste is noted by 5% to 10% of patients (196). At a plasma propafenone concentration of 900 ng/ml or higher, visual blurring, dizziness, and paresthesias may occur (205). At a level of 450 ng/ml, such effects are minimal. Poor metabolizers have increased side effects (Siddoway). Propafenone may induce generalized myasthenic symptoms in patients with ocular myasthenia (215).

Because of its beta-blocker activity, propafenone may induce severe reactive airway disease (216). Rare cases of cholestatic hepatitis have been reported. Propafenone can cause cardiac conduction abnormalities such as first-degree heart block, new left or RBBB, AV block, sinus node dysfunction, and prolonged QT interval. It may exacerbate the adverse effects of beta-adrenergic blockers and exacerbate CHF (1% to 4%). These effects are dose dependent and occur most often in patients with advanced underlying heart disease. Clinically significant prodysrhythmias may occur in 5% of patients and consist of increase in ventricular premature contractions, conversion of nonsustained to sustained VT, or new appearances of VT or VF (217). It may increase the ventricular rate in patients with atrial flutter.

Drug Interactions. Propafenone is a CYP1A2, 2D6, 3A/4 enzyme substrate and a CYP2D6 inhibitor. Drugs that may increase propafenone concentration include cimetidine, propranolol, quinidine, and ritonavir. Propafenone may increase concentrations of digoxin, cyclosporine, theophylline, and warfarin. Concurrent use of local anesthetics with propafenone may increase the risk of CNS effects. Propafenone increases metoprolol blood levels and activity (218).

DIAGNOSTIC TESTS

Acute Overdosage. Blood concentrations while taking 300 mg every 8 hours is 1000 ng/ml. CNS adverse effects are more common above 900 ng/ml. Concentrations greater than 1000 ng/ml are associated with β-adrenergic effects. Serum propafenone concentrations of 500 to 2000 ng/ml are considered to be within the therapeutic range.

Acute ingestion of 1800 to 9000 mg has been associated with plasma concentration of 1100 to 4700 ng/ml (219). Ingestion of 8.1 g of propafenone resulted in a propafenone concentration 10 hours post-ingestion of 3200 ng/ml (201). Patients who overdosed and survived had propafenone blood levels of 1888 ng/ml (220), 3000 ng/ml (214), 3185 ng/ml (221), 3449 ng/ml (197), 3737 ng/ml (222), and 4702 ng/ml (203). Reported concentrations associated with death are 7700 ng/ml (202) and 21,000 ng/ml (223).

The ECG prolongation of the PR, QT, and QRS intervals, bradycardia, AV block, and bundle branch blocks may occur (Fig. 7). ECG changes consisting of an RBBB, a posterior hemiblock, QRS duration of 190 milliseconds, and QT interval of 560 milliseconds occurred after ingestion of 3600 mg of propafenone by a 53-year-old woman. The conduction delay (QRS interval) appeared to correlate with plasma propafenone and metabolite concentrations (200).

Postmortem Considerations. Propafenone may demonstrate postmortem redistribution. Heart femoral blood concentration ratio of 2.4 has been reported (219).

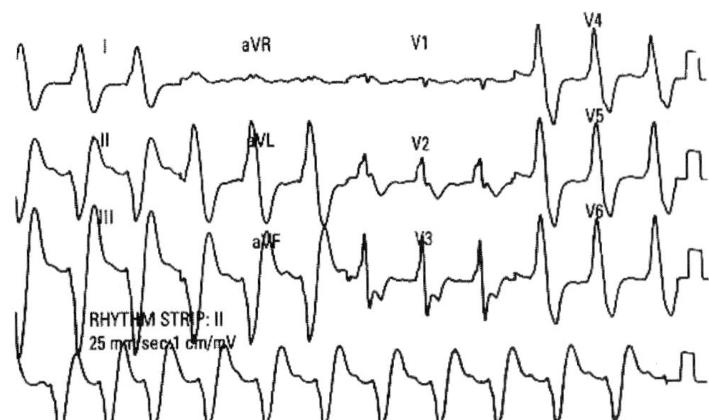

Figure 7. Propafenone toxicity electrocardiogram. (Adapted from Kerns W, English B, Ford M. Propafenone overdose. *Ann Emerg Med* 1994;24:98–103.)

TREATMENT

Gastrointestinal Decontamination. Induced emesis is contraindicated. Given the serious potential toxicity, decontamination is an appropriate intervention. Gastric lavage within 1 to 2 hours after a large ingestion and activated charcoal may be useful but have not been systematically studied.

Enhancement of Elimination. Due to its large volume of distribution and high protein binding, methods to enhance elimination are unlikely to be effective. Hemodialysis (224) and hemoperfusion (203,223) have not been useful in removing propafenone. Plasma exchange appeared useful in one case (197).

Antidotes. There is no specific antidote. Sodium loading has been proposed for wide QRS interval, but experience with hypertonic sodium bicarbonate is extremely limited. Molar sodium lactate has been used in an overdose and the patient survived (225). IV administration of molar sodium lactate (500 ml over 30 minutes) with IV potassium chloride to two propafenone overdose patients resulted in an improvement in clinical status with narrowing of the QRS (226). In other cases, sodium loading with sodium bicarbonate (214) or hypertonic saline (203) was followed by survival.

Supportive Care. All patients with potential toxicity should have supplemental oxygen, IV access, and continuous cardiac monitoring. Discontinue propafenone therapy and avoid other type I antiarrhythmic agents if possible. Hypotension should initially be treated with isotonic crystalloid fluid resuscitation followed by inotropic support if needed (Chapter 37). Pacemaker insertion should be considered early with signs of increasing bradycardia, AV block, or ventricular dysrhythmias. Cardiopulmonary bypass may be required in certain cases.

Cardiac pacing may be necessary for heart block. Intentional ingestion of 2.4 g propafenone resulted in third-degree heart block and one episode of generalized tonic-clonic seizures in an 18-year-old male. Recovery was uneventful after supportive pharmacologic management and temporary transvenous pacing (198). Bradycardia and hypotension responded to internal pacing (15 mA) and epinephrine infusion in one case (201). Isoproterenol (isoprenaline) has been reported as useful (225).

Seizures. Seizures are treated with benzodiazepines, followed by phenytoin and more invasive procedures in patients with refractory seizures (Chapter 40). Phenytoin, used in one overdose patient (204), was followed by worsening conduction defects, bradycardia, and EMD. Phenytoin has type IB antidysrhythmic properties and must be used with great caution in the presence of preexisting conduction defects.

Monitoring. Patients with evidence of hypotension, dysrhythmias, or significant conduction delay should have continuous monitoring of blood pressure and cardiac rhythm in an intensive care setting. Frequent ECGs should be obtained to assess the QT and QRS intervals and the effectiveness of therapy.

Moricizine

Moricizine hydrochloride (Ethmozine) was first released in the Soviet Union in 1971 (227) and approved by the U.S. FDA in 1990. It is also available in the United Kingdom and Ireland. Moricizine has potent local anesthetic and membrane-stabilizing properties (228). It does not fit any of the usual subclasses of the type I antidysrhythmic drugs. Moricizine suppresses abnormal automaticity, AV node and His-Purkinje conduction, and prolongs the PR and QRS intervals. Thus, it has some properties of types IA, IB, and IC. Moricizine is classified as IC by Vaughan Williams (229). It is indicated for the treatment of life-threatening ventricular dysrhythmias, such as sustained VT. It was associated with increased mortality in the Cardiac Dysrhythmia Suppression Trial. Moricizine hydrochloride is available as tablets of 200, 250, and 300 mg.

TOXIC DOSE

The *adult therapeutic dose* is 600 to 900 mg/day given in three divided doses. Patients with significant renal or hepatic dysfunction are started at doses of 600 mg or below. There is no approved dosing for children. Moricizine has a narrow therapeutic range. Ingestion of twice the therapeutic dose in an adult or a single tablet in a child should be considered potentially life threatening. Deaths have occurred after accidental or intentional overdoses of 2250 mg and 10,000 mg (230).

TOXICOKINETICS AND TOXICODYNAMICS

Moricizine is well absorbed from the GI tract. The C_{max} and T_{max} after a 300-mg dose is 0.5 μg/ml (0.2 to 1.2 μg/ml) and 1 to 2.5 hours, respectively (230). There is high first-pass metabolism, and bioavailability is only 34% to 38%. The V_d is 8 to 11 L/kg. It is highly protein bound (95%) to a_1-acid glycoprotein, albumin, and peripheral tissues.

Moricizine is extensively metabolized before elimination, mainly by sulfur oxidation, hydroxylation, *N*-dealkylation, and glucuronide or sulfate conjugation (231). Two metabolites are pharmacologically active: moricizine sulfoxide and phenothiazine-2-carbamic acid ethyl ester sulfoxide. These two metabolites represent less than 1% of the administered dose and have plasma half-lives of 3 hours. The elimination half-life of moricizine after a single oral dose is 3 to 5 hours. This increases to 6 to 13 hours with cardiac disease and 47 hours with renal failure. Approximately 56% of the drug and its metabolites are excreted in the feces and 39% in the urine, with only 0.14% excreted unchanged in the urine. Some moricizine is also recycled through the enterohepatic circulation.

PATHOPHYSIOLOGY

Moricizine has potent local anesthetic activity and myocardial membrane stabilizing effects. In controlled clinical trials, moricizine has had antidysrhythmic effects similar to those of DP, quinidine, and propranolol. Moricizine prolongs the PR interval by 20% and the QRS duration by 19%, but has little effect on the QT interval (231). The dysrhythmias sometimes associated with quinidine QT prolongation (long QT syndrome, torsade de pointes) are relatively rare with moricizine (232). Moricizine produces a dose-dependent prolongation of conduction in the atrium, AV node, His-Purkinje system, and ventricular myocardium. Its major electrophysiologic effects are a decreased maximum rate of phase 0 depolarization, increased rates of phase 2 and 3 repolarization, and decreased effective refractory period. It is structurally similar to phenothiazines but does not appear to block dopamine receptors.

PREGNANCY AND LACTATION

Moricizine is FDA pregnancy category B (Appendix I). It is not teratogenic or fetotoxic in rats and rabbits. It is excreted in human milk and has potentially adverse effects on the nursing infant (233).

CLINICAL PRESENTATION

Acute Overdosage. Deaths have occurred after accidental and intentional overdoses of 2250 and 10,000 mg. Experience is limited, but overdose may produce vomiting, lethargy, coma, syncope, hypotension, conduction disturbances, exacerbation of CHF, myocardial infarction, sinus arrest, dysrhythmias, and respiratory failure. Potential dysrhythmias include junctional bradycardia, VT, VF, and asystole.

Adverse Events. The most frequent noncardiac adverse effects are nausea and dizziness (234). Nausea, headache, palpitations, and dyspnea have been observed in 5% to 10% of patients. Drug fever, thrombocytopenia, skin rashes, and elevated liver function tests, all reversible, have been infrequently observed.

Moricizine exhibits prodysrhythmic effects in approximately 3% of patients that occurred within 10 days of initiating therapy (235). Pairs and runs of ventricular premature contractions seen in a patient on moricizine therapy are a strong indication for alternative therapy (227). It exacerbated CHF with therapeutic doses in 13% of patients with a history of CHF (236).

Drug Interactions. Moricizine may inhibit CYP1A2. Cimetidine reduces moricizine clearance to approximately one-half and increases its plasma concentration to 1.4 times its normal value. Diltiazem may also increase moricizine concentrations. Plasma theophylline half-life is decreased 19% to 33%, and its clearance is increased 44% to 66% when given with moricizine.

DIAGNOSTIC TESTS

Acute Overdosage. Antidysrhythmic and electrophysiologic effects of moricizine are not correlated with plasma concentration. Administration of 500 mg to fasting men resulted in peak plasma concentrations of 0.48 to 1.54 mg/L (237).

The ECG may show dose related increases in PR, and QRS intervals are observed with therapeutic doses. VT, VF, junctional bradycardia, and sinus arrest may occur.

Adverse Events. A few patients exhibit an increase in bilirubin or transaminase levels. Less than 1% has had evidence of renal failure.

TREATMENT

Ingestion of 100 mg or more should be observed for at least 6 hours for signs of toxicity.

Gastrointestinal Decontamination. Induced emesis is contraindicated. Given the serious potential toxicity, decontamination is an appropriate intervention. Gastric lavage within 1 to 2 hours after a large ingestion and activated charcoal may be useful but have not been systematically studied.

Enhancement of Elimination. Due to its large volume of distribution and high protein binding, methods to enhance elimination are unlikely to be effective. Activated charcoal may be able to absorb some of the enterohepatic-recycled drug and metabolites, but controlled studies have not yet been performed.

Antidotes. There is no specific antidote. Because QRS prolongation and ventricular dysrhythmias secondary to other sodium channel blockers have responded to IV sodium bicarbonate, the dysrhythmias and hypotension from moricizine may also respond, but confirmatory clinical studies have not been performed (Chapter 75).

Supportive Care. All patients with potential toxicity should have supplemental oxygen, IV access, and continuous cardiac monitoring. Discontinue moricizine therapy and avoid other type I antiarrhythmic agents if possible. Hypotension should initially be treated with isotonic crystalloid fluid resuscitation followed by inotropic support if needed (Chapter 37). Pacemaker insertion should be considered early with signs of increasing bradycardia, AV block, or ventricular dysrhythmias. Cardiopulmonary bypass may be required in certain cases.

Monitoring. Patients with evidence of hypotension, dysrhythmias, or significant conduction delay should have continuous monitoring of blood pressure and cardiac rhythm in an intensive care setting. Frequent ECGs should be obtained to assess the QT and QRS intervals and the effectiveness of therapy.

REFERENCES

1. Tujillo TC, Nolan PE. Antiarrhythmic agents: drug interactions of clinical significance. *Drug Saf* 2000;23:509–532.
2. Campbell TJ. Proarrhythmic actions of antiarrhythmic drugs: a review. *Aust N Z J Med* 1990;20:275–282.
3. Maurer HH. Identification of antiarrhythmic drugs and their metabolites in urine. *Arch Toxicol* 1990;64:218–230.
4. Pentel PR, Fifield J, Salerno DM. Lack of effect of hypertonic sodium bicarbonate on QRS duration in patients taking therapeutic doses of class IC antiarrhythmic drugs. *J Clin Pharmacol* 1990;301:789–794.
5. Jaeger A, Sauder PH, Kopferschmitt J, et al. Acute disopyramide poisoning: a multicenter study of 106 cases. *Vet Hum Toxicol* 1982;24:285(abst).
6. Powell F, Carey O, Smith P. Fatal disopyramide overdose. *J Irish Med Asso* 1978;71:552.
7. Accomero F, Pellanda A, Ruffini C, et al. Prolonged cardiac resuscitation during acute disopyramide poisoning. *Vet Hum Toxicol* 1993;35:231–237.
8. Baselt RC. *Disposition of toxic drugs and chemical in man*, 5th ed. Foster City, CA: Chemical Toxicology Institute, 2000.
9. Briggs GR, Freeman RK, Sumner JY. *Drugs in pregnancy and lactation*, 5th ed. Baltimore: Williams & Williams, 1998.
10. Ellsworth AJ, Horn JR, Raisys VA, et al. Disopyramide and *N*-monodesalkyl disopyramide in serum and breast milk. *DICP Ann Pharmacother* 1989;23:56–57.
11. Gosselin B, Matthieu D, Chopin C, et al. Acute intoxication with disopyramide: clinical and experimental study by hemoperfusion on amberlite XAD 4 resin. *Clin Toxicol* 1980;17:439–449.
12. Schattner A, Gindin J, Geltner D. Fatal torsade de pointes following jaundice in a patient treated with disopyramide. *Postgrad Med J* 1989;65:333–334.
13. Conrad ME. Agranulocytosis associated with disopyramide therapy. *JAMA* 1978;240:1857–1858.
14. Granowitz EV, Tabor KJ, Kirchhoffer JB. Potentially fatal interaction between azithromycin and disopyramide. *Pacing Clin Electrophysiol* 2000;23:1433–1435.
15. Ragosta M, Weihl AC, Rosenfeld LE. Potentially fatal interaction between erythromycin and disopyramide. *Am J Med* 1989;86:465–466.
16. Staum JM. Enzyme induction: rifampin–disopyramide interaction. *DICP Ann Pharmacother* 1990;24:701–703.
17. Orloff KG, Thompson BC, Caplan YH. Fatal dose with disopyramide. *Bull Int Assoc Forens Toxicol* 1980;15:4–5.
18. Sathyavagiswaran L. Fatal disopyramide intoxication from suicidal/accidental overdose. *J Forensic Sci* 1987;32:1813–1818.
19. Singer P, Mozayani A. An overdose fatality in a child involving disopyramide and sulindac. *J Anal Toxicol* 1995;19:529–530.
20. Anderson WH, Stafford DT, Bell JS. Disopyramide (Norpace) distribution at autopsy of an overdose case. *J For Sci* 1980;25:33–39.
21. Neuvonen PJ, Olkkola KT. Effect of dose of charcoal on the absorption of disopyramide, indomethacin and trimethoprim by man. *Eur J Clin Pharmacol* 1984;26:761–767.
22. Arimori K, Kawano H, Nakano M. Gastrointestinal dialysis of disopyramide in healthy subjects. *Int J Clin Pharmacol Ther Toxicol* 1989;27:280–284.
23. Karim A. Disopyramide dialyzability. *Lancet* 1978;2:214.
24. Yoshida K, Kimura K, Hibi, et al. A patient with disopyramide intoxication rescued by percutaneous cardiopulmonary support [in Japanese]. *J Cardiol* 1998;32:95–100.
25. Atkinson AJ, Krumlovsky FA, Huang CM, et al. Hemodialysis for severe procainamide toxicity: clinical and pharmacokinetic observations. *Clin Pharmacol Ther* 1976;20:585–592.
26. Rosansky SJ, Brady ME. Procainamide toxicity in a patient with acute renal failure. *Am J Kidney Dis* 1986;7:502–506.
27. Briggs GR, Freeman RK, Sumner JY. *Drugs in pregnancy and lactation*, 5th ed. Baltimore: Williams & Wilkins, 1998.
28. Godley PJ, Morton TA, Karbhoski JA, et al. Procainamide-induced myasthenia crisis. *Ther Drug Monit* 1990;12:411–414.
29. White SR, Dy G, Wilson JM. The case of the slandered Halloween cupcake: survival after massive pediatric procainamide overdose. *Pediatr Emerg Med* 2002;18:185–188.

30. Schwartz AB, Klausner SC, Yee S, et al. Cerebellar ataxia due to procainamide toxicity. *Arch Intern Med* 1984;144:2260.
31. Giannone L, Kugler JW, Krantz SB. Pure red cell aplasia associated with administration of sustained-release procainamide. *Arch Intern Med* 1987;147:1179–1180.
32. Putnam JB, Bolling SF, Kirsch MM. Procainamide-induced respiratory insufficiency after cardiopulmonary bypass. *Ann Thorac Surg* 1991;51:482–483.
33. Bizjak ED, Nolan PE Jr, Brody EA, et al. Procainamide-induced psychosis: a case report and review of the literature. *Ann Pharmacother* 1999;33:948–951.
34. Saal AK, Werner JA, Greene HL, et al. Effect of amiodarone on serum quinidine and procainamide levels. *Am J Cardiol* 1984;53:1264–1267.
35. Miller B, Skupin A, Rubenfire M, et al. Respiratory failure produced by severe procainamide intoxication in a patient with preexisting peripheral neuropathy caused by amiodarone. *Chest* 1988;94:663–665.
36. Bauer LA, Black D, Gensler A. Procainamide–cimetidine during interaction in elderly male patients. *J Am Geriatr Soc* 1990;38:467–469.
37. Kosoglou T, Rocci ML Jr, Vlasses PH. Trimethoprim alters the disposition of procainamide and *N*-acetyl procainamide. *Clin Pharmacol Ther* 1988;44:467–477.
38. Koch-Weser J, Klein SW. Procainamide dosage schedules, plasma concentrations and clinical effects. *JAMA* 1971;215:1454–1460.
39. Chen ML, Loo MG, Chiou WL. Pharmacokinetics of drugs in blood: III. Metabolism of procainamide and storage effects of blood samples. *J Pharm Sci* 1985;72:572–574.
40. Nguyen KPV, Thomsen G, Liem B, et al. *N*-Acetylprocainamide, torsades de pointes, and hemodialysis. *Ann Intern Med* 1986;104:283–284.
41. Heiselman DE, Litman GI. Risk factors for procainamide-induced torsade de pointes. *Clin Res* 1986;34:7A.
42. Totoritis MC, Tan EM, McNally EM, et al. Association of antibody to histone complex H2A–H2B with symptomatic procainamide induced lupus. *N Engl J Med* 1988;318:1431–1436.
43. Baselt RC. *Disposition of toxic drugs and chemicals in man*, 5th ed. Foster City, CA: Chemical Toxicology Institute, 2000.
44. Low CL, Phelps KR, Bailie GR. Relative efficacy of haemoperfusion, haemodialysis and CAPD in the removal of procainamide and NAPA in a patient with severe procainamide toxicity. *Nephrol Dial Transplant* 1996;11(5):881–884.
45. Kar PM, Kellner K, Ing TS, et al. Combined high-efficiency hemodialysis and charcoal hemoperfusion in severe N-acetylprocainamide intoxication. *Am J Kidney Dis* 1992;20:403–406.
46. Kerr F, Kenoyer G, Bilitch M. Quinidine overdose: neurological and cardiovascular toxicity in normal person. *Br Heart J* 1971;33:629–631.
47. Shub C, Gau GT, Sidell PM, et al. The management of acute quinidine intoxication. *Chest* 1978;73:173–178.
48. Woic L, Oyri A. Quinidine intoxication treated with hemodialysis. *Acta Med Scand* 1974;195:237–239.
49. Baselt RC. *Disposition of toxic drugs and chemicals in man*, 5th ed. Foster City, CA: Chemical Toxicology Institute, 2000.
50. Conrad KA, Molk BL, Chidsey CA. Pharmacokinetic studies of quinidine in patients with arrhythmias. *Circulation* 1977;55:1–7.
51. Stanek EJ, Simko RJ, DeNofrio D, et al. Prolonged quinidine half-life with associated toxicity in a patient with hepatic failure. *Pharmacother* 1997;17:622–625.
52. Finnegan TRL, Traince JR. Depression of the heart by quinidine and its treatment. *Br Heart J* 1954;16:341–350.
53. Briggs GR, Freeman RK, Sumner JY. *Drugs in pregnancy and lactation*, 5th ed. Baltimore: Williams and Williams, 1998.
54. Killeen AA, Bowers LD. Fetal supraventricular tachycardia treated with high dose quinidine: toxicity associated with marked elevation of the metabolite, 3 (*S*) -3-hydroxyquinidine. *Obstet Gynecol* 1987;70:445–449.
55. Bailey DJ. Cardiotoxic effects of quinidine and their treatment. *Arch Intern Med* 1960;105:13–22.
56. Summers WK, Allen RE, Pitts FN. Does physostigmine reverse quinidine delirium? *West J Med* 1981;135:411–412.
57. Lavie CJ, Biundo J, Quinet RJ, et al. Systemic lupus erythematosus (SLE) induced by quinidine. *Arch Intern Med* 1985;145:446–448.
58. Shalit M, Flugelman MY, Harats N, et al. Quinidine induced vasculitis. *Arch Intern Med* 1985;145:2051–2052.
59. Phillips RE, Warrell DA, White NJ, et al. Intravenous quinidine for the treatment of severe falciparum malaria: clinical and pharmacokinetic studies. *N Engl J Med* 1985;312:1273–1278.
60. Hasan MN, Hassan MA, Rawashdeh NM. Effect of oral activated charcoal on the phamacokinetics of quinidine and quinine administered intravenously to rabbits. *Pharmacol Toxicol* 1990;67:73–76.
61. Gaudreault P. Quinidine. *Clin Toxicol Rev* 1982;4(12):1–2.
62. Haapanen EJ, Pellinen TJ. Hemoperfusion in quinidine intoxication. *Acta Med Scand* 1981;210(6):515–516.
63. Prasad K. Use of glucagon in the treatment of quinidine toxicity in the heart. *Cardiovasc Res* 1977;11(1):55–63.
64. De Azevedo RM, Watanabe Y, Dreifus LS. Electrophysiologic antagonism of quinidine and bretylium tosylate. *Am J Cardiol* 1974;33:633–638.
65. Tecklenburg FW, Thomas NJ, Webb SA, et al. Pediatric ECMO for severe quinidine cardiotoxicity. *Pediatr Emerg Care* 1997;13:111–113.
66. Baselt RC. *Disposition of toxic drugs and chemicals in man*, 5th ed. Foster City, CA: Chemical Toxicology Institute, 2000.
67. Jonville AP, Barbier P, Blond MH, et al. Accidental lidocaine overdosage in an infant. *Clin Toxicol* 1990;28:101–106.
68. Armstrong DK, Bremseth DL, Lima JJ. Clinical response and total and unbound plasma concentrations after lidocaine overdose. *Ther Drug Monit* 1988;10:499–500.
69. Briggs GR, Freeman RK, Sumner JY. *Drugs in pregnancy and lactation*, 5th ed. Baltimore: Williams and Williams, 1998.
70. Poklis A, Mackell MA, Tucker EF. Tissue distribution of lidocaine after fatal accidental injection. *J Forens Sci* 1984;29:1229–1236.
71. Finkelstein F, Kreeft J. Massive lidocaine poisoning. *N Engl J Med* 1979;301:50.
72. Garrettson LK, McGee EB. Rapid onset of seizures following aspiration of viscous lidocaine. *J Toxicol Clin Toxicol* 1992;30(3):413–422.
73. Howard JJ, Mohsenufar Z, Simons SM. Adult respiratory distress syndrome following administration of lidocaine. *Chest* 1982;81:644–645.
74. O'Donohue WJ, Moss LM, Angelillo VA. Acute methemoglobinemia induced by topical benzocaine and lidocaine. *Arch Intern Med* 1980;140:1508–1509.
75. Dawling S, Flanagan RJ, Widdop B. Fatal lignocaine poisoning: report of two cases and review of the literature. *Hum Toxicol* 1989;8:389–392.
76. Edgren B, Tilelli J, Gehrz R. Intravenous lidocaine overdosage in a child. *Clin Toxicol* 1986;24:51–58.
77. Amitai Y, Whitesell L, Lovejoy FH Jr. Death following accidental lidocaine overdose in a child. *N Engl J Med* 1986;314:182–183.
78. Stargel WW, Roe CR, Toutledge PA, et al. Importance of blood-collection tubes in plasma lidocaine determinations. *Clin Chem* 1979;25:617–619.
79. Peat MA, Deyman ME, Crouch DJ, et al. Concentrations of lidocaine and monoethylglycylxylidide (MEGX) in lidocaine associated deaths. *J Forens Sci* 1985;30:1048–1057.
80. Moriya F, Hashimoto Y. Absorption of intubation-related lidocaine from the trachea during prolonged cardiopulmonary resuscitation. *J Forensic Sci* 1998;43(3):718–722.
81. Freedman MD, Gal J, Freed CR. Extracorporeal pump assistance: novel treatment for acute lidocaine poisoning. *Eur J Clin Pharmacol* 1982;22:129–135.
82. Moore DC, Crawford RD, Scurlock JE. Severe hypoxia and acidosis following local anesthetic induced convulsions. *Anesthesiology* 1980;53:259–260.
83. Noble J, Kennedy D, Latimer R, et al. Massive lignocaine overdose during cardiopulmonary bypass. Successful treatment with cardiac pacing. *Br J Anaesth* 1984;56(12):1439–1441.
84. Nelson LS, Hoffman RS. Mexiletine overdose producing status epilepticus without cardiovascular abnormalities. *Clin Toxicol* 1994;32:731–736.
85. Baselt RC. *Disposition of toxic drugs and chemicals in man*, 5th ed. Foster City, CA: Chemical Toxicology Institute, 2000.
86. Briggs GR, Freeman RK, Yaffe SJ. *Drugs in pregnancy and lactation*, 6th ed. Baltimore: Williams and Williams, 2002.
87. Jequier P, Jones R, Mackintosh A. Fatal mexiletine overdose. *Lancet* 1976;1:429.
88. Chambers SC, Milsom SM, Ikram H. Mexiletine overdose. *NZ Med J* 1982;95:898–899.
89. Blackmore RC, Oselton MD. Fatal mexiletine poisoning. *Bull Int Assoc Forens Toxicol* 1982;16(3):7–8.
90. Hruby K, Missliwetz J. Poisoning with oral antiarrhythmic drugs. *Int J Clin Pharmacol Ther Toxicol* 1985;23:253–257.
91. Kerin NZ, Aragon A, Marinescu G, et al. Mexiletine: long term efficacy and side effects in patients with chronic drug-resistant potentially lethal ventricular arrhythmias. *Arch Intern Med* 1990;150:381–384.
92. Fasola GP, D'Osvaldo F, De Pangher V, et al. Thrombocytopenia and mexiletine. *Ann Intern Med* 1984;100:162.
93. Sasaki K, Yamamoto T, Kishi M, et al. Acute exanthematous pustular drug eruption induced by mexiletine. *Eur J Dermatol* 2001;11:469–471.
94. Monk JP, Brogden RN. Mexiletine: a review of its pharmacodynamic and pharmacokinetic properties and therapeutic use in the treatment of arrhythmias. *Drugs* 1990;40:374–411.
95. Bradbrook ID, James C, Rogers HJ. A rapid method for the determination of plasma mexiletine levels by gas chromatography. *Br J Clin Pharmacol* 1977;4(3):380–382.
96. Rohrig TP, Harty LE. Postmortem distribution of mexiletine in a fatal overdose. *J Anal Toxicol* 1994;18:354–356.
97. Clarke CWF, El-Mahdi EO. Fatal oral tocainide overdosage. *BMJ* 1984;288:760.
98. Wilson JH. Breast milk tocainide levels. *J Cardiovasc Pharmacol* 1988;12:497.
99. Kreeger RW, Hammill SC. New antiarrhythmic drugs: tocainide, mexiletine, flecainide, encainide, and amiodarone. *Mayo Clin Proc* 1987;62:1033–1050.
100. Feinberg L, Travis WD, Ferrans V, et al. Pulmonary fibrosis associated with tocainide: report of a case with literature review. *Am Rev Respir Dis* 1990;141:505–508.
101. Arrowsmith JB, Creamer JI, Bosco L. Severe dermatologic reactions reported after treatment with tocainide. *Ann Intern Med* 1987;107:693–696.
102. Schuster MR, Paris PM, Kaplan RM, et al. Effect on the seizure threshold in dogs of tocainide/lidocaine administration. *Ann Emerg Med* 1987;16:749–751.
103. Cohen A. Accidental overdose of tocainide successfully treated. *Angiology* 1987;38:614.
104. Harris SC, Guerra C, Wallace JE. Assay of free and total tocainide by high performance liquid chromatography (HPLC) with ultraviolet (UV) detection. *J Forens Sci* 1989;34:912–917.

105. Sperry K, Wohlenberg N, Standefer JC. Fatal intoxications by tocainide. *J Forens Sci* 1987;32:1440–1446.
106. Koppel C, Oberdisse U, Heinimeyer G. Clinical course and outcome in class 1c antiarrhythmic overdose. *Clin Toxicol* 1990;28:433–444.
107. Pentel PR, Fifield J, Salerno DM. Lack of effect of hypertonic sodium bicarbonate on QRS duration in patients taking therapeutic doses of class IC antiarrhythmic drugs. *J Clin Pharmacol* 1990;301:789–794.
108. Ruskin JN. The Cardiac Arrhythmia Suppression Trial (CAST). *N Engl J Med* 1989;321:386–388.
109. The Cardiac Arrhythmia Suppression Trial (CAST) investigators. Preliminary report: effect of encainide and flecainide on mortality in a randomized trial of arrhythmic suppression after myocardial infarction. *N Engl J Med* 1989;321:406–412.
110. Feld GK, Chen P-S, Nicod P, et al. Possible atrial proarrhythmic effects of class IC antiarrhythmic drugs. *Am J Cardiol* 1990;66:378–383.
111. Riboulet G, Efthymiou ML, Conso F, et al. Acute intoxication by ajmaline. *Vet Hum Toxicol* 1979;2[Suppl]:91–92.
112. Hager W, Friedreich KH, Wink K, et al. Suizidversuch mit ajmalin. *Dtsch Med Wochenschr* 1968;93:1809–1812.
113. Hruby K, Missliwetz J. Poisoning with oral antiarrhythmic drugs. *Int J Clin Pharm Ther Toxicol* 1985;23:253–257.
114. Mobis A, Minz DH. Suicidal Tachmalcor poisoning—a case report [in German]. *Anaesthesiol Reamin* 1999;24:109–110.
115. Koppel C, Oberdisse V, Heinemeyer G. Clinical course and outcome in class IC antiarrhythmic overdose. *Clin Toxicol* 1990;28:433–444.
116. Lengfelder W, Senges J, Rizos I. Intraindividual comparison of intravenous ajmaline and quinidine in patients with sustained ventricular tachycardia: effects on normal myocardium and on dysrhythmia characteristics. *Eur Heart J* 1985;6:312–322.
117. Ben Schachar C, Kishon Y. Intoxication with ajmaline in an infant. *Chest* 1979;76:97–98.
118. Ikeda N, Umetsu K, Suzuki T, et al. An infant fatality involving ajmaline. *J Forens Sci* 1988;33:558–561.
119. Koppel C, Wagemann A, Martens F. Pharmacokinetics and antiarrhythmic efficacy of intravenous ajmaline in ventricular arrhythmias of recent onset. *Eur J Drug Metab Pharmacokinet* 1989;14:161–167.
120. Koppel C, Tenczer J. Mass spectral characterization of urinary metabolites of ajmaline. *Pharamcol Toxicol* 1988;65:25.
121. Bouffard Y, Roux H, Perrot D, et al. Acute ajmaline poisoning. Study of 7 cases [in French]. *Arch Mal Coeur Vaiss* 1983;76:771–777.
122. Caramella JP, Guerot C, Valere PE, et al. Cardiac toxicity of ajmaline. Comparison of acute voluntary poisoning with complications of the ajmaline test [in French]. *Arch Mal Coeur Vaiss* 1982;75:613–620.
123. Rautenburg HW, Menner K, Knothe W. Herzstillstand nach ajmaline injection bei Herz Katheterisierung unter Halothane. *Narkose Med Welt* 1962;27:2329.
124. Kallfelz HC, Rotthauwe HW. Ajmalin-intoxikation in kindesalter. *Med Klin* 1964;59:336–342.
125. Larrey D, Pessayre D, Duhamel G, et al. Prolonged cholestasis after ajmaline-induced acute hepatitis. *J Hepatol* 1986;2:81–87.
126. Haverkamp W, Monnig G, Kirchhof P, et al. Torsade de pointes induced by ajmaline. *Z Kardiol* 2001;90:586–590.
127. Hori R, Okumura K, Inui K, et al. Quinidine-induced rise in ajmaline plasma concentration. *J Pharm Pharmacol* 1984;36:202–204.
128. Kleinsorge H. Klinische untersuchungen uber die wirkungsweise des rauwolfia-alkaloids ajmaline by herzhythmusstorungen insbesondere der extrasystole. *Med Klin* 1959;54:409.
129. Batalow Z, Apostolov L. Sur certaines actions toxiques de l'ajmaline avec contribution de deux cas. *Folia Med* 1968;10:403.
130. Clarke EGC, ed. *Isolation and identification of drugs*. London: Pharmaceutical Press, 1969:177.
131. Almog C, Maidan A, Pik A, et al. Acute intoxication with ajmaline. *Isr J Med Sci* 1979;15:570–572.
132. Koppel C, Oberdisse V, Heinemeyer G. Clinical course and outcome in class IC antiarrhythmic overdose. *Clin Toxicol* 1990;28:433–444.
133. Lederle RM, Harbig K, Wermuth G, et al. Hamoperfusion mit Kunsharz-Adsorben bei schwerer Intoxikation mit *N*-Propyl-Ajmalinium-Bitartrat. *Intensivmed* 1981;18:77–82.
134. Gelbke HP, Schlicht HJ. Suicide by an overdose of *N*-propylajmalinium bitartrate. *Arch Toxikol* 1977;37:135–141.
135. Trompler AT, Woodcock BG, Bussmann WD. Pharmakokinetik und antiarrhythmische Wirkung von Prajmaliumbitartrat. *Arzneimittelforschung* 1983;33(3):436–439.
136. Aronoff G, Brier M, Mayer ML, et al. Bioavailability and kinetics of cibenzoline in patients with normal and impaired renal function. *J Clin Pharmacol* 1991;31:38–44.
137. Kostis JB, Krieger S, Moreynra A, et al. Cibenzoline for treatment of ventricular arrhythmias: a double blind placebo controlled study. *J Am Coll Cardiol* 1984;4:372–377.
138. Brazzell RK, Aogaiche K, Heber JJ, et al. Cibenzoline plasma concentrations and antiarrhythmic effect. *Clin Pharmacol Ther* 1984;35:307–316.
139. Massarella JW, Khoo K-C, Aogaichi K, et al. Effect of renal impairment on the pharmacokinetics of cibenzoline. *Clin Pharmacol Ther* 1988;43:317–323.
140. Browne KF, Prystowsky EN, Zipes DP, et al. Clinical efficacy and electrophysiologic effects of cibenzoline therapy in patients with ventricular arrhythmias. *J Am Coll Cardiol* 1984;3:857–864.
141. Nolan PE Jr. The new antiarrhythmics: cibenzoline, moricizine, and pirmenol. *Hosp Ther* 1990;15:323–331.
142. Chouty F, Funck-Brentano CF, Leenhardt A, et al. Treatment of new class I anti-arrhythmic agent poisoning with intravenous sodium molar lactate or bicarbonate. *Eur Heart J* 1989;10[Suppl]:302(abstr 1521).
143. Wyss E, Karp P, Mons P, et al. Cardiogenic shock resistant to sodium lactate during cibenzoline overdosage. *Therapie* 1990;45:455.
144. Similowski T, Straus C, Attali V, et al. Neuromuscular blockade with acute respiratory failure in a patient receiving cibenzoline.
145. Jeandel C, Preiss MA, Pierson H, et al. Hypoglycemia induced by cibenzoline. *Lancet* 1988;1:1232–1233.
146. Takada M, Fujita S, Katayama Y, et al. The relationship between risk of hypoglycemia and use of cibenzoline and disopyramide. *Eur J Clin Pharmacol* 2000;56:335–342.
147. Aoyama N, Sasaki T, Yoshida M, et al. Effect of charcoal hemoperfusion on clearance of cibenzoline succinate (cifenline) poisoning. *J Toxicol Clin Toxicol* 1999;37:505–508.
148. Massarella JW, Defeo TM, Liguori J, et al. The effects of cimetidine and ranitidine on the pharmacokinetics of cifenline. *Br J Clin Pharmacol* 1991;31:481–483.
149. Echt DS, Liebson PR, Mitchell LB, et al. Mortality and morbidity in patients receiving encainide, flecainide or placebo. The cardiac arrhythmic suppression trial. *N Engl J Med* 1991;324:781–788.
150. Pentel PR, Goldsmith SR, Salerno DM, et al. Effect of hypertonic sodium bicarbonate on encainide overdose. *Am J Cardiol* 1986;57:878–879.
151. Mortensen ME, Bolon CE, Kelley MT, et al. Encainide overdose in an infant. *Ann Emerg Med* 1992;21:998–1001.
152. Woosley RL, Wood AJJ, Roder DM. Encainide. *N Engl J Med* 1988;318:1107–1115.
153. Briggs GR, Freeman RK, Yaffe SJ. *Drugs in pregnancy and lactation*, 6th ed. Baltimore: Williams and Williams, 2002.
154. Thomas GS. Death following withdrawal of encainide. *N Engl J Med* 1989;321:393.
155. Quart BD, Gallo DG, Sami MH, et al. Drug interaction studies and encainide use in renal and hepatic impairment. *Am J Cardiol* 1986;58(5):104C–113C.
156. Pentel PR, Fifield J, Salerno DM. Lack of effect of hypertonic sodium bicarbonate on QRS duration in patients taking therapeutic doses of class IC antiarrhythmic drugs. *J Clin Pharmacol* 1990;301:789–794.
157. Salerno DM, Fifield J, Krejci J, et al. Encainide-induced hyperglycemia. *Am J Med* 1988;84:39–44.
158. Nappi JM, Anderson JL. Flecainide: a new prototype antiarrhythmic agent. *Pharmacotherapy* 1985;5:209–218.
159. Winkelmann BR, Leinberger H. Life-threatening flecainide toxicity: a pharmacodynamic approach. *Ann Intern Med* 1987;106:807–814.
160. Lovecchio F, Berlin R, Brubacher JR, et al. Hypertonic sodium bicarbonate in an acute flecainide overdose. *Am J Emerg Med* 1998;16:534–537.
161. Siegers A, Board PN. Amiodarone used in successful resuscitation after near-fatal flecainide overdose. *Resuscitation* 2002;53:105–108.
162. Forrest ARW, Marsh I, Galloway JH, et al. A rapidly fatal dose with flecainide. *J Anal Toxicol* 1991;15:41–43.
163. Crijns HJGM, Kingma JH, Viersma JW, et al. Transient giant inverted T waves during flecainide ingestion. *Am Heart J* 1987;113:214–215.
164. Hanley NA, Bourke JP, Gascoigne AD. Survival in a case of life-threatening flecainide overdose. *Intensive Care Med* 1998;24:740–742.
165. Briggs GR, Freeman RK, Yaffe SJ. *Drugs in pregnancy and lactation*, 6th ed. Baltimore: Williams and Williams, 2002.
166. Wagner X, Jouglard J, Moulin M, et al. Coadministration of flecainide acetate and sotolol during pregnancy: lack of teratogenic effects, passage across the placenta and excretion in human breast milk. *Am Heart J* 1990;119:700–702.
167. McQuinn RL, Pisani A, Wafa S, et al. Flecainide excretion in human breast milk. *Clin Pharmacol Ther* 1990;48:262–267.
168. Koppel C, Oberdisse V, Heinemeyer G. Clinical course and outcome in class IC antiarrhythmic overdose. *Clin Toxicol* 1990;28:433–444.
169. Auzinger GM, Scheinkestel CD. Successful extracorporeal life support in a case of severe flecainide intoxication. *Crit Care Med* 2001;29:887–890.
170. Palitzsch KD, Bode H, Huck K, et al. Successful multiple resuscitation in flecainide poisoning [in German]. *Dtsch Med Wochenschr* 1992;117:56–60.
171. Kennerdy A, Thomas P, Sheridan DJ. Generalized seizures as the presentation of flecainide toxicity. *Eur Heart J* 1989;10:950–954.
172. Woodburn JD Jr. Cardiac arrest from a daily newspaper article. *Ann Emerg Med* 1989;18:1375–1376.
173. Sellers TD, Di Marco JP. Sinusoidal ventricular tachycardia association with flecainide acetate. *Chest* 1984;85:647–649.
174. Rosen DM, Woosely RL. Drug therapy: flecainide. *N Engl J Med* 1986;315:36–41.
175. Holmes B, Heel RC. Flecainide: a preliminary review of its pharmacodynamic properties and therapeutic efficacy. *Drugs* 1985;29:1–33.
176. Ramhamadany E, et al. Dysarthria and visual hallucinations due to flecainide toxicity. *Postgrad Med J* 1986;62:61–62.
177. Goldman MJ, Mowry JB, Kirk MA. Sodium bicarbonate to correct widened QRS in a case of flecainide overdose. *J Emerg Med* 1997;15:183–186.
178. Xing-Sheng Y, Jing-Ping S, Guang Z. Acute flecainide toxicity. *Chin Med J* 1990;103:606–607.
179. Levine B, Chute D, Caplan YH. Flecainide intoxication. *J Anal Toxicol* 1990;14:335–336.

180. Romain N, Giroud C, Michaud K, et al. Fatal flecainide intoxication. *Forensic Sci Int* 1999;106:115–123.
181. Rogers C, Anderson DT, Ribe JK, et al. Fatal flecainide intoxication. *J Anal Toxicol* 1993;17:434–435.
182. Nitsch J, Kohler U, Luderlitz B. Inhibition of flecainide resorption by activated charcoal [in German]. *Z Kardiol* 1987;76:289–291.
183. Wurzberger R, Witter E, Avenhaus H, et al. Hamoperfusion bei flecainidintoxikation. *Klin Wochenschr* 1986;64:442–444.
184. Braun J, Kollert JR, Gessler V, et al. Failure of haemoperfusion to reduce flecainide intoxication: a case study. *Med Toxicol* 1987;2:463–467.
185. Dirks E, Gieshoff B, Stahlmann R, et al. [Successful treatment of flecainide (Tambocor) poisoning-effect of hemodialysis/hemoperfusion?]. *Z Kardiol* 1990;79:54–59.
186. Ranger S, Sheldon R, Fermini B, et al. Modulation of flecainide's cardiac sodium channel blockade actions by extracellular sodium: a possible cellular mechanism for the action of sodium salts in flecainide toxicity. *J Pharmacol Exp Ther* 1993;264:1160–1167.
187. Pentel PR, Fifield J, Salerno DM. Lack of effect of hypertonic sodium bicarbonate on QRS duration in patients taking therapeutic doses of class IC antiarrhythmic drugs. *J Clin Pharmacol* 1990;301:789–794.
188. Yasui RK, Culclasure TF, Kaufman D, et al. Flecainide overdose: is cardiopulmonary support the treatment? *Ann Emerg Med* 1997;29:680–682.
189. Corkeron MA, van Heeren PV, Newman SM, et al. Extracorporeal circulatory support in near-fatal flecainide overdose. *Anaesth Intensive Care* 1999;27:405–408.
190. Gotz D, Pohle S, Barchow D. Primary and secondary detoxification in severe flecainide intoxication. *Intensive Care Med* 1991;17:181–187.
191. Sagie A, Strasberg B, Kusniec J, et al. Rapid suppression of flecainide induced incessant ventricular tachycardia with high dose intravenous amiodarone. *Chest* 1988;93:879–880.
192. Siegers A, Board PN. Amiodarone used in successful resuscitation after near-fatal flecainide overdose. *Resuscitation* 2002;53:105–108.
193. Leclercq JF, Denjoy L, Mentere F, et al. Flecainide acetate dose concentration relationship in cardiac arrhythmias: influence of heart failure and amiodarone. *Cardiovasc Drug Ther* 1990;4:1161–1165.
194. Pritchett ELC, McCarthy EA, Wilkinson WE. Propafenone treatment of symptomatic paroxysmal supraventricular dysrhythmias: a randomized, placebo-controlled crossover trial in patients tolerating oral therapy. *Ann Intern Med* 1991;114:539–544.
195. Chow MSS, Lebsack C, Dillerman D. Propafenone: a new antiarrhythmic agent. *Clin Pharm* 1988;7:869–877.
196. Shen EN. Propafenone: a promising new antiarrhythmic agent. *Chest* 1990;98:434–441.
197. Conte F, Latini R, Meroni M, et al. Propafenone acute intoxication removed by plasma exchange. In: *Proceedings of the Fourteenth International Congress of the European Association of Poison Centers* 1990:117.
198. Eray O, Fowler J. Severe propafenone poisoning responded to temporary internal pacemaker. *Vet Hum Toxicol* 2000;42(5):289.
199. Rambourg-Schepens MO, Grossenbacher F, Buffet M, et al. Recurrent convulsions and cardiac conduction disturbances after propafenone overdose. *Vet Hum Toxicol* 1999;41(3):153–154
200. Fonck K, Haenebalcke C, Hemeryck A, et al. ECG changes and plasma concentrations of propafenone and its metabolites in a case of severe poisoning. *J Toxicol Clin Toxicol* 1998;36(3):247–251.
201. Kerns W, English B, Ford M. Propafenone overdose. *Ann Emerg Med* 1994;24:98–103.
202. Brzezinka H, Holtz J, Goenechea S. Propafenone fatality. *Bull Int Assoc Forens Toxicol* 1988;20(1):30–32.
203. Budde T, Meyer M, Breithardt G, et al. Therapie der schweren propafenonein-toxikation: eliminations versuch mittels hamoperfusion. *Z Kardiol* 1986;75:764–769.
204. McHugh TP, Perina DG. Propafenone ingestion. *Ann Emerg Med* 1987;16:437–440.
205. Siddoway LA, Roden DM, Woosley RL. Clinical pharmacology of propafenone: pharmacokinetics, metabolism and concentration response relations. *Am J Cardiol* 1984;54:9D–12D.
206. Siddoway LA, Thompson KA, McAllister CB, et al. Polymorphism of propafenone metabolism and disposition in man: clinical and pharmacokinetic consequences. *Circulation* 1987;75:785–791.
207. Giani P, Landolina M, Giudici V, et al. Pharmacokinetics and pharmacodynamics of propafenone during acute and chronic administration. *Eur J Clin Pharmacol* 1988;34:187–194.
208. Funch-Brentano C, Kroemer HK, Lee JT, et al. Propafenone. *N Engl J Med* 1990;322:518–525.
209. Connolly SJ, Kates RE, Lebsack CS, et al. Clinical efficacy and electrophysiology of oral propafenone for ventricular tachycardia. *Am J Cardiol* 1983;52:1208–1213.
210. Lee JT, Kroemer HK, Silberstein DJ, et al. The role of genetically determined polymorphic drug metabolism in the beta blockade produced by propafenone. *N Engl J Med* 1990;322:1764–1768.
211. Briggs GR, Freeman RK, Yaffe SJ. *Drugs in pregnancy and lactation*, 6th ed. Baltimore: Williams and Williams, 2002.
212. Libardoni M, Piovan D, Busato E, et al. Transfer of propafenone and 5-hydroxypropafenone to foetal plasma and maternal milk. *Br J Clin Pharmacol* 1991;32:527–528.
213. Koppel C, Oberdisse V, Heinemeyer G. Clinical course and outcome in class IC antiarrhythmic overdose. *Clin Toxicol* 1990;28:433–444.
214. Ohayon J, Colle J-P, Besse P. Intoxication volontaire a la propafenone sur coeur sain (a propos d'une observation). *Coeur* 1985;16:629–634.
215. Lecky BRF, Weir D, Chong E. Exacerbation of myasthenia by propafenone. *J Neurol Neurosurg Psychiatry* 1991;54:377.
216. Veale D, McComb JM, Gibson GJ. Propafenone. *Lancet* 1990;335:979.
217. Ravid S, Podrid PJ, Novrit B. Safety of long term propafenone therapy for cardiac arrhythmia: experience with 774 patients. *J Electrophysiol* 1987;1:580–590.
218. Wagner F, Kalusche D, Trenk E, et al. Drug interaction between propafenone and metoprolol. *Br J Clin Pharmacol* 1987;24:213–220.
219. Baselt RC. *Disposition of toxic drugs and chemicals in man*, 5th ed. Foster City, CA: Chemical Toxicology Institute, 2000.
220. Hettinger M, Siebner H. Intoxikation mit propafenone. *Mediz Welt* 1989;40:1495–1497.
221. Friocourt P, Martin C, Lozach L. Intoxication volontaire par la propafenone: a propos d'un cas. *Ann Cardiol Angeiol* 1988;37(3):133–136.
222. Olm M, Jimenez MJ, Munne P. Efficacite de la methosamine par voie veineuse los des intoxications a la propafenone. [Efficacy of intravenous methoxamine in propafenone poisoning.] *Presse Med* 1989;18:1124.
223. Bosche J, Mattern R. Todlichen vergiftungstall mid dem antiarrhythmikum propafenone. *Beitr Geriche Med* 1980;38:231–234.
224. Burgess E, Duff H, Wilkes P. Propafenone disposition in renal insufficiency and renal failure. *J Clin Pharmacol* 1989;29:112–113.
225. Dimopoulos G. A case of fatal propafenone poisoning. *Bull Int Assoc Forens Toxicol* 1987;19(3):31–32.
226. Chouty F, Funck-Brentano C, Leehardt A, et al. Intravenous sodium lactate as a treatment for class 1 anti-arrhythmic agents overdose. *Circulation* 1989;80[Suppl. II]:II–430.
227. Grubb BP. Moricizine: a new agent for the treatment of ventricular arrhythmias. *Am J Med Sci* 1991;301:298–401.
228. Vaughan Williams EM. A classification of antiarrhythmic actions reassessed after a decade of new drugs. *J Clin Pharmacol* 1984;24:129–147.
229. Vaughan Williams EM. Classification of antiarrhythmic action of moricizine. *J Clin Pharmacol* 1991;31:216–221.
230. Mann HJ. Moricizine: a new class 1 antiarrhythmic. *Clin Pharm* 1990;9:842–852.
231. Rosenshtraukh L, Anyukhovsky E, Nesterenko V. Electrophysiologic aspects of moricizine HCl. *Am J Cardiol* 1987;60:27–34.
232. Bigger T. Cardiac electrophysiologic effects of moricizine hydrochloride. *Am J Cardiol* 1990;65:15–20.
233. Briggs GR, Freeman RK, Sumner JY. *Drugs in pregnancy and lactation*, 5th ed. Baltimore: Williams and Williams, 1998.
234. Kennedy H. Noncardiac adverse effects and organ toxicity of moricizine during short term and long term studies. *Am J Cardiol* 1990;65:47–50.
235. Morganroth J, Pratt C. Prevalence and characteristics of proarrhythmia from moricizine. *Am J Cardiol* 1989;63:172–176.
236. Pratt CM, Podrid P, Greatrix B, et al. Efficacy and safety of moricizine in patients with congestive heart failure: a summary of the experience in the United States. *Am Heart J* 1990;119:1–7.
237. Whitney CC, Weinstein SH, Gaylord JC. High-performance liquid chromatographic determination of Ethmozin in plasma. *J Pharm Sci* 1981;70:462–463.

CHAPTER 119

Type II Antidysrhythmic Agents (β-Receptor Blocking Agents)

Gerald M. Brody and Michael A. McGuigan

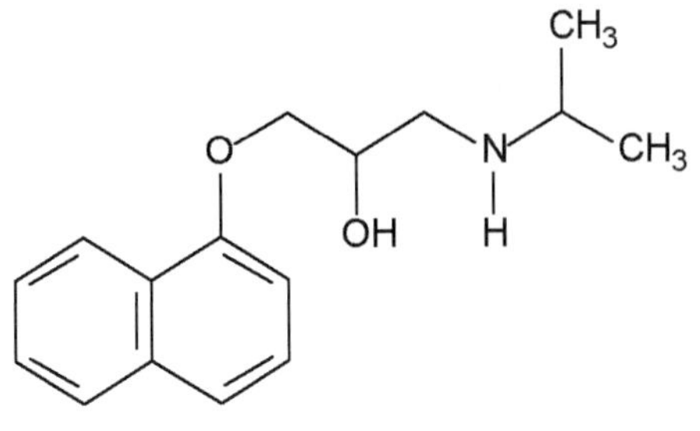

PROPRANOLOL

Compounds included:	**Acebutolol (Sectral), atenolol (Tenormin), betaxolol (Betoptic, Kerlone), bisoprolol (Zebeta), carvedilol (Coreg), esmolol (Brevibloc), labetalol (Normodyne, Trandate), metoprolol (Betabloc, Lopressor), nadolol (Corgard), pindolol (Visken), propranolol (Inderal, Prolol), timolol (Blocadren, Cosopt). Sotalol is included in Chapter 120.**
Molecular formula and weight:	**See Table 1.**
SI conversion:	**See Table 1.**
CAS Registry No.:	**See Table 1.**
Therapeutic levels:	**Not used clinically**
Special concerns:	**Propranolol is the most toxic beta-blocker.**
Target organs:	**Cardiovascular system**
Antidotes:	**β-receptor agonists, glucagon, insulin, and glucose**

OVERVIEW

The β-receptor blocking drugs competitively block the action of the β-adrenergic agonists at the β receptor (Table 2). These drugs are used for the treatment of hypertension, angina, and cardiac dysrhythmias. Because of the numerous similarities regarding the diagnostic tests and treatment of poisoning by the β-receptor antagonists, these topics are addressed for the entire group at the end of this chapter.

In a review of fatal beta-blocker ingestions from the American poison centers (1985–1995) (1), there were a total of 164 deaths; 38 of which beta-blockers were the primary cause of death. Propranolol was thought to be the cause in 71% of these deaths. Bradycardia and asystole were the most common rhythms seen. No pediatric deaths were reported despite the occurrence of 19,388 exposures.

CLASSIFICATION AND USES

Beta-blockers are classified according to the several properties (Table 1).

1. *Cardioselectivity*: Some beta-blockers (propranolol, sotalol, timolol, pindolol, oxprenolol, nadolol, labetalol) demonstrate blocking characteristics for β_1 and β_2 receptors. Others (metoprolol, atenolol, esmolol, and acebutolol) act mostly at β_1 receptors in therapeutic doses. In overdose, much of the cardioselectivity of all the agents is lost.
2. *Partial agonist activity*: Some agents (acebutolol, labetalol, pindolol) have some intrinsic agonist activity in addition to their beta-blocking effects. Overdoses with such drugs have presented with tachycardia and hypertension as well as bradycardia and hypotension (2,3). Such agonist activity is independent of their cardioselectivity.
3. *Lipid solubility*: Some agents (e.g., propranolol) are highly lipophilic and enter the central nervous system (CNS) easily. Such drugs have marked CNS effects in addition to their cardiovascular effects. Such drugs tend to be much more dangerous in overdose.
4. *Alpha activity*: Labetalol and carvedilol have both beta- and alpha-blocking activity and can cause peripheral vasodilation.
5. *Membrane stabilization effects*: Propanolol, pindolol, and acebutolol all demonstrate the ability to block the inward flow of sodium via the fast inward sodium channels, the same effect seen in Type IA antidysrhythmics. This is called *membrane-stabilizing effects or activity* and has the effect of prolonging QRS duration. These effects are not clinically significant at therapeutic doses but dramatically increase toxicity in overdose (4,5).

PATHOPHYSIOLOGY OF THE CLASS

The subtypes of β-receptors are β_1 and β_2 (Table 2). The β_1-receptor increases chromotropy, automaticity, and inotropy in the heart; increases renin production in the kidney; and increases aqueous

TABLE 1. Classification of beta-blockers

Drug	Molecular formula, molecular weight (g/mol), CAS Registry No.	SI conversion	Cardioselectivity, partial β agonist (yes/no)	Alpha blocking	Membrane stabilization	Lipid solubility
Acebutolol hydrochloride	$C_{18}H_{28}N_2O_4$,HCl, 372.9, 34381-68-5	ng/ml × 2.97 = nmol/L	β_1, yes	No	Yes	Low to moderate
Atenolol	$C_{14}H_{22}N_2O_3$, 266.3, 29122-68-7	ng/ml × 3.76 = nmol/L	β_1, no	No	No	Low
Betaxolol hydrochloride	$C_{18}H_{29}NO_3$,HCl, 343.9, 63659-19-8	ng/ml × 3.25 = nmol/L	β_1, no	No	No	Low
Bisoprolol fumarate	$(C_{18}H_{31}NO_4)_2$,$C_4H_4O_4$, 767.0, 66722-45-0	ng/ml × 3.07 = nmol/L	β_1, no	No	No	Low
Carvedilol	$C_{24}H_{26}N_2O_4$, 406.5, 72956-09-3	ng/ml × 2.46 = nmol/L	β_1/β_2, no	Yes	Yes	High
Esmolol hydrochloride	$C_{16}H_{25}NO_4$,HCl, 331.8, 81161-17-3	ng/ml × 3.39 = nmol/L	β_1, no	No	No	Low
Labetalol hydrochloride	$C_{19}H_{24}N_2O_3$,HCl, 364.9, 32780-64-6	ng/ml × 3.05 = nmol/L	β_1/β_2, no	Yes	No	Low to moderate
Metoprolol tartrate	$(C_{15}H_{25}NO_3)_2$,$C_4H_6O_6$, 684.8, 56392-17-7	ng/ml × 3.74 = nmol/L	β_1, no	No	No	Moderate
Nadolol	$C_{17}H_{27}NO_4$, 309.4, 42200-33-9	ng/ml × 3.23 = nmol/L	β_1/β_2, no	No	No	Low
Pindolol	$C_{14}H_{20}N_2O_2$, 248.3, 13523-86-9	ng/ml × 4.03 = nmol/L	β_1/β_2, yes	No	No	Moderate
Propranolol hydrochloride	$C_{16}H_{21}NO_2$,HCl, 295.8, 3506-09-0	ng/ml × 3.86 = nmol/L	β_1/β_2, no	No	Yes	High
Timolol maleate	$C_{13}H_{24}N_4O_3S$,$C_4H_4O_4$, 432.5, 26921-17-5	ng/ml × 3.16 = nmol/L	β_1/β_2, no	No	No	Low to moderate

β_1, β_1-adrenergic receptor; β_2, β_2-adrenergic receptor.
Adapted from Frishman W, Jacob H, Eisenberg E, et al. Appraisal and reappraisal of cardiac therapy: clinical pharmacology of the new β-adrenergic blocking drugs. Part 8: self-poisoning with β-adrenoreceptor blocking agents: recognition and management. *Am Heart J* 1979;98:798–811.

humor production in the eye. The cardiac effects are the most important clinically. The β_2 receptor causes bronchodilation, arteriolar dilation, glycogenolysis, gluconeogenesis, insulin release, and movement of potassium into cells.

At a cellular level, when a catecholamine binds to a β-receptor, the G protein complex in the cell membrane is phosphorylated, which catalyses the production of cyclic adenosine monophosphate. The intracellular increase in cyclic adenosine monophosphate mediates multiple intracellular actions. In the cardiac myocyte, it increases the release of calcium from the sarcoplasmic reticulum. The increase in cytosolic calcium increases the strength of myocardial contraction.

ACEBUTOLOL

Acebutolol is a selective β_1-antagonist with low lipid solubility, significant membrane stabilizing activity, and partial agonist properties. Its toxicity is related to its beta-blocking action as well as its ability to affect ventricular repolarization, prolong the QTc interval, and precipitate ventricular tachycardia and ventricular fibrillation. It is one of the most dangerous of the beta-blockers in overdose (1,3,6). Acebutolol is available in 200-mg and 400-mg capsules.

TABLE 2. Subtypes of β-adrenergic receptors

β_1-Adrenergic effects	β_2-Adrenergic effects
Eye: Increased aqueous humor	Lung: Bronchial dilation production
Kidney: Increased renin production	Vascular: Arteriolar dilation
Heart: Increased chronotropy, lipolysis, gluconeogenesis, increased inotropy, glycogenolysis, increased lactic, increased automaticity acid production	Metabolic: Increased insulin release Other: Movement of potassium into cells

Adapted from Wolf LR. β-Adrenergic blocker toxicity. In: Haddad LM, Shannon MW, Winchester JF. *Clinical management of poisoning and drug overdose*, 3rd ed. Philadelphia: WB Saunders, 1998:1032.

Toxic Dose

The *adult therapeutic dose* ranges from 200 to 1200 mg/day in divided doses. Acebutolol is not used in children. There is great variability in lethal and minimally toxic doses in acebutolol poisoning. Death has been caused by 4000 mg (2) and a patient survived a 13,600-mg ingestion (7). No pediatric fatalities in overdose have been reported. A 15-year-old child survived an ingestion of 7600 mg (7,8).

Toxicokinetics and Toxicodynamics

Acebutolol is well absorbed from the gastrointestinal (GI) tract but undergoes extensive first-pass metabolism in the liver to diacetolol, an active metabolite that accounts for most of the drug's activity. The bioavailability of acebutolol is 35%. It is 25% protein bound with a volume of distribution (V_d) of 1.2 L/kg. Peak plasma levels (T_{max}) occur at 2 to 4 hours after a therapeutic dose. The half-life of the parent drug is 2 to 4 hours and the half-life of the metabolite is 8 to 12 hours. The metabolite is excreted in the urine.

Pathophysiology

The pharmacokinetic parameters of acebutolol are provided in Table 3. It has the general properties of selective β_1-antagonists. It has low lipid solubility, significant membrane stabilizing effects, and partial agonist activity. Like sotalol, acebutolol appears to prolong the QTc interval and predispose to ventricular tachycardia and fibrillation (3).

TABLE 3. Pharmacokinetics of common beta-blockers

Drug	Absorption (%)	First-pass metabolism	Protein binding (%)	V_d (L/Kg)	Elimination route	Elimination half-life (h)
Acebutolol	95	Extensive	25	1.2	Renal/hepatic	2–4
Atenolol	50	None	<5	1	Renal	5–8
Betaxolol	100	Extensive	50–60	5–13	Hepatic	12–22
Bisoprolol	90	Small	26–33	2.9	Renal	10–12
Carvedilol	100	Significant	95–98	1.5–2.0	Hepatic	6–10
Esmolol	NA	NA	55	3.4	Red blood cell esterase	0.15
Labetalol	100	Extensive	50	9	Hepatic	8
Metoprolol	100	Extensive	10	4	Hepatic	3–4
Nadolol	20–40	None	30	2	Renal	10–20
Pindolol	95	Moderate	40–60	1.2–2.0	Hepatic/renal	3–4
Propranolol	100	Significant	90	4	Hepatic	3–5
Timolol	90	Moderate	<10	2	Hepatic/renal	2–4

NA, not applicable; V_d, volume of distribution.
Adapted from Brubacher JR. Beta adrenergic antagonists. In: Goldfrank LR, et al. *Goldfrank's toxicologic emergencies,* 6th ed. Stamford, CT: Appleton & Lange, 1998:814.

Pregnancy and Lactation

Acebutolol is U.S. Food and Drug Administration (FDA) pregnancy category B (Appendix I). There are no adequate studies of its effect in pregnancy. Acebutolol and diacetolol are concentrated in breast milk.

Clinical Presentation

ACUTE OVERDOSAGE

The major toxicity of acebutolol is hypotension and bradycardia. Heart block and conduction delays may occur. In addition, the QTc interval is often prolonged. Seizures have not been a prominent feature, but coma has occurred commonly.

ADVERSE EVENTS

Hypotension, bradycardia, heart failure, edema, fatigue, anxiety, nausea, constipation, diarrhea, vomiting, abdominal pain, impotence, frequency of urination, dyspnea, and myalgia have been reported in up to 2% to 4% of patients on acebutolol. Positive antinuclear antibodies have been seen in up to 33% of patients on therapeutic doses of acebutolol (9). Impotence, pruritus, liver function abnormalities (10), lupus syndrome, hypersensitivity, pneumonitis (11), skin rash, and pleurisy with pulmonary granulomas (12) have been reported.

ATENOLOL

Atenolol is a long-acting selective β_1-antagonist, which is not lipid soluble and has no membrane stabilizing activity or intrinsic sympathomimetic activity. Its toxicity is almost exclusively cardiac and it is thought to be significantly less toxic than other members of this class. Atenolol is used for patients with hypertension, angina, and dysrhythmias. Regular release tablets are available in 25-, 50-, and 100-mg tablets and as a 5-mg/mg solution for injection.

Toxic Dose

The *adult therapeutic dose* is 25 to 200 mg orally once a day. The intravenous (IV) dose is 2.5 mg to 10 mg. The pediatric dose is 0.3 to 2.0 mg/kg/day administered once daily.

There is great variability in the toxic dose of atenolol. Ingestions of 5000 to 6000 mg have been survived (13). Death occurred after an ingestion of 10,000 mg (14). No pediatric deaths have been reported. A 15-year-old child survived an ingestion of 500 mg (14).

Toxicokinetics and Toxicodynamics

Atenolol is approximately 50% absorbed with no significant first-pass metabolism. It is less than 5% protein bound and has a V_d of 1 L/kg. It has low lipid solubility and little penetration into the CNS. The T_{max} is 2 to 4 hours after ingestion. Approximately 50% of an atenolol dose is excreted in feces. Absorbed atenolol is excreted largely unchanged in the urine. The elimination half-life is 5 to 8 hours. The drug accumulates in renal failure and the dose is reduced for patients with creatinine clearance less than 35 ml/minute.

Pathophysiology

Atenolol has the properties of the general class of selective β_1-blockers. It has no agonist or membrane stabilizing effects and is not lipid soluble. Its β_1-selective blocking properties are probably lost in overdose. It has no significant CNS effects.

Pregnancy and Lactation

Atenolol is FDA pregnancy category D (Appendix I). It crosses the placenta. Use of atenolol in pregnancy has resulted in infants who are small for gestational age. Atenolol is excreted in breast milk and can cause clinically significant bradycardia.

Clinical Presentation

ACUTE OVERDOSAGE

The major toxicity is hypotension, bradycardia, heart block, and conduction delay. Seizures are not reported, although depression of respiration and mental status occur. Bronchospasm has also been reported. Because of its long half-life, atenolol toxicity often lasts longer than other beta-blockers.

One patient exhibited primary central hypoventilation while awake, which could be overcome by voluntary action (13). Hypothermia developed in two cases of overdose. Hypoglycemia was reported in a 15-year-old child (14).

ADVERSE EVENTS

Bradycardia, hypotension, cold extremities, dizziness, tiredness, nausea, and diarrhea are reported in 2% to 26% of patients.

Peripheral vascular disease and impotence are also seen. Rash, cutaneous vasculitis (15), elevated liver enzymes, Peyronie's disease, thrombocytopenia, and retroperitoneal fibrosis (16,17) and lupus syndrome (18) have been reported.

BETAXOLOL

Betaxolol is a long-acting β_1-selective antagonist with weak membrane stabilizing effects, low lipid solubility, and no agonist activity. It is used topically in glaucoma in addition to an oral formulation. The experience in overdose is limited. Betaxolol is used for the treatment of glaucoma, hypertension, and angina. Betaxolol is available as a 0.25% suspension, a 0.5% solution, and in 10 mg and 20 mg tablets.

Toxic Dose

The *adult therapeutic dose* is 5 to 80 mg once daily. Betaxolol is not used in children. Toxic effects have been seen after therapeutic doses of ophthalmic betaxolol. One fatality has been reported after ingestion of an unknown dose, but 65 mg were found in her stomach at autopsy and the serum concentration (36 mg/L) was much greater than therapeutic concentrations (19). No pediatric poisonings have been reported.

Toxicokinetics and Toxicodynamics

The bioavailability of betaxolol is 90%. It is 50% to 60% protein-bound with a V_d of 5 to 13 L/kg. The T_{max} is 2 to 6 hours. Betaxolol is extensively metabolized in the liver with 15% of the drug excreted unchanged in the urine. It has a half-life of 12 to 22 hours.

Pathophysiology

Betaxolol has the general properties of selective β_1-antagonists with little membrane stabilizing activity and no agonist activity.

Pregnancy and Lactation

Betaxolol is FDA pregnancy category C (Appendix I). Betaxolol rapidly crosses the placenta, and serum levels equal levels in cord blood after 4 to 6 hours. Betaxolol is concentrated in breast milk with a milk/plasma ratio of 2.5 to 3:1.

Clinical Presentation

Experience with overdose of betaxolol is quite limited. One fatality prior to medical treatment was reported with a massive overdose (19).

Adverse events during therapeutic use include (in 2% to 15% of patients): bradycardia, palpitations, headache, dizziness, fatigue, lethargy, insomnia, nausea, diarrhea, dyspepsia, dyspnea, joint pain, and myalgia. Stinging of the eyes has been reported in 30% of patients.

One case of an acute myocardial infarction was reported after instillation of one drop of betaxolol (20). There was also a report of cardiac arrest after use of ophthalmic betaxolol (21).

The following adverse reactions have also been reported: bradycardia, hypotension, heart block, nightmares, depression, exacerbation of myasthenia gravis, photophobia, anisocoria, five cases of alopecia (22), systemic lupus erythematosus (23), and toxic epidermal necrolysis (24).

BISOPROLOL

Bisoprolol is a long-acting selective β_1-antagonist without membrane stabilizing effects or intrinsic agonist activity. Bisoprolol is available in 5-mg and 10-mg tablets.

Toxic Dose

The *adult therapeutic dose* is 2.5 mg to 40 mg/day given once per day. Bisoprolol is not used in children. No deaths have been reported. A patient survived a 140-mg ingestion (25). No cases of pediatric overdose have been reported.

Toxicokinetics and Toxicodynamics

Bisoprolol has 90% oral bioavailability, an apparent V_d of 2.9 L/kg, and is 26% to 33% protein-bound. Its T_{max} is 3 to 4 hours. Bisoprolol has a small first-pass metabolism. Approximately 50% of the drug is excreted unchanged in the urine. The elimination half-life is 10.0 to 12.4 hours.

Pathophysiology

Bisoprolol has the properties of the general class of selective β_1-antagonists with no membrane stabilizing effects.

Pregnancy and Lactation

Bisoprolol is FDA pregnancy category C (Appendix I). Entry into breast milk is unknown.

Clinical Presentation

Experience in overdose is limited. Bradycardia followed the ingestion of 140 mg (25). The following adverse effects have been reported in a greater than 5% prevalence in patients taking therapeutic doses: bradycardia, cold hands, orthostatic hypotension, dizziness, fatigue, headache, and sleep disturbances. The following conditions have been reported in 1% to 5% of patients: exacerbation of peripheral vascular disease, nausea, vomiting, dementia, bronchoscopy, dyspnea, and diaphoresis. Other adverse effects reported with bisoprolol use include blurred vision, conjunctivitis, liver enzyme elevation, impotence, and Peyronie's disease.

CARVEDILOL

Carvedilol is used in congestive heart failure (CHF), coronary artery disease, and hypertension. It is a nonselective β-receptor blocker with α_1-blocking properties, moderate membrane stabilizing effects, high lipid solubility, and no intrinsic agonist activity. Carvedilol is available in 6.25-, 12.5-, and 25.0-mg tablets.

Toxic Dose

The *adult therapeutic dose* is 4.25 to 100.0 mg/day in two divided doses. The pediatric dose is 0.03 to 0.75 mg/kg/day in two divided doses. There has only been one overdose reported, in which the patient survived an ingestion of 1050 mg (26). There have been no reports of pediatric overdose.

Toxicokinetics and Toxicodynamics

Carvedilol is rapidly absorbed. The T_{max} is 1.0 to 1.5 hours. Bioavailability is 25% to 35%. The drug is 95% to 98% protein-bound and has a V_d of 1.5 to 2.0 L/kg. Carvedilol undergoes extensive first-pass metabolism in the liver. Less than 10% of the unchanged drug is excreted in the urine. The elimination half-life is 6 to 10 hours.

Pathophysiology

Carvedilol has the properties of the general class of nonselective beta-blockers. In addition it has α_1-blocking effects, moderate membrane stabilizing effects, is highly lipid soluble, and has no agonist properties. Alpha blockade may make vasodilation more of a problem than in other beta-blocker overdoses.

Pregnancy and Lactation

Carvedilol is FDA pregnancy category C (Appendix I). It is not known if the drug is excreted in milk but the drug is highly lipophilic with a large volume of distribution and therefore may accumulate in breast milk.

Clinical Presentation

Bradycardia, hypotension, and QRS prolongation may occur in overdose (26).

The following conditions have been seen in more than 5% of patients taking carvedilol: bradycardia, peripheral edema, hypotension, dizziness, GI symptoms (nausea, vomiting, diarrhea), erectile dysfunction, and visual abnormalities. The following conditions were reported in 1% to 5% of patients: thrombocytopenia, atrioventricular block, postural hypotension, insomnia, somnolence, fatigue, hyperglycemia, abdominal pain, rhinitis, and skin rashes. The incidence is typically higher in CHF patients.

One case of myoclonus has been reported (27). Two deaths from asthma were reported in patients receiving a single dose of carvedilol (28). One case of Stevens-Johnson syndrome has been reported (29).

ESMOLOL

Esmolol is an ultra short acting β_1-antagonist selective beta-blocking agent with low lipid solubility, no membrane stabilizing effects, or intrinsic agonist activity. It is only given IV. It is used to treat supraventricular dysrhythmias, hypertensive emergencies, aortic dissection, myocardial ischemia, and intraoperatively and postoperatively for dysrhythmias and hypertension. Esmolol comes as 10 mg/ml and 25 mg/ml solutions.

Toxic Dose

The *adult therapeutic dose* is 500 μg/kg as a loading dose followed by an infusion of 50 to 200 μg/kg/minute. The pediatric IV infusion dose is 300 to 1000 μg/kg/minute.

No deaths have been reported from esmolol overdosage. Up to 25% of patients receiving esmolol experience hypotension (30). Eighteen percent of patients receiving at least 200 μg/kg/ml developed adverse effects (31).

Toxicokinetics and Toxicodynamics

Esmolol is administered IV. It has a beta-blocking effect that peaks in 5 minutes. It is 55% protein bound and has a V_d of 3.43 L/kg. Esmolol is metabolized by red blood cell esterase. Its half-life is approximately 9 minutes. Approximately 20% of the dose is metabolized to methanol. Methanol levels associated with the therapeutic use of esmolol are considerably below toxic levels (32).

Pathophysiology

Esmolol is an extremely short-acting selective β_1-antagonist. Its effects are similar to other agents of this general class. It has no membrane stabilizing effects and no intrinsic agonist activity. Because of its extremely short half-life, toxic effects are ameliorated within minutes of decreasing or discontinuing the infusion.

Pregnancy and Lactation

Esmolol is FDA pregnancy category C. Its secretion into breast milk is unknown.

Clinical Presentation

The major toxic effects are hypotension and bradycardia. There are no reports of overdose. Toxicity is limited due to the extremely short half-life. Mild nausea and inflammation at the injection site are also seen. Headache, confusion, somnolence, and agitation occur in 2% to 3% of patients. There is one report of profound bradycardia and hypotension in an adult and one report of asystole in a pediatric patient after therapeutic doses of esmolol (31,33). Seizure activity has also been reported once (34).

LABETALOL

Labetalol is a nonselective combined β- and α-antagonist with moderate lipid solubility, low membrane stabilizing effects, and no agonist activity. Labetalol is available in 100-mg, 200-mg, and 300-mg tablets and a 5-mg/ml solution for injection.

Toxic Dose

The *adult therapeutic dose* is 200 to 2400 mg/day in two divided doses. The pediatric oral dose is 20 to 40 mg/kg/day in 3 to 4 divided doses. No deaths have been reported from labetalol. An adult survived an ingestion of 19 g (35).

Toxicokinetics and Toxicodynamics

Labetalol is completely absorbed and has a bioavailability of 25% to 40%. It is 50% protein-bound and has a V_d of 5.1 to 9.4 L/kg. The T_{max} is 2 to 4 hours after ingestion. Labetalol undergoes extensive first-pass metabolism in the liver. Almost no drug is excreted unchanged in the urine. The elimination half-life is 8 hours. Metabolism is highly dependent on hepatic blood flow.

Pathophysiology

Labetalol has the properties of the general class of nonselective β-antagonists. In addition, it has alpha-blocking properties. Its beta:alpha blocking properties are 3:1 after oral administration and 7:1 after parenteral administration. The drug is moderately lipid soluble with low membrane stabilizing effects. It has no intrinsic agonist activity.

Pregnancy and Lactation

Labetalol is FDA pregnancy category C (Appendix I). Hypotension, bradycardia, hypoglycemia, and respiratory depression have developed in infants of mothers who were treated with labetalol for hypertension. Small amounts (0.004%) of the maternal dose of labetalol are secreted in breast milk.

Clinical Presentation

Hypotension and bradycardia are the major toxic effects of labetalol. Heart block also occurs. Unlike overdose with other beta-blockers, acute renal failure has been reported in labetalol overdose (35,36). In addition, its alpha-blocking properties may make vasodilation more of a problem than with other beta-blocker overdoses.

Orthostatic hypotension, dizziness, fatigue, GI complaints (nausea, constipation, abdominal pain, dyspepsia, taste abnormality, vomiting, diarrhea), liver function abnormalities, and scalp tingling have been reported in more than 5% of patients using labetalol. Edema, bronchospasm, impotence, and ejaculation failure have been reported in 1% to 5% of patients taking labetalol.

Life-threatening hyperkalemia developed in a patient on dialysis receiving oral labetalol (37). Asymptomatic hyperkalemia has been reported after IV use of labetalol in dialysis patients (38). Fevers of probable immunologic origin were reported in two patients (39). Death from hepatic necrosis has been reported in one patient (40). Toxic myopathy and lupus syndromes have been reported (41,42).

METOPROLOL

Metoprolol is a selective β_1-antagonist that is moderately lipophilic with low membrane stabilizing activity and no intrinsic agonist properties. It is less toxic than propranolol and other membrane stabilizing agents (1). Metoprolol is available as 50-mg and 100-mg standard-release tablets; as 50-mg, 100-mg, and 200-mg modified-release tablets; and as a 5-mg/ml solution for injection.

Toxic Dose

The *adult therapeutic dose* is 50 to 400 mg/day orally in one or two doses or 2 to 20 mg IV. The pediatric oral dose of metoprolol is 1 to 5 mg/kg/day (maximum, 400 mg/day) in two divided doses. There is great variability in lethal and minimally toxic doses. Death has been caused by 7500 mg and a patient survived an ingestion of 50,000 mg (43,44). No pediatric deaths have been described.

Toxicokinetics and Toxicodynamics

Metoprolol is almost completely absorbed after ingestion and has a bioavailability of only 40%. It is approximately 10% protein bound and has a V_d of 4 L/kg. The T_{max} is 1 to 2 hours. Metoprolol undergoes extensive first-pass metabolism in the liver, and only 10% of the unchanged drug is excreted in the urine. The half-life is 3 to 4 hours.

Pathophysiology

Metoprolol is moderately lipid-soluble with low membrane stabilizing effects and no intrinsic agonist activity. Metoprolol has β_1-antagonist selective blocking properties that are probably lost in overdose.

Pregnancy and Lactation

Metoprolol is FDA pregnancy category C (Appendix I). The drug is excreted in small quantities in human milk (less than 1 mg/L breast milk). The American Academy of Pediatrics considers metoprolol use compatible with breast-feeding (45).

Clinical Presentation

The major toxicity of metoprolol is hypotension and bradycardia. Varying degrees of heart block may be seen but conduction delays are rare. Seizures have been reported (43,44).

Tiredness, dizziness, depression, shortness of breath, bradycardia, diarrhea, pruritus, and rash have been reported in 3% to 10% of patients. Raynaud's phenomenon, cold extremities, palpitations, CHF, peripheral edema, bronchospasm, syncope, chest pain, hypotension, and GI complaints have been reported in approximately 1% of patients.

Angioedema (46), carpal tunnel syndrome (47), retroperitoneal fibrosis (48), impotence, Peyronie's disease, and eye pain have also been reported with metoprolol.

NADOLOL

Nadolol is a nonselective beta-blocker with low lipid solubility, no membrane stabilizing activity, and no intrinsic agonist activity. Nadolol is available in 20-, 40-, 80-, 100-, 120-, and 160-mg tablets.

Toxic Dose

The *adult therapeutic dose* is 40 to 320 mg/day given once daily. The pediatric dose is 1 to 4 mg/kg/day given once daily. No deaths have been reported from nadolol and minimum toxic dose has not been reported.

Toxicokinetics and Toxicodynamics

Absorption after an oral dose is 20% to 40%. The drug is 30% protein bound with a V_d of 2 L/kg. The T_{max} is 2 to 4 hours. Nadolol is not metabolized in the liver, and the drug is excreted unchanged by the kidneys. The elimination half-life is 20 to 24 hours.

Pathophysiology

Nadolol has the properties of the general class of nonselective β-antagonists. It has no membrane stabilizing effects and no intrinsic agonist activity. It is cleared entirely by the kidneys with a long half-life; plasma levels increase in renal failure.

Pregnancy and Lactation

Nadolol is FDA pregnancy category C (Appendix I). It is excreted in breast milk.

Clinical Presentation

Hypotension, bradycardia, and first-degree AV block have been noted (49). No QRS prolongation has been reported. The following conditions are seen in 1% to 2% of patients: bradycardia, Raynaud's phenomenon, hypotension, CHF, dysrhythmias, dizziness, and fatigue. There have been case reports of hypertriglyceridemia and acute pancreatitis (50), papilledema and subsequent optic atrophy (51), and hypersensitivity pneumonitis (52).

PINDOLOL

Pindolol is a nonselective beta-blocker with high intrinsic sympathomimetic activity, moderate lipid solubility, and no membrane stabilizing effects. Its toxicity in overdose may have features of both β-receptor agonism and antagonism. Pindolol is used in hypertension and angina, especially in patients who develop symptomatic bradycardia from typical beta-blockers. Pindolol is available in 5-mg, 10-mg, and 15-mg tablets.

Toxic Dose

The *adult therapeutic dose* is 10 mg to 60 mg daily, in two divided doses. Pindolol is not used in children. No deaths have been reported. Doses of 500 mg orally have been survived (53).

Toxicokinetics and Toxicodynamics

Pindolol is 95% absorbed after oral administration. The T_{max} is 2 hours. It has 87% to 90% bioavailability, 40% to 60% protein binding, and a V_d of 1.2 to 2.0 L/kg. Approximately 60% of the drug is metabolized in the liver and 40% is excreted unchanged by the kidney. The elimination half-life is 3 to 4 hours.

Pathophysiology

Pindolol has both β-receptor blocking and intrinsic agonist properties. Its agonist properties may make the picture of overdose more variable. In addition to hypotension and bradycardia, hypertension and tachycardia may occur.

Pregnancy and Lactation

Pindolol is FDA pregnancy category B (Appendix I). It enters breast milk in measurable amounts.

Clinical Presentation

The acute toxicity of pindolol is variable because it is both an agonist and an antagonist of β-receptors. Tachycardia and hypertension have been reported as well as the more usual beta-blocker effects of hypotension and bradycardia (53–55).

Several adverse events have been reported in 5% or more of patients: edema, fatigue, insomnia, dizziness, vivid dreams, nausea and abdominal discomfort, elevated liver function tests, and joint and muscle pain. The following conditions are seen in 1% to 5% of patients: tachycardia, heart failure, palpitations, heart block, bradycardia, cold extremities, anxiety, lethargy, paresthesia, hallucinations, diarrhea, vomiting, impotence, rash, and muscle cramps.

An increase in ventricular ectopy was described in one patient after a 10-mg dose (56). There have been several reports of tremor (57–59). Hypomania and psychosis have been reported in patients with bipolar disease (60). Pulmonary fibrosis and systemic lupus erythematosus have been reported (61,62).

PROPRANOLOL

Propranolol is a nonselective β-antagonist that has high membrane stabilizing activity, is highly lipophilic, and has no intrinsic sympathomimetic activity. It is considered the most toxic beta-blocker in overdose (1,63). Propranolol is used for angina, hypertension, postmyocardial infarction, asymmetric septal hypertrophy, mitral valve prolapse, migraines, tremor, thyroid storm, and anxiety. Propranolol is available in 10-mg, 20-mg, 40-mg, 60-mg, and 80-mg regular release tablets; 60-mg, 80-mg, 120-mg, and 160-mg sustained release capsules; and as a 1 mg/ml solution for injection.

Toxic Dose

The *adult therapeutic dose* for the regular formulation is 10 to 360 mg/day orally in two to four divided doses. The dose of a modified-release formulation is 80 to 160 mg/day as a single dose. The pediatric oral dose ranges from 0.5 to 10 mg/kg/day in three or four divided doses.

Overdose toxicity of propranolol varies greatly. An overdose of 2060 mg resulted in death (64), but patients have survived ingestion of 8000 mg (65). Some authors report a rough correlation between amount ingested and symptoms, especially with respect to seizures and QRS prolongation (63,66). No pediatric deaths have been reported.

Toxicokinetics and Toxicodynamics

Propranolol is nearly completely absorbed after oral administration with 25% bioavailability. The T_{max} is 1.0 to 1.5 hours. Protein binding is 90%. The V_d is 4 L/kg. Concentrations in the CNS are 10 to 20 times plasma concentrations (67). Propranolol is metabolized in the liver and has a large first-pass metabolism. The half-life is 3 to 5 hours. Metabolites are primarily excreted in the urine.

Pathophysiology

Propranolol has the properties of the general class of non-selective beta-blockers. It has no agonist properties, has significant membrane stabilizing effects and is highly lipophilic. Propranolol is highly lipophilic with significant concentration in the CNS. In addition, it has significant membrane stabilizing effects (antidysrhythmic type 1A effects).

Pregnancy and Lactation

Propranolol is FDA pregnancy category C (Appendix I). Intrauterine growth retardation has been reported. Neonates born to mothers taking propranolol have exhibited bradycardia, hypoglycemia, and respiratory depression (68,69). Propranolol is excreted in breast milk.

Clinical Presentation

ACUTE OVERDOSAGE

Propranolol toxicity consists of cardiac, neurologic, and respiratory effects. Its cardiac effects are typical for the class as a whole and include bradycardia, hypotension, conduction delays, heart block, acute cardiomyopathy, and asystole. Neurologic effects include seizure, delirium, psychosis, depressed mental status, and coma. These effects are seen both as a manifestation of decreased cardiac output as well as a direct effect of the drug on the CNS due to its high lipophilicity and its membrane stabilizing effects. Propranolol also has a respiratory depressant effect that is separate from its hemodynamic effects. Bronchospasm may also occur.

ADVERSE EVENTS

Bradycardia, CHF, heart block, hypotension, bronchospasm, depression, fatigue, lethargy, vivid dreams, and decreased performance on neuropsychometric testing may occur with chronic use. Agranulocytosis (70), thrombocytopenia (71), rash, fever, sore throat, nausea, vomiting, ischemic colitis (72), laryngospasm, respiratory distress, lupus syndrome (73), carpal tunnel syndrome, delusions, hallucinations (74), somnolence, hypoglycemia (75,76), hyperthyroidism, retroperitoneal fibrosis (77), Raynaud's phenomenon, and Peyronie's disease have all been reported.

TIMOLOL

Timolol is a nonselective beta-blocker that has no membrane stabilizing activity, low to moderate lipid solubility, and no agonist properties. Timolol is used primarily as an ophthalmic preparation for the treatment of glaucoma. It is also used for the treatment of angina, supraventricular dysrhythmias, hypertension, and migraine. Timolol is available as an ophthalmic solution and gel of 0.25% and 0.5% and as 5-mg, 10-mg, and 20-mg tablets. Toxicity can occur after therapeutic ophthalmic use.

Toxic Dose

The *adult therapeutic dose* is 10 to 60 mg/day orally in one or two divided doses. The ophthalmic dose is 1 drop of 0.25% to 0.5% solution given 1 to 2 times per day. The gel is given once a day. The pediatric ophthalmic dose is the same as adults. Timolol is not used orally in children.

There have been no reported deaths from timolol ingestion. Toxic effects have been seen in therapeutic doses in both adults and pediatric patients from ophthalmic preparations. Survival has been seen after an ingestion of 650 mg.

Toxicokinetics and Toxicodynamics

Timolol is 90% absorbed after an oral dose. The T_{max} is 0.5 to 3.0 hours orally and 23 hours after topical application. Bioavailability is 61%. It is less than 10% protein bound with a V_d of 1.3 to 1.7 L/kg. Serum levels after intraocular instillation are low and not always detectable. Approximately 50% of an oral dose undergoes first-pass metabolism. The half-life is 2 to 4 hours; 20% of the dose is excreted unchanged in the urine.

Pathophysiology

Timolol has the properties of the general class of nonselective β antagonists without membrane stabilizing activity or intrinsic agonist properties. Timolol can be systemically absorbed from the eye and has typical beta-blocker properties.

Pregnancy and Lactation

Timolol is FDA pregnancy category C (Appendix I). It is present in human breast milk with a milk:plasma ratio of 0.8.

Clinical Presentation

Overdose after ingestion has demonstrated second- and third-degree heart block. Bronchospasm, including death and respiratory arrest, have been reported after therapeutic timolol instillation (78). Bradycardia, heart block, hypotension, CHF, and syncope have all been reported after therapeutic doses and inadvertent over-use of ophthalmic preparations (79–85).

Bradycardia is seen after oral and ophthalmic use in up to 9% of patients. Depression, confusion, headache, fatigue, and bronchospasm have all been reported in greater than 5% incidence after both oral and ophthalmic use. GI symptoms (nausea, diarrhea, and dyspepsia), impotence, and rashes have all been reported with timolol use. Alopecia has been reported with usual doses of the drug (86).

Diagnostic Tests for the Class

ACUTE OVERDOSAGE

History, physical examination, and an electrocardiogram establish the diagnosis. Continuous cardiac and respiratory monitoring is needed. Most diagnostic testing is directed at evaluation of adverse effects (complete blood count with differential, electrolytes, glucose, blood urea nitrogen, creatinine, and arterial blood gases). A chest radiograph may be used to follow heart failure. Typically, patients are in intensive care for management of significant overdose. Invasive monitoring is usually recommended in significant overdoses when high doses of sympathomimetics are being used.

Urine and serum samples for the presence of propranolol and specific levels are often drawn but typically are not helpful during the acute phase of treatment. Toxicologic analysis for the presence of other drugs and toxins is important.

ADVERSE EVENTS

Electrophysiologic studies, echocardiograms, cardiac catheterization, electrocardiograms, pulmonary function testing, and neuropsychometric testing can all be used to help differentiate between chronic toxicity and underlying disease. Hypersensitivity, agranulocytosis, and thrombocytopenia should be evaluated with the appropriate hematologic testing. Serologic testing may be required for lupus syndromes. Neurologic, psychiatric, endocrine, pulmonary, vascular, and GI evaluations may be required. Withdrawal of the drug with or without rechallenge has been used to identify drug-related syndromes.

TREATMENT STRATEGIES FOR THE CLASS

The mortality rate for acute beta-blocker overdose is low. Nearly all patients survive with appropriate supportive and symptomatic care. Endotracheal intubation or other maneuvers that increase vagal tone are potentially dangerous because β-receptor antagonists block the sympathetic activity needed to raise the heart rate. Atropine should be administered before procedures that increase vagal tone.

Decontamination

Given the potential for serious toxicity, GI decontamination may be an appropriate intervention. Induced emesis is contraindicated. Gastric lavage is generally ineffective. Activated charcoal should be administered within 1 to 2 hours after a large ingestion. Whole bowel irrigation may be used for the removal of modified-release preparations.

Enhancement of Elimination

Extracorporeal removal of beta-blockers after overdoses typically has not been effective because of the large volumes of distribution, high lipid solubility, and high degrees of protein binding. However, for some agents, it might be reasonable to consider extracorporeal removal. Successful results have been reported for atenolol (87–89), nadolol (90), and possibly acebutolol. Successful use of hemodialysis plus extracorporeal membrane oxygenation has been reported (7). Hemodialysis and peritoneal dialysis remove betaxolol. Bisoprolol is dialyzable with hemodialysis and peritoneal dialysis. Either hemodialysis or peritoneal dialysis removes less than 1% of ingested labetalol. Charcoal hemoperfusion was used in one case of poisoning with a combination of metoprolol and diltiazem, but it was unclear if a significant amount of metoprolol was removed (91). The use of multiple dose–activated charcoal significantly reduced the elimination half-lives of sotalol and nadolol (92) in volunteer studies.

Antidotes

The effectiveness of beta-blocker antidotes is difficult to judge. Clinical effectiveness may be influenced by the specific pharmacologic agent ingested, the amount of drug absorbed, and the time delay to treatment. Other modifying factors include the patient's baseline medical status and the presence of co-ingestants. In addition, multiple antidotal drugs are often used simultaneously.

Glucagon is the drug of choice for the treatment of hypotension and bradycardia due to beta-blocker overdose. The initial dose is 5 to 10 mg IV. The duration of action is 15 to 30 minutes. Repeat doses may be given but a continuous infusion may be more effective (93). Depending on response, infusion rates of 1 to 10 mg/hour are recommended. Glucagon requires reconstitution before use. The diluent that formerly came with the product contained phenol and it was recommended that glucagon be reconstituted with normal saline, sterile water, or dextrose 5% in water for use in patients with beta-blocker overdose. Glucagon has been reformulated so the diluent is now phenol-free (94). More complete information, including adverse events, is provided in Chapter 60.

Atropine should be used for bradycardia but is useful only in milder cases. Standard doses (0.5 mg to 3.0 mg) should be used (Chapter 42).

Isoproterenol, with its nearly pure β-agonist action, would seem to be the catecholamine of choice in beta-blocker overdose. In clinical practice, however, it has not been particularly effective. Further, isoproterenol can cause dysrhythmias and has the potential negative effects of peripheral beta action, which could make hypotension worse. It is clear that when sympathomimetics are used, they have to be used in significantly higher doses than usual. In healthy volunteers given labetalol, 26 times the control dose of isoproterenol was required to achieve control level hemodynamics (95). In a canine model, 15 times the standard dose of isoproterenol was required to overcome a dose of 1 mg/kg of propranolol (96). In case reports, isoproterenol doses as high as 800 μg/minute have been used to treat beta-blocker overdose (97). Physiologic parameters should guide the dose of any sympathomimetic drug (e.g., blood pressure higher than 90 mm Hg, urine output 1 to 2 ml/kg/hour) rather than absolute drug doses.

Epinephrine, with its combined α- and β-agonist properties, theoretically would be the sympathomimetic of choice. As with other sympathomimetics, large doses of epinephrine have been required (98). In a retrospective review of 39 cases of overdose involving eight different beta-blockers (99), epinephrine increased the pulse rate in four of the six patients in whom it was used and increased the blood pressure in three patients, isoproterenol increased the pulse rate in three patients in whom it was used and increased the BP in four patients, and dopamine had no effect on pulse rate but increased the BP in one of the three patients in whom it was used. Epinephrine has the added benefit of α-adrenergic stimulation that would cause some peripheral vasoconstriction.

Other β-agonists, including dopamine and norepinephrine (α- and β-agonist activity) and dobutamine (β_1-agonist), have shown mixed results. Various authors recommend using either epinephrine or isoproterenol as the initial sympathomimetic and then adding one of the other agents depending on clinical response.

Phosphodiesterase inhibitors (PDI) have also been used in the management of beta-blocker overdose. They increase intracellular concentrations of cyclic adenosine monophosphate by inhibiting its breakdown by phosphodiesterase. Agents that have been reported to be useful include amrinone, enoximone, and aminophylline. In a canine model of beta-blocker poisoning, PDIs did not show improved efficacy over the use of glucagon alone (100,101), but, in case reports, patients who did not improve with glucagon did improve with PDIs (2,102). The use of a PDI should be considered if other modalities fail.

The successful use of calcium has been reported (103,104). Beta-blockers exert their negative inotropic effects via a calcium-mediated mechanism in the heart and also decrease serum calcium. The use of calcium in a 1- to 2-g IV bolus would seem reasonable once digitalis toxicity has been ruled out. Calcium infusions have been used.

In a canine model, the use of high-dose insulin (the equivalent of 720 units/hour) and enough glucose to maintain euglycemia were shown to have at least equal efficacy to glucagon (105) (Chapter 6).

Supportive Care

The experience with the use of pacemakers has been disappointing. Although pacemakers increase the heart rate, the blood pressure does not rise concomitantly. There have been case reports of patients who failed to respond to any other therapy being successfully treated with an intraaortic balloon pump or extracorporeal circulation (7,106). These patients made full recoveries despite their extended periods of hypotension or arrest.

Seizures are treated in the usual manner with benzodiazepines, followed by phenytoin and more invasive procedures for patients with refractory seizures (Chapter 40). Bronchospasm is treated by inhaled β-agonist therapy. Use of parenteral epinephrine can also be considered. Hypoglycemia has been reported rarely in adults but seems to be significantly more common in children (107). Therapy includes the use of frequent monitoring and IV glucose. There has been one case report of a child with depressed mental status who responded to IV glucose despite having a normal serum glucose concentration (108).

Monitoring

The onset of clinical toxicity from beta-blocker overdose is less than 6 hours (108–110), typically less than 4 hours. This timeframe may not be accurate if the ingestion involves modified-release preparations or co-ingestants that reduce GI motility. If these complicating conditions are absent, patients with beta-blocker ingestions who are stable at 6 hours can be discharged from the emergency department from a medical standpoint (109).

REFERENCES

1. Love JN, Litovitz TL, Howell JM, et al. Characterization of fatal beta blocker ingestion: a review of the American Association of Poison Control Centers Data from 1985 to 1995. *Clin Toxicol* 1997;35:353–359.
2. Kollef MH. Labetalol overdose successfully treated with amrinone and alpha-adrenergic receptor agonists. *Chest* 1994;105:626–627.
3. Love JN. Acebutolol overdose resulting in fatalities. *J Emerg Med* 2000;18(3):341–344.
4. Frishman W, Jacob H, Eisenberg E, et al. Appraisal and reappraisal of cardiac therapy: clinical pharmacology of the new β-adrenergic blocking drugs. Part 8: self-poisoning with β-adrenoreceptor blocking agents: recognition and management. *Am Heart J* 1979;98:798–811.
5. Hong CY, Yang WC, Chiang BN. Importance of membrane stabilizing effect in massive overdose of propranolol: plasma level study in a fatal case. *Hum Toxicol* 1983;3:511–517.
6. Wolf LR. β-Adrenergic blocker toxicity. In: Haddad LM, Shannon MW, Winchester JF. *Clinical management of poisoning and drug overdose*, 3rd ed. Philadelphia: WB Saunders, 1998:1032.
7. Rooney M, Massey KL, Jamali F, et al. Acebutolol overdose treated with hemodialysis and extracorporeal membrane oxygenation. *J Clin Pharmacol* 1996;36:760–763.
8. Saugster B, de Wildt D, van Dijk A. A case of acebutolol intoxication. *Clin Toxicol* 1983;20:69–77.
9. Booth RJ, Wilson JD, Bullock JY. β-adrenergic-receptor blockers and antinuclear antibodies in hypertension. *Clin Pharmacol Ther* 1982;31:555–558.
10. Tanner LA, Bosco LA, Zimmerman HJ. Hepatic toxicity after acebutolol therapy. *Ann Intern Med* 1989;111:533–534.
11. Akoun GM, Herman DP, Mayaud CM. Acebutolol-induced hypersensitivity pneumonitis. *BMJ* 1983;286:266–267.

12. Leggett RJE. Pleurisy and pulmonary granulomas after treatment with acebutolol. *BMJ* 1982;285:1425.
13. Montgomery AB, Stager MA, Schoene RB. Marked suppression of ventilation while awake following massive ingestion of atenolol. *Chest* 1985;88(6):920–921.
14. Abbasi IA, Sorsby S. Prolonged toxicity from atenolol in an adolescent. *Clin Pharmacol* 1986;5:876–877.
15. Wolf R, Ophir J, Elman M, et al. Atenolol-induced cutaneous vasculitis. *Cutis* 1989;(43):231–233.
16. Doherty CC, McGeown MG, Donaldson RA. Retroperitoneal fibrosis after treatment with atenolol. *BMJ* 1978;(2):1786.
17. Johnson JN, McFarland J. Retroperitoneal fibrosis associated with atenolol. *BMJ* 1980;(280):864.
18. McGuiness M, Frye RA, b Deng J-S. Atenolol-induced lupus erythematosus. *J Am Acad Dermatol* 1997;(37):298–299.
19. Berthault F, Kintz P, Tracqui A, et al. A fatal case of betaxolol poisoning. *J Anal Toxicol* 1997;21:228–231.
20. Chamberlain TJ. Myocardial infarction after ophthalmic betaxolol. *N Engl J Med* 1989;321:1342.
21. Zabel RJ, MacDonald IM. Sinus arrest associated with betaxolol ophthalmic drops. *Am J Ophthalmol* 1987;104:431.
22. Fraunfelder FT, Meyer SM, Menacker SJ. Alopecia possibility secondary to topical ophthalmic B-blockers. *JAMA* 1990;263:1493–1494.
23. Hardee JT, Roldan CA, Du Clos TW. Betaxolol and drug-induced lupus complicated by pericarditis and large pericardial effusion. *West J Med* 1997;167:106–109.
24. Betoptic, betaxolol [package insert]. Forth Worth: Aicon Pharmaceuticals.
25. Tracqui A, Kintz D, Mangin P, et al. Self poisoning with the beta blocker bisoprolol. *Hum Exp Toxicol* 1990;9:255–256.
26. Hanston P, Lambermont SY, Simoens G, et al. Carvedilol overdose. *Acta Cardiologica* 1997;52(4):369–371.
27. Fernandez HH, Friedman JH. Carvedilol-induced myoclonus [Letter]. *Mov Disord* 1999;14(4):703.
28. Coreg (R), carvedilol [package insert]. Research Triangle Park, NC: GlaxoSmithKline (P1 revised November 2001).
29. Kowalski BJ, Cody RJ. Stevens-Johnson syndrome associated with carvedilol therapy. *Am J Cardiol* 1997;80:669–670.
30. Sung RJ, Blanski L, Kirshenbaum J, et al. Clinical experience with esmolol, a short acting beta-adrenergic blocker in cardiac dysrhythmias and myocardial infarction. *J Clin Pharmacol* 1986;26[Suppl A]:A15–A26.
31. Anderson S, Blanski L, Byrd RC, et al. Comparison of the efficacy and safety of esmolol, a short-acting beta-blocker, with placebo I the treatment of supraventricular tachyarrhythmias: the esmolol vs placebo multicenter study group. *Am Heart J* 1986;111:42–48.
32. Zarolinski J, Borgman RJ, O'Donnell JP, et al. Ultra-short acting beta-blockers: a proposal for the treatment of the critically ill patient. *Life Sci* 1982;31:899–907.
33. Litman RS, Zerngast BA. Cardiac arrest after esmolol administration: a review of beta-blocker toxicity. 1996;96(10):616–618.
34. Das G, Ferris JC. Generalized convulsions in a patient receiving ultrashort-acting beta-blocker infusion. *Drug Intel Clin Pharmacy* 1988;22:484–485.
35. Smit AJ, Mulder POM, de Jong PE, et al. Acute renal failure after overdose of labetalol. *BMJ* 1986;293:1142–1143.
36. Korzets A, Danby P, Edmunds ME, et al. Acute renal failure associated with a labetalol overdose. *Postgrad Med J* 1990;66:66–67.
37. Hamad A, Salameh M, Zihif M, et al. Life threatening hyperkalemia after intravenous labetalol injection for hypertensive emergency in a hemodialysis patient. *American J Nephrol* 2001;21:241–244.
38. Arthur S, Greenberg A. Hyperkalemia associated with intravenous labetalol therapy for acute hypertension in renal transplant recipients. *Clin Nephrol* 1990;33:269–271.
39. Stricker BH, Heijermans HSF, Braat H, et al. Fever induced by labetalol. *JAMA* 1986;256:619–620.
40. Douglas DD, Yang RD, Jensen P, et al. Fatal labetalol-induced hepatic injury. *Am J Med* 1989;87:235–236.
41. Teicher A, Rosenthal T, Kissin E, et al. Labetalol-induced toxic myopathy. *BMJ* 1982;282:1824–1825.
42. Bolli P, Waal-Manning HJ, Wood AJ, et al. Experience with labetalol in hypertension. *Br J Clin Pharmacol* 1976;3[Suppl 3]:765.
43. Shore ET, Cepin D, Davidson MJ. Metoprolol overdose. *Ann Emerg Med* 1981;10:524–527.
44. Wallin CJ, Hulting J. Massive metoprolol poisoning treated with prenalterol. *Acta Med Scand* 1983;214:253–255.
45. Anonymous. The American Academy of Pediatrics Committee on Drugs: the transfer of drugs and other chemicals into human milk. *Pediatrics* 1994;93:137–150.
46. Krikorian RK, Quick A, Tal A. Angioedema following the intravenous administration of metoprolol. *Chest* 1994;105:1922–1923.
47. Emara MK, Saadah AM. The carpal tunnel syndrome in hypertensive patients treated with beta-blockers. *Postgrad Med J* 1988;64:191–192.
48. Ahmad S. Association of metoprolol and retroperitoneal fibrosis. *Am Heart J* 1996;131:202–203.
49. Ehgartner GR, Zelinka MA. Hemodynamic instability following intentional nadolol overdose. *Arch Intern Med* 1988;148:801–802.
50. O'Donoghue DJ. Acute pancreatitis due to nadolol-induced hypertriglyceridemia. *Br J Clin Prac* 1989;43:74–75.
51. Kaul S, Wong M, Singh BN, et al. Nadolol and papilledema. *Ann Intern Med* 1982;97:454.
52. Levy MB, Fink JN, Guzzetta PA. Nadolol and hypersensitivity pneumonitis. *Ann Intern Med* 1986;105:806–807.
53. Thorpe P. Pindolol in hypertension. *Med J Australia* 1971;58:1242.
54. Langemeijer JJM, de Wildt DJ, de Groot, et al. Centrally induced respiratory arrest: main cause of death in beta-adrenoceptor antagonist intoxication [Letter]. *Hum Toxicol* 1986;5:65.
55. Weinstein RS, Cole S, Knaster HB, et al. Beta-blocker overdose with propranolol and with atenolol. *Ann Emerg Med* 1985;14:161–163.
56. Binkley PR, Lewe R, Lima J, et al. Enhanced ventricular ectopy following pindolol: an adverse effect of a beta blocker with intrinsic sympathomimetic activity. *Am Heart J* 1986;112:424–426.
57. Hod H, Kaplinsky N, Har-Zahav J, et al. Pindolol-induced tremor. *Postgrad Med J* 1980;56:346–347.
58. Koller W, Orebaugh C, Lawson, et al. Pindolol-induced tremor. *Clin Neuropharmacol* 1987;10:449–452.
59. Morgan LK. Restless legs: precipitated by beta blockers, relieved by orphenadrine. *Med J Australia* 1975;2:753.
60. Yatham LN, Lint D, Lam RW, et al. Adverse effects of pindolol augmentation in patients with bipolar depression [Letter]. *J Clin Psychopharmacol* 1999;19(4):383–384.
61. Musk AW, Pollard JA. Pindolol and pulmonary fibrosis. *BMJ* 1979;2:581–582.
62. Bensaid J, Aldigier SC, Gualde N. Systemic lupus erythematosus syndrome induced by pindolol. *BMJ* 1979;1:1603–1604.
63. Reith DM, Dawson AH, Epid D, et al. Relative toxicity of beta blockers in overdose. *Clin Toxicol* 1996;34:273–278.
64. Suarez RV, Greenwald MS, Geraghty E. Intentional overdosage with propranolol: a report of two cases. *Am J Foren Med Pathol* 1988;9:45–47.
65. Tynan F, Fisher MM, Ibels L. Self-poisoning with propranolol. *Med J Australia* 1981;1:82–83.
66. Weinstein RS, Cole S, Knaster HB, et al. Beta-blocker overdose with propranolol and with atenolol. *Ann Emerg Med* 1985;14:161–163.
67. Cruickshank JM. The clinical importance of cardioselectivity and lipophilicity in beta-blockers. *Am Heart J* 1980;100:160.
68. Briggs GG, Freeman RK, Yaffe SJ. *Drugs in pregnancy and lactation*, 5th ed. Baltimore: Williams & Wilkins, 1998.
69. Drayer JI, Zegarelli EC. Hypertension and pregnancy. *Cardiovascular Clin* 1989;19:97–111.
70. Nawabi IU, Ritz ND. Agranulocytosis due to propranolol. *JAMA* 1973;223:1376.
71. Harris A. Long term treatment of paroxysmal cardiac arrhythmias with propranolol. *Am J Cardiol* 1966;18:431–437.
72. Pettei MJ, Levy J, Abramson S. Nonocclusive mesenteric ischemia associated with propranolol overdose: implications regarding splanchnic circulation. *J Pediatr Gastroenterol Nutr* 1990;10:544–547.
73. Emara MK, Saadah AM. The carpal tunnel syndrome in hypertensive patients treated with beta-blockers. *Postgrad Med J* 1988;64:191–192.
74. Love JN, Handler JA. Toxic psychosis: an unusual presentation of propranolol intoxication. *Am J Emerg Med* 1995;13:536–537.
75. Eligs MA, Lockhart CH. Perioperative hypoglycemia in a child treated with propranolol. *Anesthesia Analg* 1984;62:1035–1037.
76. Chavez H, Ozolins D, Losek JD. Hypoglycemia and propranolol in pediatric behavioral disorders. *Pediatrics* 1999;103:1290–1292.
77. Henri L, Groleau M. Retroperitoneal fibrosis after treatment with propranolol. *Drug Intell Clin Pharmocol* 1981;15:696.
78. Botet C, Grau J, Benito P, et al. Timolol ophthalmic solution and respiratory arrest. *Ann Intern Med* 1986;105:306.
79. Adler AG, McElwain GE, Merli GJ, et al. Systemic effects of eye drops. *Arch Intern Med* 1982;142:2293–2294.
80. Britman NA. Cardiac effects of topical timolol. *N Engl J Med* 1979;300:300–566.
81. Fraunfelder FT. Ocular beta-blockers and systemic effects. *Arch Intern Med* 1986;146:1073–1074.
82. Hayes LP, Stewart CJ, Kim I, et al. Timolol side effects and inadvertent overdosing. *JAGS* 1989;37:261–262.
83. Linkewich JA, Merling IM. Bradycardia and congestive heart failure associated with ocular timolol maleate. *Am J Hosp Pharmacol* 1981;38:699–701.
84. McMahon CD, Shaffer RN, Hoskins HD, et al. Adverse effects experienced by patients taking timolol. *Am J Ophthalmol* 1979;88:736–738.
85. Nelson WL, Fraunfelde FT, Sills JM, et al. Adverse respiratory and cardiovascular events attributed to timolol ophthalmic solution, 1978–1985. *Am J Ophthalmol* 1986;102:606–611.
86. Fraunfelder FT, Meyer SM, Menacker SJ. Alopecia possibly secondary to topical ophthalmic beta blockers [Letter]. *JAMA* 1990;263:1493–1494.
87. Bouffard Y, Ritter J, Delafosse B, et al. Intoxication a l'atenolol? Etude d'une observation avec dosages plasmatiquest. *J Toxicol Med* 1984;273–277.
88. Sartz R, Williams BW, Farber HW. Atenolol induced cardiovascular collapse treated with hemodialysis. *Crit Care Med* 1991;19(1):116–118.
89. Salhanick SD, Wax PM. Treatment of atenolol overdose in a patient with renal failure using serial hemodialysis and hemoperfusion and associated electrocardiographic findings. *Vet Human Toxicol* 2000;42(4):224–225.
90. McKinney P, Lawrence L. Nadolol toxicity treated with hemodialysis. *J Toxicol Clin Toxicol* 1995;33:517(abst).
91. Anthony T, Jastremski M, Elliott W, et al. Charcoal hemoperfusion for the treatment of a combined diltiazem and metoprolol overdose. *Ann Emerg Med* 1986;15:1344–1348.
92. Anonymous. Position statement and practice guidelines on the use of multi-

dose activated charcoal in the treatment of acute poisoning. *Clin Toxicol* 1999;37(6):731–751.

93. O'Mahony D, O'Leary P, Molloy MG. Severe oxprenolol poisoning: the importance of glucagon infusion. *Human Exp Toxicol* 1990;9:101–103.
94. Burda AM, Kapustka CA. Reformulated glucagon diluent phenol-free [Letter]. *Clin Toxicol* 1999;37:127.
95. Richards DA, Prichard BNC, Boakes AJ, et al. Pharmacological basis for antihypertensive effects of intravenous labetalol. *Br Heart J* 1977;39:99.
96. Avery GJ, Spotnitz HM, Rose EA, et al. Pharmacologic antagonism of beta-adrenergic blockade in dogs: I. Hemodynamic effects of isoproterenol, dopamine, and epinephrine in acute propranolol administration. *J Thorac Cardio Surg* 1979;77:267.
97. Prichard BNC, Battersby LA, Cruickshank JM. Overdose with beta-adrenergic blocking agents. *Adverse Drug Reactions Ac Pois Rev* 1984;3:91–111.
98. Hicks PR, Rankin PN. Massive adrenaline doses in labetalol overdose. 1991;19(3):447–449.
99. Weinstein RS. Recognition and management of poisoning with beta-adrenergic blocking agents. *Ann Emerg Med* 1984;13:1123–1131.
100. Love JN, Leasure JA, Mundt DJ, et al. A comparison of amrinone and glucagon therapy for cardiovascular depression associated with propranolol toxicity in a canine model. *Clin Toxicol* 1992;30:339–412.
101. Sato S, Tsuji MH, Okubo N, et al. Combined use of glucagon and milrinone may not be preferable for severe propranolol poisoning in the canine model. *Clin Toxicol* 1995;33:337–342.
102. Hoeper MM, Boeker KHW. Overdose of metoprolol treated with enoximone [Letter]. *N Engl J Med* 1996;335:1535.
103. Henry M, Kay MM, Viccellio P. Cardiogenic shock associated with calcium-channel and beta blockers: reversal with intravenous calcium chloride. *Am J Emerg Med* 1985;3:334–336.
104. Brimacombe JR, Scully M, Swainston R. Propranolol overdose—a dramatic response to calcium chloride. *Med J Australia* 1991;155:267–268.
105. Kerns W II, Schroeder D, Williams C, et al. Insulin improves survival in a canine model of acute beta blocker toxicity. *Am J Emerg Med* 1997;29:748–757.
106. McVey FK, Corke CF. Extracorporeal circulation in the management of massive propranolol overdose. *Anaesthesia* 1991;46:744–746.
107. Hesse B, Pedersen JT. Hypoglycaemia after propranolol in children. *Acta Med Scand* 973;193:551–552.
108. Reith DM, Dawson AH, Epid D, et al. Relative toxicity of beta blockers in overdose. *Clin Toxicol* 1996;34:273–278.
109. Love JN, Howell JM, Litovitz TL, et al. Acute beta blocker overdose: factors associated with the development of cardiovascular morbidity. *Clin Toxicol* 2000;38:275–281.
110. Love JN. Beta blocker toxicity after overdose: when do symptoms develop in adults? *J Emerg Med* 1994;12:799–802.

CHAPTER 120

Class III Antidysrhythmic Agents

Amy L. Olson and Kennon Heard

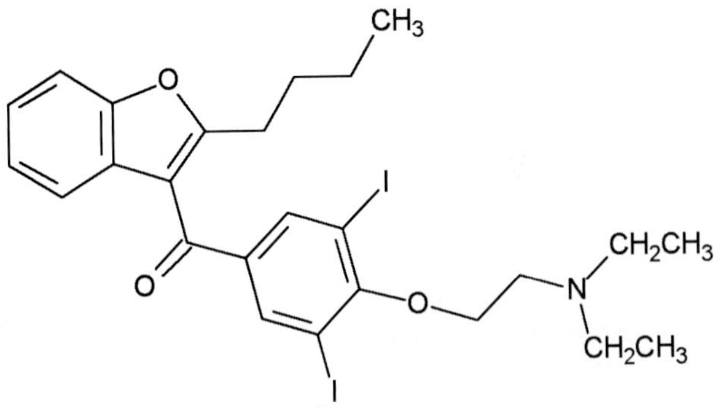

AMIODARONE

Compounds included:	**Amiodarone hydrochloride (Cordarone, Pacerone), sotalol hydrochloride (Betapace, Betapace AF)**
Molecular formula and weight:	**Amiodarone hydrochloride ($C_{25}H_{29}I_2NO_3$,HCl), 681.8 g/mol; sotalol hydrochloride ($C_{12}H_{20}N_2O_3S$,HCl), 308.8 g/mol**
SI conversion:	**Amiodarone, mg/L x 1.55 = µmol/L; sotalol, µg/ml x 3.67 = µmol/L**
CAS Registry No.:	**19774-82-4 (amiodarone); 959-24-0 (sotalol)**
Therapeutic levels:	**Amiodarone, 1.0 to 2.5 mg/L (1)**
Target organs:	**Heart (acute), lung (chronic)**
Antidotes:	**No specific antidotes; magnesium sulfate for treatment of torsade de pointes**

OVERVIEW

The class III (Vaughan-Williams classification) antidysrhythmic agents block cardiac potassium channels, prolonging the duration of the action potential by extending repolarization and the refractory period without affecting depolarization. The two medications in this class that are currently used are amiodarone and sotalol. These drugs are indicated for life-threatening, recurrent ventricular dysrhythmias. Amiodarone rarely causes life-threatening effects after acute overdose, but chronic toxicity is common. Sotalol overdose frequently results in severe cardiac toxicity.

AMIODARONE

Amiodarone hydrochloride (Cordarone) is a diiodinated benzofuran derivative. In addition to blocking cardiac potassium channels, amiodarone has weak α- and β-adrenergic antagonist activity as well as cardiac sodium and calcium-channel antagonist activity (2–4). Amiodarone is available in oral (200 mg) tablet form and in a parenteral preparation (50 mg/ml). It is effective for the treatment of atrial or ventricular dysrhythmias and tachycardia mediated via accessory pathways and is approved in the United States for life-threatening ventricular dysrhythmia that is refractory to other agents (4–6).

Toxic Dose

The adult therapeutic dose for the treatment of ventricular dysrhythmias starts with oral loading doses of 800 to 1600 mg/day for 1 to 3 weeks to establish adequate dysrhythmia control. The dose is then reduced to 600 to 800 mg/day for 1 month and then reduced further to a maintenance dose of 400 mg/day. A maintenance dose of 200 mg can be used for atrial fibrillation (7). The intravenous adult loading dose for the first 24 hours of therapy is 150 mg over the first 10 minutes followed by 360 mg over 6 hours (1 mg/minute) and then 540 mg over 18 hours (0.5 mg/minute). Then a maintenance infusion rate of 0.5 mg/minute should be continued until oral therapy is initiated (6). The safety and efficacy in pediatric patients have not been established (6).

Toxicokinetics and Toxicodynamics

The oral bioavailability is 22% to 86% (8,9). The reason for this wide range is not clear; however, it may be due in part to first-pass metabolism and the low solubility of amiodarone (8,10). The time to peak plasma levels (T_{max}) ranges from 2 to 12 hours (8). Amiodarone is 96% to 99% protein bound (11,12). The volume of distribution is 65 L/kg (13,14).

Amiodarone is eliminated by hepatic metabolism and biliary excretion (6,15). Dealkylation by the cytochrome P-450 system results in the metabolite desethylamiodarone (DEA) (11,16), which also has antidysrhythmic properties (17). Amiodarone and DEA are found in negligible amounts in the urine (18). The elimination half-life ranges from 3 to 80 hours (8). During chronic therapy, elimination half-life estimates have ranged from 13 to 107 days (8). The discrepancy in half-life estimation may be the result of initial uptake after a single oral dose into the large volume of distribution of peripheral sites and not true elimination (11,14). An alternative explanation may be that assays of plasma concentration are insensitive at the low concentrations that occur after single oral dosing and underestimate the true elimination half-life (14). During chronic therapy, the elimination half-life of DEA ranges from 20 to 118 days (13).

Amiodarone contains two iodine atoms (6,19). For every 200 mg administered, 75 mg is iodine. Approximately 10% is deiodinated to free iodine. This is a considerable amount of free iodine when compared to the average dietary iodine intake of 0.5 to 1.0 mg/day and may contribute to the development of thyroid abnormalities seen with amiodarone use (20).

Pathophysiology

Amiodarone blocks cardiac potassium channels, a class III effect. This prolongs phase 4 of the cardiac action potential and the refractory period of atrial and ventricular tissue. This effect is manifest on the electrocardiogram (ECG) by prolongation of the QT interval. Amiodarone possesses weak noncompetitive alpha- and beta-receptor blocking activity. This activity may result in bradycardia, PR prolongation, and atrioventricular (AV) heart block and can cause peripheral vasodilation. Amiodarone also has weak sodium channel–blocking properties in cardiac tissue, a class I effect, which results in a minor decrease in the upstroke velocity in phase 0 of depolarization. This effect is manifest on the ECG by prolongation of the QRS interval. Cardiac calcium-channel antagonist activity has also been reported, a class IV effect. This activity may have an effect on the sinus and AV node, causing bradycardia and AV heart block (4).

Amiodarone is structurally related to triiodothyronine (T_3) and thyroxine (T_4). Amiodarone has been shown to inhibit 5'-deiodinase activity, reducing peripheral conversion of T_4 to T_3, and may also block binding of T_3 to nuclear receptors (19). Some investigators believe that this may contribute to the antidysrhythmic properties of amiodarone (4).

Pregnancy and Lactation

Amiodarone is U.S. Food and Drug Administration pregnancy category D (Appendix I); however, it has been used in pregnancy for the treatment of maternal and fetal dysrhythmias. Amiodarone, DEA, and iodine cross the placenta, and reported adverse effects on the fetus have included congenital hypothyroidism, hyperthyroidism, mild neurodevelopmental abnormalities, intrauterine growth retardation, and fetal bradycardia (21,22). Amiodarone is excreted in human milk in significant quantities (6).

Clinical Presentation

ACUTE OVERDOSAGE

Acute toxicity from amiodarone overdosage is rare. Its poor bioavailability limits toxicity and prolongs the time to symptoms. Several case reports involve acute overdoses ranging from 2.6 to 15.0 g. No chronic sequelae or deaths were reported. The cardiovascular effects of the overdose included bradycardia, nonsustained atrial flutter, self-limiting ventricular tachycardia, and hypotension. The ECG revealed intermittent type I AV nodal conduction delay, QT prolongation, and changes mimicking an anteroseptal myocardial infarction. The onset of these effects occurred up to 2 days after ingestion (23–29).

A 67-year-old woman intentionally ingested 2.6 g amiodarone after the use of 200 mg/day for the prior week. The overdose did not produce clinical symptoms, and no dysrhythmias were noted during monitoring. A day after admission, the patient was noted to have ECG changes consistent with an anteroseptal myocardial infarction (transient loss of the R waves and T-wave inversion in leads V1 through V4) and QT-interval prolongation of 680 milliseconds. These changes reverted to baseline after hospital discharge (23). A 57-year-old woman ingested 5 g amiodarone after therapeutic use for 5 years, and prolonged hypotension developed that responded to an epinephrine infusion. Cardiac monitoring revealed a self-limited episode of atrial flutter, single ventricular premature contractions, intermittent type I AV block, and a prolonged QT interval of 500 milliseconds (24). An 18-year-old woman intentionally ingested 3.4 g, and one episode of self-limiting ventricular tachycardia developed (25).

No reports have been published of pulmonary toxicity, hypothyroidism, hyperthyroidism, hepatic toxicity, or ocular toxicity after an acute overdose. Therapeutic doses of intravenous amiodarone have reportedly caused hypotension when administered rapidly (6).

ADVERSE EVENTS

Chronic, relatively high-dose (400 mg/day) amiodarone therapy has produced numerous adverse reactions. Although up to 80% of patients have side effects due to therapy, only 10% to 15% require withdrawal of the drug because of toxicity (5). The most serious effects include amiodarone-induced pulmonary toxicity (AIPT), torsade de pointes, myxedema coma, and thyrotoxicosis. The incidence of AIPT ranges from 3% to 17% (26), and mortality ranges from 5% to 10% (20). Although the exact pathogenesis of AIPT remains unknown, it appears to be multifactorial (5). Evidence has shown that injury results from direct toxic effects of amiodarone, inflammatory processes, and immune mediated processes (27). AIPT can occur at any point in treatment, although the highest incidence occurs during the first 12 months of therapy (28). Risk factors include advanced age, lower pretreatment carbon monoxide diffusion capacity, higher maintenance dose, and higher plasma DEA concentrations during therapy (28).

AIPT has two distinct clinical forms (29). The more common form is characterized by the insidious onset of cough, dyspnea, fatigue, weight loss, pleuritic chest pain, and occasionally fevers. Chest radiographs reveal parenchymal infiltrates with a predominant interstitial pattern. The second, which occurs in approximately one-third of patients, is characterized by the acute onset of pulmonary symptoms and fever and may be caused by a hypersensitivity pneumonitis. Chest radiographs reveal patchy infiltrates with a predominant alveolar pattern. The diagnosis is one of exclusion. Two case reports have been published of fatal adult respiratory distress syndrome in patients who received amiodarone after the administration of intravenous contrast material for pulmonary angiography (30).

The incidence of cardiovascular toxicity ranges from 0% to 14% (20). Adverse reactions include bradycardia, conduction abnormalities within the AV node, and complete heart block (5). Amiodarone has been reported to be a prodysrhythmic, with an incidence of up to 5% (20); however, it is difficult to determine whether the dysrhythmia reported is caused by amiodarone or the underlying disease. The Canadian Amiodarone Myocardial Infarction Arrhythmia Trial reported a lower frequency of dysrhythmias in patients treated with amiodarone (0.3%) than those given placebo (3.0%) (31). Amiodarone may increase the threshold energy for defibrillation or cardioversion (32).

Although amiodarone does prolong the QT interval, the reported incidence of torsade de pointes is only 0% to 2.8% (33). No evidence has shown that patients with pretreatment prolonged QT intervals are predisposed to amiodarone-induced torsade de pointes; however, it does occur with increased frequency with extreme QT prolongation (600 milliseconds) (33), concurrent use of class IA antidysrhythmics, and hypokalemia (26).

Amiodarone also possesses negative inotropic action. The incidence of amiodarone-induced congestive heart failure is reported to be 1.8% in the United States and 0.2% in other countries (34). Hypotension has been reported to occur in up to 28% of patients who receive intravenous amiodarone, and it appears to be unrelated to the dose (35).

Clinically significant hypothyroidism occurs in approximately 10% of patients and has been reported to occur as early as 2 weeks and as late as 39 months after the initiation of therapy (19). Profound bradycardia may occur as a result of the additive effects of hypothyroidism and amiodarone therapy. Amiodarone-induced AV nodal block and myxedema coma have been reported (36).

Hyperthyroidism occurs in 3% of patients. It presents from 4 months to 3 years after the initiation of therapy (19). Hyperthyroidism should be suspected with clinical symptoms, recurrence of previously controlled cardiac dysrhythmias, or a resting heart rate that is greater than pretreatment heart rate. Amiodarone-induced thyrotoxicosis has been reported (37,38).

During the initial loading of amiodarone, gastrointestinal side effects are common and dose related. They include nausea, vomiting, anorexia, abdominal discomfort, constipation, and altered taste (20). Elevated aminotransferase and alkaline phosphatase levels develop in 25% of patients (5). Acute hepatitis has been reported after low cumulative doses and short treatment duration (less than 3 months). It is characterized by moderate to marked increase in serum transaminases, diversity of histologic lesions, and favorable course after discontinuation of the drug (39). Hepatic failure leading to death occurred in an 8-year-old girl (40) and three adults (two patients died after the intravenous initiation of therapy, and one patient died after 28 months of oral therapy) (41,42). Chronic liver disease is more common with high cumulative doses, and histologic changes are similar to those of alcoholic liver disease (39).

Allergic rash, photosensitivity, an unusual blue-gray skin discoloration, erythema nodosum, and alopecia have been described (5,43). Ophthalmologic symptoms occur in 0% to 14% of patients. The most common are halos around lights, as well as blurred vision, glare, dryness, and eyelid irritation (44). The most common finding is corneal microdeposits, which are universal in patients treated with amiodarone and do not cause vision loss. Optic neuropathy and optic neuritis, which has progressed to permanent blindness, have been reported (6,20).

Neurologic side effects appear to be dose related and include tremor, ataxia, peripheral neuropathy, fatigue, and weakness (5,43). Other rare effects include elevated serum creatinine (43), epididymitis (45,46), testicular dysfunction (47), thrombocytopenia (48), vasculitis (49,50), and polyserositis (50).

DRUG INTERACTIONS

Amiodarone frequently interacts with other drugs (5). Increased concentrations of digoxin, quinidine, procainamide, mexiletine, propafenone, phenytoin, and cyclosporin, and elevated prothrombin times in patients on warfarin, have been reported (20,51,52). Concurrent use of beta-blockers or calcium-channel blockers may cause significant sinus or AV nodal depression, and class I antidysrhythmics may result in drug-induced torsade de pointes (5,20). Anesthetic agents may potentiate bradycardia (53).

Diagnostic Tests

ACUTE OVERDOSAGE

Amiodarone serum levels may be useful in confirming the diagnosis but are not clinically useful. Acute overdosage has produced levels above the therapeutic range (1.0 to 2.5 mg/L) (1,54). ECG and cardiac monitoring may be necessary for 2 to 3 days after an acute ingestion. The cardiac effects of acute ingestion may occur several days after ingestion (23–25,54–57).

ADVERSE EVENTS

During therapy, plasma levels less than 1.0 mg/L were associated with recurrent dysrhythmias, and resolution of the dysrhythmia was seen in seven of eight patients after plasma levels above 1.0 mg/L were reached. Levels greater than 2.5 mg/L were associated with an increase in central nervous system effects (1), although this has not been confirmed in other studies (33). For patients on chronic therapy, plasma concentrations of amiodarone and DEA were not useful in guiding electrophysiologic, therapeutic, or toxic effects (58). However, patients in whom AIPT developed had higher plasma DEA concentrations during maintenance therapy than those patients in whom AIPT did not develop (2.34 vs. 1.92 mg/ml) (28).

Thyroid function tests should be obtained before the initiation of amiodarone therapy, every 6 months during therapy, and with any clinical symptoms suggestive of thyroid dysfunction (33). Because amiodarone inhibits 5'-deiodinase activity, reducing peripheral conversion of T_4 to T_3, and may also block binding of T_3 to nuclear receptors (19), abnormalities in thyroid function tests occur in virtually all patients (33). Thyroid function testing may reveal an elevation in T_4 and reverse T_3 and a decrease in T_3. Thyroid-stimulating hormone may initially be elevated but in most cases normalizes over time (19).

Liver function tests should be obtained at baseline and then every 6 months or with any clinical symptoms suggestive of hepatic dysfunction (26). Pulmonary function tests are recommended at baseline and then periodically to monitor for decreased carbon dioxide diffusion capacity and restrictive pathophysiology. Chest radiographs are recommended at baseline and then every 3 to 6 months, or with any clinical symptoms suggestive of AIPT (26). In chronic therapy, an ECG at baseline, 3 months, and then every 6 months is recommended (26), as monitoring may identify adverse reactions early (5).

Treatment

GASTROINTESTINAL DECONTAMINATION

As serious effects are rare after acute amiodarone ingestion, gastric emptying is not recommended. Activated charcoal may be useful. Activated charcoal (25 g) administered to volunteers 1.5 hours after ingestion reduced bioavailability of amiodarone by 50% (59).

ENHANCEMENT OF ELIMINATION

Multiple dose charcoal failed to accelerate elimination in a rodent model (60). Cholestyramine may increase elimination in chronic toxicity; however, the clinical significance of reduced half-life in chronic toxicity is unclear (61). Amiodarone is not dialyzable (6).

ANTIDOTES

No specific antidote to amiodarone toxicity is available.

MONITORING

Continuous cardiac monitoring in a cardiac care unit may be necessary for 2 to 3 days after an acute ingestion, as the toxic effects may be delayed (23–25,54–57).

SUPPORTIVE CARE

Bradycardia caused by amiodarone therapy has been reported to be resistant to atropine and is postulated to be the result of noncompetitive adrenergic antagonist activity (2). An amiodarone-induced sinus arrest was successfully treated with ephedrine and isoproterenol (53); however, temporary cardiac pacing may be required.

Hypotension should be treated with vasopressor support including dopamine and norepinephrine. Amiodarone-induced torsade de pointes is treated emergently with atrial overdrive pacing (62), isoproterenol (63), magnesium, and correction of electrolyte disturbances. A case report of amiodarone-induced torsade de pointes responded to a bolus and subsequent infusion of magnesium (64).

Because AIPT has a mortality of 5% to 10% (54), the recommended treatment is discontinuation of the drug (65). Drug withdrawal usually results in reversal of the toxicity, improved pulmonary function, and resolution of radiographic abnormalities (66). The risks and benefits of this therapeutic option must be examined, as the mortality associated with underlying dysrhythmia may be higher than that from pulmonary toxicity (67). Dose reduction may be an alternative, as there are reports of clinical improvement with this therapeutic option (65). Case reports have been published of patients with pulmonary toxicity who were maintained on amiodarone therapy and improved with the addition of steroids (65); however, this remains controversial.

Amiodarone-induced hypothyroidism responds to T_4 treatment, if amiodarone therapy must be continued. For elderly patients and those with underlying cardiovascular disease, it is recommended that one start at low replacement doses of 25 mg T_4 daily to prevent cardiac overstimulation (68). Hyperthyroidism generally responds to conventional treatment with propylthiouracil, methimazole, and propranolol (19). Thyrotoxicosis has been more challenging to treat, as the thyroid gland may be unresponsive to radioactive iodine as a result of the iodine overload of amiodarone therapy, and thyroidectomy in thyrotoxic cardiac patients may be dangerous (37). Prednisone and plasmapheresis each in combination with thionamides have been investigated as treatment strategies (38). A case report of two patients with amiodarone-induced thyrotoxicosis treated with methimazole and plasmapheresis resulted in resolution of symptoms despite elevated free T_3 and T_4 concentrations (37).

SOTALOL

Sotalol is considered a class III antidysrhythmic, as it blocks cardiac potassium channels. Sotalol also possesses β-adrenergic antagonist activity. It is a racemic mixture of the D- and the L-isomer. Both isomers have the class III antidysrhythmic property, whereas the L-isomer possesses the class II antidysrhythmic effects. Sotalol is indicated for treatment of life-threatening ventricular dysrhythmias and for maintenance of normal sinus rhythm after cardioversion of symptomatic atrial fibrillation or atrial flutter. Sotalol is available for oral use in 80-mg, 120-mg, 160-mg, and 240-mg tablets and in a parenteral preparation. Betapace and Betapace AF are both sotalol hydrochloride.

Toxic Dose

The initial adult therapeutic dose is 80 mg orally twice a day. Initiation and up-titration of therapy should be done in the hospital with cardiac monitoring. A therapeutic response is generally seen at total daily doses of 160 to 320 mg, although doses as high as 640 mg/day have been used in patients with refractory, life-threatening ventricular dysrhythmias (69). Sotalol should be dosed according to creatinine clearance, as it is primarily eliminated through renal excretion (69). Sotalol is not approved for children, but doses of 30 mg/m^2 orally three times a day titrated to a maximum dose of 60 mg/m^2 have been used.

Toxicokinetics and Toxicodynamics

The oral bioavailability of sotalol is approximately 90% to 100% (69–73). The T_{max} is 2 to 4 hours (69,74–77), and plasma concentrations are proportionally related to the dose (78,79). Sotalol is not bound to plasma proteins (70). The volume of distribution is 1.2 to 2.4 L/kg (77,78).

Sotalol is eliminated primarily through renal excretion (80–90%); a small amount is excreted in the feces (69,77,78). The renal clearance is approximately equal to the creatinine clearance. In patients with normal renal function, the clearance of sotalol is approximately 150 ml/minute (70). The clearance of sotalol is not dependent on hepatic metabolism (80). The elimination half-life ranges from 10 to 20 hours (70,72,77,78,81). The D-sotalol isomer and D,L-sotalol mixture have similar pharmacokinetics (78,82).

Pathophysiology

Both isomers of sotalol block cardiac potassium channels, a class III effect, resulting in extended repolarization, prolongation of the refractory period in atrial and ventricular tissue, and prolongation of the QT interval on the ECG. The L-isomer of sotalol also possesses nonselective β-adrenergic antagonist activity. It lacks intrinsic sympathomimetic activity and membrane-stabilizing properties. The β-adrenergic antagonist activity may cause bradycardia and AV heart block and can result in peripheral vasodilation (69,83,84).

Pregnancy and Lactation

Sotalol is U.S. Food and Drug Administration pregnancy category B (Appendix I). Sotalol crosses the placenta (69). It has been used for the treatment of fetal dysrhythmias (85). Reported adverse effects on the fetus during maternal use include low birth weight (69,79). Sotalol is excreted in human milk in significant quantities (86).

Clinical Presentation

ACUTE OVERDOSAGE

Severe intoxication with β-adrenergic antagonist drugs may result in profound bradycardia, hypotension, and low-output cardiogenic shock. Because sotalol also possesses class III antidysrhythmic effects, it can prolong the QT interval, leading to an increased susceptibility to torsade de pointes and ventricular fibrillation. Cardiovascular effects with acute intoxication include bradycardia, asystole, prolongation of the QT interval, premature ventricular contractions, torsade de pointes, ventricular tachycardia, ventricular fibrillation, and hypotension. In case reports, the amount ingested has ranged from 2.0 to 14.4 g (87–91).

Neuvonen et al. (87) reviewed six patients with acute sotalol toxicity. The dose ingested ranged from 2.4 to 8.0 g. All six patients had QT-interval prolongation at presentation, which ranged from 30 minutes to 4.5 hours after ingestion. The QT interval continued to lengthen up to 15 hours after the ingestion and then resolved over 4 days. The cardiac dysrhythmias observed included premature ventricular contractions, torsade de pointes, ventricular tachycardia, and ventricular fibrillation. The risk of severe dysrhythmia was highest from 4 hours to 20 hours after ingestion. The occurrence of dysrhythmias correlated with the prolongation of the QT interval and the serum concentration (87).

Alderfliegel et al. (89) describe the case of a 70-year-old woman who ingested 6.72 g sotalol and presented with bradycardia. The patient was initially treated with activated charcoal, glucagon, atropine, and isoproterenol; was resuscitated from two asystolic cardiac arrests; and recovered with dopamine and ventricular pacing (89).

A 47-year-old man ingested 3.2 g sotalol and presented with agitation, seizures, bradycardia with premature ventricular contractions, and hypotension. He experienced cardiac arrest, which was treated with external cardiac massage, intracardiac epinephrine, sodium bicarbonate, and tromethamine. Thereafter, he had multiple episodes of cardiac arrest and ventricular fibrillation, which became refractory to defibrillation, and died 7 hours after admission (90).

ADVERSE EVENTS

In data submitted for approval of sotalol, the overall incidence of torsade de pointes was 2.4%. In patients with a history of sustained ventricular tachycardia, the incidence of torsade de pointes was 4.1%, and the risk of torsade de pointes was related proportionally to the dose and the prolongation of the QT interval (69,92).

The most frequently reported adverse reactions leading to discontinuation of the drug were fatigue, bradycardia, dyspnea, prodysrhythmia, asthenia, and dizziness (69). No evidence of other organ toxicity has been found (92).

DRUG INTERACTIONS

No drug interactions were reported in the data submitted for the approval of sotalol (92). However, class I and other class III antidysrhythmic agents can potentially prolong the refractory period and cause tachydysrhythmias. Other drugs known to prolong the QT interval should be used with caution. Additionally, sotalol may potentiate the effects of other β-adrenergic antagonist agents (69).

Diagnostic Tests

Sotalol levels may be useful in confirming the diagnosis. A patient presented with a prolonged QT interval and torsade de pointes of unknown cause and was subsequently diagnosed with surreptitious use of sotalol after a level was obtained (93).

Serum electrolytes should be measured and corrected. In a case report, a patient ingested 13 to 14 g sotalol and was noted to have increasing prolongation of the QT interval and ventricular tachycardia despite reduction in the serum sotalol levels. The serum potassium was 3.8 mEq/L; however, the patient's condition improved after infusion of potassium, with resolution of the episodes of sustained ventricular tachycardia. This suggests that intracellular hypokalemia may potentiate ventricular dysrhythmias (94). Serial ECGs and continuous cardiac monitoring may be necessary for several days after an acute ingestion.

Postmortem Considerations

The tissue concentrations of sotalol were six times those of the plasma levels (91).

Treatment

GASTROINTESTINAL DECONTAMINATION

Gastric lavage should be considered for patients who present within 60 minutes of a large ingestion. Because of the potential for cardiovascular instability, airway management should be considered before lavage in symptomatic patients. Induced emesis should not be used. Activated charcoal binds sotalol. In a study by Karkkainen and Neuvonen (95), absorption of sotalol was reduced 99% in volunteers who ingested 160 mg sotalol, followed by immediate ingestion of 50 g activated charcoal (92).

ENHANCEMENT OF ELIMINATION

Sotalol is dialyzable (69). Hemodialysis was attempted after a sotalol overdose of 14.4 g. Multiple-dose activated charcoal has been shown to increase elimination of sotalol after a single therapeutic dose (92).

ANTIDOTES

No specific antidote is available for acute sotalol toxicity. Patients with the manifestations of bradycardia, heart block, and hypotension should be treated with standard treatment for beta-blocker toxicity, such as β-adrenergic agonists, phosphodiesterase inhibitors (milrinone), and glucagon (Chapter 119).

Patients with torsade de pointes should be treated with magnesium sulfate and overdrive pacing. Other forms of ventricular tachycardia are treated with lidocaine as the first agent. Phenytoin should be considered if ventricular dysrhythmias persist. Procainamide and disopyramide should be avoided because of the possibility of additive effects.

SUPPORTIVE CARE

Seizures are treated in the usual manner with benzodiazepines, followed by phenytoin and more invasive procedures in patients with refractory seizures (Chapter 40).

MONITORING

Serial ECGs and continuous cardiac monitoring in a cardiac care unit may be necessary for several days after an acute ingestion. Neuvonen et al. (87) found that the risk of severe dysrhythmias was highest 4 to 20 hours after ingestion.

REFERENCES

1. Haffajee CI , Love JC, Canada AT, et al. Clinical pharmacokinetics and efficacy of amiodarone for refractory tachyarrhythmias. *Circulation* 1983;67:1347–1355.
2. Charlier R, Deltour G, Baudine A, et al. Pharmacology of amiodarone, an anti-anginal drug with a new biological profile. *Arzheimittleforsch* 1968;183:1408–1417.
3. Singh BM, Vaughan Williams EM. The effect of amiodarone, a new anti-anginal drug, on cardiac muscle. *Br J Pharmacol* 1970;39:657–667.
4. Kowey PR, Marinchak RA, Rials SJ, et al. Pharmacologic and pharmacokinetic profile of class III antiarrhythmic drugs. *Am J Cardiol* 1997;80:16G–23G.
5. Podrid PJ. Amiodarone. Reevaluation of an old drug. *Ann Intern Med* 1995;122:689–700.
6. Product Information, Cordarone. Wyeth Laboratories, Inc. Revised August 1, 2000.
7. Connolly SJ. Evidence-based analysis of amiodarone efficacy and safety. *Circulation* 1999;100:2025–2034.
8. Latini R, Togono G, Kates RE. Clinical pharmacokinetics of amiodarone. *Clin Pharmacol* 1984;9:136–156.
9. Riva E, Gerna M, Latini R, et al. Pharmacokinetics of amiodarone in man. *J Cardiovasc Pharmacol* 1982;4:264–269.
10. Riva E, Gerna M, Neyroz P, et al. Pharmacokinetics of amiodarone in rats. *J Cardiovasc Pharmacol* 1982;4:270–275.
11. Freedman MD, Somberg JC. Pharmacology and pharmacokinetics of amiodarone. *J Clin Pharmacol* 1991;31:1061–1069.
12. Lalloz MRA, Byfield PGH, Greenwood RM, et al. Binding of amiodarone by serum proteins and the effects of drugs, hormones, and other interacting ligands. *J Pharm Pharmacol* 1984;36:366–372.
13. Holt DW, Tucker GT, Jackson PR, et al. Amiodarone pharmacokinetics. *Am Heart J* 1983;106:840–847.
14. Roden DM. Pharmacokinetics of amiodarone: implications for drug therapy. *Am J Cardiol* 1993;72:45F–50F.
15. Andreasen F, Agerbaek H, Bjerregaard P, et al. Pharmacokinetics of amiodarone after intravenous and oral administration. *Eur J Clin Pharmacol* 1981;19:293–299.
16. Flanagan RJ, Storey GCA, Holt DW, et al. Identification and measurement of desethylamiodarone in blood plasma specimens from amiodarone-treated patients. *J Pharm Pharmacol* 1982;34:638–643.
17. Yabek SM, Kato R, Singh BN. Effects of amiodarone and its metabolite, desethylamiodarone, on the electrophysiologic properties of isolated cardiac muscle. *J Cardiovasc Pharmacol* 1986;8:197–207.
18. Harris L, Hind CRK, McKenna WJ, et al. Renal elimination of amiodarone and its desethyl metabolite. *Postgrad Med J* 1983;59:440–442.
19. Nademanee K, Piwonka RW, Singh BN, et al. Amiodarone and thyroid function. *Prog Cardiovasc Dis* 1989;31:427–437.
20. Wilson JS, Podrid PJ. Side effects from amiodarone. *Am Heart J* 1991;121(1 Pt 1):158–171.
21. Bartalena L, Bogazzi F, Braverman LE, et al. Effects of amiodarone administration during pregnancy of neonatal thyroid function and subsequent neurodevelopment. *J Endocrinol Invest* 2001;24:116–130.
22. Magee LA, Downar E, Sermer M, et al. Pregnancy outcome after gestational exposure to amiodarone in Canada. *Am J Obstet Gynecol* 1995;172:1307–1311.
23. Oreto G, Lapresa V, Melluso C, et al. [Acute amiodarone poisoning. Description of a case.] [French]. *Arch Mal Coeur Vaiss* 1980;73:857–860.
24. Reingardene DI. [A case of acute poisoning by amiodarone.] [Russian]. *Anesteziologiaa I Reanimatologiia* 1989;4:62–63.
25. Goddard CJ, Whorewell PJ. Amiodarone overdose and its management. *Br J Clin Pract* 1989;43(5):184–186.
26. Hilleman D, Miller MA, Parker R, et al. Optimal management of amiodarone therapy: efficacy and side effects. *Pharmacotherapy* 1998;18(6 Pt 2):138S–145S.
27. Martin WJ, Rosenow EC. Amiodarone pulmonary toxicity. Recognition and pathogenesis (Pt 2). *Chest* 1988;93:1242–1248.
28. Dusman RE, Stanton MS, Miles WM, et al. Clinical features of amiodarone-induced pulmonary toxicity. *Circulation* 1990;82:51–59.
29. Martin WJ, Rosenow EC. Amiodarone pulmonary toxicity. Recognition and pathogenesis (Pt I). *Chest* 1988;93:1067–1073.
30. Woods DL, Osborn MJ, Rooke J, et al. Amiodarone pulmonary toxicity: report of two cases associated with rapidly progressive fatal adult respiratory distress syndrome after pulmonary angiography. *Mayo Clin Proc* 1985;60:601–603.
31. Cairnes JA, Connolly SJ, Roberts R, et al. Randomised trial of outcome after myocardial infarction in patients with frequent or repetitive ventricular premature depolarisations: CAMIAT. *Lancet* 1997;349:675–682.
32. Fogoros, RN. Amiodarone-induced refractoriness to cardioversion. *Ann Intern Med* 1984;100:699–700.
33. Mattioni TA. The proarrhythmic effects of amiodarone. *Prog Cardiovasc Dis* 1989;31:439–446.
34. Vrobel TR, Miller PE, Mostow ND, et al. A general overview of amiodarone toxicity: its prevention, detection, and management. *Prog Cardiovasc Dis* 1989;31:393–426.
35. Kowey PR. The IV Amiodarone Investigators: a multicentered-randomized double blind comparison of bretylium with amiodarone in patients with frequent malignant ventricular arrhythmia. *Circulation* 1993;88[Suppl 1]:I-370.
36. Mazonson PD, Williams ML, Cantley LK, et al. Myxedema coma during long-term amiodarone therapy. *Am J Med* 1984;77:751–754.
37. Aghini-Lombardi F, Mariotti S, Fosella PV, et al. Treatment of amiodarone iodine-induced thyrotoxicosis with plasmapheresis and methimazole. *J Endocrinol Invest* 1993;16:823–826.
38. Broussolle C, Ducottet X, Martin C, et al. Rapid effectiveness of prednisone and thionamides combined therapy in severe amiodarone iodine-induced thryotoxicosis. Comparison of two groups of patients with apparently normal thyroid glands. *J Endocrinol Invest* 1989;12:37–42.
39. Geneve J, Zafrani ES, Dhumeaux D. Amiodarone-induced liver disease. *J Hepatol* 1989;9:130–133.
40. Yagupsky P, Gazala E, Sofer S, et al. Fatal hepatic failure and encephalopathy associated with amiodarone therapy. *J Pediatr* 1985;107:967–970.
41. Gilinsky NH. Fatal amiodarone hepatotoxicity. *Am J Gastroenterol* 1988;83:161–163.
42. Kalantzis N, Gabriel P, Mouzas J, et al. Acute amiodarone-induced hepatitis. *Hepatogastroenterology* 1991;38:71–74.
43. Fogoros RN, Anderson KP, Winkle RA, et al. Amiodarone: clinical efficacy and toxicity in 96 patients with recurrent, drug-refractory arrhythmias. *Circulation* 1983;68:88–94.
44. Matnyjarvi M, Tuppurainen K, Ikaheimo K. Ocular side effects of amiodarone. *Surv Ophthalmol*;42:360–366.
45. Hutchinson J, Peters CA, Diamond DA. Amiodarone induced epididymitis in children. *J Urol* 1998;160:515–517.
46. Kirkali Z. Amiodarone-induced sterile epididymitis. *Urol Int* 1988;43:372–373.
47. Dobs AS, Sarma PS, Guarnieri T, et al. Testicular dysfunction with amiodarone use. *J Am Coll Cardiol* 1991;18:1328–1332.
48. Weinberger IW, Rotenberg Z, Fuchs J, et al. Amiodarone-induced thrombocytopenia. *Arch Intern Med* 1987;147:735–736.
49. Starke ID, Barbatis C. Cutaneous vasculitis associated with amiodarone therapy. *BMJ* 1985;291:940.
50. Staubli M, Zimmerman A, Bircher J. Amiodarone-induced vasculitis and polyserositis. *Postgrad Med J* 1985;61:245–247.
51. Nolan PE, Erstad BL, Hoyer GL, et al. Steady-state interaction between amiodarone and phenytoin in normal subjects. *Am J Cardiol* 1990;65:1252–1257.
52. Preuner JG, Lehle K, Keyser A, et al. Development of severe adverse effects after discontinuing amiodarone therapy in human heart transplant recipients. *Transplant Proc* 1998;30:3943–3944.
53. Navalgund AA, Alifimoff JK, Jakymec AJ, et al. Amiodarone-induced sinus arrest successfully treated with ephedrine and isoproterenol. *Anesth Analg* 1986;65:414–416.
54. Bonati M, D'Aranno V, Galletti F, et al. Acute overdosage of amiodarone in a suicide attempt. *J Toxicol Clin Toxicol* 1983;20:181–186.
55. Bouffard Y, Berger Y, Delafosse B, et al. [Acute amiodarone poisoning. Clinical and pharmacokinetic study.] [French]. *Arch Mal Coeur Vaiss* 1985;78:130–132.
56. Forunati MT, Morandi F, Santarone M, et al. [Pharmacokinetics of amiodarone in one case of acute oral intoxication.] [Italian]. *Giornale Italiano di Cardiologia* 1983;13:385–388.
57. Garson A, Gillette PC, McVey P, et al. Amiodarone treatment of critical arrhythmias in children and young adults. *J Am Coll Cardiol* 1984;4:749–755.
58. Greenberg ML, Lerman BB, Shipe JR, et al. Relation between amiodarone and desethylamiodarone plasma concentrations and electrophysiologic effects, efficacy, and toxicity. *J Am Coll Cardiol* 1987;9:1148–1155.
59. Kivisto KT, Neuvonen PJ. Effect of activated charcoal on the absorption of amiodarone. *Hum Exp Toxicol* 1991;10:327–329.
60. Laine K, Kivisto KT, Neuvonen PJ. Failure of oral activated charcoal to accelerate the elimination of amiodarone and choloroquine. *Hum Exp Toxicol* 1992;11:491–494.
61. Nitsch J, Luderitz B. Enhanced elimination of amiodarone by cholestyramine. *Dtsch Med Wochenschr* 1986;111:1241–1244.
62. Smith WM, Gallagher JJ. "Les torsades de pointes": An unusual ventricular arrhythmia. *Ann Intern Med* 1980;93:578–587.
63. Keren A, Tzivoni D, Gavish D, et al. Etiology, warning signs and therapy of torsades de pointes. *Circulation* 1981;64:1167–1174.
64. Winters SL, Sachs RG, Curwin JH. Nonsustained polymorphous ventricular tachycardia during amiodarone therapy for atrial fibrillation complicating cardiomyopathy. *Chest* 1997:111:1454–1457.
65. Pitcher WD. Southwestern Internal Medicine Conference: amiodarone pulmonary toxicity. *Am J Med Sci* 1992;303:206–212.
66. Kennedy JI. Clinical aspects of amiodarone pulmonary toxicity. *Clin Chest Med* 1990;11:119–129.
67. Dean PJ, Groshart KD, Porterfield JG, et al. Amiodarone-associated pulmonary toxicity. *Am J Clin Pathol* 1987;87:7–13.
68. Khanderia U, Jaffe CA, Theisen V. Amiodarone-induced thyroid dysfunction. *Clin Pharmacol* 1993;12:774–779.
69. Product Information, Betapace. Berlex Laboratories. Revised February 2001.
70. Anttila M, Arstila M, Pfeffer M, et al. Human pharmacokinetics of sotalol. *Acta Pharmacol Toxicol* 1976;39:118–128.
71. O'Hare MF, Leahey W, Marnaghan GA, et al. Pharmacokinetics of sotalol during pregnancy. *Eur J Clin Pharmacol* 1983;24:521–524.
72. Antonaccio MJ, Gomoll A. Pharmacology, pharmacodynamics and pharmacokinetics of sotalol. *Am J Cardiol* 1990;65:12A–21A.
73. Singh BN, Deedwania P, Nademanee K, et al. Sotalol. A review of its pharmacodynamic and pharmacokinetic properties, and therapeutic use. *Drugs* 1987;34:311–349.
74. Kahela P, Anttila M, Tikkanen R, et al. Effect of food, food constituents and fluid volume on the bioavailability of sotalol. *Acta Pharmacol Toxicol* 1979;44:7–12.

75. Kahela P, Anttila M, Sundqvist H. Antacids and sotalol absorption. *Acta Pharmacol Toxicol* 1981;49:181–183.
76. Sundquist H, Anttila M, Simon A, et al. Comparative bioavailability and pharmacokinetics of sotalol administered alone and in combination with hydrochlorothiazide. *J Clin Pharmacol* 1979;19:557–564.
77. Sundquist H. Basic review and comparison of beta-blocker pharmacokinetics. *Curr Ther Res* 1980;28[Suppl]:38S–45S.
78. Hanyok JJ. Clinical pharmacokinetics of sotalol. *Am J Cardiol* 1993;72:19A–26A.
79. O'Hare MF, Murnaghan GA, Russell CJ, et al. Sotalol as a hypotensive agent in pregnancy. *Br J Obstet Gynaecol* 1980;87:814–820.
80. Sontaniemi EA, Anttila M, Pelkonene RO, et al. Plasma clearance of propranolol and sotalol and hepatic drug-metabolizing enzyme activity. *Clin Pharmacol Ther* 1979;26:153–161.
81. Wang T, Bergstrand RH, Thompson KA, et al. Concentration-dependent pharmacologic properties of sotalol. *Am J Cardiol* 1986;57:1160–1165.
82. Poirier JM, Jaillon P, Lecocoq B, et al. The pharmacokinetics of d-sotalol and d,l-sotalol in healthy volunteers. *Eur J Clin Pharmacol* 1990;38:579–582.
83. Fourtillian JB, LeFebvre MA, Courtois P, et al. Pharmacokinetic study of sotalol after 320 mg single oral doses in healthy adults using high performance liquid chromatography. *Thérapie* 1981;36:457–463.
84. Kowey PR, Marinchak RA, Rials SJ, et al. Pharmacologic and pharmacokinetic profile of class III antiarrhythmic drugs. *Am J Cardiol* 1997;80(8A):16G–23G.
85. Oudijk MA, Michon MM, Kleinman CS, et al. Sotalol in the treatment of fetal dysrhythmias. *Circulation* 2000;101:2721–2726.
86. Hackett LP, Wojnar-Horton RE, Dusci LJ, et al. Excretion of sotalol in breast milk. *Br J Clin Pharmacol* 1990;29:277–278.
87. Neuvonen PJ, Elonen E, Vuorenmaa T, et al. Prolonged QT interval and severe tachyarrhythmia, common features of sotalol intoxication. *Eur J Clin Pharmacol* 1981;20:85–89.
88. Leatham EW, Holt DW, McKenna WJ. Class III antiarrhythmics in overdose. *Drug Safety* 1993;9:450–462.
89. Alderfliegel F, Leeman M, Demaeyer P, et al. Sotalol poisoning associated with asystole. *Intensive Care Med* 1993;19:57–58.
90. Montagna M, Groppi A. Fatal sotalol poisoning. *Arch Toxicol* 1980;43:221–226.
91. Perrot D, Bui-Xuan B, Lang J, et al. A case of sotalol poisoning with fatal outcome. *J Toxicol Clin Toxicol* 1988;26:389–396.
92. MacNeil DJ. The side effect profile of class III antiarrhythmic drugs: focus on d,l-sotalol. *Am J Cardiol* 1997;80(8A):90G–98G.
93. Link MS, Foote CB, Sloan SB, et al. Torsade de pointes and prolonged QT interval from surreptitious use of sotalol: use of drug levels in diagnosis. *Chest* 1997;112:556–557.
94. Edvardsson N, Varnauskas E. Clinical course, serum concentrations and elimination in a case of massive sotalol intoxication. *Eur Heart J* 1987;8:544–548.
95. Karkkainen S, Neuvonen PJ. Effect of oral charcoal and urine pH on sotalol pharmacokinetics. *Int J Clin Pharmacol Ther Toxicol* 1984;22:441–446.

CHAPTER 121

Class IV Antidysrhythmic Drugs (Calcium-Channel Blockers)

Andrew H. Dawson

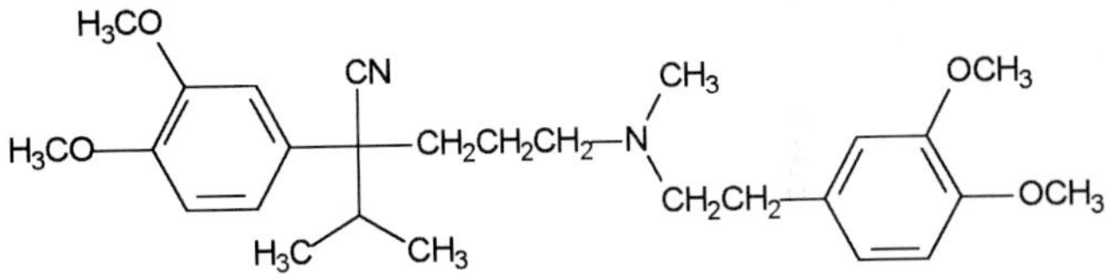

VERAPAMIL

Compounds included:	**Verapamil (Calan SR, Isoptin, Verelan, others), nifedipine (Adalat, Procardia, many others), nicardipine (Cardene, Ridene, many others), nimodipine (Nimotop), amlodipine (Amlodin, Norvasc), bepridil (Vascor), felodipine (Plendil, Renedil), isradipine (Dynacirc, Prescal); diltiazem (Cardizem, Dilator, Tiazac)**
Molecular formula and weight:	**See Table 1.**
SI conversion:	**See Table 1.**
CAS Registry No.:	**See Table 1.**
Therapeutic levels:	**Not used clinically**
Special concerns:	**Combined beta-blocker and calcium-channel blocker overdose**
Target organs:	**Heart (acute), vascular system (acute), endocrine (acute)**
Antidotes:	**Calcium chloride or gluconate, glucagon, insulin + dextrose**

OVERVIEW

Calcium-channel blockers are composed of three chemical classes: the phenylalkylamines (verapamil), the dihydropyridines (nifedipine, nicardipine, nimodipine, amlodipine, bepridil, felodipine, isradipine), and the benzothiazepines (diltiazem) (1). The dihydropyridine class drugs are used principally as peripheral vasodilators in the treatment of hypertension. Verapamil and diltiazem are also used as antihypertensives and antianginal agents. In therapeutic doses both slow sinus node firing and atrioventricular (AV) nodal conduction. This effect is most apparent with verapamil, which can be used to slow the ventricular response to supraventricular tachycardias.

Poisonings from calcium-channel blockers are over-represented in hospital deaths. Morbidity and mortality are generally due to cardiovascular collapse resulting from a combination of extreme peripheral vasodilation, myocardial depression, and impaired myocardial conduction. Extracardiac toxicity, such as hyperglycemia, lactic acidosis, seizures, and noncardiogenic pulmonary edema, is less common but implies a poorer prognosis.

TABLE 1. Calcium-channel blockers

Drug	Molecular formula, molecular weight (g/mol), CAS Registry No.	SI conversion	Therapeutic dose (mg/d)	Therapeutic blood level (mg/L)	$T_{1/2}$ (h)
Phenylalkylamines					
Verapamil hydrochloride[a]	$C_{27}H_{38}N_2O_4$,HCl, 491.1, 152-11-4	mg/L × 2.20 = µmol/L	240–480	0.2	5–12
Benzothiazepines					
Diltiazem hydrochloride[a]	$C_{22}H_{26}N_2O_4S$,HCl, 451.0, 33286-22-5	mg/L × 2.41 = µmol/L	120–480	0.4	3–5
Dihydropyridines					
Nifedipine[a]	$C_{17}H_{18}N_2O_6$, 346.3, 21829-25-4	mg/L × 2.89 = µmol/L	120	0.2	2–4
Amlodipine besilate	$C_{20}H_{25}ClN_2O_5$,$C_6H_6O_3S$, 567.1, 111470-99-6	µg/L × 2.45 = nmol/L	10	0.05	35–50
Nicardipine hydrochloride[a]	$C_{26}H_{29}N_3O_6$,HCl, 516.0, 54527-84-3	mg/L × 2.09 = µmol/L	60–120	0.5	8.6
Isradipine	$C_{19}H_{21}N_3O_5$, 371.4, 75695-93-1	mg/L × 2.69 = µmol/L	5–10	0.1	4–8
Felodipine[a]	$C_{18}H_{19}Cl_2NO_4$, 384.3, 72509-76-3; 86189-69-7	µg/L × 2.60 = nmol/L	10	0.010	10
Nisoldipine[a]	$C_{20}H_{24}N_2O_6$, 388.4, 63675-72-9	µg/L × 2.57 = nmol/L	20–40	0.010	7–12
Nimodipine	$C_{21}H_{26}N_2O_7$, 418.4, 66085-59-4	µg/L × 2.39 = nmol/L	180	0.030	9
Lercanidipine hydrochloride	$C_{36}H_{41}N_3O_6$,HCl, 648.2, 132866-11-6	mg/L × 1.63 = µmol/L	20	NR	2–5

NR, not reported; $T_{1/2}$, half-life.
[a]Available as a controlled-release formulation.

Rarer complications include pancreatitis and cerebral and bowel ischemia. Serious overdoses are more common with verapamil and diltiazem than with drugs from the dihydropyridine class such as nifedipine. Controlled-release calcium channel–blocker preparations are associated with late onset and prolonged toxicity.

TOXIC DOSE

The adult therapeutic doses of the calcium-channel blockers are provided in Table 1. Significant toxicity has occurred over a wide range of doses, particularly for verapamil and diltiazem. In a series of accidental pediatric poisonings, patients were asymptomatic if they were known to have ingested less than 12 mg/kg of a verapamil sustained-release (SR) formulation or less than 2.7 mg/kg nifedipine SR (2). These data should not be extrapolated to intentional or accidental poisonings in adults when major determinants for variability include preexisting cardiac disease and coingested medication, in particular beta-receptor blockers. The ingestion of two to three times the normal dose may cause profound toxicity in such patients. Thus, all patients need to be observed for a period that corresponds to at least the time of peak absorption.

A 33-year-old man ingested verapamil, 4.16 g, developed asystole, and died after treatment with gastric lavage, syrup of ipecac, activated charcoal, calcium chloride, atropine, naloxone, intravenous fluids, dopamine, transcutaneous pacing, intravenous potassium, and epinephrine (3). A 22-year-old ingested 7.2 to 9.6 g verapamil SR, developed respiratory depression, and died (4). A single 10-mg nifedipine capsule proved fatal in a 14-month-old child (5). A 15-year-old girl died after ingesting 140 mg amlodipine (6).

TOXICOKINETICS AND TOXICODYNAMICS

In therapeutic use, peak serum concentrations occur within 1 to 2 hours for all formulations apart from amlodipine and controlled-release formulations (6 to 12 hours) (1). Peak concentrations can be delayed in overdose up to 6 hours for standard preparations (7–9) and 22 hours for controlled release (10). All of these drugs have a high first-pass effect, causing low bioavailability in the range of 10% to 40% (1). Increased bioavailability has been demonstrated for some calcium-channel blockers in overdose, suggesting that the first-pass effect is saturable (11). The protein binding for all compounds is high (greater than 90%) with the exception of diltiazem (80%). The free fraction of verapamil may increase in overdose (12). The apparent half-life of many calcium-channel blockers appears to be longer after overdose but is generally thought to reflect a rate-limited absorption (7,9,12–14).

Peak levels of a verapamil SR preparation occurred at 22 hours after ingestion of 2.3 g. The onset of toxic effects was delayed until 16 hours after ingestion (10). Further delays in absorption can occur with the formation of pharmacobezoars of SR preparations (15). All patients with SR calcium-channel blocker overdose should be admitted to the hospital for observation, even if they are asymptomatic.

Verapamil is metabolized in the liver to norverapamil and other metabolites with less activity than the parent drug. Diltiazem is metabolized to desacetyldiltiazem, which also has lesser activity than its parent drug. The other calcium-channel blockers are metabolized to compounds with little or no activity.

PATHOPHYSIOLOGY

All calcium-channel blockers act by preventing the opening of voltage-gated calcium channels (the L type). The major actions are vasodilation (inhibiting contraction of vascular smooth muscle) and slowing of cardiac conduction, particularly the sinoatrial and AV nodes when there are no sodium gated channels and conduction is totally dependent on calcium flux. Binding of the various calcium antagonists to these channels may be use dependent as well as voltage dependent.

At therapeutic doses, nifedipine and other dihydropyridine drugs are predominantly peripheral vasodilators with little direct cardiac effect. Verapamil and diltiazem, to a lesser extent, have direct cardiac effects in addition to peripheral vasodilatation. The direct cardiac effects include decreased sinus node activity, AV conduction and myocardial contractility.

PREGNANCY AND LACTATION

All of the calcium-channel blockers are Australian pregnancy category C and U.S. Food and Drug Administration pregnancy category C (Appendix I). These drugs carry the potential to produce fetal hypoxia associated with maternal hypotension, but primarily with short-acting preparations. Nifedipine is used for threatened preterm labor.

Breast-feeding information is limited for nifedipine, diltiazem, and verapamil; nifedipine has a low excretion in breast milk and seems safe to use. No data are available for amlodipine, felodipine, and lercanidipine. They should be avoided by lactating mothers.

CLINICAL PRESENTATION

The onset of clinical toxicity is determined by the type of formulation. For standard preparations, symptoms are normally seen within 2 hours but can be delayed for up to 12 hours in controlled or SR preparations. Verapamil and diltiazem have greater toxicity in overdose than drugs from the dihydropyridine class.

Cardiac Effects

Hypotension is the most common cardiovascular finding and is caused principally by vasodilation and, with increasing drug concentration, reduced myocardial contractility. Increasing heart block typically progresses from sinus bradycardia to first-degree heart block to junctional bradycardia (with absent P waves) to a slow idioventricular rhythm and terminates with asystole. This may occur with any calcium-channel blocker, but higher degrees of block are much more common with verapamil and diltiazem (16). Cardiac and noncardiogenic pulmonary edema are reported (17). Noncardiogenic pulmonary edema can occur relatively late at a time when other cardiac parameters are improving (18). Intractable cardiogenic shock or asystole is the usual mode of death.

Other Effects

Central nervous system features include drowsiness, confusion, and, rarely, seizures. If coma occurs, it is usually secondary to cardiovascular collapse. Gastrointestinal features may include nausea and vomiting. Metabolic effects include hyperglycemia secondary to the reduced release of insulin and insulin resistance. Metabolic acidosis secondary to lactic acidosis results from poor tissue perfusion. These metabolic effects are poor prognostic features. Other complications include pancreatitis; cerebral and bowel ischemia occur rarely (19).

Adverse Events

Minor gastrointestinal and skin events and headache are relatively common with calcium-channel blockers. Rarely, bone marrow suppression or hepatitis has been reported (20). Renal insufficiency may be exacerbated by calcium-channel blockers. These effects usually resolve with discontinuation of the drug. Myoclonus is an unusual effect of several calcium-channel blockers. Gynecomastia has been reported with several agents.

DIAGNOSTIC TESTS

Routine drug testing does not detect calcium-channel blockers. Assays for specific agents may confirm ingestion but do not alter management. A digoxin level should be taken if this drug was available to the patient.

Arterial blood gases and venous blood for electrolytes, renal function, calcium, and blood glucose should be taken. They need to be repeated in symptomatic patients and in those who are receiving active treatment. No well-defined effects on electrolytes have been found. Hypocalcemia or hyperkalemia from other causes may theoretically exacerbate toxicity. Renal impairment may be associated with the accumulation of active metabolites of verapamil and diltiazem. Hyperglycemia is a consequence of calcium channel blocker–mediated impaired insulin release and increased insulin resistance and requires active treatment and ongoing monitoring. Arterial blood gases identify poor gas exchange and evidence of acidosis. Metabolic acidosis is due to multiple mechanisms, which include poor tissue perfusion and altered carbohydrate oxidation.

Electrocardiogram (ECG) abnormalities after calcium channel–blocker overdose involve prolonged conduction (QRS, PR, QT intervals), various degrees of AV block, and asystole. Patients should undergo a 12-lead ECG and continuous monitoring. In symptomatic patients who are refractory to initial treatment, other investigations such as echocardiography and monitoring of central pressures and cardiac output may be indicated. This is more likely to be helpful in patients with preexisting cardiac disease.

TREATMENT

In symptomatic patients the aim is to achieve adequate organ perfusion and to correct metabolic disturbances. This is normally achieved by combining good supportive care with the use of a number of antidotal therapies. Any symptomatic patient should be managed in an intensive care setting.

Each patient requires individual management, as response to the overdose is dependent on several variables: drug type, dose, formulation type, other medications ingested, and preexisting cardiac disease. Animal studies indicate that hypotension and bradycardia after overdose with calcium-channel blockers may be due to peripheral vasodilation (nifedipine) or a direct effect on cardiac output (diltiazem and verapamil). This indicates that different therapeutic interventions may be necessary for the management of an overdose of each subclass of calcium-channel blockers (21). Symptomatic patients should be treated aggressively. The most severe cases may require multiple simultaneous antidotal interventions as described in Supportive Care. Patients with coexistent digoxin toxicity should receive digoxin antibodies; therapeutic levels of digoxin may be protective (22).

Gastrointestinal Decontamination

Induced emesis is contraindicated due to the potential for abrupt deterioration. Gastric lavage should be considered in SR verapamil or diltiazem poisonings and patients presenting within an hour of ingestion. Patients who are bradycardic should receive atropine before lavage.

Oral activated charcoal should be given to all patients who have ingested a recent overdose of a calcium-channel blocker. Activated charcoal was shown to be significantly effective when given 2 hours after therapeutic doses of amlodipine (23). Given the delays in peak levels. it should be administered to all patients who present within 4 hours of an ingestion of a standard preparation and 12 hours for a controlled-release preparation. Multiple doses of activated charcoal are theoretically indicated for ingestion of controlled-release preparations, but in this situation whole bowel irrigation with polyethylene glycol is likely to be more efficacious (10,24).

Enhanced Elimination

The role of extracorporeal removal is poorly defined (and may be technically difficult). The existing case reports do not support its use. High biliary concentrations of verapamil have been found after overdose (18). However, multiple dose activated charcoal has not been demonstrated to enhance elimination. The high protein binding and volume of distribution of these agents indicate that hemodialysis and hemoperfusion are unlikely to be effective.

Supportive Care

In addition to the normal supportive care, intravenous access should be secured as soon as possible. All patients should receive ECG monitoring, which should continue for at least 6 hours for normal-release preparations and 12 hours for controlled-release preparations after ingestion. Intensive care is indicated for all but the most trivial poisonings.

Most patients who have hypotension without evidence of a conduction defect respond to volume expansion and should receive a bolus of an isotonic crystalloid-like normal saline (10 to 20 ml/kg) (Chapter 37). Patients whose blood pressure does not respond to such a fluid challenge should have central venous pressure monitoring. Those with continuing hypotension or with cardiac conduction defects require more intensive treatment.

Acidosis should be corrected to a pH within the normal range. Myocardial L-channel function is impaired when the pH falls outside the physiologic range. Acidosis enhances the effect of verapamil and decreases the effect of calcium (25–27). Sodium bicarbonate significantly improved myocardial contractility and cardiac output in a swine model of verapamil poisoning (28).

Calcium

Critical literature reviews support the use of intravenous calcium salts as first-line treatment of calcium antagonist poisoning (29). Their use is primarily indicated in patients with conduction defects, which are generally associated with hypotension. In practice, the majority of such patients have taken either verapamil or diltiazem. Calcium ions can be supplied by either intravenous calcium gluconate or calcium chloride (Chapter 44). The differences between them are the routes of administration and the relative amount of calcium content. Calcium chloride produces a higher concentration of calcium than calcium gluconate but should be administered by a central line. Calcium gluconate can be given through a peripheral line. The patient should initially be given 10 ml 10% calcium chloride (1 g). If no response in blood pressure or pulse rate occurs, the dose should be repeated every 3 to 5 minutes. The doses of calcium gluconate are approximately double those of calcium chloride. Large doses may be required (up to 6 g calcium gluconate as initial treatment) (9). Patients who respond to calcium should receive a continuous infusion of 1 to 2 g/hour. A doubling of serum calcium was associated with significant hemodynamic improvement in animals (30) and humans (18). An ionized serum calcium level of 2 mmol/L was effective in severe nifedipine toxicity and has been suggested as a target concentration (31).

The treatment of hypotension without conduction defects does not usually require calcium or any cardioactive medication. It is possible that high-dose calcium will be cardiotoxic in patients in this situation (particularly those who have ingested dihydropyridines) and may induce ventricular dysrhythmias. Calcium should not be used in the presence of digoxin toxicity unless such toxicity has been reversed with digoxin antibodies.

Glucagon

Glucagon has chronotropic and inotropic effects in beta-blocker overdoses, and there have been a number of reports of response in calcium channel–blocker overdose (32–36). Glucagon should be used early in the setting of combined beta-blocker and calcium channel–blocker poisoning. The binding of glucagon to its specific catecholamine-independent receptors activates adenyl cyclase and converts intracellular adenosine triphosphate to cyclic adenosine monophosphate. The intracellular cyclic adenosine monophosphate stimulates the uptake of calcium by the sarcoplasmic reticulum and plasma membrane–enriched fraction. Calcium is important for the coupling of the action potential and contraction. Increased intracellular calcium leads to increased myocardial contractility. This effect on myocardial cells appears to be influenced by the amount of circulating ionized calcium, the presence of phosphodiesterase inhibitors, and the degree of heart failure. Normal serum ionized calcium may be a prerequisite for full responsivity of myocardial cells to glucose. The use of glucagon is described in Chapter 60. A typical dose is 5 to 10 mg as a bolus injection followed by a continuous infusion of 2 to 5 mg/hour.

Insulin-Dextrose Euglycemia

Insulin-dextrose euglycemia is a technique that has been more effective in animal research than calcium, epinephrine, or glucagon (37). Efficacy has been demonstrated in a case series of clinically serious poisonings (38). Insulin infusions should be used to treat hyperglycemia or hyperkalemia. Patients with hypotension that is refractory to volume loading, correction of acidosis, and calcium salts should receive insulin-dextrose euglycemia. The suggested starting regimen is 1.0 U/kg regular insulin as a bolus followed by an infusion of 1.0 U/kg/hour for 1 hour, then reducing to 0.5 U/kg/hour (38). Patients need a glucose infusion to maintain euglycemia. Previous reports suggest glucose doses of 20 to 30 g/hour. Insulin can be weaned when clinical toxicity resolves. Glucose levels should be monitored hourly during treatment and for 6 hours after the insulin infusion ceases, as hypoglycemia is reported to occur during that time.

Atropine

Atropine should be administered in all patients with bradycardia, especially if vagal tone may be increased (nausea, endotracheal intubation, or placement of a nasogastric or orogastric tube). A response to atropine has been noted to occur only after patients have received calcium loading (18).

Other Inotropic and Vasopressors

Dopamine is an initial pressor of choice (75% response) for diltiazem overdose; it should be used in high doses (10 to 20 mg/kg/minute) (16). Isoprenolol (isoproterenol) produces a therapeutic response in 50% of patients. These agents are often ineffective chronotropes when there is a high degree of conduction block, as its action is predominantly through increasing the frequency of impulses originating in the sinoatrial node.

Inamrinone (amrinone), undiluted 0.75-mg/kg intravenous bolus, is given over 2 to 3 minutes, followed by a maintenance infusion of 5 to 10 mg/kg/minute. Based on clinical response, an additional bolus of 0.75 mg/kg can be given 30 minutes after initiation of therapy.

4-Aminopyridine is not available for general clinical use in the United States. The drug is a competitive antagonist of nondepolarizing neuromuscular blocking agents and also is a competitive antagonist of verapamil. In one anecdotal report, 4-aminopyridine restored blood pressure and cardiac rhythm in 90 minutes in a patient who was unresponsive to atropine, calcium, and Isoprenaline (39).

Electromechanical Support

Cardiac pacing is indicated for significant bradycardia and high-grade conduction blocks. The increase in heart rate alone induced by cardiac pacing can improve cardiac output. Ventricular rather than atrial pacing should be performed, as the AV node is usually blocked. The rate should not exceed 60 beats/min. Cardiac pacing (external and internal) does not always capture or improve the hemodynamic status in patients with calcium channel–blocker toxicity. Intra-aortic balloon counterpulsation directly augments cardiac output in the failing heart. Cardiac pacing can be used in concert with intra-aortic balloon counterpulsation for significant bradycardia and high-grade blocks (29).

REFERENCES

1. Martindale. *The Complete Drug Reference.* London: Pharmaceutical Press, 2002.
2. Belson MG, Gorman SE, Sullivan K, Geller RJ. Calcium channel blocker ingestions in children. *Am J Emerg Med* 2000;581–586.
3. Minella RA, Schulman DS. Fatal verapamil toxicity and hypokalemia. *Am Heart J* 1991;1810–1812.
4. MacDonald D, Alguire PC. Case report: fatal overdose with sustained-release verapamil. *Am J Med Sci* 1992;115–117.
5. Lee DC, Greene T, Dougherty T, Pearigen P. Fatal nifedipine ingestions in children. *J Emerg Med* 2000;359–361.
6. Cosbey SH, Carson DJ. A fatal case of amlodipine poisoning. *J Anal Toxicol* 1997;221–222.
7. Ferner RE, Monkman S, Riley J, et al. Pharmacokinetics and toxic effects of nifedipine in massive overdose. *Hum Exp Toxicol* 1990;309–311.
8. Jaeger A, Sauder P, Bianchetti G, et al. [Acute diltiazem poisoning: kinetic and hemodynamics study.] *J Toxicol Clin Exp* 1990;243–248.
9. Buckley CD, Aronson JK. Prolonged half-life of verapamil in a case of overdose: implications for therapy. *Br J Clin Pharmacol* 1995;680–683.
10. Buckley N, Dawson AH, Howarth D, et al. Slow-release verapamil poisoning. Use of polyethylene glycol whole-bowel lavage and high-dose calcium. *Med J Aust* 1993;202–204.
11. Toffoli G, Robieux I, Fantin D, et al. Non-linear pharmacokinetics of high-dose intravenous verapamil. *Br J Clin Pharmacol* 1997;255–260.
12. Kivisto KT, Neuvonen PJ, Tarssanen L. Pharmacokinetics of verapamil in overdose. *Hum Exp Toxicol* 1997;35–37.
13. Ferner RE, Odemuyiwa O, Field AB, et al. Pharmacokinetics and toxic effects of diltiazem in massive overdose. *Hum Toxicol* 1989;497–499.
14. Luomanmaki K, Tiula E, Kivisto KT, et al. Pharmacokinetics of diltiazem in massive overdose. *Ther Drug Monit* 1997;240–242.
15. Sporer KA, Manning JJ. Massive ingestion of sustained-release verapamil with a concretion and bowel infarction. *Ann Emerg Med* 1993;603–605.
16. Ramoska EA, Spiller HA, Winter M, et al. A one-year evaluation of calcium channel blocker overdoses: toxicity and treatment. *Ann Emerg Med* 1993;196–200.
17. Brass BJ, Winchester-Penny S, Lipper BL. Massive verapamil overdose complicated by noncardiogenic pulmonary edema. *Am J Emerg Med* 1996;459–461.
18. Howarth DM, Dawson AH, Smith AJ, et al. Calcium channel blocking drug overdose: an Australian series. *Hum Exp Toxicol* 1994;161–166.
19. Gutierrez H, Jorgensen M. Colonic ischemia after verapamil overdose. *Ann Intern Med* 1996;535.
20. Burgunder JM, Abernethy DR, Lauterburg BH. Liver injury due to verapamil. *Hepatogastroenterology* 1988;169–170.
21. Schoffstall JM, Spivey WH, Gambone LM, et al. Effects of calcium channel blocker overdose–induced toxicity in the conscious dog. *Ann Emerg Med* 1991;1104–1108.
22. Bania TC, Blaufeux B, Hughes S, et al. Calcium and digoxin vs. calcium alone for severe verapamil toxicity. *Acad Emerg Med* 2000;1089–1096.
23. Laine K, Kivisto KT, Laakso I, et al. Prevention of amlodipine absorption by activated charcoal: effect of delay in charcoal administration. *Br J Clin Pharmacol* 1997;29–33.
24. Buckley NA, Dawson AH, Reith DA. Controlled release drugs in overdose. Clinical considerations. *Drug Saf* 1995;73–84.
25. Achike FI, Dai S. Cardiovascular responses to verapamil and nifedipine in hypoventilated and hyperventilated rats. *Br J Pharmacol* 1990;102–106.
26. Achike FI, Dai S. Influence of pH changes on the actions of verapamil on cardiac excitation-contraction coupling. *Eur J Pharmacol* 1991;77–83.
27. Shahid M, Rodger IW. The inotropic effect of 4-aminopyridine and pH changes in rabbit papillary muscle. *J Pharm Pharmacol* 1989;601–606.
28. Tanen DA, Ruha AM, Curry SC, et al. Hypertonic sodium bicarbonate is effective in the acute management of verapamil toxicity in a swine model. *Ann Emerg Med* 2000;547–553.
29. Albertson TE, Dawson A, de Latorre F, et al. TOX-ACLS: toxicologic-oriented advanced cardiac life support. *Ann Emerg Med* 2001;S78–S90.
30. Hariman RJ, Mangiardi LM, McAllister RG Jr, et al. Reversal of the cardiovascular effects of verapamil by calcium and sodium: differences between electrophysiologic and hemodynamic responses. *Circulation* 1979;797–804.
31. Lam YM, Tse HF, Lau CP. Continuous calcium chloride infusion for massive nifedipine overdose. *Chest* 2001;1280-1282.
32. Doyon S, Roberts JR. The use of glucagon in a case of calcium channel blocker overdose. *Ann Emerg Med* 1993;1229–1233.
33. Fant JS, James LP, Fiser RT, et al. The use of glucagon in nifedipine poisoning complicated by clonidine ingestion. *Pediatr Emerg Care* 1997;417–419.
34. Mahr NC, Valdes A, Lamas G. Use of glucagon for acute intravenous diltiazem toxicity. *Am J Cardiol* 1997;1570–1571.
35. Stone CK, Thomas SH, Koury SI, Low RB. Glucagon and phenylephrine combination vs glucagon alone in experimental verapamil overdose. *Acad Emerg Med* 1996;120–125.
36. Stone CK, May WA, Carroll R. Treatment of verapamil overdose with glucagon in dogs. *Ann Emerg Med* 1995;369–374.
37. Kline JA, Leonova E, Raymond RM. Beneficial myocardial metabolic effects of insulin during verapamil toxicity in the anesthetized canine. *Crit Care Med* 1995;1251–1263.
38. Yuan TH, Kerns WP, Tomaszewski CA, et al. Insulin-glucose as adjunctive therapy for severe calcium channel antagonist poisoning. *J Toxicol Clin Toxicol* 1999;463–474.
39. ter Wee PM, Kremer Hovinga TK, Uges DR, et al. 4-Aminopyridine and haemodialysis in the treatment of verapamil intoxication. *Hum Toxicol* 1985;327–329.

CHAPTER 122

Digoxin and Therapeutic Cardiac Glycosides

Kennon Heard

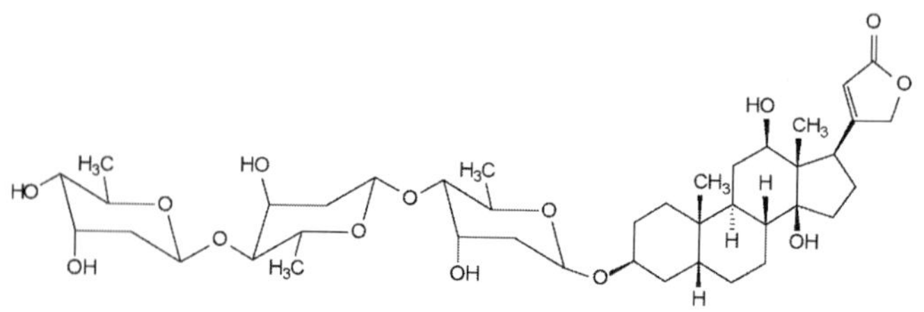

DIGOXIN

Molecular weight:	**Digoxin, 780.95 g/mol; digitoxin, 764.95 g/mol**
SI conversion:	**Digoxin, ng/ml × 1.28 = nmol/L; digitoxin, ng/ml × 1.31 = nmol/L**
Therapeutic levels:	**Digoxin, 0.8 to 2.0 ng/ml (serum); digitoxin, 15 to 25 ng/ml or higher (serum)**
Special concerns:	**Renal insufficiency or volume depletion may lead to occult chronic toxicity. Toxicity may develop with levels within therapeutic range.**
Target organs:	**Slowing or blocking of normal intracardiac conduction and increased atrial, nodal, and ventricular ectopy. Toxicity is manifested by a wide variety of dysrhythmias, most commonly bradycardia and conduction block.**
Antidote:	**Digoxin immune fragments (Fab)**

OVERVIEW

The cardiac glycosides are a diverse class of naturally occurring toxins that include digitalis, digitoxin, and structurally related plant and animal toxins. The cardiac glycosides consist of a steroid nucleus, an unsaturated lactone at the C-17 position, and a glucose moiety at the C-3 position (1). Two of these glycosides are currently used clinically: digoxin (Lanoxin, Lanoxicaps) and digitoxin (Crystodigin, Digicor, Digitaline). Digitalis and digitoxin are used for the treatment of congestive heart failure and for control of ventricular rate in atrial fibrillation and supraventricular tachycardia. Digitalis is the genus name for foxglove, and its leaf has been used therapeutically for more than 200 years. The extract of foxglove leaves contains several cardiac glycosides. Other sources of cardiac glycosides include oleander, red squill, yew berry, and *Bufo* toad poison (2–5). Plants containing cardiac glycosides are addressed in Chapter 306. Toxicity is most commonly a complication of chronic therapeutic use, but life-threatening toxicity after acute overdose also occurs.

Therapeutic Dose

The therapeutic dose of digoxin is 0.125 to 0.350 mg/day and is adjusted based on creatinine clearance (6). The therapeutic range of serum digoxin is 0.5 to 2.0 ng/ml (0.64 to 2.56 nmol/L). For digitoxin, the therapeutic dose is 0.05 to 0.30 mg/day, and the average serum level in patients without toxicity is 17 μg/L, with a range of 3 to 39 μg/L (7).

Toxic Dose

The estimated adult toxic dose after acute ingestion is 10 mg (8). Case reports suggest that toxicity from acute overdose typically occurs with serum levels above 10 ng/ml (12.8 nmol/L). A 32-year-old woman on chronic digoxin therapy developed vomiting and ventricular ectopy after ingestion of 1.75 mg of digoxin in a suicidal gesture (9). A 19-year-old woman died after ingestion of 440 μg/kg of digoxin and 1300 mg of propoxyphene (10). A 60-year-old woman with a history of moderate heart failure on chronic digoxin therapy died after acute ingestion of 10 mg of digoxin (11).

Children are generally more resistant to the effects of cardiac glycosides. Nevertheless, pediatric deaths after accidental ingestion and therapeutic errors are well described. Serious toxic effects are likely after ingestion of more than 0.1 mg/kg of digoxin (12). Death has been reported after ingestion of 10 mg in a 19-month-old child, although the management of digoxin poisoning has changed substantially since this case was reported in 1964 (13). A 2.5-year-old child developed ventricular fibrillation after ingestion of 10 mg but survived with digoxin immune Fab therapy (14).

TOXICOKINETICS AND TOXICODYNAMICS

Digoxin is concentrated in tissue (primarily skeletal muscle) and therefore has a large volume of distribution (Table 1). The volume of distribution is decreased in obese individuals and in the elderly due to loss of muscle mass, and interpatient variation is high. Time to onset of action is 0.5 to 2.0 hours for oral digoxin formulations, and peak effects are noted in 2 to 6 hours. Intravenous (IV) preparations have an onset of action within minutes, and peak effects occur in 1 to 4 hours (6). Digoxin is excreted unchanged by the kidneys (15). Unrecognized impaired renal function is one of the most common reasons for toxicity during chronic use. The elimination half-life for therapeutic levels in patients with normal renal function is 30 to 45 hours (15). Digi-

TABLE 1. Pharmacokinetic and pharmacodynamic data for digoxin and digitoxin

Parameter (reference)	Digoxin	Digitoxin
Bioavailability (%) (6,15)	Lanoxicaps: 90–100; others: 60–85	Nearly 100
Maximal drug concentration (7,15)	0.25 mg PO: mean level of 1.13 μg/L at 60 min	0.6 mg IV: mean level of 51 μg/L at 2–5 min
Time of maximal concentration (h) (15,82)	1.5–6.0	1–2
Volume of distribution (L/kg) (7,83)	Newborn: 5–10; infant: 8–16; children: 8.6–12.0; adults: 5.0–7.5	41
Route of excretion (7,15)	Renal	Hepatic
Elimination half-life (7,15)	30–45 h	4–7 d
Protein binding (%) (7,15)	20–30	97

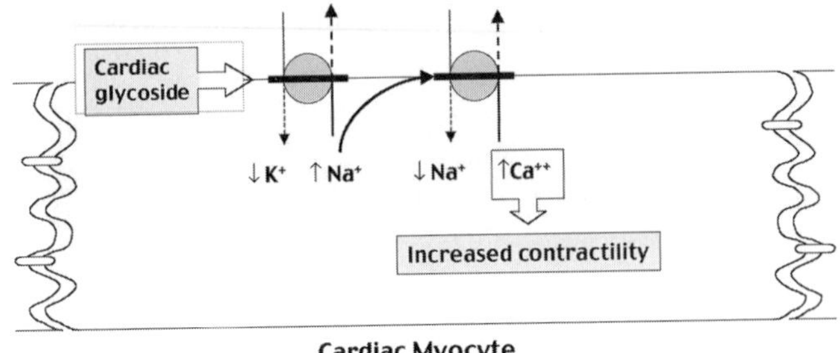

Figure 1. Mechanism of cardiac glycoside activity on the cardiac myocyte. Cardiac glycosides decrease the activity of the sodium-potassium pump. The resulting increase in sodium within the cell reduces influx of extracellular sodium. The decreased influx reduces the activity of the sodium-calcium antiport pump and thereby increases the amount of calcium within the cell. The increased calcium concentration increases the interaction of actin and myosin and produces increased contractility in failing heart cells.

toxin is extensively metabolized by the liver, primarily excreted in bile (60% to 70%) and has an elimination half-life of 4 to 7 days (7). Its primary metabolite is digoxin.

Some toxicokinetic aspects of digoxin are known. In children, the serum concentration may continue to rise well after administration has stopped (16). The volume of distribution decreases as serum concentration rises. In overdose, the elimination half-life of digoxin is reported to increase or decrease. Most reports indicate an increase in half-life.

Serum digoxin levels increase after death. In a pediatric study, digoxin levels in the first 24 hours after death averaged 5.1 ng/ml (6.5 nmol/L) higher than calculated digoxin levels at the time of death (17). Other reports have also noted markedly elevated postmortem levels (18).

PATHOPHYSIOLOGY

Cardiac glycosides have two effects that are responsible for both therapeutic and toxic effects. The first effect is inactivation of the sodium potassium–adenosine triphosphate dependent pump (Na^+,K^+-adenosine triphosphatase) on the cytoplasmic membrane of cardiac cells. The Na^+,K^+-adenosine triphosphatase exchanges extracellular potassium for intracellular sodium. After inactivation of this pump, the concentration of intracellular sodium increases, leading to decreased activity of the Na^+-Ca^{2+} antiport pump (Fig. 1). The Na^+-Ca^{2+} pump exchanges extracellular sodium for intracellular calcium; therefore, the elevation of intracellular calcium increases myocardial contractility. The elevation of intracellular calcium concentration also raises the resting membrane potential of the cell, which increases the rate of spontaneous cellular depolarization and increases myocardial automaticity (1). This effect is most pronounced in atrial tissue, the atrioventricular (AV) node, the His-Purkinje system, and in ventricular tissue (19).

The impaired sodium-potassium exchange also causes the serum potassium level to rise because potassium is moved intracellularly at a slower rate (Fig. 1). After acute poisoning with a cardiac glycoside, the serum potassium may become dangerously high (20). Interestingly, an elevated serum potassium level is actually protective in the setting of chronic digoxin toxicity because hypokalemia increases glycoside binding to the Na-K pump and worsens poisoning of the pump (1). Therefore, a temporary elevation of serum potassium is acceptable in the setting of chronic digoxin toxicity but not in the setting of acute digoxin toxicity.

A second major effect of cardiac glycosides involves the cardiac autonomic system. Digoxin increases cardiac vagal tone and decreases sympathetic nervous system activity in cardiac tissue. This prolongs the refractory period of the conducting system, decreases sinus node firing, and slows conduction through the AV node (1). In overdose, this may lead to sinus bradycardia, sinus arrest, or varying degrees of AV heart block.

The overall effect of cardiac glycoside poisoning is a combination of slowing or blocking of normal intracardiac conduction and increased atrial, nodal, and ventricular ectopy.

PREGNANCY AND LACTATION

Digoxin is U.S. Food and Drug Administration pregnancy category C (Appendix I). Digoxin is excreted in breast milk but is not contraindicated because the concentrations achieved do not cause toxicity in infants (6).

CLINICAL PRESENTATION

Acute and Subacute Overdosage

Acute toxicity most commonly follows suicidal overdose but may occur after accidental ingestion of medications or plants (Chapter 255). The primary manifestations of acute toxicity include vomiting, bradycardia, heart block, ventricular dysrhythmias, and hyperkalemia (10,21,22).

A large case series of acute digitoxin overdose reported 13% mortality with supportive treatment, including intracardiac pacing (21). Although prospective data are limited, it is likely that digoxin immune +Fab (DFab) therapy has improved survival (23). For example, survival of patients with cardiac arrest from digoxin poisoning when treated with DFab was 46%, whereas mortality before this treatment approached 100% (24).

Toxicity during Chronic Use

In older studies, up to 30% of admitted patients taking digoxin had evidence of digoxin toxicity (25). More recent studies suggest that the incidence in admitted patients and outpatients is much lower (26,27). In fact, one study reported that 20% of patients with a discharge diagnosis of digoxin poisoning had no clinical evidence of digoxin toxicity (26). Similarly, older studies suggested that mortality of patients with definite digoxin intoxication exceeded 40% (25), whereas more recent studies suggest mortality is less than 5% (26).

TABLE 2. Drugs that increase serum digoxin levels

Alprazolam	Propafenone
Amiodarone	Quinidine
Indomethacin	Spironolactone
Itraconazole	Tetracycline
Macrolide antibiotics	Verapamil

Adapted from Lanoxin. In: *Physicians' Desk Reference*, 54th ed. Oradell, NJ: Medical Economics, 2000:1225–1231.

The most clinically significant manifestations of chronic cardiac glycoside toxicity are ventricular irritability, including ventricular ectopy, bigeminy, or trigeminy, and ventricular tachycardia (22). AV block and AV nodal escape rhythms are also common (22). Gastrointestinal symptoms, such as anorexia, nausea, and vomiting, occur in approximately one-half of patients (25,28). Alteration in mental status was reported in 25% of patients (25,29). General malaise and weakness are also common and may be the most prominent symptoms (25). Visual changes, such as halos, altered color perceptions, or clouding of vision, are common. Most series report visual symptoms in 10% to 20% of toxic patients (30), but one series has reported symptoms in 95% of patients with digitoxin toxicity (31). Formal testing detected color vision alteration in 80% of digoxin-toxic patients (32).

There are three common reasons for chronic digoxin toxicity. One is alteration of the digoxin dose, either by the patient or by the caregiver. The second is alteration in digoxin clearance, most commonly by unrecognized decreased renal function. The final cause is interaction with other drugs (Table 2).

Adverse Reactions

Adverse reactions are most commonly toxic effects as described in the section Clinical Presentation: Toxicity during Chronic Use. Various psychiatric complaints, including headache, fatigue, malaise, stupor, and mild encephalopathy with electroencephalogram changes, have been described. These effects are typically associated with serum levels in the toxic range. Gynecomastia, rash, and thrombocytopenia have been noted with chronic use (6).

DIAGNOSTIC TESTS

Acute and Subacute Overdosage

An elevated serum digoxin level in the presence of toxic effects establishes the diagnosis of acute or subacute digoxin toxicity. Serum digoxin levels are commonly available and should be obtained for evaluation of acute overdose in adults and children; however, they must be interpreted carefully. Very high serum levels (greater than 10 ng/ml, 12.8 nmol/L) may be noted after acute ingestion in otherwise minimally symptomatic patients (33,34). The serum level should be drawn at least 6 hours after ingestion. Very high levels in asymptomatic patients may also occur when the measurement is performed before distribution has occurred (i.e., after IV administration). A level more than 6 hours after ingestion often is normal in these cases.

Current immunoassays for digoxin may cross-react to variable degrees with other cardiac glycosides (2,35). A positive digoxin screen in a patient with a history of ingesting cardiac glycoside helps to confirm the ingestion; however, a negative test does not exclude ingestion. One report suggests that there is a correlation between serum digoxin levels and oleandrin (the primary toxic component of oleander) levels after ingestion of pink oleander, but there is likely variation depending on the assay (36). High-performance liquid chromatography may be used to measure serum oleandrin levels (37,38).

Falsely low serum digoxin levels may be noted in patients being treated with spironolactone or canrenone (39). Newborns; pregnant women; and patients with end-stage liver disease, end-stage kidney disease, or hypothermia may have increased serum digoxin levels without toxic effect. The increased level is caused by an endogenous digoxin-like immunoreactive substance that reacts in the digoxin immunoassay (40–43).

Serum potassium is the best predictor of cardiac glycoside toxicity after acute overdose. In one large study of acute digoxin ingestion, all patients with a serum potassium level greater than 5.5 mEq/L died, whereas no patient with a serum level less than 5 mEq/L died (20). This rule is not completely reliable in clinical practice, but elevated serum potassium levels should be addressed promptly. Serum potassium has also been suggested as a useful marker of severe toxicity in toad-toxin poisoning (44).

Renal function should be evaluated because renal insufficiency has been associated with recurrent digoxin toxicity after DFab therapy (45).

The electrocardiogram is used to assess cardiac conduction effects of cardiac glycosides and to help guide therapy. Common findings include bradycardia, junctional rhythms, varying degrees of AV block, and ventricular ectopy (21).

Toxicity during Chronic Use

The serum digoxin level correlates poorly with toxicity (46,47). One older study suggested that 30% of clinically toxic patients had serum levels less than 1.7 ng/ml (48,49). A more recent study noted that many patients with toxic effects had a serum level between 1 and 2 ng/ml (26). The diagnosis of digoxin toxicity is primarily a clinical diagnosis, and only very low serum levels are helpful in excluding the diagnosis.

In addition to measurement of the serum digoxin level, serum potassium, magnesium, urea nitrogen, and creatinine should be determined. Hypokalemia and hypomagnesemia are associated with increased dysrhythmias in patients with chronic digoxin toxicity (25,47). Renal function should be determined as many cases of chronic toxicity are associated with decreased renal clearance. Furthermore, renal insufficiency may decrease clearance of the digoxin-DFab complex, which may result in recurrent toxicity after DFab treatment (45).

An electrocardiogram should be obtained and continuous cardiac monitoring initiated in all patients with suspected cardiac glycoside toxicity. Signs of myocardial irritability, such as atrial or ventricular ectopy or tachycardia, are the most common manifestations of chronic toxicity. Sinoatrial or AV blocks are also common but less so than with acute toxicity. The combination of a supraventricular tachycardia with AV block or atrial fibrillation with a nodal escape rhythm is highly suggestive of chronic digoxin toxicity (50). Other tests to evaluate the suicidal patient should be considered.

Diagnostic Pitfalls

The most common pitfall in the evaluation of possible cardiac glycoside toxicity is over-reliance on the serum digoxin level. As noted above, levels drawn before steady-state conditions after acute ingestion may be markedly elevated but result in relatively minimal toxicity (34). In contrast, patients on chronic digoxin therapy may have life-threatening toxicity with "therapeutic" serum levels.

TREATMENT

The principle of management is to treat life-threatening effects (hyperkalemia, ventricular dysrhythmia) immediately, then reduce further absorption of the drug, and finally provide meticulous supportive care during recovery. Digoxin immune antibody fragments (DFab) (DigiBind, DigiFab) have revolutionized the treatment of cardiac glycoside toxicity. Any patient with life-threatening symptoms or ingestion of a potentially life-threatening dose should be treated in a facility that has an adequate dose of DFab immediately available. Suicidal ingestion of cardiac glycoside medication should be considered life-threatening. Accidental ingestion of cardiac glycoside medication may be life-threatening, but accidental ingestion of plants that contain cardiac glycosides is rarely life-threatening.

Gastrointestinal Decontamination

Emesis is not recommended for cardiac glycoside medication ingestion, although induced emesis has theoretic usefulness in the case of deliberate ingestion of cardiac glycoside–containing plants if spontaneous vomiting has not occurred. Cardiac glycosides are well adsorbed by charcoal. Administration of charcoal should be considered in all cases that present within 1 to 2 hours of ingestion (51). There are no data to support routine administration of a cathartic with charcoal in cardiac glycoside ingestion. Similarly, there are no available data to evaluate whole bowel irrigation after cardiac glycoside ingestion, although it has theoretic usefulness in the case of deliberate plant ingestion.

Enhancement of Elimination

Multiple-dose activated charcoal is not clearly beneficial in digoxin overdose (52). Multiple-dose activated charcoal increases the clearance of digitoxin. Given the prolonged half-life of digitoxin, multiple-dose activated charcoal should be considered after digitoxin overdose (53). Hemoperfusion increases the clearance of digitoxin but is rarely used given the efficacy of digoxin immune antibody fragments. Hemodialysis and peritoneal dialysis do not increase the clearance of digoxin and are not considered clinically useful (54). Furthermore, these treatments do not appear to increase the clearance of digoxin bound to DFab (54).

Antidotes

Digoxin immune antibody fragments (DFab) were developed for the treatment of cardiac glycoside toxicity in the 1970s (Chapter 49). DFab rapidly reverses the cardiac effects of digitalis, digitoxin, oleander, yew berry, and bufotoxin, particularly in the case of acute poisoning (2,3,24,35,55). A randomized, controlled trial demonstrated effective reversal of bradycardia and hyperkalemia in patients with cardiac glycoside poisoning from yellow oleander ingestion (56). *In vitro* studies suggest DFab also binds other plant-derived cardiac glycosides (57). Effects are generally observed within 1 hour of DFab administration, and complete reversal is expected within 4 to 6 hours of administration (24). The effects of acute poisoning often reverse quickly, whereas chronic ingestion often improves slowly and partially. The beneficial effect in chronic poisoning may be difficult to ascertain because of preexisting cardiac disease.

Widely accepted indications for administration of DFab after acute digoxin ingestion include any dysrhythmia that results in hemodynamic compromise or a serum potassium level above 5 mEq/L (19). Administration is also recommended after acute ingestion of more than 4 mg in a previously healthy child and 10 mg in a previously healthy adult (8). Finally, administration is recommended if the steady-state serum digoxin level is greater than 10 ng/ml (12.8 nmol/L) (8).

The appropriate dose of DFab after acute digoxin overdose is not well established. Adult patients with hemodynamic compromise after acute cardiac glycoside ingestion should be treated with 10 to 20 vials (380 to 760 mg). Stable patients may be treated with dosing based on the ingested amount (if known) or on the steady-state serum level.

If only the amount ingested is known (Eq. 1):

$$\text{number of DFab vials} = \text{amount of digoxin ingested (mg)} \times 0.48\ \text{(mg/vial)} \qquad \text{[Eq. 1]}$$

If the serum digoxin level obtained at least 6 hours after ingestion is known (Eq. 2):

$$\text{number of DFab vials} = \frac{\text{serum digoxin level (ng/ml)} \times \text{ideal body weight (kg)}}{1000} \qquad \text{[Eq.2]}$$

It is important to note that calculating the dose of DFab using a serum level drawn before steady-state is reached (at least 6 hours after ingestion) may result in administration of a large, expensive, and unnecessary excess of DFab (34).

Patients who develop cardiac toxicity during chronic digoxin therapy usually require much less DFab than those with acute intoxication. Chronic ingestion usually requires less than five vials, whereas toxicity after acute ingestion requires more—up to 10 or 20 vials in patients with hemodynamic compromise. When a steady-state serum level is known, Equation 2 may be used to determine the dose of DFab. An alternative for stable patients with chronic poisoning is to administer two to four vials of DFab and then repeat the dose based on patient response.

Some clinicians have used an approach intended to leave some unbound digoxin present in the blood in order to maintain the desired digoxin activity. This can be accomplished theoretically using Equation 2 by substituting [serum digoxin level (ng/ml) – 1] to maintain a free digoxin level of 1 ng/ml. However, binding varies among patients, and the digoxin level varies depending on the time of serum sampling; therefore, deliberate partial reversal of patients (to maintain a therapeutic digoxin level) is likely inaccurate and cannot be recommended.

DFab is provided as a lyophilized powder. Each vial is reconstituted in 4 cc of sterile water and then may be diluted to the desired final volume in 5% dextrose or normal saline. During reconstitution the solution should be gently rolled rather than shaken to prevent foaming. DFab is administered to stable patients over 30 minutes through a 0.22 µm filter. It may be administered as a bolus to patients with hemodynamic compromise or cardiac arrest (8).

Adverse effects during or after DFab administration are rare. Because DFab is derived from animal protein, allergic reactions are the primary concern. A history of allergy to sheep products has been considered a relative contraindication to administration. No serious allergic reactions were reported in the largest multicenter study of DFab (24). A postmarketing surveillance study reported six cases of possible adverse reactions, none of which were serious (22). Patients with a history of asthma or allergy to antibiotics were found to have an increased risk of allergic reactions. Repeat DFab treatment after repeat overdose without allergic reaction has been reported (58). Other effects reported include hypokalemia (common), worsening of heart failure, and loss of ventricular rate control (rare) (24).

Atropine is a secondary antidote. Although atropine is often ineffective, several case reports and series have reported reversal of bradycardia from acute digoxin poisoning after atropine administration (10,59–62). In the setting of acute overdose, adverse effects appear to be unusual. There are some reported cases of adverse effects of atropine when given to patients with chronic digoxin toxicity (63). Atropine should be considered standard therapy (while preparing DFab for administration) for symptomatic bradycardia associated with acute digoxin overdose. The adult dose is 0.5 to 1.0 mg IV and repeated every few minutes until the heart rate increases, up to a total dose of 3 mg. The pediatric dose is 0.01 mg/kg.

Phenytoin was once considered the first-line treatment for ventricular dysrhythmias associated with digoxin toxicity. Two older case series reported successful treatment of ventricular dysrhythmias using phenytoin, although many of these patients demonstrated only ventricular ectopy. One of these series also reported successful treatment in seven of eight patients with supraventricular tachycardia. The doses used in these reports were 100 to 350 mg administered as an IV bolus (64,65). One case reported successful treatment of a patient with bradycardia and heart-block after acute overdose with repeated 25-mg IV boluses (66). Phenytoin should be administered as an IV bolus of 100 to 300 mg to patients with ventricular dysrhythmias from digoxin poisoning when DFab is not available.

Magnesium has been used for the treatment of ventricular ectopy, dysrhythmias, and cardiac arrest in the setting of chronic digoxin toxicity (67,68). The pretreatment serum magnesium levels in these case series were not reported. Successful defibrillation has been reported after magnesium administration in a case of acute digoxin overdose that did not respond to lidocaine and phenytoin (69). A case of successful magnesium therapy for ventricular dysrhythmias in a patient with acute on chronic toxicity has also been reported (70). No serious adverse effects have been reported commonly. Based on these limited data, IV administration of 2 to 4 g of magnesium sulfate appears to be helpful in the treatment of ventricular ectopy and dysrhythmias in patients with digoxin toxicity if DFab is not available. The effects are often transient, and the dose may need to be repeated.

Lidocaine is commonly recommended for digoxin-induced ventricular dysrhythmias. In one case series of eight digoxin-toxic patients with bidirectional ventricular tachycardia, seven were successfully converted to an atrial rhythm within 2.5 hours (71). The dose was two 75-mg boluses followed by a 3-mg/minute infusion. The one patient who did not respond developed ventricular fibrillation 5 minutes after the first dose. Another report noted asystole after lidocaine administration for ventricular dysrhythmias in a digoxin-toxic patient (72). Overall, the data to support the use of lidocaine for ventricular dysrhythmias associated with digoxin toxicity are limited.

Amiodarone has been used successfully to treat ventricular fibrillation in two cases of digoxin poisoning (one case in conjunction with DFab) (73,74).

Prophylactic intracardiac pacing was initially recommended (before introduction of DFab) for patients with acute digoxin ingestion and either dysrhythmias plus delayed intracardiac conduction or serum potassium over 5 mEq/L. Other indications were subsequently added: age greater than 40 years, digitoxin dose greater than 10 mg, and severe vomiting or previous organic heart disease (21). The pacer was activated for severe AV block or for ventricular ectopy. The pacer voltage is set for twice the excitability threshold, and the rate increased until ectopy resolves. Later work from this same center has demonstrated improved survival after DFab therapy compared to pacing (23). If DFab is not available, however, transvenous pacing should be instituted for patients with these indications. Transcutaneous pacing has also been used successfully during resuscitation of a patient with acute glycoside poisoning (3).

Ventricular fibrillation after cardioversion has been reported in two digoxin-toxic patients soon after electrical cardioversion introduced for tachydysrhythmias (75). Animal studies indicate that supratherapeutic digoxin doses increase the duration of ventricular tachycardia (76) and decrease the ventricular fibrillation threshold (77). Furthermore, digoxin-toxic animals that develop ventricular tachycardia or fibrillation are often recalcitrant to defibrillation (76). Overall, stepwise escalation of the energy used for cardioversion, beginning at 10 J and increasing as needed, should be used with the stable digoxin-toxic patient who requires cardioversion (75). Unstable patients may benefit from treatment with an antidysrhythmic agent before cardioversion or defibrillation, but information is limited. Patients with therapeutic digoxin levels do not appear to be at increased risk of postcardioversion dysrhythmias (78).

Potassium should be administered to patients with chronic digoxin poisoning with hypokalemia. Older studies recommend oral salt administration, although cautious IV administration may be used as well. Because hyperkalemia is a consequence of acute digoxin poisoning, potassium should not be administered after acute digoxin toxicity. After acute poisoning, DFab is considered first-line therapy for hyperkalemia. If DFab is not available, standard therapy for hyperkalemia should be used, with the exception of calcium administration. Calcium is not recommended for treatment of hyperkalemia associated with digoxin poisoning (79).

Historically, calcium disodium edetate was reported to suppress ventricular ectopy and tachycardia in the treatment of chronic digoxin toxicity, presumably due to the resultant hypocalcemia (80). However, this therapy is not currently used nor recommended.

Monitoring

The patient's vital signs, electrocardiogram, and cardiac rhythm should be monitored, usually in the intensive care unit. After administration of DFab, serum digoxin levels are often unreliable and require specific serum separation techniques to obtain meaningful results (81). Serum potassium level often falls with DFab therapy, and mild to moderate hypokalemia has been noted after DFab therapy (24).

Supportive Care

Patients with altered mental status should have early airway management and appropriate evaluation for coingestants and other causes of altered mental status. Hypotension should be treated with isotonic crystalloid fluids, DFab administration, and vasopressors, if needed. Because patients on chronic glycoside therapy have cardiac disease, patients should be monitored closely for cardiac ischemia and infarction. Patients with evidence of dehydration should receive adequate fluid resuscitation and evaluation for an underlying cause of dehydration (i.e., overuse of diuretics or underlying illness, resulting in decreased fluid intake).

Patients with typical acute toxicity present with gastrointestinal symptoms and bradycardia. However, as life-threatening effects may occur with ingestion of less than a 1-month supply of medications, patients with deliberate ingestions should be treated in a critical care setting with DFab immediately available.

Patients with chronic digoxin toxicity often present with bradycardia associated with nonspecific effects that are not life-threatening. Patients often are dehydrated, and this results in prerenal azotemia and glycoside accumulation. These patients generally do well with gentle hydration and monitoring.

As the toxic effects of digoxin are often nonspecific in older patients, the diagnosis of chronic digoxin toxicity should be entertained for older patients taking digoxin who present with an unclear etiology of their symptoms.

Management Pitfalls

The development of DFab has dramatically simplified the management of the patient with cardiac glycoside toxicity. Once the clinician determines that significant toxicity exists or is likely to occur, DFab should be administered. The most significant pitfall is failure to recognize that serious toxicity exists or will soon develop. For example, hyperkalemia may be treated without recognizing that the underlying cause is cardiac glycoside poisoning. In addition, a high-normal or elevated potassium level may not be assessed correctly in patients on chronic digoxin treatment.

REFERENCES

1. Ooi H, Colucci WS. Pharmacological treatment of heart failure. In: Hardman JG, Limbird LE, Goodman Gilman A, eds. *Goodman & Gilman's the pharmacological basis of therapeutics*, 10th ed. New York: McGraw-Hill, 2001:901–932.
2. Shumaik GM, Wu AW, Ping AC. Oleander poisoning: treatment with digoxin-specific Fab antibody fragments. *Ann Emerg Med* 1988;17:732–735.
3. Cummins RO, Haulman J, Quan L, et al. Near-fatal yew berry intoxication treated with external cardiac pacing and digoxin-specific fab antibody fragments. *Ann Emerg Med* 1990;19:38–43.
4. Tuncok Y, Kozan O, Cavdar C, et al. Urginea maritima (squill) toxicity. *J Toxicol Clin Toxicol* 1995;33:83–86.
5. Goerre S, Frohli P. [Poisoning with digitoxin-like glycosides following eating of oleander leaves]. *Schweiz Rundsch Med Prax* 1993;82:121–122.
6. Lanoxin. In: *Physicians' desk reference*, 54th ed. Oradell, NJ: Medical Economics, 2000:1225–1231.
7. Basalt RC, Cravey RH. Digitoxin. In: Basalt RC, Cravey RH, eds. *The disposition of toxic drugs and chemicals in man*, 4th ed. Foster City, CA: Chemical Toxicology Institute, 1995:244–246.
8. Digoxin immune Fab. In: *Physicians desk reference*, 54th ed. Oradell, NJ: Medical Economics, 2000:1170–1171.
9. Wharton CF. Attempted suicide by digoxin self administration and its management. *Guys Hospital Reports* 1970;119:243–251.
10. Smith TW, Willerson JT. Suicidal and accidental digoxin ingestion. Report of five cases with serum digoxin level correlations. *Circulation* 1971;44:29–36.
11. Aspland J, Edhag O, Mogensen L, et al. Four cases of massive digitalis poisoning. *Acta Med Scand* 1971;189:293–297.
12. Woolf AD, Wenger TL, Smith TW, Lovejoy FH Jr. Results of multi-center studies of digoxin-specific antibody fragments in managing digitalis intoxication in the pediatric population. *Am J Emerg Med* 1991;9:16–20.
13. Fowler RS, Rathi L, Keith JD. Accidental digoxin intoxication in children. *Pediatrics* 1964;64:188–200.
14. Zucker AR, Lacina SJ, DasGupta DS, et al. Fab fragments of digoxin-specific antibodies used to reverse ventricular fibrillation induced by digoxin ingestion in a child. *Pediatrics* 1982;70:468–471.
15. Basalt RC, Cravey RH. Digoxin. In: Basalt RC, Cravey RH, eds. *The disposition of toxic drugs and chemicals in man*, 4th ed. Foster City, CA: Chemical Toxicology Institute, 1995:246–250.
16. Koren G, Beatie D, Soldin S. Agonal elevation in serum digoxin concentrations in infants and children long after cessation of therapy. *Crit Care Med* 1988;16:793–795.
17. Koren G, Beatie D, Soldin S, et al. Interpretation of elevated postmortem serum concentrations of digoxin in infants and children. *Arch Pathol Lab Med* 1989;113:758–761.
18. Dickson SJ, Blazey ND. Post-mortem digoxin levels—two unusual case reports. *Forensic Sci* 1977;9:145–150.
19. Marchlinski FE, Hook BG, Callans DJ. Which cardiac disturbances should be treated with digoxin immune fab (ovine) antibody? *Am J Emerg Med* 1991;9:24–28.
20. Bismuth C, Gaultier M, Conso F, Efthymiou ML. Hyperkalemia in acute digitalis poisoning: prognostic significance and therapeutic implications. *J Toxicol Clin Toxicol* 1973;6:153–162.
21. Bismuth C, Motte G, Conso F, et al. Acute digitoxin intoxication treated by intra-cardiac pacemaker: experience in sixty-eight patients. *J Toxicol Clin Toxicol* 1977;10:443–456.
22. Hickey AR, Wenger TL, Carpenter VP, et al. Digoxin immune Fab therapy in the management of digitalis intoxication: safety and efficacy results of an observational surveillance study. *J Am Coll Cardiol* 1991;17:590–598.
23. Taboulet P, Baud FJ, Bismuth C, Vicaut E. Acute digitalis intoxication—is pacing still appropriate? *J Toxicol Clin Toxicol* 1993;31:261–273.
24. Antman EM, Wenger TL, Butler VP. Treatment of 150 cases of life threatening digitalis intoxication with digoxin specific Fab antibody fragments: final report of a multi-center study. *Circulation* 1990;81:1744–1752.
25. Beller GA, Hood WB Jr, Smith TW, et al. Correlation of serum magnesium levels and cardiac digitalis intoxication. *Am J Cardiol* 1974;33:225–229.
26. Mahdyoon H, Battilana G, Rosman H, et al. The evolving pattern of digoxin intoxication: observations at a large urban hospital from 1980 to 1988. *Am Heart J* 1990;120:1189–1194.
27. Steiner JF, Robbins LJ, Hammermeister KE, et al. Incidence of digoxin toxicity in outpatients. *West J Med* 1994;161:474–478.
28. Moorman JR. Digitalis toxicity at Duke hospital, 1973 to 1984. *South Med J* 1985;78:561–564.
29. Lowenthal M. Delirium due to digoxin intoxication—a reminder [Letter]. *Isr J Med Sci* 1988;24:331.
30. Robertson DM, Hollenhorst RW, Callahan JA. Ocular manifestations of digitalis toxicity. Discussion and report of three cases of central scotomas. *Arch Ophthalmol* 1966;76:640–645.
31. Lely AH, van Enter CH. Large-scale digitoxin intoxication. *BMJ* 1970;3:737–740.
32. Rietbrock N, Alken RG. Color vision deficiencies: a common sign of intoxication in chronically digoxin-treated patients. *J Cardiovasc Pharmacol* 1980;2:93–99.
33. Marcinkowska-Krolewicz M, Feldman R. Can peak serum digoxin concentration be a sign of acute poisoning severity? Analysis of two cases of digoxin poisoning. *Pol Arch Med Wewn* 1998;100:344–349.
34. Walsh FM, Sode J. Significance of non-steady-state serum digoxin concentrations. *Am J Clin Pathol* 1975;63:446–450.
35. Brubacher JR, Ravikumar PR, Bania T, et al. Treatment of toad venom poisoning with digoxin-specific fab fragments. *Chest* 1996;110:1282–1288.
36. Datta P, Dasgupta A. Interference of oleandrin and oleandrigenin in digitoxin immunoassays: minimal cross reactivity with a new monoclonal chemiluminescent assay and high cross reactivity with the fluorescence polarization assay . *Ther Drug Monit* 1997;19:465–469.
37. Namera A, Yashiki M, Okada K, et al. Rapid quantitative analysis of oleandrin in human blood by high-performance liquid chromatography. *Nippon Hoigaku Zasshi* 1997;51:315–318.
38. Tracqui A, Kintz P, Branche F, Ludes B. Confirmation of oleander poisoning by HPLC/MS. *Int J Legal Med* 1998;111:32–34.
39. Steimer W, Muller C, Eber B, Emmanuilidis K. Intoxication due to negative canrenone interference in digoxin drug monitoring [Letter]. *Lancet* 1999;354:1176–1177.
40. Seccombe DW, Pudek MR. Digoxin-like immunoreactive substances in the perinatal period. *Lancet* 1987;1:983.
41. Vinge E, Helgesen-Rosendal S, Backstrom T. Progesterone, some progesterone derivatives and urinary digoxin-like substances from pregnant women in radioimmuno- and 86Rb-uptake assays of digoxin. *Pharmacol Toxicol* 1988;63:277–280.
42. Yang SS, Korula J, Sundheimer JE, Keyser AJ. Digoxin-like immunoreactive substances in chronic liver disease. *Hepatology* 1989;9:363–366.
43. Kumar S, Saxena SK, Gahlaut DS, et al. Digoxin like substances in chronic renal failure. *J Assoc Physicians India* 1986;34:633–634.
44. Chi HT, Hung DZ, Hu WH, Yang DY. Prognostic implications of hyperkalemia in toad toxin intoxication. *Hum Exp Toxicol* 1998;17:343–346.
45. Wenger TL. Experience with digoxin immune Fab (ovine) in patients with renal impairment. *Am J Emerg Med* 1991;9:21–23.
46. Park GD, Spector R, Goldberg MJ, Feldman RD. Digoxin toxicity in patients with high serum digoxin concentrations. *Am J Med Sci* 1987;294:423–428.
47. Shapiro, W. Correlative studies of serum digitalis levels and the arrhythmias of digitalis intoxication. *Am J Cardiol* 1978;41:852–859.
48. Smith TW, Haber E. The clinical value of serum digitalis glycoside concentrations in the evaluation of drug toxicity. *Ann N Y Acad Sci* 1971;179:322–337.
49. Smith TW, Butler VP Jr, Haber E. Determination of therapeutic and toxic serum digoxin concentrations by radioimmunoassay. *N Engl J Med* 1969;281:1212–1216.
50. Chung EK. Digitalis-induced cardiac arrhythmias: a report of 180 cases *Jpn Heart J* 1969;10:409–427.
51. Chyka PA, Seger D. Position statement: single-dose activated charcoal. American Academy of Clinical Toxicology; European Association of Poisons Centres and Clinical Toxicologists. *J Toxicol Clin Toxicol* 1997;35:721–741.
52. Position statement and practice guidelines on the use of multi-dose activated charcoal in the treatment of acute poisoning. American Academy of Clinical Toxicology; European Association of Poisons Centres and Clinical Toxicologists. *J Toxicol Clin Toxicol* 1999;37:731–751.
53. Park GD, Goldberg MJ, Spector R, et al. The effects of activated charcoal on digoxin and digitoxin clearance. *Drug Intell Clin Pharm* 1985;19:937–941.
54. Caspi O, Zylber-Katz E, Gotsman O, et al. Digoxin intoxication in a patient with end-stage renal disease: efficacy of digoxin-specific Fab antibody fragments and peritoneal dialysis. *Ther Drug Monit* 1997;19:510–515.
55. Safadi R, Levy I, Amitai Y, Caraco Y. Beneficial effect of digoxin-specific Fab antibody fragments in oleander intoxication. *Arch Intern Med* 1995;155:2121–2125.
56. Eddleston M, Warrell DA. Management of acute yellow oleander poisoning. *QJM* 1999;92:483–485.
57. Cheung K, Urech R, Taylor L, et al. Plant cardiac glycosides and digoxin Fab antibody. *J Paediatr Child Health* 1991;27:312–313.
58. Bosse GM, Pope TM. Recurrent digoxin overdose and treatment with digoxin-specific fab antibody fragments. *J Emerg Med* 1994;12:179–185.
59. Duke M. Atrioventricular block due to accidental digoxin ingestion treated with atropine. *Am J Dis Child* 1972;124:754–756.
60. Navab F, Honey M. Self-poisoning with digoxin: successful treatment with atropine. *BMJ* 1967;3:660–661.
61. Citrin DL, O'Malley K, Hillis WS. Cardiac standstill due to digoxin poisoning successfully treated with atrial pacing. *BMJ* 1973;2:526–527.
62. Citrin D, Stevenson IH, O'Malley K. Massive digoxin overdose: observations on hyperkalaemia and plasma digoxin levels. *Scott Med J* 1972;17:275–277.
63. Freidberg CK, Donosco E. Arrhythmias and conduction disturbances due to digitalis. *Prog Cardiovasc Dis* 1960;2:408.

64. Bashour FA, Edmonson RE, Gupta DN, Prati R. Treatment of digitalis toxicity by diphenylhydantoin (Dilantin). *Dis Chest* 1968;53:263–270.
65. Lang TW, Bernstein H, Barbieri F, et al. Digitalis toxicity. Treatment with diphenylhydantoin. *Arch Intern Med* 1965;116:573–580.
66. Rumack BH, Wolfe RR, Gilfrich H. Phenytoin (diphenylhydantoin) treatment of massive digoxin overdose. *Br Heart J* 1974;36:405–408.
67. Eisenberg CD, Simmons HG, Mintz AA. The effects of magnesium upon cardiac arrhythmias. *Am Heart J* 1950;39:703–712.
68. Szekely P, Wynne NA. The effects of magnesium on cardiac arrhythmias caused by digitalis. *Clin Sci* 1951;10:241–253.
69. French JH, Thomas RG, Siskind AP, et al. Magnesium therapy in massive digoxin intoxication. *Ann Emerg Med* 1984;13:562–566.
70. Kinlay S, Buckley NA. Magnesium sulfate in the treatment of ventricular arrhythmias due to digoxin toxicity. *J Toxicol Clin Toxicol* 1995;33:55–59.
71. Castellanos A, Ferreiro J, Pefkaros K, et al. Effects of lignocaine on bidirectional tachycardia and on digitalis-induced atrial tachycardia with block. *Br Heart J* 1982;48:27–32.
72. Agrawal BV, Singh RB, Vaish SK, Edin H. Cardiac asystole due to lignocaine in a patient with digitalis toxicity. *Acta Cardiologica* 1974;29:341–347.
73. Maheswaran R, Bramble MG, Hardisty CA. Massive digoxin overdose: successful treatment with intravenous amiodarone. *Br Med J Clin Res Ed* 1983;287:392–393.
74. Nicholls DP, Murtagh JG, Holt DW. Use of amiodarone and digoxin specific fab antibodies in digoxin overdosage. *Br Heart J* 1985;53:462–464.
75. Lown B. Cardioversion and the digitalized patient. *J Am Coll Cardiol* 1985;5:889–890.
76. Leja FS, Euler DE, Scanlon PJ. Digoxin and the susceptibility of the canine heart to countershock-induced arrhythmias. *Am J Cardiol* 1985;55:1070–1075.
77. Lown B, Kleiger RE, Williams JS. Digitalis and cardioversion. *Proc N Engl Cardiovasc Soc* 1965;23:25.
78. Mann DL, Maisel AS, Atwood JE, et al. Absence of cardioversion-induced ventricular arrhythmias in patients with therapeutic digoxin levels. *J Am Coll Cardiol* 1985;5:882–890.
79. Ekins BR, Watanabe AS. Acute digoxin poisonings: review of therapy. *Am J Hosp Pharm* 1978;35:268–277.
80. Surawicz B. Use of the chelating agent, EDTA in digitalis intoxication and cardiac arrhythmias. *Prog Cardiovasc Dis* 1960;2:432–443.
81. Ujhelyi MR, Colucci RD, Cummings DM, et al. Monitoring serum digoxin concentrations during digoxin immune fab therapy. *DICP* 1991;25:1047–1049.
82. POISINDEX Editorial Staff. Digoxin. In: Rumack BJ, Sayer NK, Gelman CR, eds. *POISINDEX System*. Englewood, CO: Micromedex Inc, 2002.
83. Wells TG, Young RA, Kearns GL. Age-related differences in digoxin toxicity and its treatment. *Drug Saf Concepts* 1992;7:135–151.

CHAPTER 123

Phosphodiesterase Inhibitors

Andrew R. Erdman

MILRINONE

Compounds included:	**Inamrinone (Inocor), milrinone (Primacor)**
Molecular formula and weight:	**Inamrinone ($C_{10}H_9N_3O,C_3H_6O_3$), 187.2 g/mol; milrinone ($C_{12}H_9N_3O$), 211.2 g/mol**
SI conversion:	**Inamrinone, mg/ml x 5.34 = mml/L; milrinone, mg/ml x 4.73 = mmol/L**
CAS Registry No.:	**75898-90-7 (inamrinone); 78415-72-2 (milrinone)**
Therapeutic levels:	**Inamrinone, 2 to 7 mg/ml (serum)**
Special concerns:	**Hypotension, tachycardia**
Antidote:	**None**

OVERVIEW

Phosphodiesterase (PDE) is a common intracellular enzyme found in a variety of organs and tissues within the human body (1,2). It catalyzes the cytosolic breakdown of cyclic adenosine monophosphate (cAMP) and other cyclic nucleotides, which are common second messengers and potent modulators of cellular function. PDE has several different forms or isoenzymes, distinguished by their organ location and by the specific cyclic nucleotide used as a substrate. The PDE inhibitors are a diverse group of agents that have found a wide range of clinical applications in modern medicine. Most PDE inhibitors are specific for a particular PDE isoenzyme. For example, the methylxanthines, such as theophylline and aminophylline, inhibit primarily PDE 4, whereas sildenafil inhibits primarily PDE 5. This chapter focuses on drugs that inhibit PDE 3, inamrinone and milrinone.

Inamrinone and milrinone are bipyridine molecules that inhibit PDE, with particular specificity for the PDE 3 isoenzyme found in cardiac myocytes and vascular smooth muscle (1–5). This results clinically in improved cardiac contractility and peripheral vasodilation (6–14). Secondary effects include the inhibition of platelet aggregation and immunomodulation (13,15–19). Overdoses, although not well reported, may lead to an extension of the drugs' clinical effects, with excessive vasodilation causing hypotension and reflex tachycardia.

Inamrinone was the first PDE 3–specific inhibitor (20,21). It was originally called *amrinone* but was renamed due to name confusion with the drug amiodarone. Intravenous (IV) inamrinone is currently approved by the U.S. Food and Drug Administration for the short-term management of congestive heart failure (CHF) (22). Clinical trials investigating the efficacy of chronic oral PDE inhibitor administration have demonstrated an increase in the risk of hospitalization and death, and hence their chronic use has largely been abandoned in the United States (23). IV inamrinone has also been used for the short-term management of other acute low-output states, such as overdoses with negative inotropic agents (e.g., beta-blockers or calcium-channel blockers), and to help wean patients off the bypass machine after cardiac surgery. Inamrinone is also used as a "bridge" to maintain cardiac output in patients with irreversible heart failure until corrective surgery or transplantation can be undertaken. Inamrinone is available as an IV solution (5 mg/ml).

Milrinone was synthesized in the early 1980s (24). It appears to be a significantly more potent inotrope than inamrinone and causes fewer adverse effects (24,25). Like its predecessor, IV milrinone has been approved for the short-term management of CHF, but it is also used in other patients who require short-term inotropic support (26,27). Milrinone has largely replaced inamrinone (28). It is available as an IV solution (1 mg/ml). Oral preparations of inamrinone and milrinone are not commercially available in the United States.

TOXIC DOSE

The recommended adult therapeutic dose of inamrinone is an IV bolus of 0.75 mg/kg given over 2 to 3 minutes, followed by infusion of 5 to 10 mg/kg/minute, which is then titrated to effect (22). It is not approved for pediatric use, but for infants, reported doses ranging from an IV bolus of 3.0 to 4.5 mg/kg followed by infusions of 5 to 10 mg/kg/minute have been used (29–31). Oral doses of inamrinone ranging from 300 to 600 mg daily have been used in adults (32).

The adult therapeutic dose of milrinone is a loading dose of 50 mg/kg IV given over 10 minutes, followed by a maintenance infusion of 0.375 to 0.75 mg/kg/minute, titrated to effect (26). It is not approved for pediatric use, but some authors have used a 50- to 75-mg/kg IV load (repeated if necessary), followed by a maintenance infusion of 0.5 to 1.0 mg/kg/minute for pediatric patients (33,34). The dose should be reduced in patients with significant renal impairment.

The toxic doses of inamrinone and milrinone are not known, as few cases of overdose have been reported. One adult reportedly died after a dose of 840 mg inamrinone IV over 3 hours (22). In another case, a 2-year-old infant died of refractory hypotension when he received an inamrinone infusion varying between 90 and 198 mg/kg/minute for 31 hours (35). His blood inamrinone concentration reached 75.9 mg/ml. In both cases, the patients had significant underlying medical illnesses and were on multiple other medications; therefore, the causal relationship to inamrinone remains unproven. The manufacturer of inamrinone reports that infusions of up to 18 mg/kg/day have been well tolerated by adults for short periods of time. No reports of milrinone overdose could be found in the literature. Even after therapeutic doses of inamrinone or milrinone, transient hypotension and tachycardia can develop (36,37).

TOXICOKINETICS AND TOXICODYNAMICS

Oral bioavailability approaches 93% for inamrinone and 92% for milrinone (38,39). Hemodynamic effects generally occur 1 to 4 hours (peak ~3 hours) after an ingestion of a therapeutic dose of either drug (40–42). After a therapeutic IV bolus of either drug, peak blood levels occur almost immediately, followed within minutes by a hemodynamic response (the response may be delayed up to 30 minutes when a bolus is not used). The duration of clinical effects after a single therapeutic IV dose is approximately 30 minutes to 2 hours but may last much longer after overdoses.

Inamrinone has an apparent volume of distribution of 1.2 L/kg, and its protein binding ranges from 10% to 50% (22,43). Inamrinone is metabolized to varying degrees in the liver, where it is acetylated, glucuronidated, or conjugated with glutathione. The unchanged drug and its metabolites are then eliminated in the urine. The elimination half-life varies from approximately 3.6 hours in normal adult volunteers to 4.8 to 5.8 hours in patients with CHF; however, it may be as long as 15 hours in some patients (22,38,41,43,44). It is also longer in neonates and infants (10.7 and 6.1 hours, respectively) (45). Overdosage is also expected to result in a prolonged drug elimination half-life (35). Hepatic or renal impairment can significantly prolong drug elimination (46).

Milrinone has an apparent volume of distribution of 0.35 to 0.45 L/kg in adults and 0.9 L/kg in children. Approximately 70% is bound to plasma proteins (26,33). The most significant route of elimination is urinary excretion of the unchanged drug; however, small amounts of its glucuronide metabolite may also be excreted renally (26,42). Milrinone has a terminal elimination half-life in the blood ranging from 0.9 hours in healthy adults to 1.5 hours in children and up to 2.4 hours in patients with severe CHF (26,33). Hepatic or renal impairment can delay elimination significantly (42). This delay could theoretically lead to drug accumulation and toxicity or to prolonged clinical effects.

PATHOPHYSIOLOGY

Few reports of inamrinone or milrinone poisoning have been published in the literature. Clinical effects are likely to include extensions of the drugs' pharmacologic actions. This is the case in the few patients with toxicity that have been published to date (22,35).

Therapeutic doses of inamrinone and milrinone result in inhibition of the PDE 3, which is the basis for their beneficial cardiovascular effects (1–5). PDE 3 normally catalyzes the hydrolysis of cAMP (and to a lesser extent cyclic guanosine monophosphate), leading to a decrease in its intracellular concentration within the cell. Inhibitors of PDE 3 cause a buildup of intracellular cAMP. Cyclic nucleotides such as cAMP play a pivotal role as intracellular second messengers, directing or enhancing a number of functions. Alterations in their concentration can lead to a variety of cellular biochemical changes and hence a variety of physiologic changes in organ systems throughout the body. PDE 3 is found in significant concentrations in the human myocardium and vascular smooth muscle cells (1,2). It is also present to varying degrees in platelets, adipose tissue, liver and kidneys, and the penile corpora cavernosa.

In myocardial cells, PDE 3 inhibition and an increase in cAMP concentration activate protein kinase, which in turn phosphorylates a number of key intracellular proteins (Fig. 1). One of these proteins is phospholamban. When phosphorylated, phospholamban causes an increase in the activity of sarcoplasmic reticular adenosine triphosphatase, leading to increases in stored calcium within the sarcoplasmic reticulum. This enables more calcium to be released into the cytoplasm during myocyte excitation. Increases in intracellular calcium enhance myocardial contractility and increase stroke volume, without causing significant changes in heart rate (41). Another protein activated by protein kinase is the transmembranous myocyte calcium channel. Its activation allows more calcium to flow into the myocyte during depolarization, again enhancing cardiac contractility. Finally, activated protein kinase phosphorylates the con-

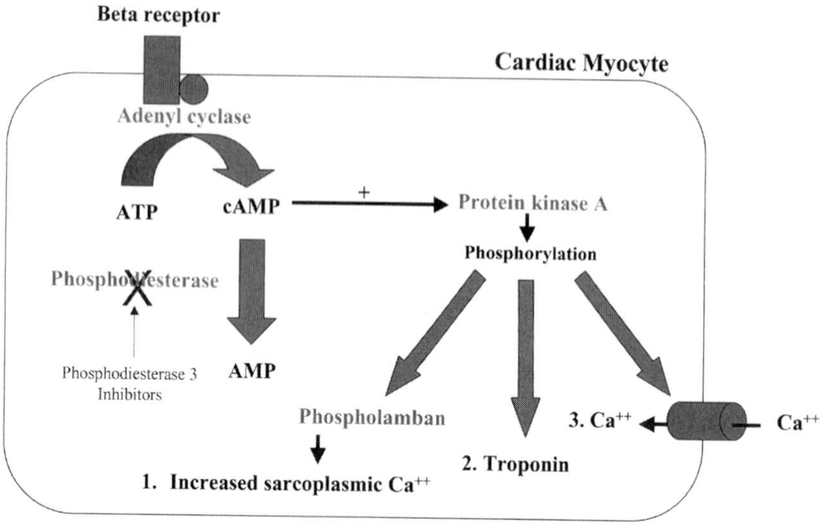

Figure 1. Pharmacologic action of phosphodiesterase 3 inhibitors on human cardiac myocytes, leading to increased contractility. cAMP, cyclic adenosine monophosphate; ATP, adenosine triphosphate.

tractile protein troponin, facilitating its unbinding after cellular contraction. The result is more effective myocardial relaxation (lusitropy) during diastole, reducing preload and enhancing myocardial filling. The clinical sum of all these biochemical effects in the heart is an improvement in cardiac output and work performance. Interestingly, myocardial oxygen consumption does not appear to increase in parallel. Overdoses of PDE 3 inhibitors are likely to result in similar increases in cardiac output. No evidence of clinical cardiotoxicity after overdoses has been shown to date.

Whether PDE 3 inhibitors affect cardiac conduction is controversial. Ventricular and supraventricular dysrhythmias have been reported with therapeutic use (22,26,47–49). However, it is difficult to assess whether the dysrhythmias were the result of a drug effect, a diseased myocardium, or both. Although animal data suggest a dysrhythmic potential, small studies in humans have found no evidence that PDE 3 inhibitors cause or contribute to dysrhythmias (50–54). Milrinone has been shown to speed conduction through the atrioventricular node, raising the possibility that it might lead to an increased ventricular response in patients with supraventricular tachycardias (26).

In vascular smooth muscle cells, increases in cAMP lead to relaxation rather than contraction (11). This effect is mediated by cAMP-dependent inhibition of myosin light-chain kinase, decreasing its ability to phosphorylate, and hence activate, myosin light chain, an essential contractile protein. The end result of PDE 3 inhibition is therefore vasodilation. Clinically, this action allows for the maintenance of blood flow to critical organ systems and, by reducing afterload, results in a further increase in cardiac output at therapeutic doses. After overdose, however, the possibility exists for excessive vasodilation and a drop in blood pressure, leading to hypotension or shock and reflex tachycardia (55–57).

In platelets, an increase in intracellular cAMP triggers calcium sequestration (58). Platelet activation, which is dependent on intracellular calcium, is therefore decreased after PDE 3 inhibition (59). This reduces platelet aggregation, improves blood flow, and lowers the risk of thrombosis. How an overdosage of a PDE 3 inhibitor might affect platelets is not clear. Instances of excessive bleeding have not been reported. Thrombocytopenia has been noted infrequently in patients treated with inamrinone and rarely milrinone (32,33,46,50,60–62). The underlying mechanism is unclear but may be related to non–immune-mediated platelet destruction associated with an acetylated drug metabolite (50,60,61). The effect of an overdose is unclear, but no cases of thrombocytopenia have been reported in association with PDE 3 inhibitor poisoning.

PREGNANCY AND LACTATION

Inamrinone and milrinone are both U.S. Food and Drug Administration pregnancy category C (Appendix I). Few data have appeared regarding the effects of inamrinone on pregnancy in humans, and animal studies are conflicting (22). With milrinone, there are also no human data, but limited animal studies have not found evidence of teratogenesis (26). The extent of inamrinone and milrinone excretion in breast milk is not known.

CLINICAL PRESENTATION

Acute Overdosage

Little is known about the clinical presentation after overdoses with a PDE 3 inhibitor because there are few published reports of poisoning. Toxicity is expected to be an extension of the drug's therapeutic actions. Excessive vasodilation may lead to hypotension (55,56). Intractable shock was the apparent cause of death in one reported overdose with inamrinone (35). In an effort to maintain normal blood pressure, a compensatory reflex tachycardia may be seen (57). Despite profound hypotension, patients can still have warm extremities and good capillary refill.

Complications of hypoperfusion, such as alterations in mentation, acidosis, cardiac ischemia, rhabdomyolysis, and oliguria or renal insufficiency, may occur (35,56). Dysrhythmias have been associated with the therapeutic use of inamrinone and theoretically could occur in cases of acute poisoning (22,26,47–49). Thrombocytopenia or other hematologic disturbances and hepatic injury have also been associated with therapeutic use and could occur after overdoses (33,63–65).

Adverse Events

Therapeutic use of PDE 3 inhibitors has been associated with dysrhythmias, thrombocytopenia, hepatic injury, and increased mortality, particularly with long-term administration (22,26,33,47–49,53,63,64). Inamrinone and milrinone have been associated with increased rates of life-threatening dysrhythmias, ventricular and supraventricular (22,26,47–49). Whether these were caused by PDE 3 inhibition or whether they are merely a manifestation of the patient's underlying medical condition remains controversial.

Chronic oral or IV inamrinone therapy leads to thrombocytopenia in approximately 2% of patients (32,46,50,60–62). Platelet counts typically begin to decline 2 to 4 days after therapy is initiated. The platelet count may continue to fall or reach a nadir and plateau. In all cases, thrombocytopenia has been reversible with cessation of therapy. Thrombocytopenia is uncommon with milrinone therapy (26,33). Other hematologic complications are rare, but pancytopenia developed in one patient during continuous IV inamrinone therapy (65).

Elevation of serum transaminase levels has been reported during inamrinone treatment but not during milrinone use (47,50,64). Dose-related hepatic injury with elevated transaminases and hepatocellular necrosis was also noted in dogs given IV inamrinone (22). Serositis, jaundice, myositis, pulmonary infiltrates, and vasculitis have also been noted during inamrinone therapy (22,23). Hypersensitivity reactions to the drugs can occur (22). The manufacturers of inamrinone and milrinone have also suggested that changes in renal blood flow due to vasodilation and increased cardiac output could potentially lead to diuresis, electrolyte changes, or renal dysfunction, but these have not been reported in the literature (22,26).

DIAGNOSTIC TESTS

Acute Overdosage

Plasma inamrinone and milrinone concentrations can be measured by high-performance liquid chromatography (66). However, these tests are not readily available in most instances, and there are no well-established toxic levels. They are unlikely to be useful in acute poisoning but may help confirm the diagnosis. Therapeutic inamrinone concentrations have been reported to range between 2 and 7 µg/ml (67).

Peak cardiovascular effects generally develop within minutes of IV administration but may be delayed after ingestion. Electrocardiography should be performed and electrocardiographic and hemodynamic monitoring should continue until any hemodynamic effects have resolved. Patients with hypotension should have serum electrolytes, acid-base status, and renal function monitored closely.

Serial complete blood counts should be followed for several days after an acute overdose to look for thrombocytopenia or pancytopenia. Patients suspected of having acute toxicity from either drug should have liver function tests, renal function tests, and serum electrolytes measured routinely and repeated regularly.

Adverse Events

Patients taking chronic inamrinone should be monitored closely for the development of thrombocytopenia. Routine monitoring of platelet counts is generally not necessary with milrinone. Liver and renal function tests should be monitored periodically in patients who take either drug.

Diagnostic Pitfalls

The greatest diagnostic pitfall lies in failure to recognize the diagnosis of PDE 3 inhibitor toxicity. These patients generally have multiple underlying medical problems, which may obscure the contribution of a PDE 3 inhibitor to hypotension.

TREATMENT

Management of overdosage should focus on supportive care and observation for potential complications. Mild hypotension associated with therapeutic doses of inamrinone or milrinone can be managed simply by decreasing the rate of infusion until symptoms resolve. Severe cases may require aggressive or invasive hemodynamic support and monitoring.

Decontamination

Gastrointestinal decontamination is unlikely to be necessary because of parenteral administration. Administration of a single dose of activated charcoal soon after ingestion would be a reasonable intervention, although decontamination measures have not been evaluated.

Enhancement of Elimination

The few case reports describing attempts at extracorporeal inamrinone removal have been conflicting in their conclusions (35,68,69). Few data have been reported on the clearance of milrinone by extracorporeal measures.

Antidotes

No antidote is available for PDE 3 inhibitor toxicity.

Supportive Care

The infusion of inamrinone or milrinone and other medications that may contribute to hypotension should be stopped. Hypotension should initially be treated with isotonic crystalloid fluid resuscitation, taking care to avoid precipitating or exacerbating pulmonary edema in patients who may have underlying impaired myocardial function. Hypotension that is unresponsive to initial fluid infusion should be managed with pressors. Because the drop in blood pressure is primarily the result of peripheral vasodilation, pressors with specific vasoconstrictive properties (e.g., phenylephrine) may be preferable to other agents. Drugs whose action is dependent on β-agonist activity (e.g., isoproterenol) are unlikely to be effective because cAMP concentrations within the cardiac myocytes are already at a maximum as the result of PDE inhibition. β-Agonists might also potentiate vasodilation and theoretically worsen hypotension. For cases of refractory hypotension, vasopressin has been reported to be effective (55,56).

Tachycardia is typically a compensatory response to excessive vasodilation, and it is rarely a clinical problem. β-Antagonist medications have been reported to control PDE 3 inhibitor–related tachycardia successfully in one patient (57). However, extreme caution is appropriate, as they may remove the body's only mechanism of maintaining cardiac output in the face of vasodilation. If they are used, a short-acting IV β-antagonist should be selected. Other dysrhythmias associated with PDE 3 inhibitor toxicity should be managed in the usual manner.

Significant thrombocytopenia, or thrombocytopenia associated with bleeding complications, should be managed by cessation of PDE 3 inhibitor therapy. Platelet counts generally begin to improve within a week. Mild, isolated drops in platelet count do not automatically require stopping therapy; however, in some cases counts begin to return toward normal even if treatment is continued.

REFERENCES

1. Beavo JA. Cyclic nucleotide phosphodiesterases: functional implications of multiple isoforms. *Physiol Rev* 1995;75(4):725–748.
2. Francis SH, Turko IV, Corbin JD. Cyclic nucleotide phosphodiesterases: relating structure and function. *Prog Nucleic Acid Res Mol Biol* 2001;65:1–52.
3. Endoh M, Yanagisawa T, Taira N, et al. Effects of new inotropic agents on cyclic nucleotide metabolism and calcium transients in canine ventricular muscle. *Circulation* 1986;73(3 Pt 2):III117–33.

4. Ito M, Tanaka T, Saitoh M, et al. Selective inhibition of cyclic AMP phosphodiesterase from various human tissues by milrinone, a potent cardiac bipyridine. *Biochem Pharmacol* 1988;37(10):2041–2044.
5. Weishaar RE, Burrows SD, Kobylarz DC, et al. Multiple molecular forms of cyclic nucleotide phosphodiesterase in cardiac and smooth muscle and in platelets. Isolation, characterization, and effects of various reference phosphodiesterase inhibitors and cardiotonic agents. *Biochem Pharmacol* 1986;35(5):787–800.
6. Colucci WS. Cardiovascular effects of milrinone. *Am Heart J* 1991;121(6 Pt 2):1945–1947.
7. Kauffman RF, Schenck KW, Utterback BG, et al. In vitro vascular relaxation by new inotropic agents: relationship to phosphodiesterase inhibition and cyclic nucleotides. *J Pharmacol Exp Ther* 1987;242(3):864–872.
8. Kishi Y, Numano F. Involvement of cyclic AMP in vasodilatation by amrinone: a comparative study with 3-isobutyl-methyl-xanthine (IBMX). *Jpn J Pharmacol* 1986;42(4):477–485.
9. De Hert SG, ten Broecke PW, Mertens E, et al. Effects of phosphodiesterase III inhibition on length-dependent regulation of myocardial function in coronary surgery patients. *Br J Anaesth* 2002;88(6):779–784.
10. Mancini D, LeJemtel T, Sonnenblick E. Intravenous use of amrinone for the treatment of the failing heart. *Am J Cardiol* 1985;56(3):8B–15B.
11. Itoh H, Sato Y, Taniguchi K, et al. Differences between vasorelaxant responses of the canine and human mesenteric arteries and veins to amrinone. *Eur J Pharmacol* 1992;218(2–3):347–349.
12. Honerjager P. Pharmacology of positive inotropic phosphodiesterase III inhibitors. *Eur Heart J* 1989;10[Suppl C]:25–31.
13. Teshima H, Tobita K, Yamamura H, et al. Cardiovascular effects of a phosphodiesterase III inhibitor, amrinone, in infants: non-invasive echocardiographic evaluation. *Pediatr Int* 2002;44(3):259–263.
14. Alousi AA, Canter JM, Montenaro MJ, et al. Cardiotonic activity of milrinone, a new and potent cardiac bipyridine, on the normal and failing heart of experimental animals. *J Cardiovasc Pharmacol* 1983;5(5):792–803.
15. Kikura M, Sato S. The efficacy of preemptive milrinone or amrinone therapy in patients undergoing coronary artery bypass grafting. *Anesth Analg* 2002;94(1):22–30.
16. Lowes BD, Tsvetkova T, Eichhorn EJ, et al. Milrinone versus dobutamine in heart failure subjects treated chronically with carvedilol. *Int J Cardiol* 2001;81(2–3):141–149.
17. Kikura M, Kazama T, Ikeda T, Sato S. Disaggregatory effects of prostaglandin E1, amrinone and milrinone on platelet aggregation in human whole blood. *Platelets* 2000;11(8):446–458.
18. Hayashida N, Tomoeda H, Oda T, et al. Inhibitory effect of milrinone on cytokine production after cardiopulmonary bypass. *Ann Thorac Surg* 1999;68(5):1661–1667.
19. Endres S, Sinha B, Fulle HJ. Amrinone suppresses the synthesis of tumor necrosis factor-alpha in human mononuclear cells. *Shock* 1994;1(5):377–380.
20. Ward A, Brogden RN, Heel RC, et al. Amrinone. A preliminary review of its pharmacological properties and therapeutic use. *Drugs* 1983;26(6):468–502.
21. Goenen M. Historical perspectives and update of amrinone. *J Cardiothorac Anesth* 1989;3[6 Suppl 2]:15–23.
22. Bedford Laboratories. Prescribing information—inamrinone injection. USP2000.
23. Nony P, Boissel JP, Lievre M, et al. Evaluation of the effect of phosphodiesterase inhibitors on mortality in chronic heart failure patients. A meta-analysis. *Eur J Clin Pharmacol* 1994;46(3):191–196.
24. Maskin CS, Sinoway L, Chadwick B, et al. Sustained hemodynamic and clinical effects of a new cardiotonic agent, WIN 47203, in patients with severe congestive heart failure. *Circulation* 1983;67(5):1065–1070.
25. Sinoway LS, Maskin CS, Chadwick B, et al. Long-term therapy with a new cardiotonic agent, WIN 47203: drug-dependent improvement in cardiac performance and progression of the underlying disease. *J Am Coll Cardiol* 1983;2(2):327–331.
26. Bedford Laboratories. Prescribing information—milrinone lactate injection. 2002.
27. Loh E, Elkayam U, Cody R, et al. A randomized multicenter study comparing the efficacy and safety of intravenous milrinone and intravenous nitroglycerin in patients with advanced heart failure. *J Card Fail* 2001;7(2):114–121.
28. Kubo SH, Cody RJ, Chatterjee K, et al. Acute dose range study of milrinone in congestive heart failure. *Am J Cardiol* 1985;55(6):726–730.
29. Allen-Webb EM, Ross MP, Pappas JB, et al. Age-related amrinone pharmacokinetics in a pediatric population. *Crit Care Med* 1994;22(6):1016–1024.
30. Lynn AM, Sorensen GK, Williams GD, et al. Hemodynamic effects of amrinone and colloid administration in children following cardiac surgery. *J Cardiothorac Vasc Anesth* 1993;7(5):560–565.
31. Sorensen GK, Ramamoorthy C, Lynn AM, et al. Hemodynamic effects of amrinone in children after Fontan surgery. *Anesth Analg* 1996;82(2):241–246.
32. Wilmshurst PT, Thompson DS, Jenkins BS, et al. Haemodynamic effects of intravenous amrinone in patients with impaired left ventricular function. *Br Heart J* 1983;49(1):77–82.
33. Ramamoorthy C, Anderson GD, Williams GD, Lynn AM. Pharmacokinetics and side effects of milrinone in infants and children after open heart surgery. *Anesth Analg* 1998;86(2):283–289.
34. Lindsay CA, Barton P, Lawless S, et al. Pharmacokinetics and pharmacodynamics of milrinone lactate in pediatric patients with septic shock. *J Pediatr* 1998;132(2):329–334.
35. Lebovitz DJ, Lawless ST, Weise KL. Fatal amrinone overdose in a pediatric patient. *Crit Care Med* 1995;23(5):977–980.
36. Benotti JR, Lesko LJ, McCue JE, et al. Pharmacokinetics and pharmacodynamics of milrinone in chronic congestive heart failure. *Am J Cardiol* 1985;56(10):685–689.
37. Bailey JM, Miller BE, Lu W, et al. The pharmacokinetics of milrinone in pediatric patients after cardiac surgery. *Anesthesiology* 1999;90(4):1012–1018.
38. Park GB, Kershner RP, Angellotti J, et al. Oral bioavailability and intravenous pharmacokinetics of amrinone in humans. *J Pharm Sci* 1983;72(7):817–819.
39. Stroshane RM, Koss RF, Biddlecome CE, et al. Oral and intravenous pharmacokinetics of milrinone in human volunteers. *J Pharm Sci* 1984;73(10):1438–1441.
40. LeJemtel TH, Keung EC, Schwartz WJ, et al. Hemodynamic effects of intravenous and oral amrinone in patients with severe heart failure: relationship between intravenous and oral administration. *Trans Assoc Am Physicians* 1979;92:325–333.
41. Benotti JR, Lesko LJ, McCue JE. Acute pharmacodynamics and pharmacokinetics of oral amrinone. *J Clin Pharmacol* 1982;22(10):425–432.
42. Larsson R, Liedholm H, Andersson KE, et al. Pharmacokinetics and effects on blood pressure of a single oral dose of milrinone in healthy subjects and in patients with renal impairment. *Eur J Clin Pharmacol* 1986;29(5):549–553.
43. Wilson H, Rocci ML Jr, Weber KT, et al. Pharmacokinetics and hemodynamics of amrinone in patients with chronic cardiac failure of diverse etiology. *Res Commun Chem Pathol Pharmacol* 1987;56(1):3–19.
44. Edelson J, LeJemtel TH, Alousi AA, et al. Relationship between amrinone plasma concentration and cardiac index. *Clin Pharmacol Ther* 1981;29(6):723–728.
45. Laitinen P, Ahonen J, Olkkola KT, et al. Pharmacokinetics of amrinone in neonates and infants. *J Cardiothorac Vasc Anesth* 2000;14(4):378–382.
46. Bottorff MB, Rutledge DR, Pieper JA. Evaluation of intravenous amrinone: the first of a new class of positive inotropic agents with vasodilator properties. *Pharmacotherapy* 1985;5(5):227–237.
47. Silverman BD, Merrill AJ Jr, Gerber L. Clinical effects and side effects of amrinone. A study of 24 patients with chronic congestive heart failure. *Arch Intern Med* 1985;145(5):825–829.
48. DiBianco R, Shabetai R, Kostuk W, et al. A comparison of oral milrinone, digoxin, and their combination in the treatment of patients with chronic heart failure. *N Engl J Med* 1989;320(11):677–683.
49. Cuffe MS, Califf RM, Adams KF Jr, et al. Short-term intravenous milrinone for acute exacerbation of chronic heart failure: a randomized controlled trial. *JAMA* 2002;287(12):1541–1547.
50. Treadway G. Clinical safety of intravenous amrinone—a review. *Am J Cardiol* 1985;56(3):39B–40B.
51. Goldstein RA, Gray EL, Dougherty AH, et al. Electrophysiologic effects of amrinone. *Am J Cardiol* 1985;56(3):25B–28B.
52. Naccarelli GV, Gray EL, Dougherty AH, et al. Amrinone: acute electrophysiologic and hemodynamic effects in patients with congestive heart failure. *Am J Cardiol* 1984;54(6):600–604.
53. Trolese-Mongheal Y, Barthelemy J, Paire M, et al. Arrhythmogenic potencies of amrinone and milrinone in unanesthetized dogs with myocardial infarct. *Gen Pharmacol* 1992;23(1):95–104.
54. Todt H, Krumpl G, Krejcy K, et al. Programmed electrical stimulation in conscious dogs: electropharmacologic testing of amrinone. *Arch Int Pharmacodyn Ther* 1990;307:32–48.
55. Gold JA, Cullinane S, Chen J, et al. Vasopressin as an alternative to norepinephrine in the treatment of milrinone-induced hypotension. *Crit Care Med* 2000;28(1):249–252.
56. Saab G, Mindel G, Ewald G, et al. Acute renal failure secondary to milrinone in a patient with cardiac amyloidosis. *Am J Kidney Dis* 2002;40(2):E7.
57. Alhashemi JA, Hooper J. Treatment of milrinone-associated tachycardia with beta-blockers. *Can J Anaesth* 1998;45(1):67–70.
58. Roevens P, de Chaffoy de Courcelles D. Cyclic AMP-phosphodiesterase IIIA1 inhibitors decrease cytosolic Ca2+ concentration and increase the Ca2+ content of intracellular storage sites in human platelets. *Biochem Pharmacol* 1993;45(11):2279–2282.
59. Pattison A, Astley N, Eason CT, et al. A comparison of the effects of three positive inotropic agents (amrinone, milrinone and medorinone) on platelet aggregation in human whole blood. *Thromb Res* 1990;57(6):909–918.
60. Ross MP, Allen-Webb EM, Pappas JB, et al. Amrinone-associated thrombocytopenia: pharmacokinetic analysis. *Clin Pharmacol Ther* 1993;53(6):661–667.
61. Ansell J, Tiarks C, McCue J, et al. Amrinone-induced thrombocytopenia. *Arch Intern Med* 1984;144(5):949–952.
62. Likoff MJ, Weber KT, Andrews V, et al. Amrinone in the treatment of chronic cardiac failure. *J Am Coll Cardiol* 1984;3(5):1282–1290.
63. Eason CT, Pattison A, Howells DD, et al. The effects of amrinone, cyclophosphamide and anti-platelet serum on platelet production in the Gunn rat. *J Appl Toxicol* 1988;8(1):29–34.
64. Gilman ME, Margolis SC. Amrinone-induced hepatotoxicity. *Clin Pharm* 1984;3(4):422–424.
65. Mattingly PM, Burnette PK, Weston MW, et al. Pancytopenia secondary to short-term, high-dose intravenous infusion of amrinone. *DICP* 1990;24(12):1172–1174.
66. Kullberg MP, Dorrbecker B, Lennon J, et al. High-performance liquid chromatographic analysis of amrinone and its N-acetyl derivative in plasma. Pharmacokinetics of amrinone in the dog. *J Chromatogr* 1980;187(1):264–270.
67. Lawless S, Burckart G, Diven W, et al. Amrinone pharmacokinetics in neonates and infants. *J Clin Pharmacol* 1988;28(3):283–284.
68. Hellinger A, Wolter K, Marggraf G, et al. Elimination of amrinone during continuous veno-venous haemofiltration after cardiac surgery. *Eur J Clin Pharmacol* 1995;48(1):57–59.
69. Lawless S, Restaino I, Azin S, et al. Effect of continuous arteriovenous haemofiltration on pharmacokinetics of amrinone. *Clin Pharmacokinet* 1993;25(1):80–82.

CHAPTER 124

Rauwolfia Alkaloids

Vikhyat S. Bebarta and Richard C. Dart

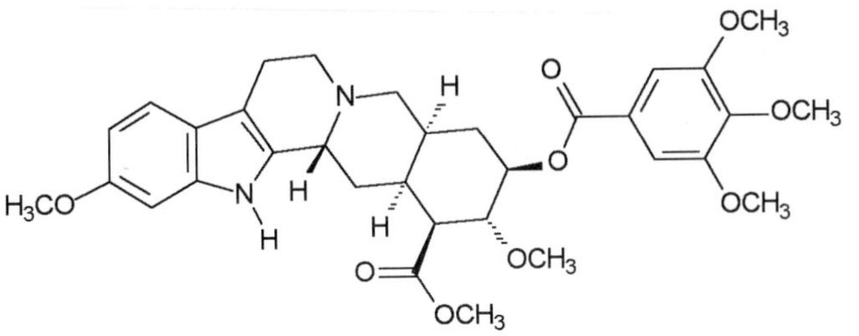

RESERPINE

Compounds included:	**Reserpine (Eskaserp, Serpasil)**
Molecular formula and weight:	$C_{33}H_{40}N_2O_9$, **608.7 g/mol**
SI conversion:	**mg/L × 1.64 = nmol/L**
CAS Registry No.:	**50-55-5**
Normal or therapeutic levels:	**10 mg/L (serum), not immediately available**
Special concerns:	**Hypotension, central nervous system depression, bradycardia, depression**
Antidote:	**None**

OVERVIEW

Reserpine (Eskaserp, Serpasil) is an alkaloid extracted from the root of *Rauwolfia serpentina*, a shrub indigenous to India. Descriptions of this medicinal plant occur throughout the Ayurvedic writings. In 1931, Sen and Bose published the first paper describing the plant's antihypertensive and sedative effects (1). Rauwolfia alkaloids were not used in western medicine until Kline (2) published his experience with the antipsychotic effects of *R. serpentina* in 1954.

Reserpine is the most common rauwolfia alkaloid used in western medicine. Only the oral form (0.1- and 0.25-mg tablets) is available in the United States. Parenteral formulations are not addressed in this chapter (3). Reserpine is typically used in combination with a thiazide as an adjunctive antihypertensive agent. The use of reserpine has been studied for many medical problems: regional pain syndrome, chorea, depression, hyperthyroidism, psychosis, Raynaud's disease, and tardive dyskinesia (3). Despite considerable use until the early 1980s, the use of reserpine and other rauwolfia alkaloids has greatly declined (4). In overdose, hypotension and central nervous system (CNS) depression predominate.

Deserpidine is another rauwolfia alkaloid derivative. It is combined with methyclothiazide and used for hypertension. *R. serpentina* itself is also used as a tranquilizer and antihypertensive.

TOXIC DOSE

The adult therapeutic dose of reserpine for hypertension is 0.5 mg/day orally for 1 to 2 weeks, then 0.1 to 0.25 mg/day (5). Although reserpine is not typically used for psychosis, the usual dose is 0.5 mg/day. The pediatric dose is 0.01 to 0.002 mg/kg/day orally, divided twice daily (3).

Two deaths secondary to respiratory failure have been reported after electroshock therapy (ECT) (6,7). In one case, 15 mg reserpine was given for 11 days before ECT; the patient died shortly after his fourth ECT (6). A case of reserpine poisoning resulting in death was reported in the Russian literature (8). Three children have had significant symptoms after ingesting up to 25 mg reserpine. Coma, absent deep tendon reflexes, and right-sided third nerve palsy developed, but they recovered completely by 48 hours (9). A 20-month-old child ingested 260 mg reserpine and was lethargic with slowed reflexes but recovered by 72 hours (10).

TOXICOKINETICS AND TOXICODYNAMICS

Reserpine is readily absorbed after oral dosing. The peak serum concentration occurs in approximately 2 hours (11,12). It is rapidly hydrolyzed to several metabolites, mostly trimethoxybenzoic acid and methylreserpate, with a small amount of reserpine acid (11,13). Urinary excretion accounts for 6% of reserpine, mainly as trimethoxybenzoic acid. Between 15% and 60% is eliminated in the feces (11). The parent compound has an elimination half-life of 11.5 days and is independent of renal function (11).

PATHOPHYSIOLOGY

Reserpine binds to storage vesicles of norepinephrine and dopamine in central and peripheral adrenergic neurons. These storage vesicles are then rendered dysfunctional, and catecholamines are leaked to the cytoplasm and destroyed by intraneuronal monoamine oxidase (14).

PREGNANCY AND LACTATION

Reserpine is U.S. Food and Drug Administration pregnancy category C (Appendix I). The drug is teratogenic in animals, but there are no studies indicating this effect in humans. It also is excreted in breast milk. In mothers who are taking reserpine for preeclampsia, neonates have developed nasal congestion and possibly increased lethargy and respiratory depression developed in neonates (15).

CLINICAL PRESENTATION

Acute Overdosage

The acute toxicity of reserpine differs from its therapeutic adverse effects. Hypotension and CNS depression dominate the clinical presentation in acute overdose. Initial hypertension and tachycardia can occur, followed by hypotension and bradycardia. Of 129 ingestions of reserpine and rauwolfia alkaloids, mostly accidental ingestions, 2 had hypotension (16). In this same group, 44% presented with CNS depression, but only one with coma (16). The CNS depression may occur 3 to 7 hours after ingestion.

Adverse Reactions

With chronic use, there are many reports of adverse reactions, including depression, sexual dysfunction, breast cancer, and nasal congestion. However, the dose of reserpine used in these cases was much higher than the doses currently used for hypertension. Most of these effects are not present at lower doses recommended by the manufacturer.

In 1954, Freis (17) first described depression in patients who received large doses of reserpine. In the next 4 years, three additional reports were published, with rates of depression of 8% to 26% and doses from 0.75 to 4.0 mg (18–20). However, at doses less than 0.2 mg (rarely is a higher dose needed for hypertension), no depression has been reported (20). In several trials of treatment for hypertension, the incidence of depression is similar to that with beta-blockers, 2% to 4% (21–23).

Sexual dysfunction and dyspepsia were initially a concern; however, these symptoms occur at similar or lower rates than with other antihypertensive drugs when using 0.25 mg or less (23,24). In the 1970s, several small studies suggested an association of breast cancer with reserpine. Two large prospective studies have dismissed this association (25,26).

Nasal congestion occurs in up to 15% of patients (27). Two cases of acute hematemesis after parenteral reserpine have been reported (28,29). One case reported the use of 5 mg intravenously and 2 mg orally. Skin flushing and miosis have been reported (10,16,30).

A case of possible reserpine withdrawal was reported after the patient discontinued reserpine at a dose of 0.1 mg/day for 20 years. Euphoria and visual hallucinations developed and resolved after the patient restarted reserpine (31).

Drug Interactions

Use of rauwolfia alkaloids is cautioned in patients who are taking digoxin or have a history of depression or sexual dysfunction (32). Several cases of cardiac dysrhythmias after administration of digoxin and parenteral reserpine have been reported (33–35). These cases are with parenteral reserpine, and the dysrhythmias could be explained by digoxin toxicity alone.

DIAGNOSTIC TESTS

Acute Overdosage

The serum level of reserpine is not helpful clinically. Reserpine binds irreversibly to its receptors so that the amount of drug in the plasma does not correlate well with the drug at the site of action (14). In addition, serum catecholamines are elevated for several days after ingestion but their measurement is also not clinically useful (5). Serum acetaminophen and salicylate levels after an overdose detect occult ingestions. Serum electrolytes, glucose, blood urea nitrogen, and creatinine are indicated to detect an occult ingestion causing acidosis such as a toxic alcohol or to evaluate for altered mental status.

An electrocardiogram is recommended to evaluate for bradycardia, conduction blocks, or signs of other cardiotoxic medications such as tricyclic antidepressants. Pulse oximetry, arterial blood gas, and chest radiography are not needed, except in the rare case of a hemodynamically unstable patient. Diagnostic interventions, such as naloxone, dextrose, thiamine, computed tomogram of the brain, and lumbar puncture should be considered to evaluate other causes of altered mental status.

TREATMENT

In general, management of an acute overdose of reserpine includes prompt decontamination, prolonged observation, and good supportive care. The threshold should be low to admit the patient for observation. Patients should be admitted if they are symptomatic or have ingested a potentially toxic dose. Symptoms are often delayed, and toxicity is prolonged. Toxic effects usually occur within 24 hours, and complete recovery is expected unless there are other complications in the care, such as hypoxia or prolonged hypotension. Patients can be discharged from the hospital if they are asymptomatic, have stable vital signs and normal mental status, and have been observed for at least 24 hours.

Decontamination

If the patient is awake and alert, one dose of activated charcoal (1 to 2 g/kg) without a cathartic should be administered if the ingestion occurred within the previous 2 hours. Charcoal can also be given if the patient's airway is protected by endotracheal intubation. Cathartics, induced emesis, and whole bowel irrigation have not been studied with reserpine poisoning and are not recommended.

Enhancement of Elimination

Reserpine is not dialyzable, partly because it is highly protein bound; thus, hemodialysis is not recommended (36). Hemoperfusion, peritoneal dialysis, and multiple dose activated charcoal have not been studied with reserpine poisoning and are not recommended.

Antidotes

No antidotes are available for toxicity from rauwolfia alkaloids.

Supportive Care

The patient should be placed on a cardiac monitor, oxygen, and continuous pulse oximetry, and intravenous access should be established. Symptomatic bradycardia is treated with atropine. Hypotension is treated with a normal saline bolus of 20 ml/kg intravenously, repeated if needed. If the patient is still hypotensive, treatment with a direct-acting vasopressor such as norepinephrine or epinephrine should be used. Dopamine may not be effective because of the mechanism to action of reserpine on presynaptic monoamines. However, it may be reasonable to initiate therapy with dopamine if it is available quickly until another vasopressor is prepared. Hypertension should be treated with a short-acting, titratable antihypertensive such as nitroprusside.

Management Pitfalls

After ingestion of reserpine of rauwolfia alkaloids, cardiac dysrhythmias and CNS depression can sometimes be delayed 3 to 7 hours and may last 48 to 72 hours. Prolonged observation on a cardiac monitor and pulse oximetry is necessary. Also, hypotension may follow the initial hypertension; therefore, only short-acting antihypertensive agents should be used.

REFERENCES

1. Sen G, Bose KC. *Rauwolfia serpentina*: a new Indian drug for insanity and high blood pressure. *Indian Medical World* 1931;11:194–201.
2. Kline NS. Use of *Rauwolfia serpentina* benth in neuropsychiatric conditions. *Ann N Y Acad Sci* 1954;59:107–132.
3. DRUGDEX Editorial Staff. Reserpine. DRUGDEX System. Edition expires 3/2003 edition. Greenwood Village, Co: MICROMEDEX.
4. Lederle FA, Applegate WB, Grimm RH Jr. Reserpine and the medical marketplace. *Arch Intern Med* 1993;153(6):705–706.
5. Becker CE. Reserpine and rauwolfia alkaloids. POISINDEX system. Edition expires 3/2003 edition. Greenwood Village, CO: MICROMEDEX.
6. Bracha S, Hes JP. Death occurring during combined reserpine-electroshock treatment. *Am J Psychiatry* 1956;13(257).
7. Foster MW, Gayle RF. *JAMA* 1955;159:1520.
8. Rogal PP, Rakitin VA, Boichak MP. Fatal reserpine poisoning. *Sud Med Ekspert* 1989;32:51–52.
9. Loggie JM, Saito H, Kahn I. Accidental reserpine poisoning: clinical and metabolic effects. *Clin Pharmacol Ther* 1967;8:692.
10. Hubbard BA. Reserpine. *JAMA* 1955;157:468.
11. Maass AR, Jenkins B, Shen Y, Tannenbaum P. Studies on absorption, excretion, and metabolism of 3H-reserpine in man. *Clin Pharmacol Ther* 1969;10(3):366–371.
12. Zsoter TT, Johnson GE, DeVeber GA, Paul H. Excretion and metabolism of reserpine in renal failure. *Clin Pharmacol Ther* 1973;14(3):325–330.
13. Stitzel RE. The biological fate of reserpine. *Pharmacol Rev* 1976;28(3):179–208.
14. Goodman LS, Hardman JG, Limbird LE, Gilman AG. *Goodman & Gilman's the pharmacological basis of therapeutics*, 10th ed. New York: McGraw-Hill, 2001.
15. Budnick IS, Leiken S, Hoeck LE. Effect in newborn infant of reserpine administered ante partum. *Am J Dis Child* 1955; 90:286–289.
16. McKown CH, Verhulst HL, Crotty JJ. Overdosage effects and dangers from tranquilizing drugs. *JAMA* 1963;185:425–430.
17. Freis ED. Mental depression in hypertensive patients treated for long periods with large doses of reserpine. *N Engl J Med* 1954;251:1006–1008.
18. Limieux G, Davignon A, Genest J. Depressive states during rauwolfia therapy for arterial hypertension: a report of 30 cases. *Can Med Assoc J* 1956;74:522–526.
19. Muller JC, Pryor WW, Gibbons JE. Depression and anxiety occurring during rauwolfia therapy. *JAMA* 1955;159:836–839.
20. Quetsch RM, Achor RWP, Litin EM, et al. Depressive reactions in hypertensive patients: a comparison of those treated with rauwolfia and those receiving no specific antihypertensive treatment. *Circulation* 1959;19:366–375.
21. Applegate WB, Carper ER, Kahn SE, et al. Comparison of the use of reserpine versus alpha-methyldopa for second step treatment of hypertension in the elderly. *J Am Geriatr Soc* 1985;33(2):109–115.
22. Gibb WE, Malpas JS, Turner P, et al. Comparison of bethanidine, alpha-methyldopa, and reserpine in essential hypertension. *Lancet* 1970; 2(7667):275–277.
23. Veterans Administration Cooperative Study Group on Antihypertensive Agents. Propranolol in the treatment of essential hypertension. *JAMA* 1977;237(21):2303–2310.
24. Materson BJ, Cushman WC, Goldstein G, et al. Treatment of hypertension in the elderly: I. Blood pressure and clinical changes. Results of a Department of Veterans Affairs Cooperative Study. *Hypertension* 1990;15(4):348–360.
25. Curb JD, Hardy RJ, Labarthe DR, et al. Reserpine and breast cancer in the Hypertension Detection and Follow-Up Program. *Hypertension* 1982;4(2):307–311.
26. Labarthe DR, O'Fallon WM. Reserpine and breast cancer. A community-based longitudinal study of 2,000 hypertensive women. *JAMA* 1980;243(22):2304–2310.
27. Participating Veterans Administration Medical Centers. Low doses v standard dose of reserpine. A randomized, double-blind, multiclinic trial in patients taking chlorthalidone. *JAMA* 1982;248(19):2471–2477.
28. Duncan DA, Fleeson W. Reserpine induced gastrointestinal hemorrhage. *JAMA* 1959;170:109–110.
29. Hollister LE. Hematemesis and melena complicating treatment with rauwolfia alkaloids. *Arch Intern Med* 1957;99:218–221.
30. Gosselin RE, Smith RP, Hodge HC. *Clinical toxicology of commercial products*, 5th ed. Baltimore: Williams & Wilkins, 1984.
31. Kent TA, Wilber RD. Reserpine withdrawal psychosis: the possible role of denervation supersensitivity of receptors. *J Nerv Ment Dis* 1982;170(8):502–504.
32. Magarian GJ. Reserpine: a relic from the past or a neglected drug of the present for achieving cost containment in treating hypertension? *J Gen Intern Med* 1991;6(6):561–572.
33. Dick HLH, McCawley EH, Fisher WA. Reserpine-digitalis toxicity. *Arch Intern Med* 1962;109:503–506.
34. Lown BL. Effect of digitalis in patients receiving reserpine. *Circulation* 1961;24:1185–1191.
35. Schreader CJ. Premature ventricular contractions due to rauwolfia. *JAMA* 1956;162(1256).
36. Bennett WM. *Drug prescribing in renal failure dosing guidelines for adults*, 2nd ed. Philadelphia: American College of Physicians, 1991.

CHAPTER 125

Vasodilators

Katherine M. Hurlbut

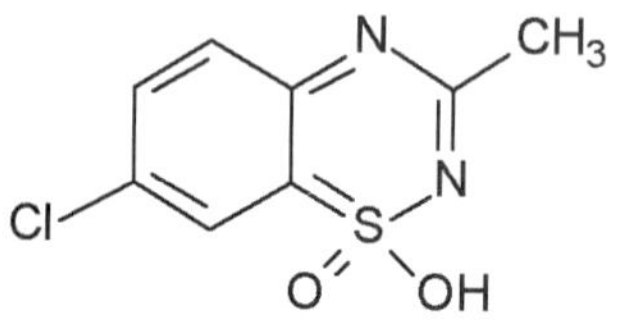

DIAZOXIDE

Compounds included:	**Cinnarizine (Glanil); diazoxide (Hyperstat, Proglycem); flosequinan (Manoplax): 239.3; flunarizine (Fluricin); guanabenz (Wytensin); guanadrel (Hylorel); guanethidine (Ismelin); hydralazine (Apresoline); minoxidil (Loniten, Rogaine); alprostadil (Caverject, Muse); dipyridamole (Persantine, Aggrenox); isoxsuprine (Vasodilan); papaverine (Pavabid); phenoxybenzamine (Dibenzyline); phentolamine (Regitine); prazosin (Minipress); terazosin (Hytrin); tolazoline (Priscoline)**
Molecular formula and weight:	**See Table 1.**
SI conversion:	**See Table 1.**
CAS Registry No.:	**See Table 1.**
Therapeutic levels:	**Not available or clinically useful**
Special concerns:	**Hypotension with potential for myocardial ischemia**
Antidote:	**α-Agonist in selected cases**

OVERVIEW

There are many different vasodilators with multiple different mechanisms of action. They are used for diverse purposes, ranging from the treatment of hypertension to the treatment of impotence. Their diagnosis and treatment are addressed for the group as a whole at the end of the chapter.

ALPROSTADIL

Toxic Dose

The *adult and pediatric therapeutic doses* are provided in Table 1. The dose of alprostadil for erectile dysfunction is generally titrated to the individual patient's response. There is limited overdose experience.

Toxicokinetics and Toxicodynamics

The onset of action is 30 to 60 minutes (1). Plasma protein binding is 81%. The elimination half-life is 5 to 10 minutes (2) (Table 2).

Pathophysiology

Alprostadil is an E class prostaglandin that causes vasodilation, inhibits platelet aggregation, and an increase in heart rate and reduction in blood pressure (3).

Pregnancy and Lactation

Alprostadil is U.S. Food and Drug Administration (FDA) pregnancy category B (Appendix I). Its entry into breast milk has not been reported.

Clinical Presentation

Parenteral administration in infants causes fever (14%), flushing (10%), bradycardia (7%), hypotension (4%), and tachycardia (3%) (4). Less common adverse effects in children include disseminated intravascular coagulation (1%), hypokalemia (1%), and diarrhea (2%). The most common adverse effect in adults using alprostadil for erectile dysfunction is penile pain (32% to 37%). Urethral burning (12%), bleeding (5%), and testicular pain (5%) are common after transurethral use (5). Intracavernosal injection can cause prolonged erection (4%) and penile fibrosis or hematoma (3%) (6).

CINNARIZINE AND FLUNARIZINE

Drowsiness, headache, and extrapyramidal reactions such as tremor, akathisia, and dyskinesia are the most common adverse effects reported (7,8). Elderly patients and those with a family history of tremor or Parkinson's disease may be at greater risk for developing extrapyramidal effects (9,10). Hallucinations, nightmares, nausea, vomiting, constipation, and weight gain are less common adverse effects (11,12).

TABLE 1. Physical characteristics and dose of the vasodilating agents

Drug	Molecular formula, molecular weight (g/mol), CAS Registry No.	SI conversion	Formulation	Therapeutic dose	
				Adult	Pediatric
Alprostadil	$C_{20}H_{34}O_5$, 354.5, 745-65-3	mg/L × 2.8 = μmol/L	10- and 20-μg syringes; 5-, 10-, 20-, and 40-μg vials; 10-, 20-, or 40-μg solutions for injection; 125-, 250-, 500-, 1000-μg urethral suppositories	125- to 1000-μg transurethral; 2.5- to 10.0-μg intracavernosal	0.05 to 0.1 μg/kg/min by IV infusion
Cinnarizine	$C_{26}H_{28}N_2$, 368.5, 298-57-7	mg/L × 2.7 = μmol/L	15-, 25-, 75-mg tablets or capsules; 75-mg/ml oral drops	30–75 mg three times daily	1 mg/kg
Diazoxide	$C_8H_7ClN_2O_2S$, 230.7, 364-98-7	mg/L × 4.3 = μmol/L	300-mg/20-ml ampule; 50-mg capsule; 50-mg/ml suspension	600–800 mg/day PO; 1–3 mg/kg IV repeated every 5–15 min as needed	1–3 mg/kg IV repeated every 5–15 min as needed
Dipyridamole	$C_{24}H_{40}N_8O_4$, 504.6, 58-32-2	mg/L × 2.0 = μmol/L	25-, 50-, 75-mg tablets; 200-mg extended release capsule	200–400 mg/d PO	NR
Flosequinan	$C_{11}H_{10}FNO_2S$, 239.3, 76568-02-0	mg/L × 4.2 = μmol/L	NR	30–75 mg/d	NR
Flunarizine hydrochloride	$C_{26}H_{26}F_2N_2$,2HCl; 477.4; 30484-77-6	mg/L × 2.1 = μmol/L	5-, 10-mg tablets	5–10 mg daily	5 mg PO
Guanabenz acetate	$C_8H_8Cl_2N_4$,$C_2H_4O_2$; 291.1; 23256-50-0	mg/L × 3.4 = μmol/L	4-, 8-mg tablets	8–32 mg/d in divided doses	NR
Guanadrel sulfate	$(C_{10}H_{19}N_3O_2)_2$,H_2SO_4; 524.6; 22195-34-2	mg/L × 1.9 = μmol/L	10-, 25-mg tablets	20–75 mg/d; maximum dose, 400 mg/d in divided doses	—
Guanethidine monosulfate	$C_{10}H_{22}N_4$,H_2SO_4; 296.4; 645-43-2	mg/L × 3.4 = μmol/L	10-, 25-mg tablets	25–50 mg/d; maximum, 50 mg twice daily	—
Hydralazine hydrochloride	$C_8H_8N_4$,HCl; 196.6; 304-20-1	mg/L × 5.1 = μmol/L	10-, 25-, 50-, 100-mg tablets	200–400 mg/d in divided doses	0.75 to 1.0 mg/kg/d in divided doses; maximum of 7.5 mg/kg/d
Isoxsuprine hydrochloride	$C_{18}H_{23}NO_3$,HCl; 337.8; 579-56-6	mg/L × 3.0 = μmol/L	10-, 20-mg tablets	10–20 mg three or four times daily	NR
Minoxidil	$C_9H_{15}N_5O$, 209.2, 38304-91-5	mg/L × 4.8 = μmol/L	2.5-, 10.0-mg tablet; 2% topical solution	5–60 mg PO daily	0.2 mg/kg/d as single dose; maximum of 0.1–0.2 mg/kg/d
Papaverine hydrochloride	$C_{20}H_{21}NO_4$,HCl; 375.8; 61-25-6	mg/L × 2.7 = μmol/L	30-mg/ml solution for injection	150 mg every 12 hours PO; 30 to 160 mg intracorporeal	1.5 mg/kg IM or IV four times daily
Phenoxybenzamine hydrochloride	$C_{18}H_{22}ClNO$,HCl; 340.3; 563-92-3	mg/L × 2.9 = μmol/L	10-mg capsules	10–40 mg PO three times daily	1 to 2 mg/kg/d in divided doses (pheochromocytoma)
Phentolamine mesylate	$C_{17}H_{19}N_3O$,CH_4SO_3; 377.5; 65-28-1	mg/L × 2.6 = μmol/L	5-mg vials	40–80 mg/d PO; 5–20 mg IV	1 mg IV (pheochromocytoma)
Prazosin hydrochloride	$C_{19}H_{21}N_5O_4$,HCl; 419.9; 19237-84-4	mg/L × 2.4 = μmol/L	1-, 2-, 5-mg capsules	6–15 mg/d in divided doses; the initial dose is 1 mg two or three times daily	5-μg/kg dose every 6 h, gradually increased to 25 μg/kg/dose[a]
Terazosin hydrochloride	$C_{19}H_{25}N_5O_4$,HCl,$2H_2O$; 459.9; 70024-40-7	mg/L × 2.2 = μmol/L	1-, 2-, 5-, 10-mg capsules	1–5 mg daily or twice daily, maximum dose, 20 mg/d; initial dose, 1 mg	NR
Tolazoline hydrochloride	$C_{10}H_{12}N_2$,HCl; 196.7; 59-97-2	mg/L × 5.1 = μmol/L	25-mg/ml ampule	25–50 mg orally four times daily	1–2 mg/kg, then 1–2 mg/kg/h (pulmonary hypertension)

NR, not reported.
[a]From Taketomo CK, Hodding JH, Kraus DM, eds. *Pediatric dosage handbook*, 4th ed. Cleveland, OH: Lexi-Comp Inc, 1998, with permission.

Toxic Dose

The *adult and pediatric therapeutic doses* are provided in Table 1. No overdose data are available.

Toxicokinetics and Toxicodynamics

Cinnarizine effects start at 3.0 to 4.5 hours and peak in 6 hours. It is rapidly absorbed; extent of absorption depends on gastric acidity. It undergoes extensive hepatic metabolism and renal excretion, 20% to 33% as metabolites (13). Fecal elimination is 40% to 67%. The elimination half-life is 3 to 6 hours (13).

Flunarizine has a time to maximum concentration (T_{max}) of 2 to 4 hours. The volume of distribution (V_d) is 43.2 L/kg, more than 90% protein bound. Hepatic metabolism is extensive. Its elimination half-life is 18 days (14) (Table 2).

Pregnancy and Lactation

Cinnarizine is FDA pregnancy category C (Appendix I). Flunarizine is not rated. The effect on the fetus during breast-feeding is unknown for both agents.

Pathophysiology

These drugs are long-acting inhibitors of potassium chloride-depolarization–induced peripheral vasoconstriction, by selectively inhibiting calcium influx into depolarized cells. This reduces the

TABLE 2. Pharmacokinetics of vasodilating drugs

Drug	Time to maximum concentration (h)	Bioavailability (%)	Protein binding (%)	Volume of distribution	Hepatic metabolism (%)	Renal elimination (%)	Half-life
Alprostadil	NR	NR	81	NR	Primarily pulmonary metabolism	90	5–10 min
Cinnarizine	2–4	Depends on gastric acidity	NR	—	Extensive	20–33 as metabolites	3–6 h
Diazoxide	3–5	NR	90	0.21 L/kg	NR	Primarily (50 as metabolites)	20–36 h
Dipyridamole	0.5–2.5	37–66	99	2.43 L/kg	Primarily	Minimal	9–13 h
Flosequinan	1–2	72	NR	NR	98	50	2 h
Flunarizine	2–4	—	90	42 L/kg	Extensive	None	18 d
Guanabenz	2–5	75	90	7.4–13.4 L/kg	Extensive	Primarily (as metabolites)	6 h
Guanadrel	1.5–2.0	Well absorbed	20	—	—	85 total; 40 unchanged	10 h
Guanethidine	NR	Variable <50	None	—	40	25–60	4–8 d
Hydralazine	1–2	38–70	88–90	NR	Significant	3–14	3–5 h
Isoxsuprine	1	Nearly complete	NR	NR	NR	Primarily	1.5 h
Minoxidil	1	90–100	Insignificant	2–3 L/kg	90	90 (mostly metabolites)	4.2 h
Papaverine	1–2	68–89 solution, 22–29 SR tablet	90	NR	Extensive	Extensive	0.5–2.0 h
Phenoxybenzamine	NR	20–30	NR	NR	Extensive	NR	24 h
Phentolamine	0.5–1.0	NR	<72	NR	Extensive	80 (10–13 unchanged)	19 min (IV), 5–7 h (PO)
Prazosin	1–3	NR	92–97	0.5 L/kg	30	3–4	2–4 h
Tolazoline	NR	90–100	NR	1.6 L/kg	Little	Extensive	3–10 h
Terazosin	1	90	90–94	25–30 L	Extensive	40 (10 unchanged)	9–12 h

NR, not reported.

free calcium available for induction and maintenance of vascular smooth muscle contraction. Cinnarizine also modifies the calcium adenosine triphosphate balance in erythrocytes by antagonizing calcium influx. This increases red blood cell flexibility and decreases blood viscosity. Cinnarizine is also an H_1 antihistamine.

Clinical Presentation

No overdose data are available.

DIAZOXIDE

Toxic Dose

The *adult and pediatric therapeutic doses* are provided in Table 1.

Toxicokinetics and Toxicodynamics

The T_{max} is 3 to 5 hours (15). Protein binding is 90% (16), and the V_d is 0.21 L/kg. It is hepatically metabolized, and then undergoes primarily renal excretion, 50% as metabolites. There is little fecal elimination. The elimination half-life is 20 to 36 hours (15) (Table 2).

Pathophysiology

Diazoxide is a direct acting vasodilator with an unclear mechanism of action.

Pregnancy and Lactation

Diazoxide is FDA pregnancy category C (Appendix I). Entry into breast milk is unknown.

Clinical Presentation

Overdose can cause hypotension, tachycardia, and dysrhythmias. Hyperglycemia and nonketotic hyperosmolar coma have developed with therapeutic use (17). The most common adverse effect is orthostatic hypotension. Severe hypotension has been reported after intravenous use; complications such as ischemic stroke and myocardial infarction have been described in a few cases (18–20). A 6-month-old child developed 2:1 atrioventricular block after receiving 5 mg/kg intravenous diazoxide (21).

DIPYRIDAMOLE

Toxic Dose

The *adult and pediatric therapeutic doses* are provided in Table 1. Little published information describing overdose is available.

Toxicokinetics and Toxicodynamics

The T_{max} is 0.5 to 2.5 hours. Bioavailability is 37% to 66%, protein binding 99%, and the V_d is 2.43 L/kg. The terminal elimination half-life is 9 to 13 hours (22). Dipyridamole has minimal renal excretion (Table 2).

Pathophysiology

Dipyridamole is a phosphodiesterase inhibitor, increasing platelet levels of cAMP and potentiating the de-aggregating effects of prostacyclin (23). Dipyridamole decreases adenosine metabolism and decreases erythrocyte uptake of adenosine; adenosine inhibits platelet aggregation and induces vasodilation. Dipyridamole increases coronary blood flow by causing selective coronary vasodilatation.

Pregnancy and Lactation

Dipyridamole is FDA pregnancy category B (Appendix I). Excretion into breast milk is unknown.

Clinical Presentation

Transient hypotension, tachycardia, dizziness, flushing, and weakness might be expected (24).

Hypotension is common with therapeutic use (25). Myocardial ischemia has been described in patients receiving intravenous dipyridamole and thallium for stress testing. It is postulated that dipyridamole-induced vasodilation reduces perfusion pressure and coronary blood flow below baseline, producing ischemia (*coronary steal*) (26). Ventricular premature contractions are fairly common in patients receiving intravenous dipyridamole and thallium for stress testing (27). Bradycardia and asystole have been reported rarely (28–31). Headache is common, developing in approximately 20% of patients (32). Patients with a history of bronchospasm can develop worsening symptoms after dipyridamole administration (33).

FLOSEQUINAN

Toxic Dose

The *adult and pediatric therapeutic doses* are provided in Table 1. No overdose data are available.

Toxicokinetics and Toxicodynamics

The onset of action is 30 to 60 minutes with a T_{max} and peak effect in 1 to 2 hours (34,35). Bioavailability is 72%. Hepatic metabolism is 98% and renal excretion is 50% (36). The elimination half-life is 2 hours (Table 2).

Pathophysiology

Flosequinan is a direct acting vasodilator, it induces cyclic guanosine monophosphate production by stimulating guanylate cyclase, and is a nonspecific phosphodiesterase inhibitor.

Pregnancy and Lactation

Flosequinan is FDA pregnancy category C (Appendix I). Its excretion in breast milk is unknown.

Clinical Presentation

Anemia, headache, postural hypotension, hypokalemia, nausea, and tachycardia are the most common adverse effects (35). Flosequinan shortens both the QT and the QRS intervals and the atrial and ventricular refractory period (37). Premature ventricular contractions and both sustained and nonsustained ventricular tachycardia have occasionally been reported. Mild, reversible elevations in hepatic transaminase levels can occur with therapeutic use.

GUANABENZ

Toxic Dose

The *adult and pediatric therapeutic doses* are provided in Table 1.

Toxicokinetics and Toxicodynamics

The onset of effect is 60 minutes, with peak effect at 2 to 4 hours and a duration 6 to 8 hours. The T_{max} is 2 to 5 hours and bioavailability is 75% (38). Protein binding is 90% and the V_d is 7.4 to 13.4 L/kg (39). Guanabenz undergoes extensive hepatic metabolism with less than 1% renal excretion as unchanged drug (39). The elimination half-life is 6 hours (Table 2).

Pathophysiology

Similar to clonidine, guanabenz reduces central sympathetic outflow by stimulating central α_2-receptors.

Pregnancy and Lactation

Guanabenz is FDA pregnancy category C (Appendix I). Excretion into breast milk is unknown.

Clinical Presentation

Overdose causes hypotension, bradycardia, somnolence, respiratory depression, and miosis. Common adverse effects include sedation, weakness, dizziness, and dry mouth (40). Atrioventricular block has been reported rarely with therapeutic use (41). An adult ingested 50 to 60 tablets containing 4 mg guanabenz each and developed somnolence, followed by bradycardia (heart rate, 38 to 45 beats/minute) and mild hypotension (100/60 mm Hg) (42). A 3-year-old (12 kg) child developed somnolence followed by hypotension and bradycardia after ingesting 12 mg. She was treated with atropine and dopamine and recovered within 24 hours (42). A 19-month-old child developed unresponsiveness with periods of apnea, as well as hypotension and bradycardia after ingesting 28 mg (42).

GUANADREL AND GUANETHIDINE

Hypotension and bradycardia are the most common effects after overdose. Orthostatic hypotension is the most common adverse effect, and may be associated with syncope or dizziness (43). Edema and weight gain are also fairly common (44).

Toxic Dose

The *adult and pediatric therapeutic doses* are provided in Table 1.

Toxicokinetics and Toxicodynamics

The bioavailability of guanethidine is less than 50% (45). It is not protein bound. Guanethidine is approximately 40% hepatically metabolized, with 25% to 60% renal excretion as unchanged drug. Fecal elimination is 40% to 50%. The elimination half-life is 4 to 8 days. Guanadrel has a T_{max} of 1.5 to 2 hours, 85% renal excretion (40% as unchanged drug), and a half-life of 10 hours. It is 20% protein bound (46) (Table 2).

Pregnancy and Lactation

Guanadrel is FDA pregnancy category B; guanethidine is category C (Appendix I). Entry into breast milk is unknown for both agents.

Pathophysiology

These drugs inhibit the release of catecholamines induced by sympathetic nerve stimulation, thus preventing vasoconstriction.

Clinical Presentation

Hypotension is the most serious effect after overdose. Clinical evidence of cerebral or myocardial ischemia may develop in patients with profound hypotension (47). Hypotension has persisted for up to 1 week after an intravenous overdose (48,49). Bradycardia, nausea, vomiting, and diarrhea may also develop after overdose.

HYDRALAZINE

Toxic Dose

The *adult and pediatric therapeutic doses* are provided in Table 1.

Toxicokinetics and Toxicodynamics

The onset of action is 1 hour with a T_{max} of 1 to 2 hours. The bioavailability is 38% to 50% for immediate release (50), and 40% to 70% for the extended release formulation (51). Protein binding is 88% to 90% (52). Hydralazine undergoes significant hepatic metabolism with 3% to 14% renal excretion (53) and 6% fecal elimination (54). The elimination half-life is 3 to 5 hours (55) (Table 2).

Pathophysiology

The exact mechanism of action is unclear. Hydralazine relaxes arterial smooth muscle by interfering with calcium movement. Vasodilation and reduced total peripheral vascular resistance causes tachycardia and an increase in stroke volume and cardiac output.

Pregnancy and Lactation

Hydralazine is FDA pregnancy category C (Appendix I). It enters breast milk in low concentrations, and breast-feeding is considered safe.

Clinical Presentation

Overdose has caused hypotension, tachycardia, hypokalemia, and ischemic changes on the electrocardiogram (ECG). An adult ingested 2 g and developed hypotension (90/48), tachycardia (148 beats/minute), hypokalemia, metabolic acidosis (pH, 7.3; bicarbonate, 11.6), and ST depression on ECG. Blood pressure normalized with intravenous fluids and she recovered (56).

Reflex tachycardia is common with therapeutic use (57). Hypotension can occur with therapeutic use. Severe hypotension has been reported when intravenous hydralazine and diazoxide are administered (58–60).

Glomerulonephritis is an uncommon adverse effect; women, slow acetylators, and patients with positive antinuclear antibody and HLA DR4 genotype are predisposed (61,62). Prolonged therapy has been associated with the development of lupus. Risk factors include female gender, slow acetylator phenotype, HLA DR4, and doses greater than 200 to 400 mg/day (63,64). Manifestations can include fever, anemia, leukopenia, thrombocytopenia, fatigue, petechiae, rash, joint pain, and swelling. In severe cases pericarditis, pneumonia, or renal failure may develop.

ISOXSUPRINE

Toxic Dose

The *adult and pediatric therapeutic doses* are provided in Table 1. There are no reports of overdose.

Toxicokinetics and Toxicodynamics

The T_{max} is 1 hour. Oral bioavailability is nearly complete. Isoxsuprine is primarily excreted in the urine (Table 2).

Pathophysiology

Isoxsuprine is a β-receptor agonist and also probably has a direct vasodilatory effect on vascular smooth muscle (65).

Pregnancy and Lactation

Isoxsuprine is FDA pregnancy category C (Appendix I). Its excretion into breast milk is unknown.

Clinical Presentation

Tachycardia and hypotension are the most common adverse effects (66). Tocolytic therapy with isoxsuprine in patients with premature rupture of membranes has been associated with a higher incidence of respiratory distress syndrome in the infant (67).

MINOXIDIL

Toxic Dose

The *adult and pediatric therapeutic doses* are provided in Table 1.

Toxicokinetics and Toxicodynamics

The onset of action is 30 to 60 minutes, with a duration of 12 to 18 hours (68). The bioavailability is 90% to 100% (1% to 4% for topical solution) (69). There is insignificant protein binding and V_d is 2 to 3 L/kg (70). Minoxidil undergoes hepatic metabolism (90%), followed by renal excretion (90%), mostly as metabolites (71). The elimination half-life is 4.2 hours (Table 2).

Pathophysiology

Minoxidil causes selective vasodilatation of the arteriolar resistance vessels by inhibiting calcium uptake into cells (72).

Pregnancy and Lactation

Minoxidil is FDA pregnancy category C (Appendix I). It is excreted in breast milk; milk concentrations are slightly lower than plasma concentrations (73).

Clinical Presentation

ACUTE OVERDOSAGE

Hypotension is the most common finding after minoxidil overdose. In a series of 224 minoxidil ingestions, 69% developed hypotension (74). After a large ingestion, hypotension may be severe and prolonged, lasting up to 72 hours (75–77). Tachycardia is also common, developing in 38% of a series of 224 patients (74). Tachycardia may persist for several days in severe cases (78).

Angina, hemorrhagic pericarditis, ischemic ECG changes (ST depression and T wave inversion), and acute myocardial infarction have been reported after minoxidil overdose but are not common (76,78,79). Patients with severe poisoning may develop central nervous system depression or coma (75). Some degree of lethargy developed in 31% of 224 minoxidil overdose patients (74).

Tachycardia was the only manifestation of poisoning in a 2-year-old child who ingested 100 mg (80). Severe hypotension, tachycardia, and coma have been reported in adults ingesting 1 g or more (75,76,78).

ADVERSE EVENTS

ECG changes are quite common with chronic therapy; approximately 90% of patients taking oral minoxidil develop ST and T wave changes, which may revert with continued therapy (81). Pericardial effusion develops in approximately 3% of patients and is more common in patients with renal failure (82,83). Edema and weight gain are also fairly common. Hypertrichosis develops in 80% to 100% of patients taking oral minoxidil and approximately 10% of patients using topical minoxidil (84,85).

PAPAVERINE

Toxic Dose

The *adult and pediatric therapeutic doses* are provided in Table 1. There are little published data regarding overdose.

Toxicokinetics and Toxicodynamics

The T_{max} is 1 to 2 hours (86). The bioavailability is 68% to 89% for the oral solution and 22% to 29% for the sustained release tablet (87). Plasma protein binding is 90%. Papaverine undergoes extensive renal secretion primarily as metabolites. The elimination half-life is 0.5 to 2.0 hours (Table 2).

Pathophysiology

Papaverine acts directly on smooth muscle cells producing relaxation and arteriolar dilatation (88). This may be secondary to phosphodiesterase inhibition increasing levels of intracellular cyclic adenosine monophosphate, which removes calcium from the cytoplasm of vascular smooth muscle cells, resulting in relaxation.

Pregnancy and Lactation

Papaverine is FDA pregnancy category C (Appendix I). Entry into breast milk is unknown.

Clinical Presentation

Tachycardia, hypotension, and metabolic acidosis have been reported. A 61-year-old woman developed lactic acidosis, respiratory alkalosis, mild hyperglycemia, hypokalemia, and elevated plasma pyruvate level after ingesting 15 g papaverine (89).

Hypotension and bradycardia may develop after intravenous or intracavernous injection (90). Priapism has been described after parenteral and oral administration (91–93). Drowsiness, vertigo, headache, nausea, vomiting, and abdominal pain are less common adverse effects (94). Reversible hepatotoxicity has been reported and is believed to be a hypersensitivity reaction (95,96).

PHENOXYBENZAMINE

Toxic Dose

The *adult and pediatric therapeutic doses* are provided in Table 1.

Toxicokinetics and Toxicodynamics

Bioavailability is 20% to 30%. It undergoes extensive hepatic metabolism and has an elimination half-life of 24 hours (97) (Table 2).

Pathophysiology

Phenoxybenzamine blocks pre- and post-synaptic α-adrenergic receptors, preventing vasoconstriction and inhibiting presynaptic norepinephrine release.

Pregnancy and Lactation

Phenoxybenzamine is FDA pregnancy category C (Appendix I). Entry into breast milk is unknown.

Clinical Presentation

Overdose can cause hypotension, dizziness, syncope, tachycardia, vomiting, and lethargy. Orthostatic hypotension is the most common adverse effect and may be associated with dizziness, syncope, or reflex tachycardia. Phenoxybenzamine also causes miosis. Sedation or drowsiness and gastrointestinal irritation occur less often with therapeutic use.

PHENTOLAMINE

Toxic Dose

The *adult and pediatric therapeutic doses* are provided in Table 1. No overdose data are available.

Toxicokinetics and Toxicodynamics

The T_{max} is 30 to 60 minutes. Protein binding is less than 72%. It undergoes extensive hepatic metabolism, 80% renal excretion (10% to 13% excreted as unchanged drug) and 20% fecal excretion. The elimination half-life is 19 minutes after intravenous administration, 5 to 7 hours after oral administration (98) (Table 2).

Pathophysiology

Phentolamine blocks α_1- and α_2-adrenergic receptors, preventing vasoconstriction and inhibiting presynaptic norepinephrine release.

Pregnancy and Lactation

Phentolamine is FDA pregnancy category C (Appendix I). It is unknown if phentolamine is excreted in breast milk.

Clinical Effects

Tachycardia, palpitations, hypotension, weakness, dizziness, nasal congestion, and headache are fairly common adverse effects. Nausea, vomiting, and diarrhea occur primarily after oral administration (98). Mild abnormalities in liver enzymes, principally alkaline phosphatase, have been reported with long-term therapy (99). Phentolamine causes mydriasis (100).

PRAZOSIN

Toxic Dose

The *adult and pediatric therapeutic doses* are provided in Table 1.

Toxicokinetics and Toxicodynamics

The T_{max} is 1 to 3 hours. Protein binding is 92% to 97% (101), and V_d is 0.5 L/kg. Hepatic metabolism is 30% (102), and renal excretion is 3% to 4%, mostly as metabolites (103). Elimination half-life is 2 to 4 hours (Table 2).

Pathophysiology

Prazosin is a selective α_1-adrenergic receptor blocker. It decreases vascular tone.

Pregnancy and Lactation

Prazosin is FDA pregnancy category C (Appendix I). It is excreted in small amounts in human milk.

Clinical Presentation

Tachycardia, mild hypotension, respiratory failure, drowsiness, and priapism have been reported after overdose. Orthostatic hypotension with palpitations, dizziness, and sometimes syncope are common adverse effects, particularly after the first dose, in patients with irregular compliance or when another antihypertensive is added to prazosin therapy (104). Headache and nausea are also fairly common adverse effects (105,106).

A 72-year-old man developed Cheyne-Stokes respirations 3 hours after ingesting 120 mg prazosin and required mechanical ventilation for 18 hours (107). A 25-year-old patient developed priapism after ingesting 150 mg of prazosin (108). A 19-year-old patient developed mild hypotension (95/60 mm Hg) and tachycardia (140 beats/minute) after ingesting 200 mg prazosin but recovered with supportive care (109). Mild hypotension (90 mm Hg systolic) was also reported in a 75-year-old patient who ingested 80 mg prazosin (110). A 2-year-old child became drowsy and had depressed reflexes but did not develop hypotension after ingesting 50 mg (104).

TERAZOSIN

Toxic Dose

The *adult and pediatric therapeutic doses* are provided in Table 1. No overdose data are available.

Toxicokinetics and Toxicodynamics

The T_{max} of terazosin is 1 hour with an onset of effect of 3 hours and a duration of 24 hours (111). The bioavailability is 90%, protein binding 90% to 94%, and the V_d is 25 to 30 L (112). After extensive hepatic metabolism, it is excreted renally (10% unchanged drug and 30% inactive metabolite). Fecal elimination is 55% to 60% (112). The elimination half-life is 9 to 12 hours (Table 2).

Pregnancy and Lactation

Terazosin is FDA pregnancy category C (Appendix I). Entry into breast milk is unknown.

Pathophysiology

Terazosin is a selective α_1-adrenergic receptor blocker. It decreases vascular tone.

Clinical Presentation

Orthostatic hypotension is common and may be associated with palpitations, dizziness, tachycardia, or syncope. Lightheadedness, weakness, fatigue, somnolence, headache, nausea, and nasal congestion are also common adverse effects (113).

TOLAZOLINE

Toxic Dose

The *adult and pediatric therapeutic doses* are provided in Table 1.

Toxicokinetics and Toxicodynamics

The bioavailability of tolazoline is 90% to 100%, and the V_d is 1.61 L/kg. It has extensive renal secretion by organic acid active transport system, producing an elimination half-life of 3 to 10 hours (114,115) (Table 2).

Pathophysiology

In addition to its α-receptor blocking effects, tolazoline is an H_2 agonist and increases gastric acid secretion.

Pregnancy and Lactation

Tolazoline is FDA pregnancy category C (Appendix I). Its excretion into breast milk is unknown.

DIAGNOSTIC TESTS FOR VASODILATING AGENTS

Therapeutic drug monitoring for these vasodilators is neither useful nor clinically available.

Diagnostic testing is directed primarily at detecting the adverse effects of therapy as well as the diagnosis of other causes of hypotension. The serum electrolytes should be measured. An ECG should be performed in patients with hypotension, bradycardia or significant tachycardia, and patients with chest discomfort. Evaluation for myocardial ischemia may be needed.

TREATMENT OF VASODILATOR TOXICITY

Decontamination

A single acute ingestion of any vasodilator is rarely life threatening, although symptomatic toxicity may occur. Decontamination procedures have not been studied for these drugs, but activated charcoal alone is expected to provide adequate decontamination.

Enhancement of Elimination

Although some of these agents are likely removed by hemodialysis, the use of hemodialysis has not been reported.

Antidotes

There are no specific antidotes for the vasodilating agents in most cases. Priapism should be treated emergently in conjunction with a urologist. Inject or irrigate with an alpha agonist such as phenylephrine: inject 2 ml of a 250-µg/ml solution into corpus cavernosum, may repeat every 5 to 15 minutes to a maximum of 3 doses.

Supportive Care

Monitor vital signs frequently, particularly pulse and blood pressure, and institute continuous cardiac monitoring. Hypotension from these agents usually responds to keeping the patient supine and administering intravenous fluids. Infusion of dopamine or norepinephrine may be required in a minority of patients with more severe hypotension (Chapter 37). Monitor urine output in patients with hypotension.

Patients who develop hypotension, persistent tachycardia, altered mental status, or evidence suggesting myocardial ischemia require admission to the intensive care unit. Patients who are asymptomatic or only develop transient mild hypotension or tachycardia can be discharged after gastrointestinal decontamination and appropriate psychiatric clearance.

REFERENCES

1. Zahka KG, Roland MA, Cutilletta AF, et al. Management of aortic arch interruption with prostaglandin E1 infusion and microporous expanded polytetrafluoroethylene grafts. *Am J Cardiol* 1980;46:1001–1005.
2. Granstrom E. On the metabolism of prostaglandin E1 in man: prostaglandins and related factors 50. *Prog Biochem Pharmacol* 1967;3:89–93.
3. Linday LA, Engle MA. Prostaglandin treatment of newborns with ductal-dependent congenital heart disease. *Pediatr Ann* 1981;10:133–138.
4. Product information: Prostin VR Pediatric(R), alprostadil. Kalamazoo, MI: The Upjohn Co, 1997.
5. Product information: MUSE(R) Urethral Suppository, alprostadil. Mountain View, CA: VIVUS, Inc, 1998.
6. Product information: Caverject(R) Sterile powder, alprostadil. Kalamazoo, MI: Pharmacia & Upjohn Co, 1999.
7. Marti-Masso JF, Obeso JA, Carrera N, et al. Aggravation of Parkinson's disease by cinnarizine. *J Neurol Neurosurg Psychiatry* 1987;50:804–805.
8. Gananca MM, Albernaz PLM, Caovilla HH, et al. Controlled clinical trial of pentoxifylline versus cinnarizine in the treatment of labyrinthine disorders. *Pharmatherapeutica* 1988;5:170–176.
9. Gimenez-Roldan S, Mateo D. Cinnarizine-induced parkinsonism. *Clin Neuropharmacol* 1991;14:156–164.
10. Negrotti A, Calzetti S, Sasso E. Calcium-entry blockers-induced parkinsonism: possible role of inherited susceptibility. *Neurotoxicology* 1992;13:261–264.
11. Navarro-Badenes J, Martinez-Mir I, Palop V, et al. Weight gain associated with cinnarizine. *Ann Pharmacother* 1992;26:928–930.
12. Volta GD, Majoni M, Cappa S, et al. Insomnia and perceptual disturbances during flunarizine treatment. *Headache* 1990;30:62–63.
13. Morrison P, Bradbrock I, Rogers H. Plasma cinnarizine levels resulting from oral administration as capsule or tablet formulation investigated by gas-liquid chromatography. *Br J Clin Pharmacol* 1979;7:349–352.
14. Holmes B, Brogden RN, Heel RC, et al. Flunarizine: a review of its pharmacodynamic and pharmacokinetic properties and therapeutic use. *Drugs* 1984;27:6–44.
15. Pruitt AW, Faraj BA, Dayton PG. Metabolism of diazoxide in man and experimental animals. *J Pharmacol Exp Ther* 1974;188:248–256.
16. Sellers EM, Koch-Weser J. Protein binding and vascular activity of diazoxide. *N Engl J Med* 1969;281:1141.
17. Lancaster-Smith M, Leigh NI, Thompson HM. Death following non-ketotic hyperglycaemic coma during diazoxide therapy and peritoneal dialysis. *Postgrad Med J* 1974;50:175–177.
18. Kumar GK, Dastoor FC, Robayo JR, et al. Side effects of diazoxide. *JAMA* 1976;235:275–276.
19. Mroczek WJ, Lee NR. Diazoxide therapy: use and risks. *Ann Intern Med* 1976;85:529.
20. Falko JM. Hazards in antihypertension therapy. *Ann Intern Med* 1977;86:111.
21. Mauer SM, Mirkin BL. Treatment of hypertension in infancy with diazoxide: report of a case with arrhythmia as a complication of therapy. *J Pediatrics* 1972;80:657–659.
22. Mahony C, Wolfram KM, Cocchetto DM, et al. Dipyridamole kinetics. *Clin Pharmacol Ther* 1982;31:330–338.
23. Harker LA, Kadatz RA. Mechanism of action of dipyridamole. *Thromb Res* 1983;4(Suppl):39–46.
24. Product information, Persantine. Ridgefield, CT: Boehringer Ingelheim Pharmaceuticals, Inc., 1998.
25. Kahn D, Argenyi EA, Berbaum K, et al. The incidence of serious hemodynamic changes in physically-limited patients following oral dipyridamole challenge before thallium-201 scintigraphy. *Clin Nucl Med* 1990;15:678–682.
26. Hansen CL, Williams E. Severe transmural myocardial ischemia after dipyridamole administration implicating coronary steal. *Clin Cardiol* 1998;21:293–296.
27. Homma S, Callahan RJ, Ameer B, et al. Usefulness of oral dipyridamole suspension for stress thallium imaging without exercise in the detection of coronary artery disease. *Am J Cardiol* 1986;57:503–508.
28. Pennell DJ, Underwood SR, Ell PJ. Symptomatic bradycardia complicating the use of intravenous dipyridamole for thallium-201 myocardial perfusion imaging. *Int J Cardiol* 1990;27:272–274.
29. Roach PJ, Magee MA, Freedman SB. Asystole and bradycardia during dipyridamole stress testing in patients receiving beta blockers. *Int J Cardiol* 1993;42:92–94.
30. Frossard M, Weiss K, Gossinger H, et al. Asystole during dipyridamole infusion in patients without coronary artery disease or beta-blocker therapy. *Clin Nucl Med* 1997;22:97–100.
31. Marwick TH, Hollman J. Acute myocardial infarction associated with intravenous dipyridamole for rubidium-82 pet imaging. *Clin Cardiol* 1990;13:230–231.
32. Johnston DL, Daley JR, Hodge DO, et al. Hemodynamic responses and adverse effects associated with adenosine and dipyridamole pharmacologic stress testing: a comparison in 2,000 patients. *Mayo Clin Proc* 1995;70:331–336.
33. Shaffer J, Simbartl L, Render ML, et al. Patients with stable chronic obstructive pulmonary disease can safely undergo intravenous dipyridamole thallium-201 imaging. *Am Heart J* 1998;136:307–313.
34. Schneeweiss A, Marmor A, Wynne RD. Flosequinan induces hemodynamic improvement in heart failure complicating acute myocardial infarction. *Herz* 1988;13:259–262.
35. Product information: Manoplax, flosequinan. Lincolnshire, IL: Boots Pharmaceuticals, 1993.
36. Wynne RD, Crampton EL, Hind ID. The pharmacokinetics and haemodynamics of BTS 49 465 and its major metabolite in healthy volunteers. *Eur J Clin Pharmacol* 1985;28:659–664.
37. Bashir Y, O'Nunain S, Paul VE, et al. The electrophysiological effects of flosequinan. *Eur Heart J* 1991;12:1288–1292.
38. Product information: Wytensin(R), guanabenz. Philadelphia: Wyeth-Ayerst Laboratories, 1995.
39. Meacham RH, Emmett M, Kyriakopoulos AA, et al. Disposition of C-guanabenz in patients with essential hypertension. *Clin Pharmacol Ther* 1980;27:44–52.
40. Walker BR, Hare LE, Deitch MW. Comparative antihypertensive effects of guanabenz and clonidine. *J Int Med Res* 1982;10:6.
41. LaRusso P, Jessup SA, Rogers FJ, et al. Sinoatrial and atrioventricular dysfunction associated with the use of guanabenz acetate. *Can J Cardiol* 1988;4:146–148.
42. Hall AH, Smolinske SC, Kulig KW, et al. Guanabenz overdose. *Ann Intern Med* 1985;102:787–788.
43. Jadad AR, Carroll D, Glynn CJ, et al. Intravenous regional sympathetic blockade for pain relief in reflex sympathetic dystrophy: a systematic review and a randomized, double-blind crossover study. *J Pain Symptom Manage* 1995;10:13–20.
44. Ronnov-Jessen V, Hansen J. Blood volume and exchangeable sodium during treatment of hypertension with guanethidine and hydrochlorothiazide. *Acta Med Scand* 1969;186:255.
45. McMartin C, Simpson P. The absorption and metabolism of guanethidine in hypertensive patients requiring different doses of the drug. *Clin Pharmacol Ther* 1971;12:73.
46. Product information: Hylorel(R), guanadrel. Rochester, NY: Fisons Corporation, 1996.
47. Goldberg AD, Raftery EB. Patterns of blood-pressure during chronic administration of postganglionic sympathetic blocking drugs for hypertension. *Lancet* 1976;2:1052.
48. Sharpe E, Milaszkiewicz R, Carli F. A case of prolonged hypotension following intravenous guanethidine block. *Anaesthesia* 1987;42:1081–1084.
49. Kalmanovitch DVA, Hardwick PB. Hypotension after guanethidine block [Letter]. *Anaesthesia* 1988;43:256.
50. Ludden TM, McNay JL Jr, Shepherd AM, et al. Clinical pharmacokinetics of hydralazine. *Clin Pharmacokinet* 1982;7:185–205.
51. Talseth T. Clinical pharmacokinetics of hydralazine. *Clin Pharmacokinet* 1977;2:317.
52. Reference deleted.
53. Talseth T, Fauchald P, Pape JF. Hydralazine slow-release: observations on serum profile and clinical efficacy in man. *Curr Ther Res* 1977;21:157–168.
54. O'Malley K, Segal JL, Israili ZH, et al. Duration of hydralazine action in hypertension. *Clin Pharmacol Ther* 1975;18:581–586.
55. Mulrow JP, Crawford MH. Clinical pharmacokinetics and therapeutic use of hydralazine in congestive heart failure. *Clin Pharmacokinet* 1989;16:86–99.
56. Smith BA, Ferguson DB. Acute hydralazine overdose: marked ECG abnormalities in a young adult. *Ann Emerg Med* 1992;21:326–330.
57. King K. Vasodilator drugs in the treatment of hypertension. *Med J Aust* 1985;142:450–453.
58. Romberg GP, Lordon RE. Hypotensive sequelae of diazoxide and hydralazine therapy. *JAMA* 1977;238:1025.
59. Mizroch S, Yurasek M. Hypotension and bradycardia following diazoxide and hydralazine therapy. *JAMA* 1977;237:2471.
60. Henrich WL, Cronin R, Miller PD, et al. Hypotensive sequela of diazoxide and hydralazine therapy. *JAMA* 1977;237:264–265.
61. Ihle BU, Whitworth JA, Dowling JP, et al. Hydralazine and lupus nephritis. *Clin Nephrol* 1984;22:230–238.
62. Almroth G, Enestrome S, Sanuelsson I, et al. Autoantibodies to leucocyte antigens in hydralazine associated nephritis. *J Intern Med* 1992;231:37–42.
63. Cameron HA, Ramsay LE. The lupus syndrome induced by hydralazine: a common complication with low dose treatment. *BMJ* 1984;289:410–412.
64. Mansilla-Tinoco R, Harland SJ, Ryan PJ, et al. Hydralazine, antinuclear antibodies, and the lupus syndrome. *BMJ* 1982;284:936–939.
65. Manley ES, Lawson JW. Effect of beta adrenergic receptor blockade on skeletal muscle vasodilation produced by isoxsuprine and nylidrin. *Arch Int Pharmacodyn Ther* 1968;175:239–250.
66. Tepperman HM, Beydoun SN, Abdul-Karim RW. Drugs affecting myometrial contractility in pregnancy. *Clin Obstet Gynecol* 1977;20:423–445.
67. Curet LB, Rao AV, Zachman RD, et al. Association between ruptured mem-

branes, tocolytic therapy, and respiratory distress syndrome. *Am J Obstet Gynecol* 1984;148:263–268.
68. Linas SL, Nies AS. Minoxidil. *Ann Intern Med* 1981;94:61–65.
69. Fiedler-Weiss VC, West DP, Buys CM, et al. Topical minoxidil dose-response effect in alopecia areata. *Arch Dermatol* 1986;122:180.
70. Gottlieb T, Chidsey C. Evaluation of relative therapeutic efficacy and pharmacokinetics of minoxidil: a new antihypertensive. *Clin Res* 1971;19:349.
71. Gottlieb TB, Thomas RC, Chidsey CA. Pharmacokinetic studies of minoxidil. *Clin Pharmacol Ther* 1972a;13:436–441.
72. Smith GH. Minoxidil. *Drug Intell Clin Pharm* 1980;14:477.
73. Valdivieso A, Valdes G, Spiro TE, et al. Minoxidil in breast milk. *Ann Intern Med* 1985;102:135.
74. Rose R, Tomaszewski C. Evaluation of minoxidil exposures reported to US poison centers. *Vet Hum Toxicol* 1993;35:347(abst).
75. McCormick MA, Forman MH, Manoguerra AS. Severe toxicity from ingestion of a topical minoxidil preparation. *Am J Emerg Med* 1989;7:419–421.
76. MacMillan AR, Warshawski FG, Steinberg RA. Minoxidil overdose. *Chest* 1993;103:1290–1291.
77. Allon M, Hall D, Macon EJ. Prolonged hypotension after initial minoxidil dose. *Arch Intern Med* 1986;146:2075–2076.
78. Farrell SE, Epstein SK. Overdose of Rogaine Extra Strength for Men topical minoxidil preparation. *J Toxicol Clin Toxicol* 1999;37:781–783.
79. Krehlik JM, Hindson DA, Crowley JJ Jr, et al. Minoxidil-associated pericarditis and fatal cardiac tamponade. *West J Med* 1985;143:527–529.
80. Isles C, MacKay A, Barton PJ, et al. Accidental overdosage of minoxidil in a child. *Lancet* 1981;1:97.
81. Traub YM, Redmond DP, Rosenfeld JB, et al. Treatment of severe hypertension with minoxidil. *Israel J Med Sci* 1975;11:991.
82. Marquez-Julio A, Uldall PR. Pericardial effusions associated with minoxidil. *Lancet* 1977;2:816–817.
83. Zarate A, Gelfand MC, Horton JD, et al. Pericardial effusion associated with minoxidil therapy in dialyzed patients. *Int J Artif Organs* 1980;2:15.
84. Headington JT, Novak E. Clinical and histological studies of male pattern baldness treated with topical minoxidil. *Curr Ther Res* 1984;6:1098.
85. Peluso AM, Misciall C, Vincenzi C, et al. Diffuse hypertrichosis during treatment with 5% topical minoxidil. *Br J Dermatol* 1997;136:118–120.
86. Koch-Weser J, Cook P, James I. Cerebral vasodilators. *N Engl J Med* 1981;305:1508–1513.
87. Drugs for ischemic peripheral arterial diseases. *Med Lett Drug Ther* 1978;20:11.
88. Hausmann H, Photiadis J, Hetzer R. Blood flow in the internal mammary artery. *Tex Heart Inst J* 1996;23:279–283.
89. Vaziri ND, Stokes J, Treadwell TR. Lactic acidosis, a complication of papaverine overdose. *Clin Toxicol* 1981;18:417–423.
90. Wespes E, Schulman CC. Systemic complication of intracavernous papaverine injection in patients with venous leakage. *Urology* 1988;31:114–115.
91. Prasad K, El-Sherif A. Priapism following ingestion of papaverine tablets. *Scand J Urol Nephrol* 1996;30:515–516.
92. Halsted DS, Weigel JW, Noble MJ, et al. Papaverine induced priapism: 2 case reports. *J Urol* 1986;136:109–110.
93. Borgstrom E. Penile ulcer as complication in self-induced papaverine erections. *Urology* 1988;32:416–417.
94. Product information: Papaverine. Indianapolis, IN: Eli Lilly and Company, 1997.
95. Ronnov-Jessen V, Tjernlund A. Hepatotoxicity due to treatment with papaverine: report of four cases. *N Engl J Med* 1969;281:1333–1335.
96. Geiger GS. Evaluations in serum transaminases and alkaline phosphatase secondary to papaverine hydrochloride. *Drug Intel Clin Pharm* 1981;15:127–129.
97. Product information: Dibenzyline, Neptune, NJ: WellSpring Pharmaceutical Corp.
98. Goldstein I, Carson C, Rosen R, et al. Vasomax for the treatment of male erectile dysfunction. *World J Urol* 2001;19:51–56.
99. Levine SB, Althof SE, Turner LA, et al. Side effects of self-administration of intravenous papaverine and phentolamine for the treatment of impotence. *J Urol* 1989;141:54–57.
100. Preis O, Nonnan L. Prolonged mydriatic effect of tolazoline in the premature infant. *Am J Dis Child* 1987;141:476.
101. Brogden RN, Heel RC, Speight TM, et al. Prazosin: a review of its pharmacological properties and therapeutic efficacy in hypertension. *Drugs* 1977;14:163.
102. Collins IS, Pek P. Pharmacokinetics of prazosin, a new antihypertensive compound. *Clin Exp Pharmacol Physiol* 1975;2:445.
103. Curtis JR, Bateman FJA. Use of prazosin in management of hypertension in patients with chronic renal failure and in renal transplant recipients. *BMJ* 1975;4:432–434.
104. Product information: Minipress(R), prazosin. New York: Pfizer, 2002.
105. Rasmussen K, Jensen HA. Prazosin in treatment of hypertension. *BMJ* 1975;4:346.
106. Bendall MJ, Baloch KH, Wilson PR, et al. Side effects due to treatment of hypertension with prazosin. *BMJ* 1975;2:727.
107. Lenz K, Druml W, Kleinberger G, et al. Acute intoxication with prazosin: case report. *Human Toxicol* 1985;4:53–56.
108. Robbins DN, Crawford D, Lackner LH. Priapism secondary to prazosin overdose. *J Urol* 1983;130:975.
109. McClean WJ. Prazosin overdose. *Med J Aust* 1976;1:592.
110. Rygnestad TK, Dale O. Self-poisoning with prazosin. *Acta Med Scand* 1983;213:157–158.
111. Abraham PA, Halstenson CE, Matzke GR, et al. Antihypertensive therapy with once-daily administration of terazosin, a new alpha1-adrenergic-receptor blocker. *Pharmacotherapy* 1985;5:285–289.
112. Sonders RC. Pharmacokinetics of terazosin. *Am J Med* 1986;80:20–24.
113. Product information: Hytrin(R), terazosin. North Chicago: Abbott Laboratories, 2002.
114. Reynolds JEF, ed. *Martindale: the extra pharmacopoeia* (electronic version). Englewood, CO: Micromedex, Inc, 1996.
115. Ward RM, Daniel CH, Kendig JW, et al. Oliguria and tolazoline pharmacokinetics in the newborn. *Pediatrics* 1986;77:307–315.

SECTION

8

Central Nervous System Agents

CHAPTER 126

Acetaminophen (Paracetamol)

Richard C. Dart and Barry H. Rumack

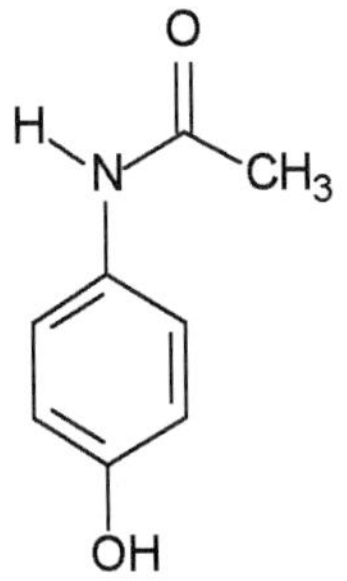

ACETAMINOPHEN

Compounds included:	**Acetaminophen, paracetamol (Tylenol, Panadol, and many others)**
Molecular formula and weight:	**$C_8H_9NO_2$, 151.2 g/mol**
SI conversion:	**mg/L × 0.00662 = mmol/L**
CAS Registry No.:	**103-90-2**
Therapeutic level:	**10 to 30 mg/L (serum)**
Target organs:	**Liver (acute and subacute), kidney (acute)**
Antidote:	***N*-acetylcysteine**

OVERVIEW

The history of acetaminophen toxicity is rich and complex. The first medical use of acetaminophen is attributed to von Mering in 1893, but Hinsberg and Treupel (1) first provided a detailed account of its clinical use. After its introduction in 1955, the first cases of hepatic damage after acetaminophen overdose were reported in 1966 (2). Mitchell et al. (3) elucidated the metabolic transformation of acetaminophen that initiates its hepatotoxicity. The work from this group led to the testing of *N*-acetylcysteine (NAC) for the treatment of hepatotoxicity. Because of its predictable efficacy and safety, acetaminophen is now the standard active comparator for studies of newer antipyretic and analgesic drugs.

Acetaminophen may be the most studied drug in toxicology. Although the seminal works of Prescott et al. (4), Mitchell et al. (3,5–9), Rumack and Matthew (10), Rumack et al. (11), Smilkstein et al. (12), and many others have described much of the toxicity for acetaminophen and its treatment, many important clinical questions remain. For example, the critical issues of acute liver failure and the evolving role of repeated supratherapeutic ingestion (RSI) remain to be investigated.

Classification and Uses

Acetaminophen is a metabolic product of acetanilide or phenacetin. It is preferred over these agents because of its superior safety profile. Benorylate is an ester of acetaminophen and acetylsalicylate that is hydrolyzed to its components *in vivo*. Propacetamol is the N,N-diethylglycine ester of paracetamol that is available in France and Belgium for intramuscular or intravenous use.

Acetaminophen is available in most countries as 325-mg and 500-mg tablets, infant drops (160 mg/ml), a suspension intended for children (160 mg/5 ml = 32 mg/ml), and chewable tablets (80 or 160 mg per tablet), as well as sprinkles in the same dosage as chewable tablets. A sustained-release tablet formulation is available in the United States (650 mg per tablet). It is also available as an adult suppository, 325 mg or 650 mg, that has caused overdose toxicity when administered to children. An effervescent form of acetaminophen is purported to be safer because its high sodium content and carbon dioxide production produce vomiting in overdose. Toxic levels have been reached after ingestion of this preparation (13).

Many combination products containing diphenhydramine or other antihistamines, pseudoephedrine or other adrenergic

TABLE 1. Toxicokinetics and toxicodynamics of acetaminophen

	Single therapeutic dose	Single overdose without severe liver injury	Presence of severe liver damage
Peak serum concentration (mg/L) at 30 min	8–32 (1000-mg dose)	NR	NR
Absorption $t_{1/2}$, adult	~30 min	~30 min route dependent	30 to >300 min route dependent
Absorption $t_{1/2}$, pediatric	4.5 min elixir, 10.3 min tablets	~30 min route dependent	30–240 min route dependent
Bioavailability, % (range)	80 (50–98)	NR	NR
V_d, L/kg, adult	0.78–1.21 with 1 accepted as standard	No change	No change
V_d as L/kg, pediatric	0.86–1.34 with 1 accepted as standard	No change	No change
Plasma protein binding (%)	5–20	24	NR
Elimination $t_{1/2}$, adult	50–160 min with 120 accepted as standard	<4 h	>4 h and rarely as high as 72 h
Elimination $t_{1/2}$, pediatric	111–148 min with 120 accepted as standard	<4 h	Greater than 4 h and as high as 14 h

NR, not reported; $t_{1/2}$, half-life; V_d, volume of distribution.

agents, and a variety of other active ingredients are available as liquids, tablets, sprinkles, or sachets. Combination products create an unusual source of poisoning because the use of multiple brand name products containing acetaminophen can lead to unintended overdose. Furthermore, the dose of acetaminophen per unit of product varies greatly.

An acute overdose in adults in terms of U.S. Food and Drug Administration (FDA)-labeled therapeutic dosing is minimally defined as a cumulative dose of acetaminophen that exceeds 4 g and is ingested over a period of 8 hours or less (some authors use a period of 4 hours). An RSI is defined as more than one episode of acetaminophen ingestion over a period exceeding 8 hours that resulted in a cumulative dose of greater than 4.0 g/day.

Toxic Dose

The maximum adult therapeutic dose is 1 g, four times a day at 4-hour intervals for adults. The pediatric dose is 10 to 15 mg/kg, four to five times a day (total of 75 mg/kg/day). Adults who were administered a single dose of 2 to 3 g (23 to 69 mg/kg) were well within the therapeutic range of 10 to 30 mg/L at 4 hours and were all below the therapeutic range at 7 hours (14). Similar data have been shown for children receiving a dose of 30 mg/kg (15).

An acute overdosage of approximately 15 g is thought to be the threshold for production of toxicity in adults. The toxic dose during RSI is controversial. Data indicate that approximately 10 g/day for 2 days is associated with liver injury in the adult (F. F. S. Daly, *unpublished data*, 2002). However, 8 g/day has been studied in human volunteers without producing liver injury (16). Additionally, cases of 12 g or greater/day without toxicity have been reported (17). Approximately 150 mg/kg/day for 2 days or more is the threshold level that may produce toxicity in children, although higher dosages are almost always required (18).

TOXICOKINETICS AND TOXICODYNAMICS

Absorption and Distribution

Pharmacokinetic and toxicokinetic data for acetaminophen are provided in Table 1. Acetaminophen is well absorbed orally but is variable among individuals. In 43 fasting hospital patients, an 80-fold difference in the plasma concentration was found at 1 hour after ingestion (19). Absorption is decreased and delayed in the presence of food, the ingestion of acetaminophen tablets that were improperly stored and are several years past their expiration date, ingestion in the morning versus evening, and the supine versus erect position, among other variables. Drugs that stimulate gastric emptying generally increase the rate of acetaminophen absorption, and drugs that delay gastric emptying generally decrease the rate of acetaminophen absorption. Absorption data may be difficult to interpret because a slower rate of absorption (and resulting lower peak serum level) may be associated with more complete absorption (increased total absorbed dose) (20). Rectal absorption is less efficient and much more variable. Acetaminophen is distributed to essentially all tissues. It crosses cell membranes passively, although a saturable component has been described (21).

Metabolism and Elimination

Although acetaminophen has more than 20 metabolites, there are three main pathways of interest clinically. The two major pathways are both phase II biosynthetic reactions, occur in the cytosol, and produce sulfate and glucuronide conjugates, which are then excreted. These pathways produce nontoxic metabolites. However, a phase I functionalization reaction mediated by CYP2E1 results in a toxic metabolite that is normally conjugated with glutathione (GSH) to produce the nontoxic mercapturic acid excreted in the urine (Fig. 1).

Approximately 5% of acetaminophen is excreted unchanged in the urine or is found as other nontoxic metabolites such as the catechol 3-hydroxy acetaminophen. In adults, glucuronidation of the phenolic hydroxy group by UDP glucuronyltransferase (UGT1A6) predominates (approximately 40% to 60%), whereas in small children, sulfation of the same phenolic position predominates (22). Both of these metabolites are nontoxic and are excreted in the urine. Although there has been some confusion in the literature because of species variation in saturation and metabolism, glucuronidation in humans is not saturable even in severely poisoned patients (23,24). These studies showed that the cat and rat were sulfate dominant, whereas the guinea pig and human were glucuronide dominant. Although there is some interindividual variability in glucuronidation, it does not exceed two- to threefold. Even after large single doses of 150 mg/kg to 214 mg/kg, the proportion of acetaminophen metabolized to the glucuronide form was the same as a therapeutic dose (25). The glucuronidation pathway is more active in the periportal region but is also found in the midzonal region of the hepatic acinus.

In contrast, the sulfation pathway normally accounts for a smaller percentage of metabolism. However, this route is limited by the availability of inorganic sulfate. In humans, a 41% to 74% reduction in sulfate was shown after acetaminophen doses

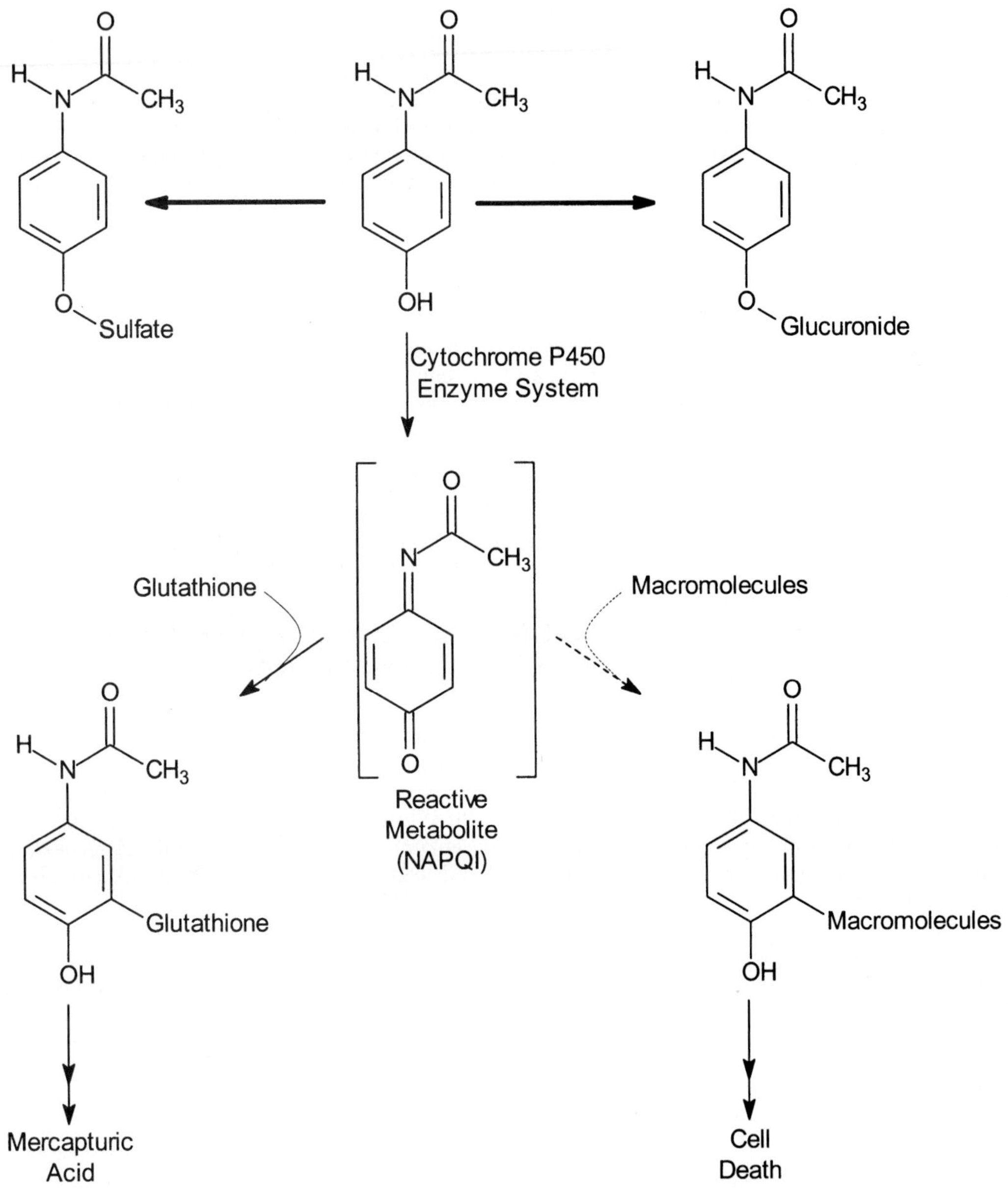

Glutathione

Macromolecules

Cytochrome P450 Enzyme System

Reactive Metabolite (NAPQI)

Sulfate

Glucuronide

Mercapturic Acid

Cell Death

Figure 1. The simplified metabolic scheme of acetaminophen.

of 32.5 to 62.5 mg/kg (26). At high doses, only 15% to 20% of acetaminophen is sulfated. The sulfation pathway is more concentrated in the periportal region of the hepatic acinus.

Propolis, a plant extract, has been shown to protect against hepatotoxicity by inhibiting phase I enzymes and inducing phase II enzymes (27). It may be an interesting model to evaluate the role of each of these phases.

Metabolism by Cytochrome P-450 System

The minor pathway of CYP2E1 metabolism accounts for a small, but important, portion of metabolism. The evidence, using intact humans with marker substances, indicates that CYP2E1 is the main source of *N*-acetyl-*p*-benzoquinone imine (NAPQI) (28). Previous publications using *in vitro* human hepatocytes, in vitro animal hepatocytes, and various animal models showed discrepant results, which must now be reconsidered in light of the *in vivo* human evidence. CYP1A2 and CYP3A4 were both previously thought to produce substantive quantities of NAPQI but now appear to play a minor role.

NAPQI is a highly reactive electrophile that reacts with nucleophiles such as reduced GSH via glutathione-*S*-transferase to form 3-(*S*-gluthathionyl) acetaminophen. This is further metabolized to 3-(*S*-cysteinyl) acetaminophen with the substitution of cysteine and finally after acetylation of the cysteine nitrogen to 3-(*S*-mercapto) acetaminophen, which is nontoxic and excreted in the urine. As NAPQI is a minor metabolite (less than 5%) with therapeutic use of acetaminophen, endogenous GSH stores are a sufficient detoxifying mechanism. In the event of acetaminophen overdose, however, endogenous GSH stores are overwhelmed and toxicity ensues. It has been established that hepatic damage occurs on 70% depletion of GSH (3). Given an average 1.5-L liver with 6 mmol GSH, 4.2 mmol would have to be depleted to reach threshold of toxicity. If approximately 4% of a dose of acetaminophen is converted to NAPQI, the dose of acetaminophen expected to produce toxicity can be calculated. Because there is 151.2 mg/mmol acetaminophen, then (4.2) (151.2)/0.04 equals 15.9 g, which would have to be absorbed in a 70-kg human to cross the threshold of toxicity (21). Furthermore, 4% of 15.9 g results in 0.635 g NAPQI produced, assuming the same molecular weight (29).

PATHOPHYSIOLOGY

Acetaminophen enters cells by passive diffusion. After cell entry, it is primarily metabolized to the nontoxic sulfate and glucuronide derivatives as described in the section Metabolism and Elimination. Toxicity results from the metabolism to NAPQI. The basic metabolic and other components that participate in this process are shown in Figure 1.

CYP2E1 and the Cytochrome P-450 Oxidation Pathway

Although present in the kidney and most other tissues, the highest concentration of CYP2E1 is located in centrilobular hepatocytes about five deep around the central vein. This area is also know as *perivenular* or *zone 3* (30). Thus, the intracellular distribution CYP2E1 and the initial hepatic injury produced by acetaminophen are the same. Although early work reported cytochrome P-450 as the responsible enzyme, further work has identified more than 500 isoenzymes as part of "P-450," of which CYP2E1 is the most important in regard to acetaminophen.

CYP2E1 is located in the endoplasmic reticulum and contains 493 amino acids with a molecular weight of 56,820. The CYP2E subfamily in humans has only one gene. It is located on chromosome 10 and spans 11,413 base pairs. It metabolizes more than 75 different compounds. It is unique among these CYP enzyme families in its ability to produce reactive oxygen radicals through reduction of dioxygen, and it is the only cytochrome isozyme that is strongly induced by ethanol (which itself is oxidized). The liver content of CYP2E1 ranges more than 20-fold from individual to individual (31). The cause of variability probably arises from a combination of variable induction by exposure to various xenobiotics, genetic inducibility, the effects of diet, and, perhaps, unrecognized factors.

Although the interindividual ranges are high, intraindividual differences appear less dramatic. For example, the induction of CYP2E1 in actively drinking alcoholic patients appears to be approximately two- to threefold (32). Some alcoholic patients seem to have no induction. Although 78% showed an increase over controls, 22% of alcoholics with similar ethanol consumption histories had no increase in CYP2E1 (33).

Induction and Inhibition of CYP2E1

Like other enzymes, induction and inhibition of CYP2E1 can occur at transcriptional, pretranslational, translational, and posttranslational points. For CYP2E1, it appears that posttranslational protein stabilization is the primary mechanism of induction. The turnover of CYP2E1 is biphasic, with half-lives of 7 and 37 hours (34). The binding of some ligands, such as acetone, ethanol, 4-methylpyrazole, pyrazole, and isoniazid, prevents the normal degradation of the enzymatic protein, thereby allowing accumulation of the enzyme (35–37). When CYP2E1 binds the ligand (acetone, ethanol), it appears that subsequent autophagocytosis of the enzyme as well as slower lysosomal degradation occurs. This process can be accelerated by glucagon or epinephrine, which activates the kinase that phosphorylates the enzyme (29).

After the use of inducers, the enzyme is increased in the same centrilobular site, indicating a local increase in the enzyme rather than development in other cells. However, when growth hormone is inhibited by hypophysectomy, recruitment of cells in zone 2 occurs and CYP2E1 can be produced, indicating transcriptional activity on the apoprotein. Additionally, growth hormone repression of CYP2E1 may be related to the levels of the enzyme seen in the young animal. At birth there is a substantially higher level of enzyme than later in life, which may correlate with increasing levels of growth hormone (38). It is important to note that recruitment in zone 1 and 2 does not occur after induction with other agents, and necrosis observed outside zone 3 is based on other mechanisms.

Several mechanisms appear to play a role in levels of CYP2E1. Acetone, ethanol, pyrazole, isoniazid, and a few others serve as an inducer and substrate for CYP2E1. Isoniazid initially inhibits and then enhances formation of NAPQI. Acetaminophen, chlorzoxazone, carbon tetrachloride, and some other compounds are substrates for the enzyme but do not induce it. Imidazole compounds (e.g., ketoconazole) are examples of agents that induce the enzyme but do not serve as a substrate. Imidazoles inhibit CYP2E1 and prevent the conversion of acetone to glucose as part of this enzyme's role in gluconeogenesis. This effect would be seen in ketotic states such as starvation or high-fat diets. In fasting, starvation, and diabetes, the indirect mediator capacity of acetone on CYP2E1 is likely. Thus, the metabolism of acetaminophen does not change unless other drugs or processes influence its metabolism. This is an important distinction during chronic therapeutic use of acetaminophen (29).

N-Acetyl-*p*-Benzoquinone Imine Production and Cellular Mechanisms of Toxicity

Figure 2 provides an overview of the mechanisms of cellular toxicity, and dual actions of some components should be noted. After absorption of an overdose of acetaminophen, a small portion is oxidized to NAPQI, which reacts with or forms adducts with more than 40 cellular components, including deoxyribonucleic acid, lipids, enzymes, and cellular organelles. This has been termed *stage I* and leads to cell necrosis (39,40). Although not fully characterized, oxidative stress, lipid peroxidation (LPO), covalent binding, and mitochondrial damage all play a role in the centrilobular necrosis.

Stage II encompasses the injury that extends beyond the centrilobular (perivenular) cells, including sinusoidal cells such as Kupffer (hepatic macrophages) and Ito (stellate) cells, and may extend outside of the liver. Stage II is extrinsic to the hepatocyte and includes chemotactic factors involving Kupffer cells, cytokine release, chemotactic factors, and various reactive oxygen species such as superoxide, as well as reactive nitrogen species such as peroxynitrite (Fig. 2). The resulting inflammatory response is an important event in the spread of cellular damage, as activation of the Kupffer and other inflammatory cells occurs. The response is also likely involved in toxicity as well as hepatocyte proliferation and hepatic regeneration. The distinction of these two stages identifies an opportunity for later treatment during the course of acetaminophen toxicity. Depending on cellular metabolic status, NAPQI can either initiate a sequence directly leading to necrosis or more indirectly by apoptosis.

During stage I, NAPQI forms adducts with several dehydrogenase enzymes primarily with cysteine and, along with other actions, produces an oxidant state in the cell. This results in a number of actions, including oxidation of GSH to GSSG, cross-linking of proteins by disulfide linkage (protein-s-s-protein), and the production of GSH protein disulfide compounds (in protein). Such disulfides change the intricate folding of these proteins and alter or prevent their activity. GSSG is known to accumulate during acetaminophen toxicity (41). If the enzyme GSH reductase is damaged, it cannot reduce GSSG back to GSH. Because mitochondria are unable to excrete GSSG, it accumulates within this organelle and decreases adenosine triphosphate production by interfering with the flow of electrons along the respiratory chain (42,43). Reactive oxygen species are pri-

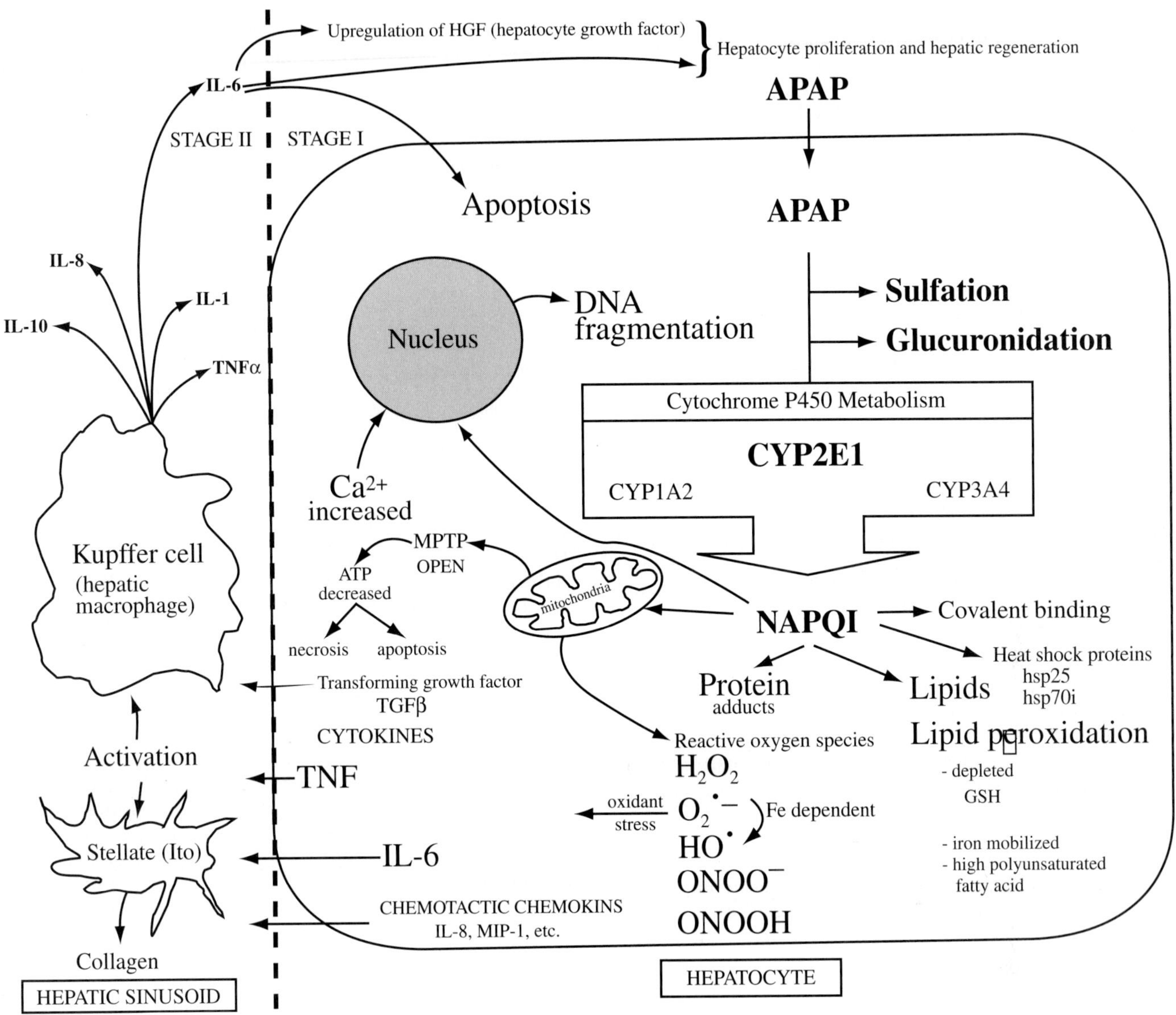

Figure 2. The liver has numerous defense mechanisms as well as repair processes such as the inflammatory response after toxic damage. This figure shows some of the relationships between events that occur after a necrogenic dose of acetaminophen. APAP, acetaminophen; ATP, adenosine triphosphate; DNA, deoxyribonucleic acid; GSH, reduced glutathione; hsp, heat shock protein; IL, interleukin; MIP, macrophage inflammatory protein; MPTP, mitochondrial permeability transport pore; NAPQI, *N*-acetyl-*p*-benzoquinone imine; TGF, tumor growth factor; TNF, tumor necrosis factor.

marily produced in the mitochondria and, along with the metabolites, can lead to an opening in the mitochondrial permeability transport pore, which can activate caspases by releasing cytochrome-*c*, resulting in apoptosis, or by terminating adenosine triphosphate production, which results in necrosis (44).

Oxidative stress refers to an excessive amount of free radicals within the cell. These include superoxide (O_2^-), hydroxyl radical ($OH^·$), hydrogen peroxide (H_2O_2), peroxynitrite ($ONOO^-$ is produced when superoxide reacts with nitric oxide), and others. The step from hydrogen peroxide to the hydroxy radical requires the oxidation of ferrous iron to ferric iron.

LPO may play some role in the toxic pathway but requires three things: active iron, vitamin E depletion, and a decrease in GSH (45). The role of iron appears critical in that the administration of deferoxamine plus NAC 1.25 hours after acetaminophen is more effective than NAC alone (46). It appears that in normal circumstances LPO is not the critical mechanism, but it may play an important role in circumstances in which vitamin E and GSH are deficient. Selenium-containing enzymes, such as GSH peroxidase and the selenium "acetaminophen binding protein" as well as the selenoprotein P scavenger, appear to play a role in toxicity, with selenium-deficient states resulting in increased toxicity (47,48). LPO may occur in stage II, which would explain some of the discrepancies as to its role in toxicity.

Injuries to hepatocytes lead to release of cytokines and other signalers that result in activation of Kupffer and other nonparenchymal cells. Once activated, the Kupffer cells produce multiple inflammatory mediators. This stage II of hepatic injury has been reduced in animals by treatment with gadolinium chloride and dextran sulfate (49). However, more recent work indicates that Kupffer cells may be a source of interleukin (IL)-10 and other hepatoprotective mediators, because administration of clodronate, which eliminates Kupffer cells, resulted in increased toxicity from acetaminophen (50). Kupffer cells are primarily located in the periportal and central areas of the lobule, where they release hydrogen peroxide, superoxide anion, and hydroxyl radicals as well as several hundred mediators, including tumor necrosis factor-α, eicosanoids, proteolytic enzymes, myeloperoxidases, IL-1a, IL-8, IL-18, and possibly IL-10 and IL-6 (51,52). Furthermore, there are differences among animal models (53). Antibodies to cytokines such as tumor necrosis factor-α reduce liver injury in some animal models but not others (54). Hyper-IL-6 has been shown to regenerate liver cells actively in the face of fulminant hepatic failure and may be of value in the treatment of patients with fulminant hepatic failure (55).

Several independent observations support the concept that cytokines are involved in the hepatic injury caused by acetaminophen; however, a coherent interpretation has yet to emerge. In animals, a toxic dose of acetaminophen induces IL-18 (56). The same authors showed a decrease in IL-6 in humans with acetaminophen hepatotoxicity. Because C-reactive protein is IL-6 dependent, the measurement of IL-6 or C-reactive protein may serve as a prognostic factor in acetaminophen overdose (57).

The observation that amphetamine pretreatment resulted in protection of hepatotoxicity of acetaminophen and bromobenzene lasting for 144 hours, but not carbon tetrachloride or cocaine, has been explained by showing the increase in two heat shock proteins (HSP): hsp25 and hsp70i (58). IL-6 may up-regulate multiple HSPs that are not inhibited by NAC; thus, adduct formation may relate to HSP induction. This class of proteins (chaperonins) appears to function by engulfing proteins that are improperly folded, unfolding them and then placing them back into the cytosol to fold normally. They can also be induced by increasing the temperature of the cell by 3° to 5°C. These functions are not fully clear but appear to be normal cellular responses to tissue damage and repair that are out of normal balance.

Drug and Disease Interactions

Drug induction and disease interactions have been proposed to increase vulnerability to acetaminophen. In each case, the fundamental issue is whether acetaminophen increases the production of NAPQI or impairs defenses to the reactive metabolite (e.g., reduces GSH).

Liver disease is thought by some to increase susceptibility to acetaminophen. The evidence is limited but indicates that the opposite is true. The level of cytochrome P-450 does not seem to be substantially decreased in most liver diseases, including various forms of hepatitis and fatty liver (Table 2). One study showed that it was decreased in cirrhosis. Furthermore, the available data indicate that GSH levels are either unchanged or increased (Table 3). It appears unlikely that hepatic diseases affect the toxicity of acetaminophen, either at therapeutic dose or in overdose.

Available data are also limited for starvation, but data to indicate increased risk are lacking as well. Although GSH levels change in starvation, that isolated fact must be examined within the knowledge that CYP2E1 is also undoubtedly reduced in concentration. In malnourished monkeys, the levels of cytochrome P-450 were substantially reduced, although the enzyme kinetics of the remaining cytochrome P-450 were normal (59). Cytochrome P-450 reductase activity and ethylmorphine-stimulated reductase were both half the levels of controls. Reduction in P-450 levels concomitantly reduces NAPQI formation, which then reduces the utilization and requirement for GSH. Humans placed on a severely calorie-restricted diet had no toxicity or any evidence of change in elimination of acetaminophen (60).

This information may help explain some of the seemingly disparate findings in patients with anorexia nervosa, although the data in this disease state are not adequate (61,62). The expectation was that patients with anorexia nervosa would have reduced quantities of GSH and would therefore be at greater risk for toxicity after an acetaminophen overdose. The fact that the reverse is true most likely indicates that the concentration of the enzyme CYP2E1 is also reduced. Lack of direct correlation between rat, mouse, and human data in this area complicates our understanding. Substantially more work remains to be done to determine dietary effects, and this should be possible *in vivo* given the probe techniques now available.

Because most reported drug interactions are based on early studies or postulated from *in vitro* or animal studies, they are unlikely to be valid. For example, phenytoin and phenobarbital have been described as agents that caused increased toxicity of acetaminophen, and in both cases that proved to be incorrect once appropriate studies were completed. Ethanol enhancement of acetaminophen toxicity has also been misunderstood, primarily because of poor understanding of the metabolic interactions. Chronic heavy alcoholics are probably at greater risk for toxicity after an overdose of acetaminophen but not from therapeutic doses.

Phenobarbital was demonstrated in the 1970s to increase the total cellular amount of cytochrome P-450 as well as other routes of hepatic metabolism. The assumption was made that aceta-

TABLE 2. Hepatic cytochrome P-450 levels present in patients with hepatic disease

Disease type	Level of cytochrome P-450 (% of control subjects)
Acute viral hepatitis	
Mild	100[a]
Moderate	118[a]
Healing	92[b]
Fatty liver	102[b]
Cirrhosis	34[b]

[a]Data from Gabrielle L, Leterrier F, Molinie C, et al. [Determination of human liver cytochrome P-450 by a micromethod using the electron paramagnetic resonance. Study of 141 liver biopsies (author's translation).] *Gastroenterol Clin Biol* 1977;1(10):775–782.
[b]Data from Schoene B, Fleischmann R, Remmer H, et al. Determination of drug metabolizing enzymes in needle biopsies of human liver. *Eur J Clin Pharmacol* 1972;4(2):65–73.
Adapted from Rumack BH. Acetaminophen hepatotoxicity: the first 35 years. *J Toxicol Clin Toxicol* 2002;41(1):3–20.

TABLE 3. Hepatic glutathione levels in hepatic disease

Disease type	Hepatic glutathione level (% of control subjects)
Hepatitis	
Toxic	231[a]
Viral	176[a]
Chronic	216[a]
Chronic active	142[b]
Cirrhosis	186[b]
	108[a]
Fatty liver	153[b]
Steatosis	78[b]

[a]Data from Poulsen HE, Ranek L, Andreasen PB. The hepatic glutathione content in liver diseases. *Scand J Clin Lab Invest* 1981;41(6):573–576.
[b]Data from Siegers CP, Bossen KH, Younes M, et al. Glutathione and glutathione-S-transferase in the normal and diseased human liver. *Pharmacol Res Commun* 1982;14(1):61–72.
Adapted from Rumack BH. Acetaminophen hepatotoxicity: the first 35 years. *J Toxicol Clin Toxicol* 2002;41(1):3–20.

minophen, being metabolized by P-450, would be induced and produce more toxicity. It is now clear that CYP2E1 does not metabolize or become induced by any of the barbiturates. Phenobarbital produces a pleiotropic response in the liver, inducing CYP2B, CYP2C, UDP-glucuronyltransferase, aldehyde dehydrogenase, and glutathione-*S*-transferase, among others. Therefore, phenobarbital does increase overall metabolism but has no effect on acetaminophen because it does not change CYP2E1. In contrast to humans, phenobarbital induction of CYP2E1 is well demonstrated in animals. The isozymes CYP2A5 in the mouse and CYP2B4 in the rabbit are inducible by phenobarbital and are capable of metabolizing carbon tetrachloride among other enzymes. It is therefore possible that isoenzymes other than CYP2E1 are related to the carbon tetrachloride mechanism because phenobarbital does not induce CYP2E1 in humans.

Phenytoin is primarily metabolized to *p*-HPPH [5-(4-hydroxyphenyl)-5-phenyhydantoin] and is then conjugated by glucuronide and excreted. The metabolism to *p*-HPPH is facilitated by CYP2C9 and CYP2C19. Phenytoin is a potent inducer of glucuronyltransferase, which facilitates the metabolism of acetaminophen to its nontoxic glucuronide metabolite as well as phenytoin to its glucuronide. Production of NAPQI from acetaminophen is not mediated by CYP2C9 or CYP2C19. It has been demonstrated *in vivo* that CYP3A4 does not play a significant role in acetaminophen metabolism, whereas it is central to the metabolism of phenytoin. CYP2E1 plays no role in phenytoin metabolism, and thus phenytoin does not enhance acetaminophen hepatotoxicity and, in fact, by increasing glucuronidation may be hepatoprotective. This explains many earlier articles that showed an increase in glucuronidation but no increase in mercapturic acid formation after administration of acetaminophen to patients who were also treated with phenytoin (29).

Ethanol has become the most interesting and important inducer, inhibitor, and substrate of CYP2E1. It was suggested as an enhancer of hepatotoxicity after acetaminophen overdose early in the acetaminophen clinical literature (63). In the first comprehensive report of the NAC protocol for acetaminophen overdose, higher bilirubin was found in patients with ethanol abuse compared to those without ethanol history as the only distinguishing feature (11). That same study reported lesser hepatic abnormalities in patients with acute ethanol consumption, as ethanol inhibition provides hepatic protection when ingested simultaneously. In a series of severe acetaminophen overdoses, the survival rates between drinkers and nondrinkers were not significantly different (64). However, a small subset of this same study looking at those who had been treated psychiatrically for alcoholism had a higher mortality, which was also associated with a larger overdose of acetaminophen, ranging from 20 to 90 g and a median of 54 g.

Ethanol induces and acts as a substrate for CYP2E1, resulting in simultaneous inhibition and induction. The two methods for the induction of CYP2E1 by ethanol appear to be concentration dependent. Below an ethanol concentration of 250 mg/dl, the activity appears to be primarily enzyme stabilization by ligand formation, which reduces degradation of the CYP2E1. In other words, ethanol prolongs the half-life of CYP2E1 within the cell. At ethanol concentrations greater than 250 mg/dl, it appears that there is *de novo* synthesis of CYP2E1 through messenger ribonucleic acid stabilization and perhaps other mechanisms, although apparently not transcriptional changes (30,65–68). Most importantly, there appears to be a maximum induction of a two- to threefold increase in NAPQI production after ethanol induction experimentally and in an adaptation of a computer model (32,69). Eighty-six percent of alcoholics have antibodies to the α-hydroxyethyl (ethanol) CYP2E1 adduct (70).

Although a great deal has been written about therapeutic doses of acetaminophen causing toxicity in alcoholics as a result of ethanol induction, a careful review of the literature does not support this view. A systematic analysis of more than 2000 reports in the literature dealing with the therapeutic use of acetaminophen in the alcoholic indicates that only retrospective series and individual case reports have implicated therapeutic doses of acetaminophen in hepatic injury in alcoholic patients. All prospective reports found no injury in these individuals (71). Why such a difference? The retrospective reports rely exclusively on the patient history and were primarily anecdotal case reports with inadequate, incomplete, or frankly conflicting data. Further review of the problems with the literature in this regard has been published (29).

A re-examination of earlier data demonstrated that acute acetaminophen overdose with chronic ethanol was associated with increased hepatotoxicity only in at-risk cases (72). Toxicity, as defined by aspartate aminotransferase (AST) and alanine aminotransferase (ALT), was worse in patients categorized in the high-risk (above the 300-mg/L study line) acetaminophen overdose. Toxicity was no different in low-risk (below the 200-mg/L line) overdoses whether or not the patients were alcoholics. This again confirms observations from England (64).

In a prospective trial using volunteers, the question was posed as to whether or not those who consume ethanol had an increase in NAPQI formation during the at-risk time shortly after ethanol is eliminated from the body (73). Acetaminophen was administered after ethanol had been metabolized. This is the most susceptible time for acetaminophen administration. The mean increase in NAPQI formation was 22%. The authors concluded that there was a small incremental increase in the risk of acetaminophen hepatotoxicity. A 22% increase in the amount going through the CYP2E1 pathway would take NAPQI production from 4.0% to 4.88%. Assuming 6 mmol GSH in the liver and the need to deplete 4.2 mmol, the single dose of acetaminophen required would decrease from 15.9 to 13.0 g acetaminophen for the threshold of toxicity to be reached. The calculation is 0.635 g NAPQI divided by 4.88% equals 13 g acetaminophen. Even considering the maximal increase of twofold in the amount of NAPQI produced after ethanol induction, there is still a considerable safety margin to reach threshold toxicity. This observation is consistent with clinical trials examining maximal therapeutic doses of acetaminophen in alcoholics.

A prospective, double-blind, randomized placebo-controlled trial of 201 alcoholics administered maximum therapeutic doses of acetaminophen (1g 4 times per day) for 2 days. No statistical difference was found in AST or ALT between alcoholics treated with acetaminophen and those treated with a placebo (74,75). The authors concluded that their study did not support a reduction of the dose of acetaminophen in alcoholics.

The entire issue of ethanol-acetaminophen interaction has been reviewed (76). Prescott states, "Finally, and most importantly, there has never been a single documented instance of any degree of acute liver damage produced by therapeutic doses of paracetamol given as a challenge in any chronic alcoholic under properly controlled conditions. If paracetamol is as dangerous in the chronic alcoholic as claimed by so many investigators, why has no such example been published?" Prescott also stated, "However convincing the numerous reports of liver damage after paracetamol overdose in chronic alcoholics may be, they are purely anecdotal and the inescapable fact remains that exactly the same severe and fatal liver damage occurs after overdosage in patients who are not chronic alcoholics."

Patients who have ethanol in their hepatic tissue at the same time as they consume acetaminophen have a hepatoprotective effect by the inhibition of CYP2E1 from ethanol (77). Ethanol consumed on a chronic basis may maximally induce CYP2E1 twofold. Some depletion of GSH may occur in alcoholics with chronic high ethanol consumption and a chronically poor diet, although a concomitant decrease in CYP2E1 under such conditions also occurs. No evidence has been found that therapeutic doses of acetaminophen cause toxicity in an ethanol-induced patient.

Other drugs (antiepileptics, antihistamines, diethylstilbestrol, ethacrynic acid, ethanol, promethazine, and still others) have been suggested as enhancers of acetaminophen toxicity. The likely explanation is that observations are coincidental, not causal, excellent examples of confounding by indication (78).

PREGNANCY AND LACTATION

Acetaminophen is FDA pregnancy category B (Appendix I). The rate of malformation in children born to mothers treated with acetaminophen is the same as the background rate (79). Maternal hepatotoxicity can produce intrauterine fetal death or miscarriage. Acetaminophen crosses the placenta and may cause hepatic injury in the fetus. Evidence in humans indicates that NAC also crosses the placenta (80,81). Acetaminophen enters breast milk, but at concentrations lower than plasma. Breastfeeding during treatment is not contraindicated.

CLINICAL PRESENTATION

Acute Overdosage

The manifestations of acute acetaminophen poisoning are well described. The course can be divided into four stages (Fig. 3). Acetaminophen produces few clinically useful findings on the physical examination, particularly during the first 12 hours, although nausea and vomiting may occur. The classic progression of illness starts with mild to moderate gastrointestinal (GI) effects, peaks with severe liver injury and possible fulminant hepatic failure, and culminates in recovery, hepatic transplant, or death (10). As hepatic injury develops over 12 to 48 hours, the patient may complain of abdominal pain and has right upper quadrant tenderness. Liver injury becomes maximal at 48 to 96 hours and is often accompanied by renal insufficiency or failure.

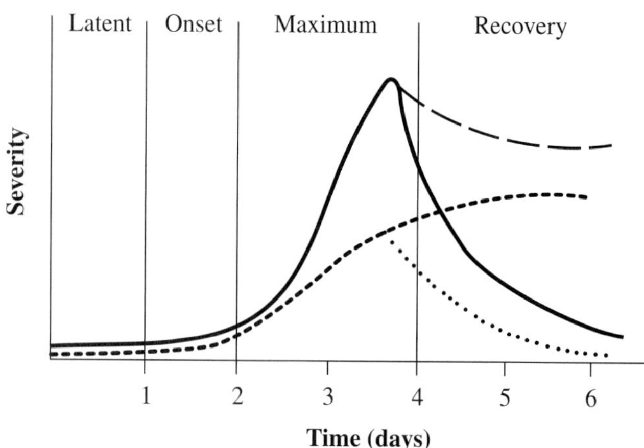

Figure 3. Clinical phases of acetaminophen toxicity. AST, alanine aminotransferase; INR, international normalized ratio; ——, AST; — —, AST in patient with severe hepatic necrosis; •, INR in patient with hepatic recovery; --, INR in patient with severe hepatic injury and no recovery. [Adapted from Rumack BH, Peterson RC, Koch GG, et al. Acetaminophen overdose: 662 cases with evaluation of oral acetylcysteine treatment. *Arch Intern Med* 1981;141(3 Spec No.):380–385.]

Jaundice and encephalopathy as well as acidosis and electrolyte disturbances may develop. Patients with more severe toxicity seem to evolve the most rapidly, whereas those with marginally hepatotoxic ingestions peak later.

Nearly all patients recover within 7 to 10 days, including those with markedly elevated aminotransferase levels. Aminotransferase levels may remain elevated for 2 weeks. Clinical and histopathologic findings return to normal in nearly all cases, although severe liver necrosis may show residual parenchymal scarring (82).

Renal injury from acetaminophen (apart from hepatorenal syndrome) occurs in fewer than 1% of patients (83). If it occurs, the serum creatinine typically begins to rise soon after the aminotransferase level has peaked. Occasionally, renal injury is reported to occur without liver injury; however, examination of these reports typically reveals that the patient simply presented very late in the course, after liver injury had resolved. It is often difficult to distinguish acetaminophen-related renal injury from hepatorenal failure. Oliguric or anuric renal failure may result from acute tubular necrosis and is sometimes accompanied by flank pain. Patients with fulminant hepatic failure developed renal complications in as many as 46% of cases, although this same center reported that to be a decrease from 60% in their studies reported 7 years previously (64).

Early Patient Presentation after Acetaminophen Ingestion

The early presenting patient offers the temptation of drawing an early acetaminophen level (before 4 hours have elapsed after ingestion). The physician may be tempted to discharge the patient earlier if the early level is zero; this temptation should be avoided. Although it seems likely that a completely undetectable acetaminophen level indicates that the patient did not ingest acetaminophen, the evidence supporting this approach is incomplete. Even more risky is the practice of trying to use an acetaminophen level drawn before 4 hours on the nomogram. This practice invites disaster. Although further research on this topic would be very useful, all patients who present before 4 hours should have their first acetaminophen level drawn at 4 hours after ingestion.

Unexpected Coma

Coma with metabolic acidosis is an unusual, but well-documented, presentation of acute severe acetaminophen poisoning. Several authors have described the presentation of a comatose patient with metabolic acidosis and a very high serum acetaminophen level (above 800 mg/L), typically with little, if any, evidence of liver injury (84). Prompt treatment with NAC can prevent liver injury in these patients.

Extended-Release Products

Extended-release formulations of acetaminophen (Tylenol Arthritis Relief, Tylenol 8 Hours) are available in the United States. These products extend the duration of action to 8 hours. The formulation is generally a 650-mg tablet composed of an immediate-release component (325 mg) and a delayed-release component (325 mg). The potential for delayed increases exist in the serum acetaminophen concentration that may cross the nomogram after 4 hours ("late crossing") (85–87). Analysis of toxicokinetics in 41 patients with overdose using the extended-release product indicated that the elimination half-life was not altered, but the onset of the elimination phase appeared delayed in some patients. This finding led to the recommendation that patients with an ingestion of the extended-release product should have at least two serum acetaminophen levels performed. These should be at least 4 to 6 hours apart (88).

Complications of Acute Overdosage

The most feared complications of liver failure are hepatic encephalopathy, hepatorenal syndrome, and sepsis. Each greatly reduces prospects for survival. Some degree of renal dysfunction develops in 46% of patients with serious liver injury (64). Renal failure is reversible if the patient survives. GI bleeding after liver failure is also common. The etiology and management of hepatic encephalopathy are addressed in Chapter 17.

Clinical Pitfalls

Many pitfalls are encountered in the assessment of the patient with acute overdose. By far the most common is basing critical decisions on the patient's history of ingestion. Patients often misidentify or understate the amount of acetaminophen that they have ingested. The time of ingestion is particularly difficult for patients to recall. Even an apparently precise history from a reliable patient may prove to be erroneous. Many reasons can be found for the inaccuracies. First, other products may have been consumed that contain acetaminophen. Second, patients' embarrassment over the episode may cause them to minimize the severity of ingestion. Whatever the cause, several patients die each year because of incomplete patient evaluation.

Repeated Supratherapeutic Ingestion

Repeated ingestion of acetaminophen is now recognized as a major cause of acetaminophen-related death. An RSI of acetaminophen is defined as more than one ingestion of acetaminophen over a period exceeding 8 hours that results in a cumulative dose of greater than 4 g/day. One study estimated that 30% of patients acquired hepatic injury after repeated ingestion of acetaminophen, rather than acute overdose (89). Unfortunately, the authors of this particular study did not acknowledge the skewed selection of accidental versus intentional misuse and mistakenly attributed the difference to ethanol (90). Others have noted the RSI problem (91).

The management of these patients has not been adequately investigated. A prospective poison center–based observational trial indicates that most patients with RSI present with liver injury that is already established. The median reported dose associated with increased aminotransferase levels showed a dose-response relationship (F. F. S. Daly, *unpublished data*, 2002). Most importantly, the use of the serum acetaminophen level and serum AST shows promise in determining which patients need treatment. A prospective observational poison center study found that no hepatic injury developed in any patient who had a normal AST at presentation and an acetaminophen level below 10 mg/L (92). These patients were typically discharged. All patients with an abnormality in either test were treated with acetylcysteine for a minimum of 12 hours. Due to a relatively small number of patients and some patients lost to follow-up, further evaluation is needed for this promising approach.

Acetaminophen RSI in children has been reported with doses well above therapeutic with mean doses of 92 mg/kg/day; changes in ALT were not substantial (93). Most authors have reported doses above 150 mg/kg/day in children with hepatic injury from repeated dosing (94).

Adverse Reactions

A wide variety of adverse reactions have been associated with acetaminophen ingestion. Because the prevalence of acetaminophen use is high in most countries, a causal relationship is unproven in many cases. Adverse effects with high probability of a causal relationship include rare allergic reactions, including anaphylactic, anaphylactoid, urticarial, and rash reactions, as well as asthma.

GI bleeding and nephrotoxicity have been attributed to acetaminophen by epidemiologic studies. They are addressed together because of the striking similarity of the evidence in both conditions. In the case of GI bleeding, numerous prospective studies involving large numbers of patients have demonstrated that GI ulceration and bleeding are not caused by acetaminophen. In contrast, a small number of large epidemiologic studies found an increased risk of GI bleeding or renal insufficiency based on patient self-reporting (95). Other large epidemiologic studies have found no relationship (96). The presence of confounding by indication likely explains the results in both cases (78). It is common for physicians to discourage the use of nonsteroidal antiinflammatory drugs and to encourage the use of acetaminophen in patients with either GI or renal disease. Furthermore, these diseases often take a prolonged period to develop. Thus, patients may have symptoms well before diagnosis and increase their use of acetaminophen.

DIAGNOSTIC TESTS

Acute and Subacute Overdosage

DETERMINING THE NEED FOR ACETYLCYSTEINE

Unlike many substances, a diagnostic tool is available to predict the risk of hepatic injury and the need for treatment with acetylcysteine. The Rumack-Matthew nomogram uses a timed plasma acetaminophen level drawn at least 4 hours after ingestion to establish the likelihood of liver injury (10). It was empirically derived from 64 patients treated at the Edinburgh poison treatment center (29). These patients had untreated acetaminophen poisoning. A line connecting a point at 200 mg/L at 4 hours after ingestion and 50 mg/L at 12 hours after ingestion was found to separate all patients with liver injury from those in whom liver injury did not develop. Because the history is often uncertain, the FDA requested that a lower line be created that was 25% below the original line to use as a treatment criterion for the initial study of NAC. Today, this is termed the *possible toxicity line* (Fig. 4). Thus, some 20% to 40% of patients with acetaminophen concentrations above the 200 mg/L "treatment line" after a single overdose (Fig. 5) escape serious hepatorenal damage even if untreated; such damage occurs only rarely in patients with concentrations below this line.

An outcome nomogram showing the results of 2540 patients, of whom 2023 met inclusion criteria for treatment with acetylcysteine and an additional 517 who did not meet inclusion criteria but received acetylcysteine treatment anyway has been published (29) (Fig. 5) Given the inaccuracy of patient histories and the dependence on time, it is not surprising that some patients whose initial plasma level was below the line showed toxicity. A small difference in historical time of ingestion can change the location on the nomogram and the likelihood of toxicity significantly in either direction.

The nomogram is used to guide the administration of acetylcysteine (Chapter 64). A serum acetaminophen level for which the time of sampling is known is simply plotted on the nomogram. In the United Kingdom, acetylcysteine treatment is started if the acetaminophen level falls above the upper 4-hour line (200 mg/L; 1323 mmol/L). In the United States, the lower

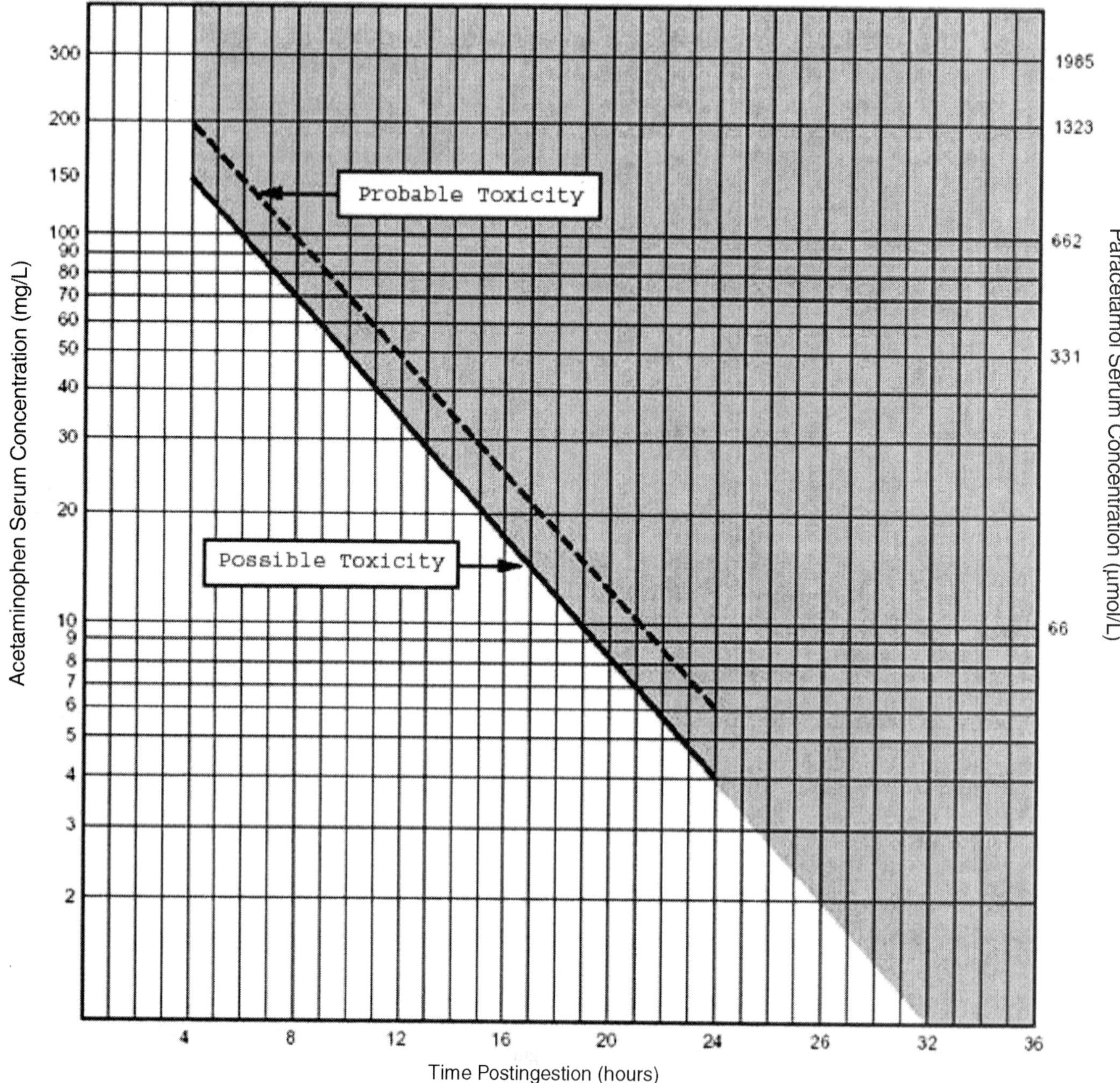

Figure 4. Rumack-Matthew nomogram. This nomogram includes the original line starting at 200 mg/ml and the additional safety line starting at 150 mg/ml as noted in the text. This nomogram should only be used after a single acute ingestion. An acetaminophen level should be obtained 4 or more hours after ingestion to assure that a peak level has occurred. Extended-release preparations should have a second level 4 hours after the first level to make certain that it is not rising. The level should be plotted in relationship to the time to determine the likelihood of toxicity and need for treatment. Caution should be used in assessing the reliability of the time of ingestion. [Adapted from Rumack BH, Matthew H. Acetaminophen poisoning and toxicity. *Pediatrics* 1975;55(6):871–876.]

line at 4 hours (150 mg/L; 993 mmol/L) is used to initiate treatment. Over the years, many variations on these treatment lines have been proposed, particularly for the patient with alcoholism. However, the available data do not support the creation of a new line (97).

ASSESSMENT OF INJURY SEVERITY

The severity of injury is monitored using repeated laboratory testing. Typical tests include serum electrolytes, ALT and AST, international normalized ratio (INR), and platelet count. In patients in whom hepatic failure develops, these tests are performed serially, acid-base status is followed closely, and serial evaluation of mental status is performed to assess prognosis and the need for liver transplant.

Several methods of assessing the severity have been developed by the liver unit at King's College in London. Listing for transplantation is recommended in patients with acute liver failure if one or more of the following is present:

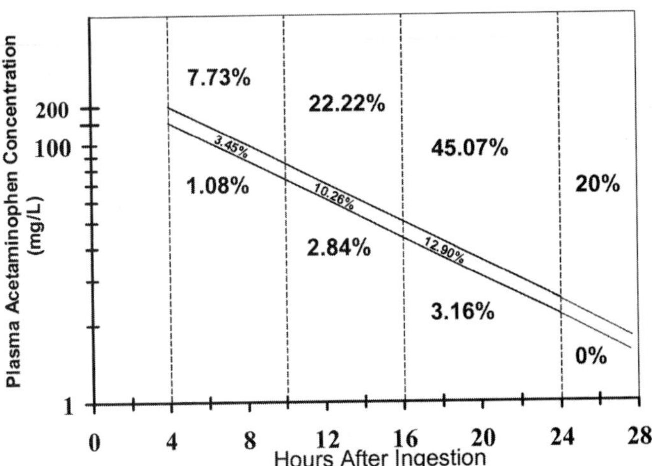

Figure 5. Outcome nomogram showing the results of 2540 patients, of whom 2023 met inclusion criteria for treatment with NAC and an additional 517 who did not meet inclusion criteria but were treated. The percentage shows the number of patients in whom an alanine aminotransferase of greater than 1000 IU/L developed. [From Rumack BH. Acetaminophen hepatotoxicity: the first 35 years. *J Toxicol Clin Toxicol* 2002;40(1):3–20, with permission.]

1. Arterial pH less than 7.3
2. Arterial lactate concentration above 3.0 mmol/L after adequate fluid resuscitation
3. Serum creatinine greater than 300 μmol/L (greater than 3.39 mg/dl)
4. INR greater than 6.5 (or partial thromboplastin time greater than 100 seconds)
5. Hepatic encephalopathy of grade 3 or 4

Furthermore, transplantation should be seriously considered if the arterial lactate concentration is above 3.5 mmol/L after early fluid resuscitation (approximately 4 hours after admission to the hospital). The addition of arterial lactate concentration to the criteria gives a positive likelihood ratio of 15, which is similar to the original King's College Hospital criteria. The negative likelihood ratio for the modified criteria was less than 2% in the validation group, which is an improvement over the original criteria (98). The addition of a serum phosphorus level to the evaluation has been proposed. Patients with low serum phosphorus had a greater chance of recovery than those with a phosphorus greater than 2.5 mEq/L. The small acetaminophen subgroup with serum phosphorus of 2.5 or greater has a 100% positive predictive value and an 82% negative predictive value (99).

DETERMINING THE ETIOLOGY OF HEPATIC NECROSIS

By definition, the serum aminotransferases and bilirubin should be increased in acute liver failure. The definition of hepatotoxicity after acetaminophen overdose has been an AST of 1000 IU/L or greater. The serum alkaline phosphatase may be increased or normal. An acetaminophen level should be obtained and the results interpreted appropriately, depending on the type of acetaminophen ingestion. A very high acetaminophen level or a positive level in the presence of known overdose is useful; however, other diagnoses should be considered, especially in patients with minimally elevated acetaminophen levels. Specific drug screening or quantitative levels of known hepatotoxins should be considered. Referral clinical laboratories may be able to test for suspected agents.

It has been asserted that very high ALT or AST levels are diagnostic of acetaminophen hepatotoxicity and exclude alcoholic and viral hepatitis. This is incorrect. The height of aminotransferase activity in the serum, even in the presence of centrilobular necrosis, is not pathognomonic of acetaminophen toxicity. AST levels as high as 11,660 IU/L have been reported in viral hepatitis, 17,050 IU/L after herpes simplex, and an ALT as high as 14,276 IU/L with hepatitis C (100–102).

An overview of the evaluation of the patient with increased liver function tests is provided in Figure 6. A complete panel of tests for viral hepatitis should be performed: hepatitis A virus, immunoglobulin M, hepatitis B virus surface antigen, and hepatitis B virus anticore immunoglobulin M serologies. Hepatitis C virus (HCV) antibody testing may be negative for several weeks or months after acute infection. Repeat testing may be necessary, but acute HCV is an uncommon cause of fulminant hepatic failure. If HCV is suspected, hepatitis C viral load should be determined. Other viral studies, such as cytomegalovirus, herpes simplex virus, or influenza A, may be helpful in the post-transplant setting or when patients are otherwise immunosuppressed. Autoimmune markers such as antinuclear antibody, antismooth muscle antibody, and a ceruloplasmin level should be obtained.

Hypotension, hypoxia, or ischemic injury produces centrilobular necrosis and high transaminase levels, most likely because of oxidative stress. The rapid rise and resolution of injury are similar to those of acetaminophen hepatotoxicity (103). In a 1-year series of patients with AST greater than 3000 IU/L, 52% were caused by acute hypotension, 12% by toxic agents, and 7% by viral hepatitis, with a 75% mortality in the hypotensive group and 33% mortality for all others (104). In another similar study of 18,000 patient admissions, 59% of all instances of AST greater than 1000 IU/L were attributed to ischemia (105). Other reports of very high transaminases have been associated with a diagnosis of obstructive sleep apnea, heat stroke, anorexia nervosa, and Epstein-Barr virus (106–109).

If the cause of liver failure is not apparent after initial evaluation, ultrasound can establish the patency and flow in the hepatic vein (to exclude Budd-Chiari syndrome), hepatic artery, and portal vein. Computed tomography or magnetic resonance imaging of the abdomen can define hepatic anatomy and help the clinician exclude other intra-abdominal processes. Head computed tomography helps identify cerebral edema and exclude intracranial mass (e.g., hematoma) that may mimic edema from fulminant hepatic failure.

Liver biopsy can narrow the diagnosis but may be contraindicated because of coagulopathy. It is rarely of clinical use during the management of ALF. A hepatologist is often helpful in establishing the diagnosis, but up to 20% of all cases of ALF remain unidentified.

TESTS TO GUIDE PATIENT MANAGEMENT

Serum electrolytes and renal function tests are used to detect and guide treatment of complications of liver failure, such as hepatorenal syndrome. Monitoring of the glucose level is important because of glycogen depletion and impaired gluconeogenesis. Serum phosphate may be low and require supplementation, although this is a good prognostic sign. The blood count may show thrombocytopenia, a common complication of ALF. Blood, urine, and other cultures are used to monitor for the common complication of sepsis.

Coagulation studies serve as a marker of liver synthetic function and help to assess prognosis. The prothrombin time or INR should be elevated and may become markedly prolonged. Individual coagulation factors become depleted, but this information is not typically used to manage patients. Factor V levels have been proposed as a prognostic indicator, among other measurements (110). A falling AST or ALT in conjunction with a rising INR indicates a poor prognosis (Fig. 3), although the King's College criteria usually have already predicted this course.

Serial evaluation of acid-base status helps determine prognosis and guides immediate management. In addition, these tests can help estimate the need for liver transplantation. The serum lactate is usually elevated due to the combination of inadequate tissue perfusion and decreased clearance by the liver. The serum ammo-

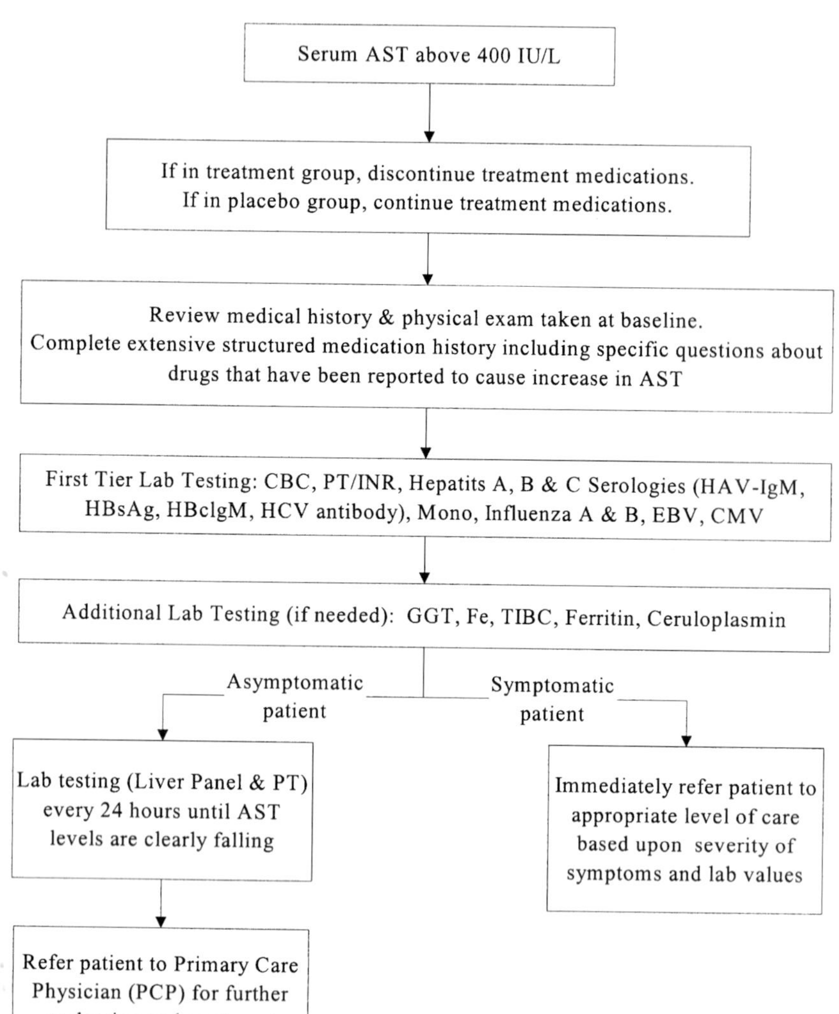

Figure 6. Evaluation of patients with elevated liver function tests. AST, aspartate aminotransferase; CBC, complete blood count; CMV, cytomegalovirus; EBV, Epstein-Barr virus; GGT, γ-glutamyltransferase; HAV, hepatitis A virus; IgM, immunoglobulin M; HBsAg, hepatitis B surface antigen; HBclgM, hepatitis B anti-core immunoglobulin M; HCV, hepatitis C virus; INR, international normalized ratio; PT, prothrombin time; TIBC, total iron-binding capacity.

nia level is generally elevated in patients with encephalopathy but is not reliable, and its use is discouraged. An electroencephalogram should be considered to exclude clinically unapparent seizures in comatose patients.

A bilirubin level above 5.0 mg/dl can produce a false-positive acetaminophen level (111). This can be important in interpretation of acetaminophen levels drawn from patients with liver failure of unknown cause.

Repeated Supratherapeutic Ingestion

The serum acetaminophen level and the serum AST or ALT levels are used to determine the need for treatment. If the AST is greater than 50 IU/L or the serum acetaminophen level is greater than 10 mg/L, the patient should be treated with acetylcysteine (Fig. 7). If both are normal, the patient can be discharged. In patients with evidence of liver injury, laboratory testing is the same as for acute overdosage.

Postmortem Considerations

The mean muscle-blood ratio for acetaminophen in six cadavers was 0.7 (112). As with other chemicals, postmortem blood levels are difficult to interpret. It appears that acetaminophen blood levels may increase after death as a result of diffusion out of the stomach, with the highest levels in the aorta, lower levels in the peripheral blood, and still lower in the liver (113).

Postmortem liver specimens demonstrate abnormalities ranging from hepatocyte swelling and cytoplasmic vacuolization to frank centrilobular eosinophilic coagulative necrosis. Fatal cases tended to have the most extensive damage and destroyed all but a rim of surviving hepatocytes around the portal tract (82,114).

Although myocardial damage has been observed in 11.6% of one series, histopathologic evidence of myocardial damage has not been found (83). The presence of cardiac effects is probably secondary to the effects of acute liver failure.

TREATMENT

The principles of management include treatment of the underlying cause combined with meticulous supportive care of liver, renal, and central nervous system injury. Survival depends on the rapid institution of aggressive medical care. Identification of disease severity is important, and timely referral to a transplant center is potentially lifesaving. Endotracheal intubation, hemodialysis, and other invasive procedures are often needed.

Decontamination

Because the treatment of acute acetaminophen poisoning is based on the serum acetaminophen level, and gastric decontamination measures have been shown repeatedly to reduce the serum concen-

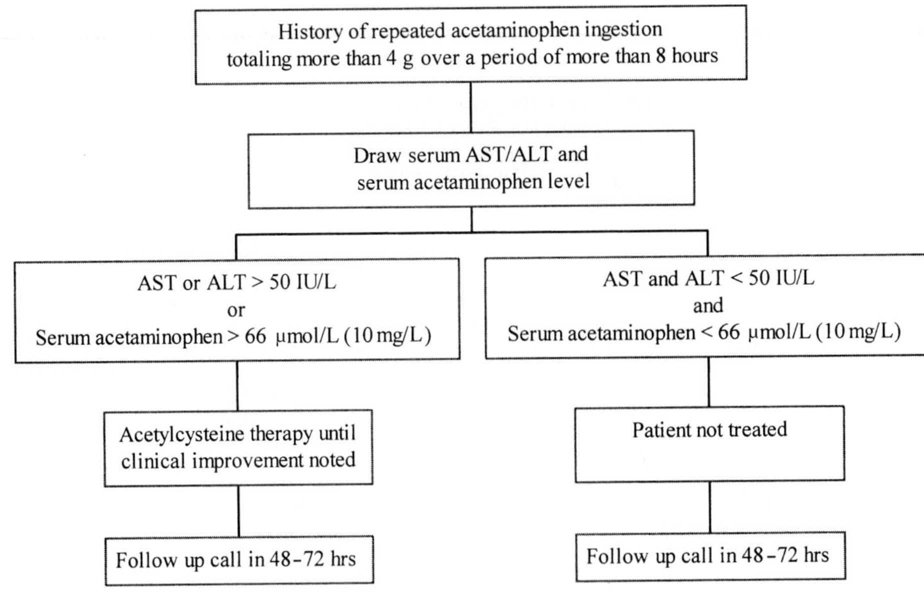

Figure 7. Management of repeated supra-therapeutic ingestion of acetaminophen. ALT, alanine aminotransferase; AST, aspartate aminotransferase; NAC, *N*-acetylcysteine.

tration, decontamination procedures have the potential to decrease the number of patients treated with acetylcysteine (Chapter 7). Activated charcoal (AC) binds acetaminophen well, and multiple volunteer and clinical studies indicate that it reduces the serum acetaminophen level (115). AC should be administered to all patients with an acute ingestion within the previous 1 to 2 hours.

Emesis also reduces the serum acetaminophen level. An advisory committee to the FDA has recommended that ipecac should no longer be available without a prescription. Induced emesis would be inappropriate in the emergency department because it delays AC administration (116). However, home use of ipecac may be useful. One study of children suggested that ipecac use may be of value and concluded that children who ingest between 140 and 200 mg/kg acetaminophen and demonstrate ipecac-induced emesis within 60 minutes can be safely managed at home (117). Under such circumstances, careful evaluation of the history and follow-up is imperative.

Acute Overdosage

Treatment consists of two categories. First, the patient who presents early is treated to reduce or prevent acetaminophen-induced injury by the early administration of acetylcysteine. The late-presenting patient is treated to limit organ injury that arises from acetaminophen toxicity.

The term *preventive* is applied to the early treatment of patients with acute overdosage. Hepatic injury can be prevented in nearly all patients treated with acetylcysteine within 8 to 10 hours of an acute ingestion, regardless of the magnitude of the acetaminophen level (12,118). Although the mortality is low (11 of 2540 patients, or 0.43%), early treatment is imperative, as no deaths occurred in this same series in patients treated before 16 hours postingestion. The data indicate that acetylcysteine also has some therapeutic effect for patients who present 10 to 24 hours after ingestion, although its efficacy diminishes as the time to treatment increases (12). Some suggestion has been made that treatment performed at even as late as 36 hours may have some benefit (119). Therefore, all patients with a single acute ingestion of acetaminophen whose serum acetaminophen level falls above the treatment line should be treated with acetylcysteine.

Acetylcysteine is a remarkably effective and low-cost antidote for acetaminophen toxicity. It is a sulfhydryl-containing tripeptide that was initially used to loosen secretions in the airway. Piperno and colleagues at McNeil laboratories developed an animal model and proved that acetylcysteine (Mucomyst) was an effective agent to protect against acetaminophen hepatotoxicity (120).

Acetylcysteine can be administered by either the oral or the intravenous route. Worldwide, the most common route of administration is intravenous. In the United States, the oral route has been used since the 1970s; however, it is likely that an intravenous preparation will be available in the United States in 2004. The dosing and administration, adverse effects, and pitfalls of acetylcysteine administration are provided in Chapter 64.

Several acetylcysteine regimens have been proposed (Table 4). The 72-hour oral NAC protocol is probably unnecessary in many cases in which acetaminophen is eliminated before the full

TABLE 4. Antidote regimens

Antidote	Route	Regimen	Total dose (mg/kg)	Length of treatment (h)
Methionine	Oral	2.5 g (36 mg/kg) 4-hourly for doses	144	12
NAC	Oral	140 mg/kg, followed 4 h later by 70 mg/kg 4-hourly for 17 doses	1300	72
NAC (20-h protocol)	IV	150 mg/kg in 200 ml 5% dextrose over 15 min; 50 mg/kg in 500 ml 5% dextrose over 4 h, and 100 mg/kg in 1 L 5% dextrose over 16 h	300	20.25
NAC (48-h protocol)	IV	140 mg/kg in 5% dextrose over 1 h, followed 4 h after initiation of treatment by 12 maintenance doses (70 mg/kg) given over 1 h in 5% dextrose, each commencing 4 h after initiation of preceding dose	980	48

NAC, *N*-acetylcysteine.
From Vale JA, Proudfoot AT. Paracetamol (acetaminophen) poisoning. *Lancet* 1995;346(8974):547–552, with permission.

acetylcysteine regimen is completed. Stopping treatment earlier may mean that some patients will have a relatively asymptomatic and a possibly, but not assuredly, modest rise in enzymes. One retrospective study terminated acetylcysteine treatment when the acetaminophen level became zero. In that study, 33 patients received truncated treatment and then had a repeat AST determination. Of these, 3 (9%) demonstrated a minor rise in the aminotransferase level (121). It is unknown whether any of the remaining patients had an increase in enzymes.

Drugs such as cimetidine that competitively inhibit CYP2E1 have been proposed as alternative antidotes. However, the addition of cimetidine therapy to standard NAC treatment did not provide additional hepatoprotection in acutely acetaminophen-poisoned patients when treatment was started later than 8 hours after the overdose (122).

It is likely that many compounds can potentially ameliorate acetaminophen toxicity, especially in stage II. Speculative antidotes are those agents that have shown to provide some benefit in animal studies (Table 5). Their use in humans has not yet been confirmed to be of value. Work on stage II (inflammatory stage) appears to indicate that some benefit may be obtained with the use of agents later in the course in addition to NAC during stage I. This area may provide useful research.

Pediatric Patient

The pediatric patient is generally considered resistant to acetaminophen toxicity. However, acute ingestion occasionally causes fulminant hepatic failure, hepatic transplant, or death. Acute ingestion by a child of any age is managed using the same approach as for adult ingestion.

Repeated Supratherapeutic Ingestion

The treatment of patients who present with repeated administration of acetaminophen over a day or more of time is still evolving. The acetaminophen nomogram cannot be used in these cases. Emerging research suggests that patients in whom liver injury is going to develop from repeated dosing already manifest that injury at the time of presentation (92). The Rocky Mountain Poison and Drug Center has followed an algorithmic approach to the management of these patients for several years (Fig. 7). In short, patients with an AST of less than 50 IU/L and a serum acetaminophen level of 10 mg/L or less are discharged from care without treatment (92). Conversely, patients with either an AST above 50 IU/L or an acetaminophen level above 10 mg/L are treated with acetylcysteine.

The issue of treatment duration remains unresolved. The authors' approach is to treat patients with a standard loading dose of acetylcysteine, followed by maintenance doses until the acetaminophen level is zero and liver functions have improved to near normal (i.e., AST and INR are both normal or are improving substantially).

TABLE 5. Speculative treatments for acetaminophen poisoning

Agent	Comments
Deferoxamine (desferrioxamine)	Although shown to be beneficial if given with NAC in animal models, no human data are available. It may be useful to consider in cases of simultaneous iron overdose, in patients who have been consuming iron supplements, or in those who have the diagnosis of hemochromatosis.
Selenium	No human data have been produced; however, patients with long-term malnutrition or states of vitamin depletion may benefit.
Gadolinium and dextran	Although it would be useful to try to ameliorate stage II toxicity, the role and benefit of these agents introduced after toxicity are unclear, and there are no data in humans.
Disulfiram	This potent CYP2E1 inhibitor may provide benefit in patients who have been receiving it chronically and then overdose with acetaminophen. Its use following acetaminophen overdose is unknown in humans.
Propolis	This well-documented folk medicine, available in Europe, may be worth investigating as a treatment but at this time has no proven benefit in humans.
Hyper-IL-6	This protein has been suggested as a way to produce hepatic regeneration in the face of fulminant hepatic failure and is currently being researched for clinical use.

IL, interleukin; NAC, *N*-acetylcysteine.

TABLE 6. Common misconceptions regarding use of the serum acetaminophen level

Reliability of the patient history: In the preclinical phase (an asymptomatic patient before any abnormal laboratory results or acetaminophen levels), diagnostic and therapeutic decisions must be based entirely on history. The usual guideline used in the triage of a patient exposed to acetaminophen is to evaluate anyone exposed to 150 mg/kg or greater. However, reliability of the history must be considered.

Agreement of patient history and serum acetaminophen level: Once the first plasma acetaminophen level (Cp) is determined, it should be correlated with the ingestion history. Because acetaminophen has a volume of distribution of approximately 1 L/kg, the body burden can be easily calculated. The plasma level times the patient's weight times 1000 provides the body burden in milligrams. For example, a Cp of 200 mg/L in a 70-kg human represents a 14,000-mg (14-g) dose. The calculation is $200 \times 1 \times 70 \times 1000$. For comparison, a therapeutic dose (1 g/70 kg) produces a 2-h Cp of approximately 10 mg/ml. Because Cp typically falls by half every 2 h, it is important to relate the time of ingestion in considering the ingestion history.

Use of estimated acetaminophen half-life: If two levels can be obtained, (three or more are preferred) a half-life can be estimated. Acetaminophen half-life after a therapeutic dose (and most overdoses) is approximately 2 h. Even after a large overdose, patients do not have an instantaneous increase in half-life, to as much as 12 h or more. Thus, if patients arrive with a prolonged half-life and the history of 4–8 h since overdose, the time of ingestion must have been much earlier or they have another reason for the increased half-life. In most patients after a large overdose, the half-life at the time of ingestion is normal and gradually increases over several days because of hepatic toxicity.

Agreement of patient history and serum aminotransferase level: ALT and AST levels take time to rise, and peak levels are not expected until 72 or 96 h after overdose. A patient who arrives with a peak level of enzyme and a history of having taken an overdose 4 h before either consumed the toxic dose considerably earlier or has some other cause for the ALT/AST elevation.

Repeated supratherapeutic ingestion: Chronic excessive consumption of acetaminophen in supratherapeutic doses is harder to quantify. The plasma level still reflects the body burden, and the half-life is helpful in determining potential toxicity.

ALT, alanine aminotransferase; AST, aspartate aminotransferase.

Monitoring

Physical examination findings are nonspecific and during phase I and phase II may demonstrate only abdominal tenderness. As phase III begins, an enlarged liver may be palpated and scleral icterus may be seen as bilirubin begins to rise. Mental status may deteriorate if liver failure occurs. Constructional dyspraxia is an easy and sensitive way to follow changes in mental status. The patient is asked to draw a house with a door, window, chimney, and walkway. The test is repeated at intervals, and deterioration of the drawing is seen consistent with worsening of hepatic function.

Laboratory monitoring studies include ALT, AST, arterial pH, arterial lactate, serum creatinine, and INR. Repeated acetaminophen levels are usually not needed. Fulminant hepatic failure may also show further changes in coagulation parameters, and disseminated intravascular coagulation may occur. Hepatorenal syndrome may develop, and kidney function must be followed. Although serum ammonia may rise in such cases, it does not correlate particularly well with the clinical condition. Serum phosphorus may be helpful in determining prognosis.

Management Pitfalls

The pharmacokinetics are not understood in many cases of acetaminophen toxicity. The normal time course and phases of toxicity were described in 1975, and a diagram was published in 1981 (10,11) (Fig. 3). Appreciation of this time course in relation to the ingestion and laboratory findings is helpful in sorting out various issues in evaluation of a case. Table 6 provides common misconceptions that can be corrected by considering acetaminophen kinetics and metabolism. Consideration of these factors as well as the remainder of the clinical picture provides a more accurate understanding of the toxicity being treated.

REFERENCES

1. Hinsberg O, Treupel, G. Ueber die physiologische Wirkung des p-Amidophenols und einiger Derivate desselben. *Naunyn Schmiedebergs Arch Exp Pathol Pharmacol* 1894;33(1):216–250.
2. Thomson JS, Prescott LF. Liver damage and impaired glucose tolerance after paracetamol overdosage. *BMJ* 1966;5512:506–507.
3. Mitchell JR, Jollow DJ, Potter WZ, et al. Acetaminophen-induced hepatic necrosis. I. Role of drug metabolism. *J Pharmacol Exp Ther* 1973;187(1):185–194.
4. Prescott LF, Roscoe P, Wright N, et al. Plasma-paracetamol half-life and hepatic necrosis in patients with paracetamol overdosage. *Lancet* 1971;1(7698):519–522.
5. Jollow DJ, Mitchell JR, Potter WZ, et al. Acetaminophen-induced hepatic necrosis. II. Role of covalent binding in vivo. *J Pharmacol Exp Ther* 1973;187(1):195–202.
6. Jollow DJ, Thorgeirsson SS, Potter WZ, et al. Acetaminophen-induced hepatic necrosis. VI. Metabolic disposition of toxic and nontoxic doses of acetaminophen. *Pharmacology* 1974;12(4–5):251–271.
7. Mitchell JR, Jollow DJ, Potter WZ, et al. Acetaminophen-induced hepatic necrosis. IV. Protective role of glutathione. *J Pharmacol Exp Ther* 1973;187(1):211–217.
8. Potter WZ, Davis DC, Mitchell JR, et al. Acetaminophen-induced hepatic necrosis. 3. Cytochrome P-450–mediated covalent binding in vitro. *J Pharmacol Exp Ther* 1973;187(1):203–210.
9. Potter WZ, Thorgeirsson SS, Jollow DJ, et al. Acetaminophen-induced hepatic necrosis. V. Correlation of hepatic necrosis, covalent binding and glutathione depletion in hamsters. *Pharmacology* 1974;12(3):129–143.
10. Rumack BH, Matthew H. Acetaminophen poisoning and toxicity. *Pediatrics* 1975;55(6):871–876.
11. Rumack BH, Peterson RC, Koch GG, et al. Acetaminophen overdose. 662 cases with evaluation of oral acetylcysteine treatment. *Arch Intern Med* 1981;141(3 Spec No.):380–385.
12. Smilkstein MJ, Knapp GL, Kulig KW, et al. Efficacy of oral *N*-acetylcysteine in the treatment of acetaminophen overdose. Analysis of the national multicenter study (1976 to 1985) [see Comments]. *N Engl J Med* 1988;319(24):1557–1562.
13. Verschuren F, Thys F, Wittebole X, et al. Effervescent paracetamol poisoning: a case report. *Eur J Emerg Med* 2002;9(4)339–341.
14. Sumida SM, Sato RL, Wong JJ, et al. Acetaminophen levels 4 and 7 hours after 2000 and 3000 mg single doses in healthy adults. *Hawaii Med J* 2003;62(1):6–9.
15. Peterson RG, Rumack BH. Age as a variable in acetaminophen overdose. *Arch Intern Med* 1981;141:390–393.
16. Gelotte C, Auiler J, Lynch J, et al. Tolerability and repeat-dose pharmacokinetics (PK) of acetaminophen (APAP) at 4, 6 and 8 g/d in healthy adults. *Toxicol Sci* 2003;72(S-1):145.
17. Blackledge HM, O'Farrell J, Minton NA, et al. The effect of therapeutic doses of paracetamol on sulphur metabolism in man. *Hum Exp Toxicol* 1991;10(3):159–165.
18. Rumack BH. Acetaminophen overdose in young children. Treatment and effects of alcohol and other additional ingestants in 417 cases. *Am J Dis Child* 1984;138(5):428–433.
19. Prescott LF. Gastrointestinal absorption of drugs. *Med Clin North Am* 1974;58(5):907–916.
20. Wojcicki J, Kazmierczyk J, Gawronska-Szklarz B, et al. Effect of papaverine and atropine on pharmacokinetics of paracetamol administered orally. *Pol J Pharmacol Pharm* 1979;31(3):239–243.
21. McPhail ME, Knowles RG, Salter M, et al. Uptake of acetaminophen (paracetamol) by isolated rat liver cells. *Biochem Pharmacol* 1993;45(8):1599–1604.
22. Miller RP, Roberts RJ, Fischer LJ. Acetaminophen elimination kinetics in neonates, children, and adults. *Clin Pharmacol Ther* 1976;19(3):284–294.
23. Gregus Z, Madhu C, Klaassen CD. Species variation in toxication and detoxication of acetaminophen in vivo: a comparative study of biliary and urinary excretion of acetaminophen metabolites. *J Pharmacol Exp Ther* 1988;244(1):91–99.
24. Prescott LF. Drug conjugation in clinical toxicology. *Biochem Soc Trans* 1984;12(1):96–99.
25. Prescott LF. Kinetics and metabolism of paracetamol and phenacetin. *Br J Clin Pharmacol* 1980;10[Suppl 2]:291S–298S.
26. Kock R, Schneider H, Delvoux B, et al. The determination of inorganic sulphate in serum and synovial fluid by high performance ion chromatography. *Eur J Clin Chem Clin Biochem* 1997;35(9):679–685.
27. Seo KW, Park M, Song YJ, et al. The protective effects of propolis on hepatic injury and its mechanism. *Phytother Res* 2003;17(3):250–253.
28. Manyike PT, Kharasch ED, Kalhorn TF, et al. Contribution of CYP2E1 and CYP3A to acetaminophen reactive metabolite formation. *Clin Pharmacol Ther* 2000;67(3):275–282.
29. Rumack BH. Acetaminophen hepatotoxicity: the first 35 years. *J Toxicol Clin Toxicol* 2002;40(1):3–20.
30. Tsutsumi M, Lasker JM, Shimizu M, et al. The intralobular distribution of ethanol-inducible P450IIE1 in rat and human liver. *Hepatology* 1989;10(4):437–446.
31. Lucas D, Berthou F, Dreano Y, et al. Comparison of levels of cytochromes P-450, CYP1A2, CYP2E1, and their related monooxygenase activities in human surgical liver samples. *Alcohol Clin Exp Res* 1993;17(4):900–905.
32. Girre C, Lucas D, Hispard E, et al. Assessment of cytochrome P4502E1 induction in alcoholic patients by chlorzoxazone pharmacokinetics. *Biochem Pharmacol* 1994;47(9):1503–1508.
33. Dupont I, Lucas D, Clot P, et al. Cytochrome P4502E1 inducibility and hydroxyethyl radical formation among alcoholics. *J Hepatol* 1998;28(4):564–571.
34. Song BJ, Veech RL, Park SS, et al. Induction of rat hepatic N-nitrosodimethylamine demethylase by acetone is due to protein stabilization. *J Biol Chem* 1989;264(6):3568–3572.
35. Eliasson E, Johansson I, Ingelman-Sundberg M. Ligand-dependent maintenance of ethanol-inducible cytochrome P-450 in primary rat hepatocyte cell cultures. *Biochem Biophys Res Commun* 1988;150(1):436–443.
36. Winters DK, Cederbaum AI. Time course characterization of the induction of cytochrome P-450 2E1 by pyrazole and 4-methylpyrazole. *Biochim Biophys Acta* 1992;1117(1):15–24.
37. Wu D, Cederbaum AI. Combined effects of streptozotocin-induced diabetes plus 4-methylpyrazole treatment on rat liver cytochrome P4502E1. *Arch Biochem Biophys* 1993;302(1):175–182.
38. Johansson I, Eliasson E, Ingelman-Sundberg M. Hormone controlled phosphorylation and degradation of CYP2B1 and CYP2E1 in isolated rat hepatocytes. *Biochem Biophys Res Commun* 1991;174(1):37–42.
39. Bessems JG, Vermeulen NP. Paracetamol (acetaminophen)-induced toxicity: molecular and biochemical mechanisms, analogues and protective approaches. *Crit Rev Toxicol* 2001;31(1):55–138.
40. Chanda S, Mehendale HM. Role of nutrition in the survival after hepatotoxic injury. *Toxicology* 1996;111(1–3):163–178.
41. Jaeschke H. Glutathione disulfide formation and oxidant stress during acetaminophen-induced hepatotoxicity in mice in vivo: the protective effect of allopurinol. *J Pharmacol Exp Ther* 1990;255(3):935–941.
42. Esposito LA, Melov S, Panov A, et al. Mitochondrial disease in mouse results in increased oxidative stress. *Proc Natl Acad Sci U S A* 1999;96(9):4820–4825.
43. Olafsdottir K, Reed DJ. Retention of oxidized glutathione by isolated rat liver mitochondria during hydroperoxide treatment. *Biochim Biophys Acta* 1988;964(3):377–382
44. Haouzi D, Lekehal M, Moreau A, et al. Cytochrome P450–generated reactive metabolites cause mitochondrial permeability transition, caspase activation, and apoptosis in rat hepatocytes. *Hepatology* 2000;32(2):303–311.
45. Younes M, Cornelius S, Siegers CP. Ferrous ion supported in vivo lipid peroxidation induced by paracetamol—its relation to hepatotoxicity. *Res Commun Chem Pathol Pharmacol* 1986;51(1):89–99.
46. Schnellmann JG, Pumford NR, Kusewitt DF, et al. A. Deferoxamine delays the development of the hepatotoxicity of acetaminophen in mice. *Toxicol Lett* 1999;106(1):79–88.
47. Peterson FJ, Lindemann NJ, Duquette PH, et al. Potentiation of acute acetaminophen lethality by selenium and vitamin E deficiency in mice. *J Nutr* 1992;122(1):74–81.
48. Schnell RC, Park KS, Davies MH, et al. Protective effects of selenium on acetaminophen-induced hepatotoxicity in the rat. *Toxicol Appl Pharmacol* 1988;95(1):1–11.
49. Michael SL, Pumford NR, Mayeux PR, et al. Pretreatment of mice with macrophage inactivators decreases acetaminophen hepatotoxicity and the formation of reactive oxygen and nitrogen species. *Hepatology* 1999;30(1):186–195.
50. Ju C, Reilly TP, Bourdi M, et al. Protective role of Kupffer cells in acetaminophen-induced hepatic injury in mice. *Chem Res Toxicol* 2002;15(12):1504–1513.
51. Decker K. Biologically active products of stimulated liver macrophages (Kupffer cells). *Eur J Biochem* 1990;192(2):245–261.

52. Decker K. The response of liver macrophages to inflammatory stimulation. *Keio J Med* 1998;47(1):1–9.
53. Chen CY, Huang YL, Lin TH. Association between oxidative stress and cytokine production in nickel-treated rats. *Arch Biochem Biophys* 1998;356(2):127–132.
54. Laskin DL. Sinusoidal lining cells and hepatotoxicity. *Toxicol Pathol* 1996;24(1):112–118.
55. Galun E, Axelrod JH. The role of cytokines in liver failure and regeneration: potential new molecular therapies. *Biochim Biophys Acta* 2002;1592(3):345–358.
56. Waksman JC, Fantuzzi G, Bogdan GM, et al. Interleukin-18 (IL18) is involved in acetaminophen (APAP) induced hepatic injury in a FAS/FAS ligand independent mechanism. *Clin Toxicol* 2001;39(5):495–496(abst 58).
57. Waksman JC, Fantuzzi G, Bogdan GM, et al. Decreased serum interleukin-6 (IL-6) following acute acetaminophen (APAP) overdose is associated with hepatic injury. *Clin Toxicol* 2001;39(5):486(abst 34).
58. Salminen WF Jr, Voellmy R, Roberts SM. Protection against hepatotoxicity by a single dose of amphetamine: the potential role of heat shock protein induction. *Toxicol Appl Pharmacol* 1997;147(2):247–258.
59. Rumack BH, Holtzman J, Chase HP. Hepatic drug metabolism and protein malnutrition. *J Pharmacol Exp Ther* 1973;186(3):441–446.
60. Schenker S, Speeg KV Jr, Perez A, et al. The effects of food restriction in man on hepatic metabolism of acetaminophen. *Clin Nutr* 2001;20(2):145–150.
61. Newman TJ, Bargman GJ. Acetaminophen hepatotoxicity and malnutrition. *Am J Gastroenterol* 1979;72(6):647–650.
62. Rumack BH. Acetaminophen overdose. *Am J Med* 1983;75(5A):104–112.
63. Wright N, Prescott LF. Potentiation by previous drug therapy of hepatotoxicity following paracetamol overdosage. *Scott Med J* 1973;18(2):56–58.
64. Makin AJ, Wendon J, Williams R. A 7-year experience of severe acetaminophen-induced hepatotoxicity (1987–1993). *Gastroenterology* 1995;109(6):1907–1916.
65. Badger TM, Huang J, Ronis M, et al. Induction of cytochrome P450 2E1 during chronic ethanol exposure occurs via transcription of the CYP 2E1 gene when blood alcohol concentrations are high. *Biochem Biophys Res Commun* 1993;190(3):780–785.
66. Badger TM, Ronis MJ, Ingelman-Sundberg M, et al. Pulsatile blood alcohol and CYP2E1 induction during chronic alcohol infusions in rats. *Alcohol* 1993;10(6):453–457.
67. Ronis MJ, Huang J, Crouch J, et al. Cytochrome P450 CYP 2E1 induction during chronic alcohol exposure occurs by a two-step mechanism associated with blood alcohol concentrations in rats. *J Pharmacol Exp Ther* 1993;264(2):944–950.
68. Takahashi T, Lasker JM, Rosman AS, et al. Induction of cytochrome P-4502E1 in the human liver by ethanol is caused by a corresponding increase in encoding messenger RNA. *Hepatology* 1993;17(2):236–245.
69. Chien JY, Thummel KE, Slattery JT. Pharmacokinetic consequences of induction of CYP2E1 by ligand stabilization. *Drug Metab Dispos* 1997;25(10):1165–1175.
70. Clot P, Albano E, Eliasson E, et al. Cytochrome P4502E1 hydroxyethyl radical adducts as the major antigen in autoantibody formation among alcoholics. *Gastroenterology* 1996;111(1):206–216.
71. Dart RC, Kuffner EK, Rumack BH. Treatment of pain or fever with paracetamol (acetaminophen) in the alcoholic patient: a systematic review. *Am J Ther* 2000;7(2):123–134.
72. Smilkstein MJ, Rumack BH. Chronic ethanol use and acute acetaminophen overdose toxicity. *Clin Toxicol* 1998;36(5):476.
73. Thummel KE, Slattery JT, Ro H, et al. Ethanol and production of the hepatotoxic metabolite of acetaminophen in healthy adults. *Clin Pharmacol Ther* 2000;67(6):591–599.
74. Kuffner EK, Dart RC, Bogdan GM, et al. Effect of maximal daily doses of acetaminophen on the liver of alcoholic patients. *Arch Intern Med* 2001;161:2247–2252.
75. Kuffner EK, Dart RC, Bogdan GM, et al. Evaluation of hepatotoxicity in alcoholic patients from therapeutic dosing of acetaminophen. *Clin Toxicol* 1999;37(5):641.
76. Prescott LF. Paracetamol, alcohol and the liver. *Br J Clin Pharmacol* 2000;49(4):291–301.
77. Slattery JT, Nelson SD, Thummel KE. The complex interaction between ethanol and acetaminophen. *Clin Pharmacol Ther* 1996;60(3):241–246.
78. Signorello LB, McLaughlin JK, Lipworth L, et al. Confounding by indication: implications for implant research. *J Long-Term Effects Medical Implants* 2003;13(1):53–58.
79. Friedman JM, Little BB, Brent RL, et al. Potential human teratogenicity of frequently prescribed drugs. *Obstet Gynecol* 1990;75(4):594–599.
80. Horowitz RS, Dart RC, Jarvie DR, et al. Placental transfer of *N*-acetylcysteine following human maternal acetaminophen toxicity. *J Toxicol Clin Toxicol* 1997;35(5):447–451.
81. Riggs BS, Bronstein AC, Kulig K, et al. Acute acetaminophen overdose during pregnancy. *Obstet Gynecol* 1989;74(2):247–253.
82. Portmann B, Talbot IC, Day DW, et al. Histopathological changes in the liver following a paracetamol overdose: correlation with clinical and biochemical parameters. *J Pathol* 1975;117(3):169–181.
83. Hamlyn AN, Douglas AP, James O. The spectrum of paracetamol (acetaminophen) overdose: clinical and epidemiological studies. *Postgrad Med J* 1978;54(632):400–404.
84. Zezulka A, Wright N. Severe metabolic acidosis early in paracetamol poisoning. *BMJ* 1982;285(6345):851–852.
85. Bizovi KE, Aks SE, Paloucek F, et al. Late increase in acetaminophen concentration after overdose of Tylenol Extended Relief. *Ann Emerg Med* 1996;28(5):549–551.
86. Douglas DR, Sholar JB, Smilkstein MJ. A pharmacokinetic comparison of acetaminophen products (Tylenol Extended Relief vs regular Tylenol). *Acad Emerg Med* 1996;3(8):740–744.
87. Stork CM, Rees S, Howland MA, et al. Pharmacokinetics of extended relief vs regular release Tylenol in simulated human overdose. *J Toxicol Clin Toxicol* 1996;34(2):157–162.
88. Cetaruk EW, Dart RC, Hurlbut KM, et al. Tylenol Extended Relief overdose. *Ann Emerg Med* 1997;30(1):104–108.
89. Schiodt FV, Rochling FA, Casey DL, et al. Acetaminophen toxicity in an urban county hospital. *N Engl J Med* 1997;337(16):1112–1117.
90. Walker, AM. Acetaminophen toxicity in an urban county hospital [Letter; Comment]. *N Engl J Med* 1998;338(8):543–545.
91. Bond GR, Hite LK. Population-based incidence and outcome of acetaminophen poisoning by type of ingestion. *Acad Emerg Med* 1999;6(11)1115–1120.
92. Daly FFS, Dart RC, Bogdan GM, et al. Repeated supratherapeutic dosing of acetaminophen (APAP): can serum transaminase levels predict the risk of hepatoxicity?(abst 189). *J Toxicol Clin Toxicol* 2000;38(5):580.
93. Kozer E, Barr J, Bulkowstein M, et al. A prospective study of multiple supratherapeutic acetaminophen doses in febrile children. *Vet Hum Toxicol* 2002;44(2):106–109.
94. Henretig FM, Selbst SM, Forrest C, et al. Repeated acetaminophen overdosing causing hepatotoxicity in children. *Clin Pediatr* 1989;28:525–528.
95. Perneger TV, Whelton PK, Klag MJ. Risk of kidney failure associated with the use of acetaminophen, aspirin, and nonsteroidal antiinflammatory drugs. *N Engl J Med* 1994;331(25):1675–1679.
96. Rexrode KM, Buring JE, Glynn RJ, et al. Analgesic use and renal function in men. *JAMA* 2001;286(3):315–321.
97. Dargan PI, Jones AL. Should a lower treatment line be used when treating paracetamol poisoning in patients with chronic alcoholism?: a case against. *Drug Saf* 2002;25(9):625–632.
98. Bernal W, Donaldson N, Wyncoll D, Wendon J. Blood lactate as an early predictor of outcome in paracetamol-induced acute liver failure: a cohort study. *Lancet* 2002;359(9306):558–563.
99. Chung PY, Sitrin MD, Te HS. Serum phosphorus levels predict clinical outcome in fulminant hepatic failure. *Liver Transpl* 2003;9(3):248–253.
100. Gordon FD, Anastopoulos H, Khettry U, et al. Hepatitis C infection: a rare cause of fulminant hepatic failure. *Am J Gastroenterol* 1995;90(1):117–120.
101. Pinna AD, Rakela J, Demetris AJ, et al. Five cases of fulminant hepatitis due to herpes simplex virus in adults. *Dig Dis Sci* 2002;47(4):750–754.
102. Yoshiba M, Dehara K, Inoue K, et al. Contribution of hepatitis C virus to non-A, non-B fulminant hepatitis in Japan. *Hepatology* 1994;19(4):829–835.
103. Biasi F, Chiarpotto E, Lanfranco G, et al. Oxidative stress in the development of human ischemic hepatitis during circulatory shock. *Free Radic Biol Med* 1994;17(3):225–233.
104. Johnson RD, O'Connor ML, Kerr RM. Extreme serum elevations of aspartate aminotransferase. *Am J Gastroenterol* 1995;90(8):1244–1245.
105. Hickman PE, Potter JM. Mortality associated with ischaemic hepatitis. *Aust NZ J Med* 1990;20(1):32–34.
106. Feranchak AP, Tyson RW, Narkewicz MR, et al. Fulminant Epstein-Barr viral hepatitis: orthotopic liver transplantation and review of the literature. *Liver Transpl Surg* 1998;4(6):469–476.
107. Furuta S, Ozawa Y, Maejima K, et al. Anorexia nervosa with severe liver dysfunction and subsequent critical complications. *Intern Med* 1999;38(7):575–579.
108. Giercksky T, Boberg KM, Farstad IN, et al. Severe liver failure in exertional heat stroke. *Scand J Gastroenterol* 1999;34(8):824–827.
109. Mathurin P, Durand F, Ganne N, et al. Ischemic hepatitis due to obstructive sleep apnea. *Gastroenterology* 1995;109(5):1682–1684.
110. Bailey B, Amre DK, Gaudreault P. Fulminant hepatic failure secondary to acetaminophen poisoning: a systematic review and meta-analysis of prognostic criteria determining the need for liver transplantation. *Crit Care Med* 2003;31(1):299–305.
111. Bertholf RL, Johannsen LM, Bazooband A, et al. False-positive acetaminophen results in a hyperbilirubinemic patient. *Clin Chem* 2003;49(4):695–698.
112. Langford AM, Taylor KK, Pounder DJ. Drug concentration in selected skeletal muscles. *J Forensic Sci* 1998;43(1):22–27.
113. Yonemitsu K, Pounder DJ. Postmortem toxico-kinetics of co-proxamol. *Int J Legal Med* 1992;104(6):347–353.
114. McCaul TF, Fagan EA, Tovey G, et al. Fulminant hepatitis. An ultrastructural study. *J Hepatol* 1986;2(2):276–290.
115. Bond GR, Requa RK, Krenzelok EP, et al. Influence of time until emesis on the efficacy of decontamination using acetaminophen as a marker in a pediatric population. *Ann Emerg Med* 1993;22(9):1403–1407.
116. Wrenn K, Rodewald L, Dockstader L. Potential misuse of ipecac. *Ann Emerg Med* 1993;22(9):1408–1412.
117. Caravati EM. Unintentional acetaminophen ingestion in children and the potential for hepatotoxicity. *J Toxicol Clin Toxicol* 2000;38(3):291–296.
118. Prescott LF, Illingworth RN, Critchley JA, et al. Intravenous *N*-acetylcystine: the treatment of choice for paracetamol poisoning. *BMJ* 1979;2(6198):1097–1100.
119. Harrison PM, Keays R, Bray GP, et al. Improved outcome of paracetamol-induced fulminant hepatic failure by late administration of acetylcysteine. *Lancet* 1990;335(8705):1572–1573
120. Piperno E, Berssenbruegge DA. Reversal of experimental paracetamol toxicosis with *N*-acetylcysteine. *Lancet* 1976;2(7988):738–739.
121. Woo OF, Mueller PD, Olson KR, et al. Shorter duration of oral *N*-acetylcysteine therapy for acute acetaminophen overdose. *Ann Emerg Med* 2000;35(4):363–368.
122. Burkhart KK, Janco N, Kulig KW, et al. Cimetidine as adjunctive treatment for acetaminophen overdose. *Hum Exp Toxicol* 1995;14(3):299–304.

CHAPTER 127A

Salicylates

Luke Yip

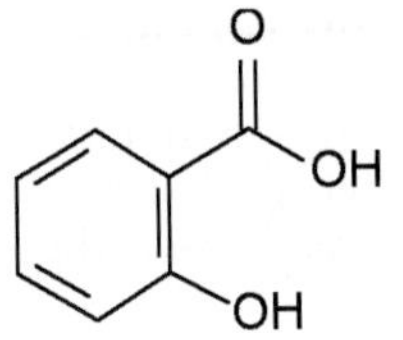

ASPIRIN

Compounds included:	**Acetylsalicylic acid, salsalate (Atisuril, Disalcid), choline salicylate (Audax, Trilisate), magnesium salicylate (Doan's Original), sodium salicylate (Pabalate)**
Molecular formula and weight:	**See Table 1.**
SI conversion:	**mg/L × 0.0072 = mmol/L**
CAS Registry No.:	**See Table 1.**
Therapeutic levels:	**15 to 30 mg/dl (serum)**
Target organs:	**Kidney, stomach, central nervous system, coagulation system**
Antidote:	**None**

OVERVIEW

Acetylsalicylic acid (aspirin) is one of the most widely used over-the-counter medications. Its analgesic and antipyretic effects have been used for more than a century. Aspirin has gained significant clinical prominence in the management of cardiovascular and cerebrovascular diseases. Salicylate-containing products have been used to treat dermatologic diseases and gastrointestinal (GI) maladies. Salicylate has also been used to provide long-term treatment of chronic inflammatory diseases.

Acute salicylate poisoning (salicylism) is one of the most common causes of poisoning death in the United States, after carbon monoxide and acetaminophen. Toxic effects after exposure are often mild to moderate. However, aspirin toxicity may be a life-threatening condition that produces multiple system organ failure requiring management in the intensive care unit. Mortality from salicylism usually occurs in patients who are inadequately treated or in whom the diagnosis is missed, usually in geriatric patients with an underlying medical illness and in the setting of chronic salicylism.

Classification and Uses

Salicylate is available in a variety of forms for oral and topical use (Table 1). Numerous brands contain aspirin alone or combination products, including narcotics, decongestants, barbiturates, caffeine, and ergotamine. Liniments and vaporizers may contain high concentrations of methyl salicylate as additives. Oil of Wintergreen is a liquid formulation containing 100% methyl salicylate. It is quickly absorbed in the GI tract, resulting in rapid onset of clinical salicylism.

TABLE 1. Physical characteristics and dosage of salicylates

Generic name; trade name	Molecular formula; molecular weight (g/mol); CAS Registry No.	Formulation	Dosage: Adult	Dosage: Pediatric
Acetylsalicylic acid (aspirin)	$C_9H_8O_4$; 180.2; 50-78-2	Multiple tablet, elixir, topical	325–650 mg every 4 h, up to 3.9 g/d	10–15 mg/kg every 4 h, up to 80 mg/kg/d
Salicylic acid	$C_7H_6O_3$; 138.12; 69-72-7	White crystalline powder	NR	NR
Salicylsalicylic acid (salsalate)	$C_{14}H_{10}O_5$; 258.2; 552-94-3	500-, 750-mg capsules and tablets	3 g/d in divided doses	10–20 mg/kg/dose every 6 hr
Choline salicylate	$C_{12}H_{19}NO_4$; 241.3; 2016-36-6	500-mg tablet	Pain or fever: 435–870 mg every 4 h Rheumatic disorders: 4.8–7.2 g/d in divided doses	50 mg/kg/d orally in divided doses
Magnesium salicylate	$C_{14}H_{10}MgO_6$,$4H_2O$; 370.6; 18917-95-8	325-, 500-, 545-, 580-mg caplets or tablets	Expressed in terms of anhydrous magnesium salicylate: Pain or fever: 300–600 mg every 4h, up to 3.5 g Arthritic disorders: 0.545–1.20 g, 3 or 4 times daily	Not approved for pediatric use
Sodium salicylate	$C_7H_5NaO_3$; 160.1; 54-21-7	1 g/ml injection; 5 grains, 10 grains, 324-mg tablets	Pain or fever: 325–650 mg every 4 h Rheumatic disorders: 3.6–5.4 g/d in divided doses	NR

NR, not recommended.

Clinical uses of aspirin include treatment of acute myocardial infarction, coronary syndromes, cerebrovascular disease, and pulmonary embolism, rheumatoid arthritis, systemic lupus erythematosus, ankylosing spondylitis, inflammatory bowel disease, fever, peptic ulcer disease due to *Helicobacter pylori*, diarrhea, indigestion, topical warts, and psoriasis.

Toxic Dose

The *adult therapeutic dosage* for analgesic, antipyretic, and antiinflammatory indications is 650 mg every 4 hours, or 1 g every 6 hours, a total of 4 g/day in divided doses. In some clinical situations (e.g., rheumatoid arthritis), larger doses of salicylate may be indicated in consultation with a physician.

The *pediatric therapeutic dose* is 10 to 15 mg/kg every 4 hours, not to exceed 80 mg/kg/day. However, some clinicians recommend up to 100 mg/kg/day for the initial treatment of Kawasaki's disease.

The *toxic dose* is typically described as ingestion of more than 150 mg/kg. Chronic ingestion of more than 100 mg/kg/day may cause toxicity. One teaspoon (5 ml) of Oil of Wintergreen contains 5 g of salicylate and is a potentially lethal dose in a child weighing less than 10 kg.

TOXICOKINETICS AND TOXICODYNAMICS

Absorption and Distribution

Absorption of aspirin from the GI tract is dependent on the amount and the formulation of the drug. Absorption of a liquid such as methyl salicylate begins within minutes, whereas enteric-coated tablets may require hours. Significant systemic absorption resulting in serious toxicity has been reported with use of topical salicylate preparations as a keratolytic on preexisting skin disease (1–6). An overdose of aspirin may be absorbed much slower than therapeutic doses, possibly due to the inhibitory effect of aspirin on gastric emptying (7) and perhaps because of the impaired dissolution of the drug in gastric fluids at high concentrations. Some preparations may coalesce and form a gelatinous, thus providing a source for continued absorption from the GI tract.

After absorption, acetylsalicylic acid is hydrolyzed to salicylic acid. The therapeutic and toxic effects of aspirin are produced by salicylic acid. The parent compound (aspirin) is responsible for the antiplatelet effect. Acetylsalicylate and salicylate are weak acids with a pK_a of 3.5 and 3.0, respectively. At a physiologic of pH 7.4, both compounds are predominately in the ionized form. The volume of distribution of salicylate is between 0.1 to 0.2 L/kg. Salicylate is primarily bound to albumin (50% to 80%). It is expected that salicylates' volume of distribution will be increased in protein deficient states or systemic acidosis.

Elimination

Metabolism and elimination of salicylate are by hepatic and renal routes. At therapeutic levels, the main pathways for hepatic salicylate metabolism are conjugation and hydroxylation, which exhibit zero order kinetics. The kidneys excrete salicylate metabolites and eliminate salicylate directly by both glomerular filtration and tubular excretion, which exhibit first-order kinetics.

Urinary elimination of salicylate is greatly influenced by the urinary pH and, to a lesser extent, by urinary flow rates (8–10). As salicylate is excreted by glomerular filtration and renal tubular secretion, nonionized molecules are reabsorbed. If the normally acidic urine is alkalinized to pH 8.0, significantly more of the salicylate molecules become ionized in the urine and thus enhance elimination (8).

As the serum salicylate concentration increases, hepatic enzymatic metabolism of salicylate is quickly saturated, and the kidneys become the major route for salicylate elimination. After an acetylsalicylic acid overdose, salicylate is excreted as salicyluric acid. It appears to be produced together with an increase in elimination as gentisic acid and salicylic acid phenolic glucuronide. This indicates progressive saturation of salicyluric acid formation and suggests the *in vivo* glycine pool may be important in salicylate elimination after an overdose (11). Renal dysfunction significantly compromises the body's ability to eliminate a salicylate burden.

PATHOPHYSIOLOGY

The toxic effects of salicylate are complex and multifactorial. Acute ingestion of large quantities of salicylate may produce nausea and vomiting as a result of local gastric irritation and stimulation of the chemoreceptor trigger zones (12). Vomiting may be severe enough to result in dehydration, adversely affecting renal salicylate elimination, and contributing to acid-base and electrolyte disturbances.

Central Nervous System Effects

Salicylate has a direct stimulatory effect on the central nervous system (CNS) medullary respiratory center (13,14) that parallels cerebrospinal fluid salicylate concentrations (15). Salicylate also affects skeletal muscles (13) by preferentially inhibiting the phosphorylation process of oxidative phosphorylation at the cellular level (16). Uncoupling of oxidative phosphorylation adversely affects cellular respiration, which includes decreased adenosine triphosphate production as a result of energy derived from the oxidative process being dissipated as heat rather than stored as adenosine triphosphate, progressive increases in carbohydrate use, oxygen consumption, and carbon dioxide production.

In an animal model of salicylate toxicity, salicylate concentration in the brain is correlated directly with mortality (17,18). At physiologic pH, almost all salicylate molecules are ionized. If the systemic pH decreases, the equilibrium shifts to favor the nonionized form of salicylate. This shift is critical because nonionized molecules readily cross cellular membranes such as the blood–brain barrier (Fig. 1). Thus, for a given serum salicylate level, brain salicylate concentration is substantially higher in the presence of acidemia than alkalemia (18–21).

Acid-Base Effects and Glucose

Both CNS respiratory stimulation and increased peripheral carbon dioxide production contribute to the respiratory alkalosis, with the former being the dominant component (13). The renal response to hypercarbia is to increase bicarbonate and potassium excretion. The urinary bicarbonate loss eventually decreases the body's bicarbonate stores and impairs its ability to buffer the metabolic acidosis of salicylate toxicity. If ventilatory compensation fails to keep pace with increased carbon dioxide production, respiratory acidosis may develop, and it compounds the metabolic acidosis.

When oxidative phosphorylation is uncoupled in salicylate toxicity, cellular respiration becomes dependent on the glycolytic pathway for adenosine triphosphate production. Because

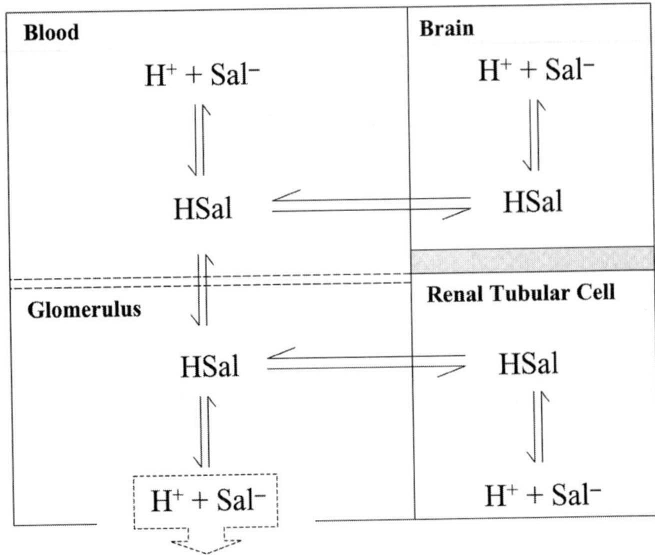

Figure 1. Effect of pH on salicylate anion distribution and elimination. Both salicylates' toxic effects and elimination can be altered by manipulating pH. Increasing blood pH increases the ionized (Sal^-) form and reduces distribution into the brain. Increasing urine pH increases Sa^- in the urine and enhances urinary excretion. H^+, hydrogen cation; Sal^-, salicylate anion; HSal, salicylate.

glycolysis is an inefficient process, much more glucose is required to produce an equivalent amount of energy as oxidative phosphorylation. This requirement depletes glycogen stores, stimulates gluconeogenesis, and causes catabolism of fats and proteins. Salicylate also inhibits fatty acid oxidation (16) and aminotransferases (22,23), which prevents alanine, the major substrate, from entering the gluconeogenesis pathway. In addition, salicylate inhibits the Krebs cycle enzymes, α-ketoglutarate dehydrogenase, and succinate dehydrogenase (24,25). The combined effects of accelerated catabolic process and disruption of metabolic pathways lead to accumulation of various metabolic intermediates, such as lactate, pyruvate, keto acids, and other organic acids, which contribute to the metabolic acidosis of salicylate toxicity (26). The acid-base disturbances associated with salicylate toxicity are respiratory alkalosis and metabolic acidosis caused by accelerated metabolism, disruption of the Krebs cycle metabolism, and the salicylate ion itself.

Salicylate affects central and peripheral glucose homeostasis. Animal studies show that a toxic dose of salicylate produces a profound decrease in brain glucose concentrations in spite of euglycemia (27,28). This suggests that the supply of glucose to the brain in salicylate intoxication may be inadequate even though the serum glucose concentration is normal.

Pulmonary Injury

Noncardiogenic pulmonary edema is well recognized as one of the manifestations of salicylate toxicity (29–39). The mechanism of salicylate-induced pulmonary edema has been investigated both *in vitro* and *in vivo* (34,40,41). Salicylate causes increased permeability of the pulmonary vasculature to fluid and protein. Pulmonary lymph flow and protein clearance increase but the pulmonary vascular pressures and cardiac performance are unaffected. Patients with severe salicylate intoxication have low pulmonary capillary wedge pressures and low cardiac filling pressures, and their bronchial transudates exhibit the same protein and electrolyte profile as serum. Other studies also support a noncardiogenic origin (30–33,35,38).

Renal Effects

The salicylate vascular injury may extend to the kidneys. Proteinuria is a prominent early finding in salicylate toxicity, starting at serum salicylate concentrations more than 30 mg/dl, and it is directly related to the salicylate concentration (34).

The kidneys become the major route for salicylate elimination as plasma salicylate concentrations reach toxic levels. The kidneys eliminate salicylate by both glomerular filtration and tubular secretion but also reabsorb salicylate in the renal tubule. Salicylate reabsorption is influenced by urinary pH and urinary flow rate. Only nonionized molecules are reabsorbed. Because salicylate is a weak acid with a pK_a of 3.5, the nonionized fraction increases as pH decreases. Under normal conditions, the urine is acidic and reabsorption is favored. Urinary alkalinization increases the amount of ionized salicylate and decreases the proportion that is reabsorbed by the renal tubule (Fig. 1) (8). Diuresis reduces salicylate reabsorption by diluting the urine salicylate concentration and by reducing the concentration gradient between urine and renal tubule cells.

Coagulation System

Although salicylates are known for their antiplatelet activity, hemorrhage is an unusual complication of chronic salicylate intoxication and is an even more rare complication of acute overdose. Metabolic studies in animals showed that salicylate produced a significant decrease in factor II, VII, and X activity; an increase in vitamin K-epoxide to vitamin K ratio (42); and did not influence vitamin K epoxide reductase activity, vitamin K–dependent carboxylase, or vitamin K epoxidase activity (43). This suggests salicylate-associated hypoprothrombinemia may be due to interruption of the vitamin K–epoxide cycle and the main effect may be vitamin K quinone reductase inhibition. Chronic administration of salicylate in large doses causes significant hypoprothrombinemia, less than 40% of normal, when the serum salicylate concentration exceeds 60 mg/dl (44).

PREGNANCY AND LACTATION

All of the salicylates are U.S. Food and Drug Administration pregnancy category C (Appendix I). Salicylate readily crosses the placenta, and the fetal to maternal salicylate ratio is 1.5 at delivery (45). Therapeutic doses of aspirin during the first trimester of pregnancy and during breast-feeding are safe; however, maternal use of aspirin within 1 week of delivery is associated with increased incidence of intracranial hemorrhage and premature closure of the ductus arteriosus in premature infants.

Transplacental salicylate poisoning from repeated maternal aspirin ingestion during late pregnancy has resulted in abnormal hemostasis (46,47), tachypnea, respiratory distress, hypotonia, metabolic acidosis, and hypoglycemia in the neonate (48,49), which may be misdiagnosed as neonatal sepsis. *In utero* fetal death has been reported of a woman with repeated aspirin overdose for 1 month (50). The use of salicylates during the first trimester of pregnancy was associated with an increased risk of gastroschisis in two epidemiologic studies (50a,50b).

Salicylate is excreted into breast milk. Adverse effects are rare, but a breast-fed infant of a mother taking daily therapeutic aspirin doses became salicylate toxic (51).

CLINICAL PRESENTATION

Acute Overdosage

Pediatric salicylate intoxication is characterized by a known history of ingestion and onset of symptoms within a few hours of ingestion (52). These patients usually present soon after the ingestion and develop mild effects, and intoxication is well tolerated (53). The typical acid-base disturbance in children 4 years or older and adults presenting to the hospital is a mixed picture of respiratory alkalosis, increased anion gap metabolic acidosis, and alkalemia (pH more than 7.42). When the duration of the intoxication was 12 to 24 hours, metabolic acidosis and acidemia (pH less than 7.38) occur primarily in children younger than 4 years, and nearly all children younger than 1 year present with acidosis (54,55). The presence of neurologic abnormalities in any age group, and in particular CNS depression, is indicative of severe intoxication.

Acute maternal salicylism during the last trimester may result in salicylate toxicity in the neonate (56) or fetal death *in utero* (57–59).

Adult salicylate intoxication is usually due to an intentional overdose by a young adult, and often the patient has a previous psychiatric or drug overdose history (29). The history is usually apparent, and typical clinical presentation includes nausea, vomiting, abdominal discomfort, tinnitus, diaphoresis, and hyperventilation, which are reported to occur when the serum salicylate concentration exceeds 30 mg/dl (60,61).

Salicylate-induced ototoxicity is characterized by a completely reversible sensorineural hearing loss, which is not idiosyncratic but rather is related to serum salicylate concentration (62). As the serum salicylate concentration exceeds 40 mg/dl, hearing loss reaches its maximum of 40 decibels (62). In volunteers with a normal baseline audiogram, the lowest salicylate concentration associated with tinnitus was 19.6 mg/dl (60). There is a linear relationship between hearing loss and unbound salicylate concentration (63).

The *acid-base* picture is usually one of mixed respiratory alkalosis and metabolic acidosis (64–66). Gabow et al. (65) reported the acid-base disturbances of adults with salicylate intoxication: 22% presented with respiratory alkalosis, 56% had respiratory alkalosis and metabolic acidosis, 20% had metabolic acidosis, and 2% had respiratory and metabolic acidosis. One-third of these patients had also ingested CNS depressant drugs, which impaired the hyperpneic response associated with salicylate intoxication and thereby altered the presenting acid-base profile. Patients ingesting a CNS depressant drug had a higher incidence of respiratory acidosis and a lower incidence of respiratory alkalosis (65).

Co-ingestion of CNS depressants should be suspected in salicylate-intoxicated adults presenting with a normal anion gap metabolic acidosis or with a respiratory acidosis. Likewise, a normal anion gap acidosis does not rule out salicylate toxicity in a patient with an unknown ingestion. To avoid missing the diagnosis of acute salicylism, it is prudent to obtain a serum salicylate concentration with the initial laboratory assessment of the patient presenting with metabolic acidosis or altered sensorium.

Uncommon features of acute adult salicylate toxicity include tetany (67), rhabdomyolysis (68–70), fever, neurologic dysfunction, renal failure, adult respiratory distress syndrome, and hypoglycemia (61). However, each of these uncommon manifestations indicates a more severe poisoning, with greater potential for morbidity and mortality. The mortality of acute salicylate toxicity has been reported to be 1% to 2% (29,61). Hyperpyrexia appears to be an adverse prognostic indicator, and death is usually preceded by a predominant metabolic acidosis disturbance and neurologic deficits (29,61,64–66). The profile of patients who die from acute salicylate toxicity includes unconscious on presentation, fever, severe acidosis, seizures, cardiac dysrhythmias, and the elderly (66).

Chronic Salicylism

Chronic pediatric salicylate toxicity, also described as *therapeutic* (repeated dose) toxicity, has a higher incidence of morbidity than acute salicylism (52,53,71). *Chronic salicylism* has been defined as ingesting more than 100 mg/kg/day for at least 2 days, or excessive repetitive administration of salicylate for more than 12 hours (53,72,73). Pediatric patients younger than 2 years of age are most often involved (74). Often, several days elapse between initial administration of salicylate and onset of symptoms (52,71). These children often have a coincidental illness that prompted salicylate administration, and they are usually more ill appearing than patients with acute intoxication (52,53). Hyperventilation, dehydration, acidosis, severe hypokalemia, and CNS disturbances are often present (52,53). Young children tend to develop hyperpyrexia, which is associated with a poor prognosis (71,75). Renal failure may be a significant complication in severe salicylate intoxication. Pulmonary edema is an unusual complication (71). In one series, all patients with chronic salicylism on admission were erroneously diagnosed as having an infection because of hyperpnea, fever, and leukocytosis (52). The delay in diagnosis may account for the more severe clinical course seen with chronic salicylism.

Severe cerebral edema has rarely been associated with chronic salicylism (76–78). In these cases, the patients were being treated with salicylate for juvenile rheumatoid arthritis, and Reye's syndrome was not part of the clinical picture.

Chronic adult salicylate toxicity (repeated ingestion of supratherapeutic dose) is characteristically seen in geriatric patients with underlying medical problems they have been treating with salicylates accidentally or in a misguided attempt to relieve their symptoms (29). Signs of intoxication include hyperventilation, tremor, asterixis, papilledema, agitation, paranoia, bizarre behavior, memory deficits, confusion, and stupor (79). Neurologic disturbances, such as agitation, confusion, hyperactivity, slurred speech, hallucinations, seizures, and coma, are more common after chronic ingestion, and may mislead physicians (29). In one report, 60% of patients underwent intensive neurologic evaluation before chronic salicylate intoxication was diagnosed, delaying the diagnosis for 6 to 72 hours after admission to the hospital (29). Chronic salicylate intoxication has been erroneously diagnosed as numerous conditions (Table 2).

Restlessness and mental aberrations, known as *salicylate jag* caused by chronic salicylism, are quite similar to alcohol intoxication (80). Chronic salicylate intoxication is frequently overlooked as a cause of noncardiogenic pulmonary edema and altered mental status (39). Sinus and atrioventricular nodal conduction disturbances and atrial dysrhythmias have been associated with chronic salicylism (81). Chronic salicylate intoxication

TABLE 2. Misdiagnosis of chronic adult salicylism

Systemic inflammatory response syndrome (165)	Organic psychosis (168)
Acute abdomen (166)	Sepsis (169,170)
Impending myocardial infarction (80)	Dementia or delirium (171,172)
Encephalopathy (29)	Diabetic ketoacidosis (80)
Alcohol withdrawal (29)	Hyperglycemia (80)
Asterixis (167)	Viral encephalitis (80)

has been reported to cause rhabdomyolysis in a patient with scleroderma and Sjögren's syndrome (82).

Adults with chronic salicylate toxicity are more likely to have complications, including pulmonary edema, seizures, and renal failure, as well as higher mortality (29). In one series, the mortality rate was 25%, which was attributed to the delay or failure to diagnose salicylate intoxication leading to delay in treatment (29). One should have a high index of suspicion for chronic salicylate intoxication in any patient with tachypnea or dyspnea, acid-base disturbances, and nonfocal neurologic or behavioral abnormalities. A serum salicylate level may be useful to assist clinicians in making the diagnosis of salicylism; however, the serum salicylate concentration, although elevated, does not appear to correlate with the severity of the intoxication. A patient with chronic salicylism may have a *therapeutic* serum salicylate concentration, whereas a level of 30 to 40 mg/dl may be lethal.

The distinction between acute and chronic salicylate intoxication may not always be clear. A patient may present many hours after an acute severe salicylate overdose, when altered mental status, acidosis, elevated prothrombin time, and serious toxicity with a *therapeutic* serum salicylate concentration are signs consistent with a chronically poisoned patient. The important aspect to remember is that significant toxicity may be evident in spite of declining or *therapeutic* serum salicylate concentrations. In these cases, the patient's clinical status is the most important parameter to assess severity of intoxication.

Adverse Events

The adverse drug events from therapeutic use of salicylate include GI discomfort, hepatitis, tinnitus, transient hearing loss, and bronchospasm. Most cases of salicylate hepatitis have occurred in children or young adults with collagen vascular diseases. Salicylate hepatitis is often asymptomatic, and 50% of patients taking salicylate in full antiinflammatory doses develop mild to moderate increase in liver aminotransferase levels with patchy necrosis and degeneration of hepatocytes (83). These changes are associated with serum salicylate concentration and are usually rapidly reversible. In a small minority of patients, particularly the young, liver damage is more severe and may be associated with liver failure, acidosis, hypoglycemia, disseminated intravascular coagulation, encephalopathy, and a fatal outcome. Many patients with Reye's syndrome have been given aspirin during the prodromal phase, and this serious condition closely resembles subacute salicylate intoxication in children.

There have also been isolated reports of chronic active hepatitis associated with the use of salicylates. However, hepatic injury is not recognized as a complication of acute aspirin poisoning.

Stevens-Johnson syndrome has been associated with therapeutic use of salicylates; however, a large international case control study indicated that the risk of this syndrome is not increased in patients that have used a salicylate-containing product in the previous week (84).

Reye's syndrome is a rare disease, and it has been associated with therapeutic use of salicylate in children 4 to 12 years old who have received aspirin in the course of a viral illness. Reye's syndrome is characterized by nausea, vomiting, fulminant hepatic failure, headache, increased intracranial pressure, stupor, coma, and death. Reye's syndrome has also been reported in adults.

The adverse drug events from chronic salicylate use include peptic ulcer disease and impaired renal function.

Drug Interactions

Patients taking aspirin may develop salicylism after dosing with acetazolamide (84a,85–87). This is a particularly important drug-drug interaction in the geriatric population who may be taking aspirin for arthritis and acetazolamide for glaucoma. Acetazolamide is a carbonic anhydrase inhibitor that sometimes produces a metabolic acidosis and facilitates the entry of salicylate into the CNS, causing toxicity at a *therapeutic* serum salicylate concentration.

DIAGNOSTIC TESTS

Acute Overdosage

Clinical chemistry tests that should be obtained in the setting of an acute intentional salicylate overdose include a serum salicylate level, electrolytes, glucose, blood urea nitrogen, and creatinine. A single serum salicylate concentration should be obtained to screen for chronic salicylism. It should be interpreted in the context of the clinical picture. A serum salicylate level should then be obtained every 1 to 2 hours until a documented decline in the patient's serial serum salicylate concentration occurs and the patient's clinical condition is improving.

Diflunisal significantly interferes with laboratory salicylate determination by Trinder, Abbott TDX, Du Pont aca, FPIA-TDx, and UV-VIS aca methods (88–93). False-positive results for serious salicylate toxicity have been reported in patients taking diflunisal.

Other tests such as a complete blood count, liver function tests, international normalized ratio, arterial blood gas, electrocardiogram, chest and abdominal radiographs, computerized tomography of the head, and lumbar puncture should be obtained, as clinically indicated.

Three *bedside salicylate screening tests* have been advocated. The ferric chloride test, Ames Phenistix tests, and Trinder reagent are qualitative tests. All positive urine results should be confirmed with serum salicylate level. There are severe limitations associated with bedside detection techniques for salicylic acid, and the author does not advocate their use in the clinical setting.

The *ferric chloride test* has been used to screen for the presence of salicylate, which uses several drops of 10% ferric chloride added to 1 ml of urine (94). A purple color develops in the presence of salicylic acid, acetoacetic acid, or phenylpyruvic acid. This test is sensitive to small quantities of salicylic acid, and a positive test result does not indicate salicylate poisoning or toxicity. False-negative results have not been reported. The qualitative ferric chloride test is not specific for salicylates and false-positive results may occur when a small quantity of urine that has been used for dipstick analysis with the N-multistix or Bili Labstix is then used for ferric chloride testing. Presumably, some impregnated chemical from the dipstick dissolves in the urine and causes a false-positive reaction.

The *Ames Phenistix* can also be used as a bedside screening test. The dipstick turns brown when either salicylic acid or phenothiazines are present in the urine or serum. Adding one drop of 20 *N* sulfuric acid to the strip bleaches out the color in the case of phenothiazines but not in the case of salicylic acid. The color change is often difficult to interpret.

The *Trinder spot test* appears to be a sensitive, but not specific bedside salicylate screening tool (95,96). The Trinder reagent can be made by combining mercuric chloride 40 g and ferric nitrate 40 g in 850 ml of type II deionized water. Concentrated hydrochloric acid (10 ml) is added to the solution. The solution is diluted to a volume of 1 L with type II deionized water. The test is performed by mixing 1 ml each of urine and Trinder reagent in a test tube. A color change in the solution is considered positive. The Trinder's colorimetric method has been reported to give false-positive serum salicylate concentrations (2.8 to 14.3

mg/dl) in premature neonates, neonates with hyperbilirubinemia, and seriously ill children (e.g., extensive burns) (97).

Chronic Salicylism

The diagnostic tests for chronic toxicity are the same as for acute toxicity, but their interpretation differs. In chronic salicylism, serious effects develop at serum salicylate concentrations lower than for acute ingestion. In the elderly, toxicity may occur at a *therapeutic* serum concentration, and seizures and death have occurred at a serum salicylate concentration of 35 mg/dl.

Diagnostic Pitfalls

The Done nomogram was created to assist in clarifying the level of salicylate intoxication that should prompt intervention, "... this (nomogram) provides only a rough guide to a single criterion of severity in previously well patients . . . it obviously does not supplant clinical judgment" (98). The nomogram was developed based on data from serial measurements of serum salicylate concentrations in six children and one adult with salicylate intoxication. The disappearance of salicylate from the serum approximated first-order kinetics with a constant fraction eliminated over time. Additional data from 13 children and four adults showed a mean salicylate half-life of 20 hours (range 15 to 29 hours). These data permitted the calculation of a theoretical time zero salicylate concentration. Done empirically defined four severity categories of salicylate intoxication based on the clinical presentation (29 children and 9 adults) and correlated the observed clinical presentation with the extrapolated salicylate concentration at time zero (98). It was found that if the initial extrapolated serum salicylate concentration was less than 50 mg/dl, the patient was not intoxicated. An initial extrapolated serum salicylate concentration of 50 to 80 mg/dl correlated with mild toxicity, 80 to 100 mg/dl indicated moderate toxicity, more than 100 mg/dl indicated severe toxicity, and more than 160 mg/dl was usually fatal.

The Done nomogram is not useful in clinical practice for several reasons. It has not been subjected to rigorous study as a diagnostic or screening tool. In practice, it frequently over- and underestimates the severity of intoxication. The nomogram is *not* useful when salicylate has been ingested over several hours or days, the preparation is an enteric-coated or a sustained-release formulation, the compound is Oil of Wintergreen, the patient has renal insufficiency, the time of ingestion is unknown or uncertain, or the patient is acidemic. It should be emphasized that the clinical picture combined with serial serum salicylate concentrations determines the patient's degree of toxicity.

Other pitfalls include the failure to anticipate worsening intoxication, which is generally due to reliance on a single serum salicylate concentration on admission, without regard to the formulation or the time of ingestion. Patients with an initial unimpressive serum salicylate level should have repeated levels to ensure that salicylate is not continuing to be absorbed. In most patients, serum salicylate levels should be obtained every 1 to 2 hours until there is serial decline in the salicylate levels and the patient's clinical condition is improving. Acidemia alters estimation of the severity of the intoxication. When the patient's serum salicylate concentration is discordant with the clinical picture, remember that salicylism requiring treatment may occur with a low serum concentration if confounding factors exist (e.g., other medications may be contributing to the clinical picture).

Anion gap metabolic acidosis and acidemia develop over time in a patient with a serious salicylate overdose. However, reliance on the development of an anion gap metabolic acidosis or acidemia as *screening tests* rather than obtaining serum salicylate concentrations may significantly delay the diagnosis and treatment of seriously salicylate poisoned patients.

The absorption of enteric-coated or sustained-release preparations may be delayed and unpredictable. These preparations are formulated to dissolve in the alkaline intestinal fluids (99,100), and minimal absorption occurs in the stomach. Peak serum salicylate concentrations may not occur until 10 to 60 hours after an overdose of an enteric-coated preparation (99–102). Some formulations of enteric-coated and sustained-release tablets are large size and cannot be removed from the stomach through a 40 French gastric lavage tube (100). This situation creates the possibility of a clear fluid return with a substantial salicylate load still in the stomach. Plain abdominal radiographs have been advocated to detect enteric-coated or sustained-release medications in the GI tract. However, the degree of radiopacity of a medication is dependent on the characteristics of the matrix used by the manufacturer (103–105). A positive radiograph can confirm the diagnosis, but a negative radiograph does not rule out the presence of enteric-coated or sustained-release medications in the GI tract.

TREATMENT

The main goals of therapy are maintenance of airway, breathing, and circulation; supportive care to correct dehydration and electrolyte and acid-base derangements induced by salicylate; and reduction of the body's salicylate burden. The treatment of salicylate poisoning is a complex, diverse, and dynamic process that requires close monitoring and prompt intervention. Anecdotally, delay in diagnosis or management can be fatal.

Decontamination

Skin decontamination involves simply wiping the salicylate product from the skin and thoroughly washing with soap and water.

GI decontamination in the prehospital setting may involve emesis with syrup of ipecac or administration of activated charcoal, if the patient is treated soon after ingestion. Gastric lavage may be appropriate in patients that have ingested a large dose within the previous 1 to 2 hours, in patients in whom delayed absorption is suspected, or in seriously ill patients.

Activated charcoal adsorbs aspirin effectively (106,107). The efficacy of activated charcoal increases with dose. An activated charcoal to aspirin ratio of 10:1 is often recommended (107). An initial dose of activated charcoal (1 to 2 g/kg) is recommended in all acute salicylate overdoses and also in patients with an acute overdose chronically taking salicylate.

Absorption of aspirin onto activated charcoal is a reversible process (107). One study on the desorption phenomena showed that 15% to 20% of absorbed salicylate is desorbed, with a time course that may extend beyond 24 hours (106). It has been speculated that improved GI decontamination could be achieved by multiple doses of activated charcoal to maintain an activated charcoal to aspirin ratio of at least 10:1. A human volunteer study indicates that three doses of activated charcoal significantly decreased urinary salicylate excretion compared with one or two doses of activated charcoal (108). The suggested repeat doses of activated charcoal are 0.25 to 0.5 g/kg every 4 to 6 hours depending on the dose and dosage form of the drug ingested. Larger doses and shorter dosing intervals may occasionally be indicated.

Whole bowel irrigation was more effective in reducing absorption of enteric-coated aspirin in volunteers than single-dose activated charcoal with sorbitol (109). Data are insufficient to determine its usefulness in clinical practice.

Enhancement of Elimination

Multiple dose activated charcoal may be beneficial (110–112). Although there are data to confirm enhanced salicylate elimination, there are no controlled studies to demonstrate clinical benefit from using multiple doses of activated charcoal (113).

Hemodialysis is typically considered the extracorporeal technique of choice because it can rapidly normalize acid-base and electrolyte abnormalities and effectively decrease the body's salicylate burden without producing the thrombocytopenia and leukopenia that frequently accompany charcoal hemoperfusion (114,115). Hemodialysis is advocated for situations that include serum salicylate concentrations more than 90 mg/dl, renal insufficiency or failure, respiratory acidosis, persistent hypotension, pulmonary edema, altered mental status, and seizure.

Although the literature discusses the use of extracorporeal methods in the management of salicylate toxicity, there is no rigorous scientific evidence on which to base recommendations concerning use of extracorporeal methods. Despite the paucity of information, there is general agreement on certain clinical indications for the use of extracorporeal detoxification. These include clinical deterioration despite supportive care (including urinary alkalinization), altered mental status, pulmonary edema, persistent acidemia, coagulopathy, renal/hepatic dysfunction, and extremes of age.

A single serum salicylate level may be helpful but should not be the sole determinant in the decision to use extracorporeal methods. A salicylate concentration of 90 mg/dl after an acute ingestion in a healthy patient may not require hemodialysis, whereas a patient with a level of 35 mg/dl in a chronic ingestion may be moribund. The literature regarding serum salicylate concentrations to guide the use of extracorporeal techniques varies widely, ranging from 40 to 200 mg/dl in acute overdose (18,72,98,116–128) and 60 to 80 mg/dl in chronic ingestion (117,122). One should err on the side of early use of hemodialysis in elderly patients, patients with chronic salicylate toxicity, patients with altered mental status or persistent acidemia, or patients with other severe underlying disease. Consultation with a nephrologist for dialysis is appropriate in patients in whom the serum salicylate concentration is increasing or if there is evidence of end-organ involvement. Anticipating the possible need for dialysis and thoughtful planning is prudent.

There is little information concerning the appropriate end point for extracorporeal procedures. Reasonable criteria for terminating hemodialysis are progressive clinical improvement, a documented serial decline in the serum salicylate concentration toward the therapeutic range, and correction of acid-base disturbances.

Hemoperfusion effectively decreases the body's salicylate burden (114), but is rarely used due to its associated complications (129) and a lack of experience with the procedure. *Continuous veno-venous hemodiafiltration* effectively decreases the body salicylate burden and has been used with success in patients with acute as well as chronic salicylism (82,130). *Peritoneal dialysis* effectively enhances salicylate elimination and may be considered in neonates or infants whose small size precludes the use of hemodialysis (125,131,132).

Double volume exchange transfusion (180 ml/kg packed red blood cells reconstituted in fresh frozen plasma) may be a safe and an effective alternative to hemodialysis in severe infant salicylism whose small size precluded the use of hemodialysis (124,133–135).

Antidotes

Sodium bicarbonate acts to reduce entry of salicylate into tissues and to enhance renal salicylate elimination. A clinical study comparing forced diuresis, forced alkaline diuresis, and urine alkalinization in an effort to maximize renal salicylate clearance showed that serum salicylate concentration decreased significantly in all three cases (10). However, the decrease in plasma salicylate concentrations with forced diuresis and forced alkaline diuresis was partially due to hemodilution effect from the intravenous fluids administered to produce the diuresis. Urinary salicylate clearance was directly proportional to urine flow rate but was logarithmically proportional to urine pH (Fig. 2) (9,10). Urine alkalinization alone is more effective than forced diuresis or forced alkaline diuresis. This is particularly important in the elderly patient with marginal cardiac reserve (10). Urine alkalinization avoids the potential complication of fluid overload that may result from forced diuresis. Urine alkalinization (target urine pH of 8 or higher) (8) should be empirically initiated in patients with signs and symptoms consistent with salicylate toxicity while awaiting the results of the initial serum salicylate level.

Urinary alkalinization has been achieved by many techniques (10,72,117,118,136–139). In practice, fluid resuscitation and urine alkalinization are initiated simultaneously. No single method of hydration or alkalinization has been proven to be superior. One animal study demonstrated that 2 mEq/kg sodium bicarbonate bolus followed by continuous infusion of sodium bicarbonate at 21 mEq/hour results in a consistent alkaline serum (140). To minimize the possibility of hypernatremia and optimize urine alkalinization, the author's approach is to give an initial sodium bicarbonate bolus of 2 mEq/kg, followed by a continuous infusion of D5W, to which 130 to 140 mEq of sodium bicarbonate have been added, starting at 1.5 to 2.0 times the maintenance rate. It is important to reassess the patient's status hourly, including fluid, electrolyte, and acid-base balance, neurologic status, and urine pH. The

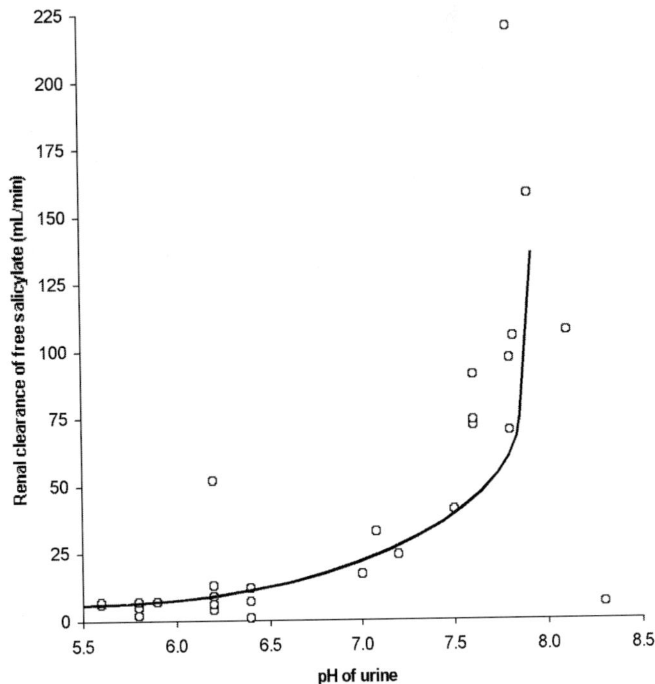

Figure 2. The effect of urinary pH on the clearance of free salicylate. (Created from data in Smith PK, Gleason HL, Stoll CG, et al. Studies on the pharmacology of salicylates. *J Pharmacol Exp Ther* 1946;87:253.)

sodium bicarbonate infusion should be increased if the urine pH is less than 7.5 and there are no contraindications to sodium bicarbonate therapy. Further information on urinary alkalinization is provided in Chapter 75.

The *discontinuation of urinary alkalinization* has not been addressed in the literature. One method is to terminate bicarbonate administration when the serum salicylate concentration falls to the therapeutic range (72). Another technique discontinues bicarbonate when the serum salicylate concentration has decreased to 35 to 40 mg/dl or symptoms have resolved (117,139). Whatever method is chosen, the patient should show progressive clinical improvement with a documented serial decline in serum salicylate concentration toward the therapeutic range and correction of fluid, acid-base, and electrolyte disturbances before discontinuing therapy.

Some patients are refractory to urinary alkalinization. It is not always possible to alkalinize the urine of pediatric patients who are severely toxic from salicylate (55). Successful sodium bicarbonate use involves patients who were not severely intoxicated or acidotic and who were treated relatively early in the course of their poisoning. Patients who were severely intoxicated routinely failed to generate alkaline urine with sodium bicarbonate therapy.

Although it is often written that urinary alkalinization is impossible until hypokalemia has been corrected (72,119,141–144), there are few clinical data supporting this conclusion. In a canine model of salicylate toxicity, profound respiratory alkalosis can be accompanied by formation of an acidic urine independent of the serum potassium concentration (145). In patients with salicylate toxicity, there does not appear to be a correlation between the serum potassium levels and the urine pH. These patients' urine remained acidic despite alkalemia and normal serum potassium concentrations (146). It is prudent to administer supplemental potassium to hypokalemic patients. However, it is inappropriate to delay sodium bicarbonate administration until normokalemia is achieved. Bicarbonate also reduces the distribution of salicylate into cells and may improve the patient's condition before alkalinizing the urine.

Hypovolemia and hypochloremia from protracted vomiting may cause difficulty in alkalinizing the urine. In a volume-depleted state, there is a decrease in glomerular filtration rate, leading to a decrease in the filtered bicarbonate load and a decrease in renal bicarbonate excretion. Fluid and electrolyte resuscitation restores the filtered bicarbonate load and facilitates bicarbonate excretion. This can be accomplished by administering intravenous normal saline solutions. Urinary alkalinization should be physiologically possible in salicylate intoxication once hypovolemia and hypochloremia have been corrected.

Adjunct Therapy

One human study of aspirin overdose suggests that oral glycine therapy increases urinary salicylate excretion (147,148), but has not yet been clinically proven.

Supportive Care

Volume depletion is a common problem of serious salicylate toxicity. Electrolyte and acid-base disturbances are also common, particularly in the later stages of intoxication. These patients require both supportive care and specific measures to enhance elimination of their salicylate burden. Fluid resuscitation should be undertaken while preparations are made for other measures.

Fluid, electrolyte, and acid-base derangements in salicylate toxicity may be similar to diabetic ketoacidosis. There are myriad recipes for the management of fluids and electrolytes in salicylate toxicity (72,75,117,137,141,149,150). In pediatric patients, fluid resuscitation similar to treatment of diabetic ketoacidosis has been recommended (149). However, a glucose-containing fluid should be used in most patients because hypoglycemia has been implicated in the pathophysiology of CNS injury from salicylate (27,28). It has been recommended that all intravenous fluids given should contain a minimum of 50 g/L (5%) glucose (149). When hypoglycemia or neurologic symptoms are evident, a minimum of 100 g/L (10%) glucose has been suggested (149). The potential benefit of administering supplemental glucose is empiric. There are no clinical data regarding the minimum glucose requirement in salicylate toxicity. A potassium deficit is usually evident. Supplemental potassium should be administered after urine output has been established.

Noncardiogenic *pulmonary edema* should be managed in the same way as adult respiratory distress syndrome from other etiologies (151). Should endotracheal intubation, mechanical ventilation, and sedation become necessary, hyperventilation should be maintained or acute deterioration may occur as a result of iatrogenic respiratory acidosis, causing a rapid shift of salicylate into the CNS (136,152). The minute volume of ventilator settings of intubated and sedated patients should be adjusted to maintain $PaCO_2$ at the patient's $PaCO_2$ before intubation.

Clinical observations indicate that pulmonary edema begins to improve concomitantly with lowering of the serum salicylate concentration (29,33). This suggests that aggressive efforts toward salicylate elimination, such as hemodialysis, might be beneficial in this subset of patients. Hemodialysis permits removal of salicylate without the volume challenge that accompanies sodium bicarbonate administration, and it avoids the possibility of aggravating pulmonary edema.

Seizures associated with salicylate toxicity should be managed as other toxic seizures with a benzodiazepine, phenobarbital, and other measures as needed to establish control (Chapter 40).

Hemorrhage is a rare complication of acute massive overdose of aspirin, despite the antiplatelet activity of acetylsalicylic acid. Chronic ingestion of salicylate in large doses causes significant hypoprothrombinemia when the serum salicylate concentration exceeds 60 mg/dl (44). However, hemorrhage rarely occurs in either animals or humans. When bleeding occurs, it does not appear to be a contributing factor in salicylate mortality. Observations in animals and humans indicate that administering large doses of vitamin K after the development of hypoprothrombinemia has little or no effect on the plasma prothrombin time when serum salicylate concentrations are high. However, the prothrombin time rapidly returns to normal after discontinuing salicylate (44).

Enteric-coated aspirin may accumulate in the stomach of patients with pyloric stenosis or spasm (153). In these rare situations, acute toxic serum salicylate concentrations have been reported after barium GI contrast study as part of the workup in these patients (154,155). Prompt evacuation of the enteric-coated aspirin tablets from the stomach is recommended (154). Gastrogavage with sodium bicarbonate (150 mEq/L) given via nasogastric tube (300 mL over 30 minutes), alternating with 30 minutes of continuous suction for 24 hours, has been reported to be an effective means of dissolving and removing enteric-coated aspirin from the stomach (156), and this may obviate the need for surgical intervention (157).

Management Pitfalls

Reliance on Done nomogram rather than the patient's clinical condition most likely results in mismanagement of the patient.

Concerns exist regarding the use of sodium bicarbonate, including worsening of alkalemia in patients who already have a respiratory alkalosis, and the possibility of inducing hypernatremia, hypokalemia, fluid overload, and congestive heart failure (55,118,128,138,139,158). Complications can be minimized by carefully maintaining the urine pH at approximately 8 and not to exceed an arterial pH of 7.55 (72,118). Hourly determination of the urine pH is necessary to assure that optimal urine pH is maintained. Use of an isotonic sodium bicarbonate solution rather than boluses of sodium bicarbonate should prevent hypernatremia.

When sodium bicarbonate is administered rapidly or in excess amounts, tetany may develop as a result of a decrease in the serum ionized calcium level (67,159). If tetany occurs, sodium bicarbonate administration should be terminated and in severe cases slow intravenous calcium gluconate (2 to 5 ml of a 10% solution) administration may be considered (67,159).

Acetazolamide is a carbonic anhydrase inhibitor that inhibits bicarbonate reabsorption in the proximal renal tubules. Acetazolamide produces an alkaline urine at the expense of systemic metabolic acidosis favoring the movement of salicylate into tissues (e.g., brain) (17,20,21,160). Animal models of salicylate toxicity have shown an overwhelming mortality associated with acetazolamide therapy when compared with control and bicarbonate treated groups (17,161). However, clinical studies reported favorable results when acetazolamide was used in combination with bicarbonate in the treatment of salicylate toxicity (9,162,163). Based on the vast clinical experience with using sodium bicarbonate and the limited expertise with administering acetazolamide, however, acetazolamide is not recommended as routine treatment of salicylate toxicity.

Clinicians should refrain from *knee jerk* responses based on the serum salicylate concentration. Although serial serum salicylate concentrations provide valuable information as to the effectiveness of the treatment being used, they are a poor substitute for conscientious bedside evaluation of the patient. Treatment options should be individualized according to the clinical status of the patient and should not depend solely on a particular serum salicylate concentration.

Monitoring

It is recommended that a patient who has overdosed on enteric-coated or sustained-release preparations of aspirin be treated regardless of initial serum salicylate concentrations, be observed for at least 24 hours, and obtain serial serum salicylate concentrations until a declining level is confirmed (100,102,164).

Invasive hemodynamic monitoring may be necessary. One of the common errors in management is lack of monitoring of the patient's response to therapy, which may allow a complication of therapy to develop or the undertreated poisoning to progress resulting in major morbidity or mortality.

REFERENCES

1. Lindsey LP. Two cases of fatal salicylate poisoning after topical application of an anti-fungal solution. *Med J Aust* 1969;1:353–354.
2. Anderson JAR, Ead RD. Percutaneous salicylate poisoning. *Clin Exp Dermatol* 1979;4:349–351.
3. Raschke R, Arnold-Capell PA, Richeson R, et al. Refractory hypoglycemia secondary to topical salicylate intoxication. *Arch Intern Med* 1991;151:591–593.
4. Pec J, Strmenova M, Palencarova E, et al. Salicylate intoxication after use of topical salicylic acid ointment by a patient with psoriasis. *Cutis* 1992;50:307–309.
5. Brubacher JR, Hoffman RS. Salicylism from topical salicylates: review of the literature. *J Toxicol Clin Toxicol* 1996;64:431–436.
6. Chiaretti A, Schembri Wismayer D, Tortorolo L, et al. Salicylate intoxication using a skin ointment. *Acta Paediatr* 1997;86:330–331.
7. Smith MJH, Irving KD. The effect of salicylate on the passage of a barium meal in the rat. *Br J Radiol* 1955;28:39–41.
8. Smith PK, Gleason HL, Stoll CG, et al. Studies on the pharmacology of salicylates. *J Pharmacol Exp Ther* 1946;87:237–255.
9. Morgan AG, Polak A. The excretion of salicylate in salicylate poisoning. *Clin Sci* 1971;41:475–484.
10. Prescott LF, Balali-Mood M, Critchley JAJH, et al. Diuresis or urinary alkalinisation for salicylate poisoning? *BMJ* 1982;285:1383–1386.
11. Patel DK, Hesse A, Ogunbona A, et al. Metabolism of aspirin after therapeutic and toxic doses. *Hum Exp Toxicol* 1990;8:131–136.
12. Smith MJH. The metabolic basis of the major symptoms in acute salicylate intoxication. *Clin Toxicol* 1968;1:387–407.
13. Tenny SM, Miller RM. The respiratory and circulatory actions of salicylate. *Am J Med* 1955;19:498–508.
14. Cameron IR, Semple SJG. The central respiratory stimulant action of salicylates. *Clin Sci* 1968;35:391–401.
15. Silva PRM, Fonseca-Costa A, Zin WA, et al. Respiratory and acid-base parameters during salicylic intoxication in dogs. *Braz J Med Biol Res* 1986;19:279–286.
16. Brody TM. Action of sodium salicylate and related compounds on tissue metabolism in vitro. *J Pharmacol Exp Ther* 1956;117:39–51.
17. Hill JB. Experimental salicylate poisoning: observations on the effects of altering blood pH on tissue and plasma salicylate concentrations. *Pediatrics* 1971;47:658–665.
18. Hill JB. Salicylate intoxication. *N Engl J Med* 1973;288:1110–1113.
19. Goldberg MA, Barlow CF, Roth LJ. The effects of carbon dioxide on the entry and accumulation of drugs in the central nervous system. *J Pharmacol Exp Ther* 1961;131:308–318.
20. Buchanan N, Rabinowitz L. Infantile salicylism—a reappraisal. *J Pediatr* 1974;84:391–395.
21. Buchanan N, Kundig H, Eyberg B. Experimental salicylate intoxication in young baboons. *J Pediatr* 1975;86:225–232.
22. Huggins AK, Smith MJM, Moses V. Effects of salicylate and 2,4-dinitrophenol on the incorporation of ^{14}C from labeled pyruvate into the soluble intermediates of isolated rat tissues. *Biochem J* 1961;79:271–275.
23. Yoshida T, Metcoff J, Kaiser E. A metabolic lesion in salicylate intoxication. *Am J Dis Child* 1961;102:511–514.
24. Kaplan EH, Kennedy J, Davis J. Effects of salicylate and other benzoates on oxidative enzymes of the tricarboxylic acid cycle in rat tissue homogenates. *Arch Biochem* 1954;51:47–61.
25. Bryant C, Smith MJH, Hines WJW. Effects of salicylate and gamma resorcylate on the metabolism of radioactive succinate and fumarate by rat-liver mitochondria and on dehydrogenase enzymes. *Biochem J* 1963;86:391–396.
26. Schwartz R, Landy G. Organic acid excretion in salicylate intoxication. *J Pediatr* 1965;66:658–666.
27. Lutwak-Mann C. The effects of salicylate and cinchophen on enzymes and metabolic processes. *Biochem J* 1942;36:706–728.
28. Thurston JH, Pollock PG, Warren SK, et al. Reduced brain glucose with normal plasma glucose in salicylate poisoning. *J Clin Invest* 1970;49:2139–2145.
29. Anderson RJ, Potts DE, Gabow PA. Unrecognized adult salicylate intoxication. *Ann Intern Med* 1976;85:745–748.
30. Andersen R, Refstad S. Adult respiratory distress syndrome precipitated by massive salicylate poisoning. *Intensive Care Med* 1978;4:211–213.
31. Thomas C. Adult respiratory-distress syndrome in salicylate intoxication. *Lancet* 1979;1:1294.
32. Heffner JE, Starkey T, Anthony P. Salicylate-induced noncardiogenic pulmonary edema. *West J Med* 1979;130:263–266.
33. Heffner JE, Sahn SA. Salicylate-induced pulmonary edema. *Ann Intern Med* 1981;95:405–409.
34. Hormaechea E, Carlson BW, Rogove H, et al. Hypovolemia, pulmonary edema and protein changes in severe salicylate poisoning. *Am J Med* 1979;66:1046–1050.
35. Hrnicek G, Skelton J, Miller WC. Pulmonary edema and salicylate intoxication. *JAMA* 1974;230:866–867.
36. Fisher CJ, Albertson TE, Foulke GE. Salicylate-induced pulmonary edema: clinical characteristics in children. *Am J Emerg Med* 1985;3:33–37.
37. Niehoff JM, Baltatzis PA. Adult respiratory distress syndrome induced by salicylate toxicity. *Postgrad Med* 1985;78:117–119,123.
38. Walters JS, Woodring JH, Stelling CB, et al. Salicylate-induced pulmonary edema. *Radiology* 1983;146:289–293.
39. Cohen DL, Post J, Ferroggiaro AA, et al. Chronic salicylism resulting in noncardiogenic pulmonary edema requiring hemodialysis. *Am J Kidney Dis* 2000;36:E20.
40. Bowers RE, Brigham KL, Owen PJ. Salicylate pulmonary edema: the mechanism in sheep and review of the clinical literature. *Am Rev Resp Dis* 1977;115:261–268.
41. Glauser FL, Egan P, Millen JE, et al. The effect of salicylate infusion on the alveolar epithelial membrane in the isolated perfused lung. *Crit Care Med* 1978;6:181–184.
42. Park BK, Leck JB. On the mechanism of salicylate-induced hypothrombinaemia. *J Pharm Pharmacol* 1981;33:25–28.
43. Hildebrandt EF, Suttie JW. The effects of salicylate on enzymes of vitamin K metabolism. *J Pharm Pharmacol* 1983;35:421–426.

44. Clausen FW, Jager BV. The relation of the plasma salicylate level to the degree of hypoprothrombinemia. *J Lab Clin Med* 1946;31:428–436.
45. Garrettson LK, Procknal JA, Levy G. Fetal acquisition and neonatal elimination of a large amount of salicylate: study of a neonate whose mother regularly took therapeutic doses of aspirin during pregnancy. *Clin Pharmacol Ther* 1975;17:98–103.
46. Haslam R, Ekert H, Gilliam GL. Hemorrhage in a neonate possibly due to maternal ingestion of salicylate. *J Pediatr* 1974;84:556–557.
47. Haslam R. Neonatal purpura secondary to maternal salicylism. *J Pediatr* 1975;86:653.
48. Buck ML, Grebe TA, Bond GR. Toxic reaction to salicylates in a newborn infant: similarities to neonatal sepsis. *J Pediatr* 1993;122:955–958.
49. Lynd PA, Andreasen AC, Wyatt RJ. Intrauterine salicylate intoxication in a newborn. *Clin Pediatr* 1976;15:912–913.
50. Palatnick W, Tenenbein M. Aspirin poisoning during pregnancy: increased fetal sensitivity. *Am J Perinatol* 1998;15:39–41.
50a. Martinez-Frias ML, Rodriguez-Pinilla E, Prieto L. Prenatal exposure to salicylates and gastroschisis: a case-control study. *Teratology* 1997;56:241–243.
50b. Torfs CP, Katz EA, Bateson TF, et al. Maternal medications and environmental exposures as risk factors for gastroschisis. *Teratology* 1996;54:84–92.
51. Clark JH, Wilson WG. A 16 day old breast-fed infant with metabolic acidosis caused by salicylate. *Clin Pediar* 1981;20:53–54.
52. Crichton JU, Elliott GB. Salicylate—a dangerous drug in infancy and childhood. *Can Med Assoc J* 1960;83:1144–1147.
53. Gaudreault P, Temple AR, Lovejoy FH. The relative severity of acute versus chronic salicylate poisoning in children: a clinical comparison. *Pediatrics* 1982;70:566–569.
54. Winters RW, White JS, Hughes MC, et al. Disturbances of acid-base equilibrium in salicylate intoxication. *Pediatrics* 1959;23:260–285.
55. Done AK. Treatment of salicylate poisoning: review of personal and published experiences. *Clin Toxicol* 1968;1:451–467.
56. Earle R. Congenital salicylate intoxication—report of a case. *N Engl J Med* 1961;265:1003.
57. Jackson AV. Toxic effects of salicylate on the foetus and mother. *J Pathol Bacteriol* 1948;60:587–593.
58. Aterman K, Holzbecher M, Ellengerger HA. Salicylate levels in a stillborn infant born to a drug-addicted mother, with comments on pathology and analytical methodology. *Clin Toxicol* 1980;16:263–268.
59. Rejent TA, Baik S. Fatal in utero salicylism. *J Forensic Sci* 1985;30:942–944.
60. Mongan E, Kelly P, Nies K, et al. Tinnitus as an indication of therapeutic serum salicylate levels. *JAMA* 1973;226:142–145.
61. Proudfoot AT. Toxicity of salicylates. *Am J Med* 1983;75[Suppl 14]:99–103.
62. Myers EN, Bernstein JM, Fostiropolous G. Salicylate ototoxicity a clinical study. *N Engl J Med* 1965;11:587–590.
63. Day RO, Graham GG, Bieri D, et al. Concentration-response relationships for salicylate-induced ototoxicity in normal volunteers. *Br J Clin Pharmacol* 1989;28:695–702.
64. Proudfoot AT, Brown SS. Acidaemia and salicylate poisoning in adults. *Br Med J* 1969;2:547–550.
65. Gabow PA, Anderson RJ, Potts DE, et al. Acid-base disturbances in the salicylate-intoxicated adult. *Arch Intern Med* 1978;138:1481–1484.
66. Chapman BJ, Proudfoot AT. Adult salicylate poisoning: deaths and outcome in patients with high plasma salicylate concentrations. *QJM* 1989;2:699–707.
67. Done AK, Temple AR. Treatment of salicylate poisoning. *Mod Treat* 1971;8:528–551.
68. Montgomery H, Porter JC, Bradley RD. Salicylate intoxication causing a severe systemic inflammatory response and rhabdomyolysis. *Am J Emerg Med* 1994;12:531–532.
69. Leventhal L, Kuritsky L, Ginsburg R, et al. Salicylate-induced rhabdomyolysis. *Am J Emerg Med* 1989;7:409–410.
70. Skjoto J, Reikvam A. Hyperthermia and rhabdomyolysis in self-poisoning with paracetamol and salicylates. Report of a case. *Acta Med Scand* 1979;205:473–476.
71. Snodgrass W. Salicylate toxicity following therapeutic doses in young children. *Clin Toxicol* 1981;18:247–259.
72. Temple AR. Acute and chronic effects of aspirin toxicity and their treatment. *Arch Intern Med* 1981;141:364–368.
73. Dove DJ, Jones T: Delayed coma associated with salicylate intoxication. *J Pediatr* 1982;100:493–496.
74. Done AK. Aspirin overdosage: incidence, diagnosis, and management. *Pediatrics* 1978;62[Suppl]:890–897.
75. Segar WE, Holliday MA. Physiologic abnormalities of salicylate intoxication. *N Engl J Med* 1958;259:1191–1198.
76. Ryder HW, Shaver M, Ferris EB. Salicylism accompanied by respiratory alkalosis and toxic encephalopathy. Report of a fatal case. *N Engl J Med* 1945;232:617–621.
77. Case records of the Massachusetts General Hospital (Case 23-1977). *N Engl J Med* 1977;296:1337–1346.
78. Bray PF, Gardiner AY. Salicylism and severe brain edema. *N Engl J Med* 1977;297:1235.
79. Greer HD III, Ward HP, Corbin KB. Chronic salicylate intoxication in adults. *JAMA* 1965;193:555–558.
80. Paul BN. Salicylate poisoning in the elderly: diagnostic pitfalls. *J Am Geriatr Soc* 1972;20:387–390.
81. Mukerji V, Alpert MA, Flaker GC, et al. Cardiac conduction abnormalities and atrial arrhythmias associated with salicylate toxicity. *Pharmarcotherapy* 1986;6:41–43.
82. Nawata Y, Kagami M, Nakajima H, et al. Chronic salicylate intoxication and rhabdomyolysis in a patient with scleroderma and Sjögren's syndrome. *J Rheumatol* 1994;21:357–359.
83. Prescott LF. Liver damage with non-narcotic analgesics. *Med Toxicol* 1986;1[Suppl 1]:44–56.
84. Kaufman DW, Kelly JP. Acetylsalicylic acid and other salicylates in relation to Stevens-Johnson syndrome and toxic epidermal necrolysis. *Br J Clin Pharmacol* 2001;51:174–176.
84a. Hurwitz GA, Wingfield W, Cowart TD, et al. Toxic interaction between salicylates and a carbonic anhydrase inhibitor: the role of cerebral edema. *Vet Hum Toxicol* 1980;22(suppl 2):42–44.
85. Anderson CJ, Kaufman PL, Sturm RJ. Toxicity of combined therapy with carbonic anhydrase inhibitors and aspirin. *Am J Ophthalmol* 1978;86:516–519.
86. Rousseau P, Fuentevilla-Clifton A. Acetazolamide and salicylate interaction in the elderly: a case report. *J Am Geriatr Soc* 1993;41:868–869.
87. Sweeney KR, Chapron DJ, Brandt JL, et al. Toxic interaction between acetazolamide and salicylate: case reports and a pharmacokinetic explanation. *Clin Pharmacol Ther* 1986;40:518–524.
88. Szucs PA, Shih RD, Marcus SM, et al. Pseudosalicylate poisoning: falsely elevated salicylate levels in an overdose of diflunisal. *Am J Emerg Med* 2000;18:641–642.
89. Adelman HM, Wallach PM, Flannery MT. Inability to interpret toxic salicylate levels in patients taking aspirin and diflunisal. *J Rheumatol* 1991;18:522–523.
90. Dalrymple RW, Stearns FM. Diflunisal interference with determination of salicylate by the Trinder, Abbott TDx, and Du Pont aca methods. *Clin Chem* 1986;32:230.
91. Duffens KR, Smilkstein MJ, Bessen HA, et al. Falsely elevated salicylate levels due to diflunisal overdose. *J Emerg Med* 1987;5:499–503.
92. Nordt SP. Diflunisal cross-reactivity with the Trinder method for salicylate determination. *Ann Pharmacother* 1996;30:1041–1042.
93. Sarma L, Wong SH, DellaFera S. Diflunisal significantly interferes with salicylate measurements by FPIA-TDx and UV-VIS aca methods. *Clin Chem* 1985;31:1922–1923.
94. Hoffman RJ, Nelson LS, Hoffman RS. Use of ferric chloride to identify salicylate-containing poisons. *J Toxicol Clin Toxicol* 2002;40;547–549.
95. King JA, Storrow AB, Finkelstein JA. Urine Trinder spot test: a rapid salicylate screen for the emergency department. *Ann Emerg Med* 1995;26:330–333.
96. Weiner AL, Ko C, McKay CA Jr. A comparison of two bedside tests for the detection of salicylates in urine. *Acad Emerg Med* 2000;7:834–836.
97. Berkovitch M, Uziel Y, Greenberg R, et al. False-high blood salicylate levels in neonates with hyperbilirubinemia. *Ther Drug Monit* 2000;22:757–761.
98. Done AK. Significance of measurements of salicylate in blood in cases of acute ingestion. *Pediatrics* 1960;26:800–807.
99. Kwong TC, Laczin J, Baum J. Self-poisoning with enteric-coated aspirin. *Am J Clin Pathol* 1983;80:888–890.
100. Henry AF. Overdose of enterophen. *Can Med Assoc J* 1983;128:1142.
101. Todd PJ, Sills JA, Harris F. Problems with overdoses of sustained-release aspirin. *Lancet* 1981;1:777.
102. Wortzman DJ, Grunfeld A. Delayed absorption following enteric-coated aspirin overdose. *Ann Emerg Med* 1987;16:434–436.
103. Handy CA. Radiopacity of oral nonliquid medications. *Radiology* 1971;98:525–533.
104. O'Brien, RP, McGeehan PA, Helmeczi AW, et al. Detectability of drug tablets and capsules by plain radiograph. *Am J Emerg Med* 1986;4:302–312.
105. Savitt DL, Hawkins HH, Roberts JR. The radiopacity of ingested medications. *Ann Emerg Med* 1987;16:331–339.
106. Filippone GA, Fish SS, Lacouture PG, et al. Reversible adsorption (desorption) of aspirin from activated charcoal. *Arch Intern Med* 1987;147:1390–1392.
107. Levy G, Tsuchiya T. Effect of activated charcoal on aspirin absorption in man. *Clin Pharmacol Ther* 1972;13:317–322.
108. Barone JA, Raia JJ, Huang YC. Evaluation of the effects of multiple-dose activated charcoal on the absorption of orally administered salicylate in a simulated toxic ingestion model. *Ann Emerg Med* 1988;17:34–37.
109. Kirshenbaum LA, Mathews SC, Sitar DS, et al. Whole-bowel irrigation versus activated charcoal in sorbitol for the ingestion of modified-release pharmaceuticals. *Clin Pharmacol Ther* 1989;46:264–271.
110. Hillman RJ, Prescott LF. Treatment of salicylate poisoning with repeated oral charcoal. *BMJ* 1985;291:1472.
111. Yeakel D, Stemple C, Dougherty J. A prospective human crossover study on single versus multiple dose charcoal in salicylate ingestion. *Ann Emerg Med* 1988;17:439.
112. Kirshenbaum LA, Mathews SC, Sitar DS, et al. Does multiple-dose charcoal therapy enhance salicylate excretion? *Arch Intern Med* 1990;150:1281–1283.
113. Bradberry SM, Vale JA. Multiple-dose activated charcoal: a review of relevant clinical studies. *J Toxicol Clin Toxicol* 1995;33:407–416.
114. Jacobsen D, Wiik-Larsen E, Bredesen JE. Haemodialysis or haemoperfusion in severe salicylate poisoning? *Human Toxicol* 1988;7:161–163.
115. James JA, Kimbell L, Read WT. Comparison of exchange transfusion, intermittent peritoneal lavage, and hemodialysis as means for removing salicylate. *Pediatrics* 1962;29:442–447.
116. Beveridge GW, Forshall W, Munro JF, et al. Acute salicylate poisoning in adult. *Lancet* 1987;1:1406–1409.

117. Ellenhorn MJ, Barceloux DH. Salicylates. In: *Medical toxicology diagnosis and treatment of human poisoning*. New York: Elsevier, 1988:561–572.
118. Gabow PA. How to avoid overlooking salicylate intoxication. *J Crit Illness* 1986;1:77–85.
119. Flomenbaum NE. Salicylates. In: Goldfrank LR, Flomenbaum NE, Lewin NA, et al., eds. *Goldfrank's toxicologic emergencies*, 7th ed. New York: McGraw-Hill, 2002:507–518.
120. Klein-Schwartz, Oderda GM. Poisoning in the elderly epidemiological, clinical and management considerations. *Drugs Aging* 1991;1:67–89.
121. Locket S. Hemodialysis in the treatment of acute poisoning. *Proc R Soc Med* 1970;63:427–430.
122. McGuigan MA. A two-year review of salicylate deaths in Ontario. *Arch Intern Med* 1987;147:510–512.
123. Krenzelok EP, Kerr F, Proudfoot AT. Salicylate toxicity. In: Haddad LM, Shannon MW, Winchester JF, eds. *Clinical management of poisoning and drug overdose*, 3rd ed. Philadelphia: WB Saunders, 1998:675–687.
124. Rentsch JB, Bradley A, Marsh SB. Two cases of salicylate intoxication successfully treated by exchange transfusion. *Am J Dis Child* 1959;98:778–784.
125. Schlegel RJ, Altstatt LB, Canales L, et al. Peritoneal dialysis for severe salicylism: an evaluation of indications and results. *J Pediatr* 1966;69:553–562.
126. Schreiner GE, Teehan BP. Dialysis of poisons and drugs—annual review. *Trans Am Soc Artif Intern Organs* 1972;18:563–599.
127. Vale A, Meredith T, Buckley B. Eliminating poisons. *BMJ* 1984;289:366–369.
128. Winchester JF, Gelfand MC, Knepshield JH, et al. Dialysis and hemoperfusion of poisons and drugs-update. *Trans Am Soc Artif Intern Organs* 1977;23:762–842.
129. Haapanen EJ. Hemoperfusion in acute intoxication. Clinical experience with 48 cases. *Acta Med Scand Suppl* 1982;668:76–81.
130. Wrathall G, Sinclair R, Moore A, et al. Three case reports of the use of haemodiafiltration in the treatment of salicylate overdose. *Hum Exp Toxicol* 2001;20:491–495.
131. Elliott GB, Crichton JU. Peritoneal dialysis in salicylate intoxication. *Lancet* 1960;2:840–842.
132. Etteldorf JN, Dobbins WT, Summitt RL, et al. Intermittent peritoneal dialysis using 5 per cent albumin in the treatment of salicylate intoxication in children. *J Pediatr* 1961;58:226–236.
133. Done AK, Otterness LJ. Exchange transfusion in the treatment of oil of wintergreen (methyl salicylate) poisoning. *Pediatrics* 1956;18:80–85.
134. Leikin SL, Emmanouilides GC. The use of exchange transfusion in salicylate intoxication. *J Pediatr* 1960;57:715–720.
135. Manikian A, Stone S, Hamilton R, et al. Exchange transfusion in severe infant salicylism. *Vet Hum Toxicol* 2002;44:224–227.
136. Yip L, Dart RC, Gabow PA. Concepts and controversies in salicylate toxicity. *Emerg Med Clinics North Am* 1994;12:351–364.
137. Curry SC. Salicylates. In: Tintinalli JE, Krome RL, Ruiz E, eds. *Emergency medicine: a comprehensive study guide*, 3rd ed. New York: McGraw-Hill, 1992:589–593.
138. Oliver TK, Dyer ME. The prompt treatment of salicylism with sodium bicarbonate. *Am J Dis Child* 1960;99:555–565.
139. Whitten CF, Kesaree NM, Goodwin JF. Managing salicylate poisoning in children. *Am J Dis Child* 1961;101:178–194.
140. Schlesinger TG, Janz TG. The efficacy of continuous bicarbonate infusion in maintaining an alkaline pH. *Ann Emerg Med* 1989;18:916.
141. Done AK. Treatment of salicylate poisoning. *Mod Treat* 1967;4:648–670.
142. Gordon IJ. Diuresis or urinary alkalinisation for salicylate poisoning? *BMJ* 1983;286:147.
143. Snodgrass WR. Salicylate toxicity. *Pediatr Clin North Am* 1986;33:381–391.
144. Rogers GC, Matyunas NJ. Salicylates. In: Behrman RE, Kliegman RM, Jenson HG, eds. *Nelson textbook of pediatrics*, 16th ed. Philadelphia: WB Saunders, 2000:2166–2167.
145. Crump CH, Murdaugh HV Jr. Studies of salicylate intoxication in dogs. *Clin Res* 1959;7:298.
146. Prescott LF, Critchley JAJH, Proudfoot AT. Diuresis or urinary alkalinisation for salicylate poisoning? *BMJ* 1983;286:147.
147. Patel DK, Ogunbona A, Notarianni LJ, et al. Depletion of plasma glycine and effect of glycine by mouth on salicylate metabolism during aspirin overdose. *Hum Exp Toxicol* 1990;9:389–396.
148. Notarianni L. A reassessment of the treatment of salicylate poisoning. *Drug Saf* 1992;7:292–303.
149. Pierce AW. Salicylate poisoning. *Pediatrics* 1974;54:342–347.
150. Riggs BS, Kulig K, Rumack BH. Current status of aspirin and acetaminophen intoxication. *Pediatr Ann* 1987;16:886–898.
151. Sørensen SC. Adult respiratory-distress syndrome in salicylate intoxication. *Lancet* 1979;1:1025.
152. Berk WA, Andersen JC. Salicylate-associated asystole: report of two cases. *Am J Med* 1989;86:505–506.
153. Baum J. Enteric-coated aspirin and the problem of gastric retention. *J Rheumatol* 1984;11:250–251.
154. Bogacz K, Caldron P. Enteric-coated aspirin bezoar: elevation of serum salicylate level by barium study. *Am J Med* 1987;83:783–786.
155. Springer DJ, Groll A. Poisoning with enteric-coated acetylsalicylic acid complicating gastric outlet obstruction. *Can Med Assoc J* 1980;122:1032–1034.
156. Sogge MR. Lavage to remove enteric-coated aspirin and gastric outlet obstruction. *Ann Intern Med* 1977;87:721–722.
157. Harris FC. Pyloric stenosis: hold up of enteric coated aspirin tablets. *BJM* 1973;60:979–981.
158. Cumming G, Dukes DC, Widdowson G. Alkaline diuresis in treatment of aspirin poisoning. *BMJ* 1964;2:1033–1036.
159. Fox GN. Hypocalcemia complicating bicarbonate therapy for salicylate poisoning. *West J Med* 1984;141:108–109.
160. Reed JR, Palmisano PA. Central nervous system salicylate. *Clin Toxicol* 1975;8:623–631.
161. Kaplan SA, del Carmen FT. Experimental salicylate poisoning: observations on the effects of carbonic anhydrase inhibitor and bicarbonate. *Pediatrics* 1958;21:762–769.
162. Schwartz R, Fellers FX, Knapp J, et al. The renal response to administration of acetazolamide (Diamox7) during salicylate intoxication. *Pediatrics* 1959;23:1103–1114.
163. Feuerstein RC, Finberg, Fleishman E. The use of acetazolamide in the therapy of salicylate poisoning. *Pediatrics* 1960;25:215–227.
164. Editorial. Poisoning with enteric-coated aspirin. *Lancet* 1981;2:130.
165. Chalasani N, Roman J, Jurado RL. Systemic inflammatory response syndrome caused by chronic salicylate intoxication. *South Med J* 1996;89:479–482.
166. Chui PT. Anesthesia in a patient with undiagnosed salicylate poisoning presenting as intraabdominal sepsis. *J Clin Anesth* 1999;11:251–253.
167. Anderson RJ. Asterixis as a manifestation of salicylate toxicity. *Ann Intern Med* 1981;95:188–189.
168. Steele TE, Morton WA. Salicylate-induced delirium. *Psychosomatics* 1986;27:455–456.
169. Pei YPC, Thompson DA. Severe salicylate intoxication mimicking septic shock. *Am J Med* 1987;82:381–382.
170. Leatherman JW, Schmitz PG. Fever, hyperdynamic shock, and multiple-system organ failure: a pseudo-sepsis syndrome associated with chromic salicylate intoxication. *Chest* 1991;100:1391–1396.
171. Lemesh RA. Accidental chromic salicylate intoxication in an elderly patient: major morbidity despite early recognition. *Vet Hum Toxicol* 1993;35:34–36.
172. Bailey RB, Jones SR. Chronic salicylate intoxication: a common cause of morbidity in the elderly. *J Am Geriatr Soc* 1989;37:556–561.

CHAPTER 127B

Nonsteroidal Antiinflammatory Drugs

Alvin C. Bronstein

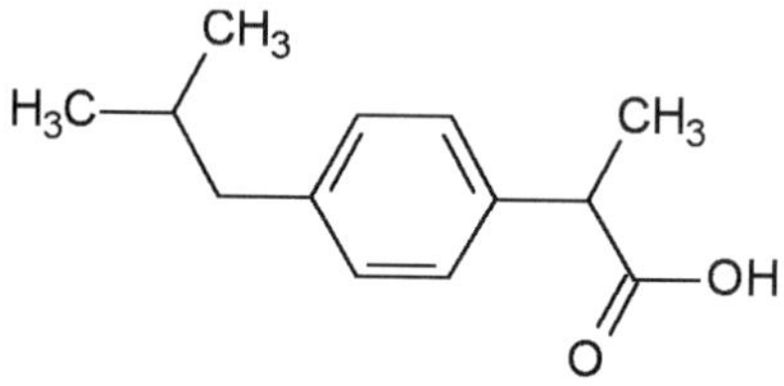

IBUPROFEN

Compounds included:	**Non-aspirin nonsteroidal antiinflammatory drugs: carprofen (Rimadyl), diclofenac (Cataflam, Voltaren), etodolac (Lodine), fenoprofen (Nalfon), ibuprofen (Motrin), indomethacin (Indocin), ketoprofen (Orudis), nabumetone (Relafen), naproxen (Naprosyn), oxaprozin (Daypro), sulindac (Clinoril), tolmetin (Tolectin); COX-2 selective drugs: Celecoxib (Celebrex), meloxicam (Mobic), rofecoxib (Vioxx), valdecoxib (Bextra)**
Molecular formula and weight:	**See Table 1.**
SI conversion:	**See Table 1.**
CAS Registry No.:	**See Table 1.**
Target organs:	**Kidneys, gastrointestinal, central nervous system**
Antidote:	**None**

OVERVIEW

Nonsteroidal antiinflammatory drugs (NSAIDs) are a ubiquitous part of modern medical prescribing practice. A large and varied therapeutic drug group, they are used acutely for fever and pain control. When administered chronically, they are effective in treating a wide array of conditions including rheumatoid arthritis. The first NSAID in pharmaceutical form was acetylsalicylic acid (aspirin). However, the non-aspirin NSAIDs (NANSAIDs) have come to dominate most applications. The NANSAIDs include ibuprofen and other nonsteroidals except aspirin (acetylsalicylic acid).

Although aspirin has been available since 1899, the use of the NANSAID drugs did not take off until the midpart of the twentieth century (1). During the 1950s, pharmaceutical companies began searching earnestly for arthritis treatment alternatives with better adverse effect profiles than aspirin. In August 1958, Stewart Adams and coworkers at Boots Pure Drug Company in the United Kingdom discovered a new class of compounds termed *phenylalkanoic acids* (2). These agents possessed antiinflammatory, antipyretic, and analgesic activity. A patent application for the new drug class was approved in 1964. One of the compounds in this group was 2-(4-isobutylphenyl) propionic acid, later named *ibuprofen* (3). Ibuprofen (Brufen) was introduced for prescription use in the United Kingdom in 1969 as a treatment for rheumatoid arthritis. In 1983, ibuprofen received over-the-counter approval in the United Kingdom under the name Nurofen. Prescription use of ibuprofen in the United States began in 1974 (3). It was approved in May 1984 (4) by the U.S. Food and Drug Administration for over-the-counter use as a 200-mg tablet formulation and marketed as Advil. Ibuprofen arginine is a new formulation of ibuprofen designed to achieve higher and earlier peak serum concentrations that may improve its efficacy for relieving pain.

The use of ibuprofen and other NSAIDs has steadily increased. In 2001, acetaminophen, ibuprofen, and aspirin ranked one, seven, and twelve, respectively, out of 1.3 billion drug mentions during ambulatory care visits in the top 20 generic medications prescription list from the National Center for Health Statistics survey (5). On the prescription medication list, Celebrex was number eight followed by Vioxx at number eleven (6). This is of interest because the selective cyclooxygenase (COX)-2 inhibitors have only been available in the United States since 1999 (7).

For the year 2001, American poison centers reported 85,577 NSAID exposures (excluding salicylates); 70% involved ibuprofen (8). Of the exposures with known outcomes (other than death), 27% had no effect, 13% mild, 4% moderate, and 1% major. For 2001, there were 1074 poisoning fatalities reported. Thirty-nine deaths involved a non-salicylate NSAID as one of the causal agents. But in only three (all adult) of the 39 deaths was ibuprofen listed as the sole drug ingested. In the remaining 36, each involving more than one ingested drug, ibuprofen was named in 17; COX-2 inhibitors in 8; naproxen in 5; indomethacin in 1; ibuprofen with hydrocodone in 1; and 4 were listed as other, not otherwise specified.

The toxicity of NSAIDs is primarily the result of COX-1 and COX-2 inhibition and the resultant diminished prostanoid synthesis. Overall NSAID toxicity is low (9). With respect to gastrointestinal (GI) damage, there may be a direct mucosal effect as well. Toxicity is dose related. Large exposures may exhibit altered mental status, coma (10,11), seizures (11), acute renal fail-

TABLE 1. Physical characteristics and dosage of non-aspirin nonsteroidal antiinflammatory agents

Generic name	Molecular formula; molecular weight (g/mol); CAS Registry No.	SI conversion	Formulation	Dosage	
				Adult	Pediatric
Acetic acids					
Diclofenac	$C_{14}H_{10}Cl_2NNaO_2$; 318.1; 15307-79-6	mg/ml × 3.1 = μmol/L	25-, 50-, 75-mg tablets; 100-mg delayed-release tablet	50–75 mg orally 2–3 times a day	Not approved for pediatric use
Etodolac	$C_{17}H_{21}NO_3$; 287.4; 41340-25-4	mg/ml × 3.5 = μmol/L	200-, 300-, 400-, 500-mg tablets and capsules; 400-, 500-, 600-mg extended-release tablets	300–1000 mg orally, 1–3 times a day	400 mg once a day for 20–30 kg child
Indomethacin	$C_{19}H_{15}ClNO_4$,$3H_2O$; 433.8; 74252-25-8	mg/ml × 2.3 = μmol/L	5-, 50-, 75-mg capsules or tablets; 25 mg/5 ml oral suspension; 50-mg suppository; 75-mg sustained-release capsule	75–200 mg/d orally in divided doses	2 mg/kg/d orally in divided doses, up to 200 mg/d
Ketorolac	$C_{19}H_{24}N_2O_6$; 376.4; 74103-07-4	mg/ml × 2.7 = μmol/L	10-mg tablet	10 mg orally every 4 hours, up to 40 mg/d	0.5–1.0 mg/kg/dose orally
Nabumetone	$C_{15}H_{16}O_2$; 228.3; 42924-53-8	mg/ml × 4.4 = μmol/L	500-, 750-mg tablets	2 g orally 1–2 times a day	Not approved for pediatric use
Sulindac	$C_{20}H_{17}FO_3S$; 356.4; 38194-50-2	mg/ml × 2.8 = μmol/L	150-, 200-mg tablets	150–200 mg orally BID	4 mg/kg/d orally in divided doses
Tolmetin	$C_{15}H_{14}NNaO_3$,$2H_2O$; 315.3; 64490-92-2	mg/ml × 3.2 = μmol/L	200-, 400-, 600-mg tablet or capsules	200–600 mg orally 3 times a day	5–30 mg/kg/d orally in divided doses
Fenamates (anthranilic acids)					
Meclofenamate	$C_{14}H_{10}Cl_2NNaO_2$,H_2O; 336.1; 6385-02-0	mg/ml × 3.0 = μmol/L	50-, 100-mg capsules	200–400 mg/d in divided doses	Not approved for pediatric use
Mefenamic acid	$C_{15}H_{15}NO_2$; 241.3; 61-68-7	mg/ml × 4.1 = μmol/L	250-mg capsule	500 mg initially, followed by 250 mg every 6 h	Not approved for ages younger than 14 yr
Oxicams					
Piroxicam	$C_{15}H_{13}N_3O_4S$; 331.3; 36322-90-4	mg/ml × 3.0 = μmol/L	10-, 20-mg tablets	20–40 mg/d orally	0.2–0.3 mg/kg/d orally, up to 15 mg/d
Propionic acids					
Carprofen	$C_{15}H_{12}ClNO_2$; 273.7; 53716-49-7	mg/ml × 3.7 = μmol/L	25-, 75-, 100-mg capsules	For veterinary use	For veterinary use
Fenoprofen	$(C_{15}H_{13}O_3)_2Ca$,$2H_2O$; 558.6; 53746-45-5	mg/ml × 1.8 = μmol/L	200-, 300-, 600-mg capsules and tablets	300–600 mg PO TID to QID, up to 3200 mg/d	Not approved for pediatric use
Flurbiprofen	$C_{15}H_{12}FNaO_2$,$2H_2O$; 302.3; 56767-76-1	mg/ml × 3.3 = μmol/L	50-, 100-mg tablets	200–300 mg/d administered in divided doses up to 300 mg	Not approved for pediatric use
Ibuprofen	$C_{13}H_{18}O_2$; 206.3; 15687-27-1	mg/ml × 4.8 = μmol/L	50-, 100-mg chewable tablet; 40-mg/ml oral drops; 100 mg/5 ml oral suspension; 200-, 300-, 400-, 600-, 800-mg tablets	1200–3200 mg/d orally in divided doses	10 mg/kg, every 6–8 h up to 40 mg/kg/d
Ketoprofen	$C_{16}H_{14}O_3$; 254.3; 22071-15-4	mg/ml × 3.9 = μmol/L	12.5-, 25-, 50-, 75-mg tablet or capsule; 200-mg controlled-release capsule; 100-, 150-mg sustained-release capsule	100–300 mg QD	Not approved for pediatric use
Naproxen	$C_{14}H_{13}NaO_3$; 252.2; 26159-34-2	mg/ml × 4.0 = μmol/L	275-, 550-mg tablet; 375-, 500- mg controlled-release tablet; 375-, 500-mg delayed-release tablet; 125 mg/5 ml oral suspension; 125-, 220-, 250-, 275-, 375-, 500-, 550-mg tablets	250–500 mg PO BID	5 mg/kg PO BID
Oxaprozin	$C_{18}H_{15}NO_3$; 293.3; 21256-18-8	mg/ml × 3.4 = μmol/L	600-mg caplets	600–1200 mg/d as a single oral dose	Not approved for pediatric use
Pyrazolones					
Phenylbutazone	$C_{19}H_{20}N_2O_2$; 308.4; 50-33-9	mg/ml × 3.2 = μmol/L	100-mg tablets	300–600 mg/d in divided doses	Not approved for pediatric use
Selective COX-2 inhibitors					
Celecoxib	$C_{17}H_{14}F_3N_3O_2S$; 381.4; 169590-42-5	mg/ml × 2.6 = μmol/L	100-, 200-mg capsules	400–600 mg/d in divided doses	Not approved for pediatric use
Meloxicam	$C_{14}H_{13}N_3O_4S_2$; 351.4; 71125-38-7	mg/ml × 2.8 = μmol/L	7.5-mg tablet	7.5–15.0 mg orally once a day	Not approved for pediatric use
Rofecoxib	$C_{17}H_{14}O_4S$; 314.4; 162011-90-7	mg/ml × 3.2 = μmol/L	12.5 mg/5 ml, 25 mg/5 ml suspension; 12.5-, 25-, 50-mg tablets	12.5–50.0 mg orally once a day	Not approved for pediatric use
Valdecoxib	$C_{16}H_{14}N_2O_3S$; 314.4; 181695-72-7	mg/ml × 3.2 = μmol/L	10-, 20-mg tablets	10 to 20 mg orally, 1–2 times a day	Not approved for pediatric use
Combination products					
Diclofenac sodium/misoprostol	Not applicable	Not applicable	50 mg/200 μg, 75 mg/200 μg tablets	50 mg/200 μg orally 2–4 times a day; 75 mg/200 μg twice a day	Not approved for pediatric use
Hydrocodone bitartrate and ibuprofen	Not applicable	Not applicable	7.5 mg/200 μg tablets	One tablet orally every 4–6 h	Not approved for pediatric use

COX, cyclooxygenase.

ure, metabolic acidosis (10,12), GI bleeding (10), shock (11), acute liver injury (10,12), acute cholestasis (6,10), and thrombocytopenia (10). Renal failure may require hemodialysis or continuous venovenous hemofiltration for support. Death is rare (9). A recent review found only seven ibuprofen deaths in the literature (13).

Classification and Uses

The NANSAID group possesses three wide-ranging medical uses: antiinflammatory, analgesic, and antipyretic. Although an oversimplification, these effects result primarily from their ability to inhibit prostaglandin synthesis by blocking the action of the COX enzyme system (14)—COX-1 and COX-2 (15–18). Based on selectivity of COX inhibition function, the NSAIDs can be grouped into two pharmacologic classes: nonspecific COX inhibitors and selective COX-2 inhibitors, the *coxibs*. Based on recent studies using the carrageenan pleurisy mode in rats, the existence of a COX-3 enzyme has been theorized. Hypothetical COX-3 may work at the end of the inflammatory cycle producing antiinflammatory prostanoids. Research continues in this area (19).

Toxic Dose

Adult and pediatric therapeutic dosages are provided in Table 1. There are no established lethal doses. Case reports of 72 and 100-g ibuprofen ingestions have survived (9,20). In adults, the reported dose ingested and the toxic effect correlate poorly (11). In an adult, 3 g was reported to be associated with mild central nervous system (CNS) depression (21). Renal injury has been reported with ingestions of more than 6 g.

For pediatric patients, a dose more than 400 mg/kg has been associated with symptoms (11,22). No symptoms were noted in the same study with an ingestion of less than 100 mg/kg. This dose has been supported by other retrospective reports (12,22–24). A 6-year-old boy in one case report developed metabolic acidosis and coma after ingesting 300 mg/kg (25). A 16-month-old child ingesting 469 mg/kg ibuprofen developed apneic episodes, aspirated, and expired due to sepsis (11).

TOXICOKINETICS AND TOXICODYNAMICS

Oral absorption is usually good (26). Ibuprofen is rapidly absorbed from the GI tract with peak concentrations achieved in 15 to 30 minutes. Although absorption is high, ibuprofen solubility is relatively low, being less than 0.1 mg/ml in water. Therefore, absorption of large ingestions may be limited because of the low solubility (9). The plasma half-life is approximately 0.9 to 2.5 hours. Like most of the propionic acids, ibuprofen is largely bound to plasma proteins. In usual doses, the liver metabolizes more than 99%. Ibuprofen has two main hepatic metabolites, which are either excreted as 2-hydroxyibuprofen and 2-carboxyibuprofen or their conjugates. The volume of distribution is 0.14 L/kg (27).

PATHOPHYSIOLOGY

Cyclooxygenases

The COX system is responsible for prostaglandin synthesis (17). Synthesis is triggered by a variety of chemical, inflammatory, mitogenic, or physical events (17,18). Arachidonic acid is the substrate for the COX enzyme system (28). The process begins with the cleavage of arachidonic acid from the cell's phospholipid membrane by the action of phospholipase A. COX exists in at least two isomeric forms: COX-1 and COX-2 (Fig. 1), also known as prostaglandin G/H synthase 1 and prostaglandin G/H synthase 2, respectively.

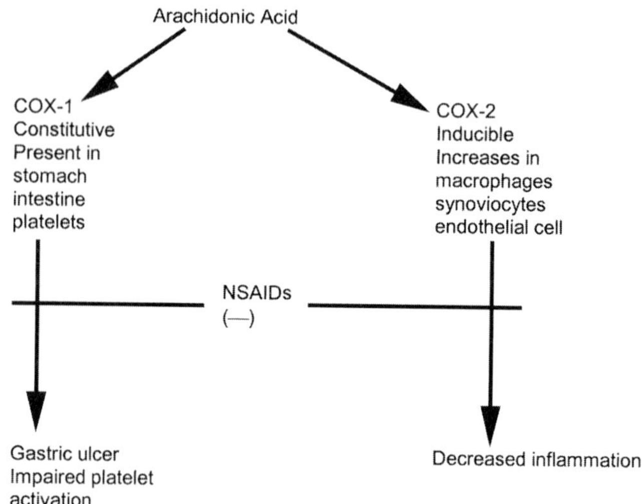

Figure 1. Simplified scheme of the role of cyclooxygenase (COX) enzymes in the effects of nonsteroidal antiinflammatory drugs (NSAIDs).

COX-1 is a constitutive cellular enzyme with a variety of *housekeeping duties* (29). These include synthesis of platelet aggregation agents, GI protection, and promotion of renal homeostasis (29). COX-1 is not thought to be inducible and is regularly present in the cell. In contrast, COX-2 is inducible (29). COX-2 cellular activity increases secondary to a variety of inflammatory stimuli. Prostanoids produced by COX-2 are part of the system's inflammatory response. For example, COX-2 is found in synovial fluid of inflamed joints. The COX-1 enzyme is part of the synthesis pathway for prostaglandin E_2 (PGE_2), PGI_2, and thromboxane A_2. The organ location of COX-1 dictates the type of prostaglandin produced.

The cyclooxygenases possess both COX and hydroxyperoxidase activities. The G/H designation stems from the enzymes' ability to catalyze the synthesis of the unstable intermediate prostaglandin G_2 (PGG_2), which is then metabolized to prostaglandin H_2 (PGH_2) via their hydroxyperoxidase function (17). PGH_2 is also unstable and rapidly metabolized by tissue-specific isomerases to multiple prostanoids such as prostacyclin (PGI_2), thromboxane A_2, prostaglandin D_2, PGE_2, and prostaglandin F_{2a}. These prostanoids stimulate their respective G-protein–coupled receptors to induce various effects ranging from GI protection to platelet-derived thromboxane A_2 causing platelet aggregation (30) and vascular smooth muscle and mast cell–derived thromboxane A_2 producing vasoconstriction and bronchoconstriction (17,31,32). The eicosanoid-derived thromboxane A_2 may also be a chemical mediator in food allergen–induced immediate hypersensitivity (33,34). Production of the gastric protective prostacyclin (PGI_2) and PGE_2 in the stomach is initialized by COX-1 activity. PGE_2 is also required for renal sodium regulation. NSAID inhibitors of COX-1 block the production of these GI protective mediators (26,35,36).

NSAIDs are reversible COX-1 and COX-2 inhibitors. This means that for the nonsalicylate NSAIDs the half-life is 6 to 10 hours depending on the specific NSAID, but the half-life for the salicylates is longer due to the time necessary for COX regeneration (26).

Gastrointestinal Toxicity

Because most NSAIDs are organic acids, local tissue damage is caused by the direct contact of dissolved drug with gastric mucosa. The NSAID increases gastric cell wall permeability resulting in cellular edema and apoptosis (37). Salicylates are the classic example of these phenomena. However, the more important ulcerogenic mechanism is NSAID inhibition of COX-1 (37). NSAID COX-1 inhibition blocks prostaglandin production. Decreased concentration of PGI_2 and PGE_2 in gastric tissue decreases mucous and bicarbonate production, promotes hydrochloric acid secretion, and decreases gastric blood flow (Fig. 1). Another risk factor may be concomitant infection with *Helicobacter pylori*. Studies to date are divided on this effect (38). The exact relationship, if any, is not clear.

Hematopoietic Effects

NSAIDs block platelet thromboxane A_2 production via COX-1 inhibition. Thromboxane A_2 is important for platelet aggregation. Thus, bleeding problems can be precipitated. Interactions with patients on anticoagulants are possible.

Renal Effects

NSAID-induced renal disease can be either acute or chronic. NSAID renal toxicity is due to COX-1 inhibition (Fig. 1). Renal prostaglandins are released to compensate for renal vasoconstriction. Prostaglandins PGE_2 and PGI_2 stimulate vasodilatation (39). NSAIDs reduce these prostaglandins by inhibiting COX-1.

PREGNANCY AND LACTATION

Most NSAIDs are classified U.S. Food and Drug Administration pregnancy category C or D (Table 2). Because of their ability to cause premature closure of the ductus arteriosus, use in pregnancy especially in the third trimester is not recommended. Nursing mothers should not use NSAIDs.

TABLE 2. U.S. Food and Drug Administration pregnancy category and breast-feeding information for the non-aspirin nonsteroidal antiinflammatory agents

Generic name, trade name	U.S. Food and Drug Administration pregnancy category (Appendix I)	Breast-feeding
Acetic acids		
Diclofenac	B	Unknown
Etodolac	C	Unknown
Indomethacin	D	Safe
Ketorolac	C	Safe
Nabumetone	C	Unknown
Sulindac	D	Not recommended
Tolmetin	C	Unknown
Fenamates (anthranilic acids)		
Meclofenamate	D	Not recommended
Mefenamic acid	C	Safe
Oxicams		
Piroxicam	C	Safe
Propionic acids		
Carprofen	C	Unknown
Fenoprofen	B, D in third trimester	Safe
Flurbiprofen	B	Unknown
Ibuprofen	B, D in third trimester	Safe
Ketoprofen	B	Unknown
Naproxen	B	Safe
Oxaprozin	C	Unknown
Pyrazolones		
Phenylbutazone	C	Safe
Selective COX-2 inhibitors		
Celecoxib	C	Unknown
Meloxicam	C	Unknown
Rofecoxib	C	Unknown
Valdecoxib	C	Unknown

COX, cyclooxygenase.

CLINICAL PRESENTATION

Acute Overdosage

Depending on the amount ingested, a patient may present with effects ranging from no symptoms to CNS depression with severe metabolic acidosis. The risk of major toxicity increases with the dose. CNS effects are relatively common with NSAID toxicity. They include changes of mood and cognition (especially in elderly persons), seizures, headaches, and hallucinations. They are most frequent after mefenamic acid overdose, but have also been reported after overdose of other highly lipid-soluble NSAIDs such as piroxicam, naproxen, and ketoprofen (40,41).

Many case reports show hepatic transaminase elevations with NSAID use and overdose (42). Fulminant hepatic failure occurs rarely.

Acute renal insufficiency is rare and usually reversible after acute ingestion. A 24-month-old boy ingesting 640 mg/kg of ibuprofen by history was reported to have a transient rise in serum creatinine with elevation to 2.1 mg/dl from baseline. Elevation began 11 hours after ingestion peaking at 27 hours post-ingestion and returned to normal by 72 hours. A 4-hour ibuprofen plasma concentration was 1724 μmol (therapeutic concentration, 50 to 250 μmol). Pediatric ingestions greater than 400 mg/kg require renal function monitoring.

Adverse Events

GI and renal injury are the most common events. NSAID use increases the risk of developing a gastric ulcer. Several large studies have shown a 2% to 4% incidence of serious GI complication requiring hospitalization in patients chronically taking NSAIDs (43,44). Other estimates are that 30% of patients on long-term NSAID experience at least one ulcer event (43). In large studies, H_2 blockers and antacids have failed to prevent the development of gastric ulcers. The combination drug diclofenac/misoprostol (misoprostol is a synthetic type E_1 prostaglandin) shows promise in being a synthetic prostaglandin but causes many other adverse events. The COX-2 inhibitors also likely decrease the frequency of gastric ulceration.

Concomitant *H. pylori* infection may potentiate gastric ulcer development, but this has not been proven unequivocally (37). NSAID effect on gastric mucosa is relatively minor compared to the COX-1 inhibitory effect. Therefore, enteric-coated NSAIDs may offer little theoretic advantage.

Gastric ulcer risk with NSAID therapy is dose dependent (45). GI adverse reactions remain the most common side effects of chronic NSAID treatment (37): 15% to 20% of patients develop ulcer disease (46). A large study of rheumatoid arthritis patients on chronic NSAID therapy revealed the following risk factors for gastric ulcer development: age older than 75 years, high-dose NSAID therapy, concomitant anticoagulant or corticosteroid use, history of peptic ulcer disease, history of GI bleeding, and history of heart disease (37,43). Other risk factors include the type of NSAID used. A metaanalysis revealed that ibuprofen and diclofenac exhibited the lowest risk for upper GI bleeding. Moderate risk was associated with indomethacin, naproxen, sulindac, and aspirin. Tolmetin, ketoprofen, and piroxicam placed patients at increased risk compared to the other NSAIDs reviewed in the study (47). A potential confounder was that lower doses of ibuprofen and diclofenac were frequently used. Risk increased with dose (47).

Nitric acid (NO)–releasing NSAIDs have been proposed to combat gastric acid risk. NO promotes ulcer healing in animal models (48,49). Because NO is a vasodilator, the mechanism of ulcer healing may be increased gastric perfusion. Modified NSAIDs, such as nitronaproxen, that release NO are being investigated in animals. In addition, the development of NSAIDs with more COX-2 specificity shows promise. Meloxicam is a new coxib. It demonstrates three times the specificity for COX-2 than COX -1.

In a prospective randomized study with 351 patients treated with either rofecoxib 25 mg/day, naproxen 220 mg/day, or placebo, the incidence of hypertension was higher in the treatment groups, probably showing the relationship of NSAID use in susceptible populations.

Drug Interactions

Many individuals take 81 mg of aspirin a day as a cardioprotective measure. Many of these same individuals also take NSAIDs (50). The concurrent ingestion of aspirin and ibuprofen may prevent the binding of aspirin to the platelet, thereby reducing its therapeutic effect (50). This was not true for rofecoxib, acetaminophen, or diclofenac.

DIAGNOSTIC TESTS

There are no specific diagnostic tests to establish the diagnosis of NSAID exposure or toxicity. Ibuprofen plasma levels are not of therapeutic benefit and correlate poorly with outcome (9). For example, a 26-year-old man has a postmortem (51) ibuprofen level of 348.3 μg/ml, whereas concentrations of 704 μg/ml have been asymptomatic (11,52). Because of the lack of correlation with plasma concentrations and clinical effect, a previously ibuprofen nomogram is primarily of historical interest (11,21).

In the patient with intentional overdose, baseline laboratory studies should include complete blood count, platelet count, international normalized ratio, activated partial thromboplastin time, serum electrolytes, including glucose, blood urea nitrogen, creatinine, as well as urinalysis, aminotransferase enzymes, and electrocardiogram as clinically appropriate. A urine pregnancy test should be obtained in women of childbearing age.

Asymptomatic children with an accidental ingestion of more than 400 mg/kg of ibuprofen may merit a baseline set of electrolytes and blood urea nitrogen and creatinine. Renal function tests are probably not required unless there is history of an adult ingesting more than 6 g (21).

Diagnostic Pitfalls

Although symptoms usually appear within 4 hours, there have been a few case reports of delayed symptoms (11).

TREATMENT

The treatment of NSAID exposure is a science of symptomatic support. There is no antidote for NSAID poisoning, and there is no substitute for a careful history. Because some NSAID overdoses can impair CNS function, attention must be paid to airway status and the possibility of aspiration.

In the nonsuicidal patient or unintentional ingestion, a baseline exposure assessment is required. In children, symptoms usually are not evident unless more than 400 mg/kg of ibuprofen has been ingested. The exact amount for other NSAIDs is unclear. Because most is absorbed in 4 to 6 hours, symptoms should be evident by that time.

Decontamination

Because most NSAIDs are rapidly absorbed, *emesis and gastric lavage* are probably not indicated and may be more hazardous than the ingestion itself. *Single dose activated charcoal* has been shown to adsorb ibuprofen and probably binds the other NSAIDs as well. Because NSAID absorption is relatively rapid, delayed use of charcoal is problematic except in intentional overdoses with massive ingestions. Charcoal may be used with or without a cathartic, as is local practice.

The comparative efficacy of activated charcoal and gastric lavage plus charcoal in reducing diazepam, ibuprofen, and citalopram absorption was evaluated in healthy adults (53). Fasting volunteers were given 5 mg diazepam, 400 mg ibuprofen, and 20 mg citalopram. They were treated with either 200 ml water (control), 25 g activated charcoal, or gastric lavage followed by 25 g charcoal in suspension given through the lavage tube. Plasma concentrations of diazepam, ibuprofen, and citalopram were determined up to 10 hours after ingestion. No difference in ibuprofen plasma concentrations was found between the lavage and charcoal groups. Activated charcoal alone may be as effective as lavage plus charcoal and is probably less risky.

Whole bowl irrigation with polyethylene glycol may be effective in limiting ibuprofen exposure. The optimal dose is not clear. In one study, adult male volunteers were given 75 mg/kg of ibuprofen. Thirty minutes after ingestion, either 3 or 8 L of polyethylene glycol solution was administered at the rate of 2 L/hour. There was no difference between groups in area under the curve, time to peak serum concentration, peak serum concentration, clearance, and volume of distribution (54). Use of whole bowel irrigation may be effective in large ingestions or ingestion of extended-release products.

Enhancement of Elimination

In most cases, the toxicity of an NSAID does not warrant an invasive procedure. Because most NSAIDs are more than 90% protein bound, hemodialysis, hemoperfusion, or peritoneal dialysis are unlikely to be beneficial. In cases of profound renal failure, hemodialysis has a support role but no use in drug removal.

Antidotes

There is no antidote for NSAID poisoning.

Supportive Care

Maintain intravenous fluid replacement as necessary.

Prevention of NSAID-induced ulcers remains problematic. Use of antacids and H_2 receptor antagonists was not found advantageous in preventing adverse GI effects in a study of 1921 patients on chronic NSAID therapy (44). Misoprostol shows some promise in chronic exposures but has a poor adverse reaction profile (37). Some recommend that proton pump inhibitors be used with chronic NSAID therapy (55).

REFERENCES

1. Vane J. The mechanism of action of anti-inflammatory drugs. *Int J Clin Pract Suppl* 2003;135:2.
2. Rainsford KD. Discovery, mechanisms of action and safety of ibuprofen. *Int J Clin Pract Suppl* 2003;135:3–8.
3. The history of ibuprofen. Available at: International Ibuprofen Foundation at http://www.ibuprofen-foundation.com/history.htm. Accessed June 18, 2003.
4. Ibuprofen. FDA electronic orange book. Available at: http://www.accessdata.fda.gov/scripts/cder/ob/docs/temptn-det.cfm?Appl_No=018989&TABLE1=OTC. Accessed June 18, 2003.
5. Cherry DK, Woodwell DA. National Ambulatory Medical Care Survey: 2000 summary advance data from vital and health statistics; no. 328. Hyattsville, MA: National Center for Health Statistics, 2002.
6. Paulo A, Lebre L, Chagas C. Celecoxib-induced cholestatic hepatotoxicity in a patient with cirrhosis. *Ann Intern Med* 2002;137:E75.
7. Crofford LJ. Specific cyclooxygenase-2 inhibitors: what have we learned since they came into widespread clinical use? *Curr Opin Rheumatol* 2002;14:225–230.
8. Litovitz TL, Klein-Schwartz W, Rodgers GC Jr, et al. 2001 annual report of the American Association of Poison Control Centers Toxic Exposure Surveillance System. *Am J Emerg Med* 2002;20:391–452.
9. Seifert SA, Bronstein AC, McGuire T. Massive ibuprofen ingestion with survival. *J Toxicol Clin Toxicol* 2000;38:55–57.
10. Lee CY, Finkler A. Acute intoxication due to ibuprofen overdose. *Arch Path Lab Med* 1986;110:747–749.
11. Hall AH, Smolinske SC, Conrad FL, et al. Ibuprofen overdose: 126 cases. *Ann Emerg Med* 1986;15:1308–1313.
12. Linden CH, Townsend PL. Metabolic acidosis after acute ibuprofen overdosage. *J Pediatr* 1987;111:922–925.
13. Volans G, Monaghan J, Colbridge M. Ibuprofen overdose. *Int J Clin Pract Suppl* 2003;135:54–60.
14. Vane JR. Towards a better aspirin. *Nature* 1994;367:215–216.
15. Dionne R. Relative efficacy of selective COX-2 inhibitors compared with over-the-counter ibuprofen. *Int J Clin Pract Suppl* 2003;135:18–22.
16. Cryer B, Feldman M. Cyclooxygenase-1 and cyclooxygenase-2 selectivity of widely used nonsteroidal anti-inflammatory drugs. *Am J Med* 1998;104(5):413–421.
17. FitzGerald GA, Patrono C. The coxibs, selective inhibitors of cyclooxygenase-2. *N Engl J Med* 2001;345:433–442.
18. Crofford LJ, Lipsky PE, Brooks P, et al. Basic biology and clinical application of specific cyclooxygenase-2 inhibitors. *Arthritis Rheum* 2000;43:4–13.
19. Willoughby DA, Moore AR, Colville-Nash PR. COX-1, COX-2, and COX-3 and the future treatment of chronic inflammatory disease. *Lancet* 2000;355:646–648.
20. Wolfe TR. Ibuprofen overdose. *Am J Emerg Med* 1995;13:375.
21. Hall AH, Smolinske SC, Stover B, et al. Ibuprofen overdose in adults. *J Toxicol Clin Toxicol* 1992;30:23–37.
22. Kim J, Gazarian M, Verjee Z, et al. Acute renal insufficiency in ibuprofen overdose. *Pediatr Emerg Care* 1995;11:107–108.
23. Primos W, Bhatnager A, Bishop P, et al. Acute metabolic acidosis due to ibuprofen overdose. *J Miss State Med Assoc* 1987;28:233–234.
24. Hall AH, Smolinske SC, Kulig KW, et al. Ibuprofen overdose—a prospective study. *West J Med* 1988;148:653–656.
25. Zuckerman GB, Uy CC. Shock, metabolic acidosis, and coma following ibuprofen overdose in a child. *Ann Pharmacother* 1995;29:869–871.
26. Roberts LJ, Morrow JD. Analgesic-antipyretics and antiinflammatory agents and drugs employed in the treatment of gout. In: Hardman JG, Limbird LE, Gillman AG, eds. *Goodman & Gillman's: the pharmacological basis of therapeutics*, 10th ed. New York: McGraw-Hill, 2001:687–731.
27. Ibuprofen. In: Basalt RC, Cravey RH. *Disposition of toxic drugs and chemicals in man*, 3rd ed. Chicago: Year Book, 1989:420–422.
28. Marnett LJ, Rowlinson SW, Goodwin DC, et al. Arachidonic acid oxygenation by COX-1 and COX-2: mechanisms of catalysis and inhibition. *J Biol Chem* 1999;274:22903–22906.
29. Gajraj NM. Cyclooxygenase-2 inhibitors. *Anesth Analg* 2003;96:1720–1738.
30. Hamberg M, Svensson J, Samuelsson B. Thromboxanes: a new group of biologically active compounds derived from prostaglandin endoperoxides. *Proc Natl Acad Sci U S A* 1975;72:2994–2998.
31. Svensson J, Strandberg K, Tuvemo T, et al. Thromboxane A2: effects on airway and vascular smooth muscle. *Prostaglandins* 1977;14:425–436.
32. Fujimura M, Sakamoto S, Saito M, et al. Effect of a thromboxane A2 receptor antagonist (AA-2414) on bronchial hyperresponsiveness to methacholine in subjects with asthma. *J Allergy Clin Immunol* 1991;87:23–27.
33. Ohtsuka T, Matsumaru S, Uchida K, et al. Pathogenic role of thromboxane A2 in immediate food hypersensitivity reactions in children. *Ann Allergy Asthma Immunol* 1996;77:55–59.
34. Grönneberg R, Dahlen S-E. Interactions between histamine and prostanoids in IgE-dependent, late cutaneous reactions in man. *J Allergy Clin Immunol* 1990;85:843–852.
35. Takeuchi K, Kato S, Ogawa Y, et al. Role of endogenous prostacyclin in gastric ulcerogenic and healing responses—a study using IP-receptor knockout mice. *J Physiol Paris* 2001;95:75–80.
36. Takeuchi K, Araki H, Umeda M, et al. Adaptive gastric cytoprotection is mediated by prostaglandin EP1 receptors: a study using rats and knockout mice. *J Pharmacol Exp Ther* 2001;297:1160–1165.
37. Bjorkman DJ. One hundred years of NSAID gastropathy: are coxibs the answer? *Rev Gastroenterol Disord* 2001;1:121–127.
38. Goggin PM, Collins DA, Jazrawi RP, et al: Prevalence of *Helicobacter pylori* infection and its effect or symptoms and non-steroidal anti-inflammatory drug induced gastrointestinal damage in patients with rheumatoid arthritis. *Gut* 1993;34:1677–1680.
39. Delmas PD. Non-steroidal anti-inflammatory drugs and renal function. *Br J Rheumatology* 1995;34[Suppl. 1]:25–28.
40. Balali-Mood M, Critchley JA, Proudfoot AT, et al. Mefenamic acid overdosage. *Lancet* 1981;1:1354–1356.
41. McKillop G, Canning GP. A case of intravenous and oral mefenamic acid poisoning. *Scott Med J* 1987;32:81–82.
42. Rodriguez LAG, Williams R, Derby LE, et al. Acute liver injury associated with nonsteroidal anti-inflammatory drugs and the role of risk factors. *Arch Intern Med* 1994;154:311–316.
43. Blower AL. Considerations for nonsteroidal anti-inflammatory drug therapy: safety. *Scand J Rheumatology* 1996;25[Suppl 105]:13–26.
44. Singh G, Ramey DR, Morfeld D, et al. Gastrointestinal tract complications of nonsteroidal anti-inflammatory drug treatment in rheumatoid arthritis. A prospective observational cohort study. *Arch Intern Med* 1996;156:1530–1536.
45. Wolfe MM. Risk factors associated with the development of gastroduodenal ulcers due to the use of NSAIDs. *Int J Clin Pract Suppl* 2003;135:32–37.
46. Armstrong CP, Blower AL. Non-steroidal anti-inflammatory drugs and life threatening complications of peptic ulceration. *Gut* 1987;28:527–532.
47. Garcia Rodriguez LA. Variability in risk of gastrointestinal complications with different nonsteroidal anti-inflammatory drugs. *Am J Med* 1998;104(3A):30S–34S.
48. Takeuchi K, Kato S, Takehara K, et al. Role of nitric oxide in mucosal blood flow response and the healing of HCl-induced lesions in the rat stomach. *Digestion* 1997;58:19–27.
49. Brzozowski T, Konturek SJ, Drozdowicz D, et al. Healing of chronic gastric ulcerations by L-arginine. Role of nitric oxide, prostaglandins, gastrin and polyamines. *Digestion* 1995;56:463–471.
50. Catella-Lawson F, Reilly MP, Muredach P, et al. Cyclooxygenase inhibitors and the antiplatelet effects of aspirin. *N Engl J Med* 2001;345:1809–1817.
51. Kunsman GW, Rohrig TP. Tissue distribution of ibuprofen in a fatal overdose. *Am J Forensic Med Path* 1993;14:48–50.
52. Court H, Streete P, Volans GN. Acute poisoning with ibuprofen. *Human Toxicol* 1983;2:381–384.
53. Lapatto-Reiniluoto O, Kivisto KT, Neuvonen PJ. Effect of activated charcoal alone or given after gastric lavage in reducing the absorption of diazepam, ibuprofen and citalopram. *Br J Clin Pharmacol* 1999;48:148–153.
54. Olsen KM, Gurley BJ, Davis GA, et al. Comparison of fluid volumes with whole bowel irrigation in a simulated overdose of ibuprofen. *Ann Pharmacother* 1995;29:246–250.
55. Chan FKL, Hung LCT, Suen BY, et al. Celecoxib versus Diclofenac and Omeprazole in reducing the risk of recurrent ulcer bleeding in patients with arthritis. *N Engl J Med* 2002;347:2104–2110.

CHAPTER 128

Opioid Medications

Steven A. Seifert

MORPHINE

Compounds included:	**See Table 1.**
Molecular formula and weight:	**See Table 1.**
SI conversion:	**See Table 1.**
CAS Registry No.:	**See Table 1.**
Therapeutic levels:	**Not used clinically**
Special concerns:	**Respiratory depression, central nervous system depression, pulmonary edema**
Antidote:	**Naloxone**

OVERVIEW

Opioid drugs are among the oldest therapeutics known, with references to the beneficial effects of the opium poppy (*Papaver somniferum*) in the Papyrus Ebers in approximately 1500 B.C. (1). Opioids are used therapeutically primarily in treating pain, pulmonary edema, anxiety, cough, and diarrhea. Drugs extracted directly from opium (the dried extract of the poppy, primarily morphine and codeine) are termed *opiates*. Other drugs with opiate-like effects are termed *opioids*, and morphine and codeine are part of this class. Semi-synthetic opioids (e.g., heroin, oxycodone) are derived directly from the opiates. Fully synthetic substances with opioid effects (e.g., meperidine, propoxyphene) have been produced. Synthetic opioids may or may not bear structural similarity to the opiates and may exhibit other pharmacologic effects as well. They may also respond variably to opioid antagonists. Although in the past *opioid* and *narcotic* were synonymous, today the term *narcotic* is used by many to identify any illegal psychoactive substance and the term *opioid* is used to describe the class.

Opioids are available in formulations for oral, subcutaneous (SQ), intramuscular (IM), intravenous (IV), intrathecal, intraarticular, transdermal, transmucosal, and inhalational administration. In 2001, opioids were responsible for 18,833 toxic exposures (0.8%), and 130 deaths (12%) reported to regional poison centers in the United States (2). The opioid drugs of abuse (e.g., heroin) are addressed in Chapter 180. Because of the shared mechanism of action, patients with toxicity from the pharmaceutic opioids are managed similarly. For that reason, the pathophysiology, diagnosis, and treatment of the opioids are addressed for the group, rather than for each agent. However, agent-specific information is also provided for individual agents.

PATHOPHYSIOLOGY OF THE DRUG CLASS

Opioids bind to a variety of receptors in the central nervous system (CNS) and elsewhere in the body. These receptors normally serve to mediate endogenous endorphin (β-endorphin and dynorphin) and dietary opioid effects. The International Union of Pharmacology Committee on Receptor Nomenclature system consists of three major classes of receptors: OP (opiate peptide) 1 to 3, corresponding to prior nomenclature of delta (OP1), kappa (OP2), and mu (OP3) receptors. There are subtypes of these three classes, represented by subscripted letters (a, b, and so forth). These receptors have been sequenced and consist of seven transmembrane segments, with amino and carboxy termini (3). The location and distribution patterns of each class of receptor, and the activated transduction mechanisms, mediate the clinical effects of opioids. There is significant overlap of function and multiple activations, and the system is not completely understood.

OP1 receptors appear to be involved in spinal and supraspinal (brain) analgesia, probably by a noncompetitive interaction with the OP3 receptor (4,5). OP1 receptors are also involved in mediating dopamine release related to amphetamine-associated motor activity (6). OP2 receptors are found primarily in the spinal cord and brain (7). Stimulation of this receptor produces miosis but not respiratory depression. Spinal analgesia and inhibition of antidiuretic hormone release are also mediated by this receptor (8). The OP3, subtype *a* receptors are the primary mediators of supraspinal analgesia. They also appear to be responsible for the psychoactive effects of opioids. OP3, subtype *b* receptors are involved in spinal analgesia and are also responsible for respiratory depression. Although there may be varying degrees of $OP3_a$ and $OP3_b$ activation with any particular drug, all opioids with activity on the OP3 receptors have at least some $OP3_b$ activity, and thus produce some degree of respiratory depression. As a general rule, equianalgesic doses of the various opioids produce about the same degree of respiratory depression. There is diminished sensitivity of the medullary chemoreceptors to hypercapnea and hypoxia (9) and hypoventilation as a result.

OP3 receptors also mediate cough, although the antitussive effect of opioids may also be related to serotonin and *N*-methyl-D-aspartate receptors (10) and are also found in the gastrointestinal (GI) tract (11,12). Other opioid receptors have been identified, although their clinical roles have not yet been elucidated (13,14).

Opioid receptor signal transduction is complex and not completely understood. Receptors are coupled to guanosine triphosphate–binding proteins (*G proteins*) (11). On activation of the opioid receptor, G protein subunits are liberated to produce an effect that may be modification of adenylate cyclase or phospholipase C, ion channel activation, or protein transport. A guanosine 5'-triphosphatase enzyme intrinsic to the alpha subunit hydrolyzes guanosine triphosphate, terminating the receptor-mediated effect (15).

TABLE 1. Physical characteristics and dosage for opioid pharmaceuticals

Compounds included	Molecular formula, molecular weight (g/mol), CAS Registry No.	SI conversion	Formulations	Typical dose	
				Adult	Pediatric
Alphaprodine hydrochloride (Nisentil)	$C_{16}H_{23}NO_2$,HCl; 297.8; 14405-05-1	ng/ml × 3.83 = nmol	NR	0.4–0.6 mg/kg over 3–4 min	0.3–0.6 mg/kg submucosally
Buprenorphine hydrochloride (Buprenex, Subutex)	$C_{29}H_{41}NO_4$,HCl; 504.1; 53152-21-9	ng/ml × 2.14 = nmol	0.3-mg/ml solution	0.3–0.6 mg IV, IM for pain; 0.2–0.4 mg SL	2–6 μg/kg
Butorphanol tartrate (Stadol)	$C_{21}H_{29}NO_2,C_4H_6O_6$; 477.5; 58786-99-5	ng/ml × 3.05 = nmol	1-, 2-mg/ml solutions; 10-mg/ml spray	0.5–2.0 mg IV every 3–4 h, 2–3 mg IM every 3–4 h as needed	Not recommended
Codeine phosphate	$C_{18}H_{21}NO_3,H_3PO_4$,1/2H_2O; 406.1; 41444-62-6	ng/ml × 3.34 = nmol	15-, 30-, 60-mg/ml solutions; 30-, 60-mg tablets	15–60 mg every 4 h	0.5 mg/kg orally
Fentanyl citrate (Actiq, Sublimaze)	$C_{22}H_{28}N_2O,C_6H_8O_7$; 528.6; 990-73-8	ng/ml × 2.97 = nmol	50-, 100-μg/ml solutions; 0.2-, 0.4-, 0.6-, 0.8-, 1.2-, 1.6-mg lozenges	50–100 μg IV; 2 sprays of 10 μg/spray; 400 μg orally; 25–100 μg/h patches	Neonates 1 μg/kg (354); infants, a bolus of 5–10 μg/kg followed by an IV infusion of 1–5 μg/kg/h is used (107); 2–12 yr, 2–3 μg/kg (100)
Hydrocodeine phosphate	$C_{18}H_{23}NO_3,H_3PO_4$; 399.4; 24204-13-5	ng/ml × 3.32 = nmol	NR	5–30 mg PO three times/d	5–10 mg three times/d for children 6 yr or older; 1 and 5 yr, the dose is 2.5–5.0 mg three times/d
Hydromorphone hydrochloride (Dilaudid, Pallidone)	$C_{17}H_{19}NO_3$,HCl; 321.8; 71-68-1	ng/ml × 3.50 = nmol	1-, 2-, 4-, 10-mg/ml solutions; 1-, 2-, 4-, 8-mg tablets; 3-mg suppository	1.0–1.5 mg every 4–6 h IV; 2–4 mg every 4 h PO	0.015 mg/kg/dose IV or IM (355); 0.05–1.0 mg/kg/dose orally (356)
Levomethadyl acetate hydrochloride (Orlaam)	$C_{23}H_{31}NO_2$; 353.5; 43033-72-3	ng/ml × 2.83 = nmol	10-mg/ml solution	20–40 mg PO 3 times/wk	Not recommended
Levorphanol tartrate (Dromoran, Levo-Dromoran)	$C_{17}H_{23}NO,C_4H_6O_6$, 2H_2O; 443.5; 5985-38-6	ng/ml × 3.89 = nmol	2-mg/ml solution; 2-mg tablet	250–500 μg IV, up to 2 mg; 2–4 mg IM or SQ[a]	Not recommended
Meperidine hydrochloride (Demerol, Pethidine)	$C_{15}H_{21}NO_2$,HCl; 283.8; 50-13-5	ng/ml × 4.04 = nmol	25-, 50-, 75-, 100-mg/ml solutions; 50-mg/ml syrup; 50-, 100-mg tablets	1.1–1.8 mg/kg parenterally; 50–150 mg every 3–4 h	1.0–1.8 mg/kg PO, IM or IV
Methadone hydrochloride (Dolophine, Physeptone)	$C_{21}H_{27}NO$,HCl; 345.9; 1095-90-5	ng/ml × 0.0032 = μmol	10-mg/ml solution; 1-, 2-mg/ml PO solutions; 5-, 10-mg tablets	2.5–10.0 mg PO every 3–4 h	0.1–0.2 mg orally
Morphine sulfate (Avinza, MS-Contin)	$(C_{17}H_{19}NO_3)_2$, H_2SO_4, 5H_2O; 758.8; 6211-15-0	ng/ml × 3.51 = nmol	Multiple	5–30 mg PO every 4 h; 2–10 mg IV	0.05–0.2 mg/kg IV; 0.125–0.225 mg/kg every 6 h (354)
Nalbuphine hydrochloride (Nubain)	$C_{21}H_{27}NO_4$,HCl; 393.9; 23277-43-2	ng/ml × 2.8 = nmol	12-, 20-mg/ml solutions	10 mg/70 kg IV, IM SQ every 3–6 h; the maximum daily dose is 160 mg	0.2 mg/kg for ages 10 mo to 14 yr (357)
Tincture of opium (10%) (Paregoric)	NR	—	10% PO liquid	60 mg, four times/d (272); 30–60 mg is given twice/d rectally (358); 5–20 mg IM or SQ (272)	0.01–0.02 ml/kg/dose every 3–4 h
Oxycodone hydrochloride (OxyContin, Oxynorm)	$C_{18}H_{21}NO_4$,HCl; 351.8; 124-90-3	ng/ml × 3.17 = nmol	5-, 10-, 15-, 20-, 30-mg tablets; 10-, 20-, 40-, 80-mg controlled release; 5-mg/ml PO solution	5–30 mg PO every 4 h; controlled-release formulation: 10–80 mg every 12 h	0.05–0.15 orally mg/kg, up to 5 mg/dose every 4–6 h
Oxymorphone hydrochloride (Numorphan)	$C_{17}H_{19}NO_4$,HCl; 337.8; 357-07-3	ng/ml × 3.32 = nmol	—	1.0–1.5 mg SQ every 4–6 h	Not recommended
Pentazocine lactate (Fortral, Talwin)	$C_{19}H_{27}NO,C_3H_6O_3$; 375.5; 17146-95-1	ng/ml × 3.50 = nmol	30-mg/ml solution; 50-mg tablets	30–60 mg IV or IM every 3–4 h; 50–100 mg orally every 3–4 h	Children aged 5–8 yr have received 15 mg and children aged 8–14 yr have received 30 mg with minor adverse reactions (359)
Propoxyphene hydrochloride (Anadin, Darvon)	$C_{22}H_{29}NO_2$,HCl; 375.9; 1639-60-7	μg/ml × 2.95 = μmol	32-, 65-mg capsule	65 mg PO every 4 h (100 mg for napsylate)	—
Sufentanil citrate (Sufenta)	$C_{22}H_{30}N_2O_2S,C_6H_8O_7$; 578.7; 60561-17-3	ng/ml × 2.95 = nmol	50-μg/ml solution	1–30 μg/kg IV	10–25 μg/kg IV, lower in neonates
Tilidine hydrochloride (Tilitrate)	$C_{17}H_{23}NO_2$,HCl,1/2H_2O; 318.8; 24357-97-9	ng/ml × 3.66 = nmol	NR	50–100 mg four times/d PO (322); 50 mg IV (360)	2.5 mg/yr of age up to four times/d, with a minimum dose of 7.5 mg (322)
Tramadol hydrochloride	$C_{16}H_{25}NO_2$,HCl; 299.8; 22204-88-2	ng/ml × 3.8 = nmol	50-mg tablet	50 mg PO; 50–100 mg IV; 100 mg rectally	0.75–1.0 mg/kg (ages 19 yr) (331)

NR, not reported.
[a]Data from Reynolds JEF, ed. Martindale: the extra pharmacopeia (CD-ROM). Micromedex, Inc, 1996.

Opioid Agonists and Antagonists

Opioid antagonists block opioid effects primarily by competitive binding to the OP receptors, although not necessarily equally. Some opioids exert both agonist and antagonist effects, activating some OP receptors and binding to, but not activating, others. OP receptor antagonists may be OP receptor class specific. Agonist/antagonist agents that stimulate OP2 receptors and block OP1 receptors produce efficacious spinal analgesia. And spinal analgesia induced by OP2 stimulation is not reversed by OP1-selective receptor antagonists (7). By an undefined mechanism, low doses of OP receptor antagonists increase the analgesic effect of OP3 receptor agonists (16). Other transmitter systems may interact with the OP receptors. Blockade of the *N*-methyl-D-aspartate receptor enhances the analgesic effect of OP3 agonists and may decrease the development of tolerance (17).

Central Nervous System Effects

The pleasurable effects of opioids appear to be modulated by the release of dopamine in the mesolimbic region (18,19). The production and strength of these effects are variable among the opioids, with some agents (e.g., pentazocine) capable of producing dysphoria. The sense of well-being and euphoria (*runner's high*) that follows strenuous exercise appears to be mediated by endogenous opioids. The effect can be blocked or reversed with naloxone (20). High-dose naloxone (approximately 4 mg/kg) can produce dysphoria in normal individuals (21). Striatal dopamine release may also be related to the development of choreoathetoid movements seen with rapid escalation of methadone dosage (22). Dopamine receptor blockade in the basal ganglia may be responsible for the truncal muscular rigidity seen with rapid IV administration of high-potency opioids (e.g., fentanyl) (23).

Other Mechanisms

Some opioids are pro-convulsant. The mechanisms are unclear. Many opioids cause nausea and vomiting, probably through stimulation at dopamine-2 receptors in the chemoreceptor trigger zone of the medulla. Slowed GI motility and constipation are mediated by the smooth muscle $OP3_b$ receptors in the intestinal wall. Oral naloxone has poor bioavailability and can thus ameliorate this effect without inducing systemic withdrawal. Priapism may result from sympatholytic effects that induce unopposed cholinergic stimulation resulting in vasorelaxation via nitric oxide pathways. In addition, alpha-blockade may be involved (24).

Abuse and Dependence

A distinction can be made between the maladaptive behavior associated with the regular use of opioids and their direct CNS effects. The former consists of opioid abuse and dependency. The latter includes the medical syndromes of opioid intoxication and withdrawal. The American Psychiatric Association has established diagnostic criteria for opioid dependency, criteria for severity of opioid dependency, and diagnostic criteria for opioid abuse (Table 2). Opioid abuse is a maladaptive pattern of opioid use that does not meet the diagnostic criteria of opioid dependence. The central feature is continued use of the drug despite persistent and recurrent social, occupational, psychological, or physical problems caused by the use of the drug.

TABLE 2. Diagnostic criteria for opioid dependence and severity of opioid dependence

Opioid dependence (at least three must be present)
- Opioids are taken in larger amounts or over a longer period than the person intended.
- A desire for the drug persists, or the patient has made one or more unsuccessful efforts to cut down or to control opioid use.
- A great deal of time is spent in activities necessary to obtain opioids (such as theft), taking the drug, or recovering from its effects.
- The patient is frequently intoxicated or has withdrawal symptoms when expected to fulfill major role obligations at work, school, or home (e.g., does not go to work, goes to school or work *high*, is intoxicated while taking care of his or her children) or when opioid use is physically hazardous (such as driving under the influence).
- Important social, occupational, or recreational activities are given up or reduced.
- Marked tolerance; needs greatly increased amounts of the drug—at least a 50% increase—to achieve the desired effect, or a notably diminished effect occurs with continued use of the same amount.
- Has characteristic withdrawal symptoms[a]
  - Either cessation or reduction of prolonged heavy use OR administration of an opioid antagonist after a period of opioid use, followed by at least three of the following (beginning within minutes to days):
    - Dysphoric mood; nausea or vomiting; muscle aches; lacrimation or rhinorrhea; pupillary dilation, piloerection, or sweating; diarrhea; yawning; fever; or insomnia
  - Symptoms cause clinically significant distress or impairment in social, occupational, or other important areas of functioning, AND the symptoms are not due to a general medical condition and are not better accounted for by another mental disorder.
- Opioids are often taken to relieve or avoid withdrawal symptoms.

In addition, some symptoms of the disturbance have persisted for at least a month or have occurred repeatedly over a longer period.

Severity of opioid dependence

Mild	Few, if any symptoms are present in excess of those required to make the diagnosis, and the symptoms result in no more than mild impairment in occupational functioning or in usual social activities or relationships with others.
Moderate	Functional impairment of symptoms is between *mild* and *severe.*
Severe	Many symptoms are present in excess of those required to make the diagnosis, and the symptoms greatly interfere with occupational functioning or usual social activities or relationships with others.
Partial remission	During the past 6 mo, there has been some use of the substance and some symptoms of dependence.
Full remission	During the past 6 mo, either there has been no use of opioids or opioids have been used and there were no symptoms of dependence.

[a]Data from *Diagnostic and statistical manual of mental disorders*, 4th ed. Washington DC: American Psychiatric Association, 1994.
From Ling W, Wesson DR. Drugs of abuse: opiates. In: *Addiction medicine* (special issue). *West J Med* 1990;152:565–572, with permission.

Drug Interactions

The administration of opioids with both agonist and antagonist properties (e.g., nalbuphine, Stadol) may induce a withdrawal syndrome in opioid-dependent patients (25). Administration of opioids with other drugs that depress CNS or respiratory function may result in potentiation of the depressant effects.

Numerous drugs induce or inhibit CYP-450 enzymes responsible for metabolism of the various opioids. Either reduced efficacy or toxicity may result. Approximately 7% of whites, 3% of blacks, and 1% of Asians are poor CYP2D6 metabolizers. If the parent drug is the most active component, poor metabolizers may have drug accumulation with increased and prolonged effects. If an active metabolite is primarily responsible for clinical effects, poor metabolizers may have decreased efficacy (26). Concomitant administration with CYP2D6 inhibitors may produce the same result. A partial list of CYP2D6 inhibitors includes amiodarone, bupropion, celecoxib, chloroquine, chlorpheniramine, chlorpromazine, cimetidine, cocaine, diphenhydramine, fluoxetine, haloperidol, imatinib, methadone, mibefradil, paroxetine, perphenazine, propafenone, propoxyphene, quinacrine, quinidine, ranitidine, ritonavir, sertraline, thioridazine, and venlafaxine.

Concomitant administration with CYP2D6 inducers may also result in increased metabolism and clearance of drug and decreased clinical efficacy. A partial list of CYP2D6 inducers includes dexamethasone and rifampin.

Opioid-dependent patients treated with risperidone developed opioid withdrawal despite regular opioid doses in-hospital. Withdrawal symptoms abated after discontinuance of risperidone (27). The mechanism for this possible interaction is not known.

ALPHAPRODINE

Alphaprodine (Nisentil) is a synthetic phenylpiperidine derivative opioid with agonist analgesic properties similar to meperidine.

Toxic Dose

A 215 lb man died after 20 mg IV. The postmortem blood concentration of alphaprodine was 0.62 mg/L (28).

Toxicokinetics and Toxicodynamics

The volume of distribution (V_d) of alphaprodine is 1.9 L/kg. It is primarily metabolized in the liver to noralphaprodine. The distribution half-life is 4.6 minutes, and the half-life of elimination is 2.2 hours. Five percent of the drug, noralphaprodine, and unidentified conjugated metabolites are excreted into the urine in dogs (28).

Pregnancy and Lactation

Alphaprodine is U.S. Food and Drug Administration (FDA) pregnancy category C. It should be considered category D if used at high doses or for a prolonged period (Appendix I) (29). Alphaprodine crosses the placenta and may produce fetal and neonatal CNS and respiratory depression (30). Alphaprodine also enters breast milk and may produce sedation in the infant (31,32).

Clinical Presentation

Acute overdosage produces signs of opioid toxicity: circulatory and CNS depression, lethargy, coma, respiratory depression, and decreased GI motility with ileus. Miosis is a variable finding, depending on the particular opioid; coingestants; and secondary effects, such as hypoxia. Apnea, hypotension, bradycardia, noncardiogenic pulmonary edema, seizures, dysrhythmias, and death may occur with severe poisoning.

Tolerance and dependence occur. In high doses of alphaprodine, seizures may occur (30), and caution should be used if there is a history of seizure disorder. There may be irritation, pruritus, and a wheal and flare reaction at the injection site (30).

Diagnostic Tests

Plasma alphaprodine levels are not clinically useful. Alphaprodine can be detected by a gas chromatography (GC) method with a detection limit of 0.03 mg/L (33).

Treatment

Acute opioid toxicity is treated with support of respiratory and circulatory function as described at the end of this chapter and may include the administration of naloxone (Chapter 65).

BUPRENORPHINE

Buprenorphine is an opioid agonist/antagonist. It is used for pain relief and has orphan drug status for the treatment of opioid dependence. It may be abused by heroin addicts during times of heroin shortage (34). Its toxicity is similar to other opioids, and it can induce withdrawal in opioid-dependent individuals.

Toxic Dose

The *adult and pediatric therapeutic dose* for analgesia is provided in Table 1. For maintenance of opioid abstinence, a typical regimen is 16 mg/70 kg/week divided into three doses (35). Alternatively, a daily dose of 4 to 8 mg/70 kg is used to prevent opioid withdrawal (36).

One patient ingested 14 to 16 mg of buprenorphine and survived (37). Psychotomimetic symptoms are experienced after total doses of 9 to 12 mg of epidural buprenorphine (38). Prolonged nausea and vomiting develop after IV buprenorphine (39). A dose of 0.8 mg sublingual (SL) for postoperative analgesia was associated in one case with late-onset, prolonged respiratory depression (40), whereas 0.4 mg of SL buprenorphine was not followed by any changes in respiratory function in one randomized double-blind, placebo study (41).

Toxicokinetics and Toxicodynamics

The time to peak serum concentration (T_{max}) is 30 to 60 minutes IM and 150 minutes SL (42,43). Buprenorphine has 90% to 100% bioavailability when given IM and 31% when given SL (42). It is highly protein bound (96%) (44). The half-life of elimination is 2.2 hours (range, 1.2 to 7.2 hours) (45). The mean duration of analgesia is 6.75 to 24 hours (46). The V_d is 97 to 187 L after IV administration (46a). Most of the drug (approximately 70%) is excreted in the feces, whereas 27% of an IM dose and 15% of an oral dose are excreted in the urine (44). Clearance is dependent on hepatic blood flow and biliary tract function (45).

Pregnancy and Lactation

Buprenorphine is FDA pregnancy category C (Appendix I). Buprenorphine is excreted into breast milk (47). Twelve of 15 neonates born to mothers maintained on buprenorphine during the latter 12 weeks of pregnancy displayed no or mild withdrawal symptoms (48). Buprenorphine enters human breast milk and is contraindicated in breast-feeding mothers.

Clinical Presentation

ACUTE OVERDOSAGE

Acute overdosage produces signs of opioid toxicity: circulatory and CNS depression, lethargy, coma, respiratory depression, and decreased GI motility with ileus. Miosis is a variable finding, depending on the particular opioid; coingestants; and secondary effects, such as hypoxia. Apnea, hypotension, bradycardia, noncardiogenic pulmonary edema, seizures, dysrhythmias, and death may occur with severe poisoning.

ADVERSE EVENTS

Nausea and vomiting are common in therapeutic use (15%) (44). Miosis occurs in only 1% to 5% of patients treated with therapeutic doses (45). Hallucinosis has been reported when the drug was given by the epidural route (38). A paradoxical pain response (increased pain) has been reported after high-dose buprenorphine. Naloxone alleviated these symptoms (49).

The incidence of physical dependence is lower than with morphine, although mild withdrawal symptoms may occur after discontinuance of moderate dose (8 mg/day), long-term (50 to 60 days) use (44). Because of its antagonist actions, withdrawal symptoms may be precipitated when buprenorphine is given to patients with opioid dependence.

Diagnostic Tests

Buprenorphine plasma levels are not clinically useful. A radioimmunoassay (RIA) method is available for quantitation of buprenorphine in urine. It has sensitivity to concentrations of 1 ng/ml (50). Buprenorphine and its major metabolite *N*-desalkylbuprenorphine can be simultaneously determined in urine by reverse-phase high-performance liquid chromatography (HPLC). The sensitivity of the assay is 0.2 ng/ml for unconjugated buprenorphine and 0.15 ng/ml for the metabolite.

Buprenorphine and its dealkylated metabolite norbuprenorphine can be detected in urine within 1 to 3 days of intake. After doses of 400, 800, 1600, or 2000 μg SL, mean total urine buprenorphine concentrations were 12.7, 14.0, 27.2, and 11.3 ng/ml, respectively (51). Adults were given 0.4-mg SL doses of buprenorphine 3 hours after a 0.3-mg IV dose. Plasma buprenorphine concentrations 2 hours after the SL dose were 450 to 840 ng/ml, decreasing to 470 ng/ml in 6.5 hours and 310 ng/ml in 10 hours (52).

Preliminary results suggest a dose-response relationship between hair concentration and administered dose (52a). Hair analysis may be useful, but data confirming this are scarce. Detection limits by coulometry are 0.01 ng/ml for norbuprenorphine and 0.02 ng/ml for buprenorphine (53).

Treatment

Acute opioid toxicity is treated with support of respiratory and circulatory function as described at the end of this chapter and may include the administration of naloxone (Chapter 65). Because of its high protein binding, extracorporeal removal of buprenorphine is not likely to be clinically useful. The respiratory depressant effects of buprenorphine are resistant to naloxone. Therapeutic doses of buprenorphine are not readily reversed by 1 mg of naloxone and only partially by 5 mg. Ten mg of naloxone reversed the effects, but the peak effect was not seen for 3 hours (54).

BUTORPHANOL

Butorphanol is a synthetic opioid agonist/antagonist. It is used as an analgesic for moderate to severe headache pain, postoperative or prepartum pain, and as an operative premedication. Toxicity and dependency are similar to other opioids.

Toxic Dose

The *adult and pediatric therapeutic doses* are provided in Table 1. A toxic dosage has not been established, but toxicity can develop after a therapeutic dose, especially in opioid-naïve patients.

Toxicokinetics and Toxicodynamics

The onset of effects after IV or IM dosing is 1 minute and 10 minutes, respectively. The peak effect is reached within 5 minutes when given IV and 30 to 60 minutes IM (55). The duration of effect is 3 to 4 hours when given parenterally (55). Bioavailability is low orally (17%), but 70% intranasally (56,57). Protein binding is 80% to 83% with a V_d of 10 to 13 L/kg (57). The drug is highly lipid soluble (58). Butorphanol is extensively metabolized in the liver and 75% excreted in the urine (57); 11% to 14% is excreted in the bile and 15% in the urine (55,59). Caution should be used in patients with impaired hepatic function (55). The elimination half-life is 4 to 7 hours (55,60).

Pathophysiology

Butorphanol is 5 to 8 times more potent as an analgesic than morphine (61). As an opioid antagonist, it is approximately 1/40 as potent as naloxone and about as potent as nalorphine (62). Butorphanol is an antagonist of the OP3 (mu) receptor, which results in a lesser degree of respiratory depression at equianalgesic doses (61).

Pregnancy and Lactation

Butorphanol is FDA pregnancy category C during therapeutic use and category D if used at high dose or for prolonged periods (Appendix I) (29). Insignificant amounts were found in the breast milk of 12 healthy, nursing mothers treated with IM butorphanol, and the drug may be used in breast-feeding mothers (63).

Clinical Presentation

ACUTE OVERDOSAGE

Acute overdosage produces the signs of the opioid toxicity: circulatory and CNS depression, lethargy, coma, respiratory depression, and decreased GI motility with ileus. Miosis is a variable finding, depending on the particular opioid; coingestants; and secondary effects, such as hypoxia. Apnea, hypotension, bradycardia, noncardiogenic pulmonary edema, seizures, dysrhythmias, and death may occur with severe poisoning.

ADVERSE EVENTS

Sedation is the most common adverse reaction (up to 40% of patients) (59). Nausea and vomiting occur in 13% (55). Use of butorphanol nasal spray for migraine treatment has been associated with hallucinations, feelings of being "extremely stoned" or "stuporous," and feelings of inability to move for hours (64). Sedation, dizziness, nausea, vomiting, insomnia, and nasal congestion have been observed (65). Hypotension, syncope, and severe hypertension may develop (66).

Cardiovascular effects of butorphanol are similar to those of pentazocine, including increased pulmonary artery, pulmonary wedge, left ventricular end diastolic, and systemic arterial pressures, and pulmonary vascular resistance (55). Tolerance and physiologic dependence may develop. A withdrawal syndrome after discontinuance or with the administration of naloxone may occur in patients taking large doses over several weeks, although drug-seeking behavior was not seen (67,68). But abuse, in combination with diphenhydramine, has been reported (69).

Diagnostic Tests

Butorphanol plasma levels are not clinically useful. Butorphanol has been analyzed in biologic fluids by RIA (70), electron-capture GC (71,72), and GC-mass spectrometry (GC-MS) (70). A 1 mg IV dose of butorphanol produced plasma butorphanol concentrations up to 1.3 μg/L within 15 minutes, declining to 0.6 μg/L by 1 hour (71). One hour after a 2 mg IV dose, the serum concentration averaged 1.5 μg/L (70). A 2 mg IM dose produced a peak plasma level of 2 μg/L in 45 minutes, declining to 1.3 μg/L by 4 hours (71). Death from cardiopulmonary arrest has followed its use in surgery (butorphanol blood level was 6 μg/L) (73).

Treatment

Acute opioid toxicity is treated with support of respiratory and circulatory function as described at the end of this chapter and may include the administration of naloxone (Chapter 65).

CODEINE

Codeine is an opiate, a component of opium, and an opioid agonist used as an analgesic, antitussive, and antidiarrheal agent. In Europe, codeine has been used in an illicit synthetic opioid mixture including hydrocodone and dihydrocodeine, called *Brown* (74). Toxicity dependence and tolerance are similar to other opioids. In 2001, there were two fatalities attributed to codeine. Both were in combination with other drugs (2).

Toxic Dose

Codeine is only approximately 60% as potent when given orally as intramuscularly (75). The dose is adjusted according to severity of renal insufficiency. The dose is decreased 25% in patients with a glomerular filtration rate (GFR) of 10 to 50 ml/minute and 50% in patients with a GFR less than 10 ml/minute (76).

In adults, ingestion of 7 to 14 mg/kg may cause death. Much higher doses may be tolerated by chronic users. Ingestion of more than 1 mg/kg of codeine in children is capable of producing symptoms, and doses more than 5 mg/kg have caused respiratory arrest. Children may exhibit increased sensitivity to the effects of codeine.

Toxicokinetics and Toxicodynamics

Oral absorption of codeine is good, but there is a significant first-pass effect. The V_d is 2.6 L/kg (75), and there is minimal protein binding. The onset of analgesic effect is 30 to 60 minutes (75), and antitussive effect is 1 to 2 hours (77). Peak effect is reached in 2 to 4 hours (75). Codeine is metabolized in the liver by glucuronidation to codeine-6-glucuronide, by *O*-demethylation to morphine via CYP2D6, and by *N*-demethylation to norcodeine via CYP3A (78), all active metabolites. There is genetic polymorphism of CYP2D6. Approximately 7% of whites, 3% of blacks, and 1% of Asians are poor CYP2D6 metabolizers. Poor metabolizers have decreased analgesic effectiveness by inhibiting conversion of codeine to morphine (79). Concomitant administration with CYP2D6 inducers may result in increased metabolism and clearance of drug and also produce decreased clinical efficacy. Examples of CYP2D6 inducers include dexamethasone and rifampin.

Between 3% and 16% is excreted unchanged in the urine, and 90% of the absorbed dose is excreted via the kidney (80). The elimination half-life of codeine is 2.5 to 3.5 hours (76) with a clinical duration of action of 4 to 8 hours because of active metabolites (75).

Pathophysiology

Codeine has 1/7 to 1/14 the analgesic potency of morphine. The increased sensitivity to CNS depression in chronic renal failure may be secondary to increased drug sensitivity (81) or to reduced clearance and increased mean residence time (82).

Pregnancy and Lactation

Codeine is FDA pregnancy category C during therapeutic use and category D if used at high dose or for prolonged periods (Appendix I) (29). Codeine enters breast milk, but in nonsignificant amounts after therapeutic dosing. Codeine crosses the placenta (77). Neonatal withdrawal has occurred in children born to dependent mothers (83) and has also been reported in children of nondependent mothers who took 350 to 500 mg/day over an 8-week period (84).

Clinical Presentation

ACUTE OVERDOSAGE

Acute overdosage produces signs of opioid toxicity: circulatory and CNS depression, lethargy, coma, respiratory depression, and decreased GI motility with ileus. Miosis is a variable finding, depending on the particular opioid; coingestants; and secondary effects, such as hypoxia. Apnea, hypotension, bradycardia, noncardiogenic pulmonary edema, seizures, dysrhythmias, and death may occur with severe poisoning.

ADVERSE EVENTS

Codeine is frequently combined with acetaminophen and other drugs, and the potential toxicity of these coingestants should be considered. In therapeutic dosing, hypersensitivity reactions have been reported. The moiety responsible for morphine allergy is believed to be the C-6 hydroxy group, which codeine does not contain (85). True type I hypersensitivity reactions to codeine are rare (86). Nausea and vomiting are common (87). Constipation is also common. Codeine is known to cause spasm of the sphincter of Oddi and may induce pancreatitis in patients with a history of cholecystectomy (88). Tolerance and both physical and psychological dependence may develop, although the incidence is less than with morphine (75). Withdrawal symptoms may occur in dependent individuals if used with opioid antagonists or agonist/antagonist agents.

DRUG INTERACTIONS

Drugs that depress CNS and respiratory function may have additive effects when combined with opioids. Withdrawal symptoms may be precipitated in dependent patients who are given naloxone or other opioid antagonists. Concomitant use of codeine and quinidine results in reduced analgesic effect because CYP2D6 inhibition prevents conversion of codeine to morphine. Other drugs that inhibit CYP2D6 may also produce this effect (89). Drugs that induce CYP2D6 and CYP3A may increase codeine conversion to morphine, with impaired analgesic control (90).

Diagnostic Tests

Plasma codeine levels are not clinically useful. The amount of codeine in commercially available poppy seeds was 78.8 ng/g of seeds (91). Ingestion of poppy seed–containing foods may result in detectable urinary opioids up to 22 hours postingestion (91–93). For the first 10 to 20 hours after an ingestion of codeine, the urinary codeine:morphine ratio is greater than 1. The presence of norcodeine indicates that codeine was taken as the primary drug. Between 20 and 40 hours after codeine ingestion, the ratio of codeine to morphine is less than 1 and norcodeine is not detectable. Three days after codeine use, the urine shows only morphine and is identical to those after heroin or morphine use (94).

Codeine, norcodeine, morphine, and normorphine with their corresponding *O*-glucuronide conjugates can be quantitated by HPLC. The detection limits for codeine, codeine-6-glucuronide, and norcodeine are 5 ng/ml in plasma and 25 ng/ml in urine. Detection limits for morphine are 5 ng/ml in plasma and 20 ng/ml in urine; for morphine-3-glucuronide, 10 ng/ml in plasma and 70 ng/ml in urine; and for morphine-6-glucuronide, 5 ng/ml in plasma and 50 ng/ml in urine (95,96).

Treatment

Acute opioid toxicity is treated with support of respiratory and circulatory function as described at the end of this chapter and may include the administration of naloxone (Chapter 65).

FENTANYL

Fentanyl is a potent opioid used primarily as an analgesic. Toxicity is similar to other opioids, with the relatively unique feature of truncal muscular rigidity in acute overdose. There is significant diversion and abuse of this drug. In 2001, there were eight deaths attributed to fentanyl reported to regional poison centers in the United States. Four involved fentanyl alone and four were in combination with other drugs. Five of the cases involved the fentanyl patch (2).

Toxic Dose

The *adult and pediatric therapeutic doses* are provided in Table 1. The dose in elderly or debilitated patients is reduced. The dose is decreased 25% in patients with a GFR of 10 to 50 ml/minute and 50% in patients with a GFR less than 10 ml/minute (76). There are protocols to convert from parenteral fentanyl to oral, intranasal, or transdermal dosing (96a,97).

Hypoventilation and other CNS effects are more likely with doses resulting in plasma concentrations more than 2 to 3 ng/ml in opioid-naïve patients (97). Six of 12 volunteers given fentanyl 15 μg/kg IV developed muscle rigidity, unconsciousness, and apnea (98). Death occurred in a 43-year-old man who cut, sucked, and chewed a 7.5 mg transdermal patch (98a). Death also occurred in a patient who injected approximately one-half the contents (2.5 mg) of a transdermal fentanyl patch (99).

Toxicokinetics and Toxicodynamics

The onset of action is related to T_{max}, which is rapid IV, 7 to 8 minutes IM, 5 to 15 minutes orally, and 12 to 24 hours transdermally (97,100). The absorption of oral transmucosal fentanyl is 11.1 μg/minute and the oral solution, 3.6 μg/minute (101). The absorption of fentanyl transdermally increases with increased temperature (97). The duration of action is 30 to 60 minutes IV, 1 to 2 hours IM (100), and 72 hours transdermally (97).

Approximately 80% to 86% of fentanyl is protein bound, with protein binding capacity affected by drug ionization. pH changes may also alter distribution between the plasma and CNS (97). Fentanyl primarily distributes to well-perfused body tissues, including fat, with a V_d of 3.2 to 6 L/kg (97,100). The drug accumulates in the fat and is slowly released back into the bloodstream (100).

The distribution half-life after an IV dose is 10 minutes (102). Fentanyl is primarily metabolized by CYP3A4 to inactive metabolites (97). Ten percent of the drug is excreted unchanged, 75% is excreted in the urine, and 9% excreted in the feces, primarily as inactive metabolites (97). Clearance is generally decreased in geriatric patients (97). The half-life of elimination is 3.65 hours after IV injection (100) and 17 hours after transdermal use (97).

Pathophysiology

Fentanyl increases intracranial pressure and decreases cerebral perfusion pressure after bolus administration (103,104). Fentanyl solution is hypotonic and may produce hemolysis if it is infused rapidly (105). Opioid use depresses serum testosterone levels, impairs sperm motility, and interrupts normal hormonal cycles in females.

Pregnancy and Lactation

Fentanyl is FDA pregnancy category C during therapeutic use and category D if used at high dose or for prolonged periods (Appendix I) (29,100). Fentanyl crosses the placenta. Fentanyl can be detected in human milk, but the concentration is not clinically significant (106,107) and fentanyl is considered compatible with breast-feeding (47).

Clinical Presentation

ACUTE OVERDOSAGE

Acute overdosage produces signs of opioid toxicity: circulatory and CNS depression, lethargy, coma, respiratory depression, and decreased GI motility with ileus. Miosis is a variable finding, depending on the particular opioid; coingestants; and secondary effects, such as hypoxia. Apnea, hypotension, bradycardia, noncardiogenic pulmonary edema, seizures, dysrhythmias, and death may occur with severe poisoning.

ADVERSE EVENTS

Death from fentanyl commonly involves pulmonary edema (108). In addition, when fentanyl is administered IV, muscular rigidity, especially of the chest wall, may develop. It may be severe enough to impair air exchange and can result in respiratory depression, apnea, hypoxia, bradycardia, and cardiac arrest, if untreated (100). Such truncal rigidity is often related to peak plasma levels and may last between 7 and 23 minutes (98). However, delayed chest wall muscle rigidity may develop up to 24 hours after administration (109) or 9 hours after ending an IV infusion (110) and may persist for hours. Masseter muscle spasm and laryngospasm may also occur (111).

It is unclear whether seizures may occur. Early reports of seizures were not related in a dose- or concentration-dependent manner, and it is thought that these may have been unrecognized episodes of truncal rigidity (112). Elevated intracranial pressures may occur (113). In general, hemodynamic instability is uncommon. Hypotension and bradycardia are reported (114,115) but are less frequent than with morphine (114). Hemolysis is reported after rapid IV infusion of fentanyl solution (105).

Common adverse reactions to the use of transdermal fentanyl are somnolence, confusion, and asthenia. Toxic delirium may occur (116). Other CNS effects of anxiety, depression, euphoria, hallucinosis, and headache are reported in between 3% and 10% of patients (97). Other adverse effects include constipation, dry mouth, nausea and vomiting, abdominal pain, anorexia, diarrhea, dyspepsia, dyspnea, and urinary retention (97).

Sexual dysfunction is common in men. Women report irregular menstrual cycles. Incapacitating myoclonus has been reported (116a). Sweating and pruritus have been reported at the site of the transdermal patch (97). Erythema, papules, and edema may develop, but less than 1% develop exfoliative dermatitis (97). Heat applied to the patches may increase fentanyl absorption and result in overdose (116b), and heat-related injury may occur (117). A 14-year-old boy developed Raynaud's disease after anesthesia induction with fentanyl and propofol. He developed recurrences of Raynaud's disease on rechallenge on two subsequent occasions (118).

Type I hypersensitivity reactions may occur and may be fatal (119,120). Cross-reactivity with other opioids may occur. Tolerance and dependence may occur. Withdrawal symptoms may occur in dependent individuals if used with opioid antagonists or agonist/antagonist agents. Inadvertent absorption secondary to improper handling of fentanyl patches can occur in health caregivers (120a).

ABUSE

Abuse of the fentanyl transdermal patch is reported. Multiple patches may be applied; the contents ingested, volatilized, and inhaled; and extracted and injected IV (99,121–124). Application of a fentanyl patch to the scrotum (125) or chewing the patch (126) resulted in coma secondary to rapid absorption and overdosage. Sufficient drug remains in the patch for abuse after 3 days of transdermal use (122,124). In addition, diversion within the health care system may occur. A 43-year-old man died after cutting, sucking, and ingesting a 7.5 mg transdermal patch. The postmortem femoral blood level was fentanyl 2.5 ng/ml and norfentanyl 4.4 ng/ml (98a).

DRUG INTERACTIONS

Drugs that depress CNS and respiratory function may have additive effects when combined with opioids. Withdrawal symptoms may be precipitated in dependent patients who are given naloxone or other opioid antagonists. Drugs that inhibit CYP3A4 may decrease fentanyl clearance and increase or prolong its effects (97,127). Drugs that induce CYP3A4 may increase fentanyl clearance and decrease and shorten its effects (97). Severe hypotension may occur when fentanyl is combined with β-adrenergic or calcium-channel blocking drugs. The combination of fentanyl and sibutramine was associated with a serotonin syndrome (128). Also, the combination of fentanyl and other opioids with monoamine oxidase (MAO) inhibitors has produced serotonin syndrome.

Diagnostic Tests

Plasma or serum fentanyl concentrations are not clinically useful. Fentanyl is quantifiable in blood and tissues by GC-MS (108). A RIA method is able to detect 0.2 ng/10 ml urine (129). A solid-phase (129a) RIA (Coat-a-Count) can detect fentanyl in blood and urine to less than 0.2 ng/ml (130). A GC method is sensitive in whole blood assays to 0.25 ng/ml (131,132).

Serum or plasma levels greater than 100 ng/ml fentanyl have been measured after IV infusion of high doses to patients (133). Death was associated with a fentanyl concentration of 17.7 ng/ml (132). The usual analgesic doses result in plasma concentrations of 0.2 to 1.2 ng/ml (Table 3) (97). Plasma concentrations up to 20 ng/ml are achieved in surgical anesthesia. Urinary norfentanyl may be detected in the urine as a marker for abuse (134).

POSTMORTEM CONSIDERATIONS

In fatalities, postmortem serum concentrations were 2.5 ng/ml (norfentanyl, 4.4 ng/ml) (98a), 4.9 ng/ml (135), and 17.7 ng/ml (132).

Treatment

Acute opioid toxicity is treated with support of respiratory and circulatory function as described at the end of this chapter and may include the administration of naloxone (Chapter 65). Acute overdoses of fentanyl should be monitored for 24 hours. Administration of between one-fourth and the full paralyzing dose of a nondepolarizing neuromuscular blocking agent may prevent or reduce the incidence of truncal muscle rigidity. The choice of nondepolarizing blocker dose depends on the dose and speed of the planned fentanyl dose (100). Naloxone has reversed truncal muscle rigidity (109,110).

TABLE 3. Therapeutic plasma levels of alfentanil, fentanyl, and sufentanil

Alfentanil[a]	Fentanyl	Sufentanil
100–200 ng/ml (superficial surgery)	1–3 ng/ml (analgesia)	0.05–1.0 ng/ml
200–400 ng/ml (intra-abdominal surgery)	4–10 ng/ml (analgesia for surgery combined with nitrous oxide) >20 ng/ml (unconsciousness, satisfactory for anesthesia if used as sole agent[b])	—

[a]Data from Larijani GE, Goldberg ME. Alfentanil hydrochloride: a new short acting narcotic analgesic for surgical procedures. *Clin Pharm* 1987;6:275–282.
[b]Data from Woods M. Opioid agonists and antagonists. In: Woods M, Wood AJJ, eds. *Drugs and anesthesia: pharmacology for anesthesiologists.* Baltimore: Williams & Wilkins 1990:151.

Based on its high degree of protein binding and fat distribution, extracorporeal measures to enhance elimination are unlikely to be of benefit (136).

MANAGEMENT PITFALLS

Because of the risk of delayed truncal rigidity, and because respiratory depression may last longer than the analgesic effect, patients who have been given IV fentanyl should be observed for a prolonged period. Epinephrine should be avoided in hypotension because unopposed β-receptor stimulation may worsen hypotension.

HYDROCODEINE

Hydrocodeine is an opiate structural congener of morphine that is used for cough suppression and as an analgesic. It is also called *dihydrocodeine* and is available in phosphate and tartrate forms. Toxicity is similar to other opioids.

Toxic Dose

The *adult and pediatric therapeutic doses* are provided in Table 1. The dose may need to be adjusted in patients with renal insufficiency as absorption, distribution, metabolism, and excretion are all affected (137,138). The dose interval should be lengthened in patients on dialysis (139).

Ingestion of 2.1 g resulted in respiratory depression 36 hours postingestion and required large doses of naloxone (46.6 mg) over a prolonged period (106 hours) (140).

Toxicokinetics and Toxicodynamics

Bioavailability is 21% (141). Absorption is rapid. The distribution half-life is 0.3 hour. The V_d is 1.1 to 1.3 L/kg (141,142). The oral T_{max} is 0.45 to 1.7 hours (143). Onset of analgesia after an oral dose is 30 minutes, with a peak response in 1.25 to 3.0 hours (143,144). The duration of action is 3 to 6 hours (144). Metabolism is primarily via the liver, followed by urinary excretion, with 31.1% of the dose excreted unchanged (145). The half-life of elimination is 3.4 to 4.5 hours (139,141,142).

Pregnancy and Lactation

Hydrocodeine is FDA pregnancy category B in therapeutic use or category D if used for prolonged periods or in high doses at term (Appendix I) (29).

Clinical Presentation

Acute overdosage produces signs of opioid toxicity: circulatory and CNS depression, lethargy, coma, respiratory depression, and decreased GI motility with ileus. Miosis is a variable finding, depending on the particular opioid; coingestants; and secondary effects, such as hypoxia. Apnea, hypotension, bradycardia, noncardiogenic pulmonary edema, seizures, dysrhythmias, and death may occur with severe poisoning.

ADVERSE EVENTS

True type I hypersensitivity reactions are rare but have been reported (146).

WITHDRAWAL

Abuse and dependence may occur (147). On discontinuation, withdrawal symptoms may occur (148). Opioid antagonists, such as naloxone, or agonist/antagonist agents, such as nalbuphine, may precipitate withdrawal symptoms in dependent individuals. In therapeutic dosing, hypersensitivity reactions have been reported, and cross-reactivity with other opioids may occur. Tolerance and both physical and psychological dependence may develop but are less common than with morphine (75). Withdrawal symptoms may occur in dependent individuals if used with opioid antagonists or agonist/antagonist agents. In Europe, there are reports of an illicit mixture, called *Brown*, which consists of codeine, hydrocodone, and dihydrocodeine. Fatalities have been reported (74).

DRUG INTERACTIONS

Drugs that induce CYP-450 enzymes involved in dihydrocodeine metabolism, such as rifampin, decrease dihydrocodeine serum levels and analgesic efficacy.

Diagnostic Tests

Plasma concentrations are not clinically useful. Dihydrocodeine may be detected in the urine by GC-MS (148a). A plasma concentration of 1 mg/L was associated with CNS depression (142).

Treatment

Acute opioid toxicity is treated with support of respiratory and circulatory function as described at the end of this chapter and may include the administration of naloxone (Chapter 65).

HYDROMORPHONE

Hydromorphone is a high potency, semisynthetic opioid used primarily as an analgesic. It is sometimes combined with methylphenidate and clonidine to enhance its analgesic effect and decrease sedation. Toxicity is similar to other opioids.

Toxic Dose

The *adult and pediatric therapeutic dose* is provided in Table 1. Hydromorphone is five to six times more potent than morphine and three times more potent than heroin. The dose may be increased by 25% to 50% every 24 to 48 hours until pain is controlled or toxicity occurs (149). Dose adjustment should be considered in patients with significant hepatic dysfunction (150).

Toxicokinetics and Toxicodynamics

Oral bioavailability is 62% (151). The V_d is 1.22 L/kg (151). Metabolism is primarily via the liver, with metabolites and unchanged drug excreted in the urine (152). The parent drug has a half-life of elimination of 2.5 hours (151). The duration of analgesic effect is 4 to 5 hours (150) and approximately 13 hours for the sustained-release formulation (153).

Pregnancy and Lactation

Hydromorphone is FDA pregnancy category B in therapeutic use or category D if used for prolonged periods or in high doses at term (Appendix I) (29). Hydromorphone is present in breast milk in only trace amounts (154).

Clinical Presentation

ACUTE OVERDOSAGE

Acute overdosage produces signs of opioid toxicity: circulatory and CNS depression, lethargy, coma, respiratory depression, and decreased GI motility with ileus. Miosis is a variable finding, depending on the particular opioid; coingestants; and secondary effects, such as hypoxia. Apnea, hypotension, bradycardia, noncardiogenic pulmonary edema, seizures, dysrhythmias, and death may occur with severe poisoning.

ADVERSE EVENTS

The incidence of all adverse effects was 18% with hydromorphone compared with 6% of morphine, 4% of methadone, and 4% of codeine recipients (155). Seizures and myoclonus have occurred with high parenteral doses (156). Nausea and vomiting are common with oral dosing (150), and constipation occurred in 40% of patients receiving it parenterally (155). Ureteral spasm is reported (150). When given by continuous SQ infusion, local edema, inflammation, and infection may occur (157). Tolerance and dependence develop. Withdrawal symptoms may occur in dependent individuals if used with opioid antagonists or agonist/antagonist agents.

DRUG INTERACTIONS

Drugs that induce CYP-450 enzymes involved in the metabolism of hydromorphone, such as rifampin and rifabutin, result in decreased serum concentrations and clinical effect (90).

Diagnostic Tests

Plasma hydromorphone concentrations are not clinically useful. Plasma concentrations of 4 ng/ml or more are needed for analgesia (158). Hydromorphone is detected by the enzyme-multiplied immunoassay technique (EMIT) immunoassay. Plasma concentrations (in normal human volunteers) reached an average peak of 0.022 ng/L 0.8 hour after a single 4-mg dose (159). An HPLC method has been used for plasma hydromorphone determination; the detection limit is 0.1 ng/ml (160).

POSTMORTEM CONSIDERATIONS

Two fatalities exhibited postmortem blood hydromorphone concentrations of 0.5 and 1.2 mg/L, respectively. Lethal blood concentrations of hydromorphone (more than 0.01 mg/dl) were present in 12 individuals who died from the IV use of Dilaudid (161).

Treatment

Acute opioid toxicity is treated with support of respiratory and circulatory function as described at the end of this chapter and may include the administration of naloxone (Chapter 65).

LEVOMETHADYL

Levomethadyl acetate (levo-alpha-acetyl-methadol, LAAM) is a long-acting opioid agonist used as an alternative to methadone for opioid maintenance. It is typically used only when other agents cannot be tolerated or are ineffective. Prescription is limited to FDA-, Drug Enforcement Administration–, and state-approved clinics and for maintenance of opioid dependence in patients hospitalized for other conditions (162). It has orphan drug status for the treatment of heroin addiction. Toxicity is similar to other opioids.

Toxic Dose

The *adult therapeutic dose* is provided in Table 1. Dose adjustments are made at 5 to 10 mg intervals, with at least 2 weeks between dose changes. Because therapeutic concentrations are reached more rapidly with methadone, patients may be started on methadone and then transitioned to LAAM. If administered daily, excessive accumulation of the drug and its metabolites is likely.

Because of extensive hepatic metabolism, dose adjustments may be needed in patients with hepatic impairment. LAAM should not be used in patients with a prolonged QT interval and therapy reconsidered if QT prolongation occurs during therapy. Ingestion of 20 mg/day of LAAM for 3 days followed by 40 mg on the fourth day in an adult resulted in respiratory failure, noncardiogenic pulmonary edema, and rhabdomyolysis (163).

Toxicokinetics and Toxicodynamics

The oral T_{max} is 2 to 4 hours. Protein binding is approximately 80%, although the metabolites nor-LAAM and dinor-LAAM are weakly and reversibly bound (163a). The V_d is 20 L/kg. The drug is metabolized in the liver by CYP3A4 to two metabolites. *N*-demethylation results in nor-LAAM. Demethylation of nor-LAAM results in dinor-LAAM. Both nor-LAAM and dinor-LAAM are more potent opioid agonists than LAAM, achieve higher plasma concentrations than the parent compound, and produce a duration of action of 48 to 72 hours. The half-life of elimination of the parent compound is 35 to 60 hours compared to 30 to 48 hours for nor-LAAM and more than 100 hours for dinor-LAAM. With three times a week dosing, steady-state concentrations are reached in 1 to 3 weeks. Excretion is in the urine and bile (162). Between 4% and 37% of a dose is recovered in the urine (164). Excretion in the bile implies the possibility of enterohepatic recirculation (165).

Pathophysiology

In addition to its opioid receptor effects, LAAM inhibits the delayed rectifier current in isolated myocytes *in vitro*, which is likely related to prolonging the QT interval (162).

Pregnancy and Lactation

LAAM is FDA pregnancy category D when used for prolonged periods or in high doses at term (Appendix I) (29). It is unknown if LAAM or its metabolites are present in breast milk.

Clinical Presentation

ACUTE OVERDOSAGE

Acute overdosage produces signs of opioid toxicity: circulatory and CNS depression, lethargy, coma, respiratory depression, and decreased GI motility with ileus. Miosis is a variable finding, depending on the particular opioid; coingestants; and secondary effects, such as hypoxia. Apnea, hypotension, bradycardia, noncardiogenic pulmonary edema, seizures, dysrhythmias, and death may occur with severe poisoning.

ADVERSE EVENTS

LAAM has caused QT prolongation and torsade de pointes. This effect is not dose-dependent. It should not be used in patients with prolonged QT intervals and should be discontinued if prolonged QT intervals develop during therapy. Constipation is reported in up to 20% of patients (162). Visual disturbances, particularly blurred vision, have been reported. Somatic complaints and sexual dysfunction are occasionally reported.

It is unclear what signs and symptoms are adverse effects and which are secondary to withdrawal. Tolerance and dependence may occur. Type I hypersensitivity reactions, but not anaphylaxis, have been reported (166). Withdrawal symptoms may occur in dependent individuals if used with opioid antagonists or agonist/antagonists (Chapter 32).

DRUG INTERACTIONS

Drugs that induce CYP3A4 may increase the metabolism and decrease the clinical efficacy of LAAM. Drugs that inhibit CYP3A4 may result in increased levels of the parent compound, prolonged elimination, and prolonged effect of the drug. Drugs known to prolong the QT interval or to cause hypokalemia or hypomagnesemia may precipitate QT prolongation (162).

Diagnostic Tests

An echocardiogram should be obtained before treatment, 12 to 14 days after beginning treatment, and periodically during therapy with LAAM. Vital signs should be monitored periodically during therapy.

Treatment

Acute opioid toxicity is treated with support of respiratory and circulatory function as described at the end of this chapter and may include the administration of naloxone (Chapter 65). Because of high lipid solubility and a large volume of distribution, hemodialysis or other extracorporeal measures are unlikely to be of clinical benefit (162).

LEVORPHANOL

Levorphanol is a synthetic opioid agonist used in the treatment of moderate to severe pain. It has similar potency to codeine and oxycodone (75). Toxicity is similar to other opioids.

Toxic Dose

The *adult and pediatric therapeutic dose* is provided in Table 1. Because the drug is primarily metabolized in the liver, the dose should be reduced in patients with significantly impaired hepatic function. There is no overdose information available.

Toxicokinetics and Toxicodynamics

The T_{max} is 30 minutes IM and 60 minutes orally. Analgesic effect begins within 20 minutes IV and 60 minutes orally. Serum protein binding is 40% to 50%. There is less first-pass hepatic metabolism compared to morphine (167). It is metabolized in the liver by glucuronide conjugation and then excreted in the urine (168). The elimination half-life is 11 hours but may be up to 30 hours with chronic dosing due to drug accumulation (168). The duration of clinical effect is 6 to 8 hours IV and up to 15 hours orally (167).

Pregnancy and Lactation

Levorphanol is FDA pregnancy category C or category D if used for prolonged periods or in high doses at term (Appendix I) (29). Its safety in breast-feeding is unknown (47).

Clinical Presentation

Tolerance and dependence can develop. Cross-reactivity with other opioids is possible. However, studies indicate that cross-reactivity is unlikely with meperidine, morphine, naltrexone, pentazocine, or propoxyphene (167). Withdrawal symptoms may occur in dependent individuals if used with opioid antagonists or agonist/antagonist agents.

Diagnostic Tests

Plasma levels are not clinically useful. A semiquantitative immunoassay has been developed for levorphanol.

Treatment

Acute opioid toxicity is treated with support of respiratory and circulatory function as described at the end of this chapter and may include the administration of naloxone (Chapter 65).

MEPERIDINE

Meperidine is a synthetic opioid used as an analgesic for moderate to severe pain, including obstetric analgesia and as a preoperative medication.

Toxic Dose

The *adult and pediatric therapeutic dose* is provided in Table 1. The dose is reduced 25% in patients with a GFR of 10 to 50 ml/minute and should be reduced 50% in patients with a GFR of less than 10 ml/minute. The dose should also be reduced in patients with significantly impaired hepatic function (169). Patients with hypothyroidism, Addison's disease, and conditions predisposing to urinary retention (prostatic hypertrophy or urethral strictures) should also receive reduced initial doses.

Daily doses of meperidine more than 25 mg/kg may be associated with seizures, especially in the presence of renal impairment or if it is administered orally. Seizures have occurred after a total dose of 3000 mg over 24 hours (170) and after 1500 mg in 12 hours (171). Infusion rates of 25 mg/kg/hour also may precipitate seizures (172).

Toxicokinetics and Toxicodynamics

The onset of analgesic effect is within 10 minutes IM or SQ and within 20 to 30 orally. Significant first-pass effect occurs, and less than 50% of the dose reaches the circulation. Protein binding is 65% to 80% (76); α_1-acid glycoprotein is the main plasma protein that binds meperidine. Plasma α_1-acid glycoprotein may be increased in patients with myocardial infarction, trauma, necrotizing enterocolitis, surgery, arthritis, Crohn's disease, and obesity, and this may affect drug protein binding. Increased meperidine protein binding in these patients may partially explain the various degrees of response to meperidine (173).

Meperidine undergoes demethylation in the liver to normeperidine, an active metabolite that causes CNS toxicity. Oral doses of meperidine result in greater amounts of normeperidine formation than equianalgesic parenteral doses (174). Neonates produce normeperidine more slowly than older age groups (175). In patients with alcoholic hepatitis and cirrhosis, multiple doses of meperidine lead to CNS excitation (176).

The distribution half-life is 4.2 minutes (177). The half-life of elimination of meperidine is 3.2 to 3.7 hours, with 53% of the dose excreted in the urine within 24 hours (178). The duration of analgesic effect is 2 to 4 hours. The half-life of elimination of normeperidine is 24 to 48 hours and it may accumulate with repeated dosing (179).

Pathophysiology

Normeperidine has CNS toxicity with excitatory and convulsive effects. Renal failure results in accumulation of normeperidine (179).

Pregnancy and Lactation

Meperidine is FDA pregnancy category B or category D if used for prolonged periods or in high doses at term (Appendix I) (29). Meperidine is considered safe for breast-feeding (29). Because of the risk for CNS depression, alternatives should be considered (180). Meperidine crosses the placenta. Post-cesarean patient-controlled analgesia with meperidine leads to accumulation of normeperidine in breast milk, which is associated with neonatal neurobehavioral depression (181).

Clinical Presentation

ACUTE OVERDOSAGE

Acute overdosage produces signs of opioid toxicity: circulatory and CNS depression, lethargy, coma, respiratory depression, and decreased GI motility with ileus. Miosis is a variable finding, depending on the particular opioid; coingestants; and secondary effects, such as hypoxia. Apnea, hypotension, bradycardia, noncardiogenic pulmonary edema, seizures, dysrhythmias, and death may occur with severe poisoning.

ADVERSE EVENTS

Miotic pupils are not seen with meperidine. Nausea and vomiting are frequent, affecting 75% of pregnant women treated during labor by the subarachnoid route (182), although constipation is seen less frequently than with morphine (67). It also has less spasmogenic effect on smooth muscles than morphine. In addition, CNS toxicity, manifested by tremors, myoclonus, and seizures, and significant drug interactions with MAO inhibitors may occur.

High doses of meperidine produce seizures because of its conversion to normeperidine. Myoclonus usually precedes convulsions (183,184). Predisposing factors for meperidine-induced seizures include doses greater than 100 mg every 2 hours for longer than 24 hours, renal failure, an alkaline urine (decreased excretion), coadministration of enzyme-inducing drugs, coadministration of phenothiazines that lower seizure threshold, and a history of seizures (185).

Tolerance and dependence may occur. Meperidine administration resulted in increased histamine levels in 31% of patients (186). Type I hypersensitivity reactions have been reported, but anaphylaxis is rare (187). Withdrawal symptoms may occur in dependent individuals if used with opioid antagonists or agonist/antagonist agents. Other neuropsychiatric manifestations of meperidine toxicity are summarized in Table 4.

TABLE 4. Neuropsychiatric manifestations of meperidine toxicity

Psychiatric symptoms	Neurologic signs
Shaky feelings	Tremor
Irritability	Muscle twitches
Auditory and visual hallucinations	Myoclonus
Psychiatric signs	Generalized seizure
Agitation	
Hypomania	
Paranoia	
Delirium	
Complex partial seizure	

Modified from Shochet RB, Murray GB. Neuropsychiatric toxicity of meperidine. *J Intensive Care Med* 1988;3:246–252.

DRUG INTERACTIONS

Drugs that inhibit hepatic metabolism of meperidine, such as cimetidine, may increase CNS depression (188). Drugs that induce hepatic metabolism of meperidine, such as phenytoin, increase meperidine clearance, decrease the half-life, and result in decreased clinical efficacy (174). Co-administration with ritonavir may increase the serum concentrations of normeperidine (189). Co-administration of meperidine with an MAO inhibitor may cause serotonin syndrome (169). There should be at least 14 days between discontinuance of MAO inhibitors and use of meperidine. A Parkinson's-like disorder occurred after IV and intranasal use of a meperidine derivative, *N*-methylphenyltetrahydropyridine (190,191).

Diagnostic Tests

Plasma levels are not clinically useful. The EMIT immunoassay detects meperidine. A minimally effective level for analgesia is 0.2 µg/ml (192), and concentrations of 0.7 µg/ml provide relief from severe pain in 95% of cases (193). Patient-controlled analgesia resulted in reduced plasma levels, compared to standard dosing regimens (193a,194). Plasma normeperidine levels and CNS irritability are significantly correlated (184,195). Toxicity is reported with mean meperidine serum concentrations of 10 to 30 µg/ml (195a) and normeperidine toxicity at 450 to 800 ng/ml (196). Twitches were seen with a mean plasma concentration of 463 ng/ml and seizures with a mean concentration of 814 ng/ml (196). Blood concentrations in six deaths ranged from 1 to 20 mg/L of meperidine and 0 to 30 mg/L of normeperidine (28).

Treatment

Acute opioid toxicity is treated with support of respiratory and circulatory function as described at the end of this chapter and may include the administration of naloxone (Chapter 65). Seizures resulting from meperidine use are usually of limited duration, respond to conventional treatment (Chapter 40), and resolve after its discontinuation. Significant resolution of normeperidine-induced neurotoxicity occurred after 4 hours of hemodialysis (197). Naloxone does not prevent or reverse meperidine-induced seizures. Serotonin syndrome is treated with drug withdrawal, supportive care, and cyproheptadine in selected cases (Chapter 24).

METHADONE

Methadone is a long-acting opioid that is used in the maintenance of opioid dependence, as part of a tapered opioid withdrawal program, and for chronic pain. Toxicity is similar to other opioids. Methadone is a Schedule II drug, available for use only through FDA-, Drug Enforcement Administration–, and state-approved treatment programs when prescribed for opioid dependency.

Toxic Dose

The *adult and pediatric therapeutic dose* is provided in Table 1. For opioid maintenance in heroin addicts, doses range up to 180 mg/day and are usually administered as an oral liquid to decrease the potential for diversion (198). A starting dose of 40 mg/day is common, with adjustment to abate opioid withdrawal symptoms. Doses of 80 to 100 mg were more successful in reducing illicit opioid use than a lower dose regimen (40 to 50 mg), but program retention rates were not different (199).

Toxicokinetics and Toxicodynamics

The oral T_{max} is 2 to 4 hours (200). Initial clinical effects begin 30 minutes to 4 hours after an oral dose (200). It has a V_d of 3.6 L/kg and is 71% to 88% bound to serum proteins (201). Metabolism is via hepatic CYP3A4 *N*-demethylation, with excretion of the parent (21%) and metabolites in the urine (202). Smaller amounts are also detectable in the bile, feces, and sweat. The steady-state half-life of elimination is 23 hours (201).

Pathophysiology

Methadone is FDA pregnancy category B, or category D if used for prolonged periods or in high doses at term (Appendix I) (29). Methadone crosses the placenta (203) and can cause a neonatal withdrawal syndrome. Withdrawal may begin within 3 hours of birth (204–206). Symptoms usually develop within 24 hours of birth and have a mean duration of 7 to 10 days (206).

Methadone enters breast milk, but in amounts that are insufficient to prevent neonatal abstinence (207). Maternal doses of 20 mg per day or less are considered safe regarding direct adverse effects (47), but one infant death was attributed to maternal methadone (208).

Clinical Presentation

ACUTE OVERDOSAGE

Acute overdosage produces signs of opioid toxicity: circulatory and CNS depression, lethargy, coma, respiratory depression, and decreased GI motility with ileus. Miosis is a variable finding, depending on the particular opioid; coingestants; and secondary effects, such as hypoxia. Apnea, hypotension, bradycardia, noncardiogenic pulmonary edema, seizures, dysrhythmias, and death may occur with severe poisoning.

ADVERSE EVENTS

Nausea and vomiting are common adverse effects during therapeutic use. Miosis occurs in adults with methadone use, but is variably present in children (209). Deaths occurring soon after initiation of methadone maintenance have been reported. In one series, ten deaths occurred 2 to 6 days after initiation of methadone maintenance (210). The mean starting dose was 53 mg. The mean blood methadone level at death was 2.1 µmol/L. When initial doses higher than 15 to 30 mg are used in an unsupervised setting, respiratory depression may ensue. Death may occur during induction of methadone maintenance when tolerance is incorrectly assessed, and during maintenance when several days' doses are combined. Death can also follow accidental ingestion (211).

Tolerance and dependence may occur. Type I hypersensitivity reactions with localized urticaria have been reported (212), but anaphylaxis is rare. Withdrawal symptoms may occur in dependent individuals if used with opioid antagonists or agonist/antagonist agents. Rapid or abrupt discontinuation of methadone frequently results in the opioid withdrawal syndrome. Withdrawal signs appear between 24 and 48 hours after drug discontinuance and, with decreasing intensity, may last up to 3 weeks (213,214).

DRUG INTERACTIONS

Concurrent administration decreases didanosine concentrations (215). The concurrent use of drugs capable of inducing CYP3A4 results in decreased methadone plasma concentrations and decreased methadone efficacy (189,216,217). Concurrent administration of drugs that inhibit CYP3A4 may result in increased plasma methadone concentrations (218).

Diagnostic Tests

Plasma levels are not clinically useful. An HPLC method for quantitation of plasma methadone levels has a detection limit of 5 ng (219). Plasma methadone concentration appears to increase by 263 ng/ml for every mg/kg of methadone consumed (220). A GC-MS assay can determine both methadone and its metabolite 2-ethyl-1-5-dimethyl-3,3-diphenylpyrrolidine in the urine (221). Good correlation exists between plasma methadone concentrations (ng/ml) and dose (mg/kg/day) at steady state over a wide dosage range (3 to 100 mg/day) (222).

The correlation between plasma levels and clinical effect is poor. A mean steady-state concentration of 0.29 μg/ml was required to produce 50% of maximal pain relief (201), but there was considerable interindividual variability (223). For opioid maintenance, trough serum concentrations of 100 ng/ml appear adequate (224), but the correlation between plasma levels and symptom complaints is poor (225). In deaths, the mean methadone plasma concentration was 0.02 to 0.45 (mean, 0.08) mg/dl, which overlaps the therapeutic dosing range (226).

Treatment

Acute opioid toxicity is treated with support of respiratory and circulatory function as described at the end of this chapter and may include the administration of naloxone (Chapter 65).

MORPHINE

Morphine is used primarily as an analgesic. It is the prototypical opiate of antiquity and the primary opioid found in sap from the opium poppy (*Papaver somniferum*). Morphine is an FDA Schedule II controlled substance. Toxicity is similar to other opioids. Blue-black poppy seeds contain 963.6 ng/g of morphine (91).

Toxic Dose

Adult and pediatric therapeutic doses are provided in Table 1. Intrathecal doses are 0.2 to 10 mg/day, and epidural doses range from 3.5 to 10 mg/day, depending on the degree of initial tolerance. Tolerance may develop during therapy, resulting in the need to increase the dose over time. Caution should be taken to avoid the use of morphine preparations with preservatives in intrathecal or epidural use.

The dose is decreased in patients with impaired hepatic function. The dose is also decreased to 75% of the normal dose (same dosing interval) in patients with a GFR of 10 to 50 ml/minute. The dose is decreased to 50% of normal in patients with a GFR less than 10 ml/minute. No dose supplementation is needed after hemodialysis (227).

Toxicokinetics and Toxicodynamics

Bioavailability is variable: 20% to 40% orally (228). The T_{max} is 1 hour after ingestion of the immediate-release drug (229) and 8.4 hours after the sustained-release product (230). Extended-release capsules have an immediate release component that rapidly achieves therapeutic concentrations (231). The V_d is 3 to 4 L/kg. Serum protein binding is 20% to 36% but decreased in renal failure (178,232). Onset of analgesia is 15 to 30 minutes when administered parenterally. Steady-state plasma concentrations are reached in 2 to 3 days with extended-release capsules (231). Morphine is metabolized in the liver by *N*-demethylation, *N*-dealkylation, O-dealkylation, glucuronidation, and hydrolysis. Codeine, normorphine, and morphine-6-glucuronide (M6G) are active metabolites, whereas morphine-3-glucuronide is inactive and antagonizes the analgesic effect of morphine (233).

M6G has greater analgesic potency than morphine. Approximately 90% of the dose is conjugated to M6G and morphine-3-glucuronide. Elimination is primarily renal, with 90% of a dose eliminated within 24 hours (232). Fecal elimination of unchanged drug is 7% to 10%, and 7% and 10% is eliminated in the bile, but, because most are inactive metabolites, there is minimal enterohepatic effect. The half-life of elimination of the parent compound is 1.5 to 4.5 hours (232). The half-lives of elimination for morphine-3-glucuronide and M6G are 31 and 33 hours, respectively (234). The duration of clinical effect is 4 to 7 hours orally and up to 24 hours when given by the intrathecal or epidural route (232). The half-life of elimination of the sustained-release formulation is 15 hours (230).

Pregnancy and Lactation

Morphine is FDA pregnancy category C (Appendix I) (235). Morphine crosses the placenta at term. Morphine is a vasoconstrictor of placental vasculature and results in absent fetal breathing movements (236). Pregnant patients in labor clear the parent compound almost twice as fast (237).

Infants younger than 1 month of age have a prolonged half-life of morphine compared to older children. The clearance of morphine approaches adult values in the second month of life (238). The milk to plasma ratio of morphine is 2.5:1. Although significant infant plasma levels may develop, breast-feeding can usually be performed safely (47). A breast-feeding infant may absorb 0.8% to 12% of the maternal dose (239).

Clinical Presentation

ACUTE OVERDOSAGE

Acute overdosage produces signs of opioid toxicity: circulatory and CNS depression, lethargy, coma, respiratory depression, and decreased GI motility with ileus. Miosis is common. Apnea, hypotension, bradycardia, noncardiogenic pulmonary edema, seizures, dysrhythmias, and death may occur with severe poisoning.

ADVERSE EVENTS

Morphine reliably produces miotic pupils. Seizures secondary to naloxone-induced withdrawal are uncommon but may occur (240). Tolerance and dependence may occur and abuse potential is high (241). Type I hypersensitivity reactions with localized urticaria have been reported, but anaphylaxis is rare. Morphine administration results in increased histamine serum levels in 10% of patients (186). Pruritus is common after administration of morphine (242). The overall incidence of adverse effects with morphine use is 6%.

Withdrawal symptoms may occur in dependent individuals if used with opioid antagonists or agonist/antagonist agents. Rapid or abrupt discontinuation of morphine may result in the opioid withdrawal syndrome: abdominal cramping, anorexia, diarrhea, generalized pain, gooseflesh, insomnia, lacrimation, restlessness, rhinorrhea, sneezing spells, yawning, and other somatic complaints. Withdrawal signs appear within hours after drug discontinuance and typically last 3 to 7 days.

Diagnostic Tests

Plasma levels are not clinically useful. Morphine and normorphine with their corresponding *O*-glucuronide conjugates can be quantitated in human plasma and urine by HPLC. The detection limits for codeine, codeine-6-glucuronide, and norcodeine are 5 ng/ml in plasma and 25 ng/ml in urine. Detection limits for morphine are 5 ng/ml in plasma and 20 ng/ml in urine; for morphine-3-glucuronide, 10 ng/ml in plasma and 70 ng/ml in urine; and for morphine-6-glucuronide, 5 ng/ml in plasma and 50 ng/ml in urine (243,244).

The minimal morphine plasma concentration required for analgesic effect is 20 to 40 ng/ml, but there is poor correlation between plasma concentration and therapeutic effect or toxicity. Because of tolerance, plasma concentrations 10 to 50 times higher may be required for analgesia. The mean morphine blood level in 10 fatalities was 0.2 to 2.3 µg/g (244a). After an overdose of morphine sulfate, a 14-year-old girl had a plasma morphine concentration of 0.5 µg/ml. She developed an atypical leukoencephalopathy (245).

Blue-black poppy seeds contain 963.6 ng/g of morphine (91). The EMIT immunoassay detects morphine with a detection limit of 0.5 µg/ml. The urine may test positively for opioids within hours after the ingestion of foods containing poppy seeds (92,246,247), and detectable levels may be found up to 24 hours postingestion (91,92). After an overdose of a sustained-release preparation, morphine and its metabolites were detectable in the urine for up to 6 days (234). To limit false-positive results, cutoff values established by the National Institute for Drug Abuse (morphine or codeine = 300 ng/ml) or the Department of Defense (morphine = 4000 ng/ml, codeine = 2000 ng/ml) should be used. Positive tests are confirmed by GC-MS. If the source of a positive result is dietary, both morphine and codeine are present, and differentiation from abuse of these agents is difficult. The ratio of codeine to morphine was not a reliable indicator of the source of opioid (248). In addition, patients on therapeutic codeine also test positively for morphine, because morphine is a codeine metabolite.

Heroin use can be included or excluded, however, by the detection or absence of its 6-monoacetylmorphine metabolite, a compound not produced by the metabolism of morphine or codeine. Past opioid use can also be detected by hair or nail analysis by RIA, HPLC, or GC-MS. A single exposure may not be reliably detected by this method (249). However, drug levels in beard hair are reasonably dose-related, and segmental analysis may allow an approximation of the time and dose of prior drug exposure (250).

Treatment

Acute opioid toxicity is treated with support of respiratory and circulatory function as described at the end of this chapter and may include the administration of naloxone (Chapter 65).

NALBUPHINE

Nalbuphine is an agonist/antagonist opioid analgesic used as a preoperative supplement to balanced anesthesia. Toxicity is similar to other opioids. It can induce withdrawal in opioid-dependent individuals.

Toxic Dose

The *adult and pediatric therapeutic doses* are provided in Table 1. Nalbuphine has approximately 0.5 to 0.9 the potency of morphine (67).

Toxicokinetics and Toxicodynamics

Absorption is rapid. The T_{max} is 0.48 to 0.63 hour after an IM dose and 0.44 to 0.48 hour after an SQ dose (251). The onset of analgesia occurs within 2 to 3 minutes after an IV dose and within 15 minutes of an IM or SQ dose (67). The V_d is 3.8 L/kg (75). Nalbuphine is metabolized in the liver to inactive metabolites (67). The plasma half-life is 5 hours, with a duration of clinical effect of 3 to 6 hours (252). Neonates whose mothers had been given nalbuphine had half-lives up to 11 hours (253). Elimination of unchanged drug and metabolites is primarily in the feces, with only 7% eliminated via the kidney (67).

Pregnancy and Lactation

Nalbuphine is FDA pregnancy category B, or category D if used for prolonged periods or in high doses at term (Appendix I) (29). Nalbuphine crosses the placenta and produces neonatal respiratory depression (252). Prolonged use during pregnancy may result in fetal dependence and subsequent withdrawal (29). It is unknown if nalbuphine is excreted into breast milk.

Clinical Presentation

ACUTE OVERDOSAGE

Acute overdosage produces signs of opioid toxicity: circulatory and CNS depression, lethargy, coma, respiratory depression, and decreased GI motility with ileus. Miosis is a variable finding, depending on the particular opioid; coingestants; and secondary effects, such as hypoxia. Apnea, hypotension, bradycardia, noncardiogenic pulmonary edema, seizures, dysrhythmias, and death may occur with severe poisoning.

ADVERSE EVENTS

Nalbuphine commonly causes sedation, reported in 36% of patients (252). Pain at the injection site is common (253a). Nausea and vomiting occurred in 6% (252). Nalbuphine has fewer adverse hemodynamic effects compared with pentazocine, butorphanol (254), and morphine (255).

Tolerance and dependence may occur, although nalbuphine is considered to have low abuse potential (252). Type I hypersensitivity reactions with localized urticaria have been reported, but anaphylaxis is rare. Withdrawal symptoms may occur in dependent individuals if used with opioid antagonists or agonist/antagonist agents. Rapid or abrupt discontinuation of nalbuphine may result in the opioid withdrawal syndrome.

DRUG INTERACTIONS

Because nalbuphine is an opioid agonist/antagonist, administration to individuals who are opioid dependent may precipitate a withdrawal syndrome.

Diagnostic Tests

Plasma levels are not clinically useful. Tests for evaluation of opioid withdrawal may be needed.

Treatment

Acute opioid toxicity is treated with support of respiratory and circulatory function as described at the end of this chapter and may include the administration of naloxone (Chapter 65).

OPIUM

Opium is the dried sap of the poppy plant, *Papaver somniferum*. Dried opium is a light brown to yellow brown powder and has a characteristic odor. The principal active pharmacologic constituents of opium are morphine (10%), codeine (0.5%), thebaine (0.2%), papaverine (1%), and noscapine (6%). Deodorized tincture of opium contains 10 mg/ml of anhydrous morphine. Paregoric is camphorated tincture of opium. Each milliliter contains 0.4 mg of anhydrous morphine. Opium is used as an analgesic and antidiarrheal. It was used in the past to treat the withdrawal of neonates born with opioid dependency but has generally been replaced by safer medications. There are numerous preparations, including raw opium, standardized opium powder, tincture of opium, camphorated opium, opium suppositories (in combination with belladonna), and papaveretum. Toxicity is similar to other opioids.

Toxic Dose

The *adult and pediatric therapeutic doses* are provided in Table 1.

Toxicokinetics and Toxicodynamics

Opium is metabolized in the liver and eliminated primarily by excretion of unchanged drug and metabolites by the kidneys (256) and, to a lesser extent, the bile (257). Patients with a defect in bilirubin glucuronyl transferase accumulate the active metabolites of morphine, which results in a prolonged effect (258).

Pregnancy and Lactation

Opium is FDA pregnancy category B, category D if used for prolonged periods or in high doses at term (Appendix I) (29). Opium is considered safe for breast-feeding.

Clinical Presentation

ACUTE OVERDOSAGE

Acute overdosage produces signs of opioid toxicity: circulatory and CNS depression, lethargy, coma, respiratory depression, and decreased GI motility with ileus. Miosis is a variable finding, depending on the particular opioid; coingestants; and secondary effects, such as hypoxia. Apnea, hypotension, bradycardia, noncardiogenic pulmonary edema, seizures, dysrhythmias, and death may occur with severe poisoning.

ADVERSE EVENTS

Tolerance and dependence may occur, and the risk of abuse is high. Type I hypersensitivity reactions with localized urticaria have been reported, but anaphylaxis is rare. Withdrawal symptoms may occur in dependent individuals if used with opioid antagonists or agonist/antagonist agents. Rapid or abrupt discontinuation may result in the opioid withdrawal syndrome: abdominal cramping, anorexia, diarrhea, generalized pain, gooseflesh, insomnia, lacrimation, restlessness, rhinorrhea, sneezing spells, yawning, and other somatic complaints.

Opium may be carcinogenic. Mutagenic activity has been shown in *Salmonella* (259), and bladder carcinomas occur in a higher proportion of opium smokers than either cigarette smokers or nonsmokers (260).

Diagnostic Tests

Plasma levels are not clinically useful. The metabolite 6-monoacetylmorphine can be quantified in serum as a good indicator of heroin intake (261). Morphine and normorphine with their corresponding *O*-glucuronide conjugates can be quantitated in human plasma and urine by HPLC with electrochemical detection. Detection limits for morphine are 5 ng/ml in plasma and 20 ng/ml in urine; for morphine-3-glucuronide, 10 ng/ml in plasma and 70 ng/ml in urine; and for morphine-6-glucuronide, 5 ng/ml in plasma and 50 ng/ml in urine (96,261a).

Treatment

Acute opioid toxicity is treated with support of respiratory and circulatory function as described at the end of this chapter and may include the administration of naloxone (Chapter 65).

OXYCODONE

Oxycodone is a semisynthetic opioid analgesic. It is available as immediate or controlled-release (OxyContin) formulations and is often combined with acetaminophen or aspirin in tablet or capsules. All formulations have become drugs of abuse. Toxicity is similar to other opioids.

Toxic Dose

The *adult and pediatric therapeutic doses* are provided in Table 1. Oxycodone is generally given orally, although it has also been used in intrabursal injection (262). Adjustments to controlled-release dosing is made to the dose, rather than the dosing interval, increasing by 25% to 50% of the current dose (263). The sustained-release formulation should be swallowed whole. Broken, crushed, or chewed sustained-released tablets may result in more rapid absorption and toxicity and may be fatal (263). Patients with impaired hepatic function should initiate therapy at one-third to one-half of the usual dose. Patients with renal impairment have increased sedation at standard doses (263). Dosing should be initiated at one-third to one-half of the usual amount in patients undergoing dialysis if they are receiving concomitant CNS depressants (263).

Toxicokinetics and Toxicodynamics

Absorption is rapid, with 60% to 87% of the immediate-release formulation and 50% to 87% of the controlled-release formulation absorbed (263,264). A high-fat meal increases peak plasma concentrations of the sustained-release formulation by 25% (263). The V_d is 2.6 L/kg (263). After oral dosing of the immediate-release formulation, the T_{max} is 1.6 hours (263). Peak pain relief occurred 1 hour after administration, with a duration of action of 3 to 4 hours. The T_{max} is 3.2 hours with the sustained-release formulation. The duration of analgesia is 12 hours (263). Metabolism occurs in the liver by CYP2D6 to the active metabolites noroxycodone and oxymorphone, with elimination of unchanged drug (19%) and metabolites (64%) in the urine (263). Approximately 7% of whites, 3% of blacks, and 1% of Asians are poor CYP2D6 metabolizers and do not obtain adequate analgesia (26). CYP2D6 inducers may increase drug metabolism and clearance and also reduce efficacy.

The half-life of elimination of immediate-release oxycodone is 3.2 hours, and 4.5 to 8.0 hours with the sustained-release formulation (265). Peak plasma concentration, area under the curve values, and elimination half-lives were 50% and 95% higher, and 2.3 hours longer, respectively, in patients with impaired hepatic function, and 50% and 60% higher, and 1 hour longer, respectively, in patients with impaired renal function.

Pathophysiology

It appears that the oxycodone is primarily responsible for the pharmacodynamic and analgesic effects, rather than the metabolite oxymorphone (266).

Pregnancy and Lactation

Oxycodone is FDA pregnancy category B, or category D if used for prolonged periods or in high doses at term (Appendix I) (29). Oxycodone enters breast milk and may induce opioid dependency in the infant.

Clinical Presentation

ACUTE OVERDOSAGE

Toxicity is similar to other opioids. The symptoms and signs of acute overdose are generally the result of predictable excessive opioid effects and include circulatory and CNS depression, lethargy, coma, respiratory depression, and decreased GI motility with ileus. Oxycodone reliably causes miosis, but miosis in an overdose setting is a variable finding, depending on the particular opioid; coingestants; and secondary effects, such as hypoxia. Apnea, hypotension, bradycardia, noncardiogenic pulmonary edema, seizures, dysrhythmias, and death may occur with severe poisoning.

ADVERSE EVENTS

Somnolence (24%), dizziness (16%), nausea (27%), vomiting (14%), constipation (26%), and pruritus (12%) are the most frequently reported adverse effects in therapeutic use. Tolerance and dependence may occur, and the risk of abuse is similar to morphine. OxyContin is an FDA schedule II controlled substance. Type I hypersensitivity reactions with localized urticaria have been reported, but anaphylaxis is rare. Withdrawal symptoms may occur in dependent individuals if used with opioid antagonists or agonist/antagonist agents. Rapid or abrupt discontinuation may result in the opioid withdrawal syndrome. In acute or chronic overdose, the major toxicity may be caused by the combined agent, resulting in acetaminophen or salicylate toxicity. In street use, the sustained-release formulation may be chewed, or crushed and snorted or injected, increasing the risk of opioid toxicity.

ABUSE

In street use, the OxyContin sustained-release formulation is often chewed, or crushed and snorted or injected, increasing the risk of opioid toxicity.

DRUG INTERACTIONS

Drugs that induce hepatic cytochromes, such as rifampin, may increase oxycodone metabolism and thereby decrease efficacy. The concomitant administration of oxycodone and the MAO inhibitor sertraline resulted in serotonin syndrome. The patient had a history of T-cell lymphoma; allogenic bone marrow transplantation; and was on numerous medications, including acyclovir, cyclosporine, fluconazole, folinic acid, oxycodone, methylprednisolone, sertraline, and trimethoprim/sulfamethoxazole. It was believed that a marked increase in the dose of oxycodone precipitated the syndrome (267).

Diagnostic Tests

The relationship between plasma concentrations and clinical effect is not clearly established. In general, higher plasma oxycodone concentrations are associated with improvement in pain scores (268). Plasma concentrations in females are up to 25% higher than in males on a body weight–adjusted basis (263). With steady state dosing, peak plasma concentrations are 15.5 and 15.1 ng/ml and trough concentrations are 7.4 and 7.1 ng/ml of the immediate-release and sustained-release formulations, respectively.

Treatment

The risk of fatality is increased when oxycodone is combined with another CNS depressant or the controlled-release formulation is crushed and inhaled or injected. Acute opioid toxicity is treated with support of respiratory and circulatory function as described at the end of this chapter and may include the administration of naloxone (Chapter 65).

OXYMORPHONE

Oxymorphone is a semisynthetic opioid used to treat moderate to severe pain and for analgesia during labor. It has 8 to 10 times the potency of morphine but lacks the antitussive effect. Toxicity is similar to other opioids.

Toxic Dose

The *adult therapeutic dose* is provided in Table 1. It is not recommended for use in children.

Toxicokinetics and Toxicodynamics

Oral bioavailability is only one-sixth, and rectal bioavailability is one-tenth that of IM administration. The initial analgesic response occurs within 5 to 10 minutes of an IM, IV, or SQ dose and 15 to 30 minutes after a rectal dose. Duration of effect is 3 to 6 hours. Metabolism is primarily in the liver, and the drug is excreted in the urine as the glucuronide conjugate (75). Rectal administration results in slower absorption, lower and delayed peak concentrations, and a longer duration of action than IM dosing (269).

Pregnancy and Lactation

Oxymorphone is FDA pregnancy category B, or category D if used for prolonged periods or in high doses at term (Appendix I) (29). There are insufficient data to establish safety in breastfeeding.

Clinical Presentation

ACUTE OVERDOSAGE

Acute overdosage produces signs of opioid toxicity: circulatory and CNS depression, lethargy, coma, respiratory depression, and decreased GI motility with ileus. Miosis is a variable finding, depending on the particular opioid; coingestants; and secondary effects, such as hypoxia. Apnea, hypotension, bradycardia, noncardiogenic pulmonary edema, seizures, dysrhythmias, and death may occur with severe poisoning.

ADVERSE EVENTS

Tolerance and dependence may occur, and the risk of abuse is similar to morphine. Oxymorphone is an FDA schedule II controlled substance. Type I hypersensitivity reactions with localized urticaria have been reported, but anaphylaxis is rare. Withdrawal symptoms may occur in dependent individuals if used with opioid antagonists or agonist/antagonist agents. Rapid or abrupt discontinuation may result in the opioid withdrawal syndrome.

DRUG INTERACTIONS

Drugs that induce hepatic cytochromes, such as rifampin, may increase oxymorphone metabolism and thereby decrease efficacy.

Diagnostic Tests

Plasma opioid concentrations are not clinically useful. Oxymorphone is detectable by GC-MS. The EMIT, TDx opiates, Abuscreen, and Coat-a-Count assays do not detect oxymorphone in urine (270). Oxymorphone is a metabolite of oxycodone.

Treatment

Acute opioid toxicity is treated with support of respiratory and circulatory function as described at the end of this chapter and may include the administration of naloxone (Chapter 65).

PENTAZOCINE

Pentazocine is an agonist/antagonist opioid analgesic. Toxicity is similar to other opioids. The oral formulation is combined with naloxone to discourage IV abuse. It also may cause leukopenia, agranulocytosis, and seizures. It has approximately the same analgesic potency as codeine and one-third to one-fifth the potency of morphine (271).

Toxic Dose

Adult and pediatric therapeutic doses are provided in Table 1. The dose should be reduced to 75% of the usual dose in patients with a GFR of 10 to 50 ml/minute and to 50% in patients with a GFR of less than 10 ml/minute (76). Bioavailability and elimination half-life are increased with hepatic impairment. Adverse reactions are observed with greater frequency and dose reduction, or lengthened dose intervals may be required (271).

Toxicokinetics and Toxicodynamics

Oral absorption is slow and incomplete. Bioavailability is less than 20% (272). The oral T_{max} is 1 to 3 hours, with a duration of effect of 3 hours (271). After epidural administration, duration of analgesia was 10.6 hours (273). Pentazocine undergoes extensive hepatic metabolism to inactive glucuronidated and oxidated metabolites. The half-life of elimination is 2.0 to 3.6 hours (271). Unchanged drug (5% to 8%) and metabolites are excreted in to the urine and, to a lesser extent, the feces.

Pathophysiology

Pentazocine is both an agonist and antagonist at OP3 (mu) receptors. It is also an agonist at sigma receptors, responsible for its psychotomimetic effects.

Pregnancy and Lactation

Pentazocine is FDA pregnancy category B, or category D if used for prolonged periods or in high doses at term (Appendix I) (29). Talwin NX is pregnancy category C (271). Pentazocine use during pregnancy has been associated with prematurity, growth retardation, and neonatal withdrawal (274). Entry into breast milk is unknown.

Clinical Presentation

ACUTE OVERDOSAGE

Acute overdosage produces signs of opioid toxicity: circulatory and CNS depression, lethargy, coma, respiratory depression, and decreased GI motility with ileus. Pentazocine does not reliably cause miosis, but miosis in an overdose setting is a variable finding, depending on the particular opioid; coingestants; and secondary effects, such as hypoxia. Apnea, hypotension, bradycardia, noncardiogenic pulmonary edema, seizures, dysrhythmias, and death may occur with severe poisoning.

ADVERSE EVENTS

Toxicity is similar to other opioids but also includes seizures, leukopenia, and agranulocytosis with chronic use. Dysphoric symptoms and encephalopathy (psychotomimetic episodes, hallucinations, paranoia, anxiety) are more frequently reported than with other opioids (271). Leukopenia and agranulocytosis usually occur with a latent period of 4 to 24 weeks during chronic therapy (148,275,276). They are usually reversible with discontinuance of the drug. Nausea and vomiting are common adverse effects of therapeutic dosing (271). There are conflicting reports regarding the ability of pentazocine to induce biliary colic (277). There is a case report of oculogyric crisis in a 39-year-old woman who was taking no other medications (278). Stevens-Johnson syndrome and toxic epidermal necrolysis occur rarely (279). Long-term parenteral use may result in local tissue necrosis (including fibrotic myopathy), sclerosis, and calcification (280).

Tolerance and dependence may occur, although the risk of abuse is less than with morphine. Pentazocine is sometimes combined with pyribenzamine in abuse (*Ts and blues*). Seizures are more common with this combination. Type I hypersensitivity reactions with localized urticaria have been reported, but anaphylaxis is rare. Parenteral use of Talwin NX may result in withdrawal in dependent individuals from the naloxone component (281). The onset of withdrawal symptoms may be within 12 hours of the last dose and may persist for up to 1 week (282).

DRUG INTERACTIONS

There is the potential for serotonin syndrome with concomitant use of pentazocine and selective serotonin reuptake inhibitors (128). Tobacco smokers metabolize pentazocine 40% more rapidly than nonsmokers.

Diagnostic Tests

Plasma drug concentrations are not clinically useful. An HPLC method rapidly quantified pentazocine in plasma. The limit of detection is 1 ng/ml of plasma (283).

Treatment

Acute opioid toxicity is treated with support of respiratory and circulatory function as described at the end of this chapter and may include the administration of naloxone (Chapter 65). Higher than usual doses of naloxone may be required to reverse pentazocine (284). If leukopenia; agranulocytosis; toxic epidermal necrolysis; Stevens-Johnson syndrome; or signs of local necrosis, fibrosis, myopathy, or calcifications develop during chronic use, the drug should be discontinued.

PROPOXYPHENE

Propoxyphene is a synthetic opioid chemically related to methadone used as an analgesic. It is frequently combined with acetaminophen or aspirin. Toxicity is similar to other opioids but also includes cardiac dysrhythmias, ototoxicity, delusions, hallucinations, confusion, and seizures. The potential for dependence and abuse is high.

Toxic Dose

Propoxyphene should be used cautiously at a reduced dose or not be administered to patients with severe hepatic dysfunction or renal failure (GFR less than 10 ml/minute) (76,285). No dose adjustment is needed for patients on hemodialysis, however. Dose intervals may need to be increased in the elderly. Toxic effects are seen with doses of 10 mg/kg, and doses of 20 mg/kg or greater are associated with fatalities.

Toxicokinetics and Toxicodynamics

Propoxyphene is readily absorbed, but there is a large first-pass effect (285,286). The T_{max} is 1 to 2 hours on an empty stomach and 2 to 4 hours when taken with food. Propoxyphene is 78% protein bound (76) and has a V_d of 12 to 26 L/kg (28). It is extensively metabolized in the liver, primarily producing the active metabolite norpropoxyphene (90%) and a number of inactive metabolites. Renal excretion is 20% to 25% of the dose (286,287). The half-life of elimination of the parent compound is 6 to 12 hours (285). The half-life of elimination of norpropoxyphene is 30 to 36 hours (285).

Pathophysiology

Norpropoxyphene has CNS toxicity, resulting in delusions, hallucinations, confusion, and seizures. Individuals who smoke tobacco may have increased propoxyphene metabolism. Three times the amount of naloxone was required to reverse propoxyphene analgesia than morphine analgesia (288).

Pregnancy and Lactation

Propoxyphene is FDA pregnancy category C, or category D if used for prolonged periods or high doses at term (Appendix I) (29). Withdrawal has been reported in neonates of mothers who were taking propoxyphene chronically before delivery (289). Small amounts of propoxyphene are excreted into breast milk. It is considered safe in breast-feeding mothers (67).

Clinical Presentation

ACUTE OVERDOSAGE

Toxicity is similar to other opioids but also includes echocardiogram effects, ototoxicity, delusions, hallucinations, confusion, and seizures at high doses. Absorption is rapid, and clinical deterioration may occur within 1 hour of overdose. Prolongation of QRS and QTc duration, heart block, and hypotension are common after significant overdose (28,290).

The symptoms and signs of acute overdose are generally the result of predictable excessive opioid effects and include circulatory and CNS depression, lethargy, coma, respiratory depression, and decreased GI motility with ileus. Pentazocine causes miosis, but miosis in an overdose setting is a variable finding, depending on the particular opioid; coingestants; and secondary effects, such as hypoxia. Apnea, hypotension, bradycardia, noncardiogenic pulmonary edema, seizures, dysrhythmias, and death may occur with severe poisoning. When the drug is injected IV, severe local sclerosis, abscesses, cellulitis, and thrombophlebitis may be seen (291). Limb ischemia and gangrene may occur with intraarterial injection (292). Nausea and vomiting rarely occur with therapeutic dosing but may be present with overdose. There are rare reports of hypoglycemia (293,294) and hepatotoxicity (295).

ADVERSE EVENTS

Tolerance and dependence may occur. The risk of abuse is less than with morphine and similar to that of codeine (198). Type I hypersensitivity reactions with localized urticaria have been reported, but anaphylaxis is rare. Withdrawal symptoms may occur in dependent individuals if used with opioid antagonists or agonist/antagonist agents. Rapid or abrupt discontinuation may result in the withdrawal syndrome.

DRUG INTERACTIONS

When given with ritonavir, serum concentrations of propoxyphene are increased (189). Concomitant administration with carbamazepine results in increased carbamazepine concentrations (296). This does not occur with oxcarbazepine (297). Concomitant administration with doxepin results in significantly increased doxepin and desmethyldoxepin concentrations (298). The prolongation of gastric emptying may result in delayed absorption of acetaminophen, resulting in delayed observation of potentially hepatotoxic concentrations (299).

Diagnostic Tests

Plasma concentrations are not clinically useful. Methods of quantitative analysis have been developed for liquid chromatography (300), mass spectrometry (301), and GC (302). The sensitivity of the EMIT immunoassay for propoxyphene in urine is 2.0 µg/ml. In a case of death after an overdose, concentrations were 9.5 mg/g in the liver, 2.8 mg/g in the kidney, 2.0 mg/g in the brain, and 7.5 mg in the bile (226).

Treatment

Acute opioid toxicity is treated with support of respiratory and circulatory function as described at the end of this chapter and may include the administration of naloxone (Chapter 65). Higher than usual doses of naloxone may be required to reverse propoxyphene. However, if there is no response to 10 mg of naloxone, the diagnosis should be questioned and coingestants or other processes should be investigated.

Toxicity of acetaminophen or aspirin is often the major factor in acute overdoses. Patients who have an uncomplicated ingestion of nonsustained release propoxyphene and who remain asymptomatic and have normal vital signs, echocardiogram, and laboratory determinations after 6 to 8 hours may be safely discharged. Hemodialysis removes a clinically insignificant amount of drug. If adverse effects occur during chronic use, the drug should be discontinued. Ototoxicity may not be reversible (303).

SUFENTANIL

Sufentanil (citrate, molecular weight, 578.68 g/mol) is a synthetic opioid chemically similar to fentanyl. Toxicity is similar to other opioids but includes truncal muscular rigidity.

Toxic Dose

The *adult and pediatric therapeutic doses* are provided in Table 1. The manufacturer recommends a reduced initial dose in elderly or debilitated patients (304). In patients weighing more than 20% of the ideal body weight, the dose should be based on lean body weight.

Toxicokinetics and Toxicodynamics

Sufentanil has a shorter time to T_{max} and a shorter elimination half-life than fentanyl, resulting in a faster onset and shorter duration of action. The onset of effect is 1 to 3 minutes with a duration of 36 minutes (305). Protein binding is 93%, largely to α_1-acid glycoprotein. Plasma α_1-acid glycoprotein may be increased in patients with myocardial infarction, trauma, necrotizing enterocolitis, surgery, arthritis, Crohn's disease, and obesity, and this may affect drug protein binding (306). Binding is also pH dependent, with an increase in plasma pH of 7.4 to 7.8 decreasing binding by 28% and a decrease in plasma pH of 7.4 to 7.0 increasing binding by 29% (307). The drug is highly lipophilic, with a V_d of 1.7 to 2.9 L/kg (308,309). Metabolism is primarily in the liver by *N*-dealkylation and O-demethylation (306). The O-demethylated metabolite has approximately 10% of the activity of the parent compound (306). The half-life of elimination is 15 to 164 minutes in adults (308,309).

Pregnancy and Lactation

Sufentanil is FDA pregnancy category C (Appendix I) (304). Entry into breast milk is unknown.

Clinical Presentation

ACUTE OVERDOSAGE

Toxicity is similar to other opioids but also includes truncal muscle rigidity, especially after rapid IV injection (304). In a rat study, toxic doses produced evidence of limbic system injury (310). The symptoms and signs of acute overdose are generally the result of predictable excessive opioid effects and include circulatory and CNS depression, lethargy, coma, respiratory depression, and decreased GI motility with ileus. It is uncertain whether sufentanil is proconvulsant. It is possible that early reports of seizures were cases of misinterpreted truncal rigidity. Seizures secondary to hypoxia from truncal rigidity may also occur. Pruritus is commonly reported (42% to 88%) (311). Sufentanil causes miosis, but miosis in an overdose setting is a variable finding, depending on the particular opioid; coingestants; and secondary effects, such as hypoxia. Apnea, hypotension, bradycardia, noncardiogenic pulmonary edema, seizures, dysrhythmias, and death may occur with severe poisoning.

ADVERSE EVENTS

Tolerance and dependence may occur. Type I hypersensitivity reactions with fatal anaphylaxis have been reported. Withdrawal symptoms may occur in dependent individuals if used with opioid antagonists or agonist/antagonist agents. Rapid or abrupt discontinuation may result in the opioid withdrawal syndrome.

Diagnostic Tests

Plasma drug concentrations are not clinically useful. Sufentanil blood and cerebrospinal fluid concentrations are quantitated by an RIA method sensitive to 0.05 ng/ml (312,313). A GC-MS method is also available (314). A bolus dose of 0.6 μg/kg epidurally, followed by a continuous epidural infusion at 2 μg/kg/day, produced peak plasma concentrations of 0.027 to 0.074 ng/ml (315).

Treatment

Acute opioid toxicity is treated with support of respiratory and circulatory function as described at the end of this chapter and may include the administration of naloxone (Chapter 65). Truncal muscular rigidity may be treated with benzodiazepines and muscle relaxants, but these may not be effective. Neuromuscular blockade and assisted ventilation may be required.

TILIDINE

Tilidine is a synthetic opioid analgesic structurally similar to meperidine. Toxicity is similar to other opioids.

Toxic Dose

In some countries, tilidine is combined with naloxone to deter abuse (316). The manufacturer suggests a reduced dose in renal insufficiency. Although tilidine is 90% excreted through the kidneys, a more recent study suggests that no uniform dose reduction schedule is needed (317). Ingestion of 1.0 g by a 20-year-old man has been reported; the patient survived (318). A 44-year-old woman was found in a semicomatose state after she ingested 750 mg of tilidine. She also ingested barbiturates. The patient died in 1 hour (319).

Toxicokinetics and Toxicodynamics

Tilidine is rapidly absorbed. Tilidine is a prodrug from which the active metabolite nortilidine is formed by demethylation (320). The mean T_{max} for plasma tilidine and nortilidine concentrations were 0.6 and 1.7 hours, respectively, after an oral dose of 1.5 mg/kg in patients with renal failure (317). Systemic availability of the parent drug is 6% and for the active metabolite nortilidine, 99% (321). The V_d of tilidine is 3.71 L/kg (320). Nortilidine and bisnortilidine are the major metabolites. The half-life of elimination of nortilidine is 3.3 hours after a single oral administration, 4.9 hours after IV administration, and 3.6 hours after multiple dosing (320). The duration of action is typically 4 to 6 hours (322). Renal elimination of unchanged drug is 1.6% of the dose after IV administration and less than 0.1% of the dose after oral administration. Total clearance is 1139 ml/minute (320).

Pregnancy and Lactation

Safety in pregnancy has not been established. Tilidine crosses into breast milk (323).

Clinical Presentation

ACUTE OVERDOSAGE

The symptoms and signs of acute overdose are generally the result of predictable excessive opioid effects and include circulatory and CNS depression, lethargy, coma, respiratory depression, and decreased GI motility with ileus. Tilidine causes miosis but with less potency than morphine (324). Apnea, hypotension, bradycardia, noncardiogenic pulmonary edema, seizures, dysrhythmias, and death may occur with severe poisoning.

ADVERSE EVENTS

Tolerance and dependence may occur. Pruritus has been described. Type I hypersensitivity reactions have occurred, but anaphylaxis is rare. Withdrawal symptoms may occur in dependent individuals if used with opioid antagonists or agonist/antagonist agents. Rapid or abrupt discontinuation may result in the opioid withdrawal syndrome.

Diagnostic Tests

Plasma drug concentrations are not clinically useful. A GC method for quantitation is available. The limit of sensitivity is approximately 1 to 2 ng/ml for tilidine and nortilidine and 5 ng/ml for bisnortilidine (320). Blood levels of tilidine in a fatal overdose were 4.3 μg/ml, with 0.30 μg/ml nortilidine and 0.6 μg/ml bisnortilidine. Tolerance is rapidly acquired in cases of abuse, and blood levels of 30 to 40 μg/ml may be measured (319).

Treatment

Acute opioid toxicity is treated with support of respiratory and circulatory function as described at the end of this chapter and may include the administration of naloxone (Chapter 65).

TRAMADOL

Tramadol is an orally active synthetic opioid agonist analgesic and an analog of codeine. Toxicity is similar to other opioids and also includes seizures and monoaminergic effects. The development of dependence and abuse appears to be less than with conventional opioids.

Toxic Dose

The *adult and pediatric therapeutic doses* are provided in Table 1. Tramadol hydrochloride 150 mg appears to be significantly more effective than the combination of 650 mg of acetaminophen and 100 mg of propoxyphene (325). Elderly patients may require lower doses and should receive no more than 300 mg/day (326).

Three to 5 g orally in an adult is potentially fatal (326). In humans, doses of 500 to 800 mg may cause seizures, respiratory depression, and coma (327,328). An accidental rectal administration of 27 mg/kg to an infant younger than 1 month of age resulted in severe CNS depression. Naloxone was required for 48 hours. The child recovered (329). A 6-month-old child was erroneously given a 100 mg tramadol suppository resulting in seizures, acidosis, and respiratory depression. The child survived with supportive therapy and naloxone (330).

Toxicokinetics and Toxicodynamics

Bioavailability is 75% after a single oral dose but increases to nearly 100% with regularly scheduled doses. The T_{max} is approximately 1.5 hours (325). Therapeutic blood levels in adults are approximately 100 to 300 ng/ml (0.1 to 0.2 μg/ml) (329). Protein binding is 20% (326). The V_d is approximately 2.7 L/kg (326). Tramadol completely penetrates the blood–brain barrier. Cerebrospinal fluid concentrations of tramadol appear to follow closely the serum elimination curve (330). Tramadol is extensively metabolized in the liver via CYP2D6 to an active O-demethylated metabolite and several inactive compounds (326). Approximately 7% of whites, 3% of blacks, and 1% of Asians are poor CYP2D6 metabolizers, which may result in difficulty with analgesic control and drug accumulation. Similar effects may be seen with concomitant administration with CYP2D6 inhibitors. CYP2D6 inducers may increase drug metabolism and clearance and reduce efficacy.

Tramadol has a plasma elimination half-life of 6.3 hours (326). Patients with severe hepatic impairment of cirrhosis had a half-life of elimination of 13 hours (326). Most excretion takes place through the kidneys (331), with 30% of the dose excreted as unchanged drug and 60% as metabolites (326).

Pathophysiology

Tramadol attaches to the OP3 (mu) receptor with low affinity and blocks norepinephrine and serotonin reuptake (325). Most of the analgesic effect of the drug may be secondary to non-opioid properties, via the central monoaminergic pathways. Naloxone only partially reduces the analgesic effect, whereas pretreatment with α_2-adrenergic antagonists significantly blocks the anti-nociceptive effect in rats (332).

Pregnancy and Lactation

Tramadol is FDA pregnancy category C (Appendix I) (326). Tramadol crosses the placenta (331). Small amounts (approximately 0.1%) of tramadol pass into the breast milk (326).

Clinical Presentation

ACUTE OVERDOSAGE

The symptoms and signs of acute overdose are generally the result of predictable excessive opioid effects and include circulatory and CNS depression, lethargy, coma, respiratory depression, and decreased GI motility with ileus. Tramadol overdose may also produce monoaminergic effects as a result of norepinephrine and serotonin reuptake inhibition, and these effects may predominate. Tramadol causes miosis, but miosis in an overdose setting is a variable finding, depending on the particular opioid; coingestants; and secondary effects, such as hypoxia. Apnea, hypotension, bradycardia, noncardiogenic pulmonary edema, seizures, dysrhythmias, and death may occur with severe poisoning.

ADVERSE EVENTS

At effective analgesic doses of 200 mg, nausea (10% to 20%), vomiting (3% to 9%), somnolence, and dizziness have been observed (333). Diaphoresis is frequent, and up to 5% of patients report anxiety, nervousness, confusion, coordination difficulty, euphoria, or sleep disturbance (326). Seizures have occurred after the first therapeutic dose, during chronic therapy, and in acute overdose. Predisposing factors, such as concomitant administration of selective serotonin reuptake inhibitors, tricyclic antidepressants, phenothiazines, a prior history of seizures, or other underlying predisposing medical condition, increase the risk (326).

Constipation occurs less frequently than with morphine (334), and no effect was seen on the bile duct sphincter (277). Other side effects occurring during therapeutic dosing include fatigue, dizziness, vertigo, headache, visual disorders, nausea, vomiting, sweating, dry mouth, constipation, premature beats, euphoria, dysphoria, hallucinations, and changed body perception (330).

Tolerance to the analgesic effect does not generally occur, but dependence may develop (335,336). Nevertheless, the abuse potential appears to be low (1 to 3 cases per 100,000 patients exposed) (335). Regional patterns of abuse may develop. In 1997, the Cincinnati Drug and Poison Information Center reported tramadol to be in the top 20 prescription drugs of abuse (337). Type I hypersensitivity reactions have occurred, but anaphylaxis is rare. Most often, these reactions occur after the first dose (326). Cross-reactivity may occur with other opioids, particularly codeine (338). Withdrawal symptoms may occur in dependent individuals if used with opioid antagonists or agonist/antagonist agents, however, minimal withdrawal signs were observed in naloxone precipitation studies (325).

DRUG INTERACTIONS

Serotonin syndrome may develop when tramadol is combined with agents known to increase brain serotonin [amitriptyline plus clomipramine, citalopram, hypericum (St. John's wort), moclobemide, and sertraline, among others] (339).

Diagnostic Tests

Plasma drug concentrations are not clinically useful. Tramadol concentrations in the cerebrospinal fluid, serum, and urine can be measured by GC-MS (330). There is also an HPLC method for quantitative determination of tramadol and metabolites (340). A serum concentration of 100 to 300 ng/ml is needed for analgesia (340a). An oral dose of 100 mg in healthy individuals resulted in a mean peak serum concentration of 280 ng/ml. Postoperative patient-controlled analgesia resulted in concentrations of 590 ng/ml (341). Administration of a 100-mg suppository to a 6-month-old child led to serum and cerebrospinal fluid concentrations of 20 μg/ml (330).

The electroencephalogram may show a flattened trace, which resolves within 1 week (330).

Postmortem Considerations

Reported postmortem concentrations in overdose fatalities have ranged from 13 to 19.7 μg/ml (336,340,342).

Treatment

Acute opioid toxicity is treated with support of respiratory and circulatory function as described at the end of this chapter and may include the administration of naloxone (Chapter 65). If serotonin syndrome occurs, tramadol should be discontinued and the patient managed with standard measures (Chapter 24). Tramadol may be combined with acetaminophen (Tramadol-N), and evaluation and management of acetaminophen toxicity should be undertaken (Chapter 126). In therapeutic dosing, nausea and vomiting have been managed with a slow titration schedule of metoclopramide (343).

DIAGNOSTIC TESTS IN OPIOID POISONING

Plasma opioid levels are not clinically useful. It is reasonable to monitor blood oxygenation, blood pressure, acid-base status and pulmonary function, and obtain a chest radiograph if there are pulmonary symptoms. Opioid overdoses may produce both a respiratory and metabolic acidosis, secondary to hypoventilation, hypoxia, hypotension, and seizures. Urinary myoglobin should be obtained if there is concern for rhabdomyolysis. Consideration should be given to possible coingestants or contaminants, especially if the overdose was with intent to cause self-harm or if street drugs were involved, and appropriate laboratory obtained for these circumstances.

The typical drugs of abuse urine toxicology screening test is an enzyme-based immunoassay. Not all opioids are detected by such assays, depending on structural similarities and drug concentrations in the urine. False-positives also occur as a result of insufficient specificity of the assay. Saliva may also be tested by immunoassay, providing a semiquantitative value for codeine (344). Dietary sources of opiates, notably poppy seeds, which are derived from a plant related to *Papaver somniferum*, may also produce a positive result on both screening tests and on follow-up testing (92,246). To limit false-positive results, cutoff values established by the Department of Defense should be used. When legal issues are involved, all positive tests should be confirmed by GC-MS. If the source of a positive result is dietary, both morphine and codeine are present, and differentiation from abuse of these agents may be difficult. The ratio of codeine to morphine was not a reliable indicator of the source of opioid (248). In addition, patients on therapeutic codeine also test positively for morphine, because morphine is a codeine metabolite. Heroin use can be included or excluded, however, by the detection or absence of its 6-monoacetylmorphine metabolite, a compound not produced by the metabolism of morphine or codeine. Past opioid use can also be detected by hair or nail analysis by RIA, HPLC, or GC-MS. A single exposure may not be reliably detected by this method (249).

TREATMENT OF OPIOID TOXICITY

The principles of managing acute opioid toxicity are support of respiratory and circulatory function and the administration of naloxone. Early use of naloxone may obviate the need for intubation.

Decontamination

Induced emesis is contraindicated because of the potential for CNS depression and seizures. Activated charcoal may be given for significant ingestions within 1 to 2 hours. When the overdose has been taken orally, consideration should be given to the administration of activated charcoal. Because of the opioid effect of slowing GI motility, activated charcoal may be effective later in the time course after an ingestion (Chapter 7).

Enhancement of Elimination

Some opioids or their metabolites (e.g., normeperidine) are amenable to enhanced removal by hemodialysis or other extracorporeal techniques and should be considered with severe toxicity with these agents, especially in the context of rhabdomyolysis or renal failure (Chapter 78).

Antidotes

Naloxone reverses most toxic effects in acute opioid overdose. The goal of naloxone therapy is return of adequate, spontaneous ventilation. Complete reversal of effects is unnecessary and may be undesirable. The typical dose is 2 mg IV in an adult and 0.02 mg/kg in a child. Higher doses may be required with massive overdose, and the effects of some synthetic opioids may be only partially antagonized. Repeat doses up to a total of 10 mg may be given, but if there is no response to this dose, higher doses are likely to be ineffective and coingestants and alternative diagnoses should be considered. If there is an insufficient response to bolus doses of naloxone, and airway compromise is still present, the patient should be intubated. However, many patients respond immediately and adequately to IV bolus naloxone. After opioid reversal, respiratory status should be observed frequently for redevelopment of toxicity and additional boluses of naloxone given as needed. Further information about naloxone is provided in Chapter 65.

If acute withdrawal is precipitated after naloxone administration, allow the effects to abate. If subsequent doses are indicated by a return of opioid toxicity, use one-half the withdrawal-inducing dose.

Most opioids of abuse have longer half-lives than naloxone. After initial opioid reversal, the need for repeat doses of naloxone does not always occur. Some opioids, such as methadone and LAAM, have long durations of effect. If symptoms of respiratory depression return rapidly or persistently, an IV infusion of naloxone is often preferable to giving multiple boluses or to using a less titratable, longer-acting opioid antagonist. The initial rate, in mg/hour, should be equal to two-thirds of the effective bolus dose and the rate adjusted as needed. If respiratory depression recurs while receiving an IV infusion, administer one-half the initial bolus and repeat until an effective reversal dose is achieved. Then, increase the IV infusion rate by 50%.

Reversal of truncal muscular rigidity induced by high-potency opioids may be accomplished by the use of opioid antagonists, but withdrawal, adverse hemodynamic effects, and reversal of pain control may occur (345). In an animal model, dopamine was effective in alleviating the rigidity (346) but not dopamine agonists, such as amantadine (347).

Naltrexone and *nalmefene* are longer-acting opioid receptor antagonists that may produce a prolonged, intractable withdrawal reaction in opioid-dependent patients and should not be used in the initial resuscitation. Their use may be considered in adults and children with short-acting opioid ingestions, who do not have opioid dependency and who do not develop withdrawal to naloxone. They should generally not be used with long-acting opioids (e.g., methadone) because of the risk of recurrent toxicity after discharge.

Supportive Care

After stabilization of the airway, seizures should be treated with benzodiazepines followed by phenobarbital and more aggressive interventions, if needed (Chapter 40). Naloxone at least partially antagonizes the proconvulsant effects of propoxyphene and meperidine and should be given for this indication. In addition, naloxone may potentiate the anticonvulsant effects of benzodiazepines and barbiturates.

Animal experiments suggest that elevated $PaCO_2$ worsens naloxone-induced pulmonary edema and that adequate ventilation before administration of naloxone may be beneficial (348,349). Ventilatory support may be required. Adequate ventilation and oxygenation with frequent monitoring of pulse oximetry and arterial blood gases should be performed. A high fraction of inspired oxygen and positive end expiratory pressures may be required to maintain oxygenation. Lower amounts of positive end expiratory pressures, small tidal volumes, and lower plateau pressures are associated with decreased barotrauma, decreased mortality, and more rapid weaning from ventilatory support (350).

Hypotension is treated by positioning in Trendelenburg, administration of isotonic crystalloid fluids, H_1 and H_2 receptor blockers (351), and pressors, if needed. A beneficial effect of opioid antagonists in reversing hypotension has not been demonstrated, but its use is often indicated by other effects of toxicity.

When a massive overdose of an opioid has been introduced intrathecally, cerebrospinal fluid aspiration and normal saline replacement have been used successfully (352). The presence of an implanted intrathecal catheter may serve as a port for the introduction of other drugs and may also result in CNS infection, granulomas, and other medical complications, which must be distinguished from opioid toxicity (353).

Ingestion of drugs to avoid arrest (*body stuffers*) or for the purpose of drug smuggling (*body packers*) is addressed in Chapter 12.

Emergency Department Disposition

When to discharge a patient who has awakened after naloxone use is based on available evidence, close observation, and practical considerations. The half-life of naloxone is approximately 20 minutes, with an effective duration of action of 1 to 2 hours. Patients who awaken to a bolus of naloxone, who do not require additional naloxone beyond 2 hours after their last bolus, who are not suicidal, and who do not have complicating medical problems may be safely discharged. Patients who have taken a long-acting opioid, who require multiple naloxone boluses or an IV infusion, who are suicidal, or who develop other complications (e.g., pulmonary edema, aspiration) should generally be admitted.

Management Pitfalls

Release of patients too quickly after revival by naloxone may result in recurrent CNS and respiratory depression.

REFERENCES

1. Bryan C. *Ancient Egyptian medicine: the papyrus Ebers*. London: Ares Publishers, Inc., 1930.
2. American Association of Poison Control Centers. 2001 Annual Report of the American Association of Poison Control Centers Toxic Exposure Surveillance System. Litovitz TL, Klein-Schwartz W, Rodgers GC, et al. *Am J Emerg Med* 2002;20(5):391–452.
3. Chen Y, Mestek A, Liu J, et al. Molecular cloning and functional expression of a μ-opioid receptor from rat brain. *Mol Pharmacol* 1993;44:8–12.
4. Rothman RB, Holaday JW, Porreca F. Allosteric coupling among opioid receptors: evidence for an opioid receptor complex. In: Herz A, Akil H, Simon EJ, eds. *Opioids I, handbook of experimental pharmacology*, vol. 104/I. Berlin, Springer-Verlag 1993:217–237.
5. Traynor JR, Elliot J. δ-Opioid receptor subtypes and cross-talk with μ receptors. *Trends Pharmacol Sci* 1993;14:84–86.
6. Jones DNC, Holtzman SG. Interaction between opioid antagonists and amphetamine: evidence for mediation by central delta opioid receptors. *J Pharmacol Exp Ther* 1992;262:638–645.
7. Millan MJ, Cslonkowski A, Lipkowski A, et al. Kappa-opioid receptor-mediated antinociception in the rat. II. Supraspinal in addition to spinal sites of action. *J Pharmacol Exp Ther* 1989;251:342–350.
8. Piercey MF, Lahti RA, Schroeder LA, et al. U-50,488, a pure κ receptor agonist with spinal analgesic loci in the mouse. *Life Sci* 1982;31:1197–1200.
9. Weil JV, McCullough BS, Kline JS, et al. Diminished ventilatory response to hypoxia and hypercapnia after morphine in normal man. *N Engl J Med* 1975;21:1103–1106.
10. Kamei J. Role of opioidergic and serotonergic mechanisms in cough and antitussives. *Pulm Pharmacol* 1996;9:349–356.
11. Minami M, Satoh M. Molecular biology of the opioid receptors: structures, functions and distributions. *Neurosci Res* 1995;23:121–145.
12. Goodman RR, Snyder SH, Kuhar MJ, et al. Differentiation of δ and μ opiate receptor localization by light microscopic autoradiography. *Proc Natl Acad Sci U S A* 1980;77:6239–6243.
13. Calo G, Guerrini R, Rizzi A, et al. Pharmacology of nociceptin and its receptor: a novel therapeutic target. *Br J Pharmacol* 2000;129:1261–1283.
14. Zagon IS, Goodman SR, McLaughlin PJ. Demonstration and characterization of zeta (z), a growth-related opioid receptor, in a neuro-blastoma cell line. *Brain Res* 1990;511:181–186.
15. Ross EM. Pharmacodynamics: mechanisms of drug action and the relationship between drug concentration and effect. In: Hardman JGJ, Limbird LE, Molinoff PB, et al., eds. *Goodman & Gilman's the pharmacologic basis of therapeutics*, 9th ed. New York, McGraw-Hill 1996:29–42.
16. Price DD, Mayer DJ, Mao J, et al. NMDA-receptor antagonists and opioid receptor interactions as related to analgesia and tolerance. *J Pain Symptom Manage* 2000;19[Suppl]:S7–S11.
17. Crain SM, Shen KF. Antagonists of excitatory opioid receptor functions enhance morphine's analgesic potency and attenuate opioid tolerance/dependence liability. *Pain* 2000;84:121–131.
18. Betz C, Mihalic D, Pinto ME, et al. Could a common biochemical mechanism underlie addictions? *J Clin Pharmacol Ther* 2000;25:11–20.
19. Nestler EJ. Under siege: the brain on opiates. *Neuron* 1996;16:897–900.
20. Davis GC. Endorphins and pain. *Psychiatr Clin North Am* 1983;6:473–487.
21. Collart L, Luthy C, Dayer P. Multimodal analgesic effect of tramadol. *Clin Pharmacol Ther* 1993;53:223.
22. Bonnet U, Banger M, Wolstein J, et al. Choreoathetoid movements associated with rapid adjustment to methadone. *Pharmacopsychiatry* 1998;31:143–145.
23. Ellenbroek B, Schwarz M, Sontag KH, et al. Muscular rigidity and delineation of a dopamine-specific neostriatal subregion: tonic EMG activity in rats. *Brain Res* 1985;345:132–140.

24. Nocchi D, D'az JE. Heroin-induced priapism (abst). *J Toxicol Clin Toxicol* 1999;37:646–647.
25. Preston KL, Bigelow GE, Liebson IA. Antagonist effects of nalbuphine in opioid-dependent human volunteers. *J Pharmacol Exp Ther* 1989;248(3):929–937.
26. Lurcott G. The effects of the genetic absence and inhibition of CYP2D6 on the metabolism of codeine and its derivatives, hydrocodone and oxycodone. *Anesth Prog* 1999;45:154–156.
27. Wines JD, Weiss RD. Opioid withdrawal during risperidone treatment. *J Clin Psychopharmacol* 1999;19(3):265–267.
28. Baselt RC. *Disposition of toxic drugs and chemicals in man*, 5th ed. Foster City, CA: Chemical Toxicology Institute, 2000.
29. Briggs GG, Freeman RK, Yaffe SJ. *Drugs in pregnancy and lactation: a reference guide to fetal and neonatal risk*, 6th ed. Philadelphia: Lippincott Williams & Wilkins, 2002.
30. Product information: Nisentil, alphaprodine. Nutley, NJ: Hoffmann-LaRoche Laboratories, 1987.
31. Pagliaro LA, Levin RH. *Problems in pediatric drug therapy*. Hamilton, Illinois: Drug Intelligence Publications, 1979.
32. White GJ, White MK. Breastfeeding and drugs in human milk. *Vet Human Toxicol* 1980;22:1–43.
33. Fung DL, Asling JH, Eisele JH, et al. A comparison of alphaprodine and meperidine pharmacokinetics. *J Clin Pharm* 1980;20:37–41.
34. Debrabandere L, Van Boven M, Daenens P. Development of a fluoroimmunoassay for the detection of buprenorphine in urine. *J Forens Sci* 1995;40:250-253.
35. Schottenfeld RS, Pakes J, O'Connor P, et al. Thrice-weekly versus daily buprenorphine maintenance. *Biol Psychiatry* 2000;47:1072–1079.
36. Petry NM, Bickel WK, Badger GJ: A comparison of four buprenorphine dosing regimens in the treatment of opioid dependence. *Clin Pharmacol Ther* 1999;66(6):306–314.
37. Banks CD. Overdosage of buprenorphine: case report. *NZ Med J* 1979;89: 255–256.
38. MacEvilly M, O'Carroll C. Hallucinations after epidural buprenorphine. *BMJ* 1989;298:928–929.
39. Fullerton T, Tinu EG, Kolski GB, et al. Prolonged nausea and vomiting associated with buprenorphine. *Pharmacotherapy* 1991;11:90-93.
40. Thorn SE, Rowal N, Wennhaer M. Prolonged respiratory depression caused by sublingual buprenorphine. *Lancet* 1988;1:179-180.
41. Tantucci C, Paoletti F, Bruni B, et al. Acute respiratory effects of sublingual buprenorphine: comparison with intramuscular morphine. *Int J Clin Pharmacol Ther Toxicol* 1992;30:202-207.
42. Bullingham RCS, McQuay HJ, Dwyer D, et al. Sublingual buprenorphine used postoperatively: clinical observations and preliminary pharmacokinetic analysis. *Br J Clin Pharmacol* 1981;12:117–122.
43. Stehling LC, Zauder HL. Double-blind comparison of butorphanol and meperidine in the treatment of post surgical pain. *J Intern Med Resp* 1978;6:306.
44. Heel RC, Brogden RN, Speight TM, et al. Buprenorphine: a review of its pharmacological properties and therapeutic efficacy. *Drugs* 1979;17:81–110.
45. Product information: Buprenex, buprenorphine hydrochloride. Richmond, VA: Reckitt & Colman Pharmaceuticals Inc.
46. Budd K. High dose buprenorphine for postoperative analgesia. *Anaesthesia* 1981;36:900–903.
46a. Bullingham RE, McQuay HJ, Moore A, et al. Buprenorphine kinetics. *Clin Pharmacol Ther* 1980;28(5):667–672.
47. Anonymous. American Academy of Pediatrics Committee on Drugs. The transfer of drugs and other chemicals into human milk. *Pediatrics* 2001;108:776–789.
48. Fischer G, Johnson RE, Eder H, et al. Treatment of opioid-dependent pregnant women with buprenorphine. *Addiction* 2000;95(2):239–244.
49. Schmidt JF, Chraemmer-Jorgensen B, Pedersen JE, et al. Postoperative pain relief with naloxone: severe respiratory depression and pain after high dose buprenorphine. *Anaesthesia* 1985;40:583–586.
50. Debrabandere L, Van Boven M, Daenens P. Analysis of buprenorphine in urine specimens. *J Forens Sci* 1991;37:82-89.
51. Hand CW, Ryan KE, Dutt Sk, et al. Radioimmunoassay of buprenorphine in urine: studies in patients and in a drug clinic. *J Anal Toxicol* 1989;33:100-104.
52. Bullingham RES, McQuay HJ, Porter EJB, et al. Sublingual buprenorphine used postoperatively: ten hour plasma drug concentration analysis. *Br J Clin Pharm* 1982;13:665-673.
52a. Kintz P, Cirimele V, Edel Y, et al. Hair analysis for buprenorphine and its dealkylated metabolite by RIA and confirmation by LC/ECD. *J Forens Sci* 1994;39:1497–1503.
53. Kintz P, Cirimele V, Edel Y, et al. Hair analysis for buprenorphine and its dealkylated metabolite by RIA and confirmation by LC/ECD. *J Forens Sci* 1994;39:1497-1503.
54. Gal TJ. Naloxone reversal of buprenorphine-induced respiratory depression. *Clin Pharmacol Ther* 1989;45:66–71.
55. Product information: Stadol, butorphanol. Princeton, NJ: Bristol-Meyers Squibb Company, 1996.
56. Shyu WC, Pittman KA, Robinson DS, et al. The absolute bioavailability of transnasal butorphanol in patients experiencing rhinitis. *Eur J Clin Pharmacol* 1993;45:559–562.
57. Pachter IJ, Evens RP. Butorphanol. *Drug Alcohol Depend* 1985;14:325–338.
58. Vandam LD. Butorphanol. *N Engl J Med* 1980;302:381–384.
59. Ameer B, Salter FJ. Drug therapy reviews: evaluation of butorphanol tartrate. *Am J Hosp Pharm* 1979;36:1683–1691.
60. Vachharajani NN, Shyu WC, Barbhaiya RH. Pharmacokinetic interaction between butorphanol nasal spray and oral metoclopramide in healthy women. *J Clin Pharmacol* 1997;37:979–985.
61. Sagraves R, Letassy NA. Obstetrics. In: Young LY, Koda-Kimble MA, eds. *Applied therapeutics the clinical use of drugs*, 4th ed. 1988.
62. Pircio AW, Gylys JA, Cavanagh RL, et al. The pharmacology of butorphanol, a 3,14-dihydroxymorphinan narcotic antagonist analgesic. *Arch Intern Pharmacodyn Ther* 1976;220:231–257.
63. Pittman KA, Smyth RD, Losada M, et al. Human perinatal distribution of butorphanol. *Am J Obstet Gynecol* 1980;138:797–800.
64. Robbins L. Stador nasal spray: treatment for migraine? *Headache* 1993;739-742.
65. *Physicians' desk reference*, 49th ed. Montvale, NJ: Medical Economics, 1994;739-742.
66. Butorphanol nasal spray for pain. *Med Lett Drugs Ther* 1993;35(909):105-106.
67. American Medical Association Department of Drugs. *Drug evaluations subscription*. Chicago: American Medical Association, 1994.
68. Jasinski DR, Pevnick JS, Griffith JD, et al. Progress Report on Studies from the Clinical Pharmacology section of the Addiction Research Center. *Problems Drug Dependence* 1976;112–120:147.
69. Smith GS, Davis WM. Nonmedical use of butorphanol and diphenhydramine. *JAMA* 1984;252:1010.
70. Pittman KA, Smyth RD, Mayol RF. Serum levels of butorphanol by radioimmunoassay. *J Pharm Sci* 1980;69:160-163.
71. Gaver RC, Vasiljer M, Wong H, et al. Disposition of parenteral butorphanol in man. *Drug Metab Disp* 1980;8:230-235.
72. Pfeffer M, Smyth RD, Pittman KA, et al. Pharmacokinetics of subcutaneous and intramuscular butorphanol in dogs. *J Pharm Sci* 1980;69:801–803.
73. Hearn WL, Rose S, Andollo W, et al. Fatality associated with enflurane and butorphanol. In: *Proceedings, American Academy of Forensic Sciences, 43rd annual meeting*, February 18-23, 1991. Abstract K35.
74. Balikova M, Maresova V. Fatal opiates overdose. Toxicological identification of various metabolites in a blood sample by GC-MS after silylation. *Forensic Sci Int* 1998;94:201–209.
75. Gilman AG, Goodman LS, Gilman A, eds. *Goodman & Gilman's the pharmacological basis of therapeutics*, 6th ed. New York: Macmillan Publishing Co, 1990.
76. Bennett WM, Aronoff GR, Golper TA, et al. *Drug prescribing in renal failure*. Philadelphia: American College of Physicians, 1994.
77. Product information: Brontex, codeine, guaifenesin. Cincinnati: Proctor & Gamble Pharmaceuticals, 1997.
78. Williams DG, Hatch DJ, Howard RF. Codeine phosphate in paediatric medicine. *Br J Anaesth* 2001;86(3):413–421.
79. Heiskanen TE, Ruismaki PM, Seppala TA, et al. Morphine or oxycodone in cancer pain? *Acta Oncol* 2000;39(8):941–947.
80. Product information: Fiorinal w/Codeine, codeine, butalbital, aspirin, caffeine. East Hanover, NJ: Sandoz Pharmaceutical Corp, 1997.
81. Matzke GR, Chan GLC, Abraham PA. Codeine dosage in renal failure. *Clin Pharm* 1986;5:15–16.
82. Guay DRP, Awni WM, Findlay JWA, et al. Pharmacokinetics and pharmacodynamics of codeine in end-stage renal disease. *Clin Pharmacol Ther* 1988;43:63–71.
83. Van Leeuwen G, Guthrie R, Stange F. Narcotic withdrawal reaction in a newborn infant due to codeine. *Pediatrics* 1965;36:635–636.
84. Mangurten HH, Benawra R. Neonatal codeine withdrawal in infants of nonaddicted mothers. *Pediatrics* 1980;65:159.
85. Voorhorst R, Sparreboom S. Four cases of recurrent pseudo-scarlet fever caused by phenanthrene alkaloids with a 6-hydroxy group (codeine and morphine). *Ann Allergy* 1980;44:116–120.
86. Gill C, Michaelides PL. Dental drugs and anaphylactic reactions: report of a case. *Oral Surg Oral Med Oral Pathol* 1980;50:30–32.
87. Product information: Codeine. Philadelphia: Wyeth Laboratories Inc, 1993.
88. Hastier P, Buckley MJM, Peten EP, et al. A new source of drug-induced acute pancreatitis: codeine. *Am J Gastroenterol* 2000;95(11):3295–3298.
89. Desmeules J, Gascon MP, Dayer P, et al. Impact of environmental and genetic factors on codeine analgesia. *Eur J Clin Pharmacol* 1991;41:23–26.
90. Product information: Mycobutin, rifabutin capsules. Columbus, OH: Adria Laboratories, 1996.
91. Struempler RE. Excretion of codeine and morphine following ingestion of poppy seeds. *J Analytical Toxicol* 1987;11:97–99.
92. Selavka CM. Poppy seed ingestion as a contributing factor to opiate-positive urinalysis results: the Pacific perspective. *J Forensic Sci* 1991;36:685–696.
93. Abelson JL. Urine drug testing: watch what you eat! [Letter] *JAMA* 1991;266:3130–3131.
94. Posey BL, Kimble SN. High-performance liquid chromatographic study of codeine, norcodeine and morphine is indication of codeine ingestion. *J Anal Toxicol* 1984;8:68–74.
95. Gjerde H, Fongen U, Gundersen H, et al. Evaluation of a method for simultaneous quantification of codeine, ethylmorphine and morphine in blood. *Forens Sci Int* 1991;51:105–110.
96. Verwez-Van Wissen CPWGM, Koopman-Kimenai PM. Direct determination of codeine, norcodeine, morphine and normorphine with their corresponding O-glucuronide conjugates by high-performance liquid chromatography with electrochemical detection. *J Chromatogr Biomed Appl* 1991;570:309–320.

96a. Kornick CA, Santiago-Palma J, Khojainova N, et al. A safe and effective method of converting cancer patients from intravenous to transdermal fentanyl (poster 762). Presented at 20th Annual Scientific Meeting of the American Pain Society; April 19–22, 2001; Phoenix, AZ.
97. Product information: Duragesic, fentanyl. Titusville, NJ: Janssen Pharmaceutical Products, L.P.
98. Streisand JB, Bailey PL, LeMaire L, et al. Fentanyl-induced rigidity and unconsciousness in human volunteers. *Anesthesiology* 1993;78(4):629–634.
98a. Gualtieri JF, Roe SJ. Schmidt CL. Lethal consequences following oral abuse of a Fentanyl transdermal patch. *J Toxicol Clin Toxicol* 2000;38(2):236.
99. Reeves MD, Ginifer CJ. Fatal intravenous misuse of transdermal fentanyl. *MJA* 2002;177(10):552–554.
100. Product information: Sublimaze, fentanyl citrate injection. Decatur, IL: Taylor Pharmaceuticals.
101. Streisand JB, Varvel JR, Stanski DR, et al. Absorption and bioavailability of oral transmucosal fentanyl citrate. *Anaesthesiology* 1991;75:223–229.
102. Koren G, Goresky G, Crean P, et al. Unexpected alterations in fentanyl pharmacokinetics in children undergoing cardiac surgery: age related or disease related? *Dev Pharmacol Ther* 1986;9(3):183–191.
103. Sperry RJ, Bailey PL, Reichman MV, et al. Fentanyl and sufentanil increase intracranial pressure in head trauma patients. *Anesthesiology* 1992;77(3):416–420.
104. Benzer A, Gottardis M, Russegger L, et al. Fentanyl increases cerebrospinal fluid pressure in normocapnic volunteers. *Eur J Anaesth* 1992;9(6):473–477.
105. Furuya H, Okumura F. Hemolysis after administration of high-dose fentanyl. *Anesth Analg* 1986;65(2):207–208.
106. Steer PL, Biddle CJ, Marley WS. Concentration of fentanyl in colostrum after an analgesic dose. *Can J Anaesth* 1992;39:321–235.
107. Leuschen MP, Willett LD, Hoie EB, et al. Plasma fentanyl levels in infants undergoing extracorporeal membrane oxygenation. *J Thorac Cardiovasc Surg* 1993;105(5):885–891.
108. Kronstrand R, Druid H, Holmgren P, et al. A cluster of fentanyl-related deaths among drug addicts in Sweden. *Forensic Sci Int* 1997;88:185–195.
109. Mirenda J, Tabatabai M, Wong K. Delayed and prolonged rigidity greater than 24 h following high-dose fentanyl anesthesia. *Anesthesiology* 1988;69(4):624–625.
110. Fahnenstich H, Steffan J, Kau N, et al. Fentanyl-induced chest wall rigidity and laryngospasm in preterm and term infants. *Crit Care Med* 2000;28:836–839.
111. Baraka A. Fentanyl-induced laryngospasm following tracheal extubation in a child. *Anaesthesia* 1995;50(4):375.
112. Benthuysen JL, Stanley TH. Concerning the possible nature of reported fentanyl seizures [Letter]. *Anesthesiology* 1985;62(2):205.
113. Tobias JD. Increased intracranial pressure after fentanyl administration in a child with closed head trauma. *Ped Emerg Care* 1994;10:89–90.
114. Zurick AM, Urzua J, Yared J-P, et al. Comparison of hemodynamic and hormonal effects of large single-dose fentanyl anesthesia and halothane/nitrous oxide anesthesia for coronary artery surgery. *Anesth Analg* 1982;61(6):521–526.
115. Russell AW. Inadvertent epidural overdose [Letter]. *Anesthesia Int Care* 1994;22:501–502.
116. Kuzma PJ, Kline MD, Stamatos JM, et al. Acute toxic delirium: an uncommon reaction to transdermal fentanyl. *Anesthesiology* 1995;83(4):869–871.
116a. Adair J, El-Nachef A, Cutler P. Fentanyl neurotoxicity (letter). *Ann Emerg Med* 1996;27(6):791–792.
116b. Rose PG, Macfee MS, Boswell MV. Fentanyl transdermal system overdose secondary to cutaneous hyperthermia. *Anesth Analg* 1993;77:390–391.
117. Newshan G. Heat-related toxicity with the fentanyl transdermal patch [Letter]. *J Pain Symptom Manage* 1998;16:277–278.
118. Bedforth N, Lockey D. Fentanyl/propofol [Letter]. *Reactions* 1995:8.
119. Konarzewski W. Unrecognised fatal anaphylactic reaction to propofol or fentanyl [Letter]. *Anaesthesia* 2001;56:497–498.
120. Bennett MJ, Anderson LK, McMillan JC, et al. Anaphylactic reaction during anaesthesia associated with positive intradermal skin test to fentanyl. *Can Anaesth Soc J* 1986;33(1):75–78.
120a. Gardner-Nix J. Caregiver toxicity from transdermal fentanyl. *J Pain Symptom Management* 2001;21:447–448.
121. DeSio JM, Bacon DR, Peer G, et al. Intravenous abuse of transdermal fentanyl therapy in a chronic pain patient. *Anesthesiology* 1993;79(5):1139–1141.
122. Marquardt KA, Tharratt RS, Musallam NA. Fentanyl remaining in a transdermal system following three days of continuous use. *Ann Pharmacother* 1995;29(10):969–971.
123. Marquardt KA, Tharratt RS. Inhalation abuse of fentanyl patch. *J Toxicol Clin Toxicol* 1994;32(1):75–78.
124. Yerasi AB, Butts JD, Butts JD. Disposal of used fentanyl patches. *Am J Health Syst Pharm* 1997;54(1):85–86.
125. Schneir AB, Offerman SR, Clark RF. Poisoning from the application of a scrotal transdermal fentanyl patch (abst). *J Toxicol Clin Toxicol* 2001;39:487–488.
126. Arvanitis ML, Satonik RC. Transdermal fentanyl abuse and misuse [Letter]. *Am J Emerg Med* 2002;20:58–59.
127. Olkkola KT, Palkama VJ, Neuvonen PJ. Ritonavir's role in reducing fentanyl clearance and prolonging its half-life. *Anesthesiology* 1999;91:681–685.
128. Product information: Meridia, sibutramine hydrochloride monohydrate. Mount Olive, NJ: Knoll Pharmaceutical Company, 1997.
129. Stiller RL, Scierka AM, Davis PJ, et al. A method to increase recovery of fentanyl from urine. *Clin Toxicol* 1989;27:101–108.
129a. Henderson GL, Harkey MR, Jones AD. Rapid screening of fentanyl (China White) powder samples by solid-phase radioimmunoassay. *J Anal Toxicol* 1990;14:172–175.
130. Henderson GL, El Shanni AS, Wilson HA, et al. Fentanyl in urine and serum by solid phase 125-I radioimmunoassay. In: Uges DRA, de Zeeuw RA, eds. *Proceedings, 25th international meeting, International Association of Forensic Toxicologists*. Groningen, 1988.
131. Watts V, Caplan Y. Determination of fentanyl in whole blood at subnanogram concentrations by dual capillary column gas chromatography with nitrogen sensitive detectors and gas chromatography/mass spectrometry. *J Anal Toxicol* 1988;12:246-254.
132. Chaturvedi AK, Rao NGS, Baird JR. A death due to self-administered fentanyl. *J Anal Toxicol* 1990;14:385–387.
133. Bovill JG, Sebel PS. Pharmacokinetics of high-dose fentanyl. *Br J Anaesth* 1980;52:795-801.
134. Silverstein JH, Rieders MF, McMullin M, et al. An analysis of the duration of fentanyl and its metabolites in urine and saliva. *Anesth Analg* 1993;76(3):618–621.
135. Levine B, Goodin JC, Caplan YH. A fentanyl fatality involving midazolam. *Forensic Sci Int* 1990;45:247–251.
136. Joh I, Sila M, Bastani B. Nondialyzability of fentanyl with high-efficiency and high-flux membranes [Letter]. *Anesth Analg* 1998;86(2):447.
137. Barnes JN, Williams AJ, Tomson MJF, et al. Dihydrocodeine in renal failure: further evidence for an important role of the kidney in the handling of opioid drugs. *BMJ* 1985;290:740–742.
138. Park GR, Shelly MP, Quinn K, et al. Dihydrocodeine—a reversible cause of renal failure? *Eur J Anaesthesiol* 1989;6:303–314.
139. Fachinformation. Paracodin, dihydrocodeine. Knoll AG, Ludwigshafen, 1996.
140. Redfern N. Dihydrocodeine overdose treated with naloxone infusion. *BMJ* 1983;287:751–2.
141. Rowell FJ, Seymour RA, Rawlins MD. Pharmacokinetics of intravenous and oral dihydrocodeine and its acid metabolites. *Eur J Clin Pharmacol* 1983;25:419–424.
142. Chan GLC, Matzke GR. Effects of renal insufficiency on the pharmacokinetics and pharmacodynamics of opioid analgesics. *Drug Intell Clin Pharm* 1987;21:773–783.
143. Webb J, Mikus G, Hofmann U, et al. Assessment of the relationship between analgesia and plasma concentrations of dihydrocodeine and dihydromorphine following dihydrocodeine administration. *Br J Clin Pharmacol* 1999;47:583P–584P.
144. Masson AHB. Sublingual buprenorphine versus oral dihydrocodeine in post-operative pain. *J Int Med Res* 1981;9:506–510.
145. Fromm MF, Hofmann U, Griese E-U, et al. Dihydrocodeine: a new opioid substrate for the polymorphic CYP2D6 in humans. *Clin Pharmacol Ther* 1995;58:374–382.
146. Assem ESK. Immunological and non-immunological mechanisms of some of the desirable and undesirable effects of anti-inflammatory and analgesic drugs. *Agents Actions* 1976;6:212–218.
147. Swadi H, Wells B, Power R. Misuse of dihydrocodeine tartrate (DF 118) among opiate addicts. *BMJ* 1990;300:1313.
148. Marks A, Abramson N. Pentazocine and agranulocytosis [Letter]. *Ann Intern Med* 1980;92:433.
148a. Balikova M, Maresova V, Habrdova V. Evaluation of urinary dihydrocodeine excretion in human by gas chromatography-mass spectrometry. *J Chromatogr* 2001;752:179–186.
149. Moulin DE, Johnson NG, Murray-Parsons N, et al. Subcutaneous narcotic infusions for cancer pain: treatment outcome and guidelines for use. *Can Med Assoc J* 1992;146(6):891–897.
150. Product information: Dilaudid, Dilaudid HP. Whippany, NJ: Knoll Pharmaceuticals, 1996.
151. Vallner JJ, Stewart JT, Kotzan JA, et al. Pharmacokinetics and bioavailability of hydromorphone following intravenous and oral administration to human subjects. *J Clin Pharmacol* 1981;21:152–156.
152. Cone EJ, Phelps BA, Gorodetzky CW. Urinary excretion of hydromorphone and metabolites in humans, rats, dogs, guinea pigs, and rabbits. *J Pharm Sci* 1977;66:1709–1713.
153. Angst MS, Drover DR, Lotsch J, et al. Pharmacodynamics of orally administered sustained-release hydromorphone in humans. *Anesthesiology* 2001;94(1):63–73.
154. Vorherr H. Drug excretion in breast milk. *Senologia* 1976;1:27–34.
155. Miller RR. Clinical effects of parenteral narcotics in hospitalized medical patients. *J Clin Pharm* 1980;20:165–171.
156. Anonymous. *FDA safety-related drug labeling changes*. August, 2001. Available at: http://www.fda.gov.medwatch/SAFETY/2001/aug01.htm. Accessed February 2003.
157. Herndon CM. Continuous subcutaneous infusion for pain management. *Am J Pain Management* 2000;10:53–59.
158. Reidenberg MM, Goodman H, Erle H, et al. Hydromorphone levels and pain control in patients with severe chronic pain. *Clin Pharmacol Ther* 1988;44:376–382.
159. Baselt RC. Two hydromorphone fatalities. *Bull Int Assoc Forens Toxicol* 1978;14(2):20.
160. Hill HF, Coda BA, Tanaka A, et al. Multiple-dose evaluation of intravenous hydromorphone pharmacokinetics in normal human subjects. *Anesth Analg* 1991;72:330–336.

161. CDS. Dilaudid R-related deaths—District of Columbia 1987. *MMWR Morb Mortal Wkly Rep* 1988;37:425-427.
162. Product information: Orlaam, levomethadyl. Columbus, OH: Roxane Laboratories, Inc, 2001.
163. Hoffman RJ, Nelson L, Hoffman RS. Life-threatening levo-alpha-acetylmethadol (LAAM) overdose. Amsterdam, The Netherlands: EAPCCT XX International Congress, May 2–5, 2000(abst).
163a. Toro-Goyco E, Martin BR, Harris LS. Binding of l-alpha-acetylmethadol and its metabolites to blood constituents. *Biochem Pharmacol* 1980;29:1897–1902.
164. Fraser AD. Clinical toxicology of drugs used in the treatment of opioid dependency. *Clin Lab Med* 1990;10:375–386.
165. Henderson GL, Wilson K, Lau DHM. Plasma l-alpha-acetylmethadol (LAAM) after acute and chronic administration. *Clin Pharmacol Ther* 1977;21:16–25.
166. Blaine JD, Renault PR, Thomas DB, et al. Clinical status of methadyl acetate (LAAM). *Ann N Y Acad Sci* 1981;362:101–115.
167. Technical information: Levo-Dromoran: comprehensive product information. Nutley, NJ: Roche Laboratories, 1982.
168. Dixon R, Crews T, Inturrisi C, et al. Levorphanol: pharmacokinetics and steady-state plasma concentrations in patients with pain. *Res Commun Chem Pathol Pharmacol* 1983;41:3–17.
169. Product information: Demerol, meperidine. New York: Sanofi Pharmaceuticals, Inc, 1997.
170. McHugh GJ. Norpethidine accumulation and generalized seizure during pethidine patient-controlled analgesia. *Anaesth Intensive Care* 1999;27(3):289–291.
171. Knight B, Thomson N, Perry G. Seizures due to norpethidine toxicity. *Aust N Z J Med* 2000;30:513.
172. Kyff JV, Rice TL. Meperidine-associated seizures in a child. *Clin Pharm* 1990;9:337–338.
173. Julius HC, Levine HL, Williams WD. Meperidine binding to isolated alpha, acid glycoprotein and albumin. *DICP Ann Pharmacother* 1989;23:568-572.
174. Pond SM, Kretschzmar KM. Effect of phenytoin on meperidine clearance and normeperidine formation. *Clin Pharmacol Ther* 1981;30:680–686.
175. Pokela ML, Olkkola KT, Koivisto M, et al. Pharmacokinetics and pharmacodynamics of intravenous meperidine in neonates and infants. *Clin Pharmacol Ther* 1992;52:342–349.
176. Danziger LH, Martin SJ, Blum RA. Central nervous system toxicity associated with meperidine use in hepatic disease. *Pharmacotherapy* 1994;14:235-238.
177. Klotz U, McHorse TS, Wilkinson GR, et al. The effect of cirrhosis on the disposition and elimination of meperidine. *Clin Pharmacol Ther* 1974;16:667–675.
178. Anderson RJ, Gambertoglio JG, Schrier RW. Clinical use of drugs in renal failure. Springfield, IL: Charles C Thomas, 1976.
179. Szeto HH, Inturrisi CE, Houde R, et al. Accumulation of normeperidine—an active metabolite of meperidine in patients with renal failure or cancer. *Ann Intern Med* 1977;86:738–741.
180. Ito S. Drug therapy for breast-feeding women. *N Engl J Med* 2000;343(2):118–126.
181. Wittels B, Scott DT, Sinatra RS. Exogenous opioids in human breast milk and acute neonatal neurobehavior: a preliminary study. *Anesthesiology* 1990;73:864-869.
182. Booth J, Lindsay DR, Olufolabi AJ, et al. Subarachnoid meperidine (pethidine) causes significant nausea and vomiting during labor. *Anesthesiology* 2000;93(2):418–421.
183. Goetting MG. Neurotoxicity of merperidine. *Ann Emerg Med* 1985;14:1007-1009.
184. Kaiko R, Foley K, Heidrich G, et al. Normeperidine plasma levels and central nervous system (CNS) irritability in cancer patients. *Fed Proc* 1978;37:568.
185. Tang R, Shimomura S, Rotblatt M. Meperidine induced seizures in sickle cell patients. *Hosp Formul* 1980;15:764-772.
186. Flacke JW, Flacke WE, Bloor BC, et al. Histamine release by four narcotics: a double-blind study in humans. *Anesth Analg* 1987;66:723–730.
187. Levy JH, Rockoff MA. Anaphylaxis to meperidine. *Anesth Analg* 1982;3:301–303.
188. Guay DRP, Meatherall RC, Chalmers JL, et al. Cimetidine alters pethidine disposition in man. *Br J Clin Pharmacol* 1984;18:907–914.
189. Product information: Norvir, ritonavir. North Chicago: Abbott Laboratories, 2002.
190. Davis GC, Williams AC, Markey SP, et al. Chronic parkinsonism secondary to intravenous injection of meperidine analogues. *Psychiatr Res* 1979;1:249–254.
191. Przedborski S, Jackson-Lewis V. Mechanisms of MPTP toxicity. *Movement Dis* 1998;13[Suppl 1]:35–38.
192. Shih AP, Robinson K, Au WY. Determination of therapeutic serum concentrations of oral and parenteral meperidine by gas liquid chromatography. *Eur J Clin Pharmacol* 1976;9:452.
193. Austin KL, Stapleton JV, Mather LE. Relationship between blood meperidine concentrations and analgesic response: a preliminary report. *Anesthesiology* 1980;53:460–466.
193a. Baumann TJ, Smythe MA, Marikis B, et al. Meperidine serum concentrations and analgesic response in postsurgical patients. *DICP* 1991;25:724–727.
194. Paech MJ, Moore JS, Evans SF. Meperidine for patient-controlled analgesia after cesarean section. *Anesthesiology* 1994;80:1268–1276.
195. Hershey LA. Meperidine and central neurotoxicity. *Ann Intern Med* 1983:98:548-549.
195a. Fochtman FW, Winek CL. Therapeutic serum concentrations of meperidine (Demerol). *J Forensic Sci* 1969;14(2):213–218.
196. Kaiko RF, Foley KM, Grabinski PY, et al. Central nervous system excitatory effects of meperidine in cancer patients. *Ann Neurol* 1983;13:180–185.
197. Hassan H, Bastani B, Gellens M. Successful treatment of normeperidine neurotoxicity by hemodialysis. *Am J Kid Dis* 2000;35:146–149.
198. American Hospital Formulary Service. American Hospital Formulary Service Drug Information 97. Bethesda, MD: American Society of Hospital Pharmacists, 1997.
199. Strain EC, Bigelow GE, Liebson IA, et al. Moderate- vs high-dose methadone in the treatment of opioid dependence: a randomized trial. *JAMA* 1999;281:1000–1005.
200. Inturrisi CE, Verebely K. The levels of methadone in the plasma in methadone maintenance. *Clin Pharmacol Ther* 1972;13:633–637.
201. Inturrisi CE, Colburn WA, Kaiko RF, et al. Pharmacokinetics and pharmacodynamics of methadone in patients with chronic pain. *Clin Pharmacol Ther* 1987;41:392–401.
202. Verebely K, Volavka J, Mule S, et al. Methadone in man: pharmacokinetic and excretion studies in acute and chronic treatment. *Clin Pharmacol Ther* 1975;18:180–190.
203. Blinick G, Inturrisi CE, Jerez E, et al. Methadone assays in pregnant women and progeny. *Am J Obstet Gynecol* 1975;121:617–621.
204. Rahbar F. Observations on methadone withdrawal in 16 neonates. *Clin Pediatr* 1975;14:369–371.
205. Pierson PS, Howard P, Kleber HD. Sudden deaths in infants born to methadone-maintained addicts. *JAMA* 1972;220:1733–1734.
206. Rajegowda BK, Glass L, Evans HE, et al. Methadone withdrawal in newborn infants. *J Pediatr* 1972;81:532–534.
207. Wojnar-Horton RE, Kristensen JH, Yapp P, et al. Methadone distribution and excretion into breast milk of clients in a methadone maintenance programme. *Br J Clin Pharmacol* 1997;44:543–547.
208. Smialek JE, Monforte JR, Aronow R, et al. Methadone deaths in children—a continuing problem. *JAMA* 1977;238:2516–2517.
209. Brooks DE, Roberge R, Spear A. Clinical nuances of pediatric methadone intoxication. *Vet Human Toxicol* 1999;41:388–390.
210. Drummer OH, Opeskin K, Syrjanen M, et al. Methadone toxicity causing death in the subjects starting on a methadone maintenance program. *Am J Forens Med Pathol* 1992;13:346-350.
211. Harding-Pink D. Methadone: one person's maintenance dose is another poison. *Lancet* 1993;341:665-666.
212. Uehlinger C, Hauser C. Allergic reactions from injectable methadone [Letter]. *Am J Psychiatry* 1999;156(6):973.
213. Finelli PF. Phenytoin and methadone tolerance [Letter]. *N Engl J Med* 1976;294:227.
214. Martin WR, Jasinski DR, Haertzen CA, et al. Methadone—a reevaluation. *Arch Gen Psychiatr* 1973;28:286–295.
215. Product information: Videx, didanosine. Princeton, NJ: Bristol-Myers Squibb Company, 2000.
216. Product information: Agenerase, amprenavir. Research Triangle Park, NC: GlaxoSmithKline, 2002.
217. Marzolini C, Troillet N, Telenti A, et al. Efavirenz decreases methadone blood concentrations. *AIDS* 2000;14(9):1291–1292.
218. Product information: Luvox, fluvoxamine. Marietta, GA: Solvay Pharmaceuticals, Inc, 1997.
219. Baselt R. *Disposition of toxic drugs and chemicals in man*, 3rd ed. Chicago: Year Book, 1989:512-516.
220. Wolff K, Sanderson M, Hay AWM, et al. Methadone concentrations in plasma and their relationship to drug dosage. *Clin Chem* 1991;37:205-209.
221. Baugh LD, Liu RH, Walia AS. Simultaneous gas chromatography/mass spectrometry assay of methadone and EDP in urine. *J Forens Sci* 1991;36:548-555.
222. Wolff K, Hay A. Methadone concentrations in plasma and their relationship to drug dosage. *Clin Chem* 1992;38:438-439.
223. Berkowitz TA. The relationship of pharmacokinetics to pharmacological activity: morphine, methadone, and naloxone. *Clin Pharmacokinet* 1976;18:180–190.
224. Bell J, Seres V, Bowron P, et al. The use of serum methadone levels in patients receiving methadone maintenance. *Clin Pharmacol Ther* 1988;43:623–629.
225. Horns WH, Rado M, Goldstein A. Plasma levels and symptoms complaints in patients maintained on daily dosage of methadone hydrochloride. *Clin Pharmacol Ther* 1975;17:636–649.
226. Irey NS, Froede RC. Evaluation of death from drug overdose: a clinicopathologic study. *Am J Clin Pathol* 1974;61:778.
227. Aronoff GR, Berns JS, Brier ME, et al., eds. Drug prescribing in renal failure, 4th ed. Philadelphia: American College of Physicians, 1999.
228. Product information: MSIR, morphine sulfate. Norwalk, CT: Purdue Frederick, 2000.
229. Hunt A, Joel S, Dick G, et al. Population pharmacokinetics of oral morphine and its glucuronides in children receiving morphine as immediate-release liquid or sustained-release tablets for cancer pain. *J Pediatr* 1999;135:47–55.
230. Booij LHDJ, Vree TB, Koppers-Hoyset H, et al. Explorative pharmacokinetic study of preoperative administration of morphine 50 mg sustained-release capsules (Kapanol(TM)) to surgical patients. *Clin Drug Invest* 1999;18(2):125–132.
231. Product information: Avinza, morphine sulfate extended-release capsules. San Diego, CA: Ligand Pharmaceuticals, Inc, 2002.

232. Product information: Duramorph, morphine sulfate. Cherry Hill, NJ: Elkins-Sinn, 2000.
233. Morley JS, Miles JB, Wells JC, et al. Paradoxical pain. *Lancet* 1992;340:1045.
234. Westerling D, Sawe J, Eklundh G. Near fatal intoxication with controlled-release morphine tablets in a depressed woman. *Acta Anaesthesiol Scand* 1998;42:586–589.
235. Product information: MS Contin. Norwalk, CT: Purdue Frederick, 2000.
236. Kopecky EA, Ryan ML, Barrett JFR, et al. Fetal response to maternally administered morphine. *Am J Obstet Gynecol* 2000;183:424–430.
237. Gerdin E, Salmonson T, Lindberg B, et al. Maternal kinetics of morphine during labor. *J Perinat Med* 1990;18:479–487.
238. Product information: Kadian, morphine sulfate. Raleigh, NC: Faulding Laboratories, 2000.
239. Robieux I, Koren G, Vandenbergh H, et al. Morphine excretion in breast milk and resultant exposure of a nursing infant. *Clin Toxicol* 1990;28:365–370.
240. Remskar M, Noc M, Leskovsek B, et al. Profound circulatory shock following heroin overdose. *Resuscitation* 1998;38:51–53.
241. Hibbs J, Perper J, Winek CL. An outbreak of designer drug-related deaths in Pennsylvania. *JAMA* 1991;265:1011–1013.
242. Larijani GE, Goldberg ME, Rogers KH. Treatment of opioid-induced pruritus with ondansetron: report of four patients. *Pharmacotherapy* 1996;16(5):958–960.
243. Bowie LJ, Kirkpatrick PB. Simultaneous determination of monoacetylmorphine, morphine, codeine and other opiates by GC/MS. *J Anal Toxicol* 1989;13:326-329.
244. Meneely KD. Poppy seed ingestion: the Oregon perspective. *J Forens Sci* 1992;37:1158-1162.
244a. Felby S, Christensen H, Lund A. Morphine concentrations in blood and organs in cases of fatal poisoning. *Forensic Sci* 1974;3:77–81.
245. Nanan R, von Stockhausen HB, Petersen B, et al. Unusual pattern of leukoencephalopathy after morphine sulphate intoxication. *Neuroradiology* 2000;42:845–848.
246. elSohly H, elSohly M, Stanford D. Poppy seed ingestion and opiates urinalysis: a closer look. *J Anal Toxicol* 1990;14:308–310.
247. Beck O, Vitols S, Stensio M. Positive urine screening for opiates after consumption of sandwich bread with poppy seed flavoring [Letter]. *Ther Drug Monit* 1990;12:585–586.
248. Cone EJ, Welch P, Paul BD, et al. Forensic drug testing for opiates, III. Urinary excretion rates of morphine and codeine following codeine administration. *J Anal Toxicol* 1991;15:161–166.
249. Staub C. Hair analysis: its importance for the diagnosis of poisoning associated with opiate addiction. *Forensic Science International* 1993;63(1–3):69–75.
250. Strang J, Marsh A, Desouza N. Hair analysis for drugs of abuse [Letter]. *Lancet* 1990;335:740.
251. Lo MW, Lee FH, Schary WL, et al. The pharmacokinetics of intravenous, intramuscular, and subcutaneous nalbuphine in healthy subjects. *Eur J Clin Pharmacol* 1987;33:297–301.
252. Product information: Nubain, nalbuphine. Manati, Puerto Rico: Du Pont Pharmaceuticals, 2002.
253. Magruder MR. Balanced anesthesia with nalbuphine hydrochloride. *Anesthesiol Review* 1980;7:25–29.
253a. Nicolle E, Devillier P, Delanoy B, et al. Therapeutic monitoring of nalbuphine: transplacental transfer and estimated pharmacokinetics in the neonate. *Eur J Clin Pharmacol* 1996;49:485–489.
254. Popio KA, Jackson DH, Ross AM, et al. Hemodynamic and respiratory effects of morphine and butorphanol. *Clin Pharmacol Ther* 1978;23:281–287.
255. Lee G, Low RI, Amsterdam EA, et al. Hemodynamic effects of morphine and nalbuphine in acute myocardial infarction. *Clin Pharmacol Ther* 1981;29:576–581.
256. USPDI: Drug information for the health care professional, vol. IB, 8th ed. United States Pharmacopeial Convention, Inc, 1988.
257. USP: Drug information for the health care professional, 8th ed. United States Pharmacopeial Convention, Inc, 1988.
258. Danks JL, Jackson AFP. Sensitivity to papaveretum in Gilbert's disease [Letter]. *Anesthesia* 1991;46:998–999.
259. Hewer T, Rose E, Ghadirian P, et al. Ingested mutagens from opium and tobacco pyrolysis products and cancer of the oesophagus. *Lancet* 1978;2(8088):494–496.
260. Sadeghi A, Behmard S, Vesselinovitch SD. Opium: a potential urinary bladder carcinogen in man. *Cancer* 1979;43:2315–2321.
261. Moeller MR, Mueller C. The detection of 6-monoacetylmorphine in urine, serum and hair by GC/MS and RIA. *Forensic Science International* 1995;70:125–133.
261a. Nakamura GR, Stoll WJ, Meeks RD. Analysis of dihydrocodeine for urine using Sep-PakR C18 cartridges for sample cleanup. *J Forens Sci* 1987;32:535–538.
262. Muittari P, Kirvela O. The safety and efficacy of intrabursal oxycodone and bupivacaine in analgesia after shoulder surgery. *Reg Anesth Pain Med* 1998;23(5):474–478.
263. Product information: OxyContin, controlled-release oxycodone. Stamford, CT: Purdue Pharmaceuticals, 2001.
264. Product information: Roxicodone, oxycodone. Columbus, OH: Roxane Laboratories, Inc, 2002.
265. Mandema JW, Kaiko RF, Oshlack B, et al. Characterization and validation of a pharmacokinetic model for controlled-release oxycodone. *Br J Clin Pharmacol* 1996;43:747–756.
266. Kaiko RF, Benziger DP, Fitzmartin RD, et al. Pharmacokinetic-pharmacodynamic relationships of controlled-release oxycodone. *Clin Pharmacol Ther* 1996;59(1):52–61.
267. Rosebraugh C, Flockhart D, Yasuda S, et al. Visual hallucination and tremor induced by sertraline and oxycodone in a bone marrow transplant patient. *J Clin Pharmacol* 2001;41:224–227.
268. Kaplan R, Parris WCV, Citron ML, et al. Comparison of controlled-release and immediate-release oxycodone tablets in patients with cancer pain. *J Clin Oncol* 1998;16(10):3230–3237.
269. Beaver WT, Feise GA. A comparison of the analgesic effect of oxymorphone by rectal suppository and intramuscular injection in patients with postoperative pain. *J Clin Pharmacol* 1977;17:276–291.
270. Smith ML, Hughes RO, Levine B, et al. Forensic drug testing for opiates. VI. Urine testing for hydromorphone, hydrocodone, oxymorphone, and oxycodone with commercial opiate immunoassays and gas chromatography-mass spectrometry. *J Anal Toxicol* 1995;19(1):18–26.
271. Product information: Talwin NX, pentazocine and naloxone. New York: Winthrop Pharmaceuticals, 1995.
272. Olin BR, ed. *Drug facts and comparisons*. St. Louis: Facts and Comparisons, 1990.
273. Kalia PK, Madan R, Saksena R, et al. Epidural pentazocine for post-operative pain relief. *Anesth Analg* 1983;62:949–950.
274. Debooy VD, Seshia MK, Tenenbein M, et al. Intravenous pentazocine and methylphenidate abuse during pregnancy. *AJDC* 1993;147:1062–1065.
275. Haibach H, Yesus YW, Doggett JJ. Pentazocine-induced agranulocytosis. *Can Med Assoc J* 1984;130:1165–1166.
276. Hoppin EC, Greenberg BR, Walter RM. Agranulocytosis secondary to pentazocine therapy. *Arch Intern Med* 1978;138:533–534.
277. Isenhower HL, Mueller BA. Selection of narcotic analgesics for pain associated with pancreatitis. *Am J Health-Syst Pharm* 1998;55:480–486.
278. Burstein AH, Fullerton T. Oculogyric crisis possibly related to pentazocine. *Ann Pharmacother* 1993;27:874–876.
279. Product information: Talacen, pentazocine, acetaminophen, New York: Sanofi Winthrop Pharmaceuticals, 1999.
280. Magee KL, Schauder CS, Drucker CR, et al. Extensive calcinosis as a late complication of pentazocine injections: response to therapy with steroids and aluminum hydroxide. *Arch Dermatol* 1991;127:1591–1592.
281. Reinhart S, Barrett SM. An acute hypertensive response after intravenous use of a new pentazocine formulation. *Ann Emerg Med* 1985;14:591–593.
282. Strain EC, Preston KL, Liebson IA, et al. Precipitated withdrawal by pentazocine in methadone-maintained volunteers. *J Pharmacol Exp Ther* 1993;267:624–634.
283. Moeller N, Dietzel K, Nuernberg B, et al. High performance liquid chromatographic determination of pentazocine in plasma. *J Chromatogr Biomed Appl* 1990;530:200-205.
284. Stahl SM, Kasser IS. Pentazocine overdose. *Ann Emerg Med* 1983;12:28–31.
285. Product information: Darvon, propoxyphene hydrochloride. Indianapolis: Eli Lilly and Company, 1997.
286. Gibson TP, Giacomini KM, Briggs WA, et al. Propoxyphene and norpropoxyphene plasma concentrations in the anephric patient. *Clin Pharmacol Ther* 1980;27:665–670.
287. Verebely K, Inturrisi CE. Disposition of propoxyphene and norpropoxyphene in man after a single oral dose. *Clin Pharmacol Ther* 1974;15:302–309.
288. Neil A, Terenius L. D-propoxyphene acts differently from morphine on opioid receptor-effector mechanisms. *Eur J Pharmacol* 1981;69:33–39.
289. Quillian WW, Dunn CA. Neonatal drug withdrawal from propoxyphene. *JAMA* 1976;235:2128.
290. Stork CM, Redd JT, Fine K, et al. Propoxyphene-induced wide QRS complex dysrhythmia responsive to sodium bicarbonate—a case report. *Clin Toxicol* 1995;33:179–183.
291. Tennant FS. Complications of propoxyphene abuse. *Arch Intern Med* 1973;132:191–194.
292. Pearlman HS, Wollowick BS, Alvarez EV. Intraarterial injection of propoxyphene into brachial artery. *JAMA* 1970;214:2055.
293. Almirall J, Montoliu J, Torras A, et al. Propoxyphene-induced hypoglycemia in a patient with chronic renal failure. *Nephron* 1989;53:273–275.
294. Wiederholt IC, Genco M, Foley JM. Recurrent episodes of hypoglycemia induced by propoxyphene. *Neurology* 1967;17:703.
295. Rosenberg W, Ryley N, Trowell J, et al. Dextropropoxyphene induced hepatotoxicity: a report of nine cases. *J Hepatol* 1993;19:470–474.
296. Allen S. Cerebellar dysfunction following dextropropoxyphene-induced carbamazepine toxicity [Letter]. *Postgrad Med J* 1994;70:764.
297. Morgensen PH, Jorgensen L, Boas J, et al. Effects of dextropropoxyphene on the steady-state kinetics of oxcarbazepine and its metabolites. *Acta Neurol Scand* 1992;85:14–17.
298. Abernethy DR, Greenblatt DJ, Steel K, et al. Impairment of hepatic drug oxidation by propoxyphene. *Ann Intern Med* 1982;97:223–224.
299. Tighe TV, Walter FG. Delayed toxic acetaminophen level after initial four hour nontoxic level. *Clin Toxicol* 1994;32:431–434.
300. Rop PP, Grimaldi F, Bresson M, et al. Simultaneous determination of dextromoramide, propoxyphene and norpropoxyphene in necropsic whole blood by liquid chromatography. *J Chromatography* 1993;615:357–364.
301. Wolen RL, Ziege EA, Gruber CM. Determination of propoxyphene and norpropoxyphene by chemical ionization mass fragmentography. *Clin Pharmacol Ther* 1975;17:15–20.

302. Karkkainen S, Neuvonen PJ. Effects of oral charcoal and urine pH on dextropropoxyphene pharmacokinetics. *J Toxicol Clin Toxicol* 1985;23:436(abst).
303. Lupin AJ, Harley CH. Inner ear damage related to propoxyphene injection. *Can Med Assoc J* 1976;114:596.
304. Product information: Sufentanil Citrate Injection, USP. Library Corner, NJ: Ohmeda Pharmaceuticals, 2000.
305. Smith NT, Dec-Silver H, Harrison WK, et al. A comparison among morphine, fentanyl and sufentanil anesthesia for open-heart surgery: induction, emergency and extubation (abst). *Anesthesiology* 1982;57(3S):A–291.
306. Rosow CE. Sufentanil citrate: a new opioid analgesic for use in anesthesia. *Pharmacotherapy* 1984;4:11–19.
307. Meuldermans WEG, Hurkmans RMA, Heykants JJP. Plasma protein binding and distribution of fentanyl, sufentanil, alfentanil and lofentanil in blood. *Arch Int Pharmacodyn Ther* 1982;257:4–19.
308. Hardman JG, Gilman AG, Limbird LE, eds. *Goodman & Gilman's the pharmacological basis of therapeutics*, 9th ed. New York: McGraw-Hill, 1996.
309. Bovill JG, Sebel PS, Blackburn CL, et al. The pharmacokinetics of sufentanil in surgical patients. *Anesthesiology* 1984;61:502–506.
310. Kofke WA, Garman RH, Janosky J, et al. Opioid neurotoxicity: neuropathologic effects in rats of different fentanyl congeners and the effects of hexamethonium-induced normotension. *Anesth Analg* 1996;83:141–146.
311. Abouleish AE, Portnoy D, Abouleish EI. Addition of dextrose 3.5% to intrathecal sufentanil for labour analgesia reduces pruritus. *Can J Anesth* 2000;47(12):1171–1175.
312. Michiels M, Hendriks R, Heykants JJ. Radioimmunoassay of the new opioid analgesics alfentanil and sufentanil. *J Pharm Pharmacol* 1983;35:86-93.
313. Hansdottir V, Hedner T, Woestenborghs R, et al. The CSF and plasma pharmacokinetics of sufentanil after intrathecal administration. *Anesthesiology* 1991;74:264-269.
314. Ferslew KE, Hagordorn AN, McCormick WF. Postmortem determination of the biological distribution of sufentanil and midazolam after an acute intoxication. *J Forens Sci* 1989;34:249-257.
315. Lejus C, Schwoerer D, Furic I, et al. Fentanyl versus sufentanil: plasma concentrations during continuous epidural postoperative infusion in children. *Br J Anaesth* 2000;85(4):615–617.
316. Reynolds JEF, ed. *Martindale: the extra pharmacopoeia* (electronic version). Denver, CO: Micromedex, Inc, 1994.
317. Seiler KU, Jahnchen E, Trenk D, et al. Pharmacokinetics of tilidine in terminal renal failure. *J Clin Pharmacol* 2001;41:79–84.
318. Klapetek J. Valoron intoxikation by selbsmod vers. *Munch Med Wochenschr* 1973;115:113-115.
319. Van Boven M, Daenens P, Bruneel N. A death case involving tilidine. *Arch Toxicol* 1976;36:121-125.
320. Vollmer K-A, Thomann P, Hengy H. Pharmacokinetics of tilidine and metabolites in man. *Arzneimmittelforschung* 1989;39(10):1283–1288.
321. Vollmer K-A, Poisson A. On the metabolism of ethyl-DL-*trans*-2-dimethylamino-1-phenyl-cyclohex-3-ene-*trans*-1-carboxylate hydrochloride (tilidine HCL). Second communication: studies with ^{14}C-labeled substances in rats and dogs. *Arzneimittelforschung* 1976;26:1827-1836.
322. Fachinformation: Valoron, tilidine. Goedecke AG, Berlin, 1996.
323. ABDA-Datenbank International. Tilidine monograph in: Mikropharm 2, electronic version. Werbe- und Vertriebsgesellschaft Deutscher Apotheker (W+V), Frankfurt/Main, 1994.
324. Jasinski DR, Preston KL. Evaluation of tilidine for morphine-like subjective effects and euphoria. *Drug Alcohol Depend* 1986;18(3):273–292.
325. Sunshine A, Olson NZ, Zighelboim I, et al. Analgesic oral efficacy of tramadol hydrochloride in postoperative pain. *Clin Pharmacol Ther* 1992;51:740-746.
326. Product information: Ultram, tramadol hydrochloride. Raritan, NJ: Ortho-McNeil Pharmaceutical, 2001.
327. Spiller HA, Gorman SE, Villalobos D, et al. Prospective multi-center evaluation of tramadol exposure (abst). *J Toxicol Clin Toxicol* 1996;34:578.
328. Spiller HA, Gorman SE, Villalobos D, et al. Prospective multicenter evaluation of tramadol exposure. *Clin Toxicol* 1997;35:361–364.
329. Bianchetti MG, Beutler A, Ferrier PE. Intoxication severe avec uoprace (tramadol) chez un nourisson de cinque semaines. *Helv Paediatr Acta* 1988;43: 241-244.
330. Riedel F, v Stockhausen H-B. Severe cerebral depression after intoxication with tramadol in a 6 month old infant. *Eur J Clin Pharmacol* 1984;26:631-632.
331. Lee CR, McTavish D, Sorkin EM. Tramadol. A preliminary review of its pharmacodynamic and pharmacokinetic properties, and therapeutic potential in acute and chronic pain states. *Drugs* 1993;46(2):313–347.
332. Kayser V, Besson JM, Guilbaud G. Evidence for noradrenergic component in the antinociceptive effect of the analgesic agent tramadol in an animal model of clinical pain, the arthritic rat. *Eur J Pharm* 1992;224:83–88.
333. Fricke JR, Minn F, Cunningham PD, et al. Tramadol HCl: dose response to pain from oral surgery. *Clin Pharmacol Ther* 1991;59:182.
334. Worz R. Control of cancer pain with analgesics acting in the central nervous system. *Recent Results Cancer Res* 1984;89:100–106.
335. Cicero TJ, Adams EH, Geller A, et al. A postmarketing surveillance program to monitor Ultram (tramadol hydrochloride) abuse in the United States. *Drug Alcohol Depend* 1999;57:7–32.
336. Michaud K, Augsburger M, Romain N, et al. Fatal overdose of tramadol and alprazolam. *Forensic Sci Int* 1999;105:185–189.
337. Krummen K, Nelson E, Tsipis G, et al. Tramadol abuse in the Cincinnati area (abst). *J Toxicol Clin Toxicol* 1999;37:647.
338. Nightingale SL. From the Food and Drug Administration: important new safety information for tramadol hydrochloride. *JAMA* 1996;275:1224.
339. ADRAC. Tramadol and serotonin syndrome. *Australian Adverse Drug Reactions Bulletin* 2001;20(4):14.
340. Lusthof KJ, Zweipfenning PGM. Suicide by tramadol overdose [Letter]. *J Anal Toxicol* 1998;22:260.
340a. Musshoff F, Madea B. Fatality due to ingestion of tramadol alone. *Forensic Sci Int* 2001;116(2–3):197–199.
341. Grond S, Meuser T, Uragg H, et al. Serum concentrations of tramadol enantiomers during patient-controlled analgesia. *Br J Clin Pharmacol* 1999;48:254–257.
342. Moore KA, Cina SJ, Jones R, et al. Tissue distribution of tramadol and metabolites in an overdose fatality. *Am J Forensic Med Pathol* 1999;20:98–100.
343. Petrone D, Kamin M, Olson W. Slowing the titration rate of tramadol HCl reduces the incidence of discontinuation due to nausea and/or vomiting: a double-blind randomized trial. *J Clin Pharm Ther* 1999;24:115–123.
344. Jehanli A, Brannan S, Moore L, et al. Blind trials of an onsite saliva drug test for marijuana and opiates. *J Forensic Sci* 2001;46:1214–1220.
345. Negus SS, Pasternak GW, Koob GF, et al. Antagonist effects of beta-funaltrexamine and naloxonazine on alfentanil-induced antinociception and muscle rigidity in the rat. *J Pharmacol Exp Ther* 1993;264:739–745.
346. Wand P, Kuschinsk K, Sontag KH. Morphine-induced muscular rigidity in rats. *Eur J Pharmacol* 1973;24:189–193.
347. Vacanti CA, Silbert BS, Vacanti FX. Fentanyl-induced muscle rigidity as affected by pretreatment with amantadine hydrochloride. *J Clin Anesth* 1992;4:282–284.
348. Mills CA, Flacke JW, Miller JD, et al. Cardiovascular effects of fentanyl reversal by naloxone and varying arterial carbon dioxide tensions in dogs. *Anesth Analg* 1988;67:730–736.
349. Mills CA, Flacke JW, Flacke WE, et al. Narcotic reversal in hypercapneic dogs: comparison of naloxone and nalbuphine. *Can J Anaesth* 1990;37:238–244.
350. Brower RG, Matthay AM, Morris A, and the Acute Respiratory Distress Syndrome Network. Ventilation with lower tidal volumes as compared with traditional tidal volumes for acute lung injury and the acute respiratory distress syndrome. *N Engl J Med* 2000;342:1301–1308.
351. Philbin DM, Moss J, Akins CW, et al. The use of H1 and H2 histamine antagonists with morphine anesthesia: a double-blind study. *Anesthesiology* 1981;55:292–296.
352. Kaiser KG, Bainton CR. Treatment of intrathecal morphine overdose by aspiration of cerebrospinal fluid. *Anesth Analg* 1987;66:475–477.
353. Burton AW, Conroy B, Garcia E, et al. Illicit substance abuse via an implanted intrathecal pump. *Anesthesiology* 1998;89:1264–1267.
354. Batagol R, ed. Drugs in pregnancy. The Royal Women's Hospital. Victoria, Australia: CSL Limited, 1993.
355. Siberry GK, Iannone R. *Formulary: hydromorphone HCl. The Harriet Lane handbook*, 15th. St. Louis: Mosby 2000:735–736.
356. Koren G, Maurice L. Pediatric uses of opioids. *Pediatr Clin North Am* 1989;36(5):1141–1156.
357. Rita L, Seleny F, Goodarzi M. Comparison of the calming and sedative effects of nalbuphine and pentazocine for paediatric premedication. *Can Anaesth J* 1980;27:546–549.
358. Product information: B & O Supprettes, powdered opium and belladonna extract. Woburn, MA: Poly Medica Pharmaceuticals (USA) Inc, 1993.
359. Waterworth TA. Pentazocine (Fortral) as postoperative analgesic in children. *Arch Dis Child* 1974;49:488–490.
360. Schlesser JL, ed. *Drugs available abroad*. Detroit: Gale Research Inc, 1991.

CHAPTER 129

Inhalational Anesthetics

Katherine M. Hurlbut

$$\mathrm{H{-}C(Cl)(Br){-}CF_3}$$

HALOTHANE

Compounds included:	**Desflurane (Suprane), enflurane (Ethrane), halothane (Fluothane), isoflurane (Forane), nitrous oxide (Entonox, Nitronox), sevoflurane (Altane)**
Molecular formula and weight:	**See Table 1.**
SI conversion:	**See Table 1.**
CAS Registry No.:	**See Table 1.**
Therapeutic levels:	**Not clinically applicable**
Special concerns:	**Acute effects involve primarily central nervous system depression and rare malignant hyperthermia. Chronic effects may include fatal hepatotoxicity.**
Antidote:	**None**

OVERVIEW

The inhalational anesthetics all cause varying degrees of mental status change, muscle relaxation, and analgesia. They are usually used as a part of so-called balanced anesthesia, in combination with other agents such as neuromuscular blockers and opioids, to maximize muscle paralysis and analgesia and to allow for rapid induction and emergence from anesthesia. Although all of these agents can be used recreationally, nitrous oxide is the most widely abused. In addition to being available as an inhalational anesthetic, nitrous oxide has been used as a propellant in whipped cream canisters, cooking oil sprays, and so forth, although it largely has been replaced by other propellants.

Because of the similarities in the management of toxicity from inhalational anesthetics, the topics of diagnostic tests and treatments are addressed for the entire class in the sections Diagnostic Tests for Inhalational Anesthetics and Treatment of the Inhalational Anesthetics.

PATHOPHYSIOLOGY OF THE INHALATIONAL ANESTHETICS

The mechanism of action of inhalational anesthetics is unknown. They may disrupt synaptic transmission by interfering with presynaptic neurotransmitter release, altering reuptake, changing postsynaptic binding, or influencing the ionic conductance change that follows neurotransmitter activation of the postsynaptic receptor (1). Because there is a high correlation between lipid solubility and anesthetic potency, it is believed that these agents have a hydrophobic site of action. It has also been postulated that inhalational anesthetics activate γ-aminobutyric acid receptors and may inhibit certain calcium channels, the release of neurotransmitters, and glutamate channels (1).

DESFLURANE

Desflurane (1,2,2,2-tetrafluoroethyl difluoromethyl ether, Suprane) is a nonflammable inhalational anesthetic. It is supplied as colorless volatile liquid of 100% concentration in a 240-ml vial. It does not react to produce byproducts in the presence of warm soda lime.

Toxic Dose

The minimum alveolar concentration (MAC) is provided in Table 1. When administered with 60% nitrous oxide, the MAC is reduced to 4% in young adults and 2.8% in older patents (2). The induction dose is 6% to 10% in oxygen or 5% to 8% in 65% nitrous oxide. Usual concentration for maintenance of anesthesia is 3% to 7% and occasionally as much as 12% (3,4).

Toxicokinetics and Toxicodynamics

The onset of anesthesia is 2 to 3 minutes (4). Desflurane has low tissue solubility with a blood-gas partition coefficient of 0.42. It undergoes minimal hepatic metabolism. The elimination half-life is 2.5 minutes (5) (Table 2).

Pregnancy and Lactation

Desflurane is U.S. Food and Drug Association (FDA) pregnancy category B (Appendix I). It is safe for use in breast-feeding mothers.

Clinical Presentation

Mild decreases in blood pressure are common with desflurane anesthesia and may be accompanied by reflex tachycardia (6–8). Postoperative nausea and vomiting develop in approximately half of the patients who receive desflurane anesthesia (5).

Initial central nervous system (CNS) excitation (struggling, purposeful movements) is fairly common during induction of anesthesia with desflurane, occurring in approximately 48% of patients who receive desflurane with oxygen and 30% of those induced with desflurane and nitrous oxide (4). With sustained inhalation, CNS depression and coma develop. Headache and vertigo are common during the immediate postoperative period, and clumsiness, impaired concentration, sedation, fatigue, and disorientation have been reported less often (2,9).

Desflurane is a respiratory irritant; coughing and increased secretions are common during induction, and breath-holding,

TABLE 1. Physical characteristics and minimum alveolar concentrations for the inhalational anesthetics

Name	Molecular formula, molecular weight (g/mol), CAS Registry No.	SI conversion	Minimum alveolar concentration (MAC)
Desflurane	$C_3H_2F_6O$, 168.0, 57041-67-5	mg/L × 5.95 = μmol/L	7.25% in young adults and 6% in older patients
Enflurane	$C_3H_2ClF_5O$, 184.5, 13838-16-9	mg/L × 5.42 = μmol/L	MAC is 1.68% in 100% oxygen and 0.57% in 70% nitrous oxide
Halothane	$CHBrClCF_3$, 197.4, 151-67-7	mg/L × 5.07 = μmol/L	MAC in 100% oxygen is 0.6–1.0%; in 65% nitrous oxide MAC is 0.3%
Isoflurane	$C_3H_2ClF_5O$, 184.5, 26675-46-7	mg/L × 5.42 = μmol/L	MAC in 100% oxygen is 1.15%, and, in 70% nitrous oxide, it is 0.50%
Nitrous oxide	N_2O, 44.01, 10024-97-2	mg/L × 2.27 = μmol/L	NR
Sevoflurane	$C_4H_3F_7O$, 200.1, 28523-86-6	mg/L × 4.99 = μmol/L	In 100% oxygen, the MAC is 3.3% in neonates, 2.6% in young adults, and 1.7% in patients 60 yr of age

NR, not reported.

apnea, and laryngospasm occur occasionally (2). Dose-related ventilatory depression is expected, with a decrease in respiratory volume and minute ventilation accompanied initially by an increase in respiratory rate (10).

Carbon monoxide has been produced by the degradation of desflurane in the presence of desiccated soda lime in absorber systems (11). Human cases of carbon monoxide poisoning have been reported rarely after desflurane anesthesia (12). Malignant hyperthermia has rarely been associated with desflurane anesthesia (13).

ENFLURANE

Enflurane [2-chloro-1-(difluoromethoxy)-1,1,2-trifluoroethane, Ethrane] is a nonflammable inhalational anesthetic. It is supplied as a colorless volatile liquid in 100% concentration. It does not react to produce byproducts in the presence of warm soda lime.

Toxic Dose

The MAC is provided in Table 1. The usual induction dose in adults is 2.0% to 4.5% in oxygen or 1.5% to 3% in 65% nitrous oxide; concentrations of 0.5% to 3% are generally used for maintenance (14). In children, concentrations of 2% to 4% are usually sufficient (15). Younger children may require higher concentrations (16).

Toxicokinetics and Toxicodynamics

The onset of anesthesia is 7 to 10 minutes, with return of consciousness generally 5 minutes after discontinuation of exposure (16). The blood-gas partition coefficient is 1.8. Hepatic metabolism is 2.5% to 10% (17). Pulmonary excretion is 80% to 90% (17); the remainder is excreted renally (Table 2).

Pregnancy and Lactation

Enflurane is FDA pregnancy category B (Appendix I). Entry into breast milk is unknown.

Clinical Presentation

ACUTE OVERDOSAGE

Enflurane abuse or misuse can cause death from respiratory failure and asphyxia (18). A 29-year-old anesthetist was found unresponsive and could not be resuscitated after apparently applying 250 ml enflurane to herpes lesions on her lip over a 4-hour period (19).

ADVERSE EVENTS

Tachycardia commonly occurs during enflurane anesthesia (20). Isorhythmic atrioventricular dissociation (gradual shortening of PR interval until it disappears into the QRS complex) has been reported in up to 15% of patients undergoing enflurane anesthesia in one study (21). Hypotension is also common with therapeutic use (22).

Coughing and laryngospasm are common, especially in children (23). Bronchospasm has been reported in patients with underlying asthma (24). Ventilatory depression is expected and increases with increasing concentration (25). Carbon monoxide has been produced by the degradation of enflurane in the presence of desiccated soda lime in absorber systems (11).

Seizures have been reported in patients after enflurane anesthesia. Seizures are more common in individuals with underlying seizure disorders and usually occur within 24 hours after surgery but may develop after a delay of several days (26,27). Myoclonus, focal seizures, generalized tonic-clonic seizures, and, rarely, status epilepticus have been reported (28–31).

Nausea and vomiting commonly occur in the postoperative period (32). Acute hepatitis is a rare hypersensitivity reaction to enflurane. It usually manifests 5 to 19 days after exposure, with fever, elevated liver enzymes, and abdominal pain; jaundice and eosinophilia may also develop, and hepatic encephalopathy and coma develop in the most severe cases (33). Most patients recover over 3 to 4 weeks, although fatalities have occurred rarely (34). Repeated exposure to enflurane increases the risk (35). Malignant hyperthermia is a rare effect of enflurane anesthesia, occurring in approximately 1 in 725,000 exposures (14).

TABLE 2. Pharmacokinetics and pharmacodynamics of the inhalational anesthetics

Parameter	Desflurane	Enflurane	Halothane	Isoflurane	Nitrous oxide	Sevoflurane
Onset (min)	2–3	7–10	1.3–3.5	7–10	Rapid	1–2
Duration (min)	5–16	5	4–16	10–14	—	4–14
Blood-gas partition coefficient	0.42	1.8	2.5	1.4	0.5	0.6–0.7
Pulmonary elimination (%)	Predominant	80–90	Up to 80	95	100	40
Hepatic metabolism (%)	Minimal	2.5–10.0	15–50	0.17	None	Yes
Renal elimination (%)	0.02 (as metabolites)	10–20	Metabolites	—	No	Metabolites
Half-life (min)	2.5	—	—	—	—	—

HALOTHANE

Halothane [(RS)-2-Bromo-2-chloro-1,1,1-trifluoroethane, Fluothane] is an inhalational anesthetic. It is supplied as colorless volatile liquid in 100% concentration. It does not react to produce byproducts in the presence of warm soda lime.

Toxic Dose

The MAC is provided in Table 1. The MAC, when combined with 65% nitrous oxide, is 0.3%. Typical concentrations range from 0.5% to 3.0% in oxygen or nitrous oxide/oxygen.

An adult who ingested 250 ml developed hypotension, coma, and respiratory failure but survived with supportive care (36). Mydriasis, vomiting, protracted coma (36 hours), and leukocytosis were reported in another adult who ingested 250 ml (37). An adult developed transient hematuria, leukocytosis, pulmonary edema, and respiratory failure after receiving 2.5 ml halothane intravenously but survived with supportive care (38).

Toxicokinetics and Toxicodynamics

The onset of action is 1.3 to 3.5 minutes (39), and the duration of action is 4 to 16 minutes (40). The blood-gas partition coefficient is 2.5. Hepatic metabolism is 15% to 50%; up to 80% is excreted unchanged in the lung. Metabolites are excreted renally (41) (Table 2).

Pregnancy and Lactation

Halothane is FDA pregnancy category C (Appendix I).

Clinical Presentation

ACUTE OVERDOSAGE

Overdose causes respiratory and CNS depression, bradycardia, and hypotension. Injection of 2.5 ml and ingestion of 250 ml have caused respiratory failure. An adult who injected 3 ml halothane intravenously initially had a transient loss of consciousness, and hypotension and respiratory distress developed 3 hours later. Myocardial depression, hypotension, and respiratory insufficiency continued to worsen despite therapy, and he died 6 days after exposure (42).

ADVERSE EVENTS

Cardiac effects include dose-dependent decreases in blood pressure, heart rate, and cardiac output (43). Reflex tachycardia may also occur. Dysrhythmias are more common with halothane than with other inhalational anesthetics (44,45). A wide variety of dysrhythmias have been reported, including atrioventricular dissociation, nodal rhythms, ventricular premature beats, ventricular tachycardia, and asystole. Halothane sensitizes the myocardium to catecholamines (43,44).

CNS depression is dose dependent. Postoperative agitation, restlessness, and delirium have been reported infrequently (46). Postoperative nausea and vomiting are not uncommon.

Hepatic enzymes (transaminases and glutathione-S-transferase) increase transiently in 25% to 30% of patients undergoing halothane anesthesia. This is also called *type I hepatotoxicity* (47). Type II hepatotoxicity is much more severe and appears to be an immune-mediated idiosyncratic reaction that occurs in between 1:2500 and 1:3500 exposures (47,48).

Clinical manifestations of type II toxicity include nausea and vomiting, abdominal pain, fever, rash, arthralgia, and jaundice, developing 10 to 14 days after exposure. With subsequent exposures the clinical manifestations may develop in 3 to 5 days (49,50). Laboratory findings include eosinophilia, marked elevations in serum transaminase concentrations, moderate elevations of alkaline phosphatase, elevated serum bilirubin levels, and coagulopathy (49). Patients may progress to acute hepatic failure, and the fatality rate ranges from 20% to 60%. Risk factors include multiple exposures to halothane, obesity, female gender, middle age, genetic predisposition, and use of cytochrome P-450 CYP2E1-inducing agents (47,49,50).

Respiratory effects include dose-related ventilatory depression, and at high doses, apnea ensues. Respiratory irritation is not common, but salivation, coughing, laryngospasm, and stridor can develop in a small minority of patients. Carbon monoxide has been produced by the degradation of halothane in the presence of desiccated soda lime in absorber systems (11). Malignant hyperthermia is a rare effect reported in susceptible individuals.

Bromism may result from prolonged exposure. Halothane contains bromine, which may lead to bromism in some individuals, particularly patients with renal insufficiency, although this is rarely reported. A 65-year-old woman who received halothane anesthesia for 46 hours developed encephalopathy (coma, then confusion and hallucinations for 12 days) and elevated bromide levels (2.4 mmol/L initially, rising to 3.4 mmol/L 4 days after halothane was discontinued) (51).

ISOFLURANE

Isoflurane [2-chloro-2-(difluoromethoxy)-1,1,1-trifluoroethane, Forane] is a nonflammable inhalational anesthetic. It is supplied as colorless volatile liquid in 100% concentration.

Toxic Dose

The MAC is provided in Table 1. The usual adult dose for induction is 3% to 4% in oxygen or 1.5% to 3.0% in 65% nitrous oxide. Anesthesia can be maintained with 1.0% to 2.5% isoflurane with nitrous oxide. In 100% oxygen, the inspired concentration is increased by 0.5% to 1% (52). In children, the MAC is 1.6% to 1.87% (53).

A fatality was reported in an adult who ingested 80 ml (54).

Toxicokinetics and Toxicodynamics

The blood-gas coefficient is 1.4. The onset of anesthesia is 7 to 10 minutes (52). It undergoes minimal hepatic metabolism (0.17%) and is eliminated primarily by the lungs (55) (Table 2).

Pregnancy and Lactation

Isoflurane is FDA pregnancy category C (Appendix I). Entry into breast milk is unknown.

Clinical Presentation

ADVERSE EVENTS

Inhalation of rapidly rising concentrations of isoflurane can cause tachycardia and mild hypertension (56). Some hypotension is common during induction, and blood pressure generally decreases as the depth of anesthesia increases (57).

Drowsiness, weakness, dizziness, headache, ataxia, disorientation, delirium, excitement, nightmares, and mood changes may develop postoperatively; symptoms may persist for several days (52,58,59). Children who were sedated with isoflurane for more than 24 hours have experienced episodes of recurrent neurologic dysfunction, agitation, hallucinations, confusion, ataxia, and CNS depression that in some cases required intubation. Ataxia persisted for as long as 72 hours (58).

Coughing and laryngospasm can occur during induction. Isoflurane causes bronchodilation and has been used in the treatment of status asthmaticus (60). Progressive ventilatory depression and apnea develop at increasing depths of anesthesia. Carbon monoxide has been produced by the degradation of isoflurane in the presence of desiccated soda lime in absorber systems (11).

Postoperative nausea and vomiting are common. Hepatitis has been reported but is uncommon, and hepatic failure is very rare (61,62). Malignant hyperthermia occurs very rarely with isoflurane anesthesia.

NITROUS OXIDE

Nitrous oxide (Entonox, Nitronox) is a nonexplosive colorless gas that is typically supplied in large metal canisters. Acute overexposure, usually secondary to recreational abuse, can cause death secondary to asphyxia. Chronic abuse can cause myelosuppression, megaloblastic anemia, and myeloneuropathy.

Toxic Dose

The usual adult dose for sedation is 25%, for analgesia 25% to 50%, and for anesthesia 70% nitrous oxide and 30% oxygen in combination with other agents (opioids, barbiturates, other inhalational agents) (63). In children, 30% nitrous oxide has been used for analgesia, and 50% nitrous oxide–50% oxygen has been used for sedation of poorly cooperative patients (64,65).

Acute inhalation of high-concentration nitrous oxide (approaching 100%) has caused acute respiratory failure and death.

Toxicokinetics and Toxicodynamics

Nitrous oxide is rapidly absorbed. The blood-gas partition coefficient is 0.5. It is eliminated almost entirely by the lungs, with a small amount eliminated through skin (Table 2).

Pregnancy and Lactation

Nitrous oxide is FDA pregnancy category A (Appendix I). Entry into breast milk has not been evaluated. Chronic occupational exposure to waste nitrous oxide has been associated with decreased fertility, increased risk of spontaneous abortion, and increased fetal anomalies in some studies (66–68).

Pathophysiology

Nitrous oxide is a partial agonist at μ, κ, and σ opioid receptors, which may be related to its emetic and addictive properties (69).

Megaloblastic anemia, myelosuppression, and neuropathy are believed to be secondary to vitamin B_{12} deficiency. Nitrous oxide oxidizes the cobalt in vitamin B_{12}, making it physiologically inactive (70–72).

Clinical Presentation

ACUTE AND CHRONIC ABUSE

Acute abuse causes excitation and euphoria followed by sedation and loss of consciousness. Asphyxia often develops in the setting of nitrous oxide abuse and can cause dysrhythmias and hypotension.

Chronic abuse can cause myeloneuropathy. Initial manifestations are usually numbness and tingling of the hands and legs. Some patients have described an electric shock–like feeling in the back that radiates down the legs when the neck is flexed (73). Hypoactive reflexes, ataxia, fatigue, loss of dexterity of the fingers, impaired gait, and equilibrium are also described (66,74–76). These effects have rarely been reported in patients with other risks for B_{12} deficiency (72,77).

Leukopenia, thrombocytopenia, and megaloblastic anemia have been reported in patients who are chronically exposed to nitrous oxide (78–80). Megaloblastic anemia was also reported after therapeutic use of nitrous oxide in an infant with unrecognized cobalamin deficiency (77) and an adult with short bowel and marginal B_{12} absorption (81). Direct inhalation of nitrous oxide from whipped cream dispensers has caused pneumomediastinum and interstitial emphysema secondary to mechanical rupture of the alveolar wall (82).

ADVERSE EVENTS

Therapeutic use can cause transient tachycardia and hypertension (83). In patients with coronary artery disease, nitrous oxide administration can cause hypotension, bradycardia, cardiac index, and stroke volume index (84). Nitrous oxide causes gaseous distention of the bowel and may produce nausea and vomiting (85).

SEVOFLURANE

Sevoflurane [1,1,1,3,3,3-hexafluoro-2-(fluoromethoxy)-propane, Altane] is a nonflammable inhalational anesthetic. It is supplied as colorless volatile liquid in 100% concentration.

Toxic Dose

The MAC is provided in Table 1. The MAC in 60% nitrous oxide is 2% in children 6 months to less than 3 years of age; in 65% nitrous oxide MAC is 1.4% in young adults and 0.9% in patients 60 years of age (86).

Toxicokinetics and Toxicodynamics

The onset of action is 1 to 2 minutes, and the duration of action is 4 to 14 minutes (87). The blood-gas partition coefficient is 0.6 to 0.7. Pulmonary excretion is 40%, with some hepatic metabolism and renal elimination (Table 2).

Pregnancy and Lactation

Sevoflurane is FDA pregnancy category B (Appendix I). Entry into breast milk is unknown.

Clinical Presentation: Adverse Events

Mild bradycardia and hypotension are common with therapeutic use but usually do not require treatment beyond lowering the inspired concentration. Prolongation of the QTc has been reported in patients undergoing surgery with sevoflurane anesthesia. Although most patients still maintain a QTc within the normal range, in one study QTc intervals of greater than 440 msec developed in 22% of 18 women (88).

Sevoflurane causes dose-related respiratory depression but little in the way of respiratory tract irritation (55). Carbon monoxide has been produced by the degradation of sevoflurane in the presence of desiccated soda lime in absorber systems (11).

CNS excitation with spontaneous or purposeful movement occurs in up to 30% of patients undergoing sevoflurane induction (87). Tonic-clonic seizures occur rarely postoperatively, and there are also rare reports of epileptiform electroencephalographic activity during sevoflurane anesthesia (90–93).

Postoperative nausea develops in about one-third of patients and vomiting in approximately 2% (94). Hepatotoxicity has been reported but is rare (86). Malignant hyperthermia has been reported rarely (95,96).

DIAGNOSTIC TESTS FOR INHALATIONAL ANESTHETICS

Respiratory and cardiac monitoring should be performed with pulse oximetry, arterial blood gases, and serial electrocardiographs. Renal function, electrolytes, and liver enzymes should be monitored after overdose. A chest radiograph should be obtained in patients with hypoxia.

TREATMENT OF THE INHALATIONAL ANESTHETICS

Treatment of acute effects is primarily supportive, involving control of the airway and waiting for the anesthetic drug to be eliminated.

Decontamination

In the unlikely event that liquid forms are ingested, activated charcoal should be administered. Endotracheal intubation should generally be performed first, as these agents cause profound CNS depression and vomiting.

Enhancement of Elimination

No reports have been published of use of these techniques in treating inhalational anesthetic toxicity. Adequate ventilation should be maintained, as these agents undergo significant elimination in exhaled air.

Antidotes

No proven antidote is available for toxicity from inhalational anesthetics. *N*-acetylcysteine pretreatment can prevent halothane-induced hepatitis in animals (97), and methionine has been used in one case of halothane hepatitis (98). No controlled human data have suggested that these agents are effective in the treatment of halothane hepatitis.

In the case of nitrous oxide–induced myelosuppression or peripheral neuropathy, supplementation may be useful. Only case report data are available, and they indicated mixed results. Given the safety of this drug, however, a course of vitamin B_{12} therapy is a reasonable intervention.

Supportive Care

Most patients survive with airway management and ventilatory support. Hypotension usually responds to administration of intravenous fluids. Vasopressors may be needed in patients with severe hypotension; these agents should be used with caution after halothane poisoning, as halothane sensitizes the myocardium to catecholamines and their use may precipitate dysrhythmias.

Malignant hyperthermia is treated by immediately discontinuing anesthesia, hyperventilating the patient with 100% oxygen, and initiating aggressive cooling measures. Intravenous fluids should be administered to maintain hydration and urine output. One should monitor for and treat hyperkalemia. Dantrolene should be administered with an initial dose of 1 mg/kg intravenously, which can be repeated as needed up to 10 mg/kg (Chapter 47).

Monitoring

Vital signs should be monitored frequently, particularly pulse and blood pressure. In patients with hypotension, urine output should be monitored. Serum levels of these agents are not widely available or useful for managing overdose. Serum electrolytes, liver and renal function, and electrocardiography should be monitored.

REFERENCES

1. Wenker OC. Review of currently used inhalation anesthetics (Pt I). *Internet J Anesthesiol* 1999;3(2).
2. Rampil IJ, Lockhart SH, Zwass MS, et al. Clinical characteristics of desflurane in surgical patients: minimum alveolar concentration. *Anesthesiology* 1991;74:429–433.
3. Ghouri AF, Bodner M, White PF. Recovery profile after desflurane-nitrous oxide versus isoflurane-nitrous oxide in outpatients. *Anesthesiology* 1991;74:419–424.
4. Van Hemelrijck J, Smith I, White PF. Use of desflurane for outpatient anesthesia. A comparison with propofol and nitrous oxide. *Anesthesiology* 1991;75:197–203.
5. Ghouri AF, White PF. Effect of fentanyl and nitrous oxide on the desflurane anesthetic requirement. *Anesth Analg* 1991;72:377–381.
6. Jones RM, Cashman JN, Mant TGK. Clinical impressions and cardiorespiratory effects of a new fluorinated inhalation anaesthetic, desflurane (I-653), in volunteers. *Br J Anaesth* 1990;64:11–15.
7. Weiskopf RB, Cahalan MK, Ionescu P, et al. Cardiovascular actions of desflurane with and without nitrous oxide during spontaneous ventilation in humans. *Anesth Analg* 1991;73:165–174.
8. Cahalan MK, Weiskopf RB, Eger EI, et al. Hemodynamic effects of desflurane/nitrous oxide anesthesia in volunteers. *Anesth Analg* 1991;73:157–164.
9. Fletcher JE, Sebel PS, Murphy MR, et al. Psychomotor performance after desflurane anesthesia: a comparison with isoflurane. *Anesth Analg* 1991;73:260–265.
10. Lockhart SH, Rampil IJ, Yasuda N, et al. Depression of ventilation by desflurane in humans. *Anesthesiology* 1991;74:484–488.
11. Wissing H, Kuhn I, Warnken U, et al. Carbon monoxide production from desflurane, enflurane, halothane, isoflurane, and sevoflurane with dry soda lime. *Anesthesiology* 2001;95(5):1205–1212.
12. Berry PD, Sessler DI, Larson MD. Severe carbon monoxide poisoning during desflurane anesthesia. *Anesthesiology* 1999;90:613–616.
13. Fu ES, Scharf JE, Mangar D, et al. Malignant hyperthermia involving the administration of desflurane. *Can J Anaesth* 1996;43:687–690.
14. Product information: Ethrane(R), enflurane. Liberty Corner, NJ: Baxter Pharmaceutical Products, 1999.
15. O'Neill MP, Sharkey AJ, Fee JPH, et al. A comparative study of enflurane and halothane in children. *Anaesthesia* 1982;37:634–639.
16. Black GW, Johnston HML, Scott MG. Clinical impressions of enflurane. *Br J Anaesth* 1977;49:857–880.
17. Chase RE, Holaday DA, Fiserova-Bergerova V, et al. The biotransformation of Ethrane in man. *Anesthesiology* 1971;35:262.
18. Jacob B, Heller C, Daldrup T, et al. Fatal accidental enflurane intoxication. *J Forensic Sci* 1989;34:1408–1412.
19. Lingenfelter RW. Fatal misuse of enflurane. *Anesthesiology* 1981;55:603.
20. Rodrigo MRC, Moles TM, Lee PK. A comparison of the incidence and nature of cardiac dysrhythmias occurring during enflurane and isoflurane anaesthesia for dental surgery. *Anaesth Intensive Care* 1987;15:179–184.
21. Chander J. Isorhythmic atrioventricular dissociation during enflurane anesthesia. *South Med J* 1982;75:945–950.
22. Morton M, Duke PC. Baroreflex control of heart rate in man awake and during enflurane and enflurane–nitrous oxide anesthesia. *Anesthesiology* 1980;52:221–223.
23. Steward DJ. A trial of enflurane for pediatric out-patient anaesthesia. *Can Anaesth Soc J* 1977;24:603–608.
24. Schwettmann RS, Casterline CL. Delayed asthmatic response following occupational exposure to enflurane. *Anesthesiology* 1976;166–169.
25. Wahba WM. Analysis of ventilatory depression by enflurane during clinical anesthesia. *Anesth Analg* 1980;59:103–109.
26. Christys AR, Moss E, Powell D. Retrospective study of early postoperative convulsions after intracranial surgery with isoflurane or enflurane anaesthesia. *Br J Anaesth* 1989;62:624–627.

27. Ohm WW, Cullen BF, Amory DW, et al. Delayed seizure activity following enflurane anesthesia. *Anesthesiology* 1975;42:467.
28. Ng AT. Prolonged myoclonic contractions after enflurane anaesthesia—a case report. *Can Anaesth Soc J* 1980;27:502–503.
29. Fahy LT. Delayed convulsions after day case anaesthesia with enflurane [Letter]. *Anaesthesia* 1987;42:1327–1328.
30. Nicoll JMV. Status epilepticus following enflurane anaesthesia. *Anaesthesia* 1986;41:927–930.
31. Parke TJ, Jago RH. Focal seizure following enflurane [Letter]. *Anesthesia* 1992;47:79–80.
32. Hovorka J, Korttila K, Erkola O. Nausea and vomiting after general anaesthesia with isoflurane, enflurane or fentanyl in combination with nitrous oxide and oxygen. *Eur J Anaesthesiol* 1988;5:177–182.
33. Gogus FY, Toker K & Baykan N: Hepatitis following use of two different fluorinated anesthetic agents. *Isr J Med Sci* 1991; 27:156-159.
34. Christ DD, Kenna JG, Kammerer W, et al. Enflurane metabolism produces covalently bound liver adducts recognized by antibodies from patients with halothane hepatitis. *Anesthesiology* 1988;69:833–838.
35. Ona FV, Patanella H, Ayub A. Hepatitis associated with enflurane anesthesia. *Anesth Analg* 1980;59:146–149.
36. Yamasita M, Matsuki A, Oyama T. Illicit use of modern volatile anesthetics. *Can Anaesth Soc J* 1984;31:76–79.
37. Curelaru I, Stanciu ST, Nicolau V, et al. A case of recovery from coma produced by the ingestion of 250 ml of halothane. *Br J Anaesth* 1968;40:283–288.
38. Sutton J, Harrison GA, Hickie JB. Accidental intravenous injection of halothane. *Br J Anaesth* 1971;43:513–519.
39. Loper K, Reitan J, Bennett H, et al. Comparison of halothane and isoflurane for rapid anesthetic induction. *Anesth Analg* 1987;66:766–768.
40. Naito Y, Tamai S, Shingu K, et al. Comparison between sevoflurane and halothane for paediatric ambulatory anaesthesia. *Br J Anaesth* 1991;67:387–389.
41. Dale O, Brown BR Jr. Clinical pharmacokinetics of the inhalational anaesthetics [Review]. *Clin Pharmacokinet* 1987;12:145–167.
42. Dwyer R, Coppel DL. Intravenous injection of liquid halothane. *Anesth Analg* 1989;69:250–255.
43. Product Information: Fluothane, halothane (liquid for vaporization). Philadelphia: Wyeth-Ayerst Laboratories, 1998.
44. Blayney MR, Malins AF, Cooper GM. Cardiac arrhythmias in children during outpatient general anaesthesia for dentistry: a prospective randomised trial. *Lancet* 1999;354:1864–1866.
45. Viitanen H, Baer G, Koivu, et al. The hemodynamic and Holter-electrocardiogram changes during halothane and sevoflurane anesthesia for adenoidectomy in children aged one to three years. *Anesth Analg* 1999;87:1423–1425.
46. Department of Drugs: AMA Evaluations Subscription. Chicago: American Medical Association, 1994.
47. Neuberger JM. Halothane and hepatitis: incidence, predisposing factors and exposure guidelines. *Drug Saf* 1990;5:28–38.
48. Sweetman S, ed. *Martindale. The complete drug reference.* London: Pharmaceutical Press, 2001:2.
49. Ray DC, Drummond GB. Halothane hepatitis. *Br J Anaesth* 1991;67:84–99.
50. Rosenak D, et al. Halothane and liver damage. *Postgrad Med J* 1989;65:129–135.
51. Echeverria M, Gelb AW, Wexler HR, et al. Enflurane and halothane in status asthmaticus. *Chest* 1986;89:152–154.
52. Product Information: Forane, isoflurane. Liberty Corner, NJ: Ohmeda, 2000.
53. Cameron CB, Robinson S, Gregory GA. The minimum anesthetic concentration of isoflurane in children. *Anesth Analg* 1984;63:418–420.
54. Dooper MM, Beerens J, Brenninkmeijer VJ, et al. Fatal intoxication after ingestion of isoflurane. *Neth J Med* 1988;33:74–77.
55. Eger EI II. The pharmacology of isoflurane. *Br J Anaesth* 1984;56:71S–99S.
56. Nakayama M, Tsuchida H, Kanaya N, et al. Effects of epidural anesthesia on the cardiovascular response to a rapid increase in isoflurane concentration. *J Clin Anesth* 2000;12:14–18.
57. Friesen RH, Lichtor JL. Cardiovascular effects of inhalation induction with isoflurane in infants. *Anesth Analg* 1983;62:111–114.
58. Kelsall AW, Ross-Russell R, Herrick MJ. Reversible neurologic dysfunction following isoflurane sedation in pediatric intensive care. *Crit Care Med* 1994;22:1032–1034.
59. Prithvi P, Tod MJ, Jenkins MT. Clinical comparison of isoflurane and halothane anesthetics. *South Med J* 1976;69:1128.
60. Johnston MD, Voseworthy TW, Friesen EG, et al. Isoflurane therapy for status asthmaticus in children and adults. *Chest* 1990;97:698–701.
61. Gelven PL, Cina SJ, Lee JD, et al. Massive hepatic necrosis and death following repeated isoflurane exposure. *Am J Forensic Med Pathol* 1996;17:61–64.
62. Scheider DM, Klygis LM, Tsang TK, et al. Hepatic dysfunction after repeated isoflurane administration. *J Clin Gastroenterol* 1993;17:168–170.
63. AMA Department of Drugs: Drug Evaluations Subscription. Chicago: American Medical Association, 1993.
64. Proudfoot J, Roberts M, Mellick LB. Providing safe and effective sedation and analgesia for pediatric patients. *Emerg Med Rep* 1993;14:207–218.
65. Gamis AS, Knapp JF, Glenski JA, et al. Nitrous oxide analgesia in a pediatric emergency department. *Ann Emerg Med* 1989;18:177–181.
66. Rowland AS, Baird DD, Weinberg CR, et al. Reduced fertility among women employed as dental assistants exposed to high levels of nitrous oxide. *N Engl J Med* 1992;327:993–997.
67. Ahlborg G, Axelsson G, Bodin L. Shift work, nitrous oxide exposure and subfertility among Swedish midwives. *Int J Epidemiol* 1996;25:783–790.
68. Cohen EN, et al. Occupational disease in dentistry and chronic exposure to trace anesthetic gases. *J Am Dent Assoc* 1980;101:21.
69. Kunkel DB. Nitrous oxide: not a laughing matter anymore. *Emerg Med* 1987;19:79–84.
70. Adonato BT. Nitrous oxide and vitamin B12 [Letter]. *Lancet* 1978;2:1318.
71. Deacon R, Lumb M, Perry J, et al: Selective inactivation of vitamin B12 in rats by nitrous oxide. *Lancet* 1978;2:1023–1024.
72. Lai NY, Silbert PL, Erber WN, et al. "Nanging": another cause of nitrous oxide neurotoxicity [Letter]. *Med J Aust* 1997;166:166.
73. Layzer RB. Myeloneuropathy after prolonged exposure to nitrous oxide. *Lancet* 1978;2:1227–1230.
74. Aston R. Drug abuse. Its relationship to dental practice. *Dent Clin North Am* 1984;28:595–610.
75. Ross AS, Riekman GA, Carley BL. Waste nitrous oxide exposure. *J Can Dent Assoc* 1984;7:561–563.
76. Brodsky JB. The toxicity of nitrous oxide. *Clin Anesthesiol* 1983;1:455–467.
77. Felmet K, Robins B, Tilford D, et al. Acute neurologic decompensation in an infant with cobalamin deficiency exposed to nitrous oxide. *J Pediatr* 2000;137:427–428.
78. Amess JAL, Burman JF, Rees GM, et al. Megaloblastic haemopoiesis in patients receiving nitrous oxide. *Lancet* 1978;2:339–342.
79. Nunn JF, Sharer NM, Gorchein A, et al. Megaloblastic haemopoiesis after multiple short-term exposure to nitrous oxide. *Lancet* 1982;1:1379–1381.
80. Sweeney B, Bingham RM, Amos RJ, et al. Toxicity of bone marrow in dentists exposed to nitrous oxide. *BMJ* 1985;291:567–569.
81. Berger JJ, Modell JH, Sypert GW. Megaloblastic anemia and brief exposure to nitrous oxide—a cause/relationship? *Anesth Analg* 1988;67:197–198.
82. LiPuma JP, Wellman J, Stern HP. Nitrous oxide abuse: a new cause for pneumomediastinum. *Radiology* 1982;145:602.
83. Kawamura R, Stanley T, English JB, et al. Cardiovascular responses to nitrous oxide exposure for two hours in man. *Anesth Analg* 1980;59:93–99.
84. Moffitt EA, Sethna DH, Gary RJ, et al. Nitrous oxide added to halothane reduces coronary flow and myocardial oxygen consumption in patients with coronary disease. *Can Anaesth Soc J* 1983;30:5–9.
85. Scheinin B, Lindgren L. Nitrous oxide and the bowel. *Surv Anesthesiol* 1991;35:119–120.
86. Product information: Ultane(R), sevoflurane. North Chicago, IL: Abbott Laboratories, 2001.
87. Smith I, Ding Y, White PF. Comparison of induction, maintenance, and recovery characteristics of sevoflurane-N2O and propofol-sevoflurane-N2O with propofol-isoflurane-N2O anesthesia. *Anesth Analg* 1992;74:253–259.
88. Kuenszberg E, Loeckinger A, Kleinsasser A, et al. Sevoflurane progressively prolongs the QT interval in unpremedicated female adults. *Eur J Anaesthesiol* 2000;17:662–664.
89. Reference deleted.
90. Schultz A, Schultz B, Grouven U, et al. Epileptiform activity in the EEGs of two nonepileptic children under sevoflurane anaesthesia. *Anaesth Intensive Care* 2000;28:205–207.
91. Kaisti KK, Jaaskelainen SK, Rinne JO, et al. Epileptiform discharges during 2 MAC sevoflurane anesthesia in two healthy volunteers. *Anesthesiology* 1999;91:1952–1955.
92. Terasako K, Ishi S. Postoperative seizure-like activity following sevoflurane anesthesia. *Acta Anaesthesiol Scand* 1996;40:953–954.
93. Adachi M, Ikemoto Y, Kubo K, et al. Seizure-like movements during induction of anaesthesia with sevoflurane. *Br J Anaesth* 1992;68:214–215.
94. Frink EJ Jr, Malan P, Atlas M, et al. Clinical comparison of sevoflurane and isoflurane in healthy patients. *Anesth Analg* 1992;74:241–245.
95. Ochiai R, Toyoda Y, Nishio I, et al. Possible association of malignant hyperthermia with sevoflurane anesthesia. *Anesth Analg* 1992;74:616–618.
96. Otsuka H, Komura Y, Mayumi T, et al. Malignant hyperthermia during sevoflurane anesthesia in a child with central core disease. *Anesthesiology* 1991;75:699–701.
97. Keaney NP, Cocking G. N-acetylcysteine protection against halothane hepatotoxicity: experiments in rats. *Lancet* 1981;2:95.
98. Windsor JA, Wynne-Jones G. Halothane hepatitis and prompt resolution with methionine therapy: case report. *N Z Med J* 1988;101:502–503.

CHAPTER 130

Anticonvulsant Medications

Donna L. Seger

PHENYTOIN

Compounds included:	**Carbamazepine (Tegretol, Teril), felbamate (Felbatol), fosphenytoin (Cerebyx, Pro-Epanutin), gabapentin (Gantin, Neurontin), lamotrigine (Lamictal), oxcarbazepine (Trileptal), phenobarbital (Luminal), phenytoin (Dilantin, Epanutin), tiagabine (Gabitril), topiramate (Topamax), valproate (Depacon), vigabatrin (Sabril), zonisamide (Zonegran)**
Molecular formula and weight:	**See Table 1.**
SI conversion:	**See Table 1.**
CAS Registry No.:	**See Table 1.**
Therapeutic levels:	**See Table 1.**
Target organs:	**Central nervous system (acute and chronic), cardiovascular (acute), renal (acute)**
Antidotes:	**Naloxone, carnitine (experimental)**

OVERVIEW

The market is exploding with new drugs to treat epilepsy, making it more important than ever for clinical toxicologists to understand the pharmacology and clinical ramifications of therapeutic and toxic ingestions of anticonvulsant drugs. Historically, anticonvulsant drug development was painstakingly slow. Phenobarbital was the first anticonvulsant, developed in 1912. This drug was not well received because it caused sedation. Phenytoin was introduced in 1938 and produced similar anticonvulsant actions but less sedation. Structurally related to the barbiturates, but with fewer side effects than either phenobarbital or phenytoin, carbamazepine gained U.S. Food and Drug Administration (FDA) approval for use as an anticonvulsant in 1974 (1).

Valproic acid was discovered serendipitously while being used in a drug-screening program. It was approved by the FDA in 1978. The following years offered little in the development of anticonvulsant drugs. When the FDA approved felbamate in 1994, it was hailed as a miracle drug. Other anticonvulsants, subsequently approved throughout the 1990s, are also currently FDA approved as first-line therapy in the treatment of mood disorders.

Epilepsy and Drug Development

A seizure is a paroxysmal transient disturbance of brain function. Seizures affect 1% of the world population. In 70% of patients with epilepsy, no specific cause of seizures is determined. When drug efficacy is defined as a 50% decrease in seizures, 75% of the epileptic population benefits from anticonvulsant therapy. This means that 25% of the epileptic population is not seizure free, which further pushes the need for new drug development (2,3). Side effects of these drugs also create the need for less toxic and more effective anticonvulsants.

The ideal anticonvulsant would be water soluble, effective for a wide range of seizure types, cause few adverse events or drug interactions, be renally excreted, and have little hepatic metabolism, a long elimination half-life that allows twice-a-day dosing, and constant interpatient pharmacokinetics. Single drug therapy is desirable as it is the best chance of seizure control with the least number of side effects. The most frequent adverse effects of anticonvulsant therapy are decreased cognition, motor slowing, and gastrointestinal (GI) symptoms (4).

Unexpected Death and Anticonvulsants

Patients with epilepsy have an increased incidence of sudden unexpected death (SUD). The mechanism is not known, but several events occur during or after seizures that may contribute to SUD: cardiac dysrhythmias and repolarization abnormalities (occur in 39% of patients with intractable partial epilepsy), central apnea followed by asystole, primary cardiac dysrhythmias of reflex neural origin, and postictal apnea (5).

In 1993, the FDA convened a panel to determine if anticonvulsant drugs contribute to or prevent SUD. The panel concluded that SUD rates in epileptic patients reflect population rates and not a specific drug effect. However, the question of whether drugs are a benefit or a risk in SUD remains unanswered. A given drug, in a given patient who experiences a sei-

TABLE 1. Physical characteristics, therapeutic dose, and concentration for the anticonvulsants

Drug	Molecular formula, molecular weight (g/mol), CAS Registry No.	Therapeutic dose		Therapeutic serum level, SI conversion
		Adult	Pediatric	
Carbamazepine	$C_{15}H_{12}N_2O$; 236.3; 298-46-4	3 mg/kg/d initially; 5–20 mg/kg/d maintenance	5 mg/kg/d, 20 to 40 mg/kg/d	4–12 μg/ml; mg/L × 4.23 = μmol/L
Felbamate	$C_{11}H_{14}N_2O_4$; 238.2; 25451-15-4	1200 mg/d initially; 3600 mg/d maintenance	15 mg/kg/d initially; 45 mg/kg/d maintenance	18–52 μg/ml; mg/L × 4.20 = μmol/L
Fosphenytoin sodium	$C_{16}H_{13}N_2Na_2O_6P$; 406.2; 92134-98-0	10–20 mg phenytoin equivalents/kg IV or IM	Same as adult	10–20 μg/ml (as phenytoin)
Gabapentin	$C_9H_{17}NO_2$; 171.2; 60142-96-3	1200 mg/d initially; 3600 mg/d maintenance	10–15 mg/kg/d in divided doses	Not used clinically; mg/L × 5.84 = μmol/L
Lamotrigine	$C_9H_7Cl_2N_5$; 256.1; 84057-84-1	50 mg/d for 2 wk, then 50 to 100 mg twice daily up to 400 mg/d	2 mg/kg/d with maintenance doses of 5 to 15 mg/kg/d (<2 years of age)	Range has not been established; mg/L × 3.90 = μmol/L
Oxcarbazepine	$C_{15}H_{12}N_2O_2$; 252.3; 28721-07-5	300 mg orally BID; up to 1200 mg/d	8–10 mg/kg orally in two divided doses; up to 600 mg/d	Range has not been established; mg/L × 3.96 = μmol/L
Phenobarbital sodium	$C_{12}H_{11}N_2NaO_3$; 254.2; 57-30-7	1–3 mg/kg/d PO	3–5 mg/kg/d PO	10–40 μg/ml; mg/L × 4.31 = μmol/L
Phenytoin sodium	$C_{15}H_{11}N_2NaO_2$; 274.2; 630-93-3	4–6 mg/kg/d PO	3–10 mg/kg/d PO	10–20 μg/ml; mg/L × 3.96 = μmol/L
Tiagabine hydrochloride	$C_{20}H_{25}NO_2S_2$,HCl; 412.0; 145821-59-6	4 mg/d initially; 64 mg/d maximum	4 mg/d initially; 32 mg/d maximum	Range has not been established; mg/L × 2.66 = μmol/L
Topiramate	$C_{12}H_{21}NO_8S$; 339.4; 97240-79-4	1 mg/kg/d initially; 3–9 mg/kg/d maintenance	1–3 mg/kg day initially; 5–9 mg/kg/d maintenance	Range has not been established; mg/L × 2.95 = μmol/L
Valproate sodium	$C_8H_{15}NaO_2$; 166.2; 1069-66-5	1000–2000 mg/d	15–60 mg/kg/d	50–125 μg/ml; mg/L × 6.93 = μmol/L
Vigabatrin	$C_6H_{11}NO_2$; 129.2; 60643-86-9	500 mg/d initially; 2–4 g/d maintenance	1–2 g/d	Range has not been established; mg/L × 7.74 = μmol/L
Zonisamide	$C_8H_8N_2O_3S$; 212.2; 68291-97-4	100 mg daily, up to 400 mg/d	2–4 mg/kg/d initially; 12 mg/kg/d maximum, up to 400 mg/d	20–30 μg/ml; mg/L × 4.71 = μmol/L

zure, may be beneficial or may contribute to SUD depending on the unique set of circumstances (5). There is much to be learned about the relationship of anticonvulsant drugs to SUD in the epileptic patient population.

Anticonvulsant Embryopathy

The syndrome of major malformation, growth retardation, and hypoplasia of the midface and fingers in newborns of mothers treated with anticonvulsants during pregnancy is called *anticonvulsant embryopathy*. Whether this embryopathy is caused by intrauterine exposure to anticonvulsant drugs or by maternal epilepsy has been questioned. A recent study revealed that infants exposed *in utero* to a single anticonvulsant drug had a significantly higher frequency of associated abnormalities than control infants. Infants whose mothers had epilepsy but took no anticonvulsant drugs during pregnancy did not have an increased incidence of abnormalities. Physical abnormalities in infants exposed to various anticonvulsant drugs vary. The occurrence of embryopathy correlated to exposure to the anticonvulsant drug, regardless of the reason the mother was taking the drug (6).

Anticonvulsant Hypersensitivity Syndrome

Anticonvulsant hypersensitivity syndrome is a rare, life-threatening syndrome that usually occurs within 8 weeks of anticonvulsant initiation. Although the true incidence is unknown due to variable presentation and inaccurate reporting, estimates of incidence are 1 in 1000 to 10,000 exposures. The aromatic anticonvulsants (phenytoin, carbamazepine, or phenobarbital) are the most frequent causes. This syndrome is not related to dosage or serum concentration of the drug. The clinical syndrome consists of fever, rash, and internal organ (most frequently liver) involvement. Fever is usually the first symptom. The cause of anticonvulsant hypersensitivity syndrome is unknown. Theories include a toxic metabolite, graft-versus-host disease, or allergic hypersensitivity reaction. Treatment is discontinuation of the anticonvulsant (7,8).

Cognitive Impairment

Although initial evidence implied that the drugs that increase γ-aminobutyrate, *GABAergic drugs* (topiramate, gabapentin, and lamotrigine), caused cognitive impairment, methodologic problems with current studies leave this question unanswered (9,10).

Visual Field Defects

Visual field defects, thought to be caused by GABA-induced retinal toxicity, have been reported in 40% to 83% of patients on vigabatrin. Other GABAergic drugs (gabapentin, topiramate, tiagabine) may also cause visual field defects (11–18). Although cases of irreversible visual field loss have been reported, most studies indicate significant reversibility (11,12,19–24). The pattern is bilateral concentric constriction. Bilateral optic disc pallor and peripheral retinal atrophy may be present on examination (25–27). The patient with visual field defects may be asymptomatic for years (17,18). Ophthalmologic examination should be considered every 3 months for patients taking vigabatrin and other GABAergic drugs.

CARBAMAZEPINE

Carbamazepine (Tegretol, Teril) was discovered in 1952 as a result of the structural similarity to imipramine and spatial similarity to phenytoin. Used as an anticonvulsant in Europe since 1962, it gained FDA approval for treatment of trigeminal neuralgia in 1960 and treatment of epilepsy in 1974 (28). Tegretol is available in 200-mg tablets, 100-mg chewable tablets, and a 100-mg/5-ml suspension.

Toxic Dose

Adult and pediatric therapeutic doses are provided in Table 1 (29). According to the package labeling, the lowest dose reported to cause death is 3.2 g in an adult (30). A dose of 1.6 g was fatal in a child who died of aspiration pneumonia (30).

Pharmacokinetics

Carbamazepine is an iminostilbene derivative that is chemically and structurally similar to imipramine, yet shares few of its pharmacologic properties (31). Absorption is slow, and peak serum concentrations usually occur within 4 to 8 hours, but may develop as late as 12 hours after ingestion. Controlled release preparations are slowly absorbed, and peak serum concentrations may be significantly delayed (32).

Plasma protein binding is 75%. The volume of distribution (V_d) is 0.79 to 1.19 L/kg. It is metabolized by CYP3A4 to an active metabolite (10,11-epoxide) with a half-life of 10 to 20 hours. In adults, the metabolite concentration is 10% to 15% of the parent compound, whereas in children the metabolite concentration is 20% of the parent compound (31). The epoxide may cause the neurotoxicity of the drug. Because carbamazepine induces its own metabolism, the half-life of the drug after an isolated single dose (35 hours) is much longer than the half-life of the drug at steady state (10 to 20 hours). The autoinduction takes approximately a month (33). Elimination of parent compound follows zero order kinetics with an elimination rate of 0.5 to 0.8 mg/L/hour (34). The epoxide is metabolized to inactive compounds, which are excreted in the urine. Three percent of parent compound is excreted unchanged in the urine (32,35).

Pathophysiology

Carbamazepine inhibits sodium channels and interferes with release of glutamate and possibly other neurotransmitters (36,37). It also inhibits muscarinic and nicotinic acetylcholine receptors, *N*-methyl-D-aspartate receptors, and central nervous system (CNS) adenosine receptors (38–41).

Pregnancy and Lactation

Carbamazepine is FDA pregnancy category D (Appendix I). Major malformations, microcephaly, and growth retardation occur more frequently in infants exposed to carbamazepine. Lumbosacral spinal bifida is most common in infants exposed to either carbamazepine or valproic acid (42,43).

Carbamazepine enters breast milk, and newborn infants have developed serum levels of 15% to 65% of the maternal level (44).

Clinical Presentation

ACUTE OVERDOSAGE

Delayed and erratic absorption due to anticholinergic properties and low water solubility can cause a cyclic clinical course. Clinical deterioration can be markedly delayed. Peak serum concentrations have occurred as long as 72 hours after ingestion of immediate release (45) and 96 hours after ingestion of controlled release carbamazepine (32). Half-life may be prolonged (39 hours) after an isolated ingestion and shorter when chronic ingestion has induced metabolism (46).

Serious complications such as coma and respiratory failure may occur. Less serious complications include ataxia, nystagmus, mydriasis, ileus, hypertonicity, increased deep tendon reflexes, and movement disorders (47). Due to the anticholinergic properties of the drug, anticholinergic toxidromes may occur.

Status epilepticus has been reported in two patients after carbamazepine overdose, but analytic testing was not comprehensive so other agents may have been ingested (48). Seizures are more likely to occur in patients with high serum concentrations and an underlying seizure disorder (49). Left ventricular dysfunction with heart failure occurred in two patients with large overdoses (50).

Liver injury resulting in hyponatremia, hyperglycemia, and transient elevation of serum liver enzymes has occurred after overdose. Cardiac dysrhythmias are rare, but first-degree and complete heart block has been reported (51–55). Animal studies reveal prolonged atrioventricular conduction and membrane depressant effect when high doses of carbamazepine are administered (51).

ADVERSE EVENTS

Cardiac conduction disturbances may occur in elderly patients taking therapeutic doses and do not appear to be dose related. Bradycardia (including complete heart block) may occur in older patients with a defective conduction system or sick sinus syndrome (56–59). Benign cardiac conduction disturbances are found in up to 57% of patients with carbamazepine toxicity (60).

Adverse effects occur in 25% of patients. Mild transient leukopenia may occur during the first month of treatment but usually resolves despite continued drug administration. This leukopenia is unrelated to aplastic anemia, which occurs in one in 575,000 patients treated with carbamazepine (61). Hematologic monitoring is recommended. Discontinuation of the drug is not required for the mild liver enzyme elevation that occurs in 10% of patients (62). Systemic lupus erythematosus–like syndrome has been reported. Serology returned to normal after carbamazepine was discontinued (63).

Any drug that inhibits the cytochrome CYP3A4 isoenzyme increases carbamazepine concentration.

Diagnostic Tests

Although serum carbamazepine concentrations do not accurately correlate with the clinical severity of the poisoning, serum concentrations more than 40 mg/L are associated with an increased risk of serious complications such as coma, seizures, respiratory failure, and cardiac conduction defects (64). The seriousness of toxicity should be judged by the clinical status of the patient, not the serum carbamazepine concentration (55).

Due to their structural similarities, carbamazepine can cause a false-positive serum tricyclic antidepressant screen. Both carbamazepine and carbamazepine epoxide are measured by standard Enzyme Multiplied Immunoassay Test. A ratio of parent compound to epoxide greater than 2.5 suggests continuing GI absorption (65).

Laboratory testing should include complete blood count to monitor bone marrow effects and liver enzymes for hepatic injury. An electrocardiogram should be performed in overdosage patients, symptomatic patients on chronic therapy, and before the initiation of therapy in patients older than 50 years of age.

Treatment

Management focuses on symptomatic and supportive treatment while monitoring for cardiac effects.

DECONTAMINATION

Gastric lavage may be considered if the patient is obtunded within 1 hour of ingestion of carbamazepine. Prolonged absorption must be considered after this overdose. Activated charcoal does bind carbamazepine, although its effect on clinical course is unknown. An initial dose within 1 to 2 hours of ingestion is reasonable.

ENHANCEMENT OF ELIMINATION

Although earlier evidence indicated that administration of multiple dose activated charcoal (MDAC) decreased half-life and increased elimination of carbamazepine (66,67), more recent evidence indicates that charcoal has no effect on the elimination of carbamazepine or the duration of coma (34). This treatment modality has not been adequately evaluated to determine if it decreases time to complete recovery or changes outcome. The benefit:risk ratio of MDAC administration in a sleepy patient or a patient that may require intubation must be assessed in each case.

Similarly, charcoal hemoperfusion has been shown to decrease the half-life of both carbamazepine and the epoxide, but the efficacy of this technique has not been compared with supportive care alone or the administration of MDAC. Complications of hemoperfusion include thrombocytopenia, hypocalcemia, and bleeding (due to heparin anticoagulation). If extracorporeal removal is considered in life-threatening overdose, hemodialysis is usually the treatment of choice as hemoperfusion cartridges are not readily available (68,69).

ANTIDOTES

Antidotal treatment with physostigmine has been considered. Its use is not recommended.

SUPPORTIVE CARE

Hypotension is treated with rapid infusion of 10 to 20 ml/kg of isotonic crystalloidal fluids, followed by the administration of vasopressors, if needed (Chapter 37).

FELBAMATE

Felbamate (Felbatol) was recommended for approval by an FDA advisory committee in 1992. The manufacturer launched the drug in 1993 with a major advertising campaign. The drug was said to have few side effects. *Time* magazine published an article entitled "Taming the Brain Storms" acknowledging the first new anticonvulsant drug in 15 years, claiming it would bring hope to more than a million Americans with uncontrolled epilepsy (70).

But the problems were only beginning. Because felbamate interacted with other anticonvulsants, an imaginative trial had been designed with placebo as comparator or low-dose valproate as *active* placebo. Although 4000 persons had been exposed to felbamate, only 900 patients had received treatment with felbamate for 6 months when it was approved. Pivotal studies did not clarify dosage and titration. Adverse events may have not been prominent because the studies were designed to evaluate efficacy rather than safety (71).

Shortly after approval, it became apparent that felbamate was not well tolerated due to GI complaints, insomnia, weight loss, dizziness, fatigue, ataxia, and lethargy (72). In 1994, it was reported that 20 cases of felbamate-induced aplastic anemia, including three fatalities, had been reported to the FDA. This incidence of aplastic anemia is 100 times higher than reported in the general population (73,74). The manufacturer notified 240,000 physicians recommending discontinuation of felbamate in all patients unless it was deemed absolutely necessary. Acute withdrawal of felbamate precipitated status epilepticus in some patients, including some fatalities (75,76). All marketing efforts were discontinued (70).

In September 1994, the FDA advisory committee voted to allow felbamate to remain on the market. In addition to the reports of aplastic anemia, eight cases of hepatic failure, including four deaths, had been associated with felbamate therapy. Yet felbamate administration decreased the number of seizures and improved the quality of life in many patients with refractory seizures (70,74). Felbamate is recommended only when other treatment regimens have failed. A patient consent explaining the risks of hepatitis and aplastic anemia accompanies the package insert. Nonetheless, patients with refractory epilepsy are willing to take the risk.

Felbamate is available as 400- and 600-mg tablets and as a 600-mg/5-ml suspension.

Toxic Dose

Adult and pediatric therapeutic doses are provided in Table 1 (29). Acute ingestion of 6.9 to 36 g has produced mild to moderate effects of somnolence, weakness, ataxia, and GI symptoms (77).

Pharmacokinetics

Felbamate is a dicarbamate derivative structurally related to meprobamate (78). Oral bioavailability is 90%. The time to peak plasma level is 1 to 4 hours and V_d is 0.75 L/kg. Plasma protein binding is 25%. The elimination half-life is 20 hours; 40% to 50% is excreted unchanged in the urine (79).

Pathophysiology

Although the mechanism of action has not been confirmed, felbamate appears to decrease the sodium current, enhance the inhibitory actions of GABA, and block *N*-methyl-D-aspartate receptors. There is no effect on benzodiazepine receptors or GABA receptor binding (79).

Pregnancy and Lactation

Felbamate is FDA pregnancy category C (Appendix I). Felbamate does enter breast milk, but its effect on the infant is unknown.

Clinical Presentation

ACUTE OVERDOSAGE

Felbamate often causes mild symptoms such as somnolence and GI disturbance (80). Massive crystalluria and acute renal failure were reported in a patient who overdosed on felbamate and valproate. The crystals were identified as containing felbamate. It is unclear if crystalluria is caused by felbamate overdose or if it was caused by the combination of felbamate with sodium valproate (81).

ADVERSE EVENTS

Fatal hepatitis and aplastic anemia are potentially life threatening and may occur with chronic use of this drug. Weight gain, weakness, malaise, influenza-like symptoms, palpitations, tachycardia, agitation, psychological disturbance, aggressive reaction, pruritus, and Stevens-Johnson syndrome have been reported (82).

Diagnostic Tests

Liver enzymes and white blood counts must be monitored while on felbamate. Although there is no recommended therapeutic range for felbamate, plasma concentrations as high as 140 μg/ml have been tolerated without significant adverse effects (83).

Treatment

Treatment is symptomatic and supportive. There is no evidence that gastric lavage or administration of single dose activated charcoal changes outcome after overdose. Felbamate is likely removed by hemodialysis; however, no reports of its use for overdose have been published.

FOSPHENYTOIN

Fosphenytoin (Cerebyx, Pro-Epanutin) is a disodium phosphate ester prodrug of phenytoin that is water-soluble and therefore does not require the presence of propylene glycol in the product. The propylene glycol–induced side effects of bradycardia and hypotension are probably less common with fosphenytoin (84,85), but an accumulating body of case reports demonstrates that fosphenytoin can cause hypotension in some patients. There is a significant cost difference between phenytoin and fosphenytoin.

Fosphenytoin is supplied as a ready-mixed aqueous solution of 50 mg/ml, buffer adjusted to pH of 8.6 to 9.0 with either hydrochloric acid or sodium hydroxide. Administration of fosphenytoin that yields 15 to 20 mg/kg phenytoin produces therapeutic serum concentrations (86).

Toxic Dose

Adult and pediatric doses are provided in Table 1. Infusion of fosphenytoin at a rate of 225 mg/minute intravenously (IV) was associated with bradycardia, hypotension, seizure, and asystole (87). Infusion of therapeutic dose is associated with mild hypotension in a small number of patients.

Pharmacokinetics

Phosphatases present in the liver, red blood cells, and other tissues cleave the phosphate molecule to convert fosphenytoin to phenytoin. After IV administration, conversion to phenytoin averages 8.4 minutes. Maximal concentration is reached within 10 to 20 minutes of starting the infusion (88,89). Therapeutic phenytoin concentrations occur within 10 minutes of a greater than 100 mg/minute infusion and within 30 minutes of infusions at less than 100 mg/minute infusion (90).

Pathophysiology

Fosphenytoin can be administered at a rate three times faster than IV phenytoin. Significant infusion-site irritation and cardiac dysrhythmias occur rarely (89,91).

Pregnancy and Lactation

Fosphenytoin is FDA pregnancy category C (Appendix I). Fosphenytoin is quickly hydrolyzed to release phenytoin, and none is expected to enter breast milk. Phenytoin is considered safe for breast-feeding.

Clinical Presentation

Fosphenytoin causes fewer local and systemic effects than phenytoin. Nystagmus, headache, ataxia, and somnolence are the most frequent symptoms (86). Paresthesias have been reported in up to 30% of volunteers. The paresthesias seem to occur at higher doses and higher infusion rates and rapidly resolve without sequelae (92).

Diagnostic Tests

Determination of fosphenytoin concentration is of no value as the drug is not clinically active (86). Phenytoin concentrations can be determined as described in the Phenytoin section later.

Treatment

The treatment of fosphenytoin toxicity is the same as for phenytoin. Administration of the drug should be discontinued and standard advanced cardiac life support provided.

GABAPENTIN

Gabapentin (Gantin, Neurontin) was approved by the FDA in December 1993. Gabapentin is available in 100, 300, and 400 mg capsules.

Toxic Dose

Adult and pediatric therapeutic doses are provided in Table 1 (29). In adults, large doses of 40 to 100 g have typically produced only drowsiness, dizziness, lethargy, and diarrhea. The combined ingestion of gabapentin 54 g and valproic acid 105 g was followed by hypotension and coma (93).

Pharmacokinetics

Gabapentin is structurally related to the neurotransmitter, GABA. Bioavailability is dose dependent due to facilitated transport during absorption by the L-amino acid transporter. The transport system becomes saturated at higher doses, limiting absorption (94). It is presumed to be transported across the blood–brain barrier in the same manner. Oral bioavailability is 60% after a 300-mg dose and decreases to 35% at a dose of 1600 mg three times a day (95). It is not metabolized or bound to plasma proteins. The elimination half-life is 5 to 7 hours. Gabapentin was the first anticonvulsant since bromide that is eliminated by the kidneys (as is vigabatrin). The dose should be adjusted in patients with renal impairment (96).

Kinetics are linear with plasma concentrations linearly related to dose. As the drug is not metabolized in the liver, it does not induce liver enzymes. Interactions with other drugs are unlikely (96).

Pathophysiology

The mechanism of action is not well understood. Gabapentin binds to a novel high affinity site, but identity of the site is unknown. Gabapentin inhibits voltage-dependent sodium currents. Structurally related to GABA, gabapentin does not bind GABA receptors but enhances the release or actions of GABA. Unlike GABA, gabapentin readily crosses the blood–brain barrier (96).

Pregnancy and Lactation

Gabapentin is FDA pregnancy category C (Appendix I). Effects on the human fetus are unknown. It is unknown if gabapentin is excreted in breast milk.

Clinical Presentation

ACUTE OVERDOSAGE

Serious toxicity has not been reported after gabapentin overdose. A 16-year-old girl ingested 48.9 g of gabapentin. The patient remained sleepy but arousable and was completely alert

18 hours after the ingestion. The initial plasma concentration was 70% of expected. At high doses, the carrier-mediated absorption pathway appears to become saturated; therefore, absorption and bioavailability decrease as the dose increases (97). Five cases of overdose without sequelae have been reported (98). Tremulousness and mild cognitive changes occurred in a patient with chronic renal failure who received extremely high doses of gabapentin for 3 weeks (99).

ADVERSE EVENTS

Side effects include dizziness, somnolence, fatigue, ataxia, headache, tremor, diplopia, nausea and vomiting, and rhinitis. Side effects are usually transient and resolve with prolonged therapy (100).

CARCINOGENICITY

Preclinical studies were stopped for a time due to increased incidence of pancreatic acinar cell tumors in male Wistar rats fed high doses of gabapentin. This did not occur in female rats, mice, or monkeys. Human pancreatic cancer tends to be ductal. Relevance of the tumors in animals to human carcinogenesis is unknown (100).

Treatment

Treatment is symptomatic and supportive. Due to the mild nature of toxicity, the risks of GI decontamination are likely to outweigh the potential benefits. Gabapentin is likely to be cleared efficiently by hemodialysis, but its use in overdose has not been reported. It is unlikely to be needed.

LAMOTRIGINE

Lamotrigine (Lamictal) was released in early 1995. It is available as 25-, 100-, 150-, and 200-mg tablets (29).

Toxic Dose

Adult and pediatric therapeutic doses are provided in Table 1. Fatalities have been reported at doses less than 15 g (102). A 17-year-old girl developed somnolence, lethargy, and ataxia and recovered after a dose of lamotrigine 2000 mg and 12,000 mg of gabapentin (103). After an 800-mg ingestion, a 2-year-old boy recovered uneventfully, despite generalized tonic-clonic seizures, ataxia, and muscle weakness (104).

Toxicokinetics and Toxicodynamics

Lamotrigine is a phenyltriazine derivative. The drug is well absorbed and bioavailability is 98%. The elimination half-life is 22 to 36 hours (105). Protein binding is 55%. It is metabolized by hepatic glucuronidation, which is a target for enzyme inducers and inhibitors. Not surprisingly, metabolism of lamotrigine is markedly increased by inducing drugs. Less than 10% is excreted unchanged (106).

Pathophysiology

Lamotrigine stabilizes presynaptic neuronal membranes by blocking voltage-dependent sodium channels and thereby prevents the release of excitatory amino acids, especially glutamate and aspartate (107). It is also a weak inhibitor of dihydrofolate reductase. Because some anticonvulsant drugs lowered folate levels, it was hypothesized that antifolate drugs may possess anticonvulsant activity. This hypothesis was never substantiated.

Hepatic drug enzyme inducers such as carbamazepine, phenytoin, and phenobarbital reduce the half-life of lamotrigine by 15 hours. Sodium valproate reduces the clearance of lamotrigine by 21% and increases its half-life to 59 hours. Lamotrigine does not induce or inhibit hepatic enzymes. Lamotrigine increases symptoms when added to carbamazepine through pharmacodynamic rather than pharmacokinetic interactions (108–110).

Pregnancy and Lactation

Lamotrigine is FDA pregnancy category C (Appendix I). It enters human breast milk, and breast-feeding is not recommended.

Clinical Presentation

ACUTE OVERDOSAGE

Serious toxicity has not been reported in adults. An ingestion of 1350 mg caused nystagmus and ataxia. Serum potassium was decreased to 3.3 mmol/L. The QRS complex widened to 112 msec but reverted to normal at 24 hours (111). Subsequent overdose patients also demonstrated ataxia and rotational nystagmus, but no electrocardiogram abnormalities were noted. In a single case report, plasma concentration time-curve was log-linear, suggesting that the pharmacokinetics are first-order after overdose (112).

More significant sequelae have been reported in children. A 2-year-old child without a history of seizure disorder experienced tonic-clonic seizures after ingesting 800 mg. Tremor, motor incoordination, and ataxia (but no nystagmus) were present but the child recovered without sequelae (104). A child who ingested more than 4000 mg was comatose for 12 hours. Coma has also occurred in other children ingesting 1000 to 3000 mg. All recovered without sequelae.

ADVERSE EVENTS

In 1997, the manufacturer issued a warning regarding the occurrence of a rash during therapeutic use of lamotrigine. Hypersensitivity reactions evidenced by multiorgan dysfunction and hepatic abnormalities, with and without the presence of the rash, were subsequently reported in patients taking lamotrigine. The majority of the cases occurred within 2 to 8 weeks of initiation of the drug, but isolated cases occurred after prolonged treatment (6 months). All patients that developed lamotrigine-associated hypersensitivity syndrome were taking concomitant anticonvulsants (114).

A variety of rashes, including Stevens-Johnson syndrome, toxic epidermal necrolysis, and hypersensitivity reaction, occur in 25% of children younger than 16 years old and in 0.3% (3/1000) of adults (115,116). Rare cases of rash-related death have been reported. Risk factors include coadministration of valproate, initial doses of lamotrigine greater than recommended, and exceeding the recommended dose escalation (117). Lamotrigine should be discontinued at the first sign of a rash. Supratherapeutic dosing of lamotrigine has also caused anticonvulsant hypersensitivity syndrome (118). Other reported side effects include headache, nausea, vomiting, dizziness, diplopia, ataxia, and tremor.

Diagnostic Tests

At therapeutic doses, trough plasma concentrations are 2 to 4 mg/L (119). The maximum reported concentration after overdose is 35.8 mg/L (112). Serum concentrations are of no clinical value after overdose.

Treatment

Treatment of lamotrigine overdose is symptomatic and supportive. There is no evidence that gastric lavage or single-dose activated charcoal changes outcome if administered after overdose.

OXCARBAZEPINE

Licensed in the United States and the United Kingdom in 2000, oxcarbazepine (Trileptal) has been in clinical use in Denmark and other countries for more than 10 years. Oxcarbazepine was developed using carbamazepine as a template in an attempt to produce a drug with an improved side effect profile (120).

Toxic Dose

Adult and pediatric therapeutic doses are provided in Table 1. A 2.4-g adult overdose recovered with supportive care (121). A 38-year-old woman inadvertently ingested 3.3 g/day (instead of 2.4 g/day) for 1 day and presented with bradycardia, hypotension, vertigo, and tinnitus. She also recovered with supportive care alone (122).

Toxicokinetics and Toxicodynamics

Oxcarbazepine is well absorbed and not affected by food. The time to peak plasma level is 4 to 6 hours. It is rapidly metabolized in the liver via a reductive pathway to an active nontoxic metabolite, 10,11 dihydro-10-hydroxy-5H-debenzolazepine-5-carboxamide, which is responsible for its pharmacologic action. Unlike carbamazepine, oxcarbazepine is not metabolized to an epoxide, which is one of the reasons for its improved side effect profile (123).

Little parent compound circulates in the plasma, and less than 1% of the drug is excreted in the urine. The metabolite is widely distributed in the brain and lipophilic tissues. It is 38% bound to plasma protein (124–126). Plasma half-life of 10,11 dihydro-10-hydroxy-5H-debenzolazepine-5-carboxamide is 8 to 10 hours, and it is not affected by other seizure medications. As the drug is excreted by the kidneys, dose may need to be reduced in patients with renal impairment (127).

Pathophysiology

Oxcarbazepine is the 10 keto analog of carbamazepine. Similar to carbamazepine, oxcarbazepine blocks voltage sensitive sodium channels causing stabilization of hyper-excited neural membranes, inhibition of repetitive neuronal firing, and inhibition of the spread of discharges. The drug also increases potassium conductance, decreases glutaminergic transmission, and modulates the calcium channel (128–130).

Pregnancy and Lactation

Oxcarbazepine is FDA pregnancy category C (Appendix I). It distributes into breast milk and is not recommended for breast-feeding mothers.

Clinical Presentation

ACUTE OVERDOSAGE

There are few data on overdose. A 2.4-g overdose by an adult recovered with supportive care (121). A 38-year-old woman inadvertently ingested 3.3 g/day (instead of 2.4 g/day) for 1 day and presented with a pulse of 27 beats/minute and a blood pressure of 60 mm Hg. Vertigo and tinnitus were also prominent. The bradycardia improved with atropine treatment (122).

ADVERSE REACTIONS

Duration and frequency of side effects are less than those of carbamazepine. Side effects include fatigue, headache, dizziness, ataxia, and nausea. Skin rash occurs in up to 10% of patients and is the main reason for discontinuation of the drug. Oxcarbazepine may be administered to patients who have developed a rash while taking carbamazepine. Cross-reactivity is approximately 25%. Mild hyponatremia, usually clinically insignificant, occurs in 20% of patients. Regular monitoring of sodium levels is not deemed necessary (124,125,131).

DRUG INTERACTIONS

One advantage of this drug is that it has few inducing properties and therefore causes few drug interactions. If oxcarbazepine is substituted for carbamazepine, deinduction can occur. One significant drug interaction is that with oral contraceptives, potentially causing contraception failure (131).

Treatment

Few data are available regarding overdose. Treatment is symptomatic and supportive.

DECONTAMINATION

The effectiveness of GI decontamination is unknown. A single dose of activated charcoal within 1 to 2 hours of ingestion is reasonable.

ENHANCEMENT OF ELIMINATION

There are no reports regarding enhancement of elimination. Because the protein binding of oxcarbazepine is low and its V_d is relatively low, it seems likely that hemodialysis removes the drug efficiently. However, there are no reports currently of illness of severity that justifies an invasive procedure.

ANTIDOTES

There is no known antidote for oxcarbazepine intoxication.

SUPPORTIVE CARE

Dystonic reactions, hyponatremia, hypothermia, and seizures are treated in the usual manner (Chapters 38 and 40).

PHENOBARBITAL

Phenobarbital (Luminal) was the main anticonvulsant for children for many years. It decreases both generalized tonic-clonic and partial seizures but is not generally useful in the control of absence seizures (132). Problems with sedation and effects on cognition decreased the use of the drug (29). Phenobarbital is available in 15-, 20-, 60-, and 100-mg tablets. There is also a 20-mg/5-cc elixir.

Toxic Dose

Adult and pediatric therapeutic doses are provided in Table 1 (29). A dose of 8 mg/kg/day can produce mild to moderate toxicity, depending on the patient's level of tolerance. In contrast, phenobarbital addicts may consume more than 1000 mg/day.

Toxicokinetics and Toxicodynamics

Phenobarbital is slowly absorbed and peak concentrations occur several hours after a single dose. Plasma protein binding is 40%

to 60%. Up to 23% of the dose is eliminated by pH-dependent renal excretion. The remainder of the drug is metabolized primarily by CYP2C9 (133).

Pathophysiology

Phenobarbital inhibits seizures by potentiation of synaptic inhibition through action on the $GABA_A$ receptor (134). Phenobarbital exerts at least two separate actions on $GABA_A$ receptors. It enhances the effects of GABA-evoked chloride currents and directly activates the receptor at supratherapeutic concentrations (135–137).

Pregnancy and Lactation

Phenobarbital is FDA pregnancy category D (Appendix I). It is contraindicated during breast-feeding and may cause adverse effects in the infant.

Clinical Presentation

ACUTE OVERDOSAGE

The CNS depressant effects of barbiturates are well-known. The reticular activating system, the cerebellum, and hypoxic drive are most sensitive to its effects (138). Vasodilation, decreased sympathetic output, and negative inotropic effects on the heart may cause hypotension (139,140). Hypothermia is caused by a direct effect on the hypothalamus (141). Clinically, the patient may have decreased consciousness, respiratory depression, hypotension, and hypothermia. Less severe toxicity may be manifest with slurred speech, ataxia, nystagmus, and confusion. The patient may appear intoxicated. Pupils may be constricted or dilated. Brainstem and deep tendon reflexes are usually depressed or absent in severe poisoning. Occasionally, focal neurologic signs may occur (142). Bullous skin lesions may also be seen.

ADVERSE EFFECTS

Impaired cognitive effects occur in both children and adults (29). In children, altered sleep, fussiness, irritability, and hyperactivity may occur.

Diagnostic Tests

The usual therapeutic serum concentration is 15 to 40 µg/ml (29). The relationship between plasma concentration and adverse effects varies with chronic use and the development of tolerance. Sedation, ataxia, and nystagmus may be present during initial therapy with this drug, but these side effects usually disappear with continued use even when serum concentrations are more than therapeutic. Concentrations more than 60 µg/ml are associated with significant toxicity in the nontolerant individual (143).

Treatment

Treatment is primarily supportive, although enhancement of elimination reduces blood concentrations.

DECONTAMINATION

Induced emesis should be avoided because of the possibility of CNS depression. Activated charcoal binds phenobarbital effectively. A single dose of 1 to 2 g/kg should be administered if the patient presents soon after an acute ingestion. Multiple doses of activated charcoal may be used as described later.

ENHANCEMENT OF ELIMINATION

Two modalities, MDAC and urinary alkalinization to a pH of 7.5 to 8.0, have been shown to increase elimination of the phenobarbital (144–146). The use of sodium bicarbonate is described in Chapter 75. Side effects of urinary alkalinization include overzealous administration of sodium bicarbonate and resultant hypernatremia, hypokalemia, and hypocalcemia (147). Although both MDAC and urinary alkalinization decrease elimination half-life, treatment with these modalities may not shorten the clinical course or change outcome (148). An underpowered study showed a trend toward shortened duration of endotracheal intubation in patients treated with MDAC but was not statistically significant (146).

Charcoal hemoperfusion or hemodialysis increases the clearance of phenobarbital, but because of the significant complication rate, it is recommended only for persistent hypotension.

ANTIDOTES

No specific antidote exists for phenobarbital toxicity.

SUPPORTIVE CARE

Hypotension is treated with rapid infusion of 10 to 20 ml/kg of isotonic crystalloidal fluids, followed by the administration of vasopressors, if needed (Chapter 37).

PHENYTOIN

First synthesized in 1908 by Blitz, phenytoin (Dilantin, Epanutin) is a hydantoin derivative that is structurally related to the barbiturates. Phenytoin is available in 50- and 100-mg capsules and tablets.

Toxic Dose

Adult and pediatric therapeutic doses are provided in Table 1 (29). Death is nearly impossible to achieve by ingestion of phenytoin alone. Adults have survived ingestion of up to 25 g (77). In the era before modern intensive care, a 7-year-old boy died after ingestion of 2 g (100 mg/kg) (149). Fosphenytoin overdosage (300 mg) caused hypotension and asystole but the patient was resuscitated (150).

Pharmacokinetics

Absorption of oral phenytoin is slow and variable. Poorly absorbed in the acidic environment of the stomach, phenytoin is primarily absorbed in the small intestine. After a 400-mg dose, peak serum concentrations occur at 8 hours, but the time to maximum concentration increases with increasing dose (151). Protein binding is 90%, and the V_d is 0.6 to 0.7 L/kg. The elimination half-life is 20 to 30 hours. Metabolism is hepatic. Metabolites [including the major metabolite 5-(*p*-hydroxyphenyl)-5-phenylhydantoin] are inactive and excreted in the urine. Only 5% of the parent drug is excreted unchanged in the urine (152–155).

Metabolism is dose dependent. At therapeutic serum concentrations, elimination is first order (rate of drug metabolism increases as the concentration of the drug increases). In the upper therapeutic and toxic serum concentrations, the hydroxylation reaction reaches maximum velocity and elimination becomes zero order (rate of metabolism is constant) (153,156).

Pathophysiology

Phenytoin causes voltage, frequency, and use-dependent block of sodium channels (157). It also inhibits calcium channels and stimulates the sodium-potassium adenosine triphosphatase pump (152,156,158).

Pregnancy and Lactation

Phenytoin is FDA pregnancy category D (Appendix I). Little enters the breast milk, and it is considered safe for breast-feeding.

Clinical Presentation

ACUTE OVERDOSAGE

Limited phenytoin solubility (dissolution rate decreases with increasing dose) and prolonged absorption caused by decreased intestinal motility cause delayed peak serum concentrations (152,159). Peak serum concentrations may occur days after ingestion of a large dose.

Symptoms follow a continuum and are related to the blood concentration. After an acute overdose, the most frequent symptoms are ocular (nystagmus) and vestibulocerebellar (ataxia). Ataxia may be the most significant symptom as the patient may sustain injuries if a fall occurs. At higher concentrations, the CNS is increasingly affected, ultimately causing coma (160). Oral phenytoin overdose does not cause cardiac toxicity. The occurrence of paradoxical seizures after overdose has not been confirmed. Life-threatening toxicity rarely occurs after ingestion of this drug alone.

ADVERSE EVENTS

Phenytoin toxicity may occur during therapeutic ingestion as a result of the following changes: small increases in maintenance doses may saturate enzyme systems and zero order kinetics ensue, protein binding of the drug is decreased (e.g., addition of another drug), or drug-induced alteration in hepatic metabolism occurs.

As serum concentrations rise, initial signs and symptoms of toxicity are primarily cerebellar (nystagmus, ataxia, and drowsiness). Higher serum concentrations (more than 20 mg/L) cause basal ganglia signs (movement disorders) (161,162). It is not known if phenytoin administration can cause cerebellar atrophy. Although computerized tomography demonstrates cerebellar atrophy and cerebellar tissue loss in patients on phenytoin, seizures can cause the same changes. However, patients with cerebellar symptoms and high serum phenytoin concentrations demonstrate symptomatic recovery when the serum concentration decreases (162–164).

Adverse effects usually occur when serum concentrations are more than 15 mg/L. Gingival hyperplasia and folic acid deficiency are dose related. Rash, acne, lupus-like syndrome, Stevens-Johnson syndrome, thyroid function inhibition, hirsutism, hypertrichosis, benign intracranial hypertension, carbohydrate intolerance, peripheral neuropathy, osteomalacia, and altered vitamin D metabolism (increased alkaline phosphatase) also occur (156). The most serious side effect is a hypersensitivity syndrome manifested by fever, rash, lymphadenopathy, hepatitis, and eosinophilia. Death occurs as a result of hepatic failure. Phenytoin should be discontinued if patients manifest signs of this syndrome (165,166). Phenytoin administration may also cause isolated elevation of serum liver enzymes. Discontinuation of the drug may not be necessary. Elevated liver enzymes should be monitored to distinguish the enzyme elevation from hypersensitivity-induced progression to hepatic failure (167).

INTRAVENOUS PHENYTOIN

Phenytoin lacks solubility and stability in unbuffered solutions. Phenytoin sodium injection preparation is a mixture of 40% propylene glycol (required to solubilize phenytoin) and 10% ethanol. The solution is adjusted to a pH of 12 with sodium hydroxide to maintain phenytoin solubility. Phenytoin should be mixed in normal saline. Phenytoin maintains solubility in concentrations of 6 to 10 mg/L. Crystallization begins to occur within an hour (168).

Rapid IV administration of phenytoin or administration of high concentrations of phenytoin can cause cardiovascular toxicity. Phenytoin concentration of 4 to 10 mg/ml in normal saline can be safely administered at a rate of 50 mg/minute in patients younger than 50 years of age. If the patient is older than 50 years of age, concentration should be 4 mg/ml and administered no faster than 25 mg/minute. Patients should be placed on a cardiac monitor. Phenytoin should not be administered to patients with marked bradycardia, second or third degree heart block, active severe atherosclerotic heart disease, or hypotension (169–171). Fatalities have occurred in elderly patients with a history of heart disease and in younger patients when the IV delivery rate or phenytoin concentration was greater than recommended (172,173). Hypotension and bradycardia have occurred in young people when phenytoin infusion concentrations were high (168).

Even if rate of delivery and concentration are appropriate, administration of more than 1 g of phenytoin may cause ataxia, dizziness, and confusion. Symptoms are caused by total dose administered (171). A constant infusion pump should monitor IV delivery. Infusion should be stopped if systemic side effects occur.

Burning and aching of the arm near the infusion site may occur due to solvent alkalinity. Decreasing the rate or concentration may alleviate the symptoms. Buffering capacity of the blood may be exceeded if the alkaline solution is infused into a small vein causing soft tissue or vascular injury. The majority of reported cases has occurred in elderly women with cardiovascular disease. To minimize the risk in the elderly, the IV catheter should be at least 20 gauge, and administration rate should not exceed 25 mg/minute (174).

Diagnostic Tests

Although the serum phenytoin concentration does not correlate well with symptoms, a progression of symptoms occurs as serum concentrations increase above the therapeutic range. Symptoms correlate better with free phenytoin concentrations, which are usually not available. Serum concentrations in the therapeutic range (10 to 20 mg/L) equate with a free phenytoin concentration of 1.0 to 2.0 mg/L. Symptoms of toxicity occur when free phenytoin concentrations are more than 5 mg/L. Conditions in which albumin is decreased or protein binding is impaired increase the free phenytoin concentration (175).

A loading dose of 15 to 18 mg/kg IV produces therapeutic serum concentrations lasting 12 to 24 hours. Distribution to the brain is rapid, and anticonvulsant activity begins within 3 to 5 minutes after IV infusion. If the serum concentration of phenytoin is known, administration of each 100 mg of IV phenytoin increases serum concentration 1.2 mg/L (176). Absorption from bone is rapid after intraosseous administration. Pharmacokinetics approximate those after IV administration (177).

Treatment

Treatment of acute or chronic phenytoin toxicity is supportive. Acute onset cardiac dysrhythmias, hypotension, and apnea are treated by immediate discontinuation of the infusion and administration of standard advanced cardiac life support.

There is no evidence that administration of single-dose activated charcoal or MDAC or any extracorporeal measures change outcome (178). There are no antidotes for phenytoin toxicity.

Prolonged elimination half-life may cause prolonged symptoms (157,179). The main concern is ataxia causing a fall and resultant injury. The patient must be in the appropriate setting for observation.

TIAGABINE

Tiagabine (Gabitril) was approved by the FDA in October 1997. Tiagabine is available in 4-, 12-, 16-, and 20-mg tablets.

Toxic Dose

Adult and pediatric therapeutic doses are provided in Table 1. A single dose of 400 mg by an adult was followed by status epilepticus, which responded to IV phenobarbital (180). In clinical trials, single doses of 800 mg in adults were followed by somnolence, agitation, confusion, dysphasia, hostility, depression, weakness, and myoclonus (180).

Toxicokinetics and Toxicodynamics

The elimination half-life is 5 to 8 hours, although it may be decreased to 3 hours by inducing drugs (181).

Pathophysiology

Tiagabine prolongs the action of GABA by selectively inhibiting GABA transporters in the glia and neurons. Tiagabine does not affect voltage-gated sodium or calcium channels (181).

Pregnancy and Lactation

Tiagabine is FDA pregnancy category C (Appendix I). Secretion into breast milk is unknown.

Clinical Presentation

Acute overdosage case reports indicate that tiagabine may precipitate seizures and nonconvulsive status (182,183). Adverse events include dizziness, headache, asthenia, and tremor. Visual field defects have been reported in patients on tiagabine (184). Whether they are completely reversible when the drug is discontinued is unclear (25–27,185–187).

Diagnostic Tests

Therapeutic monitoring of plasma concentration is not recommended, as there is no clinical correlation. The tiagabine concentration in clinical trials ranged from 1 to 234 ng/ml (183).

Treatment

The treatment of tiagabine toxicity is symptomatic and supportive. Enhanced elimination techniques have not been reported.

TOPIRAMATE

Topiramate (Topamax) has been available in the United States since early 1997, although the drug has been approved in the United Kingdom since 1995. Topiramate is available in 25-, 100-, and 200-mg tablets and as 25-mg sprinkles.

Toxic Dose

Adult and pediatric therapeutic doses are provided in Table 1. A toxic dose has not been established.

Toxicokinetics and Toxicodynamics

Topiramate is a sulfamate-substituted monosaccharide that is structurally distinct from other anticonvulsants. It is rapidly and completely absorbed from the GI tract and has minimal protein binding (9% to 17%) but is extensively bound to erythrocytes (which is saturable). The elimination half-life is 19 to 23 hours. Hepatic metabolism is low (20%), and there are no active metabolites. The drug is primarily (70%) excreted in the urine (188).

Pathophysiology

Topiramate causes a state-dependent blockade of sodium channels and potentiates GABA-mediated neuroinhibition by acting at a unique modulatory site. It enhances GABA-mediated chloride influx into neurons (similar to diazepam), increasing the frequency that GABA activates $GABA_A$ receptors but does not interact with GABA binding sites or benzodiazepine binding sites on $GABA_A$. Topiramate also causes blockade of glutamate-mediated neuroexcitation. It is a weak carbonic anhydrase inhibitor.

Pregnancy and Lactation

Topiramate is FDA pregnancy category C (Appendix I). Entry into breast milk is unknown.

Clinical Presentation

There are no data on topiramate overdose. Adverse CNS events (sedation) and cognitive side effects (trouble concentrating and word finding) are worse with rapid titration (189). Decreased appetite and weight loss, ataxia, dizziness, nystagmus, tremor, and fatigue have also been reported (190). Because the drug is a carbonic anhydrase inhibitor, there is an increased risk of metabolic acidosis and calcium phosphate stones. Reduction in carbonic anhydrase at the proximal renal tubule impairs the exchange of the hydrogen ion for the sodium ion as well as the reabsorption of bicarbonate. Metabolic acidosis can therefore develop (190,191). Carbonic anhydrase inhibitors decrease urinary citrate. Both decreased urinary citrate and acidosis increase the chance of calcium phosphate stones (191,192).

Treatment

Treatment is symptomatic and supportive. Topiramate is cleared by hemodialysis, but its use in overdose has not been reported. It is unlikely to be needed.

VALPROATE

Valproic acid was first prescribed for the treatment of absence seizures in 1978 and is currently prescribed for the treatment of all types of seizures (156). Valproate is also useful for treatment of bipolar disorder and migraine prophylaxis.

Valproic acid (Depacon, Depakene) is available in the United States as 125-, 250-, and 500-mg tablets, 125-mg sprinkles, a syrup containing 250 mg/5ml of sodium valproate (29), enteric-coated tablets, suppository, and controlled release formulations (193). Depakote contains equal proportions of valproic acid and sodium valproate. Depakote and Depakene extended release are extended-release forms of valproate and divalproex sodium, respectively. These formulations are enteric coated and must dissociate before they are absorbed. Peak concentration can occur a number of hours after ingestion (194).

Toxic Dose

Adult and pediatric therapeutic doses are provided in Table 1. Adult fatalities have been associated with doses of 2.25 g/day for multiple days (195). A 20-month-old boy died after an ingestion of 750 mg/kg (196). Although plasma levels and CNS depression correlated poorly, a series of 516 cases of acute overdosage found that unconsciousness followed ingestions of more than 200 mg/kg (197).

Toxicokinetics and Toxicodynamics

Valproate is a simple eight-carbon, branch-chained fatty acid. It is rapidly and completely absorbed with peak serum concentrations occurring 1 to 4 hours after ingestion. The drug is extensively metabolized in the liver by glucuronic acid conjugation and β-oxidation, which may be inhibited by long-term or high-dose valproate therapy (198). Protein binding changes with serum concentration: 90% binding at valproate concentrations of 40 μg/ml, and only 81% at concentrations of 130 μg/ml (199). Concentrations greater than 150 μg/ml saturate protein binding sites, and protein binding falls to less than 70% (200). The V_d is small, 0.13 to 0.23 L/kg. The half-life of valproic acid is 8 to 14 hours but may be up to 42 hours after overdose. In therapeutic concentrations and after overdose, elimination kinetics of the parent compound appear to be first order (201,202). Less than 3% of the drug is excreted unchanged in the urine and feces.

Pathophysiology

The precise mechanism of action of valproate is unclear. Valproate appears to have a number of indirect actions on the GABAergic system resulting in increased GABA concentration (203). Earlier research indicated that valproate blocked voltage-gated sodium channels to inhibit the frequency-dependent repetitive firing of neurons (204). More recent studies in rat hippocampal sections have demonstrated that this is not the primary mechanism of anticonvulsant activity (205). Valproate reduces release of GABA and blocks cell depolarization induced by *N*-Me-D-aspartate–type glutamate receptors (206). In rat brain sections, valproate increases brain endogenous opioid (207,208). Active metabolites may add to its anticonvulsant actions (209).

Pregnancy and Lactation

Valproate is FDA pregnancy category D (Appendix I). It is considered safe for breast-feeding.

Clinical Presentation

ACUTE OVERDOSAGE

If the enteric coated or controlled release formulation has been ingested, peak serum concentration may be delayed for 12 to 16 hours (201). Patients who have ingested these formulations cannot be medically cleared until the clinical picture and serum concentration are assessed at the end of this time period.

CNS depression, ranging from drowsiness to coma, is the most frequent sign after overdose. Serum concentrations more than 850 μg/ml uniformly cause coma. Respiratory depression, hypotension, and death may occur. Hypoglycemia, hypocalcemia, hypernatremia, hypophosphatemia, and anion gap metabolic acidosis may be life threatening and persist for days. Elevation in serum aminotransferases, ammonia, amylase, and lactate may also occur (210,211). Thrombocytopenia, the most common hematologic toxicity, may be clinically significant and severe.

Valproate increases renal ammonia production and blocks hepatic ammonia metabolism. Resultant hyperammonemia may increase intracellular osmolarity, which promotes influx of water into the cell and causes cerebral edema (212). Hyperammonemia (in the absence of liver failure) and cerebral edema have been reported in the overdose patient. Whether increased ammonia is the cause of cerebral edema, and resultant increased intracranial pressure, is unknown. Hyperammonemia and cerebral edema should be considered as a potential cause of agitation in a patient who has overdosed on valproate (213–215).

ADVERSE EVENTS

The serum aminotransferase increases in up to 60% of patients with therapeutic serum concentrations. Serum bilirubin increases as valproate concentrations increase. Liver enzymes normalize with dose reduction or discontinuation of the drug (216). Hepatic failure, histologically evident as microvesicular steatosis, occurs in 1 in 20,000 patients on valproate therapy (217). Valproate-induced hepatotoxicity may be either intrinsic (reversible, reproducible, and dose dependent) and benign, occurring in 44% of patients, or idiosyncratic (unpredictable, not dose dependent, long latent period). Children younger than 3 years of age who are receiving multiple antiepileptic agents and have additional medical problems are at highest risk for fatal hepatotoxicity (218) with an incidence of 1 in 500 (219,220). Liver enzymes and ammonia should be checked in children treated with valproate who demonstrate somnolence, lethargy, or even coma.

Asymptomatic hyperammonemia without hepatic damage occurs in 20% of patients taking this drug. The origin of the ammonia is hepatic, a result of impaired urea cycle function and inability to metabolize nitrogen loads. The mechanism of this impairment is unknown. Carnitine deficiency may play a role in the impaired urea production (221).

Thirty-six cases of valproate-associated pancreatitis, including nine deaths, have been reported in the medical literature. Patients on polytherapy may be at the highest risk for developing pancreatitis. The cause is unknown. Abdominal pain, lethargy, or coma may be the presenting symptoms (222,223). Thrombocytopenia, usually transient despite continuing the drug, has rarely induced bone marrow toxicity (224). Anorexia, nausea, and diarrhea occur in 15% of patients. CNS effects such as sedation ataxia and tremor also occur.

Diagnostic Tests

Serum concentration does not correlate well with either seizure control or toxicity. Therapeutic concentrations are 50 to 100 μg/ml. Incidence of adverse side effects increases at concentrations greater than 120 μg/ml. The Enzyme Multiplied Immunoassay Test assay yields higher values of serum valproate than does the gas chromatography. Serum concentrations must be consistently monitored by the same analytic method (201).

Valproate is eliminated partly as ketone bodies and may cause a false-positive test for ketones in the urine. Valproate may also decrease serum concentrations of thyroxine.

Treatment

DECONTAMINATION

There is no evidence that either gastric lavage or administration of activated charcoal changes outcome. Whole bowel irrigation should be considered if the patient ingests Depakote or an extended release preparation and presents within 6 hours of ingestion.

ENHANCEMENT OF ELIMINATION

Hemoperfusion and hemodiafiltration without hemoperfusion have been performed to treat severe valproate overdose (225–227). Although the high degree of protein binding should not make it amenable to dialysis, the hypothesis is that unbound drug is markedly increased in overdose. None of the means of extracorporeal detoxification has been compared to supportive care to determine if these measures improve outcome.

ANTIDOTES

Administration of high-dose naloxone has been reported to reverse valproate-induced CNS depression (228,229). Theories regarding the reversal of sedation by naloxone include reversal of the valproate-induced release of endogenous opioids and reversal of valproate blockade of GABA uptake by cells (230,231). Serum glucose, calcium, phosphate, and platelets must be frequently measured and treated accordingly.

The primary metabolic pathway for valproate is β-oxidation. Decreased β-oxidation metabolites have been reported after overdose. Hypocarnitinemia, which inhibits β-oxidation, has been reported after long-term valproate therapy. Clinical relevance of hypocarnitinemia in seizure patients on chronic valproate therapy or in overdose patients (if it occurs) is unknown. L-carnitine has been administered to overdose patients in an attempt to increase valproate metabolism via beta-oxidation. L-carnitine causes few adverse side effects. However, its administration is experimental (198).

MONITORING

Due to delayed peak serum concentrations, serial concentrations should be obtained. Serum ammonia concentrations should be obtained in all patients on valproate who present with an altered level of consciousness.

VIGABATRIN

Vigabatrin (Sabril) was approved by the FDA in 1997. Clinical trials with vigabatrin were cautious, as previous animal experiments revealed the development of brain microvacuoles in some animal species taking the drug. An extensive clinical monitoring program has been ongoing since 1982 throughout the United States and Europe. To date, there is no evidence of vigabatrin-related CNS vacuolation. In patients taking vigabatrin who died of causes unrelated to seizures, no vacuoles were found on autopsy (232). Vigabatrin is available in 500-mg tablets.

Toxic Dose

Adult and pediatric therapeutic dosage is provided in Table 1 (233). A 25-year-old woman developed delirium with no other clinical effects after an ingestion of 60 g (234).

Toxicokinetics and Toxicodynamics

Bioavailability is 90%, and the V_d is 0.8 L/kg. This drug is not protein bound and is primarily cleared by the kidneys. Metabolism of the drug is negligible. The elimination half-life is 5 to 7 hours (235–238). Pharmacologic half-life is much longer than elimination half-life, with the duration of action being 5 to 7 days (239).

Pathophysiology

Vigabatrin is a structural analog of GABA and an irreversible inhibitor of the enzyme (GABA transaminase) primarily responsible for GABA catabolism (240). Vigabatrin also reduces GABA reuptake activity (241). Both mechanisms increase brain GABA.

Pregnancy and Lactation

Vigabatrin has the Australian pregnancy category designation of D. Entry into breast milk is unknown.

Clinical Presentation

ACUTE OVERDOSAGE

There are few data on vigabatrin overdose. One patient experienced delirium that seemed to worsen with the administration of diazepam. The authors question if benzodiazepine administration after this overdose (in which GABA is increased) may increase delirium (234).

The most frequent symptoms after overdose include drowsiness, decreased level of consciousness, and coma. Respiratory depression, bradycardia, hypotension, agitation, irritability, confusion, and abnormal behavior have also been reported (242).

ADVERSE EVENTS

Adverse effects include mood and behavior changes such as depression, psychosis, and acute encephalopathy. Three patients were reported with vigabatrin-induced dose-dependent encephalopathy, which resolved when the drug was discontinued. All three patients had slightly elevated creatinine (1.5 to 2.4 mg/dl). Sedation, fatigue, headache, and weight gain are usually mild and short lasting.

The incidence of vigabatrin-induced psychosis is unknown. The drug should be used cautiously in patients with psychiatric disorders.

Diagnostic Tests

Plasma concentration monitoring is unnecessary because no direct correlation exists between plasma concentration and seizure control or adverse effects (233).

Treatment

Treatment is primarily symptomatic and supportive. Based on its physical characteristics, vigabatrin is likely removed by hemodialysis. However, its use in overdose has not been reported and hemodialysis is unlikely to be needed.

ZONISAMIDE

Zonisamide (Zonegran) was approved by the FDA as adjunctive therapy for partial seizures in 2000. Zonisamide is available in 100-mg capsules.

Toxic Dose

Adult and pediatric therapeutic doses are provided in Table 1 (243). Doses more than 400 mg/day are associated with lethargy, dizziness, ataxia, and mental status changes (244).

Toxicokinetics and Toxicodynamics

The C_{max} is achieved in 2.4 to 3.6 hours. In Japanese studies, linear pharmacokinetics have been reported, but in the United States, nonlinear pharmacokinetics with first-order clearance were reported (244–246). The elimination half-life is 63 hours. The drug is excreted in the urine as unchanged drug, as an acetylation product, and as the glucuronide of a metabolite. CYP3A4 isoenzyme reduces the drug (247).

Pathophysiology

Zonisamide is a sulfonamide. The drug blocks sodium channels and T-type calcium channels. It is also a weak carbonic anhydrase inhibitor (248).

Pregnancy and Lactation

Zonisamide is FDA pregnancy category C (Appendix I). It enters breast milk easily and is relatively contraindicated for nursing mothers.

Clinical Presentation

ACUTE OVERDOSAGE

There are few overdose data available. One adult overdose developed coma, bradycardia, hypotension, and respiratory depression after ingesting an unknown amount. The serum zonisamide serum level was 100.1 μg/ml at 31 hours after ingestion. Clonazepam was a coingestant. She recovered with supportive care (249).

ADVERSE EVENTS

Carbonic anhydrase inhibitors decrease urinary citrate, an inhibitor of stone formation that thereby increases the risk of calcium-containing renal stones. Nephrolithiasis was initially reported in 1.4% of patients on zonisamide in the United States, and another 6% of patients were asymptomatic but had abnormalities on ultrasound. The trials have not reported a consistent incidence of nephrolithiasis. Causality is still in question (250).

In December 2001, the manufacturer issued a letter to health care professionals warning that oligohidrosis and hyperthermia had been reported in 38 patients in Japan and two patients in the United States. An 18-year-old patient had experienced heat stroke. Decreased sweating and elevated body temperature were noted in these cases. Pediatric patients appear to be at increased risk.

There is some evidence that zonisamide contributes to psychotic episodes during polytherapy. The incidence of psychotic episodes in epileptic patients on zonisamide is higher than the prevalence of epileptic psychosis (251). Most side effects are mild and transient and usually occur during initiation of treatment. Drowsiness, (24%), ataxia (13%), anorexia, dizziness, forgetfulness, slowness of thought, and irritability have been reported (247).

Treatment

Treatment is symptomatic and supportive. The effectiveness of GI decontamination is unknown. A single dose of activated charcoal within 1 to 2 hours of ingestion is reasonable. There are no reports regarding enhancement of elimination. There is no known antidote for zonisamide intoxication. Hyperthermia, seizures, bradycardia, and hypotension are treated in the usual manner (Chapters 7, 38, and 40).

REFERENCES

1. Dichter MA. Old and new mechanisms of antiepileptic drug actions. *Epilepsy Res Suppl* 1993;10:9–17.
2. Diaz-Arrastia R, Agostini MA, Van Ness PC. Evolving treatment strategies for epilepsy. *JAMA* 2002;2917–2920.
3. Dichter MA, Brodie MJ. New antiepileptic drugs. *N Engl J Med* 1996;334:1583–1590.
4. Garnett WR. New opportunities for the treatment of epilepsy. *Am J Health Syst Pharm* 1995;52:88–91.
5. Lathers CM, Schraeder PL. Clinical pharmacology: drugs as a benefit and/or risk in sudden unexpected death in epilepsy. *J Clin Pharmacol* 2002;42:123–136.
6. Holmes LB, Harvey EA, Coull BA, et al. The teratogenicity of anti-convulsant drugs. *N Engl J Med* 2002;344:132–138.
7. Knowles SR, Shapiro LE, Shear NH. Anticonvulsant hypersensitivity syndrome. *Drug Saf* 1999;21:489–501.
8. Moss DM, Rudis M, Henderson SO. Cross-sensitivity and the anti-convulsant hypersensitivity syndrome. *J Emerg Med* 1999;17:503–506.
9. Martin R, Kuzniecky R, Ho S, et al. Cognitive effects of topiramate, gabapentin, and Lamotrigine in healthy young adults. *Neurology* 1999;52:321–327.
10. Lhatoo SD, Sander JW, Wong IC. Letter to editor. Cognitive effects of topiramate, gabapentin and Lamotrigine in healthy young adults. *Neurology* 2000;54:270–271.
11. Kalviainen R, Nousiainen I, Mantyjarvi M, et al. Vigabatrin, a gabaergic antiepileptic drug, causes concentric visual field defects. *Neurology* 1999;53:922–926.
12. Midelfart A, Midelfart E, Brodtkorb E. Visual field defects in patients taking vigabatrin. *Acta Ophthalmologica Scandinavica* 2000;78:580–584.
13. Nordmann JP, Baulac M, VanEgroo C. Concentric changes in the visual field associated with GABA-mimetic antiepileptic agents. *Journal Francais d'Ophthalmologie* 1999;22:418–422.
14. Blackwell N, Hayllar J, Kelly G. Severe persistent visual field constriction associated with vigabatrin. Patients taking vigabatrin should have regular visual field testing. *BMJ* 1997;314:1694.
15. Miller NR. Using the electroretinogram to detect and monitor the retinal toxicity of anticonvulsants. *Neurology* 2000;55:333–334.
16. Collins SD, Brun S, Kirstein YG, et al. Absence of visual field defects in patients taking tiagabine. *Epilepsia* 1998;39[Suppl 6]:146–147.
17. Manuchehri K. Visual field defect associated with vigabatrin: method of estimating prevalence was inappropriate. *BMJ* 2000;320:1403.
18. Wilton LV, Stephens MD, Mann RD. Visual field defect associated with Vigabatrin: observational cohort study. *BMJ* 1999;319:1165–1166.
19. Manuchehri K, Goodman S, Siviter L, et al. A controlled study of vigabatrin and visual abnormalities. *British Journal of Ophthalmology* 2000;84:499–505.
20. Lawden MC, Eke T, Degg C, et al. Visual field defects associated with vigabatrin therapy. *J Neurol Neurosurg Psychiatry* 1999;67:716–722.
21. Harding GFA, Wild JM, Robertson KA, et al. Electrooculography, electroretinography, visual evoked potentials, and multifocal electroretinography in patients with vigabatrin attributed visual field constriction. *Epilepsia* 2000;41:1420–1431.
22. Versino M, Veggiotti P. Reversibility of vigabatrin induced visual-field defect. *Lancet* 1999;354:486
23. Krakow K, Polizzi G, Riordan-Eva P, et al. Recovery of visual field constriction following discontinuation of vigabatrin. *Seizure* 2000;9:287–290.
24. Johnson MA, Krauss GL, Miller NR, et al. Visual function loss from Vigabatrin: effect of stopping the drug. *Neurology* 2000;50:40–45.
25. Beran RG, Currie J, Sandbach J, et al. Visual field restriction with new antiepileptic medication. *Epilepsia* 1998;39[Suppl 2]:6.
26. Beran RG, Hung A, Plunkett M, et al. Predictability of visual field defects in patients exposed to GABAergic agents, vigabatrin, or tiagabine. *Neurology* 1999;52[Suppl 2]:A249.
27. Kalviainen R, Nousiainen I, Mantyjarvi M, et al. Absence of concentric visual field defects in patients with long-term tiagabine monotherapy. *Neurology* 1999;52[Suppl 2]:A336.
28. Levy RH, Pitlick WH, Troupin AS, et al. Pharmacokinetics of carbamazepine in normal man. *Clinical Pharm and Therap* 1975;17:657–668.
29. Russell RJ, Parks B. Anticonvulsant medications. *Pediatric Annals* 1999;28:238–245.
30. Tegretol-XR, carbamazepine. Product information. East Hanover, NJ: Novartis Pharmaceutical Corp, 2000.
31. Garnett W, Carson S, Pellock J, et al. Carbamazepine and carbamazepine epoxide carbamazepine plasma levels in children following chronic dosing with Tegretol suspension and tablets. *Neurology* 1987;[Suppl. 1]:93–94.
32. Graudins A, Peden G, Dowsett RP. Massive overdose with controlled-release carbamazepine resulting in delayed peak serum concentrations and life-threatening toxicity. *Emergency Medicine* 2002;14:89–94.
33. Levy RH, Dreifuss FE, Mattson RG, et al., eds. *Antiepileptic drugs*, 3rd ed. New York: Raven Press, 1989.
34. Winnicka, RI, Lopacinski B, Szymczak WM, et al. Carbamazepine poisoning: elimination kinetics and quantitative relationship with carbamazepine 10,11-Epoxide. *J Toxicol Clin Toxicol* 2002;40:759–765.
35. Graves NM, Brundage RC, Wen Y, et al. Population pharmacokinetics of carbamazepine in adults with epilepsy. *Pharmacotherapy* 1998;18:273–81.
36. Uziel Y, Pomeranz A, Jedeikin R. Acute carbamazepine poisoning and hyponatraemia. *Child Nephrol Urol* 1988;9:87–89.
37. Lingamaneni R, Hemmings HC. Effects of anticonvulsants on Veratridine and KCL evoked glutamate release from rat cortical synaptosomes. *Neurosci Lett* 1999;276:127–130.
38. Yoshimura R, Yanagihara N, Terao T, et al. Inhibition by carbamazepine of various ion channels medicated catecholamine secretion in cultured bovine adrenal medullary cells. Naunyn-Schmiedeberg's arch. *Pharmacol* 1995;352:297–303.
39. Skerritt JH, Davies LP, Johnston GA. Interactions of the anticonvulsant carbamazepine with adenosine receptors. *Epilepsia* 1983;24:634–642.
40. Okada M, Kiryu K, Kawata Y, et al. Determination of the effects of caffeine and carbamazepine on the striatal dopamine release by in vivo microdialysis. *Eur J Pharmacol* 1997;321:181–188.
41. Lampe H, Bigalke H. Carbamazepine blocks NMDA-activated currents in cultured spinal cord neurons. *Neuroreport* 1990;1:26–28.
42. Holmes LB, Harvey EA, Coull BA, et al. The teratogenicity of anticonvulsant drugs. *N Engl J Med* 2001;344:1132–1138.

43. Rosa FW. Spina bifida in infants of women treated with carbamazepine during pregnancy. *N Engl J Med* 1991;324:647–7.
44. Wisner KL, Perel JM. Serum levels of valproate and carbamazepine in breast-feeding mother-infant pairs. *J Clin Psychopharmacol* 1998;18:167–169.
45. Sethna M, Solomon G, Cedarbaum J, et al. Successful treatment of massive carbamazepine overdose. *Epilepsia* 1989;30:1,71–73.
46. Boldy D, Heath A, Ruddock S, et al. Activated charcoal for carbamazepine poisoning. *Lancet* 1987;1 (8540):1027.
47. Lifshitz M, Gavrilov V, Sofer S. Signs and symptoms of carbamazepine overdose in young children. *Pediatr Emerg Care* 2000;16:26–27.
48. Spiller HA, Carlisle RD. Status epilepticus after massive carbamazepine overdose. *Clin Toxicol* 2002;40:81–90.
49. Weaver DF, Camfield P, Fraser A. Massive carbamazepine overdose: clinical and pharmacologic observations in five episodes. *Neurology* 1988;38:755–759.
50. Faisy C, Guerot E, Diehl JL, et al. Carbamazepine-associated severe left ventricular dysfunction. *Clin Toxicol* 2000;38:339–42.
51. Seymour JF. Carbamazepine overdose. *Drug Saf* 1993;8(1):81–88.
52. Apfelbaum J, Cavareti EM, Kerns WP, et al. Cardiovascular effects of carbamazepine toxicity. *Ann Emerg Med* 1995;256:31–35.
53. Heart block secondary to erythromycin-included carbamazepine toxicity. *Pediatrics* 1987;80:951–53.
54. Spiller HA, Krenzelok EP, Cookson E. Carbamazepine overdose: a prospective study of serum levels and toxicity. *Clin Toxicol* 1990;28(4):445–458.
55. Hojer J, Malmlund HO, Berg A. Clinical features in 28 consecutive cases of laboratory confirmed massive poisoning with carbamazepine alone. *Clin Toxicol* 1993;31(3):449–458.
56. Steiner C, Wit AL, Weis MD, et al. The antiarrhythmic actions of carbamazepine. *J Pharm Exper Ther* 1970;172:2,323–35.
57. Kenneback G, Bergfeldt L, Vallin H, et al. Electrophysiologic effects and clinical hazards of carbamazepine treatment for neurologic disorders in patients with abnormalities of the cardiac conduction system. *Am Heart J* 1981;J:1421–1429.
58. Puletti M, Iani C, Curione M, et al. Carbamazepine and the heart. *Ann Neurol* 1991;29:5,575–576.
59. Hewetson K, Ritch A, Watson R. Sick sinus syndrome aggravated by carbamazepine therapy for epilepsy. *Postgrad Med J* 1986;62:497–498.
60. Beerman B, Edhag O. Side effects of drugs. *BMJ* 1978;2(6131):171–172.
61. Apfelbaum JD, Caravati EM, Kerns WP, et al. Cardiovascular effects of carbamazepine toxicity. *Ann Emerg Med* 1994;23:631.
62. Seetharam MN, Pellock JM. Risk benefit assessment of carbamazepine in children. *Drug Saf* 1991;6(2):148–158.
63. DeGiorgio CM, Rabinowicz AL, Olivas RD. Carbamazepine-induced antinuclear antibodies and systemic lupus erythematosus-like syndrome. *Epilepsia* 1991;32:128–129.
64. Hojer J, Malmlund HO, Berg A. Clinical features in 28 consecutive cases of laboratory confirmed massive poisoning with carbamazepine alone. *Clin Toxicol* 1993;31:449–58.
65. Matos ME, Burns MM, Shannon MW, et al. False positive tricyclic antidepressant drug screening results leading to the diagnosis of carbamazepine intoxication. *Pediatrics* 2000;105:e66.
66. Neuvonen PJ, Elonen E. Effect of activated charcoal on absorption and elimination of phenobarbitone, carbamazepine and phenylbutazone in man. *Eur J Clin Pharmacol* 1980;17:51–57.
67. Stremski E, Brady W, Prasad K, et al. Pediatric carbamazepine intoxication. *Ann Emerg Med* 1995;25(5):624–630.
68. Groot G, VanHeijst A, Maes R. Charcoal hemoperfusion in the treatment of two cases of acute CBMZ poisoning. *Clin Toxicol* 1984;4:349–362.
69. Tapolyai M, Campbell M, Dailey K, et al. Hemodialysis is as effective as hemoperfusion for drug removal in carbamazepine poisoning. *Nephron* 2002;90:213–215.
70. Brodie MJ, Martin J, Pellock JM. Taming the brain storms: Felbamate updated. *Lancet* 1995;346:918–9.
71. Brodie MJ. Felbamate: a new antiepileptic drug. *Lancet* 1993;341:1445–46.
72. Leppik IE. Felbamate. *Epilepsia* 1995;36[Suppl 2]:S66–S72.
73. Wallace Laboratories. Felbamate package insert. Revised October 1994.
74. Pennell PB, Ogaily MS, MacDonald R. Aplastic anemia in a patient receiving felbamate for complex partial seizures. *Neurology* 1995;45:456–460.
75. DeGiorgio CM, Lopez JE, Zinovy NL, et al. Status epilepticus induced by Felbatol withdrawal. *Neurology* 1995;45:1021–1022.
76. Welty TE, Privitera M, Shukla R. Increased seizure frequency associated with Felbamate withdrawal in adults. *Arch Neurol* 1998;55:641–645.
77. Phenytoin. In: Toll LL, Hurlbut KM, eds. POISINDEX System. Greenwood Village, CO: MICROMEDEX (edition expires June 2003).
78. Hachad H, Ragueneau-Majlessi I, Levy RH. New antiepileptic drugs: review on drug interactions. *Ther Drug Monit* 2002;24:91–103.
79. Felbatol product information. Cranbury, NJ: Wallace Laboratories, 2000.
80. Nagel TR, Schunk JE. Felbamate overdose: a case report and discussion of a new antiepileptic drug. *Pediatr Emerg Care* 1995;11:369–371.
81. Rengstorff DS, Milstone AP, Seger DL, et al. Felbamate overdose complicated by massive crystalluria and acute renal failure. *Clin Tox* 2000;38:667–669.
82. Yuen AC, Land GS, Watherby BC, et al. Sodium valproate acutely inhibits Lamotrigine metabolism. *Br J Clin Pharmacol* 1992;33:511–513.
83. Harden C, Trifiletti R, Kutt H. Felbamate levels in patients with epilepsy. *Epilepsia* 1996;37:280–283.
84. DeToledo JC, Ramsay RE. Fosphenytoin and Phenytoin in patients with status epilepticus. *Drug Saf* 2000;22:459–466.
85. Earnest EP, Marx JA, Drury LR. Complications of IV Phenytoin for acute treatment of seizures; recommendations for usage. *JAMA* 1983;6:762–5.
86. Browne TR, Kugler AR, Eldon MA. Pharmacology and pharmacokinetics of fosphenytoin. *Neurology* 1996;46:S3–S7.
87. Leppik IO, Boucher R, Wilder BJ, et al. Phenytoin prodrug: preclinical and clinical studies. *Epilepsia* 1989;30[Suppl 2]:S22–S26.
88. Leppik IE, Boucher BA, Wilder BJ, et al. Pharmacokinetics and safety of a Phenytoin prodrug given I.V. or i.m. in patients. *Neurology* 1990;40:456–60.
89. Ramsay RE, DeToledo J. Intravenous administration of fosphenytoin: options for the management of seizures. *Neurology* 1996;46:S17–S19.
90. Kugler AR, Knapp LE, Eldon MA. Rapid attainment of therapeutic Phenytoin concentrations following administration of loading doses of fosphenytoin: a meta-analysis. *Neurology* 1996;46:A176.
91. Jamerson BD, Dukes GE, Brouwer KL, et al. Venous irritation related to intravenous administration of Phenytoin versus fosphenytoin. *Pharmacotherapy* 1994;14:47–52.
92. Broumer K, Matier, WL, Quon CY. Absolute bioavailability of Phenytoin after IV 3-phosphoryloxymethyl Phenytoin disodium. *Clin Pharmacol Ther* 1988;43:178.
93. Fernandez MC, Walter FG, Kloster JC, et al. Hemodialysis and hemoperfusion for treatment of valproic acid and gabapentin poisoning. *Vet Human Toxicol* 1996;38:438–442.
94. Fisher JH, Andrews CO, Taber JE, et al. Multidose evaluation of gabapentin pharmacokinetics in patients with epilepsy. *Epilepsia* 1995;36[Suppl 4]:121.
95. McLean MJ. Gabapentin. *Epilepsia* 1995;36:S73–S86.
96. Blum RA, Comstock TJ, Sica DA, et al. Pharmacokinetics of gabapentin in subjects with various degrees of renal function. *Int J Clinic Pharmacol Ther* 1994;56(2):154–9.
97. Fischer JH, Barr AN, Rogers SL, et al. Lack of serious toxicity following gabapentin overdose. *Neurology* 1994;44:982–3.
98. Garofale E, et al. Experience with gabapentin overdose: five case studies. *Epilepsia* 1993;34:157.
99. Verma A, St Clair EW, Radtke RA. A case of sustained massive gabapentin overdose without serious side effects. *Ther Drug Monit* 1999;21:615.
100. U.S. Gabapentin Study Group. Gabapentin as add-on therapy in refractory epilepsy: a double blind, placebo-controlled, parallel-group study. *Neurology* 1993;43:2292–8.
101. Reference deleted.
102. Lamictal, lamotrigine tablets product information. Research Triangle Park, NC: Glaxo Wellcome Co, 2000.
103. Stopforth J. Overdose with gabapentin and lamotrigine [Letter]. *S Afr Med J* 1997;87:1388.
104. Briassoulis G, Kalabalikis P, Tomiolaki M, et al. Lamotrigine childhood overdose. *Pediatr Neurol* 1998;19:239–242.
105. Russell RJ, Parks B. Anticonvulsant medications. *Pediatr Ann* 1999;28:238–45.
106. Goa KL, Ross SR, Chrisp P. Lamotrigine: a review of its pharmacological properties and clinical efficacy in epilepsy. *Drugs* 1993;46:152–176.
107. Wallace SJ. Lamotrigine—a clinical overview. *Seizure* 1994;3[Suppl A]:47–51.
108. Cohen AF, Land GS, Bremier DD, et al. Lamotrigine, a new anticonvulsant: pharmacokinetics in normal humans. *Clin Pharmacol Ther* 1987;42:535–541.
109. Yuen AWC, Land GS, Weatherby BC, et al. Sodium valproate acutely inhibits Lamotrigine metabolism. *Br J Clin Pharmacol* 1992;33:511–513.
110. Brodie MJ. Lamotrigine versus other antiepileptic drugs: a star rating system is born. *Epilepsia* 1994;35:S41–S46.
111. Jawad S, Yuen WC, Peck AW, et al. Lamotrigine: single-dose pharmacokinetics and initial 1-week experience in refractory epilepsy. *Epilepsy Res* 1987;1:194–201.
112. O'Donnell J, Bateman DN. Lamotrigine overdose in an adult. *Clin Toxicol* 2000;38:659–660.
113. Reference deleted.
114. Schlienger RG, Knowles SR, Shear NH. Lamotrigine-associated anticonvulsant hypersensitivity syndrome. *Neurology* 1998;51:1172–1175.
115. Schlumberger E, Chavez F, Palacios L, et al. Lamotrigine in treatment of 120 children with epilepsy. *Epilepsia* 1994;35:359–67.
116. Besag F, Wallace S, Dulac O, et al. Lamotrigine for the treatment of epilepsy in childhood. *J Pediatr* 1995;127:991–7.
117. Sterker M, Berrouschot J, Schneider D. Fatal course of toxic epidermal necrolysis under treatment with Lamotrigine. *Int J Clin Pharmacol Ther* 1995;33:595–597.
118. Mylonakis E, Vittorio CC, Hollik DA, et al. Lamotrigine overdose presenting as anticonvulsant hypersensitivity syndrome. *Ann Pharmacother* 1999;33:557–559.
119. Dollery C, ed. *Therapeutic drugs*. CD release 1.0, 1999.
120. Shorvon S. Oxcarbazepine: a review. *Seizure* 2000;9:75–79.
121. Trileptal, oxcarbazepine. Product information. East Hanover, NJ: Novartis Pharmaceuticals Corp, 2001.
122. Jolliff HA, Fehrenbacher N, Dart RC. Bradycardia, hypotension, and tinnitus after accidental oxcarbazepine overdose (abst). *J Toxicol Clin Toxicol* 2001;39:316–317.
123. Schutz H, Feldmann KF, Faigle JW, et al. The metabolism of 14C-oxcarbazepine in man. *Xenobiotica* 1986;19:769–778.
124. Schachter SC. Oxcarbazepine: current status and clinical applications. *Exp Options Invest Drugs* 1999;8:1–10.
125. Tecoma ES. Oxcarbazepine. *Epilepsia* 1999;40[Suppl 5]:S37–S46.
126. Rouan MC, Lecaillon MB, Godbillon J, et al. The effects of renal impairment

on the pharmacokinetics of oxcarbazepine and its metabolites. *Eur J Clin Pharmacol* 1994;47:161–167.
127. Lloyd P, Flesch G, Dielerle W. Clinical pharmacology and pharmacy and pharmacokinetics of oxcarbazepine. *Epilepsy* 1994;35[Suppl. 3]:S10–S13.
128. Kubova H, et al. Anticonvulsant action of oxcarbazepine, hydroxycarbamazepine and carbamazepine against Metrazol-induced seizures in developing rats. *Epilepsia* 1993;34:188–192.
129. Schutz M, Brugger F, Gentsch C, et al. Oxcarbazepine: preclinical profile and putative mechanism of action. *Epilepsia* 1994;35 [Suppl 3]:S5–S9.
130. McLean MJ, et al. Oxcarbazepine: mechanisms of action. *Epilepsia* 1994;35[Suppl 3]:S5–S9.
131. Dam M, Ekberg R, Loyning Y, et al. A double-blind study comparing oxcarbazepine and carbamazepine in patients with newly diagnosed, previous untreated epilepsy. *Epilepsy Res* 1989;3:70–76.
132. Painter MJ, Gavs LM. Phenobarbital: clinical use. In: Levy RH, ed. *Antiepileptic Drugs*, 4th ed. New York: Raven Press 1995:477–485.
133. McNamara JO. Antiseizure barbiturates. In: Hardman JG, Limbird, eds. *Goodman & Gilman's the pharmacological basis of therapeutics*, 10th ed. McGraw-Hill 2001:532–33.
134. McDonald RL, Barker JL. Anticonvulsant and anesthetic barbiturates: different postsynaptic actions in cultured mammalian neurons. *Neurology* 1989;29:432–47.
135. Ransom BR, Barker JL. Pentobarbital selectively enhances GABA-mediated post-synaptic inhibition in tissue cultured mouse spinal neurons. *Brain Res* 1976;114:530–5.
136. Macdonald RL, Barker JL. Enhancement of GABA-mediated post-synaptic inhibition in cultured mammalian spinal cord neurons: a common node of anticonvulsant action. *Brain Res* 1979;167:323–36.
137. Rho JM, Donevan SD, Rogawski MA. Direct activation of GABA receptors by barbiturates in cultured rat hippocampal neurons. *J Physiol* 1996;497:509–22.
138. Harris EA, Slawson KB. The respiratory effects of therapeutic doses of cyclobarbitone, triclofos and ethchlorvynol. *Br J Pharmacol* 1965;24:214–222.
139. Eckstein JW, Hamilton WK, McHammond JM. The effect of thiopental on peripheral venous tone. *Anesthesiology* 1961;22:525–528.
140. Shubin H, Weil MH. The mechanism of shock following suicidal doses of barbiturates, narcotics and tranquilizer drugs, with observations on the effect of treatment. *Am J Med* 1965;38:853–863.
141. Richter JA, Holtman JR. Barbiturates: their in vivo effects and potential biochemical mechanisms. *Prog Neurol* 1982;18:275–319.
142. Carrol BJ. Barbiturate overdosage: presentation with focal neurological signs. *Med J Aust* 1969;1:1133–1135.
143. Osborn HH, Malkevich D. Lithium. *Clin Toxicol* 2001:532–538.
144. Wakabayashi Y, Maruyama S, Hachimura S, et al. Activated charcoal interrupts enteroenteric circulation of phenobarbital. *Clin Tox* 1994;32:419–424.
145. Berg MJ, Berlinger WG, Goldberg MJ, et al. Acceleration of the body clearance of phenobarbital by oral activated charcoal. *N Engl J Med* 1982;307:642–644.
146. Pond SM, Olson KR, Osterloh JD, et al. Randomized study of the treatment of phenobarbital overdose with repeated doses of activated charcoal. *JAMA* 1994;251:3104–3108.
147. Frenia ML, Schauben JL, Wears RL, et al. Multiple-dose activated charcoal compared to urinary alkalinization for the enhancement of phenobarbital elimination. *Clin Toxicol* 1996;34:169–175.
148. Bradberry SM, Vale JA. Multiple-dose activated charcoal: a review of relevant clinical studies. *Clin Toxicol* 1995;33:407–416.
149. Schmeiser M. Todliche vergiftung mit zentropil beim kind. *Kinderarztl Prax* 1952;20:158–161.
150. Lieber BL, Snodgrass WR. Cardiac arrest following large intravenous fosphenytoin overdose in an infant (abst). *J Toxicol Clin Toxicol* 1998;36:473.
151. Jung D, Powell JR, Walson P, et al. Effect of dose on phenytoin absorption. *Clin Pharmacol Ther* 1980;28:479–485.
152. Rall T, Schlerfer L. Drugs effective in the therapy of the epilepsies. In: Gilan A, Goodman L, Rall T, et al, eds. *Goodman & Gilman's the pharmacological basis of therapeutics*. New York: Macmillan 1990:436–444.
153. Tozer T, Winter M. Phenytoin. In: Evans W, Schentag J, Jusko W, eds. *Applied pharmacokinetics*. Spokane: Appl Ther 1980:275–314.
154. Jung D, Powell R, Watson P, et al. Effect of dose on phenytoin absorption. *Clin Pharmacol Ther* 1985;28:479–485.
155. Hvidberg EF, Dan M. Clinical pharmacokinetics of anticonvulsants. *Clin Pharmacokinet* 1976;1:161–188.
156. Brodie M, Dichter M. Antiepileptic drugs. *N Engl J Med* 1996;334:168–175.
157. DeLorenzo RJ. Phenytoin: mechanisms of action. In: Levy RH, Mattson RH, Meldrum BS, eds. *Antiepileptic drugs*, 4th ed. New York: Raven Press, 1995:271–82.
158. Dichter MA. Old and new mechanisms of antiepileptic drug actions. *Epilepsy Res Suppl* 1993;10:9–17.
159. Chaikin P, Adir J. Unusual absorption profile of phenytoin in a massive overdose case. *J Clinical Pharmacol* 1987;27:70–73.
160. Mellick LB, Morgan JA, Mellick GA. Presentations of acute phenytoin overdose. *Am J Emerg Med* 1989;7:61–67.
161. Kooker J, Sumi S. Movement disorder as a manifestation of diphenylhydantoin intoxication. *Neurology* 1974;24:68–71.
162. Kokenge R, Henn, McDowell F. Neurological sequelae following Dilantin overdose in a patient and in experimental animals. *Neurology* 1964;15:823–829.
163. Masur H, Elger CE, Ludolph AC, et al. Cerebellar atrophy following acute intoxication with phenytoin. *Neurology* 1989;39:432–433.
164. McLain L, Martin T, Allen. Cerebellar degeneration due to chronic phenytoin therapy. *Ann Neurol* 1980:18–23.
165. Aaron J, Bank S, Ackert G. Diphenylhydantoin induced hepatotoxicity. *Am J Gastroenterol* 1985:200–202.
166. Flowers F, Araujo O, Hanm K. Phenytoin hypersensitivity syndrome. *J Emergency Med* 1987;5:103–108.
167. Palm R, Selsith C, Alvan G. Phenytoin intoxication as the first symptom of fatal liver damage induced by sodium valproate. *Br J Clin Pharmacol* 1984;17:597–598.
168. Barron S. Cardiac arrhythmias after small IV dose of phenytoin. *N Engl J Med* 1976;295:678.
169. Donovan P, Cline D. Phenytoin administration by constant intravenous infusion: selective rates of administration. *Ann Emerg Med* 1991;20:139–142.
170. Earnest M, Marx J, Druey L. Complications of intravenous phenytoin for acute treatment of seizures. *JAMA* 1983;249:762–765.
171. Carducci B, Hedges J, Levy R, et al. Emergency phenytoin loading by constant intravenous infusion. *Ann Emerg Med* 1984;13:1027–1031.
172. York R, Coleridge S. Cardiopulmonary arrest following intravenous phenytoin loading. *Am J Emerg Med* 1988;6:255–259.
173. Zoneraich S, Zoneraich O, Siegel J. Sudden death following intravenous sodium diphenylhydantoin. *Am Heart J* 1976;92:375–377.
174. Spengler R, Arrowsmith J, Silarski D, et al. Severe soft-tissue injury following intravenous infusion of phenytoin. *Arch Intern Med* 1988;148:1329–33.
175. Letters to the editor. The use of free phenytoin levels in adverting phenytoin toxicity. *N Y State J Med* 1990;90:39–41.
176. Wilder JB, Ramsay RE, Willmore L, et al. Efficacy of intravenous phenytoin in the treatment of status epilepticus. Kinetics of central nervous system penetration. *Ann Neurol* 1977;1:511–518.
177. Walsh-Kelly C, Berens R, Glaeser P, et al. Intraosseous infusion of phenytoin. *Am J Emerg Med* 1986;4:523–524.
178. Czajka P, Anderson W, Christoph R, et al. A pharmacokinetics evaluation of peritoneal dialysis for phenytoin intoxication. *J Clin Pharmacol* 1980;20:565–569.
179. Wyte CD, Berk WA. Severe oral phenytoin overdose does not cause cardiovascular morbidity. *Ann Emerg Med* 1991;20:508–512.
180. Gabitril product information, Tiagabine. North Chicago: Abbott Laboratories, 1997.
181. Suzdak PD, Jansen JA. A review of the preclinical pharmacology of tiagabine: a potent and selective anticonvulsant GABA uptake inhibitor. *Epilepsia* 1995;36:612–26.
182. Ostrovskiy D, Sspanaki MV, Morris GL. Tiagabine overdose can induce convulsive status epilepticus. *Epilepsia* 2002;43:773–774.
183. Viner K, Clifton JC, Hryhorczuk DO, et al. Status epilepticus following acute tiagabine overdose. *J Toxicol Clin Toxicol* 1999;36:638.
184. Kaufman KR, Lepore FE, Keyser BJ. Visual fields and tiagabine: a quandary. *Seizure* 2001;10:525–529.
185. Leach JP, Brodie MJ. Tiagabine. *Lancet* 1998;351:203–207.
186. Sills GJ, Butler E, Thompson GG, et al. Vigabatrin and tiagabine and pharmacologically different drugs. A pre-clinical study. *Seizure* 1999;8:404–411.
187. Collins SD, Brun S, Kirstein YG, et al. Absence of visual field defects in patients taking tiagabine. *Epilepsia* 1998;39[Suppl 6]:146–147.
188. Garnett WR. Clinical pharmacology of topiramate: a review. *Epilepsia* 2000;41:S61–S65.
189. Walker MC, Sander JW. Topiramate: a new antiepileptic drug for refractory epilepsy. *Seizure* 1996;5:199.
190. Stowe CD, Bollinger T, James LP, et al. Acute mental status changes and hyperchloremic metabolic acidosis with long-term topiramate therapy. *Pharmacotherapy* 2000;20:105.
191. Wilner A, Raymond K, Pollard R. Topiramate and metabolic acidosis. *Epilepsia* 1999;40:792.
192. Wasserstein AG, Rak I, Reife RA. Investigation of the mechanistic basis for topiramate-associated nephrolithiasis: examination of urinary and serum constituents. *Epilepsia* 1995;36[Suppl 3]:S153.
193. Loscher W. Valproate: a reappraisal of its pharmacodynamic properties and mechanisms of action. *Prog Neurobiol* 1999;58:31–59.
194. Ingels M, Beauchamp J, Clark R, et al. Delayed valproic acid toxicity: a retrospective case series. *Ann Emerg Med* 2002;39:616–621.
195. Tift JP. Valproic acid [Letter]. *N Engl J Med* 1980;303:394.
196. Janssen F, Rambeck B, Schnabel R. Acute valproate intoxication with fatal outcome in an infant. *Neuropediatrics* 1985;16:235–238.
197. Garnier R, Fournier E. Intoxication aigue par le valproate de sodium. *Nouv Presse Med* 1982;11:678.
198. Ishikura H, Matsuo N, Matsubara M, et al. Valproic acid overdose and L-carnitine therapy. *J Anal Toxicol* 1996;20:Jan–Feb.
199. Klotz U, Antonin KH. Pharmacokinetics and bioavailability of sodium valproate. *Clin Pharmacol Ther* 1977;21:736–743.
200. Kane SL, Constantiner M, Staubus AE, et al. High-flux hemodialysis without hemoperfusion is effective in acute valproic acid overdose. *Ann Pharmacother* 2000;34:1146–1151.
201. Dupuis R, Lichtman S, Pollack G. Acute valproic acid overdose. *Drug Saf* 1990;5(1):65–71.
202. Anderson GO, Ritland S. Life threatening intoxication with sodium valproate. *Clin Toxicol* 1995;33(3):29–284.
203. Simler S, Ciesieleski L, Maitre M, et al. Effect of sodium di-n-propylacetate on audiogenic seizures and brain y-aminobutyric acid level. *Biochem Pharmacol* 1973;22:1701–1708.

204. McLean MJ, MacDonald RL. Sodium valproate, but not ethosuximide, produces use- and voltage-dependent limitation of high frequency repetitive firing of action potentials of mouse central neurons in cell culture. *J Pharmacol Exp Ther* 1986;237:1001–1002.
205. Albus H, Williamson R. Electrophysical analysis of the action of valproate on pyramidal neurons in the rat hippocampal slice. *Epilepsia* 1998;39:124–129.
206. Loscher W. Effects of the antiepileptic drug valproate on metabolism and function of inhibitory and excitatory amino acids in the brain. *Neurochem Res* 1993;18:485–502.
207. Asai M, Talavera E, Massarini A, et al. Valproic acid-induced rapid changes of met-enkephalin levels in rat brain. Probable association with abstinence behavior and anti-convulsant activity. *Neuropeptides* 1994;227:203–210.
208. Dzoljic MR, Poel-Heisterkamp AL. The effects of GABA-ergic drugs on enkephalin-induced motor seizure phenomena in the rat. *Clin Exp Pharmacol Physiol* 1981;8:141–150.
209. Rho JM, Sankar R. The pharmacologic basis of antiepileptic drug action. *Epilepsia* 1999;40(11):1471–1483.
210. Spiller HA, Krenzelok EP, Klein-Schwartz W, et al. Multicenter case series of valproic acid ingestion: serum concentrations and toxicity. *J Toxicol Clin Toxicol* 2000;38:755–60
211. Dupuis RE, Lichtman SN, Pollack GM. Acute valproic acid overdose: clinical course and pharmacokinetic disposition of valproic acid and metabolites. *Drug Saf* 1990;5:65–70.
212. Blindauer KA, Harrington G, Morris GL, et al. Fulminant progression of demyelinating disease after valproate induced encephalopathy. *Neurology* 1998;51:292–295.
213. Bryant AE, Fritz E, et al. Valproic acid hepatic fatalities. III. U.S. experience since 1986. *Neurology* 1996;46:465–469.
214. Wen-Ling L, Chen-Chang Y, Jou-Fang D, et al. A case of severe hyperammonemia and unconsciousness following sodium valproate intoxication. *Vet Hum Toxicol* 1998;40:346–348.
215. Rawat S, Borkowski WJ, Swick HM. Valproic acid and secondary hyperammonemia. *Neurology* 1991;31:1173–1174.
216. Ralnaike R, Schapel G, Purdie G, et al. Hyperammonaemia and hepatotoxicity during chronic valproate therapy: enhancement by combination with other antiepileptic drugs. *Br J Clin Pharmacol* 1986;22:100–103.
217. Dreifuss FE, Santilli N, Langer DH, et al. Valproic acid hepatic fatalities: a retrospective review. *Neurology* 1987;37:379–385.
218. Dreifuss FE, Langer DH, Moline KA, et al. Valproic acid hepatic fatalities. US experience since 1984. *Neurology* 1989;39:201–207.
219. Dreifuss FE, Santilli N, Langer DH, et al. *Neurology* 1987;37:379.
220. Dreifuss FE, Langer DH, Moline KA, et al. *Neurology* 1989;39:201.
221. Patsalos PN, Wilson SJ, Popovik M, et al. The prevalence of valproic acid associated hyperammonaemia in patients with intractable epilepsy. *J Epilepsy* 1993;6:228–232.
222. Yazdani K, Lippmann M, Gala I. Fatal pancreatitis associated with valproic acid. *Medicine* 2002;81:305–310.
223. Binek J, Hany A, Heer M. Valproic-acid-induced pancreatitis. *J Clin Gastroenterol* 1991;13(6):690–3.
224. Glanick D, Suner T, Finley JL. Severe hematologic toxicity of valproic acid. *Am J Ped Hematol Oncol* 1990;12(1):80–85.
225. Graudins A, Aaron CK. Delayed peak serum valproic acid in massive divalproex overdose and treatment with charcoal hemoperfusion. *J Toxicol Clin Toxicol* 1996;34:335–41.
226. Tank JE, Palmer BF. Simultaneous "in series" hemodialysis and hemoperfusion in the management of valproic acid overdose. *Am J Kidney Dis* 1993;22:341–344.
227. Bowdle TA, Patel IH, Levy RH, et al. Valproic acid dosage and plasma protein binding and clearance. *Clin Pharmacol Ther* 1980;28:486–492.
228. Alberto G, Erickson T, Popiel R, et al. Central nervous system manifestations of a valproic acid overdose responsive to Naloxone. *Ann Emerg Med* 1989;18:889–891.
229. Espinoza O, Maradel I, Ramirez M, et al. An unusual presentation of opioid-like syndrome in pediatric valproic acid poisoning. *Vet Hum Toxicol* 2001;43:178–179.
230. Dingledine R, Iverson LL, Breuker E. Naloxone as a GABA antagonist: evidence from iontophoretic, receptor binding and convulsant studies. *Eur J Pharmacol* 1978;47:19–27.
231. Gruol DL, Barker JL, Smith TG. Naloxone antagonism of GABA evoked membrane polarizations in cultured mouse spinal cord neurons. *Brain Res* 1980;198:323–32.
232. Mumford JP, Cannon DJ. Vigabatrin. *Epilepsia* 1994;35:S35–S38.
233. Gidal BE, Privitera MD, Sheth RD, et al. Vigabatrin: a novel therapy for seizure disorders. *Ann Pharmacother* 1999;33:1277–86.
234. Davie MB, Cook MJ, Ng C. Vigabatrin overdose. *Med J Aust* 1996;165:403.
235. Haegele KD, Schechter PJ. Kinetics of the enantiomers of vigabatrin after an oral dose of the racemate or the active S-enantiomer. *Clin Pharmacol Ther* 1986;40:581–6.
236. Schechter PJ. Clinical pharmacology of vigabatrin. *Br J Clin Pharmacol* 1989;27:19S–22S.
237. Hoke JF, Yuh L, Antony KK, et al. Pharmacokinetics of vigabatrin following single and multiple oral doses in normal volunteers. *J Clin Pharmacol* 1993;33:458–62.
238. Rimmer EM, Richens A. Interaction between vigabatrin and phenytoin. *Br J Clin Pharmacol* 1989;27:27S–33S.
239. Guberman A. Vigabatrin. *Can J Neurol Sci* 1996;23:S13–17.
240. Lippert B, Metcalf BW, Jung MJ, et al. 4-Amino-hex-5-enoic acid, a selective catalytic inhibitor of 4-aminobutyric-acid aminotransferase in mammalian brain. *Eur J Biochem* 1977;74:441–5.
241. Leach JP, Sills GJ, Majid A, et al. Effects of tiagabine and vigabatrin and GABA uptake into primary cultures of rat cortical astrocytes. *Seizure* 1996;5:229–234.
242. Product monograph. Sabril. Canada: Hoechst Marion Roussel 1994:1–25.
243. Zonisamide approved for partial seizures. *Am J Health-Sys Pharm* 2000;57:834, 837.
244. Wilensky AJ, Friel PM, Ojemann LM, et al. Zonisamide in epilepsy: a pilot study. *Epilepsia* 1985;26:212–20.
245. Suzuki N, Seki T, Yamawaki H, et al. Treatment of paediatric epilepsy with AD-810 (Zonisamide-ZNS). *Jpn J Paediatr* 1987;40:3147–3152.
246. Wagner JG, Sackellares JC, Donofrio PD, et al. Non-linear pharmacokinetics of CI-912 in adult epileptic patient. *Ther Drug Monit* 1984;6:277–83.
247. Mimaki T. Clinical pharmacology and therapeutic drug monitoring of zonisamide. *Ther Drug Monit* 1998;20:593–597.
248. Rho JM, Sankar R. The pharmacologic basis of antiepileptic drug action. *Epilepsia* 1999;40(11):1471–1483.
249. Naito H, Itoh N, Matsui N, et al. Monitoring plasma concentrations of zonisamide and clonazepam in an epileptic attempting suicide by an overdose of the drugs. *Curr Ther Res* 1988;43:463–467.
250. Oommen KJ, Mathews S. Zonisamide: a new antiepileptic drug. *Clin Neuropharmacol* 1999;22:192–2000.
251. Miyamoto T, Kohsaka M, Koyama T. Psychotic episodes during zonisamide treatment. *Seizure* 2000;9:65–70.

CHAPTER 131

Lithium

Michael A. Miller and Kent R. Olson

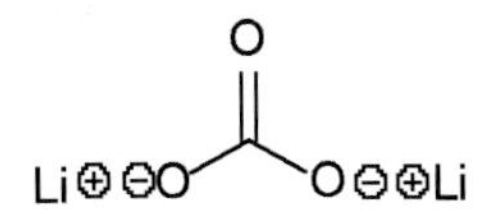

LITHIUM CARBONATE

Atomic symbol, atomic number, atomic mass:	**Li+, 3, 6.941**
Valence state:	**+1**
Molecular formula and weight:	**Li_2CO_3, 73.89 g/mol**
SI conversion:	**mg/L × 0.144 = mmol/L**
CAS Registry No.:	**7439-93-2**
Therapeutic level:	**0.6 to 1.2 mEq/L (serum; 1 mEq/L = 1 mmol/L)**
Special concerns:	**Renal insufficiency or volume depletion may lead to occult chronic toxicity.**
Target organs:	**Central nervous system: fasciculation, slurred speech, slowness to respond, confusion, hyperreflexia, coma**
Antidote:	**None**

OVERVIEW

Lithium is a monovalent metal cation with physiologic actions similar to potassium and sodium (1). In the past, lithium has been used to treat gout, as a salt substitute, and in the soft drink Seven-Up (2,3). Modern medicinal use of lithium carbonate, primarily for depression and bipolar mood disorders, gained popularity in the early 1970s. Today, lithium is also used in the treatment of schizoaffective disorders, alcoholism, and prophylaxis of cluster headaches (4). It is estimated that 0.1% of the U.S. population is treated with this agent (5) with a broad population demographic susceptible to the toxic effects of lithium (6).

The efficacy of lithium as a psychotropic agent has justified its expanded use despite a narrow therapeutic index. Patients undergoing dosing adjustments or patients in whom drug elimination is altered are at risk for developing toxicity. Common symptoms of toxicity include nausea, polyuria, somnolence, and myoclonic jerking. In severe cases, toxicity has resulted in seizures, dysrhythmias, and death (Table 1) (7–9). Lithium rarely causes death, but chronic toxicity is associated with high morbidity and prolonged hospitalization.

Available formulations include (a) regular release lithium carbonate tablets and capsules (Carbolith, Eskalith, Lithane, Lithonate, Lithizine; 150, 300, or 600 mg); (b) sustained release tablets of various types (Duralith, Eskalith CR, Lithobid; 300 to 600 mg); and (c) lithium citrate liquid (Cibalith S, LI-Liquid, 8 mEq/5 ml). Lithium carbonate 300 mg equals approximately 8 mEq of lithium.

TABLE 1. Signs and symptoms of chronic lithium toxicity

Blood lithium level >1.5 mEq/L	Blood lithium level >2.5 mEq/L
Nausea	Increasing confusion
Malaise	Ataxia
Weakness	Myoclonic movements
Blood lithium level >2.0 mEq/L	Choreoathetosis
Increasing fatigue and somnolence	Restlessness
Confusion	Blood lithium >3.0 mEq/L
Slurred speech	Coma
Nystagmus	Seizures
	Circulatory collapse

Note: Toxicity at a given blood level is variable and is influenced by the chronicity of dosing or ingestion. Levels are equilibrium levels and should be drawn more than 4 to 6 hours after the patient's last dose of lithium.

TOXIC DOSE

The typical *adult therapeutic dose* of lithium carbonate starts at 600 mg daily. The usual effective dose is 900 to 1800 mg/day. An acute single ingestion of lithium does not usually cause significant toxicity, but a single ingestion of 40 mg of lithium salt per kilogram is capable of producing a lithium blood level of 2 mEq/L (10). Therapeutic dosing can lead to significant toxicity in patients with decreased creatinine clearance or increased tubular reabsorption (11,12). Therapeutic dosing can also cause nephrogenic diabetes insipidus.

TOXICOKINETICS AND TOXICODYNAMICS

Pharmacokinetic data for lithium are provided in Table 2 (10,13–19). Lithium has a multicomponent volume of distribution. The initial volume of distribution into the circulating blood volume is small but increases over time and in overdose as it moves

TABLE 2. Pharmacokinetic parameters for lithium

Parameter	Value
Bioavailability (%)	More than 95%
Peak plasma levels	0.8–1.5 mmol/L (0.8–1.5 mEq/L)
Peak plasma level time	30 min to 2 h (2.0–5.5 h for sustained release)
Volume of distribution	0.6 L/kg
Plasma protein binding	Less than 10%
Elimination half-life	24 h (variable)
Route of elimination	Renal
Metabolism	None

intracellularly into the central nervous system (CNS) and other tissues. After overdose, the time to reach peak plasma time may reach 40 hours (20).

PATHOPHYSIOLOGY

There are several proposed mechanisms for the therapeutic effects of lithium. Lithium increases serotonin synthesis and downregulates 5-HT_{1a} receptors in the hippocampus (21,22); depletes free inositol in the CNS, an essential precursor involved in phosphoinositide second-messenger systems (23,24); and inhibits G proteins involved in the opening of ion channels (24). These mechanisms, as well as the ability of lithium to substitute for the cations potassium and sodium, may also account for the diverse neurologic manifestations of lithium poisoning (1).

The CNS is the predominant target of lithium toxicity (25). The slow distribution of lithium into and out of the CNS helps explain the delay in CNS symptoms as well as the persistence of symptoms after serum levels have dropped (25–27).

Patients chronically taking lithium often exhibit some urinary concentrating defect (Fig. 1). This defect correlates with duration of therapy and dose (28). As many as 40% of patients on chronic therapy have polyuria and 5% to 20% have frank nephrogenic diabetes insipidus (28–30). The defective responsiveness of the distal nephron to antidiuretic hormone (ADH), as well as histopathologic changes, are usually reversible with dose reduction or cessation of therapy, although persistent diabetes insipidus in the setting of interstitial nephritis has been described (31).

Serious cardiovascular effects are rare with either acute or chronic lithium poisoning, although electrocardiographic (ECG) changes, cardiac dysrhythmias, and asystole have been reported (9). A prolonged QTc interval and sinus node arrest may develop in toxic patients and occasionally in the setting of a nontoxic patient with therapeutic lithium levels (32–34). Hypotension and even cardiac arrest have been noted, although severe CNS toxicity or underlying cardiac disease is usually a comorbid condition in these reports (32–34).

Lithium may inhibit thyroid hormone synthesis, resulting in hypothyroidism (35). The risk of hypothyroidism is related to duration of therapy and dosage, with more than 20% of patients on lithium for more than 10 years having evidence of hypothyroidism (36). However, chronic lithium use can induce the full spectrum of endocrinologic thyroid disorders to include hyperthyroidism and euthyroid goiter (32,37,38).

Hypercalcemia due to hyperparathyroidism has been reported (39), but from available reports it is unclear whether lithium causes or exacerbates this condition. Lithium also stimulates

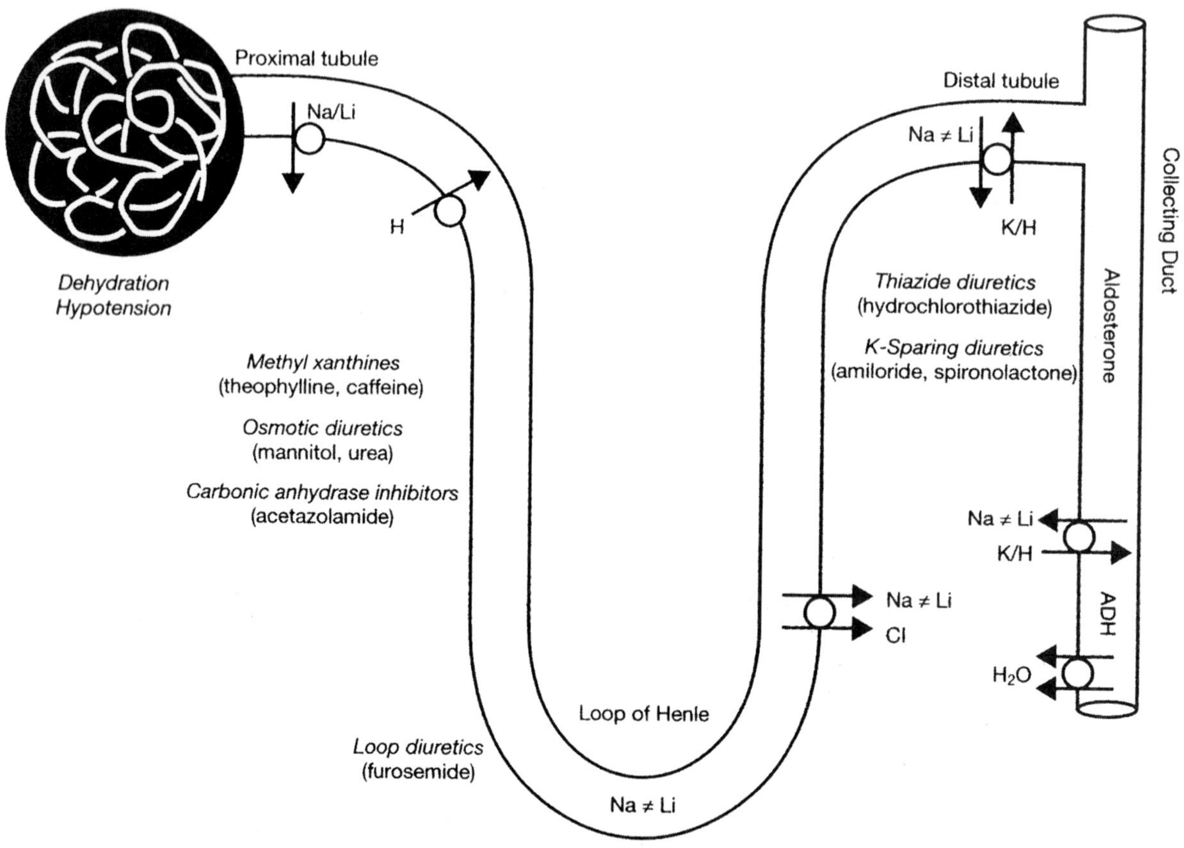

Figure 1. Renal handling of lithium. The lithium ion is freely filtered by the glomerulus. Clearance may, therefore, be influenced by various physiologic factors that reduce renal blood flow and filtration rates (e.g., dehydration or hypotension). Reabsorption of lithium occurs in parallel with sodium in the proximal tubule and, to a lesser extent, the loop of Henle. In the distal tubule and collecting duct, antidiuretic hormone (ADH) and aldosterone facilitate the reabsorption of sodium and water, but the tubular membrane appears to be impervious to lithium along the distal portion. As a result, the administration of distally acting diuretics (e.g., thiazides and spironolactone) potentiates an increase in lithium reabsorption along the proximal tubule, whereas diuretics with more proximal activity [e.g., furosemide (frusemide)] are not associated with a compensatory increase in reabsorption rates. (Adapted from Finley PR, et al. *Clin Pharmacokinet* 1995;29:172–191.)

an increase in granulocyte stem cells and neutrophil count, which has been used therapeutically to treat neutropenia (40).

PREGNANCY AND LACTATION

Lithium is U.S. Food and Drug Administration pregnancy category D (Appendix I). Early studies linked maternal lithium use with cardiac abnormalities, especially Ebstein's anomaly (32,41). Well-designed cohort studies indicate that the teratogenic potential of lithium is significantly less than previously published; however, the rates of congenital anomalies and cardiac malformations still appear to be increased (42–44). Cohort studies demonstrate a 4% to 12% rate of major congenital anomalies in infants of women taking lithium during the first trimester compared with 2% to 4% in a comparison, nonexposed group (42). Women who continue to take lithium during pregnancy should be counseled about the risks to the fetus and benefits to the mother. Fortunately, other options are now available for clinicians to treat these patients.

Lithium crosses the placenta readily, and fetal serum concentrations approximate maternal levels. Newborn lithium toxicity has been reported and may cause *floppy baby syndrome* (42,45). Lithium inhibits release of thyroid hormone and can increase thyroid-stimulating hormone production, resulting in goiter in the neonate (46). Women believed to be without a high risk of manic-depressive relapse should be tapered off lithium during pregnancy. Those considered at higher risk may be tapered off and then therapy reinstituted during the middle of the second trimester.

Lithium levels in human breast milk reach 40% of the maternal blood lithium level and may be as much as 50% higher (47–50). Toxicity in a breast-fed infant has been described (48). Lithium is relatively contraindicated during breast-feeding (51). Mothers who decide to breast-feed their children should watch for evidence of toxicity in their infant (52).

CLINICAL PRESENTATION

Lithium poisoning may occur as a result of a single acute overdose, an acute overdose in a patient chronically treated with lithium, chronic excessive overmedication, or gradual accumulation of lithium in a patient with worsening renal insufficiency (Table 1). The latter two circumstances are referred to as *chronic intoxication*.

Acute Overdosage

Acute lithium overdose, although common, is generally associated with less severe toxicity despite higher blood lithium levels (12,53,54). Signs and symptoms may be similar to chronic effects, but CNS effects are generally milder and gastrointestinal symptoms are more common (21,55). A large undertreated lithium ingestion may result in severe and prolonged toxicity. The correlation of the lithium levels with symptomatology in acute lithium overdoses is poor (53,54).

Acute overdose on chronic lithium ingestion occurs when a patient treated with lithium takes an acute ingestion. The implication is that these patients are more likely to develop clinically significant toxicity than the naïve patient who takes an acute ingestion. The clinical importance of this group arises from recognizing the increased danger. The signs and symptoms are similar to other forms of lithium intoxication.

Chronic Intoxication

Chronic lithium intoxication is often an occult illness that develops during a clinical illness leading to dehydration, especially when there is poor sodium intake, as a result of impaired excretion such as an adverse drug interaction (Table 3), or after increased intake such as a dosing change. Lithium can decrease glomerular filtration rate and thereby induce or exacerbate either acute or subacute renal failure (56). By increasing absorp-

TABLE 3. Lithium drug interactions

Drug	Lithium renal clearance: Reduced	Lithium renal clearance: Increased	Toxic at normal therapeutic lithium levels	Other
Thiazide diuretics	+			
Ibuprofen	+			
Indomethacin	+			
Phenylbutazone	+			
Diclofenac	+			
Piroxicam	+			
Mazindol	+			
Phenytoin	+			
Tetracycline	+			
Acetazolamide		+		
Theophylline		+		
Verapamil		+		
Cisplatin		+		
Sodium bicarbonate		+		
Carbamazepine			+	Neurologic toxicity signs
Methyldopa	+		+	May exacerbate central nervous system response to lithium
Neuroleptics (high doses)			+	Neuroleptic syndrome, extrapyramidal symptoms

Adapted from Groleau G, et al. *Am J Emerg Med* 1987;5:527–553.

tion and decreasing excretion, lithium contributes to its own toxicity (11,57). The signs and symptoms are variable and do not correlate well with serum or even cerebrospinal fluid levels of lithium (Table 1) (58–61). There is typically a delay of hours between peak serum levels and development of CNS effects as a result of slow CNS penetration. Mild lithium intoxication involves fatigue, tremor, and slowness to respond. As severity increases, agitation, hyperreflexia, and inability to respond develop and may progress to frank coma, seizures, and death in severe cases (8).

Adverse Events

Goiter, hypothyroidism, tremor, polyuria, and polydipsia are common adverse effects of lithium therapy (32,37,60). Nausea and vomiting are also common, but along with thirst, tremor, and polyuria, they often abate during continued therapy (62).

Drug Interactions

It is likely that any drug that decreases glomerular filtration or increases cation absorption increases the serum lithium level (Table 3). Commonly used drugs such as nonsteroidal antiinflammatory drugs may increase proximal tubule reabsorption of lithium by causing a decrease in glomerular filtration rate in the patient with elevated angiotensin or dehydration. Antibiotics such as metronidazole and tetracycline have also been implicated in decreasing lithium renal clearance. There are reports of neurotoxicity consistent with chronic lithium toxicity despite lithium levels in the therapeutic range in patients taking both neuroleptics and lithium (32,58). Serotonin syndrome has been reported in patients on combination therapy with a selective serotonin reuptake inhibitor; it is uncommon (63,64). Providers should be cognizant of this possibility and recognize it when it occurs.

DIAGNOSTIC TESTS

Suicidal ingestion should be evaluated in the typical manner. Tests specific to potential lithium intoxication include serum electrolytes, renal function, lithium level, and ECG. The serum electrolytes, blood urea nitrogen, and creatinine are used to assess renal insufficiency and may affect the decision to perform dialysis.

Therapeutic lithium levels are 0.6 to 1.2 mEq/L. Serial lithium levels are needed because of the frequent use of sustained release preparations and their use in determining the need for dialysis. Lithium levels may continue to rise for many hours, and onset of toxicity may be delayed as lithium is absorbed. Signs of toxicity may occur at levels as low as 1.5 mEq/L, but levels at which toxicity occurs vary widely (8,58,61). Signs of severe neurotoxicity have even occurred at therapeutic levels, and it appears likely that the elderly and patients on other neuroleptics are at an increased risk of this phenomenon (58,65). After acute ingestion, the lithium concentration may be quite high but symptoms minimal, especially shortly after ingestion (32,55). In patients with chronic intoxication, CNS symptoms generally provide a better measure of severity than serum levels. Erroneous markedly elevated serum levels may result from collection of serum into green top tubes, which contain lithium heparin (66).

An ECG and cardiac monitoring should be considered on any significantly intoxicated patient. Typical ECG abnormalities are nonspecific ST-T wave changes and are usually benign, though rare serious cardiovascular effects have been reported (9,32,33). Thyroid levels and thyroid-stimulating hormone should be monitored in patients on chronic therapy. If nephrogenic diabetes insipidus is suspected, obtain urine electrolytes and measure serum and urine osmolality. Elevated serum sodium and chloride levels in the setting of output of large volumes of dilute urine confirm this suspected diagnosis. Treatment consists of reestablishing adequate fluid status; sodium restriction; and the use of agents such as thiazides, amiloride, or a nonsteroidal antiinflammatory agent; and withdrawal of lithium.

Although sustained release lithium carbonate preparations may be radiopaque, the sensitivity of radiography to detect undissolved medication is unclear and should not be relied on in excluding any ingestion (67).

POSTMORTEM CONSIDERATIONS

Postmortem blood lithium appears to undergo minimal early drug redistribution in one small study, whereas whole blood specimens have yielded false-positive lithium levels in cadavers (68,69). In cattle, one study demonstrated tissue concentration on postmortem examinations, most markedly in the muscle, heart, liver, kidney, and brain (70).

TREATMENT

Treatment of lithium intoxication focuses on discontinuation of intake and increasing excretion (Table 4). Most cases can be managed by decontamination (in cases of recent acute ingestion), rehydration with isotonic crystalloid fluids, and monitoring of the lithium level. In the symptomatic patient, appropriate attention to airway, breathing, and circulation is important. The use of forced saline diuresis does not appear to increase lithium excretion, can lead to hypernatremia, and is not recommended (60).

Decontamination

Activated charcoal does not adsorb lithium but should be considered if there is a suspicion of coingestion (71–74). Although controversy exists regarding the use of gastric lavage, it may be of benefit if performed in the case of recent, acute, large ingestion to prevent the development of CNS effects (75).

TABLE 4. An approach to the lithium poisoned patient

- Assure that basic resuscitative measures have occurred, focusing on support of the patient's airway, breathing, and circulation.
- Perform gastric decontamination after acute ingestion.
  - Gastric lavage for patients presenting within 1–2 h of presentation.
  - Whole bowel irrigation for ingestions of sustained release lithium preparations.
- Clinical evaluation of the patient.
  - Consider the differential diagnosis for the patient (infections, other drug ingestions/poisonings).
  - Determine severity of poisoning (mental status, serum electrolytes, renal function, electrocardiogram, and so forth).
- Supportive care.
  - Intravascular fluid repletion with isotonic crystalloid fluid.
  - Further circulatory support as necessary with vasoactive agents.
- Enhanced elimination.
  - Hemodialysis.
    - For severe symptoms such as seizures, coma, increasing alterations in mental status.
    - For moderate symptoms such as lethargy and confusion in the setting of renal failure.
  - Continuous venovenous and arteriovenous hemodiafiltration.
    - Consider this after conventional hemodialysis to prevent *rebound* and to provide continued removal.
    - For hemodynamically unstable patients.

TABLE 5. Lithium clearance rates with and without hemodialysis

Lithium clearance	Serum half-life (h)	Renal clearance (ml/min)	Total clearance (ml/min)
Without hemodialysis	23.16 ± 9.0	17.2 ± 5.4	26.5 ± 13.3
With hemodialysis	3.6–5.7	NR	63.2–114.4

NR, not reported.
Adapted from Jaeger A, Sauder P, Kopferschmitt J, et al. When should dialysis be performed in lithium poisoning: a kinetic study in 14 cases of lithium poisoning. *J Toxicol Clin Toxicol* 1993;31:429–447.

Whole bowel irrigation has become an accepted method of gastric decontamination after ingestion of sustained release preparations. One small study of healthy volunteers demonstrated significantly reduced absorption (as estimated from area under the curve) in subjects receiving whole bowel irrigation shortly after lithium ingestion (76). It should be considered for use in patients with rising lithium levels despite treatment, the massive ingestion, or the ingestion of sustained release preparations.

Enhancement of Elimination

Due to its small size, poor protein binding, small volume of distribution, and water solubility, lithium is a good candidate for removal by hemodialysis. Indeed, hemodialysis clearance rates of 60 to 115 ml/minute have been reported (17,18). The serum half-life in the lithium toxic patient is in the range of 24 hours, whereas the use of hemodialysis reduces the elimination half-life to 3.5 to 5.7 hours (Table 5) (18). Serum lithium levels often rebound after hemodialysis, particularly in patients with chronic intoxication. More importantly, patients do not commonly show acute improvement after hemodialysis, perhaps because of slow elimination of lithium from within the intracellular space and across the blood–brain barrier. The use of hemodialysis until the lithium serum levels are less than 1.0 mEq/L, followed by a repeat serum level in 6 to 8 hours, has been advocated (18).

Valid hemodialysis criteria have not been established. The indication for dialysis after an acute, single ingestion of lithium is difficult to define, as levels of more than 8.0 mEq/L have been tolerated without development of clinically significant symptoms (18,60). Thus, the decision to hemodialyze rests on multiple variables: the clinical condition of the patient; improvement or deterioration during intravenous fluid therapy; evaluation of repeated lithium levels; and the patient's underlying renal function and physical health. The use of hemodialysis should be strongly considered with a level of more than 4.0 mEq/L after an acute ingestion (18).

In cases of chronic intoxication, common clinical criteria include evidence of severe neurologic signs or symptoms, such as agitated delirium, coma, or convulsions, and clinical deterioration or failure to improve with supportive therapy (17,18,77). One study found that hemodialysis failed to improve outcome and recommended that hemodialysis should be reserved for severe cases (7). However, the study enrolled only 18 patients who were deemed sick enough to necessitate dialysis, and only eight of those patients actually underwent this therapy. Underlying comorbidities, most important, renal failure, should also play an important role in the decision to perform hemodialysis.

Continuous venovenous and arteriovenous hemodiafiltration have been used in a small number of patients experiencing lithium toxicity (78,79). Interestingly, significant rebound of lithium levels did not occur, in contrast to the use of hemodialysis (78,79). The combination of acute hemodialysis followed by continuous venovenous hemodiafiltration has also been reported, without significant rebound of lithium levels (79). Hemoperfusion is not expected to be effective for lithium intoxication because of its poor binding by activated charcoal.

Sodium polystyrene sulfonate (SPS; Kayexalate) is a cation exchange resin used for treatment of acute hyperkalemia. Its ability to bind potassium and sodium and permit increased fecal excretion of potassium implies that it may do the same for lithium due to their chemical similarities. Animal studies have shown that SPS administration enhances lithium elimination, one study demonstrating SPS efficacy even in the setting of intravenous administration of lithium (73,80,81). A murine study used extremely large doses of SPS (10 g/kg), approximately 10 to 15 times the usual human hyperkalemia dose. Concerns have been raised about the potential adverse effects of these large doses on potassium and sodium levels (80). In small volunteer human studies using a small ingested dose of lithium, SPS did result in decreased lithium absorption (as measured by the area under the curve) of 11.6 mEq/L/hour versus 13.6 ± 1.5 mEq/L-hour without a major effect on sodium or potassium levels (82). Further studies are needed to elucidate the usefulness of SPS in lithium overdose.

Antidotes

No specific antidote exists for lithium intoxication.

Supportive Care

Correction of dehydration is important and vigilant monitoring of electrolytes is vital to avoid complications (83). After stabilization of the airway, seizures should be treated with benzodiazepines followed by more aggressive interventions if needed (Chapter 40). Hypotension is managed with normal saline, 10 to 20 ml/kg intravenously, and fluids followed by vasopressor support, if necessary (Chapter 37).

Admission Criteria

Symptomatic patients should be admitted to the hospital and given appropriate therapy. Patients who have overdosed on sustained released preparations should be observed for 24 hours with serial lithium levels performed. Patients with levels remaining below 2.0 mEq/L may be discharged home if they are asymptomatic and if factors contributing to the toxicity have been identified and corrected. Psychiatric consultation is imperative in the suicidal patient and in therapeutic decision making before discharge.

REFERENCES

1. Heng M. Lithium carbonate toxicity. *Arch Dermatol* 1982;118:246–248.
2. Aita JF, Aita JA, Aita VA. 7-Up anti-acid lithiated lemon soda or early medicinal use of lithium. *Nebr Med J* 1990;75:277–279.
3. Hanlon LW, Romaine M, Gilroy FJ, et al. Lithium chloride as a substitute for sodium chloride in the diet. *JAMA* 1949;139:688–692.
4. Kudrow L. Lithium prophylaxis for cluster headache. *Headache* 1977;17:15–18.
5. Schou M. Lithium prophylaxis in perspective. *Pharmacopsychiatry* 1992;25:7–9.
6. Friedman PB, Bekes CE, Scott WE, et al. ARDS following acute lithium carbonate intoxication. *Intens Care Med* 1992;18:123–124.
7. Bailey B, McGuigan M. Comparison of patients hemodialyzed for lithium poisoning and those for whom dialysis was recommended by PCC but not done: what lesson can we learn? *Clin Nephrol* 2000;54(5):388–392.
8. Groleau G, Barch R, Tso E, et al. Lithium intoxication: manifestations and management. *Am J Emerg Med* 1987;5:527–532.
9. Kachel F, Boning JAL. Recurrent asystole due to arrhythmic changes during treatment with lithium. *Pharmacopsychiatry* 1991;24:104.

10. Marcus S. Lithium. *Clin Toxicol Rev* 1980;2(5):1–2.
11. Amdisen A. Clinical features and management of lithium poisoning. *Med Toxicol* 1988;3:18–32.
12. Jacobsen D, Aasen G, Frederichsen P, et al. Lithium intoxication: pharmacokinetics during and after terminated hemodialysis in acute intoxications. *J Toxicol Clin Toxicol* 1987;25:81–94.
13. Anton RF, Paladino JA, Morton A, et al. Effect of acute alcohol consumption on lithium kinetics. *Clin Pharmacol Ther* 1985;38:52–55.
14. Chapron DJ. Comment on pharmacokinetics of lithium in the elderly. *J Clin Psychopharmacol* 1988;8:78.
15. Friedberg RC, Spyker DA, Herold DA. Massive overdoses with sustained release lithium carbonate preparations: pharmacokinetic model based on two case studies. *Clin Chem* 1991;37:1205–1209.
16. Hunter R. Steady state pharmacokinetics of lithium carbonate in healthy subjects. *Br J Clin Pharmacol* 1988;25:375–380.
17. Jaeger A, Sander P, Kopferschmitt J, et al. Toxicokinetics of lithium intoxication treated by hemodialysis. *J Toxicol Clin Toxicol* 1985;23:501–517.
18. Jaeger A, Sauder P, Kopferschmitt J, et al. When should dialysis be performed in lithium poisoning: a kinetic study in 14 cases of lithium poisoning. *J Toxicol Clin Toxicol* 1993;31:429–447.
19. Jermain DM, Crismon ML, Martin ES III. Population pharmacokinetics of lithium. *Clin Pharm* 1991;10:376–381.
20. Dupuis RE, Cooper AA, et al. Multiple delayed peak lithium concentrations following acute intoxication with an extended-release product. *Ann Pharmacother* 1996;30:356–360.
21. Manji HK, Hsaio JK, Risby ED, et al. The mechanism of action of lithium: effects on serotonergic and noradrenergic systems in normal subjects. *Arch Gen Psychiatry* 1991;48:505–512.
22. Odagaki Y, Koyama R, Matsubara S, et al. Effects of chronic lithium treatment on serotonin binding sites in the rat brain. *J Psychiatr Res* 1990;24:271–277.
23. Manji HK, Potter WZ, Lenox RH. Signal transduction pathways. Molecular targets for lithium's action. *Arch Gen Psychiatry* 1995;52:531–543.
24. Waldmeier PC. Mechanisms of action of lithium in affective disorders: a status report. *Pharmacol Toxicol* 1990;66[Suppl 3]:121–132.
25. Okusa MD, Crystal LT. Clinical manifestations and management of acute lithium intoxication. *Am J Med* 1994;97:383–389.
26. Sachs GS, Renshaw PF, Lafer B, et al. Variability of brain lithium levels during maintenance treatment: a magnetic resonance spectroscopy study. *Biol Psychiatry* 1995;38:422–428.
27. White K, Cohen J, Nelson R, et al. Relationship between plasma, RBC and CSF lithium concentrations in human subjects. *Int Pharmacopsychiatry* 1979;14:185–189.
28. Bendz H. Kidney function in lithium-treated patients. *Acta Psychiatr Scand* 1983;68:303–324.
29. Baylis PH, Heath DA. Water disturbances in patients treated with oral lithium carbonate. *Ann Intern Med* 1978;88:607–609.
30. Vestergaard P, Amdisen A, Hansen HE, et al. Lithium treatment and kidney function: a survey of 237 patients in long-term treatment. *Acta Psychiatr Scand* 1979;60:504–520.
31. Walker RG. Lithium nephrotoxicity. *Kidney Int* 1993;44[Suppl 42]:S93–S98.
32. Simard M, Gumbiner B, Lee A, et al. Lithium carbonate intoxication: a case report and a review of the literature. *Arch Intern Med* 1989;139:36–46.
33. Ong ACM, Handler CE. Sinus arrest and asystole due to severe lithium intoxication. *Int J Cardiol* 1991;30:364–366.
34. Wellens HJ, Cats VM, Durnen DR. Symptomatic sinus node abnormalities following lithium carbonate therapy. *Am J Med* 1975;132:529–531.
35. Santiago R, Rashkin MC. Lithium toxicity and myxedema coma in an elderly woman. *J Emerg Med* 1990;8:63–69.
36. Perrild H, Hegedus L, Basstrup P, et al. Thyroid function and ultrasonically determined thyroid size in patients receiving long-term lithium treatment. *Am J Psychiatry* 1990;147:1518–1521.
37. Chow CC, Cockram CS. Thyroid disorders induced by lithium and amiodarone: an overview. *Adv Drug React Poisoning Rev* 1990;9:207–222.
38. Oakley PW, Dawson AH, Whyte IM. Lithium: thyroid effects and altered renal handling. *J Toxicol Clin Toxicol* 2000;38(3):333–337.
39. Stancer HC, Forbath N. Hyperparathyroidism, hypothyroidism and impaired renal function after 10-20 years of lithium treatment. *Arch Intern Med* 1989;149:1042–1045.
40. Richman CM, Makki MM, Weiser PA, et al. Effect of lithium carbonate on chemotherapy induced neutropenia and thrombocytopenia. *Am J Hematol* 1984;16:313–323.
41. Weinstein MR, Goldfield MD. Cardiovascular malformations with lithium use during pregnancy. *Am J Psychiatry* 1975;132:529–531.
42. Cohen LS, Friedman JM, Jefferson JW, et al. A reevaluation of risk of in utero exposure to lithium. *JAMA* 1994;271:146–150.
43. Cunnif CM, Salm DJ, Johnson KA, et al. Pregnancy outcome in women treated with lithium. *Clin Res* 1988;36:217A.
44. Jacobson SJ, Jones K, Johnson K, et al. Prospective multicentre study of pregnancy outcome after lithium exposure during first trimester. *Lancet* 1992;339:530–533.
45. Connoley G, Menahem S. A possible association between neonatal jaundice and long-term maternal lithium ingestion. *Med J Aust* 1990;157:272–273.
46. Schou M. Lithium treatment during pregnancy, delivery, and lactation: an update. *J Clin Psychiatry* 1990;51:410–413.
47. Sykes PA, Quarrie J, Alexander FW. Lithium carbonate and breast-feeding. *Br Med J* 1976;1:878.
48. Tunnessen WW Jr, Hertz CG. Toxic effects of lithium in newborn infants: a commentary. *J Pediatr* 1972;81:804–807.
49. Iqbal M, Sohhan T, Mahmud S. The effects of lithium, valproic acid, and carbamazepine during pregnancy and lactation. *J Toxicol Clin Toxicol* 2001;39(4):381–392.
50. Schou M, Amdisen A. Lithium and pregnancy. Lithium ingestion by children breast-fed by women on lithium treatment. *BMJ* 1973;2(859):138.
51. American Academy of Pediatrics, Committee on Drugs. The transfer of drugs and other chemicals into human milk. *Pediatrics* 1994;93:137–150.
52. Linden S, Rich CL. The use of lithium during pregnancy and lactation. *J Clin Psychiatry* 1983;44:358–361.
53. Bosse GM, Arnold TC. Overdose with sustained release lithium preparations. *J Emerg Med* 1992;10:719–721.
54. Horowitz LC, Ficher GU. Acute lithium toxicity. *N Engl J Med* 1969;281: 1369–1372.
55. DePaulo J. Lithium. *Psychiatr Clin North Am* 1984;7:587–599.
56. Bendz H, Aurell M, Lanke J. A historical cohort study of kidney damage in long-term lithium patients: continued surveillance needed. *Eur Psychiatry* 2001;16(4):199–206.
57. Myers J, Morgan T, Carney S, et al. Effects of lithium on the kidney. *Kidney Int* 1980;18:601–608.
58. Bell AJ, Cole A, Eccleston D, et al. Lithium neurotoxicity at normal therapeutic levels. *Br J Psychiatry* 1993;162:689–692.
59. Agulnick PL, DiMascio A, Moore P. Acute brain syndrome associated with lithium therapy. *Am J Psychiatry* 1972;129:621–623.
60. Hansen HE, Amdisen A. Lithium intoxication: report of 23 cases and review of 100 cases from the literature. *QJM* 1978;186:123–144.
61. Marshall SM, Kesson CM. Severe lithium poisoning. *Drug Intell Clin Pharmacol* 1981;15:598–599.
62. Sansone ME, Ziegler DK. Lithium toxicity: a review of neurologic complications. *Clin Neuropharmacol* 1985;8:242–248.
63. Mekler G, Woggon B. A case of serotonin syndrome caused by venlafaxine and lithium. *Pharmacopsychiatry* 1997;30(6):272–273.
64. Faglioni A, Buysse DJ, et al. Tolerability of combined treatment with lithium and paroxetine in patients with bipolar disorder and depression. *J Clin Psychopharmacol* 2001;21(5):474–478.
65. Strayhorn JM, Nash J. Severe neurotoxicity despite "therapeutic" serum lithium levels. *Dis Nerv Syst* 1977;38:107–111.
66. Lee DC, Klachko MN. Falsely elevated lithium levels in plasma samples obtained in lithium containing tubes. *J Toxicol Clin Toxicol* 1996;34(4):467–469.
67. Tillman DJ, Ruggles DL, Leikin JB. Radiopacity study of extended-release formulations using digitalized radiography. *Am J Emerg Med* 1994;12(3):310–314.
68. Yonemitsu K, Pounder DJ. Postmortem changes in blood tranylcypromine concentration: competing redistribution and degradation effects. *Forensic Sci Int* 1993;59:177–184.
69. Green TR, Swanson JR. Detection of false lithium readings in whole-blood specimens from cadavers by flame photometry. *Clin Chem* 1996;42:1302.
70. Johnson JH, Crookshank HR, Smalley HE. Lithium toxicity in cattle. *Vet Hum Toxicol* 1980;22:249–251.
71. Favin FD, Oderda GM, Klein-Schwartz W, et al. In vitro study of lithium carbonate adsorption by activated charcoal. *J Toxicol Clin Toxicol* 1988;26:443–450.
72. Jones J, Mullen MJ, Dougherty J, et al. Repetitive doses of activated charcoal in the treatment of poisoning. *Am J Emerg Med* 1987;5:305–311.
73. Linakis JG, Lacouture PG, Eisenberg MS, et al. Administration of activated charcoal or sodium polystyrene sulfonate as gastric decontamination for lithium intoxication: an animal model. *Pharmacol Toxicol* 1989;65:387–389.
74. Spyker DA. Activated charcoal reborn. Progress in poison management. *Arch Intern Med* 1985;145:43–44.
75. Kulig K, Bar-Or D, Cantrill SV, et al. Management of acutely poisoned patients without gastric emptying. *Ann Emerg Med* 1985;14(6):562–567.
76. Smith SW, Ling LL, Haisstenson CE. Whole-bowel irrigation as a treatment for acute lithium overdose. *Ann Emerg Med* 1991;20:536–539.
77. Schou M. Long-lasting neurological sequelae after lithium intoxication. *Acta Psychiatr Scan* 1984;70:594–602.
78. Bellomo R, Kearly Y, Parkin G, et al. Treatment of life-threatening lithium toxicity with continuous arterio-venous hemodiafiltration. *Crit Care Med* 1991;19:836–837.
79. Leblanc M, Raymond M, Bonnardeaux A, et al. Lithium poisoning treated by high-performance continuous arteriovenous and venovenous hemodiafiltration. *Am J Kidney Dis* 1996;27:365–372.
80. Linakis JG, Hull KM, Lacoutre PG, et al. Sodium polystyrene sulfonate treatment for lithium toxicity. Effects on serum potassium concentration. *Acad Emerg Med* 1996;3:333–337.
81. Linakis JG, Hull KM, Lee C, et al. Effects of delayed treatment with sodium polystyrene on serum lithium concentrations in mice. *Acad Emerg Med* 1995;2:681–685.
82. Tomaszewski C, Musso C, Pearson JR, et al. Lithium absorption prevented by SPS in volunteers. *Ann Emerg Med* 1992;21:1308–1311.
83. Schonwald S. Lithium. *Clin Toxicol Rev* 1990;12(7):1–2.

CHAPTER 132
Benzodiazepines

Ian MacGregor Whyte

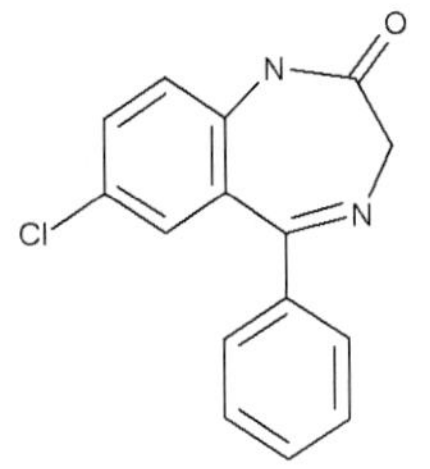

DIAZEPAM

Compounds included:	**See Table 1.**
Molecular formula and weight:	**See Table 1.**
SI conversion:	**See Table 1.**
CAS Registry No.:	**See Table 1.**
Therapeutic levels:	**See Table 1.**
Target organs:	**Central nervous system (acute)**
Antidote:	**Flumazenil**

OVERVIEW

Benzodiazepines are among the most common groups of drugs used in deliberate self-poisoning in Australia (1), Canada (2), England (3), France (4), Greece (5), United States (6), and Switzerland (7). In Sweden, benzodiazepines were used in 51% of deliberate self-poisonings, and diazepam was reported more than expected from prescription data (8). Drug screening found benzodiazepines present in 55% of fatal poisonings, and diazepam was more commonly detected in completed suicides than expected from prescription data (8). In Pakistan, where benzodiazepines are available over the counter, 84% of medication self-poisoning cases were benzodiazepine overdoses (9). They are also the commonest group in deliberate self-poisoning in China (10).

In large doses, benzodiazepines can cause coma, respiratory depression (11), and death (12). An Australian study of poisoning fatalities during 1997 found benzodiazepines present in toxic levels in 9% of cases (13). Severe toxicity is often related to coingestants, especially alcohol and opiates; advanced age is an additional risk factor for severe toxicity (11–14).

Acute overdose toxicity and risk of death has been observed more often with the short-acting benzodiazepines midazolam and triazolam and the intermediate-acting alprazolam, flunitrazepam, and temazepam than with the longer-acting diazepam, lorazepam, and nitrazepam (14–18). Death caused by benzodiazepines alone is uncommon, although it does occasionally occur (19). Death has been reported after overdose with alprazolam, bromazepam, chlordiazepoxide, diazepam, flunitrazepam, flurazepam, midazolam, nitrazepam, oxazepam, temazepam, or triazolam.

Structure, Classification, and Uses

All benzodiazepines in regular use are 1,4-benzodiazepines except for clobazam (Fig. 1), although the significance of the distinction is unclear. A practical classification of benzodiazepines uses the elimination half-life ($t_{1/2}$) of parent and active metabolites: (a) *long-acting* substances ($t_{1/2}$ up to 100 hours), including bromazepam, chlordiazepoxide, clobazam, clonazepam, clorazepate, N-desmethyldiazepam, diazepam, flurazepam, halazepam, ketazolam, nitrazepam, prazepam and quazepam (most with active metabolites); (b) *intermediate* action ($t_{1/2}$ up to 30 hours), including alprazolam, estazolam, flunitrazepam, lorazepam, oxazepam, temazepam (few active metabolites); and (c) *short-acting* substances ($t_{1/2}$ up to 8 hours), including midazolam, triazolam (few active metabolites) (20).

Indications for benzodiazepines include anxiety; panic disorder; insomnia; parasomnias (night terrors, sleepwalking); epilepsy; convulsions; acute behavioral disturbance; acute alcohol, barbiturate, and benzodiazepine withdrawal; and muscle spasm, including tetanus, premedication (anxiolytic, sedative, and amnestic effects), sedation for procedures, and in intensive care units (21).

Toxic Dose

Adult and pediatric therapeutic doses are provided in Table 2. In any discussion of toxic doses of benzodiazepines, there is always considerable variation due to interindividual differences in tolerance. Little or no information is available on toxic doses of bromazepam, clorazepate, N-desmethyldiazepam, or ketazolam.

Alprazolam produced dangerously aggressive behavior in a 34-year-old patient after ingestion of 10 mg (22). Other reactions that have been observed include mania, amnesia, agitation, depersonalization, and perceptual distortion (23). Two patients who attempted suicide with alprazolam ingested 20 to 30 mg and 60 mg, respectively (24). Neither patient demonstrated any alteration in vital signs or central nervous system (CNS) depression, and both recovered (24). In a British study the fatal toxicity index (deaths per million prescriptions) for alprazolam was 5.9 compared to 4.0 for diazepam (16). When adjusted for dose, alprazolam deliberate self-poisoning has a longer length of stay, increased need for intensive care unit admission, and ventilation and a lower Glasgow coma score (GCS) than other benzodiazepines (18).

Chlordiazepoxide was injected intraarterially and caused severe arterial spasm (25). A 45-year-old woman who ingested 5.2 g presented 4.5 days later in coma with respiratory depression thought to be due to metabolites of chlordiazepoxide. She was treated with assisted ventilation and survived (26).

Clobazam produced confusion, ataxia, and drowsiness in a 22-year-old woman who ingested 300 mg (27). *Clonazepam* produced cyclical coma in a 4-year-old boy after a dose of 14 to 32 mg (28). Doses of up to 60 mg have been well tolerated (drowsiness and ataxia only) in deliberate self-poisonings (29).

Diazepam can be tolerated in extreme doses with little adverse effect in patients with severe alcohol withdrawal [2335 mg of diazepam intravenously (IV) combined with oxazepam, 21,225

TABLE 1. Structural classification of benzodiazepines (see also Fig. 1)

Compounds included	Molecular formula, molecular weight (g/mol), CAS Registry No.	SI conversion; therapeutic, toxic concentration[a]	*United States Pharmacopeia Dictionary of Drug Names*
Alprazolam (Xanax)	$C_{17}H_{13}ClN_4$, 308.8, 28981-97-7	mg/L × 3.24 = µmol/L; 0.1 mg/L, 0.2 mg/L	8-Chloro-1-methyl-6-phenyl-4H-s-triazolo(4,3-a)(1,4)benzodiazepine
Bromazepam (Lectopam, Lexotan)	$C_{14}H_{10}BrN_3O$, 316.2, 1812-30-2	mg/L × 3.16 = µmol/L; 0.2 mg/L, 1 mg/L	7-Bromo-1,3-dihydro-5-(2-pyridinyl)-2H-1,4-benzodiazepin-2-one
Chlordiazepoxide (Librium)	$C_{16}H_{14}ClN_3O$, 299.8, 58-25-3	mg/L × 3.33 = µmol/L; 2 mg/L, 10 mg/L	7-Chloro-2-(methylamino)-5-phenyl-3H-1,4-benzodiazepine 4-oxide
Clobazam (Frisium)	$C_{16}H_{13}ClN_2O_2$, 300.7, 22316-47-8	mg/L × 3.33 = µmol/L; 1 mg/L, 5 mg/L	7-Chloro-1-methyl-5-phenyl-1H-1,5-benzodiazepine-2,4-(3H,5H)-dione
Clonazepam (Klonopin, Rivotril)	$C_{15}H_{10}ClN_3O_3$, 315.7, 1622-61-3	mg/L × 3.17 = µmol/L; 0.08 mg/L, 1 mg/L	5-(o-Chlorophenyl)-1,3-dihydro-7-nitro-2H-1,4-benzodiazepin-2-one
Clorazepate (Tranxene)	$C_{16}H_{11}ClK_2N_2O_4$, 314.7, 57109-90-7	mg/L × 3.18 = µmol/L; 0.02 mg/L, NA	7-Chloro-2,3-dihydro-2,2-dihydroxy-5-phenyl-1H-1,4-benzodiazepine-3-carboxylic acid
N-desmethyldiazepam (nordiazepam)	$C_{15}H_{11}ClN_2O$, 270.7, 1088-11-5	mg/L × 3.69 = µmol/L; 2 mg/L, 5 mg/L	7-Chloro-1,3-dihydro-5-phenyl-2H-1,4-benzodiazepin-2-one
Diazepam (Diastat, Valium)	$C_{16}H_{13}ClN_2O$, 284.7, 439-14-5	mg/L × 3.51 = µmol/L; 2 mg/L, 5 mg/L	7-Chloro-1,3-dihydro-1-methyl-5-phenyl-2H-1,4-benzodiazepin-2-one
Estazolam (Prosom)	$C_{16}H_{11}ClN_4$, 294.7, 29975-16-4	mg/L × 3.39 = µmol/L; 0.2 mg/L, NA	8-Chloro-6-phenyl-4H-s-triazolo(4,3-a)(1,4)benzodiazepine
Flunitrazepam (Rohypnol)	$C_{16}H_{12}FN_3O_3$, 313.3, 1622-62-4	mg/L × 3.19 = µmol/L; 0.02 mg/L, 0.2 mg/L	5-(o-Fluorophenyl)-1,3-dihydro-1-methyl-7-nitro-2H-1,4-benzodiazepin-2-one
Flurazepam (Dalmane)	$C_{21}H_{23}ClFN_3O{,}HCl$, 424.3, 36105-20-1	mg/L × 2.58 = µmol/L; 0.02 mg/L, 0.5 mg/L	7-Chloro-1-(2-(diethylamino)ethyl)-5-(2-fluorophenyl)-1,3-dihydro-2H-1,4-benzodiazepin-2-one
Halazepam (Paxipam)	$C_{17}H_{12}ClF_3N_2O$, 352.7, 23092-17-3	mg/L × 2.84 = µmol/L; 0.2 mg/L, NA	7-Chloro-1,3-dihydro-5-phenyl-1-(2,2,2-trifluoroethyl)-2H-1,4-benzodiazepin-2-one
Ketazolam (Anxon)	$C_{20}H_{17}ClN_2O_3$, 368.8, 27223-35-4	mg/L × 2.71 = µmol/L; 0.02 mg/L, NA	11-Chloro-8,12b-dihydro-2,8-dimethyl-12b-phenyl-4H-(1,3)-oxazino(3,2-d)(1,4)benzodiazepine-4,7(6H)dione
Lorazepam (Ativan)	$C_{15}H_{10}Cl_2N_2O_2$, 321.2, 846-49-1	mg/L × 3.11 = µmol/L; 0.3 mg/L, 1 mg/L	7-Chloro-5-(o-chlorophenyl)-1,3-dihydro-3-hydroxy-2H-1,4-benzodiazepin-2-one
Midazolam (Hypnovel, Versed)	$C_{18}H_{13}ClFN_3$, 325.8, 59467-70-8	mg/L × 3.07 = µmol/L; 0.25 mg/L, 1 mg/L	8-Chloro-6-(2-fluorophenyl)-1-methyl-4H-Imidazo(1,5-a)(1,4)benzodiazepine
Nitrazepam (Sonotrat)	$C_{15}H_{11}N_3O_3$, 281.3, 146-22-5	mg/L × 3.55 = µmol/L; 0.2 mg/L, 1 mg/L	1,3-Dihydro-7-nitro-5-phenyl-2H-1,4-benzodiazepin-2-one
Oxazepam (Alepam, Serax)	$C_{15}H_{11}ClN_2O_2$, 286.7, 604-75-1	mg/L × 3.49 = µmol/L; 1 mg/L, 5 mg/L	7-Chloro-1,3-dihydro-3-hydroxy-5-phenyl-2H-1,4-benzodiazepin-2-one
Prazepam (Centrax)	$C_{19}H_{17}ClN_2O$, 324.8, 2955-38-6	mg/L × 3.08 = µmol/L; 0.01 mg/L, NA	7-Chloro-1-(cyclopropylmethyl)-1,3-dihydro-5-phenyl-2H-1,4-benzodiazepin-2-one
Quazepam (Doral)	$C_{17}H_{11}ClF_4N_2S$, 386.8, 36735-22-5	mg/L × 2.59 = µmol/L; 0.2 mg/L, NA	7-Chloro-5-(o-fluorophenyl)-1,3-dihydro-1-(2,2,2-trifluoroethyl)-2H-1,4-benzodiazepine-2-thione
Temazepam (Euhypnos, Restoril)	$C_{16}H_{13}ClN_2O_2$, 300.7, 846-50-4	mg/L × 3.33 = µmol/L; 1 mg/L, 5 mg/L	7-Chloro-1,3-dihydro-3-hydroxy-1-methyl-5-phenyl-2H-1,4-benzodiazepin-2-one
Triazolam (Halcion)	$C_{17}H_{12}Cl_2N_4$, 343.2, 28911-01-5	mg/L × 2.91 = µmol/L; 0.02 mg/L, 0.04 mg/L	8-Chloro-6-(o-chlorophenyl)-1-methyl-4H-s-triazolo(4,3-a)(1,4)benzodiazepine

MW, molecular weight; NA, not available.
[a]From Flanagan RJ. Guidelines for the interpretation of analytical toxicology results and unit of measurement conversion factors. *Ann Clin Biochem* 1998;35(Pt 2):261–267, with permission.

mg, orally over several days]. This appears to be a receptor-site phenomenon rather than an abnormal drug disposition (30). A 54-year-old man ingested 2000 mg of bulk laboratory diazepam and was treated with activated charcoal, enhanced diuresis, and flumazenil. The patient had drowsiness, dysarthria, diplopia, and dizziness for 9 days (31). In four cases of overdose with diazepam alone, patients were minimally sedated and were discharged within 24 hours, despite diazepam doses as high as 750 mg.

However, concurrent ingestion of diazepam together with other CNS depressants like ethanol, barbiturates, analgesics, or tricyclic antidepressants produced serious intoxication regardless of the diazepam dosage (32). Two patients were hospitalized in moderately deep coma after ingestion of large doses of diazepam (500 and 2000 mg) with suicidal intent. Neither patient experienced important complications; both recovered fully and were discharged within 48 hours. Rapid clinical recovery after diazepam overdose is not attributable to rapid elimination of active compounds from the body but more likely to adaptation or tolerance to their depressant effects (33).

Estazolam (4 to 10 mg) produced coma and respiratory depression in two of ten patients in one report. One patient required assisted ventilation. All were discharged from the hospital within 4 days (34).

Flunitrazepam was reported to have caused 641 fatalities in Sweden during the period of 1992 to 1998, in which the cause of death was attributed to flunitrazepam alone (130) or in combination with other drugs or conditions (511) (35). Relating deaths due to flunitrazepam to prescription rates in Victoria, Australia, suggests that flunitrazepam may be inherently more toxic if misused than other benzodiazepines (12). A 60-year-old man was found in a deep coma after ingesting 50 mg (36). It is alleged that three 4-mg tablets of flunitrazepam mixed with food, milk, or juice can produce coma. Death has followed ingestion of seven

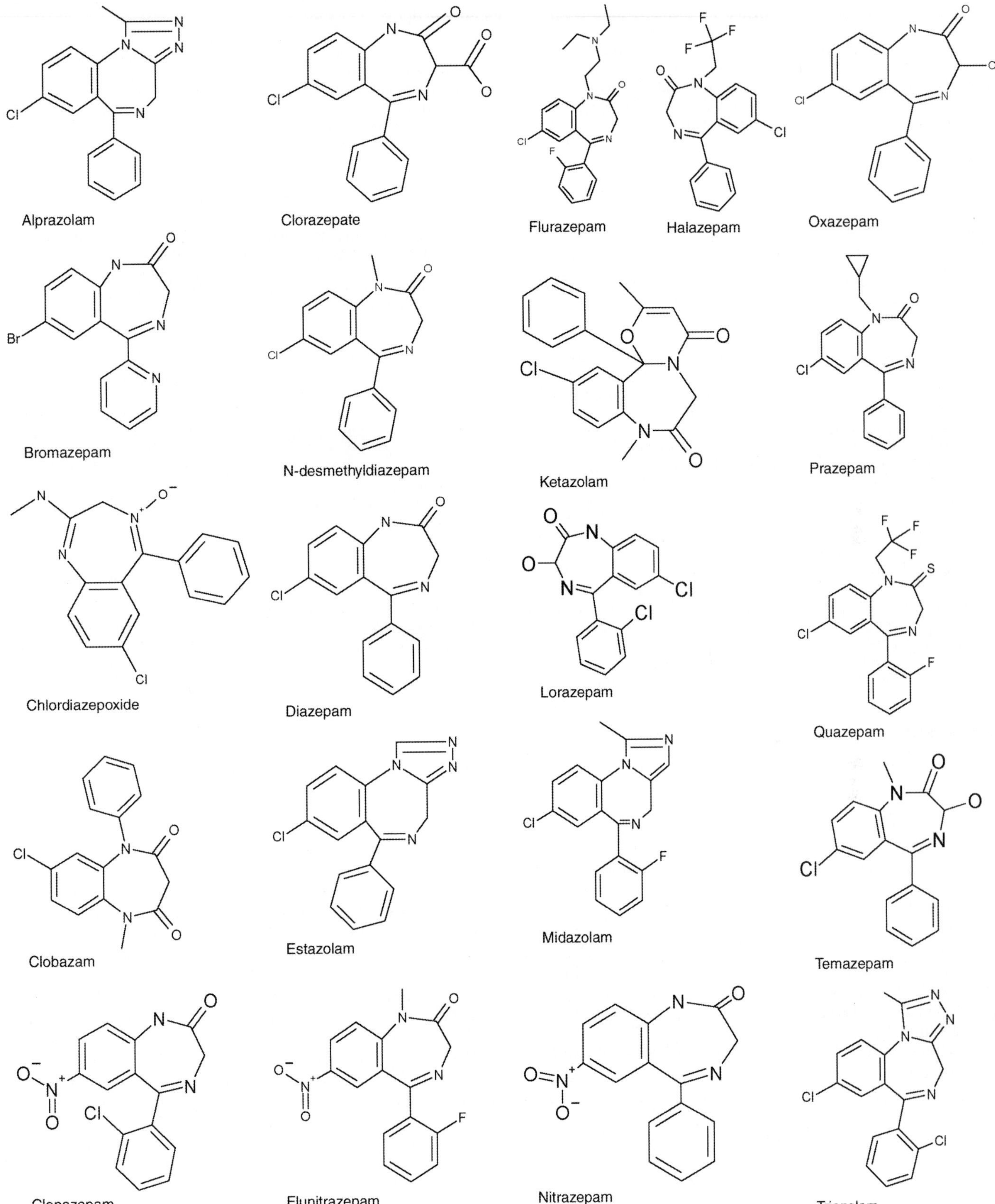

Figure 1. Structures of benzodiazepines.

TABLE 2. Primary indication and therapeutic doses of benzodiazepines

Drug	Indication	Formulation	Adult dose	Pediatric dose
Alprazolam	Anxiety	0.5-, 1.0-mg/ml solutions; 0.25-, 0.5-, 1.0-, 2.0-mg tablets	0.25–0.5 mg three times daily to a total daily dose of 3 or 4 mg	NR
Bromazepam	Anxiety	1.5-, 3.0-, 6.0-mg tablets	3–6 mg two to three times daily to a maximum of 60 mg daily	NR
Chlordiazepoxide	Anxiety	5, 10, 25 capsules and tablets; 100 mg powder for injection	Up to 30 mg daily in divided doses; in severe conditions, up to 100 mg daily	NR
Clobazam	Epilepsy	10-mg tablet	10–30 mg daily as single or divided doses to a maximum of 60–80 mg daily	NR
Clonazepam	Epilepsy	0.5, 1.0, 2.0 mg	0.5–1.0 mg at night to a maximum of 2–8 mg daily in divided doses	0.01–0.03 mg/kg in divided doses. Maximum of 0.1–0.2 mg/kg daily.
Clorazepate	Anxiety	3.75-, 7.5-, 15.0-, 22.5-mg capsules and tablets	60 mg daily, in divided doses or as a single dose at night	60 mg daily (ages 9–12 y)
N-desmethyldiazepam	Anxiety	—	Up to 15 mg daily	NR
Diazepam	Anxiety	5-mg/ml emulsion; 2.5-, 5-, 10-, 15-, 20-mg gel; 5 mg/ml; 5-, 10-mg suppository; 2-, 5-, 10-mg tablets	1–10 mg up to three times a day	0.05–0.3 mg/kg two to three times daily
Estazolam	Insomnia	1-, 2-mg tablets	1–2 mg at night	NR
Flunitrazepam	Severe insomnia	—	0.5–1.0 mg at night up to 2 mg	NR
Flurazepam	Insomnia	15-, 30-mg capsule	15–30 mg at night	NR
Halazepam	Anxiety	20-, 40-mg tablet	20–40 mg three or four times a day	NR
Ketazolam	Anxiety	—	15–60 mg daily	NR
Lorazepam	Anxiety	2-mg/ml liquid and solution; 0.5-, 1.0-, 2.0-mg SL tablet; 1-, 2-mg tablets	2–3 mg daily in divided doses up to 10 mg daily	2 mg IV has been suggested for status epilepticus in children
Midazolam	Procedural sedation	1, 2, 5 mg/ml solutions	2.5–7.5 mg (approximately 70 μg/kg) IV	0.25–0.5 mg/kg orally up to 20 mg
Nitrazepam	Insomnia	NR	5–10 mg at night	0.125 mg/kg twice daily to 0.25–0.5 mg/kg twice daily
Oxazepam	Anxiety	10-, 15-, 30-mg capsules; 15-, 30-mg tablets	7.5–15.0 mg three to four times daily up to 120 mg daily	NR
Prazepam	Anxiety	NR	30 mg daily up to 60 mg daily	NR
Quazepam	Insomnia	7.5-, 15.0-mg tablets	15 mg at night	NR
Temazepam	Insomnia	7.5-, 15.0-, 30-mg capsules	5–20 mg at night	NR
Triazolam	Insomnia	0.125-, 0.25-, 0.5-mg tablets	0.125–0.5 mg at night	NR

NR, not reported.
From Benzodiazepines. In: Rossi S, Vitry A, Hurley E, et al., eds. *Australian medicines handbook*. Adelaide: Australian Medicines Handbook Pty Ltd, 2002.; Sweetman S. *Martindale: the complete drug reference*. London: Pharmaceutical Press. Electronic ed. expires March 2003 Greenwood Village, CO: MICROMEDEX, 2003, with permission.

4-mg tablets (37). A 24-year-old woman ingested 100 mg of flunitrazepam, presented 30 minutes after ingestion with a GCS of 8, and recovered (38). The toxic dose of flunitrazepam in children is 0.29 mg/kg (39).

Flurazepam was more toxic than average (fatal toxicity index 15.0) among hypnotic benzodiazepines during the 1980s (16). An estimated overdose with more than 2400 mg resulted in death (40). A fatality was attributed to ingestion of up to 2.2 g (41). *Halazepam* produced no significant ill effects despite dosing with 1120 mg orally over 24 hours (42).

Lorazepam led to CNS depression in a study of 65 children that ingested a mean dose of 1 mg/kg (43). A 70-year-old patient ingested 100 mg of lorazepam, exhibited an alpha coma rhythm on the electroencephalogram, and recovered in 2 days (44). A 6-year-old boy ingested 30 mg of lorazepam and hallucinated 4 hours later with full recovery (45).

Midazolam in therapeutic use can produce paradoxical excitement (46,47), which may be more common in children (48) [particularly if they are autistic (49)], the elderly (50), or patients with a history of violence (51) or alcohol dependence. Inadvertent intraarterial injection of midazolam 5 mg was well tolerated in one case (52). Intramuscular injection of four times the normal dose caused no harm in two cases (53). Extreme doses of midazolam (2850 mg as a constant infusion over 5 days) can be tolerated without adverse effect in severe alcohol withdrawal (54). Death from respiratory arrest after 10 mg IV for a procedure has occurred (55).

Nitrazepam was associated with unexplained deaths in six children with a mean age of 27.8 months who received an initial dose of 0.3 to 0.6 mg/kg/day (56). Six cases of fatal overdose have been reported, one of which involved the ingestion of 250 mg of nitrazepam (57).

Oxazepam (21,225 mg orally) in combination with diazepam (2335 mg IV) can be tolerated with little adverse effect in severe alcohol withdrawal (30). Oxazepam is less sedative in overdose (14) and has a lower fatal toxicity index (2.3) than other benzodiazepines (16). Coma and skin blisters not related to pressure resulted from ingestion of 200 mg of oxazepam by a 75-year-old man (58).

Prazepam is toxic to children at doses of 7.8 to 9.0 mg/kg (59). *Quazepam* induced frequent side effects related to sleepiness at a therapeutic dose of 30 mg (60).

Temazepam is more sedative in overdose (14), has a higher fatal toxicity index (11.9) (16), and is more likely to be associated with death when taken in combination with alcohol than other benzodiazepines (17). It comprised 65.4% of all benzodiazepines overdose deaths in a Scottish study (61). Inadvertent intraarterial injection of the contents of temazepam capsules may lead to arterial spasm and digit loss (62). *Triazolam* produces toxicity in children at a dose of 0.06 to 0.07 mg/kg (63).

TOXICOKINETICS AND TOXICODYNAMICS

The pharmacokinetics of the benzodiazepine agents is provided in Table 3. Little or no information is available on the toxicokinetics and toxicodynamics of estazolam or ketazolam.

It is the development of tolerance to the benzodiazepines that determines the recovery of consciousness after overdose (rather than the clearance of the drug) (33,64). Because of tolerance and the multiple active metabolites of benzodiazepines, a poor correlation exists between concentration and effect. In subjects taking one or more benzodiazepines daily without showing excessive or adverse effects, the concentrations were below 0.5 mg/L in diazepam equivalents (65).

Alprazolam steady-state serum concentrations ranged from 0.025 to 0.055 mg/L in patients taking 1.5 to 6.0 mg/day, orally (66). After alprazolam overdose, mild symptoms were associated with a plasma concentration of 0.35 mg/L (24).

Bromazepam produced profound coma with absent brainstem reflexes and no spontaneous respiration at a serum concentration 6 mg/L (67). A 42-year-old woman was found unconscious with hypothermia (28.4°C); the blood concentration of bromazepam was 7.7 mg/L (68).

Chlordiazepoxide (5.2 g) toxicity correlated with the blood concentration of the second metabolite of chlordiazepoxide, demoxepam, but not to chlordiazepoxide itself (26). When the concentration of demoxepam fell below 10 mg/L, the patient was able to be extubated (26).

The *clobazam* mean plasma concentration after a 20-mg dose was 0.465 mg/L at 1.7 hours post dose. The mean plasma concentration of *N*-desmethylclobazam was 0.088 mg/L at 45 hours post-dose (69).

Clonazepam concentrations on chronic therapy with 6 mg/day ranged from 0.029 to 0.075 mg/L. 7-aminoclonazepam concentrations were 0.023 to 0.137 mg/L (70). Drowsiness and

TABLE 3. Pharmacokinetics of the benzodiazepines

	Bioavailability (F) (%)	T_{max} (h)	Volume of distribution (L/kg)	Clearance (L/h/kg)	Half-life (h)	Protein binding (%)	Active metabolites (half-life, h)
Alprazolam	92	1–2	0.7–1.4	0.048–0.072	11–15	70–80	1-hydroxyalprazolam (short), 4-hydroxyalprazolam (short)
Bromazepam	84	1–4	1.4	0.0456	12–32	70	—
Chlordiazepoxide	~100	1–2	0.22–0.75	0.012–0.030	5–30	94	*N*-desmethyl-chlordiazepoxide (60); demoxepam (45); *N*-desmethyldiazepam; oxazepam
Clobazam	87	1–4	0.9–1.8	0.024–0.036	17–49	85–90	*N*-desmethylclobazam (42)
Clonazepam	80–90	4	2–4	0.047	20–40	47–82	7-aminoclonazepam
Clorazepate	91	Rapidly de-carboxylated in stomach	—	—	—	—	*N*-desmethyldiazepam
N-desmethyl-diazepam	50	1	0.9–1.3	0.011	48–120	98	Oxazepam
Diazepam	98+	0.5–1.5	1–2	0.024–0.030	24–48	98–99	*N*-desmethyldiazepam; oxazepam; temazepam
Estazolam	Very high	2	0.46	0.0132	10–24	93	—
Flunitrazepam	80–90	0.5–1.0	1.1–1.4	0.214	16–35	77–80	*N*-desmethylflunitrazepam
Flurazepam	10–15; high first-pass metabolism	Rapidly metabolized to *N*-desalkyl-flurazepam	7.9[a]	2.22[a]	2–3	75–83	*N*-desalkylflurazepam (47–100); *N*-(2-hydroxyethyl)flurazepam (10–20)
Halazepam	NR	1	NR	0.343	21	NR	*N*-desmethyldiazepam; oxazepam
Ketazolam	~100	2	NR	NR	1.5	93	*N*-desmethylketazolam; *N*-desmethyldiazepam; diazepam; oxazepam
Lorazepam	90–93	2	0.8–1.6	0.048–0.078	10–20	85	—
Nitrazepam	53–94	1.5	1.5–2.8	0.07	24–30	85	—
Midazolam	31–72; high first-pass metabolism	0.3–1.0	0.8–1.7	0.240–0.488	2	96	1-hydroxymidazolam (<1)
Oxazepam	93	2–3	0.5–2.0	0.036–0.174	4–15	—	—
Prazepam	<5; very high first-pass metabolism	Precursor of *N*-desmethyl-diazepam	—	—	—	—	*N*-descyclopropylmethyl-prazepam (70); *N*-desmethyldiazepam; oxazepam
Quazepam	29–35; high first-pass metabolism	2	5.0–8.6	NR	21–40	95	2-oxoquazepam (39); N-desalkyl-2-oxoquazepam (73)
Temazepam	>95	0.5	1.32–1.53	0.060–0.084	8–15	76	—
Triazolam	61; first-pass metabolism	0.75–2.5	0.79–1.8	0.222–0.528	1.5–5.5	89	1-hydroxytriazolam (short)

NR, not reported; T_{max}, time to peak after oral dosing.
[a]Pharmacokinetics in the dog (162).
From Gaudreault P, Guay J, Thivierge RL, et al. Benzodiazepine poisoning. Clinical and pharmacological considerations and treatment. *Drug Saf* 1991;6(4):247–265; Sweetman S. *Martindale: the complete drug reference.* London: Pharmaceutical Press. Electronic ed. expires March 2003 Greenwood Village, CO: MICROMEDEX, 2003; and Dollery CT. *Therapeutic drugs.* CD-ROM DATABASE Release 1.0 ed. London: Churchill Livingstone, 1999, with permission.

ataxia are present in most patients with concentrations above 0.1 mg/L (71). Cyclical coma in a 4-year-old patient was associated with a clonazepam concentration of 0.069 mg/L (28).

Clorazepate caused prolonged sedation after routine doses for alcohol withdrawal in two patients. They required prolonged mechanical ventilation (10 days for both patients) followed by continuous flumazenil infusion (16 days for one patient and 3 days for the other) to avoid re-intubation. In both patients, *N*-desmethyldiazepam accumulation was demonstrated as the cause of the coma (72). Serum *N*-desmethyldiazepam concentrations between 0.7 and 5.1 mg/L were recorded in five cases of clorazepate-related (dose up to 300 mg) drug overdose (73).

A mean *diazepam* daily dose of 20 mg (range, 2 to 55 mg) resulted in mean steady-state plasma concentrations of 0.329 mg/L for diazepam and 0.389 mg/L for *N*-desmethyldiazepam with a mean *N*-desmethyldiazepam/diazepam ratio of 1.26 (74). Plasma diazepam concentrations ranging from 0.585 to 8.635 mg/L were found after diazepam overdose (32). In four cases of overdose with diazepam alone, patients were minimally sedated and were discharged within 24 hours, despite diazepam plasma concentrations as high as 4.8 mg/L.

The severity of poisoning after benzodiazepine overdose is determined largely by coingestion of other CNS depressants rather than its plasma concentration (32). Total serum benzodiazepine concentrations were correlated with CNS depression in 93 cases of diazepam overdose (73). Concentrations of total benzodiazepine ranged from 1 to 22 mg/L. All patients survived with supportive therapy only. Each of the 25 patients who had ingested only diazepam was awake or in grade 0 coma even when drug concentrations were tenfold greater than the accepted upper limit of the therapeutic range. None of the patients who had ingested only diazepam needed hospitalization; all were discharged from acute medical care after a period of emergency room observation. The ratios of parent drug to *N*-desmethyl diazepam averaged 3:1. This high ratio may be useful in differentiating acute overdose from high concentrations resulting from chronic therapy (73). In a 54-year-old man who ingested 2000 mg of diazepam, blood concentrations of diazepam and *N*-desmethyldiazepam were obtained for 1 month (31). The half-lives in this benzodiazepine overdose were longer than those seen with therapeutic doses although in other cases the elimination of diazepam and *N*-desmethyldiazepam seems to be dose-independent (75).

Flunitrazepam has a minimum toxic femoral blood concentration (7-aminoflunitrazepam metabolite) of 0.2 mg/L (12). During chronic therapy with 30 mg/day of *flurazepam*, *N*-desalkylflurazepam concentrations ranged from 0.033 to 0.114 mg/L. Flurazepam was not detectable (76). A *halazepam* dose of 120 mg/day produced a mean plasma concentration of 0.077 mg/L. Peak concentrations (C_{max}) of *N*-desmethyldiazepam were 1.404 to 1.657 mg/L (77).

The *lorazepam* elimination half-life after extremely high doses have been ingested is approximately the same as that found after ingestion of usual therapeutic doses (64). The plasma *midazolam* concentration required to obtain a sedative effect is approximately 0.4 mg/L (78). A midazolam-related death that occurred during endoscopy (after 10 mg IV) showed a premortem blood concentration of 2.8 mg/L and a postmortem concentration of 2.4 mg/L (55).

Nitrazepam therapeutic concentration is 0.035 to 0.084 mg/L (79). The minimum toxic femoral blood concentration of the 7-aminonitrazepam metabolite of nitrazepam has been estimated as 0.5 mg/L (12). A single 40-mg oral dose of oxazepam produced a mean peak plasma concentration of 1.06 mg/L (80).

Prazepam, 30 mg orally, has a C_{max} of 0.007 mg/L with an *N*-desmethyldiazepam concentration of 0.321 mg/L (81). After 25 mg of *quazepam* orally, C_{max} was 0.148 mg/L for quazepam, 0.046 mg/L for 2-oxoquazepam, and 0.041 mg/L for *N*-desalkyl-2-oxoquazepam (82).

The *temazepam* C_{max} after 20 mg orally averaged 0.668 mg/L (83). Varying doses of triazolam produced blood concentrations in the range of 0.002 to 0.03 mg/L, with an average concentration of 0.01 mg/L (84).

PATHOPHYSIOLOGY

Benzodiazepine Receptor

The inhibitory neurotransmitter, γ-aminobutyric acid (GABA), acts on $GABA_A$ receptors to regulate vigilance, anxiety, muscle tension, epileptogenic activity, and memory functions (85). Benzodiazepines modulate GABA-evoked chloride currents through a binding site on the $GABA_A$ receptor-operated chloride channel (Fig. 2). GABA agonists and benzodiazepine agonists simulta-

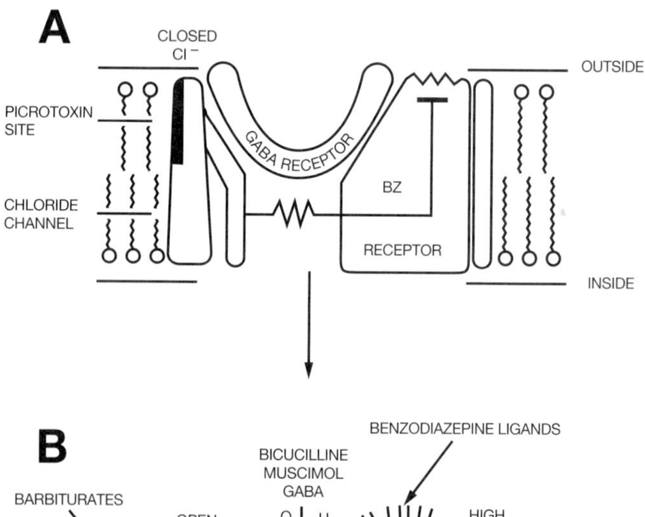

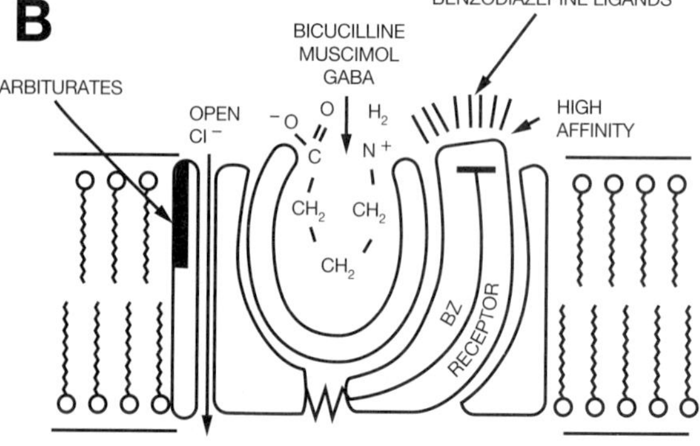

Figure 2. The γ-aminobutyric acid A ($GABA_A$) benzodiazepine receptor-chloride ion channel complex. $GABA_A$/benzodiazepine receptor–chloride ionophore complex. Receptors are depicted for GABA, barbiturates, and benzodiazepine ligands. GABA receptor agonists (e.g., GABA, muscimol) and GABA receptor antagonists (e.g., bicuculline) bind to $GABA_A$ receptors; barbiturates are thought to bind to specific recognition sites near the chloride ionophore; benzodiazepine receptor agonists (e.g., diazepam), benzodiazepine receptor antagonists (e.g., flumazenil), and benzodiazepine receptor inverse agonists (e.g., 6,7-dimethoxy-4-ethyl-3-carbomethoxy-β-carboline) bind to benzodiazepine receptors. **A:** Receptor complex in an inactivated state with the Cl^- channel closed. **B:** Receptor complex in an activated state with the Cl^- channel open. Activation is induced by GABA or GABA agonists binding to GABA receptors or by barbiturates. Activation of the receptor complex is associated with conformational changes and the opening of the Cl^- channel. Consequent entry of Cl^- into the neuron results in hyperpolarization. The frequency of chloride channel opening in the presence of GABA is increased by benzodiazepine receptor agonists. BZ, benzodiazepine. (From Amrein R, Hetzel W. Pharmacology of drugs frequently used in ICU's: Midazolam and flumazenil. *Intens Care Med* 1991;17:S1–S10, with permission.)

neously enhance the binding of the other to its receptor. Benzodiazepine binding appears to shift the GABA receptor from a low affinity state to a high affinity state and also stabilizes the receptor in a conformation that permits the ion channel to remain open. Similarly, GABA binding also enhances benzodiazepine agonist binding to its receptor via the same mechanism. Thus, GABA receptor agonists and benzodiazepine receptor agonists are positive allosteric effectors for each other (86).

The channel is not homogenous and can be assembled from multiple different combinations of α, β, and γ subunits (87). Not all of these different combinations are sensitive to benzodiazepines (88), and different combinations of subunits mediate different aspects of benzodiazepine effects (85,89). There are considerable differences in affinity for the benzodiazepine binding site amongst the benzodiazepines and their major metabolites. The most potent compound is triazolam, which has an equilibrium dissociation constant (Kd) of 0.54 nM; the least potent is chlordiazepoxide (Kd of 684 nM) (90). Stimulation of the GABA(A) receptor opens the chloride ion channel in the receptor complex and thereby increases conductance of chloride ion across the nerve cell membrane. This reduces the potential difference between the inside and outside of the cell and blocks the ability of the cell to conduct nerve impulses (91).

Tolerance and Dependence

Tolerance occurs to a number of the pharmacodynamic effects of benzodiazepines. Although tolerance usually takes a few days to develop fully, signs of acute tolerance can be demonstrated within 4 to 6 hours of a single dose of a benzodiazepine (i.e., within one dosing interval) (92). This is due to downregulation of benzodiazepine receptor binding and reduction in $GABA_A$ receptor function (93). Conversely, the discontinuation syndrome (withdrawal or rebound syndrome), which may follow the abrupt discontinuation of chronic treatment with benzodiazepines, is associated with upregulation of receptor binding and function at the $GABA_A$ receptor complex (94). The features of the discontinuation syndrome appear more rapidly (95) and may be more severe (96) after the withdrawal of the shorter-acting benzodiazepines than the longer-acting agents. The administration of a benzodiazepine antagonist alone results in upregulation of the $GABA_A$ receptor (97) and, when given with a benzodiazepine, prevents the downregulation of receptors and development of tolerance (98). In the presence of established tolerance, the administration of a benzodiazepine antagonist can precipitate withdrawal (99,100) or exacerbate existing withdrawal (101). There are also inverse agonists, agents that bind to the benzodiazepine recognition site on the $GABA_A$ receptor and produce physiologic and receptor effects that are the opposite to those of the traditional benzodiazepines (102).

Endogenous Benzodiazepine Receptors

There are benzodiazepine receptors outside the CNS, but the role of these peripheral-type receptors is unclear; it seems that they are connected with more slowly appearing drug actions, such as modulation of cell proliferation (103).

The presence of a specific receptor for benzodiazepines implies that there must be endogenous benzodiazepine-like ligands (104), which presumably have some role in modulation of anxiety and other states (105). Measurable concentrations of endogenous benzodiazepine-like substances are present in normal breast milk (106). An endogenous neuropeptide, diazepam-binding inhibitor, binds with high affinity to mitochondrial diazepam-binding inhibitor receptors in the extraneuronal glial cells (107). The diazepam-binding inhibitor receptor (also known as the *mitochondrial benzodiazepine receptor*) regulates transfer of cholesterol into glial cells where neurosteroids such as pregnenolone sulfate are synthesized (108). These neurosteroids, in turn, act as potent positive or negative allosteric modulators of $GABA_A$ receptor function (109).

PREGNANCY AND LACTATION

The pregnancy classifications from the United States and Australia are provided in Table 4. All of the benzodiazepines exhibit rapid placental transfer with significant fetal uptake (110). Clonazepam, clorazepate, diazepam, lorazepam, midazolam, nitrazepam, and oxazepam are excreted into breast milk. The levels detected in breast milk are low; therefore, the infant is unlikely to be affected. Problems may arise if the infant is premature or has been exposed to high concentrations of drug either during pregnancy or at delivery (111).

Teratogenesis

Although there are a number of studies and case reports concerning the use of benzodiazepines in human pregnancy, the data concerning teratogenicity and effects on postnatal development and behavior are inconsistent. These issues have been explored in depth in a review by McElhatton (111), from which the following is taken. There is evidence from studies in the 1970s that first trimester exposure to benzodiazepines *in utero* has resulted in the birth of some infants with facial clefts, cardiac malformations, and multiple other malformations, but no specific syndrome of defects. Diazepam and chlordiazepoxide are amongst the drugs most frequently implicated in the earlier studies. However, data from later studies provide no clear evidence of significant increase in either the overall incidence of malformations or of any particular type of defect.

Many of the women included in the earlier studies had psychiatric illness, epilepsy, or diabetes, all of which have an intrinsic risk in pregnancy. Some were on multidrug therapy. Medical, obstetric, and family histories were not always presented in the publications, which makes assessment of risk associated with benzodiazepine use difficult. Nevertheless, in most of the studies involving first trimester use of benzodiazepines, infants were normal at birth and developed normally.

Neonatal Neurologic Effects

Late third trimester use and exposure during labor seems to be associated with much greater risks to the fetus and neonate. Some infants exposed at this time exhibit either the floppy infant syndrome or marked neonatal withdrawal symptoms. Symptoms vary from mild sedation, hypotonia, and reluctance to suck, to apneic spells, cyanosis, and impaired metabolic responses to cold stress. These symptoms have been reported to persist for periods from hours to months after birth. This correlates well with the pharmacokinetic and placental transfer of the benzodiazepines and their disposition in the neonate.

The prolonged use of benzodiazepines throughout pregnancy raised the concern that there may be altered transmitter synthesis and function, leading to neurobehavioral problems in the children. In approximately 550 children who were followed for up to 4 years after birth, there was no adverse effect on either the malformation rate or neurobehavioral development and IQ. Although some of the data indicate that a small number of children were slower to develop during the first year or so, they did exhibit catchup growth, and most had developed normally by 4 years of age. Where developmental deficits persisted, it was not

TABLE 4. U.S. Food and Drug Administration risk category and breast-milk distribution of the serotonin uptake inhibitors

	U.S. Food and Drug Administration[a] (ADEC[b]) pregnancy risk category	Distribution into breast milk (milk to plasma ratio)
Alprazolam	D (B3)	0.36 ± 0.11, equivalent to approximately 3% of a maternal dose (163)
Bromazepam	NR (C)	NR
Chlordiazepoxide	D (B2)	NR
Clobazam	NR (C)	25% of the amount in the blood (range, 11–83%) (164)
Clonazepam	D (C)	Breast-milk concentrations 11–13 µg/L (165)
Clorazepate	D (C)	Breast-milk concentrations of 15 µg/L equivalent to 15–30% of maternal concentrations (166)
N-desmethyldiazepam	NR (NR)	0.13 (167)
Diazepam	D (C)	0.2 (167)
Estazolam	X (NR)	NR
Flunitrazepam	D (C)	NR
Flurazepam	X (C)	NR
Halazepam	D (NR)	NR
Ketazolam	NR (NR)	NR
Lorazepam	D (C)	<0.06, equivalent to 0.35% of the maternal dose (168)
Nitrazepam	NR (C)	0.27 ± 0.06 (169)
Midazolam	D (C)	0.15 ± 0.06 (169)
Oxazepam	D (C)	0.10 (167)
Prazepam	D (NR)	9.6 equivalent to 4% of the maternal dose (170)
Quazepam	X (NR)	4.19 equivalent to 0.11% of the maternal dose (171)
Temazepam	X (C)	0.14 (167)
Triazolam	X (C)	NR

NR, not reported.
[a]Appendix I provides definitions of U.S. Food and Drug Administration pregnancy categories.
[b]Australian Drug Evaluation Committee Pregnancy Categories.
Category A: Drugs that have been taken by a large number of pregnant women and women of childbearing age without any proven increase in the frequency of malformations or other direct or indirect harmful effects on the fetus having been observed.
Category B1: Drugs that have been taken by only a limited number of pregnant women and women of childbearing age without an increase in the frequency of malformation or other direct or indirect harmful effects on the human fetus having been observed. Studies in animals have not shown evidence of an increased occurrence of fetal damage.
Category B2: Drugs that have been taken by only a limited number of pregnant women and women of childbearing age without an increase in the frequency of malformation or other direct or indirect harmful effects on the human fetus having been observed. Studies in animals are inadequate or may be lacking, but available data show no evidence of an increased occurrence of fetal damage.
Category B3: Drugs that have been taken by only a limited number of pregnant women and women of childbearing age without an increase in the frequency of malformation or other direct or indirect harmful effects on the human fetus having been observed. Studies in animals have shown evidence of an increased occurrence of fetal damage, the significance of which is considered uncertain in humans.
Category C: Drugs that, owing to their pharmacologic effects, have caused or may be suspected of causing harmful effects on the human fetus or neonate without causing malformations. These effects may be reversible.
Category D: Drugs that have caused or are suspected to have caused or may be expected to cause an increased incidence of human fetal malformations or irreversible damage. These drugs may also have adverse pharmacologic effects.
Category X: Drugs that have such a high risk of causing permanent damage to the fetus that they should not be used in pregnancy or when there is a possibility of pregnancy.
Note: For drugs in categories B1, B2, and B3, human data are lacking or inadequate and subcategorization is therefore based on available animal data. The allocation of a B category does not imply greater safety than the C category. Drugs in category D are not absolutely contraindicated in pregnancy (e.g., anticonvulsants). Moreover, in some cases the D category has been assigned on the basis of "suspicion."

possible to prove a cause-effect relationship with benzodiazepine exposure. These children were often from families in which there was maternal illness requiring prolonged drug therapy or in which there were social problems. It is important to consider poor environmental and social factors when assessing the possible prenatal influence of the benzodiazepines on the postnatal health and development of the child (111).

Measurable concentrations of endogenous benzodiazepine-like substances are present in normal breast milk. The mean concentration of benzodiazepine-like substances in a series of 35 women was 0.0043 ± 0.0023 mg/L (range, 0 to 0.0093 mg/L) expressed as lorazepam (106).

CLINICAL PRESENTATION

Acute Overdose

Benzodiazepines are sedating drugs, which do not usually cause either profound CNS or respiratory depression or any nonsedative effects. Death may occur before hospital arrival due to sedation (particularly if combined with other CNS depressants), but the course of patients reaching hospital is generally uncomplicated. The clinical effects of benzodiazepine poisoning are due entirely to CNS depression. Severe poisoning may occasionally develop hypothermia, bradycardia, and hypotension. Respiratory and CNS depression may lead to aspiration pneumonia. However, deep coma (GCS less than 8) is unusual. Most patients are stuporous or still responsive to painful stimuli unless they have coingested other sedating drugs. Ataxia and nystagmus are common in nontolerant patients, but, if pronounced, the possibility of concomitant drug overdose should be raised (i.e., anticonvulsant).

Drug-induced coma involving benzodiazepines is characterized by snoring with flow limitation and obstructive apnea. The mechanism involves an increase in upper airway resistance and work of breathing (112), which is reversible with flumazenil (113). Cyclic coma in a 4-year-old boy followed an ingestion of clonazepam (28). Rarely, other complications have been associated with benzodiazepine overdose. An alprazolam overdose was associated with marked first-degree atrioventricular block reversed by flumazenil (114). Long-term sequelae are unusual, and patients usually recover consciousness within 12 hours, although this may take considerably longer in the elderly or patients with sedative coingestion.

Acute Withdrawal

Withdrawal from CNS depressants is addressed in Chapter 32. Suddenly stopping treatment in dependent people may produce withdrawal symptoms and signs including anxiety, dysphoria, irritability, insomnia, nightmares, sweating, memory impairment, hallucinations, hypertension, tachycardia, psychosis, tremors, and seizures (21). Acute withdrawal from benzodiazepines may present solely as a confusional state due to nonconvulsive status epilepticus. This presentation can easily be missed (101,115). A patient who received therapeutic doses of alprazolam for 8 weeks experienced a withdrawal syndrome beginning 18 hours after its abrupt discontinuation. Short-acting and minimally sedating benzodiazepines may have increased potential for withdrawal reactions (116). There is a case report of severe psychosis and seizures after abrupt discontinuation of alprazolam and then the recurrence of seizures at the end of a gradual tapering schedule. The last of these seizures appeared to be a contributing factor in the patient's death (96). Rapid development of tolerance during midazolam infusion can lead to withdrawal reactions on cessation of the infusion in adults (117,118) and children (119).

Adverse Reactions

Benzodiazepine abuse is common and occurs with all benzodiazepines. The abuse potential of individual agents is debated (120). Overall, the personal preference of patients seems more responsible for choice of a specific agent than the intrinsic pharmacologic differences between benzodiazepines (121). Changing the availability of a specific benzodiazepine on the grounds of its perceived abuse potential results in abuse of alternative benzodiazepines (122) or even other drugs with sedative-hypnotic properties (123,124).

Common adverse effects include drowsiness, oversedation, lightheadedness, memory loss, ataxia, and slurred speech. Infrequent adverse effects include headache, vertigo, hypotension, disorientation, confusion, paradoxical excitation, euphoria, aggression and hostility, anxiety, decreased libido, anterograde amnesia, pain and thrombophlebitis with IV injection, and respiratory arrest with IV use. Rare adverse effects include blood disorders, including leukopenia and leukocytosis; jaundice; transient elevated liver function tests; and allergic reactions, including rash and anaphylaxis (21).

DIAGNOSTIC TESTS

Routine quantitative benzodiazepine estimation is not indicated for clinical management. Serum bromide levels may be increased in patients who ingest bromazepam. This may be associated with a negative anion gap (125).

The blood or urine may be screened for benzodiazepines, but screening is particularly problematic because of low dosage, rapid elimination, failure to detect conjugated metabolites by immunoenzymatic reagents, and high threshold of sensitivity for certain substances (126). EMIT-tox serum benzodiazepine assay (EMIT), the Abbott ADx serum benzodiazepine fluorescence polarization immunoassay (FPIA), and a radioreceptor assay (RRA) were evaluated in 113 patients with suspected acute poisoning (127). EMIT, FPIA, and RRA can be reliably used to screen for the presence of benzodiazepines in serum, but in many cases they cannot discriminate between toxic and nontoxic concentrations (127). In screening for benzodiazepines, there is a risk of missing intoxication by benzodiazepines with low therapeutic concentration and low cross-reactivity (alprazolam, bromazepam, flunitrazepam). There is also a risk of misinterpreting a positive result for some benzodiazepines with high therapeutic range and high cross-reactivity (*N*-desmethyldiazepam), which may reflect a pharmacologically ineffective concentration (128).

Unless there are other coingested drugs or medical conditions that warrant it, there is no need for routine blood or other tests in benzodiazepine poisoning. Measurement of partial pressure of carbon dioxide ($PaCO_2$) via expired air or arterial blood gases is the best way to assess respiratory compromise from sedation.

POSTMORTEM CONSIDERATIONS

For many drugs, there is postmortem diffusion of drugs from sites of high concentration in solid organs into the blood, with resultant artefactual elevation of drug concentrations in blood (postmortem redistribution). Highest drug concentrations may be found in central vessels such as pulmonary artery and vein, and lowest concentrations are found in peripheral vessels such as subclavian and femoral veins. This creates major difficulties in interpretation and undermines the reference value of databases where the site of origin of postmortem blood samples is unknown (129). It is widely agreed, however, that the femoral vein site represents the optimum sampling site, and this site is standardized amongst forensic pathologists. Little or no postmortem information is available for chlordiazepoxide, clobazam, clorazepate, estazolam, halazepam, ketazolam, prazepam, or quazepam.

The distribution of the nitrobenzodiazepines, clonazepam, flunitrazepam, and nitrazepam and their respective 7-amino metabolites were examined in blood, serum, vitreous humor, liver, bile, and urine of decedents taking these drugs (130). Peripheral blood, serum, and liver concentrations were not significantly different. However, vitreous concentrations were one-third of blood, whereas bile concentrations were 5- to 12-fold higher. Blood, serum, and vitreous contained predominantly the 7-amino metabolites, liver contained only the metabolites, whereas bile contained significant concentrations of both the parent drug and the 7-amino metabolites (130). Urine contained only small concentrations of parent drug, but a number of metabolites were detected. There was no apparent difference in total blood concentrations of nitrobenzodiazepines when samples taken in hospital shortly before death were compared to postmortem blood. Although postmortem diffusion into peripheral blood was thought not to confound the interpretation of nitrobenzodiazepine concentrations in this study (130), others have found significant differences (see the following).

In a death attributed in part to multiple benzodiazepines, toxicologic analysis revealed the presence of flunitrazepam (heart blood of the left and right chamber 0.033 mg/L each), *N*-desmethylflunitrazepam (left heart blood 0.029 mg/L, right heart blood 0.027 mg/L), 7-amino-flunitrazepam (left heart blood 0.090 mg/L, right heart blood 0.104 mg/L), diazepam (left heart blood 0.395 mg/L, right heart blood 0.386 mg/L), *N*-desmethyldiazepam (left heart blood 0.112 mg/L, right heart blood 0.115 mg/L), and temazepam (left heart blood 0.034 mg/L, right heart blood 0.033 mg/L) (131).

Forensically relevant benzodiazepines (*N*-desmethyldiazepam, oxazepam, bromazepam, diazepam, lorazepam, flunitrazepam, alprazolam, triazolam) may be determined in human hair. The limits of detection for all benzodiazepines ranged from 1 to 20 pg/mg using a 50-mg hair sample (132). This is a useful technique in which repeated exposures have occurred (i.e., criminal sedation by a partner) (133). Bleaching influences the stability of entrapped benzodiazepines in hair with decreases in measured amounts of diazepam (39.7%), *N*-desmethyldiazepam (67.7%), and 7-aminoflunitrazepam (61.85) in bleached versus nonbleached hair (134).

An *alprazolam* blood concentration of 0.177 mg/L was determined in a case of suicidal ingestion (135). A heart blood alprazolam concentration of 2.1 mg/L has been reported (136). Blood concentrations of alprazolam, alcohol, and tramadol were 0.21 mg/L, 1.29 g/kg, and 38.3 mg/L, respectively, in a death attributed to all three agents (137). In coingestion deaths with alprazolam, postmortem blood concentrations of methadone were at the lower range or below the concentrations previously identified in methadone overdose fatalities, suggesting an increased risk from coingestion of methadone and alprazolam (138).

Bromazepam has been assayed in the fly larvae found in a putrefied corpse (139). A 60-year-old woman was found dead with a blood bromazepam concentration of 5 mg/L (140).

Flunitrazepam alone or with ethanol was associated with death in a 7-aminoflunitrazepam concentration of 0.45 mg/L and 0.16 mg/L, respectively. The presence of ethanol reduces the amount of flunitrazepam needed to cause death (19).

The *flurazepam* concentration in samples obtained from multiple ligated vessels ranged from 0.15 to 0.99 mg/L (129). In a death attributed to an ingestion of more than 2400 mg, the concentrations of flurazepam (0.51 mg/L), *N*-desalkylflurazepam (0.14 mg/L), and *N*-(2-hydroxyethyl)flurazepam (9.0 mg/L) in the blood amounted to 20 to 50 times the therapeutic concentration (40). In a fatality attributed to a 2.2-g ingestion, the concentrations of flurazepam in femoral blood, liver, bile, vitreous humor, and urine were 5.5 mg/L, 130 mg/kg, 33 mg/L, 1.3 mg/L, and 3.3 mg/L, respectively. Desalkylflurazepam was also detected in blood, liver, bile, and vitreous, but at much lower concentrations than the parent compound (41).

A *midazolam*-related death that occurred during endoscopy (after 10 mg of IV midazolam) showed a premortem blood concentration of 2.8 mg/L and a postmortem concentration of 2.4 mg/L (55).

Nitrazepam was implicated in a drowning, and blood concentrations of nitrazepam and 7-aminonitrazepam were site dependent (0.400 to 0.973 mg/L and 0.418 to 1.82 mg/L). In addition, the concentrations of the same analytes in the bile were 4.08 and 1.67 mg/L, respectively, and in the urine 0.580 and 1.09 mg/L, respectively. Accumulation of both substances was observed in various brain tissues (2.17 to 6.22 μg/g and 2.49 to 5.11 μg/g). Only small amounts of nitrazepam and 7-aminonitrazepam were detected in the liver (0.059 and 0.113 μg/g, respectively). Large differences in the observed concentrations were thought to be mainly due to dilution of arterial blood by water aspirated at the time of death. Bacterial metabolism of nitrazepam may also have contributed to the differences (141). Six cases of fatal overdose had blood concentrations of 1.2 to 1.9 mg/L (therapeutic range, 0.035 to 0.084 mg/L) (79).

Temazepam produces variable postmortem levels in skeletal muscle. It is suitable for qualitative analysis only and is not an appropriate alternative to quantitative blood levels (142).

Triazolam alone was implicated in a death with a heart blood concentration of 0.12 mg/L (143). Five fatal cases of poisoning by triazolam alone or in combination with ethanol were studied in East Denmark (84). In one case in which no ethanol was detected, a blood triazolam concentration of 0.11 mg/L was found. In the four cases in which the ethanol concentration ranged from 110 to 202 mg/100 ml, the triazolam concentration range was 0.04 to 0.22 mg/L. In contrast, the blood concentrations of living patients who had also ingested the drug were 0.002 to 0.03 mg/L (N = 28), with an average concentration of 0.01 mg/L (84).

TREATMENT

Treatment is entirely supportive with IV access and fluids and maintenance of the airway and ventilation if required. Patients with a significant sedative drug overdose should be advised not to drive until potential interference with psychomotor performance has resolved (144). For significant benzodiazepine overdose, this is at least 24 hours after discharge.

Decontamination

Oral activated charcoal is of little value in pure benzodiazepine poisoning. It may be given to patients who have recently ingested benzodiazepines with other drugs that may benefit from decontamination. Gastric lavage is not indicated.

Antidotes

The use of flumazenil is detailed in Chapter 57. Because of the rapid development of tolerance (92), patients frequently wake from their sedation or coma although high concentrations of the benzodiazepine persist (33,64). The administration of a benzodiazepine antagonist such as flumazenil in the presence of a benzodiazepine prevents the development of tolerance (98). This could theoretically result in a prolongation of the effect of the benzodiazepine manifesting as a prolonged requirement for the antagonist and hospital length of stay. This has been seen after diazepam overdose treated with flumazenil (31,145), whereas in contrast, a much shorter duration of symptoms was seen with similar doses managed before the availability of an antagonist (33). For routine management of uncomplicated benzodiazepine overdose there is no indication for the use of flumazenil.

Flumazenil (0.1 to 2.0 mg IV) has been given to unconscious patients in which the drug ingested is unknown (146,147), although this remains controversial (148). A rapid response within a minute or two is expected in pure benzodiazepine poisoning (149). The patient should have a dramatic improvement in the level of consciousness. Minor improvements may be seen with alcohol and other sedative drugs. Flumazenil may precipitate withdrawal in benzodiazepine-dependent patients (99,100) or make established withdrawal worse (101). Flumazenil should only be given if there is no evidence of proconvulsant or prodysrhythmic drug ingestion, as the removal of the benzodiazepine effect may lead to seizures, cardiac arrest, or death (150–158).

Paradoxical excitement can occur after therapeutic use of benzodiazepines (46). It responds well to small doses of flumazenil (50,159,160).

Enhancement of Elimination

Hemodialysis, hemoperfusion, hemofiltration, and forced diuresis are not indicated because they have little effect on clearance of these highly lipid soluble and widely distributed drugs (91,161).

Monitoring

Routine observation of vital signs, especially GCS and airway patency, is indicated. Measurement of partial pressure of carbon dioxide via expired air or arterial blood gases is the best way to assess respiratory compromise from sedation.

REFERENCES

1. Buckley NA, Whyte IM, Dawson AH, et al. Self-poisoning in Newcastle, 1987–1992. *Med J Aust* 1995;162(4):190–193.
2. Busto U, Kaplan HL, Sellers EM. Benzodiazepine-associated emergencies in Toronto. *Am J Psychiatry* 1980;137(2):224–227.
3. Fuller GN, Rea AJ, Payne JF, et al. Parasuicide in central London 1984–1988. *J R Soc Med* 1989;82(11):653–656.
4. Rochette A, Le Niger E, Moulins H, et al. [Voluntary drug poisoning: epidemiology, performance and limits of the emergency laboratory]. *J Toxicol Clin Exp* 1990;10(6):395–408.
5. Christakis-Hampsas M, Tutudakis M, Tsatsakis AM, et al. Acute poisonings and sudden deaths in Crete: a five-year review (1991–1996). *Vet Hum Toxicol* 1998;40(4):228–230.
6. Stern TA, Gross PL, Pollack MH, et al. Drug overdoses seen in the emergency department: assessment, disposition, and follow-up. *Ann Clin Psychiatry* 1991;3(3):223–231.
7. Velvart J. [Epidemiology of acute drug poisoning in Switzerland]. *Schweiz Med Wochenschr* 1982;112(31–32):1101–1104.
8. Alsen M, Ekedahl A, Lowenhielm P, et al. Medicine self-poisoning and the sources of the drugs in Lund, Sweden. *Acta Psychiatr Scand* 1994;89(4):255–261.
9. Khan MM, Reza H. Benzodiazepine self-poisoning in Pakistan: implications for prevention and harm reduction. *J Pak Med Assoc* 1998;48(10):293–295.
10. Wang H, Niu W, Zhang J, et al. [The application of a broad spectrum automatic rapid drug identification system in acute drug poisoning]. *Zhonghua Nei Ke Za Zhi* 2002;41(6):408–410.
11. Henderson A, Wright M, Pond SM. Experience with 732 acute overdose patients admitted to an intensive care unit over six years. *Med J Aust* 1993;158(1):28–30.
12. Drummer OH, Ranson DL. Sudden death and benzodiazepines. *Am J Forensic Med Pathol* 1996;17(4):336–342.

13. Bystrzycki A, Coleridge J. Drug- and poison-related deaths in Victoria during 1997. *Emerg Med* 2000;12:303–309.
14. Buckley NA, Dawson AH, Whyte IM, et al. Relative toxicity of benzodiazepines in overdose. *BMJ* 1995;310(6974):219–221.
15. Meier PJ, Wyss PA, Radovanovic DI. Differential acute overdose toxicity of various benzodiazepine derivatives. *Vet Hum Toxicol* 1993;35:338.
16. Serfaty M, Masterton G. Fatal poisonings attributed to benzodiazepines in Britain during the 1980s. *Br J Psychiatry* 1993;163:386–393.
17. Koski A, Ojanpera I, Vuori E. Alcohol and benzodiazepines in fatal poisonings. *Alcohol Clin Exp Res* 2002;26(7):956–959.
18. Isbister GK, O'Regan L, Sibbritt D, et al. Alprazolam is relatively more toxic than other benzodiazepines in overdose. *J Toxicol Clin Toxicol* 2003;41:715.
19. Drummer OH, Syrjanen ML, Cordner SM. Deaths involving the benzodiazepine flunitrazepam. *Am J Forensic Med Pathol* 1993;14(3):238–243.
20. Oelschlager H. [Chemical and pharmacologic aspects of benzodiazepines]. *Schweiz Rundsch Med Prax* 1989;78(27–28):766–772.
21. Benzodiazepines. In: Rossi S, Vitry A, Hurley E, et al., eds. *Australian medicines handbook*. Adelaide: Australian Medicines Handbook Pty Ltd, 2002.
22. French AP. Dangerously aggressive behavior as a side effect of alprazolam. *Am J Psychiatry* 1989;146(2):276.
23. Strahan A, Rosenthal J, Kaswan M, et al. Three case reports of acute paroxysmal excitement associated with alprazolam treatment. *Am J Psychiatry* 1985;142(7):859–861.
24. McCormick SR, Nielsen J, Jatlow PI. Alprazolam overdose: clinical findings and serum concentrations in two cases. *J Clin Psychiatry* 1985;46(6):247–248.
25. Arquilla B, Gupta R, Gernshiemer J, et al. Acute arterial spasm in an extremity caused by inadvertent intra-arterial injection successfully treated in the emergency department. *J Emerg Med* 2000;19(2):139–143.
26. Minder EI. Toxicity in a case of acute and massive overdose of chlordiazepoxide and its correlation to blood concentration. *J Toxicol Clin Toxicol* 1989;27(1–2):117–127.
27. Donlon PT, Singer JM. Clobazam versus placebo for anxiety and tension in psychoneurotic outpatients. A multicenter collaborative study. *J Clin Pharmacol* 1979;19(5–6):297–302.
28. Welch TR, Rumack BH, Hammond K. Clonazepam overdose resulting in cyclic coma. *Clin Toxicol* 1977;10(4):433–436.
29. Browne TR. Clonazepam. A review of a new anticonvulsant drug. *Arch Neurol* 1976;33(5):326–332.
30. Woo E, Greenblatt DJ. Massive benzodiazepine requirements during acute alcohol withdrawal. *Am J Psychiatry* 1979;136(6):821–823.
31. de Haro L, Valli M, Bourdon JH, et al. Diazepam poisoning with one-month monitoring of diazepam and nordiazepam blood levels. *Vet Hum Toxicol* 2001;43(3):174–175.
32. Divoll M, Greenblatt DJ, Lacasse Y, et al. Benzodiazepine overdosage: plasma concentrations and clinical outcome. *Psychopharmacology (Berl)* 1981;73(4):381–383.
33. Greenblatt DJ, Woo E, Allen MD, et al. Rapid recovery from massive diazepam overdose. *JAMA* 1978;240(17):1872–1874.
34. Dumont D, Mathe D, Piva C. Poisoning by a new benzodiazepine estazolam (France). *Med Leg Toxicol* 1980;23:257–259.
35. Druid H, Holmgren P, Ahlner J. Flunitrazepam: an evaluation of use, abuse and toxicity. *Forensic Sci Int* 2001;122(2–3):136–141.
36. Deleu D, de Keyser J. Flunitrazepam intoxication simulating a structural brainstem lesion. *J Neurol Neurosurg Psychiatry* 1987;50(2):236–237.
37. Heyndrickx B. Fatal intoxication due to flunitrazepam. *J Anal Toxicol* 1987;11(6):278.
38. Brammer G, Gibly R, Walter FG, et al. Continuous intravenous flumazenil infusion for benzodiazepine poisoning. *Vet Hum Toxicol* 2000;42(5):280–281.
39. Pulce C, Mollon P, Pham E, et al. Acute poisonings with ethyle loflazepate, flunitrazepam, prazepam and triazolam in children. *Vet Hum Toxicol* 1992;34(2):141–143.
40. Aderjan R, Mattern R. [A fatal monointoxication by flurazepam (Dalmadorm). Problems of the toxicological interpretation (author's transl)]. *Arch Toxicol* 1979;43(1):69–75.
41. McIntyre IM, Syrjanen ML, Lawrence KL, et al. A fatality due to flurazepam. *J Forensic Sci* 1994;39(6):1571–1574.
42. Fann WE, Garcia J, Richman BW. High-dose benzodiazepine therapy in hospitalized anxious patients. *J Clin Pharmacol* 1983;23(2–3):100–105.
43. Garnier R, Medernach C, Harbach S, et al. [Agitation and hallucinations during acute lorazepam poisoning in children. Apropos of 65 personal cases]. *Ann Paediatr (Paris)* 1984;31(4):286–289.
44. Guterman B, Sebastian P, Sodha N. Recovery from alpha coma after lorazepam overdose. *Clin Electroencephalogr* 1981;12(4):205–208.
45. Jeffery DI, Whitfield MF. Lorazepam poisoning [Letter]. *BMJ* 1974;4(5946):719.
46. Short TG, Forrest P, Galletly DC. Paradoxical reactions to benzodiazepines—a genetically determined phenomenon? *Anaesth Intensive Care* 1987;15(3):330–331.
47. Martinez-Telleria A, Cano ME, Carlos R. [Paradoxical reaction to midazolam after its use as a sedative in regional anesthesia]. *Rev Esp Anestesiol Reanim* 1992;39(6):379–380.
48. Massanari M, Novitsky J, Reinstein LJ. Paradoxical reactions in children associated with midazolam use during endoscopy. *Clin Pediatr (Phila)* 1997;36(12):681–684.
49. Marrosu F, Marrosu G, Rachel MG, et al. Paradoxical reactions elicited by diazepam in children with classic autism. *Funct Neurol* 1987;2(3):355–361.
50. Weinbroum AA, Szold O, Ogorek D, et al. The midazolam-induced paradox phenomenon is reversible by flumazenil. Epidemiology, patient characteristics and review of the literature. *Eur J Anaesthesiol* 2001;18(12):789–797.
51. Brown CR. The use of benzodiazepines in prison populations. *J Clin Psychiatry* 1978;39(3):219–222.
52. Marsch SC, Schafer HG. [An accidental intra-arterial injection of midazolam through a 3-way stopcock in an arterial flushing system]. *Anaesthesist* 1990;39(6):337–338.
53. Nishiyama T, Hanaoka K. Accidental overdose of midazolam as intramuscular premedication. *J Clin Anesth* 2002;14(7):543–545.
54. Lineaweaver WC, Anderson K, Hing DN. Massive doses of midazolam infusion for delirium tremens without respiratory depression. *Crit Care Med* 1988;16(3):294–295.
55. Michalodimitrakis M, Christodoulou P, Tsatsakis AM, et al. Death related to midazolam overdose during endoscopic retrograde cholangiopancreatography. *Am J Forensic Med Pathol* 1999;20(1):93–97.
56. Murphy JV, Sawasky F, Marquardt KM, et al. Deaths in young children receiving nitrazepam. *J Pediatr* 1987;111(1):145–147.
57. Baselt RC, Cravey RH. Nitrazepam. In: *Disposition of toxic drugs and chemicals in man*. Chicago: Year Book Medical Publishers, Inc, 1989:598–599.
58. Moshkowitz M, Pines A, Finkelstein A, et al. Skin blisters as a manifestation of oxazepam toxicity. *J Toxicol Clin Toxicol* 1990;28(3):383–386.
59. Pulce C, Mollon P, Pham E, et al. Acute poisonings with ethyle loflazepate, flunitrazepam, prazepam and triazolam in children. *Vet Hum Toxicol* 1992;34(2):141–143.
60. Kales A, Bixler EO, Soldatos CR, et al. Quazepam and flurazepam: long-term use and extended withdrawal. *Clin Pharmacol Ther* 1982;32(6):781–788.
61. Obafunwa JO, Busuttil A. Deaths from substance overdose in the Lothian and Borders region of Scotland (1983–1991). *Hum Exp Toxicol* 1994;13(6):401–406.
62. Feeney GF, Gibbs HH. Digit loss following misuse of temazepam. *Med J Aust* 2002;176(8):380.
63. Pulce C, Mollon P, Pham E, et al. Acute poisonings with ethyle loflazepate, flunitrazepam, prazepam and triazolam in children. *Vet Hum Toxicol* 1992;34(2):141–143.
64. Allen MD, Greenblatt DJ, Lacasse Y, et al. Pharmacokinetic study of lorazepam overdosage. *Am J Psychiatry* 1980;137(11):1414–1415.
65. Nishikawa T, Suzuki S, Ohtani H, et al. Benzodiazepine concentrations in sera determined by radioreceptor assay for therapeutic-dose recipients. *Am J Clin Pathol* 1994;102(5):605–610.
66. McCormick SR, Nielsen J, Jatlow P. Quantification of alprazolam in serum or plasma by liquid chromatography. *Clin Chem* 1984;30(10):1652–1655.
67. Rudolf J, Kaferstein H, Neveling M, et al. [Protracted course of bromazepam poisoning in advanced age]. *Dtsch Med Wochenschr* 1998;123(27):832–834.
68. Michaud K, Romain N, Giroud C, et al. Hypothermia and undressing associated with non-fatal bromazepam intoxication. *Forensic Sci Int* 2001;124(2–3):112–114.
69. Divoll M, Greenblatt DJ, Ciraulo DA, et al. Clobazam kinetics: intrasubject variability and effect of food on adsorption. *J Clin Pharmacol* 1982;22(1):69–73.
70. Naestoft J, Larsen NE. Quantitative determination of clonazepam and its metabolites in human plasma by gas chromatography. *J Chromatogr* 1974;93(1):113–122.
71. Baruzzi A, Bordo B, Bossi L, et al. Plasma levels of di-no-propylacetate and clonazepam in epileptic patients. *Int J Clin Pharmacol Biopharm* 1977;15(9):403–408.
72. Guglielminotti J, Maury E, Alzieu M, et al. Prolonged sedation requiring mechanical ventilation and continuous flumazenil infusion after routine doses of clorazepam for alcohol withdrawal syndrome. *Intensive Care Med* 1999;25(12):1435–1436.
73. Jatlow P, Dobular K, Bailey D. Serum diazepam concentrations in overdose. Their significance. *Am J Clin Pathol* 1979;72(4):571–577.
74. Greenblatt DJ, Laughren TP, Allen MD, et al. Plasma diazepam and desmethyldiazepam concentrations during long-term diazepam therapy. *Br J Clin Pharmacol* 1981;11(1):35–40.
75. Ochs HR. [Plasma levels following high diazepam doses in intensive-care medicine (author's transl)]. *Anasth Intensivther Notfallmed* 1981;16(3):143–144.
76. Kaplan SA, de Silva JA, Jack ML, et al. Blood level profile in man following chronic oral administration of flurazepam hydrochloride. *J Pharm Sci* 1973;62(12):1932–1935.
77. Chung M, Hilbert JM, Gural RP, et al. Multiple-dose halazepam kinetics. *Clin Pharmacol Ther* 1984;35(6):838–842.
78. Crevat-Pisano P, Dragna S, Granthil C, et al. Plasma concentrations and pharmacokinetics of midazolam during anaesthesia. *J Pharm Pharmacol* 1986;38(8):578–582.
79. Baselt RC. *Disposition of toxic drugs and chemicals in man*, 5th ed. Foster City, CA: Chemical Toxicology Institute, 1999.
80. Knowles JA, Ruelius HW. Absorption and excretion of 7-chloro-1,3-dihydro-3-hydroxy-5-phenyl-2H-1,4-benzodiazepin-2-one (oxazepam) in humans. Determination of the drug by gas-liquid chromatography with electron capture detection. *Arzneimittelforschung* 1972;22(4):687–692.
81. Smith MT, Evans LE, Eadie MJ, et al. Pharmacokinetics of prazepam in man. *Eur J Clin Pharmacol* 1979;16(2):141–147.
82. Zampaglione N, Hilbert JM, Ning J, et al. Disposition and metabolic fate of 14C-quazepam in man. *Drug Metab Dispos* 1985;13(1):25–29.
83. Bittencourt P, Richens A, Toseland PA, et al. Pharmacokinetics of the hypnotic benzodiazepine, temazepam. *Br J Clin Pharmacol* 1979;8(1):37S–38S.
84. Steentoft A, Worm K. Cases of fatal triazolam poisoning. *J Forensic Sci Soc* 1993;33(1):45–48.

85. Rudolph U, Crestani F, Benke D, et al. Benzodiazepine actions mediated by specific gamma-aminobutyric acid(A) receptor subtypes. *Nature* 1999; 401(6755):796–800.
86. Costa E, Auta J, Grayson DR, et al. GABA(A) receptors and benzodiazepines: a role for dendritic resident subunit mRNAs(1). *Neuropharmacology* 2002;43(6):925–937.
87. Rudolph U, Crestani F, Mohler H. GABA(A) receptor subtypes: dissecting their pharmacological functions. *Trends Pharmacol Sci* 2001;22(4):188–194.
88. Yang W, Drewe JA, Lan NC. Cloning and characterization of the human GABAA receptor alpha 4 subunit: identification of a unique diazepam-insensitive binding site. *Eur J Pharmacol* 1995;291(3):319–325.
89. Doble A. New insights into the mechanism of action of hypnotics. *J Psychopharmacol* 1999;13[4 Suppl 1]:S11–S20.
90. Richelson E, Nelson A, Neeper R. Binding of benzodiazepines and some major metabolites at their sites in normal human frontal cortex in vitro. *J Pharmacol Exp Ther* 1991;256(3):897–901.
91. Gaudreault P, Guay J, Thivierge RL, et al. Benzodiazepine poisoning. Clinical and pharmacological considerations and treatment. *Drug Saf* 1991;6(4):247–265.
92. Ingum J, Bjorklund R, Volden R, et al. Development of acute tolerance after oral doses of diazepam and flunitrazepam. *Psychopharmacology (Berl)* 1994;113(3–4):304–310.
93. Miller LG, Greenblatt DJ, Barnhill JG, et al. Chronic benzodiazepine administration. I. Tolerance is associated with benzodiazepine receptor downregulation and decreased gamma-aminobutyric acidA receptor function. *J Pharmacol Exp Ther* 1988;246(1):170–176.
94. Miller LG, Greenblatt DJ, Roy RB, et al. Chronic benzodiazepine administration. II. Discontinuation syndrome is associated with upregulation of gamma-aminobutyric acidA receptor complex binding and function. *J Pharmacol Exp Ther* 1988;246(1):177–182.
95. Lopez F, Miller LG, Greenblatt DJ, et al. Chronic administration of benzodiazepines—V. Rapid onset of behavioral and neurochemical alterations after discontinuation of alprazolam. *Neuropharmacology* 1990;29(3):237–241.
96. Haque W, Watson DJ, Bryant SG. Death following suspected alprazolam withdrawal seizures: a case report. *Tex Med* 1990;86(1):44–47.
97. Miller LG, Greenblatt DJ, Roy RB, et al. Chronic benzodiazepine administration. III. Upregulation of gamma-aminobutyric acidA receptor binding and function associated with chronic benzodiazepine antagonist administration. *J Pharmacol Exp Ther* 1989;248(3):1096–1101.
98. Brown MJ, Bristow DR. Molecular mechanisms of benzodiazepine-induced down-regulation of GABAA receptor alpha 1 subunit protein in rat cerebellar granule cells. *Br J Pharmacol* 1996;118(5):1103–1110.
99. Lopez A, Rebollo J. Benzodiazepine withdrawal syndrome after a benzodiazepine antagonist. *Crit Care Med* 1990;18(12):1480–1481.
100. Mintzer MZ, Stoller KB, Griffiths RR. A controlled study of flumazenil-precipitated withdrawal in chronic low-dose benzodiazepine users. *Psychopharmacology (Berl)* 1999;147(2):200–209.
101. Thomas P, Lebrun C, Chatel M. De novo absence status epilepticus as a benzodiazepine withdrawal syndrome. *Epilepsia* 1993;34(2):355–358.
102. Pritchard GA, Galpern WR, Lumpkin M, et al. Chronic benzodiazepine administration. VIII. Receptor upregulation produced by chronic exposure to the inverse agonist FG-7142. *J Pharmacol Exp Ther* 1991;258(1):280–285.
103. Saano V. Central-type and peripheral-type benzodiazepine receptors. *Ann Clin Res* 1988;20(5):348–355.
104. Pelissolo A. [The benzodiazepine receptor: the enigma of the endogenous ligand]. *Encephale* 1995;21(2):133–140.
105. Sand P, Kavvadias D, Feineis D, et al. Naturally occurring benzodiazepines: current status of research and clinical implications. *Eur Arch Psychiatry Clin Neurosci* 2000;250(4):194–202.
106. Dencker SJ, Johansson G, Milsom I. Quantification of naturally occurring benzodiazepine-like substances in human breast milk. *Psychopharmacology (Berl)* 1992;107(1):69–72.
107. Guidotti A, Forchetti CM, Corda MG, et al. Isolation, characterization, and purification to homogeneity of an endogenous polypeptide with agonistic action on benzodiazepine receptors. *Proc Natl Acad Sci U S A* 1983;80(11):3531–3535.
108. Papadopoulos V, Berkovich A, Krueger KE, et al. Diazepam binding inhibitor and its processing products stimulate mitochondrial steroid biosynthesis via an interaction with mitochondrial benzodiazepine receptors. *Endocrinology* 1991;129(3):1481–1488.
109. Costa E, Guidotti A. Diazepam binding inhibitor (DBI): a peptide with multiple biological actions. *Life Sci* 1991;49(5):325–344.
110. Kanto JH. Use of benzodiazepines during pregnancy, labour and lactation, with particular reference to pharmacokinetic considerations. *Drugs* 1982;23(5):354–380.
111. McElhatton PR. The effects of benzodiazepine use during pregnancy and lactation. *Reprod Toxicol* 1994;8(6):461–475.
112. Gueye PN, Lofaso F, Borron SW, et al. Mechanism of respiratory insufficiency in pure or mixed drug-induced coma involving benzodiazepines. *J Toxicol Clin Toxicol* 2002;40(1):35–47.
113. Oshima T, Masaki Y, Toyooka H. Flumazenil antagonizes midazolam-induced airway narrowing during nasal breathing in humans. *Br J Anaesth* 1999;82(5):698–702.
114. Mullins ME. First-degree atrioventricular block in alprazolam overdose reversed by flumazenil. *J Pharm Pharmacol* 1999;51(3):367–370.
115. Primavera A, Cocito L. Acute confusion in a chronic benzodiazepine patient. Withdrawal-related nonconvulsive status epilepticus misdiagnosed as acute intoxication. *Gen Hosp Psychiatry* 1995;17(6):460–462.
116. Noyes R Jr, Clancy J, Coryell WH, et al. A withdrawal syndrome after abrupt discontinuation of alprazolam. *Am J Psychiatry* 1985;142(1):114–116.
117. Mets B, Horsell A, Linton DM. Midazolam-induced benzodiazepine withdrawal syndrome. *Anaesthesia* 1991;46(1):28–29.
118. Hantson P, Clemessy JL, Baud FJ. Withdrawal syndrome following midazolam infusion. *Intensive Care Med* 1995;21(2):190–191.
119. Sury MR, Billingham I, Russell GN, et al. Acute benzodiazepine withdrawal syndrome after midazolam infusions in children. *Crit Care Med* 1989;17(3):301–302.
120. Bergman U, Griffiths RR. Relative abuse of diazepam and oxazepam: prescription forgeries and theft/loss reports in Sweden. *Drug Alcohol Depend* 1986;16(4):293–301.
121. Woods JH, Winger G. Abuse liability of flunitrazepam. *J Clin Psychopharmacol* 1997;17[3 Suppl 2]:1S–57S.
122. Lee KK, Chan TY, Chan AW, et al. Use and abuse of benzodiazepines in Hong Kong 1990–1993—the impact of regulatory changes. *J Toxicol Clin Toxicol* 1995;33(6):597–602.
123. Schwartz HI. An empirical review of the impact of triplicate prescription of benzodiazepines. *Hosp Community Psychiatry* 1992;43(4):382–385.
124. Crawford PJ, Fisher BM. Recreational overdosage of carbamazepine in Paisley drug abusers. *Scott Med J* 1997;42(2):44–45.
125. Kosnett M, Larson S, McCarthy T, et al. Investigation of an anion gap of minus 88 in a patient taking bromazepam. *Clin Chem* 1990;36:1040.
126. Boussairi A, Dupeyron JP, Hernandez B, et al. Urine benzodiazepines screening of involuntarily drugged and robbed or raped patients. *J Toxicol Clin Toxicol* 1996;34(6):721–724.
127. Verstraete AG, Belpaire FM, Leroux-Roels GG. Diagnostic performance of the EMIT-tox benzodiazepine immunoassay, FPIA serum benzodiazepine immunoassay, and radioreceptor assay in suspected acute poisoning. *J Anal Toxicol* 1998;22(1):27–32.
128. Divanon F, Debruyne D, Moulin M, et al. Benzodiazepines: toxic serum concentrations in positive enzyme immunoassay responses. *J Anal Toxicol* 1998;22(7):559–566.
129. Pounder DJ, Jones GR. Post-mortem drug redistribution—a toxicological nightmare. *Forensic Sci Int* 1990;45(3):253–263.
130. Robertson MD, Drummer OH. Postmortem distribution and redistribution of nitrobenzodiazepines in man. *J Forensic Sci* 1998;43(1):9–13.
131. Ahrens B, Rochholz G, Westphal F, et al. [Fatal outcome of poisoning with the benzodiazepines flunitrazepam and diazepam]. *Arch Kriminol* 2002;209(3–4):95–101.
132. Cirimele V, Kintz P, Ludes B. Screening for forensically relevant benzodiazepines in human hair by gas chromatography-negative ion chemical ionization-mass spectrometry. *J Chromatogr B Biomed Sci Appl* 1997;700(1–2):119–129.
133. Trestrail JH, III. *Criminal poisoning: investigational guide for law enforcement, toxicologists, forensic scientists, and attorneys.* Totowa, NJ: Humana Press, 2000.
134. Yegles M, Marson Y, Wennig R. Influence of bleaching on stability of benzodiazepines in hair. *Forensic Sci Int* 2000;107(1–3):87–92.
135. Edinboro LE, Backer RC. Preliminary report on the application of a high performance liquid chromatographic method for alprazolam in postmortem blood specimens. *J Anal Toxicol* 1985;9(5):207–208.
136. Jenkins AJ, Levine B, Locke JL, et al. A fatality due to alprazolam intoxication. *J Anal Toxicol* 1997;21(3):218–220.
137. Michaud K, Augsburger M, Romain N, et al. Fatal overdose of tramadol and alprazolam. *Forensic Sci Int* 1999;105(3):185–189.
138. Rogers WO, Hall MA, Brissie RM, et al. Detection of alprazolam in three cases of methadone/benzodiazepine overdose. *J Forensic Sci* 1997;42(1):155–156.
139. Kintz P, Tracqui A, Ludes B, et al. Fly larvae and their relevance in forensic toxicology. *Am J Forensic Med Pathol* 1990;11(1):63–65.
140. Brehmer C, Hem PX. A fatal bromazepam poisoning. *Bulletin of the International Association of Forensic Toxicology* 1992;24(4):21–22.
141. Moriya F, Hashimoto Y. Tissue distribution of nitrazepam and 7-aminonitrazepam in a case of nitrazepam intoxication. *Forensic Sci Int* 2003;131(2–3):108–112.
142. Langford AM, Taylor KK, Pounder DJ. Drug concentration in selected skeletal muscles. *J Forensic Sci* 1998;43(1):22–27.
143. Levine B, Grieshaber A, Pestaner J, et al. Distribution of triazolam and alpha-hydroxytriazolam in a fatal intoxication case. *J Anal Toxicol* 2002;26(1):52–54.
144. Baselt RC. *Drug effects on psychomotor performance.* Foster City, CA: Biomedical Publications, 2001.
145. Weinbroum A, Rudick V, Sorkine P, et al. Long-term intravenous and oral flumazenil treatment of acute diazepam overdose in an older patient. *J Am Geriatr Soc* 1996;44(6):737–738.
146. Burkhart KK, Kulig KW. The diagnostic utility of flumazenil (a benzodiazepine antagonist) in coma of unknown etiology. *Ann Emerg Med* 1990;19(3):319–321.
147. Hojer J, Baehrendtz S, Matell G, et al. Diagnostic utility of flumazenil in coma with suspected poisoning: a double blind, randomised controlled study [see comments]. *BMJ* 1990;301(6764):1308–1311.
148. Hoffman RS, Goldfrank LR. The poisoned patient with altered consciousness. Controversies in the use of a 'coma cocktail'. *JAMA* 1995;274(7):562–569.
149. Amrein R, Hetzel W, Hartmann D, et al. Clinical pharmacology of flumazenil. *Eur J Anaesthesiol Suppl* 1988;2:65–80.
150. Short TG, Maling T, Galletly DC. Ventricular arrhythmia precipitated by flumazenil. *Br Med J (Clin Res Ed)* 1988;296(6628):1070–1071.

151. Herd B, Clarke F. Complete heart block after flumazenil. *Hum Exp Toxicol* 1991;10(4):289.
152. Lheureux P, Vranckx M, Leduc D, et al. Flumazenil in mixed benzodiazepine/tricyclic antidepressant overdose: a placebo-controlled study in the dog. *Am J Emerg Med* 1992;10(3):184–188.
153. Mordel A, Winkler E, Almog S, et al. Seizures after flumazenil administration in a case of combined benzodiazepine and tricyclic antidepressant overdose. *Crit Care Med* 1992;20(12):1733–1734.
154. Derlet RW, Albertson TE. Flumazenil induces seizures and death in mixed cocaine-diazepam intoxications. *Ann Emerg Med* 1994;23(3):494–498.
155. Haverkos GP, DiSalvo RP, Imhoff TE. Fatal seizures after flumazenil administration in a patient with mixed overdose. *Ann Pharmacother* 1994;28(12):1347–1349.
156. Chern TL, Kwan A. Flumazenil-induced seizure accompanying benzodiazepine and baclofen intoxication. *Am J Emerg Med* 1996;14(2):231–232.
157. Gueye PN, Hoffman JR, Taboulet P, et al. Empiric use of flumazenil in comatose patients: limited applicability of criteria to define low risk. *Ann Emerg Med* 1996;27(6):730–735.
158. Schulze-Bonhage A, Elger CE. Induction of partial epileptic seizures by flumazenil. *Epilepsia* 2000;41(2):186–192.
159. Thurston TA, Williams CG, Foshee SL. Reversal of a paradoxical reaction to midazolam with flumazenil. *Anesth Analg* 1996;83(1):192.
160. Fulton SA, Mullen KD. Completion of upper endoscopic procedures despite paradoxical reaction to midazolam: a role for flumazenil? *Am J Gastroenterol* 2000;95(3):809–811.
161. Balogh A, Funfstuck R, Demme U, et al. Dialysability of benzodiazepines by haemodialysis and controlled sequential ultrafiltration (CSU) in vitro. *Acta Pharmacol Toxicol (Copenh)* 1981;49(3):174–180.
162. Ochs HR, Greenblatt DJ, Burstein ES, et al. Pharmacokinetics and CSF entry of flurazepam in dogs. *Pharmacology* 1988;36(3):166–171.
163. Oo CY, Kuhn RJ, Desai N, et al. Pharmacokinetics in lactating women: prediction of alprazolam transfer into milk. *Br J Clin Pharmacol* 1995;40(3):231–236.
164. Dollery CT. *Therapeutic drugs*. CD-ROM DATABASE Release 1.0 ed. London: Churchill Livingstone, 1999.
165. Fisher JB, Edgren BE, Mammel MC, et al. Neonatal apnea associated with maternal clonazepam therapy: a case report. *Obstet Gynecol* 1985;66[3 Suppl]:34S–35S.
166. Rey E, Giraux P, d'Athis P, et al. Pharmacokinetics of the placental transfer and distribution of clorazepate and its metabolite nordiazepam in the fetoplacental unit and in the neonate. *Eur J Clin Pharmacol* 1979;15(3):181–185.
167. Dusci LJ, Good SM, Hall RW, et al. Excretion of diazepam and its metabolites in human milk during withdrawal from combination high dose diazepam and oxazepam. *Br J Clin Pharmacol* 1990;29(1):123–126.
168. Humpel M, Stoppelli I, Milia S, et al. Pharmacokinetics and biotransformation of the new benzodiazepine, lormetazepam, in man. III. Repeated administration and transfer to neonates via breast milk. *Eur J Clin Pharmacol* 1982;21(5):421–425.
169. Matheson I, Lunde PK, Bredesen JE. Midazolam and nitrazepam in the maternity ward: milk concentrations and clinical effects. *Br J Clin Pharmacol* 1990;30(6):787–793.
170. Brodie RR, Chasseaud LF, Taylor T. Concentrations of N-descyclopropylmethylprazepam in whole-blood, plasma, and milk after administration of prazepam to humans. *Biopharm Drug Dispos* 1981;2(1):59–68.
171. Hilbert JM, Gural RP, Symchowicz S, et al. Excretion of quazepam into human breast milk. *J Clin Pharmacol* 1984;24(10):457–462.

CHAPTER 133

Monoamine Oxidase Inhibitors

Ian MacGregor Whyte

See Figure 1.

Compounds included:	**See Table 1.**
Molecular formula and weight:	**See Table 1.**
SI conversion:	**See Table 1.**
CAS Registry No.:	**See Table 1.**
Therapeutic levels:	**See Table 1.**
Target organs:	**Central nervous system (acute), cardiac (acute)**
Antidotes:	**Consider cyproheptadine/chlorpromazine for serotonin toxicity.**

OVERVIEW

The monoamine oxidase (MAO) inhibitors used in the management of depressive disorders consist of a group of older drugs, which tend to be nonselective and irreversible inhibitors of MAO-A and MAO-B, and a second group of compounds that reversibly inhibit MAO-A only (RIMAs). Some MAO inhibitors are selective and irreversible [e.g., clorgyline (MAO-A), rasagiline (MAO-B)]; they are not discussed here, as they are now used only experimentally (clorgyline) (1) or as an anti-Parkinson drug (rasagiline) (2). The MAO inhibitors that selectively block MAO-B [selegiline (irreversible), lazabemide (reversible)] are covered with Parkinson's disease drugs (Chapter 139).

The older, nonselective, irreversible drugs have very severe and prolonged toxicity in overdose and potentially life-threatening interactions with tyramine in food and many drugs. The newer, selective, reversible drugs have a much more benign profile in overdose and are safe with food but may still have life-threatening toxicity when combined with serotonergic drugs. The fatal toxicity index of the MAO inhibitors as a group (27 deaths per million prescriptions) in England, Scotland, and Wales between 1985 and 1989 was significantly lower than the mean of all drugs (35.6), although that of tranylcypromine was higher (3).

Structure, Classification, and Uses

Some aspects of the chemistry of these drugs are shown in Table 1, and structural diagrams are in Figure 1. Tranylcypromine is a chiral cyclopropylamine derivative that is used as a racemic mixture (4), whereas the other older MAO inhibitors (iproniazid, isocarboxazid, and phenelzine) are all hydrazine derivatives. Iproniazid is the isopropyl derivative of isoniazid (5) that was developed for use in tuberculosis (6) and has been found to be beneficial when depression complicates the disease (7). It has been withdrawn from use, even as an antidepressant, in most countries, however, because of its tendency to produce a fulminant or subfulminant autoimmune hepatitis (8). The irreversible, nonselective MAO inhibitors are primarily indicated in major depression (9) but have found use in anxiety and phobic states, panic disorder, obsessive/compulsive disorders, chronic pain, bulimia nervosa, and narcolepsy (10).

The RIMAs are less structurally related than the traditional MAO inhibitors (Table 1, Fig. 1). Nevertheless, comparative

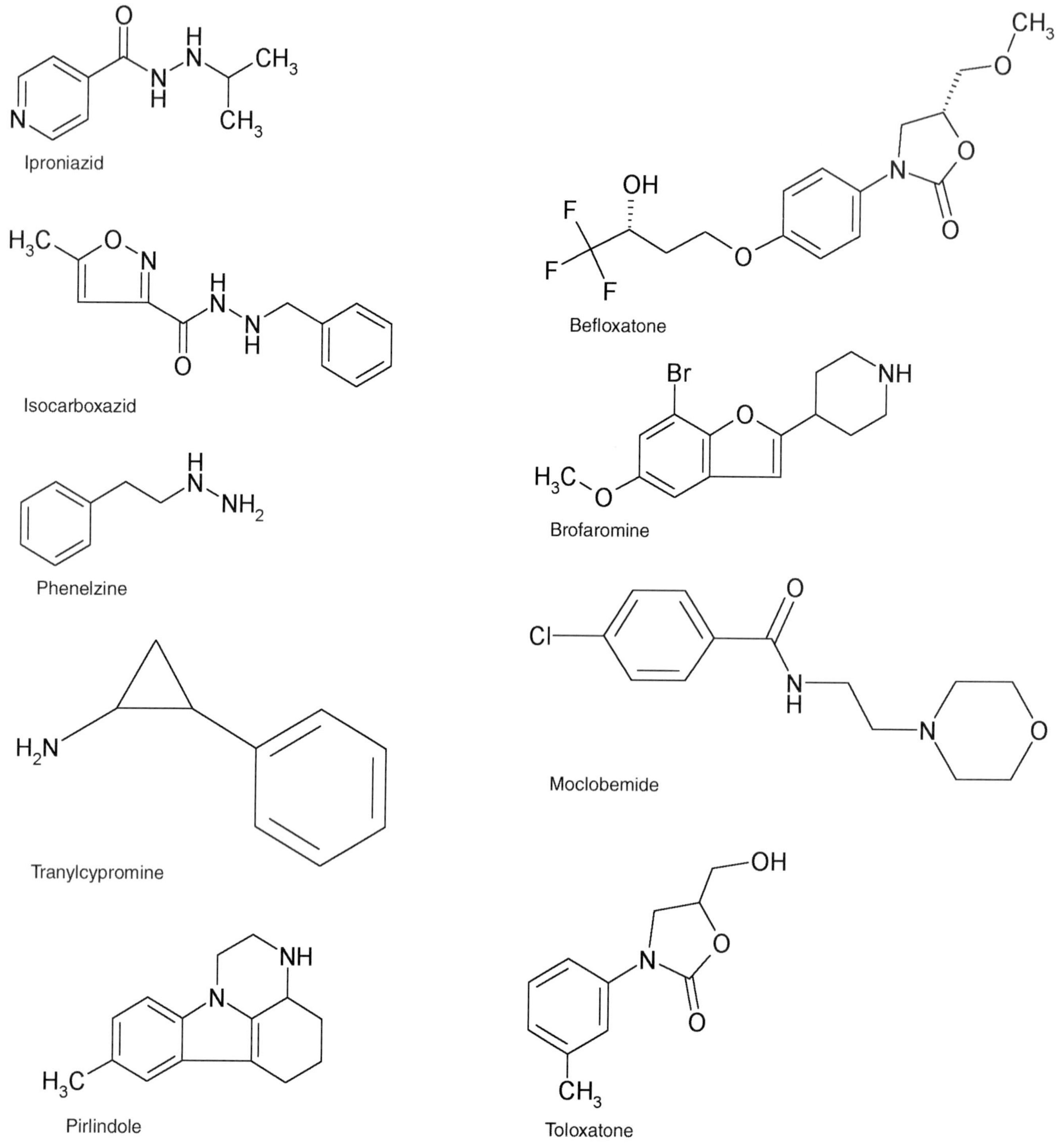

Iproniazid

Befloxatone

Isocarboxazid

Brofaromine

Phenelzine

Moclobemide

Tranylcypromine

Pirlindole

Toloxatone

Figure 1. Structures of the monoamine oxidase inhibitors.

analysis of these drugs reveals that all such inhibitors have a phenolic ring with a neighboring negatively charged nitrogen or oxygen atom; the phenol ring is an ultimate precondition for the manifestation of MAO-A inhibitory activity (11). Befloxatone and toloxatone are oxazolidinone derivatives, whereas brofaromine is a brominated piperidine derivative that bears some resemblance to the analgesic tramadol. Moclobemide is a benzamide and pirlindole a chiral pyrazinocarbazole derivative. By far, the most clinical experience has been with moclobemide, which is indicated in the treatment of depression and social phobia and has been used in post-traumatic stress disorder, panic disorder, and smoking cessation (9).

Toxic Dose

The adult and pediatric therapeutic doses for MAO inhibitors as therapy for major depression are provided in Table 2. The nonselective, irreversible MAO inhibitors have potentially fatal interactions with food containing tyramine (12–14) and some other foodstuffs (Table 3) and a variety of drugs (Table 4). Knowledge

TABLE 1. Physical characteristics of monoamine oxidase inhibitors

Compounds included	Molecular formula, molecular weight (g/mol), CAS Registry No.	SI conversion; therapeutic, toxic concentrations	*United States Pharmacopoeia Dictionary of Drug Names*
Nonselective, irreversible inhibitors			
Iproniazid (Marsilid)	$C_9H_{13}N_3O,H_3PO_4$, 179.2, 305-33-9	mg/L × 5.58 = μmol/L; 5 mg/L, N/A	2-(1-methylethyl)hydrazide-4-pyridinecarboxylic acid
Isocarboxazid (Marplan)	$C_{12}H_{13}N_3O_2$, 231.3, 59-63-2	mg/L × 4.32 = μmol/L; N/A, N/A	5-methyl-3-isoxazolecarboxylic acid 2-benzylhydrazide
Phenelzine (Nardil)	$C_8H_{12}N_2,H_2SO_4$, 136.2, 156-51-4	mg/L × 7.34 = μmol/L; 0.02 mg/L, 0.5 mg/L	(2-phenylethyl)-hydrazine
Tranylcypromine (Parnate)	$(C_9H_{11}N)_2,H_2SO_4$, 133.2, 13492-01-8	mg/L × 7.51 = μmol/L; 0.1 mg/L, 0.3 mg/L	2-phenyl-, trans-(+–)-cyclopropanamine
Selective, reversible inhibitors			
Befloxatone	$C_{15}H_{18}F_3NO_5$, 349.3, 134564-82-2	mg/L × 2.86 = μmol/L; N/A, N/A	(R)-5-(methoxymethyl)-3-(p-[(R)-4,4,4-trifluoro-3-hydroxybutoxy]phenyl)-2-oxazolidinone
Brofaromine	$C_{14}H_{16}BrNO_2$, 310.2, 63638-91-5	mg/L × 3.22 = μmol/L; N/A, N/A	4-(7-bromo-5-methoxy-2-benzofuranyl)piperidine
Moclobemide (Aurorix)	$C_{13}H_{17}ClN_2O_2$, 268.7, 71320-77-9	mg/L × 3.72 = μmol/L; 2 mg/L, 20 mg/L	p-chloro-N-(2-morpholinoethyl)benzamide
Pirlindole (Implementor)	$C_{15}H_{18}N_2$, 226.3, 60762-57-4	mg/L × 4.42 = μmol/L; N/A, N/A	2,3,3a,4,5,6-hexahydro-8-methyl-1H-pyrazino(3,2,1-jk)carbazole
Toloxatone (Umoril)	$C_{11}H_{13}NO_3$, 207.2, 29218-27-7	mg/L × 4.83 = μmol/L; N/A, N/A	5-(hydroxymethyl)-3-m-tolyl-2-oxazolidinone

N/A, not available.
From Flanagan RJ. Guidelines for the interpretation of analytical toxicology results and unit of measurement conversion factors. *Ann Clin Biochem* 1998;35(Pt 2):261–267, with permission.

of the food-drug interaction has even led to attempted suicide by cheese in a patient on an MAO inhibitor (15).

A significant overdose (greater than 1 mg/kg tranylcypromine, greater than 2 mg/kg phenelzine, or any amount of another nonreversible agent) can produce acute severe toxicity. In the context of an overdose with the MAO inhibitors (iproniazid, isocarboxazid, phenelzine, tranylcypromine, toloxatone) and another serotonergic agent, even therapeutic doses of an MAO may combine to produce life-threatening toxicity.

TABLE 2. Typical therapeutic doses of monoamine oxidase inhibitors for major depression

Drug	Formulations	Adult dose[a]
Iproniazid	NR	50–150 mg/d; some patients may respond to 25–50 mg/d or every other day
Isocarboxazid	NR	30 mg/d in single or divided doses; some patients may respond to 10–20 mg/d; one-half the normal maintenance dose may be adequate in the elderly
Phenelzine	15-mg tablet	15 mg 3 times daily; some patients may respond to 15 mg on alternate days
Tranylcypromine	10-mg tablet	10 mg in the morning and 10 mg in the afternoon; some patients may continue to respond to 10 mg/d
Befloxatone	NR	Investigational, suggested dose 20 mg/d (62)
Brofaromine	NR	50–150 mg/d
Moclobemide	NR	300 mg by mouth in divided doses; this can be increased to up to 600 mg/d according to response; in some patients, a maintenance dose of 150 mg/d may be sufficient
Pirlindole	NR	Up to a maximum of 400 mg/d
Toloxatone	NR	200 mg 3 times daily

NR, not reported.
[a]Pediatric use not reported.
From Sweetman S. Martindale: the complete drug reference. London: Pharmaceutical Press. Electronic ed. expires 3/2003. Greenwood Village, CO: MICROMEDEX, 2003, with permission.

Little information is available about iproniazid, although death has occurred (16). Isocarboxazid ingestion of 300 mg was survived by a 48-year-old woman (17). A 35-year-old woman took 1 g isocarboxazid with suicidal intent and became comatose, with poor ventilation, increasing rigidity of all muscles, and temperature rising to 41.1°C, requiring intubation and ventilation (18).

Psychotic phenomena [particularly delusional parasitosis (19,20)] can occur on therapeutic doses of phenelzine (21), as well as being a feature of phenelzine withdrawal (22). It is a feature of phenelzine withdrawal as well (22). A 2-year-old child survived ingestion of 150 to 225 mg (23), and adults have survived doses of 900 (24) to 2250 mg (25). On the other hand, overdoses of 375 to 1500 mg have resulted in death (26), leading to the suggestion that more than 2 to 3 mg/kg may be life threatening and more than 4 to 6 mg/kg may be fatal (27).

Tranylcypromine has been marketed as a combination product with trifluoperazine (Jatrosom, Parmodalin, Parstelin, Stelapar) (9). Therapy with twice the usual dose of this combination has resulted in severe neuroleptic malignant syndrome (28) (Chapter 23), and overdose of the product produces severe poisoning (29), which may be fatal in adults (30,31) and children (32). Even accidental poisoning in childhood is problematic (33).

Ingestion of 400 mg tranylcypromine resulted in only mild symptoms of intoxication (34), and regular ingestion of 440 mg (35) to 600 mg (36) tranylcypromine daily in patients with a dependence on MAO inhibitors may be tolerated without side effects until they are abruptly ceased (36). Doses of 200 to 900 mg have been survived (37–40) with varying degrees of toxicity, whereas doses of 130 to 850 mg (more than 2 to 3 mg/kg) have resulted in death (30,31,41–44). More than 1 mg/kg is likely to be a significant poisoning.

Moclobemide has produced serotonin (5-HT) toxicity and has been reported with therapeutic doses of various serotonergic

TABLE 3. Foods interacting with monoamine oxidase inhibitors

Food	Interaction
Food containing tyramine	
Avocados	Particularly if overripe.
Bananas	Reactions can occur if eaten in large amounts; tyramine levels high in peel.
Bean curd	Fermented bean curd, fermented soy bean, soy bean pastes, soy sauces, and miso soup, prepared from fermented bean curd; all contain tyramine in large amounts.
Beer and ale	Some imported brands have had high levels; nonalcoholic beer may contain tyramine and should be avoided.
Caviar	Safe if vacuum packed and eaten fresh or refrigerated only briefly.
Cheese	Reactions possible with most, except unfermented varieties such as cottage cheese; in others, tyramine concentration is higher near rind and close to fermentation holes.
Figs	Particularly if overripe.
Fish	Safe if fresh, dried products should not be eaten; caution required in restaurants; vacuum-packed products are safe if eaten promptly or refrigerated only briefly.
Liver	Safe if very fresh but rapidly accumulates tyramine; caution required in restaurants.
Milk products	Milk and yogurt appear to be safe.
Protein extracts	See also Soups; avoid liquid and powdered protein dietary supplements.
Meat	Safe if known to be fresh; caution required in restaurants.
Sausage	Fermented varieties, such as bologna, pepperoni, and salami, have a high tyramine content.
Shrimp paste	Contains large amounts of tyramine.
Soups	May contain protein extracts and should be avoided.
Soy sauce	Contains large amounts of tyramine; reactions have occurred with teriyaki.
Wines	Generally do not contain tyramine, but many reactions have been reported with Chianti, champagne, and other wines.
Yeast extracts	Dietary supplements (e.g., Marmite, contain large amounts); yeast in baked goods, however, is safe.
Food not containing tyramine	
Caffeine	A weak pressor agent; large amounts may cause reactions.
Chocolate	Contains phenylethylamine, a pressor agent that can cause reactions in large amounts.
Fava beans (broad beans, "Italian" green beans)	Contain dopamine, a pressor amine, particularly when overripe.
Ginseng	Some preparations have caused headache, tremulousness, and manic-like symptoms.
Liqueurs	Reactions reported with some (e.g., Chartreuse and Drambuie); cause unknown.
New Zealand prickly spinach	Single case report; patient ate large amounts.
Whiskey	Reactions have occurred; cause unknown.

Modified from Food interacting with MAO inhibitors. *Med Lett Drugs Ther* 1989;31(785):11–12.

drugs in combination with moclobemide. These include fluoxetine (45), meperidine (46), and citalopram (47). In one case, 5-HT toxicity with trismus developed on moclobemide alone and was fatal (48). A small series of 11 patients suggested that a serotonic reuptake inhibitor and moclobemide might be well tolerated (49). However, in a series of 50 depressed patients, moclobemide (up to 600 mg per day) was added to paroxetine or fluoxetine (20 mg/day) for 6 weeks to assess tolerability. A high rate of serotonergic adverse events occurred (50), many severe, and in the absence of convincing evidence for efficacy of such a combination there is no indication to prescribe these drugs together (51).

A review of single-drug intoxications with moclobemide at doses of up to 20.55 g revealed no deaths due solely to moclobemide overdose. All patients recovered fully within 1 to 7 days (52). In a study performed at a single toxicology treatment center, no deaths, complications, or major toxic effects occurred in 33 patients who took moclobemide alone despite a median ingested dose of 6 g (range, 0.9 to 18.0 g). In the patient who ingested 18 g, hyperreflexia, tachycardia, and a temperature of 37.4°C developed but no other significant effects (53). Death has been reported due to deliberate ingestion of moclobemide alone (54,55); in one case the estimated dose was 4.5 g (56).

Toloxatone therapy has produced fulminant and fatal hepatitis (57). In a series of 122 overdose cases, the minimal toxic dose was 2 g (58). Two of the patients died, one of whom took 6 g toloxatone together with clomipramine and lorazepam, became comatose, developed bilateral mydriasis and hyperthermia, and died in asystole (58).

TOXICOKINETICS AND TOXICODYNAMICS

The pharmacokinetics of the MAO inhibitors are provided in Table 5. Because the time course of action of the irreversible agents is dependent on the kinetics of MAO, there is no correlation between plasma concentrations and primary effect for these agents. However, some evidence has shown that some of the other effects may be correlated with plasma concentration. For example, standing systolic blood pressure is negatively correlated with plasma concentration after a dose of tranylcypromine, with the blood pressure minimum occurring at the time of peak concentration (59).

Little information is available on iproniazid or isocarboxazid. The peak plasma concentration of phenelzine after a 30-mg dose was 0.002 mg/L (60). Phenelzine concentrations of 1.5 and 2.0 mg/L were seen after overdose in two of three cases (61).

After a single oral 20-mg dose of tranylcypromine, mean peak plasma concentration in nine subjects was 0.112 mg/L (range, 0.0645 to 0.190 mg/L) (59). Tranylcypromine concentration in a case of fatal tranylcypromine-food interaction was 0.102 mg/L (14). After ingestion of 400 mg tranylcypromine, blood concentration was 0.5 mg/L, with mild symptoms of intoxication (34). In a fatal overdose estimated at 550 mg, antemortem tranylcypromine blood concentration was 0.611 mg/L (44). A befloxatone single 10-mg dose produced a peak concentration of 0.03 mg/L (62). A brofaromine single 75-mg dose produced a peak concentration of 0.37 mg/L (63).

A single 300-mg dose of moclobemide produced peak concentrations of 1.46 to 2.96 mg/L (64). In three cases of moclobemide overdose, plasma moclobemide was 2.8 mg/L at 2 hours in the first case; in case 2, 18 mg/L; and, in case 3, 60.9 mg/L at 2 hours and 4.6 mg/L 12 hours later. None of the patients showed serious effects during 24 hours of observation (65). Seizures, tachycardia, and hyperthermia occurred after a 10-g ingestion, with a plasma moclobemide concentration of 36.5 mg/L 6 hours after ingestion (66).

In five cases with estimated doses of 1.8, 3.0, 6.0, 9.0, and 12.0 g, the peak concentrations were 25, 8, 28, 30, and 50 mg/L, respectively (53). Overall, moclobemide metabolism and elimination do not appear to be saturable, even with extreme doses and very high plasma concentrations (53). Because of the considerable interindividual variation in clearance, some individuals have prolonged elimination half-lives (53,67,68) and consequently prolonged clinical effects, as these correlate with plasma moclobemide concentrations (53).

TABLE 4. Monoamine oxidase inhibitor (MAOI)–drug interactions

Drug	Interaction
Sympathomimetic agents	MAOIs potentiate the effects of all these agents, but dangerous interactions with CNS stimulation, hypertension, organ damage, or intracranial bleeding are more likely when indirect-acting drugs of this class are used.
CNS depressants	
Meperidine (Demerol), dextromethorphan (in many over-the-counter cough suppressants)	Dangerous interaction with MAOIs, characterized by hyperpyrexia, seizures, and coma
Other narcotics, other CNS depressants, anesthetics, alcohol, antihistamines, barbiturates, nonbarbiturate sedatives, benzodiazepines (e.g., diazepam), neuroleptics (e.g., haloperidol), anticonvulsants (e.g., phenytoin)	MAOIs potentiate the effects of all of these agents, leading to CNS depression and, at times, intoxication.
Antihypertensive agents	
Reserpine (Serpasil), α-methyldopa (Aldomet), guanethidine (Esimil and Ismelin)	Combination of these agents with an MAOI can lead to paradoxic hypertension and CNS excitation.
Clonidine (Catapres)	MAOIs may potentiate its effects.
Hydralazine (Apresoline)	MAOIs potentiate its effects.
Diuretics (e.g., hydrochlorothiazide)	Combination with an MAOI can lead to hypotension.
Sympathetic receptor blocking agents	
α-Antagonists (e.g., phentolamine)	MAOIs may potentiate the effects of these agents.
Beta-blockers (e.g., propranolol)	MAOI effects on these agents are unpredictable; frequently, effects are inhibited early and potentiated later.
Antidysrhythmic agents	
Bretylium (Bretylol)	Additive adrenergic effects.
Anticholinergic and antiparkinsonian agents	
Atropine, scopolamine (e.g., Donnatal)	MAOIs potentiate these agents and can lead to atropine intoxication syndrome; these agents may also decrease the metabolism of MAOIs.
L-Dopa (Dopar, Larodopa)	MAOIs potentiate its effects and can lead to unpredictable changes in blood pressure and may induce CNS excitation or intoxication.
Antibiotics	
Nitrofurans (Macrodantin)	These antimicrobial agents have MAO inhibitory activity and can cause additive toxicity, with increased or decreased blood pressure, CNS excitation, and hyperpyrexia when given to MAOI-treated patients.
Sulfisoxazole (Gantrisin)	Combination with phenelzine has led to ataxia, vertigo, tinnitus, muscle pains, and paresthesia.
Neuromuscular-blocking agents	
Succinylcholine (Anectine)	Phenelzine may reduce cholinesterase, leading to prolonged apnea.
Atracurium (Tracrium)	May cause severe hypertension when combined with tranylcypromine.
Anticoagulants	
Coumarins (e.g., warfarin)	MAOIs may potentiate their effects.
Antidiabetics	
Insulin, oral hypoglycemics (e.g., chlorpropamide)	MAOIs may potentiate effects, leading to hypoglycemia.
Chemotherapeutic agents	
Procarbazine (Matulane)	This drug has MAO inhibitory activity and can cause additive toxicity, with increased or decreased blood pressure, CNS excitation, and hyperpyrexia when given to MAOI-treated patients.
Other psychopharmacologic agents	
Tricyclic antidepressants[a] (e.g., imipramine), carbamazepine (Tegretol)	Combination of MAO inhibitory effects can lead to additive toxicity with hypertension, hypotension, CNS excitation, and hyperpyrexia.
Fluoxetine (Prozac)	Additive toxicity from serotonergic excess.
Neuroleptics (e.g., haloperidol)	Increased anticholinergic side effects and extrapyramidal side effects.

CNS, central nervous system.
[a]Safe use of tricyclic antidepressant (TCA)–MAOI combinations has been reported in treating refractory depression. TCA and MAOI must be started simultaneously or the MAOI must be added to the TCA.
Modified from Lipson RE, Stern TA. Management of monoamine oxidase inhibitor–treated patients in the emergency and critical care setting. *J Intens Care Med* 1991;6:117–125.

A pirlindole single 75-mg dose, median peak plasma pirlindole concentration was 0.045 mg/L (range, 0.017 to 0.149 mg/L) (69). A toloxatone dose of 1 mg/kg orally produced peak toloxatone concentrations of 0.384 to 0.640 mg/L (70). In acute overdose, the toxicokinetic parameters (half-life 1.5 hours, total body clearance 0.56 L/kg/hour) were not significantly different from those reported with usual therapeutic doses (71).

PATHOPHYSIOLOGY

MAO catalyzes the oxidative deamination of a number of biogenic amines in the brain and peripheral tissues by the production of hydrogen peroxide (72). Two forms of MAO are known, A and B. They are made up of different polypeptides and coded by two genes located on the X chromosome but are structurally and functionally very close (72). MAO-A preferentially metabolizes 5-HT, norepinephrine, and dopamine, and MAO-B metabolizes phenylethylamine and benzylamine, although at high substrate concentrations there is considerable cross-metabolism (72). Tyramine is deaminated by MAO-A and MAO-B; thus, inhibiting only one of the enzymes allows for continued, albeit reduced, metabolism. The three-dimensional structure of MAO is shown in Figure 2 (73).

Flavin adenine dinucleotide (FAD) is an essential cofactor for both forms of MAO and the site of action of the MAO inhibitors.

TABLE 5. Pharmacokinetics of the monoamine oxidase inhibitors

Drug	Bioavailability (%)	Time to peak after oral dosing (h)	Volume of distribution (L/kg)	Clearance (L/h/kg)	Half-life (h)	Protein binding (%)	Active metabolites
Iproniazid	NR	NR	NR	NR	NR	NR	Hydrazine (hepatotoxic)
Isocarboxazid	Probably significant first-pass metabolism	4	NR	NR	36	NR	Benzylhydrazine
Phenelzine	NR	2–4	NR	NR	1.5–4.0	NR	β-Phenylethylamine
Tranylcypromine	NR	0.7–3.5	2.71 (1.11–5.68)	0.85 (0.38–2.4)	2.45 (1.54–3.15)	NR	*N*-acetyl-tranylcypromine, *N,O*-diacetyl-*p*-hydroxy-tranylcypromine
Befloxatone (62)	NR	2	NR	NR	11.1 ± 0.8	58	*o*-Desmethyl-befloxatone (22.2 ± 2.3)
Brofaromine	90	2	3.29	0.17	14.2 (12–15)	NR	*o*-Desmethyl-brofaromine
Moclobemide	49–90 saturable first-pass metabolism	1–2	1	0.73–1.29	1.6 (0.8–2.0)	50	Ring-opened M4 and N-oxidized M5 metabolites
Pirlindole	~30	1–2	NR	NR	2.03 (0.98–6.51)	NR	Dehydropirlindole
Toloxatone (70)	50–62	0.5–1.0	1.09–1.640	0.46–0.86	1–3	50	NR

NR, not reported.
From Dollery CT. Therapeutic drugs. CD-ROM DATABASE release, 1.0 ed. London: Churchill Livingstone, 1999; and Baker GB, Urichuk LJ, McKenna KF, et al. Metabolism of monoamine oxidase inhibitors. *Cell Biol Neurobiol* 1999;19(3):4411–4426, with permission.

The irreversible inhibitors first bind reversibly to FAD; then, by the same catalytic process as for substrates, they are transformed into intermediate reactive species that bind covalently to the enzyme through a reduced form of FAD (74). Moclobemide is also transformed by the flavin cofactor into a new reactive chemical entity after forming a reversible complex with the cofactor, but the new entity is unstable and rapidly disappears (74). The other reversible inhibitors form a weak reversible charge-transfer complex with FAD that inhibits the enzyme activity (74).

Inhibition of MAO results in elevation of the relevant neurotransmitters and consequent therapeutic effect and, in excess, toxicity. Thus, the selective MAO-A inhibitors exhibit predominantly serotonergic toxicity with some features of central norepinephrine and dopamine excess, but not as much as might be expected because of remaining MAO-B activity. The nonselective agents have greater toxicity because of the lack of alternative pathways of metabolism. Phenylethylamine is increased as a result of MAO-B inhibition and may contribute to the clinical

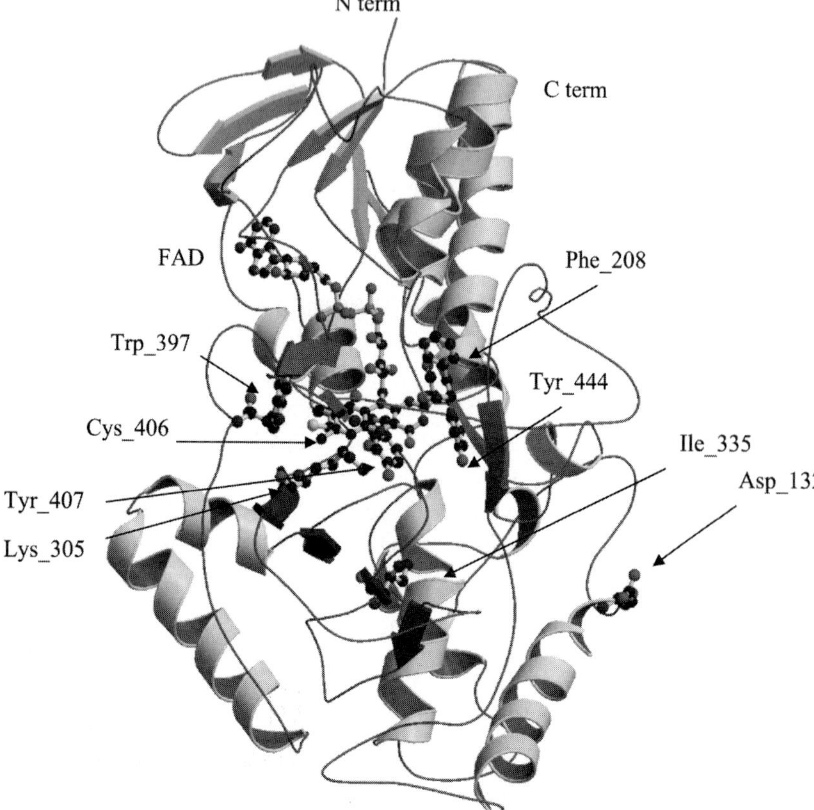

Figure 2. Three-dimensional model of human monoamine oxidase (MAO)-A and MAO-B. Secondary structures are presented using arrows for strands and cylinders for helices. The positions of the flavin adenine dinucleotide (FAD) cofactor and amino acids depicted are also given using the MAO-A numbering (73). The three-dimensional structure of human MAO-B is similar to the structure of MAO-A. The three domains of MAO are presented by broad arrows on the model: FAD noncovalent binding domain at the top, substrate binding domain at the bottom, and interface domain in the middle. [From Geha RM, Chen K, Wouters J, et al. Analysis of conserved active site residues in monoamine oxidase A and B and their three-dimensional molecular modeling. *J Biol Chem* 2002;277(19):17209–17216, with permission.]

manifestations of toxicity (40). Phenelzine is also metabolized in part to phenylethylamine (75). High concentrations of phenylethylamine, injected into mice, induce convulsions through unclear mechanisms that do not involve the benzodiazepine receptor (76).

The hepatotoxicity of iproniazid is mediated by mechanisms similar to that of isoniazid (77). Iproniazid is metabolized to isopropylhydrazine, which is further metabolized to highly reactive acylating and alkylating agents that covalently bind to liver macromolecules (78), resulting in an autoimmune hepatic injury (8) via a reactive metabolite/enzyme haptenization mechanism (79).

In addition to its effects on MAO-A, brofaromine has some 5-HT uptake inhibitory effect (80). Pirlindole inhibits 5-HT and norepinephrine uptake (81).

PREGNANCY AND LACTATION

The U.S. Food and Drug Administration pregnancy categories are provided in Table 6. For most of these drugs, no data are available on distribution into breast milk. Tranylcypromine is detectable in milk (82), but the significance of this is unknown. The small amounts of moclobemide found in breast milk suggest that the drug would be unlikely to be hazardous to infants (83).

TABLE 6. U.S. Food and Drug Administration (FDA) risk category and breast milk distribution of the monoamine oxidase inhibitors

Drug	FDA[a] (ADEC) pregnancy risk category	Distribution into breast milk
Iproniazid	NR (NR)	NR
Isocarboxazid	C (NR)	NR
Phenelzine	C (B3)	NR
Tranylcypromine	C (B2)	Detectable in breast milk, significance unknown (82)
Befloxatone	NR (NR)	NR
Brofaromine	NR (NR)	NR
Moclobemide	NR (B3)	1% of the weight-adjusted maternal daily dose (83)
Pirlindole	NR (NR)	NR
Toloxatone	NR (NR)	NR

ADEC, Australian Drug Evaluation Committee pregnancy categories; NR, not reported.
[a]Appendix I provides definitions of FDA pregnancy categories.
Category A. Drugs that have been taken by a large number of pregnant women and women of childbearing age without any proven increase in the frequency of malformations or other direct or indirect harmful effects on the fetus having been observed.
Category B1. Drugs that have been taken by only a limited number of pregnant women and women of childbearing age without an increase in the frequency of malformation or other direct or indirect harmful effects on the human fetus having been observed. Studies in animals have not shown evidence of an increased occurrence of fetal damage.
Category B2. Drugs that have been taken by only a limited number of pregnant women and women of childbearing age without an increase in the frequency of malformation or other direct or indirect harmful effects on the human fetus having been observed. Studies in animals are inadequate or may be lacking, but available data show no evidence of an increased occurrence of fetal damage.
Category B3. Drugs that have been taken by only a limited number of pregnant women and women of childbearing age without an increase in the frequency of malformation or other direct or indirect harmful effects on the human fetus having been observed. Studies in animals have shown evidence of an increased occurrence of fetal damage, the significance of which is considered uncertain in humans.
Category C. Drugs that, because of their pharmacologic effects, have caused or may be suspected of causing harmful effects on the human fetus or neonate without causing malformations. These effects may be reversible.
Category D. Drugs that have caused, are suspected to have caused, or may be expected to cause an increased incidence of human fetal malformations or irreversible damage. These drugs may also have adverse pharmacologic effects.
Category X. Drugs that have such a high risk of causing permanent damage to the fetus that they should not be used in pregnancy or when there is a possibility of pregnancy.
Note: For drugs in categories B1, B2, and B3, human data are lacking or inadequate and subcategorization is therefore based on available animal data. The allocation of a B category does not imply greater safety than the C category. Drugs in category D are not absolutely contraindicated in pregnancy (e.g., anticonvulsants). Moreover, in some cases the D category has been assigned on the basis of "suspicion."

CLINICAL PRESENTATION

Acute Overdosage

The nonselective, irreversible MAO inhibitors (iproniazid, isocarboxazid, phenelzine, tranylcypromine) produce the symptoms and signs of 5-HT toxicity (Chapter 24) with additional central nervous system and severe cardiovascular compromise (hyper- and hypotension). After a "latent" period of some hours (up to 6 to 12), restlessness, agitation, violent motor activity with moaning and grimacing, hyperreflexia and myoclonus, profuse sweating, and hallucinations may progressively develop. Other features of the central nervous system stimulation can include nystagmus, generalized hypertonia (84), jaw trismus (18), and an unusual periodic alternating gaze disturbance (alternating skew deviation) known as *ping-pong gaze* (85–87). At some stage during this process, the patient usually becomes comatose and may remain so for prolonged periods (88).

Patients may present with seriously elevated blood pressure, which may be followed by cardiovascular collapse (27) with hypotension (24) that may be unresponsive to fluids. Electrocardiographic abnormalities are unusual, although peaked T waves without hyperkalemia have been reported after tranylcypromine overdose (89). Intracranial hemorrhage may occur during the hypertensive phase. Severe, life-threatening hyperthermia (38,90) accompanied by tachycardia, tachypnea, metabolic acidosis and hypercapnia, temperatures exceeding 40°C, and muscle rigidity may peak as late as 24 hours after presentation. Multiorgan failure (16) with rhabdomyolysis and a consumptive coagulopathy, thrombocytopenia, and hemolysis (disseminated intravascular coagulation) (91) may ensue and, if so, is usually fatal (27).

Reversible inhibitors of MAO-A generally cause less severe toxicity. Little information is available on the acute toxicity of befloxatone, brofaromine, or pirlindole.

Moclobemide as a sole agent in overdose presents with a much more benign toxicity profile than that of the irreversible, nonselective MAO inhibitors even when very large doses are taken (53). Many patients are asymptomatic. Tachycardia, mild gastrointestinal symptoms, a slight increase in blood pressure, fatigue, and agitation may occur in symptomatic patients. In a series of 33 moclobemide-alone overdoses, no patients developed coma, seizures, or dysrhythmias; 21% developed a tachycardia; and 3% developed 5-HT toxicity, which was not severe (53).

In contrast, when patients coingested a serotonergic drug, 52% developed 5-HT toxicity (Chapter 24), of which half were severe (with temperature above 38.5°C and muscle rigidity interfering with ventilation requiring intubation and paralysis) (53). The incidence of 5-HT toxicity where moclobemide was taken with nonserotonergic coingestants (4%) was similar to that of moclobemide alone (53).

Case reports of severe 5-HT toxicity from moclobemide in combination with a serotonergic drug are common (92–95). The 5-HT toxicity may be severe enough to be fatal (67,96–105). Very occasionally, moclobemide alone can produce severe symptoms, such as convulsions, coma, muscle rigidity, respiratory failure, cardiovascular collapse, and hyperthermia (106), and death from moclobemide alone has been reported (54–56).

A toloxatone series of 122 cases found that the first symptoms appeared approximately 1 hour after ingestion. In most cases, only drowsiness and sinus tachycardia were observed (58). Coma, hypertonia, and myoclonic jerks occurred in a few cases with very large doses. In three cases of severe poisoning, toloxatone was taken with tricyclic antidepressants (TCAs), including clomipramine. Symptoms in these severe cases were muscular rigidity, hyperthermia, and cardiovascular collapse (58). Two of these severely poisoned patients died, one in asystole (58).

Acute Withdrawal

Symptoms associated with withdrawal of irreversible nonselective MAO inhibitors appear much sooner (hours to days) (107) than would be expected given the slow offset of the MAO inhibition. Symptoms may include anxiety, depression, confusion, hallucinations, psychosis (22), tremulousness, nausea, vomiting, diarrhea, and chills (108). Moclobemide is also associated with a withdrawal syndrome, which may present as a flu-like illness (109). The discontinuation syndrome does not respond to 5-HT uptake inhibitors (109), and moclobemide does not alleviate the discontinuation syndrome of 5-HT uptake inhibitors (110).

Adverse Reactions

MAO inhibitors may induce euphoriant-stimulating type and psychotomimetic effects in certain individuals, and the use of MAO inhibitors can be associated with dependence-tolerance (35,111). Rapid switching (with little or no antidepressant period) between irreversible MAO inhibitors may be dangerous (112), particularly if switching to tranylcypromine (113); however, others have suggested that there is no (114) or little problem (115).

Nonselective, irreversible MAO inhibitors have similar adverse effect profiles, with the exception of autoimmune hepatitis caused only by iproniazid (8). Common adverse effects of this group include orthostatic hypotension, sleep disturbances (including insomnia and, less commonly, hypersomnia), headache, drowsiness, fatigue, weakness, agitation, tremors, twitching, myoclonus, hyperreflexia, constipation, dry mouth, weight gain, impotence, loss of libido, and elevated serum transaminases (116). Infrequent effects include itch, rash, sweating, blurred vision, peripheral edema, and mania, and hypertensive crisis (tyramine or medication interactions), hepatocellular damage, leukopenia, and syndrome of inappropriate secretion of antidiuretic hormone occur rarely (116). The hypertensive crisis is characterized by severe occipital headache and a rapid and sometimes prolonged rise in blood pressure, which may result in intracranial hemorrhage or acute cardiac failure. If treatment is required, phentolamine, 2 to 5 mg intravenously (IV); nifedipine, 10 mg orally; or chlorpromazine, 50 mg IV, should be used and repeated as necessary (116).

Reversible inhibitors of MAO-A have less severe adverse effect profiles. The most frequent adverse effects reported on befloxatone were drowsiness (6.8%), headache (6.8%), and asthenia (6.8%). Nervousness and euphoria occurred in 1.5% with no complaints of insomnia (62). Brofaromine has a similar side effect profile to moclobemide, with dose-limiting side effects typically including nausea, insomnia, and tremor (117). Common adverse effects of moclobemide include nausea, dry mouth, constipation, diarrhea, anxiety, restlessness, insomnia, dizziness, and headache (116). Infrequent effects include visual disturbances, gastrointestinal complaints (feeling of fullness), rash, itch, urticaria, and flushing; sedation, hypertension, intrahepatic cholestasis, and peripheral edema occur rarely (116).

The adverse effect profile of pirlindole did not differ significantly from placebo in a small (N = 103) trial (118). Toloxatone had more sleep disturbance and anxiety but less hot flushes, dry mouth, constipation, and headache than moclobemide in a comparison trial (119).

Drug Interactions

MAO inhibitor drug interactions still occur and remain potentially fatal (120). Of particular importance is the interaction between MAO inhibitors and analgesics with serotonergic activity, such as meperidine (pethidine) (121,122), dextromethorphan (123), and tramadol (124). Drugs of abuse are also a significant problem, with a typical reaction occurring with 3,4-methylenedioxy-methamphetamine (Ecstasy) and phenelzine (125).

Concern has been raised about increased adverse effects when switching patients from a TCA to a traditional MAO inhibitor, although a limited retrospective study found no problems (126). In another retrospective study (chart review), the use of an MAO inhibitor–TCA combination in therapeutic doses appeared to be relatively safe (127). However, the efficacy of this combination has not yet been proven, and it may be particularly toxic if taken in an overdose (128). Clomipramine is the most serotonergic TCA by far and not safe to use with an MAO inhibitor (129). The therapeutic combination of clomipramine with tranylcypromine can cause severe 5-HT toxicity (130,131), which may be fatal (132). The combination in overdose is also associated with severe toxicity (85).

In contrast to the irreversible nonselective MAO inhibitors, the potential for an interaction between a RIMA and tyramine appears very small (81,133–136). Little information is available about toxic doses of befloxatone, brofaromine, or pirlindole.

The use of therapeutic doses of fluoxetine with an MAO inhibitor was accompanied by a very high incidence of adverse effects (137), especially 5-HT toxicity, and the combination of any 5-HT uptake inhibitor (138) with any MAO inhibitor cannot be recommended. Fluoxetine (and presumably other 5-HT uptake inhibitors) may precipitate 5-HT toxicity even when initiated 2 weeks after ceasing treatment with an MAO inhibitor (139). 5-HT toxicity (often life threatening) from a combination of venlafaxine with an irreversible MAO inhibitor seems a particular problem, with cases reported with isocarboxazid (140), phenelzine (141) (even after abstinence from phenelzine for more than 2 weeks) (142), and tranylcypromine (143) (even after a single therapeutic dose of venlafaxine) (144).

All major complications, including seizures and coma, in the 73 other patients who took moclobemide with a coingestant could be accounted for by the coingested drug (53). The median dose of moclobemide in the patients who coingested other drugs was 4 g (53). The combination of moclobemide with other serotonergic drugs caused 5-HT toxicity in more than half of cases and severe 5-HT toxicity in 29% of cases, necessitating intubation, paralysis, and sedation. The odds of developing 5-HT toxicity in moclobemide plus a serotonergic drug overdose was 35 times that of moclobemide-alone overdoses (53).

Despite blood concentrations of fluoxetine within the therapeutic range after an overdose, severe 5-HT toxicity ensued, later attributed to concomitant ingestion of moclobemide (145). Overdoses of paroxetine (92,93), clomipramine (94), and venlafaxine (53,95) in combination with moclobemide have resulted in severe 5-HT toxicity. Moclobemide overdose in combination with TCAs may also result in serious poisoning even when the moclobemide overdose is modest (146).

Fatalities from the combination of moclobemide taken in overdose with another serotonergic drug (96) have occurred with clomipramine (97–100), clomipramine with tramadol (101), clomipramine with fluoxetine (67), citalopram (97,100,102), paroxetine (103), sertraline (104), and, most recently, 3,4-methylenedioxy-methamphetamine (105). In the context of an overdose with another serotonergic agent, even therapeutic doses of moclobemide may combine to produce life-threatening toxicity.

DIAGNOSTIC TESTS

No diagnostic tests specific to the MAO inhibitors are available. Quantitative drug estimation is not readily available for any of these agents and is not indicated for routine management.

Blood pressure should be monitored closely and, if abnormal after a significant dose of an irreversible MAO, should be measured invasively (arterial line). Core body temperature should be assessed, as hyperthermia is common. Hepatic and renal function tests are indicated, as are tests to assess for thrombocytopenia and disseminated intravascular coagulation in more severe cases. Measurement of creatine kinase in cases of coma helps in the assessment of rhabdomyolysis. Prolonged coma with life-threatening irreversible MAO inhibitor overdose may simply be a manifestation of the poisoning, but consideration should be given to computed tomographic head scan to look for intracerebral bleeding. Measurement of arterial carbon dioxide pressure via expired air or arterial blood gases is the best way to assess respiratory compromise from sedation.

POSTMORTEM CONSIDERATIONS

Little information on postmortem examination is available after ingestion of iproniazid, isocarboxazid, befloxatone, brofaromine, pirlindole, or toloxatone. In two cases of phenelzine-related death, concentrations in blood at autopsy were 10 to 50 times greater than therapeutic concentrations (0.002 to 0.02 mg/L) (148).

Tranylcypromine blood concentrations in a human poisoning case showed preferential concentration in the liver (2.21 mg/kg) and brain stem (2.46 mg/kg). Moderate postmortem redistribution occurred with tranylcypromine concentrations that were lowest in peripheral blood (0.17 mg/L) at 0 hour and highest in central vessels at 24 hours (0.52 mg/L) (149). A femoral blood concentration of 3.7 mg/L was found in a fatality after 300 mg tranylcypromine (150). In a fatal overdose estimated at 550 mg, femoral blood tranylcypromine was 0.57 mg/L with a subclavian blood concentration twice that of the antemortem blood (suggesting postmortem redistribution) (44). Other studies have shown concentrations varying from 0.25 to 9.1 mg/L (31,43,151).

Moclobemide postmortem redistribution in a rat model showed that concentrations in the vena cava and the heart agreed with antemortem concentrations (96). In a fatality due to the combined ingestion of moclobemide, citalopram, lormetazepam, and alcohol, the results obtained for blood and urine, respectively, were 5.62 mg/L and 204 mg/L moclobemide and, 4.47 mg/L and 19.7 mg/L citalopram (102). Moclobemide (49.9 mg/L) and perazine (1.27 mg/L) were identified in a combined drug intoxication that resulted in death (152).

In a case of moclobemide overdose due to a deliberate ingestion of 4.5 g of the drug, the postmortem whole blood concentration was 15.5 mg/L (56). In a death attributed to moclobemide alone, the blood concentration of moclobemide was 137 mg/L and the liver concentration was 432 mg/kg (55).

TREATMENT

All serotonergic drugs should be withdrawn, and the use of agents with serotonergic activity is absolutely contraindicated. Intensive care admission for high-level supportive care is indicated for significant ingestions of an irreversible, nonselective MAO inhibitor poisoning (more than 1 mg/kg tranylcypromine, more than 2 mg/kg phenelzine, or any dose when combined with another serotonergic agent).

Milder 5-HT toxicity from either group of MAO inhibitors may respond to specific 5-HT antagonists, but severe 5-HT toxicity (often due to combined overdose with another serotonergic drug) has the potential for life-threatening outcomes that may require more aggressive intervention.

Decontamination

Oral activated charcoal may be of value if given early (within 1 hour) in irreversible nonselective MAO inhibitor poisoning; it is unlikely that decontamination would be of benefit in RIMA poisoning alone. The preferred treatment for RIMA poisoning is simple supportive care with venous access and fluids.

Enhancement of Elimination

The volumes of distribution for MAO inhibitors, where known, are uniformly high, and extracorporeal techniques are unlikely to be of benefit.

Antidotes

Cyproheptadine has relatively high affinity for the 5-HT_2 receptor (153) and is effective for patients with milder 5-HT toxicity secondary to 5-HT uptake inhibitor toxicity who are able to take oral medication (154–158). No experience with its use in irreversible MAO inhibitor overdose has been reported. If cyproheptadine is used, current experience suggests that the appropriate dose range is 12 mg orally or by nasogastric tube, followed by 4 to 8 mg every 4 to 6 hours (159).

For severe 5-HT toxicity, chlorpromazine, also a potent 5-HT_2 antagonist (160), has been used in 5-HT toxicity associated with irreversible MAO inhibitor drug interactions with apparent good effect (130,131). Chlorpromazine has also been used with some success in irreversible MAO inhibitor overdose (38,161,162). Current experience indicates fluid resuscitation is required before the administration of chlorpromazine and that the dose is probably in the range of 12.5 to 50.0 mg IV initially, followed by 25 to 50 mg orally or IV every 6 hours (159). Newer antipsychotic agents such as risperidone also have very potent 5-HT_2 antagonist activity (163) and may be beneficial in treating 5-HT toxicity, although there is no published experience of their use.

Supportive Care

Supportive care is focused on controlling agitation, maintaining airway, reversing hyperthermia, and symptomatic treatment. In view of the potential cardiovascular toxicity of the irreversible agents, the patient's circulatory status warrants close attention. Temperature should be monitored closely, as hyperthermia predicts worsening toxicity.

The restlessness and agitation with hyperreflexia, myoclonus, and profuse sweating with or without generalized hypertonia may be an indication for specific treatment with 5-HT antagonists such as cyproheptadine or chlorpromazine as described in the section Antidotes. Benzodiazepines may be helpful. An antipsychotic medication that does not have significant 5-HT antagonism (e.g., haloperidol) should not be used because of the effects of 5-HT on dopamine release (Chapter 135).

Hypertension may occasionally be very severe and warrant therapy in its own right. If treatment is required, phentolamine, 2 to 5 mg IV; nifedipine, 10 mg orally; or chlorpromazine, 50 mg IV, should be used and repeated as necessary (116). In the context of an overdose, treatment of the hypertension should be undertaken cautiously because of the possibility of cardiovascular collapse and hypotension. Hypotension may be very severe and should be treated initially with a 10 to 20 mL/kg bolus of 0.9% sodium chloride followed by a vasopressor (Chapter 37). Seizures are rare, but, if they occur, they should be treated with benzodiazepines as first line (Chapter 40).

Severe hyperthermia with increasing muscular rigidity heralds life-threatening toxicity. Elective intubation, neuromuscular paralysis, mechanical ventilation, and aggressive cooling measures are indicated (Chapter 38). Organ failure should be treated along standard lines.

Overdosage of a reversible MAO-A inhibitor (without coingestion of serotonergic drugs) is unlikely to be associated with severe toxicity, and the preferred treatment is simple supportive care with IV access and fluids. For cases after ingestion alone or with another serotonergic agent in which more severe features of 5-HT toxicity develop, treatment of 5-HT toxicity should be instituted as for the irreversible agents.

Monitoring

Routine observation of vital signs, especially Glasgow Coma Scale, airway patency, blood pressure, and temperature, is indicated. Frequent assessment of mental status and neuromuscular function (hyperreflexia, hypertonia, myoclonus, clonus) should be made. All patients suspected of ingesting a toxic dose of an irreversible MAO inhibitor should be observed in a monitored setting for 24 hours because of the potential for delayed onset of reactions.

Patients should be placed on special diets that are low in tyramine-containing foods. Sympathomimetic and serotonergic drugs should be avoided because of potentiation of MAO inhibitor overdose effects. Precautions for food and drug interactions should remain in effect for 1 to 2 weeks after an irreversible inhibitor is discontinued.

REFERENCES

1. Mega BT, Sheppard KW, Williams HL, et al. On the role of monoamine oxidase-A for the maintenance of the volitional consumption of ethanol in two different rat models. *Naunyn Schmiedebergs Arch Pharmacol* 2002;366(4):319–326.
2. Finberg JP, Youdim MB. Pharmacological properties of the anti-Parkinson drug rasagiline; modification of endogenous brain amines, reserpine reversal, serotonergic and dopaminergic behaviours. *Neuropharmacology* 2002;43(7):1110–1118.
3. Henry JA, Antao CA. Suicide and fatal antidepressant poisoning. *Eur J Med* 1992;1(6):343–348.
4. Spahn-Langguth H, Hahn G, Mutschler E, et al. Enantiospecific high-performance liquid chromatographic assay with fluorescence detection for the monoamine oxidase inhibitor tranylcypromine and its applicability in pharmacokinetic studies. *J Chromatogr* 1992; 584(2):229–237.
5. Bosworth DM. Iproniazid: a brief review of its introduction and clinical use. *Ann N Y Acad Sci* 1959;80:809–819.
6. Ogilvie CM. The treatment of pulmonary tuberculosis with iproniazid (1-isonicotinyl-2-isopropyl hydrazine) and isoniazid (isonicotinyl hydrazine). *Q J Med* 1955;24(94):175–189.
7. Dooneief AS, Crane GE. Iproniazid as adjunct in the treatment of debilitated patients with tuberculosis. *N Y State J Med* 1957;57(21):3477–3480.
8. Maille F, Duvoux C, Cherqui D, et al. [Auxiliary hepatic transplantation in iproniazid-induced subfulminant hepatitis. Should iproniazid still be sold in France?] *Gastroenterol Clin Biol* 1999;23(10):1083–1085.
9. Sweetman S. Martindale: the complete drug reference. London: Pharmaceutical Press. Electronic ed. expires 03/2003. Greenwood Village, CO: MICROMEDEX, 2003.
10. Dollery CT. Therapeutic drugs. CD-ROM DATABASE Release 1.0 ed. London: Churchill Livingstone, 1999.
11. Veselovsky AV, Medvedev AE, Tikhonova OV, et al. Modeling of substrate-binding region of the active site of monoamine oxidase A. *Biochemistry (Mosc)* 2000;65(8):910–916.
12. Blackwell B, Mabbitt LA. Tyramine in cheese related to hypertensive crises after monoamine-oxidase inhibition. *Lancet* 1965;62:938–940.
13. Cuthill JM, Griffiths AB, Powell DE. Death associated with tranylcypromine and cheese. *Lancet* 1964;13:1076–1077.
14. Mirchandani H, Reich LE. Fatal malignant hyperthermia as a result of ingestion of tranylcypromine (Parnate) combined with white wine and cheese. *J Forensic Sci* 1985;30(1):217–220.
15. Asensio J. Attempted suicide with cheese. *BMJ* 1964;5387:907.
16. Visfeldt J. [Iproniazid poisoning. A fatal case with liver and kidney damage.] *Ugeskr Laeger* 1961;123:1727–1728.
17. Vlahakis E. Isocarboxazid overdosage. *Med J Aust* 1964;71:506–507.
18. Nielsen K. [Hyperpyrexia following poisoning with a monoamine oxidase inhibitor.] *Ugeskr Laeger* 1989;151(12):774–775.
19. Liebowitz MR, Nuetzel EJ, Bowser AE, et al. Phenelzine and delusions of parasitosis: a case report. *Am J Psychiatry* 1978;135(12):1565–1566.
20. Aizenberg D, Schwartz B, Zemishlany Z. Delusional parasitosis associated with phenelzine. *Br J Psychiatry* 1991;159:716–717.
21. Jacobs LS, Green RA, Gillin JC, et al. Phenelzine and psychosis. *Hawaii Med J* 1976;35(4):109–111.
22. Psychosis following phenelzine discontinuation. *J Clin Psychopharmacol* 1985;5(6):360–361.
23. Greenblatt DJ, Allen MD, Koch-Weser J, et al. Accidental poisoning with psychotropic drugs in children. *Am J Dis Child* 1976; 130(5):507–511.
24. Breheny FX, Dobb GJ, Clarke GM. Phenelzine poisoning. *Anaesthesia* 1986;41(1):53–56.
25. Kaplan RF, Feinglass NG, Webster W, et al. Phenelzine overdose treated with dantrolene sodium. *JAMA* 1986;255(5):642–644.
26. Mills KC. Monoamine oxidase inhibitor toxicity. *Top Emerg Med* 1993;15:58–71.
27. Linden CH, Rumack BH, Strehlke C. Monoamine oxidase inhibitor overdose. *Ann Emerg Med* 1984;13(12):1137–1144.
28. Lappa A, Podesta M, Capelli O, et al. Successful treatment of a complicated case of neuroleptic malignant syndrome. *Intensive Care Med* 2002;28(7):976–977.
29. Carbajal CL, Raul JF. [Severe poisoning caused by tranylcypromine and trifluoperazine.] *Rev Neuropsiquiatr* 1969;32(3):180–193.
30. Mawdsley JA. "Parstelin." A case of fatal overdose. *Med J Aust* 1968;2(6):292.
31. Griffiths GJ. Overdose of Parstelin (tranylcypromine). *Med Sci Law* 1973;13(2):93–94.
32. Gamba R, Fassetta G. [On a case of fatal poisoning by a psychopharmacologic agent in childhood.] *Riv Anat Patol Oncol* 1964;25(6)[Suppl]:30.
33. Grattarola FR, Schiffer D. [Acute poisoning by a psychopharmacologic agent. Anatomo-clinical considerations on a case of accidental toxicosis caused by tranylcypromine-trifluoperazine.] *Minerva Med* 1967;58(59):2665–2669.
34. Iwersen S, Schmoldt A. One fatal and one nonfatal intoxication with tranylcypromine. Absence of amphetamines as metabolites. *J Anal Toxicol* 1996;20(5):301–304.
35. Vartzopoulos D, Krull F. Dependence on monoamine oxidase inhibitors in high dose. *Br J Psychiatry* 1991; 158:856-857.
36. Davids E, Roschke J, Klawe C, et al. Tranylcypromine abuse associated with delirium and thrombocytopenia. *J Clin Psychopharmacol* 2000;20(2):270–271.
37. Coulter C, Edmunds J, Pyle PO. An overdose of Parstelin. *Anaesthesia* 1971;26(4):500–501.
38. Robertson JC. Recovery after massive MAOI overdose complicated by malignant hyperpyrexia, treated with chlorpromazine. *Postgrad Med J* 1972;48(555):64–65.
39. Shepherd JT, Whiting B. Beta-adrenergic blockade in the treatment of M.A.O.I. self-poisoning [Letter]. *Lancet* 1974;2(7887):1021.
40. Youdim MB, Aronson JK, Blau K, et al. Tranylcypromine ('Parnate') overdose: measurement of tranylcypromine concentrations and MAO inhibitory activity and identification of amphetamines in plasma. *Psychol Med* 1979;9(2):377–382.
41. Babiak W. Case fatality due to overdosage of a combination of tranylcypromine (Parnate) and imipramine (Tofranil). *Can Med Assoc J* 1961;85:377.
42. Bacon GA. Successful suicide with tranylcypromine sulfate. *Am J Psychiatry* 1962;119:585.
43. Mackell MA, Case ME, Poklis A. Fatal intoxication due to tranylcypromine. *Med Sci Law* 1979;19(1):66–68.
44. Crifasi J, Long C. The GCMS analysis of tranylcypromine (Parnate) in a suspected overdose. *Forensic Sci Int* 1997;86(1–2):103–108.
45. Benazzi F. Serotonin syndrome with moclobemide-fluoxetine combination. *Pharmacopsychiatry* 1996;29(4):162.
46. Gillman PK. Possible serotonin syndrome with moclobemide and pethidine. *Med J Aust* 1995;162(10):554.
47. Guma M, Clemente F, Segura A, et al. [The serotoninergic syndrome: moclobemide and citalopram.] *Med Clin (Barc)* 1999;113(17):677–678.
48. Kuisma MJ. Fatal serotonin syndrome with trismus. *Ann Emerg Med* 1995;26(1):108.
49. Joffe RT, Bakish D. Combined SSRI-moclobemide treatment of psychiatric illness. *J Clin Psychiatry* 1994;55(1):24–25.
50. Hawley CJ, Quick SJ, Ratnam S, et al. Safety and tolerability of combined treatment with moclobemide and SSRIs: a systematic study of 50 patients. *Int Clin Psychopharmacol* 1996;11(3):187–191.
51. Shenfield G. Should moclobemide be used with other antidepressants? *Aust Prescrib* 1995;18(4):100–101.
52. Hilton S, Jaber B, Ruch R. Moclobemide safety: monitoring a newly developed product in the 1990s. *J Clin Psychopharmacol* 1995;15[4 Suppl 2]:76S–83S.
53. Isbister GK, Hackett LP, Dawson AH, et al. Moclobemide poisoning: toxicokinetics and occurrence of serotonin toxicity. *Br J Clin Pharmacol* 2003; *in press.*
54. Gram LF. [Antidepressive drug therapy, suicidal tendency and suicide, 2 cases reported in connection with moclobemide (Aurorix) therapy.] *Ugeskr Laeger* 1994;156(38):5542.
55. Camaris C, Little D. A fatality due to moclobemide. *J Forensic Sci* 1997;42(5):954–955.

56. Gaillard Y, Pepin G. Moclobemide fatalities: report of two cases and analytical determinations by GC-MS and HPLC-PDA after solid-phase extraction. *Forensic Sci Int* 1997;87(3):239–248.
57. Pateron D, Babany G, Hadengue A, et al. [Fatal fulminant hepatitis in 2 women taking toloxatone (Humoryl).] *Gastroenterol Clin Biol* 1990;14(5):504–506.
58. Azoyan P, Garnier R, Baud FJ, et al. [Acute toloxatone poisoning. Apropos of 122 cases.] *Therapie* 1990;45(2):139–144.
59. Mallinger AG, Smith E. Pharmacokinetics of monoamine oxidase inhibitors. *Psychopharmacol Bull* 1991;27(4):493–502.
60. Cooper TB, Robinson DS, Nies A. Phenelzine measurement in human plasma: a sensitive GLC-ECD procedure. *Commun Psychopharmacol* 1978;2(6):505–512.
61. Caddy B, Stead AH. Three cases of poisoning involving the drug phenelzine. *J Forensic Sci Soc* 1978;18(3–4):207–208.
62. Rosenzweig P, Patat A, Curet O, et al. Clinical pharmacology of befloxatone: a brief review. *J Affect Disord* 1998;51(3):305–312.
63. Schneider W, Keller B, Degen PH. Determination of the new monoamine oxidase inhibitor brofaromine and its major metabolite in biological material by gas chromatography with electron-capture detection. *J Chromatogr* 1989;488(1):275–282.
64. Mayersohn M, Guentert TW. Clinical pharmacokinetics of the monoamine oxidase-A inhibitor moclobemide. *Clin Pharmacokinet* 1995;29(5):292–332.
65. Iwersen S, Schmoldt A. Three suicide attempts with moclobemide. *J Toxicol Clin Toxicol* 1996;34(2):223–225.
66. Chen DT, Ruch R. Safety of moclobemide in clinical use. *Clin Neuropharmacol* 1993;16[Suppl 2]:S63–S68.
67. Power BM, Pinder M, Hackett LP, et al. Fatal serotonin syndrome following a combined overdose of moclobemide, clomipramine and fluoxetine. *Anaesth Intensive Care* 1995;23(4):499–502.
68. Hackett LP, Joyce DA, Hall RW, et al. Disposition and clinical effects of moclobemide and three of its metabolites following overdose. *Drug Investigation* 1993;5:281–284.
69. Ostrowski J, Theumer J, Gartner W, et al. Determination of pirlindole in plasma and urine by high-performance liquid chromatography. *J Chromatogr* 1984;309(1):115–123.
70. Benedetti MS, Rovei V, Dencker SJ, et al. Pharmacokinetics of toloxatone in man following intravenous and oral administrations. *Arzneimittelforschung* 1982;32(3):276–280.
71. Azoyan P, Garnier R, Baud FJ, Efthymiou ML. Toxicokinetics of toloxatone in overdose. Proceedings, XIVth International Congress of the European Association of Poison Centres, 1990:47.
72. Shih JC, Chen K, Ridd MJ. Monoamine oxidase: from genes to behavior. *Annu Rev Neurosci* 1999;22:197–217.
73. Geha RM, Chen K, Wouters J, et al. Analysis of conserved active site residues in monoamine oxidase A and B and their three-dimensional molecular modeling. *J Biol Chem* 2002;277(19):17209–17216.
74. Moreau F, Wouters J, Depas M, et al. Toloxatone: comparison of its physicochemical properties with those of other inhibitors including brofaromine, harmine, R40519 and moclobemide. *Eur J Med Chem* 1995;30(11):823–828.
75. Baker GB, Urichuk LJ, McKenna KF, et al. Metabolism of monoamine oxidase inhibitors. *Cell Mol Neurobiol* 1999;19(3):411–426.
76. Smith TM. [3H]-flunitrazepam binding in the presence of beta-phenylethylamine and its metabolites. *Pharmacol Biochem Behav* 1985;23(6):965–967.
77. Timbrell JA. The role of metabolism in the hepatotoxicity of isoniazid and iproniazid. *Drug Metab Rev* 1979; 10(1):125–147.
78. Nelson SD, Mitchell JR, Timbrell JA, et al. Isoniazid and iproniazid: activation of metabolites to toxic intermediates in man and rat. *Science* 1976;193(4256):901–903.
79. Pons C, Dansette PM, Gregeois J, et al. Human anti-mitochondria autoantibodies appearing in iproniazid-induced immunoallergic hepatitis recognize human liver monoamine oxidase B. *Biochem Biophys Res Commun* 1996;218(1):118–124.
80. Waldmeier PC, Glatt A, Jaekel J, et al. Brofaromine: a monoamine oxidase-A and serotonin uptake inhibitor. *Clin Neuropharmacol* 1993;16[Suppl 2]:S19–S24.
81. Bruhwyler J, Liegeois JF, Geczy J. Pirlindole: a selective reversible inhibitor of monoamine oxidase A. A review of its preclinical properties. *Pharmacol Res* 1997;36(1):23–33.
82. Product information: Parnate, tranylcypromine sulfate. Philadelphia: SmithKline Beecham Pharmaceuticals, 2003.
83. Pons G, Schoerlin MP, Tam YK, et al. Moclobemide excretion in human breast milk. *Br J Clin Pharmacol* 1990;29(1):27–31.
84. Verrilli MR, Salanga VD, Kozachuk WE, et al. Phenelzine toxicity responsive to dantrolene. *Neurology* 1987;37(5):865–867.
85. Prueter C, Schiefer J, Norra C, et al. Ping-pong gaze in combined intoxication with tranylcypromine, thioridazine, and clomipramine. *Neuropsychiatry Neuropsychol Behav Neurol* 2001;14(4):246–247.
86. Watkins HC, Ellis CJ. Ping Pong gaze in reversible coma due to overdose of monoamine oxidase inhibitor. *J Neurol Neurosurg Psychiatry* 1989;52(4):539.
87. Erich JL, Shih RD, O'Connor RE. "Ping-pong" gaze in severe monoamine oxidase inhibitor toxicity. *J Emerg Med* 1995;13(5):653–655.
88. Jourdan C, Artru F, Lamy B, et al. [Acute MAOI poisoning: report of a poisoning case with prolonged coma lasting 4 days.] *J Toxicol Clin Exp* 1988;8(6):395–400.
89. Quill TE. Peaked "T" waves with tranylcypromine (Parnate) overdose. *Int J Psychiatry Med* 1981;11(2):155–160.
90. Pennings EJ, Verkes RJ, De Koning J, et al. Tranylcypromine intoxication with malignant hyperthermia, delirium, and thrombocytopenia. *J Clin Psychopharmacol* 1997;17(5):430–432.
91. Chatterjee A, Tosyali MC. Thrombocytopenia and delirium associated with tranylcypromine overdose. *J Clin Psychopharmacol* 1995;15(2):143–144.
92. Robert P, Senard JM, Fabre M, et al. [Serotonin syndrome in acute poisoning with antidepressive agents.] *Ann Fr Anesth Reanim* 1996; 15(5):663-665.
93. FitzSimmons CR, Metha S. Serotonin syndrome caused by overdose with paroxetine and moclobemide. *J Accid Emerg Med* 1999;16(4):293–295.
94. Francois B, Marquet P, Desachy A, et al. Serotonin syndrome due to an overdose of moclobemide and clomipramine. A potentially life-threatening association. *Intensive Care Med* 1997;23(1):122–124.
95. Roxanas MG, Machado JF. Serotonin syndrome in combined moclobemide and venlafaxine ingestion. *Med J Aust* 1998;168(10):523–524.
96. Rogde S, Hilberg T, Teige B. Fatal combined intoxication with new antidepressants. Human cases and an experimental study of postmortem moclobemide redistribution. *Forensic Sci Int* 1999;100(1–2):109–116.
97. Neuvonen PJ, Pohjola-Sintonen S, Tacke U, et al. Five fatal cases of serotonin syndrome after moclobemide-citalopram or moclobemide-clomipramine overdoses. *Lancet* 1993;342(8884):1419.
98. Finge T, Malavialle C, Lambert J. [Fatal form of serotonin syndrome.] *Ann Fr Anesth Reanim* 1997;16(1):80–81.
99. Ferrer-Dufol A, Perez-Aradros C, Murillo EC, et al. Fatal serotonin syndrome caused by moclobemide-clomipramine overdose. *J Toxicol Clin Toxicol* 1998;36(1–2):31–32.
100. Hojer J, Personne M, Skagius AS, et al. [Serotonin syndrome—several cases of this often overlooked diagnosis.] *Tidsskr Nor Laegeforen* 2002;122(17):1660–1663.
101. Hernandez AF, Montero MN, Pla A, et al. Fatal moclobemide overdose or death caused by serotonin syndrome? *J Forensic Sci* 1995;40(1):128–130.
102. Dams R, Benijts TH, Lambert WE, et al. A fatal case of serotonin syndrome after combined moclobemide-citalopram intoxication. *J Anal Toxicol* 2001;25(2):147–151.
103. Singer PP, Jones GR. An uncommon fatality due to moclobemide and paroxetine. *J Anal Toxicol* 1997;21(6):518–520.
104. McIntyre IM, King CV, Staikos V, et al. A fatality involving moclobemide, sertraline, and pimozide. *J Forensic Sci* 1997;42(5):951–953.
105. Vuori E, Henry JA, Ojanpera I, et al. Death following ingestion of MDMA (Ecstasy) and moclobemide. *Addiction* 2003;98(3):365–368.
106. Pall M, Bested KM, Eriksen ND. [Poisoning with a reversible and selective monoaminooxidase inhibitor.] *Ugeskr Laeger* 1997;159(32):4859–4860.
107. Halle MH, Del Medico VJ, Dilsaver SC. Symptoms of major depression: acute effect of withdrawing antidepressants. *Acta Psychiatr Scand* 1991;83(3):238–239.
108. Baumbacher G, Hansen MS. Abuse of monoamine oxidase inhibitors. *Am J Drug Alcohol Abuse* 1992;18(4):399–406.
109. Curtin F, Berney P, Kaufmann C. Moclobemide discontinuation syndrome predominantly presenting with influenza-like symptoms. *J Psychopharmacol* 2002;16(3):271–272.
110. Coupland NJ, Bell CJ, Potokar JP. Serotonin reuptake inhibitor withdrawal. *J Clin Psychopharmacol* 1996;16(5):356–362.
111. Shopsin B, Kline NS. Monoamine oxidase inhibitors: potential for drug abuse. *Biol Psychiatry* 1976;11(4):451–456.
112. Gelenberg AJ. Switching MAO inhibitors. *Biol Ther Psychiatry* 1984;7:36.
113. Bazire SR. Sudden death associated with switching monoamine oxidase inhibitors. *Drug Intell Clin Pharm* 1986;20(12):954–956.
114. True BL, Alexander B, Carter B. Switching monoamine oxidase inhibitors. *Drug Intell Clin Pharm* 1985;19(11):825–827.
115. Szuba MP, Hornig-Rohan M, Amsterdam JD. Rapid conversion from one monoamine oxidase inhibitor to another. *J Clin Psychiatry* 1997;58(7):307–310.
116. Monoamine oxidase inhibitors. In: Rossi S, Vitry A, Hurley E, et al., eds. *Australian medicines handbook.* Adelaide: Australian Medicines Handbook Pty Ltd, 2002.
117. Lotufo-Neto F, Trivedi M, Thase ME. Meta-analysis of the reversible inhibitors of monoamine oxidase type A moclobemide and brofaromine for the treatment of depression. *Neuropsychopharmacology* 1999;20(3):226–247.
118. De Wilde JE, Geerts S, Van Dorpe J, et al. A double-blind randomized placebo-controlled study of the efficacy and safety of pirlindole, a reversible monoamine oxidase A inhibitor, in the treatment of depression. *Acta Psychiatr Scand* 1996;94(6):404–410.
119. Lemoine P, Mirabaud C. A double-blind comparison of moclobemide and toloxatone in out-patients presenting a major depressive disorder. *Psychopharmacology (Berl)* 1992;106[Suppl]:S118–S119.
120. Dawson JK, Earnshaw SM, Graham CS. Dangerous monoamine oxidase inhibitor interactions are still occurring in the 1990s. *J Accid Emerg Med* 1995;12(1):49–51.
121. Shee JC. Dangerous potentiation of pethidine by iproniazid, and its treatment. *BMJ* 1960;5197:507–509.
122. Browne B, Linter S. Monoamine oxidase inhibitors and narcotic analgesics. A critical review of the implications for treatment. *Br J Psychiatry* 1987;151:210–212.
123. Bem JL, Peck R. Dextromethorphan. An overview of safety issues. *Drug Saf* 1992;7(3):190–199.
124. Calvisi V, Ansseau M. [Clinical case of the month. Mental confusion due to the administration of tramadol in a patient treated with MAOI.] *Rev Med Liege* 1999;54(12):912–913.
125. Smilkstein MJ, Smolinske SC, Rumack BH. A case of MAO inhibitor/MDMA interaction: agony after ecstasy. *J Toxicol Clin Toxicol* 1987;25(1–2):149–159.
126. Kahn D, Silver JM, Opler LA. The safety of switching rapidly from tricyclic antidepressants to monoamine oxidase inhibitors. *J Clin Psychopharmacol* 1989;9(3):198–202.

127. Spiker DG, Pugh DD. Combining tricyclic and monoamine oxidase inhibitor antidepressants. *Arch Gen Psychiatry* 1976;33(7):828–830.
128. Peebles-Brown AE. Hyperpyrexia following psychotropic drug overdose. *Anaesthesia* 1985;40(11):1097–1099.
129. Tuck JR, Punell G. Uptake of (3H)5-hydroxytryptamine and (3H)noradrenaline by slices of rat brain incubated in plasma from patients treated with chlorimipramine, imipramine or amitriptyline. *J Pharm Pharmacol* 1973;25(7):573–574.
130. Gillman PK. Successful treatment of serotonin syndrome with chlorpromazine. *Med J Aust* 1996;165(6):345–346.
131. Graham PM. Successful treatment of the toxic serotonin syndrome with chlorpromazine. *Med J Aust* 1997;166(3):166–167.
132. Tackley RM, Tregaskis B. Fatal disseminated intravascular coagulation following a monoamine oxidase inhibitor/tricyclic interaction. *Anaesthesia* 1987;42(7):760–763.
133. Bieck PR, Antonin KH. Tyramine potentiation during treatment with MAO inhibitors: brofaromine and moclobemide vs irreversible inhibitors. *J Neural Transm Suppl* 1989;28:21–31.
134. Gieschke R, Schmid-Burgk W, Amrein R. Interaction of moclobemide, a new reversible monoamine oxidase inhibitor with oral tyramine. *J Neural Transm* 1988;26[Suppl]:97–104.
135. Patat A, Berlin I, Durrieu G, et al. Pressor effect of oral tyramine during treatment with befloxatone, a new reversible monoamine oxidase-A inhibitor, in healthy subjects. *J Clin Pharmacol* 1995;35(6):633–643.
136. Provost JC, Funck-Brentano C, Rovei V, et al. Pharmacokinetic and pharmacodynamic interaction between toloxatone, a new reversible monoamine oxidase-A inhibitor, and oral tyramine in healthy subjects. *Clin Pharmacol Ther* 1992;52(4):384–393.
137. Feighner JP, Boyer WF, Tyler DL, et al. Adverse consequences of fluoxetine-MAOI combination therapy. *J Clin Psychiatry* 1990;51(6):222–225.
138. Brannan SK, Talley BJ, Bowden CL. Sertraline and isocarboxazid cause a serotonin syndrome. *J Clin Psychopharmacol* 1994;14(2):144–145.
139. Ruiz F. Fluoxetine and the serotonin syndrome. *Ann Emerg Med* 1994;24(5):983–985.
140. Klysner R, Larsen JK, Sorensen P, et al. Toxic interaction of venlafaxine and isocarboxazide. *Lancet* 1995;346(8985):1298–1299.
141. Phillips SD, Ringo P. Phenelzine and venlafaxine interaction. *Am J Psychiatry* 1995;152(9):1400–1401.
142. Kolecki P. Venlafaxine induced serotonin syndrome occurring after abstinence from phenelzine for more than two weeks. *J Toxicol Clin Toxicol* 1997;35(2):211–212.
143. Brubacher JR, Hoffman RS, Lurin MJ. Serotonin syndrome from venlafaxine-tranylcypromine interaction. *Vet Hum Toxicol* 1996;38(5):358–361.
144. Hodgman MJ, Martin TG, Krenzelok EP. Serotonin syndrome due to venlafaxine and maintenance tranylcypromine therapy. *Hum Exp Toxicol* 1997;16(1):14–17.
145. Chambost M, Liron L, Peillon D, et al. [Serotonin syndrome during fluoxetine poisoning in a patient taking moclobemide.] *Can J Anaesth* 2000;47(3): 246–250.
146. Myrenfors PG, Eriksson T, Sandsted CS, et al. Moclobemide overdose. *J Intern Med* 1993;233(2):113–115.
147. Reference deleted.
148. Lichtenwalner MR, Tully RG, Cohn RD, et al. Two fatalities involving phenelzine. *J Anal Toxicol* 1995;19(4):265–266.
149. Yonemitsu K, Pounder DJ. Postmortem changes in blood tranylcypromine concentration: competing redistribution and degradation effects. *Forensic Sci Int* 1993;59(2):177–184.
150. Baselt RC, Shaskan E, Gross EM. Tranylcypromine concentrations and monoamine oxidase activity in tissues from a fatal poisoning. *J Anal Toxicol* 1977;1:168–170.
151. Boniface PJ. Two cases of fatal intoxication due to tranylcypromine overdose. *J Anal Toxicol* 1991;15(1):38–40.
152. Musshoff F, Varchmin-Schultheiss K, Madea B. Suicide with moclobemide and perazine. *Int J Legal Med* 1998;111(4):196–198.
153. Kapur S, Zipursky RB, Jones C, et al. Cyproheptadine: a potent in vivo serotonin antagonist [Letter]. *Am J Psychiatry* 1997;154(6):884.
154. Gillman PK. The serotonin syndrome and its treatment. *J Psychopharmacol* 1999;13(1):100–109.
155. Graudins A, Stearman A, Chan B. Treatment of the serotonin syndrome with cyproheptadine. *J Emerg Med* 1998;16(4):615–619.
156. Horowitz BZ, Mullins ME. Cyproheptadine for serotonin syndrome in an accidental pediatric sertraline ingestion. *Pediatr Emerg Care* 1999;15(5):325–327.
157. Isbister GK. Comment: serotonin syndrome, mydriasis, and cyproheptadine. *Ann Pharmacother* 2001;35(12):1672–1673.
158. McDaniel WW. Serotonin syndrome: early management with cyproheptadine. *Ann Pharmacother* 2001;35(7–8):870–873.
159. Buckley NA, Dawson AH, Whyte IM. Specific serotonin reuptake inhibitors (SSRIs). *HyperTox: assessment and treatment of poisoning*. Newcastle, Australia: MediTox Pty Ltd, 2002.
160. Tatsumi M, Jansen K, Blakely RD, et al. Pharmacological profile of neuroleptics at human monoamine transporters. *Eur J Pharmacol* 1999;368(2–3):277–283.
161. Braunlich H, Greger J, Traeger A. [The phenelzine poisoning and the possibilities of its treatment in animal experiments.] *Z Arztl Fortbild (Jena)* 1966;60(15):914–921.
162. Reid DD, Kerr WC. Phenelzine poisoning responding to phenothiazine. *Med J Aust* 1969;2(24):1214–1215.
163. Richelson E, Souder T. Binding of antipsychotic drugs to human brain receptors focus on newer generation compounds. *Life Sci* 2000;68(1):29–39.

CHAPTER 134

Cyclic Antidepressant Drugs

Andrew H. Dawson

See Figure 1.

Compounds included:	**See Table 1.**
Molecular formula and weight:	**See Table 1.**
SI conversion:	**See Table 1.**
CAS Registry No.:	**See Table 1.**
Therapeutic levels:	**See Table 8.**
Special concerns:	**Abrupt deterioration with seizures or ventricular dysrhythmias**
Antidotes:	**Sodium bicarbonate, hypertonic sodium chloride**

OVERVIEW

Cyclic antidepressants are pharmacologically *dirty* drugs: Although their primary therapeutic effect is to block presynaptic catecholamine and serotonin reuptake, most of their adverse effects and toxicity is mediated by their effects of blocking of cellular ion channels as well as α-adrenergic, histaminergic, and muscarinic receptors. Common adverse effects are sedation and anticholinergic symptoms. The group is dominated by tricyclic antidepressants (TCA) in number, clinical experience, and extent of toxicity.

Despite changes in antidepressant prescribing patterns, TCA remain a common cause for admission (1) and death from poisoning (2–4). Up to 90% of TCA suicide deaths occur outside of hospital (5,6). One-half of the in-hospital fatalities have trivial toxicity on arrival to hospital but develop major toxicity within 1 hour (5). This reflects the rapid absorption of TCA and onset of cardiac and central nervous system toxicity. Whereas a number of electrocardiogram (ECG) abnormalities are predictive of serious toxicity, a normal ECG does not exclude serious toxicity. Decontamination, management of airway, and adjustment of pH to a mild systemic alkalosis with sodium bicarbonate are the mainstays of successful management.

The primary indication for all of these drugs is depression. TCAs have also been used for panic disorder (imipramine),

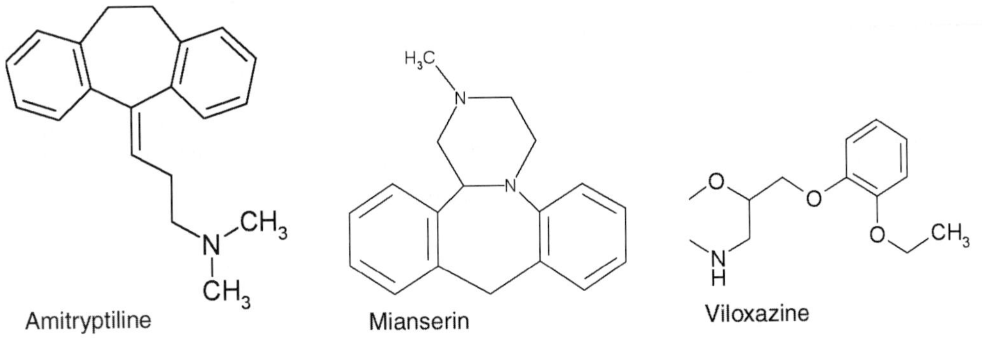

Amitryptiline Mianserin Viloxazine

Figure 1. Structures of the cyclic antidepressant drugs.

obsessive-compulsive disorders (clomipramine), cataplexy associated with narcolepsy (clomipramine), and attention deficit hyperactivity disorder (imipramine, nortriptyline). Medical uses include adjunctive treatment in pain management (amitriptyline, doxepin) and treatment of nocturnal enuresis or urge incontinence (amitriptyline, imipramine, nortriptyline) (7). Viloxazine is a bicyclic antidepressant with predominant serotonin reuptake inhibition; no deaths are reported. Mianserin and maprotiline are both tetracyclic compounds with similar indications and mechanism of action to TCAs.

TOXIC DOSE

The *adult and pediatric therapeutic dose* is provided in Table 1. The normal therapeutic dose of most TCAs in both adults and chil-

TABLE 1. Physical characteristics and dosage and elimination half-life of the cyclic antidepressants

Compounds included	Molecular formula, molecular weight (g/mol), CAS Registry No.	SI conversion	Formulation	Oral dose range (mg/d)	Elimination half-lives of drug and active metabolites[a,b] (h)
Amineptine hydrochloride (Survector)	$C_{22}H_{27}NO_2$,HCl; 373.9; 30272-08-3	ng/ml × 2.96 = nmol/L	NR	100–200	1, 2.5
Amitriptyline hydrochloride (Elavil, Laroxyl)	$C_{20}H_{23}N$,HCl; 313.9; 549-18-8	ng/ml × 3.60 = nmol/L	10 mg/ml solution; 10-, 25-, 50-, 75-, 100-, 150-mg tablets	75–150	19, 28
Amoxapine (Asendin)	$C_{17}H_{16}ClN_3O$; 313.8; 14028-44-5	ng/ml × 3.19 = nmol/L	25-, 50-, 100-, 150-mg tablets	100–300	8 (30 and 76.5)
Carpipramine hydrochloride (Prazinil)	$C_{28}H_{38}N_4O$,2HCl,H_2O; 537.6; 7075-03-8	ng/ml × 2.24 = nmol/L	NR	50–400	NR
Clomipramine hydrochloride (Anafranil)	$C_{19}H_{23}ClN_2$,HCl; 351.3; 17321-77-6	ng/ml × 3.18 = nmol/L	25-, 50-, 75-mg capsules; 10-, 25-, 50-mg tablets	75–150	20, 40
Dothiepin (Thaden)	$C_{19}H_{21}NS$,HCl; 331.9; 897-15-4	ng/ml × 3.38 = nmol/L	25-mg capsule; 75-mg tablet	75–150	25, 34
Doxepin (Sinequan, Quitaxon)	$C_{19}H_{21}NO$,HCl; 315.8; 4698-39-9	ng/ml × 3.58 = nmol/L	10, 25, 50, 75, 100, 150 capsules; 50-mg/g cream	75–150	17, 37
Imipramine hydrochloride (Tofranil)	$C_{19}H_{24}N_2$,HCl; 316.9; 113-52-0	ng/ml × 3.57 = nmol/L	12.5-mg/ml solution; 10-, 25-, 50-, 75-mg tablets	75–150	18, 22
Lofepramine hydrochloride (Tymelyt)	$C_{26}H_{27}ClN_2O$,HCl; 455.4; 26786-32-3	ng/ml × 2.39 = nmol/L	70-mg tablet; 70 mg/5 ml suspension	140–210	2
Loxapine succinate (Loxitane)	$C_{18}H_{18}ClN_3O$,$C_4H_6O_4$; 445.9; 27833-64-3	ng/ml × 3.05 = nmol/L	5-, 10-, 25-, 50-mg capsules	20–100	NR
Maprotiline hydrochloride (Ludiomil)	$C_{20}H_{23}N$,HCl; 313.9; 10347-81-6	ng/ml × 3.60 = nmol/L	10-, 25-, 50-, 75-mg tablets	75–225	51, 70
Metapramine fumarate (Timaxil)	$C_{16}H_{18}N_2$,$C_4H_4O_4$; 354.4; 93841-84-0	ng/ml × 4.20 = nmol/L	NR	150–300	4.4
Mianserin (Norval)	$C_{18}H_{20}N_2$,HCl; 300.8; 21535-47-7	ng/ml × 3.78 = nmol/L	10-, 20-, 30-mg tablets	30–90	33
Minaprine hydrochloride (Cantor)	$C_{17}H_{22}N_4O$,2HCl; 371.3; 25953-17-7	ng/ml × 3.35 = nmol/L	100-mg tablet	100–300	—
Nortriptyline hydrochloride (Aventyl, Pamelor)	$C_{19}H_{21}N$,HCl; 299.8; 894-71-3	ng/ml × 3.80 = nmol/L	10, 25, 50, 75 capsule; 10-mg/5 ml solution	75–150	28
Trimipramine maleate (Surmontil)	$C_{20}H_{26}N_2$,$C_4H_4O_4$; 410.5; 521-78-8	ng/ml × 3.40 = nmol/L	25, 50, 100 capsules; 12.5-, 25-, 50-, 100-mg tablets	75–150	23
Viloxazine (Vivalan)	$C_{13}H_{19}NO_3$,HCl; 273.8; 35604-67-2	ng/ml × 4.21 = nmol/L	NR	100	2–5

NR, not reported.
[a]The stated half-lives are generally in the middle of the range of reported values; there is considerable individual variation.
[b]Where clinically significant (40).

TABLE 2. Metabolism of antidepressants to active moieties

Parent	Metabolite
Demethylation to active metabolites	
Imipramine	Desipramine
Amitriptyline	Nortriptyline
Maprotiline	Desmethylmaprotiline
Doxepin	Desmethyldoxepin
Metapramine	*N*-desmethylmetapramine
Demethylated:parent-drug ratio 0.1–3.0	
Hydroxylation to active metabolites	
Imipramine	2-Hydroxyimipramine
Lofepramine	Desipramine
Desipramine	2-Hydroxydesipramine
Amitriptyline	10-Hydroxyamitriptyline
Nortriptyline	10-Hydroxynortriptyline
Amoxapine	8-Hydroxyamoxapine
	7-Hydroxyamoxapine
Loxapine	7-Hydroxyloxapine
	8-Hydroxyloxapine

From Ereshefsky L, Tran-Johnson T, Davis DM, et al. Pharmacokinetic factors affecting antidepressant drug clearance and clinical effect: evaluation of doxepin and imipramine: new data and review. *Clin Chem* 1988;34:863–880, with permission.

dren is 1 to 3 mg/kg given once a day. The doses for the bicyclics and tetracyclics vary (Table 1). Many TCAs have active metabolites that contribute to their therapeutic effect (Table 2).

The ingestion of 15 to 20 mg/kg or more of a TCA is potentially fatal, although there are significant differences in toxicity within the drug class (8–10). Tetracyclics and bicyclics appear to be less toxic in overdose than TCA. Small children can potentially develop life-threatening toxicity with ingestion of 1 to 2 tablets.

In a pediatric series of TCA poisonings, all single ingestions of less than 5 mg remained asymptomatic. Minor toxicity can result from ingestion of more than 5 mg/kg (11). Deaths have been reported rarely with chronic therapeutic doses (desipramine, 3.3 mg/kg/day; imipramine, 6 mg/kg/day) (12). In these cases, other factors, such as impaired metabolism due to either genetic variation, drug-induced enzyme inhibition, or preexisting cardiac conduction defects, have been implicated.

Risk for major toxicity varies within the class. Initially, a number of mortality studies examined the relative risk of death compared to prescription rates and suggested an increased fatal toxicity index (deaths per million prescriptions) for amitriptyline, dothiepin, doxepin, trimipramine, and maprotiline compared with mianserin and carpipramine (Tables 3 and 4) (13). Subsequent work demonstrated an increased risk of seizures for dothiepin compared with other TCA (9,10).

TABLE 3. Relative risk of death and antidepressant overdose

Category	Medications
Relatively safe FTI <10	Lofepramine, mianserin, fluvoxamine, fluoxetine, viloxazine
Potentially dangerous FTI >10	Clomipramine, protriptyline, trazodone
Clearly dangerous FTI >20	Phenelzine, imipramine
Very dangerous FTI >30	Maprotiline
Unacceptable risk FTI >40	Dothiepin, amitriptyline, tranylcypromine

FTI, number of reported deaths per 1 million prescriptions for the drug.
Modified from Montgomery SA, Baldwin D, Green M. Why do amitriptyline and dothiepin appear to be so dangerous in overdose? *Acta Psychiatr Scand Suppl* 1989;354:47–53.

TABLE 4. Fatal toxicity indices (1982–1986) for antidepressant drugs in England, Scotland, and Wales

Drug	Year	Fatal toxicity index (number of deaths per million prescriptions)	
Early tricyclic drugs introduced up to and including 1970			
Desipramine	1963	148.9	$p<.001$
Dothiepin	1969	59.6	$p<.001$
Amitriptyline	1961	56.1	$p<.001$
Nortriptyline	1963	42.3	NS
Doxepin	1969	40.6	NS
Imipramine	1959	30.0	$p<.05$
Trimipramine	1966	30.0	NS
Clomipramine	1970	9.9	$p<.001$
Protriptyline	1966	6.5	$p<.05$
Iprindole	1967	0.0	NS
Monoamine oxidase inhibitors			
Tranylcypromine	1960	43.8	NS
Phenelzine	1959	20.0	$p<.05$
Isocarboxazid	1960	11.0	NS
Iproniazid	1958	0.0	NS
Antidepressants introduced after 1973			
Maprotiline	1974	19.8	$p<.05$
Trazodone	1980	12.3	$p<.01$
Viloxazine	1974	0.0	NS
Butriptyline	1975	0.0	NS
Mianserin	1976	7.8	$p<.001$
Nomifensine	1977	2.4	$p<.001$
Lofepramine	1983	0.0	$p<.001$
All antidepressants		37.6	

NS, not significantly different ($p>.05$).
From Reid F, Henry JA. Lofepramine overdosage. *Pharmacopsychiatry* 1990;23[Suppl. 1]:23–27, with permission.

TOXICOKINETICS AND TOXICODYNAMICS

Absorption and Distribution

Antidepressants are highly lipid soluble and rapidly absorbed with peak levels occurring within 2 hours and extensive distribution into tissues (14). However, the anticholinergic side effects associated with symptomatic TCA poisoning may delay absorption and cause delayed peak concentrations. Delayed release formulations of amitriptyline can produce peak concentrations and delayed effects up to 42 hours after ingestion (15).

Less than 10% of a TCA circulates as free drug; the rest is bound to circulating proteins (albumin and α_1-acid glycoprotein) or dissolved in circulating free fatty acids. α_1-Acid glycoprotein has high and low affinity binding sites for TCA (16). It is more important for TCA binding than albumin; additional α_1-acid glycoprotein can reverse TCA toxicity whereas albumin has no effect (17). The *bound* fraction is sensitive to changes in pH with acidosis causing an increase in free fraction. Doses of 1000 mg/day of acetylsalicylic acid significantly increased the free fraction of imipramine (18). Alkalinization causes a significant decrease in percentage of free amitriptyline; 20% over a pH range of 7.0 to 7.4 and 42% over a pH range of 7.4 to 7.8 (19).

All the cyclic antidepressants have large volumes of distribution ranging from 5 to 20 L/kg or more. Clinical toxicity usually develops when the drugs are still in the distribution phase. As

TABLE 5. *In vitro* short-term biochemical activity of selected older and newer antidepressant drugs

	Reuptake inhibition			Receptor affinity				
Drug	NA	5-HT	D	α_1	α_2	H_1	MUSC	D_2
Older drugs								
Amitriptyline	±	++	0	+++	±	++++	++++	0
Clomipramine	±	+++	0	++	0	+	++	++
Desipramine	+++	0	0	+	0	±	+	0
Dothiepin	±	+	0	±	0	+++	+++	0
Doxepin	++	+	0	+++	0	++++	++	0
Imipramine	+	+	0	++	0	+	++	0
Nortriptyline	++	±	0	++	0	+	++	0
Trimipramine	+	0	0	+++	±	++++	++	++
Newer drugs								
Amoxapine	++	0	0	++	0	+	0	++
Lofepramine	+++	0	0	+	0	—	+	++
Maprotiline	++	0	0	++	0	+++	+	+
Mianserin	0	0	0	+++	++	++++	0	0
Trazodone	0	+	0	+++	±	±	0	0

α_1, α_1-adrenergic receptor; α_2, α_2-adrenergic receptor; D, dopamine; D_2, D_2 dopamine receptor; H_1, H_1 histamine receptor; 5-HT, 5-hydroxytryptamine (serotonin); MUSC, muscarinic (cholinergic) receptor; NA, noradrenaline (norepinephrine); 0, no effect; ±, equivocal effect; +, small effect; ++, moderate effect; +++, large effect; ++++, maximal effect.
Modified from Rudorfer MW, Manji HE, Potter WZ. Comparative tolerability profiles of the newer versus older antidepressants. *Drug Saf* 1994;10:18–42.

they are all weak bases (pK_a around 8.5), acidosis causes the fraction of ionized drug to increase. An increase in the ionized fraction could theoretically slow diffusion across membranes and prolong redistribution time.

Elimination

Clearance of cyclic antidepressants is dependent primarily on hepatic cytochrome P-450 (CYP) oxidative enzymes. Although the activities of some P-450 isoenzymes are largely under genetic control, they may be influenced by external factors, such as the concomitant use of other medications, hepatic disease, and intercurrent illness. Patient variables such as ethnicity and age also affect TCA metabolism. Metabolism of TCA, especially their hydroxylation, results in the formation of active metabolites, which contribute to both the therapeutic and the adverse effects of these compounds (Table 2). Both the parent drug and the active metabolites may undergo enterohepatic circulation. Renal excretion is low (3% to 10%). The elimination half-life averages approximately 1 day (up to 3 days for protriptyline) (14).

Zero-order kinetics can be reached at the top end of the therapeutic range in some patients (20). After overdose the P-450 enzymes responsible for TCA benzyl-hydroxylation become saturated and thus reduce TCA elimination to zero-order kinetics (21). The elimination half-life becomes significantly longer (21). Amitriptyline elimination half-life in overdose ranges from 25 to 81 hours (22).

PATHOPHYSIOLOGY

Cyclic antidepressants variably inhibit reuptake of norepinephrine and serotonin into presynaptic terminals (Table 5). Although unrelated to their therapeutic effects, TCA also block cholinergic, histaminergic, α_1-adrenergic, $GABA_A$ and serotonergic receptors. Mianserin has a tetracyclic structure and antagonizes α_2-adrenoceptors but has little anticholinergic effect. It also blocks postsynaptic serotonergic receptors. Clomipramine has a greater effect on serotonin transport than other TCA (7).

The exact mechanism of action in depression has not been clearly established but involves blocking reuptake of norepinephrine and serotonin and possibly the resetting of serotonin receptors. These effects are probably unimportant in overdose except in combined overdose with selective serotonin reuptake inhibitors.

Blockade of histamine receptors leads to sedation, α-receptor blockade leads to vasodilation, $GABA_A$ blockade may contribute to seizures, and anticholinergic effects result from muscarinic receptor blockade. Cardiac toxicity is predominantly due to rate-dependent blockade of sodium ion channels (23). The influx of sodium is the major event responsible for the zero phase of depolarization in cardiac muscle and Purkinje fibers. This initiates cardiac muscle contraction (systole). The duration of phase 0 in the heart as a whole is measured indirectly by the duration of the QRS complex on the ECG. Prolongation of the QRS is a correlate of TCA concentration (24) and is predictive of both seizures and cardiac dysrhythmias. Clinically, a widening QRS should be interpreted as increasing concentration of drug within the ion channel. In common with local anesthetic agents, the sodium channel preferentially binds ionized TCA (25); these effects can be reversed by alkalinization (26). As TCAs are weak bases, the ionized fraction increases with acidosis and the degree of block increases. As the sodium channel block is rate dependent, the QRS width increases with increasing heart rates (27). Eventually, the heart rate slows with increasing sodium channel blockade.

Other cardiac channel effects include reversible inhibition of the outward potassium channels responsible for repolarization giving a mechanism for QT prolongation and dysrhythmia generation (28). TCA demonstrate a dose-dependent direct depressant effect on myocardial contractility that is independent of impaired conduction (29). Although the mechanism is not well defined, it is known that TCA alter mitochondrial function and uncouple oxidative phosphorylation (30).

Animal models have shown direct vasoconstrictive effects on pulmonary vasculature with rupture of capillaries and alveolar epithelium causing pulmonary edema (31). These changes are linearly related to concentration over the range of 0.01 to 1.0 mM and have been demonstrated with wide range of cyclic antidepressants (32).

PREGNANCY AND LACTATION

The U.S. Food and Drug Administration and Australian pregnancy categories for all these agents are C (Appendix I), with the exception of imipramine and nortriptyline (U.S. Food and Drug Administration category D). No adverse events were found, and amitriptyline and nortriptyline blood levels were undetectable in nursing mothers treated with amitriptyline, nortriptyline, desipramine, and imipramine (33). A metaanalysis of maternal exposure (34) found no greater risk of major malformations after antidepressant exposure. A case control study found no association between TCA exposure and either congenital malformations or developmental delay (35).

CLINICAL PRESENTATION

Acute Overdosage

After overdose, there are three major components to the clinical presentation. These are anticholinergic symptoms, cardiovascular toxicity, and central nervous system toxicity. Symptoms and signs at presentation depend on the dose and the time since ingestion. The rapid absorption of TCA can cause a patient with initially trivial symptoms to deteriorate and develop life-threatening toxicity within an hour (5). Patients who are asymptomatic at 3 hours post-ingestion of normal release medication do not normally develop major toxicity (36). With good supportive care the mortality of patients presenting to hospital is less than 0.5%.

Serious complications of TCA ingestion—ventricular dysrhythmias, seizures, and severe hypotension—usually develop within 6 hours. Patients at high risk are identified by a history of high-ingested dose, early onset of deteriorating level of consciousness, and the presence of ECG conduction abnormalities. The QRS duration correlates with the unbound amitriptyline and nortriptyline concentrations in the distribution (α) phase. The level of consciousness correlated with plasma and unbound amitriptyline concentrations in both α and β (elimination) phases and with red blood cell amitriptyline concentration in the alpha phase. Generally, patients wake up within 24 hours, even after a severe TCA overdose (24). As TCA concentrations are still high, this suggests some tolerance to the sedative effects.

Two separate series of consecutive admissions to one unit included 157 dothiepin and 417 other TCA ingestions. Seizures occurred in 11.5% of the dothiepin group and 2.8% of the other TCA group (9,10). Although QRS prolongation more than 100 msec occurred in 47% of the groups, only 2.3% had life-threatening dysrhythmias (10). In the same unit, 80% of patients who presented with seizures and QRS prolongation had ingested a TCA (37).

Anticholinergic Effects

Anticholinergic effects can occur early or late in the course of TCA toxicity. Patients who present early or who have not developed unconsciousness may experience a central cholinergic syndrome and other anticholinergic effects. The pupils may be dilated but are often found to be mid range and poorly reactive to light. Paralysis of accommodation may lead to blurred vision. The other anticholinergic effects lead to a dry mouth, dry skin, tachycardia, and occasionally urinary retention. Bowel sounds may be absent. These early anticholinergic symptoms or signs are a sensitive indicator for ingestion of TCAs but are a poor predictor for life-threatening toxicity.

Severely poisoned patients commonly have an anticholinergic delirium at the time of extubation, which may persist for some days. This can occur in the relative absence of peripheral anticholinergic symptoms.

Cardiovascular Effects

Hypotension is usually due to α-receptor blockade–mediated peripheral vasodilatation and relative volume depletion. Most patients respond to volume expansion with intravenous fluids. TCAs can also cause direct myocardial depression, which is generally associated with conduction defects. Broad complex bradycardia associated with hypotension is a marker of severe toxicity. Untreated, it is likely that the patient will die within 10 minutes.

Sinus tachycardia is present in most patients with clinically significant TCA poisoning. Persistent tachycardia after regaining consciousness is most frequently due to persisting anticholinergic effect or volume depletion. Other possible etiologies that should be considered include anxiety, delirium, and drug withdrawal.

Broad complex tachycardia may develop in serious cases. It may be difficult to distinguish between a supraventricular tachycardia with QRS widening and a ventricular tachycardia. Both are poor prognostic signs as the extent of the QRS duration correlates with TCA blood levels (38). Acutely poisoned patients with QRS widening are normally unconscious. If the patient is conscious and has QRS widening at presentation, consider chronic toxicity or other cardiac disease.

Central Nervous System Effects

In most patients, a significantly impaired level of consciousness precedes cardiac complications or seizures. Patients often have a rapid onset of decreasing level of consciousness and coma because of rapid absorption. Patients should be assessed on admission to see if their deep tendon reflexes are overly reactive of if they have myoclonic jerks, which may predict subsequent seizures. A number of TCA (dothiepin, desipramine, and amoxapine) cause seizures after a smaller ingestion, with fewer ECG abnormalities and occasionally in conscious patients (9). Although seizures are often self-limited, they are associated with an increased mortality. Acidosis associated with seizure increases the risk of cardiotoxicity.

Other Clinical Effects

Pulmonary complications include aspiration, as well as cardiac and noncardiogenic pulmonary edema. Rhabdomyolysis may occur after seizures or pressure necrosis. Hyperthermia occurs rarely; the etiology is multifactorial and includes central temperature dysregulation, seizures, sepsis, and reduced heat loss (23).

Chronic Overdosage

Patients with chronic toxicity may develop the tolerance to the sedative effects and not be sedated. They can present with seizure or dysrhythmia and may have ECG changes consistent with TCA. Unlike acute poisonings, chronic poisonings show high concentrations of active metabolite (39). Chronic poisoning can occur with the continued ingestion of a high dose or the ingestion of an otherwise normal therapeutic dose in a cytochrome CYP2D6 *slow metabolizer* or in the presence of drugs that compete for the relevant cytochrome.

Adverse Events

Common adverse effects during therapeutic use include sedation, dry mouth, blurred vision, constipation, weight gain, orthostatic hypotension, urinary hesitancy or retention, reduced gastrointestinal motility, anticholinergic delirium (particularly in the elderly and in Parkinson's disease), impotence, loss of libido, other sexual adverse effects, tremor, dizziness, sweating, agitation, and insomnia (7) (Table 6).

TABLE 6. Comparative adverse effects of the antidepressants

Comparative adverse effects of tricyclic antidepressants and mianserin drug	Sedation	Anticholinergic effect	Orthostatic hypotension
Amitriptyline	+++	+++	+++
Clomipramine	++	++	++
Dothiepin	++	++	++
Doxepin	+++	+++	+++
Imipramine	++	++	++
Nortriptyline	++	+	+
Trimipramine	+++	+++	+++
Mianserin	+++	+	++

+, present; ++, +++, strongly present.
Modified from Rossi S. Tricyclic antidepressants and mianserin. In: Rossi S, ed. *Australian medicines handbook*. Adelaide: Australian Medicines Handbook Pty Ltd, 2002.

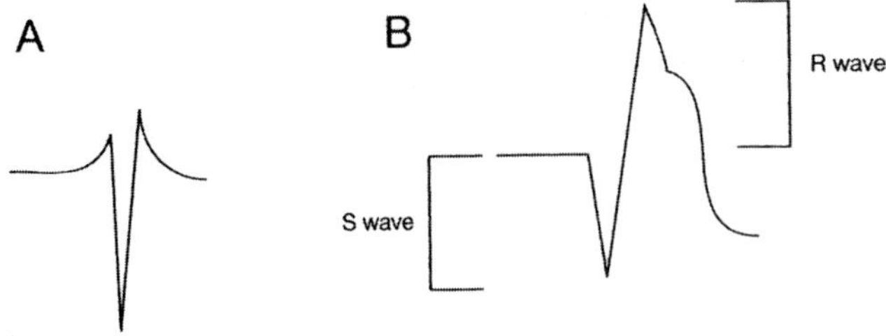

Figure 2. Electrocardiogram lead aVR in patients with tricyclic antidepressant toxicity. **A:** Normal QRS interval in lead aVR. **B:** An abnormal QRS interval as it appears in a patient with severe tricyclic antidepressant poisoning. R_{aVR} was measured as the maximal height in millimeters of the terminal upward deflection in the QRS complex, with the PQ segment used as the baseline. The S wave was measured in millimeters as the depth of the initial downward deflection. (From Liebelt EL, Francis PD, Woolf AD. ECG lead aVR versus QRS interval in predicting seizures and arrhythmias in acute tricyclic antidepressant toxicity. *Ann Emerg Med* 1995;26:195–201, with permission.)

Infrequent adverse effects include slowed cardiac conduction, T-wave inversion or flattening (particularly at high doses), dysrhythmias, sinus tachycardia, nausea, hyperglycemia, gynecomastia in men, breast enlargement and galactorrhea in women, allergic skin reactions, and manic episodes (7).

Rare adverse effects include blood dyscrasias, hepatitis, paralytic ileus, syndrome of inappropriate secretion of antidiuretic hormone with hyponatremia, seizures, and neuroleptic malignant syndrome (7). The most significant, although rare, adverse effect of tetracyclics is the development of neutropenia, which is usually reversible. Mianserin is a sedating antidepressant and may also produce a polyarthritis (40).

DIAGNOSTIC TESTS

Acute Overdosage

In conjunction with a physical examination that includes careful assessment of the level of coma, the most useful investigations are the ECG, arterial blood gas, and serum electrolytes.

Electrocardiogram

An ECG should be performed on admission and at 6 hours after the self-poisoning in asymptomatic patients. The ECG is the most accurate predictor of toxicity for the majority of TCA poisonings. Minor ECG changes are common and include an increase in the PR interval, dimpling of the T-wave, and narrow complex sinus tachycardia. The more serious changes reflect altered conduction through Purkinje fibers due predominately to sodium channel blockade (Table 7).

The majority of the studies on predicting outcome from ECG abnormalities have been too small to allow a confident estimate of sensitivity and specificity and have been weakened by the use of arbitrary cut points defined during post hoc analysis. Invariably, the prediction has not been as definitive when others have tried to replicate the findings. In addition, the observer variation (inter-rater agreement) has not been defined, particularly as it applies to these arbitrary cut points (41).

TABLE 7. Electrocardiographic changes predictive of complications in tricyclic antidepressant poisoning

Predictive measurements that have been suggested include the following:
- QRS of 100 ms or more
- Terminal 40 ms frontal plane axis greater than 120 degrees
- Height of R wave and R/S ratio greater than 0.7 in aVR

Brugada syndrome

Clinical experience indicates that the majority of patients at significant risk for developing cardiac or neurologic toxicity have a QRS complex more than 0.10 seconds or a rightward shift of the terminal 40 milliseconds of the frontal plane QRS complex vector (42). Boehnert and Lovejoy (43) described the association of a QRS duration of 100 milliseconds or more with the development of seizures and dysrhythmias. Although subsequent experience has confirmed this as a sensitive marker, it is also clear that a QRS less than 100 milliseconds cannot be used to definitely exclude major complications (44). A normal ECG does not exclude major complications (9). All patients with an abnormal ECG or altered level of consciousness require ECG monitoring.

A right axis deviation or a pattern of right bundle branch block producing a terminal 40 milliseconds frontal plane axis more than 120 degrees is often observed in TCA poisoning. The association is not absolute but appears stronger than that observed with QRS width (44). The height of the R wave and the R/S ratio in ECG lead aVR also have predictive value. The sensitivity of a R_{aVR} of 3 mm or more was 81%, and that of a R/S_{aVR} of 0.7 or more was 75% for predicting seizures or dysrhythmias (Fig. 2) (36). A group of patients who would satisfy these criteria but have additional ST segment abnormalities have been described as a TCA-induced Brugada syndrome (45). The Brugada syndrome is a genetically determined sodium-channel dysfunction. The ECG characteristically shows a right bundle-branch block and unusual ST-segment elevation in the right precordial leads. It was reported in 12 of 95 patients presenting with overdose of TCAs. The ECG changes resolved when plasma TCA concentrations dropped below 1000 ng/ml. It is not clear whether the presence of the Brugada pattern has additional prognostic importance (45).

Other Tests

Arterial blood gases assist in monitoring treatment with systemic alkalinization. In severe poisonings, a mixed respiratory and metabolic acidosis is common. Respiratory acidosis is an absolute indication for ventilation. Hypoxia may be due to a number of the pulmonary complications seen in TCA poisoning including aspiration, cardiac, and noncardiac pulmonary edema.

Urine screens confirm exposure but do not add any prognostic information to the clinical examination and ECG. Blood

TABLE 8. Suggested or expected therapeutic ranges for the antidepressant drugs available in the United States

Drug	Therapeutic range (μg/L)
Tricyclic drugs	
Imipramine desipramine	150–250
Nortriptyline	50–150
Amitriptyline nortriptyline	80–250
Desipramine	125–300
Protriptyline	70–260
Doxepin desmethyldoxepin	150–250
Trimipramine	Similar to other tricyclic drugs
Other antidepressant drugs	
Maprotiline	200–600
Amoxapine 8-hydroxyamoxapine	200–600
Trazodone	800–1600
Alprazolam	20–55
Fluoxetine	Not available

Modified from Orsulak PJ. Therapeutic monitoring of antidepressant drugs: guidelines updated. *Ther Drug Monit* 1989;11:497–507.

TABLE 9. Management of tricyclic antidepressant overdose

- Check vital signs, level of coma, 12-lead ECG, arterial blood gases
- Administer oxygen, establish IV access, and start fluids
- Intubate and ventilate
  - Ingestion of >10 mg/g with impaired consciousness if <2 h since ingestion
  - Any respiratory acidosis or failure
  - Inability to protect airway
- Decontaminate: activated charcoal in water 1 g/kg
  - All patients less than 2 h from ingestion
  - All patients who require intubation
- Treat complications
  - Acidosis
    - Uncomplicated
      - Sodium bicarbonate 1 mEq/kg bolus (or in adult 50 mEq bolus) and review
    - Complicated by hypotension or QRS >120 ms
      - Sodium bicarbonate 2 mEq/kg bolus
  - Seizures
    - Diazepam, 0.1 mg/kg IV as needed; phenobarbital infusion (15 mg/kg IV) over 30 min if refractory
    - Check the ECG and acid-base status
  - Hypotension
    - If QRS <100 ms
      - 20 ml/kg normal saline stat
      - Trendelenburg position
    - If QRS >120 ms
      - Sodium bicarbonate 2 mEq/kg bolus repeated until QRS narrows or arterial pH reaches 7.55
      - Give fluid bolus if not already done
    - Volume loading may require 3–5 L in an adult, which is best done with central venous pressure monitoring
    - Consider vasopressors
  - Broad complex tachydysrhythmias
    - With detectable output
      - Sodium bicarbonate, 2 mEq/kg bolus, repeated until QRS narrows or pH reaches 7.55
    - With no output
      - Sodium bicarbonate, 3–6 mEq/kg bolus, repeat until improvement or pH reaches 7.55
      - Standard, but prolonged ACLS resuscitation; do not stop until you have a toxicology consultation
    - Other measures
      - Consider magnesium
      - Overdrive pacing
      - Consider hypertonic saline[a]
  - Broad complex bradydysrhythmia
    - With detectable output
      - Sodium bicarbonate, 2 mEq/kg bolus, repeated until QRS narrows or pH reaches 7.55
    - With no output
      - Sodium bicarbonate, 3–6 mEq/kg bolus, repeat until improved or pH reached 7.55
      - Standard, but prolonged ACLS resuscitation; do not stop until you have a toxicology consultation
    - Other measures
      - Consider pacing or isoproterenol
      - Consider hypertonic saline[a]

ECG, electrocardiogram.
[a]Hypertonic saline: ensure you have achieved a pH of at least 7.55, and give 3 mEq of hypertonic saline as a bolus injection. The role of this treatment is not well defined. Note the clinical effects and report your findings
From Buckley NA, Dawson AH, Whyte IM. Tricyclic antidepressants. In: *HyperTox: assessment and treatment of poisoning*, v1229 ed. Newcastle, Australia: MediTox Pty Ltd, 2002, with permission.

TCA concentrations do not contribute to the acute management of most TCA poisoning. They are useful in helping to define the relative contribution of drug toxicity to neurologic dysfunction in patients who have sustained hypoxic brain injury. Therapeutic blood concentration ranges for antidepressant drugs available in the United States are listed in Table 8 (46). Patients with plasma TCA levels greater than 450 ng/ml tend to develop cognitive or behavioral toxicity (agitation, disorientation, confusion, memory impairments, fragmented speech, pacing, decreased concentration). Major toxicity and death is associated with levels above 1000 ng/ml. The ratio of parent drug to metabolite is greater than 2 in acute poisonings (47).

Postmortem Considerations

In overdose cases in which the total blood TCA concentration (parent drug and major active metabolite) exceeds 1000 ng/ml, toxicity and resulting fatality are probable (48). Postmortem blood concentrations can be substantially higher than concentrations at the time of death (49). The ratio of parent drug to major metabolite may aid in the decision process for cases in which the manner of death was ambiguous. Death soon after acute poisoning has a high parent to metabolite ratio. Postmortem blood concentrations may not reflect the drug concentration at the time of death (50). In chronic toxicity, tissue concentrations may be a better guide than plasma concentrations (51,52).

TREATMENT

Acute Overdosage

The key acute issues are airway management and correction of acidosis. A significant ingestion in a suicidal patient is generally associated with a decreasing level of consciousness that necessitates intubation to facilitate decontamination and subsequent management. Patients who are conscious at 3 hours after ingestion are unlikely to develop major toxicity. Mortality is low when patients receive good supportive care and alkalinization. An overview of management is presented in Table 9.

Decontamination

If the patient is alert, cooperative, and has potentially ingested more than 5 mg/kg, activated charcoal may be administered orally. In practice, this is only relevant for patients who present within 1 to 2 hours of ingestion. Most patients with an ingestion more than 10 mg/kg are either unconscious or have a deteriorating level of consciousness within 2 hours and should be intubated. These patients should have either a nasogastric or orogastric tube to administer charcoal. The published evidence is insufficient to support or refute orogastric lavage in this group. A trend favoring benefit of administering activated charcoal, then gastric lavage, then repeated charcoal has been reported in an underpowered study (53). If a gastric tube is inserted, it is reasonable to aspirate stomach contents before giving charcoal. There is no evidence supporting the use of cathartics or whole bowel irrigation.

Enhancement of Elimination

Repeated doses of activated charcoal increase the clearance of several TCA, but there is no evidence of improved outcome. It should not be used routinely but may be reasonable for modified-release preparations. In practice, most patients with TCA poisoning who are ventilated have an ileus, which precludes the use of multiple-dose activated charcoal.

Hemoperfusion or hemodialysis has been proposed as a treatment option for severe TCA poisoning (54). At steady state, the protein binding and volume of distribution is so high that dialysis would not be considered effective (55). Protagonists of the technique argue for benefit in the early distribution phase; however, there is no supporting clinical or animal work for this view. Calculations of the amount of TCA actually removed the amount to less than 3% of the ingested dose (56,57).

Antidotes

Magnesium sulfate may terminate persistent ventricular tachycardia; in one case a bolus followed by 7 days of continuous infusion was required (58). The use of other antidysrhythmic agents is less clear; class 1A and class 1C drugs and procainamide are contraindicated (59). Although lidocaine has been used with varying success, there is no proven efficacy for class 3 or 4 agents. Overdrive pacing should be considered for refractory ventricular tachycardia (60).

Sodium bicarbonate is the drug of choice for the treatment of all TCA-associated conduction defects, ventricular dysrhythmias, and hypotension due to TCA poisoning (59). Details regarding the use of hypertonic sodium bicarbonate are provided in Chapter 75. Sodium bicarbonate provides hypertonicity, sodium loading, and alkalinization. Sodium loading and alkalinization have been effective in reversing TCA-induced conduction defects and hypotension (61); both are supplied by hypertonic sodium bicarbonate. It should be administered by intermittent bolus injections of 1 to 3 mEq/kg body weight, not by continuous infusion. The initial treatment in critically ill patients is often titrated against clinical response with bolus injections repeated at 3- to 5-minute intervals. When the clinical situation allows it, arterial blood pH should be checked. The goal of sodium bicarbonate therapy is to narrow the QRS complex without exceeding an arterial pH of 7.50 to 7.55. Sustained elevations of pH greater than this are associated with impaired oxygen dissociation from hemoglobin. As the patient is normally ventilated, the pH can be maintained with mild hyperventilation ($Pa{CO_2}$ of 30 mm Hg).

The mechanism of the therapeutic effect is multifactorial (62). Alkalosis decreases the free drug concentration by increasing protein binding. However, pH change is effective in the absence of protein (63,64) and probably directly affects the binding affinity of TCA in the sodium channel.

Although it is common practice for patients with conduction defects to receive sodium bicarbonate in the absence of dysrhythmias or hypotension, there is little evidence to support or refute this practice (62). The pH in these patients should be carefully monitored. It is rational to give bicarbonate to any patient with a wide QRS who has had a seizure or needs to be intubated as both these situations may increase acidosis. Once patients have received sodium bicarbonate their maintenance fluid should be reassessed to avoid sodium overload.

Hypertonic saline had greater efficacy than alkalinization in improving cardiac conduction and hypotension in a swine model (61). The dose used in this study was 10 ml/kg of hypertonic saline solution in the form of a 7.5% sodium chloride solution (15 mEq/kg NaCl). The mean peak serum sodium after treatment was 157 mEq/L. This dose was selected, as it had been the maximal dose used previously in the treatment of trauma in humans.

As standard supportive care and sodium bicarbonate have been so effective, the clinical use of hypertonic saline is rarely reported. A 34-year-old man with dothiepin-induced ventricular tachycardia and hypotension responded to 170 mmol of hypertonic saline given over 5 minutes; subsequent episodes responded to bolus doses of 100 mmol (65). The administration of 200 ml of 7.5% saline over 3 minutes improved refractory hypotension and conduction defects in a 29-year-old woman (66). A 6-year-old with imipramine poisoning had no response to a slow infusion of 60 mEq of hypertonic saline (67). The role of hypertonic saline remains undefined, but it could be considered in situations of refractory hypotension and dysrhythmia. It appears that it should be administered as a bolus injection rather than an infusion. The potential risks of this treatment include fluid and sodium overload and complications of hypernatremia such as central pontine myelinolysis.

Supportive Care

Intravenous access should be established in all patients; the initial fluid should be normal saline. All patients should have assessment of the adequacy of their airway protection and ventilation. Mechanical ventilation should be provided to any patient who cannot protect his or her airway, has a respiratory acidosis, or presents within 2 hours with altered level of consciousness and ingestion of greater than 10 mg/kg. Ventilation should not be the primary method of achieving systemic alkalinization (Chapter 75). Mild hyperventilation can maintain a patient in alkalosis, but the $Pa{CO_2}$ should not fall below 25 mm Hg. Patients should have continuous ECG monitoring for at least 6 hours after ingestion.

Delirium can often be managed with reassurance but occasionally requires benzodiazepines to control agitation. Neuroleptics should be avoided as most of them have either anticholinergic activity or ion channel blocking effects. Although physostigmine is effective, the short half-life of this drug and its occasional life-threatening adverse effects (particularly in TCA overdose) make it contraindicated.

Seizures are often self-limited. If prolonged or repeated, seizures are treated with diazepam, 5 to 20 mg IV. If benzodiazepines do not control the seizures, patients may require phenobarbital, 15 to 18 mg/kg IV, and elective intubation and ventilation. If neuromuscular blockade is required for management, electroencephalogram monitoring is mandatory. The major complication of seizures is increased acidosis precipitating major cardiovascular toxicity. All patients who have seized should be assessed for the presence of indications to receive sodium bicarbonate.

Hypotension in the conscious patient is usually due to peripheral vasodilation (68) and responds to volume expansion. The initial fluid challenge should be 10 to 20 ml/kg of normal saline. As TCA concentrations increase, other factors may contribute to hypotension. This includes further volume loss into third spaces such as intestinal ileus and direct myocardial depression. Myocardial depression is commonly associated with conduction defects and should be initially treated with sodium bicarbonate (59). Most hypotension responds to these measures. Temporary pacing should also be considered for ventricular bradydysrhythmias and bifascicular block.

Refractory hypotension requires central venous pressure monitoring and correction of volume and acid-base status. If hypotension persists, drugs with α-agonist properties (e.g., epinephrine and norepinephrine) should be used cautiously (59) as they may precipitate ventricular tachycardia. Epinephrine was superior to norepinephrine when used both with and without sodium bicarbonate in an animal model (69). Glucagon was reported to be effective in one case report (70); however, it appeared that adequate correction of acidosis had not been achieved (71).

Monitoring

Monitoring consists primarily of serial evaluation of the 12-lead ECG. Patients are medically fit for discharge if they have no symptoms or signs of toxicity (including no anticholinergic features such as tachycardia) and a normal ECG performed 6 hours after the overdose (especially if they have passed a charcoal stool). A patient with persistent isolated tachycardia should generally be kept in hospital and observed. As the usual cause is volume depletion, IV fluid to ensure adequate volume replacement should be given.

A patient with a QRS complex equal to or greater than 100 millisecond should be monitored until this has returned to normal. Typically QRS duration returns to normal within 1 day but may persist for longer periods in severe poisoning (72). Reports of occasional late cardiac arrest have occurred in patients with persistently abnormal ECG. Continued drug absorption or exposure may be the cause for late deterioration in this group, and markedly delayed toxicity (greater than 24 hours) has only been reported in patients who did not receive gastrointestinal decontamination or, more recently, in modified release amitriptyline overdose.

Management Pitfalls

Flumazenil should not be administered in any patient suspected of taking a TCA even if benzodiazepines are coingested. Its use may precipitate seizures and death (73,74).

REFERENCES

1. Graudins A, Dowsett RP, Liddle C. The toxicity of antidepressant poisoning: is it changing? A comparative study of cyclic and newer serotonin-specific antidepressants. *Emerg Med (Fremantle)* 2002;14(4):440–446.
2. Crome P. The toxicity of drugs used for suicide. *Acta Psychiatr Scand Suppl* 1993;371:33–37.
3. Frey R, Schreinzer D, Stimpfl T, et al. [Fatal poisonings with antidepressive drugs and neuroleptics. Analysis of a correlation with prescriptions in Vienna 1991 to 1997]. *Nervenarzt* 2002;73(7):629–636.
4. Schreinzer D, Frey R, Stimpfl T, et al. Different fatal toxicity of neuroleptics identified by autopsy. *Eur Neuropsychopharmacol* 2001;11(2):117–124.
5. Callaham M, Kassel D. Epidemiology of fatal tricyclic antidepressant ingestion: implications for management. *Ann Emerg Med* 1985;14(1):1–9.
6. Buckley NA, Whyte IM, Dawson AH, et al. Self-poisoning in Newcastle, 1987-1992. *Med J Aust* 1995;162(4):190–193.
7. Rossi S. Tricyclic antidepressants and mianserin. In: Rossi S, et al., eds. *Australian medicines handbook*. Adelaide: Australian Medicines Handbook Pty Ltd, 2002.
8. Buckley NA, Dawson AH, Whyte IM, et al. Toxicity of dothiepin in overdose. *Lancet* 1994;343(8899):735.
9. Buckley NA, Dawson AH, Whyte IM, et al. Greater toxicity in overdose of dothiepin than of other tricyclic antidepressants. *Lancet* 1994;343(8890):159–162.
10. Whyte IM, Dawson AH, Buckley NA. Relative toxicity of venlafaxine and selective serotonin reuptake inhibitors in overdose compared to tricyclic antidepressants. *QJM* 2003;96(5):369.
11. McFee RB, Caraccio TR, Mofenson HC. Selected tricyclic antidepressant ingestions involving children 6 years old or less. *Acad Emerg Med* 2001;8(2):139–144.
12. Varley CK, McClellan J. Case study: two additional sudden deaths with tricyclic antidepressants. *J Am Acad Child Adolesc Psychiatry* 1997;36(3):390–394.
13. Cassidy S, Henry J. Fatal toxicity of antidepressant drugs in overdose. *Br Med J (Clin Res Ed)* 1987;295(6605):1021–1024.
14. Rudorfer MV, Potter WZ. Metabolism of tricyclic antidepressants. *Cell Mol Neurobiol* 1999;19(3):373–409.
15. Greene SL, Dargan PI, Antoniades H, et al. Delayed clinical effects in modified-release amitriptyline poisoning. A case report with toxicokinetic data. *J Toxicol Clin Toxicol* 2002;40(3):138.
16. Eap CB, Cuendet C, Baumann P. Binding of amitriptyline to alpha 1-acid glycoprotein and its variants. *J Pharm Pharmacol* 1988;40(11):767–770.
17. Ma Y, Henry JA. The antidotal effect of alpha(1)-acid glycoprotein on amitriptyline toxicity in cardiac myocytes. *Toxicology* 2001;169(2):133–144.
18. Juarez-Olguin H, Jung-Cook H, Flores-Perez J, et al. Clinical evidence of an interaction between imipramine and acetylsalicylic acid on protein binding in depressed patients. *Clin Neuropharmacol* 2002;25(1):32–36.
19. Levitt MA, Sullivan JB Jr., Owens SM, et al. Amitriptyline plasma protein binding: effect of plasma pH and relevance to clinical overdose. *Am J Emerg Med* 1986;4(2):121–125.
20. Ereshefsky L, Tran-Johnson T, Davis CM, et al. Pharmacokinetic factors affecting antidepressant drug clearance and clinical effect: evaluation of doxepin and imipramine—new data and review [Review] [124 refs]. *Clin Chem* 1988;34(5):863–880.
21. Jarvis MR. Clinical pharmacokinetics of tricyclic antidepressant overdose [Review] [85 refs]. *Psychopharmacol Bull* 1991;27(4):541–550.
22. Spiker DG, Biggs JT. Tricyclic antidepressants. Prolonged plasma levels after overdose. *JAMA* 1976;236(15):1711–1712.
23. Pentel PR, Benowitz NL. Tricyclic antidepressant poisoning. Management of arrhythmias. *Med Toxicol* 1986;1(2):101–121.
24. Hulten BA, Heath A, Knudsen K, et al. Severe amitriptyline overdose: relationship between toxicokinetics and toxicodynamics. *J Toxicol Clin Toxicol* 1992;30(2):171–179.
25. Narahashi T, Frazier DT. Site of action and active form of local anesthetics. *Neurosci Res (N Y)* 1971;4:65–99.
26. Ritchie JM, Greengard P. On the mode of action of local anesthetics. *Annu Rev Pharmacol* 1966;6:405–430.
27. Ansel GM, Coyne K, Arnold S, et al. Mechanisms of ventricular arrhythmia during amitriptyline toxicity. *J Cardiovasc Pharmacol* 1993;22(6):798–803.
28. Teschemacher AG, Seward EP, Hancox JC, et al. Inhibition of the current of heterologously expressed HERG potassium channels by imipramine and amitriptyline. *Br J Pharmacol* 1999;128(2):479–485.
29. Heard K, Cain BS, Dart RC, et al. Tricyclic antidepressants directly depress human myocardial mechanical function independent of effects on the conduction system. *Acad Emerg Med* 2001;8(12):1122.
30. Weinbach EC, Costa JL, Nelson BD, et al. Effects of tricyclic antidepressant drugs on energy-linked reactions in mitochondria. *Biochem Pharmacol* 1986;35(9):1445–1451.
31. Liu X, Emery CJ, Laude E, et al. Adverse pulmonary vascular effects of high dose tricyclic antidepressants: acute and chronic animal studies. *Eur Respir J* 2002;20(2):344–352.
32. Dahlin KL, Lastbom L, Blomgren B, et al. Acute lung failure induced by tricyclic antidepressants. *Toxicol Appl Pharmacol* 1997;146(2):309–316.
33. Birnbaum CS, Cohen LS, Bailey JW, et al. Serum concentrations of antidepressants and benzodiazepines in nursing infants: a case series. *Pediatrics* 1999;104(1):e11.
34. Wisner KL, Gelenberg AJ, Leonard H, et al. Pharmacologic treatment of depression during pregnancy. *JAMA* 1999;282(13):1264–1269.
35. Simon GE, Cunningham ML, Davis RL. Outcomes of prenatal antidepressant exposure. *Am J Psychiatry* 2002;159(12):2055–2061.
36. Liebelt EL, Francis PD, Woolf AD. ECG lead aVR versus QRS interval in predicting seizures and arrhythmias in acute tricyclic antidepressant toxicity. *Ann Emerg Med* 1995;26(2):195–201.
37. Buckley NA, Whyte IM, Dawson AH. Diagnostic data in clinical toxicology—should we use a Bayesian approach? *J Toxicol Clin Toxicol* 2002;40(3):213–222.
38. Amitai Y, Erickson T, Kennedy EJ, et al. Tricyclic antidepressants in red cells and plasma: correlation with impaired intraventricular conduction in acute overdose. *Clin Pharmacol Ther* 1993;54(2):219–227.
39. Swanson JR, Jones GR, Krasselt W, et al. Death of two subjects due to imipramine and desipramine metabolite accumulation during chronic therapy: a review of the literature and possible mechanisms. *J Forensic Sci* 1997;42(2):335–339.
40. *Psychotropic guidelines*, 2nd ed. Melbourne: Therapeutic Guidelines Ltd, 2000.
41. Buckley NA, O'Connell DL, Whyte IM, et al. Interrater agreement in the measurement of QRS interval in tricyclic antidepressant overdose: implications for monitoring and research. *Ann Emerg Med* 1996;28(5):515–519.
42. Harrigan RA, Brady WJ. ECG abnormalities in tricyclic antidepressant ingestion. *Am J Emerg Med* 1999;17(4):387–393.
43. Boehnert MT, Lovejoy FH Jr. Value of the QRS duration versus the serum drug level in predicting seizures and ventricular arrhythmias after an acute overdose of tricyclic antidepressants. *N Engl J Med* 1985;313(8):474–479.
44. Foulke GE, Albertson TE. QRS interval in tricyclic antidepressant overdosage: inaccuracy as a toxicity indicator in emergency settings. *Ann Emerg Med* 1987;16(2):160–163.
45. Goldgran-Toledano D, Sideris G, Kevorkian JP. Overdose of cyclic antidepressants and the Brugada syndrome. *N Engl J Med* 2002;346(20):1591–1592.
46. Orsulak PJ. Therapeutic monitoring of antidepressant drugs: guidelines updated. *Ther Drug Monit* 1989;11(5):497–507.
47. Bailey DN, Van Dyke C, Langou RA, et al. Tricyclic antidepressants: plasma levels and clinical findings in overdose. *Am J Psychiatry* 1978;135(11):1325–1328.
48. Frommer DA, Kulig KW, Marx JA, et al. Tricyclic antidepressant overdose. A review. *JAMA* 1987;257(4):521–526.
49. Apple FS, Bandt CM. Liver and blood postmortem tricyclic antidepressant concentrations. *Am J Clin Pathol* 1988;89(6):794–796.
50. Apple FS. Postmortem tricyclic antidepressant concentrations: assessing cause of death using parent drug to metabolite ratio. *J Anal Toxicol* 1989;13(4):197–198.
51. Amitai Y. Establishing a cause of death dependent upon time of postmortem. *J Toxicol Clin Toxicol* 2001;39(6):651–652.
52. Davis G, Park K, Kloss J, et al. Tricyclic antidepressant fatality: postmortem tissue concentrations. *J Toxicol Clin Toxicol* 2001;39(6):649–650.
53. Bosse GM, Barefoot JA, Pfeifer MP, et al. Comparison of three methods of gut decontamination in tricyclic antidepressant overdose. *J Emerg Med* 1995;13(2):203–209.
54. Frank RD, Kierdorf HP. Is there a role for hemoperfusion/hemodialysis as a treatment option in severe tricyclic antidepressant intoxication? *Int J Artif Organs* 2000;23(9):618–623.

55. Gwilt PR, Perrier D. Plasma protein binding and distribution characteristics of drugs as indices of their hemodialyzability. *Clin Pharmacol Ther* 1978;24(2):154–161.
56. Heath A, Wickstrom I, Martensson E, et al. Treatment of antidepressant poisoning with resin hemoperfusion. *Hum Toxicol* 1982;1(4):361–371.
57. Pentel PR, Bullock ML, DeVane CL. Hemoperfusion for imipramine overdose: elimination of active metabolites. *J Toxicol Clin Toxicol* 1982;19(3):239–248.
58. Citak A, Soysal DD, Ucsel R, et al. Efficacy of long duration resuscitation and magnesium sulphate treatment in amitriptyline poisoning. *Eur J Emerg Med* 2002;9(1):63–66.
59. Albertson TE, Dawson A, de Latorre F, et al. TOX-ACLS: toxicologic-oriented advanced cardiac life support. *Ann Emerg Med* 2001;37(4 Suppl):S78–S90.
60. Peters RW, Buser GA, Kim HJ, et al. Tricyclic overdose causing sustained monomorphic ventricular tachycardia. *Am J Cardiol* 1992;70(13):1226–1228.
61. McCabe JL, Cobaugh DJ, Menegazzi JJ, et al. Experimental tricyclic antidepressant toxicity: a randomized, controlled comparison of hypertonic saline solution, sodium bicarbonate, and hyperventilation. *Ann Emerg Med* 1998;32(3 Pt 1):329–333.
62. Blackman K, Brown SG, Wilkes GJ. Plasma alkalinization for tricyclic antidepressant toxicity: a systematic review. *Emerg Med (Fremantle)* 2001;13(2):204–210.
63. Sasyniuk BI, Jhamandas V. Mechanism of reversal of toxic effects of amitriptyline on cardiac Purkinje fibers by sodium bicarbonate. *J Pharmacol Exp Ther* 1984;231(2):387–394.
64. Wang R, Schuyler J, Raymond R. The role of the cell membrane bicarbonate exchanger in $NaHCO_3$ therapy of imipramine cardiac dysfunction. *J Toxicol Clin Toxicol* 1997;35:533.
65. Hoegholm A, Clementsen P. Hypertonic sodium chloride in severe antidepressant overdosage. *J Toxicol Clin Toxicol* 1991;29(2):297–298.
66. Rasmussen R, McKinney PE. Hypertonic saline in severe tricyclic antidepressant cardiotoxicity. *J Toxicol Clin Toxicol* 1999;37:634.
67. Dolara P, Franconi F. Hypertonic sodium chloride and lidocaine in a case of imipramine intoxication. *Clin Toxicol* 1977;10(4):395–398.
68. Langou RA, Van Dyke C, Tahan SR, et al. Cardiovascular manifestations of tricyclic antidepressant overdose. *Am Heart J* 1980;100(4):458–464.
69. Knudsen K, Abrahamsson J. Epinephrine and sodium bicarbonate independently and additively increase survival in experimental amitriptyline poisoning. *Crit Care Med* 1997;25(4):669–674.
70. Sensky PR, Olczak SA. High-dose intravenous glucagon in severe tricyclic poisoning. *Postgrad Med J* 1999;75(888):611–612.
71. Schuster-Bruce MJ. High dose intravenous glucagon in severe tricyclic poisoning. *Postgrad Med J* 2000;76(897):453.
72. Shannon MW. Duration of QRS disturbances after severe tricyclic antidepressant intoxication. *J Toxicol Clin Toxicol* 1992;30(3):377–386.
73. Mordel A, Winkler E, Almog S, et al. Seizures after flumazenil administration in a case of combined benzodiazepine and tricyclic antidepressant overdose. *Crit Care Med* 1992;20(12):1733–1734.
74. Lheureux P, Vranckx M, Leduc D, et al. Flumazenil in mixed benzodiazepine/tricyclic antidepressant overdose: a placebo-controlled study in the dog. *Am J Emerg Med* 1992;10(3):184–188.

CHAPTER 135
Serotonin Uptake Inhibitors

Ian MacGregor Whyte

See Figure 1.

Compounds included:	**Citalopram (Celexa, Cipramil), fluoxetine (Prozac), fluvoxamine (Faverin, Fluvox), paroxetine (Paxil, Seroxat), sertraline (Lustral, Zoloft)**
Molecular formula and weight:	**See Table 1.**
SI conversion:	**See Table 1.**
CAS Registry No.:	**See Table 1.**
Therapeutic levels:	**See Table 1.**
Target organs:	**Central nervous system (acute)**
Antidotes:	**Cyproheptadine, chlorpromazine**

OVERVIEW

Serotonergic dysfunction has been implicated in illnesses such as depression, anxiety, obsessive-compulsive disorder, sleep and eating disorders, schizophrenia, Alzheimer's dementia, personality disorders, alcoholism, autism, pain, aggression, and impulse disorders. Serotonin uptake inhibitors include citalopram, fluoxetine, fluvoxamine, paroxetine, and sertraline.

Serotonin uptake inhibitors (also known as *selective serotonin reuptake inhibitors*, *serotonin-specific reuptake inhibitors*, or SSRIs) selectively inhibit the presynaptic reuptake of serotonin (5-hydroxytryptamine, 5-HT). This results in increased intrasynaptic 5-HT and subsequent stimulation of postsynaptic 5-HT receptors. 5-HT_1 receptors are thought to be responsible for the antidepressant and anxiolytic effects of the SSRI, whereas many of their toxic effects are thought to be mediated by 5-HT_2 receptors (1,2).

Studies comparing one SSRI with another have failed to demonstrate any differences in efficacy in the treatment of major depression. Toxicity unrelated to serotonin excess is rare and overdose of a single SSRI is usually well tolerated. Coingestion with other serotonergic agents, such as a monoamine oxidase (MAO) inhibitor, can, however, be fatal. SSRI overdose is becoming increasingly frequent as these agents are more commonly used.

The serotonin reuptake inhibitors are a structurally diverse group of drugs (Fig. 1, Table 1). Indications for use include unipolar depression, dysthymia, bipolar depression, treatment-resistant depression, depression in the medically ill, panic disorder, obsessive-compulsive disorder, eating disorders, social phobia, and premenstrual dysphoric disorder (3).

TOXIC DOSE

The *adult and pediatric therapeutic* doses are provided in Table 2. Serotonin toxicity may develop at therapeutic doses. The addition of another serotonergic agent even in therapeutic doses can produce life-threatening serotonin toxicity (Chapter 24). In pure SSRI overdose, serotonin toxicity (syndrome) occurs in 16.3% to 19.3% of cases (4,5).

There have been remarkably few fatal overdoses reported involving ingestion of an SSRI alone (6). Moderate overdoses (up to 30 times the usual daily dose) are associated with minor symptoms, whereas ingestions of greater amounts typically result in mild serotonin toxicity with agitation, confusion, tremor, nausea, vomiting, hyperreflexia, and occasional clonus and myoclonus. At high doses (more than 75 times the common

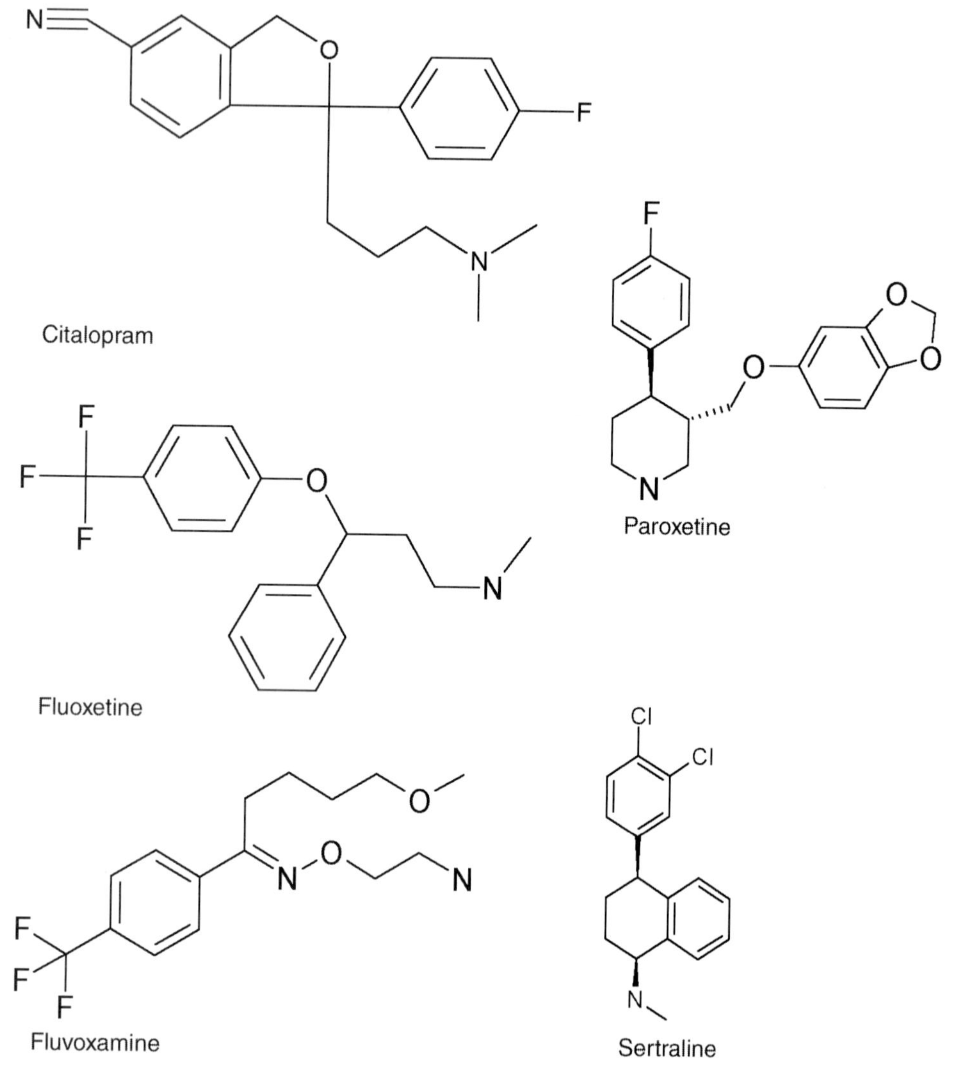

Citalopram

Paroxetine

Fluoxetine

Fluvoxamine

Sertraline

Figure 1. Structures of serotonin uptake inhibitors.

daily dose), more serious serotonin toxicity may occur, as can seizures and occasional cardiac toxicity (6). SSRI overdoses in combination with alcohol or other drugs are associated with increased toxicity, and almost all fatalities involving SSRI have involved coingestion of other substances (6). In general, SSRIs have low fatal toxicity indices (i.e., they are safer) compared with tricyclic antidepressants (7–9).

Citalopram has been associated with electrocardiographic changes (QTc interval prolongation) at a dose of 400 mg (10) and bradycardia in therapeutic doses (11,12). Long-lasting sympto-

TABLE 1. Structural classification of serotonin uptake inhibitors (see also Fig. 1)

Compound	Molecular formula, molecular weight (g/mol), CAS Registry No.	SI conversion, therapeutic, toxic concentrations[a] (mg/L)	Comments
Citalopram hydrobromide	$C_{20}H_{21}FN_2O$,HBr; 324.4; 59729-32-7	mg/L × 3.08 = μmol/L; 0.3, N/A	1-(3-(Dimethylamino)propyl)-1-(p-fluorophenyl)-5-phthalancarbonitrile; phthalane derivative
Fluoxetine hydrochloride	$C_{17}H_{18}F_3NO$,HCl; 309.3; 59333-67-4	mg/L × 3.23 = μmol/L; 0.5, 1.0	N-methyl-gamma-(4-(trifluoromethyl)phenoxy)-, (+-)-benzenepropanamine; aromatic ring phenylpropylamine derivative, bicyclic antidepressant
Fluvoxamine maleate	$C_{15}H_{21}F_3N_2O_2$,$C_4H_4O_4$; 318.3; 61718-82-9	mg/L × 3.14 = μmol/L; 0.3, 5.0	1-Pentanone, 5-methoxy-1-(4-(trifluoromethyl)phenyl)-, O-(2-aminoethyl)oxime, (E)-; one of a series of 2-aminoethyl oximethers of aralkylketones
Paroxetine hydrochloride	$C_{19}H_{20}FNO_3$,HCl, 1/2H_2O; 329.4; 78246-49-8	mg/L × 3.04 = μmol/L; 0.1, 1.0	3-[(1,3-benzodioxol-5-yloxy)methyl]-4-(4-fluorophenyl)-, (3S-trans)- piperidine
Sertraline hydrochloride	$C_{17}H_{17}Cl_2N$,HCl; 379.5; 79559-97-0	mg/L × 3.27 = μmol/L; 0.3, NA	1,2,3,4-tetrahydro-4-(3,4-dichlorophenyl)-N-methyl-, (1S-cis)-1-Naphthalenamine; a naphthylamine derivative

NA, not available.
[a]From Flanagan RJ. Guidelines for the interpretation of analytical toxicology results and unit of measurement conversion factors. *Ann Clin Biochem* 1998;35(Pt 2):261–267, with permission.

TABLE 2. Typical therapeutic doses of serotonin uptake inhibitors used for major depression

Drug	Formulation	Adult dose	Pediatric dose[a]
Citalopram	10 mg/5 ml solution; 20-, 40-mg tablets	20 mg once daily, to 60 mg daily (40 mg in the elderly); little increase in effect for doses >20 mg	NR
Fluoxetine	10-, 20-mg capsule; 20 mg/5 ml syrup; 90-mg timed-release capsule	20 mg once daily, to 60 mg daily; little increase in effect for doses >20 mg	NR
Fluvoxamine	25, 50, 100 mg capsules	50 mg once daily, to 100–300 mg daily; little increase in effect for doses >100 mg	25 mg once daily, to 200 mg daily
Paroxetine	12.5-, 25.0-mg controlled-release tablet; 10 mg/5 ml suspension; 10-, 20-, 30-, 40-mg tablet	20 mg once daily, to 50 mg daily; little increase in effect for doses >20 mg	NR
Sertraline	20 mg/ml concentrated solution; 25-, 50-, 100-mg tablets	50 mg once daily, to 200 mg daily; little increase in effect for doses >50 mg	25 mg once daily, to 50 mg daily; maximum daily dose, 200 mg

NR, not reported.
[a]Where not reported, the following may be a guide (101): children older than 12 years, use one-half the adult starting dose for 4 to 7 days, then titrate according to effect and tolerability to adult dose. Children younger than 12 years, use one-fourth of the adult starting dose for 4 to 7 days, then titrate to one-half the adult dose.

matic bradycardia occurred after an overdose of 800 mg (13). Nevertheless, at doses less than 600 mg, usually only mild symptoms are observed (14). Doses more than 600 mg have been reported to cause electrocardiographic abnormalities and convulsions (18%) in some patients, whereas doses greater than 1900 mg have been reported to cause symptoms in all patients with seizures in 47% (14). This was a poison center series, however, and a consecutive series collected at a single center suggests a much lower seizure rate of 2.5%, which was no different from other SSRIs (15). Death occurred after 840 mg in combination with low concentrations of diazepam (16); however, the citalopram concentration of 6.1 mg/kg of femoral vein blood suggests a substantially larger ingestion. An overdose of 1960 mg in the same series had a concentration of 5.2 mg/kg (16). A deliberate self-poisoning of 3920 mg without coingestants resulted in death (16), but doses of up to 5200 mg have been survived (with seizures, hypotension, and prolonged QTc) (14,17). Death has occurred in combined overdose with moclobemide (18,19), cocaine (and other drugs) (20), trimipramine (21), and a variety of other drugs (in low concentrations) (16). In a series of 358 fatal poisoning cases, citalopram was found in 22 and determined to be the cause of death in five cases (1.4%) and contributed to death in another nine cases (2.5%) (22). In another autopsy series, citalopram was also considered to have caused death as the sole agent in some cases (23).

Fluoxetine is well tolerated in overdose. Serious toxic effects do not usually appear until the dose exceeds 1500 mg (24). Symptoms in children ages 3 months to 6 years occurred in only 2.23% with accidental ingestion of doses ranging from 5 to 140 mg (25). The mean overdose in asymptomatic patients in one study was 341 mg; symptomatic patients had ingested a mean dose of 544 mg (24). Children who ingested an average of 1.76 mg/kg fluoxetine had minor symptoms (sleepiness, hyperactivity, diarrhea); all recovered (24). Relatively mild features occurred after ingestion of up to 43 mg/kg by a 4-year-old child (26). Doses of 2400 mg in an adult (27) and 1880 mg in a 12-year-old (28) child have been survived. A dose of 1200 to 2000 mg was fatal (29). Death occurred after therapeutic doses of fluoxetine in a child with confirmed genetic polymorphism of the CYP2D6 gene that resulted in impaired drug metabolism (30). A fatal case of apparent serotonin toxicity due to combined therapy with fluoxetine and selegiline has been reported (31). Deaths have occurred after overdose in combination with moclobemide and clomipramine (32), and ethanol (33).

Fluvoxamine doses up to 1000 mg have been asymptomatic (34) or resulted in minor symptoms only (35). The minimally toxic dose in a large series was 150 mg (34). Sinus bradycardia was noted with doses of less than 1000 mg, but required no treatment (35). Seizures occurred in a few cases after high doses (generally more than 1500 mg) (35). Ingestions of 3000 mg (36,37) and 4800 mg have been survived (37). Overdoses of up to 9000 mg have produced minimal symptoms and full recovery (38). Nevertheless, significant serotonin toxicity has been reported after a single 50-mg dose in an 11-year-old boy (39), and milder forms of serotonin toxicity were found in patients on therapeutic doses (40). A single dose of fluvoxamine has resulted in a psychotic reaction (41).

Paroxetine in therapeutic doses caused mild serotonin toxicity in 5 of 42 patients (42). In 16 ingestions of 10 to 120 mg in children (age 5 years or younger), all patients remained asymptomatic (43). In 12 adolescent patients who ingested 100 to 800 mg, most remained asymptomatic (43). Minimal or no effects were seen after ingestions of 10 to 1000 mg in 35 adults (44). Both overdose and therapeutic use have been associated with hyponatremia (45,46). Paroxetine alone (3600 mg) resulted in serotonin toxicity (syndrome) with full recovery (47). Fatal serotonin toxicity from a therapeutic dose (with a possible contribution from carbamazepine and trimeprazine) has been reported (48). Death has followed combined overdosage of paroxetine with moclobemide (49), ethanol and fluoxetine (50), imipramine (50), and doxepin (51).

Sertraline was taken in a mean dose of 727 ± 686 mg in a poison center study of 52 patients with overdose; there were no symptoms in 34 cases with minor toxicity in the rest (52). In another poison center study of 40 overdoses, amounts ingested ranged from 50 to 8000 mg (mean 1579 mg). Seventeen of the 40 patients ingested sertraline alone. Of this subgroup, ten had no signs or symptoms whereas the others had minor serotonergic signs (53). Severe serotonin toxicity occurred after an estimated dose of up to 8000 mg (54). During premarketing trials, 750 mg to 2600 mg were ingested alone or in combination with other medications or alcohol in four cases and produced only minimal toxicity (55). Up to 4500 mg may be tolerated without profound toxicity (56). Seizures occurred in an adolescent after ingestion of 4000 mg (57). Fatal hepatitis has occurred during therapeutic dosing (58). Deaths have occurred from combined overdose of sertraline with moclobemide and pimozide (59) and alprazolam (60), as well as sertraline alone (61,62).

TOXICOKINETICS AND TOXICODYNAMICS

The pharmacokinetics of the serotonin uptake inhibitors in therapeutic doses is provided in Table 3. Further detail on each drug is included in the following sections.

Citalopram is metabolized to desmethylcitalopram, didesmethylcitalopram, and citalopram-N-oxide, all of which are

TABLE 3. Pharmacokinetics of the serotonin uptake inhibitors

	Time to peak (h)	Volume of distribution (L/kg)	Single dose CL/F (L/h)	Half-life (h)	Protein binding (%)
Citalopram	2–4	14	26	33	50
Fluoxetine	6–8	20–42	36	1.9 d; norfluoxetine, 7 d	95
Fluvoxamine	5 (2–8)	>5	65	15	77
Paroxetine	5 (0.5–11.0)	17	167	10–16	95
Sertraline	6–8	NR	96	26; *N*-desmethylsertraline, 62–104	99

CL/F, oral clearance; F, absolute bioavailability; NR, not reported.

active serotonin uptake inhibitors (63). Fluoxetine has an active metabolite, norfluoxetine, with a much longer elimination half-life than the parent compound (64). Fluvoxamine is extensively hepatically metabolized to multiple inactive metabolites (65). The major metabolites of paroxetine are conjugates that do not compromise its selectivity nor contribute to the clinical response (66). Sertraline has a weakly active metabolite, desmethylsertraline as well as several other inactive metabolites (67).

Cytochrome P-450

The serotonin uptake inhibitors each inhibit a different cluster of cytochrome P-450 enzymes, which are of relevance to the potential for drug interactions. CYP 1A2 is inhibited by fluvoxamine and is implicated in drug interactions with theophylline, clozapine, and others. Fluoxetine, norfluoxetine, sertraline, and paroxetine are potent *in vitro* inhibitors of CYP 2D6 and are capable of causing marked elevations in plasma desipramine and nortriptyline concentrations. The selective serotonin reuptake inhibitors display the following rank order of *in vitro* potency against CYP 2D6: paroxetine greater than fluoxetine = norfluoxetine greater than or equal to sertraline greater than or equal to fluvoxamine (68). On this basis, paroxetine appears to have the greatest and fluvoxamine the least potential for drug interactions with CYP 2D6-dependent drugs. Coadministration of desipramine and fluoxetine (20 mg/day) at steady-state produced an approximately fourfold elevation in peak plasma desipramine concentrations, whereas the long half-life of the active metabolite norfluoxetine was responsible for a significant and long-lasting (approximately 3 weeks) elevation of plasma desipramine concentrations after discontinuation of fluoxetine. Similarly, coadministration of desipramine with paroxetine produced an approximately threefold increase in plasma desipramine concentration. In contrast, coadministration of desipramine and sertraline (50 mg/day) for 4 weeks resulted in a more modest (approximately 30%) elevation in plasma desipramine concentrations (68). Consistent with its minimal *in vitro* effect on CYP 2D6, fluvoxamine shows minimal *in vivo* pharmacokinetic interaction with desipramine, but does interact with imipramine (approximately three- to fourfold increase in AUC) through inhibition of CYP 3A3/4, CYP 1A2, and CYP 2C19 (68).

Fluoxetine, sertraline, and fluvoxamine are believed to inhibit CYP 2C because of observed interactions with phenytoin, diazepam, and other drugs metabolized by these enzymes. CYP 3A4 metabolizes terfenadine, astemizole, carbamazepine, alprazolam, triazolam, and other benzodiazepines. Plasma concentrations of these drugs have increased when they are administered with fluvoxamine, fluoxetine, and sertraline (69). Citalopram at therapeutic doses in humans may produce a small degree of inhibition of P-450 1A2, 2C19, and 2D6 but negligible inhibition of P-450 2C9, 2E1, and 3A (70).

In general, there is little relationship between plasma concentrations and response for serotonin uptake inhibitors (71).

Pharmacokinetic Considerations for Individual Serotonin-Specific Reuptake Inhibitors

Citalopram and its two demethylated metabolites display linear pharmacokinetics in the dose range from 10 to 60 mg/day. At doses of 20 to 60 mg/day, plasma concentrations of racemic citalopram and desmethylcitalopram range from 0.009 to 0.2 mg/L and 0.01 to 0.105 mg/L, respectively (72). In another study of therapeutic doses, the citalopram concentration in whole blood was 0.02 to 0.3 mg/kg (23).

Fluoxetine demonstrates nonlinear kinetics (73). On dosing of 20 mg per day, mean serum concentrations range from 0.089 to 0.1 mg/L for fluoxetine, 0.114 to 0.130 mg/L for norfluoxetine, and from 0.203 to 0.230 mg/L for fluoxetine plus norfluoxetine (74). There is no relationship between concentration and response (75) or relapse prevention (74) in major depression.

Fluvoxamine has nonlinear pharmacokinetics within the usual therapeutic range of 0.03 to 0.09 mg/L (73).

Paroxetine has partially saturable first-pass metabolism and nonlinear kinetics (66). The mean plasma concentration on doses of 20 to 40 mg daily was 0.0623 mg/L with no correlation between concentration and response (76). A long half-life of paroxetine (195 hours) was measured after an overdose with 2000 mg of paroxetine and 1000 mg of clorazepate in a patient who was an extensive P-450 2D6 metabolizer (77).

Sertraline has linear kinetics with therapeutic doses (78). On therapeutic doses, sertraline plasma concentrations ranged from 0.00282 to 0.1122 mg/L (mean, 0.04042 mg/L). No correlation between sertraline plasma concentration and clinical improvement or side effects was observed (79). After a dose of up to 8000 mg, the serum sertraline concentration on admission was 2.93 mg/L, and the desmethylsertraline level was 1.678 mg/L (54). The patient survived.

PATHOPHYSIOLOGY

Serotonin (5-hydroxytryptamine, 5-HT) is a neurotransmitter discovered in 1948 and thought to have a major role in multiple states, including aggression, pain, sleep, appetite, anxiety, depression, migraine, and emesis. Serotonin is derived from dietary tryptophan, which is converted to 5-hydroxytryptophan by tryptophan hydroxylase and then to 5-HT by a nonspecific decarboxylase. 5-HT is transported back into cells by a specific transport system and is degraded mainly by MAO both within the cell and after release. MAO-A is more significant than MAO-B in this process. The breakdown products are excreted in the urine as 5-hydroxyindole acetic acid.

Serotonin Receptors

Serotonin causes excitation and inhibition of central nervous system neurons depending on the neuronal subset and the anatomical localization. It also stimulates peripheral nociceptive nerve endings and has a variety of vascular effects. Serotonin increases gastrointestinal motility, both directly via an action on smooth muscle and indirectly via enteric neurons. It causes contraction of other smooth muscle as well. Peripherally, serotonin is thought to have a role in peristalsis, vomiting, platelet aggregation, and hemostasis. It may also be involved as an inflammatory mediator and in microvascular control. Centrally, serotonin is thought to be involved in the control of appetite and have important roles in sleep and mood maintenance. Serotonin excess has been associated with hallucinations and stereotypical behavior and, in normal amounts, has a role in central pain perception.

There are at least seven serotonin receptors, and several of these have subtypes (80). The most important receptor groups are 5-HT_1 and 5-HT_2. Both of these receptors are typical G-protein linked receptors with seven transmembrane domains. 5-HT_1 is thought to be important in the anxiolytic and antidepressant actions of serotonin. 5-HT_2 is a phospholipase-C–dependent receptor that is thought to be related to the hallucinogenic effects of excess serotonin and appears to be the main receptor involved in the neuroexcitatory (and thus toxic) effects of serotonin, although the nausea is most likely related to 5-HT_3 stimulation (81). The serotonin uptake inhibitors are relatively specific for the serotonin transport system and thus have few other pharmacologic effects even in toxic doses. Thus, most of the adverse effects can be explained by excessive concentrations of serotonin, particularly in the central nervous system (82).

Mechanism of Toxicity

Serotonin acts presynaptically via 5-HT_2 receptors on dopaminergic neurons to inhibit dopamine release (83,84). This explains the common reports of extrapyramidal symptoms with all of the serotonin uptake inhibitors (85). Serotonin also plays an important role in platelet function, and inhibition of platelet serotonin reuptake may result in abnormal platelet aggregation (86).

Conflicting information exists about potential cardiotoxicity of some of the serotonin uptake inhibitors. One of the metabolites of citalopram, didesmethylcitalopram may be responsible for the cardiotoxicity of citalopram (prolongation of QTc). In dogs, didesmethylcitalopram but not citalopram itself, dose-dependently prolongs the QT interval with subsequent fatal dysrhythmias (87). Didesmethylcitalopram is produced by CYP 2D6 (88) and is present in much higher concentrations in dogs than humans because of species-specific differences (87). Theoretically, ultrafast metabolizers of CYP 2D6 (89) are at higher risk of adverse cardiac events. Citalopram and fluoxetine inhibit cardiac Na^+ and Ca^{2+} channels in animal tissue (90). These electrophysiologic effects are similar to those observed for tricyclic antidepressants. The inhibition of cardiac Ca^{2+} and Na^+ channels by fluoxetine may explain most cardiac side effects observed occasionally with the drug and the mild but significant bradycardia reported during chronic treatment. These results also suggest that fluoxetine and citalopram may have antidysrhythmic (class I plus IV type) as well as prodysrhythmic properties (due to impairment of atrioventricular or intraventricular conduction and shortening of repolarization) (90).

PREGNANCY AND LACTATION

All serotonin uptake inhibitors are U.S. Food and Drug Administration pregnancy risk category C (Table 4). Milk to plasma ratios of drug vary from 0.5 to 3.0 (Table 4) (91). The mean total infant exposure varies from 1% to 7% of the weight-adjusted maternal dose. This is below the 10% national level of concern.

TABLE 4. Pregnancy risk category and breast milk distribution of the serotonin uptake inhibitors

	U.S. Food and Drug Administration[a] (ADEC[b]) pregnancy risk category	Distribution into breast milk (milk to plasma ratio)
Citalopram	C (B3)	1.2–3.0 (120)
Fluoxetine	C (C)	0.68 (95% CI, 0.52–0.84) for fluoxetine and 0.56 (95% CI, 0.35–0.77) for norfluoxetine (92)
Fluvoxamine	C (B2)	1.21 to 1.34 (91)
Paroxetine	C (C)	0.39 (range, 0.32–0.51) (121)
Sertraline	C (C)	1.93 for sertraline and 1.64 for *N*-desmethylsertraline (122)

CI, confidence interval.
[a]Appendix I provides definitions of U.S. Food and Drug Administration pregnancy categories.
[b]ADEC, Australian Drug Evaluation Committee pregnancy categories.
Category A: Drugs that have been taken by a large number of pregnant women and women of childbearing age without any proven increase in the frequency of malformations or other direct or indirect harmful effects on the fetus having been observed.
Category B1: Drugs that have been taken by only a limited number of pregnant women and women of childbearing age without an increase in the frequency of malformation or other direct or indirect harmful effects on the human fetus having been observed. Studies in animals have not shown evidence of an increased occurrence of fetal damage.
Category B2: Drugs that have been taken by only a limited number of pregnant women and women of childbearing age without an increase in the frequency of malformation or other direct or indirect harmful effects on the human fetus having been observed. Studies in animals are inadequate or may be lacking, but available data show no evidence of an increased occurrence of fetal damage.
Category B3: Drugs that have been taken by only a limited number of pregnant women and women of childbearing age without an increase in the frequency of malformation or other direct or indirect harmful effects on the human fetus having been observed. Studies in animals have shown evidence of an increased occurrence of fetal damage, the significance of which is considered uncertain in humans.
Category C: Drugs that, owing to their pharmacologic effects, have caused or may be suspected of causing harmful effects on the human fetus or neonate without causing malformations. These effects may be reversible.
Category D: Drugs that have caused or are suspected to have caused or may be expected to cause an increased incidence of human fetal malformations or irreversible damage. These drugs may also have adverse pharmacologic effects.
Category X: Drugs that have such a high risk of causing permanent damage to the fetus that they should not be used in pregnancy or when there is a possibility of pregnancy.
Note: For drugs in categories B1, B2, and B3, human data are lacking or inadequate and subcategorization is therefore based on available animal data. The allocation of a B category does not imply greater safety than the C category. Drugs in category D are not absolutely contraindicated in pregnancy (e.g., anticonvulsants). Moreover, in some cases the D category has been assigned on the basis of "suspicion."

However, there is considerable interpatient variability. The estimated infant dose for fluoxetine and in some of the patients exceeded 10% (92). Furthermore, because adverse effects have been observed in breast-fed infants and infant plasma concentrations of up to 70% of the maternal concentration have been observed, careful monitoring of infants whose mothers use fluoxetine is mandatory (92). The use of the other agents during breast-feeding is probably safe.

CLINICAL PRESENTATION

Acute Overdosage

Serotonin uptake inhibitors are generally fairly benign in single agent overdose. The most common morbidity is due to an excess of serotonergic transmission. This gives rise to a constellation of clinical signs of serotonin excess (Chapter 24). Serotonin excess (syndrome) as defined by Sternbach (93) occurs in 16.3% of patients who have taken an overdose with a serotonin uptake inhibitor (4). Nevertheless, many patients experience some signs of serotonin toxicity even if they do not fulfill all of the Sternbach criteria (93). Features of toxicity that are common to all the serotonin uptake inhibitors, due to increased serotonin, include akathisia, tremor, agitation, shivering, hyperreflexia, diaphoresis, delirium, fever, diarrhea, clonus (inducible, spontaneous, and ocular), seizures, hypertonia, myoclonus, ataxia, tachycardia, hyperactive bowel sounds, confusion, hypertension, and mydriasis.

For the individual patient, agitated delirium, tremor, clonus, fever, and hypertonia can be distressing. These symptoms and signs identify a subset of patients who are at risk of acute respiratory failure and death. The occurrence of serotonin toxicity is not necessarily an indication for specific treatment, but it does identify a group of patients who require close observation, as severe serotonin toxicity can be life threatening (Chapter 24). In this context, the occurrence of fever and respiratory failure (associated with muscle rigidity) appear to be poor prognostic features (82). Complications of serotonin toxicity include severe hyperthermia, dehydration, seizures, and respiratory failure (indicated by a rising $PaCO_2$). Severe toxicity is more likely when an SSRI is taken with other serotonergic drugs such as an MAO inhibitor (including moclobemide) (19,20,22,23,50,61,94,95).

In a series of 233 consecutive first admissions of deliberate self-poisoning with a single SSRI (including coingestants except for moclobemide, thioridazine, and tricyclic antidepressants), seizures occurred in 1.3% of patients. A Glasgow Coma Score of 10 or less was present in 2.6% of patients, serotonin toxicity was present in 19.3%, intensive care unit admission occurred in 7.3%, and the median length of hospital stay was 15.3 hours (range, 2.0 to 185.5 hours) (5).

Acute Overdosage of Specific Agents

Citalopram was the fourth most frequently found drug in fatal poisoning cases, occurring in 22 (6%) of 358 cases in one forensic medicine district in Sweden (22). According to the assessments of the forensic physicians, citalopram was the cause of death in five cases (1.4%) and contributed to death in another nine cases (2.5%) (22).

QTc prolongation to more than 440 milliseconds duration occurred in 66% of citalopram overdoses although the clinical significance of this is unclear (15). In the same study, no significant dysrhythmias, including significant bradycardia, were found in spite of the single case report of profound bradycardia after overdose (13) and occurrence in therapeutic doses (12). Seizures become more common as the dose ingested increases (14,15). Hypotension and prolonged QTc have also been noted at these doses (14,17).

Fluoxetine in overdose does not appear to have a greatly different profile to that of the group as a whole (24), although there has been the occasional report of atrial tachydysrhythmia or bradycardia in therapeutic use and overdose (96–99).

Fluvoxamine may have some additional cardiotoxicity similar to fluoxetine. Bradycardia may occur, and, in some patients, depolarization abnormalities, atrioventricular conduction disturbances, bundle branch block, and ventricular premature beats are evident (34).

Paroxetine is more likely to be associated with a withdrawal syndrome than the other agents due to its shorter half-life (100) but otherwise appears free of drug-specific toxicity.

Sertraline appears to have only group-specific toxicity.

Adverse Reactions

Common adverse effects seen with all SSRI include nausea, agitation, insomnia, drowsiness, tremor, dry mouth, diarrhea, dizziness, headache, sweating, asthenia, anxiety, weight gain or loss, sexual dysfunction, rhinitis, myalgia, and rash. Infrequent events include extrapyramidal reactions (including akathisia, tardive dyskinesia and dystonia), sedation, confusion, palpitations, tachycardia, hypotension, Syndrome of Inappropriate Secretion of Antidiuretic Hormone and abnormal platelet aggregation/hemorrhagic complications (e.g., bruising, epistaxis, purpura). Rarely, elevated liver enzymes, hepatitis, hepatic failure, galactorrhea, blood dyscrasias, and seizures (101). There are no real differences in the side effect profiles for any of the agents.

In spite of the findings of QTc prolongation with citalopram in overdose, extensive postmarketing surveillance data have failed to show any change in QTc at therapeutic doses in large numbers of patients (102). By 1996 there were 71 reports of SSRI-induced extrapyramidal symptoms in the literature. The most common side effect was akathisia (45.1%), followed by dystonia (28.2%), parkinsonism (14.1%), and tardive dyskinesia-like states (11.3%). Among patients with Parkinson's disease treated with SSRI, there were 16 cases of worsening disease (85).

Withdrawal Syndrome

An SSRI withdrawal syndrome is well described with each agent, particularly after abrupt cessation of the shorter half-life paroxetine (100). Symptoms include vertigo, lightheadedness, severe nausea, emesis, fatigue, and myalgia. Symptoms lessen after reintroduction of the drug and gradual tapering of the dose. Changing to the longer half-life fluoxetine is beneficial in some cases (103). Features attributed to SSRI withdrawal seen in neonates may be due to serotonin toxicity (104).

DIAGNOSTIC TESTS

There are no diagnostic tests specific to the serotonin uptake inhibitors. Specific drug measurements are not readily available. Plasma concentrations do not correlate well with therapeutic or adverse effects and are not indicated for management.

Most testing is directed at assessing other potential causes of CNS effects. The temperature should be measured frequently. A complete blood count and cultures of blood and cerebrospinal fluid are obtained as needed to rule out other causes of altered mental status (Chapters 14 and 24). Hepatic and renal function tests are used as indicated.

The electrocardiogram and cardiac monitoring are used for large ingestions of citalopram and fluoxetine to assess for QTc prolongation and atrial dysrhythmias. Measurement of $PaCO_2$ via expired air or arterial blood gases is the best way to assess respiratory compromise.

POSTMORTEM CONSIDERATIONS

In postmortem specimens containing agents with measurable metabolites, the likelihood of an acute overdose can be determined by estimating parent drug to metabolite ratios (21,105).

Citalopram concentrations in medicolegal samples from 92 autopsies and 27 living persons in Denmark have been described (23). In autopsy cases in which citalopram alone was considered the cause of death, concentrations ranged from 2.0 to 6.2 mg/kg whole blood. In autopsy cases in which citalopram together with other substances was considered to be the cause of death, the concentrations of citalopram ranged from 0.6 to 5.2 mg/kg whole blood. In autopsy cases, toxic but nonfatal concentrations ranged from 0.4 to 0.9 mg/kg whole blood and therapeutic concentrations from 0.03 to 0.6 mg/kg whole blood (23). In a death attributed to an overdose of 840 mg of citalopram, a concentration of 6.1 μg/g femoral vein blood was found (16). The citalopram blood concentration was 4.47 mg/L in a death due to combined overdose of citalopram and moclobemide (19). The concentration of citalopram in the femoral blood was 0.88 mg/L in a death in which nontoxic concentrations of cocaine, oxycodone, promethazine, propoxyphene, and norpropoxyphene were found (20). Femoral blood concentration of 4.81 mg/L was found in a combined overdose with trimipramine (21).

Fluoxetine concentration in blood was 6.0 mg/L and norfluoxetine was 5.0 mg/L in a death thought due to *fluoxetine* alone (29). In the absence of other risk factors, the lowest concentration determined to have resulted in death was 0.63 mg/L (95).

Fluvoxamine postmortem peripheral blood concentrations ranged from 0.5 mg/L in a suicidal shooting to 6 mg/L in a case of drug overdose. Evidence of postmortem redistribution was noted in the only case for which both central and peripheral blood were obtained (106).

Paroxetine heart blood concentration in a death attributed solely to paroxetine was 4.0 mg/L (50). In a fatality after an overdose of paroxetine, alcohol, and fluoxetine, the postmortem heart blood contained paroxetine at 3.7 mg/L (50). In a death attributed to an interaction between paroxetine and imipramine/desipramine, the postmortem heart blood contained paroxetine at 1.4 mg/L (50). In the absence of other risk factors, the lowest concentrations determined to have resulted in death was 0.4 mg/L (95). In a death in combination with moclobemide, subclavian blood contained 1.58 mg/L of paroxetine, whereas liver had 15.3 mg/kg (49). Femoral blood drug concentrations of 0.176 mg/L were found in a death from combined paroxetine and doxepin (51).

The *sertraline* blood concentration was 1.5 mg/L, the lowest concentration determined to have resulted in death in the absence of other factors (95). A sertraline concentration of 0.62 mg/L was found in a woman who died of asthma but who was presumed to have also taken an overdose of sertraline (107). The sertraline concentration was 1.0 mg/L in peripheral blood with a desmethylsertraline concentration of 0.2 mg/L in a death from overdose of sertraline and alprazolam (60). The alprazolam was present in therapeutic concentrations. In a death attributed to sertraline alone, sertraline and its desmethyl metabolite were found in the peripheral blood in concentrations of 0.15 mg/L and 0.20 mg/L (62).

TREATMENT

Most patients require only symptomatic and supportive care. Treatment is focused on controlling agitation, maintaining airway, reversing hyperthermia, and symptomatic treatment of serotonin toxicity.

Decontamination

Gastrointestinal decontamination is not essential, but activated charcoal may be considered if not more than 1 hour has elapsed since ingestion of the drug (108). In view of the potential cardiac toxicity of citalopram and possibly fluoxetine and fluvoxamine, observation for dysrhythmia is warranted. Clinical assessment for signs that may indicate impending seizure activity (hypertonicity, hyperreflexia, or myoclonic jerking) is important. Patients with altered mental status, seizure, abnormal vital signs, or dysrhythmia are typically admitted. Milder serotonin toxicity may respond to specific serotonin antagonists, but severe serotonin toxicity (often due to combined serotonergic drug overdose) has the potential for life-threatening outcomes that may require more aggressive intervention.

Supportive Care

Agitation and confusion or other distressing symptoms of serotonin excess may be an indication for specific treatment with serotonin antagonists such as cyproheptadine or chlorpromazine (see following antidotes). Benzodiazepines may be helpful, but antipsychotic medication that does not have significant serotonin antagonism (e.g., haloperidol) should not be used because of the effects of serotonin on dopamine release. Nausea and vomiting are rarely severe enough to warrant therapy, but 5-HT_3 antagonists (e.g., ondansetron) are the drugs of choice if treatment is required (81).

Hypotension is rare but if it occurs should be treated with a 10 to 20 ml/kg bolus of 0.9% sodium chloride followed by a vasopressor, if needed (Chapter 37). One case of fluoxetine-associated QRS widening showed response to sodium bicarbonate (27), but there are no data to support routine bicarbonate therapy. Prolongation of the QTc is an indication for cardiac monitoring until the QTc returns to normal. *Seizures* are treated with benzodiazepines and other anticonvulsants (Chapter 40).

Severe *serotonin toxicity* with increasing autonomic features (hyperpyrexia, sweating, and tachycardia) and rigidity heralds life-threatening toxicity. Characteristically, the neuromuscular signs are predominantly in the lower limbs but become more generalized as the toxicity becomes more severe. As the rigidity increases in truncal muscles, respiration becomes impaired and this, in conjunction with a rapidly rising temperature, indicates a need for urgent intervention. Elective intubation, neuromuscular paralysis, mechanical ventilation, and aggressive cooling measures are indicated (Chapter 38) (82).

Enhancement of Elimination

Hemoperfusion and hemodialysis are not indicated and are, in any case, unlikely to be effective in view of the high volumes of distribution of these agents.

Antidotes

Cyproheptadine has relatively high affinity for the 5-HT_2 receptor (109) and is effective for milder cases of serotonin toxicity in which patients are able to take oral medication (1,110–113). Current experience suggests that 12 mg orally or by nasogastric tube, followed by 4 to 8 mg every 4 to 6 hours, is an appropriate dose range (82). For severe serotonin toxicity, chlorpromazine, a potent 5-HT_2 antagonist (114), has been used in many cases with apparent good effect (1,115–118). Current experience indicates fluid resuscitation is needed before administration of chlorpromazine and that the dose is probably in the range of 12.5 to 50 mg IV initially, followed by 25 to 50 mg orally or IV every 6 hours (82). Newer antipsychotic agents such as risperidone also have potent 5-HT_2 antagonist activity (119) and may be beneficial in treating serotonin toxicity. Severe late-stage serotonin toxicity progresses to rigidity of the lower limbs and then truncal muscles, which can produce impairment of breathing and a rise in $PaCO_2$ requiring intubation and neuromuscular paralysis.

Monitoring

The patient should be observed and, for cases of citalopram, fluoxetine, and fluvoxamine, should have continuous cardiovascular monitoring until he or she is improving. Frequent assessment of mental status, temperature, and neuromuscular function (hyperreflexia, hypertonia, myoclonus, clonus) should be made.

REFERENCES

1. Gillman PK. The serotonin syndrome and its treatment. *J Psychopharmacol* 1999;13:100–109.
2. Nisijima K, et al. Potent serotonin (5-HT)(2A) receptor antagonists completely prevent the development of hyperthermia in an animal model of the 5-HT syndrome. *Brain Res* 2001;890:23–31.
3. Masand PS, Gupta S. Selective serotonin-reuptake inhibitors: an update. *Harv Rev Psychiatry* 1999;7:69–84.
4. Whyte IM, Dawson AH. Redefining the serotonin syndrome. *J Toxicol Clin Toxicol* 2002;40:668–669.
5. Whyte IM, Dawson AH, Buckley NA. Relative toxicity of venlafaxine and selective serotonin reuptake inhibitors in overdose compared to tricyclic antidepressants. *QJM* 2003;96:369–374.
6. Barbey JT, Roose SP. SSRI safety in overdose. *J Clin Psychiatry* 1998;59[Suppl 15]:42–48.
7. Henry JA, Antao CA. Suicide and fatal antidepressant poisoning. *Eur J Med* 1992;1:343–348.
8. Ohberg A, Vuori E, Klaukka T, et al. Antidepressants and suicide mortality. *J Affect Disord* 1998;50:225–233.
9. Buckley NA, McManus PR. Fatal toxicity of serotoninergic and other antidepressant drugs: analysis of United Kingdom mortality data. *BMJ* 2002;325:1332–1333.
10. Catalano G, Catalano MC, Epstein MA, et al. QTc interval prolongation associated with citalopram overdose: a case report and literature review. *Clin Neuropharmacol* 2001;24:158–162.
11. Favre MP, Sztajzel J, Bertschy G. Bradycardia during citalopram treatment: a case report. *Pharmacol Res* 1999;39:149–150.
12. Isbister GK, Prior FH, Foy A. Citalopram-induced bradycardia and presyncope. *Ann Pharmacother* 2001;35:1552–1555.
13. Rothenhausler HB, Hoberl C, Ehrentrout S, et al. Suicide attempt by pure citalopram overdose causing long-lasting severe sinus bradycardia, hypotension and syncopes: successful therapy with a temporary pacemaker. *Pharmacopsychiatry* 2000;33:150–152.
14. Personne M, Sjoberg G, Persson H. Citalopram overdose—review of cases treated in Swedish hospitals [published erratum appears in *J Toxicol Clin Toxicol* 1997;35(5):577]. *J Toxicol Clin Toxicol* 1997;35:237–240.
15. Isbister GK, Dawson AH, Whyte IM. Relative toxicity of citalopram and other selective serotonin reuptake inhibitors in overdose. *J Toxicol Clin Toxicol* 2002;40:275.
16. Ostrom M, Eriksson A, Thorson J, et al. Fatal overdose with citalopram. *Lancet* 1996;348:339–340.
17. Grundemar L, Wohlfart B, Lagerstedt C, et al. Symptoms and signs of severe citalopram overdose. *Lancet* 1997;349:1602.
18. Neuvonen PJ, Pohjola-Sintonen S, Tacke U, et al. Five fatal cases of serotonin syndrome after moclobemide-citalopram or moclobemide-clomipramine overdoses. *Lancet* 1993;342:1419.
19. Dams R, Benijts TH, Lambert WE, et al. A fatal case of serotonin syndrome after combined moclobemide-citalopram intoxication. *J Anal Toxicol* 2001;25:147–151.
20. Fu K, Konrad RJ, Hardy RW, et al. An unusual multiple drug intoxication case involving citalopram. *J Anal Toxicol* 2000;24:648–650.
21. Musshoff F, Schmidt P, Madea B. Fatality caused by a combined trimipramine-citalopram intoxication. *Forensic Sci Int* 1999;106:125–131.
22. Jonasson B, Saldeen T. Citalopram in fatal poisoning cases. *Forensic Sci Int* 2002;126:1–6.
23. Worm K, Dragsholt C, Simonsen K, et al. Citalopram concentrations in samples from autopsies and living persons. *Int J Legal Med* 1998;111:188–190.
24. Borys DJ, Setzer SC, Ling LJ, et al. Acute fluoxetine overdose: a report of 234 cases. *Am J Emerg Med* 1992;10:115–120.
25. Baker SD, Morgan DL. Fluoxetine exposures—are they safe for children, as believed? *J Toxicol Clin Toxicol* 2002;40:634–635.
26. Feierabend RH Jr. Benign course in a child with a massive fluoxetine overdose. *J Fam Pract* 1995;41:289–291.
27. Graudins A, Vossler C, Wang R. Fluoxetine-induced cardiotoxicity with response to bicarbonate therapy. *Am J Emerg Med* 1997;15:501–503.
28. Riddle MA, Brown N, Dzubinski D, et al. Fluoxetine overdose in an adolescent. *J Am Acad Child Adolesc Psychiatry* 1989;28:587–588.
29. Kincaid RL, McMullin MM, Crookham SB, et al. Report of a fluoxetine fatality. *J Anal Toxicol* 1990;14:327–329.
30. Sallee FR, DeVane CL, Ferrell RE. Fluoxetine-related death in a child with cytochrome P-450 2D6 genetic deficiency. *J Child Adolesc Psychopharmacol* 2000;10:27–34.
31. Bilbao GJ, Mesa PN, Castilla CV, et al. [Serotonin syndrome: report of a fatal case and review of the literature]. *Rev Clin Esp* 2002;202:209–211.
32. Power BM, Pinder M, Hackett LP, et al. Fatal serotonin syndrome following a combined overdose of moclobemide, clomipramine and fluoxetine. *Anaesth Intensive Care* 1995;23:499–502.
33. Rohrig TP, Prouty RW. Fluoxetine overdose: a case report. *J Anal Toxicol* 1989;13:305–307.
34. Azoyan PH, Garnier R, Chataigner D, et al. Toxicokinetics of fluvoxamine in overdose. In: *Proceedings, Fourteenth International Congress of the European Association of Poison Centres.* Milan, Italy 1990.
35. Garnier R, Azoyan P, Chataigner D, et al. Acute fluvoxamine poisoning. *J Int Med Res* 1993;21:197–208.
36. Banerjee AK. Recovery from prolonged cerebral depression after fluvoxamine overdose. *Br Med J (Clin Res Ed)* 1988;296:1774.
37. Lebegue B. Survivable fluvoxamine overdose. *Am J Psychiatry* 1990;147:1689.
38. Henry JA. Overdose and safety with fluvoxamine. *Int Clin Psychopharmacol* 1991;6 [Suppl 3]:41–45.
39. Gill M, LoVecchio F, Selden B. Serotonin syndrome in a child after a single dose of fluvoxamine. *Ann Emerg Med* 1999;33:457–459.
40. Kaneda Y, Ishimoto Y, Ohmori T. Mild serotonin syndrome on fluvoxamine. *Int J Neurosci* 2001;109:165–172.
41. Sim FH, Massabki RA. A single dose of fluvoxamine associated with an acute psychotic reaction. *Can J Psychiatry* 2000;45:762.
42. Hegerl U, Bottlender R, Gallinat J, et al. The serotonin syndrome scale: first results on validity. *European Archives of Psychiatry & Clinical Neuroscience* 1998;248:96–103.
43. Myers LB, Krenzelok EP. Paroxetine (Paxil) overdose: a pediatric focus. *Vet Hum Toxicol* 1997;39:86–88.
44. Myers LB, Dean BS, Krenzelok EP. Paroxetine (PAXIL): overdose assessment of a new selective serotonin reuptake inhibitor. *Veterinary & Human Toxicology* 1994;36:370.
45. Johnsen CR, Hoejlyng N. Hyponatremia following acute overdose with paroxetine. *Int J Clin Pharmacol Ther* 1998;36:333–335.
46. Odeh M, Seligmann H, Oliven A. Severe life-threatening hyponatremia during paroxetine therapy. *J Clin Pharmacol* 1999;39:1290–1291.
47. Johnson R, Velez LI, Roth B. Paroxetine as a sole cause of serotonin syndrome: a massive overdose with documented serum paroxetine levels. *J Toxicol Clin Toxicol* 2001;39:491–492.
48. Apelland T, Gedde-Dahl T, Dietrichson T. [Serotonin syndrome with fatal outcome caused by selective serotonin reuptake inhibitors]. *Tidsskr Nor Laegeforen* 1999;119:647–650.
49. Singer PP, Jones GR. An uncommon fatality due to moclobemide and paroxetine. *J Anal Toxicol* 1997;21:518–20.
50. Vermeulen T. Distribution of paroxetine in three postmortem cases. *J Anal Toxicol* 1998;22:541–544.
51. Musshoff F, Grellner W, Madea B. [Toxicologic findings in suicide with doxepin and paroxetine]. *Arch Kriminol* 1999;204:28–32.
52. Klein-Schwartz W, Anderson B. Analysis of sertraline-only overdoses. *Am J Emerg Med* 1996;14:456–458.
53. Lau GT, Horowitz BZ. Sertraline overdose. *Acad Emerg Med* 1996;3:132–136.
54. Brendel DH, Bodkin JA, Yang JM. Massive sertraline overdose. *Ann Emerg Med* 2000;36:524–526.
55. Doogan DP. Toleration and safety of sertraline: experience worldwide. *Int Clin Psychopharmacol* 1991;6[Suppl 2]:47–56.
56. Myers LB, Dean BS, Krenzelok EP. Sertraline (Zoloft): overdose assessment of a new antidepressant. *Vet Hum Toxicol* 1993;34:341.
57. Meier K, Lam R. 4 Gram sertraline [Zoloft(R)] overdose resulting in delayed seizures. *J Toxicol Clin Toxicol* 1998;36:520–521.
58. Fartoux-Heymann L, Hezode C, Zafrani ES, et al. Acute fatal hepatitis related to sertraline. *J Hepatol* 2001;35:683–684.
59. McIntyre IM, King CV, Staikos V, et al. A fatality involving moclobemide, sertraline, and pimozide. *J Forensic Sci* 1997;42:951–953.
60. Milner DA, Hall M, Davis GG, et al. Fatal multiple drug intoxication following acute sertraline use. *J Anal Toxicol* 1998;22:545–548.
61. Logan BK, Friel PN, Case GA. Analysis of sertraline (Zoloft) and its major metabolite in postmortem specimens by gas and liquid chromatography. *J Anal Toxicol* 1994;18:139–142.
62. Musshoff F, Banaschak S, Madea B. [Postmortem distribution of sertraline and desmethylsertraline in a fatality]. *Arch Kriminol* 2002;210:51–56.
63. Milne RJ, Goa KL. Citalopram. A review of its pharmacodynamic and pharmacokinetic properties, and therapeutic potential in depressive illness. *Drugs* 1991;41:450–477.
64. Lemberger L, Bergstrom RF, Wolen RL, et al. Fluoxetine: clinical pharmacology and physiologic disposition. *J Clin Psychiatry* 1985;46:14–19.
65. Claassen V. Review of the animal pharmacology and pharmacokinetics of fluvoxamine. *Br J Clin Pharmacol* 1983;15[Suppl 3]:349S–355S.
66. Kaye CM, Haddock RE, Langley PF, et al. A review of the metabolism and pharmacokinetics of paroxetine in man. *Acta Psychiatr Scand Suppl* 1989;350:60–75.
67. Doogan DP, Caillard V. Sertraline: a new antidepressant. *J Clin Psychiatry* 1988;49[Suppl]:46–51.
68. Ereshefsky L, Riesenman C, Lam YW. Antidepressant drug interactions and the cytochrome P450 system. The role of cytochrome P450 2D6. [Review]. *Clin Pharmacokin* 1995;29[Suppl 1]:10–18.
69. Nemeroff CB, DeVane CL, Pollock BG. Newer antidepressants and the cytochrome P450 system [see comments]. [Review]. *Am J Psychiatry* 1996;153:311–320.
70. von Moltke LL, Greenblatt DJ, Grassi JM, et al. Citalopram and desmethylcitalopram in vitro: human cytochromes mediating transformation, and cytochrome inhibitory effects. *Biol Psychiatry* 1999;46:839–849.
71. Baumann P. Pharmacokinetic-pharmacodynamic relationship of the selective serotonin reuptake inhibitors. *Clin Pharmacokinet* 1996;31:444–469.
72. Brosen K, Naranjo CA. Review of pharmacokinetic and pharmacodynamic interaction studies with citalopram. *Eur Neuropsychopharmacol* 2001;11:275–283.
73. Goodnick PJ. Pharmacokinetic optimisation of therapy with newer antidepressants. *Clin Pharmacokinet* 1994;27:307–330.
74. Brunswick DJ, Amsterdam JD, Fawcett J, et al. Fluoxetine and norfluoxetine

plasma concentrations during relapse-prevention treatment. *J Affect Disord* 2002;68:243–249.

75. Amsterdam JD, Fawcett J, Quitkin FM, et al. Fluoxetine and norfluoxetine plasma concentrations in major depression: a multicenter study. *Am J Psychiatry* 1997;154:963–969.
76. Baron FJ, Perez V, Puigdemont D, et al. Paroxetine plasmatic levels and clinical response in major depression. *Eur Neuropsychopharmacol* 1997;S137.
77. Hilleret H, Voirol P, Bovier P, et al. Very long half-life of paroxetine following intoxication in an extensive cytochrome P4502D6 metabolizer. *Ther Drug Monit* 2002;24:567–569.
78. Hiemke C, Hartter S. Pharmacokinetics of selective serotonin reuptake inhibitors. *Pharmacol Ther* 2000;85:11–28.
79. Mauri MC, Laini V, Cerveri G, et al. Clinical outcome and tolerability of sertraline in major depression: a study with plasma levels. *Prog Neuropsychopharmacol Biol Psychiatry* 2002;26:597–601.
80. Peroutka SJ. Molecular biology of serotonin (5-HT) receptors. *Synapse* 1994;18:241–260.
81. Ueda N, Yoshimura R, Shinkai K, et al. Characteristics of fluvoxamine-induced nausea. *Psychiatry Res* 2001;104:259–264.
82. Buckley NA, Dawson AH, Whyte IM. Specific serotonin reuptake inhibitors (SSRIs). In: *HyperTox: assessment and treatment of poisoning*, v1229 edn. Newcastle, Australia: MediTox Pty Ltd, 2002.
83. Millan MJ, Dekeyne A, Gobert A. Serotonin (5-HT)2C receptors tonically inhibit dopamine (DA) and noradrenaline (NA), but not 5-HT, release in the frontal cortex in vivo. *Neuropharmacology* 1998;37:953–955.
84. Muramatsu M, Tamaki-Ohashi J, Usuki C, et al. 5-HT2 antagonists and minaprine block the 5-HT-induced inhibition of dopamine release from rat brain striatal slices. *Eur J Pharmacol* 1988;153:89–95.
85. Leo RJ. Movement disorders associated with the serotonin selective reuptake inhibitors. *J Clin Psychiatry* 1996;57:449–54.
86. Abraham KI, Ieni JR, Meyerson LR. Purification and properties of a human plasma endogenous modulator for the platelet tricyclic binding/serotonin transport complex. *Biochim Biophys Acta* 1987;923:8–21.
87. Wijnands-Kleukers APG, Van Zoelen GA, de Vries I, et al. A prospective study on intoxications with citalopram. *J Toxicol Clin Toxicol* 2002;40:274–275.
88. Sindrup SH, Brosen K, Hansen MG, et al. Pharmacokinetics of citalopram in relation to the sparteine and the mephenytoin oxidation polymorphisms. *Ther Drug Monit* 1993;15:11–17.
89. Sachse C, Brockmoller J, Bauer S, et al. Cytochrome P450 2D6 variants in a Caucasian population: allele frequencies and phenotypic consequences. *Am J Hum Genet* 1997;60:284–295.
90. Pacher P, Ungvari Z, Nanasi PP, et al. Speculations on difference between tricyclic and selective serotonin reuptake inhibitor antidepressants on their cardiac effects. Is there any? *Curr Med Chem* 1999;6:469–480.
91. Kristensen JH, Hackett LP, Kohan R, et al. The amount of fluvoxamine in milk is unlikely to be a cause of adverse effects in breastfed infants. *J Hum Lact* 2002;18:139–143.
92. Kristensen JH, Ilett KF, Hackett LP, et al. Distribution and excretion of fluoxetine and norfluoxetine in human milk. *Br J Clin Pharmacol* 1999;48:521–527.
93. Sternbach H. The serotonin syndrome. *Am J Psychiatry* 1991;148:705–713.
94. Dalfen AK, Stewart DE. Who develops severe or fatal adverse drug reactions to selective serotonin reuptake inhibitors? *Can J Psychiatry* 2001;46:258–263.
95. Goeringer KE, Raymon L, Christian GD, et al. Postmortem forensic toxicology of selective serotonin reuptake inhibitors: a review of pharmacology and report of 168 cases. *J Forensic Sci* 2000;45:633–648.
96. Allhoff T, Bender S, Banger M. Atrial arrhythmia in a woman treated with fluoxetine: is there a causal relationship? *Ann Emerg Med* 2001;37:116.
97. Buff DD, Brenner R, Kirtane SS, et al. Dysrhythmia associated with fluoxetine treatment in an elderly patient with cardiac disease. *J Clin Psychiatry* 1991;52:174–176.
98. Friedman EH. Fluoxetine-induced bradycardia. *J Clin Psychiatry* 1991;52:477.
99. Roberge RJ, Martin TG. Mixed fluoxetine/loxapine overdose and atrial flutter. *Ann Emerg Med* 1994;23:586–590.
100. Haddad PM. Antidepressant discontinuation syndromes. *Drug Saf* 2001;24:183–197.
101. Selective serotonin reuptake inhibitors. In: *Australian medicines handbook*, 3rd ed. Adelaide, Australian: Medicines Handbook Pty Ltd, 2002.
102. Rasmussen SL, Overo KF, Tanghoj P. Cardiac safety of citalopram: prospective trials and retrospective analyses. *J Clin Psychopharmacol* 1999;19:407–415.
103. Benazzi F. SSRI discontinuation syndrome treated with fluoxetine. *Int J Geriatr Psychiatry* 1998;13:421–422.
104. Isbister GK, Dawson A, Whyte IM, et al. Neonatal paroxetine withdrawal syndrome or actually serotonin syndrome? *Arch Dis Child Fetal Neonatal Ed* 2001;85:F147–F148.
105. Spigset O, Ostrom M, Eriksson A. Death resulting from asthma associated with sertraline "overdose". *Am J Forensic Med Pathol* 2001;22:419–420.
106. Kunsman GW, Rodriguez R, Rodriguez P. Fluvoxamine distribution in postmortem cases. *Am J Forensic Med Pathol* 1999;20:78–83.
107. Carson HJ, Zweigart M, Lueck NE. Death from asthma associated with sertraline overdose. *Am J Forensic Med Pathol* 2000;21:273–275.
108. Chyka PA, Seger D. Position statement: single-dose activated charcoal. American Academy of Clinical Toxicology; European Association of Poisons Centres and Clinical Toxicologists. *J Toxicol Clin Toxicol* 1997;35:721–741.
109. Kapur S, Zipursky RB, Jones C, et al. Cyproheptadine: a potent in vivo serotonin antagonist [letter]. *Am J Psychiatry* 1997;154:884.
110. Graudins A, Stearman A, Chan B. Treatment of the serotonin syndrome with cyproheptadine. *J Emerg Med* 1998;16:615–619.
111. Horowitz BZ, Mullins ME. Cyproheptadine for serotonin syndrome in an accidental pediatric sertraline ingestion. *Pediatr Emerg Care* 1999;15:325–327.
112. Isbister GK. Comment: serotonin syndrome, mydriasis, and cyproheptadine. *Ann Pharmacother* 2001;35:1672–1673.
113. McDaniel WW. Serotonin syndrome: early management with cyproheptadine. *Ann Pharmacother* 2001;35:870–873.
114. Tatsumi M, Jansen K, Blakely RD, et al. Pharmacological profile of neuroleptics at human monoamine transporters. *Eur J Pharmacol* 1999;368:277–283.
115. Chan BS, Graudins A, Whyte IM, et al. Serotonin syndrome resulting from drug interactions. *Med J Aust* 1998;169:523–525.
116. Gillman PK. Successful treatment of serotonin syndrome with chlorpromazine. *Med J Aust* 1996;165:345–346.
117. Graham PM. Successful treatment of the toxic serotonin syndrome with chlorpromazine. *Med J Aust* 1997;166:166–167.
118. Green AR. Repeated chlorpromazine administration increases a behavioural response of rats to 5-hydroxytryptamine receptor stimulation. *Br J Pharmacol* 1977;59:367–371.
119. Richelson E, Souder T. Binding of antipsychotic drugs to human brain receptors focus on newer generation compounds. *Life Sci* 2000;68:29–39.
120. Rampono J, Kristensen JH, Hackett LP, et al. Citalopram and demethylcitalopram in human milk; distribution, excretion and effects in breast fed infants. *Br J Clin Pharmacol* 2000;50:263–268.
121. Begg EJ, Duffull SB, Saunders DA, et al. Paroxetine in human milk. *Br J Clin Pharmacol* 1999;48:142–147.
122. Kristensen JH, Ilett KF, Dusci LJ, et al. Distribution and excretion of sertraline and N-desmethylsertraline in human milk. *Br J Clin Pharmacol* 1998;45:453–457.

CHAPTER 136

Other Antidepressants

Ian MacGregor Whyte

OCH3, OH, H3C—N, H3C

VENLAFAXINE

Compounds included:	**Bupropion (Amfebutamone, Wellbutrin, Zyban), mirtazapine (Remeron, Zispin), nefazodone (Dutonin, Serzone), reboxetine (Edronax), venlafaxine (Effexor)**
Molecular formula and weight:	**See Table 1.**
SI conversion:	**See Table 1.**
CAS Registry No.:	**See Table 1.**
Therapeutic levels:	**See Table 1.**
Target organs:	**Central nervous system (acute), cardiac (acute)**
Antidotes:	**Consider cyproheptadine for serotonin toxicity.**

GENERAL

The other antidepressants are a diverse group of drugs that interact with a variety of serotonergic and adrenergic neurotransmitter systems. There is no consistent structural relationship amongst these agents (Table 1; Fig. 1), and they have different toxicologic profiles in overdose. A comprehensive review of these *atypical* antidepressants in overdose has been published (1).

Bupropion is an antidepressant with a unicyclic aminoketone structure, which is also known as *amfebutamone.* It is related to the central stimulant and indirect-acting sympathomimetic diethylpropion (2). It was widely used as an antidepressant until postmarketing studies showed an unacceptable incidence of seizures (3), particularly in patients with eating disorders (4), resulting in the drug's withdrawal from the U.S. market and subsequent re-introduction with a lower recommended maximum dose of 450 mg/day. It is also used as an aid to smoking cessation in which it is available as a sustained release product.

Mirtazapine is a tetracyclic piperazinoazepine and an analog of mianserin. It is indicated for the treatment of major depression and produces anxiety and confusion in overdose.

Nefazodone is a synthetic derivative of phenylpiperazine and a structural analog of the antidepressant trazodone. It is indicated for the symptomatic treatment of depressive illness and causes drowsiness and nausea in overdose.

Reboxetine is a bicyclic morpholine derivative, unrelated to any other antidepressants. It is a racemic mixture in which both

TABLE 1. Structural classification of miscellaneous anxiolytics, sedatives, and hypnotics

Compound	Molecular formula, molecular weight (g/mol), CAS Registry No.	SI conversion; therapeutic, toxic concentrations[a]	*U.S. Pharmacopeia Dictionary of Drug Names*
Bupropion hydrochloride	$C_{13}H_{18}ClNO,HCl$; 239.8; 31677-93-7	mg/L × 4.17 = µmol/L; 0.4 mg/L, 4 mg/L	1-(3-chlorophenyl)-2-((1,1-dimethylethyl)amino)-, (+-)-1-propanone
Mirtazapine	$C_{17}H_{19}N_3$; 265.4; 61337-67-5	mg/L × 3.77 = µmol/L; NA, NA	1,2,3,4,10,14b-hexahydro-2-methylpyrazino(2,1-a)pyrido(2,3-c)benzazepine
Nefazodone hydrochloride	$C_{25}H_{32}ClN_5O_2,HCl$; 470; 82752-99-6	mg/L × 2.13 = µmol/L; 1 mg/L, NA	2-(3-(4-(3-chlorophenyl)-1-piperazinyl)propyl)-5-ethyl-2,4-dihydro-4-(2-phenoxyethyl)-3H-1,2,4-triazol-3-one
Reboxetine mesylate	$C_{19}H_{23}NO_3,CH_4O_3S$; 313.4; 98769-82-5; 98769-84-7	mg/L × 3.19 = µmol/L; NA, NA	(+-)-(2R*)-2-((alphaR*)-alpha-(o-ethoxyphenoxy)benzyl)morpholine
Venlafaxine	$C_{17}H_{27}NO_2,HCl$; 277.4; 99300-78-4	mg/L × 3.6 = µmol/L; 0.1 mg/L, NA	(+-)-1-(2-(dimethylamino)-1-(4-methoxyphenyl)ethyl)-cyclohexanol

NA, not available.
[a]From Flanagan RJ. Guidelines for the interpretation of analytical toxicology results and unit of measurement conversion factors. *Ann Clin Biochem* 1998;35(Pt 2):261–7, with permission.

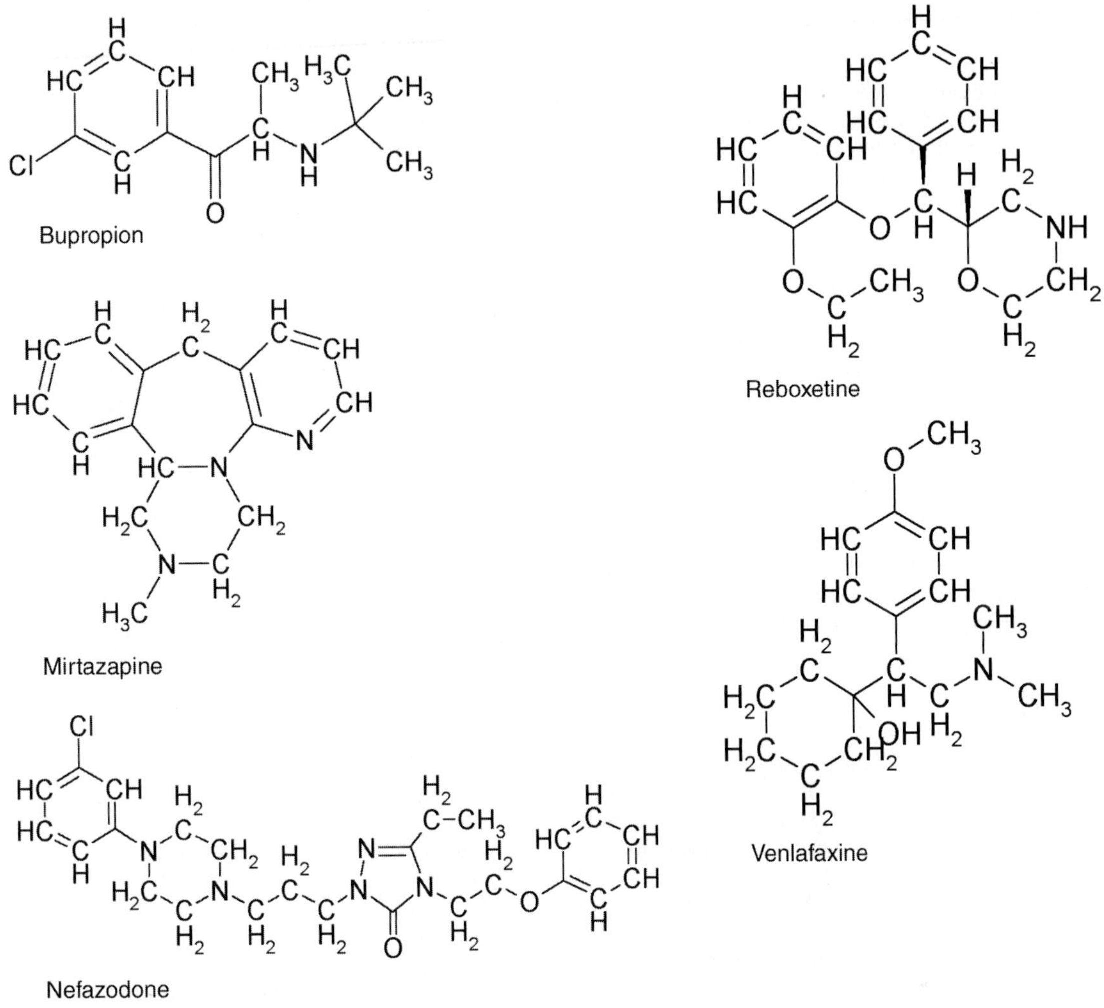

Bupropion

Reboxetine

Mirtazapine

Venlafaxine

Nefazodone

Figure 1. Structures of other antidepressants.

enantiomers are active and is indicated for the treatment of depression. It has mild adrenergic toxicity.

Venlafaxine is a hydroxycycloalkylphenylethylamine derivative bicyclic antidepressant that is structurally and pharmacologically related to the analgesic tramadol but not to any of the conventional antidepressant drugs. It is indicated for the management of depression. It may cause significant cardiac dysrhythmias.

TOXIC DOSE

The *adult therapeutic doses* for these agents are provided in Table 2.

Bupropion has a dose-related incidence of seizures within the therapeutic dose range. The incidence of seizures with bupropion doses of 450 mg/day or less ranged from 0.35% to 0.44% (3), increasing almost tenfold at a dose of 600 mg/day (5). In a study of all new onset generalized seizures over a 4-year period in subjects 16 years of age and older, 17 of 279 (6.1%) of the new-onset seizures were drug related (6). After cocaine intoxication and benzodiazepine withdrawal, bupropion (4/279 or 1.4%) was the third leading cause of drug-related seizures. Dose-related perceptual distortions (at a mean dose of 561 mg daily) (7) and dose-related acute psychoses (8) also occur at therapeutic doses.

TABLE 2. Typical therapeutic doses of other antidepressants for major depression (147,148)

Drug	Formulation	Adult dose[a]
Bupropion	75-, 100-mg tablets; 100-, 125-mg sustained-release tablets	100 mg twice daily to a maximum of 150 mg three times daily; for smoking cessation, sustained release preparation 150 mg once daily for 6 d, increasing to 150 mg twice daily
Mirtazapine	15-, 30-, 45-mg tablets	15 mg at night to a maximum of 60 mg at night
Nefazodone	50-, 100-, 150-, 200-, 250-mg tablets	50–100 mg twice daily to 150–300 mg twice daily
Reboxetine	4-mg tablet	4 mg twice a day to a maximum of 12 mg/d
Venlafaxine	37.5-, 50-, 75-, 100-mg tablets	37.5 mg twice daily, increasing to a maximum of 375 mg/d; extended-release preparation, 75 mg once daily, increasing to a maximum of 300 mg/d

[a]Pediatric use not reported.

Seizures after overdose are also dose related. In a series of 19 sustained release bupropion overdoses, the seizure rate was 18% for patients ingesting 0 to 4.5 g, 50% for 4.65 to 9 g, and all patients had one or more seizures at a dose 9 g or more (9). In a retrospective poison center series of 58 cases of immediate release tablet overdose, seizures occurred in 21% of cases with a mean dose of 3.078 g (10). In a prospective poison center series of 50 cases of sustained-release bupropion, 24% had convulsions; the dose ingested in these cases was 1.5 to 18.75 g (median, 4.7 g) (11).

Overdoses with 900 to 3000 mg of bupropion in five patients led to vomiting, confusion, hypokalemia, and nonspecific ST-T changes (12). Intraventricular conduction delay and a prolonged QTc (600 milliseconds 4 hours after ingestion) was seen after ingestion of 1.5 g (13). A 14-year-old boy developed tachycardia, delirium, and two brief seizures after ingesting 1.5 to 3 g (14). An ingestion of 9 g of bupropion (with 300 mg of tranylcypromine and an unknown amount of aspirin) resulted in seizures, sinus tachycardia without conduction abnormality, and complete neurologic recovery (15). An adult man who ingested 9 g bupropion developed neurologic toxicity as well as intraventricular conduction disturbances on electrocardiogram (ECG) (16). Two patients had prolonged convulsions and cardiac arrest after ingestion of 1.5 g and 5.4 g (11). A 31-year-old woman developed seizures, broad complex tachycardia, and required ventilation after ingestion of 13.5 g of sustained-release bupropion (17). Several of the cases of apparent cardiotoxicity involved coingestion of drugs that could explain the cardiotoxicity.

A 26-year-old man ingested 23 g of bupropion, developed seizures and hypoxia, presented in cardiac arrest, was resuscitated but died 4 days after ingestion (18). In two deaths attributed to bupropion, the doses in both cases were estimated by history to be less than 10 g (19).

Mirtazapine in therapeutic doses has been reported to cause serotonin toxicity. This has been reported with mirtazapine monotherapy (20); however, the bilateral cogwheel rigidity reported in this case is inconsistent with serotonin toxicity and much more consistent with neuroleptic malignant syndrome (Chapter 23). Serotonin toxicity has also been reported in combination therapy with fluoxetine (21); however, in this case the features were more likely those of fluoxetine withdrawal (22). A case of serotonin toxicity from a combination with fluvoxamine has also been reported (23) but again the clinical picture is more consistent with an alternative diagnosis (22), in this case, increased anxiety due to increased mirtazapine concentrations from fluvoxamine induced inhibition of CYP3A4 (24). The known pharmacology of mirtazapine indicates that serotonin toxicity is unlikely and, indeed, mirtazapine has been successfully used to treat serotonin toxicity (25). Mirtazapine and nefazodone, with intrinsic 5-HT_2 blocking effects, may be possible alternatives for persons with susceptibility to serotonin toxicity induced by serotonergic agents (22).

After ingestion of ethanol and 375 mg of mirtazapine, a 43-year-old man developed lethargy and little else (26). Overdosage up to 975 mg has caused significant sedation but no cardiovascular or respiratory effects or seizures (27). In six patients, mirtazapine doses ranged from 450 to 1350 mg with no serious adverse effects of overdose. Four patients who combined other central nervous system (CNS) depressants with mirtazapine appeared to experience more CNS depression (28). After 1200 mg mirtazapine, 20 mg lorazepam, and lying outside in cold weather, a 41-year-old woman experienced severe hypothermia and rhabdomyolysis (29). Two patients, taking 900 and 1500 mg, achieved a full recovery without complications (30).

In a retrospective poison center case series of 73 overdoses of mirtazapine alone, there were no symptoms in 31 cases with doses up to 900 mg, minor symptoms in 32 cases with doses up to 2250 mg, moderate toxicity in three cases (maximum dose, 900 mg) and severe toxicity (unidentified dysrhythmia) in 1 case at a dose of 600 mg (31). There were no fatalities, and seizures were not observed (31). A few deaths have been attributed by U.K. coroners to mirtazapine overdose. The fatal toxicity index (FTI), deaths per million prescriptions, for mirtazapine was 3.1 (95% CI, 0.1 to 17.2) (32).

Nefazodone in therapeutic doses has been reported to cause serotonin toxicity in combination with other serotonergic agents (33,34). However, none of these cases provides clear evidence of nefazodone causing clinically severe serotonin toxicity (1), a picture consistent with the drug's known pharmacology.

A series of 1338 nefazodone-alone exposures collected from American national poisoning data found no dose-response relationship. However, the doses recorded were generally small (50 mg to 13.5 g) and more than one-half of the exposures were to therapeutic doses (median dose, 250 to 300 mg) (35). In fact, the median dose was less than the average dose during therapy for depression (36). Overdoses of 1 to 11.2 g produced only nausea, vomiting, and minor sedation (37). A combined overdose of 16.8 g of nefazodone with an unknown amount of verapamil (38) resulted in CNS depression with cardiovascular findings (bradycardia and hypotension) more consistent with verapamil poisoning (39). However, hypotension and bradycardia with QT/QTc prolongation occurred in a well-documented case of ingestion of 2.4 g (40). In the years 1995 to 1999, there were no deaths recorded in the United Kingdom as due to nefazodone alone. The FTI for nefazodone was 0 (95% CI, 0 to 6.4) (32).

Reboxetine overdoses of up to 240 mg have produced minor symptoms of sympathetic overactivity (41). In the years 1995 to 1999, there were no deaths recorded in the United Kingdom as due to reboxetine alone. The FTI for reboxetine was 0 (95% CI, 0 to 21.1) (32).

Venlafaxine has been reported to produce serotonin toxicity in therapeutic doses either alone (42) or in combination with another serotonergic agent such as amitriptyline and meperidine (43), dexamphetamine (44), St. John's Wort (45), phenelzine (46), and tranylcypromine (47,48). When the other serotonergic agent is a monoamine oxidase inhibitor, the reaction can be severe and life threatening (47,48). Due to its indirect dopamine-inhibition effect, neuroleptic malignant syndrome has been reported on venlafaxine therapy alone (49) and in combination with trifluoperazine (50) and metoclopramide (51) (although both these cases are misreported as serotonin toxicity).

Seizures were reported in 0.26% of patients on therapeutic doses in premarketing trials (52). Seizures can also occur at therapeutic doses when venlafaxine is given in combination with other drugs affecting seizure threshold (53).

Serotonin toxicity can also occur after venlafaxine overdose either alone (54,55) or in combination with other serotonergic drugs such as moclobemide (56). In a single toxicology treatment center series of 51 overdoses of venlafaxine without other serotonergic drugs, serotonin toxicity occurred in 29.4% with a median ingested dose of 1000 mg (57).

Severe CNS depression occurred in a 41-year-old woman after ingestion of 4500 mg of venlafaxine, 500 mg of diphenhydramine, and 50 mg of thiothixene (58). An overdose of 1300 mg by a 40-year-old woman resulted in a single generalized seizure (59). In a single toxicology treatment center series of 51 venlafaxine overdoses, seizures occurred in 7/51 (14%) cases; all patients with seizures consumed at least 900 mg and the median dose of those with seizures was 3150 mg (57). A retrospective poison center follow-up study of 632 inquiries about venlafaxine overdose found 30 (4.8%) cases had seizures (60). The dose ingested ranged from 375 mg to 10,500 mg with doses more than 1500 mg being most associated with seizures (60).

TABLE 3. Pharmacokinetics of the other antidepressants (87,148)

Drug	Bioavailability (%)	Time to peak after oral dosing (h)	Volume of distribution (L/kg)	Clearance (L/h/kg)	Half-life (h)	Protein binding (%)	Active metabolites (half-life)
Bupropion (149)	Extensive first-pass metabolism	2; 3[a]	1.4–3.2	NR	14 (8–24)	84	Hydroxybupropion (22); threohydrobupropion (20); erythrohydrobupropion (33)
Mirtazapine (65)	50; moderate first-pass metabolism	2	1.53	0.44	20–40	85	*N*-desmethylmirtazapine (25)
Nefazodone (150)	15–23; extensive first-pass metabolism	1–3	0.22–0.87	NR	1.9–5.3[b]	99	Hydroxynefazodone (4); triazolodione (18–33); *m*-chlorophenylpiperazine (4–9)
Reboxetine (151)	93	2	0.385–0.92	0.027–0.071	13	97	None
Venlafaxine (150)	12.6; extensive first-pass metabolism	2.0–2.5; 5.5[a]	7.5	0.6–1.2	5	27	*o*-desmethylvenlafaxine (11)

NR, not reported.
[a]Sustained- and extended-release preparation.
[b]Nonlinear elimination.

Cardiac toxicity appears dose dependent, both in animal models (61) and in overdose, with life-threatening ventricular dysrhythmias appearing at doses more than 7000 mg (60,62). Death from ventricular fibrillation has occurred after ingestion of 8400 mg (63). A patient who ingested 2750 mg of venlafaxine was observed to have two generalized convulsions and a prolongation of QTc to 500 milliseconds, compared with 405 milliseconds at baseline (52). A combination of venlafaxine (1987.5 mg) and paroxetine (360 mg) resulted in hypertension, transient ECG abnormalities, and persistent myocardial damage (64). At 13.2 (95% CI, 9.2 to 18.5), the FTI for venlafaxine was substantially higher than for the other antidepressants in this group or specific serotonin reuptake inhibitors, which may reflect an intrinsic proconvulsant effect (57) and cardiac toxicity.

TOXICOKINETICS AND TOXICODYNAMICS

The pharmacokinetics of these agents are provided in Table 3.

Bupropion has a therapeutic range from 0.05 to 0.10 mg/L (5). In patients with seizures in therapeutic use, the mean concentration was 0.17 mg/L (3). After an ultimately fatal ingestion of 23 g, the 18-hour post-presentation bupropion concentration was 0.446 mg/L and the hydroxybupropion concentration was 3.212 mg/L (18).

Mirtazapine plasma concentrations range from 0.005 to 0.1 mg/L after a therapeutic dose (15 to 45 mg/day) (65). After 375 mg of mirtazapine, the serum concentration at admission was 0.53 mg/ml (26). After 1200 mg, the plasma concentration was 0.368 mg/L at 41 hours (29). Concentrations of up to 2.3 mg/L have been tolerated with minor symptoms (30).

Nefazodone and hydroxynefazodone demonstrate nonlinear pharmacokinetics at therapeutic doses (66) and in overdose (40). There is no meaningful therapeutic plasma concentration as much of the therapeutic effect resides with the metabolites (1), although concentrations of 0.3 to 0.5 mg/L have been quoted (67). After a 2.4 g ingestion, the peak nefazodone concentration was 7.5 mg/L and the elimination half-lives of nefazodone and hydroxynefazodone were 8.3 and 14.6 hours, respectively (40). There was a significant negative correlation between systolic blood pressure and concentration of the hydroxynefazodone metabolite but not the parent drug. The QT length correlated with both nefazodone and its metabolite, suggesting some potential for cardiotoxicity (40).

Reboxetine peak concentrations after 4 mg orally were 0.101 mg/L (both enantiomers) at 1.5 hours post-dose (68). There are no toxicokinetic data available.

Venlafaxine concentrations in responders to therapy with venlafaxine range from 0.025 to 0.4 mg/L (69). In two patients who took 2750 mg and 2500 mg, the resultant peak plasma concentrations of venlafaxine were 6.24 and 2.35 mg/L, and the peak plasma levels of *o*-desmethylvenlafaxine were 3.37 and 1.30 mg/L (52). A prolonged elimination half-life of venlafaxine (15.3 hours) was shown in a 33-year-old woman who ingested 3000 mg of venlafaxine and 210 mg of zolpidem (70). Other cases also support nonlinear kinetics due to saturation of metabolic pathways in overdose (71,72).

PATHOPHYSIOLOGY

The *bupropion* mechanism of antidepressant action appears to have an unusual, not fully understood, noradrenergic link (73). Bupropion inhibits neuronal reuptake of dopamine > norepinephrine >> serotonin (74). The bupropion metabolite hydroxybupropion probably plays a critical role in antidepressant activity, which appears to be predominantly associated with long-term noradrenergic effects (73). The mild CNS activating effects of bupropion appear to be due to weak dopaminergic mechanisms, and there is some evidence that dopamine may contribute to its antidepressant properties (73). Antidepressant effects of bupropion are not serotonergically mediated (73). Bupropion has minimal or no affinity for cholinergic, histaminergic (H_1), β or α_2 adrenergic, 5-HT_2, or dopamine (D_2) receptors (75). There is dose-dependent CNS toxicity in animals, but the mechanism is unclear (76).

There is some question about the potential for cardiac toxicity in bupropion overdose. Although QTc prolongation has been reported (13), there is doubt about the validity of the standard calculation of QTc using Bazett's formula (77) in the presence of tachycardia. It is generally agreed that for heart rates within the range 50 to 70 beats/minute, Bazett's formula is reasonably accurate (78). However, it has been shown repeatedly that Bazett's formula significantly overcorrects for fast heart rates and significantly undercorrects for slow heart rates (78,79). Bupropion toxicity manifests mainly as tachycardia (9) and, thus, any QTc prolongation calculated by Bazett's formula is likely to be a significant overestimation of the true QT.

Mirtazapine preferentially blocks the noradrenergic α_2-auto- and heteroreceptors that are responsible for controlling norepinephrine and serotonin release (80). The noradrenergic activation and the consequent indirect enhancement of serotonergic transmission results in marked increases in serotonin release. Mirtazapine has low affinity for serotonin 5-HT_{1A} receptors but potently blocks 5-HT_2 and 5-HT_3 receptors, thus, when serotonin is increased in the synaptic cleft, 5-HT_1–mediated transmission is enhanced (80). The blockade of 5-HT_2 and 5-HT_3 receptors prevents development of the side effects associated with nonselective 5-HT activation, in particular, the features of serotonin toxicity that appear to be primarily 5-HT_2 mediated (Chapter 24). Mirtazapine has been described as a noradrenergic and specific serotonergic antidepressant (80). Mirtazapine has potent histamine (H_1) antagonist properties as well as minor anticholinergic activity (81). The antihistamine effect is responsible for the sedation seen during therapy and in overdose.

Nefazodone is a serotonin antagonist at postsynaptic 5-HT_{2A} receptors and also blocks presynaptic serotonin reuptake (82). It has little or no affinity for cholinergic, histaminic, or α-adrenergic receptors (82). Hydroxynefazodone has similar pharmacologic properties. The metabolite, *m*-chlorophenylpiperazine, is an agonist at 5-HT_{1A} and 5-HT_{2C} receptors and an antagonist at 5-HT_{2A} and 5-HT_3 receptors (82). This combination of pharmacologic effects makes significant serotonin toxicity unlikely (Chapter 24).

Reboxetine is a potent and selective norepinephrine reuptake inhibitor with more than 125-fold selectivity for the norepinephrine transporter compared to the serotonin transporter (83). It has minimal affinity for histamine (H_1), muscarinic, or α-adrenergic receptors (83).

Venlafaxine inhibits monoamine uptake (serotonin > norepinephrine >> dopamine) (84) and has been termed a *serotonin norepinephrine reuptake inhibitor*. Stimulation of 5-HT_2 inhibitory presynaptic receptors on dopaminergic neurons can decrease dopamine release with symptoms of dopamine underactivity (85,86). Venlafaxine does not inhibit monoamine oxidase, it is not antimuscarinic, nor does it have any appreciable affinity for α-adrenergic or histaminergic binding sites (84). Its major metabolite, *o*-desmethylvenlafaxine, has similar pharmacology (87). Venlafaxine also inhibits peak inward sodium current in myocardial tissue, which likely explains its cardiac toxicity in overdose (61). Unlike most tricyclic antidepressants or conventional class I antidysrhythmic drugs, inhibition was exclusively of a tonic nature and rate-independent, suggesting it binds to the resting state of the sodium channel (61).

PREGNANCY AND LACTATION

The pregnancy risk categories for these antidepressants are shown in Table 4. Results of pregnancies in 150 women suggest that the use of venlafaxine during pregnancy does not increase the rates of major malformations above the baseline rate of 1% to 3% (88).

For mirtazapine and reboxetine, there are no data on distribution into breast milk. There is no evidence of accumulation of bupropion in the infant though bupropion and two of its metabolites accumulate in human breast milk in concentrations much higher than in maternal plasma (89). Only small amounts of nefazodone are found in breast milk but produced clinical effects in an infant, which resolved on cessation of breast-feeding (90). Venlafaxine was detected in 1 of 7 infants and *o*-desmethylvenlafaxine was detected in 4 of 7 infants in one study (91).

TABLE 4. U.S. Food and Drug Administration (FDA) risk category and breast milk distribution of the serotonin uptake inhibitors

Drug	FDA[a] (ADEC[b]) pregnancy risk category	Distribution into breast milk (milk to plasma ratio)
Bupropion	B (B2)	2.51–8.58 (89)
Mirtazapine	C (B3)	NR
Nefazodone	C (B3)	0.45% of the weight-adjusted maternal daily dose (90)
Reboxetine	NR (B1)	NR
Venlafaxine	C (B2)	2.5 (2.0–3.2), 6.4% (5.5–7.3%) of the weight-adjusted maternal daily dose (91)

NR, not reported.
[a]Appendix I provides definitions of FDA pregnancy categories.
[b]ADEC, Australian Drug Evaluation Committee (see Table 5).

TABLE 5. Australian Drug Evaluation Committee pregnancy categories

Category A
Drugs that have been taken by a large number of pregnant women and women of childbearing age without any proven increase in the frequency of malformations or other direct or indirect harmful effects on the fetus having been observed.

Category B1
Drugs that have been taken by only a limited number of pregnant women and women of childbearing age without an increase in the frequency of malformation or other direct or indirect harmful effects on the human fetus having been observed. Studies in animals have not shown evidence of an increased occurrence of fetal damage.

Category B2
Drugs that have been taken by only a limited number of pregnant women and women of childbearing age without an increase in the frequency of malformation or other direct or indirect harmful effects on the human fetus having been observed. Studies in animals are inadequate or may be lacking, but available data show no evidence of an increased occurrence of fetal damage.

Category B3
Drugs that have been taken by only a limited number of pregnant women and women of childbearing age without an increase in the frequency of malformation or other direct or indirect harmful effects on the human fetus having been observed. Studies in animals have shown evidence of an increased occurrence of fetal damage, the significance of which is considered uncertain in humans.

Category C
Drugs that, owing to their pharmacologic effects, have caused or may be suspected of causing harmful effects on the human fetus or neonate without causing malformations. These effects may be reversible.

Category D
Drugs that have caused or are suspected to have caused or may be expected to cause an increased incidence of human fetal malformations or irreversible damage. These drugs may also have adverse pharmacologic effects.

Category X
Drugs that have such a high risk of causing permanent damage to the fetus that they should not be used in pregnancy or when there is a possibility of pregnancy.

Note: For drugs in categories B1, B2, and B3, human data are lacking or inadequate and subcategorization is therefore based on available animal data. The allocation of a B category does not imply greater safety than the C category. Drugs in category D are not absolutely contraindicated in pregnancy (e.g., anticonvulsants). Moreover, in some cases the D category has been assigned on the basis of "suspicion."

CLINICAL PRESENTATION

Acute Overdose

Bupropion clinical effects in overdose include sinus tachycardia (83%), hypertension (56%), seizures (37%), gastrointestinal symptoms (37%), and agitation (32%) (9). Other common features include drowsiness or lethargy, hallucinations, delirium, and tremor (10). Bupropion-related seizures, which have been reported in 15% to 37% (9–11,92) of cases, may be multiple (93), with rare status epilepticus (94), but are usually brief and self-limiting with no apparent long-term sequelae (9). Nevertheless, seizures may rarely be followed by cardiac arrest (11,18) and death (18). Seizures may be delayed for 19 (95) to 32 hours or more (94) after ingestion of a sustained-release preparation.

Cardiac toxicity (96), including cardiac arrest, has occurred, although coingestants may have contributed. More usually, the only cardiovascular effects are tachycardia and hypertension, although occasional hypotension can also occur (10). When more significant cardiac toxicity occurs, it is usually tachycardia and conduction delays (widened QRS complex and/or prolonged QTc interval) (13,16), which resolve within 2 to 4 days after ingestion (97). However, life-threatening cardiac toxicity (17,18) (especially with coingestants) and death (18,19,98–100) may occur.

Mirtazapine overdose can cause sedation but seems to have no associated cardiovascular or respiratory effects or seizures (27). Around 40% of exposures are asymptomatic (31).

Nefazodone overdose was often asymptomatic in a large poison center series (N = 1338) (35). However, the median dose ingested was only 250 to 300 mg (36). The most common manifestations were drowsiness (17.3% of all patients), nausea (9.7%), and dizziness (9.5%). The most common serious effect was hypotension (1.6%), although bradycardia was present in 1.4%. The median onset time for symptoms was 1.75 hours. Manifestations resolved within 8 to 24 hours. No patient required intubation, mechanical ventilation, or vasopressors and none died (35). A combined overdose of nefazodone with an unknown amount of verapamil (38) resulted in CNS depression with cardiovascular findings (bradycardia and hypotension) (39). In a well-documented case of nefazodone poisoning, bradycardia, hypotension, and QT/QTc prolongation lasted for 18 hours or more (40).

Reboxetine overdosage has been rarely reported. Patients may have minor symptoms of sympathetic overactivity (tachycardia, hypertension, sweating) (41).

Venlafaxine poisonings have a toxicologic profile that is a hybrid of tricyclic antidepressant (Chapter 134) and serotonin uptake inhibitor (Chapter 135) overdose (57). In a series of 51 consecutive overdoses, the major features were QRS of 100 milliseconds or greater (36.8%), serotonin toxicity (29.4%), and seizures (13.7%). Coma occurred in 2.1% and mild tachycardia and hypertension also occurred (57). No life-threatening dysrhythmias were seen, but seizures were much more common than with TCA or specific serotonin reuptake inhibitors in the same study (57).

In preclinical trials of venlafaxine there were 14 cases of overdose, all of whom recovered without sequelae (52). One of these patients had multiple seizures and QTc prolongation (52), and more recent cases support the clinical picture of seizures (59,101–105), potentially life-threatening cardiac toxicity (101,106), and possible death (107,108) after overdose. The London Poison Center had 2954 inquiries about venlafaxine poisoning, of which they were able to follow up 632 cases (60). Most patients only had minor effects, but 30 patients (4.7%) had seizures and two had ventricular tachycardia (60). There are two cases of venlafaxine overdose that were complicated by delayed rhabdomyolysis (109).

Acute Withdrawal

Abrupt discontinuation of ethanol, benzodiazepines, and sedatives during bupropion therapy may precipitate seizure activity. In a small study, no evidence of a withdrawal syndrome from bupropion was noted (110). Mirtazapine withdrawal has been associated with symptoms including panic attack and mania (111–113). Nausea, vomiting, diarrhea, ataxia, insomnia, marked agitation, headache, and flu-like symptoms have been reported after abrupt discontinuation of nefazodone (114–117). There has been no evidence of a withdrawal syndrome from reboxetine (118,119). A withdrawal syndrome identical to that after sudden withdrawal of serotonin uptake inhibitors can follow abrupt cessation of venlafaxine (120,121). It may respond to substitution by a serotonin uptake inhibitor (122).

Adverse Reactions

Bupropion adverse effects include insomnia, nightmares, dizziness, concentration difficulties, agitation, anxiety, tremor, drowsiness, headache, fever, rash, itch, urticaria, nausea, dry mouth, and constipation (123). Infrequently, palpitations, tachycardia, hypertension, chest pain, anorexia, and confusion may occur, whereas rarely seizures, anaphylaxis, angioedema, erythema multiforme, serum sickness, depression, paresthesia, and hallucinations may be evident (123). Seizures are more frequent when a predisposing condition is present, a higher dose of bupropion is taken, and when concurrent medication lowers the seizure threshold (123).

Mirtazapine adverse effects include increased appetite, weight gain, sedation, asthenia, and peripheral edema, whereas postural hypotension, seizures, mania, and rash occur rarely (124).

Nefazodone adverse effects include nausea, sedation, dry mouth, asthenia, constipation, blurred vision, confusion, dizziness, orthostatic hypotension, and sinus bradycardia (124). Infrequently, agitation, tremor, insomnia, visual trails, or tracking can occur, whereas rare events include hepatitis, hepatic necrosis, and liver failure (124).

Reboxetine adverse effects include urinary retention, dry mouth, sweating, paresthesia, constipation, increase in diastolic blood pressure, increase in heart rate, impotence, insomnia, and headache (124).

Venlafaxine adverse effects include nausea, vomiting, anorexia, headache, sweating, rash, anxiety, dizziness, fatigue, syncope, hypertension (dose-related), orthostatic hypotension, and tremor (124). Infrequently, sexual dysfunction (e.g., impotence), loss of libido, dry mouth, insomnia, somnolence, constipation, hyponatremia, ECG changes, palpitations, hepatitis, and seizures may occur. Rarely, skin and mucous membrane bleeding has been noted (124).

DIAGNOSTIC TESTS

Routine quantitative drug estimation is not readily available for any of these agents and not indicated for routine management.

Mortality is closely related to the development of cardiac dysrhythmias. An ECG and cardiac monitoring are needed for bupropion and venlafaxine and advisable for nefazodone and reboxetine. Hepatic and renal function tests are indicated. Measurement of creatine kinase in cases of coma help in the assessment of rhabdomyolysis. Measurement of partial pressure of carbon dioxide ($PaCO_2$) via expired air or arterial blood gases is the best way to assess respiratory compromise from sedation.

POSTMORTEM CONSIDERATIONS

There are no postmortem data available for nefazodone or reboxetine.

Bupropion overdose resulted in a pharmacobezoar in a fatal bupropion sustained-release overdose (1). In two cases in which bupropion was the major toxicology finding, peripheral blood concentrations of the parent drug were 4.0 and 4.2 mg/L and total metabolite levels were 15 and 16.6 mg/L (19). In a fatality involving bupropion and ethanol, the concentrations of bupropion, hydroxybupropion, and the erythroamino and threoamino alcohol metabolites in heart blood were 4.2, 5.0, 0.6, and 4.6 mg/L, respectively. The heart blood ethanol concentration was 0.27 g/dl. In addition, bupropion was distributed as follows: subclavian blood, 6.2 mg/L; bile, 1.4 mg/L; kidney, 2.4 mg/L; liver, 1.0 mg/kg; stomach contents, 16 mg; and urine, 37 mg/L (98).

In cases in which mirtazapine was an incidental finding at postmortem and not related to death, the mean peripheral blood concentration was 0.09 mg/L (less than 0.01 to 0.14, $N = 4$) (126). In another series, femoral blood concentrations were 0.04 to 0.24 mg/L (9 cases) (127). There was no evidence of postmortem redistribution (126).

Venlafaxine postmortem tissue concentrations in each of 12 postmortem cases for venlafaxine and *o*-desmethylvenlafaxine were 0.1 to 36 and less than 0.05 to 3.5 mg/L (peripheral blood), less than 0.05 to 22 mg/kg and less than 0.05 to 9.9 mg/kg (liver), less than 0.05 to 10 mg/L and less than 0.05 to 1.5 mg/L (vitreous), less than 0.05 to 53 mg/L and less than 0.05 to 6.8 mg/L (bile), less than 0.05 to 55 mg/L and less than 0.05 to 21 mg/L (urine), respectively. Venlafaxine was typically present with other drugs, including other antidepressants, alcohol, and benzodiazepines and there were no deaths ascribed solely to venlafaxine intoxication (128).

Blood concentrations of venlafaxine in two overdose cases were 53 mg/L and 78 mg/L. Comparison of venlafaxine concentrations in blood samples taken at different times after death revealed increasing concentration over time, suggesting possible postmortem redistribution (107). The heart-blood venlafaxine and *o*-desmethylvenlafaxine concentrations in three cases were 6.6 and 31.0 mg/L, 84 and 15 mg/L, and 44 and 50 mg/L, respectively (129). Two venlafaxine-related deaths showed blood concentrations of 7.27 mg/L venlafaxine and 5.03 mg/L *o*-desmethylvenlafaxine and 89.67 mg/L venlafaxine with 3.44 mg/L of the desmethyl metabolite (130).

TREATMENT

Decontamination

Oral activated charcoal may be of value if given early (within 1 hour) in nefazodone poisoning; there is insufficient information on reboxetine overdose to make a recommendation. It may have some value if given early (within 1 hour) in mirtazapine poisoning, especially if ingested in large amounts [more than 1000 mg (1)] or with other drugs that may benefit from decontamination. Oral activated charcoal within 1 hour of ingestion is probably of value in poisoning with bupropion and venlafaxine.

Because both bupropion and venlafaxine are available in sustained- or extended-release preparations and have significant potential delayed toxicity, whole bowel irrigation may be of value in large ingestions of these drugs (131). Doses that warrant significant concern are more than 4500 mg of bupropion or 3000 mg of venlafaxine in adults.

Enhancement of Elimination

Principles of elimination enhancement are discussed in Chapter 78. Based on their volumes of distribution and plasma protein binding (132), there is no indication for extracorporeal techniques in poisoning with any of these drugs and there are no reports of their use in these poisonings.

Antidotes

Venlafaxine overdose has a high incidence of serotonin toxicity (57). Agitated, tremulous patients with hyperreflexia, clonus, and rigidity may benefit from specific drug therapy to relieve serotonin toxicity. Cyproheptadine has relatively high affinity for the 5-HT_2 receptor (133) and is effective for milder cases of serotonin toxicity in which patients are able to take oral medication (134–138). Current experience suggests that 12 mg orally or by nasogastric tube, followed by 4 to 8 mg every 4 to 6 hours, is an appropriate dose range (139). For severe serotonin toxicity, chlorpromazine, a potent 5-HT_2 antagonist (140), has been used in many cases with apparent good effect (134,141–144). However, for a proconvulsant drug like venlafaxine (57), using a drug like chlorpromazine that can lower seizure threshold may be unwise (1).

Newer antipsychotic agents such as risperidone also have potent 5-HT_2 antagonist activity (145) and may be beneficial in treating serotonin toxicity. Severe late stage serotonin toxicity progresses to rigidity of the lower limbs and then truncal muscles, which can produce impairment of breathing and a rise in $Pa{CO_2}$ requiring intubation and neuromuscular paralysis. Such treatment may be indicated if cyproheptadine therapy is unhelpful in venlafaxine overdose.

Although serotonin toxicity has been reported in therapeutic use of mirtazapine and nefazodone, it has not been reported in overdose. Given the known pharmacology of these agents, this is not surprising. In any case, if serotonin toxicity were suspected after an overdose of either of these agents, it would not be rational to use either cyproheptadine or chlorpromazine, as both agents have similar effects on serotonin receptors as do mirtazapine and nefazodone.

Supportive Care

The preferred treatment for mirtazapine, nefazodone, or reboxetine poisoning is supportive with intravenous access and fluids and maintenance of the airway and ventilation if required. In bupropion and venlafaxine poisoning, seizures are common, and cardiac toxicity in venlafaxine overdose may be fatal. If they require treatment, seizures should be managed with benzodiazepines (Chapter 40) in the first instance. The use of sodium channel blocking drugs (e.g., phenytoin, carbamazepine) to control seizures might contribute to cardiotoxicity. Therefore, high-dose benzodiazepines followed by barbiturates are the preferred agents for refractory seizures (1).

Most hypotension responds to isotonic fluid resuscitation, but, if not, inotropic agents may be required (Chapter 37). Given the proposed mechanism of cardiac toxicity of venlafaxine, it is reasonable to trial sodium bicarbonate in venlafaxine-induced dysrhythmias with a widened QRS. There is one case report in which some success was achieved with this approach (62). Dose and administration should be similar to that used in tricyclic antidepressant poisoning (Chapter 75).

Patients with a significant overdose of drugs with sedating properties (e.g., mirtazapine) should be advised not to drive until potential interference with psychomotor performance has resolved (146). For an overdose of mirtazapine with its long elimination half-life, this may be 24 to 48 hours after discharge.

Monitoring

Routine observation of vital signs, especially Glasgow coma scale, airway patency and blood pressure, is indicated. For sustained- or extended-release bupropion and venlafaxine, continuous cardiac monitoring for at least 18 hours or until the patient is asymptomatic is mandatory (1). For an asymptomatic mirtazapine, nefazodone, or reboxetine overdose, observation until 4 hours post-ingestion is indicated. For symptomatic ingestions of these drugs and immediate-release bupropion and venlafaxine, most patients clearly improve within 4 to 6 hours and are self-caring shortly after that.

REFERENCES

1. Buckley NA, Faunce TA. 'Atypical' antidepressants in overdose. *Drug Saf* 2003;26(8):539–551.
2. Kinnell HG. Bupropion for smokers: drug is almost identical in structure to diethylpropion, a controlled drug. *BMJ* 2001;322:431–432.
3. Davidson J. Seizures and bupropion: a review. *J Clin Psychiatry* 1989;50(7):256–261.
4. Horne RL, Ferguson JM, Pope HG Jr, et al. Treatment of bulimia with bupropion: a multicenter controlled trial. *J Clin Psychiatry* 1988;49(7):262–266.
5. Johnston JA, Lineberry CG, Ascher JA, et al. A 102-center prospective study of seizure in association with bupropion. *J Clin Psychiatry* 1991;52(11):450–456.
6. Pesola GR, Avasarala J. Bupropion seizure proportion among new-onset generalized seizures and drug related seizures presenting to an emergency department. *J Emerg Med* 2002;22(3):235–239.
7. Becker RE, Dufresne RL. Perceptual changes with bupropion, a novel antidepressant. *Am J Psychiatry* 1982;139(9):1200–1201.
8. Golden RN, James SP, Sherer MA, et al. Psychoses associated with bupropion treatment. *Am J Psychiatry* 1985;142(12):1459–1462.
9. Balit CR, Lynch CN, Isbister GK. Bupropion poisoning: a case series. *Med J Aust* 2003;178(2):61–63.
10. Spiller HA, Ramoska EA, Krenzelok EP, et al. Bupropion overdose: a 3-year multi-center retrospective analysis. *Am J Emerg Med* 1994;12(1):43–45.
11. Colbridge MG, Dargan PI, Jones AL. Bupropion—the experience of the National Poisons Information Service (London). *J Toxicol Clin Toxicol* 2002;40(3):398–399.
12. Wenger TL, Stern WC. The cardiovascular profile of bupropion. *J Clin Psychiatry* 1983;44(5 pt 2):176–182.
13. Shrier M, Diaz JE, Tsarouhas N. Cardiotoxicity associated with bupropion overdose. *Ann Emerg Med* 2000;35(1):100.
14. Ayers S, Tobias JD. Bupropion overdose in an adolescent. *Pediatr Emerg Care* 2001;17(2):104–106.
15. Storrow AB. Bupropion overdose and seizure. *Am J Emerg Med* 1994;12(2):183–184.
16. Paris PA, Saucier JR. ECG conduction delays associated with massive bupropion overdose. *J Toxicol Clin Toxicol* 1998;36(6):595–598.
17. Tracey JA, Cassidy N, Casey PB, et al. Bupropion (Zyban) toxicity. *Ir Med J* 2002;95(1):2324.
18. Harris CR, Gualtieri J, Stark G. Fatal bupropion overdose. *J Toxicol Clin Toxicol* 1997;35(3):321–324.
19. Friel PN, Logan BK, Fligner CL. Three fatal drug overdoses involving bupropion. *J Anal Toxicol* 1993;17(7):436–438.
20. Hernandez JL, Ramos FJ, Infante J, et al. Severe serotonin syndrome induced by mirtazapine monotherapy. *Ann Pharmacother* 2002;36(4):641–643.
21. Benazzi F. Serotonin syndrome with mirtazapine-fluoxetine combination. *Int J Geriatr Psychiatry* 1998;13(7):495–496.
22. Isbister GK, Dawson AH, Whyte IM. Comment: serotonin syndrome induced by fluvoxamine and mirtazapine. *Ann Pharmacother* 2001;35(12): 1674–1675.
23. Demers JC, Malone M. Serotonin syndrome induced by fluvoxamine and mirtazapine. *Ann Pharmacother* 2001;35(10):1217–1220.
24. Anttila AKR. Fluvoxamine augmentation increases serum mirtazapine concentrations three- to fourfold. *Ann Pharmacother* 2001;35(10):1221–1223.
25. Hoes MJ, Zeijpveld JH. Mirtazapine as treatment for serotonin syndrome. *Pharmacopsychiatry* 1996;29(2):81.
26. Velazquez C, Carlson A, Stokes KA, et al. Relative safety of mirtazapine overdose. *Vet Hum Toxicol* 2001;43(6):342–344.
27. Stimmel GL, Dopheide JA, Stahl SM. Mirtazapine: an antidepressant with noradrenergic and specific serotonergic effects. *Pharmacotherapy* 1997;17(1):10–21.
28. Bremner JD, Wingard P, Walshe TA. Safety of mirtazapine in overdose. *J Clin Psychiatry* 1998;59(5):233–235.
29. Retz W, Maier S, Maris F, et al. Non-fatal mirtazapine overdose. *Int Clin Psychopharmacol* 1998;13(6):277–279.
30. Holzbach R, Jahn H, Pajonk FG, et al. Suicide attempts with mirtazapine overdose without complications. *Biol Psychiatry* 1998;44(9):925–926.
31. Schaper A, Färber E, Ebbecke M, et al. Suicide with mirtazapine—hardly possible. *J Toxicol Clin Toxicol* 2002;40(3):343–344.
32. Buckley NA, McManus PR. Fatal toxicity of serotoninergic and other antidepressant drugs: analysis of United Kingdom mortality data. *BMJ* 2002;325(7376):1332–1333.
33. John L, Perreault MM, Tao T, et al. Serotonin syndrome associated with nefazodone and paroxetine. *Ann Emerg Med* 1997;29(2):287–289.
34. Smith DL, Wenegrat BG. A case report of serotonin syndrome associated with combined nefazodone and fluoxetine. *J Clin Psychiatry* 2000;61(2):146.
35. Benson BE, Mathiason M, Dahl B, et al. Toxicities and outcomes associated with nefazodone poisoning: an analysis of 1,338 exposures. *Am J Emerg Med* 2000;18(5):587–592.
36. Robinson DS, Marcus RN, Archibald DG, et al. Therapeutic dose range of nefazodone in the treatment of major depression. *J Clin Psychiatry* 1996;57(suppl 2):6–9.
37. Robinson DS, Roberts DL, Smith JM, et al. The safety profile of nefazodone. *J Clin Psychiatry* 1996;57(suppl 2):31–38.
38. Catalano G, Catalano MC, Tumarkin NB. Nefazodone overdose: a case report. *Clin Neuropharmacol* 1999;22(1):63–65.
39. Whyte I, Buckley N. Calcium channel blocking drugs. *Medicine (Baltimore)* 1999;27(4):28–29.
40. Isbister GK, Hackett LP. Nefazodone poisoning: toxicokinetics and toxicodynamics using continuous data collection. *J Toxicol Clin Toxicol* 2003;41(2):167–173.
41. Baldwin D, Hawley C, Szabadi E, et al. Reboxetine in the treatment of depression: Early clinical experience in the UK. *Int J Psychiatry Clin Pract* 1998;2(3):195–201.
42. Perry NK. Venlafaxine-induced serotonin syndrome with relapse following amitriptyline. *Postgrad Med J* 2000;76(894):254–256.
43. Dougherty JA, Young H, Shafi T. Serotonin syndrome induced by amitriptyline, meperidine, and venlafaxine. *Ann Pharmacother* 2002;36(10):1647–1648.
44. Prior FH, Isbister GK, Dawson AH, et al. Serotonin toxicity with therapeutic doses of dexamphetamine and venlafaxine. *Med J Aust* 2002;176(5):240–241.
45. Prost N, Tichadou L, Rodor F, et al. [St. Johns wort-venlafaxine interaction]. *Presse Med* 2000;29(23):1285–1286.
46. Kolecki P. Venlafaxine induced serotonin syndrome occurring after abstinence from phenelzine for more than two weeks. *J Toxicol Clin Toxicol* 1997;35(2):211–212.
47. Brubacher JR, Hoffman RS, Lurin MJ. Serotonin syndrome from venlafaxine-tranylcypromine interaction. *Vet Hum Toxicol* 1996;38(5):358–361.
48. Hodgman MJ, Martin TG, Krenzelok EP. Serotonin syndrome due to venlafaxine and maintenance tranylcypromine therapy. *Hum Exp Toxicol* 1997;16(1):14–17.
49. Cassidy EM, O'Kearne V. Neuroleptic malignant syndrome after venlafaxine. *Lancet* 2000;355(9221):2164–2165.
50. Nimmagadda SR, Ryan DH, Atkin SL. Neuroleptic malignant syndrome after venlafaxine. *Lancet* 2000;355(9200):289–290.
51. Fisher AA, Davis MW. Serotonin syndrome caused by selective serotonin reuptake-inhibitors-metoclopramide interaction. *Ann Pharmacother* 2002;36(1):67–71.
52. Rudolph RL, Derivan AT. The safety and tolerability of venlafaxine hydrochloride: analysis of the clinical trials database. *J Clin Psychopharmacol* 1996;16(3 suppl 2):54S–59S.
53. Schlienger RG, Klink MH, Eggenberger C, et al. Seizures associated with therapeutic doses of venlafaxine and trimipramine. *Ann Pharmacother* 2000;34(12):1402–1405.
54. Daniels RJ. Serotonin syndrome due to venlafaxine overdose. *J Accid Emerg Med* 1998;15(5):333–334.
55. Kolecki P. Isolated venlafaxine-induced serotonin syndrome. *J Emerg Med* 1997;15(4):491–493.
56. Roxanas MG, Machado JF. Serotonin syndrome in combined moclobemide and venlafaxine ingestion. *Med J Aust* 1998;168(10):523–524.
57. Whyte IM, Dawson AH, Buckley NA. Relative toxicity of venlafaxine and selective serotonin reuptake inhibitors in overdose compared to tricyclic antidepressants. *QJM* 2003;96(5):369–374.
58. Fantaskey A, Burkhart KK. A case report of venlafaxine toxicity. *J Toxicol Clin Toxicol* 1995;33(4):359–361.
59. White CM, Gailey RA, Levin GM, et al. Seizure resulting from a venlafaxine overdose. *Ann Pharmacother* 1997;31(2):178–180.
60. Colbridge MG, Volans GN. Venlafaxine in overdose—experience of the national poisons information service (London centre). *J Toxicol Clin Toxicol* 1999;37(3):383.
61. Khalifa M, Daleau P, Turgeon J. Mechanism of sodium channel block by venlafaxine in guinea pig ventricular myocytes. *J Pharmacol Exp Ther* 1999;291(1):280–284.
62. Thorsson B, Snook C, Thorgeirsson G, et al. Survival after prolonged cardiac arrest from venlafaxine. *J Toxicol Clin Toxicol* 2000;38(2):246–247.
63. Banham ND. Fatal venlafaxine overdose. *Med J Aust* 1998;169(8):445, 448.
64. Partridge SJ, MacIver DH, Solanki T. A depressed myocardium. *J Toxicol Clin Toxicol* 2000;38(4):453–455.
65. Timmer CJ, Sitsen JM, Delbressine LP. Clinical pharmacokinetics of mirtazapine. *Clin Pharmacokinet* 2000;38(6):461–474.
66. Barbhaiya RH, Shukla UA, Greene DS. Single-dose pharmacokinetics of nefazodone in healthy young and elderly subjects and in subjects with renal or hepatic impairment. *Eur J Clin Pharmacol* 1995;49(3):221–228.

67. Anderson W. Antidepressants. In: Levine B, ed. *Principles of forensic toxicology*. Chapel Hill: American Association of Clinical Chemistry, 1999.
68. Penttila J, Syvalahti E, Hinkka S, et al. The effects of amitriptyline, citalopram and reboxetine on autonomic nervous system. A randomised placebo-controlled study on healthy volunteers. *Psychopharmacology (Berl)* 2001;154(4):343–349.
69. Charlier C, Pinto E, Ansseau M, et al. Relationship between clinical effects, serum drug concentration, and concurrent drug interactions in depressed patients treated with citalopram, fluoxetine, clomipramine, paroxetine or venlafaxine. *Hum Psychopharmacol* 2000;15(6):453–459.
70. Langford NJ, Martin U, Ruprah M, et al. Alternative venlafaxine kinetics in overdose. *J Clin Pharm Ther* 2002;27(6):465–467.
71. Woo OF, Vredenburg M, Freitas P. Seizures after venlafaxine overdose: a case report. *J Toxicol Clin Toxicol* 1995;33(5):549–550.
72. Kokan L, Dart RC. Life threatening hypotension from venlafaxine overdose. *Ann Emerg Med* 1996;27(6):815.
73. Ascher JA, Cole JO, Colin JN, et al. Bupropion: a review of its mechanism of antidepressant activity. *J Clin Psychiatry* 1995;56(9):395–401.
74. Richelson E, Pfenning M. Blockade by antidepressants and related compounds of biogenic amine uptake into rat brain synaptosomes: most antidepressants selectively block norepinephrine uptake. *Eur J Pharmacol* 1984;104(3–4):277–286.
75. Ferris RM, Beaman OJ. Bupropion: a new antidepressant drug, the mechanism of action of which is not associated with down-regulation of postsynaptic beta-adrenergic, serotonergic (5-HT2), alpha 2-adrenergic, imipramine and dopaminergic receptors in brain. *Neuropharmacology* 1983;22(11):1257–1267.
76. Tucker WE, Jr. Preclinical toxicology of bupropion: an overview. *J Clin Psychiatry* 1983;44(5 pt 2):60–62.
77. Bazett H. An analysis of the time-relations of electrocardiograms. *Heart* 1920;7:353–370.
78. Malik M, Farbom P, Batchvarov V, et al. Relation between QT and RR intervals is highly individual among healthy subjects: implications for heart rate correction of the QT interval. *Heart* 2002;87(3):220–228.
79. Aytemir K, Maarouf N, Gallagher MM, et al. Comparison of formulae for heart rate correction of QT interval in exercise electrocardiograms. *Pacing Clin Electrophysiol* 1999;22(9):1397–1401.
80. de Boer T. The effects of mirtazapine on central noradrenergic and serotonergic neurotransmission. *Int Clin Psychopharmacol* 1995;10(suppl 4):19–23.
81. de Boer TH, Maura G, Raiteri M, et al. Neurochemical and autonomic pharmacological profiles of the 6-aza-analogue of mianserin, Org 3770 and its enantiomers. *Neuropharmacology* 1988;27(4):399–408.
82. Owens MJ, Morgan WN, Plott SJ, et al. Neurotransmitter receptor and transporter binding profile of antidepressants and their metabolites. *J Pharmacol Exp Ther* 1997;283(3):1305–1322.
83. Wong EH, Sonders MS, Amara SG, et al. Reboxetine: a pharmacologically potent, selective, and specific norepinephrine reuptake inhibitor. *Biol Psychiatry* 2000;47(9):818–829.
84. Muth EA, Haskins JT, Moyer JA, et al. Antidepressant biochemical profile of the novel bicyclic compound Wy-45,030, an ethyl cyclohexanol derivative. *Biochem Pharmacol* 1986;35(24):4493–4497.
85. Millan MJ, Dekeyne A, Gobert A. Serotonin (5-HT)2C receptors tonically inhibit dopamine (DA) and noradrenaline (NA), but not 5-HT, release in the frontal cortex in vivo. *Neuropharmacology* 1998;37(7):953–955.
86. Muramatsu M, Tamaki-Ohashi J, Usuki C, et al. 5-HT2 antagonists and minaprine block the 5-HT-induced inhibition of dopamine release from rat brain striatal slices. *Eur J Pharmacol* 1988;153(1):89–95.
87. Dollery CT. *Therapeutic drugs* [database on CD-ROM]. Release 1.0 ed. London: Churchill Livingstone, 1999.
88. Einarson A, Fatoye B, Sarkar M, et al. Pregnancy outcome following gestational exposure to venlafaxine: a multicenter prospective controlled study. *Am J Psychiatry* 2001;158(10):1728–1730.
89. Briggs GG, Samson JH, Ambrose PJ, et al. Excretion of bupropion in breast milk. *Ann Pharmacother* 1993;27(4):431–433.
90. Yapp P, Ilett KF, Kristensen JH, et al. Drowsiness and poor feeding in a breast-fed infant: association with nefazodone and its metabolites. *Ann Pharmacother* 2000;34(11):1269–1272.
91. Ilett KF, Kristensen JH, Hackett LP, et al. Distribution of venlafaxine and its O-desmethyl metabolite in human milk and their effects in breastfed infants. *Br J Clin Pharmacol* 2002;53(1):17–22.
92. Belson MG, Kelley TR. Bupropion exposures: clinical manifestations and medical outcome. *J Emerg Med* 2002;23(3):223–230.
93. Sigg T. Recurrent seizures from sustained-release bupropion. *J Med Toxicol* [serial online]1999;2(3):4.
94. Velez LI, Delaney KA, Rivera W, et al. Delayed status epilepticus after a sustained release bupropion overdose. *J Toxicol Clin Toxicol* 2002;40(3):323–324.
95. Falkland M, McMorrow J, McKeown R, et al. Bupropion SR in overdose: subsidized poisoning. *J Toxicol Clin Toxicol* 2002;40(3):275–276.
96. Biswas AK, Zabrocki LA, Mayes KL, et al. Cardiotoxicity associated with intentional ziprasidone and bupropion overdose. *J Toxicol Clin Toxicol* 2003;41(1):79–82.
97. Druteika D, Zed PJ. Cardiotoxicity following bupropion overdose. *Ann Pharmacother* 2002;36(11):1791–1795.
98. Ramcharitar V, Levine BS, Goldberger BA, et al. Bupropion and alcohol fatal intoxication: case report. *Forensic Sci Int* 1992;56(2):151–156.
99. Rohrig TP, Ray NG. Tissue distribution of bupropion in a fatal overdose. *J Anal Toxicol* 1992;16(5):343–345.
100. Wooltorton E. Bupropion (Zyban, Wellbutrin SR): reports of deaths, seizures, serum sickness. *Can Med Assoc J* 2002;166(1):68a.
101. Peano C, Leikin JB, Hanashiro PK. Seizures, ventricular tachycardia, and rhabdomyolysis as a result of ingestion of venlafaxine and lamotrigine. *Ann Emerg Med* 1997;30(5):704–708.
102. Durback LF, Scharman EJ. Comment: seizure resulting from venlafaxine overdose. *Ann Pharmacother* 1997;31(6):790–791.
103. Zhalkovsky B, Walker D, Bourgeois JA. Seizure activity and enzyme elevations after venlafaxine overdose. *J Clin Psychopharmacol* 1997;17(6):490–491.
104. Leaf EV. Comment: venlafaxine overdose and seizure. *Ann Pharmacother* 1998;32(1):135–136.
105. Coorey AN, Wenck DJ. Venlafaxine overdose. *Med J Aust* 1998;168(10):523.
106. Blythe D, Hackett LP. Cardiovascular and neurological toxicity of venlafaxine. *Hum Exp Toxicol* 1999;18(5):309–313.
107. Jaffe PD, Batziris HP, van der Hoeven P, et al. A study involving venlafaxine overdoses: comparison of fatal and therapeutic concentrations in postmortem specimens. *J Forensic Sci* 1999;44(1):193–196.
108. Parsons AT, Anthony RM, Meeker JE. Two fatal cases of venlafaxine poisoning. *J Anal Toxicol* 1996;20(4):266–268.
109. Oliver JJ, Kelly C, Jarvie D, et al. Venlafaxine poisoning complicated by a late rise in creatine kinase: two case reports. *Hum Exp Toxicol* 2002;21(8):463–466.
110. Remick RA, Campos PE, Misri S, et al. A comparison of the safety and efficacy of bupropion HCL and amitriptyline hcl in depressed outpatients. *Prog Neuropsychopharmacol Biol Psychiatry* 1982;6(4–6):523–527.
111. Benazzi F. Mirtazapine withdrawal symptoms. *Can J Psychiatry* 1998;43(5):525.
112. Klesmer J, Sarcevic A, Fomari V. Panic attacks during discontinuation of mirtazapine. *Can J Psychiatry* 2000;45(6):570–571.
113. MacCall C, Callender J. Mirtazapine withdrawal causing hypomania. *Br J Psychiatry* 1999;175:390.
114. Benazzi F. Nefazodone withdrawal symptoms. *Can J Psychiatry* 1998;43(2):194–195.
115. Kotlyar M, Golding M, Brewer ER, et al. Possible nefazodone withdrawal syndrome. *Am J Psychiatry* 1999;156(7):1117.
116. Lauber C. Nefazodone withdrawal syndrome. *Can J Psychiatry* 1999;44(3):285–286.
117. Rajagopalan M, Little J. Discontinuation symptoms with nefazodone. *Aust N Z J Psychiatry* 1999;33(4):594–597.
118. Mucci M. Reboxetine: a review of antidepressant tolerability. *J Psychopharmacol* 1997;11(4 suppl):S33–S37.
119. Tanum L. Reboxetine: tolerability and safety profile in patients with major depression. *Acta Psychiatr Scand Suppl* 2000;402:37–40.
120. Haddad PM. Antidepressant discontinuation syndromes. *Drug Saf* 2001; 24(3):183–197.
121. Pinzani V, Ginies E, Robert L, et al. [Venlafaxine withdrawal syndrome: report of six cases and review of the literature]. *Rev Med Interne* 2000;21(3):282–284.
122. Luckhaus C, Jacob C. Venlafaxine withdrawal syndrome not prevented by maprotiline, but resolved by sertraline. *Int J Neuropsychopharmacol* 2001;4(1):43–44.
123. Other drugs for nicotine dependence. In: Rossi S, Vitry A, Hurley E, et al., eds. *Australian medicines handbook*. Adelaide: Australian Medicines Handbook Pty Ltd, 2002.
124. Other antidepressants. In: Rossi S, Vitry A, Hurley E, et al., eds. *Australian medicines handbook*. Adelaide: Australian Medicines Handbook Pty Ltd, 2002.
125. Reference deleted.
126. Moore KA, Levine B, Smith ML, et al. Tissue distribution of mirtazapine (Remeron) in postmortem cases. *J Anal Toxicol* 1999;23(6):541–543.
127. Anderson DT, Fritz KL, Muto JJ. Distribution of mirtazapine (Remeron) in thirteen postmortem cases. *J Anal Toxicol* 1999;23(6):544–548.
128. Goeringer KE, McIntyre IM, Drummer OH. Postmortem tissue concentrations of venlafaxine. *Forensic Sci Int* 2001;121(1–2):70–75.
129. Levine B, Jenkins AJ, Queen M, et al. Distribution of venlafaxine in three postmortem cases. *J Anal Toxicol* 1996;20(6):502–505.
130. Long C, Crifasi J, Maginn D, et al. Comparison of analytical methods in the determination of two venlafaxine fatalities. *J Anal Toxicol* 1997;21(2):166–169.
131. Buckley NA, Dawson AH, Reith DA. Controlled release drugs in overdose. Clinical considerations. *Drug Saf* 1995;12(1):73–84.
132. Gwilt PR, Perrier D. Plasma protein binding and distribution characteristics of drugs as indices of their hemodialyzability. *Clin Pharmacol Ther* 1978;24(2):154–161.
133. Kapur S, Zipursky RB, Jones C, et al. Cyproheptadine: a potent in vivo serotonin antagonist [Letter]. *Am J Psychiatry* 1997;154(6):884.
134. Gillman PK. The serotonin syndrome and its treatment. *J Psychopharmacol* 1999;13(1):100–109.
135. Graudins A, Stearman A, Chan B. Treatment of the serotonin syndrome with cyproheptadine. *J Emerg Med* 1998;16(4):615–619.
136. Horowitz BZ, Mullins ME. Cyproheptadine for serotonin syndrome in an accidental pediatric sertraline ingestion. *Pediatr Emerg Care* 1999;15(5):325–327.
137. Isbister GK. Comment: serotonin syndrome, mydriasis, and cyproheptadine. *Ann Pharmacother* 2001;35(12):1672–1673.
138. McDaniel WW. Serotonin syndrome: early management with cyproheptadine. *Ann Pharmacother* 2001;35(7–8):870–873.

139. Buckley NA, Dawson AH, Whyte IM. Specific serotonin reuptake inhibitors (SSRIs). *HyperTox: assessment and treatment of poisoning*. Newcastle, Australia: MediTox Pty Ltd, 2002.
140. Tatsumi M, Jansen K, Blakely RD, et al. Pharmacological profile of neuroleptics at human monoamine transporters. *Eur J Pharmacol* 1999;368(2–3):277–283.
141. Chan BS, Graudins A, Whyte IM, et al. Serotonin syndrome resulting from drug interactions. *Med J Aust* 1998;169(10):523–525.
142. Gillman PK. Successful treatment of serotonin syndrome with chlorpromazine. *Med J Aust* 1996;165(6):345–346.
143. Graham PM. Successful treatment of the toxic serotonin syndrome with chlorpromazine. *Med J Aust* 1997;166(3):166–167.
144. Green AR. Repeated chlorpromazine administration increases a behavioural response of rats to 5-hydroxytryptamine receptor stimulation. *Br J Pharmacol* 1977;59(2):367–371.
145. Richelson E, Souder T. Binding of antipsychotic drugs to human brain receptors focus on newer generation compounds. *Life Sci* 2000;68(1):29–39.
146. Baselt RC. *Drug effects on psychomotor performance*. Foster City, California: Biomedical Publications, 2001.
147. Other anxiolytics and hypnotics. In: Rossi S, Vitry A, Hurley E, et al., eds. *Australian medicines handbook*. Adelaide: Australian Medicines Handbook Pty Ltd, 2002.
148. Sweetman S. *Martindale: the complete drug reference*. London: Pharmaceutical Press. Electronic ed. expires 03/2003. Greenwood Village, Colorado: MICROMEDEX, 2003.
149. Findlay JW, Van Wyck FJ, Smith PG, et al. Pharmacokinetics of bupropion, a novel antidepressant agent, following oral administration to healthy subjects. *Eur J Clin Pharmacol* 1981;21(2):127–135.
150. Horst WD, Preskorn SH. Mechanisms of action and clinical characteristics of three atypical antidepressants: venlafaxine, nefazodone, bupropion. *J Affect Disord* 1998;51(3):237–254.
151. Fleishaker JC. Clinical pharmacokinetics of reboxetine, a selective norepinephrine reuptake inhibitor for the treatment of patients with depression. *Clin Pharmacokinet* 2000;39(6):413–427.

CHAPTER 137

Antipsychotic Drugs (Neuroleptics)

Nicholas A. Buckley

R1 N R2 S

Cl N N N N

PHENOTHIAZINE	**CLOZAPINE**
Compounds included:	**See Table 1.**
Molecular formula and weight:	**See Table 2.**
SI conversion:	**See Table 2.**
CAS Registry No.:	**See Table 2.**
Normal levels:	**See Table 3.**
Antidote:	**None**

OVERVIEW

The antipsychotic drugs are generally used for primary psychiatric disorders, such as schizophrenia, bipolar disorder, schizoaffective disorder, and psychotic depression. They are also sometimes used for borderline personality disorder, anesthesia, behavioral disorders, alcohol withdrawal, drug-induced psychosis, Tourette's syndrome, nausea and vomiting, and hiccups (1).

Antipsychotic drugs are divided into several chemical classes (Table 2). However, grouping the drugs into low-potency, high-potency, and atypical antipsychotic drugs is probably the most useful classification. The differentiation between low-potency and high-potency drugs refers to the drug's potency in blocking dopamine (D_2) receptors. In general, drugs that are low potency are less selective and have more effects on other receptors. In particular, they have more anticholinergic and vasodilating effects in therapeutic doses and produce more sedation. The most important beneficial compensation for this is that they cause less drug-induced parkinsonism because of their anticholinergic effects (2). Most of the newer drugs have successfully reduced the problem of all extrapyramidal adverse effects. Many are also potent serotonin antagonists, but they are a diverse group, and many of their toxicity profiles are still being recognized (3,4).

Antipsychotic drugs are a relatively common cause of poisoning in most countries of the developed world (5–7). Antipsychotic effects are attributable primarily to the blockade of D_2 receptors (8). This pharmacologic action contributes significantly to adverse effects in therapeutic use. However, the major effects in overdose with any of these agents are mainly due to other effects. The toxicity of each individual agent in overdose varies considerably, although the general effects in overdose are qualitatively similar, comprising sedation, hypotension, tachycardia, and other anticholinergic effects and, in the most severe cases, dysrhythmias and seizures. These effects are similar to those seen with tricyclic antidepressant (TCA) overdose, but these drugs are generally less toxic in overdose.

TABLE 1. Compounds included

Phenothiazines	Thioxanthines
Chlorpromazine (Thorazine)	Thiothixene (Navane)
Fluphenazine (Prolixin)	Zuclopenthixol (Sedanxol)
Loxapine (Loxitane)	Atypical antipsychotic drugs
Pericyazine (Neulactil)	Amisulpride (Deniban)
Perphenazine (Trilafon)	Clozapine (Clozaril)
Promazine (Sparine)	Olanzapine (Zyprexa)
Thioridazine (Mellaril)	Quetiapine (Seroquel)
Trifluoperazine (Stelazine)	Risperidone (Risperdal)
Butyrophenones	Ziprasidone (Geodon)
Droperidol (Inapsine)	
Haloperidol (Haldol)	

TABLE 2. Chemical classification, physical characteristics, and defined daily doses of antipsychotic drugs

Drug	DDD[a] (mg/d)	Molecular formula	Molecular weight (g/mol)	SI conversion	CAS Registry No.
Aliphatic phenothiazines					
Acepromazine	100	$C_{19}H_{22}N_2OS$	326.5	—	61-00-7
Chlorpromazine	300	$C_{17}H_{19}ClN_2S$	318.9	mg/L × 3.14 = µmol/L	50-53-3
Levomepromazine (methotrimeprazine)	300	$C_{19}H_{24}N_2OS$	328.5	—	60-99-1
Prochlorperazine	100		373.9	—	
Promazine	300	$C_{17}H_{20}N_2S$	284.4	mg/L × 3.52 = µmol/L	58-40-2
Promethazine	—	$C_{17}H_{20}N_2S$	284.4	—	60-87-7
Trifluoperazine	20	$C_{21}H_{24}F_3N_3S$	407.5	µg/L × 2.45 = nmol/L	117-89-5
Triflupromazine	100	$C_{18}H_{19}F_3N_2S$	352.4	—	146-54-3
Piperazine-phenothiazines					
Acetophenazine	50	$C_{23}H_{29}N_3O_2S$	411.6	—	2751-68-0
Butaperazine	10	$C_{24}H_{31}N_3OS$	409.6	—	653-03-2
Dixyrazine	50	$C_{24}H_{33}N_3O_2S$	427.6	—	2470-73-7
Fluphenazine	10	$C_{22}H_{26}F_3N_3OS$	437.5	µg/L × 2.29 = nmol/L	69-23-8
Perazine	100	$C_{20}H_{25}N_3S$	339.5	—	84-97-9
Perphenazine	30	$C_{21}H_{26}ClN_3OS$	404.0	µg/L × 2.48 = nmol/L	58-39-9
Prochlorperazine	100	$C_{20}H_{24}ClN_3S$	373.9	—	58-38-8
Thiopropazate	60	$C_{23}H_{28}ClN_3O_2S$	446.0	—	84-06-0
Thioproperazine	75	$C_{22}H_{30}N_4O_2S_2$	446.6	—	316-81-4
Piperidine phenothiazines					
Mesoridazine	200	$C_{21}H_{26}N_2OS_2$	386.6	—	5588-33-0
Pericyazine	50	$C_{21}H_{23}N_3OS$	365.5	µg/L × 2.74 = nmol/L	2622-26-6
Pipotiazine	10	$C_{24}H_{33}N_3O_3S_2$	475.7	—	39860-99-6
Thioridazine	300	$C_{21}H_{26}N_2S_2$	370.6	mg/L × 2.70 = µmol/L	50-52-2
Butyrophenone					
Benperidol	1.5	$C_{22}H_{24}FN_3O_2$	381.4	—	2062-84-2
Bromperidol	10	$C_{21}H_{23}BrFNO_2$	420.3	—	10457-90-6
Droperidol	—	$C_{22}H_{22}FN_3O_2$	379.4	µg/L × 2.64 = nmol/L	548-73-2
Haloperidol	8	$C_{21}H_{23}ClFNO_2$	375.9	mg/L × 2.66 = µmol/L	52-86-8
Melperone	300	$C_{16}H_{22}FNO$	263.4	—	3575-80-2
Pipamperone	200	$C_{21}H_{30}FN_3O_2$	375.5	—	1893-33-0
Trifluperidol	2	$C_{22}H_{23}F_4NO_2$	409.4	—	749-13-3
Indoles					
Molindone	50	$C_{16}H_{24}N_2O_2$	276.4	—	7416-34-4
Oxypertine	120	$C_{23}H_{29}N_3O_2$	379.5	—	153-87-7
Sertindole	16	$C_{24}H_{26}ClFN_4O$	441.0	—	106516-24-9
Ziprasidone	80	$C_{21}H_{21}ClN_4OS$	467.4	mg/L × 2.42 = µmol/L	146939-27-7
Thioxanthines					
Chlorprothixene	—	$C_{18}H_{18}ClNS$	315.9	—	113-59-7
Flupenthixol	4	$C_{23}H_{25}F_3N_2OS$	434.5	—	2709-56-0
Thiothixene	30	$C_{23}H_{29}N_3O_2S_2$	443.6	mg/L × 2.25 = µmol/L	5591-45-7
Zuclopenthixol	30	$C_{22}H_{25}ClN_2OS$	473.9	mg/L × 2.49 = µmol/L	53772-83-1
Diphenylbutylpiperidine derivatives					
Fluspirilene	0.7	$C_{29}H_{31}F_2N_3O$	475.6	—	1841-19-6
Penfluridol	6	$C_{28}H_{27}ClF_5NO$	524.0	—	26864-56-2
Pimozide	4	$C_{28}H_{29}F_2N_3O$	461.6	—	2062-78-4
Benzodiazepines					
Clozapine	300	$C_{18}H_{19}ClN_4$	326.8	mg/L × 3.06 = µmol/L	5786-21-0
Loxapine	100	$C_{18}H_{18}ClN_3O$	327.8	mg/L × 3.05 = µmol/L	1977-10-2
Olanzapine	10	$C_{17}H_{20}N_4S$	312.4	mg/L × 3.20 = µmol/L	132539-06-1
Quetiapine	400	$C_{21}H_{25}N_3O_2S$	383.5	mg/L × 2.61 = µmol/L	111974-69-7
Benzamides					
Amisulpride	400	$C_{17}H_{27}N_3O_4S$	369.5	mg/L × 2.71 = µmol/L	71675-85-9
Levosulpiride	—	$C_{15}H_{23}N_3O_4S$	341.4	—	23672-07-3
Remoxipride	300	$C_{16}H_{23}BrN_2O_3$	371.3	—	80125-14-0
Sulpiride	800	$C_{15}H_{23}N_3O_4S$	341.4	—	15676-16-1
Sultopride	1200	$C_{17}H_{26}N_2O_4S$	354.5	—	53583-79-2
Tiapride	400	$C_{15}H_{24}N_2O4_S$	328.4	—	51012-32-9
Other					
Clotiapine	—	$C_{18}H_{18}ClN_3S$	343.9	—	2058-52-8
Mosapramine	—		479.1	—	89419-40-9
Prothipendyl	240	$C_{16}H_{19}N_3S$	285.4	—	303-69-5
Risperidone	5	$C_{23}H_{27}FN_4O_2$	410.5	µg/L × 2.44 = nmol/L	106266-06-2
Zotepine	200	$C_{18}H_{18}ClNOS$	331.9	—	26615-21-4

DDD, defined daily dose.
[a]DDD (oral, where available) is the assumed average maintenance dose per day for a drug used for its main indication in adults.
Data from WHO Collaborating Centre for Drug Statistics Methodology Web site. Available at: http://www.whocc.no/atcddd/. Accessed July 2003.

TABLE 3. Pharmacokinetic information and therapeutic and lethal concentrations of selected antipsychotic drugs

Drug	Elimination half-life (h; range)	Typical therapeutic blood concentrations (mg/L)	Lethal blood concentrations (mg/L)	Heart-femoral ratios mean (range)	Active metabolites
Low potency					
Chlorpromazine	7–119	0.02–3.0	1–44	4 (1–8)	Promazine
Loxapine	3–4	NR	>3.0	NR	Amoxapine
Mesoridazine	2–9	0.1–1.0	>3.0	1.3 (1.0–2.3)	Sulforidazine
Methotrimeprazine	17–78	0.05–0.14	0.8–4.1	1.3 (0.6–2.8)	Yes
Promethazine	9–16	0.006–0.1	>2.4	NR	NR
Remoxipride	3.5–7.0	1.5–3.3	>41	NR	Yes
Sulpiride	4–11	0.6–30.0	3.9	NR	NR
Thioridazine	26–36	0.14–2.60	0.8–13.0	1.4 (0.4–2.8)	Mesoridazine, sulforidazine
Moderate-high potency					
Trifluoperazine	7–18	0.0009–0.004	0.06	(0.6–1.0)	Yes
Perphenazine	8–12	0.0004–0.03	3.0	NR	NR
Haloperidol	14–41	0.005–0.05	>1.0	3.6 (1.4–10.0)	None
Atypical					
Clozapine	6–7	0.2–0.7	1.2–13.0	2.8	None
Olanzapine	21–54	0.009–0.026	1.2	NR	None
Quetiapine	5–8	0.19–0.63	0.24–4.0	NR	Minor
Risperidone	3–20	0.004–0.008	1.8	NR	9-Hydroxyrisperidone
Ziprasidone	4–10	NR	None recorded	NR	None

NR, not reported.
From Trenton A, Currier G, Zwemer F. Fatalities associated with therapeutic use and overdose of atypical antipsychotics. *CNS Drugs* 2003;17(5):307–324; and Baselt RC. *Disposition of toxic drugs and chemicals in man,* 5th ed. Foster City, CA: Chemical Toxicology Institute, 1999, with permission.

Relative Toxicity of the Neuroleptic Agents

Substantial differences are found between the neuroleptic agents in terms of their toxicity. These differences are apparent in studies of the clinical effects in overdose and in studies that examine the number of deaths due to each drug compared to measures of drug use [fatal toxicity indices (FTIs)] (9–11). The drugs that cause the most deaths per prescription are generally low-potency antipsychotic drugs such as chlorpromazine and thioridazine. Loxapine has a much higher FTI than any other antipsychotic drug, and its active metabolite amoxapine has the highest FTI of any antidepressant (10,12). This drug is less commonly used, but limited experience suggests that it is very proconvulsant in overdose (13). In clinical studies, thioridazine causes significantly more electrocardiographic (ECG) changes and cardiac dysrhythmias than other conventional antipsychotic drugs, and chlorpromazine is significantly more sedating (9). It has been proposed on the basis of a review of published case reports that quetiapine is less toxic than other atypical antipsychotic drugs (3). However, a larger series of 45 patients reports seizures, hypotension, QTc prolongation, and sedation to the point of requiring mechanical ventilation—all similar to the effects seen with clozapine and olanzapine overdose (14).

Adverse Event Profile of the Class

Substantial differences in the adverse effect profiles of the neuroleptic drug group are also found. Most importantly, this affects severe adverse idiosyncratic reactions; clozapine is more frequently implicated in agranulocytosis, seizures, myocarditis, and cardiomyopathy (2). It is also apparent in different propensity to cause QT prolongation, dysrhythmias, and sudden death, with thioridazine and, to a lesser extent, droperidol being more frequently implicated (15–17). Olanzapine, clozapine, and some low-potency conventional neuroleptics appear to cause significantly more weight gain, glucose intolerance, and hyperlipidemia (18).

Toxic Dose

The adult defined daily doses (DDDs) of the antipsychotic drugs are shown in Table 1. This is an average dose, and therapeutic doses two to three times larger than this would occasionally be used. Generally, much smaller doses are used in the elderly, who metabolize the drugs less efficiently and are more prone to extrapyramidal adverse effects.

Dose-related toxicity is common in the therapeutic range with many of these drugs. Sedation, mild hypotension, and tachycardia are commonly seen with relatively small overdoses of most of these drugs. Some drugs have a large margin of safety, whereas for others the concentrations found in therapeutic use overlap with those found in fatal overdoses(4,19) (Table 3). These give some indication of the margin of safety of the drugs. However, these figures should be interpreted conservatively, as most of the drugs would be expected to be subject to postmortem redistribution.

Occasional cases of one or two children ingesting a neuroleptic are reported. Some cases report clinical toxicity (e.g., sedation, dystonia) with ingestion of only 1 tablet by young children.(3,4,20). Little information is available on pediatric poisoning with these drugs, as there are only a few indications for them to be used in children (e.g., Tourette's syndrome). No deaths have been reported in the few pediatric ingestions of these drugs that have appeared in the literature (3,4,20). However, therapeutic use of phenothiazine antihistamines has been suspected of contributing to sudden infant death syndrome (21).

TOXICOKINETICS AND TOXICODYNAMICS

Antipsychotic drugs are generally lipid-soluble weak bases that are rapidly absorbed and have high protein binding to α_1-acid glycoprotein and large volumes of distribution. Generally, peak concentrations occur within a few hours. Anticholinergic effects associated with many of these drugs may delay absorption and

TABLE 4. Potency ($10^{-7} \times$ L/kd) at blocking D_2 receptors, muscarinic, α_1-adrenergic receptors, and direct cardiac effects

Drug[a]	D_2 potency	M_2 potency	M_2/D_2	α_1 potency	α_1/D_2	Direct cardiac effects
Quetiapine	0.13	0.071[b]	**0.55**	12	**92.3**	
Clozapine	0.47	0.714	**1.52**	15	**31.9**	
Promazine	0.625	0.238	**0.381**			
Molindone	0.83	0.0002	0.0003	0.04	0.048	
Thioridazine	3.8	1.96	**0.52**	20	**5.26**	EADs, QTc, TdP
Olanzapine	5.1	2.8[b]	**0.55**	2.3	**0.451**	
Mesoridazine	5.3	0.833	**0.16**	50	**9.43**	
Chlorpromazine	5.3	0.442	0.083	38	**7.17**	EADs, I_{Na}, QTc
Loxapine	6.1	0.132	0.022	3.6	**0.59**	
Chlorprothixene	12.5	0.769	0.062			
Prochlorperazine	14	0.0714	0.005	4.2	**0.3**	
Risperidone	27	0.0029[b]	0.0001	37	**1.37**	QTc
Sertindole	37	0.02[b]	0.0005	25	**0.676**	HERG, QTc, TdP
Trifluoperazine	38	0.0457	0.0012	4.2	**0.111**	QTc
Ziprasidone	39	0.041[b]	0.0011	38	**0.974**	
Haloperidol	39	0.0128	0.0003	5.9	**0.151**	HERG, I_{Na}, QTc, TdP
Perphenazine	71	0.0345	0.0005	10	**0.141**	QTc
Fluphenazine	125	0.0417	0.0003	11	0.088	
Pimozide	154	2.8[b]	0.018	1.2	0.0078	QTc, TdP
cis-Thiothixene	222	0.036	0.0002	9.1	0.041	

D_2, dopamine; EADs, induces early after-depolarizations *in vivo*; HERG, blocks the inward rectifying potassium channel; I_{Na}, blocks the depolarizing sodium channel; M_2, muscarinic receptor; QTc, causes significant QTc prolongation in clinical use; TdP, documented to cause torsade de pointes (any dose).
[a]Drugs are listed in ascending order of D_2 potency. Values shown in bold indicate that a pharmacologic effect is likely in some patients at therapeutic dosages.
[b]Nonspecific antimuscarinic potency.
Modified from Buckley NA, Sanders P. Cardiovascular adverse effects of antipsychotic dogs. *Drug Saf* 2000;23(3);215–228.

cause delayed peak concentrations. The initial fall in serum concentrations after overdose would be primarily due to distribution rather than clearance (3,4,20).

All of the neuroleptic drugs are metabolized in the liver. Many have active metabolites and complex metabolic pathways. The main enzymes involved in metabolism are cytochrome P-450 (CYP) enzymes; CYP1A2, CYP2D6, and CYP3A4 are the major enzymes involved (3,4,22). Many sources of variation are found in CYP metabolism. For example, 5% to 10% of whites are CYP2D6 "poor metabolizers," meaning that they do not produce a normally functioning CYP2D6 enzyme (22). CYP1A2 and CYP3A4 are inducible enzymes, which may lead to significant interactions, particularly with anticonvulsants (23). All three enzymes may be inhibited by other drug treatment. Where multiple enzymes are involved, such variations have only a relatively small effect on clearance and drug concentrations. Where an enzyme is responsible for a large proportion of a drug's metabolism, such variations can lead to much larger and clinically significant effects (24).

For example, risperidone, perphenazine, zuclopenthixol, haloperidol, and thioridazine are largely metabolized by CYP2D6. Poor metabolizers and those taking drugs that inhibit this enzyme may have drug concentrations that are up to tenfold higher than those of other individuals (22). Thus, there are a large number of potential drug interactions, although the literature contains only a few reports of clinically significant adverse outcomes (24).

Clozapine therapeutic concentrations are usually in the range of 0.2 to 0.7 mg/L. Concentrations reported in deliberate overdose are generally tenfold higher. Clozapine is metabolized by the liver through the enzymes CYP1A2 and CYP2D6. Olanzapine is also metabolized through CYP1A2 and CYP2D6 but has less potential for significant interactions, as there are also other metabolic pathways. Smoking cessation can roughly double the concentration of these drugs, as smoking induces the CYP1A2 enzyme (25). Drugs that inhibit CYP1A2, such as fluvoxamine, cimetidine, and erythromycin, can cause substantial increases in the concentrations of these drugs (24,26). Smaller increases occur with drugs that inhibit other pathways (such as fluoxetine, paroxetine, and sertraline). However, one fatality has been attributed to a fluoxetine-clozapine interaction (27).

PATHOPHYSIOLOGY

The primary pharmacologic effect of all of the antipsychotic drugs is to block D_2 receptors in the central nervous system (8). With the minor exception of acute dystonic reactions, this effect is unimportant in overdose. However, the drugs are pharmacologically "dirty," and they bind to many other receptors, including histamine (H_1, H_2), γ-aminobutyric acid–A and muscarinic receptors, α_1- and α_2-adrenoreceptors, and sodium and potassium voltage gated ion channels (3,20,28,29) (Table 4).

Seizures

Many antipsychotic drugs lower the seizure threshold. Abnormalities on electroencephalography, including spikes and generalized slowing, are very common in patients receiving regular therapeutic doses. Drug-induced seizures are much less common, occurring in fewer than 1% of patients taking most drugs (2). The mechanism for this general effect is not known and is probably multifactorial. However, a small number of these drugs are potent γ-aminobutyric acid antagonists (28). This includes clozapine, which has a much higher rate of drug-induced seizures (approximately 5%) (2). It also includes loxapine and its active metabolite amoxapine. These two drugs are very proconvulsant in overdose and, perhaps due to this, far more lethal in overdose (10,13).

Cardiac Effects

In acute overdose, the mechanism of the cardiac toxicity appears to be similar to that of the TCA drugs. Minor effects such as hypotension and tachycardia are most commonly due to α_1-adrenoreceptor blocking and anticholinergic effects. Myocardial depression and dysrhythmias are assumed to be due to "quinidine-like" blockade of sodium, potassium, and calcium ion channels. Indirect effects also occur through blockade of α_2-adrenoreceptors in the central nervous system (similar to the effect of clonidine) (30).

Adverse Events

A large number of serious idiosyncratic adverse reactions, such as neutropenia and myocarditis, are reported from some of the antipsychotic drugs (2). However, although the mechanisms underlying these adverse effects are currently unknown, they do not appear to be dose related and are rarely, if ever, reported after overdose (2,31). An immunologic mechanism is assumed to be partly responsible for many of these drug reactions. An eosinophilic infiltrate has been reported in interstitial nephritis and myocarditis (32,33), and a number of studies have linked clozapine-induced agranulocytosis with human leukocyte antigen phenotypes (34).

PREGNANCY AND LACTATION

Neuroleptic drugs are all potentially harmful in pregnancy (Table 5). Little human experience has been reported with atypical antipsychotic drugs, and low doses of high-potency conventional agents (e.g., haloperidol) are generally preferred in early pregnancy. Teratogenic effects from first-trimester exposure have not been proven with human use of any of these drugs (35). The most frequent adverse effects are neonatal extrapyramidal side effects, including generalized hypertonicity and dystonia.

These compounds achieve significant concentrations in breast milk, with milk-plasma ratios of 0.5 to 1.0 (36). Extrapyramidal adverse effects can be seen in breast-feeding infants, and breast-feeding is generally not recommended. No agents are preferred, but if there are compelling reasons for breast-feeding the infant should be observed for signs of extrapyramidal toxicity (35). High prolactin levels are a direct consequence of D_2-receptor blockade and thus occur with all these drugs. This may lead to galactorrhea and also impaired fertility (2).

TABLE 5. Reproductive risk information for antipsychotic drugs

Drug	FDA/American	ADEC/Swedish
Chlorpromazine	C	C
Prochlorperazine	C	C
Trifluoperazine	C	C
Triflupromazine	C	–
Fluphenazine	C	C
Perphenazine	C	C
Prochlorperazine	C	C
Pericyazine	–	C
Thioridazine	C	C
Droperidol	C	C
Haloperidol	C	C
Flupenthixol	C	C
Thiothixene	C	B1
Zuclopenthixol	C	C
Pimozide	C	B1
Clozapine	B	C
Olanzapine	C	B3
Quetiapine	C	B3
Amisulpride	–	B3
Risperidone	C	B3
Ziprasidone	C	–

ADEC, Australian Drug Evaluation Committee; FDA, U.S. Food and Drug Administration; –, not classified by that system.
From Rossi S, ed. *The Australian medicines handbook (AMH)*, 4th ed. Canberra: Commonwealth Department of Health and Family Services, 2003; and Briggs GG, Freeman RK, Yaffe SJ. *Drugs in pregnancy and lactation*, 6th ed. Baltimore: Williams & Wilkins, 2002, with permission.

CLINICAL PRESENTATION

Acute Overdosage

Toxicity is strongly correlated with peak serum concentrations and thus usually occurs within the first 4 to 6 hours after these rapidly absorbed drugs. Patients who present early may deteriorate rapidly, and close observation is indicated for the first few hours after presentation. A large ingested dose, decreased level of consciousness, and abnormal ECG at presentation are probably the best indicators of the most toxic ingestions. With good supportive care the mortality of patients who present to the hospital should be less than 0.5% (9).

The presentation for most of these drugs is qualitatively similar to that following TCA overdose, but in general they are less toxic. Sedation, hypotension, small pupils, anticholinergic effects, and ECG changes are the most common effects in significant overdose (3,37). The most serious effects, seizures, and dysrhythmias occur in a small proportion of presentations to the hospital. They are probably significant contributors to out-of-hospital mortality.

Cardiovascular System

Hypotension and tachycardia are both common. Hypotension may be due to a number of causes. Some neuroleptics can cause direct myocardial depression. However, in practice, the hypotension usually relates to relative volume depletion and α_1-adrenoreceptor blockade–induced vasodilation. Thus, it generally responds rapidly to intravenous (IV) fluids. Tachycardia is usually due to the anticholinergic effects of these drugs or is a reflex tachycardia from volume depletion and vasodilation. Persistent tachycardia after apparent recovery should raise the possibility of alcohol or drug withdrawal.

ECG changes are common, for example, "dimpling" of the T waves. QRS and QTc prolongation are also common, although the rate varies considerably between drugs. Thioridazine and mesoridazine cause more ECG changes and dysrhythmias than other agents. In one study thioridazine caused more ECG changes. The odds ratio for a QTc exceeding 450 milliseconds was 4.7 (95% confidence interval: 2.7 to 7.9), and the odds ratio for cardiac dysrhythmias reached infinity (95% confidence interval: 2.4 to infinity) compared to other antipsychotic drugs ingested in that hospital (including chlorpromazine, trifluoperazine, pericyazine, haloperidol, prochlorperazine, and fluphenazine) (9).

The atypical agents can also cause ECG abnormalities in overdose, but there are no comparative studies to suggest whether any agents are of particular concern (3). It has been proposed on the basis of case reports that quetiapine was less toxic than other atypical antipsychotic drugs (3). However, a larger series of 45 patients reports seizures, hypotension, QTc prolongation, and sedation to the point of requiring mechanical ventilation, all similar to the effects seen with clozapine and olanzapine overdose (14).

Broad complex tachycardia is a sign of severe cardiac toxicity. It is difficult to distinguish between the types of broad complex tachycardia in neuroleptic poisoning. These resemble (and may be) ventricular tachycardia. They may also be due to a sinus (anticholinergic effect) or supraventricular tachycardia with the prolonged QRS due to rate-dependent sodium channel blockade. In any case, it is not uncommon for the blood pressure to be reasonably well maintained during such dysrhythmias.

Bradycardia associated with an abnormal QRS width is a much more ominous marker of severe toxicity. It indicates severe conduction block, is usually associated with refractory hypotension, and often precedes death (20).

Central Nervous System

Central nervous system effects manifest first as an impaired level of consciousness. The level of consciousness may rapidly deteriorate into deep coma because of the very rapid absorption of most of these drugs.

Seizures occur in a few percent of overdoses with most of these drugs (3,20). Loxapine causes seizures much more frequently (13). Seizures are associated with an increased risk of cardiac toxicity and death. The acidosis produced by seizures causes an increase in free drug levels by reducing protein binding. In addition, acidosis affects the partitioning of basic drugs between the cell membrane and the sodium channel–binding site and increases sodium channel blockade. The increased sodium channel blockade may then lead to cardiac dysrhythmias. Patients should be assessed on admission to see if they have hyperreflexia, myoclonic jerks, or other evidence of seizure activity. In most overdoses with these drugs, the reflexes are normal or decreased, as seen with coma from other sedative drugs.

Dopamine Blocking (Extrapyramidal) Effects

Extrapyramidal effects are the most common problem in therapeutic use. They are no more common in overdose, perhaps due to competing anticholinergic effects. Dystonia, dyskinesia, or akathisia may develop in some patients. This is more common with high-potency antipsychotic drugs (i.e., butyrophenones and other drugs with a low DDD) (20).

Anticholinergic Effects

The anticholinergic effects seen in antipsychotic drug poisoning are usually much less obvious than those seen in the classic syndrome from pure anticholinergic drugs. The typical agitated delirium is uncommon, as patients are usually significantly sedated. Although the pupils may be dilated, they are more often small (3,37). Other anticholinergic effects, such as tachycardia, urinary retention, or absent bowel sounds, are less obvious but more often present. These symptoms or signs are poor predictors for life-threatening toxicity.

CLINICAL PRESENTATION

Acute Overdosage

In antipsychotic drug overdose, there are no specific diagnostic features to look for. A general examination of the unconscious patient, including vital signs and neurologic examination, should be done. Typically, patients are drowsy or unconscious, with small (but not pinpoint) pupils. Tone and reflexes are usually normal. Tachycardia and mild hypotension are also common (3,37).

Antipsychotic drugs should be considered, along with other drugs with ion channel blocking effects, in patients with seizures, QRS prolongation, or ventricular dysrhythmias. In Australia, a presentation with coma in the presence of minor anticholinergic signs usually means that either an antipsychotic drug or a TCA has been ingested (37).

Adverse Events

Adverse reactions in therapeutic use are very common and a frequent reason for poor compliance. The most common adverse effects with conventional agents are extrapyramidal side effects, tardive dyskinesia, sedation, mild cognitive impairment, orthostatic hypotension, abnormal liver function tests, anticholinergic side effects, sexual dysfunction, and weight gain. The newer atypical agents have a lower risk of extrapyramidal side effects but are also associated with sedation, cardiovascular effects, anticholinergic effects, weight gain, sexual dysfunction, abnormal liver tests, and lowered seizure threshold (2).

Drug-induced parkinsonism is much more common with high-potency drugs (e.g., haloperidol, fluphenazine, trifluoperazine, and pimozide) and less common with low-potency drugs with compensatory anticholinergic effects (e.g., chlorpromazine and pericyazine) (2). It is even less common with atypical antipsychotic drugs; clozapine has even been used successfully to treat Parkinson's disease (38). The symptoms and signs are clinically indistinguishable from Parkinson's disease.

Rabbit syndrome is a late-onset neuroleptic drug-induced extrapyramidal syndrome characterized by rhythmic 5.0 to 5.5 cycles per second involuntary movements of the oral and masticatory musculature that mimic the chewing movements of a rabbit. The high frequency of the perioral movements and the absence of lingual movements distinguish the rabbit syndrome from tardive dyskinesia. In contrast to tardive dyskinesia, it is reversible when neuroleptic drug therapy is discontinued and responds to antiparkinsonian drug therapy. It is possibly just a particular manifestation of drug-induced parkinsonism (2).

Neuroleptic malignant syndrome (NMS) is a tetrad of fever, rigidity, altered sensorium, and autonomic dysfunction (Chapter 23). The temperature in severe cases typically ranges from 38.5° to 42°C, but fever is not always present. The rigidity is typical of severe drug-induced parkinsonism, with either lead pipe or cogwheeling rigidity. Other extrapyramidal signs, such as tremor, bradykinesia, festinating gait, dystonia, opisthotonus, sialorrhea, and dysphagia, may be present. Mental status ranges from mild confusion and agitation to lethargy, stupor, and coma. Autonomic dysfunction is manifested by sweating, tachycardia, labile blood pressure, and tachypnea. Patients who present early in their course may not have all the classic features (2,39).

NMS frequently occurs 3 to 9 days after initiation of neuroleptic treatment or an increase in dose. Symptoms of NMS usually develop over 24 to 72 hours and last 5 to 10 days after the neuroleptic drug is discontinued. All D_2 antagonists in common use, including atypical antipsychotic drugs, have been associated with NMS (2,38,40,41). Withdrawal of D_2 agonists (e.g., levodopa, bromocriptine, cabergoline) has caused a similar syndrome.

The most common complication of NMS is rhabdomyolysis, which results from muscle rigidity and breakdown. Other reported complications include aspiration pneumonia, pulmonary embolism, pulmonary edema, adult respiratory distress syndrome, sepsis, disseminated intravascular coagulation, seizures, renal failure, myocardial infarction, peripheral neuropathy, and death. Periarticular ossification has also been reported following NMS and other central nervous system disturbances (39).

Tardive dyskinesia is a late-onset adverse effect that leads to involuntary movements. The face and mouth are most severely affected, but the limbs and trunk may also be involved. Lip smacking, protrusion of the tongue, chewing and jaw deviations, facial grimacing, eye blinking, and furrowing of the eyebrows are typical dyskinesias. Movements disappear during sleep, and voluntary activity of the involved muscle group markedly reduces the frequency of involuntary repetitive movements. This disorder affects a substantial proportion of long-term users of antipsychotic drugs. The incidence appears to be lower with atypical antipsychotic drugs such as olanzapine (38). Dyskinesias may appear at any time during treatment. They typically respond temporarily to dose escalation (not recommended) and get temporarily worse when doses are reduced (2).

Toxic ictal delirium (drug-induced nonconvulsive status epilepticus) is a rare syndrome, although it is probably also underdiagnosed. It presents as an acute confusional syndrome. The notable features are a fluctuating mental state, sporadic involuntary movements resembling myoclonus, and hyperreflexia. A rapid and significant response of the confusional state to benzodiazepines is also a feature that might support the diagnosis. It is triggered by increasing doses of psychotropic drugs or benzodiazepine withdrawal (42,43).

Cardiac adverse effects include myocarditis, cardiomyopathy, and sudden death. The most commonly implicated drug is clozapine, but other agents have also been reported (2). The actual incidence reported varies considerably. The highest estimate for the incidence of fatal and nonfatal myocarditis in the first month of treatment was 2.9 per 1000 patients. In this study, the median time to onset of symptoms of 15 days and biopsy evidence of eosinophilic infiltrates strongly suggested that the myocarditis was due to an acute hypersensitivity reaction (32).

Hematologic toxicity includes clozapine-induced agranulocytosis. Estimates of the incidence of this condition range between 0.2% and 1.0% (2). Hematologic toxicity has also been reported much more rarely with other antipsychotic drugs, including chlorpromazine, olanzapine, and risperidone (2). A significantly increased risk of thromboembolic disease has also been reported with clozapine (44).

DIAGNOSTIC TESTS

An ECG, electrolytes, and arterial blood gases are commonly measured. An ECG should be performed on admission and a few hours later. It may be assumed that an abnormal ECG is a predictor of dysrhythmias based on the similarity to TCA poisoning, with which such a strategy is commonly used. However, this may be an unwarranted extrapolation. Thioridazine is the only antipsychotic drug that commonly causes dysrhythmias and ECG changes (30,45), but a case-control study of patients with dysrhythmias indicated that the initial ECG was not a good indicator of risk in thioridazine overdose (46). This can be explained in a number of possible ways: QT prolongation is common in therapeutic use, thioridazine has a cardiotoxic metabolite, and dysrhythmias often occur relatively late in the course of the overdose (30). Despite these concerns, a conservative approach suggests that a patient with a significantly abnormal ECG requires monitoring for at least 24 hours. Those with an initially normal ECG should still be monitored for a few hours and have the ECG repeated.

The purpose of checking electrolytes is to identify other risk factors for dysrhythmias (e.g., hypokalemia, hypomagnesemia). Arterial blood gases are performed to determine if patients have a respiratory acidosis. It is likely that acidosis would increase the risk of dysrhythmias, as it increases free drug concentrations and may increase ion channel blocking effects. Abnormalities of other biochemical or hematologic tests are not expected and should raise the possibility of other drug ingestion. In particular, clozapine does not appear to cause agranulocytosis in overdose.

Plasma Concentrations

Blood concentrations are useful postmortem to indicate the cause of death but are generally unhelpful in clinical management. Therapeutic drug monitoring is used commonly for clozapine therapy (therapeutic range, 0.35 to 0.7 mg/L) but not for any other antipsychotic drugs. Most of these drugs have active metabolites, meaning that the parent drug concentration may poorly reflect the total pharmacologic activity. Also, the correlation between drug concentration and response appears to be poor. This may have pharmacodynamic (e.g., different receptor density or affinity, D_2 turnover) or pharmacokinetic reasons (i.e., the blood concentration does not predict the free concentration of drug at the receptor). In any case, many patients respond to quite low doses, whereas many are resistant to treatment at much higher concentrations (47).

At normal therapeutic doses of low- and high-potency drugs, D_2 receptors are more than 75% occupied. Thus, there is little rationale for further increasing doses in most clinical situations. Plasma concentrations may help to diagnose noncompliance in this situation or indicate patients with extremely rapid metabolism (47).

Postmortem Considerations

It is difficult to generalize about the antipsychotic drugs in regard to interpretation of postmortem drug concentrations. Many factors may have an impact on the blood (or plasma) concentration in therapeutic use and overdose. A summary of typical concentrations in therapeutic use and found postmortem in presumed fatal overdoses is shown in Table 3. The data are simplifications of more detailed information from a specialist text and a review (4,19). It is apparent that, for some of these drugs, there is a large margin of safety, whereas for others, concentrations in therapeutic use and fatal overdose overlap. The contribution to the overlap of postmortem redistribution may be considerable. The heart–femoral blood concentration ratios indicate that there is potential for substantial postmortem change for some drugs, a common problem with basic drugs. A full consideration of these issues is covered in specialist textbooks for these and some other antipsychotic drugs (19).

TREATMENT

The outcome with supportive care alone is generally favorable if no other more toxic drugs are ingested (9,48,49). Coingestion of a TCA may be a particular concern due to synergistic cardiac effects; combined overdoses appear to have a higher rate of dysrhythmias (46,50). A simple guide to management decisions is shown in Figure 1 (20).

Decontamination

No specific issues in gastrointestinal decontamination pertain to antipsychotic drugs, and general recommendations should apply (Chapter 7). A single dose of activated charcoal may be worthwhile in patients who present within an hour of ingesting a potentially lethal amount of one of these drugs (generally at least 10 times the DDD) (Table 1). Forced emesis, cathartics, and whole bowel irrigation are unlikely to provide any additional benefit and may be potentially harmful due to common complications, such as rapid deterioration in consciousness, seizures, dystonia, and paralytic ileus.

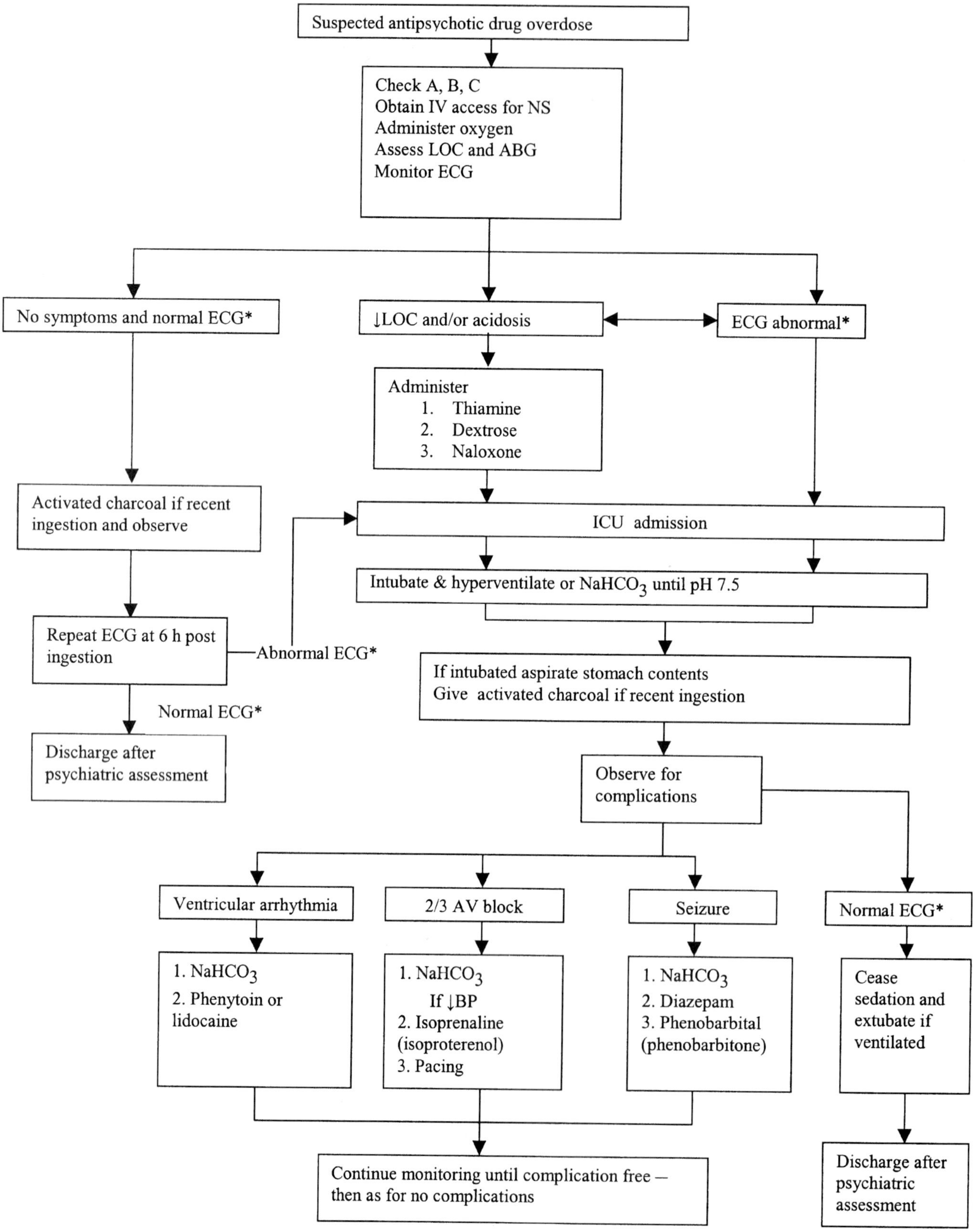

Suspected antipsychotic drug overdose

Check A, B, C
Obtain IV access for NS
Administer oxygen
Assess LOC and ABG
Monitor ECG

No symptoms and normal ECG*

↓LOC and/or acidosis

ECG abnormal*

Administer
1. Thiamine
2. Dextrose
3. Naloxone

Activated charcoal if recent ingestion and observe

ICU admission

Intubate & hyperventilate or $NaHCO_3$ until pH 7.5

Repeat ECG at 6 h post ingestion

Abnormal ECG*

Normal ECG*

Discharge after psychiatric assessment

If intubated aspirate stomach contents
Give activated charcoal if recent ingestion

Observe for complications

Ventricular arrhythmia

1. $NaHCO_3$
2. Phenytoin or lidocaine

2/3 AV block

1. $NaHCO_3$
If ↓BP
2. Isoprenaline (isoproterenol)
3. Pacing

Seizure

1. $NaHCO_3$
2. Diazepam
3. Phenobarbital (phenobarbitone)

Normal ECG*

Cease sedation and extubate if ventilated

Continue monitoring until complication free — then as for no complications

Discharge after psychiatric assessment

Figure 1. Algorithm for the treatment of patients with suspected antipsychotic drug overdose. A, B, C, airway, breathing, circulation; ABG, arterial blood gases; AV, atrioventricular block; BP, blood pressure; ECG, electrocardiogram; ICU, intensive care unit; LOC, level of consciousness; NS, normal saline; *, ECG abnormalities include dysrhythmias, QRS greater than 120 milliseconds, QTc greater than 480 milliseconds, and right bundle branch block. [Modified from Parsons M, Buckley NA. Antipsychotic drugs in overdose: practical management guidelines. *CNS Drugs* 1997;6(6):417–441.]

Enhancement of Elimination

Repeated doses of activated charcoal may increase the clearance of some antipsychotic drugs. However, it is likely that the main mechanism for falling drug concentrations is distribution rather than clearance. No evidence of clinical benefit has been shown, and many of these patients have an ileus.

The principles of elimination enhancement are discussed in Chapter 78. The volumes of distribution and the extent of protein binding for antipsychotic drugs, when known, are uniformly high, and extracorporeal techniques do not remove a significant proportion of ingested drug (51).

Antidotes

Sodium bicarbonate has been shown to be effective in reversing TCA-induced conduction defects and hypotension (Chapter 75). Little experimental or clinical data are available on its effect on cardiac toxicity due to antipsychotic drugs. Just a few cases have been reported of rapid and significant response of ECG abnormalities (52,53), and experimental evidence does not support a sustained effect in all drugs with sodium channel blocking activity (54,55). However, the antipsychotics have mechanisms of toxicity similar to those for TCA, for which sodium bicarbonate is the treatment of choice (56). Sodium bicarbonate is also relatively safe, making it the initial drug of choice for the treatment of dysrhythmias due to antipsychotic drug poisoning. Suggested specific indications are any ventricular or supraventricular dysrhythmia, heart block, or a QRS width that exceeds 120 milliseconds. The dose is 1 to 3 mEq/kg body weight by bolus injection, repeated if necessary at 3- to 5-minute intervals. The arterial blood pH should not exceed 7.55. Higher pH is associated with a range of adverse effects, and the pH should be monitored if repeated doses are used (56).

Supportive Care

Level of consciousness, airway patency, and ventilation should be assessed. Any patient who is not protecting the airway, has a respiratory acidosis, or has a Glasgow Coma score of less than 12 should be ventilated. Mild hyperventilation (pH, 7.45 to 7.55) may be beneficial in reducing cardiac toxicity. IV access should be established in all patients with significant toxicity. Patients should have continuous ECG monitoring for at least 6 hours after ingestion and until the ECG is normal.

Dysrhythmias and conduction defects are difficult to diagnose accurately, as rate-dependent QRS and QT prolongation mean that sinus or supraventricular tachycardia may have very broad complexes and P waves are often lost in the preceding T wave. The initial treatment for all dysrhythmias should be rapid plasma alkalinization with sodium bicarbonate as described in the section Antidotes.

The preferred treatment for polymorphic ventricular tachycardia (torsade de pointes) is usually magnesium sulfate (57). However, in the overdose setting the calcium channel blocking effects of magnesium may worsen hypotension and should be used only after sodium bicarbonate has been unsuccessful. The use of other antidysrhythmic agents is controversial. Class 1A (quinidine, procainamide) and class 1C (flecainide) drugs are contraindicated (56). Overdrive pacing should be considered for polymorphic or refractory ventricular tachycardia (58). This approach was successful in an overdose of haloperidol and orphenadrine (59). Temporary pacing should also be considered for refractory bradydysrhythmias such as second- and third-degree heart block (58). Class 1B antidysrhythmic drugs (lidocaine, phenytoin, mexiletine) are sodium channel blocking drugs with rapid offset kinetics. They may theoretically be useful in reducing rate-dependent sodium channel blockade from other drugs with slower offset kinetics. Experimental evidence is not conclusive, but they could be regarded as second-line drugs for the treatment of ventricular dysrhythmias (60,61).

Seizures are usually self-limited; protection of the airway is the main priority. If prolonged or multiple, they should be treated with diazepam, 5 to 20 mg IV. If benzodiazepines do not control the seizures, patients may require phenobarbital or more aggressive therapy (Chapter 40). A possible complication of seizures is cardiac dysrhythmia precipitated by the acidosis.

Hypotension is most likely to be due to vasodilation and usually responds to isotonic volume expansion with normal saline. Refractory hypotension may indicate direct myocardial depression. This is almost always associated with conduction defects and should be treated with sodium bicarbonate. Central venous pressure monitoring should be used to ensure optimal fluid replacement. If hypotension persists, pharmacologic pressure support (e.g., epinephrine, norepinephrine) can be used cautiously, but these drugs may precipitate dysrhythmias, as they further prolong the effective refractory period.

Acute dystonia and parkinsonism are mainly treated with anticholinergic drugs. They are much more useful for the treatment of acute dystonia than for chronic parkinsonism. The drug of choice for acute dystonia is benztropine, 1 to 2 mg intramuscularly or IV. A response is usual within 5 to 10 minutes. Regular oral doses of 2 to 8 mg/day in divided doses can be used for persistent dystonia (for example, that due to depot antipsychotic drugs) or for drug-induced parkinsonism. An alternative is benzhexol (trihexyphenidyl) in doses of 5 to 15 mg/day (2).

NMS is a life-threatening condition. Some patients require monitored intensive care management. The treatment is primarily supportive, with cessation of the offending drug. Most deaths are due to medical complications of the condition, such as pneumonia and other infections, pulmonary embolism, dehydration, malnutrition, and severe hyperthermia. Thus, treatment should primarily consist of attention to such issues as diagnosis and treatment of secondary infections; thromboembolic disease stockings or heparin, or both; monitoring of vital signs with aggressive treatment of severe hyperthermia; and maintenance of fluid balance (39). If the condition is slow to resolve, patients may require supplemental feeding to maintain nutrition.

Therapy with bromocriptine or dantrolene, or both, should be started immediately in severe cases and considered in less severe cases. They should be continued until the patient's condition improves clinically (typically 5 to 9 days), at which time creatinine kinase levels are usually returning to normal. Bromocriptine is generally used in patients who are able to take tablets, with dantrolene reserved for more severe cases of NMS who are unable to swallow. Suggested initial doses are bromocriptine, 2.5 to 10.0 mg orally, three or four times a day. Doses as high as 20 mg have been used in severe cases.

Dantrolene sodium is used in dosages of 1 to 3 mg/kg/day IV in four divided doses. The dosage can be increased to 10 mg/kg/day IV in four divided doses. Oral maintenance doses range from 50 to 200 mg/day. Electroconvulsive therapy has also been suggested to be of use in severe NMS. It is used as well in catatonia and psychotic depression with severe psychomotor retardation. Sometimes it may be difficult to differentiate these conditions from NMS, and electroconvulsive therapy may be particularly useful in this situation. Most patients with NMS can be cautiously retreated with antipsychotic drugs after a few weeks have elapsed (39). The use of low doses of an atypical antipsychotic drug is recommended.

REFERENCES

1. Rossi S, ed. *The Australian medicines handbook (AMH)*, 4th ed. Canberra: Commonwealth Department of Health and Family Services, 2003.
2. Simpson GM, Pi EH, Sramek JJ. Neuroleptic and antipsychotic drugs. In: Dukes MN, Aronson JK, eds. *Meyler's side effects of drugs*. Elsevier Science, 2000:139–163.
3. Burns MJ. The pharmacology and toxicology of atypical antipsychotic agents. *J Toxicol Clin Toxicol* 2001;39(1):1–14.
4. Trenton A, Currier G, Zwemer F. Fatalities associated with therapeutic use and overdose of atypical antipsychotics. *CNS Drugs* 2003;17(5):307–324.
5. Buckley NA, Whyte IM, Dawson AH, et al. Self-poisoning in Newcastle, 1987–1992. *Med J Aust* 1995;162(4):190–193.
6. Crombie IK, McLoone P. Does the availability of prescribed drugs affect rates of self poisoning? *Br J Gen Pract* 1998;48(433):1505–1506.
7. Weir P, Ardagh M. The epidemiology of deliberate self poisoning presenting to Christchurch Hospital Emergency Department. *N Z Med J* 1998;111(1063):127–129.
8. Richelson E. Preclinical pharmacology of neuroleptics: focus on new generation compounds. *J Clin Psychiatry* 1996;57[Suppl 11]:4–11.
9. Buckley NA, Whyte IM, Dawson AH. Cardiotoxicity more common in thioridazine overdose than with other neuroleptics. *J Toxicol Clin Toxicol* 1995;33(3):199–204.
10. Buckley N, McManus P. Fatal toxicity of drugs used in the treatment of psychotic illnesses. *Br J Psychiatry* 1998;172:461–464.
11. Schreinzer D, Frey R, Stimpfl T, et al. Different fatal toxicity of neuroleptics identified by autopsy. *Eur Neuropsychopharmacol* 2001;11(2):117–124.
12. Buckley NA, McManus PR. Fatal toxicity of serotoninergic and other antidepressant drugs: analysis of United Kingdom mortality data. *BMJ* 2002;325:1332–1333.
13. Peterson CD. Seizures induced by acute loxapine overdose. *Am J Psychiatry* 1981;138(8):1089–1091.
14. Balit CR, Isbister GK, Hackett LP, et al. Quetiapine poisoning: a case series. *Ann Emerg Med* 2003;(*in press*).
15. Reilly JG, Ayis SA, Ferrier IN, et al. QTc-interval abnormalities and psychotropic drug therapy in psychiatric patients. *Lancet* 2000;355(9209):1048–1052.
16. Mehtonen OP, Aranko K, Malkonen L, et al. A survey of sudden death associated with the use of antipsychotic or antidepressant drugs: 49 cases in Finland. *Acta Psychiatr Scand* 1991;84(1):58–64.
17. Working Group of the Royal College of Psychiatrists' psychopharmacology sub-group. The association between antipsychotic drugs and sudden death. Council report [CR 57]. London: Royal College of Psychiatrists, 1997.
18. Baptista T, Kin NM, Beaulieu S, et al. Obesity and related metabolic abnormalities during antipsychotic drug administration: mechanisms, management and research perspectives. *Pharmacopsychiatry* 2002;35(6):205–219.
19. Baselt RC. *Disposition of toxic drugs and chemicals in man*, 5th ed. Foster City, CA: Chemical Toxicology Institute, 1999.
20. Parsons M, Buckley NA. Antipsychotic drugs in overdose: practical management guidelines. *CNS Drugs* 1997;6(6):427–441.
21. Dyer KS, Woolf AD. Use of phenothiazines as sedatives in children: what are the risks? *Drug Saf* 1999;21(2):81–90.
22. Dahl ML. Cytochrome p450 phenotyping/genotyping in patients receiving antipsychotics: useful aid to prescribing? *Clin Pharmacokinet* 2002;41(7):453–470.
23. Meyer MC, Baldessarini RJ, Goff DC, et al. Clinically significant interactions of psychotropic agents with antipsychotic drugs. *Drug Saf* 1996;15(5):333–346.
24. Stockley IH. *Drug interactions*, 6th ed. London: Pharmaceutical Press, 2002.
25. Van Der WJ, Steijns LS, Van Weelden MJ. The effect of smoking and cytochrome P450 CYP1A2 genetic polymorphism on clozapine clearance and dose requirement. *Pharmacogenetics* 2003;13(3):169–172.
26. Heeringa M, Beurskens R, Schouten W, et al. Elevated plasma levels of clozapine after concomitant use of fluvoxamine. *Pharm World Sci* 1999;21(5):243–244.
27. Ferslew KE, Hagardorn AN, Harlan GC, et al. A fatal drug interaction between clozapine and fluoxetine. *J Forensic Sci* 1998;43(5):1082–1085.
28. Squires RF, Saederup E. Mono N-aryl ethylenediamine and piperazine derivatives are GABAA receptor blockers: implications for psychiatry. *Neurochem Res* 1993;18(7):787–793.
29. Studenik C, Lemmens-Gruber R, Heistracher P. Proarrhythmic effects of antidepressants and neuroleptic drugs on isolated, spontaneously beating guinea-pig Purkinje fibers. *Eur J Pharm Sci* 1999;7(2):113–118.
30. Buckley NA, Sanders P. Cardiovascular adverse effects of antipsychotic drugs. *Drug Saf* 2000;23(3):215–228.
31. Buur-Rasmussen B, Brosen K. Cytochrome P450 and therapeutic drug monitoring with respect to clozapine. *Eur Neuropsychopharmacol* 1999;9(6):453–459.
32. Killian JG, Kerr K, Lawrence C, et al. Myocarditis and cardiomyopathy associated with clozapine. *Lancet* 1999;354(9193):1841–1845.
33. Elias TJ, Bannister KM, Clarkson AR, et al. Clozapine-induced acute interstitial nephritis. *Lancet* 1999;354(9185):1180–1181.
34. Yunis JJ, Corzo D, Salazar M, et al. HLA associations in clozapine-induced agranulocytosis. *Blood* 1995;86(3):1177–1183.
35. Briggs GG, Freeman RK, Yaffe SJ. *Drugs in pregnancy and lactation*, 6th ed. Baltimore: Williams & Wilkins, 2002.
36. Yoshida K, Smith B, Craggs M, et al. Neuroleptic drugs in breast-milk: a study of pharmacokinetics and of possible adverse effects in breast-fed infants. *Psychol Med* 1998;28(1):81–91.
37. Buckley NA, Whyte IM, Dawson AH. Diagnostic data in clinical toxicology—should we use a Bayesian approach? *J Toxicol Clin Toxicol* 2002;40(3):213–222.
38. Tarsy D, Baldessarini RJ, Tarazi FI. Effects of newer antipsychotics on extrapyramidal function. *CNS Drugs* 2002;16(1):23–45.
39. Velamoor VR. Neuroleptic malignant syndrome. Recognition, prevention and management. *Drug Saf* 1998;19(1):73–82.
40. Kogoj A, Velikonja I. Olanzapine induced neuroleptic malignant syndrome—a case review. *Hum Psychopharmacol* 2003;18(4):301–309.
41. Karagianis JL, Phillips LC, Hogan KP, et al. Clozapine-associated neuroleptic malignant syndrome: two new cases and a review of the literature. *Ann Pharmacother* 1999;33(5):623–630.
42. van Sweden B, Mellerio F. Toxic ictal delirium. *Biol Psychiatry* 1989;25(4):449–458.
43. Primavera A, Cocito L. Acute confusion in a chronic benzodiazepine patient. Withdrawal-related nonconvulsive status epilepticus misdiagnosed as acute intoxication. *Gen Hosp Psychiatry* 1995;17(6):460–462.
44. Hagg S, Spigset O, Soderstrom TG. Association of venous thromboembolism and clozapine. *Lancet* 2000;355(9210):1155–1156.
45. Le Blaye I, Donatini B, Hall M, et al. Acute overdosage with thioridazine: a review of the available clinical exposure. *Vet Hum Toxicol* 1993;35(2):147–150.
46. Chevalier S, Buckley NA, O'Connell DL, et al. ECG predictors of arrhythmias after tricyclic and thioridazine overdose. *Aust N Z J Med* 1995;25:625.
47. Cohen BM, Waternaux C. Neuroleptic plasma levels: limitations and values. In: Marder SR, Davis JM, Janicak PG, eds. *Clinical use of neuroleptic plasma levels*. Washington, DC: American Psychiatric Press, 1993.
48. Acri AA, Henretig FM. Effects of risperidone in overdose. *Am J Emerg Med* 1998;16(5):498–501.
49. Capel MM, Colbridge MG, Henry JA. Overdose profiles of new antipsychotic agents. *Int J Neuropsychopharmacol* 2000;3(1):51–54.
50. Wilens TE, Stern TA, O'Gara PT. Adverse cardiac effects of combined neuroleptic ingestion and tricyclic antidepressant overdose. *J Clin Psychopharmacol* 1990;10(1):51–54.
51. Gwilt PR, Perrier D. Plasma protein binding and distribution characteristics of drugs as indices of their hemodialyzability. *Clin Pharmacol Ther* 1978;24(2):154–161.
52. Rivera W, Gracia R, Roth B, et al. Quinidine-like effects from quetiapine overdose with documented serum levels. *J Toxicol Clin Toxicol* 2003;41(4):508.
53. Diltoer MW, Poelmans LW, Hubloue I, et al. Combined intoxication with a tricyclic antidepressive agent and a neuroleptic. *Eur J Emerg Med* 1996;3(1):52–55.
54. Bou-Abboud E, Nattel S. Relative role of alkalosis and sodium ions in reversal of class I antiarrhythmic drug-induced sodium channel blockade by sodium bicarbonate. *Circulation* 1996;94(8):1954–1961.
55. Wang RY, Raymond RM. The effects of sodium bicarbonate on thioridazine-induced cardiac dysfunction in the isolated perfused rat heart. *Vet Hum Toxicol* 2001;43(2):73–77.
56. Albertson TE, Dawson A, de Latorre FJ, et al. TOX-ACLS: toxicologic-oriented advanced cardiac life support. *Ann Emerg Med* 2001;37[4 Suppl]:S78–S90.
57. Keren A, Tzivoni D. Magnesium therapy in ventricular arrhythmias. *Pacing Clin Electrophysiol* 1990;13(7):937–945.
58. Donatini B, Le Blaye I, Krupp P. Transient cardiac pacing is insufficiently used to treat arrhythmia associated with thioridazine. *Cardiology* 1992;81(6):340–341.
59. Henderson RA, Lane S, Henry JA. Life-threatening ventricular arrhythmia (torsades de pointes) after haloperidol overdose. *Hum Exp Toxicol* 1991;10(1):59–62.
60. Kamiya K, Kodama I, Toyama J. A combination of inactivated sodium channel blockers causes competitive interaction on dV/dtmax of single ventricular myocytes. *Cardiovasc Res* 1991;25(6):516–522.
61. Kawamura T, Kodama I, Toyama J, et al. Combined application of class I antiarrhythmic drugs causes "additive," "reductive," or "synergistic" sodium channel block in cardiac muscles. *Cardiovasc Res* 1990;24(11):925–931.

CHAPTER 138

Anorectic Agents and Respiratory and Cerebral Stimulants

E. Martin Caravati

See Figure 1.

Compounds included:	**Almitrine (Vectarion, Duxil), doxapram (Dopram), dexfenfluramine (Redux), fenfluramine (Ponderax, Pondimin), mazindol (Sanorex, Teronac, Diestet), modafinil (Provigil, Modiodal, Alertec), phendimetrazine (Bontril, Plegine, Prelu-2, Statobex), phenmetrazine (Preludin), phentermine (Fastin, Adipex-P, Ionamin), pemoline (Phenoxazole, Phenylisohydantoin, Cylert, Dynalert, others), sibutramine (Meridia)**
Molecular formula and weight:	**See Table 1.**
SI conversion:	**See Table 1.**
CAS Registry No.:	**See Table 1.**
Therapeutic levels:	**Almatrine 200 to 300 ng/ml; Pemoline 1 to 7 μg/ml**
Special concerns:	**All agents: central nervous system stimulation and agitation. Almitrine: peripheral neuropathy. Doxapram: central nervous system, cardiovascular system. Fenfluramine: pulmonary hypertension, valvular defects. Pemoline: hepatotoxicity (chronic).**
Antidote:	**Cyproheptadine for serotonin toxicity**

OVERVIEW

This chapter discusses drugs that are prescribed for their central stimulant or anorectic effects. Most are sympathomimetics and are subject to abuse. The primary indications are hyperactivity disorders, narcolepsy, respiratory depression, and obesity. The anorectic agents have varying capacities to inhibit the reuptake of dopamine, norepinephrine, or serotonin. The respiratory stimulants act on the central respiratory center. Acute toxicity is similar to amphetamine but generally less intense. Management is generally supportive, with benzodiazepines being the first-line agent for agitation, hypertension, or seizures. There are no specific antidotes.

ALMITRINE

Almitrine dismesylate (Vectarion, Duxil) is used in Europe as a respiratory stimulant for short-term treatment of patients with respiratory failure associated with chronic bronchitis and emphysema. It is reported to improve ventilation and oxygenation in these patients. Prolonged use may lead to a severe peripheral neuropathy. Intravenous (IV) use has been associated with lactic acidosis. Acute overdose may result in abdominal pain, headache, flushing, hyperventilation, or hypercapnia. Blood concentrations are not helpful in managing toxicity. It is available as 50-mg tablets and as an IV form (pH, 2 to 3) containing lyophilized almitrine bismesylate. This drug has not been approved by the U.S. Food and Drug Administration (FDA).

Toxic Dose

The adult *therapeutic dose* is provided in Table 1. The *toxic dose* is not well defined. Doses greater than 100 mg/day are associated with nausea, abdominal discomfort, headache, and flushing (1). At doses of 100 to 200 mg daily, some patients attain plasma levels well above the optimal therapeutic plasma concentration of 200 to 300 ng/ml. Elevated almitrine levels are associated with the development of peripheral paresthesias (2).

Toxicokinetics and Toxicodynamics

Almitrine is rapidly absorbed from the gastrointestinal tract with a bioavailability approximately 70% because of hepatic first-pass metabolism. It is 99% protein bound, mostly to albumin. The volume of distribution (V_d) is 14 to 15 L/kg. Almitrine undergoes hepatic oxidation to several hydroxylated inactive metabolites. Its elimination half-life is 40 to 80 hours. Steady-state elimination is 11 to 15 days. Approximately 10% of a dose appears in the urine. Pharmacokinetics in patients with chronic obstructive lung disease are similar to those in healthy subjects (1).

Pathophysiology

Almitrine bismesylate acts directly on peripheral chemoreceptors to improve ventilation and blood oxygenation. It appears to be effective in increasing PaO_2 in patients with hypoxemic chronic bronchitis and emphysema (3). Chronic almitrine

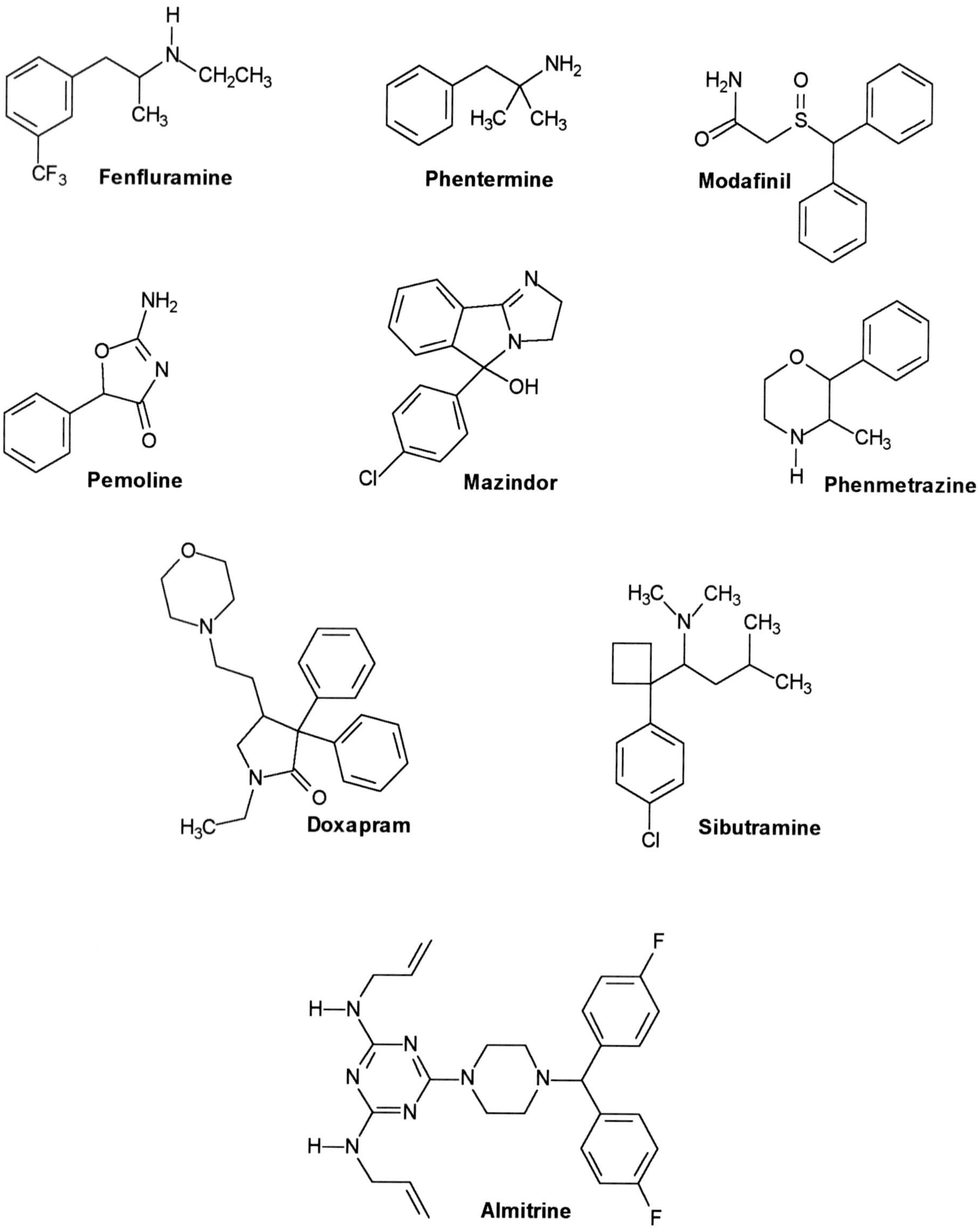

Figure 1. Structures of the anorectic agents and respiratory and cerebral stimulants.

therapy has resulted in axonal injury of predominately large myelinated fibers. Axonal regeneration may occur after withdrawal of the drug. The pathogenesis of the neuropathy is unclear (4).

Pregnancy and Lactation

There are no human data on possible teratogenic effects. It is unknown to what extent almitrine is excreted into breast milk. Breast-feeding is not recommended during treatment.

Clinical Presentation

ACUTE OVERDOSAGE

There are no published reports of acute overdose with almitrine. Based on similar agents, acute overdose may result in abdominal pain, headache, flushing, hyperventilation, or hypercapnia.

ADVERSE EVENTS

Chronic use has been associated with peripheral neuropathy. This sensory neuropathy may develop after 2 months of treatment and is

TABLE 1. Physical characteristics and dosage of the anorectic agents and respiratory and cerebral stimulants

Name	Molecular formula, molecular weight (g/mol), CAS Registry No.	SI conversion	Therapeutic dose	
			Adult	Children
Almitrine dismesylate	$C_{26}H_{29}F_2N_7,2CH_4SO_3$; 669.8; 27469-53-0	mg/L × 1.5 = μmol/L	50–100 mg/d orally; up to 3 mg/kg/d IV	1.5 mg/kg orally
Doxapram hydrochloride	$C_{24}H_{30}N_2O_2,HCl,H_2O$; 433.0; 309-29-5	mg/L × 2.3 = μmol/L	0.5–2.0 mg/kg IV, or 1.5–4.0 mg/min for respiratory failure; maximum daily dose is 3000 mg	0.25–2.50 mg/kg/h IV for neonatal apnea
Fenfluramine hydrochloride	$C_{12}H_{16}F_3N,HCl$; 267.7; 404-82-0	mg/L × 3.7 = μmol/L	20–160 mg/d orally	NR
Mazindol	$C_{16}H_{13}ClN_2O$; 284.7; 22232-71-9	mg/L × 3.5 = μmol/L	1 mg orally daily for appetite control; up to 8 mg/d for narcolepsy	1–2 mg/d for narcolepsy
Modafinil	$C_{15}H_{15}NO_2S$; 273.4; 68693-11-8	mg/L × 3.7 = μmol/L	100–400 mg/d for ADHD or narcolepsy	50–100 mg/d for ADHD
Phendimetrazine tartrate	$C_{12}H_{17}NO,C_4H_6O_6$; 341.4; 50-58-8	mg/L × 2.9 = μmol/L	35 mg regular release or 105 mg sustained release tablet daily	NR
Phenmetrazine hydrochloride	$C_{11}H_{15}NO$; 177.2; 134-49-6	mg/L × 5.6 = μmol/L	75 mg/d	NR
Phentermine hydrochloride	$C_{10}H_{15}N,HCl$; 185.7; 122-09-8	mg/L × 5.4 = μmol/L	37.5 mg/d	Not recommended
Pemoline	$C_9H_8N_2O_2$; 176.2; 2152-34-3	mg/L × 5.7 = μmol/L	37.5 daily orally; up to a maximum of 112.5 mg/d	Same as adult dose
Sibutramine	$C_{17}H_{26}ClN$; 279.8; 106650-56-0	mg/L × 3.6 = μmol/L	10–15 mg/d orally	NR

ADHD, attention deficit hyperactivity disorder; NR, not reported.

often associated with weight loss (5). The weight loss occurs more commonly in overweight patients (6). A sensory peripheral neuropathy developed in five patients treated with almitrine dimesylate, 60 to 100 mg/day for 2 to 4 months. It began in the lower extremities and was associated with a symmetric *stocking* sensory deficit. The histology suggested a distal axonopathy (7). Peripheral neuropathy began most frequently 9 to 25 months after initiation of treatment in patients taking almitrine or almitrine/raubasine combination therapy in another study (8). Recovery tends to be poor (9).

Lactic acidosis occurred in 8 out of 25 patients treated with *IV* almitrine for less than 24 hours for pneumonia or lung contusion. An increase in alanine aminotransferase and aspartate aminotransferase was also noted. Lactate and transaminase levels returned to normal after cessation of treatment (10).

Central nervous system (CNS) adverse effects include dizziness, insomnia, anxiety, irritability, agitation, and confusion. Other adverse effects include weight loss, headache, urticaria, diarrhea, chest pain, nausea, and vomiting.

Diagnostic Tests

A sensitive high-pressure liquid chromatography method has a detection limit of 5 ng/ml for almitrine and 10 to 25 mg/ml for its metabolites (11). After a single dose of 50 mg, a plasma almitrine concentration of 18.5 ng/ml is obtained in 30 to 40 minutes. A dose of 1.5 mg/kg leads to a peak plasma level of 300 ng/ml (12). Increased plasma levels (more than 30 ng/ml) are related to the occurrence of symptoms (peripheral paresthesias) (3). There is no correlation between arterial blood gas and plasma almitrine concentrations.

Treatment

Experience with almitrine overdose is limited. Patients should receive cardiac and oxygen saturation monitoring until evidence of clinical effects (i.e., tachycardia, tachypnea) resolve.

DECONTAMINATION

Administration of activated charcoal soon after oral overdose probably decreases drug absorption from the gut although there are no studies to confirm this effect.

ANTIDOTES

There are no specific antidotes.

ENHANCEMENT OF ELIMINATION

The large volume of distribution and high protein binding of almitrine prevents effective elimination enhancement.

SUPPORTIVE CARE

Benzodiazepines should be administered for agitation or combativeness (e.g., diazepam, 5 mg IV). Patients who remain symptomatic after 4 to 6 hours of observation should be admitted to the hospital for continued monitoring of vital signs. Lactic acidosis should resolve with discontinuation of the drug and IV fluids (10).

DOXAPRAM

Doxapram (Dopram) has been used as a peripheral- and central-acting respiratory stimulant since 1966. It is used in the treatment of acute respiratory failure, postoperative respiratory depression, and neonatal apnea. It is available as an IV injection (20 mg/ml) that also contains 0.9% benzyl alcohol. Acute overdose may result in tachycardia, hypertension, seizures, hyperventilation, tremor, and involuntary muscle movements. Treatment of overdose is similar to that for amphetamines.

Toxic Dose

The *adult therapeutic dose* is provided in Table 1. The *toxic dose* is not well established. A 7 mg/kg infusion resulted in extreme agitation in an adult (13).

Toxicokinetics and Toxicodynamics

The onset of action is less than 1 minute after IV administration, with duration of effect lasting 5 to 15 minutes. Doxapram is metabolized in the liver. The major metabolite is 2-ketodoxapram. Approximately 1% of an IV dose is excreted unchanged in a 24-hour urine. The V_d is 1.5 L/kg. The elimination half-life is 6 to 9 hours after IV administration.

Pathophysiology

Doxapram stimulates carotid chemoreceptors and central respiratory centers. It causes increased cardiac output that may increase blood pressure. It may also increase catecholamine release.

Pregnancy and Lactation

Doxapram is FDA pregnancy category B (Appendix I). There are no data in humans on its effects during pregnancy or with breast-feeding.

Clinical Presentation

Overdose experience with doxapram is limited. Based on similar agents, acute overdose may result in tachycardia, hypertension, seizures, hyperventilation, tremor, and involuntary muscle movements.

ADVERSE REACTIONS

Cough, bronchospasm, laryngospasm, hyperventilation, muscle fasciculation, spasticity, headache, dizziness, hyperactivity, confusion, hypertension, and seizures may occur. Extravasation of doxapram IV infusion may cause thrombophlebitis. Cardiovascular adverse effects include chest pain, palpitations, hypertension, and tachycardia.

DRUG INTERACTIONS

Concurrent administration of monoamine oxidase inhibitors or vasopressor could result in additive vasopressor effects. Cardiac dysrhythmias may occur if administered with anesthetics that sensitize the heart such as halothane, enflurane, and isoflurane.

Diagnostic Tests

Toxic effects usually occur when plasma concentrations of doxapram and metabolite reach 9 mg/L (14). An infusion of 7 mg/kg over 2 hours resulted in plasma concentrations of 2.7 to 5.2 mg/L (13).

Treatment

Treatment of overdose is similar to that for amphetamines (Chapter 174). Continuous cardiac monitoring and supplemental oxygen should be provided. Benzodiazepines are the drug of choice for agitation, muscle hypertonicity, seizures, tachycardia, and hypertension. Due to its short duration of action, enhancement of elimination is not expected to be beneficial. There are no specific antidotes.

FENFLURAMINE

Fenfluramine (Ponderax, Pondimin) and its dextro-isomer dexfenfluramine (Redux) were developed in the 1960s as appetite suppressants. They were withdrawn from the world market in 1997 due to concerns of potential cardiac valve toxicity and pulmonary hypertension. Fenfluramine is a substituted phenylethylamine structurally related to amphetamine. Unlike amphetamine, it causes CNS depression at therapeutic doses. Both agents are serotonin receptor agonists. Acute overdose may be rapidly fatal. Chronic administration has caused primary pulmonary hypertension and aortic and mitral valve disease. The treatment of overdose is primarily supportive. Patients manifesting signs of serotonin syndrome may benefit from a serotonin antagonist.

Toxic Dose

The *adult therapeutic dose* is provided in Table 1. The *toxic dose* is not well defined. Ingestion of greater than 15 mg/kg may result in coma and seizures (15). A 2.5-year-old child ingested 440 mg of fenfluramine and developed agitation and tachycardia and survived (16). A 17-year-old girl ingested 1600 mg of fenfluramine and developed cardiac dysrhythmias, seizures, and cardiac arrest within 3 hours and died (17). Ten patients experienced cardiac arrest within 4 hours of ingesting doses of 28.7 to 70 mg/kg (15). A fenfluramine dose of more than 30 mg/day for several months was associated with increased risk for valvular heart disease (18).

Toxicokinetics and Toxicodynamics

Fenfluramine is widely distributed into tissues with a V_d of 12 to 16 L/kg. It is metabolized in the liver by *N*-dealkylation to the active metabolite norfenfluramine. Less than 15% of a therapeutic dose is excreted as parent compound or active metabolite; the remainder is nonactive benzoic acid and alcohol derivatives. Excretion of the parent compound is enhanced in acidic urine. The half-life of fenfluramine is 13 to 30 hours and is urine pH dependent.

Dexfenfluramine undergoes biotransformation similar to fenfluramine producing the active metabolite nordexfenfluramine, which is also a serotonin receptor agonist. It has an elimination half-life of approximately 32 hours.

Pathophysiology

Fenfluramine is an indirect-acting sympathomimetic agent. Dexfenfluramine is believed to have little sympathomimetic activity at therapeutic doses. They usually depress rather than stimulate the CNS at therapeutic doses. Both agents are serotonin receptor agonists. They stimulate the release of serotonin and inhibit its reuptake resulting in increased CNS serotonin concentrations. The valvular lesions associated with its use are thought to be due to excess serotonin concentrations. Serotonin receptors (5-HT_{2B}) are located on mitral and aortic valves. Serotonin stimulates fibroblast growth and is thought to accelerate valve fibrosis (19).

Pregnancy and Lactation

Fenfluramine is FDA pregnancy category C (Appendix I). Six congenital malformations associated with the use of fenfluramine during pregnancy have been reported. In one study, 30 women took fenfluramine during the third trimester without adverse effects on the fetus (20). There are no reports of fenfluramine and breast-feeding but it is probably excreted into breast milk because of its low molecular weight. The use of fenfluramine is contraindicated during pregnancy and breast-feeding.

Clinical Presentation

ACUTE OVERDOSAGE

Symptoms typically begin within 60 minutes and may last several days. Acute overdose can be rapidly fatal, occurring within 1 to 4 hours after exposure (15,17). Manifestations include mydriasis, tachycardia, flushing, diaphoresis, hyperthermia, tremors, hypertonia, trismus, hyperreflexia, ankle clonus, agitation, coma, and seizures.

A 23-year-old woman ingested 1800 mg of dexfenfluramine and presented with a blood pressure of 160/88 mm Hg, pulse 162 beats/minute, respiratory rate less than 6/minute, and rectal temperature of 38.4°C. Clonus, muscle fasciculations, hyperreflexia, and muscle stiffness developed in the lower extremities only. Her urine screen was positive for stimulant amines. Creatine kinase peaked at 1122 U/L. She recovered in 48 hours with supportive care (21). Large overdoses of dexfenfluramine can produce a hyperadrenergic state and serotonin syndrome (Chapter 24).

ADVERSE REACTIONS

Chronic use of fenfluramine has been associated with primary pulmonary hypertension and valvular heart defects. The development of pulmonary hypertension was associated with prolonged (more than 3 months) or repeated therapy and may be irreversible. There is a 23-fold increased risk of pulmonary hypertension after treatment with dexfenfluramine for more than 3 months (22). It has resulted in death (23).

A 29-year-old woman took a combination of fenfluramine, 10 mg three times daily, and phentermine, 15 mg daily for 23 days, for obesity. Five months after cessation of therapy she developed shortness of breath, pedal edema, and syncope. A cardiac catheterization showed severe pulmonary hypertension and elevated pulmonary vascular resistance. Pulmonary angiography, liver function tests, abdominal ultrasonography, and antinuclear antibodies ruled out other causes of pulmonary hypertension. She died suddenly 6 weeks later. Histopathology revealed a plexiform arteriopathy of the pulmonary arteries. All other organs were normal. This anatomical finding was also present in European patients who had taken the appetite suppressant aminorex in the 1960s and 1970s (23).

Aortic and mitral valvular heart disease has also been associated with chronic use (24). As of February 1997, the FDA had received 144 reports of valvular disease associated with the use of fenfluramine or dexfenfluramine. All patients who received fenfluramine were advised to be screened with echocardiography for valvular heart disease. Aortic regurgitation occurred more commonly than mitral regurgitation (25). The valvular lesions tend not to progress over time in patients who use the drug for a short period of time (26).

Emotional instability, cognitive deficits, and depression were reported in 27 patients taking fenfluramine and dexfenfluramine chronically (27). Psychosis has been reported after use of dexfenfluramine for 2 months (28). Headache, diarrhea, dizziness, dry mouth, impotence, palpitations, anxiety, insomnia, irritability, lethargy, and CNS excitation at higher doses have been reported with therapeutic use.

DRUG INTERACTIONS

Administration of fenfluramine or dexfenfluramine with drugs that increase serotonin levels (e.g., antidepressants, monoamine oxidase inhibitors, and migraine medications) may precipitate serotonin syndrome (Chapter 24).

Diagnostic Tests

ACUTE OVERDOSAGE

An oral dose of 60 mg fenfluramine results in a peak plasma level of 0.05 to 0.07 mg/L and a T_{max} of 3 hours (29). A 30-mg oral dose of dexfenfluramine produced an average plasma concentration of 0.027 mg/L at 3 hours after ingestion (30). An overdose of fenfluramine, 440 mg, in a 2.5-year-old child resulted in plasma concentrations of 0.78 mg/L fenfluramine and 0.17 mg/L norfenfluramine (16).

Acute overdose patients should have an electrocardiogram (ECG) performed to assess cardiac rhythm. A serum creatine kinase and creatinine should be obtained on patients with muscle rigidity to evaluate for rhabdomyolysis and possible renal injury.

ADVERSE EVENTS

Patients who take the drug chronically and develop shortness of breath, chest pain, or syncopal episodes should be referred to a cardiologist and undergo echocardiography and possibly other tests to evaluate for valvular heart disease and primary pulmonary hypertension.

POSTMORTEM CONSIDERATIONS

Postmortem blood concentrations in one adult and three children ranged from 6.5 to 16 mg/L (31). A fenfluramine hair level of 14.1 ng/mg was demonstrated in an overdose fatality (32).

Treatment

Acute overdose can be rapidly fatal. The treatment is primarily supportive. All patients should have an adequate airway established, IV access, and cardiac monitoring.

DECONTAMINATION

Induction of emesis is contraindicated due to the rapid onset of symptoms and possible loss of airway control. A single dose of activated charcoal should be administered if the patient presents within a couple of hours of exposure. Whole bowel irrigation may be of benefit for ingestion of sustained release tablets although its efficacy has not been studied.

ENHANCEMENT OF ELIMINATION

There are no data on the use of elimination enhancement for fenfluramine overdose. Due to its large volume of distribution, these techniques are not expected to be of clinical benefit.

ANTIDOTES

Cyproheptadine, a serotonin receptor antagonist, has been recommended as adjunct therapy for severe serotonin syndrome (Chapter 24). Experience is only anecdotal. The initial dose is 4 to 16 mg orally and repeated every 2 to 4 hours as needed up to 0.5 mg/kg/day.

SUPPORTIVE CARE

Benzodiazepines are indicated for muscle rigidity, seizure activity, or agitation (diazepam, initial dose 5 to 10 mg IV). Hypotension should be managed with IV crystalloid fluid bolus (normal saline, 10 to 20 ml/kg) followed by vasopressors as needed.

MONITORING

Acute overdoses should be observed for symptoms for at least 6 hours. There are no reports of delayed toxicity if patients are asymptomatic after this observation period.

MAZINDOL

Mazindol (Sanorex, Teronac, Diestet) is an isoindole anorectic agent used as adjunctive therapy for obesity. Its toxic effects are similar to dexamphetamine, resulting in CNS stimulation. Blood concentrations are not helpful in managing toxicity. The treatment is the same as for amphetamines.

Toxic Dose

The *adult therapeutic dose* is provided in Table 1. The *toxic dose* is not well defined. A 25-year-old woman died after ingesting 200 mg of mazindol and an unknown amount of alcohol (33). A 20-

year-old woman who ingested 80 mg of mazindol and 9375 mg phenmetrazine developed frequent premature ventricular contractions, and survived. Children aged 1 to 4 years have ingested from 4 to 40 mg and survived (33).

Toxicokinetics and Toxicodynamics

Mazindol is slowly absorbed from the gastrointestinal tract with a T_{max} of 2 hours after a therapeutic dose. It is conjugated in the liver, and 40% to 60% of a dose is recovered in the urine. The elimination half-life is 30 to 50 hours.

Pathophysiology

Mazindol is a CNS stimulant with action similar to dexamphetamine. It inhibits the reuptake of dopamine and norepinephrine.

Pregnancy and Lactation

Mazindol is FDA pregnancy category C (Appendix I). In animals an increase in neonatal mortality has been observed. There are no data available on risk to the fetus or for breast-feeding.

Clinical Presentation

ACUTE OVERDOSAGE

The toxic effects are similar to amphetamines but tend to be less severe. The following symptoms have been observed after overdose: agitation, irritability, hyperactivity, tachycardia, tachypnea, and premature ventricular contractions.

ADVERSE EVENTS

Most common adverse effects are dry mouth, tachycardia, constipation, nervousness, and insomnia. Testicular pain was reported as an adverse effect in eight men. Psychosis has been rarely associated with chronic use.

DRUG INTERACTIONS

Lithium toxicity has been associated with concurrent administration of mazindol (34). Hypertensive crisis may result with concomitant administration of mazindol and monoamine oxidase inhibitors.

Diagnostic Tests

Therapeutic serum concentrations have not been established. An ECG should be performed to assess cardiac ischemia or infarction after overdose.

Treatment

Treatment of overdose is similar to that for amphetamines (Chapter 174). Activated charcoal probably adsorbs mazindol but studies have not been conducted. Benzodiazepines are the drug of choice for agitation, muscle hypertonicity, seizures, tachycardia, and hypertension. Nitroprusside is indicated for hypertensive emergencies (Chapter 36). There is no experience with hemodialysis for elimination enhancement. The urine should not be acidified; this increases the risk of renal injury associated with rhabdomyolysis.

Monitoring

Mazindol has a long half-life (30 to 50 hours), and monitoring of blood pressure and cardiac rhythm may be required for several days in symptomatic patients after overdose.

MODAFINIL

Modafinil (Provigil, Modiodal, Alertec) is a CNS stimulant indicated for excessive daytime sleepiness associated with narcolepsy. There is limited clinical experience with overdose, but it appears to have a large therapeutic index. Up to a tenfold overdose has resulted in non–life-threatening toxicity. Management is supportive. There is no specific antidote.

Toxic Dose

The *adult therapeutic dose* is provided in Table 1. The *toxic dose* is not well defined. A dose of 800 mg/day for 3 days resulted in tachycardia and elevated blood pressure (35). Intentional ingestion of 4000 mg and 4500 mg by two patients resulted in non–life-threatening symptoms that resolved within 24 hours (36).

Toxicokinetics and Toxicodynamics

The T_{max} is 2 to 3 hours after ingestion. Modafinil has a V_d of 0.9 L/kg and is 60% protein bound. It undergoes hepatic metabolism via CYP3A3/4 to inactive metabolites. It has an elimination half-life of approximately 10 to 15 hours. Urine acidification does not enhance elimination.

Pathophysiology

The exact mechanism of action is unclear. Its stimulant effects may result from decreased GABA-mediated neurotransmission. It binds to the dopamine reuptake site and causes an increase in extracellular dopamine but no increase in dopamine release. It does not appear to enhance the release of norepinephrine.

Pregnancy and Lactation

Modafinil is FDA pregnancy category C (Appendix I). There are no human studies evaluating teratogenicity. Several normal births have occurred in patients who have received modafinil during pregnancy. It is not known whether modafinil or its metabolites are excreted in breast milk.

Clinical Presentation

ACUTE OVERDOSAGE

Overdose experience is limited. Signs and symptoms generally consist of mild CNS stimulation and include agitation, insomnia, tremor, confusion, palpitations, tachycardia, and hypertension. There have been no fatalities reported as a result of overdose.

ADVERSE EVENTS

The most common reactions include diarrhea (8%), nausea (13%), anorexia, xerostomia (5%), nervousness, dizziness, depression, anxiety, insomnia, paresthesia, and abnormal liver function tests (3%).

DRUG INTERACTIONS

Modafinil may increase serum levels of warfarin, diazepam, phenytoin, and propranolol. It may decrease levels of oral contraceptives and cyclosporine.

Diagnostic Tests

Serum concentrations of modafinil are not readily available and do not guide management.

Treatment

Experience with modafinil overdose and its treatment are limited. Patients should receive cardiac and oxygen saturation monitoring until evidence of clinical effects (i.e., tachycardia, tachypnea) resolve. Administration of activated charcoal soon after oral overdose will probably decrease drug absorption from the gut, although there are no studies to confirm this effect. Benzodiazepines should be administered for agitation or combativeness (e.g., diazepam 5 mg IV). Patients who remain symptomatic after 4 to 6 hours of observation should be admitted to the hospital for continued monitoring of vital signs. There is no specific antidote.

PHENMETRAZINE

Phendimetrazine (Bontril, Plegine, Prelu-2, Statobex) is a phenethylamine derivative with a morpholine ring. It is a sympathomimetic amine and used as an anorectic agent. Phenmetrazine (Preludin) is the active metabolite and also available as an anorectic agent. Manifestations of overdose are similar to those of other drugs in the sympathomimetic class.

Toxic Dose

The usual *adult therapeutic doses* of phendimetrazine and phenmetrazine are provided in Table 1.

Toxicokinetics and Toxicodynamics

Phendimetrazine is metabolized in the liver by *N*-demethylation to the active metabolite phenmetrazine. Phenmetrazine is hydroxylated, conjugated, and excreted in the urine. The elimination half-life of phendimetrazine is approximately 9 hours for the sustained release and 2 hours for the regular release preparation. The half-life of phenmetrazine is approximately 8 hours. Excretion is enhanced in acidic urine.

Pathophysiology

It has sympathomimetic actions similar to other drugs in its class (amphetamine).

Pregnancy and Lactation

Phendimetrazine is FDA pregnancy category C (Appendix I). Entry into breast milk is unknown.

Clinical Presentation

ACUTE OVERDOSAGE

Manifestations of overdose are similar to those of other drugs in the sympathomimetic class. Clinical effects include tremor, fever, tachycardia, hypertension, altered mental status, confusion, seizures, hallucinations, dysrhythmias, cardiovascular collapse, and death.

ADVERSE REACTIONS

Reported adverse effects include palpitations, hypertension, tachycardia, restlessness, dizziness, insomnia, tremor, headache, dry mouth, diarrhea, and nausea. Abrupt cessation after prolonged administration of high doses may result in fatigue and depression.

DRUG INTERACTIONS

Use of phendimetrazine within 2 weeks of taking a monoamine oxidase inhibitor may result in a hypertensive crisis.

Diagnostic Tests

Phenmetrazine has been reported to cross-react with immunoassays designed for amphetamines. The average blood concentration after a 75-mg dose of phenmetrazine was 0.13 mg/L (range, 0.00 to 0.24 mg/L). The average phenmetrazine blood concentration in *drug abusers* arrested while driving was 0.5 to 4.0 mg/L. An oral dose of phendimetrazine, 35 mg, produced serum concentrations of 0.09 mg/L 1 hour after ingestion (37).

Postmortem Considerations

Fatalities from phendimetrazine have been associated with blood levels of 0.1 to 4.9 mg/L (37,38).

Treatment

Experience with phenmetrazine overdose and its treatment are limited. Patients should receive cardiac and oxygen saturation monitoring until evidence of clinical effects resolve. Administration of activated charcoal soon after oral overdose probably decreases drug absorption from the gut. Benzodiazepines should be administered for agitation or combativeness (e.g., diazepam, 5 mg IV). Patients who remain symptomatic after 4 to 6 hours of observation should be admitted to the hospital for continued monitoring of vital signs. There is no specific antidote.

PHENTERMINE

Phentermine (Fastin, Adipex-P, Ionamin, others) is the alpha-methyl derivative of amphetamine and is used as an anorectic agent. It has been prescribed in combination with fenfluramine (*fen-phen*) as a treatment for obesity. This combination has been associated with an increased incidence of valvular heart disease (39).

Toxic Dose

The *adult therapeutic dose* is provided in Table 1.

Toxicokinetics and Toxicodynamics

The V_d is 3 to 4 L/kg and the half-life is approximately 20 hours. A majority of the drug is excreted unchanged in the urine. An average of 48% of the dose is excreted in the urine in 24 hours, which increases to 84% in acidic urine.

Pregnancy and Lactation

Phentermine is FDA pregnancy category C (Appendix I). Entry into breast milk is unknown.

Clinical Presentation

Manifestations of overdose and its treatment are similar to amphetamines.

Diagnostic Tests

POSTMORTEM CONSIDERATIONS

Fatalities associated with phentermine overdose have reported postmortem blood concentrations of 1.5 to 7.6 mg/L. It may demonstrate postmortem redistribution with a heart to femoral blood concentration ratio of 1.7 (40).

Treatment

Experience with phentermine overdose and its treatment are limited. Patients should receive cardiac and respiratory monitoring until evidence of clinical effects resolves. Administration of activated charcoal soon after oral overdose probably decreases drug absorption from the gut. Benzodiazepines should be administered for agitation or combativeness. Patients who remain symptomatic after 4 to 6 hours of observation should be admitted to the hospital for continued monitoring of vital signs. There is no specific antidote.

PEMOLINE

Pemoline (Phenoxazole, phenylisohydantoin, Cylert, Dynalert, others) is an oxazolidine derivative that is structurally different from amphetamines. It is a CNS stimulant used principally in children with attention deficit disorder and in adults with memory deficit or narcolepsy. It has been withdrawn for the treatment of hyperactivity in the United Kingdom because of liver toxicity.

Toxic Dose

The initial *adult therapeutic dose* is provided in Table 1. The *toxic dose* is not well defined. Acute ingestion of 200 mg (41) and 1125 to 1350 mg (42) by adults has resulted in choreiform movements and rhabdomyolysis.

Toxicokinetics and Toxicodynamics

Pemoline is readily adsorbed from the gastrointestinal tract with peak effect occurring 4 hours after ingestion. It is approximately 50% protein bound. It is partially metabolized in the liver and excreted in the urine as unchanged pemoline and metabolites. The V_d is 0.2 to 0.6 L/kg. The elimination half-life is 7 to 9 hours in children and 11 to 12 hours in adults.

Pathophysiology

Pemoline inhibits reuptake of catecholamines in the CNS resulting in increased concentrations of norepinephrine, epinephrine, and dopamine. An increased dopaminergic tone may result in choreoathetoid movements (43).

Pregnancy and Lactation

Pemoline is FDA pregnancy category B (Appendix I). There are no reports of the use of pemoline during pregnancy. High doses were associated with stillbirth in rats (44).

Clinical Presentation

ACUTE OVERDOSAGE

Pemoline overdose may produce hyperadrenergic effects including agitation, sinus tachycardia, hypertension, hyperpyrexia, mydriasis, and seizures. Acute choreoathetoid movements (43) and hallucinations have also been reported after overdose. In children, choreoathetosis may be the predominant effect and difficult to control (43). These movements may last up to 24 hours despite treatment with benzodiazepines. Elevated creatine kinase indicating rhabdomyolysis may occur secondary to muscle hypertonicity or seizure activity. The onset of symptoms is usually within 6 hours and may last for 48 hours (45).

Twin 3-year-old boys ingested an unknown amount of pemoline and were diaphoretic, agitated, tachypneic (respiratory rate, 24 to 28 per minute), tachycardic (heart rate 120 to 145 beats/minute), and hyperpyrexic (38° to 39°C) within 30 minutes. Both patients had mydriasis and developed persistent choreoathetoid movements. They were treated with activated charcoal and IV benzodiazepines. The abnormal movements continued for 24 hours despite treatment. They recovered in 48 hours (43).

ADVERSE REACTIONS

Chronic use has induced adverse effects such as addiction, paranoid psychosis, choreoathetosis, and precipitation of Gilles de la Tourette's syndrome. It may precipitate psychosis and has a potential for drug abuse and dependency (46).

Pemoline may be associated with abnormal involuntary movements after treatment with 1.5 to 2 mg/kg/day for 3 weeks to 3 months (47–49). Acute abnormal involuntary movements occurred in 5 of 20 children given a single dose of 2 mg/kg (47).

Hepatotoxicity, which may be fatal, has occurred. Reversible elevations of serum aminotransferases have been reported in 2% of children taking pemoline for hyperactivity. Some believe that the risk of hepatotoxicity has been over estimated (50). It usually occurs at least 6 months after the initiation of therapy but may occur sooner. Manifestations range from asymptomatic elevation of hepatic transaminases to fulminant liver failure. Some patients present with a viral-like prodrome and dark urine. Liver transplantation has been performed as a result of this adverse reaction and some patients have died (51,52).

Other adverse effects that may be observed are insomnia, dizziness, irritability, seizures, hallucinations, headache, anorexia, weight loss, and abdominal pain.

DRUG INTERACTIONS

Hypertensive crisis may result if taken concurrently with monoamine oxidase inhibitors.

Diagnostic Tests

The plasma concentration after therapeutic doses ranges from 1 to 6 µg/ml (53). Due to the increased risk of hepatotoxicity, liver function tests (aspartate aminotransferase and alanine aminotransferase) should be evaluated after acute overdose or chronic overmedication.

Treatment

Treatment of overdose is similar to that for other CNS stimulants. The patient should have IV access established along with frequent monitoring of vital signs and oxygen saturation.

DECONTAMINATION

Activated charcoal should be administered to patients with recent ingestions and a protected airway.

ENHANCEMENT OF ELIMINATION

Although there is no published experience, the low protein binding and small volume of distribution of pemoline suggest that its elimination may be enhanced by hemodialysis. Acidification of the urine is not recommended to enhance elimination of the parent compound because of increased risk of renal injury from rhabdomyolysis.

ANTIDOTES

There is no specific antidote or antagonist agent for pemoline toxicity.

SUPPORTIVE CARE

Seizure precautions should be observed. A benzodiazepine (diazepam or lorazepam) is the drug of choice for treatment of agitation, tachycardia, hypertension, involuntary movements, or seizures (Chapter 40). Aggressive cooling measures should be undertaken for hyperpyrexia. Hypertensive crisis not responding to benzodiazepines may be treated with sodium nitroprusside.

MONITORING

Monitoring of liver function tests should occur every 2 weeks during treatment with pemoline.

SIBUTRAMINE

Sibutramine (Meridia) is an anorectic agent used in the treatment of obesity. It blocks the reuptake of norepinephrine, serotonin, and dopamine. Unlike fenfluramine, it does not cause the release of serotonin from neurons and has not been associated with valvular heart disease. Experience with overdose is limited. Tachycardia, dizziness, and hypertension have been the main clinical manifestations (54). Treatment is supportive.

Toxic Dose

The *adult therapeutic dose* is provided in Table 1. The *toxic dose* is not well defined. An adult ingested 400 mg and developed sinus tachycardia only. A 2-year-old child ingested 80 mg and remained asymptomatic (55).

Toxicokinetics and Toxicodynamics

Sibutramine is well absorbed orally with a T_{max} of 1 to 2 hours. It is metabolized in the liver by the cytochrome P-450 isoenzyme CYP3A4. It is demethylated to the active metabolites mono- and di-desmethylsibutraimine. These are hydroxylated, conjugated, and excreted in the urine. Protein binding is 97% and the elimination half-life is 14 to 16 hours.

Pathophysiology

Sibutramine and metabolites inhibit the reuptake of serotonin, norepinephrine, and dopamine. It does not stimulate release of neurotransmitters.

Pregnancy and Lactation

Sibutramine is FDA pregnancy category C (Appendix I). There are no published reports of use during pregnancy or data on excretion in breast milk.

Clinical Presentation

ACUTE OVERDOSAGE

The experience with overdose of sibutramine is limited. Two patients reportedly ingested between 80 to 100 mg and remained asymptomatic. A third patient ingested 400 mg and developed sinus tachycardia only (pulse, 120/minute) (55). Eight adults ingested a median dose of 30 mg and developed tachycardia, dizziness, and hypertension (54).

ADVERSE REACTIONS

Sibutramine may be associated with dry mouth, headache, insomnia, constipation, dizziness, tachycardia, elevated serum aminotransferase levels, mydriasis, and hypertension.

DRUG INTERACTIONS

There is a risk of serotonin syndrome if sibutramine is taken concurrently with selective serotonin reuptake inhibitors, sumatriptan, lithium, dextromethorphan, or within 2 weeks of stopping therapy with monoamine oxidase inhibitors.

Diagnostic Tests

Blood concentrations are not readily available and do not guide management. An ECG should be performed on patients with significant overdose to evaluate for dysrhythmias and cardiac ischemia.

Treatment

Experience with sibutramine overdose and its treatment are limited. Patients should receive cardiac and oxygen saturation monitoring until evidence of clinical effects (i.e., tachycardia) resolve. Administration of activated charcoal soon after oral overdose probably decreases drug absorption. Benzodiazepines should be administered for agitation or combativeness (e.g., diazepam, 5 mg IV). Patients who remain symptomatic after 4 to 6 hours of observation should be admitted to the hospital for continued monitoring of vital signs. There are no specific antidotes.

The blood pressure should be monitored for hypertension, the temperature for hyperthermia, and an ECG for tachycardia.

REFERENCES

1. Bardsley PA, Tweney J, Morgan N, et al. Oral almitrine in treatment of acute respiratory failure and cor pulmonale in patients with an exacerbation of chronic obstructive airway disease. *Thorax* 1991;46:493–498.
2. Howard P. Hypoxia, almitrine and peripheral neuropathy. *Thorax* 1989;44:247–250.
3. Voisin C, Howard P, Ansquard C. Almitrine bimesylate: a long-term placebo controlled double-blind study in COAD-Vectarian International Multicentre Study Group. *Bull Eur Physiopathol Respir* 1987;23[Suppl. 11]:1695–1825.
4. Gherardi R, Baudrimont M, Gray F, et al. Almitrine neuropathy. A nerve biopsy study of 8 cases. *Acta Neuropathol (Berl)* 1987;73(2):202–8.
5. Gherardi R, Belec L, Louarn F. Almitrine-induced peripheral neuropathy and weight loss. *J Neurol* 1989;236:374.
6. Tweney J. Almitrine bismesylate: current status. *Bull Eur Physiopathol Respir* 1987;23[Suppl. 1]:156–163.
7. Gherardi R, Louarn F, Benvenuti C, et al. Peripheral neuropathy in patients treated with almitrine dimesylate. *Lancet* 1985;1(8440):1247–50.
8. Bouche P, Lacomblez L, Leger JM, et al. Peripheral neuropathies during treatment with almitrine: report of 46 cases. *J Neurol* 1989;236:29–33.
9. Allen MB, Prowse K. Peripheral nerve function in patients with chronic bronchitis receiving almitrine or placebo. *Thorax* 1989;44:292–7.
10. B'Chir A, Mebazaa A, Losser MR, et al. Intravenous almitrine bismesylate reversibly induces lactic acidosis and hepatic dysfunction in patients with acute lung injury. *Anesthesiology* 1998;89(4):823–830.
11. Vidon N, Chaussade S, Jeanniot P, et al. Almitrine bismesylate disposition in the human digestive tract. *Eur J Clin Pharmacol* 1989;37:487–491.
12. Bromet N, Singlas E. Pharmacokinetique clinique de bismesylate d'almitrine. *Presse Med* 1984;13:2071–2077.
13. Baselt RC. *Disposition of toxic drugs and chemicals in man*, 6th ed. Foster City, CA: Chemical Toxicology Institute, 2002:363–4.
14. Barbe F, Hanse C, Badonnel Y, et al. Severe side effects and drug plasma concentration in preterm infants treated with doxapram. *Ther Drug Mon* 1999;21:547–552.
15. Von Muhlendahl KE, Krienke EG. Fenfluramine poisoning. *J Toxicol Clin Toxicol* 1979;14:97–106.
16. Campbell DB, Moore BWR. Fenfluramine overdosage. *Lancet* 1969;2:1306.
17. Veltri JC, Temple AR. Fenfluramine poisoning. *J Pediatr* 1975;87:119–21.
18. Graham DJ, Green L. Further cases of valvular heart disease associated with fenfluramine-phentermine. *N Engl J Med* 1997;337:635.
19. Fitzgerald LW, Burn TC, Brown BS, et al. Possible role of valvular serotonin 5-HT(2B) receptors in the cardiopathy associated with fenfluramine. *Mol Pharmacol* 2000;57:75–81.
20. Briggs GG, Freeman RK, Yaffe SJ. *Drugs in pregnancy and lactation*, 6th ed. Baltimore, MD: Williams and Wilkins, 2002:540–541.
21. LoVecchio F, Curry SC. Dexfenfluraimine overdose. *Ann Emerg Med* 1998;32:102–103.
22. Abenhaim L, Moride Y, Brenot F, et al. Appetite-suppressant drugs and the risk of primary pulmonary hypertension. International Primary Pulmonary Hypertension Study Group. *N Engl J Med* 1996;335(9):609–16.

23. Mark EJ, Patalas ED, Chang HT, et al. Fatal pulmonary hypertension associated with short-term use of fenfluramine and phentermine. *N Engl J Med* 1997;337:602–6.
24. Anonymous. Cardiac valvulopathy associated with exposure to fenfluramine or dexfenfluramine: U.S. Department of Health and Human Services interim public health recommendations, November 1997. *MMWR Morb Mortal Wkly Rep* 1997;46:1061–6.
25. Weissman NJ, Tighe JF Jr, Gottdiener JS, et al. An assessment of heart-valve abnormalities in obese patients taking dexfenfluramine, sustained-release dexfenfluramine, or placebo. Sustained-release Dexfenfluramine Study Group. *N Engl J Med* 1998;339:725–32.
26. Weissman NJ, Tighe JF Jr, Gottdiener JS, et al. Prevalence of valvular-regurgitation associated with dexfenfluramine three to five months after discontinuation of treatment. *J Am Coll Cardiol* 1999;34:2088–95.
27. McCann UD, Eligulashvili V, Ricaurte GA. Adverse neuropsychiatric events associated with dexfenfluramine and fenfluramine. *Prof Neruo-Psychopharm Biol Psych* 1998;22:1087–1102.
28. Preval H, Pakyurik AM. Psychotic episode associated with dexfenfluramine. *Am J Psychiatry* 1997;154:1624–1625.
29. Campbell DB. Gas chromatographic measurement of levels of fenfluramine and norfenfluramine in human plasma, red cells and urine following therapeutic doses. *J Chrom* 1970;49:442–447.
30. Cheymol G, Weissenburger J, Poirier JM, et al. The pharmacokinetics of dexfenfluramine in obese and non-obese subjects. *Brit J Clin Pharm* 1995;39:684–687.
31. Baselt RC. *Disposition of toxic drugs and chemicals in man*, 6th ed. Foster City, CA: Chemical Toxicology Institute, 2002:423–424.
32. Kintz P, Mangin P. Toxicological findings after fatal fenfluramine self-poisoning. *Hum Exp Toxicol* 1992;11:51–2.
33. Anonymous. Maxindol. In: *Mosby's GenRx*, 9th ed. St. Louis: Mosby, 1999:1378–1379.
34. Hendy MS, Dove AF, Arblaster PG. Mazindol-induced lithium toxicity. *BMJ* 1980;280(6215):684–5.
35. Wong YN, Simcoe D, Hartman LN, et al. A double-blind, placebo-controlled, ascending-dose evaluation of the pharmacokinetics and tolerability of modafinil tablets in healthy male volunteers. *J Clin Pharmacol* 1999;39:30–40.
36. Anonymous. Modafinil. In: *Drug facts and comparisons*. St. Louis: Wolters Kluser Health, Inc., 2003:766–769.
37. Baselt RC. *Disposition of toxic drugs and chemicals in man*, 6th ed. Foster City, CA: Chemical Toxicology Institute, 2002:838–839.
38. Hood I, Monforte J, Gault R, et al. Fatality from illicit phendimetrazine use. *J Toxicol Clin Toxicol* 1988;26:249–255.
39. Connolly HM, Crary JL, McGoon MD, et al. Valvular heart disease associated with fenfluramine-phentermine. *N Engl J Med* 1997;337:581–588.
40. Baselt RC. *Disposition of toxic drugs and chemicals in man*, 6th ed. Foster City, CA: Chemical Toxicology Institute, 2002:846–847.
41. Bonthala CM, West A. Pemoline induced chorea and Gilles de la Tourette's syndrome. *Br J Psychiatry* 1983;143:300–302.
42. Briscoe JG, Curry SC, Gerkin RD, et al. Pemoline-induced choreoathetosis and rhabdomyolysis. *Med Toxicol* 1988;3:72–76.
43. Stork CM, Cnator R. Pemoline induced acute choreoathetosis: case report and review of the literature. *J Toxicol Clin Toxicol* 1997;35:105–108.
44. Briggs GG, Freeman RK, Yaffe SJ. *Drugs in pregnancy and lactation*, 6th ed. Baltimore, MD: Williams and Wilkins, 2002:1074–5.
45. Nakamura H, Blumer JL, Reed MD. Pemoline ingestion in children: a report of five cases and review of the literature. *J Clin Pharmacol* 2002;42(3):275–82.
46. Polchert SE, Morse RM. Pemoline abuse. *JAMA* 1985;254:946–947.
47. Sallee FR, Stiller RL, Perel JM, et al. Pemoline-induced abnormal involuntary movements. *J Clin Psychopharmacol* 1989;9:125–129.
48. Merrian AE. Pemoline-induced abnormal involuntary movement. *J Clin Psychopharmacol* 1990;10:302–303.
49. Singh BK, Singh A, Chusid E. Chorea in long-term use of pemoline. *Ann Neurol* 1983;13:218.
50. Shevell M, Schreiber R. Pemoline-associated hepatic failure: a critical analysis of the literature. *Pediatr Neurol* 1997;16:14–6.
51. Marotta PJ, Roberts EA. Pemoline hepatotoxicity in children. *J Pediatr* 1998;132:894–7.
52. Adcock KG, MacElroy DE, Wolford ET, et al. Pemoline therapy resulting in liver transplantation. *Ann Pharmacother* 1998;32:422–5.
53. Baselt RC. *Disposition of toxic drugs and chemicals in man*, 6th ed. Foster City, CA: Chemical Toxicology Institute, 2002:807–808.
54. Mrvos R, Cubberley V, Krenzelok EP. A toxicity profile of sibutramine (abst). *J Toxicol Clin Toxicol* 2000;38:521–522.
55. Anonymous. Sibutamine. In: *Drug facts and comparisons*. St. Louis: Wolters Kluser Health, Inc., 2003:780–3.

CHAPTER 139

Parkinson's Disease Drugs

Stefan P. Rosenbach and Erica L. Liebelt

HO, HO, O, OH, NH_2

LEVODOPA

Compounds included:	**See Table 1.**
Molecular formula and weight:	**See Table 2.**
SI conversion:	**See Table 2.**
CAS Registry No.:	**See Table 2.**
Therapeutic levels:	**Amantadine, 0.7 to 1.0 mg/ml (serum)**
Antidote:	**Physostigmine (amantadine)**

OVERVIEW

Parkinson's disease is a neurodegenerative disease that occurs in approximately 1% of adults over 65 years. Although the precise cause of parkinsonism remains unknown, its symptoms arise from a deficiency in the function of dopamine-secreting neurons in the basal ganglia. Functional activity of the basal ganglia is determined by the balance of dopamine-secreting (inhibitory) neurons and acetylcholine-secreting (excitatory) neurons. The clinical disease emerges when dopamine is depleted to approximately 20% of normal. Therapy is aimed at either resupplying deficient dopamine or blocking the unopposed acetylcholine system (1).

Levodopa is the cornerstone in the treatment of Parkinson's disease. Acting as a dopamine precursor, levodopa crosses the blood–brain barrier and is metabolized into the pharmacologically active dopamine. Drugs that inhibit the peripheral degradation of levodopa, catechol-O-methyltransferase (COMT) inhibitors, frequently supplement levodopa use. Although this combination remains the most effective drug in the treatment of Parkinson's disease, motor complications, dyskinesias, and hallucinations are problematic.

Dopamine receptor agonists exert their effect by stimulating postsynaptic dopamine receptors. Other drugs used in the treatment of parkinsonism include amantadine, which acts to stimulate dopamine release in the basal ganglia and potentiate the effects of levodopa. The final drug class, anticholinergic drugs, exert their effect by blocking the excitatory cholinergic neurons that persist in the basal ganglia (Table 2).

TABLE 1. Compounds included

Levodopa preparations
  Levodopa/carbidopa (Sinemet)
  Carbidopa (Lodosyn)
Catechol-O-methyltransferase inhibitors
  Entacapone (Comtan)
  Tolcapone (Tasmar)
Dopamine agonists
  Bromocriptine (Parlodel)
  Pergolide (Permax)
  Ropinirole (Requip)
  Pramipexole (Mirapex)
Anticholinergics
  Benztropine (Cogentin)
  Trihexyphenidyl (Artane, Tremin) (addressed in Chapter 100)
Other
  Amantadine (Symmetrel)
  Selegiline (Eldepryl)

LEVODOPA AND CATECHOL-O-METHYLTRANSFERASE INHIBITORS

Levodopa is well established as the most effective drug for the treatment of Parkinson's disease. Its therapeutic actions result from increasing dopamine levels in the brain, thus ameliorating the symptoms of the movement disorder. Frequently, levodopa is combined with a COMT inhibitor. These drugs augment the effects of levodopa by extending the duration of action. By combining levodopa and a COMT inhibitor, the effective dose of levodopa can be reduced by 75%, with a concomitant reduction in side effects (2). Examples of COMT inhibitors include carbidopa (Lodosyn), entacapone (Comtan), and tolcapone (Tasmar).

Treatment with levodopa is associated with potential motor and psychiatric complications. The motor effects consist of involuntary writhing movements of the limbs and trunk (choreoathetosis), painful cramps (dystonia), and shortened response time to levodopa (end-of-dose-deterioration). These symptoms affect 50% of patients after 6 years of therapy (3,4).

Levodopa-induced hallucinations and other psychotic manifestations occur in approximately one-third of patients treated with dopaminergic drugs. Although the specific pathogenesis of hallucinations is not certain, abnormalities of dopaminergic and serotonergic systems are likely to play a role.

Toxic Dose

The adult therapeutic dose of levodopa is provided in Table 2. Slow-release preparations of levodopa (Sinemet CR) prolong its half-life. Sinemet CR consists of a mixture of 200 mg levodopa and 50 mg carbidopa (Sinemet 50/200) or 100 mg levodopa and 25 mg carbidopa (Sinemet CR 25/100). Frequently, controlled-release preparations are combined with standard preparations to alleviate fluctuations in clinical symptoms (5). Tolcapone, 100 mg or 200 mg, is taken three times daily, and entacapone (200 mg) is usually taken with each dose of levodopa/carbidopa (6,7).

Insufficient data exist regarding toxicity associated with acute ingestion of levodopa-containing products. One case report describes tachycardia, confusion, and excessive motor activity after ingestion of 30 levodopa/carbidopa (200-mg/50-mg) tablets (8). Another case report describes initial hypertension followed by rapidly developing hypotension and tachycardia in a patient who acutely ingested 100 g (9). Other case reports describe the development of refractory choreiform movements and rhabdomyolysis subsequent to intentional ingestion of 15 levodopa/carbidopa (1500-mg/150-mg) tablets (10).

TABLE 2. Physical characteristics, formulation, and dose of drug used for the treatment of Parkinson's disease

Drug	Molecular formula, molecular weight (g/mol), CAS Registry No.	SI conversion	Formulation	Adult therapeutic dose
Levodopa preparations				
Levodopa	$C_9H_{11}NO_4$; 197.2; 59-92-7	NA	NR	500–1000 mg/d initially in divided doses; increased by 100–750 mg/d every 3–7 d until response or total dose of 8000 mg
Levodopa/carbidopa	$C_{10}H_{14}N_2O_4,H_2O$; 244.2; 38821-49-7	NA	10- to 100-mg, 25- to 100-mg, 25-, 250-mg tablets	1 tab orally 3 times daily; increased slowly to 8 tabs daily
COMT inhibitors				
Entacapone	$C_{14}H_{15}N_3O_5$; 305.3; 130929-57-6	μg/ml × 3.28 = μmol/L	200-mg tablet	200 mg orally with each dose of levodopa
Tolcapone	$C_{14}H_{11}NO_5$; 273.2; 134308-13-7	μg/ml × 3.66 = μmol/L	100-, 200-mg tablets	100–200 mg 3 times daily
Dopamine agonists				
Bromocriptine mesylate	$C_{32}H_{40}BrN_5O_5,CH_4O_3S$; 750.7; 22260-51-1	ng/ml × 1.53 = nmol/L	5-, 10-mg capsules; 2.5-mg tablets	30–75 mg/d up to 300 mg/d has been used
Pergolide mesylate	$C_{19}H_{26}N_2S,CH_4O_3S$; 410.6; 66104-23-2	ng/ml × 3.18 = nmol/L	0.5-, 0.25-, 1-mg tablets	0.05 mg/d, increased slowly over weeks
Ropinirole hydrochloride	$C_{16}H_{24}N_2O,HCl$; 296.8; 91374-20-8	ng/ml × 3.84 = nmol/L	0.25-, 0.5-, 1-, 2-, 4-, 5-mg tabs	0.25 mg 3 times daily, increased weekly to reach a dose of 1 mg 3 times daily
Pramipexole	$C_{10}H_{17}N_3S,2HCl$; H_2O; 302.3; 191217-81-9	ng/ml × 4.73 = nmol/L	0.125-, 0.25-, 0.5-1.0-, 1.5-mg tabs and tablets	1.5–4.5 mg/d, titrated to desired effect over 3 wk
Anticholinergic agents				
Benztropine	Addressed in Chapter 100			
Trihexyphenidyl	Addressed in Chapter 100			
Other				
Amantadine hydrochloride	$C_{10}H_{17}N,HCl$; 187.7; 665-66-7	μg/ml × 6.61 = μmol/L	100-mg capsule; 50 mg/5 ml syrup	100 mg/d initially; often increased to 100 mg twice daily; occasionally, 400 mg daily in divided doses
Selegiline hydrochloride	$C_{13}H_{17}N,HCl$; 223.7; 14611-52-0	μg/ml × 5.34 = μmol/L	5-mg capsule	5 mg orally, twice daily

COMT, catechol-O-methyltransferase; NA, not applicable; NR, not reported.

TABLE 3. Pharmacokinetics/pharmacodynamics of catechol-O-methyltransferase inhibitors

	Entcapone (7)	Tolcapone (6)
Onset of effect (h)	1	2
Duration of effect	Variable	Variable
Volume of distribution (L)	8–20	9
Route of excretion	Hepatic	Hepatic
Elimination half-life (h)	1–2	Not reported
Excreted unchanged (%)	0.1–0.2	0.5
Active metabolites	Not reported	Not reported
Protein binding (%)	98	99.9

Toxicokinetics and Toxicodynamics

Pharmacokinetic/pharmacodynamic information for COMT inhibitors is displayed in Table 3. Levodopa is rapidly absorbed into the blood, where most of it is converted to dopamine. The majority of dopamine remains in the plasma and body tissue and does not cross the blood–brain barrier. The volume of distribution is 1.1 L/kg. Although only a small amount of the ingested levodopa actually enters the brain (approximately 1%), it is enough to alleviate the symptoms of parkinsonism.

Levodopa is transported across the intestinal wall by a saturable carrier system. Amino acids contained in protein meals can compete with levodopa transport across the intestinal mucosa and at the blood–brain barrier. Careful attention to protein intake is advocated by parkinsonologists to avoid erratic dopamine levels. Levodopa is primarily excreted in the urine (80%) as dopamine, norepinephrine, and homovanillic acid. The rate of clearance is 0.3 L/kg/hour.

Pathophysiology

The clinical manifestations of Parkinson's disease are secondary to a relative deficiency of dopamine. However, when dopamine is present in the plasma, it does not cross the blood–brain barrier, and therefore dopamine itself is therapeutically ineffective. Levodopa, which is the immediate metabolic precursor of dopamine, does cross the blood–brain barrier. In the central nervous system, levodopa is metabolized into dopamine by the enzyme dopa decarboxylase. Inhibition of this enzyme in the systemic circulation (but not the brain) produces decreased levels of peripheral dopamine while maintaining central levels. With the use of a COMT inhibitor, there is a concomitant reduction in side effects and no loss of therapeutic effect. Pharmacokinetic studies demonstrate that co-administration of tolcapone or entacapone increases the plasma levodopa area under the curve and its elimination half-life (11).

Pregnancy and Lactation

Levodopa is U.S. Food and Drug Administration (FDA) pregnancy category C (Appendix I). Dosages above 200 mg/kg/day have been shown to decrease fetal and postnatal growth and viability in animals. Tolcapone and entacapone are pregnancy category C and are excreted into breast milk (6,7).

Clinical Presentation

ACUTE OVERDOSAGE

The most prominent signs and symptoms associated with acute overdose are anxiety, confusion, agitation, insomnia, and hemodynamic compromise including tachycardia and hypotension. In addition, it is not uncommon to see motor abnormalities.

ADVERSE EVENTS

The most common form of clinical fluctuation, termed the *wearing-off effect*, is characterized by end-of-dose deterioration and recurrence of parkinsonian symptoms. The wearing-off effect consists of choreiform or stereotypic movements involving the head, trunk, limbs, and, occasionally, the respiratory muscles (12).

Dystonia tends to occur when central dopamine levels fall beneath a given threshold. This is usually manifested by painful flexion or extension of the toes. The most common form of dystonia in levodopa-treated patients consists of morning or nocturnal foot cramps (13). This clinical finding is consistent with early loss of dopaminergic innervation of the dorsolateral striatum, which corresponds somatotopically to the foot.

Other common central toxic effects of levodopa include psychiatric problems, particularly hallucinations, delusions, impulsivity, and hypersexuality (14). Some patients even exhibit an addictive behavior (hedonistic homeostatic dysregulation) associated with pathologic gambling and substance abuse (15). Hallucinations, mainly visual, affect about one-fourth of patients with Parkinson's disease. Unlike individuals with schizophrenia, the hallucinations associated with Parkinson's disease usually fluctuate and are initially sporadic (14). Most authors believe that these hallucinations are secondary to increased activity in the dopaminergic pathways; however, there is no universal agreement.

After the introduction of tolcapone, three cases of acute liver failure were described within a relatively short period of time. All of the patients who experienced liver failure were elderly women who previously had not had their liver function assessed (16). Patients with COMT inhibitor toxicity present similarly to those with levodopa toxicity, often exhibiting dyskinesias, visual hallucinations, and other psychiatric manifestations.

After the withdrawal of levodopa therapy, neuroleptic malignant syndrome associated with myoglobinuric renal failure has been reported. It is thought that this developed secondary to cessation of central dopaminergic stimulation (17).

DIAGNOSTIC TESTS

Plasma levels of levodopa are not routinely available. Abnormalities in alkaline phosphates, lactic dehydrogenase, and Coombs' test have been reported. It is recommended that liver function be assessed if COMT inhibitor toxicity is suspected.

TREATMENT

Treatment of acute overdosage is primarily symptomatic and supportive. Treatment of motor complications initially involves strategies that are designed to prolong and smooth out the therapeutic concentrations of levodopa. Slow-release preparations of levodopa offer the advantage of slowly releasing the levodopa with a special erodible matrix. Potential disadvantages and side effects of slow-release preparations include delayed or poor response after the morning dose (absence of "morning kick") and an exacerbation and prolongation of peak-dose dyskinesias. Clinical pharmacologic studies have demonstrated (contrary to the common practice of administering frequent small doses) that higher doses of levodopa may be more beneficial because they enhance the long-duration response without increasing dyskinesias.

Several drugs are reported to improve levodopa-induced dyskinesias without reducing the levodopa dosage. Clozapine not only may improve tremor and levodopa-related psychiatric implications but has been shown to improve dyskinesias without worsening parkinsonian symptoms (18). Fluoxetine has also been reported to have beneficial effects on levodopa-induced dyskinesias (19). Administration of propranolol to a small group of patients improved choreic and ballistic, but not dystonic, complications (20).

TABLE 4. Pharmacokinetics and pharmacodynamics of dopamine agonists

	Bromocriptine	Pergolide	Ropinirole (33)	Pramipexole (34)
Onset of effect (h)	1–2	Not reported	1–2	2
Duration of effect	Not reported	Not reported	Not reported	Not reported
Volume of distribution (L/kg)	13	Not reported	7.5	Not reported
Route of excretion	Hepatic	Renal	Hepatic	Renal
Elimination half-life (h)	6–8	Not reported	6	8
Excreted unchanged (%)	2–6	55	88	90
Active metabolites	None	Yes	None	None
Protein binding (%)	90	90	40	15

Psychiatric-induced complications can be treated by reducing the dose of the dopaminergic drug, if possible, and eliminating nonessential drugs. In addition, beta-blockers and benzodiazepines may provide an anxiolytic effect. In general, typical antipsychotics, including haloperidol, should be avoided in Parkinson's disease because they may exacerbate parkinsonian symptoms by blocking central dopamine receptors. Atypical antipsychotics offer the best strategy for controlling levodopa-induced psychosis (21). In contrast to the traditional (typical) antipsychotics, atypical antipsychotics usually control hallucinations and other psychiatric side effects without exacerbating the underlying parkinsonism. Clozapine effectively controls levodopa-induced side effects but has the potential to cause agranulocytosis (22). Olanzapine has been reported to exert an antipsychotic effect similar to clozapine without the risk of agranulocytosis. However, olanzapine was associated with exacerbation of parkinsonian motor disability (23). Quetiapine, which blocks not only D_1 and D_2 receptors but also serotonergic receptors, has been shown to be beneficial in hallucinating patients (24).

Levodopa-induced gastrointestinal side effects can be controlled with ondansetron or granisetron, 5-HT_3 receptor antagonists (25). Orthostatic hypotension usually improves with the addition of salt to a patient's diet and the use of fludrocortisone and midodrine (26).

DOPAMINE AGONISTS

After chronic levodopa therapy, many patients become less responsive to therapy. Dopamine agonists offer an alternative therapy, acting directly on dopamine receptors. Dopamine agonists have traditionally been used in a levodopa-sparing capacity, but the more recent trend has been to use them initially to delay the introduction of levodopa.

Several dopamine agonists are available: bromocriptine (Parlodel), lisuride, pergolide (Permax), ropinirole (Requip), and pramipexole (Mirapex). Apomorphine and lisuride are additional dopamine agonists that can be administered parenterally for "rescue therapy" in patients who experience sudden akinetic episodes; however, they are not currently approved in the United States. Selegiline (Eldepryl), a selective monoamine oxidase–B inhibitor, is thought to be a neuroprotective agent but provides little relief of symptoms (27,28).

Toxic Dose

The adult therapeutic dose of the dopamine agonists is provided in Table 2. Several cases of acute ingestion of bromocriptine have been documented, most resulting in nausea/vomiting, hypotension, and psychiatric manifestations (29). An ingestion of 32.5 mg in a child resulted in vomiting and diarrhea (30). In preclinical trials, ten patients ingested greater than 24 mg per day of ropinirole. These individuals reported increased dyskinesia, sedation, orthostatic hypotension, and confusion. Similarly, in preclinical trials with pergolide, several patients took toxic doses ranging from 7 to 60 mg. They experienced palpitations, hallucinations, dyskinesia, and transient hypotension (31). In both preclinical studies, these symptoms resolved after the medication was discontinued.

Toxicokinetics and Toxicodynamics

Selected pharmacokinetic and pharmacodynamic information is provided in Table 4.

Pathophysiology

Dopamine agonists act directly in postsynaptic dopamine receptors in the striatum. Unlike levodopa, no biochemical conversion is needed with dopamine agonists. Studies have shown that dopamine agonists may be neuroprotective secondary to antioxidant effects or reduced endogenous dopamine turnover (32).

The earliest dopamine agonist was bromocriptine, which is an ergot derivative that structurally resembles dopamine. Bromocriptine is a mixed D_1 agonist and antagonist, with some activity on D_2 and D_3 receptors. The efficacy of bromocriptine is often not sustained, and it is associated with adverse events. Ropinirole, pramipexole, and pergolide have been shown to be better tolerated (33,34). The agents are more potent and have a longer half-life than bromocriptine. Pramipexole and ropinirole are nonergot compounds that selectively stimulate D_2 and D_3 dopamine receptors. Unlike bromocriptine, these drugs do not significantly stimulate serotonin or adrenergic receptors.

Pregnancy and Lactation

All of the dopamine agonists are FDA pregnancy category C, except pergolide, which is category B (Appendix I). Safety for breast-feeding is unknown for pergolide and is considered unsafe for the other agents.

Clinical Presentation

ACUTE OVERDOSAGE

Limited data are available concerning manifestations of overdose with the newer dopamine agonists. Animal studies indicate that manifestations include nausea, vomiting, convulsions, hypotension, and exacerbation of central nervous system function.

Toxicity from acute ingestion of bromocriptine results from precipitous rises of dopamine levels. Several case reports describe hallucinations in patients after acute ingestion (29). Bromocriptine-induced schizophrenia has been described (35). Acute vision loss has been reported after a patient ingested 2.5

mg bromocriptine (36). The use of pramipexole has been associated with idiosyncratic sleep attacks (37). In all cases, symptoms resolved after cessation of the medication.

ADVERSE EVENTS

Other non-neurologic adverse reactions have been reported. Possible bromocriptine-induced myocardial infarction has been described. On bromocriptine rechallenge 1 month after the myocardial infarction, coronary angiography revealed severe narrowing of the right coronary at the peak of action of bromocriptine (38). Another case report describes hyponatremia in a patient treated with bromocriptine (39). Despite several case studies describing adverse effects of the dopamine agonists, at least one large study has confirmed the long-term safety in patients taking large doses of dopamine agonists (40).

Diagnostic Tests

Therapeutic drug monitoring is not used for dopamine agonists. Diagnostic testing is directed at the manifestations of toxicity, including serum electrolytes and renal function testing. Typical evaluations of myocardial ischemia or seizures may be needed if those complications occur.

Treatment

Little information is available to guide therapy. Treatment is primarily symptomatic and supportive. Decontamination procedures have not been evaluated. Given the relatively mild acute toxicity, a single dose of activated charcoal would be appropriate. Enhancement of elimination has not been assessed for these agents. No specific antidotes are available.

AMANTADINE

Amantadine (Symmetrel) is an antiviral agent that relieves the symptoms of Parkinson's disease through an unknown mechanism. It is indicated in the treatment of idiopathic Parkinson's disease, postencephalitic parkinsonism, and parkinsonism secondary to carbon monoxide toxicity. It is thought that amantadine potentiates the release of dopamine from remaining neurons within the basal ganglia. Amantadine appears to potentiate the therapeutic effects of levodopa, although such potentiation is not consistent.

Toxic Dose

The adult therapeutic dose is provided in Table 2. The dosage is decreased in patients with renal impairment. Death has been reported from overdose with amantadine. The lowest reported acute lethal dose was 2.5 g. In this case, malignant ventricular tachydysrhythmias developed in a suicidal patient after ingestion; these dysrhythmias were exacerbated by the administration of isoproterenol and dopamine (41). Similarly, the pediatric literature describes an intentional ingestion of 1.3 g resulting in ventricular dysrhythmias that were responsive to lidocaine (42).

Toxicokinetics and Toxicodynamics

Amantadine is well absorbed orally. The half-life ranges from 10 to 14 hours. The volume of distribution ranges from 3 to 8 L/kg. Amantadine is excreted renally. The clearance is significantly reduced in adult patients with renal insufficiency. The pH of the urine has been reported to influence the excretion rate of amantadine. The administration of urine-acidifying drugs increases the elimination of the drug. It is primarily excreted unchanged in the urine, but eight metabolites have been identified.

Pathophysiology

Although the precise mechanism of action is unknown, it is thought that amantadine works by augmenting release of dopamine from the presynaptic terminal. Amantadine is often used as initial monotherapy, while reserving the more powerful levodopa-carbidopa combination until needed.

Pregnancy and Lactation

Amantadine is FDA pregnancy category C (Appendix I). It is known that amantadine crosses the placenta and blood–brain barrier and is excreted in breast milk.

Clinical Presentation

ACUTE OVERDOSAGE

Toxicity from acute overdosage has been reported to result in psychosis and cardiac dysrhythmias. The literature describes several cases of patients presenting with delirium and visual hallucinations after acute ingestions (43,44). The adult and the pediatric literature describe cases of ventricular dysrhythmias secondary to acute toxicity (41,42).

ADVERSE REACTIONS

The majority of adverse reactions with amantadine are secondary to renal impairment. Amantadine neurotoxicity has been described in the pediatric and the adult literature (42,43). In both cases, the neurotoxicity resolved after cessation of amantadine.

Other case reports describe amantadine-induced lower extremity edema, refractory to diuretic therapy (45). Severe hyponatremia has been reported; when the amantadine was discontinued, complaints diminished and the hyponatremia resolved (46). Livedo reticularis is not an uncommon reported adverse effect of amantadine; one case series noted the skin finding in 10 of 18 patients who received amantadine (47). Seizures may be exacerbated in patients with a prior history of seizure disorder. Amantadine withdrawal–induced neuroleptic malignant syndrome has been reported after the sudden cessation of amantadine therapy (48).

Diagnostic Tests

Amantadine plasma levels can be obtained from reference laboratories. The therapeutic range is 0.7 to 1.0 μg/ml; toxic and potentially fatal levels range from 4 to 23 mg/ml. No reports have been published describing the usefulness of plasma levels in the acute clinical management of amantadine toxicity.

Treatment

DECONTAMINATION

A single dose of activated charcoal may be valuable.

ENHANCEMENT OF ELIMINATION

Multiple-dose charcoal has not been studied. Hemodialysis does not remove significant amounts of amantadine; in patients with renal failure, a 4-hour hemodialysis removed 7 to 15 mg after a single 300-mg dose. The pH of the urine has been reported to influence the excretion rate of amantadine. Because the excretion rate is increased when the urine is acidic, the administration of urine-acidifying drugs may increase the elimination of the drug from the body.

ANTIDOTES

No specific antidote is available for an overdose of amantadine. However, administration of intravenous physostigmine in 1- and 2-mg doses in adults at 1- and 2-hour intervals has been successful in reversing toxicity (49). A pediatric case report describes successful treatment of acute amantadine toxicity with physostigmine, 0.5 mg intravenously at 5-minute intervals (50).

Supportive Care

Supportive care includes close monitoring for seizure activity. Seizures have been treated with benzodiazepines. Plasma electrolytes, urine pH, and urine output should be closely monitored.

REFERENCES

1. Julien RM. *A primer of drug action: a concise nontechnical guide to the actions, uses and side effects of psychoactive drugs.* New York: W.H. Freeman, 1995:293.
2. Ruottine HM, Rinne UK. COMT inhibition in the treatment of Parkinson's disease. *J Neurol* 1998;245[Suppl 3]:25–342.
3. Jankovic J. Complications and limitations of drug therapy for movement disorders. *Neurology* 2000;55[Suppl 6]:S2–S6.
4. Leuqin MR, Scipioni O, Vaamonde J, et al. Levodopa-induced dyskinesias in Parkinson's disease: clinical and pharmacological classification. *Mov Disord* 1992;7:117–124.
5. Hannerstad JP, Woodward WR, Nutt JG, et al. Controlled release levodopa/carbidopa 25/100 (Sinemet CR 25/100): pharmacokinetics and clinical efficacy in untreated parkinsonian patients. *Clin Neuropharmacol* 1994;17:429–434.
6. *Tasmar.* Available at: http://www.tasmar.com/pi/index.html. Accessed June 2, 2002.
7. *Comtan.* Available at: http://www.comtan.com/content/dr_Comtan_PO_Pharma.htm. Accessed June 2, 2002.
8. Stuernberg HJ, Schoser BG. Acute overdosage and intoxication with carbidopa/levodopa can be detected in the subacute state by measurement of 3-O-methyldopa. *J Neurol Neurosurg Psychiatry* 1999;67:122–123.
9. Hoehn NM, Rutledge CO. Acute overdose with levodopa. Clinical and biochemical consequences. *Neurology* 1975;25(8):792–794.
10. Sporer KA. Carbidopa-levodopa overdose. *Am J Emerg Med* 1991;9:47–48.
11. Kakkola S, Gordin A, Mannisto P. General properties and clinical possibilities of new selective inhibitors of catechol-O-methyl transferase. *Gen Pharmacol* 1994;25:814–824.
12. Fahn S. The spectrum of levodopa-induced dyskinesias. *Ann Neurol* 2000;47[Suppl 1]:2–11.
13. Vidailhet M, Bonnet AM, Marconi N, et al. Do parkinsonian symptoms and levodopa induced dyskinesias start in the foot? *Neurology* 1944;44:1613–1616.
14. Fenelon G, Mahieux F, Huon R, et al. Hallucinations in Parkinson's disease. Prevalence, phenomenology and risk factors. *Brain* 2000;123:733–745.
15. Giovannoni GO, Sullivan JD, Turner K, et al. Hedonistic homeostatic dysregulation in patients with Parkinson's disease on dopamine replacement therapies. *J Neurol Neurosurg Psychiatry* 2000;68:423–428.
16. Watkins P. COMT inhibitors and liver toxicity. *Neurology* 2000;55[Suppl 4]:51–52.
17. Gibb WR, Griffith DN. Levodopa withdrawal syndrome identical to neuroleptic malignant syndrome. *Postgrad Med J* 1986;62(723):59–60.
18. Bonucceli U, Ceravolo R, Salvetti S, et al. Clozapine in Parkinson's disease tremor. Effects of acute and chronic administration. *Neurology* 1997;49:1587–1590.
19. Durif F, Vidailhet M, Bonnet AM, et al. Levodopa-induced dyskinesias are improved by fluoxetine. *Neurology* 1995;45:1855–1858.
20. Carpentier AF, Bonnet AM, Vidailhet M, et al. Improvement of levodopa-induced dyskinesia by propranolol in Parkinson's disease. *Neurology* 1996;46:1548–1551.
21. Friedman JH, Factor SA. Atypical antipsychotics in the treatment of drug induced psychosis in Parkinson's disease. *Mov Disord* 2000;15:201–211.
22. Rabey JM, Treves TA, Neufled MY, et al. Low-dose clozapine for the treatment of drug-induced psychosis in Parkinson's disease. *Neurology* 1995;45:432–435.
23. Ondo WG, Hunter C, Vuong KD, et al. Olanzapine treatment for dopaminergic induced hallucinations. *Mov Disord* 2000;15[Suppl 3]:127.
24. Fernandez HH, Friedman JH, Jacques C, et al. Quetiapine for the treatment of drug-induced psychosis in Parkinson's disease. *Mov Disord* 1999;14:484–487.
25. Wolde MI, Markham A. Ondansetron. A review of its pharmacology and preliminary clinical findings in novel applications. *Drugs* 1996;52:773–794.
26. Jankovic J, Gilden JL, Hiner BC, et al. Neurogenic orthostatic hypotension: a double-blind placebo-controlled study with midodrine. *Am J Med* 1993;95:38–48.
27. Olanow CW. Selegiline: current perspectives on issues related to neuroprotection and mortality. *Neurology* 1996;47:S210.
28. Olanow CW, Myllyla VV, Sontaniemi KA, et al. Effects of selegiline on mortality in patients with Parkinson's disease: an evidence-based review. *Neurology* 2002;58:11.
29. Warren DE, Nakfoor E. Acute overdose of bromocriptine. *Drug Intell Clin Pharm* 1983;17(5):374.
30. Vermund SH, Goldstein RG, Romano AA, et al. Accidental bromocriptine ingestion in childhood. *J Pediatr* 1984;105(5):838–840.
31. *Pergolide RxList monographs.* Available at: http://www.rxlist.com/cgi/generic2/pergol_cp.htm. Accessed June 2, 2002.
32. Kurlan R. International symposium on early dopamine agonist therapy of Parkinson's disease. *Arch Neurol* 1988;45:204.
33. *Ropinirole RxList monographs.* Available at: http://www.rxlist.com/cgi/generic2/ropinirole_cp.htm. Accessed June 2, 2002.
34. *Mirapex.* Available at: http://www.mirapex.com/includes/mirapexpdf. Accessed August 25, 2003.
35. Peter SA, Autz A, Jean-Simon ML. Bromocriptine-induced schizophrenia. *J Natl Med Assoc* 1993;85:700–701.
36. Couldwell WT, Weis MH. Visual loss associated with bromocriptine. *Lancet* 1992;340:1410–1411.
37. Shuster J. More on sleep attacks with pramipexole. *Hosp Pharm* 2000;35:240.
38. Larrazet F, Spaulding C, Laobreau HJ, et al. Possible bromocriptine-induced myocardial infarction. *Ann Intern Med* 1993;118:199–200.
39. Damase-Michael C, Sarrail E, Laens J, et al. Hyponatremia in a patient treated with bromocriptine. *Drug Invest* 1993;5:285–287.
40. Weil C. Safety of bromocriptine in long term use: review of literature. *Curr Med Res Opin* 1986;10:25–51.
41. Sartori M, Pratt CM, Young JB. Torsade de pointe. Malignant cardiac arrhythmia induced by amantadine poisoning. *Am J Med* 1984;77(2):388–391.
42. Pimentel L, Hughes B. Amantadine toxicity presenting with complex ventricular ectopy and hallucinations. *Pediatr Emerg Care* 1991;7(2):89–92.
43. Snoey ER, Bessen HA. Acute psychosis after amantadine overdose. *Ann Emerg Med* 1990;19(6):668–670.
44. Fahn S, Craddock G, Kumin G. Acute toxic psychosis from suicidal overdosage of amantadine. *Arch Neurol* 1971;25(1):45–48.
45. Kootsikas ME, Shahin J, Thompson JF, et al. Case report of amantadine-induced edema. *J Geriatric Drug Ther* 1990;4[Suppl 3]:69–78.
46. Lammers GJ, Roos RA. Hyponatremia due to amantadine hydrochloride and L-dopa/carbidopa. *Lancet* 1993;342:439.
47. Shealy CN, Weeth JB, Mercier DJ. Livedo reticularis in patients with parkinsonism receiving amantadine. *JAMA* 1970;212:1522–1523.
48. Bower DJ, Chalasani P, Ammons JC. Withdrawal-induced neuroleptic malignant syndrome. *Am J Psychiatry* 1994;151:451–452.
49. Casey DE. Amantadine intoxication reversed by physostigmine. *N Engl J Med* 1978;298:516.
50. Berkowitz CD. Treatment of acute amantadine toxicity with physostigmine. *J Pediatr* 1979;95:144–145.

CHAPTER 140

Miscellaneous Anxiolytics, Sedatives, and Hypnotics

Ian MacGregor Whyte

See Figure 1.	
Compounds included:	**Buspirone (Buspar), chloral hydrate (Noctec), ethchlorvynol (Placidyl), glutethimide (Doriden), hexapropymate, meprobamate (Miltown), methaqualone (Quaalude), methyprylon (Noludar), zolpidem (Ambien), zopiclone (Zimovane)**
Molecular formula and weight:	**See Table 1.**
SI conversion:	**See Table 1.**
CAS Registry No.:	**See Table 1.**
Therapeutic levels:	**See Table 1.**
Target organs:	**Central nervous system (acute), cardiac (acute) (chloral hydrate)**
Antidote:	**Consider flumazenil for zolpidem and zopiclone**

OVERVIEW

The miscellaneous anxiolytics, sedatives, and hypnotics are a diverse group of drugs that produce central nervous system (CNS) depression in overdose. Most are older drugs (chloral hydrate was synthesized in 1832) that have been superseded in clinical practice by the benzodiazepines (Chapter 132). Zolpidem and zopiclone are two newer non-benzodiazepine agents with effects on the γ-aminobutyric acid A ($GABA_A$) receptor. They were developed in the hope of producing less physical dependence than the benzodiazepines. Buspirone is unusual in this group, being an anxiolytic that is a partial agonist at serotonin $5\text{-}HT_{1A}$ receptors.

The older agents can cause a profound, prolonged and occasionally cyclical coma, respiratory depression, and death in relatively small doses, especially when cardiac dysrhythmias accompany the toxic profile as in chloral hydrate. Toxicity is even more severe with some coingestants, especially alcohol and opiates. Advanced age is an additional risk factor for severe toxicity. The therapeutic role of the older agents has been questioned (1).

Acute overdose toxicity and risk of death has been observed disproportionately with chloral hydrate, but death has been reported after overdose with all of the older agents. Zopiclone and zolpidem appear less toxic in overdose with a profile more similar to the benzodiazepines and produce mild to moderate CNS depression, although deaths have been recorded after overdose with both agents. Buspirone has a risk of serotonin toxicity when combined with other serotonergic agents (Chapter 24) but little intrinsic toxicity otherwise although a death in combination with alprazolam, diltiazem, alcohol, and cocaine has been reported.

Structure, Classification, and Uses

There is no consistent structural relationship amongst these agents (Table 1; Fig. 1). Indications include anxiety and insomnia (Table 2). Buspirone may have some benefit in dopamine-induced movement disorders (2) and tardive dyskinesia (3) although it can produce movement disorders of its own (4).

Toxic Dose

The *adult therapeutic dose* for these agents is provided in Table 2. There is considerable variation in the toxic dose due to interindividual differences in tolerance and the contribution of active metabolites.

Buspirone has caused serotonin toxicity (Chapter 24) when therapeutic doses are combined with serotonin uptake inhibitors (5–8), monoamine oxidase inhibitors (9,10), and, possibly, on its own (11), although it has been used successfully to treat serotonin uptake inhibitor adverse effects (12). Daily doses as high as 375 mg have been administered to healthy male volunteers (13). Doses up to 2400 mg daily were administered during early trials in which akathisia, tremor, and rigidity were observed (14). Deliberate self-poisoning with 250 mg (14) and up to 300 mg (15) resulted in drowsiness in approximately one-half of patients. One fatality followed ingestion of 450 mg of buspirone with alprazolam, diltiazem, alcohol, and cocaine (16).

Chloral hydrate was by far the most commonly implicated single compound in fatal overdoses in Brisbane, Australia, between 1979 and 1987 (17) and had one of the highest odds ratios for death from deliberate self-poisoning when adjusted for prescription numbers (58.1; 95% CI, 18.1 to 187.0) (18). Doses of 80 to 100 mg/kg have been given to children with sedation as the only effect (19). Paradoxical excitement occurred in 18% of children receiving a mean dose 87 mg/kg (20). A preterm infant developed severe chloral hydrate toxicity after its therapeutic administration as an adjunct to the treatment of hyaline membrane disease (21). Therapeutic doses of chloral hydrate may produce cardiac dysrhythmias when used to sedate children with stimulant ingestions (22). A 2-year-old child had a cardiorespiratory arrest after aspiration of 250 mg of chloral hydrate but survived (23). More than 1.5 to 2.0 g of chloral hydrate has produced excessive sedation in children and adults (19). Lethargy and ataxia occur in adults at doses of 2 to 3 g (13), although tolerant individuals have consumed up to 25 g/day without mishap (24).

Two cases of intravenous (IV) administration of a therapeutic dose of the oral chloral hydrate formulation resulted in CNS depression and minimal local effects (25). Ingestion of 219 mg/kg of chloral hydrate resulted in transient bigeminy; ingestion of up to 960 mg/kg caused torsade de pointes and ventricular fibrillation (25). A 5 g ingestion by a 67-year-old man resulted in tachydysrhythmia and polymorphic ventricular extrasystoles (26). Accidental repeated overdose totaling 8 g in a 42-year-old woman produced mild CNS depression with ventricular bigeminy (27). An adult ingestion of 10 g produced unconsciousness,

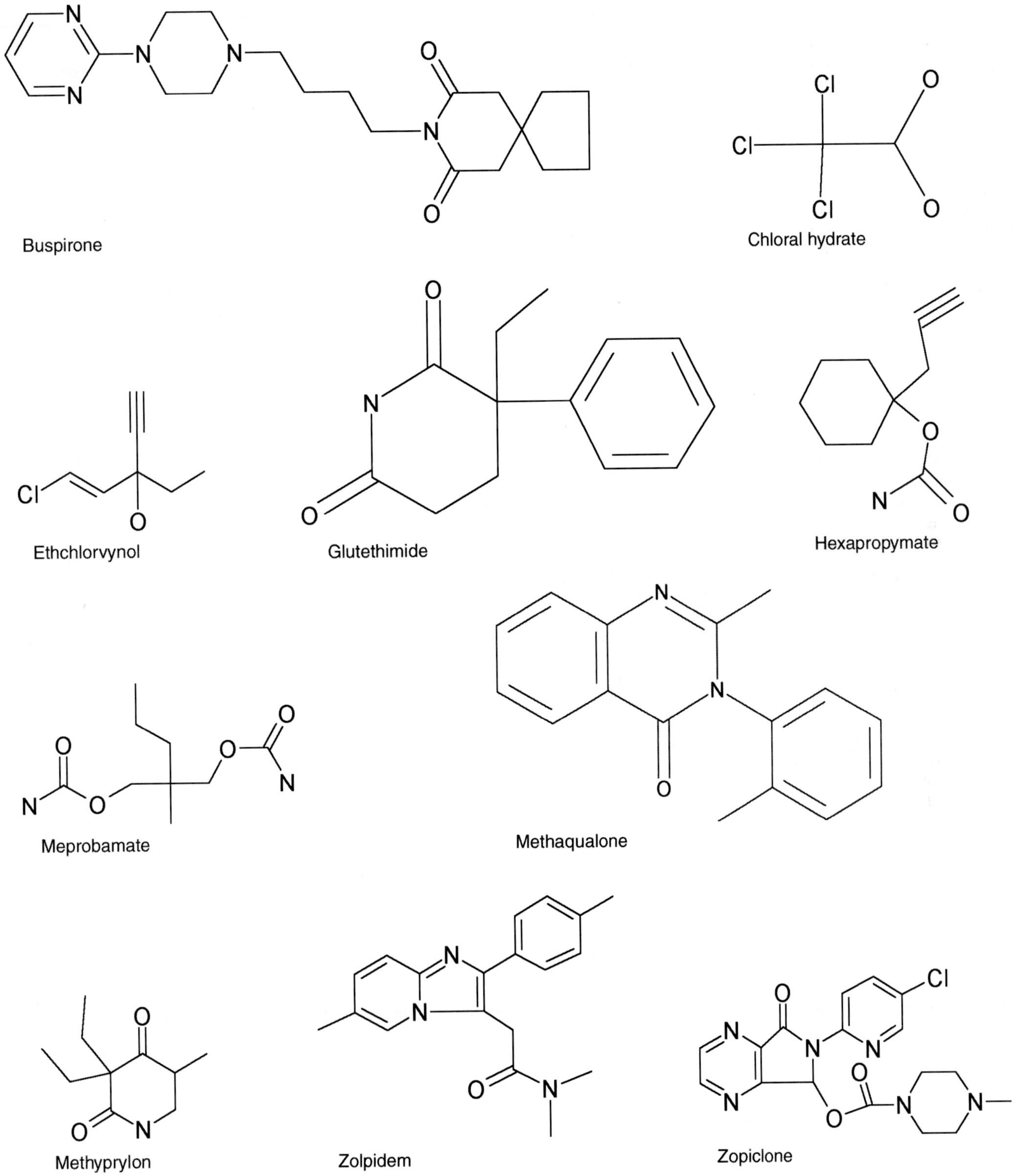

Buspirone

Chloral hydrate

Ethchlorvynol

Glutethimide

Hexapropymate

Meprobamate

Methaqualone

Methyprylon

Zolpidem

Zopiclone

Figure 1. Structures of the miscellaneous anxiolytics, sedatives, and hypnotics.

respiratory depression, and hypotension (28). Doses of 10.0 to 37.5 g (29) and 38.0 g (19) were associated with severe toxicity (coma and dysrhythmia) but ultimate survival.

Gastric perforation and gastrointestinal (GI) hemorrhage with later gastroesophageal stricture formation have been reported after doses of 30 g (30) and 18 g (31). Coma and signs of cardiac toxicity appeared 2 hours after ingestion of approximately 38 g of chloral hydrate (32). A 29-year-old man was admitted after ingestion of 70 g of chloral hydrate. He was hypotensive, hypothermic, and profoundly unconscious but survived (33).

The minimum lethal dose of chloral hydrate for an adult is unclear and has been variously quoted as 3, 4, or 5 to 10 g (13,24,34,35). A healthy young woman died after a therapeutic

TABLE 1. Structural classification of miscellaneous anxiolytics, sedatives, and hypnotics

Compound	Molecular formula, molecular weight (g/mol), CAS Registry No.	SI conversion; therapeutic levels, toxic concentrations[a]	*United States Pharmacopeia Dictionary of Drug Names*
Buspirone hydrochloride	$C_{21}H_{31}N_5O_2$,HCl; 385.5; 33386-08-2	mg/L × 2.59 = μmol/L; 0.005 mg/L, NA	8-(4-(4-(2-pyrimidinyl)piperizinyl)butyl)-8-aza-spiro(4,5)decane-7,9-dione
Chloral hydrate	$C_2H_3Cl_3O_2$; 149.4; 302-17-0	mg/L × 6.69 = μmol/L; 10 mg/L, 50 mg/L[b]	2,2,2-trichloro-1,1-ethanediol (2,2,2-trichloroethanol)
Ethchlorvynol	C_7H_9ClO; 144.6; 113-18-8	mg/L × 6.92 = μmol/L; 20 mg/L, 100 mg/L	1-chloro-3-ethyl-1-penten-4-yn-3-ol
Glutethimide	$C_{13}H_{15}NO_2$; 217.3; 77-21-4	mg/L × 4.60 = μmol/L; 5 mg/L, 30 mg/L	2-ethyl-2-phenylglutarimide
Hexapropymate	$C_{10}H_{15}NO_2$; 181.2; 358-52-1	mg/L × 5.52 = μmol/L; NA, NA	1-(2-propynyl)cyclohexanol carbamate
Meprobamate	$C_9H_{18}N_2O_4$; 218.3; 57-53-4.	mg/L × 4.58 = μmol/L; 25 mg/L, 50 mg/L	2-methyl-2-propyl-1,3-propanediol dicarbamate
Methaqualone	$C_{16}H_{14}N_2O$; 250.3; 72-44-6	mg/L × 4.00 = μmol/L; 5 mg/L, 10 mg/L	2-methyl-3-o-tolyl-4(3H)-quinazolinone
Methyprylon	$C_{10}H_{17}NO_2$; 183.3; 125-64-4	mg/L × 5.46 = μmol/L; 10 mg/L, 30 mg/L	3,3-diethyl-5-methyl-2,4-piperidinedione
Zolpidem tartrate	$(C_{19}H_{21}N_3O)_2$, $C_4H_6O_6$; 307.4; 99294-93-6	mg/L × 3.25 = μmol/L; 0.3 mg/L, 3 mg/L	N,N,6-trimethyl-2-(4-methylphenyl)-imidazo(1,2-a)pyridine-3-acetamide
Zopiclone	$C_{17}H_{17}ClN_6O_3$; 388.8; 43200-80-2	mg/L × 2.57 = μmol/L; 0.1 mg/L, NA	4-methyl-1-piperazinecarboxylic acid ester with 6-(5-chloro-2-pyridyl)-6,7-dihydro-7-hydroxy-5H-pyrrolo(3,4-b)pyrazin-5-one

NA, not available.
[a]Data from Flanagan RJ. Guidelines for the interpretation of analytical toxicology results and unit of measurement conversion factors. *Ann Clin Biochem* 1998;35(Pt 2):261–267.
[b]As trichloroethanol.

dose of chloral hydrate syrup before dental surgery (36). A 33-year-old woman died after 40 g (34) and a 35-year-old woman died after ingestion of 35 g (37).

Ethchlorvynol produced only minor symptoms at doses up to 4 g/day (38), however, death has occurred after ingestion of only 2.5 g alone (39) or in combination with alcohol (40). Deep coma occurred after ingestion of 12.5 g (41). Severe noncardiogenic pulmonary edema occurred after 25 to 40 mg/kg IV (42,43). Death occurred after ingestion of 5 g (44) and up to 49.5 g of ethchlorvynol (45), but survival of doses of 25 to 45 g has been reported (45).

Glutethimide overdose ended in death of six of 63 patients hospitalized with glutethimide overdose, including all three aged 60 years or older. Age was the major identifiable determinant of survival, regardless of other factors. An ingested dose of 10 g or more was almost always associated with deep coma (46). Relatively small doses (2.5 and 5 g) have been associated with bleeding, liver failure, and acute renal failure (47). A dose of at least 15 g resulted in cyclic and, sometimes, unilateral clinical findings that were reflected in the electroencephalogram (EEG). Complete clinical recovery resulted with supportive care (48). The minimum lethal dose for an adult is estimated as 5 g (49) although ingestion of 75 g has been survived (50).

Hexapropymate has caused respiratory depression and coma after doses as small as 3.6 g (51). Doses of 8 g or more appear to involve an increased risk of hypotension and shock (52). Patients who have ingested 16 to 40 g have survived with supportive care (53,54). A 20-year-old man who ingested 9.2 g died in 12 hours (55) and a 32-year-old man who ingested 40 g lapsed into a deep coma before he died after 3 days (56).

Meprobamate was implicated in 50 (6.5%) of 773 admissions to Massachusetts General Hospital due to psychotropic drug overdose between 1962 and 1975. Estimated doses ingested were as high as 40 g. Two patients died, one of whom ingested 12 to 20 g of meprobamate apparently with no other drugs (57). A 36-year-old woman was deeply comatose after ingestion of 40 g (58). A patient was deeply unconscious, hypotensive, and in respiratory failure 4 hours after an overdose of 30 to 40 g (59). Ingestions of 72 to 100 g have produced profound hypotension (60,61). Death has followed the ingestion of 3.6 g of meprobamate alone (62). A series of 12 fatal cases involved doses of 16 to 40 g (63).

TABLE 2. Typical therapeutic doses of miscellaneous anxiolytics, sedatives, and hypnotics for their primary indication (13,122,230)

Drug	Indication	Formulation	Adult dose	Pediatric dose
Buspirone	Anxiety	5-, 10-, 15-mg tablets	5–10 mg 3 times daily to a total daily dose of 60 mg	NR
Chloral hydrate	Insomnia	250-, 500-mg capsules; 500-mg suppository; 500 mg/5 ml syrup	500 mg to 1 g at night	50 mg/kg to a maximum dose of 1 g
Ethchlorvynol	Insomnia	200-, 500-, 750-mg capsules	500 mg at night	NR
Glutethimide	Insomnia	500-mg capsule or tablet	250–500 mg at night	NR
Hexapropymate	Insomnia	NR	400 mg at night	100–200 mg at night depending on age
Meprobamate	Anxiety	200-, 400-, 600-mg tablets	400 mg 3–4 times a day up to a maximum of 2.4 g/d	NR
Methaqualone	Insomnia	Discontinued	150–300 mg at night	NR
Methyprylon	Insomnia	Discontinued	200–400 mg at night	Children older than 12 years of age, 50 mg at night up to 200 mg at night
Zolpidem	Insomnia	5-, 10-mg tablets	5–10 mg at night	NR
Zopiclone	Insomnia	7.5-mg tablets	3.75–7.50 mg at night	NR

NR, not reported.

Methaqualone produced mild toxicity (slurred speech, ataxia, drowsiness, and nystagmus) after cumulative doses of 300 to 4900 mg in chronic users (64). Deep coma occurred after an estimated ingestion of more than 4.5 g (65). A 23-year-old man was admitted after ingestion of 4 to 5 g. On admission, he was somnolent and poorly responsive to painful stimuli and later became deeply comatose. He recovered completely (66).

Methyprylon produces prolonged coma frequently accompanied by hemodynamic, respiratory, and hepatic dysfunction in doses more than 6 g (13). Although a dose of 6 g was fatal in one patient (67), others have recovered after ingestion of up to 30 g (68).

Zolpidem in therapeutic doses has been implicated in psychotic reactions characterized by auditory and visual hallucinations as well as delusional thinking (69). In a series of 344 adult patients, the dose of zolpidem ranged from 10 to 1400 mg. Drowsiness occurred at doses of 140 to 440 mg; coma or respiratory failure was rare (70). In a series of 54 single-drug adult poisonings with zolpidem, doses up to 600 mg produced only mild symptoms. Only one patient became comatose after ingestion of 600 mg zolpidem. On the other hand, in combined intoxications with other CNS active drugs, a zolpidem dose as low as 100 to 150 mg induced coma in some patients, even if the amount of the coingested drugs would not have caused a comatose state (71). An overdose of 200 mg of zolpidem alone in a 44-year-old man resulted in coma (Glasgow coma score of 7) and respiratory failure (72). In a series of 12 pediatric ingestions, one child had no effect with 2.5 mg. As little as 5 mg caused symptoms with minor outcome in six unintentional ingestions (5 to 30 mg). Minor to moderate symptoms were reported 1 to 4 hours after intentional ingestions (12.5 to 150.0 mg) (73).

The effect of *zopiclone* (7.5 mg) is enhanced and prolonged by alcohol without increasing the plasma concentration (74). Transient first-degree atrioventricular heart block occurred after ingestion of 127.5 mg of zopiclone (with piperazine) (75). Sleepiness was the only feature after a 300-mg ingestion (76). A 72-year-old man with lung cancer died 4 to 10 hours after ingesting 90 mg of zopiclone (77). A combined alcohol and zopiclone (150 mg) ingestion resulted in the death of a 29-year-old woman (78). A 72-year-old woman with poor respiratory function died after ingesting 200 to 350 mg (79).

TOXICOKINETICS AND TOXICODYNAMICS

The pharmacokinetic parameters for the miscellaneous sedatives are provided in Table 3. In most cases, it is the development of tolerance to sedative-hypnotics that determines the recovery of consciousness after overdose rather than the clearance of the drug. In general, because of tolerance and the active metabolites of these drugs, there is a poor correlation between concentration and effect.

Buspirone has little or no information available.

Chloral hydrate (single oral dose of 1000 mg) produced a mean peak trichloroethanol concentration in blood (C_{max}) of 8.0 mg/L (range, 2 to 12) at 1 hour (80), with an elimination half-life of 8 to 12 hours (13). In chloral hydrate intoxication, there may be delayed absorption and some slowing of metabolism (81). Two hours after ingestion of 38 g, the plasma concentration of trichloroethanol in a 38-year-old woman was 330 mg/L, and the half-life was 35 hours (32).

Ethchlorvynol (500 mg orally) produced a C_{max} of 6.5 mg/L at 1 hour (82). Chronic abusers may ingest up to 4 g/day with steady state serum concentrations of up to 37 mg/L (38). Initial serum concentrations were reported at 70 mg/L in a somnolent yet totally conscious adult with evidence of tolerance (83). Admission blood concentrations in a series of 38 overdose patients ranged from 3 to 46 mg/L in ethchlorvynol alone ingestions and from 3 to 75 mg/L when combined with other agents (84). When ingested alone, ethchlorvynol concentrations more than 19 mg/L were usually associated with dysarthria, mydriasis, nystagmus, and tachycardia; when concentrations exceeded 38 mg/L, coma, areflexia, hypotension, and respiratory depression were generally noted (84).

Although serial measurements can estimate when the ethchlorvynol concentration will fall to the *therapeutic* range (85), the correlation between drug concentrations and clinical status

TABLE 3. Pharmacokinetics of the miscellaneous anxiolytics, sedatives, and hypnotics (13,122)

Drug	Bioavailability (F) (%)	Time to peak after oral dosing (h)	Volume of distribution (L/kg)	Clearance (L/h/kg)	Half-life (h)	Protein binding (%)	Active metabolites (half-life)
Buspirone	4; high first pass metabolism	1.0–1.5	5.3	1.7–3.5	2.4 (2–11)	95	1-(2-pyrimidinyl)-piperazine (2–6)
Chloral hydrate (as trichloroethanol)	Rapid conversion to trichloroethanol	0.5–1.0	0.6–1.6	NR	8–12 (parent drug, 4–5 min)	35	Trichloroethanol (8–12); trichloroacetic acid (inactive, 67)
Ethchlorvynol	NR	2	3–4	0.17	10–20	35–50	NR
Glutethimide	Erratic	1–6	2.7	NR	13.5 (8.1–17.9)	50	4-hydroxy-2-ethyl-2-phenylglutarimide (NR); 2-phenylglutarimide (NR); alpha-phenyl-gamma-butyrolactone (NR)
Hexapropymate	NR	NR	1.5–3.5	NR	2.7–8.1	NR	NR
Meprobamate	NR	1–2	0.5–0.8	NR	10 (6.4–16.6)	20	None
Methaqualone	67–97	1–2	2.4–6.4	0.081–0.15	33–43	80	2-hydroxymethyl-methaqualone (NR)
Methyprylon	NR	1–2	0.97	0.0119	9–11	60	5-methylpyrithyldione (NR); 6-oxomethyprylone (NR)
Zolpidem	70	1–2	0.54	0.014–0.016	2.4 (2–4)	92	None
Zopiclone	80	0.5–1.5	1.43	0.257	3.5–6.0	45–80	Zopiclone N-oxide (NR)

NR, not reported.

are poor (86). In a series of nonfatal (51) and fatal (38) ingestions involving ethchlorvynol over a 14-year period (1975 through 1988), the concentrations in the (nonfatal) pure and mixed ingestions were similar (3 to 115 mg/L) and were little different from the concentrations in fatal cases (5 to 258 mg/L) (87). Concentrations of 8 (45,86), 22 (45), and 85 mg/L (45) were associated with coma in nontolerant individuals.

Glutethimide (single dose of 500 mg) produced a C_{max} of 4.3 mg/L (range, 2.9 to 7.1 mg/L) (88). Balance disturbances, psychomotor retardation, and changes in consciousness with temporary excitation were observed with a concentration of 5 mg/L in the blood (89).

Some evidence for concentration-dependent toxicity was found in a series of 70 cases of glutethimide overdose (90). Mild features were seen with concentrations in the range of 5 to 56 mg/L (mean, 27 mg/L), moderate toxicity developed at concentrations of 22 to 78 mg/L (mean, 45 mg/L), and severe toxicity was present at 15 to 120 mg/L (mean, 50 mg/L) (90). Blood concentrations and clinical findings were evaluated in 26 nonfatal and 12 fatal intoxications involving the combination of glutethimide and codeine (*loads*) (91). The mean glutethimide concentration was 10 mg/L for nonfatal cases (range, 2 to 18 mg/L) and 13.9 mg/L for fatal cases (range, 4.6 to 26.4 mg/L). Six patients with serum glutethimide concentrations of 10 mg/L or more were comatose (91). In another study of 63 cases, a plasma concentration exceeding 30 mg/L was almost always associated with deep coma (46).

Normal plasma half-lives of glutethimide and the relatively small amounts in urine of unchanged drug and unconjugated metabolites indicated that drug elimination is not markedly impaired in intoxicated patients (92).

Hexapropymate serum concentrations of 5.5 mg/L or lower are regarded as nontoxic (54). In a study of six patients, maximum serum concentrations varied from 7.6 to 72.5 mg/L with no relationship between concentration and severity of clinical effects (54). Detailed analysis of the drug elimination in one patient showed a terminal elimination half-life of 21 hours, suggesting delayed absorption or dose-dependent elimination (54).

Meprobamate exhibits significant differences in arterial versus venous plasma concentrations (93). A single 400-mg dose produces a C_{max} of 7.7 mg/L at 2 hours (94). Analysis of single psychoactive drug cases and single-drug plus ethanol cases showed that the toxic blood concentration of meprobamate was decreased by an average of 50% in the presence of ethanol (95). Light coma occurred in patients with plasma concentrations of 60 to 120 mg/L whereas deep coma was associated with concentrations of 100 to 240 mg/L (96). Coma, hypotension, and hypothermia occurred in four cases of severe meprobamate intoxication with maximal plasma concentrations of 176, 180, 190, and 203 mg/L (97). All patients survived without sequelae including one patient resuscitated from cardiac arrest. Four hours after an overdose of meprobamate (30 to 40 g), a patient with a serum meprobamate concentration of 500 mg/L was deeply unconscious, hypotensive, and in respiratory failure (59). Eight hours after ingestion of 100 g of meprobamate, the plasma concentration was 460 mg/L and the patient was profoundly hypotensive (61). Twenty-five hours after admission after a meprobamate overdose, deep coma and cerebral electrical silence (flat line EEG) were observed at a time when the meprobamate plasma concentration was 250 mg/L (98). The patient recovery was uneventful.

Methaqualone (250-mg oral dose) produced a C_{max} of 2.2 mg/L (range, 1 to 4 mg/L) (99). Concentrations more than 8 mg/L have been associated with unconsciousness (100); concentrations in overdose have ranged from 2 to 230 mg/L (101). A mean serum methaqualone concentration of 5 ± 3 mg/L (mean ± SD) was seen in a series of 60 poisonings (102). Serum methaqualone concentrations did not correlate with the physical findings, except that concentrations of 9 mg/L or higher were always associated with CNS depression, whether other drugs were present (102).

Methyprylon has a therapeutic plasma concentration of 10 mg/L (13). Concentrations in excess of 30 mg/L are associated with stupor (68) or coma (103), and concentrations over 100 mg/L are said to be potentially lethal (13). Nevertheless, a patient who survived coma had a peak methyprylon concentration of 168 mg/L (104). The elimination half-life of methyprylon was 50 hours, suggesting concentration-dependent elimination (104). This was confirmed in another study that showed the decline in the concentration of plasma methyprylon was nonlinear between 66 and 30 mg/L and linear at concentrations less than 30 mg/L (105). The patient regained consciousness when the methyprylon concentration fell below 43 mg/L. Serial measurements in a 14-year-old girl after an overdose also showed much longer half-lives than the usually reported 4 hours (106).

Zolpidem (single 20-mg oral dose) produced a C_{max} of 0.192 to 0.324 mg/L at 0.75 to 2.60 hours post dose (107). Zolpidem concentrations ranged from 0.05 to 1.40 mg/L (mean 0.29 mg/L) in the blood of 29 subjects arrested for impaired driving (108). In the subjects in which zolpidem was present with other drugs or alcohol, symptoms included slow movements and reactions, slow and slurred speech, poor coordination, lack of balance, flaccid muscle tone, and horizontal and vertical gaze nystagmus (108). In five separate cases, in which zolpidem was the only drug detected (0.08 to 1.40 mg/L; mean, 0.65 mg/L), signs of impairment included slow and slurred speech, slow reflexes, disorientation, lack of balance and coordination, and *blacking out* (108). After ingestion of 300 mg of zolpidem, an initial plasma concentration above 0.5 mg/L was reported in a comatose patient (109).

Zopiclone disposition was investigated after oral administration of a single 15 mg dose of a racemic mixture (twice the therapeutic dose) in 12 adult white volunteers. Determination of concentrations of zopiclone enantiomers in plasma showed that zopiclone pharmacokinetics is stereoselective with peak concentrations of 0.0873 and 0.044 mg/L for (+)-zopiclone and (–)-zopiclone, respectively (110). After 7.5 mg, alcohol enhanced and prolonged the effects without increasing the zopiclone concentration (74). After ingestion of 300 mg of zopiclone, the plasma concentration was 1.6 mg/L at 4.5 hours after the dose and the elimination half-life was 3.5 hours (76).

PATHOPHYSIOLOGY

Buspirone is a partial agonist at the 5-HT_{1A} receptor, which is present on both presynaptic and postsynaptic neurons. The net effect of the binding of buspirone to these 5-HT_{1A} receptors is a reduction in serotonergic activity (implying greater effect on presynaptic autoreceptors than postsynaptic heteroceptors) (13). Buspirone has a direct antagonist effect on the presynaptic dopamine receptor, thus increasing dopaminergic transmission; it does not interact directly with noradrenergic receptors, but decreased serotonergic activity may lead to a secondary increase in noradrenergic activity (13). Buspirone does not interact directly with either the benzodiazepine-GABA receptor complex or with GABA receptors (111), but there is some evidence that buspirone enhances benzodiazepine receptor binding *in vivo* (112). Nevertheless, benzodiazepine antagonists (e.g., flumazenil) do not reverse buspirone effects (113) and buspirone is ineffective in ameliorating features of benzodiazepine withdrawal in humans (114). There is evidence for the development of tolerance to some of the effects of buspirone that does not seem to be due to a change in the binding properties of the 5-HT_{1A} receptor itself but may be due to a change in its coupling mechanism (115). The abuse liability of buspirone appears lower than that of the benzodiazepines (116).

Chloral hydrate produces sedation attributed to its metabolite trichloroethanol. The mechanism of action is unknown (35). The parent compound is quite irritating to mucosal surfaces (30). Trichloroethanol-mediated enhanced automaticity of supraventricular and ventricular pacemaker cells (117) with increased myocardial irritability to circulating catecholamines (118) is believed to be the mechanism of the cardiac dysrhythmias. Tolerance to the sedative effects appears rapidly and prominently with a high potential for abuse/dependence and a major withdrawal syndrome (13).

Ethchlorvynol interferes with the integrity of endothelial cells in the lung to create gaps between the cells and resultant reversible pulmonary edema (119,120). The mechanism of the CNS depression is unknown. Tolerance, dependence, and withdrawal occur (39,121). Like the barbiturates, it can precipitate acute intermittent porphyria in susceptible individuals (122).

Glutethimide causes CNS depression through an unknown mechanism of action. There is evidence of weak enhancement of GABA binding with inhibition of diazepam binding (123). Glutethimide also has some anticholinergic activity. The contribution to glutethimide toxicity of its metabolite, 4-hydroxy-2-ethyl-2-phenylglutarimide (4-hydroxyglutethimide), is unclear with some supporting evidence for a significant contribution (124) but other evidence of lack of correlation with clinical effect (125). There is also the potentially confounding issue of rapid (4 to 6 hours) tolerance developing to the parent drug and its metabolites, as occurs with benzodiazepines (126). There is evidence for toxic activity of the alpha-phenyl-gamma-butyrolactone metabolite (127) but its clinical relevance is unknown. Tolerance, dependence, and a withdrawal syndrome occur (128,129), particularly when combined with codeine (*loads*) (130–132). Glutethimide has been associated with acute attacks of porphyria and is unsafe in porphyric patients (122).

Hexapropymate produces CNS depressant effects through an unknown mechanism. There are no reports of tolerance, abuse, or dependence; however, it is likely the drug has a high potential for these effects. Hexapropymate is considered to be unsafe in patients with porphyria because it has been shown to be porphyrinogenic in *in vitro* systems (122).

Meprobamate has a CNS depressant effect similar to the barbiturates but the mechanism of action is unknown. It has no effect on the $GABA_A$ receptor-benzodiazepine receptor-chloride ion channel complex. It has some skeletal muscle relaxant effect (133). Peripheral vasodilatation appears to be the cause of significant hypotension and shock with little evidence of myocardial dysfunction except when hypothermia is present (134). Meprobamate use can result in psychological and physical dependence with a barbiturate-type withdrawal syndrome (13). Like the barbiturates, it can precipitate acute intermittent porphyria in susceptible individuals (13).

Methaqualone has an unclear mechanism of action. Some of its actions are related to effects at the $GABA_A$ receptor-benzodiazepine receptor-chloride ion channel complex (135). Serotonin appears to play a facilitatory role in the anticonvulsant activity of methaqualone (136). The physical dependence picture on methaqualone is similar to that of benzodiazepines (137). Methaqualone has been withdrawn from the market in many countries because of its abuse (122,138,139).

Methyprylon produces CNS depression through an unknown mechanism. Habituation, dependence, and tolerance may occur, similar to that seen with barbiturates (13).

Zolpidem is a $GABA_A$ agonist. The $GABA_A$ receptor-benzodiazepine receptor-chloride ion channel complex is discussed in Chapter 132. The channel is not homogenous and can be assembled from multiple different combinations of α-, β-, and γ-subunits (140). Zolpidem is a potent agonist at $GABA_A$ receptors but only those containing the α_1-subunit [corresponding to the benzodiazepine $(BZ)_1$ or Ω_1 subtype]; it is not effective at receptors containing the α_5-subunit (corresponding to one type of BZ_2 or Ω_2 receptors) (141,142). It is this selectivity for BZ_1 receptors that is thought to explain its greater potency as a sedative-hypnotic and lesser activity as a muscle relaxant and anticonvulsant (142,143). The sedative-hypnotic effects are antagonized by flumazenil (144). It has been proposed that zolpidem lacks benzodiazepine-like side effects, having minimal abuse and dependence potential. Nevertheless, there are case reports of zolpidem dependence in the literature (145,146), and a withdrawal syndrome including seizures (147) exists. Zolpidem has recently been classified as a psychotropic at risk of abuse in Europe (148).

Zopiclone is a potent agonist at binding sites that belong to the $GABA_A$ receptor–benzodiazepine receptor–chloride ion channel complex but which are not the benzodiazepine-specific sites. The $GABA_A$ receptor-benzodiazepine receptor-chloride ion channel complex is discussed in Chapter 132. Zopiclone either acts on a site distinct from the benzodiazepines or induces conformational changes different from those of the benzodiazepines (149). It is possible that zopiclone acts via the mitochondrial benzodiazepine receptor, which can result in allosteric modulation of $GABA_A$ receptor function (150). Zopiclone has no effect on other brain receptors such as the GABA receptor itself, dopamine receptors, serotonin, or noradrenergic receptors (151). The sedative-hypnotic effects are antagonized by flumazenil (107). As with zolpidem, it was initially asserted that there was little potential for tolerance, abuse, or dependence; however, all can occur (145,152), and a withdrawal syndrome, including delirium, has been reported (153).

PREGNANCY AND LACTATION

The pregnancy risk categories are shown in Table 4. In several cases, there are no data on distribution into breast milk, but small amounts of drug are expected. For those in which information is available, only small amounts appear in breast milk, and only for chloral hydrate is there likely to be significant concern for the child.

CLINICAL PRESENTATION

Acute Overdose

Buspirone typically produces mild toxicity even after large doses. Nausea, vomiting, dizziness, drowsiness (15), miosis, and gastric distress may occur at lower doses (13), whereas akathisia, tremor, and rigidity may occur at higher doses (14). Combined overdose with a serotonergic agent may produce features of serotonin toxicity (Chapter 24) (5–10). There is one case of buspirone overdose that resulted in a generalized tonic clonic seizure approximately 36 hours after ingestion (154). A combined overdose with fluvoxamine resulted in prolonged bradycardia (155). Death from buspirone alone has not been reported.

Chloral hydrate produces an acrid disagreeable pear-like odor on the breath (13,156). Typical presentation of a significant chloral hydrate ingestion is CNS depression, which rapidly progresses to profound unconsciousness with hypotension (33,118) and hypothermia (33). Patients are often found already

TABLE 4. Pregnancy risk category and breast milk distribution of the serotonin uptake inhibitors

Drug	U.S. Food and Drug Administration[a] (ADEC[b]) pregnancy risk category	Distribution into breast milk (milk to plasma ratio)
Buspirone	B (B1)	NR
Chloral hydrate (as trichloro-ethanol)	C (A)	Passes into breast milk, observe for sedation (301)
Ethchlorvynol	C (NR)	NR
Glutethimide	C (NR)	Probably safe after single doses (302)
Hexapropymate	NR (NR)	NR
Meprobamate	D (C)	Concentrations up to four times that in the mother's plasma (13), 4.1% of the weight-adjusted maternal dose (303)
Methaqualone	D (NR)	NR
Methyprylon	B (NR)	NR
Zolpidem	B (B3)	0.3, 0.004% to 0.019% of the administered dose (304)
Zopiclone	NR (C)	0.51, 1.4% of the weight-adjusted dose (305)

NR, not reported.
[a]Appendix I provides definitions of U.S. Food and Drug Administration pregnancy categories.
[b]ADEC, Australian Drug Evaluation Committee Pregnancy Categories.
Category A: Drugs that have been taken by a large number of pregnant women and women of childbearing age without any proven increase in the frequency of malformations or other direct or indirect harmful effects on the fetus having been observed.
Category B1: Drugs that have been taken by only a limited number of pregnant women and women of childbearing age without an increase in the frequency of malformation or other direct or indirect harmful effects on the human fetus having been observed. Studies in animals have not shown evidence of an increased occurrence of fetal damage.
Category B2: Drugs that have been taken by only a limited number of pregnant women and women of childbearing age without an increase in the frequency of malformation or other direct or indirect harmful effects on the human fetus having been observed. Studies in animals are inadequate or may be lacking, but available data show no evidence of an increased occurrence of fetal damage.
Category B3: Drugs that have been taken by only a limited number of pregnant women and women of childbearing age without an increase in the frequency of malformation or other direct or indirect harmful effects on the human fetus having been observed. Studies in animals have shown evidence of an increased occurrence of fetal damage, the significance of which is considered uncertain in humans.
Category C: Drugs that, owing to their pharmacologic effects, have caused or may be suspected of causing harmful effects on the human fetus or neonate without causing malformations. These effects may be reversible.
Category D: Drugs that have caused or are suspected to have caused or may be expected to cause an increased incidence of human fetal malformations or irreversible damage. These drugs may also have adverse pharmacologic effects.
Category X: Drugs that have such a high risk of causing permanent damage to the fetus that they should not be used in pregnancy or when there is a possibility of pregnancy.

in coma (157) with respiratory failure (33,157) or frank cardiorespiratory arrest (118,157). Death is usually due to the effects of cerebral hypoxia (157).

Mortality is increased if cardiac dysrhythmias are present. These manifest as supraventricular and ventricular tachydysrhythmias (29,117,158,159). The ventricular dysrhythmias vary from extrasystoles, which may be polymorphic (26), to polymorphic ventricular tachycardia (160), torsade de pointes (25,161), and ventricular fibrillation (25). These dysrhythmias also occur in children (162–164). The dysrhythmias may be precipitated by catecholamines used to treat the hypotension (33,118) and can also occur when chloral hydrate is used to treat agitation due to stimulants (22) or when flumazenil is used to reverse the sedation (165). In one case report, reversible symptomatic myocardial ischemia of 4 hours duration was attributed to chloral hydrate overdose (166).

The caustic effect of chloral hydrate can result in gastroesophageal necrosis (30), with or without perforation (167), and subsequent stricture formation (31).

Ethchlorvynol has a characteristic pungent, aromatic, *vinyl-like* odor (156). Severe poisoning produces a deep, often prolonged (86) coma with hypotension, respiratory depression, and hypothermia (45). The coma is deep enough to result in pressure necrosis, rhabdomyolysis (168), and may be accompanied by flexor or extensor posturing (169) and acute urinary retention (170). In a series of 11 ethchlorvynol-alone overdose cases, the most common physical findings were depressed level of consciousness (10 cases), dysarthria (7), mydriasis (6), nystagmus (6), areflexia (4), tachycardia (4), and hypotension, ataxia, and respiratory depression (two cases each) (84). In a series of seven patients who ingested the drug, all had severe CNS depression; three were hemodynamically unstable, and one developed noncardiogenic pulmonary edema 40 hours after admission (43).

IV injection of ethchlorvynol reproducibly causes severe noncardiogenic pulmonary edema (42,43).

Glutethimide often causes deep coma, which may be cyclical (48) due to delayed absorption related to its anticholinergic effects. Hypotension (46) can occur and features of anticholinergic toxicity are common. Hypothermia can occur, particularly in combined overdose with other sedative-hypnotics (171), as can occasional hyperthermia (172). Mortality is high (173), especially in the elderly (46). In 63 patients hospitalized with glutethimide poisoning, assisted ventilation was used in 59% of cases, and 32% developed hypotension (46). In a series of 26 nonfatal cases, depressed level of consciousness was the most common physical finding (24 cases); 18 patients were lethargic but rousable with nonpainful stimulation and six were comatose (91). Glutethimide overdose has been associated with skin lesions resembling those seen in barbiturate poisoning (174,175) and with pressure necrosis and rhabdomyolysis (176).

Occasionally, unilateral neurologic findings have been noted in pupillary responses (177) and on EEG (48), and cerebellar degeneration has been reported (178). There is a single case report of methemoglobinemia (179) and isolated reports of bleeding and hepatic and renal injury (47), although it is unclear what contribution hypoperfusion had to the organ injury. Seizures attributed to hypocalcemia have been seen after misuse of glutethimide (180), but it is unclear what contribution there was of glutethimide withdrawal.

Hexapropymate causes prolonged, deep coma (53,56) with respiratory depression (51) and hypotension (52). Death can occur in as little as 12 hours (55). In a series of eight overdose patients, initial symptoms included coma, hypotension, hypothermia, and hypoventilation (54). Maximum coma depth (Glasgow coma score) was 3 to 5 in five out of eight events, and on seven occasions, assisted ventilation was needed (for 12 hours or more in five events) (54).

Meprobamate toxicity is primarily CNS depression with rapid onset of deep coma (58,181,182) and respiratory failure (59). Hypotension of varying degrees (61,183,184) up to and including cardiogenic shock (60,185) is common and worsens the prognosis (186,187). Hypothermia may be severe (188,189) and, if present, worsens the hypotension (134).

In an unselected group of 1125 consecutively hospitalized self-poisonings in Oslo, the complication rate was highest in poisonings with opiates (60.7%), meprobamate (37.5%), and antihistamines (30.0%) (190). Meprobamate poisoning is still a problem in France (5.5% of presentations) and is most frequently involved in fatal pharmaceutical overdoses (15.3%) (191). Meprobamate was implicated in 50 (6.5%) of 773 admissions to Massachusetts General Hospital due to psychotropic drug overdose between 1962 and 1975. In 25 cases, deep coma (grade 3 or 4)

(192) was reached; 23 patients became hypotensive, and 16 required assisted ventilation. Two patients died (57). In four cases of severe meprobamate intoxication, the clinical course was complicated by coma, hypotension, and hypothermia in all patients (97). As with all cases of prolonged coma, pulmonary embolism is a potential risk (193).

The coma may be so profound that the issue of brain death is raised. The EEG in this context may show an isoelectric trace even though subsequent recovery may be complete (98,194). Ischemic muscle injury may result in rhabdomyolysis (195,196) with subsequent contractures (197), and noncardiogenic pulmonary edema has been reported (198,199). Rare complications include acute pancreatitis (200) and esophageal spasm (201).

Large oral ingestions of meprobamate may result in clumping and bezoar formation (202,203). As with many sedative drug overdoses, delirium during recovery is not uncommon and may be contributed to by withdrawal in dependent patients (204).

Methaqualone causes CNS depression. In a series of 60 cases of methaqualone ingestion from 1977 through 1980, there was CNS depression that generally responded to a brief period of supportive care (102). More severe overdose can produce early CNS excitation (occasionally) (66), followed by CNS depression and coma (205), which may be profound (65) and accompanied by convulsions (206) and hypotension (207). Necrosis of pressure areas can occur (208). If CNS excitement is present, delirium (209) or even a schizophreniform psychosis (210), increased limb reflexes (66), myoclonus (66,211), and positive pyramidal signs (66) may be present. The muscular hyperactivity may be so severe as to require drug paralysis for control (212). Flexor or extensor posturing may appear as an early and transient feature (169). Ocular movements may be absent (169) or show roving eye movements (213). Signs may occasionally be unilateral (209). Respiratory insufficiency (214), including apnea (215), and noncardiogenic pulmonary edema (66,216), which can be unilateral (217), may occur. There is one case report of hemorrhagic complications possibly due to methaqualone-induced thrombocytopenia (218) or platelet dysfunction (219).

Methyprylon poisoning produces CNS depression with respiratory depression, nystagmus, pupillary abnormalities, dysarthria, drowsiness, confusion, and coma (105,220), accompanied by hypotension (68) and hypothermia or hyperpyrexia (221). ST segment and T-wave changes on electrocardiogram have been ascribed to methyprylon overdose (221).

Zolpidem in overdose generally produces mild CNS depression with drowsiness, slow movements and reactions, slow and slurred speech, poor coordination, lack of balance, flaccid muscle tone, and horizontal and vertical gaze nystagmus (108). Occasionally, more severe CNS depression occurs with development of a profound but short-lasting coma (72,109), associated with pin-point pupils (109) and respiratory depression (72,109,222), especially if other drugs or ethanol are ingested (71) or in cases of chronic hepatic or respiratory insufficiency (223). Pulmonary edema occurs in fatal cases (224).

In a series of 244 cases of intentional overdose, half of the patients ingested other substances (psychotropic drugs and alcohol) concomitantly (70). Signs of intoxication were observed in two-thirds of the patients but could be attributed to zolpidem in only 105 cases. Signs included drowsiness ($N = 89$), vomiting ($N = 7$), coma ($N = 4$), or respiratory failure ($N = 1$). There were no electrocardiographic abnormalities that were directly related to zolpidem, and symptoms of intoxication rapidly remitted in 91% of cases (70).

In a series of 91 well-documented cases of acute zolpidem intoxication, there were 54 single-drug poisonings with zolpidem. Of these, only one patient became comatose. On the other hand, in combined ingestions with other CNS active drugs or ethanol, coma was more common even if the amount of the additionally ingested drug in itself would not have caused coma (71). In 12 pediatric zolpidem ingestions, the onset of symptoms was within 10 to 60 minutes (mean, 31.6 minutes). The duration of symptoms in the unintentional cases ranged from less than 60 minutes up to 4 hours (mean, 2.4 hours) and 6 to 10 hours (mean 7.5 hours) in the intentional exposures (73).

Zopiclone principally causes drowsiness (76), lethargy, and ataxia in overdose (13). Rarely, coma may occur (225). In a death due to respiratory failure after zopiclone overdose, it was postulated that hypoventilation due to CNS depression occurred (79). Similar to benzodiazepines, coma may be due to flow limitation and obstructive apnea via an increase in upper airway resistance and work of breathing (226). There is a single case report of first-degree heart block after zopiclone poisoning (75).

Acute Withdrawal

Withdrawal from CNS depressants is addressed in Chapter 32. Suddenly stopping treatment in dependent people may produce withdrawal symptoms and signs including anxiety, dysphoria, irritability, insomnia, nightmares, sweating, memory impairment, hallucinations, hypertension, tachycardia, psychosis, tremors, and seizures (227). The withdrawal syndromes associated with the older agents are similar to those associated with barbiturates (228); they are severe and likely to be associated with life-threatening events such as seizures. Acute withdrawal from sedative-hypnotics may present solely as a confusional state due to nonconvulsive status epilepticus (toxic ictal delirium), which can easily be missed (229).

Adverse Reactions

Buspirone commonly causes dizziness, lightheadedness, headache, nausea, nervousness, and excitement. Rare adverse effects include tachycardia, palpitations, chest pain, confusion, drowsiness, dry mouth, sweating, dystonia, akathisia, tardive dyskinesia, serotonin toxicity, and angioedema (230).

Chloral hydrate has an unpleasant taste and is a skin and mucous membrane irritant unless well diluted. The most frequent adverse effect is gastric irritation; abdominal distension and flatulence may also occur. CNS effects such as drowsiness, lightheadedness, ataxia, headache, and paradoxical excitement, hallucinations, nightmares, delirium, and confusion (sometimes with paranoia) occur occasionally (122). Paradoxical excitement can occur after therapeutic use of chloral hydrate in up to 18% of children (20).

Ethchlorvynol adverse effects include GI disturbances, dizziness, headache, unwanted sedation, and other symptoms of CNS depression such as ataxia, facial numbness, blurred vision, and hypotension. Hypersensitivity reactions include skin rashes, urticaria, and, occasionally, thrombocytopenia and cholestatic jaundice. Idiosyncratic reactions include excitement, severe muscular weakness, and syncope without marked hypotension (122).

Glutethimide causes nausea, headache, blurred vision, unwanted sedation, and other CNS effects, such as ataxia, impaired memory, and paradoxical excitement, and occasional skin rashes. Acute hypersensitivity reactions, blood disorders, and exfoliative dermatitis have been reported in rare instances (122).

Hexapropymate has little information available, but unwanted sedation and CNS depression are likely. Thrombocytopenic purpura has been reported (231).

Meprobamate frequently produces drowsiness. Other effects include nausea, vomiting, diarrhea, paresthesia, weakness, and CNS effects such as headache, paradoxical excitement, dizziness, ataxia, and disturbances of vision (122). There may be hypotension, tachycardia, and cardiac dysrhythmias. Hypersensitivity reactions occur occasionally. These may be limited to skin rashes, urticaria, and purpura or may be more severe with angioedema, bronchospasm, or anuria. Erythema multiforme or Stevens-Johnson syndrome and exfoliative or bullous dermatitis have been reported (122). Blood disorders, including agranulocytosis, eosinophilia, leukopenia, thrombocytopenia, and aplastic anemia, have occasionally been reported (122).

Methaqualone produces sedation and CNS depression. Peripheral neuropathies are a significant problem (232). Fixed drug eruptions (233) and erythema multiforme (234) are reported. Platelet aggregation can be impaired with consequent bleeding disorder (219), and the possibility of agranulocytosis has been suggested (235). Drug-induced gout has been reported with methaqualone (236).

Methyprylon frequently causes headache, dizziness, drowsiness, and vertigo. However, nightmares, anxiety, excitation, depression, ataxia, and incoordination have been described. GI complaints, such as nausea, vomiting, heartburn, and changes in bowel habit, are also recognized. Methyprylon may precipitate allergic disorders, pruritus, and skin eruptions (13).

Zolpidem causes dizziness and lightheadedness (5.2%), somnolence (5.2%), headache (3%), and GI disturbance (3.6%) (13). Memory disturbance (anterograde amnesia), nightmares, nocturnal restlessness, depressive syndrome, episodes of confusion, perceptual disturbances or diplopia, tremor, unsteady gait, and falls occurred rarely in long-term clinical trials (237). Zolpidem has been implicated in psychotic reactions characterized by auditory and visual hallucinations as well as delusional thinking (69,238).

Zopiclone commonly produces a mild metallic or bitter aftertaste (13). Less commonly, mild GI disturbances, including nausea and vomiting, or minor mental disturbances, such as irritability, confusion, and depressed mood, have occurred. Allergic manifestations are rare (13).

DIAGNOSTIC TESTS

Routine quantitative drug estimation is not readily available for any of these agents and not indicated for routine management. Core body temperature should be assessed, as hypothermia is common. Measurement of creatine kinase in cases of coma help in the assessment of rhabdomyolysis. Hepatic and renal function tests are indicated.

Electrocardiographic and cardiac monitoring are important in chloral hydrate poisoning. Measurement of partial pressure of carbon dioxide via expired air or arterial blood gases assesses respiratory compromise from sedation. Chest radiography is helpful to assess for noncardiogenic pulmonary edema in a patient with oxygen desaturation. Chloral hydrate is radio-opaque and large amounts may be seen on abdominal radiography (239).

Esophagogastroscopy may be indicated after a large ingestion of chloral hydrate to assess mucosal damage and potential for stricture formation. If bezoar formation in meprobamate poisoning is considered to be contributing to continuing toxicity, esophagogastroscopy could be considered.

Postmortem Considerations

Diffusion of a drug down its concentration gradient may occur after death, typically from sites of high concentration in solid organs into the blood, with resultant artefactual elevation of drug concentration in blood (postmortem redistribution) (240).

Chloral hydrate ingestion produced postmortem trichloroethanol blood concentrations of 119 mg/L (range, 20 to 240 mg/L) in 14 cases (241). In four cases with ingestions of 15 to 30 g, postmortem blood trichloroethanol concentrations averaged 265 mg/L (range, 100 to 640 mg/L) (242). Fatalities have been associated with trichloroethanol concentrations above 250 mg/L (243,244). A death due to chloral hydrate alone had trichloroethanol measured in blood (127 mg/L), urine (128 mg/L), and stomach contents (25 mg total) (245). The blood trichloroethanol concentration found in a case in which laboratory grade chloral hydrate was ingested was 1700 mg/L (244).

The trichloroethanol concentration in a 2-year-old boy who died after ingestion of chloral hydrate, lidocaine, and nitrous oxide was plasma, 79.0 mg/L; urine, 31.0 mg/L; gastric contents, 454.0 mg/L; bile, 111.0 mg/L; vitreous, 40.2 mg/L; cerebrospinal fluid, 68.3 mg/L; and liver, 164.0 mg/kg (246). Perimortal fixation of the GI mucosa was found in a 34-year-old man who died of chloral hydrate overdose (trichloroethanol blood concentration was 52 mg/L) (247). The phenomenon of perimortal fixation should direct suspicion to oral poisoning (247).

Ethchlorvynol postmortem blood concentrations averaged 199 mg/L (range, 14 to 400 mg/L) in 13 deaths (241). Even after embalming, a high concentration of ethchlorvynol (112 mg/L) was identifiable in the bile (248).

Glutethimide postmortem blood concentrations averaged 45 mg/L (range, 10 to 97 mg/L) in 11 cases (242). Death has been associated with a mean blood glutethimide concentration in excess of 40 mg/L (103). The blood concentration in 12 fatalities involving the combination of glutethimide and codeine (*loads*) was 13.9 mg/L (range, 4.6 to 26.4 mg/L) for glutethimide and 1.21 mg/L (range, 0.13 to 4.32 mg/L) for codeine (91).

Meprobamate postmortem blood concentrations averaged 226 mg/L (range, 142 to 346 mg/L) in 12 fatal cases involving doses of 16 to 40 g (63). In a series of 16 deaths attributed solely to meprobamate, the mean blood concentration was 95 mg/L (range, 35 to 240 mg/L) (242). Death has been associated with a mean blood meprobamate concentration of 205 mg/L (103). Postmortem concentrations have ranged from 41 to 397 mg/L (mean, 182 mg/L) (191).

In a death in which the blood concentration was 204.6 mg/L, the maximum concentration was found in the heart (708 mg/kg) suggesting postmortem redistribution (62). In a case of suicidal overdose of meprobamate and sparteine, the blood concentrations of meprobamate and sparteine were found to be 88.2 and 40.4 mg/L, respectively (249).

Methyprylon postmortem blood concentrations were 53 to 66 mg/L (mean, 59 mg/L) in four cases (250). Death has been associated with a mean blood methyprylon concentration of 117 mg/L (103).

Zolpidem postmortem concentrations were blood (subclavian), 4.5 mg/L; blood (iliac), 7.7 mg/L; vitreous humor, 1.6 mg/L; bile, 8.9 mg/L; urine, 1.2 mg/L; liver, 22.6 mg/kg; and gastric contents, 42 mg (224). In a 58-year-old woman, zolpidem concentrations were blood (iliac), 1.6 mg/L; vitreous humor, 0.52 mg/L; bile, 2.6 mg/L; liver, 12 mg/kg; and gastric contents, 0.9 mg (224). The blood/vitreous humor ratios of zolpidem were 2.81 (subclavian) and 4.81 (iliac) in the first case and 3.08 (iliac) in the second case. These ratios, along with the sampling times of blood and vitreous humor for both cases, do not establish either the presence or absence of postmortem drug redistribution (224). Zolpidem concentration in the death of an elderly woman was blood, 7.9 mg/L and urine, 4.1 mg/L (251).

After the death of a 39-year-old obese man, the zolpidem concentrations were 2.91, 1.40, and 2.13 mg/L in the heart blood, peripheral blood, and urine, respectively. The liver had zolpidem present at a concentration of 4.74 mg/kg, and the gastric contents had a total of 172 mg zolpidem. Additional drugs present included hydrocodone and morphine (unconjugated) at

0.16 and 0.04 mg/L, respectively. The cause of death was determined to be multiple drug intoxication (252). In a fatality due to ingestion of zolpidem and acepromazine, zolpidem and acepromazine blood concentrations were 3.29 and 2.40 mg/L, respectively (253). In another fatal case, a 68-year-old woman ingested at least 300 mg of zolpidem, but analyses revealed blood levels of 4.1, 19.3, and 2.3 mg/L of zolpidem, meprobamate, and carisoprodol, respectively (254).

Zopiclone showed little concentration in solid organs and relatively stable postmortem blood concentrations in a 29-year-old, 64-kg woman. Her cardiac blood ethanol was 153 mg/dl and zopiclone blood concentrations ranged from 0.9 to 2.0 mg/L in ten distinct sampling sites (78). In two other cases, the blood concentration of zopiclone was 1.4 to 3.9 mg/L in the blood, 0.81 and 8.7 mg/kg in the liver, and 13.5 and 133.0 mg in the stomach contents (255).

The zopiclone concentration was 1.9 mg/L in postmortem femoral blood after ingestion of 200 to 350 mg by a 72-year-old woman with respiratory debilitation (79). A 72-year-old man died between 4 and 10 hours after the ingestion of 90 mg of zopiclone. Zopiclone concentrations in the femoral blood, cardiac blood, vitreous humor, urine, and bile were 0.254, 0.408, 0.094, 7.33, and 114.7 mg/L, respectively (77). A patient with suicidal ingestion of zopiclone and subsequent drowning had a testicular zopiclone tissue concentration of 2.2 mg/kg (256).

After deliberate self-poisoning with multiple psychoactive drugs, toxicologic analysis demonstrated that the gastric contents contained 44.9 mg/L of zopiclone, 12.8 mg/L of phenobarbital, 10.9 mg/L of chlorpromazine, and 4.8 mg/L of promethazine. The serum contained 0.5 mg/L of zopiclone, 8.6 mg/L of phenobarbital, 0.2 mg/L of chlorpromazine, and 0.3 mg/L of promethazine, and the urine contained 43.0 mg/L of zopiclone, 8.1 mg/L of phenobarbital, 1.3 mg/L of chlorpromazine, and 1.3 mg/L of promethazine. Zopiclone was considered primarily responsible for her death (257).

TREATMENT

The preferred treatment for buspirone, zolpidem, or zopiclone poisoning is entirely supportive with IV access and fluids and maintenance of the airway and ventilation if required. More aggressive respiratory and cardiovascular support is required for the older agents.

Decontamination

Activated charcoal is unlikely to be of value in pure buspirone, zolpidem, or zopiclone poisoning. It may be given to patients who have recently ingested these drugs with other drugs that may benefit from decontamination. Oral activated charcoal within 1 hour of ingestion may be of some value in poisoning with the other drugs named in this chapter. Given the caustic nature of chloral hydrate, gastric lavage is not indicated.

Enhancement of Elimination

Principles of elimination enhancement are discussed in Chapter 78. Based on their volumes of distribution and plasma protein binding (258), there is no indication for extracorporeal techniques in buspirone, zolpidem, or zopiclone poisoning and there are no reports of their use in these poisonings.

There are numerous case reports describing a variety of techniques in ethchlorvynol (259–262), glutethimide (50,263–266), and methaqualone (101,262,267) poisoning, but there is unlikely to be significant additional elimination of these drugs with these techniques. Studies indicate that removal of ethchlorvynol from the overdosed patient by hemoperfusion is limited by extensive distribution into and slow redistribution out of body tissues (268). In a separate study, patients intoxicated with ethchlorvynol and methaqualone did not improve with charcoal hemoperfusion (269). In addition, methaqualone could not be eliminated effectively in animal trials of charcoal hemoperfusion (270), and a large series (116 patients) showed that patients could indeed be managed conservatively (271).

Glutethimide has significant enterohepatic recirculation, thus repeated doses of charcoal may be of benefit (272). The use of repeated oral activated charcoal administration has been reported to shorten half-life in two patients who presented with acute meprobamate ingestions (273) but whether this changed outcome is unclear. However, a series of 31 cases (274) and another of 70 cases (90) of glutethimide overdose also showed that patients can be successfully managed without extracorporeal elimination. Given the quality of supportive care that can be provided in centers capable of performing these techniques, there does not seem to be any indication to use extracorporeal elimination in ethchlorvynol, glutethimide, or methaqualone poisoning.

Methyprylon may have greater elimination during extracorporeal elimination than ethchlorvynol, glutethimide, or methaqualone (258). Methyprylon poisoning has been managed with a variety of extracorporeal techniques (68,106,262,275–279), but it is unclear whether there is an effect on outcome.

For chloral hydrate and meprobamate, which have relatively low plasma protein binding and volumes of distribution of less than or near 1 L/kg, there is the potential for elimination with extracorporeal techniques. There is good evidence that elimination half-lives can be significantly reduced for trichloroethanol by hemodialysis (32,81,280), resin hemoperfusion (281), and combined hemoperfusion and hemodialysis (33). In all these cases there was clinical improvement coincident with the procedure, but it is unknown whether the same outcome would have been achieved with conservative therapy.

It has been estimated that one hemodialysis or hemoperfusion removes 7% to 17% of ingested meprobamate (282). Significant reduction in meprobamate elimination half-life has been demonstrated with charcoal and resin hemoperfusion (97) and continuous arteriovenous hemoperfusion (283), indicating a possible role for these techniques.

Antidotes

The use of flumazenil is addressed in Chapter 57. There is one report of reversal of CNS sedation after chloral hydrate with flumazenil (28), but ventricular dysrhythmias have been precipitated by flumazenil in this context (165) and its use cannot be recommended. There is also one report of reversal of CNS depression by flumazenil after carisoprodol (which is metabolized to meprobamate) (284).

Flumazenil rapidly and effectively reverses sedation due to zolpidem or zopiclone. However, by analogy with the benzodiazepines, patients are likely to wake from their sedation or coma because of the rapid development of tolerance (126) rather than from clearance of the drug. The administration of a benzodiazepine antagonist such as flumazenil in the presence of a benzodiazepine prevents the development of tolerance (285). This could theoretically prolong the effect of the benzodiazepine and be manifested as a prolonged requirement for the antagonist and hospital length of stay. This has occurred after diazepam overdose treated with flumazenil (286,287). In contrast, a much shorter duration of symptoms was seen with similar doses managed before the availability of an antagonist (288). For routine management of uncomplicated zolpidem or zopiclone overdose there is no indication for the use of flumazenil.

Flumazenil (0.1 to 2.0 mg IV) has been given to unconscious patients in whom the drug ingested is unknown (289,290) although this remains controversial (291). Flumazenil should only be given if there is no evidence of proconvulsant/prodysrhythmic drug ingestion, as the removal of the effects of benzodiazepines or other similar drugs that have been coingested may lead to seizures, cardiac dysrhythmia, or death. (165,292–299).

Supportive Care

Noncardiogenic pulmonary edema should be managed along conventional lines (Chapter 33). In the face of continuing hypotension not responding to isotonic fluid resuscitation, inotropic agents may be required (Chapter 37). Adrenergic inotropes should be used with caution, if at all, in chloral hydrate poisoning because of the risk of precipitating a dysrhythmia.

Chloral hydrate–induced dysrhythmias are frequently life-threatening and often resistant to conventional antidysrhythmics (29,158–160). There is good case evidence for the routine use of an IV beta-blocker (propranolol or esmolol) in these patients (25,29,158–160).

Patients with a significant sedative drug overdose should be advised not to drive until potential interference with psychomotor performance has resolved (300). This is at least 24 to 48 hours after discharge for overdose of most of these agents.

Monitoring

Routine observation of vital signs is important, especially Glasgow coma scale, airway patency, and blood pressure. For chloral hydrate, continuous cardiac monitoring until the patient is clearly awake is mandatory. For the older agents, continuous arterial blood pressure monitoring should be considered. Measurement of $PaCO_2$ via expired air or arterial blood gases is the best way to assess respiratory compromise from sedation.

REFERENCES

1. Smith AJ, Whyte IM. New drugs for old: an issue for debate? *Med J Aust* 1988;149(11–12):581–582.
2. Bonifati V, Fabrizio E, Cipriani R, et al. Buspirone in levodopa-induced dyskinesias. *Clin Neuropharmacol* 1994;17(1):73–82.
3. Moss LE, Neppe VM, Drevets WC. Buspirone in the treatment of tardive dyskinesia. *J Clin Psychopharmacol* 1993;13(3):204–209.
4. LeWitt PA, Walters A, Hening W, et al. Persistent movement disorders induced by buspirone. *Mov Disord* 1993;8(3):331–334.
5. Baetz M, Malcolm D. Serotonin syndrome from fluvoxamine and buspirone. *Can J Psychiatry* 1995;40(7):428–429.
6. Bonin B, Vandel P, Vandel S, et al. Serotonin syndrome after sertraline, buspirone and loxapine? *Therapie* 1999;54(2):269–271.
7. Manos GH. Possible serotonin syndrome associated with buspirone added to fluoxetine. *Ann Pharmacother* 2000;34(7–8):871–874.
8. Spigset O, Adielsson G. Combined serotonin syndrome and hyponatraemia caused by a citalopram-buspirone interaction. *Int Clin Psychopharmacol* 1997;12(1):61–63.
9. Hojer J, Personne M, Skagius AS, et al. [Serotonin syndrome. Several cases of this often overlooked diagnosis]. *Lakartidningen* 2002;99(18):2054–2060.
10. Lantz MS. Serotonin syndrome. A common but often unrecognized psychiatric condition. *Geriatrics* 2001;56(1):52–53.
11. Ritchie EC, Bridenbaugh RH, Jabbari B. Acute generalized myoclonus following buspirone administration. *J Clin Psychiatry* 1988;49(6):242–243.
12. Bostwick JM, Jaffee MS. Buspirone as an antidote to SSRI-induced bruxism in 4 cases. *J Clin Psychiatry* 1999;60(12):857–860.
13. Dollery CT. *Therapeutic drugs*. CD-ROM DATABASE release 1.0 ed. London: Churchill Livingstone, 1999.
14. Tiller JW, Burrows GD, O'Sullivan BT. Buspirone overdose. *Med J Aust* 1989;150(1):54.
15. Goetz CM, Krenzelok EP, Lopez G, et al. Buspirone toxicity: a prospective study. *Ann Emerg Med* 1990;19:630.
16. Napoliello MJ, Domantay AG. Buspirone: a worldwide update. *Br J Psychiatry Suppl* 1991;(12):40–44.
17. Cantor CH. Substances involved in fatal drug overdoses in Brisbane, 1979–1987. *Acta Psychiatr Scand Suppl* 1989;354:69–71.
18. Buckley NA, Whyte IM, Dawson AH, et al. Correlations between prescriptions and drugs taken in self-poisoning. Implications for prescribers and drug regulation. *Med J Aust* 1995;162(4):194–197.
19. Pershad J, Palmisano P, Nichols M. Chloral hydrate: the good and the bad. *Pediatr Emerg Care* 1999;15(6):432–435.
20. Lipshitz M, Marino BL, Sanders ST. Chloral hydrate side effects in young children: causes and management. *Heart Lung* 1993;22(5):408–414.
21. Laptook AR, Rosenfeld CR. Chloral hydrate toxicity in a preterm infant. *Pediatr Pharmacol (New York)* 1984;4(3):161–165.
22. Seger D, Schwartz G. Chloral hydrate: a dangerous sedative for overdose patients? *Pediatr Emerg Care* 1994;10(6):349–350.
23. Granoff DM, McDaniel DB, Borkowf SP. Cardiorespiratory dysrest following aspiration of chloral hydrate. *Am J Dis Child* 1971;122(2):170–171.
24. Baselt RC, Cravey RH. Chloral hydrate. In: *Disposition of toxic drugs and chemicals in man*. Chicago: Year Book Medical Publishers, Inc., 1989:144–147.
25. Sing K, Erickson T, Amitai Y, et al. Chloral hydrate toxicity from oral and intravenous administration. *J Toxicol Clin Toxicol* 1996;34(1):101–106.
26. Fetu D, Carel N, Fossier T, et al. [Chloral hydrate poisoning]. *Ann Fr Anesth Reanim* 1994;13(5):745–748.
27. Jonville AP, Mesny J, Quillet L, et al. [Accidental chloral hydrate poisoning]. *J Toxicol Clin Exp* 1991;11(6):337–341.
28. Donovan KL, Fisher DJ. Reversal of chloral hydrate overdose with flumazenil. *BMJ* 1989;298(6682):1253.
29. Brown AM, Cade JF. Cardiac dysrhythmias after chloral hydrate overdose. *Med J Aust* 1980;1(1):28–29.
30. Vellar ID, Richardson JP, Doyle JC, et al. Gastric necrosis: a rare complication of chloral hydrate intoxication. *Br J Surg* 1972;59(4):317–319.
31. Gleich GJ, Mongan ES, Vaules DW. Esophageal stricture following chloral hydrate poisoning. *JAMA* 1967;201(4):266–267.
32. Stalker NE, Gambertoglio JG, Fukumitsu CJ, et al. Acute massive chloral hydrate intoxication treated with hemodialysis: a clinical pharmacokinetic analysis. *J Clin Pharmacol* 1978;18(2–3):136–142.
33. Ludwigs U, Divino Filho JC, Magnusson A, et al. Suicidal chloral hydrate poisoning. *J Toxicol Clin Toxicol* 1996;34(1):97–99.
34. Gerretsen M, de Groot G, van Heijst AN, et al. Chloral hydrate poisoning: its mechanism and therapy. *Vet Hum Toxicol* 1979;21[Suppl]:53–56.
35. Gauillard J, Cheref S, Vacherontrystram MN, et al. [Chloral hydrate: a hypnotic best forgotten?] *Encephale* 2002;28(3 Pt 1):200–204.
36. Jastak JT, Pallasch T. Death after chloral hydrate sedation: report of case. *J Am Dent Assoc* 1988;116(3):345–348.
37. King K, England JF. Chloral hydrate (Noctec) overdose. *Med J Aust* 1983;2(6):260.
38. Millhouse J, Davies DM, Wraith SR. Chronic ethchlorvynol intoxication. *Lancet* 1966;2(7475):1251–1252.
39. Flemenbaum A, Gunby B. Ethchlorvynol (Placidyl) abuse and withdrawal (review of clinical picture and report of 2 cases). *Dis Nerv Syst* 1971;32(3):188–192.
40. Harenko A. On special traits of acute ethchlorvynol poisoning. *Acta Neurol Scand* 1967;43[Suppl].
41. Kathpalia SC, Haslitt JH, Lim VS. Charcoal hemoperfusion for treatment of ethchlorvynol overdose. *Artif Organs* 1983;7(2):246–248.
42. Glauser FL, Smith WR, Caldwell A, et al. Ethchlorvynol (Placidyl)-induced pulmonary edema. *Ann Intern Med* 1976;84(1):46–48.
43. Schottstaedt MW, Nicotra MB, Rivera M. Placidyl abuse: a dimorphic picture. *Crit Care Med* 1981;9(9):677–679.
44. Cravey RH, Baselt RC. Studies of the body distribution of ethchlorvynol. *J Forensic Sci* 1968;13(4):532–536.
45. Teehan BP, Maher JF, Carey JJ, et al. Acute ethchlorvynol (Placidyl) intoxication. *Ann Intern Med* 1970;72(6):875–882.
46. Greenblatt DJ, Allen MD, Harmatz JS, et al. Correlates of outcome following acute glutethimide overdosage. *J Forensic Sci* 1979;24(1):76–86.
47. Krell I, Jordan T, Queck G, et al. [A contribution to acute glutethimide (Elrodorm) intoxication]. *Z Gesamte Inn Med* 1975;30(2):81–83.
48. Myers RR, Stockard JJ. Neurologic and electroencephalographic correlates in glutethimide intoxication. *Clin Pharmacol Ther* 1975;17(2):212–220.
49. Baselt RC, Cravey RH. Glutethimide. In: *Disposition of toxic drugs and chemicals in man*. Chicago: Year Book Medical Publishers, Inc., 1989:379–383.
50. Rosenbaum JL, Kramer MS, Raja R. Resin hemoperfusion for acute drug intoxication. *Arch Intern Med* 1976;136(3):263–266.
51. Noirfalise A. [5 cases of suspected hexapropymate poisoning]. *Eur J Toxicol* 1971;4(1):50–52.
52. Ellenhorn MJ, Schonwald S, Ordog G, et al. *Ellenhorn's medical toxicology: diagnosis and treatment of human poisoning*, 2nd ed. Baltimore: Williams & Wilkins, 1997.
53. Robbins G, Brown AK. Hexapropymate self-poisoning. *BMJ* 1978;1(6127):1593.
54. Gustafsson LL, Berg A, Magnusson A, et al. Hexapropymate self-poisoning causes severe and long-lasting clinical symptoms. *Med Toxicol Adverse Drug Exp* 1989;4(4):295–301.
55. Yamarellos P, Dimopoulos G. Three cases of hexapropymate (Merinax) poisoning. *Bulletin of the International Association of Forensic Toxicology* 1979;14(3):29–30.
56. Hassoun A, Van Binst R. Fatal hexapropymate intoxication. *Bull Int Assoc Forensic Toxicol* 1979;14(3):28.

57. Allen MD, Greenblatt DJ, Noel BJ. Meprobamate overdosage: a continuing problem. *Clin Toxicol* 1977;11(5):501–515.
58. Freund LG. Severe meprobamate intoxication treated by hemoperfusion over amberlite resin. *Artif Organs* 1981;5(1):80–81.
59. Lobo PI, Spyker D, Surratt P, et al. Use of hemodialysis in meprobamate overdosage. *Clin Nephrol* 1977;7(2):73–75.
60. Eeckhout E, Huyghens L, Loef B, et al. Meprobamate poisoning, hypotension and the Swan-Ganz catheter. *Intensive Care Med* 1988;14(4):437–438.
61. Pontal PG, Bismuth C, Baud F, et al. [Respective roles of gastric lavage, haemodialysis, haemoperfusion, diuresis and hepatic metabolism in the elimination of a massive meprobamate overdose (author's transl)]. *Nouv Presse Med* 1982;11(20):1557–1558.
62. Kintz P, Tracqui A, Mangin P, et al. Fatal meprobamate self-poisoning. *Am J Forensic Med Pathol* 1988;9(2):139–140.
63. Felby S. Concentrations of meprobamate in the blood and liver following fatal meprobamate poisoning. *Acta Pharmacol Toxicol (Copenh)* 1970;28(5):334–337.
64. Faulkner TP, Hayden JH, Mehta CM, et al. Dose-response studies on tolerance to multiple doses of secobarbital and methaqualone in a polydrug abuse population. *Clin Toxicol* 1979;15(1):23–37.
65. Baggish D, Gray S, Jatlow P, et al. Treatment of methaqualone overdose with resin hemoperfusion. *Yale J Biol Med* 1981;54(2):147–150.
66. Kurz RW, Hainz R, Gremmel F, et al. [Dangerous intoxication from extreme serum concentrations of methaqualone metabolites. Detection and quantification of biosynthesis with gas chromatography-mass spectrometry]. *Anaesthesist* 1995;44(12):863–868.
67. Reidt WU. Fatal poisoning with methyprylon (Noludar), a nonbarbiturate sedative. *N Engl J Med* 1956;255:231–232.
68. Xanthaky G, Freireich AW, Matusiak W, et al. Hemodialysis in methyprylon poisoning. *JAMA* 1966;198(11):1212–1213.
69. Markowitz JS, Brewerton TD. Zolpidem-induced psychosis. *Ann Clin Psychiatry* 1996;8(2):89–91.
70. Garnier R, Guerault E, Muzard D, et al. Acute zolpidem poisoning—analysis of 344 cases. *J Toxicol Clin Toxicol* 1994;32(4):391–404.
71. Wyss PA, Radovanovic D, Meier-Abt PJ. [Acute overdose of Zolpidem (Stilnox)]. *Schweiz Med Wochenschr* 1996;126(18):750–756.
72. Hamad A, Sharma N. Acute zolpidem overdose leading to coma and respiratory failure. *Intensive Care Med* 2001;27(7):1239.
73. Kurta DL, Myers LB, Krenzelok EP. Zolpidem (Ambien): a pediatric case series. *J Toxicol Clin Toxicol* 1997;35(5):453–457.
74. Kuitunen T, Mattila MJ, Seppala T. Actions and interactions of hypnotics on human performance: single doses of zopiclone, triazolam and alcohol. *Int Clin Psychopharmacol* 1990;5[Suppl 2]:115–130.
75. Regouby Y, Delomez G, Tisserant A. [First-degree heart block caused by voluntary zopiclone poisoning]. *Therapie* 1990;45(2):162.
76. Royer-Morrot MJ, Rambourg M, Jacob I, et al. Determination of zopiclone in plasma using column liquid chromatography with ultraviolet detection. *J Chromatogr* 1992;581(2):297–299.
77. Meatherall RC. Zopiclone fatality in a hospitalized patient. *J Forensic Sci* 1997;42(2):340–343.
78. Pounder DJ, Davies JI. Zopiclone poisoning: tissue distribution and potential for postmortem diffusion. *Forensic Sci Int* 1994;65(3):177–183.
79. Bramness JG, Arnestad M, Karinen R, et al. Fatal overdose of zopiclone in an elderly woman with bronchogenic carcinoma. *J Forensic Sci* 2001;46(5):1247–1249.
80. Kaplan HL, Forney RB, Hughes FW, et al. Chloral hydrate and alcohol metabolism in human subjects. *J Forensic Sci* 1967;12(3):295–304.
81. Buur T, Larsson R, Norlander B. Pharmacokinetics of chloral hydrate poisoning treated with hemodialysis and hemoperfusion. *Acta Med Scand* 1988;223(3):269–274.
82. Cummins LM, Martin YC, Scherfling EE. Serum and urine levels of ethchlorvynol in man. *J Pharm Sci* 1971;60(2):261–263.
83. Kolpek JH, Pdysr MD, Marshall ML, et al. Ethchlorvynol pharmacokinetics during long-term administration in a patient with hyperlipidemia and hypothyroidism. *Pharmacotherapy* 1986;6(6):323–327.
84. Kelner MJ, Bailey DN. Ethchlorvynol ingestion: interpretation of blood concentrations and clinical findings. *J Toxicol Clin Toxicol* 1983;21(3):399–408.
85. Pochopien DJ. Rate of decrease in serum ethchlorvynol concentrations after extreme overdosage—a case study. *Clin Chem* 1975;21(7):894–895.
86. Westerfield BT, Blouin RA. Ethchlorvynol intoxication. *South Med J* 1977;70(8):1019–1020.
87. Bailey DN, Shaw RF. Ethchlorvynol ingestion in San Diego County: a 14-year review of cases with blood concentrations and findings. *J Anal Toxicol* 1990;14(6):348–352.
88. Curry SH, Gordon JS, Riddall D, et al. Disposition of glutethimide in man. *Clin Pharmacol Ther* 1971;12(5):849–857.
89. Mankowski W, Krupinski B, Skret K. [Suicidal attempts with old (currently unused) drug]. *Przegl Lek* 2002;59(4–5):390–391.
90. Chazan JA, Garella S. Glutethimide intoxication. A prospective study of 70 patients treated conservatively without hemodialysis. *Arch Intern Med* 1971;128(2):215–219.
91. Bailey DN, Shaw RF. Blood concentrations and clinical findings in nonfatal and fatal intoxications involving glutethimide and codeine. *J Toxicol Clin Toxicol* 1985;23(7–8):557–570.
92. Kennedy KA, Ambre JJ, Fischer LJ. A selected ion monitoring method for glutethimide and six metabolites: application to blood and urine from humans intoxicated with glutethimide. *Biomed Mass Spectrom* 1978;5(12):679–685.
93. Sato S, Baud FJ, Bismuth C, et al. Arterial-venous plasma concentration differences of meprobamate in acute human poisonings. *Hum Toxicol* 1986;5(4):243–248.
94. Meyer MC, Melikian AP, Straughn AB. Relative bioavailability of meprobamate tablets in humans. *J Pharm Sci* 1978;67(9):1290–1293.
95. Dinovo EC, Gottschalk LA, McGuire FL, et al. Analysis of results of toxicological examinations performed by coroners' or medical examiners' laboratories in 2000 drug-involved deaths in nine major U.S. cities. *Clin Chem* 1976;22(6):847–850.
96. Maddock RK Jr., Bloomer HA. Meprobamate overdosage. Evaluation of its severity and methods of treatment. *JAMA* 1967;201(13):999–1003.
97. Jacobsen D, Wiik-Larsen E, Saltvedt E, et al. Meprobamate kinetics during and after terminated hemoperfusion in acute intoxications. *J Toxicol Clin Toxicol* 1987;25(4):317–331.
98. Tirot P, Hdysry P, Bouachour G, et al. [Electroencephalographic silence after intoxication with a carbamate tranquilizer]. *J Toxicol Clin Exp* 1991;11(7–8):417–420.
99. Brown SS, Goenechea S. Methaqualone: metabolic, kinetic, and clinical pharmacologic observations. *Clin Pharmacol Ther* 1973;14(3):314–324.
100. Bailey DN, Jatlow PI. Methaqualone overdose: analytical methodology, and the significance of serum drug concentrations. *Clin Chem* 1973;19(6):615–620.
101. Proudfoot AT, Noble J, Nimmo J, et al. Peritoneal dialysis and haemodialysis in methaqualone (Mandrax) poisoning. *Scott Med J* 1967;13(7):232–236.
102. Bailey DN. Methaqualone ingestion: evaluation of present status. *J Anal Toxicol* 1981;5(6):279–282.
103. Bailey DN, Shaw RF. Interpretation of blood glutethimide, meprobamate, and methyprylon concentrations in nonfatal and fatal intoxications involving a single drug. *J Toxicol Clin Toxicol* 1983;20(2):133–145.
104. Bridges RR, Peat MA. Gas-liquid chromatographic analysis of methyprylon and its major metabolite (2,4-dioxo-3,3-diethyl-t-methyl-1,2,3,4-tetrahydropyridine) in an overdose case. *J Anal Toxicol* 1979;3:21–25.
105. Contos DA, Dixon KF, Guthrie RM, et al. Nonlinear elimination of methyprylon (Noludar) in an overdosed patient: correlation of clinical effects with plasma concentration. *J Pharm Sci* 1991;80(8):768–771.
106. Pancorbo AS, Palagi PA, Piecoro JJ, et al. Hemodialysis in methyprylon overdose. Some pharmacokinetic considerations. *JAMA* 1977;237(5):470–471.
107. Salva P, Costa J. Clinical pharmacokinetics and pharmacodynamics of zolpidem. Therapeutic implications. *Clin Pharmacokinet* 1995;29(3):142–153.
108. Logan BK, Couper FJ. Zolpidem and driving impairment. *J Forensic Sci* 2001;46(1):105–110.
109. Lheureux P, Debailleul G, De Witte O, et al. Zolpidem intoxication mimicking narcotic overdose: response to flumazenil. *Hum Exp Toxicol* 1990;9(2):105–107.
110. Fernandez C, Maradeix V, Gimenez F, et al. Pharmacokinetics of zopiclone and its enantiomers in Caucasian young healthy volunteers. *Drug Metab Dispos* 1993;21(6):1125–1128.
111. De Deyn PP, Macdonald RL. Effects of non-sedative anxiolytic drugs on responses to GABA and on diazepam-induced enhancement of these responses on mouse neurones in cell culture. *Br J Pharmacol* 1988;95(1):109–120.
112. Goeders NE, Ritz MC, Kuhar MJ. Buspirone enhances benzodiazepine receptor binding in vivo. *Neuropharmacology* 1988;27(3):275–280.
113. Goldberg ME, Salama AI, Patel JB, et al. Novel non-benzodiazepine anxiolytics. *Neuropharmacology* 1983;22(12B):1499–1504.
114. Schweizer E, Rickels K. Failure of buspirone to manage benzodiazepine withdrawal. *Am J Psychiatry* 1986;143(12):1590–1592.
115. Matheson GK, Raess BU, Tunnicliff G. Effects of repeated doses of azapirones on rat brain 5-HT1A receptors and plasma corticosterone levels. *Gen Pharmacol* 1996;27(2):355–361.
116. Troisi JR, Critchfield TS, Griffiths RR. Buspirone and lorazepam abuse liability in humans: behavioral effects, subjective effects and choice. *Behav Pharmacol* 1993;4(3):217–230.
117. Gustafson A, Svensson SE, Ugander L. Cardiac dysrhythmias in chloral hydrate poisoning. *Acta Med Scand* 1977;201(3):227–230.
118. Cherian PT, Casement J, Cherian VT, et al. Management of chloral hydrate overdose. *Br J Intensive Care* 2000;10(4):136–138.
119. Fischer P, Glauser FL, Millen JE, et al. The effects of ethchlorvynol on pulmonary alveolar membrane permeability. *Am Rev Respir Dis* 1977;116(5):901–906.
120. Wysolmerski R, Lagunoff D, Dahms T. Ethchlorvynol-induced pulmonary edema in rats. An ultrastructural study. *Am J Pathol* 1984;115(3):447–457.
121. Garza-Perez J, Lal S, Lopez E. Addiction to ethchlorvynol. A report of two cases. *Med Serv J Can* 1967;23(5):775–778.
122. Sweetman S. *Martindale: the complete drug reference*. London: Pharmaceutical Press. Electronic ed. expires 03/2003. Greenwood Village, Colorado: MICROMEDEX, 2003.
123. Skerritt JH, Johnston GA. Interactions of some anaesthetic, convulsant, and anticonvulsant drugs at GABA-benzodiazepine receptor-ionophore complexes in rat brain synaptosomal membranes. *Neurochem Res* 1983;8(10):1351–1362.
124. Hansen AR, Kennedy KA, Ambre JJ, et al. Glutethimide poisoning. A metabolite contributes to morbidity and mortality. *N Engl J Med* 1975;292(5):250–252.
125. Curry SC, Hubbard JM, Gerkin R, et al. Lack of correlation between plasma 4-hydroxyglutethimide and severity of coma in acute glutethimide poison-

ing. A case report and brief review of the literature. *Med Toxicol Adverse Drug Exp* 1987;2(4):309–316.
126. Ingum J, Bjorklund R, Volden R, et al. Development of acute tolerance after oral doses of diazepam and flunitrazepam. *Psychopharmacology (Berl)* 1994;113(3–4):304–310.
127. Andresen BD, Davis FT, Templeton JL, et al. Toxicity of alpha-phenyl-gamma-butyrolactone, a metabolite of glutethimide in human urine. *Res Commun Chem Pathol Pharmacol* 1977;18(3):439–451.
128. Jones AH, Mayberry JF. Chronic glutethimide abuse. *Br J Clin Pract* 1986;40(5):213.
129. Bauer MS, Fus AF, Hanich RF, et al. Glutethimide intoxication and withdrawal. *Am J Psychiatry* 1988;145(4):530–531.
130. DiGiacomo JN, King CL. Codeine and glutethimide addiction. *Int J Addict* 1970;5(2):279–285.
131. Sramek JJ, Khajawall A. "Loads." *N Engl J Med* 1981;305(4):231.
132. Loghin F, Popa DS, Socaciu C. Influence of glutethimide on rat brain mononucleotides by sub-chronic codeine treatment. *J Cell Mol Med* 2001;5(4):409–416.
133. Ludwig BJ, Potterfield JR. The pharmacology of propanediol carbamates. *Adv Pharmacol Chemother* 1971;9:173–240.
134. Landier C, Lanotte R, Legras A, et al. [State of shock during acute meprobamate poisoning. 6 cases]. *Ann Fr Anesth Reanim* 1994;13(3):407–411.
135. Hicks TP, Kaneko T, Oka JI. Receptive-field size of S1 cortical neurones is altered by methaqualone via a GABA mechanism. *Can J Neurol Sci* 1990;17(1):30–34.
136. Leadbetter MI, Parmar SS. Serotonin as a facilitatory neurotransmitter in the anticonvulsant activity of methaqualone. *Physiol Behav* 1989;46(1):105–106.
137. Suzuki T, Koike Y, Chida Y, et al. Cross-physical dependence of several drugs in methaqualone-dependent rats. *Jpn J Pharmacol* 1988;46(4):403–410.
138. Inaba DS, Ray GR, Newmeyer JA, et al. Methaqualone abuse. "Luding out." *JAMA* 1973;224(11):1505–1509.
139. Pascarelli EF. Methaqualone abuse, the quiet epidemic. *JAMA* 1973;224(11):1512–1514.
140. Rudolph U, Crestani F, Mohler H. GABA(A) receptor subtypes: dissecting their pharmacological functions. *Trends Pharmacol Sci* 2001;22(4):188–194.
141. Doble A. New insights into the mechanism of action of hypnotics. *J Psychopharmacol* 1999;13[4 Suppl 1]:S11–S20.
142. Crestani F, Martin JR, Mohler H, et al. Mechanism of action of the hypnotic zolpidem in vivo. *Br J Pharmacol* 2000;131(7):1251–1254.
143. Depoortere H, Zivkovic B, Lloyd KG, et al. Zolpidem, a novel nonbenzodiazepine hypnotic. I. Neuropharmacological and behavioral effects. *J Pharmacol Exp Ther* 1986;237(2):649–658.
144. Patat A, Naef MM, van Gessel E, et al. Flumazenil antagonizes the central effects of zolpidem, an imidazopyridine hypnotic. *Clin Pharmacol Ther* 1994;56(4):430–436.
145. Hypnotic dependence: zolpidem and zopiclone too. *Prescrire Int* 2001;10(51):15.
146. Liappas IA, Malitas PN, Dimopoulos NP, et al. Zolpidem dependence case series: possible neurobiological mechanisms and clinical management. *J Psychopharmacol* 2003;17(1):131–135.
147. Bdysrero-Hernandez FJ, Ruiz-Veguilla M, Lopez-Lopez MI, et al. [Epileptic seizures as a sign of abstinence from chronic consumption of zolpidem]. *Rev Neurol* 2002;34(3):253–256.
148. Zolpidem: now classified as a psychotropic at risk of abuse. *Prescrire Int* 2003;12(64):60.
149. Julou L, Blanchard JC, Dreyfus JF. Pharmacological and clinical studies of cyclopyrrolones: zopiclone and suriclone. *Pharmacol Biochem Behav* 1985;23(4):653–659.
150. Costa E, Guidotti A. Diazepam binding inhibitor (DBI): a peptide with multiple biological actions. *Life Sci* 1991;49(5):325–344.
151. Blanchard JC, Boireau A, Julou L. Brain receptors and zopiclone. *Pharmacology* 1983;27[Suppl 2]:59–69.
152. Jones IR, Sullivan G. Physical dependence on zopiclone: case reports. *BMJ* 1998;316:117.
153. Harter C, Piffl-Boniolo E, Rave-Schwank M. [Development of drug withdrawal delirium after dependence on zolpidem and zoplicone]. *Psychiatr Prax* 1999;26(6):309.
154. Catalano G, Catalano MC, Hanley PF. Seizures associated with buspirone overdose: case report and literature review. *Clin Neuropharmacol* 1998;21(6):347–350.
155. Langlois RP, Paquette D. Sustained bradycardia during fluvoxamine and buspirone intoxication. *Can J Psychiatry* 1994;39(2):126–127.
156. Goldfrank L, Weisman R, Flomenbaum N. Teaching the recognition of odors. *Ann Emerg Med* 1982;11(12):684–686.
157. Gaulier JM, Merle G, Lacassie E, et al. Fatal intoxications with chloral hydrate. *J Forensic Sci* 2001;46(6):1507–1509.
158. Graham SR, Day RO, Lee R, et al. Overdose with chloral hydrate: a pharmacological and therapeutic review. *Med J Aust* 1988;149(11–12):686–688.
159. Zahedi A, Grant MH, Wong DT. Successful treatment of chloral hydrate cardiac toxicity with propranolol. *Am J Emerg Med* 1999;17(5):490–491.
160. Bowyer K, Glasser SP. Chloral hydrate overdose and cardiac dysrhythmias. *Chest* 1980;77(2):232–235.
161. Young JB, Vandermolen LA, Pratt CM. Torsade de pointes: an unusual manifestation of chloral hydrate poisoning. *Am Heart J* 1986;112(1):181–184.
162. Nordenberg A, Delisle G, Izukawa T. Cardiac dysrhythmia in a child due to chloral hydrate ingestion. *Pediatrics* 1971;47(1):134–135.
163. Wiseman HM, Hampel G. Cardiac dysrhythmias due to chloral hydrate poisoning. *BMJ* 1978;2(6142):960.
164. Paret G, Kassem R, Vardi A, et al. [Chloral hydrate—is it safe?] *Harefuah* 1996;130(1):14–5, 71.
165. Short TG, Maling T, Galletly DC. Ventricular dysrhythmia precipitated by flumazenil. *Br Med J (Clin Res Ed)* 1988;296(6628):1070–1071.
166. Bailey B, Loebstein R, Lai C, et al. Two cases of chlorinated hydrocarbon-associated myocardial ischemia. *Vet Hum Toxicol* 1997;39(5):298–301.
167. Lee DC, Vassalluzzo C. Acute gastric perforation in a chloral hydrate overdose. *Am J Emerg Med* 1998;16(5):545–546.
168. Chamberlain JM, Klein-Schwartz W, Gorman R. Pressure necrosis following ethchlorvynol overdose. *Am J Emerg Med* 1990;8(5):467–468.
169. Greenberg DA, Simon RP. Flexor and extensor postures in sedative drug-induced coma. *Neurology* 1982;32(4):448–451.
170. Voto SJ, Drake ME Jr. Acute urinary retention precipitated by ethchlorvynol overdose. *J Natl Med Assoc* 1986;78(9):896–897.
171. Fell RH, Dendy PR. Severe hypothermia and respiratory dysrest in diazepam and glutethimide intoxication. *Anaesthesia* 1968;23(4):636–640.
172. Schleissner LA. Glutethimide intoxication with prolonged coma and hyperpyrexia treated with methylphenidate. *Calif Med* 1966;105(1):41–44.
173. Kovacs T, Pall D, Abafalvi Z, et al. [Acute toxicological cases during a ten-year period in our clinic]. *Orv Hetil* 2002;143(2):71–76.
174. Burdon JG, Cade JF. "Barbiturate burns" caused by glutethimide. *Med J Aust* 1979;1(3):101–102.
175. Leavell UW Jr., Coyer JR, Taylor RJ. Dermographism and erythematous lines in glutethimide overdose. *Arch Dermatol* 1972;106(5):724–725.
176. Penn AS, Rowland LP, Fraser DW. Drugs, coma, and myoglobinuria. *Arch Neurol* 1972;26(4):336–343.
177. Brown DG, Hammill JF. Glutethimide poisoning: unilateral pupillary abnormalities. *N Engl J Med* 1971;285(14):806.
178. Valsamis MP, Mancall E. Toxic cerebellar degeneration. *Hum Pathol* 1973;4(4):513–520.
179. Filippini L. [Methemoglobinemia in Doriden poisoning]. *Schweiz Med Wochenschr* 1965;95(47):1618–1619.
180. Pedersen JG, Kristensen IH. [Hypocalcemic seizures after misuse of glutethimide (Doriden)]. *Ugeskr Laeger* 1976;138(20):1202–1204.
181. Lanzoni V. Drug-induced coma. *Surg Clin North Am* 1968;48(2):395–401.
182. Gluckman JC, Bismuth C, Frejaville JP. [Acute massive poisoning by meprobamate]. *Coeur Med Interne* 1969;8(1):97–105.
183. Hulting J, Thorstrand C. Hemodynamic effects of norepinephrine in severe hypnotic drug poisoning with arterial hypotension. *Acta Med Scand* 1972;192(5):447–453.
184. Lhoste F, Lemaire F, Rapin M. Treatment of hypotension in meprobamate poisoning. *N Engl J Med* 1977;296(17):1004.
185. Longchal J, Tenaillon A, Trunet P, et al. [Meprobamate poisoning with cardiac insufficiency. Treatment with dobutamine]. *Nouv Presse Med* 1978;7(16):1408–1409.
186. Jouglard J, Imbert M, Fogliani J. [A case of fatal poisoning by Equanil]. *Mars Med* 1970;107(3):217–224.
187. Peyriere H, Gervais C, Flangakis S, et al. [Acute voluntary poisoning with meprobamate may still be fatal: case report]. *Therapie* 1998;53(6):604–606.
188. Cosic V, Kop P, Kusic R. [Resuscitation after acute accidental hypothermia and acute drug poisoning]. *Vojnosanit Pregl* 1969;26(11):547–551.
189. Bonsing E. [Re-warming of 3 poisoned patients with profound accidental hypothermia]. *Ugeskr Laeger* 1977;139(12):706–709.
190. Jacobsen D, Frederichsen PS, Knutsen KM, et al. Clinical course in acute self-poisonings: a prospective study of 1125 consecutively hospitalised adults. *Hum Toxicol* 1984;3(2):107–116.
191. Gaillard Y, Billault F, Pepin G. Meprobamate overdosage: a continuing problem. Sensitive GC-MS quantitation after solid phase extraction in 19 fatal cases. *Forensic Sci Int* 1997;86(3):173–180.
192. Plum F, Posner JB. The diagnosis of stupor and coma. *Contemp Neurol Ser* 1972;10:1–286.
193. Gaultier M, Fournier E, Bismuth C, et al. [Acute poisoning by meprobamate. Apropos of 141 cases]. *Bull Mem Soc Med Hop Paris* 1968;119(8):675–705.
194. Mellerio F. [EEG in the prognosis of toxic coma: reflections apropos of unusual data]. *Rev Electroencephalogr Neurophysiol Clin* 1982;12(4):325–331.
195. Jeanmet A, Guyonnaud C, Duwoos H, et al. [Myocardial and muscular damage during drug poisoning]. *Coeur Med Interne* 1978;17(1):151.
196. Bertran F, de la Sayette V, Lacotte J, et al. [Acute rhabdomyolysis and meprobamate poisoning]. *Therapie* 1992;47(5):444.
197. Godtfredsen J, Poulsen J. [Volkmann's contracture after prolonged unconsciousness. A case after meprobamate and chlorprothixene poisoning]. *Ugeskr Laeger* 1968;130(6):236–237.
198. Goulon M, Barois A, Gajdos P, et al. [Physiopathologic and therapeutic problems raised by acute toxic pulmonary edema]. *Poumon Coeur* 1970;26(9):1039–1065.
199. Axelson JA, Hagaman JF. Meprobamate poisoning and pulmonary edema. *N Engl J Med* 1977;296(25):1481.
200. Bourry J, Sainty JM, Roux JJ, et al. [Acute pancreatitis in the course of meprobamate poisoning. Possible role of pressor amine therapy]. *Nouv Presse Med* 1976;5(30):1918.
201. Laaban JP, Bodenan P, Marty M, et al. Esophageal spasm in a case of drug overdose. *N Engl J Med* 1984;311(22):1443.
202. Schwartz HS. Acute meprobamate poisoning with gastrotomy and removal of a drug-containing mass. *N Engl J Med* 1976;295(21):1177–1178.
203. Meprobamate & bezoar formation. *Ann Emerg Med* 1987;16(4):472–473.
204. Lange E, Rossner M. [Delirious condition of excitation after meprobamate

intoxication—intoxication effect or inanition delirium?]. *Psychiatr Neurol Med Psychol (Leipz)* 1966;18(12):446–450.
205. Daiute PC, Martinak JF. Methaqualone coma. *J Maine Med Assoc* 1974;65(5):101–102.
206. Gaultier M, Pebay-Peyroula FC, Griffoul E, et al. [Acute poisoning due to Mandrax]. *Eur J Toxicol* 1972;5(2):144–149.
207. Jouglard J, Airaudo CB, Di Costanzo J, et al. [Acute poisoning by Mandrax. Evaluation of known cases at the Marseilles Poison Control Center (88 cases in 27 months)]. *Mars Med* 1972;109(9):565–567.
208. Ibe K. [Acute methaqualone poisoning. II. Clinical picture, pathophysiology and therapy]. *Arch Toxikol* 1966;21(5):289–309.
209. Zabransky S. [Eatan poisoning in childhood. Dyskinetic, deliriant syndrome with unilateral symptoms and cerebellar deficit]. *Anasthesiol Intensivmed Prax* 1975;10(1):105–108.
210. Roman D. Schizophrenia-like psychosis following 'Mandrax' overdose. *Br J Psychiatry* 1972;121(565):619–620.
211. Mack RB. Methaqualone intoxication. *N C Med J* 1981;42(11):796.
212. Abboud RT, Freedman MT, Rogers RM, et al. Methaqualone poisoning with muscular hyperactivity necessitating the use of curare. *Chest* 1974;65(2):204–205.
213. Pan HY, Huang CY. Alternating skew deviation associated with Mandrax overdosage. *Aust N Z J Med* 1984;14(3):265–266.
214. Thamdrup B, Jensen S, Ostergaard OV. [Methaqualone poisoning treated with hemoperfusion]. *Ugeskr Laeger* 1983;145(18):1380.
215. Johnstone RE, Manitsas GT, Smith EJ. Apnea following methaqualone ingestion. Report of a case. *Ohio State Med J* 1971;67(11):1018–1020.
216. Holmberg G, Wiklund PE. [Treatment of acute poisoning. 8. Intoxications with preparations containing methaqualone]. *Lakartidningen* 1971;68[Suppl].
217. Oh TE, Gordon TP, Burden PW. Unilateral pulmonary oedema and "Mandrax" poisoning. *Anaesthesia* 1978;33(8):719–721.
218. Trese M. Retinal hemorrhage caused by overdose of methaqualone (Quaalude). *Am J Ophthalmol* 1981;91(2):201–203.
219. Mills DG. Effects of methaqualone on blood platelet function. *Clin Pharmacol Ther* 1978;23(6):685–691.
220. Durakovic Z, Dujmic S, Dujmic L, et al. [Methyprylon poisoning]. *Arh Hig Rada Toksikol* 1985;36(2):195–199.
221. Pellegrino ED, Henderson RR. Clinical toxicity of methyprylon (Noludar). Case report and review of twenty three cases. *J Med Soc N J* 1957;54:515–518.
222. Debailleul G, Khalil FA, Lheureux P. HPLC quantification of zolpidem and prothipendyl in a voluntary intoxication. *J Anal Toxicol* 1991;15(1):35–37.
223. Hdysry P. [Acute poisoning by new psychotropic drugs]. *Rev Prat* 1997;47(7):731–735.
224. Gock SB, Wong SH, Nuwayhid N, et al. Acute zolpidem overdose—report of two cases. *J Anal Toxicol* 1999;23(6):559–562.
225. Ahmad Z, Herepath M, Ebden P. Diagnostic utility of flumazenil in coma with suspected poisoning. *BMJ* 1991;302(6771):292.
226. Gueye PN, Lofaso F, Borron SW, et al. Mechanism of respiratory insufficiency in pure or mixed drug-induced coma involving benzodiazepines. *J Toxicol Clin Toxicol* 2002;40(1):35–47.
227. Benzodiazepines. In: Rossi S, Vitry A, Hurley E, et al., eds. *Australian medicines handbook*. Adelaide: Australian Medicines Handbook Pty Ltd, 2002.
228. Coupey SM. Barbiturates. [Review] [13 refs]. *Pediatr Rev* 1997;18(8):260–264.
229. van Sweden B, Mellerio F. Toxic ictal delirium. *Biol Psychiatry* 1989;25(4):449–458.
230. Other anxiolytics and hypnotics. In: Rossi S, Vitry A, Hurley E, et al., eds. *Australian medicines handbook*. Adelaide: Australian Medicines Handbook Pty Ltd, 2002.
231. Siguier F, Godeau P, Vergoz D, et al. [Immuno-allergic thrombopenic purpura caused by hexapropymate sensitization]. *Ann Med Interne (Paris)* 1971;122(3):435–438.
232. Marks P, Sloggem J. Peripheral neuropathy caused by methaqualone. *Am J Med Sci* 1976;272(3):323–326.
233. Slazinski L, Knox DW. Fixed drug eruption due to methaqualone. *Arch Dermatol* 1984;120(8):1073–1075.
234. Parish LC, Cander L, Witkowski JA. Erythema multiforme due to methaqualone. *Acta Derm Venereol* 1981;61(1):88–89.
235. Azizi F. Letter: agranulocytosis from methaqualone? *Ann Intern Med* 1974;81(2):268–269.
236. Chan OL. Letter: drug-precipitated acute attacks of gout. *BMJ* 1975;2(5970):561.
237. Langtry HD, Benfield P. Zolpidem. A review of its pharmacodynamic and pharmacokinetic properties and therapeutic potential. *Drugs* 1990;40(2):291–313.
238. Pitner JK, Gardner M, Neville M, et al. Zolpidem-induced psychosis in an older woman. *J Am Geriatr Soc* 1997;45(4):533–534.
239. Savitt DL, Hawkins HH, Roberts JR. The radiopacity of ingested medications. *Ann Emerg Med* 1987;16(3):331–339.
240. Pounder DJ, Jones GR. Post-mortem drug redistribution—a toxicological nightmare. *Forensic Sci Int* 1990;45(3):253–263.
241. Rehling CJ. Poison residues in human tissues. *Prog Chem Toxicol* 1967;3:363–386.
242. Baselt RC, Cravey RH. A compendium of therapeutic and toxic concentrations of toxicologically significant drugs in human biofluids. *Analytical Toxicology* 1977;1:81–103.
243. Winek CL. Tabulation of therapeutic, toxic, and lethal concentrations of drugs and chemicals in blood. *Clin Chem* 1976;22(6):832–836.
244. Levine B, Park J, Smith TD, et al. Chloral hydrate: unusually high concentrations in a fatal overdose. *J Anal Toxicol* 1985;9(5):232–233.
245. Heller PF, Goldberger BA, Caplan YH. Chloral hydrate overdose: trichloroethanol detection by gas chromatography/mass spectrometry. *Forensic Sci Int* 1992;52(2):231–234.
246. Engelhart DA, Lavins ES, Hazenstab CB, et al. Unusual death attributed to the combined effects of chloral hydrate, lidocaine, and nitrous oxide. *J Anal Toxicol* 1998;22(3):246–247.
247. Sperhake J, Tsokos M, Sperhake K. Perimortem fixation of the gastric and duodenal mucosa: a diagnostic indication for oral poisoning. *Int J Legal Med* 1999;112(5):317–320.
248. Winek CL, Wahba WW, Rozin L, et al. Determination of ethchlorvynol in body tissues and fluids after embalmment. *Forensic Sci Int* 1988;37(3):161–166.
249. Mangin P, Kintz P, Tracqui A, et al. A fatal ingestion of sparteine and meprobamate: medicolegal and toxicological data. *Acta Med Leg Soc (Liege)* 1989;39(1):385–388.
250. Baselt RC, Wright JA, Cravey RH. Therapeutic and toxic concentrations of more than 100 toxicologically significant drugs in blood, plasma, or serum: a tabulation. [Review] [153 refs]. *Clin Chem* 1975;21(1):44–62.
251. Lichtenwalner M, Tully R. A fatality involving zolpidem. *J Anal Toxicol* 1997;21(7):567–569.
252. Meeker JE, Som CW, Macapagal EC, et al. Zolpidem tissue concentrations in a multiple drug related death involving Ambien. *J Anal Toxicol* 1995;19(6):531–534.
253. Tracqui A, Kintz P, Mangin P. A fatality involving two unusual compounds—zolpidem and acepromazine. *Am J Forensic Med Pathol* 1993;14(4):309–312.
254. Winek CL, Wahba WW, Janssen JK, et al. Acute overdose of zolpidem. *Forensic Sci Int* 1996;78(3):165–168.
255. Boniface PJ, Russell SG. Two cases of fatal zopiclone overdose. *J Anal Toxicol* 1996;20(2):131–133.
256. Mannaert E, Tytgat J, Daenens P. Detection and quantification of the hypnotic zopiclone, connected with an uncommon case of drowning. *Forensic Sci Int* 1996;83(1):67–72.
257. Yamazaki M, Terada M, Mitsukuni Y, et al. [An autopsy case of poisoning by neuropsychopharmaceuticals including zopiclone]. *Jpn J Leg Med* 1998;52(4):245–252.
258. Gwilt PR, Perrier D. Plasma protein binding and distribution characteristics of drugs as indices of their hemodialyzability. *Clin Pharmacol Ther* 1978;24(2):154–161.
259. Ogilvie RI, Douglas DE, Lochead JR, et al. Ethchlorvynol (Placidyl) intoxication and its treatment by hemodialysis. *Can Med Assoc J* 1966;95(19):954–956.
260. Hyde JS, Lawrence AG, Moles JB. Ethchlorvynol intoxication. Successful treatment by exchange transfusion and peritoneal dialysis. *Clin Pediatr (Phila)* 1968;7(12):739–741.
261. Welch LT, Bower JD, Ott CE, et al. Oil dialysis for ethchlorvynol intoxication. *Clin Pharmacol Ther* 1972;13(5):745–749.
262. Koffler A, Bernstein M, LaSette A, et al. Fixed-bed charcoal hemoperfusion. Treatment of drug overdose. *Arch Intern Med* 1978;138(11):1691–1694.
263. DeMyttenaere M, Schoenfeld L, Maher JF. Treatment of glutethimide poisoning. A comparison of forced diuresis and dialysis. *JAMA* 1968;203(10):885–887.
264. Ozdemir AI, Tannenberg AM. Peritoneal and hemodialysis for acute glutethimide overdosage. *N Y State J Med* 1972;72(16):2076–2079.
265. von Hartitzsch B, Pinto MH, Mauer SM, et al. Treatment of glutethimide intoxication: an in vivo comparison of lipid, aqueous, and peritoneal dialysis with albumin. *Proc Clin Dial Transplant Forum* 1973;3:102–106.
266. Vale JA, Rees AJ, Widdop B, et al. Use of charcoal haemoperfusion in the management of severely poisoned patients. *BMJ* 1975;1(5948):5–9.
267. De Broe ME, Verpooten GA, Christiaens MA, et al. Clinical experience with prolonged combined hemoperfusion-hemodialysis treatment of severe poisoning. *Artif Organs* 1981;5(1):59–66.
268. Benowitz N, Abolin C, Tozer T, et al. Resin hemoperfusion in ethchlorvynol overdose. *Clin Pharmacol Ther* 1980;27(2):236–242.
269. de Torrente A, Rumack BH, Blair DT, et al. Fixed-bed uncoated charcoal hemoperfusion in the treatment of intoxications: animal and patient studies. *Nephron* 1979;24(2):71–77.
270. Okonek S. [Hemoperfusion with coated activated charcoal for treating acute poisoning by remedies, plant protectants, and fungi. I. Remedies (author's transl)]. *Med Klin* 1976;71(26):1120–1124.
271. Matthew H, Proudfoot AT, Brown SS, et al. Mandrax poisoning: conservative management of 116 patients. *BMJ* 1968;2(597):101–102.
272. Charytan C. The enterohepatic circulation in glutethimide intoxication. *Clin Pharmacol Ther* 1970;11(6):816–820.
273. Hassan E. Treatment of meprobamate overdose with repeated oral doses of activated charcoal. *Ann Emerg Med* 1986;15(1):73–76.
274. Wright N, Roscoe P. Acute glutethimide poisoning. Conservative management of 31 patients. *JAMA* 1970;214(9):1704–1706.
275. el Badry A, Hassaballa A, el Ayadi A. Treatment of a non-barbiturate hypnotic poisoning-methyprylon- by extra-corporeal haemodialysis. *Dtsch Zahnarztl Z* 1966;21(3):605–607.
276. Yudis M, Swartz C, Onesti G, et al. Hemodilaysis for methyprylon (Noludar) poisoning. *Ann Intern Med* 1968;68(6):1301–1304.
277. Chang TM, Coffey JF, Lister C, et al. Methaqualone, methyprylon, and glutethimide clearance by the ACAC microcapsule artificial kidney: in vitro and in patients with acute intoxication. *Trans Am Soc Artif Intern Organs* 1973;19:87–91.

278. Polin RA, Henry D, Pippinger CE. Peritoneal dialysis for severe methyprylon intoxication. *J Pediatr* 1977;90(5):831–833.
279. Collins JM. Peritoneal dialysis for methyprylon intoxication. *J Pediatr* 1978;92(3):519–520.
280. Vaziri ND, Kumar KP, Mirahmadi K, et al. Hemodialysis in treatment of acute chloral hydrate poisoning. *South Med J* 1977;70(3):377–378.
281. Heath A, Delin K, Eden E, et al. Hemoperfusion with Amberlite resin in the treatment of self-poisoning. *Acta Med Scand* 1980;207(6):455–460.
282. Bismuth C, Fournier PE, Galliot M. Biological evaluation of hemoperfusion in acute poisoning. *Clin Toxicol* 1981;18(10):1213–1223.
283. Lin JL, Lim PS. Continuous arteriovenous hemoperfusion in acute poisoning. *Blood Purif* 1994;12(2):121–127.
284. Roberge RJ, Lin E, Krenzelok EP. Flumazenil reversal of carisoprodol (Soma) intoxication. *J Emerg Med* 2000;18(1):61–64.
285. Brown MJ, Bristow DR. Molecular mechanisms of benzodiazepine-induced down-regulation of $GABA_A$ receptor alpha 1 subunit protein in rat cerebellar granule cells. *Br J Pharmacol* 1996;118(5):1103–1110.
286. de Haro L, Valli M, Bourdon JH, et al. Diazepam poisoning with one-month monitoring of diazepam and nordiazepam blood levels. *Vet Hum Toxicol* 2001;43(3):174–175.
287. Weinbroum A, Rudick V, Sorkine P, et al. Long-term intravenous and oral flumazenil treatment of acute diazepam overdose in an older patient. *J Am Geriatr Soc* 1996;44(6):737–738.
288. Greenblatt DJ, Woo E, Allen MD, et al. Rapid recovery from massive diazepam overdose. *JAMA* 1978;240(17):1872–1874.
289. Burkhart KK, Kulig KW. The diagnostic utility of flumazenil (a benzodiazepine antagonist) in coma of unknown etiology. *Ann Emerg Med* 1990;19(3):319–321.
290. Hojer J, Baehrendtz S, Matell G, et al. Diagnostic utility of flumazenil in coma with suspected poisoning: a double blind, randomised controlled study [see comments]. *BMJ* 1990;301(6764):1308–1311.
291. Hoffman RS, Goldfrank LR. The poisoned patient with altered consciousness. Controversies in the use of a 'coma cocktail'. *JAMA* 1995;274(7):562–569.
292. Herd B, Clarke F. Complete heart block after flumazenil. *Hum Exp Toxicol* 1991;10(4):289.
293. Lheureux P, Vranckx M, Leduc D, et al. Flumazenil in mixed benzodiazepine/tricyclic antidepressant overdose: a placebo-controlled study in the dog. *Am J Emerg Med* 1992;10(3):184–188.
294. Mordel A, Winkler E, Almog S, et al. Seizures after flumazenil administration in a case of combined benzodiazepine and tricyclic antidepressant overdose. *Crit Care Med* 1992;20(12):1733–1734.
295. Derlet RW, Albertson TE. Flumazenil induces seizures and death in mixed cocaine-diazepam intoxications. *Ann Emerg Med* 1994;23(3):494–498.
296. Haverkos GP, DiSalvo RP, Imhoff TE. Fatal seizures after flumazenil administration in a patient with mixed overdose. *Ann Pharmacother* 1994;28(12):1347–1349.
297. Chern TL, Kwan A. Flumazenil-induced seizure accompanying benzodiazepine and baclofen intoxication. *Am J Emerg Med* 1996;14(2):231–232.
298. Gueye PN, Hoffman JR, Taboulet P, et al. Empiric use of flumazenil in comatose patients: limited applicability of criteria to define low risk. *Ann Emerg Med* 1996;27(6):730–735.
299. Schulze-Bonhage A, Elger CE. Induction of partial epileptic seizures by flumazenil. *Epilepsia* 2000;41(2):186–192.
300. Baselt RC. *Drug effects on psychomotor performance*. Foster City, CA: Biomedical Publications, 2001.
301. Lacey JH. Dichloralphenazone and breast milk. *BMJ* 1971;4(788):684.
302. Pons G, Rey E, Matheson I. Excretion of psychoactive drugs into breast milk. Pharmacokinetic principles and recommendations. *Clin Pharmacokinet* 1994;27(4):270–289.
303. Nordeng H, Zahlsen K, Spigset O. Transfer of carisoprodol to breast milk. *Ther Drug Monit* 2001;23(3):298–300.
304. Pons G, Francoual C, Guillet P, et al. Zolpidem excretion in breast milk. *Eur J Clin Pharmacol* 1989;37(3):245–248.
305. Matheson I, Sande HA, Gaillot J. The excretion of zopiclone into breast milk. *Br J Clin Pharmacol* 1990;30(2):267–271.

SECTION

9

Electrolytes and Diuretics

CHAPTER 141

Magnesium

Seth Schonwald

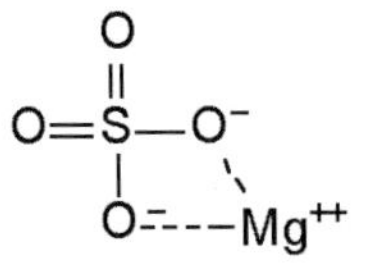

MAGNESIUM SULFATE

Atomic symbol, atomic number, and molecular weight:	**Mg, 12, 24.30 g/mol**
Valence states:	**0, +2**
CAS Registry No.:	**7439-95-4**
Normal levels:	**1.5 to 2.5 mEq/L (1.8 to 3.0 mg/dl; 0.65 to 1.10 mmol/L) (serum)**
SI conversion:	**mg/dl × 4.1 = μmol/L**
Antidotes:	**Calcium gluconate, calcium chloride**

OVERVIEW

Magnesium was discovered by Sir Humphrey Davy in 1808. Hypermagnesemia can result from ingestion (e.g., Epsom salts, magnesium citrate cathartics), impaired excretion, and excess intravenous (IV) administration. Symptoms of hypermagnesemia include nausea, vomiting, weakness, and flushing.

Magnesium is commonly used to treat preeclampsia (1,2), to stop premature labor, to treat supraventricular dysrhythmias (3), and in cathartics and laxatives (4–7). Other proposed uses include blood pressure control after cocaine ingestion, migraine treatment (8,9), and brain protection during ischemia (10,11). Magnesium has a bronchodilating effect in asthma (12–14) and is an adjunct in the treatment of dysrhythmias that develop from digoxin poisoning (15,16). Magnesium is also used to treat torsade de pointes (17).

In adults, magnesium toxicity is rare because the kidney excretes magnesium effectively. However, severe magnesium intoxication may occur through iatrogenic overdose during the treatment of preeclampsia and other conditions. Oral magnesium hydroxide laxatives and magnesium sulfate enemas administered to infants and neonates can induce symptoms of elevated serum magnesium levels and cause severe intoxication (18,19). Death occurred from a medication error involving the IV administration of 1 "amp," which resulted in infusion of a 50-ml vial of 50% magnesium sulfate instead of the usual 2-ml amp (20).

The usual daily adult intake provides 200 to 350 mg of magnesium (approximately 100 mg) (21). Magnesium metal is used in alloys to make airplanes, missiles, racing bikes, and other items that require light metals. It is also used in fireplace bricks, flashbulbs, pigments, and filters. Regulatory agencies in the United States have identified no regulatory guidelines or standards.

Iatrogenic hypermagnesemia with respiratory depression has been reported in patients with mild renal dysfunction who received doses of hemiacidrin and magnesium citrate. A patient with normal kidney function developed symptomatic hypermagnesemia (respiratory arrest, bradycardia) after receiving 90 g of magnesium sulfate over 18 hours. In contrast, 1.5 g/hour was well tolerated by a 40-weeks'-pregnant patient in the early stages of labor.

TOXICOKINETICS AND TOXICODYNAMICS

The gut rapidly absorbs approximately 30% of an oral dose. The glomerulus filters, and the proximal tubule resorbs 95% of the filtered load. Glomerular filtration rates less than 30 ml/minute predispose patients to hypermagnesemia. The kidney has a common carrier for both calcium and magnesium, in addition to separate active processes.

Magnesium is primarily an intracellular (46%) and skeletal (53%) ion; less than 1% is extracellular. Total serum magnesium concentrations reflect free or ionized (55%), chelated (12%), and protein-bound (33%) fractions. A decrease in albumin lowers total serum levels without affecting the ionized level. Alkalosis increases and acidosis decreases protein binding. Magnesium is excreted via the kidneys and the stool (22).

PATHOPHYSIOLOGY

Magnesium is a vital cation involved in cell homeostasis. In normal humans, magnesium increases cardiac output, dilates the coronary arterioles, and decreases systolic arterial pressure and systemic vascular resistance. Magnesium prolongs conduction through the sinoatrial and atrioventricular nodes and increases atrioventricular nodal refractoriness in normal humans.

Hypermagnesemia impairs neuromuscular junction transmission by decreasing acetylcholine release from the presynaptic membrane, diminishing the depolarizing action of acetylcholine at the postsynaptic junction, and impairing postsynaptic junction sensitivity to acetylcholine.

VULNERABLE POPULATIONS

Magnesium sulfate is U.S. Food and Drug Administration pregnancy risk category B. It is used widely to treat preeclampsia.

CLINICAL PRESENTATION

Cardiovascular Effects

Magnesium is a calcium antagonist. Clinically, its effects are similar to those of calcium-blocking agents. These include peripheral vasodilation, flushing, decrease in blood pressure, and decrease in strength of cardiac conduction. Bradycardia and hypotension may develop at plasma levels of 4 to 5 mEq/L. The PR, QRS, and QT intervals may increase at levels of 5 to 10 mEq/L. Myocardial injury was noted after magnesium fluorosilicate ingestion (23). Serum levels of 9 to 12 mEq/L may cause apnea and cardiovascular collapse (24).

Neurologic Effects

Hypermagnesemia typically results in loss of deep tendon reflexes at 4 to 6 mEq/L. At magnesium levels above 5 mEq/L, central nervous system depression may range from drowsiness to coma. Although concentrations greater than 10 mEq/L lead to respiratory depression in adults, this may occur at much lower levels in pediatric cases. Severe hypermagnesemia can cause parasympathetic blockade; fixed, dilated pupils; and neuromuscular blockade, mimicking a midbrain syndrome; it can also produce a pseudocomatose state (25).

Pulmonary Effects

Excess magnesium decreases neuromuscular transmission. This impairs respiratory function, an effect that is antagonized by calcium. Cardiopulmonary arrest with coma, nonreactive pupils, flaccid extremities, loss of deep tendon reflexes, and no response to painful stimulus may be observed early after magnesium overdose (26).

DIAGNOSTIC TESTS

The serum magnesium concentration may not precisely reflect total body stores of magnesium. Although a low serum magnesium concentration predicts the presence of intracellular depletion, a normal serum magnesium concentration can exist in the face of a clinically important intracellular magnesium deficiency (27,28). In addition, hypomagnesemia is often found concurrently with hypokalemia (29) and hypochloremia (30). Magnesium repletion may facilitate correction of potassium and calcium deficiencies.

The plasma magnesium level usually exceeds 4 mEq/L before signs of magnesium excess appear. The deep tendon reflexes usually decrease or disappear at blood levels of 4 mEq/L. Somnolence is observed at levels of 4 to 7 mEq/L and flaccid paralysis of voluntary muscles at 10 mEq/L or greater. Complete heart block and cardiac arrest in asystole may occur at levels of 15 mEq/L or greater.

TREATMENT

First, the administration of magnesium should be discontinued. The patient with magnesium poisoning is often critically ill and requires monitoring of serum electrolytes, calcium, phosphorus, renal function, fluid intake, and urinary output, as well as an electrocardiogram. Parenteral administration of magnesium lowers plasma calcium concentrations in both normal and hypoparathyroid patients. IV lines, oxygen, and a cardiac monitor must be available.

Activated charcoal does not absorb magnesium salts. IV fluids work by dilution of extracellular magnesium. Fluids are used with diuretics to increase excretion. If renal function is normal, IV furosemide (40 mg, adults; 1 mg/kg, infants and children) may be administered with replacement of urine volume by 0.90% saline. Exchange transfusion produced equivocal results in a neonate with severe magnesium intoxication (31).

Hemodialysis effectively removes magnesium and may be needed for hypermagnesemia in patients whose kidney function is poor or who are unable to eliminate magnesium. Pacemaker therapy may be useful in refractory hypotension.

ANTIDOTES

Calcium is a magnesium antagonist. Treatment depends on the level of magnesium and the presence of symptoms. Calcium should be reserved for patients with life-threatening symptoms, such as arrhythmia or severe respiratory depression. The mechanism of action is unknown, but calcium may displace magnesium from cell membranes. Calcium should be considered in a symptomatic patient, especially if the serum magnesium level is above 5 mEq/L. The adult dose of calcium gluconate is 10 ml of a 10% solution over several minutes. The dose may be repeated once, and then the calcium level, preferably the ionized calcium level, should be rechecked. IV calcium chloride may also be used and should be administered through a central line (Chapter 44).

REFERENCES

1. Lu JF, Nightingale CH. Magnesium sulfate in eclampsia and pre-eclampsia: pharmacokinetic principles. *Clin Pharmacokinet* 2000;38:305–314.
2. Pritchard JA, Pritchard SA. Standardized treatment of 154 consecutive cases of eclampsia. *Am J Obstet Gynecol* 1975;123:543–552.
3. Wesley RC Jr, Haines DE, Lerman BR, et al. Effect of intravenous magnesium sulfate on supraventricular tachycardia. *Am J Cardiol* 1989;63:1129–1131.
4. Walton PJ, Fraser JJ Jr, Wilhelm GW. Gastrointestinal decontamination in the emergency department. *Indian J Pediatr* 1997;64:451–455.
5. Jones J, Heiselman D, Dougherty J, Eddy A. Cathartic-induced magnesium toxicity during overdose management. *Ann Emerg Med* 1986;15:1214–1218.
6. Woodard JA, Slauson M, Lacouture PG, Woolf A. Serum magnesium concentrations after repetitive magnesium cathartic administration. *Am J Emerg Med* 1990;8:297–300.
7. Qureshi T, Melonakos TK. Acute hypermagnesemia after laxative use. *Ann Emerg Med* 1996;28:552–555.
8. Peikert A, Wilimzig C, Kohne-Volland R. Prophylaxis of migraine with oral magnesium: results from a prospective, multi-center, placebo-controlled and double-blind randomized study. *Cephalalgia* 1996;16:257–263.
9. Corbo J, Esses D, Bijur PE, et al. Randomized clinical trial of intravenous magnesium sulfate as an adjunctive medication for emergency department treatment of migraine headache. *Ann Emerg Med* 2001;38:621–627.
10. Vink R, Nimmo AJ, Cernak I. An overview of new and novel pharmacotherapies for use in traumatic brain injury. *Clin Exp Pharmacol Physiol* 2001;28:919–921.
11. Goldman RS, Finkbeiner SM. Therapeutic use of magnesium sulfate in selected cases of cerebral ischemia and seizure. *N Engl J Med* 1988;319:1224–1225.

12. Noppen M, Vanmuele L, Impens N, Schandevyl W. Bronchodilating effect of intravenous magnesium sulfate in acute severe bronchial asthma. *Chest* 1990;97:272–276.
13. Okayama H, Aikawa T, Okayama M, et al. Bronchodilating effect of intravenous magnesium sulfate in bronchial asthma. *JAMA* 1987;257:1076–1078.
14. Rowe BH, Bretzlaff JA, Bourdon C, et al. Intravenous magnesium sulfate treatment for acute asthma in the emergency department: a systematic review of the literature. *Ann Emerg Med* 2000;36:181–190.
15. Kinlay S, Buckley NA. Magnesium sulfate in the treatment of ventricular arrhythmias due to digoxin toxicity. *J Toxicol Clin Toxicol* 1995;33:55–59.
16. Reisdorff EJ, Clark MR, Walters BL. Acute digitalis poisoning: the role of intravenous magnesium sulfate. *J Emerg Med* 1986;4:463–469.
17. Tzivoni D, Keren A, Cohen AM, et al. Magnesium therapy for torsade de pointes. *Am J Cardiol* 1984;53:528–530.
18. Mofenson HC, Caraccio TR. Magnesium intoxication in a neonate from oral magnesium hydroxide laxative. *J Toxicol Clin Toxicol* 1991;29:215–222.
19. Outerbridge EW, Papageorgiou A, Stern L. Magnesium sulfate enema in a newborn. Fatal systemic magnesium absorption. *JAMA* 1973;224:1392–1393.
20. Hoffman RS, Smilkstein MJ, Rubenstein F. An "amp" by any other name: the hazards of intravenous design. *JAMA* 1989;261:557.
21. Chernow B, Bamberger S, Stroiko M, et al. Hypomagnesemia in patients in the postoperative intensive care unit. *Chest* 1989;95:391–397.
22. Dai LJ, Ritchie G, Kerstan D, et al. Magnesium transport in the renal distal convoluted tubule. *Physiol Rev* 2001;81:51–84.
23. Ortega-Carnicer J, de la Nieta DS, Alcazar R. Acute myocardial injury caused presumably by coronary spasm after magnesium fluoro-silicate ingestion. *J Electrocardiol* 2001;34:335–337.
24. McCubbin JH, Sibai BM, Abdella TN, Anderson GD. Cardiopulmonary arrest due to acute maternal hypermagnesemia. *Lancet* 1981;1:1058.
25. Szabo MD, Crosby G. Central nervous system effects of magnesium. *Anesth Analg* 1989;69:691–692.
26. Rabinerson D, Gruber A, Kaplan B, et al. Accidental cardiopulmonary arrest following magnesium sulphate overdose. *Eur J Obstet Gynecol Reprod Biol* 1994;55:149–150.
27. Fiaccadori E, Del Canale S, Coffrini E, et al. Muscle and serum magnesium in pulmonary intensive care unit patients. *Crit Care Med* 1988;16:751–760.
28. Hamill-Ruth RJ, McGory R. Magnesium repletion and its effect on potassium homeostasis in critically ill adults: results of a double-blind, randomized, controlled trial. *Crit Care Med* 1996;24:38–45.
29. Whang R, Whang D, Ryan MP. Refractory potassium repletion: a consequence of magnesium deficiency. *Arch Intern Med* 1992;152:40–44.
30. Seelig M. Cardiovascular consequences of magnesium deficiency and loss: pathogenesis, prevalence and manifestations—magnesium and chloride loss in refractory potassium repletion. *Am J Cardiol* 1989;63:4G–21G.
31. Versteegh FG, van Vught AJ, vande Walle JG, Rademaker CM. Magnesium poisoning in an infant. *Ned Tijdschr Geneeskd* 1991;135:1186–1188.

CHAPTER 142

Potassium Chloride and Potassium Permanganate

Seth Schonwald

Atomic symbol, atomic number, and molecular weight:	**Potassium: K, 19, 39.1; potassium chloride: KCl, 74.55 g/mol**
Valence state:	**+1**
CAS Registry No.:	**7447-40-7 (potassium); 7447-40-7 (potassium chloride)**
Normal levels:	**3.5 to 5.3 mEq/L, 137 to 207 mg/L (serum)**
SI conversion:	**g/L × 25.6 = mmol/L**
Antidotes:	**Calcium, sodium bicarbonate, insulin and glucose, β-adrenergic agonist**

OVERVIEW

Potassium is an essential intracellular ion involved in cellular electrical conduction. It is found in numerous chemical agents. Ingestion of potassium supplements can cause life-threatening hyperkalemia (1), but hyperkalemia due to renal disease is much more common. Patients with normal renal function rarely develop hyperkalemia.

Potassium is a component of many toxic substances [dichromate (2), traditional remedies (3,4), potassium permanganate (5,6), potassium perchlorate (7,8), potassium iodide (9,10), chloroplatinate (11), and bromate (12)]. In most of these poisons, the toxicity is related to the other constituent.

Potassium is used in making glass, soap, and lenses and as a salt substitute. It is also used to make explosives and to color fireworks in mauve. The average American diet includes 2 to 6 g/day (13). Death by lethal injection in the United States uses potassium chloride as one of its agents.

TOXIC DOSE

There are no regulatory standards for potassium. Cardiac manifestations of toxicity are frequent at potassium levels above 8.0 mEq/L and rare below 6.5 mEq/L. Oral ingestion of potassium dichromate produces a complex spectrum of complications, including renal and liver failure. It has an extremely poor prognosis and usually leads to rapid death (14).

A 53-year-old man died after ingesting 1 tablespoon of salt substitute containing 52.8% potassium (283 mmol) (15). The causes of death from rare potassium permanganate ingestion include cardiovascular collapse and hypotensive shock due to massive gastrointestinal (GI) and pancreatic hemorrhage, and respiratory obstruction (16).

Sustained-release potassium chloride overdose has been reported. A 50-year-old woman who ingested 100 potassium chloride (K-Dur) tablets (10 mEq potassium per tablet) developed a serum potassium level of 9.7 mEq/L, had life-threatening electrocardiographic (ECG) changes, and survived. A 17-year-old boy who ingested 20 to 30 potassium chloride (Klor-Con) tablets (10 mEq potassium per tablet) developed a serum potassium level of 6.1 mEq/L and had a normal ECG. In both patients, tablets were visualized on abdominal radiographs, and they were successfully decontaminated using whole bowel irrigation (3).

A 27-year-old patient who ingested 60 tablets of sustained-release potassium chloride (Slow-K) developed first degree heart block, wide QRS complexes, and tall T waves. The plasma potassium concentration was 91 mmol/L, and the patient survived (17).

A 48-year-old man drank 150 ml of a solution containing 22.5 g of potassium dichromate in a suicide attempt. He was treated with hemodialysis and calcium ethylenediaminetetraacetic acid and survived (18). An 8-week-old boy died after ingesting an unknown quantity of black potassium permanganate crystals (19).

TOXICOKINETICS AND TOXICODYNAMICS

Potassium is well absorbed in the small intestine. The half-life of potassium chloride is 16 seconds. Potassium is primarily eliminated via the kidney; some is excreted in feces and sweat. Renal potassium excretion depends on chloride ion concentration, acid-base status, and adrenal hormone secretion.

PATHOPHYSIOLOGY

Hyperkalemia is a relatively uncommon complication of poisoning. Hyperkalemia follows inhibition of Na^+,K^+–adenosine triphosphatase activity (e.g., by digoxin); increased uptake of potassium salts; disruption of intermediary metabolism (e.g., cyanide poisoning); activation of K^+ channels (e.g., fluoride poisoning); and the presence of acidosis and rhabdomyolysis, particularly if the latter is complicated by renal failure (20).

PREGNANCY AND LACTATION

Potassium chloride is U.S. Food and Drug Administration pregnancy category C. It is extremely unlikely that potassium chloride adversely affects pregnancy or breast-feeding.

CLINICAL PRESENTATION

Cardiovascular signs of hyperkalemia may include bradycardia, slowed conduction, hypotension, ventricular fibrillation, and asystole. The patient may develop serious cardiac problems without prominent early symptoms of systemic toxicity and despite modest elevations of serum potassium. *Respiratory toxicity* includes glottic edema, respiratory obstruction, and adult respiratory distress syndrome after ingestion of a concentrated potassium permanganate solution.

GI effects include nausea, vomiting, paralytic ileus, and local mucosal necrosis, which may lead to perforation. Small bowel ulcerations may follow the use of enteric-coated tablets, and local pain and inflammation may result from intravenous administration of potassium chloride. Gastric stenosis has been reported after ingestion (21). Irreversible liver damage may occur after potassium dichromate ingestion (22).

Neuromuscular signs of hyperkalemia include weakness, paresthesia, hyporeflexia, and paralysis. Chronic ingestion of potassium permanganate may result in neurologic effects (parkinsonism) similar to manganism (23). *Other effects* include toxic retinopathy after potassium iodate overdose. Methemoglobinemia and hemolysis have been reported after potassium permanganate overdose. Potassium perchlorate has been associated with aplastic anemia.

Ingestion of dilute *potassium permanganate* antiseptic solutions are usually benign, and mild irritation is self-limited. Spontaneous emesis and diarrhea may occur. A concentrated solution may cause corrosive burns on the skin and mucous membranes, and oropharyngeal, esophageal, or gastric injury may occur, resulting in ulceration, hemorrhage, and perforation. Late complications of upper GI ulceration may include esophageal stricture (24) and pyloric stenosis (25). Pancreatitis has also been reported.

DIAGNOSTIC TESTS

The sequential ECG manifestations of hyperkalemia include tall, peaked T waves; depressed ST segments; decreased amplitude of R waves; PR interval prolongation; decreased P waves; widened QRS complexes; QT prolongation; sine wave appearance; and asystole.

Potassium may be measured by atomic absorption spectrometry or by ion selective electrode. Cardiac toxicity is frequent at serum potassium levels above 8.0 mEq/L and rare below 6.5 mEq/L. Factitious hyperkalemia may result from the release of intracellular potassium stores (Chapter 35).

Abdominal radiographs may be helpful in tracking the efficacy of whole bowel lavage after sustained-release potassium chloride overdose.

TREATMENT

Potassium chloride overdose is a serious decontamination and treatment challenge. The poisoned patient may have a large dose of potassium chloride tablets in the GI tract that are absorbed in a delayed manner. Calcium chloride infusion, dextrose and insulin in water, and correction of acidosis with sodium bicarbonate are helpful in controlling acute, life-threatening cardiac dysrhythmias.

Decontamination

Gastric emptying may be needed in patients with a large ingestion of enteric-coated or controlled-release formulations of potassium. This can be difficult because of the potential to increase absorption. Whole bowel irrigation or gastric lavage with a large bore tube have been used, but the facilities to treat sudden severe hyperkalemia must be immediately available.

Enhancement of Elimination

Dialysis effectively removes potassium. Patients who cannot tolerate fluid loads or those with severe renal dysfunction may benefit from early hemodialysis after potassium overdose.

In addition to other measures, symptomatic hyperkalemia or the presence of ECG changes should be treated with potassium-binding resin. A cation exchange resin [e.g., sodium polystyrene sulfonate (Kayexalate)] removes approximately 1 mEq of potassium per gram of resin. The oral dose of sodium polystyrene sulfonate is 20 to 50 g dissolved in 100 to 200 ml of 20% sorbitol. The dose is repeated every 4 hours up to four or five daily doses until the potassium level returns to normal. It may be administered as a retention enema in a dose of 8 g and 50 g of sorbitol in 200 ml of water.

Antidotes

The treatment of hyperkalemia includes calcium salts and sodium bicarbonate as well as insulin and glucose. Details are provided in Chapter 35. These modalities do not remove excess potassium from the body. That is achieved either by using ion exchange resins or by hemodialysis (26).

Potassium Permanganate

After ingestion of crystals, tablets, or concentrated solutions, monitor the airway for swelling, and intubate if necessary. Perform endoscopy as soon as practicable for the assessment of burns. Do not induce emesis because of the risk of corrosive injury. Activated charcoal and cathartics are not effective (27).

For a significant ingestion, aspiration of stomach contents should be considered; however, the risks of hemorrhage or GI perforation are present. After ocular exposure, irrigate the eyes and skin with copious amounts of tepid water.

Corticosteroids have not been proved effective for caustic ingestion and may be harmful in the patient with perforation by masking early signs of inflammation and inhibiting resistance to infection. Antibiotics are considered in the case of severe burns and for secondary infection. The prophylactic use of antibiotics is controversial. After ingestion of potassium permanganate, the use of H_2 antagonists has been proposed, but efficacy has not been evaluated. *N*-acetylcysteine has been used in the treatment of potassium permanganate–induced hepatotoxicity, but efficacy has not been established (28).

REFERENCES

1. Su M, Stork C, Ravuri S, et al. Sustained-release potassium chloride overdose. *J Toxicol Clin Toxicol* 2001;39:641–648.
2. Picaud JC, Cochat P, Parchoux JC, et al. Acute renal failure in a child after chewing of match heads. *Nephron* 1995;57:225–226.
3. Michie CA, Hayhurst M, Knobel GJ, et al. Poisoning with a traditional remedy containing potassium dichromate. *Hum Exp Toxicol* 1991;10:129–131.
4. Wood R, Mills PB, Knobel GJ, et al. Acute dichromate poisoning after use of traditional purgatives. A report of 7 cases. *S Afr Med J* 1990;77:640–642.
5. Middleton SJ, Jacyna M, McClaren D, et al. Haemorrhagic pancreatitis—a cause of death in severe potassium permanganate poisoning. *Postgrad Med J* 1990;66:657–658.
6. Lifshitz M, Shahak E, Sofer S. Fatal potassium permanganate intoxication in an infant. *J Toxicol Clin Toxicol* 1999;37:801–802.
7. Soldin OP, Braverman LE, Lamm SH. Perchlorate clinical pharmacology and human health: a review. *Ther Drug Monit* 2001;23:316–331.
8. Barzilai D, Sheinfeld M. Fatal complications following use of potassium perchlorate in thyrotoxicosis. Report of two cases and a review of the literature. *Isr J Med Sci* 1966;2:453–456.
9. Mercurio MG, Elewski BE. Therapy of sporotrichosis. *Semin Dermatol* 1993;12:285–289.
10. Horio T, Danno K, Okamoto H, et al. Potassium iodide in erythema nodosum and other erythematous dermatoses. *J Am Acad Dermatol* 1983;9:77–81.
11. Woolf AD, Ebert TH. Toxicity after self-poisoning by ingestion of potassium chloroplatinite. *J Toxicol Clin Toxicol* 1991;29:467–472.
12. Kurokawa Y, Maekawa A, Takahashi M, Hayashi Y. Toxicity and carcinogenicity of potassium bromate—a new renal carcinogen. *Environ Health Perspect* 1990;87:309–335.
13. Hass EM. Potassium. Available at: http://www.healthy.net/asp/templates/article.asp?PageType=article&ID=2063. Accessed April 2003.
14. Stift A, Friedl J, Langle F, et al. Successful treatment of a patient suffering from severe acute potassium dichromate poisoning with liver transplantation. *Transplantation* 2000;69:2454–2455.
15. Restuccio A. Fatal hyperkalemia from a salt substitute. *Am J Emerg Med* 1992;10:171–173.
16. Ong KL, Tan TH, Cheung WL. Potassium permanganate poisoning—a rare cause of fatal self poisoning. *J Accid Emerg Med* 1997;14:43–45.
17. Steedman DJ. Poisoning with sustained release potassium. *Arch Emerg Med* 1988;5:206–211.
18. Kolacinski Z, Kostrzewski P, Kruszewska S, et al. Acute potassium dichromate poisoning: a toxicokinetic case study. *J Toxicol Clin Toxicol* 1999;37:785–791.
19. Lifshitz M, Shahak E, Sofer S. Fatal potassium permanganate intoxication in an infant. *J Toxicol Clin Toxicol* 1999;37:801–802.
20. Bradberry SM, Vale JA. Disturbances of potassium homeostasis in poisoning. *J Toxicol Clin Toxicol* 1995;33:295–310.
21. Peeters JW, van der Werf SD. Gastric stenosis after potassium chloride ingestion. *Endoscopy* 1998;30:S110.
22. Stift A, Friedl J, Laengle F. Liver transplantation for potassium dichromate poisoning. *N Engl J Med* 1998;338:766–767.
23. Holzgraefe M, Poser W, Kijewski H, Beuche W. Chronic enteral poisoning caused by potassium permanganate: a case report. *J Toxicol Clin Toxicol* 1986;24:235–244.
24. Kochhar R, Das K, Mehta SK. Potassium permanganate induced oesophageal stricture. *Hum Toxicol* 1986;5:393–394.
25. Temple WA, Smith NA. International Programme on Chemical Safety Poisons Information Monograph 409. Dunedin, New Zealand: National Toxicology Group, 1998.
26. Saxena K. Clinical features and management of poisoning due to potassium chloride. *Med Toxicol Adverse Drug Exp* 1989;4:429–443.
27. Position statement and practice guidelines on the use of multi-dose activated charcoal in the treatment of acute poisoning. European Association of Poison Centers and Clinical Toxicology and American Academy of Clinical Toxicology. *J Toxicol Clin Toxicol* 1997;35:731–751.
28. Young RJ, Critchley J, Young KK, et al. Fatal acute hepatorenal failure following potassium permanganate ingestion. *Hum Exp Toxicol* 1996;15:259–261.

CHAPTER 143

Diuretics

Seth Schonwald

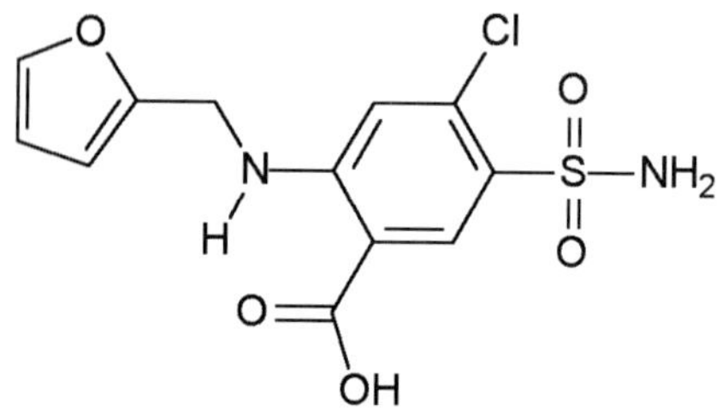

FUROSEMIDE

Compounds included:	**Thiazides (bendroflumethiazide, chlorothiazide, hydrochlorothiazide, hydroflumethiazide, methyclothiazide, polythiazide, trichlormethiazide, metolazone, indapamide); loop diuretics (bumetanide, furosemide, chlorthalidone, torsemide, ethacrynic acid); potassium-sparing diuretics (amiloride, triamterene, spironolactone); carbonic-anhydrase inhibitors (acetazolamide, dichlorphenamide, dorzolamide, methazolamide); osmotic diuretics (mannitol, urea)**
SI conversion:	**Not applicable**
Therapeutic levels:	**Not applicable**
Target organs:	**Skin (acute or chronic), electrolyte abnormalities (acute or chronic), ear (acute)**
Antidote:	**None**

OVERVIEW

Diuretics are used to treat hypertension, congestive heart failure, diabetes insipidus, calcium-containing kidney stones, and hypercalcemia. Intentional diuretic overdose is rare; however, inadvertent overuse is common in elderly patients. Patients with anorexia nervosa may abuse diuretics to promote weight loss (1,2).

TOXICOKINETICS AND TOXICODYNAMICS

The pharmacokinetics of loop, thiazide, and potassium-sparing diuretic agents are provided in Table 1 (3). In addition, acetazolamide is rapidly absorbed. The maximum serum concentration for tablets and extended-release capsules is achieved in 2 to 4 hours and 8 to 12 hours, respectively. When used for glaucoma, the onset of action for the tablets is approximately 1.5 to 2.0 hours, and the peak effect on intraocular pressure (IOP) is achieved within 2 to 12 hours. The onset of action after intravenous (IV) administration is approximately 2 minutes, reaching a peak effect in 15 minutes and lasting 4 to 5 hours. Acetazolamide is 90% plasma protein bound and widely distributed. It is eliminated renally; 90% to 100% of a dose is excreted within 24 hours. Approximately 47% of an extended-release dose is eliminated within 24 hours (4).

Mannitol is an osmotic diuretic that produces diuresis in 15 to 60 minutes, reduction of IOP in 30 to 60 minutes, and reduction of intracranial pressure within 15 minutes. Peak effect for diuresis is 1 hour, 1 to 2 hours for reduction of IOP. Duration of action for diuresis is 3 to 8 hours, reduction of IOP is 4 to 6 hours, and reduction of intracranial pressure is 3 to 8 hours (5).

PREGNANCY AND LACTATION

Potassium-Sparing Agents

Amiloride is U.S. Food and Drug Administration (FDA) pregnancy category B. First trimester exposure has resulted in an increased rate of major birth defects (6). Triamterene is pregnancy category B. It may cross the placental barrier in humans. Spironolactone is pregnancy category C and is usually compatible with breast-feeding (7).

Thiazide Diuretics

Thiazide diuretics cross the placenta, and jaundice can occur in the fetus or neonate. Hydrochlorothiazide is FDA pregnancy category D. Thiazide diuretics distribute into breast milk. Breast-feeding should be avoided during the first month of lactation because suppression of lactation has been reported.

Loop Diuretics

Furosemide and bumetanide are FDA pregnancy category C. Bumetanide is contraindicated in breast-feeding.

TABLE 1. Pharmacokinetic parameters of diuretic drugs

Diuretic	Oral bioavailability (%)	Elimination half-life (h)			
		Normal subjects	Renal insufficiency	Cirrhosis	Congestive heart failure
Thiazides					
Bendroflumethiazide	ND	2–5	ND	ND	ND
Chlorthalidone	64	24–55	ND	ND	ND
Chlorothiazide	30–50	1.5	ND	ND	ND
Hydrochlorothiazide	66–75	2.5	Increased	ND	ND
Hydroflumethiazide	73	6–25	ND	ND	6–28
Indapamide	93	15–25	ND	ND	ND
Polythiazide	ND	16	ND	ND	ND
Trichlormethiazide	ND	1–4	5–10	ND	ND
Loop					
Furosemide	10–100	1.5–2.0	2.8	2.5	2.7
Bumetanide	30–100	1	1.6	2.3	1.3
Torsemide	30–100	3–4	4–5	8	6
Potassium sparing					
Amiloride	Conflicting data	17–26	100	Negligible change	ND
Triamterene[a]	>80	2–5	Prolonged	No change	ND
Spironolactone	Conflicting data	1.5	No change	No change	ND
Active metabolites	—	>15	ND	ND	ND
Carbonic anhydrase inhibitors					
Acetazolamide	ND	4–8	26	ND	ND
Osmotic					
Mannitol	ND	1.0–1.5	ND	ND	ND

ND, not determined.
[a]Values are for active metabolite.
Modified from Brater DC. Diuretic therapy. *N Engl J Med* 1998;339:387–395.

Carbonic Anhydrase Inhibitors

Acetazolamide is FDA pregnancy category C. It has not been linked to congenital defects in humans. Because there have been reports of teratogenic effects in animals (8), however, acetazolamide is not recommended for use during the first trimester of pregnancy. Its use during breast-feeding has not been established.

Osmotic Agents

Mannitol is classified as FDA pregnancy category C.

POTASSIUM-SPARING DIURETICS

The potassium-sparing diuretics (amiloride, triamterene, spironolactone) are typically used to treat congestive heart failure and hypertension, often in conjunction with other diuretics. Spironolactone has been used to prevent amphotericin B–related hypokalemia in cancer patients (9) and in the management of neonatal chronic lung disease. Hyperkalemia has been reported with spironolactone use, often in conjunction with other drugs, such as angiotensin-converting enzyme inhibitors (10).

Pathophysiology

Amiloride acts by blocking sodium channels in the later portions of the nephron, distal tubule, and collecting duct. Secretion of potassium into urine is inhibited, and potassium is retained by interfering with the passage of sodium through this channel. Increased urinary excretion of sodium, bicarbonate, calcium, and water causes a slight diuretic effect.

Triamterene inhibits the reabsorption of sodium ions in exchange for potassium and hydrogen ions in the segment of the distal tubule under the control of adrenal mineralocorticoids (especially aldosterone) (8).

Spironolactone binds to aldosterone receptors in the distal tubules and collecting duct, thereby preventing the binding of aldosterone to its receptor and its subsequent effects. Aldosterone is a mineralocorticoid steroid hormone produced in the adrenal cortex that acts at the kidney to cause sodium (and water) retention and potassium loss in the urine.

Clinical Presentation

Diuretic overdose, although rare, can result in dehydration and electrolyte abnormalities. Manifestations of volume loss can include tachycardia, hypotension, dry mucous membranes, and, in severe cases, mental status changes.

Amiloride has caused phototoxic eczema in patients receiving amiloride in combination with thiazide diuretics (11). Chronic amiloride administration has been associated with hyperkalemic metabolic acidosis (12).

Triamterene can cause anaphylaxis and photodermatitis (13). As with all potassium-sparing diuretics, hyperkalemia may develop. Drug-induced interstitial nephritis has also been associated with triamterene (14).

Spironolactone is similar in structure to steroid compounds and can produce similar adverse effects. In men, it may cause gynecomastia (15,16), decreased libido, and impotence. Women may develop menstrual irregularities, postmenopausal bleeding, and breast tenderness. These effects are generally reversible after discontinuation of therapy.

Hepatitis from spironolactone developed in a woman being treated for alopecia (17) and in other patients treated with this agent. Bullous pemphigoid (18), lichenoid drug eruption (19), and allergic contact dermatitis (20) may be induced by spironolactone.

CARBONIC ANHYDRASE INHIBITORS

Carbonic anhydrase inhibitors are used to treat glaucoma (21,22) and pseudotumor cerebri (23) and to prevent or treat mountain sickness (24).

Pathophysiology

The enzyme carbonic anhydrase produces certain ocular fluids. Its inhibition decreases fluid production and pressure within the eye. Carbonic anhydrase inhibitors interfere with the actions of carbonic anhydrase in the renal cortex, eye, and central nervous system. They can control seizures and decrease the rate of cerebrospinal fluid formation. In the kidney, acetazolamide enhances the clearance of sodium and bicarbonate. In the distal tubule, potassium is lost in an effort to reclaim filtered sodium (25).

Clinical Presentation

Adverse effects with this type of diuretic include numbness, tingling, or burning in the hands, fingers, feet, toes, and mouth. Potassium deficiency can occur at high doses or when used simultaneously with other drugs that can cause potassium loss.

A 1-year-old girl, weighing 10 kg, developed metabolic acidosis after ingestion of between 500 and 1250 mg of acetazolamide. The maximum base deficit recorded was 11.6 mEq/L. She was treated with sodium bicarbonate and recovered completely (26). Carbonic anhydrase inhibitors can cause a normal anion gap acidosis (27).

Carbonic anhydrase inhibitors infrequently cause elevated blood sugars in diabetics. These drugs are sulfonamide derivatives and infrequently cause sulfa allergies. Numerous cases of hematopoietic toxicity due to carbonic anhydrase inhibitors have been reported. Death from aplastic anemia (28,29), thrombocytopenia, or agranulocytosis has been attributed to these agents (30).

Acetazolamide-induced central nervous system toxicity occurred in two patients during hemodialysis. Symptoms included fatigue, lethargy, and confusion, which resolved several days after discontinuing acetazolamide. Pharmacokinetic studies showed markedly elevated serum concentrations of the drug, which decreased at a slower rate compared to patients with normal renal function (31).

THIAZIDES

Thiazides are commonly used to treat high blood pressure and congestive heart failure and, occasionally, to decrease swelling and fluid retention associated with premenstrual syndrome and corticosteroid or estrogen therapy. Thiazide diuretics are also used to treat diabetes insipidus (32) and patients who form hypercalciuric stones (33).

Pathophysiology

Thiazides reduce urine volume primarily by reducing extracellular fluid volume and increasing water reabsorption at early portions of the nephron. Thiazides inhibit a protein that transports sodium chloride in the distal nephron, which results in an increased loss of sodium, chloride, and water in the urine. Thiazides can also cause increased potassium and magnesium loss and decreased calcium loss in the urine.

Clinical Presentation

Signs of electrolyte imbalance may include confusion, fatigue, dizziness, muscle cramps, headache, tingling in the hands and feet, thirst, nausea, and vomiting. Hypokalemia can cause dysrhythmias. Atrioventricular premature contractions and atrioventricular block have been reported in a patient with renal failure on high-dose hydrochlorothiazide therapy (34). Pulmonary edema has been reported after therapeutic ingestion of hydrochlorothiazide in numerous instances (35). Pancreatitis developed in a case of thiazide abuse (36).

Thiazide diuretics can cause elevated blood sugar in diabetics (37) and hyperlipidemia (38). There may be cross-sensitivity between people with allergies to sulfa antibiotics and thiazide diuretics. Thiazides can decrease excretion of uric acid by the kidney and may precipitate a gout attack in patients with this disease (39). Thiazides may increase sensitivity to the sun as well (40).

LOOP DIURETICS

Loop diuretics are used to treat edema associated with congestive heart failure, cirrhosis of the liver, and certain kidney diseases as well as moderate to severe cases of hypertension and pulmonary edema. They are occasionally used to treat hypercalcemia. Aside from subtle differences in their sites of action, furosemide, bumetanide, and torsemide are essentially interchangeable. Torsemide has a longer duration of action and can be dosed once daily. Ethacrynic acid is both chemically and pharmacologically distinct from the other loop-acting diuretics. Some clinicians feel it may be effective in acute renal failure when the other drugs are inactive. Due to adverse reactions, ethacrynic acid has fallen out of routine use.

Pathophysiology

In addition to increasing sodium elimination in the urine, loop diuretics also increase the excretion of potassium, calcium, magnesium (41), bicarbonate, ammonium, and phosphate. They must be used cautiously in combination with other drugs that cause hearing impairment or kidney damage.

Clinical Presentation

The large amount of urine produced, particularly early in treatment, can cause dehydration and mild hypotension. Symptoms include mental confusion, weakness, dizziness, muscle cramps, headache, tingling in the hands and feet, thirst, nausea, and vomiting. Syncope has been associated with fasting and high-dose IV furosemide (42). Occasionally, loop diuretics cause elevated blood sugar in diabetics. They can elevate cholesterol and triglycerides, although the long-term clinical significance of this effect is uncertain. A death due to ventricular dysrhythmias after IV furosemide has been reported (43).

Simultaneous use of nonsteroidal antiinflammatory agents may decrease the effect of loop diuretics. All of the loop diuretics except ethacrynic acid are sulfonamides. People with a sulfa allergy may have cross-sensitivity to these diuretics.

Hypokalemia (44) and hypochloremic alkalosis may follow chronic therapeutic use or abuse of thiazide and loop diuretics (45). Furosemide and ethacrynic acid can cause ototoxicity after large IV doses (46). Hearing loss is generally reversible, resolving within 24 hours (47). Bumetanide has also been associated with ototoxicity (48).

OSMOTIC DIURETICS

Urea has been touted as a treatment for Meniere's disease (49). Mannitol is administered IV to reduce intracranial pressure (50) and to increase urine flow in certain types of kidney failure, such as that induced by rhabdomyolysis (51) and hemolytic transfusion reactions. Mannitol is also used to increase urinary excretion of toxins or drugs in certain overdose cases, such as ciguatera poisoning (52).

Pathophysiology

Mannitol is an osmotic diuretic that is freely filtered at the glomerulus, undergoes limited reabsorption by the renal tubule, and is pharmacologically inert by conventional criteria. Mannitol does not undergo metabolic alteration. When renal circulation is acutely compromised, mannitol is still filtered at the glomerulus.

Clinical Presentation

Mannitol can cause hyponatremia, even in patients with normal renal function (53), and has caused fatal colonic perforation when used as a purgative (54). Acute renal failure has followed massive mannitol infusion (55). A case of subcutaneous mannitol extravasation caused swelling and multiple cutaneous bullous eruptions in the hand and forearm during craniotomy (56).

TREATMENT

Treatment of diuretic excess is directed at correction of volume loss and electrolyte abnormalities. All patients should be monitored for fluctuations in sodium and potassium and treated accordingly. Volume repletion with normal saline is generally effective in the hypotensive patient with diuretic excess. Central pontine myelinolysis, a disruption of the myelinated neurons of the pons, has been associated with rapid correction of severe hyponatremia due to diuretic abuse (57). There are no antidotes to treat diuretic excess.

REFERENCES

1. Favaro A, Santonastaso P. Self-injurious behavior in anorexia nervosa. *J Nerv Ment Dis* 2000;188:537–542.
2. Bulik CM. Abuse of drugs associated with eating disorders. *J Subst Abuse* 1992;4:69–90.
3. Brater DC. Diuretic therapy. *N Engl J Med* 1998;339:387–395.
4. The parkinsn's list drug database. Available at: http://www.parkinsons-information-exchange-network-online.com/drugdb/002.html. Accessed April 11, 2003.
5. MedicineHouse Web site. Available at: http://www.medicinehouse.com/cgi-bin/drug1.php?drug=mannitol. Accessed April 11, 2003.
6. Drugs in pregnancy and breastfeeding. Available at: http://www.perinatology.com/exposures/druglist.htm#Amiloride. Accessed April 11, 2003.
7. Phelps DL, Karim Z. Spironolactone: relationship between concentrations of dethioacetylated metabolite in human serum milk. *J Pharm Sci* 1977;66:1203.
8. Holmes LB, Kawanishi H, Munoz A. Acetazolamide: maternal toxicity, pattern of malformations, and litter effect. *Teratology* 1988;37:335–342.
9. Ugur UA, Avcu F, Cetin T, et al. Spironolactone: is it a novel drug for the prevention of amphotericin B-related hypokalemia in cancer patients? *Eur J Clin Pharmacol* 2002;57:771–773.
10. Highlights of the 22nd French pharmacovigilance meeting. *Prescrire Int* 2002;11:21–23.
11. Thestrup-Pedersen K. Adverse reactions in the skin from anti-hypertensive drugs. *Dan Med Bull* 1987;34[Suppl 1]:3–5.
12. DuBose TD Jr. Molecular and pathophysiologic mechanisms of hyperkalemic metabolic acidosis. *Trans Am Clin Climatol Assoc* 2000;111:122–134.
13. Fernandez de Corres L, Bernaola G, Fernandez E, et al. Photodermatitis from triamterene. *Contact Dermatitis* 1987;17:114–115.
14. Magil AB. Drug-induced acute interstitial nephritis with granulomas. *Hum Pathol* 1983;14:36–41.
15. Pitt B, Zannad F, Remme WJ, et al. The effect of spironolactone on morbidity and mortality in patients with severe heart failure. Randomized Aldactone Evaluation Study Investigators. *N Engl J Med* 1999;341:709–717.
16. Thompson DF, Carter JR. Drug-induced gynecomastia. *Pharmacotherapy* 1993;13:37–45.
17. Thai KE, Sinclair RD. Spironolactone-induced hepatitis. *Australas J Dermatol* 2001;42:180–182.
18. Modeste AB, Cordel N, Courville P, et al. Bullous pemphigoid induced by spironolactone. *Ann Dermatol Venereol* 2002;129:56–58.
19. Schon MP, Tebbe B, Trautmann C, et al. Lichenoid drug eruption induced by spironolactone. *Acta Derm Venereol* 1994;74:476.
20. Corazza M, Strumia R, Lombardi AR, et al. Allergic contact dermatitis from spironolactone. *Contact Dermatitis* 1996;35:365–366.
21. Kaur IP, Smitha R, Aggarwal D, et al. Acetazolamide: future perspective in topical glaucoma therapeutics. *Int J Pharm* 2002;248:1–14.
22. Goldberg I, Graham SL, Healey PR. Primary open-angle glaucoma. *Med J Aust* 2002;177:535–536.
23. Villain MA, Pageaux GP, Veyrac M, et al. Effect of acetazolamide on ocular hemodynamics in pseudotumor cerebri associated with inflammatory bowel disease. *Am J Ophthalmol* 2002;134:778–780.
24. Hackett PH, Roach RC. High-altitude illness. *N Engl J Med* 2001;345:107–114.
25. The PPA online. Available at: http://www.periodicparalysis.org/PPRC/Pharmacy/. Accessed April 11, 2003.
26. Baer E, Reith DM. Acetazolamide poisoning in a toddler. *J Paediatr Child Health* 2001;37:411–412.
27. Kreisberg RA, Wood BC. Drug and chemical-induced metabolic acidosis. *Clin Endocrinol Metab* 1983;12:391–411.
28. Shapiro S, Fraunfelder FT. Acetazolamide and aplastic anemia. *Am J Ophthalmol* 1992;113:328–330.
29. Keisu M, Wiholm BE, Ost A, Mortimer O. Acetazolamide-associated aplastic anaemia. *J Intern Med* 1990;228:627–632.
30. Fraunfelder FT, Meyer SM, Bagby GC Jr, et al. Hematologic reactions to carbonic anhydrase inhibitors. *Am J Ophthalmol* 1985;100:79–81.
31. Schwenk MH, St. Peter WL, Meese MG, et al. Acetazolamide toxicity and pharmacokinetics in patients receiving hemodialysis. *Pharmacotherapy* 1995;15:522–527.
32. Bendz H, Aurell M. Drug-induced diabetes insipidus: incidence, prevention and management. *Drug Saf* 1999;21:449–456.
33. Rivers K, Shetty S, Menon M. When and how to evaluate a patient with nephrolithiasis. *Urol Clin North Am* 2000;27:203–213.
34. Zahid M, Krumlovsky FA, Roxe D, et al. Central nervous system and cardiac manifestations of hydrochlorothiazide overdosage; treatment with hemodialysis. *Am J Kidney Dis* 1988;11:508–511.
35. Bernal C, Patarca R. Hydrochlorothiazide-induced pulmonary edema and associated immunologic changes. *Ann Pharmacother* 1999;33:172–174.
36. Spratt DI, Pont A. The clinical features of covert diuretic use. *West J Med* 1982;137:331–335.
37. Roe DA. Drug and nutrient interactions in the elderly diabetic. *Drug Nutr Interact* 1988;5:195–203.
38. Ames R. Hyperlipidemia of diuretic therapy. *Arch Mal Coeur Vaiss* 1998;91:23–27.
39. Waller PC, Ramsay LE. Predicting acute gout in diuretic-treated hypertensive patients. *J Hum Hypertens* 1989;3:457–461.
40. Allen JE. Drug-induced photosensitivity. *Clin Pharm* 1993;12:580–587.
41. Miller SJ. Drug-induced hypomagnesemia. *Hosp Pharm* 1995;30:248–260.
42. Niezgoda JA, Walter MC, Jarrard MR. Furosemide overdose and maximal allowable weight standards. *Mil Med* 1989;154:608–609.
43. Dagli AJ, Moos JS. Sudden death following injection of frusemide: case report. *Indian J Med Sci* 1983;37:49–50.
44. Wilcox CS. Metabolic and adverse effects of diuretics. *Semin Nephrol* 1999;19:557–568.
45. Greenberg A. Diuretic complications. *Am J Med Sci* 2000;319:10–24.
46. Humes HD. Insights into ototoxicity. Analogies to nephrotoxicity. *Ann N Y Acad Sci* 1999;884:15–18.
47. Rybak LP. Ototoxicity of loop diuretics. *Otolaryngol Clin North Am* 1993;26:829–844.
48. Halstenson CE, Matzke GR. Bumetanide: a new loop diuretic (Bumex, Roche Laboratories). *Drug Intell Clin Pharm* 1983;17:786–797.
49. Angelborg C, Klochoff I, Larsen HC. Hyperosmotic solutions and hearing in Ménière's Disease. *Am J Otol* 1982;3:200–203.
50. Dennis LJ, Mayer SA. Diagnosis and management of increased intracranial pressure. *Neurol India* 2001;49[Suppl 1]:S37–S50.
51. Chaikin HL. Rhabdomyolysis secondary to drug overdose and prolonged coma. *South Med J* 1980;73:990–994.
52. Chan TY, Kwok TC. Chronicity of neurological features in ciguatera fish poisoning. *Hum Exp Toxicol* 2001;20:426–428.
53. Huff JS. Acute mannitol intoxication in a patient with normal renal function. *Am J Emerg Med* 1990;8:338–339.
54. Moses FM. Colonic perforation due to oral mannitol. *JAMA* 1988;260:640.
55. Perez-Perez AJ, Pazos B, Sobrado J, et al. Acute renal failure following massive mannitol infusion. *Am J Nephrol* 2002;22:573–575.
56. Chang KA, Jawan B, Luk HN, et al. Bullous eruptions caused by extravasation of mannitol—a case report. *Acta Anaesthesiol Sin* 2001;39:195–198.
57. Copeland PM. Diuretic abuse and central pontine myelinolysis. *Psychother Psychosom* 1989;52:101–105.

CHAPTER 144

Acidifying and Alkalinizing Agents

Seth Schonwald

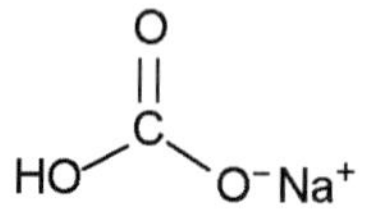

SODIUM BICARBONATE

Compounds included:	**Sodium bicarbonate, citrate, sodium lactate, tromethamine**
Molecular formula and weight:	**Sodium bicarbonate ($NaHCO_3$), 84.01; citrate ($C_6H_5Na_3O_7$), 258.1; sodium lactate ($C_3H_5NaO_3$), 112.1; tromethamine ($C_4H_{11}NO_3$), 121.1 g/mol**
SI conversion:	**1 × mEq/L = mmol/L (bicarbonate and lactate)**
CAS Registry No.:	**144-55-8 (sodium bicarbonate); 68-04-2 (sodium citrate anhydrous); 72-17-3 (sodium lactate); 77-86-1 (tromethamine)**
Normal levels:	**Serum bicarbonate, 22 to 26 mEq/L; serum lactate, 0.5 to 2.2 mEq/L**
Therapeutic levels:	**Serum citrate, 8 to 25 mg/dl**
Target organs:	**Heart (acute fluid overload), multiple organs from hypersensitivity reactions**
Antidote:	**None**

SODIUM BICARBONATE

Sodium bicarbonate is used as an alkalinizing agent to treat metabolic acidosis from all causes. It is used as an antidote to treat antidepressant overdose, diphenhydramine toxicity, chlorine gas exposure, flecainide overdose, propoxyphene overdose, and weakly acidic toxins, such as salicylates, phenobarbital, chlorpropamide, and chlorophenoxy herbicides (Chapter 75).

Bicarbonate-containing dentifrice is used to treat plaque and gingivitis. Ingestion of baking soda (30% sodium bicarbonate, cornstarch, sodium aluminum sulfate, calcium acid phosphate, and calcium sulfate) has been used for decades as a home remedy for indigestion. Excessive bicarbonate ingestion can produce a variety of metabolic derangements, including metabolic alkalosis, hypokalemia, hypernatremia, and even hypoxia. The clinical presentation is highly variable but can include seizures, dysrhythmias, and cardiopulmonary arrest (1). Gastric rupture due to excessive sodium bicarbonate ingestion has rarely been reported (2,3).

Even though hydrochloric acid and sodium bicarbonate react instantaneously, the resulting gas production is slow because carbon dioxide is produced from the dehydration of carbonic acid and is only slowly released into the gas phase (4). The approximate volume of gas produced from one teaspoon of sodium bicarbonate (12 g) is 3.4 L.

Toxic Dose

A 6-week-old infant developed life-threatening complications, including altered mental status and status epilepticus, after unintentional sodium bicarbonate intoxication (5).

Toxicokinetics and Toxicodynamics

Sodium bicarbonate dissociates to provide sodium and bicarbonate ions. Plasma concentration is regulated by the kidney through acidification of the urine when there is a deficit or by alkalinization of the urine when there is excess of bicarbonate.

Bicarbonate anion is considered "labile" because at a proper concentration of hydrogen ion it may be converted to carbonic acid and thence to its volatile form. Carbon dioxide is excreted by the lung. Normally a ratio of 1:20 (carbonic acid:bicarbonate) is present in the extracellular fluid. In a healthy adult with normal kidney function, practically all the glomerular filtered bicarbonate ion is reabsorbed; less than 1% is excreted in the urine (6).

Pathophysiology

The main effect of ingestion and chronic abuse of sodium bicarbonate is hypokalemic hypochloremic metabolic alkalosis. After sodium bicarbonate powder ingestion, gas formation and pressure buildup can play a large part in subsequent morbidity.

Pregnancy and Lactation

Sodium bicarbonate is U.S. Food and Drug Administration pregnancy category C. Rapid injection (10 ml/minute) of hypertonic sodium bicarbonate solutions into neonates and children younger than 2 years of age may produce hypernatremia, a decrease in cerebrospinal fluid pressure, and possible intracranial hemorrhage. The rate of administration in such patients should be limited to no more than 8 mEq/kg/day. Entry into breast milk has not been studied but undoubtedly occurs.

Clinical Presentation

The main effect of ingestion and chronic abuse of sodium bicarbonate is hypokalemic hypochloremic metabolic alkalosis. Other metabolic abnormalities include hypernatremia and hypocalcemia (7). Transient albuminuria; neuromuscular irritability, including hyperreflexia; and elevations in blood urea nitrogen have been observed.

Severe metabolic alkalosis in patients with unsuspected antacid overdose has been reported (8). Sodium bicarbonate (3 to 4 tablespoons/day) may be ingested by patients with anorexia nervosa to dampen their appetites (9). This may be associated with recurrent hypokalemic metabolic alkalosis. Munchausen's syndrome has been associated with sodium bicarbonate abuse (10).

Potentially large loads of sodium given with bicarbonate require that caution be exercised in the use of sodium bicarbonate in patients with congestive heart failure or other edematous or sodium-retaining states as well as in patients with oliguria or anuria (11).

The diagnostic triad for spontaneous rupture of the stomach includes surgical emphysema of the neck and a distended abdomen after sudden abdominal pain. Radiography is often unhelpful. A perforated peptic ulcer is rarely bigger than 1.5 cm, whereas gastric ruptures may be 5 cm long. The lesser curvature of the stomach is the usual site of rupture (12).

Diagnostic Tests

The aim of bicarbonate therapy is to produce a substantial correction of low total CO_2 content and blood pH, but the risks of overdosage and alkalosis should be avoided. Hence, periodic monitoring of electrolytes is recommended to minimize the possibility of overdosage.

Treatment

Follow and monitor serum sodium, electrolytes, pH, and volume status. Early surgery in cases of gastric rupture is important. Postoperative intraabdominal sepsis can be fatal. Gut decontamination after sodium bicarbonate ingestion is not recommended, as this may increase the potential for gastric rupture. These methods have not proved to be helpful in baking soda ingestion. There is no antidote.

In infants, rehydration with oral electrolyte solutions may be useful in cases of mild metabolic alkalosis from bicarbonate ingestion. Intravenous (IV) correction of electrolytes may be necessary. "Rebound hyperkalemia" may require weeks to normalize.

CITRATES

Citrates and citric acid solutions are used to correct the acidosis of certain renal tubular disorders, to treat metabolic acidosis, for long-term urinary alkalinization, for prevention and treatment of uric acid and calcium kidney stones (13), and as nonparticulate neutralizing buffers. Oral citrate salts are also used as cathartics (e.g., magnesium citrate) (14). Hypermagnesemia has been associated with their use (15–17).

Sodium citrate and citric acid are used to prevent blood clotting during blood collection and storage. Rapid infusion of blood can lead to a fall in ionized calcium. Citrate-phosphate-dextrose has been approved by the U.S. Food and Drug Administration for blood storage. Citric acid ingestion can cause life-threatening metabolic acidosis (18).

Toxic Dose

Cardiac arrest has followed IV administration of a citrate anticoagulant solution (8). However, transfusion of blood at a rate not exceeding 50 ml every 30 minutes has shown no evidence of citrate intoxication. If the rate at which citrate is infused remains below 0.5 mg/kg body weight/minute, the serum concentration of citrate ion remains below 9 mg/dl (0.5 mmol/L), and the calculated ionized calcium level remains above 0.85 mmol/L, which is within the normal range (19).

Harmful effects of citrate infusion may occur if the dosage exceeds 250 mg/kg/hour. An inadvertent injection of 400 ml of the citrate-phosphate-dextrose solution over 50 minutes led to cardiac arrest with electromechanical dissociation that responded to calcium chloride therapy. The estimated peak serum citrate level is greater than 120 mg/dl (20).

Toxicokinetics and Toxicodynamics

Citric acid is metabolized rapidly by the liver, adrenal cortex, and muscle. Approximately 20% is excreted in the urine.

Pathophysiology

Sodium and potassium citrates are metabolized to sodium bicarbonate and potassium bicarbonate and thus act as systemic alkalinizers. Citrate retards glycolysis and prevents coagulation by binding ionized calcium. Rapid infusion of blood or plasma can lead to a fall in ionized calcium. Insufficient ionized calcium may increase the irritability of muscle and may induce fasciculation, tetany, seizures, or cardiac failure if the level is reduced for more than a few seconds.

Pregnancy and Lactation

The use of citrates during pregnancy and lactation is safe.

Clinical Presentation

Citrate intoxication can occur in patients receiving blood at a rate greater than 1 unit in 5 to 10 minutes (21). Citrate also binds magnesium, which has also caused cardiac dysrhythmias (long QT syndrome, torsade de pointes) in massively transfused patients (22). In general, when blood is being transfused at a rate less than 30 ml/kg/hour (less than 8 U/hour), compensating mechanisms ensure that ionized calcium concentration remains normal (11). Patients with severe osteoporosis (decreased calcium stores) or severe liver disease (inability to mobilize citrate to bicarbonate) may be at increased risk.

Neurologic signs of citrate intoxication occur early and include perioral and acral numbness and tingling, feelings of tenseness or lightness of muscles, and a sense of "twitchiness."

Cardiac effects many include bradycardia and decreased cardiac output as well as ventricular fibrillation and cardiac asystole. Arterial hypotension may be resistant to further blood transfusion or pressor agents. These problems may be enhanced if cold blood is infused. Electrolyte effects include ionized hypocalcemia, hypomagnesemia, and hyperkalemia followed by hypokalemia.

Diagnostic Tests

Acute disturbances in *ionized* calcium homeostasis may not be apparent from *total* calcium measurement. The normal range of ionized calcium is 0.9 to 1.6 mmol (1.8 to 3.2 mEq/L). The total calcium level in the blood after the injection of citrate usually remains normal or may even increase. Serum potassium and magnesium should also be measured, particularly in patients receiving a large rapid transfusion and those with symptoms or with renal insufficiency.

Citrate may be measured via an enzymatic method. A citrate infusion of 1 ml/kg/minute produces plasma citrate levels of between 8 and 25 mg/dl. A toxic plasma citrate level of 50 mg/dl can result in a calculated plasma ionized calcium level of approximately 0.5 mmol and can lead to marked depression of myocardial function (23).

Treatment

Treatment focuses on detection of signs of hypocalcemia and prompt reduction of infusion rate and administration of calcium. Decontamination is not helpful because of parenteral administration.

There is no antidote for citrate intoxication. Skeletal stores of calcium are large, and calcium salts are not usually needed for treatment. IV infusion of calcium may cause disturbances in the cardiac rhythm and should be avoided if possible. There is a real danger of calcium overdosage with aggressive treatment of citrate-induced hypocalcemia. Cardiac monitoring and serial electrocardiograms should be followed, as calcium levels normalize in overdose.

Severe hypocalcemia and citrate toxicity have been successfully managed with exchange transfusions in newborns (24). In children, calcium replacement has led to hypercalcemia and death. The use of calcium may be helpful in the massively transfused patient with profound liver disease or acute heart failure, two situations in which metabolism of citrate may be impaired.

Monitoring

During the management of massive hemorrhage, coagulation tests and platelet counts should be monitored frequently, and aggressive correction of hypovolemia should be instituted to avoid coagulation defects associated with prolonged shock.

SODIUM LACTATE

Hypertonic sodium lactate has been used as an alkalinizing resuscitation fluid during cardiac surgery (25). As it is hypertonic, secure IV access is essential to minimize the risk of extravasation. It is also found in peritoneal dialysis solutions to help maintain acid-base balance (26) and in continuous venovenous hemofiltration as a buffer solution (27), and it has been used to induce panic disorder (28–31). Sodium lactate was also used in the past to treat poisoning from sodium channel–blocking agents, such as tricyclic antidepressants (32), antidysrhythmic drugs, cibenzoline (33), nadoxolol (34), and chloroquine.

Toxic Dose

One liter contains 167 mEq each of sodium and bicarbonate (as lactate). Dosage is determined by acidosis severity; laboratory values; and patient's age, weight, and clinical condition.

Pathophysiology

Sodium lactate is metabolized by the liver to bicarbonate in more than 1 to 2 hours. Metabolism produces alkalinization by removing both a hydrogen ion and its corresponding lactate. Lactate is metabolized to glycogen and ultimately to water and carbon dioxide in the liver. Sodium lactate delivers a high load of sodium.

Pregnancy and Lactation

The pregnancy category of sodium lactate and its use during breast-feeding have not been addressed.

Clinical Presentation

Sodium lactate may induce panic attacks (35). Extravasation may result in phlebitis and local necrosis. Overdose may yield sodium and water overload, hypokalemia, neuromuscular hyperexcitability, metabolic alkalosis, and respiratory depression (36).

Diagnostic Tests

Testing is directed at the potential adverse effects of lactate infusion: hypernatremia, undesired alkalemia, and hypokalemia. In addition, tests related to the patient's underlying disorder may be needed (e.g., hypotension, trauma).

Treatment

Frequent electrolyte determination and correction is mandated in potential cases of sodium lactate overdose. General treatment of extravasation is addressed in Chapter 16.

TROMETHAMINE

Tromethamine (THAM) is a systemic alkalizing and buffering agent used to correct the acidity of acid citrate dextrose blood in cardiac bypass surgery and for cardiac arrest during thoracic surgery. Other indications are diabetic or renal acidosis, salicylate or barbiturate intoxication, and increased intracranial pressure associated with cerebral trauma. THAM is used in cardioplegic solutions, during liver transplantation, and for chemolysis of renal calculi. Apnea, hypoglycemia, hypokalemia, alkalosis, transient hypocalcemia, venospasm, and tissue necrosis from infiltration have all been described with its use (37).

Tris(hydroxymethyl)aminomethane or THAM reverses acidemia without excretion of carbon dioxide. It has been used for the correction of metabolic acidosis in lieu of sodium bicarbonate in hypernatremic infants.

Toxic Dose

The adult therapeutic dose for acidosis during cardiac arrest is 3.6 to 10.8 g IV.

Toxicokinetics and Toxicodynamics

THAM distributes into all tissues and is excreted renally (80%). The volume of distribution ranges from 0.34 to 0.86 L/kg, and the elimination half-life is 3 to 8 hours in patients with cerebral edema.

Pathophysiology

THAM is an organic amine hydrogen ion (proton) acceptor. A weak base combines with hydrogen ions from carbonic acid to form bicarbonate and cationic buffer. Administration of THAM decreases hydrogen ion concentration, which results in a decrease in carbon dioxide concentrations and an increase in serum bicarbonate concentrations. The decrease in carbon dioxide concentration removes a potent respiratory stimulus and may result in hypoxia. THAM also increases urine output through osmotic diuresis. Excretion of electrolytes and carbon dioxide is also increased. Urine pH is raised along with the excretion of electrolytes (38).

Pregnancy and Lactation

The pregnancy category and use during breast-feeding have not been addressed.

Clinical Presentation

Adverse effects are infrequent but include hypoglycemia, respiratory depression, and hemorrhagic hepatic necrosis. Most reported adverse reactions are local and occur from the administration of an alkaline solution. Local adverse effects may include irritation at the injection site, chemical phlebitis, and venous thrombosis (39).

Diagnostic Tests

Serum bicarbonate, glucose and electrolytes, carbon dioxide, and blood pH should be monitored during infusion.

Treatment

Treatment is symptomatic and supportive. Treatment of extravasation is addressed in Chapter 16.

REFERENCES

1. Fitzgibbons LJ, Snoey ER. Severe metabolic alkalosis due to baking soda ingestion: case reports of two patients with unsuspected antacid overdose. *J Emerg Med* 1999;17:57–61.
2. Lazebnik N, Iellin A, Michowitz M. Spontaneous rupture of the normal stomach after sodium bicarbonate ingestion. *J Clin Gastroenterol* 1986;8:454–456.
3. Brismar B, Strandberg A, Wiklund B. Stomach rupture following ingestion of sodium bicarbonate. *Acta Chir Scand Suppl* 1986;530:97–99.
4. Fordtran JS, Morawski SG, Santa Ana CA, et al. Gas production after reaction of sodium bicarbonate and hydrochloric acid. *Gastroenterology* 1984;87:1014–1021.
5. Nichols MH, Wason S, Gonzalez del Rey J, et al. Baking soda: a potentially fatal home remedy. *Pediatr Emerg Care* 1995;11:109–111.
6. RxList. Sodium bicarbonate. Available at: http://www.rxlist.com/cgi/generic2/sodbic_cp.htm. Accessed 04/21/2003.
7. Thomas SH, Stone CK. Acute toxicity from baking soda ingestion. *Am J Emerg Med* 1994;12:57–59.
8. Lee BL, Auerbach PS, Olson KR, et al. Cardiac arrest following direct intravenous administration of a citrate anticoagulant solution. *Ann Emerg Med* 1986;15:1353–1356.
9. Kennedy S. Sodium bicarbonate abuse in anorexia nervosa. *J Clin Psychiatry* 1988;49:168.
10. Linford SM, James HD. Sodium bicarbonate abuse: a case report. *Br J Psychiatry* 1986;149:502–503.
11. Rutledge R, Sheldon GF, Collins ML. Massive transfusion. *Crit Care Clin* 1986;2:791–805.
12. Barna P. Sodium bicarbonate: burst stomachs and high sodium. *J Clin Gastroenterol* 1986;8:697–698.
13. Tekin A, Tekgul S, Atsu N, et al. Oral potassium citrate treatment for idiopathic hypocitruria in children with calcium urolithiasis. *J Urol* 2002;168:2572–2574.
14. Sue YJ, Woolf A, Shannon M. Efficacy of magnesium citrate cathartic in pediatric toxic ingestions. *Ann Emerg Med* 1994;24:709–712.
15. Clark BA, Brown RS. Unsuspected morbid hypermagnesemia in elderly patients. *Am J Nephrol* 1992;12:336–343.
16. Gren J, Woolf A. Hypermagnesemia associated with catharsis in a salicylate-intoxicated patient with anorexia nervosa. *Ann Emerg Med* 1989;18:200–203.
17. Jones J, Heiselman D, Dougherty J, Eddy A. Cathartic-induced magnesium toxicity during overdose management. *Ann Emerg Med* 1986;15:1214–1218.
18. DeMars CS, Hollister K, Tomassoni A, et al. Citric acid ingestion: a life-threatening cause of metabolic acidosis. *Ann Emerg Med* 2001;38:588–591.
19. Bunker JP, Dendixen HH, Murphy AJ. Hemodynamic effects of intravenously administered sodium citrate. *N Engl J Med* 1962;266:372–377.
20. Lee-Chow BL, Auerbach PS, Olson KR, et al. Cardiac arrest following direct intravenous administration of a citrate anticoagulant solution. *Vet Hum Toxicol* 1985;28:296.
21. Rudolph R, Boyd CR. Massive transfusion: complications and their management. *South Med J* 1990;83:1065–1070.
22. Scott VL, De Wolf AM, Kang Y, et al. Ionized hypomagnesemia in patients undergoing orthotopic liver transplantation: a complication of citrate intoxication. *Liver Transpl Surg* 1996;2:343–347.
23. Ludbrook J, Wynn W. Citrate intoxication: a clinical and experimental study. *Br Med J* 1985;2:523–528.
24. Nelson N, Finnstrom O. Blood exchange transfusions in newborns, the effect on serum ionized calcium. *Early Hum Dev* 1988;18:157–164.
25. Mustafa I, Leverve XM. Metabolic and hemodynamic effects of hypertonic solutions: sodium-lactate versus sodium chloride infusion in postoperative patients. *Shock* 2002;18:306–310.
26. Wolfson M, Jones MR. Nutrition impact of peritoneal dialysis solutions. *Miner Electrolyte Metab* 1999;25:333–336.
27. Heering P, Ivens K, Thumer O, et al. The use of different buffers during continuous hemofiltration in critically ill patients with acute renal failure. *Intensive Care Med* 1999;25:1244–1251.
28. Peskind ER, Jensen CF, Pascualy M, et al. Sodium lactate and hypertonic sodium chloride induce equivalent panic incidence, panic symptoms, and hypernatremia in panic disorder. *Biol Psychiatry* 1998;44:1007–1016.
29. George DT, Umhau JC, Phillips MJ, et al. Serotonin, testosterone and alcohol in the etiology of domestic violence. *Psychiatry Res* 2001;104:27–37.
30. George DT, Hibbeln JR, Ragan PW, et al. Lactate-induced rage and panic in a select group of subjects who perpetrate acts of domestic violence. *Biol Psychiatry* 2000;47:804–812.
31. Goetz RR, Klein DF, Gorman JM. Symptoms essential to the experience of sodium lactate-induced panic. *Neuropsychopharmacology* 1996;14:355–366.
32. Bismuth C, Bodin F, Pebay-Peroula F, et al. Imipramine poisoning and acute cardiac failure. Value of sodium lactate. *Presse Med* 1968;76:2277–2278.
33. Viallon A, Page Y, Lafond P, et al. Fatal voluntary poisoning with cibenzoline. Failure of conventional therapies. *Presse Med* 1998;27:1621–1625.
34. Jaeger A, Kopferschmitt J, Sauder P, et al. Acute nadoxolol poisoning. A multicentric study of 35 cases. *Toxicol Eur Res* 1982;4:163–166.
35. Otte C, Kellner M, Arlt J, et al. Prolactin but not ACTH increases during sodium lactate-induced panic attacks. *Psychiatry Res* 2002;109:201–205.
36. egora.fr. http://www.egora.fr/. Accessed 04/21/2003.
37. Neonatology on the Web. Available at: http://www.neonatology.org/ref/meds/med95.html. Accessed 04/21/2003.
38. Nahas GG, Sutin KM, Fermon C, et al. Guidelines for the treatment of acidemia with THAM. *Drugs* 1998;55:191–224.
39. McEvoy GK. Alkalinizing agents. In: McEvoy GK, ed. *American hospital formulary service drug information*. Bethesda, MD: American Society of Hospital Pharmacists, 1993:1559–1566.

CHAPTER 145

Replacement Preparations

Seth Schonwald

Compounds included:	**Iron dextran (INFeD); hydroxyethyl starch (HES; hetastarch); polygeline (Haemaccel)**
Molecular formula and weight:	**Not applicable**
SI conversion:	**Not applicable**
CAS Registry No.:	**9004-66-4 (iron dextran); 9005-27-0 (hydroxyethyl starch); 9015-56-9 (polygeline)**
Therapeutic levels:	**Not applicable**
Target organs:	**Heart (acute fluid overload), multiple organs from hypersensitivity reactions**
Antidote:	**None**

OVERVIEW

Replacement preparations are administered parenterally. Their toxicity arises from acute hypersensitivity reactions or therapeutic overuse, resulting in hypervolemia or unintended anticoagulation.

IRON DEXTRAN

Iron dextran (INFeD) is used in the treatment of microcytic hypochromic anemia, resulting from iron deficiency (1), especially in those patients in whom oral administration of iron is not feasible or ineffective. It is used extensively as part of the treatment of anemia in dialysis patients (2).

Toxic Dose

Fatal anaphylaxis after intravenous (IV) or intramuscular administration has occurred (3,4). A 32-ml dose of INFeD IV has induced meningitis symptoms (5). A child who received 1.3 g of elemental iron IV as INFeD remained asymptomatic (6). A 4-year-old child who was inadvertently given 2 g of INFeD died of sepsis (7).

Toxicokinetics and Toxicodynamics

INFeD is absorbed into capillaries and the lymphatic system after intramuscular injection. Circulating INFeD is removed from the plasma by the reticuloendothelial system, which splits the complex into its iron and dextran components. The iron is then bound to form hemosiderin or ferritin and transferrin. This iron replenishes hemoglobin and depleted iron stores (8). Dextran is a polyglucose and is either metabolized or excreted. Negligible amounts of iron are lost via the urinary or alimentary pathways after administration of INFeD. The plasma half-life of the INFeD complex is 2 to 3 days (9). Trace quantities of INFeD appear in the urine.

Pathophysiology

INFeD is a complex of ferric hydroxide with dextran of average molecular weight between 5000 and 7500 d (10). Approximately 98% of the iron in INFeD is present as a stable INFeD complex. As iron is released, free iron increases. The serum hemoglobin does not rise during the infusion. This results in abnormally high concentrations of free iron, which crosses into the cerebrospinal fluid and is responsible for meningitis symptoms.

Pregnancy and Lactation

INFeD is U.S. Food and Drug Administration (FDA) pregnancy category C (Appendix I). It is teratogenic in animals. Traces of INFeD are excreted in breast milk.

Clinical Presentation

After an overdose with INFeD, a meningitis-like syndrome characterized by muscle cramps, bilateral frontal headache, neck stiffness, opisthotonus, and photophobia may develop (11).

Arthralgias, vomiting, metabolic acidosis, bradycardia, and depressed central nervous system sensorium may be seen within hours (7).

Hypersensitivity reactions can develop, including potentially fatal anaphylactoid (12) and anaphylactic reactions. The anaphylactoid reaction manifests during the first few minutes of an infusion (13). Pulmonary edema has occurred in hemodialysis patients (14). The most common hypersensitivity reaction involves arthralgias and fever within 24 to 48 hours of parenteral therapy. These reactions are usually controlled easily with nonsteroidal antiinflammatory drugs (15). Rare systemic hypersensitivity reactions may occur 1 to 2 weeks after initiation of therapy and include lymphadenopathy, malaise, fever, elevated erythrocyte sedimentation rate, serum sickness, vasculitis (16), and splenomegaly.

Infrequent reactions to INFeD include rhabdomyolysis (17), severe generalized dermatitis (18), and systemic lupus erythematosus (19,20).

Diagnostic Tests

The INFeD complex persists in the circulation for 2 to 3 weeks. It interferes with all colorimetric iron assays and produces false-positive and abnormally elevated readings of serum iron (21). The total iron-binding capacity may be markedly increased. Transferrin-based iron, total iron-binding capacity, total iron (except hemoglobin iron), and dextran-bound iron levels can be measured by a colorimetric technique using dithionite.

Treatment

The treatment of an INFeD overdose is symptomatic and supportive. Monitoring of serum iron and total iron-binding capacity is indicated. Decontamination is not possible because it is administered parenterally. The drug removal by hemodialysis is negligible. Exchange transfusion has been useful if performed early (7).

Antidotes

Deferoxamine may decrease the side effects of INFeD treatment, but because the iron probably remains substantively bound to dextran, deferoxamine is probably ineffective.

HYDROXYETHYL STARCH

Hydroxyethyl starch refers to a class of synthetic colloids with less immunogenic potential than dextran. Different forms are available, which have different characteristics and produce different clinical effects (22). Hetastarch is the most common agent in this class. It is derived from cornstarch and has a molecular weight of 450,000 d. Hetastarch is indicated in the treatment of hypovolemia. It is not a substitute for blood or plasma.

Toxic Dose

Total therapeutic dosage and rate of infusion depend on the amount of blood or plasma lost and the resultant hemoconcentration as well as age, weight, and clinical condition of the patient. Hetastarch is administered by IV infusion only. The safety and effectiveness of hydroxyethyl starch in children have not been established. No toxic dose has been established.

Toxicokinetics and Toxicodynamics

Hetastarch molecules less than 50,000 d molecular weight are rapidly eliminated by renal excretion. A single dose of Hetastarch, 500 ml (30 g), results in urinary elimination of 33% of the dose within 24 hours. Less than 10% of the total dose is present 2 weeks after injection.

Pathophysiology

Hetastarch is composed almost entirely of amylopectin. Hydroxyethyl ether groups are introduced into the glucose units of the starch, and the resultant material is hydrolyzed to yield a high-molecular-weight compound.

Pregnancy and Lactation

Hetastarch is FDA pregnancy category C (Appendix I). Its entry into breast milk is unknown.

Clinical Presentation

In a double-blind study, children ages 1.0 to 15.5 years and scheduled for surgery were randomized to either hetastarch or albumin as a postoperative volume expander. No differences were found in the coagulation parameters or in the amount of replacement fluids required in the children receiving 20 ml/kg or less of either of the colloid replacement therapies (23).

Although volume expanders are commonly used to prevent acute tubular necrosis by correcting underlying volume depletion, these agents are associated with renal impairment (24,25). Intracranial bleeding resulting in death has occurred during the use of hetastarch injection (26).

Patients may experience severe pruritus, which can persist for months (27,28). Hypersensitivity reactions include anaphylactic/anaphylactoid reactions (29), cardiac arrest, severe hypotension, noncardiac pulmonary edema, laryngeal edema, bronchospasm (30), angioedema, wheezing, restlessness, tachypnea, stridor, fever, chest pain, bradycardia, tachycardia, chills, urticaria, pruritus, facial and periorbital edema, coughing, sneezing, flushing, erythema multiforme, rash, and death (31).

Diagnostic Tests

Clinical evaluation and periodic laboratory determinations are necessary to monitor changes in fluid balance, serum electrolyte concentrations, acid-base balance, and coagulation parameters. Large volumes of isotonic solutions containing 6% hetastarch may transiently alter the coagulation mechanism due to hemodilution and a mild direct inhibitory action on factor VIII. Hemodilution may also result in a decline of total protein, albumin, and fibrinogen levels and in transient prolongation of prothrombin, clotting, and bleeding times.

Treatment

Treatment is symptomatic and supportive. Decontamination is not possible because of parenteral administration. It is not removed by hemodialysis. There is no antidote.

HAEMACCEL

Haemaccel and Gelofusin are modified gelatins used as low viscosity colloid plasma expanders to maintain intravascular volume after heart surgery (32) and in hypovolemic resuscitation. Haemaccel contains a high concentration of Ca^{2+}, whereas Gelofusin does not (33).

Toxic Dose

The adult therapeutic dose of polygeline, 3.5% solution, is typically 500 to 1000 ml IV; the total dosage should not exceed 2500 ml/day. No toxic dose has been established.

Toxicokinetics and Toxicodynamics

Haemaccel is distributed between intravascular and extravascular compartments. Fluid is not drawn from the extravascular compartment, and the increase in intravascular volume does not exceed the volume of Haemaccel infused. The apparent volume of distribution is 8 L. The main route of excretion is renal (80%). Intestinal excretion and metabolic breakdown occur to a smaller extent. The elimination half-life is 5 to 8 hours.

Pathophysiology

Haemaccel increases the osmotic pressure with the vascular system. This increases perfusion of organs. If overused, it may over-expand the intravascular compartment. It interferes with coagulation by dilution and perhaps a decrease in the ionized calcium level.

Pregnancy and Lactation

The pregnancy category and excretion into breast milk have not been established.

Clinical Presentation

Anaphylaxis anaphylactoid reactions to Haemaccel have been reported (34,35). A severe life-threatening reaction with bronchial asthma may occur (36). A reduced quality of clot formation with Haemaccel and Gelofusin has been reported (37).

Diagnostic Tests

In addition to laboratories needed for evaluation of hypotension and organ perfusion, coagulation studies should be followed serially.

Treatment

Treatment is symptomatic and supportive. Decontamination is not possible because of parenteral administration. It is not removed by hemodialysis. There is no antidote.

REFERENCES

1. Burns DL, Pomposelli JJ. Toxicity of parenteral iron dextran therapy. *Kidney Int Suppl* 1999;69:S119–S124.
2. Johnson CA, Mason NA, Bailie GR. Intravenous iron products. *ANNA J* 1999;26:522–524.
3. Zipf RE Jr. Fatal anaphylaxis after intravenous iron dextran. *J Forensic Sci* 1975;20:326–333.
4. Becker CE, MacGregor RR, Walker KS, et al. Fatal anaphylaxis after intramuscular iron-dextran. *Ann Intern Med* 1966;65:745–748.
5. Shuttleworth D, Spence C, Slade R. Meningism due to intravenous iron dextran. *Lancet* 1983;2:453.
6. Rodgers G, Matyunas N, Ross M. Lack of toxicity following a large inadvertent dose of iron-dextran: a case report. *J Toxicol Clin Toxicol* 1995;33:475–486.
7. Davidar SM, Snodgrass WR. Fatal iron-dextran poisoning: a combined iron toxicity and dextran induced immune block. *Vet Hum Toxicol* 1989;31:34L.
8. RxList Web site. Clinical pharmacology. Available at: http://www.rxlist.com/cgi/generic3/fedex_cp.htm. Accessed April 7, 2003.
9. Wood JK, Milner PFA, Pathak UN. The metabolism of iron-dextran given as a total dose infusion to iron-deficient Jamaican subjects. *Br J Haematol* 1968;14:119–129.
10. Reynold JEF, ed. *Martindale: the extra pharmacopoeia*, 30th ed. London: Pharmaceutical Press, 1993:851–853.
11. Avasthi R, Aggarwal M, Kataria SP. Meningism following intravenous iron dextran. *J Assoc Physicians India* 1991;39:428–429.
12. Hamstra RD, Block MH, Schocket AL. Intravenous iron dextran in clinical medicine. *JAMA* 1980;243:1726–1731.
13. Furhoff AK. Anaphylactoid reaction to dextran—a report of 133 cases. *Acta Anaesthesiol Scand* 1977;21:161–167.
14. Freter S, Davidman M, Lipman M, et al. Pulmonary edema: atypical anaphylactoid reaction to intravenous iron dextran. *Am J Nephrol* 1997;17:477–479.
15. Auerbach M, Witt D, Toler W, et al. Clinical use of the total dose intravenous infusion of iron dextran. *J Lab Clin Med* 1988;111:566–570.
16. Bielory L. Serum sickness from iron-dextran administration. *Acta Haematol* 1990;83:166–168.
17. Foulkes WD, Sewry C, Calam J, et al. Rhabdomyolysis after intramuscular iron-dextran in malabsorption. *Ann Rheum Dis* 1991;50:184–186.
18. Teoh ES, Chan DP. Severe generalised dermatitis with intravenous iron-dextran (Imferon) therapy. *Med J Malaya* 1966;21:63–65.
19. Oh VM. Iron dextran and systemic lupus erythematosus. *BMJ* 1992;305:1000.
20. Harchelroad F, Rice S. Iron-dextran: treatment or overdose. *Vet Hum Toxicol* 1992;34:329.
21. Hvisman W. Interference of Imferon in colorimetric tests for iron. *Clin Chem* 1980;26:635–637.

22. Weidhase R, Faude K, Weidhase R. Hydroxyethyl starch—an interim report. *Anaesthesiol Reanim* 1998;23:4–14.
23. Brutocao D, Bratton SL, Thomas JR, et al. Comparison of hetastarch with albumin for postoperative volume expansion in children after cardiopulmonary bypass. *J Cardiothorac Vasc Anesth* 1996;10:348–351.
24. Boldt J. Hydroxyethylstarch as a risk factor for acute renal failure: is a change of clinical practice indicated? *Drug Saf* 2002;25:837–846.
25. Schortgen F, Lacherade J, Bruneel F, et al. Effects of hydroxyethylstarch and gelatin on renal function in severe sepsis: a multicentre randomised study. *Lancet* 2001;357:911–916.
26. Damon L. Intracranial bleeding during treatment with hydroxyethyl starch. *N Engl J Med* 1987;317:964–965.
27. Stander S, Szepfalusi Z, Bohle B, et al. Differential storage of hydroxyethyl starch (HES) in the skin: immunoelectronmicroscopical long term study. *Cell Tissue Res* 2001;304:261–269.
28. Murphy M, Carmichael AJ, Lawler PG, et al. The incidence of hydroxyethyl starch-associated pruritus. *Br J Dermatol* 2001;144:973–976.
29. Ebo DG, Schuerwegh A, Stevens WJ. Anaphylaxis to starch. *Allergy* 2000;55:1098–1099.
30. Takada M, Tomatsu T, Harada T, et al. Bronchospasm due to anaphylactic reaction to hydroxyethyl starch (HESPANDER). *Masui* 1997;46:397–400.
31. U.S. Food and Drug Administration. Product approval information—licensing action. Available at: http://www.fda.gov/cber/nda/hexbio033199.htm. Accessed April 7, 2003.
32. Wahba A, Sendtner E, Birnbaum DE. Fluid resuscitation with Haemaccel vs. human albumin following coronary artery bypass grafting. *Thorac Cardiovasc Surg* 1996;44:178–182.
33. Evans PA, Glenn JR, Heptinstall S, et al. Effects of gelatin-based resuscitation fluids on platelet aggregation. *Br J Anaesth* 1998;81:198–202.
34. Russell WJ, Fenwick DG. Anaphylaxis to Haemaccel and cross reactivity to Gelofusin. *Anaesth Intensive Care* 2002;30:481–483.
35. Fenwick DG, Andersen GJ, Munt PS. Anaphylactoid reaction to Haemaccel. *Anaesth Intensive Care* 1995;23:521–522.
36. Kathirvel S, Podder S, Batra YK, et al. Severe life threatening reaction to Haemaccel in a patient with bronchial asthma. *Eur J Anaesthesiol* 2001;18:122–123.
37. Mardel SN, Saunders FM, Allen H, et al. Reduced quality of clot formation with gelatin-based plasma substitutes. *Br J Anaesth* 1998;80:204–207.

CHAPTER 146

Uricosuric Agents

Seth Schonwald

PROBENECID

Compounds included:	**Probenecid (Benemid); sulfinpyrazone (Anturane)**
Molecular formula and weight:	**Probenecid ($C_{13}H_{19}NO_4S$), 285.4; sulfinpyrazone ($C_{23}H_{20}N_2O_3S$), 404.5 g/mol**
SI conversion:	**Probeneid, mg/L × 3.5 = µmol/L; sulfinpyrazone, mg/L × 2.5 = µmol/L**
CAS Registry No.:	**57-66-9 (probenecid); 57-96-5 (sulfinpyrazone)**
Normal levels:	**Not applicable**
Target organs:	**Skin (acute or chronic), gastrointestinal tract (acute), kidney (chronic)**
Antidote:	**None**

OVERVIEW

Uricosuric agents decrease the serum uric acid level by increasing renal excretion. Probenecid and sulfinpyrazone are used in patients who are considered "underexcretors" of uric acid. Uricosuric drugs should not be given to patients with a urine output of less than 1 ml/minute, a creatinine clearance of less than 50 ml/minute, or a history of renal calculi. The physiologic decline in renal function that occurs with aging limits the use of uricosuric agents (1).

PROBENECID

Probenecid is used for the treatment of hyperuricemia associated with gout (2). It is also combined with penicillin and related antibiotics to delay renal clearance of the antibiotic (3). Probenecid is recommended for allopurinol-intolerant patients with gout and "underexcretion" hyperuricemia who have normal renal function and no history of nephrolithiasis (4).

Toxic Dose

The adult therapeutic dose for gout is 500 mg orally twice per day. A typical pediatric dose is 40 mg/kg/day in divided doses. A 36-year-old man died after ingestion of approximately 75 g. Tissue concentrations of probenecid were highest in serum (710 mg/L) and liver (550 mg/kg). Probenecid was also detected in vitreous and bile. The blood ethanol was 0.13 g/100 ml (5).

Toxicokinetics and Toxicodynamics

Probenecid is completely absorbed orally. Probenecid and its oxidized metabolites are extensively bound to plasma proteins, mainly albumin. Peak plasma levels occur at 2 to 4 hours; time-to-peak uricosuric effect is 0.5 hour. Therapeutic plasma levels for uricosuric effect are 100 to 200 μg/ml (6). The half-life of probenecid in plasma (4 to 12 hours) is dose dependent. Renal excretion is the major route of elimination of the metabolites; excretion of the parent drug is minimal and is dependent on urinary pH (7).

Pathophysiology

Probenecid is a competitive inhibitor of organic acid transport. It acts on kidney tubules to increase excretion of uric acid, thus lowering blood uric acid levels. It also blocks the urinary excretion of penicillin and related antibiotics, thus prolonging their half-lives.

Pregnancy and Lactation

Probenecid is U.S. Food and Drug Administration pregnancy category B. It has been used with procaine penicillin in pregnancy without apparent adverse effect. Excretion in breast milk is unknown.

Clinical Presentation

Adverse effects of probenecid are uncommon and usually mild. In addition to causing kidney stones and precipitating acute gouty arthritis (8), it has been associated with hair loss, skin rash, headache, nausea, sore gums, and fever. In rare instances, it has caused immune hemolytic anemia (9,10). Probenecid hypersensitivity has been reported in an acquired immunodeficiency syndrome patient on cidofovir (11).

Diagnostic Tests

There are a number of analytic procedures for the assay of probenecid, including spectrophotometry, spectrofluorometry, and gas chromatography-mass spectrometry, and radioimmunoassay.

Treatment

Treatment is symptomatic and supportive. There is no specific antidote or therapy.

SULFINPYRAZONE

Sulfinpyrazone is a uricosuric agent indicated for the treatment of chronic and intermittent gouty arthritis. It also inhibits thrombosis. One study showed that sulfinpyrazone has the potential to reduce the risk of mural thrombosis after endocardial injury (12), and another study concluded that it prevented sudden cardiac death after an acute myocardial infarction (13). It is available as 100- and 200-mg tablets.

Toxic Dose

The adult therapeutic dose is 400 to 800 mg/day. The pediatric dose is 10 mg/kg/24 hours. An acute dose has not been determined.

Toxicokinetics and Toxicodynamics

Peak plasma levels are reached in 1 to 2 hours. The therapeutic plasma level for uricosuria is up to 160 μg/ml on a dose of 800 mg/day. The duration of action is 4 to 6 hours (10 hours in some patients). The elimination half-life is 3 to 8 hours. Sulfinpyrazone is hepatically metabolized; approximately 45% of the drug is excreted unchanged by the kidney, and a small amount is excreted in the feces (14).

Pathophysiology

Sulfinpyrazone increases uric acid excretion and reduces blood urate levels. It also inhibits the thrombotic processes associated with platelet adhesion, aggregation, and reduced platelet survival (15).

Pregnancy and Lactation

Sulfinpyrazone is U.S. Food and Drug Administration pregnancy category C. The safe use of sulfinpyrazone in pregnancy has not been established, although there have been no reported cases of human congenital malformation proved to be due to the use of the drug. It is not known whether sulfinpyrazone can be found in breast milk.

Clinical Presentation

The most frequently reported adverse reactions with sulfinpyrazone have been upper gastrointestinal disturbances. In these patients it is advisable to administer the drug with food, milk, or antacids. Despite this precaution, sulfinpyrazone may aggravate or reactivate peptic ulcer disease. Rash has also been reported. In most instances, this reaction did not necessitate discontinuance of therapy.

Rarely, blood dyscrasias (anemia, leukopenia, agranulocytosis, thrombocytopenia, and aplastic anemia) have been reported. One report associated the combined long-term use of sulfinpyrazone, colchicine, and other drugs with leukemia (16).

Sulfinpyrazone may precipitate urolithiasis and renal colic, especially in the initial stages of therapy. Adequate fluid intake and urinary alkalinization are recommended. In patients with renal impairment, periodic assessment of renal function is indicated. Sulfinpyrazone can cause reversible acute renal failure from acute tubular necrosis in patients with volume depletion (17). Acute nonoliguric renal failure secondary to sulfinpyrazone overdose has been reported (18).

Diagnostic Tests

No specific tests are needed after acute ingestion. In symptomatic patients on long-term therapy, monitoring for potential gastrointestinal bleeding and renal insufficiency may be needed.

Treatment

Treatment of sulfinpyrazone-induced acute tubular necrosis consists of intravascular hydration, supportive care, and withholding sulfinpyrazone.

Sulfinpyrazone is related to phenylbutazone. Because it can act as an antiplatelet drug, it should be used cautiously in patients who are anticoagulated or have bleeding problems. As sulfinpyrazone can cause gastrointestinal problems, caution should be exercised in giving this drug to patients with peptic ulcer disease (1).

REFERENCES

1. Diagnosis and management of gout. Available at: http://www.aafp.org/afp/990401ap/1799.html. Accessed April 2003.
2. Pittman JR, Bross MH. Diagnosis and management of gout. *Am Fam Physician* 1999;59:1799–1806, 1810.
3. Available at: http://www.medicine.mcgill.ca/cai/meded/drugdb/probenecid/probenecid_db.htm.

4. Fam AG. Difficult gout and new approaches for control of hyperuricemia in the allopurinol-allergic patient. *Curr Rheumatol Rep* 2001;3:29–35.
5. McIntyre IM, Crump K, Roberts AN, et al. *J Forensic Sci* 1992;37:1190–1193.
6. Probenecid. Available at: http://www.nursespdr.com/members/database/ndrhtml/probenecid.html. Accessed April 2003.
7. Cunningham RF, Israili ZH, Dayton PG. Clinical pharmacokinetics of probenecid. *Clin Pharmacokinet* 1981;6:135–151.
8. Patrone NA. Polyarticular gout induced by probenecid therapy. *N C Med J* 1986;47:401–402.
9. Kickler TS, Buck S, Ness P, et al. Probenecid induced immune hemolytic anemia. *J Rheumatol* 1986;13:208–209.
10. Sosler SD, Behzad O, Garratty G, et al. Immune hemolytic anemia associated with probenecid. *Am J Clin Pathol* 1985;84:391–394.
11. Myers KW, Katial RK, Engler RJ. Probenecid hypersensitivity in AIDS: a case report. *Ann Allergy Asthma Immunol* 1998;80:416–418.
12. Carter G, Gavin JB. Sulphinpyrazone reduces endocardial injury and mural thrombosis. *Cardiovasc Res* 1990;24:257–262.
13. Anturane Reinfarction Trial (ART) Research Group. Sulfinpyrazone in the prevention of sudden death after myocardial infarction. *N Engl J Med* 1980;302:250–256.
14. Sulfinpyrazone. Available at: http://www.nursespdr.com/members/database/ndrhtml/sulfinpyrazone.html. Accessed April 2003.
15. RXmed. Available at: http://www.rxmed.com/. Accessed April 2003.
16. Witwer MW, Schmid FR, Tesar JT. Acute myelomonocytic leukaemia and multiple myeloma after sulphinpyrazone and colchicine treatment of gout. *BMJ* 1976;2:89.
17. Walls M, Goral S, Stone W. Acute renal failure due to sulfinpyrazone. *Am J Med Sci* 1998;315:319–321.
18. Florkowski CM, Ching GW, Ferner RE. Acute non-oliguric renal failure secondary to sulphinpyrazone overdose. *J Clin Pharm Ther* 1992;17:71.

CHAPTER 147

Irrigating Solutions

Seth Schonwald

$H_3C-S(=O)-CH_3$

DIMETHYL SULFOXIDE

Molecular formula and weight:	**Acetic acid ($C_2H_4O_2$), 60.05; glycine ($C_2H_5NO_2$), 75.1; dimethyl sulfoxide (DMSO; C_2H_6OS), 78.1 g/mol**
SI conversion:	**Acetic acid, mg/dl × 1.7 = µmol/L; glycine, mg/dl × 1.3 = µmol; dimethyl sulfoxide, mg/dl × 1.3 = µmol/L**
CAS Registry No.:	**64-19-7 (acetic acid); 56-40-6 (glycine); 67-68-5 (dimethyl sulfoxide)**
Therapeutic levels:	**Not applicable**
Target organs:	**Acetic acid: gastrointestinal (acute); glycine: hyponatremia (acute), heart (acute); dimethyl sulfoxide: liver, skin (chronic)**
Antidote:	**None**

ACETIC ACID

Acetic acid is the chemical compound responsible for the odor and sour taste of vinegar (4% to 8% acetic acid). Acetic acid is used as an irrigating agent for the treatment or prevention of urinary obstruction of indwelling catheters. It has also been used to treat jellyfish stings (1), granular myringitis (2), and otitis externa; as a douching agent (3); to clean root canals (4); as a wound disinfectant (5); and to commit suicide (6). The name *glacial acetic acid* refers to the 33% concentration.

Acetic acid is widely used in the production of vinyl plastics and many other chemicals. It is also used alone in the dye, rubber, pharmaceutical, food-preserving, textile, and laundry industries and is used in the manufacture of Paris green, white lead, tint rinse, photographic chemicals, stain removers, insecticides, and plastics.

Toxic Dose

There are no occupational regulatory standards for acetic acid. The toxicity is dependent on the concentration and the duration of contact.

Toxicokinetics and Toxicodynamics

Acetate is absorbed from the gastrointestinal tract and through the lungs and is almost completely oxidized by tissues. Metabolic pathways involve the formation of ketone bodies. Acetic acid participates in the acetylation of amines and the formation of proteins of plasma, liver, kidney, gut mucosa, muscle, and brain (7).

Pathophysiology

Acetic acid, like other acids, acts by coagulation necrosis.

Vulnerable Populations

Human data are not available. Animal studies have not indicated significant reproductive or teratogenic effects.

Clinical Presentation

Acute ingestion produces toxicity with higher concentration solutions. Vinegar does not cause injury, although glacial acetic acid always causes injury. Gastrointestinal effects include bleeding. Ulcerative injury to the oropharynx and esophagus are well-recognized sequelae (8). Immediate pain, dysphagia, and drooling are often present. Late esophageal, gastric, and pyloric strictures and stenoses, which may require major surgical repair, should be anticipated. Signs of obstruction commonly appear within a few weeks but may be delayed for months (9). Massive noninflammatory periportal liver necrosis after concentrated acetic acid ingestion has been reported (10). Pancreatitis may follow acetic acid ingestion as well (11).

Hematologic effects of hemolysis and disseminated intravascular coagulopathy are well-known consequences of acetic acid ingestion in attempted suicides (12). Disseminated intravascular coagulopathy in this setting has been successfully treated with fresh frozen plasma and cryoprecipitate (13). In cases of severe hemolysis, exchange transfusion may be necessary (14).

Other effects, including oliguric renal failure, may follow acetic acid ingestion (15). A splash of vinegar (4% to 10% acetic acid solution) in the human eye causes immediate pain and conjunctival hyperemia, sometimes with injury of the corneal epithelium (16). Inhalation may result in spasm, inflammation, and edema of the larynx and bronchi; chemical pneumonitis; and pulmonary edema.

Inhalation exposure results in a burning sensation, coughing, wheezing, laryngitis, shortness of breath, headache, nausea, and vomiting (17).

Dermal exposure, if repeated or prolonged, causes skin darkening, erosion of the exposed front teeth, and chronic inflammation of the nose, throat, and bronchi.

Diagnostic Tests

Diagnostic testing is directed at the effects of toxicity. Consider laparoscopic evaluation in patients with third degree burns, as transmucosal gastric burns or perforation may be present. Emergent surgical evaluation is needed for patients with signs of perforation.

Treatment

Treatment focuses on supporting hemodynamic function and evaluating the severity of burns. Manage airway aggressively after inhalation; airway edema may develop rapidly. Acid ingestion is addressed in Chapter 201.

Decontamination for ingestion involves dilution with 4 to 8 oz of milk or water. Emesis should not be induced. Neutralization with a basic solution is not recommended, as it may cause thermal burns. Irrigate exposed mouth, skin, and eyes copiously with water. Remove patients with inhalation injury from further exposure. Do not administer activated charcoal unless toxic coingestant is involved.

Enhanced elimination with hemodialysis has been used to treat patients with severe acetic acid poisoning (18). There is no known specific antidote.

Supportive care includes oxygen for all patients with pulmonary symptoms. Significant edema and stridor may indicate the need for intubation and the use of a bronchodilator. Hypotension is treated with intravenous (IV) crystalloid, 10 to 20 ml/kg (Chapter 37). Steroids are considered in patients with second degree burns on endoscopy but are not indicated for first degree burns, as stricture formation is unlikely; steroids are generally avoided for third degree burns because they increase risk of perforation. Antibiotics are used only for suspected infection or perforation.

GLYCINE

Glycine is an amino acid used as an irrigant during urologic and gynecologic surgery.

Toxic Dose

The oral therapeutic dose is 150 to 300 mg. Solutions for bladder irrigation are 1.0% to 1.5%. A 69-year-old man received glycine irrigation during prostatic surgery. He developed abdominal distention with increasing ventilatory pressures and hyponatremia and died. Hyponatremia with markedly elevated levels of blood, urine, and body fluid glycine was demonstrated. Death was attributed to glycine toxicity after tracking of glycine through a defect in the bladder wall (19).

Toxicokinetics and Toxicodynamics

Glycine-serine interconversion contributes to maintenance of cellular tetrahydrofolate coenzymes, the primary transport mechanism of one-carbon units for the metabolism of amino acids, proteins, purines, and vitamins (20). The elimination half-life is 85 minutes.

Pathophysiology

Glycine is an essential amino acid. Like glutamic acid and γ-aminobutyric acid, glycine inhibits neurotransmitter signals in the central nervous system (21). Glycine enhances the activity of neurotransmitters in the brain that are involved in memory and cognition (22) and may play a role in maintaining the health of the prostate gland (23).

Vulnerable Populations

No information is available. Glycine is not typically used in women of reproductive age.

Clinical Presentation

Endoscopic operations in the genitourinary tract require the use of an irrigating fluid containing glycine 1.5% and expose patients to adverse events summarized as "transurethral resection reactions" or "TURP syndrome." Dilutional hyponatremia and toxicity of glycine and its metabolites explain the clinical symptoms. Hyponatremia and the osmotic gap assess the diagnosis of TURP syndrome (24,25). Transient blindness has been attributed to the TURP syndrome (26,27).

Other signs may include nausea and vomiting, hypotension, and bradycardia (28). Osmolar shifts may result in hemolytic anemia. During transcervical endometrial resection, the uterine cavity is also irrigated under pressure with 1.5% glycine solution. This solution may be absorbed, with consequent fluid and electrolyte shifts (29).

Diagnostic Tests

Diagnostic testing is directed at the adverse effects of dilutional hyponatremia as well as osmotic effects. Serial monitoring of vital signs, complete blood cell count, serum electrolytes, electrocardiogram, and other tests, as indicated by clinical effects (e.g., mental status change from cerebral edema), may be needed.

Treatment

Treatment is symptomatic and supportive. Activated charcoal may be effective in the unusual event of an oral overdose. Most treatment is directed at the toxic effect (e.g., replacement therapy for hemolysis, management of cerebral edema). Enhanced elimination has not been evaluated. There is no antidote.

DIMETHYL SULFOXIDE

Dimethyl sulfoxide (DMSO) is an intravesical agent for interstitial cystitis (30). A catheter introduces DMSO into the bladder where it is allowed to remain for approximately 15 minutes. Interstitial cystitis is the only use for DMSO that is approved by the U.S. Food and Drug Administration. Claims that DMSO is effective for treating various types of arthritis, ulcers in scleroderma, amyloidosis of the skin (31), muscle sprains and strains, bruises, infections of the skin, burns, wounds, Down syndrome (32), and mental conditions (33) remain unproven (34).

Toxic Dose

The therapeutic intravesical dose is 50 ml of a 50% solution. A dose of 606 mg/kg IV was associated with nausea and jaundice. There are no occupational guidelines or standards for DMSO exposure.

Toxicokinetics and Toxicodynamics

After topical application, DMSO is absorbed and distributed widely to tissues and body fluids. DMSO is metabolized by oxidation to dimethyl sulfone or by the reduction to dimethyl sulfide. DMSO and dimethyl sulfone are excreted in the urine and feces. Dimethyl sulfide is eliminated through the breath and skin and is responsible for the characteristic odor exuded from patients. The drug can persist in serum for more than 2 weeks after a single intravesical instillation (35).

Vulnerable Populations

Teratogenic effects have occurred in animal studies, but insufficient human information is available.

Clinical Presentation

Adverse reactions to DMSO are common but are usually minor and related to the concentration of DMSO in solution. The most frequent side effects, such as skin rash and pruritus after dermal application, intravascular hemolysis after IV infusion, and gastrointestinal discomfort after oral administration, can be avoided by using dilute solutions (36).

DMSO frequently causes a garlic-like body odor and taste in the mouth. Other reported side effects include stomach upset, sensitivity to light, visual disturbances, and headache. Skin irritation can develop at the site where DMSO is applied topically. Sulfhemoglobinemia has been reported after topical DMSO application (37).

Diagnostic Tests

In symptomatic patients, liver function, kidney function, hemoglobin, and platelet count should be monitored.

Treatment

Treatment is symptomatic and supportive. After intravesical administration, the bladder can be emptied. Most treatment is directed at the toxic effect (e.g., replacement therapy for hemolysis). Enhanced elimination has not been evaluated. There is no antidote.

REFERENCES

1. Nomura JT, Sato RL, Ahern RM, et al. A randomized paired comparison trial of cutaneous treatments for acute jellyfish (*Carybdea alata*) stings. *Am J Emerg Med* 2002;20:624–626.
2. Jung HH, Cho SD, Yoo CK, et al. Vinegar treatment in the management of granular myringitis. *J Laryngol Otol* 2002;116:176–180.
3. Monif GR. The great douching debate: to douche, or not to douche. *Obstet Gynecol* 1999;94:630–631.
4. Liolios E, Economides N, Parissis-Messimeris S, et al. The effectiveness of three irrigating solutions on root canal cleaning after hand and mechanical preparation. *Int Endod J* 1997;30:51–57.
5. Phillips D, Davey C. Wound cleaning versus wound disinfection: a challenging dilemma. *Perspectives* 1997;21:15–16.
6. Faller-Marquardt M, Bohnert M, Logemann E, et al. Combined suicide by drinking acetic acid with subsequent hanging. *Arch Kriminol* 2000;206:140–149.
7. FAO nutrition meetings. Available at: http://www.inchem.org/documents/jecfa/jecmono/40abcj37.htm. Accessed April 2003.
8. Chung CH. Corrosive oesophageal injury following vinegar ingestion. *Hong Kong Med J* 2002;8:365–366.
9. Gosselin RE, Smith RP, Hodge HC. *Clinical toxicology of commercial products*, 5th ed. Baltimore: Williams & Wilkins, 1984:II-102.
10. Kamijo Y, Soma K, Iwabuchi K, et al. Massive noninflammatory periportal liver necrosis following concentrated acetic acid ingestion. *Arch Pathol Lab Med* 2000;124:127–129.
11. Bergenfeldt M, Skold G, Borgstrom A. Acute pancreatitis after ingestion of acetic acid. *Pancreas* 1996;12:207–209.
12. Greif F, Kaplan O. Acid ingestion: another cause of disseminated intravascular coagulopathy. *Crit Care Med* 1986;14:990–991.
13. Jurim O, Gross E, Nates J, Eldor A. Disseminated intravascular coagulopathy caused by acetic acid ingestion. *Acta Haematol* 1993;89:204–205.
14. Boseniuk S, Rieger C. Acute oral acetic acid poisoning—case report. *Anaesthesiol Reanim* 1994;19:80–82.
15. Schardijn GH, Kastelein JJ, Statius van Eps LW. Kidney tubule dysfunction caused by acetic acid. *Ned Tijdschr Geneeskd* 1989;133:556–559.
16. Mackison FW, Stricoff RS, Partridge LJ, eds. NIOSH/OSHA—occupational health guidelines for chemical hazards. DHHS(NIOSH) Publication No. 81-123 (3 volumes). Washington, DC: U.S. Government Printing Office; 1981.
17. Acetic acid. Available at: http://ehs.fullerton.edu/Safety4Students/MSDS/acetic_acid.htm. Accessed April 2003.
18. Sergeeva EP, Shchebina AA, Demina LM, et al. Hemodialysis in the treatment of severe poisoning with acetic acid. *Klin Med (Mosk)* 2001;79:53–57.
19. Byard RW, Harrison R, Wells R, et al. Glycine toxicity and unexpected intraoperative death. *J Forensic Sci* 2001;46:1244–1246.
20. 13C NMR serine isotopomer analysis. Available at: http://www.ccs.uq.edu.au/medicine/RBH/RENAL/glycine.htm. Accessed April 2003.
21. Glycine. Available at: http://micro.magnet.fsu.edu/aminoacids/pages/glycine.html. Accessed April 2003.
22. File SE, Fluck E, Fernandes C. Beneficial effects of glycine (Bioglycin) on memory and attention in young and middle-aged adults. *J Clin Psychopharmacol* 1999;19:506–512.
23. Damrau F. Benign prostatic hypertrophy: amino acid therapy for symptomatic relief. *J Am Geriatr Soc* 1962;10:426–430.
24. Tauzin-Fin P. An adverse effect of glycine irrigation solution: absorption syndrome. *Therapie* 2002;57:48–54.
25. Ayus JC, Arieff AI. Glycine-induced hypo-osmolar hyponatremia. *Arch Intern Med* 1997;157:223–226.
26. Khan-Ghori SN, Khalaf MM, Khan RK, et al. Loss of vision: a manifestation of TURP syndrome. A case report. *Middle East J Anesthesiol* 1998;14:441–449.
27. Radziwill AJ, Vuadens P, Borruat FX, et al. Visual disturbances and transurethral resection of the prostate: the TURP syndrome. *Eur Neurol* 1997;38:7–9.
28. Olsson J, Nilsson A, Hahn RG. Symptoms of the transurethral resection syndrome using glycine as the irrigant. *J Urol* 1995;154:123–128.
29. McSwiney M, Myatt J, Hargreaves M. Transcervical endometrial resection syndrome. *Anaesthesia* 1995;50:254–257.
30. Lukban JC, Whitmore KE, Sant GR. Current management of interstitial cystitis. *Urol Clin North Am* 2002;29:649–660.
31. Ozkaya-Bayazit E, Baykal C, Kavak A. Local DMSO treatment of macular and papular amyloidosis. *Hautarzt* 1997;48:31–37.
32. Aspillaga MJ, Morizon G, Avendano I. Dimethyl sulfoxide therapy in severe retardation in Mongoloid children. *Ann N Y Acad Sci* 1975;243:421–431.
33. Gabourie J, Becker JW, Bateman B, et al. Oral dimethyl sulfoxide in mental retardation. *Ann N Y Acad Sci* 1975;243:449–459.
34. American Medical Association. Dimethyl sulfoxide. Controversy and current status—1981. *JAMA* 1982;248:1369–1371.
35. RXmed. Available at: http://www.rxmed.com/. Accessed April 2003.
36. Swanson BN. Medical use of dimethyl sulfoxide (DMSO). *Rev Clin Basic Pharm* 1985;5:1–33.
37. Burgess JL, Hamner AP, Robertson WO. Sulfhemoglobinemia after dermal application of DMSO. *Vet Hum Toxicol* 1998;40:87–89.

SECTION

10

Eye, Ear, Nose, and Throat Preparations

CHAPTER 148

Ear, Nose, and Throat Preparations

Richard C. Dart

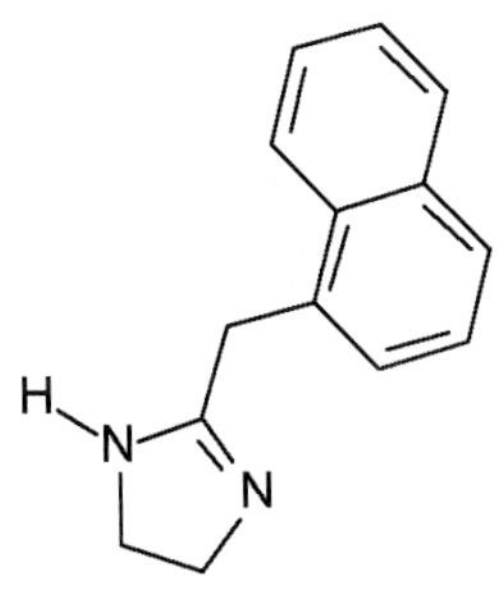

IMIDAZOLINE

Compounds included:	**Pilocarpine (Isopto Carpine, Vistacarpine); cyclopentolate (AK-Pentolate); homatropine (Isopto Homatropine); phenylephrine (AK-Dilate, Neosynephrine); scopolamine (Isopto Hyoscine); naphazoline (Clear Eyes, Vasocon); oxymetazoline (Afrin, OcuClear); tetrahydrozoline (Murine Plus, Visine)**
Molecular formula and molecular weight:	**See Table 1.**
SI conversion:	**See Table 1.**
CAS Registry No.:	**See Table 1.**
Therapeutic levels:	**Not used clinically**
Special concerns:	**Imidazoline drugs may cause hypertension followed by hypotension.**
Antidotes:	**Physostigmine, naloxone**

OVERVIEW

A wide range of medications are indicated for ear, nose, and throat conditions (Table 1). Often, the same medications are used for other conditions. Local anesthetics, antihistamines, antibiotics, antiinflammatory agents, carbonic anhydrase inhibitors, and apraclonidine are addressed in their respective chapters. This chapter addresses pilocarpine, cyclopentolate, homatropine, phenylephrine, scopolamine, and the imidazoline drugs (naphazoline, oxymetazoline, and tetrahydrozoline).

TOXIC DOSE

The *adult and pediatric therapeutic doses* are provided in Table 1. Although no fatalities have been reported for any of these products, toxicity can arise from their overuse or ingestion. The lethal adult dose of pilocarpine was estimated to be 60 mg in one case (1). In contrast, subcutaneous injection of 80 mg of pilocarpine in an adult produced cholinergic symptoms that were survived without treatment (2).

Scopolamine reportedly caused a pediatric death after 10 mg (3). In a study of 115 patients with acute poisoning, the lowest ingested dose of scopolamine associated with severe symptoms was 2 to 4 mg (4). A 0.45-mg dose has caused toxic psychosis (5). Anticholinergic poisoning may occur after absorption of four to five drops (less in children) of ocular solutions containing 0.25% scopolamine (5–7).

Imidazolines cause dose-related toxicity. A poison center review of 193 children who potentially ingested 0.05% tetrahydrozoline reported no toxicity in 54 children who ingested less than 7.5 ml, whereas six patients developed toxicity among the

TABLE 1. Physical characteristics and doses of ear, nose, and throat preparations

Preparation	Molecular formula	Molecular weight (g/mol)	SI conversion	CAS Registry No.	Formulations	Therapeutic dose	
						Adult	Pediatric
Miotics							
Pilocarpine hydrochloride	$C_{11}H_{16}N_2O_2$,HCl	244.7	mg/L × 4.1 = µmol/L	54-71-7	1%, 2%, 3%, 4% drops; 4% gel; 0.5%, 1%, 5%, 6%, 8%, 10% solutions; 5-mg tablet; 20 and 40 µg/h ocular insert	1–2 drops in eye four times a day	Dose has not been established.
Mydriatics							
Cyclopentolate hydrochloride	$C_{17}H_{25}NO_3$,HCl	327.8	mg/L × 3.1 = µmol/L	5870-29-1	0.5%, 1% solutions	1–2 drops of 0.5–2.0% solution; may repeat once	1–2 drops of 0.5–2.0% solution; may repeat once.
Homatropine hydrobromide	$C_{16}H_{21}NO_3$,HBr	356.3	mg/L × 2.8 = µmol/L	51-56-9	2%, 5% solutions	1–2 drops of 0.5–2.0% solution	1–2 drops of 0.5–2.0% solution.
Phenylephrine hydrochloride	$C_9H_{13}NO_2$,HCl	203.7	mg/L × 4.9= µmol/L	61-76-7	0.25%, 0.5%, 1% nasal drops; 0.25%, 0.5% nasal spray; 2.5%, 10% ophthalmic solution	1–2 drops of 2.5–10.0% solution; may repeat once	1–2 drops of 2.5–10.0% solution; may repeat once.
Scopolamine hydrobromide	$C_{17}H_{21}NO_4$,HBr, $3H_2O$	438.3	mg/L × 2.3 = µmol/L	6533-68-2	0.25% ocular solution	1–2 drops four times a day	Not reported.
Vasoconstrictors							
Naphazoline hydrochloride	$C_{14}H_{14}N_2$,HCl	246.7	mg/L × 4.1 = µmol/L	550-99-2	0.012% eye drops; 0.05% nasal drops; 1:2000 nasal spray; 0.02%, 0.025%, 0.1%, 1% solution	1–2 drops or sprays four times daily	0.05%, 1–2 drops or sprays four times daily.
Oxymetazoline hydrochloride	$C_{16}H_{24}N_2O$,HCl	296.8	mg/L × 3.4 = µmol/L	2315-02-8	0.025%, 0.05% drops; 0.05% spray	1–2 drops or sprays	1–2 drops or sprays of 0.025%.
Tetrahydrozoline hydrochloride	$C_{13}H_{16}N_2$,HCl	236.7	mg/L × 4.2 = µmol/L	522-48-5	0.05% drops; 0.05%, 0.1% solution; 0.1% spray	1–2 drops or sprays	1–2 drops or sprays of 0.05%.

43 patients who ingested more than 7.5 ml (8). Infants may develop sedation after nasal administration of as little as one to two drops of the 0.1% solution (9). Ingestion of 4 to 5 ml of tetrahydrozoline 0.1% was followed by lethargy, bradycardia, and hypotension in a 17-month-old child (10). Seizures followed two drops of oxymetazoline, 0.25 mm/ml, in a 5-year-old boy (11).

TOXICOKINETICS AND TOXICODYNAMICS

The pharmacokinetic data for these agents are poorly established. All of these agents are liquids that are rapidly absorbed if ingested. The time to maximum serum concentration for *pilocarpine* is 0.85 to 1.25 hours, and its elimination half-life is 0.76 to 1.35 hours (12). *Phenylephrine* undergoes hepatic metabolism to phenolic metabolites and has an elimination half-life of 2 to 3 hours (13). *Oxymetazoline* has a half-life of 5 to 8 hours (14).

PATHOPHYSIOLOGY

Pilocarpine is a postganglionic cholinergic receptor agonist that causes muscarinic effects. *Cyclopentolate, homatropine,* and *scopolamine* are antimuscarinic agents that competitively antagonize acetylcholine and produce mostly muscarinic effects. *Phenylephrine* is a potent sympathomimetic that stimulates α-adrenergic receptors. *Imidazoline* derivatives act peripherally as α_2-receptor agonists. In overdose, it is likely that crossover stimulation of α_1-receptors occurs.

PREGNANCY AND LACTATION

All agents are U.S. Food and Drug Administration pregnancy category C (Appendix I). Entry into breast milk is unknown for all the agents except phenylephrine, homatropine, and scopolamine, which are considered safe for breast-feeding (15).

CLINICAL PRESENTATION

Acute Overdosage

PILOCARPINE

A 39-year-old woman was erroneously administered 2 ml of 4% pilocarpine drops subcutaneously (80 mg pilocarpine). Diaphoresis, salivation, and nausea developed quickly and were followed by typical signs of excess. The effects resolved over 4 days without treatment (2).

IMIDAZOLINES

Hypertension followed by hypotension may occur. Naphazoline causing mild hypothermia was reported in 5 of 19 patients (26%) (16). Toxic effects develop within the first hour, peak after 8 hours, and disappear within a day or more (16). Severe cases may develop all or part of a constellation of effects, including bradycardia, hypotension, hypoventilation or apnea, and hypotonia; central nervous system (CNS) depression or coma (16,17) has been reported in both adults (18) and children (16,17,19). Bradycardia is common, especially in children (10,17,18,20). An accidental overdose (3 to 4 mg) of naphazoline during bronchoscopy resulted in hypotension, tachycardia, respiratory insufficiency, and prolonged unconsciousness that resolved over 11 hours (19).

Chronic Overdosage: Imidazolines

Mydriasis precipitating acute angle-closure glaucoma and ultimately producing blindness was reported in three patients with chronic overuse of vasoconstricting eye drops (21). A 36-year-old man developed acute ischemia of the hand after intraarterial injection of oxymetazoline (22). He ultimately developed gangrene, requiring amputation. Hallucinations were reported after therapeutic doses of oxymetazoline (11) and after chronic excessive use (23).

Adverse Events

PILOCARPINE

Acute angle closure has occurred during therapeutic use (24). Topical ocular effects include miosis (lasting 10 to 20 minutes with acetylcholine and 4 to 8 hours with pilocarpine) (25), myopia and difficulty in visual accommodation, ciliary spasm, ocular pain, and eyelid twitching. Corneal abrasion and visual impairment have been reported after the use of pilocarpine eye drops (26).

CYCLOPENTOLATE

A series of 66 healthy adults were treated with one drop of a 2% cyclopentolate solution in each eye. Ten reactions occurred: Six were mild and four moderate (tachycardia, nausea, weakness, headache, delusions, dizziness, dry mouth, lightheadedness, incoordination, and mental depression). The effects persisted from 1 hour to 3 days (27). The therapeutic use of a 2% solution in 40 children resulted in five cases of acute psychotic reactions. Patients recovered spontaneously over 1 to 5 days (28).

HOMATROPINE

The typical effects of anticholinergic toxicity may develop after therapeutic ocular use (29).

SCOPOLAMINE

Anisocoria is a common occurrence when a contaminated finger has contact with one eye.

IMIDAZOLINES

Use of nasal decongestants for several consecutive days can result in persistent nasal obstruction "rhinitis medicatosum" (30).

DIAGNOSTIC TESTS

Although the serum concentration can be measured, it is not used clinically for any of these agents. Diagnostic testing is directed at testing for and monitoring of drug effects on vital signs and toward evaluation of CNS depression. Typically, serum electrolytes, complete blood cell count, and renal function are measured. An electrocardiogram, cardiac monitoring, and pulse oximetry should be performed in symptomatic patients. Computerized tomography of the head, lumbar puncture, and bacterial cultures may be needed in unusual cases resistant to diagnosis.

TREATMENT

Treatment should focus on immediate supportive care with appropriate airway management. Most patients recover completely within a few hours.

Decontamination

Decontamination has not been evaluated for these agents. Gastric emptying is not recommended because they are liquid agents that are rapidly absorbed and can cause CNS depression. A single dose of activated charcoal soon after exposure may be helpful.

Enhancement of Elimination

Attempts at enhanced elimination of these compounds have not been reported.

Antidotes

Potential antidotes exist for imidazoline agents and anticholinergic agents. Physostigmine may be appropriate in selected cases of anticholinergic toxicity (Chapter 67). It has been reported that naloxone may reverse the effects of imidazoline toxicity, but this has never been tested in a well-controlled clinical trial.

Supportive Care: Imidazolines

Symptomatic bradycardia typically fails to respond to atropine. Hypotension should initially be treated with isotonic crystalloid fluid resuscitation followed by inotropic support, if needed (Chapter 37). Naloxone has been reported to reverse both coma and hypotension. Hypertension may occur and be followed by hypotension. Treatment of hypertension should be avoided, if possible. However, in the rare case that end-organ damage develops, a titratable and reversible antihypertensive, such as nitroprusside, should be used.

Monitoring

All patients should be monitored for respiratory and cardiovascular effects. The patient may be discharged if no effects develop within hours. Patients with bradycardia, hypotension, or persistent CNS depression should be admitted to the hospital.

Management Pitfalls

Because it can produce small pupils and altered mental status, toxicity from imidazoline drugs may be confused with opioid overdose. Transient hypertension is consistent with imidazoline toxicity and should not be over-treated.

REFERENCES

1. Cordner SM, Fysh RR, Gordon H, et al. Deaths of two hospital inpatients poisoned by pilocarpine. *BMJ* 1986;293:1285–1287.
2. Kastl PR. Inadvertent systemic injection of pilocarpine. *Arch Ophthalmol* 1987;105:28–29.
3. Thakkar M, Lasser R. Scopolamine intoxication from a non-prescription sleeping pill. *N Y State J Med* 1972;72:725–726.
4. Hooper RG, Conner CS, Rumack BH. Acute poisoning from over-the-counter sleep preparations. *JACEP* 1979;8:98–100.
5. Goldfrank L, Flomenbaum N, Lewin N, et al. Anticholinergic poisoning. *J Toxicol Clin Toxicol* 1982;19:17–25.
6. Adler AG, McElwain GE, Merli GJ et al. Systemic effects of eye drops. *Arch Intern Med* 1982;42:2293–2294.
7. Hoefnagel D. Toxic effects of atropine and homatropine eye drops in children. *N Engl J Med* 1961;264:168–171.
8. Kuffner EK, Falbo SC, Bogdan GM, et al. Dose related effects of tetrahydrozoline (THZ) ingestion in children. *J Toxicol Clin Toxicol* 1996;34:579(abst).
9. Brainerd WK, Olmsted RW. Toxicity due to the use of tyzine hydrochloride. *J Pediatr* 1956;48:157–164.
10. Jensen P, Edgren B, Hall L, et al. Hemodynamic effects following ingestion of an imidazoline-containing product. *Pediatr Emerg Care* 1989;5(2):110–112.
11. Soderman P, Sahlberg D, Wiholm BE. CNS reactions to nose drops in small children. *Lancet* 1984;1:573.

12. Salagen, pilocarpine. Product information. Minnetonka, MN: MGI Pharma, Inc., 1998.
13. Hengstmann JH, Goronzy J. Pharmacokinetics of 3H-phenylephrine in man. *Eur J Clin Pharmacol* 1982;21:335–341.
14. Oxymetazoline hydrochloride. In: Dollery C, ed. *Therapeutic drugs*. New York: Churchill Livingstone, 1991.
15. Heitland G, Hurlbut KM, eds. Reprotext database. Greenwood Village, CO: Micromedex, 2003.
16. Mahieu LM, Rooman RP, Goossens E. Imidazoline intoxication in children. *Eur J Pediatr* 1993;152:944–946.
17. Holmes JF, Berman DA. Use of naloxone to reverse symptomatic tetrahydrozoline overdose in a child. *Pediatr Emerg Care* 1999;15:193–194.
18. Lev R, Clark RF. Visine overdose: case report of an adult with hemodynamic compromise. *J Emerg Med* 1995;5:649–652.
19. Stamer UM, Buderus S, Wetegrove S, et al. Prolonged awakening and pulmonary edema after general anesthesia and naphazoline application in an infant. *Anesth Analg* 2001;93:1162–1164.
20. Higgins GL 3rd, Campbell B, Wallace K, et al. Pediatric poisoning from over-the-counter imidazoline-containing products. *Ann Emerg Med* 1991;20(6):655–658.
21. Rumelt MB. Blindness from misuse of over-the-counter eye medications. *Ann Ophthalmol* 1988;20:26–27.
22. Shukla PC. Acute ischemia of the hand following intra-arterial oxymetazoline injection. *J Emerg Med* 1995;13(1):65–70.
23. Escobar JI, Karno M. Chronic hallucinosis from nasal drops. *JAMA* 1982;247:1859–1860.
24. Mohamed Q, Fahey DK, Manners RM. Angle closure in fellow eye with prophylactic pilocarpine treatment. *Br J Ophthalmol* 2001;85:1263.
25. Rizzuti AB. Acetylcholine in surgery of the lens, iris and cornea. *Am J Ophthalmol* 1967;63(3):484–487.
26. Ocusert Pilo, pilocarpine. Product information. Palo Alto, CA: Alza Corporation, 1993.
27. Awan KJ. Adverse systemic reactions of topical cyclopentolate hydrochloride. *Ann Ophthalmol* 1976;8:695–698.
28. Awan KJ. Systemic toxicity of cyclopentolate hydrochloride in adults following topical ocular installation. *Ann Ophthalmol* 1976;8:803–806.
29. Reilly KM, Chan L, Mehta NJ, Salluzzo RF. Systemic toxicity from ocular homatropine. *Acad Emerg Med* 1996;3:868–871.
30. Capel LH, Swanston AR. Beware congesting nasal decongestants. *BMJ* 1986;293:1258–1259.

SECTION

11

Gastrointestinal Drugs

CHAPTER 149

Antacids

Michael A. McGuigan

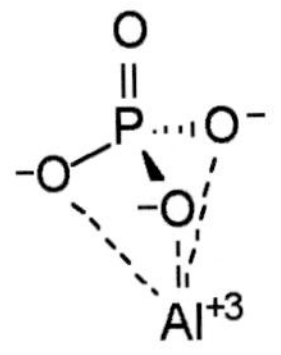

ALUMINUM PHOSPHATE

Compounds included:	**Aluminum (carbonate, hydroxide, phosphate, dihydroxyaluminum aminoacetate); calcium carbonate; magnesium (carbonate, hydroxide, oxide, trisilicate); magaldrate (aluminum magnesium hydroxide sulfate)**
Molecular formula and weight:	**See Table 1.**
SI conversion:	**See Table 1.**
CAS Registry No.:	**See Table 1.**
Therapeutic levels:	**Not applicable**
Special concerns:	**Milk-alkali syndrome may arise during the chronic use of high doses of antacids and milk products.**
Target organs:	**Kidney (calcium); neuromuscular (aluminum, magnesium)**
Antidote:	**None**

OVERVIEW

Antacids are soluble and insoluble salts used to increase the pH of gastric fluid for the symptomatic treatment of conditions caused by gastric acid. These products have few adverse effects and little acute toxicity. Chronic use of antacids by patients with compromised renal function may result in encephalopathy and bone resorption from aluminum and in cardiovascular toxicity from magnesium. Chronic use of antacids in conjunction with high calcium intake may lead to milk-alkali syndrome.

The most commonly used antacids contain aluminum, calcium (carbonate), magnesium, or combinations of these. (These products are used in the treatment of conditions, such as esophagitis, gastroesophageal reflux, gastritis, dyspepsia, ulcers, and gastrointestinal bleeding.) Due to the success of H_2 receptor–blocking agents and proton pump inhibitors, antacids are recommended only for the short-term treatment of stress gastritis and nonulcer dyspepsia (1). Sodium bicarbonate is not used as an oral antacid because of the risk of developing alkalosis.

TOXIC DOSES

Therapeutic adult doses for these agents are 15 to 30 ml or 250.0 mg to 1.5 g four times a day. The pediatric dosage is 0.5 to 5.0 ml or 150 to 250 mg/kg/day in four to six divided doses. The toxic dose of these agents is unknown. The maximum daily dose of aluminum has been estimated to be 30 mg/kg.

TOXICOKINETICS AND TOXICODYNAMICS

Antacids vary in the amount that the metal cations are absorbed. Reaction of the antacid with hydrochloric acid in the stomach produces chloride salts. Aluminum chloride and magnesium chloride are partially (15% to 30%) absorbed from the stomach (2). In the small intestine, each of the chloride salts is converted to an insoluble, poorly absorbed form, which is eliminated in the feces; aluminum-containing antacids form insoluble salts with dietary phosphate. Absorbed cations are excreted through the kidneys.

TABLE 1. Physical characteristics of antacids

Compound	Molecular formula, molecular weight (g/mol), CAS Registry No.	SI conversion
Aluminum carbonate	$Al_2(CO_3)_2$, 145.97, NR	mg/L × 6.9 = μmol/L
Aluminum hydroxide	$Al(OH)_3$, 77.99, 21645-51-2	mg/L × 12.8 = μmol/L
Aluminum phosphate	$AlPO_4$, 121.95, 7784-30-7	mg/L × 8.2 = μmol/L
Aluminum dihydroxyaluminum aminoacetate	$C_2H_6AlNO_4(+xH_2O)$, 135.1, 41354-48-7	mg/L × 7.4 = μmol/L
Calcium carbonate	$CaCO_3$, 100.1, 471-34-1	mg/L × 9.9 = μmol/L
Magnesium carbonate	$CMgO_3$, NR, 546-93-0	NA
Magnesium hydroxide	$Mg(OH)_2$, 58.32, 1309-42-8	mg/L × 17.1 = μmol/L
Magnesium oxide	MgO, 40.30, 1309-48-4	mg/L × 24.8 = μmol/L
Magnesium trisilicate	$H_4MG_2O_8SI_3$, NR, 14987-04-3	NA
Magaldrate (aluminum magnesium hydroxide sulfate)	$Al_5Mg_{10}(OH)_{31}(SO_4)_2$,$xH_2O$, 1097.3 (anhydrous), 74978-16-8	NA

NA, not applicable; NR, not reported.

PATHOPHYSIOLOGY

Systemic toxicity from antacids occurs as a result of systemic absorption and accumulation of the calcium, aluminum, or magnesium cation secondary to excessive chronic doses or decreased renal function.

Milk-alkali syndrome involves the triad of hypercalcemia, alkalosis, and renal impairment (3) caused by large doses of an absorbable alkalinizing agent (e.g., sodium bicarbonate or calcium carbonate) and calcium (e.g., milk or cream). The metabolic alkalosis is caused by absorption of the antacid; in addition, parathyroid hormone suppression and calcium increase renal tubular reabsorption of bicarbonate. High calcium intake and reduced renal excretion of calcium result in hypercalcemia. Hypercalcemia causes a reduction of parathyroid hormone secretion, which, in turn, results in renal phosphate retention. Hypercalcemia along with alkalosis encourages the precipitation of calcium in the kidney and subsequent renal failure (4,5).

PREGNANCY AND LACTATION

Antacids are U.S. Food and Drug Administration pregnancy category B (Appendix I).

CLINICAL PRESENTATION

Acute Overdosage

Acute overdosage with antacids may cause osmotic catharsis, leading to fluid and electrolyte losses. Hypermagnesemia and central nervous system depression may follow overdoses of magnesium-containing antacids (6).

Chronic Overdosage

Hypercalcemia may be associated with nausea, vomiting, mental status changes, lethargy, muscle weakness, and possibly renal calculi and electrocardiographic changes. Milk-alkali syndrome presents with symptoms of hypercalcemia (5). Common effects of moderate hypermagnesemia (less than 10 mEq/L) include nausea, weakness, hyporeflexia, bradycardia, and hypotension. Accumulation of aluminum has been associated with phosphate depletion (7,8) and encephalopathy (Chapter 211).

Adverse Reactions

Antacids may alter the dissolution, absorption, bioavailability, and renal excretion of a number of drugs by altering gastric and urinary pH (9). Chronic use of antacids contributes to a phosphate depletion syndrome and nephrolithiasis (10).

DIAGNOSTIC TESTS

Acute Overdosage

Assess fluid and electrolyte status after large overdoses with significant catharsis. Serum magnesium levels are unlikely to be significantly elevated after overdoses of magnesium-containing antacids by patients with normal renal function. An electrocardiogram may be useful in assessing patients with clinical effects of hypercalcemia or hypermagnesemia.

Chronic Overdosage

Renal function should be monitored during chronic use. Serum calcium levels should be monitored if an absorbable alkali is used with high dietary calcium intake. Serum phosphate levels should be monitored. If renal function is compromised, serum aluminum, calcium, or magnesium should be measured.

TREATMENT

Specific treatment is rarely needed in either suicidal or nonsuicidal patients. Gastrointestinal decontamination is not indicated unless toxic coingestants are suspected.

Hypermagnesemia may be treated with fluids and loop diuretics. Hemodialysis reduces plasma levels of magnesium. Aluminum may be removed with deferoxamine followed by hemodialysis (Chapter 211) (11).

REFERENCES

1. Maton PN, Burton ME. Antacids revisited. A review of their clinical pharmacology and recommended therapeutic use. *Drugs* 1999;57:855–870.
2. Fleming LW, Prescott A, Stewart WK, et al. Bioavailability of aluminum. *Lancet* 1989;1:433.
3. Sippy BW. Gastric and duodenal ulcer; medical cure by an efficient removal of gastric juice corrosion. *JAMA* 1915;64:1625–1630.
4. Walan A. Metabolic side effects of and interaction of antacids. *Scand J Gastroenterol* 1982;17:63–67.
5. Fiorino AS. Hypercalcemia and alkalosis due to the milk-alkali syndrome: a case report and review. *Yale J Biol Med* 1997;69:517–523.
6. Wilson C, Azmy AF, Beattie TJ, et al. Hypermagnesemia and progression of renal failure associated with renacidin therapy. *Clin Nephrol* 1986;25:266–267.
7. Lotz M, Zisman E, Bartter FC. Evidence for a phosphorus-depletion syndrome in man. *N Engl J Med* 1968;275:409–415.
8. Spencer H, Kramer, L, Norris C, et al. Effects of small doses of aluminum-containing antacids on calcium and phosphorus metabolism. *Am J Clin Nutr* 1982;36:32–40.
9. Brunton LL. Agents for the control of gastric acidity and treatment of peptic ulcers. In: Hardman JE, Limbird LE, eds. *Goodman & Gilman's the pharmacological basis of therapeutics*, 9th ed. New York: McGraw-Hill, 1996:901–915.
10. Harmeln DL, Martin FIR, Wark JD. Antacid induced phosphate depletion syndrome presenting as nephrolithiasis. *Austr N Z J Med* 1990;20:803–805.
11. Malluche HH, Smith AJ, Abreo KA, et al. The use of deferoxamine in the management of aluminum accumulation in bone in patients with renal failure. *N Engl J Med* 1984;311:140–144.

CHAPTER 150

Antidiarrhea Drugs

Michael A. McGuigan

DIPHENOXYLATE

Compounds included:	**Diphenoxylate, loperamide, opium derivatives (e.g., paregoric)**
Molecular formula and weight:	**Diphenoxylate ($C_{30}H_{32}N_2O_2$, HCl), 452.6; loperamide ($C_{29}H_{33}ClN_2O_2$, HCl), 477.1; opium derivatives, mixture g/mol**
SI conversion:	**Diphenoxylate, μg/L × 2.21 = nmol/L; loperamide, μg/L × 2.10 = nmol/L; morphine, mg/L × 3.51 = μmol/L**
CAS Registry No.:	**915-30-0 (diphenoxylate); 34552-83-5 (loperamide)**
Therapeutic levels:	**Diphenoxylate, 10 μg/L; loperamide, 5 μg/L; morphine (single dose), 0.05 mg/L**
Special concerns:	**Diphenoxylate products contain atropine. Initial toxic effects may be anticholinergic; opioid manifestations may be delayed and prolonged.**
Antidote:	**None**

OVERVIEW

There are three classes of antidiarrheal drugs: antimotility agents, intraluminal agents, and antisecretory agents. Antimotility agents include diphenoxylate, loperamide, and other opioid preparations. Intraluminal agents include silicates, bulk-forming fibers, and agents to alter the intestinal microflora (*Saccharomyces boulardii* and *Lactobacillus acidophilus*). Antisecretory agents (somatostatin, octreotide) are not discussed in this chapter. This chapter is limited to the antimotility agents.

The antidiarrheal drugs are widely used for the symptomatic treatment of acute uncomplicated diarrhea. These agents should be used only after infectious causes have been eliminated and oral rehydration and dietary management have been tried. The antimotility agents are opioids, produce their toxic effects by acting as agonists at the μ opioid receptor, and respond to naloxone and supportive care. *Lactobacillus* appears to have no serious toxicity. Any toxic effects from *Lactobacillus* are treated with supportive care.

DIPHENOXYLATE

Diphenoxylate is a synthetic meperidine congener used in the symptomatic treatment of acute uncomplicated diarrhea. The commercial product is combined with atropine (0.025 mg/tablet or /5 ml) to reduce its abuse potential. In overdose, diphenoxylate decreases gastrointestinal (GI) motility and also causes central nervous system (CNS) depression, respiratory depression, and miotic pupils. The atropine component produces anticholinergic effects.

Toxic Dose

The adult dose of diphenoxylate is 5 mg orally every 6 hours. The pediatric dose is 0.3 to 0.4 mg of diphenoxylate/kg/day in four divided doses for a daily maximum of 6 mg for ages 2 to 5 years, 8 mg for ages 6 to 8 years, and 10 mg for ages 9 to 12 years. The dose for children 13 to 16 years of age is 5 mg of diphenoxylate every 8 hours.

No lethal dose has been established in adults. Adult volunteers who received a single diphenoxylate dose of 32 mg demonstrated pupillary constriction (1). Diphenoxylate doses of 40 to 60 mg produce typical opioid effects (2). The pediatric lethal single dose of diphenoxylate is 2.4 mg/kg (3). With multiple dosing, 1 mg/kg given over 24 hours has been associated with death (4). The minimum toxic dose of diphenoxylate is 0.16 mg/kg (5).

Toxicokinetics and Toxicodynamics

Diphenoxylate is poorly soluble in aqueous solutions but is rapidly absorbed after ingestion. After an overdose, diphenoxylate absorption may be delayed due to decreased GI motility. Peak plasma levels occur 2 to 3 hours after an oral therapeutic dose in adults (6,7). The apparent volume of distribution is approximately 4 L/kg (7).

Diphenoxylate undergoes hydroxylation of the ester group in the liver to difenoxin, a potent active metabolite. The metabolic pathway is diphenoxylate → diphenoxylic acid (difenoxin) → hydroxydiphenoxylic acid. The elimination half-life is 2.5 hours (range, 1.9 to 3.1 hours) for diphenoxylate. The elimination half-life of difenoxin (diphenoxylic acid) has been reported to be 4.4 hours (7), 7.2 hours (6), and 12.0 hours (8). Less than 1% of diphenoxylate is excreted unchanged in the urine, approximately 14% of the dose appears in the urine as metabolites over 96 hours (7), and 50% is excreted in the feces as metabolites.

Pathophysiology

Diphenoxylate is an opioid and produces its toxic effects by acting as an agonist at the μ opioid receptor. It inhibits gut motility and prolongs intestinal transit time by decreasing contraction of smooth muscle in the gut.

Pregnancy and Lactation

Diphenoxylate is U.S. Food and Drug Administration pregnancy category C. Both atropine and difenoxin (diphenoxylic acid) enter breast milk.

Clinical Presentation

Diphenoxylate poisoning is similar to other opioids: dose-related decreased GI motility, CNS depression, respiratory depression, and miotic pupils (Chapter 126). The atropine in the commercial products causes anticholinergic effects (Chapter 10).

ACUTE OVERDOSAGE

After an overdose, anticholinergic effects due to the atropine may or may not be noticeable. If anticholinergic signs are present, it is likely that opioid effects will follow. The average time after ingestion that initial symptoms or signs were noted was 4.5 hours (range, 1 to 8 hours) (5,9). However, the development of significant opioid effects (miosis, coma, respiratory depression, apnea, lethargy) may be delayed and may last 24 hours.

ADVERSE REACTIONS

Toxic manifestations during chronic use are similar to those for acute overdose but are due to accumulation of difenoxin. Diphenoxylate use may cause dizziness, drowsiness, malaise, lethargy; abdominal discomfort, decreased bowel motility; miosis; and allergic manifestations (anaphylaxis, angioneurotic edema, urticaria, and pruritus).

The atropine component may cause tachycardia, elevated body temperature, urinary retention, skin dryness, flushing, and pruritus. Therapeutic use of diphenoxylate has not been associated with the development of addiction.

Diagnostic Tests

Diphenoxylate or difenoxin plasma levels are not clinically useful. If respiratory depression develops, tests to assess respiratory insufficiency (e.g., arterial blood gas) are needed.

Treatment

Treatment of diphenoxylate toxicity is primarily supportive, with the addition of naloxone if signs of opioid toxicity develop. The use of ipecac or lavage is not indicated due to the aspiration risk associated with CNS depression. The benefits of activated charcoal within 1 hour of ingestion must be weighed against the possibility of emesis associated with its administration to a patient who may develop CNS depression.

Urinary retention may be significant and require bladder catheterization. Enhanced elimination techniques are not useful.

ANTIDOTES

Naloxone is the primary antidote for diphenoxylate. The initial intravenous dose is 0.4 to 2.0 mg. Continuous infusion of naloxone may be useful in some cases due to the long half-life of difenoxin. Atropine-induced anticholinergic effects may respond to a benzodiazepine or to physostigmine (Chapter 67). However, severe anticholinergic delirium develops rarely.

MANAGEMENT PITFALLS

Anticholinergic effects may precede the development of opioid effects by several hours. Patients who may have ingested diphenoxylate should be observed for 8 hours. Patients with any symptoms or signs of anticholinergic or opioid effects should be admitted and carefully monitored for at least 12 hours after the initial development of any toxicity.

LOPERAMIDE

General

Loperamide is a meperidine congener with opioid effects used for the symptomatic treatment of diarrhea. The major adverse effect is abdominal cramping. Clinical toxicity after overdose is similar to other opioids.

Toxic Dose

The adult therapeutic dose is 4 mg initially followed by 2 mg after each loose stool up to a maximum of 16 mg/day. Loperamide is not approved for use in children younger than 2 years of age.

The therapeutic dose is 1 mg every 8 hours for 2- to 5-year-olds, 2 mg every 12 hours for 6- to 8-year-olds, and 2 mg every 8 hours for 9- to 12-year-old children.

No fatalities have been reported. The oral median lethal dose in guinea pigs and dogs is approximately 40 mg/kg. A single loperamide dose of 16 mg did not produce pupillary constriction in adult volunteers (1). An adult who took three 20-mg doses within 24 hours was nauseated after 40 mg and vomited after 60 mg (10).

Six of 18 children younger than 6.5 months of age (weights unspecified) died after receiving loperamide 0.8 to 4.0 mg/day for an unspecified length of time (11). No other pediatric deaths have been reported. A single dose of loperamide 0.125 mg/kg was followed by CNS depression and bradypnea in a 15-month-old (12). A total daily dose of loperamide of 0.1 mg/kg produced drowsiness, irritability, and personality changes in a 34-month-old after 3 days of therapy (13).

Toxicokinetics and Toxicodynamics

Approximately 40% of an oral dose is absorbed from the GI tract within 4 hours. Less than 0.5% of an oral dose reaches the systemic circulation due to first-pass hepatic clearance; 90% of the drug is distributed to the GI tract and the liver. Protein binding is approximately 97% (10). Peak CNS levels of loperamide occur at 4 hours.

Loperamide is partially metabolized to glucuronic acid conjugates; 30% to 50% of unchanged drug is excreted primarily in the feces. The parent compound has an elimination half-life of 11 hours (range, 7 to 15 hours), which is not lengthened in overdose (10,14).

Pathophysiology

Loperamide is an opioid agonist at the μ receptor. It acts locally in the GI tract to inhibit circular and longitudinal muscle action and slow GI motility. Loperamide may also reduce GI secretions.

Pregnancy and Lactation

Loperamide is U.S. Food and Drug Administration pregnancy category B. It is not known if loperamide enters breast milk, but a significant concentration in breast milk is unlikely given its poor systemic absorption.

Clinical Presentation

The most frequent symptoms attributed to loperamide overdose by poison centers are drowsiness or lethargy (15.7% of presumed exposures), vomiting (9.0%), abdominal pain (3.7%), nausea (2.3%), headache (2.3%), xerostomia (2.3%), and constipation (1.9%). Bradycardia, respiratory difficulty, and hypotonia occurred rarely (15).

Adverse reactions are unusual and may be difficult to separate from the effects of the underlying condition. Reported adverse reactions to loperamide include drowsiness or lethargy, disorientation, and hallucinations. An adult with ulcerative colitis developed a toxic megacolon after 2 weeks of loperamide use (16). Paralytic ileus occurred in infants younger than 6 months of age after short-term treatment with loperamide (11,17). Two older infants developed necrotizing enterocolitis after 2 days of treatment with loperamide (18).

Diagnostic Tests

No laboratory tests are indicated routinely in an acute or subacute overdose. Patients with respiratory difficulty should have a chest radiograph and arterial blood gas determination. Marked abdominal pain should be investigated radiographically to rule out paralytic ileus.

Treatment

The treatment of acute or chronic loperamide overdosage is symptomatic and supportive. Activated charcoal may be useful within 2 hours of an overdose, especially if a coingestant is possible. In the case of a large ingestion, multiple doses of activated charcoal may enhance clearance of loperamide, which undergoes significant enterohepatic recirculation. The potential benefit of this treatment must be balanced with the expectation of mild toxicity and reduced GI motility. Dialysis or perfusion is not expected to remove significant quantities of loperamide.

Antidote

Naloxone reverses the dose-related opioid effects of loperamide. The recommended initial intravenous dose is 0.4 to 2.0 mg of naloxone.

OPIUM PREPARATIONS

Opium preparations are antimotility agents that contain opium or one of its derivatives (e.g., morphine). Adverse effects and toxicity are related to the preparation's opioid effects. Paregoric (camphorated tincture of opium) is the classic example of an opium antidiarrheal preparation. It contains prepared opium, essential oils, benzoic acid (3.8 g/L), ethanol (45%), and glycerol. Each 5-ml dose contains approximately 2 mg of anhydrous morphine. Note that paregoric is *not* opium tincture: The concentration of morphine in paregoric is 0.4 mg/ml, whereas the concentration of morphine in opium tincture (also referred to as *deodorized tincture of opium*) is 10 mg/ml. More complete information on opioid medications is provided in Chapter 126.

Toxic Dose

The usual therapeutic dose of paregoric is 5 to 10 ml given one to four times per day for adults and 0.25 to 0.5 ml/kg given one to four times per day for children. Therapeutic doses of morphine depress all phases of respiration. Oral morphine doses of 100 mg or more may produce significant toxicity in a nontolerant adult or child.

The acute oral lethal dose of morphine is estimated to be 120 mg (19). An adult is alleged to have died after an oral dose of 50 mg of morphine (20). In children, no acute lethal dose of oral morphine has been established.

Toxicokinetics and Toxicodynamics

The bioavailability of oral morphine preparations is 25%. At therapeutic blood concentrations, approximately one-third of the drug is bound to plasma proteins. The apparent volume of distribution of morphine is approximately 3.5 L/kg. Morphine is conjugated with glucuronide to form a more potent metabolite, morphine-6-glucuronide, which is excreted through the kidneys. Little morphine is excreted unchanged. In individuals older than 6 months of age, the elimination half-life of morphine is approximately 2 hours, slightly longer for the glucuronide metabolite (2).

Pathophysiology

The opioid in paregoric is a μ opioid receptor agonist and depresses respiratory rate, minute volume, and tidal volume.

Pregnancy and Lactation

When used acutely or for short periods, morphine is U.S. Food and Drug Administration pregnancy category B. When used for prolonged periods or in high doses at term, morphine is category D. Morphine crosses the placenta and constricts the placental vasculature (21). Morphine use is compatible with breast-feeding (22).

Clinical Presentation

Acute and chronic toxicity is typical of opioid poisoning: respiratory depression, CNS depression, miotic pupils, decreased bowel motility. Habituation and dependence may occur.

Diagnostic Tests

Patients with significant respiratory depression should have arterial blood gas determinations performed. Serum levels of morphine or its metabolite are not clinically useful. Morphine and its metabolite can be measured in bodily fluids and tissues.

Treatment

Treatment of paregoric overdose consists of support for the respiratory and cardiovascular systems and administration of naloxone. A single dose of activated charcoal may be useful within 1 hour of ingestion, but airway must be monitored closely and protected as clinically indicated. Other interventions are not recommended because a safe and effective antidote is available.

Antidotes

Naloxone is the antidote of choice for most cases of opioid medication toxicity (Chapter 65). The recommended initial intravenous dose of naloxone is 0.4 to 2.0 mg.

REFERENCES

1. Schuermans V, Van Lommel R, Dom J, et al. Loperamide (R18553), a novel type of antidiarrheal agent. Part 6: clinical pharmacology. Placebo-controlled comparison of the constipating activity and safety of loperamide, diphenoxylate and codeine in normal volunteers. *Arzneimittel-Forschung* 1974;24:1653–1657.
2. Reisine T, Pasternack G. Opioid analgesics and antagonists. In: Hardman JE, Limbird LE. *Goodman & Gilman's the pharmacological basis of therapeutics*, 9th ed. New York: McGraw-Hill, 1996:521–555.
3. Harries JT, Rossiter M. Fatal 'Lomotil' poisoning. *Lancet* 1969;1:150.
4. Ginsberg CM, Angle CR. Diphenoxylate-atropine (Lomotil) poisoning. *Clin Toxicol* 1969;2:377–381.
5. Rumack BH, Temple AR. Lomotil (R) poisoning. *Pediatrics* 1974:495–500.
6. Jackson LS, Stafford JEH. The evaluation and application of a radioimmunoassay for the measurement of diphenoxylic acid, the major metabolite of diphenoxylate hydrochloride (Lomotil), in human plasma. *J Pharmacol Methods* 1987;18:189–197.
7. Karim A, Ranney RE, Evensen KL, et al. Pharmacokinetics and metabolism of diphenoxylate in man. *Clin Pharmacol Ther* 1972;13:407–419.
8. Brunton LL. Agents affecting gastrointestinal water flux and motility; emesis and antiemetics; bile acids and pancreatic enzymes. In: Hardman JE, Limbird LE. *Goodman & Gilman's the pharmacological basis of therapeutics*, 9th ed. New York: McGraw-Hill, 1996:917–936.
9. McCarron MM, Challoner KR, Thompson GA. Diphenoxylate-atropine (Lomotil) overdose in children: an update (report of eight cases and review of the literature). *Pediatrics* 1991;87:694–700.
10. Heel RC, Brogden RN, Speight TM, et al. Loperamide: a review of its pharmacological properties and therapeutic efficacy in diarrhea. *Drugs* 1978;15:33–52.
11. Bhutta TI, Tahir KI. Loperamide poisoning in children. *Lancet* 1990;335:363.
12. Minton NA, Smith PGD. Loperamide toxicity in a child after a single dose. *BMJ* 1987;294:1383.
13. Marcovitch H. Loperamide in "toddler diarrhea." *Lancet* 1980;1:1413.
14. Killinger JM, Weintraub HS, Fuller BL. Human pharmacokinetics and comparative bioavailability of loperamide hydrochloride. *J Clin Pharmacol* 1979;19:211–218.
15. Litovitz TL, Clancy C, Korberly B, et al. Surveillance of loperamide ingestions: an analysis of 216 poison center reports. *Clin Toxicol* 1997;35:11–19.
16. Brown JW. Toxic megacolon associated with loperamide therapy. *JAMA* 1979;241:501–502.
17. Motala C, Mann MD, Bowie MD. Effect of loperamide on stool output and duration of acute infectious diarrhea in infants. *J Pediatr* 1990;117:467–471.
18. Chow CB, Li SH, Leung NK. Loperamide associated necrotising enterocolitis. *Acta Paediatrica Scandinavica* 1986;75:1034–1036.
19. Baselt RC. *Disposition of toxic drugs and chemicals in man*, 5th ed. Foster City: Chemical Toxicology Institute, 2000.
20. *Hazard alert! Recurring confusion between tincture of opium and paregoric.* Institute for Safe Medication Practice, February 20, 2002.
21. Kopecky EA, Ryan ML, Barret JFR, et al. Fetal response to maternally administered morphine. *Am J Obstet Gynecol* 2000;183:424–430.
22. Briggs GG, Freeman RK, Yaffee SJ. *Drugs in pregnancy and lactation: a reference guide to fetal and neonatal risk*, 5th ed. Baltimore: Williams & Wilkins, 1998.

CHAPTER 151

Antiemetic Drugs

Robin B. McFee and Michael A. McGuigan

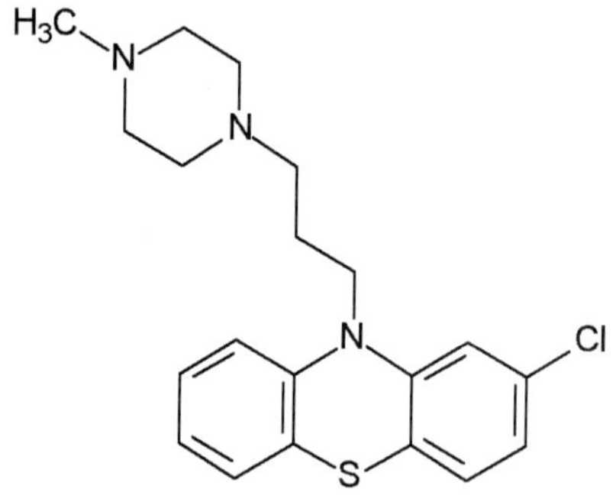

H_3C–N, N, N, Cl, S

PROCHLORPERAZINE

Compounds included:	**Cannabinoids (dronabinol); diphenidol (Cephadol); droperidol (Inapsine); prochlorperazine (Compazine); serotonin receptor antagonists: alosetron (Lotronex), dolasetron (Anzemet), granisetron (Kytril), ondansetron (Zofran), ramosetron**
Molecular formula and weight:	**See Table 1.**
SI conversion:	**See Table 1.**
CAS Registry No.:	**See Table 1.**
Normal levels:	**Not applicable**
Target organs:	**Heart (acute), central nervous system (acute)**
Antidote:	**Magnesium sulfate for torsade de pointes**

OVERVIEW

There are several categories of antiemetic drugs: cannabinoids, including marijuana or tetrahydrocannabinol; corticosteroids, such as prednisone; histamine antagonists, such as dimenhydrinate; dopamine receptor antagonists, such as droperidol; and the serotonergic receptor antagonist medications, including ondansetron (1,2). Cannabinoids, antihistamines, and metoclopramide are addressed in Chapters 178, 85, and 155, respectively.

There are few large-scale studies to compare the effectiveness of older agents to the newer serotonin (5-HT) antagonists (1–3). 5-HT antiemetics have the advantage of less sedative, dys-

TABLE 1. Physical characteristics of antiemetic drugs

Compound	Molecular formula, molecular weight (g/mol), CAS Registry No.	SI conversion
Cannabinoids (dronabinol)	$C_{21}H_{30}O_2$, 314.5, 1972-08-3	mg/L × 3.2 = µmol/L
Diphenidol (Cephadol)	$C_{21}H_{27}NO,HCl$, 345.9, 3254-89-5	mg/L × 2.9 = µmol/L
Droperidol (Inapsine)	$C_{22}H_{22}FN_3O_2$, 379.4 , 548-73-2	mg/L × 2.6 = µmol/L
Prochlorperazine (Compazine)	$C_{20}H_{24}ClN_3S$, 373.9, 58-38-8	mg/L × 2.7 = µmol/L
Serotonin receptor antagonists		
Alosetron (Lotronex)	$C_{17}H_{18}N_4O$, 294.4, 122852-42-0	mg/L × 3.4 = µmol/L
Dolasetron (Anzemet)	$C_{19}H_{20}N_2O_3,CH_4O_3S$, 420.5, 115956-13-3	mg/L × 2.4 = µmol/L
Granisetron (Kytril)	$C_{18}H_{24}N_4O,HCl$, 348.9, 107007-99-8	mg/L × 2.9 = µmol/L
Ondansetron (Zofran), ramosetron	$C_{18}H_{19}N_3O,HCl,2H_2O$, 365.9, 103639-04-9	mg/L × 3.41 = µmol/L

phoric, and extrapyramidal symptoms than antiemetics, such as droperidol and metoclopramide (1–9). 5-HT antiemetics do not seem to influence glucose levels or sleep patterns, as do glucocorticoids. The 5-HT antiemetics enjoy a wide safety margin and low toxicity risk and are increasingly used for prevention of chemotherapy-associated nausea and postoperative nausea and vomiting (PONV) in pediatric surgery (9).

PATHOPHYSIOLOGY

The physiology of nausea and vomiting involves the complex interplay of multiple neurotransmitters, including dopamine, 5-HT, and neurokinin (1,4,5). These neurotransmitters influence the activity of the chemoreceptor trigger zone (CTZ) and the vomiting center within the lateral reticular formation (5). Neuroreceptors in the gastrointestinal (GI) tract also have a role in emesis, as does histamine (1,5,6). Because of this, selected antihistamines have been used for their antiemetic effects. The nuclei of the solitary tract, the raphe nucleus, and area postrema contain glucocorticoid receptors that influence nausea and vomiting (3,5). Dexamethasone and other glucocorticoids also exert antiemetic action (1,5).

Nausea and vomiting differ in their pathophysiology and responses to pharmaceutical agents (2). There are multiple causes of emesis and the perception of nausea (1,5). Because each is dependent on multiple transmitters and multiple etiologies, an agent classified as an "antiemetic" may, in fact, be able to interrupt postoperative vomiting, while being minimally effective in preventing nausea or vomiting (7). Influences on eye movement or inner-ear receptors can trigger nausea and vomiting. There is also interindividual variation in terms of susceptibility to emesis and nausea. Influences include age; gender; obesity; and metabolic, psychogenic, and vestibular factors (1,8). There is a dynamic interplay among the oculomuscular cranial nerves, the medial longitudinal fasciculus tracts, and vestibular receptors.

CANNABINOIDS (DRONABINOL)

Cannabinoid medications continue to be used as antiemetics (10–14). In the setting of chemotherapy, cannabinoids are slightly more effective than conventional antiemetics. They may also be more toxic than other antiemetics and pose the risk for abuse (14).

Dronabinol (Marinol) is a cannabinoid and the primary psychoactive substance found in marijuana (11). It is available as 2.5-, 5.0-, and 10.0-mg gelatin capsules.

Toxic Dose

The oral antiemetic dose for children and adults is 5 mg/m^2 given 1 to 3 hours before chemotherapy, then every 2 to 4 hours for a total of 4 to 6 doses/day. The dose may be titrated up in 2.5-mg/m^2 increments until reaching a maximum of 15 mg/m^2 per dose. The therapeutic dose is 5 mg orally three or four times daily. Concurrent use of a phenothiazine, such as prochlorperazine, may improve the antiemetic effect (10,12–14).

The estimated lethal human dose of dronabinol is 30 mg/kg intravenously (IV). Central nervous system (CNS) symptoms have occurred after doses of 0.4 mg/kg and 15.0 mg/m^2 in cancer patients. The elderly may be more sensitive to the psychoactive effects. The euphoric or dysphoric effects appear to be less common in younger patients.

Toxicokinetics and Toxicodynamics

The onset of action is 30 to 60 minutes, with a duration of action of 4 to 6 hours. Tolerance may occur with chronic use (11). Absorption after oral dosing is 90% to 95%, with a first-pass metabolism resulting in systemic bioavailability of 10% to 20%. Dronabinol may be administered without regard to food intake. Protein binding is 95% to 99%. The volume of distribution (V_d) is 10 L/kg due to high lipid solubility. Using a two-compartment model, dronabinol has an initial α half-life ($t_{1/2}$) of 4 hours and a terminal β $t_{1/2}$ of 25 to 36 hours. Time to peak plasma concentration (T_{max}) is 2 to 3 hours.

Dronabinol is metabolized in the liver by microsomal hydroxylation to active and inactive metabolites with biliary elimination. Excretion is in feces and urine. Dronabinol and its principal active hydroxy metabolite are present in equal concentration in the plasma.

Pathophysiology

Although the antiemetic mechanism of action is still under investigation, the putative effect is probably inhibition or attenuation of the influence of the CTZ in the medulla. Dronabinol has sympathomimetic activity, affecting conjunctival injection, and the potential for tachycardia.

Clinical Presentation

Acute effects of severe intoxication include incoordination, lethargy, slurred speech, and hypotension. Seizures may occur in patients with underlying seizure disorders.

Adverse reactions primarily involve the following systems: cardiovascular (orthostatic hypotension, tachycardia, and hypotension), CNS effects (dizziness, drowsiness, euphoria, mood changes, anxiety, hallucinations, headache, memory lapse), and musculoskeletal (tremors, myalgia, paresthesias, and weakness). Transient elevations in liver enzymes may occur.

Drug interactions are common. Dronabinol may increase tachycardia and hypertension when coadministered with sympathomimetics, such as amphetamines, cocaine, and tricyclic antidepressants (11,12). It may also potentiate the CNS effects of sedatives, antihistamines, hypnotics, tricyclic antidepressants, alcohol, and psychomimetics. A hypomanic state is possible when the patient is using disulfiram or fluoxetine. Dronabinol decreases barbiturate clearance and increases theophylline metabolism.

Because dronabinol is highly protein bound, the potential exists for displacing other protein-bound drugs. The clinician should monitor patients for a change in dosing requirements when administering dronabinol to patients taking other highly protein-bound drugs (11,12). Dronabinol may exacerbate schizophrenia. Dronabinol has a high abuse potential.

Diagnostic Tests

Diagnostic tests are directed at the manifestations of toxicity, usually the result of adverse drug interactions.

Treatment

Symptomatic and supportive care is the mainstay of management (11,12). There is no specific antidote for dronabinol overdose. Enhanced excretion is difficult to achieve due to its lipophilicity and high degree of protein binding.

DIPHENIDOL

Diphenidol (Cephadol, Vontrol) is an antimuscarinic medication that may inhibit a common locus of motion and apomorphine emesis (15–18).

Toxic Dose

A 2.5-year-old boy ingested 15 mg/kg of diphenidol and developed recurrent seizures, hypotension, respiratory failure, and coma. He died despite aggressive supportive care (15).

Toxicokinetics and Toxicodynamics

Diphenidol is well absorbed and reaches maximal drug concentration in 1.5 to 3.0 hours after oral administration (16). It is primarily eliminated by renal excretion.

Pathophysiology

The emetic pathways through the inner ear, the visceral afferent, and the CTZ appear independent and mediated by histamine H_1 receptors, 5-HT_3 receptors, and dopamine D_2 receptors, respectively (17,18). Diphenidol may inhibit the emetic center. The exact range of receptors that it acts on is still under investigation (19).

Pregnancy and Lactation

The U.S. Food and Drug Administration (FDA) pregnancy category and entry of diphenidol into breast milk have not been determined.

Clinical Presentation

Adverse effects include drowsiness, hypotension, confusion, hallucination, restlessness, and other antimuscarinic effects (15). Serious anticholinergic toxicity, especially in children, may occur. Symptoms include facial flushing, tachycardia, seizures, dyspnea, drowsiness, mydriasis, coma, and fever.

Diagnostic Tests

Diagnostic tests are directed at the manifestations of toxicity, such as seizures and respiratory depression.

Treatment

Treatment is symptomatic and supportive. Seizures should be treated aggressively (Chapter 40). The role of physostigmine is still unclear.

DROPERIDOL

Droperidol (Inapsine) is an antipsychotic, sedative, neuroleptic, and antiemetic (21–23). It is a dopamine receptor antagonist (24). In addition to its dopamine CNS effects, it also possesses α-adrenergic–blocking and anticholinergic effects.

In 2001, the FDA issued a "Black Box" warning on droperidol due to concerns about cases of QT prolongation, torsade de pointes, and unexpected deaths that followed administration at or below normally recommended doses (21). This action has been analyzed and reveals many of the weaknesses inherent in the MedWatch program (28). Droperidol remains available in many countries.

Droperidol injectable is available in a 2.5-mg/ml (1, 2, 5, and 10 ml) solution that contains sulfites and benzyl alcohol. Patients known to be hypersensitive to sulfites may suffer an allergic reaction to some droperidol preparations (23).

Toxic Dose

The therapeutic adult dose as a premedication is 2.5 to 10.0 mg intramuscularly (IM). For nausea and vomiting, droperidol can be given, 2.5 to 5.0 mg/dose IM or IV every 3 to 4 hours. The therapeutic dose in children 2 to 12 years of age is 0.088 to 0.165 mg/kg IM as a premedication. For nausea and vomiting, the dose is 0.05 to 0.06 mg/kg/dose IM or IV every 4 to 6 hours as needed. The safety in children younger than 6 years of age has not been established. Droperidol should be infused over 2 to 5 minutes.

According to several studies, death is uncommon at recommended doses and doses less than 2.5 mg. Most reported deaths are associated with doses greater than 25 mg (21–23).

Toxicokinetics and Toxicodynamics

The onset of action is 3 to 10 minutes. Peak effects occur within 30 minutes with a duration of action averaging 2 to 4 hours but may extend to 12 hours (21,23). Droperidol is metabolized in the liver. The $t_{1/2}$ is 2.3 hours. Elimination occurs primarily in the urine.

Pathophysiology

Dopamine receptor antagonist antiemetics have been a mainstay in preventing PONV. However, this class of antiemetics has undesirable side effects, including sedation and extrapyramidal symptoms. Nonetheless, they remain a widely used class of medications for the prevention of PONV, rescue therapy for surgery-associated vomiting, and chemotherapy-associated nausea and vomiting (21–26).

Pregnancy and Lactation

Droperidol is FDA pregnancy category C (Appendix I). Excretion into breast milk is unknown.

Clinical Presentation

Acute effects include hypotension, tachycardia, QT interval prolongation, potentially life-threatening dysrhythmias, and torsade de pointes (21–23). Droperidol causes dose-dependent prolongation of the QTc interval. Orthostatic hypotension may occur, particularly in elderly patients. Respiratory effects can include laryngospasm or bronchospasm.

Adverse reactions include akathisia. Up to 50% of patients older than 60 years of age develop extrapyramidal reactions, which can include dystonic reactions, akathisia, and oculogyric crisis. Tardive dyskinesia has a prevalence rate of 40% in the elderly. This may be irreversible and proportional to cumulative dose over time. If diagnosed early, it may be reversible. Drug-induced Parkinson's syndrome also occurs. Confusion, memory loss, anxiety, dizziness, chills, psychotic behavior, and agitation occur frequently. Antipsychotic effects, including depersonalization and dysphoria, may occur.

Drug interactions include additive effects with other CNS depressant drugs, including respiratory depression, hypertension with fentanyl or other analgesics, hypotension with anesthesia or epinephrine administration, and tachycardia with atropine.

Diagnostic Tests

The FDA recommends that an electrocardiogram (ECG) be performed before administration of droperidol and the drug withheld in patients with QTc prolongation.

Treatment

Treatment is symptomatic and supportive. If torsade de pointes occurs, the standard treatment of magnesium bolus infusion, isoproterenol, and overdrive cardiac pacing should be performed.

PROCHLORPERAZINE

Prochlorperazine (Compazine) is used in the management of nausea and vomiting as well as for acute and chronic psychosis (29–31). Prochlorperazine blocks the postsynaptic mesolimbic dopaminergic receptors in the brain, including the CTZ. There is also a strong α-adrenergic blockade effect. In addition, prochlorperazine depresses the release of hypothalamic and hypophyseal hormones.

Prochlorperazine is provided as 5- and 10-mg tablets; vials containing 2 ml (5 mg/ml) and 10 ml (5 mg/ml); suppositories containing 2.5, 5.0, or 25.0 mg; and a syrup (5 mg/5 ml). Some preparations of prochlorperazine may contain sulfites or tartrazine dye that can cause hypersensitivity reactions.

Toxic Dose

The adult therapeutic dose is 5 to 10 mg orally or IM three to four times a day. The IV dose is 2.5 to 10.0 mg, repeated every 3 to 4 hours as needed. The dose by suppository is 25 mg twice daily (29,30). The pediatric dose for children more than 10 kg is 0.4 mg/kg/day in three to four divided doses. The IM dose is 0.10 to 0.15 mg/kg/dose. Adverse effects may occur at the therapeutic dose. A lethal dose has not been established.

Toxicokinetics and Toxicodynamics

The onset of action is 30 to 40 minutes orally (29,31), 10 to 20 minutes IM, and 60 minutes rectally. The duration of action is 12 hours with IM or oral extended release and 3 to 4 hours with rectal or oral immediate release. The $t_{1/2}$ is 23 hours. Metabolism is hepatic (29,31).

Pregnancy and Lactation

Prochlorperazine is FDA pregnancy category C (Appendix I). It crosses the placenta. There are no data establishing risk associated with breast-feeding. The American Academy of Pediatrics considers the use of prochlorperazine compatible with breast-feeding.

Clinical Presentation

Acute ingestion may produce extrapyramidal reactions, especially in children who are suffering from acute illness. It should be used cautiously in patients with a history of seizure disorder, as prochlorperazine may lower seizure threshold.

Adverse events include hypotension, especially after IV administration, orthostatic hypotension, tachycardia, dysrhythmias, and sudden death. CNS reactions include sedation, extrapyramidal reactions that may include dystonia, neck spasm, torticollis, opisthotonus, trismus, and mandibular tics. Signs of pseudoparkinsonism, tardive dyskinesia, and seizures may occur. Neuroleptic malignant syndrome and altered central temperature regulation have occurred.

Hematologic reactions include agranulocytosis, leukopenia (although this may occur after prolonged use of prochlorperazine), hemolytic anemia, and thrombocytopenia.

Hypersensitivity to prochlorperazine or any component of the drug may occur. Cross-sensitivity with other phenothiazines may occur. Anaphylactoid reactions have occurred. Rash, photosensitivity, hyperpigmentation, and pruritus are examples of dermatologic reactions that have been reported.

Caution should also be exercised in the presence of other CNS depressants and α-adrenergic agonists, such as epinephrine. Avoid in patients with severe liver or cardiac disease or CNS depression or coma as well as narrow angle glaucoma and bone marrow suppression (29,30).

Diagnostic Tests

Diagnostic tests are directed at the manifestations of toxicity, such as seizures and respiratory depression. Although not clinically available, a prochlorperazine blood level above 1 μg/ml is associated with toxicity.

Treatment

Treatment is symptomatic and supportive. Emesis should not be induced because a dystonic reaction of the head or neck may develop that could result in aspiration of vomitus. Seizures should be aggressively treated (Chapter 40). There is no specific antidote for prochlorperazine overdose.

Extrapyramidal reactions are treated with diphenhydramine, 1 mg/kg/dose IV. In the case of severe reactions, an antiparkinsonism agent (except L-dopa) may promote reversal. It is essential to monitor intravascular fluid volume and maintain a patent airway.

Neuroleptic malignant syndrome represents a medical emergency. The management of neuroleptic malignant syndrome includes aggressive control of body temperature and the administration of medications, such as bromocriptine (Chapter 23).

Dystonic reactions are treated with diphenhydramine, 1 mg/kg/dose IV (29–31). Maintenance should be considered for 1 to 2 days. Benztropine can also be used.

SEROTONIN RECEPTOR ANTIEMETICS

5-HT (5-hydroxytryptamine) is a biogenic amine neurotransmitter synthesized from L-tryptophan, which exerts generally inhibitory effects (32,33). Because 5-HT cannot enter the brain, the CNS absorbs L-tryptophan, subsequently synthesizing 5-HT in the cell. 5-HT plays a role in depression, thermoregulation, early-onset alcoholism, and a variety of GI functions.

5-HT may also have a role in neuroleptic-induced tardive dyskinesia due to interplay between 5-HT and dopamine (34). The 5-HT system also affects the dopaminergic system, which affects emesis. Of the 21 subtypes of 5-HT receptors, the principal types include 5-HT_1, 5-HT_2, 5-HT_3, 5-HT_4, and 5-HT_7 (35,36). The 5-HT_1 group is divided into subtypes A, B, C, D, and E. The effects relevant to GI physiology are primarily mediated through the 5-HT

1A, 1P, 3, and 4 receptors. 5-HT_1 receptors are G protein linked. 5-HT_2 receptors exist as 5-HT 2A, 2B, and 2C, also G protein linked.

5-HT is distributed in enteroendocrine cells and the enteric nervous system (35). In the GI tract, 5-HT_{1P} agonists stimulate release of nitrous oxide, thus relaxing the gastric fundus. 5-HT plays an important role in peristalsis.

The 5-HT_3 receptor plays a role in the regulation of colonic function (37). The 5-HT_3 receptor is a ligand-gated ion channel. In the brain, there is the 5-HT_{3A} receptor subunit. 5-HT_3 receptors are also located in the CTZ, which is an area associated with nausea and emesis (38). Antagonists of peripheral 5-HT_3 receptors, such as ondansetron, granisetron, and others, are used in the treatment of nausea and vomiting (39–42). They inhibit colonic motility and decrease defecation frequency in women with diarrhea-predominant irritable bowel syndrome (IBS).

The 5-HT_4 receptor is also a G protein–linked receptor. Both 5-HT_3 and 5-HT_4 receptor agonists stimulate propulsion and secretion. One of the effects of 5-HT in the stomach is the induction of nausea and vomiting associated with chemotherapy. Emetogenic regimens, such as cisplatinum, produce significant increases in 5-hydroxyindoleacetic acid, a metabolite of 5-HT. Data suggest that the optimal dose to block 5-HT_3 receptors in a vomiting patient as a result of PONV may be less than needed to block those receptors before vomiting occurs (43).

More than 60% of the 1.2 million patients diagnosed with cancer in the United States each year are older than 65 years of age (44,45). Selecting antiemetics with low risk for side effects is essential. Currently, there are three 5-HT_3 receptor antagonists available in the United States: ondansetron (Zofran), granisetron (Kytril), and dolasetron (Anzemet). Only dolasetron carries a warning that ECG interval changes can occur.

Alosetron

Alosetron (Lotronex) is a selective 5-HT_3 receptor antagonist used in the treatment of women with severe diarrhea-predominant IBS who have failed conventional therapy (46,47). It was developed for severe IBS-related diarrhea as well as rectosigmoid distention (48–50). The manufacturer withdrew alosetron after ischemic colitis, serious complications of constipation, and four deaths were reported (50,51–54). It was reintroduced in June 2002 for treatment of woman with severe IBS refractory to traditional treatment. Lotronex is available as 1-mg tablets.

TOXIC DOSE

The adult oral therapeutic dose in women is one tablet (1 mg) orally once a day for 4 weeks. The dose can be increased to 1 mg twice a day if the lower dose is well tolerated. Alosetron should be discontinued if patients do not experience adequate control of symptoms within 4 weeks. Safety and effectiveness have not been studied in pediatric patients.

There are no reports of acute toxicity. Single doses of 16 mg have not produced significant adverse events. Single oral doses at 15 mg/kg in female mice and 60 mg/kg in female rats (30 and 240 times, respectively, the human dose) produced labored respiration, subdued behavior, ataxia, tremor, convulsion, and death.

During therapeutic use, the most commonly reported symptoms are constipation, ileus, fecal impaction, obstruction, perforation, ulceration, ischemic colitis, small bowel mesenteric ischemia, headache, and rash (46–48,50).

TOXICOKINETICS AND TOXICODYNAMICS

The bioavailability of alosetron ranges from 30% to 90%. The T_{max} after a 1-mg dose in young women was 1 hour, with a maximal drug concentration of 9 ng/ml. Administration with food delays T_{max} by 15 minutes and decreases absorption by 25%. Alosetron has a V_d of 65 to 95 L. Plasma protein binding is 82%. Plasma concentrations increase proportionately with an increasing dose up to 8 mg and more than proportionately at a single oral dose of 16 mg. The elimination $t_{1/2}$ is approximately 1.5 hours, with a plasma clearance of 600 ml/minute. Renal clearance accounts for 6% of the dose; only 1% recovered in feces is unchanged drug.

Alosetron is metabolized by human CYP2C9, CYP3A4, and CYP1A2. The biologic activity of the metabolites is unknown. *In vitro* human hepatic microsome studies demonstrated that alosetron did not inhibit CYP enzymes 2D6, 3A4, 2C9, or 2C19. It did inhibit CYP1A2 and CYP2E1 at drug concentrations 27-fold greater than observed with a therapeutic dose. No effect on metabolism was observed in a drug interaction study with theophylline. Alosetron had no clinically significant effect on plasma concentrations of oral contraceptive agents (CYP3A4 substrates). No significant effects on cisapride metabolism or QT interval were noted. It is unlikely alosetron inhibits the hepatic metabolic clearance of drugs metabolized by the major cytochrome enzymes 3A4, 2D6, 2C9, 2C19, 2E1, or 1A2.

PATHOPHYSIOLOGY

Alosetron is a potent and selective 5-HT_3 receptor antagonist. The 5-HT_3 receptor is involved in the regulation of visceral pain, colonic transit time, and GI secretions related to the pathophysiology of IBS (46,50,51,55). Alosetron inhibits activation of nonselective cation channels, which results in the modulation of the enteric nervous system.

The 5-HT_3 receptor has been demonstrated in the spinal cord, vagal afferent, and supraspinal sites, such as the hippocampus, medulla, ventral striatum, and hypothalamus. Studies suggest inhibition of select circuits of the emotional motor system (amygdala, ventral striatum, hypothalamus, and brainstem) by alosetron is associated with improvement of subjective symptoms and responses to visceral stimulus (46–48,55,56).

The mechanism of ischemic colitis is unknown, and this result was unexpected (46,48,50–52,54,57). In animal studies, alosetron does not alter intestinal blood flow.

CLINICAL PRESENTATION

In the 8 months after its introduction, four deaths and nearly 200 serious adverse GI events occurred. More than 150 patients were hospitalized during chronic use. GI events with hemodynamic sequelae are the most common severe adverse events. Serious complications of constipation, including obstruction, perforation, impaction, toxic megacolon, secondary colonic ischemia, and death, have occurred during use. In IBS clinical trials, the incidence of serious complications of constipation in women was 1:1000 patients, but 10% of patients withdrew prematurely during the trial because of constipation.

Ischemic colitis has been reported both before and after introduction of the drug (46,50,52–54,57,58). The severity of colitis ranges from rectal bleeding, bloody diarrhea, and new or worsening abdominal pain to life-threatening effects. The cumulative incidence of ischemic colitis was 3:1000 patients over 6 months. There is insufficient evidence to estimate the incidence of ischemic colitis for patients taking alosetron for more than 6 months. The FDA has concluded that the "risk factors remain to be determined."

Elderly patients may be at greater risk for complications of constipation (46). In atherosclerotic monkeys, 5-HT decreases perfusion to the colon, stomach, and duodenum. In spontaneously hypertensive and diabetic rats, the vasoconstrictor effect of 5-HT is exaggerated. In diabetic rats, 5-HT enhances mesenteric arteriolar vasoconstrictor responses. Alosetron may cause severe constipation and fecal impaction, increased colonic intraluminal pressure, compression of the mucosal vessels, and decreased perfusion. Constipation is one of the factors that facilitate the development of ischemic colitis. Alosetron should be discontinued in patients who develop constipation or symptoms consistent with ischemic colitis.

TREATMENT

Symptomatic and supportive care is the mainstay of medical management. There is no specific antidote.

Dolasetron

Dolasetron mesylate (Anzemet) is an antinauseant and antiemetic (63–69). It is used primarily for the prevention of PONV. Dolasetron may be effective in preventing postanesthetic shivering, although a higher dose may be needed (70–72). Dolasetron is available as a clear, colorless solution (20 mg/ml of dolasetron mesylate and 38.2 mg of mannitol in an acetate buffer) and as a 50- or 100-mg tablet.

TOXIC DOSE

The adult therapeutic dose is 12.5 mg IV. Single doses of 5 mg/kg IV or 400 mg orally were safely administered to healthy volunteers and cancer patients. A 59-year-old man with metastatic melanoma and no known cardiac conditions developed severe hypotension and dizziness 40 minutes after receiving a 15-minute infusion of 1000 mg (13 mg/kg).

In children 2 to 16 years of age, the dose is 0.35 mg/kg with a maximum dose of 12.5 mg (63). Dolasetron solution can be mixed with juice for oral dosing. A 7-year-old boy received 6 mg/kg dolasetron mesylate orally. No symptoms occurred.

Single doses of 160 mg/kg IV in male mice and 140 mg/kg in female mice and rats (6.3 to 12.6 times the human dose) produced tremors, depression, convulsions, and death.

TOXICOKINETICS AND TOXICODYNAMICS

Dolasetron is metabolized by CYP2D6 to hydrodolasetron, an active metabolite with affinity for the 5-HT_3 receptor (63,67). *N*-oxidation of hydrodolasetron is via CYP3A and flavin monooxygenase. Hydrodolasetron is excreted unchanged in the urine. Other urinary metabolites include hydroxylated glucuronides and *N*-oxide. After IV administration, T_{max} is 0.6 hours, with a mean $t_{1/2}$ of 7.3 hours. The mean V_d is 5.8 L/kg. After oral administration, the T_{max} is 1 hour, with a $t_{1/2}$ of 8.1 hours. The apparent clearance is 13.4 ml/minute/kg but is 1.6 to 3.4 times greater in children and adolescents and decreases approximately 42% with severe hepatic impairment and 44% with severe renal impairment. Approximately 77% of hydrodolasetron is protein bound.

Because dolasetron is eliminated by multiple routes, the potential is low for clinically significant drug interactions (63,67). Blood levels of dolasetron increased 24% when cimetidine was coadministered for 7 days and decreased 28% when rifampin was coadministered for 7 days. It also decreased 27% when administered with atenolol. Drugs that prolong the QTc should be avoided during treatment with dolasetron.

PREGNANCY AND LACTATION

Dolasetron is FDA pregnancy category B (Appendix I). Excretion into breast milk has not been determined.

DIAGNOSTIC TESTS

Diagnostic tests are directed at the manifestations of toxicity, such as seizures and respiratory depression.

CLINICAL PRESENTATION

Severe hypotension, bradycardia, and syncope have been reported immediately or closely after IV administration. Local pain or burning on IV administration can occur. Peripheral ischemia, thrombophlebitis, or phlebitis rarely occurs.

Dolasetron carries a warning that ECG interval changes (PR, QTc, JT prolongation and QRS widening) can occur. The active metabolites of dolasetron may block sodium channels, independent of the effect on 5-HT_3 receptors (63,69). Adverse events have included mild and transient hepatic enzyme elevations, constipation, and headache.

TREATMENT

Management should be directed by appropriate symptomatic and supportive care. After a suspected overdose, a patient found to have a second degree or higher atrioventricular conduction defect should be monitored on cardiac telemetry (63). There is no specific antidote.

Granisetron

Granisetron (Kytril) is a selective 5-HT_3 receptor antagonist with little affinity for other receptors (73,74). It is an antiemetic used in the treatment of patients receiving cytotoxic chemotherapeutic drugs and for PONV (73,75–79). Granisetron is available in 1-ml single-dose and 4-ml multiple-dose vials.

TOXIC DOSE

The oral therapeutic dose for adults is 2 mg orally once daily or 1 mg twice daily. The IV dose for adults or children older than 2 years of age is 10 to 20 µg/kg. Single doses of 40 µg/kg have been used safely and effectively (73,79). Overdosage of up to a 38.5-mg injection has occurred without symptoms or only mild headache.

TOXICOKINETICS AND TOXICODYNAMICS

Onset of action after an IV dose is 1 to 3 minutes with a duration of action less than 24 hours (73). Granisetron metabolism involves *N*-demethylation and oxidation followed by conjugation. Clearance is primarily hepatic, with approximately 12% eliminated unchanged in the urine at 48 hours. Granisetron is widely distributed in the body with a V_d of 2 to 3 L/kg. Plasma protein binding is 65%, distributed freely between plasma and red blood cells. The $t_{1/2}$ is 10 to 12 hours in cancer patients and 3 to 4 hours in healthy volunteers. Elimination is primarily hepatic; 8% to 15% of the dose is excreted unchanged in urine. Granisetron is metabolized by hepatic cytochrome P-450 system. CYP450 inducers or inhibitors could theoretically change the clearance and $t_{1/2}$ of granisetron. Ketoconazole inhibits its major route of metabolism *in vitro*. Creatinine clearance values have no relationship to granisetron clearance.

PREGNANCY AND LACTATION

Granisetron is FDA pregnancy category B (Appendix I). Excretion into breast milk has not been reported.

DIAGNOSTIC TESTS

Diagnostic tests are directed at the manifestations of toxicity, such as seizures and respiratory depression.

CLINICAL PRESENTATION

Mild symptoms, including hypertension, hypotension, agitation, skin rashes, constipation, diarrhea, and headache, may occur (73,79). Mild transient elevations in hepatic enzymes may occur. Dysrhythmias may also occur, including atrial fibrillation. Side effects are mild and can include headache, dizziness, sedation, myalgia, and constipation. No extrapyramidal side effects have been reported.

TREATMENT

Therapy is symptomatic and supportive. There are no specific antidotes for granisetron overdose.

Ondansetron

Ondansetron (Zofran) is a 5-HT_3 antagonist used for PONV and the prevention of emesis during cytotoxic chemotherapy (80–87). Ondansetron is available as 2-mg/ml (20-ml vial) or 32-mg single-dose vials. Oral tablets are available in 4 mg and 8 mg (80,83).

Ondansetron is unstable in an alkaline environment. To prevent precipitation in the tubing of a patient receiving an alkaline IV solution, the access line should be flushed before and after the infusion. Subcutaneous infusion has been well tolerated in patients with cancer.

TOXIC DOSE

The therapeutic dose for chemotherapy in patients older than 11 years of age is 8 mg as a single dose. For adults, it may be given as an oral 16- to 24-mg single dose or 8 mg twice daily. The IV dose is 0.15 mg/kg (80,83). It has not been approved for use in children younger than 4 years of age, but doses of 1 to 4 mg three times a day have been used. The dose for prevention of PONV (80,83) is 4 mg for patients greater than 40 kg and 0.1 mg/kg for smaller patients.

No fatalities have been reported as a result of overdose. Individual doses of 145 mg and a total daily dose of 252 mg IV have been administered without serious effect. The dose of 252 mg (1.5 mg/kg) every 2 hours produced itchy nose, vague restlessness, and hot flashes. A patient received three individual 84-mg doses (1.5 mg/kg) at 2-hour intervals (ten times the normal dose) and survived. Another patient received a single dose of 40 mg without adverse effect. A patient who received 145 mg (1.5 mg/kg) experienced hot flashes and a feeling that the skin was hot. The patient also experienced a transient, mild increase in serum lactate dehydrogenase. There were no ECG changes or extrapyramidal events.

TOXICOKINETICS AND TOXICODYNAMICS

The oral bioavailability of ondansetron is 60%. Nonlinear absorption occurs with increasing oral doses. After an oral dose of 8 mg, the maximal drug concentration is 30 ng/ml, and the T_{max} is 1 hour. The protein binding of ondansetron is 70% to 76%. The V_d is approximately 1.8 L/kg in adults (80–83).

Ondansetron undergoes extensive first-pass metabolism, primarily by hydroxylation, followed by glucuronidation and sulfate conjugation. Ondansetron is a substrate for CYP1A2, CYP2D6, and CYP3A4, which is the predominant enzyme. Clearance is 0.39 to 0.50 L/hour/kg in children and 25 to 50 L/hour in adults. Adults with cancer have a clearance of 16 to 32 L/hour. The $t_{1/2}$ in children ranges from 2.6 to 3.1 hours and 4.5 hours in adults. Ondansetron does not appear to induce or inhibit the hepatic cytochrome P-450 (80). However, ondansetron has the same imidazole nucleus as cimetidine and omeprazole. Therefore, patients receiving concurrent theophylline, phenytoin, or warfarin should be followed closely. Inducers or inhibitors of CYP450 may effect its elimination.

Less than 5% of the parent drug is recovered unchanged in urine. Therefore, renal impairment is not expected to have a significant clinical impact, and dosing frequency or dose reductions do not appear warranted.

PREGNANCY AND LACTATION

Ondansetron is FDA pregnancy category B (Appendix I). Excretion into breast milk is unknown.

CLINICAL PRESENTATION

Acute overdose with ondansetron has been followed by fever (hot flashes), rash, pruritus, and restlessness, which were treated with diphenhydramine and resolved within 12 hours (80,83).

Adverse reactions include tachycardia, hypotension, or bradycardia. Rash and local injection site reactions can occur. Headache, blurred vision, diarrhea, musculoskeletal pain, tremor, and seizures have been reported. Mild transient elevations of the serum lactate dehydrogenase level may occur, as can hypokalemia (80,83). Minor prolongation of cardiac conduction intervals has occurred in small studies (80,88).

DIAGNOSTIC TESTS

Diagnostic tests are directed at the manifestations of toxicity, such as seizures and respiratory depression.

TREATMENT

The mainstay of treatment is symptomatic and supportive care. There are no specific antidotes. Hemodialysis and hemoperfusion are unlikely to be useful due to the large V_d and significant protein binding.

RAMOSETRON

Ramosetron is a new, selective 5-HT_3 receptor antagonist (97–101) that is more potent and longer acting than granisetron in the treatment of cisplatin-induced emesis (100).

TOXIC DOSE

The adult therapeutic dose is 6 μg/kg IV. The pediatric dose has not been established (97,100). There are no deaths reported from Ramosetron.

TOXICOKINETICS AND TOXICODYNAMICS

Ramosetron has higher affinity for 5-HT_3 receptors than granisetron. Its $t_{1/2}$ is 5.8 hours.

PATHOPHYSIOLOGY

Studies suggest that ramosetron may prevent PONV by acting at the area postrema and nucleus tractus solitarius, areas that contain a significant number of 5-HT_3 receptors (98,100).

DIAGNOSTIC TESTS

Diagnostic tests are directed at the manifestations of toxicity, such as seizures and respiratory depression.

CLINICAL PRESENTATION

Side effects are minimal and may include headache. No extrapyramidal effects have been reported.

TREATMENT

The mainstay of therapy is symptomatic and supportive care. There are no specific antidotes.

REFERENCES

Overview

1. Markman M. Progress in preventing chemotherapy-induced nausea and vomiting. *Cleve Clin J Med* 2002;69:609–617.
2. Kazemi-Kjellberg F, Henzi I, Tramer MR. Treatment of established postoperative nausea and vomiting: a quantitative systemic review. *BMC Anesthesiol* 2001;1:2.
3. Goksu S, Kocoglu H, Bayazit Y, et al. Antiemetic effects of granisetron, droperidol and dexamethasone in otologic surgery. *Auris Nasus Larynx* 2002;29:253–256.
4. Bijak M, Zahorodna A, Tokarski K. Opposite effects of antidepressants and corticosterone on the sensitivity of hippocampal CA1 neurons to 5-HT1A and 5-HT4 receptor activation. *Naunyn Schmiedebergs Arch Pharmacol* 2001;363:491–498.
5. Zeid HA, Al-Gahamdi A, Abdul-Hadi M. Dolasetron decreases postoperative nausea and vomiting after breast surgery. *Breast J* 2002;8:216–221.
6. Spiller R. Serotonergic modulating drugs for functional gastrointestinal diseases. *Br J Clin Pharmacol* 2002;54:11–20.
7. Domino KB, Anderson EA, Polissar NL. Comparative efficacy and safety of ondansetron, droperidol, and metoclopramide for preventing postoperative nausea and vomiting: a meta-analysis. *Anesth Analg* 1999;88:1370–1379.
8. Sirota P, Mosheve T, Shabtay H, et al. Use of the selective serotonin 3 receptor antagonist ondansetron in the treatment of neuroleptic-induced tardive dyskinesia. *Am J Psychiatry* 2000;157:2:287–289.
9. Fujii Y, Tanaka H, Ito M. Ramosetron compared with granisetron for the prevention of vomiting following strabismus surgery in children. *Br J Ophthalmol* 2001;85:670–672.

Cannabinoids (Dronabinol)

10. Markman M. Progress in preventing chemotherapy-induced nausea and vomiting. *Cleve Clin J Med* 2002;69:609–617.
11. Marinol. Product information. Marietta, GA: Unimed Pharmaceuticals, Inc., 2003.
12. Feld LG, Cimino M. *Pediatric dosing handbook, Children's Medical Center/ Atlantic Health System*. Hudson, OH: Lexi-Comp, 2000.
13. Gralla RJ, Tyson LB, Bordin LA, et al. Antiemetic therapy; a review of recent studies and a report of a random assignment trial comparing metoclopramide with delta-9-THC. *Cancer Treat Rep* 1984;68:163–172.
14. Tramer MR, Carroll D, Campbell FA, et al. Cannabinoids for control of chemotherapy induced nausea and vomiting: quantitative systemic review. *BMJ* 2001;323:1–8.

Diphenidol

15. Yang CC, Deng JF. Clinical experience in acute overdosage of diphenidol. *J Toxicol Clin Toxicol* 1998;36:33–39.
16. Reynolds JEF, ed. *Martindale: the extra pharmacopoeia*, (electronic version). Denver: Micromedex, Inc., 1997.
17. Takeda N, Hasegawa S, Morita M, et al. Neuropharmacological mechanism of emesis. I. Effects of antiemetic drugs on motion—and apomorphine—induced pica in rats. *Methods Find Exp Clin Pharmacol* 1995;17:589–590.
18. Takeda N, Hasegawa S, Morita M, et al. Neuropharmacological mechanism of emesis. I. Effects of antiemetic drugs on motion—and apomorphine—induced pica in rats. *Methods Find Exp Clin Pharmacol* 1995;17:647–652.
19. Varoli L, Angeli P, Burnelli S, et al. Synthesis and antagonistic activity at muscarinic receptor subtypes of some 2-carbonyl derivatives of diphenidol. *Bioorg Med Chem* 1999;7:1837–1844.
20. Reference deleted.

Droperidol

21. Mieckowski A, Burns M. Droperidol and the black box. *J Toxicol Clin Toxicol* 2002;40:669–670.
22. Mullins M, van Zwieten K, Blunt J. Unexpected cardiovascular deaths with droperidol: a smoking gun or just smoke and mirrors? *J Toxicol Clinical Toxicol* 2002;40:600–601.
23. Feld LG, Cimino M. *Pediatric dosing handbook, Children's Medical Center/ Atlantic Health System*. 2000. Lexi-Comp. Hudson, Ohio.
24. Goksu S, Kocoglu H, Bayazit Y, et al. Antiemetic effects of granisetron, droperidol and dexamethasone in otologic surgery. *Auris Nasus Larynx* 2002;29:253–256.
25. Domino KB, Anderson EA, Polissar NL, et al. Comparative efficacy and safety of ondansetron, droperidol, and metoclopramide for preventing postoperative nausea and vomiting: a meta-analysis. *Anesth Analg* 1999;88:1370–1379.
26. Piper SN, Triem WH, Maleck M, et al. Placebo-controlled comparison of dolasetron and metoclopramide in preventing postoperative nausea and vomiting in patients undergoing hysterectomy. *Eur J Anaesthesiol* 2001;18:251–256.
27. Reference deleted.
28. Horowitz BZ, Bizovi K, Moreno R. Droperidol—behind the black box warning. *Acad Emerg Med* 2002;9:615–618.

Prochlorperazine

29. Prochlorperazine (Compazine). Product information. Brentford, UK: GlaxoSmithKline, 2002.
30. Feld LG, Cimino M. *Pediatric dosing handbook, Children's Medical Center/ Atlantic Health System*. Hudson, OH: Lexi-Comp, 2000.
31. Hurlbut KM. Neuroleptic malignant syndrome and serotonin syndrome. In: Dart RD, ed. *The 5 minute toxicology consult*. Philadelphia: Lippincott Williams & Wilkins, 2000.

Serotonin Receptor Antiemetics

32. Ito H, Kiso T, Miyata K, et al. Pharmacological profile of YM-31636, a novel 5-HT3 receptor agonist, in vitro. *Eur J of Pharmacol* 2000;409:195–201.
33. Bijak M, Zahorodna A, Tokarski K. Opposite effects of antidepressants and corticosterone on the sensitivity of hippocampal CA1 neurons to 5-HT1A and 5-HT4 receptor activation. *Naunyn Schmiedebergs Arch Pharmacol* 2001;363:491–498.
34. Sirota P, Mosheve T, Shabtay H, et al. Use of the selective serotonin 3 receptor antagonist ondansetron in the treatment of neuroleptic-induced tardive dyskinesia. *Am J Psychiatry* 2000;157:2:287–289.
35. Spiller R. Serotonergic modulating drugs for functional gastrointestinal diseases. *Br J Clin Pharmacol* 2002;54:11–20.
36. Kiso T, Ito H, Miyata K, et al. A novel 5-HT_3 receptor agonist, YM-31636, increases gastrointestinal motility without increasing abdominal pain. *Eur J Pharmacol* 2001;431:35–41.
37. Kamm MA. Review article: the complexity of drug development for irritable bowel syndrome. *Aliment Pharmacol Ther* 2002;16:343–351.
38. Markman M. Progress in preventing chemotherapy-induced nausea and vomiting. *Cleve Clin J Med* 2002;69:609–617.
39. Zeid HA, Al-Gahamdi A, Abdul-Hadi M. Dolasetron decreases postoperative nausea and vomiting after breast surgery. *Breast J* 2002;8:216–221.
40. Fujii Y, Tanaka H, Ito M. Ramosetron compared with granisetron for the prevention of vomiting following strabismus surgery in children. *Br J Ophthalmol* 2001;85:670–672.
41. Kazemi-Kjellberg F, Henzi I, Tramer MR. Treatment of established postoperative nausea and vomiting: a quantitative systemic review. *BMC Anesthesiol* 2001;1:2.
42. Tramer MR, Reynolds DJM, Moore RA, et al. Efficacy, dose-response, and safety of ondansetron in prevention of postoperative nausea and vomiting: a quantitative systematic review of randomized placebo-controlled trials. *Anesthesiology* 1997;87:1277–1289.
43. Jokela R, Koivuranta M, Kangas-Saarela T, et al. Oral ondansetron, tropisetron or metoclopromide to prevent postoperative nausea and vomiting: a comparison in high-risk patients undergoing thyroid or parathyroid surgery. *Acta Anasthesiol Scand* 2002;46:519–524.
44. Keefe DL. The cardiotoxic potential of the 5-HT3 receptor antagonist antiemetics: is there cause for concern? *Oncologist* 2002;7:65–72.
45. National Cancer Institute. Surveillance, epidemiology and end results. 1999 estimated U.S. prevalence counts. http://www.nci.nih.gov. Accessed 12/2002.

Alosetron

46. Lotronex—alosetron hydrochloride. Product information. Brentford, UK: GlaxoSmithKline, 2002.
47. Mayer EA, Berman S, Derbyshire SW, et al. The effect of the 5-HT3 receptor antagonist alosetron, on brain responses to visceral stimulation in irritable bowel syndrome patients. *Aliment Pharmacol Ther* 2002;16:1357–1366.
48. Wolfe SG, Chey WY, Washington MK, et al. Tolerability and safety of alosetron during long-term administration in female and male irritable bowel syndrome patients. *Am J Gastroenterol* 2001;96:803–811.
49. Camilleri M, Chey WY, Mayer EA, et al. A randomized controlled clinical trial of the serotonin type 3-receptor antagonist alosetron in women with diarrhea predominant irritable bowel syndrome. *JAMA* 2001;161:1733–1740.
50. Kamm MA. Review article: the complexity of drug development for irritable bowel syndrome. *Aliment Pharmacol Ther* 2002;16:343–351.
51. Callahan MJ. Irritable bowel syndrome neuropharmacology. A review of approved and investigational compounds. *J Clin Gastroenterol* 2002;35:S58–S67.
52. Barclay L, DeNoon DJ. Lotronex back on market despite drug-related deaths MedscapeWire. Available at: http://www.medscape.com/viewarticle/436333. Accessed 2002.
53. McCarthy M. FDA allows controversial bowel drug back on to market. *Lancet* 2002;359:2095.
54. Camilleri M. Safety concerns about alosetron. *JAMA* 2002;162:100–101.
55. Spiller R. Serotonergic modulating drugs for functional gastrointestinal disease. *Br J Clin Pharmacol* 2002;54:11–20.
56. Olivier B, van Wijngaarden I, Soudijn W. 5-HT3 receptor antagonists and anxiety: a preclinical and clinical review. *Eur Neuropsycholpharmacol* 2000;10:77–95.
57. Friedel D, Thomas R, Fisher RS. Ischemic colitis during treatment with alosetron. *Gastroenterology* 2001;120:557–560.
58. Beck IT. Possible mechanisms for ischemic colitis during alosetron therapy. *Gastroenterology* 2001;121:231.
59. Reference deleted.
60. Reference deleted.
61. Reference deleted.
62. Reference deleted.

Dolasetron

63. Anzemet, dolasetron mesylate. Product information. Bridgewater, NJ: Aventis pharmaceuticals, 2003.
64. Zeid HA, Al-Gahamdi A, Abdul-Hadi M. Dolasetron decreases postoperative nausea and vomiting after breast surgery. *Breast J* 2002;8:216–221.
65. Markman M. Progress in preventing chemotherapy-induced nausea and vomiting. *Cleve Clin J Med* 2002;69:609–617.
66. Hesketh P, Navari R, Grote T, et al. Double-blind, randomized comparison of the antiemetic efficacy of intravenous dolasetron mesylate and intravenous ondansetron in the prevention of acute cisplatin-induced emesis in patients with cancer. *J Clin Oncol* 1996;14:2242–2249.
67. Balfour JA, Goa KL. Dolasetron. A review of its pharmacology and therapeutic potential in the management of nausea and vomiting induced by chemotherapy, radiotherapy or surgery. *Drugs* 1997;54:273–298.
68. Piper SN, Triem JG, Maleck WH, et al. Placebo-controlled comparison of dolasetron and metoclopramide in preventing postoperative nausea and vomiting in patients undergoing hysterectomy. *Eur J Anesthesiol* 2001;18:251–256.
69. Keefe DL. The cardiotoxic potential of the 5-HT3 receptor antagonist antiemetics: is there cause for concern? *Oncologist* 2002;7:65–72.

70. Bock M, Sinner B, Gottlicher M, et al. Dolasetron prevents postanesthetic shivering. *Anesthesiology* 1999;91:A1184(abst).
71. Piper SN, Rohm KD, Maleck WH, et al. Dolasetron for preventing postanesthetic shivering. *Anesth Analg* 2002;94:106–111.
72. Powell RM, Buggy DJ. Ondansetron given before induction of anesthesia reduces shivering after general anesthesia. *Anesth Analg* 2000;90:1423–1427.

Granisetron

73. Kytril. Product information. Basel, Switzerland: Roche Laboratories, 2003.
74. Wang JJ, Ho ST, Liu YH, et al. Dexamethasone reduces nausea and vomiting after laparoscopic cholecystectomy. *Br J Anaesth* 1999;83:772–775.
75. Kumakura H, Koyanagi J, Nishioka Y, et al. Phase I study of granisetron: pharmacokinetics of granisetron following single and repeat intravenous drips infusion in Japanese healthy volunteers. *J Clin Ther Med* 1990;5:25–34.
76. Markman M. Progress in preventing chemotherapy-induced nausea and vomiting. *Cleve Clin J Med* 2002;69:609–617.
77. Goksu S, Kocoglu H, Bayazit Y, et al. Antiemetic effects of granisetron, droperidol and dexamethasone in otologic surgery. *Auris Nasus Larynx* 2002;29:253–256.
78. Fujii Y, Toyooka H, Tanaka H. Granisetron in the prevention of nausea and vomiting after middle-ear surgery: a dose-ranging study. *Br J Anaesth* 1998;80:764–766.
79. Feld LG, Cimino M, eds. *Pediatric dosing handbook*. Hudson, OH: Lexi-comp, 2000.

Ondansetron

80. Ondansetron (Zofran). Product information. Brentford, UK: GlaxoSmith-Kline, 2002.
81. Sirota P, Mosheve T, Shabtay H, et al. Use of the selective serotonin 3 receptor antagonist ondansetron in the treatment of neuroleptic-induced tardive dyskinesia. *Am J Psychiatry* 2000;157:2:287–289.
82. Markham A, Sorkin EM. Ondansetron: an update of its therapeutic use in chemotherapy-induced and postoperative nausea and vomiting. *Drugs* 1993;45:934–952.
83. Feld LG, Cimino M, eds. Pediatric dosing handbook. Hudson, OH: Lexi-comp, 2000.
84. Ondansetron granted marketing approval. *Clin Pharmacol* 1991;10:249.
85. Derswitz M, Rosow CE, DiBiase PM, et al. Ondansetron is effective in decreasing postoperative nausea and vomiting. *Clin Pharmacol Ther* 1992;52:96–101.
86. Domino KB, Anderson EA, Polissar NL, Posner KL. Comparative efficacy and safety of ondansetron, droperidol, and metoclopramide for preventing post operative nausea and vomiting: a meta-analysis. *Anesth Analg* 1999;88:1370–1379.
87. Dundee JW, McMillan CM, Yang J, Wright PM. Is ondansetron a less effective antiemetic against moderately emetic as compared with highly emetic chemotherapy? *Br J Clin Pharmacol* 1992;33:200–201.
88. Keefe DL. The cardiotoxic potential of the 5-HT3 receptor antagonist antiemetics: is there cause for concern? *Oncologist* 2002;7:65–72.
89. Reference deleted.
90. Reference deleted.
91. Reference deleted.
92. Reference deleted.
93. Reference deleted.
94. Reference deleted.
95. Reference deleted.
96. Reference deleted.

Ramosetron

97. Kawabata Y, Sakiyama H, Muto S, et al. Clinical evaluation and pharmacokinetics of ramosetron against the nausea and vomiting induced by anticancer drugs. *Nishinihon J Urol* 1994;56:1445–1456.
98. Ito H, Kiso T, Miyata K, et al. Pharmacological profile of YM-31636, a novel 5-HT3 receptor agonist, in vitro. *Eur J Pharmacol* 2000;409:195–201.
99. Akuzawa S, Ito H, Yamaguchi T. Comparative study of [3H]Ramosetron and [3H]granisetron binding in the cloned human 5-hydroxytryptamine 3 receptors. *Jpn J Pharmacol* 1998;78:381–384.
100. Fujii Y, Tanaka H, Ito M. Ramosetron compared with granisetron for the prevention of vomiting following strabismus surgery in children. *Br J Ophthalmol* 2001;85:670–672.
101. Kumakura H, Koyanagi J, Nishioka Y, et al. Phase I study of granisetron: pharmacokinetics of granisetron following single and repeat intravenous drips infusion in Japanese healthy volunteers. *J Clin Ther Med* 1990;5:25–34.

CHAPTER 152

Cisapride

David C. Lee and Michael A. McGuigan

F
O
N
O
OCH_3
N
H
H_3CO
NH_2
Cl

CISAPRIDE

Molecular formula and weight:	**$C_{23}H_{29}ClFN_3O_4$, 466.0 g/mol**
SI conversion:	**mg/L × 2.15 = μmol/L**
CAS Registry No.:	**81098-60-4**
Therapeutic level:	**0.1 mg/L (plasma)**
Special concerns:	**Cisapride may cause ventricular dysrhythmias at therapeutic doses.**
Antidote:	**Magnesium (torsade de pointes)**

OVERVIEW

Cisapride is a substituted benzamide used as a gastrointestinal (GI) prokinetic agent. It had widespread use in the United States after its introduction in 1993. Multiple reports of its association with cardiac dysrhythmias led to its restricted use in the United States, where it is now available only as an investigational agent. It is still in use in other countries.

TOXIC DOSE

The adult therapeutic dose is 10 mg orally every 6 hours or 20 mg orally every 8 hours. The pediatric dose is 0.1 to 0.3 mg/kg every 8 hours, with a maximum of 10 mg/kg.

No dose-related fatalities have been reported in either adults or children. An adult developed mild GI toxicity after an acute ingestion of 540 mg of cisapride. Cardiac dysrhythmias may develop at therapeutic doses in patients with risk factors (other drugs causing QTc prolongation, drugs that inhibit cytochrome P-450 CYP3A4, electrolyte abnormalities, underlying cardiac disorders).

TOXICOKINETICS AND TOXICODYNAMICS

The bioavailability of cisapride after oral administration is 40%. Peak serum levels occur 1 to 2 hours after a therapeutic dose. The apparent volume of distribution is 2.4 L/kg, and 98% is bound to plasma proteins.

Cisapride has a large first-past metabolism and is extensively metabolized by CYP3A4 enzymes. Cisapride undergoes *N*-dealkylation and aromatic hydroxylation to an active metabolite, norcisapride. Norcisapride—but not cisapride—is renally excreted. In subjects who have normal liver function, elimination half-life is reported to be 7 to 10 hours for the parent compound and 27 to 75 hours for norcisapride (1).

PATHOPHYSIOLOGY

Cisapride increases gastric and intestinal motility. The primary site of action appears to be at intestinal serotonergic sites, specifically 5-hydroxytryptamine-4 receptors. Activation of these receptors causes gastric acetylcholine release at the postganglionic synapses in the myenteric plexus. An increase in gastric acetylcholine stimulates the muscarinic receptors in the gut, which increases smooth muscle contraction and peristalsis (1,2).

Another possible site of action of cisapride is through mechanisms related to the human ether-a-go-go-related gene in the GI tract. Cisapride may block potassium channels located in the GI tract or at the presynaptic nerve terminals in the myenteric plexus, causing smooth muscle depolarization (3,4).

In the heart, cisapride increases the QT interval and monophasic action potential durations. Clinically, this manifests as cardiac toxicity and ventricular dysrhythmias, specifically torsade de pointes. The conduction defects caused by cisapride are due to its ability to block one or more of the potassium channels in myocytes. The most important one of these channels is the delayed rectifier potassium channel associated with human ether-a-go-go-related gene (3,5–7). Other agents that can cause conduction delay and cardiac toxicity through this mechanism include terfenadine and astemizole.

Other possible mechanisms of toxicity are cisapride's structural similarity to procainamide and its ability to stimulate 5-hydroxytryptamine-4 receptors in the heart, causing tachycardia (8,9).

Because of its elimination pathway, cisapride may have significant drug–drug interactions. Drugs that are metabolized by CYP3A4 enzymes may interfere with cisapride metabolism, increase cisapride levels, and thereby cause toxicity.

PREGNANCY AND LACTATION

Cisapride crosses the placenta within 5 minutes of oral ingestion. It is U.S. Food and Drug Administration (FDA) pregnancy category C. Due to cisparide's high protein binding, minimal amounts (less than 0.1%) are excreted in breast milk (1).

CLINICAL PRESENTATION

There are few reported cases of acute cisapride overdose with clinical findings (10). Many of the reports are of children who had inaccurate dosing or very high therapeutic doses of cisapride. The majority of the adverse event reports focus on patients who are on cisapride chronically (1,10,11).

Acute Overdose Ingestion

An acute overdose of cisapride was followed by emesis, hyperactive bowel sounds, tachycardia, mild hyperthermia, and abnormal posturing in an 8-month-old child (1).

Electrocardiogram abnormalities associated with acute overdose include prolonged QTc, negative T waves, and U waves (10). The only death reported in an acute poisoning was associated with its treatment. A 1-month-old boy who developed third degree heart block died from a ruptured ventricle caused by a pacemaker wire insertion (10).

Adverse Events

The most common adverse reactions in patients taking a therapeutic dose of cisapride include headache, diarrhea, abdominal pain, and nausea (1).

Postmarketing surveillance of more than 36,000 patients treated with cisapride did not show an association between cisapride use and cardiac dysrhythmias. Yet the FDA has received more than 341 reported cases of ventricular dysrhythmia and 80 deaths since its introduction in 1993. It has been calculated that one adverse event was reported for every 111,000 prescriptions and one fatality for every 430,000 prescriptions (12,13).

Risk factors for cisapride toxicity include patients with altered drug kinetics (liver disease), patients with congenital (long QT syndrome) or preexisting cardiac disease, or patients taking other agents that inhibit CYP3A4 activity. Another specific at-risk group is neonates and young children. Neonates and, especially, premature neonates metabolize cisapride more slowly due to immature hepatic enzymes (14). Young children are also placed on relatively higher doses than adults (15–19).

The majority of reports of cisapride toxicity describe adverse events with chronic use. Therefore, patients may not present with overt poisoning but may present with symptoms related to cardiac toxicity, specifically palpitations or syncope (13,19).

DIAGNOSTIC TESTS

Serum cisapride levels can be measured, although it is unlikely to affect clinical management. Metabolites of cisapride can be detected in urine (2). Postmortem cisapride concentrations have not been reported.

Because of the possibility of cardiac toxicity, all patients with potential cisapride poisoning should have an electrocardiogram and cardiac monitoring. Because most acute overdoses of cisapride have a relatively benign presentation, the presence of QTc prolongation may be an early manifestation of toxicity and can easily be overlooked.

TREATMENT

The treatment of cisapride toxicity is symptomatic and supportive, except when cardiac dysrhythmia occurs during therapeutic use. In patients who present with ventricular dysrhythmias (e.g., torsade de pointes), treatments, such as cardioversion, overdrive cardiac pacing, magnesium, and lidocaine, should be considered.

GI decontamination is not recommended because of the mild effects after acute ingestion. The role of enhanced elimination of cisapride has not been evaluated. The high degree of protein binding mitigates against the use of dialysis.

Antidotes

There are no specific antidotes for cisapride. Cyproheptadine, a serotonergic antagonist, has been suggested for life-threatening serotonergic signs (1).

Management Pitfalls

Because cisapride has been promoted in neonates and young children, accidental poisoning due to inaccurate dosing or concomitant use of contraindicated medications has led to multiple reports of ventricular dysrhythmias in young children (20).

Patients who are at risk for cisapride poisoning should avoid other medications that prolong the QTc interval, especially class IA, IC, or III dysrhythmics; cyclic antidepressants; and antiinfectives, such as erythromycin and ketoconazole. Patients should also avoid other agents that may interfere with the metabolism of cisapride, specifically agents that inhibit CYP3A4 hepatic microsomal enzymes (2).

REFERENCES

1. Gibly RL, Walter FG, Kloster J, et al. Cisapride poisoning. *Vet Hum Toxicol* 1997;39:231–233.
2. Webster R, Allan G, Anto-Awuakye K, et al. Pharmacokinetic/pharmacodynamic assessment of the effects of E4031, cisapride, terfenadine and terodiline on monophasic action potential duration in dog. *Xenobiotica* 2001;31:633–650.
3. Mohammad S, Zhou Z, Gong Q, January CT. Blockage of the HERG human cardiac K+ channel by the gastrointestinal prokinetic agent cisapride. *Am J Physiol* 1997;273:H2534–H2538.
4. Wymore RS, Gintant GA, Wymore RT, et al. Tissue and species distribution of mRNA for the IKr-like K+ channel, erg. *Circ Res* 1997;80:261–268.
5. Walker BD, Singleton CB, Bursill JA, et al. Inhibition of the human ether-a-go-go-related gene (HERG) potassium channel by cisapride: affinity for open and inactivated states. *Br J Pharmacol* 1999;128:444–450.
6. Drolet B, Khalifa M, Daleau P, et al. Block of the rapid component of the delayed rectifier potassium current by the prokinetic agent cisapride underlies drug-related lengthening of the QT interval. *Circulation* 1998;97:204–210.
7. Rampe D, Roy ML, Dennis A, Brown AM. A mechanism for the proarrhythmic effects of cisapride (Propulsid): high affinity blockade of the human cardiac potassium channel HERG. *FEBS Lett* 1997;417:28–32.
8. de Ridder WJ, Schuurkes JA. Cisapride and 5-hydroxytryptamine enhance motility in the canine antrum via separate pathways, not involving 5-hydroxytryptamine1,2,3,4 receptors. *J Pharmacol Exp Ther* 1993;264:79–88.
9. Kii Y, Ito T. Effects of 5-HT4-receptor agonists, cisapride, mosapride citrate, and zacopride, on cardiac action potentials in guinea pig isolated papillary muscles. *J Cardiovasc Pharmacol* 1997;29:670–675.
10. Pezzilli R, Cavazza M, Calliva R, Barakat B. Cisapride poisoning associated with negative T waves. *Dig Liver Dis* 2000;32:648–650.
11. Ward RM, Lemons JA, Molteni RA. Cisapride: a survey of the frequency of use and adverse events in premature newborns. *Pediatrics* 1999;103:469–472.
12. Paakkari I. Cardiotoxicity of new antihistamines and cisapride. *Toxicol Lett* 2002;127:279–284.
13. Malik M, Camm AJ. Evaluation of drug-induced QT interval prolongation: implications for drug approval and labeling. *Drug Saf* 2001;24:323–351.
14. Bernardini S, Semama DS, Huet F, et al. Effects of cisapride on QTc interval in neonates. *Arch Dis Child Fetal Neonatal Ed* 1997;77:F241–F243.
15. Benatar A, Feenstra A, Decraene T, Vandenplas Y. Cisapride plasma levels and corrected QT interval in infants undergoing routine polysomnography. *J Pediatr Gastroenterol Nutr* 2001;33:41–46.
16. Treluyer JM, Rey E, Sonnier M, et al. Evidence of impaired cisapride metabolism in neonates. *Br J Clin Pharmacol* 2001;52:419–425.
17. Semama DS, Bernardini S, Louf S, et al. Effects of cisapride on QTc interval in term neonates. *Arch Dis Child Fetal Neonatal Ed* 2001;84:F44–F46.
18. Benatar A, Feenstra A, Decraene T, Vandenplas Y. Effects of cisapride on corrected QT interval, heart rate, and rhythm in infants undergoing polysomnography. *Pediatrics* 2000;106:E85.
19. Hill SL, Evangelista JK, Pizzi AM, et al. Proarrhythmia associated with cisapride in children. *Pediatrics* 1998;101:1053–1056.
20. Levy J, Hayes C, Kern J, et al. Does cisapride influence cardiac rhythm? Results of a United States multicenter, double-blind, placebo-controlled pediatric study. *J Pediatr Gastroenterol Nutr* 2001;32:458–463.

CHAPTER 153

Digestants

Michael A. McGuigan

OVERVIEW

Description, Use, Adverse Effects, and Toxicity

Pancreatin and pancrelipase (Pancrease MT, Viokase, others) are preparations of pancreatic enzymes used as digestants in pancreatic malfunction. Adverse effects include hypersensitivity, nausea, diarrhea, hyperuricemia, and mucosal irritation. Dose-related toxicity is uncommon, and acute overdose is unlikely to result in serious clinical effects.

Classification

Pancreatin (also known as *pancreatinum*) is made from porcine pancreas, whereas pancrelipase is prepared from either porcine or bovine pancreas. Both preparations contain amylase, lipase, and protease; pancrelipase has relatively more lipase. These preparations are used in the treatment of chronic pancreatitis and pancreatic insufficiency (e.g., cystic fibrosis, pancreatic duct obstruction, pancreatectomy, chronic pancreatitis) (1).

Therapeutic Dose

Doses of pancreatic supplements are titrated based on stool fat content and dietary consultation. The adult dose of pancreatin is 600 mg orally with each meal and an additional 300 to 600 mg with each snack. The pancrelipase dose is one to three enteric-coated capsules with each meal and one capsule with snacks. Each pancrelipase capsule contains lipase, 4000 units; amylase, 20,000 U; and protease, 25,000 U. In children with cystic fibrosis, the mean effective dose was pancreatin, 0.84 to 1.80 g/kg/day (2), and pancrelipase, one to three enteric-coated capsules with each meal and 1 capsule with snacks.

Toxic Dose

The adult and pediatric lethal and minimum toxic doses have not been established. Epidemiologic evidence suggests that chronic ingestion of total daily doses of enzyme supplementation greater than 2500 lipase units/kg/day may be associated with the risk of developing fibrosing colonopathy in children with cystic fibrosis (3).

PHARMACOKINETICS AND PHARMACODYNAMICS

Pancreatic enzymes are not absorbed from the gastrointestinal tract. Onset of therapeutic effects is 30 minutes (4). Peak therapeutic effect occurs in 2 to 5 hours (4).

PATHOPHYSIOLOGY

Exogenous pancreatic enzymes provide active enzymes to catalyze the hydrolysis of fat, proteins, and starch. The high purine content of the digestants may result in dose-related hyperuricemia, uric acid crystalluria, and urolithiasis (5).

Fibrosing colonopathy was first described in 1994, approximately 2 months after pediatric cystic fibrosis patients had been switched to a new "high-strength" pancreatic enzyme preparation (6). One hypothesis proposed that the new preparation delivered more active ingredients to the large bowel. A second hypothesis suggested that the methacrylate acid copolymer in the coating of the microencapsulated preparations caused dose-dependent colonic damage. This is supported by gut toxicity in animals (7,8), case reports of fibrosing colonopathy in children taking low-strength preparations containing a copolymer based on methylacrylic acid and ethyl acrylate (9,10), and reports of severe mucosal inflammations in patients taking the high-strength preparation containing the copolymer (11).

PREGNANCY AND LACTATION

Pancreatic enzyme supplements are U.S. Food and Drug Administration pregnancy category C. Pancreatic enzymes do not appear in breast milk because they are not absorbed.

CLINICAL PRESENTATION

Toxicity from Acute and Subacute Overdosage

No cases of acute or subacute overdosage have been reported. Mild self-limited mucous membrane irritation, nausea, and diarrhea may result from acute ingestion.

Toxicity during Chronic Use

Fibrosing colonopathy presents with the gradual development of abdominal pain, distention, vomiting, and constipation (12) unresponsive to standard therapy for distal intestinal obstruction.

Adverse Reactions

Side effects are rare. Asthma, bronchial hypersensitivity, and pulmonary sensitivity have been reported after occupational exposure to the powder. Skin rashes may occur. Preexisting hypersensitivity to beef or pork proteins may predispose to allergic reactions.

DIAGNOSTIC TESTS

Acute and Subacute Overdosage

No tests are typically needed.

Toxicity during Chronic Use

No tests are typically needed. Urinalysis identifies crystalluria. Plain abdominal x-ray may identify thickening of the colon wall. Ultrasound, computed tomography, or magnetic resonance imaging and biopsy can be used to confirm colonic abnormalities. Features compatible with fibrosing colonopathy are bowel wall thickening of more than 2 mm, reduced peristalsis, and free fluid adjacent to the affected areas (13,14).

Diagnostic Pitfalls

Fibrosing colonopathy may be differentiated from distal intestinal obstruction syndrome by its failure to respond to usual medical management.

Postmortem Considerations

The stenosed segments are long and associated with fibrous connective tissue in the submucosa with very little inflammatory changes. The intraluminal diameter of the colonic segment is narrowed, but the external diameter is not.

TREATMENT

Gastrointestinal decontamination and enhancement of elimination are not indicated after the ingestion of pancreatic enzyme supplements. Irritation or allergic reactions should be treated symptomatically. Surgical resection of stenotic bowel segments may be necessary. There are no antidotes for pancreatic enzymes. Supportive care includes treatment of respiratory symptoms, removal from the source in occupational powder exposure, and supplemental humidified oxygen. Antihistamines may be used to treat mild allergic reactions. In severe cases, epinephrine may be needed to treat allergic effects. Dermal or ocular exposures should be irrigated with copious amounts of water.

REFERENCES

1. Brunton LL. Agents affecting gastrointestinal water flux and motility; emesis and antiemetics; bile acids and pancreatic enzymes. In: Hardman JE, Limbird LE, eds. *Goodman & Gilman's the pharmacological basis of therapeutics*, 9th ed. New York: McGraw-Hill, 1996:917–936.
2. Beckles Willson N, Taylor CJ, Ghosal S, et al. Reducing pancreatic enzyme dose does not compromise growth in cystic fibrosis. *J Hum Nutr Dietet* 1998;11:487–492.
3. Borowitz DS, Grand DJ, Durie P, Consensus Committee. Use of pancreatic enzyme supplements for patients with cystic fibrosis in the context of fibrosing colonopathy. *Pediatrics* 1995;127:681–684.
4. Bruno MJ, Borm JJ, Hoek FJ, et al. Gastric transit and pharmacodynamics of a two-millimeter enteric-coated pancreatin microsphere preparation in patients with chronic pancreatitis. *Dig Dis Sci* 1998;43:203–213.
5. Stapleton FB, Kennedy J, Nousia-Arvanitakis S, et al. Hyperuricosuria due to high-dose pancreatic extract therapy in cystic fibrosis. *N Engl J Med* 1976;295:246–248.
6. Smyth RL. Fibrosing colonopathy in cystic fibrosis. *Arch Dis Child* 1996;74:464–468.

7. Treon JF, Signom H, Wright H, Kitzmiller KV. The toxicity of methyl and ethyl acrylate. *J Industr Hyg Toxicol* 1949;31:317–326.
8. Ghanayem BI, Maonpot RR, Matthews HB. Ethyl acrylate-induced gastric toxicity. I. Effect of single and repetitive dosing. *Toxicol Appl Pharmacol* 1985;80:323–335.
9. van Velzen D. Colonic strictures in children with cystic fibrosis on low-strength pancreatic enzymes. *Lancet* 1995;346:499–500.
10. Jones R, Franklin K, Spicer R, Berry J. Colonic strictures in children with cystic fibrosis on low-strength pancreatic enzymes. *Lancet* 1995;346:449.
11. Croft NM, Marshall TG, Ferguson A. Gut inflammation in children with cystic fibrosis on high-dose enzyme supplements. *Lancet* 1995;346:1265–1267.
12. Zerin JM, Kuhn-Gulton J, White SJ, et al. 1994: colonic strictures in children with cystic fibrosis. *Radiology* 1995;194:223–226.
13. MacSweeney EJ, Oades PJ, Buchdahl R, et al. Relation of thickening of colon wall to pancreatic enzyme treatment of cystic fibrosis. *Lancet* 1995;345:752–756.
14. Taylor CJ. Commentary: colonic strictures in cystic fibrosis. *Lancet* 1994;343:615–616.

CHAPTER 154

Proton Pump Inhibitors

Robin B. McFee and Michael A. McGuigan

OMEPRAZOLE

Compounds included:	**Esomeprazole (Nexium), lansoprazole (Prevacid), omeprazole (Prilosec), pantoprazole (Protonix), rabeprazole (Aciphex)**
Molecular formula and weight:	**See Table 1.**
SI conversion:	**See Table 1.**
CAS Registry No.:	**See Table 1.**
Therapeutic levels:	**Not applicable**
Target organs:	**Central nervous system (acute)**
Antidote:	**None**

OVERVIEW

Worldwide, peptic ulcer and other acid-related diseases affect tens of millions of people. Peptic ulcers arise secondary to an imbalance of acid secretory mechanisms and mucosal protective factors (1–3). The pathogenesis of reflux esophagitis is related to incompetent antireflux barrier, composition of the refluxate, and prolonged acid contact with the esophageal mucosa (4).

Antacids, anticholinergics, antispasmodics, and histamine receptor antagonists (e.g., cimetidine) have been the mainstay of treatment for gastrointestinal (GI) diseases. Comparative studies demonstrate that the antisecretory proton pump inhibitors (PPIs) are superior to H_2 receptor antagonists in providing pain relief, ulcer healing, and suppression of acid secretion (2). As a medication class, they are effective and safe and produce relatively few side effects or drug interactions (1–17). They have become the preferred drug class for the treatment of gastroesophageal reflux disease, Barrett's esophagus, erosive gastritis, and Zollinger-Ellison syndrome as well as other acid-related diseases, such as gastric ulcer and duodenal ulcer (1–4).

PPIs have become the most prescribed class of medications. Omeprazole (Prilosec) was introduced in 1989, followed by pantoprazole, lansoprazole, rabeprazole, and esomeprazole (5–9). All five agents have similar effectiveness (2,4,16).

Toxic Dose

In 2001, 5300 PPI-related exposures were reported to American poison centers. Most of these produced minor or no clinically significant outcomes (17). There have been few overdoses reported with PPI; mild and few clinical effects are to be expected.

Mechanism of Action

PPIs are prodrugs that belong to the chemical family of substituted benzimidazoles. These agents are weak bases that accumulate in acidic spaces with a pH less than 4, specifically the secretory canaliculus of the gastric parietal cell. Once in an acidic environment, the PPI becomes protonated, producing the activated sulfonamide form of the drug that binds with the H^+,K^+–adenosine triphosphatase enzyme and thereby inhibits irreversibly acid secretion (2). Parietal acid secretion is regulated by several major pathways

Table 1. Physical characteristics of proton pump inhibitors

Compounds	**Molecular formula, molecular weight (g/mol), CAS Registry No.**	**SI conversion**
Someprazole (Nexium)	$C_{34}H_{36}MgN_6O_6S_2$,$3H_2O$, 767.2, 217087-09-7	mg/L × 1.30 = µmol/L
Lansoprazole (Prevacid)	$C_{16}H_{14}F_3N_3O_2S$, 369.4, 103577-45-3	mg/L × 2.71 = µmol/L
Omeprazole (Prilosec)	$C_{17}H_{19}N_3O_3S$, 345.4, 73590-58-6	mg/L × 2.90 = µmol/L
Pantoprazole (Protonix)	$C_{16}H_{15}F_2N_3O_4S$, 383.4, 102625-70-7	mg/L × 2.60 = µmol/L
Rabeprazole (Aciphex)	$C_{18}H_{20}N_3NaO_3S$, 381.4, 117976-89 3	mg/L × 2.62= µmol/L

that rely on neural stimulation via the vagus nerve, endocrine stimulation from gastrin release, and paracrine stimulation from local histamine release (1). Unlike H_2 receptor antagonists and anticholinergic agents, PPIs are highly specific inhibitors of gastric acid secretion that antagonize the final mediator of acid secretion—the H^+,K^+ adenosine triphosphatase (1). They pass through the stomach intact and are absorbed in the proximal small bowel. They have a short plasma half-life from 1 to 2 hours. There are some differences among PPIs in terms of potency and time to clinical effect due to differences in the rate of activation of the prodrug, pK_a, and the drug-specific metabolic pathways.

In addition to suppressing acid secretion, PPIs inhibit the growth of *Helicobacter pylori*. Although the exact mechanism is not completely understood, the primary effect may be related to PPIs potently inhibiting *H. pylori* urease activity, which normally allows the bacterium to colonize the gastric mucosa. Concurrent use of antibiotics and a PPI appears to have a synergetic therapeutic effect (3).

Adverse Effects

PPIs are well tolerated. Their rate of adverse effects is similar to that of placebo and H_2 receptor antagonists, with an overall incidence of less than 5% (5–9). Diarrhea appears to be age and dosage related. This seems to be related to the effect of profound acid suppression on the bacterial flora of the intestine. All other side effects appear to be unrelated to age, dosage, or duration of treatment.

The time of onset of acid secretion inhibition depends on the pK_a of each drug, ranging from minutes (rabeprazole) to hours (pantoprazole). Because the parietal cell must produce new proton pumps or activate the resting pumps to resume acid secretion, which can take 50 hours, PPIs have a duration of action well in excess of their half-lives. PPIs are inactivated by metabolism hepatic CYP2C19 and CYP3A4. Clinically, the risk of significant drug interaction, even with medications such as diazepam, phenytoin, and carbamazepine, is low (1–16). Nonetheless, there are significant differences in plasma drug levels between CYP2C19 extensive metabolizers and poor metabolizers. Rabeprazole is metabolized primarily via nonenzymatic reduction (3,9,16). Omeprazole has the greatest potential for influencing cytochrome activity, whereas CYP2C19 and CYP3A4 are only partially involved in rabeprazole metabolism (2,16). Theoretically, rabeprazole should have less potential for drug interaction or alteration of drug metabolism (16). Early data suggest both pantoprazole and rabeprazole have fewer drug interactions.

Because PPIs increase gastric pH, they may alter the absorption of drugs that are weak acids or bases. The absorption of medications, such as griseofulvin, ketoconazole, itraconazole, cefpodoxime, and iron salts may be inhibited to varying degrees. Use of these drugs with a PPI should be approached cautiously due to the potential for treatment failure (1,2,5–9,13).

ESOMEPRAZOLE

Esomeprazole (Nexium) is the *S*-isomer of omeprazole (6). It is supplied as 20-mg and 40-mg delayed-release capsules.

Toxic Dose

The maximum adult therapeutic dose of esomeprazole is 40 mg/day orally. It has not been studied in children. Dosage adjustment is not required for the elderly or in patients with mild to moderate hepatic impairment. In patients with severe hepatic impairment, the maximum daily dose should not exceed 20 mg. A toxic dose has not been established, but 120 times the recommended dose has been ingested with only moderate effects. No deaths have been attributed to acute overdose.

Toxicokinetics and Toxicodynamics

After oral administration, the peak plasma level (C_{max}) occurs at approximately 1.5 hours postingestion [time-to-peak plasma concentration (T_{max})]. The C_{max} increases proportionately with increasing dose. Esomeprazole has greater bioavailability than omeprazole due to less first-pass effect and slower plasma clearance. Side effects, therapeutic window, and drug-interaction profile appear similar to omeprazole.

With repeated 40-mg once-daily dosing, the bioavailability is approximately 90%, compared with 64% after a single dose. The area under the curve (AUC) after a 40-mg dose decreases 33% to 53% with food intake. The volume of distribution at steady-state is approximately 16 L. Esomeprazole is 97% protein bound.

Esomeprazole is metabolized by CYP2C19 to inactive metabolites and by CYP3A4 to a lesser degree. CYP2C19 exhibits polymorphism. Approximately 3% of whites and 15% to 50% of Asians lack this isoenzyme and are thus referred to as "poor metabolizers." The ratio of poor metabolizers' AUCs to extensive metabolizers is approximately 2:1. Although AUC and C_{max} values are slightly higher in the elderly, dosage adjustments are not recommended.

The elimination half-life of esomeprazole is 1.0 to 1.5 hours. Less than 1% of the parent drug is excreted in the urine. Approximately 80% of an oral dose is excreted as inactive metabolites in the urine. The remainder is found as inactive metabolites in the feces.

Drug Interactions

Esomeprazole is extensively metabolized, but no clinically relevant drug interactions are expected. Coadministration of esomeprazole, 30 mg, and diazepam, which is a CYP2C19 substrate, resulted in a 45% decrease in diazepam clearance. However, plasma diazepam levels were below therapeutic, so this interaction is not likely to be clinically significant.

Pregnancy and Lactation

Esomeprazole is U.S. Food and Drug Administration (FDA) pregnancy category B (Appendix I). Excretion into breast milk has not been studied.

Clinical Presentation

In humans, large doses are required for toxic effect. A dose of 2400 mg produced confusion, drowsiness, tachycardia, nausea, blurred vision, flushing, headache, and dry mouth.

Treatment

Treatment is symptomatic and supportive. There is no antidote. Due to its extensive protein binding, it is unlikely dialysis will be effective.

LANSOPRAZOLE

Lansoprazole (Prevacid) is available as a single agent and as part of a three-medication product [lansoprazole, amoxicillin, clarithromycin (PREVPAC)] for the treatment of *H. pylori* that includes 30 mg of lansoprazole, 500 mg of amoxicillin, and 500 mg of clarithromycin. Each delayed-release capsule contains 30 mg of enteric-coated granules (7).

Toxic Dose

The adult therapeutic dose ranges from 15 to 30 mg/day orally. It is administered before eating; capsules may be opened and mixed with applesauce without affecting bioavailability. The safety and effectiveness of lansoprazole have not been established in children.

A reported overdose of 600 mg of lansoprazole was associated with no adverse clinical outcome. This correlates well with animal studies. Oral doses up to 5000 mg/kg in rats (1300 times the human dose) did not produce clinical signs.

Toxicokinetics and Toxicodynamics

In the fasting state, bioavailability is 80%, and plasma protein binding is 97%. The C_{max} of 0.75 to 1.15 mg/L is reached in 1.5 to 2.0 hours. The plasma half-life is 1.5 hours. Approximately 20% of the dose is excreted as conjugated and unconjugated metabolites in urine and bile.

Lansoprazole is metabolized in the liver by CYP2C19 and CYP3A4 to two main metabolites. There have been no reports of clinically significant interactions with drugs that are metabolized similarly, such as phenytoin and diazepam, warfarin, ibuprofen, or propranolol. When lansoprazole was administered with theophylline, a 10% increase in the clearance of theophylline was observed. According to the manufacturer, this interaction is unlikely to be of clinical consequence. Nevertheless, patients requiring theophylline and PPI therapy may need additional titration of theophylline blood levels. Sucralfate can delay absorption if taken concurrently with lansoprazole. Lansoprazole may interfere with the absorption of drugs that are gastric pH dependent in terms of bioavailability.

A single dose of lansoprazole inhibits 80% to 97% of acid secretion in healthy volunteers. The duration of activity is greater than 24 hours. The gastric acid pump inhibition effect is dose related and leads to the inhibition of both basal and stimulated gastric acid secretion.

Pregnancy and Lactation

Lansoprazole is FDA pregnancy category B (Appendix I). Excretion into breast milk has not been studied.

Clinical Presentation

The adverse effects associated with PPI are similar to placebo, but diarrhea, skin rashes, fatigue, melena, dyspepsia, headache, dizziness, and respiratory tract symptoms may occur. Increases have been observed in serum gastrin levels, mildly elevated hepatic transaminase levels, hematocrit, urinary protein excretion, and uric acid levels.

Acute overdose can produce mild tachycardia, flushing, and central nervous system and GI effects. Elevated liver function tests may occur during chronic therapy (7,12).

Treatment

Treatment is symptomatic and supportive. There are no antidotes to lansoprazole overdose. Due to the large percentage of protein binding, dialysis is not likely to be effective.

OMEPRAZOLE

Omeprazole was the first PPI approved for the treatment of acid-related GI diseases. It has been used for the treatment of stress-induced gastric mucosal hemorrhage (2,5,11,16). Omeprazole is available as 20-mg delayed-release capsules (5).

Toxic Dose

The therapeutic adult dose for gastroesophageal reflux disease is 20 mg daily for 4 to 8 weeks. A dose of 0.5 mg/kg/day (20 mg/day/1.73 m^2 body surface area) has been suggested for the treatment of refractory gastroesophageal reflux in children. Doses up to 400 mg/day have been well tolerated with no serious adverse effects reported. A pregnant woman who ingested 320 mg and a man who ingested 400 mg both survived. There have been no reports of a fatal dose.

Toxicokinetics and Toxicodynamics

The oral bioavailability is 30% to 60%. The T_{max} is 1.5 hours, and the elimination half-life is 1.0 hour. Plasma protein binding is 95%, with a volume of distribution of 0.3 L/kg. Omeprazole is metabolized by CYP2C19 and CYP3A4 isoenzymes and inhibits the oxidative metabolism of diazepam, phenazone, warfarin, and nifedipine. Clinically significant drug interactions are unlikely; however, catatonia has been reported with concomitant disulfiram administration, and ataxia has occurred when omeprazole was used with benzodiazepines.

Pregnancy and Lactation

Omeprazole is FDA pregnancy category C (Appendix I). Breast-feeding information is limited, but the peak concentration in one nursing infant was only 7% of the mother's serum level (18).

Clinical Presentation

Acute overdoses may result in drowsiness, diaphoresis, headache, blurred vision, and dry mouth. Most symptoms resolve without sequelae within 3 hours. Chronic use of omeprazole has been associated with subacute myopathy, hemolytic anemia, gynecomastia, headache, diarrhea, abdominal pain, nausea, painful erections, hepatic failure, peripheral neuropathy, gastric carcinoid tumors in patients with Zollinger-Ellison syndrome, and gastric polyposis.

Treatment

Symptomatic and supportive care is the mainstay of therapy. There is no antidote. Due to significant protein binding, dialysis is unlikely to be effective.

PANTOPRAZOLE

Pantoprazole is the only PPI approved for both intravenous (IV) and oral administration (2,8). As the only IV formulation, pantoprazole is used for the short-term treatment of hospitalized patients with gastroesophageal reflux disease (7 to 10 days) who are unable to take an oral PPI. Unlike other PPIs, pantoprazole can be administered without regard to meals.

Toxic Dose

The adult therapeutic IV dose is the same as the oral dose (40 mg). The IV dose should be administered over 2 to 15 minutes. Dosing has not been established in children. Doses up to 240 mg/day IV were given for 7 days to healthy patients without adverse effect. A patient ingested unknown doses of chloroquine and zopiclone with 560 mg of pantoprazole and subsequently died. Overdose involving doses of 400 and 600 mg has occurred without adverse effects being reported.

Toxicokinetics and Toxicodynamics

Pantoprazole is metabolized by several CYP450 isoenzymes. It is highly stable at neutral pH, has linear pharmacokinetics, and has a lower potential to interact with cytochrome P-450 enzymes than omeprazole and lansoprazole. Pantoprazole does not accumulate, and its pharmacokinetics are unaltered by multiple daily dosing. The oral bioavailability is approximately 77%. The T_{max} is 2.4 hours in patients who are extensive metabolizers. Total clearance after IV administration in extensive metabolizers is 7.6 to 14.0 L/hour. The apparent volume of distribution is 11.0 to 23.6 L. Plasma protein binding is 98%.

Pregnancy and Lactation

Pantoprazole is FDA pregnancy category B (Appendix I). Pantoprazole is excreted in the breast milk of rats but has not been studied in humans.

Clinical Presentation

Although an array of complaints ranging from musculoskeletal to cardiac have been reported, these are not appreciably different from placebo. Headache, diarrhea, and generalized GI complaints may occur. Symptoms of acute toxicity in animal studies include hypoactivity, ataxia, and tremor.

Treatment

Treatment is symptomatic and supportive. There is no specific antidote. Due to its volume of distribution and extensive protein binding, dialysis is unlikely to be an effective therapy.

RABEPRAZOLE

In contrast to other PPIs, rabeprazole forms a partially reversible bond with the proton pump and is activated at a broader range of gastric pH. As a result, it may have a more sustained acid-suppressing effect than the other PPIs.

Toxic Dose

The adult dose is 20 mg/day. Seven reports of accidental overdosage noted no clinical signs or symptoms. Patients with Zollinger-Ellison syndrome have been treated with up to 120 mg of rabeprazole daily. Single doses of rabeprazole at 786 mg/kg and 1024 mg/kg were lethal to mice and rats, respectively. A single oral dose of 2000 mg/kg was not lethal to dogs.

Toxicokinetics and Toxicodynamics

Rabeprazole has a higher pK_a than the other PPIs, allowing it to be activated over a wider pH range than other PPIs. It converts to the sulfonamide faster as well and has a faster onset of H^+,K^+ adenosine triphosphatase and acid secretion inhibition (3,9).

Absolute bioavailability for a 20-mg oral tablet (compared to IV administration) is 52%. The C_{max} occurs in 2 to 5 hours (T_{max}). The rabeprazole C_{max} and AUC are linear over the range of 10 to 40 mg. Its pharmacokinetics are not altered by multiple dosing. Rabeprazole is 96.3% bound to plasma proteins. It is extensively metabolized by CYP3A and CYP2C19 to inactive metabolites. The plasma half-life ranges from 1 to 2 hours. Studies in healthy subjects indicate that rabeprazole does not have clinically significant interactions with other drugs.

Rabeprazole may interact with compounds that are dependent on gastric pH for absorption. In normal subjects, coadministration of rabeprazole, 20 mg every day, resulted in a 30% decrease in the bioavailability of ketoconazole and increased the AUC and C_{max} of digoxin by 19% and 29%, respectively.

Pregnancy and Lactation

Rabeprazole is FDA pregnancy category B (Appendix I). Excretion into breast milk has not been reported.

Clinical Presentation

Rabeprazole is well tolerated, with side-effect rates similar to that of placebo. The most common adverse effect is headache. The major symptoms of acute toxicity are hypoactivity; labored respiration; lateral or prone position and convulsion in mice and rats; and watery diarrhea, tremor, convulsion, and coma in dogs.

Treatment

Treatment is symptomatic and supportive. No specific antidote for rabeprazole is known. Rabeprazole is extensively protein bound and is not readily dialyzable.

REFERENCES

1. Perlin DS. Ion pumps as targets for therapeutic intervention: old and new paradigms. *J Biotechnol* 1998;1:55–64.
2. Vanderhoff BT. Proton pump inhibitors: an update. *Am Fam Physician* (via FindArticles.com: http://www.findarticles.com). Accessed July, 2002.
3. Horn J. The proton-pump inhibitors: similarities and differences. *Clin Ther* 2000;22:266–280.
4. Meneghelli UG, Boaventura S, Moraes-Filho JPP, et al. Efficacy and tolerability of pantoprazole versus ranitidine in the treatment of reflux esophagitis and the influence of *Helicobacter pylori* infection on healing rate. *Dis Esophagus* 2002;15:50–56.
5. Omeprazole (Prilosec). Product information. Wayne, PA: Astra Pharmaceuticals, 2002.
6. Esomeprazole (Nexium). Product information. Wayne, PA: Astra Pharmaceuticals, 2003.
7. Lansoprazole (Prevacid). Product information. Lake Forest, IL: TAP Pharmaceuticals, 2002.
8. Pantoprazole (Protonix). Product information. Philadelphia: Wyeth-Ayerst, 2002.
9. Rabeprazole (Aciphex). Product information. Teaneck, NJ: Eisai Inc. and Titusville, NJ: Janssen Pharmaceutica, 2002.
10. Patrick M. Woster, instructor. PHA 4140—gastrointestinal and nutrition section medicinal chemistry tutorial. Available at: http://wiz2.pharm.wayne.edu/module/gastromed.html. Accessed 2/3/03.
11. Feld LG, Cimino M. *Pediatric dosing handbook, Children's Medical Center/Atlantic Health System*. Hudson, OH: Lexi-Comp, 2000.
12. Seifert SA. Omeprazole and lansoprazole. In: Dart RC, ed. *The 5 minute toxicology consult*. Philadelphia: Lippincott Williams & Wilkins, 2000:548–549.
13. Meyer UA. Interaction of proton pump inhibitors with cytochromes P450: consequences for drug interactions. *Y J Biol Med* 1996;69:203–209.
14. Steinijans VW, Huber R, Hartmann M, et al. Lack of pantoprazole drug interactions in man: an updated review. *Int J Clin Pharmacol Ther* 1996;34:243–262.
15. Radhofer Welte S. Pharmacokinetics and metabolism of the proton pump inhibitor pantoprazole in man. *Drugs Today* 1999;35:765–772.
16. Saitoh T, Fukushima Y, Otsuka H, et al. Effects of rabeprazole, lansoprazole and omeprazole on intragastric pH in CYP 2 C 19 extensive metabolizers. *Aliment Pharmacol Ther* 2002;16:1811–1817.
17. Litovitz T, Klein-Schwartz W, Rodgers GC Jr, et al. 2001 annual report of the American Association of Poison Control Centers toxic exposure surveillance system. *Am J Emerg Med* 2002;20:391–452.
18. Marshall JK, Thomson AB, Armstrong D. Omeprazole for refractory gastroesophageal reflux disease during pregnancy and lactation. *Can J Gastroenterol* 1998;12:225–227.

CHAPTER 155

Miscellaneous Gastrointestinal Drugs

Michael A. McGuigan

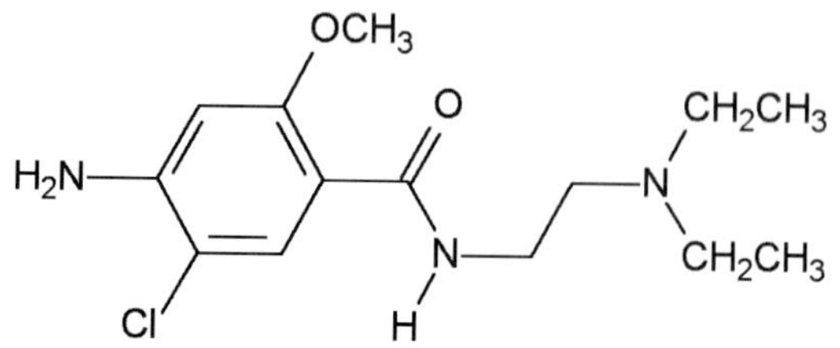

METOCLOPRAMIDE

Molecular formula and weight:	**Mesalamine ($C_7H_7NO_3$), 153.1; metoclopramide ($C_{14}H_{22}ClN_3O_2$), 299.8; misoprostol ($C_{22}H_{38}O_5$), 382.5; sucralfate, 2086.7 g/mol**
SI conversion:	**mg/L × 3.34 = μmol/L**
CAS Registry No.:	**89-57-6 (mesalamine), 54143-57-6 (metoclopramide), 59122-46-2 (misoprostol), 54182-58-0 (sucralfate)**
Therapeutic level:	**Metoclopramide, 0.15 mg/L**
Special concerns:	**Metoclopramide can cause dysphoria and dyskinesia after a single dose.**
Antidote:	**None**

MESALAMINE

Overview

Mesalamine is an antiinflammatory drug used for its local effects on the intestinal mucosa in the treatment of ulcerative colitis and Crohn's disease. Mesalamine is available in delayed-release tablets, controlled-release capsules, suspension enemas, and suppositories. Sulfasalazine contains mesalamine linked to sulfapyridine. The most common adverse effects during mesalamine therapy are headache and diarrhea. Clinical effects similar to acetylsalicylic acid toxicity may theoretically occur after overdose.

Toxic Dose

The maximum therapeutic adult dose ranges from 2.4 to 4.0 g/day orally in divided doses. Maintenance doses are lower. The pediatric oral dose is 30 to 50 mg/kg/day in divided doses (1).

The lethal and minimum toxic doses have not been established in humans. Death occurred in mice, rats, and monkeys after single oral doses of 3 to 5 g/kg of uncoated mesalamine. Pigs that received a single oral dose (formulation not stated) of 5 g/kg showed no toxicity. A 3-year-old patient ingested 2 g of oral mesalamine without adverse effect.

Toxicokinetics and Toxicodynamics

Controlled-release formulations of mesalamine are poorly absorbed from the gastrointestinal (GI) tract. Only 20% to 30% of an oral ethylcellulose controlled-release formulation was absorbed. Absorption of the immediate-release preparation occurred rapidly (2). Protein binding is 50%, and the apparent volume of distribution is 0.2 L/kg (3).

Absorbed mesalamine is acetylated in the liver to *N*-acetyl-5-aminosalicylic acid, which is excreted in the urine. Mesalamine is also acetylated in the colon wall. After an intravenous (IV) dose, the elimination half-life of mesalamine is 42 minutes; due to the controlled-release formulation, the elimination half-life after oral administration cannot be determined. Renal excretion is 20% to 30% after an oral dose; 70% is excreted in the feces.

Pathophysiology

The mechanism of action of mesalamine is unclear but is most likely topical rather than systemic activity. Therapeutic effects result from the modulation of the immune response in the intestinal wall, particularly through prostaglandins and leukotrienes. The antiinflammatory effect is due to blocking cyclooxygenase and inhibiting prostaglandin production.

Pregnancy and Lactation

Mesalamine is U.S. Food and Drug Administration (FDA) pregnancy category B. Mesalamine and its metabolite have been detected in breast milk. The clinical significance of this is unclear, and caution is advised.

Clinical Presentation

No cases of acute or subacute overdose have been reported. The most commonly reported adverse effect is headache (6.5%) (3,4). Rare adverse reactions have been reported in just about every organ system. The oligospermia and infertility associated with sulfasalazine have not been reported with oral mesalamine.

Diagnostic Tests

A plasma salicylate concentration is recommended in patients who have taken very large overdoses because of the hypothetical risk of developing salicylate toxicity. No specific laboratory tests are recommended after a mesalamine ingestion.

Treatment

Treatment of mesalamine overdose is symptomatic and supportive. GI decontamination is not routinely recommended.

Patients who ingest very large overdoses of mesalamine should receive a single dose of activated charcoal.

There are no antidotes to mesalamine. Enhancement of elimination is not recommended. Patients who have high plasma salicylate concentrations might benefit from hemodialysis (Chapter 127A).

METOCLOPRAMIDE

Overview

Metoclopramide is a dopamine D_2 receptor antagonist and a weak serotonin 5-hydroxytryptamine receptor antagonist (5). It stimulates motility of the upper GI tract, accelerates gastric emptying times, and abolishes the slowing of gastric emptying that is caused by apomorphine. It is used for the prevention of nausea and vomiting associated with chemotherapy and the prevention of postoperative nausea and vomiting as well as the treatment of gastroesophageal reflux disease.

Toxic Dose

The adult and pediatric therapeutic dose for chemotherapy-induced emesis is 1 to 2 mg/kg/dose orally or IV every 2 to 4 hours. For postoperative nausea and vomiting, the usual dose is 10 mg IV every 6 to 8 hours as needed. The pediatric therapeutic dose for postoperative nausea and vomiting is 0.1 to 0.2 mg/kg/dose IV every 6 to 8 hours as needed. Children older than 14 years of age may be given adult doses. Parenteral doses should be infused at a rate not exceeding 5 mg/minute. Dosing adjustments are necessary for patients with renal impairment.

In rodents, the oral median lethal dose (LD_{50}) range is 270 to 750 mg/kg, and the IV LD_{50} range is 33 to 50 mg/kg (6). No human dose-related metoclopramide fatalities have been reported, although acute dystonic reactions have been blamed for the deaths of patients on low-dose and high-dose metoclopramide therapy (7,8).

Two adults who ingested 360 and 800 mg developed somnolence, confusion, and traces of albumin in the urine (9). Ingestion of 4.6 to 6.6 mg/kg resulted in transient neurologic symptoms (10). Children who ingested 3.3 to 7.7 mg/kg developed transient neurologic symptoms (10). A 6-month-old infant ingested 3 mg/kg of metoclopramide over 9 hours and developed opisthotonic posturing (11).

Toxicokinetics and Toxicodynamics

Metoclopramide is rapidly absorbed from the GI tract with an onset of action of 30 to 60 minutes after ingestion. The oral bioavailability averages 80% (range, 65% to 95%). Peak concentrations increase linearly with dose; time to peak remains the same. The duration of therapeutic effect is 1 to 2 hours. Protein binding is 40%. The apparent volume of distribution is 3.5 L/kg (12).

Approximately 30% of the drug is eliminated unchanged in the urine and feces. Renal impairment affects the clearance of metoclopramide. The mean elimination half-life is 5 hours (range, 2.5 to 6.0 hours). An elimination half-life of 23 hours has been reported in a 3-week-old infant (13).

Pathophysiology

Metoclopramide is a dopamine D_2 receptor antagonist and a weak serotonin 5-hydroxytryptamine receptor antagonist (5). The antiemetic effect of metoclopramide is due to its antagonism of central and peripheral dopamine receptors, including the dopamine receptors in the chemoreceptor trigger zone. Metoclopramide appears to block L-dopa or apomorphine stimulation of the chemoreceptor trigger zone.

Pregnancy and Lactation

Metoclopramide is FDA pregnancy category B. It crosses the placenta and enters breast milk. Although evidence is limited, no congenital malformations were found in a study of 435 pregnant women taking metoclopramide during pregnancy (14,15). A nursing infant ingests 1 to 45 μg/kg/day during maternal use of 30 mg/day. This is less than the 500 μg/kg/day dose recommended for infants or the 100 μg/kg/day that has been given to premature infants (16,17). Metoclopramide appears to be safe during breast-feeding in doses of 45 mg/day or less (18).

Clinical Presentation

ACUTE OVERDOSAGE

Dose-related neurologic effects include drowsiness, fatigue, anxiety, agitation, confusion, hypertonia, convulsions, and extrapyramidal reactions. Hematologic events, such as methemoglobinemia, neutropenia, leukopenia, and agranulocytosis, may occur. Methemoglobin levels up to 25% have occurred in adults and infants after excessive or therapeutic doses (19,20). Metoclopramide-induced neuroleptic malignant syndrome has been reported (21–23).

ADVERSE REACTIONS

Rapid IV administration may be associated with a transient and intense feeling of anxiety and restlessness followed by drowsiness. Dyskinesia occurred in up to 27% of patients after IV administration of high doses of metoclopramide (24). However, extrapyramidal effects can occur after the administration of low doses to patients with renal disease (25). The overall incidence of "extrapyramidal reactions" ranges from 0.003% to 0.500% (26,27). The onset of toxicity is usually within 24 to 48 hours of the initiation of therapy. Muscle hypertonia is the most common manifestation, but other effects include muscular contractions of the face and neck, ataxia, dystonia, and opisthotonus (28). Long-term use has resulted in tardive dyskinesia lasting for 18 months (range, 6 to 36 months) after discontinuation of the drug.

Cardiovascular effects include hypertension or hypotension, tachycardia or bradycardia, and atrioventricular blockade. Dysrhythmias (supraventricular extrasystoles, supraventricular tachycardia, bigeminy associated with hypotension) have been reported in isolated cases (29–31). Metoclopramide administration may precipitate bronchospasm in patients with asthma (32,33).

Concurrent use of metoclopramide decreases absorption of cimetidine and digoxin and increases absorption of cyclosporine. L-Dopa decreases the effects of metoclopramide. There is an increased risk of hypertensive events with monoamine oxidase inhibitors. Increased neuromuscular blockade occurs with succinylcholine. The GI motility effects of metoclopramide are antagonized by anticholinergic or narcotic analgesics.

Caution should be exercised when using metoclopramide in diabetics because it can affect the delivery time of food to the intestines and, thus, the rate of absorption. Insulin dosage or timing of dosage may require adjustment. Metoclopramide should not be administered in the presence of GI hemorrhage, obstruction, or perforation, as this medication stimulates GI motility. Because the drug can cause hypertension, it should not be administered to patients with pheochromocytoma. It should also be avoided in patients with seizure disorders because extrapyramidal reactions may occur, or seizure severity can be enhanced.

Diagnostic Tests

Methemoglobin concentrations should be measured in patients who appear cyanotic or have respiratory distress. An electrocardiogram should be performed after overdose or in symptomatic patients. Patients should be monitored for methemoglobinemia and cardiac dysrhythmias.

Treatment

Symptomatic and supportive care is the mainstay of treatment unless specific toxicity (e.g., methemoglobinemia, neuroleptic malignant syndrome, or dyskinesia) occurs. GI decontamination is not routinely recommended because metoclopramide is absorbed rapidly. Enhancement of elimination is not expected to be beneficial.

Antidote

There are no antidotes to metoclopramide. Diphenhydramine may be used to treat extrapyramidal reactions.

MISOPROSTOL

Overview

Misoprostol is an analog of prostaglandin E_1 that is used to suppress gastric acid secretion. Adverse effects include seizures, headache, dizziness, fatigue, vomiting, diarrhea, abdominal pain, and uterine bleeding and rupture. Therapeutic use of misoprostol in the first trimester may cause miscarriage. Dose-related toxicity may include hypertension, tachycardia, abdominal cramps, fever, and tremor. Overdose in pregnancy has resulted in uterine contraction with fetal death.

Misoprostol prevents drug-induced gastric or duodenal ulcers. Although misoprostol is not approved for use in pregnancy by the FDA, it is used to terminate pregnancy, facilitate labor, and to reduce postpartum hemorrhage.

Toxic Dose

The usual adult therapeutic dose of misoprostol is 100 to 200 µg four times daily, although higher doses have been used. Misoprostol is not approved for use in children.

The lethal dose of misoprostol has not been established. The oral LD_{50} in mice is 27 to 138 mg/kg. Three cases of maternal death after the use of misoprostol have been due to uterine complications (34). Ingestion of 2 to 3 mg has resulted in mild to moderate toxicity (35,36). The toxic dose of misoprostol has not been established in children.

Toxicokinetics and Toxicodynamics

The oral bioavailability of misoprostol is 80%. It is rapidly absorbed from the GI tract with peak blood levels occurring in 30 minutes. Up to 90% of circulating misoprostol is bound to plasma proteins. The apparent volume of distribution is 14 L/kg.

Misoprostol is rapidly deesterified to misoprostol acid, the active metabolite. Less than 1% is excreted unchanged in the urine. The elimination half-life is 30 minutes.

Pathophysiology

Prostaglandins are one family of the lipid-derived autocoids known as *eicosanoids*. Members of the prostaglandin E group dilate blood vessels, relax bronchial smooth muscle, inhibit gastric acid secretion, increase renal blood flow, and increase circulating concentrations of many hormones (37). The mechanisms of toxicity from misoprostol have not been elucidated.

Pregnancy and Lactation

Because of its uterotonic activity, misoprostol is FDA pregnancy category X (38). The safety of misoprostol use during lactation has not been established.

Clinical Presentation

Misoprostol overdose is rare. Hyperthermia (41.4°C), tachycardia, tachypnea, hypertension or hypotension, nausea, abdominal cramps, vomiting, headache, confusion, tremor, muscle cramping, metabolic acidosis, and rhabdomyolysis have been reported after ingestion or intravaginal administration of 2000 to 6000 µg (35,36,39,40). Overdose in pregnancy has resulted in uterine contraction with fetal death (40).

Adverse Reactions

Adverse reactions are common with misoprostol use (41). Central nervous system effects include headache (0.9% to 6.0%), fatigue or malaise (1.0% to 4.5%), and dizziness (0.9%). GI effects include abdominal pain (17%), diarrhea (3% to 13%), nausea (2% to 5%), vomiting (0.9%), and constipation (0.6% to 2.0%).

Diagnostic Tests

Misoprostol blood levels have not been used in the management of acute poisoning. After a large ingestion, measurement of arterial blood gases may identify metabolic acidosis, and blood levels of creatine kinase and myoglobin identify rhabdomyolysis.

Treatment

Treatment is symptomatic and supportive. The need for vaginal decontamination should be considered. Endotracheal intubation with neuroparalytic therapy helps to control agitation and hyperthermia. GI decontamination is not routinely indicated given the rapidity of absorption. Fetal monitoring should be done when pregnant women overdose on misoprostol.

The effectiveness of enhanced elimination has not been studied. The high protein binding and molecular weight would mitigate against dialysis.

Antidotes

There are no antidotes to misoprostol.

SUCRALFATE

Overview

Sucralfate is an oral antiulcer agent that acts by forming a protective barrier over the ulcer site, thus promoting ulcer healing. Adverse effects include constipation and dry mouth. No cases of poisoning have been reported.

Toxic Dose

The adult dose of sucralfate is 1 g two to four times daily. The pediatric dose is 40 to 80 mg/kg/day in divided doses (42). No lethal or minimum toxic dose of sucralfate has been established in either adults or children. Animals survived oral sucralfate doses of 12 g/kg.

Toxicokinetics and Toxicodynamics

Only minimal amounts of sucralfate are absorbed from the GI tract (43). Approximately 5% of sucrose octasulfate and 0.005% of aluminum are absorbed (44). Sucralfate is not metabolized. Any absorbed sucrose octasulfate or aluminum is excreted unchanged in the urine. In healthy volunteers, the total urinary excretion of sucralfate was 0.5% to 2.2% of the administered dose (45). Approximately 90% of sucralfate is excreted unchanged in the feces (46).

Pathophysiology

Sucralfate is a complex formed from sucrose octasulfate and polyaluminum hydroxide. In the stomach, polymerization and cross-linking results in the formation of a sticky, yellow-white gel that combines with protein exudates in the stomach to form an adherent barrier that blocks gastric acid contact with the mucosa (47). Continued exposure to acid gradually releases the aluminum, which may result in constipation. The risk for aluminum accumulation and toxicity is increased in patients with chronic renal failure or in those receiving dialysis.

Pregnancy and Lactation

Sucralfate is FDA pregnancy category B and is generally considered safe for use during breast-feeding. Animal studies using doses that exceed the recommended human dose of sucralfate have demonstrated no evidence of teratogenicity.

Clinical Presentation

No cases of acute or subacute overdosage have been reported. Constipation attributed to the aluminum occurs in 2% of cases. Less common clinical effects include abdominal pain, nausea, diarrhea, and dry mouth. The effect of sucralfate on plasma aluminum concentrations is similar to aluminum hydroxide (Chapter 149).

Adverse Reactions

Sucralfate may inhibit the absorption of orally administered drugs, such as cimetidine, digoxin, fluoroquinolone antibiotics, ketoconazole, phenytoin, and tetracycline.

Diagnostic Tests

Plasma aluminum levels should be followed in patients with renal compromise.

Treatment

Treatment is symptomatic and supportive. GI decontamination is not recommended. Enhancement of elimination is unlikely to be needed or useful. Absorbed aluminum may be removed during hemodialysis.

REFERENCES

1. Holmes JL, Roy R. *The 2000–2001 formulary of drugs*, 19th ed. Toronto: The Hospital for Sick Children, 2000.
2. Nielsen OH, Bondesen S. Kinetics of 5-aminosalicylic acid after jejunal instillation in man. *Br J Clin Pharmacol* 1983;16:738–740.
3. Bondesen S, Rasmussen SN, Rask-Madsen J, et al. 5-Aminosalicylic acid in the treatment of inflammatory bowel disease. *Acta Med Scand* 1987;221:227–242.
4. Guarino J, Chatzinoff M, Berk T, et al. 5-Aminosalicylic acid enemas in refractory distal ulcerative colitis: long-term results. *Am J Gastroenterol* 1987;82:732–737.
5. Weddington WW Jr, Banner A. Organic affective syndrome associated with metoclopramide: case report. *J Clin Psychiatry* 1986;47:208–209.
6. Registry of toxic effects of chemical substances. National Institute for Occupational Safety and Health (CD-ROM version). Englewood, CO: Micromedex, Inc., 2001.
7. Reasbeck P, Hossenbocus A. Death following dystonic reaction to oral metoclopramide. *Br J Clin Pract* 1979;33:31–33.
8. Ryle PR. Sudden death after acute dystonic reaction to high-dose metoclopramide. *Lancet* 1984;2:460–461.
9. Bar J. A propos d'une tentative de suicide sand consequence facheuse, avec le metoclopramide. *Therapie* 1966;21:349.
10. Giger M. Toxische wirkungen von metoclopramid. *Praxis* 1975;64:930.
11. Batts KF, Munter DW. Metoclopramide toxicity in an infant. *Pediatr Emerg Med* 1998;14:39–41.
12. Bateman DN, Kahn C, Mashiter K, et al. Pharmacokinetic and concentration effect—studies with intravenous metoclopramide. *Br J Clin Pharmacol* 1978;6:401–407.
13. Kearns GC, Butler HL, Carchman SH, et al. Metoclopramide pharmacokinetics in infants. *Clin Pharmacol Ther* 1987;41:219(abst).
14. Sorensen HT, Nielsen GL, Christensen K, et al. Birth outcome following maternal use of metoclopramide. *Br J Clin Pharmacol* 2000;49:264–268.
15. Berkovitch M, Elbirt D, Addis A, et al. Fetal effects of metoclopramide therapy for nausea and vomiting of pregnancy [Letter]. *N Engl J Med* 2000;343:445–446.
16. Harrington RA, Hamilton CW, Brogden RN, et al. Metoclopramide: an update review of its pharmacological properties and clinical use. *Drugs* 1983;25:451–494.
17. Sankaran K, Yeboah E, Bingham WT, et al. Use of metoclopramide in preterm infants. *Dev Pharmacol Ther* 1982;5:114–119.
18. Briggs GG, Freeman RK, Yaffe SJ. *Drugs in pregnancy and lactation*, 5th ed. Baltimore: Williams & Wilkins, 1998.
19. Wilson CM, Bird SG, Bocash W, et al. Methemoglobinemia following metoclopramide therapy in an infant. *J Pediatr Gastroenterol Nutr* 1987;6:640–642.
20. Grant SC, Close JR, Bray CL. Methaemoglobinaemia produced by metoclopramide in an adult. *Eur J Clin Pharmacol* 1994;47:89.
21. Donnett A, Harle JR, Dumont JC, et al. Neuroleptic malignant syndrome induced by metoclopramide. *Biomed Pharmacother* 1991;45:461–462.
22. Henderson A, Longdon P. Fulminant metoclopramide induced neuroleptic malignant syndrome rapidly responsive to intravenous dantrolene. *Austr N Z J Med* 1991;21:742–743.
23. Nonino F. Neuroleptic malignant syndrome associated with metoclopramide [Letter]. *Ann Pharmacol* 1999;33:644–645.
24. Kris MG, Tyson LB, Gralla RJ, et al. Extrapyramidal reactions with high-dose metoclopramide. *N Engl J Med* 1983;309:433–434.
25. Sirota RA, Kimmel PL, Trichtinger MD, et al. Metoclopramide-induced Parkinsonism in hemodialysis patients. *Arch Intern Med* 1986;146:2070–2071.
26. Bateman DN, Rawlins MD, Simpson JM. Extrapyramidal reactions with metoclopramide. *BMJ* 1985;291:930–932.
27. Bateman DN, Darling WM, Boys R, Rawlings MD. Extrapyramidal reactions to metoclopramide and prochlorperazine. *QJM* 1989;71:307–311.
28. Miller LG, Jankowitz J. Metoclopramide-induced movement disorders. *Arch Intern Med* 1989;149:2486–2492.
29. Hughes RL. Hypotension and dysrhythmia following intravenous metoclopramide. *Anaesthesia* 1984;39:720.
30. Shaklai M, Pinkhas J, de Viries A. Metoclopramide and cardiac arrhythmia. *BMJ* 1974;2:385.
31. Bevacqua BK. Supraventricular tachycardia associated with postpartum metoclopramide administration. *Anesthesiology* 1988;68:124–125.
32. Chung MM, Chatty KG, Jerome D. Metoclopramide and asthma. *Ann Intern Med* 1985;103:809.
33. MacLaren R, Shields CA. Respiratory failure following oral administration of metoclopramide. *Ann Pharmacol* 1998;32:1017–1020.
34. Daisley H Jr. Maternal mortality following the use of misoprostol. *Med Sci Law* 2000;40:78–82.
35. Graber DJ, Meier KH. Acute misoprostol toxicity. *Ann Emerg Med* 1991;20:549–551.
36. Toerne T, Aks S. Intentional Cytotec overdose in a non-pregnant female. *J Toxicol Clin Toxicol* 1997;35:493–494(abst).
37. Campbell WB, Halushka PV. Lipid-derived autacoids. In: Hardman JG, Limbird LE, eds. *Goodman & Gilman's the pharmacological basis of therapeutics*, 9th ed. New York: McGraw-Hill, 1996:601–616.
38. Briggs GG, Freeman RK, Yaffe SJ. *Drugs in pregnancy and lactation*, 5th ed. Baltimore: Williams & Wilkins, 1998.
39. Bond GR, Van Zee A. Overdosage of misoprostol in pregnancy. *Am J Obstet Gynecol* 1994;171:561–562.
40. Austin J, Ford MD, Rouse A, Hanna E. Acute intravaginal misoprostol toxicity with fetal demise. *J Emerg Med* 1997;15:61–64.
41. Herting RL, Clay GA. Overview of clinical safety with misoprostol. *Dig Dis Sci* 1985;30:185S–193S.
42. Arguelles-Martin F, Gonzalez-Fernandez F, Gentles MG, et al. Sucralfate in the treatment of reflux esophagitis in children. *Scand J Gastroenterol* 1989;24[Suppl 156]:43–47.
43. Bighley LD, Giesing D. Mechanism of action studies of sucralfate. In: *11th International Congress of Gastroenterology*. Hamburg, Germany, 1980:380(abst H9.1).
44. Haram EM, Weberg R, Berstad A. Urinary excretion of aluminium after ingestion of sucralfate and an aluminium-containing antacid in man. *Scand J Gastroenterol* 1987;22:615–618.
45. Giesing D, Lanman N, Nunser D. Absorption of sucralfate in man. *Gastroenterology* 1982;82:1066.
46. Garnett WR. Sucralfate—alternative therapy for peptic ulcer disease. *Clin Pharmacy* 1982;1:307–314.
47. Brunton LL. Agents for control of gastric acidity and treatment of peptic ulcers. In: Hardman JG, Limbird LE, eds. *Goodman & Gilman's the pharmacological basis of therapeutics*, 9th ed. New York: McGraw-Hill, 1996:901–915.

SECTION

12

Hormones and Synthetic Substitutes

CHAPTER 156

Sex Hormones

Seth Schonwald

ESTROGEN

Compounds included:	**Oral contraceptive pills (estrogen, progestin), hormone replacement therapy, testosterone**
SI conversion:	**Not applicable**
Therapeutic levels:	**Not used clinically**
Special concerns:	**Estrogens increase the risk of thromboembolic disease as well as certain cancers with long-term use.**
Antidote:	**None**

OVERVIEW

Estrogens, progestins, and androgens are steroids used for a growing number of conditions. Oral contraceptive pills (OCs) have been widely used by women since the 1960s. In addition to providing effective contraception, OCs are sometimes used to treat menstrual irregularities and to manage premenstrual symptoms.

Most contraceptive pills contain varying degrees of estrogens and progestins. Some birth control pills contain progestin only, such as norethindrone and norgestrel. Hormone replacement therapy (HRT) is used in postmenopausal women to replace hormones as they age and also provides varying amounts of estrogens and progestins.

Testosterone, a male sex hormone or androgen, is used to treat men for conditions associated with a deficiency or absence of endogenous testosterone. Such conditions include primary hypogonadism (congenital or acquired), testicular failure due to cryptorchidism, bilateral torsion, orchitis, vanishing testis syndrome, orchiectomy, Klinefelter's syndrome, chemotherapy, or toxic damage from alcohol or heavy metals.

Anabolic steroids, or synthetic substances related to androgens, promote the growth of skeletal muscle and androgenic effects that foster the development of male sexual characteristics. They can be used to legitimately treat human immunodeficiency virus–related muscle wasting and other catabolic conditions, such as chronic obstructive pulmonary disease, severe burn injuries, and alcoholic hepatitis (1). They have also been increasingly abused to build muscles, reduce body fat, and improve sports performance. Abuse is estimated to be very high among competitive bodybuilders and may be widespread among other athletes.

ORAL CONTRACEPTIVE PILLS

OCs have undergone an evolution in content and dosage. The doses of the steroid components of combination OCs have decreased dramatically since the first formulations. Ethinyl estradiol is now used as the estrogenic component of most combination OCs. The majority of progestins currently used in combination OCs are derivatives of 19-nortestosterone (2). Estrogen- and progesterone-containing contraceptives are of low toxicity. They may cause nausea and, rarely, a withdrawal bleed in prepubertal girls.

Toxicokinetics and Toxicodynamics

Estrogens used in therapy are well absorbed through the skin, mucous membranes, and gastrointestinal tract (3). Metabolic conversion of estrogens occurs primarily in the liver (first-pass effect) but also at local target tissue sites. Metabolism and inactivation occur primarily in the liver. Some estrogens are excreted into the bile; however, they are reabsorbed from the intestine and returned to the liver through the portal venous system.

After ingestion of progesterone, the maximum serum concentration is attained within 3 hours. Progesterone is approximately 96% to 99% bound to serum proteins, primarily to serum albumin (50% to 54%) and transcortin (43% to 48%). It is metabolized primarily by the liver, largely to pregnanediols and pregnanolones. Pregnanediols and pregnanolones are conjugated in the liver to glucuronide and sulfate metabolites, which are excreted in the bile and urine. Progesterone metabolites excreted in the bile may undergo enterohepatic recycling or may be excreted in the feces.

Pathophysiology

Estrogens are important in the development and maintenance of the female reproductive system and secondary sex characteristics. They promote growth and development of the vagina, uterus, and fallopian tubes and enlargement of the breasts. Estrogen and progesterone inhibit ovulation by "fooling" the pituitary gland into producing less follicle-stimulating hormone and luteinizing hormone. By reducing these two hormones, which are required for ovulation, an OC suppresses, but does not eliminate, ovulation. Progesterone also produces local effects on the endometrium, the cervical mucus, and, possibly, the fallopian tubes. Progestins thin the endometrium, depleting it of glycogen and blood supply, and may thicken the cervical mucus, making it more difficult for sperm to travel through the cervix.

Pregnancy and Lactation

Estrogens are U.S. Food and Drug Administration pregnancy category X (Appendix I). Progestins are pregnancy category B.

Clinical Presentation

Contraceptive overdoses are rare. Numerous reports of ingestion of large doses of estrogen-containing OCs by young children indicate that acute serious ill effects do not occur. Signs and symptoms in adults may include excessive vaginal bleeding, breast tenderness, urine discoloration, rash, nausea, vomiting, headache, drowsiness, and/or mental status changes.

Dermatologic effects include melasma, moniliasis, photosensitivity (4), alopecia, and bullous eruptions, which are the most frequently reported dermatologic side effects of OCs. Other conditions reported occasionally as resulting from or being aggravated by these drugs have been acne, hidradenitis suppurativa, and seborrhea. Very rarely, erythema nodosum (5), purpura, lupus erythematosus, an increase in number of moles, and hypertrophic gingivitis have been associated (6). Beneficial effects of OCs include improvement of acne, lessening of premenstrual flaring of aphthous ulcers, and improvement of Fox-Fordyce disease with estrogenic preparations (7).

Autoimmune progesterone dermatitis is a rare condition that appears during the perimenstrual period or after progesterone treatment. Signs and symptoms include pruritus, urticaria, papulovesicular eruptions, and bullous erythema multiforme (8). Patients with autoimmune progesterone dermatitis may benefit from prophylactic treatment with danazol (9).

Neurologic effects of estrogen plus progestin include an increased risk of ischemic stroke in generally healthy postmenopausal women (10). Exacerbation of migraine headaches is a well-recognized consequence of OCs.

Hematologic effects include a fourfold increase in the risk for venous thromboembolism (11). Epidemiologic studies indicate that women who use third-generation OCs containing desogestrel, gestodene, or norgestimate have a higher risk of developing venous thrombosis than do women who use second-generation OCs containing levonorgestrel (12). OCs have been associated with central retinal vein occlusion (13).

Gastrointestinal, liver, and pancreatic effects are rare but potentially serious. Intrahepatic cholestasis induced by OCs resembles that of pregnancy. Both conditions may have a genetic predisposition involving a dose-dependent estrogen effect of decreasing bile secretion. Symptoms include pruritus with anorexia, asthenia, vomiting, and weight loss without fever, rash, or abdominal pain.

Several cases of acute pancreatitis within the first 3 months of contraceptive pill treatment have been reported in women with preexisting lipid metabolic anomalies (14). The relative risk of Budd-Chiari syndrome in OC users is estimated at 2.37. A benign tumor of the liver called *hepatic adenoma* has also been found to occur, although rarely, among OC users. These tumors do not spread, but they may rupture and cause internal bleeding (15). OCs increase the prevalence of hepatic adenomas as a function of duration of treatment. They are usually discovered fortuitously but may be revealed by vague abdominal pains.

Cancer of the cervix is associated with long-term OC use (16,17). An increased risk of some breast cancers has been linked to OCs, particularly in younger women (18); it may be related mostly to the estrogen component (19,20). Studies have consistently shown that the use of an OC reduces the risk of ovarian cancer (21,22). Researchers estimate that the risk is reduced by 5% to 10% for each additional year of use. Researchers have also found that OC users have a reduced risk of endometrial cancer (23).

At least nine case-control studies conducted in developed countries have identified an association between OCs and liver cancer. One population-based study in 1997 from developed and developing countries failed to confirm such an association, however (24).

Treatment

OC or HRT overdose is uncommon. Management is essentially symptomatic and supportive. In recent overdoses, particularly in the pediatric population, gastrointestinal decontamination with activated charcoal may be warranted. No antidote is available.

HORMONE REPLACEMENT THERAPY

HRT, consisting of estrogen-progestin combinations or individual hormones, is used to relieve the short-term symptoms of menopause, such as hot flashes, sweats, and disturbed sleep. It is also believed to be useful in preventing or alleviating an increased rate of bone loss that leads to osteoporosis. Preliminary evidence shows that HRT may be helpful in preventing colon cancer (25) and macular degeneration (age-related vision loss) (26). Conflicting studies have postulated that HRT may (27,28) or may not be useful in treating Alzheimer's disease (29).

Randomized controlled trials have failed to show a protective effect of HRT in reducing the risk of coronary artery disease and instead have revealed an increased risk of heart disease, stroke, invasive breast cancer, and venous thromboembolism (30,31). One trial of estrogen plus progestin in postmenopausal women did not have a clinically meaningful effect on health-related quality of life (32).

Toxic Dose

A 47-year-old postmenopausal woman developed eczematous lesions at the sites of application of an estradiol therapeutic transdermal system and successively at the sites of application of a gel containing estradiol. Due to the topical intolerance, the therapy was switched to oral estrogen, which caused a systemic pruritic rash (33).

Clinical Presentation

See the section Oral Contraceptive Pills regarding clinical presentations associated with sex hormone use.

The National Institutes of Health Women's Health Initiative stopped a major clinical trial in 2002 because an increased risk of invasive breast cancer from HRT with estrogen and progestin, and an increased risk of ischemic stroke, were found (10). The increased risk of breast cancer appeared after 4 years of hormone use. After 5.2 years, estrogen plus progestin use resulted in a 26% increase in the risk of breast cancer, or eight more breast cancers each year for every 10,000 women. Women who had used estrogen plus progestin before entering the study were more likely to develop breast cancer than others, indicating that the therapy may have a cumulative effect.

TESTOSTERONE AND ANDROGENS

In addition to the legitimate uses for testosterone, androgens such as testosterone may be misused and abused to improve sporting ability and to change physical appearance (i.e., increase muscle size and strength). Doses taken by abusers can be up to 100 times greater than doses used for treating medical conditions.

Side effects of androgens include acne, weight gain, mood changes (especially aggressive behavior), decreased testes size, and low sperm counts leading to infertility. Some men take chemically modified forms of testosterone, for example, 17-α-alkylated androgens, and put themselves at risk of liver disease. Alternative practitioners have increasingly used testosterone to "improve vigor" or to "prolong life."

Toxicokinetics and Toxicodynamics

Testosterone transdermal systems have been used to mimic the normal circadian variation observed in healthy young men (3). Maximum concentrations occur in the early morning hours, with minimum concentrations in the evening. In serum, testosterone is bound with high affinity to sex hormone binding globulin and with low affinity to albumin.

Inactivation of testosterone occurs primarily in the liver. Testosterone is metabolized to various 17-keto steroids through two different pathways, and the major active metabolites are estradiol and dihydrotestosterone. Approximately 90% of a testosterone dose given intramuscularly is excreted in the urine as glucuronide and sulfate conjugates of testosterone and its metabolites; about 6% is excreted in the feces, mostly in unconjugated form.

Pathophysiology

Testosterone and dihydrotestosterone, endogenous androgens, are responsible for normal growth and development of the male sex organs and for maintenance of secondary sex characteristics. These effects include the growth and maturation of the prostate, seminal vesicles, penis, and scrotum; the development of male hair distribution, such as facial, pubic, chest, and axillary hair; laryngeal enlargement; vocal cord thickening; alterations in body musculature; and fat distribution.

Toxic Dose

In one report of acute overdosage with testosterone enanthate injection, testosterone levels up to 11,400 ng/dl were implicated in a cerebrovascular accident (34). In another case, a 26-year-old male bodybuilder who used testosterone enanthate (500 mg intramuscularly twice a week), stanozolol (40 mg/day), and methylandrostenediol (30 mg/day by mouth for 5 weeks) induced toxic hepatitis with predominantly hepatocellular necrosis instead of intrahepatic cholestasis (35).

Pregnancy and Lactation

Testosterone is U.S. Food and Drug Administration pregnancy category X (Appendix I). Androgens should not be used in pregnant women.

Clinical Presentation

Gastrointestinal effects of prolonged use of high doses of orally active 17-α-alkyl androgens (e.g., methyltestosterone) have been associated with serious hepatic adverse effects (e.g., peliosis hepatitis, hepatic neoplasms, cholestatic hepatitis, and jaundice). Peliosis hepatitis can be a life-threatening or fatal complication (36). Long-term therapy with testosterone enanthate, which elevates blood levels for prolonged periods, has produced multiple hepatic adenomas (37,38). Transdermal testosterone is not known to produce these adverse effects.

Psychiatric effects of anabolic-androgenic steroid use are diverse. The available data concerning possible effets of anabolic-androgenic steroids on libido in men and in women and in the way in which they affect libido differently in men and women, however are often inconsistent and inconclusive. Anabolic-androgenic steroids may relieve as well as cause depression. Cessation or diminished use of anabolic-androgenic steroids may also result in depression (39). Psychotic symptoms have also been associated with steroid use (40).

Endocrine effects of acute high-dose methyltestosterone administration include suppression of the reproductive axis and significantly influence thyroid axis balance without a consistent effect on pituitary-adrenal hormones (41). Anabolic steroid abuse can result in reduced sperm production (42), shrinking of the testicles, impotence, and irreversible breast enlargement in boys and men. Decreased body fat and breast size, deepening of the voice, growth of excessive body hair, loss of scalp hair, and clitoral enlargement can occur in girls and women.

Treatment

Testosterone and anabolic steroid overdose is uncommon. The drug should be terminated. Management is symptomatic and supportive. In recent overdose, particularly in the pediatric population, gastrointestinal decontamination with activated charcoal may be warranted. No antidote is available.

REFERENCES

1. Shahidi NT. A review of the chemistry, biological action, and clinical applications of anabolic-androgenic steroids. *Clin Ther* 2001;23(9):1355–1390.
2. Yuzpe AA. Oral contraception: trends over time. *J Reprod Med* 2002;47[11 Suppl]:967–973.
3. The internet drug list Web Site. Available at: http://www.rxlist.com. Accessed July 2003.
4. Cooper SM, George S. Photosensitivity reaction associated with use of the combined oral contraceptive. *Br J Dermatol* 2001;144(3):641–642.
5. Winkelman RK. Erythema nodosum and oral contraceptive therapy. *JAMA* 1978;239(14):1437.
6. Chowdhury DS. Oral contraceptive and dermatology. *Calcutta Med J.* 1973;70(7–8):187–188.
7. Krueger GG, McQuarrie HG, Swinyer LJ. Desirable and undesirable cutaneous effects of oral contraceptives. *Drug Ther (N Y)* 1972,7(9):46–48.
8. Shelley WB, Shelley ED, Talanin NY, et al. Estrogen dermatitis. *J Am Acad Dermatol* 1995;32(1):25–31.

9. Shahar E, Bergman R, Pollack S. Autoimmune progesterone dermatitis: effective prophylactic treatment with danazol. *Int J Dermatol* 1997;36(9):708–711.
10. Wassertheil-Smoller S, Hendrix SL, Limacher M, et al. Effect of estrogen plus progestin on stroke in postmenopausal women: the Women's Health Initiative: a randomized trial. *JAMA* 2003;289(20):2673–2684.
11. Girolami A, Spiezia L, Vianello F. Proposal of a flow chart for thrombosis-free oral contraceptive therapy. *Clin Appl Thromb Hemost* 2003;9(1):33–37.
12. Belicova M, Lukac B, Dvorsky J, et al. Thromboembolic disease and present oral contraception. *Clin Appl Thromb Hemost* 2003;9(1):45–51.
13. Kundu AK. Oral contraceptives and central retinal vein occlusion. *J Assoc Physicians India* 2002;50:1339–1340; author reply 1340.
14. Grimaud JC, Bourliere M. Contraception and hepatogastroenterology. *Fertil Contracept Sex* 1989;17(5):407–413.
15. Tao LC. Oral contraceptive–associated liver cell adenoma and hepatocellular carcinoma. *Cancer* 1991;68:341–347.
16. Green J, Berrington de Gonzalez A, Smith JS, et al. Human papillomavirus infection and use of oral contraceptives. *Br J Cancer* 2003;88(11):1713–1720.
17. Smith JS, Green J, Berrington de Gonzalez A, et al. Cervical cancer and use of hormonal contraceptives: a systematic review. *Lancet* 2003;361(9364):1159–1167.
18. Brinton LA, Daling JR, Liff JM, et al. Oral contraceptives and breast cancer risk among younger women. *J Ntl Cancer Inst* 1995;87(13):827–835.
19. Marchbanks PA, McDonald JA, Wilson HG, et al. Oral contraceptives and the risk of breast cancer. *N Engl J Med* 2002;346:2025–2032.
20. Dumeaux V, Alsaker E, Lund E. Breast cancer and specific types of oral contraceptives: a large Norwegian cohort study. *Int J Cancer* 2003;105(6):844–850.
21. Centers for Disease Control. Oral contraceptive use and the risk of ovarian cancer: the Centers for Disease Control Cancer and Steroid Hormone Study. *JAMA* 1983;249:1596–1599.
22. Centers for Disease Control and the National Institute of Child Health and Human Development. The reduction in risk of ovarian cancer associated with oral contraceptive use: the Cancer and Steroid Hormone Study of the Centers for Disease Control and the National Institute of Child Health and Human Development. *N Engl J Med* 1987;316:650–655.
23. Centers for Disease Control. Combination oral contraceptive use and the risk of endometrial cancer: the Cancer and Steroid Hormone Study of the Centers for Disease Control and the National Institute of Child Health and Human Development. *JAMA* 1987;257(6):79.
24. Oral contraceptives and liver cancer. *Contracept Rep* 1997;8(5):4–8.
25. Gambacciani M, Monteleone P, Sacco A, et al. Hormone replacement therapy and endometrial, ovarian and colorectal cancer. *Best Pract Res Clin Endocrinol Metab* 2003;17(1):139–147.
26. Snow KK, Cote J, Yang W, et al. Association between reproductive and hormonal factors and age-related maculopathy in postmenopausal women. *Am J Ophthalmol* 2002;134(6):842–848.
27. Yoon BK, Kim DK, Kang Y, et al. Hormone replacement therapy in postmenopausal women with Alzheimer's disease: a randomized, prospective study. *Fertil Steril* 2003;79(2):274–280.
28. Kesslak JP. Can estrogen play a significant role in the prevention of Alzheimer's disease? *J Neural Transm Suppl* 2002;(62):227–239.
29. Fillit HM. The role of hormone replacement therapy in the prevention of Alzheimer disease. *Arch Intern Med* 2002;162(17):1934–1942.
30. Humphries KH, Gill S. Risks and benefits of hormone replacement therapy: the evidence speaks. *CMAJ* 2003;168(8):1001–1010.
31. Nelson HD, Humphrey LL, Nygren P, et al. Postmenopausal hormone replacement therapy: scientific review. *JAMA* 2002;288(7):872–881.
32. Hays J, Ockene JK, Brunner RL, et al. Effects of estrogen plus progestin on health-related quality of life. *N Engl J Med* 2003;348(19):1839–1854. Epub Mar 17, 2003.
33. Corazza M, Mantovani L, Montanari A, et al. Allergic contact dermatitis from transdermal estradiol and systemic contact dermatitis from oral estradiol. A case report. *J Reprod Med* 2002;47(6):507–509.
34. Testim package insert. Auxilium Pharmaceuticals, Inc, October 2002.
35. Stimac D, Milic S, Dintinjana RD, et al. Androgenic/anabolic steroid-induced toxic hepatitis. *J Clin Gastroenterol* 2002;35(4):350–352.
36. Nuzzo JL, Manz HJ, Maxted WC. Peliosis hepatis after long-term androgen therapy. *Urology* 1985;25(5):518–519.
37. Dourakis SP, Tolis G. Sex hormonal preparations and the liver. *Eur J Contracept Reprod Health Care* 1998;3(1):7–16.
38. Carrasco D, Prieto M, Pallardo L, et al. Multiple hepatic adenomas after long-term therapy with testosterone enanthate. Review of the literature. *J Hepatol* 1985;1(6):573–578.
39. Uzych L. Anabolic-androgenic steroids and psychiatric-related effects: a review. *Can J Psychiatry* 1992;37(1):23–28.
40. Pope HG Jr, Katz DL. Affective and psychotic symptoms associated with anabolic steroid use. *Am J Psychiatry* 1988;145(4):487–490.
41. Daly RC, Su TP, Schmidt PJ, et al. Neuroendocrine and behavioral effects of high-dose anabolic steroid administration in male normal volunteers. *Psychoneuroendocrinology* 2003;28(3):317–331.
42. Pena JE, Thornton MH Jr, Sauer MV. Reversible azoospermia: anabolic steroids may profoundly affect human immunodeficiency virus–seropositive men undergoing assisted reproduction. *Obstet Gynecol* 2003;101(5 Pt 2):1073–1075.

CHAPTER 157

Insulins

Katherine M. Hurlbut

Compounds included:	**Insulin, insulin aspart (Novolog), insulin glargine (Lantus), insulin human (Humulin, Novolin), insulin isophane (NPH), insulin lispro (Humalog), insulin zinc**
Molecular weight:	**See Table 1.**
SI conversion:	**μg/L × 0.172 = nmol/L**
CAS Registry No.:	**See Table 1.**
Normal levels:	**1 μg/L (25 mU/L)**
Target organs:	**Central nervous system (acute)**
Antidotes:	**Intravenous dextrose, oral glucose, and carbohydrates**

OVERVIEW

Insulin is a hormone secreted by the β cells of the pancreatic islets of Langerhans. Preparations of insulin used in clinical practice differ in purity, onset and duration of action, and species of origin. Pork insulin is extracted from pork pancreas; beef insulin is extracted from beef pancreas but is no longer available in the United States. Human insulin is made by using recombinant deoxyribonucleic acid technology or enzymatic modification of pork insulin.

Insulin is used primarily in the treatment of diabetes mellitus. Large studies of patients with type I and type II diabetes (Stockholm Diabetes Intervention Study, United Kingdom Prospective Diabetes Study, Diabetes Control and Complications Trial) have shown that regimens that result in good blood glucose control result in a decreased incidence of complications such as retinopathy, nephropathy, and neuropathy. Insulin is also used in the treatment of severe hyperkalemia, as a provocative test for growth hormone secretion, and in the regulation of blood glucose in critically ill patients (multiple organ system failure, sepsis).

The primary effect in overdose or as an adverse effect is hypoglycemia. Manifestations include hunger, fatigue, diaphoresis, nausea, palpitations, tremors, weakness, agitation, confusion, and seizures or loss of consciousness in severe cases.

TABLE 1. Selected pharmacokinetic and pharmacodynamic parameters of the insulins

Drug	Molecular weight (g/mol), CAS Registry No. (references)	Onset (h)	Peak (h)	Duration (h)
Rapid-acting insulins				
Insulin aspart	5826.38, 116094-23-6 (2,3)	0.17–0.33	1–3	3–5
Insulin lispro	5807.9, 133107-64-9 (4)	0.25–0.5	0.5–2.5	3.0–6.5
Short-acting insulins				
Insulin	9004-10-8 (4)	0.5–1.0	1–5	6–10
Intermediate-acting insulins				
Insulin zinc (Lente)	9004-21-1 (4)	1–3	6–14	16–24
Insulin isophane (NPH)	53027-39-7 (4)	1–3	6–14	16–24
Long-acting insulins				
Insulin glargine	6062.9, 160337-95-1 (4)	1.1	2–20	24
Insulin human zinc, extended (Ultralente)	99551-09-4 (4)	4–6	8–20	24–28

TOXIC DOSE

The adult and pediatric therapeutic dose of insulin is individualized for each patient using the blood glucose concentration. For patients with type I diabetes who are receiving a twice-daily insulin regimen, the morning dose (before breakfast) generally consists of one-third rapid- or short-acting insulin and two-thirds intermediate-acting insulin, and the evening dose (before supper) consists of equal amounts of rapid- or short-acting and intermediate-acting insulin. In patients receiving multiple daily subcutaneous (SQ) injections, approximately half of the daily dose is administered as intermediate- or long-acting insulin, and the remainder is given as rapid- or short-acting insulin with meals (25% breakfast, 10% lunch, 20% supper). For diabetic ketoacidosis an intravenous bolus of 0.15 U/kg is followed by an infusion of 0.1 U/kg/hour, adjusted as needed depending on clinical response.

Therapeutic doses of insulin can cause severe hypoglycemia in diabetics who decrease food intake or increase exercise. A therapeutic dose of insulin usually causes hypoglycemia in non-diabetic patients. Survival has been reported after injection of as much as 7000 U with intensive supportive care (1).

TOXICOKINETICS AND TOXICODYNAMICS

The pharmacokinetic and pharmacodynamic parameters of the insulins are provided in Table 1. The duration of effect may be greatly prolonged (several days) after a massive SQ injection (1). In general, insulin is approximately 5% protein bound, and approximately 18% of endogenous insulin is excreted renally. Insulin is not effective after oral administration.

PATHOPHYSIOLOGY

Insulin stimulates carbohydrate metabolism and facilitates transfer of glucose into cardiac muscle, skeletal muscle, and adipose tissue. Insulin facilitates conversion of glucose to glycogen. In addition, insulin inhibits lipolysis from adipose cells and stimulates lipogenesis and protein synthesis. Insulin also shifts potassium and magnesium intracellularly.

PREGNANCY AND LACTATION

Regular insulin is U.S. Food and Drug Administration pregnancy category B (Appendix I). All other insulins (insulin aspart, insulin glargine, insulin human isophane or regular) are pregnancy category C. All insulins are considered safe for breast-feeding.

CLINICAL PRESENTATION

Acute or Subacute Overdosage

Overdose causes hypoglycemia; the onset and duration depend on the type and quantity of insulin injected. Duration of hypoglycemia may be prolonged (several days) after administration of massive SQ doses of insulin (1). Early manifestations of hypoglycemia may include hunger, anxiety, fatigue, diaphoresis, nausea, palpitations, tachycardia, tremor, or headache. As the brain becomes more deprived of glucose, blurred vision, inability to concentrate, weakness, altered behavior or coordination, or somnolence may develop. In severe cases seizures, hemiplegia, and coma may develop (5).

In patients with central nervous system depression, mild hypothermia commonly develops (6). Protracted, untreated hypoglycemia may cause permanent neurologic injury or death (7). Cardiac manifestations of hypoglycemia are not as common but may include atrial fibrillation, premature ventricular contractions, hypertension, and angina (7–11). Hypokalemia is fairly common after insulin overdose; hypomagnesemia and hypophosphatemia have also been reported (12–14).

Adverse Events

Hypoglycemia may occur during chronic use, usually as a result of decreased carbohydrate intake. Increased exercise can also induce hypoglycemia. In patients with worsening renal function, hypoglycemia may also develop secondary to decreased insulin clearance. Hypoglycemia that develops during therapeutic use is usually not as prolonged as hypoglycemia that occurs after overdose, but otherwise the presentations are similar.

Drug Interactions

Substances that induce hypoglycemia exacerbate the hypoglycemic effects of insulin. These substances include drugs such as the sulfonylureas, biguanides, α-glucosidase inhibitors (acarbose, voglibose), thiazolidinedione derivatives (rosiglitazone, pioglitazone) and alternative medicines such as bitter melon, fenugreek, gymnema silvestre, aloe, glucomannan, and St. John's wort. Many other drugs may exacerbate hypoglycemia when taken with insulin, including angiotensin-converting enzyme inhibitors, allopurinol, chloramphenicol, clofibrate, ethanol, fenfluramine, methotrexate, monoamine oxidase inhibitors, pentamidine, phenylbutazone, probenecid, quinine, salicylates, sulfonamide, and trimethoprim-sulfamethoxazole. β-Adrenergic blocking agents may mask some of the clinical effects of hypoglycemia.

DIAGNOSTIC TESTS

Acute and Subacute Overdosage

The blood glucose is measured hourly, occasionally more frequently depending on the severity of poisoning and the patient's course. The serum electrolytes should be monitored, focusing on potassium, magnesium, and phosphorus in patients with large overdose or recurrent hypoglycemia. The electrocardiogram should be monitored in patients with recurrent hypoglycemia or large overdose.

Adverse Events

The blood glucose is monitored hourly. Renal function should be assessed in patients with hypoglycemic episodes without another obvious cause (increased dose or exercise, decreased carbohydrate intake, etc.).

Diagnostic Pitfalls

In patients with possible surreptitious insulin use, simultaneous serum glucose, insulin, C peptide, and proinsulin concentrations and urinary sulfonylurea concentrations should be obtained. In the setting of hypoglycemia, surreptitious insulin injection is suggested by very high plasma insulin levels, low C peptide, and absent proinsulin concentrations. A molar ratio of insulin to C peptide in peripheral blood of more than 1.0 in the setting of hypoglycemia suggests exogenous insulin administration (15).

Postmortem Considerations

The diagnosis of exogenous insulin administration can be substantiated at autopsy if postmortem levels of insulin are elevated and C peptide is low, or by using the molar ratio of insulin to C peptide (16,17).

TREATMENT

Patients with suicidal insulin overdose often inject extremely large quantities in multiple locations. Recurrent, protracted hypoglycemia is common. Patients should be admitted to an intensive care unit for frequent serum glucose monitoring, monitoring of mental status, and dextrose administration.

The nonsuicidal patient with inadvertent overdosage (the "insulin reaction") typically has much smaller amounts of insulin administered. The serum glucose and mental status should be monitored. Often, patients with inadvertent overdosage can be monitored in the emergency department and discharged if hypoglycemia resolves after feeding and intravenous dextrose. Patients with recurrent hypoglycemia, or overdose with long-acting insulin, require inpatient admission.

Decontamination

Decontamination is not needed after ingestion because insulin is degraded in the stomach. Surgical removal of SQ injected insulin has been described after large overdose (18–20), but there is no evidence that this improves outcome, and it is not recommended.

Enhancement of Elimination

Methods to enhance elimination are not useful after insulin overdose.

Antidotes

The mainstay of treatment is intravenous dextrose sufficient to maintain euglycemia. Dextrose administration is guided by frequent measurement of serum glucose levels and monitoring of mental status. In adults an intravenous bolus of 25 g dextrose (50 ml 50% dextrose in water) is usually an adequate initial dose. Patients with profound hypoglycemia may require an additional dose. In children the initial dose is 0.5 to 1.0 g/kg 25% dextrose (a 1:1 dilution of 50% dextrose and sterile water). Neonates should receive 0.5 to 1.0 g/kg 10% dextrose (a 1:4 dilution of 50% dextrose and sterile water). Once patients return to a normal mental status, they should be fed. Those with inadvertent hypoglycemia (secondary to a missed meal, increased exercise, etc.) often require no further treatment.

Patients with insulin overdose or recurrent hypoglycemia should receive an intravenous infusion of 10% dextrose titrated to maintain a blood glucose of 100 to 200 mg/dl. Hyperglycemia should be avoided, as it enhances endogenous insulin release and may cause recurrent hypoglycemia in some patients. If patients have recurrent hypoglycemia despite 10% dextrose infusion, or if volume loading is a concern, 20% dextrose may be needed; however, it should be administered via a central venous catheter to avoid venous irritation. Dextrose solutions should be titrated and slowly discontinued once the patient is eating an adequate diet and hypoglycemic episodes have stopped.

Acute hepatic steatosis (moderate increases in transaminase levels, bilirubin and lactase levels, metabolic acidosis, and mild hepatomegaly) has been reported in patients who received large amounts of intravenous dextrose (1400 g/day for 3 days) to treat recurrent hypoglycemia from insulin overdose. The abnormalities resolved rapidly once intravenous dextrose was discontinued (21).

Secondary Antidote

Glucagon can be used as a temporizing method to correct hypoglycemia. It has the advantage of being able to be used intramuscularly (IM) or SQ in the prehospital setting in a patient who cannot be given oral carbohydrates safely because of depressed mental status and in whom intravenous access cannot be established. It acts in the liver by stimulating glycogenolysis and gluconeogenesis and requires adequate glycogen stores to be effective; thus, in certain populations (children, alcoholics, otherwise malnourished patients) it may fail to reverse hypoglycemia. The usual dose in patients who weigh more than 44 lb (20 kg) is 1 mg IM or SQ. In children less than 44 lbs, the usual dose is 0.5 mg (or 20 to 30 mg/kg) SQ or IM. Patients should be given oral carbohydrates as soon as possible after mental status is restored to avoid recurrent hypoglycemia.

Monitoring

Patients with insulin overdose require frequent monitoring of blood glucose, initially at least hourly, and observation for clinical evidence of hypoglycemia such as agitation or depressed mental status.

REFERENCES

1. Roberge R, Martin TG, Delbridge TR. Intentional massive insulin overdose: recognition and management. *Ann Emerg Med* 1993;22:228–234.
2. Heinemann L, Kapitza C, Starke AAR, et al. Duration of action of the insulin analogue B28Asp in comparison to regular insulin. *Diabetes* 1996;45: 139A.
3. Heinemann L, Weyer C, Rave K, et al. Comparison of the time-action profiles of U40- and U100-regular human insulin and the rapid-acting insulin analogue B28 Asp. *Exp Clin Endocrinol Diabetes* 1997;105:140–144.
4. Insulins. In: *AHFS drug information*. 2003:2960–2968.
5. Malouf R, Brust JCM. Hypoglycemia: causes, neurological manifestations and outcome. *Ann Neurol* 1985;17:421–430.
6. Kedes LH, Field JB. Hypothermia: a clue to hypoglycemia. *N Engl J Med* 1964;271:785.
7. Cooper AJ. Attempted suicide using insulin by a non diabetic: a case study demonstrating the acute and chronic consequences of profound hypoglycemia. *Can J Psychiatry* 1994;39:103–107.
8. Collier A, Matthews DM, Young RJ, et al. Transient atrial fibrillation precipitated by hypoglycaemia: two case reports. *Postgrad Med J* 1987;63:895–897.
9. Leak D, Starr P. The mechanism of arrhythmias during insulin induce hypoglycemia. *Am Heart J* 1962;63:688–691.
10. Odeh M, Oliven A, Bussan H. Transient atrial fibrillation precipitated by hypoglycemia. *Ann Emerg Med* 1990;19:565–567.
11. Bowman CE, MacMahon DG, Mourant AJ. Hypoglycemia and angina. *Lancet* 1985;1:639–640.
12. Haskell RJ, Stapczynski JS. Intravenous glucose for the treatment of intentional insulin overdoses. *Ann Emerg Med* 1983;12:260(abst).
13. Arem R, Zoghbi W. Insulin overdose in eight patients: insulin pharmacokinetics and review of the literature. *Medicine* 1985;64:323–332.
14. Matsumura M, Nakashima A, Tofuku Y. Electrolyte disorders following massive insulin overdose in a patient with type 2 diabetes. *Intern Med* 2000;39:55–57.
15. Lebowitz MR, Blumenthal SA. The molar ratio of insulin to C-peptide. An aid to the diagnosis of hypoglycemia due to surreptitious (or inadvertent) insulin administration. *Arch Intern Med* 1993;153(5):650–655.
16. Iwase H, Kobayahsi M, Nakajima M, Takatori T. The ratio of insulin to C-peptide can be used to make a forensic diagnosis of exogenous insulin overdosage. *Forensic Sci Int* 2001;115(1–2):123–127.
17. Winston DC. Suicide via insulin overdose in nondiabetics: the New Mexico experience. *Am J Forensic Med Path* 2000;21(3):237–240.
18. Levine DF, Bulstrode C. Managing suicidal insulin overdose. *BMJ* 1982;285: 974–975.
19. McIntyre AS, Woolf VJ, Burnham WR. Local excision of subcutaneous fat in the management of insulin overdose. *Br J Surg* 1986;73:538.
20. Campbell IW, Ratcliffe JG. Suicidal insulin overdose managed by excision of insulin injection site. *BMJ* 1982;285:408–409.
21. Jolliet P, Leverve X, Pichard C. Acute hepatic steatosis complicating massive insulin overdose and excessive glucose administration. *Intensive Care Med* 2001;27(1):313–316.

CHAPTER 158

Sulfonylurea and Antihyperglycemic Drugs

Patrick E. McKinney and Steven A. McLaughlin

See Figure 1.

Compounds included:	**Acetohexamide (Dimelor), chlorpropamide (Diabinese), gliclazide (Glycemirex), glimepiride (Amaryl), glipizide (Glucotrol, Minidiab), gliquidone (Glurenorm), glyburide (Daonil, DiaBeta, Micronase, Glynase-PresTab), tolazamide (Tolinase), tolbutamide (Orinase, Rastinon)**
Molecular formula and weight:	**See Table 1.**
SI conversion:	**See Table 1.**
CAS Registry No.:	**See Table 1.**
Therapeutic and toxic levels:	**See Table 4.**
Special concerns:	**Acute and delayed-onset hypoglycemia**
Antidotes:	**Dextrose, octreotide, diazoxide, glucagon**

OVERVIEW

The sulfonylureas are sulfonamide derivatives that lower the blood glucose concentration by promoting release of preformed insulin from pancreatic β cells. As a group, they are weakly acidic drugs that are highly protein bound and have a small volume of distribution. They are metabolized by the liver, and some have active metabolites. Sulfonylureas are used alone or in combination with biguanides, α-glucosidase inhibitors, or thiazolidinediones in non–insulin-dependent (NIDDM) diabetics in whom blood sugar concentrations remain elevated despite weight loss, diet control, and exercise. Even therapeutic doses of sulfonylureas may cause hypoglycemia in nondiabetic individuals as well as in susceptible individuals with NIDDM.

Treatment priorities in patients with known exposure who present with hypoglycemia include providing supplemental glucose by intravenous (IV) bolus and appropriate gastrointestinal decontamination, if indicated. In cases in which sulfonylurea exposure is not known or suspected, identification of hypoglycemia as the cause of neurologic or sympathomimetic symptoms is critical. Because patients with sulfonylurea-induced hypoglycemia may be at risk for recurrent and prolonged hypoglycemic episodes, patients with an initial episode of significant hypoglycemia should be admitted to the hospital for monitoring. Patients with repeated episodes of hypoglycemia should be given octreotide acetate, which blocks sulfonylurea-mediated insulin release. Glucagon and diazoxide are second-line therapies for sulfonylurea-induced hypoglycemia. Chlorpropamide is also used rarely as a second-line agent in the treatment of centrally mediated diabetes insipidus.

Classification and Uses

Sulfonylureas are sulfonamide derivatives. Their hypoglycemic effects were first noted by Ruiz et al. (1) as early as 1937. These investigators were investigating a sulfonylurea known as *2254 RP* as an antibacterial agent in the treatment of typhoid fever when it was noted that some patients manifested severe signs and symptoms of hypoglycemia including death (2). Subsequent investigations by Loubatieres (3) showed that 2254 RP was an orally active hypoglycemic agent that required a functioning pancreas for its hypoglycemic action. Despite this knowledge, the sulfonylureas were not used in clinical practice as hypoglycemic agents until 1955 (4).

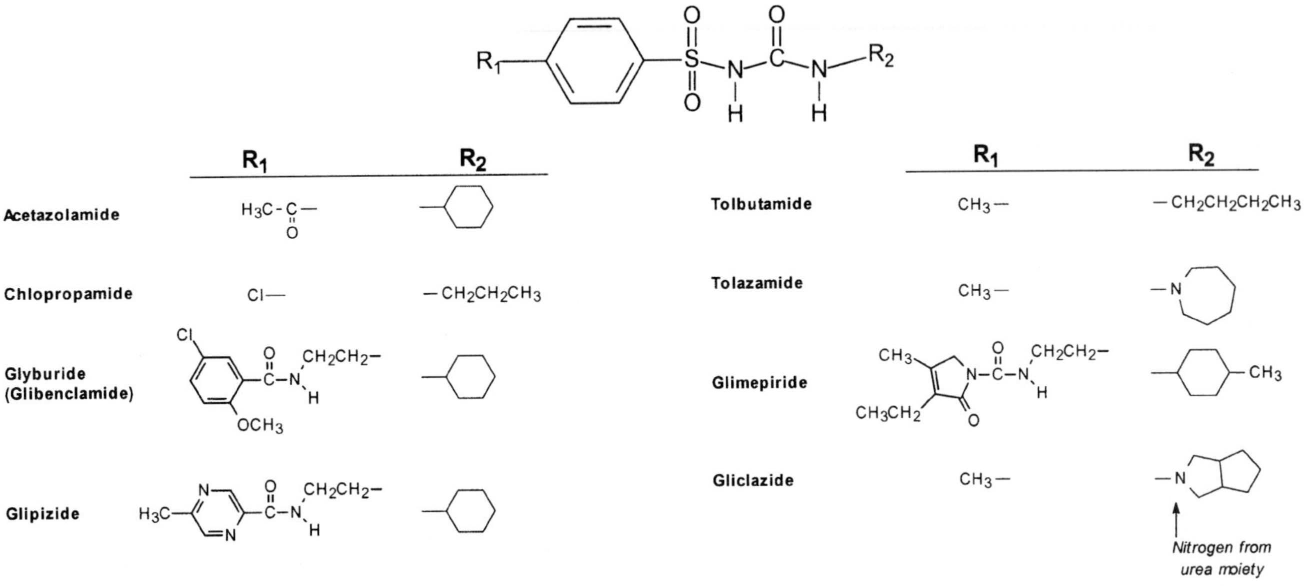

Figure 1. Structures of the oral sulfonylurea drugs.

Tolbutamide, tolazamide, chlorpropamide, and acetohexamide were the first agents to be widely used as therapy for NIDDM and are known as the first-generation sulfonylureas. The second-generation sulfonylureas include glyburide (also known as *glibenclamide*), glipizide, gliclazide, and glimepiride, among others. These agents have similar chemical and pharmacokinetic properties to the first-generation agents but are significantly more potent due to higher affinity for the sulfonylurea receptor.

Estimates suggest that 100 million patients across the globe have NIDDM and that the prevalence will rise to 200 million in 15 years (5). As sulfonylureas are the mainstay of pharmacologic therapy for NIDDM, the use of these agents is expected to continue to increase. In 1999, sulfonylureas entered the list of the top 20 product categories by prescriptions dispensed in the United States (6). In 2001, five different sulfonylureas were included on the top 200 prescriptions filled by U.S. pharmacists (7).

Sulfonylureas are adjunctive pharmacologic therapy to diet and exercise in the treatment of NIDDM (type 2) diabetes mellitus. This form of diabetes is characterized as impaired insulin secretion, peripheral insulin resistance, and overproduction of glucose by the liver. Patients who are most likely to respond to sulfonylurea therapy include those with NIDDM who develop the disease after the age of 40 years, have a duration of disease less than 5 to 10 years at the start of therapy, and have no history of ketoacidosis. Extremely obese patients or those with markedly elevated blood sugars may not respond to sulfonylurea treatment. Although many patients respond initially to sulfonylurea therapy, secondary failures may occur over time. These patients may respond to a dose increase or a change to another sulfonylurea agent or may require the addition of a second oral hypoglycemic drug of a different class or insulin. These agents lower fasting and postprandial blood sugar concentrations and glycosylated hemoglobin. Improved control of blood sugar concentrations is associated with decreased risk of microvascular complications of diabetes mellitus.

Toxic Dose

The adult therapeutic dose for the commonly available forms of sulfonylureas is provided in Table 1. Sulfonylurea therapy is usually initiated at the lowest available dose. Doses can be

TABLE 1. Physical characteristics and dosage of sulfonylurea antihyperglycemic drugs

Drug	Molecular formula, molecular weight (g/mol), CAS Registry No.	SI conversion	Available forms	Usual dose range[a]	Maximum dose	Doses/d
Acetohexamide	$C_{15}H_{20}N_2O_4S$, 324.4, 968-81-0	µg/ml × 3.08 = µmol/L	250, 500 mg	125–750 mg PO BID	1500 mg	1–2
Chlorpropamide	$C_{10}H_{13}ClN_2O_3S$, 276.7, 94-20-2	µg/ml × 3.61 = µmol/L	100, 250 mg	100–500 mg PO QD	—	1
Gliclazide	$C_{15}H_{21}N_3O_3S$, 323.4, 21187-98-4	µg/ml × 3.09 = µmol/L	NR	40–320 mg PO QD	320 mg	1
Glimepiride	$C_{24}H_{34}N_4O_5S$, 490.6, 93479-97-1	µg/ml × 2.04 = µmol/L	1, 2, 4 mg	1–4 mg PO QD	8 mg	1
Glipizide	$C_{21}H_{27}N_5O_4S$, 445.5, 29094-61-9	µg/ml × 2.24 = µmol/L	5, 10 mg; 2.5, 5, 10 mg	5–15 mg PO QD; 2.5–10.0 mg PO QD	40 mg; 20 mg	1–2
Gliquidone	$C_{27}H_{33}N_3O_6S$, 527.6, 33342-05-1	µg/ml × 1.9 = µmol/L	NR	15–180 mg PO QD	180 mg	1
Glyburide	$C_{23}H_{28}ClN_3O_5S$, 494.0, 10238-21-8	µg/ml × 2.02 = µmol/L	1.25, 5 mg; micronized: 1.5, 3, 4.5, 6 mg	1.25–20.0 mg PO QD; micronized: 1.5–12.0 mg PO QD	20 mg; micronized: 12 mg	1–2; micronized: 1
Tolazamide	$C_{14}H_{21}N_3O_3S$, 311.4, 1156-19-0	µg/ml × 3.21 = µmol/L	100, 250, 500 mg	100–1000 mg PO QD	1000 mg	1–2
Tolbutamide	$C_{12}H_{18}N_2O_3S$, 270.3, 473-41-6	µg/ml × 3.7 = µmol/L	500 mg	500–2000 mg	3000 mg	2–3

NR, not reported.
[a]At higher dose ranges, can be administered BID.

TABLE 2. Pharmacokinetics and pharmacodynamics of the sulfonylurea antihyperglycemic drugs

Drug	Onset of effect (h)	Duration of effect (h)	Volume of distribution (L/kg)	Protein binding (%)	Bioavailability (%)
Tolbutamide	1	6–24	0.1–0.15	80–99	May differ between formulations
Chlorpropamide	1–2	24–72	0.9–0.27	88–96	Good
Tolazamide	1	12–20		98	Good (peak 4–8 h)
Acetohexamide	—	12–24	0.21	65–90	Almost complete
Glyburide	0.5	16–24	0.125–0.3	99	Almost complete[a]
Glipizide	0.5	12–24	0.16	92–99	80–100
Glimepiride	—	24	0.28–0.52	99	100
Gliclazide	—	24	0.2	85–99	80–96
Gliquidone	1.0–1.5	12–24	—	99	—

[a]Micronized forms have greater bioavailability and more rapid absorption.

increased every 1 to 2 weeks if the blood glucose–lowering response is inadequate. Low doses are often given once daily. As the dose increases, many agents are given in two divided doses. Evidence shows that the upper range for sulfonylureas widely used in the United States is too high and that many patients respond better to low or intermediate doses (8). When transferring patients from one agent to another, no washout period is typically needed except for chlorpropamide, in which residual drug effect may persist for up to 2 weeks. The sulfonylureas are not approved by the U.S. Food and Drug Administration (FDA) for use in children. Nevertheless, they are sometimes used in the therapy of youth-onset NIDDM (9).

The toxic dose of a sulfonylurea is dependent on circumstances. Patients without an adequate population of functioning β cells (IDDM or resistant NIDDM) are resistant to the hypoglycemic actions of sulfonylureas. Life-threatening hypoglycemia may develop in sulfonylurea-naïve individuals (adults and children) without diabetes mellitus after ingestion of a single therapeutic dose. The duration of hypoglycemia may be 12 to 24 hours or longer in cases of large overdose, extended-release preparations, or ingestion of chlorpropamide or glyburide. In patients with NIDDM, hypoglycemia may also develop while they are taking therapeutic doses. Risk factors for hypoglycemia in these patients include advanced age, intercurrent illness, hepatic or renal dysfunction, polypharmacy, recent increase in dose, decreased dietary intake, or drug-drug interactions (10–15). Infants born to mothers who are using a sulfonylurea in the last trimester are at risk for hypoglycemia (possibly excepting glyburide).

TOXICOKINETICS AND TOXICODYNAMICS

The pharmacokinetics and pharmacodynamics of the sulfonylurea agents is provided in Tables 2 and 3. The sulfonylureas are weakly acidic drugs with small volumes of distribution and high protein binding. Protein binding may be ionic as well as nonionic. The first-generation agents bind primarily to albumin and α-globulins (16). Second-generation agent protein binding is generally nonionic (16). All currently available sulfonylureas have excellent bioavailability after oral administration. They are generally well absorbed on an empty stomach but can be taken before meals to provide optimal postprandial insulin release. All are metabolized by the liver to less active or inactive metabolites with the exception of acetohexamide. Acetohexamide is metabolized to hydroxyhexamide, which is more potent and longer lasting than the parent drug. Glimepiride, glipizide, and glyburide are metabolized in part by CYP2C9. Inhibition of this enzyme can lead to increased drug concentrations and increased risk of hypoglycemia (17–19). Drug-drug interactions are listed in Table 4.

Metabolites and small amounts of the unchanged first-generation parent drugs are excreted primarily in the urine. The urinary excretion of unchanged chlorpropamide is dependent on urinary pH. The elimination half-life of chlorpropamide was shortened from 49.7 to 12.8 hours by sodium bicarbonate (20). Second-generation drugs, such as gliclazide, glimepiride, and glicquidone, are excreted to a greater extent via bile in feces. In patients with renal insufficiency, tolazamide, acetohexamide, chlorpropamide, and glyburide should be used with caution

TABLE 3. Metabolism and excretion of the sulfonylurea antihyperglycemic drugs

Drug	Metabolism	Excretion	Excreted unchanged (%)	Elimination half-life (h)	Active metabolites	Avoid in renal failure
Tolbutamide	Liver	Renal	Minimal	4–12	Minimal	No
Chlorpropamide	Liver	Renal	10–30%[a]	24–48	Yes	Yes
Tolazamide	Liver	85% renal, 7% feces	7	4–7	Yes	Yes
Acetohexamide	Liver	Renal	Minimal	0.8–2.4, 4–6 (metab)	Yes	Yes
Glyburide	Liver	Renal	5–10	1.4–3.0[b]	Yes	Yes
Glipizide	Liver	Renal, 11% feces	3–9	1–7	No	No
Glimepiride	Liver	60% renal, 40% feces	—	5–9	Weakly	No
Gliclazide	Liver	80% renal, 20% feces	1–20	6–15	No	No
Gliquidone	Liver	5% renal, 95% biliary	—	24	Yes[c]	No

[a]Renal clearance increases 100-fold when urine pH increases from 5 to 7.
[b]Elimination half-life may be as long as 15 to 20 h.
[c]Active metabolite present in low concentrations.
From Jönnson A, Rydberg T, Ekberg G, et al. Slow elimination of glyburide in NIDDM subjects. *Diabetes Care* 1994;17:142–145, with permission.

TABLE 4. Drug interactions with sulfonylureas

Drug	Mechanism
Increased sulfonylurea effect	
Acarbose	Decreased carbohydrate availability
Antacids	Increased absorption glipizide, glyburide
Aspirin	Displace from proteins, alter carbohydrate metabolism, decreased tubular secretion
Cimetidine	Inhibit metabolism, glimepiride not affected
Ciprofloxacin, other quinolones	Inhibit metabolism
Clofibrate	Displaced protein binding
Doxepin	?
Enalapril	?
Erythromycin-sulfamethoxazole	Displaced protein binding, inhibit metabolism
Ethanol	Alter carbohydrate metabolism
Fenugreek	?
Fluconazole	Inhibit metabolism
Ginseng	?
MAOI	Increased carbohydrate metabolism?
NSAIDs	Inhibit metabolism?
Psyllium, guar gum	Decreased carbohydrate availability
Ranitidine	Inhibit metabolism glipizide, glimepiride not affected
Sulfa antibiotics	Displaced protein binding
Decreased sulfonylurea effect	
Acetazolamide	?
Diazoxide	Sulfonylurea receptor antagonism
Fosphenytoin	Increased metabolism
Hydrochlorothiazide	?
Probenecid	Decrease renal clearance
Rifabutin, rifampin	P-450 induction
Steroids	Altered carbohydrate metabolism
Other	
Cyclosporine	Cyclosporine levels may be increased
Phenytoin-fosphenytoin	Phenytoin levels may be increased

MAOI, monoamine oxidase inhibitor; NSAIDs, nonsteroidal antiinflammatory drugs.
Note: Protein binding displacement may be more important for first-generation agents.

because the parent drug, an active metabolite, or both are dependent in part on renal elimination (21).

The first-generation agents are usually dosed one to three times per day, except for chlorpropamide, which is given once a day. The second-generation agents are generally given once a day, although higher doses can be split. Increased insulin release can be detected 30 to 120 minutes after ingestion. Peak plasma drug levels are generally detected 1 to 2 hours after therapeutic doses, except in the case of tolazamide, in which peaks occur 4 to 8 hours after ingestion. Duration of hypoglycemic action varies from 12 to 24 hours in most cases after ingestion of therapeutic doses. Hypoglycemia may be prolonged after overdose to several days or even several weeks in the case of chlorpropamide (22).

PATHOPHYSIOLOGY

Sulfonylureas produce hypoglycemia by binding to the SUR1 sulfonylurea receptor on pancreatic β cells. The potency of these agents roughly parallels their binding affinity (23). This receptor is associated with adenosine triphosphate (ATP)-dependent K^+ channels (K_{ATP} channels), known as *Kir6.2* (24). Sulfonylureas bind to and then inactivate K_{ATP} channels on the membrane surface of the β cells, decreasing K^+ efflux (25,26). This is followed by depolarization of the β cell, the opening of voltage-gated Ca^{2+} channels, and subsequent release of preformed insulin (27). Pancreatic β-cell insulin release in response to elevated blood glucose concentrations is augmented.

Evidence has been shown that some sulfonylureas may be taken up into the β cell and exert their hypoglycemic action by mechanisms independent of the sulfonylurea membrane receptor. A protein kinase C–dependent mechanism may be involved (28). Sulfonylureas may also attenuate the release of glucagon in response to hypoglycemia (29). At high doses, sulfonylureas appear to inhibit glucagon secretion (30). Sulfonylureas may have extrapancreatic functions that contribute to therapeutic effect over the long term, including reduced hepatic clearance of insulin and potentiation of insulin effects on peripheral tissues (31). These mechanisms do not appear to contribute to acute toxicity relating to hypoglycemia.

Other sulfonylurea receptor subtypes (SUR2) have been found in tissues outside the pancreas (32). In the heart, sulfonylurea binding to SUR2 appears to block protective preconditioning responses in ischemic myocardium. Glyburide has been shown to increase the incidence of dysrhythmias and decrease the postischemic recovery in an experimental model (33). Sulfonylureas may increase γ-aminobutyric acid (GABA)ergic tone in the brain and may affect smooth muscle vascular tone. Glimepiride appears to have lower affinity for the SUR2 receptor subtype compared to glyburide and other older sulfonylureas (8). It is unclear whether these mechanisms play any significant role in acute toxicity or during long-term therapy (24).

PREGNANCY AND LACTATION

All sulfonylureas are rated as FDA pregnancy risk category C with the exception of glyburide, which is rated category B (Appendix I) (34–36). Standard pharmacologic and obstetric references recommend avoiding sulfonylurea agents during pregnancy and lactation because of the risk of fetal or infant hypoglycemia as well as concerns regarding teratogenesis. First-generation sulfonylurea use during pregnancy has been associated with fetal hypoglycemia persisting 4 to 10 days (37). Therapeutic levels of chlorpropamide and tolbutamide have been detected in the cord blood of infants delivered from mothers receiving these drugs (38,39). Fetal hyperglycemia (secondary to maternal hyperglycemia) and fetal exposure to sulfonylureas may result in fetal islet cell hyperplasia. Thus, persistent fetal hypoglycemia in these cases may be due to persistent sulfonylurea action or to endogenous hyperinsulinism (37).

Sulfonylureas may also be associated with teratogenic effects. Animal models inconsistently demonstrate fetal anomalies, including long bone abnormalities, growth retardation, and eye defects (40,41). Human birth defect data are confounded by the fact that hyperglycemia is associated with adverse pregnancy outcomes, and typically only mothers with poor glycemic control are considered for hypoglycemic drug therapy (42,43). Evidence suggests that glyburide does not cross the human placenta in appreciable quantities (40). A randomized trial showed that pregnant women between 11 and 33 weeks of gestation had effective glycemic control from glyburide compared to insulin. No difference was found in the incidence of fetal hypoglycemia between groups or in adverse fetal outcomes (44). Because of these data, glyburide (Micronase, Glynase-PresTab) is rated FDA pregnancy category B. However, the current consensus is that most women who require drug therapy for hyperglycemia during pregnancy should be treated with insulin, although this practice pattern may be slowly changing.

Chlorpropamide and tolbutamide have been detected in low concentrations in the breast milk of mothers who take these agents. Data for other sulfonylureas are lacking. Because of the risk of hypoglycemia in the breast-feeding infant, it is recommended that either sulfonylurea therapy or breast-feeding be stopped (American Hospital Formulary Service, 2002).

CLINICAL PRESENTATION

Acute Overdosage

The primary toxicity of all of the sulfonylurea agents when taken in overdose is hypoglycemia. Hypoglycemia can present with symptoms from a variety of different organ systems, including neurologic, gastrointestinal, cardiovascular, respiratory, and others. However, the major manifestations of hypoglycemia result from effects on the brain and autonomic nervous system.

Central nervous system findings of hypoglycemia include lethargy, confusion, coma, dizziness, slurred speech, seizures (45), syncope (46,47), and hallucinations. The incidence of hypoglycemic coma in adults following sulfonylurea overdose has been reported to be as high as 53% to 58% (46,48). In children, the reported incidence of hypoglycemia after suspected sulfonylurea ingestion ranges from 27% to 78% (48–51).

Hypoglycemia from sulfonylurea agents can be prolonged and severe and can recur after treatment with glucose (52). In five case series describing adult exposures to glipizide, glyburide, and glibenclamide, hypoglycemia recurred in 26% to 62% of patients despite glucose therapy (10,46,48,53,54). In 15% to 26% of these patients, hypoglycemia lasted for up to 60 hours (46,54). The severity of hypoglycemia may be similar in children; one study reported that persistent or recurrent hypoglycemia developed in 10% of children despite glucose therapy (49). Recurrent or rebound hypoglycemia is thought to be due to continued effect of the drug on the pancreas. Iatrogenic glucose administration stimulates additional insulin release, resulting in rebound hypoglycemia (55).

The onset of hypoglycemia can be significantly delayed. In one study of children who became hypoglycemic, 74% did so within 4 hours, 86% within 6 hours, and 93% to 96% within 8 hours of ingestion (50,51). This is consistent with the time to peak effect (approximately 8 hours) for most sulfonylurea agents (56). However, isolated cases of delayed hypoglycemia have been reported, with initial onset to detected hypoglycemia ranging from 11 to 18 hours after ingestion in children (50,51). Complicating interpretation of these cases is the fact that many patients received glucose supplementation (potentially obscuring early hypoglycemia) or did not have serum glucose levels determined early in their course (thereby allowing earlier hypoglycemia to remain undetected).

Focal neurologic findings have been reported in patients with hypoglycemia, although global findings are more common (47,57,58). Minor symptoms may include headache, paresthesia, and subjective weakness. Permanent neurologic deficits, including cognitive dysfunction, memory loss, confusion, and coma, may develop in patients with prolonged hypoglycemic coma (46,59,60). The onset, severity, and duration of hypoglycemia from sulfonylurea overdose depend on host factors, such as age, diet, and renal and hepatic function (61), as well as the specific agent and dose involved.

Cardiac effects of sulfonylurea overdose are primarily tachycardia secondary to catecholamine release from hypoglycemia (47). Other autonomic findings associated with hypoglycemia include tremor and diaphoresis (46,47).

Gastrointestinal effects, including nausea, vomiting, hunger, and epigastric pain, can occur after overdose and may precede overt hypoglycemia (62,63). These symptoms are probably related to counterregulatory hormone release secondary to falling blood glucose levels.

Adverse Events

Hypoglycemia has been reported with all agents at all doses (10). Epidemiologic studies and case series evaluating NIDDM patients with sulfonylurea-induced hypoglycemia suggest that hypoglycemic risk is increased at the initiation of therapy, in the elderly, in occasional or short-term users (15), and in those with decreased hepatic or renal function. Other risk factors in this group include polypharmacy, intercurrent illness, decreased food intake, increased activity, weight reduction (13), and recent hospitalization. Frequency estimates of hypoglycemic events in this population vary widely. Studies using a liberal definition of hypoglycemia suggest that up to 20% of patients receiving sulfonylureas will experience hypoglycemic symptoms during 6 months of therapy (64).

The incidence of more serious hypoglycemia (requiring medical care or the assistance of others) is much lower. In one retrospective study, serious hypoglycemia rates were 1.23 per 100 person-years for patients using sulfonylureas compared to 2.76 per 100 person-years for patients using insulin (14). Older case series data suggested fatality rates of up to 20% in hospitalized hypoglycemic patients, but this likely reflects reporting bias, and actual fatality rates are probably much lower (10). A retrospective study estimated the rate of catastrophic complications at 1 per 1000 patient-years of therapy (15). The long-term morbidity following severe, prolonged, or repeated episodes of hypoglycemia in this population has not been studied, although hypoglycemic episodes may produce cognitive deficits. Some evidence from primarily retrospective data has shown that chlorpropamide and glyburide may be associated with a greater risk of hypoglycemic events compared to other currently available sulfonylureas (12,14,15,46,64). It is not clear whether this increased risk is related to the longer elimination half-life of these two agents or other factors such as an intracellular action of these drugs in the β cell (15).

The objective of sulfonylurea therapy is normalization of glycemic control as measured by a decrease in glycosylated hemoglobin. However, stricter glycemic control is associated with an increased risk of hypoglycemic events. Paradoxically, in patients with diabetes who have hypoglycemic events, a blunted awareness to subsequent hypoglycemic events, so-called hypoglycemic unawareness, may also develop. Normal responses to hypoglycemia follow a hierarchy of events (63,65). At blood sugars approaching 70 mg/dl, insulin secretion is decreased in healthy young adults. When blood sugar drops to 60 to 70 mg/dl, epinephrine, glucagon, cortisol, and growth hormone secretion are increased. Autonomic symptoms, including tachycardia, sweating, and tremor, begin at glucose concentrations of approximately 50 mg/dl. Symptoms of confusion, ataxia, and agitation then follow. In patients with poorly controlled NIDDM, this sequence of events may begin at higher glucose levels (66).

In diabetic patients who are tightly controlled, however, the counterregulatory response is shifted downward such that symptoms do not develop until blood glucose concentrations reach levels that may be dangerously low. In addition, typical autonomic warning signs may be absent or blunted so that the first symptoms may reflect decreased glucose concentrations in the brain. In this scenario, the first symptom may be confusion that prevents an appropriate behavioral action on the part of the patient, such as the emergent consumption of glucose. In addition to this shift in the glucose levels necessary to initiate the counterregulatory response, patients with long-standing NIDDM may have a deficient glucagon response to hypoglycemia, adding to their compromised counterregulatory response (62). In this case, epinephrine becomes the predominant counterregulatory hormone released in response to hypoglycemia (67). This explains part of the potential danger of beta-receptor blockers in diabetic patients. The beta receptor–blocking agents may attenuate the catecholamine counterregulatory response as well as blunt the autonomic symptoms to hypoglycemia (except sweating, which is preserved) (68).

Other serious adverse reactions are unusual in patients taking sulfonylureas. Individuals with allergic reactions to one sulfonylurea may react to other members of the class. In addition, these drugs should be used with caution in patients with allergic reactions to sulfonamides or thiazides because of the risk of cross-reaction. The syndrome of inappropriate antidiuretic hormone secretion has been associated with chlorpropamide and less commonly with tolbutamide (69). Lesser degrees of hyponatremia are associated with the use of gliclazide and glyburide (70).

Disulfiram-type reactions after drinking alcohol have been reported to occur in up to 30% of patients taking chlorpropamide. The risk of this reaction is lower with tolbutamide and glyburide; it may not occur with glipizide and glimepiride (69). Hematologic reactions rarely occur but include agranulocytosis, aplastic anemia, hemolytic anemia, and thrombocytopenia (71–74). Less serious but more common side effects involve the gastrointestinal system and include nausea, vomiting, dyspepsia, diarrhea, abdominal pain, and dysgeusia. Hepatitis or cholestatic jaundice, or both, have been reported with several sulfonylureas (75,76). Photosensitization and a variety of allergic skin reactions can occur (77,78).

All sulfonylureas, with the exception of glimepiride, may bind to non–β-cell sulfonylurea receptors (SUR2), including those in the heart. A study by the University Group Diabetes Program (79) more than 30 years ago suggested that patients receiving first-generation sulfonylureas had a higher cardiac mortality than diabetics treated with diet alone. This study has been widely criticized, and the results have not been replicated. In vitro and in vivo data suggest that glyburide may reduce the frequency of reperfusion dysrhythmias (80,81). This is counterbalanced by evidence that glyburide may worsen the extent of damage during myocardial ischemia, perhaps by inhibiting the preconditioning response (80,81). Thus, the overall effect of sulfonylureas on the morbidity and mortality of cardiac disease remains speculative.

TABLE 5. Therapeutic and toxic serum concentrations of the oral sulfonylurea antihyperglycemic drugs

Drug/dose	Therapeutic range	Toxic concentration
Tolbutamide, 1000–2000 mg dose (peak)	53–96 μg/ml	Not established
Chlorpropamide		>400 μg/ml
Single dose (peak)	29 μg/ml	
250–500 mg (steady state)	76–246 μg/ml	
500–1000 mg (steady state)	102–363 μg/ml	
Tolazamide	N/A	Not established
Acetohexamide, 500–2000 mg (steady state)	21–56 μg/ml	Not established
Glyburide		Not established
(Peak)	315.7 ± 60.35 μg/ml	
(Steady state)	237 ± 237 μg/ml	
Glipizide, 5 mg single dose	41 ng/ml	Not established
Glimepiride		Not established
6 mg 24 h mean	108.8 ± 49.8 ng/ml	
2 h	295 ± 155.7 ng/ml	
8 mg (peak)	550.8 ng/ml	
Gliclazide, 160 mg (steady state)	15.0 ± 3.7 ng/ml	Not established
Gliquidone, 30 mg single dose	81 ± 7 ng/ml	Not established

N/A, not available.

DIAGNOSTIC TESTS

Glucose Determinations

The diagnosis of acute toxicity from sulfonylurea agents is made by confirming the presence of hypoglycemia. Because not all patients manifest classic autonomic and neurologic symptoms of hypoglycemia, laboratory confirmation of hypoglycemia is essential. Rapid bedside glucose determination is part of the management of any patient with altered mental status and is reliable under hospital conditions. A bedside glucose determination is made using whole blood, which may give values that are 10% to 15% lower than a serum glucose determined in the laboratory. A single normal value should not be reassuring; blood glucose concentrations should be measured frequently. Bedside glucose measurements should be made every 1 to 2 hours while the patient is awake and hourly while asleep during the initial 8 to 12 hours of hospitalization. Also, many NIDDM patients being treated with sulfonylureas have elevated baseline glucose values, and a "normal value" must be taken into the context of normal for a given patient and their degree of glycemic control. Patients with poor glycemic control may exhibit signs and symptoms of hypoglycemia when their glucose drops to "normal range."

Drug Concentrations

Therapeutic and toxic concentrations for the sulfonylureas are not well established, and blood concentrations are not typically monitored as part of therapy. Nevertheless, kinetic studies and overdose cases provide a range of concentrations that reflect therapeutic and "toxic" conditions. Ranges of plasma concentrations measured after therapeutic doses are shown in Table 5. Because hypoglycemia can occur even with administration of a single dose of the lowest therapeutic dose, any sulfonylurea concentration should be viewed as potentially "toxic" if it is measured in conjunction with hypoglycemia. Conversely, hypoglycemia does not develop in patients without functioning β cells (e.g., IDDM) even with large doses of sulfonylureas and high plasma sulfonylurea concentrations. Sulfonylurea concentrations can be measured when there is suspicion of factitious causes of hypoglycemia, malicious poisoning by others, or mistaken filling of a prescription with a look-alike or sound-alike medication (e.g., acetohexamide for acetazolamide). Sulfonylurea concentrations are generally measured by reference laboratories. Analytic techniques include gas chromatography (82), high-performance liquid chromatography with ultraviolet or fluorescence detection (83), radioimmunoassay (84), mass spectrometry with a variety of detection methods, and liquid chromatography–electrospray mass spectrometry (85).

Because sulfonylureas act by facilitating secretion of endogenous insulin, patients with sulfonylurea-induced hypoglycemia may have inappropriately elevated insulin concentrations. In addition, C peptide and proinsulin concentrations are also elevated, which is not the case when exogenous insulin has been injected.

Other Tests

The patient with documented hypoglycemia who fails to return to normal mental status after correction of blood sugar may have cerebral edema due to prolonged hypoglycemia or concurrent intracranial processes such as cerebral infarction or intracranial hemorrhage. In this case, appropriate imaging studies may be helpful. In addition, other pathophysiologic processes should be considered, including electrolyte disorders, sepsis, and adrenal or thyroid dysfunction. Prolonged immobilization may result in rhabdomyolysis, and creatine phosphokinase or urine myoglobin should be measured in these cases.

A 12-lead electrocardiogram is often useful in patients with NIDDM and an episode of hypoglycemia. The counterregulatory response in these patients activates the sympathoadrenal axis, potentially increasing myocardial workload. Many of these patients have preexisting coronary artery disease coupled with decreased awareness of cardiac ischemic pain. An initial electrocardiogram and cardiac enzyme monitoring in cases of significant hypoglycemia may be prudent.

Adverse Events

Chlorpropamide use may be associated with syndrome of inappropriate antidiuretic hormone and hyponatremia in up to one-third of patients. Newer agents are associated with smaller quantitative changes in serum sodium. Serum sodium should be monitored if hyponatremia is suspected or in patients who are receiving chlorpropamide. Liver function tests including transaminases and bilirubin should be monitored in cases of suspected hepatic injury. Sulfonylureas are rarely associated with blood cell dyscrasias. A complete blood count with differential should be obtained if these conditions are suspected.

TREATMENT

The primary clinical effect of sulfonylurea toxicity is hypoglycemia; therefore, management goals include identifying hypoglycemia in the case of an unknown overdose, initial stabilization of abnormal vital signs, and repletion of glucose. In symptomatic patients, glucose should be provided by the IV route in the form of a bolus of concentrated glucose solution as described in Antidotes. Supplemental dextrose (10%) by constant IV infusion should be provided, and the patient can be encouraged to eat, if mental status permits. For recurrent hypoglycemia despite glucose therapy, octreotide acetate should be provided by subcutaneous (SQ) injection. Other potential therapeutic agents include glucagon and diazoxide. These therapies should be regarded as second-line agents in the therapy of sulfonylurea-induced hypoglycemia. Corticosteroids are not reliably effective in this setting and are not recommended as treatment for hypoglycemia.

Decontamination

Emesis is unlikely to play a significant role in the therapy of sulfonylurea ingestion. Because pediatric patients with a potential exposure of even one tablet should be monitored in a health care setting for up to 24 hours, all of these children should be referred to a health care facility where they can receive activated charcoal, if indicated.

Activated charcoal binds all of the sulfonylurea drugs. In vitro experiments document adsorption of these agents to charcoal at pH values that are typically encountered in the stomach (86). Volunteer studies show that early charcoal administration can greatly inhibit absorption of therapeutic doses of these agents (20,87,88). The binding affinity of the second-generation agents to activated charcoal is higher than that of the first-generation agents (86). This higher binding affinity coupled with the fact that dosing forms of the second-generation agents are in milligram rather than gram amounts suggests that 50 g activated charcoal should be sufficient in most overdoses. Because the first-generation agents are often dosed in gram amounts, overdose with large amounts of these agents should be treated with as large a dose of activated charcoal as possible, when indicated.

Neither the role of cathartics nor the role of whole bowel irrigation in the treatment of sulfonylurea ingestion has not been evaluated. However, extended-release formulations are available (Glucotrol XL), suggesting the potential for delayed absorption. Whole bowel irrigation has been advocated after the ingestion of some extended-release preparations; however, it is not clear whether this therapy is superior to multiple doses of activated charcoal or whether either therapy has an impact on clinical outcome.

Enhancement of Elimination

Multiple doses of activated charcoal did not decrease the elimination half-life after a therapeutic dose of chlorpropamide in normal volunteers. Some indirect evidence suggests that gliclazide may undergo limited enterohepatic recirculation (89). Multiple doses of charcoal could theoretically interrupt this enterohepatic recycling and increase clearance, although this has not been studied. The role of multiple doses of activated charcoal in preventing delayed absorption from an extended-release sulfonylurea formulation has not been formally evaluated, but it should be considered when clinically appropriate.

Hemodialysis has not been reported as a treatment of sulfonylurea toxicity. Currently available agents have small volumes of distribution; however, they are extensively protein bound, suggesting that they would not be effectively removed by hemodialysis.

Hemoperfusion has been used after ingestion of chlorpropamide in a dialysis-dependent patient with renal failure (90). In this case, hemoperfusion was associated with a reduction of elimination half-life from 93.6 to 3.4 hours. In patients with functioning kidneys, the availability of antidotal therapy should supersede any considerations for hemoperfusion. Because the most commonly used sulfonylureas are eliminated primarily by hepatic metabolism to primarily inactive metabolites, extracorporeal drug removal should not be required, even in patients with renal failure. Antidotal therapy with glucose and octreotide should be adequate, although the treatment course may be prolonged.

Peritoneal dialysis performed on a 3-year-old after chlorpropamide ingestion did not result in increased drug clearance. Only minimal amounts of drug were recovered in the dialysate (91).

Urinary alkalinization has a dramatic impact on the urinary excretion of chlorpropamide. In a volunteer study after ingestion of a therapeutic dose of chlorpropamide, alkalinization of the urine with sodium bicarbonate resulted in a decrease of elimination half-life from 49.7 ± 7.4 hours to 12.8 ± 1.1 hours (20). The 72-hour urinary chlorpropamide excretion increased fourfold with bicarbonate therapy. An increase in urine pH from 5 to 8 resulted in a dramatic increase in drug clearance. No studies address whether this therapy has an impact on clinical outcome. If urinary alkalinization therapy is used for a patient with chlorpropamide-induced hypoglycemia, close attention should be paid to electrolyte balance, especially potassium. Urinary alkalinization is not expected to have a significant impact on urinary clearance of other sulfonylureas.

Antidotes

The primary treatment for sulfonylurea overdose is IV dextrose or oral glucose replacement to reverse hypoglycemia. The indications for dextrose therapy are blood glucose concentrations of less than 60 mg per day or clinical hypoglycemia. The initial dose of dextrose in adults is a 50-ml bolus of IV 50% dextrose, which provides 25 g carbohydrates or approximately 100 kcal. This dose should be adequate to reverse hypoglycemia in most patients. In pediatric patients, IV dextrose should be given as 25% dextrose in water at a dose of 0.5 to 1.0 g/kg. In newborns, dextrose can be provided as a 10% solution in water at the same weight-based doses. One pediatric case series suggested that hypoglycemia from sulfonylurea overdose can be managed with oral supplementation (50).

Following the initial bolus, an IV infusion of 10% to 20% dextrose can be started and titrated to the desired blood glucose concentration. Additional dextrose bolus therapy may be required if hypoglycemia recurs. Dextrose infusion may have some benefit over repeated bolus therapy by not producing high peak glucose concentrations, which may serve as strong stimuli for additional insulin secretion, leading to rebound hypoglycemia (55). Providing the patient with high calorie content food is a physiologic and safe way to provide a significant source of calories once the initial neurologic symptoms have resolved.

Potential complications of IV dextrose administration include tissue necrosis after extravasation, volume overload, hyperglycemia, and rebound hypoglycemia. Dextrose should be given only through a patent and freely running IV line by slow bolus or infusion to avoid extravasation.

Octreotide is a long-acting synthetic analog of somatostatin. It has a number of physiologic effects, including the suppression of insulin release. In sulfonylurea-poisoned patients, it has been shown to suppress insulin release to baseline levels, resulting in lower glucose requirements and fewer episodes of rebound hypoglycemia (53,55). During short-term use, octreotide is very safe, with no significant reported side effects (55,92,93). One reasonable recommended dose is 50 to 100 mg SQ. It can be repeated every 6 to 8 hours as needed. Further information is provided in Chapter 66. Octreotide alone does not rapidly return a hypoglycemic patient to euglycemia; IV dextrose must be used first to restore the blood glucose concentrations to normal. Octreotide can be given after dextrose to prevent further episodes of hypoglycemia and reduce the need for glucose supplementation (53,55). Octreotide is indicated in any patient with recurrent hypoglycemia after sulfonylurea exposure and can be considered even in patients with a single episode of hypoglycemia.

Diazoxide is a vasodilator that has been used to treat sulfonylurea-associated hypoglycemia that is refractory to other therapy (48). Like octreotide, it appears to block insulin release; however, it seems to be less effective than octreotide (55), and dosing is more complex. Diazoxide can cause postural hypotension (94). This effect is usually not seen when the drug is given by slow infusion (95). Diazoxide should be considered in patients who do not respond to other first-line therapies, including octreotide. The dose of diazoxide is 300 mg by slow IV infusion in adults and 1 to 3 mg/kg by slow IV infusion in children.

Glucagon increases gluconeogenesis and glycogenolysis in the liver through activation of cyclic adenosine monophosphate. In patients with adequate hepatic glycogen stores, glucagon administration may increase blood glucose levels. Glucagon therapy was associated with longer times to return of normal neurologic function and a greater number of treatment failures when compared to IV dextrose in the treatment of hypoglycemia (96–98). It is of limited value in treating sulfonylurea overdose except in unusual situations. If treatment with IV dextrose is not possible, intramuscular (IM) glucagon followed by oral carbohydrates may be effective. If a suspected paradoxic hypoglycemic reaction to octreotide is observed, glucagon along with dextrose may be indicated. The adult dose of glucagon is 1 mg given IV, IM, or SQ. In children over 20 kg, the dose (IM or IV) is 0.5 mg, and in children under 20 kg, the dose is 20 to 30 mg/kg. In neonates, the dose is 50 mg/kg. Glucagon administration may be associated with nausea and vomiting.

Supportive Care

Airway management, supplemental oxygen, ventilatory support, and support of the blood pressure with IV fluids, vasopressor, and inotropic agents may be indicated in severe sulfonylurea overdose. After rapid treatment of hypoglycemia with IV dextrose, consideration should be given to administration of thiamine and naloxone. In the suicidal patient, appropriate monitoring for patient safety and psychiatric evaluation are critical.

Monitoring

Because sulfonylurea overdose can be associated with delayed onset of hypoglycemia, euglycemic adult patients with suspected or confirmed overdose should be admitted for observation and serial glucose measurements for 24 hours. In pediatric patients, the optimal period of observation is controversial. One proposed approach is to perform serial blood glucose measurements every hour for 8 hours while allowing the child to eat, but providing no additional dextrose. If hypoglycemia occurs, the child should be admitted. If the child remains euglycemic for 8 hours, he or she can be discharged (50,56,99,100). This approach has been challenged by authors with data suggesting that cases of sulfonylurea-induced hypoglycemia can present later than 8 hours from ingestion (102,103). This more conservative approach recommends 24-hour observation for all pediatric sulfonylurea exposures.

Monitoring for hypoglycemia should include observation for clinical signs of hypoglycemia and periodic blood glucose measurements. The optimal interval for blood glucose measurement has not been determined. If the patient is asymptomatic and awake, the interval between measurements can be extended. During sleep, glucose measurement every 60 minutes may be reasonable. In comatose patients or those with labile hypoglycemia, glucose measurements may need to be performed more frequently.

Management Pitfalls

Hypoglycemia should be considered as a cause of neurologic symptoms, including focal deficits. Sulfonylurea overdose should be considered in all patients with hypoglycemia of unknown cause.

Each patient should be monitored for several hours after discontinuing a dextrose infusion to detect rebound hypoglycemia. Octreotide is a useful method for treating patients with rebound. Each patient must also be monitored for a substantial period to avoid missing delayed presentation of hypoglycemia.

REFERENCES

1. Ruiz CL, Silva LL, Libenson L. Contrabucion al estudio sobre la composicion quimica de la insulina. Estudio algunos cuerpos sinteticos sulfurados con action hipoglucemiante. *Rev Soc Argent Biol* 1930;6:134–141.
2. Levine R. Sulfonylureas: background and development of the field. *Diabetes Care* 1984;7[Suppl]:S3–S7.
3. Loubatieres A. Etude physiologique et pharmacodynamique des certains derives sulfonamides hypoglycemiants. *Arch Int Physiol Biochim* 1946;54:174–177.
4. Franke H, Fuchs J. Ein neues antidiabetisches prinzip. *Deutsch Med Wochenschr* 1955;80:1449–1452.
5. Cruickshank K. Epidemiology of diabetes mellitus: noninsulin dependent diabetes mellitus. In: Pickup J, Williams G, eds. *Textbook of diabetes*, 2nd ed. Oxford: Blackwell Science, 1997: 3.17–3.28.

6. Latner AW. The top 200 drugs of 1999. *Pharmacy Times* 2000;16:16–32.
7. The Internet drug index Web site. Available at: http://www.rxlist.com/top200htm. Accessed July 2003.
8. Melander A, Donnelly R, Rydberg T. Is there a concentration-effect relationship for sulphonylureas? *Clin Pharmacokinet* 1998;34:181–188.
9. Dabelea D, Pettitt DJ, Jones KL, et al. Type 2 diabetes mellitus in minority children and adolescents. *Endocrinol Metab Clin North Am* 1999;28:709–729.
10. Asplund K, Wilholm B-E, Lithner F. Glibenclamide-associated hypoglycaemia: a report on 57 cases. *Diabetologia* 1983,24:412–417.
11. Berger W. Incidence of severe side effects during therapy with sulfonylureas and biguanides. *Horm Metab Res* 1985;15[Suppl]:111–115.
12. Burge M, Sood V, Sobhy TA, et al. Sulphonylurea-induced hypoglycemia in type 2 diabetes mellitus: a review. *Diabetes Obesity Metabolism* 1999;1:199–206.
13. Paice BJ, Paterson KR, Lawson DH. Undesired effects of the sulphonylurea drugs. *Adverse Drug Reaction and Acute Poisoning Review* 1985;1:23–36.
14. Shorr RI, Ray WA, Daugherty JR, et al. Individual susceptibility and serious hypoglycemia in older people. *J Am Geriatr Soc* 1996;44:751–755.
15. van Staa T, Abenhaim L, Monette J. Rates of hypoglycemia in users of sulfonylureas. *Clin Epidemiol* 1997;50:735–741.
16. Gerich JE. Oral hypoglycemic agents. *N Engl J Med* 1989;321:1231–1245.
17. Reference deleted.
18. Niemi M, Backman JT, Neuvonen M, et al. Effects of fluconazole and fluvoxamine on the pharmacokinetics and pharmacodynamics of glimepiride. *Clin Pharmacol Ther* 2001;69:194–200.
19. Niemi M, Backman JT, Neuvonen M, et al. Effects of rifampin on the pharmacokinetics and pharmacodynamics of glyburide and glipizide. *Clin Pharmacol Ther* 2001;69:400–406.
20. Neuvonen PJ, Kärkkäinen S. Effects of charcoal, sodium bicarbonate and ammonium chloride on chlorpropamide kinetics. *Clin Pharmacol Ther* 1983;33:386–393.
21. Harrower ADB. Pharmacokinetics of oral antihyperglycaemic agents in patients with renal insufficiency. *Clin Pharmacokinet* 1996;31:111–119.
22. Ciechanowski K, Borowiak KS, Potocka BA, et al. Chlorpropamide toxicity with survival despite 27-day hypoglycemia. *J Toxicol Clin Toxicol* 1999;37:869–871.
23. Boyd AE III. Sulfonylurea receptors, ion channels and fruit flies. *Diabetes* 1988;37:847–850.
24. Ashcroft FM, Gribble FM. ATP-sensitive K^+ channels and insulin secretion: their roles in health and disease. *Diabetologia* 1999;42:903–919.
25. Gaines KL, Hamilton S, Boyd AE III. Characterization of the sulfonylurea receptor on beta cell membranes. *J Biol Chem* 1988;263:2589–2592.
26. Schmidt-Antomarchi H, De Weille J, Fosset M, et al. The receptor for antidiabetic sulfonylureas controls the activity of the ATP-modulated K^+ channel in insulin-secreting cells. *J Biol Chem* 1987;262:15840–15844.
27. Nelson TY, Gaines KL, Rajan AS, et al. Increased cytosolic calcium: a signal for sulfonylurea-stimulated insulin release from beta cells. *J Biol Chem* 1987;262:2608–2612.
28. Eliasson L, Renstrom E, Ämmälä C, et al. PKC-dependent exocytosis by sulfonylureas in pancreatic β cells. *Science* 1996;271:813–815.
29. Landstedt-Hallin L, Adamson U, Lins P-E. Oral glibenclamide suppresses glucagon secretion during insulin-induced hypoglycemia in patients with type 2 diabetes. *J Clin Endocrinol Metab* 1999;84:3140–3145.
30. Grodsky GM, Epstein GH, Fanska R, et al. Pancreatic action of sulfonylureas. *Fed Proc* 1977;36:2714–2719.
31. Lebovitz HE, Melander A. Sulfonylureas: basic aspects and clinical uses. In: Alberti KGMM, Zimmet P, DeFronzo RA, et al., eds. *International textbook of diabetes mellitus*, 2nd ed. Chichester: John Wiley and Sons, 1997:817–840.
32. Lazdunski M. Ion channel effects of antidiabetic sulfonylureas. *Horm Metab Res* 1996;28:488–495.
33. Coetzee WA. ATP-sensitive K+ channels and myocardial ischemia: why do they open? *Cardiovasc Drugs Ther* 1992;6:201–208.
34. American Diabetes Association. Gestational diabetes mellitus. *Diabetes Care* 1998;21[Suppl 1]:S60–S61.
35. ACOG. *Diabetes and pregnancy*. ACOG technical bulletin. No. 200. Washington, DC: American College of Obstetricians and Gynecologists, December 1994:359–366.
36. Reference deleted.
37. Fanelli CG, Bolli GB. Sulphonylureas and pregnancy. *Eur J Endocrinol* 1998;138:615–616.
38. Kernball ML, McIver C, Milner RDG, et al. Neonatal hypoglycemia in infants of diabetic mothers given sulphonylurea drugs in pregnancy. *Arch Dis Child* 1970;45:696–701.
39. Miller DI, Wishinsky H, Thompson G. Transfer of tolbutamide across the human placenta. *Diabetes* 1962;11[Suppl]:93–97.
40. Farquhar JW, Isles TE. Hypoglycemia in newborn infants of normal and diabetic mothers. *South Afr Med J* 1968;42:237–245.
41. Smoak IW. Embryopathic effects of the oral hypoglycemic agent chlorpropamide in cultured mouse embryos. *Am J Obstet Gynecol* 1993;169:409–414.
42. Piacquadio K, Hollingsworth DR, Murphy H. Effects of in-utero exposure to oral hypoglycaemic drugs. *Lancet* 1991;338:866–869.
43. Schiff D, Aranda JV, Stern L. Neonatal thrombocytopenia and congenital malformations associated with administration of tolbutamide to the mother. *J Pediatr* 1970;77:457–458.
44. Langer O, Conway DL, Berkus MD, et al. A comparison of glyburide and insulin in women with gestational diabetes. *N Engl J Med* 2000;343:1134–1138.
45. Fanego L, Crumple L, Edelson GW. Seizure in a polypharmacy household. *Hosp Pract* 1992;101:104.
46. Asplund K, Wilhom BE, Lundman B. Severe hypoglycemia during treatment with glipizide. *Diabetes Med* 1991;8:726–731.
47. Sener A, Gillet C, Verhelst J, et al. Factitious hypoglycemia documented by modified assay for the measurement of plasma sulfonylurea. *Diabetes Med* 1995;12:433–435.
48. Palatnick W, Meatherall RC, Tenenbein M. Clinical spectrum of sulfonylurea overdose and experience with diazoxide therapy. *Arch Intern Med* 1991;151:1859–1862.
49. Quadrani DA, Spiller HA, Widder P. Five year retrospective evaluation of sulfonylurea ingestion in children. *J Toxicol Clin Toxicol* 1996;34:267–270.
50. Spiller HA, Villalobos D, Krenzalok EP, et al. Prospective multicenter study of sulfonylurea ingestion in children. *J Pediatr* 1997;131:141–146.
51. Spiller HA, Villalobos D, Krenzalok EP, et al. Prospective multicenter study of sulfonylurea ingestion in children. *J Toxicol Clin Toxicol* 1995;33:509.
52. Goran, B, Bo B, Martin F, et al. Glipizide induced severe hypoglycemia. *Acta Endocrinol* 1981;98:13.
53. McLaughlin SA, Crandall CS, McKinney PE. Octreotide: an antidote for sulfonylurea-induced hypoglycemia. *Ann Emerg Med* 2000;36:133–138.
54. Sonneblick M, Shilo S. Glibenclamide induced prolonged hypoglycemia. *Age Ageing* 1986;15:185–189.
55. Boyle PJ, Justice K, Krentz AJ, et al. Octreotide reverses hyperinsulinemia and prevents hypoglycemia induced by sulfonylurea overdoses. *J Clin Endocrinol Metab* 1993;76:752–756.
56. Harrigan RA, Nathan MS, Beattie P. Oral agents for the treatment of type 2 diabetes mellitus: pharmacology, toxicity and treatment. *Ann Emerg Med* 2001;38:68–78.
57. Malouf R, Brust JC. Hypoglycemia: causes, neurologic manifestations and outcome. *Ann Neurol* 1985;17:421–430.
58. Vanpee D, Donckier J, Gillet JB. Hemiplegia hypoglycemia syndrome. *Eur J Emerg Med* 1999;6:157–159.
59. Kumar S, Boulton AJM. Serious, prolonged hypoglycemia with glibenclamide in a patient with Mendenhall's syndrome. *Clin Endocrinol* 1993;39:109–111.
60. Scala-Barnett DM, Donoghue ER. Dispensing error causing fatal chlorpropamide intoxication in a non-diabetic. *J Forensic Sci* 1986;31:293–295.
61. Chan JC, Cockram CS, Critchley JA. Drug-induced disorders of glucose metabolism. Mechanisms and management. *Drug Saf* 1996;15(2):135–157.
62. Cryer PE, Gerich JE. Glucose counterregulation, hypoglycemia, and intensive insulin therapy in diabetes mellitus. *N Engl J Med* 1985;313:232–241.
63. Schwartz NE, Clutter WE, Shah SD, et al. Glycemic thresholds for activation of glucose counterregulatory systems are higher than the threshold for symptoms. *J Clin Invest* 1986;79:777–781.
64. Jennings AM, Wilson RM, Ward JD. Symptomatic hypoglycemia in NIDDM patients treated with oral hypoglycemic agents. *Diabetes Care* 1989;12:203–208.
65. Cryer PE. Hierarchy of physiological responses to hypoglycemia: relevance to clinical hypoglycemia in type 1 (insulin-dependent) diabetes mellitus. *Horm Metab Res* 1997;29:92–96.
66. Boyle PJ, Schwartz NS, Shah SD, et al. Plasma glucose concentration at the onset of hypoglycemic symptoms in patients with poorly controlled diabetes and in nondiabetics. *N Engl J Med* 1988;318:1487–1492.
67. Boyle PJ, Shah SD, Cryer PE. Insulin, glucagon and catecholamines in prevention of hypoglycemia during fasting. *Am J Physiol* 1989;19:E651–E661.
68. Kerr D, MacDonald IA, Heller SR, et al. Beta-adrenoceptor blockade and hypoglycaemia. A randomised, double-blind, placebo controlled comparison of metoprolol CR, atenolol and propranolol LA in normal subjects. *Br J Clin Pharmacol* 1990;29(6):685–693.
69. Kadowaki T, Hagura R, Kajinuma H, et al. Chlorpropamide-induced hyponatremia: incidence and risk factors. *Diabetes Care* 1983;6(5):468–471.
70. Harrower AD. Comparative tolerability of sulphonylureas in diabetes mellitus. *Drug Saf* 2000;22(4):313–320.
71. Levitt LJ. Chlorpropamide-induced pure white cell aplasia. *Blood* 1987;69:394–400.
72. Nataas OB, Nesthus I. Immune haemolytic anaemia induced by glibenclamide in selective IgA deficiency. *BMJ* 1987;295:366–367.
73. Planas AT, Kranwinkel RN, Soletsky HB, et al. Chlorpropamide-induced pure RBC aplasia. *Arch Intern Med* 1980;140:707–708.
74. Väätainen N, Fräki JE, Hyvönen M, et al. Purpura with a linear epidermodermal deposition of IgA. *Acta Derm Venereol* 1983;63:169–170.
75. Goodman RC, Dean PJ, Radparvar A, et al. Glyburide induced hepatitis. *Ann Intern Med* 1987;106:837–839.
76. Lambert M, Guebel A, Rahier J, et al. Cholestatic jaundice associated with glibenclamide therapy. *Eur J Gastroenterol Hepatol* 1990;2:389–391.
77. Barnett JH, Barnett SM. Lichenoid drug reactions to chlorpropamide and tolazamide. *Cutis* 1984;34:542–544.
78. Wongpatoon V, Mills PR, Russell PI, et al. Intrahepatic cholestasis and cutaneous bullae associated with glibenclamide therapy. *Postgrad Med J* 1981;57:244–246.
79. University Group Diabetes Program. A study of the effects of hypoglycemic agents on vascular complications in patients with adult onset diabetes. *Diabetes* 1970;19[Suppl 2]:747–830.
80. Gögelein H. Inhibition of cardiac ATP-dependent potassium channels by sulfonylurea drugs. *Curr Opin Invest Drugs* 2001;2:72–80.

81. Howes LG, Sundaresan P, Lykos D. Cardiovascular effects of oral hypoglycaemic drugs. *Clin Exp Pharmacol Physiol* 1996;23:201–206.
82. Sartor G, Melander A, Scherstén B, et al. Serum glibenclamide in diabetic patients, and influence of food: the kinetics and effects of glibenclamide. *Diabetologia* 1980;18:17–22.
83. Lehr KH, Damm P. Simultaneous determination of the sulfonylurea glimepiride and its metabolites in human serum and urine by high performance liquid chromatography after pre-column derivitization. *J Chromatogr* 1990;526:497–505.
84. Ostman J, Jannson B, Weiner L. Relationship between therapeutic effect and bioavailability of glipizide in maturity onset diabetes mellitus. *Excerpta Medica International Congress* Ser 481, 1979(abst).
85. Magni F, Marazzini L, Pereira S, et al. Identification of sulfonylureas in serum by electrospray mass spectrometry. *Ann Biochem* 2000;282:136–141.
86. Kannisto H, Neuvonen PJ. Adsorption of sulfonylureas onto activated charcoal in vitro. *J Pharm Sci* 1984;73:253–256.
87. Kivistö KT, Neuvonen PJ. The effect of cholestyramine and activated charcoal on glipizide absorption. *Br J Clin Pharmacol* 1990;30:733–736.
88. Neuvonen PJ, Kannisto H, Hirvisalo EL. Effect of charcoal on absorption of tolbutamide and valproate in man. *Br J Clin Pharmacol* 1983;24:243–246.
89. Davis TME, Daly F, Walsh JP, et al. Pharmacokinetics and pharmacodynamics of gliclazide in Caucasians and Australian aborigines with type 2 diabetes. *Br J Clin Pharmacol* 2000;49:223–230.
90. Ludwig SM, McKenzie J, Faiman C. Chlorpropamide overdose in renal failure: management with charcoal hemoperfusion. *Am J Kidney Dis* 1987;10:457–460.
91. Graw RG, Clarke RR. Chlorpropamide intoxication—treatment with peritoneal dialysis. *Pediatrics* 1070;40:106–109.
92. Barrons RW. Octreotide in hyperinsulinism. *Ann Pharmacother* 1997;31:239–241.
93. Wass JAH, Popovic V, Chayvialle JA. Proceedings of the discussion, "Tolerability and safety of sandostatin." *Metabolism* 1992;41:80–82.
94. Koch-Weser J. Drug therapy: diazoxide. *N Engl J Med* 1976;294:1271–1274.
95. Johnson SF, Schade DS, Peake GT. Chlorpropamide-induced hypoglycemia. Successful treatment with diazoxide. *Am J Med* 1977;63:799–804.
96. Collier A, Steedman DJ, Patrick AW, et al. Comparison of intravenous glucagon and dextrose in treatment of severe hypoglycemia in an accident and emergency department. *Diabetes Care* 1987;10:12–15.
97. Howell MA, Guly HR. A comparison of glucagon and glucose in prehospital hypoglycemia. *J Accident Emerg Med* 1997;14:30–32.
98. Patrick AW, Collier A, Hepburn DA, et al. Comparison of intramuscular glucagon and intravenous dextrose in the treatment of hypoglycemic coma in an accident and emergency department. *Arch Emerg Med* 1990;7:73–77.
99. Burkhart KK. When does hypoglycemia develop after sulfonylurea ingestion? *Ann Emerg Med* 1998;31:771–772.
100. Spiller HA. Management of sulfonylurea ingestions. *Pediatr Emerg Care* 1999;15:227–230.
101. Reference deleted.
102. Borowski H, Caraccio T, Mofenson H. Sulfonylurea ingestion in children: is an 8-hour observation period sufficient? *J Pediatr* 1998;133:584.
103. Szlatenyi CS, Capes KF, Wang RY. Delayed hypoglycemia in a child after ingestion of a single glipizide tablet. *Ann Emerg Med* 1998;31:773–776.

CHAPTER 159

Metformin (Biguanides)

E. Martin Caravati and Henry A. Spiller

METFORMIN

Compounds included:	**Buformin hydrochloride (Silubin), metformin hydrochloride (Diabetase, Diabex, Glucophage), phenformin hydrochloride**
Molecular formula and weight:	**Buformin hydrochloride: $C_6H_{15}N_5HCl$, 157.2 g/mol; metformin hydrochloride: $C_4H_{11}N_5HCl$, 165.6 g/mol; phenformin hydrochloride: $C_{10}H_{15}N_5,HCl$, 241.7 g/mol**
SI conversion:	**mg/L × 7.74 = μmol/L**
CAS Registry No.:	**1190-53-0 (buformin hydrochloride); 1115-70-4 (metformin hydrochloride); 834-28-6 (phenformin hydrochloride)**
Therapeutic levels:	**Metformin, 1 to 2 mg/L (serum), not readily available**
Target organs:	**Lactic acidosis**
Antidote:	**None**

OVERVIEW

Biguanides are antihyperglycemic drugs that are used to treat diabetes mellitus. They include metformin, phenformin, and buformin and are sold throughout the world, including Australia, Germany, the United Kingdom, and South Africa. Metformin hydrochloride (Glucophage) is the only agent approved for use in the United States. Buformin is available in Europe, and its toxicology is expected to be the same as that of metformin. Phenformin was removed from the U.S. market in 1977 due to the relatively high incidence of lactic acidosis that occurred during therapeutic use. Although rare, lactic acidosis may also occur after overdose or with therapeutic use of metformin. This chapter focuses primarily on metformin toxicity.

Metformin is *N*-1,1-dimethylbiguanide hydrochloride. It is used primarily in the treatment of type II diabetes (non-insulin–

dependent diabetes) but also as a lipid-lowering agent and in the treatment of obesity for patients with non-insulin–dependent diabetes mellitus. Biguanides can be used alone or in combination with oral hypoglycemics or insulin. They are available as single-agent 500-mg, 850-mg, or 1000-mg oral tablets, as an extended-release 500-mg tablet (Glucophage XR), and in combination with glyburide (Glucovance).

TOXIC DOSE

The initial adult therapeutic dosage is 500 mg twice a day of the regular-release tablets or one 500-mg extended-release tablet once a day. Subsequent dosing is adjusted to patient response. The pediatric dose is the same (ages above 10 years). The minimum toxic dose is not well established. An overdose of 25 g induced lactic acidosis in an 82-year-old patient (1). After a young male adult ingested 5 to 6 g metformin, diarrhea developed but no acidosis or hypoglycemia (2). Buformin has been associated with the death of an 84-year-old diabetic woman during therapeutic use. The buformin serum concentration was 5.5 mg/L on admission (3).

A poison control center study of potential unintentional ingestion of 250 to 500 mg metformin in 29 nondiabetic children under the age of 6 years resulted in only mild gastrointestinal effects in 5 patients. An additional 12 patients potentially ingested greater than 500 mg. Symptoms of hypoglycemia or acidosis did not develop in any child (4). Ingestion of one pill by adult or child is not expected to produce effects unless a child ingests the combination product with glyburide.

TOXICOKINETICS AND TOXICODYNAMICS

Metformin oral bioavailability is 50% to 60%. Absorption is slow and complete within 6 hours. The peak plasma concentration occurs approximately 2 to 4 hours after an oral dose of regular tablets and within 7 hours for extended-release tablets (range, 4 to 8 hours). Control of plasma glucose may occur in a few days, but maximum antihyperglycemic effect may be delayed up to 2 weeks on therapeutic doses. Metformin is negligibly bound to plasma proteins. The average apparent volume of distribution is 654 L.

Metformin is primarily eliminated by renal excretion (35% to 52% unchanged). The principal plasma elimination half-life ranges from 3 to 6 hours; 90% of the drug is cleared within 24 hours by patients with normal renal function. Elimination is prolonged with renal impairment and increasing age and results in higher peak plasma concentration with repeated dosing.

PATHOPHYSIOLOGY

The biguanides exert their pharmacologic effects by a similar basic mechanism. Metformin acts in the presence of insulin to increase peripheral glucose utilization, decrease hepatic gluconeogenesis, and decrease intestinal absorption of glucose (5). Metformin requires insulin for its action but does not induce an elevation in plasma insulin levels, which explains the absence of hypoglycemia in diabetic and nondiabetic patients. The biguanides do not usually lower the blood glucose in a normal patient unless ethanol or another hypoglycemic agent is simultaneously ingested (6) or severe hepatic insufficiency is present (7). Metformin generally lowers the blood glucose only in the diabetic patient. It depresses the blood sugar level in a nutritionally starved individual but not in one who is well fed (8). In its usual dose administered to a healthy individual, metformin does not induce lactic acidosis (9).

Metformin also improves plasma lipid concentrations and promotes weight loss (10). It may also increase tissue-type plasminogen activator activity that is independent of insulin. Biguanides may induce elevations in the lactate-pyruvate ratio (normally 10:1), the hydroxybutyrate-acetoacetate ratio, the concentration of 3-β-hydroxybutyrate, the alanine-pyruvate ratio, and free fatty acids.

LACTIC ACIDOSIS

Lactic acidosis was first clearly defined and classified by Huckabee (11). Although it has been produced by all three biguanides (12), the incidence is by far the greatest after phenformin use (13). The origins of lactic acidosis are still the subject of investigation; however, phenformin may act on the cell membranes to decrease oxidative phosphorylation, produce tissue anoxia, and increase peripheral glucose uptake (Pasteur effect), leading to lactic acidosis and hypoglycemia (14,15).

PREGNANCY AND LACTATION

Metformin is U.S. Food and Drug Administration pregnancy category B (Appendix I). Metformin crosses the placenta. It has been used as monotherapy for diabetes mellitus in pregnancy with no reports of lactic acidosis or neonatal hypoglycemia. Because of its low molecular weight, it is likely excreted into breast milk, exposing the nursing infant; effects, however, are unknown (16).

CLINICAL PRESENTATION

Acute Overdosage

Acute overdosage often causes no toxicity. If it occurs, acidosis usually develops within several hours of ingestion. Nausea, vomiting, diarrhea, abdominal cramps (17), anorexia, epigastric discomfort and pain, metallic taste, abdominal distention, and hematemesis (18) have been seen in patients with phenformin and metformin poisoning.

In patients in whom severe acidosis develops, agitation, confusion, absent corneal reflexes (6), fixed dilated pupils, lethargy, seizures (6), extensor plantar reflexes, coma (19), and death have occurred. The patient may have rapid, deep respiratory efforts, and pulmonary hypertension has been observed (20). Tachycardia, hypotension (19), and myocardial infarction have occurred (21).

Rare leukocytoclastic vasculitis has been induced by metformin (22). Hemolytic anemia and jaundice associated with metformin use developed in two patients (23).

Adverse Events

Life-threatening and fatal lactic acidosis has occurred with therapeutic use. Two types of metformin-associated lactic acidosis occur. Type I is associated with high lactate and metformin levels, anuria, and low mortality. Type II is associated with tissue hypoxia, normal metformin levels, moderate lactate, and high mortality (23).

The estimated incidence of metformin-related lactic acidosis is approximately one-tenth to one-twentieth that reported with phenformin, or 0.03 cases/1000 patient-years (10). Impaired renal function is the predominant condition associated with the development of lactic acidosis. Other predisposing conditions are hepatic dysfunction, cardiac failure, and alcohol abuse. Early symptoms of lactic acidosis during therapeutic use are nausea, vomiting, diarrhea, and lower abdominal pain. The diagnosis of nonketotic metabolic acidosis may be an early indication of lactic acidosis in patients who are taking biguanides.

Biguanide-induced lactic acidosis has a high mortality (18% to 52%) (12). This rate is lessened if patients are not older than 60 years; do not have cardiovascular, hepatic, renal, or infectious disease; and have not experienced other conditions that lead to increased lactate production, such as shock, diabetic ketoacidosis, surgery, pulmonary insufficiency, alcoholism, weight reduction, or fasting. Death may occur after serum bicarbonate and pH levels have been corrected if the serum lactate level is still elevated (11).

Dose-related gastrointestinal effects, such as nausea, vomiting, diarrhea, and abdominal cramps, are common (24) and may cause dehydration. Headache, agitation, and dizziness have also been reported. Hypoglycemia does not occur with metformin alone but may be observed when the drug is given in combination with sulfonylurea or alcohol (25).

Alcohol potentiates the antihyperglycemic and hyperlactatemic effects of metformin (26). Cationic drugs (e.g., amiloride, digoxin, morphine, procainamide, quinidine, quinine, ranitidine, triamterene, trimethoprim, and vancomycin) that are eliminated by renal tubular secretion theoretically have the potential to interact with metformin by competing for common renal tubular transport systems. Certain drugs tend to produce hyperglycemia and may lead to loss of glycemic control: corticosteroids, oral contraceptives, phenytoin, nicotinic acid, sympathomimetics, calcium channel-blocking drugs, and isoniazid. Cimetidine increases peak plasma concentrations by 60%.

DIAGNOSTIC TESTS

A complete blood count, serum electrolytes (sodium, potassium, chloride, bicarbonate), creatinine, glucose, and lactate should be obtained in patients who have ingested an acute overdose or in symptomatic patients on chronic therapy. An arterial blood gas may be needed to assess blood pH. An increased anion gap metabolic acidosis may be due to lactic acidemia. Serum lactate determination is required to make the diagnosis of metformin-associated lactic acidosis. Arterial blood gases and electrolytes may reflect a high anion gap metabolic acidosis.

The therapeutic metformin plasma concentration is 1 to 2 mg/L; however, levels are not available for clinical management. Lactate and metformin concentrations are not prognostic with respect to mortality (27). No correlation has been found between plasma lactate concentration and plasma metformin concentration at therapeutic drug levels (28). Gas-liquid chromatography (29), high-pressure liquid chromatography (30), and mass fragmentography (28) are highly specific and sensitive methodologies for metformin concentration.

Metabolic acidosis with a high anion gap must be evaluated carefully (Chapter 9). Lactic acidosis should be confirmed by plasma or blood lactate concentrations and by excluding other causes of metabolic acidosis. Lactic acidosis may be either primary, secondary to diseases associated with hypoxemia, or idiopathic in onset (31). Laboratory findings may include anion gap metabolic acidosis, low serum bicarbonate and pH, elevated serum potassium, normal or depressed serum chloride, and increased blood lactate.

In biguanide-induced lactic acidosis, blood glucose concentrations may be depressed (6), normal (17), or elevated. Hypoglycemia is not seen in isolated metformin overdose (2,4). Some children and adults have had severe acidosis with normal blood sugar levels (32). Early reports indicated that phenformin could produce acidosis without warning in adult patients whose blood glucose concentrations were within normal limits and who had no glycosuria (33). A leukocytosis (20,000 to 60,000 cells/ml) is frequently observed. Thrombocytopenia may be present (20). Plasma insulin levels are usually not elevated.

Bilateral hypodensity and swelling of the lentiform nucleus (basal ganglia) have been seen on computed tomographic scan (34). This is a nonspecific finding and may also occur from methanol, carbon monoxide, and cyanide poisoning.

TREATMENT

Treatment involves termination of exposure and providing intensive supportive care. Hemodialysis may be useful in selected cases.

Decontamination

Gastric lavage or a single dose of activated charcoal may be useful in preventing absorption shortly after acute single ingestion. Neither has been systematically studied, however.

Enhancement of Elimination

No data are available demonstrating that multiple-dose activated charcoal is effective. This method would probably not enhance clearance appreciably because of its large volume of distribution. Hemoperfusion has not been evaluated in the treatment of biguanide-induced lactic acidosis.

Hemodialysis is the treatment of choice for metformin-induced severe lactic acidosis (35). Metformin is removed by hemodialysis with a clearance of up to 170 ml/minute. The decision to use hemodialysis is based on the patient's clinical condition and degree of acidosis. Forcing fluids may be counterproductive and result in fluid overload. Althoff et al. (36) dialyzed nine diabetic patients under treatment for biguanide-induced lactic acidosis, five of whom had had no prior renal disease; seven lived. They observed that hemodialysis, in addition to rapid removal of biguanide and excess lactate, permitted adequate amounts of sodium bicarbonate to be given without risking fluid overload or hypernatremia (36). Heaney et al. (37) described a 29-year-old patient with central nervous system depression, serum glucose of 0.6 mmol/L, bicarbonate of 17 mmol/L, and creatinine of 167 mmol/L after ingesting quantities of metformin, glyburide, and nabumetone. Over 3 hours, the bicarbonate decreased to 2 mmol/L, and the serum lactate increased to 31 mmol/L. No evidence of tissue hypoxia was found. Hemodialysis with a sodium bicarbonate buffer was performed for 10 hours, and the postdialysis serum lactate was 3.7 mmol/L. In this case, hemodialysis with bicarbonate dialysate allowed clearance of metformin and bicarbonate to be given without the associated risks of intravenous bicarbonate administration. The metformin serum concentration may quickly rebound secondary to redistribution (38).

Antidotes

No specific antidotes are available for metformin. Hypoglycemia secondary to concomitant sulfonylurea ingestion is treated immediately with 50 ml 50% glucose intravenously in adults. In children the initial dose is 0.5 to 1.0 g/kg 25% dextrose (a 1:1 dilution of 50% dextrose and sterile water). Glucagon, 1 mg intravenously, had no effect on increasing blood sugar in one study (39). Toxic doses of phenformin may depress hepatic gluconeogenesis, and glucagon-induced hepatic glycogenolysis to raise blood glucose levels may not occur (40).

Supportive Care

Supportive care should be provided by assuring an intact airway and correcting hemodynamic instability, electrolyte disturbances, acid-base imbalance, dehydration, and hypoxia. Underlying co-morbid disease that may have predisposed the patient to acidosis should be treated. Dehydration and hypovolemia may require placement of a central venous line.

Hypotension is treated with infusion of 10 to 20 ml/kg isotonic crystalloidal fluid. Fluids that contain lactate should be avoided. Vasopressor amines (dopamine, norepinephrine) may increase lactic acid production by producing a relative hypoxia of the skeletal muscles and should be used cautiously with blood lactate monitoring.

Lactic acidosis may respond to fluid resuscitation with normal saline if the patient is clinically dehydrated. The use of bicarbonate for acidosis is controversial because paradoxic acidification of the cerebrospinal fluid, volume overload, hypernatremia, and increased cellular membrane permeability to biguanides may occur. Supplemental sodium bicarbonate (1 to 2 mEq/kg initial bolus) is administered to correct serum pH to 7.25 to 7.5. Doses of 44 to 50 mEq every 15 minutes may be needed (41). The patient may require 200 to 400 mEq sodium bicarbonate (31).

Monitoring

Monitoring of arterial blood gases, serum sodium, chloride, potassium, creatinine, and the electrocardiogram is important when administering sodium bicarbonate. These tests should be obtained shortly after bolus bicarbonate therapy is given to detect hypernatremia, hyper- or hypokalemia, and alterations in acid-base status. Further doses of bicarbonate or the need for hemodialysis for intractable acidosis are determined by monitoring these parameters every 2 hours until the patient's condition is stable.

REFERENCES

1. McLellan J. Recovery from metformin overdose. *Diabetic Med* 1985;2:410–411.
2. Brady WJ, Carter CT. Metformin overdose [Letter]. *Am J Emerg Med* 1997;15:107-108.
3. Verdonck LF, Sangster B, Van Heifst AN, et al. Buformin concentrations in a case of fatal lactic acidosis. *Diabetologia* 1981;20(1):45-46.
4. Spiller HA, Weber JA, Winter ML, et al. Multicenter case series of pediatric metformin ingestion. *Ann Pharmacother* 2000;34(12):1385-1388.
5. Czyzyk A, Tawecki J, Sadowski J, et al. Effect of biguanides on intestinal absorption of glucose. *Diabetes* 1968;17:492–498.
6. Davidson MB, Bozarth WR, Challoner DR, et al. Phenformin hypoglycemia and lactic acidosis: report of attempted suicide. *N Engl J Med* 1966;275:886–888.
7. Fajans SS, Moorhouse JA, Doorenbos H, et al. Metabolic effects of phenethylbiguanide in normal subjects and in diabetic patients. *Diabetes* 1960;9:194–201.
8. Lyngsoe J, Trap-Jensen J. Phenformin induced hypoglycaemia in normal subjects. *BMJ* 1969;2:224–226.
9. Guttler F, Petersen FB, Kjeldsen K. Influence of phenformin on blood lactic acid in normal and diabetic subjects during exercise. *Diabetes* 1973;12:420–423.
10. DeFronzo RA, Goodman AM, Multicenter Metformin Study Group. Efficacy of metformin in patients with non-insulin-dependent diabetes mellitus. *N Engl J Med* 1995; 333:541–549.
11. Huckabee WE. Lactic acidosis. *Am J Cardiol* 1963;12:663–666.
12. Luft D, Schmulling RM, Eggstein M. Lactic acidosis in biguanide treated diabetes: a review of 330 cases. *Diabetologia* 1978;14:75–78.
13. Biron P. Metformin monitoring. *Can Med Assoc J* 1980;123:11–12.
14. Bernier GM, Miller M, Sporingate CS. Lactic acid and phenformin hydrochloride. *JAMA* 1963;184:43–46.
15. Tranquada RE, Bernstein S, Martin HE. Irreversible lactic acidosis associated with phenformin therapy. *JAMA* 1963;184:37–42.
16. Brigg GG, Freeman RK, Yaffe SJ. *Drugs in pregnancy and lactation.* Baltimore: Williams & Wilkins, 1998:687-690.
17. Dobson HL. Attempted suicide with phenformin. *Diabetes* 1965;14:811–812.
18. Pashley NRT, Felix RH. Phenformin overdose. *BMJ* 1972;1:112–113.
19. Bingle JP, Storey GW, Winter JM. Fatal self poisoning with phenformin. *BMJ* 1970;3:752.
20. Bergman U, Boman G, Wiholm B-E. Epidemiology of adverse drug reactions to phenformin and metformin. *BMJ* 1978;2:464–466.
21. UGDP. A study of the effects of hypoglycemic agents on vascular complications in patients with adult onset diabetes: V. Evaluation of phenformin therapy. *Diabetes* 1975; 24[Suppl 1]:65–184.
22. Klapholz L, Leitersdorf E, Weinrauch L. Leucocytoclastic vasculitis and pneumonitis induced by metformin. *BMJ* 1986;293:483.
23. Lin KD, Lin JD, Juang JH. Metformin-induced hemolysis with jaundice. *N Engl J Med* 1998;339:1860-1861.
24. Crofford OB. Metformin. *N Engl J Med* 1995;333:588–589.
25. Campbell IW. Metformin and the sulphonylureas: the comparative risk. *Horm Metab Res Suppl Ser* 1984;15:105–111.
26. Schaffalitsky de Muckadell OB, Mortensen H, Lyngsoe J. Metabolic effects of glucocorticoid and ethanol administration in phenformin and metformin-treated obese diabetics. *Acta Med Scand* 1979;206:269–273.
27. Lalau JD, Race JM. Lactic acidosis in metformin-treated patients. Prognostic value of arterial lactate levels and plasma metformin concentrations. *Drug Saf* 1999;20(4):377-384.
28. Sirtori CR, Franceschini G, Galli-Kienle M, et al. Disposition of metformin (*N,N*-demethyl-biguanide) in man. *Clin Pharmacol Ther* 1978;24:683–693.
29. Tucker GT, Casey C, Phillips PJ, et al. Metformin kinetics in healthy subjects and in patients with diabetes mellitus. *Br J Clin Pharmacol* 1981;12:235–246.
30. Charles BG, Jacobsen NW, Ravencroft PJ. Rapid liquid chromatographic determination of metformin P in plasma and urine. *Clin Chem* 1981;27:434–436.
31. Medical Staff Conference. Lactic acidosis. *Calif Med* 1969;110:330–336.
32. Walker RS, Lindon AL. Phenethyldiguanide: a dangerous side effect. *BMJ* 1959;2:1005–1006.
33. McGavack TH. Discussion. *Diabetes* 1958;7:91–92.
34. Mewborne JD, Ricci PE, Appel RG. Cranial CT findings in metformin (Glucophage)-induced lactic acidosis. *J Comput Assist Tomogr* 1998;22:528-529.
35. Lalau JD, Andrejak M, Moriniere P, et al. Hemodialysis in the treatment of lactic acidosis in diabetics treated by metformin: a study of metformin elimination. *Int J Clin Pharmacol Ther Toxicol* 1989;27(6):285–288.
36. Althoff P-H, Fassbinder W, Neubauer M, et al. Hamodialyse bei der Behandlung der Biguanid-induzierten Lactacidose. *Dtsch Med Wochenschr* 1978;103:61–68.
37. Heaney D, Majid A, Junor B. Bicarbonate haemodialysis as a treatment of metformin overdose. *Nephrol Dial Transplant* 1997;12:1046-1047.
38. Pearlman BL, Fenves AZ, Emmett M. Metformin-associated lactic acidosis. *Am J Med* 1996;101:109-110.
39. Marri G, Cozzolino G, Palumbo R. Glucagon in sulphonylurea hypoglycemia. *Lancet* 1968;1:303–304.
40. Taylor JR, Sherratt HSA, Davies DM. Intramuscular or intravenous glucagon for sulphonylurea hypoglycaemia. *Eur J Clin Pharmacol* 1978;14:125–127.
41. Johnson HK, Waterhouse C. Lactic acidosis and phenformin. *Arch Intern Med* 1968;122:367–370.

CHAPTER 160

Other Oral Antidiabetic Drugs

Henry A. Spiller

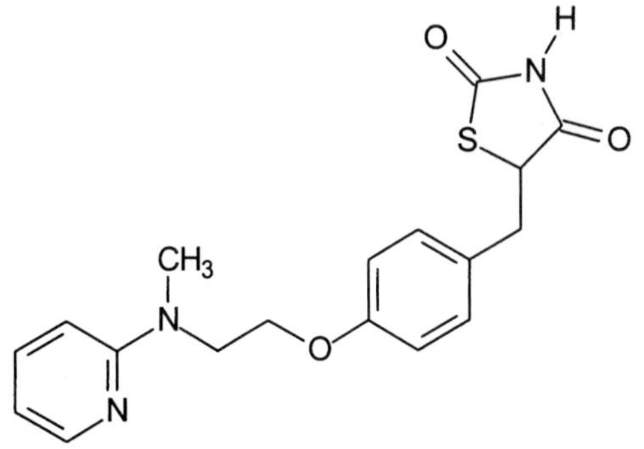

ROSIGLITAZONE

Compounds included:	**Glinides: Repaglinide (Prandin, Novonorm), nateglinide (Starlix); α-glucosidase inhibitors: acarbose (Precose, Glucobay), miglitol (Diastabol, Glyset); thiazoladinedione drugs: pioglitazone (Actos), rosiglitazone (Avandia), troglitazone**
Molecular formula and weight:	**See Table 1.**
SI conversion:	**See Table 1.**
CAS Registry No.:	**See Table 1.**
Therapeutic levels:	**Not used clinically**
Target organs:	**Glinides (pancreas), α-glucosidase inhibitors (liver injury), thiazoladinedione drugs (liver failure)**
Antidotes:	**Glinides: glucose, octreotide; α-glucosidase inhibitors: none; thiazoladinedione drugs: none**

OVERVIEW

Diabetes mellitus is generally divided into insulin-dependent diabetes mellitus (IDDM, type 1) and non-IDDM (NIDDM, type 2). It is a disorder characterized by impaired insulin secretion and insulin resistance. In general, approximately 15% of patients with diabetes have IDDM (1). Approximately 80% of patients have NIDDM, and about 5% who appear to have NIDDM may actually have a slowly progressive form of IDDM (2). The drugs that are used to treat diabetes are diverse and involve several classes. However, these drugs can be roughly separated into hypoglycemic agents, such as insulin, the sulfonylureas, and repaglinide, and antihyperglycemic agents, such as the α-glucosidase inhibitors and the glitazones. The effects seen in overdose tend to be an exacerbation of the side effects of these drugs that are seen in lower doses. The biguanide antidiabetic agents are addressed in Chapter 159.

GLINIDES

Nateglinide and repaglinide are chemically distinct amino acid derivatives that are approved for the treatment of type 2 diabetes. The glinides act on the sulfonylurea receptor, closing the potassium channel in the pancreatic β-cell and allowing depolarization of the cell membrane, opening of the voltage-sensitive calcium channel, and ultimately, release of preformed insulin. The glinides are absorbed rapidly, with short onset and short duration, making them suitable for administration prandially. They can be administered on a one-meal one-tablet, no-meal no-tablet basis. The rapid clearance and lack of accumulation are suggested to reduce the risk of between-meal and nocturnal hypoglycemia. Hypoglycemia was reported in one case of repeated surreptitious ingestion of repaglinide (3). The major risk from ingestion of one of the glinides is hypoglycemia secondary to hyperinsulinemia.

Toxic Dose

The adult and pediatric therapeutic doses are provided in Table 1. A toxic dose has not been established for adults or children. Repeated surreptitious ingestion of unknown amounts of repaglinide caused multiple episodes of hypoglycemia in an 18-year-old male, with a measured glucose concentration as low as 1 mmol/L (18 mg/dl). Serum repaglinide levels measured 4.8 to 20.7 ng/ml (3). The patient experienced lethargy, seizures, and coma during the periods of hypoglycemia.

Toxicokinetics and Toxicodynamics

After oral administration, peak repaglinide and nateglinide concentrations occur in 30 minutes to 1 hour (4), with a bioavailability of 60%. Both drugs are highly protein bound (over 98%) and extensively metabolized in the liver, primarily by CYP3A4 and CYP2C9 (5,6). Onset and duration of clinical effects are 30 minutes and less than 4 hours, respectively, for repaglinide and nateglinide. For rep-

TABLE 1. Physical characteristics and dosage of other oral antidiabetic agents

Agent	Molecular formula, molecular weight (g/mol), CAS Registry No.	SI conversion	Formulations	Therapeutic dose: Adult	Therapeutic dose: Pediatric
Glinides					
Repaglinide	$C_{27}H_{36}N_2O_4$, 452.6, 135062-02-1	mg/L × 2.2 = μmol/L	0.5-, 1.0-, 2.0-mg tablets	0.5–2.0 mg, 2–4 times daily	Dose not established
Nateglinide	$C_{19}H_{27}NO_3$, 317.4, 105816-04-4	mg/L × 3.1 = μmol/L	60-, 120-mg tablets	60–120 mg 3 times daily	Dose not established
α-Glucosidase inhibitors					
Acarbose	$C_{25}H_{43}NO_{18}$, 645.6, 56180-94-0	mg/L × 1.5 = μmol/L	25-, 50-, 100-mg tablets	25–300 mg/d, depending on weight	Dose not established
Miglitol	$C_8H_{17}NO_5$, 207.2, 72432-03-2	mg/L × 4.8 = μmol/L	25-, 50-, 100-mg tablets	25–100 mg 3 times daily	Dose not established
Thiazolidinediones					
Pioglitazone	$C_{19}H_{20}N_2O_3S{,}HCl$; 392.9; 112529-15-4	mg/L × 2.5 = μmol/L	15-, 30-, 45-mg tablets	15–45 mg/d, once a day, maximum dose 45 mg	Dose not established
Rosiglitazone	$C_{18}H_{19}N_3O_3S{,}C_4H_4O_4$; 473.5; 155141-29-0	mg/L × 2.1 = μmol/L	2-, 4-, 8-mg tablets	4–8 mg/d, once a day, maximum dose 8 mg	Dose not established
Troglitazone	$C_{24}H_{27}NO_5S$, 441.5, 97322-87-7	mg/L × 2.3 = μmol/L	Discontinued	Discontinued	Discontinued

aglinide, drugs that induce CYP3A4, such as rifampin, carbamazepine, or phenytoin, may reduce plasma drug concentrations of repaglinide as well as the clinical response to the drug (5).

Pathophysiology

The effects of glinide toxicity are essentially the same as those of the sulfonylureas with the exception of a more rapid onset and shorter duration. Repaglinide and nateglinide primarily cause serum glucose reduction by stimulating the release of preformed insulin from the pancreatic islets. In a manner similar to that of glucose and the sulfonylureas, the glinides reduce conductance through the adenosine triphosphate–sensitive potassium channel on the β-cells of the pancreatic islets (7,8). This action, in turn, causes a change in the cell membrane potential, signaling the voltage-sensitive calcium channel to open. Rapid calcium influx occurs with intracellular kinase activation and release of preformed insulin from secretory granules (Fig. 1). The central nervous system is the most sensitive organ system to the rapid drop in blood glucose, secondary to the hyperinsulinemia.

Pregnancy and Lactation

Repaglinide and nateglinide are both U.S. Food and Drug Administration (FDA) category C (Appendix I). The American College of Obstetricians and Gynecologists recommends that insulin be used for type I and type II diabetes that occurs during pregnancy if diet therapy alone is not successful for gestational diabetes.

Clinical Presentation

Limited data are available on acute overdose. An 18-year-old male experienced lethargy, coma, and seizures after multiple surreptitious ingestions of repaglinide without meals (3). The cascade of symptoms from a repaglinide or nateglinide overdose reflects the patient's hypoglycemic state. Initial symptoms may include restlessness, diaphoresis, altered mental status, combative behavior, tremors, or confusion. This may be followed by increasing central nervous system depression, seizures, and coma if the blood glucose continues to fall. Onset of symptoms is expected to be rapid (within 30 minutes) and duration short (less than 8 hours). Toxicity from chronic use is not expected because of its rapid clearance and lack of accumulation (9).

Diagnostic Tests

The blood glucose should be monitored frequently, similar to sulfonylurea overdosage. The appropriate duration of blood glucose monitoring has not been established.

The serum concentration can be measured but is not widely available. Therapeutic use of glinide agents is guided by fasting glucose levels and glycosylated hemoglobin. For repaglinide

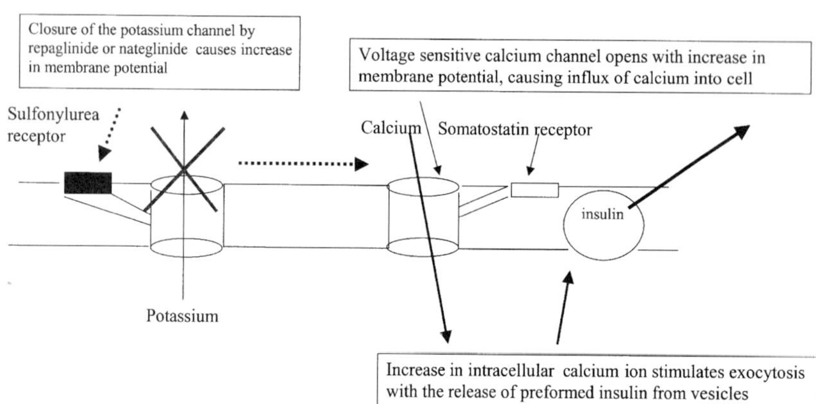

Figure 1. Mechanism of action for glinide-induced release of insulin.

peak serum levels of 15, 25, and 51 ng/ml were obtained after 0.5, 1.0, and 2.0 mg ingestion, respectively. For nateglinide, plasma levels of 3.5 mg/ml and 2.0 mg/ml were obtained after administration of 60 mg nateglinide, 10 minutes before a meal or with food, respectively.

Treatment

In the suicidal patient with a massive ingestion, onset of hypoglycemia is expected to be rapid. Initial observation of these patients for 2 to 4 hours after ingestion for onset of hypoglycemia may be warranted. Treatment is aimed primarily at restoring euglycemia. Toxicity from chronic use is not expected because of its rapid clearance and lack of accumulation (9).

DECONTAMINATION

Activated charcoal is expected to bind repaglinide and nateglinide and should be administered. Because of the rapid absorption and short duration of these drugs, charcoal would not be warranted if more than 2 to 4 hours has passed since ingestion.

ENHANCEMENT OF ELIMINATION

Data are not available, but repaglinide and nateglinide are unlikely to be amenable to extracorporeal elimination due to their high degree of protein binding.

ANTIDOTES

Oral glucose or intravenous glucose supplementation is sufficient to maintain euglycemia in the majority of cases. Occasional boluses of 25% dextrose or 50% dextrose may be necessary. In patients who are refractory to glucose supplementation, it may be necessary to reduce insulin secretion. Octreotide, a long-acting somatostatin analog, is capable of inhibiting glucose-stimulated β-cell insulin release (Chapter 66). Octreotide can be given subcutaneously or intravenously at a dose of 50 to 100 mg for adults and 1 mg/kg for children.

α-GLUCOSIDASE INHIBITORS

Acarbose is a complex pseudotetrasaccharide obtained from the fermentation processes of the microorganism *Actinoplanes utahensis* (10,11). Acarbose competitively and reversibly inhibits the α-glucosidase enzymes (glucoamylase, sucrase, maltase, and isomaltase) in the brush border in the small intestine, which delays the hydrolysis of complex carbohydrates. Judging from published reports of clinical trials and pharmacokinetic data, it seems unlikely that acarbose will cause significant injury in overdose.

Toxic Dose

The adult and pediatric therapeutic dosages are provided in Table 1. No reports of acarbose overdose have been published.

TOXICOKINETICS AND TOXICODYNAMICS

Less than 2% of acarbose is absorbed as the parent drug, possibly secondary to its large molecular size (12). Unabsorbed acarbose is metabolized extensively in the gut, with about 34% absorbed. Approximately 50% is excreted in the feces. Because acarbose acts locally, its pharmacologic effects are not dependent on systemic absorption. Reported side effects are primarily gastrointestinal in nature: bloating, flatulence, diarrhea, and abdominal pain (11,13–15). Miglitol is rapidly and completely absorbed in low doses, but at higher doses a saturation of absorption becomes evident (16). No protein binding occurs, and it is cleared renally without apparent hepatic biotransformation (16). It has an estimated half-life of 0.4 to 1.8 hours.

Pregnancy and Lactation

Acarbose and miglitol are FDA pregnancy category B (Appendix I). Entry into breast milk has not been reported for either agent.

Clinical Presentation

Toxicity from acute overdose has not been reported. In overdose diarrhea could be expected. Acarbose does not stimulate endogenous insulin release, has not caused hypoglycemia with monotherapy, and would not be expected to cause hypoglycemia in overdose (11,13,17). Like other α-glucosidase inhibitors miglitol appears to have no other clinically relevant extraintestinal effects (18,19). It appears unlikely to produce hypoglycemia in overdose, but abdominal discomfort and diarrhea may occur.

Adverse effects of acarbose during therapy include idiosyncratic liver injury (20,21). Elevation of the serum transaminase has been noted in clinical trials, and it would be prudent to check transaminases in the case of a massive overdose.

Treatment

No specific therapy should be required with overdose of the α-glucosidase inhibitors.

THIAZOLADINEDIONE AGENTS

The thiazoladinedione group is comprised of three drugs: troglitazone, which has been removed from the market due to association with fulminant hepatic failure; rosiglitazone (Avandia); and pioglitazone (Actos). Their function is that of an insulin sensitizer via stimulation of the peroxisomal proliferator-activated receptor-γ (PPAR-γ) in adipose tissue, skeletal muscle, and the liver. They are used in type II NIDDM to reduce insulin resistance as monotherapy or in combination with metformin, a sulfonylurea, or insulin. The adverse effects include weight increase, edema, myalgias, and potential hepatic injury. In overdose, hypoglycemia appears unlikely. Hepatic injury has been reported with all three drugs in this class.

Troglitazone was first introduced in Europe and the United States in 1997. It was withdrawn from Europe later that year on the grounds of liver toxicity but continued to be available in the United States. Ultimately, it caused at least 90 cases of liver failure, with 70 resulting in liver transplantation or death before its withdrawal from the U.S. market in 2000 (22).

The "glitazones" function by stimulation of PPAR-γ. Activation of these receptors modulates transcription of several insulin-responsive genes that control glucose and lipid metabolism. The glitazones are only effective in the presence of insulin.

Toxic Dose

The adult and pediatric therapeutic doses are provided in Table 1. No cases of overdosage of the glitazones have been reported. A toxic threshold has not been established.

Toxicokinetics and Toxicodynamics

Rosiglitazone is well absorbed with approximately 99% bioavailability. Pioglitazone has a bioavailability of approximately 50%. Both drugs are highly protein bound (98%). The volume of distribution of rosiglitazone and pioglitazone is 17.6 L and 0.63 L/kg, respectively. Rosiglitazone is extensively metabolized via CPY2C8 and CYP2C9. The metabolites are cleared primarily via the kidney (64%), with a smaller portion cleared via the feces (23%). Pioglitazone is metabolized to active and inactive metabolites via CYP2C8 and CYP3A4 and appears to be cleared primarily via the feces. Elimination half-life is 3 to 4 hours and 3 to 7 hours for rosiglitazone and pioglitazone, respectively.

Pathophysiology

Thiazolidinediones act by binding to the PPAR-γ in the cell nucleus that moderates diverse metabolic pathways involving lipoprotein lipase, glucose transporters, and insulin signaling pathways (23–25).

The specific mechanism for hepatotoxicity has not been fully elucidated. One suggestion has been that troglitazone contains an alpha-tocopherol moiety, which may contribute to the formation of quinone metabolites. Neither rosiglitazone nor pioglitazone contains an alpha-tocopherol moiety. This may explain the greater reported incidence of hepatic injury associated with troglitazone (26,27). The estimated incidence of troglitazone-induced liver failure is between 1 in 8000 and 1 in 20,000 patients treated (22). However, this does not fully explain the effect because hepatotoxicity has also been described in rosiglitazone and pioglitazone (28–32).

Pregnancy and Lactation

Rosiglitazone and pioglitazone are both FDA pregnancy category C (Appendix I). The American College of Obstetricians and Gynecologists recommends that insulin be used for type I and type II diabetes occurring during pregnancy if diet therapy alone is not successful for gestational diabetes.

Clinical Presentation

ACUTE OVERDOSAGE

No acute overdoses have been reported. The glitazones do not stimulate endogenous insulin release, have not caused hypoglycemia with monotherapy, and would not be expected to cause hypoglycemia in overdose.

ADVERSE EVENTS

Toxicity during chronic therapy has produced hepatic injury and failure (28–32). The patient may present with anorexia, nausea, abdominal discomfort, fatigue, scleral icterus, or shortness of breath. Laboratory results may show elevated transaminases, bilirubin, and alkaline phosphatase. An additional laboratory finding may be elevated prothrombin time and International Normalized Ratio. Coma, hypotension, and bradycardia have been reported in one case associated with hepatic failure (29).

Diagnostic Tests

No tests are needed following acute ingestion unless there are co-ingestants. The serum aminotransferases, alkaline phosphatase, bilirubin, prothrombin time, and international normalized ratio should be monitored during therapy.

Treatment

In the suicidal patient with a massive ingestion, the potential for hepatic injury is unknown but likely to be low. A single dose of activated charcoal would be warranted if the ingestion were recent. Toxicity that develops during therapy is treated with removal of the drug and supportive care.

No known antidote is available. Hemodialysis, hemoperfusion, and diuresis would be of little value because of the large volume of distribution and high protein binding.

REFERENCES

1. Eisenbarth GS. Type 1 diabetes mellitus: a chronic autoimmune disease. *N Engl J Med* 1986;314:1360–1368.
2. Oats JA, Wood AJJ. Oral hypoglycemic agents. *N Engl J Med* 1989;321:1231–1245.
3. Hirshberg B, Skarulis MC, Pucino F, et al. Repaglinide-induced factitious hypoglycemia. *J Clin Endocrinol Metab* 2001;86:475–477
4. Kikuchi M. Modulation of insulin secretion in non-insulin-dependent diabetes mellitus by two novel oral hypoglycaemic agents, NN623 and A4166. *Diabetic Med* 1996;13[Suppl]:151–155.
5. Mikko N, Backman JT, Neuvonen M, et al. Rifampin decreases the plasma concentration and effects of repaglinide. *Clin Pharmacol Ther* 2000;68:495–500.
6. Karara AH, Dunning BE, McLeod JF. The effect of food on the oral bioavailability and the pharmacodynamic actions of the insulinotropic agent nateglinide in healthy subjects. *J Clin Pharmacol* 1999;39:172–179.
7. Hu S. Interaction of nateglinide with the K(ATP) channel in beta cells underlies its unique insulinotropic action. *Eur J Pharmacol* 2002;442:163–171.
8. Dabrowski M, Wahl P, Holmes WE, et al. Effects of repaglinide on cloned beta cell, cardiac and smooth muscle types of ATP-sensitive potassium channels. *Diabetalogia* 2001;44:747–756.
9. Massi-Benedetti M, Damsbo P. Pharmacology and clinical experience with repaglinide. *Expert Opin Investig Drugs* 2000;9:885–898.
10. Bischoff H. Pharmacology of alpha-glucosidase inhibition. *Eur J Clin Invest* 1994;24:3–10.
11. Yee HS, Fong NT. A review of the safety and efficacy of acarbose in diabetes mellitus. *Phamacotherapy* 1996;16:792–805.
12. Clissold SP, Edwards C. Acarbose. A preliminary review of its pharmacodynamic and pharmacokinetic properties and therapeutic potential. *Drugs* 1988;35:214–243.
13. Hollander P, Pi-Sunyer X, Coniff RF. Acarbose in the treatment of type I diabetes. *Diabetes Care* 1997;20:248–253.
14. Coniff RF, Krol A. Acarbose: a review of US clinical experience. *Clin Ther* 1997;19:16–26.
15. Martin AE, Montgomery PA. Acarbose: an alpha-glucosidase inhibitor. *Am J Health System Pharm* 1996;53:2277–2290.
16. Ahr HJ, Boberg M, Brendel E, et al. Pharmacokinetics of miglitol. Absorption, distribution, metabolism and excretion following administration to rats, dogs and man. *Arzneimittel-Forschung* 1997;47:734–745.
17. Campbell LK, White JR, Campbell RK. Acarbose: its role in the treatment of diabetes mellitus. *Ann Pharmacother* 1996;30:1255–1262.
18. Sels JP, Nauta JJ, Menheere PP, et al. Miglitol (BAY m 1099) has no extraintestinal effects on glucose in healthy volunteers. *Br J Clin Pharmacol* 1996;42:503–506.
19. Sels JP, Kingma PJ, Wolffenbuttel BH, et al. Effect of miglitol (BAY m 1099) on fasting blood glucose in type 2 diabetes mellitus. *Neth J Med* 1994;44:198–201.
20. Carrascosa M, Pascual F, Aresti S. Acarbose-induced severe hepatotoxicity. *Lancet* 1997;349:698–699.
21. Andrade RJ, Lucena MI, Rodriguez-Mendizabel M. Hepatic injury caused by acarbose. *Ann Intern Med* 1996;124:931.
22. Gale EAM. Lesson from the glitazones: a story of the drug development. *Lancet* 2001:357:1870–1875.
23. Spencer CM, Markham A. Troglitazone. *Drugs* 1997;54:89–101.
24. Santiago JV. Troglitazone . *Comp Ther* 1997;23:560–562.
25. Kapland F, Al-Majali K, Betteridge DJ. PARRs, insulin resistance and type 2 diabetes. *J Cardiovasc Risk* 2001;8:211–217.
26. Lloyd S, Hayden MJ, Sakai Y, et al. Differential in vitro hepatotoxicity of troglitazone and rosiglitazone among cryopreserved human hepatocytes from 37 donors. *Chem Biol Interact* 2002;142:57–71.
27. Lebovitz HE, Kreider M, Freed MI. Evaluation of liver function in type 2 diabetic patients during clinical trials: evidence that rosiglitazone does not cause hepatic dysfunction. *Diabetes Care* 2002;25:815–821.
28. May LD, Lefkowitch JH, Kram MY, et al. Mixed hepatocellular-cholestatic liver injury after pioglitazone therapy. *Ann Intern Med* 2002;136:449–452.
29. Forman LM, Simmons DA, Diamond RH. Hepatic failure in a patient taking rosiglitazone. *Ann Intern Med* 2000;132:118–121.
30. Ravinuthala RS, Nori U. Rosiglitazone toxicity. *Ann Intern Med* 2000;133:658.
31. Al-Salaman J, Arjomand H, Kemp D, et al. Hepatocellular injury in a patient receiving rosiglitazone: a case report. *Ann Intern Med* 2000;132:121–124.
32. Maeda K. Hepatocellular injury in a patient receiving pioglitazone. *Ann Intern Med* 2001;135:306.

CHAPTER 161

Thyroid Hormones

Luke Yip

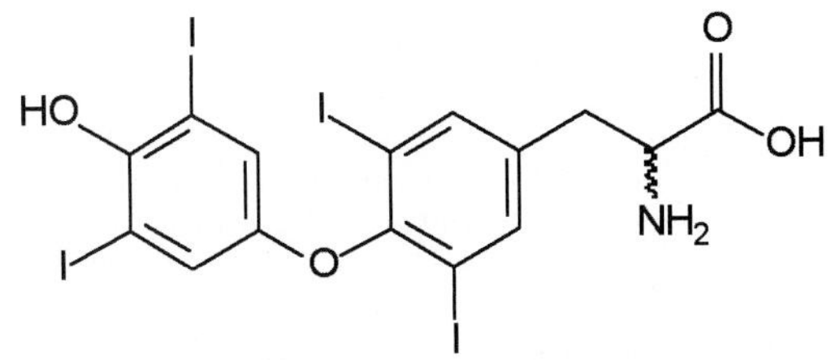

T_4 (L-3,3′,5,5′-TETRAIODOTHYRONINE

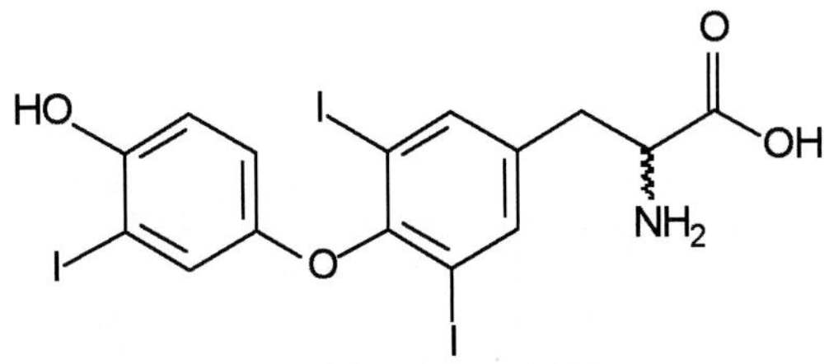

T_3 (L-3,5,3′-TRIIODOTHYRONINE)

Compounds included:	**T_4 (levothyroxine, Levothroid, Oroxine, Synthroid); T_3 (liothyronine, triiodothyronine, Cytomel, Triostat)**
Molecular formula and weight:	**T_4: $C_{15}H_{11}I_4NO_4$, 776.87 g/mol; T_3: $C_{15}H_{12}I_3NO_4$, 650.98 g/mol**
SI conversion:	**Levothyroxine: nmol/L × 0.077 = μg/dl; liothyronine: nmol/L × 65 = ng/dl**
CAS Registry No.:	**T_4: 25416-65-3; T_3: Liotrix (T_4/T_3 in ratio 4:1) 8065-29-0, thyroid extract (desiccated), thyroglobulin (Proloid) 9010-34-8**
Normal levels:	**T_4: Serum, total 5 to 12 μg/dl; free, 1 to 3 ng/dl (0.02% of total T_4); T_3: Serum total 70 to 200 ng/dl; free serum T_3: 0.2 to 0.4 ng/dl (0.2% of total T_3); rT_3: serum total 10 to 60 ng/dl; free serum 0.05 to 0.15 ng/dl (0.5% of total rT_3). There is considerable interlaboratory variation in the "normal range" for thyroid function tests.**
Special concerns:	**Signs of toxicity develop hours or days after acute ingestion. Toxic effects are primarily adrenergic in nature.**
Antidote:	**None**

OVERVIEW

The clinical uses of thyroid hormones include replacement therapy for hypothyroidism or suppressive therapy to abolish thyroid-stimulating hormone (TSH) secretion in patients with differentiated thyroid carcinoma after total thyroidectomy or with diffuse/nodular nontoxic goiter. However, thyroid hormones are also abused by patients with thyrotoxicosis factitia, a psychiatric disorder that causes surreptitious thyroid hormone ingestion (1–6). Most cases of acute thyroid hormone ingestion follow a generally benign clinical course with few signs and symptoms (7–11). In others, moderate thyrotoxicosis (e.g., flushing, tachycardia, fever, diarrhea, irritability, and insomnia) (12–15) or thyroid storm (16–18) develops. The incidence of life-threatening reactions that require treatment has been low (2,12,14,15,17,19–22), and morbidity (5,16,23–28) and mortality (24,29,30) are rarely reported after a single or repeated thyroid hormone overdose. Adverse reactions or toxicity during therapeutic use may occur (23,31–34).

The approximate equivalent dosages for the various thyroid medications are provided in Table 1.

TOXIC DOSE

The adult therapeutic dose of oral levothyroxine (T_4) is 100 to 200 μg daily. The initial daily oral T_3 dose is 10 μg every 8 hours and can be increased to 20 μg every 8 hours. The initial intravenous T_3 dose is 5 to 20 μg every 8 to 12 hours. In children, the initial daily oral dose of T_4 is 25 μg, gradually increased to 3 to 5 μg/kg per day. The initial daily oral T_3 dose is 0.2 μg/kg per dose (up to 10 μg) every 8 hours and can be increased to 0.4 μg/kg per dose (up to 20 μg) every 8 hours. The recommended initial intravenous T_3 dose is 0.1 to 0.4 μg/kg per dose (up to 5 to 20 μg) every 8 to 12 hours.

A 19-year-old female ingested an estimated 10 mg or more of T_4 16 hours before presenting with tachycardia and hand tremor (14). Her serum T_4, T_3, and reverse T_3 (rT_3) levels were elevated above the reference range. Propranolol was initiated, and the patient's hospital course was unremarkable. A 31-year-old woman ingested an estimated 10 mg T_4 and vomited 2 hours later (15). She was asymptomatic 12 hours later but had elevated serum T_4, T_3, and T_3 resin uptake (T_3RU) levels. Tremor, anxiety, tachycardia, and fever developed on day 5. Her symptoms were controlled with propranolol for the next 10 days, at which time she was chemically euthyroid.

TABLE 1. Approximate equivalent doses of thyroid medications

Agent	Approximate equivalent dose
Liothyronine sodium (T_3)	25 μg
Levothyroxine sodium (T_4)	100 μg
Liotrix: T_4-T_3 in ratio 4:1	50 μg/12.5 μg
Thyroid extract (desiccated thyroid)	60–65 μg (1 grain)
Thyroglobulin	65 μg

A 34-year-old man was initially asymptomatic after ingesting an estimated 720 mg T_4 (16). He became less energetic 2 days after ingestion, but vomiting, diaphoresis, and restlessness developed on day 4. On day 5, he became agitated and violent and stopped speaking intelligibly; on day 6, he became combative and confused. He had tachycardia, hypertension, tachypnea, and fever. Physical examination was remarkable for diaphoresis, mydriasis, hyperactive bowel sounds, hyperreflexia, and profound tremor. When the patient was discharged on day 15, he had lost 18.5 kg body weight.

Death from acute or repeated thyroid hormone overdose is rare (24,29,30). A 50-year-old woman ingested up to an estimated 800 μg per day of T_4 and presented with sharp substernal chest pain that was not relieved with sublingual nitroglycerin (30). The patient's examination was remarkable for tachypnea and atrial fibrillation, with a rapid ventricular response. Laboratory assessment was remarkable for hypokalemia and a normal ventilation/perfusion lung scan and echocardiogram. Serum T_4, T_3RU, and free T_4 index were elevated above the reference range. The patient died of refractory ventricular fibrillation on the third hospital day. Autopsy showed normal heart size and coronary arteries and no evidence of acute myocardial infarction.

A patient ingested an estimated 250 mg T_4 over 2 days, and tachycardia, fever, nervousness, insomnia, heat intolerance, asthenia, arthromyalgia, and diarrhea developed within 3 days of ingestion of the first T_4 dose (24). The patient became comatose on day 7, developed ventricular fibrillation on day 9, and subsequently died on day 27.

TOXICOKINETICS AND TOXICODYNAMICS

Absorption and Distribution

The average T_4 bioavailability is 80% after an oral therapeutic dose, and the time to maximal absorption is 2 hours. The serum T_4 level reaches its peak 4 hours after ingestion of 3 mg (35). Gastrointestinal (GI) diseases, such as sprue, diabetic diarrhea, and short bowel syndrome, and ileal jejunal bypass surgery, may reduce absorption. Cholestyramine, calcium carbonate, sucralfate, aluminum hydroxide, ferrous sulfate, soybean formula, lovastatin, and dietary fiber supplements may also impair T_4 absorption. The maximum effects of T_4 are apparent 1 to 3 weeks after initiation and persist for the same amount of time after discontinuation of the drug.

Oral absorption of T_3 is 95%. The serum T_3 level begins to rise at 1.5 to 2.5 hours (36). The serum T_3 level peaks 2 hours after ingestion of 360 mg desiccated thyroid and 4 hours after ingestion of 75 μg T_3 (35).

T_4 is distributed widely, with highest concentrations in the liver and kidneys. T_4 and T_3 are primarily bound to thyroxine binding globulin and to a lesser extent to thyroxine binding prealbumin and albumin. T_4 is more extensively and tightly bound than T_3. It is estimated that 0.04% of T_4 and 0.5% of T_3 are unbound (free) hormone, which is available to elicit a physiologic effect.

Elimination

Endogenously secreted T_4 (35%) is enzymatically monodeiodinated by type I 5'-monodeiodinase to T_3 in the peripheral tissues (e.g., liver and kidney) and accounts for 80% of total daily T_3 production. T_4 is also enzymatically monodeiodinated to rT_3. In the liver, T_4 may undergo glucuronidation and sulfation, which are eliminated in bile, some of which are hydrolyzed in the intestine and reabsorbed, and the remainder of which are hydrolyzed in the colon and eliminated unchanged in the feces. After an oral 3 mg T_4 dose, a significant increase in serum T_3 level is evident at 4 hours, and peak level is achieved between 2 and 4 days (35). The elimination half-life of T_4 is 6 to 7 days. Drugs that increase nondeiodinative T_4 clearance include rifampin, carbamazepine, and phenytoin. Selenium deficiency and amiodarone may block T_4 conversion to T_3.

One metabolic pathway for T_3 and rT_3 is peripheral monodeiodination. The half-life of T_3 is 1 to 2 days. The maximum effects of T_3 are apparent within 24 to 72 hours after initiation of oral therapy, and the effects persist for up to 72 hours after discontinuation. Urinary T_3 elimination increases linearly with the rise in urine flow rate and is doubled or tripled when urine flow rate is increased by five- to eightfold during acute hydration (37).

Toxicodynamics

In a thyroidectomized patient who had ingested an estimated 2000 μg T_4, the serum concentrations of most thyroid hormones reached a peak on the second day (38). The serum T_3 level peaked 1 day later and did not exceed the upper limit of the reference range. The serum T_4 and rT_3 levels returned to the reference range 13 to 17 days after ingestion. The serum TSH level was rapidly suppressed and reached nadir on the sixth day postingestion. The serum T_4 half-life and metabolic clearance rate were 10.4 days and 0.64 L/day, respectively. An acute single oral ingestion of a large amount of T_4 does not induce a proportional increase in the serum T_3 level in a person without a thyroid gland. The serum T_4 metabolic clearance rate is decreased, and the serum T_4 half-life is prolonged. This is consistent with D1 deiodinase activity in the thyroid being one of the major determinants in the metabolic clearance of serum T_4.

Two hours after an acute oral T_4 overdose, the serum T_4, free T_4, and free T_3 levels were 2.27, 7.17, and 2.85 times the upper limit of the reference range, respectively (39). Two hours after an acute oral triiodothyronine overdose, the serum total T_4 and T_3 levels were 1.83 and 25.0 times the upper limit of the reference range, whereas the T_3RU remained in the reference range (19).

Two previously healthy girls remained asymptomatic after ingestion of 2500 μg T_4, and treatment with ipecac, gastric lavage, propranolol, prednisone, cholestyramine, and propylthiouracil (PTU) (40). Serial serum T_4, T_3, rT_3, and thyroglobulin levels were obtained during the 20 days after ingestion. Serum T_4 serum concentrations were elevated 2 hours postingestion and returned to the reference range after 13 days. The serum TSH levels were at their nadir 14 hours after ingestion and remained low until the fourth day, after which they rose gradually. However, the TSH levels remained below their initial values at 20 days postingestion. The serum T_3 concentrations peaked 11 hours after ingestion and decreased to reference values after 3 days. T_3 production and degradation constants were significantly increased. The serum rT_3 concentration peaked on the second day postingestion and decreased to reference values on the fourth day. rT_3 production and degradation constants were below reference values. The T_3-rT_3 ratio decreased from a reference value of 3 to 1 and then increased after 13 days to as high as 8. The serum thyroglobulin concentration continuously decreased with a half-life of 1 to 5 days and began rising after 2 to 13 days.

The toxicokinetic data from 15 previously healthy patients aged 12 to 49 months, who were treated with GI decontamination within 6 hours of the overdose, showed elevation in serum T_4 concentration as early as 1 to 2 hours postingestion (8). In 71% of the patients, peak serum T_4 level was reached within 12 hours, whereas the serum T_3 concentration did not peak until after 24 hours postingestion. The mean elimination half-life of T_4

was 2.8 days (range, 1.5 to 4.5 days), and the mean elimination half-life of T_3 was 6 days (range, 2.2 to 12.3 days), which is five times longer than normal. Also, in physiologic conditions the elimination half-life of T_3 is shorter than that of T_4.

PATHOPHYSIOLOGY

The effects of thyroid hormone include regulation of the hypothalamic-pituitary-thyroid axis, regulation of growth and development, and calorigenic, metabolic, and cardiovascular effects. Exaggeration of thyroid hormone's physiologic effects in overdose produces a hyperadrenergic state that primarily affects the cardiovascular system and the central nervous system.

PREGNANCY AND LACTATION

T_4 and liothyronine are U.S. Food and Drug Administration pregnancy category A (Appendix I). Thyroid hormones do not readily cross the placenta, and maternal thyroid hormone transfer is slow. Mild hyperthyroidism has little effect on the course of pregnancy; severe and uncontrolled thyrotoxicosis is complicated by an increased frequency of abortion, premature labor, and toxemia of pregnancy. Infants may be born with a transient, neonatal hyperthyroidism (weight loss, hyperkinesis, tachycardia, diarrhea), which regresses within 3 to 4 weeks of birth.

Thyroid preparations are excreted into breast milk in low concentrations. They are considered safe when used appropriately during pregnancy.

CLINICAL PRESENTATION

Acute and Subacute Overdosage

The temporal relation between overdose and the onset of signs and symptoms is delayed by hours to days. Adult patients primarily present with cardiovascular and central nervous system effects (14–16,39). Vomiting may be evident as soon as 2 hours, tachycardia may be noted in 2 to 6 hours, and fever has been reported 6 hours postingestion. However, cardiovascular signs and symptoms usually do not become apparent until 16 hours to 4 days after ingestion, and neurologic manifestations may not occur until 2 to 6 days postingestion.

A patient may complain of having less energy, vomiting, sweating, and restlessness. He or she may appear agitated and anxious and speak unintelligibly. Diaphoresis, tachycardia, fever, hypertension, tachypnea, mydriasis, hyperactive bowel sounds, hyperreflexia, tremor, and confusion may develop. The patient may be combative or violent.

A review of 92 cases involving children 6 years or less who accidentally ingested an estimated 5 mg or less of T_4 or its equivalent suggests that a majority of acute pediatric T_4 overdose results in no toxicity (11). In eight patients (8.7%), fever, vomiting, diarrhea, increased appetite, irritability, hyperactivity, flushing, and rash developed. No significant symptoms developed in patients who ingested doses up to 3.75 mg with GI decontamination and 2.0 mg without decontamination.

Children who ingested an estimated 0.6 to 8.8 mg T_4 may present with fever, supraventricular tachycardia, diaphoresis, flushing, increased appetite, vomiting, diarrhea, abdominal pain, lethargy, irritability, hyperactivity, agitation, and rash (7–9,11). Signs and symptoms of fever, tachycardia, and agitation may be delayed 12 to 48 hours after ingestion (8).

A patient presented with severe myxedema and was treated with oral and intravenous T_4 (29). The patient became unresponsive and asystolic 15 minutes after administration of intravenous T_4. Resuscitative efforts resulted in return of sinus rhythm. Intravenous T_4 therapy was continued, and on the tenth day hypotension and bradycardia developed and the patient died.

A patient presented with mental confusion 1 hour after ingestion of an estimated 1600 μg T_3, 480 mg brompheniramine, and 200 mg clomipramine (19). The patient became diaphoretic, and sinus tachycardia developed 5 to 7 hours after ingestion. The serum total T_3 concentration was 80 nmol/L (normal, 1.4 to 3.2 nmol/L) at 2 hours postingestion. All signs and symptoms resolved over the next 12 hours.

Chronic Overdosage

Repeated ingestion of T_4 may cause palpitations, hypersalivation, nervousness, insomnia, heat intolerance, asthenia, arthromyalgia, and diarrhea 1 to 3 days after the first dose is ingested (5,24,27). Patients may also complain of weight loss, fatigability, and dyspnea on exertion. They may appear anxious, hostile, restless, apprehensive, and depressed. Patients may present with hypertension, fever, tachycardia, atrial fibrillation, agitation, and slurred speech. They may have warm moist palms, tremors, and generalized muscle weakness. Neurologic effects, such as hemipareses, aphasia, stupor, delirium, and coma, may appear at 5 to 10 days. Left ventricular failure and atrial and ventricular fibrillation may develop after 8 to 11 days. Intense laminar desquamation of the palms and soles may occur 17 to 37 days after ingestion.

Six patients aged 46 to 74 years ingested an estimated 70 to 1200 mg T_4 over 2 to 12 days (24). Tachycardia, fever, nervousness, insomnia, heat intolerance, asthenia, arthromyalgia, and diarrhea developed in all patients within 3 days of ingesting the first T_4 dose. Neurologic signs and symptoms developed in all patients between day 7 and 10 after ingestion; coma developed in five patients and stupor in one patient, and one patient had hemipareses and aphasia before being comatose. Left ventricular failure, atrial fibrillation, and ventricular fibrillation developed between day 8 and 11 in five patients. Diffuse STT-wave changes developed in one patient on electrocardiography on day 29. Intense laminar desquamation of the palms and soles developed between day 17 and 37 in five patients. The serum total T_4 and T_3 levels were above the reference range. One patient died, and all the other patients completely recovered.

Adverse Events

The adverse drug effects associated with chronic thyroid hormone therapy include tachycardia, premature atrial contractions, atrial flutter or fibrillation, coronary artery spasm, acute myocardial infarction, left ventricular hypertrophy, cardiac failure, reduced bone density and bone mass, thyroid storm, coma, and death (31–33). Tachycardia is often out of proportion to fever. Idiosyncratic or allergic reactions may occur with animal-derived products such as desiccated thyroid and thyroglobulin.

A 52-year-old man with a history of coronary bypass surgery and receiving daily thyroid hormone replacement therapy presented with unstable angina and acute myocardial infarction (34). He was hypertensive, tachycardic, and thyrotoxic. Iopanoic acid was administered. He was taken to surgery for coronary revascularization, where a thyroid storm developed. The patient was started on an esmolol infusion, which depressed his myocardial contractility. Amrinone and noradrenaline infusions were required for inotropic support. Over the following 20 hours, the patient's condition stabilized.

Drug Interactions

Patients with endogenous thyrotoxicosis have a significant increase in serum free T_4 and T_3 levels after intravenous heparin (5000 to 30,000 U) administration (41). This effect may be due to a hormonal shift from the cellular to the intravascular compartment when cellular and intravascular hormonal binding sites are blocked by heparin. The metabolic significance is unknown.

DIAGNOSTIC TESTS

Acute or Repeated Overdosage

After thyroid hormone exposure, there are no essential tests. However, serum T_4, T_3, and thyroglobulin levels may have diagnostic and prognostic value. Elevated serum T_4 and T_3 levels help to confirm ingestion of thyroid preparations. In pediatric patients, a serum T_4 concentration greater than 75 mg/dl within 7 hours after ingestion may predict toxicity (e.g., fever, tachycardia, and agitation) 12 to 48 hours postingestion (8).

In thyrotoxicosis factitia (repeated ingestion), the serum T_4-T_3 ratio and thyroglobulin concentration may help to identify patients (42). The serum T_4-T_3 ratio in those taking pharmacologic doses of T_4 is higher than in patients with endogenous thyrotoxicosis, who have marked T_3 secretion. In individuals with thyrotoxicosis from Graves' disease, the mean T_4-T_3 ratio is 28 (range, 11 to 57), whereas patients with thyrotoxicosis factitia have a mean ratio of 70 (range, 48 to 114). Thyroglobulin release is in part dependent on TSH. Patients with thyrotoxicosis factitia have either low or undetectable serum thyroglobulin levels (43).

The dynamic pattern of a patient's serial thyroid function tests may provide evidence for diagnosis of exogenous T_3 ingestion (6). The serum T_3 concentration will most likely far exceed that observed in endogenous causes of hyperthyroidism. The rapid fall in serum T_3 concentration indicates that T_3 toxicosis is a transient event rather than a sustained physiologic process. The serum T_4-T_3 ratio is expected to be consistently less than 20, which is smaller than that observed in conditions of endogenous hyperthyroidism associated with T_3 toxicosis. This ratio reflects the extreme elevation of serum T_3 concentration and the decreased T_4 concentration with T_3 suppression of TSH. Laboratory studies, such as serum electrolytes, renal tests, glucose levels, creatine kinase, cardiac enzymes, electrocardiography, computed tomography of the head, lumbar puncture, and toxicology studies should be obtained as clinically indicated.

Diagnostic Pitfalls

An increased serum T_4-T_3 ratio may be observed in thyrotoxic states other than ingestion of excess amounts of T_4. Patients receiving amiodarone therapy have elevated T_4-T_3 ratios (mean, 57.3; range, 27.5 to 119.9), and they are associated with increased serum thyroglobulin concentration (mean, 117.8 ng/dl; range, 17 to 460 ng/dl) (43).

TREATMENT

Emergent medical assessment and GI decontamination are not recommended for many patients exposed to thyroid hormone, and selected individuals can be managed as outpatients.

Decontamination

The patient with suicidal ingestion should be emergently assessed in a hospital, receive GI decontamination, and be admitted for close observation and expectant treatment. The observation period should be at least 3 to 5 days. Ipecac-induced emesis is recommended for asymptomatic children if the ingestion was 2 mg or more of T_4 and occurred within 1 hour (9,11).

GI decontamination is unnecessary for children less than 12 years old who accidentally ingest a dose of T_4 estimated as 0.5 mg (9) and may not be necessary for ingestions up to 2.0 mg (11). These patients can be observed at home pending the onset of symptoms. GI decontamination should be performed in asymptomatic patients after a significant overdose, and serial outpatient follow-up should be organized for at least 7 days postingestion.

Although it has not been well studied, a single dose of activated charcoal (with or without a cathartic) is recommended after an acute ingestion that occurred within the previous few hours. On the other hand, clinical studies have shown that cholestyramine significantly interferes with T_4 absorption from the GI tract and interrupts T_4 and T_3 enterohepatic circulation (44,45). One in vitro study showed that 50 mg cholestyramine resin is capable of irreversibly binding 3 mg T_4 (44). The typical cholestyramine dose is 50 to 150 mg/kg per dose (adult, 3 to 9 g), and this dose can be repeated every 6 to 8 hours. Neither cathartic nor whole bowel irrigation has been formally studied for thyroid hormone overdose.

Enhancement of Elimination

Case reports suggest that multiple-dose activated charcoal does not appreciably affect serum thyroid hormone levels or clinical outcome (8,22). However, multidose cholestyramine may be an effective adjunctive means of decreasing the exogenous hormone load (44,45).

Hemodialysis is ineffective because of the high protein binding and limited renal excretion of thyroid hormones. Exchange transfusion (39,46) and plasmapheresis (24,39,47) have been used in acute and nonacute thyroid hormone poisoning, but conclusive studies are lacking. Extracorporeal techniques do not remove significant amounts of thyroid hormones, and their efficacy decreases with time.

Antidotes

Antidotal treatment is directed at blocking the conversion of T_4 to T_3 or toward blocking the pathophysiologic effects of T_3. Oral iodinated radiocontrast agents (i.e., sodium ipodate and iopanoic acid) inhibit peripheral conversion of T_4 to T_3 and appear to be an effective adjunctive treatment for patients with either exogenous (8,48–50) or endogenous thyrotoxicosis (51–54). These agents markedly prolong the serum T_4 half-life with a concurrent sharp increase in serum rT_3 level and a marked decrease in serum T_3 level (48–50). The typical sodium ipodate and iopanoic acid dose is 3 g for adults and 150 mg/kg per dose for children and can be repeated for recurrence of symptoms. The dose of sodium ipodate is 250 mg/kg per dose every 3 days for 18 days followed by 500 mg/kg per dose every 3 days for 21 days. It has been successfully used to treat a patient with moderately severe neonatal Graves' disease (52).

The β-adrenergic antagonists (e.g., propranolol and esmolol) block the pathophysiologic effects of T_3 and rapidly reduce the heart rate, blood pressure, tremor, and stare in hyperthyroidism as well as relieve palpitation, anxiety, and tension (14,15,20,21, 27,34,49,55,56). The typical oral propranolol dose is 0.2 to 0.5

mg/kg per dose (10 to 40 mg for an adult) every 4 to 6 hours. The dose is titrated to response. Large doses (240 to 280 mg per day) may be required in severely toxic patients. The intravenous propranolol dose is 0.1 mg/kg (adult, 5 mg) over 10 minutes and can be repeated up to three times as clinically indicated. An esmolol infusion can be initiated by administering 0.5 mg/kg over 1 minute, then 50 μg/kg/minute for 4 minutes; if the response is inadequate, one should rebolus with 0.5 mg/kg and then 50 to 200 μg/kg/minute for up to 48 hours.

Diltiazem appears to be an effective alternative therapy in controlling thyrotoxic symptoms in patients in whom a beta-blocker may be contraindicated (57,58). The oral diltiazem dose is 1 to 3 mg/kg per dose (adult, 60 to 180 mg) every 6 to 8 hours.

Hydrocortisone (100 to 200 mg/day) should be administered if adrenal insufficiency is suspected. Dexamethasone (2 mg every 6 hours for 4 doses) alters peripheral T_4 metabolism whereby conversion from T_4 to T_3 is diminished and rT_3 is enhanced (59).

PTU appears to inhibit thyroid hormone biosynthesis by interrupting thyroid peroxidase-catalyzed inorganic iodide oxidation and thyroidal T_4 secretion. It has limited efficacy in the management of exogenous thyroid hormone toxicity. The effects of PTU are evident in hyperthyroid patients and not in iatrogenic thyrotoxicosis or most euthyroid and hypothyroid patients.

A paucity of information is available regarding acute PTU or methimazole overdose, and rare adverse drug events have been associated with their therapeutic use (61–67). Adverse effects associated with PTU include skin rash, granulocytopenia, eosinophilia, lupus-like syndrome, acute hepatitis, cholestatic hepatotoxicity, hepatic necrosis, liver failure, and death. Diagnostic laboratory studies include abnormal liver function tests, centrilobular hepatic necrosis, positive migration inhibition factor test to PTU, and PTU-induced peripheral lymphocyte transformation (63,67,68). PTU may traverse the placenta and cause neonatal hepatitis and lymphocyte sensitization (68). Management of PTU toxicity includes discontinuation of PTU, supportive care, steroid therapy, and, in cases of fulminant liver failure, orthotopic liver transplantation (62–64,69,70).

Adverse drug events associated with methimazole use include agranulocytosis, pancytopenia, plasmacytosis, serum sickness, acute hepatitis, cholestatic jaundice, granulomatous hepatitis, hepatocellular necrosis, and death (61,71,72–76). Diagnostic laboratory studies include abnormal complete blood count, abnormal liver function tests, liver biopsy, and bone marrow biopsy (71,72,74). Management includes discontinuation of methimazole, supportive care, and, in cases of severe bone marrow toxicity, reverse isolation, antibiotics, and dexamethasone (71,74).

Iodide acutely inhibits thyroid hormone biosynthesis and release and has no proven clinical utility in the treatment of exogenous thyroid hormone exposure.

Supportive Care

The patient's fluid, electrolyte, and acid-base status should be assessed and corrected as required, and urine output should be at least 1 to 2 ml/kg/hour. Hyperthermia should be managed using standard measures (Chapter 38). Case reports suggest that dantrolene may be an effective adjunct therapy for endogenous thyrotoxicosis (77–79), but its efficacy remains to be established in exogenous thyroid hormone toxicity. Hypertension requiring medical treatment is rare.

Monitoring

Patients who become symptomatic, are symptomatic, have taken a massive overdose, or have significant underlying cardiovascular disease should be admitted to the hospital for expectant treatment. Patients manifesting significant cardiovascular or neurologic signs and symptoms should be managed in an intensive care unit.

Serial thyroid function tests should be obtained in patients receiving thyroid hormone therapy who became toxic after thyroid hormone overdose. Thyroid hormone therapy can be resumed after the patient's serum (free) T_4 and TSH levels are within the reference range. Serum T_4, T_3, and thyroglobulin levels obtained within 7 hours after ingestion may have diagnostic and prognostic value (8,43).

Management Pitfalls

The initial absence or presence of minor symptoms (i.e., tachycardia) does not preclude delayed toxicity (i.e., seizures), which may manifest 7 days after ingestion (25). However, prophylactic treatment with propranolol, PTU, corticosteroid, or extracorporeal procedure is not recommended (7–11).

REFERENCES

1. Bogazzi F, Bartalena L, Scarcello G, et al. The age of patients with thyrotoxicosis factitia in Italy from 1973 to 1996. *J Endocrinol Invest* 1999;22:128–133.
2. Braunstein GD, Koblin R, Sugawara M, et al. Unintentional thyrotoxicosis factitia due to a diet pill. *West J Med* 1986;145:388–391.
3. Mariotti S, Martino E, Cupini C, et al. Low serum thyroglobulin as a clue to the diagnosis of thyrotoxicosis factitia. *N Engl J Med* 1982;307:410–412.
4. Matsubara S, Inoh M, Tarumi Y, et al. An outbreak (159 cases) of transient thyrotoxicosis without hyperthyroidism in Japan. *Intern Med* 1995;34:514–519.
5. Rose E, Sanders TP, Webbs WL Jr, et al. Occult factitial thyrotoxicosis. Thyroxine kinetics and psychological evaluation in three cases. *Ann Intern Med* 1969;71:309–315.
6. Sylvia Vela B, Dorin RI. Factitious triiodothyronine toxicosis. *Am J Med* 1991;90:132–134.
7. Golightly LK, Smolinske SC, Kulig KW, et al. Clinical effects of accidental levothyroxine ingestion in children. *Am J Dis Child* 1987;141:1025–1027.
8. Lewander WJ, Lacouture PG, Silva JE, et al. Acute thyroxine ingestion in pediatric patients. *Pediatrics* 1989;84:262–265.
9. Litovitz TL, White JD. Levothyroxine ingestions in children: an analysis of 78 cases. *Am J Emerg Med* 1985;3:297–300.
10. Tenenbein M, Dean HJ. Benign course after massive levothyroxine ingestion. *Pediatr Emerg Care* 1986;2:15–17.
11. Tunget CL, Clark RF, Turchen SG, et al. Raising the decontamination level for thyroid hormone ingestions. *Am J Emerg Med* 1995;13:9–13.
12. Funderburk SJ, Spaulding JS. Sodium levothyroxine (Synthroid) intoxication in a child. *Pediatrics* 1970;45:298–301.
13. Kirkland RT, Kirkland JL, Greger NG, et al. Thyroid hormone poisoning: therapy questioned. *Pediatrics* 1984;74:901.
14. Nystrom E, Lindstedt G, Lundberg PA. Minor signs and symptoms of toxicity in a young woman in spite of massive thyroxine ingestion. *Acta Med Scand* 1980;207:135–136.
15. Von Hofe SE, Young RL. Thyrotoxicosis after a single ingestion of levothyroxine. *JAMA* 1977;237:1361.
16. Hack JB, Leviss JA, Nelson LS, et al. Severe symptoms following a massive intentional L-thyroxine ingestion. *Vet Hum Toxicol* 1999;41:323–326.
17. Levy R, Gilger WC. Acute thyroid poisoning. Report of a case. *N Engl J Med* 1957;255:456–460.
18. Schottstaedt ES, Smoller M. "Thyroid storm" produced by acute thyroid hormone poisoning. *Ann Intern Med* 1966;64:847–849.
19. Dahlberg PA, Karlsson FA, Wide L. Triiodothyronine intoxication. *Lancet* 1979;2:700.
20. Mandel SH, Magnusson AR, Burton BT, et al. Massive levothyroxine ingestion. Conservative management. *Clin Pediatr* 1989;28:374–376.
21. Roesch C, Becker PG, Sklar S. Management of a child with acute thyroxine ingestion. *Ann Emerg Med* 1985;14:1114–1115.
22. Shilo L, Kovatz S, Hadari R, et al. Massive thyroid hormone overdose: kinetics, clinical manifestations and management. *Isr Med Assoc J* 2002;4:298–299.
23. Bergeron GA, Goldsmith R, Schiller NB. Myocardial infarction, severe reversible ischemia, and shock following excess thyroid administration in a woman with normal coronary arteries. *Arch Intern Med* 1988;148:1450–1453.
24. Binimelis J, Bassas L, Marruecos L, et al. Massive thyroxine intoxication: evaluation of plasma extraction. *Intensive Care Med* 1987;13:33–38.
25. Kulig K, Golightly LK, Rumack BH. Levothyroxine overdose associated with seizures in a young child. *JAMA* 1985;254:2109–2110.
26. Petit WA Jr, Barrett EJ. Chronic thyroxine ingestion leading to thyroid storm and accelerated thyroxine turnover. *Conn Med* 1987;51:291–292.
27. van Huekelom S, Kinderen LH, der Vingerhoeds PJ. Plasmapheresis in L-thyroxine intoxication. *Vet Hum Toxicol* 1979;[Suppl 21]:7.

28. Vlase H, Lungu G, Vlase L. Cardiac disturbances in thyrotoxicosis: diagnosis, incidence, clinical features and management. *Endocrinologie* 1991;29:155–160.
29. Bacci V, Schussler GC, Bhogal RS, et al. Cardiac arrest after intravenous administration of levothyroxine. *JAMA* 1981;245:920.
30. Bhasin S, Wallace W, Lawrence JB, et al. Sudden death associated with thyroid hormone abuse. *Am J Med* 1981;71:887–890.
31. Bartalena L, Bogazzi F, Martino E: Adverse effects of thyroid hormone preparations and antithyroid drugs. *Drug Saf* 1996;15:53-63.
32. Hiasa Y, Ishida T, Aihara T, et al. Acute myocardial infarction due to coronary spasm associated with L-thyroxine therapy. *Clin Cardiol* 1989;12:161–163.
33. Locker GJ, Kotzmann H, Frey B, et al. Factitious hyperthyroidism causing acute myocardial infarction. *Thyroid* 1995;5:465–467.
34. Redahan C, Karski JM. Thyrotoxicosis factitia in a post-aortocoronary bypass patient. *Can J Anaesth* 1994;41:969–972.
35. LeBoff MS, Kaplan MM, Silva JE, et al. Bioavailability of thyroid hormones from oral replacement preparations. *Metabolism* 1982;31:900–905.
36. Wenzel KW, Meinhold H. Evidence of lower toxicity during thyroxine suppression after a single 3 mg L-thyroxine dose: comparison to the classical L-triiodothyronine test for thyroid suppressibility. *J Clin Endocrinol Metab* 1974;38:902–905.
37. Loos U, Wagner H, Bellstedt G, et al: The influence of hydration on T3 elimination in urine. *Horm Metab Res* 1976;8:154–155.
38. Ishihara T, Nishikawa M, Ikekubo K, et al. Thyroxine (T4) metabolism in an athyreotic patient who had taken a large amount of T4 at one time. *Endocr J* 1998;45:371–375.
39. Henderson A, Hickman P, Ward G, et al. Lack of efficacy of plasmapheresis in a patient overdosed with thyroxine. *Anaesth Intensive Care* 1994;22:463–464.
40. Kaiserman I, Avni M, Sack J. Kinetics of the pituitary-thyroid axis and the peripheral thyroid hormones in 2 children with thyroxine intoxication. *Horm Res* 1995;44:229–237.
41. Herrmann J, Rudorff KH, Gockenjan G, et al. Charcoal haemoperfusion in thyroid storm. *Lancet* 1977;1:248.
42. Mariotti S, Martino E, Cupini C, et al. Low serum thyroglobulin as a clue to the diagnosis of thyrotoxicosis factitia. *N Engl J Med* 1982;307:410–412..
43. Pearce CJ, Himsworth RL. Thyrotoxicosis factitia. *N Engl J Med* 1982;307:1708–1709.
44. Northcutt RC, Stiel JN, Hollifield JW, et al. The influence of cholestyramine on thyroxine absorption. *JAMA* 1969;208:1857–1861.
45. Shakir KMM, Michaels RD, Hays JH, et al. The use of bile acid sequestrants to lower serum thyroid hormones in iatrogenic hyperthyroidism. *Ann Intern Med* 1993;118:112–113.
46. Gerard P, Malvaux P, De Visscher M. Accidental poisoning with thyroid extract treated by exchange transfusion. *Arch Dis Child* 1972;47:981–982.
47. May ME, Mintz PD, Lowry P, et al. Plasmapheresis in thyroxine overdose: a case report. *J Toxicol Clin Toxicol* 1983;20:517–520.
48. Berkner PD, Starkman H, Person N. Acute L-thyroxine overdose; therapy with sodium ipodate: evaluation of clinical and physiologic parameters. *J Emerg Med* 1991;9:129–131.
49. Brown RS, Cohen JH, Braverman LE. Successful treatment of massive acute thyroid hormone poisoning with iopanoic acid. *J Pediatr* 1998;132:903–905.
50. Lacouture PG, Lewander WJ, Silva E, et al. Pharmacokinetics of T3 and T4 after iopanoic acid. *Pediatr Res* 1987;21:249A.
51. Bal C, Nair N. The therapeutic efficacy of oral cholecystographic agent (iopanoic acid) in the management of hyperthyroidism. *J Nucl Med* 1990;31:1180–1183.
52. Karpman BA, Rapoport B, Filetti S, et al. Treatment of neonatal hyperthyroidism due to Graves' disease with sodium ipodate. *J Clin Endocrinol Metab* 1987;64:119–123.
53. Sharp B, Reed AW, Tamagna EI, et al. Treatment of hyperthyroidism with sodium ipodate (Oragrafin) in addition to propylthiouracil and propranolol. *J Clin Endocrinol Metab* 1981;53:622–625.
54. Wu SY, Shyh TP, Chopra IJ, et al. Comparison of sodium ipodate (Oragrafin) and propylthiouracil in early treatment of hyperthyroidism. *J Clin Endocrinol Metab* 1982;54:632–634.
55. Singh GK, Winterborn MH. Massive overdose with thyroxine—toxicity and treatment. *Eur J Pediatr* 1991;150:217.
56. Gorman RL, Chamberlain JM, Rose SR, et al. Massive levothyroxine overdose: high anxiety—low toxicity. *Pediatrics* 1988;82:666–669.
57. Milner MR, Gelman KM, Phillips RA, et al. Double-blind crossover trial of diltiazem versus propranolol in the management of thyrotoxic symptoms. *Pharmacotherapy* 1990;10:100–106.
58. Roti E, Montermini M, Roti S, et al. The effect of diltiazem, a calcium channel-blocking drug, on cardiac rate and rhythm in hyperthyroid patients. *Arch Intern Med* 1988;148:1919–1921.
59. Chopra IJ, Williams DE, Orgiazzi J, et al. Opposite effects of dexamethasone on serum concentrations of 3,3',5'-triiodothyronine (reverse T3) and 3,3',5-triiodothyronine (T3). *J Clin Endocrinol Metab* 1975;41:911–920.
60. Reference deleted.
61. Baker B, Shapiro B, Fig LM, et al. Unusual complications of antithyroid drug therapy: four case reports and review of literature. *Thyroidology* 1989;1:17–26.
62. Deidiker R, deMello DE. Propylthiouracil-induced fulminant hepatitis: case report and review of the literature. *Pediatr Pathol Lab Med* 1996;16:845–852.
63. Ichiki Y, Akahoshi M, Yamashita N, et al. Propylthiouracil-induced severe hepatitis: a case report and review of the literature. *J Gastroenterol* 1998;33:747–750.
64. Levy M. Propylthiouracil hepatotoxicity. A review and case presentation. *Clin Pediatr (Phila)* 1993;32:25–29.
65. Lock DR, Sthoeger ZM. Severe hepatotoxicity on beginning propylthiouracil therapy. *J Clin Gastroenterol* 1997;24:267–269.
66. Pacini F, Sridama V, Refetoff S. Multiple complications of propylthiouracil treatment: granulocytopenia, eosinophilia, skin reaction and hepatitis with lymphocyte sensitization. *J Endocrinol Invest* 1982;5:403–407.
67. Seidman DS, Livni E, Ilie B, et al. Propylthiouracil-induced cholestatic jaundice. *J Toxicol Clin Toxicol* 1986;24:353–360.
68. Hayashida CY, Duarte AJ, Sato AE, et al. Neonatal hepatitis and lymphocyte sensitization by placental transfer of propylthiouracil. *J Endocrinol Invest* 1990;13:937–941.
69. Garty BZ, Kauli R, Ben-Ari J, et al. Hepatitis associated with propylthiouracil treatment. *Drug Intell Clin Pharm* 1985;19:740–742.
70. Kirkland JL. Propylthiouracil-induced hepatic failure and encephalopathy in a child. *Drug Intell Clin Pharm* 1990;24:470–471.
71. Breier DV, Rendo P, Gonzalez J, et al. Massive plasmacytosis due to methimazole-induced bone marrow toxicity. *Am J Hematol* 2001;67:259–261.
72. Di Gregorio C, Ghini F, Rivasi F. Granulomatous hepatitis in a patient receiving methimazole. *Ital J Gastroenterol* 1990;22:75–77.
73. Fischer MG, Nayer HR, Miller A. Methimazole-induced jaundice. *JAMA* 1973;223:1028–1029.
74. Luther AL, Wade JS, Slaughter JM. Agranulocytosis secondary to methimazole therapy: report of two cases. *South Med J* 1976;69:1356–1357.
75. Schwab GP, Wetscher GJ, Vogl W, et al. Methimazole-induced cholestatic liver injury, mimicking sclerosing cholangitis. *Langenbecks Arch Chir* 1996;381:225–227.
76. Van Kuyk M, Van Laethem Y, Duchateau J, et al. Methimazole-induced serum sickness. *Acta Clin Belg* 1983;38:68–69.
77. Bennett MH, Wainwright AP. Acute thyroid crisis on induction of anaesthesia. *Anaesthesia* 1989;44:28–30.
78. Christensen PA, Nissen LR. Treatment of thyroid storm in a child with dantrolene. *Br J Anaesth* 1987;59:523.
79. Ebert RJ. Dantrolene and thyroid crisis. *Anaesthesia* 1994;49:924.

SECTION

13

Local Anesthetics

CHAPTER 162

Local Anesthetics

Christy L. McCowan and E. Martin Caravati

See Figure 1 for chemical structures.

Synonyms:	**Bupivacaine (Sensorcaine); etidocaine (Duranest); lidocaine (Xylocaine); mepivacaine (Carbocaine); prilocaine (Citanest); dibucaine (Cinchocaine); benzocaine (Americaine, Hurricaine, Orajel); chloroprocaine (Nesacaine); procaine (Novocain); proparacaine (Alcaine); tetracaine (Amethocaine); dyclonine (Cepacol)**
Molecular formula and weight:	**See Table 1.**
SI conversion:	**See Table 1.**
CAS Registry No.:	**See Table 1.**
Therapeutic levels:	**See Table 1.**
Target organs:	**Central nervous system (acute)**
Antidote:	**Methylene blue**

OVERVIEW

Local anesthetic toxicity may follow excessive intravenous (IV) anesthetic dosage, inadvertent spinal or epidural administration, intraarterial injection, or absorption of large amounts of the anesthetic through mucous membranes, damaged skin, or highly vascular areas. In general, toxicity results from exaggerated pharmacologic activity. Toxic reactions include cardiovascular collapse, respiratory depression or arrest, seizures, dysrhythmias, and death. Treatment is largely supportive and symptomatic. Methemoglobinemia may be treated with methylene blue (Chapter 63).

Local anesthetics range from odorless to slightly aromatic. They may have a numbing or bitter taste. Most solutions are acidic (pH, 4 to 7). The acidity increases water solubility and stability. The majority of local anesthetics used in clinical practice have similar chemical structures. In general, an aromatic residue is joined to an amine portion by either an ester or an amide link.

The type of chemical linkage determines the class and specific properties of the drug (Fig. 1; Table 1). Amides are metabolized by enzymatic degradation in the liver, whereas esters are hydrolyzed by plasma pseudocholinesterase. The *amide*-type agents include bupivacaine, dibucaine, etidocaine, lidocaine, mepivacaine, and prilocaine. *Ester*-type agents include benzocaine, chloroprocaine, procaine, proparacaine, and tetracaine.

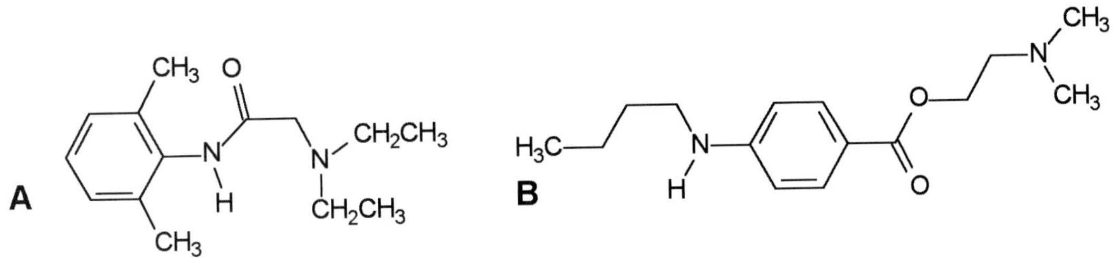

Figure 1. Examples of structures of amide and ester types of local anesthetics. **A:** Lidocaine. **B:** Tetracaine.

TABLE 1. **Physical characteristics and general dosages of local anesthetics**

Class name	Molecular formula	Molecular weight (g/mol)	SI conversion	CAS Registry No.	Therapeutic concentration	Maximum single dose[a] Adult (mg)	Maximum single dose[a] Children (mg/kg)
Amides							
Bupivacaine	$C_{18}H_{28}N_2O,HCl,H_2O$	342.9	mg/L × 2.9 = μmol/L	2180-92-9	0.25–0.50%	175 (225)	2 (3)
Etidocaine	$C_{17}H_{28}N_2O,HCl$	312.9	mg/L × 3.2 = μmol/L	36637-18-0	0.5%	300 (400)	NR
Lidocaine	$C_{14}H_{22}N_2O,HCl,H_2O$	234.3	mg/L × 4.3 = μmol/L	137-58-6	0.5–1.0%	300 (500)	4.5 (7)
Mepivacaine	$C_{15}H_{22}N_2O,HCl$	282.8	mg/L × 3.5 = μmol/L	96-88-8	0.5–1.0%	400	5–6
Prilocaine	$C_{13}H_{20}N_2O,HCl$	256.8	mg/L × 3.9 = μmol/L	721-50-6	0.5%, 1.0%, 2.0%	400 (300[b])	5
Dibucaine	$C_{20}H_{29}N_3O_2,HCl$	379.9	mg/L × 2.6 = μmol/L	61-12-1	0.5% cream; 1.0% ointment	30 g in 24 h	7.5 g in 24 h
Esters							
Benzocaine[c]	$C_9H_{11}NO_2$	165.2	mg/L × 6.1 = μmol/L	94-09-7	7.5%, 10.0%, 20.0% gel	—	—
Chloroprocaine	$C_{13}H_{19}ClN_2O_2,HCl$	307.2	mg/L × 3.3 = μmol/L	133-16-4	1.0–2.0%	800 (1000)	11
Procaine	$C_{13}H_{20}N_2O_2,HCl$	272.8	mg/L × 3.7 = μmol/L	59-46-1	0.25–0.50%	1000	15
Proparacaine	$C_{16}H_{26}N_2O_3,HCl$	330.9	mg/L × 3.0 = μmol/L	499-67-2	0.5%	NR	NR
Tetracaine	$C_{15}H_{24}N_2O_2,HCl$	264.4	mg/L × 3.8 = μmol/L	94-24-6	0.5%	20 (spinal)	NR
Other							
Dyclonine	$C_{18}H_{27}NO_2,HCl$	325.9	mg/L × 3.1 = μmol/L	536-43-6	0.5–1.0% topical preparations; 1.2–3.0 mg lozenge; 0.1% oral spray	200	NR

NR, not reported.
[a]Higher maximum doses are listed in parentheses for solutions containing epinephrine (1:200,000).
[b]If used with felypressin.
[c]Do not use in infants younger than the age of 2 years.

TOXIC DOSE

The *adult and pediatric therapeutic doses* of the local anesthetics are provided in Table 1. Toxicity associated with therapeutic doses is rare but may include allergic reactions or local irritation to tissues exposed to high drug concentrations. In general, reduced doses of local anesthetics should be used in patients with liver dysfunction and in elderly, debilitated, or young patients. Table 2 provides toxic doses after IV, intracarotid-artery, or intravertebral-artery administration. Amides are contraindicated in patients with porphyria.

Bupivacaine is not recommended for children younger than 12 years of age because of increased susceptibility to its central nervous system and cardiotoxic effects, especially children younger than the age of 1 year (1). Dibucaine caused death in two children after ingestions of 15 mg/kg and 19 mg/kg, respectively (2). Procaine administration of 4000 mg was followed by mydriasis, unreactive pupils, hypertension, sinus tachycardia, and electrocardiogram changes. The blood procaine level reached 96 μg/ml. A tetracaine dose of 60 to 160 mg to the pharynx may be followed by seizures or syncope in adults (3).

TABLE 2. **Toxic dose of local anesthetics: systemic circulation versus cerebral circulation[a]**

Local anesthetic	Minimum intravenous toxic dose in humans (mg/kg)	Estimated intravertebral artery toxic dose (mg/kg)[b]	Estimated intracarotid artery toxic dose (mg/kg)[a]
Procaine	19.2	0.288	2.592
Chloroprocaine	22.8	0.342	3.078
Tetracaine	2.5	0.038	0.337
Lidocaine	6.4	0.096	0.864
Mepivacaine	9.8	0.147	1.323
Bupivacaine	1.6	0.024	0.216
Etidocaine	3.4	0.051	0.459

[a]Adapted from Durrani Z, Winnie AP. Brainstem toxicity with reversible locked-in syndrome after intrascalene brachial plexus block. *Anesth Analg* 1991;72:249–252.
[b]Based on the cerebral circulation being 15% of the total cardiac output, and vertebral basilar circulation being 10% of the total cerebral circulation.

TOXICOKINETICS AND TOXICODYNAMICS

The absorption pharmacokinetics of the local anesthetic agents are provided in Table 3. Distribution and elimination are provided in Table 4.

PATHOPHYSIOLOGY

Local anesthetics block the transmission of nerve impulses reversibly. This is accomplished by inhibiting the sodium influx that is necessary to initiate and propagate an action potential. Sensory, autonomic, and motor nerve fibers are all affected. However, smaller diameter fibers are more susceptible to blockade. This causes a progressive blockade, which is dependent on the size of the nerve. Thus, nerve blockade develops in the following order: peripheral vasodilation, loss of pain and temperature sensation, loss of proprioception, loss of touch and pressure, and, finally, motor paralysis (4). Greater lipid solubility increases the potency and onset of action of local anesthetics. The relative potency of the various anesthetics (from increasing to decreasing) is as follows: dibucaine, tetracaine, bupivacaine, etidocaine, lidocaine, mepivacaine, prilocaine, chloroprocaine, procaine. The duration of

TABLE 3. Pharmacokinetics of local anesthetic absorption

Local anesthetic	Onset (min)	Duration	Peak plasma level	Time-to-peak blood level (min)
Bupivacaine HCl				
(Dental) 0.5%	2–10	7 h	0.45–1.25 μg/ml (after 125–150 mg)	30–45
(Epidural) 0.25–0.50%	4–17	3–7 h	0.22–6.0 μg/ml (after 10 ml of 0.5%)[a,b]	10–35[a,b]
(Epidural) 0.75%	3–16	6–9 h	—	—
(Spinal) 0.75% in 8.25% dextrose	1 (sensory) 15 (motor)	2 h 3.5 h	— —	— —
Chloroprocaine	6–12	0.5–1.0 h; 1.5 h with epinephrine	3.5–4.3 μg/ml of 2-chloro-4-aminobenzoic acid after 250 mg chloroprocaine	—
Etidocaine HCl	2–8	4.5–13.0 h	0.50–0.64 μg/ml (after 100–200 mg)	5–30
Lidocaine HCl (0.5–1.0%)	3–5	0.5–2.0 h (without epinephrine)	—	—
	—	1–3 h (with epinephrine)	0.28–0.53 μg/ml	30–60
Mepivacaine HCl (0.5–1.0%)				
(Epidural) 1–2%	5–15[c]	6–180 min[c]	—	—
(Major nerve) 1–2%	10–20[c]	3–5 h[c]	4.22 μg/ml (after 731.5 mg and epinephrine)[d]	30–60[d,e]
Prilocaine HCl (4%)	2	1–2 h	0.5–1.0 μg/ml	10–20
Procaine HCl (0.5–1.0%)	2–5	0.25–0.50 h (without epinephrine)	—	—
	—	0.5–1.5 h (with epinephrine)	—	—
Tetracaine HCl (2% gel)	30[f]	2.5 h[f]	—	—
Benzocaine				
(Gel)	7 (7.5%)[g]	3–5 h (10–20%)[h]	—	—
(Topical)	15–30 sec	12–15 min	—	—

HCl, hydrochloride.
[a]From Murat I, Montay G, Delleur MM, et al. Bupivacaine pharmacokinetics during epidural anaesthesia in children. *Eur J Anaesthesiol* 1988;5:113–120, with permission.
[b]From Thomas J, Climie CR, Mather LE. The maternal plasma levels and placental transfer of bupivacaine following epidural analgesia. *Br J Anaesth* 1969;41:1035–1040, with permission.
[c]From Concepcion M, Covino BG. Rational use of local anaesthetics. *Drugs* 1984;27:256–270, with permission.
[d]From Simon MAM, Vree TB, Gielen MJM, et al. Plasma concentrations after high doses of mepivacaine with epinephrine in the combined psoas compartment sciatic nerve block. *Reg Anesth* 1990;15:256–260, with permission.
[e]From Agostoni M, Fanelli G, Nobili F, et al. Mepivacaine plasma levels in the double block of sciatic and femoral nerves. *Minerva Anestesiol* 1992;58:281–284, with permission.
[f]From Peters H, Moll F. Pharmacodynamics of a liposomal preparation for local anesthesia. *Arzneimittelforschung* 1995;45:1253–1256, with permission.
[g]From Sveen OB, Yaekel M, Adair SM. Efficacy of using benzocaine for temporary relief of toothache. *Oral Surg Oral Med Oral Pathol* 1982;53:574–576, with permission.
[h]From Graser GN. The efficacy of topical anesthetics in reducing intraoral discomfort. *Oral Surg* 1984;58:42–46, with permission.
Adapted from Dershowitz M. In: Firestone LL, Lebowitz PW, Cook CE, eds. *Clinical anesthesia procedures of the Massachusetts General Hospital*, 3rd ed. Boston: Little, Brown, 1988.

action of local anesthetics increases with increased lipid solubility, protein binding, and vasoconstriction.

PREGNANCY AND LACTATION

The U.S. Food and Drug Administration pregnancy category is C (Appendix I) for all agents except etidocaine, lidocaine, and prilocaine, which are category B. Dibucaine has not been assigned a category. Lidocaine is considered safe during breast-feeding (4a), but safety has not been established for most local anesthetics. Bupivacaine and lidocaine are present in breast milk. Bupivacaine should not be used for obstetric paracervical–block anesthesia. Its use may cause fetal bradycardia and death.

CLINICAL PRESENTATION

Acute Overdosage

In general, the severity of toxicity is dose related and corresponds to the serum concentration. Initial symptoms include tinnitus, dizziness, and numbness of the mouth. Progression to neuromuscular signs and seizures may occur in severe cases.

TABLE 4. Pharmacokinetics of local anesthetic

Drug	Protein bound (%)	Volume of distribution (L/kg)	Half-life (adult)	Metabolism	Unchanged drug excreted (%)
Bupivacaine	82–96	0.4–1.0	1.3–5.5 h (8.1 in neonates)	L	4–10[a]
Etidocaine	94–96	1.9	1.0–2.7 h	L	<3
Lidocaine	51–80	1.1	1.5–2.0 h	L	<10
Mepivacaine	60–85	1.2	1.9 h	L	5–10
Prilocaine	55	NR	1.5 h	L	<1
Benzocaine	NR	NR	Fast hydrolysis	P	Minimal
Chloroprocaine	NR	NR	Fast hydrolysis	P	Metabolites
Tetracaine	NR	NR	Fast hydrolysis	P	Metabolites
Procaine	NR	0.3–0.8	7–8 min	P	<2

L, liver; NR, not reported; P, plasma.
[a]From Mather, 1971 Mather LE, Long GJ, Thomas J. The intravenous toxicity and clearance of bupivacaine in man. *Clin Pharm Ther* 1971;12:935–943, with permission.

Cardiac toxicity is usually preceded by central nervous system toxicity except in massive overdoses, in which cardiac arrest may be the first clinical manifestation. An initial period of physiologic stimulation is followed by generalized depression of vital signs. Miosis and tinnitus may be noticed. Mild intoxication may produce hypertension and tachycardia. Toxic doses may cause bradycardia, hypotension, atrial or ventricular dysrhythmias, asystole, or, rarely, ventricular tachycardia or fibrillation. Methemoglobinemia may occur in patients exposed to prilocaine, lidocaine, tetracaine, or benzocaine.

Respiratory effects are respiratory depression and apnea, which may be precipitous with large doses. Nausea and vomiting are common. Methemoglobinemia may occur in patients exposed to prilocaine, lidocaine, tetracaine, or benzocaine. Urticaria or angioedema can occur during a systemic allergic reaction. Vasodilation and contact dermatitis are local reactions. Muscle twitching, shivering, and weakness may occur; spinal anesthesia may cause complete motor blockade.

Neurologic effects range from mild toxicity (drowsiness, headache, dizziness, paresthesia, anxiety) to confusion, tremors, agitation, disorientation, and hallucinations. Seizures and coma may occur after rapid IV administration. Central nervous system symptoms precede cardiovascular toxicity except in the case of rapid IV injection.

Drug-Specific Considerations

Bupivacaine produces dizziness, tinnitus, hypotension, seizures, and ventricular tachycardia (5,6). It is cardiotoxic in both animal (7–10) and human studies (11,12). Toxic reactions to bupivacaine usually do not occur at plasma levels below 4 μg/ml. However, a 28-year-old woman developed convulsions with a blood level of 1.1 μg/ml (13). Bupivacaine is more cardiotoxic than other local anesthetics (8–12). Routine use of the 0.75% concentration of bupivacaine is not recommended and should be reserved for surgical procedures in which a high degree of muscle relaxation or prolonged effect is needed. Etidocaine exhibits similar cardiotoxic effects to bupivacaine (11).

Dibucaine is a topical anesthetic that is used for minor skin conditions. One of the most toxic amide anesthetics, it is no longer used for spinal anesthesia in the United States because of its toxicity. Dibucaine ointment ingestion has produced conduction delay, bradycardia, and ventricular dysrhythmias in children (1). The 1% ointment should not be used in children younger than the age of 2 years or in children weighing less than 35 lbs. Children between the ages of 2 and 12 years should use the ointment only under the direct supervision of a physician.

Lidocaine has a toxic blood level of 10 μg/ml (14). Ingestion of lidocaine solutions intended for topical anesthesia may result in signs of toxicity with serum levels of 7.3 to 12.0 μg/ml (15,16). Asystole, grand mal seizures, and a serum level of 19 μg/ml followed IV injection of 1200 mg (17). A 1-month-old child inadvertently received an IV bolus of 50 mg of lidocaine and developed respiratory arrest, seizures, and coma. The blood lidocaine level was 5.39 μg/ml (18).

Mepivacaine concentrations of 4.4 to 8.6 μg/ml after caudal administration of 5.5 to 9.4 mg/kg are associated with apprehension, confusion, muscular twitching, nausea, and vomiting (19). Neonates experiencing blood levels of up to 75 μg/ml require respiratory support and exchange transfusion. Toxic signs disappear when blood levels decrease to approximately 8 μg/ml (20). The toxic threshold for blood mepivacaine is a serum concentration of 5 to 10 μg/ml (21). However, others have not detected systemic toxicity with serum concentrations as high as 7 μg/ml (22).

Prilocaine has slower onset of action than lidocaine and a slightly longer duration of action. It has less vasodilator activity and is considered to be less toxic. It is used in combination with lidocaine (eutectic mixture of local anesthetics) as a topical anesthetic. Dose-related methemoglobinemia occurs with this medication.

Benzocaine can cause methemoglobinemia. Methemoglobinemia is more common in infants and young children (23–25) but has also been described in adults (26,27). Most cases of methemoglobinemia result from excessive use, although it has been reported after application of normal doses (28).

Chloroprocaine should not be used for regional anesthesia (Bier block) due to an increased risk of thrombophlebitis. In addition, it is not recommended for spinal anesthesia because of its potential neurotoxicity. Two patients who received epidural anesthesia with a 2% to 3% solution of chloroprocaine experienced motor paralysis. One patient had complete recovery in 72 hours, whereas the other had only partial recovery after 4 weeks (29).

Procaine is ineffective for surface application. In general, its use has been replaced by lidocaine. Peak plasma concentrations of 21 to 86 μg/ml followed administration of 18 to 55 mg/kg of procaine hydrochloride by IV infusion. Within 17 to 44 minutes, the plasma levels decreased to 1 to 13 μg/ml (30). The patient recovered after supportive treatment (31). Plasma procaine concentrations after intramuscular administration of 4.8 million U of procaine penicillin G ranged from 3.6 to 11.0 μg/ml (32).

Proparacaine is used as a topical anesthetic in ophthalmology. Rarely, severe corneal reactions or allergic contact dermatitis may occur. There have been several cases of keratitis in patients who developed an idiosyncratic reaction (33).

Tetracaine is used for topical anesthesia and spinal blocks. Its use as a local anesthetic is limited by its systemic toxicity. The application of tetracaine is contraindicated on highly vascular surfaces. Seizures and death in children have been reported with mixtures of tetracaine, epinephrine, and cocaine applied to mucous membranes (34).

Dyclonine is used for topical anesthesia on mucous membranes or skin. It can cause local irritation and should not be injected or used in the eyes. Two patients developed an allergic contact dermatitis, resembling extensive herpes simplex, after using dyclonine (35).

Adverse Events

Adverse effects associated with therapeutic dosages are rare but may include allergic reactions or local irritation of tissues exposed to high drug concentrations.

DIAGNOSTIC TESTS

Acute Overdosage

Thin-layer chromatography can qualitatively detect local anesthetics. Blood levels may be of value in lidocaine toxicity. Therapeutic levels of lidocaine are 1 to 5 μg/ml. Serious poisoning can occur with lidocaine, mepivacaine, or procaine levels more than 5 μg/ml. Bupivacaine concentrations of 1.5 to 2.3 μg/ml may cause dizziness, tinnitus, and hypotension (3).

Serum electrolytes and arterial blood gases should be followed closely in patients exhibiting symptoms of toxicity. Methemoglobin concentration should be determined in cases of cyanosis (benzocaine) (Chapter 21). An electrocardiogram is indicated in patients with tachycardia, bradycardia, hypotension, or dysrhythmias.

Postmortem Considerations

The postmortem blood dibucaine concentration was 1.3 μg/ml in a 2-year-old boy who ingested an unknown amount of 0.5% cream (2). Postmortem lidocaine blood concentrations of 5 and 9 μg/ml were found after paracervical administration of lidocaine in two adults (3). Topical administration of lidocaine for endotracheal intubation may undergo postmortem diffusion and produce significant heart blood concentrations (3). After a dose of 864 mg of prilocaine, postmortem prilocaine concentrations of 13 μg/ml were measured. The patient died in the dentist's chair within 1 hour of administration (36).

TREATMENT

Decontamination

Emesis and whole bowel irrigation are not recommended. Activated charcoal binds lidocaine and probably other anesthetics as well. Administration of activated charcoal to patients with an intact airway may be helpful in large ingestion of creams or ointments, especially if given within 1 hour of ingestion. Routine administration of a cathartic is not indicated (37). Activated charcoal is contraindicated in patients with an unstable airway or with seizures (38).

Enhancement of Elimination

Hemodialysis (39), hemofiltration (40), forced diuresis (41), and urinary acidification (42) are not useful in the management of local anesthetic toxicity. The clearance rates of hemodialysis and hemoperfusion are 100 to 200 ml/minute. Hepatic clearance of lidocaine is 1000 ml/minute in patients with normal cardiac output. Ensuring adequate cardiac output with extracorporeal pump assistance allows hepatic clearance of lidocaine (43). In one case, an asystolic arrest induced by inadvertent administration of lidocaine was successfully treated with cardiopulmonary bypass followed by inotropic support and atrial pacing (44).

Antidotes

Patients with methemoglobinemia should be treated with oxygen and possibly methylene blue. The dose of methylene blue is 1 to 2 mg/kg/dose over 5 minutes, with repeated doses every 4 hours if necessary. This treatment is contraindicated in patients with glucose 6 phosphate dehydrogenase deficiency. Details of the use of methylene blue are provided in Chapter 63.

Supportive Care

Patients should have IV access, cardiorespiratory monitoring, supplemental oxygen, and seizure precautions provided. Sodium bicarbonate (1 to 2 mEq/kg) should be considered in patients who have a severe metabolic acidosis (pH less than 7.1) (Chapter 75). Respiratory acidosis should be treated with assisted ventilation. Symptomatic bradycardia can be treated with atropine (Chapter 42). Hypotension is managed with isotonic crystalloidal IV fluids followed by vasopressor support, if necessary (Chapter 37).

After stabilization of the airway, seizures should be treated with benzodiazepines followed by more aggressive interventions if needed (Chapter 40). In general, phenytoin should be avoided in local anesthetic overdoses because of the possibility of causing or worsening cardiac dysrhythmias (45). A study using rabbit hearts exposed to bupivacaine showed that both lidocaine and phenytoin enhanced the QRS prolongation associated with bupivacaine toxicity (46). There has been one report of successful treatment of cardiac toxicity with phenytoin in neonates (47).

Monitoring

Patients should have continuous cardiac and respiratory monitoring. Oxygen saturation should be monitored with pulse oximetry. Seizure precautions should be undertaken and supplement oxygen made available for hypoxia. Serum electrolytes and arterial blood gases should be followed closely. A methemoglobin concentration should be obtained if methemoglobinemia is suspected (benzocaine).

REFERENCES

1. Dalens BJ, Mazoit JX. Adverse effects of regional anaesthesia in children. *Drug Saf* 1998;19:251–268.
2. Dayan PS, Litovitz TL, Crouch BI, et al. Fatal accidental dibucaine poisoning in children. *Ann Emerg Med* 1996;28:442–445.
3. Baselt RC. *Disposition of toxic drugs and chemicals in man*, 6th ed. Foster City, CA: Chemical Toxicology Institute, 2002:577–581.
4. Dershowitz M. Local anesthetics. In: Firestone LL, Lebowitz PW, Cook CE, eds. *Clinical anesthesia procedures of the Massachusetts General Hospital*, 3rd ed. Boston: Little, Brown, 1988.

4a. Anonymous. American Academy of Pediatrics Committee on Drugs. The transfer of drugs and other chemicals into human milk. *Pediatrics* 1994;93:137–150.

5. Hollmen A, Korhonen M, Ojala A. Bupivacaine in paracervical block—plasma levels and changes in maternal and fetal acid-base balance. *Br J Anaesth* 1969;41:603–608.
6. Moore DC, Balfour RI, Fitzgibbons D. Convulsive arterial plasma levels of bupivacaine and the response to diazepam therapy. *Anesthesiology* 1979;50:454–456.
7. Anonymous. Cardiotoxicity of local anaesthetic drugs. *Lancet* 1986;2:1192–1194.
8. Chang DH, Ladd LA, Copeland S, et al. Direct cardiac effects of intracoronary bupivacaine, levobupivacaine and ropivacaine in the sheep. *Br J Pharmacol* 2001;132:649–658.
9. Kotelko DM, Shnider SM, Dailey PA, et al. Bupivacaine-induced cardiac arrhythmias in sheep. *Anesthesiology* 1984;60:10–18.
10. Thomas RD, Behbehani MM, Coyle DE, et al. Cardiovascular toxicity of local anesthetics: an alternative hypothesis. *Anesth Analg* 1986;65:444–450.
11. Albright GA. Cardiac arrest following regional anesthesia with etidocaine or bupivacaine. *Anesthesiology* 1979;51:285–287.
12. Scott DB, Lee A, Fagan D, et al. Acute toxicity of ropivacaine compared with that of bupivacaine. *Anesth Analg* 1989;69:563–569.
13. Hasselstrom LJ, Mogensen T. Toxic reaction of bupivacaine at low plasma concentration. *Anesthesiology* 1984;61:99–100.
14. Bromage PR, Robson JG. Concentrations of lignocaine in the blood after intravenous, intramuscular, epidermal and endotracheal administration. *Anaesthesia* 1961;16:461–478.
15. Gorman RL, King JD, Oderda GM. Ingestion of topical lidocaine. It's time to stop the pain. *Vet Hum Toxicol* 1984;26:413.
16. Fruncillo RJ, Gibbons W, Bowman SM. CNS toxicity after ingestion of topical lidocaine. *N Engl J Med* 1982;306:426–427.
17. Edgren B, Tilelli J, Gehrz R. Intravenous lidocaine overdosage in a child. *J Toxicol Clin Toxicol* 1986;24:51–58.
18. Jonville AP, Barbier P, Blond MH, et al. Accidental lidocaine overdosage in an infant. *J Toxicol Clin Toxicol* 1990;28:101–106.
19. Morishima HO, Daniel SS, Finster M, et al. Transmission of mepivacaine hydrochloride (carbocaine) across the human placenta. *Anesthesiology* 1966;27:147–154.
20. Finster M, Popper PJ, Sinclair JC, et al. Accidental intoxication of the fetus with local anesthetic drug during caudal anesthesia. *Am J Obstet Gynecol* 1965;92:922–924.
21. Concepcion M, Covino BG. Rational use of local anaesthetics. *Drugs* 1984;27:256–270.
22. Buettner J, Klose R, Hoppe U, et al. Serum levels of mepivacaine-HCl during continuous axillary brachial plexus block. *Reg Anesth* 1989;14:124–127.
23. Seibert RW, Seibert JJ. Infantile methemoglobinemia induced by a topical anesthetic cetacaine. *Laryngoscope* 1984;94:816–817.
24. Tush GM, Kuhn RJ. Methemoglobinemia induced by an over-the-counter medication. *Ann Pharmacother* 1996;30:1251–1254.
25. Eldadah M, Fitzgerald M. Methemoglobinemia due to skin application of benzocaine. *Clin Pediatr (Phila)* 1993;32:687–688.
26. Linares LA, Peretz TY, Chin J. Methemoglobinemia induced by topical anesthetic (benzocaine). *Radiother Oncol* 1990;18:267–269.
27. Ferraro-Borgida MJ, Mulhern SA, DeMeo MO, et al. Methemoglobinemia from perineal application of an anesthetic cream. *Ann Emerg Med* 1996;27:785–788.
28. Olson ML, McEvoy GK. Methemoglobinemia induced by local anesthetics. *Am J Hosp Pharm* 1981;38:89–93.
29. Kane RE. Neurologic deficits following epidural or spinal anesthesia. *Anesth Analg* 1981;60:150–161.
30. Usubiaga JE, Wikinski J, Ferrero R, et al. Local anesthetic-induced convulsions in man—an electroencephalographic study. *Anesth Analg* 1966;45:611–620.
31. Wikinski JA, Usubiaga JE, Wikinski RW. Cardiovascular and neurological effects of 4,000 mg of procaine. *JAMA* 1970;213:621–623.
32. Green RL, Lewis JE, Kraus SJ, et al. Elevated plasma procaine concentrations after administration of procaine penicillin G. *N Engl J Med* 1979;91:223–226.

33. Theodore FH. Idiosyncratic reactions of the cornea from proparacaine. *Eye Ear Nose Throat Monthly* 1968;47:286–289.
34. Wong S, Hart LL. Tetracaine/adrenaline/cocaine for local anesthesia. *DICP Ann Pharmacother* 1990;24:1181–1183.
35. Purcell SM, Dixon SL. Allergic contact dermatitis to dyclonine hydrochloride simulating extensive herpes simplex labialis. *J Am Acad Dermatol* 1985;12:231–234.
36. Kaliciak HA, Chan SC. Distribution of prilocaine in body fluids and tissues in lethal overdose. *J Anal Toxicol* 1986;10:75–76.
37. Barceloux D, McGuigan M, Hartigan-Go K. Position statement: cathartics. American Academy of Clinical Toxicology; European Association of Poisons Centres and Clinical Toxicologists. *J Toxicol Clin Toxicol* 1997;35:743–752.
38. Chyka PA, Seger D. Position statement: single-dose activated charcoal. American Academy of Clinical Toxicology; European Association of Poisons Centres and Clinical Toxicologists. *J Toxicol Clin Toxicol* 1997;35:721–736.
39. Jacobi J, McGory RW, McCoy H, et al. Hemodialysis clearance of total unbound lidocaine. *Clin Pharm* 1983;2:54–57.
40. Saima S, Echizen H, Yoshimoto K, et al. Negligible removal of lidocaine during arteriovenous hemofiltration. *Ther Drug Monit* 1990;12:154–156.
41. Hillman LS, Hillman RE, Dodson WE. Diagnosis, treatment and follow-up of neonatal mepivacaine intoxication secondary to paracervical and pudendal blocks during labor. *J Pediatr* 1979;95:472–477.
42. Meffin P, Long GJ, Thomas J. Clearance and metabolism of mepivacaine in the human neonate. *Clin Pharmacol Ther* 1973;14:218–225.
43. Freedman MD, Gal J, Freed CR. Extracorporeal pump assistance—novel treatment for acute lidocaine poisoning. *Eur J Clin Pharmacol* 1982;22:129–135.
44. Noble J, Kennedy DJ, Latimer RD, et al. Massive lignocaine overdose during cardiopulmonary bypass. *Br J Anaesth* 1984;56:1439–1441.
45. Wood RA. Sinoatrial arrest: an interaction between phenytoin and lignocaine. *BMJ* 1971;20:645.
46. Simon L, Kariya N, Pelle-Lancien E, Mazoit JX. Bupivacaine-induced QRS prolongation is enhanced by lidocaine and by phenytoin in rabbit hearts. *Anesth Analg* 2002;94:203–207.
47. Maxwell LG, Martin LD, Yaster M. Bupivacaine-induced cardiac toxicity in neonates: successful treatment with intravenous phenytoin. *Anesthesiology* 1994;80:682–686.

SECTION 14

Serums, Toxoids, and Vaccines

CHAPTER 163
Serums and Toxoids

Katherine M. Hurlbut

Compounds included:	**See Table 1.**
SI conversion:	**Not applicable**
Therapeutic levels:	**Not used clinically**
Special concerns:	**All protein-containing pharmaceuticals can produce acute allergic reactions (anaphylactic and anaphylactoid reactions) as well as delayed reactions (serum sickness).**
Antidote:	**None**

OVERVIEW

Serums are composed of immune globulins derived from one of several sources, most commonly immune human serum, or serum from hyperimmunized horses or sheep. Serums are used to provide passive immunity to a variety of infectious diseases or to neutralize the effects of venoms. In the case of digoxin immune Fab the antibody is used to bind digoxin in patients with digoxin overdose (Table 2).

The immunoglobulins in serums act by binding the specific free circulating antigens (present in venoms, infecting organisms, drugs, and so forth) and preventing the interaction of those antigens with the usual targets within the body. In the case of serums against infectious agents, this allows the organism to be killed more efficiently by the patient's immune defenses without native antibodies to or previous immunization against the infecting organism. In the case of a venom, the serum binds venom components, preventing or in some cases reversing their local or systemic effects. In the case of digoxin immune Fab the serum binds free digoxin, preventing its binding to the sodium-potassium adenosine triphosphatase enzyme.

Digoxin immune Fab is also addressed in Chapter 49. The scorpion, snake, and spider antivenoms are addressed in Chapters 73, 74, and 76.

TABLE 1. Compounds included

Antivenin (Crotalidae) polyvalent
Antivenin (*Latrodectus mactans*)
Antivenin (*Micrurus fulvius*)
Crotalidae polyvalent immune Fab (CroFab)
Cytomegalovirus immune globulin (CytoGam)
Digoxin immune Fab (Digibind, DigiFab)
Diphtheria antitoxin
Hepatitis B immune globulin (BayHep B)
Immune globulin (BayGam, Sandoglobulin)
Rabies immune globulin (BayRab, Imogam Rabies-HT)
Rho(D) immune globulin (Michrogam, Rhogam)
Tetanus immune globulin (BayTet)
Varicella-zoster immune globulin

TOXIC DOSE

No toxic dose has been established for any of these agents. Allergic reactions may occur at therapeutic doses.

TOXICOKINETICS AND TOXICODYNAMICS

Pharmacokinetic information for the serums and toxoids is provided in Table 3.

PATHOPHYSIOLOGY

Immune globulins used in infectious diseases (cytomegalovirus immune globulin, rabies immune globulin, immune globulin, diphtheria antitoxin, hepatitis B immune globulin, respiratory syncytial virus immune globulin, tetanus immune globulin, varicella-zoster immune globulin) are products derived from pooled human serum with high titers of antibodies against the specific infecting organism in question. The antibodies provide passive immunization, allowing efficient killing of the infecting organism by a nonimmune host. When immune globulin is used in the therapy of autoimmune disorders much larger doses are required than those used to treat immunodeficiency states. At these large doses, immune globulins are believed to block Fc receptors in macrophages, preventing phagocytosis of platelets or cells with autoantibodies.

Antivenoms are derived from pooled serum from animals (horses or sheep) that have been hyperimmunized with venoms

TABLE 2. Physical characteristics and dosage of serums and toxoids

Product	Formulation	Dose	
		Adult	Pediatric
Antivenin (Crotalidae) polyvalent	Single vial containing lyophilized antivenom and 10-ml sterile diluent for reconstitution[a]	Initial dose of 5–20 vials by slow intravenous infusion depending on the severity of the envenomation. Subsequent doses of 5–10 vials may be needed depending on patient response.	Same as for adult.
Antivenin (Latrodectus mactans)	Single vial containing lyophilized antivenom (not less than 6000 antivenom units) and vial of 2.5-ml sterile diluent for reconstitution[a,b]	One vial by slow intravenous infusion. A subsequent vial may be administered if there is insufficient response.	Same as for adult.
Antivenin (Micrurus fulvius)	Single vial containing lyophilized antivenom and 10-ml sterile diluent for reconstitution[a,b]	Initial dose of 3–5 vials by slow intravenous infusion. This dose can be repeated if symptoms progress.	Same as for adult.
Crotalidae polyvalent immune Fab	—	Initial dose 4–6 vials by slow intravenous infusion, followed by 2 vials every 6 h for 18 h. Subsequent 2-vial doses as needed.	Same as for adult.
Cytomegalovirus immune globulin intravenously	Vials containing either 1000 mg (20 ml) or 2500 mg (50 ml) immunoglobulin	Initial dose of 150 mg/kg by slow IV infusion, subsequent doses of between 50 and 150 mg/kg depending on type of organ and time since transplant.	Not established.
Digoxin immune Fab	Single vial of 38 mg lyophilized digoxin-specific Fab	10–20 vials for severe acute unknown ingestion, 6 vials usually sufficient for chronic toxicity. Lesser amounts more commonly used depending on amount ingested or steady state serum digoxin levels.	10 vials for severe acute unknown ingestion, 1 vial is usually sufficient for chronic toxicity. Lesser amounts more commonly used for acute ingestion depending on amount ingested or serum levels.
Diphtheria antitoxin	—	40,000–120,000 U (depending on duration and severity of disease) IM or slow IV infusion.	Same as adult.
Hepatitis B immune globulin	Single-use vials of 1–5 ml, neonatal single-dose syringe of 0.5 ml	0.06 ml/kg intramuscularly.	Neonates 0.5 ml IM.
Immune globulin	Single-use vials containing 2, 10, 25, 50, 100, 200, or 250 ml; single-use vials of 0.5, 1.0, 2.5, 5.0, and 10.0 g of lyophilized immunoglobulin and sterile diluent for reconstitution	Depending on the indication and formulation, doses range from 0.02–1.3 ml/kg intramuscularly, 400 mg/kg to 2 g/kg by intravenous infusion.	Same as adult.
Rabies immune globulin	Single-use vials of 2 and 10 ml, 150 IU/ml	20 IU/kg, as much as possible is infiltrated around the bite site and the remainder administered IM.	20 IU/kg, as much as possible is infiltrated around the bite site and the remainder administered IM.
Respiratory syncytial virus immune globulin IV	50-ml vials containing 2500 mg immune globulin	NA.	750 mg/kg as an IV infusion.
Rho(D) immune globulin	Single-dose syringes, single-use vials containing 120 μg (600 IU), 300 μg (1500 IU), and 1000 μg (5000 IU)	50–300 μg IM depending on the indication. Larger doses needed for Rh incompatible transfusion.	NA.
Tetanus immune globulin	250-U prefilled syringes	250 U IM.	250 U IM (children younger than 7 yr old may receive 4 U/kg).
Varicella-zoster immune globulin	Single-use vials containing 1.25 or 6.25 ml	IM injection of 125 U for patients up to 10 kg; 250 U for patients 10.1–20.0 kg; 375 U for patients 20.1–30.0 kg; 500 U for patients 30.1–40.0 kg; 625 U for patients >40 kg.	Same as adult.

NA, not available.
[a]Contains thimerosal as a preservative.
[b]Contains phenol as a preservative.

(in the case of crotalid antivenoms the animals are immunized against several species of snakes). Crotalidae polyvalent immune Fab is derived from serum from hyperimmunized sheep that is then subject to papain digestion (to separate Fab fragments and remove the immunogenic Fc fraction) and affinity purification (to remove nonspecific Fab fragments). These procedures reduce the incidence of immediate and delayed hypersensitivity reactions. Antivenoms act by binding and neutralizing venom toxins and allowing them to be cleared by the reticuloendothelial system.

Digoxin immune Fab is derived from the serum of hyperimmunized sheep. The serum is then digested with papain, which separates the Fab fragment and allows removal of the immunogenic Fc portion. The Fab is then subjected to affinity purification to remove nonspecific Fab. These procedures reduce the incidence of immediate and delayed hypersensitivity reactions. Digoxin immune Fab acts by binding digoxin and other digitalis-like glycosides, preventing their binding to sodium potassium adenosine triphosphatase and reversing the cardiotoxic effects of digitalis overdose.

TABLE 3. Pharmacokinetics of serums and toxoids

Product	Onset	Duration	Volume of distribution	Half-life
Cytomegalovirus immune globulin intravenously	NR	NR	NR	7 days
Digoxin immune Fab	30 min or less, peak 3–4 h	Several days	0.46 L/kg	15–20 h
Hepatitis B immune globulin	Peak response 3–21 d	2 mo or more	NR	17–25 d
Crotalidae polyvalent immune Fab	Within 4 h	NR	0.3 L/kg	2.5 h
Immune globulin	T_{max} 2 days after IM dosing	NR	42 ml/kg (in neonates)	3–6 wk
Rabies immune globulin	Onset 24 h, peak 2–7 d	NR	—	21 d
Respiratory syncytial virus immune globulin intravenously	NR	NR	—	22–28 d
Rho(D) immune globulin	8 h to 2 d	30 d (for idiopathic thrombocytopenic purpura)	—	24 d IV, 30 d IM
Tetanus immune globulin	—	—	—	3–5 wk
Varicella-zoster immune globulin	—	—	—	3 wk

NR, not reported.

PREGNANCY AND LACTATION

All of the serums and toxoids are U.S. Food and Drug Administration pregnancy category C (Appendix I). Because they are large protein molecules, none of the serums and toxoids is expected to be excreted in breast milk.

CLINICAL PRESENTATION

Acute Overdosage

Acute toxicity has not been reported; however, acute allergic events may occur. The rate of allergic events ranges widely and may depend on the rate of infusion. Early (acute) hypersensitivity reactions range in severity from mild to life-threatening (1,2). An acute reaction involves flushing, pruritus, diaphoresis, and urticaria, to angioedema, bronchospasm, hypotension, anaphylactic shock, and cardiorespiratory arrest. The effects can progress rapidly (2,3). A few deaths have been attributed to snake antivenom (4,5).

There are two types of acute reactions: *anaphylactic* (type I allergic) or an *anaphylactoid* response. Anaphylactic reactions are mediated by IgE, which results in the release of histamine and other inflammatory mediators from mast cells. An anaphylactoid reaction is similar to anaphylaxis, but usually less severe. Anaphylactoid reactions are unpredictable because they require no prior exposure. They appear to be related to the rate and concentration of the infusion (6) and may arise from direct activation of complement (7). However, other studies have found that neither complement activation nor immune complexes appeared to be associated with anaphylactoid reactions (8).

Adverse Events

Nonspecific effects of protein administration are common during infusion of these products. Adverse effects include nausea, malaise, fever, muscle aches, and chills.

Serum sickness is a type III hypersensitivity reaction that is relatively common after antivenom administration (6,9). It is a flu-like illness characterized by symptoms such as fever, chills, myalgia, malaise, arthralgia, rash or flushing, urticaria, nausea, vomiting, lymphadenopathy, and pruritus. It generally develops 5 to 10 days after antivenom treatment. On rare occasions, serum sickness involves complications like bronchospasm, hypotension, glomerulonephritis or proteinuria, and pericarditis (8,10). The reaction is believed to be caused by immune complex formation (8). Administration of foreign serum stimulates an immune response and the production of host antibodies against the foreign immunoglobulins. The host and foreign immunoglobulins combine to form large complexes, which deposit throughout the body. The recipient's immune system is activated by the complexes, resulting in a variety of symptoms and sequelae. The incidence of serum sickness appears to be dose related.

The incidence of serum sickness varies markedly between antivenoms. Many studies underestimate the true incidence of serum sickness because follow-up is often problematic, especially in remote areas. A review of publication indicated the serum sickness rate for antivenin (Crotalidae) polyvalent was approximately 75% of recipients (1). Crotalidae polyvalent Fab appears to cause far fewer delayed reactions than Wyeth antivenom, with postmarketing data suggesting an incidence of approximately 7% (9).

Immune globulin has been associated with many adverse effects. Hemolysis and anemia may occur. It has also been associated with neutropenia, although adverse clinical sequelae have not been reported. Aseptic meningitis (headache, fever, nausea, vomiting, and nuchal rigidity) may develop within hours to 7 days (11). Acute renal failure may develop, primarily secondary to products that contain sucrose (12). Hepatitis has been transferred by some immune globulin products.

Rho(D) immune globulin causes hemolysis and decreased hemoglobin in Rho(D) positive patients with immune thrombocytopenic purpura. It should be used with extreme caution in patients with a hemoglobin level less than 8 g/dl (13).

DIAGNOSTIC TESTS

Acute toxicity from overdosage has not been reported. Diagnostic tests for acute hypersensitivity reactions include complete blood count and evaluation of serum electrolytes and renal function, especially in patients with prolonged or severe hypotension or tachycardia. Evaluation of respiratory function with arterial blood gases may also be needed.

Aseptic meningitis from immune globulin has shown neutrophils with mildly raised protein and depressed glucose levels in the cerebrospinal fluid.

TREATMENT

Most adverse effects (fever, rash, renal failure, aseptic meningitis) are managed with symptomatic and supportive care. Decontamination has not been evaluated and is not expected to be effective. There are no antidotes for toxicity from serums or toxoids.

Acute Allergic Reactions

Although mechanistically different, anaphylactoid and anaphylactic reactions are treated in the same manner. If signs of a reaction develop, the infusion should be stopped immediately and the patient treated as an allergic reaction. Skin reactions can usually be controlled with H_1- and H_2-blockers. Typical treatment includes diphenhydramine, 25 to 50 mg intravenously (IV), and cimetidine, 300 mg IV, or their equivalents. Bronchospasm can generally be managed with inhaled β_2-receptor agonists (e.g., metered dose inhaler or albuterol 5 mg by nebulizer). Patients with severe bronchospasm, angioedema, or anaphylaxis are treated as anaphylaxis (Chapter 34). Patients on beta-blocking agents who develop anaphylactic shock may respond to IV glucagon if epinephrine is not effective. For most acute allergic reactions, corticosteroids (e.g., methylprednisolone, 125 mg IV, or its equivalent) are recommended.

Delayed Allergic Reactions

Serum sickness can be effectively controlled with antipruritic drugs and corticosteroids (e.g., prednisone, 60 mg orally daily for 7 to 14 days) and antihistamines (e.g., diphenhydramine, 25 to 50 mg orally every 6 to 8 hours). The most common mistake is to administer corticosteroids for a short period, which allows rash and pruritus to recur.

REFERENCES

1. Corrigan P, Russell FE, Wainschel J. Clinical reactions to antivenin. *Toxicon* 1978;65[Suppl]:457–465.
2. Clark RF, McKinney PE, Chase PB, Walter FG. Immediate and delayed allergic reactions to Crotalidae polyvalent immune Fab (ovine) antivenom. *Ann Emerg Med* 2002;39(6):671–676.
3. Chippaux JP, Williams V, White J. Snake venom variability: methods of study, results and interpretation. *Toxicon* 1991;29(11):1279–1303.
4. Reid HA. Adder bites in Britain. *BMJ* 1976;2(6028):153–156.
5. Christensen PA. The treatment of snakebite. *S Afr Med J* 1969;43(41):1253–1258.
6. Sutherland SK, Lovering KE. Antivenoms: use and adverse reactions over a 12-month period in Australia and Papua New Guinea. *Med J Aust* 1979;2(13):671–674.
7. Malasit P, Warrell DA, Chanthavanich P, et al. Prediction, prevention, and mechanism of early (anaphylactic) antivenom reactions in victims of snake bites. *Br Med J (Clin Res Ed)* 1986;292(6512):17–20.
8. Nielsen H, Sorensen H, Faber V, Svehag SE. Circulating immune complexes, complement activation kinetics and serum sickness following treatment with heterologous anti-snake venom globulin. *Scand J Immunol* 1978;7(1):25–33.
9. Dart RC, Seifert SA, Boyer LV, et al. A randomized multicenter trial of Crotalidae polyvalent immune Fab (ovine) antivenom for the treatment for crotaline snakebite in the United States. *Arch Intern Med* 2001;161(16):2030–2036.
10. Cuzic S, Scukanec-Spoljar M, Bosnic D, et al. Immunohistochemical analysis of human serum sickness glomerulonephritis. *Croat Med J* 2001;42(6):618–623.
11. De Vlieghere FC, Peetermans WE, Vermylen J. Aseptic granulocytic meningitis following treatment with intravenous immunoglobulin. *Clin Infect Dis* 1994;18:1008–1010.
12. Epstein JS, Zoon KC. *Important drug warning*. Rockville, MD: United States Food and Drug Administration, Center for Biologics Evaluation and Research, September 24, 1999.
13. WinRho SDF. Rho(D) immune globulin. Product information. Boca Raton, FL: Nabi Pharmaceuticals, revised December 1999.

CHAPTER 164
Vaccines

Leslie Ann Mendoza-Temple and Steve N. Vogel

Compounds included: See Table 1.
SI conversion: Not applicable
Special concerns: Overdosage of bacillus Calmette-Guérin vaccine can cause systemic infection.
Antidotes: Antituberculous antimicrobials

OVERVIEW

A *vaccine* is defined as a suspension of live (usually attenuated) or inactivated microorganisms (e.g., bacteria or viruses) or their fractions administered to induce immunity and prevent an infectious disease or its sequelae. Some vaccines contain highly defined, complex, or incompletely defined antigens. Vaccines may be categorized as (a) live attenuated virus, (b) noninfectious inactivated virus, (c) antigenic capsular polysaccharides, subunit/recombinants, (d) cell culture–derived diploid cell vaccine, and (e) cell-free filtrates.

A *toxoid* is a modified bacterial toxin that has been made nontoxic but retains the ability to stimulate the formation of antibodies to the toxin. *Immune globulin* is a sterile solution containing antibodies, which are usually obtained from pooled human blood plasma. It is primarily indicated for routine maintenance of immunity among certain immunodeficient people and for passive protection against measles and hepatitis A.

Thimerosal is a mercury-containing preservative used to prevent bacterial contamination in several vaccines (1). Thimerosal contains 49% ethylmercury and is found in some preparations of hepatitis B recombinant, immune globulin IM, diphtheria/tetanus toxoids and acellular pertussis vaccine adsorbed, influenza vaccine, Japanese encephalitis (JE) virus vaccine, meningococcal vaccine, *Haemophilus influenza* (Hib) pneumococcal 23-valent polysaccharide vaccine, and rabies vaccine. Several vaccines have never contained thimerosal: measles, mumps, and rubella (MMR), varicella (chickenpox), and inactivated polio vaccine. The toxicity of thimerosal is addressed in Chapter 224.

Federal guidelines are meant to reduce mercury exposure to women of childbearing age who may expose their fetuses to mercury during rapid brain development and growth. However, the

TABLE 1. Compounds included

Anthrax vaccine adsorbed (Biothrax)
Bacillus Calmette-Guérin (BCG) vaccine (TICE)
Haemophilus b conjugate vaccine (Act-Hib, Hibtiter, Pedvaxhib)
Hepatitis A virus vaccine (Havrix, Vaqta)
Hepatitis A inactivated and hepatitis B recombinant vaccine (Twinrix)
Hepatitis B recombinant (Recombivax HB, Engerix-B)
Haemophilus b polysaccharide and hepatitis B vaccine combined (Comvax)
Influenza virus vaccine (FluShield, Fluzone)
Japanese encephalitis vaccine (JE-Vax)
Lyme disease vaccine (LYMErix)
Measles, mumps, and rubella virus vaccine live (MMR vaccine)
Meningococcal polysaccharide vaccine (Menomune)
Pneumococcal vaccine (Pneumovax 23, Pnu-Immune 23)
Rabies vaccines (chick embryo culture vaccine, human diploid cell vaccine, rabies vaccine adsorbed)
Rotavirus vaccine
Tick encephalitis vaccine
Typhoid vaccine (Vivotif Berna, Typhim Vi)

use of vaccines that contain thimerosal is preferable to withholding vaccination because failure to provide protection against vaccine-preventable diseases poses a greater risk to neonates and young infants. Most people do not develop reactions to the thimerosal in vaccines, even when patch or intradermal tests indicate thimerosal hypersensitivity. Most reported postvaccination thimerosal reactions are of the delayed, localized type.

The Institutes of Medicine thoroughly reviewed all studies of thimerosal and concluded that there was not enough evidence to determine whether neurodevelopmental disorders (autism, attention deficit hyperactivity disorder, and speech or language delay) can be caused by thimerosal exposure from childhood vaccines (2). A recent study conducted by the National Institute of Allergy and Infectious Diseases concluded that mercury levels in the blood of babies who received vaccines with thimerosal remained well below levels considered acceptable by the Environmental Protection Agency. Furthermore, ethylmercury (thimerosal) seems to be removed from the body quickly in feces. Research examining relationships between thimerosal and neurologic disorders (e.g., speech and language delay, tics, and attention deficit hyperactivity disorder) has not been conclusive. Studies to examine these issues are ongoing. The American Academy of Pediatrics states that infants and children who have received thimerosal-containing vaccines do not need mercury testing for hair, blood, or urine because the concentrations of mercury are likely too low to require treatment.

Extensive information resources involving all vaccines are available at the Centers for Disease Control and Prevention (CDC) Web site (3). Specific pharmaceutical information on vaccines is also available in the American Hospital Formulary Service (4).

ANTHRAX VACCINE ADSORBED

Anthrax is an infectious, zoonotic disease caused by *Bacillus anthracis*, a gram-positive, capsulated, spore-forming bacillus. Anthrax is a disease of wild and domesticated animals, transmitted to humans by contact with diseased animals or their products. The disease occurs in three forms: cutaneous (most common), inhalational (highest mortality), and gastrointestinal.

The anthrax vaccine adsorbed (Biothrax) is derived from a cell-free filtrate of *B. anthracis* culture that contains no dead or live bacteria. The current vaccine is produced in a protein-free medium, with aluminum hydroxide adjuvant and benzethonium chloride preservative. The vaccine is indicated for use in military personnel, animal workers, veterinarians, and laboratory staff exposed to contaminated animals or their products (4).

Safety and efficacy of the vaccine in children younger than 18 years of age have not been established. However, based on experience with other inactivated vaccines in this age group, the U.S. Working Group on Civilian Biodefense states that anthrax vaccine adsorbed is likely to be safe and effective in children. Safety and efficacy of the vaccine in adults older than 65 years of age have not been established, and the vaccine is not recommended for this age group (5,6).

Anthrax vaccine is contraindicated in patients with a previous history of anaphylaxis or anaphylactoid reactions and Guillain-Barré syndrome and in individuals who have recovered from anthrax. Administer with caution to individuals with latex sensitivity.

Toxic Dose

The *adult therapeutic dosage* is 0.5 ml subcutaneously (SQ) on a three-dose schedule at 0, 2, and 4 weeks. Booster doses are administered at 6, 12, and 18 months. Yearly booster is indicated if immunity is to be maintained. There are no overdose data available.

Pathophysiology

Anthrax vaccine adsorbed stimulates active immunity to *B. anthracis* infection by inducing specific antibodies against the bacterium. The vaccine induces humoral and cell-mediated responses in vaccinees (4).

Pregnancy and Lactation

Anthrax vaccine is U.S. Food and Drug Administration (FDA) pregnancy risk category C (Appendix I). Studies in pregnant mothers have produced conflicting results (7). Its use during breast-feeding has not been evaluated.

Clinical Presentation

ADVERSE EVENTS

Local site reactions (erythema, edema, pain) are most common: headache, arthralgia, asthenia, peripheral swelling, and pruritus. The rate of joint inflammation increases dramatically after immunization (8). Rates of adverse reactions have been higher in women than in men and are more intense with the second to fifth doses of vaccine. SQ vaccinations are associated more frequently with local reactions than intramuscular (IM) injections (9).

Like all vaccines, anthrax vaccine may cause soreness, redness, itching, and swelling at the injection site. A lump at the site occurs commonly, usually lasting for a few weeks before resolving spontaneously. Large local reactions are rare, occurring in less than 1% of patients. Large reactions include swelling that extends to the elbow or forearm, which can limit its movement, or a rash that is limited to the arm.

Systemic effects include fever, chills, body aches, and nausea. Anaphylaxis is extremely rare. Serious adverse effects have been reported and include cellulitis, pneumonia, pneumonitis (10), Guillain-Barré syndrome, seizures, cardiomyopathy, systemic lupus erythematosus, multiple sclerosis, collagen vascular disease, sepsis, angioedema, and transverse myelitis. To date, however, the FDA Vaccine Adverse Event Reporting System has not revealed a pattern of serious adverse events clearly associated with anthrax vaccine adsorbed.

Chronic multisymptom illness in Gulf War veterans has been identified as potentially associated with the anthrax vaccine adsorbed. However, current evidence does not support such an association.

BACILLUS CALMETTE-GUÉRIN VACCINE

Bacillus Calmette-Guérin (BCG) vaccine (TICE) is a lyophilized preparation of live, attenuated organisms of the Calmette-Guérin strain of *Mycobacterium bovis*. The vaccine is used to stimulate active immunity to tuberculosis in immunocompetent individuals. In developing countries where tuberculosis is epidemic and short-term prophylaxis with antituberculosis agents or tuberculin skin-test screening is not possible, BCG vaccine is used routinely to attempt tuberculosis control. It is not routinely recommended in the United States. BCG vaccine is also used intravesically as adjuvant therapy for the treatment of superficial bladder cancer. BCG vaccine is contraindicated in immunocompromised individuals (4).

Toxic Dose

The *therapeutic dose* for patients 1 month of age or older is 0.2 to 0.3 ml percutaneously with a multiple puncture device (United

States) or intradermal injection (outside the United States). Neonates younger than 1 month of age should receive 50% of the above dose by diluting with 2 ml instead of 1 ml of sterile water for injection. Dosing for intravesical instillation in superficial bladder cancer therapy is dependent on the strain of BCG used.

The FDA has alerted clinicians that the dose of BCG (6×10^9 viable organisms) reported in several protocols for the treatment of bladder cancer is ten times the recommended dose. Administration of this incorrect dose may result in severe adverse reactions and possibly death.

Toxicokinetics and Toxicodynamics

Intravesicular BCG is eliminated through the bladder where it is locally instilled. Percutaneously administered vaccine data are not available on absorption, protein binding, distribution, and elimination.

Pathophysiology

The Calmette-Guérin strain of *M. bovis* is immunologically similar to *Mycobacterium tuberculosis*. Vaccination with BCG simulates natural infection with *M. tuberculosis* and promotes cell-mediated immunity against tuberculosis.

The mechanism of intravesical BCG as cancer therapy has not been fully determined. However, both inflammatory effects and immune response are believed to be involved. A BCG-induced granulomatous reaction within the bladder wall leads to sloughing of the epithelium and destruction of cancer cells in superficial bladder cancer. Adherence of live, attenuated BCG organisms to the bladder mucosa and tumor cells appears to be important for the development of an antitumor immune response, which includes T-lymphocyte activation and cytokine release.

Pregnancy and Lactation

BCG vaccine is FDA pregnancy risk category C (Appendix I). BCG vaccine should be used in pregnant or lactating women only when there is an immediate, excessive risk of unavoidable exposure to infectious tuberculosis. If travel is anticipated to high-risk areas, the CDC recommends that a tuberculin skin test be performed before and after travel. The use of BCG vaccine during breast-feeding is not recommended but has not been evaluated.

Clinical Presentation

ACUTE OVERDOSAGE

If acute overdosage of BCG vaccine occurs, infection may develop. Complications generally do not occur if the patient is treated immediately with antituberculosis agents. If not treated immediately, antituberculosis agent therapy can still be successful. However, complications, such as regional adenitis, lupus vulgaris, SQ cold abscesses, and ocular lesions, can occur.

Intravascular absorption of BCG is an important contributing factor to systemic BCG infections in patients who have had surgical manipulation or traumatic transurethral catheterization. Intravesicular therapy should be initiated no sooner than 1 week after procedures to allow time for healing and reduce the risk of systemic toxicity.

ADVERSE EVENTS

Adverse effects are usually mild and infrequent in individuals vaccinated with BCG against tuberculosis. Mucocutaneous effects include ulceration or abscess at injection site, scarring, keloid formation, granulomas, persistent lupus reactions of the skin, and transient urticaria. Cases have been reported of histiocytoma, hydradenoma, erythema nodosum, erythema multiforme, and generalized eruptions after BCG vaccination. Local and dermatologic reactions to BCG tend to be more severe in those who have received previous immunization with BCG vaccine.

Systemically, lymphadenitis occurs at the site of injection, with an incidence of 1% to 10%. Lymphangitis may occur, especially when the vaccine is administered too close to the shoulder, with streaking seen from the site of injection toward regional lymph nodes. Draining fistulas may result. Osteomyelitis has been reported to occur rarely (1 case per 1 million patients), most frequently occurring in neonates. Tuberculous meningitis has occurred in at least two immunocompetent children vaccinated with BCG. Disseminated BCG infection, which can be fatal, occurs only rarely (1 to 10 cases per 10 million patients), mostly in immunodeficient children or symptomatic patients with human immunodeficiency virus (HIV) infection. Rarely, anaphylactic shock has been reported after vaccination.

The most frequent adverse local effect occurring in approximately 90% of patients receiving intravesical BCG is cystitis. The most frequent adverse systemic effect is a flu-like syndrome with low-grade fever, malaise, and chills. A 72-year-old man receiving intravesical instillations of BCG developed fatal hemolytic uremic syndrome after his eighth dose (11).

BOTULINUM ANTITOXIN

Botulism antitoxin trivalent (Equine), types A, B, and E, is a refined and concentrated preparation of horse globulins modified by enzymatic digestion. The clinical effects of botulism are addressed in Chapter 253. It is a licensed product supplied in 10-ml multidose vials. Each vial contains the following: type A, 7500 IU (equivalent to 2381 U.S. U); type B, 5500 IU (equivalent to 1839 U.S. U); type E 8500 IU (equivalent to 8500 U.S. U) (12).

In the United States, the antitoxin is available only from the CDC because of its limited use and its relatively short expiration date. The antitoxin is released for actual cases of botulinum toxin poisoning only. The antitoxin is stored at the various CDC quarantine stations at major airports around the nation for easy access from anywhere in the United States within hours. All suspected cases of botulinum poisoning and the subsequent requests for antitoxin must be initiated through state or local health departments and are released only after consultation with CDC physicians. This allows CDC and the state health departments to maintain effective botulinum surveillance and detect outbreaks as soon as possible.

HAEMOPHILUS B CONJUGATE VACCINE

Haemophilus influenzae is a gram-negative coccobacillus that enters the body through the nasopharynx. Worldwide, *Haemophilus influenzae* type b (Hib) is estimated to cause at least 3 million cases of serious disease and hundreds of thousands of deaths annually. The most important manifestations of Hib disease are seen mainly in children less than 5 years of age, particularly infants. Of the six polysaccharide capsular types of the infection, type b (Hib) causes the most systemic infections, including pneumonia, meningitis, epiglottitis, sepsis, cellulitis, septic arthritis, osteomyelitis, and pericarditis.

Haemophilus b conjugate vaccine (Act-Hib, Hibtiter, Pedvax-hib) is indicated for all children as shown in Figure 1. The vaccine is also recommended for children receiving cochlear implants and for HIV-infected children. Contraindications include a previous history of anaphylaxis or anaphylactoid reactions (4).

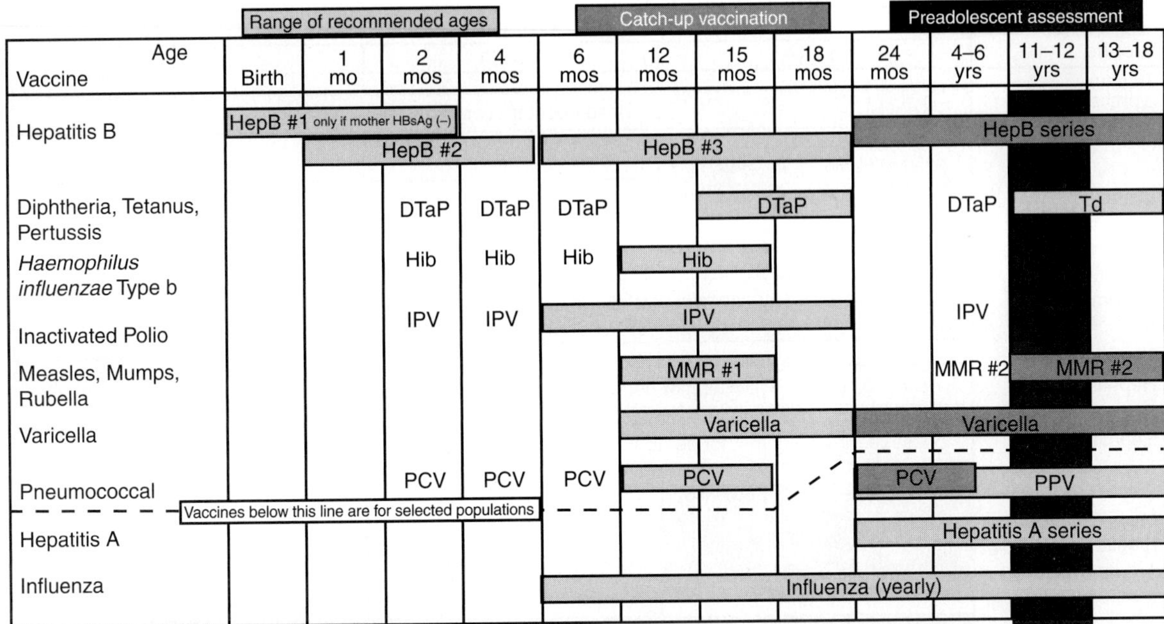

Figure 1. Recommended childhood and adolescent immunization schedule—United States, 2003. Additional information about vaccines, including precautions and contraindications for vaccination and vaccine shortages, is available at http://www.cdc.gov/nip or at the National Immunization information hotline, 800-232-2522 (English) or 800-232-0233 (Spanish). Copies of the schedule can be obtained at http://www.cdc.gov/nip/recs/child-schedule.htm. DTaP, diphtheria, tetanus, pertussis; HepB, hepatitis B; Hib, *Haemophilus influenzae* type b; IPV, inactivated polio; MMR, measles, mumps, and rubella; PCV, pneumococcal 7-valent conjugate; PPV, pneumococcal 23-valent conjugate; Td, tetanus-diphtheria. (From *MMWR Morb Mortal Wkly Rep* 2002;51:944–908, with permission.)

Toxic Dose

The *therapeutic dosing schedule* for children 6 weeks to 5 years of age is provided in Figure 1. Immunization is not recommended for patients older than 5 years of age. A toxic dose has not been established. The therapeutic dose for children 2 months to 71 months of age is 0.5 ml intramuscularly.

Pathophysiology

The vaccines currently licensed for use against Hib disease are based on Hib polysaccharide conjugated to a protein carrier (polyribosylribitol phosphate conjugated (PRP)] as diphtheria toxoid (PRP-D), a diphtheria toxoid–like protein (PRP-HbOC), tetanus toxoid (PRP-T), or meningococcal outer membrane protein (PRP-OMP). The conjugation of PRP to the protein induces a T-cell–dependent immune response to the Hib polysaccharide. These vaccines not only induce protective circulating antibodies and immunologic memory in infants but also result in decreased nasopharyngeal colonization by Hib. A herd effect is thus achieved through reduced transmission of the microorganism.

Pregnancy and Lactation

Haemophilus b conjugate vaccine is FDA pregnancy risk category C (Appendix I). It is considered safe for use during breastfeeding.

Clinical Presentation

Reported reactions to the three conjugate vaccines have been mild among both infants and children. Localized redness, tenderness, swelling, induration, urticaria, and sterile abscess at injection site have been reported with the three conjugate vaccines.

Serious adverse reactions to PRP-OMP have been rare, including temperature greater than 38.3°C within 48 hours, erythema of more than 2.5 cm in diameter, and swelling and induration of more than 2.5 cm in diameter. Adverse events after the first dose were less frequent. Severe cardiorespiratory events developed in 20% of neonates immunized with diphtheria and tetanus toxoids and pertussis/*Haemophilus influenzae* type b conjugate (13).

HEPATITIS A

Hepatitis A virus (HAV) causes a viral infection of the liver characterized by malaise, fever, nausea, vomiting, and jaundice. Transmission most commonly occurs from children to adults via contaminated food and water. Infection with HAV results in lifelong immunity.

HAV vaccine inactivated is a noninfectious, sterile suspension of a cell culture–adapted, attenuated strain of HAV. There are two inactivated-virus vaccines available for HAV: Havrix and Vaqta. Havrix contains phenoxyethanol preservative and no thimerosal. Vaqta is manufactured from a different attenuated virus strain and does not contain thimerosal or other preservatives. Hepatitis A inactivated and hepatitis B (recombinant) vaccine (Twinrix) is a combination vaccine containing Havrix and hepatitis B vaccine (recombinant) (4).

Hepatitis A vaccines are used in international travelers to high-risk areas for hepatitis A, children older than 2 years of age living in high-risk areas, men who have sex with men, people with chronic liver disease, laboratory/animal workers at risk of exposure, people with clotting-factor disorders, and food handlers in high-risk areas (5). Other groups may be considered, depending on their exposure risk: military personnel, day care workers, personnel in institutions for the developmentally disabled, people

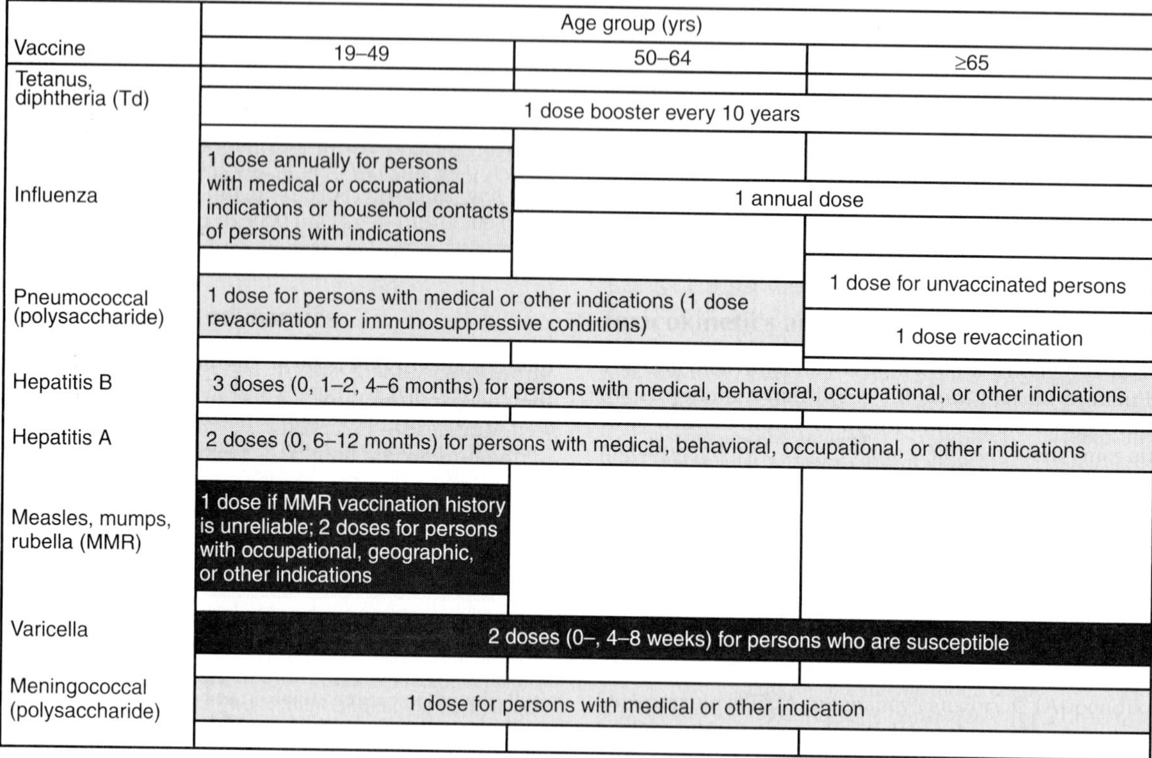

Vaccine	Age group (yrs) 19–49	50–64	≥65
Tetanus, diphtheria (Td)	1 dose booster every 10 years		
Influenza	1 dose annually for persons with medical or occupational indications or household contacts of persons with indications	1 annual dose	
Pneumococcal (polysaccharide)	1 dose for persons with medical or other indications (1 dose revaccination for immunosuppressive conditions)		1 dose for unvaccinated persons 1 dose revaccination
Hepatitis B	3 doses (0, 1–2, 4–6 months) for persons with medical, behavioral, occupational, or other indications		
Hepatitis A	2 doses (0, 6–12 months) for persons with medical, behavioral, occupational, or other indications		
Measles, mumps, rubella (MMR)	1 dose if MMR vaccination history is unreliable; 2 doses for persons with occupational, geographic, or other indications		
Varicella	2 doses (0–, 4–8 weeks) for persons who are susceptible		
Meningococcal (polysaccharide)	1 dose for persons with medical or other indication		

Figure 2. Recommended adult immunization schedule—United States, 2002–2003. (From *MMWR Morb Mortal Wkly Rep* 2002;51:944–908, with permission.)

who repeatedly contract sexually transmitted diseases, and consumers of high-risk foods (e.g., raw shellfish) (Fig. 2).

The vaccine is contraindicated in people with hypersensitivity to ingredients in the vaccine formulation. HAV vaccine inactivated is well tolerated and highly immunogenic in children 2 years of age and older. In younger children and infants, additional studies are necessary before incorporating use in regular immunization schedules.

Toxic Dose

The *adult therapeutic dose* of Havrix formulation is 1440 U (1.0 ml) via IM injection only into the deltoid muscle, with a booster dose 6 to 12 months after the primary dose. The dose of Havrix for patients aged 2 to 18 years is 720 U (0.5 ml) via IM injection only into the deltoid muscle, with one booster dose 6 to 12 months from the primary dose.

Safety and efficacy of the combination HAV and hepatitis B vaccine have not been established in children younger than 18 years of age. No overall differences in immunogenicity or safety were observed between geriatric and younger patients. However, current studies cannot exclude the possibility that patients older than 65 years of age may have increased sensitivity to the vaccine.

Pathophysiology

HAV vaccine inactivated stimulates active immunity to HAV infection. It induces production of HAV-specific immunoglobulin (Ig) G and IgM antibodies (anti-HAV). This results in humoral immunity.

Pregnancy and Lactation

Each of these HAV vaccines is FDA pregnancy risk category C (Appendix I). They are produced using inactivated toxin, so the theoretic risk to the fetus is low. However, the vaccine should be used with caution in pregnant or lactating women because animal reproduction studies have not been performed to study the effect on fetuses or reproductive capacity. The vaccine is not contraindicated in nursing women.

Clinical Presentation

Local effects are the most common adverse effects associated with Havrix or Vaqta. Soreness, pain at injection site, induration, erythema, warmth, swelling, hematoma, ecchymosis, and tenderness may occur. Vaqta is associated with a higher rate of adverse local effects in adults than in children.

Systemic effects may include urticaria, edema, pruritus, rash, and, most commonly, headache in adults. In children, fatigue, asthenia, feeding problems, fussiness, lethargy, fever, malaise, anorexia, and nausea have been most commonly reported. Anaphylaxis/anaphylactoid reactions have been reported rarely. A definite causal relationship to HAV vaccine with many other reported side effects has not been definitively established.

The hepatitis A and B combination vaccine has been associated with local effects including soreness, erythema and swelling.

HEPATITIS B (RECOMBINANT)

Hepatitis B recombinant is a noninfectious subunit viral vaccine containing hepatitis B surface antigen that stimulates active immunity to hepatitis B infection. The vaccine comes in several forms: Recombivax HB or Engerix-B (hepatitis B only), Comvax (*Haemophilus* b polysaccharide and hepatitis B vaccine combined), and Twinrix (hepatitis A and hepatitis B combined) (4).

Hepatitis B immunization is recommended for all infants and people 18 years of age and younger born in the United States (Fig. 1) and individuals at high risk from exposure to hepatitis B through occupational risk, sexual behavior or sexual abuse, intravenous drug use, blood transfusion, household contacts or extended-care facility contacts, solid organ transplantation, and hemodialysis (14). Hypersensitivity to yeast is a contraindication as well as previous history of anaphylactic reaction to the vaccine. Moderate or severe illness is considered a contraindication, and vaccination should be delayed until recovery. The adult form of the vaccine contains thimerosal.

Toxic Dose

The *adult therapeutic dosage* of Recombivax HB is 10 μg (1 ml) or 20 μg (1 ml) × 3 doses at 0, 1, and 6 months. A toxic dose has not been established.

Pathophysiology

The vaccine stimulates active immunity to hepatitis B infection.

Pregnancy and Lactation

Hepatitis B vaccine is FDA pregnancy risk category C (Appendix I). Pregnancy and lactation are not considered contraindications.

Clinical Presentation

Local effects, including soreness, pain, induration, tenderness, pruritus, erythema, ecchymosis, swelling, warmth, burning, and nodule formation, have been reported in 10% to 29% of people receiving the hepatitis B vaccine recombinant.

Systemic effects are mild and include fatigue, weakness, headache, fever, and vertigo/dizziness, reported in approximately 15% of patients receiving the vaccine. Nausea, diarrhea, pharyngitis, and upper respiratory symptoms have been reported in approximately 1% of patients. Anaphylaxis and serum sickness with delayed onset (arthralgia, arthritis, Stevens-Johnson syndrome, urticaria, ecchymoses, and erythema nodosum) have also been reported, although rare. Many adverse systemic effects have been reported, many of which have not been determined to have a definite causal relationship with the vaccine (4).

INFLUENZA

Influenza virus vaccine (FluShield, Fluzone) stimulates active immunity to influenza virus strains contained in the vaccine. The vaccine is made from highly purified, egg-grown viruses that have been made noninfectious (i.e., inactivated or killed).

The vaccine contains noninfectious, inactivated influenza virus types A and B subunits and is administered IM. A live, attenuated influenza virus vaccine is now available for intranasal administration (FluMist). The FDA Vaccines and Related Biological Products Advisory Committee determines the composition of the yearly influenza vaccine, based on antigenic analyses of recently isolated influenza viruses, epidemiologic data, and postvaccination serologic studies in humans. Vaccines from prior years should not be used for the current year (15).

The following groups should receive yearly influenza vaccinations (Fig. 2): (a) adults older than 50 years of age or anyone with certain chronic medical conditions; (b) people who live with or care for persons at high risk (e.g., health care workers and household contacts who have frequent contact with people at high risk and who can transmit influenza to people at high risk); (c) children aged 6 to 23 months; (d) children and adolescents (aged 6 months to 18 years) who are receiving long-term aspirin therapy and, therefore, might be at risk for experiencing Reye's syndrome after influenza infection; and (e) women who are in the second or third trimester of pregnancy during the influenza season (4).

Contraindications include a history of anaphylaxis to the vaccine, a proven sensitivity to eggs, or a known sensitivity to neomycin, polymyxin, gentamicin, streptomycin, sulfites, or other aminoglycosides. Most influenza vaccines contain thimerosal, with preservative-free and reduced-thimerosal vaccines available in limited supply to children starting in 2003.

Toxic Dose

The *adult therapeutic dose* is 0.5 ml IM in the deltoid muscle. The dosage for children who have never received an influenza vaccine is two injections at least 1 month apart before December: 0.25 ml each IM in the anterolateral thigh for children aged 6 to 35 months; two injections 1 month apart, 0.5 ml IM, in the anterolateral thigh or deltoid for children aged 3 to 8 years; or one injection, 0.5 ml IM, in the deltoid for children aged 9 to 12 years. A toxic dose has not been established.

Pathophysiology

Influenza virus vaccine stimulates active immunity to influenza virus strains determined on a yearly basis.

Pregnancy and Lactation

Influenza virus vaccine is FDA pregnancy risk category C (Appendix I). Women who will be beyond the first trimester of pregnancy (more than 14 weeks' gestation) during the influenza season should be vaccinated. Certain providers prefer to administer influenza vaccine during the second trimester to avoid a coincidental association with spontaneous abortion, which is common in the first trimester. Because pregnant women are at increased risk for influenza-related complications and because a substantial safety margin has been incorporated into the health guidance values for organic mercury exposure, the benefit of influenza vaccine with reduced or standard thimerosal content outweighs the potential risk, if any, for thimerosal.

Influenza vaccine does not affect the safety of mothers who are breast-feeding or their infants. Breast-feeding does not adversely affect the immune response and is not a contraindication for vaccination. The live attenuated intranasal vaccine (FluMist) should be avoided in pregnant women and used with caution in nursing women.

Clinical Presentation

The most frequent side effect of vaccination is soreness at the vaccination site (affecting 10% to 64% of patients), which lasts less than 2 days.

Fever, malaise, myalgia, and other systemic symptoms can occur after vaccination and most often affect people who have had no prior exposure to the influenza virus antigens in the vaccine (e.g., young children). These reactions begin 6 to 12 hours after vaccination and can persist for 1 to 2 days. The most frequently reported events among children were fever, injection-site reactions, and rash. Investigations to date indicate no substantial increase in Guillain-Barré syndrome associated with influenza vaccines (other than the swine influenza vaccine in 1976).

JAPANESE ENCEPHALITIS VACCINE

JE is the leading cause of encephalitis in Asia, occurring most frequently in China, Korea, India, and Southeast Asia. It is caused by a flavivirus transmitted by *Culex* mosquitoes to vertebrate hosts (pigs and wading birds), with humans as incidental hosts. The vaccine is an inactivated-virus preparation from infected mouse brains (United States) or infected hamster kidney cells. The commercially available Nakayama-NIH strain preparation in the United States was originally derived from a patient infected in 1935 (4).

JE vaccine is indicated for travelers who will spend more than 1 month in rural or endemic areas during transmission season. Laboratory workers with risk of exposure to the virus should also receive vaccination. The vaccine is contraindicated in patients with hypersensitivity to thimerosal or rodent proteins (5).

Toxic Dose

The *adult and pediatric dose* is 1 ml and 0.5 ml for children 1 to 3 years of age. The vaccine is administered on days 0, 7, and 30. A toxic dose has not been established.

Pathophysiology

The vaccine stimulates activity immunity to infection by inducing production of specific neutralizing antibodies.

Pregnancy and Lactation

JE vaccine is FDA pregnancy risk category C (Appendix I). The vaccine should not be given to pregnant patients unless the risk of acquiring infection is high. JE infection during the first or second trimester of pregnancy may result in uterine infection and fetal demise. Data are lacking on safety of the vaccine for nursing mothers.

Clinical Presentation

Pain, redness, and induration occur at the injection site in approximately 20% of vaccines. A causal relationship between the vaccine and neurologic events, such as encephalitis, seizures, encephalopathy, or peripheral neuropathy, has not been established but may occur in 1.0 to 2.3 patients per million. Rarely, JE vaccine may cause anaphylaxis/anaphylactoid reactions and should be used with great caution in people with a history of bee sting–induced urticaria. Generalized urticaria or angioedema of the extremities, face, and oropharynx may occur as well as fever, headache, myalgia, chills, dizziness, nausea, vomiting, abdominal pain, and malaise. Patients should be observed in the office for at least 30 minutes after immunization to observe for adverse reactions and should watch for adverse reactions as long as 1 week after any dose (16).

Symptomatic illness and neuroinvasive disease may be more likely in adults older than 55 years of age, so vaccination should be considered for those at risk.

LYME DISEASE VACCINE

Lyme disease is caused by the spirochete *Borrelia burgdorferi*, transmitted by infected *Ixodes* ticks, which take a blood meal on human hosts. Lyme disease is the most common vector-borne disease in the United States, most prevalent in the northeastern United States.

Lyme disease vaccine (LYMErix) is a noninfectious, sterile suspension containing outer-surface protein A of *B. burgdorferi* sensu strictu. The vaccine is indicated in people with risk for contracting Lyme disease, namely people who work or spend recreational time in high- to moderate-risk habitats of the *Ixodes* tick. The vaccine is contraindicated in people with history of treatment-resistant Lyme arthritis. Because the vaccine is given IM only, caution must be exercised in administering to people with bleeding disorders. The vaccine is not for use in people younger than 15 years of age or older than 70 years of age (4).

Toxic Dose

The *therapeutic dosage* is a three-dose regimen of 0.5 ml (IM only, preferably deltoid), recommended at 0, 1, and 12 months for at-risk people from 15 to 70 years of age. The LYMErix formulation of vaccine should not be administered to people with hypersensitivity to yeast, kanamycin, aluminum, or aluminum hydroxide. A toxic dose has not been established.

Pathophysiology

The vaccine stimulates formation of antibodies that kill Lyme disease spirochetes within the tick gut.

Pregnancy and Lactation

Lyme disease vaccine should be used in pregnant women only if clearly needed. The vaccine should be used with caution in nursing mothers.

Clinical Presentation

Pain, soreness, erythema, and swelling at the injection site are the most common adverse effects of Lyme disease vaccine. Anaphylactoid events have been reported only very rarely. Adverse musculoskeletal effects, such as arthralgia, myalgia, back pain, and stiffness, have been reported. Fatigue, headache, fever, dizziness, upper respiratory symptoms, and rash have also been reported in association with the Lyme disease vaccine (17,18).

MEASLES, MUMPS, AND RUBELLA VACCINE

Measles (rubeola) is a contagious febrile disease characterized by cough, conjunctivitis, coryza, an erythematous maculopapular rash, and Koplik's spots. Mumps is characterized by swelling of the salivary glands and may be severe if contracted in adulthood. Orchitis may develop with mumps after puberty. Rubella (German measles) is usually mild and manifests by generalized lymphadenopathy, rash, and slight fever. Congenital rubella, however, is teratogenic and can result in neonatal deafness and ophthalmic, cardiac, neurologic, hematologic, and growth disturbances.

MMR vaccine is a live, attenuated virus vaccine consisting of the three monovalent (single antigen) vaccines that contain measles (Attenuvax), mumps (Mumpsvax), and rubella vaccines (Meruvax II). The vaccines may also be given alone (4).

MMR vaccine is recommended as a routine series for children (Fig. 1). All susceptible or nonimmune adults, such as travelers, women of childbearing age, college students, childcare personnel, health care workers, and military personnel, should be immune to MMR (19).

There are several contraindications to MMR vaccine. Anaphylactic reaction to any vaccine component (e.g., neomycin, gelatin) contraindicates further use. A delayed-type hypersensitivity reaction (e.g., contact dermatitis) to neomycin or other vaccine components does *not* contraindicate the vaccine. MMR vaccine should be used with caution in children with a history of febrile seizures or with a first-degree relative history of seizures. Prophylaxis with antipyretics (except aspirin) before the expected onset of fever may reduce the risk of febrile seizures, with continuation of the antipyretics for 5 to 7 days. Individuals with anaphylactoid reactions after ingestion of eggs may receive MMR vaccine if caution is exercised, ideally in a setting with emergency equipment and medications readily available.

MMR vaccine is also contraindicated in people receiving immunosuppressive therapy, those with primary immunodeficiencies, and those with symptomatic HIV infection who are severely immunosuppressed (low $CD4^+$ T-lymphocyte count or low percentage of total lymphocytes). People receiving steroid replacement therapy for Addison's disease and asymptomatic HIV- and symptomatic HIV-infected people without evidence of severe immunosuppression may receive the MMR vaccine with caution.

Women who receive MMR or measles live virus vaccine should avoid pregnancy for at least 1 to 3 months after vaccination because of the theoretic risk of fetal infection with the live viruses. A second dose of MMR/measles vaccine live may be avoided in people who developed thrombocytopenia within 1 to 2 months after the first dose of vaccine. Serologic evidence of measles immunity may be obtained instead of vaccination.

Toxic Dose

The *therapeutic dose* for MMR vaccine is 0.5 ml administered SQ. A toxic dose has not been established.

Pathophysiology

MMR vaccine stimulates active immunity to MMR by producing disease-specific antibodies, resulting in humoral immunity. A mild or inapparent, noncommunicable infection occurs with the vaccines individually or in combination as MMR.

Pregnancy and Lactation

MMR vaccine is FDA pregnancy risk category C (Appendix I). Breast-feeding is generally not a contraindication to administration of measles virus vaccine live or MMR vaccine, but one should proceed with caution. There is no evidence that infection from organisms distributed in the milk from MMR vaccine causes adverse effects in the nursing infant. Immunizing children with pregnant mothers does not pose a risk to the pregnant mother or fetus.

Clinical Presentation

Pain, edema, induration, and rash may occur at the injection site for MMR vaccine or any of the single-antigen vaccines. These side effects tend to occur more frequently in nonimmune recipients, with only rare frequency after revaccination.

Anaphylactoid events after immunization with MMR or the single-antigen vaccines have been reported only rarely. Transient thrombocytopenia may also occur.

Atypical measles syndrome may occur in individuals who received the inactivated measles vaccine in the past and who subsequently became exposed to natural measles. These people should receive a two-dose vaccination with the live measles virus vaccine. Joint pain may also occur 1 to 3 weeks after vaccination, lasting 1 to 2 days in recipients of measles live vaccine (usually adults).

Mumps infection with parotitis, pruritus, and purpura has been rarely associated with the mumps virus vaccine live.

The rubella component may cause (rare) arthralgia and transient arthritis after vaccination. These reactions generally are mild and occur 1 to 3 weeks after vaccination, persisting 1 day to several weeks.

MENINGOCOCCAL POLYSACCHARIDE VACCINE

The gram-negative diplococcus *Neisseria meningitides* bacteria can infect cerebrospinal fluid and meninges, causing fatal meningococcemia and meningococcal meningitis. The bacteria are introduced via infected airborne droplets to the upper respiratory tract or by intimate contact (e.g., kissing or sharing eating utensils).

Meningococcal polysaccharide vaccine (Menomune) contains group-specific capsular polysaccharide antigens isolated from *N. meningitides*. A quadrivalent vaccine against serogroups A, C, Y, and W-135 is available. Some countries may have mono- or bivalent vaccines that cover only one or two of these serogroups (4).

The disease occurs at any age, most commonly occurring in children younger than 5 years of age and in adults aged 18 to 23 years. The disease is most common in poor, overcrowded areas. Outbreaks may occur in daycare centers, schools, colleges, and military institutions. People with functional/anatomic asplenia or complement deficiencies, travelers to high-risk areas (e.g., Mecca or the sub-Saharan African "meningitis belt"), and laboratory workers are at risk of exposure. Prior history of anaphylactoid reactions to the vaccine contraindicates further use. Thimerosal is a component of the Menomune formulation.

Toxic Dose

The *adult and pediatric therapeutic dose* is 0.5 ml SQ, preferably in the upper-outer triceps area. The patient should be revaccinated 3 to 5 years later if risk of exposure remains elevated. The vaccine may be given to children as young as 3 months of age when necessary. A toxic dose has not been established.

Pathophysiology

The quadrivalent vaccine (available in the United States) stimulates active immunity to infection caused by *N. meningitides* serogroups A, C, Y, and W-135. A vaccine against serogroup B is currently not available.

Pregnancy and Lactation

Meningococcal polysaccharide vaccine is FDA pregnancy risk category C (Appendix I). The vaccine should only be given to pregnant women with substantial risk of infection. It should be used with caution in nursing women.

Clinical Presentation

Erythema, pain, or induration at the injection site may occur and are usually mild, lasting 1 to 3 days. Headache, malaise, fever, chills, lethargy, pruritic rash, coryza, and gastrointestinal symptoms have been reported to occur with the quadrivalent vaccine. IgA nephropathy has been reported rarely in association with the vaccine, but no causal relationship has been established. Anaphylactoid reactions have been reported rarely as well.

PLAGUE

Plague is an infectious disease of animals and humans caused by the bacterium *Yersinia pestis*. The plague vaccine was withdrawn from the U.S. market in 1998 on FDA request. Travelers at risk for acquiring the plague should consider taking antibiotic prophylaxis, as the vaccine has not been found to protect quickly enough during an outbreak and has been found ineffective against pneumonic plague. Those at risk are individuals bitten by rodent fleas that carry the plague bacterium or those who handle or live among infected animals. Streptomycin is the antibiotic of choice for treatment of the plague. Gentamicin is used when streptomycin is not available, or tetracycline and chloramphenicol may be used.

PNEUMOCOCCAL VACCINE

Pneumococcal disease is caused by the bacterium *Streptococcus pneumoniae*, a gram-positive diplococcus. The disease is transmitted by respiratory droplets and is most common in crowded environments and during the winter and early spring. *S. pneumoniae* is the most common cause of bacterial meningitis in the United States.

Two types of vaccines are available in the United States against pneumococcal disease. The pneumococcal 7-valent conjugate vaccine (PCV, Prevnar) is indicated for routine administration in infants 2 to 23 months of age or in children as old as to 59 months of age with certain medical conditions (Fig. 1). The pneumococcal 23-valent vaccine (PPV23, Pneumovax 23, Pnu-Imune-23) is used for routine vaccination in adults 50 years of age or older or in younger adults with certain chronic medical conditions. All people with cochlear implants should receive the age-appropriate vaccine. All adults 65 years of age and older should receive the 23-valent vaccine if 5 to 6 years have passed since the last PPV23 (4).

Aside from the routine immunizations as mentioned above, the vaccine is important for use in individuals with immunocompromised conditions, chronic pulmonary disease, and functional or anatomic asplenia and in nursing home or daycare residents, Alaskan natives, or certain American Indian populations (Fig. 2).

The 7-valent vaccine is contraindicated in people with hypersensitivity to components in the formulation, including diphtheria toxoid. Care must be exercised with giving this IM-only injection to children with thrombocytopenia or bleeding disorders. The PCV vaccine does not contain thimerosal. The PPV23 contains phenol preservative.

Toxic Dose

The 7-valent vaccine is given IM only, whereas the 23-valent vaccine may be given IM or SQ. For both preparations, the dose is 0.5 ml for individuals 6 months of age and older. A toxic dose has not been established.

Pathophysiology

The capsular saccharides present in pneumococcal 7- and 23-valent conjugate vaccines promote production of specific antibodies for each type of pneumococcal capsular type in the vaccines. The antibodies enhance opsonization, phagocytosis, and death of *S. pneumonia* by leukocytes and other phagocytic cells.

Pregnancy and Lactation

Each of these agents is FDA pregnancy risk category C (Appendix I). The PCV vaccine is not for use in adults or pregnant or lactating women. PPV23 may be used with caution in pregnancy and lactation only when clearly needed.

Clinical Presentation

Tenderness, erythema, and induration at the injection site may occur with the PCV or PPV23 vaccines. Intradermal administration of PPV23 should be avoided, due to severe local reactions. Low-grade fever and myalgia may occur occasionally. Rare side effects include arthralgia, arthritis, myalgia, headache, nausea, vomiting, thrombocytopenia in people with idiopathic thrombocytopenic purpura, hemolytic anemia in people with hematologic disorders, rash, and anaphylactoid reactions.

Administration to patients infected with HIV does not cause serologic or immunologic deterioration (20). Low body weight and preterm infants have higher rates of adverse events, such as local redness and swelling, as well as systemic effects (hives) (21). Systemic cutaneous reactions occur rarely (22).

RABIES

Rabies is a viral infection of the nervous system by the RNA rhabdovirus. The virus is transmitted by the saliva of an infected animal. Direct bite exposure, contamination of preexisting open wounds or mucous membranes with infectious material (saliva or brain tissue), large quantities of aerosolized rabies virus, and organ transplants from infected donors may transmit the virus to humans. Convulsions, coma, encephalitis, and ultimately death occur with untreated rabies infection.

Three inactivated-virus cell-culture vaccines are available in the United States for preexposure immunization and postexposure prophylaxis: PCEC (chick embryo culture vaccine), HDCV (human diploid cell vaccine), and RVA (rabies vaccine adsorbed). Human rabies immune globulin (RIG) is used for postexposure treatment of individuals not previously immunized with rabies vaccine to provide rapid, passive, short-term immunity (4).

Preexposure immunization is recommended for travelers visiting high-risk areas such as Asia (except Taiwan and Japan), Africa, and Latin America. Animal and laboratory workers, spelunkers, veterinarians, and other people at occupational risk of contracting rabies should receive preexposure immunization (23).

The Semple vaccine is the original rabies vaccine, which is still available in some developing countries. It should be avoided due to severe side effects and lower efficacy. Because of the morbidity and mortality associated with rabies disease, people with a history of serious adverse reaction to rabies vaccine should still be revaccinated but with caution. Proper emergency equipment and medications should be readily available. RVA and RIG contain thimerosal, but the risks of rabies infection outweigh the relatively negligible risk posed by the thimerosal in RVA and RIG.

Toxic Dose

The *adult and pediatric dose* for PCEC and RVA is 1.0 ml IM in the deltoid. HDCV may be given intradermally, 0.1 ml. All rabies vaccines are given as a series of three injections at 0, 7, and 21 or 28 days.

Pathophysiology

The rabies vaccine stimulates production of antibody that neutralizes the rabies virus. The antibody retards the spread of the virus and inhibits its infective and pathogenic properties.

Pregnancy and Lactation

Rabies vaccines are FDA pregnancy risk category C (Appendix I). If substantial risk of rabies exposure is present, preexposure immunization with HDCV, PCEC, or RVA may be necessary during pregnancy. It is unknown whether these vaccines are distributed into milk or if transmission to the nursing infant poses any unusual risk.

Clinical Presentation

Injection site pain, swelling, induration, and rash may occur with all rabies vaccines. Headache, nausea, abdominal pain, myalgia, localized lymphadenopathy, low-grade fever, and dizziness may occur after rabies vaccination. A type III hypersensitivity (serum sickness)–like reaction has been reported in association with HDCV 2 to 21 days later. Adverse neurologic effects have also been reported with HDCV.

The original Semple vaccine, still used in India and other countries, causes encephalitis, radiculitis, and acute inflammatory demyelinating polyradiculoneuropathy (24).

ROTAVIRUS

In 1998, the FDA approved a live virus vaccine (Rotashield) for use in children. However, the Advisory Committee on Immunization Practices recommended that Rotashield no longer be recommended for infants in the United States because of data that indicated a strong association between Rotashield and intussusception (bowel obstruction) among some infants during the first 1 to 2 weeks after vaccination.

TICK-BORNE ENCEPHALITIS

Tick-borne encephalitis affects the central nervous system and is a viral infection transmitted by bites from the *Ixodes ricinus* tick or from consuming unpasteurized dairy products from infected cows, goats, or sheep. The disease is most common in western and central Europe and the European section of the former Soviet Union.

A killed virus vaccine and special Ig preparation are available in Europe. No vaccine or Ig preparation is available in the United States for prevention of tick-borne encephalitis. The Ig preparation provides protection within 24 hours and lasts approximately 4 weeks. The vaccine regimen is a three-dose course, with a booster given approximately 3 years after completion of the primary series.

TYPHOID

Typhoid fever is a life-threatening illness caused by the bacterium *Salmonella typhi.* The bacterium is spread via contaminated food or water. Travelers to Asia, Africa, and Latin America have been especially at risk. A chronic carrier state (excretion of the organism for more than 1 year) occurs in approximately 5% of infected people.

Two typhoid vaccines are available for use in the United States: (a) an oral, live, attenuated vaccine (Vivotif Berna vaccine, manufactured from the Ty21a strain of *S. typhi* by the Swiss Serum and Vaccine Institute); and (b) a Vi capsular polysaccharide vaccine (ViCPS) (Typhim Vi, manufactured by Aventis Pasteur) for parenteral use. Both vaccines have been shown to protect 50% to 80% of recipients. The parenteral heat-phenol-inactivated vaccine (manufactured by Wyeth-Ayerst) has been discontinued (4).

Typhoid vaccination is not required for international travel, but it is recommended for travelers to areas where there is a recognized risk of exposure to *S. typhi*. Risk is greatest for travelers to the Indian subcontinent and to other developing countries (those in Asia, Africa, and Central and South America). Intimate contacts of infected people with *S. typhi* and laboratory workers exposed to the bacterium are advised to get vaccinated.

Contraindications include a history of sensitivity to the oral or injectable typhoid vaccine. The oral vaccine should be avoided in people with acute gastrointestinal illness. The oral Ty21a vaccine, because it is a live attenuated bacterial vaccine, should not be used in people with immunodeficiency or in those receiving immunosuppressive therapy. These individuals should receive the injectable ViCPS vaccine instead. People with latex allergy should be given the injectable ViCPS vaccine with caution.

Sulfonamides or antibiotics active against *S. typhi* should not be used in conjunction with oral vaccination for at least 24 hours after receiving the vaccine and vice versa. The antibiotics exert a negative effect on stimulating an immune response by the oral vaccination.

Toxic Dose

The *adult and pediatric therapeutic dose* of typhoid ViCPS vaccine is 0.5 ml IM, with boosters every 2 years if continually exposed to risk of typhoid fever. The oral typhoid Ty21a vaccine capsule is taken with cool liquid every 48 hours, for a total of four doses. It is necessary to complete either oral or injectable typhoid vaccination at least 1 week before travel. The injectable ViCPS vaccine is indicated in people 2 years of age and older. The oral, live attenuated Ty21a vaccine is for people 6 years of age and older.

A toxic dose has not been established. When a minimum of five simultaneous doses were administered to healthy adults, no effects consistent with *S. typhi* infection were observed (25). It was speculated that the bacterium might be shed in the feces.

Pathophysiology

Both vaccines stimulate active immunity to *S. typhi* infection.

Pregnancy and Lactation

Vivotif Berna (Ty21a) is FDA pregnancy risk category C (Appendix I). The injectable typhoid vaccine ViCPS may be given in pregnancy only when clearly needed. The oral, live attenuated Ty21a vaccine should be avoided in pregnant women. In women of childbearing age, pregnancy should be postponed for at least 3 months after vaccination with the oral Ty21a vaccine. Breastfeeding is not a contraindication with the inactivated injectable ViCPS vaccine. The oral, live attenuated Ty21a vaccine, however, should not be used in lactating women.

Clinical Presentation

The oral vaccine Ty21a does not have any local adverse reactions. The injectable vaccine ViCPS may cause erythema, induration, and pain at the injection site. The side effects of oral typhoid vaccine Ty21a are rare and mainly consist of fever, headache, abdominal discomfort, nausea, vomiting, and rash or urticaria. The injectable vaccine ViCPS may cause malaise, headache, muscle ache, and fever.

DIAGNOSTIC TESTS FOR VACCINES

Most vaccine reactions do not require special diagnostic tests. Large local reactions do not typically require laboratory evaluation. In very rare cases, systemic effects may require evaluation of cardiovascular and respiratory systems.

Only a few vaccines created have unique diagnostic tests. *Anthrax vaccine* skin testing is available for military personnel. If the patient understands the risks and benefits of further vaccination and seeks desensitization, progressive dose challenge may be started without pretreatment initially. Serum from before and

3 to 4 weeks after the procedure may be saved to evaluate immune response later.

People who have received *HAV vaccine inactivated* and who are being evaluated for suspected HAV infection may have a positive IgM anti-HAV test if the vaccine was given less than 1 month before a suspected HAV-infection diagnosis. HAV infection does not induce a chronic carrier state.

The actual serum titer of *rabies vaccine* antibody indicating immunity has not been established. However, the definition of minimally acceptable antibody titers varies from laboratory to laboratory, ranging from 1:5 to 1:25.

TREATMENT OF VACCINE EFFECTS

Treatment is symptomatic and supportive in most cases.

Local Reactions

Local reactions are treated with high-potency topical corticosteroid cream or ointment at least two to three times per day until the local reaction has resolved. Patients rarely require oral corticosteroids (e.g., prednisone at 1 mg/kg or 50 to 60 mg/day for 3 to 4 days, tapering off by 10 to 20 mg per day over the next 2 to 4 days). Avoid unprotected sun exposure at the treated sites and use sunscreen aggressively for at least 1 to 2 weeks. For at least 3 to 4 days, avoid strenuous exercise using the arm that has received the vaccination. If itching/pruritus is present, an antihistamine should be administered. If swelling extends below the elbow, a sling may be useful. Some vaccine recipients may benefit from an ice pack within the first 24 hours. Consider cellulitis or lymphangitis in the evaluation.

A large local reaction may be reduced in patients with a previous reaction by pretreating with an antihistamine in typical dosage. Start at least 24 hours before vaccine administration, continuing for 48 to 72 hours after the injection (longer if local reaction persists or reflares).

Mild to Moderate Systemic Events

Symptomatic treatment to prevent recurrence of adverse events has been effective for many vaccines, including those receiving anthrax vaccine. Acetaminophen or ibuprofen are administered for pain or headache. Additional treatment for nausea and other symptoms may be indicated.

Severe Systemic Events

Epinephrine, antihistamines, oxygen, and supportive equipment/personnel should always be on hand in the office to deal with immediate adverse reactions to vaccines. Anaphylaxis is treated by assuring an airway and treating with epinephrine and antihistamines as indicated (Chapter 34). Vaccinees should be observed for at least 30 minutes before being allowed to return home to monitor for shortness of breath, rash, or other adverse reactions to the vaccine. Prompt transport to medical facilities equipped to handle severe reactions is essential as well.

Special Considerations

If acute overdosage of *BCG vaccine* occurs, complications generally do not occur if the patient is treated immediately with antituberculosis agents. If not treated immediately, antituberculosis-agent therapy can still be successful. However, complications, such as regional adenitis, lupus vulgaris, SQ cold abscesses, and ocular lesions, can occur. For BCG sepsis with hypotension diagnosed clinically, a regimen of isoniazid (300 mg daily), rifampin (600 mg daily), and prednisolone (40 mg daily) may be used.

Nonsteroidal antiinflammatory drugs may be used for the pain associated with cystitis in intravesicular therapy. BCG vaccine dermatologic reactions are treated by leaving the BCG skin lesion open to the air and keeping it clean and dry to facilitate healing. Application of a strong antiseptic solution or dressings to a normal scab reaction to BCG vaccine may cause dermatitis and an inflammatory reaction accompanied by ulceration or granuloma formation.

Once initiated, *rabies vaccine* should not be discontinued because of mild systemic or local adverse reactions to the vaccine. Serious systemic, neuroparalytic, or anaphylactic reactions to rabies vaccine must be weighed against the patient's risk of developing rabies disease, which has high morbidity and mortality as well.

REFERENCES

1. Leikin J, Paloucek FP. *Thimerosal. Poisoning and toxicology handbook*, 3rd ed. Hudson, Ohio: Lexi-Comp, 2002.
2. Institute of Medicine. Immunization safety review: thimerosal—containing vaccines and neurodevelopmental disorders. Washington DC: Institute of Medicine, 2001.
3. Centers for Disease Control. Travelers' health. Available at: http://www.cdc.gov/travel/vaccinat.htm. Accessed July 2003.
4. American Hospital Formulary Service Drug Information 2003—chapter on vaccines. Bethesda, MD: American Society of Hospital Pharmacists, Inc., 2003:3107–3272.
5. Thompson RF. *Travel & routine immunizations: a practical guide for the medical office*. Milwaukee, WI: Shoreline Inc., 2001.
6. Advisory Committee on Immunization Practices (ACIP). Use of anthrax vaccine in the United States. *MMWR Recomm Rep* 2000;49.
7. Wiesen AR, Littell CT. Relationship between prepregnancy anthrax vaccination and pregnancy and birth outcomes among US Army women. *JAMA* 2002;287:1556–1560.
8. Geier DA, Geier MR. Anthrax vaccination and joint related adverse reactions in light of biological warfare scenarios. *Clin Exp Rheumatol* 2002;20:217–220.
9. Sever JL, Brenner AI, Gale AD, et al. and the Anthrax Vaccine Export Committee. Safety of anthrax vaccine: a review by the Anthrax Vaccine Expert Committee (AVEC) of adverse events reported to the Vaccine Adverse Event Reporting System (VAERS). *Pharmacoepidemiol Drug Saf* 2002;11:189–202.
10. Timmer SJ, Amundson DE, Malone JD. Hypersensitivity pneumonitis following anthrax vaccination. *Chest* 2002;122:741–745.
11. Peyriere H, Klouche K, Beraud J-J, et al. Fatal systemic reaction after multiple doses of intravesical bacillus Calmette-Guérin for polyposis. *Ann Pharmacother* 2000;34:1279–1282.
12. CDC and Prevention National Center for Infectious Diseases Division of Bacterial and Mycotic Diseases. *Botulism in the United States* 1899–1996. 1998.
13. Sen S, Cloete Y, Hassan K, Buss P. Adverse events following vaccination in premature infants. *Acta Paediatr* 2001;90:916–920.
14. Rich J, et al. A review of the case for Hepatitis B vaccination of high-risk adults. *Am J Med* 2003;114:316–318.
15. Update: Influenza activity—United States and worldwide, 2002–03 season, and composition of the 2003–04 influenza vaccine. *MMWR Morb Mortal Wkly Rep* 2003;52:516–521.
16. Inactivated Japanese encephalitis virus vaccine: recommendations of the Advisory Committee on Immunization Practices (ACIP). *MMWR Recomm Rep* 1993;42.
17. Schoen RT, Deshefy-Longhi T, Van-Hoecke C, et al. An open-label, nonrandomized, single-center, prospective extension, clinical trial of booster dose schedules to assess the safety profile and immunogenicity of recombinant outer-surface protein A (OspA) Lyme disease vaccine. *Clin Ther* 2003;25:210–224.
18. Lathrop SL, Ball R, Haber P, et al. Adverse event reports following vaccination for Lyme disease: December 1998–July 2000. *Vaccine* 2002;20:1603–1608.
19. Measles, mumps, and rubella—vaccine use and strategies for elimination of measles, rubella, and congenital rubella syndrome and control of mumps: recommendations of the Advisory Committee on Immunization Practices (ACIP). *MMWR Recomm Rep* 1998;47.
20. Amendola A, Tanzi E, Zappa A, et al. Safety and immunogenicity of 23-valent pneumococcal polysaccharide vaccine in HIV-1 infected former drug users. *Vaccine* 2002;20:3720–3724.
21. Black S, Shinefield H. Safety and efficacy of the seven-valent pneumococcal conjugate vaccine: evidence from Northern California. *Eur J Pediatr* 2002;161[Suppl 1]:S127–S131.
22. Holdiness MR. Rare systemic dermatologic reactin after pneumococcal vaccine administration. *South Med J* 2003;96:64–65.
23. Compendium of animal rabies prevention and control, 2003. *MMWR Recomm Rep* 2003;52.
24. Tullu MS, Rodrigues S, Muranjan MN, et al. Neurological complications of rabies vaccines. *Indian Pediatr* 2003;40:150–154.
25. Gilman RH, Hornick RB, Woodward WE, et al. Evaluation of a UDP-glucose-4-epimeraseless mutant of *Salmonella typhi* as a live oral vaccine. *J Infect Dis* 1977;136:717–723.

SECTION

15

Skin and Mucous Membrane Agents

CHAPTER 165

Skin and Mucous Membrane Agents

Dean G. Olsen and Richard C. Dart

See Figure 1.

Compounds included:	**Bexarotene (Targretin), crotamiton (Eurax), gentian violet, isotretinoin (Accutane, Isotrex), podofilox (Condyline, Condylox), podophyllum, tacrolimus (Prograf), pimecrolimus (Elidel), terbinafine (Lamisil), urea**
Molecular formula and weight:	**See Table 1.**
SI conversion:	**See Table 1.**
CAS Registry No.:	**See Table 1.**
Special concerns:	**Toxicity for most agents is mild to moderate. Podophyllum may cause severe toxicity.**
Antidote:	**None**

OVERVIEW

Skin and mucous membrane agents comprise a small proportion of exposures or poisoning in acute care toxicology. Although overdose is rarely reported, either because of limited use or because of minimal toxicity, poisoning does occur. Often, toxicity is mild, and no specific treatment is required. The information on these agents is limited to case reports. There are few evidence-based data to guide therapy and predict outcome after large exposures to one of these medications. This chapter serves as a guide of expected clinical course of overdose and treatment recommendations of these agents based on current anecdotal evidence.

BEXAROTENE

Bexarotene (Targretin) is an antineoplastic selective retinoid X receptor ligand available for topical or oral use. No information on overdose is available. It is supplied in 75-mg capsules or 1% gel for topical use (1,2).

Toxic Dose

Adult therapeutic dosages are provided in Table 1 (1). The topical dosage for lymphoma, cutaneous T cell (stage 1A/1B), is 1% gel every other day for 1 week then at weekly intervals increase to once daily, increasing to four times daily (as tolerated) (2). A pediatric therapeutic dose has not been established.

The toxic dose for this medication has not been established. Bexarotene dosages up to 1000 mg/m^2/day have been tolerated without acute toxic effects after short-term administration to patients with advanced cancer (1). There are no reported fatalities from bexarotene overdose.

Toxicokinetics and Toxicodynamics

Information on absorption, volume of distribution, and protein binding for bexarotene has not been studied. Information on the oral bioavailability of the capsules, as well as the cream, is unavailable. Bexarotene is greater than 99% protein bound. In the serum, bexarotene is primarily metabolized by cytochrome P-450 3A4 enzyme system and eliminated via the hepatobiliary system with no appreciable amounts eliminated via urine (1). The elimination half-life of bexarotene ranges from 2 to 7 hours (1).

Pathophysiology

The mechanism of action for bexarotene is through its binding to the retinoid X receptor, which leads to the regulation of cellular growth and differentiation and the induction of programmed cell death (apoptosis) (1) as well as other cellular activities (e.g., enhanced insulin effects). Overdose information is unavailable, and mechanism of toxicity, if any, is unknown.

Pregnancy and Lactation

Bexarotene is U.S. Food and Drug Administration (FDA) pregnancy risk category X (Appendix I) (1,2). Its excretion into breast milk is unknown (1,2).

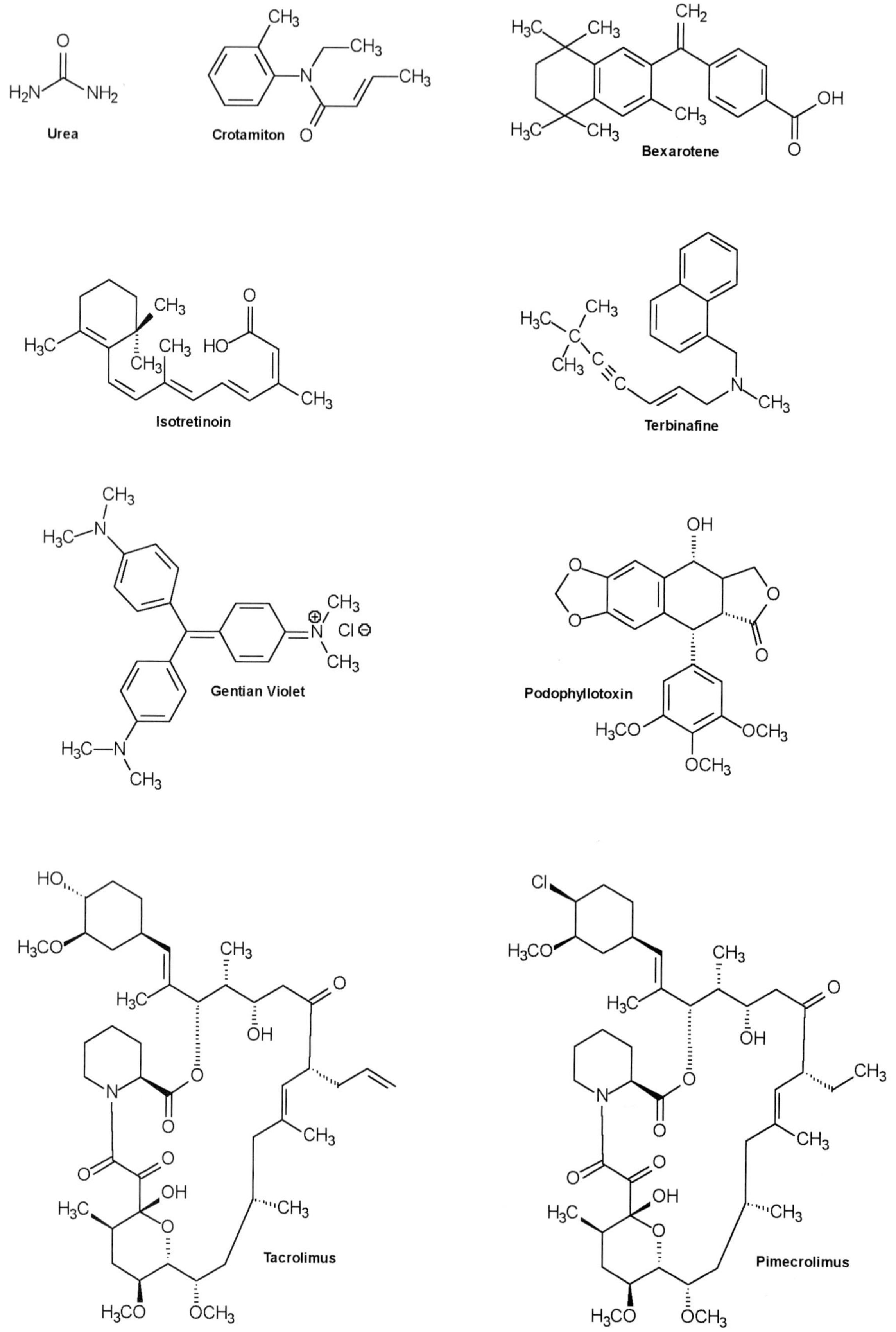

Urea

Crotamiton

Bexarotene

Isotretinoin

Terbinafine

Gentian Violet

Podophyllotoxin

Tacrolimus

Pimecrolimus

Figure 1. Chemical structures of various skin and mucous membrane agents.

TABLE 1. Physical characteristics of the miscellaneous skin and mucous membrane agents

Name	Molecular formula	Molecular weight (g/mol)	SI conversion	CAS Registry No.	Therapeutic dosage	
					Adult	Pediatric
Bexarotene	$C_{24}H_{28}O_2$	348.5	mg/L × 2.9 = μmol/L	153559-49-0	300 mg/m²/d orally.	Not recommended
Crotamiton	$C_{13}H_{17}NO$	203.3	mg/L × 4.9 = μmol/L	483-63-6	Applied topically to lesion (~30 g).	Applied topically to lesion
Gentian violet	$C_{25}H_{30}ClN_3$	408.0	mg/L × 2.4 = μmol/L	548-62-9	Applied topically daily for 2–3 d.	Not recommended
Isotretinoin	$C_{20}H_{28}O_2$	300.4	mg/L × 3.3 = μmol/L	4759-48-2	0.5–3.0 mg/kg/d orally.	Not recommended
Podofilox	$C_{22}H_{22}O_8$	414.4	mg/L × 2.4 = μmol/L	518-28-5	Apply gel or solution to wart daily for 4 d.[a]	Not recommended
Tacrolimus	$C_{44}H_{69}NO_{12}$, H_2O	822.0	mg/L × 1.2 = μmol/L	109581-93-3	0.03–0.20 mg/kg/d orally or IV in divided doses every 12 h.	0.03–0.20 mg/kg/d orally or IV in divided doses every 12 h
Terbinafine	$C_{21}H_{26}ClN$	327.9	mg/L × 3.0 = μmol/L	78628-80-5	250 mg/d orally for 6–12 wk.	No recommended dose for oral
Urea	CH_4N_2O	60.1	mg/L × 16.6 = μmol/L	57-13-6	0.5–5.0 g/kg IV, up to 120 g/d. The dose of intraamniotic urea is ~80 g.	0.5–5.0 g/kg IV, up to 120 g/d

[a]Treatment area no more than 10 cm² and no more than 0.5 g per day.

Clinical Presentation

Doses of up to approximately three and a half times the therapeutic dose have been tolerated without acute toxic effects. Adverse effects in therapeutic dosing include hyperlipidemia and leukopenia, which are the dose-limiting toxicities after therapeutic administration of bexarotene (1–6). Other common adverse effects that may occur include headaches, asthenia, hypothyroidism, and skin rashes (1,5–8). Pancreatitis, coagulopathy, photosensitivity, elevated liver enzymes, and liver failure have been infrequently reported with bexarotene therapy (1–6). It is unclear if these reactions are more likely in overdose. There are no reported fatalities from bexarotene overdose.

Diagnostic Tests

A complete blood cell count (CBC), electrolytes, serum lipid levels, liver function, and thyroid tests should all be monitored in the setting of symptomatic bexarotene overdose. A white blood cell count with differential should be monitored for several weeks after overdose. Time to onset of leukopenia is 4 to 8 weeks after therapeutic use. Serum bexarotene levels are available but not clinically useful.

Treatment

There is no antidote for the treatment of bexarotene overdose. After ingestion, activated charcoal at a dose of 1 g/kg can be administered, although the effectiveness of decontamination has not been evaluated for bexarotene. Dermal exposures should be washed with soap and water. Management is mainly symptomatic and supportive with laboratory monitoring of target organs (e.g., bone marrow, pancreas, thyroid).

CROTAMITON

Crotamiton (Eurax) is used as an alternative agent for the topical treatment of scabies. It has largely been replaced by more efficacious scabicides such as permethrin. Crotamiton has also been touted as an antipruritic, but these claims remain largely unstudied. Data on overdose and ingestion of this agent are limited to a small number of case reports.

Toxic Dose

Adult and pediatric therapeutic doses are provided in Table 1 (9). The *toxic dose* of crotamiton in humans has not been established. The highest known dose ingested of a cream was 2 g by a 1.5-year-old, and the highest known dose ingested of a lotion was 1 oz (3 g) by a 2-year-old (9). No fatalities from overdose have been reported in the literature.

Toxicokinetics and Toxicodynamics

Information on systemic absorption after ingestion or dermal application is not known. Both the mechanism of action and the mechanism of toxicity are unknown.

Pregnancy and Lactation

Crotamiton is FDA pregnancy risk category C (Appendix I) (9). Its excretion into breast milk is unknown.

Clinical Presentation

Limited data are on the clinical presentation and toxicity of crotamiton overdose. This information is based on a few case reports involving ingestion of the topical preparation. Patients who ingest crotamiton may present with somnolence, nausea and vomiting, hypotension, generalized seizures, and coma with hyperreflexia and bilateral ankle clonus (10). Methemoglobinemia has been reported after topical administration of crotamiton and responded to vitamin C therapy, but this finding was never confirmed by a methemoglobin level (11). The active agent of crotamiton is crotonyl-*N*-ethyl-*o*-toluidine (12), a molecule derived from ortho-toluidine. Ortho-toluidine is a known causative agent of methemoglobinemia (13).

A 23-year-old female developed drowsiness, hypotension, complex generalized tonic-clonic seizures, and grade III coma with marked hyperreflexia and bilateral ankle clonus after ingesting an unknown amount of crotamiton emulsion. A full toxicologic screen revealed a serum crotamiton concentration of 34 mg/L; crotamiton and several metabolites were also detected in the urine and identified by gas chromatography-mass spectrometry. The patient was discharged 6 days later after supportive care (10).

Diagnostic Tests

Serum crotamiton levels are not available or clinically useful in the management of crotamiton overdose or ingestion. In symptomatic patients, monitor the CBC, electrolytes, blood pressure, and neurologic status. A methemoglobin level should be obtained in patients who are cyanotic or have respiratory complaints.

Treatment

Management is mainly symptomatic and supportive. After ingestion, activated charcoal (1 to 2 g/kg) should be administered, although this intervention has not been evaluated. Dermal exposures should be washed with soap and water.

Hypotension should be treated with a bolus of 20 ml/kg isotonic crystalloid solution and vasopressors for patients unresponsive to fluid therapy (Chapter 37). Seizures should be treated with benzodiazepines and other measures as needed (Chapter 40). Methemoglobinemia should be treated with methylene blue and oxygen therapy (Chapter 63). No studies to date have established the effectiveness of extracorporeal elimination in the overdose of this agent. There is no antidote for the treatment of crotamiton overdose.

GENTIAN VIOLET

Gentian violet is a topical antifungal used in the treatment of mucosal candidiasis and as a skin antiseptic. Its mechanism of action is unknown. Little is known about the toxicity of this compound; however, it was implicated as a cause of occupational epistaxis in the mid-1960s among apple packers and pulp workers exposed to wood pulp trays impregnated with gentian violet for color and as a bactericide (14). Ocular exposure can cause keratoconjunctivitis. Gentian violet consists of a mixture of 96% hexamethylpararosaniline chloride (crystal violet) and 4% pentamethylrosaniline chloride (methyl violet) with tetramethylpararosaniline (brilliant green) (14). It is supplied as a 1% or 2% aqueous solution.

Toxic Dose

Adult and pediatric therapeutic dosages are provided in Table 1 (15). The toxic dose has not been established. The oral dose lethal to 50% of animals ranges from 96 to 450 mg/kg (16). There are no reported fatalities from gentian violet overdose.

Toxicokinetics and Toxicodynamics

Data on the kinetics of gentian violet in humans are not available. Animal studies indicate that gentian violet is well absorbed from the gastrointestinal (GI) tract (17).

Pathophysiology

The mechanism of action, as well as the mechanism of toxicity, if any, is unknown. Gentian violet is a skin irritant causing erythema and necrotic ulceration with prolonged exposure to 1% concentrations (18). Exposure to the eye causes keratoconjunctivitis, corneal staining, and corneal and conjunctival abrasions, sometimes with permanent scarring (19–21). The severity of dermal and ocular injury appears to be concentration dependent, with more severe injury occurring with higher concentration solutions.

Pregnancy and Lactation

Gentian violet is FDA pregnancy risk category C (Appendix I) (22). Entry into breast milk is unknown (15).

Clinical Presentation

Information on human overdose is limited. Nausea, vomiting, and diarrhea are the most common manifestations after ingestion. The vomitus, feces, and skin may be colored purple. Dermal exposure can result in erythema, purple discoloration of the skin, and necrotic ulceration of the skin (18). Ocular exposure can cause keratoconjunctivitis, corneal staining, and corneal and conjunctival abrasions manifested by pain, photophobia, and fluorescein uptake of the cornea (19–21).

Diagnostic Tests

Electrolytes should all be monitored in the setting of symptomatic gentian violet overdose, as vomiting and diarrhea may cause electrolyte abnormalities. Patients with ocular exposure should have fluorescein staining and a slit-lamp examination done to assess severity of corneal injury. Ophthalmology should be consulted on all patients with ocular complaints.

Treatment

Management is mainly symptomatic and supportive. After ingestion, activated charcoal (1 to 2 g/kg) should be administered, although this intervention has not been evaluated. Dermal exposures should be washed with soap and water. Ocular exposures should be irrigated with copious amounts of normal saline for 15 minutes. There is no antidote for the treatment of gentian violet overdose.

ISOTRETINOIN

Isotretinoin (Accutane, Isotrex) is a synthetic retinoid used in the treatment of acne, psoriasis, neoplasms, and disorders in keratinization. *Isotretinoin* is the 13-*cis* isomer of naturally occurring all-*trans*-retinoic acid (tretinoin). Its mechanism of action is not fully elucidated, but *in vitro* studies suggest that retinoids increase cellular mitotic activity, DNA and RNA synthesis, and protein synthesis. When used for the treatment of acne, isotretinoin appears to involve inhibition of sebaceous gland function and follicular keratinization (23). It has known teratogenic activity and is absolutely contraindicated in pregnancy. The toxic mechanism is not well understood. Isotretinoin is available in 10-, 20-, and 40-mg capsules that also contain parabens and soybean oil (24).

Toxic Dose

Adult and pediatric therapeutic dosages are provided in Table 1 (24). The *toxic dose* for this medication has not been established. Doses of up to 1600 mg in an adult and 63 mg/kg in a child have resulted in only mild toxicity (25,26). There are no reported fatalities from isotretinoin overdose.

Toxicokinetics and Toxicodynamics

Information on absorption, protein binding, metabolism, and excretion in overdose of isotretinoin is unstudied and not available. In therapeutic dosing after ingestion of isotretinoin, there is an apparent lag time of approximately 0.5 to 2.0 hours before the drug appears in the systemic circulation. Peak blood levels usually occur at 2 to 3 hours, and the drug is 99.9% protein bound (23,27). Isotretinoin is metabolized in the liver to its corresponding carboxylic acid, with the major metabolite being 4-oxo-isotretinoin (27). The terminal elimination half-life of isotretinoin ranges from 10 to 20 hours, and the terminal elimination half-life of 4-oxo-isotretinoin ranges from 24 to 29 hours (24,27). Isotretinoin and its metabolites are eliminated almost equally in the urine and feces (28).

Pathophysiology

The teratogenic mechanism of isotretinoin and its main metabolite, 4-oxo-isotretinoin, is believed to result from an adverse effect on the initial differentiation and migration of cephalic neural crest cells (29). It is believed that the ophthalmic toxicity associated with isotretinoin (poor night vision and excessive glare sensitivity) may be due to competition for normal retinol binding sites on cell surfaces or transport molecules (30).

Pregnancy and Lactation

Isotretinoin is FDA pregnancy risk category X (Appendix I) (24). Its excretion into breast milk is unknown (24).

Clinical Presentation

Isotretinoin overdose information is limited to a small number of case reports. Doses up to 30 times the therapeutic dose have resulted in mild symptoms, including dryness of the lips, scaly patches on the skin, mild tachypnea, mild hypertension, mild tachycardia, facial flushing (26), headache (25,31), abdominal discomfort, and hallucinations (31).

Many adverse effects have been reported with therapeutic use, including extreme severe teratogenicity and complications such as spontaneous abortions, mucutaneous abnormalities, corneal opacities, idiopathic intracranial hypertension, hyperuricemia, hypercalcemia, liver function abnormalities, and elevated triglycerides (32–35). A major problem arises in that a significant portion of the users of isotretinoin are women of childbearing age. This subset of patients should be informed of the risks of becoming pregnant while on this medication, and a reliable form of birth control should be instituted at the commencement of therapy with isotretinoin.

Diagnostic Tests

A CBC, electrolytes, and liver function tests should all be monitored in the setting of symptomatic isotretinoin overdose. A complete ocular examination should be done to assess the presence and severity of corneal opacification. Serum isotretinoin levels are available; however, it is unclear how serum levels correlate with toxicity.

Treatment

Management is mainly symptomatic and supportive. After ingestion, activated charcoal (1 to 2 g/kg) should be administered, although this intervention has not been evaluated. Dermal exposures should be washed with soap and water. Ocular exposures should be irrigated with copious amounts of normal saline for 15 minutes. There is no antidote for the treatment of isotretinoin overdose.

PODOPHYLLUM

Podofilox (Condyline, Condylox) and podophyllum resin are used topically for the treatment of external genital warts and perianal warts caused by the human papilloma virus. These agents are also used as homeopathic medications. The active ingredient in these compounds is podophyllum, which is found in the rhizomes and roots of *Podophyllum peltatum* or "mayapple," which contains 40% to 50% of the active compound podophyllotoxin (36). In addition, the substance podophyllum also contains podophyllum resin, picropodophyllin, quercetin, and pellatins (37). Podofilox is available as a 0.5% gel or 0.5% topical solution.

Toxic Dose

Adult and pediatric therapeutic dosages are provided in Table 1. The *toxic dose* of podophyllum has not been well described in the literature. Death has been reported with as little as 350 mg ingested orally (38), and survival has occurred with as much as 2.8 g in an adult (39). A 17-year-old girl died after topical application of 90 ml of 17.5% podophyllum in tincture of benzoin to condylomata (40), and as little as 3 to 8 ml of a 20% podophyllum resin mixture applied dermally has caused systemic toxicity (41). The pediatric toxic dose is not well described.

Toxicokinetics and Toxicodynamics

Podophyllum is well absorbed from the cutaneous and oral route, and its elimination half-life is estimated to be 1.0 to 4.5 hours. Detectable blood levels after topical application of 0.1 ml of solution are reported, and toxicity generally develops 12 to 24 hours after dermal exposure and within 4 to 8 hours or sooner after ingestion (42–45).

Pathophysiology

Podophyllum exerts its toxic effect by arresting cellular mitosis in metaphase. Podophyllum reversibly binds to tubulin, the protein subunit of the spindle microtubules, at a site that is the same or overlaps with the colchicine binding site, thereby preventing polymerization of tubulin into microtubules (46). As a result, podophyllum is believed to inhibit cellular mitosis at metaphase and can stimulate or arrest cell proliferation and arrest cell differentiation (46). Podophyllum also inhibits axonal transport, protein, RNA and DNA synthesis, and blocks oxidation enzymes in tricarboxylic acid cycle. When taken orally, podophyllum is extremely irritating to the intestinal mucosa and results in drastic peristalsis. The exact mechanism of toxicity has not been fully elucidated but appears to be related to mitochondrial inhibition and reduction in cytochrome oxidase activity.

Pregnancy and Lactation

Podophyllum and podofilox are FDA pregnancy risk category C (Appendix I) (47). Podophyllum resin and podophyllotoxin are FDA pregnancy risk category X (47). The excretion of these agents during lactation is unknown.

Clinical Presentation

Oral exposure or dermal application may result in toxicity. Toxicity begins 30 minutes to several hours after ingestion and 12 to 24 hours after dermal exposure. Initial signs include nausea, vomiting, abdominal pain, and diarrhea, often severe as this toxin produces vigorous peristalsis (36,42,48). Confusion, altered mental status, stupor, coma, and peripheral neuropathy may then progress, depending on the dose.

Neurologic manifestations are the hallmark of toxicity and may rapidly progress to loss of reflexes, paralysis and repository failure. Coma lasting 7 to 10 days, cardiotoxicity, ileus, metabolic acidosis, and hallucinations may also occur. Orthostatic hypotension and tachycardia may appear early in the course and last several months after poisoning (40,43,49,50).

Encephalopathy, seizures, and memory impairment have also been reported with dermal and oral overdose (51). Coma and metabolic acidosis occur in large overdoses and are usually preterminal events.

Within the first week after exposure, patients usually develop pancytopenia and hepatic dysfunction that generally resolves within 2 to 3 weeks. During the second week, a polyneuropathy may appear, manifested by paresis, areflexia, selective dorsal radiculopathy, severe sensorimotor axonal neuropathy, and diffuse myopathy, all of which persist as long-term sequelae (36,40,43,45,48,52,53).

Dermal exposure may cause local burns, as podophyllum is very irritating to skin and mucous membranes. Death has been reported after topical exposure (49).

Diagnostic Tests

Frasca et al. (54) described a high-performance liquid chromatography method for the determination of podophyllum concentrations; however, it is unclear how serum levels correlate with toxicity.

A baseline CBC, hemoglobin, electrolytes, calcium, and renal and liver function tests should be obtained for all patients suspected of podophyllotoxin exposure. Follow serial CBCs with differential and platelets for at least 1 week in symptomatic patients to assess bone marrow effects. Serum electrolytes, glucose, blood urea nitrogen, creatinine, and urinalysis are monitored to assess electrolyte abnormalities due to GI and renal injury. Monitor liver function tests and amylase levels to assess organ injury.

Podophyllum can cause a polyneuropathy. Patients with neurologic symptoms may be monitored with serial electromyograms, serial computerized tomography scans, and nerve conduction studies (52). Peripheral neuropathy generally progresses to its peak within 1 week and tends to persist for months to years.

Treatment

Any patient suspected of ingesting or being dermally exposed to amounts greater than that recommended therapeutically should be referred to a health care facility. Signs and symptoms of podophyllum toxicity are often delayed, especially after dermal application, so observation for 6 to 12 hours is advisable after ingestion and up to 24 hours for large dermal exposures.

DECONTAMINATION

Decontamination of dermal exposure consists of removal of contaminated clothing and washing affected areas with copious amounts of water. After ingestion, activated charcoal (1 g/kg) should be administered. Podophyllum is highly irritating to skin and mucous membranes; therefore, emesis is not recommended.

ENHANCEMENT OF ELIMINATION

Due to its large molecular weight, podophyllum is unlikely to be removed by hemodialysis. Charcoal hemoperfusion has been recommended by some clinicians for severe poisoning or for patients who continue to deteriorate despite intensive supportive care; however, there is no conclusive evidence regarding its usefulness.

ANTIDOTES

No antidote is available for podophyllum poisoning.

SUPPORTIVE CARE

No effective treatment is known for either oral or cutaneous exposure aside from intensive supportive care. Hypotension should be treated with a fluid bolus of 20 cc/kg of isotonic crystalloid solution followed by vasopressive agents as clinically indicated (Chapter 37). Bone marrow suppression usually reverses within 1 month and does not require specific treatment. Granulocyte colony-stimulating factor, or filgrastim, may be effective in accelerating recovery from neutropenia after podophyllum poisoning (55).

TACROLIMUS AND PIMECROLIMUS

Tacrolimus (Prograf) is a macrolide antibiotic produced by *Streptomyces tsukubaensis* (56,57). The drug is a potent immunosuppressive agent that is pharmacologically related to cyclosporine and exhibits only limited antimicrobial activity. Tacrolimus is used intravenously for the prevention of rejection of hepatic and renal allotransplantation and topically in the treatment of atopic dermatitis. The exact mechanism of immunosuppressive action is not known but appears to involve inhibition of the activation of T cells through intracellular protein binding (58). Information on acute overdose is limited to case reports, and toxicity appears to be mild. Tacrolimus is available in 0.5-, 1.0-, and 5.0-mg capsules, 0.03% and 0.1% ointment, and a 5 mg/ml solution for injection.

Pimecrolimus (Elidel) is a topical immunosuppressive agent that is an ascomycin derivative that selectively inhibits inflammatory cytokine release (59,60). Although chemically dissimilar, the mechanism of action of this agent resembles that of tacrolimus. Information on overdose is unavailable at this time. Pimecrolimus is available in a 1% cream.

Toxic Dose

Adult and pediatric therapeutic dosages are provided in Table 1 (58). The toxic dosage for these medications has not been established in humans. For tacrolimus, doses of up to 350 mg orally and 20 mg intravenously in an adult and 11 mg in an 11-kg child were administered without adverse effects (61). No fatalities have been reported as a result of tacrolimus or pimecrolimus overdose.

Toxicokinetics and Toxicodynamics

Information on absorption, volume of distribution, and protein binding in overdose for tacrolimus has not been studied. After ingestion of a therapeutic dose, absorption of tacrolimus is erratic and incomplete, with peak serum levels of tacrolimus occurring 1 to 4 hours after oral dosing. The absolute bioavailability is approximately 14% to 32%. Tacrolimus is 75% to 99% protein bound, mainly to albumin and α_1-acid glycoprotein, and the volume of distribution is 0.85 to 1.67 L/kg (58,62).

Metabolism of tacrolimus is mainly hepatic. More than 98% is metabolized by CYP 3A to ten metabolites, two of which are minimally active. Less than 1% of the drug is excreted in the urine unchanged, and metabolites are excreted via the bile (58,63). The elimination half-life (mean values) of tacrolimus is 8.7 to 11.3 hours (63). The elimination half-lives were 3.5 hours in healthy volunteers and 40 hours in patients with liver dysfunction (58,64).

Pimecrolimus oral kinetics are not studied; however, topical application twice a day for 3 weeks resulted in undetectable levels in 78% of the patients studied and very low serum concentrations in the remainder of the subjects. There was no indication of drug accumulation (65).

Pathophysiology

The mechanism of action of tacrolimus is related to its ability to inhibit the activation of T cells and cell-mediated response. The exact mechanism of this inhibition is not known but does involve binding of intracellular proteins and inhibition of the enzyme calcineurin phosphatase, which causes inhibition of release of lymphokines, such as interleukins, and gamma interferon (66). Overdose information is limited, and mechanism of toxicity, if any, is unknown.

Pregnancy and Lactation

Tacrolimus and pimecrolimus are both FDA pregnancy risk category C (Appendix I) (58,67). The excretion into breast milk is unknown for both agents (58,67).

Clinical Presentation

There is limited information on overdose in humans. In patients who have received an inadvertent overdosage of tacrolimus, no adverse reactions have been reported that differ from those of patients receiving therapeutic doses. Overdoses of just over ten times the therapeutic dose have been reported without adverse effects in adults. In a child, five times the therapeutic dose resulted in no toxic effects (61). For tacrolimus, tremor, seizures, nausea, diarrhea, and hypertension have been reported with therapeutic dosing (58,68,69). It is unclear if these reactions are more likely in larger overdoses than previously reported.

Diagnostic Tests

A CBC, electrolytes, and liver function tests should all be monitored in the setting of symptomatic tacrolimus and pimecrolimus overdosage. Serum tacrolimus and pimecrolimus levels are available but not clinically useful.

Treatment

Management is mainly symptomatic and supportive. After ingestion, activated charcoal (1 to 2 g/kg) should be administered, although this intervention has not been evaluated. Dermal exposures should be washed with soap and water. Ocular exposures should be irrigated with copious amounts of normal saline for 15 minutes.

Enhancement of elimination is unlikely to be effective because of the high degree of protein binding. There is no antidote for the treatment of tacrolimus or pimecrolimus overdose.

TERBINAFINE

Terbinafine (Lamisil) is an antifungal used in the treatment of dermal fungal infections, including onychomycosis, tinea (pityriasis) versicolor, and tinea pedis, tinea cruris, or tinea corporis. Terbinafine is an allylamine derivative and acts by inhibiting fungal sterol synthesis. This is achieved through inhibition of squalene epoxidase, a key enzyme necessary for the development of the fungal cell-wall sterol (70). Terbinafine is available in a 1% cream or 250-mg tablets (71–73). Information on overdose is limited and involves a small amount of case studies. Toxicologic manifestations are generally mild and resolve with supportive care.

Toxic Dose

Adult and pediatric therapeutic dosages are provided in Table 1 (71–73). The toxic dose for this medication has not been established. Doses of up to 5 g in an adult (20 times the therapeutic dose) have resulted in only mild toxicity (73). There are no reported fatalities from terbinafine overdose.

Toxicokinetics and Toxicodynamics

Terbinafine is 70% absorbed from the GI tract, 99% protein bound in the serum, and has a volume of distribution of 947 L (71,73). The bioavailability is 40%, and peak serum levels are reached within 2 hours in therapeutic dosing (73). Topical absorption is variable and depends on the amount applied (71,72).

Terbinafine is extensively metabolized in the liver to inactive metabolites via *N*-demethylation or hydroxylation of the alkyl side chain and oxidation to the corresponding carboxylic acids (74–76). The primary metabolites are the *N*-dimethyl and carboxy metabolites (75). Approximately 80% of terbinafine is excreted in the urine as metabolites with no renal elimination of parent drug, and approximately 20% of terbinafine is excreted in the feces (77). Terbinafine undergoes triphasic elimination, with a terminal elimination half-life ranging from 100 to 400 hours with prolonged therapy (73,75,76).

Pathophysiology

The therapeutic mechanism of action for terbinafine is inhibition of the enzyme squalene epoxidase, which is necessary for development of the fungal cell wall (70). Overdose information is limited, and mechanism of toxicity, if any, is unknown.

Pregnancy and Lactation

Terbinafine is FDA pregnancy risk category B (Appendix I) (71,73). Its use in breast-feeding is not recommended (71,73).

Clinical Presentation

Terbinafine overdose information is limited. Doses of up to 5 g have been associated with nausea, vomiting, abdominal pain, rash, headache, dizziness, and frequent urination (73). Ocular disturbances, taste impairment, thrombocytopenia and leukopenia, renal impairment, and hepatotoxicity are infrequent occurrences after therapeutic doses. Various dermal reactions, including pustular and psoriasis-like eruptions, erythema multiforme, toxic epidermal necrolysis, and Stevens-Johnson syndrome, have been reported with therapeutic dosing (78–88). It is unclear if these reactions are more likely in overdose. There are no reported fatalities from overdose.

Drug interactions may result from terbinafine's competitive inhibition of CYP 2D6 (89). Up to 10% of the population are poor metabolizers or genetically deficient in hepatic 2D6 (90). These interactions may be more severe in individuals with already decreased levels of 2D6 resulting from genetic polymorphism. At least seven CYP-450 enzymes are involved in the metabolism of terbinafine itself; however, its metabolism requires less than 5% of the total CYP-450 capacity of the liver, making a drug-drug interaction secondary to its metabolism less likely (91,92). Drug interactions have been reported with nortriptyline (93), desipramine (94), imipramine (95), warfarin (96), cimetidine (73), cyclosporine (73), rifampin (73), and terfenadine (73).

Diagnostic Tests

The CBC, electrolytes, and liver function tests should all be monitored in the setting of symptomatic terbinafine overdose. Patients may develop thrombocytopenia from chronic terbinafine therapy. Electrolyte disturbances may occur in overdose secondary to vomiting. Terbinafine is a strong inhibitor of CYP 2D6 and may cause a rise in liver function tests. Serum terbinafine levels are available but not clinically useful.

Treatment

Management is mainly symptomatic and supportive. After ingestion, activated charcoal (1 to 2 g/kg) should be administered, although this intervention has not been evaluated. Dermal exposures should be washed with soap and water. Ocular exposures should be irrigated with copious amounts of normal saline for 15 minutes. Enhancement of elimination is not expected to be useful because of the high degree of protein binding. There is no antidote for the treatment of terbinafine overdose.

UREA

Urea is the diamide of carbonic acid and is used topically in the treatment of dry skin. It is also used as a diuretic, antineoplastic, and abortifacient; in fertilizers; as an aid in wound healing; and in the processing of plastics, paper, animal feed, resins, barbituric acid, and toothpaste (97). In nearly all uses, its mechanism of action is related to its osmotic activity, creating an osmotic pressure gradient that pulls water toward the drug.

Toxic Dose

Adult and pediatric therapeutic dosages are provided in Table 1. The toxic dose for this medication has not been established. Urea is not highly toxic, and toxicity and death caused from uremic poisoning are due to a combination of factors, not from urea alone. There are no reported fatalities from urea overdose.

Toxicokinetics and Toxicodynamics

Information on kinetics in overdose is not available. Urea is rapidly absorbed orally (98) and is believed to be absorbed dermally based on a case of two infants who were noted to have increased blood urea concentrations after topical application of a cream containing urea (99). Urea readily traverses mammalian membranes (100) and is distributed approximately in total body water (101). A portion of urea is hydrolyzed to ammonia and carbon dioxide. Urea is excreted unchanged in the urine and sweat (98,101) and has a serum half-life of 1.17 hours.

Pathophysiology

Toxicity and death caused from uremic poisoning are due to a combination of factors, not from urea alone. Urea is one of the less toxic factors seen in uremic poisoning. Its toxic mechanism is related to ammonia toxicosis and not to urea itself. Ammonia appears to inhibit the citric acid cycle. Acidosis may occur, and increases are seen in anaerobic glycolysis, blood glucose, and blood lactate. One theory is that ammonia saturation of the glutamine-synthesizing system causes a backup in the citrate cycle, a decrease in its intermediates, and a decrease in energy production and cellular respiration. This may also lead to seizures (102).

Pregnancy and Lactation

Urea is FDA pregnancy risk category C (Appendix I) (103). Its excretion into breast milk is unknown.

Clinical Presentation

Information on overdose with urea is limited, and clinical presentation appears to be similar to reactions encountered with therapeutic dosing. These include a decrease in blood pressure, headache, confusion, diuresis, and hemolysis (97,104,105). It is unclear if these reactions are more likely in overdose. There are no reported fatalities from urea overdose.

Diagnostic Tests

CBC and electrolytes should be monitored in the setting of symptomatic urea overdose. Urea acts as an osmotic diuretic and may cause electrolyte disturbances secondary to renal losses with excessive diuresis. Blood urea nitrogen should be monitored. This is a standard test available in most clinical laboratories. Other clinical laboratory abnormalities have not been reported in humans.

Treatment

There is no antidote for the treatment of urea overdose. GI decontamination is generally not indicated due to the low toxicity of urea. Hydration and the replacement of fluid and electrolyte losses from diuresis are the mainstay of therapy. Other management is mainly symptomatic and supportive. Dermal exposures should be washed with soap and water.

REFERENCES

1. Targretin capsules, bexarotene. Product information. San Diego: Ligand Pharmaceuticals Inc., 2001.
2. Targretin gel, bexarotene. Product information. San Diego: Ligand Pharmaceuticals Inc., 2000.
3. Millikan L, Mustafa M, Yocum R. *RXR-selective oral retinoid bexarotene (Targretin) shows efficacy and safety in AIDS-related Kaposi's sarcoma (poster).* Presented at the Fifth Annual AIDS Malignancy Conference, Bethesda, MD, 2001 Apr 23–25.
4. Khuri FR, Rigas JR, Figlin RA, et al. Multi-institutional phase I/II trial of oral bexarotene in combination with cisplatin and vinorelbine in previously untreated patients with advanced non-small-cell lung cancer. *J Clin Oncol* 2001;19:2626–2637.
5. Duvic M, Hymes K, Heald P, et al. Bexarotene is effective and safe for treatment of refractory advanced-stage cutaneous T-cell lymphoma: multinational phase II-III trial results. *J Clin Oncol* 2001;19:2456–2471.
6. Duvic M, Martin AG, Kim Y, et al. Phase 2 and 3 clinical trial of oral bexarotene (Targretin capsules) for the treatment of refractory or persistent early-stage cutaneous T-cell lymphoma. *Arch Dermatol* 2001;137:581–593.
7. Heald PW, Duvic M. *Palliation and remission of erythrodermic cutaneous T-cell lymphoma with a novel oral RXR-selective retinoid (abstract 428).* Annual Meeting and Exposition of the American Society of Hematology, New Orleans, 1999 Dec 3–7.
8. Rizvi N, Hawkins MJ, Eisenberg PD, et al. Placebo-controlled trial of bexarotene, a retinoid X receptor agonist, as maintenance therapy for patients treated with chemotherapy for advanced non-small-cell lung cancer. *Clin Lung Cancer* 2001;2:210–215.
9. Eurax, crotamiton. Product information. Buffalo, NY: Westwood-Squibb Pharmaceuticals Inc., 1997.
10. Meredith TJ, Dawling S, McNicol MW. Crotamiton overdose [Letter]. *Hum Exp Toxicol* 1990;9:57.
11. Arditti J, Jouglard J. Percutaneous overdose of crotaminon and suspected methemoglobinemia. *Bull Med Leg Toxicol* 1978;21:661–662.
12. *MICROMEDEX healthcare series.* Greenwood Village, CO: MICROMEDEX, 2003.
13. Prilocaine-induced methemoglobinemia—Wisconsin, 1993. *MMWR Morb Mortal Wkly Rep* 1994;43:655–657.
14. Quinby GE. Gentian violet as a cause of epidemic occupational nose bleeds. *Arch Environ Health* 1968;16:485–489.
15. Gentian violet topical solution 1% or 2%. Product information. Texarkana, TX: Humco, 2000.
16. RTECS. Registry of Toxic Effects of Chemical Substances. National Institute for Occupational Safety and Health, Cincinnati (Internet version). Greenwood Village, CO: MICROMEDEX Inc., 2002.
17. McDonald JJ, North BM, Breeder CR, et al. Synthesis and disposition of (14)C-labeled gentian violet in F-344 rats and Bfc3Fl mice. *Food Chem Toxicol* 1984;22:331–336.

18. Sweetman S, ed. *Martindale: the complete drug reference*. London: Pharmaceutical Press (Internet version). Greenwood Village, CO: MICROMEDEX, Inc.
19. Pessah A, Ofosu JR, Klein BL. Conjunctival staining and corneal and conjunctival abrasions caused by 2% aqueous gentian violet solution. *Pediatr Emerg Care* 1998;14:285–286.
20. Parker WT, Binder PS. Gentian violet keratoconjunctivitis. *Am J Ophthalmol* 1979;87:340–343.
21. Dhir SP, et al. Keratoconjunctivitis sicca following instillation of gentian violet. *Indian J Ophthalmol* 1982;30:21–22.
22. Briggs GG, Freeman RK, Yaffe SJ. *Drugs in pregnancy and lactation*, 5th ed. Baltimore: Williams & Wilkins, 1998.
23. McEvoy GK. *AHFS drug information 2003*. Bethesda, MD: American Society of Health System Pharmacists, 2003.
24. Accutane, isotretinoin. Product information. Nutley, NJ: Roche Laboratories, 2001.
25. Sutton JD. Overdose of isotretinoin. *J Am Acad Dermatol* 1983;9:600.
26. Munter DW, Wilkinson JA. Isotretinoin ingestion in a pediatric patient. *J Emerg Med* 1988;6:273–275.
27. Brazzell RK, Colburn WA. Pharmacokinetics of the retinoids isotretinoin and etretinate. *J Am Acad Dermatol* 1982;6:643–651.
28. Colburn WA, Vane FM, Bugge CJL, et al. Pharmacokinetics of (14)C-isotretinoin in healthy volunteers and volunteers with biliary T-tube drainage. *Drug Metab Dispos* 1985;13:327–332.
29. Briggs GG, Freeman RK, Yaffe SJ. *Drugs in pregnancy and lactation*, 5th ed. Baltimore: Williams & Wilkins, 1998.
30. Reynolds JEF, ed. *Martindale: the extra pharmacopoeia* (CD-ROM version). Denver: MICROMEDEX, Inc., 1990.
31. Lindemayr H. Isotretinoin intoxication in attempted suicide. *Acta Derm Venereol* 1986;66:452–453.
32. FDA. Adverse effects with isotretinoin. *FDA Drug Bull* 1983;13:21–23.
33. Flynn WJ, Freeman PG, Wickboldt LG. Pancreatitis associated with isotretinoin-induced hypertriglyceridemia. *Ann Intern Med* 1987;107:63.
34. Hall JG. Vitamin A teratogenicity [Letter]. *N Engl J Med* 1984;311:797–798.
35. Hall JG. Vitamin A. A newly recognized human teratogen-harbinger of things to come? *J Pediatr* 1984;105:583–584.
36. Reynolds JEF, ed. *Martindale: the extra pharmacopoeia* (electronic version). Denver: MICROMEDEX, Inc., 2000.
37. Cassidy DE, Drewry J, Fanning JP. Podophyllum toxicity: a report of a fatal case and a review of the literature. *J Toxicol Clin Toxicol* 1982;19:35–44.
38. Dudley WH. Fatal podophyllum poisoning. *Med Rec* 1890;37:409.
39. Clark ANG, Parsonabe MJ. A case of podophyllum poisoning with involvement of the nervous system. *BMJ* 1957;2:1155.
40. Conard PF, Hanna N, Rosenblum M, et al. Delayed recognition of podophyllum toxicity in a patient receiving epidural morphine. *Anesth Analg* 1990;71:191–193.
41. Moher LM, Maurer SA. Podophyllum toxicity: case report and literature review. *J Fam Pract* 1979;9:237–240.
42. Montaldi DH, Giambrone JP, Courey NG, et al. Podophyllin poisoning associated with the treatment of condyloma acuminatum: a case report. *Am J Obstet Gynecol* 1974;119:1130–1131.
43. Stoehr GP, Peterson AL, Taylor WJ. Systemic complications of local podophyllin therapy. *Ann Intern Med* 1978;89:362–363.
44. Balucani M, Zellers DD. Podophyllin resin poisoning with complete recovery. *JAMA* 1964;189:639–640.
45. Slater GE, Rumack BH, Peterson RG. Podophylline poisoning—systemic toxicity following cutaneous application. *Obstet Gynecol* 1978;52:94–96.
46. McEvoy GK. *AHFS drug information 2003*. Bethesda, MD: American Society of Health System Pharmacists, 2003.
47. Briggs GG, Freeman RK, Yaffe SJ. *Drugs in pregnancy and lactation*, 5th ed. Baltimore: Williams & Wilkins, 1998:41.
48. O'Mahony S, Keohane C, Jacobs J, et al. Neuropathy due to podophyllin intoxication. *J Neurol* 1990;237:110–112.
49. Ward JW, Clifford WS, Monaco AR. Fatal systemic poisoning following podophyllin treatment of condyloma acuminatum. *South Med J* 1954;47:1204–1206.
50. Balucani M, Zellers DD. Podophyllin resin poisoning with complete recovery. *JAMA* 1964;189:639–640.
51. Fisher AA. Severe systemic and local reactions to topical podophyllum resin. *Curr Contact News* 1981;28:233–266.
52. Juurlink DN, Sellens C, Tompson M, et al. Danger in the doctor's office: two cases of severe neurologic sequelae after ingestion of podophyllin. *J Toxicol Clin Toxicol* 1999;37:620(abst).
53. But PPH, Cheung KO, Yong SP, et al. Adulterants of herbal products can cause poisoning [Letter]. *Br Med J* 1996;313:117; Fisher AA. Severe systemic and local reactions to topical podophyllum resin. *Curr Contact News* 1981;28:233–266.
54. Frasca T, Brett AS, Yoo SD. Mandrake toxicity. A case of mistaken identity. *Arch Intern Med* 1997;157:2007–2009.
55. *MICROMEDEX healthcare series*. Greenwood Village, CO: MICROMEDEX, 2003.
56. Goto T, Kino T, Hatanaka H, et al. Discovery of FK-506, a novel immunosuppressant isolated from *Streptomyces tsukubaensis*. *Transplant Proc* 1987;19[Suppl 6]:4–8.
57. Kino T, Hatanaka H, Hashimoto M, et al. FK-506, a novel immunosuppressant isolated from a *Streptomyces*. I. Fermentation, isolation, and physicochemical and biological characteristics. *J Antibiot* 1987;40:1249–1255.
58. Prograf, tacrolimus. Product information. Deerfield, IL: Fujisawa USA, Inc., 2002.
59. Griffiths CE. Ascomycin: an advance in the management of atopic dermatitis. *Br J Dermatol* 2001;144:679–681.
60. Wellington K, Spencer CM. SDZ ASM 981. *BioDrugs* 2000;14:409–416.
61. Mrvos R, Hodgman M, Krenzelok EP. Tacrolimus (FK 506) overdose: a report of five cases. *J Toxicol Clin Toxicol* 1997;35:395–399.
62. Fay JW, Wingard JR, Antin JH, et al. FK506 (tacrolimus) monotherapy for prevention of graft-versus-host disease after histocompatible sibling allogeneic bone marrow transplantation. *Blood* 1996;87:3514–3519.
63. Venkataramanan R, Jain A, Warty VW, et al. Pharmacokinetics of FK 506 following oral administration: a comparison of FK 506 and cyclosporine. *Transplant Proc* 1991;23:931–933.
64. Jain AB, Venkataramanan R, Cadoff E, et al. Effect of hepatic dysfunction and T tube clamping on FK 506 pharmacokinetics and trough concentrations. *Transplant Proc* 1990;22[Suppl 1]:57–59.
65. Van Leent EJ, Ebelin ME, Burtin P, et al. Low systemic exposure after repeated topical application of pimecrolimus (Elidel), (SD Z ASM 981) in patients with atopic dermatitis. *Dermatology* 2002;204:63–68.
66. McEvoy GK. *AHFS drug information 2003*. Bethesda, MD: American Society of Health System Pharmacists, 2003.
67. Elidel, pimecrolimus 1% cream. Product information. East Hanover, NJ: Novartis Pharmaceuticals, 2001.
68. Fung JJ, Abu-Elmagd K, Todo S, et al. FK 506 in clinical organ transplantation. *Clin Transplant* 1991;5:517–522.
69. Fung JJ, Todo S, Jain A, et al. Conversion from cyclosporin to FK506 in liver allograft recipients with cyclosporin-related complications. *Transplant Proc* 1990;22[Suppl 1]:6–12.
70. *MICROMEDEX healthcare series*. Greenwood Village, CO: MICROMEDEX, 2003.
71. Lamisil cream 1%, terbinafine. Product information. East Hanover, NJ: Novartis Pharmaceutical Corporation, 1997.
72. Lamisil solution 1%, terbinafine. Product information. East Hanover, NJ: Novartis Pharmaceutical Corporation, 1997.
73. Lamisil tablets, terbinafine. Product information. East Hanover, NJ: Novartis Pharmaceutical Corporation, 1997.
74. Humbert H, Cabiac MD, Denouel J, et al. Pharmacokinetics of terbinafine and of its five main metabolites in plasma and urine, following a single oral dose in healthy subjects. *Biopharm Drug Dispos* 1995;16:685–694.
75. Abdel-Rahman SM, Nahata MC. Oral terbinafine: a new antifungal agent. *Ann Pharmacother* 1997;31:445–456.
76. Sweetman S, ed. *Martindale: the complete drug reference*. London: Pharmaceutical Press (electronic version). Englewood, CO: MICROMEDEX Inc., 2001.
77. Jensen JC. Clinical pharmacokinetics of terbinafine (Lamisil). *Clin Exp Dermatol* 1989;14:110–113.
78. Dupin N, Gorin I, Djien V, et al. Acute generalized exanthematous pustulosis induced by terbinafine. *Arch Dermatol* 1996;132:1253–1254.
79. Kempinaire A, De Raeve L, Merckx M, et al. Terbinafine-induced acute generalized exanthematous pustulosis confirmed by a positive patch-test result. *J Am Acad Dermatol* 1997;37:653–655.
80. Condon CA, Downs AMR, Archer CB. Terbinafine-induced acute generalized exanthematous pustulosis [Letter]. *Br J Dermatol* 1998;138:709–710.
81. Bennett ML, Jorizzo JL, White WL. Generalized pustular eruptions associated with oral terbinafine. *Int J Dermatol* 1999;38:596–600.
82. Gupta AK, Lynde CW, Lauzon GJ, et al. Cutaneous adverse effects associated with terbinafine therapy: 10 case reports and a review of the literature. *Br J Dermatol* 1998;138:529–532.
83. Hall AP, Tate B. Acute generalized exanthematous pustulosis associated with oral terbinafine. *Australas J Dermatol* 2000;41:42–45.
84. Pauluzzi P, Boccucci N. Inverse psoriasis induced by terbinafine [Letter]. *Acta Derm Venereol* 1999;79:389.
85. McGregor JM, Rustin MHA. Terbinafine and erythema multiforme [Letter]. *Br J Dermatol* 1994;131:587–588.
86. Todd P, Halpern S, Munro DD. Oral terbinafine and erythema multiforme. *Clin Exp Dermatol* 1995;20:247–248.
87. White SI, Bowen-Jones D. Toxic epidermal necrolysis induced by terbinafine in a patient on long-term anti-epileptics [Letter]. *Br J Dermatol* 1996;134:188–189.
88. Carstens J, Wendelboe P, Sogaard H, et al. Toxic epidermal necrolysis and erythema multiforme following therapy with terbinafine. *Acta Derm Venereol (Stock)* 1994;74:391–392.
89. Vickers AE, Sinclair JR, Zollinger M, et al. Multiple cytochrome P-450s involved in the metabolism of terbinafine suggest a limited potential for drug-drug interactions. *Drug Metab Dispos* 1999;27:1029–1038.
90. Goodman Gilman A, Limberd L, Hardman J. *Goodman & Gilman's: the pharmacological basis of therapeutics*, 10th ed. McGraw Hill, 2001:15–18.
91. Abdel-Rahman SM, Marcucci K, Boge T, et al. Potent inhibition of cytochrome P-450 2D6-mediated dextromethorphan O-demethylation by terbinafine. *Drug Metab Dispos* 1999;27:770–775.
92. Balfour J, Faulds D. Terbinafine. A review of its pharmacodynamic and pharmacokinetic properties and therapeutic potential in superficial mycoses. *Drugs* 1992;43:259–284.

93. van der Kuy PHM, Hooymans PM, Verkaaik AJB. Nortriptyline intoxication induced by terbinafine. *BMJ* 1998;316:441.
94. O'Rearden JP, Hetznecker JM, Rynn MA, et al. Desipramine toxicity with terbinafine. *Am J Psychiatry* 2002;159:1067.
95. Titelbaum ML, Pearson VE. Imipramine toxicity with terbinafine. *Am J Psychiatry* 2001;158:2086.
96. Warwick JA, Corrall RJ. Serious interaction between warfarin and oral terbinafine. *Br Med J* 1998;316:440.
97. *MICROMEDEX healthcare series*. Greenwood Village, CO: MICROMEDEX, 2003.
98. Sweetman S, ed. *Martindale: the complete drug reference*. London: Pharmaceutical Press (electronic version). Greenwood Village, CO: MICROMEDEX, 2001.
99. Beverley DW, Wheeler D. *Arch Dis Child* 1986;61:696.
100. Hayes WJ Jr. *Toxicology of pesticides*. Baltimore: Williams & Wilkins, 1975.
101. LaDu BN, Mandel HG, Way EL. Fundamentals of drug metabolism and disposition. Baltimore: Williams & Wilkins, 1971.
102. Booth NH, McDonald LE, eds. *Veterinary pharmacology and therapeutics*, 5th ed. Ames, IA: Iowa State University Press, 1982.
103. Briggs GG, Freeman RK, Yaffe SJ, eds. *Drugs in pregnancy and lactation*, 4th ed. Baltimore: Williams & Wilkins, 1994.
104. Osol A, Hoover JE, eds. *Remington's pharmaceutical sciences*, 15th ed. Easton, PA: Mack Publishing Company, 1975:864.
105. Sweetman S, ed. *Martindale: the complete drug reference*. London: Pharmaceutical Press (electronic version). Greenwood Village, CO: MICROMEDEX, 2001.

SECTION

16

Smooth Muscle Relaxants

CHAPTER 166

Smooth Muscle Relaxants

E. Martin Caravati

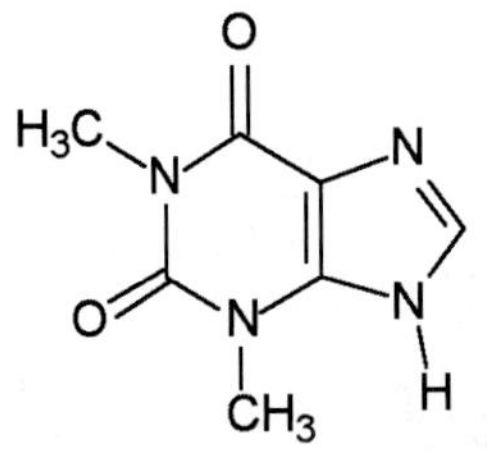

THEOPHYLLINE

Compounds included:	**Bamifylline hydrochloride (Bami-med, Trentadil); theophylline (Theo-Dur, many others); oxybutynin chloride (Ditropan)**
Molecular formula and weight:	**Bamifylline ($C_{20}H_{27}N_5O_3$, HCl), 421.9 g/mol; theophylline ($C_7H_8N_4O_2$), 180.2 g/mol; oxybutynin chloride ($C_{22}H_{31}NO_3$, HCl), 393.9 g/mol**
SI conversion:	**Theophylline, mg/L × 5.55 = µmol/L; oxybutynin, µg/L × 2.79 = nmol/L**
CAS Registry No.:	**20684-06-4 (bamifylline); 58-55-9 (theophylline)**
Normal or therapeutic levels:	**Bamifylline, 0.18 to 20.00 µg/ml; theophylline, 5 to 20 µg/ml**
Special concerns:	**Narrow therapeutic index, seizures**
Antidote:	**Physostigmine (oxybutynin)**

THEOPHYLLINE

Theophylline (1,3-dimethylxanthine, Elixophylline, Theo-Dur, Slo-bid) is a methylated xanthine. Other xanthine derivatives include caffeine and theobromine. Once a mainstay of asthma therapy, β-agonists and leukotriene antagonists have largely replaced theophylline in the treatment of asthma. It was also used to relieve dyspnea in chronic obstructive pulmonary disease. It is commonly used to treat neonatal apnea of preterm infants. The incidence of poisoning has declined dramatically in recent years. In 1991, American poison centers reported that 4470 patients were treated in health care facilities and 38 deaths occurred as a result of theophylline or aminophylline intoxication (1). In 2001, there were only 639 patients treated in health care facilities and 18 fatalities reported (2).

Theophylline is available as injection, immediate-release, sustained-release (8 to 12 hours), and time-release (12 to 24 hours) formulations. Aminophylline is the ethylenediamine salt and contains approximately 85% anhydrous theophylline. It is available as an injection and as regular-release and controlled-release preparations.

Toxic Dose

The *therapeutic dose* of aminophylline for bronchospasm is 5 to 6 mg/kg intravenously (IV) as a loading dose infused over 20 to 30 minutes. The oral loading dose is 4 to 6 mg/kg. The oral maintenance dosage ranges from 4 to 20 mg/kg/day depending on age. The highest doses are needed for 1- to 9-year-old children. The dose is reduced in adults with cardiac or liver dysfunction.

The *toxic dose* is not well defined. Acute ingestion of 10 to 12 g by an adult has resulted in death. (3). A 5-day-old, 1.3-kg premature neonate inadvertently received 180 mg of theophylline over 26 hours during treatment for bradycardia and developed tachycardia, hyperventilation, increased diuresis, central nervous system (CNS) excitation, hyperglycemia, and hypercalcemia. The child survived (4).

Toxicokinetics and Toxicodynamics

Therapeutic doses are rapidly absorbed, but overdoses of sustained-release preparations may have prolonged or delayed absorption of up to 24 hours. Time-to-peak plasma concentration (T_{max}) for a therapeutic dose is 1 to 2 hours for regular release and 5 to 6 hours for enteric-coated or sustained-release tablets. Bezoar formation can produce secondary peaks in theophylline levels (5).

The apparent volume of distribution (V_d) ranges from 0.2 to 0.7 L/kg (mean, 0.5 L/kg). Liver cirrhosis increases and obesity decreases the V_d at therapeutic doses, whereas age, gender, chronic pulmonary disease, and smoking have little effect. The elderly have a slightly smaller V_d than do young adults. Protein binding is approximately 50% at therapeutic concentrations in adults and 35% in neonates and patients with hepatic cirrhosis.

Theophylline is metabolized by hepatic oxidation, primarily by cytochrome P1A2, to 1,3-dimethylureic acid and by *N*-demethylation to 3-methylxanthine and 1-methyluric acid. In adults, approximately 77% of a therapeutic dose is renally excreted within 48 hours as unchanged drug (10%) and metabolites (90%). In the neonate, 50% is excreted unchanged. The unique difference in theophylline disposition between adults and neonates is the formation of caffeine (8.5%) in the neonate. Caffeine may be a minor urinary metabolite in adults.

At therapeutic doses, blood levels follow first-order kinetics with a half-life of 3 to 11 hours. Infants tend to have a longer half-life (7 hours), compared with older children (4 hours). Neonates have an extended half-life (30 hours) due to immature cytochrome enzymes. In overdose, mixed first- and zero-order kinetics (Michaelis-Menten) predominate. Overdose may produce a biphasic elimination pattern with a slow initial phase due either to continued absorption or to saturation of metabolic pathways (6). Viral infections in children prolong the half-life to 10 to 20 hours. In adults, the half-life is prolonged in patients with congestive heart failure (23 hours) and liver cirrhosis (65 hours).

Pathophysiology

Theophylline inhibits phosphodiesterase at high concentrations, which leads to an increase in cyclic adenine monophosphate and subsequent catecholamine release. It is also an adenosine antagonist. It promotes diaphragmatic contractility and mucociliary clearance. It causes smooth muscle relaxation; bronchodilation; diuresis; cardiac, respiratory, and CNS stimulation; and increases gastric acid secretion.

In the CNS, theophylline is an adenosine receptor antagonist and may cause seizures by antagonizing the depressant effect of adenosine in the cerebral cortex. Theophylline induces cerebral vasoconstriction and relative ischemia.

Increased catecholamine levels (epinephrine and norepinephrine) are observed after therapeutic use and overdose. The catecholamine effects of theophylline intoxication include hyperglycemia, hypercalcemia, metabolic acidosis, and prolongation of the QT interval on the electrocardiogram (ECG), which may be a cause of theophylline-induced tachydysrhythmias (7). The exact etiology of the metabolic acidosis is unclear, but it may result from a lactic acidosis secondary to catecholamine-induced glycolysis (8). The clinical effects of xanthine-induced increases in catecholamine and cyclic adenine monophosphate appear synergistic. Theophylline probably causes hypercalcemia through beta-adrenergic regulation because propranolol can reduce serum calcium levels in theophylline-poisoned patients (9).

Hypokalemia may be due to potassium loss from protracted vomiting, potassium diuresis associated with metabolic acidosis, or potassium shifts into the intracellular compartment. The shift from the extracellular compartment is secondary to hyperglycemia, hyperinsulinemia, and the catecholamine-induced stimulation of membrane-bound Na^+,K^+–adenosine triphosphate. Hypokalemia is two to three times more common after acute intoxication, compared with chronic overmedication (10). As the serum theophylline level decreases, potassium returns from the cell to the extracellular compartment.

Theophylline-induced cardiotoxicity may be due to its direct action on cardiac membrane depolarization, antagonism of the cardioprotective effects of endogenous adenosine, stimulation of plasma catecholamine activity, and the resultant increase in myocardial oxygen demand.

Pregnancy and Lactation

Theophylline is U.S. Food and Drug Administration (FDA) pregnancy category C (Appendix I). Pregnancy results in slightly decreased theophylline protein binding, increased V_d, and increased elimination half-life (262 minutes vs. 389 minutes) (11). A study of 59,931 pregnancies concluded that theophylline use during pregnancy was not associated with an increased risk of stillbirth (12). The association of some rare cardiovascular anomalies (aortic anomalies, double-outlet right ventricle, transposition of the great arteries, anomalous pulmonary venous connection, hypoplasia of the left ventricle) with theophylline exposure in animals and in an initial human study suggested that theophylline may be a cardiovascular teratogen. Fetal echocardiography may be useful in detecting any possible severe cardiac defect. Additional studies are required to confirm the validity of these observations (13).

Theophylline crosses the placenta, and newborn infants may have therapeutic serum levels. It is excreted into breast milk with a milk to serum ratio of 0.7 (14). Tachycardia, vomiting, and irritability have been observed in newborns of mothers taking theophylline. Theophylline is considered compatible with breast-feeding, although irritability may occur in the nursing infant (15).

Clinical Presentation

ACUTE VERSUS CHRONIC OVERDOSAGE

Theophylline poisoning may be acute (single exposure), chronic (maintenance therapy), or acute-on-chronic (single toxic exposure while on maintenance therapy). Patients are four to five times more likely to have major signs of toxicity from chronic overmedication, compared with acute ingestion, despite having lower serum levels. The major predictors of severe toxicity are peak serum theophylline levels greater than 100 μg/ml in acute ingestion and patient age older than 60 years in chronic overmedication (16). In chronic toxicity, the risk of a life-threatening event increases with age and is not related to peak serum theophylline concentration (17). In a prospective cohort reported to a poison center, death was three times more likely after toxicity from chronic overmedication, compared with acute ingestion (35% vs. 10%) (18).

In a prospective study of 125 pediatric patients with theophylline intoxication, approximately 10% exhibited life-threatening events (seizures, dysrhythmias). In acute, single exposures, the theophylline concentration was significantly higher in those with seizures or dysrhythmias. Patient age was not a predictive factor for major toxicity. Patients with acute intoxication also had lower serum potassium (3.04 mmol/L vs.

3.80 mmol/L) and higher serum glucose (194 mg/dl vs. 127 mg/dl) levels than did children with chronic intoxication (19). Peak theophylline concentration did not identify high-risk patients after acute-on-therapeutic or chronic intoxication. Children who experienced life-threatening events after chronic exposure were younger, however (1.6 year vs. 8.0 years) (19).

Inadvertent neonatal overdose has occurred in the treatment of apnea and bradycardia. Toxic effects include tachycardia, jitteriness, clonic posturing, emesis, diarrhea, hyperglycemia, hypercalcemia, generalized seizures, and intracranial hemorrhage. Toxicity is enhanced by the delayed elimination of theophylline in the premature infant, presumably due to immaturity of the mixed-function overdose system (4).

CLINICAL EFFECTS BY ORGAN SYSTEM

Gastrointestinal (GI) effects, such as nausea and vomiting, are prominent and early features of toxicity. Hematemesis and abdominal pain may also occur.

CNS toxicity begins with agitation and tremor. Theophylline-induced seizures are associated with a significant morbidity. In chronic overmedication, seizures may be the initial sign of toxicity. Theophylline-induced seizures may result in status epilepticus, rhabdomyolysis, and hypoxic injury. Seizures in children or adults may occur at therapeutic or mildly toxic levels. Elderly patients have a poorer prognosis after theophylline-induced seizures. Other risk factors for serious outcome in theophylline-associated seizures are previous brain injury or disease, severe pulmonary disease, and possibly a low serum albumin level (20). Ataxia and visual hallucinations have occurred in pediatric theophylline overdose cases (21).

Cardiotoxic effects may occur with theophylline intoxication or with levels in the therapeutic range (22). Dysrhythmias are five times more likely to occur after chronic overmedication than after acute overdose (18). Sinus tachycardia and complex atrial and ventricular ectopy are common with serum theophylline concentrations greater than 30 µg/ml. Sustained supraventricular or ventricular tachydysrhythmias that require treatment are rare (23,24). Ventricular tachycardia is a rare complication that tends to occur with advanced age, underlying heart disease, or very high serum theophylline concentrations. Ventricular fibrillation and cardiac arrest typically follow intentional single ingestions that result in a serum theophylline concentration greater than 100 µg/ml or after rapid central venous infusion of theophylline. These life-threatening dysrhythmias often develop in young or middle-aged patients with no known underlying heart disease (24). Hypotension resistant to vasopressor therapy has been reported.

An acute myocardial infarction followed by severe heart failure occurred in a 26-year-old woman after ingestion of 25 tablets of controlled-release theophylline (270-mg tablets). Her serum theophylline level was 32 µg/ml. She recovered after aggressive therapy (25).

Rhabdomyolysis may result from repeated seizure activity. Acute compartment syndrome occurs rarely in theophylline poisoning (26). It may follow rhabdomyolysis or repeated seizures and is exacerbated by hypokalemia, hypotension, and limb compression.

Electrolyte abnormalities include hypokalemia, hypomagnesemia, hypophosphatemia, metabolic acidosis, hyperglycemia, leukocytosis, and hypercalcemia. Hypokalemia, metabolic acidosis, and hyperglycemia are more common after acute overdose, compared with chronic overmedication (8,27).

ADVERSE EVENTS

A substantial portion of young adult patients (30% to 80%) on maintenance therapy that have serum concentrations in the toxic range (greater than 20 µg/ml) are asymptomatic (28,29). Cardiovascular adverse events include palpitations, tachycardia, chest pain, and vasodilatation. CNS effects include headache, tremor, insomnia, irritability, psychosis, and visual hallucinations. GI effects include nausea, vomiting, abdominal pain, and decreased esophageal sphincter tone.

DRUG INTERACTIONS

Many drugs *increase* the plasma concentration of theophylline: allopurinol, beta-blockers, calcium-channels blockers, carbamazepine, cimetidine, ciprofloxacin, corticosteroids, disulfiram, ephedrine, erythromycin, influenza vaccine, interferon, isoniazid, furosemide, macrolide antibiotics, mexiletine, oral contraceptives, quinolones, thyroid hormones, zafirlukast, zileuton.

Other drugs *decrease* the plasma concentration: barbiturates, carbamazepine, activated charcoal, isoniazid, isoproterenol, ketoconazole, phenobarbital, phenytoin, rifampin, St. John's wort, sulfinpyrazone, sympathomimetics.

Asthmatic patients may experience a delayed hypersensitivity reaction to the ethylenediamine component of theophylline (aminophylline). Cross-reactivity may occur with chemically related agents, including ethanolamine antihistamines (diphenhydramine, carbinoxamine, clemastine), triethanolamine-containing creams (Aspercreme, Myoflex, Sportscreme), and the piperazine antihistamine, hydroxyzine (30).

Diagnostic Tests

THEOPHYLLINE CONCENTRATION

High-performance liquid chromatography is the standard of measurement. Initial studies suggest that a commercially available theophylline assay obtained by fingerstick is able to measure theophylline concentrations within the range 0.4 to 30.0 µg/ml. This method allows multiple determinations within short periods and correlates well with high-performance liquid chromatography. Additional clinical studies need to be performed to determine its clinical usefulness (31,32).

The therapeutic concentration of theophylline is 5 to 20 µg/ml. After an acute single ingestion, mild toxicity typically occurs with peak theophylline levels of 20 to 40 µg/ml, moderate toxicity at 40 to 100 µg/ml, and severe toxicity greater than 100 µg/ml. Young adult asthma patients on chronic theophylline therapy may have levels greater than 20 mg/L without symptoms (29). Yet, several older patients have died from seizures with serum levels of 25 to 62 mg/L (33). Patients with toxicity from chronic overmedication may develop seizures or dysrhythmias with serum levels less than 70 µg/ml, whereas those with acute ingestions are unlikely to suffer life-threatening events unless serum levels exceed 100 µg/ml (27). Peak serum theophylline levels cannot predict which elderly patients with chronic theophylline intoxication will have a life-threatening effect (17).

In children, 29% of patients with levels of 25 to 50 µg/ml were asymptomatic, but those with levels greater than 50 µg/ml were always symptomatic. Vomiting and tachycardia were most common (28). Seizures or dysrhythmias occurred in acute intoxications with mean serum levels of 100 µg/ml and in chronic exposures with a mean level of 42 µg/ml. Serum concentration did not predict which patient would suffer seizures or dysrhythmias in chronic toxicity (19). Seizures have been reported in neonates 7 to 8 hours after acute intoxication with concentrations of 51 and 54 µg/ml (34).

OTHER TESTS

Serial electrolyte and anion gap evaluation is needed in symptomatic patients with either acute or chronic exposure. Hypokalemia, hyperglycemia, increased anion-gap metabolic acidosis, lactic acidosis, respiratory alkalosis, and hypercalcemia may occur.

The most common ECG abnormality is sinus tachycardia. Atrial and ventricular ectopy, atrial fibrillation, and ventricular dysrhythmias may also occur.

DIAGNOSTIC PITFALLS

The severity of intoxication should not be judged by laboratory values alone. Typically, chronic overmedication, which usually develops in the very young or the elderly, causes toxicity at lower serum theophylline levels compared to acute overdosage. Seizures and serious dysrhythmias frequently appear in those chronic overmedication cases at theophylline levels between 40 and 70 μg/ml (27,35). Patients younger than 40 years of age tend to develop serious dysrhythmias when theophylline levels exceed 50 μg/ml; older patients can display serious rhythm disturbances at levels greater than 35 μg/ml (36). Clinical manifestations of toxicity in children are variable and cannot be used to screen those who should have their serum levels monitored (28).

POSTMORTEM CONSIDERATIONS

The postmortem redistribution of theophylline is not clinically significant (33).

Treatment

The patient with major theophylline toxicity presents several therapeutic dilemmas. Many patients do well with simple termination of exposure and supportive care, whereas others develop progressively rising levels or deteriorating clinical condition.

GASTROINTESTINAL DECONTAMINATION

Induction of emesis has not been shown to be of benefit after acute ingestion. Further, it may exacerbate the vomiting inherent in theophylline toxicity. It also complicates the use of activated charcoal, which is known to decrease the serum theophylline level.

Gastric emptying shortly after ingestion followed by activated charcoal reduces theophylline absorption from the gut, reduces the serum theophylline concentration and elimination half-life, and may reduce hospital stay (37). Gastric pharmacobezoar formation has been described that resulted in delayed peak blood levels and death despite decontamination with gastric lavage and activated charcoal (38).

Activated charcoal binds theophylline and should be administered as soon as possible after ingestion. The usual dose is 50 g orally in adults and 1 g/kg in children. It may be administered orally or by nasogastric tube. Vomiting associated with acute theophylline toxicity may be prolonged and can limit the effectiveness of activated charcoal (39). Activated charcoal has been used in neonates. One report describes treatment with a single total dose of 0.6 g/kg (1 g) aqueous activated charcoal without sorbitol in a premature infant on the second day of life. This was diluted with sterile water 1:1, which was followed by sterile water every 6 hours via a nasogastric tube to facilitate passage of charcoal stool. It led to a decrease in the half-life of theophylline concentration with clinical improvement (40). Oral activated charcoal may be the treatment of choice in acute overdose with sustained-release theophylline tablets in infants. This therapy might not be feasible in neonates with absent bowel sounds or potential risk factors for necrotizing enterocolitis (19).

In approximately 25% of patients who have ingested an overdose of sustained-release theophylline, a further rise in serum theophylline concentration may occur despite conventional therapy with gastric lavage and activated charcoal. One dose of activated charcoal (50 mg in 150 ml of 70% sorbitol) may be followed by a second dose of charcoal not containing sorbitol 4 hours after the first. Serum theophylline levels, measured at 2-hour intervals for the first 12 to 24 hours, are used as a guide to further therapy (41).

Whole bowel irrigation has been used successfully in sustained-release (42) and regular-preparation (43) ingestions. It may be useful in patients with rapidly increasing serum theophylline concentrations that persist even after multiple doses of activated charcoal or extracorporeal removal. It can be used in combination with activated charcoal (e.g., 50 g of activated charcoal added to each liter of polyethylene glycol solution). Current recommendations are for administration of nonabsorbable isosmolar fluid containing polyethylene glycol via nasogastric tube at a rate of 1 to 2 L/hour in adults and 500 ml/hour in children. The irrigation is continued until the rectal effluent is clear and the abdominal radiograph is clear of radiopaque tablets. The average time for this to occur is approximately 4 hours. However, there is no clinical evidence that whole bowel irrigation provides additional benefit over activated charcoal alone in sustained-release theophylline poisoning (44). Performing whole bowel irrigation in conjunction or shortly after giving activated charcoal may decrease charcoal's ability to adsorb theophylline (45).

ENHANCEMENT OF ELIMINATION

Multiple-dose activated charcoal (MDAC) administration increases elimination of theophylline from the plasma (46,47). In the absence of a contraindication (e.g., bowel obstruction), all patients with acute or chronic poisoning should receive multiple doses of activated charcoal (without sorbitol) every 4 hours until the serum concentration is less than 20 μg/ml. Antiemetic therapy may be necessary to control vomiting. MDAC in the neonate may increase the risk for necrotizing enterocolitis and may be limited by vomiting or ileus (48).

The optimum dose for MDAC has not been established. In adults, administer 30 to 75 g initially, followed by 25 to 50 g every 4 hours. In children, administer 15 to 30 g (or 1 g/kg) initially, with repeat doses of one-half the initial dose every 4 hours. A continuous charcoal infusion of 0.25 to 0.50 g/kg/hour (maximum rate, 50 g/hour) has also been recommended for pediatric patients who cannot tolerate the bolus dosing. The activated charcoal is diluted in normal saline and infused via nasogastric tube (49).

Contraindications to MDAC include an unprotected airway, bowel obstruction, or ileus. Complications have included vomiting, aspiration pneumonitis, bowel obstruction, and pseudoobstruction (Ogilvie's syndrome). Multiple-dose oral activated charcoal and sorbitol may lead to hypernatremia and dehydration (50). Sorbitol containing activated charcoal should be avoided. Patients must be closely monitored for the possible development of fluid and electrolyte abnormalities.

Hemodialysis is used for selected cases, although its effectiveness in improving outcome has not been tested. Its recommendation for use is based on evidence that major toxicity has been associated with peak serum concentrations of greater than 100 μg/ml in acute overdose and greater than 60 μg/ml in chronic toxicity. Theophylline clearance with hemodialysis has been estimated to be 185 to 200 ml/kg/hour, which is less than that usually obtained with hemoperfusion (295 ml/kg/hour). However, hemodialysis is usually available much more quickly and is associated with fewer complications than hemoperfusion. Hemodialysis may be equally effective in preventing morbidity or mortality, compared with hemoperfusion (51). Hemodialysis should certainly be considered when hemoperfusion is not readily available and may be preferable.

The indications for hemodialysis are controversial. The early use of hemodialysis should be considered if serum theophylline levels in the moderately toxic range are rising quickly despite activated charcoal therapy. Life-threatening effects, such as seizures, ventricular dysrhythmias, or hypotension unresponsive to other therapy, are also indications for hemodialysis. A serum concentration greater than 100 μg/ml after acute overdose is associated with major toxicity, and prophylactic hemodialysis is reasonable. Other situations in which hemodialysis should be considered are chronic intoxication in a patient younger than 60 years of age, with serum concentration greater than 60 μg/ml, or in a patient older than 60 years of age, with serum concentration greater than 40 μg/ml. Hemodialysis should continue until resolution of clinical toxicity or serum level is less than 20 to 30 μg/ml.

Theophylline elimination achieved with hemodialysis approached that of hemoperfusion in one case report. A 1220-g, 8-day-old infant born at 28 weeks' gestation presented with status epilepticus after receiving oral theophylline for 24 hours. The initial peak serum concentration was 82 mg/L. Hemodialysis was performed for 3 hours with a blood flow rate of 17.5 ml/hour. After 2 hours of dialysis, the concentration was 11.8 mg/L. The calculated extraction ratio was 0.67, and the theophylline clearance during dialysis was 4.86 ml/kg/minute. The half-life during dialysis was 0.8 hours. No rebound of the theophylline level was noted (52). The high extraction ratio may be due to the low protein binding and high dialysate to blood flow rates in neonates, compared with adults. Hemodynamic instability, small patient size, and a concern about anticoagulation may limit its usefulness in this age group. Peritoneal dialysis may be effective in severe intoxication when hemodialysis is unavailable (53). It decreased the theophylline half-life to 14.8 hours in a 6-week-old infant with a peak theophylline concentration of 133 μg/ml (54).

Hemoperfusion provides a higher clearance of theophylline than hemodialysis (1.88 to 5.84 ml/kg/minute; extraction ratio, 0.82:0.95) (55). There are no clinical trials that establish improved morbidity or mortality with hemoperfusion, compared with hemodialysis. Case reports have demonstrated clinical improvement during the procedure (55). Charcoal hemoperfusion probably is more effective than resin hemoperfusion (56). Hemoperfusion has not been shown to reduce morbidity or mortality in late severe toxicity, and its prophylactic role before severe manifestations is yet to be determined.

The indications for hemoperfusion are similar to hemodialysis and include intractable seizures; persistent hypotension–unresponsive treatment; uncontrollable dysrhythmias; chronic ingestion, with serum theophylline levels greater than 60 μg/ml; and single acute ingestion, with theophylline levels exceeding 100 μg/ml (55). The goal is resolution of symptoms and a serum theophylline concentration less than 20 to 30 μg/ml. Complications encountered with hemoperfusion include hypocalcemia, hypoglycemia, thrombocytopenia, hemolysis, and leukopenia in addition to those seen with hemodialysis (57).

Hemoperfusion is not the ideal method of enhancing elimination in neonates because it requires a large priming volume (50 ml). In addition, the heparin requirements and potential thrombocytopenia increase the risk of intracranial bleeding in these patients (52).

Combined hemodialysis and hemoperfusion were used in a patient with a theophylline level of 183 μg/ml. The combined mean extraction rate was 86% during the procedure. The mean extraction rate of hemodialysis was 62%, compared with 48% for charcoal hemoperfusion (58).

Continuous arteriovenous hemodialysis produced a mean extraction rate of 25% in a patient with a blood level of 183 μg/ml. The same patient also received hemodialysis with an extraction rate of 62% (58). Continuous venovenous hemofiltration has the advantage of being tolerated by hemodynamically unstable patients for long periods of time. Continuous venovenous hemofiltration was begun 32 hours after ingestion of 22.4 g of slow-release theophylline tablets by a 53-year-old woman. The indications were a rising theophylline level and a tonic-clonic seizure. The patient's peak serum concentration was 96.4 mg/L, which declined to 6 mg/L after 24 hours of hemofiltration. The average ultrafiltration rate was 25 ml/minute, using a Gambro HFM-10 (Gambro, Stockholm, Sweden) hemofilter with a polyamide filter (1.4 m^2). She also received 50 g activated charcoal every 4 hours, 12 hours after the onset of hemofiltration. The estimated theophylline half-life was 5.9 hours during hemofiltration (59).

Exchange transfusion has limited information available. Anecdotal reports in critically ill neonates suggest that exchange transfusion may be effective (60,61). It is usually considered as a last resort in newborns who cannot tolerate hemodialysis, hemoperfusion, or repetitive oral charcoal such as premature or paralyzed infants. A single volume exchange transfusion of a 32-week gestational-age girl decreased the plasma theophylline concentration 19% and removed 13% of whole-body theophylline (62).

ANTIDOTES

There is no specific antidote for theophylline toxicity.

SUPPORTIVE CARE

All patients with potential toxicity should have supplemental oxygen, intravenous access, and continuous cardiac monitoring. Seizure precautions should be undertaken, especially for elderly patients and patients with a history of a prior seizure disorder, chronic overmedication, and acute ingestions with serum levels greater than 100 μg/ml.

Vomiting may be persistent and interfere with the administration of activated charcoal. A slow infusion of ondansetron, 8 mg in 100 ml of normal saline over 20 minutes, is reported to be effective (63). Metoclopramide (10 mg or 0.1 mg/kg IV) has also been successful. Henderson identified 38 patients with acute theophylline poisoning, 35 who had taken a sustained-release preparation. The vomiting in 17 patients was controlled by intravenous metoclopramide (10 mg), but the remaining patients required mechanical ventilation with sedation and muscle relaxation for effective delivery of nasogastric charcoal (64).

Only mild repletion of extracellular potassium is usually necessary (5 to 10 mEq KCl/hour) because the main cause is intracellular shifting of potassium. Care must be taken to avoid hyperkalemia from overzealous replacement of potassium within the first 24 hours of admission.

Hypotension should be treated with an intravenous bolus of isotonic crystalloid (10 to 20 ml/kg normal saline) and correction of acidosis and electrolyte abnormalities. Vasopressors with strong α-adrenergic properties, such as levarterenol and phenylephrine, may be needed.

Supraventricular tachycardia in young patients without hemodynamic instability or cardiac ischemia usually does well with supportive care only. Elderly patients and patients with cardiac ischemia or hypotension can have the heart rate controlled with beta-blockers or calcium-channel blockers (6). Propranolol may block the vasodilator properties of theophylline and, particularly, may improve diastolic hypotension (65). It should be administered in 1-mg doses up to a maximum of 10 mg. Although some authors have not encountered bronchospasm with the use of propranolol in the acute toxicity setting (65), the administration of propranolol to poisoned asthmatics requires careful evaluation of risks and benefits. Further beta-blocker therapy may also result in myocardial depression.

Esmolol, with its relative β_1-receptor cardioselectivity and short duration of activity, may be useful to reduce tachycardia and hypotension. A preliminary anecdotal report suggests that esmolol provided prompt resolution of theophylline-induced tachycardia and hypotension (66). The initial dose of esmolol was a 500-μg/kg intravenous bolus over 1 minute, followed by a 50-μg/kg/minute continuous infusion.

Ventricular tachycardia should be treated with lidocaine in the hemodynamically stable patient and with cardioversion if unstable.

Seizures are a hallmark of serious toxicity, and status epilepticus is a frequent cause of mortality. After stabilization of the airway, initial anticonvulsant treatment should be used with benzodiazepines followed by more aggressive interventions if needed (Chapter 40). Phenytoin does not appear to be effective in theophylline-induced seizures (67,68). General anesthesia with midazolam, propofol, or pentobarbital should be considered when continuous seizures last more than 30 minutes, despite anticonvulsant treatment in adults or children (69). Consider the early use of hemodialysis or hemoperfusion, especially if serum theophylline levels are rising into the serious toxicity range.

MONITORING

All theophylline overdoses should be observed until the peak serum concentrations have been determined. Serial theophylline levels 2 to 3 hours apart should be drawn in all significant ingestions to confirm a decreasing theophylline level. All patients with rising serum concentration greater than 20 μg/ml should be admitted for continuous monitoring. Serum electrolytes, magnesium, phosphate, calcium, creatinine, creatine kinase and acid-base balance should be monitored every 4 to 6 hours until the patient is stable.

Inpatient admission is recommended for patients with intractable vomiting, seizures, dysrhythmias, or hypotension. Patients with acute ingestion with rising serum concentrations greater than 20 μg/ml and chronic overmedication with a theophylline concentration greater than 30 μg/ml who are symptomatic, younger than 2 years of age, older than 60 years of age, or with chronic illness should be admitted for continuous monitoring.

MANAGEMENT PITFALLS

The control of nausea and vomiting with an antiemetic and the early administration of activated charcoal is crucial in order to prevent further absorption and enhance elimination of theophylline.

BAMIFYLLINE HYDROCHLORIDE

Bamifylline hydrochloride (benzetomophylline, Bami-med, Trentadil) is a methylxanthine theophylline derivative used as a bronchodilator. It is absorbed orally but does not generate theophylline in the body. Bamifylline is available as a suppository and by intramuscular or slow intravenous injection (70).

Toxic Dose

The *adult therapeutic dosage* is 600 to 900 mg twice daily. Ingestion of approximately 20 tablets was fatal in an adult (71).

Toxicokinetics and Toxicodynamics

The peak plasma level is 400 to 1700 ng/ml. The T_{max} is 1 hour. The V_d is approximately 18 L/kg. The terminal half-life is approximately 20 hours (72).

Pathophysiology

The mechanism of action and pathophysiology are similar to theophylline.

Clinical Presentation

Overdose experience is very limited. Toxicity is expected to be similar to theophylline. Bamifylline hydrochloride may induce fatal, catecholamine-induced dysrhythmias.

Diagnostic Tests

A gas chromatography–mass spectrometry method is available for confirmation of bamifylline hydrochloride in body fluids. It has a detection limit of 20 μg/ml (72).

A patient who ingested approximately 20 tablets of Bamifix had a blood bamifylline level of 205 μg/ml. The minimum active and maximum tolerated plasma levels in animals are 0.18 to 20.00 μg/ml. Clinical efficacy is observed at levels of approximately 0.18 μg/ml. The toxicity threshold is 20 μg/ml (73).

Postmortem Considerations

The postmortem serum bamifylline hydrochloride level was 205 μg/ml in one case of overdose (71).

Treatment

Treatment of bamifylline hydrochloride overdose is similar to theophylline poisoning. However, it is unlikely that hemodialysis or hemoperfusion would be effective in removing significant quantities of bamifylline hydrochloride because of its high V_d. There is no antidote.

Other Bronchodilator Drugs

DYPHYLLINE [7-(2,3-DIHYDROXYPROPYL) THEOPHYLLINE]

Dyphylline (Lufyllin, many others; molecular weight, 254.2 g/mol) is incompletely absorbed by the GI tract with an elimination half-life of 2 hours. It is approximately one-fifth as potent as theophylline as a bronchodilator. Overdose is managed in the same manner as theophylline.

ENPROFYLLINE (3-PROPYLXANTHINE)

Enprofylline (molecular weight, 194.2 g/mol) is used for the treatment of asthma in Europe and is more potent than theophylline. It has less CNS, renal, or cerebrovascular effects, but tachycardia is more prominent. It is well absorbed orally, and 90% is excreted unchanged in the urine. The elimination half-life is less than 2 hours. Overdose is managed in the same manner as theophylline.

OXTRIPHYLLINE

Oxtriphylline, 200 mg, is equivalent to 127.2 mg of anhydrous theophylline (65%).

OXYBUTYNIN CHLORIDE

Oxybutynin chloride (Ditropan) is a smooth muscle antispasmodic agent used in the treatment of urinary frequency, incontinence, and nocturnal enuresis; in uninhibited vesical hyperactivity after bladder surgery and prostatectomy; and in acute and chronic cystitis. Overdose may result in anticholinergic effects, involving primarily the CNS, eyes, skin, and heart. Treatment is supportive. There have been no fatalities. Oxybutynin chloride is available in 5-mg regular-release tablets, as syrup (5 mg/5 ml), and as 5-, 10-, and 15-mg extended-release tablets.

Toxic Dose

The *adult therapeutic dosage* is 5 mg orally two or four times daily for regular release or 5 to 15 mg once a day as extended-release formulation. The *pediatric dosage* for children older than 5 years of age is 2.5 to 5.0 mg two to three times daily. A 100-mg oral dose was ingested by a 34-year-old woman. She recovered after developing drowsiness, mydriasis, hallucinations, and urinary retention (74). Fatalities after overdose have not been reported.

Toxicokinetics and Toxicodynamics

The regular formulation of oxybutynin chloride is rapidly absorbed. The onset of action is 30 to 60 minutes, and peak effect occurs in 3 to 6 hours. The peak plasma level is approximately 8 ng/ml, and T_{max} is less than 1 hour after oral ingestion of 5 mg (75). It undergoes extensive first-pass hepatic metabolism, and the systemic availability is only approximately 6%. The V_d is 0.5 to 1.2 L/kg. Oxybutynin chloride is metabolized in the liver by CYP3A4 to *N*-desethyloxybutynin and oxybutynin-*N*-oxide. The elimination half-life is 2 to 3 hours. With high doses, the elimination half-life is probably increased, due to a dose-related increase in the V_d (75). Very little oxybutynin chloride is excreted unchanged in the urine (0.017% of a dose in 12 hours).

The extended-release formulation achieves T_{max} at 12 hours after a therapeutic dose, and levels are maintained for approximately 24 hours. The half-life is approximately 13 hours.

Pathophysiology

Oxybutynin chloride is a direct smooth muscle relaxant with antimuscarinic properties. Its primary effect is on urinary bladder, biliary tract, GI, ureter, and uterine smooth muscle. Its anticholinergic action is 20% of that seen with atropine (76). In addition, it possesses a local anesthetic and analgesic effect (74). Oxybutynin chloride has no antinicotinic effects at skeletal neuromuscular junctions or autonomic ganglia. In overdose, anticholinergic clinical effects predominate (74).

Pregnancy and Lactation

Oxybutynin chloride is FDA pregnancy category B (Appendix I). Excretion into breast milk is expected due to its low molecular weight (15).

Clinical Presentation

ACUTE OVERDOSAGE

Oxybutynin chloride overdose may produce CNS effects such as restlessness, tremor, irritability, disorientation, seizures, delirium, hallucinations, or psychotic behavior. Additional anticholinergic symptoms, such as fever, dilated pupils, dry skin and mouth, urinary retention, and coma, have been reported. Cardiovascular symptoms include flushing, tachycardia, hypertension, hypotension, and circulatory failure. Nausea and vomiting may also occur. Severe overdose may lead to paralysis, respiratory failure, coma, and death (75,77).

ADVERSE EVENTS

Therapeutic use of oxybutynin chloride produces adverse effects similar to those produced by other antimuscarinic agents. Oxybutynin may aggravate signs and symptoms of hyperthyroidism, coronary heart disease, congestive heart failure, cardiac dysrhythmias, hiatal hernia, hypertension, tachycardia, and prostatic hypertrophy. In patients with ulcerative colitis, it may enhance induction of paralytic ileus or toxic megacolon. Oxybutynin may decrease sweating and induce fever and heat stroke (78).

DRUG INTERACTIONS

Alcohol or other sedatives may increase the drowsiness observed with oxybutynin. Antihistamines, tricyclic antidepressants, phenothiazines, and atropine may enhance the anticholinergic effects of oxybutynin.

Diagnostic Tests

After a 10-mg dose, peak plasma level is 16 ng/ml (38 nmol/L). Blood levels after an overdose have not been reported. Plasma levels may be useful to confirm presence of the drug but not to guide treatment. The ECG showed sinus tachycardia for 3 hours after an overdose of 100 mg. Ventricular premature beats lasted 30 hours. Full recovery occurred in 3 days (74).

Treatment

DECONTAMINATION

Induction of emesis has not been shown to be of benefit after acute ingestion. The potential for lethargy and seizure activity after overdose increases the risk of aspiration of gastric contents. Activated charcoal probably binds oxybutynin, and a dose should be administered as soon as possible after ingestion. The usual empiric dose is 50 g orally in adults and 1 g/kg in children. Delayed gastric emptying may result from the anticholinergic effect; therefore, administration of activated charcoal may be beneficial several hours after ingestion. There are no data on the efficacy of whole bowel irrigation. However, it should be considered with a large ingestion of extended-release tablets.

ENHANCEMENT OF ELIMINATION

There are no data on the effectiveness of enhancing elimination of oxybutynin with MDAC, hemodialysis, or hemoperfusion.

ANTIDOTES

Physostigmine may be considered for patients with anticholinergic syndrome in which combative behavior, severe hallucinations, or agitation are present. The initial dose is 0.5 to 1.0 mg IV over 2 minutes and may be repeated in 20 minutes (Chapter 67).

SUPPORTIVE CARE

All patients with potential toxicity should have intravenous access and continuous cardiac monitoring. Seizure precautions should be undertaken. Hypotension should be initially treated with an intravenous bolus of isotonic crystalloid. Fever is treated with cooling measures such as cooling blankets, water mist, and fans (Chapter 38). Airway patency should be ensured at all times. Assisted ventilation may be required if paralysis of respiratory muscles occurs (77). Restlessness and delirium can be treated with a benzodiazepine or possibly physostigmine (Chapter 10). Phenothiazines can lead to additive anticholinergic effects and should be avoided (74,77).

MONITORING

Ingestion of the extended-release product may result in delayed absorption and observation for at least 6 hours after exposure is recommended. Symptomatic patients should be monitored for at least 24 hours. Observe for signs of anticholinergic effects such as fever, mydriasis, tachycardia, ileus, altered mental status, seizures, and hallucinations. Severely poisoned patients require an intensive care unit admission for treatment of hyperthermia, seizures, tachydysrhythmias, and rhabdomyolysis. Serum electrolytes, creatine kinase, acid-base status, and ECG should be monitored.

REFERENCES

1. Litovitz TB, Holm KC, Bailey KM, et al. 1991 Annual report of the American Association of Poison Control Centers National Data Collection System. *Am J Emerg Med* 1992;10:452–505.
2. Litovitz TB, Klein-Schwartz W, Rodgers GC, et al. 2001 Annual report of the American Association of Poison Control Centers Toxic Exposure Surveillance System. *Am J Emerg Med* 2002;20:391–452.
3. Helliwell M, Berry D. Theophylline poisoning in adults. *BMJ* 1979;2:1114.
4. Skopnik H, Bertl U, Heimann G. Neonatal theophylline intoxication: pharmacokinetics and clinical evaluation. *Eur J Pediatr* 1992;151:221–224.

5. Coupe M. Self-poisoning with sustained-release aminophylline: a mechanism for observed secondary rise in serum theophylline. *Hum Toxicol* 1986;5:341–342.
6. Greenberg A, Piraina BH, Kroboth PD, et al. Severe theophylline toxicity: role of conservative measures, antiarrhythmic agents, and charcoal hemoperfusion. *Am J Med* 1984;76:854–860.
7. Shannon M. Hypokalemia, hyperglycemia and plasma catecholamine activity after severe theophylline intoxication. *J Toxicol Clin Toxicol* 1994;32:41–47.
8. Sawyer WT, Caravati EM, Ellison MJ, et al. Hypokalemia, hyperglycemia and acidosis after intentional theophylline overdose. *Am J Emerg Med* 1985;3:408–411.
9. McPherson ML, Prince SR, Atamer ER, et al. Theophylline-induced hypercalcemia. *Ann Intern Med* 1986;105:52–54.
10. Shannon M, Lovejoy FH. Hypokalemia after theophylline intoxication: the effects of acute vs chronic poisoning. *Arch Intern Med* 1989;149:2725–2729.
11. Frederiksen MC, Ruo TI, Chow MJ, et al. Theophylline pharmacokinetics in pregnancy. *Clin Pharmacol Ther* 1986;40:321–328.
12. Neff RK, Leviton A. Maternal theophylline consumption and the risk of stillbirth. *Chest* 1990;97:1266–1267.
13. Park JM, Schmer V, Myers TL. Cardiovascular anomalies associated with prenatal exposure to theophylline. *South Med J* 1990;83:1487–1488.
14. Stec GP, Greenberger P, Ruo TI, et al. Kinetics of theophylline transfer to breast milk. *Clin Pharmacol Ther* 1980;28:404–408.
15. Briggs GR, Freeman RK, Yaffe, SJ. *Drugs in pregnancy and lactation*, 6th edition. Baltimore: Williams &Wilkins, 2002:1053, 1343–1346.
16. Shannon M. Predictors of major toxicity after theophylline overdose. *Ann Intern Med* 1993;119:1161–1167.
17. Shannon M, Lovejoy FH. The influence of age vs peak serum concentration on life-threatening events after chronic theophylline intoxication. *Arch Intern Med* 1990;150:2045–2048.
18. Shannon M. Life-threatening events after theophylline overdose: a 10-year prospective analysis. *Arch Intern Med* 1999;159:989–994.
19. Shannon M, Lovejoy FH Jr. Effect of acute versus chronic intoxication on clinical features of theophylline poisoning in children. *J Pediatr* 1992;121:125–130.
20. Bahls FH, Mak K, Bird TD. Theophylline-associated seizures with "therapeutic" or low toxic serum concentrations: risk factors for serious outcome in adults. *Neurology* 1991;41:1309–1312.
21. Baker MD. Theophylline toxicity in children. *J Pediatr* 1986;109:538–542.
22. Shannon M. Therapeutic theophylline levels and adverse cardiac events. *Ann Intern Med* 1994;120:891.
23. Levine JH, Michael JR, Guarnieri T. Multifocal atrial tachycardia: a toxic effect of theophylline. *Lancet* 1985;1:12–14.
24. Sessler CN, Cohen MD. Cardiac arrhythmias during theophylline toxicity: a prospective continuous electrocardiographic study. *Chest* 1990;98:672–678.
25. Hantson P, Gautier P, Vekemans MC, et al. Acute myocardial infarction in a young woman: possible relationship with sustained-release theophylline acute overdose. *Intensive Care Med* 1992;18:496.
26. Ryan MF, Vale JA. Acute compartment syndrome secondary to theophylline poisoning. *Lancet* 1990;2:882.
27. Olson KR, Benowitz NL, Woo OF, Pond SM. Theophylline overdose: acute single ingestion versus chronic repeated overmedication. *Am J Emerg Med* 1985;3:386–394.
28. Powell EC, Reynolds SL, Rubenstein JS. Theophylline toxicity in children: a retrospective review. *Pediatr Emerg Care* 1993;9:129–133.
29. Melamed J, Beaucher WN. Minor symptoms are not predictive of elevated theophylline levels in adults on chronic therapy. *Ann Allergy Asthma Immunol* 1995;75:516–520.
30. Terzian CG, Simon PA. Aminophylline hypersensitivity apparently due to ethylenediamine. *Ann Emerg Med* 1992;21:312–317.
31. Poklis A, Saady JJ, Edinboro LE. Evaluation of the Abbott Vision Analyzer for determination of theophylline and implementation of a program for on-site emergency room testing. *Clin Chem* 1990;36:1040.
32. Jones LA, Gonzalez ER, Venitz J, et al. Evaluation of the Vision theophylline assays in the emergency department setting. *Ann Emerg Med* 1992;21:777–781.
33. Baselt RC. *Disposition of toxic drugs and chemicals in man*, 6th edition. Foster City, CA: Biomedical Publications, 2002:1013–1017.
34. Gal P, Roop C, Robinson H, Erkan NV. Theophylline-induced seizures in accidentally overdosed neonates. *Pediatrics* 1980;65:547–549.
35. Zwililich CW, Sutton FD Jr, Neff TA, et al. Theophylline induced seizures in adults: correlation with serum concentration. *Ann Intern Med* 1975;82:784–787.
36. Gaudreault P, Guay J. Theophylline poisoning: pharmacological considerations and clinical management. *Med Toxicol* 1986;1:169–191.
37. Parr MJ, Anaes FC, Day AC, et al. Theophylline poisoning: a review of 64 cases. *Intensive Care Med* 1990;16:394–398.
38. Bernstein G, Jehle D, Bernaski E, et al. Failure of gastric emptying and charcoal administration in fatal sustained-release theophylline overdose: pharmacobezoar formation. *Ann Emerg Med* 1992;21:1388–1390.
39. Amitai Y, Lovejoy FH Jr. Characteristics of vomiting associated with acute release theophylline poisoning: Implications for management with oral activated charcoal. *J Toxicol Clin Toxicol* 1987;27:539–554.
40. Jain R, Tholl DA. Activated charcoal for theophylline toxicity in a premature infant on the second day of life. *Dev Pharmacol Ther* 1992;19:106–110.
41. Henderson A, Salin P, Pond SM. Rapid rise in serum theophylline concentration after overdose with sustained release theophylline. *Med J Aust* 1992;157:354–355.
42. Laggner AN, Kaik G, Lenz K, et al. Treatment of severe poisoning with slow release theophylline. *BMJ* 1985;288:1497.
43. Tenenbein M, Cohen S, Sitar DS. Whole bowel irrigation as a decontamination procedure after acute drug overdose. *Arch Intern Med* 1987;147:905–907.
44. Burkhart KK, Wuerz RC, Donovan JW. Whole bowel irrigation as adjunctive treatment for sustained-release theophylline overdose. *Ann Emerg Med* 1992;21:1316–1320.
45. Hoffman RS, Chiang WH, Howland MA, et al. Theophylline desorption from activated charcoal caused by whole bowel irrigation solution. *J Toxicol Clin Toxicol* 1991;29:191–201.
46. Lim DT, Singh P, Nourtsis S, et al. Absorption inhibition and enhancement of elimination of sustained-release theophylline tablets by oral activated charcoal. *Ann Emerg Med* 1986;15:1303–1307.
47. Berlinger WG, Spector R, Goldberg MJ, et al. Enhancement of theophylline clearance by oral activated charcoal. *Clin Pharm Ther* 1983;33:351–354.
48. Shannon M, Amitai Y, Lovejoy FH Jr. Multiple dose activated charcoal for theophylline poisoning in young infants. *Pediatrics* 1987;80:368–370.
49. Ohning BL, Reed MD, Blumer JL. Continuous nasogastric administration of activated charcoal for the treatment of theophylline intoxication. *Pediatr Pharmacol (New York)* 1986;5:241–245.
50. Gazda-Smith E, Synhavsky A. Hypernatremia following treatment of theophylline toxicity with activated charcoal and sorbitol. *Arch Intern Med* 1990;150:689–690.
51. Shannon MW. Comparative efficacy of hemodialysis and hemoperfusion in severe theophylline intoxication. *Acad Emerg Med* 1997;4:674–678.
52. Gitomer JJ, Khan AM, Ferris ME. Treatment of severe theophylline toxicity with hemodialysis in a preterm neonate. *Pediatr Nephrol* 2001;16:784–786.
53. Miceli JN, Clay B, Fleischmann LE, et al. Pharmacokinetics of severe theophylline intoxication managed by peritoneal dialysis. *Dev Pharmacol Ther* 1980;1:16–25.
54. Colonna F, Trappan A, de Vonderweid U, Nisi G. Peritoneal dialysis in a 6-weeks old preterm infant with severe theophylline intoxication. *Minerva Pediatr* 1996;48:383–385.
55. Woo OF, Pond SM, Benowitz NL, et al. Benefit of hemoperfusion in acute theophylline intoxication. *J Toxicol Clin Toxicol* 1984;22:411–424.
56. Jefferys DB, Raper SM, Helliwell M, et al. Haemoperfusion for theophylline overdose. *BMJ* 1980;280:1167.
57. Gallagher EJ, Howland M, Greenblatt H. Hemolysis following treatment of theophylline overdose with coated charcoal hemoperfusion. *J Emerg Med* 1987;5:19–22.
58. Higgins RM, Hearing S, Goldsmith DJ, et al. Severe theophylline poisoning: charcoal haemoperfusion or haemodialysis. *Postgrad Med J* 1995;71:224–226.
59. Henderson JH, McKenzie CA, Hilton PJ, et al. Continuous venovenous haemofiltration for the treatment of theophylline toxicity. *Thorax* 2001;56:242–243.
60. Shannon M, Wernovsky G, Morris C. Exchange transfusion in the treatment of severe theophylline poisoning. *Pediatrics* 1992;89:145–147.
61. Henry GC, Wax PM, Howland MA, et al. Exchange transfusion for the treatment of a theophylline overdose in a premature neonate. *Vet Hum Toxicol* 1991;33:356.
62. Osborn HN, Henry G, Wax P, et al. Theophylline toxicity in a premature neonate: elimination kinetics of exchange transfusion. *J Toxicol Clin Toxicol* 1993;31:639–644.
63. Roberts JR, Carney S, Boyle SM, Lee DC. Ondansetron quells drug-resistant emesis in theophylline poisoning. *Am J Emerg Med* 1993;11:609–610.
64. Henderson A, Wright DM, Pond SM. Management of theophylline overdose patients in the intensive care unit. *Anaesth Intensive Care* 1992;20:56–62.
65. Biberstein MP, Ziegler MG, Ward DM. Use of beta-blockade and hemoperfusion for acute theophylline poisoning. *West J Med* 1984;141:485–490.
66. Seneff M, Scott J, Friedman B, Smith M. Acute theophylline toxicity and the use of esmolol to reverse cardiovascular irritability. *Ann Emerg Med* 1990;19:671–673.
67. Goldberg MJ, Spector R, Miller G. Phenobarbital improves survival in theophylline-intoxicated rabbits. *J Toxicol Clin Toxicol* 1986;24:203–211.
68. Hoffman A, Pinto E, Gilhar D. Effect of pretreatment with anticonvulsants on theophylline-induced seizures in the rat. *J Crit Care* 1993;8:198–202.
69. Lowenstein DH, Allredge BK. Status epilepticus. *N Engl J Med* 1998;338:970–976.
70. Berti F, Magni F, Rossoni G, et al. New pharmacological data on the bronchospasmolytic activity of bamifylline. *Arzneimittelforschung* 1988;38:40–44.
71. Offidani C, Ottaviano V, Chiarotti M. Fatal case of bamifylline intoxication. *Am J Forensic Med Pathol* 1993;14:244–245.
72. Segre G, Cerretani D, Moltoni L, et al. Pharmacokinetics of bamifylline during chronic therapy. *Arzneimittelforschung* 1990;40:450–452.
73. Schiantarelli P, Acerbi D, Botta GC, et al. Evidence of pulmonary tropism of bamifylline and its main active metabolite. *Arzneimittelforschung* 1989;39:215–219.
74. Banerjee S, Routledge PA, Pugh S, Smith PM. Poisoning with oxybutynin. *Hum Exp Toxicol* 1991;10:222–226.
75. Douchamps J, Derenne F, Stockis A, et al. The pharmacokinetics of oxybutynin in man. *Eur J Clin Pharmacol* 1988;35:515–520.
76. Aaltonen L, Allonen H, Iisalo E, et al. Antimuscarinic activity of oxybutynin in the human plasma quantitated by a radioreceptor assay. *Acta Pharmacol Toxicol* 1984;55:100–103.
77. Thuroff JW, Bunke B, Ebner A, et al. Randomized double-blind multi-center trial on treatment of frequency, urgency and incontinence related to detrusion hyperactivity: oxybutynin versus propantheline versus placebo. *J Urol* 1991;125:813–817.
78. Malone-Lee J, Lubel D, Szonyi G. Low dose oxybutynin for the unstable bladder. *BMJ* 1992;304:1053.

SECTION

17

Vitamins

CHAPTER 167

Vitamin Toxicity

Brigham R. Temple

See Figure 1.	
Compounds included:	**Fat-soluble vitamins: vitamin A, vitamin D, vitamin E, vitamin K; water-soluble vitamins: ascorbic acid (vitamin C), biotin, cobalamin (B_{12}), folate (folic acid), niacin (B_3), pantothenic acid (B_5), pyridoxine (B_6), riboflavin (B_2), thiamine (B_1)**
Molecular formula and weight:	**See Table 1.**
SI conversion:	**See Table 1.**
CAS Registry No.:	**See Table 1.**
Special concerns:	**Vitamin toxicity often develops at doses that patients or their health care provider consider innocuous.**
Antidote:	**None**

OVERVIEW

Vitamins have long been considered by the public and by prescribing physicians as relatively harmless, even in high doses or "megadoses." More than 100 million Americans regularly use vitamin supplements. In the United States, consumer spending on vitamin supplements has doubled in the last 7 years, reaching $6.5 billion annually. Iron-containing vitamins are the most toxic, especially in pediatric acute ingestions (Chapter 106). Overall, 49,709 exposures to various types of vitamins were reported to American poison centers in 1998, accounting for 14 major adverse outcomes and no deaths. Of the total exposures, 39,396 occurred in children younger than 6 years of age (1).

Indications for vitamin use above the recommended dietary allowance (RDA) (2) (Table 1) for treatment of a variety of ailments, from the common cold to psychiatric illnesses to cancer treatment, continue to increase (Table 2). Furthermore, the use of megadose vitamins is touted to enhance athletic performance, facilitate weight loss, and improve cognitive performance. Nonetheless, many vitamins, when taken in excess either chronically or acutely, can cause significant toxicity.

Large doses of some water-soluble vitamins (vitamin B_6, vitamin C, and niacin) are readily excreted in the urine yet have been associated with potentially toxic side effects when taken in large doses for a prolonged period of time. However, many of the water-soluble vitamins (folate, biotin, riboflavin) have no documented severe toxic effects when taken in megadoses. Fat-soluble vitamins (A, D, E, and K) are stored in the tissues and therefore are most likely to cause adverse effects when taken in excess (Fig. 1).

VITAMIN A

Vitamin A or retinol is a fat-soluble vitamin that can be either ingested or synthesized within the body from plant carotenes. Vitamin A is essential for the normal functioning of the retina and for growth and differentiation of epithelial tissue as well as being necessary in embryonic development, reproduction, and bone growth. However, vitamin A has been shown to produce teratogenic effects in animal studies when administered in high doses. The possible teratogenic risk associated with vitamin A has come under some debate concerning the amount that will begin to produce an increased frequency of congenital malformations in human offspring exposed during gestation.

Toxic Dose

The RDA for adults and children is provided in Table 1. Acute toxicity has been reported in adults after doses of 1.5 to 2.0 million IU or after excessive consumption of animal liver and in children after doses of 75,000 to 350,000 IU.

Toxicokinetics and Toxicodynamics

The term *vitamin A* encompasses two forms: a retinoid, which is a preformed vitamin A originating from animal tissue, and β-carotene, a provitamin A compound that originates from plant food, such as carrots, meats, and dark-green leafy vegetables. β-Carotene is converted in the body to the retinol form of vitamin A. This conversion decreases substantially when large amounts of β-carotene are ingested. The most common sources of pre-

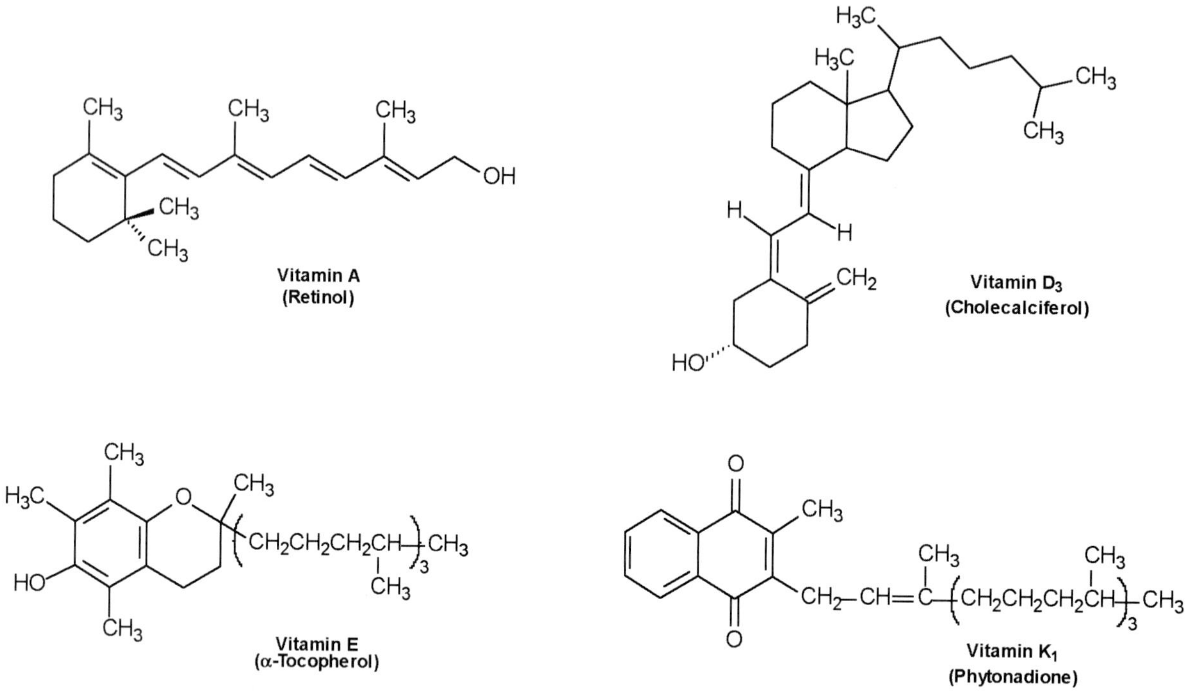

Figure 1. Structures of the fat-soluble vitamins.

formed vitamin A can be found in liver, kidney, and milk products as fatty acid esters. During digestion, the esters are hydrolyzed, absorbed in the free form, re-esterified in the intestinal mucosa, and transported to the liver in the lymphatics.

Synthesis of vitamin A occurs in the liver from carotene substrates. β-Carotene can either be absorbed intact or cleaved into retinaldehyde, which is reduced by aldehyde reductase to retinol. Retinol from whatever source is stored as retinyl esters in the liver with a total body pool of 300 to 900 mg.

Pathophysiology

Toxicity is caused by unbound vitamin A. It may occur at low serum vitamin A concentrations in patients with a lower retinol-binding protein for such disorders as liver disease, hyperlipoproteinemias, and malnutrition. The portion of vitamin A retinyl ester found in the plasma in normal individuals is 0.1% to 4.7%, whereas in hypervitaminosis A, it rises up to 67%. The pathophysiologic effects are related to effects in the central nervous system (CNS), bone, dermal tissues, and liver. The most serious manifestations result from increased intracranial pressure (3–6).

Pregnancy and Lactation

In 1987, the Centers for Disease Control and Prevention (CDC), Teratology Society, and Council for Responsible Nutrition published recommendations for use of vitamin A during pregnancy. These were made because teratogenicity appears to occur at

TABLE 1. Physical characteristics and dosage of vitamins

Drug	Molecular formula, molecular weight (g/mol), CAS Registry No.	SI conversion	Dietary reference intake	
			Adult (male/female)	Pediatric
Fat-soluble vitamins				
Vitamin A (and β-carotene)	$C_{20}H_3O$, 430.7, 11103-57-4	ng/ml × 2.32 = nmol/L	900/700 μg/d	300–600 μg/d
Vitamin D (cholecalciferol)	$C_{27}H_{44}O$, 396.66, 1406-16-2	ng/ml × 2.52 = nmol/L	5/5 μg/d	5 μg/d
Vitamin E	$C_{29}H_{50}O_2$, 430.72, 59-02-9	ng/ml × 2.32 = μmol/L	15/15 mg/d	6–11 mg/d
Vitamin K	Not specified,12001-79-5	—	120/90 μg/d	30–60 μg/d
Water-soluble vitamins				
Ascorbic acid (vitamin C)	$C_6H_8O_6$, 176.13, 50-81-7	—	90/75 mg/d	15–45 mg/d
Biotin	$C_{10}H_{16}N_2O_3S$, 244.3, 58-85-5	—	30/30 μg/d	8–12 μg/d
Cobalamin (B_{12})	$C_{62}H_{88}CoN_{13}O_{14}P$, 1329.4, 13408-78-1	—	2.4/2.4 μg/d	0.9–1.8 μg/d
Folate (folic acid)	$C_{19}H_{19}N_7O_6$, 441.4, 59-30-3	—	400/400 μg/d	150–200 μg/d
Niacin	$C_6H_5NO_2$, 123.1, 59-67-6	—	16/14 mg/d	6–12 mg/d
Pantothenic acid (B_5)	$C_9H_{17}NO_5$, 219.2, 79-83-4	—	5/7 mg/d	2–4 mg/d
Pyridoxine (B_6)	$C_8H_{11}NO_3$, 169.2, 65-23-6	—	1.3/1.3 mg/d	0.5–1.0 mg/d
Riboflavin (B_2)	$C_{17}H_{20}N_4O_6$, 376.4, 83-88-5	—	1.3/1.1 mg/d	0.9–0.9 mg/d
Thiamine (B_1)	$C_{12}H_{17}N_4OSCl$, 300.8, 59-43-8	—	1.2/1.1 mg/d	0.5–0.9 mg/d

Adapted from Institute of Medicine Web site. Available at: http://www.iom.edu. Accessed July 17, 2003.

TABLE 2. Legitimate uses of megavitamin therapy

Vitamin	Disorder treated
A	Darier's disease, ichthyosis, malabsorption
B_6	Infantile convulsive disorder, sideroblastic anemia, urinary oxalate stones, homocystinuria
B_{12}	Pernicious anemia, methylmalonic aciduria, homocystinuria, hypomethionemia
C	Acquired immunodeficiency syndrome, adjuvant chemotherapy, burn treatment, psychopharmacotherapy
D	Fanconi's syndrome, hepatic rickets, hypoparathyroidism, renal osteodystrophy, malabsorption
E	Fibrocystic breast disease, hemolytic anemias, retrolental fibroplasia, malabsorption
K	Coagulopathy induced by liver disease

some undetermined level above 8000 IU. Further, pregnant women do not seem to benefit from additional vitamin A. These groups recommended limiting intake of vitamin A from prenatal vitamins to 5000 to 8000 IU and vitamin A content of all multivitamins to 10,000 IU, therein suggesting that women should not ingest more than 10,000 IU before consulting a physician.

Case reports and anecdotal studies suggest that vitamin A intake of 25,000 IU or more during pregnancy increases the risk for congenital anomalies (7). Rothman et al. (8) undertook a study to clarify the issue of what dose of vitamin A may begin to pose an increased risk for congenital anomalies. Between October 1984 and June 1987, 22,748 pregnant women who reported taking vitamin A were identified. Of 339 babies, 121 had birth defects, characteristically arising from the cranial neural crest. The trend for the risk for musculoskeletal and urogenital tract defects was less apparent, and no discernible risk was observed for neural tube defects. The relative risk for women who consumed more than 15,000 IU preformed vitamin A to deliver infants with defects associated with cranial-neural-crest tissue was 3.5 times greater than women who consumed 5000 IU or less [95% confidence interval (CI), 1.7 to 7.3].

The prevalence ratio of these defects for women who consumed more than 10,000 IU/day compared to women who consumed less than 5000 IU/day from supplement alone was 4.8 (95% CI, 2.2 to 10.5). Malformations were observed more frequently among infants born to women who ingested large amounts of vitamin A before the seventh week of gestation. The authors concluded that approximately 1 in 57 infants were at risk for malformations attributable to vitamin A supplements at doses above 10,000 IU/day. The study by Rothman et al. (8) is controversial. Oakley and Erickson (9) noted that the mean vitamin A intake in the "more than 10,000" unit group was 21,675 IU per day; therefore, some fetuses were exposed to more than 25,000 IU/day. Specific exposure information is necessary before it is recommended that the dose-response threshold curve described in the paper by Rothman et al. be used (7,8).

Other studies have assessed the risk to a pregnancy with maternal intake of 8000 IU or less of preformed vitamin A during pregnancy. Khoury et al. (10) examined data from a large population-based case-control study of major birth defects conducted by the CDC. No increased risk was observed among vitamin A and multivitamin users or among women who took multivitamins and vitamin A supplements together (odds ratio, 0.54; 95% CI, 0.22 to 1.33). These authors also reviewed numerous case studies to assess whether specific phenotypes were associated with vitamin A use. No distinguishing patterns were observed between the two groups when looking at patterns and types of birth defects, presence of multiple congenital anomalies, and recognizable phenotypes. They did not have information on the amount of vitamin A ingested, but most multivitamins and supplements during that time period contained 8000 IU retinol. The authors state that "these data should provide reassurance that vitamin A supplements less than 8000 IU do not increase the risk for birth defects" (10).

Several studies have been reported revealing no increase in congenital anomalies after prenatal exposure to large amounts of vitamin A. These include 1203 infants exposed to 6000 IU daily during the first trimester of gestation (11) and a case-control study of 11,293 children with minor and major malformations and maternal use of 10,000 IU or more of vitamin A per day (12,13). Vitamin A in the form of isotretinoin (Accutane) has been shown to be teratogenic. β-Carotene is not mutagenic in animal studies (12).

Clinical Presentation

ACUTE OVERDOSAGE

The principal manifestations occur as a result of cerebral edema. In adults, headache, nausea, vomiting, and irritability have been reported. Ocular examination may reveal papilledema. CNS symptoms generally appear within 8 to 12 hours after single large overdoses. In children, the presenting symptoms and signs include vomiting, irritability, bulging fontanels, and elevated cerebrospinal fluid pressures.

CHRONIC TOXICITY

In adults, toxic effects may occur after ingestion of 25,000 IU/day for 8 months, with papilledema, diplopia, headaches, pseudotumor cerebri, weakness, fatigue, joint and bone pain, anoxia, headaches, muscle stiffness, weight loss, polyuria, polydipsia, urinary frequency, dry skin, desquamation, pruritus, hair loss, hepatomegaly, splenomegaly, and nasal and oral bleeding (14,15). Laboratory evidence of hepatic toxicity may be observed.

Diagnostic Tests

Peak serum levels of vitamin A retinyl esters are found 4 hours after ingestion of a therapeutic dose. Therapeutic vitamin A levels in the serum are 65 to 275 IU/dl, and liver storage levels are 300 μg/g. However, such levels are not a useful guide in clinical vitamin A overdosage.

The serum transaminase enzymes are typically increased moderately. Hypercalcemia occurs in 25% to 33% of all cases, especially in adolescents and adults. Radiographic studies of long bones reveal cortical hyperostosis and premature epiphyseal closure and hypomineralization or hypermineralization. Prothrombin times are prolonged due to hypoprothrombinemia. Intracranial pressure may be increased on lumbar puncture. Evaluation of increased intracranial pressure, including computerized tomography of the head, is needed in patients with CNS effects.

Treatment

Treatment is primarily supportive, with discontinuation of vitamin A or carotene supplements, including megavitamin use. Following acute ingestion, gastric decontamination (activated charcoal) can be initiated. Gastric emptying is probably not justified, except possibly for a recent and very large ingestion.

For patients with signs of increased intracranial pressure, mannitol and steroids may be useful (16). The dose of mannitol is 0.25 g/kg intravenously, repeated every 5 minutes as required up to 1 g/kg per dose. Plasma osmolality should be monitored. The initial dose of steroids (dexamethasone) is 0.15 mg/kg intravenously, followed by a maintenance regimen of 0.25 mg/kg/day, divided every 4 to 6 hours for 5 days. This dosage is then tapered over the next 5 days and discontinued. The blood pressure, fluids, electrolytes, and CNS status are monitored throughout treatment.

VITAMIN D

Vitamin D, calciferol, is a fat-soluble vitamin. It is found in food but also is made in the body after exposure to ultraviolet rays from the sun. Vitamin D exists in several forms, each with a different activity. Some forms are relatively inactive in the body and have limited ability to function as a vitamin. The liver and kidney help convert vitamin D to its active hormone form. Calcitriol, the most active form of vitamin D, is classified as a steroid hormone and is air and light sensitive.

The major biologic function of vitamin D is to maintain normal blood levels of calcium and phosphorus. Vitamin D aids in the absorption of calcium, helping to form and maintain strong bones. It promotes bone mineralization in concert with a number of other vitamins, minerals, and hormones. Without vitamin D, bones can become thin, brittle, soft, or misshapen. Vitamin D prevents rickets in children and osteomalacia in adults.

Vitamin D toxicity occurs commonly during the treatment of hypoparathyroidism and with the misguided use of megavitamins. Hypervitaminosis D can result from excessive intake of vitamin D supplementation, prolonged use of vitamin D–fortified infant formulas, or poorly monitored vitamin D therapy for disorders such as rickets and hypoparathyroidism (17–19). Vitamin D_3 is more stable than vitamin D_2.

Toxic Dose

The RDA for adults and children is provided in Table 1. Vitamin D, 1000 μg/day (40,000 IU/day), produces toxicity within 1 to 4 months in infants, and as little as 75 μg/day (3000 IU/day) can produce toxicity over years. Toxic effects have occurred in adults who receive 2500 μg/day (100,000 IU/day) for several months. Elevated serum calcium levels of 12 to 16 mg/dl (3 to 4 mmol/L) are a constant finding when toxic symptoms occur; normal levels are 8.5 to 10.5 mg/dl (2.12 to 2.62 mmol/L) (20,21). Hypercalcemia in infancy with failure to thrive has occurred with a daily vitamin D intake of 50 to 75 μg (2000 to 3000 IU).

Toxicokinetics and Toxicodynamics

Vitamin D is well absorbed from the gut and stored in fat deposits. Plasma 25(OH)-D_3 levels are elevated as much as 15-fold in vitamin D toxicity, whereas 1,25$(OH)_2$-D_3 levels are usually within the normal range.

Pathophysiology

The principal manifestations of hypervitaminosis D are secondary to the disruption of normal calcium and phosphorus homeostasis. Renal function is impaired, as evidenced by low urine specific gravity, proteinuria, casts, and azotemia. Metastatic calcifications may occur, particularly in the kidneys.

Hypercalcemia in infancy is usually due to an unidentified defect in vitamin D metabolism rather than to excessive intake. Williams' syndrome involves transient hypercalcemia in infancy with the triad of supravalvular aortic stenosis, mental retardation, and elfin facies. Plasma levels of 1,25$(OH)_2$-D_3 during the hypercalcemic phase are eight to ten times normal. 1,25$(OH)_2$-D_3 is 100 times more potent than vitamin D_3. When it is used to treat various disorders, possible toxic effects of long-term therapy must be monitored.

Pregnancy and Lactation

Vitamin D is U.S. Food and Drug Administration (FDA) pregnancy category C (Appendix I), and safety in nursing infants is unknown.

Clinical Presentation

A history of excessive vitamin D intake is critical for differentiating vitamin D toxicity from all other hypercalcemic states. Primary presenting symptoms are anorexia, nausea, and vomiting, followed by polyuria, polydipsia, weakness, nervousness, and pruritus (20,22).

Diagnostic Tests

In symptomatic patients, the serum electrolytes and calcium should be measured. In patients receiving large doses of vitamin D, the serum calcium should be measured frequently (weekly at first, then monthly) in all patients. Renal function should be monitored.

Treatment

Treatment consists of discontinuing the vitamin, providing a low-calcium diet, keeping the urine acidic, and giving corticosteroids (23,24). Kidney damage or metastatic calcification, if present, may be irreversible. Diuretics and forced fluids are not helpful.

VITAMIN E

Eight tocopherols with vitamin E activity occur naturally. α-Tocopherol is the most important, constituting approximately 90% of the total tocopherols in animal tissue. The standard unit of vitamin E activity is DL-α-tocopheryl acetate (1 mg = 1 IU) with RDA based on age and sex.

Toxic Dose

The RDA for adults and children is provided in Table 1. Long-term use of 400 to 800 IU/day can result in nausea, muscular weakness, fatigue, headache, and blurred vision. Doses of 2000 to 12,000 IU/day have caused gonadal dysfunction, creatinuria, and gastrointestinal upset. Conversely, relatively large doses of vitamin E have been taken by adults for extended periods without causing any apparent harm.

Toxicokinetics and Toxicodynamics

Vitamin E is 50% to 80% absorbed, transported by lipoproteins, and stored in adipose tissue, liver, and muscle.

Pathophysiology

Vitamin E is a major lipid antioxidant in cell membranes that prevents free radical attack on polyunsaturated fatty acids in membranes. Excessive use may deplete vitamin A stores and antagonize vitamin K function, leading to inhibition of prothrombin production.

Pregnancy and Lactation

Vitamin E is FDA pregnancy category A (Appendix I) and is considered safe in nursing infants.

Clinical Presentation

Long-term use of high doses may result in nausea, muscular weakness, fatigue, headache, and blurred vision. Chronic use of very large doses has caused gonadal dysfunction, creatinuria, and gastrointestinal upset. These symptoms disappear within a few weeks after discontinuation of excessive doses.

In April 1984, the CDC reported an illness in premature infants (less than 1500 g) in whom ascites developed plus some of the following: hepatosplenomegaly, cholestatic jaundice, azotemia, and thrombocytopenia. Of the 13 infants, 8 died, and all had received E-Ferol, which was subsequently recalled by the manufacturer. No intravenous form of tocopherol has been available since E-Ferol was discontinued (21,25). Drug interactions include vitamin E, which increases the effect of oral anticoagulants.

Diagnostic Tests

Normal vitamin E levels are 0.5 to 2.0 mg/dl. Adverse events generally occur above levels of 3 to 4 mg/dl. If recommended, a pharmacologic dose of 100 mg/kg/day for retrolental fibroplasias is used; plasma levels must be monitored on a weekly basis.

Abnormalities in prothrombin time and clotting time have been observed. Careful hematologic evaluations for hemolysis and platelets should be performed in neonates who receive vitamin E in high doses. A high-performance liquid chromatography method is available for determination of vitamin E levels in serum and plasma.

Treatment

Treatment should include discontinuation of large doses of vitamin E and evaluation of serum levels as clinically indicated.

VITAMIN K

Vitamin K is a fat-soluble vitamin that is used in the production of prothrombin. It is primarily given for treatment of hypoprothrombinemia and hemorrhage caused by overdosage of oral anticoagulants. Newborns are given vitamin K as prophylaxis and treatment of hemorrhagic disease. Vitamin K deficiency from poor nutrition, malabsorption, and defective hepatic synthesis is another indication for vitamin K supplementation. No U.S. RDA is given for vitamin K.

Vitamin K is readily available through dietary sources. Vitamin K for therapeutic use is available in oral tablets, liquid nutrition preparations, and solution for injection. (See Table 1 for preparation names and concentrations.)

Toxic Dose

The U.S. guidelines for dietary intake of vitamin K for adults and children is provided in Table 1.

Toxicokinetics and Toxicodynamics

Vitamin K is a fat-soluble vitamin that is readily absorbed in the gastrointestinal tract and stored in adipose tissue. It can inhibit or reverse the effect of warfarin anticoagulants (Chapter 68).

Pathophysiology

Vitamin K is used by the liver to produce clotting factors that lead to prothrombin. Vitamin K deficiency is rare but can result in hypoprothrombinemia. Deficiency typically is caused by poor nutrition, malabsorption, or defective hepatic synthesis.

Pregnancy and Lactation

Vitamin K is FDA pregnancy category C (Appendix I) and is considered safe in nursing infants. Large amounts of vitamin K in pregnancy can cause jaundice in the newborn.

Clinical Presentation

Hypersensitivity or anaphylaxis may occur after injection. In infants who are being treated for hemorrhagic diseases, vitamin K may increase hemolysis and plasma levels of unbound bilirubin, resulting in kernicterus, hemolytic anemia, and hemoglobinuria. Phytonadione has only rarely produced this result. Hemolytic effects of vitamin K are greatest in infants or adults with a glucose 6 phosphate dehydrogenase deficiency. Dietary supplements that are high in vitamin K can block the effects of oral anticoagulants.

Diagnostic Tests

Prothrombin monitoring must be instituted before, during, and after vitamin K use. Liver function and bilirubin should be monitored in newborns and infants.

Treatment

One should stop vitamin K immediately. Daily prothrombin and liver function test measurements should be obtained as clinically indicated.

ASCORBIC ACID (VITAMIN C)

Ascorbic acid is a water-soluble vitamin that is an essential dietary nutrient because it cannot be synthesized by the human body. Vitamin C can be synthesized endogenously by most animals; however, humans and many primates have an inborn error of metabolism that requires vitamin C in their diet.

Vitamin C is readily found in the diet, and the major dietary sources include citrus fruits, berries, tomatoes, potatoes, broccoli, green peppers, and other green and yellow vegetables. It is used for the prevention and treatment of scurvy, to facilitate wound healing and recovery from extensive burns or trauma, and anecdotally for the treatment of the common cold and acute treatment of methemoglobinemia.

Vitamin C preparations are sold without prescription and come in three forms: ascorbic acid, ascorbate calcium, and ascorbate sodium. Vitamin C is administered orally as tablets and in solution for injection.

Toxic Dose

The RDA for adults and children is provided in Table 1. The maximum dose for treatment of deficiency states is in the range of 250 to 500 mg/day. However, patients often take 1 to 3 g/day or more for treatment of upper respiratory infections. Burn patients are treated with 3 to 10 g/day to maximize wound-healing parameters. Megadose vitamin C therapy with doses as high as 40 to 80 g/day has been used in cancer treatment regimens, experimental psychiatric therapy, and as adjunctive treatment in patients with acquired immunodeficiency syndrome. No toxic or lethal dose has been determined.

Toxicokinetics and Toxicodynamics

Ascorbic acid is a required cofactor for the function of a number of enzymes involved in hydroxylation and amidation reactions, such as collagen and proteoglycan synthesis. It is also important in microsomal drug metabolism. It is readily absorbed from the gastrointestinal tract via active transport. At low serum concentrations, vitamin C is metabolized in the liver to several metabolites, including oxalate. At high serum concentrations, unmetabolized vitamin C is excreted in the urine, producing urine acidification.

Pathophysiology

Insufficient dietary intake of vitamin C causes scurvy, which is a disease characterized by a loss of appetite, irritability, depression, bleeding gums, and loss of teeth. Wounds fail to heal because of poor collagen production and bruises, and petechiae are common.

Excessive intake has been found to increase the urinary excretion of oxalate. Some evidence has been shown that the increased excretion of oxalate may lead to renal calcium oxalate stones, but this remains controversial (26,27). Hemolysis has been reported after administration of oral and intravenous vitamin C. The mechanism for hemolysis is unknown; however, patients at highest risk for hemolysis have glucose 6 phosphate dehydrogenase deficiency or paroxysmal nocturnal hemoglobinuria (28–31).

Pregnancy and Lactation

Vitamin C is FDA pregnancy category C (Appendix I). It is excreted in breast milk but is considered safe in nursing infants.

Clinical Presentation

Significant vitamin C toxicity is uncommon, and these patients are usually receiving doses as high as 40 to 80 g/day as part of megadose therapy. Excessive vitamin C intake most commonly causes gastrointestinal symptoms, including nausea, abdominal cramping, and diarrhea. Patients with hemolysis due to vitamin C use may present with symptoms of anemia, including fatigue and malaise or jaundice.

Diagnostic Tests

If clinical suspicion for hemolysis is present, a complete blood count with indices is warranted. Significant hemolysis causes elevation of serum lactate dehydrogenase and decreased haptoglobin levels. Evaluation of urine may reveal oxaluria, uricosuria, and hemoglobinuria.

Treatment

All sources of vitamin C should be withdrawn and treatment for gastrointestinal symptoms provided, including antiemetics. If significant hemolysis occurs, intravenous hydration to maintain urine output should be administered. Monitoring renal function should be performed, and, rarely, transfusion of packed red blood cells is required.

NIACIN (VITAMIN B_3)

Niacin, also known as nicotinic acid or vitamin B_3, is a water-soluble vitamin that is responsible for cellular oxidation-reduction reactions and is used therapeutically as a lipid-lowering agent. Niacin is also addressed in Chapter 114. Niacin is available in immediate-release and sustained-release oral preparations, elixir, and solution for injection.

At doses of 500 to 3000 mg/day, niacin is an effective agent for reducing serum concentrations of total cholesterol, very-low-density lipoprotein, low-density lipoprotein cholesterol, and triglyceride levels. The mechanism of action of niacin affecting lipoprotein metabolism includes inhibition of adipose tissue lipolysis, decreased triglyceride esterification, and increased lipoprotein lipase activity. Niacin can also rarely be used as a vasodilatory agent.

Toxic Dose

The RDA for adults and children is provided in Table 1. The maximum therapeutic adult dose is 6 g orally in two or three divided doses daily. The maintenance dose is 1 to 2 g orally two or three times per day. No pediatric dosing is given for therapeutic use of niacin.

Toxicokinetics and Toxicodynamics

Niacin is readily absorbed from the gut and converted into either nicotine adenine dinucleotide or nicotine adenine dinucleotide phosphate in the liver. Both function as important coenzymes in cellular oxidation-reduction reactions.

Pathophysiology

Niacin deficiency causes pellagra, which is characterized by dermatitis, diarrhea, and dementia. Other symptoms include irritability, loss of appetite, weakness, and dizziness. Niacin deficiency is rare in the United States but may still be seen in alcoholics, dietary cultists, and patients with malabsorption syndrome. Pellagra is cured by institution of a niacin-rich diet or niacin supplementation.

Niacin toxicity may present as an acute vasodilatory syndrome or as a subacute hepatotoxic syndrome. Niacin-induced vasodilatory symptoms are thought to be mediated through increased prostaglandin levels and are minimized or abated by use of aspirin or other nonsteroidal antiinflammatory agents while the patient is still receiving niacin therapy.

The mechanism of hepatotoxicity is unknown. The most common finding on noninvasive radiologic studies and liver biopsies is fatty liver infiltration. Cessation of niacin therapy results in resolution of fatty infiltration. Liver biopsies have also demonstrated hepatocellular death, portal fibrosis, and inflammatory changes (32–34).

Pregnancy and Lactation

Niacin is FDA pregnancy category C (Appendix I). Niacin and its metabolites have not been detected in breast milk. Safety in nursing infants is unknown.

Clinical Presentation

ACUTE TOXICITY

Following acute ingestion, the vasodilatory syndrome from histamine release is the most common presenting side effect and is more commonly seen with the immediate-release oral preparations of niacin. It can occur acutely after ingestion of as little as 100 mg immediate-release niacin. Patients usually complain of a severe flushed sensation, pruritus, nausea, headache, dizziness, and lightheadedness. These symptoms are generally self-limited and tend to occur less frequently as patients develop tolerance. Premedication with aspirin or nonsteroidal antiinflammatory drugs may lessen the manifestations.

Other acute side effects include exacerbation of asthma, abdominal pain, diarrhea, vomiting, gout exacerbation, hyperglycemia, and orthostatic hypotension when niacin is used in conjunction with other ganglionic blocking agents.

CHRONIC TOXICITY

Patients who use sustained-release niacin preparations have a higher frequency of gastrointestinal complaints as well as signs and symptoms of hepatitis, cholestatic jaundice, ascites, edema, elevated ammonia levels, hepatic encephalopathy, and, rarely, fulminant hepatic failure (35–37). Myopathy has been reported with muscle weakness, fatigue, and myalgias (38).

Diagnostic Tests

Patients with niacin-induced hepatotoxicity may have elevated serum hepatic transaminase levels, hyperbilirubinemia, hypoprothrombinemia, and acidemia. Niacin-induced myopathy may cause elevated serum creatinine phosphokinase levels from rhabdomyolysis. Hyperglycemia and hyperuricemia have been reported.

Treatment

Immediate withdrawal of niacin is the primary treatment in acute toxicity. Symptoms should resolve over several hours without sequelae. Aspirin or nonsteroidal antiinflammatory drugs can be used for symptoms.

For chronic toxicity treatment, niacin should be stopped and attention given to presenting symptoms and findings. Patients with significant hepatotoxicity may require intensive care monitoring and supportive care until liver function recovers. The management of acute liver failure is provided in Chapter 17. Treatment of rhabdomyolysis includes monitoring of renal function, urinary alkalinization, and maintenance of urinary output.

PYRIDOXINE (VITAMIN B_6)

Pyridoxine is a water-soluble vitamin that is composed of three structural forms: pyridoxine, pyridoxal, and pyridoxamine. However, the terms *vitamin B_6* and *pyridoxine* are used synonymously. Pyridoxine is widely distributed in all foods. Major dietary sources include organ meats, meat, poultry, fish, whole grain and enriched breads and cereals, legumes (dried beans), potatoes, and bananas.

Therapeutic use of pyridoxine is rare and is reserved for patients who use medications with known pyridoxine antagonist properties, such as INH (isoniazid). It is also used for pyridoxine-responsive seizures in infants who are unable to produce sufficient γ-aminobutyric acid (GABA) due to apoenzyme dysfunction (31).

Toxic Dose

The RDA for adults and children is provided in Table 1. Typical dosing in deficiency states is 5 to 15 mg/day in infants and 20 to 500 mg/day in children and adults. Similar dosing is used in the treatment of peripheral neuritis, 50 to 500 mg/day in children and adults. Doses at or above this have been reported in association with toxicity. Chronic doses of 5 to 6 g/day for 2 to 3 months have been reported to produce a distal neuropathy. No lethal dosage is known.

The maximum adult therapeutic dosage for deficiency states is 500 mg orally or by injection daily for a period of 3 weeks. Oral supplementation as an adjunct to INH therapy is 50 mg/day orally. Dosages up to 500 mg/day have been reported as a treatment for premenstrual syndrome.

Toxicokinetics and Toxicodynamics

Pyridoxine is readily absorbed, metabolized in the liver, and excreted in the urine.

Pathophysiology

Pyridoxine is an important cofactor for many enzymes in amino acid metabolism, including transaminases, synthetases, and hydroxylases. Pyridoxine is also a cofactor required for the conversion of tryptophan to serotonin, as well as dopa to dopamine. In addition, pyridoxine is essential in the synthesis of the inhibitory neurotransmitter γ-aminobutyric acid (GABA).

Pyridoxine deficiency causes decreased production of GABA in the brain, which may lead to seizure activity. INH, used for treating tuberculosis, antagonizes the action of pyridoxine, which clinically mimics a deficiency state (39). INH is initially metabolized to a hydrazone derivative that inhibits pyridoxine phosphokinase and inactivates pyridoxal 5′ phosphate. These coenzymes are essential for glutamate decarboxylase to make GABA. Pyridoxine is also depleted after forming a complex with an INH derivative, which is readily excreted in the urine. The sum effect is a decrease in GABA production and lowering of the seizure threshold. INH-induced seizures are due to a deficiency of pyridoxine and are reversed by the antidotal administration of pyridoxine. Similarly, a metabolite of gyromitrin found in *Gyromitra* mushrooms interferes with pyridoxine requiring enzymes and binds to pyridoxine (40,41).

Pregnancy and Lactation

Pyridoxine is FDA pregnancy category A (Appendix I) and is considered safe in nursing infants. One case report revealed a girl with near-total amelia of her left leg at the knee after her mother ingested 50 mg/day during the first 7 months of pregnancy.

Clinical Presentation

The predominant feature seen in acute and chronic pyridoxine toxicity is sensory neuropathy (42). The patient may complain of difficulty in walking, loss of balance, and loss of manual dexterity. Physical examination demonstrates decreased touch, proprioception, temperature, and vibratory sense. Reflexes are absent, and motor strength is preserved. Patients may be ataxic or have a wide-based gait. The Romberg test, which demonstrates an increase in ataxia when visual input is interrupted, is positive. The sensory deficits follow a "stocking-glove" distribution and in severe cases may include perioral numbness. Symptoms may persist or progress for 2 to 3 weeks after pyridoxine is discontinued. Although most patients recover completely, permanent deficits may remain.

Chronic doses of 5 to 6 g/day for 2 to 3 months have been reported to produce a distal neuropathy that predominantly affects position, vibration, and deep tendon reflexes. Chronic use of 500 mg/day has also been reported to produce neurosensory deficits, including sensory ataxia, numbness, paresthesiae, and pain (43,44).

Pyridoxine interacts with the antiparkinsonian medication levodopa. Pyridoxine antagonizes the effects of levodopa by promoting peripheral conversion to dopamine and reducing the amount available to cross the blood–brain barrier.

Diagnostic Tests

Serum pyridoxine levels can be measured if the diagnosis is unclear. Elevated levels have been measured in patients who take high-dose vitamin B_6 supplements. After discontinuation of pyridoxine, serum levels returned to normal, but sensory deficits persisted longer. Quantitative neurologic measurements showed elevation of thermal and vibratory sensory thresholds, reduction of sural nerve sensory potential amplitudes, and unchanged nerve conduction velocity.

Treatment

Treatment is limited to cessation of vitamin B_6 supplementation. No antidote to pyridoxine toxicity is available.

REFERENCES

1. Brody JE. In vitamin mania, millions take a gamble on health. In: *New York Times* October 26, 1997:1, 20.
2. Food and Nutrition Board. *Recommended dietary allowances*, 10th ed. Washington, DC: National Academy Press, 1989.
3. Fisher G, Skillern PG. Hypercalcemia due to hypervitaminosis A. *JAMA* 1974;27:1413–1414.
4. Geubel AP, de Galocsy C, Alves N, et al. Liver damage caused by therapeutic vitamin A administration: estimates of dose-related toxicity in 41 cases. *Gastroenterology* 1991;100:1701–1709.
5. Kowalski TE, Falestiny M, Furth E, et al. Vitamin A hepatotoxicity: a cautionary note regarding 25,000 IU supplements. *Am J Med* 1994;97:523–528.
6. Moskowitz Y, Leibowitz, Ronen M, et al. Pseudotumor cerebri induced by vitamin A combined with minocycline. *Ann Ophthalmol* 1993;25:306–308.
7. Rosa FW, et al. Teratogen update: vitamin A congeners. *Teratology* 1986;33(3):355–364.
8. Rothman KJ, et al. Teratogenicity of high vitamin A intake. *N Engl J Med* 1995;333:1369–1373.
9. Oakley GP Jr, Erickson JD. Vitamin A and birth defects: continuing caution is needed. *N Engl J Med* 1995;333:1414–1415.
10. Khoury MJ, Moore CA, Mulinare J. Vitamin A and birth defects. *Lancet* 1996;347:322.
11. Dudas I, Czeizel AE. Use of 6,000 IU vitamin A during early pregnancy without teratogenic effect. *Teratology* 1992;45(4):335–336.
12. Martinez-Frias ML, Salvador J. Epidemiological aspects of prenatal exposure to high doses of vitamin A in Spain. *Eur J Epidemiol* 1990;6(2):118–123.
13. Martinez-Frias ML, Salvador J. Megadose vitamin A and teratogenicity. *Lancet* 1988;1(8579):236.
14. Nesher G, Zuckner J. Rheumatologic complications of vitamin A and retinoids. *Semin Arthritis Rheum* 1995;24:291–296.
15. Russell RM, Boyer JL, Bagheri SA, et al. Hepatic injury from chronic hypervitaminosis A resulting in portal hypertension and ascites. *N Engl J Med* 1974;291:435–440.
16. Bergman SM, O'Maila J, Krane NK, et al. Vitamin A–induced hypercalcemia: response to corticosteroids. *Nephron* 1988;50:362–364.
17. Jacobus CH, Holick MF, Shoa Q, et al. Hypervitaminosis D associated with drinking milk. *N Engl J Med* 1992;326:1173–1177.
18. Nako Y, Fukushima N, Tomomasa T, et al. Hypervitaminosis D after prolonged feeding with a premature formula. *Pediatrics* 1993;92:862–864.
19. Peregrin T. Expanding vitamin D fortification: a balance between deficiency and toxicity. *J Am Diet Assoc* 2002;102(9):1214–1216.
20. Howard JE, Meyer RJ. Intoxication with vitamin D. *J Clin Endocrinol* 1948;8(11):895–910.
21. Marcus R, Coulston AM. Fat-soluble vitamins. In: Hardman JG, Limbird LE, Molinoff PB, et al., eds. *Goodman & Gilman's the pharmacological basis of therapeutics*, 9th ed. New York: McGraw-Hill, 1996:1573–1590.
22. Hirano T, Janakiraman N, Rosenthal IM. Vitaminosis D poisoning from ingestion of concentrated vitamin D used to fortify milk. *Ill Med J* 1977;151:418–420.
23. Rizzoli R, Stoermann C, Ammann P, et al. Hypercalcemia and hyperosteolysis in vitamin D intoxication: effects of clodronate therapy. *Bone* 1994;15:193–198.
24. Selby PL, Davies M, Marks JS, et al. Vitamin D intoxication causes hypercalcaemia by increased bone resorption which responds to pamidronate. *Clin Endocrinol* 1995;43:531–536.
25. Meyers DG, Maloley PA, Weeks D. Safety of antioxidant vitamins. *Arch Intern Med* 1996;156:925–935.
26. Smith LH. Risk of oxalate stones from large doses of vitamin C. *N Engl J Med* 1978;298:856.
27. Urivetzky M, Kessaris D, Smith AD. Ascorbic acid overdosing: a risk for calcium oxalate nephrolithiasis. *J Urol* 1992;147:1215–1218.
28. Campbell G, Steinberg M, Bower D. Ascorbic acid–induced haemolysis in G-6-PD deficiency. *Ann Intern Med* 1975;82:810.
29. Costello J. Re: ascorbic acid overdosing: a risk for calcium oxalate nephrolithiasis. *J Urol* 1993;149:1146.
30. Iwamoto N, Kawaguchi T, Horikawa K, et al. Haemolysis induced by ascorbic acid in paroxysmal nocturnal haemoglobinuria. *Lancet* 1994; 343:357.
31. Rees DC, Kelsey H, Richard JDM. Acute haemolysis induced by high dose ascorbic acid in glucose-6-phosphate dehydrogenase deficiency. *BMJ* 1993;306:841–842.
32. Clementz GL, Holmes AW. Nicotinic acid–induced fulminant hepatic failure. *J Clin Gastroenterol* 1987;9:582–584.
33. Coppola A, Brady PG, Nord HJ. Niacin-induced hepatotoxicity: unusual presentations. *South Med J* 1994;87:30–32.
34. Lawrence SP. Transient focal hepatic defects related to sustained-release niacin. *J Clin Gastroenterol* 1993;16(3):234–236.
35. Dalton TA, Berry RS. Hepatotoxicity associated with sustained-release niacin. *Am J Med* 1992;93:102–104.
36. McKenney JM, Proctor JD, Harris S, et al. A comparison of the efficacy and toxic effects of sustained- vs immediate-release niacin in hypercholesterolemic patients. *JAMA* 1994;271:672–677.
37. Rader JI, Calvert RJ, Hathcock JN. Hepatic toxicity and time-released preparations of niacin. *Am J Med* 1992;92:77–81.
38. Gharavi AG, Diamond JA, Smith DA, et al: Niacin-induced myopathy. *Am J Cardiol* 1994;74:841–842.
39. Biehl JP, Vilter RW. Effects of isoniazid on pyridoxine metabolism. *JAMA* 1954;156:1549–1552.
40. Nisar M, Watkin SW, Bucknall RC, et al. Exacerbation of isoniazid-induced peripheral neuropathy by pyridoxine. *Thorax* 1990;45:419–420.
41. Wason S, Lacouture PG, Lovejoy FH. Single high-dose pyridoxine treatment for isoniazid overdose. *JAMA* 1981;246:1102–1104.
42. Berger AR, Schaumberg HH, Schroeder C, et al. Dose response, coasting, and differential fiber vulnerability in human toxic neuropathy: a prospective study of pyridoxine neurotoxicity. *Neurology* 1992;42:1367–1370.
43. Albin RL, Alpers JW, Greenberg HS, et al. Acute sensory neuropathy-neuronopathy from pyridoxine overdose. *Neurology* 1987;37:1729–1732.
44. Parry GJ, Bredesen DE. Sensory neuropathy with low-dose pyridoxine. *Neurology* 1985;35:1466–1468.

SECTION 18

Bone Disorder Agents

CHAPTER 168

Bone Disorder Agents

Vikhyat S. Bebarta and Richard C. Dart

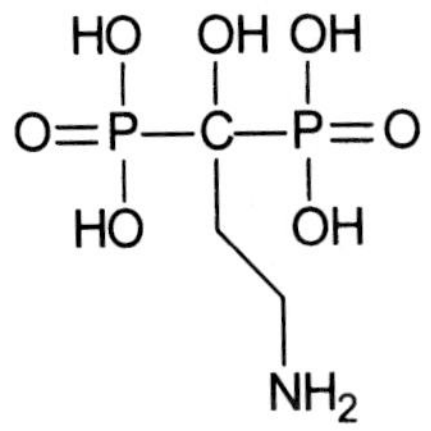

BISPHOSPHONATE

Compounds included:	**Bisphosphonates, including alendronate (Fosamax), clodronate (Bonephos, Ostac), etidronate (Didronate, Didronel), risedronate (Actonel); selective estrogen receptor modulators, including raloxifene (Evista) and tamoxifen (Nolvadex); calcitonin (Miacalcin); estrogen/progestin (multiple)**
Molecular formula and weight:	**See Table 1.**
CAS Registry No.:	**See Table 1.**
SI conversion:	**See Table 1.**
Therapeutic levels:	**Not used clinically**
Special concerns:	**Hypocalcemia, esophagitis**
Antidote:	**None**

OVERVIEW

Bone disorder agents include a group of drugs that either inhibit resorption of bone formation or increase its formation. These agents are used mostly for prevention or treatment of osteoporosis with the goal of decreasing the rate of fractures. They are also used for Paget's disease, hypercalcemia, breast cancer, multiple myeloma, and severe osteogenesis imperfecta (1). Often, these drugs are used in combination, and some are given to specific patient populations. The first- and second-line therapies for bone disorders are bisphosphonates, selective estrogen receptor modulators (SERMs), calcitonin, and hormone replacement therapy (HRT) (Table 1). Several other therapies that are uncommonly used or given as adjuvant treatment are discussed briefly in Adjuvant or Alternative Therapies. Experience with acute poisoning is very limited, and, in general, bone disorder agents are well tolerated chronically with few severe adverse effects. In addition to agents that are used to increase bone mineral density, several medications can adversely affect bone metabolism (Table 2).

BISPHOSPHONATES

Bisphosphonates are stable analogs of pyrophosphate, a naturally occurring substance that inhibits the mineralization of bone (6). These agents contain two phosphonate groups attached to one carbon atom and inhibit bone resorption by interfering with osteoclast activity (7). They are currently first-line therapy for osteoporosis and effectively decrease vertebral and nonvertebral fractures and increase bone mass (8). Bisphosphonates are also considered first line for male osteoporosis and glucocorticoid-induced bone loss (9). Oral and parenteral bisphosphonates have been used effectively to treat hypercalcemia from accidental vitamin D overdose (10,11).

The two categories of oral bisphosphonates are those that resemble pyrophosphate (clodronate and etidronate) and the more potent nitrogen-containing bisphosphonates (alendronate and risedronate). Use of etidronate has decreased because it may induce osteomalacia. Two parenteral formulations are available: pamidronate and zoledronic acid. Both intravenous preparations are approved to treat malignancy-induced hyper-

TABLE 1. Physical characteristics and dose of bone disorder agents

Agent	Molecular formula, molecular weight (g/mol), CAS Registry No.	SI conversion	Formulations	Therapeutic dose	
				Adult	Pediatric
Bisphosphonates					
Alendronate sodium	$C_4H_{12}NNaO_7P_2,3H_2O$, 325.1, 121268-17-5	mg/L × 3.1 = μmol/L	5-, 10-, 35-, 40-, 70-mg tablets	5–40 mg once daily	5 mg for body weight <20 kg, 10 mg for body weight >20 kg
Clodronate sodium	$CH_2Cl_2Na_2O_6P_2,4H_2O$, 360.9, 22560-50-5	mg/L × 2.8 = μmol/L	NR	1.6–3.2 g/d	Dose not established
Etidronate sodium	$C_2H_6Na_2O_7P_2$, 250.0, 7414-83-7	mg/L × 4.0 = μmol/L	50-mg/ml solution; 200-, 400-mg tablets	5–20 mg/kg once daily	Dose not established
Risedronate sodium	$C_7H_{10}NNaO_7P_2$, 305.1, 115436-72-1	mg/L × 3.3 = μmol/L	5-, 30-, 35-mg tablets	5–30 mg once daily	Dose not established
Selective estrogen receptor modulators					
Raloxifene	$C_{28}H_{27}NO_4S,HCl$, 510.0, 82640-04-8	mg/L × 2.0 = μmol/L	60-mg tablet	60 mg once daily	Dose not established
Tamoxifen citrate	$C_{26}H_{29}NO,C_6H_8O_7$, 563.6, 54965-24-1	mg/L × 1.8 = μmol/L	10-, 20-mg tablets	20–40 mg once daily	Dose not established
Calcitonin, salmon recombinant	$C_{145}H_{240}N_{44}O_{48}S_2$, 3431.9, 47931-85-1	mg/L × 0.3 = μmol/L	200-IU/ml solution or 200-IU/spray	100–200 IU every other day	Dose not established
Estrogen/progestin	Various	NA	Various	0.625 mg conjugated estrogen and 0–5 mg medroxyprogesterone	Not indicated

NA, not applicable; NR, not reported.

calcemia; however, they are also being investigated as a treatment of postmenopausal osteoporosis (12). Two other agents are being investigated but are not in clinical use: tiludronate and ibandronate (13,14).

Toxic Dose

The adult therapeutic doses of bisphosphonates in osteoporosis are provided in Table 1. Other dosing regimens for osteoporosis and larger doses for other diseases such as Paget's disease are available. For malignancy-induced hypercalcemia, pamidronate, 60 to 90 mg, or zoledronic acid, 4 mg, is given intravenously.

TABLE 2. Medications that adversely affect bone metabolism

Agent	Mechanism
Anticonvulsant drugs	Vitamin D deficiency from interference of metabolism and decreased gut absorption; additional causes of bone loss that are unclear
Cyclosporine	Increases bone resorption and bone loss
Glucocorticoids	Increases bone resorption and reduces bone formation by inhibiting production of insulin growth factor-I and increasing osteoblast apoptosis (2)
Heparin	Decreases bone formation, increases bone resorption, or both
Ifosfamide	Damages proximal tubules, causing renal phosphate loss and hypophosphatemic osteomalacia
Medroxyprogesterone	High doses for long periods of time may induce estrogen deficiency
Methotrexate	Increases bone resorption and inhibits bone formation
Thyroid hormone	Direct stimulation of bone resorption mediated by the T3 receptor (3,4); increased interleukin-6 may play a role by increasing osteoclast production (5)
Vitamin A	Excess doses suppress osteoblast activity and stimulate osteoclast formation
Warfarin	Inhibits γ-carboxylation of osteocalcin, major bone protein that prevents it from binding calcium

Toxicokinetics and Toxicodynamics

Toxicokinetic and toxicodynamic data are not available. Bisphosphonates have low oral bioavailability of 1% to 3% (15). They are not metabolized, and they are excreted unchanged in the urine. The plasma half-life ranges from 1 to 6 hours; however, the half-life in the bone is quite long (15). The volume of distribution is large, and bisphosphonates have significant protein binding.

Pregnancy and Lactation

The bisphosphonates are U.S. Food and Drug Administration (FDA) pregnancy category C (Appendix I). Teratology and toxicity studies performed in rats and rabbits report no adverse effects (15). Alendronate was secreted in the milk of rats after an intravenous dose (15). Because it is not known if it or other bisphosphonates are secreted in human breast milk, it is recommended that women who take this drug do not breast-feed their infants.

Clinical Presentation

ACUTE OVERDOSAGE

In general, the toxicity of bisphosphonates is mild, and severe toxicity is uncommon. Hypocalcemia has been reported in acute supratherapeutic and in therapeutic dosages. Data on acute poisoning are limited, and most of the reported cases are unintentional. An acute overdose of 4 to 6 g etidronate produced mild hypocalcemia (7.5 mg/dl) and hand paresthesia (15). Hypocalcemia has been reported in several cases of accidental supratherapeutic infusions of pamidronate that responded well to calcium without significant morbidity (15). Diarrhea and mild electrolyte imbalances developed in a 92-year-old woman after she ingested 1.5 g over 3.5 days. A patient received 285 mg pamidronate over 3 days and reported high fever and hypotension but recovered uneventfully (15). Renal failure has been reported with large acute doses of tiludronate and etidronate (16).

ADVERSE EVENTS

At therapeutic doses, several adverse drug reactions have been reported. Overall, gastrointestinal problems in women receiving oral bisphosphonates were not different from those receiving placebo (17,18). Pill-induced esophagitis and esophageal ulcers can occur and may rarely lead to esophageal stricture (19,20). This risk may be increased with concomitant use of nonsteroidal antiinflammatory drugs (21).

Hypertension may develop in patients who receive therapeutic doses of pamidronate (15). A number of adverse ocular effects have been reported with bisphosphonates. These effects include uveitis, ocular pain, conjunctivitis, photophobia, and scleritis (22). It is the only medication reported to cause scleritis (22). Clinically important hypocalcemia has been commonly reported after intravenous bisphosphonate use, but only in patients with hypoparathyroidism for oral bisphosphonates (23). Asymptomatic hypocalcemia occurs commonly with alendronate and risedronate (24).

Diagnostic Tests

Serum calcium, phosphate, hemoglobin, and renal function should be obtained in patients who have overdosed or are suspected of having bisphosphonate toxicity from chronic use. An electrocardiogram (ECG) and cardiac monitoring are necessary to monitor for dysrhythmias from QT interval prolongation with hypocalcemia. Guaiac testing for occult blood in stool or gastric aspirate is indicated for patients with gastrointestinal symptoms suggestive of bleeding. If upper gastrointestinal symptoms are persistent, consultation with a gastroenterologist for upper endoscopy is recommended. Measurement of serial blood pressure and temperatures is necessary during intravenous bisphosphonate infusion to monitor for hypertension and hyperpyrexia.

Treatment

Treatment of bisphosphonate toxicity is supportive. The likelihood of the development of serious effects is low.

DECONTAMINATION

Activated charcoal administration has not been reported with acute overdose, and it is not known whether charcoal binds bisphosphonates to any significant extent. Despite this lack of data, it is a reasonable measure in most accidental or intentional overdose patients who do not have altered mental status, particularly if coingestants are suspected.

ENHANCEMENT OF ELIMINATION

Bisphosphonates are not dialyzable. This is due to their significant protein binding, large volume of distribution, and large molecule size.

ANTIDOTES

No antidote is available for bisphosphonate toxicity.

SUPPORTIVE CARE

The risk of esophagitis can be minimized by taking the pill on an empty stomach with 8 oz of water and remaining upright for 30 minutes after ingestion. A proton pump inhibitor has been reported to improve symptoms from bisphosphonate-induced esophagitis (25).

SELECTIVE ESTROGEN RECEPTOR MODULATORS

SERMs are nonhormonal agents that bind to estrogen receptors with similar affinity to estradiol but have agonist and antagonist effects on target tissue. Raloxifene is the only approved SERM for prevention and treatment of osteoporosis. Raloxifene has estrogen agonist activity on bone and cholesterol, decreasing bone resorption and lowering cholesterol. Its antagonistic activity on breast and uterus does not increase the risk of breast or uterine cancer. Tamoxifen is another SERM that is used to treat breast cancer because of its tissue-specific estrogen antagonism.

Toxic Dose

The typical adult therapeutic dose of raloxifene is 60 mg orally given once a day (Table 1). It is administered without regard to meals. The toxic dose has not been established.

Toxicokinetics and Toxicodynamics

The onset of action is approximately 8 weeks (26). Although the oral absorption of raloxifene is 60%, the bioavailability is low at 2%; there is extensive first-pass effect (26). It is highly protein bound (greater than 95%) and has a volume of distribution of 2348 L/kg (26). Elimination half-life is approximately 30 hours. Excretion is mostly fecal; only 0.2% is eliminated in the urine (26).

Pathophysiology

The structure of the ligand that binds to the estrogen receptor determines the conformational changes in the estrogen receptor that determine interactions with protein cofactors and deoxyribonucleic acid responses (27). This ultimately determines tissue-specific estrogen agonist or antagonist activity. Estrogen causes a conformational change that induces estrogen agonist activity on bone, lipid, breast, and uterus. Raloxifene causes agonist activity only on lipid and bone.

Pregnancy and Lactation

The SERMs are all FDA pregnancy category X, contraindicated in pregnancy (Appendix I). Animal studies with tamoxifen have shown similar results to those using diethylstilbestrol and could cause genital tract abnormalities in humans (28). It is unknown whether SERMs are excreted in breast milk, and therefore breast-feeding is not recommended.

Clinical Presentation

Based on clinical trials and acute exposures of tamoxifen, the expected toxicity is low. No acute overdoses of raloxifene have been reported. Prolonged QT, tremor, hyperreflexia, unsteady gait, nausea, vomiting, and dizziness have been reported with loading doses of tamoxifen and can be expected with raloxifene (29).

In therapeutic doses, venous thromboembolism is a serious, although infrequent, adverse effect. Venous thromboembolism is reported at 1.44 events per 1000 person-years for placebo, compared to 3.32 for raloxifene (30). The rate in raloxifene is similar to that of HRT (31). Transient hepatitis was reported after 1 month of therapy (32).

Diagnostic Tests

An ECG and cardiac monitoring are necessary to monitor for prolonged QT interval and dysrhythmias. Hepatic enzymes should be monitored after acute overdose.

Treatment

Treatment is symptomatic and supportive; no antidote is available. No deaths from exposure have been reported. Gastrointestinal decontamination has not been evaluated. A single dose of activated charcoal should be administered if the patient presents recently after ingestion. Intravenous fluids and antiemetics are necessary if the patient is vomiting. Serial neurologic examinations should be performed to monitor for deteriorating neurologic status. Although not specifically evaluated, dialysis is not likely to be effective because raloxifene has a large volume distribution, significant protein binding, and minimal urinary clearance.

CALCITONIN

Calcitonin is a naturally occurring peptide hormone. Although its precise physiologic role is not well understood, at pharmacologic doses calcitonin inhibits osteoclast activity (9). Calcitonin from many different animals is effective in humans; however, recombinant salmon calcitonin is the one most widely used. It is highly potent in humans because of its high affinity (40 times that of human calcitonin) for the human calcitonin receptor and its slow rate of clearance (33). Because it is a polypeptide, it cannot be given orally and was initially administered by subcutaneous and intramuscular injection (9). The nasal spray is preferred because it provides more effective analgesia, and parenteral administration is associated with significant nausea, vomiting, and flushing (9,34). Calcitonin is typically a second-line treatment for postmenopausal women with osteoporosis and first line for pain associated with acute vertebral fractures (9).

Toxic Dose

The adult therapeutic dose is provided in Table 1. No toxic dose has been established.

Toxicokinetics and Toxicodynamics

The onset of action of the nasal spray is approximately 30 minutes, and the elimination half-life is 43 minutes (35). Bioavailability is 3% after nasal spray (35). Calcitonin does not cross the placenta (35).

Pathophysiology

Calcitonin directly inhibits osteoclastic bone resorption. Another way calcitonin plays a role in calcium homeostasis is by decreasing tubular reabsorption and promoting renal excretion of calcium (35). The mechanism for analgesia is unknown, but it is thought to be from decreased prostaglandins and stimulation of β-endorphins (36).

Pregnancy and Lactation

Calcitonin is FDA pregnancy category C (Appendix I). Excretion in breast milk is unknown, and breast-feeding is not recommended. In animal studies, calcitonin caused lower birth weight when given during pregnancy and reduced milk production during lactation (9).

Clinical Presentation

No acute overdose or death from calcitonin has been reported. Adverse effects in therapeutic trials are mild. In 30% of patients, nasal salmon calcitonin causes nasal irritation, with 15% having minor nosebleeds and fewer than 5% with nasal ulceration (9). Adverse effects are more common with the injectable calcitonin and include nausea, vomiting, flushing, and skin rash at the site of injection.

Diagnostic Tests

Serum calcium and phosphate should be evaluated.

Treatment

Treatment is supportive. After ingestion, the gastric acid would be expected to destroy the peptide hormone, although mild effects such as nausea and vomiting may occur. Gastric lavage is not recommended. Intravenous fluids and antiemetics are needed for vomiting. Epistaxis should be treated with cauterization or nasal packing.

ESTROGEN/PROGESTIN

Although previously considered first-line therapy for osteoporosis, the results of the Women's Health Initiative (WHI) demonstrated that HRT with conjugated estrogen alone or estrogen/progestin may cause untoward effects. HRT is now considered a second-line agent and should be used only when the benefits outweigh the risks (9). In general, acute and chronic toxicity is uncommon.

Toxic Dose

The adult therapeutic dose of estrogen/progestin is provided in Table 1. No toxic dose has been established.

Toxicokinetics and Toxicodynamics

Oral absorption is immediate, with peak effect in 4 to 6 hours (37). HRT is highly protein bound, metabolized in the liver, and excreted in the urine.

Pregnancy and Lactation

HRT is FDA pregnancy category X (Appendix I). Reproductive hormones enter the breast milk. Breast-feeding is not recommended. The concern with HRT in pregnancy is derived from the teratogenic effects of diethylstilbestrol that were attributed to increased fetal genitourinary abnormalities.

Clinical Presentation

Data are limited on the effects of acute overdose; however, nausea, vomiting, and mild abdominal cramping would be expected (38). Epidemiologic studies, in particular the WHI study, have shown that HRT increases the risk of coronary heart disease, breast cancer, stroke, and venous thromboembolic disease (39). Since publication of the WHI study in 2002, HRT is no longer a recommended first-line therapy and should only be used for osteoporosis if the patient cannot tolerate other bone disorder agents (9). Estrogen without progesterone is associated with an increased risk of endometrial cancer. Therapeutic doses of HRT have also been associated with pancreatitis, mild hypertension, elevated hepatic enzymes, and nasal congestion (40).

Diagnostic Tests

No specific laboratory work is needed unless clinically indicated.

Treatment

Treatment is primarily supportive, and expected toxicity is mild. Gastrointestinal decontamination is needed with activated charcoal, particularly if other coingestants are present, provided that the patient does not have an altered sensorium.

ADJUVANT OR ALTERNATIVE THERAPIES

Sodium Fluoride

Fluoride therapy is no longer recommended for osteoporosis or other bone disorders because it has not shown significant benefit in reducing fractures (41,42). In addition, the FDA has not approved it for the treatment or prevention of osteoporosis, although it is used to prevent dental caries. The predominant effect on bone is stimulation of osteoblasts (9,43).

Acute exposure of elevated sodium fluoride in a water source results in shortness of breath, weakness, headache, vomiting, low serum magnesium, and elevated liver enzymes (44). The most common toxicities at therapeutic doses are mild abdominal pain, nausea, and skeletal pain (45,46). Upper gastrointestinal injury has been seen by endoscopy at therapeutic doses (47). In studies with dogs and high doses of sodium fluoride, significant cardiac toxicity included widened QRS duration, and dysrhythmias were seen (48–50). Treatment is supportive and symptomatic. The most important treatment is to remove the exposure source.

Ipriflavone

Ipriflavone is a synthetic phytoestrogen. Phytoestrogens are weak estrogen-like chemicals produced by plants that have estrogen agonist and antagonist activity (9). Although epidemiologic studies suggest that phytoestrogens may be effective, randomized clinical trials show no benefit (51,52). Adverse effects of this treatment include epigastric pain, diarrhea, and asymptomatic lymphopenia (51,53,54).

Vitamin K

Because vitamin K has an important function in bone proteins and high blood levels have been associated with lower risk of hip fractures, it was investigated as a treatment for osteoporosis (55). Unfortunately, the trials that have been performed have been limited and not conclusive (56,57).

Parathyroid Hormone

Recombinant parathyroid hormone (teriparatide) has been approved for osteoporosis and is more effective than bisphosphonates in increasing bone mineral density and decreasing fractures (58,59). Its use has been limited thus far because it is relatively new and expensive. Although effects from acute overdose have not been reported, the most common adverse effects from therapeutic trials are dizziness, headache, leg cramps, orthostatic hypotension, and mild hypercalcemia (58,59). High doses led to an increased incidence of osteogenic sarcoma in rats (60,61).

Vitamin D and Calcitrol

Vitamin D works by increasing metabolism of calcium and intestinal absorption. Calcitrol is a vitamin D analog and is no longer universally recommended for osteoporosis or other bone-thinning diseases (62). The main toxicity of vitamin D is hypercalcemia and the symptoms associated with it, which include weakness, vomiting, hypertension, renal insufficiency, confusion, and irritability (63,64). Management consists of obtaining serum calcium and renal function tests, gastrointestinal decontamination, and an ECG. Aggressive treatment of hypercalcemia includes intravenous fluids, loop diuretics, and parenteral bisphosphonates.

REFERENCES

1. Glorieux FH, Bishop NJ, Plotkin H, et al. Cyclic administration of pamidronate in children with severe osteogenesis imperfecta. *N Engl J Med* 1998; 339(14):947–952.
2. Manolagas SC, Weinstein RS. New developments in the pathogenesis and treatment of steroid-induced osteoporosis. *J Bone Miner Res* 1999;14(7):1061–1066.
3. Abu EO, Bord S, Horner A, et al. The expression of thyroid hormone receptors in human bone. *Bone* 1997;21(2):137–142.
4. Mundy GR, Shapiro JL, Bandelin JG, et al. Direct stimulation of bone resorption by thyroid hormones. *J Clin Invest* 1976;58(3):529–534.
5. Lakatos P, Foldes J, Horvath C, et al. Serum interleukin-6 and bone metabolism in patients with thyroid function disorders. *J Clin Endocrinol Metab* 1997;82(1):78–81.
6. Ellenhorn MJ, Ellenhorn MJ. *Ellenhorn's medical toxicology: diagnosis and treatment of human poisoning*, 2nd ed. Baltimore: Williams & Wilkins, 1997.
7. Russell RG, Rogers MJ. Bisphosphonates: from the laboratory to the clinic and back again. *Bone* 1999;25(1):97–106.
8. Solomon CG. Bisphosphonates and osteoporosis. *N Engl J Med* 2002; 346(9):642.
9. Brown JP, Josse RG. 2002 Clinical practice guidelines for the diagnosis and management of osteoporosis in Canada. *Can Med Assoc J* 2002;167[10 Suppl]:S1–S34.
10. Lee DC, Lee GY. The use of pamidronate for hypercalcemia secondary to acute vitamin D intoxication. *J Toxicol Clin Toxicol* 1998;36(7):719–721.
11. Bereket A, Erdogan T. Oral bisphosphonate therapy for vitamin D intoxication of the infant. *Pediatrics* 2003;111(4 Pt 1):899–901.
12. Reid IR, Brown JP, Burckhardt P, et al. Intravenous zoledronic acid in postmenopausal women with low bone mineral density. *N Engl J Med* 2002;346(9):653–661.
13. Thiebaud D, Burckhardt P, Kriegbaum H, et al. Three monthly intravenous injections of ibandronate in the treatment of postmenopausal osteoporosis. *Am J Med* 1997;103(4):298–307.
14. Reginster JY, Lecart MP, Deroisy R, et al. Prevention of postmenopausal bone loss by tiludronate. *Lancet* 1989;2(8678–8679):1469–1471.
15. Hurlbut KM. Bisphosphonates. POISINDEX® System. Edition expires 7/2003 edition. Greenwood Village, Colorado: MICROMEDEX.
16. O'Sullivan TL, Akbari A, Cadnapaphornchai P. Acute renal failure associated with the administration of parenteral etidronate. *Ren Fail* 1994; 16(6):767–773.
17. Bauer DC, Black D, Ensrud K, et al. Upper gastrointestinal tract safety profile of alendronate: the fracture intervention trial. *Arch Intern Med* 2000;160(4):517–525.
18. Greenspan S, Field-Munves E, et al. Tolerability of once-weekly alendronate in patients with osteoporosis: a randomized, double-blind, placebo-controlled study. *Mayo Clin Proc* 2002;77(10):1044–1052.
19. de Groen PC, Lubbe DF, Hirsch LJ, et al. Esophagitis associated with the use of alendronate. *N Engl J Med* 1996;335(14):1016–1021.
20. Levine J, Nelson D. Esophageal stricture associated with alendronate therapy. *Am J Med* 1997;102(5):489–491.
21. Graham DY, Malaty HM. Alendronate and naproxen are synergistic for development of gastric ulcers. *Arch Intern Med* 2001;161(1):107–110.
22. Fraunfelder FW, Fraunfelder FT. Bisphosphonates and ocular inflammation. *N Engl J Med* 2003;348(12):1187–1188.
23. Schussheim DH, Jacobs TP, Silverberg SJ. Hypocalcemia associated with alendronate. *Ann Intern Med* 1999;130(4 Pt 1):329.
24. Roux C, Ravaud P, Cohen-Solal M, et al. Biologic, histologic and densitometric effects of oral risedronate on bone in patients with multiple myeloma. *Bone* 1994;15(1):41–49.
25. Maconi G, Porro GB. Multiple ulcerative esophagitis caused by alendronate. *Am J Gastroenterol* 1995;90(10):1889–1890.
26. Wilks J, DRUGDEX editorial staff. Raloxifene. DRUGDEX System. Greenwood Village, CO: MICROMEDEX, edition expires 6/2003 edition.
27. Riggs BL, Hartmann LC. Selective estrogen-receptor modulators—mechanisms of action and application to clinical practice. *N Engl J Med* 2003; 348(7):618–629.
28. Vancutsem P, Williams GM. Tamoxifen and teratogenicity in animals. *Lancet* 1993;342(8875):873–874.
29. Hurlbut KM, Jolliff H. Selective estrogen receptor modulators. POISINDEX® System. Greenwood Village, CO: MICROMEDEX, edition expires 6/2003 edition.
30. Cauley JA, Norton L, Lippman ME, et al. Continued breast cancer risk reduction in postmenopausal women treated with raloxifene: 4-year results

from the MORE trial. Multiple outcomes of raloxifene evaluation. *Breast Cancer Res Treat* 2001;65(2):125–134.
31. Grady D, Wenger NK, Herrington D, et al. Postmenopausal hormone therapy increases risk for venous thromboembolic disease. The Heart and Estrogen/Progestin Replacement Study. *Ann Intern Med* 2000;132(9):689–696.
32. Vilches AR, Perez V, Suchecki DE. Raloxifene-associated hepatitis. *Lancet* 1998;352(9139):1524–1525.
33. Carstens JH Jr, Feinblatt JD. Future horizons for calcitonin: a U.S. perspective. *Calcif Tissue Int* 1991;49[Suppl 2]:S2–S6.
34. Reginster JY, Franchimont P. Side effects of synthetic salmon calcitonin given by intranasal spray compared with intramuscular injection. *Clin Exp Rheumatol* 1985;3(2):155–157.
35. Tullio C, DRUGDEX editorial staff. Calcitonin. DRUGDEX System. Greenwood Village, CO: MICROMEDEX, edition expires 6/2003 edition.
36. Gennari C, Agnusdei D, Camporeale A. Use of calcitonin in the treatment of bone pain associated with osteoporosis. *Calcif Tissue Int* 1991;49[Suppl 2]:S9–S13.
37. Edwards S, Gad T, Batagol R, DRUGDEX editorial staff. Estrogens. DRUGDEX System. Greenwood Village, CO: MICROMEDEX, edition expires 6/2003 edition.
38. Hurlbut KM, Praneuk L, Rumack B. Estrogens. POISINDEX® System. Greenwood Village, CO: MICROMEDEX, edition expires 6/2003 edition.
39. Rossouw JE, Anderson GL, Prentice RL, et al. Risks and benefits of estrogen plus progestin in healthy postmenopausal women: principal results from the Women's Health Initiative randomized controlled trial. *JAMA* 2002;288(3):321–333.
40. Parker WA. Estrogen-induced pancreatitis. *Clin Pharm* 1983;2(1):75–79.
41. Eastell R. Treatment of postmenopausal osteoporosis. *N Engl J Med* 1998;338(11):736–746.
42. Kleerekoper M. Osteoporosis and the primary care physician: time to bone up. *Ann Intern Med* 1995;123(6):466–467.
43. DRUGDEX editorial staff. Sodium fluoride. DRUGDEX System. Greenwood Village, CO: MICROMEDEX, edition expires 6/2003 edition.
44. Gessner BD, Beller M, Middaugh JP, Whitford GM. Acute fluoride poisoning from a public water system. *N Engl J Med* 1994;330(2):95–99.
45. Reginster JY, Meurmans L, Zegels B, et al. The effect of sodium monofluorophosphate plus calcium on vertebral fracture rate in postmenopausal women with moderate osteoporosis. A randomized, controlled trial. *Ann Intern Med* 1998;129(1):1–8.
46. Riggs BL, Hodgson SF, O'Fallon WM, et al. Effect of fluoride treatment on the fracture rate in postmenopausal women with osteoporosis. *N Engl J Med* 1990;322(12):802–809.
47. Das TK, Susheela AK, Gupta IP, et al. Toxic effects of chronic fluoride ingestion on the upper gastrointestinal tract. *J Clin Gastroenterol* 1994;18(3):194–199.
48. Cummings CC, McIvor ME. Fluoride-induced hyperkalemia: the role of Ca2+-dependent K+ channels. *Am J Emerg Med* 1988;6(1):1–3.
49. Gaugl JF, Wooldridge B. Cardiopulmonary response to sodium fluoride infusion in the dog. *J Toxicol Environ Health* 1983;11(4–6):765–782.
50. McIvor ME, Cummings CE, Mower MM, et al. Sudden cardiac death from acute fluoride intoxication: the role of potassium. *Ann Emerg Med* 1987;16(7):777–781.
51. Alexandersen P, Toussaint A, Christiansen C, et al. Ipriflavone in the treatment of postmenopausal osteoporosis: a randomized controlled trial. *JAMA* 2001;285(11):1482–1488.
52. Scheiber MD, Rebar RW. Isoflavones and postmenopausal bone health: a viable alternative to estrogen therapy? *Menopause* 1999;6(3):233–241.
53. Agnusdei D, Camporeale A, Gonnelli S, et al. Short-term treatment of Paget's disease of bone with ipriflavone. *Bone Miner* 1992;19[Suppl 1]:S35–S42.
54. Agnusdei D, Zacchei F, Bigazzi S, et al. Metabolic and clinical effects of ipriflavone in established post-menopausal osteoporosis. *Drugs Exp Clin Res* 1989;15(2):97–104.
55. Hart JP, Catterall A, Dodds RA, et al. Circulating vitamin K1 levels in fractured neck of femur. *Lancet* 1984;2(8397):283.
56. Iwamoto I, Kosha S, Noguchi S, et al. A longitudinal study of the effect of vitamin K2 on bone mineral density in postmenopausal women: a comparative study with vitamin D3 and estrogen-progestin therapy. *Maturitas* 1999;31(2):161–164.
57. Somekawa Y, Chigughi M, Harada M, Ishibashi T. Use of vitamin K2 (menatetrenone) and 1,25-dihydroxyvitamin D3 in the prevention of bone loss induced by leuprolide. *J Clin Endocrinol Metab* 1999;84(8):2700–2704.
58. Neer RM, Arnaud CD, Zanchetta JR, et al. Effect of parathyroid hormone (1-34) on fractures and bone mineral density in postmenopausal women with osteoporosis. *N Engl J Med* 2001;344(19):1434–1441.
59. Body JJ, Gaich GA, Scheele WH, et al. A randomized double-blind trial to compare the efficacy of teriparatide. *J Clin Endocrinol Metab* 2002;87(10):4528–4535.
60. Teriparatide (forteo) for osteoporosis. *Med Lett Drugs Ther* 2003;45(1149):9–10.
61. Vahle JL, Sato M, Long GG, et al. Skeletal changes in rats given daily subcutaneous injections of recombinant human parathyroid hormone (1-34) for 2 years and relevance to human safety. *Toxicol Pathol* 2002;30(3):312–321.
62. Salter F, Ward ME, Nobili A, DRUGDEX editorial staff. Calcitrol. DRUGDEX System. Greenwood Village, CO: MICROMEDEX, edition expires 6/2003 edition.
63. Jenkins JK, Best TR, Nicks SA, et al. Milk-alkali syndrome with a serum calcium level of 22 mg/dl and J waves on the ECG. *South Med J* 1987;80(11):1444–1449.
64. Schaiff RA, Hall TG, Bar RS. Medical treatment of hypercalcemia. *Clin Pharm* 1989;8(2):108–121.

SECTION

19

Unclassified Therapeutic Agents

CHAPTER 169

Unclassified Therapeutic Agents

Katherine M. Hurlbut and Richard C. Dart

Compounds included:	**Allopurinol (Progout, Zyloprim), benzonatate (Tessalon), chymopapain (Chymodiactin), colchicine, dexrazoxane (Zinecard), gallium nitrate (Ganite), hyaluronidase (Wydase), orlistat (Xenical), sibutramine (Meridia), zipeprol**
Molecular formula and weight:	**See Table 1.**
SI conversion:	**See Table 1.**
CAS Registry No.:	**See Table 1.**
Antidote:	**None**

ALLOPURINOL

Allopurinol is an inhibitor of the enzyme xanthine oxidase that is used in the treatment of hyperuricemia from gout or antineoplastic treatment.

Toxic Dose

Adult and pediatric therapeutic doses are provided in Table 1. The toxic dose has not been established. Large overdoses have occurred without significant clinical effects (1).

Toxicokinetics and Toxicodynamics

The pharmacokinetics of allopurinol are provided in Table 2.

Pathophysiology

Allopurinol inhibits xanthine oxidase, the enzyme responsible for the conversion of hypoxanthine and xanthine to uric acid.

Pregnancy and Lactation

Allopurinol is U.S. Food and Drug Administration (FDA) pregnancy risk category C. Excretion into breast milk is unknown.

Clinical Presentation

ACUTE OVERDOSAGE

Acute overdosage has not been reported to cause acute effects. Nausea and vomiting after overdosage would be expected.

ADVERSE EVENTS

Adverse events during therapeutic use include a pruritic rash. Rarely, dermal effects have included exfoliation, urticaria, purpura. Stevens-Johnson syndrome has occurred rarely. Toxic epidermal necrolysis may develop. Fever or alopecia has been reported with or without rash.

Rarely, a phenomenon termed the *allopurinol hypersensitivity syndrome* develops (2,3). This adverse effect includes fever, chills, nausea, vomiting, and arthralgias. It appears similar to other rashes initially but also develops leukocytosis and eosinophilia and may develop vasculitis with hepatic, renal, and pulmonary involvement.

Hematopoietic adverse effects include leukocytosis, leukopenia, eosinophilia, thrombocytopenia, and bone marrow suppression, and granulocytopenia and pancytopenia (4). However, allopurinol is also used in patients with malignancies, and these effects may represent the toxicity of concomitant drugs.

Neurologic effects have included rare cases of paresthesis, peripheral neuropathy, optic neuritis, and foot drop. The peripheral neuropathy is often reversible (5). Dizziness, vertigo, depression, and confusion have also been reported (6). Cataracts have been associated with allopurinol use (7).

Diagnostic Tests

The normal peak serum allopurinol level after a 300-mg dose is 3 to 9 µg/ml. An elderly man with fatal centrilobular liver necrosis associated with allopurinol overuse had a blood concentration of 230.8 µg/ml (8).

Other tests are directed at the adverse event, such as liver function tests for hepatitis, blood counts, smears, and so forth, for bone marrow suppression.

TABLE 1. Physical characteristics, pregnancy category, and dosage of selected therapeutic agents

Compound	Molecular formula, molecular weight (g/mol), CAS Registry No.	SI conversion, therapeutic	Therapeutic dosage	
			Adult	Pediatric
Allopurinol	$C_5H_4N_4O$, 136.1, 315-30-0	mg/L × 7.35 = μmol/L	100–300 mg/dose; up to 800 mg/d	50–100 mg 3 times a day
Benzonatate	$C_{13}H_{18}NO_2(OCH_2CH_2)_nOCH_3$, where n has an average value of 8, 104-31-4	mg/L × 7.35 = μmol/L	100 mg orally 3 times a day	Same as adult for age 10 yr or more
Chymopapain	High-molecular-weight protein, 9001-09-6	NR	2000–4000 picokatal units per disk	Not approved for use
Colchicine	$C_{22}H_{25}NO_6$, 399.4, 64-86-8	μg/L × 2.50 = nmol/L	0.5–1.2 mg, then 0.5–0.6 mg every h or 1.0–1.2 mg every 2 h until symptoms abate or diarrhea occurs	0.5 mg/d
Dexrazoxane	$C_{11}H_{16}N_4O_4$, 268.3, 24584-09-6	mg/L × 3.73 = μmol/L	10 times the doxorubicin dose	Not approved for use
Dornase alfa	$C_{1321}H_{1995}N_{339}O_{396}S_9$; 29249.6, 143831-71-4; 132053-08-8	NR	2.5 mg inhaled once to twice daily	Same as adult
Gallium nitrate	$Ga(NO_3)_3,9H_2O$, 417.9, 135886-70-3	mg/L × 2.39 = μmol/L	100–200 mg/m²/d IV over 24 h for 5–7 d	Not approved for use
Hyaluronidase	Large-molecular-weight enzyme, 9001-54-1	NR	150 units and higher	150 units
Orlistat	$C_{29}H_{53}NO_5$, 495.7, 96829-58-2	mg/L × 2.02 = μmol/L	120 mg orally 3 times daily	Same as adult
Sibutramine	$C_{17}H_{26}ClN,HCl,H_2O$, 334.3, 125494-59-9	mg/L × 2.99 = μmol/L	10 mg daily, 15 mg maximum	Not approved for use
Zipeprol	$C_{23}H_{32}N_2O_3,2HCl$, 457.4, 34758-84-4	mg/L × 2.60 = μmol/L	150–300 mg/d orally	3–5 mg/kg/d orally

NR, not reported.

Treatment

No specific treatment is available for toxicity that arises from acute or chronic use of allopurinol. Treatment involves symptomatic and supportive care of rashes, bone marrow suppression, and liver, kidney, or peripheral nerve injury. Gastrointestinal decontamination is not needed unless a potentially toxic coingestant is present.

BENZONATATE

Benzonatate (Tessalon) is used to suppress cough.

Toxic Dose

Adult and pediatric therapeutic doses are provided in Table 1. Little experience with overdose from this agent has been reported. Benzonatate ingestion in a toddler has resulted in hypotension (9).

Pathophysiology

Benzonatate is chemically similar to tetracaine. Its mechanism of action is not clear, but toxic effects appear similar to those of other local anesthetic agents.

Pregnancy and Lactation

Benzonatate is FDA pregnancy category C (Appendix I). Entry into breast milk is unknown.

Clinical Presentation

A large overdose may result in CNS stimulation (seizures), which may be followed by profound CNS depression. Hypotension and dysrhythmias may occur (9). Seizures with ventricular tachycardia occurred in a 39-year-old man after ingestion of 3600 mg. The patient was successfully cardioverted and survived (10).

Local anesthesia may occur, particularly if the capsules are chewed or dissolved in the mouth. This may affect oropharyngeal mucosa and abolish the gag reflex.

Diagnostic Tests

Serum levels of benzonatate are not widely available. An electrocardiogram (ECG) should be performed to assess conduction and rhythm abnormalities.

Treatment

DECONTAMINATION

Gastrointestinal decontamination with activated charcoal (1 to 2 g/kg body weight) should be administered within 1 to 2 hours of ingestion. No data are available to evaluate gastric emptying, but the potential benefit does not appear to warrant the risk.

TABLE 2. Clinical phases of colchicine toxicity and recovery

0–24 h after ingestion
- Abdominal pain, nausea and vomiting, diarrhea, leukocytosis
- Electrolyte balance disorders, hypovolemia
- Excessive fibrinolytic activity
- Coagulation factors consumption
- Massive cytolysis

Days 2–7
- Bone marrow hypoplasia, leukopenia, thrombocytopenia
- Spontaneous hemorrhages, anemia
- Cardiac dysrhythmias
- Hepatic insufficiency
- Confusion, delirium, convulsions, coma
- Multiple organ failure and acute respiratory distress syndrome

Day 7 and later
- Beginning of alopecia
- Rebound leukocytosis

Adapted from Folpini A, Furfori P. *J Toxicol Clin Toxicol* 1995;33:71–77.

ENHANCEMENT OF ELIMINATION

Extracorporeal elimination has not been studied with benzonatate.

ANTIDOTES

No specific antidote is available for benzonatate poisoning.

SUPPORTIVE CARE

Ventricular dysrhythmias should be treated in the usual manner. Electrical cardioversion should be performed immediately in patients with hypotension and a ventricular dysrhythmia from benzonatate.

Seizures should be treated with benzodiazepines, phenobarbital, and more invasive procedures if needed (Chapter 40). Hypotension is treated initially with a bolus of isotonic crystalloid (10 to 20 ml/kg), followed by vasopressors if needed (Chapter 37).

CHYMOPAPAIN

Chymopapain (Chymodiactin) is a proteolytic enzyme related to papain that is injected to treat herniated lumbar disk disease. Adult and pediatric therapeutic doses are provided in Table 1. The adult therapeutic dose is 2000 to 4000 picokatal units per disk (1 to 2 ml). Chymopapain is FDA pregnancy category C (Appendix 1). Entry into breast milk is unknown.

Acute overdosage has not been reported. However, common adverse events include back pain, soreness, stiffness, and back spasms (11). Paraplegia or paraparesis and central nervous system (CNS) hemorrhage occur rarely (resulting from inadvertent intrathecal administration), usually occurring within a few hours of injection (12,13). In addition, transverse myelitis (occurring 2 to 3 weeks after injection) has been reported (14). Anaphylaxis has also occurred.

Treatment is symptomatic and supportive. No decontamination is needed. Techniques to increase elimination have not been attempted and would not be expected to be successful. Anaphylaxis is treated in the usual manner (Chapter 34).

COLCHICINE

Colchicine is derived from the plant *Colchicum autumnale* (autumn crocus) (Chapter 255). It is used in a wide variety of conditions for its antiinflammatory and antimitotic effects: gout, familial Mediterranean fever, hepatic cirrhosis, Paget's disease, and many others.

Toxic Dose

Adult and pediatric therapeutic doses are provided in Table 1. Colchicine has a narrow therapeutic index. A variety of doses have been associated with death, ranging from 7 mg intravenously to 0.8 mg/kg orally (15,16). Megarbane (17) analyzed and found several factors associated with a poor prognosis after acute colchicine overdose. These included the amount ingested, an increase in the prothrombin time, an increase in the blood leukocyte count to greater than 18 within 24 hours of ingestion, and the onset of cardiogenic shock within 72 hours of admission (17).

A prognostic rule was developed and quoted widely. It indicates that a history of ingestion of less than 0.5 mg/kg was associated with survival, whereas an ingestion of more than 0.8 mg/kg is always associated with death (15). Although this is a clinically reasonable rule, cases have been published that violate the rule. A single acute dose with a potential maximum of 0.4 mg/kg orally resulted in death (18).

Toxicokinetics and Toxicodynamics

Oral bioavailability is 25% to 50%, and the blood level peaks at 0.5 to 2.0 hours after ingestion of a therapeutic dose (19–21). Serum protein binding for colchicine is 10% to 31%. The volume of distribution is 2 L/kg. Colchicine reaches high concentrations in circulating leukocytes (24).

Colchicine is excreted unchanged (14% to 40%) or as metabolites (4% to 14%) within 48 hours (24–26). The elimination half-life is variable, ranging from 4.4 hours (27) in normal patients to 30 hours or more in elderly patients (21). A therapeutic dose produced a half-life of 18.8 hours in patients with renal dysfunction (27).

Pathophysiology

Although the specific mechanism for colchicine is not known, it prevents the polymerization of a and b forms of tubulin. This prevents mitosis and explains why it tends to affect organs with rapidly dividing cells first. Other cellular effects include decreased endocytosis and exocytosis, altered cell shape (tubulin structure determines cell shape), and depressed cellular motility (28). Polymorphonuclear cell chemotaxis decreases within hours of ingestion (29).

Pregnancy and Lactation

Colchicine is FDA pregnancy category D (Appendix I). It is secreted into human breast milk with concentrations similar to those in serum. However, adverse effects have not been reported in children, and colchicine is considered compatible with breast-feeding.

Clinical Presentation

ACUTE OVERDOSAGE

The phases of colchicine toxicity involve gastrointestinal symptoms initially, followed by progressive injury that causes fibrinolytic activity and injury to the liver and bone marrow. It culminates with multiple organ failure and death. The temporal phases of toxicity are provided in Table 2.

A review of 20 deaths from acute intravenous colchicine administration found that all patients received more than the recommended maximum cumulative dose of 2 to 4 mg. The toxic effects included thrombocytopenia, leukopenia, pancytopenia, anemia, acute renal failure, and disseminated intravascular coagulopathy. Death occurred within 1 to 40 days (30).

ADVERSE EVENTS

Numerous adverse events have been reported. The primary organ systems affected are those with more rapidly dividing cells and are similar to those of acute toxicity.

Hematologic effects include anemia, leukopenia, neutropenia, thrombocytopenia, nonthrombocytopenic purpura, agranulocytosis, pancytopenia, and aplastic anemia. In one case of chronic overdosage, the platelets were affected first, followed by leukocytes and then red cells (31).

Neurologic effects of long-term therapy have included a syndrome of myopathy and neuropathy (32). These effects seem more common in patients with renal insufficiency (33).

Ocular effects include delayed corneal ulcer healing in patients treated with colchicine. Healing occurred only after colchicine was discontinued (34).

Respiratory effects on therapeutic doses are rare. A 21-year-old woman died of progressive respiratory failure and acute respiratory distress syndrome after receiving a dosage of 1 mg intravenously every 8 hours. Respiratory signs became apparent after a cumulative dose of 11 mg. The patient died from progressive respiratory failure and acute respiratory distress syndrome.

Musculoskeletal effects of myopathy and myoneuropathy can develop with prolonged use. Adverse effects arise after several weeks or months of therapy and include profuse diarrhea, weight loss, intermittent fever (neutropenia), fatigue (anemia), peripheral paresthesiae, and weakness of the extremities. Laboratory findings typically reveal increases in renal insufficiency and elevated creatine kinase. The symptoms usually improve with discontinuation of colchicine (32).

Other effects include azoospermia and oligospermia. Alopecia may occur after prolonged administration or overdosage (35).

Diagnostic Tests

The serum colchicine concentration after a 1-mg oral dose was 3 to 5 ng/ml at 0.5 to 2.0 hours after dosing (18). Levels above 5 μg/L have been associated with toxicity (36).

Most diagnostic tests are directed toward the target organs of bone marrow, liver, lung, and kidney. Multiple diagnostic tests in the intensive care unit are usually needed in severe cases.

Postmortem Considerations

Histologic examination of autopsy specimens from the esophagus and bronchioles of a patient with fatal colchicine toxicity demonstrated an increase in the number of mitotic figures (37). In another case, there was diffuse sloughing of the surface epithelium of the esophagus and stomach. Centrilobular hepatic necrosis and hepatocytes in arrested mitosis as well as abnormal neutrophils in peripheral blood and blood vessels were other reported findings (38).

Postmortem blood levels of 0.3 to 0.4 μmol/L were found in an individual who died after a large colchicine ingestion (39).

Treatment

No antidotes are commercially available for colchicine toxicity. Treatment is symptomatic and supportive.

DECONTAMINATION

Because of the small mass involved, gastrointestinal decontamination is not likely to be effective unless performed very soon after ingestion. Colchicine is bound by activated charcoal. A dose of 1 to 2 g/kg body weight should be administered to patients who present within an hour of ingestion.

ENHANCEMENT OF ELIMINATION

Only a small amount of colchicine is removed by dialysis (40). Because colchicine is believed to undergo enterohepatic recirculation, multiple doses of activated charcoal have theoretic usefulness. This intervention has not been studied but would be a reasonable intervention given the serious toxicity associated with colchicine.

ANTIDOTES

An immunoglobulin G antibody to colchicine has been produced by immunizing goats. In one case, it appeared to have a remarkable beneficial effect even though administered late in the course of poisoning (41). Unfortunately, there has been no further funding for development, and the antidote is not available for clinical use.

SUPPORTIVE CARE

Granulocyte colony-stimulating factor (filgrastim) has been used to treat pancytopenia after colchicine overdose (42). It appears to elevate blood counts, but its effect on recovery after overdose is unknown.

DEXRAZOXANE

Dexrazoxane (Zinecard) is used to protect the heart when cardiotoxic antineoplastic medications are used (e.g., doxorubicin). It is an intravenous medication that is available as 250- and 600-mg vials.

Toxic Dose

Adult and pediatric therapeutic doses are provided in Table 1. No acute overdoses causing toxicity have been reported. Twice the manufacturer's recommended dose has been used therapeutically without adverse effect.

Toxicokinetics and Toxicodynamics

Protein binding is less than 2%, and the V_d is approximately 1.3 L/kg (43). Elimination is biphasic. After intravenous administration, the α (distribution) half-life is approximately 10 to 21 minutes. The terminal (β) elimination half-life is approximately 2 to 3 hours (43–45).

Pathophysiology

Dexrazoxane is believed to be hydrolyzed intracellularly and then produce its cardioprotective effect by chelating iron. The reduction of iron-doxorubicin complexes prevents free radical formation, which is thought to be at least partly responsible for the anthracycline-induced cardiotoxic effects (46). Other data suggest that dexrazoxane inhibits deoxyribonucleic acid synthesis and may act as an alkylating agent. It may also have an antimetastatic effect, which may contribute to its synergistic activity with other cytotoxic agents (47).

Pregnancy and Lactation

Dexrazoxane is FDA pregnancy category C (Appendix I). It is teratogenic in animals. Secretion into breast milk has not been reported.

Clinical Presentation

Adverse events are generally mild to moderate. Nausea and vomiting may occur, as may asymptomatic increases in amylase and hepatic enzymes (48).

Cutaneous and subcutaneous necrosis, and panniculitis, have been reported in a 42-year-old woman who received dexrazoxane by infusion into a peripheral right forearm vein followed by intravenous injection of doxorubicin through a different venous line in the same arm. Severe forearm pain developed followed by swelling and erythema (49).

Diagnostic Tests

The complete blood count and coagulation studies should be monitored in patients with overdose or during therapeutic use.

The serum calcium and liver function tests should be followed after an overdosage. Dexrazoxane increases urinary excretion of calcium, iron, and zinc. Transient asymptomatic decreases in serum calcium have been reported during therapeutic use (50). The ECG should be monitored for QTc prolongation or dysrhythmias in symptomatic patients or after overdose.

Treatment

Very little information is available concerning overdosage. Decontamination is not useful because it is administered parenterally. No specific information is available regarding extravasation. General management of extravasation is addressed in Chapter 16.

If needed, dexrazoxane would likely be eliminated effectively by hemodialysis (51). Hypocalcemia is treated in the usual manner with calcium supplementation, termination of exposure to the agent, and close monitoring until adverse events resolve.

DORNASE ALFA

Dornase alfa is a mucolytic agent used in the treatment of cystic fibrosis. It is available as a 2.5-mg/2.5-ml vial.

Toxic Dose

Adult and pediatric therapeutic doses are provided in Table 1. The toxic dose has not been established. Doses up to 20 mg twice a day have been tolerated (52).

Toxicokinetics and Toxicodynamics

Minimal systemic absorption occurs after inhalation. Onset of clinical effect is generally within 3 to 8 days, and duration is 4 days.

Pregnancy and Lactation

Dornase alfa is FDA pregnancy category B (Appendix I). It is unknown if dornase alfa is excreted in breast milk.

Clinical Presentation

Acute overdosage has not yet been reported.

Chest pain and pharyngitis are the most common adverse effects. Conjunctivitis, hoarseness, changes in voice, laryngitis, and rash also occur frequently (52,53). Bronchospasm has been reported with bovine pancreatic dornase (no longer marketed), but not with recombinant human dornase alfa. Antibodies to dornase alfa develop in approximately 2% to 4% of patients, but anaphylaxis has not yet been reported.

Diagnostic Tests

Routine diagnostic tests are not needed. If respiratory distress develops, chest radiography, pulmonary function, pulse oximetry, and arterial blood gases should be monitored.

Treatment

Treatment includes bronchospasm with inhaled β-agonists. Anaphylaxis is treated in the usual manner (Chapter 34).

GALLIUM NITRATE

Gallium nitrate (Ganite) is used to control hypercalcemia resulting from malignancy. It is available as a 25-g/ml injectable solution.

Toxic Dose

Adult and pediatric therapeutic doses are provided in Table 1. Nephrotoxicity has been the limiting toxicity at intravenous bolus doses up to 1400 mg/m^2 (54). Smaller doses up to 400 mg/m^2 by continuous infusion for 7 days are well tolerated without signs of renal toxicity.

Toxicokinetics and Toxicodynamics

The volume of distribution is 670 L/m^2, and the elimination half-life is 105 hours at a dose of 200 mg/m^2/day by continuous intravenous infusion (54). A plasma gallium concentration of approximately 1 mg/mL must be attained to achieve acute normalization of elevated serum calcium levels (55).

Pregnancy and Lactation

Gallium nitrate is FDA pregnancy category C (Appendix I). Entry into breast milk is unknown.

Clinical Presentation

ACUTE OVERDOSAGE

Acute renal failure may develop after administration of 1400 mg/m^2 (54).

ADVERSE EVENTS

Hypocalcemia, hypophosphatemia, hypomagnesemia, and decreased serum bicarbonate occur frequently with gallium nitrate therapy (56). Other reported adverse effects include lethargy, confusion, paresthesiae, anemia, leukopenia, visual and hearing impairment, nausea, vomiting, diarrhea, lower extremity edema, and skin rash. However, many patients were treated with concomitant medications for their underlying disease, which obscures the cause of these effects.

DRUG INTERACTIONS

Gallium nitrite may precipitate renal insufficiency when combined with other nephrotoxic drugs (57).

Diagnostic Tests

Serum electrolytes (calcium, magnesium, and phosphorus), renal function, and complete blood count should be monitored after overdose. The ECG should be monitored for QTc prolongation or dysrhythmias in symptomatic patients or after overdose. Other diagnostic tests such as a complete blood count or evaluation of CNS depression are needed, depending on the patient's underlying disease.

Treatment

Decontamination is not needed due to parenteral administration. Extracorporeal elimination has not been reported. Intravenous fluids sufficient to maintain urine output of at least 2 L/day should be administered (58). Use of an osmotic diuretic (e.g., mannitol) appears to decrease the risk of nephrotoxicity after bolus dosing (59,60) and may be of benefit after overdose. Hypocalcemia, hypophosphatemia, and hypomagnesemia are treated in the usual manner with supplementation, termination of exposure to the agent, and close monitoring until adverse events resolve.

HYALURONIDASE

Hyaluronidase (Wydase) is used to increase absorption and dispersion of injected drugs and to speed the resolution of extravasated drugs, hematomas, transudates, or edema (Chapter 16). The Wydase product was discontinued in 2001, but other generic providers continue to produce hyaluronidase.

Toxic Dose

Adult and pediatric therapeutic doses are provided in Table 1. Intravenous doses of up to 200,000 units have been used without toxic effects (61).

Pathophysiology

Hyaluronidase hydrolyzes mucopolysaccharides, allowing more rapid spread of injected material in tissues.

Pregnancy and Lactation

Hyaluronidase is FDA pregnancy category C (Appendix I). Entry into breast milk is unknown.

Clinical Presentation

No reports of acute overdose have been published.

Adverse effects include dizziness, chills, nausea, vomiting, and tachycardia (62). Conjunctivitis is common with subconjunctival injection (63); temporary myopia has also been reported (64). Local soft-tissue edema can develop. Angioedema and urticaria are rare complications (62). Anaphylaxis has occurred rarely (65).

Diagnostic Tests

No tests are usually needed following overdosage. Testing should be directed at adverse effects that develop (i.e., ECG for symptomatic tachycardia).

Treatment

Treatment is symptomatic and supportive. Decontamination is not needed because hyaluronidase is administered parenterally. The rare case of allergic reaction or anaphylaxis is treated in the usual manner (Chapter 34).

ORLISTAT

Orlistat (Xenical) inhibits the absorption of fats and is used in the treatment of obesity. It is available as 120-mg capsules.

Toxic Dose

Adult and pediatric therapeutic doses are provided in Table 1. Adverse effects develop at therapeutic doses, but no toxic dose has been established.

Toxicokinetics and Toxicodynamics

Orlistat is poorly absorbed, bioavailability is less than 5% (66), and an increase in fecal fat is seen within 24 to 48 hours of initiation of therapy. Time to maximum serum concentration (T_{max}) is 8 hours. *In vitro* protein binding is greater than 99% (67). The small amount that is absorbed undergoes metabolism in the intestinal wall (66).

Pathophysiology

Orlistat reversibly binds to gastric and pancreatic lipase to form an inactive complex. This prevents the breakdown of fat, which is necessary for its absorption by the gastrointestinal tract (68). Many of the adverse effects are secondary to the increase in fecal fat content.

Pregnancy and Lactation

Orlistat is FDA pregnancy category B (Appendix I). Secretion into breast milk is unknown.

Clinical Presentation

ADVERSE EFFECTS

Gastrointestinal adverse effects are common and likely related to decreased fat absorption; adverse effects are more common in patients who consume high-fat diets. Soft or liquid stool, fatty or oily stool, oily fecal spotting, flatus with discharge, and fecal urgency are all common (69).

DRUG INTERACTIONS

In patients who take high doses of orlistat, decreased serum levels of vitamin E or D may develop chronically (70,71). The addition of orlistat to a stable warfarin regimen resulted in a supratherapeutic international normalized ratio, likely secondary to a decrease in absorption of vitamin K (72).

Diagnostic Tests

No specific laboratory studies are needed.

Treatment

Gastrointestinal decontamination is not indicated, because systemic absorption of orlistat is minimal and adverse and toxic effects are secondary to decreased fat absorption in the gastrointestinal tract. Patients should avoid fat in the diet for several days after overdose to minimize gastrointestinal effects.

Supplementation of vitamins and close monitoring of warfarin may be needed during therapeutic use.

SIBUTRAMINE

Sibutramine is a nonamphetamine appetite suppressant and antidepressant. It is available as 5-, 10-, or 15-mg capsules.

Toxic Dose

Overdoses of up to 400 mg in adults and up to 210 mg in children did not result in significant clinical toxicity (73).

Toxicokinetics and Toxicodynamics

After ingestion, absorption is rapid, with a T_{max} of 1.2 hours. It is highly protein bound (97%). After hepatic metabolism with an extensive first-pass effect, it is excreted renally as metabolites (73).

Pathophysiology

Sibutramine blocks neuronal reuptake of norepinephrine, serotonin, and dopamine (74).

Pregnancy and Lactation

Sibutramine is FDA pregnancy category C (Appendix I). Entry into breast milk is unknown; its use by breast-feeding mothers is not recommended.

Clinical Presentation

ACUTE OVERDOSAGE

Hypertension and tachycardia are common after overdose (75,76). Serotonin syndrome is possible after overdose or when administered with other serotonergic drugs. Seizures are possible after overdose but have not yet been reported (73).

ADVERSE EVENTS

Mild increases in heart rate and blood pressure occur with therapeutic use. Insomnia, dry mouth, headache, constipation, and irritability are common (77,78).

Diagnostic Tests

Therapeutic drug levels are not available. An ECG and continuous cardiac monitoring should be performed in patients with significant tachycardia.

Treatment

Treatment is symptomatic and supportive. Activated charcoal should be administered after significant overdose. Serious toxicity has not been reported; gastric lavage is not warranted. Enhancement of elimination is unlikely to be effective because of the high degree of protein binding. No specific antidote is available. Mild tachycardia and hypertension generally do not require treatment. Serotonin syndrome or seizures should be treated in the standard fashion (Chapters 24 and 40, respectively).

ZIPEPROL

Zipeprol is an antitussive agent. It may have abuse potential because of its agonism of opiate receptors. It is available in several countries as 75-mg tablets, 50- and 150-mg suppositories, and a syrup of 15 mg/5 ml or 25 mg/5 ml.

Toxic Dose

Adult and pediatric therapeutic doses are provided in Table 1. In adults, toxicity has been reported after ingestion of 750 mg. Seizures are usually associated with doses of 1500 mg or greater (79), although they have occurred after ingestion of 750 mg (80). Fatalities have been reported after 1500 to 3000 mg (81). In children, toxicity develops after 15 to 20 mg/kg, and seizures are reported after ingestions of more than 25 mg/kg (79).

Toxicokinetics and Toxicodynamics

Zipeprol is rapidly absorbed, with a T_{max} of 15 minutes (82). It is extensively metabolized, primarily by the liver but also in the gut wall (83); 1% to 5% is excreted unchanged in urine (82).

Pathophysiology

Zipeprol is an antitussive with mucolytic effects. It also has antihistaminic, antiserotonin, and anticholinergic properties. Zipeprol has activity at μ, κ, and σ opioid receptors (84). Seizures are believed to occur secondary to inhibition of γ-aminobutyric acid (79).

Pregnancy and Lactation

The FDA pregnancy category has not been established. Little information is available. One case suggests that a neonatal withdrawal syndrome is possible (85).

Clinical Presentation

ACUTE OVERDOSAGE

Most toxicity has been reported with chronic recreational abuse of high doses. Tachycardia is common. Miotic pupils, dry mouth, flushed skin, hyperthermia, ataxia, dizziness, and diminished bowel sounds are also common. Coma and respiratory depression have been reported occasionally after large overdoses. Seizures may develop after acute overdose or chronic abuse of large doses (79,86). Visual and auditory hallucinations and tactile dysperceptions are common after zipeprol abuse (87). Constipation and urinary retention are frequent effects after chronic abuse (87).

A withdrawal syndrome has been reported after cessation of abuse. It manifests similarly to opioid withdrawal, with nausea, vomiting and diarrhea, mydriasis, lacrimation, sweating, arthralgia, muscle pain, yawning, twitching, agitation, nervousness, anxiety, and insomnia (85,87,88). Neonatal withdrawal has also been described (85).

Diagnostic Tests

Vital signs and mental status, as well as seizures, should be monitored. Serum zipeprol levels are not useful or widely available. The creatine kinase should be monitored in patients with prolonged coma or seizures. The ECG should be monitored during the acute course.

Treatment

Management is similar to that of opioid toxicity. Activated charcoal has not been tested but would be expected to be effective if administered early in the course. The airway is managed with the anticipation of CNS depression or seizures. Agitation and seizures are treated with benzodiazepines (Chapter 40). If hyperthermia develops, agitation or seizures should be controlled aggressively, patients' clothing should be removed, skin should be kept damp, and evaporative cooling should be promoted with fans (Chapter 38).

REFERENCES

1. Ferner RE, Simmonds HA, Bateman DN. Allopurinol kinetics after massive overdosage. *Hum Toxicol* 1988;7:293–294.
2. Vazquez-Mellado J, Vazquez SG, Barrientos JC, et al. Desensitization to allopurinol after allopurinol hypersensitivity syndrome with renal involvement in gout. *Clin Rheumatol* 2000;6:266–268.
3. Yale SH, Yale ES, Mann DS. Fever, rash, and angioedema after a course of allopurinol. *Hosp Pract* 1996;31:92–94.
4. Anon. Allopurinol ADRs in Sweden include fatal aplastic anemia. *Reactions* 2001;849:4.
5. Azulay JP, Blin O, Valentin P, et al. Regression of allopurinol-induced peripheral neuropathy after drug withdrawal. *Eur Neurol* 1993; 33:193–194.
6. Product information. Zyloprim, allopurinol. Mississauga, Ontario, Canada: Glaxo-Wellcome, 2000.
7. Garbe E, Suissa S, LeLorier J. Exposure to allopurinol and the risk of cataract exacerbation in elderly patients. *Arch Ophthalmol* 1998;116(12):1652–1656.
8. Tam S, Carroll W. Allopurinol hepatotoxicity. *Am J Med* 1989;86:357–358.
9. Sheen S, Osterhoudt K, Birenbaum D. Seizures in a toddler associated with benzonatate ingestion. *J Toxicol Clin Toxicol* 1997;35:493(abst).
10. Crouch BI, Knick KA, Crouch DJ, et al. Benzonatate overdose associated with seizures and arrhythmias. *J Toxicol Clin Toxicol* 1998; 36:713–718.
11. Anon. Diagnostic and therapeutic technology assessment (DATTA). *JAMA* 1989;262:953–956.
12. Cusick JF, Ho KC, Schamberg JF. Subarachnoid hemorrhage following chymopapain chemonucleolysis. *J Neurosurg* 1987;66:775–778.
13. Davis RJ, North RB, Campbell JN, et al. Multiple cerebral hemorrhages following chymopapain chemonucleolysis. *J Neurosurg* 1984;61:169–171.
14. Eguro H. Transverse myelitis following chemonucleolysis. *J Bone Joint Surg* 1983;65:1328–1330.
15. Bismuth C, Baud F, Dally S, et al. Standardized prognosis evaluation in acute toxicology: its benefit in colchicine, paraquat, and digitalis poisonings. *J Toxicol Clin Exp* 1986;6:33–38.

16. Rochdi M, Sabouraud A, Baud FJ, et al. Toxicokinetics of colchicine in humans: analysis of tissue, plasma and urine data in ten cases. *Hum Exp Toxicol* 1992;11:510–516.
17. Megarbane B, Back F, Resiere D, et al. Prognostic value of plasma colchicine concentrations in acute poisonings. *J Toxicol Clin Toxicol* 2001;39:258(abst).
18. Mullins ME, Carrico EA, Horowitz BZ. Fatal cardiovascular collapse following acute colchicine ingestion. *Clin Toxicol* 2000;38:51–54.
19. Ben-Chetrit E, Levy M. Colchicine prophylaxis in familial Mediterranean fever: reappraisal after 15 years. *Semin Arthritis Rheum* 1991;20:241–246.
20. Ferron GM, Rochdi M, Jusko WJ, et al. Oral absorption characteristics and pharmacokinetics of colchicine in healthy volunteers after single and multiple doses. *J Clin Pharmacol* 1996;36:874–883.
21. Rochdi M, Sabouraud A, Girre C, et al. Pharmacokinetics and absolute bioavailability of colchicine after I.V. and oral administration in healthy human volunteers and elderly subjects. *Eur J Clin Pharmacol* 1994;46:351–354.
22. Reference deleted.
23. Reference deleted.
24. Wallace S, Omokuku B, Ertel MH. Colchicine plasma level: implications as to pharmacology and mechanism of action. *Am J Med* 1970;48:443–448.
25. Carr AA. Colchicine toxicity. *Arch Intern Med* 1965;115:29–33.
26. Ertel NH, Wallace SL. Measurement of colchicine in urine and peripheral leukocytes. *Clin Res* 1971;19:348.
27. Ben-Chetrit E, Scherrmann JM, Zylber-Katz E, et al. Colchicine disposition in patients with familial Mediterranean fever with renal impairment. *J Rheumatol* 1994; 21:710–713.
28. Harris RD, Gillett MJ. Colchicine poisoning—overview and new directions. *Emerg Med* 1998;10:161–167.
29. Ehrenfeld M, Brzezinski A, Levy M, et al. Fertility and obstetric history in patients with familial Mediterranean fever on long-term colchicine therapy. *Br J Obstet Gynaecol* 1987; 94:1186–1191.
30. Bonnel RA, Villalba ML, Karwoski CB, et al. Deaths associated with inappropriate intravenous colchicine administration. *J Emerg Med* 2002;22:385–387.
31. Ferrannini E, Pentimone F. Marrow aplasia following colchicine treatment for gouty arthritis. *Clin Exp Rheumatol* 1984;2:173–175.
32. Kuncl RW, Duncan G, Watson D, et al. Colchicine myopathy and neuropathy. *N Engl J Med* 1987;316:1562–1568.
33. Older SA, Finbloom DS, Pezeshkpour GH. Colchicine myoneuropathy and renal dysfunction. *Ann Rheum Dis* 1992;51:1343–1344.
34. Alster Y, Varssano D, Loewenstein A, et al. Delay of corneal wound healing in patients treated with colchicine. *Ophthalmology* 1997;104:118–119.
35. Caraco Y, Putterman C, Rahamimov R, et al. Acute colchicine intoxication: possible role of erythromycin administration. *J Rheumatol* 1992;19:494–496.
36. Van der Naalt J, Haaxma-Reiche H, Van den Berg A, et al. Acute neuromyopathy after colchicine treatment. *Ann Rheum Dis* 1992;51:1267.
37. Gilbert JD, Byard RW. Epithelial cell mitotic arrest—a useful postmortem histologic marker in cases of possible colchicine toxicity. *Forensic Sci Int* 2002;126:150–152.
38. Weakley-Jones B, Gerber JE, Biggs G. Colchicine poisoning. Case report of two homicides. *Am J Forensic Med Pathol* 2001;22:203–206.
39. Davies HO, Hyland RH, Morgan CD, et al. Massive overdose of colchicine. *Can Med Assoc J* 1988;138:335–336.
40. Heaney D, Derghazarian CB, Pineo GF, et al. Massive colchicine overdose. A report on the toxicity. *Am J Med Sci* 1976;271:233–238.
41. Baud FJ, Sabouraud A, Vicaut E, et al. Brief report: treatment of severe colchicine overdose with colchicine-specific Fab fragments. *N Engl J Med* 1995;332:642–645.
42. Katz R, Chuang LC, Sutton JD. Use of granulocyte colony-stimulating factor in the treatment of pancytopenia secondary to colchicine overdose. *Ann Pharmacother* 1992;26:1087–1088.
43. Vogel CL, Gorowski E, Davila E, et al. Phase I clinical trial and pharmacokinetics of weekly ICRF-187 (NSC 169780) infusion in patients with solid tumors. *Invest New Drugs* 1987;5:187–198.
44. Narang PK, Hochester H, Reynolds RD, et al. Does the cardioprotectant dexrazoxane (DZR) affect doxorubicin (DOX) kinetics/dynamics? *Proc Am Soc Clin Oncol* 1992;11:126(abst).
45. Earhart RH, Tutsch KD, Koeller JM, et al. Pharmacokinetics of (+)-1,2-di(3,5-dioxopiperazin-1-yl) propane intravenous infusions in adult cancer patients. *Cancer Res* 1982;42:5255–5261.
46. Hoekman K, van der Vijgh WJF, Vermorken JB. Clinical and preclinical modulation of chemotherapy-induced toxicity in patients with cancer. Review article. *Drugs* 1999;57:133–155.
47. Poster DS, Penta JS, Bruno S, et al. ICRF-187 in clinical oncology. *Cancer Clin Trials* 1981;4:143–146.
48. Von Hoff DD. Phase I trials of dexrazoxane and other potential applications for the agent. *Semin Oncol* 1998;25:31–36.
49. Lossos IS, Ben-Yehuda D. Cutaneous and subcutaneous necrosis following dexrazoxane-CHOP therapy. *Ann Pharmacother* 1999;33:253–254.
50. Holcenberg JS, Tutsch KD, Earhart RH, et al. Phase I study of ICRF-187 in pediatric cancer patients and comparison of its pharmacokinetics in children and adults. *Cancer Treat Rep* 1986;70:703–709.
51. Product information. Zinecard, dexrazoxane. Columbus, OH: Pharmacia Inc, 1999.
52. Product information: Pulmozyme, dornase alfa. South San Francisco, CA: Genentech Inc, (PI revised 01/2001), reviewed 05/2001.
53. Ramsey BW, Astley SJ, Aitken ML, et al. Efficacy and safety of short-term administration of aerosolized recombinant human deoxyribonuclease in patients with cystic fibrosis. *Am Rev Respir Dis* 1993;148:145–151.
54. Leyland-Jones B. Pharmacokinetics and therapeutic index of gallium nitrate. *Semin Oncol* 1991;18:16–20.
55. Warrell RP, Skelos A, Alcock NW, et al. Gallium nitrate for acute treatment of cancer-related hypercalcemia: clinicopharmacological and dose response analysis. *Cancer Res* 1986;46:4208–4212.
56. Scher HI, Curley T, Geller N, et al. Gallium nitrate in prostatic cancer: evaluation of antitumor activity and effects on bone turnover. *Cancer Treat Rep* 1987;71:887–893.
57. Warrell RP, Israel R, Frisone M, et al. Gallium nitrate for acute treatment of cancer-related hypercalcemia. *Ann Intern Med* 1988;108:669–674.
58. Warrell RP, Coonley CJ, Straus DJ, et al. Treatment of patients with advanced malignant lymphoma using gallium nitrate administered as a seven-day continuous infusion. *Cancer* 1983;51:1982–1987.
59. Foster BJ, Clagett-Carr K, Hoth D, et al. Gallium nitrate: the second metal with clinical activity. *Cancer Treat Rep* 1986;70:1311–1319.
60. Krakoff IH, Newman RA, Goldberg RS. Clinical toxicologic and pharmacologic studies of gallium nitrate. *Cancer* 1979;44:1722–1727.
61. Pillwein K, Fuiko R, Slavc I, et al. Hyaluronidase additional to standard chemotherapy improves outcome for children with malignant brain tumors. *Cancer Lett* 1998;131:101–108.
62. Product information: Wydase, hyaluronidase. Philadelphia: Wyeth Laboratories, 2000.
63. Stanworth A. The ocular effects of local corticosteroid and hyaluronidase. In: Paterson G, Miller SJH, Patterson GD, eds. *Drug mechanisms in glaucoma.* London: Churchill, 1966.
64. Singh D. Subconjunctival hyaluronidase injection producing temporary myopia. *J Cataract Refract Surg* 1995;21:477–478.
65. Bilyk MA, Dudchik GK. Anaphylactic reactions after administration of lidase in patients with tuberculosis. *Klin Med* 1975;53:110–111.
66. Zhi J, Melia AT, Eggers H, et al. Review of limited systemic absorption of orlistat, a lipase inhibitor, in healthy human volunteers. *J Clin Pharmacol* 1995;35:1103–1108.
67. Product information: Xenical, orlistat. Nutley, NJ: Roche Pharmaceuticals, 2000.
68. Ransac S, Gargouri Y, Moreau H, et al. Inactivation of pancreatic and gastric lipases by tetrahydrolipstatin and alkyl-dithio-5-(2-nitrobenzoic acid): a kinetic study with 1,2-didecanoyl-sn-glycerol monolayers. *Eur J Biochem* 1991;202:395–400.
69. Davidson MH, Hauptman J, DiGirolamo M, et al. Weight control and risk factor reduction in obese subjects treated for 2 years with orlistat: a randomized controlled trial. *JAMA* 1999;281(3):235–242.
70. Tonstad S, Pometta D, Erkelens DW, et al. The effect of the gastrointestinal lipase inhibitor, orlistat, on serum lipids and lipoproteins in patients with primary hyperlipidaemia. *Eur J Clin Pharmacol* 1994;46:405–410.
71. Drent ML, Larsson J, William-Olsson T, et al. Orlistat (RO 18-0647), a lipase inhibitor, in the treatment of human obesity: a multiple dose study. *Int J Obes* 1995;19:221–226.
72. MacWalter RS, Fraser HW, Armstrong KM. Orlistat enhances warfarin effect. *Ann Pharmacother* 2003 Apr;37(4):510–512.
73. Product information: Meridia, sibutramine hydrochloride monohydrate. Mount Olive, NJ: Knoll Pharmaceutical Co, 1999.
74. Stock MJ. Sibutramine: a review of the pharmacology of a novel anti-obesity agent. *Int J Obes* 1997;21[Suppl 1]:S25–S29.
75. Mrvos R, Cubberley V, Krenzelok EP. A toxicity profile of sibutramine. *Clin Toxicol* 2000;38:521–522(abst).
76. Hanotin C, Thomas F, Jones SP, et al. Efficacy and tolerability of sibutramine in obese patients: a dose-ranging study. *Int J Obes* 1998;22:32–36.
77. Cerulli J, Lomaestro BM, Malone M. Update on the pharmacotherapy of obesity. *Ann Pharmacother* 1998;32:88–102.
78. Bray GA, Ryan DH, Gordon D, et al. A double-blind randomized placebo-controlled trial of sibutramine. *Obes Res* 1996;4(3):263–270.
79. Jouglard J. Zipeprol abuse. An opportunity for assessment of its neurotoxicity. *Newsletter of the Marseille Poison Centre* 1991:5–13.
80. Perraro F, Beorchia A. Convulsions and cerebral edema associated with zipeprol abuse [Letter]. *Lancet* 1984;2:45–46.
81. Baselt RC. *Disposition of toxic drugs and chemicals in man*, 5th ed. Foster City, CA: Chemical Toxicology Institute, 2000.
82. Crippa O, Polettini A, Avato FM. Lethal poisoning by zipeprol in drug addicts. *J Forensic Sci* 1990;35:992–999.
83. Constantin M, Pognat JF. Zipeprol metabolism in man and in the animal. *Arzneimittelforsch* 1978;28(1):64–72.
84. Acteo MD, Bowman E, Butelman E, et al. Zipeprol: preclinical assessment of abuse potential. *Drug Alcohol Depend* 1996;42:93–104.
85. Slobodkin D, Thompson D, Levin G, et al. Habituation to zipeprol hydrochloride during pregnancy. *J Substance Abuse Treatment* 1992;9:129–131.
86. Moroni C, Cerchiari EL, Gasparini M, et al. Overdosage of zipeprol, a non-opioid antitussive agent [Letter]. *Lancet* 1984;2:45.
87. Janiri L, Mannelli P, Persico AM, et al. Zipeprol is a newly abused antitussive with an opioid spectrum and hallucinogenic effects. *Drug Alcohol Depend* 1991;27:121–125.
88. Mallaret MP, Lauby VL, Cornier PH, et al. Zipeprol: primary dependence in an unaddicted patient [Letter]. *Ann Pharmacother* 1995;29:540.

SECTION

20

Immunosuppressants

CHAPTER 170

Immunosuppressants

Javier C. Waksman and João H. Delgado

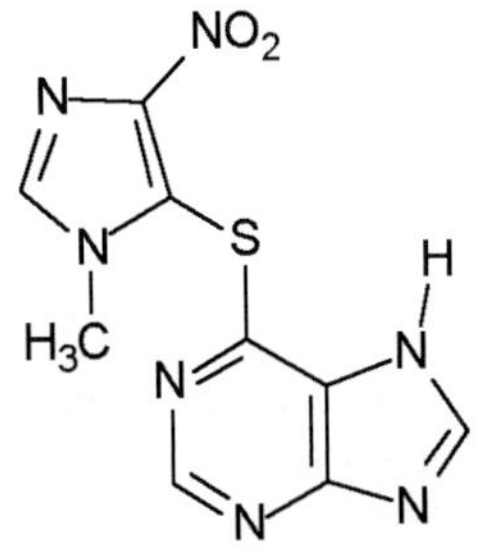

AZATHIOPRINE

Compounds included:	**Cyclosporine (Gengraf, Neoral, Sandimmune); tacrolimus (Prograf, Protopic); azathioprine (Imuran); 6-mercaptopurine (Purinethol); sirolimus (Rapamune); mycophenolate mofetil (CellCept); muromonab-CD3 (Orthoclone OKT3); daclizumab (Zenapax); basiliximab (Simulect)**
Molecular formula and weight:	**See Table 1.**
SI conversion:	**See Table 1.**
CAS Registry No.:	**See Table 1.**
Therapeutic levels:	**See Table 1.**
Target organs:	**Immune system, central nervous system, cardiovascular, kidneys, liver, hematopoietic**
Antidote:	**None**

OVERVIEW

The immunosuppressants comprise a variety of agents used in the management of solid organ and bone marrow transplantation, autoimmune diseases, and inflammatory conditions [e.g., inflammatory bowel disease (IBD)]. Their common effect is the suppression of the body's innate immune response.

These drugs can be divided into several categories: calcineurin inhibitors (cyclosporine and tacrolimus), antiinflammatory (glucocorticoids), antiproliferative agents [azathioprine, cyclophosphamide, methotrexate, and mycophenolate mofetil (MMF)], antibodies (polyclonal antithymocyte globulin, monoclonal muromonab-CD3, basiliximab, and daclizumab), and interleukin (IL)-2–mediated signal transduction inhibitor (sirolimus). The adverse effects of the glucocorticoids are well known; therefore, their toxicity is not discussed in this chapter.

CYCLOSPORINE

Cyclosporine is a cyclic polypeptide and potent immunosuppressant. It is produced by the fungus *Beauveria nivea*, among others. Along with tacrolimus (FK 506), it is classified as a calcineurin inhibitor. Its therapeutic usefulness arises from its ability to modulate T-cell activity. Cyclosporine ushered in the modern age of transplant immunosuppression and remains a mainstay of solid organ transplantation. It is used increasingly in the treatment of other conditions such as graft-versus-host disease, nephrotic syndrome, refractory granulomatous bowel disease and rheumatoid arthritis, and severe psoriasis.

Cyclosporine is available in both intravenous (IV) (Sandimmune) and oral formulations (Gengraf, Neoral, Sandimmune). The three oral formulations available do not have equivalent bioavailability.

TABLE 1. Physical characteristics and therapeutic drug levels for immunosuppressant drugs

Drug name	Molecular formula	Molecular weight (g/mol)	SI conversion	CAS Registry No.	Therapeutic level (ng/ml)
Cyclosporine	$C_{62}H_{111}N_{11}O_{12}$	1202.6	mg/L × 0.8 = μmol/L	59865-13-3	100–300[a] (whole blood)
Tacrolimus	$C_{44}H_{69}NO_{12},H_2O$	822	mg/L × 1.2 = μmol/L	109581-93-3	0.5–2.0 (plasma); 5–20 (whole blood)
Azathioprine	$C_9H_7N_7O_2S$	277.3	mg/L × 3.6 = μmol/L	446-86-6	NA
6-Mercaptopurine	$C_5H_4N_4S,H_2O$	170.2	mg/L × 5.9 = μmol/L	6112-76-1	NA
Sirolimus	$C_{51}H_{79}NO_{13}$	914.2	mg/L × 1.1 = μmol/L	53123-88-9	6–15 (whole blood)
Mycophenolate mofetil	$C_{23}H_{31}NO_7$	433.5	mg/L × 2.3 = μmol/L	115007-34-6	NA
Muromonab-CD3	NR	NR	NR	NR	800 (plasma); this is therapeutic and not trough levels
Daclizumab	—	144 kd	NR	152923-56-3	NA
Basiliximab	—	144 kd	NR	179045-86-4	NA

NA, not applicable; NR, not reported.
[a]Depends on method of analysis; therapeutic range extends greater than 500 ng/ml for some assays.

Toxic Dose

Dosing is individualized depending on the indication and target trough blood concentration. The *adult therapeutic dose* for transplantation is 15 mg/kg a few hours before the procedure that is continued postoperatively and gradually tapered over several weeks to a maintenance dose of 5 to 10 mg/kg/day. Doses of 46 mg/kg and 104 mg/kg to children have resulted in no clinically important effects (1).

Toxicokinetics and Toxicodynamics

Absorption after oral dosing is incomplete and erratic (1a). Once absorbed, 40% to 60% of drug is bound to erythrocytes and leukocytes, with most of the remaining fraction bound to lipoproteins; less than 5% of the drug remains in the plasma as free drug. Cyclosporine undergoes extensive metabolism in the liver by the cytochrome oxidase system, primarily by the CYP3A family.

Toxicokinetic data are scant. Jindal et al. reported the persistence of supratherapeutic cyclosporine levels for more than 21 days after the drug had been withdrawn in a female patient who had chronic liver rejection (2). A monoethylglycinexylidine test suggested that her P-450 activity was profoundly downregulated, probably as a result of the chronic rejection and resulting cholestasis. In contrast, half-lives as brief as 2.7 to 5.4 hours have been reported after acute 5-g oral overdoses (3,4). The largest reported single oral dose of cyclosporine (7.5 g) resulted in a trough level of 3687 ng/ml (5). The highest level reported in the literature after oral overdose is 6700 ng/ml, which occurred after a 5-g ingestion (4). Tenfold overdoses (30 mg/kg/day) of cyclosporine IV have resulted in levels ranging from 4096 to 4100 ng/ml (6,7). The half-life for cyclosporine after oral overdose has been 71 to 91 hours (8,9).

Pathophysiology

Cyclosporine inhibits primarily T cell–dependent immunity by inhibiting T-cell activation. It does this by binding to cytoplasmic receptor proteins collectively termed *cyclophilins*. This complex, in turn, binds to the phosphatase calcineurin, inhibiting its enzymatic activity. Normally, calcineurin dephosphorylates the cytosolic portion of the nuclear factor of activated T lymphocytes, which results in the translocation of the complex into the nucleus and promotion of gene transcription, including that of IL-2, a key regulator of T-cell proliferation and differentiation. Inhibition of calcineurin thus inhibits T-cell activation.

Pregnancy and Lactation

Cyclosporine is U.S. Food and Drug Administration (FDA) pregnancy category C (Appendix I). It crosses the placenta readily but does not appear to pose a major risk to the fetus. The most common finding in infants born to mothers who used cyclosporine throughout pregnancy is growth retardation (10). Teratogenicity has not been demonstrated in animals, and no specific pattern of defects has emerged in the few infants born with congenital anomalies. Cyclosporine is excreted into breast milk with reported milk to plasma ratios of 0.17:0.40 (11). Cyclosporine is considered a contraindication to breast-feeding (12).

Clinical Presentation

ACUTE OVERDOSAGE

There is limited experience with acute overdose (12a). Toxicity is relatively mild and confined primarily to abdominal pain, headache, mild encephalopathy, nausea, elevated transaminase levels, hyperbilirubinemia, and renal insufficiency (3,5,6,13). Effects are most often transient and resolve simply by withholding the drug. Other effects of acute overdose have included altered taste, biopsy-proven acute tubular necrosis, dysesthesias, peripheral edema, and thrombotic thrombocytopenia purpura (7,14,15,15a). Severe side effects, such as cerebral edema and coma, usually occur as a result of accidental IV overdose (16).

ADVERSE EVENTS

The adverse effects associated with chronic use are well documented (17,18). Although the incidence is dose related, these side effects may be seen at therapeutic levels as well. The most common adverse effects are hypertension and nephrotoxicity. The mechanism of hypertension is unknown. The renal insufficiency is believed to occur primarily as a result of arteriolopathy and interstitial fibrosis with tubular atrophy.

A variety of neurologic effects have been described: ataxia, cerebral edema, dysarthria, encephalopathy, extrapyramidal symptoms, headache, motor polyneuropathy, paresthesias, seizures, tremor, and visual hallucinations (18). Cyclosporine also causes a somewhat distinctive posterior leukoencephalopathy syndrome, which results in altered mental status, cortical blindness, and occasionally seizures. Elevated cyclosporine levels, hypocholesterolemia, and hypomagnesemia have been identified as risk factors for developing this syndrome. Brain imaging may show bilateral white matter changes, typically involving the parietooccipital lobes. This syndrome is almost always accompanied by hypertension and is usually completely reversible with cessation of the drug.

Other effects of chronic use include anaphylaxis (1a), acute respiratory distress syndrome (18a), diabetes, gingival hyperplasia, hepatitis, hyperbilirubinemia, hyperlipidemia, hypomagnesemia, myopathy, and posttransplant lymphoproliferative disorders (19–21).

DRUG INTERACTIONS

A large number of drugs can affect metabolism by inducing or inhibiting cytochrome P-450 enzymes that metabolize cyclosporine. In addition, a careful history regarding herbal supplements should be sought. Breindenbach et al. described 30 patients in whom concomitant use of St. John's wort resulted in a profound drop of cyclosporine levels (22). A recent review found 11 case reports and two case series documenting this effect (23).

Diagnostic Tests

Serum electrolytes, including magnesium; liver function tests; and renal function tests should be obtained in patients who have overdosed or are suspected of having cyclosporine toxicity from chronic use. A whole blood cyclosporine level should also be obtained. In the acute overdose setting, it helps determine the patients at risk to develop adverse effects. Renal function should be monitored for at least 2 days after an acute overdose, especially if the overdose results in a supratherapeutic trough level.

A therapeutic level is imperative in the renal transplant patient presenting with worsening renal function. Because both cyclosporine toxicity and acute rejection can present with worsening renal failure, it can be difficult to differentiate between the two. However, this distinction is crucial because the treatment for the former is to withhold therapy, whereas treatment for the latter may involve increasing the dose. Although a therapeutic level does not exclude cyclosporine nephrotoxicity, a high trough level is suggestive of this diagnosis (Table 1).

Computerized tomography or magnetic resonance imaging of the brain should be obtained in patients presenting with altered mental status or any other symptoms attributable to central nervous system pathology.

Treatment

Treatment of cyclosporine overdose is supportive. Although several treatment modalities have been proposed, the likelihood of developing serious effects is small, and none of the proposed treatments has been described in settings other than isolated case reports. Empiric IV magnesium should be considered in patients who present with seizures or other severe central nervous system symptoms because hypomagnesemia is a relatively frequent occurrence in such cases. Restarting cyclosporine therapy or substituting another immunosuppressant should only be done in consultation with a specialist familiar with the proper use of this medication.

DECONTAMINATION

After ingestion, activated charcoal has been used, but it is not known if charcoal binds cyclosporine well (4,24).

ENHANCEMENT OF ELIMINATION

Both phenytoin and phenobarbital have been used in attempts to increase P-450 metabolism of cyclosporine (2,5). There appears to be no significant advantage to using this approach. Cyclosporine is not dialyzable. Less than 1% of cyclosporine is recovered in the dialysate after a 4-hour dialysis run (25).

Kokado et al. reported a patient who accidentally received a dose of 30 mg/kg/day that resulted in severe abdominal pain and hyperbilirubinemia (6). Plasmapheresis was performed twice, 20 days apart. Although it was associated with a transient increase in cyclosporine elimination rate, this effect was modest and probably did not affect the outcome. Plasmapheresis has also been used to treat hypertriglyceridemia associated with cyclosporine (26).

TACROLIMUS

Tacrolimus (FK 506, Prograf) is a macrolide antibiotic used to prevent rejection after solid organ transplant as well as a variety of autoimmune and inflammatory conditions.

Toxic Dose

The *adult therapeutic dosage* is 0.15 mg/kg twice daily. The *pediatric dosage* is 0.15 to 0.30 mg/kg/day in two divided doses. The dose is then adjusted based on indication and target trough concentration. Two 2-year-old girls remained asymptomatic after ingesting 10 mg and 11 mg, respectively. Laboratory values were measured in one child and remained normal. A 29-year-old man ingested 90 mg, developed a creatinine of 3.9 mg/dl, and recovered. There were no other adverse effects (27).

Toxicokinetics and Toxicodynamics

Oral absorption is rapid but incomplete. In the blood, tacrolimus partitions into erythrocytes with a red blood cell to plasma ratio that exceeds 4:1. The remaining fraction is 75% to 99% protein bound, primarily to albumin and α_1-acid glycoprotein. Tacrolimus is extensively metabolized in the liver by *O*-demethylation and hydroxylation, especially via the CYP3A family of P-450 enzymes. Less than 1% of tacrolimus is excreted in urine unchanged.

Toxicokinetic data are scant. In a case involving a repeated daily tenfold overdose for 8 days, the trough blood levels remained supratherapeutic for 4 days, with a peak level on admission of 118.5 ng/ml (28). In a 4-month-old girl who underwent orthotopic liver transplantation and developed tacrolimus toxicity (peak blood concentration, 49 ng/ml), the elimination half-life ranged from 13 to 235 hours (29).

Pathophysiology

Like cyclosporine, tacrolimus is a calcineurin inhibitor. It binds to a family of intracellular protein receptors collectively termed *FK506-binding proteins*. The tacrolimus-FK506–binding protein complex inhibits calcineurin activity, which in turn prevents intranuclear translocation of the nuclear factor of activated T lymphocytes and the downstream production of IL-2 and other cytokines. The end result is the blunting of T-cell activation.

Pregnancy and Lactation

Tacrolimus is FDA pregnancy category C (Appendix I). It crosses the placenta and has been associated with hyperkalemia (29a), growth retardation, and prematurity in the infant. Tacrolimus is excreted into breast milk with a reported milk to plasma ratio of 0.5 (30).

Clinical Presentation

ACUTE OVERDOSAGE

The limited evidence indicates that acute overdosage of tacrolimus is mild (31,32). In a series of 12 acute overdoses that resulted in whole blood concentrations of 19 to 197 ng/ml (33), nausea, tremor, elevated liver enzymes, and worsened renal function occurred, nearly all of which were mild and transient. One patient developed renal failure and sepsis, but details on the amount ingested and clinical course were not provided. In a series of five patients who ingested 0.25 to 7.00 mg/kg, the only reported effect was a transient elevation of creatinine 48 hours after ingestion in a patient who was 4 years post–renal transplant (27). Hardwick and Batiuck described a patient who inadvertently received a tenfold oral overdose over an 8-day period (28). Despite a peak level of 118.5 ng/ml and the persistence of a supratherapeutic level for over 1 week, the only signs of toxicity were confusion, hypomagnesemia, hypophosphatemia, and worsened diabetes control. All of these problems resolved after tacrolimus was discontinued.

ADVERSE EVENTS

Reported effects include bone marrow suppression, diabetes, gastrointestinal (GI) symptoms, hyperkalemia, hypertension, hypertrophic cardiomyopathy, nephrotoxicity, posttransplant lymphoproliferative disorder, rhabdomyolysis, and thrombotic thrombocytopenia purpura (34–38). Neurologic effects range from tremor and headache to altered mental status, coma, demyelinating polyneuropathy, and seizures (39). Most side effects improve or resolve with dose reduction or withdrawal of the drug.

Diagnostic Tests

Electrolytes, liver function tests, and renal function tests should be considered in all patients who have overdosed or are suspected of having tacrolimus toxicity. Toxic effects may occur at therapeutic blood levels. Whole blood or serum tacrolimus levels should be followed serially until they return to a therapeutic range (Table 1).

Treatment

Treatment is supportive. Patients presenting within a few hours of an acute overdose should receive activated charcoal, although this approach has not been formally studied. Because the side effects after overdose have been relatively mild, gastric lavage should not be performed unless it involves a massive overdose of tacrolimus or a dangerous coingestant. Dialysis and plasmapheresis are not effective because of the extensive drug binding and sequestration by erythrocytes (40,41). Hemoperfusion has been proposed as an alternative, although data supporting this approach are very limited (42). Restarting tacrolimus or substituting for another drug should only be done in consultation with a physician experienced with the use of this drug who will be able to monitor the patient for the development of complications.

AZATHIOPRINE

Azathioprine (Imuran), a thiopurine agent, is the imidazole derivative of 6-mercaptopurine (6-MP). Classified as an antiproliferative agent, azathioprine inhibits the differentiation and proliferation of T and B lymphocytes by inhibiting DNA and RNA synthesis and replication. It is therefore effective in the treatment of immune-mediated diseases (42a), inflammatory diseases (e.g., IBD), and rheumatoid arthritis (43) and as an adjunct to prevent the rejection of organs in transplantation (44). Azathioprine is also used as a steroid-sparing agent and as an alternative to corticosteroids (45).

Toxic Dose

The *adult therapeutic dose* for organ transplant is 4 mg/kg for several days, then reduced to approximately 3 mg/kg (46). For IBD, the dosage ranges from 1.5 to 3.0 mg/kg/day. Azathioprine is available in IV, oral, and three colonic delivery formulations (delayed oral release, hydrophobic rectal foam, and hydrophilic rectal foam). IV administration is no longer common because the response time is not shorter than with oral administration (47). The *pediatric dosage* is 0.5 mg/kg/day orally, increased to 2 mg/kg/day in two divided doses.

A 7500-mg ingestion produced only vomiting, diarrhea, mild elevation of aspartate aminotransferase, and mild leukopenia (44), whereas ingestion of 650 mg followed by decontamination produced no effects (48).

Toxicokinetics and Toxicodynamics

Azathioprine is approximately 50% bioavailable. The bioavailability of 6-MP by the colonic route is significantly lower than after oral administration. For this reason, it is possible that ileocolonic delivery of azathioprine can reduce the systemic toxicity of the drug (49). Azathioprine is 30% protein bound. Azathioprine is converted to 6-MP, presumably in the liver, when the imidazole group is split off through nonenzymatic and enzymatic processes (44,50). 6-MP is further metabolized either to (a) the active compounds 6-thioguanine nucleotides (6-TGN) and 6-metilmercaptopurinic ribonucleotides (6-methylmercaptopurine) by the enzyme thiopurine methyltransferase (TPMT) and inosine-amino-phosphate dehydrogenase, respectively; or (b) via xanthine oxidase and TPMT to inactive metabolites 6-thiouric acid and 6-methylmercaptopurine.

The main route of elimination is the urine; 13.0% to 21.4% is excreted as 6-thioric acid, 1.3% to 2.4% as 6-MP, 0% to 2.25% unchanged, and 7% as 5-mercapto-1-methyl-4-nitroimidazole (46). Whereas elimination half-life of azathioprine is short in plasma, ranging from 1 to 2 hours, 6-TGN accumulate in erythrocytes and have a half-life of 3 to 13 days (46,49).

Pathophysiology

The main effect of azathioprine is the inhibition of purine synthesis. The cytotoxic effects of azathioprine result from the active metabolites derived from 6-MP inhibiting the production of inosinic acid, an intermediate in the biosynthesis of adenylic and guanylic acids, which leads to a metabolic disruption of DNA and RNA synthesis (49).

Pregnancy and Lactation

Azathioprine is FDA pregnancy category D (Appendix I). Azathioprine and its metabolites are excreted into breast milk.

Clinical Presentation

ACUTE OVERDOSAGE

An accidental overdose of 7500 mg of azathioprine by a renal transplant recipient was followed by vomiting and diarrhea, reversible mild elevation of aspartate aminotransferase, and bone marrow depression in the form of mild leukopenia (44). A patient who was treated with induced vomiting and activated charcoal developed no toxicity after ingestion of 650 mg of azathioprine (48).

ADVERSE EVENTS

The adverse effects can be classified into two primary groups: idiosyncratic/allergic (e.g., pancreatitis, hepatitis, skin rashes, arthralgias) and direct (nonallergic) toxicity (susceptibility to infection, hematologic toxicity, neoplastic diseases). Whereas the former group is not dose dependent, the latter group depends not only on the dose but on the drug's metabolism and the genetic disposition of the individual (51,52).

Among the dose-related effects, myelosuppression (primarily leukopenia) is the most common complication of therapy and develops within 0.5 to 132.0 months of initiation (43). Pancytopenia is rare (53). There appears to be a direct correlation between the patient's level of TPMT activity, which is controlled by a common genetic polymorphism, and the likelihood of developing acute myelosuppression. Patients with extremely low red blood cell TPMT activities (homozygous for the allele that encodes the enzyme) are more likely to develop myelosuppression (52).

The GI toxicity of azathioprine includes anorexia, oral mucositis, nausea, vomiting, diarrhea, and pancreatitis (46,54). The diarrhea may be devastating, particularly in patients with IBD (47,51,55). However, this may be minimized or abated when the drug is administered in the 6-MP form (47).

Other azathioprine-associated effects include hepatitis, interstitial pneumonitis, neoplasia, erythroid hypoplasia with accompanied macrocytosis, and inclination toward infection (46,52,56–58).

DRUG INTERACTIONS

Allopurinol, a xanthine oxidase inhibitor, may increase the toxicity of azathioprine and 6-MP by inhibiting the conversion of 6-MP to its inactive metabolites. This interaction is important given the increased incidence of hyperuricemia and gout after transplantation (59).

Diagnostic Tests

The complete blood cell count (CBC) should be monitored both after acute overdosage and during treatment. Liver function tests (including alkaline phosphatase and bilirubin), lipase, and amylase should be considered case by case. Measurements of plasma concentrations of azathioprine or 6-MP are not useful predictors of efficacy or toxicity.

Treatment

Treatment is symptomatic and supportive. The scant information available regarding the benefits of gastric emptying and activated charcoal administration limits their use in acute azathioprine overdose. These measures should be considered depending on the extent of the dose ingested and the presence of coingestants.

ENHANCEMENT OF ELIMINATION

Azathioprine and its metabolites can be removed by dialysis; however, the lack of acute severe toxicity indicates that this technique is rarely needed (60).

SUPPORTIVE CARE

When leukopenia develops, the dosage of azathioprine should be reduced or the drug discontinued depending on the leukocyte count and the patient's clinical condition. However, the rate of fall in the leukocyte count can be more important than the absolute level. If the white blood cell count falls as much as 40% in 1 day, it is recommended to promptly discontinue therapy (46). Dosage reduction minimizes the severity of adverse effects (51).

6-MERCAPTOPURINE

6-MP is the thiopurine metabolic product of azathioprine. It was seen as a powerful immunosuppressant for organ transplantation until the severity of its adverse effects was recognized. 6-MP depressed hematopoiesis, caused jaundice, and negatively affected the intestinal tract epithelium in animals. Azathioprine, the *S*-imidazole derivative of 6-MP, was adopted as the main immunosuppressive agent for renal allotransplants in humans because of lesser toxicity (46). As both drugs developed, they came to be used interchangeably, demonstrating similar efficacy and side effects. Recently, however, it has been demonstrated that severe life-threatening diarrhea can be caused by azathioprine and not 6-MP in IBD patients (47).

Toxic Dose

The *adult therapeutic dose* is 1.25 to 1.50 mg/kg body weight orally (47). The *pediatric dose* is 2.5 mg/kg daily.

Toxicokinetics and Toxicodynamics

A 6-MP standard dose has a bioavailability of just 5% to 37%. The relative bioavailability of high-dose mercaptopurine (500 mg/m^2) is 55% (37% to 77%) of the bioavailability of standard dose, and the area under the concentration-time curve (AUC) only increases fourfold. Once converted *in vivo* to active compounds (6-TGN), the metabolic process of 6-MP follows the same path as azathioprine. The half-life of 6-MP in plasma is between 1 and 2 hours, although 6-TGN accumulates in erythrocytes and has a half-life of 3 to 13 days (49).

Pathophysiology

6-MP achieves its cytotoxic similarity to azathioprine by inhibiting purine biosynthesis (49).

Pregnancy and Lactation

6-MP is FDA pregnancy category D (Appendix I). Entry into breast milk is unknown.

Clinical Presentation

ACUTE OVERDOSAGE

Ingestion of 1500 mg in a 15-year-old girl caused only minimal effects initially. Interestingly, 9.5 hours after the ingestion, 6-MP in peripheral blood cells was undetectable; however, the 6-thioinosine monophosphate level was 6.02 pg/10^6 cells and peaked to 26.3 pg/10^6 cells at 68.5 hours after the ingestion (61).

ADVERSE EVENTS

Because 6-MP is an azathioprine derivative, the toxicities of the two drugs are similar. Increased susceptibility to infection is the most serious effect of 6-MP. Other common adverse effects are pancreatitis, thrombocytopenia, normocytic and macrocytic anemia, fever, nausea, leukopenia, infection, and hepatitis (47).

The most significant clinical difference between azathioprine and 6-MP is their effect on patients with IBD. When azathioprine is converted to 6-MP *in vivo*, it also forms a nitroimidazole moiety that is cleaved from the azathioprine to form 6-MP. Researchers suggest that the imidazole derivative may be the cause of the severe diarrhea that may occur when patients are administered azathioprine but not 6-MP (47).

Diagnostic Tests

The CBC is monitored during treatment. Liver function tests (including alkaline phosphatase and bilirubin), lipase, and amylase should be considered case by case. Measurements of plasma concentrations of azathioprine or 6-MP are not useful predictors of efficacy or toxicity; hence, they are not routinely necessary.

Treatment

DECONTAMINATION

Limited data exist regarding the decontamination in acute 6-MP overdose. In the single case reported, syrup of ipecac and charcoal were administered (61). Whether the reported favorable outcome was related to these is unknown.

ENHANCEMENT OF ELIMINATION

6-MP and its metabolites can be removed by dialysis; however, the lack of acute severe toxicity indicates that this technique is rarely needed (60).

ANTIDOTE

There is no antidote for 6-MP toxicity.

SUPPORTIVE CARE

Treatment is symptomatic and supportive. As a dose-dependent agent, most of the adverse effects abate when the dosage is reduced or withdrawn (62).

SIROLIMUS

Sirolimus (rapamycin, Rapamune) is a macrocyclic lactone. Originating from a soil sample collected on Rapa Nui (Easter Island), *sirolimus* is a natural fermentation product isolated from the fungus *Streptomyces hygroscopicus*. As an alternative to calcineurin inhibitor therapy (cyclosporine and tacrolimus), it decreases the occurrence of acute rejection in renal transplant patients. It is used for other forms of transplantation as well. Sirolimus is available as an oral solution (1 mg/ml) or tablet (1 mg).

Toxic Dose

The usual *therapeutic dose* for adults after a renal transplantation is 0.2 to 5.0 mg/day and 1 mg/m^2/day in small children, with an initial loading dose three times greater than the maintenance dose (63). The dosage may have to be tapered during treatment to maintain target trough levels (64). A single overdosage of 150 mg was followed by transient atrial fibrillation in an adult (65).

Toxicokinetics and Toxicodynamics

Dosing depends on the indication and target trough blood concentration. There is strong correlation between trough concentrations and AUC estimates, so it is important to administer the drug accordingly (63). Oral bioavailability of sirolimus is 14%; the time-to-peak absorption ranges from 0.7 to 3.0 hours (66). Distribution is extensive to various tissues through a steady-state volume of distribution (V_d) of 7 to 15 L/kg and is metabolized by the CYP3A4 isozymes. The elimination half-life is 60 hours (67).

Pathophysiology

Sirolimus binds to the same enzyme substrate (FK506-binding protein 12) as cyclosporine and tacrolimus but blocks T-cell activation at a later time in the cell cycle. Unlike tacrolimus, sirolimus has no effect on calcineurin; rather, it binds to and inhibits the intracellular protein designated as the mamaliam target of sirolimus and the downstream janus tyrosine kinase, which are part of the IL-2–mediated signal transduction pathway and necessary for cytokine-induced T-cell activation. By preventing T-cell responses triggered by IL-2, IL-12, IL-7, and IL-15, sirolimus inhibits cell-cycle progression from G_1 to S phase (64,68). Additionally, sirolimus inhibits growth factor–mediated proliferation of nonimmune cells and prevents platelet-derived growth factor stimulation of smooth muscle cells (68).

Pregnancy and Lactation

Sirolimus is FDA pregnancy category C (Appendix I). Entry into breast milk is unknown.

Clinical Presentation

There is no information available for acute overdosage. The adverse events associated with the therapeutic use of sirolimus are related to the dose. The outcome of sirolimus use is a balance between under- and overdosing. Underdosing leads to acute rejection, whereas overdosing can cause thrombocytopenia, leukopenia, anemia, and hyperlipidemia (triglycerides and cholesterol) (63). Caution should be taken with concomitant use of sirolimus and CYP3A4-inhibiting drugs.

Diagnostic Tests

Monitoring the trough concentration is important in reducing adverse effects. Patients with trough sirolimus levels above 15 ng/ml have platelet counts roughly 25% lower than patients with trough levels less than 5 ng/ml. Conversely, patients with trough levels above 15 ng/ml had serum triglyceride levels 50% higher than patients with lower trough concentrations (67). Thus, it is recommended to monitor the triglyceride level, platelet count, and trough concentration. Monitoring of trough concentrations predicts inadequate immunosuppression (acute rejection) or drug-induced toxicity.

Treatment

The toxic effects of sirolimus typically resolve when the dose is reduced: Generally, halving the dose on the onset of an adverse effect leads to resolution within 1 week. If the toxicity persists for longer than 1 week, sirolimus should be discontinued until laboratory levels are normal (63). No data are available regarding the efficacy of decontamination or extracorporeal elimination in acute sirolimus toxicity.

MYCOPHENOLATE MOFETIL

MMF (CellCept) is a prodrug immunosuppressive agent. MMF is primarily used to prevent rejection of heart and kidney transplants, but recently it was introduced as an alternative treatment for IBD (69). MMF is available in oral (250- and 500-mg tablets) and IV forms (200 mg/ml).

Toxic Dose

The *adult and pediatric therapeutic dosage* is 1 g and 600 mg/m^2 twice a day. Dosage adjustment is necessary in patients with chronic renal insufficiency.

Toxicokinetics and Toxicodynamics

MMF is rapidly and completely hydrolyzed to an active metabolite, mycophenolic acid (MPA), which is then metabolized to an inactive metabolite, phenolic glucuronide. The oral bioavailability of MMF is 94%, and the V_d is 3.6 to 4.0 L/kg; protein binding of MPA is 97%. It is eliminated primarily by the kidneys. The plasma half-life of MPA is approximately 18 hours (depending on the route of administration). The AUC is dose dependent.

Pathophysiology

MMF noncompetitively inhibits inosine monophosphate dehydrogenase, thereby interfering with guanine nucleotide production and DNA replication. This pathway is required for lymphocytes to initiate purine synthesis so that MMF is able to have a selective effect on lymphocyte proliferation (68). MMF is a purine inhibitor. MPA, the active immunosuppressant form of MMF, is a specific inhibitor of *de novo* guanosine nucleotide synthesis without incorporation to the DNA. As a result of purine inhibition, both T and B lymphocytes are blocked from proliferation, and antibody production is prevented (70). MPA also inhibits leukocyte recruitment into sites of inflammation.

Pregnancy and Lactation

MMF is FDA pregnancy category C (Appendix I). Entry into breast milk is unknown.

Clinical Presentation

There is no information on acute overdosage. The adverse events after oral and IV administration are similar. The primary effects are local edema and inflammation, injection-site hemorrhage, phlebitis, and venous thrombosis among the patients who received peripheral infusion (70).

Additional effects occurring in transplant patients include bone marrow depression, nausea, hypophosphatemia, hyponatremia, renal failure, pain, hypertension, constipation, and vomiting (70–72). There is low incidence of GI effects, including hemorrhage, erosions, and perforation, in addition to vomiting and diarrhea. A small percentage of patients develop opportunistic infections (70).

Adverse effects occurring in patients with IBD consist of nausea and headache, arthralgia, and, possibly, severe GI events, including rectal bleeding, bloody diarrhea, and colonic ulceration (69).

Diagnostic Tests

The practice of therapeutic drug monitoring for MMF is still evolving. It seems that there is clinical evidence for a relationship between AUC for MPA and rates of acute rejection, which implies that therapeutic drug monitoring will become standard for MPA in the future (66). CBC monitoring and a chemistry panel are needed in patients receiving MMF.

Treatment

Most of the adverse effects caused by MMF are reversible by dose reduction or interruption. No data are available regarding the efficacy of decontamination. MMF and its metabolites are not removed by hemodialysis.

MONOCLONAL ANTIBODIES

Muromonab-CD3

Muromonab-CD3 (Orthoclone OKT3) is used primarily for acute allograft rejection treatment but is also effective as rescue treatment for transplant rejections that are resistant to conventional treatment. This immunoglobulin 2a originates through hybridoma technique in pathogen-free standard-bred mice. Muromonab-CD3 is always used with other immunosuppressive drugs such as cyclosporine or azathioprine and corticosteroids. It is available only IV.

TOXIC DOSE

The *adult therapeutic dosage* is 5 mg IV daily for 10 to 14 days. The *pediatric dosage* is 2.5 mg daily (less than 30 kg) (72).

TOXICOKINETICS AND TOXICODYNAMICS

A dosage of 5 mg/day for 14 days produced mean serum trough levels of 0.9 µg/ml (73). The V_d is 6.5 L (74). The elimination half-life is 18 hours (75).

PATHOPHYSIOLOGY

Muromonab-CD3 recognizes, binds, and blocks the CD3 complex of T-cell receptors. Specifically, it binds to one of the 20-kd glycoprotein subunits of the T-cell receptor. By doing so, it blocks the function of CD3 and prevents the generation and proliferation of effector T cells (76). After administration, there is a rapid decline of available CD3-positive cells, which reappear 2 to 7 days after completion of therapy. They reach pretreatment levels approximately 1 week after the treatment ends.

Muromonab-CD3 activates lymphocytes and monocytes, initially causing a significant cell lysis and cytokine release termed *cytokine release syndrome*. Levels of IL-2, IL-6, tumor necrosis factor (TNF), and interferon gamma rise and cause the acute clinical symptoms that accompany muromonab-CD3.

PREGNANCY AND LACTATION

Muromonab-CD3 is FDA pregnancy category C (Appendix I). Entry into breast milk is unknown.

CLINICAL PRESENTATION

The adverse effects associated with muromonab-CD3 can be divided into two primary groups: consequences of overimmunosuppression and effects that result from the activation of the immune system (cytokine release syndrome) (76). The toxicity associated with muromonab-CD3 may be dose dependent (77).

The cytokine release syndrome includes fever, chills, tachycardia, bronchospasm, pyrexia, dyspnea, chest pain and tightness, headache, vomiting, and diarrhea (72,77,78). These adverse effects usually do not occur with subsequent treatments.

Other effects, which can have a longer duration, are cytokine nephropathy, which causes deterioration of renal function; pulmonary edema, a rare but potentially very dangerous syndrome; coagulation disorders, which can lead to graft rejection; and central nervous symptom complications. The symptoms for central nervous system complications can be aseptic meningitis, meningismus, or more serious complications such as encephalopathy or typical encephalitis-complicated blindness (76).

The main toxicity of chronic use is increased risk of viral infection and development of human antimurine antibodies that could limit the effectiveness of muromonab-CD3 in future treatments or possibly cause anaphylaxis (72).

Cancer induction may result from immunosuppression, including risk of posttransplantation malignancies and lymphoproliferative disorders. It is debatable whether muromonab-CD3 alone causes this toxicity because it is always administered in conjunction with other immunosuppressives. It is clear, however, that the combination of muromonab-CD3 and cyclosporine does induce a high risk of malignancies. The other common type of adverse effect is infectious disease. Studies suggest that muromonab-CD3 enhances the occurrence of cytomegalovirus and herpes infections (76).

DIAGNOSTIC TESTS

Patients receiving muromonab-CD3 should be monitored with a CBC and renal function tests for the side effects, as previously described. The serum drug level should be maintained at the therapeutic level or above (Table 1).

TREATMENT

Research shows that most of the acute adverse effects are mediated by TNF release and can be ameliorated by premedication with hydrocortisone and antihistamines administered 0.5 hour before the initial injection of muromonab-CD3 (72). Another possible prophylactic measure is to inject a bolus injection of methylprednisolone (greater than 8 mg/kg) 1 hour before the administration of muromonab-CD3 in order to decrease TNF and interferon gamma levels. Using a monoclonal anti-TNF antibody, oral pentoxifylline, or indomethacin also reduces the occurrence and severity of cytokine release syndrome.

Daclizumab and Basiliximab

Daclizumab (Zenapax) is a humanized (10% murine, 90% human) anti–IL-2 receptor monoclonal immunoglobulin G antibody. It is used in conjunction with other immunosuppressants to prevent acute rejection after renal and liver transplant, and to treat acute graft-versus-host disease that is refractory to steroid treatment (79). It is derived from a recombinant gene, in which the hypervariable region from the mouse antibody anti-Tac has been introduced into a human framework (80).

Basiliximab (Simulect) is a chimeric monoclonal antibody (25% murine, 75% human) derived from a recombinant gene; the entire variable and constant regions are derived from mouse and human, respectively. Because of the similarity between daclizumab and basiliximab, this section focuses only on the adverse effects of daclizumab.

TOXIC DOSE

The *adult therapeutic dose* of daclizumab is 1 mg/kg IV. The drug is infused over 15 minutes every 14 days for five doses, with the first dose being given no more than 24 hours before the transplant occurs. The dose of basiliximab is 20 mg IV before transplantation, repeating the same dose 4 days afterward. In children, the dose is 12 mg/m^2, up to 20 mg/dose.

TOXICOKINETICS AND TOXICODYNAMICS

The V_d is 5.3 L/kg. The elimination half-life of daclizumab ranges from 11.4 to 20.0 days, which concurs with administration every 14 days. For the entire run of therapy (five doses over 10 weeks), the estimated duration of CD25 receptor suppression is 12 weeks (79).

PATHOPHYSIOLOGY

The IL-2 receptor (IL-2R), located on the T-cell surface, stimulates the multiplication and differentiation of those cells after exposure to a foreign antigen. The receptor is composed of three transmembrane protein chains: α (CD25), β (CD122), and γ (CD132). The α-chain is essential to form a functional receptor. Binding of IL-2 to IL-2R causes clonal expansion of the T lymphocyte, eventually leading to acute rejection of transplanted solid organs. Daclizumab selectively binds to the α-chain of IL-2R and prevents IL-2–initiated mitosis (80). The CD25 antigen is saturated by daclizumab, which blocks T-cell activation at serum levels of 5 to 10 μg/ml. At the recommended dose, this saturation is estimated to persist for 12 weeks after the initial dose (79).

PREGNANCY AND LACTATION

Daclizumab is FDA pregnancy category C (Appendix I). Basiliximab is pregnancy category B. Entry into breast milk is unknown for both agents.

CLINICAL PRESENTATION

The adverse effects (including malignancies) reported with daclizumab and basiliximab are similar to those reported with placebo. It is difficult to identify specific events because the agents are usually administered as part of a multiple immunosuppressant drug protocol. As with many protein-containing drugs, acute hypersensitivity reactions may occur. Furthermore, these agents can also cause the cytokine release syndrome as described for muromonab-CD3.

DIAGNOSTIC TESTS

Patients receiving immunosuppressant antibodies should be monitored with a CBC and renal function tests for the side effects, as previously described.

TREATMENT

GI decontamination is not needed because these drugs are administered parenterally and are proteins that are degraded if ingested. Their molecular weight is very large, making extracorporeal elimination not feasible. There are no antidotes available. Manifestations similar to cytokine release syndrome can usually be pretreated as described for muromonab-CD3.

REFERENCES

1. de Meer K, Houwen RHJ, Bijleveld CMA, et al. Blood concentrations after accidental cyclosporin overdose. *Eur J Pediatr* 1989;149:219–220.

1a. Baselt RC. Cyclosporine. In: *Disposition of toxic drugs and chemicals in man*, 5th ed. Foster City, CA: Chemical Toxicology Institute, 2000:231–232.

2. Jindal RM, Pescovitz MD, Cummings OW, et al. Persistence of cyclosporine after withdrawal of the drug in a patient with chronic liver transplant rejection. Role of the monoethylglycinexylidine test. *Transplantation* 1996;61(11):1657–1658.

3. Schroeder TJ, Wadhwa NK, Pesce AJ, et al. An acute overdose of cyclosporine. *Transplantation* 1986;41(3):406–409.

4. Honcharik N, Anthone S. Activated charcoal in acute cyclosporin overdose. *Lancet* 1985;1(8436):1051.

5. Nghiem DD. Role of pharmacologic enhancement of p-450 in cyclosporine overdose. *Transplantation* 2002;74(9):1355–1356.

6. Kokado Y, Takahara S, Ishibashi M, et al. An acute overdose of cyclosporine. *Transplantation* 1989;47(6):1096–1097.

7. Dussol B, Reynaud-Gaubert M, Saingra Y, et al. Acute tubular necrosis induced by high level of cyclosporine A in a lung transplant. *Transplantation* 2000;70(8):1234–1236.

8. Sketris IS, Onorato L, Yatscoff RW, et al. Eight days of cyclosporine overdose: a case report. *Pharmacotherapy* 1993;13(6):658–660.

9. Zylber-Katz E, Putterman C, Caraco Y. Multiple drug overdose in a kidney transplant patient. *Ther Drug Monit* 1994;16(3):327–331.

10. Cockburn I, Krupp P, Monka C. Present experience of Sandimmune in pregnancy. *Transplant Proc* 1989;21:3730–3732.

11. Briggs GG, Freeman RK, Yaffee SJ. Cyclosporine. In: *Drugs in pregnancy and lactation: a reference guide to fetal and neonatal risk*, 6th ed. Philadelphia: Lippincott, Williams & Wilkins, 2002:347–350.

12. Committee on Drugs, American Academy of Pediatrics. The transfer of drugs and other chemicals into human milk. *Pediatrics* 1994;93:137–150.

12a. Arellano F, Monka C, Krupp PF. Acute cyclosporin overdose: a review of present clinical experience. *Drug Saf* 1991;6:266–276.

13. Wallemacq PE, Lesne ML. Accidental massive IV administration of cyclosporine in man. *Drug Intell Clin Pharm* 1985;19:29–30.

14. Medina PJ, Sipols JM, George JN. Drug-associated thrombotic thrombocytopenic purpura-hemolytic uremic syndrome. *Curr Opin Hematol* 2001;8(5):286–293.

15. Baumhefner RW, Myers LW, Ellison GW, et al. Huge cyclosporin overdose with favorable outcome. *Lancet* 1987;2:332.

15a. Docci D, Baldrati L, Capponcini C, et al. Hemolytic uremic syndrome/thrombotic thrombocytopenia purpura in a patient with Behçet's disease treated with cyclosporine. *Nephron* 1997;75:356–357.

16. De Perrot M, Spiliopoulos A, Cottini S, et al. Massive cerebral edema after IV cyclosporin overdose. *Transplantation* 2000;70:1259–1260.

17. Paul LC. Overview of side effects of immunosuppressive therapy. *Transplant Proc* 2001;33(3):2089–2091.
18. Gijtenbeek JM, van den Bent MJ, Vecht CJ. Cyclosporine neurotoxicity: a review. *J Neurol* 1999;246(5):339–346.
18a. Powell-Jackson PR, Carmichael FJL, Calne RY, et al. Adult respiratory distress syndrome and convulsions associated with administration of cyclosporine in liver transplant recipients. *Transplantation* 1984;39:341.
19. Friedman LS, Dienstag JL, Nelson PW, et al. Anaphylactic reaction and cardiopulmonary arrest following intravenous cyclosporine. *Am J Med* 1985;78:343–345.
20. Goy JJ, Stauffer JC, Dervaz JP, et al. Myopathy as possible side-effect of cyclosporin. *Lancet* 1989;1:1446–1447.
21. Holman MJ, Gonwa TA, Cooper B, et al. FK 506-associated thrombotic thrombocytopenic purpura [Letter]. *Transplantation* 1993;55:205–206.
22. Breidenbach T, Kliem V, Burg M, et al. Profound drop of cyclosporin A whole blood trough levels caused by St. John's wort (*Hypericum perforatum*) [Letter]. *Transplantation* 2000;69(10):2229–2230.
23. Ernst E. St John's Wort supplements endanger the success of organ transplantation. *Arch Surg* 2002;137(3):316–319.
24. Anderson AB, Primack W. Treatment of a child with acute cyclosporine overdose [Letter]. *Pediatr Nephrol* 1992;6:222.
25. Venkataramanan R, Ptachcinski RJ, Burckart GJ, et al. The clearance of cyclosporine by hemodialysis. *J Clin Pharmacol* 1984;24(11–12):528–531.
26. Valbonesi M, Occhini D, Capra C, et al. Plasma exchange for the management of cyclosporin A-induced hypertriglyceridemia. *Int J Artif Organs* 1988;11:209–211.
27. Mrvos R, Hodgman M, Krenzelok EP. Tacrolimus (FK 506) overdose: a report of five cases. *J Toxicol Clin Toxicol* 1997;35:395–399.
28. Hardwick LL, Batiuk TD. Severe prolonged tacrolimus overdose with minimal consequences. *Pharmacotherapy* 2002;22(8):1063–1066.
29. McLaughlin GE, Rossique-Gonzalez M, Gelman B, et al. Use of phenobarbital in the management of acute tacrolimus toxicity: a case report. *Transplant Proc* 2000;32(3):665–668.
29a. Jain A, Venkataramanan R, Fung JJ, et al. Pregnancy after liver transplantation under tacrolimus. *Transplantation* 1991;52:106–110.
30. Briggs GG, Freeman RK, Yaffee SJ. Tacrolimus. In: *Drugs in pregnancy and lactation: a reference guide to fetal and neonatal risk*, 6th ed. Philadelphia: Lippincott, Williams & Wilkins, 2002:1303–1307.
31. Su M, Hoffman RS, Nelson LS. Acute tacrolimus overdose without significant toxicity. *J Toxicol Clin Toxicol* 2002;40:207–208.
32. Yeh CN, Hsieh CH, Hung CM, et al. Acute overdoses of tacrolimus. *Dig Dis Sci* 1999;44:1650–1652.
33. Curran CF, Blahunka PC, Lawrence ID. Acute overdoses of tacrolimus. *Transplantation* 1996;62:1376–1377.
34. Alessiani M, Cillo U, Fung JJ, et al. Adverse effects of FK 506 overdosage after liver transplantation. *Transplant Proc* 1993;25(1 Pt 1):628–634.
35. Atkison P, Joubert G, Barron A, et al. Hypertrophic cardiomyopathy associated with tacrolimus in pediatric transplant patients. *Lancet* 1995;345:894–896.
36. de-la-Serna-Higuera C, Marugan RB, Aviles J, et al. Tacrolimus-induced bone marrow suppression. *Lancet* 1997;350:714–715.
37. Fung JJ, Alessiani M, Abu-Elmagd K, et al. Adverse effects associated with the use of FK 506. *Transplant Proc* 1991;23(6):3105–3108.
38. Hibi S, Misawa A, Tamai M, et al. Severe rhabdomyolysis associated with tacrolimus. *Lancet* 1995;345:894–896.
39. Haviv YS, Friedlaender M, Dranitzki-Elhallel M. Chronic inflammatory demyelinating polyneuropathy possibly associated with tacrolimus. *Clin Drug Invest* 1999;18:169–172.
40. Przepiorka D, Suzuki J, Ippoliti C, et al. Blood tacrolimus concentration unchanged by plasmapheresis [Letter]. *Am J Hosp Pharm* 1994;51:1708.
41. Venkataramanan R, Jain A, Warty VS, et al. Pharmacokinetics of FK 506 in transplant patients. *Transplant Proc* 1991;23:2736–2740.
42. Hopp L, Lombardozzi S, Gilboa N, et al. *Clin Transplant* 1993;7:546.
42a. Corley CC, Lessner HE, Larsen WE. Azathioprine therapy of autoimmune diseases. *Am J Med* 1966;41:404.
43. Connell WR, Kamm MA, Ritchie JK, Lennard-Jones JE. Bone marrow toxicity caused by azathioprine in inflammatory bowel disease: 27 years of experience. *Gut* 1993;34:1081–1085.
44. Carney, Douglas M, Charles F, et al. Massive azathioprine overdose. Case report and review of the literature. *Am J Med* 1974;56:133–136.
45. Small P, Lichter M. Probable azathioprine hepatotoxicity: a case report. *Ann Allergy* 1989;62:518–520.
46. Pierce JC, Hume DM. Toxicity of azathioprine. *Laval Med* 1970;41:295–303.
47. Marbet U, Schmid I. Severe life-threatening diarrhea caused by azathioprine but not by 6-mercaptopurine. *Digestion* 2001;63:139–142.
48. Kruger C, Jungert J, Schmitt-Grohe S, et al. Azathioprine ingestion with suicidal intent by an adolescent with chronic juvenile polyarthritis. *Klinische Padietrie* 1998;210:136–138.
49. Schwab M, Klotz U. Pharmacokinetic considerations in the treatment of inflammatory bowel disease. *Clin Pharmacokinet* 2001;40:723–751.
50. Van OE, Zins BJ, Sandborn WJ, et al. Azathioprine pharmacokinetics after intravenous, oral, delayed release oral, and rectal foam administration. *Gut* 1996;39:63.
51. Martinez F, Nos P, Pastor M, et al. Adverse effects of azathioprine in the treatment of inflammatory bowel disease. *Rev Esp Enferm Dig* 2001;93:774–778.
52. Lennard L, Van Loon JA, Weinshilboum RM. Pharmacogenetics of acute azathioprine toxicity: relationship to thiopurine methyltransferase genetic polymorphism. *Clin Pharmacol Ther* 1989;46:149–154.
53. Jeurissen ME, Boerbooms AM, van de Putte LB. Pancytopenia related to azathioprine in rheumatoid arthritis. *Ann Rheum Dis* 1988;47:503–505.
54. Pozniak AL. Azathioprine-induced pancreatitis. *Arthritis Rheum* 1982;25:1149.
55. Cox J, Daneshmend TK, Hawkey CJ, et al Devastating diarrhea caused by azathioprine: management difficulty in inflammatory bowel disease. *Gut* 1988;29:686–688.
56. Bedrossian CWM, Sussman J, Conklin RH. Azathioprine-associated interstitial pneumonitis. *Am J Clin Pathol* 1984;82:148–154.
57. Kissel JT, Levy RJ, Mendell JR, Griggs RC. Azathioprine toxicity in neuromuscular disease. *Neurology* 1986;36:35–39.
58. Perreaux F, Zenaty D, Capron F, et al. Azathioprine-induced lung toxicity and efficacy of cyclosporin a in a young girl with type 2 autoimmune hepatitis. *J Pediatr Gastroenterol Nutr* 2000;31:190-192.
59. Cummings D, Sekar M, Halil O, et al. Myelosuppression associated with azathioprine-allopurinol interactions after heart and lung transplantation. *Transplantation* 1996;61:1661.
60. Bennett WM, Muther RS, Parker RA, et al. Drug therapy in renal failure: dosing guidelines for adults. Part II. *Ann Intern Med* 1980;93:286–325.
61. Hendrick D, Mirkin BL. Metabolic disposition and toxicity of 6-mercaptopurine after massive overdose. *Lancet* 1984:277.
62. Marion JF. Toxicity of 6-mercaptopurine/azathioprine in patients with inflammatory bowel diseases. *Inflamm Bowel Dis* 1998;4:116–117.
63. Kahan BD, Napoli KL, Kelly PA, et al. Therapeutic drug monitoring of sirolimus: correlations with efficacy and toxicity. *Clin Transplant* 2000;14:97–109.
64. Groth CG, Backman L, Morales J, et al. Sirolimus (rapamycin)-based therapy in human renal transplantation: similar efficacy and different toxicity compared with cyclosporine. *Transplantation* 1999;67:1036–1042.
65. Editorial staff. Tacrolimus/sirolimus. In: Toll LL, Hurlbut KM, eds. POISINDEX System. Greenwood Village, CO: Micromedex, 2003.
66. Kahan BD, Keown P, Levy GA, et al. Therapeutic drug monitoring of immunosuppressant drugs in clinical practice. *Clin Ther* 2002;24:330–350.
67. Meier-Kriesche, Herwig-Ulf, Kaplan K. Toxicity and efficacy of sirolimus: relationship to whole-blood concentrations. *Clin Ther* 2000;22[Suppl]:B93–B100.
68. Levy GA. Long-term immunosuppression and drug interactions. *Liver Transpl* 2001;7:S53–S59.
69. Skelly MM, Logan RFA, Jenkins D, et al. Toxicity of mycophenolate mofetil in patients with inflammatory bowel disease. *Inflamm Bowel Dis* 2002;8:93–97.
70. Pescovitz M, Conti D, Dunn J, et al. Intravenous mycophenolate mofetil: safety, tolerability, and pharmacokinetics. *Clin Transplant* 2000;14:179–188.
71. Catalano C, Fabbian F, Bordin V, Di Landro D. Mycophenolate mofetil toxicity in an anorexic kidney transplant patient treated with sulphinpirazone. *Nephrol Dial Transplant* 1997;12:2467–2468.
72. Jain A, Khanna A, Ernesto P, Molmenti, et al. Immunosuppressive therapy: new concepts. *Surg Clin North Am* 1999;79:59–76.
73. Orthoclone OKT3. Product information. Raritan, NJ: Ortho Biotech, 2000.
74. Goldstein G, Norman DJ, Henell KR, et al. Pharmacokinetics study of orthoclone OKT-3(R) serum levels during treatment of acute renal allograft rejection. *Transplantation* 1988;46:587–589.
75. Hooks MA, Wade CS, Millikan WJ Jr. Muromonab CD-3: a review of its pharmacology, pharmacokinetics, and clinical use in transplantation. *Pharmacotherapy* 1991;11:26–37.
76. Sgro C. Side-effects of a monoclonal antibody, muromonab Cd3/ orthoclone Okt3: bibliographic review. *Toxicology* 1995;105:23–29.
77. Parlevliet K, Fbemelman F, Yong S, et al. Toxicity of Okt3 increases with dosage: a controlled study in renal transplant recipients. *Transplant Int* 1995;8:141–146.
78. Walker RW, Brochstein JA. Neurologic complications of immunosuppressive agents. *Neurol Clin* 1988;6:261–278.
79. Berard JL, Velez RL, Freeman RB, Tsunoda SM. A review of interleukin-2 receptor antagonists in solid organ transplantation. *Pharmacotherapy* 1999;19:1127–1137.
80. Nashan B. The interleukin-2 inhibitors and their role in low-toxicity regimens. *Transplant Proc* 1999;31[Suppl 8A]:23S–26S.

CHAPTER 171

Gold

Seth Schonwald

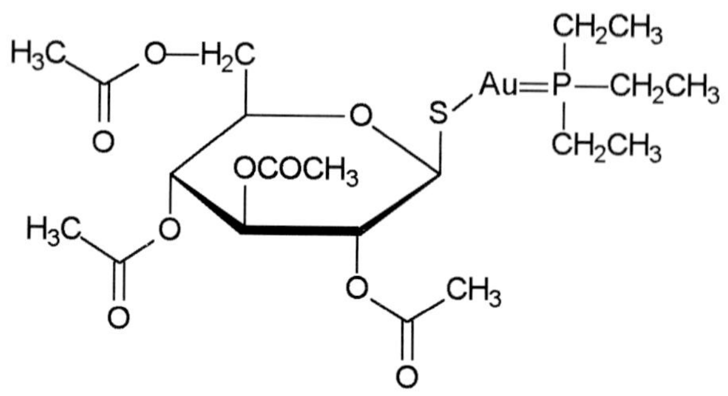

AURANOFIN

Synonyms:	**Disodium aurothiomalate (Myochrysine); aurothioglucose (Solganal); and auranofin (Ridaura)**
Molecular formula and weight:	**Aurothioglucose ($C_6H_{11}AuO_5S$), 392.2; auranofin ($C_{20}H_{34}AuO_9PS$), 678.5 g/mol**
SI conversion:	**Aurothioglucose, mg/L × 2.5 = µmol/L; auranofin, mg/L × 1.5 = µmol/L**
CAS Registry No.:	**39377-38-3 (disodium aurothiomalate); 12192-57-3 (aurothioglucose); 34031-32-8 (auranofin)**
Therapeutic level:	**Not used clinically**
Special concerns:	**Toxicity is often an iatrogenic error.**
Target organs:	**Bone marrow, gastrointestinal tract, kidney**
Antidotes:	**Dimercaprol, other chelating agents**

OVERVIEW

Gold has fascinated humans for centuries. The pharaohs of ancient Egypt used gold circa 3000 B.C., and it is mentioned several times in the Old Testament. Although most gold is used in jewelry production, it also has a variety of medical uses. Disodium aurothiomalate, aurothioglucose, and auranofin are pharmaceutical products used to treat rheumatoid arthritis. Pemphigus (1) and psoriatic arthritis (2) have also been treated with gold.

Dental amalgams containing gold are still desirable as crowns. An isotope, 198-Au, has been used to treat certain cancers (3) and as a tracer within the body (4). A fine leaf of gold is added to selected liqueurs such as Goldwasser. Certain exotic dishes are wrapped in extremely thin 99.9% pure gold leaf, and the gold is actually eaten.

Toxic Dose

The dosage of auranofin is 6 mg/day in one to two doses. The dosage of aurothioglucose is 10 mg intramuscularly (IM) the first week, then 25 mg/week for 2 weeks, then 25 to 50 mg/week until improvement or toxicity occurs (up to 1 g total dose). The maintenance dosage is 25 to 50 mg every 2 weeks for up to 20 weeks, then every 3 to 4 weeks. The dosage of gold sodium thiomalate is 10 mg IM initially, then 25 mg 1 week later, followed by 25 to 50 mg weekly until improvement or toxicity occurs (up to 1 g total).

Gold is not regulated by occupational and environmental government agencies in the United States. Ingestion of gold is harmless in small amounts; however, therapeutic doses can cause toxicity. Gastrointestinal distress can also result from excessive ingestion, but there are no reported deaths from overdose of gold-containing products. A 53-year-old man received 450 mg IM of sodium aurothiomalate. Palpebral edema and a rash were observed within 30 minutes. His gold blood level reached 2970 µg/dl without significant toxicity. The patient was treated with dimercaprol (BAL) and recovered (5).

TOXICOKINETICS AND TOXICODYNAMICS

Auranofin is 20% to 25% absorbed orally. Sodium gold thiomalate is rapidly absorbed after IM administration, and aurothioglucose is more slowly absorbed. Gold is distributed to many tissues, including erythrocytes, and is highly protein bound, mainly to albumin. It appears to concentrate in arthritic joints more than in uninvolved joints and in the liver, kidney, spleen, lymph nodes, bone marrow, and adrenal glands. Gold is excreted primarily by the kidneys (60% to 90%); 10% to 40% is excreted in the feces. The initial plasma half-life is 5.5 days; the terminal half-life is approximately 250 days. The apparent half-life in synovial fluid is 6 to 7 days.

PATHOPHYSIOLOGY

Gold plays an important role in initiation of the immune response, namely the uptake and presentation of foreign antigens. It is taken up by the macrophages and stored in the lysosomes (called *aureosomes*) where it inhibits antigen processing (6). Gold reduces lysosomal enzyme activity, decreases mast cell histamine release, and inactivates the first component of complement. It also suppresses phagocytosis by polymorphonuclear leukocytes. In patients treated with gold, decreased concentrations of rheumatoid factors and immunoglobulins are often observed. Auranofin has also been shown to inhibit chemotaxis, phagocytosis, and the inflammatory effects of prostaglandins.

PREGNANCY AND LACTATION

Auranofin, aurothioglucose, and sodium gold thiomalate are U.S. Food and Drug Administration pregnancy category C. Information on the safety of gold in pregnancy is limited (7). As lactating mothers under treatment with gold excrete significant amounts of gold into their breast milk, it has been recommended that they not breast-feed their infants.

CLINICAL PRESENTATION

Dermatologic Effects

Dermatitis is a common effect of gold therapy (8). Pruritus may warn of an impending cutaneous reaction and may occur in 10% to 15% of patients on gold therapy. Erythema and occasionally more severe reactions, such as papular, vesicular, and exfoliative dermatitis leading to alopecia and shedding of the nails, may occur. Yellow nails have been associated with gold therapy for rheumatoid arthritis (9).

Chrysiasis has been reported, especially on photo-exposed areas (10). Sunlight may aggravate gold dermatitis or cause an actinic rash. Stomatitis has also been described. A metallic taste may precede shallow ulcers on the buccal membranes; the borders of the tongue; and the palate, diffuse glossitis, or gingivitis.

Ophthalmologic Effects

Gold deposits may form in the lens or cornea. These deposits have not led to visual impairment, however, and clear within 3 to 6 months of cessation of therapy. Gold-induced interstitial keratitis has also been reported (11).

Respiratory Effects

Gold therapy can cause pneumonitis, ranging from mild to severe (12,13). "Gold lung" is a rare toxic effect that develops after a total dose of 300 to 1000 mg (14). Dyspnea appears suddenly over a period of 2 to 10 days. The chest radiograph shows diffuse bilateral pulmonary shading. Pulmonary function tests may show a restrictive defect (15). The prognosis is good after simple withdrawal of gold, but impairment may be permanent.

Allergic Effects

Allergic reactions from gold include anaphylaxis, angioneurotic edema, and the nitritoid reaction. The nitritoid reaction is a rare, unpredictable side effect of sodium aurothiomalate. It consists of a brief episode of facial flushing, nausea, dizziness, and occasionally hypotension (16). It occurs within minutes of an IM injection during the first week of treatment.

Gastrointestinal Effects

On rare occasions, gastrointestinal symptoms, such as nausea, vomiting, colic, anorexia, abdominal cramps, diarrhea, and ulcerative enterocolitis, occur during therapy (17). Gold-induced enterocolitis may follow treatment with either oral or injected gold and may involve any segment of the gastrointestinal tract. Hepatotoxicity is a rare consequence of parenteral gold therapy (18,19). Intrahepatic cholestasis with eosinophilia may be observed after gold injections (20). Hepatitis associated with neutropenia has been reported in a patient receiving injectable gold (21).

Hematologic Effects

Idiosyncratic agranulocytosis and aplastic anemia (22) may develop after gold therapy (23). Spontaneous neutrophil recovery may take 15 to 30 days after drug withdrawal. Enlarged regional lymph nodes may contain deposits of elemental gold (24). Lymphadenopathy and lymph node infarction may occur as a result of gold injections (25). Eosinophilia is commonly reported during gold therapy. Other hematologic findings include granulocytopenia, leukopenia, agranulocytosis, thrombocytopenia with or without purpura, panmyelopathy, and hemorrhagic diathesis. Thrombocytopenia from gold has been treated with cyclophosphamide (26).

Renal Effects

Renal toxicity is a well-described consequence of gold therapy (27). Proteinuria occurs in 2% to 20% of patients treated with injected gold and may cause nephrotic syndrome in 10% to 30% of those affected (28,29). Membranous glomerulonephritis may occur. Proteinuria usually resolves when the drug is stopped. Nephrotic syndrome or mild glomerulonephritis with hematuria subsides completely if recognized early and if treatment is discontinued. These may become severe and chronic if treatment is continued.

Neurologic Effects

Peripheral neuropathy and Guillain-Barré syndrome have been associated with gold therapy (30,31). Cranial nerve palsies and encephalopathy have also been reported (32,33).

DIAGNOSTIC TESTS

Gold is measured by atomic absorption spectrometry. Gold levels do not guide therapy or overdose management. "Normal" gold levels during therapy vary widely. The serum level after a single 50-mg IM dose was 255 μg/ml 168 hours after injection (34). It is estimated that auranofin, 3 mg twice daily for 12 weeks, would produce blood levels of 0.7 μg/ml (35).

A complete blood cell count, platelet count, and urinalysis should be monitored before every other injection or every 2 to 4 weeks. Liver enzyme monitoring every few weeks is also important. Proteinuria or hematuria may necessitate discontinuation of therapy. Rapid decrease in hemoglobin, white blood cell count less than 4000/mm^3, eosinophils greater than 5%, granulocytes less than 1500/mm^3, platelets less than 100,000 to 150,000/mm^3; albuminuria; hematuria, rash, dermatitis, pruritus, skin eruption, stomatitis, persistent diarrhea, jaundice, or petechiae may indicate gold toxicity.

Every candidate for gold therapy should be investigated fully to avoid administration of gold to those with gross renal or hepatic defects, diabetes, a history of blood dyscrasias, or exfoliative dermatitis. The presence of albuminuria, pruritus or rash, or eosinophilia is indication of developing toxicity, and gold therapy should be withheld for 1 to 2 weeks. When signs disappear, the course may be restarted on a smaller dosage.

TREATMENT

Acute ingestion is a rare problem that has not produced significant toxicity. Therefore, decontamination is not needed, and medical care is symptomatic and supportive. Adverse effects during treatment may have specific interventions. If signs of hematologic toxicity occur, glucocorticoids are usually used to reverse effects. A chelating agent, BAL, may be given to enhance gold excretion when glucocorticoids are ineffective.

Skin reactions are treated with systemic and topical antihistamines and steroids. If agranulocytosis, thrombocytopenia, or aplastic anemia is diagnosed, immediate treatment with BAL and corticosteroids has been advocated. More severe cases may require blood and platelet transfusions.

ANTIDOTES

Several chelating agents have been used to treat the adverse effects that appear to be caused by gold itself (rather than an immune response to gold). BAL (British antilewisite) has been used to treat overdose; however, effects have been variable (36,37). The dosage and administration are addressed in Chapter 50. Penicillamine at low dosage is an unreliable chelator of gold salts *in vivo*, and its use in the management of gold toxicity remains speculative (38). Dimercapto-propanesulfonate and *N*-(2-mercapto-2-methylpropanoyl)-L-cysteine (bucillamine) were effective antidotes in rats with gold-induced arthritis (39). Acetylcysteine has been used to remove/redistribute gold and reduce hematologic reactions. The dose was 2 to 9 g in 100 ml of crystalloid intravenous fluid infused over 2 to 6 hours. The total dose of acetylcysteine ranged from 13 to 153 g (40).

Finally, granulocyte colony-stimulating factor may be useful in reversing gold-induced absolute neutropenia. The dose is 5 µg/kg/day subcutaneously, increased to 10 µg/kg/day after 3 days (41).

REFERENCES

1. Pandya AG, Dyke C. Treatment of pemphigus with gold. *Arch Dermatol* 1998;134:1104–1107.
2. Lacaille D, Stein HB, Raboud J, Klinkhoff AV. Long-term therapy of psoriatic arthritis: intramuscular gold or methotrexate? *J Rheumatol* 2000;27:1922–1927.
3. Balat O, Edwards CL, Delclos L. Intraoperative gold grain implants for pelvic wall recurrences of various malignancies: toxicity, results, and failure analysis in 37 patients. *Eur J Gynaecol Oncol* 2000;21:472–474.
4. Hainfeld JF. Gold, electron microscopy, and cancer therapy. *Scanning Microsc* 1995;9:239–254.
5. Barelli A, Calimici A, Pala F. Gold salts acute poisoning: a case report. *Vet Hum Toxicol* 1987;29[Suppl 2]:108–110.
6. Burmester GR. Molecular mechanisms of action of gold in treatment of rheumatoid arthritis—an update. *Z Rheumatol* 2001;60:167–173.
7. Ostensen M, Ramsey-Goldman R. Treatment of inflammatory rheumatic disorders in pregnancy: what are the safest treatment options? *Drug Saf* 1998;19:389–410.
8. Suarez I, Ginarte M, Fernandez-Redondo V, Toribio J. Occupational contact dermatitis due to gold. *Contact Dermatitis* 2000;43:367–368.
9. Roest MA, Ratnavel R. Yellow nails associated with gold therapy for rheumatoid arthritis. *Br J Dermatol* 2001;145:855–856.
10. Langan SM, Harrison C, Wright GD. Unusual and memorable. Chrysiasis secondary to sodium aurothiomalate treatment. *Ann Rheum Dis* 1999;58:68.
11. Zamir E, Read RW, Affeldt JC, et al. Gold induced interstitial keratitis. *Br J Ophthalmol* 2001;85:1386–1387.
12. Sinha A, Silverstone EJ, O'Sullivan MM. Gold-induced pneumonitis: computed tomography findings in a patient with rheumatoid arthritis. *Rheumatology* 2001;40:712–714.
13. Blancas R, Moreno JL, Martin F, et al. Alveolar-interstitial pneumopathy after gold-salts compounds administration, requiring mechanical ventilation. *Intensive Care Med* 1998;24:1110–1112.
14. Richard AM. Gold lung. *N Z Med J* 1982;2:897–898.
15. Gortenuti G, Parrinello A, Vicentini D. Diffuse pulmonary changes caused by gold salt therapy. Report of a case. *Diagn Imaging Clin Med* 1985;54:298–303.
16. Healey LA, Baches MB. Nitritoid reactions and angiotensin-converting-enzyme inhibitor. *N Engl J Med* 1989;326:763.
17. Jackson CW, Habouli NY, Whorwell PJ, Schofield PF. Gold-induced enterocolitis. *Gut* 1986;27:452–456.
18. te Boekhorst PA, Barrera P, Laan RF, van de Putte LB. Hepatotoxicity of parenteral gold therapy in rheumatoid arthritis: a case report and review of the literature. *Clin Exp Rheumatol* 1999;17:359–362.
19. Koryem HK, Taha KM, Ibrahim IK, Younes LK. Liver toxicity profile in gold-treated Egyptian rheumatoid arthritis patients. *Int J Clin Pharmacol Res* 1998;18:31–37.
20. Farre JM, Peree T, Hautefemille P, et al. Cholestasis and pneumonitis induced by gold therapy. *Clin Rheumatol* 1989;8:538–540.
21. Uhm WS, Yoo DH, Lee JH, et al. Injectable gold-induced hepatitis and neutropenia in rheumatoid arthritis. *Korean J Intern Med* 2000;15:156–159.
22. Williame LM, Joos R, Proot F, Immesoete C. Gold-induced aplastic anemia. *Clin Rheumatol* 1987;6:600–605.
23. Brown SL, Hill ER. G-CSF in gold-induced aplastic anemia. *Ann Rheum Dis* 1994;53:213.
24. Rollins SO, Craig JP. Gold-associated lymphadenopathy in a patient with rheumatoid arthritis. *Arch Pathol Lab Med* 1991;115:175–177.
25. Roberts C, Batstone PJ, Goodlad JR. Lymphadenopathy and lymph node infarction as a result of gold injections. *J Clin Pathol* 2001;54:562–564.
26. Kozloff M, Votaw M, Penner JA. Gold-induced thrombocytopenia responsive to cyclophosphamide. *South Med J* 1979;72:1490–1492.
27. Schiff MH, Whelton A. Renal toxicity associated with disease-modifying antirheumatic drugs used for the treatment of rheumatoid arthritis. *Semin Arthritis Rheum* 2000;30:196–208.
28. Hall CL, Fothergill NJ, Blackwell MM, et al. The natural course of gold nephropathy: long term study of 21 patients. *BMJ* 1987;295:745–748.
29. Hall CL. The natural coma of gold nephropathy. *BMJ* 1988;296:293.
30. Weiss JJ, Thompson GR, Lazaro R. Gold toxicity presenting as peripheral neuropathy. *Clin Rheumatol* 1982;1:285–289.
31. Dick DJ, Raman D. The Guillain-Barré syndrome following gold therapy. *Scand J Rheumatol* 1982;11:119–120.
32. Fam AG, Gordon DA, Sarkozi J, et al. Neurologic complications associated with gold therapy for rheumatoid arthritis. *J Rheumatol* 1984;11:700–706.
33. Machtey I. Neurological signs in RA patients receiving gold. *Br J Rheumatol* 1996;35:804.
34. Lorber A, Atkin C, Chang CC. Antirheumatic action of gold salts observed in chrysotherapy. *Arthritis Rheum* 1970;13:333–334.
35. Berglof FE, Berglof K, Waltz DT. Auranofin: an oral chrysotherapeutic agent for the treatment of rheumatoid arthritis. *Arthritis Rheum* 1977;20:108.
36. Bunch TW. Gold overdose treated with BAL. *Arthritis Rheum* 1976;19:123–125.
37. England JM, Smith DS. Gold-induced thrombocytopenia and response to dimercaprol. *BMJ* 1972;2:748–749.
38. Davis P, Barraclough D. Interaction of D-penicillamine with gold salts: in vivo studies on gold chelation and in vitro studies on protein binding. *Arthritis Rheum* 1977;20:1413–1418.
39. Takahashi Y, Funakoshi T, Shimada H, Kojima S. The utility of chelating agents as antidotes for nephrotoxicity of gold sodium thiomalate in adjuvant-arthritic rats. *Toxicology* 1995;97:151–157.
40. Godfrey NF, Peter A, Simon TM, et al. IV N-acetylcysteine treatment of hematologic reactions to chrysotherapy. *J Rheumatol* 1982;9:519–526.
41. Collins DA, Tobias JH, Hill RP, et al. Reversal of gold-induced neutropenia with granulocyte colony-stimulating factor (G-CSF). *Br J Rheumatol* 1993;32:518–520.

SECTION

21

Over-the-Counter Products

CHAPTER 172

Over-the-Counter Products

Thomas R. Caraccio and Michael A. McGuigan

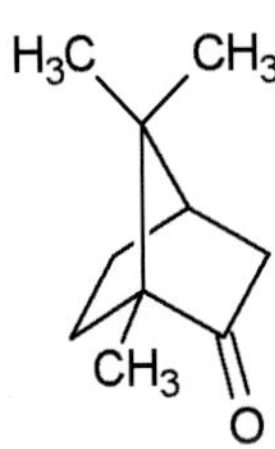

CAMPHOR

Compounds included:	**Bromide, camphor, ethanol (pediatric), fluoride, rhodamine B, sodium chloride (salt)**
Molecular formula and weight:	**Bromides, variable; camphor ($C_{10}H_{16}O$), 152.2; ethanol (C_2H_5OH), 46.1; fluoride (NaF), 19; rhodamine B, 479; sodium chloride (NaCl), 58.4 g/mol**
SI conversion:	**Bromide, mg/L × 12.52 = µmol/L; camphor, mg/L × 6.57 = µmol/L; ethanol, g/L × 21.7 = µmol/L; fluoride, mg/L × 52.6 = µmol/L; sodium, g/L × 43.5 = µmol/L**
CAS Registry No.:	**76-22-2 (camphor), 64-17-5 (ethanol), 7681-49-4 (fluoride), 81-88-9 (rhodamine), 7647-14-5 (sodium chloride)**
Normal level:	**Bromide, 0.5 to 1.0 mg/dl (0.060 to 0.125 mEq/L); ethanol, 0; fluoride, 0.01 to 0.20 mg/L (0.526 to 10.500 µmol/L); sodium chloride, 135 to 147 mEq/L**
Antidote:	**None**

BROMIDES

Bromides were introduced as anticonvulsants in 1857 by Lolock and later used as sedative-hypnotic drugs (1–3). The term *bromide* refers to the bromine ion usually in the form of various salts of the element bromine. Bromides were available as over-the-counter (OTC) preparations, such as Bromo-Seltzer, until 1971. Bromide was discontinued in some medications in 1978 because of teratogenicity concerns, and its use as a sedative was banned in 1990. Many drugs still contain a bromide ion (Table 1), but the use of these drugs does not result in bromide toxicity. Acute oral overdose of a bromide usually produces gastric irritation; chronic intoxication can result in a variety of neurologic, psychiatric, gastrointestinal (GI), and dermatologic effects. The commercial use of bromides (e.g., methyl bromide) is addressed in Chapter 251.

Bromides are found in photographic chemicals and hot tub and pool chemicals. Methyl and ethyl bromides are used as fumigant insecticides and in some fire extinguishers and refrigerants. Ethylene dibromide is a scavenger of lead in leaded fuels and a fumigant insecticide.

Toxic Dose

An ingestion of 100 g of sodium bromide over 36 hours was fatal in one adult patient (4). Carbromal, which contains an organic

TABLE 1. Medications containing bromide (Br)

Acetylcarbromal
Ammonium Br
Bromodiphenhydramine
Bromisovalum
Bromocriptine
Brompheniramine
Calcium bromogalactogluconate
Carbromal
Dexbrompheniramine
Dextromethorphan HBr
Halothane Br
Homatropine HBr
Neostigmine Br
Pamabrom
Pancuronium Br
Potassium Br
Propantheline Br
Pyridostigmine Br
Quinine HBr
Scopolamine HBr
Sodium Br
Vecuronium Br

HBr, hydrobromide.

form of bromide, has produced deaths in adults after ingestion of 10 g (5). Death due to bromide poisoning is rare.

A 50-kg adult ingesting a sodium bromide dose of 16.5 mEq/day would reach a possible toxic serum bromide level of 72 mg/dl after 8 days and a definite toxic level of 152 mg/dl after 25 days (6). Increasing the daily dose of pyridostigmine bromide from 640 to 1380 mg for 2 days in a 59-year-old woman with myasthenia gravis produced a negative anion gap and an elevated bromide concentration of 40 mg/dl (7).

Toxicokinetics and Toxicodynamics

Oral absorption is rapid and complete. The bioavailability of bromide is 96%. Peak blood concentrations occur within 2 hours but can be delayed up to 9 hours with carbromal (8). The volume of distribution is 0.35 to 0.48 L/kg. Bromide crosses the cell membrane more quickly than chloride, resulting in greater renal excretion of chloride. Reabsorption occurs in the renal tubule, with preference for bromide over chloride. The elimination half-life of bromide is 7 to 12 days but longer in renal failure (9). Chloride loading reduces the half-life of bromide to 3 days.

Pathophysiology

Once absorbed, bromide replaces chloride in cells, particularly in the brain where it stabilizes membrane function, impairing neuronal transmission and producing sedation (10). With high bromide levels, the kidneys increase the elimination of chloride ions in an attempt to maintain a constant total halide ion concentration.

Pregnancy and Lactation

Bromide passes through the placenta and enters breast milk. Fetal abnormalities, including "neonatal bromism," have been reported. Case reports suggest that prenatal exposure may cause growth retardation, craniofacial abnormalities, and developmental delay (9,11,12). Bromide enters the breast milk and may produce adverse reactions in the breast-fed infant (8).

Clinical Presentation

Acute ingestion of bromide causes nausea, vomiting, and abdominal pain in large amounts; therefore, most toxicity is due to chronic rather than acute exposure. Central nervous system (CNS) depression and coma have been reported. Constipation may occur. Tachycardia, hypotension, and possibly respiratory arrest have been reported.

Chronic oral bromide intoxication or "bromism" develops over 2 to 4 weeks and is manifested by neurologic and dermatologic changes along with elevated serum bromide levels. Neurologic features include behavioral changes (agitation, dementia, hallucinations, mental confusion, psychosis), tremor, irritability, anorexia, slurred speech, ataxia, lethargy, hyperreflexia, hypertension, and cerebral edema. There are reports of increased intracranial pressure with papilledema and increased cerebrospinal fluid protein occurring in 25% to 40% of patients. At one time, bromism was responsible for 3% to 7% of admissions to psychiatric facilities (1–3).

Dermal effects include an acneiform eruption on the face in up to 30% of cases. Granulomas of the skin, pigmentation, and bullae may be present (2). Stevens-Johnson syndrome may occur in 25% of patients. The typical bromide rash consists of pustule-studded or ecthyma-like plaques on the legs in 10% to 20% of patients. Bromoderma tuberosum manifests as tumor-like lesions. Hypertension and foul breath have been reported (2,3).

Diagnostic Tests

Bromide serum levels are reported in several different units. For conversion purposes:

$$1 \text{ mg/dl} = 0.125 \text{ mmol/L} = 0.125 \text{ mEq/L}$$

Serum bromide levels of 50 to 100 mg/dl may be associated with symptoms. *Bromism* is defined as a bromide concentration greater than 160 mg/dl (13). Bromide levels of 200 mg/dl produce toxic symptoms, and levels of 300 mg/dl may be fatal (14,15). Factors such as reduced salt intake, dehydration, diarrhea, vomiting, and renal failure may enhance bromide toxicity (10). Bromide intoxication causes a low anion gap.

Treatment

The first step is to control immediately life-threatening events (e.g., seizure) in the standard manner and then focus on increasing elimination of bromide. Further exposure should also be terminated. GI decontamination is rarely of use because acute poisoning often causes vomiting, and most poisoning arises from chronic ingestion. Activated charcoal does not adsorb inorganic bromide ions but may adsorb organic bromides.

ENHANCEMENT OF ELIMINATION

Aggressive hydration with normal saline and a diuretic may assist urinary excretion. Administer 0.9% sodium chloride intravenously (IV) at a rate sufficient to obtain a urine output of 4 to 6 ml/kg/hour. The use of furosemide or an osmotic diuretic may shorten the half-life of bromide. Therapy should be continued until the bromide level falls below 50 mg/dl (16,17). Hemodialysis is effective in removing bromide and may be useful in severe cases or in patients with renal failure.

TABLE 2. Camphor-containing products

Product	Camphor (%)
Absorbine Arthritic Pain Lotion	10
Act-On Rub Lotion	1.5
Anabalm Lotion	3
Aveeno Anti-Itch Conc. Lotion	0.3
Avalgesic[a]	—
Banalg Muscle Pain Reliever	2
Bangesic[a]	—
Ben Gay Children's Vaporizing Rub	5
Betuline Lotion[a]	—
Campho-Phenique First Aid Gel	10.8
Campho-Phenique Liquid	10.85
Campho-Phenique Powder	4.375
Counterpain Rub[a]	—
Deep Down Rub	0.5
Dencorub Cream	1
Dermal Rub[a]	—
Dermolin Liniment[a]	—
Emul-O-Balm	1.1
Heet Lotion	3
Heet Spray	3.6
Minit-Rub	3.5
Mollifene Ear Drops[a]	—
Musterole Regular	4
Panalgesic	3
Pronto-Gel	1
Save the Baby	6
Sloan's Liniment	3.35
Soltice Quick Rub	5
Suring Ointment	0.475
ThermoRub Lotion[a]	—
Vicks VapoRub	4.75
Vicks Vaposteam	6.2
Vicks Throat Drops	<0.5
Yager's Liniment[a]	—

[a]These agents list camphor as an ingredient, but the concentrations are not specified.
From Kauffman RE. Committee on drugs. *Pediatrics* 1994;94:127–128, with permission.

CAMPHOR

Camphor is a naturally occurring essential oil that was originally produced from the *Saliva officinalis* tree or the *Cinnamomum camphora* tree. Today, it is produced synthetically from turpentine. Camphor has been used as an external rubefacient; in moth balls (now removed from the market); as an aphrodisiac, cardiac stimulant, cold remedy, contraceptive, suppressor of lactation, and abortifacient; and as a topical analgesic for fever blisters and cold sores (18).

Camphor is an ingredient in many OTC products despite its classification by the U.S. Food and Drug Administration (FDA) as "not generally recognized as safe" (Table 2) (19). FDA regulations limit the camphor concentration in OTC products to less than 11%. Higher concentration products can be purchased in other countries. Camphorated oil was banned by the FDA in 1983, but camphor is still used as an herbal remedy and muscle liniment. Camphor is a rubefacient that has CNS stimulant effects, ranging from mild excitation to major motor seizures and status epilepticus (20).

Camphor has a characteristic penetrating aromatic odor and pungent aromatic taste. It produces a sensation of cold on the skin (21).

Toxic Dose

Clinically significant toxicity has not been reported with ingestions of less than 30 mg/kg and is uncommon with ingestions of less than 50 mg/kg (20). The probable adult lethal dose of liquid camphor is reported to be 50 to 500 mg/kg (20). An 84-year-old woman ingested an unknown amount of camphor moth balls and developed seizures after an attempted gastric lavage. She became hypotensive after administration of diazepam, and her respirations deteriorated. Seizures continued, and she died 40 hours after the ingestion (22).

In infants, 1 g of ingested camphor may be fatal (23). A 19-month-old child died after ingesting approximately 5 ml (1 g of camphor) of camphorated oil (24). The ingestion of more than 60 mg/kg or a single dose of 1 g in a child has resulted in syncope, cyanosis, hypotension, dysrhythmias, mental state changes, and convulsions. Rarely, death has been associated with ingestions of 60 mg/kg (25–27). Less than 10 mg/kg is unlikely to cause seizures. GI irritation and sedation may occur between 10 to 30 mg/kg (27).

Carcinogenicity tests using camphor alone have been negative (28).

Toxicokinetics and Toxicodynamics

Camphor is rapidly absorbed through the skin, mucous membranes, and GI tract. Protein binding is 61%, and the apparent volume of distribution is 2 to 4 L/kg. The absorption of camphor from the GI tract is facilitated by fatty substances or alcohol. Its onset of action is 5 to 20 minutes, with a peak effect within 90 minutes (18,24,25).

Camphor undergoes hepatic hydroxylation to the active metabolite campherol, which is oxidized to ketones and carbonic acid. Carbonic acid is conjugated with glucuronide before renal excretion. Pulmonary excretion causes a distinctive odor on the breath (18,25–27). The elimination half-life of camphor is 90 to 160 minutes.

Pathophysiology

Camphor acts as a CNS stimulant, but the underlying mechanism of toxicity is unknown.

Vulnerable Populations

Camphor is FDA pregnancy category C (29). Camphor crosses the placenta and has been involved in neonatal death (30).

Clinical Presentation

Acute camphor toxicity begins with nausea and vomiting and quickly progresses to CNS depression, seizures, respiratory failure, and death from respiratory arrest or status epilepticus (Table 3) (31). Monitor vital signs and observe carefully for the onset of convulsions. The pungent odor of camphor is usually present.

TABLE 3. Progression of severe camphor intoxication

Nausea and vomiting
Feeling of warmth, headache
Confusion, vertigo, excitement, restlessness, delirium, and hallucinations
Increased muscular excitability, tremors, and jerky movements
Tremors, progressing to epileptiform convulsions, followed by depression
Coma, central nervous system depression
Death from respiratory failure or from status epilepticus
Slow convalescence

From Koeppel C, Tenezer J, Schirop T, et al. Camphor poisoning: abuse of camphor as a stimulant. *Arch Toxicol* 1982;51:101–106, with permission.

CENTRAL NERVOUS SYSTEM EFFECTS

Classically, seizures may occur suddenly and without warning within 5 minutes of ingestion (25) and may be followed by coma. In a review of 748 patients, 42% had seizures after ingestion of 700 to 6000 mg of camphor (23). Apnea and visual hallucinations, confusion, tremors, and myoclonic jerking may occur (32,33). Other disturbances that may precede seizures include anxiety, confusion, dizziness, and facial fasciculation.

GASTROINTESTINAL EFFECTS

Initial symptoms include a feeling of warmth, thirst, nausea, spontaneous vomiting, epigastric burning, and abdominal pain. Aspiration of vomitus is a significant complication.

RENAL EFFECTS

Urinary retention, anuria, and albuminuria (transient) have been described. Elevation of the liver enzymes may occur and may mimic Reye's syndrome. The liver has shown fatty metamorphosis with no cell necrosis, inflammation, or biliary stasis (32).

Diagnostic Tests

Camphor plasma concentrations are not readily available and do not correlate well with symptoms. However, patients with a camphor plasma concentration of 1.5 μg/ml were asymptomatic, whereas those with seizures had levels of 19.5 μg/ml (19). A complete blood cell count, electrolytes, liver function tests, and renal function tests should be monitored. A chest radiograph may help in the evaluation of aspiration pneumonitis. Arterial blood gases should be evaluated as needed. Leukocytosis, albuminuria, and a transient rise in liver enzymes may occur.

Treatment

Treat seizures, twitching, or agitation with an IV benzodiazepine, such as diazepam; high doses may be required. Phenobarbital may be used for refractory seizures. In severe cases, thiopental anesthesia and a neuromuscular-blocking agent may be required.

Induced emesis is contraindicated because of the possibility of seizure (21). Activated charcoal has doubtful efficacy (18). Avoid giving fats, oils, alcohol, or milk, which increase absorption and the risk of aspiration (18).

Remove contaminated clothing, and wash exposed area thoroughly with soap and water. A physician may need to examine the area if irritation or pain persists after washing. There are no data on the effectiveness of multiple-dose–activated charcoal. Hemodialysis does not remove a significant amount of camphor due to its large volume of distribution.

There are no specific antidotes for the treatment of acute poisoning, but *N*-acetylcysteine may be effective in ameliorating liver damage in chronic poisoning (33,34).

If prolonged seizures occur, monitor arterial blood gases, body temperature, renal function, creatine kinase, and the urine for myoglobin.

Home observation without GI decontamination can be recommended for children who ingest less than 30 mg/kg of camphor (27). Medical evaluation and monitoring for symptoms (CNS depression or seizures) with seizure precautions should be considered for ingestions greater than 30 mg/kg in a child or more than 3 g in adults (25,33,35). Patients who are asymptomatic or who have only mild GI symptoms for 4 to 6 hours after ingestion are at low risk for serious complications (25,33).

ETHANOL IN CHILDREN (PEDIATRIC)

Ethanol is a two-carbon alcohol most commonly available in beverages. Perfumes, colognes, and aftershave products are the preparations most commonly involved in unintentional ethanol exposures in children younger than 6 years of age. However, alcoholic beverages produce the highest rate of emergency department visits for children as well as the highest hospital admission rates (36). Although the dose-related effects of ethanol are important, the primary concern for unintentional ethanol consumption by young children is the development of hypoglycemia.

Ethanol is present in numerous products, including beverages, colognes, perfumes, mouthwashes, antiseptics, and fuels, and in medications as a solvent (Table 4) (36,37). Except for the treatment of methanol or ethylene glycol poisoning, there are no therapeutic doses of ethanol.

Toxic Dose

The estimated lethal amount of ethanol in children is 3 g/kg (36,38). A 2-year-old child ingested 100 to 200 ml of gin and died 36 hours postingestion with a blood ethanol level of 52 mg/dl (39). One of 119 children was symptomatic after an estimated ingestion of less than 60 ml of a cologne, perfume, or aftershave product (50% to 99% ethanol); slurred speech and ataxia developed in two out of four children who ingested an estimated 60 to 105 ml of a cologne, perfume, or aftershave product (40). The minimum dose of ethanol that produces hypoglycemia has not been established.

Toxicokinetics and Toxicodynamics

Ethanol is rapidly and completely absorbed after oral ingestion. Peak levels occur in 0.5 to 3.0 hours; food impairs and delays absorption (41). Vapors are well absorbed through the lungs (41), and ethanol may be absorbed through intact skin of infants and children. Ethanol is not protein bound (41). The apparent volume of distribution is 0.6 L/kg (41).

TABLE 4. Approximate percent ethanol content of some common products

Product	Ethanol (%)
Aftershaves	15–80
Ale	3–6
Beer, lager	3–8
Colognes	40–60
Cooking wine	11–18
Cough medicine	5–25
Elixir	2–10
Fermented cider	4–7
Gasohol	10
Glass cleaners	9–10
Liqueurs (bourbon, brandy, cognac, gin, rum, scotch, tequila, vodka)	22–50
Lysol spray	68–79
Medications	0.3–68.0
Mouthwash, plaque rinse	6–27
Paint remover/stripper	25
Perfumes	25–95
Sterno (liquid fuel)	60–90
Sherry, port	6–13
Wine	10–14

Ethanol is oxidized in the liver by alcohol dehydrogenase and the mitochondrial ethanol oxidizing system (41); the rest is excreted unchanged through the lungs, sweat, and kidneys (41). The rate of elimination in children is approximately 28 mg/dl/hour (38). Details of ethanol metabolism are provided in Chapter 193.

Pathophysiology

The general mechanisms of the pathophysiology of ethanol in children are similar to those in adults (Chapter 193). The mechanisms by which ethanol induces hypoglycemia in well-nourished young children are not clear. Ethanol metabolism encourages the metabolism of pyruvate to lactate so that less pyruvate is available for gluconeogenesis in patients with depleted hepatic glycogen stores (38,42). Neither the dose of ethanol that puts a child at risk for developing hypoglycemia nor the time postingestion of the onset of hypoglycemia has been established.

Pregnancy and Lactation

Ethanol is FDA pregnancy category D; it is category X if used in large amounts or for prolonged periods (43). There is a significant, dose-related relationship between ethanol use by breastfeeding mothers and impaired motor development in their nursing infants (44).

Clinical Presentation

Acute ingestion of ethanol results in dose-related inebriation and CNS depression. Seizures may occur in young children (45). In addition, acute ingestion of ethanol may result in hypoglycemia in children (46,47).

Diagnostic Tests

Serum ethanol levels are rapidly determined by most hospital laboratories. In young children, there is reasonable correlation between blood ethanol levels and clinical presentation. No correlation has been established between the blood ethanol level at presentation and the subsequent development of hypoglycemia.

Treatment

Treatment is usually symptomatic and supportive. For most patients, the child can simply be observed for CNS depression until his or her serum ethanol level is below 50 mg/dl, and there is no evidence of hypoglycemia (36).

Emesis is not indicated because of the rapid absorption of ethanol and the potential for CNS depression. Activated charcoal does not effectively adsorb ethanol. Hemodialysis efficiently removes ethanol. There are no specific antidotes for ethanol.

FLUORIDE

Fluoride salts are used in low concentrations in toothpastes, mouth rinses, professional dental products, and dietary supplements (Table 5). Fluoride is commonly added to community drinking water and is found in small amounts in bottled water (48). Fluoride acts as a cellular poison, interfering with electrolyte balance and function of several enzymes. It binds with serum calcium and stimulates calcium uptake by bone to cause hypocalcemia, anticoagulation, and tetany. It also causes efflux of potassium from red blood cells, resulting in hyperkalemia, cardiac dysrhythmias, and sudden death. Ingested fluoride salts react with gastric acid to form hydrofluoric acid, resulting in local irritation.

TABLE 5. Fluoride product conversions from salt to fluoride ion

Fluoride compound	Amount of salt	Amount of fluoride ion
Sodium fluoride tablets	2.2 mg	1 mg
Sodium fluoride toothpaste	0.24%	1.1 mg/g
Sodium fluoride rinse	2%	9.1 mg/ml
Stannous fluoride	4.1 mg	1 mg
Stannous fluoride gel	0.4%	1 mg/ml
Stannous fluoride rinse	1.64%	4 mg/ml
Acidulated phosphate fluoride	1.23% fluorine	12.3 mg/ml
Sodium MFP	7.6 mg	1 mg
MFP toothpaste	0.76%	1 mg/g

MFP, monofluorophosphate.

Sodium fluoride is approved by the FDA for use in the prevention of dental caries. Studies indicate that fluoride may also be useful in combination with calcium and vitamin D in the treatment of osteoporosis and otosclerosis. Fluoride doses of 30 to 60 mg/day are recommended, in conjunction with calcium salts, for the treatment of osteoporosis (49). The daily dose of fluoride for preventing dental caries is 0.05 to 0.07 mg/kg/day.

Toxic Dose

A dose of 32 to 64 mg/kg of fluoride is potentially fatal in an untreated patient (50). Nausea and vomiting are associated with ingestion of 47 to 188 mg in contaminated drinking water (51). Death occurred after ingestion of 16 mg/kg of elemental fluoride by a 3-year-old boy (52).

Mild fluorosis has been seen after 0.1 mg/kg/day (53). Vomiting and abdominal pain are common with ingestions of 3 to 5 mg/kg elemental fluoride. Hypocalcemia and muscular symptoms appear after ingestions of 5 to 10 mg/kg (54).

Toxicokinetics and Toxicodynamics

Sodium fluoride and other soluble fluorides are readily and completely absorbed from the GI tract. The bioavailability of sodium fluoride and sodium monofluorophosphate dentifrices is 84% to 105% (55,56). Fluoride exists as a free ion in the plasma and is not bound to plasma proteins (57). Fluoride is bound to bone over several hours and is slowly released (58). This occurs to the extent of 50% in growing children but only 10% in adults (50). The apparent volume of distribution is 0.5 to 0.7 L/kg.

Half of ingested fluoride is excreted unchanged in the urine, 6% to 10% in feces, 13% to 23% in sweat, and the balance is retained in bone (57). An alkaline urine may hasten excretion (50). The elimination half-life normally is 1.2 to 9.0 hours but can be as long as 2 years in the presence of end-stage renal disease (59).

Pathophysiology

Sodium fluoride reacts with gastric hydrochloric acid to form hydrofluoric acid, which has direct corrosive effect on the gastric mucosa. The fluoride ion also chelates calcium (CaF_2) and stimulates calcium uptake by the bone as fluorapatite (in which four calcium ions are taken up for each two fluoride molecules), which lowers serum ionized calcium and may result in paresthesia, tetany, convulsion, coagulopathy, and cardiac dysrhythmias. Although fluoride reduces the extracellular calcium concentration, it increases the intracellular concentration of calcium and stimulates an efflux of potassium from the erythrocytes by opening the calcium-dependent potassium channels (60–62). The resulting hyperkalemia typically precedes death.

Fluoride binds with magnesium and interferes with many enzymes, particularly the cholinesterases and enzymes in which magnesium or manganese is present. Fluoride also stimulates adenyl cyclase, producing beta-adrenergic effects. Fluoride poisons the Na^+,K^+–adenosine triphosphatase on the cell surface; thus, potassium leaks out, and sodium moves into the cell. Oxidative phosphorylation also is impaired (61). Fluoride impairs the formation of collagen tissue and also has a direct action on muscle and nerve tissue that has been reported to result in neurologic disturbances (63). Fluoride poisoning also produces a metabolic acidosis (64).

Pregnancy and Lactation

Prenatal fluoride supplementation (2.2 mg NaF or 1 mg fluoride daily) during the last two trimesters of pregnancy is safe (65). Up to 25% of absorbed fluoride is excreted in breast milk, sweat, tears, and feces (64). Fluoride supplementation is recommended for breast-feeding babies (53).

Clinical Presentation

ACUTE EXPOSURE

Toxic effects typically begin within 1 hour of ingestion (66) but may be delayed up to 6 hours. An oral dose of 5 mg/kg produces GI irritation, sore tongue, sialorrhea, and a metallic taste, which may last 48 hours (66,67). Ingestion of more than 10 mg/kg is associated with more severe GI effects, such as nausea, vomiting, abdominal cramps, and hematemesis. Fluoride may produce convulsions and coma.

Cardiac disturbances include dysrhythmias and conduction disturbances, such as prolonged QT interval and peaked T waves; vasomotor instability may occur. Fluoride may produce direct myocardial depression. Pulmonary edema has been reported.

Fluoride intoxication is often associated with electrolyte abnormalities, such as hypocalcemia, hyperkalemia, hypokalemia, and hypomagnesemia. Hypocalcemia can develop very rapidly, and hyperglycemia and coagulopathies occur as a result. Musculoskeletal disturbances include tetany, muscle weakness, and respiratory paralysis. Hyperpyrexia and leukocytosis have been reported.

CHRONIC EXPOSURE

Chronic consumption of 1 parts per million fluoride in drinking water can cause mottling of the teeth. Exposure to 1.7 parts per million produces mottling in 30% to 50% of patients. Chronic poisoning may cause osteosclerosis, calcification of ligaments and tendons, bony exostoses, and renal calculi. "Fluorosis" is characterized by weakness, marked increase in bone density, and calcification of the soft tissues (64). A daily intake of 20 to 80 mg of fluoride for 29 years is required to produce chronic fluorosis (65).

Diagnostic Tests

Normal plasma fluoride concentrations range from 0.01 to 0.20 mg/L and are dependent on the fluorine concentrations in the water supply (68,69). Acute toxicity is associated with plasma fluoride levels above 2 mg/L. In acute poisoning, blood levels for fluoride are useful only within the first hour of ingestion because of rapid distribution. Urine levels may be more useful but should be obtained shortly after exposure because of rapid urine excretion. Neither plasma nor urine levels are readily or rapidly available.

Radiographs of the long bones may show evidence of fluorohydroxyapatite deposition. Radiograph evidence of aortic calcium deposits has been reported. Fluoride concentrations in bone ash from bone biopsies may be useful in confirming chronic exposure (68). Urine fluoride levels greater than 5 mg/L may indicate chronic toxicity (68).

Treatment

If the patient has a history of ingesting an OTC dental product containing fluoride in an amount less than 8 mg/kg of elemental fluoride, milk and observation at home are satisfactory (70).

If the ingestion is more than 8 mg/kg elemental fluoride or symptoms are present, administer milk immediately and refer to medical evaluation and monitoring. Maintain a protected airway and assist ventilation, if necessary. Hyperkalemia may be treated with IV calcium gluconate, sodium bicarbonate, or glucose and insulin therapy (Chapter 35). In severe cases that are refractory to treatment, consider hemodialysis. Adequate urine flow should be maintained. Neutral or slightly alkaline urine pH may enhance fluoride excretion. The patient must be monitored closely for cardiac dysrhythmias. Correction of electrolyte imbalance is crucial. Hypotension unresponsive to IV fluids and patient positioning may be treated with vasopressors, such as dopamine.

Seizures not responding to correction of electrolytes may be treated with an IV benzodiazepine, such as diazepam. Monitor electrocardiograph and serum calcium and potassium for at least 4 hours, and admit symptomatic patients to an intensive care setting.

GASTROINTESTINAL DECONTAMINATION

The use of activated charcoal, cathartics, or whole bowel irrigation is not expected to be of benefit (64). Emesis is not advised because fluoride can form hydrogen fluoride in the stomach, and emesis interferes with assessment of the toxic manifestations. Instead, administer calcium salts (e.g., calcium carbonate, calcium lactate, or milk) to minimize absorption by forming insoluble complexes with fluoride. Magnesium-containing antacids may also bind fluoride, although there are no reports of their use. Avoid calcium chloride because it can produce acidosis (67,70).

ENHANCEMENT OF ELIMINATION

Hemodialysis should be reserved for situations in which there is renal compromise, severe or refractory hyperkalemia or hypocalcemia, or life-threatening clinical toxicity. Hemodialysis may remove as much as 30% of fluoride (63). Fluoride binds rapidly to free calcium and bone, so hemodialysis may not be effective if performed late after ingestion.

There are no data indicating that charcoal hemoperfusion or peritoneal dialysis is beneficial.

ANTIDOTES

If more than 10 mg/kg of elemental fluoride has been ingested, an IV dose of 10% calcium gluconate (0.2 to 0.3 ml/kg in children or 10 to 20 ml in adults) is recommended along with electrocardiograph monitoring. If symptoms are present, follow the bolus with an infusion of 10% calcium gluconate, 150 ml/m^2/day (58). Do not use 10% calcium chloride (70).

If hypomagnesemia is present, treat with IV magnesium sulfate (1 to 2 g given over 10 to 15 minutes for adults; 5 to 50 mg/kg diluted to less than 10 mg/ml given over 10 to 15 minutes for children).

RHODAMINE B

Rhodamine B, also known as *basic violet 10*, is used as a color additive in drugs and cosmetics in the United States. This compound may be a reddish-violet powder or green crystals. Solutions are bluish red in color and fluorescent (71). Humans are exposed through some food products, cosmetics, and industrial uses. Toxicity has included mucous membrane irritation of the lungs, eyes, throat, nose, and GI tract as well as red urine. Because of potential toxic and carcinogenic effects, rhodamine B is no longer used as a food additive in the United States. There have been few human cases of overdose.

Rhodamine B is used primarily as a food additive (not in the United States), an analytic agent, a coloring agent in cosmetics, and to test for fuel leaks in various military vehicles (72–74).

Toxic Dose

No occupational standards have been established (75–77). The lethal dose and the minimum toxic dose are not known for adults or children. A 17-year-old boy ate several hundred milligrams of rhodamine in cookies without obvious toxic effect except for red urine (73).

Pathophysiology

Rhodamine appears to be an irritant and a possible carcinogen. It is carcinogenic in animals (78). When heated to decomposition, rhodamine emits chlorine, ammonia, and nitrogen oxide fumes (79).

Clinical Presentation

Seventeen patients were exposed to aerosolized rhodamine B for an average of 26 minutes (range, 2 to 65 minutes) (72). In order of frequency, symptoms were eye burning, tearing, nasal burning and itching, tightness in the chest, rhinorrhea, cough and difficulty in breathing, throat irritation, skin irritation, burning sensation in the chest, headache, and nausea. All of these symptoms resolved in 24 hours or less, and no patient developed any serious sequelae.

Various lymphomas, sarcomas, and stomach polyps have been noted in experimental animal testing (80).

Diagnostic Tests

There are no specific laboratory tests that have been shown to be of value. The urine may become fluorescent red. If pulmonary exposure is severe, a chest radiograph and other pulmonary function tests may be of diagnostic value.

Treatment

No decontamination should be needed because several hundred milligrams have been ingested without serious effect.

Remove contaminated clothing and wash exposed area thoroughly with soap and water.

Move patient to fresh air and monitor for respiratory distress. If cough or difficulty breathing develops, evaluate for respiratory tract irritation, bronchitis, or pneumonitis. Administer oxygen and assist ventilation as required. Treat bronchospasm with β_2-agonist and corticosteroid aerosols.

Irrigate exposed eyes copiously. If irritation, pain, swelling, lacrimation, or photophobia persists, the patient should be examined.

There are no antidotes or known methods for enhancing elimination of rhodamine B.

SODIUM CHLORIDE (SALT)

Sodium chloride is a ubiquitous substance. It occurs as colorless cubic crystals or white crystalline powder and is used primarily as a preservative or flavoring agent. Salt intoxication and death have occurred when hypertonic salt solutions have been inappropriately administered (81–106). Cases of abused children with acute hypernatremia have been attributed to the intentional administration of excess salt, with or without water deprivation.

Signs and symptoms of salt intoxication include vomiting, diarrhea, restlessness, thirst, dizziness, headache, seizures, coma, tachycardia, hypotension, and respiratory arrest. Sodium is responsible for more than 90% of the extracellular fluid osmolarity. Cerebral edema may occur if hypernatremia is corrected too quickly.

Toxic Dose

Because it is monovalent, 1 mEq of sodium equals 1 mmol. One g of sodium chloride equals 17.2 mEq. The bulk pour density of NaCl (table salt) is 1190 mg/ml; 1 teaspoon (5 ml) is 125 mEq NaCl.

The adult oral replacement dose is 3 to 6 g daily (107). The parenteral replacement dose varies depending on age, weight, and clinical condition of the patient (107). In children, the daily amount of sodium needed for growth is 0.5 mEq/kg from birth to 3 months of age and decreases to 0.1 mEq/kg at 6 months of age (108).

The estimated fatal dose of sodium chloride is approximately 0.75 to 3.00 g/kg (103). Death occurs with serum sodium levels above 185 mEq/L. The minimum toxic dose has not been established. The maximum tolerated sodium intake is 250 mEq/m^2/day (109). Because toxicity is closely related to serum sodium level, it is possible to calculate the potential change in serum sodium based on the ingested dose of sodium chloride:

$$\frac{\text{ingested dose (mg of NaCL)}}{\text{molecular weight of NaCl}} = \text{ingested dose of sodium (mEq)}$$

$$\frac{\text{ingested dose of sodium (mEq)}}{\text{volume of distribution (L)}} = \text{change in serum sodium (mEq/L)}$$

CNS signs are common with sodium levels above 150 mEq/L. At such levels, there is a 10% chance of seizures that increases as the sodium level reaches 160 to 185 mEq/L. Ingestion of sodium chloride in a dose of 0.5 to 1.0 g/kg (8.6 to 17.2 mEq/kg) is toxic in most patients (110).

An estimated dose of more than 400 mEq/kg resulted in brain injury and death in a 2-year-old child given a salt water solution to induce emesis (111). One level tablespoon (17.85 g) is approximately 305 mEq of sodium; if retained in a 3-year-old, 15-kg child, it would raise serum levels by 30 mEq/L.

Toxicokinetics and Toxicodynamics

Sodium is rapidly absorbed from the GI tract; it is also absorbed from rectal enemas. Intestinal wall absorption occurs via the Na^+,K^+–adenosine triphosphatase system that is augmented by aldosterone and desoxycorticosterone acetate. Sodium is not bound by plasma proteins. The volume of distribution is 0.64 L/kg (112).

The primary route of sodium excretion is the urine; additional excretion occurs in sweat and feces. The kidney filters sodium at the glomerulus, but 60% to 70% is reabsorbed in the proximal tubules along with bicarbonate and water. Another 25% to 30% is reabsorbed in the loop of Henle, along with chloride and water. In the distal tubules, aldosterone modulates the reabsorption of sodium and, indirectly, chloride. The renal threshold for sodium is 110 to 130 mEq/L. Less than 1% of the filtered sodium is excreted in the urine (113). Salt poisoning impairs the kidney's ability to excrete excess solute (114–117).

Pathophysiology

Oral administration of concentrated salt solutions causes irritation of the orogastric mucosa. Acute systemic salt poisoning produces CNS damage when brain cells become dehydrated after the acute osmotic shift of intracellular fluids to the extracellular space (118). Brain cell damage may also occur after idiogenic osmoles have been established and vigorous therapeutic hydration leads to cerebral edema. This may result in a diffuse encephalopathy with multiple small hemorrhages or thromboses.

Clinical Presentation

Acute systemic salt poisoning has been reported in many different situations. Hypernatremia has resulted from ingesting or aspirating seawater (serum sodium, 152 to 173 mEq/L). The Dead Sea in the Middle East contains 168 mEq/L of sodium, and the Great Salt Lake in Utah has a sodium concentration of 384 mEq/L (76). The inadvertent preparation of infant formula with salt instead of carbohydrate has resulted in individual and mass poisonings (87–91). In one of the first reported instances of mass salt poisoning, there were 6 fatalities out of 14 cases (87). Excessive ingestion of Karo syrup (sodium, 35 mEq/L) has produced hypernatremia (92).

The treatment of diarrhea with bouillon prepared by dissolving cubes or powder in inadequate amounts of water has caused significant hypernatremia (93). The administration of skim milk to ill infants has resulted in a subtle salt intoxication. The use of hypertonic nasal salt solutions has caused irritation of the nasal mucosa, with edema, inflammation, nasal obstruction, and respiratory distress in infants and small children (97). Overzealous use of hypertonic solutions or intraamniotic injections can result in symptomatic hypernatremia and permanent neurologic damage (98,99). Salt poisoning has occurred from the use of salt in enemas to treat high fevers, chronic constipation, and Hirschsprung's disease (100).

The GI effects of oral salt administration include swollen tongue, nausea, vomiting, diarrhea, abdominal cramps, and thirst (107).

Neurologic effects include thirst, irritability, weakness, headache, convulsions, and coma. Cerebral edema may occur, and muscle tremors may be noted. Cardiovascular manifestations of acute hypernatremia include both hypertension and hypotension. Tachycardia (107), cardiac failure, and peripheral edema may develop.

Pulmonary edema and respiratory arrest may occur (119). Renal insufficiency has been reported (119). Metabolic acidosis has been reported in an infant who received formula reconstituted with a hypertonic salt solution (sodium, 396 mEq/L) (119). Sweating may occur, and the skin may have a "doughy" consistency. Pitting edema may be noted in adults.

Diagnostic Testing

An elevated serum sodium concentration is the hallmark of acute or subacute salt poisoning and correlates with the clinical picture. When the serum sodium concentration is between 150 and 160 mEq/L, mild CNS symptoms are common, and seizures occur in approximately 10% of patients. With a concentration of 160 to 185 mEq/L, seizures occur more commonly, particularly if treatment precipitates a rapid drop in serum sodium. Fatalities occur at serum sodium concentrations greater than 185 mEq/L.

Computed axial tomography has revealed areas of hypodensity in the basal ganglion in infants with salt poisoning (118). Elevated cerebral spinal fluid protein concentration and an abnormal electroencephalogram have been associated with significant sodium chloride excess (120). Vacuolization of the renal tubular cells and acute tubular necrosis may be noted (117).

Treatment

Management should be directed at restoring normal osmolality and fluid volume. The speed of correction depends on the rate of development and the accompanying toxicity. Chronic hypernatremia requires a rate of correction of the sodium level that should not exceed 0.7 mEq/L/hour or approximately 10% of the serum sodium per day and correction of the fluid deficit over 48 to 96 hours. Rapid correction offers no advantage and may cause cerebral edema (112,116,121).

GASTROINTESTINAL DECONTAMINATION

Immediately dilute with 4 to 8 oz (120 to 240 ml) of water (not to exceed 4 oz or 120 ml in a child). Syrup of ipecac is not recommended for routine use, although it might be considered when the ingestion is caught early, and it appears that a large amount of salt might be retained. Activated charcoal does not effectively bind sodium.

ENHANCEMENT OF ELIMINATION

Indications for hemodialysis include a serum sodium level greater than 200 mEq/L, renal impairment, or moribund patient (120). The dialysate should contain a sodium concentration at least 10 mEq/L less than the serum sodium.

Although peritoneal dialysis does remove sodium, it is far less effective than hemodialysis. Peritoneal dialysis removed 53 mEq of sodium over 14 hours and reduced the serum sodium concentration from 189 mEq/L to 160 mEq/L (122). Peritoneal dialysis may require more than 24 hours of continuous exchanges to effect clinical improvement (113). Hemofiltration techniques may be useful in managing hypernatremia (120).

OTHER

The hydrating fluids need to be chosen carefully. In general, the hydrating solution should contain 20 to 60 mEq/L sodium chloride so that serum sodium is not reduced too fast (116). If the patient is acidotic, half of the sodium may be administered as sodium bicarbonate. The amount of water required to reduce the body sodium concentration should be provided slowly and the osmolality corrected over 24 to 72 hours. The usual fluid requirement is estimated at 150 ml/kg/day. The calculation of the total amount of free water for rehydration is

$$\text{water required (L)} = \frac{(\text{actual serum sodium}) - (\text{desired serum sodium})}{(\text{desired serum sodium}) \times [\text{total body water (L)}]}$$

ANTIDOTES

There are no antidotes to salt poisoning.

SUPPORTIVE CARE

Control seizures with diazepam or phenobarbital. Hypernatremic patients may have low insulin levels. If the blood glucose is above 130 mg/dl, a 2.5 % glucose solution should be used initially (121). Insulin is not used even if hyperglycemia exists because it may enhance sodium transport into the brain. To protect against tetany, calcium gluconate (10%), 10 ml in adults (0.2 to 0.3 ml/kg for children) in every 500 ml of fluid, has been recommended (116,121).

MANAGEMENT PITFALLS

Hypernatremic dehydrated infants may not appear severely dehydrated but are often febrile, lethargic, and irritable when aroused. The presence of hypernatremia with metabolic alkalosis suggests poisoning with a sodium-containing alkali. Rapid correction of hypernatremia offers no advantage over slow controlled correction and may cause cerebral edema and convulsions (112,116,121).

HOLIDAY HAZARDS

There is little question that holidays and vacations offer opportunities for unintentional exposures in young children. Parental distraction, household disruption, and the presence of unusual products all contribute to these exposures. The fact that these predisposing factors do lead to exposures has been documented by increased call volumes from parents temporally related to holiday seasons. A number of products have received considerable attention from poison centers and are reflected in public education materials. Serious poisonings are rare, however, and documentation of the true risks of poisonings is lacking.

The following discussion summarizes many of the issues that arise around a fall holiday (Halloween) and a winter holiday (Christmas). It is interesting to note that little public information has been generated regarding a spring holiday (Easter) or a summer holiday (Fourth of July), and almost nothing addresses the hazards associated with non-Christian holidays.

Halloween

If a parent suspects a tampering (e.g., torn wrapper, broken seal) and there has been no ingestion, discard the product (123,124).

If tampering is suspected and there has been an ingestion, seek emergency department evaluation.

If tampering is obvious (glass, foreign objects, razor blades) and no ingestion has occurred, the parent should report this immediately to the local police department.

The American Association of Poison Control Centers discourages hospitals from offering free x-ray screening of Halloween candy. Although radiographs of candy may show adulteration with some substances of a metallic nature, they offer no true screening to assure product safety. A negative radiograph may contribute a false sense of security that the item is fit to eat; it does not rule out contamination and is not a substitute for careful visual examination by parents.

Poison center and emergency room personnel are often asked about exposures to other common Halloween items, such as items listed below.

Dry ice: When ingested in solid form, oral burns may occur. Immediate dilution is recommended. It is not a problem in punch as long as no ice is ingested. Direct contact with the skin can also cause tissue damage. Irrigate immediately with lukewarm water.

Light sticks: Necklaces and bracelets that glow in the dark contain cyalume, a higher alcohol, which is usually not found in amounts large enough to be harmful if swallowed.

Makeup: Many types of makeup are nontoxic or contain small amounts of emollient laxatives, talc, or hydrocarbons. Treatment depends on the amount ingested, the ingredients of the specific product, and the presence of symptoms or signs.

Christmas

Potentials for harm during Christmas are summarized in Table 6.

BEVERAGES

Alcoholic beverages are often part of holiday celebrations. Children often imitate adults and drain partially filled glasses regardless of the contents. Small amounts of alcohol can be harmful or fatal to children by causing hypoglycemia and coma (see the section Ethanol in Children).

DECORATIONS

By their nature, children are attracted to decorations. They touch, taste, and manipulate these items. Be alert to the hazards associated with some of these (125,126).

Angel hair: Angel hair is made of spun glass, which can cause irritations of the eyes, skin, and digestive tract. Observe children for evidence of irritations or bleeding caused by angel hair.

Candles: Candles consist of wax and synthetic materials that are inert and not toxic. Coloring and scents are added in such small quantities that they do not present toxic problems. However, small chunks of candles may represent a foreign body risk.

Christmas tree ornaments: Christmas tree ornaments, often made of glass, metal, plastic, or foam, can be hazardous because they can act as foreign bodies, which can cut the skin, digestive tract, or air passages.

Christmas tree lights with bubbling fluid: The fluid in a single bulb contains a nontoxic amount of methylene chloride. If the contents of several bulbs are consumed, convulsions, coma, liver, and kidney damage may occur. The glass may cause internal cuts.

Fireplace colors or log colors: Fireplace colors or log colors are produced by metallic salts, which may be toxic if ingested in large quantities.

Gift wrapping: Gift wrapping often contains toxic metals. Metallic wraps should not be chewed or burned in the fireplace.

Metallic icicles or tinsel: Ingestions of these can cause intestinal irritation and can act as a foreign body. Because they usually contain lead and tin, they may be toxic with repeated ingestion.

Styrofoam: If swallowed, Styrofoam may produce irritation. Otherwise, it is not toxic.

Artificial trees: The plastic or metallic portions of artificial trees may cause GI tract irritations. Otherwise, they are not toxic.

Electrical connections: Check all electrical connections for proper insertion into outlets and contacts. Turn out tree lights when no adult is at home. Electrical fires can quickly consume trees, decorations, and packages.

Holiday Plants

Leaves, stems, flowers, and berries found on holiday plants are attractive nuisances for children (125). Some potentially toxic plants used during holiday times are boxwood, holly, mistletoe, Jerusalem cherry, and rhododendron (Chapter 255).

TABLE 6. Christmas hazards

Product	Ingredients	Hazard
Artificial Christmas tree	Aluminum, plastic	Mechanical obstruction, mucous membrane irritation
Christmas tree decorations		
Angel hair	Spun glass	Considered nontoxic in small amounts but may be irritating to mucous membranes
Icicles or tinsel	Polyvinyl chloride (metallized) aluminum coloring; some may be tin, lead, and plastic	Nontoxic but possibly may cause mechanical obstruction
Glitter or sparkles	Small pieces of plastic or glass	Nontoxic
Christmas tree ornaments	Metal, plastic, wood, glass	Nontoxic but may cause lacerations
Christmas tree lights	Glass	Nontoxic but may cause lacerations
Christmas tree bubble lights	Methylene chloride	Toxicity unlikely if small amount ingested
Christmas tree hook hanger	Metal	Possibility for choking if lodged in throat or esophagus
Homemade Christmas ornaments	Shellac, paint, polyurethane spray	Small amounts are not a problem
Snow spray or snow flock	Propellant, methylene chloride	Dry snow: nontoxic prolonged inhalation of spray; dizziness and headache may occur
Under the Christmas tree		
Crayons	Wax	Nontoxic
Candles	Wax	Nontoxic
Snow scene globes	Plastic or calcium carbonate	Potential for *Salmonella enteritis* if water is not sterile
Aftershave, perfume, toilet water, colognes	Can be up to 90% ethanol	Doubtful to see symptoms from this exposure, as children typically do not ingest more than a swallow of these products; if large ingestion does occur, may see drowsiness, ataxia, hypoglycemia
Sachets	Talc powder, essential oils	Small amounts not serious; may cause respiratory irritation or obstruction from powder
Airplane glue	Toluene, benzene, zylene	Mucous membrane irritation; inhalation can produce headache, dizziness, excitement
Disc battery	Various heavy metals, alkaline corrosive	If lodged in the GI tract, can cause erosion; location by x-ray is needed with follow-up to ensure passage
Battery	Acid or alkaline corrosive	Mucous membrane irritation or burns
Bubble bath soaps	Detergent	Vomiting
Silly putty	Silicones, glycerin, borates	Small amounts not serious; mechanical obstruction may occur with large amounts
Gift wrapping		
Ribbon and wrapping paper	—	Nontoxic
Tape	—	Nontoxic, possibility of obstruction
Ballpoint pens, felt tip pens	—	Not serious in small amounts
Watercolor paints	—	Nontoxic
Others		
Fireplace colors	Salts of metals, such as copper, selenium, lead	GI irritation; treatment depends on amount and type of salt ingested
Fireplace ashes	—	Nontoxic
Matches	Chlorates	20 wooden matches (not fireplace matches) or two books of paper matches not serious
Salt to melt ice	Sodium chloride	Hypernatremia

GI, gastrointestinal.

REFERENCES

Bromides

1. Sensenbach W. Bromide intoxication. *JAMA* 1944;125:769–772.
2. Perkins HA. Bromide intoxication: analysis of cases from a general hospital. *Arch Intern Med* 1950;85:783–794.
3. Hanes F, Yates A. Analysis of 400 cases of chronic bromide intoxication. *South Med J* 1838;31:667–671.
4. Sollmann T. *A manual of pharmacology*, 8th ed. Philadelphia: WB Saunders Co., 1957:85.
5. Baselt RC, Cravey RH. *Disposition of toxic drugs and chemicals in man*, 3rd ed. Chicago: Year-Book Medical Publishers, 1989:55.
6. Torosian G, Finger KF, Stewart RB. Hazards of bromides in proprietary medication. *Am J Hosp Pharm* 1973;30:716–718.
7. Rothenberg DM, Berns AS, Barkin R, et al. Bromide intoxication secondary to pyridostigmine bromide therapy. *JAMA* 1990;263:1121–1122.
8. Vaiseman N, Koren G, Peucharz P. Pharmacokinetics of oral and intravenous bromide in normal volunteers. *J Toxicol Clin Toxicol* 1986;24:403–413.
9. Mangurten HH, Kaye CI. Neonatal bromism secondary to maternal exposure in a photographic laboratory. *J Pediatr* 1982;100:596–598.
10. James LP, Farrar HC, Griebel ML, et al. Bromism: intoxication from a rare anticonvulsant therapy. *Pediatr Emerg Care* 1997;13:268–270.
11. Opitz JM, Grosse FR, Haneberg G. Congenital effects of bromism [Letter]. *Lancet* 1972;1:91–92.
12. Rossiter EJ, Rendle-Short TJ. Congenital effects of bromism [Letter]. *Lancet* 1972;2:705.
13. Bowers GN, Onoroski M. Hyperchloremia and the incidence of bromism in 1990. *Clin Chem* 1990;36:1399–1403.
14. Hanes FM, Yates A. Analysis of four hundred instances of chronic bromide intoxication. *South Med J* 1938;31:667–671.
15. Harenko A. Serum bromide level and its reduction in chronic bromisovalum poisoning. *Ann Med Int Fenn* 1967;56:173–176.
16. Adamson JS Jr, Flanigan WJ, Ackerman GL. Treatment of bromide intoxication with ethacrynic and mannitol diuresis. *Ann Intern Med* 1966;65:749–752.
17. Trump DL, Hochbergh MC. Bromide intoxication. *John Hopkins Med J* 1976;138:119–123.

Camphor

18. Dean BS, Burdick JD, Goetz PD. In vivo evaluation of the adsorptive capacity of activated charcoal for camphor. *Vet Hum Toxicol* 1992;34:297–299.
19. American Academy of Pediatrics Committee on Drugs. Camphor revisited: focus on toxicity. *Pediatrics* 1994;94:127–128.
20. Gleason MN, Gosselin RE, Hodge HC, et al. *Clinical toxicology of commercial products*, 4th ed. Baltimore: Williams & Wilkins, 1976:77–79.

21. Camphor monograph. In: Reynolds JEF, ed. *Martindale: the extra pharmacopeia* (CD-ROM version). Greenwood Village, CO: Micromedex Inc, 1988.
22. Nishimori S, Shimizu K, Honma, M et al. Camphor intoxication by mouth in an old female. *Nihon Kyukyu Igakukai Kanto Chihoukaishi* 1994;15:346–347.
23. Phelan WJ III. Camphor poisoning: the over-the-counter dangers. *Pediatrics* 1976;57:428–443.
24. Smith AG, Margolis G. Camphor poisoning: anatomical and pharmacologic study; report of a fatal case; experimental investigation of protective action of barbiturate. *Am J Pathol* 1954;30:857–868.
25. Geller RJ, Spyker DA, Garretson LK, et al. Camphor toxicity: development of a triage strategy. *Vet Hum Toxicol* 1984;26[Suppl 2]:8–10.
26. Siegel E, Wason S. Camphor toxicity. *Pediatr Clin North Am* 1986;33:375–379.
27. Gibson DE, Moore CP, Pfaff JA. Camphor ingestion. *Am J Emerg Med* 1989;7:41–43.
28. ACGIH. *Documentation of the threshold limit values and biological exposure indices*, 5th ed. Cincinnati: American Conference of Governmental Industrial Hygienists, 1986:75.
29. Briggs GG, Freeman RK, Yaffe SJ. *Drugs in pregnancy and lactation*, 5th ed. Baltimore: Williams & Wilkins, 1998:115.
30. Weiss J, Catalano P. Camphorated oil intoxication in pregnancy. *Pregnancy* 1973;52:713–714.
31. Koeppel C, Tenezer J, Schirop T, et al. Camphor poisoning: abuse of camphor as a stimulant. *Arch Toxicol* 1982;51:101–106.
32. Enez JF, Brown AL, Arnold WC, et al. Chronic camphor poisoning mimicking Reyes' syndrome. *Gastroenterology* 1983;84:394–398.
33. Koppel C, Martens F, Schirop T, et al. Hemoperfusion in acute camphor poisoning. *Intensive Care Med* 1988:14:431–433.
34. Riggs JR, Hamilton R, Homel S, et al. Camphorated oil intoxication in pregnancy. *Obstet Gynecol* 1965;25:255–258.
35. Goium S, Patel H. Unusual cause of seizure. *Pediatr Emerg Care* 1996:12:298–300.

Ethanol

36. Vogel C, Carracio TR, Mofenson HC, et al. Alcohol intoxication in young children. *J Toxicol Clin Toxicol* 1995:33:25–33.
37. Weller-Fahy ER, Berger LR, Troutman WG. Mouthwash: a source of acute ethanol intoxication. *Pediatrics* 1980;66:302–304.
38. Leung AK. Ethyl alcohol ingestion in children: a fifteen year review. *Clin Pediatr* 1986;25:617–619.
39. Parker CE. Ethanol poisoning: case report of coma, convulsions and death in a 2 yr old following ethanol ingestion. *Clin Pediatr (Phila)* 1967;6:686.
40. Scherger DL, Wruk KM, Kulig KW, et al. Ethyl alcohol (ethanol) containing cologne, perfume, and after shave ingestions in children. *Am J Dis Child* 1988:142:630–632.
41. Hollord NH. Clinical pharmacokinetics of ethanol. *Clin Pharmacokinet* 1987;12:272–292.
42. Rice LR, Hoffman SA. Ethanol induced hypoglycemia coma in a child. *Ann Emerg Med* 1982;11:202–204.
43. Briggs GG, Freeman RK, Yaffe SJ. *Drugs in pregnancy and lactation*, 5th ed. Baltimore: Williams & Wilkins, 1998:220.
44. Little RE, Anderson KW, Ervin CH, et al. Maternal alcohol use during breast-feeding and infant mental and motor development at one year. *N Engl J Med* 1989;321:425–430.
45. Ragan FA, Samuels MS, Hite SA. Ethanol ingestion in children: a five year review. *JAMA* 1979;242:2787–2788.
46. Leung AK. Acute alcohol toxicity following mouthwash ingestion. *Clin Pediatr (Phila)* 1985;24:470.
47. Leung AK. Ethanol-induced hypoglycemia from mouthwash. *Drug Intell Clin Pharm* 1985;19:480–481.

Fluoride

48. McGuire S. Fluoride content of bottled water. *N Engl J Med* 1989;321:836–837.
49. Richmond V. Thirty years of fluoridation: a review. *Am J Clin Nutr* 1985;41:125–138.
50. Heifetz SB, Horowitz HS. The amounts of fluoride in self-administered dental products: safety considerations for children. *Pediatrics* 1986;77:876–882.
51. Vogt RL, Witherell L, LaRue D, et al. Acute fluoride poisoning associated with an on-site fluoridator in a Vermont elementary school. *Am J Public Health* 1982;72:1168–1169.
52. Eichler HG, Lenz K, Fuhrmann M, et al. Accidental ingestion of NaF tablets by children. Report of a poison control center and one case. *Int J Clin Pharmacol Ther Toxicol* 1982;20:334–338.
53. AAP Committee on Nutrition. Fluoride supplementation. *Pediatrics* 1986;77:758–761.
54. Spoerke Vogt RL, Witherell L, LaRue D, et al. Acute fluoride poisoning associated with an on-site fluoridator in a Vermont elementary school. *Am J Public Health* 1982;72:1168–1169.
55. Trautner K, Einwag J. Human plasma fluoride levels following intake of dentifrices containing aminefluoride or monofluorophosphate. *Arch Oral Biol* 1988;33:543–546.
56. Drummond BK, Curzon ME, Strong M. Estimation of fluoride absorption from swallowed fluoride toothpastes. *Caries Res* 1990;24:211–215.
57. Ekstrand J, Alvan G, Boreus LO, et al. Pharmacokinetics of fluoride in man after single and multiple oral doses. *Eur J Clin Pharmacol* 1977;12:311–317.
58. Yolken R, Konecny P, McCarthy P. Acute fluoride poisoning. *Pediatrics* 1976;58:90–93.
59. McIvor ME. Acute fluoride toxicity: pathophysiology and management. *Drug Saf* 1990:41:129–138.
60. Baltazar RF. Acute fluoride poisoning leading to fatal hyperkalemia. *Chest* 1980;78:660–663.
61. McIvor M, Baltazar RF, Beltram J. Hyperkalemia and cardiac arrest from fluoride exposure during hemodialysis. *Am J Cardiol* 1983;51:901–902.
62. Cummings CC, McIvor ME. Fluoride-induced hyperkalemia: the role of calcium-dependent potassium channels. *Am J Emerg Med* 1988;6:1–3.
63. Berman I, Travis D, Mitra S, et al. Inorganic fluoride poisoning treatment by hemodialysis. *N Engl J Med* 1973;289:922.
64. McIver ME. Acute fluoride toxicity. *Drug Saf* 1990;5:79–85.
65. Glenn FB, Glenn WD, Duncan RC. Fluoride tablet supplementation during pregnancy for caries immunity: a study of the offspring produced. *Am J Obstet Gynecol* 1982;141:560–564.
66. Mack RB. Fluoride ingestion—cavity emptor. *Contemp Pediatr* 1988:5:115–124.
67. Augenstein WL, Spoerke DG, Kulig KW, et al. Fluoride ingestion in children: a review of 87 cases. *Pediatrics* 1991;88:907–912.
68. Hodge HC, Smith FA. Occupational fluoride exposure. *J Occup Med* 1977;19:12–39.
69. Fluoride. *Science* 1990;248:681.
70. Fluoride. In: Rodgers GA, ed. *AAP Handbook Pediatric Poisoning*. Elk Grove Village, IL: American Academy of Pediatrics, 1994:86.

Rhodamine B

71. Budavari S, ed. *The Merck index*, 12th ed. Whitehouse Station, NJ: Merck & Co Inc, 1996:320.
72. Dire DJ, Wilkinson JA. Acute exposure to rhodamine B. *J Toxicol Clin Toxicol* 1987;25:603–607.
73. Kelner MJ. Rhodamine B ingestion as a cause of fluorescent red urine. *West J Med* 1985;143:523–524.
74. IARC. *IARC monographs on the evaluation of the carcinogenic risks of chemicals to man.* Lyon, France: World Health Organization International Agency for Research on Cancer, 1978;16:221–231.
75. OSHA. *List of highly hazardous chemicals, toxics and reactives (mandatory)*. 29 CFR 1910.119, appendix A. Washington, DC: Occupational Safety and Health Administration, 1996.
76. NIOSH. *Pocket guide to chemical hazards. National Institute for Occupational Safety and Health* (CD-ROM version). Englewood, CO: Micromedex, Inc, 1996.
77. Webb JM, Hansen WH. Studies of the metabolism of rhodamine B. *Toxicol Appl Pharmacol* 1961;3:86–95.
78. RTECS. *Registry of toxic effects of chemical substances. National Institute for Occupational Safety and Health* (CD-ROM version). Englewood, CO: Micromedex, Inc, 1991.
79. Sax NI, Lewis RJ. *Hawley's condensed chemical dictionary*, 11th ed. New York: Van Nostrand Reinhold Co, 1987.
80. Hansen WH, Fitzhugh OG, Williams WM. Subacute oral toxicity of nine D&C coal tar colors. *J Pharmacol Exp Ther* 1959;122:29A(abst).

Sodium Chloride

81. DeGenaro F, Nyhan WL. Sal—a dangerous antidote. *J Pediatr* 1971;78:1048–1049.
82. Barer J, Hill LL, Hill RM, et al. Fatal poisoning from salt used as an emetic. *Am J Dis Child* 1973;125:889–890.
83. Laurence BH, Hokins BE. Hypernatremia following a saline emetic. *Med J Aust* 1969;1:1301–1303.
84. Roberts CJ, Nooks MJ. Fatal outcome from administration of a salt emetic. *Postcard Med* 1974;50:513–515.
85. Carter RF, Fotheringham BJ. Fatal salt poisoning due to gastric lavage with hypertonic saline. *Med J Aust* 1971;1:539–541.
86. Porath A, Mosseri M, Harman I, et al. Dead sea water poisoning. *Ann Emerg Med* 1989;18:187–191.
87. Finberg L, Kiley J, Luttrell CN. Mass accidental poisoning in infancy. *JAMA* 1963;184:187–190.
88. Rostad R, Blystad W, Knuturd O. Sodium chloride intoxication in newborn infants. *Clin Pediatr* 1964;3:1.
89. Hansted C. Alimentary salt poisoning. *Arch Pediatr* 1960;77:457.
90. Calvin ME, Knepper R, Robertson WO. Hazards to health: salt poisoning. *N Engl J Med* 1964;270:625–626.
91. Saunders N, Balfe JW, Laski B. Severe salt poisoning in an infant. *J Pediatr* 1976;88:258–261.
92. Hopp R, Woodruff C. Sodium overload from Karo Syrup. *J Pediatr* 1978;93:883–884.
93. Nomura FM Jr. Broth edema in infants. *N Engl J Med* 1966;274:1077.

94. Fujiwara P, Berry M, Hauger P, et al. Chicken-soup hypernatremia [Letter]. *N Engl J Med* 1985;313:1161–1162.
95. Fuchs S, Listernick R. Hypernatremia and metabolic alkalosis as a consequence of the therapeutic misuse of baking soda. *Pediatr Emerg Care* 1987;3:242–243.
96. Puczynski MS, Cunningham DG, Mortimer JC. Sodium intoxication caused by the use of baking soda as a home remedy. *Can Med Asoc J* 1983;128:821–822.
97. Utin LS, Bartlett GL Jr. Iatrogenic acute nasal obstruction in an obligate nasal breather. *JAMA* 1980;243:1657.
98. Frost AC. Death following intrauterine injection of hypertonic saline solution with hydatidiform mole. *Am J Obstet Gynecol* 1968;101:342.
99. Cameron JM, Dayan AD. Association of damage with therapeutic abortion induced by amniotic fluid replacement: report of 2 cases. *BMJ* 1966;1:1010–1013.
100. Moseley PK, Segar WE. Fluid and electrolyte disturbances as a complication of enemas in Hirshsprung's disease. *Am J Dis Child* 1968;115:714.
101. Pickel S, Anderson C, Holliday MA, et al. Thirsting and hypernatremic dehydration—a form of child abuse. *Pediatrics* 1970;45:54–59.
102. Rodgers D, Tripp D, Bentouim A, et al. Non-accidental poisoning: an extended syndrome of child abuse. *BMJ* 1976;1:793.
103. Baugh JR, Krug EF, Weir MR. Punishment by salt poisoning. *South Med J* 1983;76:540–541.
104. Dockey WK. Fatal intentional salt poisoning associated with radiopaque mass. *Pediatrics* 1991;87:964–965.
105. Smith EJ, Palevsky S. Salt poisoning in a 2 year old child. *Am J Emerg Med* 1990;8:571–572.
106. Meadow R. Salt poisoning in children. *Arch Dis Child* 1993;68:448–452.
107. Committee on Nutrition American Academy of Pediatrics. *Pediatric nutrition handbook*. Elk Grove Village, IL: 1985:23.
108. Habbick BF, Hill A, Tchang SP. Computerized tomography in an infant with salt poisoning: relationship of hypodense areas in the basal ganglia to serum sodium concentration. *Pediatrics* 1984;74:1123–1125.
109. Bennett DR. Daily dose of sodium bicarbonate. *JAMA* 1978;239:2385.
110. DeGenaro F, Nyhan WL. Salt—a dangerous antidote. *J Pediatr* 1971;78:1048–1049.
111. Hey A, Hickling KG. Accidental salt poisoning. *N Z Med J* 1982;95:864.
112. Sodium chloride monograph. In: Reynolds JEF, ed. *Martindale: the extra pharmacopeia* (CD-ROM version). Englewood, CO: Micromedex Inc, 1989.
113. Finberg L, Rush BF Jr, Chueng CS. Renal excretion of sodium in hypernatremia. *Am J Dis Child* 1964;107:483.
114. Simpson FO. Sodium intake, body sodium, and sodium excretion. *Lancet* 1988;1:25–28.
115. Feig PU. Hypernatremia and hypertonic syndromes. *Med Clin North Am* 1981;65:271–290.
116. Elton NW, Elton WJ, Nazareno JP. Pathology of acute salt poisoning in infants. *Am J Pathol* 1963;39:252.
117. Habbick BF, Hill A, Tchang SPK. Computed tomography in an infant with salt poisoning: relationship of hypodense areas in basal ganglia to serum sodium concentration. *Pediatrics* 1984;74:1123–1125.
118. Paut O, Andre N, Fabre P, et al. The management of extreme hypernatremia secondary to salt poisoning in an infant. *Paediatr Anaesthes* 1999;9:171–174.
119. El-Dahr S, Gomez A, Campbell FG, et al. Rapid correction of acute salt poisoning by peritoneal dialysis. *Pediatr Nephrol* 1987;1:602–604.
120. Oh MS, Carroll HJ. Disorders of the sodium metabolism: hypernatremia and hyponatremia. *Crit Care Med* 1992;20:95–103.
121. Moder KG, Hurley DL. Fatal hypernatremia from exogenous salt intake: report of a case and review of the literature. *Mayo Clin Proc* 1990;65:1587–1594.
122. Finberg L. Hypernatremia (hypertonic) dehydration in infants. *N Engl J Med* 1973;289:196.

Holiday Hazards

123. Mofenson HC, Caraccio TR. Tips to keep Halloween safe. *Long Island Regional Poison Information Center Newsletter*, 2001.
124. Janco N. Seasonal topics. Halloween hazards. *Rocky Mountain Poison Center Bulletin* 1988;7:6–7.
125. Mofenson HC, Caraccio TR. Dangers of holiday decorations and plants. *Long Island Regional Poison and Drug Information Center*, 2001.
126. *Rocky Mountain Poison Center Bulletin* 1990:9 and 1988:4.

PART

III

Drugs of Abuse

CHAPTER 173

Introduction: Drugs of Abuse

Jeffrey Bernstein

Those who cannot remember the past are condemned to repeat it.

—Santayana

Substance abuse is the use of psychoactive substance in a manner detrimental to the individual or society but not meeting criteria for substance or drug dependence. The abuse potential of a drug is defined as that property of a substance that, by its physiologic or psychological effects, or both, increases the likelihood of an individual's abusing or becoming dependent on that substance. An *addict* is defined as a person who is physically dependent on one or more psychoactive substances, whose long-term use has produced tolerance, who was lost control over his or her intake, and who would manifest with withdrawal phenomena if discontinuance were to occur. *Misuse* of a drug is defined as any use of a drug that deviates from a socially or medically acceptable use (1–3).

Abuse of a drug must be understood not only in medical terms but in social and political terms as well. We know that wine was used by the early Egyptians and remains in use in religious ceremonies in many cultures. The religious use of small amounts of alcohol would not be considered misuse despite the lack of medical indication. The use of opiates can be traced back to 4000 B.C., and medicinal uses for marijuana have been traced back to 2737 B.C. The sixth-century Peruvians had religious and cultural uses for cocaine. Traces of cocaine dating back to the year 1100 suggest that the Incas used cocaine for ritual trephination (4,5).

The golden age of drug abuse occurred during the nineteenth century concurrent with the ability to isolate specific chemicals from plants or other substances with abuse potential. Until that time, drugs were only available in plant form (e.g., cocaine and morphine). The advent of organic chemistry changed the availability of these drugs. During this time, addiction could occur via several avenues. Physicians either dispensed or wrote prescriptions for opiates, cocaine, and marijuana. Even without a physician's prescription, one could obtain these substances from a drugstore or a grocery store or even by mail order. In addition, because no law existed to require truth in advertising, one could become addicted from one of the many patent medicines on the market or from a medicine sold by a traveling tinker (6). This latter route to addiction remained in place until the Pure Food and Drug Act of 1906.

OPIOIDS AND COCAINE

Opium

Opium was brought to China in 1772 by Warren Hastings, the Governor of Bengal. Although the use of opium was illegal in China, Bengal merchants had been able to bribe local officials until 1839, when the emperor of China tried again to enforce a ban on open imports. Allied with Bengal, Great Britain declared war against the Chinese in 1842 to win the right to export opium to China (6).

In the United States, opium became associated with Chinese laborers who had immigrated during the building of the transcontinental railroad. Because the wives and families of these laborers were not permitted to immigrate, opium continued to play a large role in Chinese culture in the United States. Later when the job market became tight, sentiment against the Chinese laborers was linked to the use of opium. Propagandist media fanned the flames by printing reports that the idle rich were taking up opium smoking and that upper-class white women were being seduced into addiction by the opium den. This association was one of the earliest examples of a powerful theme in the American perception of drugs: linkage between the drug and a feared or rejected group within society (7–9). This sentiment led to the Chinese Exclusion Act of 1882 and eventually the total banning of the import of opium into the United States by the state of California in 1909.

A number of patent medicines containing opium or morphine could be bought in the United States without a prescription, including Ayer's Cherry Pectoral, Mrs. Winslow's Soothing Syrup, and Darby's Carminative. Godfrey's Cordial, a mixture of opium, molasses, and sassafras, was especially popular in England, and laudanum was used extensively to quiet crying babies. In the mid nineteenth century in Coventry, 10 gallons of Godfrey's Cordial (12,000 doses) was sold weekly and was administered to 3000 infants under 2 years of age (10–12).

The introduction of the hypodermic syringe into British medical practice in approximately 1860 contributed to the prevalence of addiction. Because pain could be controlled with less morphine when injected, it was presumed that this procedure was less likely to cause addiction (7).

In 1868, the Pharmacy Act made it illegal for anyone other than a registered chemist to sell opium (13). In 1898, Bayer synthesized aspirin and heroin and advertised both substances widely (13). By 1906, it was estimated that 13.5 million Chinese, or 27% of men, smoked opium.

A second wave of opiate addiction occurred in the 1930s and 1940s associated with the "beatnik" subculture of jazz musicians. The Vietnam War was another landmark time for the use of heroin: 40% of American soldiers in Vietnam admitted to the use of heroin. This information helped to drive the aggressive drug abuse policies of the Nixon administration. However, a survey 12 months after their return home showed that only 7% were still on drugs, suggesting that drug addiction was a surmountable disease (9).

In the late 1980s and throughout the 1990s, heroin saw a dramatic increase as a result of better methods of production and a change in the route of administration. The stigma of the needle was gone, and addicts could get the same high from nasal insufflation. A wave of movies produced by Hollywood and independent films glamorized the "opiate lifestyle" and helped to promote the trend (*Trainspotting*, *Shallow Grave*, and others) (14). Indicators from the Drug Enforcement Agency (DEA) (15) and the research from the National Institute on Drug Abuse (NIDA) (16–19) show that heroin availability and abuse represent a serious problem in the United States. In 2000, heroin/morphine was the second most frequently mentioned illegal drug reported to the Drug Abuse Warning Network (DAWN).

Currently, the National Drug Intelligence Center (NDIC) (15) and the DEA list controlled-release oxycodone (OxyContin) as the most commonly prescribed schedule II drug in the United States. However, poison center data indicate that hydrocodone produces the greatest number of contacts regarding drug abuse, followed by immediate-release oxycodone, methadone, and controlled-release oxycodone (20). Law enforcement reports indicate that prescription opioid drugs are attractive to the addict for their reliable strength and dosage levels. Often, an insurance provider covers the cost of the drug. In 2001, NDIC reported that doctor shopping was the most widely used technique of diversion, followed by improper prescribing practices and pharmacy diversion. The DEA reports that diversion of oxycodone has become one of their main priorities for the immediate future; however, it is clear that all abused prescription drugs (including benzodiazepines) are in need of intervention.

Cocaine

Cocaine was isolated in 1860 by Albert Neimann. Once its extraction had been refined, multiple products with cocaine became popular in Europe. The most notable was Vin Mariani, a coca wine produced in France by Angelo Mariani. The wine developed a loyal following throughout Europe and America and was marketed with enthusiastic endorsements from celebrities such as Anatole France, Henrik Ibsen, Jules Verne, Alexander Dumas, Sir Arthur Conan Doyle (21–23), Robert Louis Stevenson, Queen Victoria, King George I of Greece, King Alphonse XIII of Spain, the Shah of Persia, President William McKinley of the United States, and Dr. Gilles de la Tourette (7). Pope Leo XIII awarded Mariani with a gold medal for wine. Sigmund Freud published his major work *Uber Coca* (24) in 1884 and advocated the medical uses of cocaine, including a cure for morphine addiction. Replicas of the Mariani wine spread to the United States and Europe. One version of the wine was brought to America by an Atlanta pharmacist, J. S. Pemberton. As the temperance movement against the use of alcohol gained momentum, Pemberton was forced to remove the ethanol from his wine. The resultant bitter mixture was sweetened with a cola nut, imported from Africa and believed to have aphrodisiac and other properties. The resultant mixture was later renamed *Coca-Cola*. The J. S. Pemberton Chemical Company was later bought by two entrepreneurs, and the name of the company changed to the Coca-Cola Bottling Company. The cocaine in Coca-Cola was replaced with caffeine in 1903.

The works of Sir Arthur Conan Doyle reflected the attitude of society toward drug use. In 1890, he wrote, "'…for me,' said Sherlock Holmes, 'there remains the cocaine bottle and….'" Just a few years later, in 1896, Dr. Watson expresses concern for the drug mania that is threatening the career of his friend, Sherlock Holmes, in *The Adventure of the Missing Three-Quarter*. By 1887, even Freud had recanted his enthusiasm for cocaine as a wonder drug in his paper entitled "The Nervous System, Remarks on Craving for and Fear of Cocaine." In 1885, Robert Louis Stevenson wrote his masterpiece, *The Strange Case of Dr. Jekyll and Mr. Hyde*. The instant success of this work may reflect a society that was becoming alarmed about drugs such as cocaine (23).

Like opiates, cocaine had also been used for political agenda. In parts of the South on cotton plantations, railroad work camps, and construction sites, cocaine was believed to give black workers superhuman strength and to make them violent (7,25).

The late 1970s showed a resurgence of cocaine use as "coke" became the status drug associated with the fast lane (4). In the mid-1980s, crack cocaine, a purified, smokable form of cocaine selling for $5 a rock, brought cocaine to the working class. Cocaine continues to be the "number one drug threat" in the United States according to NDIC and DEA statistics (26).

MARIJUANA

Marijuana was brought to the United States by the Jamestown settlers, who grew the hemp plant for its fibrous properties and used it to make rope. During the nineteenth century, marijuana plants flourished in Mississippi, Georgia, California, South Carolina, Nebraska, New York, and Kentucky and was a major source of revenue for the United States. Between 1850 and 1937, marijuana was widely used as a medicinal drug and could easily be purchased in cough and cold remedies. The Mexican Revolution of 1910 brought a large wave of immigration into the United States and, with it, the habit of smoking marijuana. A significant rise in marijuana abuse occurred in 1920 with the Volstead Act, which raised the price of alcohol and made other drugs more attractive (7,26).

During the 1920s, larger numbers of workers migrated from Mexico to the United States to work in agriculture (7). As the Great Depression of the 1930s worsened, so did the job market, and the laborers became unwelcome and were blamed for the rise of violence in the larger cities. In 1931, New Orleans officials attributed many of the region's crimes to marijuana, which they believed was also a dangerous sexual stimulant (13). Drug use was no longer seen as the unfortunate consequence of a physician's prescription. Drugs were now associated with foreigners and racial minorities, popular attitudes that persist today.

Exaggeration became part of the strategy against drug addiction. In 1936, an article in the *American Journal of Nursing* reported that the user of marijuana "will suddenly turn with murderous violence upon whomever is nearest to him. He will run amuck with knife, axe, gun or anything else that is close at hand, and will kill or maim without any reason" (27).

Many products containing marijuana were available, particularly cough and cold preparations. Nevertheless, its prevalence for smoking "reefer" was low because the political climate did not favor abuse as it did during the introduction of opiates and cocaine (17).

The Marijuana Tax Act of 1937 imposed a transfer tax on marijuana. The federal government now had the authority to deny transfer stamps to individuals (6,28). It was not until the 1960s that marijuana use became prevalent again, when it became a symbol of protest against the established order of the parental generation and of the Vietnam War. Few people believed the extremist warnings of the dangers of drug use, and many witnessed firsthand the lack of deleterious effects. The credibility of the overstated warnings of the government were questioned as half of the nation's youth admitted to using marijuana.

In 1970, Richard Nixon created the National Commission on Marijuana and Drug Abuse. In 1972, the commission issued their report: "Marijuana: A Signal of Misunderstanding," that reliance on the criminal justice system was an ineffective approach to decreasing the use of marijuana. Realizing that it would not be practical to jail half of the nation's youth, the commission called for the decriminalization of marijuana. That same year the National Organization for the Reform of Marijuana Laws was founded. Lobbying throughout the 1970s was fruitful for National Organization for the Reform of Marijuana Laws decriminalization of marijuana for those caught with less than 1 oz, but in 1986 the Anti-Drug Abuse Act reinstated mandatory minimums and federal penalties for possession and distribution. Ten years later, the State of California legalized marijuana for use in the treatment of anorexia associated with acquired immunodeficiency syndrome and cancer (Proposition 215). Arizona followed suit later that same year (28).

PHENCYCLIDINE AND KETAMINE

Phencyclidine (PCP) was created in 1926 but remained unused until Parke-Davis marketed it in the late 1950s as a prototype dissociative anesthetic with little respiratory depression. Its medical use was abandoned early due to an unacceptably high incidence of side effects, notably postoperative psychomimetic effects (29). By 1967, its medical use was restricted to veterinary applications, but in the drug culture of San Francisco at that time it became popular as the "Peace Pill." Because of the dysphoria associated with its use, its popularity declined steadily until the early 1970s, when its use resurged. It became popular as a combined agent often associated with gang members looking to develop the reputation for taking the hardest possible drug. Another explanation for the resurgence during the 1970s was a change in the route of administration. Beginning in 1972, the drug was taken in pill form; however, in the 1970s, it became common to smoke the drug, usually in a marijuana cigarette (often called *angel dust*). This way the user could titrate the dosage easier and the incidence of unwanted side effects could be decreased (30).

A similar drug, ketamine, was synthesized in the 1960s and first given to a volunteer in 1966. The manufacturer described the drug as a rapid-acting induction agent suitable for use as a sole anesthetic for short procedures. Like PCP, its use has been limited by an unacceptably high incidence of emergence delirium (31). An upsurge of ketamine use occurred in the 1990s associated with the rave club scene, where the incidence of adverse events appears to be lower, perhaps secondary to lower dosage or oral route (31).

AMPHETAMINES

Phenylisopropylamine, the basic structure of amphetamine, was first synthesized in Germany in 1887. It was not until the 1920s that its potential use in asthma was explored (32,34). In 1932, an amphetamine (Benzedrine) inhaler was marketed as an over-the-counter treatment for allergic rhinitis and asthma. The use of amphetamines increased as the use of cocaine declined, particularly after a 1936 report of increased intellectual performance during amphetamine use. During World War II, amphetamines were used extensively in the military forces of the United States and Europe. In Japan, intravenous methamphetamine abuse reached epidemic proportions immediately after World War II, when military stockpiles became available to the public (36). The abuse potential for amphetamines was readily apparent, and large numbers of legal drugs, mostly used for the treatment of obesity, were diverted.

In 1965, Drug Abuse Control Amendments were enacted to deal with problems caused by abuse of depressants, stimulants, and hallucinogens. Amphetamines began to decline in use as a result of tighter scrutiny by the U.S. Food and Drug Administration (FDA). A resurgence of cocaine use developed as amphetamines became more difficult to obtain. In 1970, the Comprehensive Drug Abuse Prevention and Control Act categorized drugs based on abuse potential as compared to their therapeutic value. For the first time drugs were placed into schedules based on their abuse potential (Table 1) (37). The circulation of amphetamines became restricted, and legal production diminished. A loophole in the Comprehensive Drug Abuse Prevention and Control Act allowed for minor alterations to an amphetamine to result in a not yet classified and, therefore, legal drug. The mid 1970s and early 1980s saw a proliferation of "designer drugs" that had not yet been placed into a schedule. Most of these drugs were not being newly discovered. Methamphetamine, discovered by Ogata (38) in 1919, is easily manufactured from either amphetamine or even ephedrine, by adding a methyl group to the amino group of phenylisopropylamine. The product is phenylisopropylmethylamine. Methylenedioxymethamphetamine (MDMA; Ecstasy) was patented by Merck in 1914 (39).

The concept of a designer drug was not limited to amphetamines. Modifications of PCP, fentanyl, meperidine, and mescaline were produced, which yielded similar drugs to the parent compound. The loophole was closed with the Controlled Substances Analogue Enforcement Act of 1986, but the production of designer drugs continues because of the high demand and high profit margin of recreational drugs (40–42).

The 1990s again showed a resurgence of methamphetamine use when a smokable form of amphetamine, crystal methamphetamine, or "ice," entered the market. Today, the production of MDMA continues at epidemic numbers to supply the demand created by frequenters of raves and nightclubs.

TABLE 1. Summary of narcotic schedules created by the United States Controlled Substances Act

The drugs that come under the jurisdiction of the Drug Enforcement Agency (DEA), formerly the Bureau of Narcotics and Dangerous Drugs (BNDD), and the Controlled Substances Act are divided into five schedules.

Schedule I substances

Schedule I substances have no accepted medical use in the United States and have a high abuse potential. Some examples include heroin, marijuana, lysergic acid diethylamine (LSD), peyote, mescaline, psilocybin, tetrahydrocannabinols, ketobemidone, levomoramide, racemoramide, benrylmorphine, dihydromorphine, nicocodeine, nicomorphine, and others.

Schedule II substances

Schedule II substances have a high abuse potential with psychic or physical dependence liability. Schedule II controlled substances include certain narcotic, stimulant, and depressant drugs: opium, morphine, codeine, hydromorphone (Dilaudid), methadone (Dolophine), Pantopon, meperidine (Demerol), cocaine, oxycodone (Percodan), anileridine (Leritine), and oxymorphone (Numorphan). Also in schedule II are amphetamine (Benzedrine, Dexedrine) and methamphetamine (Desoxyn), phenmetrazine (Preludin), methylphenidate (Ritalin), amobarbital, pentobarbital, secobarbital, methaqualone, etorphine hydrochloride, diphenoxylate, and phencyclidine.

Schedule III substances

Schedule III substances have an abuse potential less than those in schedules I and II and include compounds that contain limited quantities of certain narcotic drugs and nonnarcotic drugs, such as derivatives of barbituric acid, except those that are listed in another schedule, glutethimide (Doriden), methyprylon (Nodular), chlorhexadol, sulfondiethylmethane, sulfomethane, nalorphine, benzphetamine, chlorphentermine, clortermine, mazindol, phendimetrazine, and paregoric.

Schedule IV substances

Schedule IV drugs have an abuse potential less than those listed in schedule III, including barbital, phenobarbital, methylphenobarbital, chloral betaine (Beta-Chlor), chloral hydrate, ethchlorvynol (Placidyl), ethinamate (Valmid), meprobamate (Equanil, Miltown), paraldehyde, methohexital, fenfluramine, diethylpropion, phentermine, chlordiazepoxide (Librium), diazepam (Valium), oxazepam (Serax), clorazepate (Tranxene), flurazepam (Dalmane), clonazepam (Klonopin), prazepam (Verstran), lorazepam (Ativan), mebutamate, and dextropropoxyphene (Darvon).

Schedule V substances

Schedule V drugs have an abuse potential less than those listed in schedule IV and consist of preparations that contain limited quantities of certain narcotic drugs, generally for antitussive and antidiarrheal purposes.

Methylphenidate (Ritalin) remains high on the NDIC list of drugs of diversion and abuse. The drug can be legally obtained and continues to be prescribed for hyperactivity and attention deficit disorders.

HALLUCINOGENS

Hallucinogens have been used since ancient times, for religious ceremonies as well as recreational abuse. The earliest hallucinogens were naturally occurring plants and fungi such as *Amanita muscaria* and psilocybin-containing mushrooms and ayahuasca (yage), a root indigenous to South America (39,43). Drug experimentation abounded in the United States and Europe during the 1960s as the culture attempted to get in touch with its spirituality. Romanticized by writers such as Castaneda in *A Yaqui Way of Knowledge* (44), people experimented with mescaline and Jimson weed (*Datura* species). The most commonly used synthetic compounds in the contemporary drug culture are MDMA, PCP, and ketamine (39).

Lysergic acid diethylamine (LSD) was discovered in 1943 by Albert Hofmann, a Swiss chemist working for Sandoz Laboratories. He was attempting to develop a new analeptic and subsequently described the first "acid trip" after topical exposure. The drug was tested for possible psychiatric uses as well as a truth serum by the U.S. military and the Central Intelligence Agency (40,43). The drug was abandoned in favor of other agents. Nontherapeutic use continued throughout the 1950s and 1960s. By the time that LSD became officially illegal in 1966, it was the most widely available psychedelic drug in the United States (45). Writers of the early 1960s (Kesey, Huxley, and Ginsberg) romanticized the drug, and LSD became linked to the counterculture made popular by the media coverage of the 1967 tribal "Be-in" in San Francisco's Golden Gate Park. The summer of 1967 became known as the "Summer of Love" in San Francisco. Although its popularity waned somewhat during the 1970s and 1980s, LSD made a resurgence in the 1990s, particularly among the rave culture. Its ease of manufacture assures that its production in clandestine laboratories will continue (46–50).

Raves

The rave phenomenon has been a major element in the resurgence of psychedelic drug use (39). Raves originated in Europe in the 1980s as secretive after-hours clubs, only open to a select group of people. They were known as *acid houses* in England and spread quickly to Germany (51). Often the location was not disclosed until several hours, or minutes, before the event. Partygoers would meet at a "map point" to receive further directions to the designated location. Raves became more commercialized in the 1990s, and they became less secretive. Entrepreneurs and business people have exploited raves, often renting out huge clubs or stadiums and charging $7 to $20 to enter the party. Pamphlets are passed out by the sponsors warning partygoers of the dangers of drug use and encouraging large quantities of water to be ingested (which are also for sale, marked up several times). Vitamins and juices are also sold to prevent the toxicity caused by the depletion of essential amino acids by MDMA. Raves have become associated with characteristic paraphernalia (40,52). Dealers who have drugs for sale often wear backpacks typically laden with PCP, MDMA, LSD, γ-hydroxybutyrate (GHB), ketamine, or rohypnol. Partygoers (ravers) who plan on using drugs, particularly stimulants, dress in multiple layers of lightweight loose-fitting clothing, intended to be stripped off as their temperatures rise from continuous vigorous dancing. Glow sticks are believed to enhance the visual perception changes associated with MDMA and LSD, and menthol vapor rub is inhaled to "enhance" the high from MDMA. Blow-pop lollipops are sold, and pacifiers are worn around the neck to combat the bruxism associated with amphetamine use.

So-called harm-reduction organizations have sprung up that are specifically associated with the rave culture. These organizations (http://www.dancesafe.org) purport to promote safety within the rave community. Stationed at the front of the rave location or nearby, they use home test kits to test purity of drug samples brought to the party. Most sell drug kits for home use, purchasable on their Web site.

EMERGING DRUGS OF ABUSE

Under the 1958 Food Additive Amendments to the Federal Food, Drug, and Cosmetic Act, the FDA is charged with making sure that food additives, including dietary supplements, are safe. However, with passage of the Dietary Supplements Health and Education Act of 1994, Congress amended the Food, Drug, and Cosmetic Act to include several provisions that apply only to dietary supplements and dietary ingredients of supplements (53,54). As a result of these provisions, dietary ingredients used in dietary supplements are no longer subject to the premarket safety evaluations required of other new food ingredients or for new uses of old food ingredients. This amendment opened the door for yet another epidemic of drug abuse that continues today.

GHB was originally synthesized in 1960 as an anesthetic agent (55,56). Its use was mostly abandoned due to lack of analgesia and presence of petit mal–type epilepsy in animal models. In the mid 1980s, the body-building community, fueled by the misinformation that GHB released growth hormone from the pituitary, created a market for GHB sold in nutrition stores. The abuse potential for GHB became readily apparent; soon it was marketed as everything from a sleep aid to "herbal Ecstasy." Because of increasing numbers of auto accidents and sexual assaults ("date rape"), the FDA called for the recall of all products containing GHB. As the products became scarce in food and nutrition stores, the internet market soared. A number of GHB analogs and prodrugs were produced in an attempt to circumvent the law. Gamma-butyrolactone, 1,4-butanediol, gamma-hydroxyvalerate, and gamma-valerolactone are just a few of these products. On February 18, 2000, the Hillory J. Farias and Samantha Reid Date-Rape Prohibition Act of 1999 (Public Law 106-172) was signed into law, legislating GHB as a schedule I controlled substance. Under this same law, rohypnol (flunitrazepam) was made schedule I in many states despite its legitimate use as a preanesthetic in many countries.

Other "nutraceuticals" and over-the-counter medications have evaded oversight by the FDA. Spurred by a multibillion-dollar industry, many over-the-counter drugs continue to be marketed for abuse. Ephedra and other stimulant products continue to be sold as diet aids, and sports supplements are marketed under the guise of being the "natural" herbs ma huang, guarana, and white willow. These supplements have been slow to regulate despite increasing reports of myocarditis (57–59) associated with ephedra and withdrawal of phenylpropanolamine from the market in 2000 for association with strokes.

Additionally, new products appear to be marketed specifically for abuse. In 2002, products that isolate dextromethorphan were marketed. More than one bar opened in the state of Florida in 2002 to serve kava to minors who are unable to purchase alcohol legally, apparently free from regulation because of the nutraceutical label that the herb carries.

NARCOTERRORISM

In the wake of September 11, 2001, the Office of National Drug Control Policy (ONDCP) and the DEA linked drug use to terrorism (60). Immediately after September 11, newsreels could be seen of Afghan farmers harvesting poppies for production of heroin. The DEA uses the following rationalization:

> It is clear that at times there have been connections between the drug trade and terrorist activities. The first connection is geographical. Terrorists and drug traffickers both search for bases in countries where the rule of law is weak. The second connection is money. There is a huge amount of money in international drug trafficking. Terrorists need a steady source of money to finance their operations, and they have often found it in drug trafficking. The third connection is violence. Both drug traffickers and terrorists use many of the same methods to achieve their evil ends.

However, the DEA keeps track of major heroin arrests, and, in the *National Drug Threat Assessment 2002* published by the NDIC (19), 60% of heroin analyzed in 1999 under the DEA Heroin Signature Program was found to be derived from South America, most prominently Colombia. Mexico, Southeast Asia, and Southwest Asia account for 24%, 10%, and 6% of heroin seizures, respectively. No specific mention of Afghanistan or other terrorist countries is made.

WAR ON DRUGS

In 1906, the Food and Drugs Act was passed. This act prohibited the interstate commerce in misbranded and adulterated foods, drinks, and drugs. Manufacturers of drugs could no longer make misleading statements about the content or ingredient of a medication, thus diminishing the risk of addiction from an undisclosed proprietary medication. Two years later, the Sherley Amendment prohibited not only the mislabeling of medications but also the labeling of medications with false therapeutic claims (61). This standard has been difficult to enforce, even today.

In 1914, Congress adopted the Harrison Narcotic Act. It required prescriptions by a physician or a pharmacist for products that exceeded the recommended quantity of narcotics. It also mandated record keeping by the physician and the pharmacist. For the first time in history, physicians' records were scrutinized. In 1919, the U.S. Supreme Court ruled that providing morphine to addicts without the intention of curing them violated the Harrison Narcotic Act (62,63).

In 1927, the U.S. Food, Drug, and Insecticide Administration was formed as an entity of the Bureau of Chemistry and was subsequently shortened to the FDA in 1930. At that time, what is known today as the *DEA* was located in the Department of the Treasury. From 1915 to 1927, it was in the Bureau of Internal Revenue, and it was moved to the Bureau of Prohibition from 1927 to 1930. In 1930, still under the Department of the Treasury, it became the Bureau of Narcotics, where it remained for the next 38 years. In 1968, the FDA Bureau of Drug Abuse Control and Treasury Department Bureau of Narcotics were transferred to the Department of Justice to form the Bureau of Narcotics and Dangerous Drugs and consolidate efforts against abused drugs. The reorganization of several federal health programs that same year placed the FDA in the Public Health Service. On July 1, 1973, Richard Nixon created the DEA by merging the Bureau of Narcotics and Dangerous Drugs, the Office for Drug Abuse Law Enforcement, the Office of National Narcotics Intelligence, elements of the U.S. Customs Service that worked in drug-trafficking intelligence and investigations, and the Narcotics Advance Research Management Team (http://www.justice.gov/jmd/mps/mission.htm). The primary mission of the DEA is the enforcement of the Controlled Substances Act.

In 1970, the Comprehensive Drug Abuse Prevention and Control Act categorized drugs based on abuse potential as compared to their therapeutic value. This "controlled substances act" has become the legal foundation for the government's fight against the illegal use of drugs of abuse. It places all substances that are regulated under existing federal law into one of five schedules (Table 1). This placement is based on the substance's medicinal value, harmfulness, and potential for abuse or addiction. Schedule I is reserved for the most dangerous drugs that have no recognized medical use, whereas schedule V is the classification used for the least dangerous drugs.

The White House ONDCP was established by the Anti–Drug Abuse Act of 1988. The ONDCP differs from the DEA and the NDIC in that the latter two agencies are located within the Department of Justice. The FDA, along with the Substance Abuse and Mental Health Services Administration (SAMHSA), the Centers for Disease Control and Prevention, and the National Institutes of Health (NIH), are located under the Department of Health and Human Services (HHS). The ONDCP, often referred to as the *Drug Czar*, reports directly to the President of the United States. The principal purpose of ONDCP is to establish policies, priorities, and objectives for the nation's drug control program. The goals of the program are to reduce illicit drug use, manufacturing, and trafficking; drug-related crime and violence; and drug-related health consequences. To achieve these goals, the director of ONDCP is charged with producing the National Drug Control Strategy. This strategy directs the nation's antidrug efforts and establishes a program, a budget, and guidelines for cooperation among federal, state, and local entities (http://whitehousedrugpolicy.gov) (60).

SAMHSA is an agency of the U.S. Department of HHS. It serves as the umbrella under which substance abuse and mental health service centers are housed, including the Center for Mental Health Services, the Center for Substance Abuse Prevention, and the Center for Substance Abuse Treatment. SAMHSA also houses the Office of the Administrator, the Office of Applied Studies, and the Office of Program Services.

DRUG ABUSE RESOURCES

Indices of Drug Abuse

The University of Michigan publishes *Monitoring the Future* through a grant from the NIDA. The report is a long-term survey of American adolescents, college students, and adults through age 40 (64). The results have been published yearly since 1975. In 2001, 44,300 students in grades 8, 10, and 12 from 424 schools participated in the study. A random subsample of twelfth graders is chosen each year for longitudinal follow-up. A standard set of three questions is used for each of the drugs surveyed, such as, "On how many occasions have you used LSD (acid) a. in your lifetime? b. in the past 12 months? c. in the last 30 days?"

In 2001, *Monitoring the Future* reported a continued increase in MDMA and anabolic steroid use, whereas a decline or trend toward decline was noted for inhalant use, cocaine, LSD, and alcohol. Heroin was also found to be trending downward; however, its use remains high, having reached all-time peaks in the late 1990s. Drugs that have held steady are marijuana, hallucinogens other than LSD, narcotics other than heroin, heroin with a needle, amphetamines, methamphetamine, crystal methamphetamine (ice), barbiturates, and the so-called club drugs: GHB, rohypnol, and ketamine.

Sources of Information

The Center for Substance Abuse Prevention is one of the SAMHSA centers. It houses the National Clearinghouse for Alcohol and Drug Information. It provides reference materials for the public and runs a 24/7 hotline (1-800-729-6686) for questions about drug abuse (http://www.health.org). A second center of SAMHSA, the Center for Substance Abuse Treatment (http://www.samhsa.gov/centers/csat2002/csat_frame.html), contracts the National Evaluation Data Services, the Treatment Improvement Exchange, a Substance Abuse Treatment Facility Locator, the Division of Pharmacologic Therapies, and the National Treatment Plan.

The Office of Applied Statistics serves as the data collection component of SAMHSA and performs several ongoing studies:

1. *DAWN* is an ongoing drug abuse data collection system sponsored by the SAMHSA Office of Applied Studies. It collects data from hospital emergency departments (ED) and medical examiners (http://www.samhsa.gov/oas/dawn.htm). The DAWN ED component relies on a nationally representative sample of hospitals to produce information on the number and characteristics of drug abuse–related visits to each ED in the coterminous United States and in 21 metropolitan areas. The DAWN mortality component produces information on drug abuse–related deaths, based on reports from participating medical examiners. DAWN cases (drug-related ED visits or deaths) include detailed information about the abuse of illegal drugs or legal drugs used for nonmedical purposes.
2. The *National Household Survey on Drug Abuse* started in 1971 and reports annually based on interviews with 70,000 people over the age of 12 from all states in the United States (http://www.samhsa.gov/oas/nhsda.htm).

The Drugs and Alcohol Services Information System has three components:

1. The *Inventory of Substance Abuse Treatment Services (I-SATS)* is a listing of all known public and private substance abuse treatment facilities in the United States and its territories (http://wwwdasis.samhsa.gov/dasis2/nssats.htm). Before 2000, the I-SATS was known as the National Master Facility Inventory.
2. The *National Survey of Substance Abuse Treatment Services (N-SSATS)* is an annual survey of all facilities in the I-SATS that collects information on location, characteristics, services offered, and utilization. Information from the N-SSATS is used to compile and update the National Directory of Drug and Alcohol Abuse Treatment Programs and the online Substance Abuse Treatment Facility Locator (http://findtreatment.samhsa.gov). The N-SSATS includes a periodic survey of substance abuse treatment in adult and juvenile correctional facilities. Before 2000, the N-SSATS was known as the *Uniform Facility Data Set*.
3. *The Treatment Episode Data Set* is a compilation of data on the demographic and substance abuse characteristics of admissions to substance abuse treatment (http://www.icpsr.umich.edu:8080/SAMHDA-SERIES/00056.xml). Information on treatment admissions is routinely collected by state administrative systems and then submitted to SAMHSA in a standard format.

SAMHSA also subcontracts several clearinghouses for the dissemination of drug and mental health information. The NDIC was established in 1993 as a component of the U.S. Department of Justice and serves as an intelligence-gathering agency for the DEA, the Federal Bureau of Investigation, and the ONDCP. The NDIC publishes the annual National Drug Threat Assessment, State Drug Threat Assessments, Bulletins and Briefs, and Drug Type Threat Assessments (http://www.usdoj.gov/ndic/).

The NIH within HHS contains 27 institutes and centers. Two of them concern drug abuse and alcoholism. NIDA publishes an ongoing monograph series that can be found in most university libraries, a number of basic research articles that can be purchased online, and a research report series (http://www.nida.nih.gov). Established by NIDA in 1976, the Community Epidemiology Work Group is a network composed of researchers from major metropolitan areas of the United States and selected foreign countries that meets semiannually to discuss the current epidemiology of drug abuse. The primary mission of the Work Group is to provide ongoing community-level surveillance of drug abuse through analysis of quantitative and qualitative research data. Through this program the Community Epidemiology Work Group provides current descriptive and analytical information regarding the nature and patterns of drug abuse, emerging trends, characteristics of vulnerable populations, and social and health consequences (http://www.nida.nih.gov/about/organization/CEWG/CEWGHome.html). The second institute under the NIH is the National Institute on Alcohol Abuse and Alcoholism.

The DEA publishes "Briefs and Background" reports with descriptions of various drugs of abuse. State fact sheets are similar to those published by NDIC but with emphasis on tracing the drug of abuse back to the country from which it was imported. Intelligence reports of various drug trends, descriptions of DEA operations listed by code name, lists of DEA wanted fugitives, and scheduling information from the Controlled Substances Act can also be found on the DEA Web site.

The ONDCP is an appointed position by the President of the United States. It differs from the U.S. Department of Justice and the U.S. Department of HHS in that it is not a cabinet level position. The National Drug Control Strategy is the President's policy on drug abuse and delineates the federal budget allocated for the fight against drug abuse in any given year. The "strategy" pools information from various sources, notably the 2000 National Household Survey on Drug Abuse, Columbia University's National Center on Addiction and Substance Abuse, and the University of Michigan's Monitoring the Future Survey. The strategy proposes 2- and 5-year goals that jointly aim to reduce the current use of illegal drugs in the teenage and adult population by 10% and 25%, respectively. The strategy represents a multidisciplinary plan that includes local, state, federal, and international cooperation. This collaboration strives to thwart the production, distribution, and sale of illegal drugs (http://www.whitehousedrugpolicy.gov).

REFERENCES

1. Rinaldi RC, Steindler EM, Wilford BB, Goodwin D. Clarification and standardization of substance abuse terminology. *JAMA* 1988;259:555–557.
2. Abel EL. *A dictionary of drug abuse terms and terminology.* Westport, CT: Greenwood Press, 1984:4–5, 46, 53, 157.
3. Jaffe JH. *Encyclopedia of drugs and alcohol,* vol 1. Macmillan Library Reference USA. New York: Simon & Schuster Macmillan, 1995:18–23.

4. Krug SE. Cocaine abuse: historical, epidemiologic, and clinical perspectives for pediatricians. *Adv Pediatr* 1989;36:369–399.
5. Springfield AC, et al. Cocaine and metabolites in the hair of ancient Peruvian coca leaf chewers. *Forensic Sci Int* 1993;63:269–275.
6. Brecher EM, and the Editors of *Consumer Reports Magazine*. The Consumers Union report on licit and illicit drugs. 1972. Available at: http://www.druglibrary.org/schaffer/library/studies/cu/cu1.html. Accessed June 2003.
7. Musto DF. Opium, cocaine and marijuana in American history. *Sci Am* 1991;265:40–47.
8. Edwards G. Opium and after. *Lancet* 1980;1:351–354.
9. White WL. Themes in chemical prohibition from *Drugs in perspective*. National Institute on Drug Abuse, 1979. Available at: http://www.druglibrary.org/schaffer/History/ticp.html. Accessed June 2003.
10. Brockington CF. Public health in the nineteenth century. London: E & S Livingstone, 1965:225–226.
11. Towns CB. The peril of the drug habit. *Century Magazine* 1912;84:580–587.
12. Terry CE, Pellens M. *The opium problem*. New York: Committee on Drug Addictions, Bureau of Social Hygiene, Inc, 1928:18.
13. Golding AMB. Two hundred years of drug abuse. *J R Soc Med* 1993;86:282–286.
14. Roberts DF, Henrickson L, Christenson P. Substance use in popular music and movies. 1999. *Reference morbid cravings: the emergence of addiction*. Catalog of an exhibition held in conjunction with the centenary meeting of the Society for the Study of Addiction, October 22, 1984 to 25 and January 1985. London: Wellcome Institute for the History of Medicine, 1984:19.
15. DEA history. Available at: http://www.usdoj.gov/dea/deamuseum/museum_deahistory.html. Accessed June 2003.
16. Johnston LD, et al. *Monitoring the Future national results on adolescent drug use*. Bethesda, MD: National Institute on Drug Abuse, 2002:1–56.
17. Musto DF. Cocaine's history, especially the American experience. *Cocaine: scientific and social dimensions*. Ciba Foundation Symposium 166. Chichester: Wiley, 1992:7–19.
18. OxyContin diversion and abuse. *National Drug Intelligence Center information bulletin US Department of Justice*. No. 2001-L0424-001, 2001.
19. NDIC-USDOS. National drug threat assessment 2002. Product 2002-Q0317-001. December 2002.
20. Hughes AA, Bogdan GM, Bond R, Dart RC. *J Toxicol Clin Toxicol* 2002;40:656.
21. Schoenberg BS. Coke's the one: the centennial of the "ideal brain tonic" that became a symbol of America. *South Med J* 1988;81(1):69–74.
22. Das G. Cocaine abuse in North America: a milestone in history. *J Clin Pharmacol* 1993;33:296–310.
23. Bailey BJ. Looking back at a century of cocaine—use and abuse. The retrospectoscope. *Laryngoscope* 1996;106:681–683.
24. Classics revisited. Uber Coca. By Sigmund Freud. *J Subst Abuse Treat* 1984;1(3):206–217.
25. Niehaus MR. History of chemical abuse in America by Addictions and More. 1997–2002. Available at: http://www.addictions.net/history1.htm. Accessed June 2003.
26. *A social history of America's most popular drugs*. Available at: http://www.pbs.org/wgbh/pages/frontline/shows/drugs/buyers/socialhistory.html. Accessed June 2003.
27. Lewitus V. Mariahuana. *Am J Nurs* 1936;36(7):677–678.
28. National Clearinghouse for Alcohol and Drug Information. *A short history of the drug laws*. Available at: http://mir.drugtext.org/druglibrary/schaffer/LIBRARY/shrthist.htm
29. Greifenstein Fe, Devault M, Yoshitake J, et al. A study of a 1-aryl cyclo hexyl amine for anesthesia. *Anesth Analg* 1958;37(5):283–294.
30. Crider R. Phencyclidine: changing abuse patterns. *NIDA Res Monogr* 1986;64:163–173.
31. Dundee JW. Twenty-five years of ketamine. *Anaesthesia* 1990;45:159–160.
32. Anderson RJ, Reed WG, Hillis LD, et al. History, epidemiology, and medical complications of nasal inhaler abuse. *J Toxicol Clin Toxicol* 1982;19(1):95–107.
33. Buchanan JF, Brown CR. 'Designer drugs'. A problem in clinical toxicology. *Med Toxicol Adverse Drug Exp* 1988;3(1):1–17.
34. McDowell DM, Herbert DK. MDMA: its history and pharmacology. *Psychiatr Ann* 1994;24(3):127–130.
35. Reference deleted.
36. Amphetamines. Available at: http://www.a1b2c3.com/drugs/amp01.htm. Accessed June 2003.
37. Controlled Substances Act. Available at: http://www.usdoj.gov/dea/pubs/csa.html. Accessed June 2003.
38. Snyder SH. A short history of amphetamines from "Drugs and the brain." Available at: http://www.druglibrary.org/schaffer/cocaine/amphhis.htm. Accessed June 2003.
39. Millman RB, Beeder AB. The new psychedelic culture: LSD, Ecstasy, "rave" parties and the Grateful Dead. *Psychiatr Ann* 1994;24:148–150.
40. Hoffman A. History of the discovery of LSD. In: Pletschon A, Ladewis D, eds. *50 years of LSD: current status and perspective of hallucinogens*. New York: Praflovon, 1994:7–16.
41. MDMA in New England. *National Drug Intelligence Center information bulletin US Department of Justice*. No. 2001-L0424-006, 2001.
42. Methamphetamine and OxyContin. *National Drug Intelligence Center information bulletin US Department of Justice*. No. 2001-L0424-009, 2001.
43. Schultes RE. Hallucinogens of plant origin. *Science* 1969;163:245–254.
44. Castaneda C. *A Yaqui way of knowledge*. Berkeley: University of California Press, 1968.
45. Smith DE, Seymour RB. LSD: history and toxicity. *Psychiatr Ann* 1994;24:145–147.
46. Fawcett. Stimulants, hallucinogens, and the generation gap. *Psychiatr Ann* 1994;24(3):122–123.
47. Froede R. Drugs of abuse: legal and illegal. *Hum Pathol* 1972;3(1):23–36.
48. Erickson TB, et al. Drug use patterns at major rock concert events. *Ann Emerg Med* 1996;28(1):22–26.
49. Gold MS. The epidemiology, attitudes, and pharmacology of LSD use in the 1990s. *Psychiatr Ann* 1994;24(3):124–126.
50. Giannini A. Inward the mind's I: description, diagnosis, and treatment of acute and delayed LSD hallucinations. *Psychiatr Ann* 1994;24(3):134–136.
51. Miller NS, Gold MS. LSD and Ecstasy: pharmacology, phenomenology, and treatment. *Psychiatr Ann* 1994;24:131–133.
52. Narconon Southern California & Stop Meth Addiction.com. Meth, meth addiction and treatment. 2001. Available at: http://www.stopmethaddiction.com/history-of-meth.htm. Accessed June 2003.
53. Dietary Supplement Health and Education Act of 1994. December 1995. Available at: http://vm.cfsan.fda.gov/~dms/dietsupp.html. Accessed June 2003.
54. Drug abuse legislative history. Available at: http://www.gwu.edu/~pretrial/jer1a.htm. Accessed June 2003.
55. Graeme KA. New drugs of abuse. *Pharmacol Adv Emerg Med* 2000;18(4):625–636.
56. GHB Analogs GBL, BD, GHV, and GVL. *National Drug Intelligence Center information bulletin US Department of Justice*. No. 2002-L0424-003, 2002.
57. Leikin JB, Klein L. Ephedra causes myocarditis. *J Toxicol Clin Toxicol* 2000;38(3):353–354.
58. Kurt TL. Hypersensitivity myocarditis with ephedra use. *J Toxicol Clin Toxicol* 2000;38(3):351.
59. Zaacks SM, Klein L, Tan CD, et al. Hypersensitivity myocarditis associated with ephedra use. *J Toxicol Clin Toxicol* 1999;37(4):485–489.
60. White House. National drug control strategy. 2002:1–117.
61. U.S. Food and Drug Administration Web site. Milestones in U.S. Food and Drug Law history. Available at: http://www.fda.gov/opacom/backgrounders/miles.html. Accessed June 2003.
62. Blendon RJ, Young JT. The public and the war on illicit drugs. *JAMA* 1998;279(11):827–832.
63. Berridge V. Opium and the historical perspective. *Lancet* 1977;2:78–80.
64. Johnston LD, O'Malley PM, Bachman, JG. *Monitoring the Future national results on adolescent drug use: overview of key findings*. NIH Publication No. 02-5105. Bethesda, MD: National Institute on Drug Abuse, 2002.

CHAPTER 174

Amphetamines and Designer Drugs

Richard C. Lynton and Timothy E. Albertson

See Figure 1.

Compounds included:	**See Table 1.**
Molecular formula and weight:	**See Table 2.**
SI conversion:	**Methamphetamine, mg/L × 6.70 = mmol/L**
CAS Registry No.:	**See Table 2.**
Therapeutic levels:	**Methamphetamine, 20 to 30 ng/ml**
Target organs:	**Amphetamine and its derivatives affect nearly all organ systems acutely. Target organs of chronic exposure are primarily central nervous system and myocardium.**
Antidote:	**None**

OVERVIEW

Amphetamines are a class of noncatechol sympathomimetic amines that produce central nervous system stimulation (Fig. 1). Amphetamine was first synthesized by Edelano in 1877. The D-isomer is three to four times more potent than the L-isomer (1). A remarkable variety of amphetamine derivatives have been produced. A partial list of drugs and their intended uses are provided in Table 2. This chapter focuses on two commonly abused amphetamine derivatives: methamphetamine and methylenedioxymethamphetamine (MDMA; Ecstasy) and briefly describes some of the numerous related compounds. Because of their similarities, the diagnosis and treatment of the toxicity of amphetamine and its derivatives are addressed as a group at the end of this chapter (see Other Pharmaceutical Agents).

Amphetamines were given to World War II soldiers to improve alertness and performance. The use of stimulants by athletes to enhance performance is well known and persistent (2). The typical oral amphetamine dose for enhancement is

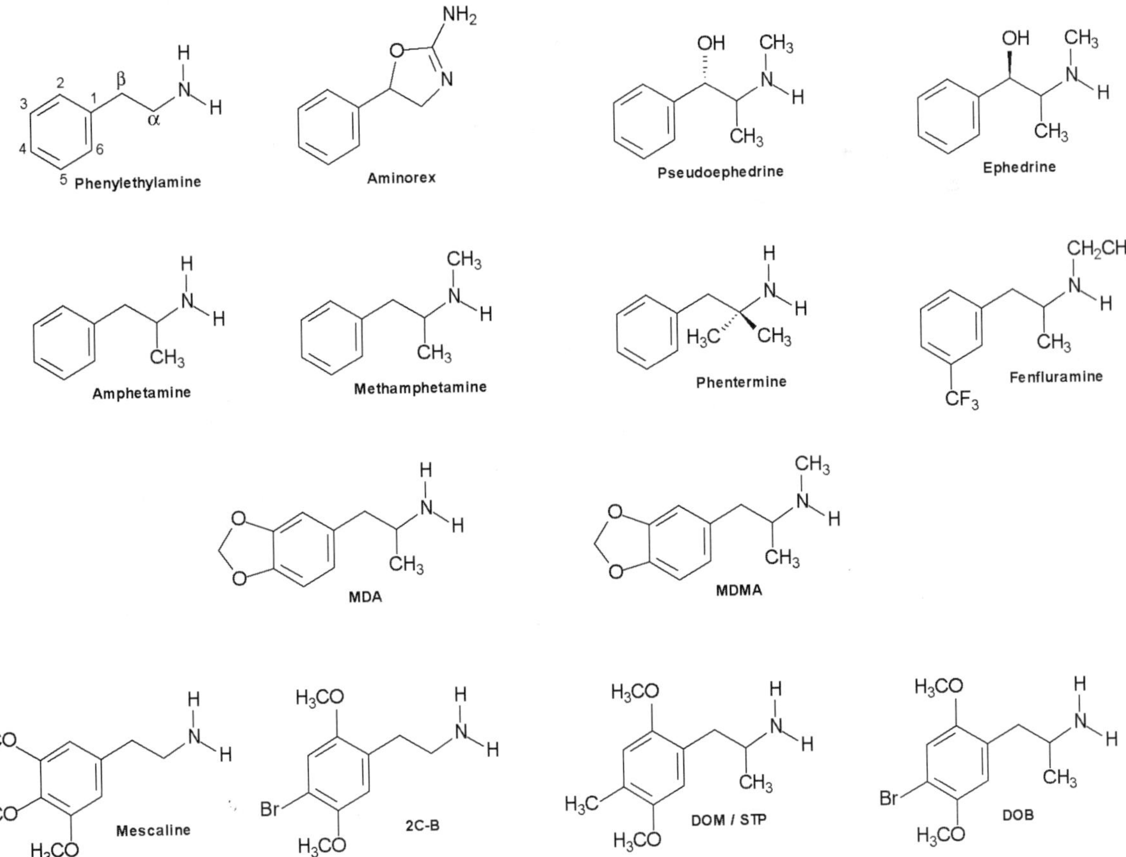

Figure 1. Chemical structures of phenethylamine derivatives. 2C-B, 4-bromo-2,5-dimethoxyphenylethylamine; DOB, 4-bromo-2,5-dimethoxyamphetamine; DOM/STP, 2,5-dimethoxy-4-methylamphetamine; MDA, 3,4-methylenedioxyamphetamine; MDMA, 3,4-methylenedioxymethamphetamine.

TABLE 1. Compounds included

Aminorex
Amphetamine
Benzphetamine
4-Bromo-2,5-dimethoxyphenylethylamine (2C-B, Venus)
Clobenzorex
D-desoxyephedrine
Dexfenfluramine
Dextroamphetamines
Diethylpropion
Ephedra (ma huang)
Fenfluramine
Khat (cathinone)
Mescaline
Methamphetamine
Methcathinone (Jeff)
Methylenedioxymethamphetamine (MDMA, Ecstasy, many others)
3,4-Methlenedioxyamphetamine (MDA)
3,4-Methylenedioxyethamphetamine (MDEA, Eve)
Methylphenidate (Ritalin)
4-Methylaminorex (4-MAX)
Methyl-2,5-dimethoxyamphetamine (DOM, STP)
Methylephedrine
4-Bromo-2,5-dimethoxyamphetamine (DOB, LSD-25)
4-Methylthioamphetamine (4-MTA, Flatliner)
Paramethoxyamphetamine (PMA)
Phendimetrazine
Phentermine
2,4,5-Trimethoxyamphetamine (TMA)

between 5 and 20 mg. A portion of these users become daily users of 20 to 40 mg. Tolerance can develop, leading to the use of doses of 50 to 150 mg or more a day. When these users try to quit, they typically become depressed and lethargic, prompting continued use (3).

MODES OF AMPHETAMINE ABUSE

Intravenous use produces a more intense "rush" in amphetamine abusers. In an effort to achieve this high continually, abusers have used up to 1000 mg methamphetamine at a time. This behavior can become cyclic and compulsive. Users known as *speed freaks* have an initial "action" phase that can last from 1 to 10 days. During this phase the abuser uses the drug constantly, often without sleeping or eating. Classic signs include skin picking, head banging, pacing, extreme suspiciousness, and paranoid psychosis. This phase is followed by the reaction phase, in which exhaustion, fatigue, and sleep ensue for 1 to 2 days. Patients may then have a ravenous appetite followed by depression. This often starts the cycle over again.

The smokable form of methamphetamine is also known as *ice*, a hydrochloride salt. The average "hit" is 100 mg smoked methamphetamine, and the effects can last up to 15 hours (4). Because the bioavailability is approximately 50%, it takes more to achieve the same effect as an intravenous dose (5–7). However, inhalation still has a similar immediate clinical euphoria as a result of the rapid absorption from the lungs (8). Chronic psy-

TABLE 2. Amphetamines

Compound (reference)	Molecular formula, molecular weight (g/mol), CAS Registry No.	Uses	Associated toxicity	Comments
4-Methylaminorex (4-MAX, "ice," or "U4Euh") (50,239,240)	NR, NR, 3568-94-3	Appetite suppression, abused stimulant	Pulmonary hypertension, seizures (250)	Removed from U.S. market
Aminorex (desmethyl form of 4-MAX) (50)	$C_9H_{10}N_2O$, 162.2, 2207-50-3	Appetite suppression, abused stimulant	Pulmonary hypertension	Removed from U.S. market
Amphetamine (18)	$C_9H_{13}N$, 135.2, 300-62-9	Bronchial dilation, appetite suppression, stimulant	See Table 3	—
Benzphetamine hydrochloride	$C_{17}H_{21}N$,HCl, 275.8, 5411-22-3	Appetite suppression	Fewer cardiovascular effects than amphetamine	—
Clobenzorex (204,241)	$C_{16}H_{18}ClN$,HCl, 296.2, 5843-53-8	Appetite suppression	Dilated cardiomyopathy (242)	Adulterant in Chinese herbal preparations (243)
D-desoxyephedrine	$C_{10}H_{15}N$,HCl, 185.7, 51-57-0	Attention deficit hyperactivity disorder	—	—
Dexfenfluramine (244,245)	$C_{12}H_{16}F_3N$,HCl, 267.7, 3239-45-0	Appetite suppression	Valvular heart disease, pulmonary hypertension (249)	Removed from U.S. market in 1997
Dextroamphetamine	$C_9H_{13}N_2$,H_2SO_4, 368.5, 51-63-8	Attention deficit hyperactivity disorder	Cardiomyopathy (38)	—
Diethylpropion	$C_{13}H_{19}NO$,HCl, 241.8, 134-80-5	Appetite suppression	—	—
Fenfluramine (244,245)	$C_{12}H_{16}F_3N$,HCl, 267.7, 404-82-0	Appetite suppression	Valvular heart disease, pulmonary hypertension	Removed from U.S. market in 1997
L-desoxyephedrine (L-methamphetamine)	$C_{10}H_{15}N$, 149.2, 33817-09-3	Bronchodilator	—	Fewer central stimulant properties
Methylphenidate (180)	$C_{14}H_{19}NO_2$,HCl, 269.8, 298-59-9	Attention deficit hyperactivity disorder	Agitation, hallucination, psychosis	—
Phendimetrazine (246–248)	$C_{12}H_{17}NO$,$C_4H_6O_6$, 341.4, 7635-51-0	Appetite suppression	Ischemic stroke, peripheral vasculopathy, nephropathy, acute interstitial nephritis	—
Phentermine (246–248)	$C_{10}H_{15}N$,HCl, 185.7, 1197-21-3	Appetite suppression	Ischemic stroke, peripheral vasculopathy, nephropathy, acute interstitial nephritis	—

NR, not reported.

chosis has also been documented (9). Snorting methamphetamine can lead to increased tooth wear and alterations in the anterior maxillary sinus (10).

Oral abuse of amphetamines may be increasing in some parts of the world, such as in Asia. Case reports of death after oral ingestion have been described (11,12). Death is usually seen with blood methamphetamine concentrations greater than 0.5 mg/L but have been noted with levels as low as 0.05 mg/L with co-ingestions (13).

Benzedrine was an over-the-counter amphetamine inhaler removed from the market after its abuse potential was discovered. It contained 250 mg racemic amphetamine. It was replaced by Benzedrex, an inhaler with 250 mg propylhexedrine. Also known as *peanut butter methamphetamine*, it can be extracted from the inhaler by soaking it in hydrochloric acid and then heating it to remove other chemicals such as methanol. Erythema, ulceration, and corrosion of the skin have been noted at injection sites. Patients present with tachycardia, hypertension, severe headache, diplopia, psychosis, and findings of brain stem dysfunction (14). It also has been associated with ventricular hypertrophy, cor pulmonale, foreign body granulomas, pulmonary fibrosis, and pulmonary hypertension (15–17).

METHAMPHETAMINE

Methamphetamine was first synthesized by a Japanese pharmacologist in 1893 (18). Illicit production now is widespread (Fig. 2). Today the most common clandestine manufacture process uses ephedrine or pseudoephedrine in a reduction process that involves hydriodic acid and red phosphorus to form both the D- and L-isomers of methamphetamine. Another process uses metal lithium and anhydrous ammonia. The traditional "P2P" method uses phenyl-2-propanone but is used less commonly now. α-Benzyl-n-methylphenethylamine is a metabolite of a common byproduct of P2P synthesis dibenzylketone. The presence of α-benzyl-n-methylphenethylamine has been suggested as a marker for assessing illegal production of methamphetamine (19,20). Lead poisoning has also occurred from precursor products used in the manufacture of phenyl-2-propanone (21).

Chloroephedrine has been identified as an important contaminant in illicit manufacture using ephedrine. In one study chloroephedrine in combination with methamphetamine produced more tachycardia than either substance alone. At larger doses vagal stimulation also occurred (22). Phosphine exposure has also been reported during the red phosphorus–hydriodic acid method of amphetamine production. Phosphine gas with a garlic odor may be produced when red phosphorus is heated with hydriodic acid. Gastrointestinal symptoms can occur rapidly, whereas significant pulmonary toxicity may be delayed. Respiratory symptoms can persist for weeks, and deaths from phosphine exposure during methamphetamine manufacture have occurred (23,24).

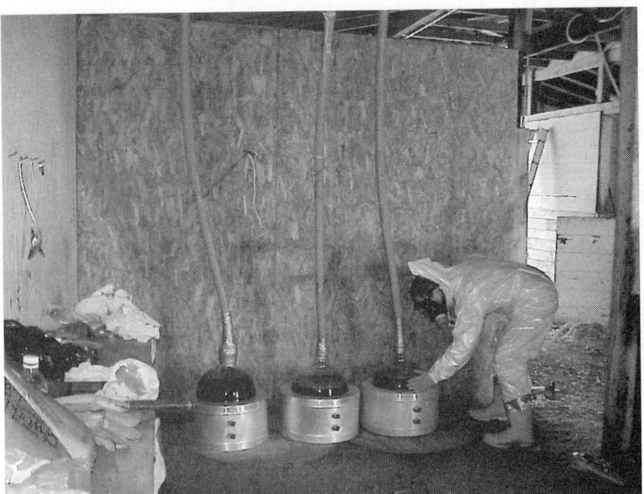

Figure 2. Clandestine methamphetamine production. (Courtesy Sacramento District Attorney Crime Laboratory.)

TABLE 3. Characteristic profiles of methamphetamine users (injection vs. noninjection)

	Injection users (N = 55)	Noninjection users (N = 372)	Analysis X^2
Ethnicity			
White	80%	82%	NS
Hispanic and other	15%	16%	NS
African American	4%	1%	NS
History of psychological problems	38.5%	25.4%	3.90[a]
Depression	80.0%	64.1%	5.38[a]
Suicidal ideation	32.7%	18.8%	5.66[a]
Hallucinations	46.3%	32.3%	4.08[a]
Body part disconnect	26.4%	12.4%	7.41[b]
Sex problems	27.3%	12.9%	4.85[a]
Loss of consciousness	18.2%	6.9%	7.82[b]
HIV+	5.5%	0.20%	13.93[a]
Felony	37.1%	17.8%	7.23[b]
Parole	46.1%	18.7%	4.53[a]
Probation	53.8%	70.3%	4.53[a]
Heavy MA use (mean years ± SD)	5.58 ± 5.40	3.06 ± 3.15	33.75[b,c]
Unemployed (%)	81	59	29.94[b,c]

HIV, human immunodeficiency virus; MA, methamphetamine; NS, not significant; SD, standard deviation.
[a]p <.05.
[b]p <.01.
[c]By t-test.
Adapted from Domier CP, Simon SL, Rawson RA, et al. A comparison of injecting and noninjecting methamphetamine users. *J Psychoactive Drugs* 2000;32(2):229–232.

Epidemiology

The typical methamphetamine user is a young, white man with a high school education (25). Intravenous methamphetamine users have a higher incidence of human immunodeficiency virus (HIV), felony violations, depression, and sex problems than do nonintravenous users (26) (Table 3). A study by the National Collegiate Athletic Association found that alcohol was the most commonly abused substance and that amphetamines and ephedrine were more popular than cocaine (27).

The "rave scene" has reintroduced amphetamines and their designer derivatives to a new generation of teenagers (28). Designer amphetamines and other "club" drugs, such as γ-hydroxybutyrate (GHB), cocaine, and marijuana, are commonly used together by club rave participants (29). An animal study has investigated the effects of noise from rave music in combination with methamphetamine exposure. Rats exposed to rave music compared to white noise had greater stereotypic locomotion, more seizures, higher mortality, and a greater preference for middle squares in an open field (30).

The D-isomer of methamphetamine has more central nervous system stimulant effects than the L-isomer, which has been used as a decongestant in nasal inhalers. Methamphetamine has many clinical cardiovascular effects. The most common side effects are tachycardia, palpitations, and hypertension (31). Smoking crystal methamphetamine, or "ice," has been associated with cardiac pulmonary edema and dilated cardiomyopathy (32). The sudden rapid increase in blood pressure has also been associated with vision loss from intraretinal hemorrhages (33).

Toxic Dose

The adult therapeutic dose of methamphetamine is 2.5 to 5.0 mg orally. The toxic dose varies widely. A dose as low as 1.3 mg/kg has been fatal (34).

Toxicokinetics and Toxicodynamics

Methamphetamine is rapidly absorbed orally and within seconds of inhalation. Its volume of distribution is 3.2 to 3.7 L/kg (35). It is metabolized to amphetamine (4% to 7%) and hydroxymethamphetamine (15%). In normal patients, 43% of the dose is excreted renally but increases to 76% in an acid urine and decreases to 2% in an alkaline urine (36). The elimination half-life is 12 to 34 hours.

Pathophysiology

The basic mechanism for most cardiovascular effects of amphetamines involves release of norepinephrine, dopamine, and serotonin from nerve terminals. Amphetamines also mildly inhibit monoamine oxidase (MAO) but do not affect fast sodium channels (37). The release of large amounts of catecholamines causes destruction of heart and skeletal myofibers with cellular infiltration, mitochondrial swelling, sarcoplasmic fragmentation, foci of hypereosinophilic myocytes, myocytolysis, myofiber contraction bands, edema, and spotty fibrosis with chronic use (38–40). Binge methamphetamine use leads to cardiovascular consequences, including mononuclear inflammatory infiltrates, disrupted architecture, and occasional myofibril necrosis in the heart. In addition, a significant alteration in the Bezold-Jarisch reflex has been reported (41).

Neurotoxic effects of methamphetamine are thought to be related to changes in neurotransmitter concentration, receptor availability, and direct toxic effect in various region cell types of the brain. Methamphetamine predominantly affects serotonin and dopamine neurotransmitters, with resultant impairment of serotonergic and dopaminergic adenosine triphosphate production, activation of adenosine diphosphate polymerase, decrease in tryptophan hydroxylase, and loss of dopamine transporters (42). Tryptamine-4,5-dione, a metabolite of serotonin, may contribute to this toxicity as an irreversible inhibitor of tryptophan hydroxylase (43). Repeated high-dose methamphetamine use has been associated with glucose depletion in the extrapyramidal system, the hippocampus, and the dorsal raphe nucleus of rats (44). It also has been suggested as a mechanism for long-term psychosis.

Dopamine depletion, perhaps related to cytochrome oxidase effects, can occur with methamphetamine and is predominantly seen in the basal ganglia in the substantia nigra. Animal models have suggested that this effect may have long-term consequences (45,46).

Even after long-term abstinence from methamphetamine, positron emission tomography scans have shown persistent decreases in dopamine transporter density and dopamine levels in the caudate nucleus and putamen. The extent of the decrease is not as significant as that seen in Parkinson's disease, and Parkinson's disease did not develop in any of the subjects (47). Other research has shown recovery of the dopamine transporter system. However, no improvement was shown on neuropsychological testing after methamphetamine was stopped (42,48).

Sexual differences to these effects also seem to be present, with male mice showing more depletion than female mice. These differences imply that ovarian hormones can modulate methamphetamine neurotoxicity (49). Estrogen and testosterone have neuroprotective effects on nigrostriatal dopamine depletion from methamphetamine toxicity (50,51). This protective effect is nullified by the estrogen antagonist tamoxifen (52,53). Apomorphine may have a protective effect against methamphetamine nigrostriatal dopamine depletion. Apomorphine is a nonselective dopamine receptor agonist used in the treatment of Parkinson's disease. It is also a free radical scavenger and antioxidant that may protect against methamphetamine-induced toxicity (54).

Apoptosis has been suggested as a mechanism in cell death possibly caused by cytokines. Rats that lack interleukin-6 showed minimal gliosis and dopamine or serotonin depletion after being given methamphetamine (55). Additional genes are thought to modulate methamphetamine-programmed cell death, including the bc12, a proto-oncogene found in B-cell lymphoma, and p53, a tumor suppressor gene seen in several forms of cancer (56,57). Reactive oxygen species such as hydrogen peroxide, superoxide, and hydroxyl radicals may also be involved in this process (57–59). Selenium, another antioxidant, has been shown to attenuate this effect (60,61). Brain cells treated with methamphetamine were shown to produce decreased levels of the antioxidant glutathione and also to induce certain transcription genes that may induce tumor necrosis factor-α production. This could directly promote toxicity and also could ultimately affect the blood–brain barrier (62).

Pregnancy and Lactation

The effect of methamphetamine on pregnancy includes increased fetal and newborn deaths (63). After one dose of methamphetamine, fetal sheep cardiovascular effects lasted for approximately 2 hours with levels detected in the umbilical blood, suggesting significant placental transfer to the fetus (64). Reduced birth rates in rats after a single dose of methamphetamine have also been reported (65).

Clinical Presentation

The remarkable spectrum of clinical effects is provided in Table 4. Neurologic symptoms include hemorrhagic and ischemic stroke. Almost half of the patients have systemic hypertension (66). Elevated blood pressure has been seen in most cases; however, cerebral vasculitis has also been implicated as a mechanism for stroke (67,68). These same effects are likely to contribute to cases of ruptured berry aneurysms (69). Synergistic neurotoxicity has been suggested with methamphetamine and infection by HIV. Estrogen may protect against this synergism (70). Cognitive deficits from methamphetamine use include impaired memory, decreased psychomotor speed, and decreased concentration (71). A paranoid hallucinatory state causing psychosis can occur and is thought to be due to increased norepinephrine levels seen during flashbacks (72).

The hypertensive effects of amphetamine drugs and their derivatives are well known, but methamphetamine has also been shown to cause hypotension and bradycardia (73). The

TABLE 4. Major signs and symptoms of amphetamine toxicity

Sign/symptom	Frequency
Cardiac	
Chest pain	+++
Myocardial infarction	+
Palpitations	++
Arrhythmia	++
Cardiomyopathy	+
Myocarditis	+
Hypertension	++
Sudden death	+
Valve thickening	+++
Neurologic	
Headache	+
Seizure	++
Cerebral infarcts/stroke	++
Cerebral edema	++
Mydriasis	+
Cerebral hemorrhage	++
Subarachnoid	++
Intraventricular	+++
Intracerebral	++
Psychiatric	
Anxiety	+++
Depression	++
Paranoia	++
Delirium/hallucination	+++
Psychosis	+++
Suicide	++
Aggressive behavior	++
Euphoria/hyperactivity	++
Irritability	++
Respiratory	
Pulmonary edema	+
Dyspnea	++
Bronchitis	+
Pulmonary hypertension	+++
Hemoptysis	+
Pleuritic chest pain	++
Asthma exacerbation	+
Pulmonary granuloma	+
Other	
Ulcers	++
Hyperpyrexia	++
Renal failure	+
Ischemic colitis	+
Obstetric complications	++
Anorexia/weight loss	+++
Rhabdomyolysis	++
Nausea/vomiting	+
Disseminated vasculitis	+

Estimated frequency of events: +, reported rare cases; ++, commonly reported; +++, frequently seen or reported with chronic use or overdose.
Adapted from Albertson TE, Derlet RW, Van Hoozen BE. Methamphetamine and the expanding complications of amphetamines. *West J Med* 1999;170(4):214–219.

effect of methamphetamine on baroreceptors, depletion of catecholamines, the formation of false adrenergic transmitters, and depression of central vasomotor functions have been suggested mechanisms (73). Hypotension may be more common after chronic administration (74).

Pulmonary sequelae include noncardiogenic pulmonary edema and pulmonary hypertension caused by endothelial injury, direct spasm, and dysregulation of mediators of vascular tone (15). Other consequences of methamphetamine exposure include rhabdomyolysis and severe metabolic acidosis in overdoses and in trauma patients (75–77). A review of 84 autopsies of patients who died from acute aortic dissection found that 7 had positive drug tests for methamphetamine. Although the overall mean age was 52 years, the mean age was 41 years for the seven methamphetamine-positive cases (78).

Drug Interactions

Fatal interactions between the protease inhibitor ritonavir and methamphetamine have been reported (79,80). Ritonavir inhibits CYP2D6 (81), which is the same cytochrome that metabolizes methamphetamine. This can cause increased levels of methamphetamine (82). Ethanol has been shown to enhance the toxic cardiovascular effects of methamphetamine in humans (83,84).

3,4-METHYLENEDIOXYMETHAMPHETAMINE

MDMA was first synthesized by the Merck Chemical Company in 1914 from safrole (85). Illicit MDMA or "Adam" (Fig. 3) first started to be abused in the United States in 1968, and its use has steadily increased with the popularity of raves (86). MDMA use

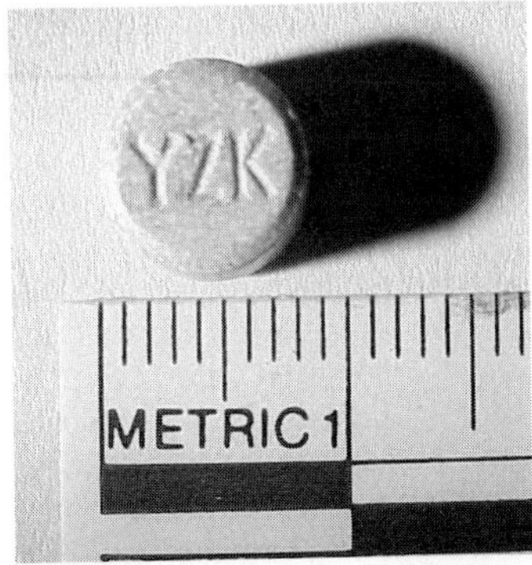

Figure 3. Methylenedioxymethamphetamine (MDMA) tablet. This tablet also contained methamphetamine, ketamine, and caffeine in addition to MDMA. (Courtesy of Sacramento County District Attorney Crime Laboratory.)

has been identified with risk-taking behaviors such as sexual promiscuity and with increased risk of domestic violence. Other markers of use include younger age, being less educated, having a greater risk for HIV, and increased concomitant use of other illicit drugs (87,88).

Toxic Dose

The usual dose is 100 mg MDMA per tablet but can vary from 50 mg or less to 250 mg. One pill has been associated with death from hypertension and aortic dissection (89).

Toxicokinetics and Toxicodynamics

Onset of action is within 30 minutes, and peak serum levels occur in 1 to 3 hours. The elimination half-life is 7 hours (90). The toxic dose is variable, with near fatal and fatal ingestions having been reported with blood levels between 0.11 mg/L to 2.1 mg/L (91,92). Survival has also been reported after MDMA blood levels of 4.3 mg/L drawn 13 hours after ingestion (93). The compound 4-hydroxy-3-methoxymethamphetamine is the major metabolite of MDMA metabolism and can be found in plasma or in urine (94,95).

Pathophysiology

MDMA affects the $5HT_{2A}$ serotonin receptor (96). Reduced density of serotonin transporters have been shown after MDMA. This has been implicated as the cause for mild serotonin syndrome, with evidence of mental confusion, trismus, hyperactivity, and hyperthermia seen in MDMA users (97).

Pregnancy and Lactation

Exposure to MDMA *in utero* may be associated with an increased risk of congenital defects (15.4%) (98).

Clinical Presentation

Acute toxic effects of MDMA include hyperthermia, muscle rigidity, metabolic acidosis, disseminated intravascular coagulation, and rhabdomyolysis (99–101). These effects can lead to multiorgan failure and death (99,102–104). The level of hyperthermia predicts the potential for survival (93,105,106). MDMA produces cardiovascular effects similar to those seen with methamphetamine, including an increase in blood pressure and heart rate (107) (Table 4).

Several reports of pneumomediastinum associated with MDMA abuse suggest a mechanical cause such as vigorous Valsalva's maneuvers or excessive physical activity during rave parties (108–112). Bilateral gluteal compartment syndrome requiring fasciotomy is a rare complication of this effect (113).

MDMA has been implicated as a cause of amnesic syndrome associated with severe ataxia (114). Chronic use of MDMA has been implicated in sleep disorders and mood changes. The failure to phase shift circadian rhythms in response to changes in light and dark after a serotonin agonist was given to a user of MDMA implies serotonin receptor depletion (115).

Cognitive deficits such as memory recall were also seen in users of MDMA even after 6 months of abstinence (116). A positron emission tomography study done in human MDMA users has also shown decreased glucose use in the caudate and putamen. The effect was more severe in those patients who had started MDMA use before age 18 (117).

Serious sequelae can occur from electrolyte abnormalities seen in MDMA abuse and overdose. Hyponatremia from inappropriate antidiuretic hormone production and increased free water intake has been described in several case reports of significant cerebral edema and subsequent death (118–120). The mechanism is poorly understood, but there is some evidence to suggest that high levels of serotonin brought on by MDMA may cause increased secretion of antidiuretic hormone (121–125).

Urinary retention occurs with MDMA abuse and may relate to its effect on the adrenergic system (126,127). Priapism may be an uncommon MDMA toxicity, possibly through serotonin receptor activity (128). Acute hepatotoxicity has been described as a consequence of MDMA use (91,129–131). An acute hepatitis pattern with lymphocytic infiltration of hepatic parenchyma is seen. Liver injury attributed to MDMA should be a diagnosis of exclusion.

Eye pathology, including retinal hemorrhage with blurred vision, has been described with the use of MDMA (132). Central serous chorioretinopathy has also been reported with MDMA use (133). These effects tended to resolve spontaneously and may be mediated by the sudden increase in blood pressure that occurs after MDMA. Similar to data with methamphetamine, an antioxidant (lipoic acid) has been shown to prevent serotonergic depletion and neurotoxicity (134).

Drug Interactions

The isoenzyme CYP2D6 has also been implicated in the metabolism of MDMA and is absent in 5% to 9% of the white population (135,136). Poor metabolizers may also be at increased risk for MDMA toxicity (135). Patients who also take MAO inhibitor antidepressants are at particular risk if they ingest MDMA. Severe hypertension, altered mental status, hypertonicity, and diaphoresis can develop after use of MDMA (137). Ethanol coadministration with MDMA resulted in longer-lasting euphoria and fewer sedative effects from alcohol but continued psychomotor impairment (138).

MESCALINE

Mescaline (3,4,5-trimethoxyamphetamine; Fig. 1) is derived from the peyote cactus (*Lophophora williamsii*) found in Mexico. Structurally similar to many of the designer amphetamines (139), it is a known hallucinogen at doses of 200 to 500 mg. It has a half-life of 6 hours and duration of effect of 12 hours. In addition to its psychedelic effect, it commonly causes nausea, vomiting, abdominal cramps, and diarrhea, mimicking acute gastroenteritis (140). Mescaline has been used for centuries, based on samples taken from archeological sites in Mexico and the southwestern United States (141).

OTHER METHOXYLATED AMPHETAMINES

Paramethoxyamphetamine

Paramethoxyamphetamine is a hallucinogen reported to be about five times more potent than mescaline (142). Levels of 0.5 mg/L appear to be associated with serious toxicity and potential lethality (143). It first became popular in the 1970s and has been mistaken for Ecstasy. It is ten times more active in elevating brain serotonin levels than MDMA and is also a potent inhibitor of MAO (144). Multiple deaths have been associated with paramethoxyamphetamine use in Canada and Australia (143,145). The clinical features include hyperthermia, tachycardia, coma, seizures, and cardiac dysrhythmias (146). Infrequent episodes of hypoglycemia and hyperkalemia have also been noted (147).

2,4,5-Trimethoxyamphetamine

Trimethoxyamphetamine was the first designer drug synthesized in 1947. It is also structurally related to mescaline and therefore shares similar psychoactive and hallucinogenic properties. It is reportedly twice as potent as mescaline (148).

Methyl-2,5-dimethoxyamphetamine

Methyl-2,5-dimethoxyamphetamine, or STP (serenity, tranquility, and peace), was first introduced around 1963 (Fig. 1). At low doses (less than 3 mg), its effects are similar to those of mescaline. With higher doses, nausea, tremor, diaphoresis, and hallucinations can occur. The duration of action is approximately 8 hours (148).

4-Bromo-2,5-dimethoxyamphetamine

4-Bromo-2,5-dimethoxyamphetamine (DOB; "LSD-25" or "golden eagle") is a potent hallucinogen and sympathomimetic (Fig. 1). It is a $5HT_{2A/2C}$ receptor agonist (149,150). It is more potent than mescaline, with a delayed onset of action of approximately 3 to 4 hours and a duration of 24 hours. Like lysergic acid diethylamide, it can be impregnated onto blot paper and sold as 1-cm squares. The dose varies depending on original concentration and the amount of migration on the paper (149). Significant morbidity and mortality are associated with DOB use (151). One case report describes a man who presented with vomiting, diarrhea, and paresthesias of extremities; visual hallucinations; and psychosis after drinking wine laced with DOB. Symptoms resolved with supportive care (152). DOB has also been implicated as a cause of peripheral arterial spasm with paresthesias, cold extremities, and hand pain (153).

4-Bromo-2,5-dimethoxyphenylethylamine

The compound 4-bromo-2,5-dimethoxyphenylethylamine is also structurally related to mescaline (Fig. 1). Its street names include "Venus," "Bromo," "MFT," "Erox," and "Nexus." As with most of the other methoxylated derivatives, it has been found as a contaminant in illicit MDMA pills. Its dose is 4 to 30 mg. Symptoms include euphoria and visual, auditory, tactile, and olfactory sensations mediated by its affinity on central serotonin receptors. The duration of action is between 4 and 8 hours (139,154,155).

3,4-Methylenedioxyamphetamine

3,4-Methylenedioxyamphetamine (MDA), or "love drug," was first synthesized in 1910 (156). It can be relatively easily manufactured from safrole and oil found in nutmeg. The product is a mixture of D- and L-isomers, the former producing its amphetamine-like effects and the latter its hallucinogenic effects (157). Low doses cause mild intoxication, empathy, and euphoria. High doses produce agitation, delirium, and hallucinations. Several case reports of death have been published (156,158). MDA is abused orally or intravenously at doses of 50 to 250 mg. The minimal lethal dose is thought to be 500 mg. Onset of effect is usually within 30 to 60 minutes, with a duration of action of 6 to 20 hours. It is a metabolite of MDMA and of 3,4-methylenedioxyethamphetamine (MDEA) and is metabolized to the hypotensive agent α-methyldopamine, although large amounts of MDA have been found in urine samples unchanged (148).

3,4-Methylenedioxyethamphetamine

MDEA was first synthesized between 1986 and 1987 (159). MDEA, or "Eve," has similar effects to MDMA and has also been found in tablets that were supposed to contain MDMA. Several cases have been reported of psychosis and death from hyperthermia, rigor, rhabdomyolysis, and disseminated intravascular coagulation with this chemical (159–161). Characteristic effects of MDEA include relaxation and peacefulness at low doses and a rise in blood pressure, moderate rise in temperature, and increases in cortisol and prolactin levels at higher exposures (162). Other common effects after acute intoxication include anxiety, dissociative feelings, depression, and paranoia (161).

4-Methylthioamphetamine

4-Methylthioamphetamine (4-MTA), or p-methioamphetamine, is a relatively new compound known on the street as "flatliner" for its flat half-scored tablet. 4-MTA has dose-dependent serotonin effects that do not appear to produce neurotoxicity (163). In an animal model, 4-MTA was shown to be a reversible inhibitor of MAO-A (164). Blood concentrations of 0.2 to 0.6 mg/L are thought to be moderately toxic. Concentrations greater than 1.5 mg/L have been fatal (165,166).

N-methyl-1-(3,4-methylenedioxyphenyl)-2-butanamine

N-methyl-1-(3,4-methylenedioxyphenyl)-2-butanamine (MBDB) is the alpha-ethyl homologue of MDMA, first synthesized in 1986. Tablets contain 50 to 200 mg (140). MBDB is metabolized to 3,4-(methylenedioxyphenyl)-2-butanamine, which can be found in urine, sweat, and saliva (167). The use of MBDB has been increasing in Europe and North America. It is a selective serotonin-releasing agent with almost no dopaminergic or hallucinogenic properties (168). MBDB is reported to enhance understanding, communicativeness, and empathy. It has been suggested that this designer amphetamine should be placed in a new class of agents called *entactogens* (169,170).

METHCATHINONE

Methcathinone was first patented in the United States in 1957 by Parke-Davis but was never commercially introduced because of its adverse effects (171). In the 1970s, it became popular in Russia, where it was known as ephedrine or "Jeff." Its use became popular in the rural Midwest in the early 1990s (172). The most common illicit production uses L-ephedrine as the precursor molecule. Cyclic binge use causes paranoid psychosis, auditory hallucinations, weight loss, hyperreflexia, antisocial behavior, and tremor (171) Methcathinone use has resulted in a loss of dopamine transmitter function and density similar to that often seen with methamphetamine. This effect persists even after prolonged abstinence (47).

HERBAL PRODUCTS

Ma huang is the herb *Ephedra vulgaris* that has been used in China for centuries. The active natural ingredient is the L-isomer of ephedrine. Most plants contain approximately 1% ephedrine, and commercial preparations contain anywhere from 4% to 8%. It is now one of the most common precursor molecules used to manufacture methamphetamine. It can also be found in weight loss products, food supplements, and energizer drinks. The half-life is 5.0 to 7.5 hours, and it has a volume of distribution of 2.6 to 3.1 L/kg. The majority of ephedrine is excreted unchanged, with a small portion undergoing n-demethylation to norephedrine (140). Ephedrine has a toxic profile similar to that of amphetamine. Abuse of ephedrine-containing products has been described as a cause of congestive heart failure due to cardiomyopathy (173).

Methylephedrine is another in this class of ephedra alkaloids found in over-the-counter cough and cold medications, especially in Japan. It is rapidly absorbed after oral administration, with clinical effects similar to those of ephedrine in addition to hallucination and paranoia. The majority of methylephedrine is eliminated unchanged with approximately 8% being metabolized (174).

Khat is obtained from the African plants subbare kat or muktaree kat. Historically, the leaves have been chewed. Khat leaves contain approximately 1 mg cathinone, 0.9 mg norpseudoephedrine, and 0.5 mg norephedrine per gram of fresh leaves (140). The active ingredient is cathinone or 2-amino-1-phenyl-1-propanone. It has a structure very similar to that of amphetamine and is about one-third as potent as amphetamine. The half-life is 2.7 to 6.0 hours. It increases blood pressure and temperature and has positive inotropic and chronotropic effects. Cathinone is rapidly converted to cathine, which is much less potent. Other effects of cathinone include acute psychosis, reactive depression, malnutrition, gastritis, impotence, and low birth weight (175,176).

Khat chewing is common in African and Arab countries for recreational and medicinal purposes. In Somalia and Yemen, as much as one-third of the family income can be spent on khat, and 80% of the population uses khat. To achieve maximum effect users typically continue to chew for up to 6 hours at a time (177). Its use has been associated with acute liver fluke infection (178). In conjunction with alcohol and tobacco use, khat may be a cause of oral malignancy (179).

OTHER PHARMACEUTICAL AGENTS

Methylphenidate is an amphetamine that has been used as adjunctive therapy for attention deficit hyperactivity disorder (ADHD). Twice-a-day oral doses of 5 mg are administered and titrated upward until the desired effect is achieved. It has a half-life range of 1.4 to 4.2 hours and a large volume of distribution of 11 to 33 L/kg. It is metabolized to ritalinic acid and 6-oxo-ritalinic acid (140). Side effects include nervousness, headaches, insomnia, and anorexia. Acute overdoses can produce agitation, hallucinations, and psychosis (180).

Dextroamphetamine (the D-isomer of amphetamine) is also used orally to treat ADHD and narcolepsy. Cardiomyopathy has been described with its use. A case report described a patient who took dextroamphetamine for narcolepsy for 12 years and developed congestive heart failure, which paradoxically got worse when attempts to withdraw the drug were made (38). High doses have been associated with lethargy or hyperexcitability, psychosis, tachycardia, and ataxia (181).

D-desoxyephedrine is the D-isomer of methamphetamine and is used for the short-term treatment of obesity and as an adjunct in ADHD (182). Similar to other amphetamines, it undergoes n-demethylation to D-amphetamine (140). The half-life ranges from 6 to 15 hours depending on urine pH. It has a volume of distribution of 3.0 to 7.0 L/kg.

The Vicks inhaler contains L-desoxyephedrine (L-methamphetamine) for its peripheral sympathomimetic activity. It has fewer central stimulant properties. It has been used in nonprescription inhalers, which contain 50 mg of the L-isomer of methamphetamine. The L-isomer undergoes a similar metabolism as the D-isomer at a slower rate to L-amphetamine. Attempts have been made to extract the contents of the inhalers to manufacture methamphetamine illicitly (140).

Fenfluramine has a half-life between 13 and 30 hours depending on urine pH, with acidic urine pH decreasing the half-life. It has a volume of distribution of 12 to 16 L/kg. Its metabolites include norfenfluramine, m-trifluoromethylbenzoic acid, and glycine conjugates. Dexfenfluramine is the D-isomer of fenfluramine. It has a half-life of 17 to 20 hours and a volume of distribution of 12 L/kg (140).

Phentermine has a half-life of 19 to 24 hours and a volume of distribution of 3 to 4 L/kg. Approximately 84% is eliminated unchanged, with the remainder undergoing p-hydroxylation and n-oxidation (140).

Pemoline, although not structurally related to amphetamine, has similar pharmacologic effects and is used to treat ADHD. It has been implicated in hepatic injury, rhabdomyolysis, and choreoathetosis (182a–182f).

DIAGNOSTIC TESTS

Differential Diagnosis

Pediatric patients who are inadvertently exposed to methamphetamine can present with inconsolable irritability, agitation, vomiting, and abdominal pain (183). In children, envenomation with the *Centruroides sculpturatus* scorpion can present with similar symptoms, and differentiating between the two syndromes may be difficult (183–185). Differences between the two syndromes include hypersalivation, tongue fasciculation, involuntary eye movements, and purposeless motor movements after scorpion envenomation (186).

A tetanus-like syndrome has been described in a patient with an oral ingestion of amphetamine and alcohol. Severe opisthotonus and risus sardonicus that required intubation developed in this patient (187).

GHB is another drug used at raves, where it is known as *liquid Ecstasy* or *liquid e*. Although GHB overdose does not have a similar presentation to amphetamines, GHB withdrawal may present with tachycardia, increased blood pressure, hallucinations, altered mental status, and tremors. Hyperthermia is not a major component of this syndrome (90).

The cardiovascular effects of amphetamine overdoses are similar to those of other clinical syndromes of catecholamine excess, including cocaine and phencyclidine abuse. Pheochromocytoma has been shown in one case to have been confused with methamphetamine overdose (188).

Malignant hyperthermia, neuroleptic malignant syndrome, and anticholinergic syndrome can produce temperature abnormalities similar to those of amphetamine overdoses (Chapters 10 and 23). Several drugs, including lysergic acid diethylamide and psilocybin, can cause similar hallucinations and paranoid behavior (Chapter 177). Seizures can occur in amphetamine overdose and in a multitude of other drug overdoses (e.g., cocaine) or withdrawal syndromes (e.g., alcohol).

Laboratory Principles

Most screening tests of urine for amphetamine-related compounds use an immunoassay technique (189). Confirmation is performed by a gas chromatography and mass spectroscopy (GC-MS) analysis (190). Methamphetamine isomer cross-reactivity on screening immunoassays has been described (191) but can be differentiated by GC-MS. Many amphetamine screening tests are further hampered by a low positive predictive value (192). Amphetamine can remain present in the urine for greater than 48 hours and is affected by factors such as pH and hydration status (193). An MDMA identification and quantitation method for saliva has been described and may have utility for simple noninvasive testing (194).

Multiple drugs and chemicals can interfere with amphetamine identification. Buflomedil is a vasodilator used for cerebrovascular and peripheral artery disease that interferes with the enzyme-multiplied immunoassay (EMIT) monoclonal assay for methamphetamine (195). Trazodone has been reported to cause a false-positive result (196). Histamine (H_2)-blockers such as ranitidine are a common cause of false-positive screening results (197–199). Ritodrine, a β-sympathomimetic amine used for the management of preterm labor, and phenothiazine derivatives such as chlorpromazine and promethazine have also been implicated (200–202). Selegiline is metabolized to L-amphetamine and L-methamphetamine and causes a positive screen and confirmatory test. Quantitative isomer analysis can resolve this issue (203). Clobenzorex, an anorectic drug prescribed in Mexico, is metabolized to amphetamine, giving positive results by GC-MS (204).

Mebeverine, an antispasmodic, has been reported to cause a false-positive amphetamine test in a fluorescent polarization assay (205). Doxepin, and specifically its metabolite n-desmethyldoxepin, in high concentrations can cause a false-positive methamphetamine test (206). Perazine can cause a false-positive amphetamine screening result (207). Benzathine, a salt used for the phenoxymethyl penicillin preparation, has been shown to cause a false-positive test with the Syva EMIT I polyclonal amphetamine/methamphetamine preparation (208). The compound 3-amino-1-phenylbutane, a metabolite of labetalol, can cause a false-positive test with several immunoassays and by thin-layer and gas chromatography (209).

Newer detection approaches include infrared transmission spectroscopy. This also can be used to differentiate methamphetamine enantiomers (210). Hair analysis has also been suggested as a means of identifying amphetamines and derivatives (211–213), but its use is not recommended for common clinical practice given lack of standardization (214). Nonaqueous capillary electrophoresis-fluorescence spectroscopy has been evaluated as a rapid detection method for MDMA, and a portable high-pressure liquid chromatography method for MDMA has been evaluated for use at rave parties to identify the exact content of tablets of designer amphetamines (215,216). A visual panel detection method for pediatric and adolescent populations as a means to rapidly screen patients who may have been exposed to drugs of abuse when presenting to an emergency department was found to have a positive predictive value of only 53% for amphetamines (217).

Postmortem Considerations

When attempting to collect postmortem blood specimens, it is recommended that peripheral blood rather than blood from the heart be used because of redistribution of methamphetamine to the heart, resulting in higher levels from heart blood compared to peripheral blood (218).

TREATMENT

Acute treatment is based mainly on controlling the stimulant effects of amphetamine compounds. Studies of the composition of MDMA tablets have routinely found other compounds, such as GHB, caffeine, acetaminophen, and ketamine. The dose of MDMA varied significantly, and other derivatives of amphetamine were commonly found (219,220).

Decontamination

The patient should receive activated charcoal for decontamination after recent drug ingestion. Gastric lavage has been recommended after massive designer amphetamine ingestion, especially when other drugs are involved (105).

Enhancement of Elimination

The utility of multiple dose–activated charcoal for the purpose of removing systemic drugs was not demonstrated in a rat model after intravenous methamphetamine (221). Urinary acidification can increase excretion of methamphetamine but is not recommended due to its potentially deleterious effects and the lack of evidence indicating efficacy. Peritoneal and hemodialysis also enhance elimination slightly but do not seem to have a beneficial clinical effect, probably because the drug is eliminated rapidly through other routes as well.

Antidotes

No specific antidotes for methamphetamine poisoning are available.

Supportive Care

Hyperthermia may quickly become life-threatening, and treatment should be instituted as early as possible. Treatment of hyperthermia includes wet soaks, fans, cold-water immersion, and pharmacologic control of muscle activity (Chapter 38). The role of dantrolene remains controversial (222–229).

The use of physical restraints can increase the risk for muscle injury, and "chemical restraints" should be considered (230,231). Atypical antipsychotics, such as risperidone and olanzapine, have been used in treating methamphetamine psychosis (232,233). To treat acute agitation, psychosis, and violent behavior, benzodiazepines and neuroleptics have been used to control symptoms. A comparative study in methamphetamine-toxic patients found droperidol to have increased efficacy over a longer period of time than lorazepam (234).

Addiction is a key component of the methamphetamine problem in society. Novel agents that may help in preventing addiction have been studied. It is known that the ability of methamphetamine to gain access to nerve terminals occurs through biogenic amine transporter, which allows the drug to release catecholamines. Indatraline, a reuptake inhibitor with high affinity for norepinephrine, dopamine, and serotonin transporter, is an agent that has been shown to block the ability of methamphetamine and MDMA to release neurotransmitters in nerve terminals (235). Dexedrine, the D-isomer of amphetamine, has been used as a substitute in patients with amphetamine dependence in Europe (236). Compliance to abstinence by determining the amphetamine isomer ratios has been described (237). Cognitive behavioral treatment is also becoming more important in treating the addiction to methamphetamine (238).

REFERENCES

1. Masand PS, Tesar GE. Use of stimulants in the medically ill. *Psychiatr Clin North Am* 1996;19(3):515–547.
2. Karch S. Drug abuse handbook. In: Segura J, ed. *Sports.* Boca Raton, FL: CRC, 1998.
3. Cohen S. Amphetamine abuse. *JAMA* 1975;231(4):414–415.
4. Mack RB. The iceman cometh and killeth: smokable methamphetamine. *NC Med J* 1990;51(6):276–278.
5. Beebe DK, Walley E. Smokable methamphetamine ("ice"): an old drug in a different form. *Am Fam Physician* 1995;51(2):449–453.
6. Perez-Reyes MR, White WR, McDonald S, et al. Pharmacologic effects of methamphetamine vapor inhalation (smoking) in man. *NIDA Res Monogr* 1991;105:575–577.
7. Perez-Reyes M, White WR, McDonald SA, et al. Clinical effects of methamphetamine vapor inhalation. *Life Sci* 1991;49(13):953–959.
8. Guharoy R, Medicis J, Chol S, et al. Methamphetamine overdose: experience with six cases. *Vet Hum Toxicol* 1999;41(1):28–30.
9. Buffenstein A, Heaster J, Ko P. Chronic psychotic illness from methamphetamine. *Am J Psychiatry* 1999;156(4):662.
10. Richards JR, Brofeldt BT. Patterns of tooth wear associated with methamphetamine use. *J Periodontol* 2000;71(8):1371–1374.
11. Sribanditmongkol P, Chokjamsai M, Thampitak S. Methamphetamine overdose and fatality: 2 case reports. *J Med Assoc Thai* 2000;83(9):1120–1123.
12. Logan BK, Weiss EL, Harruff RC. Case report: distribution of methamphetamine in a massive fatal ingestion. *J Forensic Sci* 1996;41(2):322–323.
13. Logan BK, Fligner CL, Haddix T. Cause and manner of death in fatalities involving methamphetamine. *J Forensic Sci* 1998;43(1):28–34.
14. Fornazzari L, Carlen PL, Kapur BM. Intravenous abuse of propylhexedrine (Benzedrex) and the risk of brainstem dysfunction in young adults. *Can J Neurol Sci* 1986;13(4):337–339.
15. Schaiberger PH, Kennedy TC, Miller FC, et al. Pulmonary hypertension associated with long-term inhalation of "crank" methamphetamine. *Chest* 1993;104(2):614–616.
16. White L, DiMaio VJ. Intravenous propylhexedrine and sudden death. *N Engl J Med* 1977;297(19):1071.
17. Perez J, Burton BT, McGirr JG. Airway compromise and delayed death following attempted central vein injection of propylhexedrine. *J Emerg Med* 1994;12(6):795–797.
18. Anglin MD, Burke C, Perrochet B, et al. History of the methamphetamine problem. *J Psychoactive Drugs* 2000;32(2):137–141.
19. Moore KA, Lichtman AH, Poklis A, et al. Alpha-benzyl-n-methylphenethylamine (BNMPA), an impurity of illicit methamphetamine synthesis: pharmacological evaluation and interaction with methamphetamine. *Drug Alcohol Depend* 1995;39(2):83–89.
20. Moore KA, Ismaiel A, Poklis A. Alpha-benzyl-n-methylphenethylamine (BNMPA), an impurity of illicit methamphetamine synthesis: III. Detection of BNMPA and metabolites in urine of methamphetamine users. *J Anal Toxicol* 1996;20(2):89–92.
21. Allcott JV 3rd, Barnhart RA, Mooney LA. Acute lead poisoning in two users of illicit methamphetamine. *JAMA* 1987;258(4):510–511.
22. Varner KJ, Hein ND, Ogden BA, et al. Chloroephedrine: contaminant of methamphetamine synthesis with cardiovascular activity. *Drug Alcohol Depend* 2001;64(3):299–307.
23. Burgess JL. Phosphine exposure from a methamphetamine laboratory investigation. *J Toxicol Clin Toxicol* 2001;39(2):165–168.
24. Willers-Russo LJ. Three fatalities involving phosphine gas, produced as a result of methamphetamine manufacturing. *J Forensic Sci* 1999;44(3):647–652.

25. Wolkoff DA. Methamphetamine abuse: an overview for health care professionals. *Hawaii Med J* 1997;56(2):34–36, 44.
26. Domier CP, Simon SL, Rawson RA, et al. A comparison of injecting and noninjecting methamphetamine users. *J Psychoactive Drugs* 2000;32(2):229–232.
27. Green GA, Uryasz FD, Petr TA, et al. NCAA study of substance use and abuse habits of college student-athletes. *Clin J Sport Med* 2001;11(1):51–56.
28. Schwartz RH, Miller NS. MDMA (ecstasy) and the rave: a review. *Pediatrics* 1997;100(4):705–708.
29. Arria AM, Yacoubian GS Jr, Fost E, et al. The pediatric forum: Ecstasy use among club rave attendees. *Arch Pediatr Adolesc Med* 2002;156(3):295–296.
30. Morton AJ, Hickey MA, Dean LC. Methamphetamine toxicity in mice is potentiated by exposure to loud music. *Neuroreport* 2001;12(15):3277–3281.
31. Chan P, Chen JH, Lee MH, et al. Fatal and nonfatal methamphetamine intoxication in the intensive care unit. *J Toxicol Clin Toxicol* 1994;32(2):147–155.
32. Hong R, Matsuyama E, Nur K. Cardiomyopathy associated with the smoking of crystal methamphetamine. *JAMA* 1991;265(9):1152–1154.
33. Wallace RT, Brown GC, Benson W, et al. Sudden retinal manifestations of intranasal cocaine and methamphetamine abuse. *Am J Ophthalmol* 1992;114(2):158–160.
34. Zalis EG, Parmley LF. Fatal amphetamine poisoning. *Arch Intern Med* 1963;112:822–826.
35. Cook CE, Jeffcoat AR, Hill JM, et al. Pharmacokinetics of methamphetamine self-administered to human subjects by smoking S-(+)-methamphetamine hydrochloride. *Drug Metab Dispos* 1993;21:717–723.
36. Beckett AH, Rowland M. Urinary excretion kinetics of amphetamine in man. *J Pharm Pharmacol* 1965;17:628–639.
37. Ghuran A, Nolan J. Recreational drug misuse: issues for the cardiologist. *Heart* 2000;83(6):627–633.
38. Smith HJ, Roche AH, Jausch MF, et al. Cardiomyopathy associated with amphetamine administration. *Am Heart J* 1976;91(6):792.
39. Haft JI. Cardiovascular injury induced by sympathetic catecholamines. *Prog Cardiovasc Dis* 1974;17(1):73–86.
40. He SY, Matoba R, Fujitani N, et al. Cardiac muscle lesions associated with chronic administration of methamphetamine in rats. *Am J Forensic Med Pathol* 1996;17(2):155–162.
41. Varner KJ, Ogden BA, Delcarpio J, et al. Cardiovascular responses elicited by the "binge" administration of methamphetamine. *J Pharmacol Exp Ther* 2002;301(1):152–159.
42. Volkow ND, Chang L, Wang GJ, et al. Loss of dopamine transporters in methamphetamine abusers recovers with protracted abstinence. *J Neurosci* 2001;21(23):9414–9418.
43. Wrona MZ, Dryhurst G. A putative metabolite of serotonin, tryptamine-4,5-dione, is an irreversible inhibitor of tryptophan hydroxylase: possible relevance to the serotonergic neurotoxicity of methamphetamine. *Chem Res Toxicol* 2001;14(9):1184–1192.
44. Huang YH, Tsai SJ, Su TW, et al. Effects of repeated high-dose methamphetamine on local cerebral glucose utilization in rats. *Neuropsychopharmacology* 1999;21(3):427–434.
45. Chapman DE, Hanson GR, Kesner RP, et al. Long-term changes in basal ganglia function after a neurotoxic regimen of methamphetamine. *J Pharmacol Exp Ther* 2001;296(2):520–527.
46. Cass WA, Manning MW. Recovery of presynaptic dopaminergic functioning in rats treated with neurotoxic doses of methamphetamine. *J Neurosci* 1999;19(17):7653–7660.
47. McCann UD, Wong DF, Yokoi F, et al. Reduced striatal dopamine transporter density in abstinent methamphetamine and methcathinone users: evidence from positron emission tomography studies with [11c]win-35,428. *J Neurosci* 1998;18(20):8417–8422.
48. Harvey DC, Lacan G, Tanious SP, et al. Recovery from methamphetamine induced long-term nigrostriatal dopaminergic deficits without substantia nigra cell loss. *Brain Res* 2000;871(2):259–270.
49. Yu L, Liao PC. Estrogen and progesterone distinctively modulate methamphetamine-induced dopamine and serotonin depletions in c57bl/6j mice. *J Neural Transm* 2000;107(10):1139–1147.
50. Gao X, Dluzen DE. The effect of testosterone upon methamphetamine neurotoxicity of the nigrostriatal dopaminergic system. *Brain Res* 2001;892(1):63–69.
51. Dluzen DE. Neuroprotective effects of estrogen upon the nigrostriatal dopaminergic system. *J Neurocytol* 2000;29(5–6):387–399.
52. Gao X, Dluzen DE. Tamoxifen abolishes estrogen's neuroprotective effect upon methamphetamine neurotoxicity of the nigrostriatal dopaminergic system. *Neuroscience* 2001;103(2):385–394.
53. Dluzen DE, McDermott JL, Anderson LI. Tamoxifen diminishes methamphetamine-induced striatal dopamine depletion in intact female and male mice. *J Neuroendocrinol* 2001;13(7):618–624.
54. Fornai F, Battaglia G, Gesi M, et al. Dose-dependent protective effects of apomorphine against methamphetamine-induced nigrostriatal damage. *Brain Res* 2001;898(1):27–35.
55. Ladenheim B, Krasnova IN, Deng X, et al. Methamphetamine-induced neurotoxicity is attenuated in transgenic mice with a null mutation for interleukin-6. *Mol Pharmacol* 2000;58(6):1247–1256.
56. Imam SZ, Itzhak Y, Cadet JL, et al. Methamphetamine-induced alteration in striatal p53 and bcl-2 expressions in mice. *Brain Res Mol Brain Res* 2001;91(1–2):174–178.
57. Frost DO, Cadet JL. Effects of methamphetamine-induced neurotoxicity on the development of neural circuitry: a hypothesis. *Brain Res Rev* 2000;34(3):103–118.
58. Maragos WF, Jakel R, Chesnut D, et al. Methamphetamine toxicity is attenuated in mice that overexpress human manganese superoxide dismutase. *Brain Res* 2000;878(1–2):218–222.
59. Kita T, Matsunari Y, Saraya T, et al. Evaluation of the effects of alpha-phenyl-n-tert-butyl nitrone pretreatment on the neurobehavioral effects of methamphetamine. *Life Sci* 2000;67(13):1559–1571.
60. Imam SZ, Ali SF. Selenium, an antioxidant, attenuates methamphetamine-induced dopaminergic toxicity and peroxynitrite generation. *Brain Res* 2000;855(1):186–191.
61. Kim H, Jhoo W, Shin E, et al. Selenium deficiency potentiates methamphetamine-induced nigral neuronal loss; comparison with MPTP model. *Brain Res* 2000;862(1–2):247–252.
62. Lee YW, Hennig B, Yao J, et al. Methamphetamine induces ap-1 and nf-kappab binding and transactivation in human brain endothelial cells. *J Neurosci Res* 2001;66(4):583–591.
63. Stewart JL, Meeker JE. Fetal and infant deaths associated with maternal methamphetamine abuse. *J Anal Toxicol* 1997;21(6):515–517.
64. Stek AM, Fisher BK, Baker RS, et al. Maternal and fetal cardiovascular responses to methamphetamine in the pregnant sheep. *Am J Obstet Gynecol* 1993;169(4):888–897.
65. Yamamoto Y, Yamamoto K, Hayase T. Effect of methamphetamine on male mice fertility. *J Obstet Gynaecol Res* 1999;25(5):353–358.
66. Yen DJ, Wang SJ, Ju TH, et al. Stroke associated with methamphetamine inhalation. *Eur Neurol* 1994;34(1):16–22.
67. Perez JA Jr, Arsura EL, Strategos S. Methamphetamine-related stroke: four cases. *J Emerg Med* 1999;17(3):469–471.
68. Kase CS. Intracerebral hemorrhage: non-hypertensive causes. *Stroke* 1986;17(4):590–595.
69. Davis GG, Swalwell CI. Acute aortic dissections and ruptured berry aneurysms associated with methamphetamine abuse. *J Forensic Sci* 1994;39(6):1481–1485.
70. Turchan J, Anderson C, Hauser KF, et al. Estrogen protects against the synergistic toxicity by HIV proteins, methamphetamine and cocaine. *BMC Neurosci* 2001;2(1):3.
71. Simon SL, Domier C, Carnell J, et al. Cognitive impairment in individuals currently using methamphetamine. *Am J Addict* 2000;9(3):222–231.
72. Yui K, Goto K, Ikemoto S, et al. Methamphetamine psychosis: spontaneous recurrence of paranoid-hallucinatory states and monoamine neurotransmitter function. *J Clin Psychopharmacol* 1997;17(1):34–43.
73. Schindler CW, Zheng JW, Tella SR, et al. Pharmacological mechanisms in the cardiovascular effects of methamphetamine in conscious squirrel monkeys. *Pharmacol Biochem Behav* 1992;42(4):791–796.
74. Vidrio H, Pardo EG. Antihypertensive effects of sympathomimetic amines. *J Pharmacol Exp Ther* 1973;187(2):308–314.
75. Richards JR, Johnson EB, Stark RW, et al. Methamphetamine abuse and rhabdomyolysis in the ED: a 5-year study. *Am J Emerg Med* 1999;17(7):681–685.
76. Horiguchi T, Hori S, Shinozawa Y, et al. A case of traumatic shock complicated by methamphetamine intoxication. *Intensive Care Med* 1999;25(7):758–760.
77. Burchell SA, Ho HC, Yu M, et al. Effects of methamphetamine on trauma patients: a cause of severe metabolic acidosis? *Crit Care Med* 2000;28(6):2112–2115.
78. Swalwell CI, Davis GG. Methamphetamine as a risk factor for acute aortic dissection. *J Forensic Sci* 1999;44(1):23–26.
79. Henry JA, Hill IR. Fatal interaction between ritonavir and MDMA. *Lancet* 1998;352(9142):1751–1752.
80. Hales G, Roth N, Smith D. Possible fatal interaction between protease inhibitors and methamphetamine. *Antivir Ther* 2000;5(1):19.
81. Barry M, Mulcahy F, Merry C, et al. Pharmacokinetics and potential interactions amongst antiretroviral agents used to treat patients with HIV infection. *Clin Pharmacokinet* 1999;36(4):289–304.
82. Lin LY, Di Stefano EW, Schmitz DA, et al. Oxidation of methamphetamine and methylenedioxymethamphetamine by cyp2d6. *Drug Metab Dispos* 1997;25(9):1059–1064.
83. Mendelson J, Jones RT, Upton R, et al. Methamphetamine and ethanol interactions in humans. *Clin Pharmacol Ther* 1995;57(5):559–568.
84. Molina NM, Jejurikar SG. Toxicological findings in a fatal ingestion of methamphetamine. *J Anal Toxicol* 1999;23(1):67–68.
85. Shulgin AT. The background and chemistry of MDMA. *J Psychoactive Drugs* 1986;18(4):291–304.
86. Siegel RK. MDMA. Nonmedical use and intoxication. *J Psychoactive Drugs* 1986;18(4):349–354.
87. Klitzman RL, Greenberg JD, Pollack LM, et al. MDMA ("ecstasy") use, and its association with high risk behaviors, mental health, and other factors among gay/bisexual men in New York City. *Drug Alcohol Depend* 2002;66:115–125.
88. von Sydow K, Lieb R, Pfister H, et al. Use, abuse and dependence of ecstasy and related drugs in adolescents and young adults—a transient phenomenon? Results from a longitudinal community study. *Drug Alcohol Depend* 2002;66:147–159.
89. Duflou J, Mark A. Aortic dissection after ingestion of "ecstasy" (MDMA). *Am J Forensic Med Pathol* 2000;21:261–263.
90. Doyon S. The many faces of ecstasy. *Curr Opin Pediatr* 2001;13(2):170–176.
91. Henry JA, Jeffreys KJ, Dawling S. Toxicity and deaths from 3,4-methylenedioxymethamphetamine ("ecstasy"). *Lancet* 1992;340(8816):384–387.

92. Forrest AR, Galloway JH, Marsh ID, et al. A fatal overdose with 3,4-methylenedioxyamphetamine derivatives. *Forensic Sci Int* 1994;64(1):57–59.
93. Regenthal R, Kruger M, Rudolph K, et al. Survival after massive "ecstasy" (MDMA) ingestion. *Intensive Care Med* 1999;25(6):640–641.
94. de la Torre R, Farre M, Roset PN, et al. Pharmacology of MDMA in humans. *Ann NY Acad Sci* 2000;914:225–237.
95. Segura M, Ortuno J, Farre M, et al. 3,4-Dihydroxymethamphetamine (HHMA). A major in vivo 3,4-methylenedioxymethamphetamine (MDMA) metabolite in humans. *Chem Res Toxicol* 2001;14(9):1203–1208.
96. Reneman L, Endert E, de Bruin K, et al. The acute and chronic effects of MDMA ("ecstasy") on cortical 5-HT(2a) receptors in rat and human brain. *Neuropsychopharmacology* 2002;26(3):387–396.
97. Parrott AC. Recreational ecstasy/MDMA, the serotonin syndrome, and serotonergic neurotoxicity. *Pharmacol Biochem Behav* 2002;71(4):837–844.
98. McElhatton PR, Bateman DN, Evans C, et al. Congenital anomalies after prenatal ecstasy exposure. *Lancet* 1999;354:1441–1442.
99. Walubo A, Seger D. Fatal multi-organ failure after suicidal overdose with MDMA, "ecstasy": case report and review of the literature. *Hum Exp Toxicol* 1999;18(2):119–125.
100. Callaway CW, Clark RF. Hyperthermia in psychostimulant overdose. *Ann Emerg Med* 1994;24(1):68–76.
101. Murthy BV, Wilkes RG, Roberts NB. Creatine kinase isoform changes following ecstasy overdose. *Anaesth Intensive Care* 1997;25(2):156–159.
102. Hall AP, Lyburn ID, Spears FD, et al. An unusual case of ecstasy poisoning. *Intensive Care Med* 1996;22(7):670–671.
103. Logan AS, Stickle B, O'Keefe N, et al. Survival following "ecstasy" ingestion with a peak temperature of 42 degrees C. *Anaesthesia* 1993;48(11):1017–1018.
104. Cadier MA, Clarke JA. Ecstasy and whizz at a rave resulting in a major burn plus complications. *Burns* 1993;19(3):239–240.
105. Ramcharan S, Meenhorst PL, Otten JM, et al. Survival after massive ecstasy overdose. *J Toxicol Clin Toxicol* 1998;36(7):727–731.
106. Shannon M. Methylenedioxymethamphetamine (MDMA, "ecstasy"). *Pediatr Emerg Care* 2000;16(5):377–380.
107. Mas M, Farre M, de la Torre R, et al. Cardiovascular and neuroendocrine effects and pharmacokinetics of 3,4-methylenedioxymethamphetamine in humans. *J Pharmacol Exp Ther* 1999;290(1):136–145.
108. Rezvani K, Kurbaan AS, Brenton D. Ecstasy induced pneumomediastinum. *Thorax* 1996;51(9):960–961.
109. Quin GI, McCarthy GM, Harries DK. Spontaneous pneumomediastinum and ecstasy abuse. *J Accid Emerg Med* 1999;16(5):382.
110. Pittman JA, Pounsford JC. Spontaneous pneumomediastinum and ecstasy abuse. *J Accid Emerg Med* 1997;14(5):335–336.
111. Levine AJ, Drew S, Rees GM. "Ecstasy" induced pneumomediastinum. *J R Soc Med* 1993;86(4):232–233.
112. Ryan J, Banerjee A, Bong A. Pneumomediastinum in association with MDMA ingestion. *J Emerg Med* 2001;20(3):305–306.
113. Ferrie R, Loveland RC. Bilateral gluteal compartment syndrome after "ecstasy" hyperpyrexia. *J R Soc Med* 2000;93(5):260.
114. Kopelman MD, Reed LJ, Marsden P, et al. Amnesic syndrome and severe ataxia following the recreational use of 3,4-methylene-dioxymethamphetamine (MDMA, "ecstasy") and other substances. *Neurocase* 2001;7(5):423–432.
115. Biello SM, Dafters RI. MDMA and fenfluramine alter the response of the circadian clock to a serotonin agonist in vitro. *Brain Res* 2001;920(1–2):202–209.
116. Morgan MJ, McFie L, Fleetwood H, et al. Ecstasy (MDMA): are the psychological problems associated with its use reversed by prolonged abstinence? *Psychopharmacology (Berl)* 2002;159(3):294–303.
117. Obrocki J, Schmoldt A, Buchert R, et al. Specific neurotoxicity of chronic use of ecstasy. *Toxicol Lett* 2002;127:285–297.
118. O'Connor A, Cluroe A, Couch R, et al. Death from hyponatraemia-induced cerebral oedema associated with MDMA ("ecstasy") use. *N Z Med J* 1999;112(1091):255–256.
119. Parr MJ, Low HM, Botterill P. Hyponatraemia and death after "ecstasy" ingestion. *Med J Aust* 1997;166(3):136–137.
120. Holden R, Jackson MA. Near-fatal hyponatraemic coma due to vasopressin over-secretion after "ecstasy" (3,4-MDMA). *Lancet* 1996;347(9007):1052.
121. Brownfield MS, Greathouse J, Lorens SA, et al. Neuropharmacological characterization of serotoninergic stimulation of vasopressin secretion in conscious rats. *Neuroendocrinology* 1988;47(4):277–283.
122. Hall AP. Hyponatraemia, water intoxication and "ecstasy." *Intensive Care Med* 1997;23(12):1289.
123. Ajaelo I, Koenig K, Snoey E. Severe hyponatremia and inappropriate antidiuretic hormone secretion following ecstasy use. *Acad Emerg Med* 1998;5(8):839–840.
124. Gomez-Balaguer M, Pena H, Morillas C, et al. Syndrome of inappropriate antidiuretic hormone secretion and "designer drugs" (ecstasy). *J Pediatr Endocrinol Metab* 2000;13(4):437–438.
125. Henry JA, Fallon JK, Kicman AT, et al. Low-dose MDMA ("ecstasy") induces vasopressin secretion. *Lancet* 1998;351(9118):1784.
126. Bryden AA, Rothwell PJ, O'Reilly PH. Urinary retention with misuse of "ecstasy." *BMJ* 1995;310(6978):504.
127. Worsey J, Goble NM, Stott M, et al. Bladder outflow obstruction secondary to intravenous amphetamine abuse. *Br J Urol* 1989;64(3):320–321.
128. Dubin NN, Razack AH. Priapism: Ecstasy related? *Urology* 2000;56(6):1057.
129. Lawler LP, Abraham S, Fishman EK. 3,4-Methylenedioxymethamphetamine (ecstasy)-induced hepatotoxicity: multidetector CT and pathology findings. *J Comput Assist Tomogr* 2001;25(4):649.
130. Ellis AJ, Wendon JA, Portmann B, et al. Acute liver damage and ecstasy ingestion. *Gut* 1996;38(3):454–458.
131. Andreu V, Mas A, Bruguera M, et al. Ecstasy: a common cause of severe acute hepatotoxicity. *J Hepatol* 1998;29(3):394–397.
132. Jacks AS, Hykin PG. Retinal haemorrhage caused by "ecstasy." *Br J Ophthalmol* 1998;82(7):842–843.
133. Hassan L, Carvalho C, Yannuzzi LA, et al. Central serous chorioretinopathy in a patient using methylenedioxymethamphetamine (MDMA) or "ecstasy." *Retina* 2001;21(5):559–561.
134. Aguirre N, Barrionuevo M, Ramirez MJ, et al. Alpha-lipoic acid prevents 3,4-methylenedioxy-methamphetamine (MDMA)-induced neurotoxicity. *Neuroreport* 1999;10(17):3675–3680.
135. Tucker GT, Lennard MS, Ellis SW, et al. The demethylation of methylenedioxymethamphetamine ("ecstasy") by debrisoquine hydroxylase (CYP2D6). *Biochem Pharmacol* 1994;47(7):1151–1156.
136. Gonzalez FJ, Meyer UA. Molecular genetics of the debrisoquin-sparteine polymorphism. *Clin Pharmacol Ther* 1991;50:233–238.
137. Smilkstein MJ, Smolinske SC, Rumack BH. A case of MAO inhibitor/MDMA interaction: agony after ecstasy. *J Toxicol Clin Toxicol* 1987;25(1–2):149–159.
138. Hernandez-Lopez C, Farre M, Roset PN, et al. 3,4-Methylenedioxymethamphetamine (ecstasy) and alcohol interactions in humans: psychomotor performance, subjective effects, and pharmacokinetics. *J Pharmacol Exp Ther* 2002;300(1):236–244.
139. Giroud C, Augsburger M, Rivier L, et al. 2c-b: A new psychoactive phenylethylamine recently discovered in ecstasy tablets sold on the Swiss black market. *J Anal Toxicol* 1998;22(5):345–354.
140. Baselt RC. *Disposition of toxic drugs and chemicals in man*, 5th ed. Foster City, CA: Chemical Toxicology Institute, 2000.
141. Bruhn JG, De Smet PA, El-Seedi HR, et al. Mescaline use for 5700 years. *Lancet* 2002;359(9320):1866.
142. Shulgin AT, Sargent T, Naranjo C. Structure-activity relationships of one-ring psychotomimetics. *Nature* 1969;221(180):537–541.
143. Felgate HE, Felgate PD, James RA, et al. Recent paramethoxyamphetamine deaths. *J Anal Toxicol* 1998;22(2):169–172.
144. Green AL, El Hait MA. P-methoxyamphetamine, a potent reversible inhibitor of type-a monoamine oxidase in vitro and in vivo. *J Pharm Pharmacol* 1980;32(4):262–266.
145. Cimbura G. PMA deaths in Ontario. *Can Med Assoc J* 1974;110(11):1263–1267.
146. James RA, Dinan A. Hyperpyrexia associated with fatal paramethoxyamphetamine (PMA) abuse. *Med Sci Law* 1998;38(1):83–85.
147. Ling LH, Marchant C, Buckley NA, et al. Poisoning with the recreational drug paramethoxyamphetamine ("death"). *Med J Aust* 2001;174(9):453–455.
148. Ropero-Miller JD, Goldberger BA. Recreational drugs. Current trends in the 90s. *Clin Lab Med* 1998;18(4):727–746.
149. Misane I, Johansson C, Ogren SO. Analysis of the 5-HT1a receptor involvement in passive avoidance in the rat. *Br J Pharmacol* 1998;125(3):499–509.
150. Arvanov VL, Liang X, Russo A, et al. LSD and DOB: interaction with 5-HT2a receptors to inhibit NMDA receptor-mediated transmission in the rat prefrontal cortex. *Eur J Neurosci* 1999;11(9):3064–3072.
151. Winek CL, Collom WD, Bricker JD. A death due to 4-bromo-2,5-dimethoxyamphetamine. *Clin Toxicol* 1981;18(3):267–271.
152. Toennes SW, Ohlmeier M, Schmidt K, et al. [explanation of an unclear neurologic syndrome by toxicologic investigation]. *Dtsch Med Wochenschr* 2000;125(30):900–902.
153. Bowen JS, Davis GB, Kearney TE, et al. Diffuse vascular spasm associated with 4-bromo-2,5-dimethoxyamphetamine ingestion. *JAMA* 1983;249(11): 1477–1479.
154. Glennon RA, Titeler M, Lyon RA. A preliminary investigation of the psychoactive agent 4-bromo-2,5-dimethoxyphenethylamine: a potential drug of abuse. *Pharmacol Biochem Behav* 1988;30(3):597–601.
155. Shulgin AT, Carter MF. Centrally active phenethylamines. *Psychopharmacol Commun* 1975;1(1):93–98.
156. Lukaszewski T. 3,4-Methylenedioxyamphetamine overdose. *Clin Toxicol* 1979;15(4):405–409.
157. Glennon RA, Young R. MDA: an agent that produces stimulus effects similar to those of 3,4-DMA, LSD and cocaine. *Eur J Pharmacol* 1984;99(2–3):249–250.
158. Simpson DL, Rumack BH. Methylenedioxyamphetamine. Clinical description of overdose, death, and review of pharmacology. *Arch Intern Med* 1981;141(11):1507–1509.
159. Arimany J, Medallo J, Pujol A, et al. Intentional overdose and death with 3,4-methylenedioxymethamphetamine (MDMA; "Eve"): case report. *Am J Forensic Med Pathol* 1998;19(2):148–151.
160. Weinmann W, Bohnert M. Lethal monointoxication by overdosage of MDEA. *Forensic Sci Int* 1998;91(2):91–101.
161. Tsatsakis AM, Michalodimitrakis MN, Patsalis AN. MDEA related death in Crete: a case report and literature review. *Vet Hum Toxicol* 1997;39(4):241–244.
162. Gouzoulis-Mayfrank E, Thelen B, Habermeyer E, et al. Psychopathological, neuroendocrine and autonomic effects of 3,4-methylenedioxyethylamphetamine (ME), psilocybin and d-methamphetamine in healthy volunteers. Results of an experimental double-blind placebo-controlled study. *Psychopharmacology (Berl)* 1999;142(1):41–50.
163. Huang X, Marona-Lewicka D, Nichols DE. P-methylthioamphetamine is a potent new non-neurotoxic serotonin-releasing agent. *Eur J Pharmacol* 1992;229(1):31–38.

164. Elliott SP. Analysis of 4-methylthioamphetamine in clinical specimens. *Ann Clin Biochem* 2001;38(Pt 4):339–347.
165. Elliott SP. Fatal poisoning with a new phenylethylamine: 4-methylthioamphetamine (4-MTA). *J Anal Toxicol* 2000;24(2):85–89.
166. Decaestecker T, De Letter E, Clauwaert K, et al. Fatal 4-MTA intoxication: development of a liquid chromatographic-tandem mass spectrometric assay for multiple matrices. *J Anal Toxicol* 2001;25(8):705–710.
167. Kintz P. Excretion of MBDB and BDB in urine, saliva, and sweat following single oral administration. *J Anal Toxicol* 1997;21(7):570–575.
168. Kronstrand R. Identification of n-methyl-1-(3,4-methylenedioxyphenyl)-2-butanamine (MBDB) in urine from drug users. *J Anal Toxicol* 1996;20(6):512–516.
169. Maurer HH. On the metabolism and the toxicological analysis of methylenedioxyphenylalkylamine designer drugs by gas chromatography–mass spectrometry. *Ther Drug Monit* 1996;18(4):465–470.
170. Nichols DE. Differences between the mechanism of action of MDMA, MBDB, and the classic hallucinogens. Identification of a new therapeutic class: entactogens. *J Psychoactive Drugs* 1986;18(4):305–313.
171. Calkins RF, Aktan GB, Hussain KL. Methcathinone: the next illicit stimulant epidemic? *J Psychoactive Drugs* 1995;27(3):277–285.
172. Emerson TS, Cisek JE. Methcathinone: a Russian designer amphetamine infiltrates the rural Midwest. *Ann Emerg Med* 1993;22(12):1897–1903.
173. To LB, Sangster JF, Rampling D, et al. Ephedrine-induced cardiomyopathy. *Med J Aust* 1980;2(1):35–36.
174. Kunsman GW, Jones R, Levine B, et al. Methylephedrine concentrations in blood and urine specimens. *J Anal Toxicol* 1998;22(4):310–313.
175. Halbach H. Medical aspects of the chewing of khat leaves. *Bull World Health Organ* 1972;47(1):21–29.
176. Pantelis C, Hindler CG, Taylor JC. Use and abuse of khat (catha edulis): a review of the distribution, pharmacology, side effects and a description of psychosis attributed to khat chewing. *Psychol Med* 1989;19(3):657–668.
177. Salib E, Ahmed AG. The khat-chewing elderly. *Int J Geriatr Psychiatry* 1998;13(7):493–494.
178. Cats A, Scholten P, Meuwissen SG, et al. Acute fasciola hepatica infection attributed to chewing khat. *Gut* 2000;47(4):584–585.
179. Kassie F, Darroudi F, Kundi M, et al. Khat (catha edulis) consumption causes genotoxic effects in humans. *Int J Cancer* 2001;92(3):329–332.
180. Klein-Schwartz W. Abuse and toxicity of methylphenidate. *Curr Opin Pediatr* 2002;14(2):219–223.
181. Baggott M, Heifets B, Jones RT, et al. Chemical analysis of ecstasy pills. *JAMA* 2000;284(17):2190.
182. McEvoy GK. *AHFS drug information.* ASHP, 2002.
182a. Rothman RB, Baumann MH, Savage JE, et al. Evidence for possible involvement of 5-HT(2b) receptors in the cardiac valvulopathy associated with fenfluramine and other serotonergic medications. *Circulation* 2000;102(23):2836–2841.
182b. Hanson GR, Jensen M, Johnson M, et al. Distinct features of seizures induced by cocaine and amphetamine analogs. *Eur J Pharmacol* 1999;377(2–3):167–173.
182c. Adcock KG, MacElroy DE, Wolford ET, et al. Pemoline therapy resulting in liver transplantation. *Ann Pharmacother* 1998;32(4):422–425.
182d. Marotta PJ, Roberts EA. Pemoline hepatotoxicity in children. *J Pediatr* 1998;132(5):894–897.
182e. Stork CM, Cantor R. Pemoline induced acute choreoathetosis: case report and review of the literature. *J Toxicol Clin Toxicol* 1997;35(1):105–108.
182f. Zhang Y. Dextromethorphan: enhancing its systemic availability by way of low-dose quinidine-mediated inhibition of cytochrome. *Clin Pharmacol Ther* 1991;51:647–655.
183. Kolecki P. Inadvertent methamphetamine poisoning in pediatric patients. *Pediatr Emerg Care* 1998;14(6):385–387.
184. Curry SC, Vance MV, Ryan PJ, et al. Envenomation by the scorpion *Centruroides sculpturatus. J Toxicol Clin Toxicol* 1983;21(4–5):417–449.
185. Nagorka AR, Bergeson PS. Infant methamphetamine toxicity posing as scorpion envenomation. *Pediatr Emerg Care* 1998;14(5):350–351.
186. Suchard JR, Curry SC. Methamphetamine toxicity. *Pediatr Emerg Care* 1999;15(4):306.
187. Humphreys A, Tanner AR. Acute dystonic drug reaction or tetanus? An unusual consequence of a "whizz" overdose. *Hum Exp Toxicol* 1994;13(5):311–312.
188. Lynton RC, Marquardt K, Albertson T, et al. Pheochromocytoma masked as suspected methamphetamine abuse. *J Toxicol Clin Toxicol* 2002;40:393.
189. Lekskulchai V, Mokkhavesa C. Evaluation of Roche Abuscreen online amphetamine immunoassay for screening of new amphetamine analogues. *J Anal Toxicol* 2001;25(6):471–475.
190. Valentine JL, Middleton R. GC-MS identification of sympathomimetic amine drugs in urine: rapid methodology applicable for emergency clinical toxicology. *J Anal Toxicol* 2000;24(3):211–222.
191. Poklis A, Moore KA. Response of emit amphetamine immunoassays to urinary desoxyephedrine following Vicks inhaler use. *Ther Drug Monit* 1995;17(1):89–94.
192. Skelton H, Dann LM, Ong RT, et al. Drug screening of patients who deliberately harm themselves admitted to the emergency department. *Ther Drug Monit* 1998;20(1):98–103.
193. Smith-Kielland A, Skuterud B, Morland J. Urinary excretion of amphetamine after termination of drug abuse. *J Anal Toxicol* 1997;21(5):325–329.
194. Navarro M, Pichini S, Farre M, et al. Usefulness of saliva for measurement of 3,4-methylenedioxymethamphetamine and its metabolites: correlation with plasma drug concentrations and effect of salivary pH. *Clin Chem* 2001;47(10):1788–1795.
195. Papa P, Rocchi L, Mainardi C, et al. Buflomedil interference with the monoclonal emit d.A.U. Amphetamine/methamphetamine immunoassay. *Eur J Clin Chem Clin Biochem* 1997;35(5):369–370.
196. Roberge RJ, Luellen JR, Reed S. False-positive amphetamine screen following a trazodone overdose. *J Toxicol Clin Toxicol* 2001;39(2):181–182.
197. Dietzen DJ, Ecos K, Friedman D, et al. Positive predictive values of abused drug immunoassays on the Beckman synchron in a veteran population. *J Anal Toxicol* 2001;25(3):174–178.
198. Grinstead GF. Ranitidine and high concentrations of phenylpropanolamine cross react in the emit monoclonal amphetamine/methamphetamine assay. *Clin Chem* 1989;35(9):1998–1999.
199. Kelly KL. Ranitidine cross-reactivity in the emit D.A.U. Monoclonal amphetamine/methamphetamine assay. *Clin Chem* 1990;36(7):1391–1392.
200. Nice A, Maturen A. False-positive urine amphetamine screen with ritodrine. *Clin Chem* 1989;35(7):1542–1543.
201. Smith-Kielland A, Olsen KM, Christophersen AS. False-positive results with emit ii amphetamine/methamphetamine assay in users of common psychotropic drugs. *Clin Chem* 1995;41(6 Pt 1):951–952.
202. Olsen KM, Gulliksen M, Christophersen AS. Metabolites of chlorpromazine and brompheniramine may cause false-positive urine amphetamine results with monoclonal EMIT D.A.U. Immunoassay. *Clin Chem* 1992;38(4):611–612.
203. Meeker JE, Reynolds PC. Postmortem tissue methamphetamine concentrations following selegiline administration. *J Anal Toxicol* 1990;14(5):330–331.
204. Tarver JA. Amphetamine-positive drug screens from use of clobenzorex hydrochlorate. *J Anal Toxicol* 1994;18(3):183.
205. Kraemer T, Wennig R, Maurer HH. The antispasmodic drug mebeverine leads to positive amphetamine results by fluorescence polarization immunoassay (FPIA)—studies on the toxicological analysis of urine by FPIA and GC-MS. *J Anal Toxicol* 2001;25(5):333–338.
206. Merigian KS, Browning R, Kellerman A. Doxepin causing false-positive urine test for amphetamine. *Ann Emerg Med* 1993;22(8):1370.
207. Schmolke M, Hallbach J, Guder WG. False-positive results for urine amphetamine and opiate immunoassays in a patient intoxicated with perazine. *Clin Chem* 1996;42(10):1725–1726.
208. Berthier M, Bonneau D, Mura P, et al. Benzathine as a cause for a false-positive test result for amphetamines. *J Pediatr* 1995;127(4):669–670.
209. Gilbert RB, Peng PI, Wong D. A labetalol metabolite with analytical characteristics resembling amphetamines. *J Anal Toxicol* 1995;19(2):84–86.
210. Chappell JS. Infrared discrimination of enantiomerically enriched and racemic samples of methamphetamine salts. *Analyst* 1997;122(8):755–760.
211. Nakahara Y, Kikura R. Hair analysis for drugs of abuse. XVIII. 3,4-Methylenedioxymethamphetamine (MDMA) disposition in hair roots and use in identification of acute MDMA poisoning. *Biol Pharm Bull* 1997;20(9):969–972.
212. Rohrich J, Kauert G. Determination of amphetamine and methylenedioxyamphetamine derivatives in hair. *Forensic Sci Int* 1997;84(1–3):179–188.
213. Kronstrand R, Grundin R, Jonsson J. Incidence of opiates, amphetamines, and cocaine in hair and blood in fatal cases of heroin overdose. *Forensic Sci Int* 1998;92(1):29–38.
214. Kintz P, Cirimele V. Interlaboratory comparison of quantitative determination of amphetamine and related compounds in hair samples. *Forensic Sci Int* 1997;84(1–3):151–156.
215. Fang C, Chung YL, Liu JT, et al. Rapid analysis of 3,4-methylenedioxymethamphetamine: a comparison of nonaqueous capillary electrophoresis/fluorescence detection with GC/MS. *Forensic Sci Int* 2002;125(2–3):142–148.
216. Meyer V. HPLC on the dance floor. *Anal Chem* 2000;72(23):735A–736A.
217. Valentine JL, Komoroski EM. Use of a visual panel detection method for drugs of abuse: clinical and laboratory experience with children and adolescents. *J Pediatr* 1995;126(1):135–140.
218. Barnhart FE, Fogacci JR, Reed DW. Methamphetamine—a study of postmortem redistribution. *J Anal Toxicol* 1999;23(1):69–70.
219. Sherlock K, Wolff K, Hay AW, et al. Analysis of illicit ecstasy tablets: implications for clinical management in the accident and emergency department. *J Accid Emerg Med* 1999;16(3):194–197.
220. Spruit IP. Monitoring synthetic drug markets, trends, and public health. *Subst Use Misuse* 2001;36(1–2):23–47.
221. Hutchaleelaha A, Mayersohn M. Influence of activated charcoal on the disposition kinetics of methamphetamine enantiomers in the rat following intravenous dosing. *J Pharm Sci* 1996;85(5):541–545.
222. Campkin NJ, Davies UM. Treatment of "ecstasy" overdose with dantrolene. *Anaesthesia* 1993;48(1):82–83.
223. Watson JD, Ferguson C, Hinds CJ, et al. Exertional heat stroke induced by amphetamine analogues. Does dantrolene have a place? *Anaesthesia* 1993;48(12):1057–1060.
224. Webb C, Williams V. Ecstasy intoxication: appreciation of complications and the role of dantrolene. *Anaesthesia* 1993;48(6):542–543.
225. Roberts L, Wright H. Survival following intentional massive overdose of "ecstasy." *J Accid Emerg Med* 1994;11(1):53–54.
226. Wake D. Ecstasy overdose: a case study. *Intensive Crit Care Nurs* 1995;11(1):6–9.
227. Dowsett RP. Deaths attributed to "ecstasy" overdose. *Med J Aust* 1996;164(11):700.
228. Gillman PK. Ecstasy, serotonin syndrome and the treatment of hyperpyrexia. *Med J Aust* 1997;167(2):109, 111.

229. Singarajah C, Lavies NG. An overdose of ecstasy. A role for dantrolene. *Anaesthesia* 1992;47(8):686–687.
230. Deschamp C. Calming the demon within. Chemical vs. physical restraint. *J Emerg Med Serv JEMS* 1994;19(10):49–53.
231. Sullivan-Marx EM. Physical and chemical restraints: meeting the challenge. *Dimens Crit Care Nurs* 1994;13(2):58–59.
232. Misra L, Kofoed L. Risperidone treatment of methamphetamine psychosis. *Am J Psychiatry* 1997;154(8):1170.
233. Misra LK, Kofoed L, Oesterheld JR, et al. Olanzapine treatment of methamphetamine psychosis. *J Clin Psychopharmacol* 2000;20(3):393–394.
234. Richards JR, Derlet RW, Duncan DR. Methamphetamine toxicity: treatment with a benzodiazepine versus a butyrophenone. *Eur J Emerg Med* 1997;4(3):130–135.
235. Rothman RB, Partilla JS, Baumann MH, et al. Neurochemical neutralization of methamphetamine with high-affinity nonselective inhibitors of biogenic amine transporters: a pharmacological strategy for treating stimulant abuse. *Synapse* 2000;35(3):222–227.
236. Fleming PM, Roberts D. Is the prescription of amphetamine justified as a harm reduction measure? *J R Soc Health* 1994;114(3):127–131.
237. George S, Braithwaite RA. Using amphetamine isomer ratios to determine the compliance of amphetamine abusers prescribed dexedrine. *J Anal Toxicol* 2000;24(3):223–227.
238. Huber A, Ling W, Shoptaw S, et al. Integrating treatments for methamphetamine abuse: a psychosocial perspective. *J Addict Dis* 1997;16(4):41–50.
239. Kankaanpaa A, Ellermaa S, Meririnne E, et al. Acute neurochemical and behavioral effects of stereoisomers of 4-methylaminorex in relation to brain drug concentrations. *J Pharmacol Exp Ther* 2002;300(2):450–459.
240. Bunker CF, Johnson M, Gibb JW, et al. Neurochemical effects of an acute treatment with 4-methylaminorex: a new stimulant of abuse. *Eur J Pharmacol* 1990;180(1):103–111.
241. Valtier S, Cody JT. Metabolic production of amphetamine following administration of clobenzorex. *J Forensic Sci* 1999;44(1):17–22.
242. Cornaert P, Camblin J, Graux P, et al. [congestive cardiomyopathy in addiction to clobenzorex, an anorexigenic drug]. *Arch Mal Coeur Vaiss* 1986;79(4):515–518.
243. Ku YR, Chang YS, Wen KC, et al. Analysis and confirmation of synthetic anorexics in adulterated traditional Chinese medicines by high-performance capillary electrophoresis. *J Chromatogr A* 1999;848(1–2):537–543.
244. Gardin JM, Schumacher D, Constantine G, et al. Valvular abnormalities and cardiovascular status following exposure to dexfenfluramine or phentermine/fenfluramine. *JAMA* 2000;283(13):1703–1709.
245. Steffee CH, Singh HK, Chitwood WR. Histologic changes in three explanted native cardiac valves following use of fenfluramines. *Cardiovasc Pathol* 1999;8(5):245–253.
246. Kokkinos J, Levine SR. Possible association of ischemic stroke with phentermine. *Stroke* 1993;24(2):310–313.
247. Jefferson HJ, Jayne DR. Peripheral vasculopathy and nephropathy in association with phentermine. *Nephrol Dial Transplant* 1999;14(7):1761–1763.
248. Markowitz GS, Tartini A, D'Agati VD. Acute interstitial nephritis following treatment with anorectic agents phentermine and phendimetrazine. *Clin Nephrol* 1998;50(4):252–254.

CHAPTER 175

Cocaine

Judd E. Hollander

$Cl^{\ominus}$ CH_3 O H—$N^{\oplus}$ —OCH_3 O O

COCAINE HYDROCHLORIDE

Molecular formula and weight:	**$C_{17}H_{21}NO_4$, 303.4 g/mol**
SI conversion:	**mg/L × 3.30 = mmol/L**
CAS Registry No.:	**50-36-2**
Therapeutic levels:	***Not used clinically***
Target organs:	**Central nervous system (acute and chronic), cardiovascular system (acute and chronic), multiple other effects**
Antidote:	**None**

OVERVIEW

Erythroxylon coca, the shrub from which cocaine is derived, grows indigenously in South America. Sixth-century inhabitants of Peru chewed or sucked on the leaves as an ancient ritual. Cocaine was first identified as the active alkaloid in the coca leaf in 1857. Although twelfth-century Incas used cocaine-filled saliva as local anesthesia for ritual trephinations (1), it was not identified medically as a local anesthetic until 1884 (2). In the early twentieth century, cocaine was used briefly as an ingredient in Coca-Cola. In 1906, the United States began to control cocaine use, and in 1914, the Harrison Narcotic Act labeled cocaine as a narcotic. It was designated a schedule II drug. Since 1975, recreational cocaine use has increased and reports of side effects have grown exponentially. As of 1999, 25 million U.S. residents had used cocaine at least once, with 1.5 million people using cocaine in the past month (3).

"Crack" is the direct precipitate of "free base" cocaine that results from alkalinization of aqueous cocaine hydrochloride.

Medical Use

Cocaine is still used as topical anesthesia (4–10% solutions) for intranasal, bronchoscopic, or ophthalmologic procedures. A mixture of tetracaine, epinephrine, and cocaine is used as a topical anesthetic in children with scalp and facial lacerations. However, systemic toxicity including seizure and death has been reported (4–7). In general, cocaine is not recommended for standard medical care, and its use should be limited to situations in which alternative agents are contraindicated.

TABLE 1. Differential cocaine effects depending on the route of administration

Administration							
Route	Mode	Initial onset of action (sec)	Duration of "high" (min)	Average acute dose (mg)	Peak plasma level (ng/ml)	Purity (%)	Bioavailability (% absorbed)
Oral	Coca leaf chewing	300–600	45–90	20–50	150	0.5–1.0	
Oral	Cocaine HCl	600–1800		100–200	150–200	20–80	20–30
Intranasal	"Snorting" cocaine HCl	120–180	30–45	5–30	150	20–80	20–30
Intravenous	Cocaine HCl	30–45	10–20	25–50	300–400	7–100	100
				>200	1000–1500		
Smoking	Coca paste	8–10	5–10	60–250	300–800	40–85	6–32
	Free base			250–1000	800–900	90–100	
	Crack				?	50–95	

Toxic Dose

The maximal "safe" total dose of cocaine is 1 to 3 mg/kg body weight. The toxic dose is highly variable and is affected by characteristics of the user, the drug, and the route of administration. For the user, physiologic tolerance, previous history of cocaine use, and individual susceptibility (e.g., cardiovascular disease, pseudocholinesterase deficiency) all affect the response to a cocaine dose. For the drug, concomitant drug use (illicit or licit) and adulterants may alter the toxicity profile. Finally, the route of administration and time between administration and death affect cocaine concentrations in plasma (Table 1). Smoked cocaine and intravenous cocaine appear to produce similar increases in heart rate, blood pressure, and subjective effects at similar venous plasma cocaine levels. The potency of smoked cocaine is approximately 60% that of intravenous cocaine; that is, a 50-mg dose of smoked cocaine has effects similar to those of a 32-mg dose of intravenous cocaine. Plasma cocaine levels may reach 425 ng/ml approximately 20 minutes after a 32-mg intravenous dose and 380 ng/ml after a 50-mg dose of smoked cocaine (8). High plasma concentrations are rarely seen because of the short half-life of cocaine.

Fatalities have followed mucous membrane application of 25 mg (9) or nasal topical use of 400 mg (10). Tracheobronchial use of 200 mg or less in six cases was fatal (10).

TOXICOKINETICS AND TOXICODYNAMICS

Absorption

Cocaine is rapidly absorbed through nasal mucosa, gastrointestinal mucosa, pulmonary alveoli, and by direct intravenous injection; all result in toxicity (Table 1). Oral administration has a lag phase of about 30 minutes but reaches peak concentration in approximately 60 minutes. Effects from buccal (chewing) and nasal insufflation begin almost immediately but are variable due to local vasoconstriction. Peak concentrations are reached within 30 to 60 minutes. Intravenous and inhalational routes of cocaine use produce near immediate distribution of cocaine to the systemic circulation and central nervous system (CNS).

Distribution

The biologic half-life of cocaine is 0.5 to 1.5 hours, the volume of distribution is 2 L/kg, and the systemic clearance is 2 L per minute. Benzoylecgonine (BE) and ecgonine methyl ester (EME), the major metabolites of cocaine, have half-lives of 5 to 8 hours and 3.5 to 6.0 hours, respectively (11).

Metabolism

Cocaine is hydrolyzed rapidly by liver and plasma esterases to EME, which accounts for 30% to 50% of the parent product. Nonenzymatic hydrolysis results in the formation of the other major metabolite, BE (approximately 40% of the parent product). Minor metabolites, norcocaine, and ecgonine account for the other degradation products. The activity of plasma cholinesterase in an individual may have an impact on the degree of cocaine toxicity.

The relative contributions of cocaine and its metabolites to the clinical effects remain somewhat unclear. Early studies suggested that cocaine and norcocaine accounted for a majority of the vascular effects of cocaine (12). However, more recent studies demonstrate an active role for many of the metabolites. Cocaine, norcocaine, ecgonine, and BE produce cerebrovascular vasoconstriction when suffused over the brain surface (13) and when introduced into the cerebral circulation (14). Intravenous administration of cocaine or BE leads to cerebral vasoconstriction (15). Most *in vitro* and animal studies suggest that cocaine and norcocaine are the most potent vasoconstrictors, with BE and ecgonine having a smaller effect. Some studies suggest that EME may result in mild cerebral vasodilation (14,16). Cocaine and norcocaine are the most potent proconvulsant metabolites, but BE and EME administration may also lead to seizures (17,18). Sodium channel antagonist effects occur with cocaine and norcocaine but do not occur with BE or EME (19).

The activity of plasma cholinesterase determines the relative concentrations of the various metabolites. Serum from patients with plasma cholinesterase deficiency produce lower concentrations of EME (20). A similar effect is described in animals and demonstrates a shift of the metabolite profile largely toward an increase in BE, with a smaller increase in norcocaine (21). Patients with endogenous pseudocholinesterase deficiency may experience greater toxicity than those with normal pseudocholinesterase activity (22–24). These observations form the basis for the hypothesis that butyl cholinesterase (BCHE) administration may alter the metabolism of cocaine in humans. Administration of exogenous plasma cholinesterase can theoretically reduce the toxicity of cocaine by shunting degradation away from BE and norcocaine to less toxic metabolites (25). However, the clinical relevance of this finding is not clear. The need for rapid administration of this treatment to patients with severe life-threatening cocaine toxicity shortly after the use of cocaine might greatly limit its use as a therapeutic agent.

Cocaethylene is a unique metabolite that results from the combined use of alcohol and cocaine (26). It is equipotent to cocaine with regard to resultant behavioral effects in animal studies. Cocaethylene is, however, more likely to result in lethality. In clinical studies, cocaethylene produces milder subjective effects (27) and comparable hemodynamic effects to cocaine. Cocaethylene has a direct myocardial depressant effect (28) that is independent of coronary artery vasoconstriction (29). The permeability of human endothelial cells to low-density lipoproteins is increased by cocaine and by cocaethylene (30).

Elimination

Relatively little cocaine is excreted unchanged in the urine (1% to 5%) (31). BE and EME are excreted in the urine. Due to the long elimination half-life of BE, urinary assays for cocaine and cocaine metabolites generally are positive for up to 48 to 72 hours following use, perhaps longer with chronic use.

PATHOPHYSIOLOGY

Cocaine has diverse actions in humans. It directly blocks fast sodium channels, stabilizing the axonal membrane, with a resultant local anesthetic effect. Blockade of myocardial fast sodium channels causes cocaine to have type I antidysrhythmic properties (32,33). Cocaine interferes with the uptake of neurotransmitters, such as epinephrine, norepinephrine, and dopamine, at the nerve terminal. Cocaine functions as a vasoconstrictive agent. These three properties account for the majority of toxicity seen in the clinical setting.

The most prominent effect of cocaine is CNS stimulation, which occurs in a rostral-to-caudal fashion (11). The cortex is stimulated first and results in restlessness, excitement, and increased motor activity. Later, lower motor center stimulation may result in tonic-clonic seizures. The initial effect of cocaine on the medullary response centers is an increase in respiratory rate. Subsequently, respiration becomes depressed, with resulting respiratory failure. The vomiting center may also be initially stimulated, but these emetic effects are most often self-limited.

The initial effect of cocaine on the cardiovascular system is a transient bradycardia, secondary to stimulation of the vagal nuclei. Tachycardia typically ensues, predominantly from increased central sympathetic stimulation. Cocaine has a cardiostimulatory effect through sensitization to epinephrine and norepinephrine. It prevents neuronal reuptake of these catecholamines and increases the release of norepinephrine from adrenergic nerve terminals (11), leading to enhanced sympathetic effects. The vasopressor effects of cocaine are mostly mediated by norepinephrine of sympathetic neural origin, and the tachycardic effects of cocaine are mostly mediated by epinephrine of adrenal medullary origin (34).

The psychostimulant effects of cocaine are mediated, in part, through inhibition of dopamine reuptake in the nucleus accumbens (35). Human volunteers experience a subjective "high" when more than 47% of dopamine transporters are blocked and typical doses of cocaine (0.3 to 0.6 mg/kg) block more than this proportion of dopamine transporters (36). Animals without dopamine transporters do not experience the psychostimulatory effects of cocaine (37). Dopamine-1 and dopamine-2 receptor agonists have opposite effects on cocaine-seeking behavior. The dopamine-2 agonists lead to cocaine-seeking behavior, whereas dopamine-1 agonists diminish the craving for cocaine (38). In human volunteers, a selective dopamine antagonist blocked euphoria but not the cardiovascular effects of cocaine (39).

Cocaine increases the concentrations of the excitatory amino acids, aspartate and glutamate, in the nucleus accumbens (40). The excitatory amino acids increase the extracellular concentrations of dopamine. Excitatory amino acid antagonists attenuate the effects of cocaine on extracellular dopamine (41) and block cocaine-induced convulsions and death (42).

TABLE 2. Conditions with increased incidence in pregnant women exposed to cocaine

Spontaneous abortion
Placenta previa
Abruptio placentae
Fetal death
Prematurity (preterm labor, delivery)
Congenital malformations
Placental infarcts
Intrauterine growth retardation
Birth of small-for-gestation age infant (smaller head circumference, decreased birth length)
Low birth weight
Ischemic infarct of bowel (necrotizing enterocolitis)
Multiple intestinal atresias

PREGNANCY AND LACTATION

As a medication, cocaine is U.S. Food and Drug Administration category C. As an abused drug, it is category X (Appendix I). Cocaine abuse may injure the fetus and newborn infant during pregnancy, at birth, during lactation, and by passive exposure to cocaine smoke during infancy and childhood (43–56). Pregnant women who use cocaine are at increased risk for maternal and fetal complications (Table 2). Although a specific teratogenic syndrome has not been identified, multiple fetal and neonatal abnormalities are associated with cocaine use (Table 3).

Cocaine is excreted in breast milk and can induce cocaine intoxication in the breast-fed infant (57,58). Apnea and seizures have been induced in an infant from the direct ingestion of cocaine used as a topical anesthetic for nipple soreness (59). Cessation of cocaine exposure early in pregnancy by social cocaine users does not appear to be associated with any subsequent adverse pregnancy outcomes (60).

CLINICAL PRESENTATION

Cocaine affects nearly every organ system. The effects may vary depending on the route of administration.

TABLE 3. Teratogenic effects reported in the offspring of women who used cocaine during pregnancy

Body area	Anomalies
Cranial–spinal	Exencephaly, hydrocephaly, porencephaly, cephalomalacia, encephalocele, myelomeningocele, hypoplastic corpus callosum, parietal lobe cleft, heterotopias
Facial	Unilateral oro-orbital cleft, cleft lip, cleft palate, facial diplegia, blepharophimosis, ptosis, skin tags, cutis aplasia, Pierre Robin syndrome
Cardiovascular	Atrial septal defect, ventricular septal defect, transposition of the great arteries, pulmonary artery stenosis, hypoplastic right heart syndrome, biventricular hypertrophy, cardiomegaly
Gastrointestinal and genitourinary tracts	Ileal atresia, inguinal hernia, prune belly syndrome, renal agenesis, multicystic kidneys, hydronephrosis, hydroureter, hypospadias, undescended testis, hydrocele
Extremities	Limb reduction defects, phocomelia, polydactyly, syndactyly

From Young SL, Vosper HJ, Phillips SA. Cocaine: its effects on maternal and child health. *Pharmacotherapy* 1992;12:2–17, with permission.

Head, Ears, Nose, and Throat Effects

Reactive hyperemia of nasal mucosa causes a persistent rhinitis in patients who insufflate cocaine. Erosions and nasal perforation complicate chronic use (61). Attempts at rhinoplasty in such users may lead to surgical complications, including septal collapse, delayed mucosal healing, and inadequate correction of septal defect (62). Pain, photophobia, and decreased visual acuity associated with an iritis may develop a few hours after the use of intranasal cocaine (63). Deep inhalation may deposit adulterants near the ethmoid sinuses, leading to sinusitis (64). Bilateral optic neuropathy with decreased visual acuity and optic nerve head swelling may occur secondary to osteolytic sinusitis (65). In long-term cocaine snorters rebound nasal stuffiness develops after intranasal use that is often self-treated with nasal inhalers, sprays, and drops containing phenylephrine, oxymetazoline, beclomethasone, and flunisolide, all drugs that can contribute to nasal mucoperichondrial necrosis and septal perforations (66). After nasal insufflation of cocaine, material may be drawn into the nasopharynx and from there into the mouth, resulting in a mixture of cocaine with saliva. The end product is an acid capable of dissolving the predominant dental mineral, calcium phosphate hydroxyapatite, from enamel and dentin (67).

Hyperthermia

Cocaine augments heat production and retention through a direct effect on thermoregulatory centers in the hypothalamic area, increased psychomotor activity, and decreased heat dissipation due to vasoconstriction. Cocaine-induced hyperthermia is of the utmost clinical relevance and is directly related to an increased mortality. One study compared the effects of hypertension and tachycardia, pH, acidosis, seizures, and hyperthermia on cocaine lethality. Only those agents that corrected hyperthermia improved survival (68). Clinically, cocaine-related deaths are more common when the ambient environmental temperatures are higher (69).

Neurologic Effects

Cocaine-intoxicated patients are often anxious or agitated. Although anxiety and agitation can be transient effects, they may also reflect underlying cerebrovascular complications (70–80) (Table 4). Cocaine is associated with a sevenfold increased risk of stroke in women (70). Most patients with neurologic catastrophes secondary to cocaine do not have predisposing cerebrovascular disease (81,82). Therefore, a search for underlying pathology (e.g., aneurysm or arteriovenous malformation) should be conducted when appropriate. The pathophysiology of cerebrovascular ischemia is analogous to that of coronary ischemia (83) and includes hypercoagulability, impaired cerebrovascular autoregulation from increased cerebrovascular resistance (73), vasospasm or vasoconstriction (84), particulate matter embolism, and arteritis/vasculitis (80,85). Immunologic mechanisms may also play a role, because an increased prevalence of anticardiolipin antibodies in cocaine users has been detected (86).

TABLE 4. Neurologic manifestations of cocaine

Seizure	Dystonic reaction
Subarachnoid hemorrhage	Toxic leukoencephalopathy
Intracerebral hemorrhage	Migraine-type headache syndromes
Cerebral infarction	Anterior spinal artery syndrome
Transient ischemic attack	Psychiatric disorders
Cerebral vasculitis	

Data from references 70–79.

Seizures may occur alone or in conjunction with underlying organic pathology. Most cocaine-induced seizures are single, generalized, and not associated with persistent deficits. Multiple or focal seizures suggest concomitant drug use, underlying seizure disorder, or possibly a massive overdose.

A decreased level of consciousness and profound lethargy characterize the cocaine "washed-out" syndrome (87,88). This syndrome is also characterized by depressed mental status ranging from lethargy to near coma. It typically occurs after a binge of stimulant use and presumably arises from depletion of CNS catecholamines. These patients are similar to those with a prolonged postictal period except that they have a normal mental status when aroused. Patients can be very difficult to arouse for up to 24 hours after cocaine use. Individuals with the cocaine washed-out syndrome assume normal sleep postures and can be aroused to full orientation. These features contrast with lethargic patients who have intracranial catastrophes such as subarachnoid hemorrhage.

Cardiovascular Effects

Cocaine-induced acute coronary syndromes (myocardial ischemia and infarction) occur secondary to cocaine use and possibly cocaine withdrawal (89–97), because spontaneous episodes of ST-segment elevation have occurred for up to 6 weeks after withdrawal of cocaine (97). The risk of myocardial infarction (MI) is increased 23.9-fold in the hour following cocaine use (98). Cocaine-induced MI typically occurs in patients 19 to 60 years old. These patients often do not have "classic" chest pain syndromes. The chest pain can be delayed for hours to days after their most recent use of cocaine, although cocaine MI usually occurs within 24 hours of last use (89,92,98–100). The electrocardiogram (ECG) is less sensitive and specific for MI in patients who have recently used cocaine than in those without recent cocaine use (100–102).

Cocaine induces vasoconstriction in coronary arteries (103). Either Q-wave or non–Q-wave infarction may occur (2,89,104). The pathophysiology of cocaine-related myocardial ischemia is complex (91). Acutely, cocaine use leads to coronary artery vasoconstriction, tachycardia, hypertension, increased myocardial oxygen demand, platelet aggregation, and thrombus formation (91). In patients with chronic cocaine use, premature atherosclerosis and left ventricular hypertrophy develop. Both of these conditions may enhance oxygen supply-demand mismatch. Cocaine-induced MI can also occur in patients without any underlying atherosclerotic disease (2,91,96,105,106).

Higher doses of cocaine are associated with virtually all types of tachydysrhythmias. Atrial fibrillation, atrial flutter, supraventricular tachycardia, ventricular premature contractions, accelerated idioventricular rhythms, ventricular tachycardia, torsade de pointes, and ventricular fibrillation may occur as a result of cocaine. High doses of cocaine lead to infranodal and intraventricular conduction delays and lethal ventricular dysrhythmias secondary to prolonged QRS and QT intervals (107,108). Prolonged QT intervals have been noted in patients with recent cocaine use who have not had dysrhythmias (102). These effects are most likely mediated by the local anesthetic effect of sodium channel blockade. In addition to the sodium channel effect, dysrhythmias may occur as a result of cocaine-induced acute coronary syndrome (32,109). Low doses of cocaine can result in a transient bradycardia.

Chronic cocaine use leads to a dilated cardiomyopathy, possibly from recurrent or diffuse ischemia with subsequent "stunned" myocardium (110). Alternatively, it may have a direct effect on myocardial contractility. Increasing doses of cocaine also appear to have a direct myocardial-depressant effect (32,111,112). Direct infusion of cocaine into human coronary arteries increases left ventricular end-diastolic pressures and end-systolic volume, as well as decreases left ventricular ejection fraction (113). Left ventricular function may improve when cocaine use is halted (114).

Infection Risks

Abusers who inject cocaine intravenously are at increased risk of human immunodeficiency virus (HIV) infection through needle sharing, perhaps because of the frequency of injection during binges of cocaine use—up to 15 to 25 times in a single day. In South America, HIV infection is now found in 36% to 57% of cocaine injectors (115). Those who smoke crack are also at higher risk of HIV infection (and sexually transmitted diseases) from sex-for-drug transactions (115). In the sex-for-drugs group, increases in rates of syphilis and congenital syphilis have been observed (116,117).

An increased risk of upper extremity deep vein thrombosis (118,119) and bacterial endocarditis (120) occurs after intravenous cocaine use. This risk of endocarditis from intravenous cocaine use is higher than that of intravenous heroin use. This finding has been attributed to the increased injection frequency in cocaine users, although direct effects of cocaine on endovascular tissues and the immune system may also play a role (121).

Aortic Dissection

Cocaine use can result in aortic dissection and rupture (122). Most patients with cocaine-induced aortic dissection were chronic cocaine users and had a history of hypertension. Dissection and rupture probably result from the increased shearing forces of cocaine-induced hypertension, vasoconstriction, tachycardia, and vascular damage to medial wall (122).

Pulmonary Effects

A wide spectrum of acute pulmonary effects or upper airway complications has been attributed to cocaine (123–138) (Table 5). Chronic effects of cocaine on the lung appear to be related to the route of use, with crack smoking having the highest risk (139). Chronic cocaine users have not been found to have significant impairment of lung mechanics (140–143). Heavy users of inhaled cocaine do not have abnormal spirometry; however, a small decrease in the carbon monoxide–diffusing capacity (DL_{CO}) has been observed, and this is a physiologic marker of the integrity of the alveolar capillary membrane (143). Early changes in the bronchial epithelium have been noted (144). Whether or not these early changes increase the risk of subsequent lung cancer remains unknown. Crack cocaine, but not intravenous cocaine, results acutely in airway bronchoconstriction, suggesting that inhaled foreign materials mediate this effect through irritation or thermal injury (145).

TABLE 5. Acute respiratory effects of cocaine

Asthma
Pneumothorax
Pneumomediastinum
Acute lung injury
Diffuse alveolar hemorrhage
Recurrent pulmonary infiltrates with eosinophilia
Goodpasture's syndrome and bronchiolitis obliterans with organizing pneumonia
Pulmonary vascular abnormalities
Upper airway burns
Upper airway abscess
Pulmonary edema
Pulmonary hypertension

Data from references 120–134.

Ophthalmic Effects

Cocaine has local and systemic effects on the eye. Direct topical application of cocaine denudes the corneal epithelium (146). Particulate matter in smoke produces corneal abrasions and ulcerations ("crack eye") (147). Vascular effects can occur through central retinal artery occlusion or cerebral insufficiency (148,149).

Rhabdomyolysis

Cocaine may lead to severe rhabdomyolysis with massive elevation of creatine phosphokinase levels, acute renal failure, profound hypotension, and hyperthermia (24,150–156). Cocaine probably causes skeletal muscle ischemia through the same mechanisms by which it affects other vascular beds. Renal failure may result from myoglobinuria and renal ischemia (157).

Uteroplacental and Perinatal Effects

Maternal cocaine use decreases the likelihood of term deliveries, adversely affects fetal growth and development (158–162), and may cause spontaneous abortion, abruptio placentae, fetal prematurity, and intrauterine growth retardation (Tables 2 and 3). Cocaine results in dose-dependent increases in maternal blood pressure with corresponding decreases in uterine blood flow (163,164). Neonatal withdrawal usually begin within 24 to 48 hours of birth. Infants display jitteriness, irritability, poor eye contact, and vigorous sucking. *In utero* cocaine exposure is associated with small head circumference and low birth weight. The long-term consequences of the decreased responsiveness and attentiveness in cocaine-exposed neonates are not clear (165). It appears that prenatal cocaine exposure is not an additive risk for deficits in school-aged children with multiple other risk factors for slow development (166).

Other Medical Effects

The intestinal blood supply is sensitive to catecholamines. Acute mucosal ischemia occurs after cocaine use (167–170) and is a serious issue in body packers (170). Clinical presentations are varied, ranging from mild colitis to severe complications of intestinal perforation (171,172). Cocaine is hepatotoxic in mouse models, but isolated hepatotoxicity in humans is uncommon. Hepatotoxicity usually manifests as elevations of aspartate aminotransferase and alanine aminotransferase in the setting of hyperthermia or severe cardiovascular instability.

A callus on the ulnar side of the right thumb can follow repeated contact of the thumb with the serrated wheel that ignites the lighter used to ignite crack cocaine in a paper (173).

Thyrotoxicosis has been observed in chronic cocaine users (174). Hypocalcemia (to calcium levels as low as 3.6 mg/dl), hyperuricemia, and elevated serum creatine phosphokinase levels (as high as 763,000 IU/L), with evidence of severe rhabdomyolysis, may be seen in intravenous cocaine recreational users (175).

Cocaine may be "cut" with compounds containing arsenic. The occurrence of nausea, vomiting, and diarrhea and the presence of a sensorimotor neuropathy in a crack cocaine abuser may indicate arsenic intoxication (176).

Psychiatric Effects

Tolerance and physical and psychological addiction to cocaine are well-known effects. Some patients experience "cocaine bugs," a crawling sensation under the skin with resultant self-excoriation, leading to irregular scratches and ulcers (Magnan's sign).

The stimulant abstinence syndrome follows a three-phase pattern of crash, withdrawal, and extinction. The crash is associated with intense depression, agitation, and anxiety. Withdrawal is marked by decreased energy, limited interest in the environment, and limited ability to experience pleasure. Craving appears greatest in the 24 hours before admission and is associated with intense psychological depression. No definite crash may be observed. Mood states, craving, and sleep disturbances gradually improve during the initial 4 weeks (177). This cocaine abstinence syndrome is usually medically benign and requires little medication for detoxification in an inpatient setting.

DIAGNOSTIC TESTS

Acute and Subacute Exposure

Patients manifesting cocaine toxicity should receive a complete evaluation, including a history of cocaine use, recognition of signs and symptoms consistent with sympathetic nervous system excess, and evaluation of organ-specific complaints. It is imperative to determine whether signs and symptoms are due to cocaine itself, underlying unrelated structural abnormalities, or cocaine-induced structural abnormalities. Friends or family of patients with altered cognition should be questioned about events before presentation. Many patients deny cocaine use. Urine drug testing can be helpful in establishing recent cocaine use.

When the history is clear and symptoms are mild, laboratory evaluation is usually unnecessary. If the patient has severe toxicity, laboratory evaluation is directed at evaluation of the target organs of cocaine: complete blood count, electrolytes, glucose, blood urea nitrogen, creatinine, arterial blood gas analysis, creatine kinase (CK), and cardiac marker determinations and urinalysis. Excess sympathetic stimulation often results in hyperglycemia and hypokalemia. Lack of fluid intake combined with sweating and increased activity may cause electrolyte abnormalities. Elevated CK occurs with rhabdomyolysis and dehydration.

Cardiac markers are elevated in cocaine-induced MI. However, false elevations of CK-MB fraction are common (178–181). Additionally, in the setting of an elevated absolute CK-MB, one should not rely on the CK-MB relative index. The CK-MB relative index may be falsely low when concurrent MI and skeletal muscle rhabdomyolysis occur. Cardiac troponin I is preferred to identify true positive CK-MB determinations (180).

Pulmonary evaluation includes a chest radiograph in patients with cardiopulmonary complaints (Table 5). An ECG should be obtained in patients with chest pain or cardiovascular complaints. The initial ECG is not as useful as in patients with chest pain that is unrelated to cocaine. Young cocaine-using patients may have ST-segment elevation in the absence of acute MI (AMI) because of early repolarization changes (100,102). Conversely, most patients with AMI do not have ST-segment elevation on their initial ECG.

Neurologic evaluation may involve radiography. A brief cocaine-induced seizure in an otherwise healthy person should be evaluated with computed tomography. Further work-up in an otherwise asymptomatic patient is not necessary (178). Patients with headache or other neurologic manifestations may necessitate lumbar puncture after computerized tomography to rule out serious pathology.

Analytic Considerations

Cocaine or its metabolites can be detected in multiple body fluids. Nasal swabs, serum tests, or urine analysis for cocaine can be performed. Laboratory tests include gas chromatography and thin-layer chromatography (BE in the serum or urine), as well as enzyme-multiplied immunoassay techniques and gas chromatography–mass spectrometry (GC-MS). Urine immunoassays for cocaine metabolites are screening tests that generally detect BE at concentrations above 300 ng/ml. Cocaine or its metabolites can be detected for 48 to 72 hours following use (179), although cocaine metabolites have been detected for up 22 days after last use, using more sensitive methods (GC-MS) (182). Analytic methods for cocaine determination are summarized in Table 6 (183–189).

Salivary cocaine and BE concentrations are 5.0 and 2.5 times higher, respectively, than in the serum of individuals who have used cocaine in the previous 24 hours. Simultaneous measurement of cocaine and BE in saliva is useful in screening for recent cocaine use (190).

Cocaine, BE, and EME can be analyzed in human hair by GC-MS (191–193) and radioimmunoassay. This technique has been used as an adjunct to the usual analyses performed or to document exposure to drugs in situations in which traditional specimens, such as blood and urine, have not been collected in a timely fashion (194). Scalp hair cocaine analysis may be useful in confirming the presence of cocaine either in an adult or in an infant whose mother is a possible cocaine user. Pyrolysis of crack results in accumulation of cocaine, but not its BE metabolite, in the hair of persons in the area. After admitted systemic use of cocaine, both species are detectable in hair. External contamination with crack smoke is washable, whereas systemic exposure is not (195). Although hair cocaine may sometimes be positive when a urine test is negative, cocaine use occurring only in recent days would not yet be detectable by hair analysis. Analysis of hair from the neonate provides information regard-

TABLE 6. Laboratory assays for cocaine and benzoylecgonine

Laboratory assay	Specimen	Metabolite	Cocaine	BE sensitivity
Enzyme-multiplied immunoassay technique (EMIT)	Urine	BE	—	200–300 ng/ml
Radioimmunoassay (RIA)	Urine/ blood	BE	>50	5–100 ng/ml
Thin-layer chromatography (TLC)	Urine	BE, EME	—	500–1000 ng/ml
Gas chromatography (GC)	Serum/ urine	BE, EME	5–50 ng/ml serum	200–300 ng/ml
High-pressure liquid chromatography (HPLC)	Serum/ urine	BE, EME	50 ng/ml serum	200–300 ng/ml
Gas chromatography–mass spectrometry (GC-MS)	Serum/ urine	BE, EME	5 ng/ml serum	200–300 ng/ml

BE, benzoylecgonine; EME, ecgonine methyl ester.

ing long-term rather than recent cocaine use. The results remain positive for 5 to 6 months until the infant fetal hair is shed (196).

Cocaine can be detected in neonatal urine for 12 to 24 hours after delivery if the drug was consumed within 2 days preceding delivery. BE can be detected for up to 5 days. Urine testing is negative if cocaine use was terminated several days before delivery. Meconium may be positive for up to 3 days after delivery (197).

Postmortem Changes

Cocaine and its metabolites are present postmortem. One study found that there was no consistent pattern of direction or magnitude of change of these analytes after death. The authors concluded that postmortem concentrations of these compounds are not necessarily reflective of perimortem concentrations and should not be used to determine the cause of death (198).

TREATMENT

The initial treatment of cocaine-toxic patients should focus on airway, breathing, and circulation. Specific treatments are based on the specific sign, symptom, or organ system affected (Table 7). Because of the direct relationship between the neuropsychiatric and other systemic complications, management of neuropsychiatric manifestations has an impact on the systemic manifestations of cocaine toxicity.

Decontamination

Decontamination is rarely needed because abuse occurs by inhalation or injection. Body stuffers and packers present special concerns (Chapter 12).

Enhancement of Elimination

Elimination does not currently play a clinically significant role in the management of cocaine toxicity.

Antidotes

Cocaine poisoning has no true antidote. It has been hypothesized that exogenous BCHE could be used to alter the metabolic pathways of cocaine from more toxic to less toxic metabolites. Lower than normal levels of plasma cholinesterase have been noted in patients experiencing cocaine-associated adverse effects. Om et al. (24) found lower levels of BCHE in patients with cardiovascular complications than normal volunteers or cocaine addicts in a detoxification program. Hoffman et al. (23) found that patients with life-threatening toxicity from cocaine had lower levels of BCHE than did patients with non–life-threatening toxicity. These observations form the basis for the theory that BCHE administration might alleviate cocaine toxicity.

Animal data, but no human data, support the use of BCHE for the treatment of cocaine intoxication. Hoffman et al. (25) found that administration of BCHE before the use of cocaine reduced the likelihood of death or seizures from cocaine. Mattes et al. (199) found that pretreatment with BCHE reduced the blood pressure effects of cocaine in rats. Lynch et al. (200) pretreated rats with BCHE and demonstrated reduced blood pressure, dysrhythmogenesis, and lethality from cocaine. These studies cannot be extrapolated directly to patients who typically experience cocaine-related complications for several hours before an antidote can be administered.

A few animal studies have given BCHE after cocaine. Lynch et al. (200) administered BCHE to conscious rats 3 minutes after

TABLE 7. Treatment summary for specific cocaine-related medical conditions

Medical condition	Treatments
Cardiovascular complications	
Dysrhythmias	
Sinus tachycardia	Observation; oxygen; diazepam, 5 mg IV, or lorazepam, 2–4 mg IV titrated to effect
Supraventricular tachycardia	Oxygen; diazepam, 5 mg IV, or lorazepam, 2–4 mg IV; consider diltiazem, 20 mg IV, or verapamil, 5 mg IV; adenosine, 6 mg or 12 mg IV; cardioversion if hemodynamically unstable
Ventricular dysrhythmias	Oxygen; sodium bicarbonate, 1–2 mEq/kg; lidocaine, 1.5 mg/kg IV bolus followed by 2-mg/min infusion; defibrillation if hemodynamically unstable; diazepam, 5 mg IV, or lorazepam, 2–4 mg IV
Acute coronary syndrome	Oxygen; diazepam, 5–10 mg IV, or lorazepam, 2–4 mg IV; soluble aspirin, 325 mg; nitroglycerin, 1/150 sublingual × 3 every 5 min followed by an infusion titrated to a mean arterial pressure reduction of 10% or relief of chest pain; morphine sulfate, 2 mg IV every 5 min titrated to pain relief; phentolamine, 1 mg IV, repeated in 5 min; verapamil, 5–10 mg IV; heparin, 80-U/kg bolus followed by 18 U/kg/hr; percutaneous intervention (angioplasty and stent placement); glycoprotein IIb/IIIa inhibitors; fibrinolytic therapy
Hypertension	Observation; diazepam, 5–10 mg IV, or lorazepam, 2–4 mg IV titrated to effect; phentolamine, 1 mg IV, repeated in 5 min; nitroglycerin or nitroprusside continuous infusion titrated to effect
Pulmonary edema	Furosemide (Lasix), 20–40 mg IV; morphine sulfate, 2 mg IV every 5 min titrated to effect; nitroglycerin infusion titrated to blood pressure; consider phentolamine or nitroprusside
Hyperthermia	Sedation with benzodiazepines; tepid water with fans, cool water, or ice baths
Neuropsychiatric symptoms	
Anxiety and agitation	Diazepam, 5–10 mg IV, or lorazepam, 2–4 mg IV titrated to effect
Seizures	Diazepam, 5–10 mg IV, or lorazepam, 2–4 mg IV titrated to effect; phenobarbital, 25–50 mg/min up to 10–20 mg/kg
Intracranial hemorrhage	Neurosurgery consultation
Rhabdomyolysis	IV hydration with isotonic crystalloid to maintain urine output at 3 ml/kg/hr; hemodialysis, as necessary for renal failure
Cocaine washed-out syndrome	Supportive care
Body packers	Activated charcoal; whole bowel irrigation; admission to monitored setting even if asymptomatic; laparotomy or endoscopic retrieval for obstruction or cocaine-related symptoms

Adapted from Hollander JE, Hoffman RS. Cocaine. In: Goldfrank LR, Flomenbaum NE, Lewin NA, et al., eds. *Goldfrank's toxicologic emergency*, 6th ed. Stamford, CT: Appleton & Lange, 1998:1071–1089.

a large dose of cocaine. Rats with BCHE treatment were less likely to seize and die than were rats without such treatment. Mattes et al. (199) gave BCHE 1 minute after completion of a cocaine infusion. BCHE caused a 15% narrowing of the QRS complex that was not statistically different from when they did not get BCHE (199). Treatment within this time frame would not be possible in the clinical setting. Thus, there are no animal studies demonstrating that BCHE has a positive effect that mimics the clinical setting where treatment with BCHE follows the onset of symptomatic cocaine intoxication.

Based on current data, it is not possible to determine whether or not administration of BCHE could improve the outcome in patients with cocaine intoxication. The observation of low BCHE levels in patients with cocaine-associated medical complications certainly raises the possibility of treatment with BCHE. To theorize about the success of BCHE, one needs to have a better understanding of the role of various cocaine metabolites. It is clear that cocaine and norcocaine cause serious complications. Data have confirmed that BE can result in serious medical complications. The precise role of EME is ill defined. However, EME and BE have been demonstrated to be increasing at the time of coronary artery narrowing in humans (201). Thus, increasing concentrations of EME with BCHE have the theoretic potential to worsen this condition.

Another reason that BCHE may not work in the clinical setting involves the concentration of cocaine at the time of treatment. Fewer than half of patients with AMI present within 4 hours (93). The median time to presentation for patients with chest pain is 5 hours (100). The half-life of cocaine is 30 to 90 minutes, meaning that 90% to 99% of the drug has already been eliminated by the time of presentation (5 hours). Thus, even if BCHE is effective in removing cocaine, little cocaine remains, and it is unclear what role it might have in clinical practice.

Supportive Care

Hyperthermia and agitation are the major causes of cocaine-related death. Hyperthermia is treated with cooling measures and sedation. Aggressive measures to decrease the body temperature are warranted (Chapter 38). Sedative-hypnotics are usually successful for the treatment of cocaine toxicity (68,202,203). Sedation with a benzodiazepine is based on experimental efficacy (68,202,203) and experience with their use in other clinical conditions associated with severe agitation and catecholamine excess. In animal studies, phenothiazines are not as effective as benzodiazepines and may worsen the outcome.

Patients with *rhabdomyolysis* as evidenced by elevation of CK or myoglobinuria (rhabdomyolysis) should be treated with aggressive hydration using isotonic crystalloidal fluids such as normal saline to maintain a urine output of at least 3 ml/kg/hour. Assessment of fluid balance may be difficult. These patients are often volume depleted due to marked insensible losses and decreased oral intake. However, volume resuscitation in the patient with acute renal failure can later develop volume overload. If renal failure occurs, hemodialysis may be necessary.

Hypertension and tachycardia due to cocaine rarely require specific treatment. Effective treatment of anxiety, agitation, and ischemia often leads to resolution of the hypertension and tachycardia. When necessary, treatment directed toward the central effects of cocaine, such as benzodiazepines, usually reduce blood pressure and heart rate. Occasionally, sedation is unsuccessful and hypertension can be managed with short-acting agents such as sodium nitroprusside, nitroglycerin, or intravenous phentolamine (204,205).

Acute coronary syndromes in cocaine toxicity are treated based on studies in the cardiac catheterization laboratory. In these studies, adults without prior cocaine use were given 2 mg/kg intranasal cocaine. An increase in heart rate, blood pressure, and coronary vascular resistance developed. Coronary arterial diameter narrowed by 13% (205). With administration of phentolamine the coronary arterial diameter returned to baseline (205), suggesting usefulness for treatment of cocaine-induced ischemia. Based on these data and retrospective reports, the International Guidelines for Emergency Cardiovascular Care recommend α-adrenergic antagonists (phentolamine) for the treatment of cocaine-associated acute coronary syndrome (206).

Studies in the cardiac catheterization laboratory demonstrate that nitroglycerin also reverses cocaine-induced vasoconstriction (204). Case series have confirmed that nitroglycerin is associated with relief of cocaine-induced chest pain (207). As a result of their salutary effect on the hyperdynamic effects of cocaine, benzodiazepines also relieve chest pain, and their effect on cardiac dynamics and left ventricular function is similar to that of nitroglycerin (208).

The precise role of calcium-channel blockers for the treatment of cocaine toxicity is unclear. Cocaine-intoxicated animals pretreated with calcium-channel blockers have had favorable effects with respect to survival, seizures, and cardiac dysrhythmias in some studies but not in others (202,209–214). Using the human cardiac catheterization as a model, verapamil reverses cocaine-induced coronary artery vasoconstriction (215). However, multicenter clinical trials in more than 5000 patients with myocardial ischemia unrelated to cocaine did not find beneficial effects of calcium-channel blockers on important outcomes such as survival. Thus, the role of calcium-channel blockers in cocaine-induced acute coronary syndrome has not yet been defined.

Coronary artery vasoconstriction is exacerbated by the administration of propranolol and has been found to produce anginal symptoms and ST-segment elevation (216). In theory, β-adrenergic blockade produces "unopposed α-adrenergic receptor stimulation," which leads to vasoconstriction and an increased blood pressure (217–219). These human observations have also been found in multiple experimental models, in which the use of β-adrenergic antagonists leads to decreased coronary blood flow, increased seizure frequency, and high fatality (68,203,214,220,221). The use of short-acting β-adrenergic antagonists such as esmolol has resulted in significant increases in blood pressure in up to 25% of patients (222,223). Given the availability of other effective agents, therefore, the use of β-adrenergic antagonists for the treatment of cocaine toxicity is contraindicated (91,206,224–226).

Labetalol does not appear to offer any advantages over propranolol. It has substantially more β-adrenergic antagonism than α-adrenergic antagonist effects (227). Labetalol increases the risk of seizure and death in animal models of cocaine toxicity (214) and does not reverse coronary artery vasoconstriction in humans (228). Nitroprusside, nitroglycerin, or phentolamine is considered a better option to achieve vasodilation.

Cocaine injures the vascular endothelium, increases platelet aggregation, and impairs normal fibrinolytic pathways (61,229–232). As a result, the use of aspirin, heparin or low-molecular-weight heparin, and thrombolytic agents makes theoretic sense in the setting of vascular ischemia (91,92,233). With respect to thrombolytic therapy for AMI, many young patients have benign early repolarization and very few patients with cocaine-associated chest pain and J-point/ST-segment elevation are actually sustaining an acute infarction (102). Case reports document adverse outcomes following thrombolytic administration in cocaine-using patients (234–236). The use of thrombolytic therapy should be reserved for individuals who are definitely having an MI, cannot receive percutaneous intervention, fail to respond to medical management, and have low risk for bleeding catastrophe (233). Glycoprotein IIb/IIIa antagonists may be useful in patients with cocaine-associated acute coronary syndromes, but they have not been well studied (237).

Cardiac dysrhythmias are associated with cocaine toxicity. Most atrial tachydysrhythmias respond to sedative-hypnotics or control of the central sympathetic stimulus. When they do not, verapamil or diltiazem may be indicated. The treatment of ventricular dysrhythmias depends on the time between cocaine use, dysrhythmia onset, and initiation of treatment. Ventricular dysrhythmias that occur soon after cocaine use should be presumed to occur from the local anesthetic (type I antidysrhythmic) effects on the myocardium. These wide complex rhythms may respond to the administration of sodium bicarbonate, similar to dysrhythmias associated with other type IA and type IC agents (33,238) (Chapter 75). In addition, one animal model suggested that lidocaine exacerbated cocaine-induced seizures and dysrhythmias as a result of similar effects on sodium channels (239); however, this finding has not been confirmed in other animal models (33,240,241). Bicarbonate therapy may be preferable and has been used effectively (242).

Ventricular dysrhythmias that occur several hours after the last use of cocaine are often the result of myocardial ischemia. Standard management for ventricular dysrhythmias, including lidocaine, is indicated and appears safe (109). No data are available concerning the efficacy of amiodarone in clinical cocaine intoxication. Torsade de pointes is a rare complication of cocaine use (243) and should be managed in the standard manner with intravenous magnesium sulfate and overdrive pacing. The other cardiovascular end-organ manifestations of cocaine toxicity may necessitate specific intervention for managing the individual medical complications of catecholamine excess, myocardial ischemia, and hypertension (Table 7).

Ischemia of noncardiovascular organs may also occur. Cocaine-induced constriction of the cerebral (84,85), ophthalmic (146), pulmonary (131,132), mesenteric (165,167), and musculoskeletal vascular beds is well described. These effects are presumed to occur by mechanisms similar to those of cocaine-induced coronary vasoconstriction, and a similar approach to management should be initiated in patients with clinical signs and symptoms of vasoconstriction in other vascular beds.

Neurologic manifestations of agitation and seizures are treated with an emphasis on expeditious control of motor activity and the patient's airway. Respiratory depression should be treated with intubation and ventilation. Oxygen should be routinely administered. Transient use of restraints may be essential to initiate intravenous access but should be avoided whenever possible. Treatment of hypoglycemia and hypoxia is necessary. Bedside glucose testing should be performed. A benzodiazepine should be used intravenously to achieve sedation. Diazepam, 10 to 20 mg, or lorazepam, 2 to 8 mg, is used acutely and repeated as needed with continuous cardiorespiratory monitoring until the effects of the cocaine and the sedative cease. Lorazepam is often initially administered intramuscularly to very combative patients. Much larger doses of diazepam may be needed for control of the extremely combative patient (244). Flumazenil may precipitate seizures. Sedatives with butyrophenones (such as haloperidol and droperidol) or phenothiazines (such as chlorpromazine) are not recommended. These agents are anticholinergic atropine-like drugs that can cause a patient to become hot, worsen hyperthermia, and lower the seizure threshold (68,203,245,246).

Diazepam or lorazepam should be used for initial management of seizures. If generous doses of a benzodiazepine are ineffective, barbiturates are theoretically preferable over phenytoin because they are sedating and generally more effective for toxin-induced convulsions. If seizures remain resistant to therapy, nondepolarizing neuromuscular blockade and general anesthesia may be necessary. When possible, succinylcholine should be avoided because it is a depolarizing neuromuscular-blocking agent that may increase the risk of hyperkalemia in the setting of rhabdomyolysis. Plasma cholinesterase is responsible for the metabolism of succinylcholine and cocaine, so that, theoretically, if these agents are used simultaneously, prolonged clinical effects of either agent might result.

Cocaine-induced constriction of the cerebral vessels is presumed to occur by mechanisms similar to those described for cocaine-induced coronary vasoconstriction. As a result, the treatment strategies used for patients with cocaine-associated myocardial ischemia may be applicable to individuals with strokes or transient ischemic attacks. No studies have been reported of fibrinolytic agents for treatment of cocaine-induced stroke. Treatment of patients with intracerebral catastrophes secondary to cocaine is otherwise similar to treatment of individuals with the same syndromes that are unrelated to cocaine.

Body packers and stuffers may present management challenges (Table 8; Chapter 12). "Body packers" carefully wrap large amounts of highly pure drug that is less likely to disrupt and spill their contents into the gastrointestinal lumen. Cocaine body packers typically present asymptomatic, having been discovered by customs officers while trying to enter the country. The most common clinical decisions are the method of evacuation and confirmation that the package is out of the gastrointestinal system. These patients should be monitored in an intensive care unit setting until the cocaine bags have been eliminated, even if they are asymptomatic. Whole bowel irrigation with radiologic verification of passage of all packages is warranted. If patients present with symptoms or symptoms of cocaine toxicity develop, rapid deterioration and severe toxicity may occur because of exposure to huge doses of cocaine. Immediate surgical removal of the ruptured package may be life saving (247,248).

Surgical removal may be necessary for bowel obstruction or cocaine toxicity in approximately 3% of cases (249). Obstruction at the ileocecal valve or splenic flexure may necessitate laparotomy

TABLE 8. Body packers versus body stuffers

	Body packers	Body stuffers
Background	Hired specifically to smuggle drugs (e.g., heroin or cocaine)	User or seller, on verge of arrest, swallows the evidence
Wrapping	Carefully wrapped (latex, sometimes condoms, with or without covering of aluminum foil)	May not be carefully wrapped or in aluminum foil; may be in an open porous container, such as a sandwich bag, glass, or plastic "crack vials"; sometimes swallowed
Detection	Most escape detection	—
Toxicity	Few toxic effects	Initially asymptomatic; later may be seizing, comatose, or dead in a jail cell
Radiograph	Carefully wrapped package with air or liquid trapped in packaging material (useful in 75–80% of cases)	Rarely useful; number of ingested containers small; little liquid or air in packaging material
History	Inaccurate	Inaccurate
Co-ingestants	Usually not; most are not drug abusers, transport one drug	Present (users, street sellers)
Treatment	Gastric emptying, activated charcoal, whole bowel irrigation	Gastric emptying, hazardous; careful induction of emesis; activated charcoal with whole bowel irrigation
Surgery	If severely symptomatic	If severely symptomatic risk of obstruction is less
Endoscopy	Encourage gastrointestinal transit	Empty bags pass through on normal gastrointestinal transit

Adapted from Pollack CV, Biggers DW, Carlton FB Jr, et al. Two crack cocaine body stuffers. *Ann Emerg Med* 1992;21:1370–1380.

with enterotomy. In cases of gastric outlet obstruction, surgery and endoscopic techniques have been used successfully (247).

Body stuffers may be seen before symptoms have developed. They are unlikely to be diagnosed by radiography (250). Body stuffers who manifest clinical signs of toxicity should be treated similarly to other cocaine-intoxicated patients. Additionally, gastrointestinal decontamination with activated charcoal should be administered (251). Assessment for additional unruptured cocaine packages should be considered. Whole bowel irrigation with subsequent radiologic verification of passage of all drug-filled containers may be necessary (247).

Management Pitfalls

Underuse of benzodiazepines as a first-line agent in treating cocaine-related toxicities is a common problem. Benzodiazepines beneficially affect several aspects of toxicity from adrenergic agents and should be one of the first interventions administered.

Another concern is the failure to consider cocaine intoxication in the differential diagnosis of patients with chest pain, seizures, agitation, altered mental status, and dysrhythmias. Conversely, attribution of all signs and symptoms to cocaine intoxication without a search for underlying structural or non–cocaine-related explanations of symptoms can also create a missed diagnosis.

Delayed therapy may result from failure to recognize the limitations of the ECG in the evaluation of cocaine-related chest pain as well as the differences in management of chest pain from traditional coronary artery disease compared to cocaine-related causes. Similarly, hyperthermia may be overlooked initially.

REFERENCES

1. Haddad LM. 1978: Cocaine in perspective. *JACEP* 1979;8:374–376.
2. Hollander JE, Hoffman RS. Cocaine induced myocardial infarction: an analysis and review of the literature. *J Emerg Med* 1992;10:169–177.
3. SAMHSA. 1999 National household survey on drug abuse summary findings. Available at: http://www.samhsa.gov/oas/oasftp.htm. Accessed June 2003.
4. Dailey RH. Fatality secondary to misuse of TAC solution. *Ann Emerg Med* 1988;17:159–160.
5. Daya MR, Burton BT, Schleiss MR, et al. Recurrent seizures following mucosal application of TAC. *Ann Emerg Med* 1988;17:646–648.
6. Dronen SC. Complications of TAC [Letter]. *Ann Emerg Med* 1983;12:333.
7. Grant SA, Hoffman RS. Use of tetracaine, epinephrine and cocaine as a topical anesthetic in the emergency department. *Ann Emerg Med* 1992;21:987–997.
8. Foltin RW, Fischman MW. Smoked and intravenous cocaine in humans: acute tolerance, cardiovascular and subjective effects. *J Pharmacol Exp Ther* 1991;257:247–261.
9. Gay GR. Clinical management of acute and chronic cocaine poisoning. *Ann Emerg Med* 1982;11:562–572.
10. Henderson RL, Johns ME. The clinical use of cocaine. *Drug Ther* February 1977:8–14.
11. Hollander JE, Hoffman RS. Cocaine. In: Goldfrank LR, Flomenbaum NE, Lewin NA, eds. *Goldfrank's toxicologic emergencies*, 7th ed. New York: McGraw-Hill, 2002.
12. Borne RF, Bedford JA, Buelke JL, et al. Biological effects of cocaine, derivatives I: improved synthesis and pharmacologic evaluation of norcocaine. *J Pharm Sci* 1977;66:119–129.
13. Kurth CD, Monitto C, Albuquerque ML, et al. Cocaine and its metabolites constrict cerebral arterioles in newborn pigs. *J Pharmacol Exp Ther* 1993;265:587–591.
14. Schreiber MD, Madden JA, Covert RF, Torgerson LJ. Effects of cocaine, benzoylecgonine and cocaine metabolites on cannulated pressurized fetal sheep cerebral arteries. *J Appl Physiol* 1994;77:834–839.
15. Covert RF, Schreiber MD, Tebbett IR, Torgerson LJ. Hemodynamic and cerebral blood flow effects of cocaine, cocaethylene and benzoylecgonine in conscious and anesthetized fetal lambs. *J Pharmacol Exp Ther* 1994;270:118–126.
16. Madden J, Powers R. Effect of cocaine and cocaine metabolites on cerebral arteries in vitro. *Life Sci* 1990;47:1109–1114.
17. Konkol RJ, Erickson BA, Doerr JK, et al. Seizure induced by the cocaine metabolite benzoylecgonine in rats. *Epilepsia* 1992;33:420–427.
18. Mets B, Virag L. Lethal toxicity from equimolar infusions of cocaine and cocaine metabolites in conscious and anesthetized rats. *Anesth Analg* 1995;81:1033–1038.
19. Crumb WJ, Clarkson CW. Characterization of sodium channel blocking properties of the major metabolites of cocaine in single cardiac myocytes. *J Pharmacol Exp Ther* 1992;261:910–917.
20. MacGregor SN, Keith LG, Chasnoff IJ, et al. Cocaine use during pregnancy: adverse perinatal outcome. *Am J Obstet Gynecol* 1987;157:686–690.
21. Kambam J, Mets B, Hickman RM, et al. The effects of inhibition of plasma cholinesterase and hepatic microsomal enzyme activity on cocaine, benzoylecgonine, ecgonine methyl ester, and norcocaine blood levels in pigs. *J Lab Clin Med* 1992;120:323–328.
22. Devenyi P. Cocaine complications and pseudocholinesterase [Letter]. *Ann Intern Med* 1989;110:167–168.
23. Hoffman RS, Henry GL, Weisman RS, et al. Association between life-threatening cocaine toxicity and plasma cholinesterase activity. *Ann Emerg Med* 1991;21:247–253.
24. Om A, Ellahham S, Ornato JP, et al. Medical complications of cocaine: possible relationship to low plasma cholinesterase enzyme. *Am Heart J* 1993;125:1114–1117.
25. Hoffman RS, Morasco R, Goldfrank LR. Administration of purified human plasma cholinesterase protects against cocaine toxicity in mice. *J Toxicol Clin Toxicol* 1996;34:259–266.
26. Brookoff D, Rotondo MF, Shaw LM, et al. Cocaethylene levels in patients who test positive for cocaine. *Ann Emerg Med* 1996;27:316–320.
27. Perez-Reyes M. Subjective and cardiovascular effects of cocaethylene in humans. *Psychopharmacology* 1993;113:144–147.
28. Henning RJ, Wilson LD, Glauser JM. Cocaine plus ethanol is more cardiotoxic than cocaine or ethanol alone. *Crit Care Med* 1994;22:1896–1906.
29. Pirwitz MJ, Willard JE, Landau C, et al. Influence of cocaine, ethanol, or their combination on epicardial coronary arterial dimensions in humans. *Arch Intern Med* 1995;155:1186–1191.
30. Kolodgie FD, Wilson PS, Mergner WJ, Virmani R. Cocaine induced increase in the permeability function of human vascular endothelial cell monolayers. *Exp Mol Pathol* 1999;66:109–122.
31. Jatlow PI. Drug of abuse profile: cocaine. *Clin Chem* 1987;33:66b–71b.
32. Bauman JL, Grawe JJ, Winecoff AP, et al. Cocaine-related sudden cardiac death: a hypothesis correlating basic science and clinical observations. *J Clin Pharmacol* 1994;34:902–911.
33. Winecoff AP, Hariman RJ, Grawe JJ, et al. Reversal of the electrocardiographic effects of cocaine by lidocaine (Pt 1). Comparison with sodium bicarbonate and quinidine. *Pharmacotherapy* 1994;14:698–703.
34. Tella SR, Schindler CW, Goldberg SR. Cocaine: cardiovascular effects in relation to inhibition of peripheral neuronal monoamine uptake and central stimulation of the sympathoadrenal system. *J Pharmacol Exp Ther* 1993;267:153–162.
35. Heikkila RE, Orlansky H, Cohen G. Studies on the distinction between uptake inhibition and release of dopamine in rat brain tissue slices. *Biochem Pharmacol* 1975;24:847–852.
36. Volkow ND, Wang GJ, Fischman MW, et al. Relationship between subjective effects of cocaine and dopamine transported occupancy. *Nature* 1997;386:827–830.
37. Giros B, Jaber M, Jones S, et al. Hyperlocomotion and indifference to cocaine and amphetamine in mice lacking the dopamine transporter. *Nature* 1996;379:606–612.
38. Self DW, Barnhart WJ, Lehman DA, Nestler EJ. Opposite modulation of cocaine seeking behavior by D1 and D2 like dopamine receptor antagonists. *Science* 1996;271:1586–1589.
39. Romach MK, Glue P, Kampman K, et al. Attenuation of the euphoric effects of cocaine by the dopamine D1/D5 antagonist ecopipam (SCH 39166). *Arch Gen Psychiatry* 1999;56:1101–1106.
40. Smith JA, Mo Q, Guo H, et al. Cocaine increases extraneuronal levels of aspartate and glutamate in the nucleus accumbens. *Brain Res Bull* 1995;683:264–269.
41. Pap A, Bradberry CW. Excitatory amino acid antagonists attenuate the effects of cocaine on extracellular dopamine in the nucleus accumbens. *J Pharmacol Exp Ther* 1995;274:127–133.
42. Rockhold RW, Oden G, Ho IK, et al. Glutamate receptor antagonists block cocaine induced convulsions and death. *Brain Res Bull* 1991;27:721–723.
43. Handler A, Kiston N, Davis F, Ferri C. Cocaine use during pregnancy: perinatal outcomes. *Am J Epidemiol* 1991;133:818–825.
44. Collins E, Hardwich RJ, Jeffrey H. Perinatal cocaine intoxication. *Med J Aust* 1989;150:331–334.
45. Chasnoff I, Griffith DR, MacGregor S, et al. Temporal patterns of cocaine use in pregnancy: perinatal outcome. *JAMA* 1989;261:1741–1744.
46. Hadeed AJ, Siegel SR. Maternal cocaine use during pregnancy: effect on the newborn infant. *Pediatrics* 1989;84:205–210.
47. Rosenak D, Diamont YZ, Haffe H, et al. Cocaine: maternal use during pregnancy and its effect on the mother, the fetus, and the infant. *Obstet Gynecol Surv* 1990;45:348–359.
48. Telsey AM, Merrit A, Dixon SD. Cocaine experience in a term neonate: necrotizing enterocolitis as a complication. *Clin Pediatr* 1988;27:547–550.
49. Spinazzola R, Kenigsberg K, Usmani SS, Harper RG. Neonatal gastrointestinal complications of maternal cocaine abuse. *N Y State J Med* 1992;92:22–23.
50. Van den Anker JN, Cohen-Overbeek TE, Wladimiroff JW, Sauer PJJ. Prenatal diagnosis of limb reduction defects due to maternal cocaine use. *Lancet* 1991;338:1332.

51. Hoyme HE, Lyons Jones K, Dixon SD, et al. Prenatal cocaine exposure and fetal vascular disruption. *Pediatrics* 1990;85:743–747.
52. Lyons Jones K. Developmental pathogenesis of defects associated with prenatal cocaine exposure: fetal vascular disruption. *Clin Perinatol* 1991;18:139–146.
53. Hannig VL, Phillips JA III. Maternal cocaine abuse and fetal anomalies: evidence for teratogenic effects of cocaine. *South Med J* 1991;84:498–499.
54. Spires MC, Gordon EF, Choudhuri M, et al. Intracranial hemorrhage in a neonate following prenatal cocaine exposure. *Pediatr Neurol* 1989;5:324–326.
55. Maynard EC, Dreyer SA, Oh W. Prenatal cocaine exposure and hyaline membrane disease (HMD). *Pediatr Res* 1989;24:223A.
56. Zuckerman B, Maynard EC, Cabral H. A preliminary report of prenatal cocaine exposure and respiratory distress syndrome in premature infants. *Am J Dis Child* 1991;145:695–698.
57. Chasnoff IJ, Lewis DE, Squires L. Cocaine intoxication in a breast fed infant. *Pediatrics* 1987;80:836–838.
58. Giacoia GP. Cocaine in the cradle: a hidden epidemic. *South Med J* 1990;83:947–951.
59. Chaney NE, Franke J, Wadlington WB. Cocaine convulsions in a breast-feeding baby. *J Pediatr* 1988;112:134–135.
60. Graham K, Dimitrakoudis D, Pellegrini E, Koren G. Pregnancy outcome following first trimester exposure to cocaine in social users in Toronto, Canada. *Vet Hum Toxicol* 1989;31:143–148.
61. Vilensky W. Illicit and licit drugs causing perforation of the nasal septum. *J Forensic Sci* 1982;27:958–962.
62. Slavin SA. The cocaine user: the potential problem patient for rhinoplasty. *Plast Reconstr Surg* 1990;86:436–442.
63. Wang SJ. Cocaine-induced iritis. *Ann Emerg Med* 1991;20:192–193.
64. Cohen S. Cocaine: acute medical and psychiatric complications. *Psychiatr Ann* 1984;14:747–749.
65. Newman NM, DiLoreto DA, Ho JT, et al. Bilateral optic neuropathy and osteolytic sinusitis: complications of cocaine abuse. *JAMA* 1988;259:72–74.
66. Schweitzer VG. Osteolytic sinusitis and pneumomediastinum: deceptive otolaryngological complications of cocaine abuse. *Laryngoscope* 1985;96:206–210.
67. Krutchkoff DJ, Eisenberg E, O'Brien JE, et al. Cocaine induced dental erosion. *N Engl J Med* 1990;322:408.
68. Catravas JD, Waters IW. Acute cocaine intoxication in the conscious dog: studies on the mechanism of lethality. *J Pharmacol Exp Ther* 1981;217:350–356.
69. Marzuk PM, Tardiff K, Leon AC, et al. Ambient temperature and mortality from unintentional cocaine overdose. *JAMA* 1998;279:1795–1800.
70. Petitti DB, Sidney S, Quesenberry C, et al. Stroke and cocaine or amphetamine use. *Epidemiology* 1998;9:956–1600.
71. Lichtenfeld PJ, Rubin DB, Feldman RS. Subarachnoid hemorrhage precipitated by cocaine snorting. *Arch Neurol* 1984;41:223–224.
72. Schwartz KA, Cohen JA. Subarachnoid hemorrhage precipitated by cocaine snorting [Letter]. *Arch Neurol* 1984;41:705.
73. Levine SR, Brust JCM, Futrell N, et al. Cerebrovascular complications of the use of the "crack" form of alkaloidal cocaine. *N Engl J Med* 1990;323:699–704.
74. Mody CK, Miller BL, McIntyre HB, et al. Neurologic complications of cocaine abuse. *Neurology* 1988;38:1189–1193.
75. Catalano G, Catalano MC, Rodriguez R. Dystonia associated with crack cocaine use. *South Med J* 1997;90:1050–1052.
76. Maschke M, Fehlings T, Kastrup O, et al. Toxic leukoenchalopathy after intravenous consumption of heroin and cocaine with unexpected clinical recovery. *J Neurol* 1999;246:850–851.
77. Satel SL, Gawin FH. Migraine like headache and cocaine use. *JAMA* 1989;261:2995–2996.
78. Choy-Kwong M, Lipton RB. Seizures in hospitalized cocaine users. *Neurology* 1989;39:425–427.
79. Kaye BR, Fainstat M. Cerebral vasculitis associated with cocaine abuse. *JAMA* 1987;258:2104–2106.
80. Krendel DA, Ditter SM, Frankel MR, et al. Biopsy-proven cerebral vasculitis associated with cocaine abuse. *Neurology* 1990;40:1092–1094.
81. Henderson CE, Torbey M. Rupture of intracranial aneurysm associated with cocaine use during pregnancy. *Am J Perinatol* 1988;5:142–143.
82. Wojak JC, Flamm ES. Intracranial hemorrhage and cocaine use. *Stroke* 1987;18:712–715.
83. Wallace EA, Wisnieksi G, Zubal G, et al. Acute cocaine effects on absolute cerebral blood flow. *Psychopharmacology* 1996;128:17–20.
84. Kaufman MJ, Levin JM, Ross MH, et al. Cocaine induced cerebral vasconstriction detected in humans with magnetic resonance imaging. *JAMA* 1998;279:376–380.
85. Caplan LR, Hier DB, Banks G. Current concepts of cerebrovascular disease: stroke and drug abuse. *Stroke* 1982;13:869–872.
86. Fritsma GA, Leikin JB, Maturen AJ, et al. Detection of anticardiolipin antibody in patients with cocaine abuse. *J Emerg Med* 1991;9:37–43.
87. Dart RC. Cocaine "washed-out" syndrome. In: Dart RC, Hurlbut KM, Kuffner EK, et al., eds. *The 5 minute toxicology consult.* Philadelphia: Lippincott Williams & Wilkins, 2000.
88. Sporer KA, Lesser SH. Cocaine washed out syndrome. *Ann Emerg Med* 1992;21:112.
89. Amin M, Gabelman G, Karpel J, et al. Acute myocardial infarction and chest pain: syndromes after cocaine use. *Am J Cardiol* 1990;66:1434–1437.
90. Del Aguila C, Rosman H. Myocardial infarction during cocaine withdrawal [Letter]. *Ann Intern Med* 1990;112:712.
91. Hollander JE. Management of cocaine associated myocardial ischemia. *N Engl J Med* 1995;333:1267–1272.
92. Hollander JE, Carter WC, Hoffman RS. Use of phentolamine for cocaine induced myocardial ischemia [Letter]. *N Engl J Med* 1992;327:361.
93. Hollander JE, Hoffman RS, Burstein J, et al. Cocaine associated myocardial infarction. Mortality and complications. *Arch Intern Med* 1995;155:1081–1086.
94. Lange RA, Hillis RD. Cardiovascular complications of cocaine use. *N Engl J Med* 2001;345:351–358.
95. Levine MAH, Nishakawa J. Acute myocardial infarction associated with cocaine withdrawal. *Can Med Assoc J* 1991;144:1139–1140.
96. Minor RL, Scott BD, Brown DD, et al. Cocaine induced myocardial infarction in patients with normal coronary arteries. *Ann Intern Med* 1991;115:797–806.
97. Nademanee K, Gorelick DA, Josephson MA, et al. Myocardial ischemia during cocaine withdrawal. *Ann Intern Med* 1989;111:876–880.
98. Mittleman MA, Mintzer D, Maclure M, et al. Triggering of myocardial infarction by cocaine. *Circulation* 1999;99:2737–2741.
99. Hollander JE, Hoffman RS, Gennis P, et al. Cocaine associated chest pain: one year follow-up. *Acad Emerg Med* 1995;2:179–184.
100. Hollander JE, Hoffman RS, Gennis P, et al. Prospective multicenter evaluation of cocaine associated chest pain. *Acad Emerg Med* 1994;1:330–339.
101. Gitter MJ, Goldsmith ER, Dunbar DN, et al. Cocaine and chest pain: clinical features and outcome of patients hospitalized to rule out myocardial infarction. *Ann Intern Med* 1991;115:277–282.
102. Hollander JE, Lozano M Jr, Fairweather P, et al. "Abnormal" electrocardiograms in patients with cocaine-associated chest pain are due to "normal" variants. *J Emerg Med* 1994;12:199–205.
103. Vongpatanasin W, Lange RA, Hillis LD. Comparison of cocaine induced vasoconstriction of left and right coronary arterial systems. *Am J Cardiol* 1997;79:492–493.
104. Hollander JE, Burstein JL, Shih RD, et al. Cocaine associated myocardial infarction: clinical safety of thrombolytic therapy. *Chest* 1995;107:1237–1241.
105. Howard RE, Hueter DC, Davis GJ. Acute myocardial infarction following cocaine abuse in a young woman with normal coronary arteries. *JAMA* 1985;254:95–96.
106. Pasternack PF, Colvin SB, Baumann FG. Cocaine-induced angina pectoris and acute myocardial infarction in patients younger than 40 years. *Am J Cardiol* 1985;55:847.
107. Parker RB, Beckman KJ, Hariman RJI, et al. The electrophysiologic and arrhythmogenic effects of cocaine. *Pharmacotherapy* 1989;9:176(abst).
108. Schwartz AB, Janzen D, Jones RT, et al. Electrocardiographic and hemodynamic effects of intravenous cocaine in the awake and anesthetized dog. *J Electrocardiol* 1989;22:159–166.
109. Shih RD, Hollander JE, Hoffman RS, et al. Clinical safety of lidocaine in cocaine associated myocardial infarction. *Ann Emerg Med* 1995;26:702–706.
110. Weiner RS, Lockhart JT, Schwartz RG. Dilated cardiomyopathy and cocaine abuse. *Am J Med* 1986;81:699–701.
111. Hale SL, Alker KJ, Rezkalla S, et al. Adverse effects of cocaine on cardiovascular dynamics, myocardial blood flow, and coronary artery diameter in an experimental model. *Am Heart J* 1989;118:927–933.
112. Perreault CL, Allen PD, Hague AN, et al. Differential mechanisms of cocaine-induced depression of contractile function in cardiac versus vascular smooth muscle. *Circulation* 1989;80[4 Suppl 2]:15(abst).
113. Pitts WR, Vongpatannasin W, Cigoarroa JE, et al. Effects of intracoronary infusion of cocaine on left ventricular systolic and diastolic function in humans. *Circulation* 1998;97:1270–1273.
114. Chokshi SK, Moore R, Pandian NG, et al. Reversible cardiomyopathy associated with cocaine intoxication. *Ann Intern Med* 1989;111:1039–1040.
115. Farrell M. Cocaine and HIV. *BMJ* 1991;303:330.
116. Nanda D, Feldman J, Delke I, et al. Syphilis among parturients at an inner city hospital: association with cocaine use and implications for congenital syphilis rates. *N Y State J Med* 1990;90:448–490.
117. Minkoff HL, McCalla S, Delke I, et al. The relationship of cocaine use to syphilis and human immunodeficiency virus infections among inner city parturient women. *Obstet Gynecol* 1990;163:521–526.
118. Lisse JR, Davis CP, Thurmond-Anderle ME. Cocaine abuse and deep venous thrombosis [Letter]. *Ann Intern Med* 1989;110:571–572.
119. Lisse JR, Davis CP, Thurmond-Anderle ME. Upper extremity deep venous thrombosis: increased prevalence due to cocaine abuse. *Am J Med* 1989;87:457–458.
120. Chambers HF, Morris DL, Tauber MG, et al. Cocaine use and the risk for endocarditis in intravenous drug users. *Ann Intern Med* 1987;106:833–836.
121. Weiss SH. Links between cocaine and retroviral infection. *JAMA* 1989;261:607–608.
122. Rashid J, Eisenberg MJ, Topol EJ. Cocaine induced aortic dissection. *Am Heart J* 1996;132:1301–1304.
123. Haim DY, Lippman ML, Goldberg SK, et al. The pulmonary complications of crack cocaine. A comprehensive review. *Chest* 1995;107:233–240.
124. Thadani PV. NIDA conference report on cardiopulmonary complications of crack cocaine use—clinical manifestations and pathophysiology. *Chest* 1996;110:1072–1076.
125. Leitman BS, Greengart A, Wasser HJ. Pneumomediastinum and pneumopericardium after cocaine abuse. *AJR Am J Roentgenol* 1988;151:614.
126. Shesser R, Davis D, Edelstein S. Pneumomediastinum and pneumothorax after inhaling alkaloidal cocaine. *Ann Emerg Med* 1981;10:213–215.

127. Cucco RA, Yoo OH, Gregler L, et al. Non-fatal pulmonary edema after freebase cocaine smoking. *Am Rev Respir Dis* 1987;136:179–181.
128. Hoffman CK, Goodman PC. Pulmonary edema in cocaine smokers. *Radiology* 1989;172:463–465.
129. Kline JN, Hirasuna JD. Pulmonary edema after freebase cocaine smoking—not due to an adulterant. *Chest* 1990;97:1009–1010.
130. Murray RJ, Albin RJ, Mergner W, et al. Diffuse alveolar hemorrhage temporally related to cocaine smoking. *Chest* 1988;93:427–429.
131. O'Donnell AE, Mappin G, Sepo TJ, et al. Interstitial pneumonitis associated with "crack" cocaine abuse. *Chest* 1991;100:1155–1157.
132. Garcia-Rostan Y, Perez GM, Bragado FG, et al. Pulmonary hemorrhage and antiglomerular basement membrane antibody mediated glomerulonephritis after exposure to smoked cocaine (crack). A case report and review of the literature. *Pathol Int* 1997;47:692–697.
133. Patel RC, Dutta D, Schoenfeld SA. Free base cocaine use associated with bronchiolitis obliterans organizing pneumonia. *Ann Intern Med* 1987;107:186–187.
134. Delaney K, Hoffman RS. Pulmonary infarction associated with crack cocaine use in a previously healthy 23 year old woman. *Am J Med* 1991;91:92–94.
135. Smith GT, McClaughry PL, Purkey J, et al. Crack cocaine mimicking pulmonary embolism on pulmonary ventilation perfusion scan. A case report. *Clin Nucl Med* 1995;20:65–68.
136. Nadel DM, Lyons KM. "Shotgunning" crack cocaine as a potential cause of retropharyngeal abscess. *Ear Nose Throat J* 1998;77:47–50.
137. Ettinger NA, Albin RJ. A review of the respiratory effects of smoking cocaine. *Am J Med* 1989;87:664–668.
138. Murray RJ, Simialek J, Golle M, et al. Pulmonary artery medial hypertrophy in cocaine users without foreign particle microembolization. *Chest* 1989;96:1050–1053.
139. Albertson TE, Walby WF, Derlet RW. Stimulant induced pulmonary toxicity. *Chest* 1995;108:1140–1149.
140. Itkonen J, Schnoll S, Glassroth J. Pulmonary dysfunction in "freebase" cocaine users. *Arch Intern Med* 1984;144:2195–2197.
141. Suhl J, Gorelick DA. Pulmonary function in male freebase cocaine users. *Am Rev Respir Dis* 1988;137:A488(abst).
142. Tashkin DP, Khalsa ME, Gorelick D, et al. Pulmonary status of habitual cocaine users. *Am Rev Respir Dis* 1992;145:92–100.
143. Tashkin DP, Kleerup EC, Hoh CK, et al. Effects of "crack" cocaine on pulmonary alveolar permeability. *Chest* 1997;112:327–335.
144. Barsky SH, Roth MD, Kleerup ED, et al. Histopathologic and molecular alterations in bronchial epithelium in habitual smokers of marijuana, cocaine and/or tobacco. *J Natl Cancer Inst* 1998;90:1198–1205.
145. Tashkin DP, Kleerup EC, Koyal SN, et al. Acute effects of inhaled and IV cocaine on airway dynamics. *Chest* 1996;110:904–910.
146. Ravin JG, Ravin LC. Blindness due to illicit use of topical cocaine. *Ann Ophthalmol* 1979;11:863–864.
147. McHenry JG, Zeiter JH, Madion MP, et al. Corneal epithelial defects after smoking crack cocaine. *Am J Ophthalmol* 1989;108:732.
148. Devenyi P, Schneiderman JF, Devenyi RG, et al. Cocaine-induced central retinal artery occlusion. *Can Med Assoc J* 1988;138:129–130.
149. Hoffman RS, Reimer BI. "Crack" cocaine–induced bilateral amblyopia. *Am J Emerg Med* 1993;11:35–37.
150. Anand V, Siami G, Stone WJ. Cocaine-associated rhabdomyolysis and acute renal failure. *South Med J* 1989;82:67–69.
151. Brody SL, Wrenn KD, Wilber MM, et al. Predicting the severity of cocaine associated rhabdomyolysis. *Ann Emerg Med* 1990;19:1137–1143.
152. Menashe PI, Gottlieb JE. Hyperthermia, rhabdomyolysis, and myoglobinuric renal failure after recreational use of cocaine. *South Med J* 1988;81:379–381.
153. Merigian KS, Roberts JR. Cocaine intoxication: hyperpyrexia, rhabdomyolysis and acute renal failure. *J Toxicol Clin Toxicol* 1987;25:135–148.
154. Roth D, Alarcon FJ, Fernandez JA, et al. Acute rhabdomyolysis associated with cocaine intoxication. *N Engl J Med* 1988;319:673–677.
155. Rubin RB, Neugarten J. Cocaine-induced rhabdomyolysis masquerading as myocardial ischemia. *Am J Med* 1989;86:551–553.
156. Welch RD, Todd K, Krause GS. Incidence of cocaine associated rhabdomyolysis. *Ann Emerg Med* 1991;20:154–157.
157. Sharff JA. Renal infarction associated with intravenous cocaine use. *Ann Emerg Med* 1984;13:1145–1147.
158. Acker D, Sachs BP, Tracey KJ. Abruptio placentae associated with cocaine use. *Am J Obstet Gynecol* 1983;146:220–221.
159. Chavez GF, Mulinare J, Cordero JF. Maternal cocaine use during early pregnancy as a risk factor for congenital urogenital anomalies. *JAMA* 1989;262:795–798.
160. Doberczak TM, Shanzer S, Senie RT, et al. Neonatal neurologic and electroencephalographic effects of intrauterine cocaine exposure. *J Pediatr* 1988;113:354–358.
161. MacGregor SN, Keith LG, Chasnoff IJ, et al. Cocaine use during pregnancy: adverse perinatal outcome. *Am J Obstet Gynecol* 1987;157:686–690.
162. Ness RB, Grisso JA, Hirschinger N, et al. Cocaine and tobacco use and the risk of spontaneous abortion. *N Engl J Med* 1999;340:333–339.
163. Moore TR, Sorg J, Miller L, et al. Hemodynamic effects of intravenous cocaine on the pregnant ewe and fetus. *Am J Obstet Gynecol* 1986;155:883–888.
164. Woods JR, Plessinger MA, Clark KE. Effect of cocaine on uterine blood flow and fetal oxygenation. *JAMA* 1987;257:957–961.
165. Eyler FD, Behnke M, Conlon M, et al. Birth outcome from a prospective, matched study of prenatal crack/cocaine use: II. Interactive and dose effects on neurobehavioral assessment. *Pediatrics* 1998;101:237–241.
166. Wasserman GA, Kline JK, Bateman DA, et al. Prenatal cocaine exposure and school-age intelligence. *Drug Alc Depend* 1998;50:203–210.
167. Endress C, Kling GA. Cocaine-induced small-bowel perforation. *Am J Radiol* 1990;154:1346–1347.
168. Freudenberger RS, Cappell MS, Hutt DA. Intestinal infarction after intravenous cocaine administration. *Ann Intern Med* 1990;113:715–716.
169. Grafia A, Valverde JL, Borondo JC, et al. Vascular lesions in intestinal ischemia induced by cocaine-alcohol abuse: report of a fatal case due to overdose. *J Forensic Sci* 1990;35:740–745.
170. Nalbandian H, Sheth N, Dietrich R, et al. Intestinal ischemia caused by cocaine ingestion: report of two cases. *Surgery* 1985;97:374–376.
171. Fishel R, Hamamoto G, Barbul A, et al. Cocaine colitis: is this a new syndrome? *Dis Colon Rectum* 1985;28:264–266.
172. Lee HS, LaMaute HR, Pizzi WF, et al. Acute gastrointestinal perforations associated with use of crack. *Ann Surg* 1990;211:15–17.
173. Larkin RF. The callus of crack cocaine. *N Engl J Med* 1990;323:685.
174. Burton KR, Marin CA, Murray FT, et al. Hyperthyroidism in a cocaine-dependent patient. *J Clin Psychiatry* 1989;50:305–306.
175. Goetz C, Harchelroud F. Severe hypocalcemia associated with cocaine-induced rhabdomyolysis. *Vet Hum Toxicol* 1991;33:387.
176. Lombard J, Levin IH, Weiner WJ. Arsenic intoxication in a cocaine abuser. *N Engl J Med* 1989;320:869.
177. Miller NS, Summers GL, Gold MS. Cocaine dependence: alcohol and other drug dependence and withdrawal characteristics. *J Addict Dis* 1993;12:25–35.
178. Holland RW, Marx JA, Earnest MP, et al. Grand mal seizures temporally related to cocaine use: clinical and diagnostic features. *Ann Emerg Med* 1992;21:772–776.
179. Ambre J. The urinary excretion of cocaine and metabolites in humans: a kinetic analysis of published data. *J Anal Toxicol* 1985;9:241–245.
180. Hollander JE, Levitt MA, Young GP, et al. The effect of cocaine on the specificity of cardiac markers. *Am Heart J* 1998;135(2):245–252.
181. Tokarsky GF, Paganussi P, Urbanski R, et al. An evaluation of cocaine-induced chest pain. *Ann Emerg Med* 1990;19:1088–1092.
182. Weiss RD. Protracted elimination of cocaine metabolites in long term high dose cocaine abuse. *Am J Med* 1988;85:879–880.
183. Wallace JE, Hamilton HE, Christenson JG, et al. An evaluation of selected methods for determining cocaine and benzoylecgonine in urine. *J Anal Toxicol* 1977;1:20–25.
184. Budd RD, Mathis DF, Yang FC. TLC analysis of urine for benzoylecgonine and norpropoxyphene. *Clin Toxicol* 1980;16:1–5.
185. Rafla FK, Epstein RL. Identification of cocaine and its metabolites in human urine in the presence of ethyl alcohol. *J Anal Toxicol* 1979;3:59–63.
186. Kogan MJ, Verebey KG, De Pace AC, et al. Quantitative determination of benzoylecgonine and cocaine in human biofluids by gas–liquid chromatography. *Anal Chem* 1977;49:1965–1969.
187. Wallace JE, Hamilton HE, King DE, et al. Gas–liquid chromatographic determination of cocaine and benzoylecgonine in urine. *Anal Chem* 1976;48:34–48.
188. Masoud AN, Knipski DM. High performance liquid chromatographic analysis of cocaine in human plasma. *J Anal Toxicol* 1980;4:305–310.
189. Jatlow P. Cocaine: analysis, pharmacokinetics and metabolic disposition. *Yale J Biol Med* 1988;61:105–113.
190. Schramm W, Craig PA, Smith RH, Berger GE. Cocaine and benzoylecgonine in saliva, serum and urine. *Clin Chem* 1993;39:481–487.
191. Harkey MR, Henderson GL, Zhou C. Simultaneous quantitation of cocaine and its major metabolites in human hair by gas chromatography/chemical ionization mass spectrometry. *J Anal Toxicol* 1991;15:260–265.
192. Cone EJ, Youselnejad D, Darwin WD, et al. Testing human hair for drugs of abuse: II. Identification of unique cocaine metabolites in hair of drug abusers and evaluation of decontamination procedures. *J Anal Toxicol* 1991;15:250–255.
193. Reuschel SA, Smith FP. Benzoylecgonine (cocaine metabolite) detection in hair sample of jail detainees using radioimmunoassay (RIA) and gas chromatography/mass spectrometry (GC/MS). *J Forensic Sci* 1991;36:1179–1185.
194. Martz R, Donnelly B, Fetterolf D, et al. The use of hair analysis to document a cocaine overdose following sustained survival period before death. *J Anal Toxicol* 1991;15:279–281.
195. Koren GB, Klein J, Forman R, Graham K. Hair analysis of cocaine: differentiation between systemic exposure and external contamination. *J Clin Pharmacol* 1992;32:671–675.
196. Szeti HH. Kinetics of drug transfer to the fetus. *Clin Obstet Gynecol* 1993;36:246–254.
197. Callahan CM, Grant TM, Phipps P, et al. Measurement of gestational cocaine exposure: sensitivity of infants' hair, meconium and urine. *J Pediatr* 1992;120:763–768.
198. Logan BD, Smirnow D, Gullverg RG. Lack of predictable site-dependent differences and time-dependent changes in postmortem concentration of cocaine, benzoylecgonine, and cocaethylene in humans. *J Anal Toxicol* 1997;21:23–31.
199. Mattes CE, Lynch TJ, Singh A, et al.. Therapeutic use of butyrylcholinesterase for cocaine intoxication. *Toxicol Appl Pharmacol* 1997;145:372–380.
200. Lynch TJ, Mattes CE, Singh A, et al. Cocaine detoxification by human plasma butyrylcholinesterase. *Toxicol Appl Pharmacol* 1997;145:363–371.

201. Brogan WC, Lange RA, Glamann B, et al. Recurrent coronary vasoconstriction caused by intranasal cocaine: possible role for metabolites. *Ann Intern Med* 1992;116:556–561.
202. Derlet RW, Albertson TE. Diazepam in the prevention of seizures and death in cocaine-intoxicated rats. *Ann Emerg Med* 1989;18:542–546.
203. Guinn MM, Bedford JA, Wilson MC. Antagonism of intravenous cocaine lethality in nonhuman primates. *Clin Toxicol* 1980;16:499–508.
204. Brogan WC, Lange RA, Kim AS, et al. Alleviation of cocaine-induced coronary vasoconstriction by nitroglycerin. *J Am Coll Cardiol* 1991;18:581–586.
205. Lange RA, Cigarroa RG, Yancy CW, et al. Cocaine-induced coronary-artery vasoconstriction. *N Engl J Med* 1989;321:1557–1561.
206. American Heart Association in Collaboration with the International Liaison Committee on Resuscitation (ILCOR). Guidelines for Cardiopulmonary Resuscitation and Emergency Cardiovascular Care. *Circulation* 2000;102:I89.
207. Hollander JE, Hoffman RS, Gennis P, et al. Nitroglycerin in the treatment of cocaine associated chest pain: clinical safety and efficacy. *J Toxicol Clin Toxicol* 1994;32:243–256.
208. Baumann BM, Perrone J, Hornig SE, et al. Randomized controlled double blind placebo controlled trial of diazepam, nitroglycerin or both for treatment of patients with potential cocaine associated acute coronary syndromes. *Acad Emerg Med* 2000;7(8):878–885.
209. Billman GE, Hoskins RS. Cocaine-induced ventricular fibrillation: protection afforded by the calcium antagonist verapamil. *FASEB J* 1988;2:2990–2995.
210. Nahas G, Trouve R, Demus JF, et al. A calcium channel blocker as antidote to the cardiac effects of cocaine intoxication [Letter]. *N Engl J Med* 1985;313:519.
211. Trouve R, Nahas GG, Maillet M. Nitrendipine as an antagonist to the cardiac toxicity of cocaine. *J Cardiovasc Pharmacol* 1987;9[Suppl 4]:S49–S53.
212. Derlet RW, Albertson TE. Potentiation of cocaine toxicity with calcium channel blockers. *Am J Emerg Med* 1989;7:464–468.
213. Hale SL, Alker KJ, Rezkalla SH, et al. Nifedipine protects the heart from the acute deleterious effects of cocaine if administered before but not after cocaine. *Circulation* 1991;83:1437–1443.
214. Smith M, Garner D, Niemann JT. Pharmacologic interventions after an LD50 cocaine insult in a chronically instrumented rat model: are beta blockers contraindicated? *Ann Emerg Med* 1991;20:768–771.
215. Negus BH, Willard JE, Hillis LD, et al. Alleviation of cocaine induced coronary vasoconstriction with intravenous verapamil. *Am J Cardiol* 1994;73:510–513.
216. Lange RA, Cigarroa RG, Flores ED, et al. Potentiation of cocaine-induced coronary vasoconstriction by beta-adrenergic blockade. *Ann Intern Med* 1990;112:897–903.
217. Ramoska E, Sacchetti AD. Propranolol-induced hypertension in treatment of cocaine intoxication. *Ann Emerg Med* 1985;14:112–113.
218. Rappolt RT, Gay G, Inaba DS. Use of Inderal (propranolol-Ayerst) in 1-a (early stimulative) and 1-b (advanced stimulative) classification of cocaine and other sympathomimetic reactions. *Clin Toxicol* 1978;13:325–332.
219. Rappolt TR, Gay G, Inaba DS, Rappolt NR. Propranolol in cocaine toxicity [Letter]. *Lancet* 1976;2:640–641.
220. Spivey WH, Schoffstall JM, Kirkpatrick R, et al. Comparison of labetalol, diazepam, and haloperidol for the treatment of cocaine toxicity in a swine model. *Ann Emerg Med* 1990;19:467–468.
221. Vargas R, Gillis RA, Ramwell PW. Propranolol promotes cocaine induced spasm of porcine coronary artery. *J Pharmacol Exp Ther* 1991;257:644–646.
222. Pollan S, Tadjziechy M. Esmolol in the management of epinephrine and cocaine induced cardiovascular toxicity. *Anesth Analg* 1989;69:663–664.
223. Sand IC, Brody SL, Wrenn KD, et al. Experience with esmolol for the treatment of cocaine associated cardiovascular complications. *Am J Emerg Med* 1991;9:161–163.
224. Haynes S, Stork CM, Hoffman RS, Goldfrank L. Beta-adrenergic blockade in cocaine toxicity [Letter]. *J Emerg Med* 1995;13:537–538.
225. Hollander JE. Beta-adrenergic blockade in cocaine toxicity [Letter]. *J Emerg Med* 1995;13:538–539.
226. Albertson TE, Dawson A, de Latorre F, et al. TOX-ACLS: toxicologic-oriented advanced cardiac life support. *Ann Emerg Med* 2001;37:S78–S90.
227. Sybertz EJ, Sabin CS, Pula KK, et al. Alpha and beta adrenoreceptor blocking properties of labetalol and its R,R-isomer, SCH 19927. *J Pharmacol Exp Ther* 1981;218:435–443.
228. Boehrer JD, Moliterno DJ, Willard JE, et al. Influence of labetalol of cocaine-induced coronary vasoconstriction in humans. *Am J Med* 1993;94:608–610.
229. Moliterno DJ, Lange RA, Gerard RD, et al. Influence of intranasal cocaine on plasma constituents associated with endogenous thrombosis and thrombolysis. *Am J Med* 1994;96:492–496.
230. Rezkalla S, Mazza JJ, Kloner RA, et al. The effect of cocaine on human platelets. *Am J Cardiol* 1993;72:243–246.
231. Rinder HM, Ault KA, Jatlow PI, et al. Platelet alpha granule release in cocaine users. *Circulation* 1994;90:1162–1167.
232. Togna G, Tempesta E, Togna AR, et al. Platelet responsiveness and biosynthesis of thromboxane and prostacyclin in response to in vitro cocaine treatment. *Haemostasis* 1985;15:100–107.
233. Hoffman RS, Hollander JE. Thrombolytic therapy in cocaine-induced myocardial infarction [Editorial]. *Am J Emerg Med* 1996;14:693–695.
234. Bush HS. Cocaine associated myocardial infarction: a word of caution about thrombolytic therapy. *Chest* 1988;94:878.
235. Hollander JE, Wilson LD, Leo PJ, Shih RD. Complications from the use of thrombolytic agents in patients with cocaine associated chest pain. *J Emerg Med* 1996;14:731–736.
236. LoVecchio F, Nelson L. Intraventricular bleeding after the use of thrombolytics in a cocaine user. *Am J Emerg Med* 1996;14:663–664.
237. Franogiannis NG, Farmer JA, Lakkis NM. Tirofiban for cocaine induced coronary artery thrombosis. A novel therapeutic approach. *Circulation* 1999;100:1939.
238. Beckman KJ, Parker RB, Hariman RJ, et al. Hemodynamic and electrophysiological actions of cocaine: effects of sodium bicarbonate as an antidote in dogs. *Circulation* 1991;83:1799–1807.
239. Derlet RW, Albertson TE, Tharratt RS. Lidocaine potentiation of cocaine toxicity. *Ann Emerg Med* 1991;20:135–138.
240. Grawe JJ, Hariman RJ, Winecoff AP, et al. Reversal of the electrocardiographic effects of cocaine by lidocaine, 2. Concentration-effect relationships. *Pharmacotherapy* 1994;14:704–711.
241. Heit J, Hoffman RS, Goldfrank LR. The effects of lidocaine pretreatment on cocaine neurotoxicity and lethality in mice. *Acad Emerg Med* 1994;1:438–442.
242. Kerns W, Garvey L, Owens J. Cocaine induced wide complex dysrhythmia. *J Emerg Med* 1997;15:321–329.
243. Schrem SS, Belsky P, Schwartzman D, et al. Cocaine-induced torsades de pointes in a patient with idiopathic long QT syndrome. *Am Heart J* 1990;120:980–984.
244. Hoffman B, Derlet R. Cocaine intoxication considerations, complications and strategies: point and counterpoint. *Emerg Med* 1992;1:1–6.
245. Derlet RW, Albertson TE, Rice P. The effect of haloperidol in cocaine and amphetamine intoxication. *J Emerg Med* 1989;7:633–637.
246. Witkin JM, Godberg SR, Katz JL. Lethal effects of cocaine are reduced by the dopamine-1 receptor antagonist SCH 23390 but not by haloperidol. *Life Sci* 1989;44:1285–1291.
247. Hoffman RS, Smilkstein MJ, Goldfrank LR. Whole bowel irrigation and the cocaine "bodypacker": a new approach to a common problem. *Am J Emerg Med* 1990;8:523–527.
248. McCarron MM, Wood JD. The cocaine body packer syndrome. *JAMA* 1983;250:1417–1420.
249. Aldrighetti L, Paganelli M, Giacomelli M, et al. Conservative management of cocaine-packet ingestion: experience in Milan, the main Italian smuggling center of South American cocaine. *Panminerva Med* 1996;38:111–116.
250. Hoffman RS, Chiang WK, Weisman RS, et al. Prospective evaluation of "crack-vial" ingestions. *Vet Hum Toxicol* 1990;32:164–166.
251. Tomaszewski C, McKinney P, Phillips S, et al. Prevention of toxicity from oral cocaine by activated charcoal in mice. *Ann Emerg Med* 1993;22:1804–1806.

CHAPTER 176

γ-Hydroxybutyrate, γ-Butyrolactone, and 1,4-Butanediol

Jo Ellen Dyer and Christine A. Haller

HO–CH₂–CH₂–CH₂–C(=O)–OH

γ-HYDROXYBUTYRATE

Compounds included:	**γ-Hydroxybutyrate, γ-butyrolactone, butadiene**
SI conversion:	**γ-Hydroxybutyrate, mg/L × 11.6 = μmol/L; 1,4-butanediol, mg/L × 11.1 = μmol/L**
Molecular formula and weight:	**See Table 1.**
CAS Registry No.:	**See Table 1.**
Normal levels:	**Endogenous γ-hydroxybutyrate levels in blood, less than 2 ng/ml; endogenous γ-hydroxybutyrate levels in urine, less than 10 μg/ml**
Special concerns:	**Abrupt deterioration of mental status may lead to respiratory arrest.**
Antidotes:	**No proven antidotes**

OVERVIEW

γ-Hydroxybutyrate (GHB; sodium oxybate) is a short-chain, carboxylic acid that freely crosses the blood–brain barrier and depresses consciousness. It is both a drug of abuse and a pharmaceutical preparation. The pharmaceutical preparation of GHB is named *Xyrem* in the United States and *Alcover* in Italy. Initially, GHB was investigated as an anesthetic agent during the 1960s. The lack of analgesia and difficulty controlling depth and duration of anesthesia, along with adverse events such as myoclonus, emergence delirium, and seizures in animals, prevented drug approval in the United States as an anesthesia adjunct. More recently, research into the therapeutic uses of GHB has included investigations for the treatment of alcoholism in Europe and cataplexy for narcoleptic patients in the United States.

Because of increased abuse, anabolic steroids were regulated under the federal Controlled Substances Act in 1989. That year GHB emerged as a steroid substitute for bodybuilders. Despite being touted as an "undetectable steroid," GHB has not been demonstrated to have anabolic activity (1). GHB itself became a federal controlled substance in March 2000. The chemical analogs γ-butyrolactone (GBL) and 1,4-butanediol (BD) are now sold as alternatives to GHB.

Sometimes termed a "club drug," the dreamy, altered sensorium from GHB is the desired effect in the settings of rave parties and dance clubs. Emergency department admissions for GHB-related overdoses have increased dramatically over the past 10 years. Federal reporting data on emergency department admissions due to drug abuse now list GHB as a more frequently encountered drug than another popular club drug, ecstasy (methylenedioxymethamphetamine) (2). GHB is also promoted as a sex-enhancing drug with claims to heighten sexual arousal and diminish inhibitions. These effects, along with anterograde amnesia and reduced level of consciousness, have led to exploitation of GHB as an agent to facilitate sexual assault.

Vulnerable user populations are the targets of advertising and promotional materials on the Internet and in bodybuilding magazines. GHB products are promoted to the elderly as a "fountain-of-youth" product, restoring muscle tone, and sleep and sexual function changes related to aging. A preliminary publication describing promising effects of human growth hormone in men older than 60 years of age is often cited (3). These claims are extended to underweight or cachectic individuals, such as those with cancer or human immunodeficiency virus, in addition to bodybuilders.

Profound coma, myoclonus, and bradycardia are recognized as hallmark features of GHB overdose. The onset of effect is rapid, and symptoms persist for an unusually short time, given the depth of coma produced. Prolonged use results in tolerance, dependence, and a withdrawal syndrome with abstinence.

Chemical and Physical Properties

Illicit dietary supplement products use chemical synonym names on the label, obscuring their identity as GHB or an analog substance (Table 1). GHB is a water-soluble, white-powder salt of the carboxylic acid. GHB is manufactured easily by base hydrolysis of the lactone ring of GBL. The addition of excess base produces a dangerously alkaline solution that has resulted in mucosal and gastrointestinal burns when ingested. GBL, an oily liquid, is miscible in water and soluble in alcohol. BD is soluble in water and alcohol and may solidify at temperatures less than 19.0°C (66.2°F).

Endogenous GHB results from γ-aminobutyric acid (GABA) metabolism in humans and other mammals (Fig. 1) (4–6). Although the trace physiologic levels in blood are frequently below detection limits, endogenous urine levels as high as 14 μg/ml have occasionally been detected (7,8). Endogenous levels of BD have also been identified in rat brain and liver and in human cortex and cerebellum, although the metabolic source is not known (9–11). GBL has not been identified as an endogenous substance in humans (12).

GBL occurs naturally as a vapor in the aroma of coffee and the volatile flavor of roasted filberts. The chemical is a food additive "generally regarded as safe." GBL is added in low concentrations (20 μg/ml) to flavor soups, cheeses, breakfast cereal, beverages, or tobacco (13,14). GBL may be a constituent of paint removers, textile aids, and drilling oils. In the electronics industry, GBL-EL (electronics grade) is currently used in the manufacture of printed circuit boards and as a developer in solder mask and conformal coatings as well as a degreasing and semiaqueous defluxing agent. GBL has been suggested as a less toxic substitute for chlorinated hydrocarbons (15,16). GBL is also a

TABLE 1. Chemical names for γ-hydroxybutyric acid–related compounds

γ-Hydroxybutyric acid	γ-Butyrolactone	1,4-Butanediol
Molecular formula		
$C_4H_8O_3$	$C_4H_6O_2$	$C_4H_{10}O_2$
Molecular weight		
104.11 g/mol	86.09 g/mol	90.1 g/mol
CAS Registry No.		
502-85-2	96-48-0	110-63-4
Chemical names		
γ-Hydroxybutanoic acid	1,2-Butanolide	1,4-Butylene glycol
	1,4-Butanolide	1,4-Dihydroxybutane
γ-Hydroxybutyrate	3-Hydroxybutyric acid lactone	1,4-Tetramethylene glycol
γ-Hydroxybutyric acid	Alpha-butyrolactone	Butane-1,4-diol
	Blon	Butanediol, BD, BDO
	Butyric acid lactone	Butylene glycol
	Butyric acid, 4-hydroxy-gamma-lactone	Diol 1-4 B
		Sucol B
	Butyrolactone	Tetramethylene 1,4-diol
	Butyryl lactone	
	Dihydro-2(3H)-furanone	Tetramethylene glycol
	γ-BL	
	γ-Butanolide	
	γ-Butyrolactone	
	γ-Deoxytetronic acid	
	γ-Hydroxybutanoic acid lactone	
	γ-Hydroxybutyric acid cyclic ester	
	γ-Hydroxybutyric acid lactone	
	γ-Hydroxybutyric acid, gamma-lactone	
	γ-Hydroxybutyrolactone	
	γ-Lactone 4-hydroxybutanoic acid	
	Gamma-6480	
	Nci-c55875	
	Tetrahydro-2-furanone	

From *Allured's flavor and fragrance materials. 1998 edition addendum.* Carol Stream, IL: Allured Publishing Corporation, 1998; *Merck index.* 12th ed. Whitehouse Station, NJ: Merck Research Laboratories, 1996; and MSDS 1,4-butanediol. Available at: http://www.ispcorp.com/products/industrial/ind_ref.html. Columbus, OH: International Specialty Products, ISP, Fine Chemicals Industrial Reference Guide Performance-Enhancing Products for Industrial Markets, 1999, with permission.

household solvent for acrylics and may be found in removal products for paint, glue, synthetic fingernails, fingernail polish, and cyanoacrylate products.

Other sources of GHB are the dietary supplement products that contain GHB and claim to be effective for insomnia, sexual enhancement, weight loss, and bodybuilding. These products are persuasively promoted and sold on the Internet, in gyms, and in "health and fitness" magazines. Table 2 lists various names of GHB-containing pharmaceutical products, precursors, and illicitly sold dietary supplements. There are likely other new precursors yet to be identified that may have additional toxicities that will be revealed with initiation of widespread use. GHB is a Food and Drug Administration–approved, schedule III therapeutic agent (Xyrem) available as a 500-mg/ml solution.

Toxic Dose

The *adult therapeutic dosage* for cataplexy is 6 to 9 g/night in two to three divided doses. For anesthesia, the dose is 50 to 100 mg/kg intravenously (IV) (17,18). The *pediatric dose* as an anesthesia adjunct is 66 to 88 mg/kg orally (19) or 70 to 80 mg/kg IV (20,21). GBL is an adjunct to anesthesia, with a dose of 66 mg/kg orally (19).

GHB has a narrow safety margin. GHB doses of 10 to 20 mg/kg induce muscle relaxation and possible anterograde amnesia. Loss of consciousness may occur at a dose of 50 to 60 mg/kg (22,23). Accidental overdoses account for most episodes of toxicity. Coma may result when an intended 30 mg/kg-"euphoric" dose is doubled to 60 mg/kg. Further complicating the response is the individual variability in dose response due to factors such as capacity-limited absorption and elimination, fasting, tolerance, and coingestion of other central nervous system (CNS) depressant drugs.

Fatalities related to GHB intoxication are associated with respiratory compromise due to aspiration of gastric contents, positional asphyxia, and pulmonary edema. Some deaths result from traumatic injury or accident, possibly due to the abrupt loss of consciousness seen with GHB. GHB levels in fatal cases without detectable coingestions have ranged from 170 to 344 mg/L in blood and 1840 to 2839 mg/L in urine (24). GBL and GHB levels in urine were detected in a fatal case at 69 mg/L and 1840 mg/L, respectively (24). BD levels after a fatal ingestion by a 32-year-old man were BD, 845 mg/L, and GHB, 5430 mg/L, in urine. The blood GHB level was 432 mg/L. In a second reported fatality involving a 42-year-old woman, the blood level of BD and GHB were 220 mg/L and 837 mg/L, respectively. The urine levels were BD, 1756 mg/L, and GHB, 1161 mg/L (25).

A BD dose, 6.3 to 8.4 g, was ingested by a 22-year-old man who presented to the emergency department with a Glasgow Coma Score (GCS) of 3, bradycardia, hypothermia, and emesis. He required endotracheal intubation and mechanical ventilation. Successful extubation was achieved 4 hours later, and he made a full recovery. The urine GHB level was 415 mg/L, and BD was undetectable (25).

A 15-year-old boy ingested an unknown quantity of GHB at a rave party. Shortly after ingestion, he vomited, lapsed into coma, and never regained consciousness. At autopsy, pathologic findings included severe pulmonary congestion, intra-alveolar hemorrhage, and edema. There was mild cerebral edema and visceral organ congestion. His GHB blood level was 375 mg/L, and no other substances were detected (24).

GHB oral doses of 66 to 88 mg/kg given as surgical premedication produced profound sleep in 41% of children. Less than 1 hour after accidental ingestion of an unknown concentration of GHB in a soft drink, a 9-year-old boy was found unconscious and apneic, lying in vomitus, with a GCS of 6 and a heart rate of 20 beats/minute. His hospital course included mild metabolic acidosis resolving within 5 hours, tension pneumothorax, and aspiration pneumonia followed by full recovery (26).

Ingestion of GBL at 66 mg/kg orally produced profound sleep in 34% of children, with a more rapid onset and equivalent sedative action to GHB at a 66 to 88 mg/kg dose. Salivary secretions and bradycardia were significant. Emesis occurred in 19% of the children around the time of onset of marked drowsiness (15 to 60 minutes) and occasionally recurred during anesthesia (19). A 2-year-old boy was unresponsive 40 minutes after oral exposure to less than 1 oz of Bullet (GBL; 1 oz equals 33.6 g), a solvent for methacrylate fingernails. The patient experienced flaccid coma, with bradycardia and apnea over 6 hours, after which he awoke and breathed spontaneously (27).

TOXICOKINETICS AND TOXICODYNAMICS

GHB exhibits capacity-limited (zero order) absorption and elimination. The time-to-peak level is delayed at higher doses and by food. Average time-to-peak levels increased from 23 minutes at 12.5 mg/kg to 45 minutes at 50.0 mg/kg (28). Food increased the

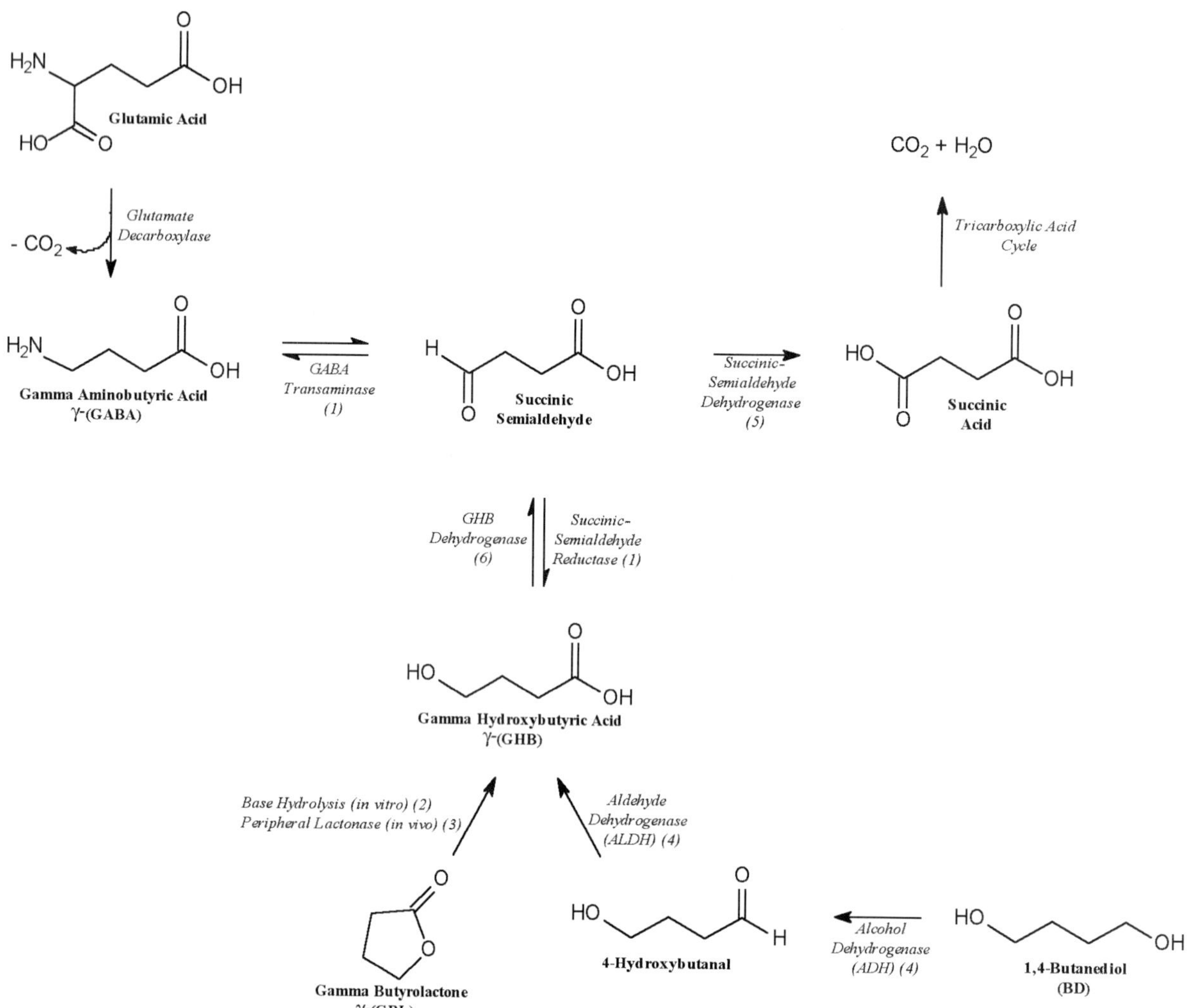

Figure 1. Synthetic and metabolic pathways of GHB. Generation of GHB is as follows: (1) transamination of GABA followed by reduction of succinic semialdehyde with succinic-semialdehyde reductase; (2) *in vitro* basic hydrolysis (saponification) of GBL; (3) *in vivo* hydrolysis of GBL by lactonase; and (4) *in vivo* oxidation of BD by ADH followed by oxidation of GHB by aldehyde dehydrogenase. Inborn error of GABA oxidative metabolism is as follows: (5) Succinic-semialdehyde dehydrogenase deficiency results in increased levels of GHB, GABA, and GHB aciduria. Metabolism of GHB occurs as follows: (6) oxidation of GHB to succinic semialdehyde by GHB dehydrogenase followed by oxidation of succinic semialdehyde by succinic-semialdehyde dehydrogenase to form succinic acid, which is taken into the tricarboxylic acid cycle and converted to carbon dioxide and water, which are eliminated.

peak absorption time from 45 minutes to 2 hours after a high-fat meal. The total amount of GHB absorbed is also diminished 37% by a high-fat meal (29). Plasma protein binding is less than 1%.

The synthetic and metabolic pathways for GHB, GBL, and BD are interrelated (Fig. 1). GHB is synthesized from GBL by base or converted after oral ingestion by a lactonase enzyme in plasma and hepatocytes. The half-life of conversion is less than 1 minute (12,30). BD is oxidized by alcohol dehydrogenase to γ-hydroxybutyraldehyde and, in a second step, by aldehyde dehydrogenase to GHB, primarily in the liver (31,32). Importantly, the first reaction is inhibited by ethanol, which competitively binds to alcohol dehydrogenase. Alternatively, ethanol taken after 1,4-butanediol conversion to GHB potentiates the CNS-depressant effects of GHB. The conversion intermediate is an aldehyde, which is potentially toxic, although the conversion is so extensive and proceeds so rapidly that toxicity has not been detected.

GHB is primarily metabolized by GHB dehydrogenase in two steps, to succinate, then through the tricarboxylic acid cycle to carbon dioxide and water. Elimination undergoes a biphasic decay with initial rapidly falling levels followed by a second phase slower rate of elimination. This is attributed to a pronounced distribution phase and nonlinear kinetics (28). GHB elimination pathways become unsaturated with levels falling below 50 mg/L, showing a more rapid terminal elimination half-life of less than 30 minutes (28,33,34). The portion of GHB eliminated unchanged in the urine is approximately 5% (35). Recently, an inborn error of GABA metabolism has been described (36,37). A deficiency in the enzyme succinate-semialdehyde dehydrogenase results in increased serum and cerebrospinal fluid levels of GABA and GHB and produces γ-hydroxybutyric aciduria. Clinically, symptoms of hypotonia, ataxia, mental retardation, speech delay, hyperkinesis, and epilepsy of differing degrees are observed (38).

PATHOPHYSIOLOGY

GHB is believed to act as a neuromodulator in the CNS where high-affinity binding to a specific GHB receptor occurs. Effects of this binding at physiologic levels remain unclear, and peripheral

TABLE 2. Dietary supplement products, medical products, and slang names for γ-hydroxybutyrate (GHB) and related drugs

γ-Hydroxybutyrate	γ-Butyrolactone	1,4-Butanediol	Slang names
Gamma hydrate	Blast	AminoFlex	Cherry meth
GHB	BLO	Biocopia PM	Easy lay
Natural sleep 500	Blow	BlueRaine	Fantasy
Oxy sleep	Blue Moon	Borametz	G
Somatomax PM	Blue Nitro Vitality	Butylene glycol	G caps
Vita G	Dihydro-2(3H)-furanone	BVM	Georgia home boy
Pharmaceutical products (country where available)	Eclipse	Dormir	GHB
Alcover (Italy)	Firewater	Enliven celluplex	Ghbers
Gamma OH (Europe)	Furanone Extreme	FX Cherry Bomb	Grievous bodily harm
Sodium oxybate	Gamma G	FX Lemon Drop	G-riffick
Somsanit (Germany)	GBL	FX Orange	Liquid E
Xyrem (USA)	GenX	FX Rush	Liquid ecstasy
	GH Gold (GHG)	GHRE (GH Releasing Extract)	Liquid X
	GH Release	Inner G	Organic quaalude
	GH Relief	NeuroMod	Salty water
	GH Revitalizer	NRG3 Weight Belt Cleaner	Scoop
	Insom-X	Omega-G	Soap
	Invigorate	Pine Needle Extract	Water
	Jolt	Pro G	
	Knock out	Promusol	
	Liquid Libido	Rejuv@night	
	ReActive	Rest-Q	
	Regenerize	Revitalize Plus	
	Remforce	Serenity	
	RenewTrient	Soma Solutions	
	RenewTrient caps	SomatoPro caps	
	Rest-eze	Sucol B	
	Revivarant	Tetramethylene glycol	
	Revivarant-G	Thunder	
	V-3	Thunder Nectar	
	Verve	Ultradiol, 1gm/oz	
		White Magic	
		X-12	
		Zen	

activity is not known. GHB has also been shown to be a weak agonist at the GABA-B receptor, and exogenous GHB activity is mediated by GHB and GABA-B receptors (39). There are other GHB analogs that may act directly at the GHB receptor or be metabolized to GHB. γ-Valerolactone may convert to γ-hydroxyvalerate and bind to the GHB receptor with reduced potency. Other GHB analogs are anticipated and may have unexpected toxicity that becomes evident after widespread use. Butyrate, for example, was initially evaluated as an anesthetic, but in therapeutic doses, it was associated with ketone formation (40).

PREGNANCY AND LACTATION

The use of GHB in pregnancy and lactation has not been evaluated. However, GHB does cross the placenta, and use of GHB as an anesthetic adjunct for 94 women in labor resulted in lowered Apgar scores (average, 6.7) due to sleepy babies (40).

CLINICAL PRESENTATION

Acute Overdosage

The prominent symptoms of GHB overdose are coma, myoclonus, and bradycardia. Coma is typically profound, often graded as a GCS of 3, the deepest level of coma. The characteristic toxidrome begins with altered mental status—even coma—within 15 minutes. The unusually short duration of effects allows most comatose patients to recover consciousness within 5 hours (41). The depressed mental status may be abrupt in onset, often resulting in injury from falls, and frequently self-limited myoclonus occurs with this sudden loss of consciousness. For these reasons, the onset of symptoms of GHB overdose may be reported as witnessed seizure activity. Status epilepticus has not been reported in GHB overdose, but the possibility of seizure activity in this syndrome remains controversial. Early anesthesia studies report rare generalized clonic activity with cyanosis (17). GHB is used to induce nonfocal seizures in animal models, although similar electroencephalogram phenomena have not been seen in humans at therapeutic doses (42).

Delirium may accompany emergence from deep coma. Usually a brief period of agitation and combativeness occurs for approximately 30 minutes as the patient is awakening, especially when stimulated (18). Pupil size is a variable finding in GHB overdose. Pupils are small during deep GHB-induced coma and increase in diameter as the level of consciousness increases. However, coingested stimulants and depressants may also affect pupil size, making this an unreliable sign of GHB overdose.

Airway obstruction by a flaccid tongue or vomitus may occur with the loss of airway protective reflexes, and respiratory arrest is a potential cause of death in GHB overdose. Pulmonary edema has also been noted and is a finding at autopsy (20,24,43). Central depression of respiratory drive can result from GHB alone but is more commonly described when ethanol and GHB are coingested. Periodic (Cheyne-Stokes) respirations are seen in deep coma from GHB, although increased tidal volume often compensates for the reduced rate. Endotracheal intubation is needed to protect the airway when gag or cough reflexes are absent or when respiratory depression leads to significant hypoxemia. A review of GHB overdose cases found that endotracheal intubation and mechanical ventilation were used in only 13% of cases. Ventilatory management did not correlate directly with the GCS score: Only 8 of 25 patients with a GCS of 3 were intubated. Two of these were discharged directly from the emergency department after rapid recovery, and the remaining patients were released within 24 hours. Respiratory acidosis with arterial blood gas pH in the range of 7.22 to 7.43 and $PaCO_2$ ranging from 32 to 56 mm Hg was documented (41).

In overdose, GHB typically causes sinus bradycardia that is most often asymptomatic. Coingestion of ethanol may cause hypotension. In three cases, atrial fibrillation has been described that spontaneously converted to sinus rhythm (41,44). During early investigations of GHB in surgical anesthesia, a low but concerning incidence of unpredictable hypertension occurred (40,45). Vomiting has been shown to occur during the induction phase and occurs in 30% of cases during emergence. Urinary or fecal incontinence less frequently occurs. Other common findings are hypothermia and diaphoresis.

Chronic Exposure

Toxicity from chronic exposure results in tolerance and dependence (Chapter 32). Patients with succinic semialdehyde dehydrogenase deficiency, an inborn error of metabolism, are chronically exposed to high GHB levels and present with mental, motor, or language delay; hypotonia; or seizures of unknown cause (38).

Adverse effects seen after accidental overdose reflect what is documented in research into the anesthetic use of GHB. Induction occurs with CNS depression in 30 to 45 minutes. Adverse events included myoclonus, emergence delirium, incontinence, Cheyne-Stokes respiration, and vagally mediated effects such as diaphoresis, salivation, and bradycardia (46). Rarely, pulmonary edema occurred (20). The lack of analgesia left the autonomic response to incision intact, and blood pressure elevated significantly, lasting the duration of the procedure (18).

Drug Interactions

GHB drug interactions have been demonstrated with depressant therapeutic agents. GHB potentiates the anesthetic effect of ethanol, thiopental, and hexenal by a factor of 2:3 in mice and less potently affects chloral hydrate (47,48). Ethanol is commonly reported as a coingestion in overdoses and fatalities. The synergistic depressant effect of GHB and alcohol taken in combination may increase the risk of an adverse outcome.

Carcinogenesis

BD has not been evaluated for chronic toxicity or carcinogenicity, as studies at the National Toxicology Program determined that the toxicity of BD was similar to that of GBL due to rapid and extensive conversion to the same active metabolite GHB. GBL has been evaluated in 2-year rat and mouse studies and has no chronic toxicity or carcinogenic potential, although acute, chemical-related mortality occurred at high doses (35). It was surmised that there was a high likelihood that BD would also be negative in a similar study.

DIAGNOSTIC TESTS

Acute Overdosage

Evaluation of coma, a common presenting sign after GHB overdose, requires a thorough diagnostic evaluation, including physical examination, laboratory studies (including serum glucose and electrolytes), pulse oximetry, and electrocardiogram. Prolonged coma may necessitate brain imaging and lumbar puncture to rule out infection, trauma, or other CNS causes.

Serum levels after a 25 to 50 mg/kg oral dose of GHB in eight human subjects yielded serum levels of 35 to 98 mg/L and mild transient dizziness, drowsiness, and nausea (28). In a study involving administration of 75 to 100 mg/kg orally to 12 adults, serum GHB levels rapidly decreased from peak levels of 90 to 120 mg/L at 1.5 to 2.0 hours to undetectable amounts 12 hours later (49). A 50 mg/kg IV dose produced a mean peak level of 182 mg/ml; 100 mg/kg gave a mean peak level of 306 mg/ml, and 165 mg/kg gave a mean peak level above 416 mg/ml. These levels correlated with level of consciousness.

GHB levels above 260 mg/L produced coma unresponsive to noxious stimuli and abolished pharyngeal and laryngeal reflexes, although the autonomic reflex to surgical incision remained intact. A serum level of 156 to 260 mg/L allowed spontaneous blinking and response to tactile pressure. A level of 52 to 156 mg/L demonstrated occasional eye opening and spontaneous movement; with levels falling below 52 mg/L, there was awakening (50).

Fifteen GHB overdose patients, with a GCS of less than 8 but with spontaneous respirations, had GHB present in serum and urine on presentation to the emergency department. The GHB serum level ranged from 45 mg/L to 245 mg/L, and urine levels ranged from 432 mg/L to 2407 mg/L. Quantitative serum GHB levels did not correlate with degree of coma, time to awakening, or respiratory status. Multiple-drug use was common, with ethanol being the most prevalent coingestant.

Urine and serum tests for GHB and analogs are not routinely available but may be useful in confirming the diagnosis in forensic cases. Reference laboratories can detect levels of 1 to 2 μg/ml, although the time window for detection is short. Blood levels decline rapidly to become undetectable within 6 hours. Urine testing also demonstrates a rapid decrease in GHB concentrations over several hours but typically is detectable for 8 to 12 hours (26,49,51,52). Urine drug concentration depends on fluid intake and voiding frequency after ingestion and may not directly correlate with serum levels or level of consciousness. Nonetheless, the higher concentrations of GHB and longer duration of detection in the urine make this the specimen of choice for testing.

Diagnostic Pitfalls

Because GHB is not detected on routine urine toxicology screens, a sedative drug overdose may erroneously be ruled out in cases of GHB-related coma.

Postmortem Considerations

Postmortem analysis of suspected GHB-related deaths revealed serum levels ranging from 11.5 to 170.0 mg/L (53–55). Other data from a small descriptive surveillance study of GHB-related fatalities described deaths resulting from respiratory compromise due to aspiration of gastric contents, positional asphyxia, and pulmonary edema. Some deaths were a result of traumatic injury or accident, possibly due to abrupt loss of consciousness seen with GHB. Cardiac enlargement was a finding in one-third of cases.

Postmortem GHB levels in cases without detectable coingestions have ranged from 170 to 344 mg/L in blood and 1840 to 2839 mg/L in urine (24). These levels contrast with what has been detected in non-GHB–related deaths with presumed postmortem generation. Postmortem blood in non-GHB–related deaths has contained GHB in concentrations from 1 to 168 mg/L and 0 to 14 mg/L in urine (8,56). Postmortem GHB levels should be interpreted with an understanding that there is some endogenous production of GHB detectable in serum after death.

TREATMENT

Most often, acute GHB overdose has a dramatic clinical presentation with a rapid onset of profound coma and bradycardia, preceded by reported "jerking" movements, vomiting, and sudden collapse. Because symptoms typically resolve within a few hours, treatment of GHB toxicity involves primarily supportive care, which focuses on immediate attention to the airway and respiratory status.

Decontamination

Because GHB is typically consumed as a small quantity of liquid that is rapidly absorbed, the utility of administering activated charcoal is minimal. In cases of known or suspected coingestion, or in situations of large overdoses, the use of activated charcoal may be warranted in the context of appropriate airway protection.

Enhanced Elimination

Because of the rapid clearance and short duration of action of the drug, elimination techniques are not expected to improve the clinical course.

Antidotes

There is no specific antidote to reverse the clinical effects of GHB, but empiric use of naloxone to any patient with a depressed level of consciousness in the setting of possible drug overdose is appropriate. Naloxone administration has been shown to reverse some of the central effects of GHB (57), although the mechanism does not appear to be mediated via opioid receptor antagonism, and naloxone has not been clinically effective to reverse coma after accidental overdose in humans.

Physostigmine is another potential antidote for the treatment of GHB toxicity (58,59). Although the mechanism is unclear, physostigmine has been reported to reverse GHB-induced sedation during anesthesia (60), and two small case series have described improvement in the level of consciousness in five of six patients administered 1 to 2 mg of IV physostigmine after GHB overdose (61,62). At this point, there is insufficient scientific evidence to support the routine use of physostigmine for GHB toxicity; however, this agent may offer some therapeutic effect in cases of known GHB-induced coma.

Flumazenil is a selective benzodiazepine receptor antagonist that has been demonstrated to antagonize the anxiolytic effects of GHB (63) and block its actions on growth hormone secretion (64). However, there is no clinical evidence that it reverses the sedative effects of GHB; therefore, empiric use of flumazenil is not indicated in cases of GHB-induced coma.

Supportive Care

As with other sedative-hypnotic agents, loss of airway protective mechanisms, including cough and gag reflexes, may be seen in overdoses of GHB. Airway obstruction by a hypotonic tongue and vomitus has been implicated as a cause of death related to GHB use (24). Endotracheal intubation and mechanical ventilation may be required in deeply comatose patients for airway protection as well as respiratory depression. The degree of respiratory compromise does not always correlate with the GCS. In a review of 88 cases of GHB overdose, one-third of patients with a GCS of 3 were intubated (41). Central depression of respiratory drive is most commonly observed when GHB and ethanol are coingested.

Because of their severely depressed level of consciousness, patients may be hypothermic on arrival in the emergency department, necessitating gentle rewarming (Chapter 38). Bradycardia associated with GHB use is most often asymptomatic and does not require treatment. In hypotensive patients, atropine should be administered along with IV fluid therapy. In three cases, atrial fibrillation has been reported that spontaneously converted to sinus rhythm without medical intervention (41,44).

Jerking movements of the extremities have been described in association with GHB toxicity, but whether this represents true seizure activity or abrupt loss of muscle tone due to lapse in consciousness has not been established. As with other drug-induced seizures, benzodiazepines are the first-line therapy but should be used with caution in GHB overdoses because of respiratory and CNS depressant effects. IV valproic acid has been proposed as a potential therapy for GHB-induced seizures because of its inhibitory actions at GABA-B receptors (65).

GHB-induced coma is self-limited, and patients awaken suddenly in several hours, often accompanied by a brief period of agitation, delirium, and combativeness. This "emergence phenomenon" typically lasts 30 minutes and may require the use of physical restraints to prevent self-extubation or injury to the patient or staff. Pharmacologic sedation should be avoided, if possible, in order to assess changes in level of consciousness as the patient transitions from coma to a normal state. Patients who are fully awake and breathing adequately on their own may be extubated and released after a brief period of observation.

Treatment of GHB withdrawal syndrome is described in Chapter 32.

REFERENCES

1. Addolorato G, Capristo E, Gessa GL, et al. Long-term administration of GHB does not affect muscular mass in alcoholics. *Life Sci* 1999;65:L191–L196.
2. DAWN. The DAWN Report: club drugs September 2001 update. Rockville, MD: Office of Applied Studies, SAMHSA, Drug Abuse Warning Network; 2001.
3. Rudman D, Feller AG, Nagraj HS, et al. Effects of human growth hormone in men over 60 years old. *N Engl J Med* 1990;323:1–6.
4. Roth RH, Giarman NJ. Evidence that central nervous system depression by 1,4-butanediol is mediated through a metabolite, gamma-hydroxybutyrate. *Biochem Pharmacol* 1968;17:735–739.
5. Roth RH. Formation and regional distribution of gamma-hydroxybutyric acid in mammalian brain. *Biochem Pharmacol* 1970;19:3013–3019.
6. Bessman SP, Fishbein WN. Gamma-hydroxybutyrate, a normal brain metabolite. *Nature* 1963;200:1207–1208.
7. Snead OC 3rd, Brown GB, Morawetz RB. Concentration of gamma-hydroxybutyric acid in ventricular and lumbar cerebrospinal fluid. *N Engl J Med* 1981;304:93–95.
8. Anderson DT, Kuwahara T. Endogenous gamma hydroxybutyrate (GHB) levels in postmortem specimens. CAT/NWAFS/SWAFS/SAT combined meeting. Las Vegas; 1997.
9. Vayer P, Mandel P, Maitre M. Gamma-hydroxybutyrate, a possible neurotransmitter. *Life Sci* 1987;41:1547–1557.

10. Barker SA, Snead OC, Poldrugo F, et al. Identification and quantitation of 1,4-butanediol in mammalian tissues: an alternative biosynthetic pathway for gamma-hydroxybutyric acid. *Biochem Pharmacol* 1985;34:1849–1852.
11. Sprince H, Josephs JA, Wilpizeski CR. Neuropharmacological effects of 1,4-butanediol and related congeners compared with those of gamma-hydroxybutyrate and gamma-butyrolactone. *Life Sci* 1966;5:2041–2052.
12. Fishbein WN, Bessman SP. Purification and properties of an enzyme in human blood and rat liver microsomes catalyzing the formation and hydrolysis of gamma-lactones. II. Metal ion effects, kinetics, and equilibra. *J Biol Chem* 1966;241:4842–4847.
13. *Allured's flavor and fragrance materials. 1998 edition.* Carol Stream, IL: Allured Publishing Corporation, 1998.
14. *Allured's flavor and fragrance materials. 1998 edition addendum.* Carol Stream, IL: Allured Publishing Corporation, 1998.
15. *Merck index.* 12th ed. Whitehouse Station, NJ: Merck Research Laboratories, 1996.
16. Lyondell. MSDS gamma butyrolactone. Houston: Lyondell Chemical Company; 2002. Available at: http://www.lyondell.com/html/products/products/gbl.shtml. Accessed June 2003.
17. Appleton PJ, Burn JM. A neuroinhibitory substance: gamma hydroxybutyric acid. Preliminary report of first clinical trial in Britain. *Anesth Analg* 1968;47:164–170.
18. Solway J, Sadove MS. 4-Hydroxybutyrate: a clinical study. *Anesth Analg* 1965;44:532–539.
19. Root B. Oral premedication of children with GHB. *Anaesthesiology* 1965;26:259.
20. Brown TC. Gammahydroxybutyrate in paediatric anaesthesia. *Aust N Z J Surg* 1970;40:94–99.
21. Hunter AS, Long WJ, Ryrie CG. An evaluation of gamma-hydroxybutyric acid in paediatric practice. *Br J Anaesth* 1971;43:620–628.
22. Vickers MD. Gammahydroxybutyric acid. *Int Anesthesiol Clin* 1969;7:75–89.
23. Mamelak M, Escriu JM, Stokan O. The effects of gamma-hydroxybutyrate on sleep. *Biol Psychiatry* 1977;12:273–288.
24. Dyer JE, Haller CA. GHB related fatalities. *J Toxicol Clin Toxicol* 2001;39:518.
25. Zvosec DL, Smith SW, McCutcheon JR, et al. Adverse events, including death, associated with the use of 1,4-butanediol. *N Engl J Med* 2001;344:87–94.
26. Suner S, Szlatenyi CS, Wang RY. Pediatric gamma hydroxybutyrate intoxication. *Acad Emerg Med* 1997;4:1041–1045.
27. Higgins TF Jr, Borron SW. Coma and respiratory arrest after exposure to butyrolactone. *J Emerg Med* 1996;14:435–437.
28. Palatini P, Tedeschi L, Frison G, et al. Dose-dependent absorption and elimination of gamma-hydroxybutyric acid in healthy volunteers. *Eur J Clin Pharmacol* 1993;45:353–356.
29. Mani RB. Consideration of (NDA) 21-196, Xyrem (sodium oxybate, Orphan Medical, Inc.), proposed to reduce the incidence of cataplexy and to improve the symptom of daytime sleepiness for persons with narcolepsy. A main focus of the deliberations will be on risk management issues. In: FDA briefing information safety review. NDA 21-196 Xyrem, Orphan Medical, Inc.; 2001. Available at: http://www.fda.gov/ohrms/dockets/ac/01/briefing/3754b1.htm. Bethesda, MD: FDA Peripheral and Central Nervous System Drugs Advisory Committee, 2001:16.
30. Roth R, Giarman N. Gamma-butyrolactone and gamma-hydroxygutyric acid I: distribution and metabolism. *Biochem Pharmacol* 1966;15:1333–1348.
31. Poldrugo F, Barker S, Basa M, et al. Ethanol potentiates the toxic effects of 1,4-butanediol. *Alcohol Clin Exp Res* 1985;9:493–497.
32. Maxwell R, Roth RH. Conversion of 1,4-butanediol to -hydroxybutyric acid in rat brain and in peripheral tissue. *Biochem Pharmacol* 1972;21:1521–1533.
33. Vree TB, Baars AM. Capacity-limited elimination of 4-hydroxybutyrate (gamma OH), ethanol and vinylbital. *Pharmaceutish Weekblad* 1975;110:1257–1262.
34. Lettieri J, Fung HL. Improved pharmacological activity via pro-drug modification: comparative pharmacokinetics of sodium gamma-hydroxybutyrate and gamma-butyrolactone. *Res Commun Chem Pathol Pharmacol* 1978;22:107–118.
35. Irwin RD. National Toxicology Program summary report on the metabolism, disposition, and toxicity of 1,4 butanediol. National Toxicology Program, NIH Publication No. 96-3932; 1996.
36. Jakobs C, Jaeken J, Gibson KM. Inherited disorders of GABA metabolism. *J Inherit Metab Dis* 1993;16:704–715.
37. Gibson KM, Hoffmann GF, Hodson AK, et al. 4-Hydroxybutyric acid and the clinical phenotype of succinic semialdehyde dehydrogenase deficiency, an inborn error of GABA metabolism. *Neuropediatrics* 1998;29:14–22.
38. Gibson KM, Christensen E, Jakobs C, et al. The clinical phenotype of succinic semialdehyde dehydrogenase deficiency (4-hydroxybutyric aciduria): case reports of 23 new patients. *Pediatrics* 1997;99:567–574.
39. Carai MAMC, Brunetti G, Melis S, et al. Role of GABA-B receptors in the sedative/hypnotic effect of gamma-hydroxybutyric acid. *Eur J Pharmacol* 2001;428:315–321.
40. Geldenhuys FG, Sonnendecker EW, De Klrk MC. Experience with sodium-gamma-4-hydroxybutyric acid (gamma-OH) in obstetrics. *J Obstet Gynaecol Br Commonw* 1968;75:405–413.
41. Chin RL, Sporer KA, Cullison B, et al. Clinical course of gamma-hydroxybutyrate overdose. *Ann Emerg Med* 1998;31:716–722.
42. Entholzner E, Mielke L, Pichlmeier R, et al. EEG changes during sedation with gamma-hydroxybutyric acid. *Anaesthesist* 1995;44:345–350.
43. Piastra M, Barbaro R, Chiaretti A, et al. Pulmonary oedema caused by "liquid ecstasy" ingestion. *Arch Dis Child* 2002;86:302–303.
44. Hardy CJ, Slifman NR, Klontz K, et al. Adverse events reported with the use of gamma butyrolactone products marketed as dietary supplements. *J Toxicol Clin Toxicol* 1999;37:649–650.
45. Tunstall ME. Gamma-OH in anesthesia for caesarean section. *Proc R Soc Med* 1968;61:827–829.
46. Cole WH. Observations on the pharmacology of gamma hydroxy sodium butyrate, with special reference to microsurgery of the larynx. *Med J Aust* 1970;1:372–375.
47. Serebryakov LA. Effect of sodium gamma-hydroxybutyrate combined with anesthetics. *Farmakologiya* 1964;27:275–277.
48. McCabe ER, Layne EC, Sayler DF, et al. Synergy of ethanol and a natural soporific—gamma hydroxybutyrate. *Science* 1971;171:404–406.
49. Hoes MJ, Vree TB, Guelen PJ. Gamma-hydroxybutyric acid as hypnotic. Clinical and pharmacokinetic evaluation of gamma-hydroxybutyric acid as hypnotic in man. *Encephale* 1980;6:93–99.
50. Helrich M, McAslan TC, Skolnik S, Bessman SP. Correlation of blood levels of 4-hydroxybutyrate with state of consciousness. *Anesthesiology* 1964;25:771–775.
51. Dyer JE, Isaacs SM, Keller KH. Gamma hydroxybutyrate (GHB)-induced coma with serum and urine drug levels. *Vet Hum Toxicol* 1994;36:348.
52. Stephens BG, Baselt RC. Driving under the influence of GHB? *J Anal Toxicol* 1994;18:357–358.
53. Timby N, Eriksson A, Bostrom K. Gamma-hydroxybutyrate associated deaths. *Am J Med* 2000;108:518–519.
54. Ferrara SD, Tedeschi L, Frison G, Rossi A. Fatality due to gamma-hydroxybutyric acid (GHB) and heroin intoxication. *J Forensic Sci* 1995;40:501–504.
55. Gamma hydroxy butyrate use—New York and Texas, 1995–1996. *MMWR Morb Mortal Wkly Rep* 1997;46:281–283.
56. Fieler EL, Coleman DE, Baselt RC. Gamma-hydroxybutyrate concentrations in pre- and postmortem blood and urine [Letter]. *Clin Chem* 1998;44:692.
57. Feigenbaum JJ, Howard SG. Naloxone reverses the inhibitory effect of gamma-hydroxybutyrate on central DA release in vivo in awake animals: a microdialysis study. *Neurosci Lett* 1997;224:71–74.
58. Nattel S, Bayne L, Ruedy J. Physostigmine in coma due to drug overdose. *Clin Pharmacol Ther* 1979;25:96–102.
59. Di Liberti J, O'Brien ML, Turner T. The use of physostigmine as an antidote in accidental diazepam intoxication. *J Pediatr* 1975;86:106–107.
60. Henderson RS, Holmes CM. Reversal of the anaesthetic action of sodium gamma-hydroxybutyrate. *Anaesth Intensive Care* 1976;4:351–354.
61. Yates SW, Viera AJ. Physostigmine in the treatment of gamma-hydroxybutyric acid overdose. *Mayo Clin Proc* 2000;75:401–402.
62. Caldicott DG, Kuhn M. Gamma-hydroxybutyrate overdose and physostigmine: teaching new tricks to an old drug? *Ann Emerg Med* 2001;37:99–102.
63. Schmidt-Mutter C, Pain L, Sandner G, et al. The anxiolytic effect of gamma-hydroxybutyrate in the elevated plus maze is reversed by the benzodiazepine receptor antagonist, flumazenil. *Eur J Pharmacol* 1998;342:21–27.
64. Gerra G, Caccavari R, Fontanesi B, et al. Flumazenil effects on growth hormone response to gamma-hydroxybutyric acid. *Int Clin Psychopharmacol* 1994;9:211–215.
65. Okun MS, Boothby LA, Bartfield RB, Doering PL. GHB: an important pharmacologic and clinical update. *J Pharm Pharm Sci* 2001;4:167–175.

CHAPTER 177

Hallucinogenic Drugs

E. Martin Caravati

See Figure 1.

Compounds included:	**L-lysergic acid diethylamide (LSD); *N,N*-dimethyltryptamine; phencyclidine; ketamine hydrochloride (Ketalar, Ketaject, Ketanest)**
Molecular formula and weight:	**LSD ($C_{20}H_{25}N_3O$), 323.4; *N,N*-dimethyltryptamine ($C_{12}H_{16}N_2$), 188.3; phencyclidine ($C_{17}H_{25}N$), 279.8; ketamine hydrochloride ($C_{13}H_{16}ClNO$, HCl), 274.2 g/mol**
SI conversion:	**LSD, mg/L × 3.1 = µmol/L; phencyclidine, mg/L × 3.6 = µmol/L; ketamine hydrochloride, mg/L × 3.6 µmol/L**
CAS Registry No.:	**50-37-3 (LSD); 61-50-7 (*N,N*-dimethyltryptamine); 77-10-1 (phencyclidine); 1867-66-9 (ketamine hydrochloride)**
Therapeutic or normal levels:	**Not applicable**
Target organs:	**Central nervous system (acute and chronic), heart**
Antidote:	**None**

OVERVIEW

Hallucinogenic drugs, or "psychedelics," are abused for their ability to produce distortions of reality. They have been used for centuries as part of religious, ritual, and spiritual experiences. In the United States, their popularity rose during the "drug culture" revolution of the 1960s and decreased during the 1980s. Hallucinogenic drugs are distinguished from other drugs that may also produce hallucinations by their highly reliable capacity to induce altered feelings, thoughts, and perceptions as their primary effect. Common psychedelic effects include heightened sensory input, passive observer of events (a "spectator ego"), lack of boundaries between the self and the environment, and a sense of union with the "cosmos." In addition to the psychedelic effects, they produce varied dose-dependent physiologic alterations, depending on the class of the agent.

The major hallucinogenic drugs are classified as indoleamines [lysergic acid diethylamide (LSD), *N,N*-dimethyltryptamine (DMT), and psilocybin] and phenethylamines (mescaline, dimethoxy-methylamphetamine, methylenedioxyamphetamine, and 3,4-methylenedioxy-methamphetamine) (Table 1). Both groups have a relative high affinity for 5-hydroxytryptamine (5-HT)-2 receptors, and LSD is the most potent. The arylcycloalkylamines, phencyclidine (PCP), and ketamine are also frequently abused for their hallucinogenic potential. Each hallucinogen produces behavioral effects related to its serotonergic, dopaminergic, or adrenergic activity. LSD acts on serotonin 5-HT_2 receptors with effects primarily in the cerebral cortex and locus ceruleus. PCP is a noncompetitive antagonist of *N*-methyl-D-aspartate–type glutamate receptors. A *flashback* is a recurrence of imagery associated with hallucinogen use that occurs after the acute effects of the drug have worn off. They have been described with LSD, mescaline, PCP, and marijuana use and may occur months to years after cessation of use. Reassurance and the reduction of sensory stimuli are the most important aspects of management.

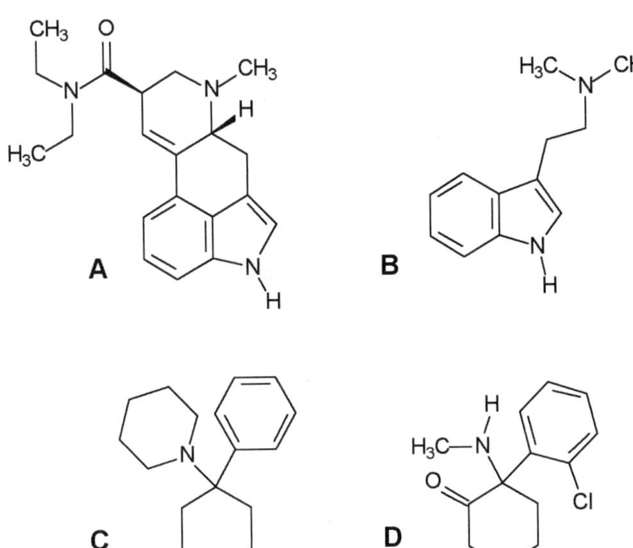

Figure 1. Chemical structures of the hallucinogens. **A:** Lysergic acid diethylamide. **B:** *N,N*-dimethyltryptamine. **C:** Phencyclidine. **D:** Ketamine.

LYSERGIC ACID DIETHYLAMIDE

LSD is a potent hallucinogenic indoleamine abused for its ability to consistently produce alterations of perception. Its popularity began in the 1960s but waned during the 1980s. In the early 1990s, LSD made a comeback in the United States among middle-class high school and college students with an approximate 25% increase in the use of LSD (Table 2) (1). The number of LSD-related emergency department (ED) visits by adolescents increased, and LSD-related violence, including suicide, homicide, and accidental death, was higher than in the previous 5-year period. LSD, from the German name *Lyserg-Säure-Diäthylamid*, remains available in large quanti-

TABLE 1. Chemical classification of hallucinogens

Common name	Chemical name
Indole alkaloid derivatives	
Psilocin	Dimethyl-4-hydroxytryptamine
Psilocybin	Dimethyl-4-phosphoryitryptamine
Harmine	7-Methoxy-1-methyl-9*H*-pyridol-[3,4b]-indole
Ibogaine	12-Methoxyibogamine
LSD	Lysergic acid diethylamide
DMT	Dimethyltryptamine
DPT	Dipropyltryptamine
AMT	α-Methyltryptamine
DET	Diethyltryptamine
Bufotenine	Dimethyl-5-hydroxytryptamine
Piperidine (arylcyclohexylamine) derivatives	
Phencyclidine (PCP)	1-(1-Phencyclohexyl) piperidine
Ketamine	2-(*O*-Chlorophenyl-2-methylamino)cyclohexanone
Phenylethylamine derivatives	
Mescaline	3,4,5-Trimethoxyphenylethylamine
DOM or "STP"	2,5-Dimethoxy-4-methylamphetamine
DOE	2,5-Dimethoxy-4-ethylamphetamine
DOB	2,5-Dimethoxy-4-bromoamphetamine
MDA	Methylenedioxyamphetamine
DOET	Dimethoxyethylamphetamine
MMDA	3-Methoxy-4,5-methylenedioxyamphetamine
PMA	*p*-Methoxyamphetamine
TMA	3,4,5-Trimethoxyamphetamine

Adapted from Leikin JB, Krantz AJ, Zell-Kanter M, et al. Clinical features and management of intoxication due to hallucinogenic drugs. *Med Toxicol Adverse Drug Exp* 1989;4:324–350.

ties in almost every state. Its production is concentrated on the West Coast, particularly in San Francisco, Northern California, and the Pacific Northwest. The vast majority of users are middle-class high school and college students. In 1998, the Drug Enforcement Administration seized only one clandestine LSD laboratory.

LSD is synthesized from lysergic acid, which is derived from a wheat or rye fungus (ergot). It is a clear or white, odorless, water-soluble crystal that is usually crushed into a powder. This powder can be used to produce tablets known as *microdots* or thin gelatin squares called *window panes*. It is often diluted and applied to sheets of colored paper with small square dosage units and referred to as *blotter acid* (Fig. 2). The postage stamp–size papers contain from 50 to 300 μg of drug, sometimes more.

Toxic Dose

LSD is the most potent hallucinogenic drug known. Doses of 25 to 50 μg orally can produce psychedelic effects for 6 to 12 hours. A dose of 100 μg orally consistently produces perceptual distortions. There are no deaths directly attributable to the pharmacologic effects of LSD. Fatalities have occurred shortly after exposure due to trauma or drowning. An 8-month-old boy ingested 5 blotters of LSD and developed tachycardia. The neurologic examination was normal. He was discharged in 24 hours after intravenous (IV) fluids were administered. Gastric aspirate and urine were positive for LSD (2).

Toxicokinetics and Toxicodynamics

The route of administration is usually oral, although it may be smoked or injected. The onset of effects is 30 to 90 minutes after ingestion and peaks in 2 to 4 hours. The typical duration of action is 6 to 8 hours. Psychotropic effects may last days in some cases. Metabolism is by hepatic hydroxylation. The serum half-life is 2.5 hours, and volume of distribution (V_d) is 0.27 L/kg.

TABLE 2. History of lysergic acid diethylamide (LSD)

Year	Event
1938	Albert Hoffman synthesized LSD for medical research.
1943	Hoffman accidentally discovered hallucinogenic properties of LSD.
1961	LSD observed to interact with brain serotonin.
1966	Hallucinogens banned in the United States.
1970	Psychedelic drugs placed in schedule I of the U.S. Controlled Substances Act.
1970s and 1980s	Young people using lower doses; more ritualized use.
1988–1990	Increase in emergency department admissions for bad experience with LSD.
1993	LSD sold in large quantities.

Tolerance develops rapidly among patients given LSD. An initial dose of 50 μg, with weekly or twice-weekly administration, often leads to an eventual dose of 400 μg or even 800 μg within a few weeks (3). LSD also produces tolerance for other hallucinogenic drugs that act on serotonin receptors such as psilocybin and mescaline. The tolerance is short-lived and is lost after several days of nonuse. There is no evidence of physical withdrawal.

Pathophysiology

LSD is a potent agonist at brain 5-HT_{1A} receptors on raphe cell bodies, which results in a decreased firing rate of serotonergic neurons. It also acts as a partial or full agonist at 5-HT_{2A}, 5-HT_{2C}, and many other 5-HT receptors. It has an affinity for postsynaptic 5-HT_2 receptors in the locus ceruleus and the cerebral cortex. Most 5-HT_2 receptors in the brain are located in the cerebral cortex, where hallucinogens exert an effect on perceptual and cognitive functions.

Pregnancy and Lactation

LSD is U.S. Food and Drug Administration (FDA) pregnancy category C (Appendix I). Its low molecular weight suggests that it crosses the human placenta. There is no significant evidence to suggest that LSD is a teratogen. There is no evidence that it produces clinically significant chromosomal damage in the fetus. In case reports of congenital abnormalities associated with LSD, other drugs of abuse or medications were also consumed by the mother. LSD may theoretically pass into breast milk, but there are no reports of effects in breast-fed infants. Its use during breast-feeding is contraindicated (4).

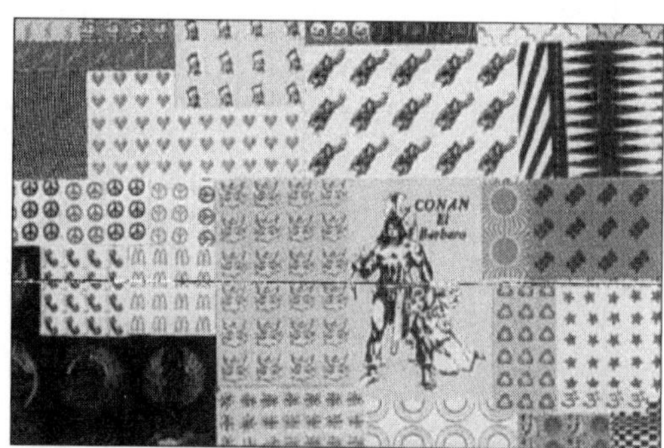

Figure 2. LSD blotter paper. (From U.S. Drug Enforcement Agency, with permission.)

Clinical Presentation

ACUTE EXPOSURE

There is a large variation in the clinical effect and experiences among individuals abusing LSD. The most common effect is altered visual perception. They may also be hypersensitive to sound. Sensory perceptions may blend, in which the user "feels colors" and "sees sound" (synesthesia). Mood swings, depression, depersonalization, and body image distortion may occur. Rapid mood alterations may occur, ranging from euphoria to fear. Anxiety, despair, suicidal thoughts, and panic characterize a "bad trip." It may include feelings of insanity, losing control, or death.

Sympathomimetic effects include mydriasis, flushing, tremor, hyperreflexia, hyperthermia, tachycardia, increased blood pressure, piloerection, diaphoresis, and ataxia. Nausea and vomiting may occur, and severe toxicity can result in coma, seizures, and respiratory arrest. Neuroleptic malignant syndrome may occur after LSD use. Muscle biopsy may show myoedema, focal necrosis, and glycogen and lipid depletion.

CHRONIC REACTIONS

A distinctive chronic visual complication of use was described in three patients who experienced prolonged afterimages (palinopsia) during LSD intoxication and continued to be symptomatic up to 3 years after they stopped using the drug (5). Prolonged psychotic reactions that are similar to schizophrenia appear to occur most often in people with preexisting psychological difficulties. Psychedelic drug-induced personality disorders can be severe and prolonged. Appropriate treatment often requires antipsychotic medication and residential care in a mental health facility followed by outpatient counseling.

Four chronic reactions were reported in the 1960s: (a) prolonged psychotic reactions, (b) depression and suicidal ideation, (c) flashbacks, and (d) exacerbation of preexisting psychiatric illness (6). Since then, another diagnostic category has been described: hallucinogen persisting perception disorder (HPPD).

The term "flashbacks" and HPPD are sometimes used interchangeably. They occur most commonly after LSD use. HPPD consists of the reexperiencing of one or more of the perceptual symptoms and causes significant distress or impairment. HPPD may be extremely debilitating. Individuals may experience a persistent perceptual disorder that includes fleeting perception on peripheral visual fields, color flashes, and positive afterimages. This represents a permanent alteration of the visual system. This perceptual disorder is aggravated by use of any psychoactive drug, including alcohol or marijuana; stress; fatigue; and anxiety. It is accompanied by an unpleasant dysphoric effect. Individuals with HPPD do not have a disturbed psychiatric history before the onset of psychedelic drug use. HPPD can occur even after a single dose and may persist for months to years. It is distinguished from flashbacks, which are episodic, nondistressing, reversible, and often accompanied by a pleasant effect (7).

DRUG INTERACTIONS

Patients taking fluoxetine and lithium in therapeutic doses may develop seizures after taking LSD for recreational use (8). Patients with a history of LSD use may experience flashbacks or hallucinatory episodes if they use selective serotonin reuptake inhibitor drugs such as sertraline or paroxetine (9). The proposed mechanism is the similarity in neuroreceptor physiology for both LSD and serotonin. Three patients with HPPD had an exacerbation of LSD-like panic and visual symptoms after taking risperidone (10).

Diagnostic Tests

Screening large numbers of urine samples for drugs of abuse is typically done with immunoassays that allow for processing large numbers of samples without the requirement of sample preparation. Until fairly recently, screening of LSD in urine samples could only be accomplished by the use of radioimmunoassay (RIA). Nonisotopic immunoassays have also been developed for screening of urine samples for LSD. These assays are rapid, high-volume, automated analyses compared with RIA procedures (11). Gas chromatography-mass spectrometry is useful in confirming positive LSD urine levels to a lower limit of 5 pg/ml. LSD can be detected in the urine by RIA 3 days after exposure at the 0.1-ng/ml cutoff level.

LSD concentrations in serum or urine specimens are of limited value except to confirm the presence of LSD. The availability of this test among hospital clinical toxicology laboratories is limited. McCarron and colleagues analyzed the serum and urine specimens of patients with suspected LSD intoxication by both RIA (limit of detection, 0.1 ng/ml) and high-pressure liquid chromatography (HPLC; limit of detection, 0.5 ng/ml). RIA tends to give higher readings than HPLC because the RIA cross-reacts with LSD metabolites. The average quantitative LSD serum value by HPLC was 1.2 ng/ml; urine values averaged 2.9 ng/ml. Specimens for RIA may be collected and stored frozen for batch analysis at a convenient time (12).

Basic laboratory tests, such as complete blood cell count, serum electrolytes, liver and renal function, and urine drug screening may be needed, especially in altered patients without a known cause.

Diagnostic Pitfalls

Overdoses of cocaine, amphetamines, anticholinergic agents, dextromethorphan, and other hallucinogens (mescaline, psilocybin) may mimic LSD intoxication. In addition, withdrawal from alcohol or other sedative-hypnotic agents shares similar features such as agitation, diaphoresis, tachycardia, hypertension, and hallucinations. The differential diagnosis should also include primary psychiatric disorders, head trauma, hypoxia, hypoglycemia, hyponatremia, sepsis, meningitis, encephalitis, hyperthermia, thyroid storm, and neuroleptic malignant syndrome.

Treatment

The mainstay of treatment is to provide a nonthreatening environment and benzodiazepines for anxiety or agitation and to monitor vital signs until the patient is oriented and ambulatory.

GASTROINTESTINAL DECONTAMINATION

Gastrointestinal (GI) decontamination is unnecessary unless there are coingestants involved. LSD is rapidly absorbed, and decontamination procedures may intensify behavior abnormalities.

ENHANCEMENT OF ELIMINATION

Because of the short half-life and few serious medical complications, hemoperfusion, hemodialysis, and peritoneal dialysis have not been used for LSD intoxication.

ANTIDOTES

There are no specific antidotes for LSD intoxication. If signs of neuroleptic malignant syndrome develop, dantrolene may reduce fever and muscle rigidity and improve the level of consciousness (Chapter 47) (13). Phenothiazines are not antidotes and may cause serious adverse effects such as diminishing the threshold for seizure.

SUPPORTIVE CARE

The patient should be placed in a quiet, darkened room, preferably with a friend or family member who can provide reassurance. Administer a benzodiazepine (e.g., diazepam, 5 to 10 mg orally or IV) for anxiety, agitation, or dysphoria. Haloperidol may be administered as a second-line drug if the above measures fail to calm the patient and continued agitation represents an increased medical risk. Avoid the use of physical restraints if possible. Vital signs and mental status should be monitored periodically. Most patients can be managed in an ED or observation unit. The patient should be referred for substance abuse counseling when medically stable and oriented.

Acute Psychotic Reactions. Neuroleptic drugs should be administered cautiously in this setting because they may intensify the experience. Phenothiazine use has been associated with hypotension, sedation, potentiation of anticholinergic effects, decreased seizure threshold, and extrapyramidal reactions. Frequently, the actual psychedelic drug involved is not known, and phenothiazines can potentiate drugs with anticholinergic effects. The use of chlorpromazine in 2,5-dimethoxy-4-methylamphetamine ingestions reportedly caused several cases of cardiovascular collapse (14). Most visual hallucinations are actually illusions rather than true hallucinations, and the patients understand that what they are seeing is drug induced. When antipsychotic drugs are necessary, haloperidol probably is the safest neuroleptic agent.

Hallucinogen Persisting Perception Disorder. Pharmacologic agents, such as clonidine, perphenazine, and clonazepam, have been shown to ameliorate this syndrome in some individuals. Clonazepam administered 2 mg/day orally was successful in reducing symptoms in one study (15).

MANAGEMENT PITFALLS

Failure to consider alternative diagnoses, such as encephalitis, hyponatremia, and hypoglycemia, can result in delayed treatment and increased morbidity.

N,N-DIMETHYLTRYPTAMINE

DMT is 3-[2-(dimethylamino)ethyl]indole and a tryptamine hallucinogenic drug of abuse. It can be synthesized or obtained from the seeds and leaves of *Piptadenia peregrina* (Mimosaceae), the yopo tree (*Anadenanthera peregrina*), and other South American plants. It may be present in the tropical legume *Mucuna pruriens.* Street names include businessman's trip, DMT, fantasia, and Dimitri.

IV dimethyltryptamine fumarate is a hallucinogen at doses of 0.2 mg/kg and 0.4 mg/kg. Effects are felt almost instantaneously, peak within 2 minutes, and resolve within 30 minutes. Effects include visual hallucinatory phenomena, dissociated state, extreme shifts in mood, and auditory effects.

There are several other hallucinogenic tryptamines.

5-Methoxy-*N,N*-dimethyltryptamine ($C_{13}H_{18}N_2O$, 5-MeO-DMT): Street names are "methoxy" and "foxy-methoxy." The addition of a 5-methylhydroxy group to DMT increases lipid solubility and central nervous system (CNS) penetration. The dried venom of *Bufo alvarius* (Colorado River Toad) contains this compound. A typical dose is 5 to 10 mg IV or smoked.

α-Methyltryptamine: Street names are alpha, alpha-ET, and AMT.

Psilocin (4-hydroxy-dimethyltryptamine, $C_{12}H_{16}N_2O$): Street names are Alice, boomers, magic mushrooms, and shrooms.

Psilocybin (4-phosphoryloxy-dimithyltryptamine, $C_{11}H_{15}N_2O_4P$): Street names are Alice, boomers, magic mushrooms, shrooms.

Bufotenine (5-hydroxy-dimethyltryptamine): commonly known as toad, toady, and yopo.

Toxic Dose

Dimethyltryptamine fumarate, 0.2 to 0.4 mg/kg IV (20 to 50 mg), produces visual hallucinations and a brief "rush," which is followed by a dissociated state. Lower doses, 0.05 mg/kg and 0.1 mg/kg, are not hallucinogenic. At 0.05 mg/kg, no auditory or visual effects are experienced. At doses of 0.4 mg/kg, visual imagery predominates. The threshold dose for hallucinogenic effects is 0.2 mg/kg (16,17).

Toxicokinetics and Toxicodynamics

Routes of absorption are injection and smoking. Effects peak within 2 minutes after injection and resolve quickly within 20 to 30 minutes (16).

Pathophysiology

Tryptamine hallucinogens are agonists or partial agonists at serotonin (5-HT) receptors, specifically at 5-HT_2, 5-HT_{1A}, and 5-HT_{1C} subtypes (16). The hyperthermic effect of DMT is probably mediated by the 5-HT_2 subtype. DMT doses of up to 0.4 mg/kg produce elevations of β-endorphin, cortisol, corticotropin, growth hormone, and prolactin (17).

Clinical Presentation

DMT produces pupillary dilation, tachycardia, and elevated blood pressure and temperature. Visual hallucinations are usually present at abuse doses, and brightly colored, rapidly moving images are typical. Auditory hallucinations occur less commonly. A dissociated state may ensue, but effects usually only last for 30 minutes (16,17). Negative experiences reported include anxiety, panic, difficulty speaking, mood depression, and disturbing visual images.

Diagnostic Tests

A method for determination of DMT by gas chromatography with surface ionization detection is possible with a detection limit of 0.5 ng/ml (18). Peak values range from 32 to 200 ng/ml 2 minutes after injection of 0.4 mg/kg. Plasma DMT concentrations are not readily available and do not influence treatment. It may be useful for forensic or drug abuse monitoring purposes.

Treatment

GI decontamination with activated charcoal is useful only in massive oral overdose. This drug is typically used IV or smoked. Due to the short duration of action, enhancement of elimination is not warranted. There are no specific antidotes for DMT.

The patient should be placed in a quiet, dark room and given verbal reassurance. Try to avoid physical restraints because they may exacerbate panic and combativeness. Agitation or anxiety should be treated with benzodiazepines (e.g., diazepam, 5 to 10 mg orally or IV). Monitor for tachycardia or hypertension. Admission to the hospital is rarely required. Most patients can be managed in an ED or observation unit. The patient should be referred for substance abuse counseling when medically stable and oriented.

PHENCYCLIDINE

PCP was initially developed as a general anesthetic in the 1950s but was abandoned due to side effects of postoperative halluci-

TABLE 3. Street names for phencyclidine

Angel dust	Mint weed
Angel hair	Mist
Angel mist	Monkey dust
Animal tranquilizer	PCP
Cadillac	Peace
C.J.	Peace pill
Crystal joint	Rocket fuel
Cyclones	Scuffle
Dust	Selma
Elephant tranquilizer	Sherman
Embalming fluid	Snorts
Goon	Soma
Gorilla biscuits	Supercools
Hog	Superweed
Horse tranquilizers	Surfer
Jet fuel	T
Kay Jay	TAC
K.J.	TIC
Killer weed	Tranks
Krystal joint	Whacky weed
K.W.	Zombie dust
Lovely	

Modified from Milhorn HT Jr. Diagnosis and management of phencyclidine intoxication. *Am Fam Physician* 1991;43:1293–1302.

TABLE 4. Phencyclidine additives

Active
Phenylpropanolamine
Benzocaine
Procaine
Ephedrine
Caffeine
Piperidine
PCC (1-piperidinocyclohexanecarbonitrile)
TCP (1-[1-(2-thienyl)cyclohexyl]piperidine)
PCE (cyclohexamine)
PHP (phenylcyclohexylpyrrolidine)
Ketamine
Inert
Magnesium sulfate
Ammonium chloride
Ammonium hydroxide
Phenyllithium halide
Phenylmagnesium halide
Volatile
Ethyl ether
Toluene
Cyclohexanol
Isopropanol

From Shesser R, Jotte R, Olshaker J. The contribution of impurities to the acute morbidity of illegal drug use. *Am J Emerg Med* 1991;9:336–342, with permission.

nations and delirium. In the 1970s, it was discovered as a drug of abuse. During the late 1980s and early 1990s, crack cocaine replaced the demand for PCP. More recently, however, reports suggest that PCP abuse is increasing slightly in many cities. The Drug Enforcement Administration seized three clandestine PCP laboratories in 1998.

PCP causes distortion of perception and produces a feeling of detachment or "dissociation" from the user's surroundings and self. It is not a classic "hallucinogen" but better described as a "dissociative" agent or anesthetic. The most common physical findings are nystagmus and hypertension.

PCP is an arylcycloalkylamine dissociative anesthetic. It has no medical indication and is manufactured for its abuse potential. Common street names for PCP are listed in Table 3 (19). PCP is a white crystalline powder with a bitter taste. It is soluble in water or alcohol. It is available as a tablet, capsule, or powder on the illicit market. It can be snorted, smoked, or ingested. It is often applied to parsley, oregano, cigarettes ("sherms"), or marijuana for smoking. Active, inert, and volatile additives found in PCP are summarized in Table 4 (20).

Analogs of PCP that are abused include PHP (rolicyclidine, phenylcyclohexylpyrrolidine), PCC (1-piperidinocyclohexanecarbonitrile), PCE (*N*-ethyl-1-phenylcyclohexylamine), TCP (1-[1-(2-thienyl)cyclohexyl]piperidine), and PCPP.

Toxic Dose

Catatonic posturing, emotional withdrawal, and bizarre behavior are seen at doses of 0.05 mg/kg. A dose of 0.1 mg/kg causes alteration of body image and a feeling of unreality. A dose of 10 mg causes total disorientation and catatonic stupor (21). Typical abuse doses are 1 to 3 mg IV, smoked, or snorted and 2 to 6 mg by ingestion.

Toxicokinetics and Toxicodynamics

Routes of exposure include ingestion, IV injection, and inhalation by smoking and insufflation. PCP elimination from plasma is consistent with first-order kinetics with a half-life of 7 to 26 hours. The duration of effect is usually 4 to 6 hours but may be much longer in overdose. The V_d is 6.2 L/kg. It is highly lipid soluble and accumulates in adipose tissue and in the brain. Plasma protein binding is approximately 65%. It undergoes oxidative metabolism to inactive metabolites that are conjugated and excreted in the urine. An initial rapid decrease in urine PCP levels during the first 9 days is followed by a more gradual decline. Renal clearance is increased in the presence of acidic urine.

Pathophysiology

PCP is a noncompetitive antagonist of *N*-methyl-D-aspartate–type glutamate receptors in the cerebral cortex and limbic system. It stimulates α-adrenergic receptors, causing sympathomimetic effects. It also causes cerebral vasospasm.

Pregnancy and Lactation

PCP is FDA pregnancy category X (Appendix I). PCP crosses the human placenta and has been found in the urine of neonates for up to 3 days after birth. Irritability, hypertonicity, poor feeding, and abnormal neurobehavior have been reported in newborns of PCP-abusing mothers (22). PCP concentrates in breast milk, and breast-feeding is contraindicated (4).

Clinical Presentation

Patients may present with various combinations of CNS stimulation and depression, cholinergic and anticholinergic effects, and adrenergic effects. The most common physical findings are nystagmus (horizontal, vertical, or rotatory) and hypertension (23). Respiratory depression and aspiration may also occur. Some patients display evidence of nystagmus, ataxia, loss of muscle coordination, and vital sign abnormalities without obvious signs of behavioral toxicity. Incidental intoxication has been documented in a chronically depressed elderly woman who lived above a clandestine PCP laboratory (24).

CENTRAL NERVOUS SYSTEM EFFECTS

PCP causes confusion, disorientation, auditory and visual hallucinations, and delusions. Patients are alert but display bizarre behavior, agitation, or violence. Acute PCP intoxication can produce a psychosis indistinguishable from acute schizophrenia. Patients may develop catatonia, with unusual posturing, mutism, and staring. A patient who appears calm one minute may be agitated or violent the next. Symptoms often resolve within hours, although some patients have symptoms lasting days or even weeks. Recovery from psychosis may be very gradual over weeks to months.

The level of consciousness ranges from fully alert to comatose. Coma may occur suddenly but often develops after a period of bizarre or violent behavior. It may be of relatively short duration but can last up to 1 week. Some patients with prolonged coma have been found to have continued drug absorption from ruptured packets of ingested PCP (25). On emergence from coma, agitation and psychosis are common.

Nervous system effects include seizures, stupor, coma, cerebral ischemia, subarachnoid hemorrhage, amaurosis fugax, and muscle rigidity. The muscle rigidity, along with agitation, can result in acute rhabdomyolysis and myoglobin-induced renal failure. Myoclonic, choreoathetoid, and dystonic movements, including opisthotonus and torticollis, may be seen.

Children have become intoxicated by ingesting the butts of used PCP-impregnated cigarettes or from passive inhalation of sidestream smoke. Children aged 5 years and younger often present with lethargy, severe depression of consciousness, ataxia, nystagmus, and staring episodes. Presenting signs may also include apnea, seizures, opisthotonus, and choreoathetosis. Miosis may be present. In children, unexplained stupor or coma, seizures, ataxia, nystagmus, strange behavior, staring spells, or unusual posturing can indicate possible PCP intoxication (26).

A withdrawal syndrome from PCP has been observed in monkeys. It is characterized by somnolence, tremors, seizures, diarrhea, piloerection, and bruxism. Psychological dependence has occurred in humans (27).

OTHER EFFECTS

Cardiovascular effects include tachycardia and hypertension. Hypertension-induced complications are rare. Tachycardia occurs in approximately one-third of patients. Cholinergic effects include diaphoresis, miosis, bronchospasm, and salivation. Anticholinergic effects that may occur are fever, tachycardia, mydriasis, and urinary retention.

FATALITIES

Most deaths in PCP-intoxicated patients occur because of its behavioral effects. The bizarre and violent behavior along with analgesic effects and lack of muscular coordination may cause drowning or significant trauma. Nontraumatic causes of death include cardiopulmonary arrest after status epilepticus or hyperpyrexia, primary respiratory arrest, and intracranial hemorrhage.

Diagnostic Tests

PCP blood levels do not correlate well with clinical findings and do not guide clinical management. A "body stuffer" of PCP developed muscle rigidity, diaphoresis, and a temperature of 41.3°C. His serum PCP concentration was 1879 ng/ml, and the cerebrospinal fluid concentration was 245 ng/ml. Thirteen days after ingestion, he passed two plastic bags per rectum, one of which was ruptured. He recovered (25). People arrested for driving under the influence of PCP have blood levels ranging from 0.012 to 0.118 mg/L (28). Positive blood PCP levels were reported in law enforcement officers who handled PCP confiscated during drug raids (29).

As part of the U.S. National Institute on Drug Abuse guidelines for laboratories performing federal workplace drug testing, laboratories are required to detect, identify, and quantitate PCP urine concentrations of 25 ng/ml. The initial and confirmatory test cutoff level is 25 ng/ml. On average, urine samples are positive for 2 weeks, and most samples are PCP negative by 30 days (30).

Ketamine, diphenhydramine, and dextromethorphan may cause urine drug screens to test positive for PCP. Diphenhydramine in urine concentrations of 50 to 1200 μg/L may cause a urine specimen to test positive for PCP, with apparent concentrations up to 32 to 37 μg/L by fluorescence polarization immunoassay (31). Intoxication from dextromethorphan may result in a false-positive urine screen for PCP using HPLC or immunoassays (32).

Other tests should be obtained in order to evaluate for other diagnoses or potential complications of PCP intoxication. These include serum electrolytes, glucose, creatinine, creatine kinase, urinalysis, and toxicology screen for stimulants, cocaine, and opiates. In addition, bacterial and other cultures may be needed for evaluation of coma or altered mental status.

Diagnostic Pitfalls

Overdoses of cocaine, amphetamines, anticholinergic agents, dextromethorphan, and other hallucinogens (LSD, mescaline, psilocybin) may mimic PCP intoxication. In addition, withdrawal from alcohol or other sedative-hypnotic agents shares similar features, such as agitation, diaphoresis, tachycardia, hypertension, and hallucinations. The differential diagnosis should also include primary psychiatric disorders, head trauma, hypoxia, hypoglycemia, hyponatremia, sepsis, meningitis, encephalitis, hyperthermia, thyroid storm, and neuroleptic malignant syndrome.

Treatment

GASTROINTESTINAL DECONTAMINATION

Because of the small amounts ingested, GI decontamination is unlikely to be helpful unless coingestants are involved.

ENHANCEMENT OF ELIMINATION

Urinary acidification has been recommended to achieve "ion trapping" and enhance urinary PCP excretion. Although the amount of PCP excreted in the urine can be increased by this method, urinary acidification is not indicated. Only a small percentage of PCP is excreted in the urine. Acidification does not affect liver metabolism, the major route of drug elimination, and thus does not significantly increase the overall removal of the drug. Induction of metabolic acidosis may cause complications. Rhabdomyolysis is a potential complication of PCP intoxication, and acidic urine increases the risk of myoglobinuric renal failure.

Charcoal hemoperfusion removed only 2% of the administered dose in a dog model and did not affect the clinical outcome (33). Due to the high lipid solubility and V_d, hemodialysis and hemoperfusion are not expected to be effective in removing PCP from humans.

ANTIDOTES

There is not a specific PCP antagonist available for human use. An anti-PCP monoclonal Fab fragment has been developed and tested in animals. It has been shown to remove PCP from the brain and reverse locomotor activity in a dose-dependent manner. It also reversed the effects of PCP analogs, suggesting it may be effective for "designer" drugs in this class (34). Animal studies suggest that antipsychotic drugs can block PCP receptor–mediated behavioral effects (35). This requires confirmation in human studies (36).

SUPPORTIVE CARE

Place the patient in a quiet, dark room with minimal stimuli. Agitation may be treated with benzodiazepines (e.g., diazepam, 5 to 10 mg orally or IV). Seizures caused by PCP should also be treated with IV benzodiazepines. Phenobarbital is the agent of choice if benzodiazepines fail to control seizure activity. The use of other anticonvulsants has not been evaluated.

Prolonged psychosis may be treated with haloperidol. Because PCP has anticholinergic activity, neuroleptics with significant anticholinergic effects, such as chlorpromazine, should be avoided. Rhabdomyolysis is treated by correcting volume depletion with crystalloid IV fluids (e.g., normal saline). Metabolic acidosis may be treated with sodium bicarbonate.

Patients should be observed until their mental status has remained normal for several hours. Patients with mild to moderate symptoms improve rapidly and can be discharged from the ED or observation unit. Indications for hospitalization include seizures, rhabdomyolysis, hyperthermia, persistent psychosis, or significant injuries. Pediatric patients who are symptomatic from PCP exposure should be admitted. The patient should be referred for substance abuse counseling when medically stable and oriented.

Twenty-four PCP abusers underwent withdrawal over a 1-month period. Buspirone (10 mg three times a day) was effective in controlling symptoms over placebo after 2 weeks of treatment (37). Desipramine has also been shown to help alleviate abstinence symptoms in patients who were combined cocaine free-base and PCP users ("space base") (38).

MANAGEMENT PITFALLS

Failure to consider alternative diagnoses, such as encephalitis, hyponatremia, encephalitis, head trauma, and hypoglycemia, can result in delayed treatment and increased morbidity.

KETAMINE

Ketamine (Ketalar, Ketaject, Ketanest) is a synthetic chemical that was developed in the 1960s because of dissatisfaction with PCP as a surgical anesthetic drug. It induces sedation, immobility, amnesia, analgesia, and an unusual trance-like cataleptic state, where the patient appears to be "dissociated" from his or her environment but not necessarily asleep. Ketamine is used for induction anesthesia, primarily for short-term painful diagnostic or surgical procedures in children, where it maintains anesthesia and analgesia while preserving pharyngeal reflexes and respiratory function. It is also used for anesthesia in the Third World and in military campaigns where extensive anesthetic equipment is unavailable. It is subject to drug abuse and may result in death (39). Illicit abuse of ketamine was first observed in San Francisco and Los Angeles in 1971 (40) and also occurs in the United Kingdom (41). Overdose produces sedation and respiratory depression. Tachycardia, hypertension, muscle rigidity and delirium may also occur.

Ketamine is normally a white crystalline powder but may have a green crystalline appearance. The green color results from its mixture with vitamin B_{12}, which is thought to minimize adverse reactions (42). It may be taken intranasally, orally, or by injection. Street names for ketamine solutions include K, Jet, Super Acid, and 1980. Powders are called Green, Purple, Mauve, Special LA, Coke, Super C, and Special K. Commercial preparations are available in solutions of 10, 50, and 100 mg/ml for IV or intramuscular injection.

Toxic Dose

The *adult therapeutic dose* for induction of anesthesia is 1 to 4.5 mg/kg IV given over one minute or 6.5 to 13 mg/kg intramuscularly (IM) for dissociation. A dose of 0.5 mg/kg in adults results in analgesia with minimal alteration in consciousness; 1.5 to 2.0 mg/kg results in incoherent conversation in 50% of patients. The *pediatric dose* is a minimum of 4 mg/kg IM to consistently produce dissociation.

The dose for abuse is in the range of 1 to 2 mg/kg IM or IV. The typical adult abuse dose is 100 to 200 mg IM or subcutaneously (43). Repeated usage results in increasing dosages required for clinical effects, as high as 67 mg/kg has been reported (44).

A total dose of 900 mg led to a fatality in an adult (45). Almost all deaths associated with ketamine are due to trauma or are associated with co-ingestants such as opiates, cocaine, and amphetamines (46). Inadvertent overdoses ranging from 20 to 56 mg/kg IM and 10 to 50 mg/kg IV (5 to 100 times the intended dose) resulted in prolonged sedation and occasional respiratory depression (47).

Toxicokinetics and Toxicodynamics

Ketamine is not well absorbed orally and undergoes first-pass metabolism (bioavailability, 20%). Protein binding is 12%, and the V_d is 2 to 4 L/kg. The half-life is 2.5 hours in adults and 1 to 2 hours in children. It is highly lipid soluble and readily crosses the blood–brain barrier. After an IV induction dose, the dissociation effect occurs within 15 seconds. Unconsciousness ensues within 30 seconds and lasts 10 to 15 minutes. The duration of action after 10 mg/kg IM is 12 to 25 minutes. Most abusers report a duration of effect of less than 1 hour. It undergoes hepatic *N*-demethylation by microsomal cytochrome P-450 (CYP3A4) to the active metabolite norketamine. Other metabolic pathways include hydroxylation and conjugation with glucuronic acid, with metabolites excreted in the urine.

Pathophysiology

Ketamine is a noncompetitive antagonist of *N*-methyl-D-aspartate receptors, similar to PCP. The primary site of action is the cerebral cortex and limbic system. It causes electrophysiologic dissociation between the limbic and cortical systems. It also inhibits the reuptake of catecholamines, resulting in increased sympathetic activity and hypertension and tachycardia. Cerebral blood flow, metabolic rate, and intracranial pressure are increased. Other sites of action include muscarinic and opiate receptors. Increases in pulmonary arterial pressure, coronary perfusion, and myocardial oxygen consumption may occur.

Pregnancy and Lactation

Ketamine is FDA pregnancy category B (Appendix I). Ketamine crosses the placenta. It has been used for obstetric anesthesia. It causes dose-related maternal hypertension, tachycardia, and increased uterine tone and contractions. High doses (1.5 to 2.2 mg/kg) have been associated with low neonatal APGAR scores, increased neonatal muscle tone, and apnea. These effects can be avoided with lower doses. There are no data on the effects of ketamine use during early pregnancy. There are no data on ketamine in breast milk. Based on the plasma half-life, it should be safe to breast feed 12 hours after a dose of ketamine (4).

Clinical Presentation

ACUTE OVERDOSAGE

Ketamine induces a clinical state of "dissociative anesthesia" during which the patient is dissociated from his or her environment but not necessarily asleep. At induction doses, amnesia may last for 1 to 2 hours after the injection. Increased muscle tone, purposeless movements, and irrational responses to stimuli may occur. The cough reflex may be suppressed, but pharyngeal reflexes are maintained.

Cardiovascular effects include hypertension, pulmonary hypertension, sinus tachycardia, and supraventricular tachycardia (48). Respiratory effects are laryngospasm (rare), coughing, increase in pharyngeal secretions, transient apnea, pulmonary edema (39), and respiratory depression.

The CNS effects include ataxia, visual distortions and illusions, slurring of speech, and dystonic reactions. Reports of seizure activity are extremely rare. Nystagmus, increased intraocular pressure, and blurred vision are common. Nystagmus is often absent in recreational users (43). Increased muscle tone, sudden jerking movements, and myoclonus are common. Hallucinations, alterations in perception of body image, and unpleasant dreams may occur. Recurrence of hallucinations without additional use of the drug may occur in drug abusers (49). GI effects include nausea and vomiting and hypersalivation.

Unintentional overdose in children undergoing ketamine induction has been reported in 20 children (47). Doses ranged from 20 to 56 mg/kg IM and 10 to 50 mg/kg IV (5 to 100 times the intended dose). Transient respiratory depression occurred in the majority of cases. Oxygen desaturation occurred in a few patients but was corrected with assisted ventilation and supplemental oxygen. Normal spontaneous respirations resumed after 2 to 10 minutes. Prolonged sedation occurred in all patients (3 to 9 hours after IV and 4 to 24 hours after intramuscular administration). There was no cardiovascular toxicity or seizure activity reported. No complications or long-term sequelae were noted.

CHRONIC ABUSE

Frequent recreational users of ketamine have been found to have impaired memory 3 days after their last dose, compared with infrequent users (50). Flashbacks have also been reported. Frequent use results in tolerance and the need to increase the dose in order to maintain similar effects. A withdrawal syndrome has not been described.

ADVERSE REACTIONS

Up to 50% of adults and 10% of children exhibit excitement or delirium or have visual hallucinations on awakening. This reaction may recur days or weeks later. The incidence of this "emergence phenomenon" can be reduced with benzodiazepine pretreatment. Risk factors are age older than 10 years, female gender, rapid IV injection, excessive noise during recovery, prior personality disorder, or prior history of frequent dreams (44).

Nausea and vomiting (3% to 12% in children) may occur, usually during the recovery phase when patients are alert. The incidence of laryngospasm is very low with clinical use (0.02% to 0.90%) and increases fivefold with concurrent laryngeal infection (44). Respiratory depression and apnea may occur with high doses, with rapid infusion, or in infants younger than 3 months of age.

Other adverse reported effects include increased heart rate, blood pressure, and muscle tone; depressed respiratory response to hypercarbia; hypersalivation; increased intraocular pressure and cerebrospinal fluid pressure; muscle hypertonicity; myoclonus; and rigidity. At doses of 14 to 19 mg/kg, opisthotonus has occurred. Intracranial pressure may increase approximately 20 mm Hg in adults. Ataxia, disequilibrium, transient erythematous rash, and recovery agitation (19% in children) are also reported (51).

DRUG INTERACTIONS

Coadministration of benzodiazepines or barbiturates prolongs the half-life of ketamine by competing for its metabolic pathway.

Diagnostic Tests

ACUTE OVERDOSAGE

Blood concentrations are not helpful in the management of adverse reactions or overdose. Ketamine and dextromethorphan can result in a false-positive PCP urine drug screen. Because the extent of cross-reactivity between PCP and ketamine is unknown, the PCP drug screen should not be used to test for the presence of ketamine. The serum creatine kinase may be elevated due to muscle hypertonicity or agitation.

DIAGNOSTIC PITFALLS

The differential diagnosis includes intoxication with PCP, LSD, amphetamines, hallucinogenic mushrooms, marijuana, or anticholinergic agents. Psychotic disorders, encephalitis, temporal lobe seizures, and head trauma should also be considered.

POSTMORTEM CONSIDERATIONS

A fatality involving ketamine and ethanol (blood ethanol, 170 mg/dl) had the following postmortem ketamine tissue concentrations: blood, 1.8 mg/L; urine, 2.0 mg/L; brain, 4.3 mg/L; liver, 4.9 mg/L; and spleen, 6.1 mg/L (52). In another fatality, the ketamine tissue concentrations were blood, 27.4 mg/L; urine, 8.51 mg/L; bile, 15.2 mg/L; brain, 3.24 mg/L; liver, 6.6 mg/L; and kidney, 3.38 mg/L (39).

Treatment

GASTROINTESTINAL DECONTAMINATION

There are no data on the ability of activated charcoal to bind ketamine. The oral bioavailability of ketamine is low (20%), and onset of effect is rapid. The risk of CNS depression, vomiting, and aspiration outweighs the possible benefit of gastric emptying and probably activated charcoal as well. Activated charcoal may be indicated if coingestants are involved.

ENHANCEMENT OF ELIMINATION

Due to its large V_d and high lipid solubility, ketamine is poorly eliminated during hemodialysis (10% of dose) or hemofiltration (4% of dose) (48).

ANTIDOTES

There is no specific antidote. Naloxone is not effective is reversing its analgesic properties. Clonidine (2.5 to 5.0 μg/kg orally) has been effective in attenuating the hypertension, tachycardia, salivation, and nightmares associated with IV ketamine given for anesthesia (53,54). Verapamil and benzodiazepines have also been shown to block cardiovascular stimulation (55).

Hypersalivation after ketamine use can be minimized with concurrent atropine (0.01 mg/kg; maximum total dose, 0.5 mg) or glycopyrrolate (0.005 mg/kg; maximum total dose, 0.25 mg) (44). Dystonic reactions are managed with diphenhydramine (25 to 50 mg IV).

SUPPORTIVE CARE

Patients should be placed in a quiet, darkened room until they recover. Diazepam may be given for panic attacks, vivid dreams, or hallucinations. In the absence of other mind-altering drugs, adult patients presenting to the ED after abuse are typically stable and ready for discharge in less than 5 hours (43).

Patients with respiratory depression should have ventilatory support, initially with a bag-valve mask, and supplemental oxygen. If respiratory depression persists for more than 10 minutes, endotracheal intubation may be required for continued ventilation and airway protection.

MONITORING

Mild disequilibrium may persist for 1 to 4 hours after ketamine administration. Close observation should be maintained during this period. Periodic vital sign measurement and continuous cardiac and respiratory monitoring or oximetry should be performed during unconsciousness or deep sedation.

MANAGEMENT PITFALLS

If symptoms do not improve within 2 hours of observation after recreational use of ketamine, prompt evaluation for other causes or coingestants should be undertaken. The absence of nystagmus is common among patients presenting to the ED for ketamine abuse and does not rule out this diagnosis (43).

REFERENCES

1. Schwartz RH. LSD. Its rise, fall, and renewed popularity among high school students. *Pediatr Clin North Am* 1995;42:403–413.
2. Maslanta AM, Scott SK. LSD overdose in an eight-month-old boy. *J Emerg Med* 1992;10:481–483.
3. Madden JS. LSD and post-hallucinogen perceptual disorder. *Addiction* 1994;89:762–763.
4. Briggs GR, Freeman RK, Yaffe, SJ. *Drugs in Pregnancy and lactation*, 6th ed. Baltimore: Williams & Wilkins, 2002:748–752, 817–823, 1094–1095.
5. Kawasaki A, Purvin V. Persistent palinopsia following ingestion of lysergic acid diethylamide (LSD). *Arch Ophthalmol* 1996;114:47–50.
6. Smith DE, Seymour RD. LSD: history and toxicity: today, there is group concern over long-term post hallucinogenic disorder. *Psychiatr Ann* 1994;24:145–147.
7. Lerner AG, Gelkopf M, Skladman I, et al. Flashback and hallucinogen persisting perception disorder: clinical aspects and pharmacological treatment approach. *Isr J Psychiatry Relat Sci* 2002;39:92–99.
8. Jackson TW, Hornfeldt CS. Seizure activity following recreational LSD use in patients treated with lithium and fluoxetine. *Vet Hum Toxicol* 1991;33:387.
9. Markel H, Lee A, Holms RD, Domino EF. LSD flashback syndrome exacerbated by selective serotonin reuptake inhibitor antidepressants in adolescents. *J Pediatr* 1994;125:817–819.
10. Abraham HD, Mamen A. LSD-like panic from risperidone in post-LSD visual disorder. *J Clin Psychopharmacol* 1996;16:238–241.
11. Cody JT, Valtier S. Immunoassay analysis of lysergic acid diethylamide. *J Anal Toxicol* 1997;21:459–464.
12. McCarron MM, Walberg CB, Baselt RC. Confirmation of LSD intoxication by analysis of serum and urine. *J Anal Toxicol* 1990;14:165–167.
13. Behan WMH, Bakheit AMO, Behan PO, More IAR. The muscle findings in the neuroleptic malignant syndrome associated with lysergic acid diethylamide. *J Neurol Neurosurg Psychiatry* 1991;54:741–743.
14. Solursh LP, Clement WR. Hallucinogenic drug abuse: manifestations and management. *Can Med Assoc J* 1968;98:407–413.
15. Lerner AG, Gelkopf M, Skladman I, et al. Clonazepam treatment of lysergic acid diethylamide-induced hallucinogen persisting perception disorder with anxiety features. *Int Clin Psychopharmacol* 2003;18:101–105.
16. Strassman RJ, Qualls CR. Dose–response study of *N,N*- dimethyltryptamine in humans: I. Neuroendocrine, autonomic and cardiovascular effects. *Arch Gen Psychiatry* 1994;56:85–97.
17. Strassman RJ, Qualls CR. Dose–response study of *N,N*-dimethyltryptamine in humans: II. Subjective effects and preliminary results of a new rating scale. *Arch Gen Psychiatry* 1994;56:98–108.
18. Ishii A, Seno H, Suzuki O, et al. A simple and sensitive quantitation of N,N-dimethyltryptamine by gas chromatography with surface ionization detection. *J Anal Toxicol* 1997;21:36–40.
19. Milhorn HT. Diagnosis and management of phencyclidine intoxication. *Am Fam Physician* 1991;43:1293–1302.
20. Shesser R, Jotte R, Olshaker J. The contribution of impurities to the acute morbidity of illegal drug use. *Am J Emerg Med* 1991;9:336–342.
21. Aniline O, Pitts FN. Phencyclidine (PCP): a review and perspectives. *CRC Crit Rev Toxicol* 1982;10:145–177.
22. Strauss AA, Modaniou HD, Bosu SK. Neonatal manifestations of maternal phencyclidine (PCP) abuse. *Pediatrics* 1981;68:550–552.
23. McCarron MM, Schulze BW, Thompson GA, et al. Acute phencyclidine intoxication: incidence of clinical findings in 1,000 cases. *Ann Emerg Med* 1981;10:237–242.
24. Aniline O, Pitts FN, Allen RE, et al. Incidental intoxication with phencyclidine. *J Clin Psychiatry* 1980;41:393–394.
25. Jackson JE. Phencyclidine pharmacokinetics after a massive overdose. *Ann Intern Med* 1989;111:613–615.
26. Schwartz RH, Einhorn A. PCP intoxication in seven children. *Pediatr Emerg Care* 1986;2:238–241.
27. Gorelick DA, Wilkins JN, Wong C. Outpatient treatment of PCP abusers. *Am J Drug Alcohol Abuse* 1989;15:367–374.
28. Kunsman GW, Levine B, Costantino A, et al. Phencyclidine blood concentrations in DRE cases. *J Anal Toxicol* 1997;21:498–502.
29. Pitts FN Jr, Allen RE, Aniline O, et al. Occupational intoxication and long-term persistence of phencyclidine (PCP) in law enforcement personnel. *J Toxicol Clin Toxicol* 1981;18:1015–1020.
30. Simpson GM, Khajawall AM, Alatorre E, et al. Urinary phencyclidine excretion in chronic abusers. *J Toxicol Clin Toxicol* 1982/1983;19:1051–1059.
31. Levine BS, Smith ML. Effects of diphenhydramine or immunoassay of phencyclidine in urine. *Clin Chem* 1990;36:1258.
32. Budai B, Iskandar H. Dextromethorphan can produce false positive phencyclidine testing with HPLC. *Am J Emerg Med* 2002;20:61–62.
33. Allen WR, O'Barr TP, Corby DG. Hemoperfusion of phencyclidine in the dog. *Int J Artif Organs* 1985;8:101–104.
34. Hardin JS, Wessinger WD, Proksch JW, et al. Pharmacodynamics of a monoclonal antiphencyclidine Fab with broad selectivity for phencyclidine-like drugs. *J Pharmacol Exp Ther* 1998;285:1113–1122.
35. Valentine JL, Mayersohn M, Wessinger WD, et al. Antiphencyclidine monoclonal Fab fragments reverse phencyclidine-induced behavioral effects and ataxia in rats. *J Pharmacol Exp Ther* 1996;278:709–716.
36. Farber NB, Price MT, Labruyer J, et al. Antipsychotic drugs block phencyclidine receptor-mediated neurotoxicity. *Biol Psychiatry* 1993;34:119–121.
37. Giannini AJ, Loiselle RH, Graham BH, Folts DJ. Behavioral response to buspirone in cocaine and phencyclidine withdrawal. *J Subst Abuse Treat* 1993;10:523–527.
38. Giannini AJ, Loiselle RH, Giannini MC. Space-based abstinence: alleviation of withdrawal symptoms in combinative cocaine-phencyclidine abuse. *J Toxicol Clin Toxicol* 1987;25:493–500.
39. Licata M, Pierini G, Popoli G. A fatal ketamine poisoning. *J Forensic Sci* 1994;39:1314–1320.
40. Seigel RK. Phencyclidine and ketamine intoxication. A study of four populations of recreational users. National Institute of Drug Abuse Research Monograph series. 1978;21:119–147.
41. Jansen KLR. Non-medical use of ketamine. *BMJ* 1993;306:601–602.
42. Felser JM, Orban DJ. Dystonic reaction after ketamine abuse. *Ann Emerg Med* 1982;11:673–675.
43. Weiner Al, Vieira L, McKay CA, et al. Ketamine abusers presenting to the emergency department: a case series. *J Emerg Med* 2000;18:447–451.
44. Green SM, Johnson NE. Ketamine sedation for pediatric procedures: part 2: review and implications. *Ann Emerg Med* 1990;19:1033–1046.
45. Peyton SH, Couch AT, Bost RO. Tissue distribution of ketamine: two case reports. *J Anal Toxicol* 1988;12:268–269.
46. Gill JR, Stajic M. Ketamine in non-hospital and hospital deaths in New York City. *J Forensic Sci* 2000;45:655–658.
47. Green SM, Clark R, Hostetler MA, et al. Inadvertent ketamine overdose in children: clinical manifestations and outcome. *Ann Emerg Med* 1999;34:494–497.
48. Koppel C, Arndt I, Ibe K. Effects of enzyme induction, renal and cardiac function on ketamine plasma kinetics in patients with ketamine long-term analgosedation. *Eur J Drug Metab Pharmacokinet* 1990;15:259–263.
49. Fine J, Firestone SC. Sensory disturbances following ketamine anesthesia: recurrent hallucinations. *Anesth Analg* 1973;52:428–430.
50. Curran HV, Monaghan L. In and out of the K-hole: a comparison of the acute and residual effects of ketamine in frequent and infrequent ketamine users. *Addiction* 2001;96:749–760.
51. Green SM, Rothrock SG, Lynch EL, et al. Intramuscular ketamine for pediatric sedation in the emergency department: safety profile in 1,022 cases. *Ann Emerg Med* 1998;31:688–697.
52. Moore KA, Kilbane EM, Jones R, et al. Tissue distribution of ketamine in a mixed drug fatality. *J Forensic Sci* 1997;42:1183–1185.
53. Handa F, Tanaka M, Nishikawa T, Toyooka H. Effects of oral clonidine premedication on side effects of intravenous ketamine anesthesia: a randomized, double-blind, placebo-controlled study. *J Clin Anesth* 2000;12:19–24.
54. Tanaka M, Nishikawa T. Oral clonidine premedication attenuates the hypertensive response to ketamine. *Br J Anaesth* 1994;73:758–762.
55. Reich DL, Silvay G. Ketamine: an update on the first twenty-five years of clinical experience. *Can J Anaesth* 1989;36:186–197.

CHAPTER 178

Marijuana and Other Cannabinoids

E. Martin Caravati

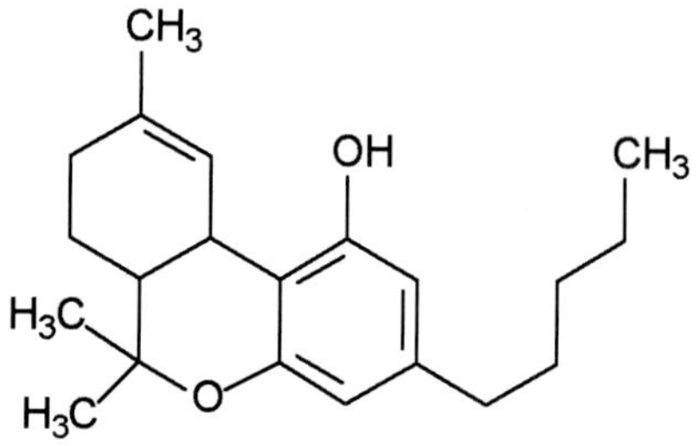

Δ-9-TETRAHYDROCANNABINOL

Compounds included:	**Marijuana (tetrahydrocannabinol); dronabinol (Marinol); nabilone (Cesamet)**
Molecular formula and weight:	**Marijuana, dronabinol ($C_{21}H_{30}O_2$), 314.47; nabilone ($C_{24}H_{36}O_3$), 372.5 g/mol**
SI conversion:	**Marijuana and dronabinol, mg/L × 3.2 = μmol/L; nabilone, mg/L × 2.7 = μmol/L**
CAS Registry No.:	**8063-14-7 (cannabis); 1972-08-3 (dronabinol); 51022-71-0 (nabilone)**
Therapeutic or normal levels:	**Not applicable**
Special concerns:	**Cognitive impairment**
Antidote:	**None**

OVERVIEW

Marijuana is the most commonly used illicit drug. It consists of dried, chopped plant parts of *Cannabis sativa,* the hemp plant. The principal psychoactive agent is Δ-9-tetrahydrocannabinol (THC), which constitutes up to 20% of the plant material.

Dronabinol (Marinol) is a synthetic pharmaceutical preparation of Δ-9-THC that is approved for the treatment of nausea and vomiting associated with cancer chemotherapy in patients who fail to respond to conventional antiemetic therapy and for the treatment of anorexia associated with weight loss in patients with acquired immunodeficiency syndrome. Dronabinol is formulated in sesame oil and supplied as round, soft gelatin capsules containing 2.5, 5.0, or 10.0 mg.

Nabilone (Cesamet) is a synthetic cannabinoid with antiemetic and anxiolytic properties that is marketed in Ireland, Canada, and the United Kingdom. Its indications, pathophysiology, clinical effects, and adverse reactions are similar to dronabinol. Dronabinol has antiemetic efficacy similar to prochlorperazine but less than that of metoclopramide. The results of small clinical trials suggest that nabilone can reduce tremor and spasticity in some patients with multiple sclerosis (1). Large amounts may induce seizures (2).

More than 83 million Americans (37%) aged 12 years and older have tried marijuana at least once. In 2001, 20% of eighth graders and 50% of twelfth graders reported that they had used marijuana. Marijuana was a contributing factor in more than 110,000 emergency department visits in 2001 (3). A survey of university students in the United Kingdom found that approximately 60% had tried cannabis and 20% reported regular use (4). Individual usage varies from one-time experimentation to daily use of multiple "joints."

Multiple-drug abuse (alcohol, amphetamines, benzodiazepines, cocaine, and opiates) continues to be a problem with marijuana users. Trauma and inadequate methadone maintenance are associated with abuse (5,6). Phencyclidine (PCP) may be intentionally combined with marijuana ("superweed") to obtain a more intense hallucinogenic experience (7).

In 1989, the U.S. Drug Enforcement Administration (DEA) rejected a petition to reschedule marijuana in smoked form from schedule I (prohibited) to schedule II (available only by prescription) status under the Controlled Substances Act (8–10). The DEA issued a final order in 1992, stating that the plant marijuana had no accepted medical use and would remain a schedule I controlled substance (11). The U.S. Public Health Service also concluded that smoked marijuana is potentially more harmful than helpful to patients with compromised immune systems (12). Nevertheless, in early 1994, a sharp increase in the use of marijuana among eighth graders and high school students was reported (13).

Classification and Uses

Cannabinoid is the collective term for the psychoactive compounds derived from *C. sativa.* They are aryl-substituted monoterpenes that are unique to this plant genus. The most potent psychoactive agent is Δ-9-THC. Other cannabinoids include Δ-8-THC, cannabinol, and cannabidiol. They are present in the stalks, leaves, flowers, and seeds.

Marijuana (marihuana) refers to any part of the plant or its extract that is used to induce psychotomimetic or therapeutic effects. Synonyms include pot, Mary Jane, MJ, weed, grass, reefer, puff, hagga, macohna, and numerous others. It is a greenish-gray mixture of dried, shredded leaves, stems, and flowers of *C. sativa.* It is usually smoked but also may be mixed into foods. Over time, the potency has greatly increased due to improved cultivation techniques from approximately 10 to 150 mg of THC per joint (14). In addition to cannabinoids, the plant contains other constituents similar to tobacco except for nicotine.

Marijuana "blunts" are fat, 5-in., inexpensive cigars. Because their wrappers are easily resealed, the cigars can be filled with marijuana, crack cocaine, or other drugs. Young adults, teenagers, and even younger children slice the cigars open and pack them with the drug. The combination also can stretch the use of small quantities of cheap marijuana. The harsh stench of the cheap cigar is prized for its ability to mask the sweet smell of marijuana.

Hashish is the natural product of the dried resin collected from flower tops of *C. sativa* and contains varying concentrations of THC up to 20%. *Hashish oil* is a dark viscous organic solvent extract that contains 15% to 30% THC. *Sinsemilla* is a seedless (unpollenated female) plant grown widely that accounts for a majority of domestic production. It typically has a high THC content.

Toxic Dose

The *adult therapeutic dosage* for dronabinol is 2.5 mg twice a day to a maximum dose of 20 mg/day. The average daily dose is 5 to 20 mg. Doses of 5 to 15 mg/m^2 are used in the management of emesis in chemotherapy. The adult dose of nabilone is 1 to 2 mg orally 1 to 3 hours before and every 8 to 12 hours after chemotherapy. The dose of nabilone should not exceed 6 mg/day.

The adult dose for intentional abuse of marijuana is typically 5 to 15 mg of THC to produce the desired psychoactive effects. No specific toxic dose has been established, but 30 mg/kg is estimated as a lethal dose (15). The estimated lethal human dose of intravenous dronabinol is 30 mg/kg (2100 mg/70 kg). Significant central nervous system (CNS) symptoms have followed oral doses of 0.4 mg/kg (28 mg/70 kg) (16).

TOXICOKINETICS AND TOXICODYNAMICS

The pulmonary absorption of THC during inhalation is approximately 20% to 30% of a cannabis cigarette. Absorption is rapid, with onset of effect within minutes. Due to first-pass metabolism, the bioavailability is greatly reduced if ingested (6% to 10%). The acute effects begin in 1 to 3 hours. The duration of effect is 1 to 4 hours after inhalation and up to 8 hours after ingestion. THC is rapidly distributed to the brain and other tissues. Cannabinoids are highly lipid soluble and accumulate in fatty tissue where peak concentration is reached in 4 to 5 days.

The major active compound is Δ-9-THC. It is 98% protein bound and has a volume of distribution of 10 L/kg. THC is metabolized by hepatic hydroxylation, with a half-life of 25 to 57 hours. There are many active and inactive metabolites that have half-lives of several days. The major inactive metabolite is 11-nor-THC-9-carboxylic acid. Less than 1% of THC is excreted unchanged.

Clinical studies have reported that heavy cannabis users show positive urinary cannabinoid levels for many weeks after discontinuation from the drug. This prolonged excretion could be explained by accumulation of THC in deep tissue compartments, such as fat, followed by return of THC to plasma with subsequent elimination. The average terminal elimination half-life of THC in plasma and urine is approximately 5 days (range, 1 to 12 days) in frequent marijuana users (17). Repeated usage results in accumulation of high levels of cannabinoids in the body.

Dronabinol is slowly absorbed from the gastrointestinal tract. It undergoes first-pass metabolism, and its bioavailability after oral administration is 10% to 20%. It is 97% to 99% bound to plasma proteins. The volume of distribution is approximately 10 L/kg. Dronabinol is metabolized to 11-hydroxydronabinol (11-OH-Δ-9-THC), which is similar in activity to the parent compound. Biliary excretion is the major route of elimination. Less than 5% of an oral dose is recovered unchanged in the feces. It has a terminal half-life of 25 to 36 hours.

PATHOPHYSIOLOGY

Cannabinoid receptors are found in the brain and peripheral nerves (CB_1 receptors) and in macrophages and other immune cells (CB_2 receptors). The CB_1 receptors are distributed in the cerebral cortex, hippocampus, amygdala, basal ganglia, cerebellum, thalamus, and brain stem (14). THC has been shown to increase the release of dopamine in the brain. It has central sympathomimetic activity that results in sinus tachycardia. Marijuana's effect on the hippocampus results in impaired short-term memory. Chronic THC exposure may hasten the age-related loss of hippocampal neurons.

Dronabinol is a centrally acting sympathomimetic drug that acts at cannabinoid receptor sites in the brain. Orthostatic hypotension is associated with initial treatment. It has dose-related, reversible effects on mood, cognition, memory, and coordination. Tolerance to the cardiovascular and CNS effects develops within 2 weeks.

PREGNANCY AND LACTATION

THC itself is not classified. The pharmaceutical form (dronabinol) is U.S. Food and Drug Administration pregnancy category C (Appendix I). A prospective study of marijuana use in pregnancy suggested that infants whose mothers had positive urine assays for marijuana exhibited impaired fetal growth (lower birth weight, decrease in length) when compared with infants of nonusers (18). The study did not demonstrate a causal relationship. Data from the Ottawa Prenatal Prospective Study showed no significant reduction in birth weight or head circumference in babies of marijuana users (19). Richardson and colleagues later concluded that there is no increased risk of spontaneous abortion, effects on birth weight or head circumference, or effects on the rate of minor or major physical anomalies as a result of prenatal marijuana use. There do not appear to be significant effects on the neurobehavioral outcome of newborns (20). Long-term development and behavioral effects remain to be determined.

An initial unconfirmed case-control study suggests that there is a tenfold increased risk of leukemia in the offspring of mothers who smoked marijuana just before or during pregnancy (21).

THC is secreted into breast milk. The long-term effects of this exposure are unknown, and the use of marijuana during breastfeeding is contraindicated (19).

CLINICAL PRESENTATION

Acute Overdosage

Acute intoxication may result in tachycardia (heart rates up to 160 beats/minute), conjunctival injection, and ataxia. The effects of naturally occurring cannabinoids and synthetic forms are similar in overdose, with the exception of toxicity arising from routes other than ingestion (e.g., pneumomediastinum from Valsalva's maneuver).

The pupils are unchanged, and sensorium is often clear. Nystagmus is not present. Postural hypotension and syncope may occur. Euphoria, anxiety, increased appetite, dry mouth, and time-space distortions are common. Occasionally, fear, distrust, dysphoria, or panic occurs after use. Impaired short-term memory, judgment, and attention spans also occur. Hallucination may occur with high doses. The use of Valsalva's maneuvers during cannabinoid smoking has rarely caused pneumothorax, pneumomediastinum, and pneumopericardium (22). Symptoms and signs of severe intoxication include decreased motor coordination, lethargy, slurred speech, and postural hypotension.

Effects on cognition and psychomotor performance are dose related and additive with other CNS depressants such as alcohol. Manifestations include slowing of reaction time, motor incoordination, difficulty in concentrating, and impaired performance of complex tasks that require divided attention such as driving an automobile or flying an airplane. Aircraft pilot performance after the smoking of one cigarette containing 20 mg of THC can be impaired for as long as 24 hours after smoking. The user may be unaware of the drug's influence (23).

Pediatric toxicity usually follows ingestion. In children, cannabis ingestion can result in coma. It should be suspected if a combination of the following clinical signs is present and particularly if siblings develop symptoms simultaneously: rapid onset of drowsiness, moderate pupillary dilation, marked hypotonia, lid lag, presence of small dark particles (e.g., granules, leaves, or resin) in the mouth, and the absence of a history and symptoms indicative of trauma, CNS, or seizures (24).

Hashish resin ingestion in children in amounts ranging from 0.25 to 1.00 g has led to a rapid onset of obtundation (30 to 75 minutes). Some children have developed opisthotonic-like movements alternating with hypotonia, and others may have meningismus. Approximately one-third of children experience tachycardia (greater than 150 beats/minute) after exposure. Occasional cyanosis, right bundle-branch block, and apnea with bradycardia may be observed. All children usually recover 10 to 36 hours after ingestion without sequelae. The acute ingestion of cannabinoids is potentially life-threatening. Acute supportive care and decontamination may be required (25).

Acute psychosis associated with the use of marijuana was reported in U.S. soldiers during the Vietnam War, one of whom shot an individual on guard duty (26). Suicidal ideation, anxiety, and paranoia accompanied the organic psychosis, which lasted 1 to 11 days. The development of acute psychosis after chronic use remains controversial because of questions about the contribution of premorbid personalities and multiple-drug use (e.g., PCP) (27). Undifferentiated manic, schizophreniform, and confusional psychoses have been reported in heavy marijuana users admitted to psychiatric hospitals (28). Comparison between psychotic men with high urinary cannabinoid levels and negative control groups suggests that high THC intake is associated with a rapidly resolving psychosis characterized by hypomania and occasionally schizophrenic symptoms (29). Flashbacks can occur.

Chronic Use

Pulmonary effects of smoking marijuana include a nearly fivefold greater increment in the blood carboxyhemoglobin level and an approximately threefold increase in the amount of tar inhaled and retained in the respiratory tract. These observations may account for previous findings that smoking only a few marijuana cigarettes a day (without tobacco) has the same effect on the prevalence of acute and chronic respiratory toxicity and the extent of tracheobronchial epithelial histopathology as smoking more than 20 tobacco cigarettes a day (without marijuana) (30). Chronic cannabis smoking is associated with bronchitis and emphysema.

Dronabinol causes psychological and physiologic dependence in healthy individuals after chronic use. True addiction is uncommon but may follow prolonged high-dose administration.

Aspergillosis may be a complication of marijuana use. Illegally obtained marijuana may be contaminated with *Aspergillus* species, most often *Aspergillus flavus* and *Aspergillus fumigatus*. *Aspergillus* spores easily pass through contaminated marijuana that is smoked (31). Whereas immunocompetent individuals are unlikely to be affected, immunocompromised patients may develop invasive pulmonary aspergillosis (32). *Aspergillus* can be eliminated by baking marijuana at a minimum temperature of 150°C (300°F) 15 minutes before smoking. Similar conditions do not degrade THC (33).

Digital clubbing has been reported in chronic users. The cause is believed to be chronic elevation of catecholamine levels causing vasodilation of peripheral arteries that results in digital clubbing (34).

Cognitive impairment may affect chronic cannabis users, including impaired attention, memory, and ability to process complex information even when not intoxicated. This can last for weeks to months after cessation of usage (35).

Daily doses of 180 mg of THC (two joints per day) for 2 to 3 weeks is sufficient to produce tolerance and a physical withdrawal after cessation. Symptoms include restlessness, insomnia, anxiety, tremor, and autonomic effects such as "hot flashes," rhinorrhea, loose stools, and anorexia (36). Symptoms abate over 48 hours.

Carcinogenesis

Cancer of the mouth and larynx appear increased in patients using marijuana regularly (37,38). Marijuana smoking may also be associated with an increased risk for the development of respiratory tract malignancy (39). Several cases have been reported of respiratory tract malignancy (tongue, tonsil, piriform sinus, paranasal sinus, larynx, lung) in young, long-term marijuana smokers (39). The smoking of one marijuana cigarette leads to the deposition in the lower respiratory tract of approximately a fourfold greater quantity of insoluble smoke particulates (tar) than smoking a filtered tobacco cigarette of comparable weight (30).

Adverse Events

Dronabinol's adverse effects in clinical trials consisted primarily of asthenia, palpitations, tachycardia, facial flushing, anxiety, confusion, depersonalization, dizziness, euphoria, paranoia, somnolence, and abnormal thinking. The most common adverse effects of nabilone include vertigo, dizziness, drowsiness, dry mouth, and difficulty in concentration. Nabilone increases the psychomotor impairment produced by diazepam, alcohol, and codeine (40).

Drug Interactions

Additive effects on psychomotor performance may follow concomitant use of marijuana and ethanol. Combinations of cocaine and marijuana appear to increase heart rates above levels seen with either drug alone. Increases in mean arterial pressure after combinations of cocaine and marijuana are equivalent to those produced by cocaine alone (41).

DIAGNOSTIC TESTS

Urine Screening for Tetrahydrocannabinol

Urine screening for 11-nor-THC-9-carboxylic acid is usually performed by enzyme-multiplied immunoassay test (EMIT) and radioimmunoassay. The reliable detection limit is 50 ng/ml. False-negatives can be produced by dilution, lemon juice, vinegar, salt, bleach, tetrahydrozoline (Visine), potassium nitrite, or detergent additives. False-positive screening tests may be caused by ibuprofen, naproxen, fenoprofen, efavirenz, and hemp seed oil. Gas chromatography-mass spectrometry is the most sensitive and specific method to confirm drug identity and detects concentrations at 5 ng/ml.

Laboratory tests do not differentiate acute from chronic intoxication. Prescription use of dronabinol can be distinguished from the abuse of marijuana by the presence of Δ-9-tetrahydrocannabivarin, which is only present in the plant material (42).

Plasma THC concentrations do not correlate well with the level of intoxication due to rapid distribution. Plasma levels greater than 10 ng/ml are associated with impairment. Peak plasma THC concentrations range from 46 to 188 ng/ml in adults who smoke marijuana cigarettes containing 8 to 16 mg of THC over a period of approximately 10 minutes. The plasma levels declined rapidly (42).

Urine metabolites of THC are detectable in urine at 1 hour after smoking marijuana. Cannabinoids are detectable for an average of 1 to 2 days and as long as 7 days after a single marijuana cigarette. Smoking an additional marijuana cigarette extends the detection time 1 to 2 days. Chronic users may have detectable metabolites present for 1 to 2 months. Testing by EMIT (EMIT-dau: sensitivity, 20 ng/ml) detected urine cannabinoids for an average of 27 days (maximum, 46 days) after cessation of chronic marijuana use (43). Urine cannabinoid levels fluctuate, and as many as 77 days were required before these levels dropped below the detectable level for 10 consecutive days. A combination of screening by EMIT (specificity, 90%; sensitivity, 95%) and confirmation by gas chromatography-mass spectrometry (specificity, greater than 99.9%, sensitivity, greater than 99.9%) yields almost 100% accuracy in testing for marijuana (44). Ingestion of hemp seed food products, such as snack bars, cookies, and hemp oil, may result in urine that is positive for marijuana at 20 ng/ml using an EMIT (45,46).

Passive inhalation of marijuana smoke is unlikely to result in a positive cannabinoid urine screening test except for heavy prolonged exposure (e.g., the equivalent of 16 marijuana cigarettes in a small room for 1 hour on 6 consecutive days) (47). Nonsmoking subjects who were confined to a room or a car did not develop psychotomimetic symptoms at maximum levels of tolerable smoke (48). It is unlikely that passive inhalation produces a urine concentration of 50 ng/ml. A study of 31 attendees at a rock concert in an enclosed area where marijuana was heavily used did not reveal any positive urine samples for cannabinoids at a detection limit of 50 ng/ml by EMIT drug-abuse urine test (49). Passive inhalation has resulted in 11-carboxy-THC urine levels as high as 39 ng/ml (42).

The five drug classes monitored by the U.S. Substance Abuse and Mental Health Services Administration for the civilian drug-testing program are cocaine, marijuana, amphetamines, PCP, and opiates. The initial testing cutoff for urine cannabinoids is 50 μg/L. The procedure is provided in Table 1.

TABLE 1. U.S. government standards for urine testing of cannabinoids

Initial test

The initial test shall use an immunoassay that meets the requirements of the Food and Drug Administration for commercial distribution. The initial cutoff levels shall be used when screening specimens to determine whether they are negative for these five drugs or classes of drugs.

These cutoff levels are subject to change by the Department of Health and Human Services as advances in technology or other considerations warrant identification of these substances at other concentrations.

Confirmatory test

All specimens identified as positive on the initial test shall be confirmed using gas chromatography-mass spectrometry techniques at the cutoff levels listed for each drug. All confirmations shall be by quantitative analysis. Concentrations that exceed the linear region of the standard curve shall be documented in the laboratory record as "greater than highest standard curve value."

These cutoff levels are subject to change by the Department of Health and Human Services as advances in technology or other considerations warrant identification of these substances at other concentrations. Positive urine tests indicate only the likelihood of prior use and do not correlate with psychomotor impairment. The urine cannabinoid concentration is at best a poor guide to the amount actually taken, as a low level may result from either a large dose taken a long time previously or a small dose taken recently.

Blood Levels and Driving

The major urinary metabolite is 11-nor-Δ-9-carboxy-THC (THC-COOH). THC-COOH has been most often measured to determine the presence and involvement of marijuana in traffic fatalities; however, THC-COOH is not pharmacologically active. Measurement of THC and 11-hydroxy-THC in blood is therefore more likely to be a better indicator of impairment than measurement of THC-COOH in blood or urine. The mean concentrations of THC and 11-hydroxy-THC in the blood of 13 drivers were 5.4 ng/ml and 18 ng/ml, respectively. Plasma levels of THC have been shown to fall rapidly within 1 hour of smoking to approximately 10% of peak concentration and, after 3 to 4 hours, are typically less than 1 ng/ml. The metabolite THC-COOH reportedly appears in blood in higher concentrations for a number of hours after smoking marijuana but well after the psychoactive effects of marijuana have worn off (50).

Acute Overdosage

Prompt urine screening for the presence of cannabinoids and rapid reporting of results may obviate the need for invasive measures such as lumbar puncture, expensive biochemical studies, and computerized tomography. An unexplained coma in a child requires a full work-up, which should not be delayed inappropriately; a broad toxic screen is advised to rule out other toxic agents (24).

A 4-year-old child developed euphoria, nausea, hypotonia, and increasing drowsiness. The Glasgow coma score was 6 of 15. The toxicology screen showed cannabinoids in the blood and urine. An 18-month-old child who had been eating hashish developed coma. Cannabinoids (11-nor-Δ-7-THC-9-carboxylic acid) were present in the blood (41 ng/ml) and urine (332 ng/ml). Both children recovered (51).

Chronic Use

Δ-9-THC is stored largely in adipose tissue and may accumulate faster than it can be eliminated in persistent users. After using three or more joints per day, an individual who then stops smoking marijuana completely and adopts an excessive fitness program mobilizing body fat tests positive for urinary THC at 50 to 100 ng/ml for more than 2 months. Passive inhalation of marijuana smoke by nonusers occasionally results in a urine concentration of 20 ng/ml and rarely as high as 40 ng/ml (44).

TREATMENT

Decontamination

There are no data on the ability of activated charcoal to bind cannabinoids. Because THC toxicity is rarely life-threatening, the risk of gastric emptying outweighs the potential benefit. Ingested marijuana plant material may remain in the gut for a prolonged period of time, and the administration of activated charcoal may be beneficial in preventing absorption of the psychoactive compounds.

Enhancement of Elimination

Due to the large volume of distribution and high protein binding, THC and metabolites are not prone to enhancement of elimination.

Antidotes

There are no specific antidotes for marijuana toxicity.

Supportive Care

Marijuana intoxication is not life-threatening. Agitation, anxiety, and dysphoria may be treated with benzodiazepines. Patients complaining of chest pain should be given supplemental oxygen and evaluated for pulmonary and cardiac complications such as pneumothorax or pneumopericardium. Other drugs of abuse, such as PCP, cocaine, or amphetamine, may have concurrently been used and warrant consideration in the evaluation.

Patients experiencing depressive, hallucinatory, or psychotic reactions should be placed in a quiet room and offered reassurance. Benzodiazepines may be used for the treatment of agitation or anxiety. Hypotension should be treated with Trendelenburg position and intravenous isotonic fluid administration.

REFERENCES

1. Martyn CN, Illis LS, Thom J. Nabilone in the treatment of multiple sclerosis. *Lancet* 1995;345:579.
2. Bhargava HN. Potential therapeutic application of naturally occurring and synthetic cannabinoids. *Gen Pharmacol* 1978;9:195–213.
3. National Institute on Drug Abuse. Marijuana Abuse. Research Report Series. NIH Publication Number 02-3859. Washington, DC; 2002.
4. Webb E, Ashton CH, Kelly P, et al. Alcohol and drug use in UK university students. *Lancet* 1996;348:922–925.
5. Soderstrom CA, Trifillis AL, Shankar DS, et al. Marijuana and alcohol use among 1,023 trauma patients. *Arch Surg* 1988;123:733–737.
6. Du Pont RL, Saylor KE. Marijuana and benzodiazepines in patients receiving methadone treatment. *JAMA* 1989;2611:3409.
7. Lanska DJ, Lanska MJ. PCP use among adolescent marijuana users. *J Pediatr* 1988;113:950–951.
8. Young FL. Opinion and recommended ruling, marijuana rescheduling petition. Washington, DC: Department of Justice, Drug Enforcement Administration, Sep 1988: Docket 86-22.
9. Department of Health and Human Services. Marijuana scheduling petition: denial of petition remand. *Federal Register* 1992;57:10503.
10. Grinspoon L, Bakalar JB, Doblin R. Marijuana, the AIDS wasting syndrome and US government. *N Engl J Med* 1995;333:670–671.
11. U.S. Department of Justice, Drug Enforcement Administration. Marijuana scheduling petition: final order. *Federal Register* 1992;57:10499–10508.
12. U.S. Public Health Service. Denying new requests for medicinal marijuana. *Int Med News Cardiol News* 1992;25:31.
13. Treaster JB. Survey finds marijuana use is up in high schools. *New York Times* 1994 Feb 1.
14. Ashton CH. Pharmacology and effects of cannabis: a brief review. *Br J Psychol* 2001;178:101–106.
15. Editorial Staff. Marijuana. In: Toll LL, Hurlbut KM, eds. *POISINDEX system*. Greenwood Village, CO: Micromedex, 2003.
16. Schwartz RH, Hawks RI. Laboratory detection of marijuana use. *JAMA* 1985;254:788–792.
17. Johansson E, Halldin MM, Agurell S, et al. Terminal elimination plasma half-life of delta^9-tetrahydrocannabinol (delta^9-THC) in heavy users of marijuana. *Eur J Clin Pharmacol* 1989;37:273–277.
18. Zuckerman R, Frank DA, Kingson R, et al. Effects of material marijuana and cocaine use on fetal growth. *N Engl J Med* 1989;320:767–768.
19. Briggs GR, Freeman RK, Yaffe, SJ. *Drugs in pregnancy and lactation*, 6th ed. Baltimore: Williams & Wilkins, 2002:830–840.
20. Richardson GA, Day NL, McGaughey PJ. The impact of prenatal marijuana and cocaine use on the infant and child. *Clin Obstet Gynecol* 1993;36:302–328.
21. Robison LL, Buckley JD, Daigle AE, et al. Maternal drug use and risk of childhood non-lymphoblastic leukemia among offspring: an epidemiologic investigation implicating marijuana (a report from the Children's Cancer Study Group). *Cancer* 1989;63:1904–1910.
22. Birrer RB, Calderon J. Pneumothorax, pneumomediastinum and pneumopericardium following Valsalva's maneuver during marijuana smoking. *N Y State J Med* 1984;84:619–620.
23. Leirer VO, Yesavage JA, Morrow DG. Marijuana carry-over effects on aircraft pilot performance. *Aviat Space Environ Med* 1991;62:221–227.
24. MacNab A, Anderson E, Susak L. Ingestion of cannabis: a cause of coma in children. *Pediatr Emerg Care* 1989;5:238–239.
25. Johnson D, Convadi A, McGuigan M. Hashish ingestion in toddlers. *Vet Hum Toxicol* 1991;33:393.
26. Talbot JA, Teague JW. Marihuana psychosis: acute toxic psychosis associated with the use of cannabis derivatives. *JAMA* 1969;210:299–302.
27. Halikas JA, Goodwin DW, Gage SB. Marijuana use and psychiatric illness. *Arch Gen Psychiatry* 1972;27:162–165.
28. Carney MWP, Bacelle L, Robinson B. Psychosis after cannabis use. *BMJ* 1984;288:1047.
29. Rottanburg D, Robins AH, Ben-Arie O, et al. Cannabis-associated psychosis with hypomanic features. *Lancet* 1982;2:1364–1366.
30. Wu T-C, Tashkin DP, Djahed B, Rose JE. Pulmonary hazards of smoking marijuana as compared with tobacco. *N Engl J Med* 1988;318:347–351.
31. Kagen SL, Kurup VP, Sohnle PG, Fink JN. Marijuana smoking and fungal sensitization. *J Allergy Clin Immunol* 1983;71:389–393.
32. Chesid MJ, Gelfand JA, Nutter C, Fauci AS. Pulmonary aspergillosis, inhalation of contaminated marijuana smoke, a chronic granulomatosis disease. *Ann Intern Med* 1975;82:682–683.
33. Levitz SM, Diamond RD. Aspergillosis and marijuana. *Ann Intern Med* 1991;115:578–579.
34. Baris YI, Tan E, Kalyoncu F, et al. Digital clubbing in hashish addicts. *Chest* 1990;98:1545–1546.
35. Hall W, Solowij N. Adverse effects of cannabis. *Lancet* 1998;352:1611–1615.
36. Kouri EM, Harrison G, Pope G, et al. Changes in aggressive behavior during withdrawal from long-term marijuana use. *Psychopharmacology* 1999;143:302–308.
37. Caplan GA. Marijuana and mouth cancer. *J R Soc Med* 1991;84:386.
38. Taylor FM. Marijuana as a potential respiratory tract carcinogen: a retrospective analysis of a community hospital population. *South Med J* 1988;81:1213–1216.
39. Tashkin DP. Is frequent marijuana smoking harmful to health? *West J Med* 1993;158:635–636.
40. Rubin A, Lemberger L, Warrick P, et al. Physiologic disposition of nabilone, a cannabinol derivative, in man. *Clin Pharmacol Ther* 1977;22:85–91.
41. Foltin RW, Fischman MW, Pedroso JJ, Pearlson GD. Marijuana and cocaine interactions in humans: cardiovascular consequences. *Pharmacol Biochem Behav* 1987;28:459–464.
42. Baselt RC. *Disposition of toxic drugs and chemical in man*, 6th ed. Foster City, CA: Biomedical Publications, 2002:1004–1007.
43. Ellis BM Jr, Mann MA, Judson BA, et al. Excretion patterns of cannabinoid metabolites after last use in a group of chronic users. *Clin Pharmacol Ther* 1985;38:572–578.
44. Stein IN. Marijuana testing. *West J Med* 1988;148:78.
45. Fortner N, Fogerson R, Lindman D, et al. Marijuana-positive urine test results from consumption of hemp seeds in food products. *J Anal Toxicol* 1997;21:476–481.
46. Struempler RE, Nelson G, Urry FM. A positive cannabinoids workplace drug test following the ingestion of commercially available hemp seed oil. *J Anal Toxicol* 1997;21:283–285.
47. Cone EJ, Johnson RE. Contact highs and urinary cannabinoid excretion after passive exposure to marijuana smoke. *Clin Pharmacol Ther* 1986;40:245–256.
48. Morland J, Bugge A, Shuterud B, et al. Cannabinoids in blood and urine after passive inhalation of cannabis smoke. *J Forensic Sci* 1985;30:997–1002.
49. Toussi A. Side-stream inhalation of marijuana: the Grateful Dead experience. *Ann Emerg Med* 1996;27:816–817(abst).
50. Gerostamoulos J, Drummer OH. Incidence of psychoactive cannabinoids in drivers killed in motor vehicle accidents. *J Forensic Sci* 1993;38:649–656.
51. Rubio F, Quintero S, Hernandez A, et al. Flumazenil for coma reversal in children after cannabis. *Lancet* 1993;341:1028–1029.

CHAPTER 179

Inhalant Abuse

Gerald F. O'Malley

See Figure 1.

Compounds included:	**Toluene, amyl nitrite, butyl nitrite, methylene chloride**
Molecular formula and weight:	**Toluene ($C_6H_5CH_3$), 92.138; amyl nitrite ($C_5H_{11}NO_2$), 117.1; butyl nitrite ($C_4H_9NO_2$), 103.1; methylene chloride ($ClCH_2Cl$), 84.93 g/mol**
SI conversion:	**Toluene, mg/L × 10.9 = μmol/L; amyl nitrite, mg/L × 8.5 = μmol/L; butyl nitrite, mg/L × 9.7 = μmol/L; methylene chloride, mg/L × 11.8 = μmol/L**
CAS Registry No.:	**108-88-3 (toluene); 463-04-7 (amyl nitrite); 544-16-1 (butyl nitrite); 75-09-2 (methylene chloride)**
Normal levels:	**Not applicable**
Therapeutic levels:	**Not applicable**
Target organs:	**Central nervous system (acute and chronic), heart (acute), hemoglobin (acute and chronic), kidney (chronic), bone marrow (chronic), peripheral nervous system (chronic), liver (chronic)**
Antidotes:	**Methylene blue, oxygen**

OVERVIEW

Virtually any volatile substance may be inhaled either accidentally or intentionally (Table 1). These substances are contained in an equally diverse array of products (Table 2). The term *inhalant abuse* is used when referring to the recreational use of volatile substances that are not normally ingested by any other route for the purpose of achieving an alteration in mental status (1). This chapter focuses on the inhalational abuse aspects of toluene, inhaled nitrites, and related agents. Inhaled anesthetic agents are addressed in Chapter 129. Methanol is addressed in Chapter 191. Undoubtedly, every chemical that is gaseous under normal conditions has been experimented with by humans.

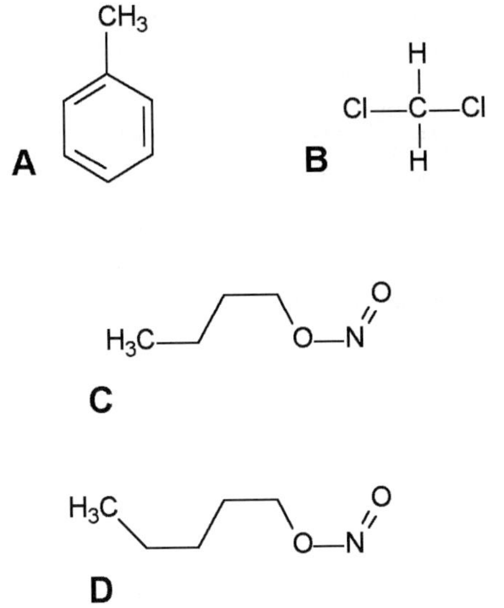

Figure 1. Chemical structures of the abused inhalants. **A:** Toluene. **B:** Methylene chloride. **C:** Butyl nitrite. **D:** Amyl nitrite.

CLASSIFICATION AND USES

One useful classification system divides abused inhalants into four categories:

Volatile solvents include liquids that vaporize at room temperature such as gasoline, kerosene, nail polish, nail polish remover, paint thinner, typewriter correction fluid, felt-tip markers, rubber cement, and shoe polish. Carburetor cleaner contains various combinations of methanol, methylene chloride, and toluene.

Aerosols are sprays that contain propellants and solvents, including spray paints, hair spray, fabric protector spray, vegetable oil spray.

Gases include medical anesthetics as well as gases used in household and commercial products such as chloroform, halothane, and nitrous oxide, which is found in whipped-cream dispensers, butane lighters, and refrigerants.

Nitrites are considered a special class of inhalant because of the unique vasodilator and muscle relaxation effects that are absent from the other classes, which have primarily central nervous system (CNS) effects. Nitrites are used primarily as sexual stimulants, including cyclohexyl nitrite, which is found in room deodorizers; isoamyl (amyl) nitrite; and isobutyl (butyl) nitrite.

Inhalants may be abused in a variety of ways. When an individual pours a liquid substance into a bag or piece of cloth, such as a sock, and then holds the liquid-soaked material up to the face and inhales deeply, it is termed *huffing*. When the substance is sprayed or poured into a bag and the bag placed over the head, the term is *bagging*. Substances may be "sniffed" or "snorted" directly from containers, as is done with nitrous oxide from whipped-cream containers or butane from lighters. Bal-

TABLE 1. Chemicals used for inhalational abuse

Aliphatic hydrocarbons
- Acetylene
- *n*-Butane
- Isobutane (2-methylpropane)
- *n*-Hexane
- Propane

Alicyclic/aromatic hydrocarbons
- Cyclopropane (trimethylene)
- Toluene (toluol, methylbenzene, phenylmethane)
- Xylene (xylol, dimethylbenzene)

Mixed hydrocarbons
- Petrol (gasoline)
- Petroleum ethers

Halogenated compounds
- Bromochlorodifluoromethane (BCF)
- Carbon tetrachloride (tetrachloromethane)
- Chlorodifluoromethane (Halon 22, Propellant 22, Freon 22)
- Chloroform (trichloromethane)
- Dichlorodifluoromethane (Halon 12, Propellant 12, Freon 12)
- Dichloromethane (methylene chloride)
- 1,2-Dichloropropane (propylene dichloride)
- Enflurane (2-chloro-1,1,2-trifluoroethyl difluoromethyl ether)
- Ethyl chloride (monochloroethane)
- Halothane (2-bromo-2-chloro-1,1,1-trifluoroethane)
- Isoflurane (1-chloro-2,2,2-trifluoroethyl difluoromethyl ether)
- Methoxyflurane (2,2-dichloro-1,1-difluoroethyl methyl ether)
- Tetrachloroethylene (perchloroethylene)
- 1,1,1-Trichloroethane (methylchloroform, Genklene)
- Trichloroethylene (trike, Trilene)
- Trichlorofluoromethane (Halon 11, Propellant 11, Freon 11)
- 1,1,2-Trichlorotrifluoroethane (Halon 113)

Nitrites
- Amyl nitrite
- Butyl nitrite
- Cyclohexyl nitrite

Oxygenated compounds
- Acetone (dimethyl ketone)
- Butanone (butan-2-one, methyl ethyl ketone, MEK)
- Diethyl ether (ethoxyethane)
- Dimethyl ether (DME, methoxymethane)
- Ethyl acetate
- Methyl acetate
- Methyl isobutyl ketone (MIBK, isopropyl acetone)
- Methyl-*tert*-butyl ether (MTBE)
- Nitrous oxide (dinitrogen monoxide, laughing gas)

[a]Adapted from Flanagan RJ, et al. *Drug Saf* 1990;5:359–383.

loons may be filled with nitrous oxide and sold for a dollar apiece for consumption by concert- and partygoers (2,3).

Recreational inhalation of volatile chemical vapors is a common problem, particularly among adolescents (4,5). Substances that are commonly abused as inhalants are inexpensive, easily available, legal, easy to conceal, require no complicated paraphernalia, and are perceived erroneously by abusers as relatively harmless (2). There is evidence that abuse of inhalants may lead to the recreational use of other "hard" drugs such as cocaine or heroin (6–8). Inhalant abuse has been reported in virtually every part of the world (1,9–15).

TOXICOKINETICS AND TOXICODYNAMICS

Abused inhalants are always well absorbed by inhalation. Toluene is 50% absorbed after inhalation, with peak blood concentrations at 15 to 30 minutes (16,17). It is absorbed by dermal exposure as well. It is metabolized in the liver with an extraction ratio approaching 1.0; 80% is metabolized to benzoic acid. The benzoic acid conjugates with glycine to form hippuric acid, which is excreted in the urine (18). Approximately 20% of a dose is exhaled unchanged. The terminal elimination half-life is 15 to 72 hours (19).

TABLE 2. Selected products that may be abused by inhalation

Product	Major volatile components
Adhesives	
Balsa wood cement	Ethyl acetate
Contact adhesives	Toluene, hexane, esters
Cycle tire repair adhesive	Toluene and xylenes
PVC cement	Trichloroethylene
Aerosols	
Air freshener	Halons, butane, or dimethyl ether
Deodorants, antiperspirants	Halons, butane, or dimethyl ether
Fly spray	Halons, butane, or dimethyl ether
Hair lacquer	Halons, butane, or dimethyl ether
Paint	Halons, butane, and esters
Anesthetics/analgesics	
Gaseous	Nitrous oxide, cyclopropane
Liquid	Diethyl ether, halothane, enflurane, isoflurane
Local	Halons 11 and 12, ethyl chloride
Commercial dry-cleaning and degreasing agents	1,1,1-Trichloroethane, tetrachloroethylene, trichloroethylene (rarely carbon tetrachloride, 1,2-dichloropropane)
Domestic spot removers and dry cleaners	1,1,1-Trichloroethane, tetrachloroethylene, trichloroethylene
Fire extinguishers	Bromochlorodifluoromethane, Halons 11 and 12
Fuel gases	
Cigarette lighter refills	*n*-Butane, isobutane, propane
Butane	*n*-Butane, isobutane, propane
Propane	Propane, butanes
Nail varnish/nail varnish remover	Acetone, esters
Paints/paint thinners	Butanone, esters, hexane, toluene, xylene
Paint stripper	Dichloromethane, toluene
Surgical plaster/chewing gum remover	Trichloroethylene
Typewriter correction fluids/thinners	1,1,1-Trichloroethane

Modified from Flanagan RJ, et al. *Drug Saf* 1990;5:359–383.

PATHOPHYSIOLOGY

The etiology of the brain injury in volatile solvent inhalant abuse is not fully understood. Injury to the cerebral cortex is believed to be caused by perivascular myelin loss with degeneration of white matter, leading to loss of memory and concentration and personality changes (20). Similar to the pathophysiologic changes seen in the cerebral cortex, cerebellar damage and atrophy are probably due to loss of myelin. Cerebellar injury is reported to cause nystagmus, opsoclonus, and ataxia (21).

Hypoperfusion is believed to play an important role in all aspects of solvent-induced brain injury. Brain perfusion (single-photon emission computerized tomography) scanning from ten teenage patients who were long-term (mean, 48 months) abusers of toluene, benzene, and acetone demonstrated nonhomogeneous ^{99m}Tc-hexamethylpropyleneamine oxime uptake and hypoperfusion areas in all patients, compared with control patients of the same age (22).

PREGNANCY AND LACTATION

Toluene, trichloroethylene, and other volatile solvents and hydrocarbons are very lipid soluble and should cross the placenta easily (23). Exposure *in utero* increases the risk of preeclampsia and spontaneous abortion and may result in a number of fetal abnormalities (24). Fetal solvent syndrome is similar to fetal alcohol syndrome and is characterized by small palpebral fissures, a thin upper lip, micrognathia, ear abnormalities, down-turned corners of the mouth, and hypoplasia of the philtrum and nose (25–27). Infants regularly exposed to solvents during gestation may demonstrate an abstinence phenomenon similar to ethanol withdrawal during the first weeks of life (28).

CLINICAL PRESENTATION

Acute Exposure

"Accidental" death may occur during inhalant abuse via asphyxiation from repeated inhalations that displace oxygen in the alveoli. Similarly, a patient may lose consciousness after placing a solvent-filled bag over the head and suffocate or vomit and aspirate (29). People may also be killed or injured by falling, drowning, or crashing a car while intoxicated by inhalants. Several patients have suffered thermal injuries to the face and respiratory tract due to the concomitant use of volatile inhalants and cigarettes (30).

Inhalation of solvents and aerosols causes intense irritation to the skin of the face and oral and nasal mucosa (31). Respiratory dysfunction may range from mild mucous membrane swelling with congestion and bronchospasm to noncardiogenic pulmonary edema and requirement for assisted ventilation (32).

Sudden sniffing death occurs after the inhalation of butane, propane, fluorocarbon propellants, or trichloroethane (33–36). Initial descriptions of this phenomenon hypothesized that the rapid hemodynamic disruption was caused by irregular rapid cardiac dysrhythmias induced by sensitization of the myocardium to endogenous catecholamines (33). This theory is supported by the observation that sudden death after huffing is often precipitated by a sudden fright or while running to elude capture (35,37). Subsequent case series and animal experiments implicate profound respiratory depression and a direct depressant effect on the sinoatrial node as also having a significant contribution to the sudden sniffing death syndrome (38,39).

Acute inhalational intoxication from toluene primarily affects the CNS, causing a wide variety of effects. The desired effect of inhaling solvents is to achieve an alteration in cognitive functioning that clinically resembles intoxication with ethanol or other sedative-hypnotic compounds. General impairment of psychomotor function, as measured by reaction time, manual dexterity, coordination, and body balance, results after acute exposure to volatile solvents (20). Patients are disinhibited, lethargic, and ataxic, with slurred speech and an inappropriate affect (20). These may be followed in severe cases by confusion, depression of mentation, headache, hallucinations, seizures, ataxia, tinnitus, stupor, and coma. Like other hydrocarbons, toluene may sensitize the myocardium to catecholamine-induced dysrhythmia, which can be lethal. Pulmonary effects include bronchospasm, asphyxia, and aspiration pneumonitis.

Chronic Toxicity

Recurrent inhalant abuse of solvents, aerosols, and gases may result in significant harmful effects on a variety of organ systems. The most devastating effects are to the nervous system. Peripheral nervous system changes are characterized by a stocking-glove sensorimotor neuropathy with prolonged terminal latency and slowed nerve conduction (40,41). Patients who huff and abuse hexane containing glues or other aliphatic compounds or methyl butyl ketone are particularly at risk for the development of peripheral neuropathy, as these compounds are metabolized to toxic intermediates (35).

CNS injury is associated with chronic inhalation of aromatic compounds and is characterized by cranial neuropathies, particularly cranial nerves V and VII (42), and cerebellar destruction as well as injury to the cerebral cortex (43). The CNS is lipophilic and is susceptible to injurious effects of hydrocarbons and other volatile solvents, most of which are highly lipophilic (20). The clinical spectrum of injury varies from mild, reversible personality changes to Parkinson's disease and severe dementia (44).

Long-term exposure to aviation jet fuels, even at low doses, has been associated with the development of pulmonary interstitial fibrosis characterized by reduced lung volumes, decreased diffusing capacity of carbon monoxide, hypoxemia, and respiratory alkalosis. A causative association has not been proved (45).

The most important and common type of renal injury is seen with abuse of toluene-containing glues, paints, and solvents. The proposed mechanism of renal injury is interference with hydrogen ion transport, which causes a type I (distal) renal tubular acidosis (46). Severe hypokalemia due to potassium wasting, hypomagnesemia, hypocalcemia, hypophosphatemia, and a hyperchloremic metabolic acidosis is a common pattern of electrolyte abnormality. In severe cases, patients may develop amino-acid and glucose wasting, rhabdomyolysis, and acute tubular necrosis (32,47).

Hepatic injury in the form of acute chemical hepatitis is associated with abuse of halogenated hydrocarbon–containing inhalants. Chloroform, halothane, and carbon tetrachloride are all known hepatotoxins that are found in commonly abused inhalants (48–50). Multiple studies have failed to demonstrate a consistent pattern of hepatic injury caused by toluene (51). Occupational studies of groups of individuals chronically exposed to a variety of aliphatic and aromatic hydrocarbons describe a pattern of hepatic enzyme elevation and liver biopsy characterized by steatosis, enlarged portal tracts with fibrosis, and necrosis (32,52–54).

Hematologic injury includes several derangements of the blood and bone marrow. The type of derangement may be due to a secondary or tertiary component of the inhaled substance, and it is for this reason that it is important to identify the product accurately. Exposure to nitrate inhalants may cause enough oxidative stress to result in the formation of methemoglobin (Chapter 21) (48). A potentially serious accumulation of carboxyhemoglobin may occur after prolonged exposure to high concentrations of methylene chloride, a component of many paint strippers, degreasers, and solvents (48). The methylene chloride is absorbed and metabolized by the liver to carbon monoxide, so symptoms may be delayed for several hours after exposure (55).

Exposure to benzene during chronic solvent abuse has been associated with bone marrow depression and neoplasia. Acute myelocytic leukemia and multiple myeloma have been reported in chronic benzene exposure in the occupational setting and could be expected to result from chronic exposure during solvent abuse (56). Toluene has, in large part, replaced benzene in many volatile solvents (51). Short- and long-term inhalation of nitrous oxide produces bone marrow depression and megaloblastic hematopoiesis (57).

Immunosuppression may result from chronic inhalation of nitrites by animals or humans, including immunomodulation to predispose to the development of acquired immunodeficiency syndrome and Kaposi's sarcoma (58–61). Brief, intermittent exposure to isobutyl nitrite leads to increased tumor growth in mice (62).

Withdrawal

Chronic inhalant abuse of solvents results in the development of tolerance and psychological addiction (43). There are data to suggest the development of physical addiction, and sudden abstinence may result in a withdrawal syndrome similar to alcohol withdrawal (35,63). Because most volatile inhalants cause CNS depression and inebriation, withdrawal from them is expected to cause symptoms similar to ethanol abstinence with chills, headache, abdominal pain, and muscle cramps. The syndrome may rarely progress to delirium tremens (53).

TREATMENT

Acute Exposure

The patient who presents after the acute inhalation of a volatile anesthetic requires primarily supportive care with attention to the maintenance of a patent airway, adequate breathing, and ventilation (2,35).

Decontamination

Decontamination is not needed except to remove the patient from the source of fumes.

Enhancement of Elimination

Because they are volatile, these drugs are typically eliminated quickly through respiration and in the urine. Attempts to enhance exertion with extracorporeal techniques have not been reported.

Antidotes

There are no specific antidotes to acute or chronic inhalational toxicity. Oxygen or methylene blue may be appropriate for carbon monoxide (Chapter 62) and methemoglobinemia (Chapter 63), respectively.

Supportive Care

Patients who present in cardiac arrest secondary to sudden sniffing death syndrome should be treated the same as any other overdose arrest. At this time, there are inadequate data on the usefulness of alternate therapies in the circumstance of hemodynamic collapse due to volatile solvent exposure to recommend deviation from the standard pharmacologic management of cardiac arrest (63).

Hypotension should initially be treated with isotonic crystalloid fluid resuscitation followed by inotropic support if needed (Chapter 37). Intravascular volume expansion alone has been successful in restoring and maintaining blood pressure.

The decision to administer supplemental bicarbonate, potassium, calcium, and phosphorus is somewhat controversial. In general, the renal defect simply allows the administered electrolytes to be excreted and does not affect the patient's course appreciably.

Chronic Exposure

Several new pharmacologic therapies, such as risperidone, have been used in recent years in the treatment of chronic, recurrent inhalant dependence with mixed results (64). CNS injury, such as nystagmus, postural tremor, dysarthria, ataxia, visual acuity, and handwriting legibility, has reportedly improved after the introduction of amantadine (65). Objective measurements of solvent-induced parkinsonian-type CNS dysfunction similarly improved after surgical ablative therapy (thalamotomy) (66).

REFERENCES

1. Edwards RW, Oetting ER. Inhalant use in the United States. In: Kozel N, Sloboda Z, De La Rosa M, eds. *Epidemiology of inhalant abuse: an international perspective.* National Institute on Drug Abuse Research Monograph 148. DHHS Publication No. NIH 95-3831. Washington, DC: US Government Printing Office; 1995; 8–28.
2. Weiss H. Inhalants & poisons: they're right under your nose. Presented at the North American Congress of Clinical Toxicology Annual Conference. St. Louis: Sep 1997.
3. Done AK. Sniffing, bagging and huffing. *Emerg Med* 1979;9:187–195.
4. Hogan MJ. Adolescent medicine. Diagnosis and treatment of teen drug use. *Med Clinic North Am* 2000;84:927–966.
5. Neumark YD. The epidemiology of adolescent inhalant drug involvement. *Arch Pediatr Adolesc Med* 1998;152:781–786.
6. Davies B, Thorley A, O'Connor D. Progression of addiction careers in young adult solvent misusers. *BMJ* 1985;290:109–110.
7. Young SJ. Inhalant abuse and the abuse of other drugs. *Am J Drug Alcohol Abuse* 1999;25:371–375.
8. Altenkirch H, Kinderman W. Inhalant abuse and heroin addiction: a comparative study on 574 opiate addicts with and without a history of sniffing. *Addict Behav* 1986;11:93–104.
9. Wright SP, Pottier ACW, Taylor JC, et al. *Trends in deaths associated with volatile substances 1971–1989.* London: St. George's Hospital Med School 1991;337:548.
10. Lerner R, Ferrando D. Inhalants in Peru. *NIDA Res Monogr* 1995;148:191–204.
11. Obot JS. Epidemiology of inhalant abuse in Nigeria. *NIDA Res Monogr* 1995;148:175–189.
12. Medina-Mora ME, Berenzon S. Epidemiology of inhalant abuse in Mexico. *NIDA Res Monogr* 1995;148:136–174.
13. Katona E. Inhalant abuse: a Hungarian review. *NIDA Res Monogr* 1995;148:100–120.
14. Baldivieso LE. Inhalant abuse in Bolivia. *NIDA Res Monogr* 1995;148:50–63.
15. Kin F, Navaratnam V. An overview of inhalant abuse in selected countries of Asia and the Pacific Region. *NIDA Res Monogr* 1995;148:29–49.
16. Flanagan RJ, Ruprah M, Meredith TJ, et al. An introduction to the clinical toxicology of volatile substances. *Drug Saf* 1990;5:359–383.
17. Bergman K. Whole-body autoradiography and allied tracer techniques in distribution and elimination studies of some organic solvents: benzene, toluene, xylene, styrene, methylene chloride, chloroform, carbon tetrachloride and trichloroethylene. *Scand J Work Environ Health* 1979;5[Suppl 1]:29–53.
18. Ameno K, Fuke C, Ameno S, et al. A fatal case of oral ingestion of toluene. *Forensic Sci Int* 1989;41:255–260.
19. Brugnone F. Toluene concentrations in the blood and alveolar air of workers during the workshift and the morning after. *Br J Ind Med* 1986;43:56–61.
20. NIOSH (1987). Current intelligence bulletin 48: organic solvent neurotoxicity Publication No. 87-104. Cincinnati: U.S. Department of Health, Education and Welfare, Public Health Service, Center for Disease Control, National Institute for Occupational Safety and Health, DHEW (NIOSH).
21. Rosenberg NL, Kleinschmidt-DeMasters BK, Davis KA, et al. Toluene abuse causes diffuse central nervous system white matter changes. *Ann Neurol* 1988;23:611–614.
22. Kucuk NO, Kilie EO, Ibis E. Brain SPECT findings in long-term inhalant abuse. *Nucl Med Commun* 2000;21:769–773.
23. Danielson BRG, Ghantous H, Denker L. Distribution of chloroform and methyl chloroform and their metabolites in pregnant mice. *Biol Res Preg* 1986;7:77.
24. Wilkins-Haug L, Gabow PA. Toluene abuse during pregnancy: obstetric complications and perinatal outcomes. *Obstet Gynecol* 1991;7:504.
25. Jones HE, Balster RL. Inhalant abuse in pregnancy. *Obstet Gynecol Clin North Am* 1997;25:153–167.
26. Jones HF, Balster RL. Neurobehavioral consequences of intermittent prenatal exposure to high concentrations of toluene. *Neurotoxicol Teratol* 1997;19:305–313.
27. Toutant C, Lippman S. Fetal solvents syndrome. *Lancet* 1979;1:1356.
28. Tenenbein M, Casiro O, Seshia MM, et al. Neonatal withdrawal from maternal volatile substance abuse. *Arch Dis Child* 1996;74:F204.
29. Williams NR, Whittington RM. Death due to inhalation of industrial acetylene. *J Toxicol Clin Toxicol* 2001;39:69–71.
30. Kurbat RS, Pollack CV Jr. Facial injury and airway threat from inhalant abuse: a case report. *J Emerg Med* 1998;16(2):167–169.
31. Brouette T, Anton R. Clinical review of inhalants. *Am J Addict* 2001;10:79–94.
32. Flanagan RJ, Ruprah M, Meredith TJ, et al. An introduction to the clinical toxicology of volatile substances. *Drug Saf* 1990;5:359–383.
33. Bass M. Sudden sniffing death. *JAMA* 1970;212:2075–2079.
34. Ramsey J, Anderson HR, Bloor K, Flanagan RJ. An introduction to the practice, prevalence and chemical toxicology of volatile substance abuse. *Hum Toxicol* 1989;8:261–269.
35. Flanagan RJ, Ives RJ. Volatile substance abuse. United Nations International Drug Control Programme. *Bull Narc* 1994;46:49—78.
36. King GS, Smialek JE, Troutman WE. Sudden death in adolescents resulting from the inhalation of typewriter correction fluid. *JAMA* 1986;253:1604–1606.
37. Wason S, Gibler WB, Hassan M. Ventricular tachycardia associated with non-freon aerosol propellants. *JAMA* 1986;256:78–80.
38. Taylor GJ, Harris WS. Glue sniffing causes heart block in mice. *Science* 1970;170:866–868.

39. Cronk SL, Barkley DEH, Farrell MF. Respiratory arrest after solvent abuse. *BMJ* 1984;290:897–898.
40. Ashton CH. Solvent abuse: little progress after 20 years. *BMJ* 1990;300:135–136.
41. Dittmer DK, Jhamandas JH, Johnson ES. Glue-sniffing neuropathies. *Can Fam Physician* 1993;39:1965–1971.
42. Hormes JT, Filley CM, Rosenberg JL. Neurologic sequelae of chronic solvent vapor abuse. *Neurology* 1986;36:698–702.
43. Balster RL. Neural basis of inhalant abuse. *Drug Alcohol Depend* 1998;51:207–214.
44. Uitti RJ, Snow BJ, Shinotoh H, et al. Parkinsonism induced by solvent abuse. *Ann Neurol* 1994;35:617–619.
45. McKay CA, Hart K, Siddiqi M, et al. Case report: pulmonary interstitial fibrosis associated with inhalation exposure to aviation fuels. *Int J Med Toxicol* 2001;4:20.
46. Patel R, Benjamin J. Renal disease associated with toluene inhalation. *J Toxicol Clin Toxicol* 1986;24:213–223.
47. Carlisle EJF, Donnelly SM, Vasuvattakul S. Glue-sniffing and distal renal tubular acidosis: sticking to the facts. *J Am Soc Nephrol* 1991;1:1019–1027.
48. National Institute on Drug Abuse (NIDA) Research Report: inhalant abuse. NIH Publication No. 3618; 1994, revised July 2000.
49. Kaplan HG, Bakken J, Quadracci L, Schubach W. Hepatitis caused by halothane sniffing. *Ann Intern Med* 1979;90:797–798.
50. Hutchens KS, Kung M. "Experimentation" with chloroform. *Am J Med* 1985;78:715–718.
51. ATSDR (1993). Case studies in environmental medicine 21: toluene toxicity. Atlanta: U.S. Department of Health and Human Services, Public Health Service, 1993.
52. Marjot R, McLeod AA. Chronic non-neurological toxicity from volatile substance abuse. *Hum Toxicol* 1989;8:301–306.
53. Henretig F. Inhalant abuse in children and adolescents. *Pediatr Ann* 1996;25:47–52.
54. Engstrand DA, England DM, Huntington RW. Pathology of paint sniffers' lung. *Am J Forensic Med Pathol* 1986;7:232–236.
55. Shusterman D, Quinlan P, Lawengart R, et al. Methylene chloride intoxication in a furniture refinisher. *J Occup Med* 1990;32:451–454.
56. Aksoy M. Benzene as a leukemogenic and carcinogenic agent. *Am J Ind Med* 1985;8:9–20.
57. Skacel PO, Hewlett AM, Lewis JD, et al. Studies on the hematopoietic toxicity of nitrous oxide in man. *Br J Haematol* 1983;53:189–200.
58. Soderberg LS, Roy A, Flick JT, Barnett JB. Nitrite inhalants spontaneously liberate nitric oxide, which is not responsible for the immunotoxicity in C57BL/6 mice. *Int J Immunopharmacol* 2000;22:151–157.
59. Soderberg LS. Immunomodulation by nitrite inhalants may predispose abusers to AIDS and Kaposi's sarcoma. *J Neuroimmunol* 1998;83:157–161.
60. Haverkos HW. The search for cofactors in AIDS, including an analysis of the association of nitrite inhalant abuse and Kaposi's sarcoma. *Prog Clin Biol Res* 1990;325:93–102.
61. Haverkos HW. Nitrite inhalant abuse and AIDS-related Kaposi's sarcoma. *J Acquir Immune Defic Syndr* 1990;3[Suppl 1]:S47–S50.
62. Soderberg LS. Increased tumor growth in mice exposed to inhaled isobutyl nitrite. *Toxicol Lett* 1999;101:35–41.
63. Ashton CH. Solvent abuse. *BMJ* 1990;300:135–136.
64. Misra LK, Kofoed L, Fuller W. Treatment of inhalant abuse with risperidone. *J Clin Psychiatry* 1999;60:620.
65. Deleu D, Hanssens Y. Cerebellar dysfunction in chronic toluene abuse: beneficial response to amantadine hydrochloride. *J Toxicol Clin Toxicol* 2000;38:37–41.
66. Miyagi Y, Shima F, Ishido K, et al. Tremor induced by toluene misuse successfully treated by a Vim thalamotomy. *J Neurol Neurosurg Psychiatry* 1999;66:794–796.

CHAPTER 180

Heroin, Fentanyl, and Street Opioids

Steven A. Seifert

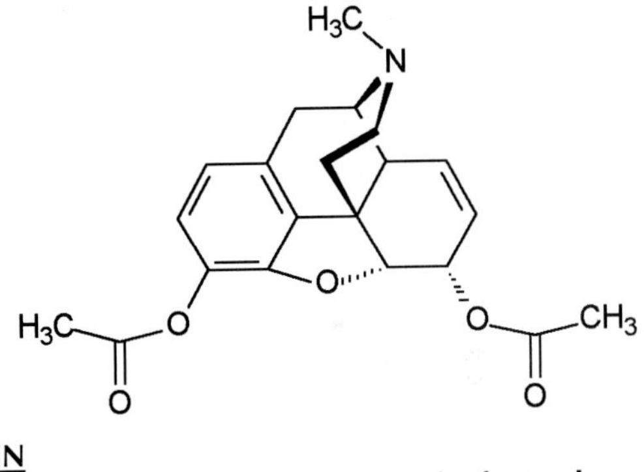

HEROIN

Compounds included:	**Heroin, fentanyl**
Molecular formula and weight:	**Heroin ($C_{21}H_{23}NO_5$,HCl), 423.9; fentanyl ($C_{22}H_{28}N_2O$), 336.5 g/mol**
SI conversion:	**Heroin, mg/L × 2.4 = µmol/L; fentanyl, mg/L × 3.0 = µmol/L**
CAS Registry No.:	**1502-95-0 (heroin); 437-38-7 (fentanyl)**
Therapeutic levels:	**Not used clinically**
Special concerns:	**Users often have sequelae of parenteral drug abuse (e.g., infection, trauma).**
Antidote:	**Naloxone**

OVERVIEW

Street opioids include nonpharmaceutical drugs that are abused for their opioid effects. The most common opioids, heroin and fentanyl derivatives, are addressed in this chapter, whereas prescription drug abuse of opioids is addressed in Chapter 128. Although heroin is the prototypic street opioid, other opioids are abused as street drugs as well. "China White" was originally the name used to describe highly purified heroin but now may be used to describe α-methyl fentanyl. Other fentanyl derivatives, such as 3-methyl fentanyl and para-fluorofentanyl) are also used (1). Counterfeit drugs, manufactured or packaged to look like a legitimate pharmaceutical, may not contain the advertised product in the stated dose and have all of the potential risks of nonpharmaceuticals.

The process of using opioids as drugs of abuse on the street often involves nonsterile subcutaneous, intravenous (IV), and inadvertent intraarterial injection with syringes and needles that may be contaminated with particulates, bacteria, or human blood. Each of these factors carries a health risk that individually and cumulatively results in major morbidity and mortality. Bacterial infections with clostridial species (*Clostridium botulinum, Clostridium tetani, Clostridium novyi*) and injectional anthrax can occur (2–5). Common bacterial infections may occur at the injection site or at remote sites by seeding. Endocardial and cardiac valvular damage can occur. Infection with hepatitis B and C virus, human immunodeficiency virus, or other blood-borne pathogens may be acquired by unsanitary practices. Needle exchange programs are a publicly supported (6) and cost-effective (7,8) way to reduce some of these hazards but suffer from selection effect, inherent or drug-related risk-taking behavior, and philosophic differences in program design and function (9). There is substantial political opposition that takes the view of substance abuse as a criminal act rather than medical illness (8).

Regional epidemic deaths may occur, often in association with higher-than-usual purity or more potent opioid derivatives (10–12). In early 1994, there was resurgence in the use of heroin in the United States. The product became more easily available and of sufficient purity to be used by snorting, similar to cocaine. This was perceived as a safe alternative to injection. However, even when using these drugs orally or by insufflation or inhalation, significant uncertainties and health risks remain regarding dose, drug-drug interactions, underlying medical conditions, polysubstance use, and social and legal risks of illicit drug use.

Heroin users may inadvertently be exposed to a variety of inert or active additives (Table 1). Adulterants are usually benign substances designed to increase profit by dilution of the drug and may include cornstarch, dextrose, and other substances with a similar appearance to the base product. Talc or other powders that are unsuitable for IV use may be used. Contaminants may result from the manufacturing process or are introduced into the drug to mimic the taste or effects of heroin, to counteract some heroin effects, or add desired additional psychoactive effects. Examples include quinine, strychnine, caffeine, and barbiturates (13). Variability and imprecision regarding the identification of substances taken as well as unfamiliar or changing street names for substances may pose data acquisition challenges for clinicians. Patterns regarding the choice of adulterants and contaminants change over time. In recent years, for example, quinine has not been found in survey analyses of street drugs in Denmark or the United Kingdom (13,14).

TABLE 1. Substances detected as heroin additives

Alkaloids	Procaine
Acetylcodeine	Promazine
Narceine	Quinine
Noscapine	Scopolamine
Thebaine	Strychnine
Papaverine	Sulfonamide
Active nonalkaloids	Tolmetin
Acetaminophen	Inert
Allobarbital	Barium sulfate
Aminopyrine	Calcium carbonate
Amphetamine[a]	Calcium tartrate
Arsenic	Dextrin
Caffeine	Dextrose
Chloroquine	Lactose
Cocaine[a]	Magnesium sulfate
Dextromoramide	Silicon dioxide
Diazepam	Sodium carbonate
Diphenhydramine	Starch
Doxepin	Sugar
Fentanyl	Sucrose
Glutethimide	Vitamin C
Indomethacin	Volatile
Lidocaine	Acetaldehyde
Methamphetamine[a]	Acetic acid
Methaqualone	Acetone
Naproxen	Chloroform
Nicotinamide	Diethyl ether
N-phenyl-2-naphthylamine	Ethanol
Phenacetin	Rosin
Phenobarbital	Toluene
Phenolphthalein	Methanol
Piracetam	

[a]Considered frequent additives/coinjectants; absolute frequency unknown.
Modified from Shesser R, Jotte R, Olshaker J. The contribution of impurities to the acute morbidity of illegal drug use. *Am J Emerg Med* 1991;9:336–342.

HEROIN

> Heroin beckons like the sweet seductive calls of Ulysses' sirens. . . . Once experienced [it] is not easy to escape. . . (15).

Heroin is 3,6-diacetylmorphine (diamorphine). It was first synthesized in 1874 (16). Its toxicity is similar to other opioids, and it may also cause myoclonus and seizures. Dependence and abuse potential is high. It is a U.S. Food and Drug Administration (FDA) schedule I substance, determined to have no therapeutic benefit, and is not available in the United States. It is available in the United Kingdom for the treatment of cancer pain and as a maintenance drug of opioid dependency.

Classification and Uses

As a street drug, heroin has no quality control regarding purity, sterility, or dose. Two distinct forms are produced. The drug may be taken by IV, intramuscular (IM), subcutaneous, epidural, inhalation, or oral routes. The hydrochloride salt is a white or beige powder that is highly water soluble (13). Heroin base, the more prevalent form, is often brown or black ("black tar heroin"), is insoluble in water, and requires heating until it liquefies for IV administration. Alternatively, a pyrolysate is generated by heating heroin base on aluminum foil, which is then inhaled ("chasing the dragon"). Heroin users may inadvertently be exposed to a variety of inert or active additives (Table 1), including quinine, strychnine, caffeine, barbiturates, and others (13). Street users may intentionally combine heroin with other psychoactive agents (e.g., cocaine or amphetamine plus heroin, known as a *speedball*). In early 1994, there was resurgence in the use of heroin in the United States. The product became more easily available and of sufficient purity to be used by snorting, similar to cocaine. Two decades ago, the average purity of heroin in the United States was 7%. In 2000, the nationwide average was 36.8%. The availability of South American heroin in the northeastern United States, where purity exceeds 80%, has driven this increase (17).

Illicit laboratories in New Zealand have produced morphine and heroin from commercially available codeine-based pharmaceutical preparations. The codeine demethylation procedure is based on the use of pyridine hydrochloride. The recipe using simple laboratory equipment and reagents requires no chemistry background. The process yields a characteristic product known as *homebake* (18).

Overdosage is prevalent in IV heroin users, with 23% of recent-onset users self-reporting an overdose and 48% reporting being present when an overdose occurred (19). Almost two-thirds of long-term (more than 10 years) heroin users report having self-overdosed (20). Fluctuation in drug purity (21,22) and possibly decreased tolerance secondary to variable periods of voluntary or enforced abstinence (23) increase the risk of overdose. Polydrug use is common, and the combination of drugs with additive central nervous system (CNS) depression, such as ethanol (24), may contribute to morbidity and mortality, as can underlying medical conditions such as hepatic dysfunction and undiagnosed pneumonia, a frequent finding in heroin fatalities (25).

Nonfatal overdoses are common, with 1797 cases reported to regional poison centers in 2001 (26). In Australia, nonfatal heroin overdose resulted in Emergency Medical Services involvement in 59% of cases; 33% required hospital treatment, and 14% required admission (27). Overdoses are frequent in subjects who have used heroin with alcohol, benzodiazepines, cannabis, or amphetamines. In 2001, there were 24 heroin-related fatalities reported to regional poison centers. Seventeen of those cases involved heroin alone and seven in combination with other drugs (26). Heroin laced with phencyclidine (Angel Dust) has led to deaths in New York (28). In New York, symptoms of agitation, hallucinations, paranoia, sinus tachycardia, mild hypertension, dilated pupils, dry skin and mucous membranes, and diminished bowel sounds have followed insufflation of heroin sold as "point on point" and "sting" containing scopolamine (29).

Toxic Dose

The *adult therapeutic dose* of heroin is 2.5 to 10.0 mg IV, IM, or subcutaneously. Epidural doses of 2.5 to 5.0 mg have been used. In neonates, a continuous IV infusion at 50 μg/kg over 30 minutes followed by 15 μg/kg/hour has been used (30). A toxic dose is determined by the concentration of heroin in the product, the route of administration, and the tolerance of the individual to opioids.

TOXICOKINETICS AND TOXICODYNAMICS

Toxicokinetic data for fentanyl and its derivatives are provided in Table 2. Heroin is a prodrug. After IV administration, it is rapidly converted to 6-acetylmorphine (6-AM) and then more slowly to morphine. The plasma half-life is 3 minutes for heroin and 0.6 hour for 6-AM. The half-life of free morphine is 3.6 hours and that of total morphine is 7.9 hours. With oral administration, first-pass metabolism results in only morphine being produced (31). Onset of effects is rapid, with IV users describing a rush of euphoria that is a desired effect. Heroin and 6-AM are lipid soluble and readily penetrate into the brain (31). The volume of distribution is 25 L/kg (32). Inhalation of heroin base pyrrolate produces kinetics similar to IV administration (33). Elimination is primarily by the kidneys, with 70% of the dose excreted in the urine as morphine with small amounts of 6-AM (1%) and parent drug (0.1%). Additional metabolism of morphine results in the active metabolite morphine-6-glucuronide and the inactive metabolites normorphine-3-glucuronide, normorphine, and normorphine glucuronide.

TABLE 2. Toxicokinetic data for the fentanyl derivatives

Analog	Half-life (min) α	Half-life (min) β	Clearance (ml/min)	Volume of distribution (L/kg)
Fentanyl	13–28	90–360	150–575	60–300
Alfentanil	16	100	178–560	40–70
Sufentanil	17	150	730	150

Adapted from Poklis A. Fentanyl: a review for clinical and analytical toxicologists. *J Toxicol Clin Toxicol* 1995;33:439–447.

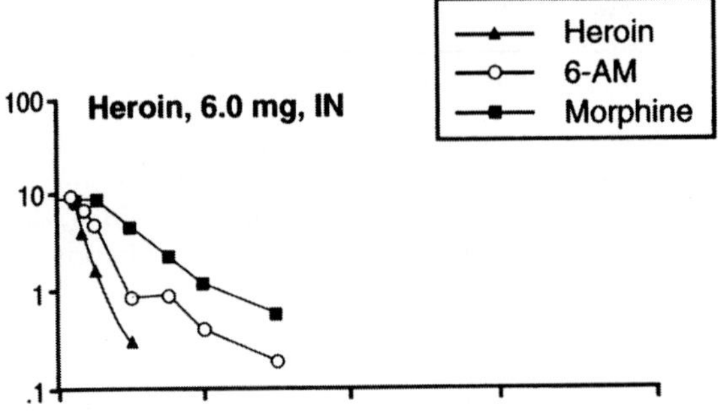

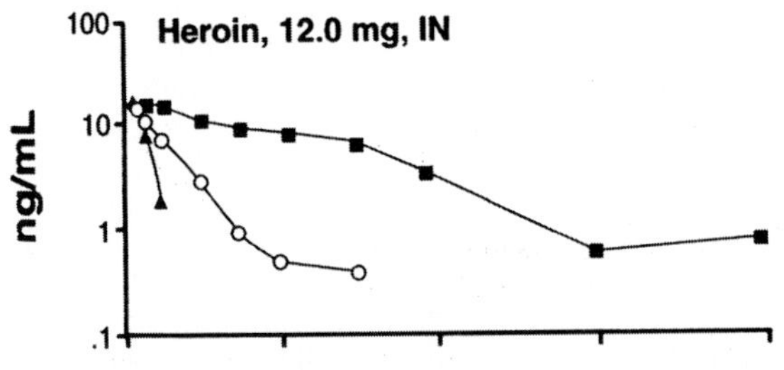

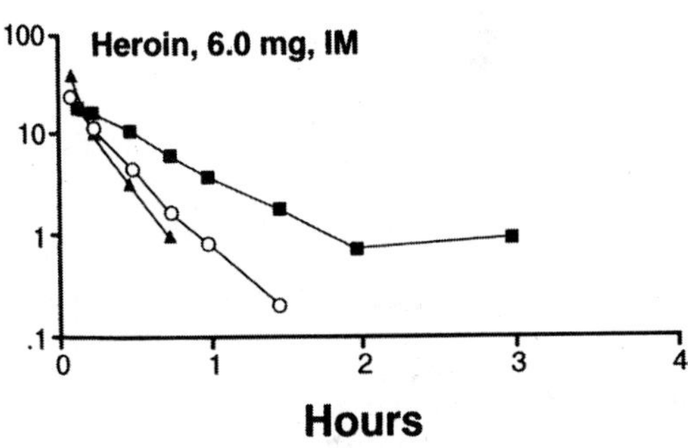

Figure 1. Mean blood concentrations of heroin, 6-acetylmorphine (6-AM), and morphine after administration of heroin hydrochloride by the intranasal (IN) and intramuscular (IM) routes. (From Cone EJ, Holicky BA, Gran TM, et al. Pharmacokinetics and pharmacodynamics of intranasal "snorted" heroin. *J Anal Toxicol* 1993;17:327–337, with permission.)

A recent shift from IV injection to intranasal use ("snorting") has been observed among heroin addicts. Peak levels of heroin, similar to those observed after IM administration, are attained with intranasal administration of 6 mg of heroin (Fig. 1). Physiologic, behavioral, and performance effects after the intranasal route are similar to those after IM use. Intranasal heroin is approximately one-half as potent as IM heroin (34).

PATHOPHYSIOLOGY

The primary toxicity of opiates is mediated through opioid receptors. The types and effects of opioid receptor stimulation and inhibition are provided in Chapter 128.

PREGNANCY AND LACTATION

Heroin is FDA pregnancy category B (Appendix I) (35). It enters breast milk and can produce physiologic dependence in the infant (35).

CLINICAL PRESENTATION

Acute Overdosage

The toxicity of heroin is similar to other opioids (Chapter 128), with CNS and respiratory depression, miotic pupils, and possibly pulmonary edema. Miosis is a variable finding, depending on coingestants and secondary effects such as hypoxia. In addition, heroin may present with myoclonus, seizures, and the additional sequelae of illicit drug use. Seizures are uncommon and may be related to hypoxia or to naloxone use (36). Patients with reactive airway disease can have exacerbations in response to inhalational use (37,38).

Occasionally, no heroin is present in the product, and other drugs are substituted. Agents that have been substituted in the past include pentazocine combined with tripelennamine and dextromethorphan combined with terfenadine (resulting in a fatality) (39). Individuals have used various implanted access ports for illicit drug injection, which may result in a variety of complications related to the type of access (e.g., IV, intrathecal) (40).

The adulterant can also cause an epidemic of adverse reactions, as happened when a batch of heroin was adulterated with scopolamine, producing severe anticholinergic toxicity (29). Cadmium, copper, iron, and zinc have all been found as contaminants in illicit heroin (41) and can contribute their toxicity to the clinical picture. Acetylcodeine, an impurity of illicitly manufactured heroin, elicits seizures, antinociceptions, and locomotor stimulation in mice (42).

Type I hypersensitivity reactions with localized urticaria have been reported, but anaphylaxis is rare. Morphine is a major metabolite of heroin and increases histamine serum levels in 10% of patients (43). Pruritus is common after administration of morphine (44). Cross-reactivity with other opioids is possible.

A delayed encephalopathy may become evident after an overdose. Magnetic resonance imaging a few weeks later may disclose bilateral infarcts in the putamen and caudate. Initial physical and radiographic findings may not predict the outcome (45–47). A cluster of spongiform leukoencephalopathy was reported in the 1980s and was associated with the process of inhalation of heroin pyrolysate (chasing the dragon) (48). Symptoms occurred after as little as 2 weeks of use, and in those who died (approximately 25% of victims), progression occurred over several weeks. Computerized tomography (CT) scanning showed symmetric cerebellar and cerebral white matter destruction (48). In survivors, slow resolution of symptoms is possible. Although numerous contaminants were suspected and sought, the cause has not been determined.

Complications of Drug Abuse

Local infection at injection sites is common. Wound botulism is reported with black tar heroin use (4), and injectional anthrax has been reported (2). Compartment syndrome may occur from prolonged compression secondary to coma (49). Blood-borne diseases may be acquired from the sharing of syringes or needles, including hepatitis B and C and human immunodeficiency virus. Endocarditis and valvular injury may occur secondary to particulates and bacterial contamination.

Natural killer cell activity is reduced in parenteral heroin abusers who are human immunodeficiency virus negative, compared with methadone maintenance patients. This suggests that abnormalities of cellular immunity in parenteral heroin abusers may be normalized by long-term methadone treatment (50).

Heroin is produced in subtropical countries from plants and may be susceptible to contamination by aflatoxins. Urine from IV heroin users may contain aflatoxins. Users risk direct systemic exposure to aflatoxin B, a consequence of which may be suppression of cell-mediated immunity (51).

Body Packers

Heroin body packers are drug smugglers or "mules" who transport large amounts of concentrated heroin from foreign centers by swallowing wrapped packages or inserting packages into the rectum or vagina (Chapter 12). The danger of death from heroin intoxication is the major concern in heroin body packing. McCarron and colleagues studied 14 body packers carrying 2 to 112 heroin packages (52). Nine swallowed the packets, and five inserted them rectally. Three of 20 body packers reported in the medical literature died, probably from absorption of heroin from ruptured packages. Heroin packages may be as large as 3.0 cm × 1.5 cm or 5.0 cm × 2.5 cm. The larger packages may lead to obstruction, initially at the pylorus or later at the ileocecal valve. Patients may have no symptoms, or they may exhibit diffuse abdominal tenderness and a distended abdomen with palpable packages. Simple manual examination, anoscopy, and rectal lavage usually disclose rectally inserted packs of drugs and often indicate smuggling for personal use. Professional smugglers are more liable to swallow packages, in which case the method of choice is plain abdominal radiography or abdominal CT. Magnetic resonance imaging is not generally useful. In uncertain cases, examination of the patient's stool over a period of a few days may be necessary.

Withdrawal Syndrome

Tolerance and dependence may occur, and abuse potential is similar to that of morphine (53).

A withdrawal syndrome is a common feature of the rapid or abrupt discontinuation of heroin and is a marker for physiologic heroin dependence (Chapter 32). Withdrawal signs appear within hours of drug discontinuance and typically last 3 to 7 days. Withdrawal symptoms may also occur in dependent individuals if opioid antagonists or agonist/antagonist agents are given. Withdrawal is generally characterized by drug craving and adrenergic excess. The syndrome is characterized by abdominal cramping, anorexia, diarrhea, generalized pain, gooseflesh, insomnia, lacrimation, restlessness, rhinorrhea, sneezing spells, yawning, and other somatic complaints. In children and adults, withdrawal may produce significant physiologic stress but is only potentially fatal in neonates, in whom seizures may also occur, especially when withdrawal is induced by the use of opioid antagonists.

DIAGNOSTIC TESTS

Analytic Considerations

Plasma drug concentrations are not clinically useful. The fentanyl derivatives pose special diagnostic difficulties because they are not detected by standard immunoassay opioid screening tests (54). In heroin intoxication, the total plasma morphine concentration appears to correlate better with the patient's clinical condition than with the plasma level of free morphine (55). A gas chromatography-mass spectrometry (GC-MS) assay method for quantitation of urinary 6-AM, free morphine, and total morphine is available. The limit of sensitivity for 6-AM is 0.81 ng/ml. After administration of morphine and codeine, no 6-AM is detected by GC-MS above the 0.81 ng/ml detection limit of the assay. Presence of 6-AM in the urine indicates that heroin or 6-AM was administered within 24 hours of specimen collection and that the 6-AM in the urine is not due to morphine or codeine administration (56).

O-6-monoacetylmorphine (6-MAM) is rapidly produced by hepatic catabolism of heroin (diacetylmorphine), and small amounts are excreted in the urine. 6-MAM has not been detected in the urine after the ingestion of codeine, morphine, or poppy seeds (57,58). Therefore, its presence in urine may be considered as a legally defensible evidence of heroin use or of 6-MAM itself (57). Detection of 6-MAM in urine is important for ruling out poppy seed ingestion as a cause of a false-positive result in immunoassay screens for opiates. 6-MAM is not present in poppy seeds or in urine after the ingestion of poppy seeds (59). Codeine is metabolized to morphine. The use of prescription and nonprescription medicine containing codeine can lead to positive immunoassay screening results. Between 20 and 40 hours after codeine ingestion, the ratio of codeine to morphine is less than 1, and norcodeine is not detectable. Three days after codeine use, the urine shows only morphine and is identical to those after heroin or morphine use. Simultaneous determination of 6-MAM, morphine, codeine, and other opiates by GC-MS is sensitive for all components to approximately 10 ng/ml (58).

The blood level of 6-MAM is usually very low or not detectable; stomach content can be used as a substitute in heroin detection (60). The detection of 6-MAM in blood or urine shows recent but single drug use. After more frequent or chronic heroin use, 6-MAM can be detected in hair. Analysis of hair for 6-AM can be used to differentiate heroin users from users of other opiates (e.g., poppy seed, licit morphine, and codeine) (61). Fingernail clippings may also be used to detect past heroin use. Positive radioimmunoassay results were obtained in 25 of 26 users (62), whereas positive high-performance liquid chromatography results were found in 22 of 26 heroin users. GC-MS and radioimmunoassay are the preferred analytic methods. GC-MS detection of 6-MAM in the urine supports the conclusion that heroin was ingested. Because it is so rapidly metabolized, the absence of detectable levels of 6-MAM does not exclude the possibility of heroin ingestion (63).

In a series of deaths suspected to be heroin related, conjugated morphine was found in the blood in all cases (64). In a series of five fatal heroin overdoses, the minimum blood concentration of morphine was 0.021 μg/ml (65). The presence of free morphine in blood indicates a recent heroin injection. Detection of conjugated morphine in blood indicates that life was sustained over a longer period. In most cases of fatal heroin overdoses, 6-MAM has been identified (65).

Body Packers

Plain abdominal radiographs are indicated for suspected body packers (66), but false-negatives can occur (52). CT reliably identifies drug packets (67). Serial examinations may be necessary to document passage of all drug packets.

Heroin urine tests are usually negative in body packers. Urine toxicology may identify the involved drug, but a positive result may not be indicative of the drug being smuggled, and a negative urine toxicologic screen does not exclude the possibility of body packing as, in an otherwise nondrug-using individual, it is only positive if a packet has ruptured. Therefore, it is not possible to determine whether a heroin body packer with heroin detectable in the urine has simply used heroin recently or is absorbing heroin from the packages. The development and severity of a toxidrome may assist in correlating urine toxicology results.

TREATMENT

Treatment of acute toxicity (Chapter 128) and withdrawal is similar to that for other opioids (Chapter 32). The principles of managing acute opioid toxicity are support of respiratory and circulatory function and the administration of naloxone (Chapter 65). Early use of naloxone may obviate the need for intubation. It is wise to anticipate and be prepared for uncooperative and potentially violent behavior after naloxone administration. Higher doses and longer duration of naloxone therapy may be required in neonates (68). Seizures are managed in the standard manner (Chapter 40). The possibilities of self-injurious ideation/action and coingestants should be considered. In addition, the practitioner should evaluate the patient for health risks related to street drug use.

Decontamination

Induced emesis is contraindicated because of the potential for CNS depression and seizures. Activated charcoal may be given for significant ingestion within 1 to 2 hours. A single dose of activated charcoal enhanced systemic clearance of morphine after IV administration in rabbits (69).

Body packers create unique management issues. Gastric emptying should not be used for patients who have ingested heroin packages because of the large size of the packages. Vomiting may cause package obstruction of the proximal esophagus. Endoscopic removal of packages in the stomach should be considered if packages are not progressing into the small bowel. This may produce heroin intoxication, however, if the snare used for removal causes a package to break. Any signs of heroin toxicity should be treated with naloxone (Chapter 65) (57,58).

If foreign bodies are located in the colon, whole bowel irrigation with polyethylene glycol should be considered, although there are insufficient data to support or exclude the use of whole bowel irrigation in this context (Chapter 7) (68). Contraindications include bowel obstruction, perforation, ileus, hemodynamic instability, or a compromised, unprotected airway (68). If used, it should be continued until all packets have passed (70). The first bundle obtained is opened to examine the wrappings and test the core material for heroin and cocaine. Metoclopramide, 10 mg every 8 hours, is used to encourage gastric emptying but is contraindicated in bowel obstruction. Unlike rupture of cocaine drug packets, which require surgical intervention, rupture of heroin drug packets can usually be managed by naloxone.

Indications for surgical consultation are repeated bouts of heroin toxicity, radiologic evidence of retention of packages in the stomach, bowel obstruction, and rupture of cocaine packets. A surgical consult should be obtained early. Urine toxicology screens are performed on all patients and should be repeated periodically if there is suspicion of packet rupture. Patients are not discharged until all packages are accounted for and negative plain abdominal radiographs or abdominal CT are obtained (71).

Disposition

When to discharge a patient who has awakened after naloxone use is based on available evidence, close observation, and practical considerations. The half-life of naloxone is approximately 20 minutes, with an effective duration of action of 1 to 2 hours. Discharge is appropriate for nonsuicidal patients who awaken after a bolus of naloxone, do not require additional naloxone beyond 2 hours after their last bolus, and do not have complicating medical problems. Patients who have taken a long-acting opioid, require multiple naloxone doses or an IV infusion, are suicidal, or develop other complications (e.g., pulmonary edema, aspiration) should generally be admitted.

Withdrawal

Treatment of withdrawal is generally symptomatic and supportive. If precipitated by the administration of naloxone, the patient should be observed until symptoms abate. Management of protracted withdrawal secondary to the use of a long-acting opioid antagonist in the dependent individual is also symptomatic and supportive (Chapter 32). The administration of additional opioids is contraindicated. The use of anxiolytics, clonidine, antiemetics, and other supportive and symptomatic medications may be considered.

Withdrawal symptoms in neonates born to heroin-dependent mothers should be anticipated. Naloxone is contraindicated. Titration of substitution opioids and careful dose tapering can reduce the incidence of complications of withdrawal in neonates (72).

Long-term treatment of opioid dependence is controversial, and there are frequent treatment failures and relapses. In one review, more than 17 different types of treatment approaches were identified (73). Patients may be maintained on a long-acting opioid agonist/antagonist, such as methadone or L-alpha-acetyl methadol, or slowly tapered while on such therapy to minimize the discomfort of withdrawal. Patients stay in treatment longer with methadone regimens than with management of withdrawal with α_2-adrenergic agonists (74).

Methadone maintenance suppresses opioid withdrawal and blocks and attenuates the effects of heroin (75). It is used for long-term maintenance of opioid dependency and in tapered withdrawal programs. A dose of 120 mg methadone completely suppressed withdrawal and fully attenuated the effects of heroin, whereas doses of 30 mg and 60 mg failed to fully block heroin's effects, perhaps helping to explain the frequent co-use of heroin in lower-dose methadone maintenance regimens (75). Buprenorphine is an alternative agent for opioid replacement and withdrawal and was used successfully to withdraw a 4-month-pregnant patient from heroin (76).

Management Pitfalls

Release of patients too quickly after revival by naloxone may result in recurrent CNS and respiratory depression.

REFERENCES

1. Ziporyn T. A growing industry and menace: makeshift laboratory's designer drugs. *JAMA* 1986;256:3061–3063.
2. Ringertz SH, Hoiby EA, Jensenius M, et al. Injectional anthrax in a heroin skin-popper. *Lancet* 2000;356:1574–1575.
3. Cherubin CE. Epidemiology of tetanus in narcotic addicts. *N Y State J Med* 1970;70:267–271.
4. Passaro DJ, Werner SB, McGee J, et al. Wound botulism associated with black tar heroin among injecting drug users. *J Am Med Assoc* 1998;279:859–863.
5. Ahmed S, Gruer L, McGuigan C, et al. Update: clostridium novyi and unexplained illness among injecting-drug users—Scotland, Ireland, and England, April–June 2000. *MMWR Morb Mortal Wkly Rep* 2000;49:543–545.
6. Orner MB, Meehan T, Brooks DR, et al. Support for condom availability and needle exchange programs among Massachusetts adults, 1997. *AIDS Educ Prev* 2001;13:365–376.
7. Laufer FN. Cost-effectiveness of syringe exchange as an HIV prevention strategy. *J Acquir Immune Defic Syndr* 2001;28:273–278.
8. Yoast R, Williams MA, Deitchman SD, Champoin HC. Report of the Council on Scientific Affairs: methadone maintenance and needle-exchange programs to reduce the medical and public health consequences of drug abuse. *J Addict Dis* 2001;20:15–40.
9. Strike CJ, Myers T, Millson M. Needle exchange: how the meanings ascribed to needles impact exchange practices and policies. *AIDS Educ Prev* 2002;14:126–137.
10. Kram TC, Cooper DA, Allen AC. Behind the identification of China White. *Anal Chem* 1981;3:1379A–1386A.
11. Hibbs J, Perper J, Winek CL. An outbreak of designer drug-related deaths in Pennsylvania. *JAMA* 1991;265:1011–1013.
12. Martin M, Hecker J, Clark R, et al. China White epidemic: an eastern United States emergency department experience. *Ann Emerg Med* 1991;20:158–164.
13. Kaa E. Impurities, adulterants and diluents of illicit heroin. Changes during a 12-year period. *Forensic Sci Int* 1994;64:171–179.
14. O'Neil PJ, Pitts JE. Illicitly imported heroin products (1984–1989): some physical and chemical features indicative of their origin. *J Pharm Pharmacol* 1992;44:1–6.
15. Cyngler C. The heroin addict! A personal view. *Aust Fam Physician* 2002;31:371–373.
16. Sovner R, Wolfe J. Interaction between dextromethorphan and monoamine oxidase inhibitor therapy with isocarboxazid. *N Engl J Med* 1988;319:1671.
17. Drug Enforcement Administration. Drug trafficking in the United States. http://www.usdoj.gov/dea/pubs/state_factsheets.html.
18. Treaster JB. With supply and purity up heroin use expands. *New York Times* 1993 Aug 1.
19. Gossop M, Griffiths P, Powis B, et al. Frequency of non-fatal heroin overdose: survey of heroin users recruited in non-clinical settings. *BMJ* 1996;313:402.
20. Darke S, Ross J, Hall W. Overdose among heroin users in Sydney, Australia. I: prevalence and correlates of non-fatal overdose. *Addiction* 1995;91:405–411.
21. Darke S, Hall W, Weatherburn D, et al. Fluctuations in heroin purity and the incidence of fatal heroin overdose. *Drug Alcohol Depen* 1999;754:155–161.
22. Risser D, Uhl A, Stichenwirth M, et al. Quality of heroin and heroin-related deaths from 1987 to 1995 in Vienna, Austria. *Addiction* 2000;95:375–382.
23. Seaman SR, Brettle RP, Gore SM. Mortality from overdose among injection drug users recently released from prison: database linkage study. *BMJ* 1998;316:426–428.
24. Ruttenber AJ, Kalter HD, Santinga P. The role of ethanol abuse in the etiology of heroin-related death. *J Forensic Sci* 1990;35:891–900.
25. Warner-Smith M, Darke S, Lynskey M, et al. Heroin overdose: causes and consequences (review). *Addiction* 2001;96:1113–1125.
26. Litovitz TL, Klein-Schwartz W, Rodgers GC, et al. 2001 Annual report of the American Association of Poison Control Centers Toxic Exposure Surveillance System. *Am J Emerg Med* 2002;20(5):391–452.
27. Warner-Smith M, Darke S, Day C. Morbidity associated with non-fatal heroin overdose. *Addiction* 2002;97:963–967.
28. Treaster JB. 7 Hospitalized in Bronx after using heroin mix: police warn users of potent new blend. *New York Times* 1995 Mar 18.
29. Hamilton RJ, Perrone J, Hoffman R, et al. A descriptive study of an epidemic of poisoning caused by heroin adulterated with scopolamine. *J Toxicol Clin Toxicol* 2000;38:597–608.
30. Elias-Jones AC, Barrett DA, Rutter N, et al. Diamorphine infusion in the preterm neonate. *Arch Dis Child* 1991;66:1155–1157.
31. Inturrisi CE, Max MB, Foley KM, et al. The pharmacokinetics of heroin in patients with chronic pain. *N Engl J Med* 1984;310:1213–1217.
32. Baselt RC. *Disposition of toxic drugs and chemicals in man*, 5th ed. Davis, CA: Biomedical Publications, 2000.
33. Jenkins AJ, Keenan RM, Henningfield JE, Cone EJ. Pharmacokinetics and pharmacodynamics of smoked heroin. *J Anal Toxicol* 1994;18:317–330.
34. Cone EJ, Holicky BA, Grant TM, et al. Pharmacokinetics and pharmacodynamics of intranasal "snorted" heroin. *J Anal Toxicol* 1993;17:327–337.
35. Briggs GG, Freeman RK, Yaffe SJ. *Drugs in pregnancy and lactation: a reference guide to fetal and neonatal risk*, 6th ed. Philadelphia: Lippincott Williams & Wilkins, 2002.
36. Remskar M, Noc M, Leskovsek B, et al. Profound circulatory shock following heroin overdose. *Resuscitation* 1998;38:51–53.
37. Cygan J, Trunsky M, Corbridge T. Inhaled heroin-induced status asthmaticus. Five cases and a review of the literature. *Chest* 2000;117:272–275.
38. Prachand N, Krantz A, Franklin C, et al. Severe asthma associated with heroin insufflation. *J Toxicol Clin Toxicol* 1999;37:646(abst).
39. Kintz P, Mangin P. Toxicological findings in a death involving dextromethorphan and terfenadine. *Am J Forensic Med Pathol* 1992;13:351–352.
40. Burton AW, Conroy B, Garcia E, et al. Illicit substance abuse via an implanted intrathecal pump. *Anesthesiology* 1998;89:1264–1267.
41. Infante F, Dominguez E, Trujillo D, et al. Metal contamination in illicit samples of heroin. *J Forensic Sci* 1999;44:110–113.
42. O'Neal CL, Poklis A, Lichtman AH. Acetylcodeine, an impurity of illicitly manufactured heroin, elicits convulsions, antinociception, and locomotor stimulation in mice. *Drug Alcohol Depend* 2001;65:37–43.
43. Flacke JW, Flacke WE, Bloor BC, et al. Histamine release by four narcotics: a double-blind study in humans. *Anesth Analg* 1987;66:723–730.
44. Larijani GE, Goldberg ME, Rogers KH. Treatment of opioid-induced pruritus with ondansetron: report of four patients. *Pharmacotherapy* 1996;16(5):958–960.
45. McDonald FW, Cienki JJ, Horowitz, et al. Delayed encephalopathy after heroin use. *J Toxicol Clin Toxicol* 1995;33:478–485(abst).
46. Chen CY, Lee KW, Lee CC, et al. Heroin-induced spongiform leukoencephalopathy: value of diffusion MR imaging. *J Comp Assist Tomogr* 2000;24:735–737.
47. Hill MD, Cooper PW, Perry JR. Chasing the dragon—neurological toxicity associated with inhalation of heroin vapour: case report. *Can Med Assoc J* 2000;162:236–238.
48. Wolters ECH, van Wijngaarden GK, Stam FC. Leucoencephalopathy after inhaling "heroin" pyrolysate. *Lancet* 1982;2:1233–1237.
49. Franc-Law JM, Rossignol M, Vernec A, et al. Poisoning-induced acute atraumatic compartment syndrome. *Am J Emerg Med* 2000;18(5):616–621.
50. Novick DM, Ochshorn M, Ghali V, et al. Natural killer cell activity and lymphocyte subsets in parenteral heroin abusers and long-term methadone maintenance patients. *J Pharmacol Exp Ther* 1989;250:606–610.

51. Hendrickse RG, Maxwell SM, Young R. Aflatoxins and heroin. *BMJ* 1989;299:492–493.
52. McCarron MM, Wood JD. The cocaine body packer syndrome. *JAMA* 1983;250:1417–1420.
53. Kaiko RF, Wallenstein SL, Rogers AG, et al. Analgesic and mood effects of heroin and morphine in cancer patients with postoperative pain. *N Engl J Med* 1981;304:1501–1505.
54. Brittain JL. China White: the bogus drug. *J Toxicol Clin Toxicol* 1983;19:1123–1126.
55. Gutierrez-Cebollada, Cami J, de la Torre R. Heroin intoxication: the relation between plasma morphine concentration and clinical status at admission. *Eur J Clin Pharmacol* 1991;40:635.
56. Cone EJ, Welch P, Mitchell JM, Paul BD. Forensic drug testing for opiates: 1. Detection of 6-acetylmorphine in urine as an indication of recent heroin exposure: drug and assay considerations and detection times. *J Anal Toxicol* 1991;15:1–7.
57. Mofenson HC, Caraccio TR. Continuous infusion of intravenous naloxone. *Ann Emerg Med* 1987;16:600.
58. Goldfrank L, Weisman RS, Errick JK, Lo M-W. A dosing nomogram for continuous infusion intravenous naloxone. *Ann Emerg Med* 1986;15:566–570.
59. Wang M-L, Lin JL, Liau S-J, Bullard RJ. Heroin in lung: report of two cases. *J Formosa Med Assoc* 1994;93:170–172.
60. Havier RG, Lin R-L. Confirmation of heroin use by stomach content analysis. In: Proceedings, 46th Annual Meeting, American Academy of Forensic Sciences; 1994 Feb 14:188.
61. Goldberger BA, Caplan YH, Maguire T, Cone IJ. Testing human hair for drugs of abuse: III. Identification of heroin and 6-acetylmorphine as indicators of heroin use. *J Anal Toxicol* 1991;15:222–231.
62. Lemos NP, Anderson RA, Valentini R, et al. Analysis of morphine by RIA and HPLC in fingernail clippings obtained from heroin users. *J Forensic Sci* 2000;45:407–412.
63. United States Department of Transportation Employers' Guide to 49 CFT. Part 40: procedures for transportation workplace drug testing programs; 1989 Oct.
64. Lora-Tomayo C, Tena T, Tena G. Concentrations of free and conjugated morphine in blood in twenty cases of heroin-related deaths. *J Chromatogr Biomed Appl* 1987;422:267–273.
65. Kintz P, Mangin P, Lugnier AA, et al. Toxicological data after heroin overdose. *Hum Toxicol* 1989;8:487–489.
66. Hieholzer J, Cordes M, Tantow J, et al. Drug smuggling and ingested cocaine filled packages: conventional x-ray and ultrasound. *Abdom Imaging* 1995;20:333–338.
67. Meyers MA. The inside dope: cocaine, condoms and computed tomography. *Abdom Imaging* 1995;20:339–340.
68. Tenenbein M. Position statement: whole bowel irrigation. American Academy of Clinical Toxicology; European Association of Poisons Centres and Clinical Toxicologists. *J Toxicol Clin Toxicol* 1997;35:753–762.
69. El-Sayed YM, Hasan MM. Enhancement of morphine clearance following intravenous administration by oral activated charcoal in rabbits. *J Pharm Pharmacol* 1990;42:538–541.
70. Olmedo R, Nelson L, Chu J, Hoffman RS. Is surgical decontamination definitive treatment of "body-packers"? *Am J Emerg Med* 2001;19:593–596.
71. Utrecht MJ, Stone AF, McCarron MM. Heroin body packers. *J Emerg Med* 1993;11:33–40.
72. Suresh S, Anand KJ. Opioid tolerance in neonates: mechanisms, diagnosis, assessment, and management. *Semin Perinatol* 1998;22:425–433.
73. Gowing LR, Ali RL, White JM. Systematic review processes and the management of opioid withdrawal. *Aust N Z J Public Health* 2000;24:427–431.
74. Gowing L, Ali R, White J. Opioid antagonists with minimal sedation for opioid withdrawal. *Cochrane Database Syst Rev* 2002:CD002021.
75. Donny EC, Walsh SL, Bigelow GE, et al. High-dose methadone produces superior opioid blockade and comparable withdrawal suppression to lower doses in opioid-dependent humans. *Psychopharmacology (Berl)* 2002;161:202–212.
76. Marquet P, Chevrel J, Lavignasse P, et al. Buprenorphine withdrawal syndrome in a newborn. *Clin Pharmacol Ther* 1997;62(5):569–571.

PART

IV

Chemicals

SECTION

1

Respiratory Toxicology

CHAPTER 181

Toxicology of the Lung

João H. Delgado and Scott D. Phillips

OVERVIEW

The lung is a potential target for injury due to its large surface area, volume of air intake (approximately 10,000 L/day), and high blood cardiac output (approximately 7000 L/day) (1). The lung may be affected directly by inhalation of substances injurious to the respiratory tract or from absorption of toxic agents through another route (dermal absorption, ingestion, injection) that ultimately targets the lung for injury. The lung may also serve as a route of absorption for substances that have nonrespiratory effects.

ANATOMY AND PHYSIOLOGY OF THE LUNG

Structure

The intrapulmonary respiratory tract can be conceptualized as consisting of three sections (Fig. 1) (2). The *cartilaginous airways* (trachea and bronchi) are relatively rigid and nondistensible tubes lined with ciliated epithelium. They serve to conduct air to and from the gas-exchange zones of the lung and are responsible for most of the airway resistance in the normal lung. They also serve a defensive function by trapping particulates in the mucus layer and transporting them proximally to the oropharynx where they are swallowed or expectorated (the so-called mucociliary escalator). The *membranous airways* are composed of the respiratory bronchioles, which serve the dual purpose of gas conduction and gas exchange. They lead to *alveolar ducts and sacs*, which are the main areas of gas exchange in the lung.

The pulmonary vasculature parallels the organization of the airways. With each successive branching of the airways, there are branchings of arterial vessels as well. The pulmonary arteries carry deoxygenated systemic blood from the right side of the heart to the gas-exchange region of the lung. The venous return similarly parallels the airways and returns oxygenated blood to the left atrium via the pulmonary veins. The blood supply of the conducting airway cells comes from the bronchial circulation, which arises directly from the aorta or from intercostal branches. The pulmonary circulation itself provides the blood supply for the airway cells distal to the terminal bronchioles.

The lymphatic vessels serve a key role both in fluid homeostasis of the lung and immunologic defense. Excess fluid is collected by capillary lymphatic vessels, transported proximally, and ultimately returned to systemic venous circulation via the thoracic duct. Drainage of lymph into regional lymph nodes of the hila, trachea, and bronchi serves an important function in immunosurveillance.

Respiratory Tract Cell Types

More than 40 different types of respiratory tract cells have been identified. The five major cell populations of the lung include the type I and type II alveolar epithelial cells, capillary endothelial cells, alveolar macrophages, and interstitial cells. These cells form the basic structures underlying gas exchange in the lung. Two other cell types, Clara cells and neuroendocrine cells, are of particular interest to the toxicologist because they appear to play important roles in xenobiotic metabolism and carcinogenesis (3).

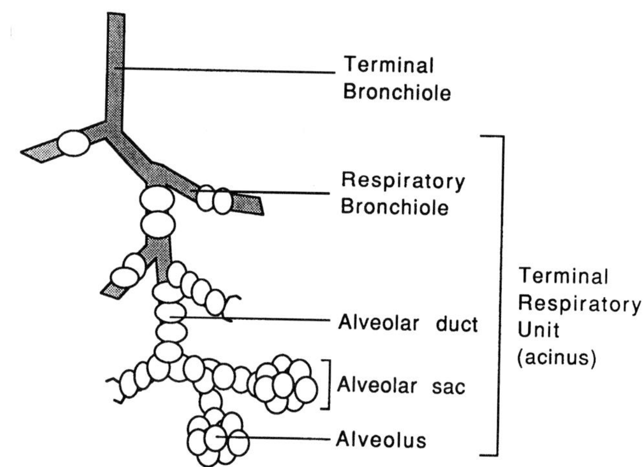

Figure 1. Anatomy of the gas-exchange zone of the lung. Gas exchange begins at the level of the respiratory bronchiole. (From Newman LS. Clinical pulmonary toxicology. In: Sullivan JB, Krieger GR, eds. *Clinical environmental health and toxic exposures*, 2nd ed. Philadelphia: Lippincott Williams & Wilkins, 2001:207, with permission.)

The respiratory tract serves an important function in xenobiotic metabolism. Phase I enzymes, which catalyze oxidation reactions, include cytochrome P-450 monooxygenases and reductases, epoxide hydrolases, and flavin-containing monooxygenases. Phase II enzymes, which catalyze conjugation reactions, include dehydrogenases, esterases, and numerous transferases (4). These enzymes are found to varying degrees in the different cell populations of the respiratory tract. Although the metabolism of a xenobiotic usually results in detoxification, metabolism (particularly by phase I enzymes) may result in bioactivation with potential tissue injury.

Alveolar type I epithelial cells comprise 8% of the parenchymal cell population and cover more than 90% of the alveolar surface. They form a thin layer of epithelial lining across which gas can diffuse efficiently to and from capillaries. Compared with other pulmonary cell types, type I cells expose the largest percentage of their surface to inhaled substances. In addition, their relative lack of cytoplasmic organelles and the long distance between their cytoplasmic processes and cell nucleus contribute to their vulnerability to injury by inhaled and blood-borne agents. Injury to the pulmonary epithelial cells by various toxic agents is summarized in Table 1.

Alveolar type II epithelial cells are cuboidal cells that cover 7% of the alveolar surface and represent 16% of the total cell population. They synthesize and secrete surfactant, a key determinant of lung compliance. In addition to producing surfactant, type II cells are able to differentiate into type I cells and replace damaged cells.

Interstitial cells (fibroblasts, lymphocytes, interstitial macrophages, mast cells, pericytes, and plasma cells) occupy the interstitial space and represent approximately 37% of the lung cell population. Some substances induce fibroblast proliferation and an increase in collagen production, resulting in interstitial pulmonary fibrosis. This may follow lung damage induced by airborne substances, including oxidant gases, dusts, and fibers (asbestos, silica), or blood-borne agents such as antineoplastic drugs.

Capillary endothelial cells are the largest single cell population in the lung, comprising 30% of all human lung cells. They form the first line of defense against blood-borne toxicants.

Alveolar macrophages serve a crucial role in the clearance of inhaled foreign substances that reach the alveoli as well as defense against pathogenic organisms. When their function is compromised by certain inhaled substances, there may be increased susceptibility to infections. They are also involved in the development and pathogenesis of chronic lung disease, such as silicosis and asbestosis, through the release of cytokines (5).

TABLE 1. Pulmonary epithelial cell injury

Agent	Target cell
Inhalants	
Nitrogen dioxide	Endothelium, type I epithelium
Oxygen (hyperoxia)	Endothelium
Ozone	Endothelium
Drugs	
Amiodarone	Endothelium
Bleomycin	Type I and II epithelium
Doxorubicin	Type I and II epithelium
Nitrofurantoin	Type I and II epithelium
Other	
Endotoxemia	Endothelium
Paraquat	Type I and II epithelium
X-irradiation	Endothelium

Adapted from Smith LL, et al. *Arch Toxicol* 1986;58:214-218.

Clara cells (nonciliated bronchiolar cells) have a substantial agranular cytoplasmic reticulum and function as the primary secretory cell type in the conducting airway of the centriacinar region (terminal bronchioles). The Clara cell is able to replicate itself or differentiate into a ciliated cell. It is the primary site of cytochrome P-450 monooxygenase activity within the lungs. Naphthalene, 4-ipomeanol, 3-methylfuran, methylindole, and carbon tetrachloride may induce toxicity in the Clara cells after metabolic activation by the cytochrome P-450 monooxygenase system (5).

Neuroendocrine cells are also known as *APUD cells* (amine precursor uptake and decarboxylation) or *Kulchitsky's cells*. They are found in the mucosa lining the airways or in the pulmonary parenchyma and proliferate in response to hyperoxia (6).

Physiology

The lung has three major functions. *Ventilation* is the process of moving air through the respiratory tract to the gas-exchange zone. This involves a complex process that requires coordination between diaphragm and thoracic cage muscles and is dependent on the elastic properties of the lung and thoracic cage. Ventilation abnormalities can arise from mechanical obstruction of the airways (e.g., sloughing of necrotic epithelium), derangement of the normal elastic properties of lung and thoracic cage (e.g., high-dose fentanyl), and impairment of central respiratory drive (e.g., opioids).

Gas exchange involves oxygenation of blood and removal of carbon dioxide that accumulates as a result of the body's various metabolic processes. The barrier to physiologic gas exchange is comprised of the alveolar epithelium, the interstitium, and the capillary endothelium. Substances that affect any one of these components may result in significant impairment of gas exchange. Because carbon dioxide has a greater diffusion capacity than oxygen, hypoxia typically precedes hypercarbia after parenchymal lung injury.

Nonventilatory functions include removal of inhaled substances or particles, biotransformation, secretion of hormones and other mediators, and removal of vasoactive peptides.

PATHOPHYSIOLOGY OF LUNG INJURY

A detailed discussion of the various mechanisms of lung injury is beyond the scope of this chapter. However, because of their importance in the initiation and propagation of lung injury, inflammation and oxidant stress are briefly reviewed.

Inflammation

Inflammation is normally a localized physiologic response to injury that serves to eliminate the source of injury and facilitate the organism's repair mechanisms (7). More specifically, the response of vascularized tissue to injury has three major components: increased blood flow to the injured area as a result of vasodilation, increased vascular permeability that results in extravasation of plasma proteins and leukocytes, and migration of leukocytes from the vasculature to the site of injury (8). This initial response is aimed at removing the inciting stimulus but also sets the stage for the reparative processes that follow. The early neutrophilic infiltrate that characterizes most acute inflammation reactions is gradually replaced by macrophages and mononuclear cells over time. Eventually, the native tissue is regenerated or replaced by connective tissue.

Cytokines are a group of relatively small proteins (6 to 30 kd) that serve as communication signals between cells and are key regulators of inflammation. For example, tumor necrosis factor-α has been implicated in the pathogenic response in the lung associated with a variety of substances, including asbestos, beryllium, coal dust, ozone, and quartz, among others. Although a number of cells can produce the cytokine, alveolar macrophages are probably the most important source within the lung (7). Tumor necrosis factor-α increases the expression of adhesion molecules in vascular endothelium as well as the secretion of interleukin (IL)-1, IL-6, platelet-derived growth factor, and transforming growth factor-β. It also stimulates the production of other inflammatory mediators such as prostaglandins and reactive oxygen species (ROS). One way in which cytokines mediate the propagation of the inflammatory response is through the recruitment of leukocytes. For example, transforming growth factor-β and platelet-derived growth factor are potent chemoattractants for monocytes and neutrophils, respectively. Finally, some cytokines are also involved in the resolution of the inflammatory response through their antiinflammatory effects. A number of such cytokines have been identified and include IL-4, IL-6, IL-10, IL-11, and IL-1 receptor antagonists (7).

Oxidant Stress

Free radicals are atoms or molecules that contain one or more unpaired electrons, making them highly reactive. Much of the free-radical production within the lung originates with molecular oxygen. In biologic systems, oxygen is typically reduced to water. Partial reduction results in formation of the highly reactive superoxide anion (O_2^-), which itself can lead to the formation of other reactive nucleophiles such as hydrogen peroxide (H_2O_2) and the hydroxyl radical (OH^-). Collectively, these molecules are termed *ROS* and are particularly important sources of injury in the lung because of the relatively high oxygen tension present within the respiratory tract.

Under normal physiologic conditions, the most important source of intracellular ROS is electron "leak" from nicotinamide adenine dinucleotide dehydrogenase and from the ubiquinone Q–cytochrome-*b* complex within the mitochondria. Extracellularly, most ROS are generated by alveolar macrophages and other immune cells, although cells lining the respiratory tract and microvascular endothelial cells also contribute to the process. In addition to this physiologic oxidative burden, a large number of inhaled substances are capable of augmenting the constitutive production of ROS, thereby inducing oxidative stress.

Oxidants may interact with various cellular components, leading to lipid peroxidation, protein oxidation, and DNA adduct formation and strand breakage. Oxidants also alter extracellular biomolecules. An important example is the inactivation of α_1-antitrypsin by cigarette smoke, which may lead to endogenous protease damage of the lung parenchyma. Over time, the unregulated activity of these proteolytic enzymes results in the destruction of the alveolar architecture, leading to emphysema. Finally, oxidative stress alters cellular function by inducing the production of several proinflammatory cytokines such as nuclear factor κB and IL-8 (9).

The lung has a highly developed system to cope with oxidative stress. The fundamental overall mechanism is to transform highly reactive species to less reactive or nontoxic species before they interact with other biomolecules and cause injury. When ROS production increases beyond the antioxidant capacity or when antioxidant defenses are depressed, cells become vulnerable to oxidative injury. The ensuing dysregulation of intracellular homeostatic processes can result in rapid progression of irreversible cellular injury. Detoxification of ROS includes enzymatic (catalase, glutathione-*S*-transferase, superoxide dismutase) and nonenzymatic (glutathione; vitamins A, C, and E) processes and may occur intra- or extracellularly. A critical component of this antioxidant protective system is glutathione, which is the major low-molecular-weight thiol of both plants and animals. It is present in high concentrations in the epithelial lining fluid of the lung and serves a key protective role by participating in both enzymatic and nonenzymatic detoxification of ROS.

Hyperoxic lung injury is an example of an instance in which the major mechanism of toxicity is related to excessive oxidative stress. Although hyperoxia is associated with a number of physiologic alterations, the increased production of ROS within mitochondria and intravascular accumulation of neutrophils are believed to be critical mediators of cellular injury (10). These effects result in significant intracellular and extracellular oxidative stress, respectively. Although the lung's native antioxidant defenses are augmented during periods of prolonged oxidative stress, as in the case of hyperoxia, this response is not sufficient to overcome the increased oxidative burden, resulting in parenchymal injury (11). Emphysema related to tobacco smoke is another example of a disease process in which oxidative stress plays a key role in its pathophysiology. Smokers have more than twice the number of alveolar macrophages than nonsmokers (12). In addition, the macrophages obtained from the lungs of smokers produce several-fold more oxidative species spontaneously than those obtained from nonsmokers (12). This high oxidative burden injures cells directly but also inactivates α_1-antitrypsin, which in turn makes the airway vulnerable to endogenous proteolytic attack.

INHALATIONAL TOXICOLOGY

The ability of a substance to cause pulmonary injury is dependent on its ability to reach the various parts of the respiratory tree, its reactivity in biologic tissues, and the physiologic response elicited by its presence in the lung. These characteristics are influenced by a variety of factors discussed below. Examples of substances causing pulmonary toxicity are found in Tables 2 and 3.

Physical State

In general, substances reach the alveoli in one of two forms: gases or aerosols. A *gas* is defined as a substance that is entirely

TABLE 2. Mechanisms of potential toxicity from inhaled substances

Mechanism	Examples
Respiratory	
Simple asphyxia	Carbon dioxide, hydrogen, noble gases (argon, helium, neon, xenon), short-chain aliphatic hydrocarbons (methane, ethane, propane, butane), nitrogen
Direct cellular injury	
Moderate to high water solubility	Ammonia, chloramine, chlorine, hydrochloric acid, sulfur dioxide
Low water solubility	Oxides of nitrogen, ozone, phosgene
Nonrespiratory	
Cellular asphyxia	Carbon disulfide, carbon monoxide, hydrogen cyanide, hydrogen sulfide
Central nervous system depression	Alcohols, volatile hydrocarbons, nitrous oxide
Other systemic effects	Arsenic, amphetamines, cocaine, heroin, hydrofluoric acid, lead, manganese, mercury, nickel carbonyl, nitriles, phencyclidine

TABLE 3. Inhaled substances with potential non–respiratory tract effects

Substance	Effects
Alcohol	Acidosis, CNS depression
Arsenic	Anemia, cancer, hyperpigmentation, hyperkeratosis, neuropathy, peripheral vascular disease
Arsine gas	Hemolysis
Barium	Hypokalemia
Cadmium	Acute tubular necrosis, cancer, osteomalacia
Carbon disulfide	Neurotoxicity (axonopathy, optic neuritis), cardiovascular disease, parkinsonism
Carbon monoxide	Inhibition of cellular respiration
Chromium	Dermatitis, nephrotoxicity, skin ulceration
Cocaine	Hypertension, myocardial infarction, tachycardia, vasculitis
Cyanide	Inhibition of cellular respiration
1,2-Dibromo-3-chloropropane	Azoospermia, oligospermia
Ethylene dibromide	Hepatotoxicity
Hydrazine	Cancer, leukemia
Hydrocarbons	CNS depression, cardiotoxicity
Hydrofluoric acid	Hypocalcemia, hypomagnesemia, hyperkalemia
Hydrogen sulfide	Inhibition of cellular respiration
Lead	Anemia, encephalopathy, hypertension, neurocognitive dysfunction, renal insufficiency
Manganese	Parkinsonism
Methyl bromide	Neurotoxicity (narcosis, respiratory depression, seizures)
Monomethylhydrazine	Ataxia, seizures, tremor
Mercury	Neuropsychiatric dysfunction, renal insufficiency, tremor
Nickel carbonyl	Cancer, dermatitis, hepatotoxicity
Opiates/opioids	Depression of central respiratory drive
Phosphine	Cardiovascular collapse, hepatotoxicity, myocardial infarction
Phosphorus	Anemia, hepatotoxicity, mandibular necrosis ("phossy jaw")
Platinum/platinoids	Hypersensitivity reactions, leukopenia, nephrotoxicity, neurotoxicity (peripheral neuropathy, ototoxicity), thrombocytopenia
Sulfuryl fluoride	CNS depression, paresthesias

CNS, central nervous system.

in its vapor phase at room temperature and 1 atm of pressure. An *aerosol* refers to a relatively stable suspension of liquid droplets or solid particles suspended in a gaseous medium (13). The term *particle* is generally used to describe any substance that may become airborne. For example, dusts are fine particles of dry solid material suspended in air. These are typically from the breakdown of rocks, metals, coal, or organic materials such as fibers, wood, and grains. *Vapors* refer to chemicals that normally exist as liquids at room temperature but are volatile.

Temperature

Temperature not only influences the physical state of substances but can also have its own effects. Inhalation of cold air may precipitate an asthma exacerbation in a susceptible individual, whereas inhalation of steam can result in direct thermal injury to the airway epithelium.

Size

The main determinants of particle deposition within the respiratory tract are particle size and density (Fig. 2) (2). Large (10 to 50 μm) or heavy particles are usually not well suspended in the air

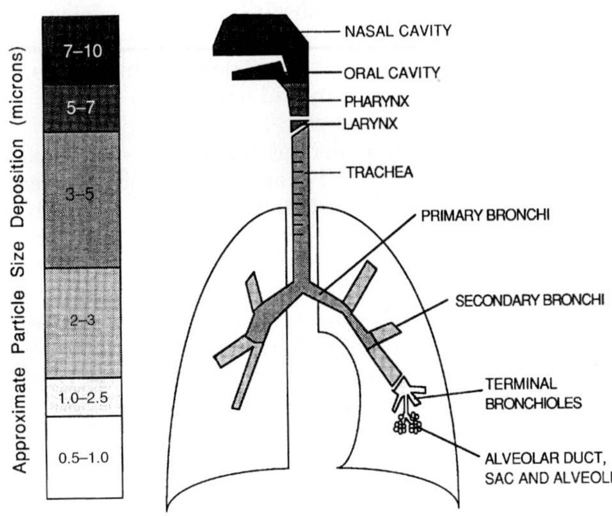

Figure 2. Schematic illustration of respiratory tract anatomy and approximate pattern of particle deposition. (From Newman LS. Clinical pulmonary toxicology. In: Sullivan JB, Krieger GR, eds. *Clinical environmental health and toxic exposures*, 2nd ed. Philadelphia: Lippincott Williams & Wilkins, 2001:206, with permission.)

column and tend to lodge in the upper respiratory tract, from which they can be cleared by the mucociliary elevator system. This may be altered depending on the minute ventilation of the individual. Very small particles (less than 0.01 μm) also deposit within the nasal airway (14). The term *respirable particle* generally refers to those particles of a particular size, mass, and shape that can be inhaled or exhaled, reaching the terminal bronchioles and alveoli. The diameters vary with different substances, but in general, such particles have diameters between 0.5 and 10.0 μm.

In industrialized countries, power generation, combustion of wood and fossil fuels, and roads account for the majority of particulate emissions. Historically, the important particulate size for regulatory purposes has been the PM_{10} fraction (particulate matter with an aerodynamic diameter less than 10 μm). However, a growing body of evidence indicates that $PM_{2.5}$ (particulate matter less than 2.5 μm diameter) is a more important determinant of adverse health effects (15).

Chemical Properties

The chemical properties of particulates include both the surface chemistry of the particle and the intrinsic particle characteristics. For example, the particle core may be comprised of carbon, silica, or organic material, each of which is associated with different lung disorders. In industrialized countries, the $PM_{2.5}$ consists primarily of particles with a carbonaceous core such as residual oil fly ash or diesel exhaust particles, whereas the $PM_{2.5-10.0}$ fraction consists primarily of inorganic minerals (15). The particle surface characteristics may involve acidity (see below), electrical charge, and adsorbed substances, such as allergens, metals, and hydrocarbons, all of which influence the health effects of particles.

Acid aerosols are particles suspended in air that contain primarily sulfur and nitrogen acids. Sulfur dioxide results mostly from the combustion of fossil fuels, and its oxidation in the atmosphere results in sulfuric acid and other sulfur-containing acids. These species dissolve in atmospheric water, which may create acid rain and fog or adsorb to particulate matter. As with sulfur dioxide, the main source of oxides of nitrogen emissions is combustion of fossil fuels. Oxidation by ultraviolet radiation in the atmosphere leads to the production of a number of nitrogen-containing acids. High concentrations of these acidic species in the atmosphere, as occurs with certain atmospheric conditions in polluted cities, has resulted in increased morbidity and mortality in patients with underlying pulmonary conditions.

Water solubility is an important determinant of pulmonary injury because it influences the depth of penetration of a particular substance. In general, substances with high water solubility (e.g., ammonia) cause irritation of the eye and nasopharynx, which usually limits further exposure. These substances tend to cause upper-airway injury with relative sparing of the distal airways. However, if the exposure occurs in an enclosed space or involves a high concentration, deeper injury may occur. Substances with low water solubility (e.g., phosgene), on the other hand, tend to penetrate more deeply and may cause severe delayed toxicity with relatively mild irritation symptoms.

Physiologic Response

The physiologic responses to the presence of a substance within the respiratory tract can be quite variable, depending on the substance and underlying host factors. Occupational asthma is an example of an immunologically mediated response. Numerous substances capable of sensitizing the respiratory tract in this manner have been identified (Chapter 11). Occupational beryllium exposure also results in sensitization through a type IV sensitization reaction that ultimately results in a clinical picture resembling sarcoidosis with progressive pulmonary fibrosis and lymphadenopathy. Some substances result in progressive lung dysfunction because of their persistence in the parenchyma and the chronic inflammatory reaction they produce. Asbestos is a well-recognized cause of such dysfunction. Finally, some substances may elicit physiologic responses within the airway cells at concentrations that are far less than those capable of causing cellular injury. Examples include the irritants formaldehyde and sulfur dioxide (16).

Reactivity

Reactivity refers to the ability of particular substances to cause direct cellular injury to respiratory tract cells. An important determinant of potential toxicity in this respect involves properties of the respiratory tract itself. For example, in the high water vapor pressure environment of the respiratory tract, ammonia reacts with water to form NH^{4+} and OH^-, both of which are directly injurious to epithelial cells. Oxidant-mediated injury is also a common phenomenon within the lung because of the relatively high oxygen tension (see earlier).

Systemic Toxicity

The lung serves as a route of absorption for a large number of substances. This property can be exploited therapeutically, as with delivery of anesthetic gases or drug administration during cardiac arrest. However, certain substances can cause significant adverse nonrespiratory effects after they have been inhaled and absorbed. Table 3 provides some examples of such substances.

Airway Particle Deposition

Most inhaled substances and particles are deposited along the conducting airways, thus filtering them before they reach the gas-exchange regions of the lung. The most important deposition mechanisms for particles larger than 0.5 µm in diameter are impaction and gravitational sedimentation (17). Impaction occurs when a suspended particle is carried by its own momentum out of the air stream into the lining of the airway. This

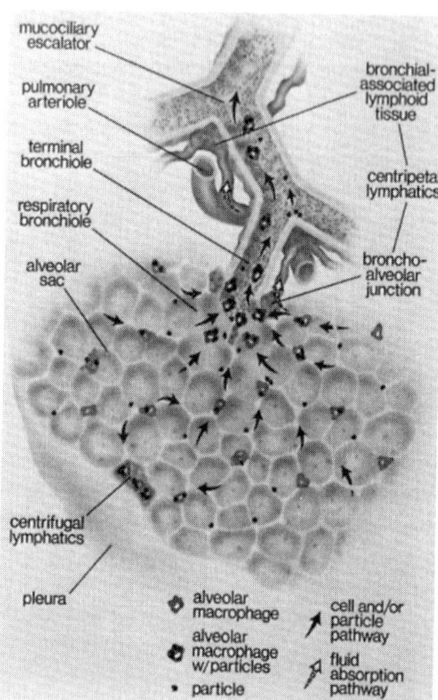

Figure 3. Alveolar particle clearance routes. (From Green GM, Jakab GJ, Low RB, et al. Defense mechanisms of the respiratory membrane. *Am Rev Respir Dis* 1977;115:479, with permission.)

occurs either at turns of the airways or at bifurcations. Gravitational sedimentation is the settling of particles onto the airway surface as a result of gravitational forces. Impaction occurs primarily in the large conducting airways, where the air velocity is highest, whereas sedimentation is a more prominent mechanism in the gas-exchange regions. Air turbulence arising from the irregular surface of the airways and the abrupt air-flow changes that occur between inspiration and expiration also influence particle deposition, particularly in the upper airways. For particles with a diameter smaller than 0.5 µm, random motion, or deposition by Brownian diffusion, becomes a more important mechanism. As with sedimentation, deposition by diffusion occurs mostly in the terminal bronchioles and alveoli, where the airway velocities are low.

Particle Clearance

The mechanisms of particle clearance depend on where the particle deposits within the respiratory tract. For example, mechanical clearance via the mucociliary escalator is prominent within the conducting airways, whereas in the nonciliated alveoli, phagocytosis by alveolar macrophages is the major mechanism. Figure 3 illustrates the main clearance mechanisms operative within the alveoli (18).

For substances that reach the alveoli, the most important mechanism is phagocytosis by alveolar macrophages. After the particle is phagocytosed, it is cleared via two main routes: The macrophage may translocate proximally so that it is swept up the mucociliary escalator, or it may move into the interstitium, where it may gain access to the lymphatic system or persist indefinitely within the interstitial connective tissue. Naked particles can similarly be cleared via either route. Some particles are completely digested and inactivated by the enzymes released by respiratory epithelial cells and macrophages, whereas others are processed by the macrophage and presented to immunocompetent cells, triggering specific immunologic responses.

The extracellular lining fluid (ELF) of the lung is also critical to the clearance of foreign substances, be they bacteria, viruses, or particles. This fluid is derived both from the transudation of plasma constituents and local secretions. The composition of ELF and its viscoelastic properties are quite different between the conducting airways and gas-exchange regions of the lung. Alveolar ELF is characterized by the presence of surfactant, which is critical in maintaining the high compliance of the alveoli. Surfactant is comprised of surface tension–reducing phospholipids and is synthesized by type II alveolar cells. Alveolar ELF also contains a number of other phospholipids, enzymes, immunoglobulins (Igs), proteins, and complement.

The fluid lining the tracheobronchial tree is approximately 95% water, 2% to 3% mucins, and 2% to 3% other constituents and is arrayed as a sol phase and a gel phase (17). The cilia of the respiratory epithelium beat within the low viscosity sol layer in a metachronous (wave-like) fashion, propelling the overlying gel layer. The *mucins* are long-chain glycoproteins secreted by submucosal mucus glands and goblet cells that are concentrated in the gel layer, imparting its viscous properties. Other components of tracheobronchial ELF include proteins (albumin, haptoglobin, lactoferrin, transferrin), enzymes (α_1-antitrypsin, chymotrypsin, lysozyme), and Igs (primarily IgA and IgG). Substances deposited on the gel layer may follow one of several possible fates: enzymatic degradation, binding and neutralization by Igs, mechanical transport out of the airways, or phagocytosis by epithelial lining cells after penetration through the gel layer.

The velocity of particle transport within the gel layer varies from 10 μm/minute in the smallest airways to 2 cm/minute in the large conducting airways. Substances deposited along the tracheobronchial tree are propelled to the posterior pharynx where they are swallowed, whereas those that are deposited in the anterior nasopharynx are propelled toward the anterior nares.

TABLE 4. Substances potentially causing pulmonary injury or dysfunction through noninhalational routes

Agent	Effect
Amiodarone	Fibrosis
Amphetamines	Pulmonary hypertension
Amphotericin	Noncardiogenic pulmonary edema
Beta-blockers	Bronchospasm
Bleomycin	Alveolitis, fibrosis
Carbamates	Bronchorrhea, bronchospasm
Carmustine	Fibrosis
Cocaine	Vasculitis
Colchicine	Acute lung injury, respiratory muscle myopathy
Cyclophosphamide	Fibrosis
Dapsone	Pulmonary eosinophilia
Ergot alkaloids	Fibrosis, pleural effusion
Ethchlorvynol	Noncardiogenic pulmonary edema
Fenfluramine	Fibrosis
Glutethimide	Thickened pulmonary secretions
Gold	Interstitial pneumonitis, fibrosis
Heroin	Noncardiogenic pulmonary edema
Hydrocarbons	Pneumonitis (intravenous administration)
Hydrogen peroxide	Gas embolism
Ifosfamide	Fibrosis
Iron	Acute lung injury
Lipopolysaccharide	Acute lung injury
Melphalan	Fibrosis
Methotrexate	Pneumonitis
Nitrofurantoin	Hypersensitivity pneumonitis
Opioids	Noncardiogenic pulmonary edema
Organophosphates	Bronchorrhea, bronchospasm
Paraquat	Alveolitis, fibrosis
Pennyroyal oil	Pulmonary necrosis
Phenformin	Pulmonary hypertension
Phosphorus	Noncardiogenic pulmonary edema
Pyrrolizidine alkaloids	Pulmonary hypertension
Procarbazine	Interstitial pneumonitis
Protamine	Noncardiogenic pulmonary edema
Salicylates	Noncardiogenic pulmonary edema
Strychnine	Respiratory muscle paralysis
Sulfa drugs	Hypersensitivity pneumonitis

RESPIRATORY TRACT RESPONSES TO INJURY

The human respiratory tract has a number of responses to injury that are not unique to specific toxicants. These responses may occur after respiratory or nonrespiratory exposure (Table 4). At the cellular level, these responses include apoptosis, fibrosis, inflammation, hypertrophy, hyperplasia, metaplasia, and neoplasia. Clinically, responses to injury range from relatively mild (e.g., cough) to life-threatening responses [e.g., acute lung injury (ALI)].

Bronchitis

Cough and mucus secretion are the most common physiologic responses to airway irritation. The cough reflex may be activated directly by stimulation of afferent nerve fibers within the airways or indirectly through the elaboration of inflammatory mediators. A wide variety of inhaled substances are capable of stimulating mucus secretion. Repeated stimulation over time results in hypersecretion of mucus as a result of goblet cell hyperplasia and submucosal gland hypertrophy (19). The term *industrial bronchitis* refers to the chronic cough and mucus hypersecretion demonstrated by workers exposed to irritants at low concentrations. This adaptive response to chronic irritation has been associated with persistent long-term sequelae such as airflow obstruction (20).

Bronchoconstriction and Airway Hyperactivity

Bronchoconstriction is a common response to airway injury and serves to limit exposure of the lung parenchyma to noxious stimuli. It should be emphasized that wheezing after exposure to an irritant does not necessarily indicate the presence of asthma. The term *asthma* refers to a specific chronic inflammatory disorder of the airways characterized by airway hyperresponsiveness to a variety of stimuli (Chapter 11). It usually involves repeated exposure to certain substances that result in sensitization of the airways. An exception to this rule is the reactive airways dysfunction syndrome, which occurs after a single exposure to very high concentrations of an airborne irritant (21). Although nonspecific airway hyperresponsiveness is a feature of this disorder, it is different from asthma in that it is transient and does not involve a sensitization mechanism.

Edema

Edema is a nonspecific response to airway injury that may result from a variety of mechanisms.

Edema occurs when there is an imbalance between fluid accumulation and removal within the pulmonary microvasculature. Alterations in hydrostatic pressure, osmotic pressure, permeability characteristics, and the capillary volume available for filtration influence pulmonary fluid homeostasis (22). In very general terms, a distinction can be made between pulmonary edema that occurs as a result of imbalances between hydrostatic and osmotic pressure (e.g., myocardial dysfunction from a calcium channel–blocker overdose) and that which occurs as a result of the breakdown of the endothelial permeability barrier (e.g., paraquat). The former is a protein-poor transudative fluid, whereas the latter is typically a protein-rich exudative fluid. Because alterations in permeability usually occur as a result of cellular injury, the pulmonary edema associated with this type of dysfunction tends to be more severe and the recovery period more prolonged. Regardless of origin, the flooding of alveoli with fluid impairs oxygenation and can be life-threatening.

Acute Lung Injury

ALI refers to the pathophysiologic manifestations of alveolar injury. The adult respiratory distress syndrome is the most severe manifestation of this broad spectrum of disorders. Although there have been several definitions and classification schemes proposed, the most widely accepted definition is that of the American-European Consensus Conference Committee: acute onset of respiratory failure, bilateral infiltrates on chest radiography, absence of cardiogenic pulmonary edema, partial pressure of arterial oxygen to fraction of inspired oxygen (PaO_2:FiO_2) ratio less than or equal to 300 for ALI, and PaO_2:FiO_2 ratio less than or equal to 200 for adult respiratory distress syndrome (23).

This pattern of lung injury may arise from exposure to inhaled substances (e.g., hydrocarbons) or from systemic disease (e.g., sepsis). There is no specific treatment for ALI at the present time, although specific approaches to its treatment have resulted in improved recovery rates. The most significant factor that has positively impacted outcomes is the limiting of excessive airway pressures to those required to maintain adequate oxygenation, even if it results in hypercarbia (permissive hypercapnia). Better understanding of appropriate ventilator management for these patients, as well as better supportive care, has led to improved survival (24).

Emphysema

Emphysema refers to the disorder associated with destruction of the alveolar septa and chronic airflow obstruction. Clinically, this results in progressive dyspnea, hypoxia, and wheezing. The most common environmental exposure associated with emphysema is tobacco smoke, although a number of other exposures, particularly in occupational settings, have also been associated with this disorder.

Fibrosis

Fibrosis refers to the replacement of the normal interstitial components with fibroblasts and collagen. Replacement of these normal structures results in impairment of gas diffusion and decreased elasticity of the lung. Clinically, fibrosis is characterized by progressive dyspnea, impaired pulmonary function, and diffuse interstitial infiltrates on chest radiography. The process is not reversible. Fibrosis related to inhaled substances is most often a result of prolonged occupational exposure.

TABLE 5. Industrial processes and industries associated with respiratory tract cancer

Asbestos mining	Mining (radon, silica)
Aluminum production	Pigment industry (chromium, lead)
Beryllium processing	Polymer industry (vinyl chloride)
Chemical plants	Rubber industry
Coal gasification	Smelting (arsenic, cadmium, nickel)
Coke production	Stone cutting (silica)
Insulation and heating (asbestos)	Uranium mining (radon)
Iron and steel founding	Woodworking and cabinetmaking

TABLE 6. Chemicals and substances associated with respiratory tract cancer

Acrylonitrile	Mustard gas
Arsenates, arsenites, arsenic trioxide	Nickel and nickel compounds
Asbestos	Polycyclic aromatic hydrocarbons
Beryllium	Radon
Cadmium	Soots
Chloroethers	Talc
Chromium (hexavalent compounds)	Tobacco smoke
Coal tars	Vinyl chloride
Coal tar pitches	

Cancer

Inhalation is the major route of exposure for respiratory tract carcinogens. Most lung cancer–related deaths are associated with tobacco smoke, with the risk of developing lung cancer in lifetime smokers being approximately 10%. In addition to its own risk, tobacco smoke may have a synergistic effect with other carcinogens such as asbestos and radon (25,26).

Neoplastic transformation is a complex process but can be conceptualized as arising from the accumulation of mutations. One way in which xenobiotics contribute to this process is by attacking electron-rich areas within DNA, producing DNA adducts (4). Any such alterations to the genome that elude enzymatic repair lead to errors in replication and downstream gene dysregulation. Ultimately, cells lose their normal growth and differentiation characteristics, such as contact inhibition and senescence, giving rise to tumors. Tables 5 and 6 list some industries, industrial processes, and chemicals that have been associated with respiratory tract cancers.

REFERENCES

1. Wheeldon EB. Mechanism of lung toxicity. *Hum Exp Toxicol* 1993;12:419.
2. Newman LS. Clinical pulmonary toxicology. In: Sullivan JB, Krieger GR, eds. *Clinical environmental health and toxic exposures*, 2nd ed. Philadelphia: Lippincott Williams & Wilkins, 2001:207.
3. Witschi H, Oreffo V, Pinkerton KE. Cell types and their importance in pulmonary toxicology. In: Volans GN, Sims J, Sullivan FM, et al., eds. *Basic science in toxicology*. London: Taylor & Francis, 1990.
4. Bogdanffy MS, Keller DA. Metabolism of xenobiotics by the respiratory tract. In: Gardner DE, Crapo JD, McClennan RO. *Toxicology of the lung*, 3rd ed. Philadelphia: Taylor & Francis, 1999:85–123.
5. Hansen K, Mossman B. Generation of superoxide from alveolar macrophages exposed to asbestiform and non fibrous particles. *Cancer Res* 1987;47:1681–1686.
6. Moldeus P, Cotgreave I. Mechanisms of endothelial lung damage. In: Volans GN, Sims J, Sullivan FM, Turner P, eds. *Basic science in toxicology*. London: Taylor & Francis, 1990:242–249.
7. Driscoll KE. Cytokines and regulation of pulmonary inflammation. In: Gardner DE, Crapo JD, McClennan RO, eds. *Toxicology of the lung*, 3rd ed. London: Taylor & Francis. 1999:149–172.
8. Kotran RS. *Robbins pathologic basis of disease*, 6th ed. Philadelphia: WB Saunders, 1999:50–88.
9. Carraway MS, Piantadosi CA. Acute lung injury in response to toxicologic exposures. In: Gardner DE, Crapo JD, McClennan RO. *Toxicology of the lung*, 3rd ed. Philadelphia: Taylor & Francis, 1999:125–147.
10. Crapo JD, Barry BE, Foscue HA, et al. Structural and biochemical changes in rat lungs occurring during exposures to lethal and adaptive doses of oxygen. *Am Rev Respir Dis* 1980;122:123–143.
11. Ho Y, Dey MS, Crapo JD. Antioxidant enzyme expression during hyperoxia. *Am J Physiol; Lung Cell Mol Physiol* 1996;27:L810–L818.
12. Hubbard RC, Ogushi F, Fells GA, et al. Oxidants spontaneously released by alveolar macrophages of cigarette smokers can inactivate the site of alpha1-antitrypsin, rendering it ineffective as an inhibitor of neutrophil elastase. *J Clin Invest* 1987;80:1289–1295.
13. McClellan RO. Particle interactions with the respiratory tract. In: Gehr P, Heyder J, eds. *Particle lung interactions*. New York: Marcel Dekker, 2000:3–63.
14. Cheng YS, Yamada T, Yeh HC, et al. Differential deposition of ultrafine aerosols in a human nasal cast. *J Aerosol Sci* 1988;19:741–751.
15. Phillips SD, Brent J. Outdoor air pollution and issues of quality. In: Green-

berg MI, Hamilton RJ, Phillips SD, eds. *Occupational, industrial, and environmental toxicology*. St. Louis: Mosby-Year Book. 1997:419–426.

16. Balmes JR. Acute pulmonary injury. In: Sullivan JB, Krieger GR, eds. *Clinical environmental health and toxic exposures*, 2nd ed. Philadelphia: Lippincott Williams & Wilkins, 2001:223–233.
17. Lippman M. Particle deposition and pulmonary defense mechanisms. In: Rom WN, ed. *Environmental and occupational medicine*, 3rd ed. Philadelphia: Lippincott-Raven Publishers, 1998:245–260.
18. Green GM, Jakab GJ, Low RB, et al. Defense mechanisms of the respiratory membrane. *Am Rev Respir Dis* 1977;115:479.
19. Reid L. An experimental study of hypersecretion of mucus in the bronchial tree. *Br J Exp Pathol* 1963;44:437–445.
20. Kennedy SM. Agents causing chronic airflow obstruction. In: Harber P, Schenker M, Balmes J, eds. *Occupational and environmental respiratory disease*. St. Louis: Mosby-Year Book, 1996:433–449.
21. Brooks SM, Weiss MA, Bernstein IL. Reactive airways dysfunction syndrome (RADS): persistent asthma syndrome after high level irritant exposure. *Chest* 1985;88:376–384.
22. Bernard GR, Pou NA, Coggeshall JW, et al. Comparison of the pulmonary dysfunction caused by cardiogenic and noncardiogenic pulmonary edema. *Chest* 1995;108(3):798–803.
23. Bernard GR. Artigas A, Brigham KL, et al. The American-European Consensus Conference on ARDS: definitions, mechanisms, relevant outcomes, and clinical trial coordination. *Am J Respir Crit Care Med* 1994;149:818–824.
24. Ware LB, Matthay MA. The acute respiratory distress syndrome. *N Engl J Med* 2000;342:1334–1349.
25. Selikoff IJ, Churg J, Hammond E. The occurrence of asbestosis among insulation workers in the United States. *Ann N Y Acad Sci* 1965;132:139.
26. Harley N, Samet JM, Cross FT, et al. Contribution of radon and radon daughters to respiratory tract cancer. *Environ Health Perspect* 1986;70:17–21.

CHAPTER 182

Air Pollution

Mark A. Kostic and Scott D. Phillips

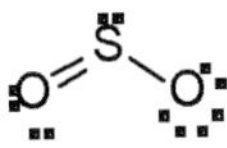

SULFUR DIOXIDE

Compounds included:	**Carbon monoxide (CO), nitrogen dioxide (NO_2), sulfur dioxide (SO_2), ozone (O_3), lead (Pb), particulate matter less than 10 μm in diameter (PM_{10}), particulate matter less than 2.5 μm in diameter ($PM_{2.5}$)**
SI conversion:	**Not applicable**
Special concerns:	**Exacerbation of asthma, increased risk of cancer**
Antidote:	**Oxygen (CO)**

OVERVIEW

A dramatic illustration of the human impact on the environment occurred in London in 1952. Approximately 4000 excess deaths, many due to respiratory illness, were temporally related to a severe temperature inversion (1). Later reassessments have estimated the related death toll to be closer to 12,000 excess deaths over the 2 to 3 months after the inversion (2). The cause has been suggested to be the substantial accumulation of the byproducts of fossil fuel combustion, namely sulfur dioxide (SO_2) and particulate matter, which were trapped in the lower atmosphere by the thermal inversion. The "London fog incident" remains a sentinel event in the history of air pollution management. Fortunately, such large-scale air pollution catastrophes occur rarely, at least in the United States, more because of advances in coal-burning technology than as a result of legislation.

Classification and Uses

Air pollution is a complex mixture of gases and fine particles, each with its own inherent, and possibly synergistic, toxicity. The United States has seen a significant decline in the concentration of air pollutants in the past few decades. However, large segments of the population continue to be routinely exposed to potentially harmful levels of these gases and particulates. For instance, those living in areas with high traffic volume in conjunction with the stagnant air created by frequent thermal inversions, such as Los Angeles, Denver, Phoenix, and Salt Lake City, are frequently exposed to potentially harmful concentrations of pollutants.

During these inversions, in which a layer of warmer air lies above the relatively cooler air near the ground, pollutants are trapped near the surface as normal atmospheric mixing is attenuated. Fog may form because water vapor cannot rise above the inversion. The term *smog* was first used to describe the mixture of smoke and fog produced during thermal inversions. Currently, smog refers more commonly to the results of sunlight acting on atmospheric gases derived mainly from automobile exhaust. These include oxides of nitrogen, hydrocarbons, oxides of sulfur, and carbon monoxide (CO). Ozone is a major product of these photochemical reactions, which most commonly occur in areas with large amounts of traffic and frequent thermal inversions.

Primary pollutants are emitted directly from a source and include SO_2, CO, nitrogen oxides (NO_x), volatile organic compounds, and other hazardous air pollutants (HAPs). Automobile exhaust, industrial emissions, agricultural erosion, and wood burning are potential sources of particulate matter, which are also considered primary pollutants. Secondary pollutants are the result of a chemical or photochemical reaction in the atmosphere. An example is the production of ozone from the reaction of volatile organic compounds and NO_x on clear, sunny, warm days.

Standards and Legislation

In the United States, the first federal legislative endeavor to improve air quality was the Air Pollution Control Act of 1955. Due to concerns over encroaching on states' rights, this act was narrow in scope and potential. The Clean Air Act was first

TABLE 1. National Ambient Air Quality Standards criteria pollutants

Pollutant	Ambient air quality standard
Carbon monoxide	9.0 ppm (8 h); 35.0 ppm (1 h)
Nitrogen dioxide	0.053 ppm (annual average)
Ozone	0.08 ppm (8 h); 0.12 ppm (1 h)
Sulfur dioxide	0.03 ppm (annual average); 0.14 ppm (24 h)
Lead	1.5 μg/m^3 (quarterly average)
Particulate matter <10 μm diameter	50 μg/m^3 (annual average); 150 μg/m^3 (24 h)
Particulate matter <2.5 μm diameter	15 μg/m^3 (annual average); 65 μg/m^3 (24 h)

ppm, parts per million.

enacted in 1963 and has been amended several times. It provided for increased research, grants for pollution control, federal authority over interstate air pollution, control over air pollution at federal facilities, and reviewing of motor vehicle pollution. Most noteworthy, it provided for the development of the National Ambient Air Quality Standards (NAAQS) and for the development of methods to remove sulfur from fuels.

The Motor Vehicle Air Pollution Control Act of 1965 further recognized the importance of automotive emissions (3,4) and, based on what was already in place in California, set the first national standards for hydrocarbon and CO exhaust. The automotive industry agreed to meet these standards by 1968. The Air Quality Act of 1967 attempted to specify "air quality control regions" and air quality criteria. This program was never implemented according to the required time schedule, and new legislation was proposed in 1970.

The Clean Air Act Amendments of 1970, now administered by the Environmental Protection Agency (EPA), established the two categories of pollutants to be regulated. These were the criteria air pollutants (Table 1), governed by the NAAQS, and the HAPs, regulated under National Emission Standards for Hazardous Air Pollutants. Among other things, it provided greater regulation of industry and tougher fines for violations. It initiated the study of aircraft emissions. It also proposed a 90% reduction in hydrocarbon, CO, and NO_x emissions. Lead was added as a criteria pollutant in 1976. The hydrocarbon standard was withdrawn in 1983. The standard of particulate matter less than 10 μm in diameter (PM_{10}) was instituted in 1987, followed by that for particulate matter less than 2.5 μm in diameter ($PM_{2.5}$) in 1997.

PATHOPHYSIOLOGY OF THE CLASS

As with all airborne toxicants, the size and solubility of the pollutant are the determining factors in the extent of delivery to the respiratory tract. The upper airway filters out large particulates, whereas smaller ones penetrate deeper. Water-soluble substances typically cause more proximal effects, such as the upper airway irritation seen with SO_2. The distal airways are more vulnerable to the lipid-soluble chemicals, such as ozone, which penetrate more deeply. This rule does not always apply, however. Under conditions of mouth-breathing and heavy exertion, the increased minute ventilation overcomes the surface solubility issues, and a greater proportion of the water-soluble substances can be delivered to the distal airway. This has been best studied in firefighters (5,6). Although each pollutant has its own effect on the respiratory system, they also act in concert. For example, a gas can attach to a particulate that is small enough to help deliver it deeper into the lungs (7). The toxic effect, therefore, should be considered individually and as a whole.

The major health concerns of air pollution are related to exacerbation of preexisting asthma and other respiratory diseases and a possible association with lung cancer. Of the criteria pollutants, only CO and lead have been shown to have no effect on airway reactivity (8). Inhaled pollutants can affect the activity of fibroblasts, β-lymphocytes, alveolar macrophages, and airway epithelial cells.

Due to their role as the first line of defense, the epithelial cells are likely the most affected. Several effects may be exerted by pollutants on these cells, including decreased ciliary activity and increased permeability. This allows decreased clearance and increased accessibility not only of pollutants but also of more routine airborne allergens to subepithelial tissue. Proinflammatory cytokines and inflammatory cells, such as mast cells, eosinophils, and lymphocytes, would then be activated. Cell membrane integrity may be further eroded by the depletion of antioxidants such as glutathione (9).

The interaction between air pollutants and inhaled antigens may be a more significant mechanism in the production of increased airway reactivity. For example, clinical studies of the effect of ozone on asthmatics have been controversial. Yet ozone exposures in asthmatics can increase bronchial reactivity to subsequent antigen challenges (10–12). Similar effects have been noted after exposure to nitrogen dioxide (13,14), particulate matter (15), and particles (16). Most likely, the mechanism of increased airway responsiveness with air pollutants is a complex interaction of increased allergen exposure, epithelial cell damage, and inflammatory cell activation (17).

The Harvard Six Cities Study collected 14- to 16-year mortality data on 8111 adults in six U.S. cities. The study controlled for individual risks, including demographics, smoking history, educational level, age, body mass index, occupational exposure to dust and fumes, and environmental factors other than air pollution. Air concentrations of pollutants were monitored in each city. Cigarette smoking exhibited the strongest association with mortality. After adjusting for this and other factors, there was a positive correlation of death from lung cancer and cardiopulmonary disease with air pollution. A statistically significant, although relatively weak, association was found between the adjusted mortality ratio for the most polluted compared with the least polluted cities (1.26, 95% confidence interval of 1.08 to 1.47). This was most strongly associated with ambient levels of fine particulates and sulfates (18).

DIAGNOSIS AND TREATMENT OF THE CLASS

The main challenge comes in recognizing patients who are at risk on days of poor air quality. These individuals include not only those with preexisting asthma but also those with other respiratory or cardiovascular diseases. Certain occupations may result in greater exposures to air pollutants. Individuals in any occupation that involves outdoor exertion, especially in proximity to automobile traffic (e.g., firefighters, police, tunnel workers, construction workers), would be expected to receive a higher relative dose of pollutants as well.

Presenting signs and symptoms of patients exposed to elevated levels of airborne toxicants include those typically seen with other airborne irritants: eye irritation, lacrimation, rhinitis, sore throat, cough, wheeze, chest pain or tightness, shortness of breath, hypoxia, and agitation. With the exception of CO poisoning, the evaluation and treatment of individuals who react to air pollutants are the same as for any patient with reactive airways. These include oxygen, β-agonist aerosols, ipratropium, and steroids.

CARBON MONOXIDE

The incomplete combustion of a carbon-based fuel produces CO. Up to 60% of ambient CO is emitted by motor vehicles. In urban areas, this may be as high as 95%. The city of New York estimates the daily emissions of CO to be 4140 tons per day per square mile, compared with 560 tons per day of hydrocarbons and 106 tons per day of oxides of nitrogen (19). An EPA study from 1983 to 1984 found automobile driving to be the greatest source of exposure to CO in nonsmokers. Travel time averaged 2 hours per day, at an average ambient air concentration of 5 parts per million (ppm) (20). Over the past 20 years, the advent of cleaner-burning more efficient vehicles, oxygenated fuels, and clean air legislation has diminished that degree of exposure, despite an increase in the number of vehicle miles traveled. Between 1980 and 1999, the average national concentration of CO decreased by 57%. The number of violations of the NAAQS has also decreased by 98%. Other sources of CO include cigarette smoking, industry, wildfires, power equipment, barbecuing, and space heating.

Whereas the other criteria pollutants exert primarily local effects on the upper and lower respiratory system, CO acts systemically. It affects the cardiovascular and neurologic systems. The rate of accumulation of CO is dependent on the inspired concentration of the gas, the subject's minute ventilation, and the diffusing capacity into the bloodstream. Studies have demonstrated a relationship between the ambient CO levels and increased cardiovascular symptoms in patients with angina and increased hospitalizations for congestive heart failure (21,22). By binding more avidly than oxygen to hemoglobin, CO reduces oxygen delivery to tissues. In occupations that require significant time in and about automobile traffic or near combustion sources, chronic low-level CO poisoning may occur. Although this may lower the angina threshold, the long-term neuropsychiatric sequelae are unknown at this time. The management of CO poisoning is presented in Chapter 184.

OXIDES OF NITROGEN

NO_x are primarily derived from the combustion of fossil fuels in automobiles and power plants and include nitric oxide, nitrogen dioxide, and nitrogen tetroxide. The reddish-brown layer often observed in polluted air is a result of nitrogen dioxide. Nitrogen dioxide is a main reactant in the formation of ground level ozone in photochemical smog and contributes to acid rain through its conversion to nitrous and nitric acids. Ambient air concentrations of nitrogen dioxide in the United States have been significantly reduced since 1980.

Nitric and nitrous acids form in the lungs on inhalation of NO_x. Mostly through lipid peroxidation, nitrogen dioxide promotes free radical production and local oxidative injury (23). Immune response in the lung may be modified, but results have been inconsistent (24). Due to its lipid solubility, mucosal irritative effects in the upper airways are not typically seen in chamber studies looking specifically at nitrogen dioxide. Several studies have looked specifically at the effects of NO_x on lung function in asthmatics. An increase in airway hyperreactivity has been found in some (25–29). Likely a result of differences in methodology and among asthmatics themselves, other studies have failed to show any effect of NO_x on lung function in these individuals (30–32).

Overall, the data imply that for all individuals, asthmatic or not, a short-term exposure to nitrogen dioxide at concentrations below 4000 parts per billion at most results in a small change in bronchial responsiveness (24). By way of comparison, a 1991 pollution epidemic in London reported maximum hourly nitrogen dioxide concentrations of 423 parts per billion (33). Long-term exposure may lead to an increase in respiratory symptoms and respiratory infections in the general population, particularly in children (34,35).

OZONE

UV

$$NO_2 \rightarrow NO^* + O^*$$

$$O^* + O_2 \rightarrow O_3$$

$$O_3 + NO^* \rightarrow NO_2$$

Figure 1. Photochemical generation cycle of ozone by the action of ultraviolet (UV) radiation on nitrogen dioxide (NO_2). O*, oxygen radical.

OZONE

Ozone, the major constituent of photochemical smog, is a potent respiratory irritant and oxidant. Requirements for the formation of ozone include NO_x, volatile organic carbons, and sunlight (Fig. 1). Automobile exhaust, being a major source of NO_x, is the most significant source of ozone. Ambient ozone concentrations tend to be highest in the summer (late morning, early afternoon) because the reactions are promoted by high temperatures and sunlight. The city of Los Angeles was the first to recognize ozone as a major air pollutant in the 1950s after a sharp rise in automobile traffic. Ironically, as stratospheric concentrations of ozone are depleting, low-level ambient concentrations remain a persistent problem. In the United States, ozone standards are the most consistently violated among criteria pollutants.

Pathophysiology

Due to its low water solubility, the effects of ozone are mainly exerted on the lower airways. Ozone plays a role in pulmonary inflammation by causing the release of inflammatory mediators from the macrophages and epithelial cells lining the respiratory tract (36–38). Using bronchoalveolar lavage as a sampling tool, studies have demonstrated a greater influx of neutrophils and eosinophils in the airways of asthmatics exposed to ozone (8,39). Ozone may also modulate the immune response and hinder the function of natural killer lymphocytes (40).

Clinical Presentation

The data regarding the effects of ozone in patients with and without pulmonary disease have been conflicting. Progressive reductions in airflow and increases in airway resistance have been noted in all populations after exposure to elevated ozone levels (41). Short-term exposure (2 to 7 hours) to 0.08 to 0.2 ppm ozone in healthy subjects is associated with shortness of breath, pleuritic chest discomfort, and lung inflammation (42,43). Ozone levels of 0.16 and 0.25 ppm have been associated with increased responsiveness to inhaled allergens (8,44,45).

Ozone-induced respiratory symptoms occur at, or below, the current NAAQS standard of 0.12 ppm (46,47). A study of summertime visits by children for asthma symptoms to an inner city emergency department found a significantly higher number of visits on days when the 1-hour maximum ozone level exceeded 0.11 ppm

(48). A cohort study of children from southern California found a correlation between the development of asthma in individuals in areas with high ozone levels who played outdoor sports versus those in the same areas who were not as active outside (49). Tachyphylaxis to these effects occurs with repeated exposures (50).

An epidemiologic study of mortality found a 6.6% increase in death from respiratory diseases during times of elevated ambient ozone concentrations (51). Despite the difficulty in consistently attaining the current NAAQS standard for ozone of 0.12 ppm (as a 1-hour maximum concentration), the data suggest that such a standard is likely still too high. It should also be noted that elevated ozone levels are not without environmental impact. This would include reduced seedling survivability with increased susceptibility to pests and inclement weather, leading to reductions in farm production and forest growth.

The effects of long-term exposure to ozone are gradually coming into light. Animal and human data suggest a permanent decline in pulmonary function due to chronic exposure to ozone (52,53). A study of healthy college students found that those who had grown up in high ozone areas scored, on average, 3% to 8% lower on pulmonary function testing than their counterparts from less polluted areas (54).

OXIDES OF SULFUR

Fossil fuels contain significant amounts of sulfur. Combustion of these fuels, mainly in power plants and industrial settings, leads to the release of SO_2. SO_2 may travel long distances and undergo oxidation to sulfuric and sulfurous acids. These acid aerosols can attach to particles forming sulfates, which are usually less than 1 μm in diameter. SO_2 or its products may also dissolve in fog droplets in the 10-μm diameter range. This results in "acid fog" or "acid rain," which, due to its size and high water solubility, might deposit in the upper airway (55).

In the United States, the environmental effects of acid rain are most obvious in the Northeast, a result of SO_2 emissions from industry in the Midwest. Health effects, however, have been more difficult to isolate. Water-soluble acids may adsorb onto particles, forming "acid particulates." These types of particles are important in that the particle becomes a "delivery system" for the acid.

The dissociation of sulfurous acid yields bisulfite, which is a bronchoconstrictor (56). In an asthmatic, low-level exposure to SO_2 can induce bronchoconstriction and chest tightness (57). This usually requires concentrations greater than 1 ppm for an asthmatic, 0.25 ppm for an exercising asthmatic, and greater than 5 ppm for a nonasthmatic. Continuous exposure of animals to low-level SO_2 has resulted in enhanced airway responses when challenged by other triggers (58). The same also appears to be true in humans (57). Epidemiologic studies have found a paradoxic inverse relationship between hospital admissions and elevated SO_2 levels. They also suggest that a "lag" period exists between exposure and hospital admission. Although not confirmed, one explanation put forth is that exposure to SO_2 results in an inflammatory process that takes time to be clinically evident (59). Because of alterations in bronchial clearance capabilities, sulfur oxides have also been postulated to contribute to the development of chronic bronchitis (60). Preliminary data from a Chinese cohort study suggest that SO_2, along with particulates, may contribute to an excess risk of preterm labor (61).

LEAD

A great public health success story has been the dramatic decline in pediatric blood lead concentrations since the abolishment of lead from gasoline and residential paint in the United States. However, leaded gasoline is still available for agricultural equipment and is used extensively in countries outside the United States. It is also still commonly used in many industries, such as those involving leaded batteries, automobile radiators, and firing ranges, to name a few. Average blood lead levels correlate well with ambient lead levels (62). At least in the developed world, lead has, for the most part, ceased to be a major contributor to outdoor air pollution. The toxicology of lead is addressed in Chapter 221.

PARTICULATE MATTER

Particulate air pollution is a complex mixture of substances. Carbon particles from fossil fuel combustion, such as diesel fuel, are major contributors, along with solid dust and acid aerosols. The most common acid aerosols in the eastern United States are acidic sulfates.

Classification and Uses

Size is a major determinant on the health effects of inhaled particulates and determines how deeply they will penetrate into the respiratory tract. PM_{10} tend to be filtered out in the upper respiratory tract. These nonrespirable particles tend to come from erosion and abrasion of nonpoint sources such as dirt roads and agricultural tilling. PM_{10} may be inhaled into the alveoli, where there is slow mucociliary clearance. These respirable particles occur from stationary (e.g., power plants) and from mobile (e.g., diesel fuel combustion) sources. These particles also tend to be acidic, affecting their toxicity.

Standards

In 1997, the EPA created more stringent NAAQS for $PM_{2.5}$. This was due to a growing, though controversial, body of evidence suggesting that such particles are inherently more dangerous due to their ability to penetrate more easily to the airways and alveoli of the lungs.

Pathophysiology

The toxic effects of elevated levels of particulate air pollution are typically aimed at the respiratory and cardiovascular systems. The inflammatory effects of particulates may be either local or systemic. In the lung, alveolar macrophages and bronchial epithelial cells are responsible for the local inflammatory reaction to inhaled particulates. Particulates are phagocytosed, and inflammatory mediators such as tumor necrosis factor and interleukin cytokines are produced (63). A review has looked at the importance of stimulation of the bone marrow and the resulting systemic inflammatory response to elevated levels of ambient particulate matter (63). Animal and human data presented in this review indicate that inflammatory mediators produced in the lungs in response to particulates stimulate the bone marrow to release leukocytes and platelets. These authors go on to postulate that it is this systemic inflammatory response that augments lung inflammation and induces a phenotypic change in atherosclerotic plaques, making them more vulnerable to rupture.

Mobile and stationary combustion of fossil fuels has added to ambient concentrations of ultrafine particles (with diameters of less than 0.1 μm) as well. This type of particulate matter is prevalent in areas such as southern California, where the chemical composition of such particles is primarily organic compounds along with varying combinations of trace metals, elemental carbon molecules, sulfates, nitrates, and ammonium ion (64). Animal studies demonstrate that ultrafine particles elicit a greater inflammatory response per given mass than do larger particles. Several factors may contribute to this enhanced toxic effect. Ultrafine particles have the ability to be inhaled and deposited as singlet rather than aggregate particles. This allows for a larger surface area per given mass to act as a catalyst within the cells. These particles are also small enough to elude alveolar macrophage surveillance, allowing easier access to the pulmonary interstitium (65).

Clinical Presentation

Epidemiologic data are mounting relating particulate air pollution to mortality. A study of 20 U.S. cities showed consistent relative increases in death rates from all causes, especially from cardiovascular and respiratory illnesses. This was true for PM_{10} concentrations well below the current 24-hour standard of 150 $\mu g/m^3$. For each increase in the PM_{10} level of 10 $\mu g/m^3$, there was a 0.68% increase in mortality from cardiovascular and respiratory disease in those cities. Levels of other pollutants were not found in this study to be significantly related to mortality (66). Excess death rates were also found in association with elevated levels of particulate matter in an earlier study of pollution and mortality in six U.S. cities (18). Although the relative effects of particulate air pollution are greater for respiratory disease, the actual numbers of deaths associated with particulates are much larger for cardiovascular causes (67).

Although particulate air pollution has not been found to cause hypoxemia (68), an increase in heart rate of 5 to 10 beats/minute has been found to be related to an increase of 100 $\mu g/m^3$ PM_{10} on the previous day (67). An 18 $\mu g/m^3$ increase in 5-day mean $PM_{2.5}$ is associated with a 22% increase in the probability of a discharge from an implantable cardiac defibrillator (67). At levels that never exceeded 70% of the NAAQS for PM_{10}, researchers in Seattle found a significant association between emergency department visits for persons under the age of 65 and the PM_{10} levels over the previous 4 days (69). Researchers have shown that fine particle concentrations in the 4 hours before ambulatory electrocardiographic monitoring were associated with decreased heart rate variability (a finding associated with age, illness, and poor cardiovascular prognosis) (70). This finding has also been reported in relation to the elderly by the U.S. EPA (71).

HAZARDOUS AIR POLLUTANTS

The Clean Air Act identified 188 HAPs that are known or suspected to have potentially adverse health effects. Data pertaining to these recommendations, when available, were based mainly on animal and occupational studies. Although not researched or governed to the degree of the criteria pollutants, these substances are receiving increased attention. The major emphasis in risk assessment for these compounds was on carcinogenicity, mutagenicity, and teratogenicity, with cancer risk being the most commonly used. Noncancer risks, such as respiratory, neurotoxic, and reproductive, are also used.

Compared with the criteria pollutants, much less is known regarding threshold concentrations and lifetime risks of disease associated with chronic exposure to HAPs (17).

Classification and Uses

Thirty-three HAPs were identified in 1999 as posing the greatest threat to public health as part of the EPA's Integrated Urban Air Toxics Strategy (Table 2). By specifically focusing on emissions of these compounds from stationary and mobile sources, the EPA hopes to meet its goal of a 75% reduction in the incidence of cancer, and a substantial decrease in noncancer effects, attributable to these compounds. Seventy percent of the increase in the median individual cancer risk over a lifetime has been attributed to four pollutants: polycyclic organic matter, 1,3-butadiene, formaldehyde, and benzene (72).

TABLE 2. Urban hazardous air pollutants for the Integrated Urban Air Toxics Strategy

Acetaldehyde	1,2-dichloropropane	Polychlorinated biphenyls (PCBs)
Acrolein	1,3-dichloropropene	Polycyclic organic matter
Acrylonitrile	Ethylene dichloride	Quinoline
Arsenic compounds	Ethylene oxide	2,3,7,8-tetrachlorodibenzo-p-dioxin
Benzene	Formaldehyde	Tetrachloroethylene (perchloroethylene)
Beryllium compounds	Hexachlorobenzene	1,1,2,2-tetrachloroethane
1,3-butadiene	Hydrazine	Trichloroethylene
Cadmium compounds	Lead compounds	Vinyl chloride
Carbon tetrachloride	Manganese compounds	
Chromium compounds	Mercury compounds	
Chloroform	Methylene chloride	
Coke oven emissions	Nickel compounds	
1,2-dibromoethane		

Polycyclic organic matter comprises a large class of compounds, including polycyclic aromatic hydrocarbons and nitropolycyclic aromatic hydrocarbons. These are known carcinogens and mutagens found in the particulate and gas phases of outdoor air (73). The primary source of polycyclic organic matter is the combustion of fossil fuels. Other sources may be more related to indoor air pollution, such as wood and tobacco smoke.

1,3-Butadiene is a volatile organic compound used in the rubber industry that has been classified as a probable human carcinogen. Inhalation of 1,3-butadiene in animal models has been linked with tumors at multiple sites, including the lungs. Epidemiologic data of occupationally exposed workers has shown an association with hematopoietic cancers (73).

Animal studies and occupational-based epidemiologic studies have linked chronic formaldehyde exposure to an excess rate of nasopharyngeal cancer. It has been classified as a probable human carcinogen (74). The combustion of fuels is the main source of aldehydes in an urban environment (3).

Based on occupational-based epidemiologic data and animal data, benzene is classified as a known human carcinogen (75). Chronic exposure has been linked with acute myeloblastic leukemia and aplastic anemia (76,77). Benzene is an aromatic hydrocarbon most commonly used as a solvent and as a gasoline additive. Natural sources include volcanoes and forest fires.

REFERENCES

1. Logan WPD. Mortality in the London fog incident, 1952. *Lancet* 1953:264:336–338.
2. Bell ML, Davis DL. Reassessment of the lethal London fog of 1952: novel indicators of acute and chronic consequences of acute exposure to air pollution. *Environ Health Perspect* 2001;109[Suppl 3]:389–394.
3. Health Effects Institute. *Research priorities for mobile air toxics.* HEI Communication No 2. Cambridge MHEI1.
4. IARC. Occupational exposures to mists and vapours from strong inorganic acids, and other industrial chemicals. In: *IARC monographs on the evaluation of carcinogenic risks to humans*, vol 54. Lyon: International Agency for Research on Cancer, 1992.
5. Sparrow D, Bosse R, Rosner B, et al. The effect of occupational exposure on pulmonary function: a longitudinal evaluation of fire fighters and nonfire fighters. *Am Rev Respir Dis* 1982;125(3):319–322.

6. Taskin DP, et al. Respiratory status of Los Angeles fireman: one-month follow-up after inhalation of dense smoke. *Chest* 1977;71:445.
7. Ormstad H, Hohansen BV, Gaarder PI. Airborne house dust particles and diesel exhaust particles as allergen carriers. *Clin Exp Allergy* 1998;28:702–708.
8. Peden DB. Air pollution in asthma: effect of pollutants on airway inflammation. *Ann Allergy Asthma Immunol* 2001;87[6 Suppl 3]:12.
9. Devalia JL, Bayram H, Rusznak C, et al. Mechanisms of pollution-induced airway disease: in vitro studies in the upper and lower airways. *Allergy* 1997;52[38 Suppl]:45–51; discussion 57–58.
10. Molfino NA, Wright SC, Katz I, et al. Effect of low concentrations of ozone on inhaled allergen responses in asthmatic subjects. *Lancet* 1991;338:199–203.
11. Jorres R, Nowak D, Magnussen H. The effect of ozone exposure on allergen responsiveness in subjects with asthma or rhinitis. *Am J Respir Crit Care Med* 1996;153(1):56–64.
12. Holtz O, Jorres RA, Timm P, et al. Ozone-induced airway inflammatory changes differ between individuals and are reproducible. *Am J Respir Crit Care Med* 1999;159:776–784.
13. Strand V, Svartengren M, Rak S, et al. Repeated exposure to an ambient level of NO_2 enhances asthmatic response to a nonsymptomatic allergen dose. *Eur Respir J* 1998;12:6–12.
14. Jenkins HS, Devalia JL, Mister RL, et al. The effect of exposure to ozone and nitrogen dioxide on the airway response of atopic asthmatics to inhaled allergen: dose and time-dependent effects. *Am J Respir Crit Care Med* 1999;160:33–39.
15. Gavett SH, Koren HS. The role of particulate matter in exacerbation of atopic asthma. *Int Arch Allergy Immunol* 2001;124:109–112.
16. Nordenhall C , Pourazar J, Ledin MC, et al. Diesel exhaust enhances airway responsiveness in asthmatic subjects. *Eur Respir J* 2001;17:909–915.
17. Leikauf GD. Hazardous air pollutants and asthma. *Environ Health Perspect* 2002;110[Suppl 4]:505–526.
18. Dockery DW, Pope CA, Xu X, et al. An association between air pollution and mortality in six U.S. cities. *N Engl J Med* 1993;329(24):1753–1759.
19. Johnson KL, Dworetzky LH, Heller AN. Carbon monoxide and air pollution from automobile emissions in New York City. *Science* 1968;160(823):67–68.
20. Akland GG, Hartwell TD, Johnson TR, et al. Measuring human exposure to carbon monoxide in Washington D.C., and Denver, Colorado, during the winter of 1982–1983. *Environ Sci Technol* 1985;19(10):911–918.
21. Allred EN, Bleecker ER, Chaitman BR, et al. Short-term effects of carbon monoxide exposure on the exercise performance of subjects with coronary artery disease. *N Engl J Med* 1989;321(21):1426–1432.
22. Burnett RT, Dales RE, Brook JR, et al. Association between ambient carbon monoxide levels and hospitalizations for congestive heart failure in the elderly in 10 Canadian cities. *Epidemiology* 1997;8(2):162–167.
23. Mustafa MG, Tierney DF. Biochemical and metabolic changes in the lung with oxygen, ozone, and nitrogen dioxide toxicity. *Am Rev Respir Dis* 1978;118:1061.
24. Tattersfield AE. Air pollution: brown skies research. *Thorax* 1996;51(1):13–22.
25. Salome CM, Brown NJ, Marks GB, et al. Effect of nitrogen dioxide and other combustible products on asthmatic subjects in a home like environment. *Eur Respir J* 1996;9(5):910–918.
26. Smith BJ, Nitschke M, Pilotto LS, et al. Health effects of daily indoor nitrogen dioxide exposure on people with asthma. *Eur Respir J* 2000;16(5):879–885.
27. Baur MA, Utell MJ, Morrow PE, et al. Inhalation of 0.30 ppm nitrogen dioxide potentiates exercise-induced bronchospasm in asthmatics. *Am Rev Respir Dis* 1986;134(6):1203–1208.
28. Moshenin V. Airway responses to nitrogen dioxide in asthmatic subjects. *J Toxicol Environ Health* 1987;22:371.
29. Orehek J, Massari JP, Gayrard P, et al. Effect of short-term, low-level nitrogen dioxide exposure on bronchial sensitivity of asthmatic patients. *J Clin Invest* 1976;57(2):301–307.
30. Bylin G, Lindvall T, Rehn T, et al. Effects of short-term exposure to ambient nitrogen dioxide concentrations on human bronchial reactivity and lung function. *Eur J Respir Dis* 1985;66(3):205–217.
31. Hazucha MJ, Ginsberg JF, Mcdonnell WF, et al. Effects of 0.1 ppm nitrogen dioxide on airways of normal and asthmatic subjects. *J Appl Physiol* 1983;54(3):730–739.
32. Klinman MT, et al. Effects of 0.2 ppm of nitrogen dioxide on pulmonary function and response to bronchoprovocation in asthmatics. *J Toxicol Environ Health* 1983;12:815.
33. Department of Health. Advisory Group on the Medical Aspects of Air Pollution Episodes. *Fourth report: health effects of exposures to mixtures of air pollutants.* London: HMSO, 1995.
34. Mathieu-Nolf M. Poisons in the air: a cause of chronic disease in children. *J Toxicol Clin Toxicol* 2002;40(4):483–491.
35. Nitschke M, Smith BJ, Pilotto LS, et al. Respiratory health effects of nitrogen dioxide exposure and current guidelines. *Int J Environ Health Res* 1999;9:39–54.
36. Hunter JA, Finkbeiner WE, Nadel JA, et al. Predominant generation of 15-lipoxygenase metabolites of arachidonic acid by epithelial cells from human trachea. *Proc Natl Acad Sci U S A* 1985;82(14):4633–4637.
37. Salari H, Wong A. Generation of platelet activating factor (PAF) by a human lung epithelial cell line. *Eur J Pharmacol* 1989;175:253.
38. Standiford TJ, Kunkel SL, Basha MA, et al. Interleukin-8 gene expression by a pulmonary epithelial cell line. A model for cytokine networks in the lung. *J Clin Invest* 1990;86(6):1945–1953.
39. Peden DB, Boehlecke B, Horstman D, et al. Prolonged acute exposure to 0.16 ppm ozone induces eosinophilic airway inflammation in asthmatic subjects with allergies. *J Allergy Clinic Immunol* 1997;100:802–808.
40. Jakab GJ, Spannhake EW, Canning BJ, et al. The effects of ozone on immune function. *Environ Health Perspect* 1995;103[Suppl 2]:77–89.
41. Kreit JW, Gross KB, Moore TB, et al. Ozone-induced changes in pulmonary function and bronchial responsiveness in asthmatics. *J Appl Physiol* 1989;66(1):217–222.
42. Hortsman DH, Folinsbee LJ, Ives PJ, et al. Ozone concentration and pulmonary response relationships for 6.6 hour exposures with five hours of moderate exercise to 0.08, 0.10, and 0.12 ppm. *Am Rev Respir Dis* 1990;142:1158–1163.
43. Devlin RB, McDonnell WF, Mann R, et al. Exposure of humans to ambient levels of ozone for 6.6 hours causes cellular and biochemical changes in the lung. *Am J Respir Cell Mol Biol* 1991;4:72–81.
44. Peden DB. Controlled exposures of asthmatics to air pollutants. In: Holgate S, Samet J, Koren HS, et al, ed. *Air pollution and health.* San Diego: Academic Press, 2001:865–880.
45. Peden DB. Indoor and outdoor air pollution. In: Middleton E, ed. *Allergy: principles and practice.* Update series. St. Louis: Mosby, 2001:1–12.
46. Raizenne ME, Burnett RT, Stern B, et al. Acute lung function responses to ambient acid aerosol exposures in children. *Environ Health Perspect* 1989;79:179–185.
47. Speizer FE. Studies of acid aerosols in six cities and in a new multicity investigation: design issues. *Environ Health Perspect* 1989;79:61.
48. Koenig JQ, Pierson WE, Covert DS, et al. The effects of ozone and nitrogen dioxide on lung function in healthy and asthmatic adolescents. Research Report, Health Effects Institute. 1988;14:5–24.
49. McConnell R, Berhane K, Gilliland F, et al. Asthma in exercising children exposed to ozone: a cohort study [Comment] [Erratum appears in *Lancet* 2002;359(9309):896]. *Lancet* 2002;359(9304):386–391.
50. Farrell BP. Adaptation in human subjects to the effects of inhaled ozone after repeated exposure. *Am Rev Respir Dis* 1979;119:725.
51. Goldberg MS, Burnett RT, Brook J, et al. Associations between daily cause-specific mortality and concentrations of ground-level ozone in Montreal, Quebec. *Am J Epidemiol* 2001;154(9):817–826.
52. Euler GL, Abbey DE, Hodgkin JE, et al. Chronic obstructive pulmonary disease symptom effects of long-term cumulative exposure to ambient levels of total oxidants and nitrogen dioxide in California Seventh-Day Adventist residents. *Arch Environ Health* 1988;43(4):279–285.
53. Rieser KM, et al. Long-term consequences of exposure to ozone. II. Structural alterations in lung collagen of monkeys. *Toxicol Appl Pharmacol* 1987;89:314.
54. Kunzli N, Lurmann F, Segal M, et al. Association between lifetime ambient ozone exposure and pulmonary function in college freshmen—results of a pilot study. *Environ Res* 1997;72:8–23.
55. US Environmental Protection Agency. Environmental Protection Agency report on the health effects of acid rain. Washington, DC: Environmental Protection Agency, 1996.
56. Fine JM, Gordon T, Shepard D. The roles of pH and ionic species in sulfur dioxide– and sulfite-induced bronchoconstriction. *Am Rev Respir Dis* 1987;136:1122.
57. Sheppard D. Sulfur dioxide and asthma—a double edged sword. *J Allergy Clin Immunol* 1988;82:961.
58. Riedel F, Kramer M, Scheibenbogen C, et al. Effects of SO_2 exposure on allergic sensitization in the guinea pig. *J Allergy Clin Immunol* 1988;82(4):527–534.
59. Tseng RYM, Li CK. Low level atmospheric sulfur dioxide pollution and childhood asthma. *Ann Allergy* 1990;65:379–383.
60. Goyer RA, Bachmann J, Clarkson TW, et al. Potential human health effects of acid rain: report of a workshop. *Environ Health Perspect* 1985;60:355–368.
61. Xu X, Ding H, Wang X. Acute effects of total suspended particles and sulfur dioxides on preterm delivery: a community-based cohort study. *Arch Environ Health* 1995;50:407.
62. Mahaffey KR, Annest JL, Roberts J, et al. National estimates of blood lead levels: United States, 1976–1980: association with selected demographic and socioeconomic factors. *N Engl J Med* 1982;307:573–579.
63. van Eeden SF, Hogg JC. Systemic inflammatory response induced by particulate matter air pollution: the importance of bone-marrow stimulation. *J Toxicol Environ Health* (Pt A) 2002;65(20):1597–1613.
64. Cass GR, Hughes LA, Bhave P, Kleeman MJ, Allen JO, Salmon LG. The chemical composition of atmospheric ultrafine particles. *Philos Trans R Soc Lond* (Series A, Mathematical and Physical Sciences) 2000;358:2581–2592.
65. Oberdorster G. Pulmonary effects of inhaled ultrafine particles. *Int Arch Occup Environ Health* 2001;74(1):1–8.
66. Samet JM, Dominici F, Curriero FC, et al. Fine particulate air pollution and mortality in 20 U.S. cities, 1987–1994. *N Engl J Med* 2000;343(24):1742–1749.
67. Dockery DW. Epidemiologic evidence of cardiovascular effects of particulate air pollution [Review]. *Environ Health Perspect* 2001;109[Suppl 4]:483–486.
68. Pope CA, Dockery DW, Kanner RE, et al. Daily changes in oxygen saturation and pulse rate associated with particulate air pollution and barometric pressure. *Am J Respir Crit Care Med* 1999;159:365–372.
69. Schwartz J, Slater D, Larson TV, et al. Particulate air pollution and hospital emergency room visits for asthma in Seattle. *Am Rev Respir Dis* 1993;147(4):826–831.

70. Gold DR, Litonjua A, Schwartz J, et al. Ambient pollution and heart rate variability. *Circulation* 2000;101:1267–1273.
71. Liao D, Creason J, Shy C, et al. Daily variation of particulate air pollution and poor cardiac autonomic control in the elderly. *Environ Health Perspect* 1999;107(7):521–525.
72. Morello-Frosch RA, Woodruff TJ, Axelrad DA, et al. Air toxics and health risks in California: the public health implications of outdoor concentrations. *Risk Analysis* 2000 Apr;20(2):273–291.
73. Cohen AJ. Outdoor air pollution and lung cancer. *Environmental Health Perspectives*. 2000;108[Suppl 4]:743–750.
74. IARC. Wood dust and formaldehyde, vol 62. In: *IARC monographs on the evaluation of carcinogenic risks to humans*. Lyon: International Agency for Research on Cancer.
75. Landrigan PJ. Benzene and blood: one hundred years of evidence. *Am J Indus Med* 1996;29:225–226.
76. Snyder R, Hedli CC. An overview of benzene metabolism. *Environ Health Perspect* 1996;104[Suppl 6]:1165–1171.
77. Yin SN, Hayes RB, Linet MS, et al. A cohort study of cancer among benzene-exposed workers in China—overall results. *Am J Indust Med* 1996;29:227–235.

CHAPTER 183

Respiratory Irritants

Richard C. Dart and Katherine M. Hurlbut

```
       O
       ||
HO—S—OH
       ||
       O
```

SULFURIC ACID

Compounds included:	**Ammonia, Portland cement (concrete, clinker), sulfuric acid, zinc chloride, and many others (Table 1)**
Molecular formula and weight:	**See Table 2.**
SI conversion:	**See Table 2.**
CAS Registry No.:	**See Table 2.**
Normal level:	**Ammonia, 80 to 110 mg/dl**
Special concerns:	**Acute bronchoconstriction, asthma (chronic)**
Antidotes:	**β-receptor agonists**

OVERVIEW

The list of respiratory irritants is nearly endless. The list includes many acids (formic, hydrochloric, phosphoric, sulfuric, and others) as well as compounds that are generally considered relatively benign (e.g., sodium hypochlorite). This chapter focuses on the clinical aspects of the strong irritants. Many of these compounds have noninhalation health effects that are addressed in the chapter regarding the specific substance (e.g., ingestion of sulfuric acid). The topics of diagnostic tests and treatment are very similar for this group and are addressed for the entire group in the sections Diagnostic Tests and Treatment.

Most of the respiratory compounds are acids, aldehydes, or other aqueous substances that dissociate into an acid on contacting the mucous lining of the airways (Table 1). Ammonia is a water-soluble alkaline volatile liquid. Ammonia sprays may be used in cases of criminal assault, during which victims are temporarily immobilized by ammonia solution squirted into their eyes. The preparation used can be household ammonia (9.5% to 35.0%). Ammonia inhalants are mild stimulants used to treat syncope, weakness, or threatened collapse and are common components of first-aid kits. Each glass capsule, enclosed in a fiber mesh, may contain 0.33 ml of a mixture of 18% ammonia and 36% alcohol. High-concentration ammonia (anhydrous) is used as a fertilizer and in manufacturing and is usually shipped by railcar (Table 3). Household-strength ammonia is addressed in Chapter 203.

Portland cement is a mixture of complex silicates that is used to bind the solid components of concrete and mortar. In its dry form, cement easily forms a respirable dust of fine particulates.

Sulfuric acid is a common chemical that is an irritant in weak solutions and a frankly caustic agent in more concentrated solutions. It is used to manufacture multiple other chemicals, fertilizers, and other products. Fuming sulfuric acid is a solution of sulfur trioxide in sulfuric acid.

Zinc chloride is a white opaque compound. It is a component of fume from smoke bombs and various other products. It is also used in chemical manufacturing and as a disinfectant, soldering

TABLE 1. Selected strong respiratory irritant chemicals

Acetic acid	Cyclohexanone	Nitric acid
Allylamine	Dichloroisocyanuric acid	Oxalic acid
Alum, aluminum sulfate	Diethanolamine	Phenol
Ammonia	Diethylene glycol	Phosphoric acid
Benzethonium chloride	Dimethyl sulfide	Portland cement
Bichloride of mercury	Ethylene diamine	Potassium permanganate
Boric acid	Ethylene dichloride	Pyrogallol
Butyl alcohol	Ferric chloride	Silver nitrate
Calcium carbide	Formaldehyde	Sodium bisulfate granules
Cobalt chloride	Formic acid	Sodium carbonate
Calcium hydroxide (dry)	Gasoline	Sodium chlorate
Calcium hypochlorite (granules)	Glycolic acid	Sodium hydroxide
Calcium oxide	Hydrochloric acid	Sodium hypochlorite
Chlorinated lime	Hydrofluoric acid	Sodium metasilicate
Copper carbonate	Hydrogen peroxide	Sodium silicate
Copper chloride	Methyl chloroformate	Sulfamic acid
Copper sulfate	Methyl ethyl ketone	Sulfuric acid
Cresylic acid (Cresol)	Methylene chloride	Tetraethylene pentamine
	Naphthalene	Triethylene tetramine
	Nickel ammonium sulfate	Trisodium phosphate
		Zinc chloride
		Zinc sulfate

TABLE 2. **Physical characteristics of selected strong respiratory irritant chemicals**

Compound, molecular weight, molecular formula (g/mol), CAS Registry No.	SI conversion	Water solubility (g/100 ml)	Agency	Description	Concentration, mg/m³ (ppm)
Ammonia, NH_3, 17.04, 7664-41-7	µg/dl × 0.587 = µmol/L	34	OSHA	PEL-TWA	35 (50)
			ACGIH	TLV-TWA	18 (25)
				STEL	35 (50)
			NIOSH	REL-TWA	18 (25)
				STEL	27 (35)
				IDLH	209 (300)
Portland cement, 65997-15-1	NR	NR	OSHA	PEL-TWA	10 (total dust), 5 (respirable fraction)
			ACGIH	TLV-TWA	10
Sulfuric acid, HSO_4, 98.08, 7664-93-9	mg/L × 10.20 = µmol/L	High	OSHA	PEL-TWA	1 (0.24)
			ACGIH	TLV-TWA	1 (0.24)
				STEL	3 (0.75)
			NIOSH	REL-TWA	1 (0.24)
				STEL	
				IDLH	15 (3.74)
Zinc chloride, $ZnCl_2$, 136.3, 7646-85-7	mg/L × 7.34 = µmol/L	432	OSHA	PEL-TWA	1 (0.18)
			ACGIH	TLV-TWA	1 (0.18)
				STEL	2 (0.36)
			NIOSH	REL-TWA	1 (0.18)
				STEL	2 (0.36)
				IDLH	50 (9)

ACGIH, American Conference of Governmental Industrial Hygienists; IDLH, immediate danger to life or health; NIOSH, National Institute for Occupational Safety and Health; NR, not reported; OSHA, U.S. Occupational Safety and Health Administration; PEL, permissible exposure limit; ppm, parts per million; REL, recommended exposure limit; STEL, short-term exposure limit; TLV, threshold limit value; TWA, time-weighted average.

flux, and moss killer (1). Formaldehyde is addressed in Chapter 195.

TOXIC DOSE

The health effects of respiratory irritants depend on concentration. The regulatory standards for each of these compounds is provided in Table 2. The severity of clinical effects is related to the concentration and duration of exposure to the inhaled compound. Lower concentrations and shorter periods of exposure produce less severe injury.

Levels of ammonia below its threshold limit value and short-term exposure limit can induce asthma in susceptible persons. Burnisher's asthma may follow ammonia exposure during polishing of silverware (2). A sulfuric acid concentration of 5 mg/m³ produced cough and impaired lung capacity (3).

PATHOPHYSIOLOGY

The lungs are exposed to the external environment with each breath. As a result of the enormous exposure to environmental toxins, the respiratory system has developed defense mechanisms, such as cough, to reduce exposure to inhaled injurious substances.

The potential for lung injury is dependent on a variety of factors, including the intensity and duration of exposure, the physical properties of the substances involved, and preexisting lung disease. In general, it is useful to categorize substances according to their water-solubility characteristics. Substances that have high water solubility, such as ammonia, typically have good warning properties because they cause immediate mucous membrane irritation. As a result, individuals who are exposed to these substances reflexively attempt to limit further exposure, which decreases the risk of injury. Although the full

TABLE 3. **Historic ammonia accidents**

Location	Year	Source	Scenario	Area	Quantity (Te)	Fatalities	Casualties	Evacuees
Lievin, France	1968	Road tanker	Tank failed	Urban	19	6	15	
Crete, NE, U.S.	1969	Rail tanker	Collision	Urban	90	8	35	
Blair, NE, U.S.	1970	Storage	Overflow	Rural	160			(3-km cloud)
Potchefstroom, So. Africa	1973	Storage	Embrittlement/rupture	Urban	38	18	65	
Houston, TX, U.S.	1976	Road tanker	Collision	Highway/urban	19	5	150	(Local)
Deer Park, TX, U.S.	1976	Road tanker	Skid/crash	Highway	19	6	200	
Cartagena, Colombia	1976	Fertilizer plant	Explosion	Urban		21	30	
Cuernevaca, Mexico	1977	Pipeline	Failure	Urban		2	90	
Pensacola, FL, U.S.	1977	Rail tankers (2)	Derailed	Urban		2	46	1000
Crestview, FL, U.S.	1979	Rail tankers (10)	Derailed	Urban			14	5000
Los Pajaritos, Mexico	1984	Pipeline	Failure	Urban (slum)		4	46	

Adapted from Vilain J. In: Bourdeau P, Green G, eds. *Methods for assessing and reducing injury from chemical accidents.* Chichester: John Wiley and Sons, 1989:252–290.

extent of injury may take hours to days to develop, the onset of significant pulmonary symptoms is evident relatively soon after exposure to a water-soluble substance. In contrast, inhalation of substances with low water solubility, such as ozone (0.00003 g/dl H_2O), may result in the development of delayed pulmonary edema.

DIAGNOSTIC TESTS

Many patients improve quickly after exposure has ended. Patients with persistent signs or symptoms should have pulse oximetry and peak expiratory flow measured. Spirometry may also be helpful. Generally, peak expiratory flow rate values over 80% of predicted (based on height and gender) are considered to be normal or to indicate mild obstruction. Values between 60% and 80% represent moderate obstruction, whereas a value of less than 60% represents severe obstruction.

In rare cases, an exposure to a respiratory irritant is associated with the subsequent development of asthma. The diagnosis of asthma requires detailed diagnostic evaluation as described in Chapter 11.

Spirometry results must be interpreted within clinical context. Many conditions can cause obstruction. Obstruction to airflow alone does not conclusively make the diagnosis of asthma. Conversely, asthmatic patients may not have a demonstrable airflow limitation at the time of testing. In such cases it is necessary to pursue further confirmatory testing. In workplaces with onsite spirometry, pre- and postshift testing can be useful (4). A decline in forced expiratory volume in 1 second of 20% over the workday with a progressive decline over the workweek are highly suggestive of occupational asthma.

POSTMORTEM CONSIDERATIONS

Fatal ammonia inhalation exposures produced pulmonary and femoral blood ammonia levels (0.26 mg/ml and 0.65 mg/ml) in one decedent (371 times and 928 times higher than normal, respectively). The second decedent had the pulmonary and femoral blood ammonia levels of 0.51 mg/ml and 0.43 mg/ml (5).

CLINICAL PRESENTATION

Acute Exposure

Each of the respiratory irritants rapidly produces mucosal irritation, including eye irritation, lacrimation, rhinitis, sore throat, cough, wheeze, chest pain or tightness, shortness of breath, hypoxia, and agitation. In severe cases, mucosal edema and ulceration of the airways may develop. Interstitial edema and noncardiogenic pulmonary edema may also occur.

Ammonia in high concentration (especially anhydrous) can produce caustic injury to the mucous airways and other mucous membranes. Portland cement has also been claimed to cause more serious, chronic effects such as pneumoconiosis in addition to the early irritant effects; however, a causal relationship to other conditions has not been established.

Sulfuric acid mist exposure has led to emphysema after long-term exposure (6). Zinc chloride has caused laryngeal, tracheal, and bronchial mucosal edema and ulceration; interstitial fibrosis; alveolar obliteration; interstitial edema; and bronchiolitis obliterans, which have been associated with inhalation of zinc chloride smoke (7).

Repeated Exposure

Because the respiratory irritants produce obvious immediate effects in nearly all patients, it has often been thought that they must have long-term effects. The effects of concern are reactive airway disease, initiation of asthma, fibrosis, and carcinogenesis. Little evidence has suggested that any of these conditions are related to recurrent exposures to these agents, at least within the guidelines set by regulatory agencies.

Portland cement has mixed evidence regarding cancer. Although studies have related Portland cement exposure with lung cancer and stomach cancer, other studies have found no effect (8,9). This may be a relatively insensitive epidemiologic method, however, and did not take into account possible regional differences in mortality.

DIAGNOSTIC TESTS

Patients who recover promptly after exposure probably need no diagnostic tests. More serious signs or persistent effects should be evaluated with spirometry, arterial blood gases, and chest radiography. An electrocardiogram may be needed if symptoms of myocardial ischemia develop. If zinc chloride exposure is suspected as a cause of pulmonary injury, the urine zinc level may be elevated (10). Measurement of ammonia concentrations is not recommended.

TREATMENT

Initial management involves removal from the exposure and provision of supplemental oxygen as needed to maintain adequate oxygenation.

Decontamination

The principle of decontamination is to remove the patient from the exposure. The rescuers must protect themselves as well. Mucous membrane effects from an irritant are treated with copious water irrigation.

Ammonia can cause an immediate and serious ocular chemical burn. Within a few seconds of injury, it may diffuse through the cornea into the anterior chamber. Permanent impairment of vision and even blindness may follow. Treatment should include prolonged (30 minutes or longer until the eye reaches neutral pH as tested in the conjunctival sac), immediate irrigation with water.

When the aromatic ammonia "smelling salts" are bitten into by children, vomiting, drooling, dysphagia, cough, and oral pharyngeal burns may ensue. Endoscopy has usually not indicated any esophageal burns. Treatment is symptomatic. Endoscopy is reserved only for those children with clinical evidence suggestive of upper airway involvement, such as stridor, dysphagia, or drooling (11–13).

Enhancement of Elimination

Respiratory irritants produce relatively low or nonexistent systemic levels and are not expected to be amenable to enhancement of elimination.

Antidotes

No antidotes are available for these pulmonary irritants. Inhalation of nebulized sodium bicarbonate has been used for chlorine inhalation, although its efficacy for chlorine or for these agents has not been clearly established. Some irritants may also cause methemoglobinemia, which is treated with methylene blue (Chapter 21).

Supportive Care

In severe cases, mechanical ventilation may be required. Ventilator settings should be adjusted so as to minimize secondary injury resulting from barotrauma. In some cases, the substance involved may also result in significant systemic toxicity that should be treated accordingly. Examples include arsenic, hydrocarbons, hydrofluoric acid, hydrogen sulfide, manganese, mercury, nickel carbonyl, nitriles, and smoke inhalation (carbon monoxide, cyanide). For eye injuries, topical antibiotics and topical steroids have been used, but their efficacy is unproven.

Monitoring

Concentrated inhalation exposure may produce delayed acute lung injury. Monitoring of pulmonary functions (arterial blood gas, peak expiratory flow rate, chest radiograph) should be performed serially on symptomatic patients.

REFERENCES

1. Knapp JF, Kennedy C, Wasserman GS, et al. Case 01-1994: a toddler with caustic ingestion. *Pediatr Emerg Care* 1994;10:54–58.
2. Lee HS, Chan CC, Tan KT, et al. Burnisher's asthma—a case due to ammonia from silverware polishing. *Singapore Med J* 1993;34:565–566.
3. Hathaway GJ, Proctor NH, Hughes JP, et al. *Chemical hazards of the workplace*, 4th ed. New York: Van Nostrand Reinhold, 1996.
4. Cote J, Kennedy S, Chan-Yeung MB. Quantitative versus qualitative analysis of peak expiratory flow in occupational asthma. *Thorax* 1993;48:48–51.
5. Chao TC, Lo DS. Ammonia gassing deaths—a report on two cases. *Singapore Med J* 1996;37:147–149.
6. Sittig M. *Handbook of toxic and hazardous chemicals and carcinogens*, 2nd ed. Park Ridge, NJ: Noyes Publications, 1985:815–817.
7. Pettila V, Takkunen O, Tukiainen P. Zinc chloride smoke inhalation: a rare cause of severe acute respiratory distress syndrome. *Intens Care Med* 2000;26:215–217.
8. McDowall ME. A mortality study of cement workers. *Br J Ind Med* 1984;41:179–182.
9. Rafnsson V, Johannesdottir SG. Mortality among masons in Iceland. *Br J Ind Med* 1986;43:522–525.
10. Proctor NH, Hughes JP. *Chemical hazards of the workplace*. Philadelphia: JB Lippincott Co, 1978.
11. Lopez GP, Dean BS, Krenzelok EP. Oral exposure to ammonia inhalants. A report of 8 cases. *Vet Hum Toxicol* 1988;30:350.
12. Wallace DE. Consequence of exposure to aromatic ammonia solution in 15 patients. *Vet Hum Toxicol* 1989;31:399.
13. Wason S, Stephan M, Breide C. Ingestion of aromatic ammonia "smelling salts" capsules. *Am J Dis Child* 1990;144:139–140.

CHAPTER 184

Carbon Monoxide

Lindell K. Weaver

$^{+}C{\equiv}O^{-}$

CARBON MONOXIDE

Molecular formula and weight:	**Carbon monoxide (CO), 28.01; methylene chloride (CH_2Cl_2), 84.93 g/mol**
SI conversion:	**Methylene chloride, mg/L × 11.8 = μmol/L**
CAS Registry No.:	**630-08-0 (carbon monoxide); 75-09-2 (methylene chloride)**
Normal levels:	**Blood, 2% to 3%; up to 10% or slightly higher in smokers**
Target organs:	**Brain, heart**
Antidote:	**Hyperbaric oxygen**

OVERVIEW

Carbon monoxide (CO) poisoning is the most common poisoning in the United States (1,2) as well as the most common cause of poisoning-related deaths (3). This toxic gas is ubiquitous in industrialized and nonindustrialized societies. Approximately 40,000 emergency department visits annually are due to CO poisoning (4,5). Raising society and health care worker awareness of CO poisoning, as well as its prevention, is important. Treatment for CO poisoning is 100% oxygen and occasionally hyperbaric oxygen therapy (HBO_2). Despite oxygen therapy, cognitive and affective sequelae are common after CO poisoning. However, there are no biochemical or genetic markers that predict outcome.

Methylene chloride (dichloromethane) is a volatile liquid used as a degreaser, solvent, extraction medium, and paint remover. It has mild central nervous system depressant properties that are less pronounced than those of chloroform and carbon tetrachloride. Exposure to methylene chloride vapors for 2 to 3 hours produces arterial carboxyhemoglobin (COHb) levels between 5% and 15%, leading to CO poisoning or complicating concomitant CO exposure. Pankow provides a thorough review of dichloromethane and its metabolism to CO as well as its combined toxicity (6). The use of a paint remover in a poorly ventilated setting has been implicated in a fatal myocardial infarction (7).

Sources

Common sources of CO include faulty furnaces, hot water heaters, and ovens; exhaust from automobiles, boats, or machinery (or any other internal combustion engine); cooking indoors with charcoal; and paint remover (methylene chloride). CO is also produced physiologically, arising as an end product of erythropoiesis as well as serving as a neurotransmitter.

Most people in developing countries still depend on biomass fuels, such as agricultural wastes, dried animal dung, wood, or charcoal, that are burned in traditional cook stoves without a chimney (8). It is estimated that at least 300 to 400 million people, mostly women, are exposed to such smoke. Data from India suggest that exposure to biomass smoke from cooking increases COHb levels to approximately 13% (9).

CO poisoning is a cause of "warehouse workers' headache" (10) and has caused mass poisoning in schools (11,12), at ice rinks (13,14), and during winter ice storms (15,16). Riding in the back of pick-up trucks can result in CO poisoning (17), and recreational boating can cause CO poisoning (18). Numbers of CO-related deaths in swimmers have occurred, with CO accumulating from generator exhaust from houseboats (19). Cooking indoors with charcoal can also result in CO poisoning (20).

Carbon Monoxide Alarms

According to Underwriter's Laboratories (UL), UL-listed CO alarms are required to sound an alarm signal before most people experience adverse effects due to CO exposure (see http://ulstandardsinfonet.ul.com/scopes/2034.html; also see Table 38.1 and Figure 38.1 in the UL2034 standard). Under the revised UL 2034 standard, a UL-listed alarm is required to activate an 85 dB alarm within 189 minutes if 70 ppm CO is present; 50 minutes at 150 parts per million (ppm); and 15 minutes at 400 ppm. UL-listed CO alarms (as of October 1, 1998) are required to not alarm in the presence of low-level concentrations of CO (i.e., 30 ppm for at least 30 days or 70 ppm CO or less for at least 1 hour). The UL-listed alarms are required to have a manually operated reset/silence button. If a CO level of 70 ppm is present after resetting the alarm, the alarm will activate again in 6 minutes.

It is estimated that CO alarms would have prevented one-half of CO-related fatalities in New Mexico over a 15-year period (21). All homes that contain a source of CO should have alarms. However, the CO alarm is merely a warning. Annual furnace inspections, health care provider comments to their patients, and public campaigns to raise awareness of the sources and dangers of CO exposure are mandatory.

Toxic Dose

Regulatory guidelines and standards for methylene chloride and CO are provided in Table 1. At equilibrium, atmospheric CO levels of 50, 100, and 200 ppm produce average COHb levels of 8%, 16%, and 30%, respectively (22). Reduced cognitive performance was observed in college students exposed for 1.5 to 2.5 hours to CO concentrations of 17 to 100 ppm, with COHb levels from 2% to 10% (23). CO toxicity is potentially worsened by a reduced alveolar oxygen partial pressure (e.g., high altitude exposure) (24), increased alveolar ventilation (e.g., increased activity or a high metabolic rate) (25), preexisting cardiovascular and cerebral vascular disease, reduced cardiac output, increased affinity of hemoglobin for CO (e.g., fetal hemoglobin has an oxygen dissociation curve to the left of adult hemoglobin; fetal hypoxia may be greater for similar degrees of CO exposure), anemia, hypovolemia, and increased rate of endogenous CO production.

TABLE 1. U.S. regulatory guidelines and standards

Agency	Description	Concentration (mg/m^3) (ppm)	
		Methylene chloride[a]	Carbon monoxide[b]
OSHA (air)	PEL-TWA	87 (25)	55 (50)
	Action level	43.0 (12.5)	None
	PEL-STEL	434 (125)	None
ACGIH (air)	TLV-TWA	174 (50)	(25)
	STEL	None	None
NIOSH (air)	REL-TWA	None	40 (35)
	REL-Ceiling	None	229 (200)
	IDLH	8000 (2300)	1380 (1200)

ACGIH, American Conference of Governmental Industrial Hygienists; IDLH, immediate danger to life or health; NIOSH, National Institute for Occupational Safety and Health; OSHA, U.S. Occupational Safety and Health Administration; PEL, permissible exposure limit; ppm, parts per million; REL, recommended exposure limit; STEL, short-term exposure limit; TLV, threshold limit value; TWA, time-weighted average.
[a]Conversion equation: ppm × 3.47 = mg/m^3.
[b]Conversion equation: ppm × 1.15 = mg/m^3.

An 8-hour exposure to 150 ppm methylene chloride produced COHb levels similar to those produced by exposure to 35 ppm CO. An 8-hour exposure to 250 ppm methylene chloride caused the COHb level to exceed 8% (26). Severe, acute methylene chloride exposures have resulted in COHb levels as high as 50% (27). Physical exercise and cigarette smoking produced an additive effect on the COHb level (28).

TOXICOKINETICS AND TOXICODYNAMICS

Carbon Monoxide

The lungs rapidly absorb CO, which avidly combines with hemoglobin at 200 to 240 times greater affinity than does oxygen (1). Small amounts of CO are metabolized by oxidation to carbon dioxide (29). Approximately 85% of absorbed CO combines with hemoglobin; the remainder attaches to myoglobin and blood proteins.

Elimination occurs predominantly through the lungs; the half-life of COHb in room air is 3 to 4 hours depending on minute ventilation. Administration of 100% oxygen shortens the COHb half-life to 30 to 126 minutes depending on whether the subject was experimentally exposed to CO or was poisoned with CO (22,30,31). In 93 patients with acute CO poisoning, the COHb half-life ranged from 26 to 146 minutes, with a mean value of 74 minutes and a standard deviation of 25 minutes (31). Isocapneic hyperventilation accelerated CO elimination in healthy subjects (25). In two healthy individuals, hyperbaric oxygen (100% O_2 at 2.5 atm) reduced the COHb half-life to 23 minutes (22). The COHb half-life of fetal hemoglobin is longer than that of adult hemoglobin—approximately 7 hours with the maternal inspiration of air (32).

Methylene Chloride

Methylene chloride is well absorbed by the lung (55% retention in rats, 35% in humans). Toxicity has also resulted from ingestion. Methylene chloride can be absorbed by intact skin but probably not in quantities sufficient to cause systemic toxicity (33). The lungs exhale most of the absorbed dose of methylene chloride unchanged. The body metabolizes between one-fourth and one-third of the absorbed dose to CO and the remainder to carbon dioxide (34,35). The COHb elimination half-life after methylene chloride ingestion is longer than that after direct CO inhalation.

PATHOPHYSIOLOGY

CO toxicity results from impaired oxygen delivery and use, which lead to cellular hypoxia, dysfunction, and death. Areas of poorly developed anastomotic vessels with high metabolic activity (e.g., brain and heart) are particularly susceptible. CO affects several different sites within the body, but the exact contribution of each pathophysiologic effect remains unclear.

CO replaces oxygen on the hemoglobin molecule, leading to a relative functional anemia. The body requires 5 ml of oxygen per 100 ml of blood; the remaining 3 ml of oxygen per 100 ml blood (3% volume) comes from the release of oxygen from hemoglobin. Impairment of oxyhemoglobin formation by CO can result in cellular hypoxia.

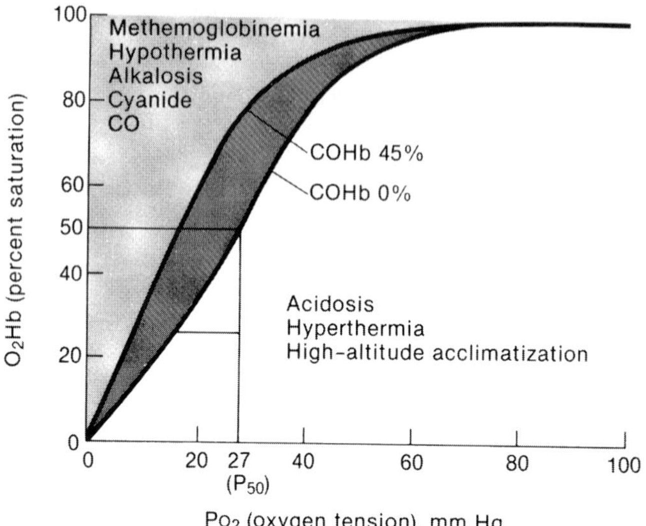

Figure 1. Factors that shift the oxygen/hemoglobin dissociation curve. CO, carbon monoxide; COHb, carboxyhemoglobin; O_2Hb, oxyhemoglobin; P_{50}, oxygen half-saturation pressure of hemoglobin. (Adapted from Goldfrank L, Lewin N, Kirstein R, et al. *Hosp Physician* 1981;17:50.)

An elevated COHb level impairs the release of oxygen from hemoglobin by increasing the affinity of hemoglobin for oxygen. When CO binds two of the four oxygen molecule binding sites, an allosteric alteration of the hemoglobin moiety occurs, and oxygen release is impaired (1). The result is a shift of the oxyhemoglobin dissociation curve to the left, which reduces unloading of oxygen in the tissues (Fig. 1). Exercise (acidosis, hypoxia, and hyperthermia) moves the oxyhemoglobin dissociation curve to the right, and elevated COHb levels move the curve to the left. It has been speculated that treating acidemia with bicarbonate during concomitant CO poisoning with elevated COHb levels might decrease oxygen delivery to tissues because acidemia should mitigate the CO-induced rightward shift of the oxyhemoglobin dissociation curve (36).

CO binds to cytochrome oxidase *in vitro*; however, the affinity of oxygen for cytochrome oxidase is greater than that of CO; therefore, binding of CO to cytochrome oxidase *in vivo* may be small. However, if cardiac performance is impaired by CO (i.e., COHb and CO myoglobin), oxygen delivery to the brain may be compromised, resulting in hypoxia to cytochromes and facilitating CO interactions (1). Piantadosi states ". . .CO hypoxia increases the reduction level of cytochrome c oxidase, which favors binding of the CO molecule to the enzyme. . . . This process occurs in the brain at COHb values of 50% or more, and it is reversed slowly after CO hypoxia. It is not yet clear whether or not there is a lower limit for this effect; however, it is worth emphasizing that elevated levels of COHb can produce sufficient tissue hypoxia for CO to bind to the enzyme noncompetitively—this is, during local anoxia" (37). In addition, others have shown that sheep exposed to CO increase brain oxygen delivery but have reduced brain activity, indicating that CO exerts a deleterious effect in the brain despite adequate oxygen delivery (38).

CO saturates myocardial myoglobin in three times higher concentration than skeletal muscle (39). The resultant myocardial depression and hypotension cause ischemia and potentiate the hypoxia induced by impaired oxygen delivery.

CO causes oxidative stress, including brain lipid peroxidation through activation and release of oxygen radicals by neutrophils (1,40,41). Furthermore, through interactions with nitric oxide released by platelets, peroxynitrate is formed, contributing to extensive endovascular oxidative stress, after relatively low-level CO exposures (42).

CO causes accelerated cellular death by apoptosis within specific regions of the brain, including the hippocampus (43,44).

Persistent and Delayed Neurologic Deterioration

Patients can improve after acute CO poisoning to normal function, or they may have persistent dysfunction. Some manifest delayed neurologic deterioration, usually within a few days after CO poisoning, but can present after 40 days or more (45). Other precipitating causes of delayed neurologic deterioration include drug overdose, strangulation, and seizures (46). Any type of brain anoxia can result in delayed sequelae (47), although this syndrome may be more common after CO poisoning (45).

VULNERABLE POPULATIONS

The fetus is particularly vulnerable to CO poisoning because of increased accumulation of CO in fetal blood (10% to 15% higher than maternal levels) and lower initial fetal arterial oxygen levels (20 to 30 mm Hg, compared with 100 mm Hg in adults) (32,48). Furthermore, the fetal hemoglobin dissociation curve lies to the left of the adult curve, decreasing release of oxygen from hemoglobin and resulting in greater tissue hypoxia at similar COHb levels. Animal studies suggest that maternal CO exposures as low as 125 ppm over 4 to 18 days may affect fetal growth (49).

Neonates are more susceptible to the adverse effects of CO than adults because fetal hemoglobin constitutes 20% of their total hemoglobin at 3 months (50). Some co-oximeters overestimate the COHb level (51–53), so newborns should have their COHb level measured by co-oximeters that can accurately measure COHb in the presence of fetal hemoglobin, as described in laboratory testing below (54).

Acute nonlethal maternal intoxication may result in fetal demise (55–57) or permanent neurologic sequelae (e.g., cerebral palsy) (58). A comatose woman delivered an apparently normal infant (4-month neurologic check-up was normal) despite an initial COHb level of 58.2% (59). However, others have noted that a single maternal COHb level cannot be used to estimate fetal COHb if the exposure pattern is unknown and the maternal symptoms at the time of exposure seemed to predict the risk of associated morbidity to the fetus (56). A prospective, multicenter study documented outcome of 31 patients with CO poisoning during pregnancy. The study found that severe CO poisoning posed serious short- and long-term fetal risk, whereas mild poisoning (mother alert, oriented, but could have headache, dizziness, or nausea with COHb levels less than 20%) was likely to result in normal fetal outcome. Treatment with HBO_2 may decrease fetal hypoxia and improve outcome (60). Prolonged exposure to low doses (5% to 15% COHb in smoking mothers) is associated with smaller babies and elevated neonatal mortality (61). In addition to elevated COHb levels, fetal cord blood from the smoking mother demonstrates a dose-related decreased pH and arterial oxygen tensions as well as increased arterial carbon dioxide levels (62).

CLINICAL PRESENTATION

Acute Exposure

Approximately 75% of patients with acute CO poisoning complain of headache (63,64). Other common effects include weakness, fatigue, nausea, vomiting, confusion, apathy, and distractibility

(63–65). Combinations of the five most common symptoms in patients without loss of consciousness (headache, nausea, dizziness, vomiting, and weakness) did not aid in diagnostic accuracy (64). Transient loss of consciousness occurs relatively frequently. If ambient CO levels are sufficiently elevated, unconsciousness can be prolonged and can result in death.

Predictably, weather cold enough to require the use of a furnace increases the number of accidental poisonings. The symptoms and signs of acute CO poisoning are often misdiagnosed as headache or viral infection. Mistaken diagnoses often occur after CO poisoning (Table 2) (66). Clues to a diagnosis of acute CO poisoning include groups of patients with similar complaints, especially if fever is absent. For example, occult CO exposure was believed to be the cause of 18.9% of patients presenting to the emergency department with the complaint of headache (67).

Any organ can be affected by CO poisoning: retinal hemorrhage (68), Parkinson's dyskinesia (69), mutism (70), urinary incontinence (71), pulmonary injury (72), bowel ischemia (73), myocardial infarction (74,75), rhabdomyolysis (76), hearing loss (77), diaphragmatic paralysis (78), and peripheral neuropathy (71,79,80).

Cardiovascular effects involve acute worsening of ischemic manifestations. The presence of ischemic symptoms (chest pain, syncope, dyspnea, diaphoresis, nausea) depends on the existence of preexisting cardiovascular disease and COHb concentration. Conduction defects, premature ventricular contractions, and atrial fibrillation may also occur in these patients. Although occasionally overlooked by attending physicians, occult CO exposure has resulted in coronary care unit admission for unstable angina (81). Sudden death has occurred in workers with severe arteriosclerotic heart disease when their COHb levels exceeded 20% (82). Hypotension results from myocardial depression, even in healthy patients, when COHb levels exceed 60% but may occur with lower COHb levels. Myocardial infarction can occur, including in young patients without coronary artery disease (75). Hospital admissions for the elderly are associated with increased air CO levels (83).

TABLE 2. Some possible mistaken diagnoses in patients with carbon monoxide poisoning

Misdiagnosis	Cause
Neurologic	
Cerebrovascular accident	Cerebral ischemic accident due to carbon monoxide poisoning
Migraine, tension headache	Headache
Epilepsy	Anoxic convulsions
Meningitis, encephalitis	Vomiting, headache, bizarre neurologic symptoms
Parkinsonism	Late-onset parkinsonian symptoms
Psychiatric	
Depression	Lethargy, somatic symptoms
Anxiety state	Hyperventilation, headache, malaise
Hyperventilation syndrome	Hyperventilation
Acute confusional state	Confusion, hallucinations
Cardiac	
Myocardial infarction	Critical coronary artery lesion decompensated through hypoxia
Cardiac dysrhythmias	Conduction system hypoxia
Pharmacologic or toxicologic	
Drug overdose	Hypoxic coma, nontraumatic rhabdomyolysis
Ethylene glycol poisoning	Coma and renal failure
Ethanol intoxication	Vomiting, ataxia, slurred speech, coma
Drug abuse	Agitation, confusion, hallucinations
Infections	
Influenza and other viral infections	Muscle aches, tachypnea, headache, exhaustion
Postviral syndrome	Lethargy, myalgia
Gastroenteritis and food poisoning	Nausea, vomiting
Pneumonia	Dyspnea, delirium
Sinusitis	Headache, malaise
Other	
Cholecystitis and other acute abdominal conditions	Abdominal pain, nausea, vomiting

Adapted from Lowe-Ponsford FL, Henry JA. Clinical aspects of carbon monoxide. *Adverse Drug React Acute Pois Rev* 1989;8:212–220.

Patients with cardiovascular disease are particularly sensitive to CO cardiotoxicity and develop increased exertional angina at COHb levels as low as 2% to 10% (74). As expected, high altitude exposure in unacclimatized individuals exposed to relatively low levels of CO (COHb level, 4%) reduced exercise capacity and time to angina, compared with sea level (81,84). Evidence is conflicting regarding if low-level CO exposure (COHb level of 3% to 5%) at sea level reduces cardiac performance (84–86). However, the preponderance of evidence indicates that elevated COHb levels in patients with coronary artery disease aggravate angina, especially with concomitant exercise (87–89).

Some patients may have an acute CO exposure due to a single poisoning circumstance, whereas others may have an acute event arising from a longer, chronic background exposure. Chronic, lower-level exposures also occur. Some believe that the chronic exposures result in more morbidity than the acute exposures, although no study to date has systematically validated this hypothesis.

Ilano and Raffin have presented criteria for mild, moderate, and severe CO poisoning (90). However, categorizing patients into "mild, moderate, or severe" poisoning can be misleading. Even patients with "mild" poisoning can have an unfavorable long-term outcome (91–93), and patients with "severe" poisoning can have a normal functional and cognitive recovery (94). However, no marker exists that can accurately predict immediate or long-term outcome.

The levels of COHb can be dissimilar in individuals simultaneously exposed to the same source. The symptoms manifested by the individuals and long-term outcome can be dissimilar despite similar COHb levels for reasons that are unknown.

Methylene Chloride

Because methylene chloride inhalation elevates blood COHb levels, symptoms of CO poisoning may occur, especially in patients with cardiopulmonary disease or workers who are exposed to other CO sources. Epidemiologic studies have not identified an increased mortality among methylene chloride workers (95), but workers with cardiovascular disease may be more susceptible to methylene chloride vapor. Symptoms may persist longer than COHb levels predict because of continuing *in vivo* COHb production (96).

DIAGNOSTIC TESTS

Diagnostic tests are directed at confirming the diagnosis with a COHb level and assessing the degree of end-organ injury.

Arterial Blood Gases

An arterial blood gas provides information about the COHb level and adequacy of oxygenation and ventilation (i.e., carbon dioxide elimination) as well as the presence and degree of metabolic acidosis. However, if the patient appears stable, it may be appropriate to confirm CO exposure by measuring the venous COHb level, which correlates with the arterial COHb level (97). The arterial oxygen tension may be normal or elevated if the patient is breathing supplemental oxygen. The oxyhemoglobin saturation is decreased due to an elevated COHb. It is important that the laboratory measures the COHb level with a co-oximeter. In the absence of actual COHb measurements, the laboratory may calculate the oxyhemoglobin saturation from arterial oxygen measurements, which are inaccurate and misleading if the COHb level is actually elevated. Metabolic acidosis reflects both ischemia and hypoxia.

Depending on the co-oximeter, fetal hemoglobin can interfere with COHb determinations by falsely elevating COHb in direct proportion to fetal hemoglobin (51–53). The CCD270 (Ciba Corning Diagnostics, Medfield, MA) is not subject to this interference (54), whereas the IL 282 (Instruments Laboratory, Lexington, MA) falsely elevated the COHb in direct proportion to the fetal hemoglobin content (53).

Pulse oximetry does not discriminate COHb from oxyhemoglobin (98), so the actual oxyhemoglobin can only be determined by measuring it by co-oximetry. Because the COHb level falls relatively rapidly with inhalation of high-flow supplemental O_2 (30,31,99), pulse oximetry can be valuable after the COHb level normalizes.

Cardiac Tests

An electrocardiogram should be performed in most adult patients with symptomatic CO poisoning. The electrocardiogram is a sensitive test for the presence of myocardial damage in adults (74). Ischemic changes range from ST depression and T-wave flattening or inversions to ST elevation indicative of myocardial infarction. Dysrhythmias range from frequent premature ventricular contractions to atrial fibrillation and ventricular tachydysrhythmias. Sinus tachycardia is the most common abnormality, but nonspecific STT wave changes occur frequently. If there is clinical suspicion of myocardial involvement, cardiac enzymes (creatinine kinase and troponin I) should be measured.

Other Tests

In suicide attempts, appropriate urine and blood toxicology studies should be performed. If concomitant smoke inhalation has occurred, cyanide levels should be measured (Chapter 190). Muscle necrosis may result in elevated serum creatine kinase and lactate dehydrogenase levels and myoglobinemia. Elevated creatinine levels may result from either myoglobinemia- or ischemia-induced acute tubular necrosis. Patients with significant CO poisoning may exhibit hypokalemia, hyperglycemia, and hemoconcentration that may be a result of elevated catecholamine levels as a response to acute cellular hypoxia. Elevated lactic acid levels may predict more severe CO poisoning (100).

Imaging

Chest radiographs may show evidence of aspiration in comatose patients. In severe CO poisoning, chest radiographs may display ground-glass appearance, perihilar haze, peribronchial cuffing, and intraalveolar edema (72). Brain computerized tomography (CT) imaging is usually normal initially in patients with acute CO poisoning. A positive CT (e.g., low-density globus pallidus lesions) predicts neurologic sequelae within 24 hours, but not all patients with neurologic impairment have an abnormal scan (101). In severe poisoning, especially if associated with cardiac arrest, brain edema, including herniation, may develop within a few hours of poisoning.

CO causes cytotoxic edema and demyelination. White matter and basal ganglia are commonly damaged. These findings are nonspecific and may be associated with barbiturate intoxication; hypoglycemia; and cyanide, disulfiram, and hydrogen sulfide poisoning. Magnetic resonance imaging (MRI) is more sensitive than CT scans in detecting tissue edema caused by demyelination (102). One study compared CT, clinical MRI, quantitative MRI, and technetium-99m hexamethylpropylen amine oxime (HMPAO) spectroscopy with neuropsychological tests in CO-poisoned patients. A clinical MRI conducted 21 months (range, 4 to 45 months) after poisoning was abnormal in 40%, and quantitative MRI was abnormal in 67%, although all patients were abnormal by neuropsychological testing (103). In a prospective study of 73 patients with acute CO poisoning, MRI scans were performed within 1 day of poisoning and at 2 and 6 weeks after poisoning. This study demonstrated that white matter hyperintensities occurred in 12% of poisoned patients, compared with 5% in a controlled, nonpoisoned cohort. Only one patient had globus pallidus lesions, which were present at 2 weeks but not at 6 months after CO poisoning (104).

Methylene Chloride

Laboratory evaluation of serious methylene chloride exposures should include complete blood cell count, serum aminotransferase levels, creatinine, urinalysis, urine myoglobin, and blood COHb level. Exposure to approximately 1000 ppm methylene chloride for several hours has resulted in COHb levels as high as 15%. The COHb level of the average worker exposed to 183 ppm (8-hour time-weighted average) ranges from 4.5% to 9.0% (105). COHb produced by methylene chloride metabolism has a half-life almost twice as long as equivalently inhaled CO because of continuing COHb formation after cessation of exposure. Methanol, exercise, and concomitant CO exposures, such as smoking, elevate COHb levels. Serious poisonings from methylene chloride exposure may occur without significant elevation of COHb levels (106).

Biologic monitoring exposure measurements include blood methylene chloride and COHb levels as well as air sampling. For average, sedentary, nonsmoking workers, maximum allowable exposures (200 ppm) produce methylene chloride levels of 80 ppm in expired air and 0.18 mg/100 ml in blood and COHb levels of 6.8% (34).

TREATMENT

Stabilization and Decontamination

Immediate removal from the contaminated environment, airway management, support of breathing with ventilation, administration of 100% oxygen, and the institution of intravenous lines and cardiac monitoring are the initial priorities. If rescue takes more than a few moments, rescuers must use protective equipment to avoid poisoning themselves. Fire victims should be evaluated for airway obstruction from thermal or chemical injury, pulmonary edema, trauma, concomitant toxin inhalation (e.g., cyanide and methemoglobin formers), and cerebral edema.

Enhancement of Elimination

Oxygen increases the elimination of CO and is addressed in the section Antidotes. Enhanced elimination of methylene chloride has not been reported.

Antidotes

The antidote of CO is oxygen, which both ameliorates its toxic effects and enhances its excretion. Both normobaric oxygen (administered at ambient pressure) and HBO_2 (administered at 2 or more times the atmospheric pressure) are used in treatment.

Normobaric Oxygen Therapy

High concentration oxygen (1,63,90,107–109) should be delivered through a tight-fitting, nonrebreathing, reservoir facemask or an endotracheal tube. Such a mask can deliver a fractional inspired concentration of oxygen (FiO_2) of 0.7 to 0.9 but not 100% oxygen (110,111). An FiO_2 of 1.0 can be achieved with a continuous positive pressure mask, aviator mask, or by endotracheal tube. However, it is unknown if clinical outcomes are improved with delivery of an FiO_2 of 1.0, compared with 0.7.

The half-life of COHb is reduced from 5 to 6 hours to a mean of 36 to 137 minutes by administration of 100% oxygen (11,22,30,31,99,112,113). The COHb half-lives calculated from patients with CO poisoning treated with 100% normobaric oxygen range from 72 minutes (31) to 137 minutes (11). If the patient has normal pulmonary function, 100% oxygen inhalation increases dissolved oxygen from 0.3 ml oxygen per 100 ml blood to 2 ml oxygen per 100 ml blood. Oxygen should be continued until the COHb level falls below 5% (90).

Hyperbaric Oxygen Therapy

Hyperbaric oxygen increases the amount of dissolved oxygen in plasma (109) and enhances the elimination of COHb (22,30,99). Results from animal investigations support the efficacy of HBO_2 for acute CO poisoning (1,37,41,114–123). Results from clinical trials are conflicting (91,93,124–126). However, a recent double-blind, randomized clinical trial with a 6-week follow-up rate of 97% and a rigorous trial design demonstrated that cognitive sequelae at 6 weeks after poisoning was reduced from 46% to 25% ($N = 152$; $p = .007$) (126). This clinical trial enrolled patients who were symptomatic from acute CO poisoning, older than 15 years of age, not pregnant, and received HBO_2 within 24 hours of the end of their exposure. The mean COHb level was 25%, and 50% of the patients had lost consciousness. Three hyperbaric sessions were given in 24 hours, although 10% of patients randomized to HBO_2 failed to complete all three prescribed HBO_2 treatments. Prechamber cerebellar dysfunction was associated with cognitive sequelae at 6 weeks (odds ratio = 5.71; $p = .005$). Prospective follow-up at 6 and 12 months after CO poisoning of 118 of the 152 enrolled patients in this randomized trial (126), demonstrated a continued difference in cognitive sequelae favoring HBO_2 (18%), compared with patients treated with normobaric oxygen (34%) ($p = .03$) (126,127). The majority of biochemical, animal, and clinical trial data indicate a favorable role for HBO_2 for acute CO poisoning.

The risk of HBO_2 is low (114), as is the risk of transport to a chamber, if using an experienced transport team. The incidence of reversible hyperoxic seizures is 1% in CO-poisoned patients (128), compared with a seizure incidence of 0.02% in non–CO-poisoned patients treated with HBO_2 (114). Critically ill patients should be transported to a hyperbaric facility that accepts critically ill patients. Monoplace (single person) hyperbaric chambers can also be used to treat critically ill patients if they are appropriately configured and staffed (129). The Divers Alert Network, Duke University Medical Center, Durham, NC, provides a 24-hour hotline (919-684-8111) for diving emergencies and can provide information about the location of hyperbaric oxygen chambers for acute CO poisoning. When readily available, HBO_2 should be considered for patients with acute CO poisoning. However, which patients require HBO_2 and the optimal dosing of HBO_2 for patients with acute CO poisoning remain challenges. Pending results from further trials designed to address selection criteria and recommendations for HBO_2 are proposed in Table 3.

TABLE 3. Proposed indications for hyperbaric oxygen therapy of patients with carbon monoxide poisoning

History of loss of consciousness even if brief.
A COHb level above 20%, although the COHb level does not correlate well with symptoms or outcome.
Evidence of major end-organ dysfunction (e.g., myocardial ischemia, confusion, metabolic acidosis).
Abnormal cerebellar examination because this abnormality was associated with cognitive sequelae in one study (126).
Pregnancy (60,139).
- Fetal distress (e.g., fetal tachycardia; decreased beat-to-beat variability; late decelerations, which are consistent with the COHb levels and carbon monoxide exposure history).
- Maternal COHb is above 20%.
- Any maternal neurologic signs regardless of the COHb level.
- If the patient continues to demonstrate neurologic signs or if signs of fetal distress, additional hyperbaric oxygen treatments may be necessary (60,139).

COHb, carboxyhemoglobin.

HBO_2 may be futile in patients who have regained cardiac function after cardiac arrest (130). If brain death is confirmed, the individual may be a candidate for cardiac (131,132) or liver donation (133) despite lethal CO poisoning.

Supportive Care

The decision to admit the patient to the hospital involves the degree of expression of signs and symptoms as well as individual comorbidities. Recognizing the lack of prospective data available, proposed indications for hospital admission are provided in Table 4.

During hospitalization, the patient's cardiac and respiratory status is monitored. Obtain a baseline electrocardiogram and cardiac enzymes (myocardial muscle creatine kinase isoenzyme and troponin I) in patients with underlying coronary arterial disease, chest pain, or with an altered mental status. Monitor for

TABLE 4. Proposed indicators for hospital admission of patients exposed to carbon monoxide

The magnitude of the initial COHb level is not the sole criterion for hospital admission. The following patients may need to be admitted to the hospital or observed for 12 to 24 hours in an observation setting depending on the patient's age, symptoms, proximity to the hospital, whether hyperbaric oxygen was used, and the patient's social support structure:
- Pregnant patients with COHb levels greater than 10% (recommend consultation with obstetrics/fetal medicine).
- Patients with myocardial ischemia by electrocardiogram or cardiac enzyme elevations.
- Patients who remain symptomatic from their poisoning after several hours of 100% normobaric oxygen therapy.
- Patients with suicide attempts need to be evaluated by a psychiatrist for disposition once medically "cleared."

COHb, carboxyhemoglobin.

hypercapnia in chronic lung disease patients [not due to suppression of the so-called hypoxic-drive but rather due to higher inspired concentrations of oxygen worsening ventilation-perfusion inequalities (134,135)].

In patients with smoke inhalation, consider cyanide toxicity, especially if the patient has a large metabolic acidosis, and treat for cyanide poisoning (Chapter 185).

Monitor for the development of cerebral edema with serial neurologic exams, CT scans, and funduscopic examination. Obtain a neurologic consultation when the diagnosis of cerebral edema is suspected. Corticosteroids have no proven role at preventing neurologic sequelae or improving CO-induced cerebral edema. Hyperventilation ($Pa{CO_2}$ tension of 25 to 30 mm Hg), head elevation (35 degrees), and mannitol (0.25 to 1.0 g/kg of a 20% solution over 30 minutes) constitute the initial treatment of elevated intracranial pressure. However, none of these therapies offers any therapeutic advantage for cytotoxic edema, and hyperventilation or hypovolemia (due to mannitol) may be harmful. Induced hypothermia might be helpful based on data from randomized clinical trials in post–cardiac arrest patients (136,137), although inferences drawn from post–cardiac arrest literature (136,137) to CO poisoning–related brain injury are limited.

Supplemental normobaric (100%) oxygen therapy may be stopped when the patient becomes asymptomatic or the COHb level falls below 5% (90). Four to 6 hours of 100% oxygen should be sufficient if the patient does not receive HBO_2. High-flow oxygen after an initial HBO_2 treatment is unnecessary. However, patients with concomitant aspiration pneumonitis may need supplemental oxygen to maintain an arterial saturation of oxygen greater than 90%.

Metabolic acidosis should not be treated aggressively unless the acidosis itself contributes to toxicity (i.e., pH less than 7.15). Acidosis increases the unloading of oxygen in tissues and therefore has a theoretic advantage in CO poisoning where the oxyhemoglobin dissociation curve shifts leftward (36).

For methylene chloride, the usual measures suffice, with primary attention given to the extent of hepatorenal toxicity and the COHb level. Follow-up measurements of hepatic aminotransferase levels should be scheduled within 1 week of exposure. At least two patients had a favorable outcome after HBO_2 treatment (138).

Pregnancy

Pregnant patients with acute CO poisoning should be treated with normobaric 100% up to five to seven times longer than in the nonpregnant CO-poisoned patients due to the longer half-life of fetal COHb (48,139). Effectively, the pregnant female should be treated with 12 to 24 hours of 100% normobaric oxygen depending on initial COHb and symptoms or evidence of fetal distress (60). In addition, the recommended indications for HBO_2 are altered for the pregnant patient (Table 3).

Outcome

Physical activity should be guided by the patient's abilities, but it is common for the patient to express physical limitations, ranging from a few days to weeks after poisoning. For prolonged weakness and fatigue, a neurologic and cardiologic evaluation is reasonable.

Differing results exist regarding long-term outcome after CO poisoning. The incidence of neurocognitive sequelae after acute CO poisoning ranges from 2.75% to 50.00% (1,45,63,65,69–71,91,108,109,114,124,140–148). Dramatic neurologic dysfunction after CO poisoning includes apathy, dementia, amnesia, disorientation, hypokinesia, mutism, gait disturbance, focal neurologic signs, Parkinson-like syndrome, and cortical blindness (45,70,71,148). In a prospective neuropsychological outcome study at 6 and 12 months after CO poisoning, 30% of poisoned patients had cognitive sequelae at both 6 and 12 months, and 40% of patients had new affective problems related to the poisoning (143). Loss of consciousness is not necessary for developing CO-related sequelae (23,91–93,141,143,149). Also, patients treated with HBO_2 can develop cognitive sequelae (45,63,91,109,124,146).

No known marker predicts who will or will not develop cognitive sequelae, including the initial COHb or the severity of poisoning. Therefore, CO-poisoned patients need to have routine follow-up, particularly if they remain symptomatic days or weeks after poisoning. Appropriate follow-up resources include neuropsychologists, neurologists, and psychiatrists (because affective problems are also common sequelae). Efforts at preventing further brain injury should also be emphasized (e.g., CO detectors in the home, avoidance of workplace exposure, wearing a helmet if participating in activities associated with closed head injuries).

ACKNOWLEDGMENTS

I appreciate Rachelle Taylor's assistance with preparation of this chapter. I am indebted to Susan Churchill, NP, for critically reviewing this chapter.

REFERENCES

1. Piantadosi CA. Diagnosis and treatment of carbon monoxide poisoning. *Respir Care Clin North Am* 1999;5:183–202.
2. Winter PM, Miller JN. Carbon monoxide poisoning. *JAMA* 1976;236:1502–1504.
3. Cobb N, Etzel RA. Unintentional carbon monoxide-related deaths in the United States, 1979 through 1988. *JAMA* 1991;266:659–663.
4. Hampson NB. Emergency department visits for carbon monoxide poisoning in the Pacific Northwest. *J Emerg Med* 1998;16:695–698.
5. Weaver LK, Mobasher H, Hopkins RO, et al. Emergency department visits for CO poisoning in Utah in 1996. *Undersea Hyperb Med* 1999;26[Suppl]:51(abst).
6. Pankow D. Carbon monoxide formation due to metabolism of xenobiotics. In: Penney DG, ed. *Carbon monoxide*. Boca Raton, FL: CRC Press, Inc., 1996:25–43.
7. Ratney RS, Wegman DH, Elkins HB. In vivo conversion of methylene chloride to carbon monoxide. *Arch Environ Health* 1974;28:223–236.
8. Mavalankar DV. Indoor air pollution in developing countries. *Lancet* 1991;1:358–359.
9. Behera D, Dash S, Malik SK. Blood carboxyhaemoglobin levels following acute exposure to smoke of biomass fuel. *Indian J Med Res* 1988;88:522–524.
10. Fawcett TA, Moon RE, Fracica PJ, et al. Warehouse worker's headache. Carbon monoxide poisoning from propane-fueled forklifts. *J Occup Med* 1992;34:12–15.
11. Burney RE, Wu S, Nemiroff MJ. Mass carbon monoxide poisoning: clinical effects and results of treatment in 184 victims. *Ann Emerg Med* 1982;11:394–399.
12. Klasner AE, Smith SR, Thompson MW, et al. Carbon monoxide mass exposure in a pediatric population. *Acad Emerg Med* 1998;5:992–996.
13. Wrenn K, Conners GP. Carbon monoxide poisoning during ice storms: a tale of two cities. *J Emerg Med* 1997;15:465–467.
14. Daley WR, Smith A, Paz-Argandona E, et al. An outbreak of carbon monoxide poisoning after a major ice storm in Maine. *J Emerg Med* 2000;18:87–93.
15. Anonymous. From the Centers for Disease Control and Prevention. Carbon monoxide poisoning at an indoor ice arena and bingo hall—Seattle, 1996. *JAMA* 1996;275:1468–*1469.
16. Paulozzi LJ, Satink F, Spengler RF. A carbon monoxide mass poisoning in an ice arena in Vermont. *Am J Public Health* 1991;81:222.
17. Hampson NB, Norkool DM. Carbon monoxide poisoning in children riding in the back of pickup trucks. *JAMA* 1992;267:538–540.
18. Silvers SM, Hampson NB. Carbon monoxide poisoning among recreational boaters. *JAMA* 1995;274:1614–1616.
19. Anonymous. From the Centers for Disease Control and Prevention. Houseboat-associated carbon monoxide poisonings on Lake Powell—Arizona and Utah, 2000. *JAMA* 2001;285:530–532.
20. Hampson NB, Kramer CC, Dunford RG, et al. Carbon monoxide poisoning from indoor burning of charcoal briquets. *JAMA* 1994;271:52–53.

21. Yoon SS, Macdonald SC, Parrish RG. Deaths from unintentional carbon monoxide poisoning and potential for prevention with carbon monoxide detectors. *JAMA* 1998;279:685–687.
22. Peterson JE, Steward RD. Absorption and elimination of carbon monoxide by inactive young men. *Arch Environ Health* 1970;21:165–171.
23. Amitai Y, Zlotogorski Z, Golan-Katzav V, et al. Neuropsychological impairment from acute low-level exposure to carbon monoxide. *Arch Neurol* 1998;55:845–848.
24. McGrath JJ. The interacting effects of altitude and carbon monoxide. In: Penney D, ed. *Carbon monoxide toxicity*. Boca Raton, FL: CRC Press, 2000:135–156.
25. Takeuchi A, Vesely A, Rucker J, et al. A simple "new" method to accelerate clearance of carbon monoxide. *Am J Respir Crit Care Med* 2000;161:1816–1819.
26. Lawwerys RR, ed. *Industrial chemical exposure: guidelines for biological monitoring*. Davis, CA: Biomedical Publications, 1983:83.
27. Fagin J, Bradley J, Williams D. Carbon monoxide poisoning secondary to inhaling methylene chloride. *BMJ* 1980;281:1461.
28. Di Vincenzo GD, Kaplan CJ. Effect of exercise or smoking on the uptake, metabolism and excretion of methylene chloride vapor. *Toxicol Appl Pharmacol* 1981;59:141–148.
29. Vreman HJ, Wong RJ, Stevenson DK. Carbon monoxide in breath, blood, and other tissues. In: Penney D, ed. *Carbon monoxide toxicity*. Boca Raton, FL: CRC Press, 2000:19–60.
30. Pace N, Strajman E, Walker E. Acceleration of carbon monoxide elimination in man by high pressure oxygen. *Science* 1950;111:652–654.
31. Weaver LK, Howe S, Hopkins R, et al. Carboxyhemoglobin half-life in carbon monoxide-poisoned patients treated with 100% oxygen at atmospheric pressure. *Chest* 2000;117:801–808.
32. Longo LD. Carbon monoxide effects on oxygenation of the fetus in utero. *Science* 1976;194:523–525.
33. Stewart RD, Dodd HC. Absorption of carbon tetrachloride, trichloroethylene, tetrachloroethylene, methylene chloride and 1,1,1-trichloroethane through the human skin. *Am Ind Hyg Assoc J* 1964;25:439–446.
34. Di Vincenzo GD, Kaplan CJ. Uptake, metabolism and elimination of methylene chloride vapors by humans. *Toxicol Appl Pharmacol* 1981;59:130–140.
35. Steward RD, Fisher TN, Hosko MJ, et al. Carboxyhemoglobin elevation after exposure to dichloromethane. *Science* 1972;176:295–296.
36. Peirce EC. Treating acidemia in carbon monoxide poisoning may be dangerous. *J Hyperbaric Med* 1986;1:87–97.
37. Piantadosi CA. Toxicity of carbon monoxide: hemoglobin vs. histotoxic mechanisms. In: Penney DG, ed. *Carbon monoxide*. Boca Raton, FL: CRC Press, 1996:163–186.
38. Langston P, Gorman D, Runciman W, et al. The effect of carbon monoxide on oxygen metabolism in the brains of awake sheep. *Toxicology* 1996;114:223–232.
39. Coburn RF. The carbon monoxide body stores. In: Coburn RF, ed. Biological effects of carbon monoxide. *Ann N Y Acad Sci* 1970;174:11.
40. Thom SR. Carbon monoxide mediated brain lipid peroxidation in the rat. *J Appl Physiol* 1990;68:997–1003.
41. Zhang J, Piantadosi CA. Mitochondrial oxidative stress after CO hypoxia in the rat brain. *J Clin Invest* 1992;90:1193–1199.
42. Thom SR, Zu YA, Ischiropoulous H. Vascular endothelial cells generate peroxynitrite in response to carbon monoxide exposure. *Chem Res Toxicol* 1997;10:1023–1031.
43. Turcanu V, Dhouib M, Gendrault JL, et al. Carbon monoxide induces murine thymocyte apoptosis by a free radical-mediated mechanism. *Cell Biol Toxicol* 1998;14:47–54.
44. Piantidosi CA, Zhang J, Levin ED, et al. Apoptosis and delayed neuronal damage after carbon monoxide poisoning in the rat. *Exp Neurol* 1997;147:103–104.
45. Choi S. Delayed neurologic sequelae in carbon monoxide intoxication. *Arch Neurol* 1983;40:433–435.
46. Opeskin K, Drummer OA. Delayed death following carbon monoxide poisoning, a case report. *Am J Forensic Med Pathol* 1994;15:36–39.
47. Plum R, Posner JB, Haini RH. Delayed neurological deterioration after anoxia. *Arch Intern Med* 1962;110:56–63.
48. Longo LD. The biological effects of carbon monoxide on the pregnant woman, fetus, and newborn infant. *Am J Obstet Gynecol* 1977;129:69–103.
49. Singh J, Scott LJ. Threshold for carbon monoxide induced fetotoxicity. *Teratology* 1984;30:253–257.
50. Venning H, Robertson D, Milner AD. Carbon monoxide poisoning in an infant. *Br Med J* 1982;284:651.
51. Perrone J, Hoffman RS. Fetal hemoglobin interference with carboxyhemoglobin determination. *J Toxicol Clin Toxicol* 1995;33:475–486 (abst).
52. Perrone J, Hoffman RS. Falsely elevated carboxyhemoglobin levels secondary to fetal hemoglobin. Letter to the editor. *Acad Emerg Med* 1996;3:287–288.
53. Vreman HJ, Ronquillo RB, Ariagno RL, et al. Interference of fetal hemoglobin with the spectrophotometric measurement of carboxyhemoglobin. *Clin Chem* 1988;34:975–977.
54. Vreman HJ, Stevenson DK. Carboxyhemoglobin determined in neonatal blood with a co-oximeter unaffected by fetal oxyhemoglobin. *Clin Chem* 1994;40:1522–1527.
55. Goldstein DP. Carbon monoxide poisoning in pregnancy. *Am J Obstet Gyencol* 1965;9:526–528.
56. Caravati EM, Adams CJ, Joyce SM, et al. Fetal toxicity associated with maternal carbon monoxide poisoning. *Ann Emerg Med* 1988;17:714–717.
57. Muller GL, Graham S. Intrauterine death of the fetus due to accidental carbon monoxide poisoning. *N Engl J Med* 1995;252:1075–1078.
58. Cramer CR. Fetal death due to accidental maternal carbon monoxide poisoning. *J Toxicol Clin Toxicol* 1982;19:297–301.
59. Margulies JL. Acute carbon monoxide poisoning during pregnancy. *Am J Emerg Med* 1986;4:516–519.
60. Koren G, Sharav T, Pastuszak A, et al. A multicenter, prospective study of fetal outcome following accidental carbon monoxide poisoning in pregnancy. *Reprod Toxicol* 1991;5:397–403.
61. De Haas JH. Parental smoking. Its effect on fetus and child health. *Eur J Obstet Gynecol Reprod Biol* 1975;5:283–296.
62. Harrison KL, Robinson AG. The effect of maternal smoking on carboxyhemoglobin levels and acid-base balance of fetus. *J Toxicol Clin Toxicol* 1981;18:165–168.
63. Weaver LK. Carbon monoxide poisoning. *Crit Care Clin* 1999;15:297–317.
64. Hampson NB, Ball LB, Macdonald SC. Are symptoms helpful in the evaluation of patients with acute carbon monoxide poisoning? *Undersea Hyper Med* 1999;26[Suppl]:50–51(abst).
65. Thorpe T. Chronic carbon monoxide poisoning. *Can J Psychiatry* 1994;39:59–61.
66. Lowe-Ponsford FL, Henry JA. Clinical aspects of carbon monoxide. *Adverse Drug React Acute Pois Rev* 1989;8:212–220.
67. Heckerling PS. Occult carbon monoxide poisoning: a cause of winter headache. *Am J Emerg Med* 1987;5:201–204.
68. Kelley JS, Sophocleus GJ. Retinal hemorrhages in subacute carbon monoxide poisoning. Exposures in homes with blocked furnace flues. *JAMA* 1978;239:1515–1517.
69. Choi IS. Parkinsonism after carbon monoxide poisoning. *Eur Neurol* 2002; 48:30–33.
70. Min SK. A brain syndrome associated with delayed neuropsychiatric sequelae following acute carbon monoxide intoxication. *Acta Psychiatr Scand* 1986;73:80–86.
71. Choi IS, Cheon HY. Delayed movement disorders after carbon monoxide poisoning. *Eur Neurol* 1999;42:141–144.
71. Choi IS. Carbon monoxide poisoning: systemic manifestations and complications. *J Korean Med Sci* 2001;16:253–261.
72. Sone S, Higoshihari T, Kotake T, et al. Pulmonary manifestations in acute carbon monoxide poisoning. *AJR Am J Roentgenol* 1974;120:865–871.
73. Balzan M, Cacciottolo JM, Casha S. Intestinal infarction following carbon monoxide poisoning. *Postgrad Med J* 1993;69:302–303.
74. Anderson R, Allensworth DC, De Groot WJ. Myocardial toxicity from carbon monoxide poisoning. *Ann Intern Med* 1967;67:1172–1182.
75. Marius-Nunez AL. Myocardial infarction with normal coronary arteries after acute exposure to carbon monoxide. *Chest* 1990;97:491–494.
76. Florkowski CM, Rossi ML, Carey MP, et al. Rhabdomyolysis and acute renal failure following carbon monoxide poisoning: two case reports with muscle histopathology and enzyme activities. *J Toxicol Clin Toxicol* 1992;30:443–454.
77. Makishima K, Keane WM, Vernose GV, et al. Hearing loss of a central type secondary to carbon monoxide poisoning. *Trans Am Acad Ophthalmol Otolaryngol* 1977;84:452–457.
78. Joiner TA, Sumner JR, Catchings TT. Unilateral diaphragmatic paralysis secondary to carbon monoxide poisoning. *Chest* 1990;97:498–499.
79. Snyder RD. Carbon monoxide intoxication with peripheral neuropathy. *Neurology* 1970;20:177–180.
80. Eltorai IM, Strauss MB, Hart GB, et al. Carbon monoxide neural toxicity with report of a clinical case. *Ariz Med* 1984;41:729–734.
81. Leaf DA, Kleinman MT. Urban ectopy in the mountains: carbon monoxide exposure at high altitude. *Arch Environ Health* 1996;51:283–290.
82. Balzan MV, Cassiottolo JM, Mifsud S. Unstable angina and exposure to carbon monoxide. *Postgrad Med J* 1994;70:699–702.
83. Schwartz J. Air pollution and hospital admissions for heart disease in eight U.S. counties. *Epidemiology* 1999;10:17–20.
84. Kleinman MT, Leaf DA, Kelly E, et al. Urban angina in the mountains: effects of carbon monoxide and mild hypoxemia on subjects with chronic stable angina. *Arch Environ Health* 1998;53:388–397.
85. Hinderliter AL, Adams KF Jr, Price CJ, et al. Effects of low-level carbon monoxide exposure on resting and exercise-induced ventricular arrhythmias in patients with coronary artery disease and no baseline ectopy. *Arch Environ Health* 1989;44:89–93.
86. Sheps DS, Adams KF Jr, Bromberg PA, et al. Lack of effect of low levels of carboxyhemoglobin on cardiovascular function in patients with ischemic heart disease. *Arch Environ Health* 1987;42:108–116.
87. Aronow WS. Aggravation of angina pectoris by two percent carboxyhemoglobin. *Am Heart J* 1981;101:154–157.
88. Allred EN, Bleecker ER, Chaitman BR, et al. Short-term effects of carbon monoxide exposure on the exercise performance of subjects with coronary artery disease. *N Engl J Med* 1989;321:1426–1432.
89. Kleinman MT, Davidson DM, Vandagriff RB, et al. Effects of short-term exposure to carbon monoxide in subjects with coronary artery disease. *Arch Environ Health* 1989;44:361–369.
90. Ilano AL, Raffin TA. Management of carbon monoxide poisoning. *Chest* 1990;7:165–169.
91. Raphael JD, Elkharrat D, Jars-Guincestre MC, et al. Trial of normobaric and hyperbaric oxygen for acute carbon monoxide intoxication. *Lancet* 1989;2:414–419.
92. Hopkins RO, Weaver LK, Larson-Lohr V, et al. Loss of consciousness (LOC) is not required for neurological sequelae due to CO poisoning. *Undersea Hyperb Med* 1995;22[Suppl]:14–15(abst).

93. Mathieu D, Wattel F, Mathiue-Nolf M, et al. Randomized prospective study comparing the effect of HBO versus 12 hours NBO in non-comatose CO poisoned patients: results of the interim analysis. *Undersea Hyperb Med* 196;23[Suppl]:7–8(abst).
94. Weaver LK, Hopkins RO, Larson-Lohr V. Neuropsychologic and functional recovery from severe carbon monoxide poisoning without hyperbaric oxygen therapy. *Ann Emerg Med* 1996;27:736–740.
95. Friedlander BR, Hearne T, Hall S. Epidemiologic investigation of employees exposed to methylene chloride. Mortality analysis. *J Occup Med* 1973;20:657–666.
96. Langehennig PL, Seeler RA, Berman E. Paint removers and carboxyhemoglobin. *N Engl J Med* 1976;295:1137.
97. Touger M, Gallagher EJ, Tyrell J. Relationship between venous and arterial carboxyhemoglobin levels in patients with suspected carbon monoxide poisoning. *Ann Emerg Med* 1995;25:481–483.
98. Hampson NB. Pulse oximetry in severe carbon monoxide poisoning. *Chest* 1998;114:1036–1041.
99. Jay GD, Tetz DJ, Hartigan CF, et al. Portable hyperbaric oxygen therapy in the emergency department with the modified Gamow bag. *Ann Emerg Med* 1995;26:707–711.
100. Sokal JA, Kralkowska E. The relationship between exposure duration, carboxyhemoglobin, blood glucose, pyruvate and lactate and the severity of intoxication in 39 cases of acute carbon monoxide poisoning in man. *Arch Toxicol* 1985;57:196–199.
101. Sawada Y, Takahashi M, Ohashi N, et al. Computerized tomography as an indication of long term outcome after acute carbon monoxide poisoning. *Lancet* 1980;1:783–784.
102. Kanaga N, Imaizumi H, Nakayana M, et al. The utility of MRI in acute stage of carbon monoxide poisoning. *Intensive Care Med* 1992;18:371–372.
103. Gale SD, Hopkins RO, Weaver LK, et al. MRI, quantitative MRI, SPECT, and neuropsychological findings following carbon monoxide poisoning. *Brain Injury* 1999;13:229–243.
104. Parkinson RB, Hopkins RO, Cleavinger HB, et al. White matter hyperintensities and neuropsychological outcome following carbon monoxide poisoning. *Neurology* (*in press*).
105. Stewart RD, Hake CC. Paint remover hazard. *JAMA* 1976;235:398–401.
106. Hall AH, Mountain R, Kulig KW, et al. Methylene chloride poisoning without significantly elevated carboxyhemoglobin level. *Vet Hum Toxicol* 1986;28:482–483(abst).
107. Jain KK. General principles of management of carbon monoxide poisoning. In: Jain KK, ed. *Carbon monoxide poisoning*. St. Louis: Warren H. Green, 1990:138–146.
108. Ernst A, Zibrak JD. Carbon monoxide poisoning. *N Engl J Med* 1998;339:1603–1608.
109. Tibbles PM, Edelsberg JS. Hyperbaric-oxygen therapy. *N Engl J Med* 1996;34:1642–1648.
110. Burkhart JE Jr, Stoller JK. Oxygen and aerosolized drug delivery: matching the device to the patient. *Cleve Clin J Med* 1998;65:200–208.
111. Jackson RM. Oxygen. In: Webb A, Shapiro M, Singer M, Suter PM, eds. *Oxford textbook of critical care*. Oxford, UK: Oxford University Press, 1999:1265–1269.
112. Myers RAM, Jones DW, Britten JS. Carbon monoxide half-life study. In: Kindwall EP, ed. *Proceedings of the Eighth International Congress on Hyperbaric Medicine*. Flagstaff, AZ: Best Publishing, 1987:263–266.
113. Peirce EC II, Bensky WH. Carbon monoxide poisoning in New York City: treatment with hyperbaric oxygen. In: *Proceedings of the Ninth International Congress on Hyperbaric Medicine*. Flagstaff, AZ: Best Publishing, 1987:109–114.
114. Hampson NB, ed. *Hyperbaric oxygen therapy: 1999 committee report revised*. Kensington, MD: Undersea and Hyperbaric Medical Society, 1999.
115. End E, Long C. Oxygen under pressure in carbon monoxide poisoning—effect on dogs and guinea pigs. *J Ind Hygiene Toxicol* 1942;24:302–306.
116. Peirce EC, Zacharias A, Alday JM Jr, et al. Carbon monoxide poisoning: experimental hypothermic and hyperbaric studies. *Surgery* 1972;72:229–237.
117. Brown SD, Piantadosi CA. Reversal of carbon monoxide-cytochrome c oxidase binding by hyperbaric oxygen in vivo. *Adv Exp Med Biol* 1989;248:747–754.
118. Thom SR. Antagonism of carbon monoxide-mediated brain lipid peroxidation by hyperbaric oxygen. *Toxicol Appl Pharmacol* 1990;105:340–344.
119. Tomaszewski C, Rudy J, Wathen J, et al. Prevention of neurologic sequelae from carbon monoxide by hyperbaric oxygen in rats. *Ann Emerg Med* 1992;21:631–632.
120. Thom SR. Functional inhibition of leukocyte B2 integrins by hyperbaric oxygen in carbon monoxide-mediated brain injury in rats. *Toxicol Appl Pharmacol* 1993;123:248–256.
121. Jiang J, Tyssebotn I. Cerebrospinal fluid pressure changes after acute carbon monoxide poisoning and therapeutic effects of normobaric and hyperbaric oxygen in conscious rats. *Undersea Hyperb Med* 1997;24:245–254.
122. Jiang J, Tyssebotn I. Normobaric and hyperbaric oxygen treatment of acute carbon monoxide poisoning in rats. *Undersea Hyperb Med* 1997;24:107–116.
123. Thom SR. Learning dysfunction and metabolic defects in globus pallidus and hippocampus after CO poisoning in a rat model. *Undersea Hyperb Med* 1997;24[Suppl]:20.
124. Scheinkestel CD, Bailey M, Myles PS, et al. Hyperbaric or normobaric oxygen for acute carbon monoxide poisoning: a randomised controlled clinical trial. *Med J Aust* 1999;170:203–210.
125. Ducasse JL, Celsis P, Marc-Vergnes JP. Non-comatose patients with acute carbon monoxide poisoning: hyperbaric or normobaric oxygenation? *Undersea Hyperb Med* 1995;22:9–15.
126. Weaver LK, Hopkins RO, Churchill S, et al. Hyperbaric oxygen for acute carbon monoxide poisoning. *N Engl J Med* 2002;347:1057–1067.
127. LK Weaver, RO Hopkins, S Churchill, KJ Chan. 6 and 12-month outcome of acute carbon monoxide poisoning treated with hyperbaric or normobaric oxygen. *Undersea Hyperb Med* 2002(abst) (*in press*).
128. Hampson N, Simonson SG, Kramer CC, et al. Central nervous system oxygen toxicity during hyperbaric treatment of patients with carbon monoxide poisoning. *Undersea Hyperb Med* 1996;23:215–219.
129. Weaver LK. Management of critically ill patients in the monoplace hyperbaric chamber. In: Kindwall EP, ed. *Hyperbaric medicine practice*, 2nd ed. Flagstaff, AZ: Best Publishing, 1999:245–294.
130. Hampson NB, Zmaeff JL. Outcome of patients experiencing cardiac arrest with carbon monoxide poisoning treated with hyperbaric oxygen. *Ann Emerg Med* 2001;38:36–41.
131. Koerner MM, Tenderich G, Minami K, et al. Extended donor criteria: use of cardiac allografts after carbon monoxide poisoning. *Transplantation* 1997;63:1358–1360.
132. Luckraz H, Tsui SS, Parameshwar J, et al. Improved outcome with organs from carbon monoxide poisoned donors for intrathoracic transplantation. *Ann Thorac Surg* 2001;72:709–713.
133. Verran D, Chui A, Painter D, et al. Use of liver allografts from carbon monoxide poisoned cadaveric donors. *Transplantation* 1996;62:1514–1515.
134. Crossley DJ, McGuire GP, Barrow PM, Houston PL. Influence of inspired oxygen concentration on dead space, respiratory drive, and Pa_{CO_2} in intubated patients with chronic obstructive pulmonary disease. *Crit Care Med* 1997;25:1522–1526.
135. Hoyt JW. Debunking myths of chronic obstructive lung disease. *Crit Care Med* 1997;25:1450–1451.
136. Bernard SA, Gray TW, Buist MD, et al. Treatment of comatose survivors of out-of-hospital cardiac arrest with induced hypothermia. *N Engl J Med* 2002;346:557–563.
137. The Hypothermia after Cardiac Arrest Study Group. Mild therapeutic hypothermia to improve the neurologic outcome after cardiac arrest. *N Engl J Med* 2002;346:549–556.
138. Rioux JP, Myers RA. Hyperbaric oxygen for methylene chloride poisoning: report on two cases. *Ann Emerg Med* 1989;18:691–695.
139. Van Hoesen KB, Camporesi EM, Moon RE, et al. Should hyperbaric oxygen be used to treat the pregnant patient for acute carbon monoxide poisoning? A case report and literature review. *JAMA* 1989;261:1039–1043.
140. Thom SR, Taber RL, Mendiguren II, et al. Delayed neuropsychologic sequelae after carbon monoxide poisoning: prevention by treatment with hyperbaric oxygen. *Ann Emerg Med* 1995;25:474–480.
141. Myers RA, Snyder SK, Emmett TA. Subacute sequelae of carbon monoxide poisoning. *Ann Emerg Med* 1985;14:1163–1167.
142. Yang ZD. Observation of hyperbaric oxygen in 160 patients with later manifestations after acute carbon monoxide poisoning. *Undersea Biomed Res* 1986;1[Suppl]:188–189.
143. Weaver LK, Hopkins RO, Howe S, et al. Outcome at 6 and 12 months following acute CO poisoning. *Undersea Hyperb Med* 1996;23[Suppl]:9–10(abst).
144. Haberstock D, Hopkins RO, Weaver LK, et al. Prospective longitudinal assessment of symptoms in acute carbon monoxide (CO) poisoning. *Undersea Hyperb Med* 1998;25[Suppl]:48(abst).
145. Hopkins RO, Weaver LK, Bigler ED. Psychological/emotional changes following carbon monoxide poisoning. *Undersea Hyperb Med* 1997;24[Suppl]:20(abst).
146. Gorman DF, Runciman WB. Carbon monoxide poisoning. *Anaesth Intensive Care* 1991;19:506–511.
147. Myers R, Thom S. Carbon monoxide and cyanide poisoning. In: Kindwall EP, Whelan HT, eds. *Hyperbaric medicine practice*. Flagstaff, AZ: Best Publishing, 1999:509–548.
148. Smith JD, Brandon S. Morbidity from acute carbon monoxide poisoning at three-year follow-up. *BMJ* 1973;1:318–321.
149. Ryan CM. Memory disturbances following chronic, low-level carbon monoxide exposure. *Arch Clin Neuropsychol* 1990;5:59–67.

CHAPTER 185

Cyanide

Andrew R. Erdman

H—C≡N

HYDROGEN CYANIDE

Compounds included:	**See Table 1.**
Molecular formula and weight:	**See Table 1.**
SI conversion:	**mg/L × 38.5 = μmol/L**
CAS Registry No.:	**See Table 1.**
Normal level:	**0.02 to 0.20 μg/ml; slightly higher in smokers**
Toxic level:	**Greater than 0.5 μg/ml (whole blood)**
Special concerns:	**Cyanide can knock down patients after just a few breaths.**
Target organs:	**Brain, heart**
Antidotes:	**Cyanide Antidote Kit (amyl nitrite, sodium nitrite, sodium thiosulfate), hydroxocobalamin**

OVERVIEW

Cyanide (CN^-) is an extremely toxic and rapidly acting agent that can be found in a variety of chemical compounds (Tables 1 and 2). Cyanide was first isolated and identified in the late 1700s. Since then, it has gained widespread notoriety as a result of its significant toxicity and its use in a number of well-publicized incidents. Hydrogen cyanide (HCN) gas was used as a chemical warfare agent in World Wars I and II, and HCN-penetrated pellets (Zyklon B) were used to commit genocide in the Nazi concentration camps during the Holocaust. Potassium cyanide was mixed with fruit punch in the 1978 Jonestown mass suicide in Guyana, resulting in the deaths of more than 900 people. Deliberate tampering incidents in which various over-the-counter medications or foodstuffs have been laced with cyanide salts have poisoned and killed a number of people in North America—for example, acetaminophen (Tylenol) in 1982 and pseudoephedrine (Sudafed) in 1991 (1–4). In the United States, HCN gas continues to be used in "gas chambers" for judicial executions.

TABLE 1. Common cyanide-containing or cyanide-liberating chemical compounds and U.S. regulatory guidelines and standards

Compound	Molecular formula	Molecular weight (g/mol)	CAS Registry No.	Agency	Description	Concentration (mg/m^3) (ppm)
Inorganic cyanide compounds						
Hydrogen cyanide	HCN	27.03	74-90-8	OSHA (air)	PEL-TWA	11 (10)
				ACGIH (air)	TLV-TWA	None
					Ceiling	5.0 (4.7)
				NIOSH (air)	REL-TWA	None
					STEL	5.0 (4.7)
					IDLH	55 (50)
Cyanide salts						
Potassium cyanide	KCN	65.12	151-50-8	OSHA (air)	PEL-TWA	Not listed
				ACGIH (air)	TLV-TWA	None
					Ceiling	5.0 (4.7) as CN
				NIOSH (air)	REL-TWA	None
					Ceiling	5.0 (4.7) as CN
					IDLH	25 (23)
Sodium cyanide	NaCN	49.01	143-33-9, 13998-03-3	OSHA (air)	PEL-TWA	Not listed
				ACGIH (air)	TLV-TWA	None
					STEL	5.0 (4.7) as CN
				NIOSH (air)	REL-TWA	None
					Ceiling	5.0 (4.7) as CN
					STEL	25 (23)
Calcium cyanide	$Ca(CN)_2$	92.11	592-01-8	OSHA (air)	PEL-TWA	Not listed
				ACGIH (air)	TLV-TWA	None
					STEL	5.0 (4.7) as CN
				NIOSH (air)	REL-TWA	Not listed
Metal cyanides						
Potassium silver cyanide	C_2AgN_2,K	199.01	506-61-6	OSHA	PEL-TWA	Not listed
				ACGIH	TLV-TWA	Not listed
				NIOSH	REL-TWA	Not listed
Gold (I) cyanide	AuCN	223	506-65-0	OSHA	PEL-TWA	Not listed
				ACGIH	TLV-TWA	Not listed
				NIOSH	REL-TWA	Not listed

(continued)

TABLE 1. (*continued*)

Compound	Molecular formula	Molecular weight (g/mol)	CAS Registry No.	Agency	Description	Concentration (mg/m³) (ppm)
Mercury cyanide	$Hg(CN)_2$	252.6	592-04-1	OSHA	PEL-TWA	Not listed
				ACGIH	TLV-TWA	Not listed
				NIOSH	REL-TWA	Not listed
Zinc cyanide	$Zn(CN)_2$	117.4	557-21-1	OSHA	PEL-TWA	Not listed
				ACGIH	TLV-TWA	Not listed
				NIOSH	REL-TWA	Not listed
Lead cyanide	$Pb(CN)_2$	259.2	592-05-2	OSHA	PEL-TWA	Not listed
				ACGIH	TLV-TWA	Not listed
				NIOSH	REL-TWA	Not listed
Metal cyanide salts						
Sodium cyanoaurite	Not reported	Not reported	Not reported	OSHA	PEL-TWA	Not listed
				ACGIH	TLV-TWA	Not listed
				NIOSH	REL-TWA	Not listed
Cyanogen halides						
Cyanogen chloride	CClN	61.47	506-77-4	OSHA (air)	PEL-TWA	Not listed
				ACGIH (air)	TLV-TWA	None
					Ceiling	0.6 (0.3)
				NIOSH (air)	REL-TWA	None
					Ceiling	0.6 (0.3)
					IDLH	None
Cyanogen bromide	CBrN	105.92	506-68-3	OSHA	PEL-TWA	Not listed
				ACGIH	TLV-TWA	Not listed
				NIOSH	REL-TWA	Not listed
Cyanogens						
Cyanogen	$(CN)_2$	52.04	460-19-5	OSHA (air)	PEL-TWA	Not listed
				ACGIH (air)	TLV-TWA	20 (10)
					STEL	None
				NIOSH (air)	REL-TWA	20 (10)
					STEL	None
					IDLH	None
Aliphatic nitriles						
Acetonitrile	C_2H_3N	41.05	75-05-8	OSHA (air)	PEL-TWA	70 (40)
				ACGIH (air)	TLV-TWA	34 (20)
					STEL	None
				NIOSH (air)	REL-TWA	34 (20)
					STEL	None
					IDLH	840 (500)
Acrylonitrile	C_3H_3N	53.06	107-13-1	OSHA (air)	PEL-TWA	Not listed
				ACGIH (air)	TLV-TWA	4.5 (2.0)
					STEL	None
				NIOSH (air)	REL-TWA	2.2 (1.0)
					Ceiling	22 (10)
					STEL	None
					IDLH	185 (85)
Butyronitrile	C_4H_7N	69.11	109-74-0	OSHA (air)	PEL-TWA	Not listed
				ACGIH (air)	TLV-TWA	Not listed
				NIOSH (air)	REL-TWA	22 (8)
					STEL	None
					IDLH	None
Propionitrile	C_3H_5N	55.08	107-12-0	OSHA (air)	PEL-TWA	Not listed
				ACGIH (air)	TLV-TWA	Not listed
				NIOSH (air)	REL-TWA	14 (6)
					STEL	None
					IDLH	None
Cyanogenic glycosides						
Amygdalin[a]	$C_{20}H_{27}NO_{11}$	457.4	29883-15-6	—	—	—
Linamarin[a]	$C_{10}H_{17}NO_6$	247.24	—	—	—	—

ACGIH, American Conference of Governmental Industrial Hygienists; IDLH, immediate danger to life or health; NIOSH, National Institute for Occupational Safety and Health; OSHA, U.S. Occupational Safety and Health Administration; PEL, permissible exposure limit; ppm, parts per million; REL, recommended exposure limit; STEL, short-term exposure limit; TLV, threshold limit value; TWA, time-weighted average.

[a]OSHA, ACGIH, and NIOSH guidelines and standards are not listed because compounds are not used occupationally.

While cyanide-containing compounds are rare in most homes, they are used in a number of common industrial and commercial processes; therefore, the potential for exposure is great among a wide range of occupations (Table 2). In addition, cyanide poisonings in the United States also occur with inhalation exposures to smoke. Rarely, they result from intentional ingestion by chemists or other workers with access to cyanide or from malicious tampering incidents. Few U.S. household prod-

TABLE 2. Sources of cyanide exposure

Industries and occupations
- Firefighting
- Rubber manufacturing
- Plastics manufacturing
- Leather manufacturing
- Mining
- Metal extraction/leaching
- Electroplating
- Metal polishing
- Metal hardening
- Welding
- Chemical synthesis
- Chemists and laboratory personnel
- Pharmaceutical manufacturing
- Photography
- Fumigation
- Pesticide workers
- Dyeing
- Paper production
- Synthetic fiber manufacturing
- Aerospace industry

Other potential sources of cyanide exposure
- Artificial nail remover (containing acetonitrile)
- Solvents (e.g., aliphatic nitriles)
- Hospitalized patients on nitroprusside
- Smoke inhalation
- Herbal medicines, fruit pits or seeds containing amygdalin or laetrile
- Malicious tampering

ucts contain cyanide, but imported or commercial products and certain cyanogenic compounds may still be found in some homes. In 2000, American poison centers reported approximately 300 cyanide exposures, which resulted in 38 cases of moderate to severe toxicity and six deaths. There were also nearly 3000 reports of exposure to cyanogenic plants, but none of these resulted in severe toxicity or death. Cyanide poisonings are probably more common outside the United States due to less stringent regulations on its use.

Classification and Uses

Cyanide (more specifically the CN^- anion) can be found in a wide variety of chemical and biologic compounds in a number of different forms (Table 1). The primary sources of medical significance include HCN, the inorganic cyanide salts and metallic cyanides, and organic cyanogenic compounds. Exposures to cyanogen gas, a cyanide dimer [CNNC or $(CN)_2$], can also lead to cyanide toxicity.

HCN is used in a number of industries (Table 2), and it may also be formed as the byproduct of certain reactions or processes (5–7). It is used as a fumigant for ships or buildings, an intermediate in the synthesis of various resins (e.g., acrylate, methacrylate), and in electroplating (8). HCN may also be released when cyanide salts are mixed with mineral acids or water (unless the aqueous solution is stabilized with the addition of a base) (7). HCN has a boiling point of approximately 78°F; therefore, it may be found either as a gas or a liquid depending on environmental conditions (6). HCN gas is also liberated with the combustion of certain plastics (e.g., polyurethanes, nitrocellulose) and other natural or synthetic materials (e.g., wool, nylon, silk) (9–11). Hence, it is commonly found in the smoke from household or industrial fires, blast furnaces, and the manufacture of coke and coal (12–14). The gaseous form of HCN is colorless and often described as having an almond-like odor when air concentrations exceed 1 parts per million (ppm). It is rapidly absorbed by inhalation and is extremely toxic even at relatively low air concentrations (15). Liquid HCN is colorless or slightly blue and has an odor similar to the gas. Dermal and mucous membrane exposures, combined with the inhalation of any evaporated HCN, can result in toxicity.

Inorganic cyanide salts and cyanide salt solutions are used in the extraction of precious metals from ore or other wastes (e.g., circuit boards), in steel hardening, electroplating, metal cleaning, cement stabilizing, rubber and plastic synthesis, the paper and photography industries, as fumigant powders in agriculture, and as laboratory reagents. Household use of such compounds is rare due to restrictions on their sale, but certain products, such as metal cleaning solutions and rodenticides, have been used in the past or may be imported from abroad, so they are still encountered occasionally in U.S. households (16,17).

The inorganic cyanide salts [KCN, $Ca(CN)_2$, NaCN, among others] are generally whitish crystalline solids (6). They can be easily mixed into aqueous solutions. Cyanide salt solutions can liberate HCN gas spontaneously, particularly in an acidic milieu, which can be a problem for workers who enter storage tanks containing such solutions without appropriate precautions (7). Cyanide salt solutions are typically kept at an alkaline pH (more than 12) to prevent off-gassing of HCN. Cyanide also forms strong complexes with many metals. Metal cyanides, such as copper, ferric, or silver cyanide, are whitish or colored solids (depending on the metal) with variable water solubility.

Poisoning from cyanide salts, metals, or their solutions usually occurs by way of ingestion (18–21). There are scattered reports of toxicity after dermal or mucous membrane exposure and intravenous injection, but other routes of exposure may have played a role in these cases (e.g., inhalation of HCN gas formed spontaneously from cyanide salt solutions) (7,22,23).

Cyanogens are complex organic compounds that can release cyanide after *in vivo* biotransformation. The aliphatic nitriles, such as acetonitrile, acrylonitrile, butyronitrile, and propionitrile, are synthetic cyanogens consisting of a hydrocarbon chain attached to a CN group. After ingestion or inhalation, they are oxidized *in vivo* by cytochrome P-450, which liberates the cyanide moiety and may result in toxicity (24–33). The aliphatic nitriles are used in various synthetic processes and as organic solvents. Acetonitrile may be found in some household and commercial artificial nail removers. Most of the aliphatic nitriles are clear, colorless liquids with a sweet, ether-like odor.

Naturally occurring cyanogens include amygdalin (D-mandelonitrile-β-*d*-glucoside), a cyanogenic glycoside. It is found in the seeds or pits of certain fruits (e.g., apricot pits, cherry pits, apple seeds); the foliage, stems, or roots of certain plants (e.g., bamboo, almonds, lima beans); and in a number of "herbal" remedies. Toxicity can result because amygdalin is broken down in the intestine to cyanide and other byproducts, primarily due to the action of the enzyme β-glucosidase (34–37). Laetrile is a semisynthetic derivative of amygdalin that has been touted (and disproved) as a cancer cure. It has caused fatal cyanide poisoning after ingestion (38–42). Laetrile may be found in a solid form for ingestion, or dissolved in solution for parenteral injection. Cassava root is a significant source of food in Africa, Asia, and South America that contains cyanogens, particularly linamarin, which can cause cyanide toxicity (43).

Sodium nitroprusside, a commonly used intravenous antihypertensive agent, contains five molecules of cyanide per molecule of nitroprusside and releases cyanide *in vivo*. After excessive or prolonged infusions, patients may develop signs of cyanide toxicity (Chapter 187).

The *isocyanates* (e.g., methyl isocyanate, toluene diisocyanate) have sometimes mistakenly been lumped together with cyanide compounds, but their toxicity does not appear to be related to the release of cyanide (Chapter 188).

Toxic Dose

The exact toxic dose of cyanide is difficult to quantify and depends on the chemical form, the route and duration of exposure, and patient-specific factors such as individual susceptibility, differences in metabolism, or underlying medical problems (44). Regulatory standards and guidelines for selected cyanide compounds are provided in Table 1.

HCN gas can result in immediate collapse and death after inhalation. Toxicity primarily depends on the air concentration of HCN and the duration of exposure. Other factors, such as minute ventilation, respiratory protection, and dermal exposure, can affect the development of toxicity. Death has been reported after exposures to as little as 200 to 300 ppm of HCN (7,45). An addendum to a paper by Dudley presents a table listing the concentration of HCN immediately fatal to humans as 270 ppm (46). It also states that concentrations from 110 to 135 ppm can be fatal after 30 to 60 minutes, whereas concentrations of 45 to 54 ppm can generally be tolerated for a similar time period without significant effects. It is unclear, however, on what evidence these limits were based. The odor threshold for HCN has been reported as 1 ppm, but many people are genetically unable to detect the odor even at high levels (47).

The average fatal ingested dose for *inorganic cyanide salts, cyanide metal compounds, and their solutions* has been calculated from human case reports to be approximately 1.5 mg/kg (45). The lowest fatal dose reported in the literature is approximately 0.56 mg/kg. There are other reported cases of significant toxicity or death after ingestion of 1 to 3 g (a teaspoonful or a single tablet) of sodium or potassium cyanide (19,20,48–54). Numerous authors have suggested that oral doses of 50 to 100 mg of HCN or 200 to 300 mg of sodium or potassium cyanide should be considered potentially lethal (47,55). Ingestion of as little as 8 ml of a 5% cyanide solution was fatal in one case (56). The likelihood of toxicity after ingestion may be less than after inhalation or parenteral injection due to delayed absorption by the oral route and partial detoxification during first-pass metabolism through the liver (which contains a large proportion of the body's crucial rhodanese stores) (57).

The toxic dose of *cyanogens* is less well defined. Ingestion of 6 g of laetrile has caused serious toxicity in one case (42). Parenteral administration of laetrile is much less toxic than oral administration because of intestinal bacteria or ingested foodstuffs required to express β-glucosidase activity, which enzymatically liberate cyanide. The acidic milieu of the stomach may enhance this breakdown. Intravenous exposures to laetrile or amygdalin do not appear to result in cyanide toxicity because they bypass this environment.

Aliphatic nitriles can cause severe poisoning after ingestion of as little as several ml in an adult (26). The toxic threshold for inhalation or dermal exposures is not known. The aliphatic nitrile compounds vary in their ability to release cyanide *in vivo*. Some agents, such as propionitrile and butyronitrile, appear to liberate a greater amount of cyanide than the other nitriles (58–60). Individual metabolic differences may also play a role.

TOXICOKINETICS AND TOXICODYNAMICS

The final common pathway for all cyanide compound exposures is the absorption or liberation of HCN followed by its rapid distribution to all organs. Much of total body burden appears to reside in the erythrocyte, bound to endogenous methemoglobin and, to a lesser extent, normal hemoglobin (61,62). However, cyanide is detectable in virtually every organ after significant exposures, particularly those organs with high blood flow (48,63,64). It has an estimated volume of distribution of 0.075 to 0.500 L/kg (65–67).

The blood elimination half-life of cyanide varies widely, from a few minutes to up to 66 hours, depending on many factors (9,23,27,65,66,68–70). Larger cyanide exposures and higher blood levels can result in longer elimination half-lives, compared with smaller doses, suggesting that endogenous mechanisms of metabolism are quickly overwhelmed. Antidotal treatment reduces the blood half-life. Ongoing absorption or metabolic liberation may also result in longer blood elimination half-lives. With higher blood levels, cyanide may exhibit a biphasic elimination pattern with a rapid initial phase of declining levels over the first hour (representing redistribution and the effects of treatment or endogenous metabolism) followed by a longer terminal elimination phase (70–72). Animal studies suggest that chronic cyanide exposures do not lead to significant accumulation in the blood or tissues (73,74).

The body has several endogenous mechanisms capable of eliminating small amounts of cyanide, but these systems are easily overwhelmed. Under normal homeostatic conditions, minute amounts of cyanide are absorbed from the environment and generated by the body. The majority (60% to 80%) of this cyanide is detoxified by rhodanese, a mitochondrial trans-sulfurase enzyme found primarily in the liver and skeletal muscle (47,75–78). Rhodanese catalyzes the transfer of CN^- to the sulfur group of thiosulfate to form thiocyanate, a less toxic metabolite that can be easily removed by renal excretion. However, the body's thiosulfate supply represents the major rate-limiting step for this reaction, and endogenous stores of thiosulfate are typically quite limited.

A second enzyme, β-mercaptopyruvate-cyanide sulfurtransferase, can transfer a sulfur group from mercaptopyruvate to cyanide, again forming thiocyanate. However, in humans, this latter system probably accounts for only a small proportion of normal cyanide elimination. In addition to the action of these enzymes, a small amount of cyanide may combine with cystine to be converted to 2-aminothizoline-4-carboxylic acid for elimination (75). A minute fraction is eliminated unchanged through the lungs by exhalation. Some cyanide may react with the salts or esters of various amino acids (alpha-ketoglutarate, oxaloacetate, or pyruvate), and some binds avidly to the cobalt ions in endogenous hydroxocobalamin (vitamin B_{12a}) to form cyanocobalamin (vitamin B_{12}), which can then be excreted in the urine or bile (63).

Thiocyanate, the principal metabolite of cyanide, has a volume of distribution of 0.25 L/kg and is renally excreted, with an elimination half-life of 3 days (61).

PATHOPHYSIOLOGY

Inhibition of Cytochrome Oxidase

HCN is a weak acid and exists primarily in its nonionized (HCN) form at a physiologic pH of approximately 7.4. This allows HCN to cross cellular and mitochondrial membranes easily, where the CN^- anion can dissociate and bind to cations, metalloproteins, and other enzymes. It binds particularly avidly to the ferric ions of cytochrome-a_3, an integral component of the third and final cytochrome oxidase enzyme in the mitochondrial electron transport chain (79–82). Once bound, the enzyme becomes inactivated, and oxidative phosphorylation is blocked. Cells are thus deprived of their major energy source.

The inhibition of oxidative phosphorylation results in widespread metabolic derangements. Adenosine triphosphate (ATP) is consumed by active cells, but very little can be produced. Tissues quickly exhaust their supply of ATP. Furthermore, hydrogen ions that are generated by ATP hydrolysis begin to accumulate because they can no longer be recycled back into the process of ATP formation. Metabolic acidosis ensues. Pyruvate and nicotinamide adenine dinucleotide both accumulate as well. Cells attempt to compensate by converting pyruvate to lactate, which generates a small amount of ATP and regenerates the oxidized form of nicotinamide adenine dinucleotide. The resulting elevation in lactate levels serves as a good indicator of the degree of overall cellular metabolic impairment. Concomitant respiratory depression from central nervous system (CNS) dysfunction or hypotension from direct cardiovascular toxicity may contribute to the development of acidosis.

The result of these intracellular derangements (known as *cellular asphyxia* or *histotoxic hypoxia*) is cellular dysfunction and ultimately cell death if cytochrome inhibition persists. The most sensitive tissues are those with the highest metabolic demands such as the brain and heart. Hence, cyanide toxicity is dominated by CNS and cardiovascular manifestations along with acidosis and lactate accumulation as already described.

Other Mechanisms

Although most of cyanide's effects can be attributed to the inhibition of cytochrome oxidase, it also inhibits a number of other enzymes that may contribute to its toxicity. For example, cyanide impairs the function of glutamate decarboxylase, which results in a drop in CNS γ-aminobutyric acid levels and may lower the seizure threshold (83). It binds to succinate dehydrogenase, catalase, peroxidase, xanthine oxidase, aldolase, phosphatase, and carbonic anhydrase, although the clinical effects of such binding are uncertain (6,45,84). Cyanide has also been shown to alter carbohydrate metabolism, which might exacerbate cellular metabolic dysfunction (85).

Central Nervous System Injury

Cyanide causes neurotoxicity, primarily manifested by clinical CNS dysfunction, alterations in electrical activity, and histopathologic evidence of cellular necrosis and demyelination (86–88). Its effects have a predilection for areas of the brain such as the basal ganglia, hippocampus, substantia nigra, and deep white matter structures. Much of the toxicity may simply be due to the loss of oxidative phosphorylation, which impairs the energy-dependent enzymes and ion pumps required for normal neuronal function, homeostasis, and cellular integrity (89,90). There is also evidence, however, that lipid peroxidation and oxidative injury may play a role (84,91,92). Cyanide may cause direct nucleophilic attack, resulting in further damage to important cellular constituents. Alterations in cerebral blood flow have also been demonstrated (93). Finally, cyanide has been shown to cause the release of the excitatory neurotransmitter glutamate, which activates *N*-methyl-D-aspartate receptors in the brain, and cyanide has also been demonstrated to stimulate *N*-methyl-D-aspartate receptors directly on its own (94,95). Both mechanisms may exacerbate its neurologic effects and further lower the seizure threshold.

Thiocyanate

The metabolism of cyanide to thiocyanate can lead to excessive thiocyanate accumulation, particularly in patients with renal dysfunction or renal failure. Although thiocyanate is much less toxic than cyanide itself, high levels have been associated with abdominal discomfort, vomiting, rash, and neurologic dysfunction in some patients (61,96–99). The pathophysiology of these effects is not clear.

Sequelae of Acute Exposure

Occasionally, survivors of acute cyanide toxicity develop prolonged or permanent neurologic sequelae. Several cases of basal ganglia injury after acute poisoning have been reported (49,50). It is not clear whether cyanide itself is responsible (e.g., direct cellular toxicity or cellular asphyxia) or whether the secondary manifestations of cyanide poisoning, such as respiratory depression or hypotension, are to blame.

VULNERABLE POPULATIONS

There are currently no data to suggest that either children or elderly patients are at increased risk for cyanide toxicity; however, it is not unlikely that patients with preexisting conditions, such as cerebral or coronary vascular disease, or chronic respiratory insufficiency, might have a greater likelihood for complications. Individuals with acquired protein deficiency, such as malnourished or postsurgical patients, may be at increased risk for cyanide toxicity due to inadequate levels of the normal detoxification enzymes. Patients with acquired vitamin B_{12} deficiency may also be at some risk, although this is not clear.

Certain patients may be genetically predisposed to toxicity because of hereditary deficiencies or dysfunctions (e.g., from polymorphisms) in the enzymes involved in cyanide detoxification.

The reproductive effects of cyanide are based on animal studies alone, and the results are conflicting. Some studies found no effect on fetal development (100). Others found effects only in the presence of obvious maternal clinical toxicity (101). Still others noted developmental abnormalities, such as microcephaly, limb defects, growth retardation, encephalocele, or rib abnormalities, even in the absence of maternal symptoms (37,102,103).

The effects of cyanide on breast-feeding have not been well studied. However, in certain animal species, cyanide has been shown to be passed from lactating mothers to their young (100,104,105).

CLINICAL PRESENTATION

Acute cyanide toxicity may be difficult to recognize because the clinical signs of poisoning are protean and nonspecific. The "classic" presentation is that of an industrial worker (or someone with access to cyanide) who either collapses in the field or is found down with a triad of severe CNS effects, shock, and profound lactic acidosis. Clues to the diagnosis include the rapidity of onset, the severity of effects, and a history of work with or access to chemicals or cyanide-containing products. The presence of an almond-like odor or a cherry-red skin color may also be helpful if present but is neither sensitive nor specific.

Onset of Effects

Cyanide toxicity produces myriad clinical effects (Table 3). However, the presentation and time course of symptom development vary depending on the chemical form of cyanide, the route of exposure, and the dose. Certain patient-specific factors and cointoxicants may also affect the picture. Most patients with significant cyanide toxicity have obvious manifestations by the time of hospital presentation, although patients may continue to deteriorate as absorption or metabolic liberation continues.

Inhalation produces the most rapid onset of effects. Lower levels of HCN (i.e., less than 50 ppm) can lead to manifestations,

TABLE 3. Clinical signs and symptoms of acute cyanide poisoning

Cardiovascular
- Hypertension (initially)
- Tachycardia
- Hypotension
- Bradycardia
- Electrical conduction abnormalities
- Dysrhythmias
- Cardiac arrest

Neurologic
- Headache
- Fatigue
- Nausea
- Agitation
- Confusion
- Somnolence
- Hyporeflexia
- Mydriasis
- Collapse
- Coma
- Seizures
- Respiratory depression

Metabolic
- Increased anion gap acidosis
- Tachypnea
- Hyperlactatemia
- Reddish skin discoloration
- Decreased arterial-venous oxygen gap (arteriolization of venous blood gases)
- Hyperglycemia

Other
- Vomiting
- Almond-like odor
- Cyanosis
- Pulmonary edema

such as nausea, vomiting, headache, weakness, shortness of breath, drowsiness, and chest discomfort, after exposure times ranging from minutes to several hours (15,44,48). Inhalation of higher HCN concentrations can result in more severe clinical toxicity or even death within seconds to minutes (8,106,107).

Ingestion of an inorganic cyanide compound (e.g., cyanide salts, metal cyanides) is generally followed by the onset of clinical effects within 30 minutes (17,18,50,53–55,108–110). Powders and solutions are more readily absorbed than pellets or tablets and are more likely to result in a faster onset of toxicity. Food in the stomach or agents that decrease gastric motility may delay absorption and the onset of effects. Clinical effects may also be delayed somewhat or be more insidious in onset when a smaller dose of cyanide is ingested (18,53).

After ingestion of cyanogenic glycosides or exposure to any of the aliphatic nitriles, clinical effects may not develop for up to 24 hours because both absorption and metabolic liberation of the cyanide ion are required (24,27,111–114). Coingestions of agents that block the cytochrome P-450 system may delay the onset of toxicity even further (24). However, massive exposures can cause much more rapid development of effects.

With *dermal* exposures to HCN or inorganic cyanide compounds, absorption and toxicity may be delayed somewhat, but large enough exposures can still result in symptoms that develop within minutes (115).

Neurologic Effects

Neurologic manifestations initially include headache, nausea, vomiting, difficulty concentrating, dizziness, confusion, weakness, somnolence, or lethargy (15,18,44,53,107,115–117). With larger exposures, coma, respiratory depression, and seizures may rapidly develop (8,18,19,53,54,107,117–119). Many patients with significant exposures are found unconscious or witnessed to collapse (7,8,19,41,54,56,107,108,118–124). Occasionally, an initial but transient period of CNS excitation occurs (7,107,123).

Depending on the degree of neurologic impairment, reflexes may be decreased or abnormal, posturing can be present, muscle tone may be flaccid, and pupils dilated with decreased reactivity (5,65,118,119,124,125). Twitching and rigidity have occasionally been reported, but these may actually represent underlying seizure activity (120). With aliphatic nitrile exposures, the neurologic effects may initially resemble those of ordinary hydrocarbon poisoning, characterized by lethargy, stupor, confusion, or coma in the absence of any cardiovascular or metabolic manifestations. As cyanide is metabolically liberated, its effects begin to intervene.

Cardiorespiratory Effects

Dyspnea, palpitations, or a bounding pulse may be noted initially (15,20,49,51,117,125). With more severe toxicity, hypotension, tachycardia, bradycardia, dysrhythmias, tachypnea, irregular or depressed respirations, and cardiorespiratory arrest may occur (7,18,20,23,106,117,120,126). The patient's heart rate and blood pressure depend on the degree and stage of poisoning. Initially, or with low-level toxicity, a mild bradycardia with sinus pauses and hypertension may be observed (106). With the development of more severe poisoning, hypotension and tachycardia typically occur (18,20,126). With severe or premorbid toxicity, bradycardia associated with profound hypotension may be seen and generally presages imminent cardiac arrest (106).

Pulmonary edema is a less common complication of cyanide poisoning, and frothing at the mouth, or rales and rhonchi on pulmonary auscultation, may be evident in such cases (16,17,51). Inhalation of cyanide compounds has been reported to cause respiratory and mucous membrane irritation (127).

Acid-Base Effects

Metabolic effects of cyanide poisoning invariably include metabolic acidosis and hyperlactatemia (18,23,42,117). Usually, these are severe and serve as good indicators as to the degree of cellular impairment (16,18,22,41,128,129).

Gastrointestinal Effects

Nausea, vomiting, and abdominal discomfort are common after cyanide ingestions, but they may also develop with systemic poisoning from inhalation or dermal exposures (8,15,20,44,51,107,117,120,124,126). Cyanide salt and metal solutions are typically maintained at an alkaline pH to limit the spontaneous formation of HCN gas. The ingestion of such solutions can result in corrosive injury to the gastrointestinal (GI) tract, with all of its incumbent clinical manifestations (vomiting, abdominal pain, diarrhea, bleeding, perforation).

Dermal Manifestations

Redness or flushing of the skin has been described due to an elevated venous oxygen content from decreased tissue use (7,8,18,108,109,118,125). This finding may be particularly striking in the face of a patient with otherwise significant cardiovascular compromise. Such "arteriolization" of the venous blood is sometimes best detected on ophthalmoscopy by looking at the color of the retinal veins (126). However, neither the dermal nor retinal venous coloration is a reliable finding. Pallor or cyanosis has also been reported with significant poisonings (19,56,108).

Dermal burns may occur after skin exposures to certain compounds, particularly the cyanide salts or metal cyanides and their solutions (7,130).

Other Findings

Patients may or may not note the distinctive almond-like odor of cyanide. Its presence cannot be relied on as a marker of cyanide exposure for several reasons: A significant percentage of the population is genetically unable to detect the smell; odor fatigue may occur, making it difficult to detect increases in concentration or prolonged exposures; and because in high enough concentrations, only one breath of HCN may be sufficient to cause serious injury (15,68,131). Medical personnel may occasionally recognize the odor on poisoned patients, their clothing, or contaminated body fluids, but the same caveats apply (7,19,20,55,109).

Smoke Inhalation

Patients with cyanide poisoning from smoke inhalation exhibit signs and symptoms similar to others with cyanide poisoning. However, concomitant carbon monoxide exposure may exacerbate the effects. In addition, some victims display other physical manifestations of smoke inhalation such as singed nasal hair, oropharyngeal burns or soot, and evidence of pulmonary burn injury on auscultation. Smoke inhalation is addressed in Chapter 190.

Evolution and Duration of Clinical Effects

Symptom evolution varies, but clinical deterioration is rapid in most cases (18,108,129). After inhalation, patients typically manifest peak toxicity at the time of removal from the exposure. Patients with dermal exposures or ingestions may continue to deteriorate for minutes or sometimes even several hours after the initial onset of symptoms (18,53,108). With exposures to the various cyanogens, patients typically exhibit a slowly worsening course over many hours (42).

The duration of clinical effects varies. Most patients who receive antidotal treatment respond with a rapid improvement in cardiovascular, neurologic, and metabolic effects (132). Untreated or inadequately treated patients may require several hours or days to fully recover depending on the agent, dose, and route of exposure (18,41,115,133). Ongoing absorption or metabolic liberation of cyanide can result in prolonged toxicity.

Recrudescence of clinical effects may occur after antidotal therapy either because the beneficial effects of treatment have begun to wear off or due to the further absorption or metabolic liberation of cyanide (26). Even patients with inhalational HCN exposures can develop recurrence of symptoms (21). It is not clear whether this is the result of CN^- dissociating from circulating methemoglobin or due to tissue redistribution.

Sequelae of Acute Exposure

Mortality after significant cyanide exposures is high, ranging from 11% to 95% in hospitalized patients (117). Prompt decontamination, antidotal treatment, and good supportive care may significantly lower this rate (117).

Patients who survive a severe episode of cyanide toxicity may exhibit persistent or delayed neurologic sequelae. Both parkinsonian (e.g., tremor, rigidity, masked facies, slowed speech and gait) and dystonic symptoms have been described, implying susceptibility of dopaminergic neurons to cyanide-induced injury (49,50). However, long-term cerebellar, cognitive, and neuropsychiatric effects have also been reported (21). These neurologic effects may be evident immediately on recovery of the individual after the acute poisoning episode, or they may develop after a delay of several days to weeks. Postacute neurologic sequelae may vary in severity from subtle to severe. Imaging studies (e.g., computerized tomography or magnetic resonance imaging) of the brain typically reveal basal ganglia lesions, but radiographic findings may lag behind the development of clinical effects, so repeat testing may be needed several months later (50). The effects may be progressive, persistent, or improve spontaneously over time. Treatment with antiparkinsonian agents may offer some symptomatic improvement, but the response to medications is often suboptimal.

Chronic Exposure Toxicity

Chronic skin contact with cyanide compounds can lead to an irritative or corrosive chemical dermatitis, with varying degrees of pruritus, redness, discomfort or rash (45,134,135). Similarly, persistent low-level exposure to airborne cyanide compounds may cause chronic mucous membrane or respiratory irritation (45,134,135).

Whether chronic low-level exposures to cyanide compounds can cause significant systemic toxicity is somewhat controversial. A few reports have indicated an association with memory problems, neuropsychiatric symptoms, and subjective complaints such as weakness, nausea, vomiting, dyspnea, chest pains, palpitations, and headaches (134–136). The air levels of cyanide in these studies ranged from between 4 to 15 ppm. However, the effects are mainly subjective and difficult to quantify, and because the exposures occurred in an industrial setting, coexposure to other toxic agents may have contributed to any toxicity. More data are needed to establish and elucidate a causal relationship.

Increased hemoglobin and lymphocyte counts have been reported in some cyanide workers (134). Thyroid dysfunction has also been reported in patients with chronic exposures, presenting either as an enlarged thyroid gland on physical examination or with subclinical abnormalities in thyroid function or radioactive iodine uptake studies (134,135,137).

Several rare syndromes have also been associated, at least in part, with the effects of chronic cyanide; however, causation has yet to be proved. Tobacco amblyopia is an extremely rare disorder with progressive bilateral loss of vision in male smokers who may also report bilateral, symmetric scotomata and other visual disturbances such as altered color vision (138–144). The syndrome has been attributed to low levels of cyanide in inhaled cigarette smoke, causing a toxic injury to the optic nerve or retina. Certain patients with an underlying deficiency in cyanide detoxification capacity, possibly the result of decreased vitamin B_{12} or folate, or an altered methionine metabolism, may be at risk. Ophthalmoscopic findings vary based on the stage of illness but may reveal abnormal retinal vasculature, temporal pallor, or atrophy of the optic nerve; however, in other patients, the examination may be unremarkable. Visual evoked potentials are often decreased in amplitude. Leber's hereditary optic neuropathy is a rare genetic syndrome consisting of progressive visual dysfunction similar to patients with tobacco amblyopia (145). It may be related to a hereditary deficiency in the cyanide-detoxifying enzyme rhodanese. Tropical ataxic neuropathy is a demyelinating syndrome associated with the consumption of large amounts of cassava roots (146–148). Cassava contains linamarin, a cyanogenic glycoside, and is a staple of the diet in certain developing nations such as Nigeria. The disease is typically characterized by the development of distal, symmetric sensory symptoms such as paresthesias, bilateral neurosensory hearing loss, visual dysfunction from optic nerve atrophy, and ataxia (148).

DIAGNOSTIC TESTS

Cyanide Concentrations in Acute Poisoning

Cyanide can be quantified in plasma, red blood cells, whole blood, or urine using a variety of methods (47). Quantitative blood levels are the most useful and correlate best with the acute clinical effects of poisoning. Results may be available in some hospitals within a couple of hours; however, patients with significant cyanide toxicity invariably require antidotal therapy before the results are available. Blood cyanide levels should be drawn in any suspected case of cyanide poisoning—they can help confirm the diagnosis and may assist in guiding further treatment or decontamination measures.

Most of the cyanide in blood is bound to methemoglobin and to a much lesser extent to hemoglobin. Consequently, quantitative cyanide determinations in whole blood or red blood cell samples typically exceed those measured in plasma (47,149,150). Whole blood cyanide levels may overestimate the actual concentration due to the acidification process used in most analyses; therefore, some authors recommend plasma or red cell measurements as the methods of choice (6).

The timing of sampling is important because levels can drop quickly after removal from the exposure or after antidotal treatment has been instituted. Conversely, early in the course of poisoning, cyanide levels can continue to rise if ongoing absorption or metabolic liberation continues. After inhalation exposures to HCN, blood levels probably peak within seconds to minutes. After ingestions of inorganic cyanide-containing compounds, peak levels typically occur within minutes to several hours depending on the form and the presence of food. After exposures to cyanogenic compounds, blood cyanide may not peak for many hours (e.g., 7 hours later) (42).

Quantitative cyanide determinations can also be performed on gastric fluid samples to demonstrate a recent ingestion.

Correlation of Clinical Effects and Cyanide Concentration

The correlation between cyanide levels and clinical toxicity is not firmly established. The *normal blood cyanide level* averages approximately 0.015 to 0.030 μg/ml in nonsmokers and approximately 0.03 to 0.08 μg/ml in smokers (47,98,151). Another study revealed a mean level of 0.2 μg/ml, but both smokers and nonsmokers were included in the analysis (9).

A *toxic blood cyanide level* is generally considered to be greater than 0.5 μg/ml. Blood levels ranging from 2.1 to 16.3 μg/ml have been reported in cases of serious clinical toxicity, most of which appear to have been drawn on initial presentation (41,42,50,53, 120,121,123,128,152). Levels in reported fatalities have ranged from 2.2 to 34.6 μg/ml (7,19,41, 108,124,133). Baselt, on the other hand, quotes an average blood level of 12.4 μg/ml in human cyanide fatalities, with a range between 1.1 to 53.0 μg/ml (47). Clinical toxicity may be evident at lower levels in victims of smoke inhalation because of the additive effects of carbon monoxide.

Thiocyanate levels can be quantified in blood or urine, usually by colorimetry (47). Blood thiocyanate levels peak later (by several hours) than do levels of cyanide. However, they are not available any faster than blood cyanide levels, and even less is known about their correlation with the clinical effects of acute toxicity. As a result, blood thiocyanate determinations are not generally recommended for evaluation of an acute cyanide exposure. However, urine thiocyanate levels may remain elevated for several days after an acute cyanide exposure. Hence, significantly elevated levels may help in confirming a recent exposure. However, urine levelscannot be used to estimate its severity. Normal plasma thiocyanate levels range between 1 and 4 mg/L (3 to 12 mg/L in smokers), and urinary concentrations typically range between 1 and 4 mg/L (7 to 17 mg/L in smokers) (47).

Clinical Chemistry Tests

Certain routine laboratory abnormalities can establish a provisional diagnosis of acute cyanide poisoning. A serum electrolyte panel, renal function tests, blood gases, serum lactate level, baseline blood count, and an electrocardiogram should be performed.

Metabolic acidosis with an elevated anion gap is nearly always present in patients with significant cyanide poisoning (18,23,42,117). The blood pH may drop as low as 6.8 to 6.9 in severe cases (18,22,42,128). Blood lactate levels are generally elevated in conjunction, and they can serve as a good marker for the degree of cellular anoxia (16,18,41,128). Unlike other causes of acidosis, the acidosis due to cyanide toxicity is unlikely to respond to fluid resuscitation, pressors, or supplemental oxygen.

Arterial blood gas measurements also reveal varying degrees of respiratory compensation. Unless hypoventilation has already developed (e.g., from CNS depression), the blood oxygen content is usually elevated, as extraction at the tissue level decreases markedly with the inhibition of cellular respiration. The decrease in peripheral oxygen extraction can also be detected on venous blood gas as a decrease in the arteriovenous oxygen gap—that is, a decrease in the normal difference between arterial and venous blood oxygen pressures (117,126). This phenomenon is often referred to as *arteriolization* of venous gases.

Hyperglycemia is a common finding in patients with severe acute cyanide poisoning (18,22,42,52). In some cases, it may be the result of prehospital dextrose administration; however, it may also represent the impairment of cellular substrate use in poisoned tissues. A baseline complete blood cell count usually reveals little more than a nonspecific leukocytosis, but the hemoglobin level may be useful in guiding the dose of antidotal therapy (see later) (7,18,42,53). Electrolyte abnormalities are occasionally present in acute toxicity, but they are rarely severe (16,18,53,126).

The *electrocardiogram* may show a variety of nonspecific changes consistent with hypoxia (7,19,20,41,52,106,126). One change that has been reported with severe poisonings is a progressive shortening of the ST segment to the point that the T wave occurs almost on the R wave.

A *creatine kinase* level should be measured in patients with significant toxicity to look for evidence of cardiac ischemia or rhabdomyolysis. *A chest radiograph* should be performed if pulmonary aspiration or edema is suspected or if smoke inhalation may have occurred. *Liver and kidney function* should be performed in patients with suspected end-organ injury as the result of significant hypotension or ischemia. In victims of smoke inhalation, a *carbon monoxide level* is essential.

If the patient has ingested a cyanide substance with significant caustic potential, upper *endoscopy* should be seriously considered to evaluate the extent of GI injury even in patients without significant GI symptoms. Caustic ingestions are addressed in Chapters 201 and 202.

Computerized tomography of the brain may help rule out other conditions and may be helpful in evaluating for evidence of anoxic damage (16,18,52). If neurologic sequelae persist or develop after an acute exposure (e.g., parkinsonian syndrome), brain imaging should be performed as well as evaluation to rule out other potential causes. A computerized tomographic scan may be less sensitive than magnetic resonance imaging in detecting any changes. Radiographic effects may take several weeks or months to develop despite the presence of clinical effects (50). Neuropsychiatric testing may also reveal nonspecific impairment.

Chronic Toxicity

The biologic monitoring of patients with chronic cyanide exposures is not well established, and the very phenomenon of chronic cyanide toxicity remains controversial. The American Council of Governmental Industrial Hygienists makes no specific recommendations for the biologic monitoring of workplace cyanide exposures.

Because cyanide does not accumulate in the body, quantitative blood cyanide levels are not likely to be helpful unless an acute exposure is suspected. End-of-shift blood cyanide levels may reflect, to a limited extent, the day's exposure level in some workers. Such levels were found to be elevated in one study of factory employees with excessive exposures (151). However, the range of values in this paper was great, and smoking affected the results. More importantly, there are no well-established levels that correlate with clinical toxicity, and daily phlebotomy is impractical in most cases.

Thiocyanate has a long elimination half-life, making it a potentially useful marker of chronic exposure. However, diet and smoking can influence quantitative measurements, and there are no well-established toxic levels. Nonetheless, several studies have demonstrated elevated urinary thiocyanate concentrations in workers with larger cyanide exposures (134,151).

Environmental sampling at the workplace is probably the best and easiest method for evaluating cyanide exposure. Continuous or sequential air monitoring can detect even low levels of HCN or airborne particulate cyanide.

Postmortem Considerations

Postmortem blood cyanide levels may be significantly lower than premortem levels due to evaporation, thiocyanate formation, or tissue binding (47,153). Conversely, significant amounts of cyanide can also be formed by certain tissues, potentially increasing postmortem levels (47,154). Postmortem determinations in fire victims revealed a range of 0.01 to 4.36 μg/ml in two separate studies (47,155). These investigations are difficult to interpret, however, given the potential role of carbon monoxide and concomitant thermal injuries. Postmortem blood levels in patients who died solely of acute cyanide poisoning have been reported from 1.1 to 53.0 μg/ml after ingestions and 1.0 to 15.0 μg/ml after inhalations (47). Cyanide can also be measured in a variety of other postmortem tissue samples (110).

TREATMENT

The successful management of acute cyanide poisoning depends on a timely diagnosis, or consideration of the diagnosis, and the rapid institution of supportive measures and antidotal therapy. The sooner treatment is instituted, the more rapid and complete the recovery appears to be. Patients in extremis or cardiac arrest can make an immediate and near-total recovery with aggressive medical care and antidotal therapy (8,124).

In rare cases, patients with cyanide poisoning have been reported to improve simply by removing them from the exposure (15,115). However, such cases should be interpreted with caution, as they usually involve relatively brief inhalation exposures and are the exception rather than the rule. There are other scattered reports of patients surviving significant poisonings with supportive measures alone (15,18,41). However, resolution may take longer, may require the use of significant resources (e.g., prolonged ventilatory support or intensive care unit monitoring), and may subject patients to potentially significant complications, compared with those who receive antidotal treatment.

Decontamination

Prehospital workers must be extremely careful to avoid exposure. Protective gear and airborne cyanide monitors should be used because high air concentrations of HCN can cause immediate unconsciousness. Gas-impervious suits with self-contained breathing units should be used when concentrations exceed 200 ppm.

Medical personnel must also avoid self-contamination. The appropriate personal protective equipment should be used, and patient care should take place in a room with adequate ventilation. Contaminated clothing should be removed and disposed of immediately and irrigation performed before moving a patient into a room to limit off-gassing of HCN.

The recommended method of decontamination depends on the type of exposure, the chemical form of cyanide, and the time since exposure. After inhalations, removing the patient from the environment and providing fresh air or oxygen may be sufficient. After cutaneous exposures, contaminated clothing should be removed and treated as hazardous waste. All exposed areas should then be irrigated with copious amounts of water or saline. Vigorous scrubbing is to be avoided. GI decontamination should be performed after ingestions. Gastric lavage may be warranted in cases of recent, potentially large ingestions with a solid material (e.g., cyanide tablets or powders or laetrile). Liquid products may be removed by nasogastric suction. Instillation of activated charcoal should be considered in all patients. Although cyanide does not bind extremely well to charcoal *in vitro*, any resultant *in vivo* reduction in its bioavailability might be clinically important, and the risks of its administration are minimal (156). Indeed, limited animal studies have shown charcoal to be effective in increasing survival after cyanide overdose (157). The usual dose of 1 g/kg should be given orally or by nasogastric tube.

In patients with ingestions of corrosive cyanide compounds (e.g., cyanide salt solutions), the potential benefits of gastric decontamination must be weighed against the possibility of a concomitant corrosive injury and the risks that subsequent decontamination measures might entail. For example, charcoal might induce vomiting and exacerbate any corrosive injury, or it might obscure endoscopy; lavage carries the risk of perforation. In most cases, the potential for significant systemic cyanide absorption will outweigh the risks of local injury. Ipecac is contraindicated in all cases of suspected cyanide toxicity because of the risk of rapid coma or seizures.

Enhancement of Elimination

Antidotal therapy is technically a form of enhanced cyanide elimination (see later). Other than antidotal therapy, however, there are no proven effective measures to improve cyanide's removal. There is no evidence to support the use of multiple doses of charcoal, and it should only be considered in the rare instance that ongoing GI absorption is suspected. One case of hemodialysis with a temporal relation to patient improvement has been reported in a patient with cyanide toxicity, but the patient also received nitrite and thiosulfate treatment along with supportive care at the same time (128). The clearance of cyanide was reported as 38 ml/minute in this particular study. The use of hemoperfusion has also been reported, but again, the patient received multiple concomitant treatments (16). The value of hemodialysis and hemoperfusion remains unproven.

Antidotes

There are a variety of antidotes that have either been proposed or reported for the treatment of cyanide toxicity. The two most commonly used today include the Cyanide Antidote Package and hydroxocobalamin. Although there have been no randomized controlled trials demonstrating their efficacy in humans, both antidotes improve survival and increase the median lethal dose of cyanide in animal studies (66,81,158–165). In addition, successful human case reports and case series abound. Some of these anecdotal reports are quite compelling, with otherwise moribund patients or patients in cardiac arrest awakening and stabilizing within minutes of treatment (8,51,65,109,117,119,122–125,166–168). Furthermore, a comparison with historical controls suggests that the morbidity and mortality from cyanide poisoning have decreased appreciably in parallel with the widespread use of antidotal treatment. Survival has also been demonstrated with much larger exposures and with higher blood cyanide levels than before the introduction of specific antidotes. Although there are scattered reports of patients who do not respond favorably to one antidote or another, the overall literature supports their use in patients with significant toxicity.

Cyanide Antidote Package

The Cyanide Antidote Package is the only antidote approved by the U.S. Food and Drug Administration (previously marketed as the Cyanide Antidote Kit by Eli Lilly, IN). More details regarding the mechanism of action, method of administration, and contraindications of this antidote are available in Chapter 46. The package consists of three separate, but synergistic, agents: amyl nitrite, sodium nitrite, and sodium thiosulfate. The components can be administered separately but are typically given in combination. The nitrites (amyl and sodium) primarily work by inducing a modest methemoglobinemia, which binds cyanide and pulls it away from the target tissues. The resultant cyanomethemoglobin is then detoxified by the body's endogenous rhodanese, a process enhanced by administration of the substrate thiosulfate, the second part of the kit.

Indications for treatment with the full Cyanide Antidote Package include severe acidosis; CNS effects such as coma or seizures; cardiovascular effects such as hypotension, dysrhythmias, or arrest; and patients who continue to deteriorate clinically despite supportive measures. The full package should not be administered to asymptomatic patients with cyanide exposures, but the thiosulfate portion alone can be given to such patients if clinical deterioration is anticipated. For patients with clinical effects consistent with poisoning but without a good history of exposure or in cases in which the suspicion for cyanide toxicity is low, only the thiosulfate portion of the kit may be given.

Some authors have also recommended treating victims of smoke inhalation with only the thiosulfate portion of the kit, given the risks of generating methemoglobinemia in a patient with potential concomitant respiratory injury or carbon monoxide poisoning. Others have argued that methemoglobin levels rarely exceed 10% with the normal recommended doses and appropriate use of nitrites, and that these agents may be of significant immediate benefit. Given these opposing views, the decision to administer nitrates in fire victims should be individualized based on the likelihood of cyanide poisoning, the patient's clinical condition, and a consideration for the risks of inducing small amounts of methemoglobinemia. The thiosulfate portion should be given in all such cases.

TABLE 4. Cyanide Antidote Package administration

Amyl nitrite
- Break open one pearl and administer by inhalation for 30 sec out of every minute, with 100% supplemental oxygen in between.
- Break open a fresh pearl every 3–5 min.
- Switch to sodium nitrite once IV access has been established.

Sodium nitrite
- *Adults*: Administer 300 mg (10 ml of a 3% solution) IV over 3–5 min.
- *Children (hematocrit unknown)*: Administer 10 mg/kg (0.33 ml/kg of a 3% solution) IV over 3–5 min.
- Should be followed as soon as possible by sodium thiosulfate administration.

Sodium thiosulfate
- *Adults*: Administer 12.5 g (50 ml of a 25% solution) IV.
- *Children*: Administer 400 mg/kg (1.65 ml/kg of a 25% solution) IV.

Monitoring
- Monitor blood pressure and heart rate closely for hypotension after nitrite therapy.
- Monitor methemoglobin levels at 30 and 60 min after administration of nitrites (sooner if effects of excessive methemoglobinemia develop); if methemoglobin levels exceed 30% or signs of significant methemoglobin toxicity develop, withhold further nitrite treatment and consider administration of methylene blue (1 mg/kg IV).
- Monitor for signs of persistent or recurrent cyanide toxicity; sodium nitrite, sodium thiosulfate, or both may be repeated as needed in such cases at full or half doses.

The method and dose of administration are summarized in Table 4 and described in more detail in Chapter 46. In patients who might not tolerate even a modest methemoglobinemia or in those patients who have already received a significant amount of amyl nitrite, the dose can be reduced or infused over a longer period of time. The recommended dose of sodium nitrite in children has traditionally been tailored to the patient's baseline hematocrit (Chapter 46). However, treatment should not be delayed while waiting for a blood cell count, and in such cases, an empiric pediatric dose of 0.33 ml/kg of a 3% solution, or approximately 10 mg/kg intravenously, should be infused over several minutes (169). The final portion of the kit consists of sodium thiosulfate as a 25% solution. The recommended dose is 12.5 g intravenously in adults and 400 mg/kg (or approximately 1.65 ml/kg of a 25% solution) in children.

The nitrites can cause hypotension and excessive methemoglobinemia. Methemoglobin levels and clinical status should therefore be monitored closely after administration of the package. Patients receiving nitrites should have methemoglobin levels measured at 30 and 60 minutes after administration, or sooner if signs of significant methemoglobinemia develop (e.g., bluish skin discoloration or worsening acidosis, tachycardia, hypotension, or mental status). Traditionally, the goal for nitrite therapy has been the establishment of a methemoglobin level between 20% and 30%. However, this recommendation was not based on data, and in actuality, methemoglobin levels probably do not need to be that high for clinical efficacy (121,161). It is not the resultant methemoglobin level that is important but rather the degree of clinical improvement. In most cases, the recommended doses of nitrites only produce a methemoglobin level of approximately 8% to 13% (13). Should excessive or clinically deleterious methemoglobinemia occur, it can usually be managed successfully with supplemental oxygen and methylene blue, 1 mg/kg intravenously (Chapter 63) (8,19,170).

If clinical signs of cyanide toxicity persist or recur after treatment, the nitrite and sodium thiosulfate components should be repeated. Some recommend re-treatment at only one-half the original dose for sodium nitrite, but there are few downsides to readministering a full dose of sodium thiosulfate. Persistence or recurrence of mild or moderate toxicity can sometimes be treated with sodium thiosulfate alone. Caution should be used when giving repeated doses of thiosulfate to patients with renal impairment, as thiocyanate can accumulate and cause toxicity.

Patients with significant cyanide poisoning may demonstrate dramatic clinical improvement within 15 to 30 minutes of antidotal administration; however, in other patients, recovery may progress more slowly (8,51,65,109,119,121–125,166,171,172). There are a few reported cases of treatment failure, but these may have been complicated by coingestants or anoxic sequelae (21,110,117,122,173). In general, patients with uncomplicated cyanide poisoning should be expected to improve significantly within several hours of treatment.

Occasionally, patients may redevelop effects of cyanide toxicity after the initial benefits of antidotal treatment wane. This is particularly likely in patients with cyanogen exposures or ongoing cyanide absorption and so patients should be monitored closely even after improvement.

Hydroxocobalamin

Hydroxocobalamin (vitamin B_{12a}) is the most promising alternative to the Cyanide Antidote Package, and it is the treatment of choice in France for patients with cyanide toxicity. Cyanide ions have high affinity for the cobalt moiety in hydroxocobalamin (174–176). The two react to form cyanocobalamin (vitamin B_{12}), a nontoxic, water-soluble metabolite that can be easily excreted in the urine or bile (177–180). Hydroxocobalamin is often given in combination with sodium thiosulfate. Based on animal data and human case reports, it appears to have a level of efficacy similar to the Cyanide Antidote Package (174,180–187). The potential advantage of hydroxocobalamin, however, is that it has fewer side effects than the methemoglobin-forming and potentially hypotensive nitrites. More detail regarding its use is provided in Chapter 61. It is not currently approved or commercially available in the United States in a form sufficient for treating cyanide poisoning. However, given its efficacy and improved risk profile, there has been a recent push to have the drug reformulated and approved for use.

Other Antidotes

4-Dimethylaminophenol and *hydroxylamine* are oxidizing agents that have been used in Europe as alternatives to the nitrites for methemoglobin induction (19,159,188). Like the nitrites, they are typically given in combination with sodium thiosulfate. They offer no clear advantages over traditional nitrite therapy, however, and at least one study in animals has suggested they may be inferior (159,189). In addition, they do not induce methemoglobin as reliably or predictably as nitrites. Cases of excessive, even life-threatening, methemoglobinemia (i.e., 70%) have been reported with their use (19).

Dicobalt ethylenediaminetetraacetic acid acts by combining with cyanide to form an innocuous cyanide-cobalt complex, which can then be renally excreted. However, there are little data regarding its use, and its efficacy appears quite variable based on the few existing anecdotal reports (7,22,55,108,120). Even more concerning are reports of angioedema and severe allergic or anaphylactoid reactions associated with its use (22,55).

Stroma-free methemoglobin and alpha-ketoglutarate also bind cyanide, and their exogenous administration has been investigated in animal models (190,191).

Hyperbaric oxygen (HBO) therapy has also been used for patients with cyanide poisoning, in a few anecdotal cases, with varying degrees of success, although the mechanism underlying any potential benefit remains unclear (123,130,173). The reports of its efficacy are far from compelling (e.g., many patients received multiple treatments in conjunction with HBO or may have recovered with time). Furthermore, animal studies have found HBO to be ineffective. Other potential drawbacks include its cost, labor requirements, poor regional availability, and the need for patient transport. For these reasons, HBO therapy is not recommended for most patients. One possible exception is the treatment of combined cyanide and carbon monoxide poisoning among patients with significant smoke inhalation.

Supportive Care

After removal from the exposure, a patent airway and adequate ventilation should be ensured. The patient's minute ventilation must compensate for severe metabolic acidosis. Patients who do not require intubation either for airway protection or for maintenance of ventilation should still receive 100% oxygen by mask until their symptoms resolve. In theory, additional oxygen should not overcome or circumvent the blockade in cytochrome oxidase. However, there is some evidence to suggest that oxygen may be clinically beneficial, particularly in combination with other cyanide antidotes (192–195). Continuous cardiac and oximetry monitoring should be instituted in all patients. Hypotension should be managed with antidotal therapy in addition to fluids and pressors in the usual fashion (Chapter 37). Seizures should also be managed by antidotal administration along with the usual anticonvulsive agents such as benzodiazepines or barbiturates (Chapter 40). Dysrhythmias are managed in typical advanced cardiac life support fashion after the administration of antidotes.

The treatment of patients with delayed or persistent neurologic sequelae after acute cyanide poisoning is symptomatic. Patients with parkinsonian symptoms sometimes respond to treatment with antiparkinsonian agents, but the response is often suboptimal (21,49,50). The neurologic sequelae may be progressive, persistent, or improve spontaneously over time.

Monitoring

Given the potential for precipitous deterioration and life-threatening effects, all patients with cyanide poisoning should be observed in an intensive care setting and have frequent clinical and laboratory reexaminations. After an inhalation exposure to HCN, patients can usually be discharged as soon as it has been determined that there is no clinical or laboratory evidence of toxicity. After dermal or oral exposure, asymptomatic patients should be observed for at least 6 hours (after adequate decontamination) for the onset of clinical or laboratory sequelae. Patients with inhalation, dermal, or oral exposures to any of the cyanogens (e.g., laetrile or the aliphatic nitriles) should be observed for at least 24 hours, even if asymptomatic, due to the slow metabolic liberation of cyanide and the risk for delayed toxicity. Patients who develop evidence of toxicity at any time should be admitted until well after the clinical effects have resolved.

In general, patients with uncomplicated cyanide poisoning should improve significantly within several hours and even sooner with appropriate antidotal therapy. Regular assessments of a patient's level of consciousness or awareness should be made; frequent measurements of vital signs and oxygenation should be performed; and acid-base status should be monitored. Patients occasionally redevelop symptoms of cyanide toxicity after an initial improvement, particularly in cases of cyanogen exposure or inadequate decontamination. Patients should therefore be observed for at least 6 hours after the resolution of toxicity with antidotal treatment. Patients with cyanogen exposures who respond to treatment should be observed until asymptomatic and antidote free for at least 24 hours. Consideration may be given to monitoring serial blood cyanide levels in such cases until they decline or approach baseline.

Patients who recover should be followed up and screened for the development of long-term neurologic sequelae. Industrial or occupational exposures should be investigated by the appropriate authorities or a qualified industrial hygienist.

Chronic Toxicity

The management of patients with suspected chronic toxicity is not well established. The treatment of systemic, nonspecific symptoms is symptomatic and supportive. The most important intervention is a removal from the exposure to cyanide or at least a significant reduction through the institution of various workplace measures. Antidotal treatment with the Cyanide Antidote Package is not recommended. Hydroxocobalamin has been used in such patients but is unlikely to provide significant benefit and has not been well studied.

The respective management of tobacco amblyopia, Leber's hereditary optic neuropathy, and tropical ataxic neuropathy is not well established. Once the diagnosis has been made and distinguished from other similar syndromes, some authors recommend measures such as smoking cessation, improved nutrition, and, occasionally, hydroxocobalamin or vitamin B_{12} supplementation (138,139,142–144,196–198). Many patients respond favorably to such measures, but complete resolution is rare (144). In all cases, consultation with an experienced ophthalmologist is advised.

Management Pitfalls

The greatest pitfall in managing patients with cyanide toxicity is awaiting the results of specific confirmatory tests before initiating treatment. Specific antidotes should be started as soon as the diagnosis is suspected.

The inappropriate use of some antidotes is another potential pitfall. Nitrites can induce hypotension and excessive methemoglobinemia, particularly if used improperly. They should be administered only when indicated, and close monitoring of blood pressure and methemoglobin levels should always be undertaken with their use.

Discharging patients who may deteriorate later is another potential pitfall. Patients with large tablet ingestions, inadequate initial decontamination, or cyanogen (e.g., laetrile, aliphatic nitrile) exposures may develop delayed toxicity, sometimes many hours after the initial exposure. Such patients should be hospitalized and observed in a monitored setting for at least 24 hours.

REFERENCES

1. Logan B, Howard J, Kiesel EL. Poisonings associated with cyanide in over the counter cold medication in Washington State, 1991. *J Forensic Sci* 1993;38:472–476.
2. Brahams D. "Sudafed" capsules poisoned with cyanide. *Lancet* 1991;337:968.
3. Beck M, Monroe S. The Tylenol scare: the death of seven people who took the drug triggers a nationwide alert—and a hunt for a madman. *Newsweek* 1982 Oct:100:32–36.
4. Wolnik KA, Fricke FL, Bonnin E, et al. The Tylenol tampering incident—tracing the source. *Anal Chem* 1984;56:466A–470A, 474A.
5. Bonsall JL. Survival without sequelae following exposure to 500 mg/m^3 of hydrogen cyanide. *Hum Toxicol* 1984;3:57–60.
6. Curry SC, LoVecchio FA. Hydrogen cyanide and inorganic cyanide salts. In: Sullivan JB, Krieger GR, eds. *Clinical environmental health and toxic exposures*, 2nd ed. Philadelphia: Lippincott Williams & Wilkins, 2001:705–716.
7. Singh BM, Coles N, Lewis P, et al. The metabolic effects of fatal cyanide poisoning. *Postgrad Med J* 1989;65:923–925.
8. Chen KK, Rose CL. Treatment of acute cyanide poisoning. *JAMA* 1956;162:1154–1155.
9. Baud FJ, Barriot P, Toffis V, et al. Elevated blood cyanide concentrations in victims of smoke inhalation. *N Engl J Med* 1991;325:1761–1766.
10. Terrill JB, Montgomery RR, Reinhardt CF. Toxic gases from fires. *Science* 1978;200:1343–1347.
11. Yamamoto K, Yamamoto Y. On the acute toxicities of the combustion products of various fibers, with special reference to blood cyanide and Po_2 values. *Z Rechtsmed* 1978;81:173–179.
12. Jones J, McMullen MJ, Dougherty J. Toxic smoke inhalation: cyanide poisoning in fire victims. *Am J Emerg Med* 1987;5:317–321.
13. Kirk MA, Gerace R, Kulig KW. Cyanide and methemoglobin kinetics in smoke inhalation victims treated with the cyanide antidote kit. *Ann Emerg Med* 1993;22:1413–1418.
14. Clark CJ, Campbell D, Reid WH. Blood carboxyhaemoglobin and cyanide levels in fire survivors. *Lancet* 1981;1:1332–1335.
15. Peden NR, Taha A, McSorley PD, et al. Industrial exposure to hydrogen cyanide: implications for treatment. *Br Med J (Clin Res Ed)* 1986;293:538.
16. Krieg A, Saxena K. Cyanide poisoning from metal cleaning solutions. *Ann Emerg Med* 1987;16:582–584.
17. Mascarenhas BR, Geller AC, Goodman AI. Cyanide poisoning, medical emergency. *N Y State J Med* 1969;69:1782–1784.
18. Brivet F, Delfraissy JF, Duche M, et al. Acute cyanide poisoning: recovery with non-specific supportive therapy. *Intensive Care Med* 1983;9:33–35.
19. van Heijst AN, Douze JM, van Kesteren RG, et al. Therapeutic problems in cyanide poisoning. *J Toxicol Clin Toxicol* 1987;25:383–398.
20. De Busk RF, Seidl LG. Attempted suicide by cyanide. A report of two cases. *Calif Med* 1969;110:394–396.
21. Peters CG, Mundy JV, Rayner PR. Acute cyanide poisoning. The treatment of a suicide attempt. *Anaesthesia* 1982;37:582–586.
22. Dodds C, McKnight C. Cyanide toxicity after immersion and the hazards of dicobalt edetate. *Br Med J (Clin Res Ed)* 1985;291:785–786.
23. DiNapoli J, Hall AH, Drake R, et al. Cyanide and arsenic poisoning by intravenous injection. *Ann Emerg Med* 1989;18:308–311.
24. Boggild MD, Peck RW, Tomson CR. Acetonitrile ingestion: delayed onset of cyanide poisoning due to concurrent ingestion of acetone. *Postgrad Med J* 1990;66:40–41.
25. Caravati EM, Litovitz TL. Pediatric cyanide intoxication and death from an acetonitrile-containing cosmetic. *JAMA* 1988;260:3470–3473.
26. Michaelis HC, Clemens C, Kijewski H, et al. Acetonitrile serum concentrations and cyanide blood levels in a case of suicidal oral acetonitrile ingestion. *J Toxicol Clin Toxicol* 1991;29:447–458.
27. Mueller M, Borland C. Delayed cyanide poisoning following acetonitrile ingestion. *Postgrad Med J* 1997;73:299–300.
28. Scolnick B, Hamel D, Woolf AD. Successful treatment of life-threatening propionitrile exposure with sodium nitrite/sodium thiosulfate followed by hyperbaric oxygen. *J Occup Med* 1993;35:577–580.
29. Bismuth C, Baud FJ, Djeghout H, et al. Cyanide poisoning from propionitrile exposure. *J Emerg Med* 1987;5:191–195.
30. Ahmed AE, Patel K. Acrylonitrile: in vivo metabolism in rats and mice. *Drug Metab Dispos* 1981;9:219–222.
31. Feierman DE, Cederbaum AI. Role of cytochrome P-450 IIE1 and catalase in the oxidation of acetonitrile to cyanide. *Chem Res Toxicol* 1989;2:359–366.
32. Freeman JJ, Hayes EP. Microsomal metabolism of acetonitrile to cyanide. Effects of acetone and other compounds. *Biochem Pharmacol* 1988;37:1153–1159.
33. Losek JD, Rock AL, Boldt RR. Cyanide poisoning from a cosmetic nail remover. *Pediatrics* 1991;88:337–340.
34. Humbert JR, Tress JH, Braico KT. Fatal cyanide poisoning: accidental ingestion of amygdalin. *JAMA* 1977;238:482.
35. Newmark J, Brady RO, Grimley PM, et al. Amygdalin (Laetrile) and prunasin beta-glucosidases: distribution in germ-free rat and in human tumor tissue. *Proc Natl Acad Sci U S A* 1981;78:6513–6516.
36. Hill HZ, Backer R, Hill GJ 2nd. Blood cyanide levels in mice after administration of amygdalin. *Biopharm Drug Dispos* 1980;1:211–220.
37. Frakes RA, Sharma RP, Willhite CC. Comparative metabolism of linamarin and amygdalin in hamsters. *Food Chem Toxicol* 1986;24:417–420.
38. Sadoff L, Fuchs K, Hollander J. Rapid death associated with laetrile ingestion. *JAMA* 1977;1978:1532.
39. Braico KT, Humbert JR, Terplan KL, et al. Laetrile intoxication. Report of a fatal case. *N Engl J Med* 1979;300:238–240.
40. Beamer WC, Shealy RM, Prough DS. Acute cyanide poisoning from laetrile ingestion. *Ann Emerg Med* 19831;12:449–451.
41. Vogel SN, Sultan TR, Ten Eyck RP. Cyanide poisoning. *J Toxicol Clin Toxicol* 1981;18:367–383.
42. Hall AH, Linden CH, Kulig KW, Rumack BH. Cyanide poisoning from laetrile ingestion: role of nitrite therapy. *Pediatrics* 1986;78:269–272.
43. Akintonwa A, Tunwashe OL. Fatal cyanide poisoning from cassava-based meal. *Hum Exp Toxicol* 1992;11:47–49.
44. Barcroft J. The toxicity of atmospheres containing hydrocyanic acid gas. *J Hyg* 1931;31:1–34.
45. Harper C, Goldhaber S. *Toxicological profile for cyanide*. Atlanta: U.S. Department of Health and Human Services, Public Health Service, Agency for Toxic Substances and Disease Registry, 1997.

46. Dudley HC, Sweeney TR, Miller JW. Toxicology of acrylonitrile (vinyl cyanide) II: studies of effects of daily inhalation. *J Ind Hyg Toxicol* 1942;24.
47. Cyanide. In: Baselt RC, ed. *Disposition of toxic drugs and chemicals in man*, 6th ed. Foster City, CA: Biomedical Publications, 2002:264–268.
48. Gettler AO, Baine JO. The toxicology of cyanide. *Am J Med Sci* 1938;195:182–198.
49. Uitti RJ, Rajput AH, Ashenhurst EM, et al. Cyanide-induced parkinsonism: a clinicopathologic report. *Neurology* 1985;35:921–925.
50. Rosenberg NL, Myers JA, Martin WR. Cyanide-induced parkinsonism: clinical, MRI, and 6-fluorodopa PET studies. *Neurology* 1989;39:142–144.
51. Wood GC. Acute cyanide intoxication: diagnosis and management. *Clin Tox Consult* 1982;4:140–149.
52. Litovitz TL, Larkin RF, Myers RA. Cyanide poisoning treated with hyperbaric oxygen. *Am J Emerg Med* 1983;1:94–101.
53. Hall AH, Rumack BH. Hydroxycobalamin/sodium thiosulfate as a cyanide antidote. *J Emerg Med* 1987;5:115–121.
54. Carden E. Hyperbaric oxygen in cyanide poisoning. *Anaesthesia* 1970;25:442–443.
55. Naughton M. Acute cyanide poisoning. *Anaesth Intensive Care* 1974;2:351–356.
56. Peters CG, Mundy JV, Rayner PR. Acute cyanide poisoning. The treatment of a suicide attempt. *Anaesthesia* 1982;37:582–586.
57. Evans CL. Cobalt compounds as antidotes for hydrocyanic acid. *Br J Pharmacol* 1964;23:455–475.
58. Silver EH, Kuttab SH, Hasan T, et al. Structural considerations in the metabolism of nitriles to cyanide in vivo. *Drug Metab Dispos* 1982;10:495–498.
59. Froines JR, Postlethwait M, LaFuente EJ, et al. In vivo and in vitro release of cyanide from neurotoxic aminonitriles. *J Toxicol Environ Health* 1985;16:449–460.
60. Willhite CC. Inhalation toxicology of acute exposure to aliphatic nitriles. *J Toxicol Clin Toxicol* 1981;18:991–1003.
61. Schulz V. Clinical pharmacokinetics of nitroprusside, cyanide, thiosulphate and thiocyanate. *Clin Pharmacokinet* 1984;9:239–251.
62. Farooqui MY, Ahmed AE. Molecular interaction of acrylonitrile and potassium cyanide with rat blood. *Chem Biol Interact* 1982;38:145–159.
63. Ansell M, Lewis FA. A review of cyanide concentrations found in human organs. A survey of literature concerning cyanide metabolism, "normal," non-fatal, and fatal body cyanide levels. *J Forensic Med* 1970;17:148–155.
64. Finck PA. Postmortem redistribution studies of cyanide. Report of three cases. *Med Ann Dist Columbia* 1969;38:357–358.
65. Hall AH, Doutre WH, Ludden T, et al. Nitrite/thiosulfate treated acute cyanide poisoning: estimated kinetics after antidote. *J Toxicol Clin Toxicol* 1987;25:121–133.
66. Sylvester DM, Hayton WL, Morgan RL, et al. Effects of thiosulfate on cyanide pharmacokinetics in dogs. *Toxicol Appl Pharmacol* 1983;69:265–271.
67. Schulz V, Gross R, Pasch T, et al. Cyanide toxicity of sodium nitroprusside in therapeutic use with and without sodium thiosulphate. *Klin Wochenschr* 1982;60:1393–1400.
68. Graham DL, Laman D, Theodore J, et al. Acute cyanide poisoning complicated by lactic acidosis and pulmonary edema. *Arch Intern Med* 1977;137:1051–1055.
69. Kirk MA, Gerace R, Kulig KW. Cyanide and methemoglobin kinetics in smoke inhalation victims treated with the cyanide antidote kit. *Ann Emerg Med* 1993;22:1413–1418.
70. Mannaioni G, Vannacci A, Marzocca C, et al. Acute cyanide intoxication treated with a combination of hydroxycobalamin, sodium nitrite, and sodium thiosulfate. *J Toxicol Clin Toxicol* 2002;40:181–183.
71. Bright JE, Marrs TC. Pharmacokinetics of intravenous potassium cyanide. *Hum Toxicol* 1988;7:183–186.
72. Lundquist P, Rosling H, Sorbo B, et al. Cyanide concentrations in blood after cigarette smoking, as determined by a sensitive fluorimetric method. *Clin Chem* 1987;33:1228–1230.
73. Howard JWHRF. Chronic toxicity for rats of food treated with hydrogen cyanide. *Agricultural Food Chem* 1955;3:325–329.
74. Leuschner J, Winkler A, Leuschner F. Toxicokinetic aspects of chronic cyanide exposure in the rat. *Toxicol Lett* 1991;57:195–201.
75. Wood JL, Cooley SL. Detoxification of cyanide by cystine. *J Biol Chem* 1956;218:449–457.
76. Westley J, Adler A, Westley L, et al. The sulfur transferases. *Fundam Appl Toxicol* 1983;3:377–382.
77. Devlin DJ, Smith RP, Thron CD. Cyanide metabolism in the isolated, perfused, bloodless hindlimbs or liver of the rat. *Toxicol Appl Pharmacol* 1989;98:338–349.
78. Janse van Rensburg L, Schabort JC. Rhodanese from *Cercopithecus aethiops* (Vervet monkey) liver. II. Aspects of enzyme kinetics and mechanism of action. *Int J Biochem* 1984;16:547–551.
79. Albaum HG, Tepperman J, Bodansky O. The in vivo inactivation by cyanide of brain cytochrome oxidase and its effect on glycolysis and on the high energy phosphorus compounds in the brain. *J Biol Chem* 1946;64:45–51.
80. Keilin D, Hartree EF. Cytochrome and cytochrome oxidase. *Proc R Soc London B Biol Sci* 127:167–191.
81. Piantadosi CA, Sylvia AL, Jobsis FF. Cyanide-induced cytochrome a,a3 oxidation-reduction responses in rat brain in vivo. *J Clin Invest* 1983;72:1224–1233.
82. van Buuren KJ, Nicholis P, van Gelder BF. Biochemical and biophysical studies on cytochrome aa 3. VI. Reaction of cyanide with oxidized and reduced enzyme. *Biochim Biophys Acta* 1972;256:258–276.
83. Tursky T, Sajter V. The influence of potassium cyanide poisoning on the aminobutyric acid level in rat brain. *J Neurochem* 1962;9:519–523.
84. Ardelt BK, Borowitz JL, Isom GE. Brain lipid peroxidation and antioxidant protectant mechanisms following acute cyanide intoxication. *Toxicology* 1989;56:147–154.
85. Isom GE, Liu DHW, Way JL. Effect of sublethal doses of cyanide on glucose catabolism. *Biochem Pharmacol* 1975;24:871–875.
86. Lessell S. Experimental cyanide optic neuropathy. *Arch Ophthalmol* 1971;86:194–204.
87. Burrows GE, Liu DHW, Way JL. Effect of oxygen on cyanide intoxication: V. Physiologic effects. *J Pharmacol Exp Ther* 1973;184:739–748.
88. Cope C. The importance of oxygen in the treatment of cyanide poisoning. *J Am Med Assoc* 1961;175:1061–1064.
89. Johnson JD, Meisenheimer TL, Isom GE. Cyanide induced neurotoxicity: role of neuronal calcium. *Toxicol Appl Pharmacol* 1986;84:464–469.
90. Adams DJ, Takeda K, Umbach J. A. Inhibitors of calcium buffering depress evoked transmitter release at the giant squid synapse. *J Physiol* 1985;369:145–159.
91. Johnson JD, Conroy WG, Burris KD, Isom GE. Peroxidation of brain lipids following cyanide intoxication in mice. *Toxicology* 1987;46:21–28.
92. Ardelt BK, Borowitz JL, Maduh EU, et al. Cyanide-induced lipid peroxidation in different organs: subcellular distribution and hydroperoxide generation in neuronal cells. *Toxicology* 1994;89:127–137.
93. Aitken PG, Braitman DJ. The effects of cyanide on neural and synaptic function in hippocampal slices. *Neurotoxicology* 1989;10:239–248.
94. Patel MN, Yim GKWGE. Blockade of N-methyl-D-aspartate receptors prevents cyanide-induced neuronal injury in primary hippocampal cultures. *Toxicol Appl Pharmacol* 1992;115:124–129.
95. Patel MN, Yim GKWGE. N-methyl-D-aspartate receptors mediate cyanide-induced cytotoxicity in hippocampal cultures. *Neurotoxicology* 1993;14:35–40.
96. Curry SC, Arnold-Capell P. Toxic effects of drugs used in the ICU. Nitroprusside, nitroglycerin, and angiotensin-converting enzyme inhibitors. *Crit Care Clin* 1991;7:555–581.
97. Pahl MV, Vaziri ND. In-vivo and in-vitro hemodialysis studies of thiocyanate. *J Toxicol Clin Toxicol* 1982;19:965–974.
98. Cailleux A, Subra JF, Riberi P, et al. Cyanide and thiocyanate blood levels in patients with renal failure or respiratory disease. *J Med* 1988;19:345–351.
99. Barnett HJM, Jackson MV, Spaulding WB. Thiocyanate psychosis. *JAMA* 1951;147:1554–1555.
100. Tewe OO, Maner JH. Performance and pathophysiological changes in pregnant pigs fed cassava diets containing different levels of cyanide. *Res Vet Sci* 1981;30:147–151.
101. Willhite CC. Congenital malformations induced by laetrile. *Science* 1982;215:1513–1515.
102. Frakes RA, Sharma RP, Willhite C. Developmental toxicity of the cyanogenic glycoside linamarin in the golden hamster. *Teratology* 1985;31:241–246.
103. Singh JD. The teratogenic effects of dietary cassava on the pregnant albino rat: a preliminary report. *Teratology* 1981;24:289–291.
104. Soto-Blanco B, Gorniak SL. Milk transfer of cyanide and thiocyanate: cyanide exposure by lactation in goats. *Vet Res* 2003;34:213–220.
105. Miller KW, Anderson JL, Stoewsand GS. Amygdalin metabolism and effect on reproduction of rats fed apricot kernels. *J Toxicol Environ Health* 1981;7:457–467.
106. Wexler J, Whittenberger JL, Dumke PR. The effect of cyanide on the electrocardiogram in man. *Am Heart J* 1947;34:163–173.
107. Bonsall JL. Survival without sequelae following exposure to 500 mg/m^3 of hydrogen cyanide. *Hum Toxicol* 1984;3:57–60.
108. Hilmann B, Bardham KD, Bain JTB. The use of dicobalt edetate (Kelocyanor) in cyanide poisoning. *Postgrad Med J* 1974;50:171–174.
109. Hirsch FG. Cyanide poisoning. *Arch Environ Health* 1964;8:622–624.
110. Lee-Jones M, Bennett MA, Sherwell JM. Cyanide self-poisoning. *BMJ* 1970;4:780–781.
111. Turchen SG, Manoguerra AS, Whitney C. Severe cyanide poisoning from the ingestion of an acetonitrile-containing cosmetic. *Am J Emerg Med* 1991;9:264–267.
112. Caravati EM, Litovitz TL. Pediatric cyanide intoxication and death from an acetonitrile-containing cosmetic. *JAMA* 1988;260:3470–3473.
113. Muraki K, Inoue Y, Ohta I, et al. Massive rhabdomyolysis and acute renal failure after acetonitrile exposure. *Intern Med* 2001;40:936–939.
114. Geller RJ, Ekins BR, Iknoian RC. Cyanide toxicity from acetonitrile-containing false nail remover. *Am J Emerg Med* 1991;9:268–270.
115. Drinker P. Hydrocyanic acid gas poisoning by absorption through the skin. *J Indust Hyg* 1932;14:1–2.
116. Yen D, Tsai J, Wang LM, et al. The clinical experience of acute cyanide poisoning. *Am J Emerg Med* 1995;13:524–528.
117. Yen D, Tsai J, Wang LM, et al. The clinical experience of acute cyanide poisoning. *Am J Emerg Med* 1995;13:524–528.
118. De Busk RF, Seidl LG. Attempted suicide by cyanide. A report of two cases. *Calif Med* 1969;110:394–396.
119. DiNapoli J, Hall AH, Drake R, Rumack BH. Cyanide and arsenic poisoning by intravenous injection. *Ann Emerg Med* 1989;18:308–311.
120. Bain JT, Knowles EL. Successful treatment of cyanide poisoning. *BMJ* 1967;2:763.
121. Johnson WS, Hall AH, Rumack BH. Cyanide poisoning successfully treated without "therapeutic methemoglobin levels." *Am J Emerg Med* 1989;7:437–440.

122. Krieg A, Saxena K. Cyanide poisoning from metal cleaning solutions. *Ann Emerg Med* 1987;16:582–584.
123. Litovitz TL, Larkin RF, Myers RA. Cyanide poisoning treated with hyperbaric oxygen. *Am J Emerg Med* 1983;1:94–101.
124. Stewart R. Cyanide poisoning. *J Toxicol Clin Toxicol* 1974;7:561–564.
125. Potter L. The successful treatment of two recent cases of cyanide poisoning. *Br J Industr Med* 1950;7:125–130.
126. Johnson RP, Mellors JW. Arteriolization of venous blood gases: a clue to the diagnosis of cyanide poisoning. *J Emerg Med* 1988;6:401–404.
127. McNemey JM, Schrenk HH. The acute toxicity of cyanogen. *Am Ind Hyg Assoc J* 1960;21:121–124.
128. Wesson DE, Foley R, Sabatini S, et al. Treatment of acute cyanide intoxication with hemodialysis. *Am J Nephrol* 1985;5:121–126.
129. Baud FJ, Borron SW, Bavoux E, et al. Relation between plasma lactate and blood cyanide concentrations in acute cyanide poisoning. *BMJ* 1996;312:26–27.
130. Trapp WG. Massive cyanide poisoning with recovery: a boxing-day story. *Can Med Assoc J* 1970;102:517.
131. Bonnichsen R, Maehly AC. Poisoning by volatile compounds. 3. Hydrocyanic acid. *J Forensic Sci* 1966;11:516–528.
132. Wurzburg H. Treatment of cyanide poisoning in an industrial setting. *Vet Hum Toxicol* 1996;38:44–47.
133. Graham DL, Laman D, Theodore J, Robin ED. Acute cyanide poisoning complicated by lactic acidosis and pulmonary edema. *Arch Intern Med* 1977;137:1051–1055.
134. El Ghawabi SH, Gaafar MA, El-Saharti AA, et al. Chronic cyanide exposure: a clinical, radioisotope, and laboratory study. *Br J Ind Med* 1975;32:215–219.
135. Blanc P, Hogan M, Mallin K, et al. Cyanide intoxication among silver-reclaiming workers. *JAMA* 1985;253:367–371.
136. Hardy HL, Jeffries WM, Wasserman MM, et al. Thiocyanate effect following industrial cyanide exposure. *N Engl J Med* 1950;242:968–972.
137. Banerjee KK, Muthu PM. Effect of cigarette smoking on thyroid hormone homeostasis. *Indian J Med Res* 1996;99:74–76.
138. Samples JR, Younge BR. Tobacco-alcohol amblyopia. *J Clin Neuroophthalmol* 1981;1:213–218.
139. Rizzo JF 3rd, Lessell S. Tobacco amblyopia. *Am J Ophthalmol* 1993;116:84–87.
140. Knox DL. Neuro-ophthalmology. *Arch Ophthalmol* 1970;83:103–125.
141. Heaton JM. Tobacco amblyopia: a clinical manifestation of vitamin B12 deficiency. *Lancet* 1958;2:286.
142. Chisholm IA, Bronte-Stewart J, Foulds WS. Hydroxocobalamin versus cyanocobalamin in the treatment of tobacco amblyopia. *Lancet* 1967;2:450–451.
143. Foulds WS, Cant JS, Chisholm IA, et al. Hydroxocobalamin in the treatment of Leber's hereditary optic atrophy. *Lancet* 1968;1:896–897.
144. Krumsiek J, Kruger C, Patzold U. Tobacco-alcohol amblyopia neuro-ophthalmological findings and clinical course. *Acta Neurol Scand* 1985;72:180–187.
145. Berninger TA, Bird AC, Arden GB. Leber's hereditary optic atrophy. *Ophthalmic Paediatr Genet* 1989;10:211–227.
146. Osuntokun BO, Langman MJ, Wilson J, et al. Controlled trial of hydroxocobalamin and riboflavine in Nigerian ataxic neuropathy. *J Neurol Neurosurg Psychiatry* 1970;33:663–666.
147. Osuntokun BO. Cassava diet, chronic cyanide intoxication and neuropathy in the Nigerian Africans. *World Rev Nutr Diet* 1981;36:141–173.
148. Oluwole OS OALHRH. Persistence of tropical ataxic neuropathy in a Nigerian community. *J Neurol Neurosurg Psychiatry* 2000;69:96–101.
149. Vesey CJ, Wilson J. Red cell cyanide. *J Pharm Pharmacol* 1978;30:20–26.
150. McMillan DE, Svoboda AC. The role of erythrocytes in cyanide detoxification. *J Pharmacol Exp Ther* 1982;221:37–42.
151. Chandra H, Gupta BN, Bhargava SK, et al. Chronic cyanide exposure—a biochemical and industrial hygiene study. *J Anal Toxicol* 1980;4:161–165.
152. Pasch T, Schulz V, Hoppelshauser G. Nitroprusside-induced formation of cyanide and its detoxication with thiosulfate during deliberate hypotension. *J Cardiovasc Pharmacol* 1983;5:77–85.
153. Curry AS. Cyanide poisoning. *Acta Pharm Toxicol* 1963;20:291–294.
154. Curry AS, Price DE, Rutter ER. The production of cyanide in post-mortem material. *Acta Pharm Toxicol* 1967;25:339–344.
155. Wetherell HR. The occurrence of cyanide in the blood of fire victims. *J Forensic Sci* 1966;11:167–173.
156. Andersen AH. Experimental studies on the pharmacology of activated charcoal. I. Adsorption power of charcoal in aqueous solutions. *Acta Pharmacol* 1946;2:69–78.
157. Lambert RJ, Kindler BL, Schaeffer DJ. The efficacy of superactivated charcoal in treating rats exposed to a lethal dose of potassium cyanide. *Ann Emerg Med* 1988;17:595–598.
158. Chen KK, Rose C, Clowes HA. Methylene blue, nitrites, and sodium thiosulphate against cyanide. *Proc Soc Exp Biol Med* 1933;31:250–253.
159. Kruszyna R, Kruszyna H, Smith RP. Comparison of hydroxylamine, 4-dimethylaminophenol and nitrite protection against cyanide poisoning in mice. *Arch Toxicol* 1982;49:191–202.
160. Chen KK, Rose CL. Nitrite and thiosulfate therapy in cyanide poisoning. *JAMA* 1952;149:113–115.
161. Vick JA, Froehlich HL. Studies of cyanide poisoning. *Arch Int Pharmacodyn Ther* 1985;273:314–322.
162. Vick JA, Froehlich H. Treatment of cyanide poisoning. *Mil Med* 1991;156:330–339.
163. Klimmek R, Krettek C. Effects of amyl nitrite on circulation, respiration and blood homoeostasis in cyanide poisoning. *Arch Toxicol* 1988;62:161–166.
164. Burrows GE. Cyanide intoxication in sheep; therapeutics. *Vet Hum Toxicol* 1981;23:22–28.
165. Burrows GE, Way JL. Cyanide intoxication in sheep: enhancement of efficacy of sodium nitrite, sodium thiosulfate, and cobaltous chloride. *Am J Vet Res* 1979;40:613–617.
166. Hall AH, Linden CH, Kulig KW, Rumack BH. Cyanide poisoning from laetrile ingestion: role of nitrite therapy. *Pediatrics* 1986;78:269–272.
167. Johnson WS, Hall AH, Rumack BH. Cyanide poisoning successfully treated without "therapeutic methemoglobin levels." *Am J Emerg Med* 1989;7:437–440.
168. Johnson RP, Mellors JW. Arteriolization of venous blood gases: a clue to the diagnosis of cyanide poisoning. *J Emerg Med* 1988;6:401–404.
169. Berlin CM Jr. The treatment of cyanide poisoning in children. *Pediatrics* 1970;46:793–796.
170. Mascarenhas BR, Geller AC, Goodman AI. Cyanide poisoning, medical emergency. *N Y State J Med* 1969;69:1782–1784.
171. Johnson RP, Mellors JW. Arteriolization of venous blood gases: a clue to the diagnosis of cyanide poisoning. *J Emerg Med* 1988;6:401–404.
172. Mueller M, Borland C. Delayed cyanide poisoning following acetonitrile ingestion. *Postgrad Med J* 1997;73:299–300.
173. Carden E. Hyperbaric oxygen in cyanide poisoning. *Anaesthesia* 1970;25:442–443.
174. Evans CL. Cobalt compounds as antidotes for hydrocyanic acid. *Br J Pharmacol* 1964;23:455–475.
175. Houeto P, Borron SW, Sandouk P, et al. Pharmacokinetics of hydroxocobalamin in smoke inhalation victims. *J Toxicol Clin Toxicol* 1996;34:397–404.
176. Kaczka EA, Wolf DE, Kuehl FA, et al. Vitamin B12: reactions of cyano-cobalamin and related compounds. *Science* 1950;112:354–355.
177. Houeto P, Hoffman JR, Imbert M, et al. Relation of blood cyanide to plasma cyanocobalamin concentration after a fixed dose of hydroxocobalamin in cyanide poisoning. *Lancet* 1995;346:605–608.
178. Forsyth JC, Mueller PD, Becker CE, et al. Hydroxocobalamin as a cyanide antidote: safety, efficacy and pharmacokinetics in heavily smoking normal volunteers. *J Toxicol Clin Toxicol* 1993;31:277–294.
179. Williams HL, Johnson DJ, McNeil JS, et al. Studies of cobalamin as a vehicle for the renal excretion of cyanide anion. *J Lab Clin Med* 1990;116:37–44.
180. Mushett CW, Kelley KL, Boxer GE, et al. Antidotal efficacy of vitamin B12a (hydroxo-cobalamin) in experimental cyanide poisoning. *Proc Exp Biol Med* 1952;81:234–237.
181. Cottrell JE, Casthely P, Brodie JD, et al. Prevention of nitroprusside-induced cyanide toxicity with hydroxocobalamin. *N Engl J Med* 1978;298:809–811.
182. Rose CL, Worth RM, Chen KK. Hydroxo-cobalamine and acute cyanide poisoning in dogs. *Life Sci* 1965;4:1785–1789.
183. Posner MA, Tobey RE, McElroy H. Hydroxocobalamin therapy of cyanide intoxication in guinea pigs. *Anesthesiology* 1976;44:157–160.
184. Posner MA, Rodkey FL, Tobey RE. Nitroprusside-induced cyanide poisoning: antidotal effect of hydroxocobalamin. *Anesthesiology* 1976;44:330–335.
185. Friedberg KD, Shukla UR. The efficiency of aquocobalamine as an antidote in cyanide poisoning when given alone or combined with sodium thiosulfate. *Arch Toxicol* 1975;33:103–113.
186. Hall AH, Rumack BH. Hydroxycobalamin/sodium thiosulfate as a cyanide antidote. *J Emerg Med* 1987;5:115–121.
187. Bismuth C, Baud FJ, Djeghout H, et al. Cyanide poisoning from propionitrile exposure. *J Emerg Med* 1987;5:191–195.
188. Weger NP. Treatment of cyanide poisoning with 4-dimethylaminophenol (DMAP)—experimental and clinical overview. *Fundam Appl Toxicol* 1983;3:387–396.
189. Smith L, Kruszya H, Smith RP. The effect of methemoglobin on the inhibition of cytochrome c oxidase by cyanide, sulfide, or azide. *Biochem Pharmacol* 1977;26:2247–2250.
190. Bhattacharya R, Rao PV, Vijayaraghavan R. In vitro and in vivo attenuation of experimental cyanide poisoning by alpha-ketoglutarate. *Toxicol Lett* 2002;128:185–195.
191. Hume AS, Mozingo JR, McIntyre B, et al. Antidotal efficacy of alpha-ketoglutaric acid and sodium thiosulfate in cyanide poisoning. *J Toxicol Clin Toxicol* 1995;33:721–724.
192. Burrows GE, Way JL. Cyanide intoxication in sheep: therapeutic value of oxygen or cobalt. *Am J Vet Res* 1977;38:223–227.
193. Way JL, Gibbon SL, Sheehy M. Cyanide intoxication: protection with oxygen. *Science* 1966;152:210–211.
194. Sheehy M, Way JL. Effect of oxygen on cyanide intoxication. 3. Mithridate. *J Pharmacol Exp Ther* 1968;161:163–168.
195. Isom GE, Burrows GE, Way JL. Effect of oxygen on the antagonism of cyanide intoxication—cytochrome oxidase, in vivo. *Toxicol Appl Pharmacol* 1982;65:250–256.
196. Leighton DA, Bhargava SK, Shail G. Tobacco amblyopia: the effect of treatment on the electroretinogram. *Doc Ophthalmol* 1979;46:325–331.
197. Syme IG, Bronte-Stewart J, Foulds WS, et al. Clinical and biochemical findings in Leber's hereditary optic atrophy. *Trans Ophthalmol Soc U K* 1983;103:556–559.
198. Chew SJ. Leber's hereditary optic atrophy: an atypical case with response to hydroxycobalamine therapy. *Singapore Med J* 1990;31:293–294.

CHAPTER 186

Hydrogen Sulfide

E. Martin Caravati

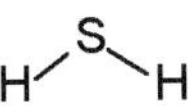

HYDROGEN SULFIDE

Synonyms:	**Hydrosulfuric acid, sewer gas, stink damp, hepatic acid, sour gas, sulfureted hydrogen, sulfur hydride**
Molecular formula and weight:	**H_2S, 34.1 g/mol**
SI conversion:	**1 mg/m^3 = 0.717 ppm**
CAS Registry No.:	**7783-06-4**
Normal levels:	**Whole blood sulfide less than 0.05 mg/L**
Target organs:	**Cellular hypoxia, central nervous system, lungs, mucous membranes, eyes**
Antidote:	**Oxygen**

OVERVIEW

Hydrogen sulfide (H_2S) is a toxic gas commonly associated with the "rotten egg" smell of homemade "stink bombs," but in the workplace, it is one of the leading causes of sudden death. A review of the U.S. Occupational Safety and Health Administration (OSHA) investigation records from 1984 to 1994 revealed 80 fatalities from hydrogen sulfide in 57 incidents, with 19 fatalities and 36 injuries among coworkers attempting to rescue fallen workers. OSHA issued citations for violation of respiratory protection and confined space standards in 60% of the fatalities. The use of hydrogen sulfide detection equipment, air-supplied respirators, and confined space safety training would have prevented most of the fatalities (1).

The most important determinants of clinical toxicity are gas concentration and duration of exposure. Hydrogen sulfide's excellent olfactory warning properties are lost at high concentrations, leading to insidious exposures and serious toxicity. Exposure to levels exceeding 1000 parts per million (ppm) results in coma, respiratory paralysis, and hypoxia. Death occurs unless the victim is quickly removed from the exposure and effective artificial ventilation is established. Although the exact mechanics of toxicity are unknown, hydrogen sulfide produces both local irritation and cellular asphyxia, probably by binding to the iron in cytochrome oxidase-a_3. Pulmonary edema is a common complication of serious toxicity, whereas upper respiratory tract irritation, keratoconjunctivitis, and nonspecific complaints (e.g., headache, nausea, dizziness) develop at lower exposure levels.

Most fatalities occur at the scene. Patients who have vital signs on arrival at the hospital usually survive, provided severe hypoxic encephalopathy is not present. The mainstay of treatment is supplemental oxygen and cardiovascular support. Nitrite-induced methemoglobinemia and hyperbaric oxygen (HBO) have been proposed as possibly efficacious based on the pathophysiology of hydrogen sulfide and anecdotal case reports.

Chemical and Physical Properties

Hydrogen sulfide is a colorless gas that is heavier than air (vapor density, 1.19). It has a strong "rotten egg" odor detectable at 0.02 to 0.77 ppm. It burns with a blue flame, decomposing to water, sulfur dioxide, and elemental sulfur. At physiologic pH, approximately one-third of hydrogen sulfide exists as the undissociated form (H_2S) and the remainder as hydrosulfide anion (HS^-). Very little of hydrogen sulfide exists as sulfide anion (S^2) (2). Blackened coins may be found in the pockets of patients poisoned by hydrogen sulfide (3).

Classification and Uses

Hydrogen sulfide is a byproduct of organic decomposition (e.g., sewers), the petroleum industry, tanning, rubber vulcanizing, and heavy water production. It is present in coal pits, gas wells, sulfur springs, and decaying organic matter. Serious toxicity and fatalities have been reported in poorly ventilated spaces after agitation of underground liquid manure tanks (4), addition of sulfuric acid to a drain (5) and hydrochloric acid to a well (6), cleaning of a propane tank (7), and entry of both patients and rescuers into a sewer (8) and ship holds containing fish meal (9).

The addition of dilute sulfuric or hydrochloric acid to iron sulfide or the reaction of hydrogen with elemental sulfur produces hydrogen sulfide gas. Natural sources include subterranean emission (e.g., caves), volcanoes, and bacterial decomposition of sulfur in soil and the gastrointestinal tract (minor amounts). Decay of organic sulfur-containing products (e.g., fish, sewage, manure, septic tanks) and pouring of acid on sewage liberate hydrogen sulfide. Toxic gases released from the decomposing environment include hydrogen sulfide, carbon monoxide, sulfur dioxide, carbon dioxide, methane, ammonia, and amines (trimethylamine, diethylamine, *N*-butylamine).

Common commercial exposures involve hydrogen disulfide as the manufacturing byproduct of viscose rayon; silk; petroleum and tanning; paper mills; damp mines; geothermal energy and hot sulfur springs; roofing asphalt tanks; burning of wool, hair, meals, and hides; production of heavy water for nuclear reactors; metal refining; and vulcanization of sulfur-containing rubber. Agitation of solutions containing hydrogen sulfide may dramatically increase ambient air hydrogen sulfide levels (7). Occupations subject to exposure to hydrogen sulfide are listed in Table 1.

Toxic Dose

Governmental standards and limits have been established for hydrogen sulfide. The OSHA permissible exposure limit–time-weighted average has not been established. The permissible exposure limit–ceiling limit is 20 ppm for 15 minutes and 50 ppm for 10 minutes. The American Conference of Governmental Industrial Hygienists has established the threshold limit value–

TABLE 1. Occupations with potential for exposure to hydrogen sulfide (National Institute for Occupational Safety and Health, 1977)

Animal fat and oil processors	Fishing and fish-processing workers	Pyrite burners
Animal manure removers	Fur dressers	Rayon makers
Artificial flavor makers	Geothermal power drilling and production workers	Refrigerant makers
Asphalt storage workers	Glue makers	Rubber and plastics processors
Barium carbonate makers	Gold ore workers	Septic tank cleaners
Blast furnace workers	Heavy metal precipitators	Sewage treatment workers
Brewery workers	Heavy water manufacturers	Sewer workers
Bromide-brine workers	Hydrochloric acid purifiers	Sheep dippers
Cable splicers	Landfill workers	Silk makers
Caisson workers	Lead ore sulphidizers	Slaughterhouse workers
Carbon disulphide workers	Lithographers	Smelting workers
Cellophane makers	Lithophone makers	Soap makers
Chemical laboratory workers, students, teachers	Livestock farmers	Sugar beet and cane workers
Cistern cleaners	Manhole and trench workers	Sulphur spa workers
Citrus root fumigators	Metallurgists	Sulphur products processors
Coal gasification workers	Miners	Synthetic fiber makers
Coke oven workers	Natural gas production and processing workers	Tank gaugers
Copper ore sulphidizers	Painters using polysulfide caulking compounds	Tannery workers
Depilatory makers	Paper makers	Textile printers
Dye makers	Petroleum production and refinery workers	Thiophene makers
Excavators	Phosphate purifiers	Tunnel workers
Felt makers	Photoengravers	Well diggers and cleaners
Fermentation makers	Pipeline maintenance workers	Wool pullers
Fertilizer makers		

Adapted from Prior MG, et al., eds. *Proc Int Conf on Hydrogen Sulfide Toxicity*. Banff, Canada, 1989.

time-weighted average at 10 ppm (14 mg/m^3), with a short-term exposure limit of 15 ppm (21 mg/m^3) and an immediate danger to life or health of 300 ppm. The National Institute of Safety and Health standards are 10 ppm ceiling for 10 minutes and evacuate the work area at 50 ppm.

The toxic effects of hydrogen sulfide are dose related (Table 2). An odor may be detectable at 0.02 to 0.03 ppm, and a definite odor appears at 3 to 10 ppm. Exposure to 10 ppm for 15 minutes during exercise had no effect on respiratory function in 19 healthy adults (10). At 50 to 100 ppm, eye irritation is the most commonly reported effect. Olfactory paralysis develops between 100 and 150 ppm. Between 150 and 300 ppm, respiratory tract and eye irritation is prominent (blepharospasm, keratoconjunctivitis, blurred vision, colored halos around lights [gas eyes]), accompanied by mucous membrane irritation, bronchitis, and pulmonary edema.

Severe systemic toxicity develops at more than 500 ppm and consists of headache, nausea, vomiting, weakness, disorientation, and coma within 30 minutes of exposure. At more than 700 ppm, cardiorespiratory arrest occurs, and death is imminent. One reason for the insidious toxicity of hydrogen sulfide is the unpredictability of its presence and concentration, which lead to unexpected accidents.

TOXICOKINETICS AND TOXICODYNAMICS

Hydrogen sulfide gas is rapidly absorbed by the lungs. Cutaneous absorption is negligible. The toxicokinetics of hydrogen sulfide have not been studied in humans. In animals, respiratory excretion of hydrogen sulfide is minimal after parenteral administration (2). Elimination occurs via methylation, oxidation to sulfate, and reaction with metalloproteins or disulfide-containing proteins. Detoxification of hydrogen sulfide occurs rapidly, with the red blood cells and liver mitochondria being the primary sites. The major metabolic pathway is hepatic oxidation of sulfide to sulfate and subsequent elimination in the urine (Fig. 1). Eighty-five percent of a lethal dose is eliminated per hour in animals. Lung sulfide concentrations increased during hydrogen sulfide exposure and rapidly returned to endogenous levels within 15 minutes after the cessation of a 3-hour, 400-ppm exposure in rats (11). Con-

TABLE 2. Physiologic effects of human exposure to hydrogen sulfide

Concentration (ppm)	Physiologic effect
0.02	Odor threshold.
0.13	Detectable, minimum perceptible odor.
0.77	Faint, weak odor, readily perceptible.
3–5	Offensive, moderately intense odor.
10	Obvious and unpleasant odor, threshold limit value–time weighted average, "sore eyes."
20	Maximum allowable concentration for daily 8-h exposure.
20–30	Strong and intense odor but not intolerable.
50	Conjunctival irritation is first noticeable.
50–100	Mild irritation to the respiratory tract and especially to the eyes after 1 h of exposure.
100	Loss of smell in 3–15 min, may sting eyes and throat, olfactory fatigue level.
150	Olfactory nerve paralysis.
~200	Less intense odor, olfactory paralysis.
250	Prolonged exposure may cause pulmonary edema.
300–500	Pulmonary edema, imminent threat to life.
500	In 0.5–1.0 h causes excitement, headache, dizziness, and staggering followed by unconsciousness and respiratory failure.
500–1000	Acts primarily as a systemic poison causing unconsciousness and death through respiratory paralysis.
700	Unconscious quickly, death results if not rescued promptly.
5000	Imminent death.

ppm, parts per million.
Adapted from Beauchamp RD Jr, Bus JS, Popp JA, et al. *CRC Crit Rev Toxicol* 1984;13:40.

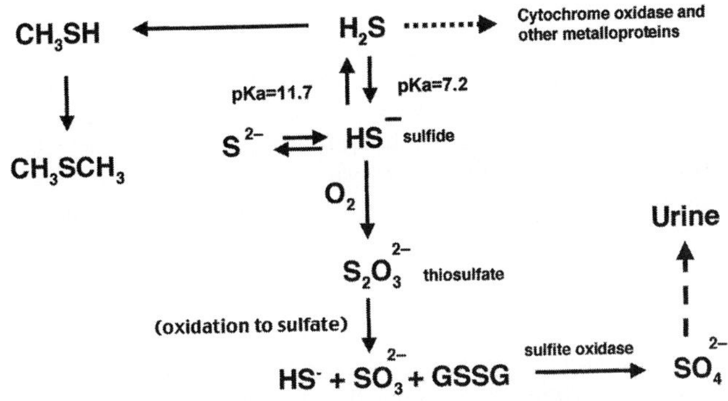

Figure 1. Metabolism of hydrogen sulfide. GSSG, oxidized glutathione; pKa, measure of acid strength. (From Dorman DC, Moulin FJ, McManus BE, et al. Cytochrome oxidase inhibition induced by acute hydrogen sulfide inhalation: correlation with tissue sulfide concentrations in the rat brain, liver, lung, and nasal epithelium. *Toxicol Sci* 2002;65:18–25, with permission.)

sequently, hydrogen sulfide is not a cumulative poison, and low concentrations (i.e., less than 20 ppm) are often tolerated without adverse effects. Endogenous sulfide is mostly oxidized to thiosulfate, with a smaller portion excreted unchanged by the lungs and urine.

Sulfhemoglobin is not produced by hydrogen sulfide poisoning (12). Inorganic sulfides are present in the body only in small quantities (0.05 mg/L).

PATHOPHYSIOLOGY

Hydrogen sulfide is a mucous membrane irritant and an asphyxiant. It is an intracellular toxin that directly inhibits cytochrome oxidase and disrupts electron transport (11). It is a more potent inhibitor of the cytochrome oxidase system than cyanide (13). The resulting anaerobic metabolism causes lactate accumulation and metabolic acidosis. Concentration-dependent toxicity occurs to the nervous, respiratory, and cardiovascular systems. At lower doses, hydrogen sulfide is a mucous membrane and respiratory irritant (200 ppm), but at high doses (1000 ppm), it causes direct respiratory depression. Death usually results from respiratory arrest and hypoxia.

PREGNANCY AND LACTATION

Exposure of pregnant rats to 100 ppm for 6 hours per day did not result in any fetal toxicity (14).

CLINICAL PRESENTATION

Acute Exposure

Hydrogen sulfide is an irritant to the eyes and respiratory tract at low concentrations. In high doses, the central nervous system is the primary target organ. A short exposure to a high concentration (750 to 1000 ppm) can produce "knockdown," a phenomenon that is characterized by sudden, brief loss of consciousness followed by complete recovery (assuming exposure is terminated). Abrupt collapse may produce traumatic injuries (7% of cases in one series) (15). Pulmonary edema is common after exposures to 250 ppm for a prolonged period. Symptoms of severe exposure in one large series were, in the order of frequency: loss of consciousness, dizziness, nausea, vomiting, headache, sore throat, conjunctivitis, weakness of extremities, dyspnea, seizures, pulmonary edema, cyanosis, and hemoptysis (16). Almost 5% of patients were dead on arrival at the hospital.

Central nervous system effects include headache, lethargy, vertigo, agitation, horizontal or vertical nystagmus (17), weakness, seizures, and coma. The combination of vomiting and central nervous system depression may lead to aspiration pneumonia. Rapid loss of consciousness and respiratory paralysis occurs at 1000 ppm. Neurologic recovery is variable. Some patients have complete recovery, whereas others manifest permanent deficits. Spasticity, cerebellar ataxia, tremor, and exacerbation of exercise-induced angina were reported in a patient rendered unconscious and cyanotic by a 30-minute hydrogen sulfide exposure (3).

Cardiac effects include dysrhythmias, bradycardia, myocardial depression, conduction defects, abnormal ventricular repolarization, and hypotension.

Gastrointestinal effects include nausea, vomiting, abdominal pain, and diarrhea and occur with subacute toxic exposure.

Respiratory effects include rhinitis, pharyngitis, bronchitis, and pneumonitis with prolonged exposures to more than 50 ppm. Symptoms include sore throat, cough, hoarseness, runny nose, and chest tightness. Pulmonary edema, bronchiolitis, reactive airway disease, bronchiolitis obliterans, and pulmonary interstitial fibrosis (18) have also been reported. Pulmonary edema may result from prolonged exposure to 250 ppm. It occurs in 4% to 16% of acute exposures (19).

Ocular effects include conjunctivitis, eye pain, lacrimation, photophobia, keratoconjunctivitis ("gas eye"), and corneal erosions with exposures to more than 50 ppm. Conjunctivitis and "sore eyes" have been observed at concentrations as low as 5 ppm.

Olfactory effects include a rotten-egg odor at 0.02 to 0.13 ppm. Olfactory fatigue occurs at approximately 100 ppm and paralysis at 150 ppm. Thus, odor is not a reliable warning sign at high concentrations.

Delayed and Chronic Complications

Long-term adverse effects are unusual in patients who are promptly resuscitated (16). A patient developed interstitial pulmonary fibrosis 4 years after an acute inhalation exposure to hydrogen sulfide (18). Occupational exposures may result in chronic olfactory deficits (20).

Permanent neurologic sequelae have occurred after severe exposures, probably as a result of cerebral anoxia (21). Neuropsychiatric disorders and abnormal brain evoked responses have been associated with exposure to relatively low concentrations of hydrogen sulfide (22). Further research is needed to better define potential chronic complications and disability from exposures.

Chronic Exposure

Headache, weakness, nausea, vomiting, and weight loss occur in chronic exposure and may appear for several months after acute exposure. Chronic exposure to at least 0.6 ppm of hydrogen sulfide for almost 1 year was associated with truncal ataxia, choreoathetosis, and dystonia with bilateral lucent areas in the basal ganglia in a 20-month-old child. Removal from the source of the gas resulted in clinical recovery with resolution of the basal ganglia abnormalities (23).

DIAGNOSTIC TESTS

Biologic Monitoring and Health Surveillance

Most adverse effects occur from brief exposure to high concentrations; therefore, routine biologic monitoring is not of value.

Sulfide is detoxified to thiosulfate, which can be measured in the urine. The normal urinary thiosulfate concentration is 0.4 to 5.4 μmol/mmol creatinine. Volunteers exposed to 18 ppm hydrogen sulfide for 30 minutes had peak urinary thiosulfate concentrations of 30 μmol/mmol creatinine at 15 hours, which decreased to normal at 17 hours after exposure. Elevated urine thiosulfate is associated with ingesting food or water high in sulfur and can confound the results (19). Medical surveillance examinations should be performed to assess the worker's ability to use respiratory protection.

Acute Exposure

The normal whole blood sulfide is less than 0.05 mg/L. Sulfide was detected in the blood of two patients who died of an acute hydrogen sulfide exposure at 0.13 and 0.11 mg/L. Sulfide concentrations can be determined by gas dialysis/ion chromatography or ion-selective electrode analytic techniques.

Thiosulfate is a metabolite of sulfide and can be detected in the blood and urine after exposure. The normal urine thiosulfate is less than 8 mg/L; it is normally undetectable in blood. A serum thiosulfate greater than 1.3 mg/L is associated with toxicity. In two fatalities, the urine thiosulfate was 0.9 mg/L in one patient. Thiosulfate was not detected in the plasma of a survivor but was present in the urine at 29.3 mg/L. Urine thiosulfate may be the only indication of a hydrogen sulfide exposure in survivors of an acute exposure (24).

Other Tests

All seriously poisoned patients should have a chest radiograph, serum lactate, electrolytes, and arterial blood gas performed to evaluate for evidence of aspiration pneumonia, pulmonary edema, metabolic acidosis, and electrolyte disturbances. If nitrites have been administered, blood methemoglobin concentrations should be monitored. Early widening of the alveolar-arterial oxygen gradient suggests the development of pulmonary edema or pneumonia.

Evaluation for other agents capable of producing unexpected collapse in an occupational setting, such as cyanide or simple asphyxiants, should be evaluated.

Myocardial ischemia, infarction, and cardiac dysrhythmias have been observed after acute exposure (5,25).

Bilateral symmetric lucent areas within the cerebral hemispheres, which probably correspond to the lentiform nucleus, have been observed on computerized tomography of the brain (26). Such lesions are consistent with focal brain lesions produced by hypoxia or hypotension.

Postmortem Considerations

Autopsies demonstrate nonspecific findings such as visceral congestion, scattered petechiae, and hemorrhagic pulmonary edema. Greenish discoloration of gray matter, viscera, and bronchial secretions have been reported in documented hydrogen sulfide–related fatalities (27) but may disappear after the injection of formalin (8). A sulfide smell may be present on the slicing of tissue, and autolysis of tissue may be accelerated (28). Most autopsy cases demonstrate pulmonary edema.

Sulfide ion levels measured soon after hydrogen sulfide–induced death ranged from 1.70 to 3.75 mg/L (29). Postmortem confirmation of toxic levels is complicated by the rapid endogenous destruction of the sulfide ion, formation of sulfide from protein degradation postmortem, and deterioration of the sulfide ion in storage (30).

TREATMENT

Immediate supportive care is the most important phase of treatment because most fatalities occur at the scene. However, rescuers must be very cautious when entering areas that potentially contain hydrogen sulfide. Entering closed areas (e.g., inside storage tanks) requires self-contained breathing apparatus, safety lines, and outside observation. Evacuate the immediate area and monitor hydrogen sulfide levels with Draeger tubes. Be sure to move the victim to an area without toxic hydrogen sulfide levels because would-be rescuers have lost consciousness while applying mouth-to-mouth resuscitation (31).

After protection of the rescuer, the most important priority is the establishment of adequate ventilation and circulation. Supportive care and supplemental oxygen may be sufficient to treat the victim without the need to use nitrites (32). All patients who lose consciousness yet recover promptly should be admitted for observation of potential aspiration pneumonitis or pulmonary edema.

Decontamination and First Aid

Decontamination is not useful because only pulmonary exposure occurs. Skin decontamination is not necessary due to poor cutaneous absorption.

Enhancement of Elimination

The use of extracorporeal measures to enhance elimination has not been reported and is not expected to be successful.

Antidotes

Two antidotal interventions have been proposed: the induction of methemoglobinemia and treatment with HBO. Neither is likely to have a major clinical impact because the toxicity of hydrogen sulfide is manifested and death occurs within the first minutes of exposure.

The induction of methemoglobinemia has been proposed as an antidote because the toxic mechanism of hydrogen sulfide is similar to cyanide. Mice pretreated with sodium nitrite demonstrated increased survival, whereas those treated with 100% oxygen did not, compared with room air controls (33). However, the efficacy of this treatment is not well established in humans. Nitrites produce methemoglobin, which in turn potentially attracts sulfide from the cytochrome oxidase to form sulfmethemoglobin and thus reactivates aerobic metabolism. Sulfmethemoglobin undergoes rapid spontaneous detoxification in the body. The induction of methemoglobin by nitrites is relatively slow. The lifetime of sulfide in oxygenated blood is short, and induction of methemoglobin more than 10 to 15 minutes postexposure may not aid the victim. The use of nitrites in serious cases may be effective only if given within minutes of exposure (34).

The use of an antidote must not delay the establishment of adequate ventilation and oxygenation. The dosages of nitrites are similar to those used in cyanide poisoning. An amyl nitrite pearl is broken and inhaled for 30 seconds every minute. Adults should receive sodium nitrite, 300 mg (10 ml of 3% sodium nitrite solution), intravenously over 4 minutes immediately after access is established (35). No absolute guidelines are available for the use of nitrites in hydrogen sulfide poisoning in the hospital setting because most hospital inpatients survive with supportive care only and nitrites have inherent toxicity. Thiosulfate is not required because the body spontaneously detoxifies sulfmethemoglobin. The use of the Cyanide Antidote Package and its adverse effects are described in Chapter 46.

HBO increases oxyhemoglobin and oxygen delivery to the tissues. Increased oxygen delivery may compete with sulfide for cytochrome oxidase and relieve tissue hypoxia. Two anecdotal case studies suggest that HBO therapy may be useful for severe hydrogen sulfide toxicity (36,37). One patient had no response to nitrite therapy but 10 hours after exposure received HBO and became more alert (37). In another report, HBO did not improve the patient's status (38). Although unproven, an HBO treatment in patients unresponsive to supportive care and nitrite therapy may be reasonable.

Supportive Care

Symptomatic patients should have intravenous access, frequent blood pressure, cardiac rhythm, and oxygen saturation monitoring. Patients should receive high-flow supplemental oxygen by nonrebreathing face mask or be intubated if necessary to protect the airway and provide maximum oxygen delivery (100% oxygen concentration). Hypotension should be treated with intravenous fluids (e.g., 10 to 20 ml/kg bolus of normal saline) and vasopressors, such as dopamine or norepinephrine, if necessary (Chapter 37). Seizures should be treated with intravenous benzodiazepines (Chapter 40).

Monitoring

All symptomatic patients should be admitted to the hospital and monitored for lactic acidosis, electrolyte disturbances, aspiration pneumonia, pulmonary edema, and cardiac ischemia. If nitrites are used, monitor methemoglobin levels.

REFERENCES

1. Fuller DC, Suruda AJ. Occupationally related hydrogen sulfide deaths in the United States from 1984 to 1994. *J Occup Environ Med* 2000;42:939–942.
2. Beauchamp RO Jr, Bus JS, Popp JA, et al. A critical review of the literature on hydrogen sulfide toxicity. *CRC Crit Rev Toxicol* 1984;13:25–97.
3. Hurwitz LJ, Taylor GI. Poisoning by sewer gas with unusual sequelae. *Lancet* 1954;1:1110–1111.
4. Morse DL, Woodbury MA, Rentmeester K, et al. Death caused by fermenting manure. *JAMA* 1981;245:63–64.
5. Peters JW. Hydrogen sulfide poisoning in a hospital setting. *JAMA* 1981;246:1588–1589.
6. Thoman M. Sewer gas: hydrogen sulfide intoxication. *J Toxicol Clin Toxicol* 1969;2:383–386.
7. Vannatta JB. Hydrogen sulfide poisoning: report of four cases and brief review of the literature. *J Okla Med Assoc* 1982;75:29–32.
8. Adelson L, Sunshine I. Fatal hydrogen sulfide intoxication: report of three cases occurring in a sewer. *Arch Pathol* 1966;81:375–380.
9. Dalgaard JB, Dencker F, Fallentin B, et al. Fatal poisoning and other health hazards connected with industrial fishing. *Br J Ind Med* 1972;29:307–316.
10. Bhambhani Y, Burnham R, Snydmiller G, et al. Effects of 10-ppm hydrogen sulfide inhalation on pulmonary function in healthy men and women. *J Occup Environ Med* 1996;38:1012–1017.
11. Dorman DC, Moulin FJ, McManus BE, et al. Cytochrome oxidase inhibition induced by acute hydrogen sulfide inhalation: correlation with tissue sulfide concentrations in the rat brain, liver, lung, and nasal epithelium. *Toxicol Sci* 2002;65:18–25.
12. Smith RP, Gosselin RE. Hydrogen sulfide poisoning. *J Occup Med* 1979;21:93–97.
13. Nicholls P. The effect of sulphide on cytochrome a_3, isosteric and allosteric shifts of the reduced alpha peak. *Biochim Biophys Acta* 1975;396:24–35.
14. Saillenfait AM, Bonnet P, deCeaurriz J. Effects of inhalation exposure to carbon disulfide and its combination with hydrogen sulfide on embryonal and fetal development in rats. *Toxicol Lett* 1989;48:57–66.
15. Arnold IMF, Dufresne RM, Alleyne BC, et al. Health implication of occupational exposures to hydrogen sulfide. *J Occup Med* 1985;27:373–376.
16. Burnett WW, King EG, Grace M, et al. Hydrogen sulfide poisoning: review of 5 years experience. *CMAJ* 1977;117:1277–1280.
17. Stine RJ, Slosberg B, Beacham BE. Hydrogen sulfide intoxication. A case report and discussion of treatment. *Ann Intern Med* 1976;85:756–758.
18. Duong TX, Suruda AJ, Maier LA. Interstitial fibrosis following hydrogen sulfide exposure. *Am J Ind Med* 2001;40:221–224.
19. Milby TH, Baselt RC. Hydrogen sulfide poisoning: clarification of some controversial issues. *Am J Ind Med* 1999;35:192–195.
20. Hirsch AR, Zavala G. Long-term effects on the olfactory system of exposure to hydrogen sulphide. *Occup Environ Med* 1999;56:284–287.
21. Snyder JW, Safir EF, Summerville GP, et al. Occupational fatality and persistent neurological sequelae after mass exposure to hydrogen sulfide. *Am J Emerg Med* 1995;13:199–203.
22. Hirsch AR. Hydrogen sulfide exposure without loss of consciousness: chronic effects in four cases. *Toxicol Ind Health* 2002;18:51–61.
23. Gaitonde VB, Sellar RJ, O'Hare AE. Long term exposure to hydrogen sulphide producing subacute encephalopathy in a child. *BMJ* 1987;294:614.
24. Kage S, Kashimura S, Ikeda H, et al. Fatal and nonfatal poisoning by hydrogen sulfide at an industrial waste site. *J Forensic Sci* 2002;47:652–655.
25. Kemper FD. A near fatal case of hydrogen sulfide poisoning. *CMAJ* 1966;94:1130–1131.
26. Matsuo F, Cummins JW, Anderson RE. Neurological sequelae of massive hydrogen sulfide inhalation. *Arch Neurol* 1979;36:451–452.
27. Winek CL, Collom WD, Wecht CH. Death from hydrogen sulphide fumes. *Lancet* 1968;1:1096.
28. Simson RE, Simpson GR. Fatal hydrogen sulphide poisoning associated with industrial waste exposure. *Med J Aust* 1971;1:331–334.
29. McAnalley BH, Lowry WT, Oliver RD, et al. Determination of inorganic sulfide and cyanide in blood using specific ion electrodes. Application to the investigation of hydrogen sulfide and cyanide poisoning. *J Anal Toxicol* 1979;3:111–114.
30. Evans L. The toxicity of hydrogen sulphide and other sulphides. *Q J Exp Physiol* 1967;52:231–248.
31. Milby TH. Hydrogen sulfide intoxication: review of the literature and report of unusual accident resulting in two cases of nonfatal poisoning. *J Occup Med* 1962;4:431–437.
32. Ravizza AG, Carugo D, Cerchiari EL, et al. The treatment of hydrogen sulfide intoxication: oxygen versus nitrites. *Vet Hum Toxicol* 1982;24:241–242.
33. Smith RP, Kruszyna R, Kruszyna H. Management of acute sulfide poisoning. Effects of oxygen, thiosulfate, and nitrite. *Arch Environ Health* 1976;31:166–169.
34. Beck JF, Bradbury CM, Connors AJ, et al. Nitrite as antidote for acute hydrogen sulfide intoxication? *Am Ind Hyg Assoc J* 1981;42:805–809.
35. Hoidal CR, Hall AH, Robinson MD, et al. Hydrogen sulfide poisoning from toxic inhalations of roofing asphalt fumes. *Ann Emerg Med* 1986;15:826–830.
36. Whitcraft DD III, Bailey TD, Hart GB. Hydrogen sulfide poisoning treated with hyperbaric oxygen. *J Emerg Med* 1985;3:23–25.
37. Smilkstein MJ, Bronstein AC, Pickett HM, et al. Hyperbaric oxygen therapy for severe hydrogen sulfide poisoning. *J Emerg Med* 1985;3:27–30.
38. Al-Mahasneh OM, Cohle SK, Haas E. Lack of response to hyperbaric oxygen in a fatal case of hydrogen sulfide poisoning. *Vet Hum Toxicol* 1989;31:353(abst).

CHAPTER 187

Nitrates and Nitrites

Steven A. Seifert

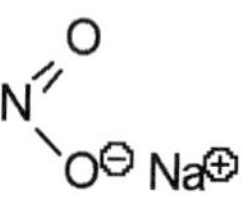

SODIUM NITRITE

Compounds included:	**Nitrates: ammonium nitrate; nitrites: amyl nitrite, butyl nitrite, tert-butyl nitrite, ethyl nitrite, isobutyl nitrite, cyclohexyl nitrite, potassium nitrite, sodium nitrite, silver nitrite**
Molecular formula and weight:	**Ammonium nitrate (NH_4NO_3), 80.06; amyl nitrite ($C_5H_{11}NO_2$), 117.1; butyl nitrite ($C_4H_9NO_2$), 103.1; sodium nitrite ($NaNO_2$), 69.0 g/mol**
SI conversion:	**Ammonium nitrate, mg/dl × 1.2 = μmol/L; amyl nitrite, mg/L × 8.5 = μmol/L; butyl nitrite, mg/L × 9.7 = μmol/L; sodium nitrite, mg/dl × 1.4 = μmol/L**
CAS Registry No.:	**6484-52-2 (ammonium nitrate); 7632-00-0 (sodium nitrite)**
Normal levels:	**Normal level of methemoglobin is less than 10%.**
Special concern:	**Methemoglobinemia**
Antidote:	**Methylene blue**

OVERVIEW

Humans are exposed to nitrates and nitrites in their diet, environment, work, and medications (Tables 1 and 2). Because they may be interconverted, the nitrates and nitrites have similar diagnostic and treatment considerations, which are addressed for the group as a whole in the sections Diagnostic Tests for Nitrates and Nitrates and Treatment. Acute toxicity is a result of excessive vasodilation and hypotension and the development of methemoglobinemia. The treatment of hypotension is by fluid expansion and pressors as needed. The treatment of methemoglobinemia is by methylene blue.

NITRATES

Nitrates are commonly found in environmental, occupational, and therapeutic settings and include fertilizers, nitrogen-containing plants, contaminated well water, and nitrate-containing pharmaceuticals. They are used therapeutically for angina pectoris and as a preload reducer in the treatment of congestive heart failure and hypertension. The toxicity of nitrates is secondary to their *in vivo* conversion to nitrites.

Depending on growth conditions or processing treatment, plant and food sources may include beets, carrots, corn (foliage only), cured meats, *Datura* species, goldenrod, *Solanum* species, spinach, sunflowers, sweet clover, and wheat (1). Some nitrates are stable in boiling water for up to 24 hours (2). Epidemic outbreaks are possible because of potential contamination of food and water sources and occupational exposures (3).

Organic nitrate pharmaceuticals include isosorbide dinitrate, isosorbide mononitrate, nitroglycerin, sodium nitrate, and sodium nitroprusside. Ammonium nitrate is found in cold packs, containing up to 234 g per pack (4).

Toxic Dose

The initial *therapeutic dosage* of *isosorbide dinitrate* is 5 to 30 mg four times a day up to 320 mg a day. The dosage of a sustained-release formulation is 40 mg every 6 to 12 hours (5). *Isosorbide mononitrate* has a dosage of 20 mg twice a day. A sustained-release formulation is dosed at 30 to 240 mg once a day. *Nitroglycerin* is usually administered as a sublingual tablet, 0.15 to 0.60 mg, or as a translingual spray (0.4 mg) every 5 minutes until relief or up to three doses. A sustained-release formulation is dosed at 2.5 mg three or four times a day. Nitroprusside is administered as an intravenous infusion. The usual adult and pediatric (older than 3 months of age) dose of nitroprusside is 0.5 to 10.0 μg/kg/minute, with a maximum cumulative dose of 70 mg/kg within 14 days. Neonates should not exceed 3 μg/kg/minute. Caution should be used in the presence of severe hepatic impairment (6).

The minimal toxic dose of a nitrate varies among individuals. The rapid development of tolerance also prevents the determination of toxic doses. The maximum allowable chronic ingestion of nitrates is no greater than 5 mg/kg/day. The most common cause of induced methemoglobinemia in infants younger than 6 months of age is nitrate-contaminated drinking water. The maximum allowable level of nitrates in drinking water is 45 parts per million (ppm) (7). For water used in hemodialysis units, a standard of 2-ppm nitrates has been suggested (7). Infants younger than 6 months of age are more susceptible to develop methemo-

TABLE 1. Occupational sources of nitrites and nitrates

Occupation/activity	Source of nitrite/nitrate
Case hardener	Cyanogens, sodium dichromate or nitrite
Cartridge maker	Lead, mercury, nitrites
Explosives maker	Acetone, ammonia amyl acetate, mercury, nitrites, nitroglycerin, picric acid, TNT
Fertilizer producer/user	Ammonia, arsenic, calcium cyanamide, carbon dioxide, castor bean pomace, cyanogens, fluoride, hydrogen sulfide, lime, magnesium, manganese, nitrates, nitric acid, phosphates, sulfur oxides, sulfuric acid
Gunsmith/hunter/marksman (see also explosives maker)	Cyanide, kerosene, lead, magnesium, mercury, nickel, nitrites, nitrobenzene, solvents
Bluing	Chlorate, mercury, methanol, nitrite, selenium
Ink maker	Ammonia, arsenic, benzene, benzine, chromates, cobalt, formaldehyde, lead, mercury, nitrites, other solvents, silver
Tanner	Acetates, acids, aniline, arsenic, benzene, carbon dioxide, chromates, cyanide, diethylamine, dyes, formaldehyde, hydrogen sulfide, mercury, nitrites, oxalate, picric acid, sodium sulfide, tannin
Lithographer	Acids, aniline, arsenic, benzene, benzine, chromates, lead, mercury, methanol, nitric acid, nitrites, oxalate, tetrachloroethane, turpentine
Petroleum refiner	Acetone, ammonia, arsenic, benzene, benzine, gasoline and other petroleum distillates, hydrofluoric acid, hydrogen sulfide, nitrites, solvents, sulfur oxides

globinemia because of decreased levels of methemoglobin reductase and greater oxidation potential of fetal hemoglobin (8).

Sodium nitrate is a frequent cause of nitrate poisoning in China, where at least 2 g are ingested at each meal. Building workers are frequently exposed (9). The ingestion of one hundred 0.4-mg nitroglycerin tablets over 2 days caused a fatal 7% methemoglobinemia in an elderly adult with severe cardiovascular disease (10). Methemoglobin concentrations of 9% were associated with the extension of a recent myocardial infarction in a cardiac patient receiving high-dose intravenous nitroglycerin (11). Isosorbide-5-mononitrate is the principal acetone metabolite of *isosorbide dinitrate*.

A 15-year-old girl ingested 80 isosorbide-5-mononitrate tablets (1.6 g) and 20 nitroglycerin tablets (20 mg). She developed severe headache, nausea, and vomiting. The skin was flushed and hot and dry. Symptoms disappeared in 24 hours (12).

Nitroprusside resulted in profound hypotension and death when a 50-kg patient with renal failure was given 13 mg over 90 minutes (13). The risk of cyanide toxicity in terms of dose is not well established. *Ammonium nitrate* produces toxicity with as little as 24 g, including symptomatic methemoglobinemia. Ingestion of up to 234 g produced only mild methemoglobinemia in one series (4).

Toxicokinetics and Toxicodynamics

Nitrates may be given sublingually, orally, transdermally, or intravenously. They are moderately well absorbed orally. Oral bioavailability of isosorbide dinitrate is 19% to 93%, depending on the formulation (14,15). Peak levels by the oral route are achieved within 40 to 45 minutes (16) and within 5 minutes by the sublingual route (17). Absorption in toxic amounts is also possible through burned skin (18). Nitrates are converted to nitrites by the action of bacteria in the gastrointestinal tract and are excreted in the urine. The duration of effect varies by agent and formulation.

TABLE 2. Reported inducers of methemoglobinemia

Agent	Source
Inorganic nitrates/nitrites	Contaminated well water, meat preservatives, vegetables/carrot juice, spinach, silver nitrate burn therapy, industrial salts, contaminants of nitrous oxide canisters for anesthesia
Organic nitrites	
Butyl/isobutyl nitrite	Room deodorizer propellants
Amyl nitrite	Inhalant in cyanide antidote kit
Nitroglycerine	Oral, sublingual, or transdermal pharmaceuticals for treatment of angina

Isosorbide dinitrate is rapidly absorbed and distributed. The distribution half-life is 8.7 minutes (14). The volume of distribution is 3.1 L/kg, and protein binding is low. The half-life of elimination is 1 to 4 hours and 4 hours for the active metabolite, isosorbide-4-mononitrate. The duration of effect of sublingual isosorbide dinitrate is 1 to 2 hours and of oral, 4 to 6 hours.

Isosorbide mononitrate is a long-acting metabolite of isosorbide dinitrate. It has nearly complete oral bioavailability (19). The volume of distribution is 0.6 to 0.7 L/kg, and protein binding is low (20). The distribution half-life is 8.6 minutes (20). The drug has a half-life of elimination of 6.2 to 6.6 hours (20), and it is denitrated to inactive metabolites (21). The immediate-release formulation has a duration of action of 6 hours (22) and the sustained-release formulation, approximately 12 hours.

Nitroglycerin is rapidly absorbed and distributed. Oral and transdermal absorption of nitroglycerin is up to 75% of the dose. It has up to 60% protein binding and a volume of distribution of 3 L/kg (23). The half-life of elimination is 19 to 33 minutes, with a duration of effect of up to 1 hour for immediate-release, up to 12 hours for transdermal, and up to 8 hours for sustained-release formulations (24,25). There is extensive hepatic metabolism, with excretion of inactive metabolites and 22% of the parent compound by the kidney.

Nitroprusside has a nearly immediate onset of action with institution of an intravenous infusion. The half-life of elimination is 3 to 4 minutes, and the effects terminate within minutes after discontinuation of the infusion. Nitroprusside is metabolized in the red blood cell. The ferrous ion in nitroprusside reacts with sulfhydryl compounds in the red blood cell, resulting in the liberation of cyanide. Cyanide is further metabolized in the liver by the enzyme rhodanese, which combines cyanide with endogenous thiosulfate to form thiocyanate, which is excreted by the kidney.

Pathophysiology

Vasodilating organic nitrates are reduced to organic nitrite, which is then converted to nitric oxide. Nitric oxide is then converted to an *S*-nitrosothiol derivative by the addition of a sulfhydryl group. This activates guanylcyclase, thereby producing cyclic guanosine monophosphate (cGMP), the mediator for relaxation of vascular smooth muscle. Vasodilation occurs in both arterial and venous vessels. Hypotension, low systemic vascular resistance, an increase in vascular volume, and a reduced sensitivity to vasoconstrictors may follow (26–28).

Tolerance to the effects of inhaled nitrites is reported and may be a function of the depletion of intracellular cysteine and other sulfhydryl group sources. Workers in a munitions plant had fewer nitrite-induced headaches with increased exposure and a recurrence when returning to work after an absence (29). Depletion of sulfhydryl group donors is possibly one mechanism for tolerance to the organic nitrates in patients with angina pectoris. Such tolerance may be reversed by sulfhydryl group donors such as *N*-acetylcysteine (30). Such tolerance reversal has not, however, been demonstrated in healthy patients after use of glyceryl trinitrate skin patches with concurrent administration of N-acetylcysteine (31).

Nitroglycerin is known to decompose to nitric oxide in biologic systems (26). There is no evidence at present that nitrogen dioxide is endogenously formed from nitric oxide. Bacteria in the mouth also convert nitrates to nitrites. When there are high loads of nitrates, recycling through the oral cavity also increases conversion to nitrites (32).

Ammonium nitrate is a strong oxidizing agent that reacts violently with reducing agents, strong acids, powdered metals, and organic materials. Nitrogen oxides and ammonia are generated during combustion (33).

Chronic administration of *nitroprusside* (more than 2 μg/kg/minute) may result in the production of cyanide in excess of the endogenous systems' (methemoglobin, rhodanese enzyme) ability to detoxify. Patients with a relative deficiency of endogenous thiosulfate (malnutrition, recent surgery, or the use of diuretics) have a decreased ability to detoxify cyanide (34). The presence of renal failure may result in thiocyanate accumulation. Sudden withdrawal of nitroprusside may result in sudden, severe increases in blood pressure (35). The mechanism of tachyphylaxis is not known (6).

Pregnancy and Lactation

Nitrate pharmaceuticals are U.S. Food and Drug Administration (FDA) pregnancy risk category C (Appendix I) (36). Although nitroprusside has been used during pregnancy, it should be considered a treatment of last resort (37).

Clinical Presentation

ACUTE OVERDOSAGE

Nitrates can cause dizziness, syncope, giddiness, hypotension, cerebral ischemia, headache, reflex tachycardia, increased intraocular pressure, confusion, headache, nausea, vomiting, methemoglobinemia, hemolysis, seizures, myocardial ischemia, coma, cardiovascular collapse, and asphyxia and can be fatal in overdose. Patients with underlying cardiovascular medical conditions may be at greater risk (38).

Too rapid administration of *nitroprusside* may result in profound hypotension. Prolonged administration has resulted in cyanide toxicity (Chapter 185) (39,40). Resistance and tachyphylaxis have been reported (41). Methemoglobinemia is uncommon at typical therapeutic doses (24).

ADVERSE EVENTS

Confusion between a tube of *nitroglycerin ointment*, 2%, and a look-alike tube of lanolin skin lubricant made by the same manufacturer resulted in episodes of flushing, headache, presyncope, and hypotension (42). Another patient placed a nitroglycerin patch over a superficial laceration and developed headaches, dizziness, and weakness (43). A transient methylene-blue responsive methemoglobinemia may occur in infants younger than 3 months of age, who then develop cyanosis, diarrhea, and metabolic acidosis (44). *Intravenous nitroglycerin* has an ethanol component to the formulation that may increase serum uric acid and lead to gouty flares in predisposed patients (45).

Disposable *ammonium nitrate* cold packs are widely used in emergency departments instead of ice bags (Table 3) (4). Chronic ingestion of 6 to 12 g/day may cause gastritis, acidosis, isosmotic diuresis, and nitrite toxicity manifested by hemoglobinemia or vasodilation. Five patients tore open the cold packs and ingested from 6 to 234 g of ammonium nitrate in a single dose. None developed severe toxicity, although three had symptoms of gastritis, three had slight methemoglobinemia, and two had mild hypotension. A decrease in anion gap was observed in one asymptomatic patient who ingested a commercial ice pack mixture containing ammonium nitrate. The decreased anion gap was due to an increase in CO_2. The instrument (Ektachem, Kodak) that measured the total CO_2 used a method that cross-reacts positively with nitrate (46). Cross-reactivity also occurs with the Ektachrom 700 instrument (47).

Lacrimation and pulmonary irritation are observed after exposure to *peroxyacetyl nitrate*. Hypersensitivity reactions may occur with nitrates.

Chronic effects include an association with the development of cancer-causing nitrosamines (48) and a higher incidence of childhood diabetes with higher nitrate levels in drinking water (49). An increased incidence of stomach cancer was reported in workers with an occupational exposure to *nitrate fertilizer* (50).

Occupational exposure to nitrates may result in withdrawal symptoms during periods away from work, including the development of angina and myocardial infarction (51).

Thiocyanate, generated by the metabolism of nitroprusside, is potentially toxic, producing tinnitus, miosis, and hyperreflexia at serum levels of 1 mmol/L (60 mg/L) and potentially life-threatening with levels of 3.3 mmol/L (200 mg/L) (6,13). Thiocyanate also inhibits the iodide-concentrating capacity of the thyroid gland, resulting in reversible hypothyroidism.

Ammonium nitrate is an oxidizer, irritating to the eyes, nose, throat, and mucous membranes, that may cause severe burns and death. It may also be systemically absorbed through the skin (52).

DRUG INTERACTIONS

Severe hypotension has been reported when sildenafil is combined with organic nitrates. Sildenafil inhibits phosphodiesterase type 5, resulting in increased intracellular cGMP. Concomitant use is considered contraindicated (53).

TABLE 3. Contents of common ammonium nitrate cold packs

Brand name	Manufacturer	Ammonium nitrate (g)			Other
		Small size	Medium size	Large size	
American Instant Cold Pack	American Hospital Supply Co.	127	—	234	Binasol, water
Disposable Instant Cold Pack	Cramer	—	—	210	Water (plastic cover)
Reditemp-C Cold Pack	Wyeth Company	127	—	234	Water, modified starch
Zee Instant Ice Pack	Zee Medical Company	86	—	200	Water
Kwick Kold Instant Ice Pack	American Pharmaceuticals	57	113	218	Water
Instant Cold Pack	Jack Frost Company	50	150	—	Water

Adapted from Challone KR, McCarron MM. *J Emerg Med* 1988;6:289–293.

NITRITES

Nitrites are divided into organic and inorganic forms and may further be classified regarding volatility. They have occupational and pharmaceutical uses and are also drugs of abuse. Nitrites are used therapeutically for their vasodilation activity and also as an antidote for cyanide toxicity. In evaluating a possible nitrite or nitrate toxicity, because of the possibility of glucose 6 phosphate dehydrogenase (G6PD) deficiency or familial methemoglobin reductase deficiency, history is crucial and may include a past episode in the same patient or in a family member, drug exposure, source of drinking water, use of home remedies, diarrhea, pica, specific foods, and occupations or hobbies of child/parents.

Included in the class are the organic nitrites: amyl nitrite, butyl nitrite, tert-butyl nitrite, ethyl nitrite, and isobutyl nitrite; cyclohexyl nitrite; and the inorganic nitrites: barium nitrite, potassium nitrite, sodium nitrite, and silver nitrite. Amyl, butyl, and cyclohexyl nitrites are alkyl nitrites, which are esters of nitrous acid (54). Amyl nitrite is a rapidly acting vasodilator that was once widely used for the relief of angina pectoris and is part of the antidotal treatment of cyanide toxicity. It may also be used to prevent erections postoperatively (55) and to promote uterine relaxation in difficult deliveries (56).

Butyl nitrite and isobutyl nitrite preparations are found in room deodorizers and liquid scents. These agents are not considered drugs by the FDA and, thus, are available without a prescription. Volatile nitrites are also drugs of abuse [called *poppers* as well as a variety of other slang and trade names (Table 4)] for their effects as enhancers of sexual pleasure and the belief that they expand creativity (57,58). Acute toxicity is a result of excessive vasodilation and hypotension, and the development of methemoglobinemia. The treatment of hypotension is by fluid expansion and pressors as needed. The treatment of methemoglobinemia is by methylene blue.

Toxic Dose

The *therapeutic dose* of *amyl nitrite* is inhalation of 1 perle (0.3 ml) of amyl nitrite crushed and inhaled for one to six breaths, which reportedly produces 3% to 5% methemoglobinemia. It may be repeated in 3 to 5 minutes (24). The shelf-life of amyl nitrite is 1 year. The therapeutic dose of *sodium nitrite,* 3% (as an antidote for cyanide toxicity), is 10 ml (300 mg) intravenously over 4 minutes. This produces 20% methemoglobinemia in adults. The initial pediatric dose is 0.33 ml/kg of the 3% solution at 2.5 ml/minute, up to a maximum of 10 ml. The shelf-life of sodium nitrite is 5 years.

TABLE 4. Slang and trade names of commonly abused volatile nitrites

Bang	Natural Brutes[b]
Bolt	Odor of Man[b]
Bullet	Oz
Climax	Poppers[a]
Discoroma	Quick Silver
Flash (street name)	Ram[a]
Hardware	Rush
HiBall	Satan's Secret
Jungle Juice[a]	Snappers (street name)
Lightning Bolt[b]	Sweat
Locker Room	Thrust (slang)
Mama Poppers	

[a]Sarvesvaran ER, Fysh R, Bowen DAL. Amyl nitrite related deaths. *Med Sci Law* 1992;32:267–269.
[b]Schwartz RH. When to suspect inhalant abuse. *Patient Care* 1989;23:39–64.
From Nitrates. Greenwood Village, CO: POISINDEX, 2003.

The minimal toxic dose of nitrites varies among individuals. The acceptable daily intake of nitrites in individuals older than 6 months of age is 0.4 mg/kg (59). Cyanosis appears at methemoglobin levels of 15%. Symptoms usually do not appear until the level reaches 20% to 40% (60). Methemoglobin levels above 70% are likely to be fatal. Infants younger than 6 months of age are more susceptible to the effects of nitrites because of decreased levels of methemoglobin reductase and oxidation potential of fetal hemoglobin (8).

An ingestion of 700 mg of sodium nitrite in contaminated drinking water produced a methemoglobin level of 49%, with cyanosis and sinus tachycardia (61). A fatality occurred (methemoglobin level of 38%) after ingestion of an unknown amount of amyl nitrate (62). A fatality occurred after the ingestion of 9.5 ml of butyl nitrite (63). Ingestion of less than 15 ml of isobutyl nitrite was fatal in a 15-month-old child (64) and in two young adults (64,65).

Toxicokinetics and Toxicodynamics

Aliphatic nitrites are volatile liquids and rapidly absorbed from the lungs. Amyl nitrite is rapidly absorbed (approximately 30 seconds), with a duration of action of 5 minutes. Approximately 60% of the nitrite ion of *sodium nitrite* is metabolized, with ammonia as a primary metabolite (66). Approximately 40% is excreted unchanged in the urine (66,67). *Butyl nitrite* is hydrolyzed to the nitrite ion and its corresponding alcohol, with a half-life of 2 to 3 seconds. Elimination is by first order kinetics (54).

Pathophysiology

In general, absorption is rapid via parenteral or inhalation routes and slower by ingestion or dermal absorption. Inhalation or ingestion of a therapeutic dose produces systemic vasodilation. Systolic blood pressure decreases by 40 mm Hg and diastolic by 20 mm Hg, although cerebral (68) and myocardial (69) blood flow is increased. Because of the reduction of afterload, the workload of the heart is also decreased (69,70). When amyl nitrite is inhaled just before orgasm, the experience is reported to be perceived as more intense and prolonged (70).

Nitrites induce methemoglobinemia by oxidation of the iron molecules in hemoglobin (conversion from Fe^{2+} to Fe^{3+}). Cyanosis appears at methemoglobin levels of 15%, but symptoms usually do not appear until the level reaches 30% to 40%. The lethal methemoglobin level is 70%. The metabolism of nitroprusside may result in cyanide toxicity.

The rate at which methemoglobin develops is dependent on the route of exposure and whether conversion from a nitrate to nitrite form is required. Exposure by the inhalation route produces methemoglobin more rapidly than those that must be absorbed across the skin or from the intestine (71). Drugs that must be converted to nitrite by metabolic processes may exhibit a significant delay in toxicity.

Nitric oxide is formed endogenously in humans from L-arginine and has been found in macrophages, endothelial cells (endothelium-derived relaxing factors), and the central nervous system. Vasodilating organic nitrates are reduced to organic nitrite, which is then converted to nitric oxide. Nitric oxide is then converted to an *S*-nitrosothiol derivative by the addition of a sulfhydryl group. This activates guanylcyclase, thereby producing cGMP, the mediator for relaxation of vascular smooth muscle.

Hypotension, low systemic vascular resistance, and a reduced sensitivity to vasoconstrictors may follow (26–28). Tolerance to the effects of inhaled nitrites is reported. Workers in a munitions plant had fewer nitrite-induced headaches with increased exposure and a recurrence when returning to work after an absence (29).

Depletion of sulfhydryl group donors is possibly one mechanism for tolerance to the organic nitrates in patients with angina pectoris. Such tolerance may be reversed by sulfhydryl group donors such as *N*-acetylcysteine (30). Such tolerance reversal has not, however, been demonstrated in healthy patients after use of glyceryl trinitrate skin patches with concurrent administration of *N*-acetyl-L-cysteine (31). Nitroglycerin, a vasodilator, is known to decompose to nitric oxide in biologic systems (26). There is no evidence at present that nitrogen dioxide is endogenously formed from nitric oxide.

The protective effect of dietary vitamin E and selenium may be their ability to reduce the production of the highly reactive peroxynitrite (72).

Pregnancy and Lactation

Amyl nitrite is FDA pregnancy risk category C (Appendix I) (36). Sodium nitrite is FDA pregnancy risk category C (36). Sodium nitrite crosses the placenta and can induce methemoglobinemia in the fetus (73).

Clinical Presentation

Nitrites can cause dizziness, syncope, giddiness, hypotension, cerebral ischemia, headache, reflex tachycardia, increased intraocular pressure, confusion, headache, nausea, vomiting, methemoglobinemia, hemolysis, seizures, myocardial ischemia, coma, cardiovascular collapse, and asphyxia and can be fatal in overdose. Patients with underlying cardiovascular medical conditions may be at greater risk (38). Fatalities have also been reported with sodium nitrite, both as accidental poisoning (74) and as a complication of the treatment of presumed cyanide toxicity (75,76).

Patients with underlying cardiovascular or cerebrovascular disease are at greater risk of adverse effects. Preexisting hypovolemia or concurrent ethanol ingestion also potentiates hypotensive effects. Sodium nitrite may exacerbate the hypotension of cyanide toxicity (11).

Methemoglobinemia may be caused by nitrates or nitrites (13) among other causes (Table 2) (3). A methemoglobinemia level up to 68% has been reported in occupational exposures to methyl nitrite (77).

Hemolytic anemia may also occur acutely after nitrite exposure. A 60-year-old human immunodeficiency virus–positive man who used amyl nitrite recreationally in large doses several times a day for weeks presented with a hemoglobin of 8.9 g/dl and evidence of acute hemolysis (78). Hemolytic anemia with Heinz bodies has been demonstrated in patients after abuse of amyl and butyl nitrites over prolonged periods of time (13).

Somatic symptoms in healthy volunteers who inhaled amyl nitrite included palpitations, dizziness, headache, and difficulty breathing, compared with controls (68). Transient flushing of the skin occurs secondary to vasodilation (70). Cyclohexyl nitrite use is associated with anemia and leukopenia in mice (79). The vapors of amyl and isobutyl nitrite may be irritating and cause lacrimation and a stinging sensation of the eyes (80,81). Splash contact is also irritating and may cause corneal damage. *Sodium nitrite* appears to have carcinogenic potential in animal studies (82,83).

The formation of carcinogenic *N*-nitroso compounds by the use of the nitrosation agents *amyl and butyl nitrite* may play a role in Kaposi's sarcoma development. Inhalation exposure to the nitrites produces a nonspecific cytotoxicity, depleting many cells of the immune system. Inhalation of the nitrites also impairs a variety of humoral and cell-mediated immune mechanisms. In addition, inhalant-increased macrophage production of cytokine tumor necrosis factor-α can directly stimulate human immunodeficiency virus replication and the growth of Kaposi's sarcoma cells (84).

Drug Interactions

Severe hypotension has been reported when sildenafil is combined with organic nitrates. Although it is not known whether a similar reaction occurs with nitrites, it is possible that combined use would produce increased cGMP levels, and concomitant use is considered contraindicated (53).

DIAGNOSTIC TESTS FOR NITRATES AND NITRITES

Plasma concentrations of nitrites or nitrates are not clinically useful. In nitrite/nitrate poisoning, rapid tests may confirm the diagnosis. These include the diphenylamine blue test (DTA test), the sulfanilic acid–1 naphthylamine test (SA-INA test), and the "cooking test." (The cooking test consists of a clotted blood sample placed in a boiling water bath. After cooking and cooling, a blood sample containing nitrite is salmon pink; a normal blood sample is chocolate brown.) Commercial urine reagent strips (used for detection of urinary tract infections due to nitrite-producing bacteria) may be more rapid and more sensitive (85). An intense pink color develops in the presence of nitrites.

Standard laboratory tests in symptomatic patients should include a complete blood cell count, an arterial blood gas, and a quantitative methemoglobin. A 12-lead electrocardiogram with continuous monitoring should be performed in patients with a significant degree of methemoglobinemia or underlying disease. Pulse oximetry is usually inaccurate in the presence of methemoglobin.

Other tests that may be considered include a G6PD screen, quantitative hemoglobin electrophoresis in citrate agar and cellulose acetate, quantitative G6PD if deficient, stool culture, toxicology screen, and quantitation of suspect drugs. After an ingestion of isosorbide-5-mononitrate (1.6 g), plasma levels were 2993 ng/ml (at 4 hours) and 3140 ng/ml (at 6 hours) (12). After methylene blue treatment of methemoglobinemia, repeat methemoglobin levels should be obtained 1 to 2 hours after therapy. The complete blood cell count and reticulocyte counts should also be followed posttreatment for evidence of hemolysis.

Ammonium nitrate may produce a falsely decreased anion gap because of a potential cross-reactivity and incorrect measurement of total CO_2 by the Ektachem (46) and Ektachrom 700 (47) instruments. Ingestion of potassium nitrate may result in hyperkalemia, falsely elevated CO_2 levels, and a negative anion gap (47).

When using *nitroprusside* for prolonged periods, monitoring of blood thiocyanate is appropriate. Thiocyanate concentrations greater than 5 to 10 mg/dl are associated with toxicity (86). Blood cyanide levels above 0.015 mg/dl are associated with toxicity, but tissue cyanide levels are not well correlated (87). The development of an anion gap metabolic acidosis or elevated serum lactate may indicate cyanide toxicity but is not always present (88), especially in the first hour after endogenous cyanide detoxification systems are exhausted (6). Patients on long-term therapy should also have baseline and periodic thyroid function tests.

Information of the assessment of methemoglobinemia is provided in Chapter 21. In asymptomatic patients, a quantitative methemoglobin may be obtained on venous blood. Because the degree of blood oxygenation does not affect the amount of methemoglobin production, arterial and venous methemoglobin levels are equal. With clinically significant methemoglobinemia, a "chocolate brown" color of the blood is seen, and the gross impression of the patient is that of cyanosis. Blood should be analyzed rapidly, as endogenous methemoglobin reductase decreases the amount of methemoglobin over time.

The total CO_2 may be falsely elevated when measured by the Ektachem (46) and Ektachrom 700 (47) instruments. Ingestion of potassium nitrate may result in hyperkalemia, falsely elevated CO_2 levels, and a negative anion gap (47).

TREATMENT

Suspect methemoglobinemia in cyanotic patients who do not improve with adequate oxygenation and ventilation.

Decontamination

External decontamination is crucial in dermal exposures. The exposed area should be washed with soap and water. Ipecac-induced emesis is contraindicated because of the risk of seizures and rapid loss of consciousness and protective airway reflexes. Inhalant agents (amyl nitrite, butyl nitrite, or isobutyl nitrite) that are ingested are rapidly absorbed, and the usefulness of activated charcoal diminishes rapidly.

Most nitrates/nitrites bind to activated charcoal, and they should be administered in significant ingestions, presenting within 1 to 2 hours (1 g/kg without cathartic). Inhalant agents that are ingested are absorbed rapidly, and the usefulness of activated charcoal may decrease rapidly.

Elimination Enhancement

Hemodialysis may be of value in enhancing the removal of long-acting nitrates (89). Hemodialysis, forced diuresis, and hemoperfusion are not effective for pure methemoglobinemia. Clearance of isosorbide mononitrite was increased by hemodialysis in a study of ten patients, with a maximum plasma concentration reduced by 20%, the area under the curve decreased by 30%, and a half-life shortened by 21% (89).

Exchange transfusion or the transfusion of packed red blood cells should be considered for methylene blue failures or for patients with known G6PD or nicotinamide adenine dinucleotide phosphate methemoglobin reductase deficiencies. Large blood volumes may be required in adults, limiting its application.

Antidotes

Intravenous methylene blue (tetramethylthionine chloride) is the antidote of choice for serious methemoglobinemia, as described in Chapter 63. The indication for methylene blue is symptomatic patients with a methemoglobin level greater than 30% or with a level below 30% in the presence of anemia, pulmonary disease, or processes that reduce coronary or cerebral perfusion. Cyanosis alone is not an indication for treatment without symptomatic evidence of hypoxia.

Increased nutritional intake of vitamin E and selenium appears to be associated with decreased nitrite and nitrate toxicity (72).

Supportive Care

In symptomatic patients, 100% oxygen and assisted ventilation should be supplied as required. Seizures are treated by the administration of oxygen and benzodiazepines, followed by phenobarbital and more aggressive measures if needed (Chapter 40).

Hypotension should be managed by placement in Trendelenburg position, administering intravenous isotonic fluids at 10- to 20-ml/kg bolus and as required thereafter, and pressors (dopamine, norepinephrine) as needed. The hypotensive effects induced by sodium nitrite therapy may be prevented by diluting the sodium nitrite dose in 50 to 100 ml of normal saline, beginning administration as a slow drip with frequent blood pressure and methemoglobin monitoring, and then increasing the infusion rate to the most rapid rate tolerated (90).

Hyperbaric oxygen therapy may be of some benefit by increasing dissolved oxygen in the blood and bypassing the need for functional hemoglobin (91). If used, it should be considered a temporary, adjunctive therapy before exchange transfusion or other, more definitive, management.

Gout prophylaxis should be considered for patients who are predisposed to gout and who will be receiving *intravenous nitroglycerin* (45).

The treatment of acute cyanide toxicity is addressed in Chapter 185. If cyanide toxicity is suspected, the infusion should be discontinued. Gradual reduction of the infusion rate prevents hypertensive rebound and initiation of other blood-pressure control measures. Coinfusion of sodium thiosulfate with nitroprusside results in much higher thiocyanate levels and decreased cyanide toxicity (34).

Monitoring

Patients with decreasing methemoglobin levels, stable vital signs, and no signs of secondary organ injury may be discharged after approximately 6 hours of observation.

REFERENCES

1. Benowitz NL. Nitrite and nitrate poisoning. *San Francisco Bay Area Regional Poison Cntr Newsletter* 1982;4:1–4.
2. Dalefield RR, Oehme FW. Stability of water nitrate levels during prolonged boiling. *Vet Hum Toxicol* 1997;39:313.
3. Askew GL, Finell L, Genese CA, Sorhage FE, et al. Boilerbaisser. An outbreak of methemoglobinemia in New Jersey in 1992. *Pediatrics* 1994;94:381–384.
4. Challoner KR, McCarron MM. Ammonium nitrate cold pack ingestion. *J Emerg Med* 1988;6:200–201.
5. Sorbitrate, isosorbide dinitrate. Product information. Wilmington, DE: Zeneca Pharmaceuticals, 2000.
6. *Drug facts and comparisons. Nitroprusside sodium.* St. Louis: Wolters Kluwer Co., 2003:525–527.
7. Fan AM, Willhite CC, Book SA. Evaluation of the nitrate drinking water standard with reference to infant methemoglobinemia and potential reproductive toxicity. *Regul Toxicol Pharmacol* 1987;7:135–148.
8. Dusdieker LB, Dungy CI. Nitrates and babies: a dangerous combination. *Contemp Ped* 1996;13:91–102.
9. Lu G, Yan-Sheng G. Acute nitrate poisoning. A report of 80 cases. *Am J Emerg Med* 1991;9:200–201.
10. Marshall JB, Eckland RE. Methemoglobinemia from overdose of nitroglycerin. *JAMA* 1980;244:330.
11. Gibson GR, Hunter JB, Raabe DS, et al. Methemoglobinemia produced by high dose intravenous nitroglycerin. *Ann Intern Med* 1982;96:615–616.
12. Sobrino JM, Fernandez N, Martinez A, et al. Massive ingestion of isosorbid-5-mononitrate and nitroglycerin: suicide attempt by an adolescent girl without previous heart disease. *Eur Heart J* 1992;13:145.
13. Reynolds JEF, ed. *Martindale: the extra pharmacopoeia* (electronic version). Englewood, CO: Micromedex Inc., 1998.
14. Straehl P, Galeazzi RL. Isosorbide dinitrate bioavailability, kinetics, and metabolism. *Clin Pharmacol Ther* 1985;38:140–149.
15. Morrison RA, Wiegand UW, Jahnchen E, et al. Isosorbide dinitrate kinetics and dynamics after intravenous, sublingual and percutaneous dosing in angina. *Clin Pharmacol Ther* 1983;33:747–756.
16. Cortas NK, Wakid NW. Pharmacokinetic aspects of inorganic nitrate ingestion in man. *Pharmacol Toxicol* 1991;68:192–195.
17. Willis WH, Russell RO Jr, Mantle JA, et al. Hemodynamic effects of isosorbide binitrate versus nitroglycerin in patients with unstable angina. *Chest* 1976;69:15.

18. Mozingo DW, Smith AA, McManus WF, et al. Chemical burns. *J Trauma* 1988;28:642–647.
19. Hutt V, Bonn R, Fritschi E, et al. Evaluation of the pharmacokinetics and absolute bioavailability of three isosorbide-5-mononitrate preparations in healthy volunteers. *Arzneimittelforschung* 1995;45:142–145.
20. Straehl P, Galeazzi RL, Soliva M. Isosorbide 5-mononitrate and isosorbide 2-mononitrate kinetics after intravenous and oral dosing. *Clin Pharmacol Ther* 1984;36(4):485–492.
21. Chasseaud LF. Isosorbide 5-mononitrate pharmacokinetics. *Cardiology* 1987;74[Suppl 1]:6–11.
22. Rabinowitz B, Hod H, Chouraqui P, et al. Hemodynamic effects of oral isosorbide-5-mononitrate and dinitrate in ischemic heart failure. *Clin Cardiol* 1987;10:603–608.
23. Product information. Nitrostat. Morris Plains, NJ: Parke-Davis, Division of Warner-Lambert Co. 07950 USA, 2000.
24. *Drug facts and comparisons. Nitroglycerin.* St. Louis: Wolters Kluwer Co., 2003:457.
25. Product information. Nitrol Ointment, nitroglycerin. Melville, NY: Savage Laboratories, 2000.
26. Marletta MA. Nitric oxide, nitrovasodilators, and L-arginine—an unusual relationship. *West J Med* 1991;154:107–109.
27. Vallance P, Moncada S. Hypodynamic circulation in cirrhosis: a role for nitric oxide? *Lancet* 1991;337:776–778.
28. Griffith T, Randall M. Nitric oxide comes of age. *Lancet* 1989; 2:875–876.
29. Cohen S. The volatile nitrites. *JAMA* 1979;241:2077–2078.
30. Svendsen JH, Klarlund K, Aldershrile J, et al. *N*-acetylcysteine modifies the acute effects of isosorbid-5-mononitrate in angina pectoris patients evaluated by exercise testing. *J Cardiovasc Pharmacol* 1989;13:320–323.
31. Hogan JC, Lewis MJ, Henderson AH. N-acetylcysteine fails to attenuate haemodynamic tolerance to glyceryl trinitrate in healthy volunteers. *Br J Clin Pharmacol* 1989;28:421–426.
32. Burrows GE. Nitrate intoxication. *J Am Vet Med Assoc* 1990;177:82–83.
33. NFPA. *Fire protection guide to hazardous materials*, 10th ed. Quincy, MA: National Fire Protection Association, 1991.
34. Curry SC, Arnold-Capell P. Toxic effects of drugs used in the ICU. Nitroprusside, nitroglycerin, and angiotensin-converting enzyme inhibitors. *Crit Care Clin* 1991;7(3):555–581.
35. Shah PK. Ventricular unloading in the management of heart disease: role of vasodilators (two parts). *Am Heart J* 1977;93:256, 403.
36. Briggs GG, Freeman RK, Yaffe SJ. *Drugs in pregnancy and lactation*, 4th ed. Baltimore: Williams & Wilkins, 1994.
37. Anonymous. National high blood pressure education program working group report on high blood pressure in pregnancy. *Am J Obstet Gynecol* 1990;163:1689–1712.
38. Bradberry SM, Whittington RM, Parry DA, et al. Fatal methemoglobinemia due to inhalation of isobutyl nitrite. *J Toxicol Clin Toxicol* 1994;32:179–184.
39. Humphrey SHN, Nash DA. Lactic acidosis complicating sodium nitroprusside therapy. *Ann Intern Med* 1978;88:58.
40. MacRae WR, Owen M. Severe metabolic acidosis following hypotension induced with sodium nitroprusside. *Br J Anesth* 1974;46:795.
41. Davies DW, Greiss L, Kadar D, et al. Sodium nitroprusside in children: observations on metabolism during normal and abnormal responses. *Can Anesth Soc J* 1975;22:553–560.
42. Ehrenpreis ED, Young MA, Leikin JB. Symptomatic nitroglycerin toxicity from erroneous use of topical nitroglycerine. *Vet Hum Toxicol* 1990;32:138–139.
43. Abrams J. Pharmacology of nitroglycerin and long-acting nitrates. *Am J Cardiol* 1985;56:12A–18A.
44. Yano SS, Danish EH, Hsia YE. Transient methemoglobinemia with acidosis in infants. *J Pediatr* 1982;100:415.
45. Shergy WJ, Gilkeson GS, German DC. Acute gouty arthritis and intravenous nitroglycerin. *Arch Intern Med* 1988;148:2505–2506.
46. Daoud EW, McClellan AC, Scott MG. Positive interferences with the Ektachem total CO_2 assay from therapy with topical cerous nitrate. *Clin Chem* 1990;36:1521–1522.
47. Sporer KA, Mayer AP. Salt pepper ingestion. *Am J Emerg Med* 1991;9:164–165.
48. Carmella SG, Borukhova A, Desai D, Hecht SS. Evidence for endogenous formation of tobacco-specific nitrosamines in rats treated with tobacco alkaloids and sodium nitrite. *Carcinogenesis* 1997;18:587–592.
49. Parslow RC, McKinney PA, Law GR, et al. Incidence of childhood diabetes mellitus in Yorkshire, northern England, is associated with nitrate in drinking water: an ecological analysis. *Diabetologia* 1997;40:550–556.
50. Zandjani F, Hogsaet B, Andersen A, et al. Incidence of cancer among nitrate fertilizer workers. *Int Arch Occup Environ Health* 1994;66:189–193.
51. Ben-David A. Cardiac arrest in an explosives factory worker due to withdrawal from nitroglycerin exposure. *Am J Ind Med* 1989;15(6):719–722.
52. Hall AH, Rumack BH. Methemoglobinemia inducers. MEDITEXT Management. In: TOMES PLUS Information System. Englewood, CO: Micromedex Inc., 1990.
53. Viagra, sildenafil citrate. Product information. New York: Pfizer Inc., 2000.
54. Haverkos HW, Dougherty J. Health hazards of nitrite inhalants. *Am J Med* 1988;84:479–482.
55. Burnakis TG. Amyl nitrite for the treatment of penile tumescence. *Hosp Pharm* 1991;26:343.
56. Hendricks SK, Ross B, Colvard MA, et al. Amyl nitrite: use as a smooth muscle relaxant in difficult preterm cesarean section. *Am J Perinatol* 1992;9:289–292.
57. Sigell LT, Kapp FT, Fusaro GA, et al. Popping and snorting volatile nitrites: a current fad for getting high. *Am J Psychiatry* 1978;135:1216–1218.
58. Lockwood B. Poppers: volatile nitrite inhalants. *Pharm J* 1996;257:154–155.
59. WHO. Technical Report No. 309. World Health Organization, 1965: 25.
60. Shih RD, Marcus SM, Genese CA, et al. The boiler room blues: two separate epidemics of methemoglobinemia due to contamination of potable water from boiler additives. *J Toxicol Clin Toxicol* 1995;33:507–508(abst).
61. Bradberry SM, Gazzard B, Vale JA. Methemoglobinemia caused by the accidental contamination of drinking water with sodium nitrite. *J Toxicol Clin Toxicol* 1994;32:173–178.
62. Sarvesvaran ER, Fysh R, Bowen DAL. Amyl nitrite related deaths. *Med Sci Law* 1992;32:267–269.
63. Wood RW, Cox C. Acute oral toxicity of butyl nitrite. *J Appl Toxicol* 1981;1:30–31.
64. Dixon DS, Reisch RF, Santinga PH. Fatal methemoglobinemia resulting from ingestion of isobutyl nitrite, a "room odorizer" widely used for recreational purposes. *J Forensic Sci* 1981;26:587–593.
65. O'Toole JB, Robbins GB, Dixon DS. Ingestion of isobutyl nitrite, a recreational chemical of abuse, causing fatal methemoglobinemia. *J Forensic Sci* 1987;32:1811–1812.
66. Sweetman S, ed. *Martindale. The complete drug reference.* London: Pharmaceutical Press. Internet version, Englewood, CO: Micromedex, Inc., 2003.
67. Baselt RC. *Disposition of toxic drugs and chemicals in man*, 5th ed. Foster City, CA: Chemical Toxicology Institute, 2000.
68. Mathew RJ, Wilson WH, Tant SR. Regional cerebral blood flow changes associated with amyl nitrite inhalation. *Br J Addict* 1989;84:293–299.
69. Murad F. Drugs used for the treatment of angina: organic nitrates, calcium channel blockers, and beta-adrenergic antagonists. In: Gilman AG, Rall TW, Nies AS, et al., eds. *Goodman and Gilman's the pharmacological basis of therapeutics*, 8th ed. New York: Pergamon Press, 1990.
70. Lowry TP. Neurophysiological aspects of amyl nitrite. *J Psychodelic Drugs* 1980;12:73–74.
71. Wax PM, Hoffman RS. Methemoglobinemia: an occupational hazard of phenylpropanolamine production. *J Toxicol Clin Toxicol* 1994;32:299–303.
72. Chow DK, Hong CB. Dietary vitamin E and selenium and toxicity of nitrite and nitrate. *Toxicology* 2002;180:195–207.
73. Gruener N, Shuval HI, Behroozi K, et al. Methemoglobinemia induced by transplacental passage of nitrites in rats. *Bull Environ Contam Toxicol* 1973;9:44–48.
74. Kaplan A, Smith C, Promnitz DA, et al. Methaemoglobinaemia due to accidental sodium nitrite poisoning. Report of 10 cases. *S Afr Med J* 1990;77:300–301.
75. Hall AH, Kulig KW, Rumack BH. Suspected cyanide poisoning in smoke inhalation: complications of sodium nitrite therapy. *J Toxicol Clin Exp* 1989;9:3–9.
76. Berlin CM. The treatment of cyanide poisoning in children. *Pediatrics* 1970;46:793–796.
77. Ger J, Kao H, Shih TS, et al. Fatal toxic methemoglobinemia due to occupational exposure to methyl nitrite. *Chin Med J (Taipei)* 1996;57:S78(abst).
78. Costello C, Pourgourides E, Youle M. Amyl nitrite induced acute haemolytic anaemia in HIV-antibody positive man. *Int J STD AIDS* 2000;11:334–335.
79. Soderberg LSF, Flick JT. Acute blood toxicity of the abused inhalant, cyclohexyl nitrite. *Int J Immunopharmacol* 1997;19:305–310.
80. Grant WM. *Toxicology of the eye*, 4th ed. Springfield, IL: Charles C Thomas, 1993.
81. Covalla JR, Strimlan CV, Lech JG. Severe tracheobronchitis from inhalation of an isobutyl nitrite preparation. *Drug Intell Clin Pharm* 1981;15:51–52.
82. Yamamoto K, Nakajima A, Eimoto H, et al. Carcinogenic activity of endogenously synthesized N-nitrosobis(2-hydroxypropyl)amine in rats administered bis(2-hydroxy-propyl)amine and sodium nitrite. *Carcinogenesis* 1989;10:1607–1611.
83. Robbiano L, Carlo P, Finollo R, et al. DNA damage induced in rats by oral administration of chlordiazepoxide plus sodium nitrite or of N-nitrosochlordiazepoxide. *Toxicol Appl Pharmacol* 1990;102:186–190.
84. Soderberg LS. Immunomodulation by nitrite inhalants may predispose abusers to AIDS and Kaposi's sarcoma. *J Neuroimmunol* 1998;83:157–161.
85. Rodriguez FS, Santiyan MPM, Zamorano JDP. Evaluation of reagent strips for the rapid diagnosis of nitrite poisoning. *J Anal Toxicol* 1992;16:63–64.
86. Ahearn DJ, Grim CE. Treatment of malignant hypertension with sodium nitroprusside. *Arch Intern Med* 1974;133:187.
87. Winek CL. Tabulation of therapeutic, toxic, and lethal concentrations of drugs and chemicals in blood. *Clin Chem* 1976;22:832–836.
88. Patel CB, Laboy V, Venus B, et al. Use of sodium nitroprusside in post-coronary bypass surgery: a plea for conservatism. *Chest* 1986;89:663–667.
89. Evers J, Bonn R, Boertz A, et al. Pharmacokinetics of isosorbide-5-nitrate during haemodialysis and peritoneal dialysis. *Eur J Clin Pharmacol* 1987;32:503–505.
90. Baskurt OK. Acute hematologic and hemorheologic effects of sulfur dioxide inhalation. *Arch Environ Health* 1988;43:345–348.
91. Hall AH. Systemic asphyxiants: cyanide and cyanogens hydrogen sulfide, methemoglobin inducers. In: Rippe JM, et al., eds. *Intensive care medicine*, 2nd ed. Boston: Little, Brown & Co., 1991:1248–1258.

CHAPTER 188

Miscellaneous Chemical Agents

Richard C. Dart

See Figure 1.

Compounds included:	**Asphyxiants (carbon dioxide, helium, hydrogen, methane, several others), carbon disulfide; isocyanates: Methylene diphenyl diisocyanate, toluene diisocyanate**
Molecular formula and weight:	**See Table 1.**
SI conversion:	**Not applicable**
CAS Registry No.:	**See Table 1.**
Special considerations:	**None**
Antidote:	**None**

ASPHYXIANTS

The simple asphyxiants include carbon dioxide, helium, methane, and any other gas that acts mainly by displacing oxygen from the atmosphere, thereby producing hypoxia. Carbon dioxide, helium, and methane are colorless gases that can replace oxygen in the atmosphere. Carbon dioxide is the most common cause of asphyxiant effects. As a byproduct of human respiration, it is a common cause of indoor air pollution.

Carbon dioxide has caused large-scale disasters. In 1986, Lake Nyos released a large amount of a gas thought to be carbon dioxide. The gas covered a large area and suffocated many victims (1,2).

Toxic Doses

Regulatory standards and guidelines for carbon dioxide are provided in Table 2. There are no regulatory guidelines for helium, hydrogen, or methane; however, the level of oxygen in inspired air must be maintained above 18%.

The physical effects of carbon dioxide begin to occur when it reaches a 3% concentration in the atmosphere [30,000 parts per million (ppm)]. However, its toxicity at this level depends on a reduction of oxygen: no ill effects were noted in humans at 3%, unless the concentration of inspired oxygen was decreased to 15% to 17% (3). Death has been reported at carbon dioxide air levels of 15% to 30% (4). With any agent, signs develop when the atmospheric oxygen concentration falls below 15% with unconsciousness and death at 6% to 8% (5,6).

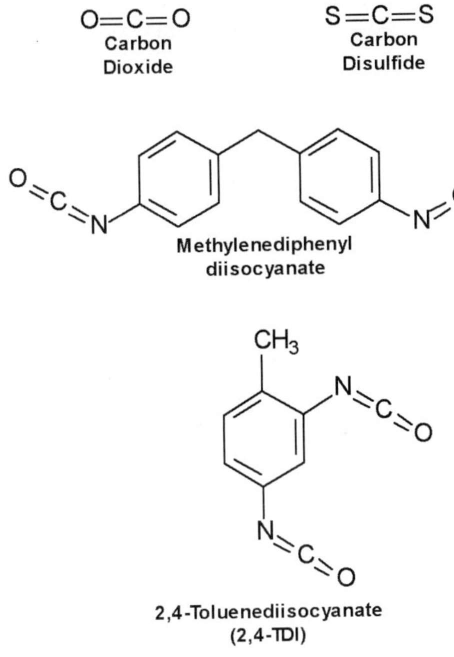

O=C=O
Carbon Dioxide

S=C=S
Carbon Disulfide

Methylenediphenyl diisocyanate

2,4-Toluenediisocyanate (2,4-TDI)

Figure 1. Chemical structure of selected chemicals.

Pathophysiology

The mechanism of toxicity is unclear. The most common hypothesis is that rising levels of the asphyxiant gas displaces oxygen and leads to hypoxic effects. Organs with high oxygen extraction, such as heart and brain, are affected first.

Vulnerable Populations

No reports specific to the simple asphyxiants have been published. In general, severe hypoxia and anoxia are associated with fetal loss rather than teratogenic effects.

The effects of increased carbon dioxide are noticed first by patients with compromised cardiopulmonary function such as congestive heart failure, chronic obstructive pulmonary disease, or decreased oxygen carrying capacity (e.g., anemia).

Clinical Presentation

ACUTE EXPOSURE

The initial effects of increased carbon dioxide concentration are compensatory: increased respiratory rate and pulse. As the carbon dioxide level persists or worsens, the patient may note shortness of breath, dizziness, fatigue, decreased visual acuity, and headache. Occasionally, the patient develops euphoria or belligerence, poor judgment, and memory loss. Notably, these effects may impair the individual's ability to escape from the toxic environment. In a severe exposure, the patient's mental status continues to deteriorate. The typical manifestations of hypoxia may occur, such as seizure, loss of consciousness, and death.

TABLE 1. Physical characteristics of selected chemicals

Compound	Molecular formula	Molecular weight (g/mol)	CAS Registry No.
Carbon dioxide	CO_2	44.01	124-38-9
Carbon disulfide	CS_2	76.14	75-15-0
Isocyanates			
Methyl isocyanate	C_2H_3NO	57.05	624-83-9
Toluene 2,4-diisocyanate	$CH_3C_6H_3(NCO)_2$	174.16	584-84-9

TABLE 2. United States regulatory guidelines and standards

Agency	Description	Concentration mg/m³ (ppm)			
		Carbon dioxide	Carbon disulfide	Methylene diphenyl diisocyanate	Toluene 1,4-diisocyanate
OSHA (air)	PEL-TWA	9000 (5000)	62 (20)	0.05 (0.02)	0.14 (0.02)
	PEL-ceiling	None	93 (30)	—	—
ACGIH (air)	TLV-TWA	9000 (5000)	(31) 10	0.05 (0.02)	0.04 (0.005)
	STEL	54,000 (30,000)	None	None	0.14 (0.02)
NIOSH (air)	REL-TWA	9000 (5000)	3 (1)	0.05 (0.02)	None
	REL-STEL	54,000 (30,000)	31 (10)	None	None
	IDLH	(72,000) 40,000	1550 (500)	7 (3)	17.8 (2.5)
		ppm × 1.8 = mg/m³	ppm × 3.1 = mg/m³	ppm × 2.33 = mg/m³	ppm × 7.1 = mg/m³

ACGIH, American Conference of Governmental Industrial Hygienists; IDLH, immediate danger to life or health; NA, not applicable; NIOSH, National Institute for Occupational Safety and Health; OSHA, U.S. Occupational Safety and Health Administration; PEL, permissible exposure limit; ppm, parts per million; REL, recommended exposure limit; STEL, short-term exposure limit; TLV, threshold limit value; TWA, time-weighted average.

Diagnostic Tests

Ambient carbon dioxide levels are easily measured. A concentration of more than 800 ppm in indoor air indicates inadequate fresh air supply (7). The American Society of Heating, Refrigeration and Air-Conditioning Engineers recommend that indoor carbon dioxide should not exceed 1000 ppm (8).

Other diagnostic tests are directed at the target organs of brain, heart, and lungs. Common tests like complete blood count, serum electrolytes, bacterial cultures, and others are needed to evaluate other potential causes of altered mental status. Serial arterial blood gases are followed to assure that hypercarbia resolves. The electrocardiogram and cardiac monitoring are used to assess cardiac injury.

A chest radiograph may be needed in some cases. In severe poisoning, computed tomography or magnetic resonance imaging of the brain may be needed to evaluate sequelae of injury.

Treatment

Treatment consists of termination of exposure and intensive cardiorespiratory care. The patient should be removed immediately from the source of exposure and ventilation provided. The asphyxiant gas is quickly excreted with increased ventilation. No other enhancement of elimination is needed.

There is no antidote for carbon dioxide toxicity. The immediate problem of carbon dioxide intoxication is easily treated by providing oxygen and increasing respiration. Hypoxic injury may have occurred in some patients. Supportive care hypoxic injury includes close monitoring and supportive care of cardiac and central nervous system injury.

CARBON DISULFIDE

Carbon disulfide (carbon bisulfide, carbon sulfide) is a colorless liquid with a foul odor unless purified. It was initially developed as a medical therapeutic agent and anesthetic. Its primary applications, however, have been as a solvent in the production of a wide variety of products, particularly *cold* vulcanization of rubber and viscose rayon. Carbon disulfide is highly soluble in organic solvents and only slightly soluble in water.

Classification and Uses

Carbon disulfide is used as a chemical intermediate for rayon, cellophane, carbon tetrachloride, xanthogenates, soil disinfectants and herbicides, carbonyl sulfide, adhesives, and other compounds (9). It is used as a solvent for phosphorus, selenium, bromine, iodine, fats, and resins and in the manufacturing of electronic tubes and optical glass. It has also been used as a fumigant, to inhibit corrosion, as a vinyl chloride polymerization inhibitor, and in a variety of activities that involve metals (cleaning, extracting, removing from waste water, regenerating metal catalysts) (9).

Toxic Doses

Regulatory standards and guidelines are provided in Table 2. The effects of carbon disulfide are dose related. Exposure to an air concentration less than 400 ppm causes few symptoms, but toxic effects increase in proportion to air concentration. An air concentration more than 4800 ppm is thought to be lethal within 30 minutes (10).

Toxicokinetics and Toxicodynamics

Carbon disulfide is well absorbed by all routes of exposure, including dermal. The proportion absorbed during inhalation decreases as the concentration of carbon disulfide increases (11). It is lipid soluble and enters essentially all tissues, especially red blood cells. Metabolism accounts for 70% to 95% of carbon disulfide elimination; the rest is excreted by the lungs primarily (11,12). The half-life in blood is less than 1 hour. Accumulation in adipose tissue with repeated or prolonged exposure is expected (13).

Pathophysiology

Two toxic mechanisms have been described (Fig. 2) (13). Carbon disulfide reacts amines and thiols (e.g., glutathione) and thereby alters their activity. This reaction also is likely to produce metabolites that further inactivate intracellular compounds, such as metalloenzymes, and react with proteins (14). In the peripheral nerve, this action could account for the *dying-back* axonopathy. The hepatotoxic effect may be caused by the formation of electrophilic species caused by the metabolism of carbon disulfide through the cytochrome P-450 system, a mechanism common to many hepatotoxins (15).

Vulnerable Populations

Carbon disulfide is associated with multiple reproductive effects. A study of synthetic fiber workers found that prolonged

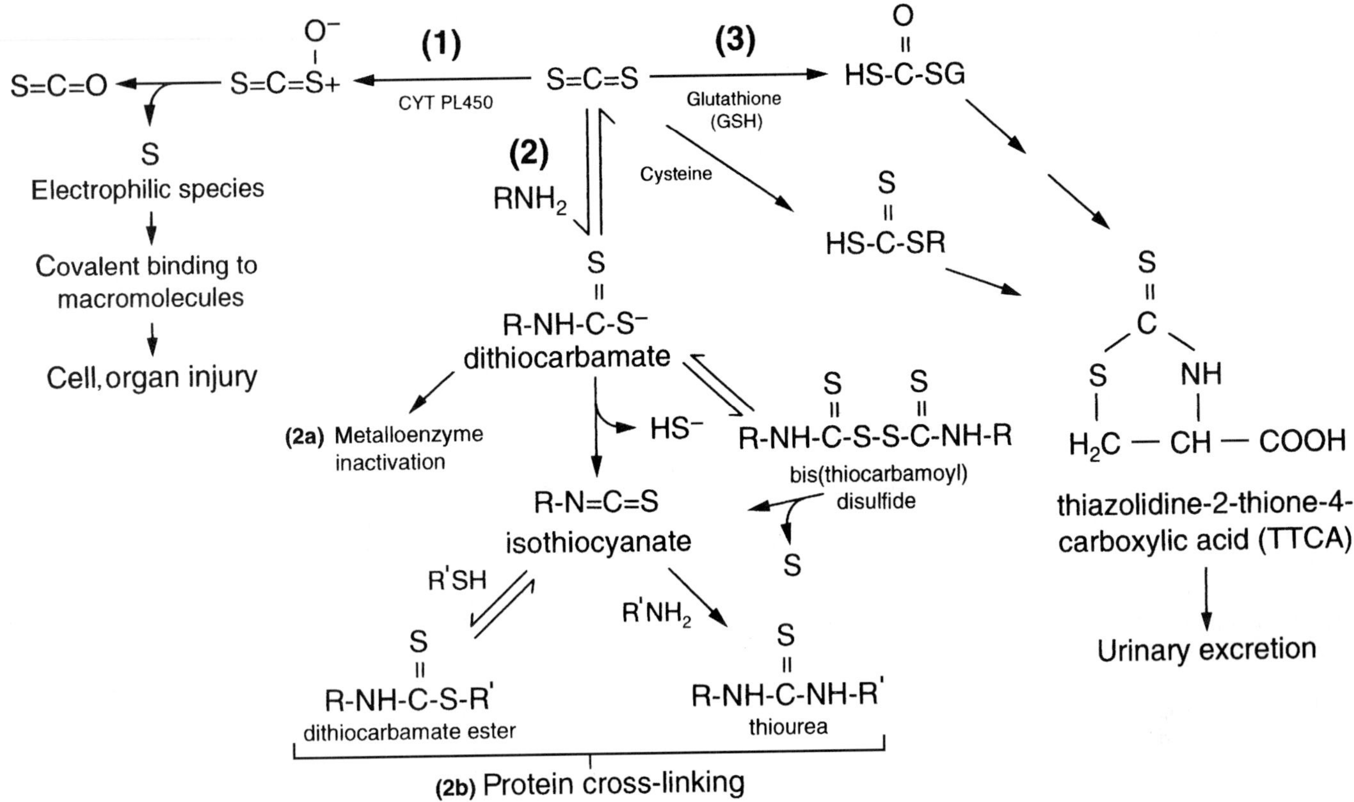

Figure 2. Major pathways of carbon disulfide metabolism: (1) oxidative metabolism by hepatic cytochrome P-450 (CYT P450), resulting in the generation of reactive species capable of causing cell and organ injury; (2) dithiocarbamate adduct formation, resulting in (a) direct effects on metalloenzyme activity and (b) protein cross-linking; (3) reductive conversion via glutathione and cysteine moieties to metabolites (e.g., thiazolidine-2-thione-4-carboxylic acid) that undergo renal elimination. (From Sullivan JB Jr, Krieger GR, eds. *Clinical environmental health and toxic exposures,* 2nd ed. Philadelphia: Lippincott Williams & Wilkins, 2001:1207, with permission.)

exposure during or before pregnancy was associated with an increased incidence of birth defects (16). Animal studies provide supportive evidence of reproductive toxicity (17). Carbon disulfide can cross the placenta and is present in the breast milk from exposed nursing mothers (18).

Clinical Presentation

Carbon disulfide toxicity can occur after inhalation, dermal contact, and ingestion.

ACUTE EXPOSURE

The acute effects of carbon disulfide involve primarily local irritation of the eyes, mucous membranes, and upper airway (19). Repeated occupational exposure to low levels can produce nausea, vomiting, headache, dizziness, irritability, confusion, disorientation, tinnitus, vertigo, insomnia, syncope, and pulmonary abnormalities (20). Hallucinations, irritability, and hand tremor that resolved when exposure was terminated have been reported (21).

The *dermal* effects of carbon disulfide include erythema and pain, which may progress to full thickness burns when high concentrations or more prolonged contact occurs. It is a known defatting agent. Dermal exposure has been followed by nausea, dizziness, cardiac dysrhythmias, and coma.

After *ingestion*, a variety of neurologic, cardiac, and pulmonary effects may develop, including tremor, convulsions, coma, dyspnea, cyanosis, respiratory failure, and cardiovascular collapse (20). *Inhalation* of high concentrations has caused delirium, hallucinations, convulsions, and coma (19).

CHRONIC EXPOSURE

Long-term exposure to carbon disulfide can cause each of the acute effects previously described. In addition, it has been associated with loss of libido, memory loss, hypertension, ischemic cardiovascular disease, as well as retinopathy and retinal nerve damage. Also striking are extreme behavioral aberrations, including extreme irritability and uncontrollable anger with mania and suicidal tendencies, marked memory loss, severe nightmares, and insomnia. A study of U.S. workers who were exposed to carbon disulfide as a grain fumigant had evidence of atypical parkinsonism, cerebellar dysfunction, and hearing loss (22).

Disulfiram-like reactions were noted in rubber workers that consumed ethanol, leading eventually to the use of disulfiram in the treatment of alcoholism (23,24).

Neurologic toxicity both centrally and peripherally has been reported. Huang et al. performed computed tomography scans in four viscose rayon workers with stroke and documented long-term exposure to carbon disulfide (25). Brain computed tomography scans showed low-density lesions in the basal ganglia in two patients, cortical atrophy in one, and was normal in one. Brain magnetic resonance image studies found multiple lesions in the corona radiata and basal ganglia in three patients and cortical atrophy. Despite moving to jobs free of carbon disulfide, two patients developed a subsequent acute episode of stroke with hemiparesis. Studies in these two patients revealed new lesions in the basal ganglia and corona radiata. Carotid Doppler scan, transcranial Doppler scan, and cerebral angiography did not show any prominent stenosis or occlusion in the major intracranial large arteries.

Carbon disulfide may also cause a peripheral neuropathy, which may be evident on physical examination or only by electrophysiologic testing (at lower exposures) (26). Huang et al. documented the natural course of the polyneuropathy in six rayon workers (27). The patients' neurologic signs persisted during the 3-year follow-up period. Nerve conduction velocity remained persistently abnormal. Biopsy from one patient, 2 years after diagnosis, showed degeneration of both axon and myelin and a predominant loss of large myelinated fibers. A remyelination process was also noted.

Cardiovascular effects include increased mortality from heart disease in carbon disulfide workers (28). The mechanism of this effect is unclear. Acceleration of typical atherosclerotic heart disease has been proposed, but others have suggested a direct cardiotoxic effect and perhaps a thrombotic effect (29,30). Reduction of workplace air levels has been associated with a reduction in mortality among workers.

Ophthalmologic effects of chronic carbon disulfide exposure include optic nerve injury. The retinal pathology is described as microvascular aneurysms and hemorrhages but has been observed only in viscose rayon workers (21,31).

Reproductive effects involve both female and male workers. Menstrual abnormalities, spontaneous abortions, and premature births have been associated with carbon disulfide exposure. Studies are mixed regarding semen quality with the most recent studies finding no effect on semen quality (32–34).

Diagnostic Tests

BIOLOGIC MONITORING AND HEALTH SURVEILLANCE

Carbon disulfide is reduced by glutathione to thiazolidine-2-thone-4-carboxylic acid, which can be monitored in the urine (35,36). A thiazolidine-2-thone-4-carboxylic acid spot urine of carbon disulfide before a shift above 0.95 mmol/mole of creatinine appears to be a reliable indicator of recent exposure at an 8-hour time-weighted average level of 10 ppm (13). Other markers are under development for long-term exposure (37).

ACUTE EXPOSURE

Diagnostic testing focuses on the acute neurologic and pulmonary effects. Typical testing in symptomatic cases includes pulse oximetry, serum electrolytes, and arterial blood cases. If neurologic effects are present, head computed tomography or magnetic resonance image may be needed to differentiate the cause.

CHRONIC EXPOSURE

The low-density lipoprotein concentration is directly related to the intensity of carbon disulfide exposure (38). Chronic exposure may also increase coagulability of the blood (39). Retired patients with high long-term carbon disulfide occupational exposure were found to have more frequent cerebral lacunae (40).

Treatment

OVERVIEW

Treatment involves removal of the patient from the source of exposure and supportive care.

DECONTAMINATION AND FIRST AID

In dermal exposure, the skin should be washed and irrigated. After ingestion, ipecac should be avoided. Gastric aspiration may be effective if performed soon after acute ingestion. Activated charcoal should be administered within 1 to 2 hours of ingestion, if possible.

ENHANCEMENT OF ELIMINATION

Extracorporeal elimination has not been studied.

ANTIDOTES

There is no antidote for carbon disulfide toxicity.

SUPPORTIVE CARE

Seizures are treated with benzodiazepines and phenobarbital, followed by more invasive measures if resistant to treatment (Chapter 40). Respiratory failure is treated in the usual manner (Chapter 28). Burns are treated as thermal burns.

ISOCYANATES

A variety of isocyanates are used in the manufacture of plastic products including urethane and polyurethane. The two compounds most commonly associated with health effects are methylene diphenyl diisocyanate and toluene diisocyanate (TDI). Since the early 1950s, manufacturers have used isocyanates primarily as starting materials in the manufacture of a variety of plastic products, including rigid and flexible polyurethane foams, urethane-based coatings (e.g., paints and electrical wire insulation), and elastomers and spandex fibers.

The main health effects of isocyanates involve the lungs, but other organ systems may be affected. Most reported toxic effects have been due to toluene diisocyanate because of its widespread use. Although slightly different in their properties, other isocyanates cause similar problems under appropriate conditions.

Classification and Uses

TDI is used in the creation of flexible foams used in the production of mattresses, cushions, automobile seats, and packaging materials. Methylene diphenyl diisocyanate is used more frequently to produce rigid foams used for insulation (i.e., refrigerators). Polyurethanes are used as electrical insulators for wiring and in various finishes and paints. The myriad other uses for isocyanates include adhesives, printing rolls, shoe soles, coated fabrics, and spandex fibers. Methyl isocyanate is used in the manufacture of carbamate pesticides and was the cause of the 1984 Bhopal, India, tragedy. An unintended release caused more than 2000 deaths.

Toxic Doses

Regulatory guidelines and standards for the isocyanates are provided in Table 2.

Toxicokinetics and Toxicodynamics

The isocyanates are reactive molecules and are thought to react with nucleophiles before being distributed throughout the body.

Pathophysiology

Although the precise mechanism of isocyanate health effects is unproven, they appear to cause immunologic effects. Isocyanates are reactive chemicals that may act as haptens and create immunogenic antigens. These allow a typical immunoglobulin E (IgE)–mediated hypersensitivity reaction such as asthma. IgE antibodies have been demonstrated in the blood of workers, although they have been found in both symptomatic and asymptomatic workers (41).

A role for cellular mechanisms has been shown through the production of a leukocyte inhibitory factor by lymphocytes from sensitized individuals (42). Eosinophils and T lymphocytes have been found in bronchoalveolar lavage and bronchial biopsies (43). Delayed reactions to TDI and airway hyperresponsiveness may be caused by airway inflammation (44).

TDI rapidly deplenishes intracellular glutathione *in vitro* in human bronchoepithelial cells at doses as low as 20 parts per billion, the current permissible exposure limit (45).

Vulnerable Populations

Teratogenesis and reproductive effects have not been reported for humans.

Clinical Presentation

ACUTE EXPOSURE

The acute effects of isocyanates are primarily direct irritants. The acute *dermal effects* include erythema and may evolve into blistering. *Respiratory effects* of TDI include cough, shortness of breath, nocturnal wheezing, and chest pain. These may worsen with continued exposure. Physical examination shows the usual effects of respiratory irritants such as wheezing. An intense exposure may result in chemical pneumonitis and pulmonary edema.

Mucous membrane irritation and skin irritation also occur. Eye, nose, and throat burning or irritation is common. Severe skin exposure may produce blisters.

CHRONIC EXPOSURE

Dermal and mucous membrane effects include primarily irritant effects such as erythema, edema, and blistering. Exposure to aerosols may cause ocular irritation, rhinitis, and sore throat.

Pulmonary effects include chemical bronchitis, or isocyanate-induced asthma, hypersensitivity pneumonitis, and chronic nonspecific airway disease (42). Changes in lung function seem to improve within 1 to 2 years in most cases, although they may persist. Chronic bronchitis also has been reported to be more frequent in workers exposed to high concentrations or exposed repeatedly to low concentrations of TDI (46).

The phenomenon of isocyanate asthma has been long recognized (47). Isocyanate asthma causes the usual signs of wheezing, cough, and shortness of breath, often at night. Isocyanate asthma tends to improve when exposure ceases (e.g., vacations). The estimated rates of isocyanate asthma have ranged from 5% to 30% of exposed workers (42) and it is the most common cause of occupational asthma (43). Isocyanate asthma often develops within the first few months of exposure. Asthma has followed low- or high-level exposures and persists for months or years (48). Sudden death has been reported in sensitized workers that become exposed to relatively low concentrations of TDI (42).

Acute nonspecific airway disease may also occur. Workers exposed to TDI may develop asymptomatic airflow obstruction during their work shift (42). Exposure to low levels of TDI has been shown to cause a dose-related acute loss of pulmonary function. At the same dose, chronic deterioration in forced expiratory volume in one second (FEV_1) has been seen.

Chronic nonspecific airway disease involves chronic persistent airflow obstruction in patients exposed to isocyanates. Wegman showed that occupational TDI exposure decreased the mean FEV_1 in workers who were exposed to 0.002 ppm for more than 2 years (49) found that exposure to low levels of isocyanates in a polyurethane manufacturing plant produced a dose-response decrease in FEV_1 when exposed for more than 2 years to 0.002 ppm of TDI. The severity of effect was directly related to the concentration and occurred at concentrations below the U.S. permissible exposure limit.

Similarly, workers in a TDI manufacturing plant were found to have frequent excursions exceeding 0.02 ppm. Workers that spent at least 15% of their time working in conditions of at least 0.005 ppm TDI showed a greater decline in FEV_1 than other subjects. Nonsmokers had an annual excess loss of 38 ml of FEV_1, equal to a total loss of 1.5 L over a 40-year working lifetime. Smoking and TDI effects on lung function were found not to be additive. Current or previous smokers experienced no effect (23).

Hypersensitivity pneumonitis or extrinsic allergic alveolitis has been associated with isocyanate exposure. Generally, symptoms of hypersensitivity pneumonitis include fever, chills, malaise, dyspnea, and a nonproductive cough.

Acute asthma has followed hypersensitivity pneumonitis. Exposure to TDI also has been reported to cause chronic restrictive pulmonary disease (50).

CARCINOGENESIS

TDI is considered an animal carcinogen by the International Agency for Research on Cancer (IARC). However, these studies were performed by gavage rather than inhalation exposure. National Institute for Occupational Safety and Health has considered TDI to be a potential occupational carcinogen (51). The mechanism of carcinogenesis in animals is unknown but is presumed to arise from a chemical adduct formed by TDI or methylene diphenyl diisocyanate (52).

Diagnostic Tests

BIOLOGIC MONITORING AND HEALTH SURVEILLANCE

Medical surveillance should be provided to all potentially exposed workers. Preplacement examinations should emphasize preexisting respiratory conditions, smoking, and should include baseline chest radiography and spirometry (53). The worker also must be judged fit to use a respirator. Annual periodic examinations consisting of interim medical and work histories, a physical examination, and spirometric assessments before and after the work shift or workweek should be performed (54). However, preplacement assessment is not able to predict which employees will develop TDI-induced lung disease. Atopy and asthma do not predispose to isocyanate asthma, and not all subjects who have a documented TDI sensitivity have increased nonspecific bronchial hyperreactivity (54). Methacholine testing is not likely to identify those who will develop TDI asthma (48).

ACUTE EXPOSURE

Tests for acute exposure are rarely needed. In patients with pulmonary symptoms, pulse oximetry, chest radiography, and pulmonary function testing should be performed and compared with baseline values. Specific IgE antibodies to monofunctional isocyanates have been reported in sensitized workers, but specific IgE antibodies to diisocyanate conjugates have not been identified (42).

CHRONIC EXPOSURE

The serial measurement of the FEV_1 is a useful means of identifying acute and long-term effects of isocyanates. The acute and chronic effects of TDI are well correlated. Thus, acute monitoring may identify individuals who are at risk of developing long-term declines in FEV_1 (42). Aging alone produces an annual FEV_1 decrement of 0.020 L in an adult nonsmoker. Work shift decrements of 0.3 L or greater and annual decrements of 5% or 0.2 L should be cause for evaluation and more frequent testing (54).

Spirometry testing may be normal or abnormal in workers with isocyanate asthma. Inhalation challenge may produce immediate, late, or dual asthmatic reactions. Challenge testing may be indicated in carefully selected cases, although some risk is involved (54). A diagnosis of isocyanate asthma usually can be made without the need to perform such a challenge. The diagnosis is made if the worker has reversible airflow obstruction associated with exposure to low levels of isocyanates.

Hypersensitivity pneumonitis is associated with chest radiographs that are normal or show diffuse patchy infiltrates or discrete nodules. Pulmonary function testing may show a restrictive pattern and impaired diffusion capacity.

Treatment

Treatment of acute or chronic effects of the isocyanates is symptomatic and supportive. Acute bronchospasm is treated in the usual manner. Chronic effects are treated by removal from exposure and medications typical for asthma. Workers who are found to be sensitized to isocyanates must be moved to jobs in which no further isocyanate exposure occurs.

DECONTAMINATION

Eye or skin exposures should be treated with immediate saline or water irrigation. The use of soap and water and then alcohol is recommended for the skin. There are no data evaluating gastric decontamination. Dilution with 4 to 8 oz of liquid is commonly recommended. Gastric aspiration of the liquid is reasonable soon after a large ingestion. Activated charcoal is also indicated.

ENHANCEMENT OF ELIMINATION

Enhanced elimination has not been studied. Because isocyanates are thought to react quickly with tissues, it is unlikely that this can be helpful.

ANTIDOTES

There is no antidote for isocyanate toxicity. Some practitioners have erroneously thought that cyanide may be involved in toxicity and therefore considered the cyanide kit an antidote. Cyanide is not part of the pathophysiology of the disease, and the induction of methemoglobinemia has no beneficial effects in isocyanate toxicity.

SUPPORTIVE CARE

Acute bronchospasm is treated in the typical manner with bronchodilators (Chapter 11). Prednisone or high-dose inhaled beclomethasone is used to prevent late asthmatic episodes and the increase in nonspecific bronchial hyperreactivity induced by TDI.

Hypersensitivity pneumonitis is treated with steroids and avoidance of continued exposure.

REFERENCES

1. Freeth S. The deadly cloud hanging over Cameroon. *New Scientist* 1992;August 15:23–27.
2. Wagner GN, Clark MA, Kownigsberg EJ, et al. Medical evaluation of the victims of the 1985 Lake Nyos disaster. *J Forensic Sci* 1988;33:899–909.
3. American Conference of Governmental Industrial Hygienists. *Documentation of the threshold limit values and biological exposure indices*, 5th ed. Cincinnati, OH: American Conference of Governmental Industrial Hygienists, Inc, 1986.
4. Brighten P. A case of industrial carbon dioxide poisoning. *Anaesthesia* 1976;31:406–409.
5. Editorial staff. Simple asphyxiants. In: Toll LL, Hurlbut KM, eds. POISINDEX system. Greenwood Village, CO: MICROMEDEX (edition expires September 2003).
6. Kizer KW. Toxic inhalations. *Emerg Med Clin North Am* 1984;2:649–666.
7. Sullivan JB, Van Ert M, Krieger GR, Brooks BO. Indoor environmental quality and health. In: *Clinical environmental health and toxic exposures*. Philadelphia: Lippincott, Williams & Wilkins, 2001:669–704.
8. Stricker S. Physiological responses to elevated carbon dioxide levels in buildings. *Indoor Built Environ* 1997;6:301–308.
9. US Department of Labor, Occupational Safety and Health Administration. Industrial exposure and control technologies for OSHA-regulated hazardous substances: carbon disulfide. Doc. no. PB89-210199. Washington: US Occupational Safety and Health Administration, 1989:366–369.
10. Bingham E, Chorssen B, Powell CH, eds. *Patty's toxicology*, 5th ed. New York: John Wiley and Sons, 2001.
11. Teisinger J, Sloucek B. Absorption and elimination of carbon disulfide in man. *J Ind Hyg* 1949;31:67.
12. Davidson M, Feinleib M. Carbon disulfide poisoning: a review. *Am Heart J* 1972;83:100–114.
13. Riihimaki V, Kivisto H, Peltonen K, et al. Assessment of exposure to carbon disulfide in viscose production workers from urinary 2-thiothiazolidine-4-carboxylic arid determinations. *Am J Ind Med* 1992;22(1):85–97.
14. Graham DG, Amarnath V, Valentine WM, et al. Pathogenetic studies of hexane and carbon disulfide neurotoxicity. *Crit Rev Toxicol* 1995;25:91–112.
15. Rojas MM, Oehme FW. A review of the acute effects of carbon disulphide on lipid liver metabolism. *Vet Hum Toxicol* 1982;24:337–342.
16. Bao YS, Cai S, Zhao SF, et al. Birth defects in the offspring of female workers occupationally exposed to carbon disulfide in China. *Teratology* 1991;43:451–452.
17. RTECS: Registry of Toxic Effects of Chemical Substances (CD-ROM version). Cincinnati, OH: National Institute for Occupational Safety and Health. Englewood, CO: Micromedex, Inc. (expires October 31, 2000).
18. HSDB. Hazardous Substances Data Bank (CD-ROM version). Bethesda, MD: National Library of Medicine. Englewood, CO: Micromedex, Inc. (expires October 31, 2000).
19. Spyker DA, Gallanosa AG, Suratt PM. Health effects of acute carbon disulfide exposure. *J Toxicol Clin Toxicol* 1982;19:87–93.
20. van Hoome M, de Douck A, de Bacquer D. Epidemiological study of eye irritation by hydrogen sulfide and/or carbon disulfide in viscose rayon workers. *Ann Occup Hyg* 1995;39:307–315.
21. Braceland F. Mental symptoms following carbon disulfide absorption and intoxication. *Ann Intern Med* 1942;16:246–261.
22. Peters HA, Levine R, Matthews CG, Chapman U. Extrapyramidal and other neurologic manifestations associated with carbon disulfide fumigant exposure. *Arch Neurol* 1988;45:537–540.
23. Williams EE. Effects of alcohol on workers with carbon disulfide. *JAMA* 1937;109:1472.
24. Martensen-Larsen O. Treatment of alcoholism with a sensitizing drug. *Lancet* 1948;2:1004.
25. Huang CC, Chu CC, Chu NS, Wu TN. Carbon disulfide vasculopathy: a small vessel disease. *Cerebrovascular Diseases* 2001;11(3):245–250.
26. Chu C, Huang C, Chen R, Shih T. Polyneuropathy induced by carbon disulphide in viscose rayon workers. *Occup Environ Med* 1995;52:404–407.
27. Huang CC, Chu CC, Wu TN, et al. Clinical course in patients with chronic carbon disulfide polyneuropathy. *Clin Neurol Neurosurg* 2002;104(2):115–120.
28. Kristensen TS. Cardiovascular diseases and the work environment. *Scand J Work Environ Health* 1989;15:245–264.
29. Kruppa K, Hietanen E, Klockars M, et al. Chemical exposures at work and cardiovascular morbidity. *Scand J Work Environ Health* 1984;10:381–388.
30. Sweetnam PM, Taylor SWC, Elwood PC. Exposure to carbon disulphide and ischaemic heart disease in a viscose rayon factory. *Br J Ind Med* 1987;44:220–227.
31. Sugimoto K, Goto S, Taniguchi H. Ocular fundus photography of workers exposed to carbon disulfide: a comparative epidemiological study between Japan and Finland. *Int Arch Occup Environ Health* 1977;39:97–101.
32. Meyer CR. Semen quality in workers exposed to carbon disulfide compared to a control group from the same plant. *J Occup Med* 1981;23:435–439.
33. Schrag SD, Dixon R. Occupational exposures associated with male reproductive dysfunction. *Am Rev Pharmacol Toxicol* 1985;25:567–592.
34. van Hoorne M, Comhaire F, de Bacquer D. Epidemiological study of the effects of carbon disulfide on male sexuality and reproduction. *Arch Environ Health* 1994;49(4):273–278.
35. Cox C, Shane S, Hee Q, Tolos W. Biological monitoring of workers exposed to carbon disulfide. *Am J Ind Med* 1998;33:48–54.
36. Ghittori B, Maestri L, Contardi I, et al. Biological monitoring of workers exposed to carbon disulfide (CS_2) in a viscose rayon fibers factory. *Am J Ind Med* 1998;33:478–484.
37. Valentine WK, Graham DC, Anthony DC. Covalent cross-linking of erythrocyte spectrin by carbon disulfide in vivo. *Toxicol Appl Pharmacol* 1992;121:71–77.
38. Harbison RM. *Hamilton and Hardy's industrial toxicology*, 5th ed. St. Louis, MO: Mosby, 1998.
39. Stanosz S, Kuligowska E, Kuligowski D. Coefficient of linear correlation between levels of fibrinogen, antithrombin III, thrombin-antithrombin complex and lipid fractions in women exposed chronically to carbon disulfide. *Med Pr* 1998;49:51–57.
40. Cho SK, Kim RH, Yim SH, et al. Long-term neuropsychological effects and MRI findings in patients with CS2 poisoning. *Acta Neurol Scand* 2002;106(5):269–275.
41. Butcher BT, O'Neil CE, Reed MA, Salvaggio JE. Radioallergosorbent testing with *p*-tolyl monoisocyanate in toluene diisocyanate workers. *Clin Allergy* 1983;13:31–34.
42. Musk AW, Peters JM, Wegman DH. Isocyanates and respiratory disease: current status. *Am J Ind Med* 1988;13:331–349.
43. Bernstein JA. Overview of diisocyanate occupational asthma. *Toxicology* 1996;111:181–189.
44. Chan-Yeung M. Occupational asthma. *Chest* 1990;98[Suppl]:148s–161s.

45. Lantz RC, Lemus R, Lange RW, et al. Rapid reduction of intracellular glutathione in human bronchial epithelial cells exposed to occupational levels of toluene diisocyanate. *Toxicol Sci* 2001;60:348–355.
46. McKerrow CB, Davies HJ, Jones AP. Symptoms and lung function following acute and chronic exposure to tolylene diisocyanate. *Proc R Soc Med* 1970;63:376–378.
47. Fuchs S, Valade P. Etude clinique et experimentale sur quelques cas d'intoxication par le desmodur T (diisocyanate de tolylene 1-24 et 1-2-6). *Arch Mal Prof* 1951;12:191–196.
48. Mapp CE, Corona PC, Fabbri L. Persistent asthma due to isocyanates. *Am Rev Respir Dis* 1988;137:1326–1329.
49. Wegman DH, Peters JM, Pagnotto L, et al. Chronic pulmonary function loss from exposure to toluene diisocyanate. *Br J Ind Med* 1977;34:196–200.
50. International Agency for Research on Cancer. Some chemicals used in plastics and elastomers. *IARC Monogr Eval Carcinog Risks Hum* 1986;39:287–323.
51. National Institute for Occupational Safety and Health. *Toluene diisocyanate (TDI) and toluenediamine (TDA): evidence of carcinogenicity*. DHHS publication no. NOSH 90-101; current intelligence bulletin no. 53. Cincinnati, OH: US Department of Health and Human Service, Centers for Disease Control, 1990.
52. Bolognesi C, Baur X, Narczynsk B, et al. Carcinogenic risk of toluene diisocyanate and 4,4′-methylenediphenyl diisocyanate: epidemiological and experimental evidence. *Crit Rev Toxicol* 2001;31:737–772.
53. US Department of Health, Education and Welfare/National Institute for Occupational Safety and Health. *Criteria for a recommended standard: occupational exposure to diisocyanates*. DHEW/NIOSH publication no. 78-21. Washington: US Government Printing Office, 1978.
54. Phillips KK, Peters JM. Isocyanates. In: Sullivan JB, Krieger GR, eds. *Clinical environmental health and toxic exposures*, 2nd ed. Philadelphia: Lippincott, Williams & Wilkins, 2001:994–998.

CHAPTER 189

Occupational Lung Disease

Scott D. Phillips and João H. Delgado

OVERVIEW

The inhalation of different materials in the workplace may lead to a variety of acute and chronic pulmonary diseases (Table 1). A given substance may be associated with several different pulmonary manifestations. Conversely, a given disease may be associated with or caused by different occupational exposures. Many factors affect the development of disease and its severity. These can be broadly divided into circumstances of exposure-related and patient-related (patient susceptibility) factors. Important exposure-related factors include concentration, duration, and route of exposure; the presence of coexposures; the type of product and its physical chemistry; the presence and adequacy of various engineering controls; respiratory protective equipment; and environmental factors (wind, humidity, structures, etc.). Patient-related susceptibility factors include genetic polymorphisms, differences in metabolism or immunologic response, predisposing medical conditions, or personal habits such as diet and smoking.

Workplace Evaluation

An occupational etiology should be considered in any working or retired person who presents with a respiratory illness of undetermined etiology. Identification of an occupational origin for such diseases is important for several reasons: Measures can be implemented to remove or ameliorate the exposure, which alone may lead to clinical improvement; identification may help prevent illness in other workers; and the illness (and resulting disabilities) may be compensable. In most cases, a thorough evaluation by the astute physician leads to the correct diagnosis and points to an etiology.

The major components of any evaluation include a detailed history, with emphasis on identification and estimation of the degree of current or past occupational and environmental exposures; a thorough physical examination; radiographic imaging; and pulmonary function testing (PFT). Additional specialized testing, such as bronchoscopy or immunologic testing, is typically done in consultation with a pulmonologist, ideally one with expertise in occupational lung diseases.

Historic features that suggest a heavier respiratory exposure include working in enclosed spaces, especially without ventilation or appropriate respiratory protection; workplaces with visible smoke, dust, vapor, or other evidence of airborne matter; and work involving grinding, blasting, spraying, friction, or heat. Historic features that imply an association between work and illness include symptom improvement on weekends or vacations and reappearance or worsening of symptoms on return to work. In addition to a thorough history, clinicians should obtain and review the Material Safety Data Sheets for all relevant products in the patient's environment and any available industrial hygiene data from the workplace, such as air sampling or wipe specimens. It is important to remember that there may be a significant delay between exposure and development of clinical effects for certain substances. A detailed avocational history should also be obtained because many hobbies can lead to exposures similar to those in the workplace. Indeed, because they are not subject to the same safety regulations and often occur in the absence of appropriate engineering controls or personal protective equipment, exposures from a patient's hobbies might actually be much higher than those that occur in the workplace.

The site visit is indispensable to the occupational health assessment process and allows the evaluator to scrutinize actual site conditions. Ideally, the site visit should be performed in conjunction with a certified industrial hygienist. The evaluators should

TABLE 1. Categories of lung disease associated with occupational exposures

Irritation (rhinitis, laryngitis, tracheitis, bronchitis, bronchiolitis)
Asthma (Chapter 11)
Obstructive disease (chronic obstructive pulmonary disease)
Interstitial lung disease
Fibrotic lung disease
Granulomatous disease
Inhalational fevers
Lung cancer

TABLE 2. Measures to reduce occupational lung exposure

Eliminating the harmful substances by substitution
Enclosing the process so that workers are not exposed
Removing the substance by exhaust ventilation
Diluting any fugitive emissions by improved general ventilation
Providing personal protection for workers by means of respirators
Changing work location or duty of a particular individual so as to reduce exposure

examine the exterior of the facility and the work area in question. It is important to make note of the current activities, industrial processes, and land use of the entire plant, as well as coworker and public accessibility to the site. It is also worthwhile to note the demographic characteristics of the community surrounding the site. If possible, the site in question should be observed for the specific industrial processes and product stream with which the worker(s) in question are involved. Heating, ventilation, and air conditioning; adjacent processes; and piping should be noted. A complete exposure assessment may require industrial hygiene sampling to document the presence and extent of exposure to specific substances. Some facilities have environmental sampling logs that may assist in this assessment process.

Management Principles

The management of occupational lung diseases is often the same as for the nonoccupational form of the disease. A primary aim is the reduction or removal of the exposure (Table 2). With the patient's permission, the employer should be contacted so that measures to reduce exposure can be performed, for the individual at hand and for other workers, and so that appropriate exposure monitoring can be instituted if necessary. In certain cases it may be appropriate for the employer, employee, or physician to contact the U.S. Occupational Safety and Health Administration (OSHA) or the National Institute of Occupational Safety and Health, particularly if a significant ongoing hazard is suspected. Physicians in many states are required to report certain occupationally acquired lung diseases to their respective state health departments.

This chapter focuses on some of the more common occupational toxicologic diseases that involve either the lungs or whereby the lungs play a major role in the pathophysiology. Substances and exposures associated with respiratory tract irritation and asthma are covered in Chapter 28 and are discussed only briefly.

PNEUMOCONIOSES

The term *pneumoconiosis* refers to a nonmalignant, fibrotic disease of the lungs caused by the inhalation of a broad range of inorganic dusts, including asbestos, beryllium, silica, and coal dust. Since 1950, the International Labour Office (ILO) in Geneva, Switzerland, has periodically proposed classifications of the radiographic appearance of various pneumoconioses. Guidelines for the use of the ILO classification and sample radiographs are available from this organization.

Asbestos-Related Disease and Asbestosis

OVERVIEW AND PATHOPHYSIOLOGY

Asbestos is not a single substance but rather a group of naturally occurring, hydrated magnesium silicates that form long, thin, microscopic fibers, generally between 0.1 and 10.0 μm in length. Asbestos is obtained by mining asbestos-bearing rock, crushing it, and then separating out the fibers and washing them (a process known as *milling*). Asbestos has been widely used in various industries for its useful physicochemical properties that include heat and acid resistance, high tensile strength, flexibility, and weavability. Several varieties of asbestos are available, categorized according to their chemical composition or crystalline structure. They include chrysotile, amosite, anthophyllite, crocidolite, tremolite, and actinolite.

Asbestos fibers are classified as serpentine or amphibole according to their microscopic appearance. Serpentine fibers appear wavy and intertwined on microscopic examination and are relatively flexible. Amphibole fibers appear straight and needle-like and are more brittle. The only serpentine form is chrysotile asbestos, and it constitutes 99% of all the asbestos used in the United States. All other forms are classified as amphibole.

Workers who may be at risk for exposures include those engaged in asbestos mining and milling, insulation and fireproofing manufacture and installation, shipbuilding, construction, plumbing and pipe fitting, and brake or cement work (1–5). The risk of acquiring asbestos-related disease is much less common today than at its peak in the 1940s to 1970s due to widespread awareness of the hazards of asbestos, implementation of workplace controls and respirators, and bans on certain uses. Asbestos-related diseases occur in workers regularly exposed to these fibers, particularly those who do not use appropriate respiratory protection. No evidence has been shown that they occur in the general population (i.e., those not specifically working with asbestos) (1). Implementation and use of appropriate engineering controls, work practices, and personal protective equipment in the workplace generally prevent asbestosis. OSHA has classified various jobs that come into contact with asbestos into four classes, based on their hazard and risk of asbestos exposure (6). The current American Conference of Governmental Industrial Hygienists (ACGIH) airborne exposure threshold limit value (TLV) time-weighted average (TWA) level for all forms of asbestos is 0.1 respirable fibers per cubic centimeter (f/cc) (7). A respirable fiber is defined as one with a length greater than 5 μm and an aspect ratio (ratio of length to width) of at least 3:1. The OSHA permissible exposure limit (PEL) TWA is also 0.1 f/cc, and airborne asbestos concentrations may not exceed 1 f/cc at any time, averaged over a 30-minute period (8).

The risk of exposure to asbestos, still present in certain older schools and buildings, is exceedingly low unless significant amounts of friable asbestos-containing materials are present and their job places individuals in close and regular contact with such materials (9–11). Minute levels of asbestos fibers can be found in outdoor ambient air and are not a significant health risk (11,12).

Inhalation is the primary route of clinically significant exposure in humans. Asbestos fibers can be released into the air as dust from various materials. Skin contact does not result in adverse health effects. Some epidemiologic studies have found an association between oral asbestos exposure and gastrointestinal malignancies; however, data are currently inadequate to establish a definitive link (5,13–16). Cumulative occupational inhalation exposures between 5 and 1200 fiber-years per milliliter have been associated with several pulmonary diseases, including diffuse interstitial fibrosis (asbestosis), various nonmalignant pleural diseases, mesothelioma, and lung cancer (5,17–26). The incidence of asbestosis and lung cancer correlates with the cumulative asbestos exposure. An association between airborne asbestos exposure and laryngeal cancer has been suggested by some, but a review of the literature argues against such an association (27). Generally, a latency period of 10 to 30 years occurs from initial exposure to disease development, depending on the particular disease manifestation and the exposure intensity.

The pattern of fiber deposition in the lung parenchyma depends on the fiber size and shape (28). Thinner fibers (less than 3 μm in diameter) are most likely to reach the alveoli (29). After lodging in the alveoli, asbestos fibers face several potential fates (5,30,31). They may persist in the alveoli, be engulfed by alveolar macrophages, and penetrate through the alveolar walls and into the interstitial space, where they eventually make their way into regional lymphatics and lymph nodes, or they may penetrate through the parenchyma entirely to be deposited in the pleural, pericardial, or peritoneal space. Although asbestos is chemically inert, all fiber types are fibrogenic. Chrysotile fibers are thought to be less injurious because they are more easily degraded by macrophages than are amphibole fibers (21,32). Additionally, although all fiber sizes are potentially harmful, larger fibers (greater than 5 to 10 μm long) tend to be more fibrogenic because they are more difficult to degrade (33).

Macrophages that unsuccessfully attempt to digest the asbestos fibers may die and leave an iron-rich proteinaceous coating, what are known as "ferruginous or asbestos bodies" on histopathologic specimen. Their number and prevalence in lung tissue generally reflect the severity of exposure. Small numbers of these bodies can be found in normal adults without any history of occupational exposure (34,35). Asbestos fibers stimulate acute and chronic inflammatory reactions in the lung tissues (33,36–40). Initially, this consists primarily of macrophages but is typically followed by recruitment of neutrophils and eosinophils, particularly in the peribronchial regions of the terminal bronchioles and their adjacent alveoli. Various proinflammatory mediators are released and contribute to disease pathogenesis (41). Fibrosis develops over time as the inflammatory infiltrate becomes organized and fibroblasts are recruited. Initially, only small, irregular areas of the lung are involved, mainly in the interstitial and subpleural spaces. With disease progression, the fibrotic process becomes more diffuse, obliterating or distorting air spaces and blood vessels. Pulmonary hypertension occurs from the compromise of the pulmonary microvasculature and alveolar hypoxia and may ultimately lead to right-sided heart failure.

Asbestosis. Asbestosis is an interstitial fibrotic disease of the lung parenchyma that can develop after heavy exposures to asbestos (17–20). Factors such as fiber type inhaled and intensity and duration of exposure and patient factors such as age, genetic susceptibility, underlying medical history, and smoking all play a role in its pathophysiology. Amphibole fibers, particularly crocidolite, appear to be the most injurious, although asbestosis may result from exposure to any type. Smoking increases the risk of asbestosis. The degree of fibrosis varies and is primarily dependent on the magnitude and duration of exposure. Often there is a latency period of 10 to 30 years from initial exposure to disease development, less after larger exposures. The disease can continue to progress even after removal from the exposure, especially if the exposure was heavy (42). Asbestosis is associated with increased mortality. Most, but not all, excess risk is attributable to lung cancer (21). Patients with asbestosis are also at increased risk for development of respiratory infections (43).

Lung Cancer. Several studies have found that patients with moderate or heavy cumulative exposures to asbestos may be at higher risk for development of bronchogenic carcinoma, after a variable latent period of approximately 20 to 30 years (21–24,44–46). The International Agency for Research on Cancer (IARC) considers asbestos to be a definite human carcinogen. The magnitude of risk is dependent on a number of variables, including intensity and duration of asbestos exposure, fiber type and size, and patient age and smoking history. Most studies suggest that lung cancer only develops in patients who also have underlying asbestosis and that the risk in those with exposures without parenchymal disease is no greater than the baseline population (3,47–49). Low-dose cumulative exposures do not appear to increase the risk of lung cancer. It has been estimated that asbestos exposure accounts for approximately 5% of all lung cancers in the United States. Smoking appears to act synergistically, with the combination of the two resulting in a far greater risk than either agent alone (50).

Mesothelioma. Inhalational asbestos exposures have been associated with the development of mesothelioma in some patients. Mesothelioma is an aggressive type of pleural or peritoneal malignancy, leading to death within several months to a year (24,25,51). This rare cancer may, under certain circumstances, be related to prior significant asbestos exposure. The latency of this disease may be slightly longer than for asbestos-related bronchogenic carcinoma.

Pleural Abnormalities. Asbestos exposure has also been linked to at least four types of nonmalignant pleural disease; benign pleural plaques, pleural thickening, pleural effusions, and progressive pleural fibrosis (26,52,53). More than one pleural abnormality may be present in a single individual. Like asbestosis, pleural abnormalities tend to develop only after a latent period of many years and do not necessarily indicate underlying parenchymal disease or predict its future development. Similarly, they do not appear to be associated with an increased risk of lung cancer in the absence of underlying parenchymal fibrosis (48,54,55). As a result, pleural sequelae should be considered a separate disease entity.

Pleural plaques are smooth, discrete, elevated, rounded lesions that typically occur on the lower aspect of the posterolateral parietal pleura. They are composed primarily of collagenous tissue covered by mesothelial cells (26,56). They may contain small numbers of submicroscopic asbestos fibers. Pleural plaques progress very slowly and occasionally calcify, but they generally do not cause any significant clinical problems.

Pleural thickening is a localized or diffuse thickening of the visceral pleura (57,58). It varies in thickness from a thin, whitish discoloration that is only visible on gross specimens to a thick rind that can be seen on chest radiographs. Pleural thickening is less common than plaques or effusions and typically results from heavy exposures. Occasionally, patients may become symptomatic if pulmonary function is impaired.

Pleural effusions related to asbestos exposure tend to be transient, lasting from months to a year, but they can recur. In a minority of patients, they may result in progressive pleural fibrosis. The effusion is typically exudative and can be either unilateral or bilateral. It is rarely the first sign of a developing mesothelioma.

Progressive fibrosis is also an uncommon complication, often beginning as an effusion and progressing to bilateral fibrotic involvement over the course of several years. Of those with isolated pleural abnormalities, this group is the most likely to develop deterioration in respiratory function.

DIAGNOSIS

Asbestosis. After a variable latent period, asbestosis usually presents with clinical signs of restrictive lung disease, including dyspnea, cough, exercise intolerance, chest discomfort, crackles, hypoxia, cyanosis, and clubbing (42,59,60). Evidence of cor pulmonale may be present in more advanced cases.

Similar to other interstitial lung diseases, radiographic features include a linear or reticular pattern of opacification, more prominent in the lower lobes and the periphery (61–63). As the disease progresses, the abnormalities become more diffuse, and frank "honeycombing" may be evident. Pleural abnormalities may or may not be seen in conjunction with the parenchymal abnormalities. When present, they are helpful in suggesting the diagnosis of asbestosis. Standards for grading the radiographic appearance have been developed by the ILO and are useful for following disease progression. High-resolution computed tomography (CT) scanning of the chest is a more sensitive indicator of early disease. PFTs usually reveal varying degrees of restrictive lung disease characterized by a reduction in lung volumes (especially inspiratory capacity and vital capacity), loss of lung compliance, impaired gas exchange, and a preservation of the forced expiratory volume in 1 second to forced vital capacity ratio (64–66).

In most cases, the diagnosis can be made clinically based on an occupational history of exposure with typical clinical or radiographic findings, or both. No single factor is diagnostic. Lung biopsy may be useful in equivocal cases but is not routinely indicated. Asbestosis must be distinguished from other causes of interstitial pulmonary fibrosis. Establishing the correct diagnosis may be particularly difficult in the presence of other pulmonary or cardiac diseases, such as smoking-related obstructive pulmonary disease or congestive heart failure. Efforts to quantify the direct, cumulative exposure for each patient may be useful. Workplace air-sampling records and consultation with an industrial hygienist may be helpful in this regard.

If lung biopsy is performed, the pathologic diagnosis depends on the presence of uncoated asbestos fibers, ferruginous bodies, and interstitial fibrosis in the peribronchiolar areas of respiratory bronchioles (67). A number of samples from different areas of the lung may be necessary. The diagnosis of asbestosis is reserved for individuals with fibrosis and with identifiable asbestos fibers on biopsy. The severity of asbestosis should be graded using well-established criteria (68).

Lung Cancer. Bronchogenic carcinoma associated with asbestos is histopathologically indistinguishable from other causes, making the establishment of causality difficult in patients with multiple risk factors. Hemoptysis, chest pain, and cough can be the presenting symptoms, but they are difficult to distinguish from the symptoms of the underlying asbestosis. Occasionally, patients present with signs of metastatic spread. The diagnosis may initially be made on chest radiographs, based on the finding of a nodule or pleural effusion. Although CT scans may detect lesions at a slightly earlier stage, early detection does not appear to reduce mortality. In fact, no screening tests have been shown to improve survival. The diagnosis is confirmed by histologic analysis from tissue obtained by transbronchial or open lung biopsy.

Pleural Abnormalities

Pleural plaques and effusions are generally asymptomatic and most often found with routine chest radiography (16,69). CT scan may be necessary to distinguish pleural plaques from parenchymal or rib lesions. Patients with pleural thickening occasionally develop respiratory symptoms, which can be difficult to differentiate from underlying parenchymal disease (70). Pleural thickening is usually best noted in the fissures, although radiographic diagnosis may be difficult in the early stages. With disease progression, diffuse thickening or pleural calcifications can be visualized. Progressive pleural fibrosis may also present with signs and symptoms of restrictive pulmonary impairment, although, again, these symptoms may simply indicate coexistent asbestosis rather than pleural disease. PFTs may reveal restrictive physiology with severe pleural involvement. However, diffusion capacity should be normal in these cases unless asbestosis is present.

MANAGEMENT

Asbestosis. No known treatment is available for asbestosis, either to reverse its effects or prevent its progression. Patients should be removed from the exposure or have proper protective equipment, and workplace measures should be instituted. Early recognition and withdrawal from exposure may lead to mild clinical improvement in some (71). In a good proportion of patients with asbestosis, the disease does not progress to become severe, and many of these subjects face only mild clinical impairment in normal activities. However, in some the disease continues to progress despite removal from the exposure (72).

The usual symptomatic and supportive respiratory care should be provided: oxygen supplementation for hypoxemia, bronchodilators for wheezing or evidence of reversible bronchoconstriction, treatment of any superinfections with antibiotics, and pneumococcal and influenza vaccination. Corticosteroids have not been demonstrated to be useful for most patients. Patients should be removed from all other potentially harmful respiratory exposures. Finally, any other factors that contribute to respiratory disease should be addressed, particularly smoking, because it may contribute to the progression of fibrosis, increase the risk of lung cancer, and exacerbate the symptoms of underlying disease.

Pleural Abnormalities. No specific treatment is available for patients with pleural abnormalities other than reducing or removing the exposure and monitoring for the development of asbestosis and cancer. A pleural effusion may be the first sign of mesothelioma in a few patients, but given the poor prognosis of this cancer, an aggressive or invasive work-up does not appear to be worthwhile in most cases. Because symptoms generally do not develop in patients with lone pleural abnormalities, treatment is not required. In the rare case of progressive fibrosis causing respiratory impairment, pleurectomies do not appear to result in significant improvement (26).

Lung Cancer and Mesothelioma. Patients with asbestos-related bronchogenic carcinoma should be treated in the usual fashion. The management of mesothelioma is beyond the scope of this chapter, but aggressive management with a multimodality regimen of surgery, radiation, and chemotherapy may increase survival in selected patients (73,74).

Man-Made Mineral Fibers

OVERVIEW AND PATHOPHYSIOLOGY

Man-made mineral fibers (MMMF), also known as *man-made vitreous fibers* or *synthetic vitreous fibers*, are made by spraying, spinning, or extruding molten glass, rock, clay, or furnace slag. This process forms long, thin microscopic fibers of three general types: fiberglass, mineral wool (including rock and slag wools), and refractory ceramic fibers. Because of their properties, MMMF are used widely as insulating materials in residential and industrial structures. In certain settings, such as construction or demolition workers, airborne particles of MMMF may be released. Particles of respirable size may lead to acute respiratory irritation when inhaled, whereas skin or eye contact may cause dermal or ocular irritation, respectively.

The dermal, ocular, and respiratory tract effects are the result of simple mechanical irritation from the sharp, pointed ends of the fibers (75). No evidence has been found of an allergic component, although some patients appear to be more susceptible than others to their irritative effects.

A long-held concern has been that, with repeated exposures, MMMF may act in a similar way to asbestos fibers, inducing chronic inflammation and possible fibrosis or cancer. Human data on this issue are limited to scattered epidemiologic studies, most of which have focused on lung cancer (76,77). To date, there have been no reports suggesting a significant increase in the risk of fibrosis or mesothelioma in populations exposed to MMMF. Several large investigations have reported that mortality from lung cancer was significantly increased in workers from the rock wool/slag wool industries, particularly in groups exposed over 30 years, before industry dust control measures had been implemented (78,79). The risk of lung cancer deaths appears to be less pronounced among workers in the glass fiber industries, although the adequacy of these data has been questioned (80,81). This difference in pathogenicity between asbestos and glass fibers is thought to relate to two main factors. First, most MMMF have large diameters, making them less likely to reach the alveoli. Second, glass fibers can be mechanically broken down into shorter pieces, thus allowing alveolar macrophages to clear them more easily than asbestos fibers. The mineral wool fibers, such as rock and slag wool, have smaller diameters and a greater persistence in the lungs. Refractory ceramic fibers are currently classified as possible human carcinogens by IARC, whereas most other types of MMMF have been listed as unclassifiable.

The ACGIH airborne exposure TLV (TWA) for synthetic vitreous fibers is 1 respirable f/cc for continuous filament glass, glass wool, rock wool, slag wool, and special-purpose glass fibers. It is 0.2 f/cc for refractory ceramic fibers. The OSHA PEL (TWA) is 1 f/cc for fiberglass and mineral wool.

DIAGNOSIS

Dermal exposures generally present with pruritus and signs of dermal irritation. Eye irritation, itching, pain, or a foreign body sensation typically develops in patients with ocular exposures. Respiratory exposures generally present with irritation, burning, or pain in the throat or nose, chest discomfort, coughing, or wheezing.

MANAGEMENT

Dermal and ocular symptoms usually resolve with removal from the exposure and performance decontamination measures such as washing or thorough irrigation. Respiratory symptoms can be managed by removal from the immediate exposure and performance of symptomatic care (e.g., bronchodilators for wheezing).

Berylliosis

OVERVIEW

Beryllium is a lightweight metal with high tensile strength and electrical and thermal conductivity. These properties are transferred when it is alloyed with other metals, making it attractive for use in the ceramics, nuclear, aerospace, electronics, computer, fluorescent light, and power industries. Beryllium is obtained from mined beryl ore, which contains beryllium aluminum silicate. Inhalation of dust or fumes containing beryllium or beryllium oxide has been associated with two distinct types of pulmonary injury. Acute, intense exposures can cause a chemical pneumonitis. Chronic, low- to moderate-level exposures have been associated with a granulomatous inflammatory disorder of the lungs, resembling sarcoidosis. Acute beryllium disease has all but been eliminated in the United States due to the institution of workplace standards and controls (82). The incidence of chronic beryllium disease varies between 2% and 16% of exposed workers, depending on the group and occupation (82–85).

Beryllium's association with lung cancer in humans is controversial (86–91). Based on the available human and animal data, it has been designated a class 1 human carcinogen by the IARC and a probable human carcinogen by the Environmental Protection Agency.

The ACGIH TLV for beryllium is 0.002 mg/m^3 as a TWA and 0.01 mg/m^3 as a short-term exposure limit. The OSHA PEL is 0.002 mg/m^3 as a TWA, 0.005 mg/m^3 as a ceiling level not to be exceeded for more than 30 minutes, and 0.025 mg/m^3 as a level that should never be exceeded.

PATHOPHYSIOLOGY

Acute. Inhalation of high concentrations (greater than 0.1 mg/m^3) of beryllium particles may lead to a rapidly evolving chemical pneumonitis from direct irritation and nonspecific inflammation of the respiratory tract and mucous membranes (92,93). Death may occur as a result of severe pulmonary edema.

Chronic. Repeated inhalational exposures to beryllium or beryllium oxide particles sensitize certain individuals and may result in a delayed-type (type IV) hypersensitivity reaction in the lung parenchyma (94–99). Beryllium is taken up by antigen-presenting cells in the lungs, after which it is presented to T lymphocytes in conjunction with major histocompatibility complex class II molecules (100,101). In susceptible individuals, this results in cytokine release, cellular proliferation, and ultimately the formation of granulomas and progressive fibrosis (102,103). Histopathologic lesions may include interstitial, noncaseating granulomas with lymphocytic and mononuclear cellular infiltrates and interstitial fibrosis (104). Regional lymph nodes may also display granulomatous changes. Although unusual, extrapulmonary involvement of the skin, liver, kidneys, spleen, and salivary glands with granulomatous inflammation has also been reported (104). Evidence is mounting that genetic susceptibility plays a crucial role in determining in which exposed patients berylliosis eventually develops (101,105).

DIAGNOSIS

Acute. Patients present with dyspnea, cough, and chest discomfort that typically develop within hours of an exposure and may progress rapidly (93). A physical examination may reveal varying degrees of respiratory distress, tachypnea, hypoxemia, tachycardia, and crackles on auscultation. Chest radiographs generally demonstrate diffuse infiltrates. Respiratory distress may become severe, and deaths have been reported. Most cases resolve uneventfully; however, a few have progressed to chronic berylliosis (106).

Chronic. Insidious onset and progression of dyspnea, cough, chest discomfort, weight loss, exercise intolerance, and fatigue generally develop (94,99). Typically, there is a latent period of months up to decades from the time of exposure to the development of clinical disease. Symptoms may develop years after exposure has ceased. A physical examination may reveal respiratory difficulty and crackles on auscultation. Signs of extrapulmonary involvement include lymphadenopathy, skin lesions, or hepatosplenomegaly. Chest radiographs generally reveal bilateral reticular, nodular, or reticulonodular infiltrates, most commonly in the upper lung regions, and associated with varying degrees of mediastinal or hilar adenopathy (107–109). Chest CT is more sensitive than plain radiography in detecting early disease. Typical findings include thickening of the septa, nodules, ground-glass opacities, and adenopathy (110). PFTs may demonstrate evidence of obstruction, restriction, or both (111–114). Bronchoalveolar lavage (BAL) generally reveals a lymphocytosis (111,115).

The diagnosis of chronic berylliosis is made based on a detailed history, in combination with a physical examination, radiography, spirometry, and histopathologic findings on transbronchial biopsy. To distinguish the diagnosis from sarcoidosis and other granulomatous disorders of the lung, a lymphocyte proliferation test (LPT or BeLPT) should be performed with lymphocytes obtained from BAL or a peripheral blood specimen to test for sensitization to the agent (98,116). However, false positives may occur with BeLPT. Beryllium can also be identified in histopathologic lesions using a special type of mass spectrometry (117).

MANAGEMENT

The management of acute beryllium pneumonitis is supportive. After recovery, measures should be undertaken to reduce the potential for further exposures.

Patients with chronic berylliosis are also treated supportively, with oxygen for hypoxemia, diuretics if necessary for right heart failure, inhaled bronchodilators for wheezing, and regular immunization against influenza and pneumococcal infections. Patients should be removed from any exposure to beryllium, although evidence that such measures affect outcome is lacking. The overall clinical course of chronic beryllium disease is variable. Some remain stable for years without significant progression or even improve slightly with removal from exposure (118). In others, the disease continues to progress in an indolent fashion. In a few, a rapidly progressive and debilitating course may lead to respiratory failure within several years. Symptomatic patients, particularly those with pulmonary function deficits, may respond favorably to a course of corticosteroids. However, because it is not known whether corticosteroids alter the progression of disease, their use must be weighed against the side effects associated with long-term treatment. Once corticosteroids are begun patients may require lifelong therapy. Other immunosuppressive drugs may also prove helpful if patients do not tolerate steroids or steroid-sparing agents. All patients, including sensitized individuals (those with a positive BeLPT) in whom evidence of clinical disease has not yet developed, should be followed regularly for disease progression, even after removal from the exposure.

Silica-Related Disease and Silicosis

OVERVIEW AND PATHOPHYSIOLOGY

Free silica or silicon dioxide (SiO_2) is ubiquitous in the earth's upper crust and is a common component of most rock and sand. Disease related to silica inhalation is a cause of morbidity and mortality among workers worldwide. It is important to distinguish between silicon (the element), silica (the mineral SiO_2), and silicone (a manmade synthetic polymer). Another term, *silicates,* refers to the minerals formed when free silica combines with cations, such as magnesium and aluminum, to form such substances as talc, kaolin, vermiculite, or mica. Free silica exists in nature in either amorphous or crystalline silica.

Disease in humans is primarily associated with inhalation of the crystalline forms, which can be divided into alpha quartz, cristobalite, and tridymite. Among these, alpha quartz is the most common mineral of commercial importance. It is a major constituent of igneous rocks such as granite and pegmatite but is also found in sandstone and sedimentary deposits such as slate and shale. The inhalation of SiO_2 has been associated with a variety of pulmonary diseases, including chronic bronchitis, emphysema, various types of silicosis, mycobacterial pulmonary diseases, and possibly lung cancer. Extrapulmonary illnesses have also been described and include nephropathy, scleroderma, systemic sclerosis, and other rheumatic and connective tissue diseases (119–124). Amorphous silica is much less injurious than crystalline silica.

Workers at risk for silica exposures include sandblasters, miners, tunnel drillers, stone carvers, masons, abrasives workers, flour workers, ceramics workers, glassmakers, and quarry and foundry workers. Measures such as engineering and ventilation controls, water suppression of dust, and respirators can reduce or prevent workers' exposure to silica.

Inhaled silica dust particles of respirable size induce the formation of fibrosis and silicotic nodules. Particles of respirable size (0.5 to 3.0 μm) reach the alveoli, where they are phagocytosed by alveolar macrophages. After ingestion, the macrophages elaborate cytokines and inflammatory mediators, activating T cells and a subsequent immunologic cascade that ultimately results in fibroblast recruitment and collagen deposition in the lungs (125). Histopathologic examination of affected individuals reveals distinctive peribronchiolar silicotic nodules, fibrotic arrangements of birefringent silica particles, layers of collagen and reticulin, and macrophages. These nodules and fibrotic areas can distort or obliterate the normal airspaces, bronchioles, and vascular structures. Exposure to crystalline silica has been associated with three major types of pulmonary disease: chronic silicosis, accelerated (or subacute) silicosis, and acute silicosis, depending on the intensity and duration of exposure. Silicosis typically follows a progressive course even in the absence of ongoing exposure.

The ACGIH TLV (TWA) for amorphous silica is 3 mg/m^3 (respirable fraction) as diatomaceous earth, 10 mg/m^3 as precipitated silica and silica gel, 2 mg/m^3 as silica fume, and 0.1 mg/m^3 as fused silica; for crystalline silica the TLV (TWA) is 0.05 mg/m^3 as cristobalite, quartz, or tridymite and 0.1 mg/m^3 as quartz tripoli. The OSHA PEL (TWA) for amorphous silica depends on its SiO_2 content and is (80 mg/m^3)/% SiO_2 for all forms; for crystalline silica the TLV (TWA) is (10 mg/m^3)/(% SiO_2 + 2) for the respirable fraction of quartz forms and (5 mg/m^3)/(% SiO_2 + 2) for the respirable fraction of cristobalite and tridymite forms.

Silicates, such as mica, talc, and soapstone, are less fibrogenic than silica but may cause characteristic lesions after heavy, prolonged exposures. The ACGIH TLV (TWA) for mica is 3 mg/m^3 for the respirable fraction; for talc without asbestos fibers, it is 2 mg/m^3 for the respirable fraction; for Portland cement it is 10 mg/m^3 for the respirable fraction; and for soapstone it is 3 mg/m^3 for the respirable fraction. The OSHA PEL (TWA) for mica, talc, and soapstone is 20 million parts per cubic feet (mppcf), and for Portland it is 50 mppcf.

Chronic silicosis, the most common form of silicosis, results from low to moderate levels of inhalation exposure for 20 years or more (126–130). Silica particles appear to stimulate the formation of nodules in the lung parenchyma and hilar lymph nodes. The upper lobes are most often affected. A considerable latent period may occur between exposure and the development of clinical or radiographic disease, and it may continue to progress despite removal from the exposure (131,132). Over a relatively short time, the nodules may coalesce into fibrotic masses that can distort or obliterate airspaces and blood vessels, a process called *progressive massive fibrosis* (PMF) (133–135).

Accelerated silicosis is similar to chronic silicosis, in clinical, radiographic, and histopathologic features, except that it generally develops over a shorter time period (after 2 to 8 years) and in response to higher levels of silica exposure or dusts with a higher percentage of quartz content (e.g., 40% to 80%) (136–138). It is uncommon but tends to progress rapidly and has a higher incidence of associated PMF than chronic silicosis. Accelerated silicosis is typically fatal within several years of the diagnosis.

Acute silicosis, sometimes called *silicoproteinosis*, is a rare, rapidly progressing condition associated with very intense exposures to free silica dust of small particle sizes, as may occur with sandblasting. It is thought that the freshly fractured quartz may be more potent in causing tissue injury (139). Silicoproteinosis appears to be fundamentally different in pathophysiology than the other forms of silicosis, and histologically it resembles idiopathic alveolar proteinosis (140,141). Along with interstitial fibrosis, the parenchymal airspaces become filled with a lipoproteinaceous exudate, desquamated cells, macrophages, and silica particles. Progressive restriction and impairment in gas exchange lead, in most cases, to death within several years.

Patients with silicosis may also have an increased risk for development of tuberculosis (silicotuberculosis) and other mycobacterial or fungal infections (e.g., *Aspergillus*, coccidiomycetes, *Sporothrix*, blastomycetes, or *Cryptococcus*) (142–144). In fact, before the development of modern antitubercular drugs, tuberculosis was a leading cause of death in patients with silicosis. Mycobacterial superinfection must be ruled out whenever patients with silicosis have radiographically evident disease progression or deterioration in respiratory function.

The association between silicosis and lung cancer had been controversial, primarily because of insufficient human evidence. However, there does appear to be an association between certain types of silica exposure, namely quartz and cristobalite, and an increase in the incidence of bronchogenic carcinoma (122,145–148). Based on the available data, the IARC has classified silica as a class 1 human carcinogen. It remains unproven whether silica exposure in the absence of chronic fibrotic silicosis increases the risk of cancer (149). In addition to silicosis, chronic inhalation exposures to silica have been associated with obstructive airways disease such as chronic bronchitis and emphysema (124,150,151).

DIAGNOSIS

Three criteria are required to make the diagnosis of silicosis: an appropriate history of exposure, radiologic (e.g., nodular or reticulonodular pattern) and spirometric (e.g., restrictive impairment) findings consistent with silicosis, and the absence of a likely alternative diagnosis. The ILO classification grades for silicosis range from category 0 (normal or nearly normal) to category 3 (severely abnormal).

Chronic Silicosis. Radiographic abnormalities usually precede the development of symptoms; thus, the diagnosis is often made on a routine chest x-ray (126–130). Nodular opacities with upper lung zone predominance are the typical radiographic findings. In simple silicosis the opacities are discrete and rounded, ranging from 1 to 10 mm in diameter and not associated with interstitial fibrosis (152,153). The degree of radiographic involvement is a poor predictor of clinical function. When clinical findings are present early, they are generally attributable to concomitant cigarette smoking or industrial bronchitis. As the disease progresses, however, decrements in pulmonary function become more apparent, particularly in smokers. Patients usually experience varying degrees of cough, dyspnea, and hypoxia. Clubbing and bibasilar crackles on auscultation are common findings with advanced disease (126). PFTs may show varying degrees of restriction and impairment in gas exchange. Chest radiography in these more advanced stages of disease may reveal an increased number of nodules and hilar adenopathy, occasionally with a characteristic peripheral ("eggshell") calcification.

Accelerated Silicosis. Accelerated silicosis typically presents similarly to chronic silicosis but progresses more rapidly (136–138). Radiographic findings include diffuse, reticulonodular opacities, especially in the middle zones of the lung.

PMF typically presents with more rapidly progressive symptoms and severe deteriorations in pulmonary function and gas exchange, eventually resulting in signs and symptoms of cor pulmonale (133–135). The radiographic appearance of PMF is large (greater than 10 mm) or coalescing opacities. PFTs may reveal severe restrictive impairment or, less often, a mixed obstructive and restrictive picture accompanied by limitation of gas exchange.

Acute Silicosis. Acute silicosis generally presents with rapidly progressing symptoms of respiratory insufficiency, typically over a span of 1 to 3 years (140,141,154). Initially, it may be mistaken for pneumonia. In patients with acute silicoproteinosis, x-ray films of the chest reveal diffuse airspace disease or an alveolar ground-glass appearance, findings that mimic pulmonary edema.

Laboratory findings in patients with silicosis are nonspecific. A moderate elevation in the angiotensin-converting enzyme concentration and various immunologic abnormalities are common. Positive antinuclear antibody titers are found in 26% to 44% of patients (154a). An increased prevalence of rheumatoid factor and elevated levels of immunoglobulins and immune complexes has also been described. In addition, scleroderma, rheumatoid arthritis, rheumatoid lung nodules, and glomerulonephritis have been reported.

MANAGEMENT

Silicosis has no specific treatment, and nothing has been shown to reverse the degree of fibrosis. Removal from the exposure arrests the disease in most patients, and thus their prognosis is good if it is recognized early enough. However, the fibrosis can continue to progress even after removal from exposure, particularly in those with PMF.

Management should include the usual symptomatic and supportive respiratory care, oxygen supplementation for hypoxemia, bronchodilators for wheezing or evidence of reversible bronchoconstriction, treatment of any superinfections with antibiotics, and periodic influenza and pneumococcal vaccination. Corticosteroids have not been shown to be useful for most patients. Patients should be removed from all other potentially harmful respiratory exposures and counseled on smoking cessation. Yearly tuberculosis screening should be instituted, and patients with evidence of active infection or exposure should be treated appropriately.

Coal Worker's Pneumoconiosis

OVERVIEW AND PATHOPHYSIOLOGY

Coal is broadly defined as a type of carbonaceous rock formed from the fossilization of plant matter. The chronic inhalation of coal may result in coal worker's pneumoconiosis (CWP), or black lung (155–157). Several types of coal exist, each of which is classified according to carbon and quartz silica content. Anthracite contains the most carbon and poses the greatest risk for the development of CWP. Coal miners and coal workers are among those whose occupation places them at high risk for CWP. In contrast to asbestosis and silicosis, smoking does not appear to affect the risk or progression of the disease. CWP develops only after decades of chronic exposure.

Inhaled coal dust particles of respirable size become deposited in the terminal bronchioles and alveoli of the lungs. They are subsequently engulfed by alveolar macrophages, stimulating the local release of various inflammatory mediators, reactive oxygen species, proteolytic enzymes, and growth factors. This inflammatory process, which itself causes cellular injury, results in the recruitment of neutrophils, causing further injury. In addition, this cascade leads to the recruitment of fibroblasts and the deposition of collagen and reticulin (158). The end result of this

TABLE 3. Hypersensitivity pneumonitis (extrinsic allergic alveolitis): reported associations

Disease	Antigen	Source of particles
Farmer's lung	Thermophilic actinomycetes	"Moldy" hay, grain, silage
Bird fancier's, breeder's, or handler's lung	Parakeet, budgerigar, pigeon, chicken, turkey proteins	Avian droppings or feathers
Humidifier or air-conditioner lung (ventilation pneumonitis)	*Aureobasidium pullulans* or other microorganisms	Contaminated water in humidification and forced-air air-conditioning systems
Chemical worker's lung	Isocyanates	Polyurethane foam, varnishes, lacquer, foundry casting
Bagassosis	Thermophilic actinomycetes	"Moldy" bagasse (sugar cane)
Malt worker's lung	*Aspergillus fumigatus* or *A. clavatus*	Moldy barley
Mushroom worker's lung	Thermophilic actinomycetes, other	Mushroom compost
Sequoiosis	*Aureobasidium, Graphium* spp.	Redwood sawdust
Maple bark disease	*Cryptostroma corticale*	Maple bark
Woodworker's lung	Wood dust, *Alternaria*	Oak, cedar, and mahogany dusts; pine and spruce pulp
Cheese washer's lung	*Penicillium casei*	Moldy cheese
Suberosis	Cork dust mold	Cork dust
Sauna taker's lung	*Aureobasidium* spp., other	Contaminated sauna water
Pituitary snuff taker's lung	Animal proteins	Heterologous pituitary snuff
Coffee worker's lung	Coffee bean dust	Coffee beans
Miller's lung	*Sitophilus granarius* (wheat weevil)	Infested wheat flour
Fish meal worker's lung	Fish meal dust	Fish meal
Furrier's lung	Animal fur dust	Animal pelts
Lycoperdonosis	Puffball spores	Lycoperdon puffballs
Familial HSP	*Bacillus subtilis*	Contaminated wood dust in walls
Compost lung	*Aspergillus*	Compost
Wood trimmer's disease	*Rhizopus* spp., *Mucor* spp.	Contaminated wood trimmings
Thatched roof disease	*Saccharomonospora viridis*	Dried grasses and leaves
Streptomyces albus HSP	*Streptomyces albus*	Contaminated fertilizer
Cephalosporium HSP	*Cephalosporium*	Contaminated basement (sewage)
Detergent worker's disease	*Bacillus subtilis* enzymes	Detergent
Japanese summer house HSP	*Trichosporon cutaneum*	House dust?, bird droppings
Potato riddler's lung	Thermophilic actinomycetes, *M. faeni, T. vulgaris, Aspergillus* spp.	"Moldy" hay around potatoes
Tobacco worker's disease	*Aspergillus* spp.	Mold on tobacco
Hot tub lung	*Cladosporium* spp.	Mold on ceiling
Wine grower's lung	*Botrytis cinerea*	Mold on grapes
Laboratory worker's HSP	Male rat urine	Laboratory rat
Tap water lung	Unknown	Contaminated tap water
Pauli's HSP	Pauli's reagent	Laboratory reagent
Woodman's disease	*Penicillium* spp.	Oak and maple trees

HSP, hypersensitivity pneumonitis.
Adapted from Richerson HB, et al. *J Allergy Clin Immunol* 1989;84:839–844.

chronic exposure and inflammation is the development of pulmonary fibrosis and scarring. Histopathologic lesions, termed *coal dust macules*, consisting of coal dust–laden macrophages with varying degrees of associated fibrosis, are characteristically found around the respiratory bronchioles. Localized alveolar destruction, emphysema, and interstitial fibrosis are also common. In some patients, particularly those with intense or prolonged exposures, a condition known as *complicated CCWP* can occur. This is analogous to the PMF associated with silicosis (159). In such cases, coal dust macules coalesce to form large fibrotic nodules, which are more prominent in the upper lungs and are occasionally filled with a black fluid.

The ACGIH TLV (TWA) for coal dust is 0.4 mg/m^3 (respirable fraction) for the anthracite form and 0.9 mg/m^3 (respirable fraction) for the bituminous form. The OSHA PEL (TWA) for coal dust depends on the SiO_2 content and is 2.4 mg/m^3 (respirable fraction) for dust with less than 5% SiO_2 and (10 mg/m^3)/(% SiO_2 + 2) for respirable dust with greater than 5% SiO_2.

DIAGNOSIS

Simple CWP is typically asymptomatic and usually diagnosed on routine chest radiography. In more advanced cases, dyspnea and cough (often productive of black sputum) may develop, although in some patients this represents the effects of smoking rather than coal dust (160,161). Spirometry may reveal varying degrees of obstructive impairment and small airways disease.

MANAGEMENT

CWP has no specific treatment. Management rests instead on supportive and symptomatic care, including bronchodilators for wheezing or evidence of reversible bronchoconstriction, and treatment of any superinfections with antibiotics. Corticosteroids have not been demonstrated to be useful. Workplace measures should be introduced to reduce inhalation of coal dust. Evidence of CWP should prompt a complete removal from any coal dust exposure. The prognosis for most patients is good, although some, particularly those with PMF, may continue to progress even after removal from exposure.

HYPERSENSITIVITY PNEUMONITIS

Overview and Pathophysiology

Hypersensitivity pneumonitis (HSP), or allergic extrinsic alveolitis, is an immunologically mediated inflammation of the lung that results from the repeated inhalation of respirable particles from a variety of etiologic agents (162–169) (Tables 3 and 4). Sensitization

TABLE 4. Agents implicated in hypersensitivity pneumonitis

Agent	Disease	Exposure
Thermophilic actinomycetes		
Micropolyspora faeni	Farmer's lung	Mold compost
Thermoactinomyces sacchari	Bagassosis	Moldy sugar cane
Thermoactinomyces vulgaris	Mushroom worker's lung	Moldy compost
Thermoactinomyces viridis	Mushroom worker's lung	Moldy compost
Thermoactinomyces candidus	Ventilation pneumonitis	Contaminated forced-air systems
Fungi		
Alternaria spp.	Woodworker's lung	Moldy wood chips
Pullularia pullulans	Sequoiosis	Moldy redwood dust
Aspergillus clavatus	Malt worker's lung	Moldy malt
Penicillium frequentans	Suberosis	Moldy work dust
Penicillium caseii	Cheese worker's lung	Moldy cheese
Penicillium roqueforti	Cheese worker's lung	Moldy cheese
Phoma spp.	Shower curtain	Moldy shower curtain
Mucor stolonifer	Paprika splitter's lung	Paprika dust
Cryptostroma corticale	Maple bark stripper's lung	Moldy maple bark

Adapted from Levy MB, Fink JN. *Ann Allergy* 1985;54:168.

and re-exposure to these inhaled antigens induce a lymphocytic alveolitis. However, because only a small percentage of those who are exposed go on to develop the disease, it has been suspected that underlying host factors, such as an inability to down-regulate the immune response appropriately, may play a significant role. HSP appears less likely to develop in smokers. The disease has acute, subacute, and chronic forms. Farmer's lung is a specific form of HSP that occurs in agricultural workers who are exposed to certain types of allergens in inhaled organic dusts (170–172).

HSP is characterized by the presence of activated T lymphocytes in BAL fluid and an interstitial mononuclear cell infiltrate. In addition to this mononuclear alveolitis, a granulomatous pneumonitis may also occur, involving a combination of immune complex, humoral, and cell-mediated immune reactions to the inhaled offending antigen.

Examination of BAL fluid in symptomatic HSP patients typically reveals activated T lymphocytes, with a predominance of $CD8^+$ cells, although occasionally a predominance of $CD4^+$ cells may be noted (173–176). Certain macrophage-derived factors that exhibit chemotactic activity for lymphocytes (including interleukin-1 and interleukin-8) may contribute to the entry of sensitized $CD8^+$ cells in the lungs of these individuals. Some authors suggest that $CD8^+$ T cells modulate granuloma formation through production of Th1- or Th2-like cytokines (177). The activated cells release fibronectin and other matrix proteoglycans and have been associated with the transformation of the interstitial matrix and ultimately lung fibrosis seen in chronic forms of HSP (178,179).

Diagnosis

Acute HSP is the more common form of the disease and resembles an influenza-like illness. It usually develops several hours (2 to 9 hours) after a relatively intense exposure to the particular antigen. Systemic symptoms can occur and include fever, chills, myalgias, and malaise (162–169,180). Respiratory symptoms such as cough and dyspnea are common but not universal. Symptoms generally peak between 6 and 24 hours and last from several hours to a few days. Acute HSP can recur with re-exposure to the antigen. Examination findings typically include fever, an overall ill appearance, and bibasilar crackles. Leukocytosis, with associated neutrophilia and lymphopenia, and hypoxemia, are common laboratory findings. Typically, significant peripheral eosinophilia is not seen. Chest radiographs may be normal, even in symptomatic patients. More often, x-rays of symptomatic patients show a diffuse reticulonodular pattern. Occasionally, a more localized pattern, with sparing of the lung apices or bases, may be seen. A diffuse or patchy interstitial infiltrate may also be seen. PFTs generally reveal restriction, with variable impairment of gas exchange. BAL usually demonstrates alveolar lymphocytes and neutrophils. Lung biopsy may show granulomatous interstitial pneumonitis with an infiltrate of neutrophils, macrophages, eosinophils, and foreign body giant cells (181).

Subacute HSP occurs with repeated, less intense exposures to the antigen. Symptoms such as cough and dyspnea develop gradually over several days to weeks. Occasionally, the syndrome progresses to severe dyspnea and hypoxemia, necessitating urgent hospitalization. Examination and radiographic findings are similar to those of the acute form.

Chronic HSP is a form of progressive interstitial fibrosis that develops with recurrent exposures. Symptoms progress insidiously over a period of months, with increasing cough, dyspnea, fatigue, and weight loss. Physical examination may reveal clubbing of the fingers and crackles with pulmonary auscultation. Chest radiographs generally reveal diffuse interstitial markings, particularly in the peripheral lung fields, and sometimes reduced lung volumes. Abnormalities rarely seen in HSP include pleural effusion or thickening, hilar adenopathy, calcification, cavitation, atelectasis, and coin lesions. PFTs typically show evidence of restrictive disease and impaired gas exchange, although obstructive and mixed patterns are occasionally seen as well.

The diagnosis of HSP can often be made with a careful history of episodic respiratory symptoms, particularly if they can be related to specific exposures to an offending antigen, and the presence of compatible radiographic and spirometric abnormalities. Resolution of symptoms on withdrawal from exposure and recurrence with re-exposure are also helpful clues.

Serologic tests may offer additional confirmatory evidence for sensitization, particularly those that demonstrate antibodies to a known panel of HSP triggers by precipitin reactions in agar (182–184). The demonstration of such antibodies in the patient, combined with compatible historic and clinical findings, is very useful in establishing the diagnosis. However, a negative result does not exclude the diagnosis. It may only mean that the correct antigen was not tested. Currently, there is no role in the routine diagnostic work-up for measures of cell-mediated immune responses (e.g., antigen- or mitogen-induced blastogenesis or release of lymphokines). Skin testing is generally not helpful. Routine use of inhalational challenge testing is not recommended. BAL is useful in the diagnostic work-up of patients with suspected HSP by determining T-cell surface markers.

To make a definitive diagnosis in patients without sufficient clinical criteria, transbronchial lung biopsy may be indicated, particularly in chronic or progressive cases, to rule out other diseases that require specific treatment. Open lung biopsy is reserved for instances in which transbronchial biopsy does not yield enough tissue to confirm the diagnosis.

Management

The acute disease is generally self-limited, and only supportive measures are usually necessary. One randomized trial exhibited a more rapid symptomatic improvement from the acute illness with the use of corticosteroids (185,186). Their role in the treatment of chronic disease is less clear, and they may potentially cause harm by masking symptoms of acute exposures or disease progression. Steroids should be considered for patients with severe acute HSP or progressive chronic disease. Therapy should be continued until significant improvement has been made. Removal of the causative agent from the patient's environment, or the patient from the environment, is generally followed by improvement of the subacute or chronic forms and may help to confirm the diagnosis.

ORGANIC DUST TOXIC SYNDROME

Overview and Pathophysiology

Organic dust toxic syndrome (ODTS) is a nonallergic, noninfectious, febrile illness caused by inhalation of large amounts of respirable organic dusts from a variety of sources, including moldy silage, hay, or other agricultural products (187,188). It is also sometimes called *silo-unloader's syndrome* because of the situations in which it often occurs and because the exposures generally involve contaminated organic matter. The exact etiologic agents of ODTS have not been defined, although inhaled fungal material or bacterial endotoxins have both been suggested. It is fairly common among agricultural or farm workers and typically occurs after activities that generate high concentrations of airborne organic dust particles, such as working with or handling hay, grain, wood chips, or feed, especially if these products are moldy (189–192). The exact pathophysiology also is uncertain, although it appears that the dusts in some way stimulate the release of cytokines by alveolar macrophages and activate the complement system (187). Lung biopsies in affected individuals have shown inflammation of terminal bronchioles and alveolar areas, exudates of neutrophils and macrophages, and, on occasion, fungal spores (193). Like HSP, ODTS is characterized by increased numbers of neutrophils in the BAL fluid and appears to be more common in nonsmokers (194). However, ODTS differs from HSP and classic *farmer's lung* in that prior sensitization by the antigen is not required and because acute pulmonary sequelae, such as infiltrates and significant hypoxia, and chronic pulmonary sequelae, such as fibrosis or recurrent attacks, do not generally occur (195). Byssinosis, humidifier fever, and grain fever may all be subtypes or variants of ODTS (189).

The ACGIH TLV (TWA) for grain dust is 4 mg/m^3; for wood dust it is 1 mg/m^3 for certain hard woods and 5 mg/m^3 for soft wood; for other particulates it is 3 mg/m^3 (respirable fraction). The OSHA PEL (TWA) for particulates not otherwise regulated is 5 mg/m^3 (respirable fraction).

Diagnosis

Symptoms include fever, chills, malaise, myalgias, cough, chest discomfort, dyspnea, headache, and nausea that generally begin several hours after a heavy exposure (188,190,193,194). Examination findings may include fever, tachycardia, and an ill appearance. Occasionally, scattered rales or rhonchi have been noted, but significant hypoxemia typically does not occur. Peripheral leukocytosis is common. Chest radiographs are generally unremarkable. PFTs may be normal or reveal mild restriction or mild impairments, or both, in diffusion capacity. Serologic tests for common HSP allergens are usually negative (188). Differentiation from HSP may be difficult.

Management

The illness is self-limited, and symptoms typically resolve within 24 hours. Unlike some patients with HSP, no significant long-term sequelae are associated with ODTS (195). No specific treatment is available other than supportive care. Steroids have not specifically been studied for ODTS, but, given their benefit in acute cases of HSP and the similarities between the two illnesses, they may be of benefit. Patients should be cautioned about the etiology and instructed on proper respiratory precautions and work conditions. Dust masks may help prevent the disease (189).

BYSSINOSIS

Overview and Pathophysiology

Byssinosis is a pulmonary disease of textile workers caused by the inhalation of dust from cotton, flax, or hemp (196,197). Exposures typically occur among workers involved in the processes of carding, ginning, or milling. The term *byssinosis* technically refers only to the chest tightness experienced by textile workers on returning to work after a break and does not include many of the other symptoms. Mill fever is a related illness that refers to the systemic symptoms that may develop after identical exposures. Both are forms of ODTS, but its ultimate pathophysiology may differ slightly, and chronic effects may occur. The illness is thought to be caused primarily by the inhalation of endotoxin from the cell walls of gram-negative bacteria that commonly colonize cotton plants in the field and which are often found in significant levels in the dust. Various other components of plants, molds, or bacteria may also play a role (198). Their inhalation leads to an inflammatory response in the lungs, with the recruitment of alveolar macrophages and the release of various inflammatory mediators, such as histamine, prostaglandins, and other cytokines, resulting in bronchoconstriction, an obstructive deficit, and occasionally systemic symptoms.

The ACGIH TLV (TWA) for raw cotton dust is 0.2 mg/m^3. The OSHA PEL (TWA) for cotton dust is 1 mg/m^3.

Diagnosis

Initially, chest tightness, cough, and dyspnea develop, most notably on the first day of the workweek ("Monday chest tightness") (199). The symptoms are generally accompanied by a modest, reversible decrement in forced expiratory volume in 1 second. Systemic symptoms such as fever and malaise may occur in some. A physical examination may reveal evidence of wheezing on auscultation. These effects typically subside as the week progresses. With repeated exposures over the course of many years, chronic and irreversible pulmonary dysfunction may occur, with either restrictive or obstructive impairment (196,200). In such cases, symptoms become more severe and may persist throughout the workweek and after removal from the exposure.

Management

Treatment is symptomatic. A trial of inhaled bronchodilators should be given to symptomatic patients. Workplace measures to reduce or eliminate the exposure should be undertaken. Occasionally, patients with evidence of chronic or progressive disease may need to be removed from the exposure.

FUME FEVERS

Metal Fume Fever

OVERVIEW AND PATHOPHYSIOLOGY

Metal fume fever (MFF) is an acute, systemic, self-limited, flu-like illness that develops after the inhalation of various metal oxides (201). Zinc oxide appears to be the most common cause of MFF. Welders, particularly those who work with galvanized steel, and bronze workers, are among those commonly exposed (202). Iron, copper, nickel, manganese, chromium, and other metals have also been associated with MFF. These exposures usually occur in the context of smelting, cutting, or welding, particularly in enclosed or poorly ventilated spaces (203,204).

The mechanism of disease is not clear but probably results from nonspecific pulmonary inflammation. The systemic effects are caused by the release of various inflammatory mediators and cytokines in response to stimulation by inhaled metal oxides (202,205,206). The inflammatory response appears to correlate with the inhaled dose of zinc oxide. Previous sensitization or exposure is not required.

The ACGIH TLV for zinc oxide fumes is 5 mg/m^3 as a TWA and 10 mg/m^3 as a short-term exposure limit; for welding fumes not otherwise specified, the TWA is 5 mg/m^3. The OSHA PEL (TWA) for zinc oxide fumes is 5 mg/m^3.

DIAGNOSIS

MFF is often confused with a nonspecific viral syndrome. The diagnosis may be obscured due to delay between exposure and the development of symptoms. However, the diagnosis can be made by a careful history and clinical examination. No specific diagnostic tests are available, and measurements of the metals involved are generally not necessary, unless the exposure is likely to result in significant systemic metal poisoning (e.g., mercury). Cadmium fume inhalation should be considered and ruled out in all such patients because its initial symptoms resemble those of MFF but it can progress to severe pulmonary injury (see the section Cadmium Fume Pneumonitis).

Clinical features of MFF include fever, malaise, myalgias, chills, headache, metallic taste, cough, and chest discomfort that typically begin 2 to 12 hours after an exposure. Spontaneous recovery generally occurs within 12 hours to several days after onset. Pulmonary function abnormalities are usually minimal, but a few reports of airflow obstruction after inhalation of metal oxide fumes have been published (202,207). Systemic leukocytosis is not uncommon. With repeated exposures, episodes of MFF may diminish in severity, indicating some adaptability or tachyphylaxis.

MANAGEMENT

Treatment of MFF is primarily symptomatic, with antipyretics, analgesics, and/or antiinflammatory agents. The use of steroids has not been evaluated. Complete resolution without permanent or long-term sequelae is the rule. Education and avoidance of the exposure prevent recurrences.

Polymer Fume Fever

OVERVIEW AND PATHOPHYSIOLOGY

Fluoropolymer plastics, such as polytetrafluoroethylene (PTFE, or Teflon), perfluoroalkoxyethylene resins, and fluorinated ethylene-propylene, are used commonly in a variety of industries and household products, such as lubricants, heat-resistant coatings, and fabric treatments. Excessive heating of these compounds can generate pyrolysis products, the inhalation of which can result in respiratory irritation and a self-limited flu-like syndrome similar to MFF. This syndrome is generally referred to as *polymer fume fever (PFF)* (208). It occurs in plastics production workers engaged in the overheating of any of these specific compounds, especially PTFE (209,210). Additionally, it may occur by smoking cigarettes contaminated with the plastic, which is then pyrolyzed and inhaled (211,212). Exposures have also occurred from overheated frying pans, burning of plastic compounds, and welding near PTFE.

As with MFF, the exact etiology is unclear but appears to be a result of inhaling fumes from various fluorinated polymers that have been heated or burned, generally at temperatures exceeding 350° to 500°C. Thermal decomposition liberates fumes that contain carbonyl fluoride and other irritant products (213). The former can react with water in the lungs and respiratory tract to form hydrofluoric acid, which may lead to direct injury of the pulmonary parenchyma (208). In addition, respirable particulate matter may cause oxidative lung damage via formation of free radicals (214). Human studies are limited, but animal data have demonstrated areas of pulmonary hemorrhage, edema, epithelial necrosis, and sloughing (215). Given the similarity to MFF, it is likely that cytokines and inflammatory cells have a significant role. Although there are currently no ACGIH TLVs or OSHA limits for fluoropolymer decomposition products, exposure levels should be kept as low as possible.

DIAGNOSIS

The diagnosis can be made based on history and clinical examination. No specific diagnostic tests are available. Urinary fluoride levels may reflect chronic fluoropolymer exposure, but they are not helpful in either diagnosing acute exposures or guiding management. Symptoms generally begin several hours after exposure, with fever, chills, headache, chest discomfort, dyspnea, cough, eye or throat irritation, and myalgias. Fever, tachycardia, tachypnea, and rales may be noted on physical examination. Resolution generally occurs spontaneously over a period of 24 to 48 hours. Rarely, symptoms may persist for several days. Peripheral leukocytosis is common. Occasionally, high-intensity exposures may result in a frank chemical pneumonitis and subsequent noncardiogenic pulmonary edema. In these cases, pulmonary involvement may take up to 1 week to resolve. Chest radiographs may be normal or may show varying degrees of diffuse, bilateral infiltration (Fig. 1). No consistent pattern of PFT abnormalities has been identified.

MANAGEMENT

No specific treatment is available for PFF. Management is supportive and symptomatic, with antipyretics, analgesics, and/or antiinflammatory agents being adequate for most, and occasionally oxygen or ventilatory support for those with significant pulmonary effects. Inhaled bronchodilators should be given for any signs of bronchospasm. Corticosteroids have not been evaluated clinically. Patients should be observed for 24 to 48 hours to be

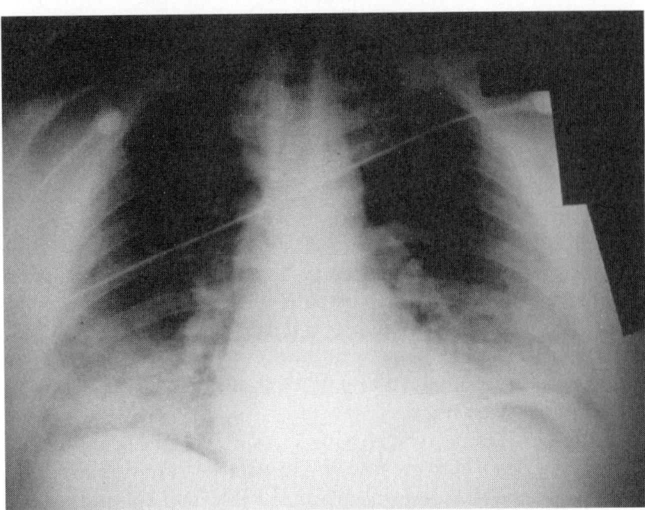

Figure 1. Chest x-ray after inhalation of fluorocarbon containing waterproofing agent.

certain significant pulmonary effects do not develop that require closer monitoring.

Cadmium Fume Pneumonitis

OVERVIEW AND PATHOPHYSIOLOGY

Inhalation of cadmium oxide or cadmium chloride fumes can cause a severe acute chemical pneumonitis that can be fatal (216–218). Such fumes may be generated during processes such as smelting, brazing, cutting, electroplating, or refining with cadmium or its alloys. Initially, symptoms of exposure resemble those of MFF, but severe interstitial pneumonitis appears to be a much more common sequela than with MFF or PFF (219). The pneumonitis related to cadmium develops 1 to 3 days after exposure and may take weeks to resolve (216). Because of its more severe course, cadmium fume inhalation should be considered a separate disease entity from MFF and PFF. Permanent fibrosis or loss of airspaces, or both, leading to obstructive or restrictive respiratory dysfunction may also occur as a result of either acute or chronic exposures to inhaled cadmium fumes (216,220–224). Renal insufficiency in association with acute cadmium fume poisoning has been reported (225). Chronic inhalation of cadmium fumes has been associated with an increased incidence of lung cancer and renal injury (226,227).

Exposures of cadmium fumes are rarely of sufficient magnitude to cause respiratory injury unless the patient has been exposed in an enclosed or poorly ventilated area (216). Although the injury is presumed to be a type of chemical pneumonitis, the pathophysiology has not been well studied. Autopsy studies show severe tracheobronchitis and parenchymal consolidation with alveolar hemorrhage and alveolar macrophages (218).

The ACGIH TLV (TWA) for respirable cadmium is 0.002 mg/m^3 cadmium. The OSHA PEL for cadmium fumes is 0.1 mg/m^3 as a TWA and 0.3 mg/m^3 as a ceiling concentration.

DIAGNOSIS

Symptoms of cadmium pneumonitis may initially resemble those of MFF. They include dyspnea, cough, wheezing, chest pain, and occasionally hemoptysis later in the course (218,228). Deaths from severe pulmonary edema and respiratory failure have been reported (216,218).

The diagnosis can be difficult. It may be mistaken for a nonspecific viral syndrome, atypical pneumonia, MFF, or other causes of noncardiogenic pulmonary edema or chemical pneumonitis. Unfortunately, the history may not be particularly useful because workers may not be aware that the metal they were working with contained cadmium. Furthermore, there are no readily available tests to distinguish cadmium fume pneumonitis from other similar syndromes. Analysis of the fumes is difficult to obtain and not likely to be available in the acute setting. Determination of cadmium levels in various biologic samples is also possible and may serve to corroborate the exposure and diagnosis. Such analyses are unlikely to be available in a clinically relevant time frame. Blood levels are more useful after acute exposures, whereas urine levels are better representatives of chronic exposure (216). If the patient has any respiratory complaints after a known or suspected cadmium inhalation exposure, a chest x-ray should be obtained for evidence of an interstitial infiltrate and the patient should be admitted to the hospital for observation.

Long-term respiratory impairment after chronic or acute cadmium exposures may present with dyspnea, cough, and restrictive or obstructive impairments on PFTs (221–224). Interstitial changes or signs of emphysema, or both, may be evident on a chest radiograph.

MANAGEMENT

Cadmium fume pneumonitis has no specific treatment. Symptomatic and supportive care should be provided. Inhaled bronchodilators should be administered for wheezing or any evidence of reversible bronchoconstriction. Supplemental oxygen and mechanical ventilatory support may be required in more severe cases. Steroids are recommended by some but have not been systematically evaluated for this indication (218,228). Patients suspected of having cadmium fume inhalation should be observed for at least 24 hours to watch for the development of severe respiratory involvement. Some have recommended bed rest or activity limitation in exposed patients to prevent or ameliorate the development of pulmonary edema, but this remains unproven (218). Chelation of cadmium with BAL or ethylenediaminetetraacetic acid is not recommended because it remains unproven and has its own associated risks (228). Unlike MFF or PFF, the pneumonitis associated with cadmium fume inhalation may lead to long-term restrictive respiratory dysfunction, although some improvement generally occurs with time (216,217,224).

Treatment for chronic respiratory dysfunction associated with cadmium fume inhalation is also symptomatic and supportive, with removal from exposure being the most important step.

IRRITANT-INDUCED PNEUMONITIS

The number of substances that have been reported to result in pneumonitis is legion. The potential for lung injury is dependent on a variety of factors, including the intensity and duration of exposure, the physical properties of the substance(s) involved, and preexisting lung disease. In general, it is useful to categorize substances according to their water-solubility characteristics. Substances that have high water solubility, such as ammonia (89.9 g/dl H_2O), typically have good warning properties because they cause immediate mucous membrane irritation. As a result, individuals who are exposed to these substances reflexively attempt to limit further exposure, which decreases the risk of injury. Although the full extent of injury may take hours to days to develop, the onset of significant pulmonary symptoms is evident relatively quickly after exposure to a water-soluble substance. Inhalation of substances with low water solubility, such as ozone (0.00003 g/dl H_2O), on the other hand, may result in the development of delayed pulmonary edema. Workers who present for evaluation after significant inhalational exposure to a substance with low water solubility should be monitored for several hours after the exposure. Asymptomatic patients can be discharged with instructions to return at the first sign of any respiratory problems. Symptomatic patients should be admitted for close monitoring of respiratory function.

Initial management is straightforward and involves removal from the exposure and provision of supplemental oxygen as needed to maintain adequate oxygenation. In severe cases, mechanical ventilation may be required. Ventilator settings should be adjusted so as to minimize secondary injury resulting from barotrauma and volutrauma (229). In some cases, the substance involved may also result in significant systemic toxicity that should be treated accordingly. Examples include arsenic, hydrocarbons, hydrofluoric acid, hydrogen sulfide, manganese, mercury, nickel carbonyl, nitriles, and smoke inhalation (carbon monoxide, cyanide).

OCCUPATIONAL ASTHMA

Overview

Occupational asthma accounts for approximately 2% to 15% of adult asthma (230). Chapter 11 provides a more detailed discussion on the evaluation and treatment of asthma as well as a list of potential causative agents. It is important to distinguish between preexisting asthma that may be exacerbated by workplace exposure from occupational asthma caused by the workplace environment. This distinction has implications for treatment as well as potential compensation for disability. It is also important to determine if the aggravation of symptoms results from simple irritants or from allergens, so that appropriate recommendations can be provided to workers regarding the advisability of their continued employment.

Exacerbation of Preexisting Asthma

Exposure to any number of irritants in the workplace, such as dusts, fumes, and smoke, may exacerbate preexisting asthma. Individuals with asthma exacerbated by simple irritants can often continue to work, provided that the exposure to irritants is limited and the asthma medication regimen is optimized so that symptoms are well controlled. Efforts to limit exposure may range from the personal respiratory protection to more elaborate engineering and ventilation controls. Exacerbations caused by an allergen may require complete removal of the exposure, either by relocating to a different section of the workplace, changing job duties, or changing jobs altogether.

Allergen-Induced Asthma

Asthma resulting from sensitization is the more common form of occupational asthma. Once an individual is sensitized to a particular substance, even minute exposure may provoke symptoms. In these cases, engineering controls and limiting exposure by changing job duties may not be sufficient to mitigate symptoms, and it may be necessary for the patient to change workplaces. Despite the inconvenience such changes may impose on the employee or employer, it should be emphasized that persistent airway inflammation can result in the permanent loss of function and progressive impairment over time.

Irritant-Induced Asthma

Irritant-induced asthma, or reactive airways dysfunction syndrome (RADS), occurs after a high-dose exposure to a respiratory irritant (231). The bronchospasm associated with this syndrome is typically transient but may persist for months or even years. Limitation of further exposure to irritants and standard asthma management should be used in these cases. The diagnosis of RADS can be made by provocation challenge testing. This may be either a specific challenge in a controlled chamber or to nonspecific bronchospasmogens such as methacholine. A properly performed negative methacholine challenge test tends to rule out RADS. Controversy exists regarding a single large exposure versus repeated exposures at somewhat lower levels. Contributing factors and preexisting bronchospasm must be considered in the evaluation of these patients.

LUNG CANCER

A detailed discussion of lung cancer and its causes is beyond the scope of this chapter. A list of probable and confirmed human occupational lung carcinogens, as classified by IARC, is included in Table 5. The diagnosis and management of lung cancers that are thought to be occupationally related are the same as for other forms of lung cancer.

TABLE 5. Definite and probable occupational/environmental lung carcinogens, as classified by International Agency for Research on Cancer

Definite	Probable
Arsenic, arsenates, arsenites	Acrylonitrile
Asbestos	Diesel exhaust
Bis-chloro-methyl-ether, chlorethers	Silica
Beryllium	
Cadmium	
Coke oven and coal gasification fumes	
Chromium	
Nickel	
Radon, radon daughters	
Soot	
Tobacco smoke	

Adapted from Steenland K, Loomis D, Shy C, et al. Review of occupational lung carcinogens. *Am J Ind Med* 1996;29(5):474–490.

REFERENCES

1. American Thoracic Society. Medical Section of the American Lung Association: the diagnosis of nonmalignant diseases related to asbestos. *Am Rev Respir Dis* 1986;134(2):363–368.
2. Wagner GR. Asbestosis and silicosis. *Lancet* 1997 May; 349(9061):1311–1315.
3. Jones RN, Hughes JM, Weill H. Asbestos exposure, asbestosis, and asbestos-attributable lung cancer. *Thorax* 1996;51[Suppl 2]:S9–S15.
4. National Institute of Occupational Safety and Health (NIOSH) CfDCC. *Work-related lung disease surveillance report.* Cincinnati: NIOSH, 1999.
5. Agency for Toxic Substances and Disease Registry (ATSDR). *Asbestos: toxicological profile.* Springfield, VA: ATSDR, 2001.
6. Occupational Safety and Health Administration (OSHA) DoL. *Asbestos standards for the construction industry.* Washington, DC: OSHA, 2002.
7. American Conference of Governmental Industrial Hygienists (ACGIH). *Threshold limit values for chemical substances and physical agents and biological exposure indices.* Cincinnati: ACGIH, 2001.
8. Occupational Safety and Health Administration (OSHA). Occupational safety and health standards—toxic and hazardous substances; standards 29 CFR 1910.1000, Tables Z-1, 2, and 3. Washington, DC.
9. Health Effects Institute (HEI)—Asbestos Research. *Asbestos in public and commercial buildings: a literature review and synthesis of current knowledge.* Cambridge, MA: HEI, 1991.
10. Hughes JM, Weill H. Asbestos exposure—quantitative assessment of risk. *Am Rev Respir Dis* 1986;133(1):5–13.
11. Lee RJ, Van Orden DR, Corn M, et al. Exposure to airborne asbestos in buildings. *Regul Toxicol Pharmacol* 1992;16(1):93–107.
12. Camus M, Siemiatycki J, Meek B. Nonoccupational exposure to chrysotile asbestos and the risk of lung cancer. *N Engl J Med* 1998;338(22):1565–1571.
13. Gamble JF. Asbestos and colon cancer: a weight-of-the-evidence review. *Environ Health Perspect* 1994;102(12):1038–1050.
14. Report on cancer risks associated with the ingestion of asbestos. DHHS Committee to Coordinate Environmental and Related Programs. *Environ Health Perspect* 1987;72:253–265.
15. Frumkin H, Berlin J. Asbestos exposure and gastrointestinal malignancy review and meta-analysis. *Am J Ind Med* 1988;14(1):79–95.
16. Kanarek MS. Epidemiological studies on ingested mineral fibres: gastric and other cancers. *IARC Sci Publ* 1989;(90):428-437.
17. Nicholson WJ, Selikoff IJ, Seidman H, et al. Long-term mortality experience of chrysotile miners and millers in Thetford Mines, Quebec. *Ann N Y Acad Sci* 1979;330:11–21.
18. Henderson VL, Enterline PE. Asbestos exposure: factors associated with excess cancer and respiratory disease mortality. *Ann N Y Acad Sci* 1979;330:117–126.
19. Dave SK, Ghodasara NB, Mohanrao N, et al. The relation of exposure to asbestos and smoking habit with pulmonary function tests and chest radiograph. *Ind J Public Health* 1997;41(1):16–24.
20. Wollmer P, Eriksson L, Jonson B, et al. Relation between lung function, exercise capacity, and exposure to asbestos cement. *Br J Ind Med* 1987;44(8):542–549.
21. McDonald AD, Fry JS, Woolley AJ, et al. Dust exposure and mortality in an American chrysotile textile plant. *Br J Ind Med* 1983;40(4):361–367.
22. Liddell FD, McDonald AD, McDonald JC. The 1891–1920 birth cohort of Quebec chrysotile miners and millers: development from 1904 and mortality to 1992. *Ann Occup Hyg* 1997;41(1):13–36.
23. Enterline PE, Hartley J, Henderson V. Asbestos and cancer: a cohort followed up to death. *Br J Ind Med* 1987;44(6):396–401.
24. Finkelstein MM. Mortality among long-term employees of an Ontario asbestos-cement factory. *Br J Ind Med* 1983;40(2):138–144.

25. Albin M, Horstmann V, Jakobsson K, et al. Survival in cohorts of asbestos cement workers and controls. *Occup Environ Med* 1996;53(2):87–93.
26. Hillerdal G. Non-malignant asbestos pleural disease. *Thorax* 1981;36(9):669–675.
27. Browne K, Gee JB. Asbestos exposure and laryngeal cancer. *Ann Occup Hyg* 2000;44(4):239–250.
28. Morgan A. Deposition of inhaled asbestos and man-made mineral fibres in the respiratory tract. *Ann Occup Hyg* 1995;39(5):747–758.
29. Timbrell V. Deposition and retention of fibres in the human lung. *Ann Occup Hyg* 1982;26(1–4):347–369.
30. Manning CB, Vallyathan V, Mossman BT. Diseases caused by asbestos: mechanisms of injury and disease development. *Int Immunopharmacol* 2002;2(2–3):191–200.
31. Kamp DW, Weitzman SA. Asbestosis: clinical spectrum and pathogenic mechanisms. *Proc Soc Exp Biol Med* 1997;214(1):12–26.
32. Bellmann B, Muhle H, Pott F, et al. Persistence of man-made mineral fibres (MMMF) and asbestos in rat lungs. *Ann Occup Hyg* 1987;31(4B):693–709.
33. Davis JM, Jones AD. Comparisons of the pathogenicity of long and short fibres of chrysotile asbestos in rats. *Br J Exp Pathol* 1988;69(5):717–737.
34. Dodson RF, Greenberg SD, Williams MG Jr, et al. Asbestos content in lungs of occupationally and nonoccupationally exposed individuals. *JAMA* 1984;252(1):68–71.
35. Roggli VL, Greenberg SD, Seitzman LH, et al. Pulmonary fibrosis, carcinoma, and ferruginous body counts in amosite asbestos workers. A study of six cases. *Am J Clin Pathol* 1980;73(4):496–503.
36. Davis JM. The long term fibrogenic effects of chrysotile and crocidolite asbestos dust injected into the pleural cavity of experimental animals. *Br J Exp Pathol* 1970;51(6):617–627.
37. Quinlan TR, Berube KA, Marsh JP, et al. Patterns of inflammation, cell proliferation, and related gene expression in lung after inhalation of chrysotile asbestos. *Am J Pathol* 1995;147(3):728–739.
38. Chang LY, Overby LH, Brody AR, et al. Progressive lung cell reactions and extracellular matrix production after a brief exposure to asbestos. *Am J Pathol* 1988;131(1):156–170.
39. Miller K. The effects of asbestos on macrophages. *CRC Crit Rev Toxicol* 1978;5(4):319–354.
40. Pinkerton KE, Pratt PC, Brody AR, et al. Fiber localization and its relationship to lung reaction in rats after chronic inhalation of chrysotile asbestos. *Am J Pathol* 1984;117(3):484–498.
41. Geist LJ, Powers LS, Monick MM, et al. Asbestos stimulation triggers differential cytokine release from human monocytes and alveolar macrophages. *Exp Lung Res* 2000;26(1):41–56.
42. Finkelstein M. Pulmonary function in asbestos cement workers: a dose-response study. *Br J Ind Med* 1986;43(6):406–413.
43. Balmes J, Cullen MR, Gee JB. What infections occur in patients with occupational lung disease? *Clin Chest Med* 1981;2(1):111–120.
44. Selikoff IJ, Hammond EC, Seidman H. Mortality experience of insulation workers in the United States and Canada, 1943–1976. *Ann N Y Acad Sci* 1979;330:91–116.
45. Browne K. A threshold for asbestos related lung cancer. *Br J Ind Med* 1986;43(8):556–558.
46. Wilkinson P, Hansell DM, Janssens J, et al. Is lung cancer associated with asbestos exposure when there are no small opacities on the chest radiograph? *Lancet* 1995;345(8957):1074–1078.
47. Kipen HM, Lilis R, Suzuki Y, et al. Pulmonary fibrosis in asbestos insulation workers with lung cancer: a radiological and histopathological evaluation. *Br J Ind Med* 1987;44(2):96–100.
48. Hughes JM, Weill H. Asbestosis as a precursor of asbestos related lung cancer: results of a prospective mortality study. *Br J Ind Med* 1991;48(4):229–233.
49. Sluis-Cremer GK, Bezuidenhout BN. Relation between asbestosis and bronchial cancer in amphibole asbestos miners. *Br J Ind Med* 1989;46(8):537–540.
50. Hammond EC, Selikoff IJ, Seidman H. Asbestos exposure, cigarette smoking and death rates. *Ann N Y Acad Sci* 1979;330:473–490.
51. Hasan FM, Nash G, Kazemi H. The significance of asbestos exposure in the diagnosis of mesothelioma: a 28-year experience from a major urban hospital. *Am Rev Respir Dis* 1977;115(5):761–768.
52. Ehrlich R, Lilis R, Chan E, et al. Long term radiological effects of short term exposure to amosite asbestos among factory workers. *Br J Ind Med* 1992;49(4):268–275.
53. Boutin G, Viallat JR, Steinbauer J, et al. Bilateral pleural plaques in Corsica: a marker of non-occupational asbestos exposure. *IARC Sci Publ* 1989;(90):406–410.
54. Harber P, Mohsenifar Z, Oren A, et al. Pleural plaques and asbestos-associated malignancy. *J Occup Med* 1987;29(8):641–644.
55. Weiss W. Asbestos-related pleural plaques and lung cancer. *Chest* 1993;103(6):1854–1859.
56. Andrion A, Colombo A, Mollo F. Lung asbestos bodies and pleural plaques at autopsy. *Ric Clin Lab* 1982;12(3):461–468.
57. Rosenstock L, Hudson LD. The pleural manifestations of asbestos exposure. *Occup Med* 1987;2(2):383–407.
58. Bohlig H, Hain E. Clinical and radiological observations on asbestos-related pathology. *IARC Sci Publ* 1980;(30):497–506.
59. Selikoff IJ, Churg J, Hammond EC. The occurrence of asbestosis among insulation workers in the United States. *Ann N Y Acad Sci* 1965;132(1):139–155.
60. Kleinfeld M, Messite J, Kooyman O, et al. Effect of asbestos dust inhalation on lung function. *Arch Environ Health* 1966;12(6):741–746.
61. Gefter WB, Conant EF. Issues and controversies in the plain-film diagnosis of asbestos-related disorders in the chest. *J Thorac Imaging* 1988;3(4):11–28.
62. Aberle DR, Gamsu G, Ray CS. High-resolution CT of benign asbestos-related diseases: clinical and radiographic correlation. *AJR Am J Roentgenol* 1988;151(5):883–891.
63. Jones RN, McLoud T, Rockoff SD. The radiographic pleural abnormalities in asbestos exposure: relationship to physiologic abnormalities. *J Thorac Imaging* 1988;3(4):57–66.
64. Becklake MR, Fournier-Massey G, Rossiter CE, et al. Lung function in chrysotile asbestos mine and mill workers of Quebec. *Arch Environ Health* 1972;24(6):401–409.
65. Murphy RL Jr, Gaensler EA, Ferris BG, et al. Diagnosis of "asbestosis." Observations from a longitudinal survey of shipyard pipe coverers. *Am J Med* 1978;65(3):488–498.
66. Miller A, Lilis R, Godbold J, et al. Spirometric impairments in long-term insulators. Relationships to duration of exposure, smoking, and radiographic abnormalities. *Chest* 1994;105(1):175–182.
67. Hourihane DO, McCaughey WT. Pathological aspects of asbestosis. *Postgrad Med J* 1966;42(492):613–622.
68. Green FH, Attfield M. Pathology standards for asbestosis. *Scand J Work Environ Health* 1983;9(2 Spec No):162–168.
69. Lilis R, Lerman Y, Selikoff IJ. Symptomatic benign pleural effusions among asbestos insulation workers: residual radiographic abnormalities. *Br J Ind Med* 1988;45(7):443–449.
70. Algranti E, Mendonca EM, DeCapitani EM, et al. Non-malignant asbestos-related diseases in Brazilian asbestos-cement workers. *Am J Ind Med* 2001;40(3):240–254.
71. Begin R, Cantin A, Masse S, et al. Contributions of experimental asbestosis in sheep to the understanding of asbestosis. *Ann N Y Acad Sci* 1991;643:228–238.
72. Becklake MR, Liddell FD, Manfreda J, et al. Radiological changes after withdrawal from asbestos exposure. *Br J Ind Med* 1979 Feb;36(1):23–28.
73. Ho L, Sugarbaker DJ, Skarin AT. Malignant pleural mesothelioma. *Cancer Treat Res* 2001;105:327–373.
74. Sugarbaker DJ, Garcia JP. Multimodality therapy for malignant pleural mesothelioma. *Chest* 1997;112[4 Suppl]:272S–275S.
75. Stokholm J, Norn M, Schneider T. Ophthalmologic effects of man-made mineral fibers. *Scand J Work Environ Health* 1982;8(3):185–190.
76. Berrigan D. Respiratory cancer and exposure to man-made vitreous fibers: a systematic review. *Am J Ind Med* 2002;42(4):354–362.
77. Lippmann M. Man-made mineral fibers (MMMF): human exposures and health risk assessment. *Toxicol Ind Health* 1990;6(2):225–246.
78. Simonato L, Fletcher AC, Cherrie J, et al. The man-made mineral fiber European historical cohort study. Extension of the follow-up. *Scand J Work Environ Health* 1986;12[Suppl 1]:34–47.
79. Enterline PE, Marsh GM, Henderson V, et al. Mortality update of a cohort of U.S. man-made mineral fibre workers. *Ann Occup Hyg* 1987;31(4B):625–656.
80. Miettinen OS, Rossiter CE. Man-made mineral fibers and lung cancer. Epidemiologic evidence regarding the causal hypothesis. *Scand J Work Environ Health* 1990;16(4):221–231.
81. Doll R. Symposium on MMMF, Copenhagen, October 1986: overview and conclusions. *Ann Occup Hyg* 1987;31(4B):805–819.
82. Eisenbud M, Lisson J. Epidemiological aspects of beryllium-induced non-malignant lung disease: a 30-year update. *J Occup Med* 1983;25(3):196–202.
83. Kreiss K, Mroz MM, Newman LS, et al. Machining risk of beryllium disease and sensitization with median exposures below 2 micrograms/m^3. *Am J Ind Med* 1996;30(1):16–25.
84. Kreiss K, Mroz MM, Zhen B, et al. Epidemiology of beryllium sensitization and disease in nuclear workers. *Am Rev Respir Dis* 1993;148(4 Pt 1):985–991.
85. Kriebel D, Sprince NL, Eisen EA, et al. Beryllium exposure and pulmonary function: a cross sectional study of beryllium workers. *Br J Ind Med* 1988;45(3):167–173.
86. Levy PS, Roth HD, Hwang PM, et al. Beryllium and lung cancer: a reanalysis of a NIOSH cohort mortality study. *Inhal Toxicol* 2002;14(10):1003–1015.
87. Mancuso TF. Mortality study of beryllium industry workers' occupational lung cancer. *Environ Res* 1980 Feb;21(1):48–55.
88. MacMahon B. The epidemiological evidence on the carcinogenicity of beryllium in humans. *J Occup Med* 1994;36(1):15–24; discussion 25–26.
89. Infante PF, Wagoner JK, Sprince NL. Mortality patterns from lung cancer and nonneoplastic respiratory disease among white males in the beryllium case registry. *Environ Res* 1980 Feb;21(1):35–43.
90. Wagoner JK, Infante PF, Bayliss DL. Beryllium: an etiologic agent in the induction of lung cancer, nonneoplastic respiratory disease, and heart disease among industrially exposed workers. *Environ Res* 1980 Feb;21(1):15–34.
91. Meyer KC. Beryllium and lung disease. *Chest* 1994;106(3):942–946.
92. VanOrdstrand HS, Hughes R, DeNardi JM, et al. Beryllium poisoning. *JAMA* 1945;129:1084–1090.
93. Eisenbud M, Berghout CF, Steadman LT. Environmental studies in plants and laboratories using beryllium: the acute disease. *J Ind Hyg Toxicol* 1948;30:281–285.
94. Newman LS, Kreiss K, King TE Jr, et al. Pathologic and immunologic alterations in early stages of beryllium disease. Re-examination of disease definition and natural history. *Am Rev Respir Dis* 1989;139(6):1479–1486.

95. Cotes JE, Gilson JC, McKerrow CB, et al. A long-term follow-up of workers exposed to beryllium. *Br J Ind Med* 1983 Feb;40(1):13–21.
96. Hardy HL, Tabershaw IR. Delayed chemical pneumonitis occurring in workers exposed to beryllium compounds. *J Ind Hyg Toxicol* 1946;28:197–211.
97. Cullen MR, Kominsky JR, Rossman MD, et al. Chronic beryllium disease in a precious metal refinery. Clinical epidemiologic and immunologic evidence for continuing risk from exposure to low level beryllium fume. *Am Rev Respir Dis* 1987;135(1):201–208.
98. Stange AW, Hilmas DE, Furman FJ, et al. Beryllium sensitization and chronic beryllium disease at a former nuclear weapons facility. *Appl Occup Environ Hyg* 2001;16(3):405–417.
99. Kreiss K, Mroz MM, Zhen B, et al. Risks of beryllium disease related to work processes at a metal, alloy, and oxide production plant. *Occup Environ Med* 1997;54(8):605–612.
100. Saltini C, Winestock K, Kirby M, et al. Maintenance of alveolitis in patients with chronic beryllium disease by beryllium-specific helper T cells. *N Engl J Med* 1989;320:1103–1109.
101. Fontenot AP, Torres M, Marshall WH, et al. Beryllium presentation to CD4+ T cells underlies disease-susceptibility HLA-DP alleles in chronic beryllium disease. *Proc Natl Acad Sci U S A* 2000;97(23):12717–12722.
102. Bost TW, Riches DWH, Schumacher B, et al. Alveolar macrophages from patients with beryllium disease and sarcoidosis express increased levels of mRNA for TNF-α and IL-6 but not IL-1β. *Am J Respir Cell Mol Biol* 1994;10:506–513.
103. Tinkle SS, Schwitters PW, Newman LS. Cytokine production by bronchoalveolar lavage cells in chronic beryllium disease. *Environ Health Perspect* 1996;104:969–971.
104. Freiman DG, Hardy HL. Beryllium disease. The relation of pulmonary pathology to clinical course and prognosis based on a study of 130 cases from the U.S. beryllium case registry. *Hum Pathol* 1970;1(1):25–44.
105. McConnochie K, Williams WR, Kilpatrick GS, et al. Chronic beryllium disease in identical twins. *Br J Dis Chest* 1988;82(4):431–435.
106. Sprince NL, Kazemi H, Hardy HL. Current (1975) problem of differentiating between beryllium disease and sarcoidosis. *Ann N Y Acad Sci* 1976;278:654–664.
107. Stoeckle JD, Kazemi H, Chamberlin R. Exposure, complaints, chest film abnormalities and lung function tests among beryllium workers: preliminary report. *J Occup Med* 1973;15(3):301.
108. Stoeckle JD, Hardy HL, Weber AL. Chronic beryllium disease. Long-term follow-up of sixty cases and selective review of the literature. *Am J Med* 1969;46(4):545–561.
109. Aronchick JM, Rossman MD, Miller WT. Chronic beryllium disease: diagnosis, radiographic findings, and correlation with pulmonary function tests. *Radiology* 1987;163(3):677–682.
110. Newman LS, Buschman DL, Newell JD Jr, et al. Beryllium disease: assessment with CT. *Radiology* 1994;190(3):835–840.
111. Rossman MD, Kern JA, Elias JA, et al. Proliferative response of bronchoalveolar lymphocytes to beryllium. A test for chronic beryllium disease. *Ann Intern Med* 1988;108(5):687–693.
112. Beryllium disease among workers in a spacecraft-manufacturing plant—California. *MMWR Morb Mortal Wkly Rep* 1983;32(32):419–420, 425.
113. Pappas GP, Newman LS. Early pulmonary physiologic abnormalities in beryllium disease. *Am Rev Respir Dis* 1993;148(3):661–666.
114. Andrews JL, Kazemi H, Hardy HL. Patterns of lung dysfunction in chronic beryllium disease. *Am Rev Respir Dis* 1969;100(6):791–800.
115. Epstein PE, Dauber JH, Rossman MD, et al. Bronchoalveolar lavage in a patient with chronic berylliosis: evidence for hypersensitivity pneumonitis. *Ann Intern Med* 1982;97(2):213–216.
116. Deubner DC, Goodman M, Iannuzzi J. Variability, predictive value, and uses of the beryllium blood lymphocyte proliferation test (BLPT): preliminary analysis of the ongoing workforce survey. *Appl Occup Environ Hyg* 2001;16(5):521–526.
117. Williams WJ, Wallach ER. Laser microprobe mass spectrometry (LAMMS) analysis of beryllium, sarcoidosis and other granulomatous diseases. *Sarcoidosis* 1989;6(2):111–117.
118. Sprince NL, Kanarek DJ, Weber AL, et al. Reversible respiratory disease in beryllium workers. *Am Rev Respir Dis* 1978;117(6):1011–1017.
119. Rustin MH, Bull HA, Ziegler V, et al. Silica-associated systemic sclerosis is clinically, serologically and immunologically indistinguishable from idiopathic systemic sclerosis. *Br J Dermatol* 1990;123(6):725–734.
120. Sluis-Cremer GK, Hessel PA, Hnizdo E, et al. Relationship between silicosis and rheumatoid arthritis. *Thorax* 1986;41(8):596–601.
121. Steenland NK, Thun MJ, Ferguson CW, et al. Occupational and other exposures associated with male end-stage renal disease: a case/control study. *Am J Public Health* 1990 Feb;80(2):153–157.
122. Adverse effects of crystalline silica exposure. American Thoracic Society Committee of the Scientific Assembly on Environmental and Occupational Health. *Am J Respir Crit Care Med* 1997 Feb;155(2):761–768.
123. Ziskind M, Jones RN, Weill H. Silicosis. *Am Rev Respir Dis* 1976;113(5):643–665.
124. Cowie RL, Hay M, Thomas RG. Association of silicosis, lung dysfunction, and emphysema in gold miners. *Thorax* 1993;48(7):746–749.
125. Davis GS. The pathogenesis of silicosis. State of the art. *Chest* 1986;89[3 Suppl]:166S–169S.
126. Koskinen H. Symptoms and clinical findings in patients with silicosis. *Scand J Work Environ Health* 1985;11(2):101–106.
127. Ng TP, Chan SL. Lung function in relation to silicosis and silica exposure in granite workers. *Eur Respir J* 1992;5(8):986–991.
128. Ziskind M, Weill H, Anderson AE, et al. Silicosis in shipyard sandblasters. *Environ Res* 1976;11(2):237–243.
129. Hnizdo E, Sluis-Cremer GK. Risk of silicosis in a cohort of white South African gold miners. *Am J Ind Med* 1993;24(4):447–457.
130. Cowie RL, Mabena SK. Silicosis, chronic airflow limitation, and chronic bronchitis in South African gold miners. *Am Rev Respir Dis* 1991;143(1):80–84.
131. Hughes JM, Jones RN, Gilson JC, et al. Determinants of progression in sandblasters' silicosis. *Ann Occup Hyg* 1982;26(1–4):701–712.
132. Hnizdo E, Murray J, Sluis-Cremer GK, et al. Correlation between radiological and pathological diagnosis of silicosis: an autopsy population based study. *Am J Ind Med* 1993;24(4):427–445.
133. White NW, Chetty R, Bateman ED. Silicosis among gemstone workers in South Africa: tiger's-eye pneumoconiosis. *Am J Ind Med* 1991;19(2):205–213.
134. Joyce BW, Mejia E, Puruckherr M, Roy TM. Progressive massive fibrosis in a zinc miner. *J Ky Med Assoc* 1996;94(4):144–147.
135. Ng TP, Allan WG, Tsin TW, et al. Silicosis in jade workers. *Br J Ind Med* 1985;42(11):761–764.
136. Jiang CQ, Xiao LW, Lam TH, et al. Accelerated silicosis in workers exposed to agate dust in Guangzhou, China. *Am J Ind Med* 2001;40(1):87–91.
137. Ehrlich RI, Gerston KF, Lalloo UG. Accelerated silicosis in a foundry shotblaster. A case report. *S Afr Med J* 1988;73(2):128–130.
138. Seaton A, Legge JS, Henderson J, et al. Accelerated silicosis in Scottish stonemasons. *Lancet* 1991 Feb;337(8737):341–344.
139. Vallyathan V, Castranova V, Pack D, et al. Freshly fractured quartz inhalation leads to enhanced lung injury and inflammation. Potential role of free radicals. *Am J Respir Crit Care Med* 1995;152(3):1003–1009.
140. Marchiori E, Ferreira A, Muller NL. Silicoproteinosis: high-resolution CT and histologic findings. *J Thorac Imaging* 2001;16(2):127–129.
141. Xipell JM, Ham KN, Price CG, et al. Acute silicoproteinosis. *Thorax* 1977 Feb;32(1):104–111.
142. Snider DE Jr. The relationship between tuberculosis and silicosis. *Am Rev Respir Dis* 1978;118(3):455–460.
143. Sherson D, Lander F. Morbidity of pulmonary tuberculosis among silicotic and nonsilicotic foundry workers in Denmark. *J Occup Med* 1990;32(2):110–113.
144. Cowie RL. The epidemiology of tuberculosis in gold miners with silicosis. *Am J Respir Crit Care Med* 1994;150(5 Pt 1):1460–1462.
145. Dubrow R, Wegman DH. Cancer and occupation in Massachusetts: a death certificate study. *Am J Ind Med* 1984;6(3):207–230.
146. Siemiatycki J, Gerin M, Dewar R, et al. Silica and cancer associations from a multicancer occupational exposure case-referent study. *IARC Sci Publ* 1990;(97):29–42.
147. Lynge E, Kurppa K, Kristofersen L, et al. Silica dust and lung cancer: results from the Nordic occupational mortality and cancer incidence registers. *J Natl Cancer Inst* 1986;77(4):883–889.
148. Chiyotani K, Saito K, Okubo T, et al. Lung cancer risk among pneumoconiosis patients in Japan, with special reference to silicotics. *IARC Sci Publ* 1990;(97):95–104.
149. Weill H, McDonald JC. Exposure to crystalline silica and risk of lung cancer: the epidemiological evidence. *Thorax* 1996;51(1):97–102.
150. Ng TP, Phoon WH, Lee HS, et al. An epidemiological survey of respiratory morbidity among granite quarry workers in Singapore: chronic bronchitis and lung function impairment. *Ann Acad Med Singapore* 1992;21(3):312–317.
151. Holman CD, Psaila-Savona P, Roberts M, et al. Determinants of chronic bronchitis and lung dysfunction in Western Australian gold miners. *Br J Ind Med* 1987;44(12):810–818.
152. Lee HS, Phoon WH, Ng TP. Radiological progression and its predictive risk factors in silicosis. *Occup Environ Med* 2001;58(7):467–471.
153. Cowie RL. The influence of silicosis on deteriorating lung function in gold miners. *Chest* 1998;113(2):340–343.
154. Suratt PM, Winn WC Jr, Brody AR, et al. Acute silicosis in tombstone sandblasters. *Am Rev Respir Dis* 1977;115(3):521–529.
154a. Jones RN, Turner-Warwick M, Ziskind M, et al. High prevalence of antinuclear antibodies in sandblasters' silicosis. *Am Rev Resp Dis* 1976;113:393–396.
155. Fairman RP, O'Brien RJ, Swecker S, et al. Respiratory status of surface coal miners in the United States. *Arch Environ Health* 1977;32(5):211–215.
156. Bates DV, Pham QT, Chau N, et al. A longitudinal study of pulmonary function in coal miners in Lorraine, France. *Am J Ind Med* 1985;8(1):21–32.
157. Seixas NS, Robins TG, Attfield MD, et al. Longitudinal and cross sectional analyses of exposure to coal mine dust and pulmonary function in new miners. *Br J Ind Med* 1993;50(10):929–937.
158. Schins RP, Borm PJ. Mechanisms and mediators in coal dust induced toxicity: a review. *Ann Occup Hyg* 1999;43(1):7–33.
159. Musk AW, Cotes JE, Bevan C, et al. Relationship between type of simple coalworkers' pneumoconiosis and lung function. A nine-year follow-up study of subjects with small rounded opacities. *Br J Ind Med* 1981;38(4):313–320.
160. Henneberger PK, Attfield MD. Respiratory symptoms and spirometry in experienced coal miners: effects of both distant and recent coal mine dust exposures. *Am J Ind Med* 1997;32(3):268–274.
161. Henneberger PK, Attfield MD. Coal mine dust exposure and spirometry in experienced miners. *Am J Respir Crit Care Med* 1996;153(5):1560–1566.

162. Solley GO, Hyatt RE. Hypersensitivity pneumonitis induced by *Penicillium* species. *J Allergy Clin Immunol* 1980;65(1):65–70.
163. van Assendelft A, Forsen KO, Keskinen H, et al. Humidifier-associated extrinsic allergic alveolitis. *Scand J Work Environ Health* 1979;5(1):35–41.
164. Nakazawa T, Tochigi T. Hypersensitivity pneumonitis due to mushroom *(Pholiota nameko)* spores. *Chest* 1989;95(5):1149–1151.
165. Yoshizawa Y, Ohtsuka M, Noguchi K, et al. Hypersensitivity pneumonitis induced by toluene diisocyanate: sequelae of continuous exposure. *Ann Intern Med* 1989;110(1):31–34.
166. Dykewicz MS, Laufer P, Patterson R, et al. Woodman's disease: hypersensitivity pneumonitis from cutting live trees. *J Allergy Clin Immunol* 1988;81(2):455–460.
167. Huuskonen MS, Husman K, Jarvisalo J, et al. Extrinsic allergic alveolitis in the tobacco industry. *Br J Ind Med* 1984;41(1):77–83.
168. Nicholls MG, Gratten MJ, Taylor BW, et al. Pigeon breeder's disease: two case reports. *NZ Med J* 1973;77(490):160–162.
169. Campbell JA, Kryda MJ, Treuhaft MW, et al. Cheese worker's hypersensitivity pneumonitis. *Am Rev Respir Dis* 1983;127(4):495–496.
170. Nakagawa-Yoshida K, Ando M, Etches RI, et al. Fatal cases of farmer's lung in a Canadian family. Probable new antigens, *Penicillium brevicompactum* and *P. olivicolor*. *Chest* 1997;111(1):245–248.
171. Barrowcliff DF, Arblaster PG. Farmer's lung: a study of an early acute fatal case. *Thorax* 1968;23(5):490–500.
172. Patterson R, Sommers H, Fink JN. Farmer's lung following inhalation of *Aspergillus flavus* growing in moldy corn. *Clin Allergy* 1974;4(1):79–86.
173. Leatherman JW, Michael AF, Schwartz BA, et al. Lung T cells in hypersensitivity pneumonitis. *Ann Intern Med* 1984;100(3):390–392.
174. Semenzato G, Agostini C, Zambello R, et al. Lung T cells in hypersensitivity pneumonitis: phenotypic and functional analyses. *J Immunol* 1986;137(4):1164–1172.
175. Brummund W, Kurup VP, Resnick A, et al. Immunologic response to *Faenia rectivirgula (Micropolyspora faeni)* in a dairy farm family. *J Allergy Clin Immunol* 1988;82(2):190–195.
176. Cormier Y, Belanger J, Laviolette M. Prognostic significance of bronchoalveolar lymphocytosis in farmer's lung. *Am Rev Respir Dis* 1987;135(3):692–695.
177. Drent M, Grutters JC, Mulder PG, et al. Is the different T helper cell activity in sarcoidosis and extrinsic allergic alveolitis also reflected by the cellular bronchoalveolar lavage fluid profile? *Sarcoidosis Vasc Diffuse Lung Dis* 1997;14(1):31–38.
178. Teschler H, Thompson AB, Pohl WR, et al. Bronchoalveolar lavage procollagen-III-peptide in recent onset hypersensitivity pneumonitis: correlation with extracellular matrix components. *Eur Respir J* 1993;6(5):709–714.
179. Bensadoun ES, Burke AK, Hogg JC, et al. Proteoglycans in granulomatous lung diseases. *Eur Respir J* 1997;10(12):2731–2737.
180. Fink JN. Clinical features of hypersensitivity pneumonitis. *Chest* 1986;89[3 Suppl]:193S–195S.
181. Sutinen S, Reijula K, Huhti E, et al. Extrinsic allergic bronchiolo-alveolitis: serology and biopsy findings. *Eur J Respir Dis* 1983;64(4):271–282.
182. Wenzel FJ, Gray RL, Roberts RC, et al. Serologic studies in farmer's lung. Precipitins to the thermophilic actinomycetes. *Am Rev Respir Dis* 1974;109(4):464–468.
183. Ojanen T. Class specific antibodies in serodiagnosis of farmer's lung. *Br J Ind Med* 1992;49(5):332–336.
184. Kaukonen K, Savolainen J, Viander M, et al. IgG and IgA subclass antibodies against *Aspergillus umbrosus* in farmer's lung disease. *Clin Exp Allergy* 1993;23(10):851–856.
185. Kokkarinen J, Tukiainen H, Terho EO. Mortality due to farmer's lung in Finland. *Chest* 1994;106(2):509–512.
186. Carlsen KH, Leegaard J, Lund OD, et al. Allergic alveolitis in a 12-year-old boy: treatment with budesonide nebulizing solution. *Pediatr Pulmonol* 1992;12(4):257–259.
187. Von Essen S, Robbins RA, Thompson AB, et al. Organic dust toxic syndrome: an acute febrile reaction to organic dust exposure distinct from hypersensitivity pneumonitis. *J Toxicol Clin Toxicol* 1990;28(4):389–420.
188. Emanuel DA, Wenzel FJ, Lawton BR. Pulmonary mycotoxicosis. *Chest* 1975;67(3):293–297.
189. Von Essen S, Fryzek J, Nowakowski B, et al. Respiratory symptoms and farming practices in farmers associated with an acute febrile illness after organic dust exposure. *Chest* 1999;116(5):1452–1458.
190. May JJ, Stallones L, Darrow D, et al. Organic dust toxicity (pulmonary mycotoxicosis) associated with silo unloading. *Thorax* 1986;41(12):919–923.
191. Rask-Andersen A. Organic dust toxic syndrome among farmers. *Br J Ind Med* 1989;46(4):233–238.
192. Malmberg P, Rask-Andersen A, Palmgren U, et al. Exposure to microorganisms, febrile and airway-obstructive symptoms, immune status and lung function of Swedish farmers. *Scand J Work Environ Health* 1985;11(4):287–293.
193. Pratt DS, May JJ. Feed-associated respiratory illness in farmers. *Arch Environ Health* 1984;39(1):43–48.
194. Lecours R, Laviolette M, Cormier Y. Bronchoalveolar lavage in pulmonary mycotoxicosis (organic dust toxic syndrome). *Thorax* 1986;41(12):924–926.
195. May JJ, Marvel LH, Pratt DS, et al. Organic dust toxic syndrome: a follow-up study. *Am J Ind Med* 1990;17(1):111–113.
196. Rylander R. Health effects of cotton dust exposures. *Am J Ind Med* 1990;17(1):39–45.
197. Bouhuys A, Heaphy LJ Jr, Schilling RS, et al. Byssinosis in the United States. *N Engl J Med* 1967;277(4):170–175.
198. Castellan RM, Olenchock SA, Kinsley KB, et al. Inhaled endotoxin and decreased spirometric values. An exposure-response relation for cotton dust. *N Engl J Med* 1987;317(10):605–610.
199. McKerrow CB, McDermott M, Gilson JC, et al. Respiratory function during the day in cotton workers: a study in byssinosis. *Br J Ind Med* 1958;15:75–83.
200. Tockman MS, Baser M. Is cotton dust exposure associated with chronic effects? *Am Rev Respir Dis* 1984;130(1):1–3.
201. Kaye P, Young H, O'Sullivan I. Metal fume fever: a case report and review of the literature. *Emerg Med J* 2002;19(3):268–269.
202. Blanc P, Wong H, Bernstein MS, et al. An experimental human model of metal fume fever. *Ann Intern Med* 1991;114(11):930–936.
203. Armstrong CW, Moore LW Jr, Hackler RL, et al. An outbreak of metal fume fever. Diagnostic use of urinary copper and zinc determinations. *J Occup Med* 1983;25(12):886–888.
204. Stoke J. Metal fume fever in ferro-chrome workers. *Cent Afr J Med* 1977;23(2):25–28.
205. Kuschner WG, D'Alessandro A, Hambleton J, et al. Tumor necrosis factor-alpha and interleukin-8 release from U937 human mononuclear cells exposed to zinc oxide in vitro. Mechanistic implications for metal fume fever. *J Occup Environ Med* 1998;40(5):454–459.
206. Kuschner WG, D'Alessandro A, Wong H, et al. Early pulmonary cytokine responses to zinc oxide fume inhalation. *Environ Res* 1997;75(1):7–11.
207. Malo JL, Cartier A. Occupational asthma due to fumes of galvanized metal. *Chest* 1987;92(2):375–377.
208. Shusterman DJ. Polymer fume fever and other fluorocarbon pyrolysis-related syndromes. *Occup Med* 1993;8(3):519–531.
209. Sprout WL. Polymer-fume fever. *J Occup Med* 1988;30(4):296, 300.
210. Harris DK. Polymer-fume fever. *Lancet* 1951;2:1008–1011.
211. Lewis CE, Kerby GR. An epidemic of polymer-fume fever. *JAMA* 1965;191:103–106.
212. Wegman DH, Peters JM. Polymer fume fever and cigarette smoking. *Ann Intern Med* 1974;81(1):55–57.
213. Arito H, Soda R. Pyrolysis products of polytetrafluoroethylene and polyfluoroethylenepropylene with reference to inhalation toxicity. *Ann Occup Hyg* 1977;20(3):247–255.
214. Pryor WA, Nuggehalli SK, Scherer KV Jr, et al. An electron spin resonance study of the particles produced in the pyrolysis of perfluoro polymers. *Chem Res Toxicol* 1990;3(1):2–7.
215. Zook BC, Malek DE, Kenney RA. Pathologic findings in rats following inhalation of combustion products of polytetrafluoroethylene (PTFE). *Toxicology* 1983;26(1):25–36.
216. Barnhart S, Rosenstock L. Cadmium chemical pneumonitis. *Chest* 1984;86(5):789–791.
217. Beton DC, Andrews GS, Davies HJ, et al. Acute cadmium fume poisoning. Five cases with one death from renal necrosis. *Br J Ind Med* 1966;23(4):292–301.
218. Blejer HP, Caplan PE, Alcocer AE. Acute cadmium fume poisoning in welders—a fatal and a nonfatal case in California. *Calif Med* 1966;105(4):290–296.
219. Johnson JS, Kilburn KH. Cadmium induced metal fume fever: results of inhalation challenge. *Am J Ind Med* 1983;4(4):533–540.
220. Hendrick DJ. Occupational and chronic obstructive pulmonary disease (COPD). *Thorax* 1996;51(9):947–955.
221. Smith TJ, Petty TL, Reading JC, et al. Pulmonary effects of chronic exposure to airborne cadmium. *Am Rev Respir Dis* 1976;114(1):161–169.
222. Sakurai H, Omae K, Toyama T, et al. Cross-sectional study of pulmonary function in cadmium alloy workers. *Scand J Work Environ Health* 1982;[8 Suppl 1]:122–130.
223. Davison AG, Fayers PM, Taylor AJ, et al. Cadmium fume inhalation and emphysema. *Lancet* 1988;1(8587):663–667.
224. Anthony JS, Zamel N, Aberman A. Abnormalities in pulmonary function after brief exposure to toxic metal fumes. *Can Med Assoc J* 1978;119(6):586–588.
225. Ando Y, Shibata E, Tsuchiyama F, et al. Elevated urinary cadmium concentrations in a patient with acute cadmium pneumonitis. *Scand J Work Environ Health* 1996;22(2):150–153.
226. Oberdorster G. Airborne cadmium and carcinogenesis of the respiratory tract. *Scand J Work Environ Health* 1986;12(6):523–537.
227. De Silva PE, Donnan MB. Chronic cadmium poisoning in a pigment manufacturing plant. *Br J Ind Med* 1981;38(1):76–86.
228. Dunphy B. Acute occupational cadmium poisoning. A critical review of the literature. *J Occup Med* 1967;9(1):22–26.
229. Brower RG, Rubenfeld GD. Lung-protective ventilations strategies in acute lung injury. *Crit Care Med* 2003;31[4 Suppl]:S312–S316.
230. Draper A. Occupational asthma. *J Asthma* 2002;39(1):1–10.
231. Brooks SM, Weiss MA, Bernstein IL. Reactive airways dysfunction syndrome. Case reports of persistent asthma syndrome after high level irritant exposure. *Chest* 1985;88:376–384.

CHAPTER 190

Smoke Inhalation Injury

Geoffrey L. Bauer and Rick A. Gimbel

Compounds included:	**Simple asphyxiants (carbon dioxide, methane, many others), chemical asphyxiants (carbon monoxide, cyanide, methemoglobin), chemical irritants (chlorine, phosgene, various aldehydes and acids)**
SI conversion:	**Not applicable**
Special concerns:	**Most exposures involve complex mixtures of smoke and chemicals. Life-threatening effects may have delayed onset.**
Antidotes:	**Oxygen, cyanide antidote kit, methylene blue**

OVERVIEW

The deadly effects of smoke inhalation have been recognized for many years. It was reported by Pliny the Elder that prisoners were executed during the second Punic War by suspending them in cages above green wood fires (1). In a classic description of the 1942 Coconut Grove nightclub fire in Boston, treating physicians recognized the most challenging aspect of care to be lung injury. Presumed to be due to both thermal and chemical insults, the damage was likened to that "resulting from inhalation of certain war gases" (2). The Dellwood Nursery fire is another early reported example of the lethality of smoke inhalation (3). In 1980, fire raged through the MGM Grand Hotel in Las Vegas killing 84 people, the vast majority due to inhalation injury rather than burns (4,5). Nearly one-half of patients presenting to emergency departments in the aftermath of the September 11, 2001, terrorist attack on the World Trade Center were treated for inhalation injury (6). With eerie similarities to the Coconut Grove incident, a Rhode Island night club fire killed 99 people in February 2003, many with inhalation injury (7,8). Although smoke inhalation may resolve uneventfully with little medical intervention, it can also be rapidly life-threatening.

Classification and Uses

Smoke inhalation injury is a term that defines the spectrum of respiratory and systemic complications sustained after exposure to superheated gases, irritants, and toxins created by fire and incomplete combustion of natural and synthetic materials. It is caused by thermal and irritant chemical insults as well as toxins with direct metabolic effects. It is difficult to predict the exact nature of the injury, as every fire contains different substances. Numerous substances promote asphyxia by decreasing both the amount of oxygen available as well as limiting the delivery of oxygen to end-organ tissues. *Simple asphyxiants* cause hypoxemia by displacing oxygen and decreasing fraction of inspired oxyven (FiO_2). Examples include carbon dioxide, methane, helium, nitrogen, and nitrous oxide (9). *Chemical asphyxiants,* such as carbon monoxide, cyanide, hydrogen sulfide, and arsine gas, lead to hypoxia by interrupting the transport or use of oxygen. Other substances, such as acrolein, ammonia, sulfur dioxide, hydrogen chloride, chlorine gas, and phosgene, are irritants and cause inflammation, bronchospasm, and pulmonary tissue destruction (10).

Inhalation injury has been estimated to cause 80% of the 10,000 fire-related fatalities in the United States annually (4,11–15). Careful fluid resuscitation combined with aggressive burn-wound care has resulted in improved survival for isolated burn injuries (12,16,17). However, inhalation injury remains a highly morbid condition (4,18). Mortality estimates of fire-related inhalation injury range from 45% to 78% (15,18–21). Inhalation injury is present in 10% to 20% of all thermal burns admitted to burn centers (16,18) and in up to one-third of all patients of burns involving more than 20% body surface area (12,17). In general, the larger the surface area of burned skin, the higher the probability of smoke inhalation injury (18,22). The presence of smoke inhalation injury greatly increases burn mortality (12,18,20, 22,23) and has been shown to be a better predictor of mortality than percent body surface area of burn (18). Isolated inhalation injury has a much lower mortality (3%) than when present with cutaneous burns (20,24).

PATHOPHYSIOLOGY

The pathophysiology of smoke inhalation injury represents a complex interplay of multiple factors. Primary in importance is the nature of the exposure itself, which is defined by the materials burned as well as the unique characteristics of the patient. To understand the effects of this exposure, it is helpful to describe the pathophysiology of inhalation injury in terms of three basic mechanisms (Table 1). Early in a fire, the effects of asphyxia and hypoxia play a major role in mortality. Thermal energy is responsible for dermal burns but is also an important mode of injury to the airway. Finally, the chemical products generated as a result of the fire cause pulmonary irritation.

TABLE 1. Mechanisms of inhalation injury and primary site of action

Mechanism	Primary site of action
Hypoxia and asphyxia	
Simple asphyxiants	Systemic effects (heart and central nervous system)
Chemical asphyxiants	
Carbon monoxide	
Cyanide	
Methemoglobin	
Thermal injury	Upper airway
Chemical injury	
High water solubility	Upper airway
Low water solubility	Lower airways
Particulate deposition	Size dependent

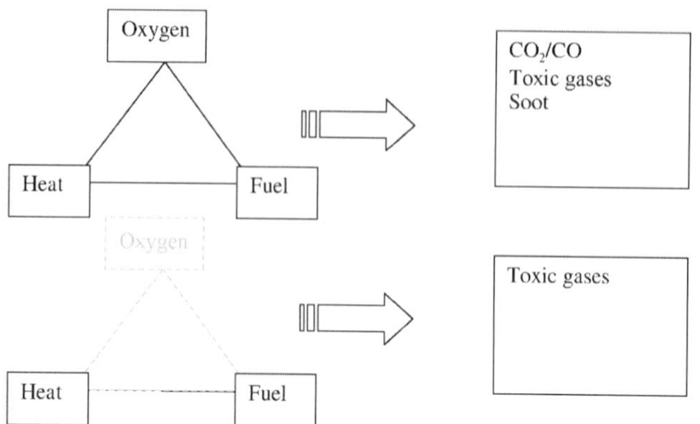

Figure 1. Combustion and pyrolysis (5). See text for explanation.

Defining the Exposure

It has been noted that every fire is different and that even the same fire is heterogeneous in space and time. Oxygen supply, temperature of the fire, and the burning substrate are just a few important variables that may differ from one part of a fire to the next and from moment to moment (5,25,26).

When heat, oxygen, and fuel are present, oxidative degradation yields carbon dioxide and carbon monoxide plus breakdown products of the original fuel. When oxygen is abundant, carbon dioxide is the primary gas produced; however, as oxygen is depleted, carbon monoxide becomes more prevalent. This process is termed *combustion* (5,26). When oxygen is completely depleted, a process called *pyrolysis* can ensue (Fig. 1). With extreme temperatures, heat can affect a change in the fuel directly and produce distinct toxic products (5). Polyvinyl chloride, for example, has been shown to yield some 75 different compounds through this process (5).

Table 2 lists some common materials and the toxic products liberated from their combustion or pyrolysis. Modern construction increasingly contains synthetic materials that yield dangerous toxins when burned (26). Polyvinyl chloride yields carbon monoxide, hydrogen chloride, chlorine, and phosgene (13,21). Polyurethane and polyacrylonitrile generate cyanide (13,21,27). Even natural products yield potentially harmful compounds. Wood produces carbon monoxide, acrolein, formaldehyde, and acetaldehyde (21). Natural fabrics (cotton, wool, silk) can generate cyanide, carbon monoxide, ammonia, and hydrogen sulfide (21). The potential number of toxins can be in the hundreds for any given fire (5,25). Fortunately, toxic products of combustion can be classified into three general categories: pulmonary irritants, simple asphyxiants, and systemic (or chemical) asphyxiants. The actions of each of these are discussed further below.

TABLE 2. Common toxic products of combustion or pyrolysis

Material	Toxic combustion/pyrolysis products
Wool	CN, CO, phosgene, chlorine
Wood	CO, aldehydes (acrolein), methane, formic acid
Cotton	Acetaldehyde, formaldehyde, methane, formic acid
Wool, silk	Ammonia, CO, CN, hydrogen sulfide, nitrogen oxides
Nylon	CN, ammonia
Paper	CN
Plastics	CN, HCl, ammonia, phosgene, chlorine
Polyvinyl chloride	CO, HCl, phosgene, chlorine
Polyurethane	CN, isocyanates
Melamine resin	CN, ammonia
Rubber	CN, sulfur dioxide
Fire retardants	CN, HCl
Nitrogen polymers	CN, nitrogen oxides

CN, cyanide; CO, carbon monoxide; HCl, hydrogen chloride.
Data from Witten ML, Quan SF, Sobonya RE, et al. New developments in the pathogenesis of smoke inhalation-induced pulmonary edema. *West J Med* 1988;148:33–36; Kirk MA, Gerace R, Kulig KW. Cyanide ad methemoglobin kinetics in smoke inhalation victims treated with the cyanide antidote kit. *Ann Emerg Med* 1993;22:1413–1418; Lee-Chiong TL. Smoke inhalation injury. *Postgrad Med* 1999;105:55–62; Leikin JB, Aks SE, Andrews S, et al. Environmental injuries. *Dis Mon* 1997;43:809–916; Barillo DJ, Goode R, Esch V. Cyanide poisoning in victims of fire: analysis of 364 cases and review of the literature. *J Burn Care Rehabil* 1994;15:46–57; Shusterman D, Alexeeff G, Hargis C, et al. Predictors of carbon monoxide and hydrogen cyanide exposure in smoke inhalation patients. *J Toxicol Clin Toxicol* 1996;34:61–71; and Silverman ST, Purdue GF, Hunt JL, et al. Cyanide toxicity in burned patients. *J Trauma* 1988;28:171–177.

In addition to knowing the relevant toxins that may be generated during the fire, it is important to consider the length of exposure. It has been suggested that a smoke-filled room may obscure vision and prevent rapid escape (5,27–30). Furthermore, as the environment becomes progressively more oxygen deficient, the ability to escape can be hampered by the effects of hypoxia (5,21,26–31). When a rapidly dwindling oxygen supply does not interfere, it has been shown that alcohol or other social drugs may impair the normal flight response (32). Lack of adequate and clearly marked exits or overcrowding at the site may also lead to prolonged exposure (33).

The location of the person with respect to the flames may help predict potential toxic mechanisms. For the person in close proximity to the flame, the combined effects of heat and hypoxia are believed to be causes of immediate mortality. Carbon monoxide, cyanide, and irritants play a more significant role in people found away from the primary fire (34).

Finally, a patient's underlying medical condition plays a role in defining the extent of injury sustained in smoke inhalation. Chronic pulmonary or cardiac medical problems may diminish reserve and leave the patient more prone to the toxic effects of irritant gases, hypoxia, and systemic asphyxia (31,35). Those patients with diminished mobility or any condition that impairs recognition and proper decision-making regarding a fire threat might be expected to suffer longer exposures (34).

Mechanism of Injury

Thermal injury is caused by the intense heat of the fire. The area of the hypopharynx above the glottis is most susceptible to direct thermal injury. As superheated air and gases are inhaled, they can transfer their heat to the mucosa of the upper airway. Unless steam is inhaled, thermal injury below the glottis is rare, as dry air has a relatively low heat capacity (13,21,35). Animal studies show that when dry air temperatures up to 500°C are measured in the larynx, distal trachea temperatures are only approximately 100°C (20). Furthermore, in the conscious patient, reflex closure of the glottis due to irritants is an additional protection (12,35). The more distal airways are not subjected to the same thermal burns as the larynx and skin. Exceptions to limited thermal injury occur with the inhalation of steam, explosive gases, and aspiration of liquids (36). Because steam has nearly 4000 times the heat capacity of dry air, it is likely to burn the distal airways (12,20).

Thermal injury results in progression of airway edema within minutes to hours (12,20). This is most notable in the supraglottic area where the mucosa is loosely adherent to the underlying supportive tissue (20). Edema may become massive, resulting in loss of airway patency.

Hypoxia and asphyxia can be caused by a low fraction of inspired oxygen or by inhibition of effective oxygen use. As a fire burns, it consumes oxygen available to the lungs and generates both toxic and nontoxic gases. Many of these gases are referred to as *simple asphyxiants*, as they displace any remaining breathable oxygen from the environment yet do not have prominent irritating or systemic toxic effects (15,37). Common examples of such gases include carbon dioxide, nitrogen, and methane, but any gas can act as an asphyxiant if present in substantial quantity. In models of fire simulation in small spaces, consumption of oxygen and production of CO_2 pushed the FiO_2 rapidly to 3% (38). In the setting of a room suddenly bursting into flames, the FiO_2 may drop from 21% to 15% within seconds (1).

Carbon monoxide and hydrogen cyanide (HCN) may also be produced. Unlike simple asphyxiants, they act at the cellular level as chemical asphyxiants (15). They exert their effects on oxygen transport and aerobic metabolism, effectively depriving cells of the energy derived from oxygen. Both carbon monoxide and HCN gases are commonly encountered together in the fire environment (14,29,39,40). They are believed to be major causes of immediate fire-related death, although their individual contribution cannot be readily determined (12,17,26,29,40). A detailed discussion of carbon monoxide and cyanide poisoning is provided in Chapters 184 and 185, respectively.

Carbon monoxide is the most prevalent toxic gas implicated in smoke inhalation injury and early death (5,12,15,34,41). The odorless, colorless gas is produced from the incomplete combustion of hydrocarbons. Carbon monoxide is rapidly absorbed from the lungs and binds to hemoglobin with an affinity 200 to 250 times greater than oxygen (12,26,41,42). As a result, carbon monoxide shifts the oxygen-hemoglobin dissociation curve leftward, impairing oxygen release to hypoxic tissues (42). Elevated temperatures may exacerbate the effect of carbon monoxide, perhaps by stimulating respiration (26). The most metabolically active tissues (i.e., brain and heart) are most susceptible to carbon monoxide exposure (5,26). It is also believed to act as a direct myocardial suppressant (4,31,43).

HCN gas is produced from the combustion or pyrolysis of many materials, including wool, synthetic rubber, polyurethanes, nylon, silk, nitrogen-containing polymers, paper, and fire retardants (5,14,29,40). HCN is rapidly absorbed through bronchial and alveolar mucosa (40). Once absorbed into the blood stream, it distributes to all body tissues where it eventually binds to the terminal component of the cytochrome oxidase system [ferric (Fe^{3+}) iron on cytochrome-a_3], effectively shutting down cellular respiration (39). This forces the body to shift to anaerobic metabolism, which produces lactic acid. The most metabolically active tissues (i.e., brain and heart) are most sensitive to the resulting chemical asphyxia (5,26,40).

Methemoglobin is a chemical asphyxiant that occurs due to heat denaturation of hemoglobin, oxidation of nitrogen, or exposure to nitrites (31). It is less frequently reported, compared with carbon monoxide or HCN (44). Methemoglobin is an oxidized form of hemoglobin that has a low affinity for oxygen and thus produces a functional anemia. Similar to carbon monoxide, methemoglobinemia decreases the oxygen-carrying capacity of the blood and shifts the oxyhemoglobin dissociation curve to the left. This could theoretically further impair oxidative metabolism in the smoke inhalation patient. Methemoglobin has been detected in the blood of burn patients, although the magnitude of its role remains undefined (45).

Closed-space fires are considered high-risk exposures for smoke inhalation; without ventilation, oxygen levels fall while the levels of asphyxiants (as well as other toxins) rise (35). In a fire, fraction of inspired oxygen may be reduced to 10%, and carbon monoxide may only be present at 0.1%, although in combination, this proves to be rapidly lethal (4,5,12,34). Simple and chemical asphyxiants are believed to be the major reason for early fire-related deaths (5,12).

Chemical injury is the final mode of injury when other irritating toxins are elaborated by fire and subsequently inhaled (Table 2). The distal airways are generally not prone to direct thermal injury (in the absence of steam). At this level of the respiratory tree, chemical irritants are much more important mediators of epithelial damage (20). Polyvinyl chloride is used widely in modern construction. It produces significant quantities of hydrogen chloride gas, phosgene, and chlorine gas when burned (12,13,20). Other plastic products yield ammonia and sulfur dioxide (12). Ammonia produces alkaline injury. Sulfur dioxide and chlorine gas create acid injury. Wood smoke contains large amounts of aldehydes, including acrolein, which has been implicated in causing increased airway resistance and in higher doses causes pulmonary edema and respiratory failure (13,20).

The location of injury from a chemical irritant is determined primarily by its water solubility (15,21,26,35). Irritants that are highly water soluble (e.g., ammonia, hydrogen sulfide) dissolve in the upper airways (15,21,35). Gases with poor water solubility (e.g., chlorine, phosgene, aldehydes, nitrogen oxides) remain in the gas phase and reach the distal airways and alveoli (15,21,35). Those irritants that are more water soluble tend to create intense irritation that is readily noticed by the patient and facilitates recognition and avoidance of possible further inhalation injury (15,21,35).

In addition to gases, many chemicals are carried to the more distal airways adsorbed on soot particles and deposited on the moist epithelial lining (35,46). This particulate mechanism may play a more damaging role than direct gas-phase exposure (47). Once deposited, these chemicals dissolve according to their relative solubility in mucus, yielding various acids and alkali (12,13,20). The mucociliary system is both directly damaged and overwhelmed by sloughing dead cells and soot (4,13,17,20). The particles also serve as a continuous source of exposure, as they are not easily cleared in the setting of airway edema, obstruction, and ciliary dysfunction (13).

Chemical irritation may cause an initial bronchospasm (13,46). As mucosal edema and bronchial epithelial sloughing continues, smaller airways become obstructed (13). This results in increased airway resistance, atelectasis, and intrapulmonary shunting (13,46).

In addition to extensive damage to the smaller airways, it has also been noted that surfactant activity is diminished, which contributes to atelectasis (13,20,35,48). Noncardiogenic pulmonary edema may also be seen, although this usually occurs days later (20,47). When present, pulmonary edema is likely due to multiple causes, including increased permeability of the alveolar membrane from direct injury, systemic release of inflammatory cytokines, and decreased oncotic pressure within capillaries due to protein losses from extensive cutaneous burns (18,20,49).

DIAGNOSIS

The assessment of smoke inhalation remains an essentially clinical one that rests on a high initial index of suspicion. The smoke inhalation patient should be viewed as a trauma patient. A primary survey focusing on immediate life-threatening issues should begin immediately. Second, a focused history reviewing the most common symptoms and signs of smoke inhalation should be obtained. Finally, a secondary survey, including past medical history, review of systems, and thorough physical examination, can be completed. However, most aspects of the history and physical examination are not reliably sensitive or specific in diagnosing smoke inhalation injury (12).

History

Important historical clues at the scene include a closed-space setting of fire, loss of consciousness, and impaired mental status.

These place a patient at higher risk for significant inhalation exposure. Prominent respiratory symptoms, such as a sense of shortness of breath, hoarseness, change in voice, or complaints of sore throat or painful swallowing, suggest a more severe prognosis (12,14,17,31,50).

Physical Examination

Examination findings traditionally believed to represent likely inhalation injury include facial and pharyngeal burns, singed nasal hairs, carbonaceous sputum, hoarseness, and wheezing (12,17,50,51). Carbonaceous sputum should be considered a marker of severe exposure that may warrant intubation (44). Patients with facial burns have a 59% incidence of respiratory injury, compared with a 22% incidence in patients with no or peripheral facial burns (52). Pneumonia also correlates with the presence of facial burns (53). A large percentage of skin involvement suggests inability to escape flame and prolonged exposure, a risk factor for respiratory complications (44). It is also important to consider the extent of cutaneous burns, as risk of inhalation injury directly correlates with percent body surface area burn (12,18,22). Burns involving more than 20% surface area should be considered high risk for concomitant inhalation injury, with one study finding its presence in 20% of cases (18). Finally, other signs of trauma, including injury to the head, chest, abdomen, pelvis, and extremities, should be carefully evaluated.

Evaluation of the suspected smoke inhalation patient should also include a targeted review of systems based on common suspected toxins. Three conditions cause clinically similar effects in the smoke inhalation patient. Most of the effects of carbon monoxide (Chapter 184) or cyanide poisoning (Chapter 185) or the development of methemoglobinemia (Chapter 21) causes the signs of hypoxia. Central nervous system and myocardial depression occur. Changes in the electrocardiogram and symptoms of ischemia may develop. Hypotension may develop as cardiac output decreases. Hypoxia and decreased cardiac output both contribute to worsening neurologic function (31). All three conditions may coexist and therefore should be considered in smoke inhalation patients with the clinical findings of hypoxia (31).

One additional physical finding in the case of methemoglobinemia is cyanosis. A methemoglobin concentration of 1.5 g/dl produces cyanosis (approximately 10% methemoglobinemia). A similar degree of cyanosis occurs with a deoxyhemoglobin concentration of 5 g/dl (54). Patients may present with cyanosis out of proportion to pulse oximetry or respiratory rate (31).

Diagnosis of smoke inhalation injury relies on a high index of suspicion combined with a careful history and examination. Although no one test exists to establish or refute the diagnosis, judicious use of ancillary studies can be used to support a suspected diagnosis.

Evaluation of Oxygenation

Pulse oximetry and the arterial blood gas (ABG) can be used to measure the level of oxygen in the blood. Pulse oximetry is a useful, rapid bedside test but has several important limitations (55–58). Carboxyhemoglobin is erroneously measured as oxyhemoglobin, giving a falsely elevated oxygen saturation. Methemoglobinemia shows a depressed saturation, but this does not reliably predict the degree of methemoglobinemia. Levels of methemoglobin greater than 30% create a constant saturation of 85% even if true levels are significantly lower.

The measurement of ABG with co-oximetry determines the true blood oxygen partial pressure and saturation as well as levels of oxyhemoglobin, deoxyhemoglobin, carboxyhemoglobin, and methemoglobin. An alveolar to arterial oxygen gradient may be calculated. An elevated alveolar to arterial oxygen gradient suggests pulmonary or cardiac shunting from an acute or chronic source. Another indicator, the PO_2 to FiO_2 ratio, can be used as an indicator of lung injury. A PO_2:FiO_2 level of 400 or more is normal; less than 300 suggests pulmonary injury, and less than 250 requires urgent intervention (19,31). Carboxyhemoglobin levels greater than 10% support the diagnosis of inhalation injury (43). An elevated carbon monoxide level may also suggest significant exposure to other toxins that cannot be readily measured (e.g., cyanide) (14,29,39,40). It should be remembered, although, that levels can be misleading, as they may rapidly normalize depending on how long the patient has been breathing 100% oxygen before sampling (40).

Laboratory Tests

Blood chemistries are used to evaluate for acidosis as well as screen for end-organ pathology, including rhabdomyolysis. Electrolytes are useful as a screen for renal function (blood urea nitrogen and creatinine) and to evaluate for anion gap acidosis. The anion gap is used in conjunction with the ABG to determine the degree and type of acidosis. Lactic acid is the most common form of acidosis in inhalation injury. Lactate levels greater than 10 mmol/L have been shown to be a sensitive indicator of cyanide levels greater than 1 μg/ml (29), but it should be recognized that levels may be elevated due to hypoperfusion.

Creatinine phosphokinase, serum myoglobin, and urine microscopy are useful in the diagnosis of acute rhabdomyolysis. A positive urine dipstick test for blood in the urine should suggest possible myoglobin in the urine, as myoglobin cross-reacts with the detection of blood. Absence of red blood cells on microscopy further suggests possible myoglobinuria. Urine myoglobin and creatinine phosphokinase can be sent if rhabdomyolysis is suspected (31).

Imaging

A chest radiograph should be obtained in intubated patients and in those with respiratory complaints. However, plain radiography is not adequately sensitive to reliably detect inhalation injury at initial presentation (4,15,24,59,60), with a false-negative rate as high as 92% (56). Common initial findings are nonspecific and include peribronchial cuffing, patchy consolidation, and pulmonary edema (61,62). If the larynx is included in the frontal view, subglottic edema, when present, may be more indicative of inhalation injury (61). Chest radiographs can be used later to follow the progression of lung injury, especially in patients later shown to develop acute respiratory distress syndrome, pulmonary edema, or pneumonia.

Radionuclide scans have also been used. Both xenon or technetium are cleared rapidly by normal lungs, compared with lungs damaged by smoke inhalation (44). These studies, however, are unavailable at community hospitals and are cumbersome or confounded by underlying pulmonary disease (4,16,50). The sensitivity and specificity of these tests have not been established.

Chest computed tomography plays a role in patients admitted to the hospital for further evaluation. The chest computed tomography identifies tracheal stenosis, empyema, bronchiolitis obliterans, or bronchiolitis (44). It is more sensitive than xenon scans or chest radiography for determining atelectasis (56). The role of chest computed tomography in the acute smoke inhalation patient has not been established.

Pulmonary function testing may reveal obstruction from airway inflammation, edema, and sloughed cells. A restrictive pattern may be seen if significant chest wall burns are present. The usefulness of pulmonary function testing has not been well defined in diagnosing acute smoke inhalation injury (4).

Direct Visualization

Bronchoscopy is generally considered to be the gold standard for confirming inhalation injury (4,17,31). Direct visualization may identify injuries undetected on physical examination that require emergent intubation. Findings consistent with inhalation injury include carbonaceous debris, mucosal pallor, mucosal edema, and ulcerations (4,15,16). Bronchoscopy does not provide any information regarding parenchymal damage, although the presence of a normal upper endoscopy greatly decreases the likelihood of lower airway injury. However, agents, such as chlorine, isocyanates, oxides of nitrogen, and phosgene, all carry a higher incidence of lower airway injury due to their intermediate to low solubility (31).

Bronchoscopy allows for diagnostic and therapeutic maneuvers such as lavage or emergent intubation (4). Bronchial alveolar lavage has been used to monitor chemical and cellular events of smoke inhalation, although the information has not proved to be clinically useful (63). A fiberoptic bronchoscope can act as a guide wire to assist in endotracheal intubation. Bronchoscopy can identify tracheal or bronchial stenosis and acquire biopsy specimens to help identify inflammatory processes such as bronchiolitis obliterans and diffuse lung injury unrelated to smoke inhalation (31). Bronchoscopy is generally not available early during care of the smoke inhalation patient, although flexible laryngoscopes and endoscopes are becoming more common in the emergency department setting.

Diagnostic Pitfalls

Smoke inhalation injury is a complex systemic illness with multiple potential complications. Patients with smoke inhalation injury are also vulnerable to the complications of their other injuries, including mechanical trauma and cutaneous burns. Loss of airway is perhaps the greatest early complication in the smoke inhalation–injured patient. Thermal injury can result in rapid progression of airway edema, potentially compromising patency. This may become dramatic once fluid resuscitation begins (12). Early recognition of a potentially compromised airway and prompt intubation are essential to a good outcome.

Subglottic stenosis, bronchiectasis, pulmonary edema (4% to 9%), bronchopneumonia (3% to 23%), atelectasis (2.6% to 11.0%), pleural effusion (2%), pulmonary embolism (1% to 2%), and pneumothorax (1% to 5%) are all potential complications that increase morbidity (56,64).

Pneumonia remains the major complication in treating smoke inhalation–injured patients and accounts for the majority of deaths in the successfully resuscitated and stabilized patient (65). Approximately one-half of patients with inhalation injury can be expected to develop pulmonary infection (16,65). Inhalation injury appears to decrease bacterial clearance rates (20,66). Pneumonia appears much earlier in burn patients with inhalation injury than without (4 days vs. 2 weeks) (4,16,20). Despite increased incidence of pneumonia, prophylactic antibiotics have not been shown to be effective (4,22).

TREATMENT

Initial Stabilization

Management of suspected smoke inhalation injury focuses on stabilizing the patient and addressing immediate life threats as in any trauma patient. Use of the traditional mnemonic ABCDE is helpful in guiding the primary survey. For the patient arriving from a fire scene with suspected smoke inhalation, the airway is of paramount concern. Thermal injury to the soft tissue above the glottis can create significant edema (12,16). Early intubation should be performed for any of the following reasons (16,67):

1. Smoke inhalation accompanied by decreased level of consciousness
2. Posterior pharyngeal edema
3. Full-thickness nasolabial burns
4. Circumferential neck burns
5. Stridor

Intubation should also be considered before transfer of the patient to another facility for definitive treatment or whenever leaving direct observation for a protracted period of time.

Endoscopic evaluation should be considered in those patients at high risk for inhalation injury who have not already required intubation. A 96% correlation has been noted between positive bronchoscopic findings and the clinical triad of closed-space fire, carboxyhemoglobin greater than 10%, and carbonaceous sputum. Therefore, if any of these three clinical findings are noted, bronchoscopy should be used (31).

Children deserve special mention as their airway is anatomically narrower and thus more prone to compromise from developing edema (16). In the patient with significant burns to the neck, escharotomy may be indicated to protect the airway.

Once the airway is secured, breathing (respiratory status) must be assessed with respect to respiratory rate, oxygen saturation, and quality-of-breath sounds. All patients with suspected smoke inhalation injury should be given 100% oxygen. In addition to improving hypoxia, oxygen also reduces the half-life of carbon monoxide from approximately 5 hours to 75 minutes (41,42,68), which can rapidly reverse the effects of chemical asphyxia. Humidified oxygen has been used to prevent the drying of nasopharyngeal secretions (31).

Bronchodilators (β_2-receptor agonists) may be useful for bronchospasm (4,16,31). The effectiveness of bronchodilators is not well documented. Nebulized β-agonists can be used and discontinued if no improvement is noted (69). More benefit may be seen in patients with underlying asthma or chronic obstructive pulmonary disease (44). Steroids have not been shown to improve airway inflammation except in those patients with underlying disease responsive to steroids (e.g., asthma, chronic obstructive pulmonary disease) (12,22,35). In fact, they may lead to greater morbidity, as evidenced by increased rates of infectious complications (4,12).

Circulation follows airway and breathing. Circulation is assessed with respect to blood pressure, heart rate, and pulses. Intravenous access (preferably two large bore peripheral lines) for fluid resuscitation and drug administration must be obtained. Fluid resuscitation should be initiated according to burn protocols. It has been shown, however, that the presence of inhalation injury significantly increases fluid requirements beyond what is predicted by standard nomograms (46). Studies suggest smoke inhalation may require 30 cc/kg/day or 2 cc/kg/% body surface area of additional fluid (4,70). Urine output and central venous pressure should be monitored to ensure adequate fluid resuscitation.

Aggressive hydration has been implicated in causing pulmonary edema and worsening airway edema in smoke inhalation patients (12,20,66). However, this is noted in isolated burn patients as well (20). Diffuse capillary leak is present in large burns and contributes to worsening airway edema (16,66). Pulmonary edema is also noted to be worse in patients with cutaneous burns (49). Fluid resuscitation itself does not cause edema and should not be withheld on these grounds. Instead, supportive measures should be initiated (66).

Finally, the smoke inhalation patient should be fully exposed to search for other possibly life-threatening injuries, as well as burning or caustic clothing, and to fully assess the extent of cutaneous burns. Strong consideration should be given to possible cervical spine injury. Cervical spine films should be obtained on any patient with complaints of neck pain or tenderness and in any patient with altered mental status. The Glasgow Coma Scale or another similar brief neurologic assessment should be made.

Once this primary survey is completed, a more thorough history and examination can be made. Imaging and laboratory testing as discussed above can also be obtained. An electrocardiogram should be done to rule out cardiac ischemia in at-risk patients because hypoxia and asphyxia combined with the metabolic stress of injury place an added burden on the heart (26).

Treatment of Carbon Monoxide Poisoning

The initial treatment of potential carbon monoxide poisoning is empiric 100% oxygen (Chapter 184). Carboxyhemoglobin levels can be readily measured with standard co-oximeters on a venous or arterial blood sample (14). It is important to remember that standard pulse oximeters can read a falsely normal oxygen saturation in the presence of very high carboxyhemoglobin concentrations (71). In some cases, hyperbaric oxygen may be indicated (Chapter 62) (72,73).

Hyperbaric oxygen remains a controversial treatment modality for carbon monoxide toxic patients. Criteria for consideration include the following:

1. Change in mental status
2. Neurologic signs or symptoms
3. Cardiovascular insufficiency or complaints
4. Pulmonary edema
5. Severe acidosis
6. Loss of consciousness
7. Carboxyhemoglobin level greater than 25%
8. Pregnancy with symptoms or carboxyhemoglobin level greater than 15%

Although isolated carbon monoxide poisoning is often referred to the nearest hyperbaric chamber facility, this is not as easily accomplished in the burn and smoke-injury patient. These patients are by nature less stable and may not be able to be safely transported to another facility (4,15,41). Continuous 100% oxygen is the best approach to treating carbon monoxide poisoning if hyperbaric therapy is unavailable or deemed unsafe (4).

Treatment of Suspected Cyanide Poisoning

The difficult aspect of cyanide toxicity is the inability to distinguish it from that due to carbon monoxide. The signs of anxiety, flushing, dizziness, and headache are nonspecific and similar to symptoms of carbon monoxide toxicity (74). Cyanide toxicity during fire exposure is common (78% to 100%), but there is conflicting evidence as to the correlation between cyanide and carboxyhemoglobin levels (29,31,40,75–77).

Although cyanide is common and important to consider in the fire inhalation patient, it is unlikely to be present in the absence of carbon monoxide poisoning (26). Although cyanide testing does exist, it is not yet widely available on an emergent basis, and treatment decisions have to be made before a cyanide level can be known (15,78). A narrow arteriovenous oxygen content gradient, as determined by simultaneous venous and ABG samples, is highly suggestive of cyanide poisoning in the smoke inhalation patient (15,79). An elevated (greater than 10 mmol/L) serum or whole blood lactate has also been shown to correlate well with elevated cyanide levels (29). It should be noted that an absolute "lethal" cyanide level has not been defined (29). Traditionally, a level of 3 mg/L has been considered lethal, but patients have survived with higher levels and died at lower levels (25,40). Other sources recommend administering cyanide antidote for any patient who is seriously ill or with a persistent metabolic acidosis despite adequate fluid resuscitation (14,25). Empiric treatment is ideal; however, no ideal antidote exists. The treatment using the standard cyanide antidote kit generates a significant methemoglobinemia, which limits oxygen-carrying capacity (14). In patients with elevated carboxyhemoglobin levels, further reducing oxygen-carrying capacity is potentially harmful. Further detail regarding the indications, contraindications, and method of administration for the cyanide antidote kit are provided in Chapter 46.

The cyanide antidote kit consists of three separate drugs: amyl nitrite inhalation capsules, sodium nitrite intravenous, and sodium thiosulfate intravenous. The major side effect of the nitrites is hypotension, which is hazardous in burn patients who should be considered volume depleted (14,39). The sodium thiosulfate component enhances metabolism of cyanide, is excreted through the kidney, and has few side effects in therapeutic doses (25). The adult dose of sodium thiosulfate is 50 ml of 25% solution (12.5 g). For smoke inhalation patients, some references suggest that only the sodium thiosulfate portion of the standard kit be given (14,26,29,39).

One prospective paper suggests the ability to give the three-drug cyanide kit to smoke inhalation patients without obvious adverse sequelae. Methemoglobin levels peaked at a mean of 50 minutes, by which time the carboxyhemoglobin levels would theoretically be decreasing if treated with hyperbaric oxygen (14). The absence of a control group compromises the ability of this paper to assess benefit.

Management of Methemoglobinemia

Significant methemoglobinemia in smoke inhalation patients is relatively rare unless generated by treatment of the patient for cyanide toxicity. Indications for treatment of methemoglobinemia include mental status changes, acidosis, electrocardiogram changes, or ischemic chest pain (31). Similar to cyanide toxicity, these symptoms are nonspecific and overlap with symptoms of carbon monoxide toxicity and cyanide toxicity. Methemoglobin levels can be rapidly obtained via co-oximetry on a venous or arterial sample. However, there is no readily available test for cyanomethemoglobinemia; therefore, true methemoglobin levels may be higher than measured if cyanide is also present.

Methemoglobinemia is treated with methylene blue. Further detail regarding the indications, contraindications, and method of administration for the cyanide antidote kit are provided in Chapter 63. Methemoglobin levels less than 30% may not require treatment, depending on the patient's cardiac and respiratory status as well as the presence of any coexisting anemia (31). Concomitant poisoning with carbon monoxide or cyanide is typically more important and should be treated first.

Monitoring

The smoke inhalation patient should be monitored for at least 4 hours in the emergency department (31). Admission should be considered for patients with a history of closed-space exposure greater than 10 minutes, arterial PO_2 less than 60 mm Hg, serum bicarbonate less than 15 mmol/L, carbonaceous sputum, carboxyhemoglobin levels above 15%, arteriovenous oxygen difference (on 100% oxygen therapy) greater than 100 mm Hg, abnormal chest radiograph, or bronchospasm (77,80). Admission to the intensive care unit should be considered for those with hypoxemia, tachypnea, rales, or worsening acidosis (31). Once stabilized, patients with significant smoke inhalation injury should be transferred to a facility experienced in managing smoke inhalation and its potential complications.

A limited number of studies have looked at the long-term effects of smoke inhalation injury. Follow-up evaluations of those who survived the Coconut Grove fire revealed nearly all patients to be doing well (20). However, long-term sequelae have been reported, including chronic bronchitis, tracheal stenosis, bronchiectasis, pulmonary fibrosis, and subclinical airflow obstruction (20,81,82). Hyperreactive airways are present for at least 6 months, although it is unclear if this is of any practical importance (83–85). Lingering effects may be more significant in those patients with the most severe initial injuries (20). There are, however, no clear factors to predict which patients will develop chronic complications.

Long-term neuropsychiatric complications may also develop due to carbon monoxide poisoning (41,42,48). These may include cognitive and personality changes, parkinsonism, psychosis, and incontinence (42).

Management Pitfalls

Failure to secure airway before development of significant edema can lead to precipitous deterioration. Early management should address respiratory injury: Cutaneous burns are unlikely to cause early morbidity. Similarly, concomitant traumatic injuries must be detected and addressed.

The lack of classic physical findings (carbonaceous sputum) should not deter the evaluation of suspected inhalation injury in burn patients.

The requirement for fluid resuscitation is usually increased in the setting of significant inhalation injury.

REFERENCES

1. Dressler DP. Laboratory background on smoke inhalation. *J Trauma* 1979;19:913–922.
2. Cope O. Management of the Cocoanut Grove burns at the Massachusetts General Hospital. *Ann of Surg* 1943;117:801–802.
3. Cox ME, Heslop BF, Kempton JJ, et al. The Dellwood fire. *BMJ* 1955;16:942–946.
4. Ruddy RM. Smoke inhalation injury. *Pediatr Clin of North Am* 1994;41:317–336.
5. Beritic T. The challenge of fire effluents. Poisonous gases are potential killers. *BMJ* 1990;300:696–698.
6. Centers for Disease Control and Prevention. Rapid assessment of injuries among survivors of the terrorist attack on the World Trade Center—New York City, September 2001. *JAMA* 2002;287:835–838.
7. Zezima K. Set for fire site. *The New York Times* 2003 Mar 22.
8. Wielawski I. Post-9/11 training helped save lives at club fire. *The New York Times* 2003 Mar 13.
9. Bresnitz EA. Simple asphyxiants and pulmonary irritants. In: Goldfrank LR, et al., eds. *Goldfrank's toxicologic emergencies*, 5th ed. East Norwalk, CT: Appleton & Lange, 1994.
10. Kirk MA. Smoke inhalation. In: Goldfrank LR, et al., eds. *Goldfrank's toxicologic emergencies*, 5th ed. East Norwalk, CT: Appleton & Lange, 1994.
11. Hart GB, Strauss MB, Lennon PA, et al. Treatment of smoke inhalation by hyperbaric oxygen. *J Emerg Med* 1985;3:211–215.
12. Robinson L, Miller RH. Smoke inhalation injuries. *Am J Otolaryngol* 1986;7:375–380.
13. Witten ML, Quan SF, Sobonya RE, et al. New developments in the pathogenesis of smoke inhalation-induced pulmonary edema. *West J Med* 1988;148:33–36.
14. Kirk MA, Gerace R, Kulig KW. Cyanide ad methemoglobin kinetics in smoke inhalation victims treated with the cyanide antidote kit. *Ann Emerg Med* 1993;22:1413–1418.
15. Lee-Chiong TL. Smoke inhalation injury. *Postgrad Med* 1999;105:55–62.
16. Sheridan RL. Airway management and respiratory care of the burn patient. *Int Anesthesiol Clin* 2000;38:129–145.
17. Ramzy PI, Barret JP, Herndon, DN. Environmental emergencies. Thermal injury. *Crit Care Clin* 1999;15:333–352.
18. Thompson PB, Herndon DN, Traber DL, et al. Effect on mortality of inhalation injury. *J Trauma* 1986;26:163–165.
19. Heimbach DM, Waeckerle JF. Inhalation injuries. *Ann Emerg Med* 1988;17:1316–1320.
20. Haponik EF, Summer WR. Respiratory complications in burned patients: pathogenesis and spectrum of inhalation injury. *J Crit Care* 1987;2:49–74.
21. Leikin JB, Aks SE, Andrews S, et al. Environmental injuries. *Dis Mon* 1997;43:809–916.
22. Monafo WW. Current concepts: initial management of burns. *N Engl J Med* 1996;335:1581–1586.
23. Alpard SK, Zwischenberger JB, Weike T, et al. New clinically relevant sheep model of severe respiratory failure secondary to combined smoke inhalation/cutaneous flame burn injury. *Crit Care Med* 2000;28:1469–1476.
24. Hanston P, Butera R, Clemessy J, et al. Early complications and value of initial clinical and paraclinical observations in victims of smoke inhalation without burns. *Chest* 1997;111:671–675.
25. Barillo DJ, Goode R, Esch V. Cyanide poisoning in victims of fire: analysis of 364 cases and review of the literature. *J Burn Care Rehabil* 1994;15:46–57.
26. Prien T. Toxic smoke compounds and inhalation injury—a review. *Burns* 1988;14:451–460.
27. Shusterman D, Alexeeff G, Hargis C, et al. Predictors of carbon monoxide and hydrogen cyanide exposure in smoke inhalation patients. *J Toxicol Clin Toxicol* 1996;34:61–71.
28. Purser D. Behavioural impairment in smoke environments. *Toxicology* 1996;115:25–40.
29. Baud FJ, Barriot P, Toffis V, et al. Elevated blood cyanide concentrations in victims of smoke inhalation. *N Engl J Med* 1991;325:1761–1766.
30. Hartzell GE. Overview of combustion toxicology. *Toxicology* 1996;115:7–23.
31. Bizovi KE, Leikin JD. Smoke inhalation among firefighters. *Occup Med* 1995; 10:721–733.
32. Gill JR, Goldfeder LB, Stajic M. The happy land homicides: 87 deaths due to smoke inhalation. *J Forensic Sci* 2003;48:161–163.
33. Rowland C. R.I. club's exits at issue in fire probe. *Boston Globe* 2003 Mar 10.
34. Alarie Y. Toxicity of fire smoke. *Crit Rev Toxicol* 2002;32:259–289.
35. Rabinowitz PM, Siegel MD. Acute inhalation injury. *Clin Chest Med* 2002;23:707–715.
36. Harwood B, Hall JR. What kills in fires: smoke inhalation or burns? *Fire J* 1989;84:29–34.
37. Genovesi MG, Tashkin DP, Chopra S, et al. Transient hypoxemia in firemen following inhalation of smoke. *Chest* 1977;71:441–444.
38. Morkawa T, Yanai E, Nishina T. Toxicity evaluation of fire effluent gases from experimental fires in building. *J Fire Sci* 1987;5:248–271.
39. Hall AH, Rumack BH. Hydroxycobalamin/sodium thiosulfate as a cyanide antidote. *J Emerg Med* 1987;5:115–121.
40. Silverman ST, Purdue GF, Hunt JL, et al. Cyanide toxicity in burned patients. *J Trauma* 1988;28:171–177.
41. Tomaszewski CA, Thom SR. Use of hyperbaric oxygen in toxicology. *Emerg Med Clin North Am* 1994;12:437–453.
42. Ernst A, Zibrak JD. Carbon monoxide poisoning. *N Engl J Med* 1998;339:1603–1608.
43. Heimbach D. What's new in general surgery: burns and metabolism. *J Am Coll Surg* 2002;194:156–164.
44. Haponik EF. Clinical smoke inhalation injury: pulmonary effects. *Occup Med State Art Rev* 1993;8:431–467.
45. Hoffman RS, Sauter P. Methemoglobinemia resulting from smoke inhalation. *Vet Hum Toxicol* 1989;31:168–170.
46. Dries D. More than smoke with fire. *Crit Care Med* 2002;30:2159–2160.
47. Lalonde C, Demling R, Brain J, Blanchard J. Smoke inhalation injury in sheep is caused by the particle phase, not the gas phase. *J Appl Physiol* 1994;77:15–22.
48. Wang C, Li A, Yang Z. The pathophysiology of carbon monoxide poisoning and acute respiratory failure in a sheep model with smoke inhalation injury. *Chest* 1990;97:736–742.
49. Soejima K, Schmalstieg FC, Sakurai H, et al. Pathophysiological analysis of combined burn and smoke inhalation injuries in sheep. *Am J Physiol Lung Cell Mol Physiol* 200;280:1233–1241.
50. Sheridan RL. Comprehensive treatment of burns. *Curr Probl Surg* 2001;38:657–756.
51. Haponik EF, Summer WR. Respiratory complications in burned patients: diagnosis and management of inhalation injury. *J Crit Care* 1987;2:121–143.
52. Philips AW, Cope O. Burn therapy III: beware the facial burn! *Ann Surg* 1962;156:759–766.
53. Wroblewski DA, Bower FC. The significance of facial burns in acute smoke inhalation. *Crit Care Med* 1979;7:335–338.
54. Price D. Methemoglobinemia. In: Goldfrank LR, et al., eds. *Goldfrank's toxicologic emergencies*, 5th ed. East Norwalk, CT: Appleton & Lange, 1994:1169–1180.
55. Buckley RG, Aks SE. The pulse oximetry gap in carbon monoxide intoxication. *Ann Emerg Med* 1994;24:252–255.
56. Sharar SR, Hudson LD. Toxic gas, fume and smoke inhalation. In: Parillo JE, Bone RC, eds. *Critical care medicine*. St. Louis: Mosby-Yearbook, 1994:849–863.

57. Touger M, Gallagher EJ, Tyrell. Relationship between venous and arterial carboxyhemoglobin levels in patients with suspected carbon monoxide poisoning. *Ann Emerg Med* 1995;25:281.
58. Vegfors M, Lenmarken C. Carboxyhaemoglobinemia and pulse oximetry. *Br J Anaesth* 1991;66:625–626.
59. Lee MJ, O'Connell DJ. The plain chest radiograph after acute smoke inhalation. *Clin Radiol* 1988;39:33–37.
60. Teixidor HS, Rubin E, Alonso DR. Smoke inhalation: radiologic manifestations. *Radiology* 1983;149:383–387.
61. Lee MJ, O'Connell DJ. The plain chest radiograph after acute smoke inhalation. *Clin Radiol* 1988;39:33–37.
62. Teixidor HS, Rubin E, Alonso DR. Smoke inhalation: radiologic manifestations. *Radiology* 1983;149:383–387.
63. Clark CJ, Reid WH, Pollock AJ, et al. Role of pulmonary alveolar macrophage activation in acute lung injury after burns and șmoke inhalation. *Lancet* 1988;2:872–874.
64. DiVincenti FC, Pruit, Reckler JM. Inhalation injuries. *J Trauma* 1971;11:109–117.
65. Shirani KZ, Pruitt BA Jr, Mason AD Jr. The influence of inhalation injury and pneumonia on burn mortality. *Ann Surg* 1987;205:82–87.
66. Holm C, Tegeler J, Mayr M, et al. Effect of crystalloid resuscitation and inhalation injury on extravascular lung water. *Chest* 2002;121:1956–1962.
67. Desai MH, Rutan RL, Herndon DN. Managing smoke inhalation injuries. *Postgrad Med* 1989;8:69–76.
68. Weaver LK, Howe S, Hopkins R, Chan KJ. Carboxyhemoglobin half-life in carbon monoxide-poisoned patients treated with 100% oxygen at atmospheric pressure. *Chest* 2000;117:801–808.
69. Clark WR. Smoke inhalation: diagnosis and treatment. *World J Surg* 1992;6:24–29.
70. Inoue T, Okabayashi K, Ohtani M, et al. Effect of smoke inhalation injury on fluid requirement in burn resuscitation. *Hiroshima J Med Sci* 2002; 51:1–5.
71. Barker SJ, Tremper KK. The effect of carbon monoxide inhalation on pulse oximetry and transcutaneous PO_2. *Anesthesiology* 1987;66:677–679.
72. Shusterman D. Clinical smoke inhalation injury: systemic effects. *Occup Med State Art Rev* 1993;8:469–503.
73. Tomaszewski CA. Carbon monoxide. In: Goldfrank LR, et al., eds. *Goldfrank's toxicologic emergencies*, 5th ed. East Norwalk, CT: Appleton & Lange, 1994:1199–1214.
74. Yen D, Tsai J, Wang LM, et al. The clinical experience of acute cyanide poisoning. *Am J Emerg Med* 1995;13:524–528.
75. Lindquist P, Rammer L, Sorbo B. The role of hydrogen cyanide and carbon monoxide in fire casualties: a prospective study. *Forensic Sci Int* 1989;43:9–14.
76. Jones J, McMullen MJ, Doughterty J. Toxic smoke inhalation: cyanide poisoning in fire victims. *Am J Emerg Med* 1987;5:318–321.
77. Clark CJ, Campbell D, Reid WH. Blood carboxyhaemoglobin and cyanide levels in fore survivors. *Lancet* 1981;2:1332–1335.
78. Calafat AM, Stanfill SB. Rapid quantitation of cyanide in whole blood by automated headspace gas chromatography. *J Chromatogr B Analyt Technol Biomed Life Sci* 2002;772:131–137.
79. Johnson RP, Mellors JW. Arteriolization of venous blood gases: a clue to the diagnosis of cyanide poisoning. *J Emerg Med* 1988;6:401–404.
80. Liu D, Olson KR. Smoke inhalation: contemporary management in critical care. In: Hoffman RS, Goldfrank LR, eds. *Critical care toxicology*. New York: Churchill Livingstone, 1991: 203–224.
81. Moisan TC. Prolonged asthma after smoke inhalation: a report of three cases and a review of the previous reports. *J Occup Med* 1991;33:458–461.
82. Tasaka S, Kanazawa M, Mori M, et al. Long-term course of bronchiectasis and bronchiolitis obliterans as late complication of smoke inhalation. *Respiration* 1995;62:40–42.
83. Park GY, Park JW, Jeong DH, et al. Prolonged airway and systemic inflammatory reactions after smoke inhalation. *Chest* 2003;123:475–480.
84. Large AA, Owens GR, Hoffman LA. The short-term effects of smoke exposure on the pulmonary function of firefighters. *Chest* 1990;97:806–809.
85. Tashkin DP, Genovesi MG, Chopra S, et al. Respiratory status of Los Angeles firemen. One month follow-up after inhalation of dense smoke. *Chest* 1977;71:445–449.

SECTION

2

Toxic Alcohols and Their Derivatives

CHAPTER 191

Ethanol, Isopropanol, and Methanol

Marco L. A. Sivilotti

See Figure 1.

Compounds included:	**Ethanol (ethyl alcohol), isopropanol (isopropyl alcohol), methanol (methyl alcohol)**
Molecular formula and weight:	**See Table 1.**
SI conversion:	**See Table 1.**
CAS Registry No.:	**See Table 1.**
Special concerns:	**Alcohols cause inebriation initially, but effects from their metabolic products are delayed for several hours.**
Antidotes:	**Ethanol, fomepizole, tetrahydrofolate**

OVERVIEW

The term *alcohol* can have several meanings. For most lay people and in forensic applications, it is synonymous with ethanol. For the organic chemist, an alcohol is any compound that contains a hydroxyl group connected to an aliphatic carbon atom. For the toxicologist, several of these alcohols are of particular interest and can be classified chemically (Fig. 1).

A primary alcohol contains a single hydroxyl group on the terminal carbon [e.g., methanol (methyl alcohol), benzyl alcohol (phenylmethanol), ethanol (ethyl alcohol)]. In secondary alcohols, the hydroxyl group is attached to a carbon atom, which in turn is attached to other carbon atoms [e.g., isopropanol (isopropyl alcohol, or 2-propanol)]. A glycol (diol) contains two hydroxyl groups [e.g., ethylene glycol (1,2-ethanediol), propylene glycol (1,2-propanediol)]. The glycols are addressed in Chapter 192. When another alcohol chain forms an ether link with ethylene glycol, a glycol ether results, several of which of these are of industrial importance. The cellusolves are a class of compounds in which an aliphatic chain is etherized. When two ethylene glycol subunits are joined by an ether link, diethylene glycol results. Combining multiple ethylene glycol subunits generates polyethylene glycols of increasing molecular weight.

Products of natural fermentation, ethanol and traces of methanol have been consumed since antiquity. Ethanol is used by a large proportion of the population for purposes that range from the socially acceptable to the criminal and from the beneficial to the noxious or indeed lethal. It is certainly the most popular drug of abuse across history and societies. The other alcohols are widely used in industry as solvents, antifreezes, brake fluids, paints, resins, and fuels. Exposure to these substances usually occurs when they are abused as ethanol substitutes or for self-harm, after transferring products from their original container or otherwise failing to store products safely in the home, and chronically in the industrial setting. Contamination of the food supply, drinking water, or pharmaceutical agents has resulted in a number of notorious poisoning epidemics.

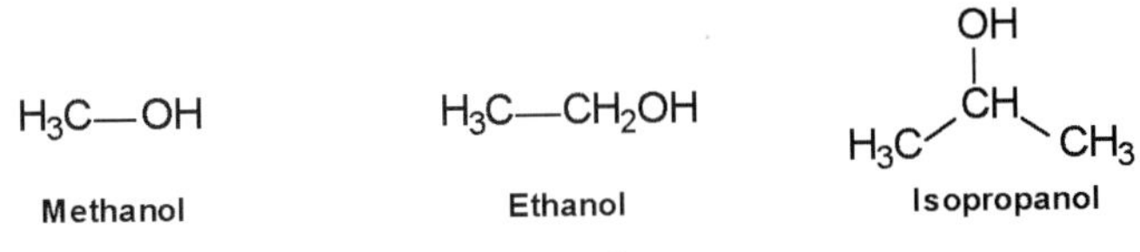

$H_3C{-}OH$ (Methanol) $H_3C{-}CH_2OH$ (Ethanol) $H_3C{-}CH(OH){-}CH_3$ (Isopropanol)

Figure 1. Chemical structure of alcohols.

ETHANOL

Undoubtedly, ethanol is the most serious drug of abuse from a public health perspective in modern society. Abstinence is

TABLE 1. Physical properties and toxic concentrations of the alcohols

Name	Molecular formula, molecular weight (g/mol), CAS Registry No.	Potentially toxic blood concentration	SI conversion
Benzyl alcohol	$(C_6H_5)CH_2OH$, 108.1, 100-51-6	Not reported, normal concentration is 0	g/L × 9.25 = mmol/L
Ethanol	CH_3CH_2OH, 46.07, 64-17-5	Toxic effects begin at ~50 mg/dl	g/L × 21.7 = mmol/L
Isopropanol	$CH_3CHOHCH_3$, 60.10, 67-63-0	Toxic effects begin at ~50 mg/dl	g/L × 16.63 = mmol/L
Methanol	CH_3OH, 32.04, 67-56-1	20–25 mg/dl	g/L × 31.25 = mmol/L

uncommon in most societies, and the prevalence of alcoholism is estimated to be 6% to 9% of the adult population. Alcohol abuse is estimated to kill 100,000 Americans per year and to be the third leading preventable cause of death (1). The economic costs directly related to ethanol exceed $200 billion annually in the United States, where 20% of health care expenditures are estimated to be ethanol related. One in seven adults self-reports a drinking binge (greater than five drinks per day) in the preceding month, a trend that is increasing in the United States (1).

Ethanol is used as a solvent in a variety of medicinal preparations and is used therapeutically as a topical antimicrobial, nerve block agent, and antidote for methanol and ethylene glycol poisoning (Chapter 56). Ethanol is also found at concentrations of up to 95% in a variety of cosmetic products, such as perfumes, colognes, mouthwashes, and industrial solvents. The most common sources are beer and ale (3% to 6% ethanol volume/volume), wine (10% to 18%), and distilled spirits (40% to 50%). Denatured ethanol has been rendered unsafe to drink (and thus exempt from taxation) by the addition of various denaturants, including benzene, methanol, kerosene, ether, camphor, terpineol, or sulfuric acid.

Toxic Dose

The toxic dose ranges widely because of the substantial tolerance that develops in habitual drinkers. Many countries define ethanol intoxication in terms of the blood concentration: 0.05%, 0.08%, or 0.10% depending on the jurisdiction. A serum concentration of 450 mg/dl may be fatal in naïve patients, whereas survival has been reported after a concentration of 1500 mg/dl (2). The approximate LD_{50} (median lethal dose) is 5 to 8 g/kg in casual drinkers and 3 to 6 g/kg in children.

Toxicokinetics and Toxicodynamics

ABSORPTION AND DISTRIBUTION

The pharmacokinetics of ethanol have been studied extensively (3,4). When ingested, ethanol is rapidly absorbed, especially in the fasting state. Ethanol distributes readily into total body water, with an apparent V_d of 0.54 ± 0.05 L/kg (young adult males, plasma data) and negligible protein binding or fat solubility. It readily crosses the blood–brain barrier. The extent of first-pass metabolism attributable to hepatic metabolism and to class IV (σ_2) alcohol dehydrogenase (ADH) activity in the gastric mucosa appears to have been overstated in the literature. Estimates of first-pass metabolism using area-under-the-curve methods are inflated during zero-order elimination and do not reflect true bioavailability (5). Under optimal conditions, 80% to 90% of an ingested dose is absorbed within 30 to 60 minutes of ingestion.

Women have a lower body mass and lower proportion of body water, resulting in higher peak circulating ethanol concentrations than men. Other influences on peak concentration include type of beverage, coingestion of food, body composition, age, rate of gastric emptying, and time of day (6).

ELIMINATION

The elimination of ethanol is an important example of zero-order drug elimination. In fact, dual Michaelis-Menton elimination, corresponding to the two main metabolizing enzyme families, describes ethanol elimination after intravenous (IV) loading of 0.3 to 0.8 g/kg (7) (Fig. 2). These enzymes are the cytosolic, NAD^+ (nicotinamide adenine dinucleotide)-dependent ADH family (largely class I, composed of α, β, and γ subunits, with K_m less than 20 mg/dl) and the microsomal ethanol oxidizing system (largely CYP2E1 but also 3A4 and 1A2) (8). The very low K_m of hepatic ADH for ethanol results in time-dependent elimination of ethanol beginning at the lower end of the clinically relevant range of serum ethanol concentrations. At higher concentrations, and with induction after habitual consumption, CYP2E1 assumes greater importance in ethanol metabolism.

Peroxisomal catalase is no longer considered to play a significant role in ethanol oxidation *in vivo* due to dependence on H_2O_2. A minor, nonoxidative pathway is mediated by fatty acid ethyl ester synthase. Direct elimination in the urine, sweat, and breath accounts for less than 10% of ethanol elimination after ingestion.

Substantial interindividual variation is found in ethanol metabolism, mostly due to genetic variation in ADH isoenzymes (mainly polymorphism of β and γ subunits) and to CYP2E1 induction (6,9,10). Coingestion of food can increase ethanol metabolism marginally, whereas IV fluids, dextrose, and fructose have no appreciable effect (3,8,11).

The pharmacodynamic effects of ethanol are characterized by substantial tolerance. Acute or within-session tolerance (Mellanby effect) is demonstrated by diminished physiologic or behavioral effects for any given blood ethanol concentration, as concentrations are falling rather than rising (12). Chronic tolerance develops with repeat dosing and may persist during times of abstinence. Finally, cross-tolerance to barbiturates and benzodiazepines develops.

Pathophysiology

The molecular sites of action for ethanol are uncertain. Historically, changes in membrane fluidity and other physicochemical alterations of membrane function were presumed to account for the effect of the alcohols and anesthetics on cellular function. This theory was consistent with the linear increase in sedation and ataxia observed as one progressed from methanol to 1-hexanol. More recently, molecular biology techniques have indicated that the alcohols and anesthetics interact with a specific site on neurotransmitter receptors (13,14). Specifically, a target within the transmembrane domains of the γ-aminobutyric acid (GABA)-A and glycine receptors appears necessary for ethanol to exert its effects. The essential role of the GABA-A receptor is also supported by the cross-tolerance to other GABA-A agonists and their central role in treating withdrawal (15,16).

Another large body of work demonstrates that inhibitory effects on the glutamate NMDA (N-methyl-D-aspartate) receptor may account for certain central effects of ethanol, such as the amnestic effect in the hippocampus (17). Effects of ethanol on the serotonin $5HT_3$ (serotonin) receptor may account for the psychosis, hallucinations, and cravings observed in ethanol-dependent individuals. Other putative targets for ethanol include the glycine, nicotinic acetylcholine, and adenosine 2X receptors, as well as L-type calcium channels.

With chronic use, ethanol has myriad effects. CYP2E1 is induced largely by post-transcriptional stabilization. As a result, additional oxidative stress results from metabolism of ethanol, fatty acids, and other xenobiotics by this enzyme (18). Alcoholics are at risk for malabsorption of essential dietary factors, even when they have access to a nutrient-rich diet. Multiple derangements result from the substitution of ethanol (7.1 kcal/g) as the primary fuel for metabolism. Indeed, when more than one-third of the caloric intake is from ethanol (approximately 2 g/day), characteristic changes of steatosis occur, even with an otherwise adequate diet (19). Deficiencies of protein, folate, thiamine, and other micronutrients potentiate these changes.

Ethanol oxidized by CYP2E1 does not directly generate NADH for ATP production, and therefore ethanol contains truly "empty calories." Ethanol interferes with nutrient activation, such as the conversion of methionine to S-adenosyl-L-methionine, which is required by phosphatidylethanolamine methyltransferase to generate phosphatidylcholine and maintain normal

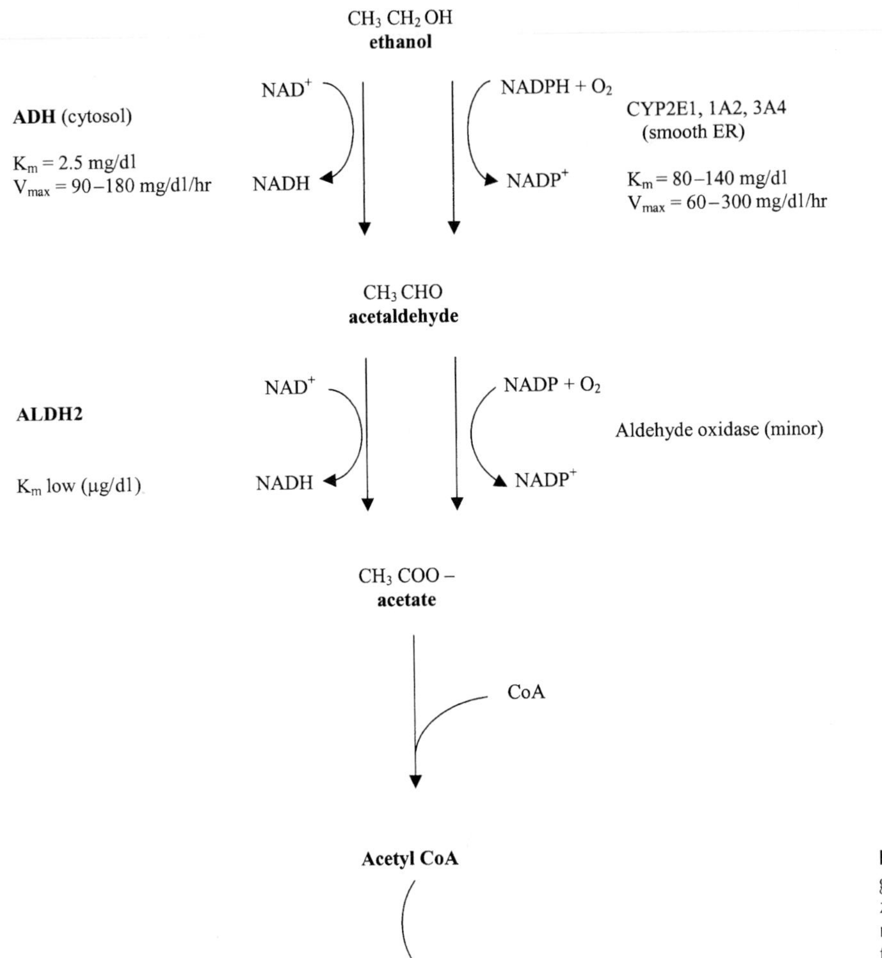

Figure 2. Ethanol oxidation. ADH, alcohol dehydrogenase; ALDH, aldehyde dehydrogenase; CoA, coenzyme A; ER, endoplasmic reticulum; NAD, nicotinamide adenine dinucleotide; NADH, reduced form of nicotinamide adenine dinucleotide; NADP, adenine dinucleotide phosphate.

cell membranes. Thiamine deficiency results in Wernicke-Korsakoff syndrome and wet beriberi. Pyridoxine deficiency results in neurologic, hematologic, and dermatologic disease. The acetaldehyde generated by oxidation of ethanol has been implicated as the toxin relevant to upper aerodigestive cancers (20). It may also cause microtubular impairment, lipid peroxidation, pyridoxine depletion, inhibition of deoxyribonucleic acid repair, and other effects. Others suggest that formic acid, which results from methanol accumulation due to ADH inhibition, is the neurotoxin of prime importance. The molecular mechanisms that underlie physical dependence, whereby ethanol ingestion is necessary to prevent withdrawal, are incompletely characterized.

Pregnancy and Lactation

Ethanol is FDA pregnancy category D, category X if used in large amounts or for prolonged periods (Appendix I). Ethanol readily crosses the placenta. Intrauterine exposure to high levels of ethanol has long been recognized to result in a characteristic pattern of pre- and postnatal growth restriction, microcephaly, adverse neurodevelopmental sequelae, and facial dysmorphism, termed the *fetal alcohol syndrome*. The prevalence of fetal alcohol syndrome is between 0.5 and 2.0 per 1000 live births in the United States, making ethanol the most significant teratogen (21). Exposure has also been associated with a range of neurobehavioral disturbances without the craniofacial malformations. Accordingly, current nomenclature includes the terms *fetal alcohol spectrum disorder*, or *alcohol-related neurodevelopmental disorder*.

Changes in brain structure and function, including decreased psychomotor, psychosocial, and cognitive performance, have been reported in subjects of all ages in association with maternal ethanol consumption (22). A threshold to these effects has not been identified, although some studies report changes at a dose of three drinks per day (23). It is possible that exposure to ethanol during the vulnerable period of synaptogenesis (brain growth spurt period) triggers a wave of apoptotic neurodegeneration (24). A variety of other candidate mechanisms have been suggested (25). Frequent binge drinking in women with childbearing potential, which is associated with unplanned pregnancy and thus exposure before pregnancy is recognized, is of concern (26).

Ethanol appears in the breast milk. The dose ingested by nursing infants can be calculated to be a small fraction (less than 3% weight-adjusted) of the typical maternal ingested dose.

Clinical Presentation

ACUTE EXPOSURE

The acute effects of ethanol concentration are summarized in Table 2. Coma is unusual at serum ethanol concentrations below 200 mg/dl. Death can occur at concentrations of 450 mg/dl in casual drinkers. Tolerance can substantially affect the concentration at which the effects of ethanol become clinically evident.

CHRONIC EXPOSURE

Chronic, heavy ingestion of ethanol over years results in toxicity to virtually every organ system and derangements in metabolic func-

TABLE 2. Clinical effects of ethanol in inexperienced drinkers

Serum ethanol concentration (mg/dl)	Clinical effects
20–50	Disinhibition, paradoxic excitation, emotional lability, gregariousness, garrulousness, euphoria
50–100	Increased reaction time, diminished judgment, fine motor incoordination, dysarthria
100–200	Diplopia, violence, disorientation, confusion, ataxia, vasodilatation, stupor
200–400	Respiratory depression, loss of protective airway reflexes, hypothermia, incontinence, hypotension, coma
>400	Cardiovascular collapse, death

TABLE 4. Selected causes of disulfiram-like ethanol reaction

Metronidazole
Cefoperazone, cefotetan, cefamandole, and other cephalosporins
Chlorpropamide and other sulfonylureas
Griseofulvin
Carbon disulfide
Calcium carbamide
Trichloroethylene
Tetramethylthiuram disulfide
Coprinus and other mushrooms
Aldehyde dehydrogenase class 2*2 phenotype (prevalent in Japanese and other Asians)

tion (20,27) (Table 3). Interestingly, there is abundant epidemiologic evidence of an association between light to moderate, regular drinking and the reduction in coronary heart disease, stroke, and overall mortality. Thus, ethanol shows a J-shaped dose-response curve for these outcomes. Regular consumption of wine at meals is believed to account for the "French paradox" of reduced cardiovascular mortality despite an atherogenic diet in certain Mediterranean countries. This protective effect on coronary heart disease relative to abstention is detectable by one drink per week and is maximal at one to two drinks per day on 5 to 6 days per week (relative risk 0.66, men) (28). It is mitigated in women, binge drinkers, and when all-cause mortality is the response (29). The mechanisms are believed to involve favorable effects on lipid profile, platelet function, fibrinolytic activity, blood pressure, insulin levels, and stress, and likely vary among individuals.

Alcoholic ketoacidosis is a condition that develops in chronic alcoholic patients that involves impaired gluconeogenesis and increased fatty acid and ketone formation. It typically develops after binge drinking, followed by vomiting and forced abstinence. As the vomiting continues and severe abdominal pain develops, the patient decides to seek medical attention. Laboratory tests usually show ketoacidosis with normal to low glucose. The ethanol concentration is low or zero. It is potentiated by malnutrition or depletion of central cofactors.

DRUG INTERACTIONS

Numerous drug interactions occur with ethanol. A reduction in mitochondrial aldehyde dehydrogenase class 2 (ALDH2) activity causes accumulation of aldehyde during ethanol metabolism, resulting in facial flushing, dyspnea, nausea, urticaria, headache, tachycardia, and hypotension. This aversive reaction after ethanol ingestion is the basis for chronic disulfiram therapy for alcoholism, although the evidence for efficacy is dubious (7). Disulfiram and its metabolites diethyldithiocarbamate and carbon disulfide irreversibly inhibit ALDH2, as well as ALDH1, CYP2E1, dopamine β-hydroxylase, and a variety of other metalloenzymes. A number of other conditions and drugs can cause a similar reaction after ethanol ingestion (Table 4).

Chronic ingestion of ethanol produces cross-tolerance to some sedative and hypnotic drugs. The alcohol interaction with acetaminophen is complex and is addressed in Chapter 126.

TABLE 3. Clinical effects of chronic ethanol ingestion

Organ system	Reported effects
Endocrine	Hypogonadism, osteoporosis, steatosis, hypoglycemia
Malnutrition	Pellagra, stomatitis, scurvy, folate deficiency
Electrolytes	Hypomagnesemia, hypophosphatemia, hypocalcemia, hypokalemia, hypoglycemia
Neuropsychiatric	Wernicke's syndrome, Korsakoff's syndrome, dementia, peripheral neuropathy, cerebellar degeneration, Marchiafava-Bignami syndrome
Cardiovascular	Cardiomyopathy, atrial fibrillation/flutter, wet beriberi
Psychiatric	Depression, hallucinations, delusions, suicide
Gastrointestinal	Esophagitis, gastritis, peptic ulcer disease, portal hypertension, esophageal varices, malabsorption, gastrointestinal bleeding, pancreatitis, alcoholic hepatitis, cirrhosis
Hematologic	Coagulopathy, thrombocytopenia, anemia, hemolysis, leukopenia, immunosuppression, hypersplenism
Malignancy	Oral mucosa, pharynx, larynx, esophagus, liver, breast, colorectal

Diagnostic Tests

ACUTE ETHANOL INTOXICATION

Ethanol can be detected in virtually any biologic fluid specimen, including blood, urine, saliva, and exhaled breath. The bladder contents are not in equilibrium with blood but may be a useful source at times. Serum osmometry is not specific for ethanol, as other alcohols depress the freezing point. Osmometry also overestimates ethanol concentrations because of the supramolar (20% to 25%) contribution of ethanol as described in Osmol Gap. More current enzymatic techniques involving ADH are fairly specific for ethanol. For example, the rate of dehydrogenation of methanol or ethylene glycol is negligible, and the rate of dehydrogenation of isopropanol is approximately 6% that of ethanol. The preferred methodology in common use is gas chromatography, which can speciate the alcohols and has a low limit of detection.

A distinction is made between serum ethanol concentrations, commonly obtained in clinical practice, and blood ethanol concentrations, which are used as the limits for drinking-driving. Most jurisdictions have enacted legislation that makes it an offense to drive with a blood ethanol concentration of 50 or 80 mg/dl (range, 20 to 150 mg/dl). Because the average water content for blood is approximately 85% weight per volume (vs. 95% for plasma), whole blood ethanol concentrations are approximately 10% lower (95% confidence interval 3% to 14%) than the corresponding plasma concentration. When mass/mass units are used, one must correct for the specific density of blood: 1.055 (i.e., 100 mg/dl = 94.7 mg/100 g).

Testing of breath samples is rapid and assumes a serum-alveolar gas ratio of approximately 2300:1 (2100:1 in forensic applications), following Henry's law. Intra- and interindividual variation is seen in this ratio (6) Most current breath ethanol detectors use the characteristic infrared absorption spectrum of the function hydroxyl group and measure absorption at selected discriminatory wavelengths. Potential interferents including other primary alcohols can be detected based on the exact methodology used. Traces of ethanol in the oral mucosa due to ingestion or emesis just before testing can falsely elevate readings. Fatty acid ethyl esters persist in adipose tissue after the disappearance of ethanol and are therefore a potential marker of recent ingestion or chronic use.

Clinically, one observes an elimination rate of 20 ± 6 mg/dl/hour in emergency department patients at serum ethanol concentrations of 20 to 400 mg/dl (30). The extremes of the range 10 to 25 mg/dl/hour have been recommended for providing a confidence interval when back-extrapolating a single serum ethanol concentration (10). Interestingly, fomepizole, which inhibits ADH and CYP2E1, has only a minor effect on ethanol elimination (31).

ALCOHOLISM

Suggested serum markers for alcoholism include mean corpuscular volume, platelet count, γ-glutamyltransferase, uric acid, serum transaminases, carbohydrate-deficient transferrin, 5-hydroxytryptophol, β-hexosaminidase, and acetaldehyde adducts (32). The clinical diagnosis of alcoholism is facilitated using validated screening tests such as the CAGE questionnaire and the Brief Michigan Alcoholism Screening Test, based largely on the behavioral and social stigmata of this disease.

POSTMORTEM CONSIDERATIONS

Putrefaction can result in changes in ethanol concentrations in postmortem tissue (33). The vitreous humor and the bladder are preferred sources for testing when necropsy is delayed (34), although urine fermentation can occur in diabetics when glucose and *Candida* are present (35). Approximately one-third of alcoholics do not have detectable ethanol at autopsy.

Treatment

Treatment is supportive, including IV access and fluids and maintenance of the airway and ventilation if required.

DECONTAMINATION

Oral activated charcoal should not be administered for pure ethanol intoxication. It should be considered if coingestants are present. The role of gastric emptying is unclear. Ipecac is contraindicated because of the potential for altered mental status. Aspiration of gastric contents may be reasonable if a very recent large ingestion has occurred. However, ethanol is absorbed rapidly, and lavage quickly becomes ineffective.

ENHANCEMENT OF ELIMINATION

Ethanol is easily removed by hemodialysis. In rare cases, the use of hemodialysis may be reasonable. In most cases, the minimal benefits of lowering the alcohol level quickly are outweighed by the risks of the procedure.

ANTIDOTES

No antidote is available for ethanol intoxication. Sporadic reports of improved mental status in response to flumazenil have been reported, but the response is rare, inconsistent, and short lasting. Its use cannot be recommended.

SUPPORTIVE CARE

The treatment of disulfiram reactions is largely supportive. In severe cases, hypotension is treated in the typical manner (Chapter 37). A direct α-agonist such as norepinephrine should be added due to inhibition of dopamine β-hydroxylase, also a metalloenzyme.

Alcoholic ketoacidosis is treated with an IV infusion of 5% glucose in 0.9% sodium chloride solution, with added thiamine and other water-soluble vitamins and with potassium replacement as required. The ketoacidosis and gastrointestinal (GI) symptoms usually respond rapidly. The use of insulin is appropriate in patients in whom there is any question of atypical diabetic ketoacidosis.

MONITORING

Routine observation of vital signs, especially Glasgow coma scale and airway patency, is indicated. Measurement of partial pressure of carbon dioxide via expired air or arterial blood gases is the best way to assess respiratory compromise from sedation.

ALCOHOLISM

Detailed treatment of chronic alcoholism is beyond the scope of this chapter. Evidence has been found to support the efficacy of brief interventions initiated at a "teachable moment" (36). Disulfiram and naltrexone are FDA approved for alcohol dependence (37). Calcium carbamide, acamprosate, and tiapride are approved in other jurisdictions. Nalmefene, serotonin agonists, carbamazepine, bromocriptine, and γ-hydroxybutyrate are being investigated (38–40).

MANAGEMENT PITFALLS

One should avoid ascribing altered mental status to ethanol when it is actually due to another process (head injury, stroke, seizure, psychosis, hypothermia, hypoglycemia, or sepsis). To avoid this pitfall, one should expect an improving level of consciousness with serial observation in any patient in whom ethanol is the cause of depressed consciousness. Also, ethanol concentrations should be measured on all patients with altered mental status that is believed to be due to ethanol.

Failing to take advantage of the teachable moment or initiate other interventions for ethanol-related illness is another management pitfall.

ISOPROPANOL

Isopropanol (2-isopropanol) is widely used in rubbing alcohol (70% concentration) and as a disinfectant, antifreeze, and window cleaner. It is also abused as an inexpensive ethanol substitute. Being a secondary alcohol, isopropanol is oxidized to a ketone rather than an aldehyde and cannot be oxidized further (41). Accordingly, no carboxylic acid metabolite is formed, and isopropanol is considerably less toxic than methanol or ethylene glycol. Its toxicity results largely from the properties of the parent compound, and this toxicity is of the same order of magnitude as ethanol. As a result, ADH inhibition therapy is unnecessary, and hemodialysis is rarely indicated for isopropanol poisoning.

Toxic Dose

The LD_{50} in animals ranges from 4500 to 8000 mg/kg. Although a dose of 240 to 250 ml has been proposed as lethal to humans (44), children and adults have survived much greater doses. For example, ingestion of 1 L 70% isopropyl alcohol solution was survived with hemodialysis (45). Children have survived isopropanol blood levels of up to 500 mg/dl (46).

Toxicokinetics and Toxicodynamics

Isopropanol is rapidly and completely absorbed after ingestion (47–52). Dermal exposure in infants and adults is known to result in toxicity (53–58). Isopropanol is metabolized by ADH to acetone, one of the endogenous ketone bodies (47,59). It is also excreted by the kidneys and more slowly by the lung.

The affinity of ADH for isopropanol is about one-tenth that for ethanol. The serum elimination half-life ranges from 2.5 to 8.0 hours, depending on habitual ethanol consumption, but may be up to 16 hours if ethanol is coingested (42,50,51,60–63). Acetone is cleared much more slowly, with a variable half-life of over 10 hours (50,51,60,63–65). Accordingly, acetone accumulates, further slowing isopropanol oxidation. Isopropanol is rapidly cleared by dialysis.

Pathophysiology

Like ethanol, isopropanol is primarily a CNS depressant (61). It is slightly more potent then ethanol (66), and its slower elimination from the serum contributes to prolonged toxicity after massive ingestion. Like the other alcohols, it commonly causes vasodilation, hypotension, gastritis, pulmonary edema, and GI hemorrhage (67,68).

Vulnerable Populations

Increased skeletal malformation and decreased birth weight have been reported in animals only at doses that produce maternal toxicity.

Clinical Presentation

The classic presentation is CNS depression and ketonemia without acidemia, due to its metabolism to acetone. The onset of toxicity is within 2 hours of ingestion and may be precipitous (50,52,61,69). A fruity breath odor may be perceptible. Patients may present with hypotension and coma, which should prompt the clinician to undertake rapid evaluation and anticipatory therapy (47,69,70). Hemorrhagic gastritis and mild hypothermia may be present (58,63).

Diagnostic Tests

Confirmatory serum isopropanol concentrations can be obtained using the same gas chromatography procedures that are used to test for other toxic alcohols. A high osmolal gap is present due to isopropanol and acetone, and serum and urine ketone testing are strongly positive (62). The onset of ketonemia may be delayed for up to 4 hours (61).

The serum creatinine can be falsely elevated due to the presence of acetone (71–75). Breath analysis for ethanol based on infrared absorbance can also detect isopropanol (76). The presence of a significant anion gap acidosis is rare and suggests tissue hypoperfusion or a coingestion. Isopropanol may be detectable in the serum of patients with severe diabetic or alcoholic ketoacidosis (77). Glucose testing is important to exclude hypoglycemia.

POSTMORTEM CONSIDERATIONS

Small quantities of isopropanol and acetone may be detected postmortem in patients who are not exposed to isopropanol antemortem (blood isopropanol, 1 to 29 mg/dl; liver, 7 to 59 mg/dl; brain, 2 to 12 mg/dl; kidney, 6 to 26 mg/dl) (78).

DIAGNOSTIC PITFALLS

A metabolic acidosis should be fully evaluated. Isopropanol causes a minor metabolic acidosis at most.

Treatment

Supportive care is the mainstay of therapy, with hemodialysis reserved for severely poisoned patients with cardiovascular instability despite IV fluid resuscitation.

DECONTAMINATION

Although activated charcoal adsorbs isopropanol and acetone in vitro when a 20:1 ratio is achieved, the rapid absorption across the GI tract and the large amount of activated charcoal required severely limit the clinical significance of this observation (79). Gastric aspiration may be useful in the unusual case of a large ingestion occurring just before presentation to health care.

ENHANCED ELIMINATION

Hemodialysis should be considered in any patient with a level greater than 400 mg/dl who is comatose and hemodynamically unstable despite IV fluid resuscitation (47,68–70). The endpoint of dialysis is clinical recovery rather than a target isopropanol concentration and is usually obtained after a few hours of hemodialysis (68–70).

ANTIDOTES

No antidote is available for isopropanol toxicity. Blockade of ADH with ethanol or fomepizole therapy is not needed because the metabolite does not cause toxicity (41,80).

SUPPORTIVE CARE

Supportive care is the same as for ethanol intoxication, as described in the previous section. Supportive care of the airway and blood volume allows isopropyl alcohol to be eliminated and recovery to occur within 24 hours.

METHANOL

Methanol (methyl alcohol, wood spirits, wood alcohol, carbinol) is widely available in concentrated forms, accounting for its frequent accidental and intentional ingestion. It is used as an antifreeze (especially gas line and windshield fluid, 30% to 95% concentration), fuel (small hobby engines, camp stoves, plate warmers), solvent (paints, varnishes, shellacs, cleaning solutions), and photocopy fluid. It occurs in trace quantities in fruit juices and fermented beverages (83–88), but its low boiling point (65°C vs. ethanol at 79°C) allows it to become concentrated relative to ethanol in home distillation misadventures (89). Accidental ingestion also occurs because of the use of methanol as an ethanol denaturant (intended to render ethanol solutions unsafe to drink and thus exempt from taxation). Most fatalities occur in adult males who consume methanol with suicidal intent or as an ethanol substitute (90). Methanol has no therapeutic uses.

Although methanol is mildly inebriating, the major toxicity results from metabolism to formic acid, which causes acidosis, blindness, and eventually death (91–94). Considerable interindividual variation exists with regard to these effects, presumably as a result of the coingestion of ethanol and variation in the rate of methanol oxidation and formic acid elimination (95,96).

Toxic Dose

The minimum dose reported to cause blindness is 8 g (10 ml × 100%) and, to cause death, 10 g (30 ml × 40% solution), but 40 g or 1 g/kg is generally regarded as a lethal adult dose in the absence of treatment (97–99). In children, a dose of 0.25 ml/kg 100% methanol has been associated with blindness and 0.5 ml/kg with death (Poisindex). It is important to remember that larger ingestions are survivable without sequela when treatment is timely (96,100,101).

Toxicokinetics and Toxicodynamics

ABSORPTION AND DISTRIBUTION

Methanol is rapidly and completely absorbed from the GI tract, with peak serum levels 30 to 90 minutes after ingestion (103–104). Absorption is also possible via skin and lungs, and rare cases of poisoning have occurred via these routes of exposure (95,105–111). The volume of distribution approximates body water (0.6 to 0.7 L/kg) (91,104,112). As a result, the accidental ingestion of less than 2 ml concentrated methanol can result in a serum concentration of 25 mg/dl in a toddler and therefore indicate antidotal therapy.

METABOLISM AND ELIMINATION

Methanol is mostly oxidized by ADH to formaldehyde. The rate of this reaction can only be approximated from the few available reports of untreated humans. It may become saturated at 8.5 mg/dl/hour (113) or display first-order kinetics, with a half-life of 8 to 28 hours (95,114–116). At very low concentrations (serum methanol less than 10 mg/dl), elimination is first order, with a half-life of 3 hours (117–123). Other elimination pathways (primarily pulmonary and renal excretion) are considerably slower, as demonstrated by the effect of the ADH inhibitors on methanol elimination half-life (80,124). Using pooled human data from 11 subjects receiving fomepizole for serious methanol poisoning, this elimination half-life was 54 hours (125). This value is comparable to the 30 to 52 hours observed during ethanol therapy (126). Hemodialysis effectively clears methanol, with an elimination half-life of 2.8 ± 0.4 hours and clearance of 260 ± 30 ml/minute (125).

Formic Acid

Formaldehyde disappears from the circulation with a half-life of less than 1 minute, becoming further oxidized to formic acid (127,128). In primates, the metabolism of formic acid is considerably slower than in lower orders, accounting for the accumulation of formic acid and blindness in monkeys and humans after methanol ingestion (99,114,120,129,130). Formic acid must combine with tetrahydrofolate to become completely oxidized to carbon dioxide (119). Reduced availability of tetrahydrofolate therefore potentiates formic acid accumulation and toxicity. Limited data exist on formic acid elimination, but in eight patients given fomepizole and folic acid for methanol poisoning, the elimination was found to be first order, with a half-life of 3.4 ± 1.5 hours before hemodialysis and 2.5 ± 0.6 hours during hemodialysis (131). Before the initiation of therapy, however, formic acid elimination must be slower than methanol oxidation (132,133). Formate is also excreted by the kidneys, with some proximal tubular reabsorption via a chloride-formate exchanger (91).

Formic acid (pK_a 3.75) is mostly ionized at physiologic pH (formate). The profound acidemia associated with severe methanol poisoning increases the ratio of nonionized formic acid to formate and enhances diffusion into target end organs such as the retina and mitochondrion (91). It is assumed that correction of the acidemia by IV administration of sodium bicarbonate and by hemodialysis can therefore reduce the intracellular burden of formate based on the principle of ion trapping (134,135).

Pathophysiology

Methanol toxicity affects primarily the CNS and the eye. Methanol itself is a CNS depressant, although it is less potent than ethanol in terms of producing sedation and ataxia. Like the other alcohols, it can cause vasodilatation, hypotension, and reduced cardiac output (136).

Metabolism to formic acid is primarily responsible for the retinal toxicity (93,137–141). Local production of formate within retinal tissue may be an important source of the toxic metabolite. Histologically, the axonal and glial cells demonstrate disruption in oxidative phosphorylation, suggesting that formate is a mitochondrial poison (92,142). This effect appears to be particularly devastating in the photoreceptor and the Müller neuroglial cells, both of which have highly active oxidative metabolism (122). The specific target may be inhibition of cytochrome aa_3 (91,143–145). Optic disk hyperemia and edema result, as well as ischemic and hemorrhagic changes in the basal ganglia (146–151).

Pregnancy and Lactation

Methanol is a proven teratogen in animals (skeletal, genitourinary, and cardiovascular in rats; CNS, face, eye in mice) (152,153). Its effect is exacerbated by maternal folate deficiency (154). Methanol would be expected to cross the placenta and appear in breast milk in proportion to body water. Antepartum bradycardia, severe and persistent acidemia, and ultimately intraventricular hemorrhage and death have been reported in an infant delivered at 28 weeks' gestation from a mother who presents with acidemia after methanol ingestion (155). In another case, a mother at her thirty-eighth week of pregnancy presented with a serum methanol concentration of 230 mg/dl and formate of 33.6 mg/dl and was treated with ethanol, bicarbonate, and hemodialysis, with no detectable sequelae in the infant born 6 days later (156,157). No data are available on ADH activity and formate elimination in the fetus.

Clinical Presentation

The delay between the ingestion and presentation and the coingestion of ethanol are the two most important parameters affecting the clinical presentation. Shortly after methanol ingestion (0.5 to 4.0 hours), the patient may exhibit mild disinhibition, sedation, or ataxia attributable to methanol itself. This phase rarely leads one to seek medical attention and may be relatively mild in an ethanol-tolerant individual or difficult to appreciate in a toddler. Therefore, its absence cannot exclude a significant ingestion (97). After a latent phase of many hours, patients may complain of headache, vomiting, vertigo, or abdominal pain (158). The symptom of breathlessness and the sign of hyperpnea with Kussmaul-Kien respirations are generally present but not readily apparent unless specifically ascertained. Patients typically complain of central scotomata, blurred vision, tunnel vision, or diplopia (159,160). Nystagmus is uncommon (161).

More severely exposed patients who present late may have coma, seizures, blindness, GI hemorrhage, and pancreatitis (96,97,134,160,162). Findings on funduscopy range from hyperemic optic disks to papilledema, retinal hemorrhages, and fixed mydriasis (159,163,164). This final sign is a marker of severe toxicity and poor prognosis (145,163). Putaminal hemorrhage and infarcts, and cerebral herniation, occur in severe cases (146–150,165–171).

Parkinsonism has been reported as a late sequela of methanol poisoning (172–177). Other long-term neurologic sequelae include cognitive deficits, transverse myelitis, and pseudobulbar palsy (178–180).

Diagnostic Tests

SERUM METHANOL CONCENTRATION

The diagnostic test of choice is a specific serum methanol concentration, generally determined using gas chromatography. Diet and endogenous metabolism result in serum methanol concentrations of up to 0.3 mg/dl, or higher after ingestion of fermented or distilled beverages that contain mostly ethanol (84,87,88,181,182). Unfortunately, serum methanol concentrations are not widely available outside of regional toxicology referral centers and may not be available in a timely manner even at tertiary care centers (183).

CLINICAL CHEMISTRY TESTS

Decisions regarding initiation of antidotal therapy and extracorporeal removal of methanol are often made empirically on the basis of a history of exposure and visual signs and symptoms, as well as testing of blood gases, anion gap, and osmolal gap. Each of these tests individually or in combination suffers from important limitations (184–190), and consultation with a medical toxicologist is recommended in all cases of suspected or confirmed exposure. The anion gap and osmolal gap are addressed separately in Chapters 9 and 25, respectively.

The arterial pH, serum bicarbonate, anion gap, and base deficit all correlate with serum formate concentration (100). In two series of 11 patients each, arterial pH and serum bicarbonate each correlated strongly with formate at presentation (correlation coefficient, r^2, 0.83 to 0.93) (131,141). Because serum formate levels are not easily obtained (191), the initial pH can serve as surrogate of formate and is also prognostic (135,158,188,192,193). If a simultaneous serum lactate is low in the presence of an anion gap metabolic acidosis, methanol poisoning is an important diagnostic consideration. Conversely, a normal serum bicarbonate and pH 6 hours after exposure to methanol, in the absence of ethanol or fomepizole, would be expected to rule out a significant methanol ingestion. This strategy is particularly useful when definitive testing for methanol will take longer than 6 hours or require transfer of an otherwise asymptomatic individual.

OSMOLAR GAP

Serum osmometry by freezing point depression is readily available in many centers, accounting for the reliance by many clinicians on osmolar gaps to diagnose the presence or absence of a toxic alcohol. This test, however, is particularly fraught with pitfalls (184–186,194–197). The osmolal gap calculation is predicated on several assumptions of questionable validity. It assumes that serum behaves as an ideal solution (infinitely dilute, no interactions between solutes). Most equations use $[Na^+]$ as the only measured cation in solution. Furthermore, error propagation through the formula results in a generous standard deviation for the final osmolal gap. Moreover, the contribution of ethanol to the osmolal gap, generally assumed to be equimolar (again based on the ideal solution assumption), should be inflated by a factor of 20% to 25% to avoid false elevations in the osmolal gap (196,197). Last, because formic acid exists as formate in circulation and is therefore charged, it will be captured by the $[Na^+]$ term in the calculation and does not generate an excess osmolal gap.

Mindful of these limitations, the calculated osmolal gap can provide some information to the knowledgeable clinician. Specifically, a very small osmolal gap (less than 5 mOsm) rules out a large, recent methanol ingestion but cannot exclude a small amount of unmetabolized methanol or a large amount of formate in the serum. Conversely, a large osmolar gap, after accounting for the supramolar contribution of ethanol and for ketonemia, is presumptive evidence in the appropriate clinical setting of a toxic alcohol (194). Unfortunately, the common clinical practice of relying on an osmolal gap less then 10 mOsm to categorically rule out methanol or ethylene glycol exposure is not justifiable (187,198–203).

OTHER TESTS

Proton nuclear magnetic resonance spectroscopy can also be used to detect methanol, ethylene glycol, isopropanol, and metabolites (204,205). Their infrared absorption spectrum is similar to that of ethanol and, thus, interferent (206,207). An alcohol oxidase dipstick intended for the detection of ethanol in saliva can also detect methanol but is insensitive to ethylene glycol and isopropanol (208).

DIAGNOSTIC PITFALLS

The diagnosis of a toxic methanol ingestion should not be excluded on the basis of a small osmolal gap, especially in the setting of a high anion gap metabolic acidosis.

Time to onset of toxicity is variable, as determined by the variable rates of bioactivation and elimination. Because methanol itself is a mild CNS depressant, an early period of inebriation and sedation occurs, followed many hours later by the acidemia and visual symptoms. In outbreaks of methanol ingestion poisoning and with ethanol coingestion, this latent period can last for up to 30 hours (160).

Treatment

Treatment for methanol poisoning can be considered along four major complementary components, analogous to ethylene glycol poisoning. These components are (a) supportive care, (b) extracorporeal removal, (c) ADH inhibition, and (d) cofactor therapy.

DECONTAMINATION

Induced emesis or activated charcoal has no role after methanol ingestion, and nasogastric aspiration should be restricted to patients who present shortly after ingestion (194).

ENHANCEMENT OF ELIMINATION

Extracorporeal removal, usually via hemodialysis, plays a fundamental role in the optimal management of seriously poisoned patients (Table 5). In fact, for the patient who presents with acidemia and end-organ dysfunction, hemodialysis should be undertaken as quickly as possible, primarily to reduce the burden of formate and acidemia as well as removing any remaining unmetabolized methanol (192). Such patients should be dialyzed until the serum pH is normal and serum methanol concentrations are undetectable (209,210). Patients with large body burdens of methanol (greater than 100 mg/dl) may demonstrate small rebounds of 10% to 20% in serum methanol in the first few hours after the completion of hemodialysis and may require three or more rounds of hemodialysis (211).

Formate elimination during hemodialysis is very efficient, with a half-life of approximately 1 hour (113,212). Methanol

TABLE 5. Indications for hemodialysis in suspected methanol poisoning

The presence of any *one* of the following is an indication for hemodialysis:
- Significant metabolic acidosis (pH <7.25–7.30), unresponsive to therapy
- Abnormalities of vision
- Deteriorating vital signs despite intensive supportive therapy
- Renal failure
- Electrolyte imbalance that is unresponsive to conventional therapy
- Serum methanol >50 mg/dl (relative indication; see text)

Adapted from Barceloux DG, Krenzelok EP, Olson K, et al. American Academy of Clinical Toxicology Practice Guidelines on the Treatment of Ethylene Glycol Poisoning. Ad Hoc Committee. *J Toxicol Clin Toxicol* 1999;37(5):537–560; and Barceloux DG, Bond GR, Krenzelok EP, et al. American Academy of Clinical Toxicology Practice Guidelines on the Treatment of Methanol Poisoning. *J Toxicol Clin Toxicol* 2002;40(4):415–446.

clearance during hemodialysis is also very efficient and flow limited (209), ranging from 140 to 280 ml/minute with standard hemodialysis or even greater with high-flux methods (125,210,213). Hemodialysis is superior to peritoneal dialysis for this indication (160,193,214).

Only for the nonacidemic patient is it appropriate to consider the serum methanol concentration per se as an indication for hemodialysis. Once the generation of formate has been blocked by either ethanol or fomepizole, such patients may need to undergo hemodialysis solely for the purpose of removing the parent alcohol, thereby shortening the duration of antidotal therapy. Because the serum half-life of methanol is approximately 2 days during complete ADH blockade (124–126), it is usually advisable to perform hemodialysis to remove intermediate concentrations of methanol. The alternative would involve prolonged administration of ethanol, which is not benign, or fomepizole, for which there is limited experience beyond 3 days of therapy. Allowing "controlled burns" of methanol at a rate just below that of formate elimination (half-life 3.5 hours) is a theoretically feasible but impractical strategy. In these nonacidemic patients who are free of end-organ toxicity, the endpoint for hemodialysis is a serum methanol concentration below 15 to 25 mg/dl.

ANTIDOTES

The inhibition of ADH is necessary to block further biotransformation of the parent alcohol to its toxic metabolites. Two competitive inhibitors are currently in clinical use: ethanol and fomepizole, which are addressed individually in Chapters 56 and 59, respectively.

Ethanol has traditionally been used for this indication (161). Its use was predicated on the greater affinity of ADH for its usual substrate. In fact, the affinity is approximately fourfold greater, on a mol-mol basis (215), and therefore a serum ethanol concentration of 100 mg/dl would be expected to slow formate generation for serum methanol concentrations as high as 300 mg/dl. Furthermore, as a competitive inhibitor, it is inappropriate to describe a "therapeutic" concentration for ethanol of 100 mg/dl without consideration of the serum methanol level. Very high serum methanol concentrations should need higher concentrations of ethanol, and the converse is also true (118,140,216).

The main advantages of ethanol are that it is relatively inexpensive, widely available, and familiar to practitioners. Ethanol suffers from some important disadvantages (194,217). The time needed to obtain and prepare pharmaceutical grade ethanol for IV administration is often longer than anticipated. Its complex dosing and infrequent use can easily lead to medication dosing errors (Chapter 56). A wide interindividual variation is found in ethanol elimination, necessitating frequent monitoring of serum concentrations and adjustments in infusion rates (218). Its behavioral and CNS depressant actions can complicate patient care or intrafacility transfer. It is not uncommon for patients to require intubation and mechanical ventilation shortly after ethanol loading due to these concerns. Finally, phlebitis or gastritis, depending on the route of administration, and difficulties with fluid management are further disadvantages of ethanol as an antidote.

Fomepizole (4–methylpyrazole) does not share these disadvantages and is considered to be a superior antidote (134,138,194,217,219–222). Its primary disadvantage is the higher acquisition cost relative to ethanol (223,224). It has a wide therapeutic index, and the recommended dosing results in serum concentration well above the minimum effective concentration of approximately 10 mmol (225–228).

The dose of fomepizole is 15 mg/kg IV as a loading dose, diluted to at least 100 ml normal saline or 5% dextrose and infused over 30 minutes. The loading dose is followed by maintenance doses of 10 mg/kg IV every 12 hours for four doses. Administration beyond the first five doses should be 15 mg/kg IV every 12 hours. If used as monotherapy, fomepizole administration should be continued until methanol concentrations are below 20 mg/dl and the patient is asymptomatic. In patients with continuing symptoms (acidosis, visual symptoms) or who presented with end-organ injury, it may be desirable to continue fomepizole until the methanol concentrations are undetectable. The fomepizole dose is increased during hemodialysis. Further details of its administration are provided in Chapter 59.

Monitoring serum concentrations of fomepizole is unnecessary. Reported adverse events are infrequent and include headache, nausea, dizziness, nystagmus, and eosinophilia (138,217,220,221,229–232). After oral fomepizole administration for 5 days in healthy volunteers, mild reversible elevation of hepatic transaminases has been observed (219).

Because of the differences in antidote safety and cost, there can be disagreement regarding the threshold to initiate antidotal therapy, especially in the absence of confirmatory methanol concentrations. Table 6 contains consensus guidelines for the initiation of antidotal therapy. Antidotal therapy should be continued until the arterial pH is normal and serum methanol concentration is less than 20 mg/dl (100,160). Consultation with a medical toxicologist is strongly recommended for all patients who are suspected of having ingested methanol.

COFACTOR THERAPY

Because the availability of tetrahydrofolate is rate limiting in the elimination of formic acid, all patients who receive ADH inhibitor therapy should also be given 50 mg folinic acid (leucovorin) followed by 50 mg folic or folinic acid every 4 to 6 hours until ADH-inhibitor therapy is discontinued (129,131,139,194,233–235).

SUPPORTIVE CARE

Attention must be directed toward supporting and correcting derangements in the major organ systems affected by methanol poisoning, namely, neurologic, metabolic, and GI. Airway protection may necessitate endotracheal intubation, in which case it is important to provide mechanical ventilation commensurate with the degree of metabolic acidosis. Metabolic acidemia (arterial pH less than 7.3) should be treated with IV sodium bicarbonate, to reduce the deleterious systemic consequences of acidemia and potentially to reduce the tissue burden of formate (135,194). Fluid and electrolytes lost or displaced due to vomiting, third spacing, and pancreatitis should be corrected.

TABLE 6. Indications for the use of fomepizole or ethanol for suspected methanol exposure

Inhibition of ADH should be performed under the following conditions:
Any *one* of the following is present
- Serum methanol >20 mg/dl
- Documented recent ingestion and residual osmolar gap >10 mOsm
- Suspected ingestion and at least *two* of the following:
  - Arterial pH <7.3
  - Serum bicarbonate <20 mmol/L
  - Osmolar gap >10 mOsm

ADH, alcohol dehydrogenase.
Adapted from Barceloux DG, Bond GR, Krenzelok EP, et al. American Academy of Clinical Toxicology Practice Guidelines on the Treatment of Methanol Poisoning. *J Toxicol Clin Toxicol* 2002;40(4):415–446.

SPECIAL CONSIDERATIONS

Because of methanol's predilection for neurologic toxicity, severely poisoned patients may remain hemodynamically intact but lack CNS activity after hemodialysis has removed all detectable methanol ("brain death"). Such patients should be considered as viable candidates for solid organ and tissue donation (236–241).

MANAGEMENT PITFALLS

Hemodialysis should not be delayed in a patient with acidemia and end-organ toxicity (vision, mental status changes) pending confirmatory methanol levels.

The dose of ethanol or fomepizole must be increased during hemodialysis (Chapters 56 and 59). The possibility of other victims should be considered when the methanol ingestion is unintentional or recreational.

MONITORING

Patients suspected of having ingested methanol should have frequent vital sign and acid-base determinations pending methanol levels. Patients who receive ethanol therapy should be admitted to the intensive care unit due to the need for frequent monitoring, phlebotomy, and adjustments in therapy. Patients who receive fomepizole or hemodialysis should be admitted to a level of nursing care consistent with their level of consciousness.

REFERENCES

1. Naimi TS, Brewer RD, Mokdad A, et al. Binge drinking among US adults [Comment]. *JAMA* 2003;289(1):70–75.
2. Johnson RA, Noll EC, Rodney WM. Survival after a serum ethanol concentration of 1 1/2%. *Lancet* 1982;2(8312):1394.
3. Jones AW. Aspects of in-vivo pharmacokinetics of ethanol [Review]. *Alcohol Clin Exp Res* 2000;24(4):400–402.
4. Matsumoto H, Fukui Y. Pharmacokinetics of ethanol: a review of the methodology [Review]. *Addiction Biol* 200;27(1):5–14.
5. Levitt MD, Levitt DG. Appropriate use and misuse of blood concentration measurements to quantitate first-pass metabolism [Review]. *J Lab Clin Med* 2000;136(4):275–280.
6. Norberg A, Jones AW, Hahn RG, et al. Role of variability in explaining ethanol pharmacokinetics: research and forensic applications [Review]. *Clin Pharmacokinet* 2003;42(1):1–31.
7. Shoaf SE. Pharmacokinetics of intravenous alcohol: two compartment, dual Michaelis-Menten elimination [Review]. *Alcohol Clin Exp Res* 2000;24(4):424–425.
8. Ramchandani VA, Bosron WF, Li TK. Research advances in ethanol metabolism [Review]. *Pathol Biol* 2001;49(9):676–682.
9. Agarwal DP. Genetic polymorphisms of alcohol metabolizing enzymes [Review]. *Pathol Biol* 2001;49(9):703–709.
10. Lands WE. A review of alcohol clearance in humans [Review]. *Alcohol* 1998;15(2):147–160.
11. Li J, Mills T, Erato R. Intravenous saline has no effect on blood ethanol clearance [Comment]. *J Emerg Med* 1999;17(1):1–5.
12. Mellanby E. Alcohol: its absorption into and disappearance from the blood under different conditions. *MRC Special Report Series* 1919;15:1–48.
13. Campagna JA, Miller KW, Forman SA. Mechanisms of actions of inhaled anesthetics [Review]. *N Engl J Med* 2003;348(21):2110–2124.
14. Ueno S, Harris RA, Messing RO, et al. Alcohol actions on GABA(A) receptors: from protein structure to mouse behavior [Review]. *Alcohol Clin Exp Res* 2001;25[5:Suppl ISBRA):81S.
15. Chester JA, Cunningham CL. GABA(A) receptor modulation of the rewarding and aversive effects of ethanol [Review]. *Alcohol* 2002;26(3):131–143.
16. Kosten TR, O'Connor PG. Management of drug and alcohol withdrawal [Review]. *N Engl J Med* 2003;348(18):1786–1795.
17. Allgaier C. Ethanol sensitivity of NMDA receptors [Review]. *Neurochem Int* 2002;41(6):377–382.
18. Lieber CS. Microsomal ethanol-oxidizing system (MEOS): the first 30 years (1968–1998)—a review [Review]. *Alcohol Clin Exp Res* 1999;23(6):991–1007.
19. Lieber CS. Alcohol: its metabolism and interaction with nutrients [Review]. *Annu Rev Nutr* 2000;20:395–430.
20. Seitz HK, Matsuzaki S, Yokoyama A, et al. Alcohol and cancer [Review]. *Alcohol Clin Exp Res* 2001;25[5:Suppl ISBRA]:143S.
21. May PA, Gossage JP. Estimating the prevalence of fetal alcohol syndrome. A summary [Review]. *Alcohol Res Health* 2001;25(3):159–167.
22. Mattson SN, Schoenfeld AM, Riley EP. Teratogenic effects of alcohol on brain and behavior. [Review] [32 refs]. *Alcohol Res Health* 2001;25(3):185–191.
23. Jacobson JL, Jacobson SW. Prenatal alcohol exposure and neurobehavioral development: where is the threshold? *Alcohol Health Res World* 1994;18:30–36.
24. Olney JW, Wozniak DF, Farber NB, et al. The enigma of fetal alcohol neurotoxicity [Review]. *Ann Med* 2002;34(2):109–119.
25. Goodlett CR, Horn KH. Mechanisms of alcohol-induced damage to the developing nervous system [Review]. *Alcohol Res Health* 2001;25(3):175–184.
26. Naimi TS, Lipscomb LE, Brewer RD, et al. Binge drinking in the preconception period and the risk of unintended pregnancy: implications for women and their children. *Pediatrics* 2003;111(5:Pt 2):art-41.
27. Klatsky AL. Alcohol and cardiovascular diseases: a historical overview [Review]. *Ann N Y Acad Sci* 2002;957:7–15.
28. Mukamal KJ, Conigrave KM, Mittleman MA, et al. Roles of drinking pattern and type of alcohol consumed in coronary heart disease in men. *N Engl J Med* 2003;348(2):109–118.
29. Agarwal DP. Cardioprotective effects of light-moderate consumption of alcohol: a review of putative mechanisms [Review]. *Alcohol Alcoholism* 2002;37(5):409–415.
30. Gershman H, Steeper J. Rate of clearance of ethanol from the blood of intoxicated patients in the emergency department [Comment]. *J Emerg Med* 1991;9(5):307–311.
31. Wax P, Cobaugh D, McMartin K, et al. Effect of fomepizole (4MP) on ethanol elimination in ethylene glycol (EG) and methanol poisoned patients. *J Toxicol Clin Toxicol* 1998;36(5):512(abst).
32. Sharpe PC. Biochemical detection and monitoring of alcohol abuse and abstinence [Comment] [Review]. *Ann Clin Biochem* 2001;38(Pt:6):6–64.
33. O'Neal CL, Poklis A. Postmortem production of ethanol and factors that influence interpretation: a critical review [Review]. *Am J Forensic Med Pathol* 1996;17(1):8–20.
34. Pounder D. Dead sober or dead drunk? [Comment]. *BMJ* 1998;316(7125):87.
35. Alexander WD, Wills PD, Eldred N. Urinary ethanol and diabetes mellitus. *Diabetic Med* 1988;5(5):463–464.
36. D'Onofrio G, Degutis LC. Preventive care in the emergency department: screening and brief intervention for alcohol problems in the emergency department: a systematic review. *Acad Emerg Med* 2002;9(6):627–638.
37. Swift RM. Drug therapy for alcohol dependence [Review]. *N Engl J Med* 1999;340(19):1482–1490.
38. Colombo G, Agabio R, Carai MA, et al. Characterization of the discriminative stimulus effects of gamma-hydroxybutyric acid as a means for unraveling the neurochemical basis of gamma-hydroxybutyric acid actions and its similarities to those of ethanol [Review]. *Alcohol* 2000;20(3):237–245.
39. Gessa GL, Agabio R, Carai MA, et al. Mechanism of the antialcohol effect of gamma-hydroxybutyric acid [Review]. *Alcohol* 2000;20(3):271–276.
40. Krystal JH, Cramer JA, Krol WF, et al. Naltrexone in the treatment of alcohol dependence. *N Engl J Med* 2001;345(24):1734–1739.
41. Su M, Hoffman RS, Nelson LS. Error in an emergency medicine textbook: isopropyl alcohol toxicity. *Acad Emerg Med* 2002;9(2):175.
42. Reference deleted.
43. Reference deleted.
44. Lewis RJ. *Sax's dangerous properties of industrial materials*, 9th ed. New York: Van Nostrand Reinhold, 1996.
45. Freireich AW, Cinque TJ, Xanthaky G, et al. Hemodialysis for isopropanol poisoning. *N Engl J Med* 1967;277:699–700.
46. Visudhiphan P, Kaufman H. Increased cerebrospinal fluid protein following isopropyl alcohol intoxication. *NY State J Med* 1971;71:887–888.
47. Lacouture PG, Heldreth DD, Shannon M, et al. The generation of acetonemia/acetonuria following ingestion of a subtoxic dose of isopropyl alcohol. *Am J Emerg Med* 1989;7(1):38–40.
48. Haviv YS, Safadi R, Osin P. Accidental isopropyl alcohol enema leading to coma and death. *Am J Gastroenterol* 1998;93(5):850–851.
49. Jerrard D, Verdile V, Yealy D, et al. Serum determinations in toxic isopropanol ingestion. *Am J Emerg Med* 1992;10(3):200–202.
50. Pappas AA, Ackerman BH, Olsen KM, et al. Isopropanol ingestion: a report of six episodes with isopropanol and acetone serum concentration time data. *J Toxicol Clin Toxicol* 1991;29(1):11–21.
51. Parker KM, Lera TA Jr. Acute isopropanol ingestion: pharmacokinetic parameters in the infant. *Am J Emerg Med* 1992;10(6):542–544.
52. Stremski E, Hennes H. Accidental isopropanol ingestion in children. *Pediatr Emerg Care* 2000;16(4):238–240.
53. Leeper SC, Almatari AL, Ingram JD, et al. Topical absorption of isopropyl alcohol induced cardiac and neurologic deficits in an adult female with intact skin. *Vet Hum Toxicol* 2000;42(1):15–17.
54. Lewin GA, Oppenheimer PR, Wingert WA. Coma from alcohol sponging. *JACEP* 1977;6:165–167.
55. Martinez TT, Jaeger RW, deCastro FJ, et al. A comparison of the absorption and metabolism of isopropyl alcohol by oral, dermal and inhalation routes. *Vet Hum Toxicol* 1986;28(3):233–236.
56. McFadden SW, Haddow JE. Coma produced by topical application of isopropanol. *Pediatrics* 1969;43(4):622–623.
57. Mydler TT, Wasserman GS, Watson WA, et al. 1993. Two-week-old infant with isopropanol intoxication. *Pediatr Emerg Care* 9(3):146–148.
58. Vivier PM, Lewander WJ, Martin HF, et al. Isopropyl alcohol intoxication in a neonate through chronic dermal exposure: a complication of a culturally-based umbilical care practice. *Pediatr Emerg Care* 1994;10(2):91–93.
59. Clewell HJ III, Gentry PR, Gearhart JM, et al. Development of a physiologically based pharmacokinetic model of isopropanol and its metabolite acetone. *Toxicol Sci* 2001;63(2):160–172.

60. Daniel DR, McAnalley BH, Garriott JC. Isopropyl alcohol metabolism after acute intoxication in humans. *J Anal Toxicol* 19815(3):110–112.
61. Gaudet MP, Fraser GL. Isopropanol ingestion: case report with pharmacokinetic analysis. *Am J Emerg Med* 1989;7(3):297–299.
62. Monaghan MS, Ackerman BH, Olsen KM, et al. The use of delta osmolality to predict serum isopropanol and acetone concentrations. *Pharmacotherapy* 1993;13(1):60–63.
63. Natowicz M, Donahue J, Gorman L, et al. Pharmacokinetic analysis of a case of isopropanol intoxication. *Clin Chem* 1985;31(2):326–328.
64. Jones AW. Elimination half-life of acetone in humans: case reports and review of the literature [Review]. *J Anal Toxicol* 2000;24(1):8–10.
65. Vicas IM, Beck R. Fatal inhalational isopropyl alcohol poisoning in a neonate. *J Toxicol Clin Toxicol* 1993;31(3):473–481.
66. Wallgren H. Relative intoxicating effects on rats of ethyl, propyl and butyl alcohols. *Acta Pharmacol Toxicol* 16:217–222.
67. Alexander CB, McBay AJ, Hudson RP. Isopropanol and isopropanol deaths—ten years' experience. *J Forensic Sci* 1982;27(3):541–548.
68. Rosansky SJ. Isopropyl alcohol poisoning treated with hemodialysis: kinetics of isopropyl alcohol and acetone removal. *J Toxicol Clin Toxicol* 1982;19(3):265–271.
69. King LH Jr, Bradley KP, Shires DL Jr. Hemodialysis for isopropyl alcohol poisoning. *JAMA* 1970;211(11):1855.
70. Freireich AW, Cinque TJ, Xanthaky G, et al. Hemodialysis for isopropanol poisoning. *N Engl J Med* 1967;277(13):699–700.
71. Blijenberg BG, Brouwer HJ. The accuracy of creatinine methods based on the Jaffe reaction: a questionable matter. *Eur J Clin Chem Clin Biochem* 1994;32(12):909–913.
72. Hawley PC, Falko JM. 1982. "Pseudo" renal failure after isopropyl alcohol intoxication. *South Med Assoc J* 75(5):630–631.
73. Linden CH. Unknown alcohol [Letter; Comment]. *Ann Emerg Med* 1996;28(3):371.
74. Nanji AA, Campbell DJ. Falsely-elevated serum creatinine values in diabetic ketoacidosis—clinical implications. *Clin Biochem* 1981;14(2):91–93.
75. Rich J, Scheife RT, Katz N, et al. Isopropyl alcohol intoxication [see Comments] [Review]. *Arch Neurol* 1990;47(3):322–324.
76. Logan BK, Gullberg RG, Elenbaas JK. Isopropanol interference with breath alcohol analysis: a case report. *J Forensic Sci* 1994;39(4):1107–1111.
77. Jones AE, Summers RL. Detection of isopropyl alcohol in a patient with diabetic ketoacidosis. *J Emerg Med* 2000;19(2):165–168.
78. Davis PL, Dal Cortivo LA, Maturo J. Endogenous isopropanol: forensic and biochemical implications. *J Anal Toxicol* 1984;8(5):209–212.
79. Burkhart KK, Martinez MA. The adsorption of isopropanol and acetone by activated charcoal. *J Toxicol Clin Toxicol* 1992;30(3):371–375.
80. Bekka R, Borron SW, Astier A, et al. Treatment of methanol and isopropanol poisoning with intravenous fomepizole. *J Toxicol Clin Toxicol* 2001;39(1):59–67.
81. Reference deleted.
82. Reference deleted.
83. Francot P, Geoffroy P. Le méthanol dans les jus de fruits, les boissons fermentées, les alcools et spiriteux. *Rev Ferment Ind Aliment* 1956;11:279.
84. Lindinger W, Taucher J, Jordan A, et al. Endogenous production of methanol after the consumption of fruit. *Alcohol Clin Exp Res* 1997;21(5):939–943.
85. Stegink LD, Brummel MC, McMartin K, et al. Blood methanol concentrations in normal adult subjects administered abuse doses of aspartame. *J Toxicol Environ Health* 1981;7(2):281–290.
86. Taucher J, Lagg A, Hansel A, et al. Methanol in human breath. *Alcohol Clin Exp Res* 1995;19(5):1147–1150.
87. Tintinalli JE. Serum methanol in the absence of methanol ingestion [see Comments]. *Ann Emerg Med* 1995;26(3):393.
88. Wargotz ES, Werner M. Asymptomatic blood methanol in emergency room patients. *Am J Clin Pathol* 198787(6):773–775.
89. Foley B, Rogers IR. Fatal methanol poisoning following home distillation of methylated spirits. *Emerg Med* 1999;11:287–289.
90. Liu JJ, Daya MR, Mann NC. Methanol-related deaths in Ontario. *J Toxicol Clin Toxicol* 1999;37(1):69–73.
91. Liesivuori J, Savolainen H. Methanol and formic acid toxicity: biochemical mechanisms [Review]. *Pharmacol Toxicol* 1991;69(3):157–163.
92. Martin-Amat G, Tephly TR, McMartin KE, et al. Methyl alcohol poisoning. II. Development of a model for ocular toxicity in methyl alcohol poisoning using the rhesus monkey. *Arch Ophthalmol* 1977;95(10):1847–1850.
93. McMartin KE, Ambre JJ, Tephly TR. Methanol poisoning in human subjects. Role for formic acid accumulation in the metabolic acidosis. *Am J Med* 1980;68(3):414–418.
94. McMartin KE, Makar AB, Martin G, et al. Methanol poisoning. I. The role of formic acid in the development of metabolic acidosis in the monkey and the reversal by 4-methylpyrazole. *Biochem Med* 1975;13(4):319–333.
95. Brent J, Lucas M, Kulig K, et al. Methanol poisoning in a 6-week-old infant [see Comments]. *J Pediatr* 1991;118[4:(Pt 1)]:t-6.
96. Scrimgeour EM. Outbreak of methanol and isopropanol poisoning in New Britain, Papua New Guinea. *Med J Aust* 1980;2(1):36–38.
97. Bennett IL, Cary FH, Mitchell GL, et al. Acute methyl alcohol poisoning: review based on experiences in an outbreak of 323 cases. *Medicine* 1953;32:431.
98. Girault C, Tamion F, Moritz F, et al. Fomepizole (4-methylpyrazole) in fatal methanol poisoning with early CT scan cerebral lesions. *J Toxicol Clin Toxicol* 1999;37(6):777–780.
99. Roe O. Species differences in methanol poisoning [Review]. *Crit Rev Toxicol* 1982;10(4):275–286.
100. Mahieu P, Hassoun A, Lauwerys R. Predictors of methanol intoxication with unfavourable outcome. *Hum Toxicol* 1989;8(2):135–137.
101. Martens J, Westhovens R, Verberckmoes R, et al. Recovery without sequelae from severe methanol intoxication. *Postgrad Med J* 1982;58(681):454–456.
102. Reference deleted.
103. Becker CE. Methanol poisoning. *J Emerg Med* 1983;1:51.
104. Graw M, Haffner HT, Althaus L, et al. Invasion and distribution of methanol. *Arch Toxicol* 2000;74(6):313–321.
105. Aufderheide TP, White SM, Brady WJ, et al. Inhalational and percutaneous methanol toxicity in two firefighters. *Ann Emerg Med* 1993;22(12):1916–1918.
106. Downie A, Khattab TM, Malik MI, et al. A case of percutaneous industrial methanol toxicity. *Occup Med (Oxford)* 1992;42(1):47–49.
107. Frenia ML, Schauben JL. Methanol inhalation toxicity. *Ann Emerg Med* 1993;22(12):1919–1923.
108. Harpin V, Rutter N. 1982. Percutaneous alcohol absorption and skin necrosis in a preterm infant. *Arch Dis Child* 57(6):477–479.
109. Kahn A, Blum D. Methyl alcohol poisoning in an 8-month-old boy: an unusual route of intoxication. *J Pediatr* 1979;94(5):841–843.
110. Kudo Y, Kubo T, Nakamura I, et al. Methanol-induced health disturbance in a worker engaged in antimold spraying. *Int Arch Occup Environ Health* 1996;68(6):513–515.
111. McCormick MJ, Mogabgab E, Adams SL. Methanol poisoning as a result of inhalational solvent abuse. *Ann Emerg Med* 1990;19(6):639–642.
112. Jacobsen D, Jansen H, Wiik-Larsen E, et al. Studies on methanol poisoning. *Acta Med Scand* 1982;212(1–2):5–10.
113. Jacobsen D, Webb R, Collins TD, et al. Methanol and formate kinetics in late diagnosed methanol intoxication. *Med Toxicol* 1988;3(5):418–423.
114. Wu AH, Kelly T, McKay C, et al. Definitive identification of an exceptionally high methanol concentration in an intoxication of a surviving infant: methanol metabolism by first-order elimination kinetics. *J Forensic Sci* 1995;40(2):315–320.
115. Mani JC, Pietruszko R, Theorell H. Methanol activity of alcohol dehydrogenases from human liver, horse liver, and yeast. *Arch Biochem Biophys* 1970;140(1):52–59.
116. Kane RL, Talbert W, Harlan J, et al. A methanol poisoning outbreak in Kentucky. A clinical epidemiologic study. *Arch Environ Health* 1968;17(1):119–129.
117. Batterman SA, Franzblau A, D'Arcy JB, et al. Breath, urine, and blood measurements as biological exposure indices of short-term inhalation exposure to methanol. *Int Arch Occup Environ Health* 1998;71(5):325–335.
118. Haffner HT, Banger M, Graw M, et al. The kinetics of methanol elimination in alcoholics and the influence of ethanol. *Forensic Sci Int* 1997;89(1–2):129–136.
119. Haffner HT, Besserer K, Graw M, et al. Methanol elimination in non-alcoholics: inter- and intraindividual variation. *Forensic Sci Int* 1997;86(1–2):69–76.
120. Horton VL, Higuchi MA, Rickert DE. Physiologically based pharmacokinetic model for methanol in rats, monkeys, and humans. *Toxicol Appl Pharmacol* 1992;117(1):26–36.
121. Jones AW, Sternebring B. Kinetics of ethanol and methanol in alcoholics during detoxification. *Alcohol Alcoholism* 1992;27(6):641–647.
122. Klaasssen C. In: Klaassen C, ed. *Casarett and Doull's toxicology: the basic science of poisons.* New York: McGraw-Hill, 2001:735.
123. Osterloh JD, D'Alessandro A, Chuwers P, et al. Serum concentrations of methanol after inhalation at 200 ppm. *J Occup Environ Med* 1996;38(6):571–576.
124. Burns MJ, Graudins A, Aaron CK, et al. Treatment of methanol poisoning with intravenous 4-methylpyrazole. *Ann Emerg Med* 1997;30(6):829–832.
125. Sivilotti ML, Burns MJ, McMartin K, et al. *Pharmacokinetics of ethylene glycol and methanol during fomepizole therapy; results of the META trial.* 1998(abst).
126. Palatnick W, Redman LW, Sitar DS, et al. Methanol half-life during ethanol administration: implications for management of methanol poisoning. *Ann Emerg Med* 1995;26(2):202–207.
127. Eells JT, McMartin KE, Black K, et al. Formaldehyde poisoning. Rapid metabolism to formic acid. *JAMA* 1981;246(11):1237–1238.
128. McMartin KE, Martin-Amat G, Noker PE, et al. Lack of a role for formaldehyde in methanol poisoning in the monkey. *Biochem Pharmacol* 1979;28(5):645–649.
129. McMartin KE, Martin-Amat G, Makar AB, et al. Methanol poisoning. V. Role of formate metabolism in the monkey. *J Pharmacol Exp Ther* 1977;201(3):564–572.
130. Medinsky MA, Dorman DC, Bond JA, et al. Pharmacokinetics of methanol and formate in female cynomolgus monkeys exposed to methanol vapors. *Research Report—Health Effects Institute* 1997;(77):1–30.
131. Kerns W, Tomaszewski C, McMartin K, et al., META Study Group. Methylpyrazole for Toxic Alcohols. Formate kinetics in methanol poisoning. *J Toxicol Clin Toxicol* 2002;40(2):137–143.
132. Shahangian S, Robinson VL, Jennison TA. Formate concentrations in a case of methanol ingestion. *Clin Chem* 1984;30(8):1413–1414.
133. Jacobsen D, Ovrebo S, Sejersted OM. Toxicokinetics of formate during hemodialysis. *Acta Med Scand* 1983;214(5):409–412.
134. Jacobsen D, McMartin KE. Antidotes for methanol and ethylene glycol poisoning [see Comments] [Review]. *J Toxicol Clin Toxicol* 1997;35(2):127–143.
135. Liu JJ, Daya MR, Carrasquillo O, et al. Prognostic factors in patients with methanol poisoning. *J Toxicol Clin Toxicol* 1998;36(3):175–181.
136. DeFelice A, Wilson W, Ambre J. Acute cardiovascular effects of intravenous methanol in the anesthetized dog. *Toxicol Appl Pharmacol* 1976;38(3):631–638.
137. Eells JT. Methanol-induced visual toxicity in the rat. *J Pharmacol Exper Thera* 1991;257(1):56–63.
138. Brent J, McMartin K, Phillips S, et al., Methylpyrazole for Toxic Alcohols Study Group. Fomepizole for the treatment of methanol poisoning. *N Engl J Med* 2001;344(6):424–429.
139. Jacobsen D, McMartin KE. Methanol and ethylene glycol poisonings. Mech-

anism of toxicity, clinical course, diagnosis and treatment [Review]. *Med Toxicol* 1986;1(5):309–334.
140. Martin-Amat G, McMartin KE, Hayreh SS, et al. Methanol poisoning: ocular toxicity produced by formate. *Toxicol Appl Pharmacol* 1978;45(1):201–208.
141. Sejersted OM, Jacobsen D, Ovrebo S, et al. Formate concentrations in plasma from patients poisoned with methanol. *Acta Med Scand* 1983;213(2):105–110.
142. Seme MT, Summerfelt P, Neitz J, et al. Differential recovery of retinal function after mitochondrial inhibition by methanol intoxication. *Invest Ophthalmol Visual Sci* 2001;42(3):834–841.
143. Nicholls P. The effect of formate on cytochrome aa3 and on electron transport in the intact respiratory chain. *Biochim Biophys Acta* 1976;430(1):13–29.
144. Keyhani J, Keyhani E. EPR study of the effect of formate on cytochrome C oxidase. *Biochem Biophys Res Comm* 1980;92(1):327–333.
145. Sullivan-Mee M, Solis K. Methanol-induced vision loss. *J Am Optom Assoc* 1998;69(1):57–65.
146. Feany MB, Anthony DC, Frosch MP, et al. August 2000: two cases with necrosis and hemorrhage in the putamen and white matter. *Brain Pathol* 2001;11(1):121–122.
147. Gaul HP, Wallace CJ, Auer RN, et al. MR findings in methanol intoxication. *AJNR Am J Neuroradiol* 1995;16(9):1783–1786.
148. Kuteifan K, Oesterle H, Tajahmady T, et al. Necrosis and haemorrhage of the putamen in methanol poisoning shown on MRI. *Neuroradiology* 1998;40(3):158–160.
149. Roberge RJ, Srinivasa NS, Frank LR, et al. Putaminal infarct in methanol intoxication: case report and role of brain imaging studies. *Vet Hum Toxicol* 1998;40(2):95–98.
150. Rubinstein D, Escott E, Kelly JP. Methanol intoxication with putaminal and white matter necrosis: MR and CT findings. *AJNR Am J Neuroradiol* 1995;16(7):1492–1494.
151. Sharma M, Volpe NJ, Dreyer EB. Methanol-induced optic nerve cupping. *Arch Ophthalmol* 1999;117(2):286.
152. Nelson BK, Brightwell WS, MacKenzie DR, et al. Teratological assessment of methanol and ethanol at high inhalation levels in rats. *Fundam Appl Toxicol* 1985;5(4):727–736.
153. Rogers JM, Mole ML, Chernoff N, et al. The developmental toxicity of inhaled methanol in the CD-1 mouse, with quantitative dose-response modeling for estimation of benchmark doses. *Teratology* 1993;47(3):175–188.
154. Fu SS, Sakanashi TM, Rogers JM, et al. Influence of dietary folic acid on the developmental toxicity of methanol and the frequency of chromosomal breakage in the CD-1 mouse. *Reprod Toxicol* 1996;10(6):455–463.
155. Belson M, Baker J, Morgan B. *Methanol toxicity in a newborn infant*. 2002(abst).
156. Hantson P, Lambermont JY, Mahieu P. Methanol poisoning during late pregnancy [see Comments]. *J Toxicol Clin Toxicol* 1997;35(2):187–191.
157. Tenenbein M. Methanol poisoning during pregnancy—prediction of risk and suggestions for management [Letter; Comment]. *J Toxicol Clin Toxicol* 1997;35(2):193–194.
158. Teo SK, Lo KL, Tey BH. Mass methanol poisoning: a clinico-biochemical analysis of 10 cases. *Singapore Med J* 1996;37(5):485–487.
159. Ingemansson SO. Clinical observations on ten cases of methanol poisoning with particular reference to ocular manifestations. *Acta Ophthalmol* 1984;62(1):15–24.
160. Swartz RD, Millman RP, Billi JE, et al. Epidemic methanol poisoning: clinical and biochemical analysis of a recent episode. *Medicine* 1981;60(5):373–382.
161. Roe O. Methanol poisoning: its clinical course, pathogenesis and treatment. *Acta Med Scand* 1946;126:1–253.
162. Hantson P, Mahieu P. Pancreatic injury following acute methanol poisoning. *J Toxicol Clin Toxicol* 2000;38(3):297–303.
163. Benton CJ, Calhour F Jr. The ocular effects of methyl alcohol poisoning: report of a catastrophe involving 320 persons. *Am J Ophthalmol* 1953;36:1677–1685.
164. Sivilotti ML, Burns MJ, Aaron CK, et al. Reversal of severe methanol-induced visual impairment: no evidence of retinal toxicity due to fomepizole. *J Toxicol Clin Toxicol* 2001;39(6):627–631.
165. Anderson CA, Rubinstein D, Filley CM, et al. MR enhancing brain lesions in methanol intoxication. *J Comput Assist Tomogr* 1997;21(5):834–836.
166. Chen JC, Schneiderman JF, Wortzman G. Methanol poisoning: bilateral putaminal and cerebellar cortical lesions on CT and MR. *J Comput Assist Tomogr* 1991;15(3):522–524.
167. Faris CS, Williams VL, Gutmann L, et al. Methanol and the brain. *Neurology* 2000;54(6):1239.
168. Ganguly G, Banerjee A, Mukherjee S, et al. Bilateral basal ganglia haemorrhage—uncommon manifestation of methanol poisoning. *J Assoc Physicians India* 1996;44(11):834–835.
169. Glazer M, Dross P. Necrosis of the putamen caused by methanol intoxication: MR findings. *AJR Am J Roentgenol* 1993;160(5):1105–1106.
170. Hantson P, Duprez T, Mahieu P. Neurotoxicity to the basal ganglia shown by magnetic resonance imaging (MRI) following poisoning by methanol and other substances. *J Toxicol Clin Toxicol* 1997;35(2):151–161.
171. Phang PT, Passerini L, Mielke B, et al. Brain hemorrhage associated with methanol poisoning. *Crit Care Med* 1988;16(2):137–140.
172. Davis LE, Adair JC. Parkinsonism from methanol poisoning: benefit from treatment with anti-Parkinson drugs. *Mov Disord* 1999;14(3):520–522.
173. LeWitt PA, Martin SD. Dystonia and hypokinesia with putaminal necrosis after methanol intoxication. *Clin Neuropharmacol* 1988;11(2):161–167.
174. Ley CO, Gali FG. Parkinsonian syndrome after methanol intoxication. *Eur Neurol* 1983;22(6):405–409.
175. Verslegers W, Van Den KM, Crois R, et al. Methanol intoxication. Parkinsonism and decreased met-enkephalin levels due to putaminal necrosis. *Acta Neurol Belg* 1988;88(3)163–171.
176. Mozaz MJ, Wyke MA, Indakoetxea B. Parkinsonism and defects of praxis following methanol poisoning. *J Neurol Neurosurg Psychiatry* 1991;54(9):843–844.
177. Quartarone A, Girlanda P, Vita G, et al. Oromandibular dystonia in a patient with bilateral putaminal necrosis after methanol poisoning: an electrophysiological study. *Eur Neurol* 2000;44(2):127–128.
178. Anderson TJ, Shuaib A, Becker WJ. Neurologic sequelae of methanol poisoning. *Can Med Assoc J* 1987;136(11):1177–1179.
179. McLean DR, Jacobs H, Mielke BW. Methanol poisoning: a clinical and pathological study. *Ann Neurol* 1980;8(2):161–167.
180. Naraqi S, Dethlefs RF, Slobodniuk RA, et al. An outbreak of acute methyl alcohol intoxication. *Aust N Z J Med* 1979;9(1):65–68.
181. Sivilotti ML. Methanol intoxication [Letter; Comment.]. *Ann Emerg Med* 2000;35(3):313–314.
182. Zuba D, Piekoszewski W, Pach J, et al. Concentration of ethanol and other volatile compounds in the blood of acutely poisoned alcoholics. *Alcohol* 2002;26(1):17–22.
183. Kearney J, Rees S, Chiang W. *Availability of serum methanol and ethylene glycol levels: a national survey*. 1997(abst).
184. Aabakken L, Johansen KS, Rydningen EB, et al. Osmolal and anion gaps in patients admitted to an emergency medical department. *Hum Exp Toxicol* 1994;13(2):131–134.
185. Demedts P, Theunis L, Wauters A, et al. Excess serum osmolality gap after ingestion of methanol: a methodology-associated phenomenon? *Clin Chem* 1994;40(8):1587–1590.
186. Glaser DS. Utility of the serum osmol gap in the diagnosis of methanol or ethylene glycol ingestion [see Comments]. *Ann Emerg Med* 1996;27(3):343–346.
187. Haviv YS, Rubinger D, Zamir E, et al. Pseudo-normal osmolal and anion gaps following simultaneous ethanol and methanol ingestion. *Am J Nephrol* 1998;18(5):436–438.
188. Jacobsen D, Bredesen JE, Eide I, et al. Anion and osmolal gaps in the diagnosis of methanol and ethylene glycol poisoning. *Acta Med Scand* 1982;212(1–2):17–20.
189. Palmisano J, Gruver C, Adams ND. Absence of anion gap metabolic acidosis in severe methanol poisoning: a case report and review of the literature [Review]. *Am J Kidney Dis* 1987;9(5):441–444.
190. Walker JA, Schwartzbard A, Krauss EA, et al. The missing gap. A pitfall in the diagnosis of alcohol intoxication by osmometry. *Arch Intern Med* 1986;146(9):1843–1844.
191. Fraser AD, MacNeil W. Gas chromatographic analysis of methyl formate and application in methanol poisoning cases. *J Anal Toxicol* 1989;13(2):73–76.
192. Meyer RJ, Beard ME, Ardagh MW, et al. Methanol poisoning. *NZ Med J* 2000;113(1102):11–13.
193. Pappas SC, Silverman M. Treatment of methanol poisoning with ethanol and hemodialysis. *CMAJ Can Med Assoc J* 1982;126(12):1391–1394.
194. Barceloux DG, Bond GR, Krenzelok EP, et al. American Academy of Clinical Toxicology practice guidelines on the treatment of methanol poisoning. *J Toxicol Clin Toxicol* 2002;40(4):415–446.
195. Hoffman RS, Smilkstein MJ, Howland MA, et al. Osmol gaps revisited: normal values and limitations [see Comments]. *J Toxicol Clin Toxicol* 1993;31(1):81–93.
196. Purssell RA, Pudek M, Brubacher J, et al. Derivation and validation of a formula to calculate the contribution of ethanol to the osmolal gap. *Ann Emerg Med* 2001;38(6):653–659.
197. Sivilotti ML, Collier CP, Choi SB. Reply to derivation and validation of a formula to calculate the contribution of ethanol to the osmolal gap [Letter]. *Ann Emerg Med* 2002;40(6):656–657.
198. Darchy B, Abruzzese L, Pitiot O, et al. Delayed admission for ethylene glycol poisoning: lack of elevated serum osmol gap. *Intensive Care Med* 1999;25(8):859–861.
199. DeLeacy EA, Moxon LN, Ellis VM, et al. A report of accidental ethylene glycol ingestion in two siblings. *Pathology (Phila)* 1995;27(3):273–276.
200. Lewis LD, Smith BW, Mamourian AC. Delayed sequelae after acute overdoses or poisonings: cranial neuropathy related to ethylene glycol ingestion. *Clin Pharmacol Ther* 1997;61(6):692–699.
201. Purssell RA, Lynd LD, Brubacher J, et al. *The osmolal gap as a screening test for toxic alcohol poisoning*. 2002(abst).
202. Scherger DL, Wruk K, Linden CH, et al. *Emerg Nurs* 1983;9(2):71–73.
203. Steinhart B. Case report: severe ethylene glycol intoxication with normal osmolal gap—"a chilling thought." *J Emerg Med* 1990;8(5):583–585.
204. Monaghan MS, Olsen KM, Ackerman BH, et al. Measurement of serum isopropanol and the acetone metabolite by proton nuclear magnetic resonance: application to pharmacokinetic evaluation in a simulated overdose model. *J Toxicol Clin Toxicol* 1995;33(2):141–149.
205. Wahl A, Azaroual N, Imbenotte M, et al. Poisoning with methanol and ethylene glycol:1H NMR spectroscopy as an effective clinical tool for diagnosis and quantification. *Toxicology* 1998;128(1):73–81.
206. Jones AW. Observations on the specificity of breath-alcohol analyzers used for clinical and medicolegal purposes. *J Forensic Sci* 1989;34(4):842–847.
207. Laakso O, Haapala M, Jaakkola P, et al. FT-IR breath test in the diagnosis and control of treatment of methanol intoxications. *J Anal Toxicol* 2001;25(1):26–30.
208. Hack JB, Chiang WK, Howland MA, et al. The utility of an alcohol oxidase reaction test to expedite the detection of toxic alcohol exposures. *Acad Emerg Med* 2000;7(3):294–297.
209. Hirsch DJ, Jindal KK, Wong P, et al. A simple method to estimate the required dialysis time for cases of alcohol poisoning. *Kidney Int* 2001;60(5):2021–2024.
210. McMurray M, Carty D, Toffelmire EB. Predicting methanol clearance dur-

ing hemodialysis when direct measurement is not available. *J CAANT* 2002;12(1):29–38.
211. Harchelroad F, Kossoff D. Tissue redistribution of methanol following hemodialysis. *Vet Hum Toxicol* 1993;35:364(abst).
212. Osterloh JD, Pond SM, Grady S, et al. Serum formate concentrations in methanol intoxication as a criterion for hemodialysis. *Ann Intern Med* 1986;104(2):200–203.
213. Mowry JB, Judge BS, Bloch R, et al. *Rapid methanol clearance with high-flux hemodialysis*. 2002(abst).
214. Keyvan-Larijarni H, Tannenberg AM. Methanol intoxication. Comparison of peritoneal dialysis and hemodialysis treatment. *Arch Intern Med* 1974;134(2):293–296.
215. Makar AB, Tephly TR, Mannering GJ. Methanol metabolism in the monkey. *Molec Pharmacol* 1963;4:471–483.
216. Davis DP, Bramwell KJ, Hamilton RS, et al. Ethylene glycol poisoning: case report of a record-high level and a review [Review]. *J Emerg Med* 1997;15(5):653–667.
217. Barceloux DG, Krenzelok EP, Olson K, et al. American Academy of Clinical Toxicology Practice Guidelines on the Treatment of Ethylene Glycol Poisoning. Ad Hoc Committee. *J Toxicol Clin Toxicol* 1999;37(5):537–560.
218. O'Neill B, Williams AF, Dubowski KM. Variability in blood alcohol concentrations. Implications for estimating individual results. *J Stud Alcohol* 1983;44(2):222–230.
219. Jacobsen D, Sebastian CS, Barron SK, et al. Effects of 4-methylpyrazole, methanol/ethylene glycol antidote, in healthy humans. *J Emerg Med* 1990;8(4):455–461.
220. Jacobsen D, Sebastian CS, Blomstrand R, et al. 4-Methylpyrazole: a controlled study of safety in healthy human subjects after single, ascending doses. *Alcohol Clin Exp Res* 1988;12(4):516–522.
221. Megarbane B, Borron SW, Trout H, et al. Treatment of acute methanol poisoning with fomepizole. *Intensive Care Med* 2001;27(8):1370–1378.
222. Shannon M. Toxicology reviews: fomepizole—a new antidote. *Pediatr Emerg Care* 1998;14(2):170–172.
223. Dart RC, Goldfrank LR, Chyka PA, et al. Combined evidence-based literature analysis and consensus guidelines for stocking of emergency antidotes in the United States [Review]. *Ann Emerg Med* 2000;36(2):126–132.
224. Sivilotti ML, Eisen JS, Lee JS, et al. Can emergency departments not afford to carry essential antidotes? *Can J Emerg Med* 2002;4:23.
225. Blomstrand R, Ostling-Wintzell H, Lof A, et al. Pyrazoles as inhibitors of alcohol oxidation and as important tools in alcohol research: an approach to therapy against methanol poisoning. *Proc Natl Acad Sci U S A* 1979;76(7):3499–3503.
226. Jacobsen D, Hewlett TP, Webb R, et al. Ethylene glycol intoxication: evaluation of kinetics and crystalluria. *Am J Med* 1988;84(1):145–152.
227. McMartin KE, Hedstrom KG, Tolf BR, et al. Studies on the metabolic interactions between 4-methylpyrazole and methanol using the monkey as an animal model. *Arch Biochem Biophys* 1980;199(2):606–614.
228. Sivilotti ML, Burns MJ, McMartin KE, et al. Toxicokinetics of ethylene glycol during fomepizole therapy: implications for management. For the Methylpyrazole for Toxic Alcohols Study Group [see Comments]. *Ann Emerg Med* 2000;36(2):114–125.
229. Baud FJ, Bismuth C, Garnier R, et al. 4-Methylpyrazole may be an alternative to ethanol therapy for ethylene glycol intoxication in man. *J Toxicol Clin Toxicol* 1986;24(6):463–483.
230. Borron SW, Megarbane B, Baud FJ. Fomepizole in treatment of uncomplicated ethylene glycol poisoning [see Comments]. *Lancet* 1999;354(9181):831.
231. Benitez JG, Swanson-Biearman B, Krenzelok EP. Nystagmus secondary to fomepizole administration in a pediatric patient. *J Toxicol Clin Toxicol* 2000;38(7):795–798.
232. Brent J, McMartin K, Phillips S, et al. Fomepizole for the treatment of ethylene glycol poisoning. Methylpyrazole for Toxic Alcohols Study Group [see Comments]. *N Engl J Med* 1999;340(11):832–838.
233. Eells JT, Gonzalez-Quevedo A, Santiesteban FR, et al. [Folic acid deficiency and increased concentrations of formate in serum and cerebrospinal fluid of patients with epidemic optical neuropathy] [Spanish]. *Rev Cubana Med Trop* 2000;52(1):21–23.
234. Johlin FC, Fortman CS, Nghiem DD, et al. Studies on the role of folic acid and folate-dependent enzymes in human methanol poisoning. *Molec Pharmacol* 1987;31(5):557–561.
235. Johlin FC, Swain E, Smith C, et al. Studies on the mechanism of methanol poisoning: purification and comparison of rat and human liver 10-formyltetrahydrofolate dehydrogenase. *Molec Pharmacol* 1989;35(6):745–750.
236. Bentley MJ, Mullen JC, Lopushinsky SR, et al. Successful cardiac transplantation with methanol or carbon monoxide–poisoned donors. *Ann Thorac Surg* 2001;71(4):1194–1197.
237. Caballero F, Cabrer C, Gonzalez-Segura C, et al. Short and long-term success of organs transplanted from donors dying of acute methanol intoxication. *Transplant Proc* 2000;31(6):2591–2592.
238. Chari RS, Hemming AW, Cattral M. Successful kidney pancreas transplantation from donor with methanol intoxication [see Comments]. *Transplantation* 1998;66(5):674–675.
239. Friedlaender MM, Rosenmann E, Rubinger D, et al. Successful renal transplantation from two donors with methanol intoxication. *Transplantation* 1996;61(10):1549-1552.
240. Hantson P, Kremer Y, Lerut J, et al. Successful liver transplantation with a graft from a methanol-poisoned donor. *Transplant Int* 1996;9(4):437.
241. Lopez-Navidad A, Caballero F, Gonzalez-Segura C, et al. Short- and long-term success of organs transplanted from acute methanol poisoned donors [Review]. *Clin Transplant* 2002;16(3):151–162.

CHAPTER 192

Ethylene Glycol

Heath A. Jolliff and Marco L. A. Sivilotti

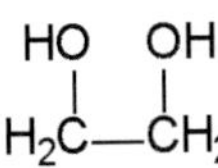

ETHYLENE GLYCOL

Molecular formula and weight:	**$C_2H_6O_2$; 62.07 g/mol**
SI conversion:	**g/L × 16.1 = mmol/L**
CAS Registry No.:	**107-21-1**
Toxic concentration:	**Serum 20 mg/dl**
Special concerns:	**Ethylene glycol causes metabolic acidosis and renal failure. Onset of these effects is delayed for several hours after ingestion.**
Antidotes:	**Ethanol, fomepizole, tetrahydrofolate**

OVERVIEW

Ethylene glycol (1,2-ethanediol) is a colorless, odorless, sweet-tasting, viscous liquid. It is primarily used as an automobile radiator antifreeze. Other uses include de-icing solutions, brake fluid, and as a solvent.

Ingestion can cause intoxication, central nervous system (CNS) depression, metabolic acidosis, cardiovascular collapse, and renal failure. In 1999, the American Association of Poison Control Centers reported 6281 exposures to ethylene glycol, resulting in 25 deaths (1). The delayed onset of toxicity after ethylene glycol ingestion, attributable to the biotransformation and accumulation of the toxic metabolite, resembles methanol, although the latency is generally shorter. Early recognition and management of ethylene glycol toxicity reduces morbidity and mortality (Table 1).

TABLE 1. Indications for hemodialysis in suspected ethylene glycol poisoning

The presence of any one of the following is an indication for hemodialysis:
- Metabolic acidosis (pH <7.25 or 7.30) with increased anion gap
- Deteriorating vital signs despite intensive supportive therapy renal failure
- Electrolyte imbalance unresponsive to conventional therapy
- Serum ethylene glycol concentration >50 mg/dl (relative indication; see text)

TOXIC DOSE

Ethylene glycol has low vapor pressure, and inhalation does not cause intoxication. The American Council of Government Industrial Hygienists has established a threshold limit value (ceiling) for aerosol exposure of 100 mg/m^3. There are no other regulatory standards for occupational exposure in the United States.

Ingestion of 1.5 cc/kg of 95% ethylene glycol has been reported to be lethal (1.56 g/kg and 398 mg/kg) (2); however, this amount is not well validated (3). As with methanol, early aggressive treatment allows for survival after much larger ingestions.

No minimum toxic dose has been confirmed in humans. However, a potential minimum dose needed to obtain a toxic level can be calculated using the following formula (in which V_d is volume of distribution):

$$\text{Serum level (mg/dl)} = [\text{amount ingested (ml)} \times \text{concentration of ethylene glycol (\%)} \times \text{specific gravity of solution (g/ml)}]/[V_d\ (\text{L/kg}) \times \text{weight of patient (kg)}]$$

In the case of a 70-kg patient and using 20 mg/ml as a lowest toxic serum level, this calculation indicates that at least 11 ml of ethylene must be ingested to attain a potentially toxic serum level. Using this formula, it is clear how a simple "sip" can potentially lead to very high serum ethylene glycol level, especially in a child.

TOXICOKINETICS AND TOXICODYNAMICS

Absorption and Distribution

Ethylene glycol toxicity does not result from dermal or inhalational exposure (4–7). However, aerosol absorption can occur in unusual circumstances. Ethylene glycol is absorbed within 30 minutes of ingestion. It is not protein bound and has an apparent V_d of 0.5 to 0.8 L/kg (8–10).

Metabolism and Elimination

Hepatic metabolism occurs through successive oxidations by the enzyme alcohol dehydrogenase (ADH; Fig. 1) (11–13). The elimination half-life ($t_{1/2}$) of ethylene glycol in the absence of ADH inhibitors is 2.5 to 3.0 hours (11,14,15). If ADH inhibitor therapy is instituted before the development of renal insufficiency, the elimination $t_{1/2}$ lengthens to approximately 17 hours, mostly via normal renal elimination (10,11,16–20). In the presence of fomepizole, the elimination $t_{1/2}$ is increased to approximately 20 hours (18,20,21).

Like methanol, ethylene glycol itself is minimally toxic but is oxidized to more toxic acid metabolites (Fig. 1). Glycolate oxidation becomes rate limiting, and evidence suggests that this metabolite is primarily responsible for toxicity (12,13,22–24). Glyoxylate can be metabolized via alternate routes, which require the presence of certain cofactors. The most prevalent pathway leads to oxalate as a metabolic end product. Glycolate kinetics are dependent on delay to treatment and remaining renal function also and have been observed to have a $t_{1/2}$ ranging from 2.3 to 19.0 hours (25). From first principles, for glycolate to accumulate, its elimination rate must be slower than its formation from ethylene glycol. During conventional hemodialysis, both ethylene glycol and glycolate are effectively cleared, with elimination $t_{1/2}$ of 2.7 ± 0.2 hours and 2.6 ± 0.7 hours, respectively (12,20).

PATHOPHYSIOLOGY

Unmetabolized ethylene glycol is not toxic. After ingestion, ethylene glycol is oxidized to glycoaldehyde, glycolic acid, glyoxylic acid, and oxalate, which produce toxic effects such as renal injury. The ability of ethylene glycol to injure the organ responsible for its excretion leads to a vicious circle of delayed elimination and ongoing production of toxic metabolites. The roles of the various metabolites of ethylene glycol in producing toxicity are debated (23,27). Perfusion of isolated rodent proximal tubule cells with pH-buffered glycolic acid suggests that glycolate is the primary renal toxin (28). Oxalate can crystallize in the presence of calcium, and these crystals are found in the urine, kidney, myocardium, and other tissues at autopsy (29,30). *In vivo*, this may lead to both hypocalcemia and obstruction of the tubular lumen. The complete oxidation of ethylene glycol also depresses the oxidized form of nicotinamide adenine dinucleotide to nicotinamide adenine dinucleotide ratio, inhibiting the citric acid cycle and generating lactate.

Besides the kidneys, other target organs include CNS (cerebral edema and herniation), respiratory (pulmonary edema, hemorrhage, pneumonitis), heart (myocarditis), muscles (myositis, rhabdomyolysis), and liver (31,32).

CNS inebriation is caused by the parent compound (33,34). CNS depression and coma are due to the metabolite, glycolic acid, and the combination of severe metabolic acidosis and electrolyte imbalance (3,35–40). Seizures may occur secondary to severe metabolic acidosis and hypocalcemia (32,41,42).

Cardiovascular effects, such as dysrhythmias and myocardial depression, occur secondary to severe metabolic acidosis and hypocalcemia (36–38,43,44).

The primary metabolic effect is an anion gap metabolic acidosis that occurs from the formation of glycolic and lactic acids (23,39,40,45–48). Hypocalcemia occurs secondary to binding of calcium to the oxalate metabolite (31,42,49).

Acute oliguric and anuric renal failure occur due to the deposition of calcium oxalate in the proximal renal tubules. This may also cause hydronephrosis and acute tubular necrosis (36,41,50).

PREGNANCY AND LACTATION

Ethylene glycol causes skeletal, craniofacial, and neural tube defects in rats and mice (51,52); glycolate appears to be the proximate teratogen in rats (53). No data regarding human carcinogenic effects have been reported. Ethylene glycol is not mutagenic in the Ames test (54).

CLINICAL PRESENTATION

Toxicity has been described as occurring in three stages (36,56). Although these stages are useful for education, they may overlap one another without obvious separation. Strict monitoring of the patient is very important. One should not be secure in a patient's condition based on time from ingestion only.

Stage 1 (neurologic effects) occurs from 0.5 to 12.0 hours postingestion. During this stage, intoxication occurs and may be confused with ethanol intoxication. Unless ethanol was ingested

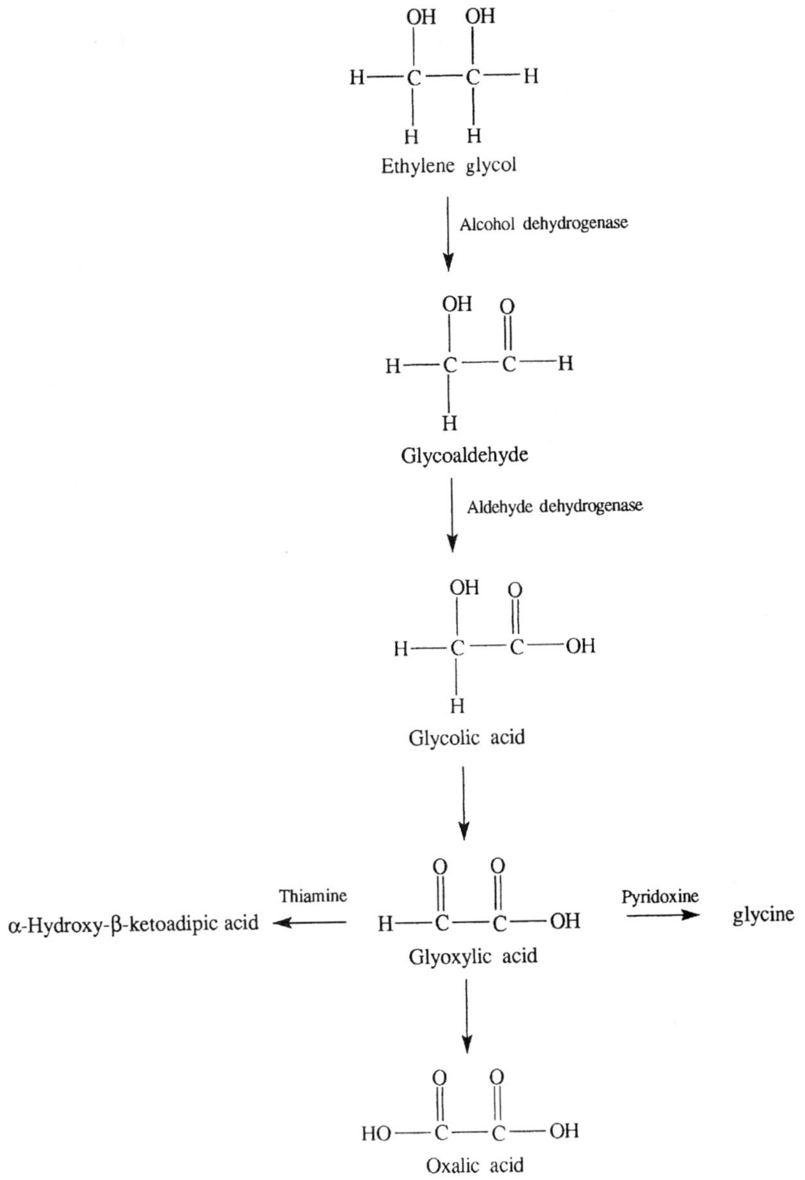

Ethylene glycol

Alcohol dehydrogenase

Glycoaldehyde

Aldehyde dehydrogenase

Glycolic acid

α-Hydroxy-β-ketoadipic acid ← Thiamine — Glyoxylic acid — Pyridoxine → glycine

Oxalic acid

Figure 1. Metabolism of ethylene glycol. (From Sullivan JB, Kreiger GR, eds. *Clinical environmental health and toxic exposures,* 2nd ed. Philadelphia: Lippincott Williams & Wilkins, 1205, with permission.)

along with the ethylene glycol, the odor of ethanol should be absent. These effects are probably due to the parent form of ethylene glycol itself. Once the ethylene glycol is metabolized, a metabolic acidosis develops and may cause CNS depression and coma. This occurs 4 to 12 hours after ingestion (3). If the poisoning is severe, coma may be accompanied by hypotonia, hyperreflexia, seizures, cerebral edema, and papilledema.

Stage 2 (cardiopulmonary effects) occurs from 12 to 24 hours postingestion. Hypertension and tachycardia are common due to the severe metabolic acidosis (3,57,58). To compensate for this acidosis, hyperventilation occurs. Hypoxia, congestive heart failure, and adult respiratory distress syndrome have all been reported during this stage (59). Multisystem organ failure and death are common at this time (60).

Stage 3 (renal effects) spans 24 to 72 hours postingestion. Renal insufficiency, as evidenced by an elevated serum creatinine, can be present as early as 16 hours postingestion, and overt renal failure is usually established by 48 hours (21). Flank pain with oliguria, hematuria, calcium oxaluria, and anuria are characteristic (19,34). Calcium oxalate crystals may appear in the urine of the patient during this stage. These crystals contribute to the acute tubular necrosis, oliguria, and anuria caused by ethylene glycol. Hematuria and crystalluria may be seen early in severe poisonings; however, the absence of these findings does not rule out ingestion. Hemodialysis is usually required at this stage. Renal function often returns to baseline, but long-term dialysis may be needed (29,50,61).

Other effects include hypocalcemia with QT prolongation, myoclonus, and tetany as well as generalized seizures (34,42). Rhabdomyolysis and pulmonary edema may also occur (34,59,62). Bone marrow suppression and pancytopenia have been reported (37,62). Patients who present late after ingestion may demonstrate cranial nerve palsies (63–66).

Severely poisoned patients may present with seizures and coma and succumb to multiorgan failure or CNS herniation (32,37,38,59,67).

DIAGNOSTIC TESTS

Serum Ethylene Glycol Concentration

Determination of serum ethylene glycol concentration, usually by gas chromatography (GC), is the preferred diagnostic procedure (3,68). Serum ethylene glycol concentrations are even less available than methanol despite the ability to assay for both substances using a single GC procedure. Propylene glycol may be mistaken for ethylene glycol on certain chromatography columns (57). This can be clinically relevant in patients receiving parenteral diazepam or phenytoin containing propylene glycol or when propylene glycol is used as the internal chromatographic standard. False positives for ethylene glycol by GC have also been caused by 2,3-butanediol, resulting from oxidation of 2-butanone in certain alcoholic beverages (69). Rarely, an inborn error of metabolism can cause a false-positive ethylene glycol result by GC (70). False positives are more common with enzymatic methods (69,71,72).

Glycolate concentrations can be assayed by GC (73–75), or high pressure liquid chromatography (46), but few laboratories perform this analysis. Serum glycolate levels at presentation correlate with pH, anion gap and serum bicarbonate (13,47,76), although the correlation with anion gap may be more reliable (12). Glycolate can be an interferent for oxidase electrodes used to assay lactate (77–79). Lactate itself can also be present at concentrations up to 7 mmol/L, and its presence should not be used to exclude the possibility of ethylene glycol when a clinician is investigating an anion gap metabolic acidosis (23,42).

Clinical Chemistry Tests

Serum calcium testing and electrocardiogram monitoring are both indicated when managing an ethylene glycol–poisoned patient. The anion gap or blood gases can be used as surrogates of accumulated glycolate and are prognostic (21,76,80,81).

Serum electrolytes, glucose, blood urea nitrogen, and creatinine should be measured. The initial serum creatinine provides a measure of end-organ toxicity (20). An anion gap should be calculated and metabolic acidosis evaluated. A serum calcium level may be obtained to rule out hypocalcemia in a severe overdose.

As ethanol can block the metabolism of ethylene glycol, a serum or breath ethanol level should also be obtained in all adult or potential suicidal exposures. A serum osmolality may be obtained and the osmolar gap calculated (Chapter 25). This may be useful when confronted with an unknown ingestion. Ethylene glycol should elevate the patient's osmolar gap (3,82). In the comatose patient with metabolic acidosis and an increased osmolar gap, ethylene glycol toxicity should be suspected. However, lack of an osmolar gap does not rule out ethylene glycol ingestion (47,83–87). In the suicidal patient, a serum aspirin and acetaminophen level should also be obtained to rule out potential ingestion and toxicity.

Other Tests

An electrocardiogram is needed to rule out the cardiac effects of ethylene glycol toxicity. A computerized tomography scan may show lesions of the CNS or cerebral edema from ethylene glycol toxicity.

Check the urine each hour for at least 5 hours after ingestion before ethylene glycol intoxication is ruled out for consideration. A urinalysis often reveals blood and protein, although the absence of these findings does not rule out ethylene glycol toxicity. The urinalysis may show calcium monohydrate or dihydrate crystals when viewed by experienced laboratory technicians (Figs. 2 and 3). Fluorescence of the urine may be helpful to document exposure, but the lack of either crystals or fluorescence does not rule out ethylene glycol ingestion or toxicity (3,88–90). If urine oxalate crystals are seen and a second 1-hour urine specimen also shows calcium oxalate crystals, begin intravenous (IV) alcohol and hemodialyze.

Some commercial ethylene glycol antifreeze products contain sodium fluorescein as a colorant to aid in the detection of automobile cooling system leaks. The urine of a patient suspected of an antifreeze ingestion may disclose visually detectable fluorescein under a Wood's lamp in the first several hours after ingestion. This observation must be confirmed by appropriate quantitative tests.

In anuric patients, irrigation of the urinary bladder with 50 to 100 ml of saline, centrifugation of the irrigant, and examination of the sediment for calcium oxalate crystals may increase the chances of detection of calcium oxalate crystalluria in a suspected ethylene glycol ingestion (38).

Pediatric "Sip"

The evaluation of a child who has potentially taken a sip of a product containing ethylene glycol is a surprisingly difficult exercise. A teaspoon of a product with a high concentration of ethylene glycol

A,B

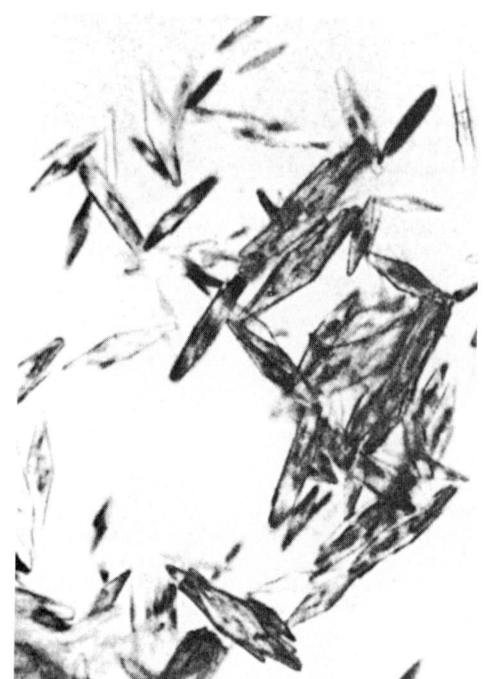

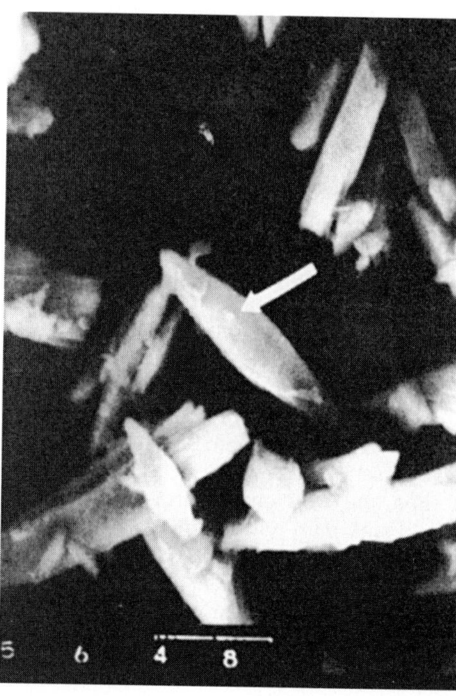

Figure 2. Calcium monohydrate crystals. **A:** ×400. **B:** Scanning electron micrograph, ×1200. White arrow indicates a point of x-ray fluorescence. (From Terlinsky AS, Growchowski J, Geoly KL, et al. *Am J Clin Pathol* 1981;76:224–225, with permission.)

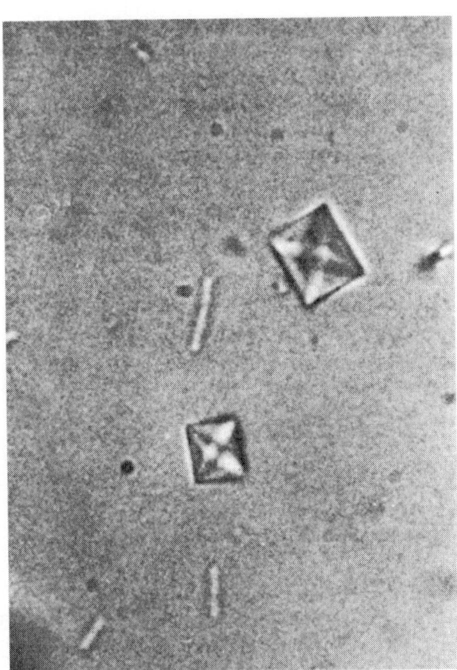

Figure 3. Calcium dihydrate crystals, ×400. (From Terlinsky AS, Growchowski J, Geoly KL, et al. *Am J Clin Pathol* 1981;76:224–225, with permission.)

may produce a toxic ethylene glycol level. It should not be assumed that ingestion is nontoxic because it was "just a sip." A serum ethylene glycol level is the only way to definitively rule out a toxic ingestion. However, a serum level may not be available in some cases. Because ethylene glycol leads to profound metabolic acidosis, serial serum bicarbonate levels can also be followed to detect occult ingestions. If a toxic ingestion has occurred, the serum bicarbonate level should fall within 4 to 6 hours. Therefore, one approach to management is to obtain baseline serum creatinine and bicarbonate levels and then repeat these tests every hour. If a metabolic acidosis does not develop within this time period (and ADH has *not* blocked from a concurrent ingestion of ethanol), a toxic amount of ethylene glycol was probably not ingested. One systematic literature analysis has supported this approach; however, no prospective studies have been performed (45).

Diagnostic Pitfalls

The diagnosis of an ethylene glycol ingestion should not be excluded on the basis of a small osmolal gap, especially in the setting of a high anion gap metabolic acidosis (Chapter 25), nor should the presence or absence of crystals or fluorescence on urinalysis to diagnose or exclude ethylene glycol exposure.

It is not uncommon for a laboratory to offer a "toxic alcohol screen" but to test only for ethanol, methanol, and isopropanol alcohol. This could have disastrous consequences for the unwary clinician who relies on a negative "screen" to rule out an ethylene glycol exposure.

TREATMENT

The diagnosis and treatment of ethylene glycol toxicity is challenging. There are multiple opportunities for missed diagnosis and therapeutic error. Severe poisoning requires advanced intensive care support for optimal outcome. To prevent delays in diagnosis and treatment, the laboratory, pharmacy, and nephrology department should be notified or consulted when the diagnosis becomes apparent. Patients with ethylene glycol toxicity should be admitted to a center where antidotes and hemodialysis are available. It is best to transfer a patient early in the course of the disease if the initial center does not have the appropriate facilities or expertise available.

Decontamination

Activated charcoal binds ethylene glycol minimally and is not expected to be effective in preventing its toxic effects (91). It should be considered if there are coingestants present. The role of gastric emptying is unclear. Ipecac is contraindicated because of the potential for altered mental status. Aspiration of gastric contents may be reasonable if a very recent large ingestion has occurred.

Enhancement of Elimination

As activated charcoal has not been shown to bind to ethylene glycol effectively, multidose charcoal should be avoided.

Hemodialysis effectively removes ethylene glycol and its metabolites from the blood. The clearance rate for ethylene glycol is 145 to 230 ml/minute (20,23,57,92). The $t_{1/2}$ of ethylene glycol during hemodialysis is 2.5 to 3.5 hours. The osmolar and anion gap decrease as the concentrations of ethylene glycol and its metabolites decrease (3,23).

Hemodialysis should be considered in the patient with severe metabolic acidosis (pH less than 7.3), in the suicidal patient with a history of a large ingestion, and in those patients with renal insufficiency or failure (Table 1). Traditionally, it has been suggested to dialyze the patient when the ethylene glycol level is greater than 50 mg/dl (3). If the patient is not acidotic, has no renal failure, and has a level above 50 mg/dl, it is possible to manage this patient with ADH blockade only (38,93,94).

The presence of renal insufficiency after ethylene glycol exposure is also an important indication for hemodialysis. Acutely, this reflects end-organ toxicity, and hemodialysis is intended to remove glycolate and other toxic metabolites in addition to the parent glycol (11,23). A serum glycolate level greater than 8 mmol/L has been proposed, but this level is usually not immediately available, and clinical experience is incomplete (76).

Once hemodialysis is initiated, the goal of therapy is to decrease the ethylene glycol level to below 20 mg/dl (3). In addition, the patient should have normal serum pH and serum bicarbonate level after dialysis. It is important to adjust the dosage of ethanol or fomepizole during dialysis as described below. Delays in turn-around time for serum ethylene glycol levels may require long periods of ADH blockade. Their concentrations therefore are lowered during dialysis, and dosage adjustments must be made to ensure adequate ADH blockade. Severely poisoned patients may require long-term hemodialysis until renal function recovers, but such recovery is typical (29,61,67).

Hemoperfusion has not been shown to adequately treat or remove ethylene glycol and its metabolites (96). Peritoneal dialysis eliminates ethylene glycol and metabolites but is much slower and requires a prolonged period of ADH blockade. It offers little advantage over ADH blockade alone and is not recommended.

Antidotes

The *inhibition of ADH* is necessary to block further biotransformation of the parent alcohol to its toxic metabolites. Two competitive inhibitors are currently in clinical use: ethanol and fomepizole. It is important to remember that ethanol and fomepizole are both dialyzable; thus, therapy must be adjusted during hemodialysis.

Ethanol has been the traditional antidote for ethylene glycol toxicity (97). Indications for ADH blockade have been proposed (Table 2) (3). Details of the dose, method of administration, and adverse effects of ethanol as an antidote are provided in Chapter

TABLE 2. Indications for use of ethanol for fomepizole for suspected ethylene glycol exposure

Inhibition of alcholol dehydrogenase should be performed when any *one* of the following are present:
- Plasma ethylene glycol levels >20 mg/dl
- Recent history of a large ingestion of ethylene glycol with an osmolar gap >10 mOsm/L

History or strong clinical suspicion of ethylene glycol poisoning and at least *two* of the following:
- Arterial pH <7.3
- Serum bicarbonate <20 mEq/L
- Osmolar gap >10 mOsm/L
- Urinary oxalate crystals present

Modified from Barceloux DG, Krenzelok EP, Olson K, Watson W. American Academy of Clinical Toxicology Practice Guidelines on the Treatment of Ethylene Glycol Poisoning. Ad Hoc Committee. *J Toxicol Clin Toxicol* 1999;37:537–560.

56. Ethanol has been shown to effectively block the formation of toxic metabolite formation during ethylene glycol toxicity (97,98). An IV infusion of ethanol should be used to prevent the metabolism of ethylene glycol and its resulting acidosis. In most cases, a serum ethanol level of 100 to 130 mg/dl is needed to effectively block ADH from metabolizing ethylene glycol. A loading dose is administered to attain this level. Once the loading dose is complete, a serum or breath ethanol level should be obtained to assure the appropriate dose was infused and the maintenance infusion started. Serum or breath ethanol levels are obtained every 1 to 2 hours to ensure ongoing, adequate ADH blockade (Chapter 56). Occasionally, a nephrologist may also choose to substitute ethanol into the dialysate to achieve the same ethanol level.

Oral dosing is not recommended but may be used to achieve the initial loading dose until IV ethanol or fomepizole can be obtained. An nasogastric tube may ensure full dosing and compliance. Ethanol is not approved by the U.S. Food and Drug Administration (FDA) for the treatment of ethylene glycol toxicity (3). It is relatively inexpensive but requires intensive-care monitoring of the patient's condition and ethanol levels.

Fomepizole (4-methylpyrazole; Antizol) is a potent ADH inhibitor. Fomepizole has been shown in animal and human studies to prevent the metabolism of ethylene glycol by ADH to its toxic metabolites (21,93). Fomepizole is approved by the FDA for the treatment of ethylene glycol poisoning and toxicity (99). It has advantages over ethanol administration in that it causes no CNS depression or hypoglycemia, it is easier to administer, it has a longer duration of action, and serum levels do not have to be followed during its use (3,100–102). However, the initial cost of the drug is much higher than ethanol and is approximately $1000 per dose.

Indications for the use of fomepizole are the same as ethanol (Table 2). It is potentially more favorable for use in the pediatric patient who may have ingested ethylene glycol, as it does not have the same adverse effects as ethanol. One loading dose can protect the patient from the toxic effects of ethylene glycol for 12 hours, while a serum ethylene glycol level is being obtained.

No head-to-head trials have been performed comparing ethanol to fomepizole. Case reports have been published with patients being solely treated with fomepizole alone and without hemodialysis. Because fomepizole therapy is relatively simple and patients with normal renal function excrete ethylene glycol with a $t_{1/2}$ of less than 18 hours, selected patients may be candidates for fomepizole monotherapy (i.e., no hemodialysis) (10,16,20). Such a patient must have a normal pH, normal creatinine and renal function, normal level of alertness, and no signs of other end-organ toxicity (3,93,94,103). In such cases, fomepizole inhibition of ADH should safely allow the patient to eliminate unmetabolized ethylene glycol via renal excretion. Although patients with ethylene glycol levels as high as 574 mg/dl have been managed with fomepizole monotherapy (19,93,104,105) and the toxicokinetics appear sound, this strategy has not been formally tested in a clinical trial and may involve the administration of fomepizole for several days, for which there is little collective experience.

Fomepizole does not eliminate the metabolites of ethylene glycol once they are formed. In patients who are already acidotic or have renal insufficiency, combined treatment with ADH blockade and hemodialysis is warranted. Fomepizole is dialyzable, and adjustments in dosing must be made (106,107). Details of the dose, method of administration, and adverse effects of fomepizole are provided in Chapter 59. During hemodialysis, the maintenance dose must be administered every 4 hours to account for the elimination of fomepizole by hemodialysis. The endpoint of treatment should be an ethylene glycol level less than 20 mg/dl, with resolution of acidosis, and the patient should be improving clinically.

Cofactor Therapy

Cofactors, such as pyridoxine and thiamine, are involved in the metabolism of ethylene glycol (3,23). No human trials have been completed to show the effectiveness of supplementing the treatment of the ethylene glycol–poisoned patient with these agents. These cofactors may be avoided in the otherwise healthy patient; however, in the alcoholic or vitamin-deficient patient, these cofactors should be used (3).

Supportive Care

As ethylene glycol toxicity results in inebriation and CNS depression, careful attention to the patient's airway is a must. IV access should be obtained early during the initial evaluation of the patient. Hypoglycemia should be ruled out in the patient with CNS depression. If chronic ethanol abuse is suspected, thiamine should be administered. Careful attention to fluid status is important, as the patient may have renal failure. Early determination of the patient's urine output and renal function is important.

Seizures are initially treated with IV benzodiazepines followed by phenobarbital and other measures as clinically indicated (Chapter 40). Systemic acidosis manifested as a low serum bicarbonate level or serum pH may be supplemented with IV sodium bicarbonate. However, the severe acidosis manifested by ethylene glycol toxicity does not respond to bicarbonate therapy alone. Hypocalcemia does not usually require supplemental calcium. If the patient develops cardiac dysrhythmias and is hypocalcemic, supplemental calcium may be administered.

Cranial nerve palsies are transient and usually present 4 to 18 days after ethylene glycol ingestion (65,66). These do not require any form of special treatment.

Monitoring

Cardiac monitoring and frequent reevaluations of the patient's mental and respiratory status are important. Laboratory testing, including serum electrolytes, glucose, blood urea nitrogen, creatinine, ethanol, acetaminophen, and aspirin levels, should be obtained. Depending on the severity of illness, acid-base status should be checked every 1 or 2 hours.

Management Pitfalls

Do not wait for symptoms to appear before treatment. Time elapsed between ingestion (fatalities reported if longer than 12 hours) and treatment and the dose ingested are major predictive factors of morbidity fatality (32).

It is important to obtain a serum or breath ethanol level on these patients, as ethanol can prevent ethylene glycol from being metabolized and serum acidosis does not occur until after the ethanol is metabolized.

Do not delay hemodialysis in a patient with acidemia and end-organ effects (renal insufficiency, mental status changes) pending confirmatory ethylene glycol levels.

It is important to compensate for increased clearance of antidotal ethanol or fomepizole during hemodialysis.

REFERENCES

1. Litovitz TL, Klein-Schwartz W, White S, et al. 199 annual report of the American Association of Poison Control Centers toxic surveillance system. *Am J Emerg Med* 2000;18:517–574.
2. Clayton GD, Clayton FE, eds. *Patty's industrial hygiene and toxicology,* 4th ed. New York: John Wiley & Sons, 1994:2F.
3. Barceloux DG, Krenzelok EP, Olson K, Watson W. American Academy of Clinical Toxicology Practice Guidelines on the Treatment of Ethylene Glycol Poisoning. Ad Hoc Committee. *J Toxicol Clin Toxicol* 1999;37:537–560.
4. Driver J, Tardiff RG, Sedik L, et al. In vitro percutaneous absorption of [^{14}C] ethylene glycol. *J Exposure Anal Environ Epidemiol* 1993;3:277–284.
5. Hodgman MJ, Wezorek C, Krenzelok EP. Toxic inhalation of ethylene glycol: a pharmacological improbability. *J Toxicol Clin Toxicol* 1997;35:109.
6. Wezorek C, Hodgman MJ, Dean BS, et al. Inadvertent ethylene glycol inhalation resulting in a toxic level. *J Toxicol Clin Toxicol* 1995;33:553(abst).
7. Wills JH, Coluston F, Harris ES, et al. Inhalation of aerosolized ethylene glycol by man. *J Toxicol Clin Toxicol* 1974;7:463–476.
8. Jacobsen D, Hewlett T, Webb R, Brown S. Ethylene glycol intoxication: evaluation of kinetics and crystalluria. *Am J Med* 1988;84:145–152.
9. Ford MD, Sivilotti MLA. Alcohols and glycols. In: Irwin RS, Cerra FB, Rippe JM, eds. *Intensive care medicine,* 4th ed. Philadelphia: Lippincott-Raven, 1999:1478–1493.
10. Baud FJ, Galliot M, Astier A, et al. Treatment of ethylene glycol poisoning with intravenous 4-methylpyrazole. *N Engl J Med* 1988;319:97–100.
11. Peterson CD, Collins AJ, Himes JM, et al. Ethylene glycol poisoning: pharmacokinetics during therapy with ethanol and hemodialysis. *N Engl J Med* 1981;304:21–23.
12. Moreau CL, Kerns W 2nd, Tomaszewski CA, et al. Glycolate kinetics and hemodialysis clearance in ethylene glycol poisoning. META Study Group. *J Toxicol Clin Toxicol* 1998;36:659–666.
13. Jacobsen D, Ovrebo S, Ostborg J, Sejersted OM. Glycolate causes the acidosis in ethylene glycol poisoning and is effectively removed by hemodialysis. *Acta Med Scand* 1984;216:409–416.
14. Winek CL, Shingleton DP, Shanor SP. Ethylene and diethylene glycol toxicity. *J Toxicol Clin Toxicol* 1978;13:297–324.
15. Jacobsen D, Sebastian CS, Blomstrand R, et al. 4-Methylpyrazole: a controlled study of safety in healthy human subjects after single, ascending doses. *Metab Clin Exp Res* 1988;12:516–522.
16. Baud FB, Bismuth C, Garnier R, et al. 4-Methylpyrazole may be an alternative to ethanol therapy for ethylene glycol intoxication in man. *J Toxicol Clin Toxicol* 1986;24:463–483.
17. Cheng J-T, Beysolow TD, Kaul B, et al. Clearance of ethylene glycol by kidneys and hemodialysis. *J Toxicol Clin Toxicol* 1987;25:94–108.
18. Harry P, Turcant A, Bouachour G, et al. Efficacy of 4-methylpyrazole in ethylene glycol poisoning: clinical and toxicokinetic aspects. *Hum Exp Toxicol* 1994;13:61–64.
19. Hantson P, Hassoun A, Mahieu P. Ethylene glycol poisoning treated by intravenous 4-methylpyrazole. *Intensive Care Med* 1998;24:736–739.
20. Sivilotti MLA, Burns RS, McMartin K, et al. Toxicokinetics of ethylene glycol during fomepizole therapy: implications for management. *Ann Emerg Med* 2000;36:114–125.
21. Brent J, McMartin K, Phillips S, et al. Fomepizole for the treatment of ethylene glycol poisoning. Methylpyrazole for Toxic Alcohols Study Group. *N Engl J Med* 1999;340:832–838.
22. McChesney EW, Golberg L, Parekh CK, et al. Reappraisal of the toxicology of ethylene glycol. II. Metabolism studies in laboratory animals. *Food Cosmetic Toxicol* 1971;9(1):21–38.
23. Gabow PA, Clay K, Sullivan JB, Lepoff R. Organic acids in ethylene glycol intoxication. *Ann Intern Med* 1986;105:16–20.
24. Garibotto G, Paoletti E, Acquarone N. Glyoxylic acid in ethylene glycol poisoning. *Nephron* 1988;48(3):248–249.
25. Reference deleted.
26. Reference deleted.
27. Jacobsen D, McMartin KE. Antidotes for methanol and ethylene glycol poisoning. *J Toxicol Clin Toxicol* 1997;35(2):127–143.
28. Poldelski V, Johnson A, Wright S, et al. Ethylene glycol-mediated tubular injury: identification of critical metabolites and injury pathways. *Am J Kidney Dis* 2001;38(2):339–348.
29. Collins JM, Hennes DM, Holzgang CR, et al. Recovery after prolonged oliguria due to ethylene glycol intoxication. the prognostic value of serial percutaneous renal biopsy. *Arch Intern Med* 1970;125:1059–1062.
30. Introna F Jr, Smialek JE. Antifreeze (ethylene glycol) intoxications in Baltimore. Report of six cases. *Acta Morphologica Hungarica* 1989;37(3–4):245–263.
31. Jacobsen D, McMartin KE. Methanol and ethylene glycol poisonings. Mechanism of toxicity, clinical course, diagnosis and treatment. *Med Toxicol* 1986;1(5):309–334.
32. Morgan BW, Ford MD, Follmer R. Ethylene glycol ingestion resulting in brainstem and midbrain dysfunction. *J Toxicol Clin Toxicol* 2000;38:445–451.
33. Buell JF, Sterling R, Mandava S, et al. Ethylene glycol intoxication presenting as a metabolic acidosis associated with a motor vehicle crash: case report. *J Trauma* 1998;45:811–813.
34. Parry MF, Wallach R. Ethylene glycol poisoning. *Am J Med* 1974;57:143–150.
35. Mair W. Cerebral computed tomography of ethylene glycol intoxication. *Neuroradiology* 1983;24:175–177.
36. Berman LB, Schreiner GE, Feys J. The nephrotoxic lesions of ethylene glycol. *Ann Intern Med* 1957;46:611–619.
37. Bobbitt WM, Williams RM, Freed CR. Severe ethylene glycol intoxication with multisystem failure. *West J Med* 1986;144:225–228.
38. Jobard E, Harry P, Turcant A, et al. 4-Methylpyrazole and hemodialysis in ethylene glycol poisoning. *J Toxicol Clin Toxicol* 1996;34:373–377.
39. Ford M, Price M, Tomaszewski CA. Ethylene glycol-induced neurotoxicity in patients with delayed or inadequate treatment. *J Toxicol Clin Toxicol* 1998;36:514(abst).
40. Clay KMR. On the metabolic acidosis of ethylene glycol intoxication. *Toxicol Appl Pharmacol* 1977;39:39–49.
41. Friedman EA, Greenberg JB, Merrill JP, et al. Consequences of ethylene glycol poisoning. *Am J Med* 1962;32:891.
42. Scully RE, Galdabini JJ, McNeely BU. Case records of the Massachusetts General Hospital, case 38-1979. *N Engl J Med* 1979;301:650–657.
43. Donovan JW, Burkhart K, Cienki J, et al. Removal of ethylene glycol and 4-methylpyrazole with continuous venovenous hemofiltration. *J Toxicol Clin Toxicol* 1997;35:538.
44. Denning DW, Berendt A, Chia Y, et al. Myocarditis complicating ethylene glycol poisoning in the absence of neurological features. *Postgrad Med J* 1988;64:867–870.
45. Jolliff HA, Dart RC, Bogdan GM, et al. Can the diagnosis of ethylene glycol (EG) toxicity be made without serum EG and osmolality values? *J Toxicol Clin Toxicol* 2000;38:539–540(abst).
46. Hewlett TP, McMartin KE, Lauro AJ, et al. Ethylene glycol poisoning. The value of glycolic acid determinations for diagnosis and treatment. *J Toxicol Clin Toxicol* 1986;24:389–402.
47. Darchy B, Abruzzese L, Pitiot O, et al. Delayed admission for ethylene glycol poisoning: lack of elevated serum osmol gap. *Intensive Care Med* 1999;25:859–861.
48. Blakeley KR, Rinner SE, Knochel JP. Survival of ethylene glycol poisoning with profound acidemia. *N Engl J Med* 1993;328:515–516.
49. Frommer JP, Ayus JC. Acute ethylene glycol intoxication. *Am J Nephrol* 1982;2:1–5.
50. Rasic S, Cengic M, Golemac S, et al. Acute renal insufficiency after poisoning with ethylene glycol. *Nephron* 1999;81:119–120.
51. Price CJ, Kimmel CA, Tyl RW, et al. The developmental toxicity of ethylene glycol in rats and mice. *Toxicol Appl Pharmacol* 1985;81:113–127.
52. Lamb JC, Maronpot RR, Gulati DK, et al. Reproductive and developmental toxicity of ethylene glycol in the mouse. *Toxicol Appl Pharmacol* 1985;81:100–112.
53. Carney EW, Liberacki AB, Bartels MJ, et al. Identification of proximate toxicant for ethylene glycol developmental toxicity using rat whole embryo culture. *Teratology* 1996;53(1):38–46.
54. IARC. Monographs on the evaluation of carcinogenic risks to humans-overall evaluations of carcinogenicity: an updating of IARC monographs volumes 1 to 42, supplement 7. Lyon, France: World Health Organization, 1987.
55. Reference deleted.
56. Kahn HS, Brotchner RJ. A recovery from ethylene glycol (antifreeze) intoxication; A case of survival and two fatalities from ethylene glycol including autopsy findings. *Ann Intern Med* 1950;32:284–294.
57. Eder AF, McGrath CM, Dowdy YG, et al. Ethylene glycol poisoning: toxicokinetic and analytical factors affecting laboratory diagnosis. *Clin Chem* 1998;44:168–177.
58. Walder AD Tyler CK. Ehtylene glycol antifreeze poisoning. Three case reports and a review of the literature. *Anaesthesia* 1994;49:964–967.
59. Catchings TT, Beamer WC, Lundy L, et al. ARDS secondary to ethylene glycol ingestion. *Ann Emerg Med* 1985;14:594–596.
60. Gordon HL, Hunter JM. Ethylene glycol poisoning. A case report. *Anaesthesia* 1982;37:332–338.
61. Jacobsen D, Mcmartin KE. Methanol and ethylene glycol poisoning. Mechanisms of toxicity, clinical course, diagnosis and treatment. *Med Toxicol* 1986;1:309–334.
62. Piagnerelli M, Lejeune P, Vanhaeverbeek M. Diagnosis and treatment of an unusual cause of metabolic acidosis: ethylene glycol poisoning. *Acta Clin Belg* 1999;54:351–356.
63. Berger JR, Ayyar DR. Neurological complications of ethylene glycol intoxication. Report of a case. *Arch Neurol* 1981;38:724–726.
64. Mallya KB, Mendis T, Guberman A. Bilateral facial paralysis following ethylene glycol ingestion. *Can J Neurol Sci* 1986;13:340–341.
65. Spillane L, Roberts JR, Meyer AE. Multiple cranial nerve deficits after ethylene glycol poisoning. *Ann Emerg Med* 1991;20:208–210.
66. Lewis LD, Smith BW, Mamourian AC. Delayed sequelae after acute overdoses or poisonings: cranial neuropathy related to ethylene glycol ingestion. *Clin Pharmacol Ther* 1997;61:692–699.

67. Hylander B, Kjellstrand CM. Prognostic factors and treatment of severe ethylene glycol intoxication. *Intensive Care Med* 1996;22:546–552.
68. Fraser A. Clinical toxicologic implications of ethylene glycol and glycolic acid poisoning. *Ther Drug Monit* 2002;24:232–238.
69. Jones AW, Nilsson L, Gladh SA, et al. 2,3-Butanediol in plasma from an alcoholic mistakenly identified as ethylene glycol by gas-chromatographic analysis. *Clin Chem* 1991;37(8):1453–1455.
70. Shoemaker JD, Lynch RE, Hoffmann JW, Sly W. Misidentification of propionic acid as ethylene glycol in a patient with methylmalonic acidemia. *J Pediatr* 1992;120:417–421.
71. Blandford DE, Desjardins PR. A rapid method for measurement of ethylene glycol. *Clin Biochem* 1994;27:25–30.
72. Malandain H, Cano Y. Interferences of glycerol, propylene glycol, and other diols in the enzymatic assay of ethylene glycol. *Eur J Clin Chem Clin Biochem* 1996;34:651–654.
73. Fraser AD, MacNeil W. Colorimetric and gas chromatographic procedures for glycolic acid in serum: the major toxic metabolite of ethylene glycol. *J Toxicol Clin Toxicol* 1993;31:397–405.
74. Yao HH, Porter W. Simultaneous determination of ethylene glycol and its major toxic metabolite, glycolic acid, in serum by gas chromatography. *Clin Chem* 1996;42:292–297.
75. Porter WH, Rutter PW, Yao HH. Simultaneous determination of ethylene glycol and glycolic acid in serum by gas chromatography-mass spectrometry. *J Anal Toxicol* 1999;23:591–597.
76. Porter WH, Rutter PW, Bush BA, et al. Ethylene glycol toxicity: the role of serum glycolic acid in hemodialysis. *J Toxicol Clin Toxicol* 2001;39:607–615.
77. Shirey T, Sivilotti. Reaction of lactate electrodes to glycolate. *Crit Care Med* 1999;27:2305–2307.
78. Morgan TJ, Clark C, Clague A. Artifactual elevation of measured plasma L-lactate concentration in the presence of glycolate. *Crit Care Med* 1999;27: 2177–2179.
79. Porter WH, Crellin M, Rutter PW, et al. Interference by glycolic acid in the Beckman synchron method for lactate: a useful clue for unsuspected ethylene glycol intoxication. *Clin Chem* 2000;46:t–5.
80. Sabeel AI, Kurkus J, Lindholm T. Intensified dialysis treatment of ethylene glycol intoxication. *Scand J Urol Nephrol* 1995;29:125–129.
81. Ammar KA, Heckerling P. Ethylene glycol poisoning with a normal anion gap caused by concurrent ethanol ingestion: importance of the osmolal gap. *Am J Kidney Dis* 1996;27:130–133.
82. Jaeger A, Kopferschmitt J, Berton C, et al. The importance of osmolal gap. Paper presented at: European Association of Poisons Centres and Clinical Toxicologists Scientific Meeting, Birmingham, UK, 1993.
83. Aabakken L, Johansen KS, Rydningen EB, et al. Osmolal and anion gaps in patients admitted to an emergency medical department. *Hum Exp Toxicol* 1994;13:131–134.
84. Glaser DS. Utility of serum osmol gap in the diagnosis of methanol or ethylene glycol ingestion. *Ann Emerg Med* 1996;27:343–346.
85. Glasser L, Sternglanz PD, Combie J, et al. A serum osmolality and its applicability to drug overdose. *Am J Clin Pathol* 1973;60:695–699.
86. Kruse JA, Cadnapaphornchai P. The serum osmole gap. *J Crit Care* 1994;9:185–197.
87. Hoffman R MJ, Howland M, et al. Osmolar gaps revisited: normal values and limitations. *J Toxicol Clin Toxicol* 1993;31:81–93.
88. Turk J, Morrell L, Avioli LV. Ethylene glycol intoxication. *Arch Intern Med* 1986;146:1601–1603.
89. Winter ML, Ellis MD, Snodgrass WR. Urine fluorescence using a Wood's lamp to detect fluorescein: a qualitative adjunct test in suspected ethylene glycol ingestions. *Ann Emerg Med* 1990;19:663–667.
90. Casavant MJ, Shah MN, Battels R. Does fluorescent urine indicate antifreeze ingestion by children? *Pediatrics* 2001;107:113–114.
91. American Academy of Clinical Toxicology and European Association of Poisons Centres and Clinical Toxicologists. Position statement: single-dose activated charcoal. *J Toxicol Clin Toxicol* 1997;35:721–741.
92. Jacobsen D, Ostby N, Bredesen JE. Studies on ethylene glycol poisoning. *Acta Med Scand* 1982;212:11–15.
93. Borron SW, Megarbane B, Baud FJ. Fomepizole in treatment of uncomplicated ethylene glycol poisoning. *Lancet* 1999;354:831.
94. Watson WA. Ethylene glycol toxicity: closing in on rational, evidence-based treatment. *Ann Emerg Med* 2000;36:139–141.
95. Reference deleted.
96. Sangster B, Prenen JA, de Groot G. Case 38-1979: ethylene glycol poisoning. *N Engl J Med* 1980;302:465.
97. Wacker WE, Haynes H, Druyan R, et al. Treatment of ethylene glycol poisoning with ethyl alcohol. *JAMA* 1965;194:1231–1233.
98. Kowalczyk M, Halvorsen S, Ovrebo S, et al. Ethanol treatment in ethylene glycol poisoned patients. *Vet Hum Toxicol* 1998;40:225–228.
99. Antizol, fomepizole. Product information. Minnetonka, MN: Orphan Medical, Inc., 1997.
100. Baud FJ, Lambert C, Bismuth C. Safety of oral or intra-venous 4 methylpyrazole (4 MP) in suspected ethylene-glycol (EG) intoxications. Paper presented at: EAPCCT XV, Istanbul., Turkey, 1992(abst).
101. McMartin K, Jacobsen D, Sebastian CS, et al. Safety and metabolism of 4-methylpyrazol in human subjects. *Vet Hum Toxicol* 1987;29:471(abst).
102. Jacobsen D, Sebastian CS, Barron SK, et al. Effects of 4-methylpyrazole, methanol/ethylene glycol antidote, in healthy humans. *J Emerg Med* 1990;8:455–461.
103. Najafi CC, Hertko LJ, Leikin JB, et al. Fomepizole in ethylene glycol intoxication. Ann Emerg Med 2001;37:358–359.
104. Donovan JW, Burkhart K, McMartin K. A comparison of fomepizole with hemodialysis vs fomepizole alone in therapy of severe ethylene glycol toxicity. *J Toxicol Clin Toxicol* 1998;36:451.
105. Boyer EW, Mejia M, Woolf A, et al. Severe ethylene glycol ingestion treated without hemodialysis. *Pediatrics* 2001;107:172–173.
106. Faessel H, Houze P, Baud FJ, et al. 4-Methylpyrazole monitoring during haemodialysis of ethylene glycol intoxicated patients. *Eur J Clin Pharmacol* 1995;49:211–213.
107. Jacobsen D, Ostensen J, Bredesen L, et al. 4-Methylpyrazole (4-MP) is effectively removed by hemodialysis in the pig model. *Vet Hum Toxicol* 1992;34:362(abst).

CHAPTER 193

Other Alcohols, Glycols, and Glycol Ethers

Luke Yip

See Figure 1.

Compounds included:	**Benzyl alcohol, diethylene glycol, ethylene glycol monomethyl ether, ethylene glycol monobutyl ether, polyethylene glycol, propylene glycol**
Molecular formula and weight:	**See Table 1.**
SI conversion:	**Not applicable**
CAS Registry No.:	**See Table 1.**
Special concerns:	**Delayed onset metabolic acidosis and renal injury with some agents**
Antidotes:	**Ethanol, fomepizole**

BENZYL ALCOHOL

Benzyl alcohol is a colorless liquid with a faint aromatic odor. It is used as a bacteriostatic agent and is commonly added to pharmaceuticals (e.g., etoposide, amiodarone, diazepam, bacteriostatic water, and sodium chloride) intended for intravenous (IV) administration. The amount of benzyl alcohol in pharmaceuticals may be 0.9% to 2.0% (1–3), and a significant amount of benzyl alcohol may be inadvertently administered to a patient during continuous (repeated) drug infusion or when bacteriostatic water or sodium chloride is used to flush IV lines. Benzyl alcohol toxicity has been reported in both pediatric (4–9) and adult patients (10–12).

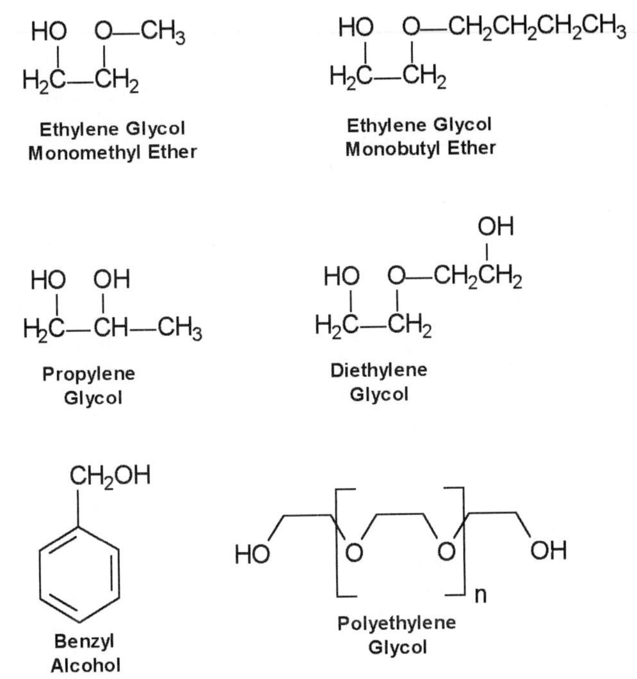

Ethylene Glycol Monomethyl Ether

Ethylene Glycol Monobutyl Ether

Propylene Glycol

Diethylene Glycol

Benzyl Alcohol

Polyethylene Glycol

Figure 1. Structures of selected alcohols.

Toxic Dose

Based on animal data, rapid infusion of benzyl alcohol, 5.4 mg/kg, may be safe for adults (13).

A 53-year-old African-American man with non-Hodgkin's lymphoma developed seizures and respiratory arrest 2 hours after completing an infusion of etoposide (3 g/m^2). The dose of benzyl alcohol was 90 mg/kg (12). Laboratory studies showed acute hemolysis and severe anion gap metabolic acidosis; glucose 6 phosphate dehydrogenase deficiency was negative.

In premature neonates, toxicity is associated with a cumulative daily dose exceeding 99 mg/kg IV (5,6). A 5-year-old girl developed hypotension, hypernatremia, and increased anion gap metabolic acidosis after receiving 180 mg/kg/day of benzyl alcohol (8).

Epidural or intrathecal injection of 7.5 mg or more benzyl alcohol as a diluent has been followed by paraparesis and flaccid paraplegia (10,11). Residual symptoms may be present 26 months after the initial injury.

Pathophysiology

Benzyl alcohol is rapidly oxidized by hepatic alcohol dehydrogenase (ADH) to benzoic acid, which is conjugated with glycine and excreted as hippuric acid in the urine (14). The livers of premature infants have a greater capacity to metabolize benzyl alcohol than term infants but have a reduced capacity to convert benzoic acid to hippuric acid (4,15). When benzoic acid production exceeds the conjugating capacity of the immature liver, benzoic acid accumulates, and anion gap metabolic acidosis develops (4–6).

Exposure to benzyl alcohol is strongly associated with development of kernicterus and intraventricular hemorrhage in premature neonates (7,16). Intrathecal benzyl alcohol diluent injection has been reported to cause demyelination of the nerve roots, matting of the cauda equina, and fibrosis of its perineurium (11). In acute and chronic animal studies, when nerve roots are exposed to benzyl alcohol in commercially used concentrations, benzyl alcohol has a local anesthetic effect on nerve fibers and causes demyelination and wallerian degeneration (11).

In vitro studies suggest that the damage to red blood cells by benzyl alcohol is time, dose, and temperature dependent (17–19). In contrast to the rapid cellular uptake that is temperature independent, benzyl alcohol binding to membranes gradually increases with time and is primarily dependent on the temperature. Hemolysis is dependent on benzyl alcohol binding to erythrocyte membranes. There appears to be a critical hemolytic level of 500 nmol/mg of protein. Benzyl alcohol elimination is dependent on ADH. ADH2 has three allelic variants (ADH*1, ADH 2*2, ADH2*3) that exhibit ethnic polymorphism and different Michaelis-Menten–constant (K_m) values. ADH2*3 has a high K_m for alcohol and is expressed in 20% of African-Americans (20). Patients with the ADH2*3 allele may be predisposed to decreased benzyl alcohol metabolism and clearance, resulting in increased serum concentrations and associated hemolysis (12).

Vulnerable Populations

Premature neonates are at high risk of toxicity as described in this chapter.

Clinical Presentation

Benzyl alcohol toxicity is a clinical diagnosis and may be confirmed by serum or urine benzyl alcohol, benzoic acid, and hippuric acid levels. The temporal relation between parenteral benzyl alcohol exposure and progressive anion gap metabolic acidosis, respiratory distress, altered central or peripheral nervous system function, seizures, and hemolysis is highly suggestive of the diagnosis.

Progressive anion gap metabolic acidosis precedes the onset of the symptoms, which occur around the second to fourth day of exposure and include hypoactivity, hypotonia, depression of sensorium, respiratory distress, apnea, progressive bradycardia, seizures, progressive unresponsiveness, and coma. Marked skin breakdown may be evident. Hypotension and renal failure herald cardiovascular collapse and death.

One striking clinical feature of benzyl alcohol toxicity in neonates is gasping respiration, "gasping syndrome," which is characterized by unremitting gasps that occur continuously at a rate of 20 per minute, despite high ventilatory settings, and last several hours to 1 week (6). Termination of benzyl alcohol exposure in neonates appears to be associated with a decrease in neonatal kernicterus and intraventricular hemorrhage but not mortality (7).

Paraparesis and flaccid paraplegia after epidural or intrathecal administration of more than 7.5 mg of benzyl alcohol as a diluent are suggestive of benzyl alcohol toxicity.

Bronchitis associated with chronic inhalation of nebulized bacteriostatic saline diluent is characterized by chest tightness,

TABLE 1. Physical properties and toxic concentrations of the alcohols

Name	Molecular formula	Molecular weight (g/mol)	CAS Registry No.
Benzyl alcohol	C_7H_8O	108.14	100-51-6
Diethylene glycol	$C_4H_{10}O_3$	106.12	111-46-6
Ethylene glycol monomethyl ether	$C_3H_8O_2$	76.10	109-86-4
Ethylene glycol monobutyl ether	$C_6H_{14}O_2$	118.18	111-76-2
Propylene glycol	$C_3H_8O_2$	76.10	57-55-6

wheezing, coughing, rhinorrhea, and purulent sputum. A blinded, controlled study in healthy volunteers who were treated with 3 ml of saline with or without benzyl alcohol (9 mg/ml) found that the benzyl alcohol group had bronchitis with erythema, tracheobronchial mucosal edema, metaplasia, denudation of cilia, and mucosal lymphocytic infiltration on bronchoscopy (20a).

Hypersensitivity reactions may occur after parenteral (21–25) or dermal exposure (26–31) to benzyl alcohol. Acute reactions include urticaria, erythema, palpable edema, fatigue, nausea, diffuse angioedema, maculopapular rash, and fever. A delayed hypersensitivity reaction characterized by erythema, edema, and vesiculation may appear 2 to 3 days after an immediate reaction to a single benzyl alcohol challenge in the same patient (23,27,32). Patients allergic to benzyl alcohol may show cross-sensitivity with balsam of Peru, benzyl paraben, and benzyl cinnamate (26).

Diagnostic Tests

Laboratory studies show leukopenia, thrombocytopenia, direct hyperbilirubinemia, hyperammonemia, intracranial hemorrhage, and abnormal electroencephalogram. Urinary organic acid profile shows large quantities of benzyl alcohol and benzoic and hippuric acid.

A 5-year-old girl on a diazepam infusion for 36 hours received 180 mg/kg/day of benzyl alcohol (8). She developed hypotension (70/40 mm Hg), hypernatremia (sodium, 158 mmol/L), anion gap (37 mmol/L), and metabolic acidosis (pH, 7.17; bicarbonate, 8 mmol/L). Her serum benzoate concentration was 18 mg/dl, and her urine benzoate concentration was 120 mg/dl. When the diazepam infusion was decreased to 0.7 mg/kg/hour, hypernatremia and metabolic acidosis resolved within 18 hours.

The diagnosis of benzyl alcohol allergy may be confirmed by skin testing patients with suspected allergy.

Treatment

The main treatment for benzyl alcohol toxicity is discontinuation of the exposure and supportive care.

ENHANCEMENT OF ELIMINATION

Hemodialysis may enhance the elimination of benzyl alcohol and its metabolites and may also be useful to help correct severe metabolic acidosis. However, most cases involve prolonged repeated infusion, and the usefulness of dialysis is unknown.

ANTIDOTES

There is no proven antidote for benzyl alcohol poisoning. Because it is metabolized by ADH, a trial of ADH blockade may be reasonable. This has not been tested because toxicity has generally developed after multiple doses and was already present at presentation.

SUPPORTIVE CARE

Metabolic acidosis may be resistant to sodium bicarbonate therapy (6,8). Blood product and volume exchange transfusions do not appear to alter the overall clinical course (6).

It has been reported that the clinical course after intrathecal benzyl alcohol injection may be improved by rinsing the cerebrospinal fluid (CSF) space (11). The procedure involves placement of a lumbar drain and 100 ml of normal saline plus methylprednisolone, 40 mg, exchanged for CSF.

Bacteriostatic saline should not be used as a nebulizer diluent. Benzyl alcohol–free solutions should be used to flush IV lines or reconstitute medications for administration and terminate all sources of benzyl alcohol exposure when toxicity is suspected.

MONITORING

Laboratory studies should include close monitoring of the patient's respiratory, cardiovascular, neurologic, hematologic, acid-base, and electrolyte status and serum benzyl alcohol or benzoate level, especially when continuous or high-dose medications containing benzyl alcohol are being administered.

DIETHYLENE GLYCOL

Diethylene glycol (DEG) is used as a solvent, plasticizer, antifreeze, liquid fuel, and humectant; it may be found in brake fluid and has been used as a wine sweetener. Although sporadic human DEG poisonings have been reported (33–36), it has most frequently been observed in outbreaks (37–39) and usually has been associated with contaminated pharmaceutical products (40–47). The Elixir Sulfanilamide disaster of 1937 was one of the most consequential mass poisonings of the twentieth century. This tragedy occurred shortly after the introduction of sulfanilamide, the first sulfa antimicrobial drug, when DEG was used as the diluent in the formulation of a liquid preparation of sulfanilamide known as *Elixir Sulfanilamide*. One hundred five patients died from its therapeutic use (48).

Toxic Dose

In a case series, 85 of 87 children died after ingestion of DEG-contaminated paracetamol. The median estimated DEG dose was 1.34 ml/kg (range, 0.22 to 4.42 ml/kg). An estimated maximum DEG dose less than 1 ml/kg was ingested by 12 children. Children ranged in age from 1 month to 13 years, with 80% of the children younger than 5 years of age (44).

A man reportedly drank 240 ml of 100% DEG along with an unknown amount of ethanol and developed anion gap metabolic acidosis, renal failure, and hepatitis 2 days later (49). Despite 4-methylpyrazole therapy and hemodialysis, he died 13 days after ingestion.

After ingestion of 2 to 3 cups of 100% DEG as an ethanol substitute, three men presented with delayed onset of symptoms (vomiting after 2 days and acute renal failure after 6 days). Despite peritoneal dialysis, all three men died 9 to 18 days after ingestion (50).

Pathophysiology

The pathophysiology of human DEG remains to be fully elucidated. Animal studies indicate that DEG is rapidly and almost completely absorbed after ingestion. It is rapidly distributed into tissues in proportion to blood flow (i.e., kidneys more than brain more than spleen more than liver more than muscle) (51). DEG is metabolized in the liver by two consecutive oxidized form of nicotinamide adenine dinucleotide–dependent reactions. First, DEG is metabolized by ADH to (2-hydroxyethoxy)acetaldehyde, which is then rapidly metabolized by aldehyde dehydrogenase (ALDH) to (2-hydroxyethoxy)acetate (51,52).

DEG oxidation is accompanied by lactate accumulation and an increase of the lactate to pyruvate ratio, enhancing the metabolic acidosis. The ether linkage of DEG is not cleaved, and (2-hydroxyethoxy)acetate does not undergo further oxidation to diglycolate. It has been suggested that (2-hydroxyethoxy)acetate forms a cyclic compound (i.e., 1,4-dioxanone) under acid conditions and is not oxidized by either ADH or ALDH (53). The formation of (2-hydroxyethoxy)acetate is reduced by either pyrazole or diethyldithiocarbamate. Pretreatment with pyrazole protected against the LD_{50} dose of DEG but did not protect animals receiving 25% more than the LD_{50} dose (52,54). This suggests DEG and (2-hydroxyethoxy)acetate are both toxic, and (2-hydroxyethoxy)acetate may enhance DEG toxicity.

After an oral DEG dose, 40% to 70% is recovered unchanged in the urine (52,55), and DEG accelerates its renal elimination by inducing osmotic diuresis (51). DEG is nephrotoxic in animals at doses of 700 mg/kg and greater (56,57). Maximal nephrotoxic effects are measured at 48 hours and may persist for 3 to 4 days (57). Animals were able to compensate for the metabolic acidosis after administration of 1 to 5 ml/kg of DEG but were unable to tolerate 10 ml/kg and died in uremic coma (51).

Vulnerable Populations

There are no studies of DEG on human reproduction.

Clinical Presentation

The patient usually does not present for evaluation until after symptoms become evident. Adults commonly present with nausea and vomiting, oliguria or anuria, altered mental status or coma, abdominal or costovertebral pain, edema, diarrhea, headache, drowsiness, dizziness, malaise, and cutaneous pallor (35,36,42,58–61). Patients may be hyperpneic (57,61).

Pediatric patients commonly present with anuria or oliguria, edema, abdominal pain, altered mental status or coma, vomiting, hematemesis, respiratory distress, diarrhea, hepatomegaly, crepitations, pallor, dehydration, seizures, headache, jaundice, and melena (33,40,43–47,59,62). Patients may develop hypertension, tachycardia, tachypnea, and have subnormal temperature (33,43,45,47,58–60). Less common findings include anorexia, bradycardia, epistaxis, cranial nerve VI palsy, pupil dilation, optic neuritis, papillitis, shock, and unilateral facial paralysis (40,44,46,57,59,62).

The onset of symptoms usually heralds rapid deterioration. Oliguria or anuria is usually evident after 2 to 6 days of DEG exposure (35,36,42,58–61); death usually occurs within 2 to 7 days from the onset of anuria and on average of 7 days (range, 1 to 24 days) of hospitalization (45,47,61). Occasionally, a patient may show apparent clinical improvement with supportive care and then die from unexpected cardiopulmonary arrest (36,40,46). The mortality rate is 70% to 100%, and intensive care, including hemodialysis, may not significantly alter the mortality rate (43–45,47). Patients with renal injury who survive usually recover to their baseline renal function.

Diagnostic Tests

DEG poisoning is a clinical diagnosis and requires a high index of suspicion. There is no reliable laboratory marker, and rarely are serum DEG levels available to assist with patient management. However, the presence of DEG or its metabolites in the serum or urine may confirm the diagnosis. The temporal relation among DEG exposure, progressive renal dysfunction, and multiorgan toxicity is highly suggestive of the diagnosis. Initially, routine laboratory studies may be deceptively unremarkable. Unlike methanol and ethylene glycol poisoning, severe metabolic acidosis is characteristically absent until renal failure becomes evident or the patient is moribund.

In adults, laboratory studies may reveal increases in blood urea nitrogen (BUN) and creatinine, proteinuria, leukocytosis, anemia, hematuria, hepatitis, pyuria, and anion gap metabolic acidosis (35,36,42,58–61). Renal biopsy findings may be similar to the pediatric cases.

In children, laboratory studies may be remarkable for leukocytosis, increased BUN and creatinine, hyperkalemia, hypoglycemia, hepatitis, pancreatitis, increased anion gap acidosis, anemia, hematuria, osmolal gap, elevated lactate level, and elevated CSF protein (33,40,43–47,59,62). Renal biopsy may show acute tubular necrosis and regeneration (40,47).

Histopathology

The combination of proximal renal tubular hydropic degeneration and hepatic centrilobular necrosis strongly suggests DEG or dioxane toxicity.

The kidneys appeared enlarged, swollen, and edematous, with pale cortices and congested medullae and a striking demarcation between cortices and medullae (37,40,42,45,60). Microscopic examination showed cortical infarction or necrosis with hemorrhage at the corticomedullary border. There was degeneration, necrosis, and disintegration of the epithelial lining of the secretory portion of the tubules; the glomeruli were intact. The characteristic lesion was severe vacuolation of the epithelium of the convoluted tubules ("hydropic degeneration"). This profound swelling produces complete obliteration of the lumens and mechanical obstruction of urine flow.

The liver appears yellowish and enlarged with pale, bulging soft surfaces macroscopically. The cut surface is mottled with a pronounced lobular pattern. There were raised, whitish areas surrounding small areas that were depressed and congested. Histologic lesions in the liver showed sharply demarcated centrilobular hydropic degeneration, the cells being swollen and rounded with pyknotic nuclei (35,37,40,45,58,60,61).

Other findings include adrenal medullary and gastrointestinal (GI) tract hemorrhages and pulmonary and cerebral edema (36,45,59).

Treatment

There is no specific antidote and no proven therapeutic approach to DEG poisoning. GI decontamination soon after an acute ingestion may be beneficial.

ENHANCEMENT OF ELIMINATION

Although there is limited experience in humans, early dialysis is recommended for all symptomatic DEG exposures, especially in patients with acidosis or renal dysfunction (49).

ANTIDOTES

The ADH inhibitor, 4-methylpyrazole, has been used as an adjunct treatment of DEG poisoning (33,34,49).

SUPPORTIVE CARE

The patient should be resuscitated with isotonic crystalloidal fluids, and acidosis should be corrected. Early treatment with a competitive ADH inhibitor (e.g., 4-methylpyrazole or ethanol), hemodialysis, and supportive care offer the best hope for patient recovery.

A patient with severe DEG toxicity was reported to have made an uneventful recovery after surgical decapsulation of the kidneys (36). At operation, the kidneys were enlarged, congested, and blue. The tension within the capsule caused the kidney to markedly bulge on incision of the capsule, the capsule stripped without assistance, and the color on the kidney surface immediately became redder.

MANAGEMENT PITFALLS

There may be a deceptively quiescent period after DEG exposure. Delayed onset of symptoms (vomiting 2 days postingestion and acute renal failure 6 days postingestion) has been reported in several fatalities (49,50).

TABLE 2. United States regulatory guidelines and standards

Agency	Description	Concentration (mg/m^3) (ppm)	
		Ethylene glycol monomethyl ether[a]	Ethylene glycol monobutyl ether[b]
OSHA	PEL-TWA	80 (25)	240 (50)
(air)	PEL-STEL	None	None
ACGIH	TLV-TWA	15 (5)	97 (20)
(air)	STEL	None	None
NIOSH	REL-TWA	0.3 (0.1)	24 (5)
(air)	REL-STEL	None	3380 (700)
	IDLH	600 (200)	—

ACGIH, American Conference of Governmental Industrial Hygienists; IDLH, immediate danger to life or health; NIOSH, National Institute for Occupational Safety and Health; OSHA, U.S. Occupational Safety and Health Administration; PEL, permissible exposure limit; ppm, parts per million; REL, recommended exposure limit; STEL, short-term exposure limit; TLV, threshold limit value; TWA, time-weighted average.
[a]Conversion equation: ppm × 3.11 = mg/m^3.
[b]Conversion equation: ppm × 4.83 = mg/m^3.

GLYCOL ETHERS

The glycol ethers (cellosolves) are a family of organic solvents used in industrial and household products. These chemicals are extensively used as major components of photoresist solvent systems. The miscibility of glycol ethers in both water and most organic solvents has been exploited as ideal "coupling" agents in many solvent systems. They are inflammable, noncarcinogenic, nonmutagenic, have low vapor pressure, and high potential for dermal absorption. There are many different glycol derivatives, and information on human exposure resulting in toxicity is limited to ethylene glycol monomethyl ether (EGME) and ethylene glycol monobutyl ether (EGBE).

Toxic Dose

Regulatory standards and guidelines for EGME and EGBE are provided in Table 2. Ingestion of 8 oz of EGME (with ethanol) by an adult resulted in death (63).

Toxicokinetics and Toxicodynamics

Glycol ethers are rapidly absorbed after respiratory, oral, and dermal exposure (64–67). Pulmonary absorption increases linearly with increasing concentration and ventilatory rate. Dermal absorption decreases with increasing molecular weight; EGME is three times more readily absorbed than EGBE (68). The volume of distribution has been estimated to be 0.7 L/kg (66).

The ethylene glycol monoalkyl ethers are metabolized by ADH and ALDH to their respective alkoxyacetic acids (64,69–76). The elimination half-life of EGBE was 210 minutes after ingestion of EGBE and ethanol (elimination half-life was 20 minutes) (64). It has been speculated that EGME and EGBE may undergo hydrolysis to yield ethylene glycol, which is metabolized to diacids, based on the observation that metabolic acidosis has been associated with peak oxaluria in patients with EGME and EGBE toxicity (76,77). However, the ether linkage in glycol ethers appears to be quite stable, and there is no direct evidence to support this proposition.

Pathophysiology

In animals, the toxicology of the glycol ethers includes hemolysis with hemoglobinemia, bone marrow toxicity, and testicular degeneration (70,78–82). In an animal model of EGBE toxicity, acute exposure to glycol ethers results in hemolysis, hemoglobinuria, decreased white blood cell count, and hypocellular bone marrow (70,79,81). Inhibition of ADH prevents hemolysis, whereas inhibition of ALDH provides partial protection against hemolysis (71).

The effects in humans have not been well described. Metabolic acidosis has primarily been attributed to the formation of methoxyacetic acid in EGME toxicity and butoxyacetic acid, and lactic acid EGBE toxicity (64,69,72,75,76).

In vitro, both EGBE and its metabolite butoxyacetic acid cause hemolysis, with the latter being the more effective hemolytic agent (70,83). However, human erythrocytes are much less susceptible to the hemolytic effects of EGBE than animal erythrocytes (70,83,84).

Clinical Presentation

ETHYLENE GLYCOL MONOMETHYL ETHER

After ingestion of EGME [or prolonged or repeated dermal (85) or inhalational exposure (86–89)], patients may present with somnolence, apathy, personality changes, impaired comprehension, memory impairment, impaired hearing, loss of appetite, fatigue, anxiety, headache, dyspnea on exertion, dyspraxia, weakness, nausea, vomiting, eye pain, blurred vision, weight loss, disorientation, constipation, dysgeusia, nocturia, and impotency. Physical findings may include tremors, cerebellar dysfunction, exaggerated reflexes, generalized hypertonia, mental retardation, psychomotor retardation, dysarthria, confusion, mydriasis, conjunctivitis, and anisocoria. Signs and symptoms progress with time, and convalescence may be prolonged and incomplete after termination of the exposure.

A 41-year-old man gradually became agitated, confused, and disoriented with marked motor restlessness 8 hours after EGME ingestion (77). He developed tachycardia, tachypnea, hyperpnea, restlessness, and cyanosis 20 hours postingestion. Laboratory studies were remarkable for severe anion gap metabolic acidosis with respiratory compensation, renal dysfunction, hypocalcemia, aciduria, proteinuria, and oxaluria. Treatment included ethanol, sodium bicarbonate, and mannitol. The patient developed dermatitis and partial hair loss before making a slow and uneventful recovery.

A 23-year-old man developed progressive muscular weakness and confusion 18 hours after EGME ingestion (77). He was tachycardic, tachypneic, hyperpneic, hypertensive, and febrile. Laboratory studies were remarkable for severe anion gap metabolic acidosis with respiratory compensation, renal dysfunction, hypocalcemia, aciduria, proteinuria, and oxaluria. The patient made a slow and uneventful recovery with treatment that included IV ethanol, sodium bicarbonate, and mannitol.

A 44-year-old man presented in coma with hypertension and hyperpnea after EGME ingestion (63). Laboratory studies were remarkable for a hemoglobin of 8.4 g/dl, BUN of 17.9 mg/dl, and proteinuria. The patient died without regaining consciousness 5 hours after admission. Autopsy showed microscopic degenerative and toxic changes in the renal tubules.

ETHYLENE GLYCOL MONOBUTYL ETHER

An 18-year-old man presented within 3 hours of ingesting 360 to 480 ml of a solution containing 22% EGBE (72). Physical examination was unremarkable. Laboratory studies were arterial pH, 7.34; PCO_2, 36.4 mm Hg; serum bicarbonate, 19.5 mmol/L; and serum osmolality, 297 mOsm/kg H_2O. Laboratory studies at 16 hours postingestion showed an arterial pH of 7.46; PCO_2, 6.4 mm Hg; serum bicarbonate, 4.3 mmol/L; creatinine, 136.6 µmol/L; serum alanine aminotransferase, 75 U/L; serum lactate, 0.65 mmol/L; and normal serum osmolality. The patient continued to deteriorate, and hemodialysis and ethanol therapy were initiated 24 hours postingestion. Treatment also included thiamine, 100 mg every 12 hours; folate, 50 mg every 12 hours; and pyridoxine, 50 mg every 6 hours. The patient was alert, oriented, and hemodynamically stable 4 hours after dialysis. Liver and renal function tests normalized. The patient was readmitted 10 days later with an ingestion of 480 ml of the same solution. At 6 hours postingestion, his laboratory studies were arterial pH, 7.4; PCO_2, 31.5 mm Hg; serum bicarbonate, 19.3 mmol/L; and creatinine, 114.9 μmol/L. He received empiric ethanol therapy and hemodialysis at 8 hours postingestion as well as thiamine, folate, and pyridoxine. He developed no significant toxic effects.

A 53-year-old man was tachycardic, hypotensive, and comatose 10 hours after EGBE ingestion (91). Gastrointestinal decontamination was performed, and laboratory studies were remarkable for hypoxia, anion gap metabolic acidosis with respiratory compensation, hypokalemia, and proteinuria; serum lactate, 5.3 mmol/L; AST, 105 U/L; bilirubin, 8.5 μmol/L; ammonia, 83 μmol/L; and PT, 15.5. He had transient polyuria (2.5 L in 2 hours). Chest radiograph showed diffuse pulmonary edema, and it was confirmed to be ARDS by hemodynamic studies. Supportive care included endotracheal intubation and mechanical ventilation with positive-end expiratory pressure, IV colloids, vasopressor, sodium bicarbonate, and ethanol therapy. Hemodialysis was initiated 12 hours after admission. The patient's hospital course was remarkable for a nonhemolytic hypochromic anemia and thrombocytopenia, but he made a gradual and full recovery.

A 23-year-old woman was bradycardic, hypotensive, and comatose 1 hour after EGBE ingestion (64). She was orotracheally intubated, gastrointestinal decontamination was performed, and forced diuresis (11.7 mL/kg/hour) and dopamine therapy was initiated. She was fully awake and was extubated 6 hours postingestion. One hour later, she developed a severe anion gap metabolic acidosis with respiratory compensation, there was no osmolal gap, and serum lactate was 7.12 mmol/L. Hemodialysis was initiated because of refractory metabolic acidosis. The patient remained fully conscious throughout this time. On the second hospital day the patient's hemoglobin dropped 2 g, and hematuria was evident. There was no evidence of oxaluria. The patient's renal function remained normal, and she had an otherwise uneventful hospital course.

A 50-year-old woman was comatose 12 hours after EGBE ingestion (76). Laboratory studies were remarkable for metabolic acidosis, hypokalemia, renal dysfunction, and oxaluria. Acid-base derangements quickly resolved with supportive care. Urine output was maintained with diuretics. Hemoglobinuria was evident on the third hospital day. The patient made a gradual recovery.

Two patients, aged 14 months and 2 years, reportedly ingested 30 ml and 300 ml, respectively, of a glass cleaner containing less than 10% EGBE, underwent gastric decontamination, and had an uneventful 24-hour hospital admission (90).

A 51-year-old woman presented with tachypnea and tachycardia 1.7 hours after EGBE ingestion (75). GI decontamination was performed, and laboratory studies were remarkable for hyperchloremic acidosis. IV ethanol therapy was initiated 2.3 hours after admission, and she became obtunded and hypotensive. The hyperchloremic acidosis persisted over 44 hours. The patient had an otherwise uneventful hospital course.

A 19-year-old man developed vomiting, lethargy, hypotension, and coma within 1 hour of ingestion (69). GI decontamination was performed. The patient was deeply comatose, had fixed dilated pupils, no corneal reflexes, positive Babinski's reflexes, and a tonic-clonic seizure 3.5 hours postingestion. Laboratory studies were remarkable for anion gap metabolic acidosis with respiratory compensation, hyperkalemia, hypocalcemia, serum lactate of 5 mmol/L, and disseminated intravascular coagulopathy. Chest radiograph was consistent with severe aspiration pneumonia. The patient significantly improved over the next 24 hours but remained acidotic and underwent hemodialysis. Hematuria and diffuse cerebral edema developed on the second day, hematocrit fell 53% on the fourth day, and thrombocytopenia occurred on the fifth day postingestion. The patient's hepatic and renal function remained normal but was slow to recover from severe neurologic deficits.

Diagnostic Tests

The diagnosis of glycol ether toxicity should be considered in the appropriate clinical setting when acute encephalopathy is characterized by agitation, confusion or coma, evidence of an anion gap metabolic acidosis, bone marrow dysfunction, hemolysis with or without hematuria and hemoglobinuria, proteinuria, renal dysfunction, elevated serum lactate level, and occasionally oxaluria.

A sensitive method for detecting butoxyacetic acid in blood and urine has been developed for use in clinical studies (92–94). However, laboratory diagnosis by measuring glycol ethers and its metabolites in body fluids is not available, but it may be useful in confirming the diagnosis or in forensic cases. Although glycol ethers and their metabolites produce a linear increase in plasma osmolality with increasing plasma concentration, the osmolal gap may be insignificant to be clinically useful as a surrogate maker in cases of acute human poisoning (95).

The glycol ether toxicity has been associated with anemia and granulocytopenia, leukocytosis, macrocytic anemia, increased neutrophilic granulocytes, decreased platelets, hypocellular marrow with decreased erythroid elements, glucose intolerance, increased intracranial pressure, and CSF protein concentration.

Treatment

The patient should be removed from the source of exposure and provided with supportive care. A small retrospective poison center study suggests that healthy patients aged 7 months to 9 years who ingest 15 ml or less (estimated) of a glass/window cleaner solution containing less than 10% EGBE and remain asymptomatic may be managed at home with simple dilution (90).

DECONTAMINATION

GI decontamination soon after an acute ingestion may be beneficial.

ENHANCEMENT OF ELIMINATION

Extracorporeal techniques may be helpful in managing patients with ethylene glycol monoalkyl ether toxicity, particularly patients with refractory acidosis or renal dysfunction (65,70). Hemodialysis has been successfully used to treat patients with EGBE toxicity and severe acidosis (64,69,72,91).

ANTIDOTES

Competitive ADH inhibitors (e.g., ethanol or 4-methylpyrazole) inhibit ethylene glycol monoalkyl ether metabolism in animals and have been used as adjunct treatment in patients with EGME and EGBE toxicity (71,72,75,77,91). Their efficacy on clinical outcome after ethylene glycol monoalkyl ether intoxication remains to be determined.

SUPPORTIVE CARE

Hypotension may require vasopressor support (Chapter 37). Metabolic acidosis may not respond to IV sodium bicarbonate therapy (64).

MONITORING

Laboratory studies should include close monitoring of the patient's electrolytes, fluids, acid-base status, and renal and liver functions.

POLYETHYLENE GLYCOL

Polyethylene glycols (PEGs; "Carbowax" compounds) are a group of compounds with molecular weights ranging from 150 to 10,000 g/mol. Each group is a mixture of several polymers, the average molecular weight of which is appended to the trade name as a means of distinguishing the individual members of the series. For example, commercially available products, such as GoLytely, are solutions of PEG 3350 combined with electrolytes [PEG electrolyte lavage solution (PEG-ELS)]. At room temperature, PEGs with molecular weights less than 600 are clear, viscous liquids with a bitter taste, and those with molecular weights greater than 1000 are solids with variable consistency and hardness. They are stable compounds soluble in water, ethanol, acetone, and aromatic hydrocarbons and used as excipients in pharmaceuticals and cosmetics.

Pharmaceuticals, such as lorazepam, contain 18% PEG 400 (96,97), and some burn creams contain 99.8% PEG 300 (98). A toxic amount of PEG may be inadvertently administered to a patient during continuous IV drug administration (96,97,99–101) or absorbed through damaged skin after topical administration (98,102).

Toxic Dose

The toxicity of PEG appears to be dependent on its molecular weight as well as the dose and duration of administration (103,104). In animals, toxicity from intraperitoneal PEG injection increased with increasing molecular weight, but the reverse relation was found with oral PEG administration. *In vitro*, 10% or more concentrated PEG solutions clump the cellular elements of human blood. All animals survived a dose of 10 g/kg IV of PEG 300, 1000, 1500, 1540, 4000, and 6000. Blood PEG concentrations ranged from 5 to 10 mg/ml, whereas urine PEG concentrations were greater than 90 mg/ml. Cloudy swelling of the renal tubular epithelium was evident in some animals that received PEG 4000 and 6000.

Acute oral toxicity in animals can be demonstrated after large single doses of PEG 200, 300, 400, 1000, 1500, 1540, 4000, 6000, or 10,000. Autopsy showed cloudy swelling of liver parenchyma and renal lesions similar to those resulting from ethylene and DEGs (103). The LD_{50} for PEGs 200 to 400 is 33 to 36 g/kg and for PEGs with molecular weights 1000 or more is greater than 42 g/kg. With PEG 1500, 1540, and 4000, there were no deaths at a dose less than 32 g/kg. Some animals developed renal and hepatic cloudy swelling at dosages greater than 20 g/kg.

Toxicokinetics and Toxicodynamics

Human volunteer studies indicate that after administration of PEG 1000 and 6000, 1 g IV, 85% of PEG 1000 and 96% of PEG 6000 were recovered in the urine within the first 12 hours (105). PEG was not recovered in the urine after a 10-g oral dose of PEG 6000, whereas 8% of a 10-g dose of PEG 1000 was recovered in the urine within the first 24 hours. PEG 3500 and PEG-ELS are oral solutions that are not absorbed to any appreciable extent and do not cause significant water and electrolyte shifts (106–108).

Pathophysiology

The presence of hydroxyglycolic acid and diglycolic acid homologs in the serum and urine of PEG-treated animals and burn patients suggests PEG metabolism involves sequential oxidation by ADH and ALDH (109). Appreciable serum ethylene glycol concentration (1.3 mmol/L) (98) and renal oxalate crystals (102) have been detected in PEG-toxic patients. *In vitro*, ADH catalyzes oxidation of PEG homologs ($N = 1$ to $N = 8$), and it is inhibited by 4-methylpyrazole (110). The K_m of ADH decreases as the homolog number increases, and the maximal velocity progressively decreases through the series.

It is postulated that serum hyperosmolality, primarily due to PEG and accumulation of its mono- and diacid metabolites, is responsible for the anion gap metabolic acidosis (98,111). Diacid metabolites are avid calcium chelators (112) and may decrease the serum ionized calcium level. In turn, parathyroid hormone may increase, resulting in an increased total serum calcium level (98,111). PEG metabolites are reactive compounds similar to ethylene glycol metabolites and appear to be highly toxic to renal tubular cells (113).

Clinical Presentation

INGESTION

No clinically significant adverse events were reported from a mean dosage of 0.8 g/kg/day (11.2 ml/kg/day) of PEG 3500 for 8 days in children 1.5 to 12.0 years of age with constipation or from 44.3 L of PEG-ELS over 5 days in a 33-month-old boy during whole bowel irrigation (106,114). However, supraventricular tachycardia, ventricular ectopy, ventricular tachycardia, and asystole have been reported during peroral PEG-ELS administration to patients older than 65 years of age (115,116). A 54-year-old woman developed Kussmaul's respiration, anion gap metabolic acidosis, and coma 5 hours after ingesting 2 L of PEG 400 (117).

A 65-year-old man presented with altered mental status, lethargy, tachycardia, tachypnea, and fever 12 to 24 hours after ingestion of the contents of a Lava light [microcrystalline wax (6%), kerosene (7%), PEG 200 (13%), chlorinated paraffin (36%), and water (38%)] (118). Laboratory studies were remarkable for anion gap metabolic acidosis, acidemia, and acute renal failure. Over the next 3 days, the patient's renal function deteriorated, which required hemodialysis. The patient was discharged to home with residual renal insufficiency.

Aspiration has occurred during administration of PEG-ELS by nasogastric tube. This may produce gag, cough, vomit, abdominal discomfort, tachycardia, tachypnea, hypertension, dyspnea, stupor, respiratory acidosis, hypoxia, cyanosis, acute respiratory distress syndrome, pulmonary edema, and death (119–122).

Hypersensitivity reactions may occur after ingestion of pharmaceuticals containing PEG 4000, 8000, and 20,000 (123,124). These reactions range from a generalized pruritic, urticarial, cutaneous rash to hypotension, unconsciousness, and grand mal seizures.

INTRAVENOUS ADMINISTRATION

High-dose, prolonged, or repeated administration of pharmaceuticals containing PEG 300 to 400 may result in hyperosmolar anion gap metabolic acidosis, stupor, oliguria and azotemia, and death (96,97,100,101). IV nitrofurantoin (10 mg/kg/day) infusion containing PEG 300 for 2 days was associated with severe metabolic acidosis and death in patients with normal renal function (101). Acute oliguric renal tubular necrosis has been attributed to lorazepam (1 ml contains 0.18 ml of PEG 400, 80% propylene glycol, and 2% benzyl alcohol) administration for 43 days. The cumulative lorazepam dose was 4089 mg, equivalent to 220 ml of PEG 400 (96).

DERMAL EXPOSURE

A syndrome of hyperosmolar anion gap metabolic acidosis, hypercalcemia with decreased ionized calcium, acute renal failure, and death has been reported in patients with 20% to 75% body surface burns who were treated with repeated topical PEG 300–based (98%) antimicrobial cream (98,102). In addition, appreciable ethylene glycol (monomer) levels were detected in these patients (98).

Immediate or delayed contract allergy has been caused by PEG 300, 400, 1500, 3000, 3350, and 6000 (125–128). Delayed eczematous contact allergy to PEG may occur (126,127). Cross-reactivity among PEGs with different molecular weights has been reported (125,128).

Diagnostic Tests

The diagnosis of PEG toxicity should be considered in the appropriate clinical setting and when laboratory studies show an anion gap metabolic acidosis, osmolal gap, renal dysfunction or failure, calcium gap (i.e., difference between the serum total calcium and ionized calcium), and an otherwise unexplainable serum ethylene glycol level.

After aspiration, chest radiography may be consistent with near drowning, fluid overload, or congestive heart failure (120,121).

Autopsy on patients who died from PEG toxicity showed extremely swollen kidneys, severe vacuolation of the convoluted tubule epithelium ("hydropic degeneration"), proximal tubule necrosis, and sometimes oxalate crystals (98,99,102).

Treatment

There is no specific antidote and no proven therapeutic approach to PEG poisoning.

DECONTAMINATION

Most cases cannot benefit from decontamination because IV administration or repeated oral administration is involved. Gastric aspiration soon after an acute ingestion may be beneficial.

ENHANCEMENT OF ELIMINATION

Extracorporeal techniques may be helpful in managing patients with PEG toxicity, particularly patients with renal or hepatic dysfunction (96,97,118). Hemodialysis has been used to treat a patient with PEG 400 toxicity and was associated with correction of metabolic acidosis and rapid neurologic recovery within 48 hours (117). However, recovery may be slow and patients may be left with residual oliguric renal insufficiency (118).

ANTIDOTES

Competitive ADH inhibitor therapy may inhibit PEG metabolism (Chapters 56 and 59) (97). However, its efficacy on clinical outcome after PEG intoxication is unknown.

SUPPORTIVE CARE

When PEG toxicity is suspected, the exposure should be terminated and IV replacement therapy provided (containing little or no PEG) along with supportive care. The target urine output should be 2 to 3 ml/kg/hour. Metabolic acidosis may require sodium bicarbonate therapy (101,117). Patients have been reported to recover with supportive care (99,101).

Acute anaphylactic reactions associated with PEG administration are managed as anaphylaxis from other causes (Chapter 34). Hypersensitive contact dermatitis reaction to PEG is best managed by terminating contact with the offending agent, decontaminating the affected area, and avoiding rechallenge with the same agent. Steroid and antihistamine therapy may be useful.

Aspiration pulmonary edema may require supplemental oxygen and mechanical ventilation with positive end-expiratory pressure. Bronchoalveolar lavage, steroids, diuretics, and nitroglycerin have also been used as adjunct therapy (119–122).

MONITORING

Patients receiving continuous infusion, repetitive, or high doses of pharmaceuticals containing PEG should have serum electrolytes, osmolality, and liver and renal function tested periodically.

PROPYLENE GLYCOL

Propylene glycol (1,2-propanediol) is a colorless, odorless fluid that is commonly used as a solvent (e.g., laundry stain removers), diluent for injectable and topical pharmaceuticals, de-icing agent, major constituent of antifreeze and hydraulic fluids, and as a component in food and cosmetic preparation. A large number of pharmaceuticals contain propylene glycol, ranging from 10% to 80% (Table 3) (129,130). A toxic amount of propylene glycol may be inadvertently administered to a patient during continuous (repeated) IV drug administration or absorbed through damaged skin after topical administration.

Toxic Dose

The permissible daily propylene glycol consumption is 25 mg/kg (131).

Toxicokinetics and Toxicodynamics

Propylene glycol is readily absorbed from the GI tract and readily crosses the blood–brain barrier (132,133). It is detected in the serum and CSF within 1 hour of oral or IV administration. Animal studies show that 55% of a propylene glycol dose is metabolized by hepatic ADH to pyruvate, lactate, and acetate, with the remainder excreted unchanged in the urine (134). Propylene glycol and its metabolites may accumulate when they exceed the endogenous hepatic and renal elimination capacity or when hepatic metabolism or renal excretion is impaired (135,136).

In people with normal liver and renal function, the propylene glycol terminal elimination half-life is 1.4 to 3.3 hours (137). Toxicokinetic data show that the propylene glycol elimination half-life is 10.8 to 30.5 hours (138,139). Lactate is increased in both serum and CSF, accounts for more than 85% of the total acid content, and significantly correlates with the corresponding serum propylene glycol concentrations (132). Acutely, L-lactate may appear shortly after propylene glycol administration, and D-lactate may be the predominant species after chronic propylene glycol intoxication and responsible for anion gap metabolic acidosis (140).

Pathophysiology

The mechanism of central nervous system toxicity remains to be elucidated. In animal studies, L-propylene glycol is more rapidly cleared from the blood than its D-isomer, perhaps due to stereospecific mammalian ADH and ALDH affinity for L-propylene glycol (141–143). Neurologic dysfunction may result from hyperosmolality and accumulation of D-propylene glycol and D-lactate (144,145).

Propylene glycol has been demonstrated to be acutely and subacutely toxic to cultured human proximal renal tubule cells (146,147). D-Propylene glycol appears to be the more toxic isomer in acute toxicity based on glucose transport and chromium, lactate dehydrogenase, and lactate release assays (146). Renal biopsy may show extensive renal tubule dilation and swollen epithelial cells with vacuolated cytoplasm on light microscopy, and the swollen cells may occlude tubular lumens (148). Electron microscopy may show swollen mitochondria and vacuoles containing debris.

TABLE 3. Propylene glycol content of pharmaceutical products

Trade name	Manufacturer	Dose	Route	Amount of propylene glycol: Volume per volume (%)	Amount of propylene glycol: Weight per volume (mg/ml)	Alternative
Amidate	Abbott	2 mg/ml	IV	35	362.6	None
Apresoline	Ciba	20 mg/ml	IM, IV	10	103.6	None
Ativan	Wyeth-Ayerst	2 mg/ml	IM, IV	80	828.8	None
Ativan	Wyeth-Ayerst	4 mg/ml	IM, IV	—	828.8	None
Bactrim	Roche	TMP, 16 mg/ml, SMX, 80 mg/ml	IV	40	414.4	None
Berocca PN	Roche	2 ml	IV	25	259	MVI Pediatric, MVI-12 lyophilized
Brevibloc	DuPont	250 mg/ml	IV	25	259	None
Dilantin	Parke-Davis	50 mg/ml	IM, IV	40	414.4	None
Dramamine	Searle	50 mg/ml	IM, IV	50	518	None
Dramocen	Central	50 mg/ml	IM, IV	50	518	None
Embolex	Sandoz	0.7 ml	SQ	44	460	None
Konakion	Roche	10 mg/ml	IM	20	207	Aqua-Mephyton
Konakion	Roche	2 mg/ml	IM	20	207	Aqua-Mephyton
Lanoxin	Burroughs Wellcome	0.25 mg/ml	IM, IV	40	414.4	None
Lanoxin Pediatric	Burroughs Wellcome	0.1 mg/ml	IM, IV	40	414.4	None
Librium	Roche	50 mg/ml	IM, IV	20	207	None
Loxitane	Lederle	50 mg/ml	IM	70	725.2	None
Luminal Sod	Winthrop	130 mg/ml	IV	67.8	702.4	Phenobarbital sodium (Lilly)
MCV9 Plus	Lyphomed	10 ml	IV	30	310.8	MVI Pediatric; MVI-12 lyophilized
MVI-12	Armour	10 ml	IV	30	310.8	MVI Pediatric, MVI-12 lyophilized
Nitro-Bid	Marion	5 mg/ml	IV	4.3	45	Nitrol
Nembutal	Abbott	50 mg/ml	IM, IV	40	414.4	None
Nitrostat	Parke-Davis	5 mg/ml	IV	30	310.8	Nitrol
Nitroglycerin	Abbott	5 mg/ml	IV	50	518	Nitrol
Pentobarbital	Wyeth	50 mg/ml	IM, IV	40	414.4	None
Phenobarbital	Elkin-Sinns	130 mg/ml	IM, IV	67.8	702.4	Phenobarbital sodium (Lilly)
Phenobarbital	Wyeth	130 mg/ml	IM, IV	67.8	702.4	Phenobarbital Sodium (Lilly)
Phenytoin	Lyphomed	50 mg/ml	IM, IV	30	310.8	None
Phenytoin	Elkin-Sinns	50 mg/ml	IM, IV	40	414.4	None
Septra	Burroughs Wellcome	TMP, 16 mg/ml, SMX, 80 mg/ml	IV	40	414.4	None
Tridil	American Critical Care	0.5 mg/ml	IV	30	310.8	Nitrol
Valium	Roche	5 mg/ml	IM, IV	40	414.4	None

SMX, sulfamethoxazole; TMP, trimethoprim.
Adapted from Smolinske SC. *Handbook of food, drug and cosmetic excipients.* Boca Raton, FL: CRC Press, 1992.

In vitro studies suggest damage to red blood cells by propylene glycol is concentration dependent, and hemolysis is consistently observed when propylene glycol concentration exceeds 30% (149).

Clinical Presentation

ACUTE OVERDOSAGE

Acute propylene glycol ingestion may result in lethargy, drowsiness, stupor, anion gap metabolic acidosis, and acidemia and an increase in serum osmolality and lactate and pyruvate levels (150–152). The manifestations of propylene glycol toxicity are dependent on the route, dose, and rate of administration and may occur within 5 minutes (153–158) or more than 24 hours after drug administration (130,136,139,148,159–166). There is considerable difference in individual susceptibility to propylene glycol–induced central nervous system toxicity.

High-dose, prolonged, or repeated IV administration of pharmaceuticals containing 30% to 80% propylene glycol may result in anion gap metabolic acidosis; elevation in serum osmolality, BUN, creatinine, and lactate levels; seizures; hypotension; tachypnea; hyponatremia; acute renal failure; hemoglobinuria; and hemolysis with associated intracerebral hemorrhage (130,135,136,139,148,159–162,164–173).

Phenytoin in 40% propylene glycol has been implicated as the etiologic agent for adverse drug events during IV phenytoin administration; phenytoin, 100 to 250 mg over 2 to 5 minutes, has been associated with opisthotonic posture with extended extremities, apnea, sinus dysrhythmia, nodal rhythm, widened QRS, complete heart block, idioventricular rhythm, ventricular fibrillation, asystole, and death (153–158). Sinus bradycardia, hypotension, syncope, apnea, second degree atrioventricular block, asystole, and death have been associated with phenytoin, 250 to 875 mg IV at 30 to 40 mg/minute (174,175).

Toxicity may also result (rarely) from acute propylene glycol inhalation (176).

REPEATED EXPOSURE

Prolonged or repeated ingestion of substances containing propylene glycol may result in toxicity (163,177–179). Signs and symptoms include tachypnea, tachycardia, diaphoresis, drowsiness, slurred speech, confusion, lethargy, dizziness, fatigue, coma, hot flashes, flushing, diplopia, tinnitus, neuropathy, menorrhagia, sinus dysrhythmias, hypoglycemia, hyperosmolality, acidosis, acidemia, central nervous system and respiratory depression, seizures, and abnormal electroencephalogram. Onset may be delayed for days.

Continuous IV nitroglycerin infusion containing 96% propylene glycol in a patient with renal dysfunction resulted in headache, vomiting, papilledema, disorientation, stupor, coma, hyponatremia, increase in serum osmolality and lactate levels, and abducens nerve palsy (136,180,181). Hemolysis may occur when red blood cells and medication containing more than 50% propylene glycol are administered through the same IV line (136). Preparing a propylene glycol solution that is less than 30% with 0.9% sodium chloride or water may eliminate the hemolytic effect (134).

Hyperosmolality, azotemia, lactic and metabolic acidosis, lethargy, coma, apnea, cardiopulmonary arrest, and death have occurred in patients with more than 35% body surface area burns receiving repeated topical silver sulfadiazine or nitrofurazone therapy, which contains 77% to 97% propylene glycol (138,182–184).

Hypersensitive contact dermatitis reaction to propylene glycol as a pharmaceutical vehicle may result in an erythematous, edematous, and vesicular, pruritic, macular, and papular eruption (185–189). Application of high concentrations of propylene glycol under occlusive dressings may give rise to a primary skin irritant reaction that resembles an allergic reaction (190). Patients with established epicutaneous allergy to propylene glycol may develop an extensive exanthem within 3 to 16 hours of an oral propylene glycol challenge, and it usually subsides without medical intervention in 24 to 48 hours (191).

Diagnostic Tests

Propylene glycol toxicity is usually a diagnosis based on the appropriate clinical setting and serum propylene glycol level, if available. When serum propylene glycol levels are unavailable in real time, osmolal gap and anion gap metabolic acidosis with or without lactic acidosis may serve as surrogate markers. However, its sensitivity and specificity remain to be determined. The serum propylene glycol level can be estimated from the osmolal gap, and formulas have been determined from linear regression analysis of experimentally derived data: propylene glycol (mg/dl) = 47.5 + (osmolal gap × 9.2); r = 0.96 or 84.6 + (osmolal gap × 7.8); r = 0.99 (138,192). The Systeme International conversion for propylene glycol is mg/L × 3.86 = µmol/L.

Propylene glycol can cause false-positive readings for ethylene glycol when measured by the colorimetric method of Russell or gas chromatography using an OV-17 but not an OV-1 column (193).

Treatment

The management of propylene glycol toxicity is symptomatic and supportive. There is no specific antidote.

DECONTAMINATION

Most patients do not benefit from decontamination because IV administration or repeated oral administration is involved. Aspiration of gastric contents soon after an acute ingestion may be beneficial.

ENHANCEMENT OF ELIMINATION

Extracorporeal techniques may be helpful in managing patients with propylene glycol toxicity, particularly patients with renal or hepatic dysfunction. Hemodialysis decreases the elimination half-life of propylene glycol and metabolites and corrects acid-base derangements (135). Hemodialysis has been successfully used to treat patients with severe propylene glycol toxicity (130,136,166). To avoid a sudden decrease in serum osmolality, hemodialysis should be performed while hypertonic saline is being administered (136). Continuous venovenous hemofiltration with dialysis is generally effective in clearing small molecules such as propylene glycol. However, it may not prevent or preclude propylene glycol toxicity during continuous IV administration of pharmaceuticals containing high concentrations of propylene glycol (e.g., lorazepam) (194).

ANTIDOTES

Competitive ADH inhibitor (e.g., 4-methylpyrazole or ethanol) therapy effectively inhibits propylene glycol metabolism. However, its efficacy on clinical outcome after propylene alcohol intoxication remains to be determined.

SUPPORTIVE CARE

When propylene glycol toxicity is suspected, terminate the infusion or remove topical application containing propylene glycol; provide IV therapy that contains little or no propylene glycol. The target urine output should be 2 to 3 ml/kg/hour. Patients usually recover with supportive care (148,151,159,162,164,167,170,176), but complete recovery may take days (138,168,169,184). Hypotension may require vasopressors (165,166), and metabolic acidosis may require sodium bicarbonate therapy.

Hypersensitive contact dermatitis reaction to propylene glycol is best managed by terminating contact with the agent, decontaminating the affected area, and avoiding rechallenge. Occasionally, steroid therapy may be necessary (191).

MONITORING

The risk of propylene glycol toxicity may be minimized by avoiding all propylene glycol–containing solutions in critically ill patients, especially those with a creatinine clearance less than 30 ml/minute (135,136). Patients receiving continuous infusion and repetitive or high doses of pharmaceuticals containing propylene glycol should have periodic laboratory studies that include serum propylene glycol level, electrolytes, osmolality, and liver and renal function.

REFERENCES

1. Griffith RA. Benzyl alcohol poisoning. *Am J Dis Child* 1983;137:805.
2. Reynolds P, Wilton N. Inadvertent benzyl alcohol administration in neonates: do we contribute? *Anesth Analg* 1989;69:855–856.
3. Weissman DB, Jackson SH, Heicher DA, et al. Benzyl alcohol administration in neonates. *Anesth Analg* 1990;70:673–674.
4. Anderson CW, Ng KJ, Andresen B, et al. Benzyl alcohol poisoning in a premature newborn infant. *Am J Obstet Gynecol* 1984;148:344–346.
5. Brown WJ, Buist NR, Gipson HT, et al. Fatal benzyl alcohol poisoning in a neonatal intensive care unit. *Lancet* 1982;1:1250.
6. Gershanik J, Boecler B, Ensley H, et al. The gasping syndrome and benzyl alcohol poisoning. *N Engl J Med* 1982;307:1384–1388.
7. Jardine DS, Rogers K. Relationship of benzyl alcohol to kernicterus, intraventricular hemorrhage, and mortality in preterm infants. *Pediatrics* 1989;83:153–160.
8. Lopez-Herce J, Bonet C, Meana A, et al. Benzyl alcohol poisoning following diazepam intravenous infusion. *Ann Pharmacother* 1995;29:632.
9. Menon PA, Thach BT, Smith CH, et al. Benzyl alcohol toxicity in a neonatal intensive care unit. Incidence, symptomatology, and mortality. *Am J Perinatol* 1984;1:288–292.
10. Craig DB, Habib GG. Flaccid paraparesis following obstetrical epidural anesthesia: possible role of benzyl alcohol. *Anesth Analg* 1977;56:219–221.
11. Hahn AF, Feasby TE, Gilbert JJ. Paraparesis following intrathecal chemotherapy. *Neurology* 1983;33:1032–1038.
12. Smith AL, Haider K, Schachtner JM, et al. Fatal hemolysis after high-dose etoposide: is benzyl alcohol to blame? *Pharmacotherapy* 2001;21:764–766.
13. Kimura ET, Darby TD, Krause RA, et al. Parenteral toxicity studies with benzyl alcohol. *Toxicol Appl Pharmacol* 1971;18:60–68.
14. Diack SL, Lewis HB. Studies in the synthesis of hippuric acid in the animal organism. VIII. A comparison of the rate of elimination of hippuric acid after the ingestion of sodium benzoate, benzyl alcohol, and benzyl esters of succinic acid. *J Biol Chem* 1928;77:89–95.
15. LeBel M, Ferron L, Masson M, et al. Benzyl alcohol metabolism and elimination in neonates. *Dev Pharmacol Ther* 1988;11:347–356.
16. Hiller JL, Benda GI, Rahatzad M, et al. Benzyl alcohol toxicity: impact on mortality and intraventricular hemorrhage among very low birth weight infants. *Pediatrics* 1986;77:500–506.
17. Chabanel A, Abbott RE, Chien S, et al. Effects of benzyl alcohol on erythro-

cyte shape, membrane hemileaflet fluidity and membrane viscoelasticity. *Biochim Biophys Acta* 1985;816:142–152.
18. Ogiso T, Iwaki M, Yamamoto M. Hemolysis induced by benzyl alcohol and effect of the alcohol on erythrocyte membrane. *Chem Pharm Bull* 1983;31:2404–2415.
19. Ohmiya Y, Nakai K. Interaction of benzyl alcohol with human erythrocytes. *Jpn J Pharmacol* 1978;28:367–373.
20. Chen CC, Lu RB, Chen YC, et al. Interaction between the functional polymorphisms of the alcohol-metabolism genes in protection against alcoholism. *Am J Hum Genet* 1999;65:795–807.
20a. Reynolds RD, Smith RM. Nebulized bacteriostatic saline as a cause of bronchitis. *J Fam Pract* 1995;40:35–40.
21. Grant JA, Bilodeau PA, Guernsey BG, et al. Unsuspected benzyl alcohol hypersensitivity. *N Engl J Med* 1982;306:108.
22. Lagerholm B, Lodin A, Genttle H. Hypersensitivity to phenylcarbinol preservative in vitamin B_{12} for injection. *Acta Allergol* 1958;12:295–298.
23. Shmunes E. Allergic dermatitis to benzyl alcohol in an injectable solution. *Arch Dermatol* 1984;120:1200–1201.
24. Verecken P, Birringer C, Knitelius AC, et al. Sensitization to benzyl alcohol: a possible cause of "corticosteroid allergy." *Contact Dermatitis* 1998;38:106.
25. Wilson JP, Solimando DA Jr, Edwards MS. Parenteral benzyl alcohol-induced hypersensitivity reaction. *Drug Intell Clin Pharm* 1986;20:689–691.
26. Corazza M, Mantovani L, Maranini C, et al. Allergic contact dermatitis from benzyl alcohol. *Contact Dermatitis* 1996;34:74–75.
27. Edwards EK Jr. Allergic reactions to benzyl alcohol in a sunscreen. *Cutis* 1981;28:332–333.
28. Guin JD, Goodman J. Contact urticaria from benzyl alcohol presenting as intolerance to saline soaks. *Contact Dermatitis* 2001;45:182–183.
29. Li M, Gow E. Benzyl alcohol allergy. *Australas J Dermatol* 1995;36:219–220.
30. Shoji A. Allergic reaction to benzyl alcohol in an antimycotic preparation. *Contact Dermatitis* 1983;9:510.
31. Wurbach G, Schubert H, Phillipp I. Contact allergy to benzyl alcohol and benzyl paraben. *Contact Dermatitis* 1993;28:187–188.
32. Fisher AA. Allergic paraben and benzyl alcohol hypersensitivity relationship of the "delayed" and "immediate" varieties. *Contact Dermatitis* 1975;1:281–284.
33. Borron SW, Baud FJ, Garnier R. Intravenous 4-methylpyrazole as an antidote for diethylene glycol and triethylene glycol poisoning: a case report. *Vet Hum Toxicol* 1997;39:26–28.
34. Brophy PD, Tenenbein M, Gardner J, et al. Childhood diethylene glycol poisoning treated with alcohol dehydrogenase inhibitor fomepizole and hemodialysis. *Am J Kidney Dis* 2000;35:958–962.
35. Wilkinson DP. Diethylene glycol poisoning. *Med J Aust* 1967;2:403–404.
36. Wordley E. Diethylene glycol poisoning: report of two cases. *J Clin Pathol* 1947;1:44–46.
37. Drut R, Quijano G, Jones MC, et al. [Pathologic findings in diethylene glycol poisoning]. *Medicina* 1994;54:1–5.
38. van der Linden-Cremers PM, Sangster B. [Medical sequelae of the contamination of wine with diethylene glycol]. *Ned Tijdschr Geneeskd* 1985;129:1890–1891.
39. van Leusen R, Uges DR. [A patient with acute tubular necrosis as a consequence of drinking diethylene glycol-treated wine]. *Ned Tijdschr Geneeskd* 1987;131:768–771.
40. Bowie MD, McKenzie D. Diethylene glycol poisoning in children. *S Afr Med J* 1972;46:931-934.
41. Calvery HO, Klumpp TG. The toxicity for human beings of diethylene glycol with sulfanilamide. *South Med J* 1939;32:1105–1109.
42. Cantarell MC, Fort J, Camps J, et al. Acute intoxication due to topical application of diethylene glycol. *Ann Intern Med* 1987;106:478–479.
43. Hanif M, Mobarak MR, Ronan A, et al. Fatal renal failure caused by diethylene glycol in paracetamol elixir: the Bangladesh epidemic. *BMJ* 1995;311:88–91.
44. O'Brien KL, Selanikio JD, Hecdivert C, et al. Epidemic of pediatric deaths from acute renal failure caused by diethylene glycol poisoning. Acute Renal Failure Investigation Team. *JAMA* 1998;279:1175–1180.
45. Okuonghae HO, Ighogboja IS, Lawson JO, et al. Diethylene glycol poisoning in Nigerian children. *Ann Trop Paediatr* 1992;12:235–238.
46. Pandya SK. An unmitigated tragedy. *BMJ* 1988;297:117–119.
47. Singh J, Dutta AK, Khare S, et al. Diethylene glycol poisoning in Gurgaon, India, 1998. *Bull World Health Organ* 2001;79:88–95.
48. Wax PM. Elixirs, diluents and the passage of the 1938 Federal Food, Drug and Cosmetic Act. *Ann Intern Med* 1995;122:456–461.
49. Rollins YD, Filley CM, McNutt JT, et al. Fulminant ascending paralysis as a delayed sequela of diethylene glycol (Sterno) ingestion. *Neurology* 2000;59:1460–1463.
50. Doyle CR, Win N, Hodgman M, et al. Diethylene glycol abuse with resultant multiple fatalities. *J Toxicol Clin Toxicol* 1998; 36:516–517(abst).
51. Heilmair R, Lenk W, Lohr D. Toxicokinetics of diethylene glycol (DEG) in the rat. *Arch Toxicol* 1993;67:655–666.
52. Wiener HL, Richardson KE. Metabolism of diethylene glycol in male rats. *Biochem Pharmacol* 1989;38:539–541.
53. Braun WH, Young JD. Identification of beta-hydroxyethoxyacetic acid as the major urinary metabolite of 1,4-dioxane in the rat. *Toxicol Appl Pharmacol* 1978;39:33–38.
54. Wiener HL. Ethylene and diethylene glycol metabolism, toxicity and treatment. PhD Dissertation. Columbus, OH: The Ohio State University, 1986.
55. Haag HB, Ambrose AM. Studies on the physiological effect of diethylene glycol. II. Toxicity and fate. *J Pharmacol Exp Ther* 1937:93–100.
56. Freundt KJ, Weis N. Transient renal impairment in rats after oral exposure to diethylene glycol. *J Appl Toxicol* 1989;9:317–321.
57. Kraul H, Jahn F, Braunlich H. Nephrotoxic effects of diethylene glycol (DEG) in rats. *Exp Pathol* 1991;42:27–32.
58. Geiling EHK, Cannon PR. Pathological effects of elixir of sulfanilamide (diethylene glycol) poisoning. A clinical experience and experimental correlation: final report. *JAMA* 1938;111:919–926.
59. Hagebusch OE. Special article from the American Medical Association chemical laboratory. Elixir of sulfanilamide-Massengill. Chemical, pharmacologic, pathologic, and necropsy report: preliminary toxicity report on diethylene glycol and sulfanilamide. VI. Necropsies of four patients following administration of elixir of sulfanilamide-Massengill. *JAMA* 1937;109:1537–1539.
60. Lynch KM. Diethylene glycol poisoning in the human. *South Med J* 1938;31:134–137.
61. Ruprecht HA, Nelson IA. Special article from the American Medical Association chemical laboratory. Elixir of sulfanilamide-Massengill. Chemical, pharmacologic, pathologic, and necropsy report: preliminary toxicity report on diethylene glycol and sulfanilamide. V. Clinical and pathologic observations. *JAMA* 1937;109:1537.
62. Scalzo AJ. Diethylene glycol toxicity revisited: the 1996 Haitian epidemic. *J Toxicol Clin Toxicol* 1996;34:513–516.
63. Young GE, Woolner LB. A case of fatal poisoning from 2-methoxy-ethanol. *J Industr Hyg Toxicol* 1946;28:267–268.
64. Gijsenbergh FP, Jenco M, Veulemans H, et al. Acute butylglycol intoxication: a case report. *Hum Toxicol* 1989;8:243–245.
65. Groeseneken D, Veulemans H, Masschelein R. Respiratory uptake and elimination of ethylene glycol monoethyl ether after experimental human exposure. *Br J Ind Med* 1986;43:544–549.
66. Johanson G, Kronborg H, Naslund PH, et al. Toxicokinetics of inhaled 2-butoxyethanol (ethylene glycol monobutyl ether) in man. *Scand J Work Environ Health* 1986;12:594–602.
67. Nakaaki K, Fukabori S, Tada O. An experimental study on percutaneous absorption of some organic solvents. *J Sci Labor* 1980;56:1–9.
68. Dugard PH, Walker M, Mawdsley SJ, et al. Absorption of some glycol ethers through human skin in vitro. *Environ Health Perspect* 1984;57:193–197.
69. Burkhart KK, Donovan JW. Hemodialysis following butoxyethanol ingestion. *J Toxicol Clin Toxicol* 1998;36:723–725.
70. Carpenter CP, Pozzani UC, Weil CS, et al. The toxicity of butyl cellosolve solvent. *AMA Arch Ind Health* 1956;14:114–131.
71. Ghanayem BI, Burka LT, Matthews HB. Metabolic basis of ethylene glycol monobutyl ether (2-butoxyethanol) toxicity: role of alcohol and aldehyde dehydrogenases. *J Pharmacol Exp Ther* 1987;242:222–231.
72. Gualtieri JF, DeBoer L, Harris CR, et al. Repeated ingestion of 2-butoxyethanol: case report and literature review. *J Toxicol Clin Toxicol* 2003;41:57–62.
73. Jonsson AK, Pedersen J, Steen G. Ethoxyacetic acid and N-ethoxyacetylglycine: metabolites of ethoxyethanol (ethylcellosolve) in rats. *Acta Pharmacol Toxicol* 1982;50:358–362.
74. Jonsson AK, Steen G. n-Butoxyacetic acid, a urinary metabolite from inhaled n-butoxyethanol (Butylcellosolve). *Acta Pharmacol Toxicol* 1978;42:354–356.
75. McKinney PE, Palmer RB, Blackwell W, et al. Butoxyethanol ingestion with prolonged hyperchloremic metabolic acidosis treated with ethanol therapy. *J Toxicol Clin Toxicol* 2000;38:787–793.
76. Rambourg-Schepens MO, Buffet M, Bertault R, et al. Severe ethylene glycol butyl ether poisoning. Kinetics and metabolic pattern. *Hum Toxicol* 1988;7:187–189.
77. Nitter-Hauge S. Poisoning with ethylene glycol monomethyl ether. Report of two cases. *Acta Med Scand* 1970;188:277–280.
78. Hardin BD. Reproductive toxicity of the glycol ethers. *Toxicology* 1983;27:91–102.
79. Kalf GF, Post GB, Snyder R. Solvent toxicology: recent advances in the toxicology of benzene, the glycol ethers, and carbon tetrachloride. *Ann Rev Pharmacol Toxicol* 1987;27:399–427.
80. Grant D, Sulsh S, Jones HB, et al. Acute toxicity and recovery in the hemopoietic system of rats after treatment with ethylene glycol monomethyl and monobutyl ethers. *Toxicol Appl Pharmacol* 1985;77:187–200.
81. Miller RR, Carreon RE, Young JT, et al. Toxicity of methoxyacetic acid in rats. *Fundam Appl Toxicol* 1982;2:158–160.
82. The glycol ethers, with particular reference to 2-methoxyethanol and 2-ethoxyethanol: Evidence of adverse reproductive effects. Current Intelligence Bulletin #39. Washington, DC, US Dept of Health and Human Services publication No. (NIOSH) 83-112, 1983.
83. Bartnik FG, Reddy AK, Klecak G, et al. Percutaneous absorption, metabolism, and hemolytic activity of n-butoxyethanol. *Fundam Appl Toxicol* 1987;8:59–70.
84. Ghanayem BI, Blair PC, Thompson MB, et al. Metabolic and cellular basis of 2-butoxyethanol-induced hemolytic anemia in rats and assessment of human risk in vitro. *Biochem Pharmacol* 1989;38:1679–1684.
85. Ohi G, Wegman DH. Transcutaneous ethylene glycol monomethyl ether poisoning in the work setting. *J Occup Med* 1978;20:675–676.
86. Donley DE. Toxic encephalopathy and volatile solvents in industry. *J Industr Hyg Toxicol* 1936;18:571–577.
87. Greenburg L, Mayers MR, Goldwater LJ, et al. Health hazards in the manufacture of "fused collars." I. Exposure to ethylene glycol monomethyl ether. *J Industr Hyg Toxicol* 1938;20:134–147.

88. Parsons CE, Moore Parsons ME. Toxic encephalopathy and "granulopenic anemia" due to volatile solvents in industry: report of two cases. *J Industr Hyg Toxicol* 1938;20:124–133.
89. Zavon MR. Methyl cellosolve intoxication. *Industr Hyg J* 1963;24:36–41.
90. Dean BS, Krenzelok EP. Clinical evaluation of pediatric ethylene glycol monobutyl ether poisonings. *J Toxicol Clin Toxicol* 1992;30:557–557.
91. Bauer P, Weber M, Mur JM, et al. Transient non-cardiogenic pulmonary edema following massive ingestion of ethylene glycol butyl ether. *Intensive Care Med* 1992;18:250–251.
92. Johanson G. Analysis of ethylene glycol ether metabolites in urine by extractive alkylation and electron-capture gas chromatography. *Arch Toxicol* 1989;63:107–111.
93. Johanson G, Michel I, Norback D, et al. Biological monitoring of exposure to ethylene glycol ethers. *Arch Toxicol Suppl* 1989;13:108–111.
94. Johanson G, Johnsson S. Chromatographic determination of butyoxyacetic acid in human blood after exposure to 2-butoxyethanol. *Arch Toxicol* 1991;65;433–435.
95. Browning RG, Curry SC. Effect of glycol ethers on plasma osmolality. *Hum Exp Toxicol* 1992;11:488–490.
96. Laine GA, Hamid Hossain SM, Solis RT, et al. Polyethylene glycol nephrotoxicity secondary to prolonged high-dose intravenous lorazepam. *Ann Pharmacother* 1995;29:1110–1114.
97. Tayar J, Jabbour G, Saggi SJ. Severe hyperosmolar metabolic acidosis due to a large dose of intravenous lorazepam. *N Engl J Med* 2002;346:1253–1254.
98. Bruns DE, Herold DA, Rodeheaver GT, et al. Polyethylene glycol intoxication in burn patients. *Burns Incl Therm Inj* 1982;9:49–52.
99. McCabe WR, Jackson GG, Grieble HG. Treatment of chronic pyelonephritis. *Arch Intern Med* 1959;104:710–719.
100. Tayar J, Saggi SJ. Hyperosmolar metabolic acidosis and intravenous lorazepam. *N Engl J Med* 2002;347:857–858.
101. Sweet AY. Fatality from intravenous nitrofurantoin. *Pediatrics* 1958;22:1204.
102. Sturgill BC, Herold DA, Bruns DE. Renal tubular necrosis in burn patients treated with topical polyethylene glycol. *Lab Invest* 1982;46:81A.
103. Smyth HF Jr, Carpenter CP, Weil CS. The toxicology of the polyethylene glycols. *J Am Pharm Assoc* 1950;39:349–354.
104. Smyth HF Jr, Carpenter CP, Weil CS. The chronic oral toxicity of the polyethylene glycols. *J Am Pharm Assoc* 1955;44:27–30.
105. Shaffer CB, Critchfield FH. The absorption and excretion of the solid polyethylene glycols ("Carbowax" compounds). *J Am Pharm Assoc* 1947;36:152–156.
106. Pashankar DS, Bishop WP. Efficacy and optimal dose of daily polyethylene glycol 3350 for treatment of constipation and encopresis in children. *J Pediatr* 2001;139:428–432.
107. Schiller LR, Santa Ana CA, Porter J, et al. Validation of polyethylene glycol 3350 as a poorly absorbable marker for intestinal perfusion studies. *Dig Dis Sci* 1997;42:1–5.
108. Tuggle DW, Hoelzer DJ, Tunell WP, et al. The safety and cost-effectiveness of polyethylene glycol electrolyte solution bowel preparation in infants and children. *J Pediatr Surg* 1987; 22:513–515.
109. Hunt DF, Giordani AB, Rhodes J, et al. Mixture analysis by triple quadrupole mass spectrometry: metabolic profiling of urinary carboxylic acids. *Clin Chem* 1982;28:2387–2392.
110. Herold DA, Keil K, Bruns DE. Oxidation of polyethylene glycols by alcohol dehydrogenase. *Biochem Pharmacol* 1989;38:73–76.
111. Herold DA, Rodeheaver GT, Bellamy WT, et al. Toxicity of topical polyethylene glycol. *Toxicol Appl Pharmacol* 1982;65:329–335.
112. Ancillotti E, Boschi G, Perago G, et al. Calcium binding capacity of carboxylic acids with an ethereal function. *J Chem Soc Dalton Trans* 1977;9:901–905.
113. McMartin KE, Cenac TA. Toxicity of ethylene glycol metabolites in normal human kidney cells. *Ann N Y Acad Sci* 2000;919:315–317.
114. Kaczorowski JM, Wax PM. Five days of whole-bowel irrigation in a case of pediatric iron ingestion. *Ann Emerg Med* 1996;27:258–263.
115. Gholson CF. Ventricular ectopy during colonic lavage. *Gastrointest Endosc* 1987;33:334.
116. Marsh WH, Bronner MH, Yantis P, et al. Ventricular ectopy during colonic lavage. *Gastrointest Endosc* 1987;33:334.
117. Belaiche J, Vesin P, Cattan D, et al. Acidotic coma after colonic preparation using polyethylene glycol. *Gastroenterol Clin Biol* 1983;7:426–427.
118. Erickson TB, Aks SE, Zabaneh R, et al. Acute renal toxicity after ingestion of Lava light liquid. *Ann Emerg Med* 1996;27:781–784.
119. Argent A, Hatherill M, Reynolds L, et al. Fulminant pulmonary oedema after administration of a balanced electrolyte polyethylene glycol solution. *Arch Dis Child* 2002;86:209.
120. Marschall HU, Bartels F. Life-threatening complications of nasogastric administration of polyethylene glycol-electrolyte solutions (Golytely) for bowel cleansing. *Gastrointest Endosc* 1998;47:408–410.
121. Paap CM, Ehrlich R. Acute pulmonary edema after polyethylene glycol intestinal lavage in a child. *Ann Pharmacother* 1993;27:1044–1047.
122. Pichlmeier R, von Hundelshausen B, Tempel G, et al. Lung edema following intestinal irrigation with Golytely solution. *Anasth Intensivther Notfallmed* 1990;25:295–296.
123. Brullett E, Moron A, Calvet X, et al. Urticarial reaction to oral polyethylene glycol electrolyte lavage solution. *Gastrointest Endosc* 1992;38:400–401.
124. Kwee YN, Dolovich J. Anaphylaxis to polyethylene glycol (PEG) in a multivitamin tablet. *J Allergy Clin Immunol* 1982;69:138.
125. Bajaj AK, Gupta SC, Chatterjee AK, et al. Contact sensitivity to polyethylene glycols. *Contact Dermatitis* 1990;22:291.
126. Daly BM. Bactroban allergy due to polyethylene glycol. *Contact Dermatitis* 1987;17:48–49.
127. Fisher AA. Immediate and delayed allergic contact reactions to polyethylene glycol. *Contact Dermatitis* 1978;4:135–138.
128. Maibach HI. Polyethylene glycol: allergic contact dermatitis potential. *Contact Dermatitis* 1975;1:247.
129. Smolinske SC. *Handbook of food, drug and cosmetic excipients.* Boca Raton, FL: CRC Press, 1992.
130. Parker MG, Fraser GL, Watson DM, et al. Removal of propylene glycol and correction of increased osmolar gap by hemodialysis in a patient on high dose lorazepam infusion therapy. *Intensive Care Med* 2002;28:81–84.
131. World Health Organization. Toxicological evaluation of certain food additives with a review of general principles and of specifications: 17th report of the Joint/WHO Expert Committee on Food Additives. Technical report series; No 539. Geneva: World Health Organization, 1974.
132. Kelner MJ, Bailey DN. Propylene glycol as a cause of lactic acidosis. *J Anal Toxicol* 1985;9:40–42.
133. Yu DK, Elmquist WF, Sawchuk RJ. Pharmacokinetics of propylene glycol in humans during multiple dosing regimens. *J Pharm Sci* 1985;74:876–879.
134. Ruddick JA. Toxicology, metabolism, and biochemistry of 1,2-propanediol. *Toxicol Appl Pharmacol* 1972;21:102–111.
135. Demey HE, Daelemans RA, Verpooten GA, et al. Propylene glycol-induced side effects during intravenous nitroglycerin therapy. *Intensive Care Med* 1988;14:221–226.
136. Demey H, Daelemans R, De Broe ME, et al. Propyleneglycol intoxication due to intravenous nitroglycerin. *Lancet* 1984;1:1360.
137. Speth PA, Vree TB, Neilen NF, et al. Propylene glycol pharmacokinetics and effects after intravenous infusion in humans. *Ther Drug Monit* 1987;9:255–258.
138. Fligner CL, Jack R, Twiggs GA, et al. Hyperosmolality induced by propylene glycol. A complication of silver sulfadiazine therapy. *JAMA* 1985;253:1606–1609.
139. Glasgow AM, Boeckx RL, Miller MK, et al. Hyperosmolality in small infants due to propylene glycol. *Pediatrics* 1983;72:353–355.
140. Christopher MM, Eckfeldt JH, Eaton JW. Propylene glycol ingestion causes D-lactic acidosis. *Lab Invest* 1990;62:114–118.
141. Huff E. The metabolism of 1,2-propanediol. *Biochim Biophys Acta* 1961;48:506–517.
142. Miller ON, Bazzano G. Propanediol metabolism and its relation to lactic acid metabolism. *Ann N Y Acad Sci* 1965;119:957–973.
143. Pietruszko R, Voigtlander K, Lester D. Alcohol dehydrogenase from human and horse liver—substrate specificity with diols. *Biochem Pharmacol* 1978;27:1296–1297.
144. Uribarri J, Oh MS, Carroll HJ. D-Lactic acidosis. A review of clinical presentation, biochemical features, and pathophysiologic mechanisms. *Medicine* 1998;77:73–82.
145. Yu DK. Pharmacokinetics of propylene glycol in the rabbit. PhD dissertation. Minneapolis: University of Minnesota, 1984.
146. Morshed KM, Jain SK, McMartin KE. Acute toxicity of propylene glycol: an assessment using cultured proximal tubule cells of human origin. *Fundam Appl Toxicol* 1994;23:38–43.
147. Morshed KM, Jain SK, McMartin KE. Propylene glycol-mediated cell injury in a primary culture of human proximal tubule cells. *Toxicol Sci* 1998;46:410–417.
148. Yorgin PD, Theodorou AA, Al-Uzri A, et al. Propylene glycol-induced proximal renal tubular cell injury. *Am J Kidney Dis* 1997;30:134–139.
149. Randolph TG, Mallory OT. The effect of in vitro propylene glycol on erythrocytes. *J Lab Clin Med* 1944;29:197–202.
150. Brooks DE, Wallace KL. Acute propylene glycol ingestion. *J Toxicol Clin Toxicol* 2002;40:513–516.
151. Glover ML, Reed MD. Propylene glycol: the safe diluent that continues to cause harm. *Pharmacotherapy* 1996;16:690–693.
152. McKinney P, Phillips S, Gomez HF, et al. Acute propylene glycol ingestion: 2 cases. *Vet Hum Toxicol* 1994;34:338.
153. Gellerman GL, Martinez C. Fatal ventricular fibrillation following intravenous sodium diphenylhydantoin therapy. *JAMA* 1967;200:337–338.
154. Goldschlager AW, Karliner JS. Ventricular standstill after intravenous diphenylhydantoin. *Am Heart J* 1967;74:410–412.
155. Russell MA, Bousvaros G. Fatal results from diphenylhydantoin administered intravenously. *JAMA* 1968;206:2118–2119.
156. Unger AH, Sklaroff HJ. Fatalities following intravenous use of sodium diphenylhydantoin for cardiac arrhythmias. *JAMA* 1967;200:335–336.
157. Voigt GC. Death following intravenous sodium diphenylhydantoin (Dilantin). *Johns Hopkins Med J* 1968;123:153–157.
158. Zoneraich S, Zoneraich O, Siegel J. Sudden death following intravenous sodium diphenylhydantoin. *Am Heart J* 1976;91:375–377.
159. Arbour RB. Propylene glycol toxicity related to high-dose lorazepam infusion: case report and discussion. *Am J Crit Care* 1999;8:499–506.
160. Arbour R, Esparis B. Osmolar gap metabolic acidosis in a 60-year-old man treated for hypoxemic respiratory failure. *Chest* 2000;118:545–546.
161. Cawley MJ. Short-term lorazepam infusion and concern for propylene glycol toxicity: case report and review. *Pharmacotherapy* 2001;21:1140–1144.
162. D'Ambrosio JA, Phelps PB, Nolen JG, et al. Propylene glycol-induced lactic acidosis secondary to a continuous infusion of lorazepam. *Pharmacotherapy* 1993;13:274.
163. Martin G, Finberg L. Propylene glycol: a potentially toxic vehicle in liquid dosage form. *J Pediatr* 1970;77:877–878.

164. Reynolds HN, Teiken P, Regan ME, et al. Hyperlactatemia, increased osmolar gap, and renal dysfunction during continuous lorazepam infusion. *Crit Care Med* 2000;28:1631–1634.
165. Seay RE, Graves PJ, Wilkin MK. Comment: possible toxicity from propylene glycol in lorazepam infusion. *Ann Pharmacother* 1997;31:647–648.
166. Wilson KC, Reardon C, Farber HW. Propylene glycol toxicity in a patient receiving intravenous diazepam. *N Engl J Med* 2000;343:815.
167. Bedichek E, Kirschbaum B. A case of propylene glycol toxic reaction associated with etomidate infusion. *Arch Intern Med* 1991;151:2297–2298.
168. Ezidinma NP, Fish JT, Wandschneider HL, et al. Propylene glycol associated renal toxicity from lorazepam infusions. *Crit Care Med* 1999;27[Suppl]:A123.
169. Huggon I, James I, Macrae D. Hyperosmolality related to propylene glycol in an infant treated with enoximone infusion. *BMJ* 1990;30:19–20.
170. Levy ML, Aranda M, Zelman V, et al. Propylene glycol toxicity following continuous etomidate infusion for the control of refractory cerebral edema. *Neurosurgery* 1995;37:363–369.
171. MacDonald MG, Getson PR, Glasgow AM, et al. Propylene glycol: increased incidence of seizures in low birth weight infants. *Pediatrics* 1987;79:622–625.
172. McConnel JR, Ong CS, McAllister JL, et al. Propylene glycol toxicity following continuous etomidate infusion for the control of refractory cerebral edema. *Neurosurgery* 1996;38:232–233.
173. Van de Wiele B, Rubinstein E, Peacock W, et al. Propylene glycol toxicity caused by prolonged infusion of etomidate. *J Neurosurg Anesth* 1995;7:259–262.
174. Barron SA. Cardiac arrhythmias after small IV dose of phenytoin. *N Engl J Med* 1976;295:678.
175. York RC, Coleridge ST. Cardiopulmonary arrest following intravenous phenytoin loading. *Am J Emerg Med* 1988;6:255–259.
176. Cate JC 4th, Hedrick R. Propylene glycol intoxication and lactic acidosis. *N Engl J Med* 1980;303:1237.
177. Arulanantham K, Genel M. Central nervous system toxicity associated with ingestion of propylene glycol. *J Pediatr* 1978;93:515–516.
178. Lolin Y, Francis DA, Flanagan RJ, et al. Cerebral depression due to propylene glycol in a patient with chronic epilepsy—the value of the plasma osmolal gap in diagnosis. *Postgrad Med J* 1988;64:610–613.
179. Sawchuk RJ, Pepin SM, Leppik IE, et al. Rapid and slow release phenytoin in epileptic patients at steady state: comparative plasma levels and toxicity. *J Pharmacokinet Biopharm* 1982;10:365–382.
180. Alexander J, Kaplan K, Davison R, et al. Intravenous nitroglycerin-induced abducens nerve palsy. *Am Heart J* 1983;106:1159.
181. Demey HE, Bossaert LL. Propylene glycol intoxication and nitroglycerin therapy. *Crit Care Med* 1987;15:540.
182. Bekeris L, Baker C, Fenton J, et al. Propylene glycol as a cause of an elevated serum osmolality. *Am J Clin Pathol* 1979;72:633–636.
183. Kulick MI, Lewis NS, Bansal V, et al. Hyperosmolality in the burn patient: analysis of an osmolal discrepancy. *J Trauma* 1980;20:223–228.
184. Peleg O, Bar-Oz B, Arad I. Coma in a premature infant associated with the transdermal absorption of propylene glycol. *Acta Paediatr* 1998;87:1195–1196.
185. Angelini GL, Meneghini CL. Contact allergy from propylene glycol. *Contact Dermatitis* 1981;7:197–198.
186. Catanzaro JM, Smith JG. Propylene glycol dermatitis. *J Am Acad Dermatol* 1991;24:90–95.
187. Corazza M, Virgili A, Mantovani L, et al. Propylene glycol allergy from acyclovir cream with cross-reactivity to hydroxypropyl cellulose in a transdermal estradiol system? *Contact Dermatitis* 1993;29:283–284.
188. Eun HC, Kim YC. Propylene glycol allergy from ketoconazole cream. *Contact Dermatitis* 1989;21:274–275.
189. Fisher AA. Use of glycerin in topical minoxidil solutions for patients allergic to propylene glycol. *Cutis* 1990;45:81–82.
190. Nater JP, Baar AJ, Hoedemaeker PJ. Histological aspects of skin reactions to propylene glycol. *Contact Dermatitis* 1977;3:181–185.
191. Hannuksela M, Forstrom L. Reactions to peroral propylene glycol. *Contact Dermatitis* 1978;4:41–45.
192. Glasgow AM, Boeckx RL, Miller MK, et al. Propylene glycol plasma level. *Pediatrics* 1985;76:654.
193. Robinson CA Jr, Scott JW, Ketchum C. Propylene glycol interference with ethylene glycol procedures. *Clin Chem* 1983;29:727.
194. Al-Khafaji AH, Dewhirst WE, Manning HL. Propylene glycol toxicity associated with lorazepam infusion in a patient receiving continuous venovenous hemofiltration with dialysis. *Anesth Analg* 2002;94:1583–1585.

SECTION

3

Antiseptics and Disinfectants

CHAPTER 194

Ethylene Oxide

Thomas R. Caraccio and Michael A. McGuigan

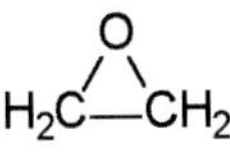

ETHYLENE OXIDE

Molecular formula and weight:	**C_2H_4O, 44.05 g/mol**
SI conversion:	**ppm × 1.8 = mg/m³**
CAS Registry No.:	**75-21-8**
Normal levels:	**Undetectable**
Special concerns:	**Toxicity may be delayed after exposure.**
Target organs:	**Acute—eyes, skin, lungs, central nervous system; chronic—central nervous system, peripheral nervous system, reproductive, mutagenic**
Antidote:	**None**

OVERVIEW

Ethylene oxide is a gas used to chemically sterilize heat-sensitive materials in the hospital setting (1,2). It is also used in the production of ethylene glycol, polyesters, and detergents. Ethylene oxide is irritating to the eyes, skin, and mucous membranes. Dermal contact with liquid ethylene oxide can cause blistering, severe chemical burns, and frostbite.

Ethylene oxide is an extremely flammable, highly reactive, colorless gas at room temperature and normal pressure. At 10°C, it is a stable, clear liquid that may polymerize violently. Ethylene oxide has an ether-like odor, also described as a sweet, olefinic odor (3–6).

Sources of Exposure

Ethylene oxide is typically supplied to U.S. hospitals in compressed gas cylinders that contain Freon (88%) and ethylene oxide (12%) or in single-dose cartridges of pure ethylene oxide (7). In 1983, approximately 62,370 workers were directly exposed to ethylene oxide, and 25,000 others may have been incidentally exposed in U.S. hospitals. There are 7700 ethylene-oxide sterilizers in operation in 6300 hospitals in the United States (7). Unless good engineering and good work practices are used, workers in central supply and surgical suites who use ethylene oxide during instrument sterilization are at risk of exposure. Workers may encounter relatively high concentrations of ethylene oxide over relatively brief periods. Data suggest the need to control short-term peak exposures to ethylene oxide.

Toxic Dose

The U.S. regulatory guidelines and standards for ethylene oxide are provided in Table 1. The odor threshold is 50 parts per million (ppm) (9). The lethal human dose for ethylene oxide has not been delineated. Severe hypersensitivity reactions have occurred in hemodialysis patients (ethylene oxide is used to dry sterilize the

TABLE 1. U.S. regulatory guidelines and standards for ethylene oxide

Agency	Description	Concentration [mg/m³ (ppm)]
OSHA	Metal and soluble compounds	
(air)	PEL-TWA	1.8 (1.0)
	Action level TWA	0.9 (0.5)
	Excursion limit (15-min TWA)	9.0 (5.0)
ACGIH		
(air)	TLV-TWA	1.8 (1.0)
	STEL	None
NIOSH		
(air)	REL-TWA	<0.18
	STEL	None
	Ceiling (10 min/d)	9.0 (5.0)
	IDLH	(800)

ACGIH, American Conference of Governmental Industrial Hygienists; IDLH, immediate danger to life or health; NIOSH, National Institute for Occupational Safety and Health; OSHA, U.S. Occupational Safety and Health Administration; PEL, permissible exposure limit; ppm, parts per million; REL, recommended exposure limit; STEL, short-term exposure limit; TLV, threshold limit value; TWA, time-weighted average.

artificial kidney), plateletpheresis donors (ethylene oxide–sterilized kits used), and hemophiliacs (10).

Brief exposure to concentrated vapors causes significant symptoms (11). Chronic exposure of 2.4 ppm for 10 years resulted in cognitive impairment and subclinical sensory neuropathy (12). In humans, exposures of 500 to 700 ppm for 2 to 3 minutes resulted in nausea, vomiting, headache, disorientation, and fluid in the lungs, followed by seizures. Volunteers breathing 2500 ppm experienced slight irritation; at 12,500 ppm, they experienced respiratory tract irritation within 10 seconds (13).

In human volunteers, 40% to 60% solutions produced second-degree burns in less than 1 minute. A 1% solution produced no effects after 20 to 25 minutes, and second-degree burns were produced after 75 minutes or more. Undiluted ethylene oxide evaporates rapidly and results in thermal injury. Three of eight volunteers developed skin sensitization (14).

TOXICOKINETICS AND TOXICODYNAMICS

Ethylene oxide is absorbed orally and by inhalation (3). Workers exposed to 0.11 to 12.30 ppm absorbed 75% to 80% of the ethylene oxide at steady-state. After exposure to 1 ppm for 8 hours, 7.2 to 7.7 mg of ethylene oxide was absorbed (5). Ethylene oxide is widely distributed throughout the body (11).

Ethylene oxide reacts with glutathione to form cysteine derivatives, forms ethylene glycol by epoxide hydrolase with subsequent metabolism of the glycol, and reacts with chloride to form 2-chloroethanol (5). The relative importance of these pathways is undefined. Ethylene glycol glutathione conjugates are metabolites of ethylene oxide (15). When ethylene oxide was administered to rats, 35% was eliminated in the urine over 24 hours (16). The elimination half-life is estimated at 40 to 55 minutes in humans (15).

PATHOPHYSIOLOGY

Ethylene oxide acts as an alkylating agent and reacts directly and irreversibly with most organic substances, such as amino acids, proteins and nucleoproteins, DNA, and histidine found in hemoglobin (17).

VULNERABLE POPULATIONS

Ethylene oxide is fetotoxic and teratogenic in animals (18). Changes in the live birth index were noted when male or female rats were given ethylene oxide (18). Nervous system and musculoskeletal abnormalities have been reported in the offspring of laboratory animals.

A higher frequency of spontaneous abortions was found in pregnant hospital workers exposed to ethylene oxide in sterilizing operations. The adjusted rate was 16.1% in the exposed group versus 7.8% in the nonexposed group (19). An increase in abortions was reported in production plant workers exposed to ethylene oxide (20). Dental hygienists who used ethylene oxide gas to sterilize instruments while pregnant had an increase in spontaneous abortions (5).

CLINICAL PRESENTATION

Acute Exposure

Symptoms may not occur for hours after inhalation. Ocular irritation and conjunctivitis may be seen on splash contact with the eyes (21). Irritation of eyes, nose, and throat and a peculiar taste are the early symptoms of exposure (21).

Cardiovascular effects do not develop until respiratory injury produces hypoxia (5). *Pulmonary* irritation is common after inhalation. Severe exposure may result in cyanosis (4). Pulmonary edema may be seen with severe acute exposure (22). Pneumonia or secondary lung infection can occur as a complication of ethylene oxide exposure (5). Reactive airway dysfunction syndrome may follow a single high-dose exposure (23).

Neurologic effects include convulsive movements, twitching, malaise, lethargy, headache, seizures, and dizziness (13,14,24). Serious exposure may result in coma (24). *Other effects* include nausea, vomiting, and diarrhea (11,13,14). Severe cases of ethylene oxide exposure may result in renal damage (22).

In the case of *skin exposure*, pure anhydrous ethylene oxide does not injure dry skin, but solutions have a vesicant action (21). Exposure to the liquid or gas may cause irritation or burns to moist skin (22). Ethylene oxide may also cause contact dermatitis, allergic contact dermatitis, thermal burns, frostbite, edema, erythema, vesiculation, blebs, and desquamation (5,14,21). Skin effects may be delayed for several hours.

Chronic Exposure

Chronic exposure to ethylene oxide can result in headache, numbness of the extremities, muscular weakness, impaired gait, skin sensitization, numbing of the sense of smell and taste, staggering, increased fatigability, and an increased susceptibility for respiratory infection; these symptoms usually clear within months of terminating exposure. Long-term exposure has also been linked to increased rates of leukemia (3,5,14,16,19). Ethylene oxide has been implicated as a causal agent for the formation of cataracts (5).

Factory workers with chronic ethylene oxide poisoning have developed symptoms of multiple neuropathy. The neuropathy is described as a sensory disturbance of the legs and feet, a diminished sense of vibration in the feet, and irregular gait, spreading gradually to other parts of the body. These signs cleared when the workers were removed from exposure (3,19).

Teratogenesis and Carcinogenesis

Ethylene oxide is mutagenic, teratogenic, and carcinogenic. It is classified as Group 1 (carcinogenic to humans) by the International Agency for Research on Cancer based on limited evidence in humans and sufficient evidence in animals (25). Occupational exposure to ethylene oxide has been linked with leukemia; stomach, brain, and pancreatic cancer; lymphatic cancer; hematopoietic cancer; non-Hodgkin's lymphoma; and Hodgkin's disease (3,6,14,25). The evidence for carcinogenicity and genotoxicity has been extensively reviewed (26).

A retrospective mortality study of 18,254 U.S. workers exposed to ethylene oxide at 14 plants demonstrated a trend toward an increased risk of death from hematopoietic cancer, with increasing lengths of time since the first exposure to ethylene oxide (27). There was no significant increase in mortality in the cancer of stomach, leukemia, pancreas, and brain. Although there was an increase in non-Hodgkin's lymphoma among men, there was no dose-response relationship, no specific job category association, and no increase in non-Hodgkin's lymphoma among women. The authors concluded that the increase was not due to ethylene oxide (28).

TABLE 2. Monitoring examination for ethylene oxide

Organ or system	Suspicious symptoms
Skin	Rashes, cracking, burns, blisters
Eyes	Swelling or irritation
Respiratory system	Breathing difficulty, nose or throat irritation, prolonged or dry cough, chest pains, wheezing
Neurologic system	Drowsiness, numbness or tingling of hands or feet, weakness or lack of coordination, headaches
Reproductive system	Spontaneous abortions, birth defects

DIAGNOSTIC TESTS

Biologic Monitoring and Health Surveillance

Determination of the level of 2-hydroxyethyl adducts to the *N*-terminal valines in hemoglobin can serve as a suitable biomonitor (1,29). Alveolar breath concentrations should not exceed 0.5 mg/m^3 for individuals exposed to the threshold limit value of 1 ppm (30). Employers should obtain preemployment baseline evaluation of the eyes, skin, blood, and respiratory tract. Periodic examinations thereafter should include several organs and systems (Table 2) (31).

Acute Exposure

Blood levels of ethylene are not available. Evaluation of ataxia or seizures may include basic blood chemistries as well as computed tomography of the brain. Pulmonary effects are evaluated with arterial blood gases and pulse oximetry; chest radiograph may be useful in patients with respiratory manifestations. Evaluation for peripheral neuropathy may include serial physical examinations as well as electromyogram and nerve conduction velocity.

Chronic Exposure

Testing for chronic effects typically involves the peripheral nervous system, cataracts, and reproductive tests. A neurobehavioral evaluation may also be needed depending on the patient's manifestations.

TREATMENT

Establish and maintain vital functions. Rescuers should use self-contained breathing apparatus and personal protective skin covering. After removal from the contaminated environment, remove clothing, wash exposed areas, and irrigate eyes. Administer warm humidified oxygen and bronchodilators, if needed. Treat cardiac dysrhythmias and control convulsions with standard treatments. Monitor for several hours after exposure. Significant exposure usually causes effects that indicate hospital admission.

If liquid is spilled on the skin, allow ethylene oxide to vaporize before washing with water. Dermal exposure should be washed with copious amounts of free-flowing water. Ethylene oxide burns are treated as a chemical burn and may take weeks to heal.

If irritation, pain, swelling, lacrimation, or photophobia persists, the patient should be seen in a health care facility. There is no specific antidote for ethylene oxide.

REFERENCES

1. NIOSH. Current intelligence bulletin 35: ethylene oxide, DHHS (NIOSH) Pub. no. 81-130, 1981.
2. Estrin WJ, Bowler RM, Lash A, et al. Neurotoxicological evaluation of hospital sterilizer workers exposed to ethylene oxide. *J Toxicol Clin Toxicol* 1990;28:1–20.
3. ACGIH. *Documentation of the threshold limit values and biological exposure indices*, 6th ed. Cincinnati: American Conference of Governmental Industrial Hygienists, Inc., 1991:617–626.
4. Budavari S, ed. *The Merck index*, 12th ed. Whitehouse Station, NJ: Merck & Co, Inc., 1996:647.
5. Bingham E, Cohrssen B, Powell CH, eds. *Patty's toxicology*, Vol. 6, 5th ed. New York: John Wiley & Sons, 2001:320.
6. Stellman JM, ed. *International Labour Office: encyclopaedia of occupational health and safety*, Vol. 1–4, 4th ed. Geneva, Switzerland: International Labour Office, 1998:280.
7. NIOSH. Guidelines for protecting the safety and health of health care workers. Washington, D.C.: U.S. Department of Health and Human Services, NIOSH, 1988.
8. Reference deleted.
9. CHRIS. CHRIS hazardous chemical data. U.S. Department of Transportation, U.S. Coast Guard, Washington, DC. (CD-ROM version). Denver: Micromedex, Inc., 1990.
10. Vermylen J, Janssens S, Ceuppens J, Vermylen C. Transfusion reactions in haemophiliac caused by sensitization to ethylene oxide. *Lancet* 1988;1:594.
11. Clayton GD, Clayton FE, eds. *Patty's industrial hygiene and toxicology*, Vol. 2A. *Toxicology*, 4th ed. New York: John Wiley & Sons, 1993:338–348.
12. Crystal HA, Schaumburg HH, Grober E, et al. Cognitive impairment and sensory loss associated with chronic low-level ethylene oxide exposure. *Neurology* 1988;38:567–569.
13. Sittig M. *Handbook of toxic and hazardous chemicals and carcinogens*, 3rd ed. Park Ridge, NJ: Noyes Publications, 1991:270.
14. Hayes WJ Jr, Laws ER Jr, eds. *Handbook of pesticide toxicology*, Vol. 2. San Diego: Academic Press, Inc., 1991:663–668.
15. Baselt RC. *Disposition of toxic drugs and chemicals in man*, 5th ed. Foster City, CA: Chemical Toxicology Institute, 2000:180.
16. Zenz C. *Occupational medicine*, 3rd ed. St. Louis: Mosby–Year Book, Inc., 1994:300.
17. Sheikh K. Adverse health effects of ethylene oxide and occupational exposure limits. *Am J Ind Med* 1984;6:117–127.
18. RTECS. Registry of Toxic Effects of Chemical Substances. National Institute for Occupational Safety and Health, Cincinnati, OH (Internet version). Greenwood Village, CO: Micromedex, Inc., 2001.
19. Hathaway GJ, Proctor NH, Hughes JP, et al. *Chemical hazards of the workplace*, 4th ed. New York: Van Nostrand Reinhold Company, 1996:260.
20. Schardein JL. *Chemically induced birth defects*, 2nd ed. New York: Marcel Dekker, Inc., 1993:280.
21. Fisher AA. Ethylene oxide dermatitis. *Cutis* 1984;34:20–24.
22. Lewis RJ. *Hawley's condensed chemical dictionary*, 13th ed. New York: John Wiley & Sons, Inc., 1997:190.
23. Goldfrank LR. *Goldfrank's toxicological emergencies*, 6th ed. New York: McGraw-Hill, 1998:310.
24. Grant WM. *Toxicology of the eye*, 4th ed. Springfield, IL: Charles C. Thomas, 1993:270.
25. IARC. Monographs on the evaluation of carcinogenicity of chemicals to humans. Ethylene oxide [75-21-8]. Geneva: World Health Organization, International Agency for Research on Cancer, 1994.
26. Thier R, Bolt HM. Carcinogenicity and genotoxicity of ethylene oxide: new aspects and recent advances. *Crit Rev Toxicol* 2000;30:595–608.
27. Steenland K, Stayner L, Greife A, et al. Mortality among workers exposed to ethylene oxide. *N Engl J Med* 1991;324:1402–1407.
28. Wong O, Trent LS. An epidemiological study of workers potentially exposed to ethylene oxide. *Br J Ind Med* 1993;50:308–316.
29. Fost U, Hallier E, Ottenwalder H, et al. Distribution of ethylene oxide in human blood and its implications for biomonitoring. *Hum Exp Toxicol* 1991;10:25–31.
30. Baselt RC. *Biological monitoring methods for industrial chemicals*, 3rd ed. Littleton, MA: PSG Publishing Company, 1997:230.
31. Ellenhorn MJ. Antiseptics and disinfectants. In: Ellenhorn MJ, Schonwald S, Ordog G, et al., eds. *Textbook of medical toxicology*, 2nd ed. Baltimore: Williams & Wilkins, 1997:1214.

CHAPTER 195

Formaldehyde and Glutaraldehyde

Thomas R. Caraccio and Michael A. McGuigan

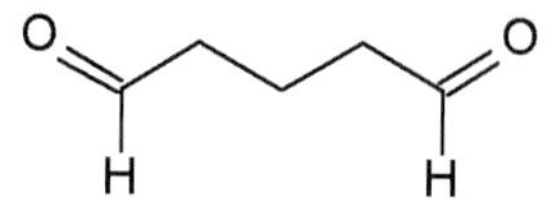

GLUTARALDEHYDE 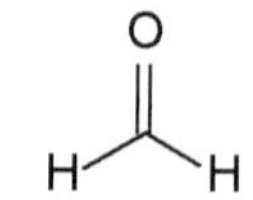 / FORMALDEHYDE

Synonyms:	**Formaldehyde (methyl aldehyde, methylene oxide); glutaraldehyde (1,3-diformylpropane, glutaric dialdehyde, pentanedial)**
Molecular formula and weight:	**Formaldehyde (HCHO), 30.03; glutaraldehyde ($C_5H_8O_2$) 100.1 g/mol**
SI conversion:	**Formaldehyde, ppm × 1.24 = mg/m^3; glutaraldehyde, ppm × 4.09 = mg/m^3**
CAS Registry No.:	**50-00-0 (formaldehyde); 111-30-8 (glutaraldehyde)**
Normal levels:	**Not applicable**
Target organs:	**Mucous membranes, lung, gastrointestinal tract (acute); skin [immune system (chronic formaldehyde)]**
Antidotes:	**Ethanol or fomepizole, if methanol level warrants**

OVERVIEW

Formaldehyde is a colorless, flammable gas with a pungent, irritating odor (1). It is produced endogenously in the body and is present in many foods (2). It is used in chemical processes and in the production of particleboard, plywood, glues and adhesives, permanent-press or crease-resistant fabrics, tissue preservative, embalming fluid (formalin), carpets, cosmetics, disinfectants, and feedstock for synthetic chemical processes (Table 1). Formaldehyde is a contact irritant (3–6), forms formic acid when metabolized, and is a possible human carcinogen (1). At room temperature, formaldehyde is a colorless gas with a pungent, irritating odor detectable at approximately 0.5 ppm. Commercially available formalin is a clear, colorless, aqueous solution of formaldehyde (37% to 50%) and methanol (6% to 15%).

TABLE 1. Sources of formaldehyde and glutaraldehyde

Source	Formaldehyde	Glutaraldehyde
Consumer products	Particleboard Plastics Dyestuff Textiles Fertilizer Polyurethane foam (during heating)	Cooling towers and air conditioners Wart remover (5–10% solutions)
Occupational and industrial	Manufacture of urea formaldehyde foam Paint pigment Plastic molding Textiles Foundry and tanning industries Tissue fixative and embalming agent	Tanning industry Tissue fixative and embalming agent (25% solution)
Medical	Disinfectant Antiseptic	Disinfectant Instrument sterilization Radiographic solution

Formaldehyde is a major oxidation byproduct of combustion processes, including tobacco smoking. Formaldehyde exposure appears to be in the range of 1.50 to 1.95 parts per million (ppm)/puff. The cumulative daily dose from cigarette smoke is approximately 188 to 2400 μg (7). Urea formaldehyde foam insulation consists of polymers of urea and formaldehyde as well as other chemicals. Formaldehyde may be released during the initial reaction and through decomposition, depending on temperature, humidity, and acid content of the foam. The free formaldehyde level in homes with urea formaldehyde foam insulation is 0.049 ppm compared with 0.034 ppm in control homes, but the level decreases to control values over 1 to 3 years (8).

Glutaraldehyde is used as a tissue fixative, to sterilize medical instruments, as a cross-linking material in chemical reactions, in the tanning industry, in embalming fluid, as a pharmaceutical, and in x-ray solutions.

FORMALDEHYDE

Toxic Dose

Occupational standards and guidelines for formaldehyde are provided in Table 2. An adult death was associated with 30 ml of 37% formaldehyde (3); 60 to 90 ml of 100% formaldehyde is considered the usual potentially fatal amount (3,4).

After ingestion of an unknown amount of formalin, a 55-year-old woman and a 34-year-old man developed extensive gastrointestinal (GI) injury, shock, and metabolic acidosis from formic acid and lactic acid as well as respiratory and renal insufficiency (9). Both died weeks later from acute respiratory distress syndrome after multiple complications, including gastrectomy in the man.

TABLE 2. U.S. regulatory guidelines and standards for formaldehyde and glutaraldehyde

		Concentration [mg/m³ (ppm)]	
Agency	Description	Formaldehyde	Glutaraldehyde
OSHA	Vapor or gas		
	PEL-TWA	0.930 (0.750)	—
	STEL	2.500 (2.000)	—
ACGIH	Vapor or gas		
	TLV-Ceiling	0.370 (0.300)	0.20 (0.05)
NIOSH	Vapor or gas		
	REL-TWA	0.020 (0.016)	0.80 (0.20)
	Ceiling (15 min)	0.124 (0.100)	—
	IDLH	24.800 (20.000)	None

ACGIH, American Conference of Governmental Industrial Hygienists; IDLH, immediate danger to life or health; NIOSH, National Institute for Occupational Safety and Health; OSHA, U.S. Occupational Safety and Health Administration; PEL, permissible exposure limit; ppm, parts per million; REL, recommended exposure limit; STEL, short-term exposure limit; TLV, threshold limit value; TWA, time-weighted average.

TABLE 3. Progression of symptoms caused by airborne formaldehyde

Formaldehyde air level (ppm)	Health effect
0.1–0.3	Lowest level causing mucous membrane irritation
0.8	Odor threshold
1–2	Irritation threshold; mild irritation of mucous membranes
2–3	Irritation of eyes, nose, and throat
4–5	Increasing irritation of mucous membranes; lacrimation becomes prominent
10–20	Profuse tearing, severe burning sensation, cough; can be tolerated for only a few minutes
50–100	Causes serious injury in 5–10 min

ppm, parts per million.

Ingestion of 120 ml of an unspecified formaldehyde "concentrated" solution and of 120 ml of a 10% solution resulted in extensive stomach tissue injury (10,11). Dermal exposure to solutions of 2% to 10% may result in blisters, fissures, and urticaria (12).

Toxicokinetics and Toxicodynamics

Formaldehyde is rapidly absorbed. Delayed absorption of methanol might occur after ingestion of formalin if the formaldehyde causes fixation of the stomach lining (3). Formaldehyde is metabolized to formic acid primarily by hepatic aldehyde dehydrogenase and to a lesser extent in erythrocytes, brain, kidney, and muscle. The conversion of formaldehyde to formic acid has a half-life of 1.5 minutes. Formic acid either is excreted in the urine or is metabolized to carbon dioxide and water via a folate-dependent enzymatic pathway (3). The half-life of formate is 80 to 90 minutes but depends on urine pH and folic acid stores.

Pathophysiology

Formaldehyde causes precipitation of proteins and coagulation necrosis of exposed tissue. The gas is highly water soluble, and inhalation produces immediate local irritation of the upper respiratory tract and has been reported to cause spasm and edema of the larynx. Formic acid may accumulate and produce a metabolic acidosis.

Vulnerable Populations

Formaldehyde has not been shown to be teratogenic in animals and probably presents little or no risk as a human teratogen (13). Menstrual disorders, birthweight abnormalities, and spontaneous abortions have been reported in women occupationally exposed to formaldehyde, but these results are controversial (14).

Clinical Presentation

ACUTE EXPOSURE

Acute airborne exposure to formaldehyde causes predictable effects (Table 3). Acute ingestion can cause metabolic acidosis and shock. Tachypnea may develop in patients with metabolic acidosis (15). Hypothermia may develop (16).

The eyes, nose, and throat are often irritated by formaldehyde or fumes from urea formaldehyde foam and adhesive resins (17). After a splash exposure to the eye, toxic effects range from transient discomfort and irritation to corneal opacification and loss of vision (18,19).

Cardiovascular effects include hypotension and cardiovascular collapse after a large ingestion (3). Pulmonary inhalation produces effects ranging from upper respiratory tract irritation and coughing to bronchitis, pulmonary edema, or pneumonia, depending on concentration and duration (9,20). Reactive airways may develop in susceptible individuals (9). Respiratory distress and acute respiratory distress syndrome have occurred after ingestion or transdermal absorption of formaldehyde-containing compounds (21). Neurologic effects, including lethargy and coma, may occur after large ingestions or marked inhalation exposure (15).

GI effects include nausea, vomiting, and severe abdominal pain after ingestion. Corrosive gastritis, hematemesis, edema, and ulceration of the esophagus may occur and result in complications of perforation or stricture (22). Hepatotoxicity has been associated with inhalation exposure in animals and suggested in humans (23). Hyperbilirubinemia has been reported after ingestion (9).

Renal toxicity leading to nephritis and acute renal failure may occur (9). An anion gap metabolic acidosis can occur after ingestion of formaldehyde (24). The hematologic effect of intravascular hemolysis has occurred in hemodialysis patients receiving doses of formaldehyde during treatment (25). Skin sensitization after a single large exposure has resulted in contact dermatitis (26).

CHRONIC EXPOSURE

Dermatologic effects include occupational dermatitis after use of urea formaldehyde resin (27) and para-tertiary-butylphenol-formaldehyde resin (28). Hardening and roughness due to superficial coagulation of the keratin layer may occur after contact with aqueous solutions (29).

Immunologic effects include antibody formation to formaldehyde. Reactions ranging from irritation to severe hypersensitivity have occurred (30). Type IV reactions may result in allergic contact dermatitis. Immunologic reactions may be delayed by hours to months (31). Asthma-like signs and symptoms have been reported (32). Evidence of formaldehyde sensitization or allergy causing true asthma is inconclusive. Respiratory effects do not consistently correlate with the development of formaldehyde-specific immunoglobulins. (33). Membranous nephropathy has been associated with immunologic reaction to suspected formaldehyde exposure in four patients living in newly built homes (31).

CARCINOGENESIS

Formaldehyde is a probable human nasopharyngeal carcinogen based on limited evidence in humans and sufficient evidence in animals (International Agency for Research on Cancer 2A) (34,35). Occupational exposure to formaldehyde is associated with buccal and nasopharyngeal metaplasia/neoplasia and, to a lesser extent, cancers of the nasal cavities (35–37). Formaldehyde reacts with hydrogen chloride to form bis (chloromethyl) ether, a known human carcinogen. Formaldehyde's role in lower respiratory tract cancer etiology has not been substantiated.

A retrospective cohort mortality study of 11,030 permanent-press garment factory workers exposed to a time-weighted average of 0.15 ppm of formaldehyde for at least 3 months in 1981 and 1986 showed a statistically significant excess in mortality from cancer of the buccal cavity and connective tissue (36). Mortality from cancers of the buccal cavity, leukemia, and other lymphopoietic neoplasms increased with duration of formaldehyde exposure and was also highest among workers first exposed during a time period of high potential formaldehyde exposures in this industry (1955 to 1962).

Diagnostic Tests

BIOLOGIC MONITORING AND HEALTH SURVEILLANCE

A sampling method consisting of drawing air through a solid solvent tube containing silica gel impregnated with 20% sodium bisulfite (38) may be useful in monitoring exposures. Urinary formic acid levels were shown to be subject to 30-fold inter- and intraindividual variation and did not correlate with known exposures to formaldehyde. Formic acid is not a suitable biomarker for formaldehyde exposure (39).

ACUTE EXPOSURE

Monitor acid-base status, complete blood cell count, serum electrolytes, and renal function tests in symptomatic patients. If respiratory irritation or depression is evident, consider pulse oximetry, arterial blood gases, chest radiograph, and pulmonary function tests.

The hematocrit and hemoglobin concentration should be monitored in dialysis patients repeatedly exposed parenterally to formaldehyde. Blood methanol levels should be monitored after significant formalin ingestion. Formaldehyde plasma levels are not widely available but may be useful for confirmation of exposure and monitoring in environmental settings. Formic acid levels are available from specialty laboratories.

Pulmonary function testing and nasal and bronchial provocation tests may be useful in patients with reactive airways dysfunction after inhalation of formaldehyde.

Treatment

Treatment may be needed for formaldehyde alone or for methanol as well after ingestion of formalin (Chapter 191).

DECONTAMINATION AND FIRST AID

Rescuers should wear self-contained breathing apparatus and appropriate chemical protective clothing if handling a heavily contaminated patient. The patient should be removed from the area of exposure. Exposed areas should be washed with soap and water after removing contaminated clothing.

INGESTION

Milk or water in small amounts should be administered immediately. Emesis should not be induced because of risk of corrosive injury. The role of gastric aspiration within 1 hour of ingestion is controversial. Activated charcoal adsorbs formalin but obscures endoscopic findings. Consider endoscopy to assess esophageal and gastric damage in patients with GI signs or if a concentrated formalin solution has been ingested.

Sodium bicarbonate is administered intravenously (IV) to treat acidemia. Administer folic acid or leucovorin, 1 mg/kg/dose (up to 50 mg), every 4 hours IV in acute formaldehyde ingestions if methanol levels are within a toxic range. Treat bronchospasm with an inhaled β_2-receptor agonist bronchodilator.

EYE EXPOSURE

Irrigate exposed eyes with copious tepid water or saline; perform fluorescein examination to rule out corneal injury if pain and lacrimation are present.

ENHANCEMENT OF ELIMINATION

There are no data supporting the use of multiple-dose activated charcoal. Hemodialysis is effective in removing methanol and formate and in correcting severe metabolic acidosis. Indications for hemodialysis include severe acidosis or a methanol level above 50 mg/dl. Neither hemoperfusion nor peritoneal dialysis is useful for treating formaldehyde poisoning.

ANTIDOTES

Treatment of concurrent methanol poisoning with fomepizole or ethyl alcohol may be indicated if the methanol level exceeds 20 mg/dl.

GLUTARALDEHYDE

Glutaraldehyde is a biocide commonly used in a 2% concentration for cold sterilization (disinfection) of surgical and dental equipment and for several other uses (Table 1). Dilute solutions may cause GI irritation. Concentrated solutions may cause abdominal pain, vomiting, diarrhea, shock, and central nervous system depression. Topical application is irritating to the skin and mucous membranes. Prolonged contact may cause skin ulceration.

Insufficient rinsing of a 2% glutaraldehyde solution from flexible sigmoidoscopes appeared to be responsible for an outbreak of fever and GI toxicity (abdominal cramps, bloody diarrhea, nausea, and vomiting) in patients undergoing sigmoidoscopy (40).

Glutaraldehyde is an aliphatic dialdehyde (41). At room temperature, it is a colorless liquid with a pungent odor. It is miscible in water and organic solvents. Glutaraldehyde is available in 99%, 50%, 25%, 10%, and 2% solutions or in a 50% biologic solution (42). It is commonly available in 2% solutions buffered with sodium bicarbonate to a pH of 7.5 to 8.5 (43).

Toxic Dose

Occupational standards and guidelines for glutaraldehyde are provided in Table 2. Complete immersion in the solution for 10 to 20 minutes is sufficient for rapid disinfection of thoroughly cleaned instruments, but 10 hours may be necessary for sterilization (44). A 5% or 10% solution or a 10% gel has been used for the treatment of warts but should not be used for facial or anogenital warts (45). It also has been used topically for treating hyperhidrosis of the palms and soles (46).

The probable oral lethal dose of glutaraldehyde for humans ranges from 50 mg/kg to 5 g/kg (47). The odor threshold concentration is 0.04 ppm. Eye and respiratory irritation are noted at a level of 0.3 ppm (48). In a rodent study, the clinical effects, time course, and postmortem findings were similar to formaldehyde (49). In another study, a 2% glutaraldehyde solution and an 8% formaldehyde solution applied to the skin of rabbits were associated with no systemic effects. The glutaraldehyde solution produced some yellow and brown skin staining. When equally bactericidal solutions of glutaraldehyde and formaldehyde solutions were allowed to evaporate in a closed system, the glutaraldehyde produced no symptoms in 4 hours, whereas the formaldehyde produced respiratory tract irritation and pulmonary damage. When the concentrations of both compounds were increased, the clinical effects became equally severe.

Toxicokinetics and Toxicodynamics

Glutaraldehyde is readily absorbed by oral, IV, and inhalation routes. It is absorbed dermally to a lesser extent. Glutaraldehyde is either metabolized by aldehyde dehydrogenase to yield an acid or inactivated by a reaction with sulfhydryl groups using glutathione. Conditions that deplete glutathione or inhibit aldehyde dehydrogenase (e.g., disulfiram treatment) may result in more serious toxicity. In rats, glutaraldehyde is eliminated in the urine and expired gases (50).

Pathophysiology

The irritant potency of a glutaraldehyde solution depends on its concentration: 2% solutions are weak irritants, whereas 20% solutions may be caustic. Its biocidal effects result from interactions with elements of the bacterial cell wall, causing partial sealing and contraction of the outer cell envelope. Glutaraldehyde polymerizes at a pH greater than 9 (49).

Vulnerable Populations

There are no human data on the effects of glutaraldehyde in pregnancy or lactation. A high dose of glutaraldehyde (5 ml/kg of a 2% acidic solution) administered during organogenesis increased malformations in pregnant mice. At this dose, significant maternal and fetal toxicity were seen. Because of clustering of the malformations within one litter, it was concluded that glutaraldehyde was not teratogenic (51).

Clinical Presentation

ACUTE EXPOSURE

Glutaraldehyde vapor or mist can be a strong irritant or corrosive to the eyes, nose, throat, and lungs (52). Inhalation of glutaraldehyde vapor may cause sudden headache (53). Ingestion may cause a burning sensation in the chest, severe abdominal pain and cramping, vomiting, diarrhea, anuria, vascular collapse, and coma (54). Glutaraldehyde penetrates the skin of experimental animals poorly and penetrates human skin to a lesser extent (55).

The no effect level for ocular irritation in rabbits was 0.1% (55). Direct contact with a concentrated solution may cause permanent corneal opacity. Failure to rinse glutaraldehyde from colonoscopic equipment resulted in proctocolitis in humans (44,56).

CHRONIC EXPOSURE

Glutaraldehyde is a potent skin sensitizer (57) and can cause dermatoses (58) and allergic contact dermatitis (59). Seven percent of funeral workers exposed to glutaraldehyde were found to have allergic contact hypersensitivity as determined by patch testing (60). Glutaraldehyde may induce an occupational asthma (61). Daily application of a 20% solution of glutaraldehyde for treatment of plantar warts was implicated in necrosis of the pad of a toe in a 7-year-old child; necrosis was evidently due to the caustic, rather than the allergenic, activity of glutaraldehyde (62). In long-term experimental studies, glutaraldehyde caused liver damage in mice (53).

Diagnostic Tests

Monitor acid-base status, complete blood cell count, serum electrolytes, liver tests, and renal function tests in symptomatic patients. If respiratory tract irritation or respiratory depression is evident, consider monitoring pulse oximetry, arterial blood gases, chest radiograph, and pulmonary function tests.

High-performance liquid chromatography has been used for the determination of glutaraldehyde in samples (63), but such testing may not have clinical relevance.

Treatment

The treatments of glutaraldehyde and formaldehyde are similar. Glutaraldehyde appears to be slightly less toxic than formaldehyde except for IV or ocular exposures. Because of its lower vapor pressure, pulmonary effects are less likely with glutaraldehyde. Treatment should be aimed at recognition and management of GI hemorrhage, ulceration, and perforation and any systemic effects, such as central nervous system depression and hypotension. If no respiratory compromise is present, dilute immediately with water.

DECONTAMINATION

Emesis is contraindicated because of the potential for caustic injury or central nervous system depression. Activated charcoal is not recommended because of the risk of producing emesis and obscuring endoscopy findings. The use of whole bowel irrigation is not recommended.

ENHANCEMENT OF ELIMINATION

There are no data available to indicate that extracorporeal techniques enhance elimination of glutaraldehyde.

ANTIDOTES

There are no antidotes to glutaraldehyde.

REFERENCES

Formaldehyde

1. Council on Scientific Affairs. Formaldehyde. *JAMA* 1989;2261:1183–1187.
2. Clary JJ, Sullivan JB. *Formaldehyde hazardous material toxicology*. Sullivan JB, Kreiger GR, eds. Baltimore: Williams & Wilkins, 1992:974–980.
3. Burkhart KK, Kulig KK, McMartin KE. Formate levels following a formalin ingestion. *Vet Hum Toxicol* 1990;32:135–137.
4. Frigas E. Bronchial challenge with formaldehyde gas: lack of bronchoconstriction in 13 patients suspected of having formaldehyde-induced asthma. *Mayo Clin Proc* 1984;59:295–299.
5. Richie IM, Lehnen RG. Formaldehyde-related health complaints of residents living in mobile and conventional homes. *Am J Public Health* 1987;77:323–328.
6. Harris JC, Rumack BH, Aldrich FD. Toxicology of urea formaldehyde and polyurethane foam insulation. *JAMA* 1981;245:243.
7. Godish T. Formaldehyde exposure from tobacco smoke: a review. *Am J Pub Health* 1989;79:1044–1045.
8. Report of the National Testing Survey on urea formaldehyde foam insulation. Ottawa: Department of Consumer and Corporate Affairs, 1981.
9. Koppel C, Baudisch H, Schneider V, et al. Suicidal ingestion of formalin with fatal complications. *Intensive Care Med* 1990;16:212–214.
10. Bartone NF, Grieco RV, Herr BS. Corrosive gastritis due to ingestion of formaldehyde without esophageal impairment. *JAMA* 1968;203:50–51.
11. Kline BS. Formaldehyde poisoning with report of a fatal case. *Arch Intern Med* 1925;36:220–228.

12. Casteel SW, Vernon RJ, Bailey EM. Formaldehyde: toxicology and hazards. *Vet Hum Toxicol* 1987;29:31–33.
13. AMA Council on Scientific Affairs. *Effects of toxic chemicals on the reproductive system*. Chicago: American Medical Association, 1985:190.
14. Schardein JL. *Chemically induced birth defects*, 2nd ed. New York: Marcel Dekker, Inc., 1993:240.
15. Allen RE, Thoshinsky MJ, Stallone RJ, et al. Corrosive injuries of the stomach. *Arch Surg* 1970;100:409–413.
16. HSDB. *Hazardous substances data bank*. Bethesda, MD: National Library of Medicine (CD-ROM version). Englewood, CO: Micromedex, Inc., 1999.
17. Weber R, Budmiger H, Siegenthaler W. Die chronische formaldehydimmission—ein verkantes Krankheitsbild. *Schweiz Med Wschr* 1988;118:457–461.
18. EPA. *EPA chemical profile on formaldehyde*. Washington, DC: Environmental Protection Agency, 1985.
19. Grant WM, Schuman JS. *Toxicology of the eye*, 4th ed. Springfield IL: Charles C Thomas, 1993:210.
20. Malaka T, Kodama AM. Respiratory health of plywood workers occupationally exposed to formaldehyde. *Arch Environ Health* 1990;45:288–294.
21. Cohen N, Modai D, Khahil A, et al. Acute resin phenol-formaldehyde intoxication. A life threatening occupational hazard. *Hum Toxicol* 1989;8:247–250.
22. Hawley CK, Harsch HH. Gastric outlet obstruction as a late complication of formaldehyde ingestion: a case report. *Am J Gastroenterol* 1999;94:2289–2291.
23. Beall JR, Ulsamer AG. Formaldehyde and hepatotoxicity: a review. *J Toxicol Environ Health* 1984;14:1–21.
24. Eells JT, McMartin KE, Black K, et al. Formaldehyde poisoning. Rapid metabolism to formic acid. *JAMA* 1981;246:1237–1238.
25. Sauder LR, Green DJ, Chatham MD, et al. Acute pulmonary response of asthmatics to 3.0 ppm formaldehyde. *Toxicol Ind Health* 1987;3:569–578.
26. Kanerva L, Tarvainen K, Pinola A, et al. A single accidental exposure may result in a chemical burn, primary sensitization and allergic contact dermatitis. *Contact Dermatitis* 1994;31:229–235.
27. Vale PT, Ryckroft RJ. Occupational contact dermatitis from fibreboard containing urea-formaldehyde resin. *Contact Dermatitis* 1988;19:62.
28. Fisher AA. Para-tertiary-butylphenol formaldehyde resin. Part I: leather watch straps and shoes. *Cutis* 1987;39:183–184.
29. Morgan DP. *Recognition and management of pesticide poisonings*, 4th ed. Environmental Protection Agency, EPA-540/9-88-0015. Washington, DC: Government Printing Office, 1989:220.
30. Thrasher JD, Madison R, Broughton A, et al. Building-related illness and antibodies to albumin conjugates of formaldehyde, toluene diisocyanate and trimellitic anhydride. *Am J Ind Med* 1989;15:187–195.
31. Breysse P, Couser WG, Alpers CE, et al. Membranous nephropathy and formaldehyde exposure. *Ann Intern Med* 1994;120:396–397.
32. Burge PS, Harries MG, Lam WK, et al. Occupational asthma due to formaldehyde. *Thorax* 1985;40:255–260.
33. Wantke F, Demmer CM, Tappler P, et al. Exposure to gaseous formaldehyde induces IgE-mediated sensitization to formaldehyde in school-children. *Clin Exp Allergy* 1996;26:276–280.
34. Roush GC, Walrath J, Stayner LT, et al. Nasopharyngeal cancer, sinonasal cancer, and occupations related to formaldehyde: a case-control study. *J Natl Cancer Inst* 1987;79:1221–1224.
35. EPA. *Formaldehyde health risk assessment fact sheet*. Washington, DC: Environmental Protection Agency, 1987.
36. Stayner LT, Elliott L, Black L, et al. A retrospective cohort mortality study of workers exposed to formaldehyde in the garment industry. *Am J Ind Med* 1988;13:667–681.
37. Sterling TD, Weinkam JJ. Reanalysis of lung cancer mortality in a National Cancer Institute Study on mortality among industrial workers exposed to formaldehyde. *J Occup Med* 1988;30:895–901.
38. Gaertner RRW. Solid sorbent media for collection of formaldehyde in air. *Appl Ind Hyg* 1988;3:258–262.
39. Schmid K, Schaller KH, Angerer J, et al. [Investigations on the importance of the formic acid excretion in urine from an environmental and occupational medical point of view] (German). *Zbl Hyg Umweltmed* 1994;196:139–152.

Glutaraldehyde

40. Durante L, Zulty J, Israel E, et al. Investigation of an outbreak of bloody diarrhea: association with endoscopic cleaning solution and demonstration of lesions in an animal model. *Am J Med* 1992;92:476–480.
41. Budavari S, ed. *The Merck index*, 12th ed. Whitehouse Station, NJ: Merck & Co, Inc., 1996:761.
42. Sweetman S. Glutaraldehyde monograph. In: *Martindale: the complete drug reference*. London: Pharmaceutical Press (electronic version). Greenwood Village, CO: MICROMEDEX, 2002.
43. Harbison RD. Glutaraldehyde. In: Harbison RD, ed. *Hamilton & Hardy's industrial toxicology*, 5th ed. St. Louis: Mosby, 1998:350.
44. Ryan CK, Potter GD. Disinfectant colitis: rinse as well as you wash. *J Clin Gastroenterol* 1995;21:6–9.
45. Warts Sterling JC. Guidelines for the management of cutaneous warts. *Br J Dermatol* 2001;144:4–11.
46. Collin J, Whatling P. Treating hyperhidrosis. *BMJ* 2000;320:1221–1222.
47. HSDB. *Hazardous substances data bank*. National Library of Medicine (Internet version). Greenwood Village, CO: MICROMEDEX, 2001.
48. Symptoms of irritation associated with exposure to glutaraldehyde—Colorado. *MMWR Morb Mortal Wkly Rep* 1987;36:190–191.
49. Stonehill AA, Krop S, Borick PM. Buffered glutaraldehyde—a new chemical sterilization solution. *Am J Hosp Pharm* 1963;20:458–465.
50. Ranly DM, Horn D, Hubbard GB. Assessment of the systemic distribution and toxicity of glutaraldehyde as a pulpotomy agent. *Pediatr Dent* 1989;11:8–13.
51. Marks TA, Worthy WC, Staples RE. Influence of formaldehyde and Sonacide (potentiated acid glutaraldehyde) on embryo and fetal development in mice. *Teratology* 1980;22:51–58.
52. Pryor P. NIOSH report no. HETA-83-074-1525, 1984:16.
53. ACGIH. *Documentation of the threshold limit values and biological exposure indices*, 6th ed. Cincinnati: American Conference of Governmental Industrial Hygienists, Inc., 1992:703–704.
54. HSDB. Hazardous substances data bank. National Library of Medicine. Greenwood Village, CO: MICROMEDEX, 2001.
55. Andersen FA. Final report on the safety assessment of glutaral. *J Am Coll Toxicol* 1996;15:98–139.
56. Dolce P, Gourdeau M, April N, et al. Outbreak of glutaraldehyde-induced proctocolitis. *Am J Infect Control* 1995;23:34–39.
57. Benson WG. Exposure to glutaraldehyde. *J Soc Occup Med* 1984;34:63–64.
58. Hansen RS. Glutaraldehyde occupational dermatitis. *Contact Dermatitis* 1983;9:81–82.
59. Jordan WP, Dahl MV, Albert HL. Contact dermatitis from glutaraldehyde. *Arch Dermatol* 1972;105:94–95.
60. Ballantyne B, Berman B. Dermal sensitizing potential of glutaraldehyde: a review and recent observations. *J Toxicol Cutan Ocular Toxicol* 1984;3:251–262.
61. Hathaway GJ, Proctor NH, Hughes JP, et al. *Chemical hazards of the workplace*, 3rd ed. New York: Van Nostrand Reinhold Company, 1991:312–313.
62. Prigent F, Iborra C, Meslay C. Glutaraldehyde-induced cutaneous necrosis after topical treatment of a wart. *Ann Dermatol Venereol* 1996;123:644–646.
63. Binding N, Witting U. Exposure to formaldehyde and glutaraldehyde in operating theatres. *Int Arch Occup Environ Health* 1990;62:233–238.

CHAPTER 196

Hexachlorophene

Thomas R. Caraccio and Michael A. McGuigan

HEXACHLOROPHENE

Synonyms:	**pHisoHex, Bilevon, Dermadex, Exofene, Gamophen, Surgi-Cen, Surofene, and many others**
Molecular formula and weight:	**$C_{13}H_{14}OH_2Cl_6$, 406.92 g/mol**
SI conversion:	**mg/L × 2.46 = μmol/L**
CAS Registry No.:	**70-30-4**
Normal levels:	**Not applicable**
Target organs:	**Gastrointestinal (acute), central nervous system (acute)**
Antidote:	**None**

OVERVIEW

Hexachlorophene (2,4,6-trichlorophenol) is a chlorinated derivative of phenol that is used in germicidal soaps, as a topical anti-infective, and in veterinary medicine (1). It has been used as a feed and water additive for the treatment of food-producing animals (2). Because of potential human neurotoxicity, the use of hexachlorophene and most preparations containing higher concentrations of hexachlorophene is limited to prescription (1,2).

Hexachlorophene has been available as a 3.00% or 0.75% milky white emulsion and as a powder (0.33% and 0.50%) and has been a component of bar soaps and other commercial products. Since 1974, U.S. Food and Drug Administration (FDA) regulations have limited hexachlorophene in cosmetics to less than 0.1%. In the United States, products containing more than 0.75% hexachlorophene require a prescription (3).

TOXIC DOSE

There are no occupational standards for hexachlorophene. Hexachlorophene should not be used routinely for bathing infants. Applications of concentrated (more than 3%) preparations to neonatal or damaged skin may result in significant toxicity or death. Acute ingestion of large amounts or repeated ingestion of small amounts may also cause toxicity or death.

The lethal dose in adults after acute ingestion or repeated skin application is not well defined but is estimated to be 43 mg/kg or 1 to 10 g (4). A woman accidentally ingested 200 ml of a detergent emulsion containing 3% hexachlorophene before abdominal surgery. The patient vomited and subsequently became febrile, lethargic, and confused and died. Her hexachlorophene blood level was 35 μg/ml (5). An adult became comatose after ingesting 20 mg/kg/day for 3 days (6).

An ingestion of 250 mg/kg by a 6-year-old child resulted in hypotension, convulsions, and death (7). Gastrointestinal disorders occur after ingestion of 10 to 20 mg/kg (8). A neonate who ingested 100 mg/kg developed lethargy, jitteriness, and exaggerated startle responses but no long-term sequelae (9).

TOXICOKINETICS AND TOXICODYNAMICS

Hexachlorophene is rapidly absorbed after ingestion. Skin absorption is also effective. The maximum serum concentration occurs 6 to 10 hours after application (10). Hexachlorophene has a high lipid-water partition coefficient and rapidly redistributes into lipoid tissues, including the central nervous system. Myelin preferentially binds hexachlorophene. Hexachlorophene is metabolized in the liver, although it apparently displays first-order (linear) kinetics (4). The half-life is 24 hours (range, 6 to 44 hours) (4,10). Hepatic dysfunction, low birth weight, and prematurity can increase the elimination half-life.

PATHOPHYSIOLOGY

The mechanism of toxicity is unclear. Neurologic symptoms in neonates after acute exposure probably result from cerebral edema (11). Pathologic lesions consist of spongiform changes confined to the myelinated white matter. Characteristic empty vacuoles formed by the splitting and separation of the myelin lamellae give this lesion the name *vacuolar encephalopathy*. The rostrocaudal distribution of the vacuolation appears age related, with the medullary portion of the reticular activating system involved primarily in premature infants and the mesencephalic portion involved primarily in full-term infants (12). Although children display vacuolation of diffuse areas of the cerebellum and cerebrum, autopsies of adult patients revealed no cerebral lesions (13).

PREGNANCY AND LACTATION

Hexachlorophene is FDA pregnancy category C (Appendix I) (15). It crosses the placenta in mice and accumulates in neural tissue (11). An epidemiologic study of occupationally exposed women found an increased incidence of congenital abnormalities (14). Hexachlorophene enters human breast milk (16).

CLINICAL PRESENTATION

Acute Exposure

The signs and symptoms of toxicity depend on the length and type of exposure as well as the age of the patient. Young patients are more susceptible. Gastrointestinal distress and an encephalopathy characterize hexachlorophene toxicity.

Acute ingestion produces nausea, vomiting, and diarrhea, which may progress to dehydration and hypotension within several hours of a toxic ingestion (8). Later, neurologic signs, including lethargy, facial twitching, fever, blurred vision, blindness, hyperreflexia, convulsions, and coma, appear and peak within 12 to 18 hours (6,8). Cardiac dysrhythmias, apnea, and cardiac arrest have occurred 48 to 60 hours postingestion (11).

Dermal exposure causes nausea, vomiting, irritability, diplopia, hypertonicity, anorexia, weakness, and fever. In severe cases, papilledema, retinal hemorrhages, convulsions, coma, and death occur. Small (less than 1200 g), premature (less than 35 weeks' gestation) infants and those with damaged skin or hepatorenal dysfunction are particularly susceptible to dermal toxicity after daily 3% hexachlorophene baths.

Chronic Exposure

The chronic dermal application of 3% hexachlorophene emulsion to neonates with severe skin defects (burns, severe ichthyosis) has been fatal (13,17). Infants exposed to 6.3% hexachlorophene-contaminated diaper talc developed an erythematous, ulcerative groin rash that corresponds to the skin lesion produced by high-dose hexachlorophene in rats (18).

DIAGNOSTIC TESTS

Follow fluid and electrolyte status as needed in symptomatic patients. Follow arterial blood gases and respiratory rate closely in severe poisonings. Severely poisoned patients should be monitored for several days in an intensive care setting to monitor for cardiac dysrhythmias, hypotension, and apnea.

The clinical value of hexachlorophene levels is uncertain because correlation between plasma levels and clinical effects is poor. Death has been reported with plasma hexachlorophene levels as low as 0.78 μg/ml in a child, but adults have remained asymptomatic with plasma levels of 2.16 μg/ml (19). Rat studies have reported effects on nerve myelin and lipid synthesis at plasma hexachlorophene levels of 0.5 μg/ml (20).

TREATMENT

Prudence suggests that patients who have ingested hexachlorophene at a dose exceeding 0.5 mg/kg (0.015 ml/kg of 3% hexachlorophene) should be referred to a health care facility for gastrointestinal decontamination and evaluation. Asymptomatic patients with limited dermal exposure can probably be managed without referral to a health care facility with skin decontamination. Seizures, respiratory depression, and hypotension are the immediate life-threatening problems. They are treated in the usual manner (Chapters 33, 37, and 40). Hypotension may respond to fluid and electrolyte replacement.

Gastrointestinal Decontamination

After ingestion, emesis is not recommended because of the potential for seizures. Although controversial, activated charcoal may be useful after a potentially toxic ingestion (21). The use of cathartics or whole bowel irrigation is not expected to be effective.

In the case of extensive skin exposure, initial soap and water washing can be followed by topical cleansing with a vehicle such as isopropanol, olive oil, or castor oil that can help dissolve hexachlorophene.

Enhancement of Elimination

No data are available regarding multiple-dose activated charcoal. Hemodialysis is probably not effective due to rapid distribution into body lipid stores. It is considered only if renal impairment is present. Hexachlorophene is not significantly cleared by peritoneal dialysis (4). Based on a rat study, urinary alkalinization may favorably alter hexachlorophene tissue distribution and enhance its renal excretion (22), but there are no human data that support this intervention.

Antidotes

There are no specific antidotes for hexachlorophene.

REFERENCES

1. Budavari S, ed. *The Merck index*, 11th ed. Rahway, NJ: Merck & Co, Inc., 1989:740.
2. Sax NI, Lewis RJ. *Dangerous properties of industrial materials*, 7th ed. New York: Van Nostrand Reinhold Company, 1989:1856–1857.
3. RTECS. *Registry of toxic effects of chemical substances.* National Institute for Occupational Safety and Health, Cincinnati, OH (CD-ROM version). Englewood, CO: Micromedex, Inc., 1997.
4. Boehm RM, Czajka PA. Hexachlorophene poisoning and the ineffectiveness of peritoneal dialysis. *J Toxicol Clin Toxicol* 1979;14:257–262.
5. Henry LD, DiMaio VJ. Hexachlorophene. *Mil Med* 1974;139:41.
6. Kimbrough RD. Review of recent evidence of toxic effects of hexachlorophene. *Pediatrics* 1973;51:391–394.
7. Lustig FW. A fatal case of hexachlorophene ("pHisoHex") poisoning. *Med J Aust* 1963;1:737.
8. Liu J, Wang CN, Yu JH, et al. Hexachlorophene in the treatment of clonorchiasis sinensis. *China Med J* 1963;82:702–711.
9. Herskowitz J, Rosman NP. Acute hexachlorophene poisoning by mouth in a neonate. *J Pediatr* 1979;94:495–496.
10. Tyrala EE, Hillman LS, Hillman RE, et al. Clinical pharmacology of hexachlorophene in newborn infants. *J Pediatr* 1977;91:481–486.
11. Martinez AJ, Boehm R, Hadfield MG. Acute hexachlorophene encephalopathy: clinico-neuropathological correlation. *Acta Neuropathol* 1974;28:93–103.
12. Shuman RM, Leech RW, Alvord ED. Neurotoxicity of hexachlorophene in the human. I. A clinicopathologic study of 248 children. *Pediatrics* 1974;54:689–695.
13. Mullick FG. Hexachlorophene toxicity—human experience at the Armed Forces Institute of Pathology. *Pediatrics* 1973;51:395–399.
14. Halling H. Suspected link between exposure to hexachlorophene and malformed infants. *Ann N Y Acad Sci* 1979;320:426–435.
15. Briggs GG, Freeman RK, Yaffe SJ. *Drugs in pregnancy and lactation*, 5th ed. Baltimore: Williams & Wilkins, 1998.
16. West RW. Hexachlorophene concentration in human milk. *Bull Environ Contam Toxicol* 1975;13:167–169.
17. Henry LD, DiMaio VJ. A fatal case of hexachlorophene poisoning. *Mil Med* 1974;139:41–43.
18. Martin-Bouyer G, Toga M, Lebreton R, et al. Outbreak of accidental hexachlorophene poisoning in France. *Lancet* 1982;1:91–95.
19. Lockhart JD. How toxic is hexachlorophene? *Pediatrics* 1972;50:229–235.
20. Pleasure D. The pathogenesis of hexachlorophene neuropathy: in vivo and in vitro studies. *Neurology* 1974;24:1068–1075.
21. Chyka PA, Seger D. Position statement: single-dose activated charcoal. American Academy of Clinical Toxicology; European Association of Poisons Centres and Clinical Toxicologists. *J Toxicol Clin Toxicol* 1997;35:721–736.
22. Flanagan RJ, Ruprah M, Strutt AV, et al. Effect of urinary alkalinisation and acidification on the tissue distribution of hexachlorophene in rats. *Hum Exp Toxicol* 1995;14:795–800.

CHAPTER 197

Hydrogen Peroxide

Thomas R. Caraccio and Michael A. McGuigan

H–O–O–H

HYDROGEN PEROXIDE

Molecular formula and weight:	**H_2O_2, 34.02 g/mol**
SI conversion:	**mg/dl × 2.9 = μmol/L**
CAS Registry No.:	**7722-84-1**
Therapeutic levels:	**Not applicable**
Target organs:	**Gastrointestinal, cardiac, brain (acute embolization)**
Antidote:	**None**

OVERVIEW

Hydrogen peroxide is an oxidizing agent that liberates oxygen on contact with water. Low concentrations of hydrogen peroxide (3%) are mildly irritating to mucous membranes; gastric injury is rare after unintentional ingestion (1,2). Higher concentrations of hydrogen peroxide (greater than 10% industrial strength or 35% "food grade" solutions) are strong oxidizers and are corrosive, causing burns to mucous membranes, gastrointestinal mucosa, skin, and eyes. Complications of ingestion include ruptured viscus, coma, seizures, and gas embolization, with subsequent shock and cardiac arrest (3–11). Ocular exposures may result in severe burns with corneal ulceration or perforation. Corneal injury can be delayed (12).

The effects of hydrogen peroxide mist or spray range from mild ocular and respiratory irritation to severe mucous membrane irritation and inflammation, pulmonary edema, and systemic poisoning with shock, coma, and seizures (13), depending on the concentration.

Rare reports of gas emboli have been described after surgical irrigation with 3% hydrogen peroxide due to the formation of microbubbles (6,9).

Hydrogen peroxide is a clear, colorless, odorless liquid with a bitter taste (14,15). Household-strength hydrogen peroxide is marketed as a low-concentration aqueous solution (3% to 6% by weight) (14). Hydrogen peroxide (Hydrogen Peroxide USP) is 3% (2.5% to 3.5% hydrogen peroxide by weight) (14). Common commercial strengths of hydrogen peroxide are more than 10% (15). Most industrial applications use hydrogen peroxide in concentrations of 35% to 70% by weight (16). "High-strength" hydrogen peroxide contains more than 52% peroxide (17).

TOXIC DOSE

Occupational guidelines and standards are provided in Table 1. Household-strength hydrogen peroxide (3% to 6%) is mildly irritating, and ingestions are usually inconsequential. Industrial strength (10% to 20%) may be toxic, and concentrations of 20% to 40% (pH, 5.0) have been fatal (3–7,24,28).

Death or permanent damage resulted when arterial gas embolization caused brain infarcts in three patients after exposures to 30 ml or less of 35% hydrogen peroxide: One patient was a 44-year-old man who initially complained of the inability to move his arms or legs and died 2 days after exposure without regaining consciousness; the second was an 84-year-old patient with persistent hemiparesis; and the third was a 4-year-old child who developed permanent spastic quadriplegia (20).

A 40-year-old woman ingested 60 ml of 35% hydrogen peroxide solution and developed gastritis and portal vein embolism but recovered without serious sequelae (11). A 63-year-old man ingested 3 cups of 35% hydrogen peroxide and developed vomiting, decreased mental status, and hypertension 45 minutes postingestion. Radiographic studies showed the presence of intraabdominal free air. Endoscopy showed diffuse gastric hemorrhage of the gastric mucosa without perforation. A magnetic resonance image of the brain showed multiple enhancement lesions, which resolved (21).

There have been at least six pediatric fatalities from ingestion of hydrogen peroxide. Emboli have been seen in the portal, gastric, and superior mesenteric venous systems as well as in multiple organs (21). An 11-month-old infant developed a gas embolus after wound irrigation with 15 ml of 3% hydrogen peroxide (22). The infant became apneic within 30 seconds, and gas was confirmed radiologically in the abdominal wall along with pulmonary edema. The infant recovered without sequelae after cardiac massage, hydrocortisone, and sodium bicarbonate.

Ingestion of low-concentration (3%) hydrogen peroxide does not produce embolism. However, if access to the vascular system occurs (e.g., wound irrigation), embolism may occur with surprisingly small amounts of hydrogen peroxide. Extrapolation from animal data suggests that 2 ml of 3% hydrogen peroxide could release 20 ml of oxygen microbubbles and that a 10-kg infant may only require 2 ml/kg of gas (20 ml) to sustain a cardiac arrest (22).

PATHOPHYSIOLOGY

Hydrogen peroxide is an unstable oxidizing agent. Gastric catabolism of hydrogen peroxide occurs in the presence of tissue catalase, producing rapid molecular decomposition and liberat-

TABLE 1. U.S. regulatory guidelines and standards for hydrogen peroxide

Agency	Description	Concentration [mg/m^3 (ppm)]
OSHA	Vapor or gas	
	PEL-TWA	1.4 (1.0)
	STEL	None
ACGIH	Vapor or gas	
	TLV-TWA	1.4 (1.0)
	STEL	None
NIOSH	Vapor or gas	
	REL-TWA	1.4 (1.0)
	STEL	None
	IDLH	75.0

ACGIH, American Conference of Governmental Industrial Hygienists; IDLH, immediate danger to life or health; NIOSH, National Institute for Occupational Safety and Health; OSHA, U.S. Occupational Safety and Health Administration; PEL, permissible exposure limit; ppm, parts per million; REL, recommended exposure limit; STEL, short-term exposure limit; TLV, threshold limit value; TWA, time-weighted average.

ing oxygen and water. When large amounts of oxygen are liberated, distention develops in closed body cavities. Mechanical distention can cause gastric or intestinal perforation as well as venous or arterial gas embolization. One ml of 3% hydrogen peroxide liberates 10 ml of oxygen at standard temperature and pressure, and 60 ml of 35% hydrogen peroxide solution has the potential to liberate 6.1 L of oxygen.

CLINICAL PRESENTATION

Acute Ingestion or Injection

Symptoms and signs involve the caustic effects of direct exposure to high concentrations of hydrogen peroxide and the sequelae of oxygen gas embolization. Severe embolization may produce hypotension and apnea.

GASTROINTESTINAL EFFECTS

Serious complications have resulted from the ingestion of concentrated solutions or the use of dilute peroxide solutions as an enema. Ingestion of a 3% solution may result in spontaneous vomiting; mild irritation to mucosal tissue; burns in the mouth, throat, esophagus, and stomach; colitis; enteritis; and tenesmus.

Gastric ulcers developed in a child who ingested 2 to 4 oz of 3% hydrogen peroxide (26). Gastric distention and rupture of the colon secondary to liberation of oxygen may occur after unintentional ingestion of the household concentration (1,2,26). Exposure to concentrated (greater than 10%) solutions causes more severe injury, including hemorrhagic gastritis; burns of the mouth, throat, esophagus, and stomach; rupture of the colon; fulminant acute ulcerating colitis, resulting in death; and potentially fatal gas embolization (1,2,26). Sepsis may develop as a complication of using a hydrogen peroxide enema.

CARDIOVASCULAR EFFECTS

Systemic embolization has occurred, resulting in electrocardiographic changes and, rarely, cardiac arrest and death (24).

NEUROLOGIC EFFECTS

Cerebral edema, cerebral gas embolism, cerebral infarction, and seizures may occur after ingestion of 35% solutions (6). Death has been reported as a result of embolic cerebrovascular injury. After ingestion or instillation into a body cavity, gas may develop and progress to gas embolism (28,29).

Inhalation and Mucous Membrane Exposure

Eye exposure to 3% hydrogen peroxide may result in immediate eye pain and irritation, although severe injury is rare. Ocular exposure to hydrogen peroxide solutions (greater than 10% concentration) may result in corneal ulceration or perforation (23). Inhalation of vapors of concentrated solutions may result in severe pulmonary irritation. Interstitial lung disease and respiratory arrest have also been reported after massive exposure (25).

Dermal exposure to 3% solutions generally results in a bleaching of the affected area in association with a tingling sensation that lasts 2 to 3 hours. Dermal exposure to concentrated solutions has resulted in burns and gangrene (27).

DIAGNOSTIC TESTS

Ingestion

No routine laboratory tests are needed after a small ingestion of 3% hydrogen peroxide. After a large-volume or high-concentration ingestion, abdominal and upright chest radiographs may reveal radiolucent gas in the gastrointestinal tract; right ventricle; mediastinum; pleural space; mesenteric, gastric, splenic, and inferior venae cava; and, most commonly, the portal venous systems. Arterial blood gases and an electrocardiogram are obtained to assess the effects of embolization.

Ingestion of high-concentration hydrogen peroxide may require gastrointestinal endoscopy to assess lower- or upper-tract caustic injury.

Inhalation

Chest radiography is often needed to assess pulmonary complaints. Slit-lamp and fluorescein examinations are indicated for ocular complaints.

TREATMENT

Ingestion

Administer water to dilute the solution. Gastric emptying is not indicated, and vomiting should not be induced. Asymptomatic patients who have ingested small amounts of 3% hydrogen peroxide may be observed. Symptomatic patients with more than one vomiting episode, bloody emesis, or abdominal distention or pain should be medically evaluated.

Endoscopy may be needed if symptoms or high concentrations are ingested (11). Gastric distention may require gastric decompression via nasogastric tube. A careful examination should be performed to detect any gas formation. Trendelenburg positioning should be avoided because it may trap air in the apex of the right ventricle and cause obstruction of blood flow.

Dermal Exposure

After skin exposure, remove contaminated clothing, and wash exposed area thoroughly with soap and water. A physician may need to examine the area if irritation or pain persists. After respiratory exposure, monitor for respiratory tract irritation and hypoxia after severe exposure.

Ocular Exposure

Ocular exposure to 3% solutions usually requires little more than thorough irrigation because serious complications are rare. Ocular exposure to an industrial-strength (greater than 10%) solution requires irrigation and should be evaluated in a health care facility because of the possibility of corneal ulceration or perforation.

Other

There are no antidotes to hydrogen peroxide. Multiple-dose activated charcoal, hemodialysis, hemoperfusion, or peritoneal dialysis is not recommended. Hyperbaric oxygen has been used in severe embolization cases (10).

REFERENCES

1. Dickenson KF, Caravati EM. Hydrogen peroxide exposure—325 exposures reported to a regional poison control center. *J Toxicol Clin Toxicol* 1994;32:705–714.
2. Gonzolas TA, Vance M, Helpern M, et al. *Legal medicine, pathology and toxicology*. New York: Appleton-Century-Crofts, 1954:201.
3. Humberston CL, Dean BS, Krenzelok EP. Ingestion of 35% hydrogen peroxide. *J Toxicol Clin Toxicol* 1990;28:95–100.

4. Christensen DW, Fraught WE, Black RE. Fatal oxygen embolization after hydrogen peroxide ingestion. *Crit Care Med* 1992;20:543–544.
5. Gervish SP. Gas embolism due to hydrogen peroxide. *Anesthesia* 1985;40:1244.
6. Tsai SK, Lee TY, Mok MS. Gas embolism produced by hydrogen peroxide irrigation of fistula during anesthesia. *Anesthesiology* 1985;63:316–317.
7. Cina SJ, Downs JC, Conradi SE. Hydrogen peroxide: a source of lethal oxygen embolism. *Am J Forensic Med Pathol* 1994;15:44–50.
8. Shaw A, Cooperman A, Fusco J. Gas embolism produced by hydrogen peroxide. *N Engl J Med* 1967;277:238–241.
9. Bassan MM, Daudai M, Shalev O. Near fatal systemic oxygen embolism due to wound irrigation with hydrogen peroxide. *Postgrad Med J* 1982;58:448–450.
10. Luu TA, Kelley MT, Strauch JA, et al. Portal vein gas embolism from hydrogen peroxide ingestion. *Ann Emerg Med* 1992;21:1391–1393.
11. Sherman SJ, Boyer LV, Sibley WA. Cerebral infarction immediately after ingestion of hydrogen peroxide solution. *Stroke* 1994;25:1065.
12. Tripathi BJ, Tripathi RC. Hydrogen peroxide damage to human corneal epithelial cells in vitro. *Arch Ophthalmol* 1989;107:1516–1519.
13. Kaelin RM, Kapanci Y, Tschopp JM. Diffuse interstitial lung disease associated with hydrogen peroxide inhalation in a dairy worker. *Am Rev Respir Dis* 1988;137:1233–1235.
14. Budavari S, ed. *The Merck index*, 11th ed. Rahway, NJ: Merck & Co, Inc., 1989:550.
15. Lewis RJ. *Hawley's condensed chemical dictionary*, 12th ed. New York: Van Nostrand Reinhold Company, 1993:616–617.
16. Freeman HM, ed. *Standard handbook of hazardous waste treatment and disposal*. New York: McGraw-Hill, 1989.
17. CHRIS. *CHRIS hazardous chemical data*. U.S. Department of Transportation, U.S. Coast Guard, Washington, DC (CD-ROM version). Englewood, CO: Micromedex, Inc., 1996.
18. Reference deleted.
19. Reference deleted.
20. Ashdown BC, Stricof DD, May ML, et al. Hydrogen peroxide poisoning causing brain infarction: neuroimaging findings. *Am J Roentgenology* 1998;170:1653–1655.
21. Cina SJ, Downs JC, Conradi SE. Hydrogen peroxide—a source of lethal oxygen embolism—case report and review of the literature. *Am J Forensic Med Pathol* 1994;15:44–50.
22. Schwab C, Dilworth K. Gas embolism produced by hydrogen peroxide abscess irrigation in an infant. *Anaesth Intensive Care* 1999;27:418–420.
23. Grant WM. *Toxicology of the eye*, 3rd ed. Springfield, IL: Charles C. Thomas, 1986:302.
24. Giberson TP, Kern JD, Pettigrew DW, et al. Near-fatal hydrogen peroxide ingestion. *Ann Emerg Med* 1989;18:778–779.
25. Kaelin RM, Kapanci Y, Tschopp JM. Diffuse interstitial lung disease associated with hydrogen peroxide inhalation in a dairy worker. *Am Rev Respir Dis* 1988;137:1233–1235.
26. Henry MC, Wheeler J, Mofenson HC, et al. Hydrogen peroxide 3% exposure. *J Toxicol Clin Toxicol* 1996;34:323–327.
27. Wade A, Reynolds JEF, eds. *Martindale: the extra pharmacopoeia*, 27th ed. London: The Pharmaceutical Press, 1977:475.
28. Sleigh JW, Litter JP. Hazards of hydrogen peroxide. *BMJ* 1985:291:1786.
29. Rackoff WR, Menton DF. Gas embolism after the ingestion of hydrogen peroxide. *Pediatrics* 1990;85:593–594.

CHAPTER 198

Benzalkonium Chloride

Thomas R. Caraccio and Michael A. McGuigan

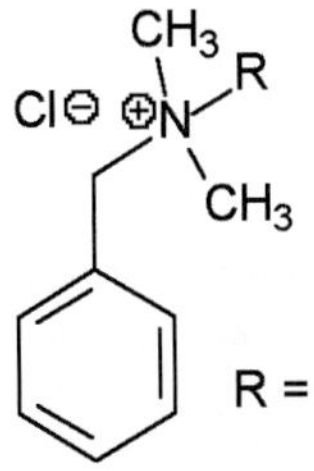

R = various alkyl chains

BENZALKONIUM CHLORIDE	
Molecular formula and weight:	**$C_9H_{18}NRCl$, 360 g/mol**
SI conversion:	**mg/L × 2.8 = µmol/L**
CAS Registry No.:	**8001-54-5**
Therapeutic levels:	**Not applicable**
Target organs:	**Gastrointestinal tract (acute), cornea (acute), central nervous system (acute)**
Antidote:	**None**

OVERVIEW

Benzalkonium chloride is a mixture of quaternary alkyldimethylbenzyl ammonium chlorides. It is a cationic bactericidal agent used in various pharmaceutical preparations, as a topical disinfectant, and as a preservative. Allergic reactions to benzalkonium chloride are common. Skin ulceration has been reported in dermal exposure, and ocular exposure causes mild discomfort of the eye. Sore throat, diarrhea, dehydration, hypotension, hypoxemia, hepatic enzyme elevation, and metabolic acidosis have been reported after oral ingestion.

Benzalkonium chloride is used as a bacteriocidal disinfectant for preoperative skin preparation; for irrigation of body cavities, mucous membranes, and wounds; and for sterile storage of surgical instruments and utensils (1). It also is used as an antimicrobial preservative in various ophthalmic and topical preparations and as a bacteriocidal agent in pharmaceutical preparations, such as beclomethasone dipropionate, metaproteronol, and ipratropium bromide nebulizer solutions.

TOXIC DOSE

The concentration of benzalkonium chloride in products used by adults is shown in Table 1. Benzalkonium chloride should not be used in pediatric products. Ingestion of 40 ml of a 33.3% solution resulted in central nervous system depression with esophageal and gastric burns (4). An 84-year-old woman ingested less than 50 ml of a 10% benzalkonium chloride solution (96 mg/kg). She experienced vomiting and erythema of the lips, tongue, mouth, pharynx, larynx, esophagus, and stomach and died 3 hours after the ingestion (2). Death has occurred in adults who ingested 100 to 400 mg of benzalkonium chloride solution in concentrations of 15.0% to 17.4% (3).

Sore throat and skin irritation were reported in two children who had a 17% solution of benzalkonium chloride applied to

TABLE 1. Concentration and application of products containing benzalkonium chloride

Concentration	Application
1:500	Disinfecting catheters and other adsorbent items
1:750	Preoperative skin preparation, treatment of minor wounds and lacerations, surgical scrub, sterilizing metallic instruments
1:1000–1:2000	Breast and nipple hygiene
1:2000–1:5000	Vaginal douches, oozing and open infections
1:3000–1:20,000	Disinfecting deep infected wounds
1:5000–1:7500	Preservative in ophthalmic solutions
1:5000–1:10,000	Irrigation of denuded skin, mucous membranes, eyes
1:5000–1:20,000	Bladder and urethral irrigation
≤1:5000	Wet dressings
1:20,000–1:40,000	Bladder retention lavage

their mouth (4). No pediatric fatalities have been attributed to benzalkonium chloride.

TOXICOKINETICS AND TOXICODYNAMICS

The human toxicokinetics of benzalkonium chloride have not been established.

PATHOPHYSIOLOGY

Benzalkonium chloride precipitates and denatures protein. It is irritating to the tissues and possesses keratolytic and corrosive action (5). It can produce hemolysis, which is thought to be due to its tendency to solubilize cholesterol, phospholipids, and the proteins in cell membranes. It also has a ganglionic-blocking effect and curare-like action, which can result in paralysis of the neuromuscular junction of striated muscles.

PREGNANCY AND LACTATION

Human data are unavailable. In a postnatal mouse screening test, benzalkonium chloride caused excessive maternal mortality (6). Excretion in human breast milk has not been studied.

CLINICAL PRESENTATION

Acute Exposure

Mild discomfort of the eye has been associated with ocular exposure (7), and severe corneal damage can occur, depending on the concentration and duration of contact.

Ingestion is followed by diarrhea, dehydration, hypotension, hypoxemia, hepatic enzyme elevation, and metabolic acidosis (4,8). Ingestion of a high-concentration solution can produce caustic injury, including ulceration, burns, and perforation. Severe exposures may cause cardiac arrest (8).

Skin ulceration and severe pustular or bullous reactions have been produced by benzalkonium chloride exposures (9,10).

Chronic Exposure

Occupational asthma has been reported (10). Deleterious effects on the tear film and corneoconjunctival surface have been noted in patients receiving eye drops preserved with benzalkonium chloride (11,12). Benzalkonium chloride is not suitable for use in storing and washing hydrophilic soft contact lenses, as it can bind to the lenses and may later produce ocular toxicity when the lenses are worn (15).

Adverse Reactions

Benzalkonium chloride used on children's lips has caused sore throat and skin ulcerations (4). A hypersensitivity reaction to benzalkonium chloride in nose drops was confirmed by a challenge test (16). As a preservative in nebulized solutions of antiasthma drugs, it may cause dose-related bronchoconstriction, especially in asthmatic patients (17). Respiratory arrest occurred in one patient (18).

DIAGNOSTIC TESTS

In severe cases, monitor complete blood cell count, fluid and electrolyte status, acid-base status, liver transaminases, and electrocardiogram. Monitor hepatic transaminases because elevations may occur (4). Metabolic acidosis has been reported in severe cases (4). Consider endoscopic evaluation if drooling, dysphagia, stridor, abdominal pain, bloody vomitus, or ingestion of caustic amounts is involved. Diarrhea and dehydration should be monitored (4). Benzalkonium chloride blood levels are not available and not clinically useful.

Gastrointestinal and esophageal necrosis and pulmonary and cerebral edema have been noted on postmortem examination (3).

TREATMENT

Ingestion

Immediately dilute with milk or water after acute ingestion. Emesis is not recommended because of potential corrosive effects. It is unknown if activated charcoal binds benzalkonium chloride. It should be avoided if endoscopy may be needed. Because benzalkonium chloride is a liquid, whole bowel irrigation is not effective.

A typical toxic patient may need management with fluids, parenteral nutrition, and oxygen therapy. Maintain ventilation and provide assisted ventilation if necessary. Manage pulmonary edema with standard care. If endoscopy reveals caustic injury, treatment should be based on clinical assessment. Seizure, hypotension, or pulmonary edema is treated in the standard manner (Chapters 33, 37, and 40). Enhancement of elimination is not expected to be useful. There is no antidote for benzalkonium chloride.

Ocular Exposure

If an eye exposure occurs, flush the eyes with water for 15 minutes. Ophthalmologic evaluation is needed if symptoms or signs persist.

Monitoring

Significant exposures should be monitored for the following manifestations: seizures, hypotension, pulmonary edema, mucosal lesions, corneal opacity, and chemical burns in the mouth.

REFERENCES

1. Benzalkonium chloride monograph. *Drugdex Martindale*, Vol. 113 (electronic version). Greenwood Village, CO: Micromedex, 2002.
2. Hitosugi M, Maruyama K, Takatsu A. A case of fatal benzalkonium chloride poisoning. *Int J Legal Med* 1998;111:265–266.

3. Tiess D, Nagel KH. [Beitrag Zur morphologic and analytic investigation]. *Toxicol J* 1967;22:333–348.
4. Van Berkel M, De Wolff FA. Survival after acute benzalkonium chloride poisoning. *Hum Toxicol* 1988;7:191–193.
5. Gloxhueber CH. Toxicological properties of surfactants. *Arch Toxicol* 1974;32:245–270.
6. Oral health care products for OTC human use; establishment of monograph. *Fed Regist* 1982:47:22760.
7. Swan KC. Reactivity of ocular tissues to wetting agent. *Am J Ophthalmol* 1944;27:1118–1122.
8. Mathielholf M, Mathieu D, Leblanc JH, et al. Poisoning with the antiseptics from quaternary ammonium class. Are they always benign? *J Toxicol Clin Exp* 1985;5:406(abst).
9. Innocenti A. Occupation asthma due to benzalkonium chloride. *Med Law* 1978;69:713–715.
10. Wahlberg JE, Wrangs JK, Hietasalo A. Skin irritancy for nonanoic acid. *Contact Dermatitis* 1985;13:266–269.
11. Herreras JM, Pastor JC, Calonge M, Asensio VM. Ocular surface alteration after long-term treatment with an antiglaucomatous drug. *Ophthalmology* 1992;99:1082–1088.
12. Kuppens EV, de Jong CA, Stolwijk TR, et al. Effect of timolol with and without preservative on the basal tear turnover in glaucoma. *Br J Ophthalmol* 1995;79:339–342.
13. Reference deleted.
14. Reference deleted.
15. Gasset AR. Benzalkonium chloride toxicity to the human cornea. *Am J Ophthalmol* 1977;84:169–171.
16. Hillerdal G. Adverse reaction to locally applied preservatives in nose drops. *ORL J Otorhinolaryngol Relat Spec* 1985;47:278–279.
17. Committee on Drugs, American Academy of Pediatrics. "Inactive" ingredients in pharmaceutical products: update. *Pediatrics* 1997;99:268–278.
18. Boucher M, Roy MT, Henderson J. Possible association of benzalkonium chloride in nebulizer solutions with respiratory arrest. *Ann Pharmacother* 1992;26:772–774.

SECTION

4

Explosives

CHAPTER 199

Explosives

Yedidia Bentur and Daniel C. Keyes

Compounds included: **Trinitrotoluene (TNT, 1-methyl-2,4,6-trinitrobenzene, sym-trinitrotoluene, α-trinitrotoluol, trotyl); dinitrotoluene (DNT, dinitrotoluol, methyl-dinitrobenzene, dinitrophenyl-methane, binitrotoluene); 1,3-dinitrobenzene (DNB, meta-dinitrobenzene, dinitrobenzene, 2,4-dinitrobenzene, 1,3-dinitrobenzol). Structures are provided in Figure 1**

Molecular formula and weight: **See text.**

CAS Registry No.: **See text.**

Normal levels: **Not applicable**

Target organs: **Lung (acute); skin (acute and chronic); cardiovascular (acute and chronic); hematologic (chronic); liver (acute and chronic); and central nervous system (acute and chronic)**

Antidote: **None**

OVERVIEW

The first explosive used was probably black powder (gunpowder, which is a mixture of charcoal, sulfur, and potassium nitrate) developed by the Chinese in the tenth century. Nitroglycerin (NG) was discovered by Ascanio Sobrero in 1846. Alfred Nobel made NG safer to use in 1867 by incorporating it into dynamite (a combination of NG, ammonium nitrate, and Fuller's earth or wood pulp). In 1890, severe throbbing headache was first described after occupational exposure to NG in dynamite. Frequent reports followed and described the phenomenon as NG head and powder headache.

Trinitrotoluene (TNT) was discovered in 1902, and its toxicity in munitions workers has been reported since World War I. Ethylene glycol dinitrate (EGDN) was discovered in 1870 and was brought into commercial use in 1930 as an addition to NG in dynamite manufacturing. In 1934, sudden unexplained deaths were observed in dynamite workers. These deaths were found to be associated with EGDN in the early 1950s. Subsequently, safety and cost considerations have resulted in the substitution of dynamite by a mixture of fuel-sensitized ammonium nitrate (1–11).

From the time gunpowder was developed, many explosives with different chemical compositions were produced for civilian and military purposes. New applications resulted in development of safer, more effective and economical explosives. In addition to their destructive military use, explosives have various civilian uses

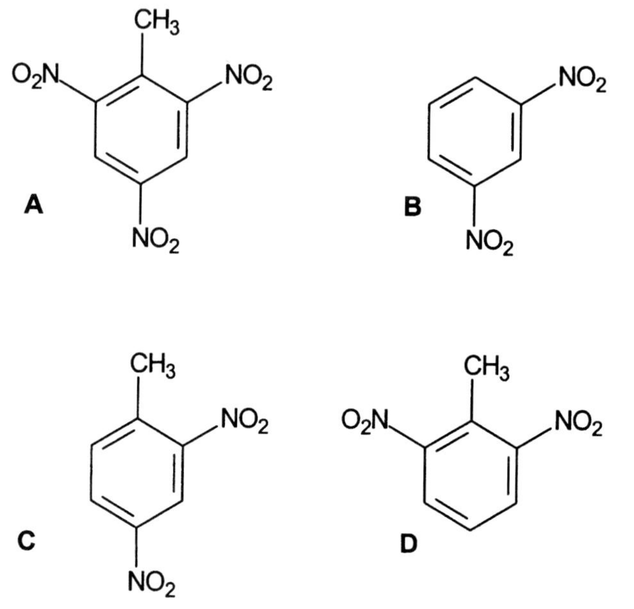

A: CH_3, O_2N, NO_2, NO_2
B: NO_2, NO_2
C: CH_3, NO_2, NO_2
D: CH_3, O_2N, NO_2

Figure 1. Physical structure of selected explosive compounds. **A:** 2,4,6-Trinitrotoluene. **B:** 1,3-Dinitrobenzene. **C:** 2,4-Dinitrotoluene. **D:** 2,6-Dinitrotoluene.

including construction projects (such as tunnels, dams, roads, and demolitions); mining metallic ores, fossil fuels, and rocks; metal forming, welding, and cladding; and high-pressure transformations that yield valuable products (e.g., fine diamonds) (2). Terrorist and criminal activities constitute the illegitimate use of explosives.

Explosives are *stable* solid or liquid substances that can undergo rapid decomposition to produce sudden large volumes of rapidly expanding gas and intense heat from different types of reactions (2,12). The Department of Transportation defines explosives as any material whose function is destruction by detonation (13). The rapid increase in pressure by the expanding gas causes an explosion. Only those substances that are intended to produce explosion are categorized as such (1). Explosives may be mixtures of combustible and oxidizing agents as in black powder or single substances such as NG (2).

The gases generated by an explosion can include carbon monoxide, carbon dioxide, nitrogen, oxygen, oxides of nitrogen, and hydrogen sulfide. The voluminous quantities of combustion products are expected to be toxic in a confined space and less so in the open air (1,3). This toxicity is superimposed on the injuries resulting from the tremendous release of heat and high pressure.

Various properties of explosives ranging from the slow propellant action of deflagrating explosives to shattering or shock effects of detonating explosives are achieved by different chemical compositions (2). These types of explosives have been classified by the Department of Transportation (3):

> *Class A explosives* can detonate by flame, spark, or shock (high explosives). *Class B explosives* are rapidly combustible materials that can explode under extreme temperatures (low explosives). *Class C explosives* offer a minimum explosion hazard. In 1991, explosives were reclassified:
>
> Division 1.1: Explosives with a mass explosion hazard (former Class A)
> Division 1.2: Explosives with a projection hazard (former Class A and B)
> Division 1.3: Explosives with predominantly a fire hazard (former Class B)
> Division 1.4: Explosives with no significant blast hazard (former Class C)
> Division 1.5: Insensitive explosives; blasting agents
> Division 1.6: Extremely insensitive detonating articles

High explosives detonate causing a rapid and tremendous release of heat and a large volume of gases producing high pressure. The detonation rate can reach 4 miles/second. Ammonium nitrate; cyclotrimethylenetrinitramine [cyclonite, hexogen, Royal Demolition Explosive (RDX)]; TNT; NG; pentaerythritol tetranitrate (PETN); tetryl picric acid; and dynamite (various compositions) are some widely used high explosives.

Detonating explosives can be divided into *primary* and *secondary explosives*. Primary explosives are sensitive to heat, shock, or friction. They develop a detonation wave in a short period of time and are used as detonators and fuses to initiate another explosive. Primary explosives that have been used as initiating materials in shells, cartridges, or blasting caps include lead azide, lead styphnate, and mercury fulminate. All these are forbidden for transport when dry because they are unstable and decompose explosively.

Secondary explosives require a booster or an initiating form of detonation to explode. Examples of secondary explosives include tetryl and RDX.

Low energy explosives react much slower than high explosives. These materials ignite and burn rapidly rather than detonate. Their detonation rate is approximately 900 feet/second, much slower than that of high explosives. The major effect of low explosives is the force produced by the rapidly expanding gases. Examples of these agents include nitrocellulose, black powder, some solid rocket fuels, and fireworks (1–3,12,13).

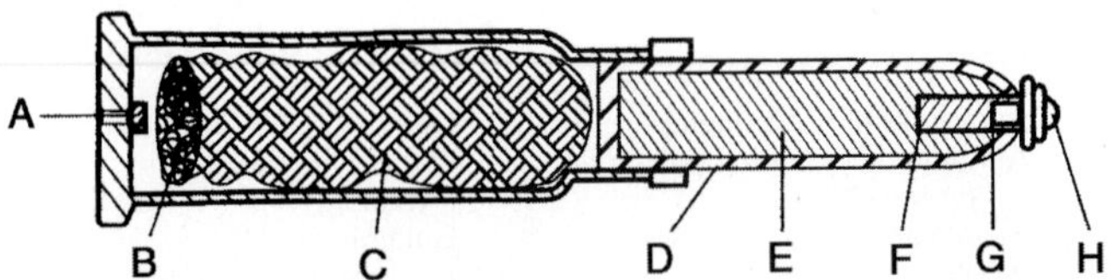

Figure 2. Diagram of an explosive shell. **A:** Primer (sensitive explosive). **B:** Igniter—black powder. **C:** Propellant charge (nitrocotton). **D:** Projectile. **E:** Bursting charge (trinitrotoluene Amatol). **F:** Booster (tetryl). **G:** Detonator (sensitive explosive). **H:** Fuse (sensitive explosive). (Adapted from Schwartz L. *JAMA* 1944;125:186–190, with permission.)

A diagram of a shell showing some of the uses of explosives is depicted in Figure 2 (14).

Forensic analysis of explosives is multifaceted and includes identification of an unexploded explosive, which is needed to prove possession or its intended use; postexplosive identification used to assist the police investigation; and trace analysis of explosives on suspects' hands and on items and premises related to them. Various analytic methods have been used for the analysis of explosives including chemical tests (color reaction), thin-layer chromatography (TLC), column chromatography, gas chromatography (GC), high-pressure liquid chromatography (HPLC), capillary electrophoresis, ion chromatography, as well as spectral methods like infrared, nuclear magnetic resonance, mass spectrometry (MS), scanning electron microscopy-energy dispersive x-ray spectroscopy, x-ray diffraction, and in-line combinations (e.g., GC/MS, HPLC/MS). The procedure chosen depends on whether the identification required involves intact explosives, postexplosion, or trace analysis (15).

Table 1 contains the list of explosive materials as prepared by the Bureau of Alcohol, Tobacco, and Firearms (16).

TRINITROTOLUENE

TNT [$CH_3C_6H_2(NO_2)_3$, molecular weight (MW) 227.1 g/mol; CAS Registry No. 118-96-7] is an aromatic nitro compound discovered in 1902. Data on its toxicity came to a large extent from U.S. and British munitions industries. In World War I, there were 17,000 cases of TNT poisoning with 475 deaths within a 7.5-month period. Between 1941 and 1945, 22 deaths were reported as a cause of aplastic anemia and toxic hepatitis (3,11,17). The British reported 24 cases of aplastic anemia due to TNT between 1939 and 1946 (18). A better health record in the TNT industry during World War II is believed to be due to the removal of tetranitromethane, a toxic and irritating impurity of crude TNT, and improvement in work conditions (17). TNT is a comparatively safe high explosive. Its relative safety and its high explosive power made it one of the most widely used explosives. It is used in all types of bursting charges in the manufacture of detonator fuses and can be used alone or with ammonium nitrate (Amatol) or barium nitrate (Baratol) (1,19–21).

Physicochemical Properties

TNT is produced by nitration of toluene. The final pure product is a colorless to pale yellow, odorless solid, or crushed flakes (21–23). In a commercial grade it may appear as yellow to dark brown crystals (13,23). Bitter taste may be apparent on exposure to the dust (14).

TNT is insoluble in water (0.01%), soluble in ethyl ether, and soluble in acetone and benzene. Its melting point is 82°C and boiling point 240°C, around which it detonates (3,21–23). TNT has a low sensitivity to impact and friction and is not susceptible to spontaneous decomposition. It is flammable and burns when

TABLE 1. U.S. Department of Transportation list of explosive materials

- Acetylides of heavy metals
- Aluminum-containing polymeric propellant
- Aluminum ophorite explosive
- Amatex
- Amatol
- Ammonal
- Ammonium nitrate explosive mixtures (cap sensitive)
- Ammonium nitrate explosive mixtures (non–cap sensitive)*
- Ammonium perchlorate composite propellant
- Ammonium perchlorate explosive mixtures
- Ammonium picrate (picrate of ammonia, Explosive D)
- Ammonium nitrate-fuel oil*
- Ammonium salt lattice with isomorphously substituted inorganic salts
- Aromatic nitro-compound explosive mixtures
- Azide explosives
- Baranol
- Baratol
- BEAF [1,2-bis (2,2-difluoro-2-nitro-acetoxyethane)]
- Bis (trinitroethyl) carbonate
- Bis (trinitroethyl) nitramine
- Black powder
- Black powder–based explosive mixtures
- Blasting agents, nitro-carbo-nitrates, including non–cap sensitive slurry and water gel explosives*
- Blasting caps
- Blasting gelatin
- Blasting powder
- 1,2,4-Butanetriol trinitrate
- Bulk salutes
- Butyl tetryl
- Calcium nitrate explosive mixture
- Cellulose hexanitrate explosive mixture
- Chlorate explosive mixtures
- Composition A and variations
- Composition B and variations
- Composition C and variations
- Copper acetylide
- Cyanuric triazide
- Cyclo-1,3,5,7-tetramethylene 2,4,6,8-tetranitramine; octogen
- Cyclonite (cyclotrimethylenetrinitramine)
- Cyclotetramethylenetetranitramine
- Cyclotol
- Cyclotrimethylenetrinitramine
- Diaminotrinitrobenzene
- Diazodinitrophenol
- Diethyleneglycol dinitrate
- Detonating cord
- Detonators
- Dimethylol dimethyl methane dinitrate composition
- Dinitroethyleneurea
- Dinitroglycerine (glycerol dinitrate)
- Dinitropentano nitrile
- 2,2-Dinitropropyl acrylate
- Dinitrophenol
- Dinitrophenolates
- Dinitrophenyl hydrazine
- Dinitroresorcinol
- Dinitrotoluene-sodium nitrate explosive mixtures
- Dipicramide; diaminohexanitrobiphenyl
- Dipicryl sulfone
- Dipicrylamine
- Display fireworks
- Dynamite
- Ednatol
- Ethylene diamine dinitrate
- Ethylenedinitramine
- Erythritol tetranitrate explosives
- Esters of nitro-substituted alcohols
- Ethyl-tetryl
- Ethyl 4,4-dinitropentanoate
- Ethylene glycol dinitrate
- Explosive conitrates
- Explosive gelatins
- Explosive liquids
- Explosive mixtures containing oxygen-releasing inorganic salts and hydrocarbons
- Explosive mixtures containing oxygen-releasing inorganic salts and nitro bodies
- Explosive mixtures containing oxygen-releasing inorganic salts and water-insoluble fuels
- Explosive mixtures containing oxygen-releasing inorganic salts and water-soluble fuels
- Explosive mixtures containing sensitized nitromethane
- Explosive mixtures containing tetranitromethane (nitroform)
- Explosive nitro compounds of aromatic hydrocarbons
- Explosive organic nitrate mixtures
- Explosive powders
- Flash powder
- Fulminate of mercury
- Fulminate of silver
- Fulminating gold
- Fulminating mercury
- Fulminating platinum
- Fulminating silver
- Gelatinized nitrocellulose
- Gem-dinitro aliphatic explosive mixtures
- Guanyl nitrosamino guanyl tetrazene
- Guanyl nitrosamino guanylidene hydrazine
- Guncotton
- Heavy metal azides
- Hexamethylenetriperoxidediamine
- Hexanite
- Hexanitrodiphenylamine
- Hexanitrostilbene
- Hexogen
- Hexogene or octogene and a nitrated *N*-methylaniline
- Hexolites
- Hydrazinium nitrate/hydrazine/aluminum explosive system
- Hydrazoic acid
- Igniter cord
- Igniters
- Initiating tube systems
- Lead azide
- Lead mannite
- Lead mononitroresorcinate
- Lead picrate
- Lead salts, explosive
- Lead styphnate (styphnate of lead, lead trinitroresorcinate)
- Liquid nitrated polyol and trimethylolethane
- Liquid oxygen explosives
- Magnesium ophorite explosives
- Mannitol hexanitrate
- Methyl 4,4-dinitropentanoate
- Mercuric fulminate
- Mercury oxalate
- Mercury tartrate
- Metriol trinitrate
- Minol-2 (40% trinitrotoluene, 40% ammonium nitrate, 20% aluminum)
- Monoethanolamine nitrate
- Monomethylamine nitrate; methylamine nitrate
- Mononitrotoluene-nitroglycerin mixture
- Monopropellants
- Nitrate explosive mixtures
- Nitrate sensitized with gelled nitroparaffin
- Nitrated carbohydrate explosive
- Nitrated glucoside explosive
- Nitrated polyhydric alcohol explosives
- Nitric acid and a nitro aromatic compound explosive
- Nitric acid and carboxylic fuel explosive
- Nitric acid explosive mixtures
- Nitro aromatic explosive mixtures
- Nitro compounds of furane explosive mixtures
- Nitrocellulose explosive
- Nitroderivative of urea explosive mixture
- Nitrogelatin explosive
- Nitrogen trichloride
- Nitrogen triiodide
- Nitroglycerine (nitro, glyceryl trinitrate, trinitroglycerin)
- Nitroglycide
- Nitroglycol (ethylene glycol dinitrate)
- Nitroguanidine explosives
- Nitroisobutametriol trinitrate
- Nitronium perchlorate propellant mixtures
- Nitroparaffins explosive grade and ammonium nitrate mixtures
- Nitropentaerythrite, pentaerythrite tetranitrate, pentaerythritol, tetranitrate (PETN)
- Nitrostarch
- Nitro-substituted carboxylic acids
- Nitrourea
- Octogen
- Octol [75% cyclo-1,3,5,7-tetramethylene 2,4,6,8-tetranitramine, 25% trinitrotoluene]
- Organic amine nitrates
- Organic nitramines
- Pellet powder
- Penthrinite composition
- Pentolite
- Perchlorate explosive mixtures
- Peroxide based explosive mixtures
- Picramic acid and its salts
- Picramide
- Picrate explosives
- Picrate of potassium explosive mixtures
- Picratol
- Picric acid (manufactured as an explosive)
- Picryl chloride
- Picryl fluoride
- Plastic bonded explosives
- PLX (95% nitromethane, 5% ethylenediamine)
- Polynitro aliphatic compounds
- Polyolpolynitrate-nitrocellulose explosive gels
- Potassium chlorate and lead sulfocyanate explosive
- Potassium dinitrobenzo-furoxane
- Potassium nitrate explosive mixtures
- Potassium nitroaminotetrazole
- Pyrotechnic compositions
- 2,6-Bis(picrylamino)-3,5-dinitropyridine
- Cyclonite, hexogen, T4, cyclo-1,3,5,-tri methylene-2,4,6,-trinitramine; hexahydro-1,3,5-trinitro-*S*-triazine
- Safety fuse
- Salts of organic amino sulfonic acid explosive mixture
- Salutes (bulk)
- Silver acetylide
- Silver azide
- Silver fulminate
- Silver oxalate explosive mixtures
- Silver styphnate
- Silver tartrate explosive mixtures
- Silver tetrazene
- Slurried explosive mixtures of water, inorganic oxidizing salt, gelling agent, fuel, and sensitizer (cap sensitive)
- Smokeless powder
- Sodatol
- Sodium Amatol
- Sodium azide explosive mixture
- Sodium dinitro-ortho-cresolate
- Sodium nitrate explosive mixtures
- Sodium nitrate–potassium nitrate explosive mixture
- Sodium picramate
- Special fireworks
- Squibs
- Styphnic acid explosives
- Tacot (tetranitro-2,3,5,6-dibenzo-1,3a,4,6a tetrazapentalene)
- Tetranitrocarbazole
- Tetrazene [tetracene, tetrazine, 1(5-tetrazolyl)-4-guanyl tetrazene hydrate]
- Tetryl (2,4,6 tetramitro-*N*-methylaniline
- Tetrytol
- Thickened inorganic oxidizer salt slurried explosive mixture
- Torpex
- Triacetonetriperoxide
- Triaminotrinitrobenzene
- Tridite
- Triethylene glycol dinitrate
- Trimethylolethane trinitrate
- Trimethylol ethyl methane trinitrate composition
- Trimethylolethane trinitrate-nitrocellulose
- Trimonite
- Trinitroanisole
- Trinitrobenzene
- Trinitrobenzoic acid
- Trinitrocresol
- Trinitroethyl formal
- Trinitroethylorthocarbonate
- Trinitroethylorthoformate
- Trinitro-meta-cresol
- Trinitronaphthalene
- Trinitrophenetol
- Trinitrophloroglucinol
- Trinitroresorcinol
- Trinitrotoluene (trotyl, trilite, triton)
- Tritonal
- Urea nitrate
- Water-bearing explosives having salts of oxidizing acids and nitrogen bases, sulfates, or sulfamates (cap sensitive)
- Water-in-oil emulsion explosive compositions
- Xanthamonas hydrophilic colloid explosive mixture

Note: This revised list supersedes the List of Explosive Materials dated September 14, 1999 (notice no. 880, 64 FR 49840; correction notice of September 28, 1999, 64 FR 52378), and was effective on April 26, 2002.

TABLE 2. United States regulatory guidelines and standards for trinitrotoluene, dinitrotoluene, and 1,3-dinitrobenzene

		Concentration mg/m³ (ppm)		
Agency	Description	Trinitro-toluene	Dinitro-toluene	1,3-Dinitrobenzene
OSHA (air)	PEL-TWA	1.5 (0.16)	1.5 (0.2)	1 (0.15)
ACGIH (air)	TLV-TWA	0.1 (0.001)	0.2 (0.03)	1 (0.15)
	STEL	—	None	—
NIOSH (air)	REL-TWA	0.5 (0.005)	1.5 (0.02)	1 (0.15)
	IDLH	500 (54)	—	50 (7.3)
Conversion factor		ppm × 9.23 = mg/m³	ppm × 7.45 = mg/m³	ppm × 6.87 = mg/m³

ACGIH, American Conference of Governmental Industrial Hygienists; IDLH, immediately dangerous to life or health; NIOSH, National Institute for Occupational Safety and Health; OSHA, U.S. Occupational Safety and Health Administration; PEL, permissible exposure limit; ppm, parts per million; REL, recommended exposure limit; STEL, short-term exposure limit; TLV, threshold limit value; TWA, time-weighted average.

contacted with flames, producing toxic combustion products of nitrogen oxides. Sudden heating, high pressure, or strong shock conditions result in detonation. It can react with strong oxidizers, ammonia, strong alkalis, and combustible materials (3,21,22).

Toxic Dose

Occupational standards and guidelines are provided in Table 2. In the past, the standard for exposure to TNT was 1.5 mg/m³. However, air levels below that were associated with numerous toxic effects, including liver damage and possible aplastic anemia. Mild effects were noted at 0.2 mg/m³.

An ambient water quality standard of 135 µg/L TNT was proposed for consumption of contaminated water and fish and 140 µg/L for consumption of water alone (24). A lifetime health advisory criterion for TNT in water recommended by the U.S. Environmental Protective Agency (EPA) is 2 µg/L (25).

Toxicokinetics and Toxicodynamics

TNT is readily absorbed through the skin, especially when the skin is exposed and moist with sweat. It is also absorbed by inhalation and ingestion (3,14,17,21). Direct absorption through the cornea was suggested, but this is probably insignificant (26). The relative importance of the routes of exposure is variable and probably depends on the physical state of the TNT, nature of work, and personal hygiene of the worker.

The major biotransformation reaction is nitroreduction and, to a lesser extent, oxidation. The main metabolite formed by nitroreduction seems to be 4-amino-2,6-dinitrotoluene (4-ADNT). Other metabolites include 2-amino-4,6-dinitrotoluene (2-ADNT), 2,4-diamino-6-nitrotoluene, and 2,6-diamino-4-nitrotoluene. The metabolites are excreted in the urine as glucuronide conjugates and in the free form (27–31). Ring oxidation products of TNT such as trinitrobenzylalcohol, trinitrobenzoic acid, and simultaneous oxidation and reduction metabolites such as 2,6-dinitro-4-aminobenzylalcohol and 2,6-dinitro-4-amino-m-cresol are of less importance (32). Untransferred TNT is also excreted in the urine but to a much lesser extent than the two major metabolites 4-ADNT and 2-ADNT (27–31). Wide variations in urine ADNT and TNT concentrations were found in workers of explosives factories (28). 4-ADNT excretion was reported to be complete within 3 to 4 days after exposure (33). However, another study reported detectable urine concentrations of ADNT in explosives workers even after 17 days away from the workplace (28).

Pathophysiology

Animal studies have suggested covalent binding between TNT and macromolecular proteins including serum albumin, hemoglobin (Hb), hepatic and renal proteins, and possibly lens protein. The Hb adduct was dose dependent. Macromolecular binding is likely to be correlated with toxic effects; however, it is unclear if a cause and effect relationship can be established (33). Formation of organic nitro radicals was also hypothesized based on hemolysis in glucose 6 phosphate dehydrogenase (G6PD)–deficient TNT workers. G6PD is a limiting factor in the maintenance of cellular glutathione, which protects against oxidative damage (27). TNT was also found to be oxidized oxyhemoglobin, resulting in methemoglobin formation (34).

Clinical Presentation

Most data on the clinical effects of TNT come from occupational exposures of munitions workers. Its toxicity is similar to that of other nitro compounds.

DERMATOLOGIC EFFECTS

TNT stains the hands, arms, and face orange and yellow and the hair reddish blond. This is believed to be a sign of absorption and should not be confused with jaundice (14,17,20,21). Dermatitis from TNT can occur after exposure at every stage of the production process. It can manifest as early as 5 days of exposure. The hands, wrists, and forearms are most commonly affected, followed by points of friction (e.g., collar line, belt line, and ankles). Facial or generalized dermatitis is rare. The lesions begin on the hands, especially between the fingers and on the thenar eminence, and are accompanied by edema. A coalescing papular eruption with erythema is seen in other parts of the body. In 7 to 14 days, the edema subsides and desquamation, which may be severe, takes place leading to complete exfoliation of the hands and feet. Irritation is intense and small *powder* holes are seen (14,20). Allergic contact dermatitis with eczematous eruption and erythema multiforme-like eruption (without classic histologic findings) has also been reported (35–37).

HEMATOLOGIC EFFECTS

Minor degrees of cyanosis are frequent, due to methemoglobinemia in the range of 1.5% to 8.6%. Although often asymptomatic, it may be accompanied by dyspnea, nausea, fatigue, lassitude, and chest pain (3,20,21,38,39). Sulfhemoglobin of 0.9% to 4.93% was also documented in some workers (39). Acute Coombs' negative hemolytic anemia was reported in G6PD-deficient patients in 2 to 4 days after start of exposure. Lowest Hb levels ranged between 4.0 and 10.2 g/dl, reticulocytes rose to 4% to 26%, and bilirubin increased to 2.6 to 5.1 mg/dl. In some of these patients the hemolytic episode was the first in their lives and the only one in 5 to 9 years of follow-up. The delayed onset of the hemolysis was attributed to the rate of TNT metabolism. A dose-response relationship in developing hemolysis was postulated, but environmental measurements and biomonitoring of TNT were not done (38,39).

Aplastic anemia has been described (11,18,20,40). Early symptoms include weakness, loss of appetite and weight, mild cough, and nose bleeding. This complication has a high fatality rate. TNT-induced aplastic anemia occurs in sensitive or susceptible workers with exposures of 1 to 10 mg/m³. As work conditions improved after World War I, the incidence has declined (41). Reduction of exposure to below 1.5 mg/m³ has nearly eliminated the problem (41).

Other reported hematologic abnormalities include anemia, usually normochromic with reticulocytosis, leukopenia, leukocytosis, and eosinophilia (40,41).

TNT is known to cause toxic hepatitis that is often associated with aplastic anemia. Although this is a rare complication, it carries a 30% mortality. Severe hepatic injury can be manifested by jaundice, which can be considered a late sign. This is often appreciated only in the conjunctiva because the skin of these workers may already be dyed yellow by the TNT itself. Nausea, vomiting, and enlargement of the liver may accompany the jaundice (3,17,20,21). This grave outcome was observed after exposure to high levels of TNT, in the range of 6 mg/m^3 (40). Lower levels of exposure of 0.6 to 0.8 mg/m^3 resulted in significant increases in glutamic oxalacetic transaminase and lactic dehydrogenase (42). These abnormalities were suggested to be reversible (41). A dose-response relationship was found between occupational TNT liver damage and the amount and the frequency of drinking alcohol. No relationship was found with smoking (43). It was hypothesized that combined depression of hepatic glutathione by ethanol and TNT might be responsible for this finding.

OPHTHALMOLOGIC EFFECTS

TNT causes retrobulbar neuritis and punctate and flame-shaped retinal hemorrhages with papillitis followed by hemorrhage into the vitreous. However, the most common effect is cataract formation, first described in 1953 (44). Harkonen described bilateral symmetric, equatorial continuous, or annular opacities in 6 out of 12 TNT workers. The cataracts did not interfere with visual acuity or vision fields. TNT air concentrations ranged from 0.14 to 0.58 mg/m^3. The authors postulated TNT induced peroxidation damage of the more vulnerable lens periphery with newly formed fiber constituents in the equatorial area (26). Other studies found cataracts in 34.6% to 54.7% of workers, reaching 88.4% in those exposed more than 20 years. The youngest subject was 22 years old, and the shortest latent period was 3 years (45,46). The characteristic lens finding included peripheral circular or cuneiform gray-yellow dot opacities; central circular, discal, or petaline opacities; and a transparent zone between the circular shadow and the lens equator (45). It was assumed that lens changes depended on duration of exposure and on TNT body concentration (46). Once exposure ceased, progression of cataracts could be halted but not reversed (26).

In a recent study, 63% of 61 U.S. explosives plant workers were found to have asymptomatic anterior cortical opacifications of the crystalline lens in a pattern of peripheral flecks. Air levels were generally below 0.5 mg/m^3. Workers exposed to TNT were 18 times more likely to have flecks than the control group (p <.001). Duration of exposure was associated with the development of lenticular changes. Cataracts were not associated with other known risk factors. It is of interest that the prevalence of lenticular damage seems to increase with the increase in TNT-Hb adduct level. No cataract was found in workers with TNT-Hb adduct level below 140 ng/g Hb, even for employment of up to 20 years. It was hypothesized that an eye lens adduct with TNT can also be formed. A long life span of eye lens protein could explain why TNT cataract is irreversible or persistent (33).

OTHER EFFECTS

Less serious or less frequently encountered toxic effects of TNT include gastritis (with nausea, anorexia, vomiting, and epigastric pain); constipation; peripheral neuritis; headache; myocardial irregularities; and upper respiratory complaints (irritation, sneezing, cough) (17,20,21,41,47,48).

MUTAGENICITY

Urine of workers occupationally exposed to TNT was found to be mutagenic in *Salmonella typhimurium* strains. Bacterial nitroreductase activity was not significantly responsible for the mutagenicity. 4-ADNT, but not TNT, concentrations correlated significantly with urinary mutagenicity (27). The less important TNT metabolite 2,4-diamino-6-nitrotoluene was not mutagenic in *Escherichia coli* (49). The Salmonella fluctuation test showed both TNT and its metabolites to be mutagenic (50). Mammalian assays of genotoxicity are contradictory with positive results in mouse lymphoma assay and negative results in micronucleus assay in mouse bone marrow and unscheduled DNA synthesis in rat liver (51,52).

CARCINOGENICITY

Limited carcinogenicity testing of TNT was negative (41). A case-control study of a German community with an increased risk of acute myelogenous leukemia and chronic myelogenous leukemia did not find an association with local TNT contamination of soil and water (53).

REPRODUCTIVE

Three Chinese studies performed in two plants investigated the male reproductive hazard of TNT. Compared to control group, TNT-exposed workers complained more of impotence, loss of libido, and sexual hypoesthesia. The volume of semen and percentage of motile spermatozoa were significantly decreased, and sperm malformations increased. Serum testosterone levels were decreased whereas levels of luteinizing hormone and follicle-stimulating hormone were increased. In addition, lower semen concentrations of several metals were found in the exposed group. TNT concentrations in these plants exceeded 1 mg/m^3 (54–56).

Diagnostic Testing

BIOLOGIC MONITORING AND HEALTH SURVEILLANCE

Urine concentrations of TNT, 4-ADNT, and 2-ADNT metabolites in exposed workers ranged from 4 to 43 μg/L, 14 to 16,832 μg/L, and 24 to 5787 μg/L, respectively (30). Lower levels of urine ADNT metabolites were found postshift in 219 workers of an explosives factory, mean 9.7 ± 7.9 mg/L (standard deviation) (28). Another study in TNT employees found a mean urine TNT concentration of 0.15 μmol/mol creatinine, and mean 4-ADNT and 2-ADNT concentrations of 25.8 μmol/mol creatinine and 5.55 μmol/mol creatinine (27). The differences among the studies probably reflect different exposures.

End-of-shift methemoglobin level of 1.5% was suggested as a biologic exposure index, but it is not specific (57). Blood TNT-Hb adduct level below 140 ng/g Hb was not associated with cataract even for long duration of exposure, up to 20 years. Increasing levels of TNT-Hb adducts were associated with increased prevalence of cataracts (33).

Because urine metabolites were too high in comparison with the environmental levels, it seems that biomonitoring of workers is preferable to assessing occupational exposure by environmental monitoring (58). This could be accomplished by measurement of urine TNT metabolites and blood TNT-Hb adducts.

Trinitrotoluene and Metabolites. Methods for the determination of TNT and metabolites in urine include GC ^{63}Ni-electron capture detection, micro liquid chromatography/MS, and GC/MS selected ion monitoring (29–31,59). In most cases the highest concentrations are found in postshift urine samples. A substantial day-to-day variation in urinary concentrations of ADNT metabolites was observed on postshift samples. In some cases, higher concentrations of the metabolites were seen in the morning after exposure compared to postshift samples. Preshift urine ADNT concentrations at the beginning of a workweek were low (28). No correlation was found between urine and air concentration of TNT. Calculation of uptake through inhalation gave a much lower figure than the total uptake estimated from urine concentrations of ADNT metabolites. This indicates the importance of dermal absorption of TNT and the need to set a biologic exposure limit (27).

TNT residue can be detected on hands after contact using an enzyme-linked immunosorbent assay. This enables detection of 50 pg of TNT (60). Two colorimetric assays exist for the detection of TNT metabolites in the urine, but neither test correlates with severity of intoxication and they may provide false-negative results (32,40).

Trinitrotoluene-Hemoglobin Adducts. Human exposure to carcinogens can be detected by using DNA or Hb adducts as dosimeters. TNT binds covalently with macromolecular proteins, including Hb. The use of TNT-Hb adduct as a biomarker for monitoring human exposure to TNT was studied in 117 workers. Inhaled TNT and skin exposure was used to determine external exposure. Blood TNT-Hb adduct levels correlated with external exposure. Only trace amounts of TNT-Hb adduct were found in control subjects.

The prevalence of lenticular damage seemed to increase with the increase of TNT-Hb adduct level (33). Other researchers used GC/MS with negative ion chemical ionization for the determination of TNT-Hb adducts (58). There are several advantages of using blood TNT-Hb adduct as a biomarker for TNT exposure: the life span of Hb adduct is 18 weeks and it can be detected long after exposure, it correlates with exposure level, and it reflects all routes of exposure (33).

ACUTE OR CHRONIC EXPOSURE

Assessment of TNT toxicity should involve the following tests: complete blood count (CBC; including white blood cells, differential count and peripheral blood smear for signs of red blood cell destruction), liver enzymes, bilirubin, blood urea nitrogen, creatinine, arterial blood gases (ABG; to assess acid-base status and hypoxemia), and methemoglobin (40,41). Oxygen saturation reading by pulse oximeter could be inaccurate in the presence of methemoglobin, and a co-oximeter should be used.

G6PD levels may be determined before employment or after a hemolytic episode. Bone marrow aspiration or biopsy should be considered when aplastic anemia is suspected. Ophthalmologic evaluation includes transillumination and slit-lamp examination or slit-lamp biomicroscopy and direct ophthalmoscopy after maximal pupillary dilation (26,44,45).

Treatment

Treatment of TNT intoxication should include immediate removal of the patient from the source of exposure coupled with symptomatic and supportive measures. Contaminated skin or eye contact should be promptly treated with irrigation with large amounts of water. Methemoglobinemia should be treated with methylene blue if patients are symptomatic, at high risk (e.g., anemia, chronic obstructive pulmonary disease, and coronary heart disease), and in any case in which the methemoglobin level exceeds 20% to 30% (Chapter 63). Caution should be exercised in using methylene blue in G6PD-deficient patients.

Exchange transfusion and hyperbaric oxygen can be considered in refractory cases or when a contraindication to methylene blue exists (Chapter 21). Bone marrow transplantation is an option in patients with TNT-induced aplastic anemia, but experience is lacking.

It is important to institute preventive measures: protective clothing, eye and respiratory protection, daily change of clothes, cleansing showers, exhaust ventilation with wet scrubbers, adequate ventilation, routine medical examinations, and biologic monitoring (14,21,22).

DINITROTOLUENE

Dinitrotoluene [DNT; $CH_3C_6H_3(NO_2)_2$, MW 182.14 g/mol; CAS Registry No. 25321-14-6 (DNT), 121-14-2 (2,4-DNT)] is an aromatic nitro compound. It is used in the munitions industry in the manufacture of explosives, in the chemical synthesis of TNT, as a modifier for smokeless gunpowder, and as a gelatinized and waterproofing agent in military and explosives compositions. Other major uses are the production of toluene diisocyanate and toluenediamine for the formulation of dyes (57,61,62). There are six isomers of DNT: 2,3-DNT, 2,4-DNT, 2,5-DNT, 2,6-DNT, 3,4-DNT, and 3,5-DNT. The most important isomer is 2,4-DNT (22,57,61).

Physicochemical Properties

DNT is manufactured by nitration of toluene. Pure DNT isomers are orange-yellow crystalline solid with a characteristic odor. The isomeric mixture is an oily liquid. DNT is slightly soluble in water (0.27 g/L), soluble in alcohol and ether, and soluble in acetone. The boiling point is 250°C. Boiling and melting points of 2,4-DNT are 300°C and 71°C, respectively. Contact of DNT with strong oxidizers may cause fire and explosion. It reacts with caustics and metals such as tin and zinc. When heated to decomposition, DNT emits toxic fumes of oxides of nitrogen. Decomposition products also include carbon monoxide and carbon dioxide. In addition, closed containers may explode when heated (22,57,61).

Toxic Dose

Occupational standards and guidelines are provided in Table 2.

Toxicokinetics and Toxicodynamics

DNT is readily absorbed, mainly percutaneously and less by ingestion and inhalation (63,64). In an *in vitro* study of human and rat liver under aerobic conditions, subcellular fractions showed that the major 2,6-DNT metabolite formed by hepatic microsomes was 2,6-dinitrobenzylalcohol, and under anaerobic conditions mainly 2-amino-6-nitrotoluene was formed. The microsomal metabolism was probably mediated by cytochrome P-450. Liver cytosolic fractions were also found to metabolize 2,6-DNT, a process supported by hypoxanthine, the reduced form of nicotinamide adenine dinucleotide phosphate, and the reduced form of nicotinamide adenine dinucleotide (65). Urine from exposed workers contained 2,4- and 2,6-DNT as well as the metabolites 2,4- and 2,6-dinitrobenzoic acid, 2,4- and 2,6-dinitrobenzyl glucuronide, 2-amino-4-nitrobenzoic acid, and 2-(*N*-acetyl)amino-4-nitrobenzoic acid. 2,4-Dinitrobenzoic acid and 2-amino-4-nitrobenzoic acid are the main metabolites, accounting for 76% to 86% of DNT metabolites detected (66). 2,4-Diaminotoluene is formed by anaerobic metabolism of 2,4-DNT by human fecal material or rodent cecal microflora via nitroso-intermediates (67). The highest levels of urine DNT metabolites were found in end-of-shift samples with considerable variations (63,64). Females appeared to excrete more dinitrobenzyl glucuronide (64). Most urinary metabolites related to exposure during an 8-hour shift are excreted by the start of work the following day (64). The calculated half-time for elimination of total DNT-related material detected in the urine was

1.0 to 2.7 hours. Half-lives for individual metabolites ranged from 0.8 to 4.5 hours (66).

Pathophysiology

DNT causes methemoglobinemia by oxidizing Hb. Methemoglobinemia is the main acute toxic effect of DNT (17,61,67).

Several experimental studies are suggestive of other possible mechanisms of toxicity. Repeated *in vivo* exposure of rats to 2,4- or 2,6-DNT was associated with dysplasia and rearrangement of aortic smooth muscle (68). *In vitro* exposure of rat aortic smooth muscle cells to DNT metabolites 2,4- or 2,6-diaminotoluene inhibited DNA synthesis, a response comparable to that seen in medial smooth muscle cells isolated from DNT-treated animals (69). Rats given 14 or 35 mg/kg/day DNT in their diet developed degenerative and proliferative changes in the hepatocytes (61). 2,6-DNT was a mild sensitizer in guinea pigs, whereas the other 5 DNT isomers were inactive (61).

Ingestion of alcohol may increase the susceptibility to DNT (70).

Clinical Presentation

HEMATOLOGIC EFFECTS

Methemoglobinemia is the main acute toxic effect. It can occur after dermal, inhalation or oral exposure and results in nausea, vomiting, dyspnea, chest pain, headache, irritability, dizziness, drowsiness, metabolic acidosis, unconsciousness, respiratory depression, and death. Cyanosis is apparent at a methemoglobin level of approximately 10% to 15%. The onset of methemoglobinemia can be delayed for several hours (57,61,67,70,71). The severity of the manifestations depends on the degree of methemoglobinemia and presence of underlying conditions such as anemia and heart and lung diseases.

CARDIOVASCULAR EFFECTS

Tachycardia, chest pain, and hypotension can occur as a result of methemoglobinemia, depending on its severity and the presence of risk factors. Exposure to DNT in two cohorts of 156 and 301 munitions workers was associated with increased mortality from ischemic heart disease. In addition, a 15-year latency and a relationship with duration and intensity of exposure were reported (72). However, this finding was not confirmed in a later retrospective cohort mortality study of 4989 workers exposed to DNT. Mortality from ischemic heart disease was close to that expected, and mortality from cerebrovascular disease was slightly lower than that expected (73).

NEUROLOGIC EFFECTS

Acute neurologic manifestations are generally attributed to methemoglobinemia. Neuropathy manifested as tingling and numbness of the toes was observed in a worker exposed to DNT during its manufacture. Symptoms began after a year, worsened over 2 more years, and improved a year after cessation of work (74). Seizures occurred in mice exposed to lethal doses of DNT (75). Repeated administration of DNT to dogs resulted in tremor, extensor rigidity, and abnormal cerebellar histopathologic changes (61,62).

HEPATIC EFFECTS

DNT was reported to cause acute toxic hepatitis in men (73). Degenerative and proliferative hepatocyte changes were found in rats with repeated oral exposure (61).

OPHTHALMOLOGIC EFFECTS

Vision acuity deteriorated in a worker employed in nitration of mononitrotoluene to DNT for 3 years and improved after a year without exposure (74). There are conflicting data about the ocular irritancy potential of DNT (57,61).

DERMATOLOGIC EFFECTS

On patch testing, DNT gave an allergic reaction in workers from the explosives industry (76). Some isomers of DNT were skin irritants or sensitizers in rabbits and guinea pigs, respectively. The main isomer, 2,4-DNT, was neither irritant nor sensitizer (61,62).

OTHER EFFECTS

Repeated or prolonged exposures to DNT can result in hemolytic anemia with Heinz bodies (62). Renal injury is possible after hemolysis.

GENOTOXICITY

Technical grade DNT gave positive results in unscheduled DNA synthesis in rats (mainly 2,6-DNT), *S. typhimurium* (all isomers), and mouse lymphoma cells (mainly 2,4-DNT) (61,75,77,78). The only isomer active for binding to DNA is 2,6-DNT, requiring reductive metabolism (61,67). Negative results were obtained in induction of mutations in cultured Chinese hamster ovary cell and in induction of dominant lethal mutations in male rats (61,78). Induction of sex-linked recessive mutations in *Drosophila* and induction of sister chromatid exchange in cultured Chinese ovary cells gave mixed results (61). Mixed and isolated isomers of DNT did not cause morphologic transformation in Syrian embryo cells (79).

CARCINOGENICITY

Several experimental studies showed mainly 2,6-DNT, but also 2,4-DNT, to cause cancers of liver, gallbladder and kidneys, and benign tumors of connective tissues (69). However, several oncogenicity assays yielded conflicting results on DNT hepatocarcinogenicity, probably related to pronounced differences in the activity of DNT isomers used (80).

In humans, one study failed to demonstrate a carcinogenic effect in two small cohorts of munitions workers (72). However, larger epidemiologic studies found an association with cancer. Standardized mortality ratio of hepatobiliary cancer of 4989 workers exposed to dynamite was 2.67 [95% confidence interval (CI), 0.98 to 5.83] and 3.88 (95% CI, 1.04 to 14.4) based on comparison with the U.S. population and the unexposed control group, respectively. No exposure-response relationship could be demonstrated between duration of exposure to DNT and hepatobiliary cancer mortality. The study was limited by the small number of workers with long duration of exposure to DNT and lack of quantitative data on exposure to DNT and other chemicals (81).

A German study revealed six cases of urothelial cancer and 14 cases of renal cell cancer in a group of 500 copper mining workers with high exposures to technical DNT. The incidence of these cancers was higher by 4.5 and 14.3, respectively, than that anticipated based on the German cancer registry. Genotyping of these patients revealed them to be slow acetylators (82). In 1996, the International Agency for Research of Cancer classified 2,4- and 2,6-DNT as possibly carcinogenic to humans (group 2B), based on inadequate evidence in humans and sufficient evidence in experimental animals. 3,5-DNT was not classifiable as to its carcinogenicity in humans, as there was inadequate evidence in humans and animals (83).

REPRODUCTIVE

Nonfunctioning ovaries were seen in female mice orally exposed to technical grade DNT (61). No teratogenicity or embryotoxicity was observed in several rat studies (67,84,85). Two studies on spontaneous abortion in 30 wives of exposed workers and 20 workers gave positive and negative results, respectively (61,62). It should be remembered that DNT workers are at risk for methemoglobinemia. The fetus is at larger risk because of the longer half-life of fetal methemoglobin and its susceptibility to hypoxic insult.

Although reduced sperm count was found in nine workers, male fertility was not found to be affected in follow-up studies (61,62). Among 84 workers exposed to DNT and toluene diamine in the production of toluene diisocyanate and polyurethane plastics, no difference was found in urogenital examination, reproductive and fertility questionnaire, testicular volume, serum follicle-stimulating hormone and sperm count, and morphology compared to nonexposed workers (86). Experimental studies on male reproduction showed testicular toxic insults with decreased or absent sperm counts and decreased fertility (63,67,87).

Diagnostic Testing

BIOLOGIC MONITORING AND HEALTH SURVEILLANCE

Methemoglobin concentration of 1.5% was set as the Biologic Exposure Indices (BEI) for methemoglobin-inducing agents (88). Levels of 2,4-DNT and 2,6-DNT in urine of workers from an ammunition dismantling shop were found to be 2 to 9 μg/L (30). Employees of a DNT manufacturing facility had urine DNT and metabolite concentrations greater than 38 μg/L (87). The range of urinary 2,4-dinitrobenzoic acid (the main DNT metabolite) concentrations in workers for an explosives disposal area was 1 to 95 μg/L (89).

DNT and its metabolites can be detected in urine using spectrophotometric analysis and GC/MS methods (30,89,90). The urinary biomarkers α_1-microglobulin, glutathione-*S*-transferase α and glutathione-*S*-transferase π were suggested to be indicative of tubular damage in DNT-exposed miners in a dose-dependent fashion (91).

ACUTE OR CHRONIC EXPOSURE

Measurement of 2,4-DNT and its metabolites can be used in the occupational setting but has no role in treating the acutely intoxicated patient. In the latter situation, repeated methemoglobin levels and ABG for the assessment of acid-base status and hypoxemia are needed (Chapter 21). Other laboratory tests include CBC and kidney and liver function tests. Ancillary tests include electrocardiogram (ECG) and chest radiograph in symptomatic patients or in those with underlying disease.

Treatment

Exposed victims should be moved from the toxic environment. Contaminated clothing should be removed at once and the skin be washed with copious amounts of water and soap. It should be emphasized that DNT is dermally absorbed and can cause systemic toxicity. Exposed eyes should be irrigated. Support of respiratory and cardiovascular functions must be initiated immediately.

In case of ingestion, induction of emesis is not recommended because of the potential for central nervous system (CNS) depression. Gastric lavage and administration of activated charcoal may be considered soon after ingestion, provided airways are protected.

Methemoglobinemia may be treated with methylene blue in symptomatic patients, methemoglobin levels exceeding 20% to 30% or lower in patients with predisposing conditions such as anemia, and respiratory and heart diseases (Chapter 21). Hyperbaric oxygen or exchange transfusion may be considered in refractory patients or when contraindication to administration of methylene blue exists (e.g., G6PD deficiency) (Chapter 63).

Prevention of exposure is needed and important. Protective measures are similar to those suggested with TNT.

1,3-DINITROBENZENE

1,3-Dinitrobenzene [1,3-DNB; $C_6H_4(NO_2)_2$, MW 168.12 g/mol; CAS Registry No. 99-65-0] is another aromatic nitro compound. It is the economically important isomer of three DNB isomers. 1,3-DNB caused poisoning in munitions workers at the end of the nineteenth century and during World War I (92). It is used as an intermediate in the production of explosives such as TNT, aniline dyes, aramid fibers, and spandex fibers. Other uses include reagent for the detection of 17-ketosteroids and for selective weed control (57).

Physicochemical Properties

1,3-DNB is manufactured by a two-stage nitration process. The final product is a yellowish to pale white crystalline solid. 1,3-DNB is insoluble in water (0.02%) and soluble in ether, acetone, hot benzene, and pyridine. Boiling point is approximately 300°C, and melting point is 80° to 90°C. The substance is combustible and reacts with strong oxidizers, caustics, and metals such as zinc and tin. Prolonged exposure to fire and heat may result in an explosion due to spontaneous decomposition. Exposure to shock may also result in explosion (22,23,57,75).

Toxic Dose

Occupational standards and guidelines are provided in Table 2. The lowest published toxic dose reported in humans was 2 mg/kg/day, dermally, causing cyanosis. The lowest lethal human dose was 28 mg/kg orally (57). Testicular lesions were readily apparent in rats at 25 mg/kg, but none were observed in hamsters at 50 mg/kg (93).

Toxicokinetics and Toxicodynamics

1,3-DNB is readily absorbed orally, dermally, and by inhalation (17,57,92,94). Extensive first-pass metabolism was found in an isolated vascularly perfused rat small intestine study (95). Experimental studies showed that the compound is metabolized by nitroreduction. The reduced form of nicotinamide adenine dinucleotide phosphate–cytochrome P-450 reductase was responsible for the reduction in microsomal incubations of isolated perfused rat duodenum and rat liver. This step is followed by hydroxylation of the benzene ring. Major metabolites formed include 2,4-diaminophenol, 1,3 diaminobenzene, 3-nitroaniline, and 2-amino-4-nitrophenol. Some of these metabolites undergo glucuronidation and to a lesser extent sulfation. Other metabolites found in much smaller quantities include 2,4-dinitrophenol, 4-amino-2-nitrophenol, 3-nitrosonitrobenzene, 3-nitrophenylhydroxylamine, and 3,3-dinitroazooxybenzene. Replacement of a nitro group by glutathione is not an important route for metabolism of 1,3-DNB but rather for 1,2- and 1,4-DNB (57,96–99). A Russian rabbit study from 1945 suggested that the kidneys convert DNB to m-nitroaniline before excreting both compounds, in addition to rapid conversion of DNB by the liver (100). It is unclear what isomers of DNB were used in this study.

After administration of 1,3-DNB to rabbits, 65% to 93% of the dose was eliminated in the urine over 2 days as free and conjugated metabolites. Feces contained between 0.3% and 5.2% of the dose (57). Other studies with radiolabeled 1,3-DNB in rats found that urine excretion accounted for 60% to 85% of the dose, and 18% of the dose was excreted in the feces (96,101). In rats, elimination half-life was approximately 10 hours after a single oral dose (57).

It seems that peak blood concentrations of 1,3-DNB were lower and declined more slowly as animal age increased. This was suggested to indicate a slower rate of metabolism and a possible increase in volume of distribution (102). It should be noted that biotransformation of DNB varies between the different isomers and different animal species (96,103).

Pathophysiology

As other aromatic nitro compounds, DNB oxidizes oxyhemoglobin to form methemoglobin (57). DNB is 20 times more potent than TNT as a methemoglobin producer (17).

1,3-DNB was reported to be a neurotoxin producing selective brain lesions. Experimental studies showed the primary cellular targets to be astrocytes, oligodendrocytes, and vascular elements with secondary neuronal involvement. It was suggested to interfere with intracellular redox mechanisms resulting in impaired glucose oxidation and generation of free radicals (104,105). *In situ* nitroreduction of 1,3-DNB may be responsible for its neurotoxicity, or this may be the result of a direct effect on brain endothelial cells (106,107). Neurotoxicity seemed to increase with reduced brain glutathione. Both concentration and time of exposure thresholds need to be exceeded for such toxicity to occur (108,109).

1,3-DNB is also a potent testicular toxicant. Varying degrees of testicular DNB reductive capacity and DNB-induced adenosine triphosphate depletion were found. This may explain species differences in susceptibility to DNB-induced testicular toxicity (110). DNB also caused apoptosis of testicular tubules, but this could be a late manifestation (111).

Clinical Presentation

HEMATOLOGIC EFFECTS

Methemoglobinemia is the major acute toxic effect of 1,3-DNB. It is manifested by headache, dyspnea, chest pain, dizziness, confusion, difficulty in concentration, and cyanosis (17,92,112–114). Methemoglobin levels after occupational exposure to p-DNB ranged from 3.8% to 41.2% (114). Hemolytic anemia with Heinz body formation followed by reticulocytosis has been reported after acute or occupational exposure. Blood morphology indicated erythropoietic damage and included megaloblastosis, karyorrhexis, atypical mitosis of normoblasts, and increases in siderocytes and sideroblasts. Recovery from the anemia was prolonged (17,92,115,116).

CARDIOVASCULAR EFFECTS

Tachycardia, palpitations, chest pain, and hypotension could result from methemoglobinemia, depending on its severity and underlying conditions such as anemia and cardiorespiratory disorders.

DERMATOLOGIC EFFECTS

Yellowish discoloration of the skin was noted after surface contact in workers (17,112).

OPHTHALMOLOGIC EFFECTS

Most of the data on the ocular toxicity of DNB originated in reports from the early 1900s. Vision disturbances from DNB appear after long occupational exposure and are often precipitated by a brief increase in intensity of exposure. This is characterized by retrobulbar neuritis manifested by marked reduction in visual acuity, central scotomas (particularly for red and green), and slight contraction of the vision fields. Occasional findings include partial optic atrophy and retinal hemorrhage. Discontinuation of exposure can result in gradual recovery of the vision. It should be noted that this type of toxicity is not characteristic for nitrobenzene or trinitrobenzene. Surface contact may dye the conjunctiva and cornea yellowish (92,112).

NEUROLOGIC EFFECTS

Neurologic manifestations such as headache, dizziness, impaired concentration, and confusion are usually the result of methemoglobinemia. Chronic poisoning with DNB was also reported to cause burning pain and paresthesia of the feet, ankles, hands, and forearms. No motor involvement was seen in this peripheral nerve neuropathy (92,112). After discontinuation of exposure, general improvement was noted in one patient (92). Seizures associated with methemoglobinemia were observed in one patient exposed to p-DNB (114).

Animal studies provide most of the information on the neurotoxicity of 1,3-DNB. It is possible that the doses used in these studies exceeded doses encountered in occupational human exposure, thus explaining the paucity of human reports of toxicity. Exposure of rats to 1,3-DNB caused ataxia and brain stem lesions (104,108,117). Histologic findings consisted of symmetric vacuolated lesions of cerebellar roof, vestibular and superior olivary nuclei, and the inferior colliculi. These lesions were associated with petechial hemorrhages (104,118). 1,3-DNB typically produced astrocyte swelling as well as blood–brain barrier breakdown (107,117,118). Lesions could be produced within 2 days of repeated administration of 10 mg/kg 1,3-DNB orally (104,118). Gliovascular lesions in the rat brain stem may involve the nuclei of the auditory pathway resulting in functional deficit (119).

HEPATIC EFFECTS

Exposure to DNB and TNT was associated with toxic hepatitis and jaundice during munitions production in both world wars (17,92). Liver damage along with anemia and CNS disorders was produced in dogs. Liver histopathologic findings consisted of structural changes, atrophy, necrosis, and fatty degeneration (120).

MUTAGENICITY

Conflicting results were reported on the mutagenicity of 1,3-DNB in different *S. typhimurium* strains (57,121,122).

CARCINOGENICITY

1,3-DNB has not been classified (57).

REPRODUCTIVE

1,3-DNB is a well-known animal testicular toxin. It was shown to produce marked testicular damage, infertility, and possibly sterility from a single exposure (123). Damage consists of reduced testicular and epididymal weight, degeneration, atrophy, necrosis, germ cell formation, vacuolation, and abnormalities of spermatogenesis (123–125). Sperm velocity decreased significantly and correlated with a decline in sperm fertility (126). The effect of 1,3-DNB on the testes was direct and not through alterations in leuteinizing hormone, follicle-stimulating hormone, and gonadotropin-releasing hormone (127). Recovery from the toxicologic insult on the testes was slow and incomplete (128). Species differences exist, the hamster being less susceptible than the rat (93). In contrast to 1,3-DNB, the two other isomers of DNB did not demonstrate testicular toxicity (129).

Diagnostic Testing

BIOLOGIC MONITORING AND HEALTH SURVEILLANCE

Blood levels of 1,3-DNB can be determined by polarographic method, enzyme-linked immunosorbent assay, HPLC with ultraviolet (UV) and radiochemical detection, and capillary GC (130–132). The latter method was also used for determination of 1,3-DNB metabolites (132). GC/MS selected ion monitoring was used for urine detection of 1,3-DNB (5). Blood and urine levels of DNB are not readily available and are not clinically useful. As for other methemoglobin-producing agents, methemoglobin level of 1.5% during or at end of shift is suggested as BEI (57).

ACUTE OR CHRONIC EXPOSURE

Other laboratory evaluations should include CBC, blood methemoglobin, liver enzymes, bilirubin, blood urea nitrogen, and creatinine (57). An ECG and chest radiograph may be useful in symptomatic patients, especially those with methemoglobinemia or underlying cardiorespiratory diseases. Other ancillary tests may include ophthalmologic and neurologic evaluations. An electromyogram should be considered if peripheral neuropathy is suspected.

TABLE 3. United States regulatory guidelines and standards for nitroglycerin, ethylene glycol dinitrate, and 1,3-dinitrobenzene

		Concentration mg/m³ (ppm)		
Agency	Description	Nitroglycerin	Ethylene glycol dinitrate	Cyclonite
OSHA (air)	PEL-Ceiling	0.2 (2)	1 (0.2)	Not listed
ACGIH (air)	TLV-TWA	0.5 (0.05)	0.3 (0.05)	0.5 (0.005)
	STEL	None	None	None
NIOSH (air)	REL-TWA	—	—	1.5 (0.16)
	REL-STEL	0.1 (0.01)	0.1 (0.16)	3 (0.32)
	IDLH	75 (8)	75 (12)	None
Conversion factor		ppm × 9.29 = mg/m³	ppm × 6.22 = mg/m³	ppm × 9.25 = mg/m³

ACGIH, American Conference of Governmental Industrial Hygienists; IDLH, immediately dangerous to life or health; NIOSH, National Institute for Occupational Safety and Health; OSHA, U.S. Occupational Safety and Health Administration; PEL, permissible exposure limit; ppm, parts per million; REL, recommended exposure limit; STEL, short-term exposure limit; TLV, threshold limit value; TWA, time-weighted average.

Treatment

Treatment of exposure to 1,3-DNB is similar to that provided in other aromatic nitro compounds such as TNT and DNT.

NITROGLYCERIN

NG (1,2,3-propanetriol trinitrate, glyceryl trinitrate, glycerol nitric acid triester, nitroglycerol, trinitroglycerol, trinitroglycerin; $CH_2NO_3CHNO_3CH_2NO_3$, MW 227.1 g/mol; CAS Registry No. 55-63-0) is a highly explosive organic nitrate compound discovered in 1846. Dynamite was created to reduce the instability of NG. To form dynamite, NG is mixed with a substance such as sawdust, pulpwood, or Fuller's earth to reduce its sensitivity to detonation. NG or dynamite may also be mixed with oxidizers (e.g., ammonium nitrate and sodium nitrate) and EGDN, which lowers its freezing point. To make gelatin dynamite, it is mixed with nitrocellulose gel. NG was used extensively in the manufacture of industrial explosives but its use has gradually declined. In medicine, NG has been used as a vasodilator for the relief of anginal pain of coronary artery disease, management of acute pulmonary edema, and for the relief of esophageal spasm.

The first report on the health hazard of NG appeared in 1890, followed by several other reports (1–4,14,57,133). Kantha hypothesized that NG poisoning was an aggravating factor that contributed to Alfred Nobel's premature death at the age of 63 years (134).

Physicochemical Properties

NG is a highly explosive substance. It is an ester of glycerol produced by nitration of anhydrous glycerol with a mixture of nitric acid and fuming nitric acid (23,57,133). NG is a pale yellow, clear, oily liquid with a sweet, burning taste. It crystallizes in two forms, one of which is labile and the other stable (3,22,23,133). The compound is slightly soluble in water (0.1%), soluble in ethyl alcohol, and miscible with ethyl ether, acetone, benzene, and chloroform (22,57,133). The melting point is 2.8°C and 13.5°C for the labile and stable forms, respectively, and it begins to decompose at 50° to 60°C (22,23). NG is sensitive to mechanical shock, and it is readily detonated by heat or spontaneous chemical reaction. In commercial explosives, its sensitivity is reduced by the addition of an adsorbent such as wood pulp and chemicals such as EGDN and ammonium nitrate (3,22,57,133). On explosion, harmless gases are expected to be produced (23).

Toxic Dose

Occupational standards and guidelines are provided in Table 3. The mean maximal plasma NG level during constant infusion, transcutaneous, or sublingual administration was 1.6 ± 0.6 ng/ml (standard error of the mean) (135). Discussion of therapeutic blood levels of NG is of little use because of the development of tolerance to its hemodynamic effect (136). Doses of NG as low as 8 µg/kg orally, which are in the therapeutic range, were reported to be associated with toxicity (75). Forty mg over a 36-hour period was associated with fatality in an 80-year-old patient (137). The federal drinking water guideline set by the U.S. EPA is 5 µg/L (57).

Airborne concentration of NG in a Swedish explosives plant where excess cardio-cerebrovascular mortality was found ranged between 0.2 to 1.1 mg/m³. Highest levels were found among cartridge fillers and mix house workers (138).

Toxicokinetics and Toxicodynamics

NG is readily absorbed through the skin, by inhalation, and from the sublingual mucosa (3,14,57,139). It is well absorbed orally but is subjected to an extensive first-pass metabolism (57,140). An average plasma concentration of 2.3 mg/ml was found 1 hour after dermal application of 2% NG ointment over an area of 40 cm² (135). Peak plasma NG level was reached 4 minutes and 40 minutes after its sublingual and oral administration, respectively (57,140,141). Protein binding is 11% to 60%, and the volume of distribution is 3 L/kg or 179.6 L according to another report (136,142). NG undergoes denitration in the liver forming 1,2- and 1,3-glyceryl dinitrate metabolites that are slightly active. The glyceryl dinitrate metabolites are then degraded by the same liver enzymes to glyceryl mononitrate (140,141,143). Biotransformation is the result of reductive hydrolysis catalyzed by hepatic glutathione-organic nitrate reductase (57,141,143). Absorption and metabolism of NG was suggested to be nonlinear and variable (144). An *in vitro* study suggested that vascular glutathione-S-transferase of the μ class possesses high metabolic activity toward NG, but the clinical relevance is unknown (145). The main metabolites excreted in the urine include glyceryl mononitrate, glycerol, and 1,2- and 1,3-glyceryl dinitrate (146). The elimination half-life of NG and its metabolites is 1 to 4.4 minutes and 40 minutes, respectively (140–142).

Pathophysiology

NG is converted in smooth muscle to nitric oxide, which interacts with and activates guanylate cyclase. Cyclic guanosine monophosphate (cGMP) is then formed stimulating protein kinase and leading to dephosphorylation of myosin and relaxation of smooth muscle. Reduced sulfhydryl groups are a necessary cofactor (57,67,136,141,147,148). At low doses NG is mainly a ventilator, and at higher doses it produces arterial and arteriolar vasodilation. This leads to varying degrees of reduced venous return, left ventricular end-diastolic volume and pressure, and systemic vascular resistance resulting in a fall in blood pressure and a compensatory increase in heart rate (141,149). Coronary vasodilation induced by NG increases coronary blood flow and ameliorates myocardial ischemia (136,141). *In vitro*, NG was shown to cause relaxation of norepinephrine-contracted vascular smooth muscle (150). Other sites where NG causes relaxation of smooth muscles include meningeal blood vessels, bronchi, biliary tract, gastrointestinal tract, and possibly also the urethra and uterus (141).

Tolerance to vasodilation by NG commonly occurs after prolonged exposure. This is believed to be associated with cellular depletion of sulfhydryl groups and reduced cGMP elevations (136,147,151). On the other hand, sudden discontinuation of chronic exposure to NG may cause unopposed compensatory vasoconstriction resulting in coronary vasospasm with angina, myocardial infarction, and even sudden death (152).

Ethanol may have a synergistic effect with NG causing hypotension and severe intoxication (4,9,57). NG can also cause methemoglobinemia (137).

Clinical Presentation

NG toxicity is seen after occupational exposure by inhalation or dermal routes or after therapeutic intravenous, sublingual, or dermal administration.

CARDIOVASCULAR EFFECTS

NG commonly causes hypotension. Hypotension is initially orthostatic and is frequently associated with reflex tachycardia with palpitations (4,9,57,149,153,154). However, bradycardia due to central α_2-adrenergic effect or in patients with sick sinus node syndrome or in those taking beta-blocking drugs has been reported (149,153). The hypotensive effect may be accentuated by alcohol (141). Accompanying symptoms include weakness, prostration, drowsiness, and diaphoresis (4,57,133).

Anginal pain, acute myocardial infarction, and sudden death were reported in explosives workers after withdrawal from exposure to NG or EGDN. This usually occurs 30 to 65 hours after interruption of exposure in workers continuously exposed for a number of years. Autopsy findings could not explain the sudden death, and the phenomena can be attributed to nonocclusive coronary artery disease due to coronary vasospasm (4,57,150,154–159). Excess cardiac mortality was found among male dynamite workers, with a risk ratio of 2.7 (95% confidence intervals, 1.4 to 5.4) (160).

Most workers employed in the manufacture of explosives adapt to the hypotension, headache, dizziness, and postural weakness within several days. Some workers never adapt and have to be removed from exposure. However, discontinuation of exposure for 2 days may interrupt this adaptation and workers may be subjected to resumed toxicity manifesting itself as the classic *Monday morning headache* (4,14,57,133). Some workers have tried to avoid this by placing NG in their hat bands (14). Tolerance is also observed during therapeutic use of NG, and its magnitude is a function of dosage and frequency of administration (141).

NEUROLOGIC EFFECTS

NG frequently causes a severe throbbing headache known as *NG head*. The headache usually lasts for several hours but can continue for 3 to 4 days (4,7,9,14,22,39,161–163). Dizziness and even syncope may occur due to the vasodilatory effect of NG (3,57,149,154). Prolonged exposure to NG may result in a variety of neuropsychiatric abnormalities. These include tremor, drowsiness, insomnia, confusion, nervousness, pugnaciousness, hallucinations, depression, and acute psychosis. In severe cases, stupor, delirium, seizures, and coma have been reported (9,57,133,157,161). Recovery from depression was reported after 3 years in one patient acutely exposed to poorly packed dynamite containing NG. In a pharmacy technician exposed for 2 years, the symptoms worsened and he committed suicide (161). Peripheral neuropathy was also reported after chronic exposure (4). The risk ratio for mortality from cerebrovascular disease among dynamite workers was 2.4 in one study (95% confidence interval, 0.9 to 6.4) (160).

HEMATOLOGIC EFFECTS

Methemoglobinemia may develop after acute or chronic exposure (3,149–151). Although not a common phenomenon, it may have been a contributory factor in a fatal case (151). An insignificant rise of methemoglobin to a maximum of 1.6% was observed after administration of 4.8 mg NG sublingually to healthy volunteers (164). Leukopenia was reported after chronic exposure to NG and nitroglycol (9).

GASTROINTESTINAL EFFECTS

Nausea, vomiting, anorexia, epigastric pain, and liver function abnormalities have been reported (4,7,57,133,149,161).

DERMATOLOGIC EFFECTS

NG has local irritant action, and it may well act as a sensitizer. Dermal manifestations in workers include irritation at the site of application, skin eruptions of the palms and interdigital spaces, and ulceration of the fingertips and under the nails. The skin may also appear flushed due to venodilation (9,57,133,157,161). Allergic contact dermatitis has occurred rarely after topical application of ointment and transdermal drug delivery systems, and after occupational exposure (76,165). Erythema multiforme due to an NG patch was reported in one patient (166). Cyanosis may be present in the presence of methemoglobinemia.

MUTAGENICITY

NG was found to produce mutations in the *S. typhimurium* assay. No genotoxic effects were found in rats and dogs (75).

CARCINOGENICITY

In experimental animals, NG is an equivocal tumorigenic agent. In rats, liver and testicular tumors were induced after 2-year oral exposure (75). No International Agency for Research of Cancer evaluation of NG carcinogenicity was found.

REPRODUCTIVE

Several reports on the use of NG to induce uterine relaxation or inhibit labor in pregnant women did not find an adverse effect on the fetus or neonate (167–170). The infusion of NG was associated with fetal bradycardia, which was eliminated by a dose reduction (171). No adverse fetal effects were reported in rats and rabbits. Abortions were found in rats after dermal application of 1.4 g/kg and 7 g/kg during organogenesis (172). Other studies reported preimplantation and developmental abnormalities in rats after intraperitoneal injections of 11 mg/kg and 220 mg/kg, respectively (75).

Diagnostic Testing

BIOLOGIC MONITORING AND HEALTH SURVEILLANCE

NG levels can be determined in blood using gas-liquid chromatography with electron capture detector (ECD) and HPLC with thermal energy analyzer detection (135,142,173). Capillary GC methods can simultaneously detect NG and its dinitrate metabolites (139,174). GC/ECD was found to be accurate and sensitive for determining NG on hands (139). The BEI for methemoglobin inducers is 1.5% methemoglobin in blood (88).

ACUTE EXPOSURE

Measurement of NG or its metabolites is not clinically useful. Laboratory evaluation includes methemoglobin level by cooximeter and ABG to assess acid-base status. Other laboratory tests include CBC and liver function tests. ECG and chest radiography are suggested in symptomatic patients or patients with cardiovascular or respiratory diseases.

Treatment

The principle of treatment is to assist ventilation if necessary, maintenance of blood pressure with intravenous crystalloid fluids and vasopressors, and correction of methemoglobinemia (see Trinitrotoluene section and Chapter 21). The airway must be protected as CNS depression or abrupt seizures may ensue in a large overdose.

DECONTAMINATION

Inhalation and dermal exposure to NG should be treated by moving the patient out of the toxic environment, removing contaminated clothing, and thorough irrigation of the skin with soap and water. Exposed eyes should be irrigated and followed by an ophthalmologic examination. Ingestion of a potentially toxic amount can be treated with gastric lavage or activated charcoal. Ingestion of sustained-release preparations may result in a delayed onset of toxicity. Decontamination is not needed for intravenous or sublingual exposure.

Appropriate occupational safety measures, periodic medical examinations, and biologic and environmental monitoring are essential to prevent exposure and protect the workers (133).

ETHYLENE GLYCOL DINITRATE

EGDN (1,2-ethanediol dinitrate, 1,2-dinitroethanediol, ethylene dinitrate, ethylene nitrate, glycol dinitrate, nitroglycol, dinitroglycol; $O_2NOCH_2CH_2ONO_2$; MW 152.06 g/mol; CAS Registry No. 628-96-6) is an aliphatic nitro ester high explosive. It was discovered in 1870 and has been in commercial use since the 1930s to lower the freezing point of NG, thus making it safer. These compounds are the major constituents of dynamite, cordite, and blasting gelatin. Dynamite is made from a mixture of NG and 20% to 90% EGDN. The proportion of EGDN depends on the climate and the season as it is much more volatile than NG with increasing temperatures (57,175). Most exposures to EGDN are occupational (explosives manufacturing, blasting works), usually with a concomitant exposure to NG. Several years after its introduction, unexplained sudden deaths were noted. In 1952, the association with EGDN occupational exposure (with NG) was made (175,176). This phenomenon was called *Monday morning death*. The increasing use of ammonium nitrate–fuel oil and slurry explosives to replace dynamite has greatly decreased the demand for EGDN (57).

Physicochemical Properties

EGDN is produced by nitrating a mixture of glycerin and ethylene glycol in the same reactor in the presence of sulfuric acid (175). It is an odorless, colorless to yellow, oily liquid. EGDN is almost insoluble in water (0.52%) and soluble in ethyl alcohol, ethyl ether, and other nonpolar solvents. The boiling point is 197°C and melting point is –22.3°C. Its vapor pressure rises rapidly with temperature: 0.038 mm Hg at 20°C and 22 mm Hg at 100°C (152- and 44-fold higher than NG, respectively). It is reactive and incompatible with acids and alkalis. EGDN is comparable to NG in explosive energy, but it is less sensitive and more stable. It can detonate at high and low velocities (8000 and 100 to 3000 m/second, respectively) (22,57,175).

Toxic Dose

Occupational standards and guidelines are provided in Table 3. An occupational Swedish study revealed combined EGDN and NG air concentrations of less than 5 mg/m^3 to be associated with symptoms in 276 explosives workers (177). Mean 8-hour time-weighted average (TWA) concentrations of nitrate esters ranging from 0.2 to 1.1 mg/m^3 were associated with excess mortality from cardio-cerebrovascular disease among dynamite workers. Highest levels were found in cartridge fillers and mix house workers (138).

Volunteers exposed to a mixture of NG and EGDN (2 mg/m^3) had an immediate drop in blood pressure and a marked headache. Exposure to 7 mg/m^3 for 25 minutes also caused lowered blood pressure and a slight headache (57).

EGDN blood levels in dynamite production workers were undetectable before work and ranged between 0 to 145 ng/ml after work. Highest levels were noted after frequent skin exposure. During the workweek no persistent trend in blood EGDN concentrations was noted but urine concentrations tended to be higher in the afternoon, in the morning, and in the second half of the week (178).

Toxicokinetics and Toxicodynamics

EGDN is readily absorbed through skin, lungs, and gastrointestinal tract (57,178–180). Skin is the major route of occupational exposure (181). In experimental animals, it penetrates skin more readily than NG (182). In humans, approximately 3 mg of EGDN was absorbed through the skin in 7 hours from a 100-mg dose of EGDN-containing explosive mixture.

EGDN undergoes rapid metabolism to ethylene glycol mononitrate, inorganic nitrites, inorganic nitrates, and ethylene glycol in the liver and blood (57,175,183,184). The metabolic process involves stepwise detachment of organic nitrate groups from the carbon skeleton (179). Reduced glutathione is involved in a reaction catalyzed by organic nitrate reductase (179,185). EGDN does not seem to affect NG metabolism in rats and dogs (186).

Inorganic nitrates are the major compound found in the urine, followed by ethylene glycol mononitrate, EGDN, and little inorganic nitrite or ethylene glycol (57,143,178,179,184). No EGDN could be detected in exhaled air of workers with high skin exposure (181).

After repeated subcutaneous injection of EGDN to experimental animals, its blood level peaked at 30 to 60 minutes and was zero at 8 hours. Inorganic nitrite reached maximum level within 1 to 3 hours and fell to zero within 12 hours. Peak and minimum levels of organic nitrates were found at 3 to 5 hours and 12 hours, respectively (143,186). Ethylene glycol reaches its peak in blood in 2 to 3 hours (57). The rate of disappearance of EGDN from human blood *in vitro* was one-half over 20 hours from a sample that contained 0.18 ppm EGDN and gradually decreased to 2 hours in a sample that contained 0.04 ppm (57).

Pathophysiology

EGDN relaxes smooth muscle resulting in vasodilation that is believed to be mediated by cGMP (187,188). Nitrovasodilators are known to act by releasing NO, which is important for regulation of vascular tone through activation of guanylate cyclase and production of cGMP. Thiol-containing compounds are prerequisite for the liberation of NO (188,189).

Vasodilation causes a decrease in blood pressure and reflex tachycardia, as well as an increase in cardiac output and coronary and femoral blood flows (178,190). As EGDN dose increases, coronary blood flow decreases (180). In rats, EGDN was shown to have negative inotropic effect on left and right atria and positive ionotropic effect on right ventricle muscle (191). On the other hand, a rat *in vivo* study showed no effect on cardiac function but increased cardiac sensitivity to exogenous epinephrine (192). A less pronounced decrease in blood pressure was produced by ethylene glycol mononitrate (190).

Repeated exposures of rat aortic strips to EGDN were shown to induce tolerance, probably by interfering with arterial muscle sensitivity to noradrenaline (193). Experimental studies did not demonstrate altered EGDN metabolism after its repeated administration, thus hypothesizing that tolerance is due to a physiologic compensatory mechanism or, less likely, due to undetected changes of metabolism at the cellular level (186). Oxidation of essential sulfhydryl-containing compounds or their cellular depletion may be the reason for nitrate tolerance (189).

Methemoglobinemia may be caused by EGDN, as other nitro compounds (185,194). No effect of EGDN on monoamine oxidase activity was found in rats (195).

Consumption of alcohol may enhance EGDN toxicity in humans (57). Hyperthyroidism increases the acute toxicity of EGDN in rats, whereas hypothyroidism reduces toxicity (57).

Clinical Presentation

Most of the data on the clinical effects of EGDN come from occupational exposures, which, in many cases, also involve NG.

CARDIOVASCULAR EFFECTS

EGDN-induced vasodilation cause a fall in systolic and diastolic blood pressure, reduction in pulse pressure, tachycardia, palpitations, and anginal chest pain (154,179,183,196). Later, diastolic pressure can increase as a result of compensatory vasoconstriction (57). Cardiac dysrhythmias were also noted during occupational exposure (57,197). These manifestations are usually evident at the beginning of employment and at the beginning of the workweek. Tolerance then develops and the rest of the week is relatively free of symptoms.

Chronically exposed workers are seriously threatened by withdrawal from exposure, a phenomenon known as *Monday morning death*. After 6 to 10 years of employment, workers who are no longer exposed to EGDN and NG mixtures may complain of sudden anginal chest pain or even die suddenly. This usually occurs on a Monday or a Tuesday morning, 30 to 64 hours after termination of exposure. It may happen during sleep, just before awakening, or during the first physical efforts on return to work after a holiday or a weekend. An ECG is often misleading and administration of coronary vasodilators, especially NG, ineffective. Autopsies have not revealed the cause of death (154,155,175,176,198–200).

Several mechanisms have been proposed for the sudden death in chronic EGDN exposure: coronary vasospasm occurring after resolution of the vasodilation; sensitization to cardioinhibitory reflexes or a sudden release in catecholamines leading to dysrhythmia or coronary spasm; chronic hypoxemia caused by reduced myocardial oxygen consumption and methemoglobinemia, which is aggravated when coronary vasodilation ceases; and a direct effect on actomyosin (57,154,176,196).

Epidemiologic studies revealed increased risk and excess mortality from chronic cardio-cerebrovascular disease among explosives workers exposed to EGDN and NG (138,201–203). Excess mortality from ischemic heart disease was found mainly among blasting and propellants workers aged 15 to 49 years (201).

NEUROLOGIC EFFECTS

Headache, which can be severe and throbbing, is common. It can begin as a dull pain in the forehead and is often accompanied by dizziness, nausea, vomiting, weakness, and syncope (154,175,177,179,183,196). Tolerance usually develops within several days. Like the cardiovascular effects, these neurologic effects appear at the beginning of employment or after a weekend leave, with common names such as *Monday head* or *nitrate head* (175,186,204). In many of these cases exposure also involves NG. Alcohol may enhance the headache (196).

Mixed high occupational exposure for more than 16 years was found to be associated with a twofold increase in mortality from cerebrovascular disease in propellants workers aged 50 to 64 years (201). Other neurologic effects reported in workers include hyperactivity, nervousness, and peripheral paresthesia (154,175,196). The latter phenomenon appears mainly at night and is attributed to peripheral neuropathy or arteriolar spasm (175). Convulsions were seen in animals administered lethal doses of EGDN (143).

HEMATOLOGIC EFFECTS

Methemoglobinemia and anemia with Heinz body formation have been reported (57,175,182). However, one study of EGDN-exposed workers did not reveal anemia in any of the 485 subjects; four of them had slightly high reticulocytosis and only one out of 342 had Heinz bodies (205). The duration of exposure was unclear in these workers. Chronic experimental poisoning was also associated with bone marrow hyperplasia (57).

OTHER EFFECTS

EGDN can cause skin sensitization as evidenced by allergic reaction on patch testing in humans (76,175). Fatty changes in the liver, kidneys, and heart muscle were observed in experimental animals chronically poisoned with EGDN (57). A single injection of EGDN to rats resulted in a marked increase in plasma corticosterone, probably due to EGDN-induced systemic hypotension leading to pituitary stimulation. Repeated EGDN injections result in a decreased corticosterone response (206).

CARCINOGENICITY

Excess lung cancer was suggested in blasting workers highly exposed to EGDN and NG (201). However, at this point no determination can be made as to EGDN's carcinogenic potential.

Diagnostic Testing

BIOLOGIC MONITORING AND HEALTH SURVEILLANCE

EGDN or its mononitrate metabolite can be determined in blood by a colorimetric method or by GC/ECD. GC and TLC have been used for urine analysis (175,184,207,208). EGDN residues on skin can also be detected by TLC (209). Air EGDN can be determined by field ionization MS (210).

Measurement of urinary EGDN was suggested as a means for assessment of its absorption and monitoring exposure, but its feasibility has not been evaluated (178,179). A blood methemoglobin level of 1.5% during or at end of shift is accepted as a BEI for methemoglobin-producing agents (88).

ACUTE EXPOSURE

Measurement of EGDN and its metabolites may have a role in monitoring occupational exposures, but they are not helpful in acute treatment. Other useful laboratory evaluation tests include CBC, ABG (for evaluation of acid-base status and hypoxemia), and blood methemoglobin level by co-oximeter. ECG and chest radiography should be considered in patients with an underlying cardiorespiratory disease.

Treatment

Treatment of EGDN poisoning is similar to that outlined for NG. Again, prevention of exposure using personal and environmental protective measures, monitoring and medical preemployment, and periodic examinations are extremely important (57,175,183). It should be noted that rubber gloves may absorb a considerable amount of EGDN and let it pass into the skin and blood. Rubber gloves with inner cotton gloves seem to offer some protection if they are changed once or twice an hour (181).

CYCLOTRIMETHYLENETRINITRAMINE

Cyclotrimethylenetrinitramine [cyclonite, hexogen, trimethylenetrinitramine, 1,3,5-trinitrohexahydro-S-triazine, hexahydro-1,3,5-trinitro-1,3,5-triazine, sym-trimethylenetrinitramine, 1,3,5-triazacyclohexane, T4; $N(NO_2)CH_2N(NO_2)CH_2N(NO_2)CH_2$; MW 222.26 g/mol; CAS Registry No. 121-82-4] is a powerful secondary high explosive. The British use it under the name RDX, which is the military name used in the United States. It was discovered in 1879 and was first used on a large scale in World War II. It is used by the military as a base charge for detonators and as an ingredient of bursting charges and plastic explosives. Cyclonite has more shattering power than TNT. It is mixed to form a castable mixture (usually 60% cyclonite: 40% RDX). Cyclonite and TNT mixtures are often found in aerial bombs, mines, and torpedoes. Because it is easily initiated by mercury fulminate, it may be used as a booster. Cyclonite is also used in smokeless powder and as a rat poison (2,3,23,57,61, 211,212). C-4 is a plastic explosive containing 91% cyclonite, 2.1% polyisobutylene, 1.6% motor oil, and 5.3% di-(2-ethylhexyl) sebacate used in the Vietnam War. With ingestion, it can produce an ethanol-like effect and has also been used as cooking oil when other sources were unavailable (213,214). *Semtex* is a plastic explosive containing cyclonite and PETN (57).

Physicochemical Properties

The most common method of manufacturing of cyclonite involves reacting hexamethylenetetramine with ammonium nitrate, concentrated nitric acid, glacial acetic acid, and acetic anhydride. The cyclonite formed in this process is known as *type B* and contains cyclotetramethylenetetranitramine (HMX) as impurity, to contrast it with cyclonite type A, which does not have this impurity. It can also be made by direct nitrolysis of hexamethylenetetramine (2,23,57). Cyclonite forms a white crystalline powder or colorless crystals. It is practically insoluble in water, ethanol, carbon tetrachloride, and carbon disulfide; slightly soluble in ether, ethylacetate, methanol, and glacial acetic acid; and soluble in acetone, hot aniline, phenol, and warm nitric acid. Its melting point is 203° to 206°C (2,23,57). Cyclonite is incompatible with oxidizing materials and combustibles. It can be detonated by sudden heat, shock, or contact with mercury fulminate. When heated to decomposition, cyclonite releases toxic fumes of nitrogen oxides (215).

Toxic Dose

Occupational standards and guidelines are provided in Table 3. Calculated range of no observed adverse effect level of cyclonite based on animal toxicologic studies was 0.03 to 0.3 mg/m^3 (216). Eight-hour TWA exposure in munitions plants where no health effects were found was 0.28 mg/m^3, range 0.01 to 1.57 mg/m^3 (217).

Oral doses of 25 to 180 g of cyclonite-containing C-4 plastic explosive resulted in severe intoxications including seizures in adults (213). Muscle spasms, but not seizures or CNS depression, were observed in an adult worker who intentionally ingested one tablespoon of cyclonite (218). An 18-year-old male developed seizures from inhalation of fumes liberated from C-4 used for cooking and from the small amounts that adhered to the knife used to cut it (214). Seizures were reported in a 3-year-old child who ingested cyclonite in a dose pharmacokinetically estimated to be 84.82 mg/kg (219).

In rats, oral doses as low as 10 to 12 mg/kg induced seizures. Significant seizure incidence was induced by 25 mg/kg and 50 mg/kg, which corresponded to plasma levels of 5.34 and 8.28 μg/ml, respectively (220). The no observable effect level of TNT and cyclonite mixture (1.0:0.62) in dogs was 0.5 mg/kg given over 90 days (221). In another rat study, intraperitoneal injection of 500 mg/kg cyclonite resulted in plasma levels of 5.2 μg/ml at seizure and 13.8 μg/ml at death (222).

An ambient water quality criterion of 103 μg/ml cyclonite was proposed by the EPA for drinking water and aquatic foodstuffs. A criterion of 105 μg/ml was proposed for drinking water alone (223). A lifetime health advisory for cyclonite was calculated by the EPA to be 2 μg/ml (224).

Toxicokinetics and Toxicodynamics

Cyclonite is slowly absorbed orally and from inhalation, and is poorly absorbed dermally (225,226). However, rapid oral absorption may be suggested by the development of seizures in humans 30 to 60 minutes after consumption of food cooked in bowls previously containing cyclonite and other chemicals (227).

The estimated volume of distribution in rats is 2.2 L/kg. Concentration of cyclonite in rats is greatest in the kidneys, most variable in the liver, and no accumulation has been found in the brain. In miniature swine, cyclonite was found in brain, heart, liver, kidneys, and fat (222).

In repeated dosing to rats, there was no accumulation in plasma or any tissue. Most of the cyclonite dose was excreted as exhaled CO_2 and as unidentified metabolites in the urine (228). Another rat study showed that excretion occurred primarily in the feces for up to 21 days and only 1% to 2% was excreted in the urine (219). Metabolism in rats was suggested to depend on hepatic microsomal enzymes (219,229). After a single oral dose, the liver and urine contained large amounts of cyclonite metabolites. After 4 days, 90% of the radioactivity was recovered, 34% in the urine, 43% as exhaled CO_2, 3% in the feces, and 10% in the carcass (222). The disappearance of cyclonite in the rat was biphasic with distribution and elimination half-lives of 6.32 minutes and 10.1 hours, respectively (222).

A toxicokinetic study in a 3-year-old child who ingested cyclonite showed detectable serum and stool levels over 120- and 144-hour periods, respectively. Apparent peak serum levels occurred within 24 hours after ingestion (10.74 mg/L), at approximately 48 hours for urine (38.41 mg/L) and at 96 hours for feces (4.49 mg/g). It has been suggested that cyclonite is concentrated and more slowly excreted in the feces than in the urine (219). Twenty-four–hour cerebrospinal fluid level was 8.94 mg/L with cerebrospinal fluid:serum ratio of 0.832, indicating passage through blood–brain barrier. The elimination half-life was 15.06 hours. Disposition was best described by a linear, one compartment open model, although the data could adequately fit into a two compartment open model (219).

Pathophysiology

The exact mechanism by which cyclonite induces toxicity, especially neurotoxicity, is unknown. The high cerebrospinal fluid:serum cyclonite ratio found in a 3-year-old child suggests extensive distribution and accumulation in the brain (219). Experimental data suggest that limbic structures may participate in cyclonite-induced seizures (220). Acute cyclonite intoxication in rats produced nonspecific vascular changes in the spinal cord and brain stem, but cerebral vessels were minimally affected. Chronic intoxication was associated with more apparent fibrous degeneration in the CNS (230). The convulsant properties of cyclonite are not thought to be due to its metabolites because, in animals, seizures are observed within seconds of infusion (212).

Other pathologic changes in animals include cloudy swelling and degeneration of renal tubular cells and fatty degeneration of the liver (225,231). Cyclonite is also an ocular dermal and respiratory tract irritant (3,212).

Cyclonite is not considered to be a clinically significant methemoglobin-producing agent and does not produce hemolysis (212,218,225). However, methemoglobin levels of up to 4% have been measured in acutely intoxicated patients (213).

Clinical Presentation

Intoxication from cyclonite may occur in three settings. First, manufacturing exposure involves mainly inhalation of dust during processing; fine dust with small particle size is associated with earlier onset of adverse effects and more severe toxicity. Second, battlefront exposure may allow ingestion or inhalation. Finally, non-wartime unintentional exposure may occur (pediatric and adult ingestion) (212,219,232).

NEUROLOGIC EFFECTS

Initial clinical manifestations include headache, nausea, vomiting, malaise, dizziness, sleeplessness, and confusion. These manifestations were reported in occupational exposures and after ingestion of cyclonite. Seizures may follow, but they may also appear without warning, especially after ingestion of a large amount of cyclonite. Onset of seizures is 30 minutes to 12 hours after exposure. The seizures are generalized tonic-clonic or myoclonic and last minutes to several hours. Seizures can recur over 24 to 60 hours and may be resistant to treatment. Between or after seizures, patients can experience confusion, amnesia, lethargy, nausea, vomiting, stupor, hyperirritability, muscle twitching, myalgia, and hyperactive deep reflexes. Some patients may have tachycardia and low-grade fever. Resolution of clinical manifestations is usually seen after 24 hours, but abnormal memory, orientation and attention span, headache, and inability to do simple arithmetic may persist for weeks.

Analysis of cerebrospinal fluid reveals no abnormalities. An electroencephalogram (EEG) done at the time of myoclonic attacks showed bilaterally synchronous and symmetric spike and wave complexes at 2 to 3 per second maximal on the frontal areas at time with multiple spikes, with background frequency of diffuse or random slow transients. An EEG done within 8 days after seizures had stopped still showed the abnormal slow background frequency, but without the bilaterally synchronous spike and wave complexes. The EEG usually normalizes in 1 to 3 months. Computerized tomography and magnetic resonance imaging of the brain did not disclose pathologic findings (212–214,218,219,227,230,232,233).

RENAL EFFECTS

Reversible oliguria, renal insufficiency, proteinuria, and hematuria were observed in some patients. Kidney biopsy in one patient demonstrated mild vacuolation in the proximal tubules with normal glomeruli. These changes could be the result of acute tubular necrosis or administration of mannitol (213,233).

MUSCULAR EFFECTS

Muscle injury due to seizures was suggested by the presence of myalgias, muscle tenderness, and elevated serum aminotransferase levels though muscle biopsy was normal in one patient. The absence of hepatomegaly, absence of other liver enzyme abnormalities, and normal liver biopsy do not support hepatic involvement (213,214,216).

DERMATOLOGIC EFFECTS

A florid petechial rash over the face and trunk similar to that seen with meningococcal infection was reported in one patient. After ruling out meningosepticemia, this was attributed to the tonic phase of severe cyclonite-induced grand mal seizure, which involved a Valsalva-like maneuver (232). Irritant and allergic contact dermatitis of the face and eyelids of workers in cyclonite production appeared to be related to fumes, although the chemical identity was unknown (226). A patch test with moistened cyclonite did not produce irritation (225).

HEMATOLOGIC EFFECTS

Leukocytosis with neutrophilia and mild anemia has occurred in several patients (213,233). Bone marrow aspiration in one patient revealed erythroid hypoplasia and normal marrow iron content consistent with toxic depression of the erythroid series (213). Methemoglobin levels of up to 4% occur rarely (213).

OTHER EFFECTS

A cross-sectional occupational epidemiologic study failed to demonstrate an excess of autoimmune disease or abnormalities of the hematologic, hepatic, or renal systems (217).

MUTAGENICITY

Several studies failed to show cyclonite or aqueous extract of soil contaminated with cyclonite and TNT to be mutagenic (50,234,235). An extract of soil contaminated with cyclonite and TNT was mutagenic in the *S. typhimurium* assay (234).

CARCINOGENICITY

Cyclonite is not classifiable as a human carcinogen (57,75). The EPA classified it as a possible human carcinogen based on hepatocellular adenomas and carcinomas in female mice, but no oncogenic effects were observed in a 2-year rat study using oral doses up to 40 mg/kg. Human carcinogenicity data are lacking (57).

REPRODUCTIVE

Reproductive studies reported in an abstract did not show adverse effects in rats or rabbits (3,57,75). Fetotoxicity was reported in other studies (75).

Diagnostic Tests

BIOLOGIC MONITORING AND HEALTH SURVEILLANCE

Cyclonite levels in human biologic fluids can be analyzed by an HPLC with UV detection (219,236). The lowest detection limit for GC/MS was achieved when the positive ion chemical ionization detection method was used (237). Capillary GC with ECD was used to determine concentrations of cyclonite in drinking water (238).

ACUTE EXPOSURE

Determination of blood and urine cyclonite levels is not clinically useful. Laboratory evaluation should include kidney and liver function tests, electrolytes, creatine kinase, lactate dehydrogenase, CBC, ABG, serum lactate, blood methemoglobin level, and urinalysis. ABG are generally normal, but combined respiratory and metabolic acidosis was reported in a patient with repeated seizures and respiratory arrest (213). Urine myoglobin should be assayed in repeated seizures. Ancillary tests such as ECG, EEG, brain computed tomography, and magnetic resonance imaging should be considered according to the clinical manifestations and the course of intoxication (212,213,219,233).

Treatment

The management of cyclonite intoxication includes respiratory and cardiovascular support. In cases of inhalation, patients should be immediately moved from exposure. Clothes contaminated with cyclonite dust should be removed and the skin thoroughly washed with soap and water. On ingestion, ipecac-induced emesis is not recommended because of the risk of seizures and potential aspiration. Gastric lavage and administration of activated charcoal can be considered, although there is no evidence to support their routine use.

Control of seizures and oxygenation are of utmost importance. Benzodiazepines (diazepam and lorazepam), phenobarbital, and possibly also phenytoin are used to treat seizures (Chapter 40). Maintenance of normal fluid and electrolyte balance is important (212,213,219,233). Some authors have suggested the use of furosemide or mannitol to treat oliguria in well-hydrated patients (213).

There is no antidote for cyclonite, and hemodialysis is not expected to remove significant quantities as the substance is highly lipid soluble (213). Hemodialysis may be required in patients with acute renal failure (214).

Maintenance of adequate occupational hygiene, environmental monitoring, and periodic medical evaluations as outlined in the previous sections of this chapter are needed to protect the workers.

CYCLOTETRAMETHYLENETETRANITRAMINE

HMX (1,3,5,7-tetrazocine actahydro-1,3,5,7-tetranitro, 1,3,5,7-tetranitro-1,3,5,7-tetraazacyclooctane, octogen, β-HMY; $C_4H_8N_8O_8$; MW 296.2 g/mol; CAS Registry No. 2691-41-0) has been used in the manufacture of explosives, as burster charge for artillery shells, component of plastic-bonded explosives, solid fuel rocket propellants, and to achieve critical mass by imploding fissionable material in nuclear devices. Small amounts are formed during the production of a related compound, cyclonite. Wastewater may contain it as a contaminant from munitions plants.

Physicochemical Properties

HMX is produced by a modified Bachman process. The final product is a colorless and odorless solid crystal. Its melting point is 276° to 286°C. HMX is poorly soluble in water (5 mg/L at 25°C) and soluble in dimethylsulfoxide, acetone, cyclohexanone, and acetic anhydride. HMX explodes violently at high temperatures (more than 279°C) (57,239).

Toxic Dose

Occupational standards and guidelines have not been defined. Federal drinking water guideline of 400 μg/L for a lifetime exposure was set by the EPA (57,239). The Agency for Toxic Substances and Disease Registry has derived an acute oral minimal risk level of 0.1 mg/kg/day for HMX. This is based on lowest observed adverse effect level of 100 mg/kg/day for neurologic effects in mice. An intermediate minimal risk level of 0.05 mg/kg/day was derived from no observed adverse effect level of 50 mg/kg/day for hepatic effects in rats exposed for 13 weeks. The lowest observed adverse effect level for skin exposure is 165 mg/kg (239).

Toxicokinetics and Toxicodynamics

There are no available human studies. HMX is poorly absorbed after oral administration in animals. It is unknown whether HMX is absorbed by inhalation or dermally. Peak plasma levels were reached in 6 to 10 hours. The small fraction absorbed (less than 5%) is distributed to the lungs, heart, and kidneys and metabolized to unidentified polar metabolites. Excretion is in the urine (3% to 4%) and in expired air (0.5% to 1.0%). Most of an oral dose is excreted in the feces. Biliary excretion does not seem to contribute significantly.

After parenteral administration to animals, the highest levels were found in the lungs followed by the heart, liver, and kidneys. The lowest levels were found in the fat, testes, and brain. Urine excretion accounted for 61% of the dose, and 6% was expired (239).

Pathophysiology

The mechanism of HMX toxicity is unclear. Generation of toxic metabolites has been proposed. Experimental methemoglobin formation and cardiovascular collapse after exposure to HMX are possibly related to nitrate formation. Possible hydrazine formation was speculated to explain its neurologic and hepatic effects in animals (239).

Clinical Presentation

The toxicity of HMX in humans has not been well studied. A single study in munitions workers exposed to HMX and cyclonite did not find evidence of hematologic, hepatic, or renal toxicity, nor the prevalence of antinuclear antibodies in comparison with a control group. Although cyclonite air levels were measured (up to 1.57 mg/m^3; mean, 0.28 mg/m^3), HMX levels were not determined (217).

Animal studies indicate that HMX causes mainly hepatic and neurotoxicity. Liver effects include hepatocyte hyperplasia, cytoplasmic eosinophilia, mottled appearance, and centrilobular degeneration. Hyperkinesia, hypokinesia, and convulsions may occur after a large oral exposure (more than 1500 mg/kg). Less prominent effects include nephrotoxicity, decreased Hb, and methemoglobinemia. Most toxicity was induced by higher oral doses, although dermal exposure also caused some neurotoxicity. HMX is also a mild skin irritant (75,239).

MUTAGENICITY AND CARCINOGENICITY

HMX was not mutagenic *in vitro* (50,57,239,240). The EPA has determined that HMX is not classifiable as to human carcinogenicity based on lack of cancer bioassays or epidemiologic studies (57,239).

REPRODUCTIVE

Ovaries or testes of mice exposed to HMX orally for 13 weeks showed no gross or histopathologic lesions. Reproductive studies could not be located (239).

Diagnostic Testing

BIOLOGIC MONITORING AND HEALTH SURVEILLANCE

HMX can be analyzed in plasma, urine, and feces by a reverse-phase HPLC with UV detection. TLC has also been used for analysis of HMX in urine and feces. Determination of HMX in water and soil samples is done primarily by an HPLC method, but GC and TLC have also been used (57,238,239,241).

ACUTE EXPOSURE

Analysis of HMX levels has no acute clinical role. It is suggested that laboratory evaluation of exposed individuals should include CBC, liver and kidney functions, and urinalysis. ABG, blood methemoglobin, ECG, and chest radiograph can be considered according to the clinical manifestations.

Treatment

Basic principles of removal from exposure, decontamination, and supportive therapy as well as adequate occupational hygiene should be used in the treatment of exposed and intoxicated patients.

PENTAERYTHRITOL TETRANITRATE

PETN (2.2-Bis [(nitrooxy)-methyl]-1,3-propanediol dinitrate (ester), 1,3-propanediol, 2,2,-bis [(nitrooxy)methyl-,dinitrate (ester)], nitropentaerythritol, pentaerythrityl tetranitrate, pentaerythrite tetranitrate; $C(CH_2NO_3)_4$; MW 316.15 g/mol; CAS Registry No. 78-11-5) is more powerful than TNT and almost as powerful as cyclonite. It is used in the manufacture of detonating fuses, as a demolition explosive, and in blasting caps. When mixed with TNT it is used for loading small caliber projectiles, grenades, and booster charges. It can also be mixed with cyclonite as a plastic-bonded explosive to form Semtex. When combined with TNT, it forms another explosive, pentolite (2,3,23,57,242–245). PETN is used medically as an oral nitrate vasodilator for long-term management of angina pectoris (2,3,57,136,246,247).

Physicochemical Properties

PETN is produced by esterification of pentaerythritol (PE) with nitric acid (2,23,57). It is a white to ivory crystal powder with faint and mild odor. Its boiling point is 180°C at 50 mm Hg and its melting point is 140°C. PETN is practically insoluble in water, sparingly soluble in alcohol and ether, and soluble in benzene and acetone. It explodes on percussion and it is more sensitive to shock than TNT. It detonates at 210°C; may explode when heated strongly, even when dissolved; and decomposes above 150°C. Decomposition products include NO (47.7%), CO (21.0%), NO_2 (11.8%), N_2O (9.5%), CO_2 (6.3%), H_2 (2.0%), and N_2 (1.6%) (2,23,24,242).

For medicinal purposes, PETN is diluted with an inert ingredient, usually lactose or mannitol, to prevent accidental explosions (23,57).

Toxic Dose

Occupational standards and guidelines have not been defined. A threshold limit value–TWA value of 10 mg/m^3 was set for PE (88). As an antianginal drug, PETN can be administered orally in doses of 10 to 40 mg three to four times daily up to 240 mg/day (136,246). The oral median lethal dose in rats is 1660 mg/kg (75).

Toxicokinetics and Toxicodynamics

PETN is readily absorbed from the gastrointestinal tract and to some extent from the oral mucosa. It is also absorbed by inhalation but not appreciably through the skin (57,136,248). Onset of hemodynamic effects was noted 20 to 60 minutes after administration of PETN in tablet form, and it lasted for 4 to 5 hours (57,136).

In rodents, PETN undergoes extensive liver metabolism by glutathione-organic nitrate reductase to PE-trinitrate, PE dinitrate (PEDN), PE mononitrate (PEMN), and PE. PETN and PE-trinitrate were not detected in blood after oral administration whereas PEDN, PEMN, and PE accounted for 33%, 42%, and 20% to 25% of the radioactivity in the blood, respectively. The PE-nitrates are converted to glucuronides, which then undergo further denitration by glutathione-organic nitro reductase. A 2-hour urine collection contained PEDN, PEMN, and PE, but only the latter two were present at 18 hours (143).

After oral administration of 20 or 40 mg ^{14}C-PETN to ten human healthy volunteers, radioactivity was detected in the blood within 15 minutes with peak concentrations at 4 to 8 hours. PETN and PE-trinitrate were not detected in the blood, PEDN was in trace amounts, and PEMN and PE were the major compounds detected. The latter two compounds were the major urinary metabolites and accounted for 50% to 60% of the dose, respectively. Urinary excretion of PETN is first order and dose-dependent. The ratio of PE to PEMN in the urine was 1:1 and 1:3 after a 20-mg and 40-mg dose, respectively. This may suggest a limited capacity of deesterification of PEMN to PE (57,143,249–254). After a single dose of PETN and glyceryl trinitrate to volunteers, 19% of PETN was excreted in the urine as conjugated metabolites in 24 hours (255). Another study showed PEMN to have an elimination half-life of 10 to 11 hours (256). Thirty-two percent to 41% of the dose was eliminated in the feces, partly as unchanged tetranitrate. This suggests partial hydrolysis in the intestine before absorption (57). Glutathione-dependent organic nitrate ester reductase activity of human small intestine extract was four times higher than liver activity for PETN, suggesting biotransformation could occur at the absorption site (257).

After oral or sublingual administration of ^{14}C-PE-trinitrate to humans, it did not appear in the blood. The PEDN was briefly present, and the major circulating form was PE (143). The plasma half-life of PE-trinitrate was suggested to be 10 minutes (258). PE-trinitrate was shown to have one-fifth of the coronary vasodilatory potency of NG and has been used clinically as an antianginal agent (143). It was suggested by another study to possess greater vasodilatory activity than PETN (246,251). The three agents PEDN, PEMN, and PE had 1/50, 1/100, and none of the PE-trinitrate potency, respectively (143).

Pathophysiology

As other antianginal nitrates, PETN causes venous and arterial vasodilation. These lead to decreased venous return with reduced ventricular volume and myocardial tension (preload reduction), and to a decrease in peripheral vascular resistance with reduced blood pressure and ventricular outflow resistance (afterload reduction). The net result is reduced myocardial oxygen requirement (57,136,246,259). PETN has slower onset of action than NG but a much longer duration of action (136,246,247). It is believed that PETN is converted in vascular smooth muscle to NO, which activates adenylate cyclase, leading to production of cGMP and vasodilation (136,247).

Treatment with PETN was not shown to cause tolerance and was not associated with increased free radical production (260). However, cross-tolerance to the vasodilatory effect of NG develops after PETN therapy (57,261). The prolonged antianginal effect of PETN was attributed to its PE-trinitrate metabolite or to strong binding to plasma and erythrocyte components that could decrease its availability to enzymatic conversion (246,251,262).

Clinical Presentation

CARDIOVASCULAR EFFECTS

Administration of PETN orally or sublingually can cause vertigo, headache, nausea, vomiting, syncope, blanching, and cold moist skin and orthostatic hypotension, often within minutes. Recovery occurs gradually over 12 to 16 hours (57,251). Alcohol may enhance the hypotensive effect PETN (136). Headache may be severe and may occur in the absence of demonstrable hemodynamic effects (259). The nitrate effects of PETN are less apparent than those associated with the use of NG or EGDN (245).

An animal study showed that an acute oral dose of 5 mg/kg PETN induced a 28% decrease in arterial blood pressure, an increase in venous pressure, and little effect on heart rate. Spinal pressure increased as did respiratory rate and minute volume. NG exerted similar but increased toxicity (263).

DERMATOLOGIC EFFECTS

Cutaneous sensitivity manifesting as erythematous rash with desquamation was reported after combined exposure to PETN and NG (264). However, patch tests did not give evidence of skin irritation or sensitization (57).

OPHTHALMOLOGIC EFFECTS

Although nitrates can increase intraocular pressure, this was not found in glaucoma patients treated with PETN for angina pectoris (57,259,265). Lens opacification was observed in workers exposed to TNT and PETN (44). This has not been reported during therapeutic use.

HEMATOLOGIC EFFECTS

PETN is a potential methemoglobin producer, but this has not been encountered clinically. No untoward effect on growth, blood picture, lungs, liver, kidney, spleen, and brain was observed in rats exposed orally to 2 mg/kg for 1 year (266).

MUTAGENICITY AND CARCINOGENICITY

PETN induced gene mutations in *E. coli* but not in *S. typhimurium*. It caused sister chromated exchanges but not chromosomal aberrations in Chinese hamster ovary cells. The metabolite PE did not induce gene mutations (57,75). PETN is classified as an equivocal tumorigenic agent (75). A 2-year study in rats and mice exposed to up to 10,000 ppm of PETN showed no neoplastic or nonneoplastic lesions that could be clearly attributed to PETN (267).

Diagnostic Testing

PETN can be determined in plasma and urine using colorimetric, TLC, GC with ECD, GC/MS with chemical ionization in the negative mode, and HPLC with UV detection or thermal energy analyzer methods (253,255,268–273). Measurement of PETN is not generally available, and toxic levels have not been determined; thus, it has no role in the treatment of the intoxicated patient.

Treatment

Treatment is symptomatic and supportive, directed mainly toward oxygenation, ventilation, and correction of hypotension. Good housekeeping and adequate control measures are needed to prevent explosions and injuries in workers.

REFERENCES

1. Stewart CE, Sullivan JB Jr. Military munitions and antipersonnel agents. In: Sullivan JB Jr, Krieger GR, eds. *Hazardous materials toxicology, clinical principles of environmental health.* Baltimore: Williams & Wilkins, 1992:986–1014.
2. Winneg CH, Banery DK. Explosives industry. In: Parmeggiani L, ed. *Encyclopedia of occupational health and safety*, 3rd ed. Geneva: International Labour Office, 1983:806–809.
3. Sullivan JB Jr. Cryogenics, oxidizers, reducing agents, and explosives. In: Sullivan JB Jr, Krieger GR, eds. *Hazardous materials toxicology, clinical principles of environmental health.* Baltimore: Williams & Wilkins, 1992:1192–1201.
4. Daum S. Nitroglycerin and alkyl nitrates. In: Rom WN, ed. *Environmental and occupational medicine.* Boston: Little, Brown and Company, 1983:639–648.
5. Darlington T. The effects of the products of high explosives, dynamite and nitroglycerin on the human system. *Med Rec* 1890;38:661–662.
6. Anonymous. The effects of nitroglycerin upon those who manufacture it. *JAMA* 1989;31:793–794.
7. Laws CE. Nitroglycerin head. *JAMA* 1910;54:793.
8. Ebright GE. The effects of nitroglycerin on those engaged in its manufacture. *JAMA* 1914;62:201–202.
9. Rabinowitch IM. Acute nitroglycerin poisoning. *Can Med Assoc J* 1944;50:199–202.
10. Schwartz AM. The cause, relief and prevention of headaches arising from contact with dynamite. *N Engl J Med* 1946;235:541–544.
11. McConnell WJ, Flinn RH. Summary of twenty-two trinitrotoluene fatalities in World War II. *Ind Hyg Toxicol* 1946;28:76–86.
12. Explosives, oxidizers and radioactive materials. In: Isman W, Carlson G. *Hazardous materials.* Encino, CA: Glenco Publishing, 1980:61–88.
13. Myer E. *Chemistry of hazardous materials—twelve chemical explosives.* Englewood Cliffs, NJ: Tintus Hall, 1977:306–327.
14. Schwartz L. Dermatitis from explosives. *JAMA* 1944;125:186–190.
15. Tamiri T. Explosives. In: Siegel JM, Saukko PJ, Knupfer GC, eds. *Encyclopedia of forensic science.* London: Academic Press, 2000:729–745.
16. Department of the Treasury, Bureau of Alcohol, Tobacco and Firearms. Commerce in explosives: list of explosive materials. Washington: US Government Printing Office, 2002.
17. Aromatic nitro and amino compounds. In: Finkel AJ, ed. *Hamilton and Hardy's industrial toxicology.* Boston: John Wright PSG Inc, 1983:256–261.
18. Crawford MAD. Aplastic anemia due to trinitrotoluene intoxication. *Br Med J* 1954;2:430–437.
19. Sax I. *Dangerous properties of industrial materials*, 5th ed. New York: Van Nostrand Reinhold, 1979:1065–1066.
20. Hilton J, Swanston CN. Clinical manifestations of tetryl and trinitrotoluene. *Br Med J* 1941;2:509–510.
21. Paterson JD. Trinitrotoluene. In: Parmeggiani L, ed. *Encyclopedia of occupational health and safety*, 3rd ed. Geneva: International Labor Office, 1983:2218–2219.
22. NIOSH pocket guide. In: *Chemknowledge*, vol. 53 [book on CD-ROM]. Englewood, CO: Micromedex Inc, 2002.
23. Budavari S, ed. *The Merck index. An encyclopedia of chemicals, drugs and biologicals*, 11th ed. Rahway, NJ: Merck & Co, 1989.
24. Ryon MG, Ross RH. Water quality criteria for 2,4,6-trinitrotoluene. *Regul Toxicol Pharmacol* 1990;11:104–113.
25. Ross RH, Hartley WR. Comparison of water quality criteria and health advisories for 2,4,6-trinitrotoluene. *Regul Toxicol Pharmacol* 1990;11:114–117.

26. Harkonen H, Karki M, Lahti A, et al. Early equatorial cataracts in workers exposed to trinitrotoluene. *Am J Ophthalmol* 1983;95:807–810.
27. Ahlborg G Jr, Einisto P, Sorsa M. Mutagenic activity and metabolites in the urine of workers exposed to trinitrotoluene (TNT). *Br J Ind Med* 1988;45:353–358.
28. Woollen BH, Hall MG, Craig R, et al. Trinitrotoluene: assessment of occupational absorption during manufacture of explosives. *Br J Ind Med* 1986;43:465–473.
29. Yinon J, Hwang DG. Metabolic studies of explosives. 5. Detection and analysis of 2,4,6-trinitrotoluene and its metabolites in urine of munition workers by micro liquid chromatography/mass spectrometry. *Biomed Chromatogr* 1986;1:123–125.
30. Bader M, Goen T, Muller J, et al. Analysis of nitroaromatic compounds in urine by gas chromatography-mass spectrometry for the biological monitoring of explosives. *J Chromatogr B Biomed Sci Appl* 1998;710:91–99.
31. Coombs M, Schillack V. Determination of trinitrotoluene and metabolites in urine by means of gas-chromatography with mass detection. *Int Arch Occup Environ Health* 1998;71[Suppl]:S22–S25.
32. Channon HJ, Mills GT, Williams RT. The metabolism of 2,4,6-trinitrotoluene (alpha-TNT). *Biochem J* 1944;38:70–85.
33. Liu YY, Yao M, Fang JL, et al. Monitoring human risk and exposure to trinitrotoluene (TNT) using haemoglobin adducts as biomarkers. *Toxicol Lett* 1995;77:281–287.
34. Maroziene A, Kliukiene R, Sarlauskas J, et al. Methemoglobin formation in human erythrocytes by nitroaromatic explosives. *Z Naturforsch [C]* 2001;56:1157–1163.
35. Goh CL, Rajan VS. Contact sensitivity to trinitrotoluene. *Contact Dermatitis* 1983;9:433–434.
36. Goh CL. Allergic contact dermatitis from tetryl and trinitrotoluene. *Contact Dermatitis* 1984;10:108.
37. Goh CL. Erythema multiforme-like eruption from trinitrotoluene allergy. *Int J Dermatol* 1988;27:650–651.
38. Djerassi LS, Vitany L. Haemolytic episode in G6 PD deficient workers exposed to TNT. *Br J Ind Med* 1975;32:54–58.
39. Djerassi L. Hemolytic crisis in G6PD-deficient individuals in the occupational setting. *Int Arch Occup Environ Health* 1998;71[Suppl]:S26–S28.
40. Voegtlin C, Hooper CW, Johnson JM. Trinitrotoluene poisoning—its nature, diagnosis and prevention. *J Indust Hyg* 1921;3:239–254, 280–292.
41. Hathaway JA. Trinitrotoluene: a review of reported dose-related effects providing documentation for a workplace standard. *J Occup Med* 1977;19:341–345.
42. Morton AR, Ranadive MV, Hathaway JA. Biological effects of trinitrotoluene from exposure below the threshold limit value. *Am Ind Hyg Assoc J* 1976;37:56–60.
43. Li J, Jiang QG, Zhong WD. Persistent ethanol drinking increases liver injury induced by trinitrotoluene exposure: an in-plant case-control study. *Hum Exp Toxicol* 1991;10:405–409.
44. Lewis-Younger CR, Mamalis N, Egger MJ, et al. Lens opacifications detected by slitlamp biomicroscopy are associated with exposure to organic nitrate explosives. *Arch Ophthalmol* 2000;118:1653–1659.
45. Zhou AS. A clinical study of trinitrotoluene cataract. *Pol J Occup Med* 1990;3:171–176.
46. Zlateva V, Pavlova S. The impact of trinitrotoluene on eyes in miners [in Russian]. *Med Tr Prom Ekol* 1998;2:26–29.
47. Jacob JC, Maroun FB. Peripheral neuropathy in a person sensitive to dynamite. *Can Med Assoc J* 1969;101:102–104.
48. Soboleva LP. State of the myocardium during chronic trinitrotoluene intoxication. *Gig Tr Prof Zabol* 1969;13:47–48.
49. Karamova NS, Mynina II, Garaeva GG, et al. 2,4,6-trinitrotoluene and 2,4-diamino-6-nitrotoluene: the absence of recA-dependent mutagenesis [in Russian]? *Genetika* 1995;31:617–621.
50. Lachance B, Robidoux PY, Hawari J, et al. Cytotoxic and genotoxic effects of energetic compounds on bacterial and mammalian cells in vitro. *Mutat Res* 1999;444:25–39.
51. Ashby J, Burlinson B, Lefevre PA, et al. Non-genotoxicity of 2,4,6-trinitrotoluene (TNT) to the mouse bone marrow and the rat liver: implications for its carcinogenicity. *Arch Toxicol* 1985;58:14–19.
52. Styles JA, Cross MF. Activity of 2,4,6-trinitrotoluene in an in vitro mammalian gene mutation assay. *Cancer Lett* 1983;20:103–108.
53. Kilian PH, Skrzypek S, Becker N, et al. Exposure to armament wastes and leukemia: a case-control study within a cluster of AML and CML in Germany. *Leuk Res* 2001;25:839–845.
54. Li Y, Jiang QG, Yao SQ, et al. Effects of exposure to trinitrotoluene on male reproduction. *Biomed Environ Sci* 1993;6:154–160.
55. Wu LP, Chang YX, Jiang QG. Effects of exposure to TNT on sex hormones in male workers [in Chinese]. *Zhonghua Yu Fang Yi Xue Za Zhi* 1994;28:162–163.
56. Liu HX, Qin WH, Wang GR, et al. Some altered concentrations of elements in semen of workers exposed to trinitrotoluene. *Occup Environ Med* 1995;52:842–845.
57. Hazardous Substances Data Bank. In: *Chemknowledge*, vol. 53 [book on CD-ROM]. Englewood, CO: Micromedex Inc, 2002.
58. Sabbioni G, Wei J, Liu YY. Determination of hemoglobin adducts in workers exposed to 2,4,6-trinitrotoluene. *J Chromatogr B Biomed Appl* 1996;682:243–248.
59. Almog J, Kraus S, Basch A. Determination of TNT metabolites in urine. *Arch Toxicol* 1983;[Suppl 6]:351–353.
60. Fetterolf DD, Mudd JL, Teten K. An enzyme-linked immunosorbent assay (ELISA) for trinitrotoluene (TNT) residue on hands. *J Forensic Sci* 1991;36:343–349.
61. ACGIH: documentation of the threshold limit values and biological exposure indices, vol. 1, 6th ed. Cincinnati: American Conference of Governmental Industrial Hygienists, Inc, 1991.
62. Hathaway GJ, Proctor NH, Hughes JP, et al. *Chemical hazards in the workplace*, 3rd ed. New York: Van Nostrand Reinhold Co, 1991:258–259.
63. Woollen BH, Hall MG, Craig R, et al. Dinitrotoluene: an assessment of occupational absorption during the manufacture of blasting explosives. *Int Arch Occup Environ Health* 1985;55:319–330.
64. Levine RJ, Turner MJ, Crume YS, et al. Assessing exposure to dinitrotoluene using a biological monitor. *J Occup Med* 1985;27:627–638.
65. Chapman DE, Michener SR, Powis G. Metabolism of 2,6-dinitro[3-3H]toluene by human and rat liver microsomal and cytosolic fractions. *Xenobiotica* 1992;22:1015–1028.
66. Turner MJ Jr, Levine RJ, Nystrom DD, et al. Identification and quantification of urinary metabolites of dinitrotoluenes in occupationally exposed humans. *Toxicol Appl Pharmacol* 1985;80:166–174.
67. Clayton GD, Clayton FE, eds. *Patty's industrial hygiene and toxicology*, vol. IIB. *Toxicology*, 4th ed. New York: John Wiley & Sons, 1994.
68. Ramos K, McMahon KK, Alipui C, et al. Modulation of smooth muscle cell proliferation by dinitrotoluene. In: Witmer CM, Snyder RR, Jallow DJ, et al., eds. *Biologic reductive intermediates*, vol. V. New York: Plenum Publishing, 1990:805–807.
69. Ramos KS, Chacon E, Acosta D Jr. Toxic responses of the heart and vascular systems. In: Klaassen CD, ed. *Casarett and Doull's toxicology. The basic science of poisons*, 5th ed. New York: McGraw-Hill, 1996:487–527.
70. Sittig M. *Handbook of toxic and hazardous chemicals and carcinogens*, 2nd ed. Park Ridge, NJ: Noyes Publications, 1985:380–381.
71. Proctor NH, Hughes JP, Fischman ML. *Chemical hazards of the workplace*, 2nd ed. New York: Van Nostrand Reinhold, 1980:218–219.
72. Levine RJ, Andjelkovich DA, Kersteter SL, et al. Heart disease in workers exposed to dinitrotoluene. *J Occup Med* 1986;28:811–816.
73. Stayner LT, Dannenberg AL, Thun M, et al. Cardiovascular mortality among munitions workers exposed to nitroglycerin and dinitrotoluene. *Scand J Work Environ Health* 1992;18:34–43.
74. Hamilton AS, Nixon CE. Optic atrophy and multiple neuritis developed in the manufacture of explosives (Binitrotoluene). *JAMA* 1918;70:2004–2006.
75. Registry of toxic effects of chemical substances. Cincinnati: National Institute of Occupational Safety and Health. In: *Chemknowledge*, vol. 53 [book on CD-ROM]. Englewood, CO: Micromedex Inc, 2002.
76. Kanerva L, Laine R, Jolanki R, et al. Occupational allergic contact dermatitis caused by nitroglycerin. *Contact Dermatitis* 1991;24:356–362.
77. Mirsalis JC, Butterworth BE. Induction of unscheduled DNA synthesis in rat hepatocytes following in vivo treatment with dinitrotoluene. *Carcinogenesis (London)* 1982;3:241–245.
78. Abernethy DJ, Couch DB. Cytotoxicity and mutagenicity of dinitrotoluenes in Chinese hamster ovary cells. *Mutat Res* 1982;103:53–59.
79. Holen I, Mikalsen SO, Sanner T. Effects of dinitrotoluenes on morphological cell transformation and intercellular communication in Syrian hamster embryo cells. *J Toxicol Environ Health* 1990;29:89–98.
80. Rickert DE, Butterworth BE, Popp JA. Dinitrotoluene: acute toxicity, oncogenicity, genotoxicity, and metabolism. *Crit Rev Toxicol* 1984;13:217–234.
81. Stayner LT, Dannenberg AL, Bloom T, et al. Excess hepatobiliary cancer mortality among munitions workers exposed to dinitrotoluene. *J Occup Med* 1993;35:291–296.
82. Bruning T, Chronz C, Thier R, et al. Occurrence of urinary tract tumors in miners highly exposed to dinitrotoluene. *J Occup Environ Med* 1999;41:144–149.
83. International Agency for Research on Cancer. 2,4-Dinitrotoluene, 2,6-dinitrotoluene and 3,5-dinitrotoluene. IARC monograph, vol. 65. Lyon: International Agency for Research on Cancer, 1996.
84. Price CJ, Tyl RW, Marks TA, et al. Teratologic evaluation of dinitrotoluene in the Fischer 344 rat. *Fundam Appl Toxicol* 1985;5:948–961.
85. Wolkowski-Tyl R, Jones-Price C, Ledoux TA, et al. Teratogenicity evaluation of technical grade dinitrotoluene in the Fischer-344 rat. *Teratology* 1981;23:70a.
86. Hamill PV, Steinberger E, Levine RJ, et al. The epidemiologic assessment of male reproductive hazard from occupational exposure to TDA and DNT. *J Occup Med* 1982;24:985–993.
87. Reader SC, Foster PM. The in vitro effects of four isomers of dinitrotoluene on rat Sertoli and Sertoli-germ cell cocultures: germ cell detachment and lactate and pyruvate production. *Toxicol Applied Pharmacol* 1990;106:287–294.
88. 2001 TLVs and BEIs. Threshold limit values for chemical substances and physical agents & biologic exposure indices. Cincinnati: American Conference of Governmental Industrial Hygienists, 2001.
89. Smith EF 2nd, Smith HJ, Kuchar EJ. Monitoring of dinitrotoluene and its metabolites in urine by spectrophotometry of their coupled aryidiazonium salts. *Am Ind Hyg Assoc J* 1995;56:1175–1179.
90. Angerer J, Weismantel A. Biological monitoring of dinitrotoluene by gas chromatographic-mass spectrometric analysis of 2,4-dinitrobenzoic acid in human urine. *J Chromatogr B Biomed Sci Appl* 1998;713:313–322.
91. Bruning T, Thier R, Mann H, et al. Pathological excretion patterns of urinary proteins in miners highly exposed to dinitrotoluene. *J Occup Environ Med* 2001;43:610–615.

92. Capellini A, Zanotti GG. A case of occupational chronic poisoning with dinitrobenzene. *Medicina del Lavoro* 1946;37:265–270.
93. Obasaju MF, Katz DF, Miller MG. Species differences in susceptibility to 1,3-dinitrobenzene-induced testicular toxicity and methemoglobinemia. *Fundam Appl Toxicol* 1991;16:257–266.
94. Ishihara N, Kanaya A, Ikeda M. m-Dinitrobenzene intoxication due to skin absorption. *Int Arch Occup Environ Health* 1976;36:161–168.
95. Adams PC, Rickert DE. The absorption and first-pass metabolism of [14C]-1,3-dinitrobenzene in the isolated vascularly perfused rat small intestine. *Biopharm Drug Dispos* 1996;17:675–698.
96. Rickert DE. Metabolism of nitroaromatic compounds. *Drug Metab Rev* 1987;18:23–53.
97. Cossum PA, Rickert DE. Metabolism of dinitrobenzenes by rat isolated hepatocytes. *Drug Metab Dispos* 1985;13:664–668.
98. Adams PC, Rickert DE. Metabolism of [14C]1,3-dinitrobenzene by rat small intestinal mucosa in vitro. *Drug Metab Dispos* 1995;23:982–987.
99. Reeve IT, Miller MG. 1,3-Dinitrobenzene metabolism and protein binding. *Chem Res Toxicol* 2002;15:352–360.
100. Beloborodova NL. Detoxifying functions of the liver and other organs in dinitrobenzene poisoning. *Farmakologiia I Toksikologiia* 1945;8:32–36.
101. Nystrom DD, Rickert DE. Metabolism and excretion of dinitrobenzenes by male Fischer-344 rats. *Drug Metab Dispos* 1987;15:821–825.
102. Brown CD, Forman CL, McEuen SF, et al. Metabolism and testicular toxicity of 1,3-dinitrobenzene in rats of different ages. *Fundam Appl Toxicol* 1994;23:439–446.
103. McEuen SF, Miller MG. Metabolism and pharmacokinetics of 1,3-dinitrobenzene in the rat and the hamster. *Drug Metab Dispos* 1991;19:661–666.
104. Philbert MA, Nolan CC, Cremer JE, et al. 1,3-Dinitrobenzene-induced encephalopathy in rats. *Neuropathol Appl Neurobiol* 1987;13:371–389.
105. Romero IA, Lister T, Richards HK, et al. Early metabolic changes during m-dinitrobenzene neurotoxicity and the possible role of oxidative stress. *Free Radic Biol Med* 1995;18:311–319.
106. Hu HL, Bennett N, Lamb JH, et al. Capacity of rat brain to metabolize m-dinitrobenzene: an in vitro study. *Neurotoxicology* 1997;18:363–370.
107. Romero IA, Rist RJ, Chan MW, et al. Acute energy deprivation syndromes: investigation of m-dinitrobenzene and alpha-chlorohydrin toxicity on immortalized rat brain microvessel endothelial cells. *Neurotoxicology* 1997;18:781–791.
108. Hu HL, Bennett N, Holton JL, et al. Glutathione depletion increases brain susceptibility to m-dinitrobenzene neurotoxicity. *Neurotoxicology* 1999;20:83–90.
109. Xu J, Nolan CC, Lister T, et al. Pharmacokinetic factors and concentration-time threshold in m-dinitrobenzene-induced neurotoxicity. *Toxicol Appl Pharmacol* 1999;161:267–273.
110. Jacobson CF, Miller MG. Species difference in 1,3-dinitrobenzene testicular toxicity: in vitro correlation with glutathione status. *Reprod Toxicol* 1998;12:49–56.
111. Strandgaard C, Miller MG. Germ cell apoptosis in rat testis after administration of 1,3-dinitrobenzene. *Reprod Toxicol* 1998;12:97–103.
112. Grant WM, Schuman JS. *Toxicology of the eye*, vol. I, 4th ed. Springfield, IL: Charles C. Thomas Publisher, 1993:579–581.
113. Laure P, Stierle F. Methaemoglobinaemia: an unusual case report [Letter]. *Intensive Care Med* 1993;19:124.
114. From the MMWR. Methemoglobinemia due to occupational exposure to dinitrobenzene—Ohio, 1986. *Arch Dermatol* 1988;124:1171–1172.
115. David A, Srbova J, Hykes P, et al. Acute aniline and nitrobenzene intoxication—a contribution to the diagnosis of morphological and biochemical blood changes during the course of their intoxication [in Slovak]. *Casopis Lekaru Ceskych* 1964;103:1251–1256.
116. Okubo T, Shigeta S. Anemia cases after acute m-dinitrobenzene intoxication due to an occupational exposure. *Ind Health* 1982;20:297–304.
117. Philbert MA, Billingsley ML, Reuhl KR. Mechanisms of injury in the central nervous system. *Toxicol Pathol* 2000;28:43–53.
118. Romero I, Brown AW, Cavanagh JB, et al. Vascular factors in the neurotoxic damage caused by 1,3-dinitrobenzene in the rat. *Neuropathol Appl Neurobiol* 1991;17:495–508.
119. Mulheran M, Ray DE, Lister T, et al. The effect of 1,3-dinitrobenzene on the functioning of the auditory pathway in the rat. *Neurotoxicology* 1999;20:27–39.
120. Kiese M. Pharmacological investigations of m-dinitrobenzene-III. Chronic poisoning with m-dinitrobenzene [in German]. *Naunyn-Schmoedeberg's Arch Exp Pharmacol* 1949;206:505–527.
121. McGregor DB, Riach CG, Hastwell RM, et al. Genotoxic activity in microorganisms of tetryl, 1,3-dinitrobenzene and 1,3,5-trinitrobenzene. *Environ Mutagen* 1980;2:531–541.
122. Ozturk K, Durusoy M. The detection and comparison of the genotoxic effects of some nitro aromatic compounds by the umu and SOS chromotest systems. *Toxicol Lett* 1999;108:63–68.
123. Linder RE, Hess RA, Perreault SD, et al. Acute effects and long-term sequelae of 1,3-dinitrobenzene on male reproduction in the rat. I. Sperm quality, quantity, and fertilizing ability. *J Androl* 1988;9:317–326.
124. Linder RE, Strader LF, Barbee RR, et al. Reproductive toxicity of a single dose of 1,3-dinitrobenzene in two ages of young adult male rats. *Fundam Appl Toxicol* 1990;14:284–298.
125. Irimura K, Yamaguchi M, Morinaga H, et al. Collaborative work to evaluate toxicity on male reproductive organs by repeated dose studies in rats. Detection of 1,3-dinitrobenzene-induced histopathological changes in testes and epididymides of rats with 2-week daily repeated dosing. *J Toxicol Sci* 2000;25:251–258.
126. Peiris LD, Moore HD. Evaluation of effects of 1,3-dinitrobenzene on sperm motility of hamster using computer assisted semen analysis (CASA). *Asian J Androl* 2001;3:109–114.
127. Rehnberg GL, Linder RE, Goldman JM, et al. Changes in testicular and serum hormone concentrations in the male rat following treatment with m-dinitrobenzene. *Toxicol Appl Pharmacol* 1988;95:255–264.
128. Hess RA, Linder RE, Strader LF, et al. Acute effects and long-term sequelae of 1,3-dinitrobenzene on male reproduction in the rat. II. Quantitative and qualitative histopathology of the testis. *J Androl* 1988;9:327–342.
129. Blackburn DM, Gray AJ, Lloyd SC, et al. A comparison of the effects of the three isomers of dinitrobenzene on the testis in the rat. *Toxicol Appl Pharmacol* 1988;92:54–64.
130. Roubal J, Tuhy K. m-Dinitrobenzene in the blood: determination by the polarographic method and its observed changes [in Slovak]. *J Czech Phys* 1946;29:1001–1013.
131. Miller MG, McEuen SF, Nasiri M, et al. Application of ELISA techniques to metabolic disposition studies for 1,3-dinitrobenzene: comparison with HPLC and radiochemical methods. *Chem Res Toxicol* 1991;4:324–329.
132. Bailey E, Peal JA, Philbert M. Determination of 1,3-dinitrobenzene and its metabolites in rat blood by capillary gas chromatography with electron-capture detection. *J Chromatogr* 1988;425:187–192.
133. Yamaguchi S. Nitroglycerin. In: Parmeggiani L, ed. *Encyclopedia of occupational health and safety*, 3rd ed. Geneva: International Labour Office, 1983:1459–1461.
134. Kantha SS. Could nitroglycerine poisoning be the cause of Alfred Nobel's anginal pains and premature death? *Med Hypotheses* 1997;49:303–306.
135. Wei JY, Reid PR. Quantitative determination of trinitroglycerin in human plasma. *Circulation* 1979;59:588–592.
136. Drugdex. In: Healthcare series, vol. 113. Greenwood Village, CO: Thomson Micromedex, 2002.
137. Marshall JB, Ecklund RE. Methemoglobinemia from overdose of nitroglycerin. *JAMA* 1980;244:330.
138. Hogstedt C, Davidsson B. Nitroglycol and nitroglycerine exposure in a dynamite industry 1958–1978. *Am Ind Hyg Assoc J* 1980;41:373–375.
139. Twibell JD, Home JM, Smalldon KW, et al. Transfer of nitroglycerine to hands during contact with commercial explosives. *J Forensic Sci* 1982;27:783–791.
140. Noonan PK, Benet LZ. The bioavailability of oral nitroglycerin. *J Pharm Sci* 1986;75:241–243.
141. Robertson RM, Robertson D. Drugs used for the treatment of myocardial ischemia. In: Hardman JG, Limbrid JE, eds. *Goodman & Gilman's the pharmacological basis of therapeutics*, 9th ed. New York: McGraw-Hill, 1996:759–779.
142. Armstrong PW, Armstrong JA, Marks GS. Blood levels after sublingual nitroglycerin. *Circulation* 1979;59:585–588.
143. Needelman P. Organic nitrate metabolism. *Annual Rev Pharmacol Toxicol* 1976;16:81–93.
144. Nakashima E, Rigod JF, Lin ET, et al. Pharmacokinetics of nitroglycerin and its dinitrate metabolites over a thirtyfold range of oral doses. *Clin Pharmacol Ther* 1990;47:592–598.
145. Haefeli WE, Srivastava N, Kelsey KT, et al. Glutathione S-transferase mu polymorphism does not explain variation in nitroglycerin responsiveness. *Clin Pharmacol Ther* 1993;53:463–468.
146. Baselt RC, Cravey RH. *Disposition of toxic drugs and chemicals in man*, 4th ed. Chicago: Year Book Medical Publishers, 1995.
147. Cottrell JE, Turndoff H. Intravenous nitroglycerin. *Am Heart J* 1978;96:550–553.
148. Nishikawa Y, Kanki H, Ogawa S. Differential acts of N-acetylcysteine on nitroglycerin- and nicorandil-induced vasodilation in human coronary circulation. *J Cardiovasc Pharmacol* 1998;32:21–28.
149. Schlafer KR, Stork CM. Dermal application of nitroglycerin ointment in place of Nystatin ointment results in fatality. *Int J Med Toxicol* 2000;3:5.
150. Gough ED, Dyer DC. Responses of isolated human uterine arteries to vasoactive drugs. *Am J Obstet Gynecol* 1971;110:625–629.
151. Molina CR, Andresen JW, Rapoport RM, et al. Effect of in vivo nitroglycerin therapy on endothelium-dependent and independent vascular relaxation and cyclic GMP accumulation in rat aorta. *J Cardiovasc Pharmacol* 1987;10:371–378.
152. Benowitz NL. Cardiotoxicity in the workplace. *Occup Med* 1992;7:465–478.
153. Khan AH, Carleton RA. Nitroglycerin-induced hypotension and bradycardia. *Arch Intern Med* 1981;141:984.
154. Lafranchi A, Beraud P. Chronic intoxication by nitrated compounds in workers of explosives plants. *Presse Medicale* 1969;77:795–796.
155. Carmichael P, Lieben J. Sudden death in explosives workers. *Arch Env Health* 1963;7:424–439.
156. Klock JC. Nonocclusive coronary disease after chronic exposure to nitrates: evidence for physiologic nitrate dependence. *Am Heart J* 1975;89:510–513.
157. Przybojewski JZ, Heyns MH. Acute myocardial infarction due to coronary vasospasm secondary to industrial nitroglycerin withdrawal. A case report. *S Afr Med J* 1983;64:101–104.
158. Ben-David A. Cardiac arrest in an explosives factory worker due to withdrawal from nitroglycerin exposure. *Am J Ind Med* 1989;15:719–722.
159. Lund RP, Haggendal J, Johnsson G. Withdrawal symptoms in workers exposed to nitroglycerin. *Br J Ind Med* 1968;25:136–138.

160. Hogstedt C, Axelson O. Mortality from cardio-cerebrovascular diseases among dynamite workers—an extended case-referent study. *Ann Acad Med Singapore* 1984;13[2 Suppl]:399–403.
161. Martimor E, Cavigneaux A, Nicolas-Charles JP. Mental disorders caused by occupational poisoning with nitroglycerin [in French]. *Archives des Maladies Professionelles, de Medicine du Travail et de Securite Social* 1958;19:574–580.
162. Meyjohann D, Zell L, Buchter A. Nitrate headache in blasting work [in German]. *Med Klin* 2001;96:295–297.
163. Trainor DC, Jones RC. Headaches in explosive magazine workers. *Arch Environ Health* 1966;12:231–234.
164. Paris PM, Kaplan RM, Stewart RD, et al. Methemoglobin levels following sublingual nitroglycerin in human volunteers. *Ann Emerg Med* 1986;15:171–173.
165. Rosenfeld AS, White WB. Allergic contact dermatitis secondary to transdermal nitroglycerin. *Am Heart J* 1984;108:1061–1062.
166. Silvestre JF, Betlloch I, Guijarro J, et al. Erythema-multiforme-like eruption on the application site of a nitroglycerin patch, followed by widespread erythema multiforme. *Contact Dermatitis* 2001;45:299–300.
167. Craig S, Dalton R, Tuck M, et al. Sublingual glyceryl trinitrate for uterine relaxation at caeserean section—a prospective trial. *Aust N Z J Obstet Gynaecol* 1998;38:34–39.
168. David M, Halle H, Lichtenegger W, et al. Nitroglycerin to facilitate fetal extraction during cesarean delivery. *Obstet Gynecol* 1998;91:119–124.
169. Dufour P, Vinatier D, Puech F. The use of intravenous nitroglycerin for cervico-uterine relaxation: a review of the literature. *Arch Gynecol Obstet* 1997;261:1–7.
170. Smith GN, Brien JF. Use of nitroglycerin for uterine relaxation. *Obstet Gynecol Surv* 1998;53:559–565.
171. Cotton DB, Longmire S, Jones MM, et al. Cardiovascular alterations in severe pregnancy-induced hypertension: effects of intravenous nitroglycerin coupled with blood volume expansion. *Am J Obstet Gynecol* 1986;154:1053–1059.
172. Shepard's catalogue of teratogenic agents. In: *Chemknowledge*, vol. 53 [book on CD-ROM]. Englewood, CO: Micromedex Inc, 2002.
173. Woodward AJ, Lewis PA, Rudman AR, et al. Determination of nitroglycerin and its dinitrate metabolites in human plasma by high-performance liquid chromatography with thermal energy analyzer detection. *J Pharm Sci* 1984;73:1838–1840.
174. Lee FW, Watari N, Rigod J, et al. Simultaneous determination of nitroglycerin and its dinitrate metabolites by capillary gas chromatography with electron-capture detection. *J Chromatogr* 1988;426:259–266.
175. Parmeggiani L. Ethylene glycol dinitrate. In: Parmeggiani L, ed. *Encyclopedia of occupational health and safety*, 3rd ed. Geneva: International Labour Office, 1983:796–797.
176. Symanski H. Schwere gesundheits schadingungen durch berfliche nitroglykoleinwirkung. *Arch Hyg (Berlin)* 1952;136:139–158.
177. Fossman S, Masreliez N, Johansson G, et al. Medical examination of workers engaged in the manufacture of nitroglycerin and ethylene glycol dinitrate in the Swedish explosives industry. *Proc 12th Int Congress Occup Health* 1957;3:254–258.
178. Fukuchi Y. Nitroglycol concentrations in blood and urine of workers engaged in dynamite production. *Int Arch Occup Environ Health* 1981;48:339–346.
179. Hogstedt C. Ethylene glycol dinitrate. In: Aitio A, Riihimaki V, Vainio H, eds. *Biological monitoring and surveillance of workers exposed to chemicals*. Washington: Hemisphere Publishing Co, 1984:187–192.
180. Fukuchi Y. The effects of nitroglycol at low concentrations [in Japanese]. *Hokkaido Igaku Zasshi* 1981;56:245–247. [Author's translation.]
181. Hogstedt C, Stahl R. Skin absorption and protective gloves in dynamite work. *Am Ind Hyg Assoc J* 1980;41:367–372.
182. Gross E, Bock M, Hellrung F. Toxicology of nitroglycol in comparison with that of nitroglycerin [in German]. *Archiv fur Experimentelle Pathologie and Pharmakologie* 1942;200:271–304.
183. Diseases caused by nitroglycerin and other nitric acid esters. In: *Early detection of occupational diseases*. Geneva: World Health Organization 1986:142–145.
184. Englund A, Ehrner-Samuel H, Kylin B, et al. On the metabolism of nitroglycol in mice. *Proc 15th Int Congress Occup Health* 1966;3:207–209.
185. Zitting A, Savolainen H. Effects of nitroglycerin and ethylene glycol dinitrate mixture (blasting oil) on rat brain, liver and kidney. *Res Commun Chem Pathol Pharmacol* 1982;37:113–121.
186. Clark DG, Litchfield MH. Metabolism of ethylene glycol dinitrate (ethylene dinitrate) in the rat following repeated administration. *Br J Ind Med* 1969;26:150–155.
187. Axelsson KL, Andersson RG, Wikberg JE. Correlation between vascular smooth muscle relaxation and increase in cyclic GMP induced by some organic nitro esters. *Acta Pharmacol Toxicol (Copenh)* 1981;49:270–276.
188. Axelsson KL, Andersson C, Ahlner J, et al. Comparative in vitro study of a series of organic nitroesters: unique biphasic concentration-effect curves for glyceryl trinitrate in isolated bovine arterial smooth muscle and lack of stereoselectivity for some glyceryl trinitrate analogues. *J Cardiovasc Pharmacol* 1992;19:953–957.
189. Noack E. Mechanisms of nitrate tolerance—influence of the metabolic activation pathways. *Z Kardiol* 1990;79[Suppl 3]:51–55.
190. Clark DG, Litchfield MH. Metabolism of ethylene glycol dinitrate and its influence on the blood pressure of the rat. *Br J Industr Med* 1967;24:320–325.
191. Tai T, Tsuruta H. The effects of nitroglycol on rat isolated cardiac muscles. *Ind Health* 1997;35:515–518.
192. Clark DG. The supersensitivity of the rat cardiovascular system to epinephrine after repeated injections of ethylene glycol dinitrate. *Toxicol Appl Pharmacol* 1970;17:433–442.
193. Johansson P, Ehrenstrom F, Ungell AL. Study on adrenergic function after development of tolerance to ethylene glycol dinitrate (EGDN) in rats. *Pharmacol Toxicol* 1987;61:172–181.
194. Clark DG, Litchfield MH. Role of inorganic nitrite in methaemoglobin formation after nitrate ester administration to the rat. *Br J Pharmacol* 1973;48:162–168.
195. Kalin M, Kylin B, Malmfors T. The effect of nitrate explosives on adrenergic nerves. *Arch Environ Health* 1969;19:32–35.
196. Hanova M. Electrocardiographic changes induced by ethylene glycol dinitrate and glyceryl trinitrate [in Slovak]. *Bratisl Lek Listy* 1965;45:220–224.
197. Bergert KD, Friedrich K, Geschke U, et al. Cardiovascular diseases in exposure to the saltpeter acid ester ethylene glycol dinitrate [in German]. *Z Gesamte Inn Med* 1987;42:581–583.
198. Sakoda A. A clinical study on nitroglycol poisoning. *Jpn J Industr Health* 1962;4:583.
199. Barsoti M. Attachi stnocardici nei lavoratori addetti alla produzioni delle dinanite con nitroglicole. *Med d Lavoro* 1954;45:544–548.
200. Yamaguchi M, Sakabe H, Kajita A, et al. Nitroglycol poisoning in an explosives plant. *Bull Nat Inst Industr Health* 1980;4:54–71.
201. Craig R, Gillis CR, Hole DJ, et al. Sixteen year follow up of workers in an explosives factory. *J Soc Occup Med* 1985;35:107–110.
202. Kristensen TS. Cardiovascular diseases and the work environment. A critical review of the epidemiologic literature on chemical factors. *Scand J Work Environ Health* 1989;15:245–264.
203. Fine LJ. Occupational heart disease. In: Rom WN, ed. *Environmental and occupational medicine*, 2nd ed. Boston: Little, Brown and Company, 1992:593–600.
204. McGuiness BW, Harris EL. "Monday head," an interesting occupational disorder. *Br Med J* 1961;2:745–747.
205. Pelnar P, Srobua J. The effect of ethylene glycol dinitrate from mine explosives [in Slovak]. *Pracovni Lekarstvi* 1961;13:469–474.
206. Clark DG. Effects of ethylene glycol dinitrate on pituitary-adrenocortical function in the rat. *Toxicol Appl Pharmacol* 1972;21:355–360.
207. Ehrner-Samuel H. Gas chromatographic determination of nitroglycerin, nitroglycol and propylene glycol dinitrate in blood with an electron capture detector. *Proc 15th Int Congress Occup Health* 1966;3:201–205.
208. Litchfield MH. The determination of the di- and mononitrates of ethylene glycol and 1,2-propylene glycol in blood by colorimetric and gas-chromatographic methods. *Analyst* 1968;93:653–659.
209. Kempe CR, Tannert WK. Detection of dynamite residues on the hands of bombing suspects. *J Forensic Sci* 1972;17:323–324.
210. St John GA, McReynolds JH, Blucher WG, et al. Determination of the concentration of explosives in air by isotope dilution analysis. *Forensic Sci* 1975;6:53–66.
211. Hathaway GJ, Proctor NH, Hughes JP. *Chemical hazards of the workplace*, 4th ed. New York: Van Nostrand Reinhold Company, 1996.
212. Testud F, Glanclaude JM, Descotes J. Acute hexogen poisoning after occupational exposure. *J Toxicol Clin Toxicol* 1996;34:109–111.
213. Stone WJ, Paletta TL, Heiman EM, et al. Toxic effects following ingestion of C-4 plastic explosive. *Arch Intern Med* 1969;124:726–730.
214. Ketel WB, Hughes JR. Toxic encephalopathy with seizures secondary to ingestion of composition C-4. A clinical and electroencephalographic study. *Neurology* 1972;22:871–876.
215. Lewis RJ. *Sax's dangerous properties of industrial materials*, 9th ed. New York: Van Nostrand Reinhold Company, 2000.
216. James RC, Roberts SM, Williams PL. Evaluation of the adequacy of the threshold limit value for cyclonite. *Appl Occup Environ Hyg* 1994;9:485–492.
217. Hathaway JA, Buck CR. Absence of health hazards associated with RDX manufacture and use. *J Occup Med* 1977;19:269–272.
218. Kaplan AS, Berghout CF, Peczenika A. Human intoxication from RDX. *Arch Environ Health* 1965;10:877–883.
219. Woody RC, Kearns GL, Brewster MA, et al. The neurotoxicity of cyclotrimethylenetrinitramine (RDX) in a child: a clinical and pharmacokinetic evaluation. *J Toxicol Clin Toxicol* 1986;24:305–319.
220. Burdette LJ, Cook LL, Dyer RS. Convulsant properties of cyclotrimethylenetrinitramine (RDX): spontaneous audiogenic, and amygdaloid kindled seizure activity. *Toxicol Appl Pharmacol* 1988;92:436–444.
221. Dilley JV, Tyson CA, Spanggord RJ, et al. Short-term oral toxicity of a 2,4,6-trinitrotoluene and hexahydro-1,3,5-trinitro-1,3,5-triazine mixture in mice, rats, and dogs. *J Toxicol Environ Health* 1982;9:587–610.
222. Schneider NR, Bradley SL, Andersen ME. Toxicology of cyclotrimethylenetrinitramine: distribution and metabolism in the rat and the miniature swine. *Toxicol Appl Pharmacol* 1977;39:531–541.
223. Etnier EL. Water quality criteria for hexahydro-1,3,5-trinitro-1,3,5-triazine (RDX). *Regul Toxicol Pharmacol* 1989;9:147–157.
224. Etnier EL, Hartley WR. Comparison of water quality criterion and lifetime health advisory for hexahydro-1,3,5-trinitro-1,3,5-triazine (RDX). *Regul Toxicol Pharmacol* 1990;11:118–122.
225. von Oettinger WF, Donahue DD, Yagoda H, et al. Toxicity and potential dangers of cyclotrimethylenetrinitramine (RDX). *J Ind Hyg Toxicol* 1949;31:21–31.

226. Stockinger HE. Aliphatic nitro compounds and nitrates. In: Clayton GD, Clayton FE, eds. *Patty's industrial hygiene and toxicology*, 3rd ed., vol. 2-C, Toxicology. New York: John Wiley and Sons, 1982.
227. Tsa MT, Lee J. Food poisoning caused by hexogen: a report of eight cases. *Chin J Prev Med* 1982;16:229–231.
228. Schneider NR, Bradley SL, Andersen ME. The distribution and metabolism of cyclotrimethylenetrinitramine (RDX) in the rat after subchronic administration. *Toxicol Appl Pharmacol* 1978;46:163–171.
229. French JE, Bradley SL, Schneider NR, et al. Cyclotrimethylenetrinitramine (RDX)-induced ultrastructural changes in rat liver and kidney. *Toxicol Appl Toxicol* 1976;37:122.
230. Barsotti M, Crotti G. Epileptic attacks as manifestations of industrial intoxication caused by trimethylenetrinitramine (T_4). *Med Lavoro* 1949;40:107–112.
231. Slanskaya RM, Pozharsky FI. Toxicity of hexogen. *Chemical Abstracts* 1945;39:3073.
232. Goldberg DJ, Green ST, Nathwani D, et al. RDX intoxication causing seizures and a widespread petechial rash mimicking meningococcaemia. *J R Soc Med* 1992;85:181.
233. Harrell-Bruder B, Hutchins KL. Seizures caused by ingestion of composition C-4. *Ann Emerg Med* 1995;26:746–748.
234. Berthe-Corti L, Jacobi H, Kleihauer S, et al. Cytotoxicity and mutagenicity of a 2,4,6-trinitrotoluene (TNT) and hexogen contaminated soil in S. typhimurium and mammalian cells. *Chemosphere* 1998;37:209–218.
235. George SE, Huggins-Clark G, Brooks LR. Use of a Salmonella microsuspension bioassay to detect the mutagenicity of munitions compounds at low concentrations. *Mutat Res* 2001;490:45–56.
236. Turley CP, Brewster MA. Liquid chromatographic analysis of cyclotrimethylenetrinitramine in biological fluids using solid-phase extraction. *J Chromatogr* 1987;421:430–433.
237. Sigman ME, Ma CY. Detection limits for GC/MS analysis of organic explosives. *J Forensic Sci* 2001;46:6–11.
238. Hable M, Stern C, Asowata C, et al. The determination of nitroaromatics and nitramines in ground and drinking water by wide-bore capillary gas chromatography. *J Chromatogr Sci* 1991;29:131–135.
239. ATSDR: Agency for Toxic Substances and Disease Registry. Toxicologic profile for HMX. Atlanta: U.S. Department of Health and Human Services, 1997.
240. Tan EL, Ho CH, Griest WH, et al. Mutagenicity of trinitrotoluene and its metabolites formed during composting. *J Toxicol Environ Health* 1992;36:165–175.
241. Glover DJ, Hoffsommer JC. Thin-layer chromatography analysis of HMX in water. *Bull Environ Contam Toxicol* 1973;10:302–304.
242. Yinon J. *Toxicity and metabolism of explosives*. Boca Raton, FL: CRC Press, 1991:165–170.
243. Sutton WL. Aliphatic nitro compounds, nitrates, nitrites. In: Patty FA, ed. *Industrial hygiene and toxicology*, vol. 2, 2nd ed. New York: Interscience, 1963:2097.
244. Sax NI. *Dangerous properties of industrial materials*, 5th ed. New York: Van Nostrand Reinhold, 1979:889.
245. Finkel AJ, ed. Esters. In: *Hamilton's and Hardy's industrial toxins*. Boston: John Bright PSG Inc, 1983:219–224.
246. Reynolds JFE, ed. *Martindale: the extra pharmacopoeia*, 13th ed. London: The Pharmaceutical Press, 1993:1025.
247. Drugs affecting renal and cardiovascular function. In: Hardman JG, Limbrid JE, eds. *Goodman & Gilman's the pharmacological basis of therapeutics*, 9th ed. New York: McGraw-Hill, 1996:760–767.
248. Lawton AH, Yagoda H, von Oettingen WF. Absorption of erythritol tetranitrate and PETN from gastro-intestinal tract. In: *Toxicity and potential dangers of penta-erythritol-tetranitrate (PETN)*. Washington: US Public Health Service, 1944:19–21. Public Health Bulletin no. 282.
249. Krantz JC Jr, Leake CD. The gastrointestinal absorption of organic nitrates. *Am J Cardiol* 1975;36:407–408.
250. Davidson IW, Miller HS Jr, DiCarlo FJ. Pharmacodynamics and biotransformation of pentaerythritol tetranitrate in man. *J Pharm Sci* 1971;60:274–277.
251. Davidson IWF, Rollins FO, DiCarlo FJ, et al. The pharmacodynamics and biotransformation of pentaerythritol trinitrate in man. *Clin Pharmacol Ther* 1971;12:972–981.
252. Davidson IWF, Miller HS Jr, DiCarlo FJ. Absorption, excretion and metabolism of pentaerythritol tetranitrate by humans. *J Pharmacol Exp Ther* 1970;175:42–50.
253. Di Carlo FJ, Crew MC, Brusco LS, et al. Metabolism of pentaerythritol trinitrate. *Clin Pharmacol Ther* 1977;22:309–315.
254. Di Carlo FJ, Crew MC, Sklow NJ, et al. Metabolism of pentaerythritol tetranitrate by patients with coronary artery disease. *J Pharmacol Exp Ther* 1966;153:254–258.
255. Neurath GB, Dunger M. Blood levels of the metabolites of glyceryl trinitrate and pentaerythritol tetranitrate after administration of a two-step preparation. *Arzneimittelforschung* 1977;27:416–419.
256. Weber W, Michaelis K, Luckow V, et al. Pharmacokinetics and bioavailability of pentaerythrityl tetranitrate and two of its metabolites. *Arzneim Forsch* 1995;45:781–784.
257. Posadas del Rio FA, Jaramillo Juarez F, Camacho Garcia R. Biotransformation of organic nitrate esters in vitro by human liver, kidney, intestine, and blood serum. *Drug Metab Dispos* 1988;16:477–481.
258. McEvoy GK, ed. *AHFS drug information 92*. Bethesda: American Society of Hospital Pharmacists, 1992:1022.
259. Reichek N. Long-acting nitrates in the treatment of angina pectoris. *JAMA* 1976;236:1399–1402.
260. Jurt U, Gori T, Ravandi A, et al. Differential effects of pentaerythritol tetranitrate and nitroglycerin on the development of tolerance and evidence of lipid peroxidation: a human in vivo study. *J Am Coll Cardiol* 2001;38:854–859.
261. Lasagna L, Schelling JL. A study of cross-tolerance to circulatory effects of organic nitrates. *Clin Pharmacol Ther* 1967;8:256–260.
262. Di Carlo FJ, Coutinho CB, Sklow NJ, et al. Binding of pentaerythritol tetranitrate and its metabolites by rat blood plasma and erythrocytes. *Proc Soc Exp Biol Med* 1965;120:705–709.
263. von Oettingen WF, Donahue DD. Acute toxic manifestations of PETN. In: *Toxicity and potential dangers of penta-erythritol-tetranitrate (PETN)*. Washington: US Public Health Service, 1944:23–30. Public Health Bulletin no. 282.
264. Ryan FP. Erythroderma due to peritrate and glyceryl trinitrate. *Br J Dermatol* 1972;87:498–500.
265. Whitworth CG, Grant WM. The use of nitrate and nitrate vasodilators by glaucomatous patients. *Arch Ophthalmol* 1964;71:492–496.
266. Donahue DD. Chronic toxic manifestations of PETN. In: *Toxicity and potential dangers of penta-erythritol-tetranitrate (PETN)*. Washington: US Public Health Service, 1944:30–39. Public Health Bulletin no. 282.
267. Bucher JR, Huff J, Haseman JK, et al. No evidence of toxicity or carcinogenicity of pentaerythritol tetranitrate given in the diet to F344 rats and B6C3F1 mice for up to two years. *J Appl Toxicol* 1990;10:353–357.
268. Yagoda H. Determination of aliphatic nitrate esters—a colorimetric method. *Ind Eng Chem* 1943;15:27–29.
269. Stalleicken D, Kuntze U, Schmid B, et al. Quantitative determination of pentaerythrityl tetranitrate and its metabolites in human plasma by gas chromatography/mass spectrometry. *Arzneimittelforschung* 1997;47:347–352.
270. Gelber L, Papas AN. Validation of high-performance liquid chromatographic methods for analysis of sustained-release preparations containing nitroglycerin, isosorbide dinitrate, or pentaerythritol tetranitrate. *J Pharm Sci* 1983;72:124–126.
271. Bighley LD, Wurster DE, Cruden-Loeb C, et al. High-performance liquid chromatographic determination of pentaerythritol in plasma. *J Chromatogr* 1975;110:375–380.
272. Yu WC, Goff EU. Measurement of plasma concentrations of vasodilators and metabolites by the TEA analyzer. *Biopharm Drug Dispos* 1983;4:311–319.
273. Yu WC, Goff EU. Determination of vasodilators and their metabolites in plasma by liquid chromatography with a nitrosyl-specific detector. *Anal Chem* 1983;55:29–32.

SECTION

5

Hobbies, Arts, and Crafts

CHAPTER 200

Hobbies, Arts, and Crafts

John M. Boe

Topics included:	**Aquaria; ceramics; chemistry sets; children, hobbies, and art materials; coin collecting; etching; firing ranges; glassworking; insect collecting; gemstone work; metalworking; modeling; painting; performing arts; photography; printmaking; woodworking and furniture refinishing**
Special concerns:	**The potential for toxic exposure from common arts and crafts products is often unrecognized.**
Antidote:	**None**

OVERVIEW

Millions of people throughout the world are involved in hobbies, arts, and crafts that may subject them to health hazards of which they may not be aware. The clinician should recognize the sources of exposure and be prepared to introduce measures to diminish the possible toxic effects that may result from hazardous hobbies (Table 1). Hazardous exposure derives from metals, woods, dust, chemicals, and physical agents (Table 2). Guidelines for an industrial hygiene survey and for studios used for design materials, printmaking, and metal sculpture have been proposed (1). Southern Illinois University has developed a hazardous waste management program for the disposal of hazardous wastes (2).

Arts Crafts and Theater Safety provides a free listing of many publications providing professional information on hazards posed by toxic materials and dangerous equipment used in arts, crafts, and theater settings (http://ACTS@caseweb.com). A detailed listing of available publications is provided online at http://www.caseweb.com/acts.

GENERAL PRECAUTIONS

There are several simple precautions people can take to work safely with art materials. More detailed information on these precautions can be found by consulting the references listed at the end of this chapter, especially The Artists Complete Health and Safety Guide by Monona Rossol. A list of recommended readings regarding toxicity prevention is provided in Table 3.

Choose the Safest Materials Possible

Whenever possible, replace solvent-containing materials with water-based materials to eliminate solvent inhalation problems. Buy wet materials, such as prepared clay, aqueous dye solutions, and water-based glazes, rather than dry powders. Avoid materials that contain chemicals that can cause cancer or adverse reproductive effects. Individuals who are at high risk, such as disabled individuals, pregnant women, children, and people with certain illnesses, should check to see if their art materials might be particularly dangerous to them. If so, safer substitutes, better ventilation, or other more stringent precautions might be needed. For pregnant women in particular, unless the art materials are known to be safe during pregnancy, the materials should be avoided.

Read Labels Carefully

Most labels only list the acute or immediate hazards. Labels with the CL (certified label) seal of the Arts and Crafts Materials Institute also have the chronic or long-term hazards listed. You should also request Material Safety Data Sheets on your products from the distributor or manufacturer. Interactive Learning Paradigms, Inc., has a complete online listing of Web sites providing Material Safety Data Sheets (3). This listing can be found at http://www.ilpi.com/msds.

TABLE 1. Where the hazards lie

Ingredient	Source	Toxic effects
Lead	A wide range of arts and crafts materials, including ceramic glazes, stained-glass materials, and pigments—especially those used in printmaking	Abdominal pain, anemia, reproductive disorders, nephritis, CNS and peripheral nervous system damage, and others
Cadmium	Silver solders, pigments, ceramic glazes, and fluxes	Suspected carcinogen and teratogen; lung and kidney dysfunction, high blood pressure, nervous system disorders, and anemia
Chromium	Oil and acrylic paint pigments and ceramic colorants	Dermatitis, allergy, skin ulcerations, and bronchial cancer
PCBs	Contaminant of certain oil and acrylic paint pigments	Suspected carcinogen and possible teratogen; adverse long-term effects, including liver damage, unusual eye discharge, digestive disturbances, and chemical acne, may not appear for months after initial exposure
Manganese dioxide	Ceramic colorants and oil and acrylic paint pigments such as Mars brown, raw umber, and burnt umber	With chronic poisoning, Parkinson-like symptoms and damage to lungs, liver, kidneys, and CNS
Cobalt	Oil and acrylic paint pigments such as cerulean blue, cobalt blue, and ultramarine blue	Suspected carcinogen and neoplastigen; allergy and cardiac damage
Formaldehyde	Preservative in many acrylic paints and photographic hardeners and stabilizers	Skin, eye, and mucous membrane irritation; allergy; and asthma
Asbestos	Contaminant in talc used in ceramics and lithography and in soapstone, serpentine, and greenstone	Known carcinogen
Solvents	Ubiquitous in arts and crafts and used for a multitude of purposes	—
Aromatic hydrocarbons	Resin solvents, paint and varnish removers, fluorescent dye solvent, silk screen cleanup, lacquer thinners, aerosol sprays, and permanent markers	Toluene and xylene linked to CNS depression, dermatitis, and respiratory tract irritation; benzene associated with aplastic anemia, liver damage, and reproductive effects
Chlorinated hydrocarbons	Ink removers, lithographic solvents, rubber cements, paint strippers, aerosol sprays, and varnish removers	Liver function abnormalities, blood-clotting changes, cardiac irregularities, and dermatitis; methylene chloride is a suspected carcinogen and causes pulmonary edema, narcosis, CNS depression, dermatitis, and heart attack; severe liver and kidney damage with small amounts of carbon tetrachloride and large amounts may result in unconsciousness and death, especially in the presence of alcoholic beverages; may be absorbed through the skin
Petroleum distillates	Paint thinners, rubber cement thinners, spray adhesives, silk screen inks, and cleanup	Mild narcotic effect and lung irritation; pulmonary edema if ingested; peripheral neuropathy with chronic inhalation of *n*-hexane; permanent CNS damage when large amounts are inhaled
Glycol ethers and acetates	Photoresists, color photography, lacquer thinners, paints, and aerosol sprays	Anemia and kidney damage; birth defects, miscarriages, testicular atrophy, and sterility in animals

CNS, central nervous system; PCBs, polychlorinated benzenes.
Adapted from *Emerg Med* 1986;18:6.

Children's art materials are of particular concern. The nontoxic label on children's art materials legally means that the art material passes the acute toxicity tests of the Federal Hazardous Substances Act. The Labeling of Hazardous Art Materials Act (Public Law 100-695, 15 U.S.C. #1277) deals with the hazards of chronic exposure to arts and crafts materials. Parents and others buying art materials, school supplies, and toys such as crayons,

TABLE 2. Hazardous materials used in arts and crafts

Metals	**Woods**	Peroxide
Arsenic	**Dusts**	Plastics
Cadmium	**Chemicals**	Styrene
Chromium	Acids, alkalis	Turpentine
Cobalt	Acrylics	Vinyls
Copper	Benzene	**Physical hazards**
Lead	Carbon tetrachloride	Infrared radiation
Manganese	Epoxides	Noise
Mercury	Epoxy foams	Ultraviolet radiation
Nickel	Methanol	
Silver	Methyl butyl ketone	
Tin	Methyl cellosolve acetate	
Titanium	Methylene chloride	
Zinc		

TABLE 3. Resources for the prevention of toxicity in arts, crafts, and hobbies

Clark N, Cutter T, McGrane J-A. *Ventilation. A practical guide.* New York: Center for Occupational Hazards, 1984.
McCann M. *Artist beware: the hazards and precautions in working with art and craft materials,* 2nd ed. Guilford, CT: The Globe Pequot Press, 1992.
McCann M. *Health hazards manual for artists,* revised 4th ed. New York: Lyons & Buford, 1990.
[a]NCECA. *Keeping clay work safe and legal.* National Council on Education for the Ceramic Arts (http://www.nceca.net) publication, accessed 08/06/2003.
[b]Rossol M. *The artists complete health and safety guide.* New York: Allworth Press, 1996.
[b]Rossol M. *The health and safety guide for film, TV & theater.* New York: Allworth Press.
[b]Rossol M. *Stage fright: health and safety in the theater.* New York: Allworth Press, 2001.
Seeger N. *Alternatives for the artist,* revised ed. Chicago: School of the Art Institute of Chicago, 1984.
[a]Shaw S, Rossol M. Overexposure: health hazards in photography, 2nd ed. New York. Allworth Press, 1997.

[a]Available from Arts Crafts and Theater Safety [(212) 777-0062].
[b]Available from Allworth Press [(800) 491-2808].

paint sets, or modeling clay should be alert and purchase only those products that are accompanied by the statement "Conforms to ASTM D-4236" (4). Products with the CP or AP (certified or approved product) seal of the Arts and Crafts Materials Institute are recommended. Children's art materials with these seals have had their formulations approved by a toxicologist with expertise in children's art materials.

Set Up a Studio Carefully

Whenever possible, do not have a studio in the home. If the work must be done at home, set up the studio in a separate room—not in the living areas. Store art materials safely where children cannot reach them. Do not store materials in containers such as orange juice containers and soda bottles because of the danger of accidental ingestion.

There are two types of ventilation for control of toxic contaminants: dilution ventilation and local exhaust ventilation. Dilution ventilation involves bringing clean air into the room where the work is performed to mix the contaminated air and dilute it to a lower and safer concentration and then exhaust it to the outside with an exhaust fan. This type of ventilation is good when working with small amounts of solvents or gases that are not very toxic. For example, a window exhaust fan is adequate dilution ventilation for oil painting, in which a maximum of approximately 1 cup of turpentine per day is used. Similarly, dilution ventilation is good for black-and-white photographic darkrooms. Dilution ventilation is not good for large amounts of solvents, such as printing with solvent-based silk screen inks; highly toxic solvents, such as those in lacquer thinners; or dusts.

Local exhaust ventilation, on the other hand, uses items such as hoods and spray booths to capture the contaminants where they are generated before they can get into the general room air. The contaminants are then exhausted to the outside through a duct. Local exhaust ventilation is preferred. For further information on ventilation of art studios, see *Ventilation: A Practical Guide*, by Nancy Clark, Thomas Cutter, and Jean-Ann McGrane (4a).

Protect Against Fire

Do not smoke or have open flames, sparks, or static electricity near flammable liquids or gases. Store flammable and combustible liquids in safety cans and keep only amounts on hand needed for a few days. Large amounts of flammable and combustible liquids should be stored in a flame-resistant storage cabinet. Have smoke alarms and the right type of fire extinguisher. If ordinary combustibles, flammable liquids, and electrical equipment are used, have a class ABC fire extinguisher. Know how to use the fire extinguisher. If flammable liquids are used, the exhaust systems must be explosion proof.

Clean Up Carefully

Always clean up spills immediately. For dusts, wet mop or vacuum; never sweep, which stirs up dust. For clay and other highly toxic dusts, the vacuum cleaner should be equipped with a special [HEPA (high-efficiency particulate air)] filter.

Dispose of Art Materials Safely

Do not pour solvents down the sink. Small amounts less than 1 pint can be disposed of safely by evaporation inside a local exhaust hood or outdoors. For large amounts, contact a waste disposal service. Nonpolluting materials dissolved in water can be poured down the sink one at a time with lots of water. Acids and alkalis should be neutralized first.

Have Good Personal Work Practices

Do not eat, drink, or smoke in the studio. Wash chemical splashes off the skin with lots of water. In case of eye contact, rinse with water for at least 20 minutes and call a doctor; an eyewash fountain is recommended. If concentrated acids and alkalis are used, have an emergency shower available. Do not wash hands with solvents; use soap and water. To remove oil paints, use baby oil and then soap and water. Have a first-aid kit available.

Wear proper personal protective clothing and equipment. Wear special work clothes (e.g., smocks, hair coverings) and wash separately from other clothing. Use the right type of gloves, goggles, hearing protectors, respirators, and so forth. Make sure they are approved for the chemicals being used and that they fit properly. Respirators, in particular, should be approved by the National Institute for Occupational Safety and Health (NIOSH; http://www.cdc.gov/niosh) for the particular contaminant.

Several types of respirators exist. All respirators require training to be used properly. Escape respirators are only for emergency use and should serve only to escape from a dangerous area to a safe area. Particulate respirators are designed only to protect against particles and offer no chemical protection. These are the inexpensive and commonly used N-95 masks. Chemical cartridge or gas mask respirators clean both chemical gases and particles from the air. These masks require that you select the proper type of cartridge for the gas involved (5).

Avoid physical and electrical hazards. Keep or put machine guards on all machinery. Do not wear loose, long hair, loose sleeves, or necklaces around machinery. Keep equipment and electrical wiring in good repair. Ground electrical equipment and do not overload the wiring.

Seek Medical Assistance

If symptoms might be connected with an art hobby, expert medical assistance should be sought. A family physician might not have this expertise because specialized training is needed to understand both the toxic effects of chemicals and the special medical problems of performing artists. In fact, the latter area is now becoming known as *arts medicine*.

SAFETY LABELING

The Labeling of Hazardous Art Materials Act directs the U.S. Consumer Product Safety Commission to set up guidelines for determining whether arts and crafts materials present chronic health hazards. The law mandates a voluntary Standard ASTM D-4236-88 as a mandatory labeling standard for arts and crafts materials. Artists, safety and health professionals, and the art materials industry developed this labeling standard, which took effect November 18, 1990. The law applies to many children's toy products such as crayons, chalk, paint sets, modeling clay, coloring books, pencils, and any other products used by children to produce a work or visual or graphic art. The labels must provide (a) a warning statement of the hazards, (b) identification of the hazardous ingredients, and (c) guidelines for safe use. The standard requires labels for all arts and crafts materials determined to present a chronic hazard, including solvents, spray paints, silk screen inks, adhesives, and any other substance marketed or represented as suitable for use in any phase of the creation of any work of visual or graphic art of any medium.

The Commission believes that under the broad statutory definition of art material three general categories exist (6):

1. Those products that actually become a component of the work of visual or graphic art, such as paint, canvas, inks, crayons, chalk, solder, brazing rods, flux, paper, clay, stone, thread, cloth, and photographic film.
2. Those products that are closely and intimately associated with the creation of the final work of art, such as brush cleaners, solvents, ceramic kilns, brushes, silk screens, molds or mold-making material, and photo-developing chemicals.
3. Those tools, implements, and furniture that are used in the process of the creation of a work of art but do not become part of the work or art. Examples are drafting tables and chairs, easels, picture frames, canvas stretchers, potter's wheels, hammers, chisels, and air pumps for air brushes.

Ideally, labels should also contain information on the type of hazard the materials present, including the following:

1. An estimate of the relative toxicity of the chemicals
2. Precautions and detailed instructions on how to work with a chemical safely (e.g., type of ventilation, protective clothing)
3. Currently recommended first-aid instructions

PREGNANCY AND LACTATION

A summary of possible adverse reproductive effects of chemical and physical agents involved in hobbies, arts, and crafts is found in Table 4. Many substances used by arts, crafts, and hobby enthusiasts are potential mutagens (e.g., lead, formaldehyde, trichloroethane). Women in the childbearing years should be counseled regarding exposure to materials that may pass the placental barrier and possibly lead to birth defects (e.g., lead; other heavy metals such as cadmium, azo dyes, benzene, and chlorinated hydrocarbon solvents; and nonchlorinated hydrocarbon solvents such as toluene and xylene). Instruct women to avoid such materials, at least during the first 3 months of pregnancy; in later pregnancy, ensure sufficient control over the environment to minimize or eliminate access to toxic chemicals (e.g., heavy metals, solvents, dyes, toxic dusts, and gases).

Breast-feeding during use of such materials described may expose the infant to toxic substances in the mother's milk supply. Suggested recommendations for pregnant and nursing artists compiled by The Center for Safety in the Arts are presented in Table 5. These are general guidelines and must be supplemented by consultation with a physician for additional specific prenatal and postnatal advice. Additional references to pregnancy and lactation exposure to many of these chemicals are available (1).

CLINICAL PRESENTATION

History of Exposure

Hobby and craft exposures largely parallel those in industrial exposures. The largest number of cases have dermatologic reactions, followed in descending order by respiratory and general poisoning reactions. Finally, there are smaller numbers of teratogenic, mutagenic, and carcinogenic problems.

The patient should be asked (a) to list all the solids, liquids, and gases used in the activity; (b) what processes are used; (c) the number of hours per week and the number of years of exposure to the activity; (d) the work environment (outdoors or indoors, small closed room or ventilated area, alone or with others); (e) leisure time activities; and (f) smoking habits. Correlate these answers to the patient's complaints (e.g., weakness, numbness, and tingling in the extremities; peripheral neuropathy) (Table 6).

Physical Examination

Examine the patient's hands, face, and exposed chest for skin problems (industrial solvents, detergents, cutting oils, photographic chemicals, oils, and solvents used in refinishing furniture). A complete neurologic examination may indicate problems related to lead or mercury exposure. When necessary, re-examine the patient immediately after a specific period of exposure to the hobby or work (e.g., pulmonary function tests and careful chest examination after exposure to a dust-promoting material).

DIAGNOSTIC TESTS

Monitoring tests for some substances used in arts and crafts are presented in Table 7.

AQUARIA

Tropical aquariums have become increasingly popular since the early 1990s. Approximately 10% of homes in the United States have aquaria, and purchases of live ornamental fish for aquaria and ponds amount to more than $600 million a year in the United States (7).

Reef or mini-reef aquariums, which attempt to re-create a small section of a coral reef, have also seen a surge in popularity. Reef keepers use a large variety of additives to maintain the water quality of their tanks. These additives may include calcium hydroxide in powder form (called *kalkwasser* in the aquarium industry), strontium chloride, magnesium chloride, potassium iodide or Lugol's solution, and various buffering solutions that may contain magnesium or borate salts. The test kits used in this type of aquaria also represent potential chemical exposures. Kits for determining ammonia levels in water may contain sodium hydroxide and sodium hypochlorite. Test kits for nitrate may contain hydrazine, a potent cellular toxin (8).

The salt mixes used to create marine water have the potential to cause respiratory irritation on mixing and inhalation of the aerosolized powder as well as a contact dermatitis from repeated exposure during routine aquarium maintenance (9).

CERAMICS

Approximately 2 million Americans are hobby ceramicists; 95% of them are women, and 70% are between the ages of 30 and 50 years. Approximately 80% of hobby glazing is done in educational studios run by distributors of hobby glazes. Hobby glazes are made up of frits (pre-fired mixtures of metal oxides, silica, aluminum, and alkalis), ceramic pigments (metal oxide–containing crystalline materials formed at high temperatures), clays, flint (fine quartz), feldspars, water, and other additives. Glazes that are certified as food safe release less than 1 ppm lead when a standard 8-oz cup fired with such a glaze is tested by a U.S. Food and Drug Administration method.

TABLE 4. Adverse reproductive effects of chemical and physical agents

Chemical name	Art process/material	Affects male[a]	Affects female[b]	Fetal death[c]	Affects newborn[d]
Metals					
Antimony	Ceramics and enameling, metalworking, pewter	H/A	H/A	H/A	H/A
Arsenic	Glassblowing, patinas, wood preservative	—	H/A	A	A
Cadmium	Pigments, silver soldering, ceramics and enameling	H/A	A	A	H/A
Chromium	Pigments, ceramics and enameling, photochemicals	A	—	—	A
Cobalt	Pigments, ceramics and enameling	A	—	—	A
Copper	Metalworking, ceramics and enameling	A	A	—	A
Gold salts	Photochemicals and electroplating	—	—	—	A
Lead	Pigments, soft solders, ceramics and enameling, stained glass, lead casting	H/A	H/A	H/A	H/A
Lithium	Ceramics and enameling	—	—	—	H/A
Manganese	Pigments, metalworking, ceramics and enameling	H/A	H/A	A	A
Mercury	Pigments, photochemicals, neon sculpture	H/A	H/A	A	H/A
Nickel	Electroplating, metalworking, ceramics and enameling	A	—	—	A
Selenium	Pigment, photochemicals	H/A	H/A	H/A	H/A
Zinc	Pigment, metalworking, solder, flux, ceramics and enameling	A	—	—	A
Solvents					
Acetone	Strippers, lacquers, thinners, plastics solvent	—	—	A	A
Benzene	Old paint strippers and old rubber cements, gasoline	H/A	H/A	—	H/A
Benzyl alcohol	Photochemicals, solvent	—	—	—	H/A
Ethyl alcohol	Shellac-denatured alcohol	H/A	H/A	H/A	H/A
Ethylene dichloride	Plastics solvent	—	H/A	A	A
Glycol ethers	Photochemicals, solvent, photoresists, lacquers, aerosol sprays	H?[e]/A	H?[e]/A	A	A
Isopropyl alcohol	Rubbing alcohol	—	—	—	A
Methyl alcohol	Shellac, French dyes, duplicating fluid, paint strippers	—	—	A	A
Methyl chloroform	Aerosol sprays, etching grounds, film cleaners	—	—	—	H[f]
Methylene chloride	Paint strippers, aerosol sprays, plastics cement	—	—	—	A
Methyl ethyl ketone	Lacquers, thinners, plastics solvent	—	—	—	H[f]
Organic solvents mixture	Wide variety of art materials	—	H/A	H/A	H/A
Perchloroethylene	Degreasing, printmaking	—	A	—	H[f]/A
Refined petroleum solvents	Paint thinner, lacquer, silk screen inks, aerosol sprays, rubber cements	—	H	—	—
Toluene	Lacquer thinners, silk screen inks, aerosols	—	H/A	H/A	H/A
Turpentine	Varnishes, painting	—	—	—	A
Xylene	Lacquer thinners, printmaking, aerosol sprays	—	H	A	H/A
Miscellaneous chemicals					
Bromides	Photochemicals	—	—	—	H
Carbon monoxide	Gas-fired kilns and furnaces, carbon arcs	H/A	H/A	H/A	H/A
Cyanides	Electroplating, photochemicals, plastics decomposition	—	A	A	A
Fluorine and compounds	Glass etching, silver solder flux and welding, ceramics and enameling	—	—	—	H/A
Formaldehyde	Preservative, photochemicals, certain glues and resins, plywood, particle board	—	H	—	A
Glycidyl ethers	Epoxy resins and glues	A	—	—	A
Hydrogen sulfide	Decomposition of sulfide toners and sulfide metal colorants	—	A	—	A
Nitrogen dioxide	Etching, arc welding, carbon arcs	—	A	A	A
Pentachlorophenol	Wood preservative	A	A	H/A	H/A
Phthalate esters	Plastics plasticizer, plastic resin hardener	A	—	A	A
Styrene	Polyester resin	A	H/A	—	—
Textile dyes	Fabric dyeing	—	—	—	A
Physical agents					
Heat	Kilns and furnaces	H/A	H/A	—	H/A
Ionizing radiation	Ceramic and pottery glazes and enamels, photochemicals	H/A	H/A	—	H/A
Noise and vibration	Wood and metalworking machinery, abrasive blasting, pneumatic tools	H/A	H/A	—	H/A

—, no studies or insufficient data; A, positive animal studies; H, positive human studies.
[a]Includes reduced fertility, cancer of the reproductive organs, abnormal or reduced sperm, testicular damage, and so forth.
[b]Includes reduced fertility, cancer of reproductive organs, menstrual changes and disorders, sterility, and so forth.
[c]Includes miscarriage, stillbirth, and spontaneous abortion.
[d]Includes low birth weight, birth defects, premature birth, growth retardation, and so forth.
[e]Based on inconclusive data that are suggestive but incomplete.
[f]Studies indicate appearance in breast milk after exposure of the mother.

TABLE 5. Recommendations for pregnant and nursing artists

Art process	Material	Recommendation
Pastels	Pigment dust	Avoid during pregnancy and nursing. Use oil pastels as substitutes.
	Spray fixative	Use only in explosion-proof spray booth or outdoors.
Photography		
Black and white	Developers, intensifiers	Do not mix dry chemicals.
	Toners (sulfide, selenium)	Use only with local exhaust ventilation.
Color	Solvents, formaldehyde	Use only with local exhaust ventilation.
Blue printing	Carbon arcs	Do not use carbon arcs. Use sunlight or other ultraviolet source.
Relief printing	Solvents	Use water-based inks only.

TABLE 6. Questionnaire for obtaining information about arts, crafts, and hobby activities

List and describe your arts, crafts, or hobby activities.
Approximately how many hours per week do you do this work?
Do you use any protective equipment when you work (e.g., gloves, coverall/apron, glasses/goggles, hearing protection)?
When you work, are you exposed to any of the following?
- Solvents (e.g., turpentine, paint thinner).
- Aerosols or sprays.
- Dusts (e.g., wood, clay, stone).
- Smoke metal fumes.
- Metals or other chemicals.

Where do you do this work?
- At home? If so, how near to the kitchen or bedroom do you work?
- In an individual studio, garage, or outbuilding?
- In a group studio or school? If so, what other chemicals and hazards are you exposed to from other workers?
- If you have any physical ailments or health problems, do others in the school or studio have similar problems?

Does your workspace have good ventilation? Describe.
Have you worked in other arts or crafts in the past?
- If so, what have you done and on what approximate dates?

Modified from McCunney RJ, et al. *Am Fam Physician* 1987;36:145–153.

TABLE 7. Health effects and appropriate monitoring tests for substances used in arts and crafts

Substance	Hobby/use	Health effect	Test
Solvents			
Benzene	Paint remover; solvent for waxes, oils	Aplastic anemia, skin irritation and dryness, headache, nausea, vertigo, coagulopathies	Complete blood cell count
Methanol	Solvent in paints and varnishes	Ocular toxicity, central nervous system depression, metabolic acidosis	Urine methanol level, urine formic acid level
Methylene chloride	Paint and varnish remover, cleaning fluid	Fatigue, weakness, lightheadedness, paresthesias, eye irritation, toxic encephalopathy	Carboxyhemoglobin level
Toluene	Paint thinner; solvent in paints, lacquers; glues	Headache, fatigue, memory impairment, ataxia, euphoria, confusion, dilated pupils	Urine hippuric acid level
1,1,1-Trichloroethane	Paints, glues	Ataxia, lightheadedness, liver and kidney damage	Blood and urine trichloroethane levels
Xylene	Paints, lacquers	Dizziness, lethargy, ataxia, anorexia, mucous membrane irritation	Urine methyl hippuric acid level
Fixatives			
n-Hexane	Lacquers, solvent in quick-drying ink and cements	Central nervous system depression, peripheral neuropathy, respiratory irritation	Nerve conduction studies
Stones and clay			
Asbestos	Clays, papier-mâché, glazes, sculpture stones, French chalk used in graphics	Asbestosis	Chest film, pulmonary function tests
Silica	Clays, glazes, sculpture dust, jewelry-buffing compound	Silicosis	Chest film, pulmonary function tests
Metals			
Cadmium	Silver soldering alloys	Pulmonary edema, fibrosis, renal disease	Blood and urine cadmium levels
Chromates (lead and zinc)	Paint pigments	Carcinogenic (suspected), respiratory irritation	Chest film, pulmonary function tests
Lead	Solders, paints, metal alloys, enamels	Neurologic complaints, abdominal pain, fatigue, anemia	Complete blood cell count, blood lead level, zinc protoporphyrin
Lithium	Drying agent, metallurgy	Anorexia, nausea, tremors, central nervous system changes	Blood and urine lithium levels
Mercury	Paint preservative	Nervousness, fatigue, tremors, bleeding gums	Blood and urine mercury levels
Other chemicals			
Benzidine	Dyes, paints	Urinary tract and bladder cancer	Urinary cytology
Formaldehyde	Acrylic paints, certain glues, resins, kiln fumes	Mucous membrane irritation, cough, bronchospasm, contact dermatitis	Urine formic acid level
Pentachlorophenol (PCP)	Wood preservative	Delirium, weakness, hyperpyrexia, tachycardia, tachypnea	Blood and urine pentachlorophenol levels
Selenium	Decolorizer in ceramic glazes	Metallic taste, garlic odor of breath, headache, sore throat, fume fever, mucous membrane irritation	Urine selenium level

Adapted from McCunney RJ, et al. *Am Fam Physician* 1987;36:145–153.

TABLE 8. Clay components and associated pulmonary diseases

Clay component	Disease
Alumina	Aluminosis (lung disease)
Asbestos (contaminant of talc)	Asbestosis, cancer of several sites
Barium carbonate	Central nervous system disease, baritosis (benign pneumoconiosis)
Diatomaceous earth (raw material for clay)	Silicosis
Feldspar	Pneumoconiosis
Iron oxide	Siderosis
Kaolin (raw material for china clay)	Kaolinosis
Talc (raw material for porcelain)	Talcosis, lung cancer

Adapted from Fuortes LJ. *Postgrad Med* 1989;85:133–136.

Clays

Many of the raw materials in clays commonly used by ceramic artists are fibrogenic and may lead to pneumoconiosis when inhaled. Little acute toxicity is experienced. Chronic exposure to fibrogenic clay compounds is associated with a number of pulmonary diseases (Table 8). Such diseases often go undetected until they have reached an advanced stage. Subclinical stages of these diseases can be detected by radiography, lung volume determinations, and testing of gas diffusion capacity (Chapter 189).

Glazes

Lead is no longer used in pottery glazes in the United States; however, potters in underdeveloped countries still commonly use lead glazes. Lead poisoning and even death have been reported. Acidic foods and liquids have the greatest propensity for leaching lead from these objects. Heavy metals used in glazes in the United States include arsenic, antimony, and cadmium (Table 9) (10).

Kiln emissions may be poorly exhausted, causing airborne contamination because of a desire of the artist to place the kiln in a state of reduction (relative oxygen depletion), being fired under lead pressure, to bring out subtle colors of various glazes (Table 10). Sulfur dioxide, which is emitted during the initial firing of clay, can produce pulmonary disease (11).

TABLE 9. Common glaze components and associated hazards

Glaze component	Hazard
Antimony trioxide	Heavy metal poisoning
Arsenic trioxide	Heavy metal poisoning, cancer
Beryllium	Pneumonitis, pneumoconiosis
Boric acid	Skin irritation, CNS depression
Cadmium oxide	Heavy metal poisoning
Calcium carbonate	Nonspecific
Cobalt	Sensitization of skin and lung, cardiomyopathy
Copper	Nontoxic unless in form of copper sulfate verdigris
Chromates (nickel, iron, potassium)	Sensitization (dermatitis, asthma, pulmonary fibrosis), cancer
Lead	Heavy metal poisoning
Lithium carbonate	CNS and renal toxicities
Manganese dioxide	CNS toxicities (parkinsonism)
Nickel oxide	Sensitization, cancer
Tin oxide	Benign pneumoconiosis
Titanium dioxide	Benign pneumoconiosis
Zinc oxide	Dermatitis, metal fume fever

CNS, central nervous system.
Adapted from Fuortes LJ. *Postgrad Med* 1989;85:133–136.

TABLE 10. Threshold limit values of kiln emissions

Emission	Threshold limit value
Carbon monoxide: byproduct of incomplete combustion; significant exposure possible during reduction phase of firing	35 ppm
Chlorine gas: byproduct of salt glaze process	1 ppm
Hydrochloric acid vapor: byproduct of salt glaze process	5 ppm
Infrared radiation: significant exposure when cones are inspected through ports	NA
Nitrogen dioxide: byproduct of natural gas combustion	6 mg/m^3
Nitric oxide: byproduct of natural gas combustion	30 mg/m^3
Smoke and soot: byproduct of raku and smoke pit firings	NA
Sulfur dioxide: byproduct of bisque firing, especially of high-sulfur clay	2 ppm
Vaporized glaze constituents	NA
Various metal fumes	—
Various hydrocarbons: aldehydes (formaldehyde), mercaptans	1.5 mg/m^3

NA, not available; ppm, parts per million.
Adapted from Fuortes LJ. *Postgrad Med* 1989;85:133–136.

Precautions for using glazes are as follows (12):

- Glazes should be stored in liquid or slurry form to minimize dust exposure and should be applied by dipping or brushing, not spraying.
- Replace the more toxic glaze substances (heavy metals and chromates) with nontoxic materials (12,13).
- Glazing should be done only in a room suitably equipped for the purpose.
- Because the danger of lead poisoning is greatest where lead or its compounds are inhaled, processes that are likely to give rise to these compounds in dust form in the air should not be allowed unless there is efficient exhaust ventilation or a suitable respirator is used. Where a spray is used, there should be a separate booth with an efficient exhaust fan. These processes are normally confined to establishments of further education (trade schools).
- Ventilation of the work area should be sufficient to exhaust away from the area all local production of toxic substances and to ensure proper functioning and exhaustion of kilns.
- Anyone who has carried out the processes should wash their hands and use a nailbrush immediately afterward.
- All benches and work surfaces should be washed down after use, and splashes of glaze should be removed from floors and walls. Clean up dust in the work area with a wet vacuum or damp mop.
- Stringent personal hygiene should be performed, such as frequent hand washing and no smoking, eating, or storing food in the areas used for pottery making. Keep work clothes in the work area. Wash them often.
- Use personal protective clothing and devices, including gloves, overalls or aprons, and respirators. An apron with a bib of impervious materials should be worn by anyone while actually engaged in glaze dipping and should be washed after use.
- Do not work and live in the same quarters.
- Art material suppliers should inform hobbyists and artisans of potential hazards. Proper labeling and storage of toxic substances should avert mishaps.
- Safety programs should be included in the studio-art curriculum.

TABLE 11. Potentially toxic chemicals

Name	Quantity (g)	Quantity (mg/kg)	Potentially toxic dose
Ammonium chloride	12.73	1061	>2000 mg total
Azurite	8.36	697	>1 g total (Cu)
	4.60 (Cu)	385 (Cu)	
Magnesium sulfate	13.68	1140	500 mg/kg
Phenolphthalein	2.00	167	>2000 mg
Potassium chloride	18.29	1524	238 mg/kg
Sodium borate$_{(-H_2O)}$	5.10	425	170 mg/kg
Sodium thiosulfate	21.82	1818	>12 g total
Strontium nitrate	24.85	2071	2750 mg/kg
Sulfur	10.42	868	>10 g total
Sodium bisulfite	16.91	1409	6 mg/kg

Note: Based on Oral LD-50 (rats).
Adapted from Everson GW, et al. *Vet Hum Toxicol* 1988;30:589–592.

CHEMISTRY SETS

Chemistry sets remain popular educational toys. Although their safety has been questioned in the past, most now advertise childproof caps, high-impact plastic containers, and special droppers to transfer chemicals. Past literature has shown multiple examples of poisonings involving acute cobalt intoxication (14,15). A 19-month-old child who ingested approximately 1 oz of a chemistry-set container of cobalt chloride died within a few hours (15). An analysis of three chemistry sets showed them to contain 28, 14, and 9 chemicals, respectively. Fifty-three percent of the chemicals contained quantities sufficient to be potentially toxic to a 2-year-old, 12-kg child; 13% contained chemicals in potentially lethal quantities; and 18% were considered nontoxic. Of the three analyzed, only one set used child-resistant closures (13). Thirty-five percent of the chemicals had incorrect or missing warning information (Tables 11, 12, and 13).

CHILDREN, HOBBIES, AND ART MATERIALS

Arts and crafts are common activities in children's educational settings (Table 14). Both types of activities may expose children to materials that could pose a serious health risk. The type and severity of the exposure may be related to the child's age group. For example, younger children may be less able to follow safety instructions and also may be more sensitive to a smaller exposure than an adult because of his or her smaller size. Exposure generally occurs by three routes: inhalation, ingestion, and skin contact, with the latter being the most common. The Labeling of Hazardous Art Material Act of 1988 requires that all art materials be reviewed to determine the potential of causing a chronic hazard and that appropriate warning labels be put on products found to pose a chronic hazard. The law applies to many children's toy products such as crayons, chalk, paint sets, modeling clay, coloring books, pencils, and any other products used by children to produce a work of visual or graphic art (10,16).

TABLE 12. Potentially lethal chemicals

Name	Quantity (g)	Quantity (mg/kg)	Potentially lethal dose (mg/kg)
Cobalt chloride hexahydrate	14.24	1187	766
Copper sulfate	12.35	1030	300
Ferric ammonium sulfate	14.19	—	—
(Elemental Fe)	(1.85)	154	60
Ferrous sulfate hexahydrate	5.72	—	—
(Elemental Fe)	(1.14)	95	60
Tannic acid	8.36	697	500

Adapted from Everson GW, et al. *Vet Hum Toxicol* 1988;30:589–592.

TABLE 13. Potentially caustic/corrosive chemicals

Name	Quantity (g)
Aluminum sulfate	14.77
Ammonium carbonate	6.97
Calcium hydroxide	4.36
Calcium oxide	4.90
Sodium bisulfate	19.88
Sodium carbonate	7.90
Sodium ferrocyanide	5.53
Sodium silicate	11.77
Calcium chloride	6.23
Calcium oxychloride	5.95

Adapted from Everson GW, et al. *Vet Hum Toxicol* 1988;30:589–592.

COIN COLLECTING

Although few serious coin collectors clean their coins, dilute nitric acid is sometimes used. A 77-year-old man developed a case of acute nitrogen dioxide toxicity after cleaning his collection of pennies at home. Nitric acid reacted with the copper in the pennies to form copper nitrate and nitrogen dioxide gas, which was inhaled. The man presented with severe dyspnea and pulmonary edema in evidence on chest radiograph (17).

ETCHING

Dutch mordant is 10% hydrochloric acid in water with potassium chlorate added. This is a reactive explosive that reacts with organic compounds, sulfur compounds, and sulfuric acid as well as with dirt and clothing (18).

FIRING RANGES/GUN SPORTS

Exposure to lead in indoor firing ranges is a well-documented occupational- and hobby-related hazard. Airborne lead is generated by the action of hot propellant gases against the base of the bullet, by the friction of bullets against the gun barrel, when leaded bullets strike the target area, and by the combustion of lead-priming compounds (19). The combustion of the primer for the powder charge in a bullet also significantly contributes to the amount of aerosolized lead (20). Most exposures related to firing ranges result from lack of adequate ventilation. However, at least one study has shown an elevation in blood lead levels in instructors in an outdoor shooting range (21). Analysis of blood lead levels in four employees of a privately owned shooting range revealed evidence of chronic and acute lead exposure. Increasing time worked at the range was associated with elevation of blood lead levels (22).

GLASSWORKING

Glassworking includes hot glass, both blown and casted; neon art; and stained glass.

TABLE 14. Art materials: recommendations for children younger than 12 years of age

Do not use	Substitutes
Dusts and powders	
Clay in dry form. Powdered clay, which is easily inhaled, contains free silica and possible asbestos. Do not sand dry clay pieces or do other dust-producing activities.	Order talc-free, premixed clay (e.g., Amaco white clay). Wet mop or sponge surfaces thoroughly after using clay.
Ceramic glazes or copper enamels.	Use water-based paints instead of glazes. Artwork may be water proofed with acrylic-based mediums.
Cold water, fiber-reactive dyes, or other commercial dyes.	Use vegetable and plant dyes (e.g., onion skins, tea, flowers) and food dyes.
Instant papier-mâché. This creates inhalable dust, and some may contain asbestos fibers, lead from pigments in colored printing inks, and so forth.	Make papier-mâché from black-and-white newspaper and library or white paste, or use approved papier-mâché.
Powdered tempera colors. They create inhalable dusts, and some contain toxic pigments, preservatives, and so forth.	Use liquid paints or paints the teacher premixes.
Pastels, chalks, or dry markers that create dust.	Use crayons, oil pastels, or dustless chalks.
Solvents	
Solvents (e.g., turpentine, shellac, toluene, rubber cement thinner) and solvent-containing materials (solvent-based inks, ? paints, rubber cement).	Use water-based products only.
Solvent-based silk screen and other printing inks.	Use water-based silk screen inks, block printing, or stencil inks containing safe pigments.
Aerosol sprays.	Use water-based paints with brushes or spatter techniques.
Epoxy, instant glue, airplane glue, or other solvent-based adhesives.	Use white glue, school paste, and preservative-free wheat paste.
Permanent felt-tip markers that may contain toluene or other toxic solvents.	Use only water-based markers.
Toxic metals	
Stained-glass projects using lead came, solder, flux, and so forth.	Use colored cellophane and black paper to simulate lead.
Arsenic, cadmium, chrome, mercury, lead, manganese, or other toxic metals that may occur in pigments, metal objects, metal enamels, ceramic glazes, metal casting, and so forth.	Do not use these ingredients. Use approved materials only.
Miscellaneous	
Photographic chemicals.	Use blueprint paper and make sun grams, or use Polaroid cameras.
Casting plaster. This creates dust, and casting hands and body parts has resulted in serious burns.	Teacher can mix plaster in a separate ventilated area or outdoors for plaster casting.
Acid etches and pickling baths.	Should not use techniques with these chemicals.
Scented felt-tip markers. These teach children bad habits about eating and sniffing art materials.	Use water-based markers.

Adapted from Babo A, Peltz PA, Rossol M. *Children's art supplies can be toxic.* New York: Center for Safety in the Arts, 1989.

Glassblowing has been associated with a chronic cough and reduction in both vital capacity and forced expiratory volume with increase of total lifetime hours exposed (23). Glassblowers are also subject to optical radiation from the superheated glass in such proximity to their eyes and are at an increased risk for the development of cataracts (24).

Neon art involves the manipulation of glass tubes into a desired shape and form. Hazards include exposure to mercury, which is used to flush the tubes, and ozone created by the electrical arc used to fire the neon or other noble gas (10).

Stained-glass workers are at risk of exposure to lead from the lead strips called *caming* used to hold together the stained glass. Exposures usually occur through neglect of basic hygiene (25).

INSECT COLLECTING

Insect collectors use all manner of poisons in killing jars to quickly subdue their specimens. Recommended volatile compounds on various Web sites include potassium or sodium cyanide, carbon tetrachloride, ethyl acetate, and isopropyl alcohol (26).

GEMSTONE WORK

Stone sculptors in lapidaries who process tiger's eyes, rose quartz, amethyst, or quartz crystals are at risk for silicosis (27). These cases are seen mainly in South Africa and wherever stone sculptors work.

METALWORKING

Major medical problems associated with metalworking usually are related to cutting or welding and the subsequent inhalation of metal fumes and gases. The gases released by welding may include fluoride, ozone, phosgene, carbon monoxide, carbon dioxide, and nitrogen dioxide. Welding of stainless steel nickel plus heat produces nickel carbonyl, which may cause headaches, dizziness, neurologic disorders, pulmonary edema, and possibly allergic bronchial asthma; the nickel fume may cause lung cancer. Toxic metal fumes produced by cutting or grinding may include beryllium, cadmium, chromium, lead, and molybdenum. Exposure to the toxic fumes from melting bronze and brass can cause metal fume fever (Chapter 20). Patients with metal fume fever have a flu-like illness with a 4- to 6-hour onset of symptoms, usually beginning the evening after exposure to the fumes. Symptoms may include fever, chills, fatigue, myalgias, cough, dyspnea, thirst, a metallic taste in the mouth, salivation, rhinitis, and conjunctivitis. Resolution of the symptoms usually occurs 36 hours after the exposure (28).

Welding, soldering, and brazing can produce toxic fumes and gases (e.g., carbon monoxide, nitrogen oxides, ozone). Metal dusts (cadmium, nickel, chromium, brass) may induce skin sensitization. Welding near chlorinated solvents can produce nickel carbonyl. Welding can produce electrical shock and burns. Exposure to infrared, visible, ultraviolet radiation can cause conjunctivitis and cataracts with long-term use. Skin burns and tumors are also possible.

Oxyacetylene torches produce carbon dioxide, carbon monoxide, and acetylene.

Metal welding produces nitrogen oxides and ozone.

Near-degreasing solvents may release phosgene, which evolves from the effect of ultraviolet radiation on chlorinated hydrocarbon.

Vaporization of metals, metal alloys, and electrodes releases metal fumes, copper, zinc, lead, tin, cadmium, nickel, titanium, and chromium.

Welding of stainless steel releases nickel carbonyl—nickel plus heat produces nickel carbonyl (headaches, dizziness, neurologic disorders, pulmonary edema, possible allergic bronchial asthma); nickel fume industry may cause possible lung cancer.

Coatings may include lead paint, mercury-containing antifouling paint, and cadmium plating.

Soldering and brazing involve the use of a third metal of lower melting point to join two metals.

The hazards involved include zinc chloride gases, cadmium fumes, and fluoride fumes. Brazing (hard or silver soldering) involves higher temperature use.

MODELING

Building plastic models using solvent-based glues has waned in popularity since the early 1990s. Most of the glues used in modeling of this sort contain toluene and represent potential abuse for sniffing or huffing as well as the hazard of chronic low-level exposure (Chapter 179). Most manufacturers recommend that model glue be used in only well-ventilated areas.

PAINTING

In painting, artists use colors such as bright yellow (arsenic, cadmium, lead), red, white, green, blue (mainly copper, cobalt, aluminum, and manganese), and violet (manganese, cobalt) (Table 15) (29,30). Cobalt colors used by artists in the twentieth century were often contaminated with arsenic. Earth colors, such as yellow and red ochre, madder red, olive green, and brown, consist of relatively harmless iron compounds. Olive green and madder red also contain lesser amounts of silicon and aluminum.

There is a case report in the literature of a 22-year-old male painter who presented twice to the emergency department with complaints of fatigue and weight loss over several months. An expanded history on his second visit included occupational contact with oil paints. Laboratory analysis later revealed the painter had manganism or locura manganica. Symptoms resolved on discontinuation of the environmental exposure (31).

TABLE 15. Hazards to photographers and painters

Substance	Hazard	
	Photographers	Painters
Metals	Borate, bromides, chromates, iodine, lead, mercury, silver, tellurium, uranium, vanadium	Arsenic barium chromates, cadmium, lead, manganese, mercury, magnesium, titanium, zinc
Solvents	Aminophenols, amyl acetate, benzene, ethylene glycol, formaldehyde, methanol, trichloroethylene	Acetone, benzene, carbon tetrachloride, methanol, turpentine
Others	Acids and alkalis, cyanide, hydroquinone oxylate, sodium bisulfate, sodium hypochrome, sodium sulfide, sodium thiosulfite	Acids and alkalis, carbon disulfide, methylene chloride, nitrogen oxides

Adapted from Lesser SH, Weiss SJ. *Am J Emerg Med* 1995;13:451–458.

Artist colors consist of linseed oil, small amounts of aluminum stearate, and up to 80% pigment. Circa 8000 B.C., Egyptians used cinnabar (mercury sulfide); brilliant blues and greens (organic copper); bright yellows (arsenic sulfide); red, yellow, and brown ochre (iron compounds); and madder red (plant extract). Between the Roman Empire period and the Renaissance, new colors were added: white lead carbonate, yellow lead oxide, antimonate and stannate, and blue aluminum sulfosilicates and barium manganate. During the 19th century, more pigments based in heavy metals began to be used: blue cobalt aluminates, yellow (cadmium sulfide and chromium oxide), red cadmium sulfide, green chromic oxide, and violets (cobalt arsenate and manganese ammonium phosphate).

Artists frequently did not wash their hands before smoking and eating; they often licked their brushes. Impoverished artists often lived, cooked, and ate in their studios. Water and food were easily contaminated by toxic heavy metals from pigments. Heat from a stove into which cloths soaked in old paint and discarded paintings were burned would have been a cheap source of heat and could have produced toxic metal fumes.

Artists today use less toxic pigments, paints carry warning labels, and artists know they should not lick brushes or burn colors indoors. Cigarettes are rarely hand-rolled, drinking water comes from taps and not buckets, and food is kept in refrigerators.

Toxic Pigments

Lead, arsenic, antimony, cadmium, chromium, cobalt, manganese, and mercury can be ingested by contamination of hands, fingernails, food, cups, and cigarettes and by holding paint brushes in the mouth (Table 16). When mixing paints from dry powdered pigments, airborne dust is generated.

White lead or flake white (basic lead carbonate cadmium pigments), chrome yellow (lead chromate), and zinc yellow (zinc chromate) may cause lung cancer. Lamp black and carbon black may contain impurities that cause skin cancer. Chromatic pigments—chrome yellow (lead chromate) and zinc yellow (zinc chromate)—may cause skin ulcerations and allergic skin reactions.

Solvents

Toxic solvents are used in oil paints, as paint removers, and in varnishes. They are found in adhesives, fixatives to keep paint from smearing, permanent markers, lacquers, and thinners. Solvents include toluene, xylene, hexane, cyclohexane, methanol, methyl ethyl ketone, acetone, mineral spirits, methylene chloride, turpentine, alcohols, glycols, ethers, and others.

Water-Based Paints

Acrylic paints contain ammonia and formaldehyde. Casein paints include ammonium hydroxide. All water-based paints have preservatives (e.g., phenylmercuric acetate).

Non–Water-Based Paints

Non–water-based paints contain solvents, turpentine, and mineral spirits.

Airbrush, Spray Cans, and Spray Guns

Toxic components include solvents, pigments, and propellants (isobutane, propanes) that may be flammable.

Liquid Drawing Media

Liquid drawing media products include solvent-based pen and ink and felt-tip markers containing xylene and propyl alcohol.

TABLE 16. Toxic pigments

Highly toxic pigments (known or probable carcinogens)
- Antimony white (antimony trioxide)
- Barium yellow (barium chromate)
- Burnt umber or raw umber (iron oxides, manganese silicates or dioxide)
- Cadmium red or orange (cadmium sulfide, cadmium selenide)
- Cadmium barium colors (cadmium colors and barium sulfate)
- Cadmium barium yellow (cadmium sulfide, cadmium selenide, barium sulfate, zinc sulfide)
- Cadmium yellow (cadmium sulfide)
- Chrome green (Prussian blue, lead chromate)
- Chrome orange (basic lead carbonate)
- Chrome yellow (lead chromate)
- Cobalt violet (cobalt arsenate or cobalt phosphate)
- Cobalt yellow (potassium cobaltinitrate)
- Lead or flake white (basic lead carbonate)
- Lithol red (sodium, barium, and calcium salts of soluble azo pigment)
- Manganese violet (manganese ammonium pyrophosphate)
- Molybdate orange (lead chromate, lead molybdate, lead sulfate)
- Naples yellow (lead antimonate)
- Strontium yellow (strontium chromate)
- Vermilion (mercuric sulfide)
- Zinc sulfide
- Zinc yellow (zinc chromate)

Moderately toxic pigments/slightly toxic pigments
- Alizarin crimson (lakes of 1,2-dihydroxyanthraquinone or insoluble anthraquinone pigment)
- Carbon black (carbon)
- Cerulean blue (cobalt stannate)
- Cobalt blue (cobalt stannate)
- Cobalt green (calcined cobalt, zinc and aluminum oxides)
- Chromium oxide green (chromic oxide)
- Manganese blue (barium manganate, barium sulfate)
- Prussian blue (ferric ferrocyanide)
- Toluidine red (insoluble azo pigment)
- Toluidine yellow (insoluble azo pigment)
- Viridian (hydrated chromic oxide)
- Zinc white (zinc oxide)

Adapted from Balin A. *Art Hazards News* 1991;14:3–6.

Paint Removers

Paint removers contain methylene chloride, toluene, methanol, ethanol, acetone, and mineral spirits (30). Toxic effects include irritation to upper respiratory tract, dermatitis, renal and hepatic damage, acute central nervous system depression, and chronic brain damage—behavioral changes, loss of memory, decreased intellectual abilities, confusion, and seizures.

Treatment

Protection from exposure is required in the form of local or exhaust ventilation and use of a glove box or an approved respirator. The artist must wash his or her hands and nails thoroughly after mixing paints and refrain from eating, drinking, or smoking in the studio.

Other helpful measures include substitution with the least toxic materials, use of dilution and local exhaust ventilation, control of storage areas, disposal of solvent-soaked rags in covered containers, minimizing skin exposure, and use of respirators and other personal protective equipment (32).

PERFORMING ARTS

A wide variety of activity sites are involved in the performing arts: dance studios, art rooms, classrooms, night clubs, discos, movie houses, orchestra halls, civic centers, fine arts centers, shops, arenas, lofts, big and little theaters, outdoor drama structures, stages, dressing rooms, costume and fabric shops, makeup areas, amusement parks, television and movie studios, carnivals, and rock shows.

Performers may be exposed to aerosols of methyl ethyl ketone, asbestos, acrylics, plastics for scenery, costumes, masks, armor, and props and to acetone, dyes, photographic chemicals, sawdust, metal filings, gases, vapors, fiber from hemp, dust, and machine oil (33).

PHOTOGRAPHY

Although film use has declined with the advent of digital photography, traditional film is still used for many artistic and industrial applications (10). There are a myriad of chemicals used by photographers in film development. Both industrial and amateur photographers use three sequential chemical baths to produce prints. These are a developer, a stop bath, and a fixer. The developer solution is perhaps the most dangerous, containing substantial amounts of toxic hydrocarbons. The different pigmenting and developing systems used in fine art photography should also be considered when assessing risks.

Photographic developer contains hydroquinone, metol, and other components. Hydroquinone (skin reactions, allergic reaction, eye problems) is a mutagen and a possible cancer risk. Metol (monomethyl *p*-aminophenol sulfate) may induce skin reactions and an allergic reaction. Some developers are toxic by inhalation of powders and, due to ingestion, cause methemoglobinemia and cyanosis. Developers are dissolved in a strongly alkaline solution, often containing sodium hydroxide, which can cause skin irritation and burns.

Stop bath is a weak solution of acetic acid. Glacial acetic acid, used to make up the stop bath, can induce severe skin burns; inhalation can irritate the upper and lower respiratory tract.

Stop hardener is potassium chrome alum, which can cause skin and nasal ulceration and allergies.

Fixer contains sodium sulfate, sodium bisulfite, sodium thiosulfate (hypo), boric acid, and potassium alum. Hypo and the mixture of sodium sulfite and acids can produce sulfur dioxide gas, which is irritating to eyes and the respiratory tract, especially in asthmatics.

Hardener contains potassium alum, which is a weak sensitizer and causes skin ulceration and dermatitis.

Toxic gases are created during the photographic process—sulfur dioxide, chlorine, formaldehyde, ammonia, and hydrogen cyanide (when reducers, such as potassium cyanide and potassium ferrocyanide, are heated, mixed with acids, or exposed to ultraviolet light).

Treatment

The topic of respiratory irritant gases is addressed in Chapter 183, and caustic agents are addressed in Chapters 201 and 202.

Precautions: The potential toxicity of the chemical must be recognized. The chemical must be handled and stored properly. Often, a less toxic chemical can be used. The darkroom should have 10 to 20 air exchanges per hour. Materials should be handled with protective gloves and photographic tongs. Chemical should be labeled and stored individually.

Advanced Black-and-White Processing

Intensification (bleaches) contain potassium dichromate and hydrochloric acids—in two-component chrome intensifiers. Each component can cause burns. Together, they produce chromic acid (Chapter 218). Vapors are corrosive and may cause lung cancer. Potassium chlorochromate produces chlorine gas when heated or treated with acid.

Mercuric chloride powder can be absorbed through the skin and cause mercury poisoning. It should not be used. *"Farmer's Reducer"* is potassium ferrocyanide. When in contact with heat, acids, or ultraviolet radiation, hydrogen cyanide gas can be released.

Toners may include selenium, uranium, sulfides, gold and platinum, and oxalic acid.

Hardeners and stabilizers often contain formaldehyde, which is irritating to the eyes, skin, and upper respiratory tract and possibly carcinogenic.

Color Processing

This process uses the same chemicals as in black-and-white processing, but, in addition, dye couplers, organ solvent, and formaldehyde may be involved. Color processing is more likely to produce sulfide dioxide fumes (34).

PRINTMAKING

Silk Screening

Solvent exposure may occur by inhalation, skin absorption, and ingestion. Excessive solvent exposure causes drowsiness, fatigue, and inattention. Exposure occurs when prints are dried on racks in an open studio. Xylene, toluene, and carbon blacks are contaminated with polycyclic aromatic hydrocarbons.

Many pigments are used in paintings such as lead pigments (chrome yellow: lead chromate; chrome green: lead chromate; Milori green: lead chromate and potassium ferrocyanide; molybdate orange: lead chromate, lead molybdate, and lead sulfate).

The drying of prints on racks in an open studio can produce dermatitis, central nervous system damage (e.g., dizziness, lightheadedness, fatigue, nausea, lack of coordination, headaches), eye irritation, and adverse reproductive hazards.

TABLE 17. Constituents of products marketed for lithography

Organic chemicals or mixtures	Naphtha
Acetone	Pitch
Benzene	Toluene
Benzoyl peroxide	1,1,1-Trichloroethane
Cyclohexane	Turpentine
Ethyl benzene	Xylene
Ethylene dichloride	Other chemicals (e.g., acids, oils)
Ethylene oxide	Acetic acid
Heptane	Castor oil
Hexane	Flaxseed oil
Hexylene glycol	Linseed oil
Isopropanol	Mineral oil
Kerosene	Nitric acid
Methanol	Sodium hydroxide
Methyl ethyl ketone	Sulfuric acid
Methyl methacrylate	Water
Mineral spirits	

Adapted from Fuchs R, McCann M. *Silkscreen printing.* New York: Center for Safety in the Arts, 1988.

TABLE 18. Toxic woods

Wood	Reaction	Site	Potency	Source	Incidence
Bald cypress	S	RE	+	D	R
Balsam fir	S	E, SK	+	LB	C
Beech	S, NC	E, SK, RE	++	LB, D	C
Birch	S	RE	++	W, D	C
Black locust	I, N	E, SK	+++	LB	C
Blackwood	S	E, SK	++	D, W	C
Boxwood	S	E, SK	++	D, W	C
Cashew	S	E, SK	+	D, W	R
Cocobolo	I, S	E, SK, RE	+++	D, W	C
Dahoma	I	E, SK	++	D, W	C
Ebony	I, S	E, SK	++	D, W	C
Elm	I	E, SK	+	D	R
Goncalo alves	S	E, SK	++	D, W	R
Greenheart (from Surinam)	S	E, SK	+++	D, W	C
Hemlock	NC	RE	?	D	U
Iroko	I, S, P	E, SK, RE	+++	D, W	C
Mahogany (*swietenia*)	S, P	SK, RE	+	D	U
Mansonia	I, S	E, SK	+++	D, W	C
	N	—	+	D	—
Maple (*Cryptostroma corticale* mold)	S, P	RE	+++	D	C
Mimosa	N	—	?	LB	U
Myrtle	S	RE	++	LB, D	C
Oak	S	E, SK	++	LB, D	R
	NC	—	?	D	U
Obeche	I, S	E, SK, RE	+++	D, W	C
Oleander	DT	N, CA	++++	D, W, LB	C
Olivewood	I, S	E, SK, RE	+++	D, W	C
Opepe	S	RE	+	D	R
Padauk	S	E, SK, N	+	D, W	R
Pau ferro	S	E, SK	+	D, W	R
Peroba rosa	I	RE, N	++	D, W	U
Purpleheart	—	N	++	D, W	C
Quebracho	I	RE, N	++	D, LB	C
	NC	—	?	D	U
Redwood	S, P	RE, E, SK	++	D	R
	NC	—	?	D	U
Rosewoods	I, S	RE, E, SK	++++	D, W	C
Sassafras	S	RE	+	D	R
	DT	N	+	D, W, LB	R
	NC	—	?	D	U
Satinwood	I	RE, E, SK	+++	D, W	C
Sequoia	I	RE	+	D	R
Snakewood	I	RE	++	D, W	R
Spruce	S	RE	+	D, W	R
Walnut, black	S	E, SK	++	D, S	C
Wenge	S	RE, E, SK	++	D, W	C
Western red cedar	S	RE	+++	D, LB	C
Willow	S	RE, N	+	D, W, LB	U
Teak	S, P	E, SK, RE	++	D	C
Yew	I	E, SK	++	D	C
	DT	N, CA	++++	D, W	C
Zebrawood	S	E, SK	++	D, W	—

+, least toxic; ++, +++, intermediate toxicities; ++++, most toxic; C, common; CA, cardiac; D, dust; DT, direct toxin; E, eyes; I, irritant; LB, leaves, bark; N, nausea, malaise; NC, nasopharyngeal cancer; P, pneumonitis, alveolitis (hypersensitivity pneumonia); R, rare; RE, respiratory; S, sensitizer; SK, skin; U, unknown; W, wood.
Adapted from Woodcock R. Toxic woods. *Art Hazards News* 1990;13.

Precautions include the use of ventilated drying rack enclosure or slotted tabletop exhaust. The least hazardous materials should be used. Solvent-soaked rags should be stored in covered containers. Personal protective equipment (selected gloves according to chemicals used) should be used.

Intaglio Hazards

Etching grounds contain asphalt in an oil or solvent. Many contain carcinogens. Rosins used in aquatinting may be allergens when inhaled. Solvents are used to clean paints. Inorganic acid is used to etch plates. Plates dipped in nitric acid can release nitrogen oxides. Dutch mordant (hydrochloric acid, potassium chlorate, and water) can liberate chlorine gas and be explosive if mixed with organics.

Lithography

In lithography, a drawing is made on stone, and then the stone is chemically treated with gum arabic and acid. Ink is applied (Table 17) (35). The stone and paper are run through a lithography press to create the image. Talc is used to dust the stones, creating potential asbestos exposure. Acids, such as nitric, phosphoric, and tannic, are used. Dichromates may cause dermatitis, allergy, and ulcerations of hands and nose. Precautions include control of dangling clothing, hair, and jewelry.

The following hazards are encountered:

- Improper storage of materials
- No metal cabinets for flammable solvent storage
- Working in a cluttered environment
- Not sweeping after sculpture or wood carving
- Not capping solvent cans when stored
- Failing to extinguish flame when not welding or soldering
- Little attention to label warnings
- No local exhaust ventilation
- No designated areas for curtain operations
- No personal protective equipment

Relief Printing

Relief printing can cause exposure to caustic soda, solvents, glues, and possibly methyl methacrylate (36,37).

WOODWORKING AND FURNITURE REFINISHING

Hazards include inhalation of dust produced in the process of working with wood; methylene chloride, which is commonly used as a paint stripper; and the compounds used to preserve the wood itself (38–40). Tables 18 and 19 give lists of toxic woods and timbers commonly used by hobbyists and in the industry. Most adverse reactions are either respiratory or cutaneous.

Woods may contain alkaloids, stains, aldehydes, quinines, flavonoids, tropolones, oils, cardiotoxic steroids, stilbenes, and resins. Wood preservatives may include copper chromated arsenate, potassium dichromate, ethyl triethanolamine, glycol humectant, naphthenate, creosote, pentachlorophenol, wood glues, and epoxy adhesives. Nasal adenocarcinomas may be associated with exposure to wood dust (41). There is one case report in the literature of suicide by ingestion of copper chromated arsenate (42).

Methylene chloride is an organic solvent that has found a wide range of uses in the industry, including degreaser, paint remover, aerosol propellant, a blowing agent for polyurethane foams, a solvent in food processing, photographic film produc-

TABLE 19. Principal toxic timbers

Trade name	Botanical name	Dermatitis (D), mucosal irritation (M), asthma (A), general symptoms (G)	Active substances
Arbor vitae	*Thuja standishii*	M, A	Tropolones
Ayan	*Distemonanthus benthamianus*	D	Oxyayanins
Blackwood, African	*Dalbergia melanoxylon*	D	Dalbergiones
Boxwood, Knysna	*Gonioma kamassi*	M, A, G	Quebrachamine ?
Cedar, western red	*Thuja plicata*	(D), M, A	Tropolones
Cocobolo	*Dalbergia retusa* et spp.	D	Dalbergiones
Cocus	*Brya ebenus*	D	Quinones ?
Dahoma	*Piptadeniastrum africanum*	M	?
Ebony	*Diospyros* spp.	D, M	Quinones
Guarea	*Guarea thompsonii* et spp.	M	?
Ipé (lapacho)	*Tabebuia ipe* et spp.	D, M, G	Desoxylapachol
Iroko	*Chlorophora excelsa*	D, (M, A)	Stilbene
Katon	*Sandoricum indicum*	M, G	?
Liverworts and lichens on bark	*Frullania* and others	D	Sesquiterpene lactones
Mahogany, African	*Khaya ivorensis* et spp.	D, (M)	Anthothecol
Mahogany, American	*Swietenia macrophylla* et spp.	D	?
Makoré	*Tieghemella heckelii*	D, M	Saponin
Mansonia	*Mansonia altissima*	(D), M, G	Mansonones (quinones), glycosides
Obeche	*Triplochiton scleroxylon*	(D), M, A	?
Opepe	*Nauclea trillesii*	D, M	?
Peroba rosa	*Aspidosperma peroba*	D, M, G	Alkaloids
Peroba, white	*Paratecoma peroba*	D, M	Desoxylapachol ?
Ramin	*Gonystylus bancanus*	D	?
Rosewoods	*Dalbergia* spp., *Machaerium* spp.	D	Dalbergiones
Satinwood, Ceylon	*Chloroxylon swietenia*	D	Alkaloid ?, furocoumarins ?
Satinwood, West Indian (and African)	*Fagara flava* et spp.	D	Alkaloid ?, furocoumarins ?
Sequoia	*Sequoia sempervirens*	M, G	?
Stavewood	*Dysoxylum muelleri*	M, G	?
Teak	*Tectona grandis*	D	Desoxylapachol

Adapted from Woods B, Calnan CD. *Br J Dermatol* 1976;95[Suppl 13]:1–97.

tion, and plastic manufacturing (Chapter 209). Its source of toxicity is its conversion to carbon monoxide *in vivo*. The amount of exposure to methylene chloride in the acute setting can be determined by measuring serum carboxyhemoglobin levels. Toxic effects are those of carbon monoxide (43).

REFERENCES

1. Lucas AD, Salisbury SA. Industrial hygiene survey in a university art department. *J Environ Pathol Toxicol Oncol* 1992;11:21–27.
2. Meister JF, Ogle JL. A waste disposal program for a university art department. *J Environ Pathol Toxicol Oncol* 1992;11:33–37.
3. Rob Torecki. ILPI Web site. Available at http://www.ilpi.com. Accessed October 2003.
4. Consumer Product Safety Commission. Document #5016.

4a. Clark N, Cutter T, McGrane JA. *Ventilation: a practical guide*. New York: Nick Lyons Books, 1984.

5. NIOSH. What you should know in deciding whether to buy escape hoods, gas masks, or other respirators for preparedness at home and work. National Institute for Occupational Safety and Health, 2003.
6. Center for Safety in the Arts. *Arts hazard news*. 1993;16.
7. Findings, conclusions, and recommendations of the Intentional Introductions Policy Review. In: *Aquatic Nuisance Species Task Force report to Congress under Nonindigenous Aquatic Nuisance Prevention and Control Act of 1990*. Washington, DC: Fish and Wildlife Service, 1994.
8. Tong D. Skin hazards of the marine aquarium industry. *Int J Dermatol* 1996;35:153–158.
9. Tong D. Salt dermatitis in the aquarium industry. *Contact Dermatitis* 1996;34:59–60.
10. Lesser SH, WSJ. Art hazards. *Am J Emerg Med* 1995;13:451–458.
11. Fischbein A, et al. Lead poisoning from art restoration and pottery work: unusual exposure source and household risk. *J Environ Pathol Toxicol Oncol* 1992;11:7–11.
12. Education, MO, Administrative Memorandum No. 517: restrictions on the use of certain type of glazes in the teaching of pottery. London, 1973.
13. McCann MF. *Ceramics. Artist beware*. New York: Lyons & Burford, 1992.
14. Everson GW, Normann SA, CJP. Chemistry set chemicals: an evaluation of their toxic potential. *Vet Hum Toxicol* 1988;30(6):589–592.
15. Jacobziner H, Raybin HW. Accidental cobalt poisoning. *Arch Pediatr* 1961;78:200–205.
16. McCann MF. *Children and arts materials. Health hazards manual for artists*. New York: Lyons & Burford, 1985.
17. Sriskandan K, PKW. "Numismatist's pneumonitis." A case of acute nitrogen dioxide poisoning. *Postgrad Med J* 1985;61:819–821.
18. Letts N. Dutch mordant and etching hazards. *Art Hazards News* 1990.
19. Lee S. Reducing airborne lead exposure in indoor firing ranges. *FBI Law Enforcement Bulletin*, 1986:15–18.
20. Svensson B, et al. Lead exposure in indoor firing ranges. *Occup Environ Health* 1992;64:219–221.
21. Goldberg LR, et al. Lead exposures at uncovered outdoor firing ranges. *J Occup Med* 1991;33:718–719.
22. Novotny T, et al. Lead exposure in a firing range. *Am J Public Health* 1987;77:1225–1226.
23. Braun SR, Tsiatis A. Pulmonary abnormalities in art glassblowers. *J Occup Med* 1979;21:487–489.
24. Oriowo OM, Chou BR, Cullen AP. Eye exposure to optical radiation in the glassblowing industry: an investigation in southern Ontario. *Can J Public Health* 2000;91:471–474.
25. Pant BC, et al. Exposure to lead in a stained glass work. An environmental evaluation. *Sci Total Environ* 1994;141:11–15.
26. Nguyen N. *Collecting insects*. 2002.
27. White NW, Chetty R, Bateman ED. Silicosis among gemstone workers in South Africa: tiger's-eye pneumoconiosis. *Am J Ind Med* 1991;19:205–213.
28. Weiss SJ, LSH. Hazards associated with metalworking by artists. *South Med J* 1997;90:665–671.
29. Pederson LM, Permin H. Rheumatic disease, heavy metal pigments and the great masters. *Lancet* 1988;1:1267–1269.
30. Fuchs R, Babin A, Rossol M. *Paint removers*. Center for Safety in the Arts, 1988.
31. McCann MF. Occupational and environmental hazards in art. *Environ Res* 1992;59:139–144.
32. Babin A. Art painting and drawing. *Art Hazard News* 1991;14(6):3–6.
33. Davidson R. Health hazards in the performing arts. In: McCann MF, ed. *Health hazards manual for artists*. New York: Lyons & Burford, 1990.
34. McCann MF. Photographic processing hazard in schools. *Art Hazard News* 1990;13:1–3.
35. Fuchs R, McCann MF. *Silk screen printing*. New York: Center for Safety in the Arts, 1988.
36. Lucas AD. Health hazards associated with cyanotype printing process. *J Environ Pathol Toxicol Oncol* 1992;11:18–20.
37. McCann MF. Proceedings 50th Conference on Health Hazards in the Arts and Crafts. In: *Society of Occupational and Environmental Health*. Washington, DC.
38. Woodcock R. Toxic woods. *Art Hazard News* 1989;13.
39. Woods B, Calnan CD. Toxic woods. *Br J Dermatol* 1976;95[Suppl 13]:1–97.
40. Borm PJ, et al. Respiratory symptoms, lung function, and nasal cellularity in Indonesian wood workers: a dose response analysis. *Occup Environ Med* 2002;59:338–344.
41. Wills JH. Nasal adenocarcinoma in woodworkers: a review. *J Occup Med* 1982;24:526–530.
42. Hay E, et al. Suicide by ingestion of a CCA wood preservative. *Selected topics in toxicology*. 2000:159–162.
43. Shusterman D, et al. Methylene chloride intoxication in a furniture refinisher. *J Occup Med* 1990;32:451–454.

SECTION

6

Household Products

CHAPTER 201

Acids

E. Martin Caravati

See Figure 1.

Compounds included:	**Acids as a group, acetic acid, carbolic acid (phenol), formic acid, hydrochloric acid (muriatic acid), monochloroacetic acid (MCA), nitric acid, oxalic acid, phosphoric acid, sulfuric acid**
Molecular formula and weight:	**See Table 1.**
SI conversion:	**Not applicable**
CAS Registry No:	**See Table 1.**
Special concerns:	**Skin, mucous membrane, and gastrointestinal injury on contact; pulmonary edema after inhalation; metabolic acidosis; renal failure; hypocalcemia with oxalic or phosphoric acid; hyperphosphatemia with phosphoric acid**
Antidotes:	**None proved; folinic acid for formic acid; *N*-acetylcysteine experimental for monochloroacetic acid**

OVERVIEW

Acids are prevalent throughout the home and workplace. They are used for multiple purposes, including general household cleaning, industrial and manufacturing processes, and cosmetics. Acids are used as oven cleaners, rust removers, toilet bowl cleaners, drain cleaners, engraving agents, and in car batteries. The type of acid and concentrations varies by its intended use (Table 2). This chapter addresses selected household and workplace acids. Due to the similarities of clinical management, all the corrosive acids are addressed as a group. However, specific information for selected agents is provided in the second half of this chapter. Chromic acid and hydrofluoric acid are addressed in Chapters 218 and 207, respectively.

Strong acids also have been used as defensive and assault weapons. Sulfuric acid from car batteries is carried in small containers by assailants. Its use as a weapon has led to an increase in chemical burns in some countries such as Jamaica (1). The ubiquitous nature of acid products is reflected in the large number of human exposures that occur each year. In 2001, approximately 25,000 exposures to acid products were voluntarily reported to U.S. poison control centers (2).

Determinants of Injury

The *type of substance ingested* has a substantial effect on tissue injury (3). Generally, substances with a pH below 2 are strong corrosives; however, pH alone is not the only determinant of severity. Lemon juice has a pH of approximately 2 and is not irritating. Important factors that increase the corrosive properties of an acid include concentration, molarity, and complexing affinity for hydroxyl ions. The more concentrated the solution, the greater the probability of serious injury regardless of other factors. A higher-molarity sulfuric acid (18 *M*) produces more damage, compared with the stronger hydrochloric acid at lower molarity (12 *M*). In addition, the greater the amount of base required to neutralize the acid, the greater the tissue damage.

Large volumes increase the area of injury. Ingestion of large volumes predisposes the patient to vomiting. This reexposes esophageal and laryngeal tissue to damage.

As the *contact time* increases, tissue damage is likely to be more severe. Areas of slowing in the gastrointestinal (GI) tract (e.g., cricopharyngeus, pyloric sphincter, diaphragmatic hiatus, aortic arch) increase contact time and therefore predispose the area to corrosive damage. Crystal formulations tend to produce intense localized upper esophageal lesions, whereas liq-

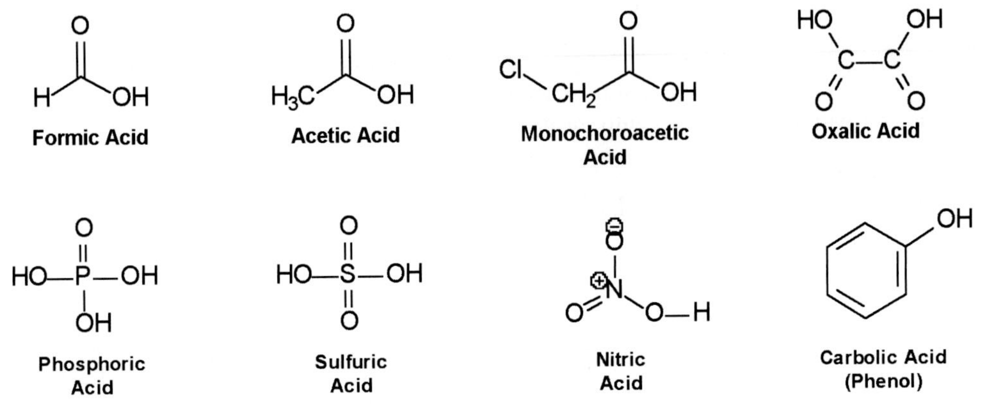

Formic Acid

Acetic Acid

Monochoroacetic Acid

Oxalic Acid

Phosphoric Acid

Sulfuric Acid

Nitric Acid

Carbolic Acid (Phenol)

Figure 1. Structures of acids.

uid preparations produce severe, circumferential, and more distal lesions.

The *volume of liquid and material in the stomach* can reduce injury. Fluid dilutes the corrosive agent and washes crystals off the mucosa. A full stomach is less susceptible to injury, and the corrosive effect may be more diffuse and superficial.

Pyloric spasm prevents gastric emptying and prolongs contact time with the gastric mucosa.

Location of Injury

Ingestion of concentrated acid results in burns throughout the GI tract. In a prospective study of 41 patients who ingested corrosive acids, 88% were found to have esophageal lesions, 85% had gastric lesions, and 34% had duodenal injury (4). Depending on the type and concentration of acid ingested, an esophageal lesion occurs in 40% to 95% of patients. The most common sites of injury are at the anatomic narrowing sites of the cricopharyngeus, the aortic arch, and the cardia. Limited esophageal damage may result from rapid esophageal transit and limited penetrating ability rather than from any special protective properties of the columnar epithelium.

The stomach, primarily the antrum, lesser curve, and pylorus, is a commonly injured site. A common pathway directs the rapid transit of fluid along the lesser curvature to the pylorus. A stomach that contains food before acid ingestion may have predominantly pyloric damage and lesser curvature damage, although the hydrophilic nature of acid tends to produce a diffuse damage. In the empty stomach, the lesser curvature is more upright and contracted so that prolonged acid contact occurs in the antrum and midgastric regions. Gastric perforation may occur (5). Relaxation of the pyloric sphincter allows the antegrade progression of acid and the production of small-bowel injury and potential perforation.

TABLE 1. Physical properties of medically important acids

Name	CAS Registry No.	Molecular formula	Molecular weight (g/mol)
Acetic acid	64-19-7	$C_2H_4O_2$	60.1
Carbolic acid	108-95-2	C_6H_6O	94.1
Formic acid	64-18-6	CH_2O_2	46
Hydrochloric acid	7647-01-0	HCl	36.5
Monochloroacetic acid	79-11-8	$C_2H_3ClO_2$	95.5
Nitric acid	7697-37-2	HNO_3	63.01
Oxalic acid	144-62-7	$C_2H_2O_4$	90
Phosphoric acid	7664-38-2	H_3O_4P	98
Sulfuric acid	7664-93-9	H_2O_4S	98.1

PATHOPHYSIOLOGY OF THE CLASS

Strong acids desiccate and denature proteins in superficial tissue, which results in coagulation necrosis. Consequently, a coagulum or eschar forms that limits the penetrating ability of acids, compared with the liquefaction necrosis of alkali ingestions. Hydrofluoric acid exposure is the major exception: The fluoride anion (not the hydrogen ion) produces a liquefaction necrosis by combining with calcium and magnesium in the tissues.

Three pathophysiologic phases characterize both acid and alkali ingestions (6).

The *acute inflammatory phase* (first 4 to 7 days) involves vascular thrombosis and cellular necrosis with destruction of the columnar epithelium, submucosa, and muscularis. This injury peaks in the first 24 to 48 hours; the necrotic mucosa sloughs by the third or fourth day, and an ulcer forms.

The *latent granulation phase* begins at approximately the middle of the first week as fibroplasia develops and fresh granula-

TABLE 2. Acid product formulations

Use	Agent	Concentration (%)
Household uses		
Toilet bowl cleaners	Sulfuric acid	8–10
	Hydrochloric acid	10–25
	Oxalic acid	2
	Sodium bisulfate	70–100
Drain cleaners	Sulfuric acid	95–99
Metal cleaners and anti-rust compounds	Phosphoric acid	5–80
	Oxalic acid	1
	Hydrochloric acid	5–25
	Sulfuric acid	10–20
	Chromic acid	5–20
Gun bluing agents	Selenious acid	—
Soldering fluxes	Zinc chloride	10–35
	Hydrochloric acid	5–25
Automobile battery fluid	Sulfuric acid	25–30
Industrial uses		
Multiple uses	Acetic acid	6–60
	Carbolic acid (phenol)	NR
Multiple uses	Chromic acid	99.9
	Formic acid	60
Multiple uses	Hydrochloric acid	NR
Engraver's acid	Nitric acid	63
	Oxalic acid	NR
Metal cleaner	Phosphoric acid	85–90
Multiple uses	Hydrofluoric acid	5–20
Multiple uses	Sulfuric acid	25–98

NR, not reported.

tion tissue fills the sloughed area of mucosa. Collagen starts to replace the granulation tissue by the end of the first week. Perforation is most likely during this phase, which lasts 2 weeks after injury.

The *chronic cicatrization phase* refers to the formation of excessive scar tissue around the submucosa and the muscularis. This dense fibrous tissue begins to form 2 to 4 weeks after injury at a rate that may be either rapid or slowly progressive. The primary goal of management is to prevent stricture.

CLINICAL PRESENTATION

Ingestion

Initial symptoms reflect the corrosive properties of strong acids: severe pain on tissue contact associated with dysphagia, drooling, vomiting, hematemesis, substernal and abdominal pain, and melena. There is no correlation between the presence or absence of oral burns and the presence of esophageal or gastric burns (7,8).

Aspiration Pneumonitis

A 4% to 5% incidence of aspiration pneumonia was found within 24 hours of ingestion in a retrospective study of 370 hydrochloric acid ingestions. Compared to patients without pneumonitis, these patients were older (52 vs. 42 years of age), more likely to develop a decreased level of consciousness (50% vs. 18%), and more frequently underwent nasogastric suction (36% vs. 6%). Aspiration pneumonia was associated with a higher mortality rate (9).

Clinical Grading and Esophageal Stricture

The clinical grading system for caustic injury to the GI tract is similar to that used for skin burns. First-degree (grade 1) burns are associated with superficial mucosal injury, mild erythema, and edema. Second degree (grades 2A and 2B) is transmucosal injury with severe erythema, white exudates, and ulceration. Grade 2B burns are differentiated from 2A by the presence of deep isolated or circumferential lesions and are more prone to stricture formation than grade 2A. Third-degree (grade 3) injury is full-thickness transmural necrosis. It is dusky or black in appearance with possible obliteration of the lumen and associated with stricture formation, perforations, and bleeding (4,7).

In one study, all patients with grade 3 injury ($N = 20$) and 5 of 8 patients with grade 2B injury developed esophageal or gastric cicatrization. Patients with grade 1 or 2A lesions recovered without complication (4). Chronic gastric stricture formation may result in pyloric obstruction, antral stenosis, or an hourglass-type deformity.

Esophageal Intramural Pseudodiverticulosis

Diverticula of the esophageal wall were found in 24% of patients with esophageal stricture from acid ingestion. They were best demonstrated on contrast barium examination. They tended to form at the site of initial contact of the acid with the esophageal mucosa. Dilation of the stricture led to partial or complete reduction of the diverticula (10).

Tracheal Stenosis

Stenosis of the distal trachea has been reported after aspiration of 35% hydrochloric acid. The signs of obstructive pulmonary disease (dyspnea, wheezing) developed approximately 6 weeks after exposure and were initially mistaken for reactive airway dysfunction syndrome. A computerized tomography scan of the chest revealed the tracheal stenosis. The patient was treated with tracheal stenting (11).

DIAGNOSTIC TESTS

Endoscopy

Endoscopy of the upper GI tract is indicated after ingestion of strong corrosive agents to determine the presence and severity of injury. Symptoms are not a reliable predictor of esophageal or gastric injury (4,7,8,12). Endoscopic evaluation should be done within 24 hours of exposure to avoid an increased risk of perforation if performed later. The risk of perforation is increased beginning a few days after exposure and continues for the next 2 weeks. The endoscope should not be advanced beyond an area of severe burns (7). Grading of the injury helps determine when oral feedings may begin and provides an estimation of the risk of perforation or stricture formation (7). Documented absence of esophageal burns allows early discharge of the patient.

Radiography

An upright chest radiograph should be obtained to detect free air from esophageal, gastric, or intestinal perforation or for evidence of pulmonary aspiration.

Other

There are no laboratory tests that predict or detect GI burns. Significant bleeding due to GI mucosal injury or perforation may be detected in the stool or emesis. Extensive bowel necrosis may result in metabolic acidosis and elevated serum lactate. The patient's acid-base status, serum electrolytes, renal function, complete blood cell count, and coagulation parameters should be monitored depending on the clinical manifestations.

TREATMENT

All ingestions of strong acids should be evaluated in a health care facility. The patient should have intravenous access established. Airway problems may arise from inhalation exposure and laryngeal edema. Respiratory distress may require cricothyroidotomy if endotracheal intubation is complicated by excessive swelling.

Decontamination and First Aid

Skin exposure patients should have all contaminated clothes removed and the exposed skin irrigated copiously with water. All solids should be removed from the skin.

Ocular exposures should be irrigated immediately at the scene, continuing for at least 20 to 30 minutes. All symptomatic eye exposures should be evaluated for corneal burns and foreign bodies at a health care facility. Thorough irrigation requires retraction of the eyelids so that the conjunctival cul-de-sacs are well washed. Topical ophthalmic anesthetic agents (proparacaine, tetracaine) and eyelid retractors are used as necessary. Be sure to remove all particulate matter. Irrigation should continue for at least 20 to 30 minutes and until the eye fluid pH is 7.

Repeated topical ophthalmic anesthetic and insertion of a Morgan lens relieves pain and allows continuous irrigation until a neutral pH is obtained. Neutralizing solutions or any other additives should not be used. Several liters of saline irrigation may be required. Caustic injuries require a complete eye examination, preferably with a slit lamp, to detect the extent of corneal injury after decontamination. The examination should include assessment of visual acuity. Fluorescein staining can be used to detect corneal and conjunctival abrasions and ulcerations. Do not use fluorescein if a corneal perforation is suspected. In such cases, shield the eye and contact an ophthalmologist.

Cycloplegic drops, antibiotic drops, or artificial tears may be indicated depending on the severity of symptoms. Steroid eye drops should be given in consultation with the consulting ophthalmologist. Although most acid exposures are less severe than alkali exposures, hydrogen fluoride exposure is an exception. All such exposures should be treated as alkali exposures, and an ophthalmologist should be consulted immediately after decontamination. All significant corneal burns should be followed by an ophthalmologist.

Ingestion of acid is treated with immediate milk or water dilution within 30 minutes of ingestion. The goal is to remove the corrosive agent from the esophagus. Do not attempt to neutralize the acid with weak bases. Dilution with water or milk was effective in decreasing injury severity in an *in vitro* rat esophagus model of acid burns (13). Other *in vitro* studies indicate that water dilution is ineffective in reducing pH and that buffering agents (e.g., antacids) produce significant exothermic reactions without significantly altering the pH (14).

Because reexposure of the mucosa to acid is harmful, be careful to avoid further vomiting and limit oral fluids to 8 oz for adults and 4 oz for children. Syrup of ipecac is contraindicated because reexposure of the esophagus to corrosive material may cause further injury. Activated charcoal also has no place in the management of acid ingestion because it is ineffective and obscures the endoscopic field.

Gastric lavage or nasogastric tube irrigation has been proposed but does not have positive studies to support them. The risks include inducing vomiting and reexposure of the esophagus to the acid, perforation, and aspiration. However, the removal of acids with lethal systemic toxicity, such as hydrofluoric acid, may outweigh the risk of perforation. There is also a potential risk of causing esophageal or gastric perforation if a nasogastric tube is inserted, although this has not been specifically studied. A retrospective review of 370 patients with hydrochloric acid ingestion found an increased use of nasogastric irrigation in patients who developed an aspiration pneumonitis (36% vs. 6%) (9).

Supportive Care

Patients should not be fed orally until endoscopy has established the extent of injury. Patients with only first-degree burns may begin oral liquids when stable, usually the first day of exposure. Second-degree burn patients should not be fed orally for 2 to 3 days. Patients with severe burns (grade 3) require a surgically placed jejunostomy tube for feeding.

Corticosteroids have been shown to decrease the incidence of stricture formation in animal models (15,16). In rabbits, rapid postburn administration of dexamethasone, but not prednisolone, was associated with significant reductions in the frequency and severity of burns and strictures, compared with controls (16).

The benefit of systemic steroids for caustic esophageal burns in humans is controversial. A controlled trial of prednisolone in children with caustic (primarily alkaline corrosives) esophageal injury did not show a decrease in stricture formation with treatment. The steroid treatment group ($N = 31$) received 2.0 to 2.5 mg/kg/day of prednisolone for 3 weeks followed by a 2- to 3-week taper. The incidence of stricture formation in the control group ($N = 29$) was 38%, compared with 32% in the steroid group (17). One limitation of the study is the small sample size and its inability to detect a small benefit if present (type II error). In another small study, children with second- or third-degree esophageal burns were treated with either dexamethasone (1 mg/kg/day) or prednisolone (2 mg/kg/day). Strictures developed in 12 (66.7%) of the children in the prednisolone-treated group ($N = 18$) and only 7 (38.9%) of the children in the dexamethasone-treated group ($N = 18$). Burn healing was significantly better in the dexamethasone-treated group. Steroid administration has typically been delayed many hours after exposure in these studies. The potential benefits of steroid administration within 1 to 2 hours of exposure have not been studied in humans. Steroids have been implicated in the obscuration of developing peritoneal signs after an acid ingestion (18,19). Another complication of systemic steroids is increased vulnerability to infection.

Antibiotics should be reserved for documented infections. If systemic steroids are administered, prophylactic antibiotics are often given concurrently.

Skin burns are treated as thermal burns with débridement, topical antibiotic ointment, nonadherent sterile gauze, and wrapping. Deep second-degree burns may benefit from topical silver sulfadiazine. Deep second- or third-degree burns and burns of the hands, face, or perineum should be evaluated by a physician with extensive experience in burn care.

Monitoring

Grade 1 and 2A esophageal injuries usually can be admitted to a general medical ward. Grade 2B and grade 3 burns should be admitted to an intensive care unit. Initial observation should be directed toward detecting perforation by serial abdominal examinations, complete blood cell counts, and, if indicated, radiographs and water-soluble contrast studies. Follow fluid and electrolyte balance carefully, including calcium, phosphorus, and protein levels in hydrogen fluoride and oxalic acid poisoning.

Hospitalized patients should be followed after discharge for the development of gastric outlet obstruction. Patients should return if signs of obstruction develop (progressive anorexia, weight loss, early satiety, nausea). A routine upper GI series 3 to 4 weeks after exposure detects early contractures.

Obtain a follow-up esophagram and upper GI series to evaluate the presence or absence of secondary scarring or stricture formation approximately 2 to 4 weeks after ingestion.

ACETIC ACID

Acetic acid (ethanoic acid, ethylic acid, methane carboxylic acid, vinegar acid, glacial acetic acid, methane carboxylic acid, TCLP extraction fluid 2, vinegar) is a colorless liquid with a pungent vinegar-like odor. Glacial acetic acid is 99% acetic acid. The 60% acetic acid solution appears in hat making, printing, dyeing, and rayon manufacturing. In some countries of Eastern Europe, high concentration acetic acid is sold to consumers in bottles that appear similar to drink containers.

Acetic acid is widely used as a chemical feedstock for the products of vinyl plastics, acetic anhydride, acetone, acetanilide, acetyl chloride, ethyl alcohol, ketone, methyl ethyl ketone, acetate esters, and cellulose acetates. It is used alone in the dye, rubber, pharmaceutical, food-preserving, textile, and laundry industries. It is also used in the manufacture of Paris green, white lead, tint rinse, photographic chemicals, stain removers, insecticides, and plastics. Dilute solutions (6% to 40%) are disin-

TABLE 3. U.S. regulatory guidelines and standards for acids

		Concentration (mg/m³) (ppm)							
Agency	Description	Acetic acid[a]	Carbolic acid[b]	Formic acid[c]	Hydrochloric acid[d]	Nitric acid[e]	Oxalic acid[f]	Phosphoric acid[f]	Sulfuric acid[f]
OSHA (air)	PEL-TWA	25 (10)	19.0 (5.0)	9.0 (5.0)	7.0 (5.0)	5.0 (2.0)	1	1	1
	STEL	—	—	—	—	—	2	—	—
ACGIH (air)	TLV-TWA	25 (10)	19.0 (5.0)	9.0 (5.0)	7.0 (5.0)	5.0 (2.0)	1	1	1
	STEL	—	—	—	—	10.0 (4.0)	2	3	—
NIOSH (air)	REL-TWA	37 (15)	19.0 (5.0)	9.0 (5.0)	7.0 (5.0)	5.0 (2.0)	1	1	1
	REL-STEL	None	None	—	—	10.0 (4.0)	2	3	—
	REL-Ceiling	None	60.0 (15.6)	—	—	—	—	—	—
	IDLH	123 (50)	962.5 (250.0)	56.4 (30.0)	74.5 (50.0)	64.5 (25.0)	500	1000	15

ACGIH, American Conference of Governmental Industrial Hygienists; IDLH, immediate danger to life or health; NIOSH, National Institute for Occupational Safety and Health; OSHA, U.S. Occupational Safety and Health Administration; PEL, permissible exposure limit; ppm, parts per million; REL, recommended exposure limit; STEL, short-term exposure limit; TLV, threshold limit value; TWA, time-weighted average.
[a]Conversion equation: 1 ppm = 2.46 mg/m³.
[b]Conversion equation: 1 ppm = 3.85 mg/m³.
[c]Conversion equation: 1 ppm = 1.88 mg/m³.
[d]Conversion equation: 1 ppm = 1.49 mg/m³.
[e]Conversion equation: 1 ppm = 2.58 mg/m³.
[f]Conversion equation not reported.

fectants and hair-wave neutralizers. Household vinegar contains 4% to 5% acetic acid and is often used as a condiment on salads and vegetables.

Toxic Dose

Regulatory standards and guidelines are provided in Table 3. Rectal administration of 50 ml of 9% acetic acid resulted in necrosis of the colon, hemicolectomy, and hepatic dysfunction (20). Ingestion of 200 ml of 90% acetic acid by an adult resulted in extensive corrosive injury, periportal liver necrosis, coagulopathy, and death within 39 hours (21).

Pathophysiology

In addition to its corrosive properties, ingestion of 90% acetic acid has resulted in periportal hepatic necrosis, coagulopathy, and severe corrosive injury (21).

Clinical Presentation

Local effects of acetic acid vapor include irritation and damage of the eyes, nose, throat, and lungs. Bronchopneumonia, pulmonary edema, and reactive airway dysfunction syndrome may follow acute inhalation overexposure (22). Contact with concentrated acetic acid may lead to severe skin damage and eye damage sufficient to cause a loss of sight. Repeated or prolonged exposure to acetic acid may cause skin darkening, erosion of the exposed front teeth, and chronic inflammation of the nose, throat, and bronchi (6). Acetic acid ingestion may result in pharyngeal, esophageal, and GI burns, bleeding, and volume depletion. Rectal administration of 9% acetic acid has resulted in extensive necrosis of the colon (20).

Systemic effects include hemolysis, hepatic dysfunction, hypotension, renal failure, and disseminated intravascular coagulation after ingestion of 90% to 100% acetic acid (21,23,24).

A *Chinese folk remedy* consists of swallowing vinegar to "dissolve" fish bones that may become lodged in the throat as a result of eating seafood (25). Direct contact of vinegar with the mucosa of the throat and GI tract can be mildly irritating. However, there are a few case reports of second-degree burn injury to the esophagus from ingesting tablespoon amounts (25). A 39-year-old woman drank 1 tablespoon of white vinegar in order to "soften" a crab shell she believed was stuck in her throat. Foreign body sensation and pain persisted, and she sought evaluation the next day. She did not vomit. Endoscopy revealed inflammation of the oropharynx and second-degree caustic injury of the esophagus extending to the cardia. No foreign body was identified. She was treated with antacids and was asymptomatic at her 1-week follow-up evaluation. This case confirmed that vinegar can cause ulcerative injury to the oropharynx and esophagus (25).

First-degree burns occurred in a newborn after vinegar was applied to the skin as a fever reducer (26).

Diagnostic Tests

For ingestion of large amounts of highly concentrated solutions, obtain a complete blood cell count, prothrombin time, and liver function tests to evaluate for hemolysis, disseminated intravascular coagulation, and liver dysfunction.

Treatment

Decontaminate and treat tissue injury as outlined for acids. A case of disseminated intravascular coagulopathy after ingestion of 100% acetic acid was successfully treated with fresh frozen plasma and cryoprecipitate (23).

CARBOLIC ACID

Pure carbolic acid (phenol, monohydroxybenzene, carbolic acid, hydroxybenzene, monophenol, oxybenzene, phenyl alcohol, phenic acid, phenyl hydrate, phenyl hydroxide, phenylic acid, phenyl hydroxide, phenylic alcohol) is colorless and used in the manufacture of phenolic resins, plastics, explosives, fertilizers, paints, rubber, textiles, adhesives, pharmaceuticals, paper, soap, and wood preservatives. Phenolic disinfectants [Meytol, Dettol, Creolin (26% phenol), others] are widely used for domestic purposes.

Toxic Dose

Regulatory standards and guidelines are provided in Table 3. Workplace biologic exposure index is 250 mg/g creatinine in end-of-shift urine and indicates excessive exposure.

Toxicokinetics and Toxicodynamics

Carbolic acid is readily absorbed via inhalation, ingestion, and dermal contact, causing both local and systemic toxicity. The elimination half-life ranges from 1 to 14 hours (27,28). It is eliminated in the urine as sulfate and glucuronate conjugates.

Pathophysiology

Phenol causes cell-wall disruption, precipitation, and denaturation of proteins; coagulation necrosis; and central nervous system (CNS) and respiratory stimulation.

Clinical Presentation

Systemic symptoms begin within minutes to hours of exposure. They include confusion, vertigo, faintness, lethargy, seizures, coma, tachycardia, hypotension, ventricular premature beats, atrial fibrillation, tachypnea, pulmonary edema, metabolic acidosis, hepatic and renal injury, and dark green urine. Swelling, blue-black discoloration, hypalgesia, and hypoesthesia of the skin may occur (28).

A 47-year-old man spilled 90% phenol on his left shoe and foot [3% total body surface area (BSA)]. After a prolonged contact time of 4.5 hours, he developed dizziness, confusion, hypotension, premature ventricular beats, atrial fibrillation, dark green urine, and marked swelling of his distal lower extremity. The peak serum phenol concentration was 21.6 mg/L. The phenol elimination half-life was 14 hours. He recovered with supportive care within 24 hours (28).

Diagnostic Tests

Serum phenol levels are not routinely available but can be obtained from referral laboratories. Prolonged contact with 90% phenol over 3% total BSA resulted in a serum concentration of 21.6 mg/L (28). Facial application of 50% phenol solution resulted in a serum concentration of 6.8 mg/L at 1 hour after exposure (29). Serum concentrations associated with death range from 4.7 to 130.0 mg/L (27,28).

Treatment

Skin exposures should be copiously irrigated with water for 15 to 20 minutes. Experimentally, polyethylene glycol (PEG) 400 solution has demonstrated some benefit over water irrigation alone. Porcine skin was exposed to 89% phenol solution for 1 minute, then washed with PEG 400 solution for 1 minute alternated with 1-minute water irrigation. This technique was superior to water alone in reducing skin damage. PEG 400 and water irrigation also reduced percutaneous absorption of phenol in this model.

Decontamination with 70% isopropanol was also effective in limiting skin damage and preventing absorption of phenol (30). In another porcine study, skin decontamination with PEG or isopropyl alcohol was more efficacious than water alone (31). A patient who suffered 20% total BSA burns and a serum concentration of 17.4 mg/L was treated with immediate and repeated decontamination with PEG and silver sulfadiazine and survived (32).

FORMIC ACID

Formic acid (methanoic acid, formylic acid, hydrogen carboxylic acid) is a colorless liquid with a pungent, penetrating odor and is soluble in water. It is used as a component of proprietary descaling agents and in stain-removing fluids. It is also used in dyeing colorfast wool, electroplating, coagulating latex rubber, regenerating old rubber, and dehairing and tanning leather; for the manufacture of acetic acid, airplane dope, allyl alcohol, cellulose formate, phenolic resins, and oxalate used in laundry; and in the textile, insecticide, refrigeration, and paper industries. In the United Kingdom, it has been marketed as "Kleenoff" (55%), "Ataka" (44%), Descale (55%), and Kilrock (60%) (33).

Ingestion may result in death after a prolonged (several weeks) course of classic acid-induced GI damage. Other complications include severe metabolic acidosis, intravascular hemolysis, and disseminated intravascular coagulation (33–35). In Europe, it is a well-known, if relatively infrequent, vehicle for suicide (33,36). Formic acid skin burns may result in systemic toxicity (37).

Toxic Dose

Regulatory standards and guidelines are provided in Table 3. Ingestions of less than 10 g in children have led to superficial oropharyngeal burns; the children recovered (33). Ingestions of 5 to 30 g in adults may cause minor superficial oropharyngeal burns, some abdominal pain, dyspnea, and dysphagia; a few patients may exhibit hematemesis, pneumonitis, or esophageal stricture. No fatalities are usually seen in this group.

Ingestions of 30 to 45 g of formic acid often produce hematemesis, hepatotoxicity, ulcerations, hemorrhage, and perforation in the GI tract. Some patients may experience a reversible disseminated intravascular coagulation or acute renal failure; many develop esophageal strictures. Occasional deaths have been reported.

Ingestion of 45 to 200 g causes reversible disseminated intravascular coagulation, pneumonitis, acute renal failure, and esophageal stricture in the few who recover. Most develop corrosive perforations of the abdominal viscera, GI hemorrhage, and in some cases acute renal failure. Death occurs at this dose level in the majority of patients within 36 hours after ingestion.

Toxicokinetics and Toxicodynamics

Formic acid is rapidly absorbed after ingestion. It undergoes saturable first-order kinetics. It interacts with tetrahydrofolate to produce 10-formyl-tetrahydrofolate, which is metabolized to nontoxic compounds. Its volume of distribution is 0.5 L/kg. It is reabsorbed by the kidneys in the proximal tubules by a chloride-formate exchanger. The elimination half-life of formic acid in one case was approximately 2.5 hours (36).

Pathophysiology

Formic acid directly damages clotting factors, leading to an increase in bleeding time and hemorrhage. It causes coagulative necrosis of the GI tract and destroys the normal histology down to the muscularis mucosa. Hematemesis may lead to hypovolemia. Formic acid has a direct hemolytic effect on red blood cells (36). Hemolysis plus the effect of formic acid on the renal parenchyma may lead to acute renal failure (38). Necrotic tissue fragments probably trigger the disseminated intravascular coagulation.

Formic acid produces a primary metabolic acidosis. Formate inhibits cytochrome oxidase and cellular respiration, which produces a lactic acidosis. Systemic acidosis may increase undissociated acid that crosses cell membranes and decreases renal excretion by increasing proximal tubular resorption (39).

Clinical Presentation

Ophthalmologic effects after ingestion include mydriasis and hyperemic conjunctivae. The visual loss associated with methanol ingestion (formic acid is the toxic metabolite) has not been observed with formic acid exposure.

GI effects include burning pain in the mouth and pharynx; salivation; hyperemic, edematous mucosae; ulcerations of the buccal mucosa and pharynx; nausea; vomiting; abdominal pain; upper GI bleeding; abdominal rigidity; pancreatitis; hemorrhagic esophagitis; and ulcerations of the stomach.

Dermatologic effects include erythema, blisters, and deep burns.

CNS effects include drowsiness, weakness, and coma.

Respiratory effects after inhalation exposure include dyspnea, aspiration pneumonitis, bilateral coarse rhonchi, "shock lung," acute respiratory distress syndrome, reactive airway dysfunction syndrome respiratory arrest, and pulmonary edema.

Hematologic effects include methemoglobinemia, intravascular hemolysis, and disseminated intravascular coagulation. *Metabolic effects* include metabolic acidosis and respiratory acidosis.

Complications include severe GI bleeding, pneumonia, acute tubular necrosis, acute respiratory distress syndrome, peritonitis, sepsis, disseminated intravascular coagulation, hemolysis, abscesses of the liver, shock, and death.

Diagnostic Tests

The formic acid concentration 2 hours after ingestion of approximately 100 g of formic acid (200 ml 50% formic acid) was 348 mg/L (7.6 mmol/L) and declined exponentially, with an elimination half-life of approximately 2.5 hours (35). Ingestion of 50 ml of formic acid led to a serum formic acid level of 180 mg/L in 6 hours (40).

Endoscopy may reveal lesions of the esophagus, stomach, and duodenum. Laboratory abnormalities encountered include elevations in the prothrombin time, fibrin degradation products, lactic acid dehydrogenase, aminotransferases, amylase, glucose, lactate, and creatinine. There may be an increase in free hemoglobin, methemoglobin, and the white blood cell and platelet counts. The hematocrit and fibrinogen levels may be within normal limits. Arterial blood gases will often reflect a severe metabolic acidosis. The chest radiograph may be normal or exhibit bilateral patchy consolidation.

Treatment

Decontaminate and treat tissue injury as outlined for acids. Patients who have ingested formic acid should be hospitalized for treatment in an intensive care facility. Airway compromise may result from laryngeal edema. The patient should receive cardiac monitoring and intravenous access. A supply of 100% oxygen should be available.

ELIMINATION ENHANCEMENT

Urinary alkalinization can decrease lipophilicity of formic acid and enhance urinary elimination of formate. Urinary alkalinization may also increase hemoglobin solubility and decrease the rate of acute tubular necrosis associated with hemolysis. Intravenous furosemide, 20 mg every 4 hours, blocks the formate-chloride exchanger and prevents renal tubular reabsorption of formate, thus enhancing elimination (39).

Hemodialysis has an unclear role in formic acid toxicity. Hemodialysis removes formate and has been used in methanol poisoning (Chapter 191). Most cases of formic acid poisoning can probably be managed without dialysis if renal function is normal, and the acidosis can be corrected with intravenous fluids and supplemental bicarbonate.

A 3-year-old girl suffered a 35% total BSA burn with 90% formic acid. She developed profound acidosis (pH, 6.85; serum bicarbonate, 6 mEq/L) and an initial serum formic acid level of 400 mg/L. After 2.5 hours of hemodialysis, the serum formic acid level was 51 mg/L. Her clinical course included intravascular hemolysis, increased hepatic enzymes, prolonged prothrombin time, and hemoglobinuria. She was also treated with blood products, mechanical ventilation, skin grafts, and supportive measures and survived (37).

ANTIDOTES

High-dose intravenous folinic acid (1 mg/kg bolus intravenously followed by 6 dosages of 1 mg/kg intravenously at 4-hour intervals until clinical improvement) may enhance formate metabolism by the liver (39).

HYDROCHLORIC ACID

Bleaching agents contain dilute (less than 10%) hydrochloric acid (chlorohydric acid, hydrogen chloride, muriatic acid, spirits of salts). Concentrated solutions (36%) are involved in dye and chemical synthesis, metal refining, and the plumbing industry. Concentrated solutions (24% to 32%) are available in Spain as domestic cleaners (Salfumant, Salfuman).

Toxic Dose

Regulatory standards and guidelines are provided in Table 3. Ingestion of more than 60 ml is associated with a high fatality rate (41).

Clinical Presentation

In one series, 21 patients who drank hydrochloric acid in self-harm attempts developed extensive necrosis of the upper GI tract (41). The amounts ingested ranged from 80 to 200 ml of a 24% to 32% HCl solution. All patients demonstrated metabolic acidosis on presentation. Physical signs of peritonitis were not present on admission. Fourteen patients died. Duodenal necrosis was uniformly fatal.

Treatment

Decontaminate and treat tissue injury as outlined for acids.

MONOCHLOROACETIC ACID

Monochloroacetic acid (MCA; α-chloroacetic acid, chloroacetic acid) is corrosive and stronger than acetic acid (42). MCA is extremely toxic both via the dermal and inhalation routes (43). It is used in the production of carboxymethylcellulose, phenoxyacetates, pigments, and drugs. It is also used as a wart remover and herbicide.

Toxic Dose

MCA is not listed by regulatory agencies.

Toxicokinetics and Toxicodynamics

MCA is readily absorbed after ingestion and after skin contact. The half-life of plasma MCA was approximately 2 hours in one case (42).

Pathophysiology

MCA reacts with the sulfhydryl groups of essential enzymes. It inhibits acetate oxidation in the tricarboxylic acid cycle (Krebs cycle). Thiodiacetic acid, glycolic acid, and oxalic acid are proposed metabolites (42).

Clinical Presentation

Vomiting and diarrhea are common early signs. Other manifestations of poisoning include malaise, cardiovascular shock, and seizures. CNS features include excitability with disorientation, delirium, and seizures followed by CNS depression and coma with cerebral edema. Cardiovascular effects include myocardial depression with shock and nonspecific electrocardiographic changes. Progressive rhabdomyolysis, renal failure, hypokalemia, and severe metabolic acidosis are observed. Hypocalcemia may be delayed for 1 to 2 days (42).

Acetylating agents, such as glacial acetic acid, acetic anhydride, MCA, and dichloroacetic acid, can cause a bullous dermatitis that may be delayed in onset and associated with extensive desquamation.

A 38-year-old man was splashed with 80% MCA solution (25% to 30% BSA) and immediately showered with water for 20 minutes. One hour after exposure, he had developed superficial skin burns and was slightly disoriented. Within 2 hours, systemic symptoms included disorientation, agitation, hypotension (systolic blood pressure, 60 mm Hg), and coma. Severe metabolic acidosis, hypokalemia, rhabdomyolysis, renal insufficiency, and cerebral edema with uncal herniation resulted in his death 8 days after exposure. The plasma MCA concentration 4 hours after exposure was 33 mg/L. Treatment consisted of intravenous fluids, buffering agents, vasopressors, ethanol (as an acetate donor), and acetylcysteine (as a sulfhydryl donor). Autopsy findings included lung congestion, liver congestion, cerebral edema, acute tubular necrosis, and skeletal muscle necrosis (42).

Diagnostic Tests

The serum MCA concentration 4 hours after a skin splash of 80% MCA on 25% to 30% of the body surface in an adult was 33 mg/L (42). After an inadvertent administration of 5 to 6 ml of an 8% MCA wart remover (Verzone), a 5-year-old child died and exhibited a postmortem MCA level of 100 mg/L (43).

Hypokalemia and elevated creatine kinase, aspartic aminotransferase, and amine aminotransferase concentrations may be observed (42). Hypocalcemia may be delayed for 1 to 2 days. Myoglobinuria can appear due to rhabdomyolysis (43).

Treatment

Decontaminate and treat tissue injury as outlined for acids.

ENHANCEMENT OF ELIMINATION

Hemodialysis may be of benefit in eliminating MCA and its metabolites, although there are no clinical studies to support it (42).

ANTIDOTE

There is no specific antidote. Ethanol and glyceryl monoacetate have been advocated both for fluoroacetate poisoning and for MCA poisoning, but there is little clinical evidence to support its use (42). MCA is bound to glutathione and other sulfhydryl-containing substances; therefore, acetylcysteine could be administered as a sulfhydryl donor. Therapy with ethanol and acetylcysteine was not successful in preventing severe toxicity and death in the case study presented above (42).

SUPPORTIVE CARE

If more than 1% of the body surface is exposed to liquid MCA, hospitalize the patient for supportive therapy, including fluids, correction of acid-base and electrolyte disturbances, alkalinization of the urine to prevent myoglobin deposition in the renal tubules, inotropic support (dopamine or dobutamine) as indicated for hemodynamic compromise, and controlled hyperventilation to prevent and treat cerebral edema (42).

NITRIC ACID

Nitric acid (aquafortis, azotic acid, hydrogen nitrate, nital, nitryl hydroxide) is a colorless, yellow, or red fuming liquid with an acrid, suffocating odor detectable at levels less than 5 parts per million. Engraver's acid is 63% nitric acid. Other commercial users include soda makers, metal refiners, electroplaters, and fertilizer manufacturers. Nitric acid decomposes to nitric oxide and nitrogen dioxide after contact to air or organic matter.

Toxic Dose

Regulatory standards and guidelines are provided in Table 3.

Clinical Presentation

Nitric acid is extremely corrosive to tissues. Inhalation of high concentrations causes pneumonitis and pulmonary edema. Initial symptoms include cough, chest pain, and shortness of breath. Skin exposures to concentrated solutions cause deep burns and ulcers and stain the skin a yellow or yellowish-brown color. Chronic exposure to low concentrations may cause chronic bronchitis.

Inhalation of nitric acid fumes by three pulp mill workers resulted in delayed pulmonary edema and death (44). Another patient died from acute pulmonary edema after inhaling nitric acid fumes while cleaning a copper chandelier (45).

Treatment

Decontaminate and treat tissue injury as outlined for acids. Monitor inhalation exposures for pneumonitis and pulmonary edema.

OXALIC ACID

Oxalic acid (ethanedioic acid, ethane-1,2-dioic acid) is a colorless, odorless powder or granular solid. It is used in the manufacture of dyes, inks, bleaches, paint removers, varnishes, wood and metal cleaners, dextrin, cream of tartar, celluloid, oxalates, tartaric acid, purified methyl alcohol, glycerol, and stable hydrogen cyanide. It is also used in the photographic, ceramic, metallurgic, rubber, leather, engraving, pharmaceutical, paper, and lithographic industries.

Oxalates are present in sorrel *(Rumex crispus)* and rhubarb, in which its content is high in the leaves and low in the stalk. It occurs in plants in a partly insoluble form as acid oxalate and free oxalic acid and in a partly insoluble form as calcium oxalate. Ingestion of oxalic acid from sorrel or rhubarb may lead to extensive renal damage and death.

Toxic Dose

Regulatory standards and guidelines are provided in Table 3. The oral lethal dose of oxalic acid for adults is 15 to 30 g. Intravenous injection of 1.2 g resulted in the death of a 16-year-old girl (27). The normal oxalate level in human blood is 1.4 to 2.4 mg/L.

Toxicokinetics and Toxicodynamics

Oxalic acid is poorly absorbed, with a bioavailability of 2% to 5%. It is excreted unchanged in the urine. Normal urinary oxalic acid excretion ranges from 8 to 40 mg/day.

Pathophysiology

Target organs for oxalic acid poisoning include the skin, eyes, respiratory system, and kidneys. Oxalic acid has a corrosive effect on the digestive tract. Once absorbed, it reacts with calcium in plasma to form insoluble calcium oxalate that tends to precipitate in the kidneys, blood vessels, heart, lungs, and liver. This reaction may also lead to hypocalcemia (46).

A patient suffered oliguric renal failure after ingestion of oxalate. Histopathologic examination of the renal biopsy specimen revealed degeneration of the renal tubular epithelial cells associated with intracellular calcium oxalate crystal deposition. Most of the renal tubules were patent despite the intraluminar crystal deposition. These findings suggest that dysfunction of the renal tubular epithelial cell plays a more important role than tubular obstruction in developing acute renal failure (47).

Clinical Presentation

Local effects of liquid oxalic acid involve irritation of the skin, eyes, and mucous membranes. Prolonged contact with hands or feet may result in localized pain, cyanosis, and possibly gangrenous changes secondary to localized vascular damage.

Chronic exposure may lead to chronic inflammation of the upper respiratory tract. Oliguric renal failure (47) and hypocalcemia (46,48) have been reported.

A 53-year-old man ingested soup containing 500 g of sorrel *(R. crispus)*. The ingested dose of oxalic acid was approximately 6 to 8 g. He developed vomiting, diarrhea, coma, respiratory depression, kidney and liver failure, severe metabolic acidosis, and hypocalcemia. Within 2 hours, he developed ventricular fibrillation and died (46). A 4-year-old child ate rhubarb leaves, became drowsy, vomited, and lapsed into a coma. An oxalic acid test of the urine was strongly positive. The child died 1.5 hours after exposure. No typical oxalate crystals were observed in the urine (48).

Chronic occupational exposure to oxalic acid fumes caused headache, vomiting, lower back pain, anemia, and fatigue (49).

Diagnostic Tests

Urinary oxalate that exceeds the normal upper limit of 40 to 50 mg/24 hours is indicative of excess oxalic acid or oxalate exposure at work. Ethylene glycol, ascorbic acid, and certain dietary plants may also increase urinary oxalate. Oxalate crystals may be present in the urine. Hypocalcemia may occur as a result of calcium oxalate formation.

Treatment

Decontaminate and treat tissue injury as outlined for acids. An electrocardiogram and serum calcium monitoring are required. Hypocalcemia should be corrected with intravenous calcium gluconate. Renal failure may require hemodialysis.

PHOSPHORIC ACID

The 85% to 90% solution of phosphoric acid (orthophosphoric acid, white phosphoric acid) is involved in metal cleaning, rustproofing, and superphosphate production. The dilute 10% solution is a disinfectant.

Toxic Dose

Regulatory standards and guidelines are provided in Table 3.

Clinical Presentation

Phosphoric acid mist is irritating to the eyes and upper respiratory tract.

Acute ingestion causes mucosal burns of the upper GI tract. Metabolic effects may include metabolic acidosis, hyperphosphatemia, and hypocalcemia (50).

A 64-year-old man ingested 90 to 120 ml of a 20% phosphoric acid solution diluted in 4 oz of "Kool-Aid" in a suicide attempt. He had throat burning, abdominal pain, hematemesis, and diarrhea. Mucosal burns were on the posterior pharynx. He developed an anion gap metabolic acidosis (serum bicarbonate, 9 mEq/L; anion gap, 23 mEq/L) and hyperphosphatemia (serum phosphate, 22 mg/dl). Eight hours after admission, the serum calcium was 6.6 mg/dl. Esophagogastroduodenoscopy revealed mild partial thickness burns of the distal esophagus and his Billroth II anastomosis. The serum phosphate returned to normal within 24 hours after treatment with oral aluminum hydroxide gel suspension (30 ml every 6 hours), a phosphate binder. The acidosis was treated with intravenous bicarbonate, 50 mEq. The hypocalcemia resolved with intravenous fluid administration only (50).

Treatment

Decontaminate and treat tissue injury as outlined for acids. Monitor for metabolic acidosis, hyperphosphatemia, and hypocalcemia. Hyperphosphatemia may be treated with phosphate binders (aluminum hydroxide). Intravenous glucose decreases serum phosphate by moving it intracellularly with the phosphorylation of glucose (51). Hydration with normal saline increases urinary excretion of phosphate. Phosphate is cleared by hemodialysis at 50 to 100 ml/minute.

SULFURIC ACID

Sulfuric acid (acid mist, dipping acid, BOU, hydrogen sulfate, oil of vitriol, sulfur acid, vitriol brown oil) is a colorless liquid. Chemical, munitions, and fertilizer manufacturers use the 95% to 98% solution. The more dilute 25% to 30% solution is used in machinery and batteries. Toilet bowl cleaners contain an 8% to 10% solution. Highly concentrated solutions of sulfuric acid are available to unclog drains.

Toxic Doses

Regulatory standards and guidelines are provided in Table 3. Lethal oral dose may be as low as 3.5 to 7.0 ml (52).

Pathophysiology

Sulfuric acid produces a coagulation necrosis of the gastric mucosa and submucosa that may involve the entire thickness of the gastric wall, with subsequent ulceration and fibrosis (53).

Clinical Presentation

Dermal exposure to highly concentrated sulfuric acid drain cleaner can produce full-thickness cutaneous burns (54).

Inhalation of low concentrations of sulfuric acid (5 mg/m^3) results in cough. Inhalation of concentrated sulfuric acid fumes can cause pulmonary edema. Sequelae include pulmonary fibrosis, chronic bronchitis, and emphysema. Chronic exposure (months to years) to sulfuric acid mist produces dental erosions. Chronic exposure to sulfuric acid mists may increase the risk of laryngeal cancer (55).

Ingestion of battery acid (sulfuric acid, 30%) resulted in esophageal burns in 55% of patients. The gastric antrum was also commonly affected. There was no correlation between severity of symptoms and degree of GI injury (12).

Pyloric and duodenal obstruction developed in an 8-year-old child who unintentionally ingested sulfuric acid (53). The onset of gastric outlet obstruction can be delayed 17 days to 5 years.

Treatment

Decontaminate and treat tissue injury as outlined for acids.

REFERENCES

1. Branday J, Arscott GD, Smoot EC, et al. Chemical burns as assault injuries in Jamaica. *Burns* 1996;22:154–155.
2. Litovitz TL, Klein-Schwartz W, Rodgers GC, et al. 2001 Annual Report of the American Association of Poison Control Centers Toxic Exposure Surveillance System. *Am J Emerg Med* 2002;20:391–452.
3. Klein-Schwartz W, Oderda GM. Management of corrosive ingestions. *Clin Toxicol Consult* 1983;5:39–55.
4. Zargar SA, Kochhar R, Nagi B, et al. Ingestion of corrosive acids. Spectrum of injury to upper gastrointestinal tract and natural history. *Gastroenterology* 1989;97:702–707.
5. Gun F, Abbasoglu L, Celik A. Acute gastric perforation after acid ingestion. *J Pediatr Gastroenterol Nutr* 2002;35:360–362.
6. Friedman EM, Lovejoy FH. The emergency management of caustic ingestions. *Emerg Med Clin North Am* 1984;2:77–80.
7. Zargar SA, Kochhar R, Mehta S, Mehta SK. The role of fiberoptic endoscopy in the management of corrosive ingestion and modified endoscopic classification of burns. *Gastrointest Endosc* 1991;37:165–169.
8. Nuutinen M, Uhari M, Karvali T, et al. Consequences of caustic ingestions in children. *Acta Paediatr* 1994;83:1200–1205.
9. Tseng YL, Wu MH, Lin MY, et al. Outcome of acid ingestion related aspiration pneumonia. *Eur J Cardiothorac Surg* 2002;21:638–643.
10. Kochhar R, Mehta SK, Nagi B, et al. Corrosive acid-induced esophageal intramural pseudodiverticulosis. A study of 14 patients. *J Clin Gastroenterol* 1991;13:371–375.
11. Rubin AE, Wang KP, Liu MC. Tracheobronchial stenosis from acid aspiration presenting as asthma. *Chest* 2003;123:643–646.
12. Wormald PJ, Wilson DA. Battery acid burns of the upper gastrointestinal tract. *Clin Otolaryngol* 1993;18:112–114.
13. Homan CS, Maitra SR, Lane BP, et al. Histopathologic evaluation of the therapeutic efficacy of water and milk dilution for esophageal acid injury. *Acad Emerg Med* 1995;2:587–591.
14. Maull KI. Liquid caustic ingestions: an in vitro study of the effects of buffer, neutralization, and dilution. *Ann Emerg Med* 1985;14:1160–1162.
15. Haller JA, Bachman K. The comparative effect of current therapy on experimental caustic burns of the esophagus. *Pediatrics* 1964;34:236–245.
16. Bautista A, Tojo R, Varela R, et al. Effects of prednisolone and dexamethasone on alkali burns of the esophagus in rabbit. *J Pediatr Gastroenterol Nutr* 1996;22:275–283.
17. Anderson KD, Rouse TM, Randolph JG. A controlled trial of corticosteroids in children with corrosive injury of the esophagus. *N Engl J Med* 1990;323:637–640.
18. Nicosia JR, Thornton JP, Folk FA. Surgical management of corrosive gastric injuries. *Ann Surg* 1974;180:139–143.
19. Kirsh MM, Ritter F. Caustic ingestion and subsequent damage to the oropharyngeal and digestive passages. *Ann Thorac Surg* 1976;21:74–82.
20. Kawamata M, Fujita S, Mayumi T, et al. Acetic acid intoxication by rectal administration. *J Toxicol Clin Toxicol* 1994;32:333–336.
21. Kamijo Y, Soma K, Iwabuchi K, et al. Massive noninflammatory periportal liver necrosis following concentrated acetic acid ingestion. *Arch Pathol Lab Med* 2000;124:127–129.
22. Kern DG. Outbreak of the reactive airways dysfunction syndrome after a spill of glacial acetic acid. *Am Rev Respir Dis* 1991;144:1058–1064.
23. Jurim O, Gross E, Nates J, et al. Disseminated intravascular coagulopathy caused by acetic acid ingestion. *Acta Haematol* 1993;89:204–205.
24. Hall S, Saliares R, Arrigoni J, et al. Systemic acidosis, hemolysis and hemoglobinuria renal failure from acetic acid ingestion. *Vet Hum Toxicol* 1985;28:291.
25. Chung CH. Corrosive oesophageal injury following vinegar ingestion. *Hong Kong Med J* 2002;8:365–366.
26. Korkmaz A, Sahiner U, Yurdakok M. Chemical burn caused by topical vinegar application in a newborn infant. *Pediatr Dermatol* 2000;17:34–36.
27. Baselt RC. *Disposition of toxic drugs and chemicals in man*, 6th ed. Foster City, CA: Biomedical Publications, 2002.
28. Bentur Y, Shoshani O, Tabak A, et al. Prolonged elimination half-life of phenol after dermal exposure. *J Toxicol Clin Toxicol* 1998;36:707–711.
29. Litton C. Chemical face peeling. *Plast Reconstr Surg* 1962;29:371–380.
30. Monteiro-Riviere NA, Inman AO, Jackson H, et al. Efficacy of topical phenol decontamination strategies on severity of acute phenol chemical burns and dermal absorption: in vitro and in vivo studies in pig skin. *Toxicol Ind Health* 2001;17:95–104.
31. Hunter DM, Timerding BL, Leonard RB, et al. Effects of isopropyl alcohol, ethanol, and polyethylene glycol/industrial methylated spirits in the treatment of acute phenol burns. *Ann Emerg Med* 1992;21:1303–1307.
32. Horch R, Spilker G, Stark GB. Phenol burns and intoxications. *Burns* 1994;20:45–50.
33. Naik RB, Stephens WP, Wilson DJ, et al. Ingestion of formic acid-containing agents—report of three fatal cases. *Postgrad Med J* 1980;56:451–456.
34. Rajan N, Rabim R, Kumar SK. Formic acid poisoning with suicidal intent: a report of 53 cases. *Postgrad Med J* 1985; 61:35–36.
35. Verstraetz AG, Vogelaers DP, Van den Bogaerde JF, et al. Formic acid poisoning. Case report and in vitro study of the hemolytic activity. *Ann J Emerg Med* 1989;7:286–290.
36. Rosewarne FA. Self-poisoning with formic acid. *Anaesthesia* 1983;38:1104–1105.
37. Chan TC, Williams SR, Clark RF. Formic acid skin burns resulting in systemic toxicity. *Ann Emerg Med* 1995;26:383–386.
38. Penner GE. Acid ingestion: toxicology and treatment. *Ann Emerg Med* 1980;9:374–379.
39. Moore DF, Bentley AM, Dawling S, et al. Folinic acid and enhanced renal elimination in formic acid intoxication. *J Toxicol Clin Toxicol* 1994;32:199–204.
40. Wiernikowski A, Guzik E. Ostre zatrucie Kwasem mrowkowyn. (Acute poisoning from formic acid). *Przeglad Lekarski* 1973;30:395–396.
41. Munoz Munoz E, Garcia-Domingo MI, Rodriguez Santiago J, et al. Massive necrosis of the GI tract after ingestion of hydrochloric acid. *Eur J Surg* 2001;167:195–198.
42. Kulling P, Andersson H, Bostrom K, et al. Fatal systemic poisoning after skin exposure to monochloroacetic acid. *J Toxicol Clin Toxicol* 1992;30: 643–652.
43. Feldhaus K, Hudson D, Rogers D, et al. Pediatric fatality associated with accidental oral administration of monochloroacetic acid (MCA). *Vet Hum Toxicol* 1993;35:344.
44. Hajela R, Janigan KI, Landrigan PL, et al. Fatal pulmonary edema due to nitric acid fume inhalation in three pulp-mill workers. *Chest* 1990;97:487–489.
45. Bur A, Wagner A, Roggla M, et al. Fatal pulmonary edema after nitric acid inhalation. *Resuscitation* 1997;35:33–36.
46. Farre M, Xirgu J, Salgado A, et al. Fatal oxalic acid poisoning from sorrel soup. *Lancet* 1989;2:1524.
47. Konta T, Yamaoka M, Tanida H, et al. Acute renal failure due to oxalate ingestion. *Intern Med* 1998;37:762–765.
48. Tallqvist H, Vaananen. Death of a child from oxalic acid poisoning due to eating rhubarb leaves. *Ann Paediatr Fenn* 1960;60:144–147.
49. Howard CD. Chronic poisoning by oxalic acid: with report of a case and results of a study concerning the volatilization of oxalic acid from aqueous solution. *J Ind Hyg* 1932;14:283–290.
50. Caravati EM. Metabolic abnormalities associated with phosphoric acid ingestion. *Ann Emerg Med* 1987;16:904–906.
51. Pollock N. Serum and muscle phosphate changes following glucose injection. *Am J Physiol* 1983;105:79.
52. Mills SW, Okoye MI. Sulfuric acid poisoning. *Am J Forensic Med Pathol* 1987;8:252–255.
53. Tamisani AM, Di Noto C, Di Rovasenda E. A rare complication due to sulfuric acid ingestion. *Eur J Pediatr Surg* 1992;2:162–164.
54. Bond SJ, Schnier GC, Sundine MJ, et al. Cutaneous burns caused by sulfuric acid drain cleaner. *J Trauma* 1998;44:523–526.
55. Soskolne CL, et al. Laryngeal cancer and occupational exposure to sulfuric acid. *Am J Epidemiol* 1984;120:358–369.

CHAPTER 202

Alkali

E. Martin Caravati

See Figure 1.

Compounds included:	**Alkalis as a group, ammonia, calcium carbonate, calcium hydroxide, potassium hydroxide, sodium hydroxide, sodium hypochlorite**
Molecular formula and weight:	**See Table 1.**
SI conversion:	**Not applicable**
CAS Registry No.:	**See Table 1.**
Target organs:	**Skin, mucous membranes, and gastrointestinal injury on contact**
Antidote:	**None**

OVERVIEW

Ingestion of caustic substances by children is a common occurrence. In 2001, more than 110,000 exposures to alkali products were voluntarily reported to U.S. poison centers (1). A 10-year retrospective analysis of childhood exposures in Galicia, Spain, found that the most common product ingested was household bleach, followed by caustic soda, then dishwasher powder. The most harmful substance was dishwasher powder, resulting in a 59% incidence of esophageal burns, whereas only 11% of bleach ingestions resulted in burns. The risk of esophageal burns was greater with ingestion of a solid (39% of cases), compared with a liquid (19% of cases), preparation. In 75% of cases, the product was not in its original container (2).

Classification and Uses

Drain cleaners contain sodium or potassium hydroxide and are used to clear plugged drains and cut grease buildup. Red Devil Drain Opener and Red Devil Lye (96% to 100% sodium hydroxide) have a pH of 14. Crystalline Drano (57% sodium hydroxide) has a pH of 14. Both Liquid Drano (10% sodium hydroxide) and Liquid Plumber (5% sodium hydroxide) also have a pH of 14. Some drain cleaners have been reformulated to contain 1,1,1-trichloroethane, which is a hydrocarbon rather than a caustic.

Household ammonia contains ammonium hydroxide concentrations, ranging from 3% to 10%. Weaker 3% solutions are mild irritants, but higher concentrations may be significantly corrosive (3). Volatile ammonia solutions can produce inhalation injuries and systemic symptoms. An 8.8% ammonia solution has a pH of 12.5 (4).

Automatic dishwasher detergents contain builders (e.g., sodium tripolyphosphate, sodium metasilicate, sodium silicate, and sodium carbonate) that produce corrosive lesions. The pH ranges from 10.5 to 13.0 (5).

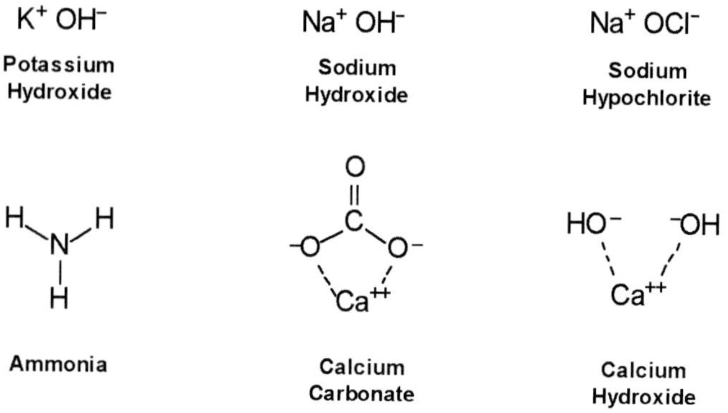

$K^+ OH^-$ Potassium Hydroxide — $Na^+ OH^-$ Sodium Hydroxide — $Na^+ OCl^-$ Sodium Hypochlorite — NH_3 Ammonia — $CaCO_3$ Calcium Carbonate — $Ca(OH)_2$ Calcium Hydroxide

Figure 1. Individual alkali bases.

Clinitest tablets contain copper sulfate (20 mg), citric acid (300 mg), sodium hydroxide (232.5 mg), and sodium carbonate (80 mg). Injury occurs both by direct corrosive action and by an exothermic heat reaction. Commonly damaged sites include the proximal esophageal mucosa and, occasionally, the gastric and duodenal mucosa (6). Esophageal stricture has resulted from ingestion of this product by children (7). These exposures have become rare because home blood glucose monitoring has become available.

Oven cleaners often contain sodium hydroxide.

Household bleach products (e.g., Clorox) usually contain 3% to 6% sodium hypochlorite and have a pH of up to 11. Some bleaches (e.g., Purex) contain silicate (15% to 17%) and sodium carbonate (60%) and have a pH of approximately 10.5.

Swimming pool sanitizers consist of concentrated calcium or sodium hypochlorite (70%).

Hair relaxer products may contain dilute concentrations of sodium hydroxide or potassium hydroxide combined with guanidine carbonate to form guanidine hydroxide with a pH of 12.5 to 13.0.

Cement contains calcium oxide, which forms calcium hydroxide when mixed with water. Prolonged contact with the skin may result in a caustic burn. It can produce full-thickness burns that require surgery after prolonged skin contact (8,9).

Other alkaline corrosives include potassium permanganate and nonphosphate detergents (sodium carbonate), and some metal cleaners, paint removers, and washing powders can produce alkali injuries. Malfunctioning automobile air-bag inflation systems may release sodium hydroxide powder, a byproduct in the chemical conversion of sodium azide to nitrogen gas that inflates the auto air bags. Chemical skin and eye burns require symptomatic treatment (10).

Toxic Doses

Regulatory standards and guidelines are provided in Table 2.

TABLE 1. Physical properties and regulatory standards of medically important alkali

Name	Molecular formula	Molecular weight (g/mol)	CAS Registry No.
Ammonia	NH_3	17.03	7664-41-7
Calcium carbonate	$CaCO_3$	100.10	471-34-1
Calcium hydroxide	$Ca(OH)_2$	74.09	1305-62-0
Potassium hydroxide	KOH	56.11	1310-58-3
Sodium hydroxide	NaOH	39.90	1310-73-2
Sodium hypochlorite	NaOCl	74.40	7681-52-9

TABLE 2. U.S. regulatory guidelines and standards for acids

Agency	Description	Concentration (mg/m³) (ppm) Ammonia	Calcium carbonate	Calcium hydroxide	Potassium hydroxide	Sodium hydroxide	Sodium hypochlorite
OSHA (air)	PEL-TWA	35 (50)	15 total dust; 5 respirable particle	15 total dust; 5 respirable particle	None	2	None
ACGIH	TLV-TWA	17 (25)	10	5	None	2	None
(air)	STEL	None	None	None	None	None	None
	Ceiling	None	None	None	2	None	None
NIOSH	REL-TWA	35 (50)	10 total dust; 5 respirable particle	5	2	2	None
(air)	REL-STEL	None	None	None	None	None	None
	REL-Ceiling	210 (300)	None	None	None	None	None
	IDLH	None	None	None	None	10	None

ACGIH, American Conference of Governmental Industrial Hygienists; IDLH, immediate danger to life or health; NIOSH, National Institute for Occupational Safety and Health; OSHA, U.S. Occupational Safety and Health Administration; PEL, permissible exposure limit; ppm, parts per million; REL, recommended exposure limit; STEL, short-term exposure limit; TLV, threshold limit value; TWA, time-weighted average.

Titratable Acid/Alkali Reserve

Titratable acid/alkali reserve is defined as the number of ml of a 0.1 M solution of HCl or NaOH required to titrate 100 ml of a 1% solution test product to a pH of 8, expressed as the mean of three determinations. An animal study suggests that the titratable acid/alkali reserve correlated better than pH with the production of caustic esophageal injury. Determining the usefulness of this procedure in prognosticating the danger of potentially caustic household agents requires additional clinical confirmation (11).

Pathophysiology

Alkaline agents cause injury to tissue by liquefaction necrosis. It can be rapidly progressive and result in extensive penetrating tissue damage. Saponification of fats and solubilization of proteins allow deep penetration into tissues. Thrombosis of vessels also occurs. Sloughing of mucosa and granulation tissue formation begin a few days after exposure and continue during the first week. The peak risk for perforation occurs during the second or third week, but perforation may occur earlier. Dense fibrous tissue and stricture develop over weeks to years.

Severe esophageal damage is caused by alkali agents with a pH as low as 11.8, and ulceration may occur with agents that have a pH of 12 or greater. Other contributing factors include volume ingested, viscosity, presence or absence of food in the stomach, and contact time (12,13). The anatomic locations at greatest risk for injury are the cricopharyngeus, aortic arch, and diaphragmatic areas of the esophagus.

Clinical Presentation

OPHTHALMIC EFFECTS

Ocular exposure to an alkali produces eye pain, tearing, foreign body sensation, conjunctival erythema, corneal ulceration and opacification, decreased visual acuity, eyelid burns, and edema.

GASTROINTESTINAL EFFECTS

Ingestion of alkali produces drooling, dysphagia, odynophagia, spontaneous vomiting, hematemesis, and abdominal pain. Most patients with esophageal injury complain of pain, but the symptoms do not localize the area of greatest mucosal injury (14). Whether all patients with significant esophageal injury have symptoms has not been resolved. Although Gaudreault (15) found no significant relationship between the presence of any symptom and injury in 378 children, Crain (16) found a positive correlation between the presence of two of three symptoms (drooling, vomiting, stridor) and esophageal injury in a series of 79 consecutive patients, ages 20 years and younger. Another study of 336 alkali ingestions (pH greater than 12) found that no single or group of initially reported signs and symptoms could identify all patients with potentially serious esophageal burns (17).

Other signs of chemical injury include erythema/ulceration of oropharynx and occasionally shock and respiratory distress. Severe signs indicate severe injury, but not all patients with significant esophageal damage have external signs of injury. Extensive alkali mucosal burns present as gray or gray-black pseudomembranes covering the buccal mucosa or palate. Approximately one-third of patients with oral burns have significant esophageal injury, whereas 2% to 15% of patients with esophageal injuries have no oral burns (18). Automatic dishwasher detergents often produce esophageal and gastric erosion without evidence of oral burns, although esophageal strictures are rare (19). Clinitest tablet ingestions differ from liquid alkali ingestions in the higher frequency of accidental adult ingestions. Compared with other alkali exposures, esophageal strictures are more proximal and less severe. Gastric and duodenal erosion are common, but oropharyngeal burns are rare from Clinitest tablets (20).

The complications of alkali injury include acute and subacute airway compromise from upper airway edema, perforation of the esophagus and the stomach, sepsis, and gastrointestinal (GI) hemorrhage. In addition, vocal cord dysfunction, pyloric stenosis, esophageal stricture formation (weeks to years), and esophageal malignancy (40 to 50 years) may occur (21). In one study, factors associated with the development of esophageal strictures included hematemesis, serum lactic dehydrogenase greater than 600 U/L, grade 3 lesions, and involvement of the entire esophagus (22).

GRADING OF ESOPHAGEAL OR GASTRIC INJURY

The clinical grading system for caustic injury to the GI tract is similar to that used for skin burns. First-degree (grade 1) burns are associated with superficial mucosal injury, mild erythema, and edema. Second degree (grade 2A and 2B) is transmucosal injury with severe erythema, white exudates, and ulceration. Grade 2B burns are differentiated from 2A by the presence of deep, isolated or circumferential lesions and are more prone to stricture formation than grade 2A. Third-degree (grade 3) injury is full-thickness transmural necrosis. It is dusky or black in appearance with possible obliteration of the lumen and associated with stricture formation, perforations, and bleeding (23).

Patients with grade 1 or 2A burns tend to recover without sequelae; grade 2B and 3 burns frequently result in significant scarring and stricture formation (24).

BLEACHES

Household bleaches are mild to moderate mucosal irritants. Products with a pH less than 12.5 do not cause serious burns, but failure to remove moderately alkaline liquids (e.g., bleaches with a pH of 11 to 12) from these areas may produce deep, partial-thickness chemical burns, especially after large, intentional ingestions.

Of all household cleaning products, bleaches produce the highest percentage of nausea, vomiting, and abdominal pain. Industrial-strength hypochlorite bleaches (15% to 20% solutions) may induce caustic injuries. Massive suicidal ingestions may produce fatal hyperchloremic metabolic acidosis or aspiration pneumonitis.

Sodium hypochlorite solutions may release small amounts of hypochlorous acid and chlorine gas, but usually the concentrations of these toxic gases are too low to cause damage. Mixing solutions of ammonia and sodium hypochlorite produces monochloramine (NH_2Cl) and dichloramine ($NHCl_2$) fumes. The release of chloramine fumes in a confined space can cause chemical pneumonitis. Prolonged inhalation of chloramine fumes can produce obstructive pulmonary deficits, chest infiltrates, and acute pulmonary edema.

CARCINOGENESIS

Squamous cell carcinoma of the esophagus has been reported to occur 40 to 50 years after corrosive alkali injury (21,25).

Diagnostic Tests

ENDOSCOPY

Endoscopy of the upper GI tract is indicated after ingestion of strong corrosive agents (e.g., lye). Patient symptoms are not reliable predictors of esophageal or gastric injury (17,23,24). Children with drooling, vomiting, or stridor are at increased risk for esophageal injury and need endoscopic evaluation (16).

The use of esophagoscopy for asymptomatic patients is controversial and requires consideration of time lapsed since ingestion, type of corrosive involved, and extent of exposure. Asymptomatic children are at very low risk of esophageal injury (26). Unintentional asymptomatic ingestion of household bleach or hair relaxer (27) does not require endoscopy, but intentional, symptomatic ingestion of more than 1 ml/kg may benefit from endoscopy. In addition, patients who are unable to tolerate oral fluids after a period of observation may benefit from endoscopy.

When a flexible fiberoptic scope is used within the first 24 to 48 hours, the risk of perforation is low. The exact timing of esophagoscopy within the first 48 hours depends on availability, edema, and the patient's general condition. The issue of whether to pass the first site of injury is controversial due to the possibility of perforation. Contraindications to endoscopy are upper airway obstruction, signs and symptoms of perforation, and more than 48 hours since exposure (relative).

The use of flexible scopes has decreased this risk, and examination of the stomach is often important. In a prospective study of 31 patients who ingested sodium or potassium hydroxide, the esophagus was injured in all patients, the stomach in 94%, and the duodenum in 30% (24). The risk of perforation is increased beginning 2 to 4 days after exposure and continues for the next 2 weeks due to tissue sloughing (23). Grading of the injury helps determine when oral feedings may begin and provides an estimation of the risk of perforation or stricture formation (23). Documented absence of esophageal burns may allow early discharge of the patient. Esophageal findings can be classified into three categories—superficial (grade 1), transmucosal (grade 2A and 2B), and transmural (grade 3)—which have therapeutic significance.

OTHER TESTS

There are no laboratory tests that predict or detect GI burns. Significant bleeding due to GI mucosal injury or perforation may be detected in the stool or emesis. Extensive bowel necrosis may result in metabolic acidosis and elevated serum lactate. The patient's acid-base status, serum electrolytes, renal function, and coagulation parameters should be monitored.

RADIOGRAPHY

An upright chest radiograph should be obtained to detect free air from esophageal, gastric, or intestinal perforation or for evidence of pulmonary aspiration.

Contrast studies are useful to detect delayed complications such as stricture formation or gastric outlet obstruction. A routine barium swallow at 3 weeks postinjury is suggested for evaluation of stricture formation unless symptoms dictate an earlier study. An upper GI series is useful for evaluating the pylorus and duodenum when endoscopy is not helpful. The routine series is necessary to identify complications, such as scarring and outlet obstruction, at the end of the first month. Water-soluble contrast media should be used whenever perforation is a possibility.

DIAGNOSTIC PITFALLS

The absence of oral burns after ingestion of a strong liquid alkali does not rule out significant esophageal or gastric injury. Endoscopy should be performed within 48 hours of exposure when indicated.

Treatment

All patients who ingest a strong alkali should be evaluated in a health care facility. The patient should have intravenous access established. Airway problems may arise from laryngeal edema and inhalation exposure. Respiratory distress may require cricothyroidotomy if endotracheal intubation is complicated by excessive swelling. The presence of shock suggests perforation and requires intravenous fluid administration and surgical evaluation.

DECONTAMINATION AND FIRST AID

Skin exposure is treated with removal of all contaminated clothes and irrigation of the exposed skin with water. All solids should be removed from the skin.

Ocular exposures should be irrigated immediately at the scene, continuing for at least 20 to 30 minutes. All symptomatic eye exposures should be evaluated for corneal burns and foreign bodies at a health care facility. Thorough irrigation requires retraction of the eyelids so that the conjunctival cul-de-sacs are well washed. Topical ophthalmic anesthetic agents (proparacaine, tetracaine) and eyelid retractors are used as necessary. Be sure to remove all particulate matter. Irrigation should continue for at least 20 to 30 minutes and until the conjunctival fluid pH is 7.

Repeated topical ophthalmic anesthetic and insertion of a Morgan lens relieve pain and allow continuous irrigation until a neutral pH is obtained. Do not use neutralizing solutions or any other additives. Several liters of saline irrigation may be required. Caustic injuries require a complete eye examination, preferably with a slit lamp, to detect the extent of corneal injury after decontamination. The examination should include assessment of visual acuity. Fluorescein staining can be used to detect corneal and conjunctival abrasions and ulcerations. Do not use fluorescein if a corneal perforation is suspected. In such cases, shield the eye and contact an ophthalmologist. All corneal burns should be referred to an ophthalmologist within 24 hours.

Cycloplegic drops, antibiotic drops, or artificial tears may be indicated depending on the severity of symptoms. Steroid eye drops should be given only with the approval of the consulting ophthalmologist. Eye patching has not been shown to improve healing.

Ingestion of alkali is treated with immediate milk or water dilution within 30 minutes of ingestion. The goal is to remove the corrosive agent from the esophagus. Dilution more than 1 hour after injury probably is not efficacious. Do not attempt to neutralize the alkali with weak acids. Dilution with water or milk was effective in decreasing injury severity in an *in vitro* rat esophagus model of alkali burns (12). Other *in vitro* studies indicate that water dilution is ineffective in reducing pH and that buffering agents (e.g., antacids) produce significant exothermic reactions without significantly altering the pH (28).

Because reexposure of the mucosa to alkali is harmful, be careful to avoid further vomiting and limit oral fluids to 8 oz for adults and 4 oz for children. Syrup of ipecac is contraindicated because reexposure of the esophagus to corrosive material may cause further injury. Activated charcoal also has no place in the management of alkali ingestion because it is ineffective and obscures the endoscopic field.

GASTRIC LAVAGE OR NASOGASTRIC TUBE IRRIGATION

There are no studies to support the use of gastric lavage or nasogastric tube irrigation in caustic ingestion. The risks include inducing vomiting and reexposure of the esophagus to the alkali and pulmonary aspiration. There is a potential risk of causing esophageal or gastric perforation if a nasogastric or lavage tube is inserted, although this has not been specifically studied. Insertion of nasogastric tube should be done only under endoscopic guidance.

SUPPORTIVE CARE

Patients should not be fed orally until endoscopy has established the extent of injury. Patients with only first-degree burns may begin oral liquids when stable, usually the first day of exposure. Second-degree burn patients should not be fed orally for 2 to 3 days. Patients with severe burns (grade 3) require a surgically placed gastrostomy or jejunostomy tube for feeding.

Corticosteroids have been shown to decrease the incidence of stricture formation in animal models (29,30). In rabbits, rapid postburn administration of dexamethasone, but not prednisolone, was associated with significant reductions in the frequency and severity of burns and strictures, compared with controls (30).

In humans, the administration of steroids is controversial. A controlled trial of prednisolone in children with caustic (primarily alkaline corrosive) esophageal injury did not show a decrease in stricture formation with treatment. The steroid treatment group ($N = 31$) received 2.0 to 2.5 mg/kg/day of prednisolone for 3 weeks followed by a 2- to 3-week taper. The incidence of stricture formation in the control group ($N = 29$) was 38%, compared with 32% in the steroid group (not statistically significant) (31). One limitation of the study is the small sample size and its inability to detect a small benefit if present (type II error).

A retrospective study of 246 patients found no difference in stricture formation with the use of methylprednisolone, compared with historical controls (32). In another study, children with second- or third-degree esophageal burns were treated with either dexamethasone (1 mg/kg/day) or prednisolone (2 mg/kg/day). Strictures developed in 12 (66.7%) of the children in the prednisolone-treated group ($N = 18$) and only 7 (38.9%) of the children in the dexamethasone-treated group ($N = 18$). Burn healing was significantly better in the dexamethasone-treated group (33). In a review of the literature, Howell suggested that steroid administration may be beneficial in limiting stricture formation after second- and third-degree injuries (34). A retrospective study of 235 children with caustic burns also suggested that steroid administration was beneficial in reducing stricture formation (35).

Steroid administration has typically been delayed many hours after exposure in these studies. The potential benefits of steroid administration within 1 to 2 hours of exposure have not been studied in humans. Grades 1 and 2A injuries usually do not result in stricture formation, and systemic steroids probably would not be beneficial in these patients. Most patients with third-degree burns develop esophageal strictures regardless of therapy (34). Thus, grade 2B lesions are most likely to benefit from any antiinflammatory action steroids may offer. Steroids may be effective in patients with dyspnea, stridor, hoarseness, or other evidence of respiratory compromise. Steroids may decrease laryngotracheal edema and may lessen respiratory dysfunction (36). Steroids have been blamed for obscuring peritoneal signs after an acid ingestion (37,38). Another complication is increased vulnerability to infection.

Some authors have used esophageal stents with good results and abandoned the use of steroids (39).

ANTIBIOTICS

Antibiotics should be reserved for documented infections. If systemic steroids are administered, prophylactic intravenous broad-spectrum antibiotics are often given concurrently.

SKIN BURNS

Treat chemical burns as thermal burns with débridement, topical antibiotic ointment, nonadherent sterile gauze, and wrapping. Deep second-degree burns may benefit from topical silver sulfadiazine. Deep second- or third-degree burns and burns of the hands, face, or perineum should be evaluated by a physician with extensive experience in burn care.

MONITORING

Grade 1 to 2 burns usually can be admitted to a general medical ward. Patients with grade 2 to 3 burns or patients with unstable vital signs, GI bleeding, metabolic acidosis, or signs of perforation should be admitted to an intensive care unit. Initial observation should be directed toward detecting GI perforation or hemorrhage by serial abdominal examinations, complete blood cell counts, and, if indicated, radiographs and water-soluble contrast studies. Follow fluid and electrolyte balance carefully. Monitor for development of complications such as sepsis, mediastinitis, and peritonitis.

Hospitalized patients should be followed after discharge for the development of esophageal stricture and gastric-outlet obstruction. Patients should return if signs of obstruction develop such as progressive anorexia, weight loss, early satiety, nausea, dysphagia, or vomiting. Obtain a follow-up esophagram and upper GI series to evaluate for secondary scarring or stricture formation approximately 2 to 4 weeks after ingestion.

MANAGEMENT PITFALLS

Esophageal and gastric injury from strong alkali ingestion may be initially underestimated because oral burns and initial symptoms may not correlate with the extent of injury. Patients should be admitted and early endoscopy considered. The patient should be asymptomatic and able to tolerate oral fluids before discharge if endoscopy is withheld. Unintentional ingestion of household bleach or hair relaxer by children typically does not require endoscopy. There is conflicting evidence concerning the benefit of systemic steroids in preventing stricture formation.

AMMONIA

Ammonium hydroxide concentration ranges from 3% to 10%. Weaker 3% solutions are mild irritants, but higher concentrations may be significantly corrosive (3). Volatile ammonia solutions can produce inhalation injuries and systemic symptoms. An 8.8% ammonia solution has a pH of 12.5 (4).

SODIUM HYDROXIDE

Sodium (Augus Hot Rod, caustic soda, caustic lye, sodium hydrate soda lye, white caustic) or potassium hydroxide clears plugged drains and cuts grease buildup. Red Devil Drain Opener and Red Devil Lye (96% to 100% sodium hydroxide) have a pH of 14. Crystalline Drano (57% sodium hydroxide) has a pH of 14. Both Liquid Drano (10% sodium hydroxide) and Liquid Plumber (5% sodium hydroxide) also have a pH of 14. Some drain cleaners have been reformulated to contain 1,1,1-trichloroethane, which is a hydrocarbon rather than a caustic.

Liquid lye ingestion produces a more severe injury than that produced by powder or granular alkaline agents or by nonalkaline corrosive liquids. Solid lye tends to stick to the mucosa and rarely injures the GI tract beyond the proximal esophagus unless ingested as a tablet or put in a capsule in a suicide attempt. Liquid alkaline agents quickly cover the surface of the esophagus and move on to the stomach, producing a liquefaction necrosis (40).

SODIUM HYPOCHLORITE

Household bleach products (e.g., Clorox) usually contain 3% to 6% sodium hypochlorite (Antiformin, bleach, Carrel-Dakin solution, Chloros, Chlorox, Clorox, Dakin's solution, Hychlorite, Modified Dakin's solution, sodium oxychloride) and have a pH of up to 11. Some bleaches (e.g., Purex) contain silicate (15% to 17%) and sodium carbonate (60%) and have a pH of approximately 10.5.

Household bleaches may produce erosions but penetrate the submucosa to cause esophageal strictures only in unusual cases. Granular and commercial bleaches may contain higher concentrations of hypochlorite or carbonate, leading to greater tissue destruction. Granular bleaches are considered more toxic because the granules prolong mucosal contact and because solid bleaches tend to be more concentrated. Commercial bleaches contain other bleaching agents (e.g., sodium peroxide, sodium perborate, sodium carbonate, oxalic acid), and proper therapy requires accurate identification. Only minor first-degree burns have been reported in children ingesting household bleach. Most children have no GI tract injury (41). Intentional ingestion of large amounts of bleach may result in hematemesis and electrolyte disturbances.

HAIR RELAXER

Hair relaxer products may contain dilute concentrations of sodium hydroxide or potassium hydroxide combined with guanidine carbonate to form guanidine hydroxide with a pH of 12.5 to 13.0. They may produce caustic injury when ingested. They usually do not produce severe esophageal injury but can cause extensive superficial burns of the skin, pharynx, and larynx. No esophageal strictures have been reported as a result of ingesting hair relaxer. A retrospective review of 59 children who ingested hair relaxers revealed initial symptoms that ranged from none to drooling and vomiting. Two patients had second-degree oral cavity bums. First-degree burns of the lip were noted in 33 patients. Fifty-six patients (95%) underwent endoscopy, which revealed normal esophageal mucosa in 53, mild erythema of the distal esophagus in 2, and mild esophagitis in 1 patient.

Based on the absence of significant esophageal burns in this and other case series, it has been recommended that selective endoscopy be used. Patients who are asymptomatic, tolerate oral fluids, and have reliable parents may be managed as outpatients without endoscopy. All other patients should be admitted for observation and further evaluation. Endoscopy should be considered for patients unable to tolerate oral fluids or who have chest pain or abdominal pain (27).

REFERENCES

1. Litovitz TL, Klein-Schwartz W, Rodgers GC, et al. 2001 Annual Report of the American Association of Poison Control Centers Toxic Exposure Surveillance System. *Am J Emerg Med* 2002;20:391–452.
2. Bautista Casasnovas A, Estevez Martinez E, Varela Cives R, et al. A retrospective analysis of ingestion of caustic substances by children. Ten-year statistics in Galicia. *Eur J Pediatr* 1997;156:410–414.
3. Ernst RW, Leventhal M, Luva R, et al. Total esophagogastric replacement after ingestion of household ammonia. *N Engl J Med* 1963;208:815–816.
4. Vancura EM, Clinton JE, Ruiz E, et al. Toxicity of alkaline solutions. *Ann Emerg Med* 1980;9:118–122.
5. Muhlendal KE, Oberoisse V, Krienke EG. Local injuries by accidental ingestion of corrosive substances by children. *Arch Toxicol* 1978;39:299–314.
6. Warren JB, Griffin DJ, Olson RC. Urine sugar reagent tablet ingestion causing gastric and duodenal ulceration. *Arch Intern Med* 1984;144:161–162.
7. Burrington JD. Clinitest burns of the esophagus. *Ann Thorac Surg* 1975;20:400–404.
8. Early SH, Simpson RL. Caustic burns from contact with wet cement. *JAMA* 1985;254:528–529.
9. Spoo J, Elsner P. Cement burns: a review 1960–2000. *Contact Dermatitis* 2001;45:68–71.
10. Hadley CM, Laubacher MA, Watson PD. Dermal and inhalation burns caused by the automotive air bag inflation system. *Vet Hum Toxicol* 1993;35:358.
11. Hoffman RS, Howland MA, Kamerow HN, Goldfrank LR. Comparison of titratable acid/alkaline reserve and pH in potentially caustic household products. *J Toxicol Clin Toxicol* 1989;27:241–261.
12. Homan CS, Maitra SR, Lane BP, et al. Therapeutic effects of water and milk for acute alkali injury of the esophagus. *Ann Emerg Med* 1994;24:14–20.
13. Smilkstein MJ. Should we add an acid to an alkali injury? For now, let's remain neutral! *Acad Emerg Med* 1995;2:945–946.
14. Grenga TE. A new risk of lye ingestion by children. *N Engl J Med* 1983;308:156–157.
15. Gaudreault P, Parent M, McGuigan M, et al. Predictability of esophageal injury from signs and symptoms: a study of caustic ingestions in 378 children. *Pediatrics* 1983;71:767–770.
16. Crain EF, Gershel JC, Mezey AP. Caustic ingestions: symptoms as predictors of esophageal injury. *Am J Dis Child* 1984;138:863–865.
17. Gorman RL, Khin-Maung-Gyi MT, Klein-Schwartz W, et al. Initial symptoms as predictors of esophageal injury in alkaline corrosive ingestions. *Am J Emerg Med* 1992;10:189–194.
18. Knopp R. Caustic ingestions. *JACEP* 1979;8:329–336.
19. Krenzelok EP, Clinton JE. Caustic esophageal and gastric erosion without evidence of oral burns following detergent ingestion. *JACEP* 1979;8:194–196.
20. Mallory A, Schaefer JW. Clinitest ingestion. *Br Med J* 1977;2:105–107.
21. Hopkins RA, Postlethwait RW. Caustic burns and carcinoma of the esophagus. *Ann Surg* 1981;194:146–148.
22. Nunes AC, Romaozinho JM, Pontes JM, et al. Risk factors for stricture development after caustic ingestion. *Hepatogastroenterology* 2002;49:1563–1566.
23. Zargar SA, Kochhar R, Mehta S, Mehta SK. The role of fiberoptic endoscopy in the management of corrosive ingestion and modified endoscopic classification of burns. *Gastrointest Endosc* 1991;37:165–169.
24. Zargar SA, Kochhar R, Nagi B, et al. Ingestion of strong corrosive alkalis: spectrum of injury to upper gastrointestinal tract and natural history. *Am J Gastroenterol* 1992;87:337–341.
25. Appelquist P, Salmo M. Lye corrosion carcinoma of the esophagus: a review of 63 cases. *Cancer* 1980;45:2655–2658.
26. Lamireau T, Rebouissoux L, Denis D, et al. Accidental caustic ingestion in children: is endoscopy always mandatory? *J Pediatr Gastroenterol Nutr* 2001;33:81–84.
27. Ahsan S, Haupert M. Absence of esophageal injury in pediatric patients after hair relaxer ingestion. *Arch Otolaryngol Head Neck Surg* 1999;125:953–955.
28. Maull KI. Liquid caustic ingestions: an in vitro study of the effects of buffer, neutralization, and dilution. *Ann Emerg Med* 1985;14:1160–1162.

29. Haller JA, Bachman K. The comparative effect of current therapy on experimental caustic burns of the esophagus. *Pediatrics* 1964;34:236–245.
30. Bautista A, Tojo R, Varela R, et al. Effects of prednisolone and dexamethasone on alkali burns of the esophagus in rabbit. *J Pediatr Gastroenterol Nutr* 1996;22:275–283.
31. Anderson KD, Rouse TM, Randolph JG. A controlled trial of corticosteroids in children with corrosive injury of the esophagus. *N Engl J Med* 1990;323:637–640.
32. Ulman I, Mutaf O. A critique of systemic steroids in the management of caustic esophageal burns in children. *Eur J Pediatr Surg* 1998;8:71–74.
33. Bautista A, Varela R, Villanueva A, et al. Effects of prednisolone and dexamethasone in children with alkali burns of the oesophagus. *Eur J Pediatr Surg* 1996;6:198–203.
34. Howell JM, Dalsey WC, Hartsell FW, Batzin CA. Steroids for the treatment of corrosive esophageal injury. A statistical analysis of past studies. *Am J Emerg Med* 1992;10:421–425.
35. Keskin E, Okur H, Koltuksuz U, et al. The effect of steroid treatment on corrosive oesophageal burns in children. *Eur J Pediatr Surg* 1991;1:335–338.
36. Wijburg FA, Heymans HSA, Urbanus NAM. Caustic esophageal lesions in childhood: prevention of stricture formation. *J Pediatr Surg* 1989;24:171–173.
37. Nicosia JR, Thornton JP, Folk FA. Surgical management of corrosive gastric injuries. Ann Surg 1974;180:139–143.
38. Kirsh MM, Ritter F. Caustic ingestion and subsequent damage to the oropharyngeal and digestive passages. *Ann Thorac Surg* 1976;21:74–82.
39. Berkovits RN, Bos CE, Wijburg FA, Holzki J. Caustic injury of the oesophagus. Sixteen years experience, and introduction of a new model oesophageal stent. *J Laryngol Otol* 1996;110:1041–1045.
40. Meredith JW, Kon ND, Thompson JN. Management of injuries from liquid lye ingestion. *J Trauma* 1988;28:1173–1180.
41. Kiristioglu I, Gurpinar A, Kilic N, et al. Is it necessary to perform an endoscopy after the ingestion of liquid household bleach in children? *Acta Paediatr* 1999;88:233–234.

CHAPTER 203

Household Products: Miscellaneous

S. Rutherfoord Rose

Compounds included:	**Nontoxic ingestions, baking soda, bezoars, cleaning products (soaps, detergents, household shampoo, general purpose cleaners, bleach, ammonia, disinfectants and deodorizers), clove cigarettes, coins, denatonium benzoate, medication-induced esophageal injury, mothballs, paraphenylenediamine, personal care products (cosmetics, dental products, hair care products, mouthwash, nail polish and nail polish removers, perfume/cologne/aftershave), pica**
SI conversion:	**Not applicable**
Special concerns:	**It is often unrecognized that household products may produce significant toxicity.**
Antidote:	**None**

NONTOXIC INGESTION

In 1970, Mofenson and Greensher (1) defined a *nontoxic ingestion* as that which occurs after an individual consumes a nonedible product that usually does not produce symptoms.

Table 1 details some of the most frequently ingested household items considered "usually nontoxic." Qualifications exist for many categories, so the extent of symptoms may depend on actual circumstances (e.g., specific product, quantity, host).

Consulting lists, such as those in Table 1, may not be sufficient without careful investigation as below:

1. The name—spelled out carefully—of the item.
2. Details of the package labeling, if any.
3. Name and address of the manufacturer.
4. Date on the label.
5. Date purchased.
6. Consultation with a current reference source or the manufacturer to determine current ingredients in the preparations. Package labels are most accurate and should be used if available.

Problems also may result from inaccurate historical information about the ingestion. Some questions that might be considered in responding include the following:

1. How certain are you that only a single dose was ingested?
2. Were any other substances ingested simultaneously?
3. Have there been any symptoms?
4. Is there a history of repeated ingestions of "nontoxic" substances?
5. Does the patient have any significant medical history: allergies, liver or kidney problems, adverse drug reactions?

Factors that mitigate against an oversimplified evaluation by the poison information professional include the following:

1. The information obtained may be incorrect and misleading. Repetitive questioning and insistence on details may minimize such errors.
2. The constantly changing chemical composition of items.
3. Agents formerly believed to be "nontoxic" may cause damage.

TABLE 1. Criteria and examples of nontoxic ingestions

Criteria
Absolute identification.
Time and amount of ingestion is known.
Amount ingested relative to patient's weight is less than smallest amount known or predicted to induce toxicity.
Time elapsed since ingestion is greater than the longest predicted interval between ingestion and peak toxicity.
Detailed history includes no symptoms or signs of toxicity.

Ingestions usually considered nontoxic (unless very large quantities)

Adhesives	Dog food	Pastes
A&D Ointment	Erasers	Pencil lead (graphite)
Air fresheners	Etch-A-Sketch	Petroleum jelly (Vaseline)
Antacids	Felt-tip markers and pens	Photographs
Antibiotic ointments	Fish bowl additives	Plastics
Antiperspirants	Glade Plug In	Plaster (non–lead containing)
Ashes (wood, fireplace)	Glitter glues and pastes	Play-Doh
Baby-product cosmetics	Glowstick/jewelry	Polaroid picture coating
Baby wipes	Golf ball core (may cause mechanical injury)	Porous tip ink marking pens
Ballpoint pen inks	Grease	Potting soil
Bathtub floating toys	Gums	Putty (small amounts)
Bath oil (castor oil and perfume)	Gypsum	Rouge
Body conditioners	Hand lotions and creams	Rust
Bubble bath soaps	Indelible markers	Rubber cement
Calamine lotion	Ink (blue, black)	Saccharin
Candles	Iodophor (not iodide or iodine)	Shampoo (nonmedicated)
Cat food	Kaolin	Shaving cream
Caulk	Kitty litter	Shoe polish
Caps (for toy pistols)	Lanolin	Silica gel
Chalk (calcium carbonate)	Laxatives (single dose)	Silly putty
Charcoal, charcoal briquettes	Lipstick, lip balm	Soaps and soap products
Cigarettes (less than one)	Lubricants	Starch
Cigarette ashes	Magic marker	Styrofoam
Clay (modeling)	Magnesium silicate	Sunscreen and tan preparations
Contraceptive pills (without iron)	Makeup (eye, liquid facial)	Super glue
Corticosteroids (single dose)	Mascara (domestic)	Sweetening agents
Cold packs (a swallow)	Matches (book type, three books)	Teething rings (fluid may have bacteria)
Crayons (AP, CP, CS-140)	Massengill disposable douches	Thermometers (mercury, phthalate alcohol)
Crayola markers	Miracle-Gro plant food	Toothpaste (even fluoride)
Crazy glue (cyanoacrylate)	Mineral oil	Vaseline
Cyclamate	Mylar balloons	Vitamins (without iron)
Dehumidifying packets (silica or charcoal)	Newspaper	Warfarin (single dose)
Deodorants (spray and refrigerator)	Nutrasweet	Watercolor paint
Disposable diapers	PAAS Easter egg dyes (after 1980)	Zinc oxide
Dishwashing liquid soap (not automatic electric dishwasher)	Paints (indoor latex acrylic)	Zirconium oxide

4. The litigious climate in which we live can be chilling to the "off-the-cuff" answer.

Poison control centers are uniquely positioned to evaluate exposures to household products and determine risk for toxicity. The successful triage of (potentially) nontoxic exposures reduces unnecessary anxiety, ambulance dispatch, emergency room visits, and hospital admissions (2).

BAKING SODA

Baking soda contains sodium bicarbonate and is available as a 100% powder and as an ingredient in some mouthwashes, toothpastes, tooth powders, and carpet deodorizers.

Clinical Presentation

Significant toxicity after acute ingestion is rare, particularly in healthy adults. Chronic exposures or acute exposures in the elderly or children can result in nausea, vomiting, and generalized weakness. Serious toxicity results from hypernatremia, hypokalemia, hypochloremic metabolic alkalosis, and hypocalcemia (3,4). Secondary effects may include paresthesias, muscle tetany, seizures, dysrhythmias, and coma. Severe metabolic alkalosis may result in respiratory failure.

Treatment

Most patients do well with simple oral dilution and observation. Ipecac-induced emesis may be useful in the home or prehospital setting as directed by a poison center. Activated charcoal is not indicated unless coingestants dictate its use. Symptomatic patients should undergo evaluation of serum electrolytes and electrocardiogram. Intravenous administration of 0.25 N hydrochloric acid has been used to correct blood pH.

BEZOARS

The word *bezoar* means antidote, and it is believed to derive either from the Hebrew word Beluzaar, the Arabic word Bedzehr, or the Persian word Padzahr (5). Bezoars were, at various times, believed to cure a variety of ailments, neutralize poisons, and rejuvenate the aged (6).

Classification

Phytobezoars consist of vegetable products or concretions of citrus fruit. Persimmons, fruit stones, raisins, grape skins, oranges, peaches, apples, bran, figs, husks of oats or psyllium, and peanuts are the foods most commonly found (7). This group constitutes as many as 40% of all bezoars. They are largely afflictions of men and are more frequent because of the increased incidence of gastric resection and vagotomy for peptic ulcer disease (8).

Trichobezoars (hair balls) are the second most common type and are concretions of human or animal hairs or synthetic or natural fibers that are found usually in the stomach or small intestine. Patients frequently are females between the ages of 15 and 20 years with long hair who are either mentally retarded, have psychiatric problems, or engage in trichotillomania (6).

Mixed bezoars are combinations of hair and vegetable matter.

Concretions are industrial exposures or ingested medications forming a gastric mass. Medications may include vitamin C or antacid tablets, liquid antacid gels, cholestyramine, hydroscopic bulk laxatives, aspirin, iron, glutethimide, meprobamate, and sucralfate (9).

Lactobezoars are undigested milk concretions that develop and are reported usually within the first year of life and follow feedings of incorrectly prepared powdered formula, ingestion of undiluted concentrated formula, and ingestion of 24 calories/oz low-birth-weight infant formulas (10–12). Factors that accelerate bezoar formation are provided in Table 2 (13).

Clinical Presentation

Patients often present with an epigastric mass, pain, nausea and vomiting, hematemesis, weight loss, lethargy, diarrhea, or constipation (also anemia, halitosis, anorexia, flatulence, and presence of foreign material in the vomitus). There may be no symptoms (5).

Complications include bleeding, obstruction with metabolic abnormalities, perforation complicated by peritonitis, and gastrocutaneous or colocutaneous fistulas (5).

Diagnosis

Gastric dilation and an intraluminal gastric mass with irregular surface contours separate from the gastric mucosa may be seen on a contrast study of the upper gastrointestinal (GI) tract. Gastroscopy with biopsy, echography, and an analysis of stool contents is also useful. Esophageal bezoars may be visualized by endoscopy.

Treatment

Esophageal bezoars are treated with bougienage and endoscopic manipulation (9,14).

TABLE 2. Factors contributing to bezoar formation

Bizarre dietary habits
Lack of teeth
Incomplete chewing
Dehydration
Gastric outlet obstruction
Vagotomy
Altered gastric mucosa and secretion (e.g., achlorhydria)
Anticholinergic or narcotic drugs (reduce peristalsis)

Modified from Delpre G, et al. *J Clin Gastroenterol* 1984;16:231–237.

Gastric bezoars are treated primarily by endoscopy. Irrigation of stomach with 0.9% sodium chloride solution and irrigation with papain (e.g., Adolph's Meat Tenderizer, Cheseborough-Pond, Inc.) in 1 to 3 teaspoonfuls in 8 oz of water before each meal have also been attempted (15). Caution must be exercised in using Adolph's Meat Tenderizer in view of a report of hypernatremia and confusion in a 65-year-old patient after its use for the treatment of a phytobezoar (16).

Cellulase (Kanulase, Dorsey Laboratories) in capsules is used to prevent bezoar formation or as an irrigant (instillation of 1.0 L of a 0.5 g/100.0 ml solution over 24 hours) (17). Metoclopramide, up to 10 mg three or four times daily, may be useful. Limited experience suggests that acetylcysteine may enhance dissolution of gastric mucus, which may encase cellulose bezoars (18).

Small bowel bezoars may require enterotomy (19).

Rectal bezoars may require rectal dilation under anesthesia, anoscopy, and proctoscopy.

Surgery can be useful when bleeding, obstruction, or perforation has occurred. If a large bezoar is present, gastrotomy, enterotomy, or bowel resection may be the treatment of choice.

CLEANING PRODUCTS

Household cleaners include soaps, detergents, household shampoo, general purpose cleaners, bleach, ammonia, disinfectants, and deodorizers. These products are among the most frequently ingested substances reported to poison control centers (2). Exposures in children result from improper storage or occur while a product is in use when caregivers are temporarily distracted. Serious complications are very rare.

Soaps

Soaps are the salts of long chain fatty acids produced by the action of alkali on naturally occurring fats and oils. Some heavy-duty soaps contain inorganic builders that alter pH and inactivate hard-water minerals.

CLINICAL PRESENTATION

Soaps are mild GI and mucous membrane irritants that occasionally produce nausea, vomiting, diarrhea, and abdominal pain. Deodorant bars contain some photosensitizing agents (e.g., biocides, perfumes, detergents). Most other ingredients (e.g., hexachlorophene) are present in concentrations too low to produce toxicity, other than hypersensitivity reactions.

TREATMENT

Ipecac-induced emesis is not required.

Irrigate all symptomatic ocular exposure with saline (water is an acceptable alternative if saline is unavailable). Minor ocular irritation may benefit from a soothing agent (e.g., a vasoconstrictor solution containing naphazoline) *after* thorough irrigation. Local ophthalmic anesthetic agents (e.g., tetracaine) should not be prescribed for outpatient use.

Administer clear liquids and antiemetic if needed for GI symptoms.

Patients can usually be managed at home with symptomatic treatment.

Detergents

Toxicity of liquid detergents is generally less than that of granular detergents. In a dose of 3 tablespoons in 8 oz of water, liquid dishwashing detergent products (not laundry or electric dishwashing detergents) have been recommended as a substitute emetic when syrup of ipecac is unavailable. However, some liquid laundry and automatic dishwasher detergents may possess sufficient alkalinity to cause caustic injury.

SURFACTANTS

Detergents contain synthetic, organic, surface-active agents called *surfactants*, which are derived from petroleum product precursors. Surfactants are designed to lower surface tension of water to reduce insoluble precipitates. The net electrical charge determines the ionic characteristic of a surfactant.

Anionic surfactants are commonly used in commercial detergent products. Examples include alkyl sodium sulfate, sodium lauryl sulfate, sodium aryl-alkyl sulfate, dioctyl sodium sulfosuccinate, sodium oleate, linear alkyl benzene, and tetrapropylene benzene sulfonates. Anionic surfactants possess irritant properties, with the major exception of electric dishwasher products in which builders enhance alkalinity.

Nonionic surfactants include electrically neutral medium- to long-chain polyether sulfates, alcohols, or sulfonates (e.g., alkylaryl polyether sulfates, alkyl ethoxylate, alkyl phenoxy polyethoxy ethanols, polyethylene glycol stearate). Nonionic surfactants produce less local irritation than anionic ones. Most household detergents contain anionic or nonionic surfactants.

Cationic surfactants include quaternary ammonium compounds: benzalkonium chloride, benzethonium chloride, cetylpyridinium chloride, and alkyl dimethyl 3,4-dichlorobenzene ammonium chloride. Concentrated cationic solutions (10% to 15%) are caustic, and even dilute solutions (0.1% to 0.5%) can produce significant mucosal irritation. Large ingestions may produce central nervous system (CNS) symptoms. Fabric softeners, automatic dishwasher detergents, and mildew removers commonly contain cationic surfactants.

Amphoteric surfactants contain both anionic and cationic surface-active molecules and occur more commonly in industrial cleaning products.

BUILDERS

Manufacturers add inorganic "builder" to detergents to improve their wetting and emulsifying properties, which are inhibited by hard-water minerals such as calcium. Most heavy-duty detergents contain builders and include inorganic salts such as phosphates, carbonates, silicate, sodium citrate, and aluminosilicates. Complex phosphate-containing detergents were reformulated to low-phosphate, biodegradable detergents in the 1960s due to their persistence in the environment and subsequent sudsing and enhanced algae production in lakes. Death has occurred after intentional ingestion of a low-phosphate detergent.

ADDITIVES

Detergents contain a variety of additives (e.g., bleaches, bactericidal agents, enzymes, perfumes, colorants, whitening agents, softeners), but their concentrations are too low to produce primary irritation. However, these additives may cause a contact dermatitis by sensitizing certain individuals.

CLINICAL PRESENTATION

Most exposures to household cleaning products reported to poison control centers do not result in symptoms. Symptomatic patients most often exhibit mild, self-limiting GI symptoms (nausea, vomiting, diarrhea). Granular laundry detergents, liquid laundry detergents, and fabric softeners produce more nausea, vomiting, and diarrhea than other household detergents and soaps. Cationic detergents may produce systemic toxicity and, in rare circumstances, severe upper airway compromise or death (fatal adult dose estimated between 1 and 3 g).

Cationic detergents are more potent irritants than anionic or nonionic detergents.

TREATMENT

Most detergents and soap ingestions require only dilution with water or milk. Patients should be observed at home several hours in the upright position for spontaneous vomiting.

Cationic detergent [quaternary ammonium compounds such as benzalkonium chloride (Zephiran Chloride), cetylpyridinium chloride, benzethonium chloride (Phemerol chloride)] ingestions require airway evaluation before decontamination. Emesis or gastric lavage is not indicated due to risk of caustic effects. For solutions less than 5%, activated charcoal may be administered as soon as possible. Ingestion of agents containing more than 5% to 10% cationic detergent should be treated as caustic ingestions (immediate dilution plus esophagoscopy as needed). Transient contact with cationic detergent requires only dilution.

Eye exposures should be irrigated copiously with saline for 20 minutes. Be sure to retract the eyelids to search for granules in the fornices of the conjunctiva. Each patient should receive an eye examination, including fluorescein staining to detect corneal abrasions.

Hypocalcemia and tetany are rare complications of ingestion of phosphate-containing detergents.

Published evidence that weak soap solutions bind quaternary ammonia compounds to prevent absorption is lacking. Because most soaps now contain anionic surfactants, the recommended use of soap for these ingestions is not warranted.

Household Shampoos

Some liquid shampoos contain alkyl sodium sulfate, which has more mucosal irritant properties than nonionic surfactants. Dry shampoos may contain methanol or isopropanol. Industrial-strength rug shampoos and carpet-cleaning products may contain potentially toxic compounds, especially when the products are not properly diluted. Potentially toxic compounds include sodium carbonate, sodium perborate, sodium phosphate, ammonia compounds, borax, pine oil, trichloroethylene, tetrachloroethylene, naphtha, naphthalene, kerosene, petroleum solvents, alkyl benzene sulfonate, and alkyl-aryl sodium sulfonate.

CLINICAL PRESENTATION

Carpet and upholstery cleaners are more toxic than personal shampoos. Household shampoos usually produce mild GI tract irritation. A rug shampoo caused a respiratory illness characterized by cough, headache, sore throat, awareness of unusual odor, dyspnea, fatigue, nausea, and other GI complaints. The duration of illness was 2 to 17 days with a 5-day average (20).

TREATMENT

Symptomatic treatment, including milk or water dilution and several hours of observation for spontaneous vomiting, usually suffices in most household shampoo exposures. Heavy-duty or industrial-strength solution exposures may require evaluation for caustic injury or specific treatment for toxic ingredients (e.g., methanol). Respiratory symptoms in rug shampoo exposures respond to improved ventilation and removal from the source.

General-Purpose Cleaners

General-purpose cleaners may contain ingredients that are potentially more toxic than detergents and soaps. Examples include sodium metasilicate (alkaline corrosive), sodium carbonate, calcium carbonate, sodium citrate, alcohols, butyl ethers, bleach, ammonia, and pine oil. *Pine oil* is a mixture of highly lipophilic unsaturated cyclic hydrocarbons (cyclic terpene alcohols, monoterpenes) that is one-fifth as toxic as turpentine in animals. *Turpentine* is a natural solvent composed of pine oils, camphenes, and terpenes. The volatile components of turpentine (α-pinene, β-pinene, γ_3-carene) are significant pulmonary aspiration hazards. Abrasive cleaners contain pumice or silica, which have minimal toxicity. A few powdered cleaners contain borates. Mildew removers generally contain hypochlorites and cationic detergents and should be treated as potentially alkaline corrosive. Furniture polishes usually contain petroleum distillate hydrocarbons, silicones, and nonionic surfactants; spray formulations may contain hydrocarbon propellants.

CLINICAL PRESENTATION

Pine oil may be lethal at a dose of 60 to 120 g, although survival without sequelae after an ingestion of 400 to 500 g has been reported. Pine oil produces primarily GI irritation (less than 20% concentration) and CNS depression with higher concentrations (21,22). Renal failure may occur, but death is rare. All patients who ingest pine oil in a hydrocarbon vehicle are at risk for aspiration and chemical pneumonitis.

Turpentine oil is absorbed from the GI tract and can produce systemic toxicity. Quantities in excess of 2 ml/kg should be considered toxic and removed by gut decontamination. As little as 15 ml of turpentine may produce symptoms in children; 120 to 180 ml is a potentially lethal adult dose. This compound is a local irritant, CNS depressant, and pulmonary aspiration hazard, similar to other volatile oils such as camphor, sassafras, eucalyptus, and wintergreen; however, acute turpentine toxicity is less severe than that of these volatile oils. Casual exposures may produce mucosal irritation, mild respiratory tract inflammation, and urinary tract irritation. In large intentional doses, coma and convulsions may occur. Pulmonary aspiration of turpentine produces a hemorrhagic pulmonary edema.

Household ammonia contains ammonium hydroxide in concentrations ranging from 5% to 10%. Weaker 3% solutions are mild irritants, but higher concentrations may be significantly corrosive. An 8.8% ammonia solution has a pH of 12.5 (23). Accidental ingestion or exposure to vapors of household ammonia can be irritating to eyes and mucous membranes. Intentional ingestion of even low concentrations, however, can result in significant caustic injury (24,25). Volatile ammonia solutions can produce inhalation injuries and systemic symptoms. Additional information is available in Chapter 183.

Bleach [household bleach (e.g., Clorox)] contains less than 5% sodium hypochlorite, which causes mild mucosal irritation. Granular bleaches are considered more toxic because the granules prolong mucosal contact and because solid bleaches tend to be more concentrated. Some bleaches that contain calcium hypochlorite may be more irritating than those with comparable concentrations of sodium hypochlorite. Commercial bleaches contain other bleaching agents (e.g., sodium peroxide, sodium perborate, sodium carbonate, oxalic acid), and proper therapy requires accurate identification. Products with a pH below 12.5 do not cause serious burns, but large volumes and prolonged contact may result in corrosive injury (26).

Of all household cleaning products, bleaches produce the highest rates of nausea, vomiting, and abdominal pain. Industrial-strength hypochlorite bleaches (15% to 20% solutions) may induce caustic injuries. Massive suicidal ingestions may produce fatal hyperchloremic metabolic acidosis or aspiration pneumonitis. Sodium peroxide decomposes in the stomach by releasing oxygen and may cause a gastritis. Sodium perborate is metabolized to peroxide and borate, which has moderate mucosal-irritating properties and systemic effects.

Sodium hypochlorite solutions may release small amounts of hypochlorous acid and chlorine gas, but usually the concentrations of these toxic gases are too low to cause damage. Mixing solutions of ammonia and sodium hypochlorite produces monochloramine (NH_2Cl) and dichloramine ($NHCl_2$) fumes. On contact with moist mucous membranes, these fumes form hydrochlorous acid and nascent oxygen, which are potent oxidizing agents. In contrast, hypochlorite solutions mixed with acids, such as hydrochloric acid found in some toilet bowl cleaners, produce chlorine fumes. Inhalation of chloramine or chlorine fumes in a confined environment can result in significant mucous membrane irritation, bronchospasm, or chemical pneumonitis (27). Prolonged inhalation of chloramine fumes can produce obstructive pulmonary deficits, chest infiltrates, and acute pulmonary edema. Patients with preexisting lung disease are at increased risk for pulmonary toxicity.

TREATMENT

Most accidental ingestions of household cleaners (including hydrocarbons) require only dilution with milk or water to reduce mucosal-irritant properties (28). Turpentine ingestions should be treated like toluene exposures, and gut decontamination measures should be used only when the ingestion exceeds approximately 2 ml/kg. Patients who ingest concentrated pine oil products (more than 20% to 30% concentration) should be decontaminated by nasogastric suction or activated charcoal. Be sure to check product contents to determine the appropriateness of decontamination measures. Observe all patients for signs or symptoms of aspiration.

For topical exposures, decontaminate both skin and eyes with copious saline irrigation. Be sure to remove all contaminated clothing (e.g., diapers in chlorine bleach exposure). Check exposed eyes for corneal abrasions with fluorescein staining.

Most symptoms resulting from transient exposures to household fumes of ammonia, bleach, chloramine, or chlorine resolve with fresh air and topical decontamination. Some patients benefit from humidified oxygen. Patients with continued dyspnea or bronchospasm should be admitted and observed for pulmonary edema and adult respiratory distress syndrome. Severe chlorine and chloramine exposures require evaluation of acid-base status.

Disinfectants and Deodorizers

LIQUID DISINFECTANTS

These products may contain acids, alkali, alcohol, pine oil, phenol, glycols, or cationic detergents such as quaternary compounds (e.g., Zephiran). Combination cleaners with pine oil and phenol are the most toxic compounds in this group.

DEODORIZERS

Cake deodorizers are commercial products for garbage pails, diaper pails, and bathrooms and usually contain *p*-dichlorobenzene (Chapter 206), which is relatively nontoxic in small doses. A few older products still contain the more toxic naphthalene or camphor.

Wick deodorizers contain petroleum distillate hydrocarbons, essential oils, camphor, or, rarely, methyl salicylate. Amyl and isobutyl nitrites have been marketed as room deodorizers ("Locker Room," "Sweat"), which have been abused by young adults (Chapter 179).

Carpet and room deodorizers in powder form contain sodium bicarbonate, sodium sulfate, talc, and fragrance.

CLINICAL PRESENTATION

The clinical effects and treatment for *p*-dichlorobenzene and naphthalene are discussed in the section Mothballs. Most other deodorizers cause mucosal irritation and GI distress. CNS depression may occur from hydrocarbon vehicles or essential oils.

TREATMENT

Treatment is primarily supportive after airway assessment and immediate dilution. Treat as a caustic ingestion if the solution pH exceeds 12. Irrigate exposed skin or eyes copiously with saline and check for corneal abrasions with fluorescein staining.

Determine the product contents to search for toxic constituents (e.g., nitrites, naphthalene, pine oil). Emesis or lavage is indicated for ingestion of nitrites, substantial amounts of pine oil (more than several swallows of a greater than 30% concentrate), and large amounts of *p*-dichlorobenzene (several mothballs or a whole cake). The presence of low-viscosity hydrocarbon and turpentines dictates caution to prevent aspiration pneumonitis. Ingestion of a single naphthalene mothball should undergo gut decontamination in a small child presenting within 2 hours of exposure. Antiemetics and demulcents, such as antacids, may be necessary.

CLOVE CIGARETTES

Clove cigarettes are imported from Southeast Asia, principally from Indonesia, and are composed of approximately one-third shredded cloves and two-thirds tobacco (29). The type of tobacco in a clove cigarette delivers approximately twice as much tars, nicotine, and carbon monoxide as does tobacco in ordinary American cigarettes (30). In addition, substantial amounts of eugenol, an anesthetic agent, are found in cloves and in the smoke of clove cigarettes (30,31).

Clinical Presentation

In 1984 and 1985, the U.S. Centers for Disease Control and Prevention received 11 case reports of acute respiratory system injury in adolescents and young adults, including two deaths that occurred in close temporal association with smoking clove cigarettes (32). The acute pulmonary effects included hemoptysis, bronchospasm, hemorrhagic and nonhemorrhagic pulmonary edema, pleural effusion, respiratory insufficiency, respiratory infection, and aspiration of foreign material. The long-term dangers from the inhalation of eugenol and other chemicals in the cloves are not known. Another area of concern is the possible association of clove cigarette smoking and subsequent marijuana use. Because the eugenol in the clove cigarette acts as a topical anesthetic to the posterior oropharynx, it reduces the noxious elements of smoking. Thus, it may facilitate the learning of smoking techniques.

Treatment

Treatment is supportive. Observe for pulmonary complications.

COINS

Coins are the foreign bodies most frequently ingested by children and adolescents (33,34), with more than 3600 exposures reported to U.S. poison centers in 2001 (2). All toxicity associated with acute ingestion is related to the coins as a foreign body. Systemic toxicity has been rarely reported after intentional ingestion in adult patients with metal pica.

The formulations of common U.S. coins are provided in Table 3.

TABLE 3. Composition and size of United States coins

Content	Penny	Nickel	Dime	Quarter
Copper (%)	2.5	75	90	90
Nickel (%)	—	25	10	10
Zinc (%)	97.5	—	—	—
Diameter (mm)	19.05	21.21	17.91	24.26

Clinical Presentation

Most ingested coins pass through the GI tract without complication. Accordingly, most patients remain asymptomatic. Coins that do not pass spontaneously usually lodge in the upper esophagus, less frequently in the lower, and least commonly in the middle portion of the esophagus (35–38). Larger coins in smaller children are more likely to get lodged (39).

Symptoms associated with coin ingestion include pain in the throat or chest, foreign-body sensation localized to area of coin, choking, cough, drooling, dysphagia, vomiting, and stridor (35,38–40). However, symptoms are a poor predictor of coin location; one-third of patients with esophageal coins may be asymptomatic (35,39,40), compared with three-fourths of patients with coins passed beyond the esophagus (39,40). Children with prolonged coin retention (up to 6 months) may complain of neck pain, food intolerance, coughing, or episodic wheezing. Complications of prolonged coin impaction include esophageal ulceration and perforation (41,42). Adults with metal pica can ingest dozens to more than 100 coins, resulting in gastric bezoars, anemia, and copper deficiency or toxicity (5,43,44).

Treatment

All patients with foreign-body ingestion must be initially assessed for airway compromise, although this is a rare complication of coin ingestion. Management of asymptomatic patients with acute coin ingestion is controversial. Many physicians and poison centers observe these patients, without evaluation, until the coin is passed spontaneously. Coins usually pass within several days but may take up to 3 to 4 weeks.

However, the risk of esophageal impaction with lack of symptoms suggests that all patients should undergo evaluation for coin localization (38,40). Patients with coins passed out of the esophagus may be discharged for home observation. Esophageal coins should be removed, although some authors recommend that asymptomatic patients, without a history of esophageal disease or surgery, be given oral fluids and observed for spontaneous passage for up to 24 hours before attempting removal (35,36,39).

The presence of ingested coins can be detected by handheld metal detectors, routine radiography, or barium swallow radiography. Several recent studies have observed excellent sensitivity and specificity using metal detectors to localize coins, even by inexperienced users (33–35,37,45). Metal detectors are easy to use, relatively inexpensive, and prevent exposure to radiation.

Esophageal coins may be removed or pushed into the stomach. Removal may be accomplished with a Foley catheter under fluoroscopic guidance (46,47) or endoscopy (48,49). Patients with recent ingestion (less than 24 hours) and upper-esophageal coin location may be the best candidates for Foley catheter removal. Advancement of a coin into the stomach is the goal of esophageal bougienage (50), which has been shown in one study to be safe and effective when performed by trained emergency physicians (51). There are insufficient data to recommend pharmacologic intervention with intravenous glucagon. The method of choice depends on the size and health of the patient, the size of the coin, coin location, duration of impaction, and the expertise and experience of the clinician.

DENATONIUM BENZOATE

A number of aversive agents (quassin, brucine, bitter aloes, sucrose octaacetate, sucrose benzoate) have been used in the past to deter ingestions of dangerous substances. Denatonium benzoate, which may be the bitterest substance available, was discovered in 1958 when a series of *N*-substituted lidocaine derivatives was prepared in a search for new local anesthetics. Its chemical name is *benzyl diethyl* [(2,6 xylyl carbamoyl) *methyl*] *ammonium benzoate*, and it is marketed as Bitrex. It is an inert, odorless material that can be detected by taste at 10 parts per billion and is recognizably bitter at 50 parts per billion.

Denatonium benzoate is now used as an alcohol denaturant, in windscreen washes, for oil and tallow denaturing, as an animal repellent, in anti–nail-biting formulations, in finger paints (Germany), as a bird-repellent seed dressing, and in rodenticides. It is being considered as an additive to toxic household and other commercial products to aid in limiting the amount of such substances ingested by young children (52–56). The role of denatonium benzoate in preventing serious poisoning has yet to be defined. The American Association of Poison Control Centers has published a policy statement on the use of aversive agents as a deterrent to accidental poisoning (http://www.aapcc.org).

MEDICATION-INDUCED ESOPHAGEAL INJURIES

Medication-induced esophageal injury (MIEI) was first described in 1970 (57). Medications that have been reported to induce esophageal injury are summarized in Table 4.

Risk factors for MIEI include abnormal esophageal transit, habit of drug ingestion (reclining after drug ingestion), form of drug (e.g., anhydrous pill), and taking drugs with little or no fluid. Structural or motility abnormalities of the esophagus, such as stricture, Schatzki's ring, esophageal tumor, hiatal hernia, extrinsic compression, and esophagitis, increase the risk of esophageal obstruction (58). Older age, male gender, left atrial enlargement, ingestion of sustained-release formulations, and prior esophageal structural abnormality may be risk factors for stricture development (59). A pH less than 3 is corrosive in the human esophagus (60).

Pathophysiology

Mechanisms of injury by drugs in MIEI that have been proposed include a caustic or acidic effect, hyperosmotic effect, heat production, gastroesophageal reflux, impaired esophageal clearance of acid, and accumulation of drug within the basal layer of squamous epithelium (61).

Clinical Presentation

MIEI must be suspected in all patients who present with unexplained esophageal symptoms (62). Symptoms present initially may include heartburn, nausea and vomiting, odynophagia, continuous retrosternal pain, dysphagia, weight loss, abdominal pain, hematemesis, fever, and dehydration.

The most common site of MIEI is the mid-esophagus at the level of the aortic arch or the area adjacent to the left atrium (62). The proximal third of esophagus is involved in 26% of pill-induced esophageal strictures; 52% are found in the middle third, and 22% of patients experience distal-third, pill-induced strictures in the esophagus (59). A variety of complications have been reported (Table 5) (62)

TABLE 4. Medications reported to induce medication-induced esophageal injury

Ampicillin
Anhydrous pills
Apocillin
Aspirin
Centrum Jr. tablets
Clindamycin
Cloxacillin
Cocaine
Decagesic (dexamethasone, aspirin, aluminum hydroxide gel)
Dextropropoxyphene/acetaminophen
Dicloxacillin
Dietary fiber
Doxycycline
Emepronium bromide
Erythromycin
Indomethacin
Iron
Lincomycin
Mexiletine
Minocycline
Oxytetracycline
Paraflex (aspirin, dextropropoxyphene, chlorzoxazone)
Percogesic (phenyltoloxamine citrate, 30 mg; acetaminophen, 325 mg)
Per diem (82% psyllium, 18% senna)
Phenoxymethylpenicillin
Piroxicam
Pivmecillinam
Potassium chloride (slow release, enteric coated)
Quinidine
Sodium meclofenamate
Sulindac
Tetracycline
Tinidazole
Trimethoprim-sulfamethoxazole
Zidovudine

TABLE 5. Medication-induced esophageal injury—effect of drugs

Indirect
- Stevens-Johnson syndrome: sulfa drugs.
  - Esophageal stricture.
- *Candida* esophagitis.
  - Antibiotic therapy.
  - Immunosuppressive drugs.
  - Cancer chemotherapeutic agents.
- Drugs may lower esophageal sphincter pressure and promote gastroesophageal reflux disease.

Direct
- Mucosal injury: after prolonged contact; pH may play some role.
- Local vascular injury, thrombosis: ulcerogenic lesions produced by potassium chloride in the small bowel.
- Aspirin may disrupt the normal cytoprotective barrier in the mucosa of the esophagus and stomach.
- Obstruction or delayed esophageal transit.
  - Slow-release or metric formulations of drugs enhance likelihood of esophageal injury.
- Adherence to esophageal mucosa: drugs that are hygroscopic.

Adapted from Bott S, et al. *Am J Gastroenterol* 1987;82:758–763.

Diagnosis

The diagnosis of MIEI can often be suspected by the clinical history alone (62). Flexible fiberoptic endoscopy is probably the most reliable method for diagnosing MIEI, but endoscopic findings are not by themselves diagnostic. Multiple ulcers at the mid-esophageal region are an important clue to MIEI. Definitive endoscopic evidence of MIEI must include debris of the drug at the ulcer base, but this is not common (63). Single contrast barium swallow is not sufficiently sensitive in detecting esophageal ulcers (63), but double contrast barium swallows may be more useful (64).

Esophagoscopy findings may include discrete ulcers (pinpoint to circumferential lesions 6 cm in length). Some patients have inflammation without ulcerations (antibiotics, antiinflammatory drugs, emepronium bromide), smooth or ulcerated strictures, mucosal edema, nodularity, and profuse exudates (potassium chloride, quinidine).

Treatment

Patients should remain standing at least 90 seconds after taking medication. Tablets should be swallowed with at least 100 ml of fluid. Large tablets should preferably be oval and not round. Capsules of a high density are easier to swallow than light ones. Patients who are bedridden or have difficulty in swallowing should be given liquid medication. Material may be removed with normal saline irrigation, suction, and optical peanut forceps (65). Repeat esophagoscopy should be performed 7 to 10 days later (65). Symptoms resolve and endoscopic healing is evident in 3 days to 6 weeks. Continuation of the medication may result in worsening of symptoms and even death.

MOTHBALLS

Mothball ingestions, particularly in children, are frequently reported to poison control centers, but significant toxicity is rare (2). Most household moth repellents contain paradichlorobenzene; others contain naphthalene or camphor.

Naphthalene

Naphthalene is an aromatic hydrocarbon with the odor of coal tar. In addition to its use as a deodorizer or moth repellent, naphthalene is used industrially in dye production, veterinary medicine, and historically as an antiseptic and antihelmintic.

Humans absorb naphthalene by pulmonary, GI, and cutaneous routes. Absorption from the GI tract may be enhanced in the presence of milk or fatty foods. Naphthalene is extensively metabolized in the liver, by oxidation to naphthols and naphtholquinones, and by conjugation with glutathione (66). Urinary metabolites may be used to confirm an acute exposure (not clinically practical) or monitor industrial exposures (67). Naphthalene and its metabolites may also be retained in adipose tissue.

CLINICAL PRESENTATION

Toxicity most often occurs after ingestion. Clinical effects include nausea, vomiting, abdominal pain, headache, confusion, restlessness, and lethargy. The oxidative metabolite α-naphthol can precipitate acute hemolysis and methemoglobinemia, particularly in children with glucose 6 phosphate dehydrogenase deficiency (68–70). Naphthalene mothballs put such children at risk for life-threatening anemia, which may not occur for up to 3 to 5 days. Death has occurred after intentional ingestion (71). Naphthalene vapors are irritating to eyes and mucous membranes, and repeated exposures can result in corneal ulceration and cataracts. Dermal exposure may cause a hypersensitivity dermatitis.

DIAGNOSTIC TESTS

1-Naphthol is found in the urine of industrial workers exposed to naphthalene (67). It is analyzed by spectrophotometry, thin-layer chromatography, and gas chromatography. Elevated plasma levels of hepatic enzymes may be observed.

TREATMENT

Ingestion of only one naphthalene mothball is potentially toxic to a child. Avoid milk or fatty foods for 4 hours after ingestion. Activated charcoal may be useful. Protect the respiratory tract. Hemolysis may require blood transfusion, packed red blood cell transfusions, or exchange transfusion, particularly in infants. Significant methemoglobinemia may be treated with methylene blue.

Paradichlorobenzene

Most mothballs contain paradichlorobenzene compressed into a solid ball, occasionally with added essential oils and fragrances. Paradichlorobenzene is less toxic than naphthalene, exhibiting fewer hematologic (hemolytic anemia, methemoglobinemia) and nervous system effects.

However, serious toxic effects have occurred (72). Inhalant abuse of unspecified mothballs has been associated with neuropathy and renal failure (73). Further information is provided in Chapter 206.

Methods to differentiate naphthalene from paradichlorobenzene mothballs may be used at home or in the emergency department. Naphthalene mothballs reportedly float in salt water, and those with paradichlorobenzene sink (74). Abdominal radiography may also differentiate paradichlorobenzene (strongly radio-opaque) from naphthalene (radiolucent) (75).

PARAPHENYLENEDIAMINE

Paraphenylenediamine (PPD) (Table 6) is used as an oxidizable hair dye, in the dyeing of furs, and in the photochemical and tire-vulcanizing industries (76). The most frequently used types of hair dyes are the oxidized "para-dyes" such as PPD. In the Middle East and some African countries, PPD is often used as a poisoning agent.

PPD is a derivative of paranitroaniline. It is an aromatic diamine related to aniline. The dyeing action of PPD depends on its oxidation by the addition of hydrogen peroxide, forming a base that is allergenic, mutagenic, and highly toxic. The metabolic products are oxidized to a quinone structure that may be nephrotoxic. Methemoglobinuria and hemolysis probably result in the acute renal failure observed.

Clinical Presentation

An oral dose of approximately 7 g is followed within 4 to 6 hours by edema of the head and neck, respiratory difficulty, drowsiness, vomiting, and dysplasia (77). Acute renal failure, shock, increased muscle tone, rhabdomyolysis, and death may follow within 24 hours (78). Permanent blindness may be observed. Anemia, leukocytosis, hemoglobinuria, and hemoglobinemia are common.

Treatment

Treatment is mainly supportive. Early asphyxia followed by renal failure requires an early tracheostomy. Renal dialysis is required when oliguria develops. Most such patients survive

TABLE 6. Paraphenylenediamine (PPDA) compared with glyceryl monothioglycolate (GMTG)

Product	Use	Dermatitis	Protective gloves	Treated hair	Cross-reactions
PPDA	Most common hair dye	Allergic	All types; protective vinyl recommended	PPDA-treated hair not sensitizing	Local anesthetics (procaine, Novocain), sulfonamides, PPDA, sunscreens
GMTG	Most common permanent wave chemical	Irritant and allergic	Thick, heavy rubber gloves that are not practical, investigative "4H" Danish glove	GMTG-treated hair sensitizing for 3 mo	Very rarely cross-reacts to ammonium thioglycolate

Adapted from Fisher AA. *Cutis* 1989;43:316–318.

and make a full recovery. The role of intravenous corticosteroids and antihistamines has yet to be determined.

PERSONAL CARE PRODUCTS

Cosmetics can include any of more than 5000 different ingredients (Table 7).

Personal shampoos contain anionic and nonionic surfactants and possibly fragrances. Dandruff shampoos may also contain zinc pyrithione, selenium sulfide, or coal-tar solution.

Permanent hair colors contain an oxidizer, which usually is 6% hydrogen peroxide, and a dye intermediate (*p*-phenylenediamine, resorcinol, aminophenols along with water, ammonia glycerin, isopropanol, and propylene glycol). Semipermanent hair colors (for covering gray) contain propylene glycol, isopropanol, fatty acids, fragrance, alkanolamines, and dyes. Some formulations (e.g., Grecian Formula) contain lead.

Hair waving lotions possess thioglycolic acids and ammonia sulfides, whereas most wave neutralizer solutions contain hydrogen peroxide, sodium bromate, or perborate in mildly acidic solutions. Some permanent wave fixatives contain 2% to 8% (weight per volume) mercuric chloride, and the accidental ingestion of 125 ml of a 2% mercuric chloride solution caused severe mercury poisoning in an adult. Bromate salts (e.g., potassium) are extremely toxic and are capable of causing serious poisonings (deafness, renal failure) at doses between 240 and 500 mg/kg.

Hair straighteners may contain highly caustic sodium hydroxide used in the 1% to 3% solution (pH 13). Ingestion by children results in drooling, vomiting, lip swelling and redness, and skin blisters. Most remain asymptomatic or develop only mild effects. Esophagoscopies are noncontributory (79,80).

Hair sprays contain ethanol solvents with resin polymers (e.g., vinyl acetate, acrylamide, methyl vinyl ether).

Hair conditioners contain synthetic cationic surfactants, perfumes, and alcohols and therefore are potentially more toxic than shampoos, although only mild effects, if any, usually occur from casual exposures.

Bath preparations: Bubble bath usually contains the mildly toxic anionic and nonionic surfactants along with alcohols and preservatives. The presence of trisodium phosphate builders enhances causticity. Bath salts may contain borax, which causes boric acid poisoning in large ingestions in addition to mucosal irritation. Bath oils contain vegetable and mineral oils. The volatile essential oils may produce systemic complaints after large ingestions of concentrated solutions.

Makeup products contain innocuous ingredients and are sold in small packages; these compounds are essentially nontoxic, except for local hypersensitivity reactions.

Nail polish contains hydrocarbon solvents (xylene, toluene, acetone), alcohol solvents (methanol, ethanol), plasticizers, and resins such as nitrocellulose.

TABLE 7. Cosmetic ingredients

Moisturizers that function as a moisture barrier or attract moisture from the environment
- Cetyl alcohol (fatty alcohol) to keep oil and water from separating, also a foam booster
- Dimethicone (silicone skin conditioner and antifoam ingredient)
- Isopropyl lanolate, myristate, and palmitate
- Lanolin and lanolin alcohols and oil (used in skin and hair conditioners)
- Octyl dodecanol (skin conditioner)
- Oleic acid (olive oil)
- Panthenol (vitamin B–complex derivative; hair conditioner)
- Stearic acid and stearyl alcohol

Preservatives and antioxidants (including vitamins) to prevent product deterioration
- Trisodium and tetrasodium edetate
- Tocopherol (vitamin E)

Antimicrobials that fight bacteria
- Butyl, propyl, ethyl, and methyl parabens
- DMDM hydantoin
- Methylisothiazolinone
- Phenoxyethanol (also rose ether fragrance component)
- Quaternium-15

Thickeners and waxes used in stick products such as lipsticks and blushers
- Candelilla, carnauba, and microcrystalline waxes
- Carbomer and polyethylene (thickeners)

Solvents used to dilute
- Butylene glycol and propylene glycol
- Cyclomethicone (volatile silicone)
- Ethanol (alcohol)
- Glycerin

Emulsifiers that break up and refine
- Glyceryl monostearate (also pearlescent agent)
- Lauramide DEA (also foam booster)
- Polysorbates

Color additives [synthetic organic colors derived from coal and petroleum sources (not permitted for use around the eye)]
- D&C Red No. 7 Calcium Lake (lakes are dyes that do not dissolve in water)

Inorganic pigments approved for general use in cosmetics, including for the area of the eye
- Iron oxides
- Mica (iridescent)

Hair dyes [phenol derivatives used in combination with other chemicals in permanent (two-step) hair dyes]
- Aminophenols

pH adjusters that stabilize or adjust acids and bases
- Ammonium hydroxide (in skin peels and hair waving and straightening)
- Citric acid (adjusts pH)
- Triethanolamine (pH adjuster used mostly in transparent soap)

Others
- Magnesium aluminum silicate (absorbent, anti-caking agent)
- Silica (silicon dioxide; absorbent, anti-caking, abrasive)
- Sodium lauryl sulfate (detergent)
- Stearic acid (cleansing, emulsifier)
- Talc (powdered magnesium silicate; absorbent, anti-caking)
- Zinc stearate (used in powder to improve texture, lubricates)

From Foulke JE. *FDA Consumer* 1994;28:21, with permission.

Nail polish removers are solvents such as acetone or ethanol. Acetone-free removers contain ethyl or butyl acetate. On a weight basis, nail polish and nail polish remover are similar in toxicity, but the smaller volumes of nail polish bottles limit their toxicity.

Colognes, perfumes, and toilet waters contain ethanol in concentrations ranging from 50% to 95%.

Dental products (toothpastes, tooth powders, and tooth liquids) contain nontoxic constituents such as calcium phosphates, alumina, abradants, and anionic surfactants. Fluoride concentrations are too small to cause systemic toxicity. Mouthwashes and breath fresheners usually contain alcohol, flavoring, and sweeteners. Toxicity depends on the ethanol content. Denture cleaners contain bicarbonates, borates, phosphates, and carbonates, some of which may be caustic. The methyl methacrylate constituent of acrylic denture material may produce a contact dermatitis in health care professionals who mix this substance, even when gloves are worn.

Deodorants contain aluminum and zinc but have limited toxicity because of packaging and formulations.

Potassium bromate is a clear odorless, tasteless compound ($KBrO_3$) and is an extremely toxic agent that produces nausea, vomiting, diarrhea, deafness, acute renal failure, hypotension, CNS depression, and hemolysis. GI symptoms usually begin within 30 minutes of ingestion. Both the otic symptoms and renal impairment may be permanent. Renal biopsies indicate primarily tubular damage, which can progress to interstitial fibrosis and glomerular sclerosis.

Volatile or essential oils (sage, eucalyptus, turpentine, pine, pennyroyal, and cinnamon) are colorless liquids that contain cyclic hydrocarbons, ethers, alcohols, esters, and ketones. Pennyroyal is also addressed in Chapter 258. Essential oils are moderate mucosal irritants, leading to GI distress and salivation. Concentrated formulations of essential oils produced convulsions in adults and CNS depression in doses as low as 10 ml. Chemical pneumonitis results from aspiration, but high viscosity limits toxicity to a chemical lipoid pneumonia. Perfumes, colognes, mouthwashes, and toilet water may contain substantial amounts of ethanol and produce intoxication. Hypoglycemia may complicate ethanol intoxication, especially in children.

Hydrogen peroxide is addressed in Chapter 197. Sodium borate is addressed in Chapter 204.

Clinical Presentation

Most accidental exposures result in no symptoms or, at worst, minor GI upset. Systemic symptoms are unusual. In clinical studies, hair dyes produce no evidence of systemic effect or teratogenesis. Skin care products, hair preparations (including colors), and facial makeup are the cosmetic products most often associated with contact dermatitis. Fragrances, preservatives (quaternium-15, formaldehyde, imidazolidinyl urea, parabens), *p*-phenylenediamine, and glycerol monothioglycolate are the most frequent skin sensitizers. Triethanolamine and diethanolamine produce mild skin irritation only in concentrations greater than 5%; little skin sensitization develops.

Treatment

Because most cosmetics ingested are nontoxic, only supportive care and perhaps dilution are required. The decision to decontaminate the GI tract depends on the product toxicity, quantity ingested, time since exposure, patient's weight, and presence of symptoms. Most ingestions of cosmetics do not require treatment, assuming no foreign-body obstruction. Cationic-surfactant, perborate, and substantial essential-oil ingestions that exceed one to two swallows of pure solution may benefit from removal via nasogastric aspiration or activated charcoal. Children who ingest products containing ethanol may be given prophylactic sugar or sweets because hypoglycemia may not correlate with blood alcohol concentration. Children who ingest more than 1 ml/kg of (100%) ethanol should be referred for observation. Gastric decontamination should be considered for ingestion of hydrocarbons containing glues (e.g., toluene, xylene) when the total dose of hydrocarbon exceeds 1 to 2 ml/kg.

Potassium bromate exposures are potentially serious. Toxicity does not correlate with serum bromide levels. The usual gut decontamination measures (ipecac or lavage) may be administered if the patient presents within the first hour or so after ingestion. Lavage with 2% sodium bicarbonate solution and the intravenous administration of 10 to 50 ml of 10% sodium thiosulfate solution (1.5 to 3.0 ml/kg) at a maximum rate of 3 ml/minute are theoretically advantageous to reduce the bromate to the less toxic bromide ion, but clinical efficacy has not been proved. An alternative intravenous solution is 100 to 500 ml of 1% sodium thiosulfate. All symptomatic patients should be observed in the hospital for the development of renal and otic damage. The role of early dialysis in the prevention of nephrotoxicity and ototoxicity remains unproven, and its use depends on clinical judgment of the severity of toxicity.

TABLE 8. Risk factors for pica

Family disorganization	Poverty
Poor nutrition (including iron deficiency)	Cultural trait
	Mental retardation

Adapted from Sheahan K, et al. *Am J Forensic Med Pathol* 1988;9:51–53.

PICA

The word *pica* derives from the Latin for magpie, a bird of fickle appetite that steals and consumes almost anything. The term encompasses the eating of clay, laundry starch, ashes, sand, coffee grounds, oyster shells, matches, ice, newspapers, and cigarette butts (81). It may occur in one-half of patients with iron deficiency (82–84). Patients usually conceal the problem from the physician. Oral iron therapy may lead to remission of the pica (83,85). It is especially prevalent in Africa, Australia (among Aborigines), and in the southern states of the United States (86,87). Controversy surrounds the cause or effect relationship with both iron and zinc (88). Some risk factors for pica development are found in Table 8. Examples of pica are found in Table 9. *Cissa* is a craving for

TABLE 9. Examples of pica

Cause	Effect
Starch eaters (93,94)	Iron deficiency anemia
Magnesium carbonate (95)	Iron deficiency anemia (iron absorption interference)
Clay ingestion (geophagy) (93,96,97)	Hypokalemia, hyperkalemia (in chronic renal failure) (98); diminished iron absorption (99)
Paint chips from old walls or cribs	Lead poisoning (infants, children)
Ice eating (pagophagia) metabolism (100)	Disorder of iron
Food pica	Symptoms of iron deficiency? parasitic infestation
Sand, stones	Anemia, possible celiac disease

unusual or unwholesome articles of food, such as the unusual longings of pregnancy.

Food pica is a common symptom of iron deficiency. The patient compulsively eats one kind of food. Celery, potato chips, carrots, peanut butter, sunflower seeds, parsley, soda crackers, pickles, orange juice, chocolate ice cream, lettuce, Life Savers, chewing gum, and pretzels have been ingested. Food pica may terminate fatally (86).

Paper pica is not uncommon, especially in the mentally retarded, and can cause intestinal obstruction, intestinal perforation, and lead poisoning (89). Glossy paper is produced by the addition of varnish, commonly ethyl cellulose, during manufacture and may lead to a paper bezoar (90). Mercurial compounds used as antifungal agents in the pulp and paper industry may lead to mercury poisoning in paper pica (tissue box, cigarette package, paperback books) devotees (85).

Geophagy is the deliberate consumption of earth substances and is classified as a form of pica. It groups together aberrant behaviors such as the consumption of starch, ice, paint, cigarette butts, and burnt matches (91). It has been implicated both as a cause and a result of particular nutritional deficiencies in humans (92) and is practiced all over the world, especially in developing nations among poor blacks, the pregnant, and children (81). Australian Aborigines have used clay for stomach discomfort and diarrhea. An abdominal radiograph may show clay opacities. The children of clay-eating, starch-eating women eat dirt, pieces of paper, flakes of paint and plaster, or whatever comes to hand (82).

Treatment

Geophagy or pica for ice (pagophagia) in some patients may rapidly resolve after iron therapy (82). Parenteral iron can stop pagophagia and food pica in some patients in 1 week; oral iron stops it in 2 weeks (88). Other consequences, such as lead poisoning, are treated as they arise. The management of bezoars is addressed in the section Bezoars.

REFERENCES

1. Mofenson HC, Greensher J. The non-toxic ingestion. *Pediatr Clin North Am* 1970;17:583–590.
2. Watson WA, Litovitz TL, Rodgers GC, et al. 2002 annual report of the American Association of Poison Control Centers toxic exposure surveillance system. *Am J Emerg Med* 2003;21:353–421.
3. Mennen M, Slovis CM. Severe metabolic alkalosis in the emergency department. *Ann Emerg Med* 1988;17:354–357.
4. Thomas SH, Stone CK. Acute toxicity from baking soda ingestion. *Am J Emerg Med* 1994; 12:57–59.
5. Yelin G, Taff ML, Sadowski GE. Copper toxicity following massive ingestion of coins. *Am J Forensic Med Pathol* 1987;8:78–85.
6. DeBakey M, Ochsner A. Bezoars and concretions. A comprehensive review of the literature with an analysis of 303 collected cases and a presentation of 8 additional cases. *Surgery* 1938;4:934–963, 1939;5:132–160.
7. Eshel G, Broide E, Azizi E. Phytobezoar following raisin ingestion in children. *Pediatr Emerg Care* 1988;4:192–193.
8. Deal DR, Vitale Q, Raffin SB. Dissolution of a postgastrectomy bezoar by cellulose. *Gastroenterology* 1973;64:467–470.
9. Carrougher JG, Barrilleaux CN. Esophageal bezoars: the sucralith. *Crit Care Med* 1991;19:837–839.
10. Singer JI. Lactobezoar causing an abdominal triad of colicky pain, emesis and mass. *Pediatr Emerg Care* 1988;4:194–196.
11. Schreiner RL, Brady MS, Franken EA. Increased incidence of lactobezoars in low birth weight infants. *Am J Dis Child* 1979;133:936–940.
12. Reddy ER, Joseph S. Lactobezoars in the low birth weight neonate. *Can Med Assoc J* 1985;133:297.
13. Delpre G, Glanz I, Neeman A, et al. New therapeutic approach in postoperative phytobezoars. *J Clin Gastroenterol* 1984;16:231–237.
14. Schneider RP. Perdiem causes esophageal impaction and bezoars. *South Med J* 1989;82:1449–1450.
15. DePiro JT, Bowden TA Jr. Treatment of gastric bezoars. *Clin Pharm* 1989;8:181–182.
16. Zarling EJ, Moeller DD. Bezoar therapy. Complication using Adolph's Meat Tenderizer and alternatives from literature review. *Arch Intern Med* 1981;141:1669–1670.
17. Andrus CH, Ponsky JL. Bezoars: classification, pathophysiology and treatment. *Am J Gastroenterol* 1988;83:476–478.
18. Schlang HA. Acetylcysteine in removal of bezoar. *JAMA* 1970;214:1329.
19. Cooper SG, Tracey EJ. Small-bowel obstruction caused by oat bran bezoar. *N Engl J Med* 1989;320:1148–1149.
20. Respiratory illness associated with carpet cleaning at a hospital clinic, Virginia. *MMWR Morb Mortal Wkly Rep* 1983;32:378, 383–384.
21. Brook MP, McCarron MM, Mueller JA. Pine oil cleaner ingestion. *Ann Emerg Med* 1989;18:391–395.
22. Conrad F, Wruk KM, Spoerke DG, et al. Pine oil cleaner ingestions: a prospective study. *Vet Hum Toxicol* 1986;28:484(abst).
23. Vancura EM, Clinton JE, Ruiz E, et al. Toxicity of alkaline solutions. *Ann Emerg Med* 1980;9:118–122.
24. Ernst RW, Leventhal M, Luva R, et al. Total esophagogastric replacement after ingestion of household ammonia. *N Engl J Med* 1963;208:815–816.
25. Klein J, Olson KR, McKinney HE. Caustic injury from household ammonia. *Am J Emerg Med* 1985;3:320.
26. Jakobsson SW, Rajs J, Jonsson JA, et al. Poisoning with sodium hypochlorite solution; report of a fatal case, supplemented with an experimental and clinico-epidemiological study. *Am J Forensic Med Pathol* 1991;12:320–327.
27. Tanen DA, Graeme KA, Raschke R. Severe lung injury after exposure to chloramine gas from household cleaners. *N Engl J Med* 1999;341:848–849.
28. Kiristioglu I, Gurpinar A, Kilic N, et al. Is it necessary to perform an endoscopy after the ingestion of liquid household bleach in children? *Acta Paediatr* 1999;88:233–234.
29. Pruitt AW, Jacobs EA, Schydlower M, et al. Committee on Substance Abuse. Hazards of clove cigarettes. *Pediatrics* 1991;88:395–396.
30. Guidotti TL, Laing L, Prakash UBS. Clove cigarettes—the basis for concern regarding health effects. *West J Med* 1989;151:220–228.
31. AMA Council on Scientific Affairs. Evaluation of the health hazard of clove cigarettes. *JAMA* 1988;260:3641–3644.
32. Illnesses possibly associated with smoking clove cigarettes. *MMWR Morb Mortal Wkly Rep* 1985;34:297–299.
33. Doraiswamy NV, Baig H, Hallam L. Metal detector and swallowed metal foreign bodies in children. *J Accid Emerg Med* 1999;16:123–125.
34. Seikel K, Primm PA, Elizondo BJ, et al. Handheld metal detector localization of ingested metallic foreign bodies. *Arch Pediatr Adolesc Med* 1999;153:853–857.
35. Bassett KE, Schunk JE, Logan L. Localizing ingested coins with a metal detector. *Am J Emerg Med* 1999;17:338–341.
36. Soprano JV, Fleisher GR, Mandl KD. The spontaneous passage of esophageal coins in children. *Arch Pediatr Adolesc Med* 1999;153:1073–1076.
37. Biehler JL, Tuggle D, Stacy T. Use of the transmitter-receiver metal detector in the evaluation of pediatric coin ingestions. *Pediatr Emerg Care* 1993;9:208–210.
38. Hodge D, Tecklenburg F, Fleisher G. Coin ingestion: does every child need a radiograph? *Ann Emerg Med* 1985;14:443–446.
39. Caravati EM, Bennett DL, McElwee NE. Pediatric coin ingestion—a prospective study on the utility of routine roentgenograms. *Arch Dis Child* 1989;143:549–551.
40. Schunk JE, Corneli H, Bolte R. Pediatric coin ingestions—a prospective study of coin location and symptoms. *Arch Dis Child* 1989;143:546–548.
41. Savitt DL, Wason S. Delayed diagnosis of coin ingestion in children. *Am J Emerg Med* 1988;6:378–381.
42. Nahman BJ, Mueller CF. Asymptomatic esophageal perforation by a coin in a child. *Ann Emerg Med* 1984;13:627–629.
43. Hassan HA, Netchvolodoff C, Raufman JP. Zinc-induced copper deficiency in a coin swallower. *Am J Gastroenterol* 2000;95:2975–2977.
44. Kumar A, Jazieh AR. Case report of sideroblastic anemia caused by ingestion of coins. *Am J Hematol* 2001;66:126–129.
45. Ros SP, Cetta F. Successful use of a metal detector in locating coins ingested by children. *J Pediatr* 1992;120:752–753.
46. Harned RJ, Strain JD, Hay TC, et al. Esophageal foreign bodies: safety and efficacy of Foley catheter extraction of coins. *AJR Am J Roentgenol* 1997;168:443–446.
47. Kelley JE, Leech MH, Carr MG. A safe and cost-effective protocol for the management of esophageal coins in children. *J Pediatr Surg* 1993;28:898–900.
48. Binder L, Anderson WA. Pediatric gastrointestinal foreign body ingestions. *Ann Emerg Med* 1984;13:112–117.
49. Bendig DW. Removal of blunt esophageal foreign bodies by flexible endoscopy without general anesthesia. *Am J Dis Child* 1986;140:789–790.
50. Bonadio WA, Jona JZ, Glicklich M, et al. Esophageal bougienage technique for coin ingestion in children. *J Pediatr Surg* 1988;23:917–918.
51. Emslander HC, Bonadio W, Klatzo M. Efficacy of esophageal bougienage by emergency physicians in pediatric coin ingestion. *Ann Emerg Med* 1996;27:726–729.
52. Berning CK, Griffith JF, Wild JE. Research on the effectiveness of denatonium benzoate as a deterrent to liquid detergent ingestion in children. *Fund Appl Toxicol* 1982;2:44–48.
53. Lawless HT, Hammer LD, Corina MD. Aversions to bitterness and accidental poisonings among preschool children. *J Toxicol Clin Toxicol* 1982–83;19:951–964.
54. Klein-Schwartz W. Denatonium benzoate. Review of efficacy and safety. *Vet Hum Toxicol* 1991;33:545–547.
55. Sibert JR, Frude N. Bittering agents in the prevention of accidental poisoning: children's reaction to denatonium benzoate (Bitrex). *Arch Emerg Med* 1991;8:1–7.

56. Hansen SR, Janssen C, Beasley VR. Denatonium benzoate as a deterrent to ingestion of toxic substance: toxicity and efficacy. *Vet Hum Toxicol* 1993:234–236.
57. Pemberton J. Oesophageal obstruction and ulceration caused by oral potassium therapy. *Br Heart J* 1970;32:267–268.
58. Nandi P, Ong GR. Foreign body in the oesophagus—review of 2394 cases. *Br J Surg* 1978;65:5–9.
59. McCord GS, Clouse RE. Pill-induced esophageal strictures: clinical features and risk factors for development. *Am J Med* 1990;88:512–518.
60. Minocha A, Greenbaum DS. Pill-esophagitis caused by nonsteroidal antiinflammatory drugs. *Am J Gastroenterol* 1991;86:1086–1089.
61. Ovartlarnporn B, Kulwichit W, Hiranniramol S. Medication-induced esophageal injury. Report of 17 cases with endoscopic documentation. *Am J Gastroenterol* 1991;86:748–750.
62. Bott S, Prokash C, McCallum RW. Medication-induced esophageal injury—survey of the literature. *Am J Gastroenterol* 1987;82:758–763.
63. Kikendall JW, Friedman AC, Oyewole MA, et al. Pill-induced esophageal injury—case reports and review of the medical literature. *Dig Dis Sci* 1983;28:174–182.
64. Amendola MA, Spera TD. Doxycycline-induced esophagitis. *JAMA* 1985;253:1009–1011.
65. Perry PA, Dean BS, Krenzelok EP. Drug-induced esophageal injury. *Vet Hum Toxicol* 1988;30:349.
66. Hibbs BF, Shore CO, Donahue JM, et al. Toxicological profile for naphthalene (update). Agency for Toxic Substances Disease Registry 1995 Aug.
67. Bieniek G. The presence of 1-naphthol in the urine of industrial workers exposed to naphthalene. *Occup Environ Med* 1994;5:357–359.
68. Mackell JV, Rieders MS, Brieger H, et al. Acute hemolytic anemia due to ingestion of naphthalene mothballs. *Pediatrics* 1951;7:722–728.
69. Chusid E, Fried CT. Acute hemolytic anemia due to naphthalene ingestion. *Am J Dis Child* 1955;86:612–614.
70. Ojwang PJ, Ahmed-Jushuf IH, Abdullah MS. Naphthalene poisoning following ingestion of moth balls. Case report. *East Afr Med J* 1985;62:72–73.
71. Gupta R, Singhal PC, Muthusethupathy MA, et al. Cerebral oedema and renal failure following naphthalene poisoning. *J Assoc Physicians India* 1979;27:347–348.
72. Hallowell M. Acute haemolytic anemia following the ingestion of paradichlorobenzene. *Arch Dis Child* 1959;34:74–75.
73. Weintraub E, Gandhi D, Robinson C. Medical complications due to mothball abuse. *South Med J* 2000;93:427–429.
74. Koyama K, Yamashita M, Ogura Y, et al. A simple test for mothball component differentiation using water and a saturated solution of table salt: its utilization for poison information service. *Vet Hum Toxicol* 1991;33:425–427.
75. Woolf AD, Saperstein A, Zauvin J, et al. Radiopacity of household deodorants, air fresheners and moth repellents. *J Toxicol Clin Toxicol* 1993;31:418–428.
76. Fisher AA. Management of hairdressers sensitized to hair dyes or permanent wave solutions. *Cutis* 1989;43:316–318.
77. Ashraf W, Dawling S, Farrow LJ. Systemic paraphenylenediamine poisoning: a case report and review. *Hum Exp Toxicol* 1994;13:167–170.
78. Averbuch A, Modai D, Leonov Y. Rhabdomyolysis and acute renal failure induced by paraphenylenediamine. *Hum Toxicol* 1989;8:345–348.
79. Mrvos R, Dean B, Krenzelok E. Hair relaxers: lack of morbidity despite high pH. *J Toxicol Clin Toxicol* 1995;33:514(abst).
80. Cox AJ, Eisenbeis JF. Ingestion of caustic hair relaxer: is endoscopy necessary? *Laryngoscope* 1997;107:897–902.
81. Editorial. Clay eating. *Lancet* 1978;2:614–615.
82. Crosby WH. Pica. *JAMA* 1976;235:2765.
83. Crosby WH. Pica: a compulsion caused by iron deficiency. *Br J Hematol* 1976;34:341–342.
84. Callinan V, O'Hare JA. Cardboard chewing: cause and effect of iron deficiency anemia. *Am J Med* 1988;85:449.
85. Olynyk F, Sharpe DH. Mercury poisoning in paper pica. *N Engl J Med* 1982;306:1056–1057.
86. Sheahan K, Page DV, Kemper T, et al. Childhood sudden death secondary to accidental aspiration of black pepper. *Am J Forensic Med Pathol* 1988;9:51–53.
87. Vermeer DE, Frate DA. Geophagia in rural Mississippi: environmental and cultural contexts and nutritional implications. *Am J Clin Nutr* 1979;32:2129–2135.
88. Korman SH. Pica as a presenting symptom in celiac disease. *Am J Clin Nutr* 1990;51:139–141.
89. Keeling PJ, Ransay J, Shand WS. Pica, paper and pseudoporphyria. *Lancet* 1987;2:1095.
90. Uretsky BF. Paper bezoar causing intestinal obstruction. *Arch Surg* 1974;109:123.
91. Johns T, Duquette M. Detoxification mineral supplementation as function of geophagy. *Am J Clin Nutr* 1991;53:448–456.
92. Halstead JA. Geophagia in man: its nature and nutritional effects. *Am J Clin Nutr* 1968;21:1384–1393.
93. Roselle HA. Association of laundry starch and clay ingestion with anemia in New York City. *Arch Intern Med* 1979;125:57–61.
94. Warshauer SE. Starch eater's anemia. *South Med J* 1966;59:538–540.
95. Leming PD, Reed DC, Martello DJ. Magnesium carbonate pica: an unusual case of iron deficiency. *Ann Intern Med* 1981;94:660.
96. Gonzalez JJ, Owens W, Ungaro PC, et al. Clay ingestion—a rare cause of hypokalemia. *Ann Intern Med* 1982;97:65–66.
97. Severance HW Jr, Holt T, Patrone NA, et al. Profound muscle weakness and hypokalemia due to clay ingestion. *South Med J* 1988;81:272–274.
98. Gelfand MC, Zarate A, Knepshield JH. Geophagia: a cause of life-threatening hyperkalemia in patients with chronic renal failure. *JAMA* 1975;234:738.
99. Minnich V, Okcuoglu A, Tarcon Y, et al. Pica in Turkey. II. Effect of clay upon iron absorption. *Am J Clin Nutr* 1968;21:78–86.
100. Coltman CAJ. Pagophagia and iron lack. *JAMA* 1969;207:513–516.

CHAPTER 204

Boron Compounds

E. Martin Caravati

See Figure 1.

Compounds included:	**Boron (B), boric acid (boron oxide, boron trioxide, borax, BNa_3O_3); sodium tetraborate anhydrous (sodium borate, $B_4Na_2O_7$); pentaborane (B_5H_9)**
Molecular formula and weight:	**See Table 1.**
SI conversion:	**μg/L × 92.6 = nmol/L (Boron)**
CAS Registry No.:	**See Table 1.**
Normal levels:	**Serum borate or boric acid; adults, 0 to 2.5 mg/L**
Toxic level:	**More than 20 mg/L**
Special concerns:	**Repeated vomiting leading to dehydration, shock, and central nervous system excitation.**
Antidote:	**None**

OVERVIEW

Boron is present naturally in soil and water in the form of borates, such as boric acid, boron oxide, and borate salts. Borates (BO_3^{-3}, $B_4O_7^{-2}$) are also manufactured to produce glass and for use in fire retardants, leather tanning, cosmetics, antiseptics, and cleaners. Poisoning has followed ingestion, parenteral injection, enemas, and lavage of tissue cavities. Toxicity has been produced by excessive topical use in surgical wounds, burns, ulcers, and diaper dermatitis. Fatalities have resulted from unintentional administration of boric acid to infants (1) and from acute ingestions (2).

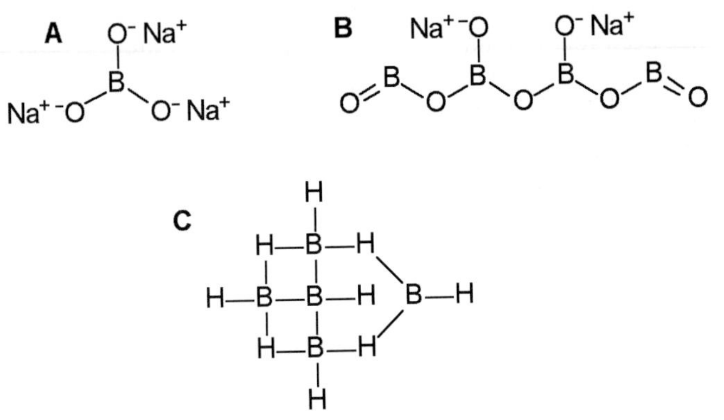

A O^-Na^+ / Na^+ ^-O–B–O^-Na^+

B Na^+ ^-O ... O^-Na^+ ; O=B–O–B–O–B–O–B=O

C Pentaborane structure (H, B atoms)

Figure 1. Structures of boron compounds. **A:** Sodium borate. **B:** Sodium tetraborate. **C:** Pentaborane.

The toxic dose is variable and depends on patient age and duration of exposure. Initial clinical manifestations are gastrointestinal followed by altered mental status, erythroderma, renal failure, and hypotension. Serum concentrations do not correlate well with toxicity. Boric acid elimination is enhanced by hemodialysis. There is no specific antidote or chelating agent.

Classification and Uses

The concentration of boron in seawater is approximately 4.5 mg/L and in the soil (United States) is 26 mg/kg. The average dietary intake for adults is approximately 1 mg/day, mostly from fruit, vegetables, coffee, wine, and milk.

Sodium borate, sodium diborate, sodium pyroborate, and sodium tetraborate (in borax cleaners) contain 21.5% boron by weight. A teaspoon of 100% boric acid crystals contains approximately 2.9 to 4.4 g of boric acid. Sodium borate solution (Dobill's Solution) contains 1.5 g of sodium borate, 1.5 g of sodium bicarbonate, and 0.3 ml of liquefied phenol. Boric anhydride, boron oxide, boron trioxide, boric oxide, boron sesquioxide, borax, tincal, and tinkal are 33% boron by weight. Sodium perborate (oxidizer in tooth powders and toothpastes) is 7.03% boron by weight, sodium metaborate is 16.44% boron, and magnesium perborate is 14% boron. Saturated solutions of boric acid contain 5.55% boron.

Other sources of boron include Harris Famous Roach Tablets, Roach-Pruf, Boraxo Powdered Hand Soap, contact lens solutions, topical preparations (5% to 10% boric acid), and otic solutions (2.75% boric acid, Swim-Ear, others). A 3.3% boric acid solution has a pH of 3.8 to 4.8. Boron is also available as a dietary supplement (Boron Extra Strength, Tri-Boron, others) in 3 mg and 6 mg tablets or capsules.

Boron-reducing agents including boron hydride (B_2H_6, diborane), decaborane ($B_{10}H_{14}$), pentaborane (B_5H_9), boron tribromide (BBr_3), and boron trifluoride (BF_3) are used in industry as reducing agents. Their reactivity makes them extremely hazardous compounds.

TABLE 1. Physical characteristics and regulatory guidelines for boron compounds

Compound, molecular weight (g/mol), molecular formula, CAS Registry No.	Agency	Description	Concentration mg/m³ (ppm)
Boron: B; 10.8; 7440-42-8	OSHA	PEL-TWA	NR
	ACGIH	TLV-TWA	NR
	NIOSH	REL-TWA	NR
Boric acid: BNa_3O_3; 127.8; 11113-50-1, 1333-73-9 (boric acid), 12447-40-4 (borax)	OSHA	PEL-TWA	15 (5.3)
	ACGIH	TLV-TWA	10 (3.5)
		STEL	None
	NIOSH	REL-TWA	10 (3.5)
		IDLH	2000 (702)
Sodium tetraborate anhydrous: $B_4Na_2O_7$; 201.2; 1330-43-4	OSHA	PEL-TWA	NR
	ACGIH	TLV-TWA	NR
	NIOSH	REL-TWA	NR
Pentaborane: B_5H_9; 63.1; 19624-22-7s	OSHA	PEL-TWA	.01 (0.005)
		STEL	'0.04 (0.015)
	ACGIH	TLV-TWA	.01 (0.005)
		STEL	'0.04 (0.015)
	NIOSH	REL-TWA	.01 (0.005)
		STEL	'0.04 (0.015)
		IDLH	2.75 (1)

ACGIH, American Conference of Governmental Industrial Hygienists; IDLH, immediate danger to life or health; NA, not applicable; NIOSH, National Institute for Occupational Safety and Health; NR, not reported; OSHA, U.S. Occupational Safety and Health Administration; PEL, permissible exposure limit; ppm, parts per million; REL, recommended exposure limit; TLV, threshold limit value; TWA, time-weighted average.

Toxic Dose

The *regulatory guidelines and standards* for boron compounds are provided in Table 1. The maximum allowed content of boron by the Environmental Protection Agency in cottonseed oil is 30 parts per million (ppm) and in citrus fruits is 8 ppm. The maximum allowed amount of boron as a food additive by the U.S. Food and Drug Administration is 310 ppm.

The *acute toxic dose* has not been established. Admission for observation is suggested for ingestion of more than 6 g in adults and more than 200 mg/kg in children. Systemic poisoning in humans has resulted from the ingestion of as little as 200 mg/kg of boric acid (3,4). The risk of clinical toxicity appears increased in chronic exposure compared to acute ingestion.

Single acute ingestions are frequently asymptomatic. A 28-year-old patient ingested 297 g in a suicide attempt. The only toxicity was spontaneous emesis 1 hour after ingestion (5). Fatalities have been reported in adults after use of 15 to 30 g (6). A 77-year-old man ingested 30 g of boric acid powder with water for hiccups. He developed vomiting, diarrhea, and generalized erythema, renal failure, and hypotension within 24 hours. His serum boric acid level was 37.7 mg/L 30 hours post-ingestion. He developed refractory hypotension despite hemodialysis, charcoal hemoperfusion, fluid resuscitation and vasopressor, and died 63 hours post-ingestion (2).

Infants have survived acute ingestion of 1.95 to 20.0 g (1,5,7). A 24-day-old (4.8 kg) infant was fed 2.6 g of boric acid diluted in formula and developed irritability, mild diarrhea, and perineal erythema. A 14-month-old (11.2 kg) boy was fed 1.95 g and was asymptomatic except for a facial erythematous rash (7). A 14-month-old child ingested 20 g but developed no adverse clinical effects. A 2-year-old child ingested 10 g and had only spontaneous vomiting for 3 hours (5). The fatal dose in five infants was reported to be 4.5 to 14.0 g (1). As little as 1 g has been fatal in an infant (1).

Chronic pediatric poisoning occurred after ingestions of 4 to 30 g over a 4- to 10-week period and resulted in seizures (8). Ingestion of 4 to 5 g/day of boric acid for 3 to 4 weeks or 6 to 20 g of borax ($Na_2B_4O_7$ $10H_2O$) daily for several months resulted in toxicity (9).

TOXICOKINETICS AND TOXICODYNAMICS

Inorganic borates are absorbed as boric acid by the gastrointestinal tract, mucous membranes, and abraded skin. It diffuses rapidly into tissues and concentrates in bone, teeth, and nails.

Boric acid is not metabolized. It is eliminated unchanged in the urine. Its volume of distribution is 0.17 to 0.5 L/kg. A mean half-life of 13.4 hours (range, 4 to 28 hours) was reported in nine human cases of poisoning (10). Serum boric acid half-lives were approximately 10 hours and 8 hours in two infants who were fed diluted boric acid–contaminated formula (7).

PATHOPHYSIOLOGY

The biochemical mechanism of boron is not known. It may play a role in cell-membrane functions or as a metabolic regulator in enzyme systems. Boric acid has weak bacteriostatic properties. Boric acid, boron salts, and boron hydrides are mucous membrane irritants. Pentaborane has caused liver necrosis. The etiology of renal insufficiency is unclear; it may be the result of severe dehydration or a direct toxic effect on the kidney (11). The cause of death is cardiovascular collapse (2,11).

PREGNANCY AND LACTATION

Boron has caused developmental toxicity in the rat fetus at 13.3 mg boron/kg/day (12). There are no reports of human fetal toxicity.

CLINICAL PRESENTATION

Acute Overdosage

Initial symptoms are gastrointestinal, followed in 1 to 2 days by generalized erythroderma, and central nervous system irritability. Renal insufficiency is common after chronic or subacute poisoning either from a direct toxic effect or dehydration and shock. Severe toxicity tends to occur more often in neonates after chronic exposure. In a retrospective review of 784 acute boric acid exposures reported to poison control centers, 88% were asymptomatic (10).

Gastrointestinal effects include persistent nausea, vomiting, and diarrhea in children that lead to acute dehydration and shock. Nausea, vomiting, diarrhea and epigastric pain, hematemesis, and blue-green discoloration of feces and vomitus characterize adult boron intoxication.

Central nervous system effects include hyperexcitability, irritability, restlessness, opisthotonus, tremors, convulsions, delirium, coma, weakness, lethargy, headaches, excitement, and depression.

Renal effects include renal tubular damage, oliguria, and elevated serum creatinine. Hepatic effects are rare, but elevated transaminases and jaundice have been reported. Cardiovascular effects include tachycardia and hypotension. Death results from circulatory collapse in severe poisonings.

A 45-year-old man dissolved boric acid crystals in water and ingested it in a suicide attempt. He developed nausea, vomiting, and green diarrhea. He presented to the hospital 2 days after ingestion with lethargy, dehydration, hypotension, renal failure, metabolic acidosis, and generalized erythematous rash. Despite treatment with intravenous fluids and vasopressors, he developed atrial fibrillation, then pulseless electric activity, and died 17 hours after admission. His whole blood boric acid concentration was 420 mg/L 52 hours after ingestion (11).

Chronic Use

Chronic toxicity is usually seen in children who have been treated with a boric acid preparation for diaper rash. Cutaneous findings develop regardless of the route of poisoning. Alopecia has been reported after chronic exposure in adults (13). Renal toxicity includes oliguria, anuria, and renal tubular necrosis, which may occur after several days of exposure. Seven infants developed seizures as a result of chronic administration of a borax and honey mixture (8). Death is more common in infants than adults (1,9,10).

Dermatologic effects are more common after chronic or subacute exposures. Skin changes may develop after boric acid ingestion or applications of a boric acid powder (14). Erythema and desquamation occurs in 1 to 2 days. Exfoliation that is generalized or localized to the hands, feet, or face may occur and has been termed the *boiled lobster* syndrome (5,15). Erythema may be prominent on the buttocks and scrotum.

Boron Hydrides

Pentaborane is a volatile liquid and the most toxic of the boron hydrides. Symptoms may be delayed 24 to 48 hours. Initial symptoms are headache, dizziness, tremors, hiccups, and ataxia. This may progress to coma, seizures, and rhabdomyolysis. Three patients exposed to pentaborane gas (B_5H_9) developed respiratory irritation within 20 minutes and seizures within 15 to 45 minutes. Severe acidosis and hypotension occurred in two patients. All had elevated aminotransferase levels and rhabdomyolysis with an elevation in creatine kinase. One died and one remained unconscious for more than 2 weeks (16). Psychiatric symptoms of stress reaction and minimal brain dysfunction may persist for at least 4 to 12 weeks after exposure (17).

Decaborane ($B_{10}H_{14}$) poisoning is similar to pentaborane. Diborane, boron tribromide, and boron trifluoride are highly reactive agents and extremely irritating to mucous membranes. Exposure can cause eye and nose irritation, cough, dyspnea, and pulmonary edema.

DIAGNOSTIC TESTS

Boric Acid (Borate) Levels

Serum boric acid levels should be obtained 2 to 4 hours after acute ingestions of more than 200 mg/kg (children) or 6 g (adults). Serum concentrations are usually reported as boric acid but may be reported as boron. The formula for conversion of a boron level to boric acid is

Boric acid concentration (mg/dl) = boron (mg/dl) × 5.72 (11)

Normal serum boric acid levels average 1.4 mg/L in children and 0.6 mg/L in adults (range, 0 to 7 mg/L) (18). Serum and urine boric acid levels do not correlate well with adverse clinical effects. Symptoms of toxicity generally occur when blood levels exceed 20 to 150 µg/ml, although blood levels of 56 and 147 µg/ml produced only mild irritability, diarrhea, and perianal erythema in two neonates (1,7). In one series with a median age of 2 years, blood borate concentrations as high as 340 mg/L were not associated with significant toxicity. Of seven patients with boric acid concentrations more than 70 µg/ml, four were asymptomatic and three developed nausea or vomiting (10). Serum concentrations of 80 to 580 mg/L from acute ingestion have caused only vomiting and diarrhea (5), whereas *chronic administration* over several weeks with borate levels of 15 to 49 mg/L have caused seizures in infants (8).

Acute ingestion of 2.6 g of boric acid resulted in a 10-hour serum boric acid level of 147 mg/L in a 24-day-old infant. A 1.95-g ingestion resulted in a serum boric acid level of 56 mg/L at 3.5 hours post-ingestion in a 24-month-old infant (7).

Lethal serum concentrations are not well defined. *Fatalities* have been reported with serum concentrations between 22 and 1600 mg/L (1,7,11).

Most laboratories are not equipped to do accurate blood boron or boric acid levels. The U.S. Borax and Chemical Corporation can analyze blood samples. Send 10 ml heparinized blood (in a polyethylene bottle) and a case summary, by airmail, to

U.S. Borax Laboratories
412 Crescent Way
Anaheim, CA 92803
Telephone: 714-774-2673

Other Tests

Dehydration may lead to electrolyte (Na, K, Ca, Mg) abnormalities. Elevated blood urea nitrogen and serum creatinine levels reflect renal damage. Liver function tests (aspartate and alanine aminotransferases) may be elevated.

Diagnostic Pitfalls

An outbreak of an illness in a newborn nursery consisting of vomiting, diarrhea, dehydration, and exfoliative dermatitis was mistakenly thought to be due to an infectious agent because *Staphylococcus aureus* was cultured from the nose, throat, and feces in two patients. The clinical picture was similar to Ritter's disease. However, because *S. aureus* was not found in other hospital cultures, boric acid toxicity was subsequently considered. It was discovered as a contaminant of the infant formula. Three infants died (19).

Postmortem Considerations

A postmortem urine boron concentration was 29.4 mg/dl 4 days after ingestion of boric acid (11). Brain and liver concentrations in fatal pediatric cases ranged from 126 to 540 mg/kg (18). High concentrations of boric acid are found in the brain and liver postmortem.

TREATMENT

Observation and no decontamination is recommended for acute ingestions of less than 200 mg/kg boric acid in children (less than 30 kg body weight) or less than 6 g in adults (10). Acute ingestion of more than 200 mg/kg or 6 g should have intravenous access established and blood sent for serum electrolytes, creatinine, and boric acid concentration. Administer crystalloid fluids to correct dehydration and consider hemodialysis for manifestations of severe toxicity or massive ingestions, particularly if renal impairment is present. There is no specific antidote.

Decontamination

After *ingestion* of more than 200 mg/kg (children) or 6 g (adult), patients who present within 1 to 2 hours should undergo gastric lavage with a large-bore tube. The airway should be protected either by suction in an alert and cooperative patient or by endotracheal intubation if compromised. Activated charcoal has not been shown to be of value and probably does not absorb boron well (20).

After *skin exposure*, wash exposed areas several times with mild soap and water. Remove all powder or crystals from skin.

Eye exposure should be irrigated copiously with water for at least 20 minutes. If irritation or pain persists, obtain an ophthalmologic consultation.

Enhancement of Elimination

Boric acid is excreted unchanged in the urine and some tubular resorption occurs under normal conditions. A case report suggests that urinary excretion may be enhanced *with forced saline diuresis* when renal function is intact. An adult ingested 36 g of boric acid and presented 14 hours later with altered mental status, erythema, and fever. She received 3.25 l of intravenous fluid and 100 mg of furosemide over 4 hours and produced 3640 ml of urine during this time. The half-life of the serum boric acid was 3.3 hours during that period. The elimination rate of boric acid obtained with diuresis was similar to that obtained with hemodialysis on a previous occasion when the same patient attempted suicide with boric acid (21).

Based on isolated case reports, forced diuresis may be useful if the kidneys are able to excrete the borates before irreversible damage to the renal tubular epithelium occurs. Administration of 0.45% saline in D_5W intravenously with a diuretic (furosemide, 1 mg/kg up to 40 mg per dose) may be useful. Urine output should be maintained at 3 to 6 ml/kg body weight per hour. The risks of forced diuresis include volume overload, electrolyte imbalances, and pulmonary edema. Hemodialysis may be a safer and more efficient method of elimination enhancement in severely poisoned patients.

Hemodialysis has been shown to enhance the elimination of boric acid in a limited number of patients. It significantly shortened the half-life compared with pre- and post-dialysis half-lives in three patients. The boric acid half-life during dialysis was 3 hours compared to 20 hours predialysis (10). The indications for hemodialysis are not well defined. It is most useful in the presence of renal failure. Patients with boric acid serum levels of 340 to 2320 mg/L shortly after an acute ingestion have had only minor symptoms and recovered without hemodialysis (5,10).

A 26-year-old woman developed altered mental status, vomiting, fever, and flushing 7 hours after ingestion of approximately 21 g of boric acid. Her serum boric concentration was 465 mg/L. The predialysis half-life of boric acid was 13.46 hours, which was shortened to 3.76 hours during hemodialysis. The total body clearance was 0.99 L/hour and increased to 3.53 L/hour by hemodialysis. The additional removal of boric acid by hemodialysis was estimated to be approximately 5 g (22).

A 12-month-old girl ingested 3 g of boric acid and developed vomiting, tremor, and seizures. The plasma half-life of boric acid was 7.0 hours and decreased to 3.6 hours and 4.4 hours during the two hemodialysis sessions. The total body clearance of boric acid increased from 21 ml/minute to 41 and 34 ml/minute. The *in vitro* boric acid clearance of the dialyzer was 18 ml/minute (23).

Peritoneal dialysis does not appear to enhance the elimination of boric acid. A 24-day-old infant with an initial serum boric acid level of 147 mg/L underwent peritoneal dialysis for 25 hours (3575-ml dialysate). The half-life before and during dialysis was 10 hours (7). Peritoneal dialysis for 54 hours was associated with a decrease in serum borate concentration from 303 mg/L to 32 mg/L in an infant poisoned from chronic boric acid powder for diaper rash. The peritoneal clearance of boric acid was 1.2 to 1.7 ml/minute. The total amount of boric acid recovered in the dialysate after the first 10 hours was 295 mg (15).

Antidotes

There are no proven antidotes for boron toxicity. Administration of *N*-acetylcysteine to rats poisoned with boron was associated with increased urinary excretion of boron and reversal of the oliguria associated with the intoxication (24). There are no studies in humans to confirm this finding.

Supportive Care

All patients with a significant exposure should have intravenous access established and isotonic fluids administered if clinically dehydrated. Administer isotonic fluids initially for hypotension (Chapter 37). Seizures may result from chronic toxicity and should be treated with an intravenous benzodiazepine such as diazepam (Chapter 40).

Management Pitfalls

Patients may have minimal or no symptoms despite high serum levels of boric acid after acute ingestions. The presence of a high serum boric acid level alone is not an indication for hemodialysis.

REFERENCES

1. Wong LC, Heimbach MD, Truscott DR, Duncan BD. Boric acid poisoning: report of 11 cases. *Can Med Assoc J* 1964;90:1018–1023.
2. Ishii Y, Fujizuka N, Takahashi T, et al. A fatal case of acute boric acid poisoning. *J Toxicol Clin Toxicol* 1993;31(2):345–352.
3. Martin GI. Asymptomatic boric acid intoxication. *N Y Stat J Med* 1971;71:1842–1844.
4. Schillinger BM, Berstein M, Goldberg LA, Shalita AR. Boric acid poisoning. *J Am Acad Dermatol* 1982;7:667–673.
5. Linden CH, Hall AH, Kulig KW, et al. Acute ingestions of boric acid. *Clin Toxicol* 1986;24:269–279.
6. Ross CA, Conway JF. The dangers of boric acid: its use as an irrigant and report of a case. *Am J Surg* 1943;60:386–395.
7. Baker MD, Bogema SC. Ingestion of boric acid by infants. *Am J Emerg Med* 1986;4:358–361.
8. O'Sullivan K, Taylor M. Chronic boric acid poisoning in infants. *Arch Dis Child* 1983;58(9):737–739.
9. Valdes-Dapena MA, Arey JB. Boric acid poisoning: three fatal cases with pancreatic inclusions and a review of the literature. *J Pediatr* 1962;61:534–546.
10. Litovitz TL, Klein-Schwartz W, Oderda GM, Schmitz BP. Clinical manifestations of toxicity in a series of 784 boric acid ingestions. *Am J Emerg Med* 1988;6:209–213.
11. Restuccio A, Mortensen ME, Kelley MT. Fatal ingestion of boric acid in an adult. *Am J Emerg Med* 1992;10:545–547.
12. Price DJ, Strong PL, Marr MC, et al. Developmental toxicity NOAEL and postnatal recovery in rats fed boric acid during gestation. *Fundam Appl Toxicol* 1996;32:179–193.
13. Beckett WS, Oskvig R, Gaynor ME, et al. Association of reversible alopecia with occupational topical exposure to common borax-containing solutions. *J Am Acad Dermatol* 2001;44(4):599–602.
14. Stein KM, Odom RB, Justice GR, et al. Toxic alopecia from ingestion of boric acid. *Arch Dermatol* 1973;108:95–97.
15. Balaih T, MacLeish H, Drummond KN. Acute boric acid poisoning: report of an infant successfully treated by peritoneal dialysis. *Can Med Assoc J* 1969;101:166–168.
16. Zolet DI, Miller T, Yarborough B, et al. Pentaborane poisoning causing extreme acidosis and death. *Vet Hum Toxicol* 1982;24:277–278(abst).
17. Silverman JJ, Hart RP, Garrettson LK, et al. Posttraumatic stress disorder from pentaborane intoxication. Neuropsychiatric evaluation and short-term follow-up. *JAMA* 1985;254:2603–2608.
18. Baselt RC. Borate. In: *Disposition of toxic drugs and chemicals in man*, 6th ed. Foster City, CA: Biomedical Publications, 2002:112–114.
19. Rubenstein AD, Musher DM. Epidemic boric acid poisoning simulating staphylococcal toxic epidermal necrolysis of the newborn infant: Ritter's disease. *J Pediatr* 1970;77:884–887.
20. Oderda GM, Klein-Schwartz W, Insley BM. In vitro study of boric acid and activated charcoal. *Vet Hum Toxicol* 1985;28(4):314(abst).
21. Teshima D, Taniyama T, Oishi R. Usefulness of forced diuresis for acute boric acid poisoning in an adult. *J Clin Pharm Ther* 2001;26:387–390.
22. Teshima D, Morishita K, Ueda Y, et al. Clinical management of boric acid ingestion: pharmacokinetic assessment of efficacy of hemodialysis for treatment of acute boric acid poisoning. *J Pharmacobiodyn* 1992;15:287–294.
23. Egfjord M, Jansen JA, Flachs H, et al. Combined boric acid and cinchocaine chloride poisoning in a 12-month-old infant: evaluation of haemodialysis. *Hum Toxicol* 1988;7(2):175–178.
24. Banner W Jr, Koch M, Capin DM, et al. Experimental chelation therapy in chromium, lead, and boron intoxication with N-acetylcysteine and other compounds. *Toxicol Appl Pharmacol* 1986;83(1):142–147.

CHAPTER 205

Disc Batteries

João H. Delgado and Richard C. Dart

Compounds included:	**Disc (*button*) batteries**
SI conversion:	**Not applicable**
Special concerns:	**Caustic injury common in airways or esophagus**
Antidote:	**None**

OVERVIEW

Disc batteries, or button batteries, are found in small electronic devices, such as calculators, handheld computer games, hearing aids, small toys, and watches. Because of their small size, they can lodge in the airway or gastrointestinal (GI) tract and cause symptoms from simple mechanical obstruction. As important, they pose the additional risk of caustic injury, especially if they lodge within the esophagus.

Disc battery ingestions are a relatively frequent occurrence. Based on reports to the National Button Battery Ingestion Hotline, it is conservatively estimated that the annual incidence in the United States is at least 2100 cases per year (1). For the most part, the incidence mirrors the overall incidence of poisoning, with children younger than 5 years of age accounting for the majority of cases. The incidence of major effects (life-threatening symptoms or permanent disability) in this database was less than 0.1%. However, severe effects, such as esophageal perforation, esophageal strictures, tracheoesophageal fistulas, and even death, have been reported (1–4).

CHEMICAL AND PHYSICAL PROPERTIES

Disc batteries are shaped like shallow cylinders and range in diameter from 6.8 to 25 mm. (For comparison, the U.S. dime measures 17 mm in diameter and the quarter 23 mm.) The batteries are composed of a negative terminal (anode) and a positive terminal (cathode) that are separated by an electrolyte soaked membrane internally (Fig. 1). Externally, the anode and cathode are separated by a plastic seal. These batteries may contain a variety of caustic chemicals (Table 1).

CLINICAL PRESENTATION

Local Effects

Although the injury observed from disc batteries may be partly attributable to pressure necrosis, the most significant mechanism of mucosal injury results from their corrosive effects. This occurs when the plastic ring ruptures allowing the contents of

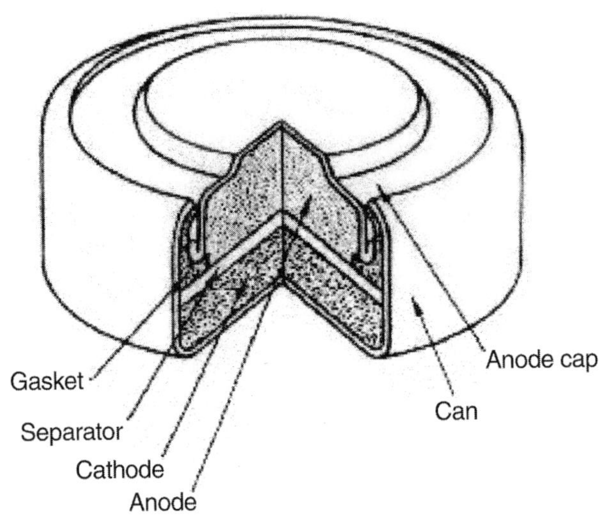

Figure 1. Schematic diagram of a disc battery.

the battery to leak or from the *in situ* formation of caustic species as the battery discharges and generates an electrical current (4). It appears that the most severe injury occurs on the anode side, especially along the plastic seal. As a result, the orientation of the battery may be of some use in predicting potential complications. Local effects range from mild superficial injury to transmural necrosis resulting in esophageal perforation, stricture formation, and even death (5,6). Lodgment of batteries in the nose and ear canal can also lead to significant local tissue injury and should be removed promptly to minimize permanent injury.

Systemic Effects

Elevated blood and urine mercury levels have been documented after rupture of mercuric oxide batteries (1,7,8). In general, the concentrations reported are not expected to produce systemic effects. The lone exception is a 2-year-old child with a blood mercury level of 34 μg/L and a urine level of 600 μg/L. The patient was treated with dimercaprol and did not develop signs of mercury toxicity (8). In this case the child underwent surgical removal of the battery, which had already fragmented, and radiopaque material was present in the small bowel. In addition, the postoperative course was complicated by a small bowel obstruction, which is a known risk factor for systemic mercury absorption. Based on these few case reports, if a battery known to contain mercuric oxide ruptures and radiopaque droplets are visible, it seems prudent to follow mercury levels until the battery is eliminated in the stool.

A rash has been reported in a small percentage of cases. This effect is probably related to nickel sensitivity (1). Other reported systemic effects are usually mild and include abdominal pain, dark-colored stools, malaise, nausea, and vomiting. Severe systemic effects occur as a result of airway obstruction, GI obstruction, or perforation. In their absence, significant systemic effects are not expected.

TABLE 1. Potential caustic chemicals found in disc batteries

Cadmium oxide	Mercuric oxide	Silver oxide
Lithium hydroxide	Nickel hydroxide	Sodium hydroxide
Manganese dioxide	Potassium hydroxide	Zinc oxide

Patient Age

Battery transit times tend to be longer in younger patients (1). In general, this does not result in increased complication rates. Young age in combination with larger battery size is associated with likelihood of significant effects.

Battery Size

Most ingested batteries are less than 15 mm in diameter. This is because they are easier to swallow than larger batteries and because they are the most common sizes available. Batteries more than 15 mm are associated with more severe effects because they are more likely to lodge in the esophagus or fail to progress beyond the pylorus, especially in children younger than 5 years of age. Batteries that lodge in the esophagus can result in the rapid progression of corrosive injury, whereas batteries that lodge in the stomach are associated with a higher rate of fragmentation than batteries that lodge elsewhere in the GI tract. The potential for corrosive injury is also increased in the stomach, as compared to the more alkaline small intestine, because the acidic environment promotes more efficient electrical discharge of the battery. Once the battery passes beyond the pylorus, intestinal transit time does not correlate with battery size.

Battery Composition

Mercuric oxide batteries are more likely to fragment than other types (1). The reason for this is not known. Lithium cells seem to be associated with a disproportionate number of adverse effects. This is probably because of their large size and higher voltage compared to other cell systems.

DIAGNOSTIC TESTS

Disc batteries may be radiographically differentiated from coins or other cylindrical radiopaque objects (9). When viewed en face, the presence of an inner ring distinguishes the disc battery from a coin, which is of uniform density (Fig. 2). On the lateral view, the disc battery usually has a bulge on one side whereas the coin is symmetric. These features are dependent on the orientation of the battery, its size, and the thickness of the casing. For example, the inner ring is obscured if the battery is oriented obliquely or if the case is thick. Therefore, the

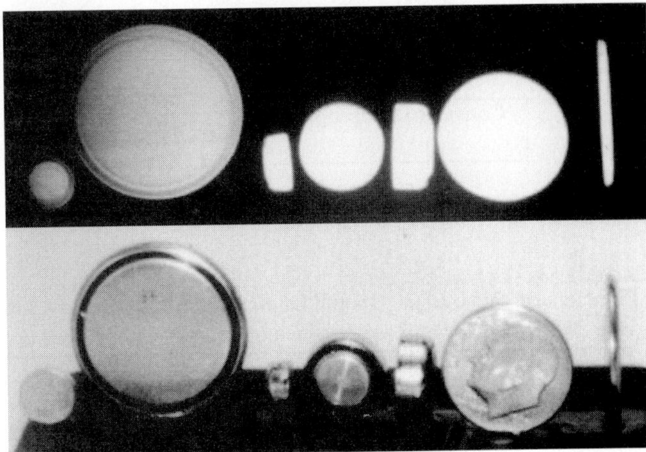

Figure 2. Radiographic appearance of several disc batteries and a U.S. dime.

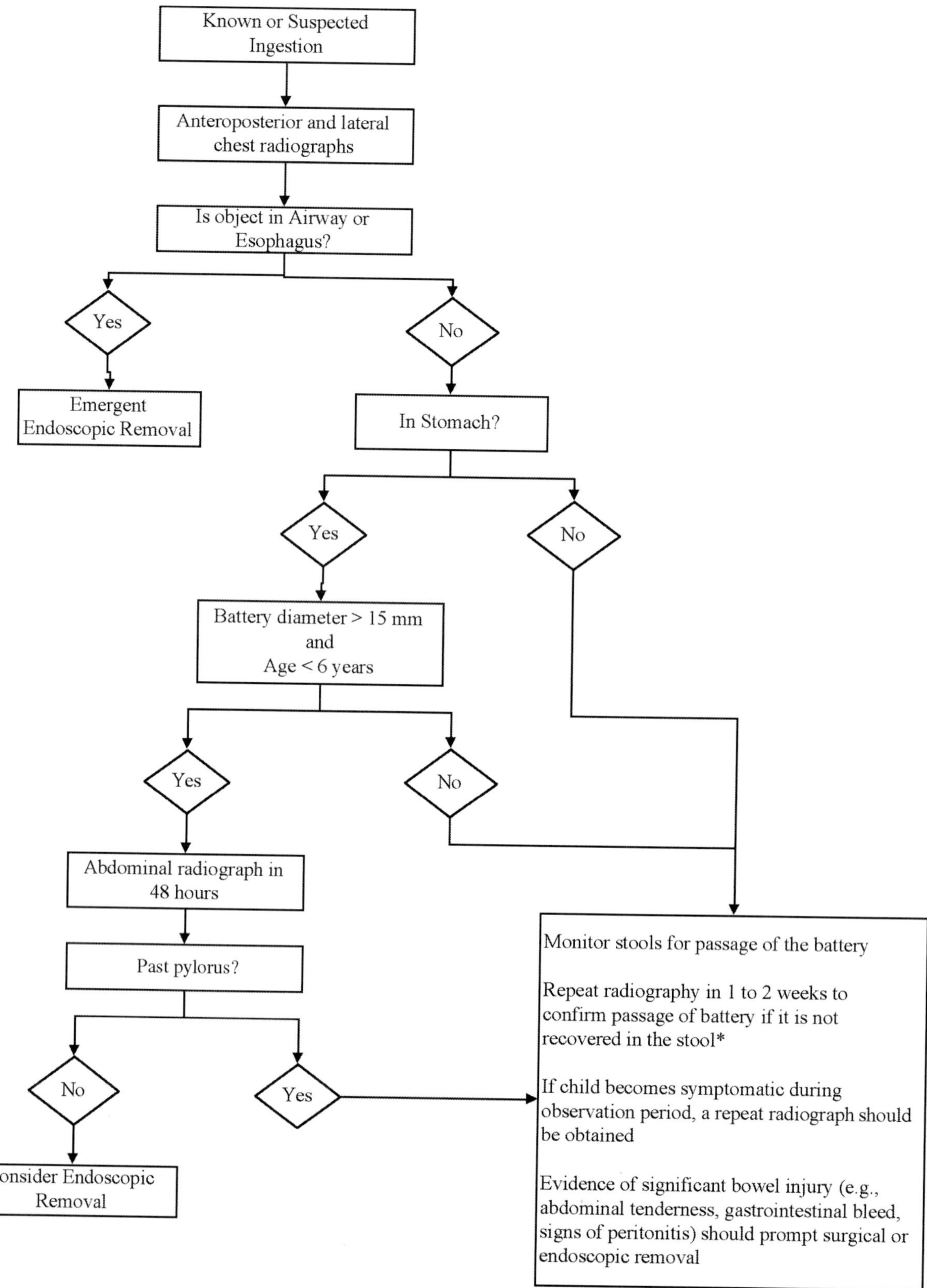

Figure 3. Treatment algorithm for disc battery ingestions.

absence of these findings should not be used to exclude the presence of a button battery.

TREATMENT

The key management issues are whether the battery is in the airway or in the GI tract. If it is in the GI tract, it must be determined whether it is in the esophagus. Anteroposterior and lateral radiographs that show the pharynx, chest, and upper abdomen are important in any case involving known or suspected ingestion of disc batteries. If the battery lodges in the airway or in the esophagus, emergent endoscopic removal is indicated. Esophageal burns have been documented within 4 hours of ingestion and esophageal perforation within 6 hours of ingestion (1). In general, because significant corrosive injury can occur so rapidly, endoscopic removal is preferred because it is the modality with the highest rate of success and it allows for direct inspection of the mucosa after battery retrieval.

If endoscopy is not immediately available and the ingestion is known to have occurred less than 4 hours prior, indirect methods such as Foley catheter or magnetized catheter removal may be attempted with or without fluoroscopic assistance. These methods should not be considered first line because they are frequently unsuccessful and because they do not allow for direct inspection of the affected area for evidence of corrosive injury.

Confirmation of battery location by radiography or fluoroscopy should be performed immediately before attempting endoscopic removal. Retrieval failure frequently results from distal migration of the battery. This is especially important in the case of esophageal location, in which early migration may obviate the need for endoscopy and its attendant risks of sedation, aspiration, and injury to the GI tract. A treatment algorithm is shown in Figure 3.

Efforts to induce emesis should never be used. They are ineffective and pose the unnecessary additional risks of corrosive injury from reflux of stomach acid as well as retrograde propulsion of the battery back into the esophagus. Pharmacologic therapy to promote movement into the stomach of a battery lodged in the esophagus, such as glucagon or nifedipine, has not been adequately studied and cannot be recommended.

PITFALLS

Failure to obtain a radiograph after a known or suspected ingestion; attempting to induce emesis; and delay in removing batteries lodged in the esophagus, nose, or ear canal are to be avoided. Similarly, overaggressive attempts to remove batteries that have moved beyond the esophagus are to be condemned because the vast majority transit the intestinal tract uneventfully.

REFERENCES

1. Litovitz T, Schmitz BF. Ingestion of cylindrical and button batteries: an analysis of 2382 cases. *Pediatrics* 1992;89:747–757.
2. Sigalet D, Lees G. Tracheoesophageal injury secondary to disc battery ingestion. *J Pediatr Surg* 1988;23:996–998.
3. Rivera EA, Maves MD. Effects of neutralizing agents on esophageal burns caused by disc batteries. *Ann Otol Rhinol Laryngol* 1987;96:362–366.
4. Yamashita M, Saito S, Hattori H, Ogata T. Esophageal electrochemical burn by button-type alkaline batteries in dogs. *Vet Hum Toxicol* 1987;29:226–230.
5. Blantnik DS, Toohill RJ, Lehman RH. Fatal complication from an alkaline battery foreign body in the esophagus. *Ann Otol Rhinol Laryngol* 1977;86:611–615.
6. Shabino CL, Feinberg AN. Esophageal perforation secondary to alkaline battery ingestion. *JACEP* 1979;8:360–362.
7. Kulig K, Rumack CM, Rumack BH. Disk battery ingestion: elevated urine mercury levels and enema removal of battery fragments. *JAMA* 1983;249:2502–2504.
8. Mant TG, Lewis JL, Mattoo TK, et al. Mercury poisoning after disc battery ingestion. *Hum Toxicol* 1987;6:179–181.
9. Maves MD, Lloyd TV, Carithers JS. Radiographic identification of ingested disk batteries. *Pediatr Radiol* 1986;16:154.

SECTION 7

Hydrocarbons

CHAPTER 206

Hydrocarbon Products

Richard Y. Wang

Compounds included:	**Petroleum distillates, dibromochloropropane, dimethyl sulfate, dimethylsulfoxide, methanethiol, monooctanoin, trimellitic anhydride, trimethylamine, halogenated hydrocarbons, dichlorobenzene, polyhalogenated biphenyls, polychlorinated dibenzofuran, polychlorinated dibenzo-p-podioxinpolycyclic aromatic hydrocarbons, creosotes, tetrahydrofuran, cyclohexanone, and hydroquinone. Representative structures are provided in Figure 1.**
Molecular formula and weight:	**See text.**
CAS Registry No.:	**See text.**
Normal levels:	**Not applicable**
Target organs:	**Lung (acute)**
Antidote:	**None**

ALIPHATIC HYDROCARBONS—PETROLEUM DISTILLATES

Hydrocarbon ingestions account for approximately 2.4% of all calls reported to poison centers in the United States. Petroleum distillates represent the most common hydrocarbon exposure. In order of decreasing frequency, the most common agents involved in calls to a poison control center concerning hydrocarbons were gasoline (34%), fluorocarbon/propellant (12%), mineral spirits/varsol (7%), lubricating oil/motor oil (6%), lighter fluid/naphtha (6%), kerosene (4%), and toluene/xylene (4%) (1).

Petroleum ether (benzin or benzine) consists primarily of *n*-pentane and *n*-hexane (but not benzene or true ethers), which are produced at boiling points from 35° to 80°C. *Petroleum naphtha* includes various mixtures of aliphatic hydrocarbons C_5 to C_{13} produced at boiling points between 30° and 238°C and may refer to any fractionalization more volatile than kerosene. Occasionally, the term is misused as a synonym for petroleum ether. *Rubber solvent* consists chiefly of C_5 to C_9 aliphatic hydrocarbons distilled between 38° and 149°C; this product is less volatile than petroleum ether. *Stoddard solvent* (mineral spirits, white spirits) is a higher boiling fraction of petroleum naphtha (at 152° to 219°C) that contains straight- and branched-chain hydrocarbons (C_9 to C_{12}), naphthalene, and higher aromatic hydrocarbons. Varnish maker and painter's naphtha and mineral spirits consist chiefly of C_7 to C_{10} aliphatic hydrocarbons refined between 94° and 175°C.

Gasoline is a mixture of C_5 to C_{12} aliphatic hydrocarbons obtained by "cracking" heavy fractions in the boiling range of 40° to 225°C. Appreciable amounts of aromatic hydrocarbons (e.g., xylene) are found in some commercial fuels, especially those with high octane ratings. Tetraethyl lead and alcohols may be added to boost the octane rating. *Kerosene* consists chiefly of C_{10} to C_{16} aliphatic hydrocarbons obtained in the boiling range of 175° to 325°C. Small amounts of unsaturated (e.g., xylene) and saturated (naphthalene) aromatics appear in these products. *Diesel oil* and *fuel oil* are complex mixtures of C_9 and higher hydrocarbons that are slightly less volatile but more viscous than kerosene.

Mineral seal oil is a light petroleum fraction obtained between boiling points 200° and 370°C. It consists mainly of saturated, higher-molecular-weight aliphatic hydrocarbons compared with gasoline and kerosene. *Turpentine* is an oleoresin solvent derived from the steam distillation of pine resin. Although technically not a petroleum distillate, it is an aromatic hydrocarbon with similar properties, toxic effects, and uses.

Chemical and Physical Properties

The physical properties of viscosity, surface tension, and volatility determine the risk of aspiration and therefore have the greatest effect on toxicity (Table 1) (2). Hydrocarbons may also become drugs of abuse (Chapter 179). The metabolism of some volatile substances is summarized in Table 2.

TABLE 1. **Physical properties and pharmacokinetic data of some volatile hydrocarbon compounds**[a]

Compound	MWt (g/mol)	BPt (°C)	OEL (ppm)	Inhaled dose absorbed (%)	Proportion of absorbed dose: Eliminated unchanged (%)	Proportion of absorbed dose: Metabolized (%)	$t_{1/2}$ (h)	Brain:blood distribution ratio from postmortem investigation	Blood:gas partition coefficient (37°C)
Acetone	58.1	56	1000	—	—	—	3–5	—	243–300
Benzene	78.1	79.5	10	46	12	80	9–24	3–6	6–9
Bromochlorodifluromethane	165.3	–4	—	—	—	—	—	—	—
n-Butane	58.1	–0.5	1000[b]	30–45	—	—	—	—	—
Isobutane	58.1	–12	1000[b]	—	—	—	—	—	—
Butanone	72.1	80	200	—	—	—	—	—	—
Carbon disulfide	76.1	46	10	40	8–20	50–90	<1	—	2.4
Carbon tetrachloride	153.8	76–78	5	—	?50	?50	48	—	1.6
Chloroform	119.4	61	10	—	20–70 (8 h)	>30	1.5	4	8
Cyclopropane	42.1	–34.5	—	—	99	0.5	—	1.5–3.6	0.56
Dichloromethane	84.9	39	200	—	?50	<40	0.7	0.5–1	5–10
Diethyl ether	74.1	34–36	400	—	>90	—	—	1.1	12
Dimethyl ether	46.1	–23.6	—	—	—	—	—	—	—
Enflurane	184.5	56–58	—	90+	>80 (5 d)	2.5	36	—	1.9
Ethyl acetate	88.1	77	400	—	—	—	—	—	—
Halon 11	137.4	23.7	1000	92	89	<0.2	1.5	2.5	0.87
Halon 12	120.9	–29.8	1000	35	99	<0.2	—	1.4	0.15
Halon 22	86.4	–41	1000	—	—	—	—	1.9	—
Halothane	197.4	50	—	90+	60–80 (24 h)	<20	0.5	2–3	2.4
n-Hexane	86.2	69	100	—	—	—	—	—	—
Methoxyflurane	165.0	103–108	—	—	19 (10 d)	>44	—	2–3	11
Methyl isobutyl ketone	100.2	117	50	—	—	—	—	—	—
Nitrous oxide	44.0	–88.5	—	—	?>99	—	—	1.1	0.47
Propane	44.1	–42.5	1000[b]	—	—	—	—	—	—
Styrene	104.2	146	100	—	1–2	>95	13	—	32
Tetrachloroethylene	165.9	118–122	100	60+	>90	1–2	72	9–15	9–18
Toluene	92.1	111	100	53	<20	80	7.5	1–2	8–16
1,1,1-Trichloroethane	133.4	71–81	350	—	60–80 (1 wk)	2	10–12	2	1–3
Trichloroethylene	131.4	85–88	100	50–65	16	>80	30–38	2	9.0
Xylene	106.2	136–142	100	64	5	>90	20–30	—	42.1

MWt, molecular weight; BPt, boiling point at atmospheric pressure; OEL, occupational exposure unit; ppm, parts per million; $t_{1/2}$, terminal half-life.
[a]Adapted from Flanagan RJ, Ruprah M, Meredith TJ, et al. An introduction to the clinical toxicology of volatile substances. *Drug Safe* 1990;5:359–389, with permission.
[b]As components of liquefied petroleum gas.

TABLE 2. Summary of the metabolism of some volatile substances

Compound	Principal metabolites (% absorbed dose)	Notes
Acetone	Intermediary metabolites (largely excreted unchanged at higher concentrations)	Endogenous compound produced in large amounts in diabetic or fasting ketoacidosis. Acetone is also the major metabolite of propan-2-ol in humans.
Benzene	Phenol 51-87, catechol (6), hydroquinone (2)	Excreted in urine as sulfate and glucuronide conjugates. Urinary phenol excretion has been used to indicate exposure but is variable and subject to interference.
Carbon disulfide	2-Mercapto-2-thiazotin-5-one, 2-thiothiazolidine-4-carboxylic acid, thiourea, inorganic sulfate, others	2-Mercapto-2-thiazolin-5-one glycine conjugates and 2-thiothiazolidine-4-carboxylic acid glutathione conjugates of carbon disulfide. Urinary 2-thiothiazolidine-4-carboxylic acid excretion reliable indicator of exposure.
Carbon tetrachloride	Chloroform, carbon dioxide, hexachloroethane, others	Trichloromethyl free radical (reactive intermediary) probably responsible for the marked hepatorenal toxicity of this compound.
Chloroform	Carbon dioxide (up to 50), diglutathionyl dithiocarbonate	Phosgene (reactive intermediate) depletes glutathione and is probably responsible for hepatorenal toxicity.
Dichloromethane	Carbon monoxide	Carbon monoxide half-life 13h (5h post-inhalation). Blood carboxyhemoglobin measurement useful indicator of chronic exposure.
Ethyl acetate	Alcohol, acetic acid	Rapid reaction catalyzed by plasma esterases.
Halothane	Chlorotrifluoroethane, chlorodifluoroethylene, trifluoroacetic acid, inorganic bromide, others	The formation of reactive metabolites may be important in the etiology of the hepatotoxicity (*halothane hepatitis*), which may occur in patients exposed to halothane.
n-Hexane	2-Hexanol (as glucuronide), 2,5-hexanedione, others	2-5-Hexanedione thought to cause neurotoxicity. Methyl a-butyl ketone also neurotoxic and also metabolized to 2.5.
Styrene	Mandelic acid (85), phenylglyoxylic acid (10), hippuric acid may be minor metabolite	Urinary mandelic acid excretion indicates exposure (8); alcohol inhibits mandelic acid excretion.
Tetrachloroethylene	Trichloroacetic acid (<3)	Urinary trichloroacetic acid excretion serves only as qualitative index of exposure.
Toluene	Benzoic acid (80), *o*-, *m*-, and *p*-cresol (1)	Benzoate largely conjugated with glycine giving hippuric acid, which is excreted in urine (half-life 2–3 h). Not ideal index of exposure because there are other (dietary) sources of benzoate.
1,1,1-Trichloroethane	2,2,2-Trichloroethanol (2), trichloroacetic acid (0.5)	Urinary metabolites serve as qualitative index of exposure only (compare tetrachloroethylene)
Trichloroethylene	2,2,2-Trichloroethanol (45), trichloroacetic acid (32)	Trichloroethanol (glucuronide) and trichloroacetic acid excreted in urine (half-lives around 12 and 100 h). Trichloroacetic acid excretion can indicate exposure.
Xylene	Methylbenzoic acids (95), xylenols (2)	Methylbenzoic acids conjugated with glycine and urinary methylhippurate excretion used as index of exposures—no dietary sources of methylbenzoates.

Adapted from Flanagan RJ, Ruprah M, Meredith TJ, et al. An introduction to the clinical toxicology of volatile substances. *Drug Safe* 1990;5:359–389, with permission.

Viscosity, the tendency to resist flow or change form, provides the best estimate of the aspiration potential (3). Low viscosity allows penetration of the hydrocarbon into the distal airways. *Surface tension* is the cohesiveness of the molecules on a liquid's surface. Reduced surface tension allows the substance to spread rapidly from the mouth to the trachea. *Volatility* is the tendency of a liquid to become a gas. Highly volatile hydrocarbons displace alveolar oxygen when aspirated, producing transient hypoxia.

Petroleum distillates with low surface tension and viscosity are serious aspiration hazards. The most viscous byproducts are the higher-molecular-weight hydrocarbon mixtures, which are usually nontoxic (e.g., lubricating oil, paraffin wax, asphalt, tar, petrolatum).

Composition

Shoe polish contains chlorinated hydrocarbons and toluene. *Liquid furniture polish* contains mineral seal oil (especially red-colored polish). *Solvents* and *thinners* contain petroleum ether, Stoddard solvent (may contain 10% to 20% aromatic hydrocarbons), and varnish maker and painter's naphtha. These products also contain various concentrations of toxic aromatic hydrocarbons (benzene, toluene, xylene) or halogenated hydrocarbons (carbon tetrachloride; acetate; methylcellulose; trichloroethylene; 1,1,1-trichloroethane). *Lighter fluid* contains petroleum naphtha and kerosene. *Gasoline* is almost exclusively a fuel. Additives such as organic lead and cresyl phosphates usually are not acute ingestion hazards. Benzene content of U.S. domestic gasoline is lower (0.8% to 2.0%) than that of some foreign gasoline (up to 5%). *Kerosene* is used for curing tobacco, heating, cooling, and jet fuel. *Turpentine* is used as a solvent for oil-based paints.

The potential for aspiration is the main determinant of petroleum distillate toxicity. One empirical measure of viscosity is Saybolt Universal Seconds units. Hydrocarbons differ in viscosity (defined as the rate of flow of the liquid through an orifice of standard diameter). For example, a Saybolt Universal Seconds units value of 35 indicates high aspiration potential (e.g., gasoline); 60 Saybolt Universal Seconds units have moderate aspiration potential (e.g., mineral seal oil); and 75.1 to 86.2 indicates low aspiration potential (e.g., light mineral oil in baby oil) (4).

Hydrocarbons are also used as a vehicle for more toxic substances (e.g., camphor, pesticides, heavy metals); in these cases, the particular toxic substance involved determines the severity of response. Most additives (e.g., tetraethyl lead) are present at subtoxic levels for acute ingestions. Hydrocarbons can be classified into three groups based on potential clinical effects (5).

Group 1: High aspiration potential with little central nervous system (CNS) toxicity (i.e., mineral seal oil, furniture oil polishes).

Group 2: Significant CNS toxicity and potential aspiration hazard (i.e., methylene chloride, carbon tetrachloride, toluene, xylene, benzene, gasoline, charcoal lighter fluid, mineral spirits, turpentine).

Group 3: Nontoxic in usual doses ingested but may lead to lipoid pneumonia on aspiration (i.e., lubricants, motor oil, mineral and baby oils, fuel and diesel oil, suntan lotion, petrolatum).

Toxic Dose

Although often difficult to assess, ingestion of most petroleum distillates in an amount below 1 to 2 ml/kg does not cause systemic toxicity. Substantially larger quantities may be necessary to produce CNS depression. Small amounts (a few milliliters) of petroleum distillates intratracheally produce severe pulmonary injury, whereas only large intragastric quantities produce CNS symptoms. In the rare case of intravenous (IV) injection, small amounts may also cause severe pulmonary injury.

Pathophysiology

The primary target organ in petroleum distillate ingestion is the lung, where toxicity occurs by aspiration rather than by hematogenous spread. Aspirated hydrocarbons inhibit surfactant, leading to alveolar instability, early distal airway closure, ventilation/perfusion mismatches, and subsequent hypoxemia. Direct pulmonary capillary damage produces injury ranging from chemical pneumonitis and hemorrhagic bronchopneumonia to noncardiogenic pulmonary edema. Initially, cyanosis may result from the replacement of oxygen by vaporized hydrocarbons. Subsequent hypoxemia occurs from surfactant loss and direct alveolar injury. Bronchospasm may contribute to ventilation/perfusion defects. Histopathologic changes of the lung include interstitial inflammation, atelectasis, hyperemia, vascular thrombosis, bronchial and bronchiolar necrosis, intraalveolar hemorrhage, edema, and polymorphonuclear exudate.

High-viscosity petroleum distillates (e.g., heavy lubricants, mineral oil, liquid paraffin) produce a lipoid pneumonia that is more localized and less inflammatory than that produced by low-viscosity petroleum distillates such as kerosene or mineral seal oil (6).

Inhalational abuse of petroleum distillate (e.g., gasoline sniffing) usually does not produce a chemical pneumonitis. Neurologic abnormalities reported to be associated with chronic gasoline sniffing include behavioral changes and movement disorders (resting and action tremor, myoclonus, chorea, and ataxia), as well as extrapyramidal signs and seizures. An organic lead encephalopathy has been described with nausea, vomiting, excitement, irritability, hallucinations, disorientation, and a clouded conscious state.

Clinical Presentation

Pulmonary toxicity is similar for most low-viscosity petroleum distillates. Death from petroleum distillates almost always results from pulmonary injury. Symptoms of respiratory distress from aspiration usually appear within 30 minutes of exposure. Gasping, coughing, and choking are presumptive evidence of aspiration, although transient symptoms may occur immediately after exposure because of volatilization of the petroleum distillate. Persistent cough usually indicates aspiration. Signs and symptoms may progress over the first 24 hours but usually resolve by the third day. Death occurs most commonly within the first 24 hours. Signs range from cough and dyspnea to retractions and cyanosis (Table 3) (7). Moderate fever (38° to 39°C) often is present and does not correlate with clinical symptoms. Most admitted patients have a temperature higher than 38°C on admission, but 75% of them defervesce within 24 hours (7).

TABLE 3. Signs of pulmonary hydrocarbon aspiration

Severity	Signs
Mild	Coughing, choking, tachypnea, irritability, drowsiness, rales, rhonchi
Moderate	Grunting, lethargy, flaccidity, bronchospasm
Severe	Tachypnea with grunting respirations, cyanosis, coma, seizures

CNS effects most commonly occur from aspiration-induced hypoxia. Large intentional ingestions or toxic additives (e.g., aromatic hydrocarbons, insecticides, nitrobenzene, aniline) may also cause seizures or altered mental status. Coma is uncommon (less than 3% of hospitalized cases), and convulsions are even rarer (less than 1%) unless insecticides are involved (Chapter 236).

Gastrointestinal (GI) symptoms are frequent but usually minor, especially after large ingestions. Local irritation of the mouth and pharynx occurs (burning of mouth, sore throat, nausea, vomiting). Diarrhea, hematemesis, and melena are rare. Furniture polish more often causes GI symptoms than other petroleum distillates.

Cardiovascular system involvement is rare after acute ingestion. Sudden deaths secondary to dysrhythmias occur during solvent abuse, perhaps as a result of sensitization of the myocardium to endogenous catecholamines (Chapter 179).

Other organ dysfunction is rare but may involve the liver, kidney, and spleen. Death or permanent hepatic or renal sequelae have not been reported as a result of acute petroleum distillate exposures, although temporary dysfunction may occur.

Diagnostic Tests

BIOLOGIC MONITORING

Blood levels for hydrocarbons are not helpful in patient management but do document exposure. Blood, breath, and urine levels of either parent compound or metabolite can be used to monitor work-related exposure to these chemicals (8).

ACUTE EXPOSURE

Leukocytosis is common during the first 48 hours. Intravascular hemolysis, acute renal failure, elevated hepatic aminotransferases, and consumptive coagulopathy develop rarely in massive gasoline aspiration (9). Urinalysis is usually normal.

Diagnostic testing is directed at the hydrocarbon organ effects, especially the lung. *Chest radiography* correlates poorly with clinical symptoms. Infiltrates often appear within 30 minutes but may develop 12 hours after exposure. Up to 75% of patients hospitalized for suspected hydrocarbon aspiration have chest radiographic abnormalities. Asymptomatic patients may have an abnormal chest radiograph, but these changes usually clear without symptoms. Symptomatic patients may have a normal chest radiograph, especially within the first several hours. Most radiographic abnormalities are mild and do not progress (7). Radiographic changes peak 72 hours after exposure and clear within several days, although occasionally the changes persist for several months (10). Radiographic changes tend to lag behind clinical improvement.

Arterial blood gases reflect hypoxemia resulting from ventilation/perfusion mismatching (low PaO_2, low $PaCO_2$) rather than alveolar hypoventilation (high $PaCO_2$). Methemoglobinemia is a rare effect of aniline or nitrobenzene exposure (Chapter 21). Carboxyhemoglobinemia can occur after exposure to methylene chloride.

Treatment

STABILIZATION

The primary threat from petroleum distillate ingestion is respiratory failure. Patients should be quickly evaluated for respiratory signs (e.g., cyanosis, tachypnea, intercostal retractions) and given oxygen. Patients with inadequate tidal volume or poor arterial blood gases should be intubated. Because dysrhythmias complicate some hydrocarbon ingestions and electrocardiographic (ECG) evidence of myocardial injury has been reported (11), IV lines and cardiac monitors should be established in symptomatic patients. A chest radiograph should be taken immediately after stabilization of breathing and circulation to document aspiration and detect the presence of pneumothorax.

Continuous positive airway pressure or positive end expiratory pressure and intubation may be necessary in severe cases to maintain adequate oxygenation, but careful observation for the development of pneumothorax must be made during therapy. Epinephrine is not recommended for treatment of bronchospasm, because of potential myocardial sensitization to catecholamines. Inhaled cardioselective bronchodilators (e.g., albuterol, salbutamol) are the preferred bronchodilator agents.

DECONTAMINATION

All contaminated clothing should be removed, and contaminated skin areas washed with green soap (lipophilic) and water. GI decontamination in accidental petroleum distillate ingestions is not generally recommended because of the aspiration hazard and the low incidence of systemic toxicity after ingestion. Decontamination may be indicated when a toxic additive is present. The preferred method is simply aspiration using a small nasogastric tube. Syrup of ipecac is not recommended, especially in the following cases: (a) ingestion of highly viscous petroleum distillates with poor GI absorption, including asphalt or tar, mineral oil (e.g., household and automotive oils), home fuel oils, and diesel fuel oil; (b) ingestion of highly volatile petroleum distillates with minimal GI absorption, including mineral seal oil, furniture polish, and signal oil; (c) significant spontaneous vomiting.

Although activated charcoal does not bind to petroleum distillate products and may induce vomiting, *in vitro* studies suggest that large quantities of activated charcoal bind significant amounts of kerosene and turpentine (12,13). Activated charcoal may be useful when the patient has ingested a toxic additive.

ELIMINATION ENHANCEMENT

No known methods exist to enhance the elimination of hydrocarbon products.

ANTIDOTES

No known antidotes exist. Calcium disodium edetate and dimercaprol appear to increase urinary lead excretion. The effect on morbidity and mortality remains to be elucidated (14). The use of steroids in mild to moderate hydrocarbon aspiration pneumonia did not improve outcome in a double-blind, controlled human study (15).

SUPPORTIVE CARE

Serial evaluation of the blood count, acid-base status, fluid and electrolyte balance, renal and liver function, and arterial blood gases is needed for patients with serious pulmonary involvement. To avoid precipitating noncardiogenic pulmonary edema, IV fluid administration should be limited to normal replacement volume. Antibiotics should be reserved for documented bacterial pneumonia or increasing infiltrates, leukocytosis, and fever after the first 24 to 48 hours. Long-term follow-up care and pulmonary function testing should be established to detect the presence of obstructive pulmonary disease, which may be seen in asymptomatic children with a history of hydrocarbon aspiration pneumonitis (16).

Extracorporeal membrane oxygenation has been used as a temporary treatment for reversible acute pulmonary insufficiency to improve oxygenation when mechanical ventilator support is inadequate. Patients who do better with extracorporeal membrane oxygenation are those with earlier institution of treatment and younger children compared to older children (17,18). Extracorporeal membrane oxygenation is a potentially lifesaving option when a patient shows no response to conventional therapy (4).

HOSPITALIZATION

Immediate hospital admission is recommended for some patients: (a) symptomatic children who have abnormal initial chest x-rays, (b) patients with suicidal intent or massive ingestion, (c) hypoxic or obtunded patients regardless of radiographic findings, (d) patients with a substantially abnormal chest radiograph.

Admission after an observation period of 6 hours may be necessary in some cases: (a) asymptomatic children with a mildly abnormal chest radiograph who develop symptoms during the observation period; (b) asymptomatic patients who develop symptoms because of toxic additives (e.g., camphor, halogenated hydrocarbons); (c) mildly symptomatic children who have a normal chest radiograph but whose symptoms do not improve; (d) all patients for whom follow-up cannot be closely established.

Many patients may be discharged after a 6-hour observation period: (a) asymptomatic children with a normal chest radiograph and (b) asymptomatic children with a mildly abnormal chest radiograph who do not develop symptoms during the observation period.

DIBROMOCHLOROPROPANE

1,2-Dibromo-3-chloropropane [$C_3H_5Br_2Cl$; molecular weight (MW) 236.3 g/mol; CAS Registry No. 96-12-8] has not been used as a pesticide in the United States since 1979. It may still be available in other countries, from U.S. distributors for research purposes, or as chemical intermediates for the synthesis of brominated flame-retardant chemicals [tris(2,3-dibromopropyl) phosphate] (19,20).

Vulnerable Populations

Animal studies indicate no teratogenic effect or adverse effect on gestation. However, human effects have included azoospermia, without maternal adverse effect.

Clinical Presentation

In July 1977, pesticide production workers exposed to 1,2-dibromo-3-chloropropane were found to have a marked reduction in sperm density; 13% were azoospermic (21). These workers had more than 100 hours of estimated exposure in production. The seminiferous tubules were the site of damage (22). Men exposed for 10 to 90 hours were normospermic. The outcome of pregnancies fathered by the exposed men disclosed no evidence of an increase in spontaneous abortion, infant or fetal deaths, or congenital malformations (23). Permanent destruction of the germinal epithelium occurred in most of the sterile men (24). Many of the patients remained oligospermic or azoospermic on follow-up 11 years later. Testicular atrophy was observed with azoospermia and the testicles subsequently increased in size among those azoospermic subjects who returned to normospermic levels (25).

DIMETHYLAMINE

Dimethylamine ($C_{12}H_{18}N_2O_2$; MW 222.3 g/mol; CAS Registry No. 124-40-3) is used as an intermediate for the production of various chemicals, including solvents, surfactants, and pesticides. Measurement of urine levels provides an indication of body exposure to this amine. Dimethylamine is a short-chain aliphatic amine and is probably, like trimethylamine, a degradation product of trimethylamine *N*-oxide. Its pathophysiologic role is unclear. It is well absorbed (bioavailability 72%); 5% is demethylated to methylene, but 95% is secreted unchanged in the urine. The half-life is 6 to 7 hours. The plasma clearance is 190 ml/minute (26).

DIMETHYL SULFATE

Dimethyl sulfate (DMS; $C_2H_6O_4S$; MW 126.1 g/mol; CAS Registry No. 77-78-1) is an industrial chemical that can produce severe ocular reactions and delayed potentially fatal respiratory tract reactions. It is widely used as a methylating agent for the organic synthesis of chemicals, especially in the manufacture of pharmaceuticals, dyestuffs, perfume, and pesticides (27). DMS may be present in the environment because of industrial processes. It may be formed during the combustion of sulfur-containing fossil fuels. Efforts should be made to use enclosed systems in processes using DMS (28).

Toxic Dose

Regulatory standards and guidelines are provided in Table 4. One patient licked the finger to taste DMS and experienced immediate irritation of the soft palate, laryngeal constriction, and increased salivation that improved on treatment. Unexpectedly, sudden onset of edema of the glottis developed 24 hours later and death ensued. At autopsy, acute corrosive changes were seen in the upper GI tract with edema of the glottis and emphysema of the lungs (29).

Pathophysiology

When DMS comes in contact with a moist mucosal surface, it is hydrolyzed slowly into sulfuric acid, methanol, and methyl hydrogen sulfate. The methanol may be absorbed into the circulation, leading to neurotoxic effects; the sulfuric acid and methyl hydrogen sulfate induce severe irritation, anesthetic, and erosive effects on the mucosa (27).

TABLE 4. U.S. Regulatory Guidelines and Standards for dimethyl sulfate, leaded gasoline, and trimethylamine

		Concentration mg/m³ (ppm)		
Agency	**Description**	**Dimethyl sulfate**	**Gasoline tetraethyl leaded**	**Trimethyl-amine**
OSHA	PEL-TWA	5 (1)[a]	0.075 (.006)[a]	12 (5)
	STEL	None	None	36 (15)
ACGIH	TLV-TWA	0.5 (0.1)	0.1 (.007)	12 (5)
	STEL	None	None	36 (15)
NIOSH	REL-TWA	0.5 (0.1)	0.075 (.006)	24 (10)
	Ceiling	None	None	36 (15)
	IDLH	36 (7 ppm)	40 (3) as Pb	Not listed
Conversion factors		ppm × 5.16 = mg/m³	ppm × 13.2 = mg/m³	ppm × 2.42 = mg/m³

[a]Skin designation.
ACGIH, American Conference of Governmental Industrial Hygienists; IDLH, immediate danger to life or health; NIOSH, National Institute for Occupational Safety and Health; OSHA, U.S. Occupational Safety and Health Administration; PEL, permissible exposure limit; REL, recommended exposure limit; STEL, short-term exposure limit; TLV, threshold limit value; TWA, time-weighted average.

Vulnerable Populations

DMS was embryotoxic in rodent studies.

Clinical Presentation

DMS can induce chemical burns on a wet epithelium; it is a strong irritant to the eyes and respiratory mucosa where it may cause desquamation and necrosis (27). Intoxication is usually through accidental inhalation of the vapor or contamination of skin and mucosa by liquid or vapor. Acute exposure may be fatal (30,31).

Clinically, the usual manifestations include skin burns, corneal irritation with photophobia, lacrimation and blurring of vision, oropharyngeal edema and hoarseness of the voice, nasal septal necrosis, cough, and dyspnea (30). Mortality results from respiratory failure after mucosal inflammation, edema of major airways, and noncardiogenic pulmonary edema (30,32). Other systemic effects include convulsions; delirium; coma; and renal, hepatic, and cardiac failure (33,34). Irreversible loss of vision has been reported (28).

Clinical signs include fever (37.5° to 49°C), tachycardia, and tachypnea. Abnormal breath sounds, including wheezing, dry rales, and moist rales, may be heard. Congestion and edema of the eyes, pharynx, and uvula are observed. After 3 to 14 days, desquamation of the tracheal and bronchial mucosa occurs.

There is a mean latent period of 3 hours (range, 20 minutes to 12 hours) between exposure and onset of symptoms. DMS is particularly hazardous because of its delayed effects, lack of color, and minimal odor.

DMS is considered to be probably carcinogenic to humans by the International Agency for Research on Cancer and as reasonably anticipated to be a human carcinogen by the U.S. Department of Health and Human Services (35,36).

Diagnostic Tests

ENVIRONMENTAL MONITORING

A sensitive gas chromatography/mass spectrometry technique has been developed (37), and a fully automated gas chromatography method is available for the routine determination of DMS in the industrial setting (38).

ACUTE EXPOSURE

No abnormalities are usually seen in routine urinalyses, red blood cell count, or serum chemistries. Elevated white blood cell counts (10,500 to 24,000/mm^3) are observed. The ECG shows an inversion of T waves and elevation or depression of ST segments, especially in patients with bronchopneumonia, noncardiogenic pulmonary edema, and myocardial damage. Clinical studies of blood methanol or formate levels are not available but are indicated within the first 24 hours if there is evidence of neurotoxicity (39).

Lung function tests show a restrictive pattern when forced expiratory volume in 1 second, forced vital capacity, forced expiratory volume in 1 second/forced vital capacity, and diffusing capacity of lung for carbon monoxide studies are performed. Periodic chest radiography indicates peribronchitis, bilateral pulmonary infiltrates, and pulmonary edema (interstitial or alveolar). Pathologic examination of the sputum from severe cases often reveals fibrin, degenerated bronchial epithelium, and ruptured inflammatory cells.

Treatment

Because of its delayed effects, early clinical monitoring and treatment during the first 24 to 72 hours are important. Patients exposed to DMS should be treated as a medical emergency.

TABLE 5. Proposed criteria for grading and disposition of patients with dimethyl sulfate intoxication

Irritative reactions

A history of dimethyl sulfate exposure, with symptoms and signs of mucosal irritation in the eyes, nose, and pharynx. No systemic signs of intoxication. Normal chest radiographs; no leukocytosis. These patients may be released after symptomatic treatment and medical observation for 24–72 h.

Mild intoxication

In addition to the irritative reactions, signs of respiratory tract irritation and corrosive effect (congestion of pharynx, larynx, and uvula; abnormal breath sounds) and positive findings on more than one test (leukocytosis or chest radiographic films showing peribronchitis or electrocardiogram demonstrating myocardial damage). With treatment, patients usually recover in 3–7 d and resume their ordinary work.

Moderate intoxication

In addition to the manifestations of mild intoxication, necrosis and desquamation of the respiratory mucosa occurs, with more than two positive clinical findings (leukocytosis, electrocardiogram demonstrating myocardial damage, chest radiographic films showing pneumonia or interstitial pneumonia,) and no other complications. After treatment and rest, these patients may recover and resume ordinary work.

Severe intoxication

In addition to the manifestations of moderate intoxication, the patients may exhibit significant laryngeal edema, noncardiogenic pulmonary edema or shock, encephalopathy, or myocardial damage. Local and systemic supportive treatment is required, with use of glucocorticoids and antibiotics.

Modified from Ying W, Jing X, Qin-Wai W. Clinical report on 62 cases of acute dimethyl sulfate intoxication. *Am J Ind Med* 1988;13:455–462.

DECONTAMINATION

Induced emesis can be dangerous because of re-exposure of the esophagus to corrosive material and because of the danger of aspiration pneumonia and respiratory tract damage. Gastric lavage can be performed, preferably within 1 hour of ingestion with appropriate tracheal protection. Endoscopy determines the extent of esophageal and gastric injury.

Oral exposure is managed as a corrosive acid ingestion (Chapter 201). Eye exposure is treated with copious irrigation with water or normal saline for at least 20 to 30 minutes. For skin exposure, all contaminated clothing should be removed and exposed skin washed thoroughly with water or saline.

ELIMINATION ENHANCEMENT

There have been no clinical studies on DMS elimination. If neurotoxic effects consistent with methanol poisoning appear, the use of ethanol or hemodialysis should be considered.

ANTIDOTE

There are no antidotes for DMS exposure.

SUPPORTIVE MEASURES

Systemic treatment depends on the severity of exposure (Table 5). All patients exposed to DMS should be admitted to a hospital for observation for at least 24 hours.

Ocular exposures are treated with topical steroid and antibiotic medications for the prevention and treatment of inflammation. Caution must be exercised when using steroids in the presence of corneal injury. Most cases of mild corneal and conjunctival injury resolve within 24 hours (27). Careful ophthalmologic follow-up is indicated for all patients with eye injuries.

Respiratory injury is treated with antibiotics and humidified oxygen (34). Repeated aerosol inhalations have been administered to patients with respiratory tract injury (dexamethasone 5 mg, aminophylline 0.25 g, and streptomycin 0.5 g or gentamicin 80,000 U in 50 ml normal saline; 10 to 20 ml/time, to 6 hours/time, 2 to 8 times/day). For those who have inhaled high concentrations of DMS, early administration of hydrocortisone (300 to 1100 mg IV) or dexamethasone (15 to 55 mg) in short courses (2 to 6 days) may prove beneficial. In addition, antibiotics, atropine, and postural drainage have been administered. Isolation procedures may be indicated. Adult respiratory distress syndrome caused by chemical pneumonitis has been treated by the previously mentioned measures without tracheotomy. Continuous, intermittent, positive pressure oxygen inhalation has been given for 10 to 16 hours until hypoxia was corrected.

Patients who have been exposed to DMS should have periodic follow-up studies to include visual, respiratory tract, and ECG examinations. Most resume suitable work.

SAFETY AND HEALTH MEASURES

All operations using DMS should be carried out in fully enclosed systems with arrangements made for removing spillage. Workers should be supplied with respiratory protective equipment, chemical eye protective wear, protective clothing, and rubber gloves. Workers should be instructed not to attempt to do a hasty cleanup of massive spillage in the event of a container breakage (33). Workers with disease of the CNS, lungs, kidneys, or liver should be precluded from working with DMS.

DIMETHYL SULFOXIDE

Dimethyl sulfoxide (DMSO; Rims 50, Dermasorb, DMS-70, DMS-90, Dromisol, Gamasol 90, Hyadur, Infiltrina, Somnipront, Syntexan; C_2H_6OS (40); MW 78.13 g/mol; CAS Registry No. 67-68-5) is a synthetic chemical capable of inducing renal, hepatic, hematopoietic, or CNS dysfunction after IV administration. Few controlled human studies have been performed.

DMSO is widely used as an industrial solvent for organic and inorganic chemicals (41). Thus, it is necessary to evaluate the patient for exposure to the dissolved chemical as well. In the United States, a 50% weight/weight aqueous solution is available clinically for intravesical instillation used for interstitial cystitis (42). DMSO has been used as a vehicle for other drugs and has been tried for various cutaneous and musculoskeletal disorders but without proven efficacy (41). DMSO has been used to protect living cells during cold storage (43). In mice, DMSO exerts a protective effect against acetaminophen-induced hepatotoxicity (44,45). Clinical studies are under way on 10% DMSO as a treatment for intractable cerebral edema (46,47).

Toxic Dose

Topical application of 80% DMSO daily for 12 weeks did not result in ocular toxicity (48). Instillation of 7.5% to 60% DMSO in tetrahydrozoline for 1 to 15 months in patients with ocular problems did not induce ocular toxicity (49). Daily injection of 10% to 40% DMSO for 3 days at a dose of 1 g/kg IV resulted in a dose-dependent hemolysis with hemoglobinuria (50,51). The lethal dose has not been established in humans.

Toxicokinetics and Toxicodynamics

Ingestion of 1 g/kg DMSO resulted in a peak serum concentration of approximately 1000 to 3000 μg/ml within 4 hours. The dimethyl sulfone ($DMSO_2$) concentration peaked 72 to 96 hours after administration with values of 300 to 600 g/ml (52). Dermal application of 1 g/kg of DMSO produced a maximum serum level of $DMSO_2$ of 500 μg/ml within 4 to 8 hours. Serum DMSO levels become maximal at 300 to 500 μg/ml after 36 to 72 hours

(52). Eight hours after the cutaneous application of 2 g of 90% DMSO, 20% remained at the application site. Within 24 hours, 10% to 15% of the total dose appeared in the urine (53).

The elimination half-life of oral DMSO is 20 hours; $DMSO_2$ has a half-life of 72 hours. At 120 hours, 50% of an oral dose was excreted in the urine as DMSO and 9.6% as $DMSO_2$ (52). The half-life of dermal DMSO is approximately 11 to 14 hours; the $DMSO_2$ half-life is 60 to 70 hours (52). DMSO is metabolized in humans by oxidation to $DMSO_2$ or by reduction to dimethyl sulfide. DMSO and $DMSO_2$ are excreted in the urine and feces. Dimethyl sulfide is eliminated through the breath and skin and is responsible for the characteristic odor (42). $DMSO_2$ can persist in the serum for more than 2 weeks after a single intravesical installation (42).

Drug Interactions

DMSO has been shown to enhance the absorption of heparin, insulin, sodium salicylate, Evans blue dye, sulfadiazine, aminophylline, and thiotepa in animals (54). Other drugs include iron chloride, tertiary and quaternary ammonium compounds, glucocorticoids, local anesthetics, and antifungal, antibacterial, and anticholinesterase agents (55).

Pathophysiology

DMSO appears to penetrate cell membranes due to its ability to form hydrogen bonds and to displace water (56). It has also been reported to have antiinflammatory, local analgesic, diuretic, vasodilatory properties, and to dissolve collagen (57).

Vulnerable Populations

DMSO is U.S. Food and Drug Administration pregnancy category C (42). Teratogenic effects have been found in animals. Excretion in breast milk is unknown. Safety and effectiveness in children has not been established.

Clinical Presentation

Intravesical administration may produce a garlic-like taste that may remain for 72 hours. Transient chemical cystitis follows its use. *Dermal application* has resulted in pruritus, urticaria, erythema, eosinophilia, a garlic odor to the breath, fatigue, headache, nausea, dizziness, eye irritation, exfoliation, and pigmentation at sites of chronic use (58). A 63-year-old arthritic patient applied 90% DMSO topically and experienced mixed sensorimotor peripheral neuropathy and segmental demyelination (59).

IV use is associated with dose-dependent intravascular hemolysis, bilirubinemia, and hemoglobinuria (50,51). When used as a carrier for other drugs, DMSO may enhance their toxic effects (41). Abnormalities in renal function tests, hepatic enzymes, and coagulation parameters have been observed (60,61). Transient encephalopathy, dysarthric speech, disorientation, hypoactive reflexes, and altered consciousness have been described (60–63). Symptoms may not clear for a week. Acute tubular necrosis followed two 100 g IV infusions of 20% DMSO (60).

Diagnostic Tests

DMSO and $DMSO_2$ have been measured by flame-ionization or electrocapture gas chromatography after solvent extraction or protein precipitation (64).

IV administration of DMSO led to serum concentrations of DMSO (1600 μg/ml) and $DMSO_2$ (3000 μg/ml), which were associated with a severe garlic odor, disorientation, and dysarthric speech (62).

After dermal applications, infrequent elevations of renal function tests and hepatic enzymes may occur (63); eosinophilia has been observed. Creatine kinase levels may increase (60). Prothrombin and partial thromboplastin times may decrease (60,61).

Treatment

DECONTAMINATION

Excess amounts of DMSO on the skin require vigorous irrigation with water or saline. Oral overdose with DMSO has not been reported. An attempt should be made to empty the gastric contents with tracheal protection. Emetic agents have not been evaluated.

Use protective clothing, including gloves and head, foot, and body protection, to minimize skin contact. Use goggles and face shield when danger of splashing exists. Avoid breathing a spray, mist, or high-concentration vapors of DMSO.

An overdose of DMSO during intravesical use may result in chemical cystitis. Bladder antispasmodics and analgesic medications may be useful.

INTRAVENOUS USE

There may be an enhanced possibility of developing signs and symptoms of CNS, renal, hepatic, or hematopoietic dysfunction after IV use. Treatment is supportive and symptomatic. Renal failure, unresponsive to conservative management, may respond to extracorporeal treatment measures. A paucity of toxicokinetic data does not provide a guide for the clinician. Clinical judgment based on severity of symptoms and laboratory parameters must form the basis for initiating hemodialysis or hemoperfusion.

ANTIDOTES

There are no antidotes for DMSO.

GASOLINE, JET FUEL, AND STODDARD SOLVENT

Gasoline (65–67) is a refined petroleum product that is highly flammable and potentially explosive. It contains more than 250 hydrocarbons and small quantities of additives and blending agents. The composition of gasoline varies by geographic region, season, performance requirements, and blending stocks. The typical hydrocarbon content of gasoline (percent volume) is approximately 60% to 70% alkanes (straight chain, branched chain, and cyclic), 5% to 10% alkenes (straight chain and branched chain), and 25% to 30% aromatics. Benzene, a known hematotoxic agent, constitutes approximately 1% of gasoline in the United States but can be as high as 5% in European formulations.

Leaded gasoline contains more than 0.05 g lead/g of gasoline. Organic lead is added to enhance a fuel's octane rating. The use of leaded gasoline in the United States ceased in 1997. However, organic lead compounds are still added to gasoline in other parts of the world. Replacements for organic lead antiknock agents include ethanol, methanol, methyl tertiary butyl ether, and tertiary butyl ether, which are typically added in concentrations of 5% to 15%.

Self-service gasoline customers typically experience short exposures (2 minutes) to hydrocarbons during refueling of approximately 200 parts per million (ppm) and less than 1 ppm benzene. These exposures are far below occupational limits. Refinery workers and people involved in removal and maintenance of underground storage tanks are at greatest risk of exposure.

Exposure to liquid gasoline also occurs by unintentional or intentional ingestion, accidental skin contact, or by misuse of the solvent. Misuse of gasoline, especially to clean and degrease floors, tools, and machine parts, represents the single most important health risk from gasoline for the general public. Persons who ingest gasoline while siphoning and those who intentionally inhale gasoline vapors to obtain euphoric effects risk serious health consequences.

Toxic Dose

Occupational standards and guidelines are provided in Table 4. Single oral doses of approximately 10 ml/kg body weight (or approximately 700 ml for an adult) may be fatal. Smaller amounts, if aspirated into the lungs, may lead to lipoid pneumonitis.

Toxicokinetics and Toxicodynamics

Gasoline can be absorbed by inhalation, ingestion, and dermal exposure routes. The hydrocarbon components with higher blood/gas partition coefficients in the lungs (e.g., xylene, benzene, toluene) have a higher absorption rate during inhalation than components with lower coefficients (e.g., cyclohexane, ethane, ethylene) (Table 6). Dermal absorption is low compared with absorption after ingestion. Aromatic hydrocarbons such as benzene have higher skin penetration than the alkanes.

After ingestion, the highest gasoline concentrations are in the liver, gastric wall, and lungs. Service station attendants (dermal contact as well as inhalation exposure) have elevated blood levels of hydrocarbons such as benzene, toluene, pentane, and hexane.

Mixed-function oxygenase activity is accelerated by gasoline. Some gasoline hydrocarbons are oxidized by liver microsomal-enzyme systems to products that are readily excreted in the urine. Alkanes are stable, saturated compounds that are not metabolized. Most of what is systemically absorbed is excreted unchanged through the lungs. Urinary phenol, a biological indicator of benzene exposure, is elevated in gasoline-pump workers (average, 40 mg/L) compared with persons with no occupational exposure to gasoline (less than 20 mg/L).

Pathophysiology

Tetraethyl and tetramethyl lead are rapidly absorbed through inhalation and skin contact. These organic lead compounds are rapidly dealkylated by the liver to trialkyl metabolites that are toxic. The trialkyl metabolites, which are water soluble, can accumulate in the brain and are slowly metabolized to inorganic lead.

Ingestion of large amounts of gasoline can result in absorption of methanol sufficient to produce methanol toxicity. Methanol toxicity in humans is rarely attributed to gasoline inhalation exposure. Depending on the dose and exposure route, 20% to 70% of the absorbed methyl tertiary butyl ether is rapidly exhaled. When metabolized, methyl tertiary butyl ether is oxidized to formaldehyde and demethylated to tertiary butyl alcohol, which may then be further oxidized to 2-methyl-1,2-propanediol and alpha-hydroxyisobutyric acid. These oxidation products are excreted in the urine.

TABLE 6. U.S. Regulatory Guidelines and Standards for aromatic hydrocarbons

Agency	Description	Concentration [mg/m³ (ppm)] Benzene	Toluene	Xylene
OSHA	PEL-TWA	32 (10)	750 (200)	435 (100)
	STEL	None	None	None
	Ceiling (10 min)	80 (25)	1125 (300)	None
	Peak above ceiling	160 (50)	1875 (500)	—
ACGIH	TLV-TWA	1.6 (0.5)	187.5 (50)	435 (100)
	STEL	8 (2.5)	None	652 (150)
NIOSH	STEL-TWA	0.3 (0.1)	375 (100)	435 (100)
	Ceiling	0.3 (0.1)	560 (150)	652 (150)
	IDLH	1595 (500)	1875 (500)	3915 (900)
Conversion factor		mg/m³ = ppm × 3.19	mg/m³ = ppm × 3.75	mg/m³ = ppm × 4.35

ACGIH, American Conference of Governmental Industrial Hygienists; IDLH, immediate danger to life or health; NIOSH, National Institute for Occupational Safety and Health; OSHA, U.S. Occupational Safety and Health Administration; PEL, permissible exposure limit; ppm, parts per million; STEL, short-term exposure limit; TLV, threshold limit value; TWA, time-weighted average.

Clinical Presentation

ACUTE EXPOSURE

Inhalation is the most common route of exposure. The CNS is the major target organ. High-concentration exposure by any route causes confusion, tinnitus, disorientation, headache, drowsiness, weakness, seizures, and coma. Inhalation may produce respiratory tract irritation, resulting in dyspnea, tachypnea, and rales that may progress rapidly to massive noncardiogenic pulmonary edema; a burning sensation in the chest may be present. Pulmonary congestion, edema, acute exudative tracheobronchitis, and intrapulmonary hemorrhage have also been observed.

Ingestion causes pain and irritation of the mucous membranes, resulting in nausea, vomiting, abdominal pain, and diarrhea. Irritation and dermatitis can occur after skin contact, and conjunctivitis can occur after eye contact. Prolonged contact with liquid gasoline can defat the skin and cause irritation and dermatitis.

CHRONIC EXPOSURE

Exposures to gasoline and its constituents, including benzene, *n*-hexane, and 1,3-butadiene during refueling of motor vehicles are not a serious health hazard for consumers. Organic lead compounds can produce chronic neurologic toxicity, particularly in countries without exposure limits. Ethanol, methanol, and other additives in gasoline pose potential exposure risks, particularly through unintentional ingestion or suicide attempts. Long-term exposure to gasoline vapor may lead to blood dyscrasias such as anemia, hypochromia, thrombocytopenia, and neutropenia thought to be due to the benzene component.

CHRONIC ABUSE

The intentional abuse (e.g., sniffing or *huffing*) of gasoline can result in death from acute exposure. Chronic abuse of leaded gasoline may cause a range of neurologic effects, including encephalopathy, ataxia, and tremor. Chronic sniffers of leaded gasoline may show neurologic effects with elevated blood lead levels. Chronic abuse of gasoline through sniffing can cause cardiac dysrhythmias and tachycardia.

CARCINOGENICITY

Epidemiologic studies have not substantiated the carcinogenic effects observed in experimental animals. The International Agency for Research on Cancer categorizes gasoline as a possible human carcinogen.

Diagnostic Tests

ACUTE EXPOSURE

Acute exposure is evaluated with a careful pulmonary evaluation, including a baseline chest radiograph to assess possible spiration. A follow-up chest radiograph should be obtained in pproximately 6 hours if pulmonary symptoms develop. Pulse ximetry or arterial blood gas analyses may be needed to assess xygenation. After severe, acute overexposure to gasoline, egenerative changes may occur in the liver and kidneys; these ffects should be evaluated through routine laboratory testing.

CHRONIC EXPOSURE

Chronic exposure evaluation in the patient with neurologic signs and symptoms includes neurobehavioral testing and electroencephalography.

Treatment

Treatment largely involves the symptomatic and supportive care of the effects of aspiration or dermal exposure. Supportive care includes management of depressed mental status and mild dermal effects. Respiratory compromise may require supplemental oxygen and tracheal intubation in rare cases. The patient should be monitored several hours for emerging signs of aspiration.

After ingestion, vomiting should not be induced because of the risk of pulmonary aspiration. Activated charcoal is of limited use. If skin or hair has been in contact with liquid gasoline, remove clothing and flush skin and hair with water for 2 to 3 minutes. Wash with mild soap; rinse thoroughly with water. If eye contact has occurred, the eye should be flushed with water for at least 5 minutes or until pain resolves.

In most cases of chronic exposure, cessation usually leads to complete recovery, even for patients who have evidence of CNS toxicity.

No specific antidotes exist for gasoline.

JET FUELS

Aviation fuel causes acute and chronic effects (68–71). It consists of straight-chain and branched-chain alkanes (paraffins), cyclic alkanes (naphthenes), alkenes (olefins), and aromatic hydrocarbons. Jet propellants (JP), JP-4, JP-5, JP-7, and JP-8, are grades of jet propulsion fuel. Components include benzene, xylene, and toluene.

Acute exposure causes CNS depression, dizziness, nausea, and vomiting. Chronic exposure is associated with neuropsychiatric disorders and peripheral sensory neuropathy, as well as dermatitis. Tests of liver function are usually normal. Inhalation may cause respiratory tract irritation. Ingestion may lead to coughing, dyspnea, tachypnea, rapidly developing pulmonary edema, and potentially fatal aspiration pneumonitis. The carcinogenic effects are unknown.

Treatment is the same as for gasoline. There is no specific treatment for chronic jet fuel toxicity. Recovery occurs within a few days after exposure.

STODDARD SOLVENT

Stoddard solvent is the name adopted by the National Association of Dryers and Cleaners to honor W.J. Stoddard for his work with petroleum distillates used in the dry cleaning industry. Stoddard solvent is a distillation fraction of crude petroleum [distilling between approximately 300°F (149°C) and 400°F (204°C)] that contains at least 200 products, predominantly C_7 through C_{12} hydrocarbons. The mixture typically consists of 30% to 40% alicyclic and 10% to 20% aromatic hydrocarbons. (Benzene, toluene, and xylene each represent less than 1% of the total mixture.) Although the toxicity of Stoddard solvent is not attributable to any one type of constituent, the aromatic components are considered to be more toxic than the paraffin or naphthalene components. Stoddard solvent is a colorless, flammable liquid that is insoluble in water. The odor threshold for Stoddard solvent is less than 1 ppm. However, odor is not a reliable indicator of dangerous concentrations because the olfactory sense fatigues after a few minutes and Stoddard solvent is no longer detected by smell.

Stoddard solvent is a solvent used in industry primarily as a dry cleaning solvent, metal degreaser, and extractant. Consumers may be exposed to Stoddard solvent through inhalation or dermal contact with cleaning products, paints, paint thinners, furniture refinishers, pesticides, or residues on dry cleaned products (72,73).

Toxic Dose

Acute exposure to Stoddard solvent at air concentrations below the odor threshold produces no adverse health effects.

Toxicokinetics and Toxicodynamics

Stoddard solvent is metabolized in the liver, thus preexisting liver disease (e.g., hepatitis, cirrhosis) decreases the rate of metabolism and increases the amount of Stoddard solvent in the blood. Excretion occurs by the lungs and kidneys; persons with lung impairment (e.g., chronic obstructive pulmonary disease) or renal insufficiency may retain Stoddard solvent or its metabolites, thereby increasing their risk of toxicity.

Vulnerable Populations

Petroleum solvents can enter breast milk.

Clinical Presentation

The major effect associated with inhalation of paraffin-like solvents is CNS excitation followed rapidly by CNS depression. Reported symptoms of acute exposure to Stoddard solvent include lightheadedness, dizziness, visual disturbances, and drowsiness. Although case reports have been published of persons who were exposed to Stoddard solvent and subsequently experienced liver, kidney, or hematologic injury, a causal relationship has not been firmly established. Cardiac dysrhythmias have not been reported in humans after exposure to Stoddard solvent (72,73).

ACUTE EXPOSURE

Acute exposure to high concentrations of Stoddard solvent can irritate mucous membranes and cause upper respiratory tract irritation. Acute ingestion and attendant aspiration of hydrocarbon mixtures similar to Stoddard solvent have resulted in chemical pneumonitis that mimics adult respiratory distress syndrome. Complications of severe overexposure by the aspiration route may also include noncardiogenic pulmonary edema, pulmonary emphysema, pneumothorax, pleuritis, pleural effusion, empyema, and pneumatoceles. Stoddard solvent is a skin irritant.

CHRONIC EXPOSURE

Chronic exposure to Stoddard solvent has been associated with headaches, fatigue, intermittent episodes of inebriation, and memory deficits that generally resolve on discontinuation of exposure.

CARCINOGENESIS

Carcinogenic effects from dermal exposure in experimental animals and inhalation exposure in humans have not been conclusively demonstrated.

Diagnostic Tests

Blood gas analyses, chest radiography, ECG monitoring, and baseline liver and kidney function tests should be considered in serious overexposures. No specific hydrocarbon in the plasma or tissues is a reproducible index of exposure.

Treatment

After acute exposure, the patient should be removed immediately from the source of exposure. Decontamination includes removal of contaminated clothing and washing of exposed areas with mild soap and shampoo. Direct eye splashes should be treated by irrigation with saline or water for 15 minutes or until pain resolves. Supplemental oxygen should be administered as needed. Gastric decontamination is not recommended in most cases. Corticosteroids and prophylactic antibiotics are not necessary for chemical pneumonitis. Patients who are asymptomatic after 6 hours of observation may be discharged from the hospital.

In cases of chronic exposure with persistent neurologic symptoms, neuropsychologic testing may be useful for diagnostic purposes and to establish baseline function.

METHANETHIOL

Methanethiol (Methyl mercaptan; CH_3SH; MW 48.11 g/mol; CAS Registry No. 74-93-1) is derived from the breakdown of methionine or the methylation of hydrogen sulfide. It is produced by decaying matter and can be found around marshes, sewage, and pulp mills. It is metabolized by oxidation to disulfides such as dimethyl disulfide ($CH_3S\text{-}SCH_3$) to sulfate, methylation to dimethyl sulfide (CH_3SCH_3), acetylation to thiolesters, and glucuronylation to thioglucuronides (74). It may be one of the endogenous factors involved in the pathogenesis of hepatic encephalopathy (75). Methanethiol and dimethyl sulfide have been found in the urine of patients with fulminant hepatic failure. The odor on the breath of patients with cirrhosis given methionine is caused by dimethyl sulfide (76). Somnolence and disorientation in cirrhotic patients are probably caused by methanethiol from which dimethyl sulfide is derived (74).

Clinical Presentation

Occupational exposure to methanethiol may induce headache, nausea, vomiting, eye irritation, chest tightness and wheezing, dizziness, diplopia, and a productive cough (77).

Laboratory

Methanethiol may be quantified by gas chromatography and mass spectrometry (74).

Treatment

Treatment is the same as for dimethyl sulfide.

MONOOCTANOIN

Monooctanoin has been used to dissolve cholesterol gallstones by intrabiliary perfusion. Rapid perfusion may result in respiratory compromise and cardiac arrest. It is a mixture of glycerol esters, principally glycerol monooctanoate (Capmine 8210, Moctanin; $C_{19}H_{22}O_4$, MW 218.3 g/mol, CAS Registry No. 26402-26-6 (78,79).

Toxic Dose

Monooctanoin is used therapeutically by continuous perfusion through a catheter inserted into the common bile duct for 7 to 21 days (78). Fatal cardiac arrest followed 0.4 ml injected through a central venous catheter (80).

Clinical Presentation

Abdominal pain, nausea, vomiting, and diarrhea occur frequently in patients treated with monooctanoin, especially with rapid infusion. There have been two associated deaths: one patient died from blood loss caused by a duodenal ulcer, and the other died from pancreatitis (79–83). Dyspnea, hypoxemia, and respiratory compromise have followed intrabiliary monooctanoin use.

A 57-year-old patient was accidentally given less than 1 ml of monooctanoin through a central venous catheter. The patient experienced respiratory and cardiac arrest. Nine hours later the patient experienced ventricular fibrillation and died. Autopsy confirmed the cause of death as respiratory failure secondary to lung infiltration of monooctanoin (80,84).

Treatment

Treatment is symptomatic and supportive. If symptoms develop, the monooctanoin is terminated. There is no known antidote.

TRIMELLITIC ANHYDRIDE

Trimellitic anhydride (anhydrotrimellitic acid, 1,2,4-benzenene tricarboxylic acid anhydrone; TMA; $C_9H_4O_5$; MW 192.1 g/mol; CAS Registry No. 552-30-7) is a white crystalline solid. It is used as a curing agent for epoxy and other resins and as a vinyl plasticizer. It is also found in anticorrosive surface coatings, polymers, paints, dyes, and pharmaceuticals. These products find applications in high-temperature plastics, wire insulation, gaskets, and automobile upholstery.

Toxic Dose

American Conference of Governmental Industrial Hygienists' ceiling limit is 0.04 mg/m^3. National Institute for Occupational Safety and Health 10-hour time-weighted average is 0.04 mg/m^3 (0.005 ppm).

Clinical Presentation

TMA induces four clinical syndromes in humans (85,86), three of which are thought to be immunologically related (85–88). The first is an immunoglobulin E (IgE)–mediated allergic rhinitis; the second is a late respiratory systemic syndrome characterized by cough, dyspnea, myalgia, fever, and chills that occur 4 to 12 hours after TMA inhalation. This is correlated with high levels of IgG, IgM, and IgA antibody to trimellitic-substituted human proteins. The third syndrome is a pulmonary disease–anemia syndrome that is characterized by dyspnea, cough, hemoptysis, and symptoms related to anemia. This syndrome may lead to respiratory failure; associated clinical findings are restrictive lung disease, infiltrates on a chest roentgenogram, and hypoxemia. Pulmonary hemosiderosis may be found on biopsy.

A fourth nonimmunologic, irritant syndrome reflects upper airway irritation in response to high concentrations of TMA dust or fumes. Treatment is symptomatic and supportive (85–88).

TRIMETHYLAMINE

Trimethylamine (*N-N*-dimethylmethaneamine; $(CH_3)_3N$; MW 59.1 g/mol; CAS Registry No. 75-50-3) is a colorless gas used as an insect attractant, as a warming agent for natural gas, and in organic synthesis. It may be an irritant to the eyes, mucous membranes, and lungs (89). The fish odor syndrome, recessively inherited, is probably due to trimethylamine in the sweat. Acidic soaps and body lotions convert trimethylamine to an odorless oxide (90,91).

Occupational guidelines and standards are provided in Table 4. The odor threshold for trimethylamine is 0.44 ppm.

HALOGENATED HYDROCARBONS—HALOGENATED SOLVENTS

The halogenated hydrocarbons are a diverse class of chemicals that are used widely in industry. They can cause profound CNS and cardiovascular toxic effects because of their halogen substitutions. They also cause eye and skin irritation and are systemically absorbed through the lungs and skin. Some of these chemicals are banned or restricted because of their health hazards.

Most halogenated hydrocarbons are clear and colorless liquids that are flammable and have chloroform or ether-like odors. This latter property arises from their low boiling points, which allows them to vaporize readily. Most of these chemicals contain impurities, such as other halogenated hydrocarbons, which result from the synthesis of these chemicals. The pyrolysis of certain chlorinated compounds (e.g., carbon tetrachloride, chlorinated fluorocarbons, chloroform, vinyl chloride) can lead to the production of phosgene and hydrochloric acid, which can cause respiratory irritation.

There are a wide variety of uses for these chemicals, including solvent, chemical intermediates, propellants, fumigants, degreasers, paint and varnish remover. In homes, products that can contain these chemicals include spot removers, aerosol products, water repellents, and furniture polishes. Table 7 lists commercial uses of halogenated solvents.

TABLE 7. Uses of halogenated hydrocarbons

1,1-Dichloroethane	Cleansing agent; degreaser; solvent for plastics, oils, and fats; grain fumigant; chemical intermediate.
1,2-Dichloroethane	Manufacture of ethyl glycol, polyvinyl chloride, nylon, viscose rayon, styrene-butadiene, rubber; solvent; degreaser; extracting agents; fumigant.
1,2-Dichloroethylene	Solvent for waxes, resins, and ethylcellulose; extract of rubber; refrigerant; manufacture of pharmaceuticals.
Dichloromethane (methylene dichloride)	Solvent, paint remover, manufacture of photographic fixant, aerosol propellants, urethane foam, degreaser.
Dichloropropane (propylene dichloride)	Degreasing, dry cleaning, soil fumigant, manufacture of cellulose plastics, metal degreasing, stain remover, chemical intermediates.
Tetrabromoethane (acetylene tetrabromide)	Gauge fluid, solvent, refractive index liquid in microscopy.
Tetrachloromethane (carbon tetrachloride)	Manufacture of fluorocarbon propellants (Freon 2, Freon 11, Freon 12); solvent for oils, fats, lacquers, varnishes, and resins; degreasing and cleaning agents; grain fumigant. Synthesis of fluorocarbons, dry cleaning agents, fire extinguisher agents.
1,1,1-Trichloroethane	Solvent for adhesives (including food packaging adhesives), metal degreasing, pesticides, textile processing, vapor degreasing, aerosols, coating, and inks. Used primarily for cold-cleaning, dip cleaning, bucket cleaning.
Trichloroethylene	Vapor degreasing of fabricated metal parts, chemical intermediates, general solvent, refrigerant, typewriter correction fluids, paint removers/stuffers, adhesives, rug cleaning fluids, spot removers.
Tetrachloroethylene	Solvent, chemical intermediate (for synthesis of fluorocarbon 113), dry cleaning and textile processing, industrial metal cleaning, vapor and liquid degreasing agent, anthelminthic, pesticide, intermediate.
1,1,2,2-Tetrachloroethane	Feed stock, in the production of trichloroethylene, tetrachloroethylene, and 1,2-dichloroethylene solvent, cleaning and degreasing metals in paint removers.
1,1,2-Trichloro-1,2,2-trifluoroethane (Fluorocarbon 113, Freon 113)	Solvent for cleaning electronic equipment and degreasing of machinery, refrigerant, fire extinguishers, dry cleaning, polymer intermediates.

Toxic Dose

Occupational standards and guidelines are provided in Table 8. Many of these chemicals can be absorbed through the skin. The toxic dose is described by various means because they can be absorbed by dermal, GI, and inhalational routes. For example, carbon tetrachloride causes headaches, dizziness, and drowsiness at approximately 2000 ppm for 5 to 10 minutes. An exposure of 10,000 ppm for several minutes causes slurred speech and stupor, and death can occur at 20,000 ppm (92). Orally, the estimated fatal adult dose is 90 to 100 ml, but wide variability results from ingestion, and as little as 5 to 10 ml has been reported to cause death (93).

Death occurred after extensive dermal contact with a 0.1% solution of ethylene dibromide for 20 to 60 minutes (94). Methylene chloride is metabolized to carbon monoxide. An 8-hour exposure to 150 ppm of methylene chloride produced carboxyhemoglobin levels similar to those produced by exposure to 35 ppm of carbon monoxide.

Toxicokinetics and Toxicodynamics

Oral absorption is rapid but less complete than pulmonary absorption. Skin absorption is insignificant, except in patients with skin breakdown (e.g., burns, ulcers, severe ichthyosis) (95,96). Increased metabolic rate can lead to greater inhalational absorption as well. Peak blood levels occur soon after inhalation but occur in 1 to 2 hours after oral administration. The chemicals distribute to tissues with high blood flow (e.g., brain, heart, liver, kidney) and then to adipose tissue, where the highest chemical concentrations are typically found.

Halogenated hydrocarbons are metabolized in the liver by cytochrome P-450 oxidation. Partial glutathione conjugation may occur. Halogenated solvents can be excreted unchanged through the lungs. Elimination half-lives can be increased because of either prolonged exposure or hepatic dysfunction. Prolonged exposure allows more chemical to be stored in the adipose tissue, which serves as a source of continued release.

Methylene chloride undergoes oxidative metabolism to yield carbon monoxide and carbon dioxide (97). The carboxyhemoglobin elimination half-life after methylene chloride ingestion is longer than after direct carbon monoxide inhalation.

Pregnancy and Lactation

Halogenated solvents cross the placenta and are found in the cord blood (79a). Tetrachloroethylene was measured in breast

TABLE 8. U.S. Regulatory Guidelines and Standards for halogenated hydrocarbons

Agency	Description	Concentration [mg/m³ (ppm)]				
		Carbon tetrachloride	Chloroform[a]	Ethylene dibromide	Methylene chloride	Trichloroethylene
OSHA	PEL-TWA	63 (10)	240 (50, ceiling)	154 (20)	87 (25)	537 (100)
	STEL	157 (25, ceiling)	None	230 (30, ceiling)	434 (125)	1074 (200, ceiling)
	Peak (in 4-h period)	1258 (200)	None	384 (50)	—	1611 (300)
ACGIH	TLV-TWA	31 (5)	50 (10)	None	174 (50)	268 (50)
	STEL	63 (10)	None	—	None	537 (100)
NIOSH	PEL-TWA	12.6 (2)	9.8 (2)	0.35 (0.045)	87 (25)	134 (25)
	Ceiling	None	None	1 (0.13)	None	10.7 (2)
	IDLH	1258 (200)	2440 (500)	768 (100)	7981 (2300)	5370 (1000)
Conversion factors		ppm × 6.29 = mg/m³	ppm × 4.88 = mg/m³	ppm × 7.68 = mg/m³	ppm × 3.47 = mg/m³	ppm × 5.37 = mg/m³

ACGIH, American Conference of Governmental Industrial Hygienists; IDLH, immediate danger to life or health; NIOSH, National Institute for Occupational Safety and Health; OSHA, U.S. Occupational Safety and Health Administration; PEL, permissible exposure limit; ppm, parts per million; STEL, short-term exposure limit; TLV, threshold limit value; TWA, time-weighted average.

[a]Skin designation.

milk after maternal exposure, and obstructive jaundice developed in the breast-fed infant (98).

Pathophysiology

Carbon tetrachloride is a hepatotoxin that causes acute fatty degeneration of the liver. Formation and release of low-density lipoproteins are significantly blocked, resulting in the rapid accumulation of fat. Although the exact mechanism of hepatic necrosis has not been entirely elucidated, cleavage of the carbon-chlorine bond produces trichlormethyl and monatomic chlorine-free radicals, which leads to lipid peroxidation (99). Energy processes and protein synthesis in the endoplasmic reticulum are disrupted. Covalent binding of radicals to cell organelles as well as lipid peroxidation contributes to the hepatic damage. However, not all compounds that protect against carbon tetrachloride toxicity are antioxidants, and nonhepatic tissue damage occurs in the rat model without an increase in lipid peroxidation (100). Aliphatic alcohols including methanol, ethanol, and isopropanol increase carbon tetrachloride hepatorenal toxicity in animals and humans (101), perhaps by mechanisms that include enzyme induction (104).

Clinical Presentation

ACUTE EXPOSURE

Acute exposures present initially with CNS depression followed by organ injury. Inhalation induces CNS depression within minutes. Early symptoms include lightheadedness, headache, and malaise that progresses to ataxia, stupor, and coma. Depending on the chemical and the duration of exposure, symptoms usually resolve within 24 hours (105). Alterations in psychomotor performance occur. Cranial neuropathies have been observed.

Elevated hepatic enzymes and hepatic failure can result from certain halogenated hydrocarbons. In the setting of carbon tetrachloride–induced hepatotoxicity, GI symptoms develop initially. Hepatic aminotransferase enzymes often elevate in the first day and liver dysfunction reaches a maximum within 3 days of exposure, with death from hepatic failure occurring within the first week. Recovery is usually complete with no long-term sequelae, and the appearance of jaundice after the fourth day is a good prognostic sign (106). GI bleeding may result from decreased production of clotting factors.

Hypotension and dysrhythmias are associated with toxic exposures to halogenated hydrocarbons. Of 110 sudden deaths in glue sniffers, 28% were associated with trichloroethane (107). Trichloroethane given to dogs in anesthetic doses produces hypotension, with an initial uncompensated vasodilation and later a decreased heart rate, stroke volume, and myocardial contractility, thus accounting for the hemodynamic changes (108), Large doses of halothane can cause vasodilation, bradycardia, and direct myocardial depression. Decreased sympathetic nervous system activity augments hypotension. Ventricular dysrhythmias exacerbated by hypoxia and epinephrine complicate anesthetic cases.

Upper respiratory tract irritation can result from exposure to halogenated hydrocarbons. Direct alveolar damage is uncommon. Combustion of methylene chloride may produce pulmonary edema by producing phosgene, which can cause a delayed noncardiogenic pulmonary edema (109).

CHRONIC EXPOSURE

Neurologic Effects. A prospective, case-referred study reported that occupational solvent exposure plus alcohol intake may be an important cause of organic brain damage (110). An anecdotal study indicates that individuals with a history of 10 years or more of regular occupational exposure to solvents in confined space may present with a spectrum of neurologic disease resembling that seen in solvent abusers (111,112).

Due to study design flaws and inadequate neuropsychiatric testing procedures, convincing evidence of chronic neurologic toxicity has not been established. Painter's syndrome (headaches, fatigue, difficulties in concentrating, short-term memory impairment, irritability, depression, and alcohol intolerance) is an occupational disease and accepted for premature retirement in the Scandinavian countries. However, critical literature reviews (113,114) have reported that flawed methodology and inattention to confounding variables may have led to the erroneous conclusion that chronic solvent exposure causes organic CNS damage. Potential confounders include age, sex, intelligence, alcohol ingestion, occupational exposure to other neurotoxins, and health status (115).

Dermal Effects. *Dermal effects* include a defatting dermatitis with erythema, fissures, and desquamation. Prolonged contact can lead to significant dermal injury (116). The ingestion of ethanol during exposure to trichloroethylene (a degreaser for metal parts) leads to patchy erythroderma known as *degreaser's flush.* This involves vasodilation of superficial skin vessels, commonly affecting the face, neck, and back. The event is self-limiting and can resolve in approximately 1 hour (117).

Renal Effects. *Renal effects* of the halogenated solvents have not been clearly established. Anecdotal studies have suggested an association between exposure to occupational organic solvents and kidney diseases—particularly malignancy and glomerulonephritis (118–120). Two case-referral studies on renal cancer and glomerulonephritis did not confirm any relation with solvent exposure (119). Indicators of renal dysfunction that might assess the integrity of the glomerulus (albuminuria, glomerular basement membrane antigens in blood and urine, circulating anti–glomerular basement membrane antibodies) and tubular function (low-molecular-weight proteinuria, hyperphosphatemia, acetyl glucosaminidase, tubular antigen excretion, prostaglandin excretion) have seen limited use in industrial studies (121).

Carcinogenesis. The National Toxicology Program of the U.S. Department of Health and Human Services (http://ehp.niehs.nih.gov/roc/toc10.html) lists several solvents as reasonably anticipated carcinogens: carbon tetrachloride, chloroform, chloroprene, ethylene dibromide, ethylene dichloride, methylene chloride, tetrachloroethylene, and trichloroethylene.

Diagnostic Tests

BIOLOGIC MONITORING

Exposure measurements are available for certain halogenated hydrocarbons. For the average sedentary, nonsmoking worker, maximum allowable exposure (200 ppm) produces methylene chloride levels of 80 ppm in expired air and 0.18 mg/dl in blood as well as carboxyhemoglobin levels of 6.8% (97). Breath samples of trichloroethylene correlate with exposure. An 8-hour exposure to 100 ppm produces exhaled air trichloroethylene levels of 25 ppm immediately and 1 ppm 16 hours after exposure. After a 1-week exposure to 100 ppm of trichloroethylene for 8 hours/day, urinary trichloroacetic acid should range from 150 to 200 mg trichloroacetic acid/g of creatinine (122). Tetrachloroethylene concentrations greater than 4 ppm in a worker's breath 16 hours after exposure suggest that the 100-ppm time-weighted average was exceeded (123).

Gas chromatography with electron capture analysis of the blood headspace can be used to determine the concentration of halogenated solvents in biological samples (124).

Trichloroethylene, tetrachloroethylene, and trichloroethane metabolism may lead to the presence of trichloroacetone and trichloroacetic acid in the urine. Other chemicals such as chloral hydrate may also be metabolized to trichloroacetic acid. Trichloroethanol levels in exposed air, blood, and urine may be increased after trichloroethylene exposure.

ACUTE AND SUBACUTE EXPOSURE

Hepatotoxicity associated with hepatorenal failure may be indicated by elevated serum hepatic aminotransferase, bilirubin, alkaline phosphatase, ammonia, creatinine, and lactate level. In addition, a prolonged prothrombin time and hypoglycemia may develop. Tests usually return to normal in several weeks. Renal dysfunction may be associated with a rise in serum creatinine and reduced urine volume.

In severely intoxicated patients, the following additional studies should be considered: arterial blood gas, chest radiograph (for pulmonary edema or aspiration pneumonia), abdominal radiograph (to detect radio-opaque chemicals such as carbon tetrachloride), carboxyhemoglobin levels for methylene chloride exposures (125), and ECG with continuous cardiac monitoring.

POSTMORTEM CONSIDERATIONS

Histologic changes are characterized by a classical yellow fatty liver picture, with discrete damage concentrated in the midzonal and centrilobular regions.

Treatment

Treatment is largely supportive. Watch for respiratory depression and dysrhythmias. Obtain arterial blood gases. Administer oxygen if there is evidence of altered mental status or dyspnea. Treat hypotension with volume expansion and vasopressors. Use lidocaine or beta-adrenergic blockers for ventricular dysrhythmias.

DECONTAMINATION

Remove contaminated clothing for *dermal exposure*. Wash affected area with soap and copious amounts of water. For *ocular exposure*, irrigate the eye for 15 to 20 minutes. Obtain ophthalmic consultation if symptoms persist. After *ingestion*, simple aspiration with a nasogastric tube may be effective because these compounds are liquid. Activated charcoal is probably ineffective (126). For *inhalation exposure*, move patient away from the contaminated area. Provide a source of oxygen and prepare for mechanical ventilation.

ENHANCEMENT OF ELIMINATION

Hemodialysis or hemoperfusion is not likely to be useful because of the lipophilic properties of these solvents. Hyperbaric oxygen is experimental. Methyl bromide intoxication is characterized by acute, resistant, myoclonic convulsions and severe and permanent mental and neurologic damage for which supportive treatment has been the mainstay of management. An anecdotal, uncontrolled report suggests the use of hemodialysis to remove the bromide from the blood (Chapter 238) (127).

ANTIDOTES

Acetylcysteine may restore glutathione stores depleted by the production of free radicals; however, its role in limiting carbon tetrachloride-induced hepatotoxicity remains investigational (128,129).

SUPPORTIVE CARE

Watch for cardiac dysrhythmias, aspiration pneumonitis, hepatotoxicity, and hypoxic encephalopathy. Monitor for dysrhythmias for at least 24 hours and for hepatorenal failure for approximately 3 days. Obtain a chest radiograph, arterial blood gas, ECG, serum creatinine, and hepatic aminotransferase. Check electrolyte imbalance daily. Treat renal failure with dialysis and hepatic failure with fresh frozen plasma, vitamin K, a low-protein diet, neomycin, and lactulose. Watch fluid and electrolyte balance.

AROMATIC HYDROCARBONS—*P*-DICHLOROBENZENE; DICHLOROBENZENE

Dichlorobenzene (DCB; 1,4-dichlorobenzene) is used in mothballs and to make deodorant blocks used in restrooms. It is also used in the manufacture of certain resins, in the pharmaceutical industry, and as a general insecticide in farming. It needs to be differentiated from naphthalene, which is also used as a moth repellent but can cause methemoglobinemia more readily.

Toxic Dose

The toxic dose has not been established. The Occupational Safety and Health Administration permissible exposure limit is 75 ppm (450 $\mu g/m^3$).

Toxicokinetics and Toxicodynamics

p-DCB has been found in human blood, fatty tissue, and breast milk (130,130a). The major route of elimination appears to be in the urine. 2,5-Dichlorophenol is the major urinary metabolite of *p*-DCB (131).

Clinical Presentation

In a case of an unintentional exposure by ingestion of an unknown quantity of *p*-DCB crystals by a 3-year-old boy, analysis of urine specimens yielded four unidentified phenols as well as 2,5-dichlorophenol. These were shown to be conjugated with glucuronic and sulfuric acid (131). Methemoglobinemia, hyperchromic anemia, and acute hemolytic anemia have also been described.

Treatment

Treatment is mainly symptomatic and supportive (132).

POLYHALOGENATED BIPHENYLS

Polychlorinated biphenyls (PCB) were widely produced in the early 1970s for their insulating and nonflammable properties. However, their environmental and health effects led to the discontinuation of their production. There are several chemical congeners that comprise the PCB chemical class. An exposure occurs to a mixture and not to individual chemicals. The health effects associated with PCB exposure vary by the number and position of the chlorine atoms on the aromatic ring structure. Health effects include skin changes (e.g., chloracne), liver disorders (elevated hepatic enzymes), elevated lipids and cholesterol, immune suppression, neurobehavioral developmental delay, and cancers (GI and skin).

Polybrominated biphenyls (PBB) are used as flame-retardants. Their toxic effects were recognized when cattle feed was contaminated with the chemical (132a). Infants and adults were exposed through meat and milk. Their effects included chloracne, arthralgia, headache, and myalgia.

There are 209 congeners of PCB available (Aroclor, Askarel, Eucarel, Pyranol, Dykanol, Clorphen, Asbestol, Diaclor, Nepolin, EEC-18, and others). The coplanar PCBs are important because they have similar toxicologic effects to the dioxins. The International Union of Pure and Applied Chemists nomenclature for these chemicals is frequently used because it is succinct and avoids confusion. These chemicals are resistant to degradation and persist in the environment. In general, the greater the number of chlorine atoms, the more persistent is the chemical. PCBs with a higher number of chlorine atoms leach less from soil. However, on heating they transform into dioxins and furans, which have increased toxicity. Thus, it is important to be able to identify which chemicals are present when health effects are being attributed.

PCBs have been used as head exchange and dielectric fluids in transformers and capacitors, hydraulic and lubricating fluids, diffusion pump oils, plasticizers, extenders for pesticides, and as ingredients of caulking compounds, paints, adhesives, and flame retardants. They have also been used in inks and carbonless paper. The U.S. Environmental Protection Agency halted PCB production in 1971 but did not require their removal from existing transformers or capacitors. Commercial PCB mixtures are described by the percentage of chlorine present. For example, Aroclor 1254 indicates 54% chlorine saturation. PBBs are used as flame-retardants.

Source of Exposure

The common source of PCB exposure for the general population is through the diet. Environmental PCBs accumulate in the food chain and are found in higher concentrations in fatty foods. Occupations entailing risk of PCB exposure include electric cable repair, electroplating, emergency response, firefighting, hazardous waste hauling/site operating, heat exchange equipment repair, maintenance cleaning, metal finishing, paving and roofing, pipefitting/plumbing, timber products manufacturing, transformer/capacitor repair, and waste oil processing (133).

TABLE 9. U.S. Regulatory Guidelines and Standards for polychlorinated biphenyls

Agency	Description	PCB	Concentration [μg/m³]
OSHA	PEL-TWA	Aroclor 1242[a]	1
		Aroclor 1254[a]	0.5
ACGIH	TLV-TWA	Aroclor 1242	1
	TLV-TWA	Aroclor 1254	0.5
NIOSH	STEL-TWA	Aroclor 1242 and 1254	1
	IDLH	Aroclor 1242	10
	IDLH	Aroclor 1254	5

ACGIH, American Conference of Governmental Industrial Hygienists; IDLH, immediate danger to life or health; NIOSH, National Institute for Occupational Safety and Health; OSHA, U.S. Occupational Safety and Health Administration; PCB, polychlorinated biphenyl; PEL, permissible exposure limit; ppm, parts per million; STEL, short-term exposure limit; TLV, threshold limit value; TWA, time-weighted average.
[a]Skin designation.
Modified from Sullivan JB, Krieger G, eds. *Clinical environmental health and toxic exposures*. Philadelphia: Lippincott Williams & Wilkins, 2001, with permission.

Toxic Dose

Regulatory standards and guidelines are provided in Table 9.

Toxicokinetics and Toxicodynamics

PCB absorption occurs through the lungs, skin, and GI tract. Chloracne is a marker of systemic as well as cutaneous absorption. Distribution occurs primarily into fat. PCB metabolism has not been studied in humans. Biotransformation of PCB is slow and depends on the chlorine content (i.e., highly chlorinated compounds are metabolized and excreted slowly) (133a). A PCB with six or more chlorine atoms or adjacent unsubstituted carbons at the ortho or meta position is eliminated most slowly from patients exposed to contaminated rice oil (mean terminal half-life 6.7 to 9.8 months) (134). The estimated half-life of Aroclor 1242 was 6 to 7 months compared with that of the more chlorinated compound Aroclor 1260, 33 to 34 months (135).

Pregnancy and Lactation

PCBs and PBBs are excreted in breast milk. In women who were exposed to PBB, their breast milk contained an average PBB concentration of 68 μg/L (range, 0 to 1200 μg/L) (135a). The average PCB concentration in breast milk in Michigan was 1 to 2 mg/L (range, trace to 5.1 mg/L).

Clinical Presentation

ACUTE EXPOSURE

The acute effects of PCB exposure are mild and include eye and skin irritation. Exposures from the release of overheated transformer mist (contains both PCB and their products of pyrolysis) resulted in nausea, eye irritation, sore throat, chest tightness, and headache. Resolution occurred in 1 day. Polychlorinated dibenzofurans (PCDF) and polychlorinated dibenzo-*p*-dioxins were documented in the air of this transformer accident (136).

CHRONIC EXPOSURE

Chloracne is the only overt effect of PCB exposure in humans, but absence of chloracne does not rule out exposure. Chloracne typically develops weeks or months after exposure and is characterized by straw-colored, cystic lesions, comedones, and inflamed pustules. These lesions appear in the head, neck, and trunk (sparing the nasal area), are often refractory to treatment, and can last for years. The Yusho (Japan) and Yu-Cheng (Taiwan) events resulted from the exposure of people to contaminated rice oil. The Yusho event involved Kanechlor-400, consisting of a mixture of PCB, PCDF, and polychlorinated quinones. In the Yu-Cheng event, blood PCB levels of 66 affected persons ranged from 11 to 720 μg/L (mean, 49 μg/L) at approximately 9 to 12 months after their exposure. Although PCB was found in the oil, the toxicant associated with the adverse health effects was the more toxic PCDF (137,138).

CARCINOGENICITY

The International Agency for Research on Cancer classifies PCB as probable human carcinogens (139). The U.S. Department of Health and Human Services lists PCB as reasonably anticipated to be human carcinogens (140). The U.S. Environmental Protection Agency classifies PCB as probable human carcinogens (141). Epidemiologic evidence supporting this association is limited by the inability to isolate the effects of individual PCB chemicals, and the presence of chemicals other than PCBs (e.g., dioxins, furans, alcohol).

PCB mixtures induce hepatocellular carcinoma in animals. Although epidemiologic studies suggest an increased incidence of cancer in occupationally exposed workers, the long-term effect of acute and chronic exposures remains unknown (142). A 15-year study did not reveal any excess mortality or cancer incidence in 142 Swedish capacitor-manufacturing workers (143).

Diagnostic Tests

BIOLOGIC MONITORING

The most prevalent congeners detected in serum lipids in the U.S. general population from 1999 to 2000 included PCBs 118, 126, and 180 (143a). At the ninety-fifth percentile, these levels were 42.4 ng/g, 82.4 ng/g, and 79 ng/g, respectively. Occupationally exposed workers had plasma PCB levels averaging 172 μg/L and ranging up to 2530 μg/L (143b). Serum PCB levels probably are the best indicator of exposure, but current knowledge of dose-response characteristics is inadequate to correlate acute or chronic effects with a serum level. Earlier measurements of serum PCB levels were conducted on a whole weight basis, which was subject to variation from changes in blood lipid concentration (143c). The current approach is to express serum PCB measurements as lipid-adjusted levels. A survey of workers from an electrical capacitor manufacturing plant that had stopped PCB use 5 years earlier had a mean serum PCB level of 18.2 μg/L (range 0 to 424 μg/L) (143d). There was no evidence of adverse health effects in these people. Follow-up levels in patients poisoned with PCB-contaminated cooking oil did not correlate with reported symptoms or signs of headache, dizziness, or sensory neuropathy (143e). This discrepancy may reflect the presence of more toxic contaminants such as the dibenzofurans.

Treatment

Management is supportive. In the event of an eye splash, irrigate with tepid water immediately for at least 15 minutes. Ophthalmic evaluation may be needed if symptoms persist. Remove contaminated clothing and discard properly. Gently wash affected skin with soap and warm water for at least 15 minutes.

If PCB-containing substances have been ingested recently, gastric decontamination may be reasonable. Activated charcoal has not been proven beneficial, but is not contraindicated.

There is no specific treatment for PCB toxicity. Initial treatment of chloracne is based on cessation of exposure, good skin hygiene, and use of dermatologic measures commonly used for acne vulgaris.

Because there are no known methods of reducing reserves of PCB in lipid tissues, attempts to purge the body of PCBs should not be undertaken. Saunas and nutritional therapies remain unproven. Crash diets risk PCB mobilization from fat. Patients should avoid exposure to other hepatotoxins such as medications with known hepatotoxicity. Serum PCB levels, chloracne, and elevated serum aminotransferase levels can assist in detecting high-risk groups.

POLYCHLORINATED DIBENZOFURANS

PCDF have no industrial application. They are the byproducts of PCB, trichlorophenol, 2,4,5-trichlorophenoxyacetic acid, and pentachlorophenol production. Several congeners comprise the PCDF chemical class. The health effects associated with PCDF exposure are similar to polychlorodibenzodioxins. Toxic effects vary by the number and position of the chlorine atoms on the aromatic ring structure: 2,3,7,8-Tetrachlorodibenzofuran is the most toxic PCDF. The health effects of concern include chloracne, eye irritation, anemia, hepatitis, bronchitis, neurosensory disorders, and neurobehavioral deficits in children born to exposed women. Epidemiologic evidence supporting this association is limited by the inability to isolate the effects of the individual chemical, the involvement of other chemicals, and inability to quantify the exposure.

PCDF is an organic compound that contains two benzene rings fused to a central furan ring (Fig. 1). PCDFs are a class of organic compounds in which one to eight chlorine atoms are attached to the benzene ring positions of a dibenzofuran structure. There are eight PCDF homologues (mono- through octachlorinated). Each homologous group contains one or more isomers. Because of molecular asymmetry, PCDFs have 135 congeners, compared with 75 for polychlorodibenzodioxins (144), including 4 mono-chlorodibenzofurans (CDF), 16 di-CDF, 28 tri-CDF, and one octa-CDF.

Compounds with chlorine atoms in positions 4 and 6 as well as 2, 3, 7, 8, particularly 2,3,4,7,8-penta-CDF and 1,2,3,4,7,8-hexa-CDF, have longer half-lives because they are difficult to metabolize. The increased number of chlorine atoms is also associated with increased protein binding.

The general population is exposed to PCDF from contaminated foods. Accidental fires or breakdowns involving capacitors, transformers, and other electrical equipment (e.g., fluorescent light fixtures) that contain PCBs are the main known environmental sources of PCDF. PCDF also enter into the environment from burning of coal, wood, or oil for home heating and production of electricity. Many of these sources are being slowly phased out or strictly controlled. At 1112°F to 1202°F polychlorinated dibenzo-*p*-dioxins and PCDF can be formed from PCB. A fire involving PCB transformers contaminated the state office building in Binghamton, New York, with PCDF.

In Japan and Taiwan, where PCBs were used as a heat exchanger fluid for processing rice oil, PCB contaminated with

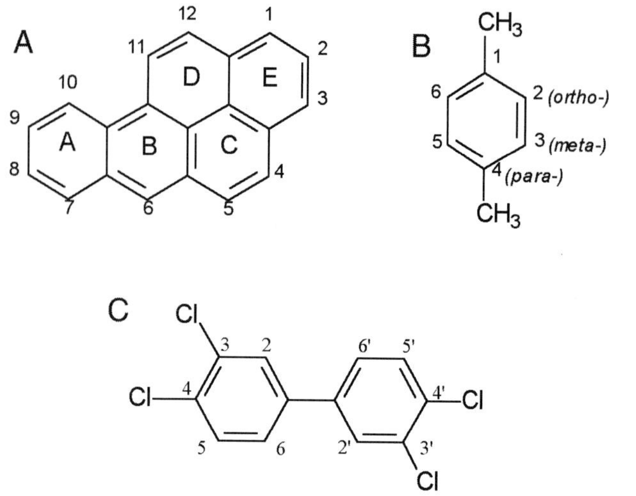

Figure 1. Chemical structures of (A) the polycyclic aromatic hydrocarbon, benzo[a]pyrene, (B) the petroleum distillate, p-xylene, and (C) the polychlorinated biphenyl congener, 3,3',4,4'-tetrachlorobiphenyl. Numbers on the structures indicate position numbers.

PCDF accidentally leaked into the oil causing *Yusho* or *Yu-Cheng* (oil disease) in approximately 4000 people. PCDFs are also byproducts of chemical manufacturing and consumer products such as wood-treatment chemicals, some metals, and paper products. Waterways become contaminated when the wastewater, sludge, or solids from these processes are released into waterways or into dumpsites. PCDFs also enter into the environment from municipal and industrial waste incinerators. Automobile exhaust from leaded gasoline releases small amounts into the environment.

Toxic Dose

The estimated average total PCDF intake in the Yusho incident was 3.3 mg, and the average daily intake was 0.9 mg/kg/day (144a). The two major PCDFs in the Yusho incident were 2,3,4,7,8-penta-CDF and 1,2,3,4,7,8-hexa-CDF.

Toxicokinetic and Toxicodynamics

PCDFs are lipid soluble and stored in adipose tissue. The elimination half-life for 2,3,4,7,8-penta-CDF and 1,2,3,4,7,8-hexa-CDF is 2 to 2.5 years from the Yu-Cheng patients and 10 years in the Yusho patients (144b).

Vulnerable Populations

Children born to mothers exposed to the contaminated rice oil in the Yu-Cheng and Yusho incidents were smaller in birth weight, developed dermal lesions, developed neurobehavioral disorders, and died (144c–144k).

Clinical Presentation

The common manifestations of the exposed people from the Yusho and Yu-Cheng events included chloracne, discharge from the meibomian glands of the eyelid, eye irritation, anemia, increases in serum triglyceride and liver enzymes, peripheral neuropathy, and bronchitis. Neurobehavioral deficits have been reported from fetal exposure (144k,144l).

Diagnostic Tests

The most prevalent PCDF congeners detected in serum lipids in the U.S. general population from 1999–2000 included 1,2,3,4,6,7,8-hepta-CDF and 2,3,4,7,8-penta-CDF (143a). At the ninety-fifth percentile, these levels were 19.1 pg/g and 15.9 pg/g, respectively. Routine testing for PCDFs is not recommended because of the expense, the expertise required by the laboratory to perform the analysis, and lack of clinical correlation.

Treatment

Treatment is symptomatic and supportive.

POLYCYCLIC AROMATIC HYDROCARBONS

The polycyclic aromatic hydrocarbons (PAH) are a class of chemicals that are produced during the combustion of fossil fuel. The workplace and the home are common sites of exposure. Home exposure occurs predominantly through heating, cooking, and food sources. Cancer is the primary concern.

PAHs consist of three or more fused benzene rings in varying arrangements that contain only carbon and hydrogen (Fig. 1). The compounds include benz[*a*]anthracene benzo[*a*]pyrene, benzo[*b*]fluoranthene, benzo[*j*]fluoranthene, benzo[*k*]fluoranthene, indeno[1,2,3,-*c,d*]pyrene, dibenz[*a,h*]anthracene, chrysene, and pyrene. Although naphthalene contains only two rings, it is commonly included in the discussion of PAHs because it is a coal tar constituent.

The primary environmental sources of PAH are forest fires and combustion of fossil fuel, in which high temperatures convert organic substances to PAH. Seafood and agricultural products contain PAH because of sedimentation from air into water. Crude coconut oil, heavily smoked ham, roasted coffee, tea, and charcoal-broiled meat contain up to 20 to 40 μg/kg of PAH.

The science of occupational medicine began with Percival Pott's 1775 report (145) of an unusually high incidence of scrotal cancer in chimney sweeps, which was ultimately attributed to benzo[*a*]pyrene and dibenz[*a,h*]anthracene in coal tar. Coke oven, coal tar, pitch, asphalt fume, and carbon black workers all have PAH exposure. The carcinogenic form of PAH results from their oxidation by the mixed-function oxidase system to diol-epoxide derivatives. These compounds contain highly reactive *bay regions* that probably bind covalently to deoxyribonucleic acid.

Residential PAH exposure occurs from contaminated foods (e.g., smoked, roasted), environmental tobacco smoke, kerosene heaters, wood stoves, and coal ovens. The primary source of PAH in the air is the combustion of wood, petroleum, and diesel fuels (145a). The PAH content of broiled meat is 20 to 40 μg/kg. Of the various pathways for PAH exposure by the general population, air and food are the greatest contributors. Dermal and inhalational routes contribute most to occupational PAH exposure. The estimated average for PAH exposure in the general population is 0.207 mg from air, 0.027 mg from water, and 0.16 to 1.6 mg from food. Smokers and people who live near industrial sites have higher exposures.

Acenaphthene, acenaphthylene, and anthracene are produced in the United States. Aside from being used for research purposes, these chemicals are also used as chemical intermediates for the production of dyes, plastics, pesticides, and synthetic fibers (145b,145c).

TABLE 10. U.S. Regulatory Guidelines and Standards for polycyclic nuclear aromatic hydrocarbons, styrene, cyclohexanone, and tetrahydrofuran

		Concentration [mg/m³ (ppm)]				
Agency	Description	Coke-oven emissions	Coal-tar pitch volatiles	Styrene	Cyclohexanone	Tetrahydrofuran
OSHA	PEL-TWA	0.15	0.2	426 (100)	200 (50)	590 (200)
	Ceiling	None	None	852 (200)	None	—
	Peak above ceiling	None	None	2556 (600)	None	—
ACGIH	TLV-TWA	None	0.2	85.2 (20)	100 (25)	590 (200)
	STEL	None	None	170 (40)	None	735 (250)
NIOSH	REL-TWA	0.5–0.7	0.1	215 (50)	100 (25)	590 (200)
	STEL	None	None	425 (100)	None	735 (250)
	IDLH	None	None	2982 (700)	(700)	5900 (2000)
Conversion factor		Not applicable	Not applicable	$mg/m^3 = ppm \times 4.26$	$mg/m^3 = ppm \times 4.02$	$mg/m^3 = ppm \times 2.95$

ACGIH, American Conference of Governmental Industrial Hygienists; IDLH, immediate danger to life or health; NIOSH, National Institute for Occupational Safety and Health; OSHA, U.S. Occupational Safety and Health Administration; PEL, permissible exposure limit; ppm, parts per million; REL, recommended exposure limit; STEL, short-term exposure limit; TLV, threshold limit value; TWA, time-weighted average.

Toxic Dose

Occupational standards and guidelines are provided in Table 10.

Toxicokinetics and Toxicodynamics

PAHs are absorbed passively by inhalational, GI, and dermal routes. The common routes of absorption for workers are inhalational and dermal. Oily media can facilitate the GI absorption (145d). Air particulates can adsorb PAH and then be inhaled and absorbed. Workers commonly absorb PAH dermally. PAHs are primarily metabolized in the liver by the microsomal cytochrome P-450 system to various oxides, which then leads to dihydrodiols, phenols, and quinones. Distribution is to fatty tissues. PAHs are eliminated in the feces or urine.

Pathophysiology

The reactive bay region epoxide diol metabolites of PAH are believed to be the active carcinogens. They are easily converted to reactive carbonium ions, which covalently bind to deoxyribonucleic acid to initiate mutagenesis and carcinogenesis. The bay region is the cup-shaped region between carbons 10 and 11 of benzo[*a*]pyrene or 1 and 12 of benz[*a*]anthracene. Diol epoxide intermediates of PAH are considered to be the carcinogen for the PAH (145e).

Vulnerable Populations

No information exists about PAH effects in humans; however, these chemicals can pass across the placenta and into fetal blood (145f).

Clinical Presentation

Acute toxicity is rare. *Chronic exposure* (146) is associated with dermal effects: erythema, burns, and warts on sun-exposed areas with progression to cancer. Toxic effects of coal tar are enhanced by exposure to ultraviolet light. Ocular irritation and photosensitivity may occur. In the monitoring of rubber manufacturing workers who were exposed to air containing a maximum of 66.0 $\mu g/m^3$ of total suspended particulate matter and 10.94 ng/m^3 of benzo[a]pyrene for periods ranging from 6 months to more than 6 years, the health effects identified included reduced lung function, abnormal chest radiographs, cough, bloody vomitus, and throat and chest irritation (146a). Respiratory effects include cough, bronchitis, and bronchogenic cancer. The GI system may develop leukoplakia, buccal-pharyngeal cancer, and cancer of the lip.

Carcinogenesis has been found for several PAHs (Table 11). Skin and lung absorption results in increased rates of skin and lung cancer. Certain PAHs are considered carcinogenic, whereas others are not (e.g., anthracene and phenanthrene). Coke oven emissions are complex mixtures of coal and coke material that include PAH. An epidemiologic study of exposed coke oven workers indicated increased rates of lung and urinary tract cancer. An epidemiologic study of workers exposed to soot, tars, and creosote found increased rates of skin, lung, bladder, and GI cancer. Benzo[*a*]anthracene, benzo[*a*]pyrene, and dibenzo[*a,h*]pyrene are suspected carcinogens based on studies in animals that show increased incidences of skin, lung, and liver cancer. Leukemia

TABLE 11. Polycyclic aromatic hydrocarbons that are listed as carcinogens

Agency (reference)	Categorization
IARC (IARC monograph Web site): http://monographs.iarc.Fr/htdocs/indexes/vol03index.htm	*Possible*: Benzo[b]fluoranthene, benzo[j]fluoranthene, benzo[k]fluoranthene, and indeno[1,2,3,-c,d]pyrene *Probable*: Benz[a]anthracene and benzo[a]pyrene
U.S. DHHS-NTP (10th Report on Carcinogens by the National Toxicology Program, DHHS)	*Reasonably anticipated* to be human carcinogens: benz[*a*]anthracene, benzo[*b*]fluoranthene, benzo[*j*]fluoranthene, benzo[*k*]fluoranthene, benzo[*a*]pyrene, dibenz[*a,h*]acridine, dibenz[a,j]acridine, dibenz[a,h]anthracene, 75H-dibenzo[c,g]carbazole, 7H-dibenzo[*a,e*]pyrene, dibenzo[*a,i*]pyrene, dibenzo[*a,h*]pyrene, dibenzo[*a,l*]pyrene, indeno[1,2,3-*c,d*]pyrene, and 5-methylchrysene.
U.S. EPA (Available at: http://www.epa.gov/ngispgm3/iris)	*Probable*: benz[*a*]anthracene, benzo[*a*]pyrene, benzo[*b*]fluoranthene, benzo[*k*]fluoranthene, chrysene, dibenz[*a,h*]anthracene, indeno[1,2,3-*c,d*]pyrene

IARC, International Agency for Research on Cancer; NTP, National Toxicology Program; U.S. EPA, U.S. Environmental Protection Agency; U.S. DHHS, U.S. Department of Health and Human Services.

(inconclusive) and lymphoma as well as hematuria, kidney, and bladder cancers have been reported.

Diagnostic Tests: Biologic Monitoring and Health Surveillance

Benzo[*a*]pyrene is often measured as an indicator of PAH exposure. Measurement of its serum protein adduct concentration appears to be a useful method for biologic monitoring (147). Benzo[*a*]pyrene is metabolized to the reactive metabolite, 7b,8a-dihydroxy-(9a,10a)-epoxy-7,8,9,10-tetrahydrobenzo[*a*]pyrene. The deoxyribonucleic acid adducts formed by this metabolite represent carcinogenic effects and have a longer window of monitoring than metabolites (147a–147c).

Urinary 1-hydroxypyrene can be used as an environmental marker of exposures to PAH as well. The median urinary 1-hydroxypyrene levels in non-smokers of general population groups from several countries range from 0.03 μmol/mol creatinine to 0.27 μmol/mol creatinine. Smokers from the same studies had urinary 1-hydroxypyrene levels that were about 2 fold higher than non-smokers. Workers in aluminum production and coke oven factories can achieve urinary 1-hydroxypyrene levels that are greater than the general population by a factor of 2. After a high PAH meal, it appears in the urine with a half-life of 4.4 hours. Maximum concentrations are found in 6.3 hours. 1-Hydroxypyrene is useful as a marker of exposure to PAHs but not as a marker for associated health effects because its parent chemical, pyrene, is not classified as a carcinogen.

Treatment

In *acute exposure*, contaminated clothing should be removed as soon as possible. The skin is cleaned by gently scrubbing with soap and water. Ocular exposure should be treated with irrigation and a complete eye examination. Ventilatory support should be available in the event of an acute inhalation exposure.

Chronic exposure patients should have periodic evaluation if they have been significantly exposed to PAHs, even in the absence of symptoms. This is recommended to facilitate early diagnosis and intervention should a malignancy develop.

CREOSOTES

Creosote (coal tar oil, coal tar creosote; CAS Registry No. 8021-39-4) is a complex mixture of hydrocarbon compounds, including PAH. It has been used as a disinfectant and treatment for cough. Skin cancer has been observed in workers exposed to creosote for long periods during timber treatment. The only products now routinely treated with creosotes are commercial wood products such as railroad ties and marine piers. Its use as a cough medicine is not recommended (149–151).

Coal tar creosote is used in industry as a wood preservative and can be found on railroad tracks. Workers may be exposed through inhalation or eye and dermal contact during the application of the creosote or using wood treated with the chemical. In the past, Beechwood creosote was used as a cough medicine (contains phenol, cresols, and guaiacol). It may still be found in herbal remedy shops and in other countries.

Toxic Dose

A *toxic dose* is approximately 0.1 g/kg body weight. Regulatory standards and guidelines have not been listed for creosote.

Clinical Presentation

Acute exposure causes irritation of the skin, mucous membranes, and conjunctiva. The skin may become red, papular, vesicular, or ulcerative. Photosensitization has been observed. After ingestion of creosote, GI irritation (nausea, vomiting, salivation, and abdominal discomfort) and cardiovascular instability (tachycardia, hypotension, respiratory distress, cyanosis, and pupillary changes) may occur.

Chronic exposure creates the same effects as PAH, as previously described in Polycyclic Aromatic Hydrocarbons.

Treatment

Treatment is entirely symptomatic and supportive.

CYCLIC ETHERS—TETRAHYDROFURAN

Tetrahydrofuran (THF; cyclotetramethylene oxide, diethylene oxide, tetramethylene oxide, 1,4-epoxybutane; MW 72.1; CAS Registry No. 109-99-9) is a colorless organic solvent liquid belonging to a group of cyclic ethers with an odor similar to acetone (152). It dissolves many plastics (polyvinyl chloride, polyurethane, epoxy compounds, and cellulosics) and a wide range of organic products. Its main applications include the manufacture of glues, paints, varnishes, inks, and wetting and dispersing agents in textile processing. It is also used as an iron oxide coating agent in the production of audio and videotapes. THF forms explosive peroxides when exposed to air.

Toxic Dose

Inhalation of 25,000 ppm results in anesthesia.

Toxicokinetics and Toxicodynamics

THF is readily absorbed after ingestion or inhalation. It can cross the skin in toxic amounts (153,154). Metabolic products may include γ-butyrolactone, which possesses convulsive properties (154,155). THF is subject to oxidative metabolism (156).

Pathophysiology

THF is an inhibitor of a number of cytochrome P-450–dependent, mixed-function oxidase activities, with particular affinity for the alcohol-induced enzyme CYP2E1 (157).

Clinical Presentation

Symptoms after exposure include nausea, headache, blurred vision, dizziness, fatigue, tinnitus, chest pain, and cough. Irritation of skin and mucous membranes may develop. THF is an upper respiratory tract irritant. At high concentrations it is a CNS depressant. THF may have contributed to the development of status epilepticus or awakening from an enflurane anesthesia in a patient occupationally exposed to solvent (158). One patient developed a peripheral neuropathy after exposure (158).

The two primary signs of intoxication are sedation and hepatocellular dysfunction, both occurring at doses of approximately one-half the lethal dose in animals. An adult ingested THF and developed abdominal pain, nausea, and vomiting. The vomitus and breath had an unusual odor. The patient developed jaundice, oliguria, a high fever, and loss of consciousness and died after 5 days. Lesions of the GI tract and kidney (glomeruli) were observed (159).

Diagnostic Tests

BIOLOGIC MONITORING

Analysis of the breath, blood, and urine is accomplished with the use of gas chromatography. Measurement of THF concentration in the urine is a sensitive, specific method for monitoring exposure (160).

ACUTE EXPOSURE

Hepatic aminotransferases may be considerably elevated. The chest radiograph and ECG are normal. The blood count and renal function tests (serum creatinine, blood urea nitrogen) are usually normal. Muscle acetylcholinesterase appeared to be increased in animal studies (156).

Treatment

Treatment is symptomatic and supportive. Decontamination is performed as for other hydrocarbons: moving patient to fresh air, removing clothing, and cleaning skin of dermal exposures and GI decontamination if patient presents early in course.

KETONES—CYCLOHEXANONE

Cyclohexanone [anone, hexanone, ketohexamethylene, nadone, pimelic ketone, pimelin ketone (161), $CO(CH_2)_4CH_2$, MW 98.16 g/mol; CAS Registry No. 108-94-1] is a cyclic six-carbon ketone. It is a colorless to slightly yellow liquid with a peppermint odor that is slightly soluble in water. Cyclohexanone dissolves most plastics, resins, and rubber. It may react with oxidizing agents and nitric acid to cause fires and explosions. Its odor threshold is 0.88 ppm.

Cyclohexanone is a commonly used industrial solvent for cellulose acetate natural resins, vinyl resins, rubber, waxes, and fats. It is also used as a solvent sealer for polyvinyl chloride in medical devices (162). It has been found as a contaminant of IV dextrose and a parenteral feeding solution used in a newborn special care unit, where it was considered to be leached into infusion fluids from administration sets (163).

Toxic Dose

Occupational standards and guidelines are provided in Table 10. In humans, exposure to 25 ppm of cyclohexanone vapor for 5 minutes did not cause side effects, but 75 ppm resulted in eye, nose, and throat irritation (164).

Toxicokinetics and Toxicodynamics

Cyclohexanone appears to be reduced to cyclohexanol at a pH of 7.0 by human liver alcohol dehydrogenase (165), an enzyme demonstrated to be present in human fetal liver as early as 2 months of gestation (166). Cyclohexanol is metabolized further by mixed-function oxidases and is excreted in human urine as *trans* 1,2- and *trans* 1,3-cyclohexanediol, the main metabolites, and *trans* 1,4-cyclohexandeliol with cyclohexane (excreted unchanged in small amounts, approximately 3.5%). Cyclohexanol disappears from the urine after 24 hours. Excretion of cyclohexanediol may continue for at least 10 days (167). A 1-kg preterm newborn baby receiving 150 ml of dextrose (contaminated with cyclohexanone) pumped through an infusion set over 24 hours can receive up to 1 mg of cyclohexanone daily (0.74 to 0.98 mg; 7.5 to 10.0 μmol) (167).

Cyclohexanone metabolites have been excreted by premature babies who received parenteral nutrition (167). Although cyclohexanone has been associated with CNS depression and hepatotoxicity in adults, its toxicity in neonates has not been evaluated.

Vulnerable Populations

Little information is available on the neonatal toxicity of cyclohexanone. Foreign compounds that compete with bilirubin and drugs for blood transport proteins and with glucuronosyltransferase in liver cells may increase the risk of kernicterus or of drug toxicity.

Clinical Presentation

A 46-year-old man ingested 50 ml of a plastic catalyst containing methyl ethyl ketone and cyclohexanone peroxides in dimethyl phthalate. He collapsed, became comatose, and exhibited severe erosion of the mucosa of the posterior pharynx, oliguria, hepatotoxicity, and an erosive gastritis preceding death (168).

A 55-year-old patient drank approximately 100 ml of liquid cement for polyvinyl chloride resin containing acetone, methyl ethyl ketone, cyclohexanone, and polyvinyl chloride. He was lavaged, treated with plasma exchanges and hemoperfusion, developed a transient hyperglycemia and hepatotoxicity, and recovered. The largest component of the ingested liquid was cyclohexanone. Cyclohexanol was detected in the urine. The comatose state was considered to be caused mainly by cyclohexanol (162).

Diagnostic Tests: Biologic Monitoring

Urinary cyclohexanol concentrations correlate well with the time-weighted-average concentration of cyclohexanone at the workplace. The detection limit for urinary cyclohexanol is 0.4 mg/L, which can detect cyclohexanol in urine for those who are exposed below the current cyclohexanone exposure limit of 25 ppm. A sensitive method for determining urinary cyclohexanol involves hydrolysis and gas chromatography with flame ionization detection (169). Cyclohexanediol is assayed by gas chromatography and mass spectrometry (165).

Treatment

Management is primarily symptomatic and supportive. However, the report of caustic effect of some mixture indicates that oral exposure should be managed as a corrosive acid ingestion (Chapter 201). Eye exposure is treated with copious irrigation with water or normal saline for at least 20 to 30 minutes. For skin exposure, all contaminated clothing should be removed. Wash and irrigate all exposed skin thoroughly with water or saline.

HYDROQUINONE

Hydroquinone (1,4 dihydroxybenzene; 1,4-benzenediol; alpha hydroquinone; beta-quinol, *p*-benzenediol, *p*-dihydroxybenzene, *p*-dioxobenzene, *p*-dioxybenzene, *p*-hydroquinone, *p*-hydroxyphenol, benzohydroquinone, benzoquinol, hydroquinol; MW 110.1 g/mol; CAS Registry No. 123-31-9) ingestion in low doses may be relatively asymptomatic (170). In higher doses it can induce an acute gastroenteritis-like syndrome. Ingestion of 5 to 12 g causes hemolysis, renal and hepatic failure, and death. Treatment is symptomatic and supportive.

Hydroquinone is a reducing agent. It is used as a photographic developer in black-and-white photography; an antioxidant or stabilizer; a polymerization inhibitor for vinyl acetate and acrylic monomers; a stabilizer in paints, varnishes, motor fuels, and oils; an intermediate for rubber-processing chemicals;

TABLE 12. Occupations with exposure to tetrahydrofuran

Antioxidant makers	Paint makers
Bacteriostatic-agent makers	Photographic-developer makers
Drug makers	Plastic-stabilizer workers
Fur processors	Stone-coating workers
Motor-fuel blenders	Styrene-monomer workers
Organic-chemical synthesizers	

and a source of the production of its mono- and dialkyl ethers (170). Many of its derivatives are used as bacteriostatic agents, and others [e.g., 2,5-bi (ethyleneimino) hydroquinone] may be antimitotic and tumor-inhibiting agents (171). Several occupations have exposure to hydroquinone (Table 12).

Hydroquinone exists in a free state in pear leaves. Arbutin, a glucoside of hydroquinone, occurs widely in the leaves, bark, buds, and fruit of many plants, especially the *Ericaceae* (170). Hydroquinone has been detected in cigarette smoke, and in the effluents from photo processing, coal tar production, and the paper industry.

Toxic Dose

The daily ingestion of 300 to 500 mg of hydroquinone for 3 to 5 months by 19 volunteers caused no observable alterations in the blood and urine (172). *Health teas* prepared from the leaves of blueberry, red whortleberry, cranberry, or bearberry may contain hydroquinone in excess of 1%. They are capable of causing irritation of the GI mucosa and inducing systemic poisoning (173). A 36-year-old man ingested 12 g of hydroquinone, developed cyanosis, and survived (174). Two other patients ingested 5 to 6 g of hydroquinone, developed cyanosis and icterus, and died (174).

Toxicokinetics and Toxicodynamics

Hydroquinone is readily absorbed from the GI tract and is excreted in the urine as sulfate and glucuronide conjugates (170,175).

Pathophysiology

In aqueous solutions (e.g., tears), hydroquinone is oxidized by air, especially rapidly in alkaline solutions in the presence of light, to form a brown color partly due to conversion to 1,4-benzoquinone (176). Hydroquinone is known to be converted by human myeloperoxidase to 1,4-benzoquinone, a toxic compound (177).

Clinical Presentation

Ingestion produces a chemical gastroenteritis. The crew of a military vessel developed an illness characterized by acute nausea, vomiting, abdominal cramps, and diarrhea; complete resolution occurred within 12 to 36 hours. The white blood cell count was elevated. The drinking water had been contaminated with photographic developer (178). Fatal cases have ingested 5 to 12 g of hydroquinone (174). These doses induced tinnitus, dyspnea, cyanosis, extreme somnolence, a dark color to the urine, scleral icterus, and bile-stained urine. Two deaths were presumed to be due to extensive hemolysis, and renal and hepatic failure (179). Death appears to follow massive hemolysis with renal and hepatic failure (174).

Ocular contamination with particles of hydroquinone (10 to 30 mg of vapor or dust of hydroquinone/m^3 air) (180,181) can cause immediate eye irritation. Chronic, low-grade, and long-time exposure may result in corneal ulceration and dark brown discoloration, distortion, and opacification of the cornea (176). The eye changes appear irreversible.

Dermal application of skin-lightening preparations containing hydroquinone may produce severe and irreversible damage (182,183). The effects begin with a darkening and coarsening of the skin, followed by a hyperpigmented papular change, an exogenous ochronosis (184).

Diagnostic Testing

Liquid chromatographic analysis has been used to quantitate serum hydroquinone levels (178). High-performance liquid chromatography can be used for the detection of hydroquinone in water samples (170).

Acutely ill patients with GI symptoms after hydroquinone ingestion had serum levels higher than 0.1 µg/ml (178). Ingestion of 12 g of hydroquinone led to a black-colored urine that tested positive for phenol (174).

Blood should be drawn for a complete blood count, serum aminotransferases, alkaline phosphatase, bilirubin (total and indirect), glucose, creatinine, and blood urea nitrogen. Arterial blood gases and serum electrolytes should be obtained periodically. Hypoglycemia, hypercholesterolemia, leukocytosis, hemoglobinemia, and granular and hyaline casts in the urine have been observed after large ingestions (174).

Treatment

Ingestion of hydroquinone is treated with symptomatic and supportive care. Induction of emesis and gastric lavage has been used (185). Typical measures are used for hepatic and renal failure. *Ocular* contamination is treated with immediate irrigation for 15 minutes; an ophthalmologic consultation is often needed (185). *Dermal* contact is decontaminated with soap and water (185). No antidote exists for hydroquinone toxicity.

REFERENCES

1. Litovitz TL, Klein-Schwartz W, White S, et al. 2000 annual report of the American Association of Poison Control Centers toxic exposure surveillance system. *Am J Emerg Med* 2001;19(5):337–395.
2. Flanagan RJ, Ruprah M, Meredith TJ, et al. An introduction to the clinical toxicology of volatile substances. *Drug Safe* 1990;5:359–389.
3. Gerarde HW. Toxicological studies in hydrocarbons vs kerosene. *Toxicol Appl Pharmacol* 1959;1:462–474.
4. Scalzo AJ, Weber TR, Jaeger RW, et al. Extracorporeal membrane oxygenation for hydrocarbon aspiration. *Am J Dis Child* 1990;144:867–871.
5. Chellino MA. Petroleum distillate hydrocarbons. *San Francisco Poison Control Center Newsletter* 1980;2(2):2.
6. Beerman B, Christensson T, Moller P, et al. Lipoid pneumonia. An occupation hazard of fire-eaters. *BJM* 1984;289:1728–1729.
7. Anas N, Namasonthia V, Ginsburg CM. Criteria for hospitalizing children who have ingested products containing hydrocarbons. *JAMA* 1981;246:840–843.
8. Lauwerys RR, Hoet P. *Industrial chemical exposure: guidelines for biological monitoring*, 3rd ed. Boca Raton, FL: Lewis Publishers, 2001.
9. Banner W, Walson PD. Systemic toxicity following gasoline aspiration. *Am J Emerg Med* 1983;3:292–294.
10. Eade NR, Taussig LM, Marks MI. Hydrocarbon pneumonitis. *Pediatrics* 1974;54:351–357.
11. James FW, Kaplan S, Benzing G. Cardiac complications following hydrocarbon ingestion. *Am J Dis Child* 1971;121:431–433.
12. Decker WJ. Adsorption of solvents by activated charcoal, polymers and mineral sorbents. *Vet Hum Toxicol* 1981;23[Suppl 1]:44–46.
13. Ng RC, Darwish H, Stewart PA. Emergency treatment of petroleum distillate and turpentine ingestion. *CMAJ* 1974;111:537–538.
14. Burns CR, Currie B. The efficacy of chelation therapy and factors influencing mortality in lead intoxicated petrol sniffers. *Aust NZ J Med* 1995;25:197–203.
15. Marks MI, Chicoine L, Legere G, et al. Adrenocorticosteroid treatment of hydrocarbon pneumonia in children—a cooperative study. *J Pediatr* 1972;81:366–369.
16. Gurwitz D, Kattan M, Levison H, et al. Pulmonary function abnormalities in asymptomatic children after hydrocarbon pneumonitis. *Pediatrics* 1978;62:789–794.

17. Green TP, Moler FW, Goodman DM. Probability of survival after prolonged extracorporeal membrane oxygenation in pediatric patients with acute respiratory failure. *Crit Care Med* 1995;23:1132–1139.
18. Banner W. Risks of extracorporeal membrane oxygenation: is there a role for the use in the management of the acutely poisoned patient? *Clin Toxicol* 1996;34(4):365–371.
19. OPD. *OPD chemical buyers directory*, 76th ed. New York: Schnell Publishing Co. Inc., 1989:235, 696.
20. Verschueren K. *Handbook of environmental data on organic chemicals.* New York: Van Nostrand Reinhold Co., 1983: 464–465.
21. Milby TH, Wharton D. Epidemiological assessment of occupationally related, chemically induced sperm count suppression. *J Occup Med* 1980;22:77–82.
22. Wharton D, Milby TH, Krauss RM, et al. Testicular function in DBCP exposed pesticide workers. *J Occup Med* 1979;21:161–166.
23. Goldsmith JR, Potashnik G, Israeli R. Reproductive outcome in families of DBCP-exposed men. *Arch Environ Health* 1984;39:85–89.
24. Eaton M, Schenker M, Wharton MD, et al. Seven-year follow-up of workers exposed to 1,2-dibromo-3-chloropropane. *J Occup Med* 1986;28:1145–1150.
25. Olson GW, Lanham JM, Bodner KM, et al. Determinants of spermatogenesis recovery among workers exposed to 1,2-dibromo-3-chloropropane. *J Occup Med* 1990;32:979–984.
26. Zhang AQ, Mitchell SC, Barrett T, et al. Fate of dimethylamine in man. *Xenobiotica* 1994;24(4):379–387.
27. Ying W, Jing X, Qin-Wai W. Clinical report on 62 cases of acute dimethyl sulfate intoxication. *Am J Ind Med* 1988;13:455–462.
28. *Dimethyl sulfate. Environmental health criteria 48.* Geneva: World Health Organization, 1985:1–55.
29. von Nida S. Fatal edema of the glottis following inflammation of the upper digestive tract due to dimethyl sulfate. *Klin Wochenschr* 1947;24/25:633–634.
30. Ip M, Wong K-L, Wong K-F, et al. Lung injury in dimethyl sulfate poisoning. *J Occup Med* 1989;31:141–143.
31. Moeschlin S. *Poisoning. Diagnosis and treatment.* New York: Grune & Stratton, 1965: 1–707.
32. Kleinfeld M. Acute pulmonary edema of chemical origin. *Arch Environ Health* 1965;10:942–946.
33. International Labour Office. Dimethyl sulfate. In: *Encyclopedia of occupational health and safety*, vol. 1. New York: McGraw-Hill, 1971:388–389.
34. Littler TR, McConnell RB. Dimethyl sulfate poisoning. *Br J Ind Med* 1955;12:54–56.
35. International Agency for Research on Cancer. Monograph on the evaluation of the carcinogenic risk of chemicals to humans. Supplement 4. 1987. IARC Press, Lyon, France.
36. Environmental Health Perspectives Web site. Available at: http://ehp.niehs.nih.gov/roc/ninth/rahc/dimethylsulfate.pdf. Accessed April 24, 2003.
37. Ellgehausen D. Determination of volatile toxic substances in the air by means of a coupled gas chromatograph–mass spectrometer system. *Anal Lett* 1975;8:11–23.
38. Ellgehausen D. A gas chromatographic monitor for dimethyl sulfate in air. In: *The monitoring of hazardous gases in the working environment*. London: The Chemical Society, 1977:27–28.
39. Dimethyl sulfate. Environmental Health Criteria 48. Geneva: World Health Organization, 1985:1–55.
40. Willhite CC, Katz PI. Dimethyl sulfoxide. *J Appl Toxicol* 1984;4:155–160.
41. Reynolds JEF. *Martindale: the extra pharmacopoeia*, 29th ed. London: The Pharmaceutical Press, 1989:1426–1427.
42. *Physicians desk reference*, 46th ed. Montvale, NJ: Medical Economics Company, 1992:1836–1837.
43. McGann LE, Walterson ML. Cryoprotection by dimethyl sulfoxide and dimethyl sulfone. *Cryobiology* 1987;24:11–16.
44. Arndt K, Haschok WM, Jeffrey EH. Mechanism of dimethyl sulfoxide protection against acetaminophen hepatotoxicity. *Drug Metab Rev* 1989;20:261–269.
45. Park Y, Smith RD, Combs AB, et al. Prevention of acetaminophen-induced hepatotoxicity by dimethyl sulfoxide. *Toxicology* 1988;52:165–175.
46. Waller FT, Tanabe CT, Paxton HD. Treatment of elevated intracranial pressure with dimethyl sulfoxide. *Ann NY Acad Sci* 1983;411:286–292.
47. Karaca M, Bilgin UY, Akar M, et al. Dimethyl sulfoxide lowers ICP after closed head trauma. *Eur J Clin Pharmacol* 1991;40:113–114.
48. Hull FW, Wood DC, Brobyn RD. Eye effects of DMSO. Report of negative results. *Northwest Med* 1969;68:39–41.
49. Gordon DM. Dimethyl sulfoxide in ophthalmology with special reference to possible toxic effects. *Ann N Y Acad Sci* 1967;141:392–401.
50. Bennett WM, Munther RS. Lack of nephrotoxicity in intravenous dimethyl sulfoxide. *Clin Toxicol* 1981;18:615–618.
51. Munther RS, Bennett WM. Effects of dimethyl sulfoxide on renal function in man. *JAMA* 1980;244:2081–2083.
52. Hucker HB, Miller JK, Hochberg A, et al. Studies on the absorption, excretion and metabolism of dimethyl sulfoxide (DMSO) in man. *J Pharm Exp Ther* 1967;155:309–317.
53. Kolb KH, Janicke G, Kramer M, et al. Absorption, distribution and elimination of labeled dimethyl sulfoxide in man and animals. *Ann N Y Acad Sci* 1967;141:85–95.
54. Jacob SW, Bischell M, Herschler RJ. Dimethyl sulfoxide (DMSO). A new concept in pharmacotherapy. *Curr Ther Res* 1964;6:134–135.
55. Rubin LF. Toxicity of dimethyl sulfoxide, alone and in combination. *Ann N Y Acad Sci* 1975;243:98–103.
56. Szmant HH. Physical properties of dimethyl sulfoxide and its function in biological systems. *Ann N Y Acad Sci* 1975;243:20–23.
57. Wood DC, Wood J. Pharmacological and biochemical considerations of dimethyl sulfoxide. *Ann N Y Acad Sci* 1975;234:7–19.
58. Kligman AM. Topical pharmacology and toxicology of dimethyl sulfoxide—part II. *JAMA* 1965;193:923–928.
59. Reinstein L, Mahon R Jr, Russo GL. Peripheral neuropathy after concomitant dimethyl sulfoxide and sulindac therapy. *Arch Phys Med Rehabil* 1982;63:581–584.
60. Yellowlees P, Greenfield C, McIntyre N. Dimethyl sulfoxide induced toxicity. *Lancet* 1980;2:1004–1006.
61. Greenfield C. Dimethyl sulfoxide toxicity. *Lancet* 1981;1:276–277.
62. Bond GR, Curry SC, Dahl DW. Dimethyl sulfoxide-induced encephalopathy. *Lancet* 1989;1:1134–1135.
63. Boby RB. The human toxicology of dimethyl sulfoxide. *Ann N Y Acad Sci* 1975;243:497–506.
64. Garretson SE, Aitchison P. Comparison of dimethyl sulfoxide levels in whole blood and serum using an auto sampler–equipped gas chromatography. *Ann N Y Acad Sci* 1983;411:328–331.
65. Logan D, Dart R. Gasoline toxicity. In: *Case studies in environmental medicine*, 31. Agency for Toxic Substances and Disease Registry; 1993.
66. Edminster SC, Bayer MJ. Recreational gasoline sniffing. Acute gasoline intoxication and latent organolead poisoning. *J Emerg Med* 1985;3:365–370.
67. Weaver NH. The petroleum industry. *State Art Rev Occup Med* 1988;3(5).
68. Dabney BJ, Brent J. Jet fuel toxicity. In: *Case studies in environmental medicine*, 32. Agency for Toxic Substances and Disease Registry; 1993.
69. Davies NE. Jet fuel intoxication. *Aerospace Med* 1964;35:481–482.
70. Ritchie GD, Still KR, Alexander WK, et al. A review of the neurotoxicity risk of selected hydrocarbon fuels. *J Toxicol Environ Health B Crit Rev* 2001;4(3):223–312.
71. Pleil JD, Smith LB, Zelnick SD. Personal exposure to JP-8 jet fuel vapors and exhaust at air force bases. *Environ Health Perspect* 2000;108(3):183–92.
72. Cocchiarella L, Hryhorczuk D, Garrettson LK. Stoddard solvent toxicity. *Case studies in environmental medicine*, 33. Agency for Toxic Substances and Disease Registry; 1993.
73. McDermott HJ. Hygienic guide series: Stoddard solvent (mineral spirits, white spirits). *Am Ind Hyg Assoc J* 1975;36:553–558.
74. Zreve L, Nagasawa HT. Methanethiol and derivatives in hepatic failure. *J Lab Clin Med* 1988;111:595–597.
75. Blom HJ, van den Elzen JPAM, Yap SH, et al. Methanethiol and methylsulfide formation for 3-methylthiopropionate in human and rat hepatocytes. *Bioch Biophys Acta* 1988;972:131–136.
76. Chen S, Zieve L, Mahadevan V. Mercaptans and dimethyl sulfide in the breath of patients with cirrhosis of the liver. *J Lab Clin Med* 1970;75:628–635.
77. Garrettson LK, Warren DA. Chronic methanethiol poisoning. *Vet Hum Toxicol* 1990;32:365.
78. Reynolds JEF, ed. *Martindale: the extra pharmacopoeia*, 30th ed. London: The Pharmaceutical Press, 1993:1390.
79. Monooctanoin for gallstones. *Med Lett Drugs Ther* 1987;29:52.
80. Hejka AG, Poquett M, Wiebe DA, et al. Fatal intravenous injection of monooctanoin. *Am J Forensic Med Pathol* 1990;11:165–170.
81. Minuk GY, Hoofnagle JH, Jones EA. Systemic site effects from the intrabiliary infusion of monooctanoin for the dissolution of gallstones. *J Clin Gastroenterol* 1982;4:133–135.
82. Shustak A, Noseworthy TW, Johnston RG, et al. Noncardiogenic pulmonary edema during intrabiliary infusion of monooctanoin. *Crit Care Med* 1986;14:659–660.
83. *Physicians' desk reference*, 41st ed. Oradell, NJ: Medical Economics, 1987:924–925.
84. Litovitz TL, Schmitz BF, Holm KC. 1988 annual report of the American Association of Poison Control Centers National Data Collection System. Case 436. *Am J Emerg Med* 1989;7:495–545.
85. Zeiss CR, Wolkonsky P, Pruzansky JJ, et al. Clinical and immunologic evaluation of trimellitic anhydride workers in multiple industrial settings. *J Allergy Clin Immunol* 1982;70:15–18.
86. Patterson R, Zeiss CR, Pruzansky JJ. Immunology and immunopathology of trimellitic anhydride pulmonary reactions. *J Allergy Clin Immunol* 1982;70:19–23.
87. Leach CL, Hatoum NS, Ratajczak HV, et al. Evidence of immunologic control of lung injury induced by trimellitic anhydride. *Am Rev Respir Dis* 1988;137:186–191.
88. Zeiss CR, Leach CL, Smith LJ, et al. A serial immunologic and histopathologic study of lung injury and histopathologic study of lung injury induced by trimellitic anhydride. *Am Rev Respir Dis* 1988;137:191–196.
89. Hathaway GJ, Proctor NH, Hughes JP, et al., eds. *Proctor and Hughes' chemical hazards of the workplace*, 3rd ed. New York: Van Nostrand Reinhold, 1991:568–569.
90. Wilcken B. Acid soaps in the fish odor syndrome. *BMJ* 1993;307:1497.
91. Ayesh R, Mitchell SC, Zhang A, et al. The fish odour syndrome: biochemical, familial and clinical aspects. *BMJ* 1993;307:655–657.
92. Bergman K. Whole-body autoradiography and allied tracer techniques in distribution and elimination studies of some organic solvents: benzene, toluene, xylene, styrene, methylene chloride, chloroform, carbon tetrachloride and trichloroethylene. *Scand J Work Environ Health* 1979;5[Suppl 1]:1–263.
93. Stewart RD, Boettner EA, Southworth RR, et al. Acute carbon tetrachloride intoxication. *JAMA* 1963;183:994–997.
94. Letz GA, Pond SM, Osterloh JD, et al. Two fatalities after acute occupational exposure to ethylene dibromide. *JAMA* 1984;252(17):2428–31.

95. Henry LD, DiMaio VJ. A fatal case of hexachlorophene poisoning. *Mil Med* 1974;139(1):41–2.
96. Mullick FG. Hexachlorophene toxicity. Human experience at the Armed Forces Institute of Pathology. *Pediatrics* 1973;51(2):395–9.
97. Di Vincenzo GD, Kaplan CJ. Effect of exercise or smoking on the uptake, metabolism, and excretion of methylene chloride vapor. *Toxicol Appl Pharmacol* 1981;59(1):141–8.
97a. Dowty BJ, Laseter JL, Storer J. The transplacental migration and accumulation in blood of volatile organic constituents. *Pediatr Res* 1976;10(7):696–701.
98. Bagnell PC, Ellenberger HA. Obstructive jaundice due to a chlorinated hydrocarbon in breast milk. *Can Med Assoc J* 1977;117:1047–1048.
99. Gordis E. Lipid metabolites of carbon tetrachloride. *J Clin Invest* 1969;48(1): 203–9.
100. Anonymous. Postoperative hepatic failure and halothane. *N Engl J Med* 1968;279(15):830–1.
101. Cornish HH, Adefuin J. Potentiation of carbon tetrachloride toxicity by aliphatic alcohols. *Arch Environ Health* 1967;14(3):447–9.
102. Reference deleted.
103. Reference deleted.
104. Traiger GJ, Plaa GL. Relationship of alcohol metabolism to the potentiation of CCl 4 hepatotoxicity induced by aliphatic alcohols. *J Pharmacol Exp Ther* 1972;183(3):481–8.
105. Hill RN, Clemens TL. Genetic control of chloroform toxicity in mice. *Science* 1975;190(4210):159–161.
106. Stewart RD, Boettner EA, Southworth RR, et al. Acute carbon tetrachloride intoxication. *JAMA* 1963;183:994–997.
107. Bass M. Sudden sniffing death. *JAMA* 1970;212(12):2075–9.
108. Herd PA, Lipsky M, Martin HF. Cardiovascular effects of 1,1,1-trichloroethane. *Arch Environ Health* 1974;28(4):227–33.
109. Gerritsen WB, Bruschmenn CH. Phosgene poisoning caused by the use of chemical paint removers containing methylene chloride in ill ventilated rooms heated by kerosene stoves. *Br J Ind Med* 1960;17:187–189.
110. Cherry NM, Labreche FP, McDonald JC. Organic brain damage and occupational solvent exposure. *Br J Ind Med* 1992;49:776–781.
111. Seaton A, Jellinek EH, Kennedy P. Major neurological disease and occupational exposure to organic solvents. *QJM* 1992;84:707–712.
112. Seedorff L, Olsen E. Exposure to organic solvents. I. A survey on the use of solvents. *Ann Occup Hyg* 1990;34:371–378.
113. Grasso P, Sharra M, Davies DM, et al. Neurophysiological and psychological disorders and occupational exposure to organic solvents. *Ed Chem Toxicol* 1984;22:819–852.
114. Errebo-Knudsen EO, Olsen F. Organic solvents and presenile dementia (the painter's syndrome). A critical review of the Danish literature. *Sci Total Environ* 1986;48:45–67.
115. Bolla KI, Schwartz BX, Agnew J, et al. Subclinical neuropsychiatric effects of chronic low-level solvent exposure in US pain manufacturers. *J Occup Med* 1990;32:676–677.
116. Wells GG, Waldron HA. Methylene chloride burns. *Br J Ind Med* 1984;41(3):420.
117. Stewart RD, Hake CL, Peterson JE. "Degreaser's flush" dermal response to trichloroethylene and ethanol. *Arch Environ Health* 1974;29:1–5.
118. Daniell WE, Couser WG, Rosenstock L. Occupational solvent exposure and glomerulonephritis. A case report and review of the literature. *JAMA* 1988;259:2280–2283.
119. Narvarte J, Saba SR, Ramirez G. Occupational exposure to organic solvents causing chronic tubulointerstitial nephritis. *Arch Intern Med* 1989;149:155–158.
120. Nelson NA, Robins TG, Port FK. Solvent nephrotoxicity in humans and experimental animals. *Am J Nephrol* 1990;10:10–20.
121. Harrington JM, Whitby W, Gray CN, et al. Renal disease and occupation exposure to organic solvents: a case report approach. *Br J Ind Med* 1989;46:643–650.
122. Droz PO, Fernandez JG. Trichloroethylene exposure. Biological monitoring by breath and urine analyses. *Br J Ind Med* 1978;35(1):35–42.
123. Fernandez J, Guberan E, Caperos J. Experimental human exposures to tetrachloroethylene vapor and elimination in breath after inhalation. *Am Ind Hyg Assoc J* 1976;37(3):143–50.
124. Ramsey JD, Flanagan RJ. Detection and identification of volatile organic compounds in blood by headspace gas chromatography as an aid to the diagnosis of solvent abuse. *J Chromatogr* 1981;240:423–444.
125. Chang YL, Yang CC, Deng JF, et al. Diverse manifestations of oral methylene chloride poisoning: report of 6 cases. *J Toxicol Clin Toxicol* 1999;37(4):497–504.
126. Laass W. Therapy of acute oral poisonings by organic solvents. Treatment by activated charcoal in combination with laxatives. *Arch Toxicol Suppl* 1980;4:406–409.
127. Moosa MR, Jansen J, Edelstein CL. Treatment of methyl bromide poisoning with hemodialysis. *Postgrad Med J* 1994;20:733–735.
128. Ruprah M, Mant TG, Flanagan RJ. Acute carbon tetrachloride poisoning in 19 patients: implications for diagnosis and treatment. *Lancet* 1985;1(8436):1027–9.
129. Mathieson PW, Williams G, MacSweeney JE. Survival after massive ingestion of carbon tetrachloride treated by intravenous infusion of acetylcysteine. *Hum Toxicol* 1985;4(6):627–31.
130. Mes J, Davies DJ, Turton D, et al. Levels and trends of chlorinated hydrocarbon contaminants in the breast milk of Canadian women. *Food Addit Contam* 1986;3(4):313–322.
130a. Jan J. Chlorobenzene residues in human fat and milk. *Bull Environ Contam Toxicol* 1983;30(5):595–599.
131. Occupational Safety and Health Association. Occupational Safety and Health Standards. Part 1910. Subpart Z—Toxic and Hazardous Substances 695 to 702-0-30. Washington, DC: Occupational Safety and Health Association, 1998.
132. Ducatman AM. Prader-Willi syndrome and paternal hydrocarbon exposure. *Lancet* 1988;1:646.
132a. Anderson HA, Wolff MS, Lilis R, et al. Symptoms and clinical abnormalities following ingestion of polybrominated-biphenyl-contaminated food products. *Ann N Y Acad Sci* 1979;320:684–702.
133. Wabeke R, Weinstein R, Letz G. Polychlorinated biphenyl toxicity. *Case studies in environmental medicine*. 12. Atlanta: Agency for Toxic Substances and Disease Registry; 1990.
133a. Mathews HB, Anderson MW. Effect of chlorination on the distribution and excretion of polychlorinated biphenyls. *Drug Metab Dispos* 1975;3(5):371–380.
134. Chen PH, Luo ML, Wong CK, et al. Comparative rates of elimination of some individual polychlorinated biphenyls from the blood of PCB-poisoned patients in Taiwan. *Food Chem Toxicol* 1982;20(4):417–25.
135. Steele G, Stehr-Green P, Welty E. Estimates of the biologic half-life of polychlorinated biphenyls in human serum. *N Engl J Med* 1986;314(14):926–7.
135a. Brilliant LB, Wilcox K, Van Amburg G, et al. Breast-milk monitoring to measure Michigan's contamination with polybrominated biphenyls. *Lancet* 1978;2:643–646.
136. Sherrell K, Meyerheim RF, Rodgers SA, et al. Polychlorinated biphenyl transformer incident—New Mexico. *MMWR Morb Mortal Wkly Rep* 1985;34:557–559.
137. Masuda Y, Kuroki H, Haraguchi K, et al. PCB and PCDF congeners in the blood and tissues of yusho and yu-cheng patients. *Environ Health Perspect* 1985;59:53–8.
138. Hsu ST, Ma CI, Hsu SK, et al. Discovery and epidemiology of PCB poisoning in Taiwan: a four-year followup. *Environ Health Perspect* 1985;59:5–10.
139. International Agency for Research on Cancer. IARC monograph, vol. 18, Suppl. 7; 1987. IARC Press, Lyon, France
140. ehpWeb site. Available at: http://ehp.niehs.nih.gov/roc/toc10.html. Accessed April 2003.
141. Integrated Risk Information System. US EPA/600/P-96/001F. Environmental Protection Agency Web site. Available at: http://www.epa.gov/iris/subst/index.html. Accessed April 2003.
142. Brown DP, Jones M. Mortality and industrial hygiene study of workers exposed to polychlorinated biphenyls. *Arch Environ Health* 1981;36(3):120–9.
143. Gustavsson P, Hogstedt C, Rappe C. Short-term mortality and cancer incidence in capacitor manufacturing workers exposed to polychlorinated biphenyls (PCBs). *Am J Ind Med* 1986;10(4):341–4.
143a. Second National Report on Human Exposure to Environmental Chemicals. Department of Health and Human Services. Centers for Disease Control and Prevention. Atlanta: National Center for Environmental Health 30341. NCEM Pub No. 02-0716. Revised March 2003.
143b. Fischbein A, Rizzo JN, Solomon SJ, et al. Oculodermatological findings in workers with occupational exposure to polychlorinated biphenyls (PCBs). *Br J Ind Med* 1985;42(6):426–430.
143c. Phillips DL, Pirkle JL, Burse VW, et al. Chlorinated hydrocarbon levels in human serum: effects of fasting and feeding. *Arch Environ Contam Toxicol* 1989;18(4):495–500.
143d. Acquavella JF, Hanis NM, Nicolich MJ, et al. Assessment of clinical, metabolic, dietary, and occupational correlations with serum polychlorinated biphenyl levels among employees at an electrical capacitor manufacturing plant. *J Occup Med* 1986;28(11):1177–1180.
143e. Chia LG, Chu FL. A clinical and electrophysiological study of patients with polychlorinated biphenyl poisoning. *J Neurol Neurosurg Psychiatry* 1985;48(9):894–901.
144. Agency for Toxic Substances and Disease Registry. *Toxicological profile for chlorinated dibenzofurans draft*. Washington, DC: U.S. Department of Health and Human Services; 1992.
144a. Hayabuchi H, Yoshimura T, Kuratsune M. Consumption of toxic rice oil by 'yusho' patients and its relation to the clinical response and latent period. *Food Cosmet Toxicol* 1979;17(5):455–461.
144b. Ryan JJ, Levesque D, Panopio LG, et al. Elimination of polychlorinated dibenzofurans (PCDFs) and polychlorinated biphenyls (PCBs) from human blood in the Yusho and Yu-Cheng rice oil poisonings. *Arch Environ Contam Toxicol* 1993;24(4):504–512.
144c. Funatsu I, Yamashita F, Ito Y, et al. Polychlorbiphenyls (PCB) induced fetopathy. I. Clinical observation. *Kurume Med J* 1972;19(1):43–51.
144d. Gladen BC, Taylor JS, Wu YC, et al. Dermatological findings in children exposed transplacentally to heat-degraded polychlorinated biphenyls in Taiwan. *Br J Dermatol* 1990;122(6):799–808.
144e. Hsu S-T, Ma C-I, Hsu SKS, et al. Discovery and epidemiology of PCB poisoning in Taiwan: a four-year followup. *Environ Health Perspect* 1985;59:5–10.
144f. Lan SJ, Yen YY, Yang CH, et al. [A study on the birth weight of transplacental Yu-Cheng babies.] *Gaoxiong Yi Xue Ke Xue Za Zhi* 1987;3(4):273–282.

144g. Rogan WJ, Gladen BC, Hung KL, et al. Congenital poisoning by polychlorinated biphenyls and their contaminants in Taiwan. *Science* 1988;241(4863):334–336.
144h. Taki I, Hisanaga S, Amagase Y. [Report on Yusho (chlorobiphenyls poisoning) pregnant women and their fetuses.] *Fukuoka Igaku Zasshi* 1969;60:471–474.
144i. Kuratsune M, Yoshimura T, Matsuzaka J, et al. Yusho, a poisoning caused by rice oil contaminated with polychlorinated biphenyls. *HSMHA Health Rep* 1971;86(12):1083–1091.
144j. Yu ML, Hsu CC, Gladen BC, et al. In utero PCB/PCDF exposure: relation of developmental delay to dysmorphology and dose. *Neurotoxicol Teratol* 1991;13(2):195–202.
144k. Kuratsune M. Yusho, with reference to Yu-Cheng. In: Kimbrough RD, Jensen A, eds. *Halogenated biphenyls, terphenyls, naphthalene, dibenzodioxins and related products*, 2nd ed. Amsterdam: Elsevier Science, 1989:381–400.
144l. Rogan WJ, Miller RW. Prenatal exposure to polychlorinated biphenyls. *Lancet* 1989;2(8673):1216.
145. Pott P. *Chirurgical observations relative to the cataract, the polyps of the nose, the cancer of the scrotum, the different kinds of ruptures, and the mortification of the toes and feet.* London: Hawkes, Clark and Collins, 1775.
145a. Perwak J, Byrne M, Coone S, et al. An exposure and risk assessment for benzo[a]pyrene and other polycyclic aromatic hydrocarbons. Volume IV. Benzo[a]pyrene, acenaphthylene, benz[a]anthracene, benzo[b]fluoranthene, benzo[k]fluroanthene, benzo[g,h,i]perylene, chrysene, dibenz[a,h]anthracene, and indeno[1,2,3-c,d]pyrene. Washington, D.C.: US Environmental Protection Agency, Office of Water Regulations and Standards. EPA 440/4-85-020-V4, 1982.
145b. Hawley GG. *The condensed chemical dictionary*. New York: Van Nostrand Reinhold, 1987.
145c. Windholz M. *The Merck index*, 10th ed. Rahway, NJ: Merck and Co., 1983.
145d. Kawamura Y, Kamata E, Ogawa Y, et al. The effect of various foods on the intestinal absorption of benzo-a-pyrene in rats. *J Food Hyg Soc Jpn* 1988;29:21–25.
145e. Jerina DM, Sayer JM, Thakker DR, et al. Carcinogenicity of polycyclic aromatic hydrocarbons: the bay-region theory. In: Pullman B, Ts'O POP, Gelboin H, eds. *Carcinogenesis: fundamental mechanisms and environmental effects*. Hingham, MA: D. Reidel Publishing, 1980:1–12.
145f. Madhavan ND, Naidu KA. Polycyclic aromatic hydrocarbons in placenta, maternal blood, umbilical cord blood and milk of Indian women. *Hum Exp Toxicol* 1995;14(6):503–506.
146. Brudzewski J, Shusterman D. *Polynuclear aromatic hydrocarbons (PAH) toxicity*. Agency for Toxic Substances and Disease Registry. Atlanta: U.S. Department of Health and Human Services; 1990.
146a. Gupta P, Banerjee DK, Bhargava SK, et al. Prevalence of impaired lung function in rubber manufacturing factory workers exposed to benzo(a)pyrene and respirable particulate matter. *Indoor Environ* 1993;2:26–31.
147. Sherson D, Sabro P, Sigsgaard T, et al. Biological monitoring of foundry workers exposed to polycyclic aromatic hydrocarbons. *Br J Ind Med* 1990;47:448–453.
147a. Harris J, Perwak J, Coon S. Exposure and risk assessment for benzo(a)pyrene and other polycyclic aromatic hydrocarbons. Volume 1. Summary:123–135.
147b. Haugen A, Becher G, Benestad C, et al. Determination of polycyclic aromatic hydrocarbons in the urine, benzo(a)pyrene diol epoxide-DNA adducts in lymphocyte DNA, and antibodies to the adducts in sera from coke oven workers exposed to measured amounts of polycyclic aromatic hydrocarbons in the work atmosphere. *Cancer Res* 1986;46(8):4178–4183.
147c. Uziel M, Ward RJ, Vo-Dinh T. Synchronous fluorescence measurement of benzo(a)pyrene metabolites in human and animal urine. *Anal Lett* 1987;20:761–776.
148. Reference deleted.
149. Landrigan PJ. Health risks of creosotes. *JAMA* 1993;209:1309.
150. Karlehagen S, Andersen A, Ohlson C-G. Cancer incidence among creosote exposed workers. *Scand J Work Environ Health* 1992;18:26–29.
151. Agency for Toxic Substances and Disease Registry. *Toxicological profile for creosote*. Atlanta: Department of Health and Human Services, Public Health Service; 1990. Publication TP 90-09.
152. Juntumen J, Kaste M, Markovan H. Cerebral convulsions after enflurane anaesthesia and occupational exposure to tetrahydrofuran. *J Neurol Neurosurg Psychiatry* 1984;47:1258–1259.
153. Garnier R, Rosenberg N, Puissant JM, et al. Tetrahydrofuran poisoning after occupational exposure. *Br J Ind Med* 1989;46:677–678.
154. Viader F, Lechevalier B, Morin P. Polynevrite toxique chez un travailleur du plastique. Role possible du methyl-ethyl-cetone. *Presse Med* 1975;4:1813–1815.
155. Stoughton RW, Robbins BH. The anesthetic properties of tetrahydrofuran. *J Pharmacol Exp Ther* 1936;58:171–173.
156. Klunk WE, McKeon AC, Covey DF, et al. Alpha substituted gamma-butyrolactones: new class of anticonvulsant drugs. *Science* 1982;217:1040–1042.
157. Moody DE. The effect of tetrahydrofuran on biological system: does a hepatotoxic potential exist? *Drug Chem Toxicol* 1991;14:319–342.
158. Elovaara E, Pfaffli P, Savolainen H. Burden and biochemical effects of extended tetrahydrofuran vapour inhalation of three concentration levels. *Acta Pharmacol Toxicol* 1984;54:221–226.
159. Nagata T, Hara M, Kageura M, et al. A fatal case of tetrahydrofuran poisoning. In: Maes RAA, ed. *Topics in forensic and analytic toxicology*. Amsterdam: Elsevier Science, 1984:33–37.
160. Ong CN, Chia SE, Phoon WH, et al. Biological monitoring of occupational exposure to tetrahydrofuran. *Br J Ind Med* 1991;48:616–621.
161. Occupational Safety and Health Guidelines for Chemical Hazards. *Cyclohexanone*. Cincinnati: U.S. Department of Health and Human Services. DHHS (NIOSH) Publication no. 89-104, Supplement II-OHG.
162. Sakata M, Kikuchi J, Haga M. Disposition of acetone, methyl ethyl ketone and cyclohexanone in acute poisoning. *Clin Toxicol* 1989;27:67–77.
163. Mills GA, Walker V. Urinary excretion of cyclohexanediol, a metabolite of solvent cyclohexanone, by infants in a special care unit. *Clin Chem* 1990;36:870–874.
164. Proctor NH, Hughes JP, Fischman ML. *Chemical hazards of the workplace*, 2nd ed. New York: Van Nostrand Reinhold, 1989:171–172.
165. Deetz JS, Luehr CA, Vallee BL. Human liver alcohol dehydrogenase isozymes: reduction of aldehydes and ketones. *Biochemistry* 1984;23:6822–6828.
166. Stave U. Liver enzymes. In: Stave U, Weech AA, eds. *Perinatal physiology*. New York: Plenum Publishing, 1978:499–521.
167. Flek J, Sedivec V. Identification and determination of metabolites of cyclohexanone in human urine. *Prac Lek* 1989;41:259–263.
168. Burger LM, Chandor SB. Fatal ingestion of plastic resin catalyst. *Arch Environ Health* 1971;23:402–404.
169. Ong CN, Sia GL, Chia SE, et al. Determination of cyclohexanol in urine and its use in environmental monitoring of cyclohexanone exposure. *J Anal Toxicol* 1991;15:13–16.
170. Devillers J, Boule P, Vasseur P, et al. Environmental and health risks of hydroquinone. *Ecotoxicol Environ Safety* 1990;19:327–354.
171. Key MM, Henschel AF, Butler J, et al., eds. *Occupational diseases. A guide to their recognition*, revised ed. Washington, DC: U.S. Government Printing Office, 1977:249–250. DHEW (NIOSH) Publication no. 77-181.
172. Carlson AJ, Brewer NR. Toxicity studies on hydroquinone. *Proc Soc Exp Biol* 1953;84:684–688.
173. Deichmann WB, Keplinger ML. Phenols and phenolic compounds. In: Patty FA, ed. *Industrial hygiene and toxicology*, 2nd revised ed. Vol. II. New York: Interscience, 1958:1380–1383.
174. Zeidman I, Deutl R. Poisoning by hydroquinone and monomethyl-paramiophenol sulfate. Report of 2 cases with autopsy findings. *Am J Med Sci* 1945;210:328–333.
175. Harbison KG, Belly RT. The biodegradation of hydroquinone. *Environ Toxicol Chem* 1982;1:9–15.
176. Grant WM. *Hydroquinone in toxicology of the eye*, 2nd ed. Springfield, IL: Charles C Thomas Publisher, 1974:564–567.
177. Subrahmanyam UV, Kolachana P, Smith MT. Metabolism of hydroquinone by human myeloperoxidase: mechanisms of stimulation by other phenolic compounds. *Arch Biochem Biophys* 1991;286:76–84.
178. Centers for Disease Control and Prevention. Hydroquinone poisoning aboard a navy ship. *MMWR Morb Mortal Wkly Rep* 1978:237–243.
179. Occupational Safety and Health Standards. *Support Z—toxic and hazardous substances*. Washington, DC: Occupational Safety and Health Administration. Code of Federal Regulations. Title 29, Section 1910.1000 air contaminants.
180. Anderson B. Corneal and conjunctival pigmentation among workers engaged in manufacture of hydroquinone. *Arch Ophthalmol* 1947;38:812–826.
181. Anderson B, Oglesby F. Corneal changes from quinone-hydroquinone exposure. *Arch Ophthalmol* 1958;59:495–501.
182. Scarpa A, Guerci A. Depigmenting procedures and drugs employed by melanoderm populations. *J Ethnopharmacol* 1987;19:17–66.
183. Schulz EJ, Summers B, Summers RS. Inappropriate treatment of cosmetic ochronosis with hydroquinone. *S Afr Med J* 1988;73:59–60.
184. Williams H. Skin lightening creams containing hydroquinone. The case for a temporary ban. *BMJ* 1992;305:963.
185. Anonymous. *Hydroquinone. Dangerous properties of industrial materials*. 1988:51–60. Report no. 3518820 000 8. Van Nostrand: Reinhold, NY.

SECTION

8

Hydrogen Fluoride

CHAPTER 207

Hydrogen Fluoride and Ammonium Fluorides

D. Eric Brush and Cynthia K. Aaron

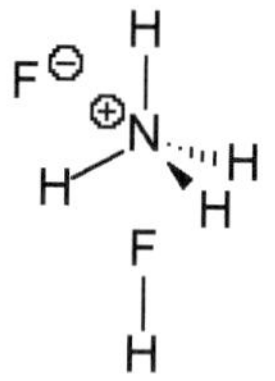

AMMONIUM BIFLUORIDE

Synonyms:	**Hydrofluoric acid [hydrogen fluoride (HF)], ammonium fluoride, ammonium bifluoride**
Molecular formula and weight:	**Hydrogen fluoride (HF), 20.01; ammonium fluoride (NH_4F), 37.04; ammonium bifluoride (NH_4HF_2), 57.04 g/mol**
SI conversion:	**Hydrogen fluoride, ppm × 0.818 = mg/m^3; serum fluoride, mg/L × 52.6 = µg/L**
CAS Registry No.:	**7664-39-3 (hydrogen fluoride); 1341-49-7 (ammonium bifluoride)**
Normal levels:	**10 to 55 µg/dl (fluoride ion, serum)**
Target organs:	**Skin (acute), gastrointestinal (acute), heart (acute), lungs (acute)**
Antidotes:	**Calcium and magnesium salts**

OVERVIEW

Fluorides comprise a group of compounds ranging from the highly corrosive hydrofluoric acid used in the petrochemical industry to sodium fluoride added to municipal drinking water and toothpaste for prevention of dental caries. The degree and mode of toxicity depend on the extent, route, and acuity of the exposure as well as the particular cation associated with the fluoride anion. Although the greatest toxicity stems from exposures to hydrofluoric acid, toxicity from ammonium fluoride and ammonium bifluoride has also caused death. In this chapter, the toxicity for all three compounds is considered similar unless otherwise specified. Sodium fluoride is addressed in Chapter 172.

Hydrogen fluoride (HF) is a highly water-soluble gas that dissolves in water to form hydrofluoric acid. The concentration in products varies from less than 10% to more than 99% (anhydrous hydrogen fluoride). The liquid form is clear and colorless, fumes at a concentration greater than 48%, and has an irritating odor. Dilute formulations are commonly available as rust removers containing from 2% to 12% HF. More concentrated solutions in the range of 20% to 99% are available for glass etching, semiconductor manufacturing, brick cleaning, and as catalysts in the production of high-octane fuels. Toxicity ranges from mild mucous membrane and upper respiratory tract irritation to third degree burns, pulmonary edema, systemic hypocalcemia, hypomagnesemia, and ventricular fibrillation.

Ammonium fluoride and *ammonium bifluoride* are closely related to HF. Ammonium fluoride is used in printing and dyeing textiles, glass etching, and wood preserving. Ammonium bifluoride is used also to etch glass, serves as a wood preservative, and removes rust. Ammonium fluoride and ammonium bifluoride exist in combination in automobile aluminum wheel cleaners and rust removers with concentrations less than 16%. Like HF, these compounds exert their toxicity from the dissociated fluoride ion. Ammonium bifluoride is potentially more toxic than ammonium fluoride because it dissociates in water, releasing both a fluoride ion and a molecule of

TABLE 1. U.S. regulatory guidelines and standards for hydrogen fluoride

Agency	Description	Concentration [mg/m³ (ppm)]
OSHA	Vapor or gas	
	PEL-TWA	2.5 (3)
	STEL	5.0 (6)
ACGIH	Vapor or gas	
	TLV-ceiling	2.5 (3)
NIOSH	Vapor or gas	
	REL-TWA	2.5 (3)
	Ceiling (15-min)	5.0 (6)
	IDLH	25.0 (30)

ACGIH, American Conference of Governmental Industrial Hygienists; IDLH, immediate danger to life or health; NIOSH, National Institute for Occupational Safety and Health; OSHA, U.S. Occupational Safety and Health Administration; PEL, permissible exposure limit; ppm, parts per million; REL, recommended exposure limit; STEL, short-term exposure limit; TLV, threshold limit value; TWA, time-weighted average.

HF. Ammonium fluoride may cause some chemical burns; however, its potential for significant dermal injury is far less than that of either hydrofluoric acid or ammonium bifluoride.

TOXIC DOSE

Occupational standards and guidelines are provided in Table 1. Exposure to hydrofluoric acid caused at least 14 deaths between 1984 and 1994 (1). With one exception, all exposures involved a highly concentrated solution splashing the face, neck, or large surface area or coincided with inhalational injury. One death in that series of patients occurred with ingestion of dilute HF in rust remover (1). The smallest dermal exposure associated with death was 2.5% total body surface area (BSA). The burn was located on the face, and evidence of upper airway irritation was noted on autopsy (2). A 14-month-old child suffered hypocalcemia and recurrent ventricular tachycardia after an 11%-BSA burn from a mixture of 8% hydrofluoric acid and 23% hydrochloric acid (3).

Although the exact amount and concentration of HF required to cause significant toxicity remains unknown, 7 ml of anhydrous HF is capable of binding all the free calcium in a normal-sized adult (4). For airborne exposure, the Health and Safety Executive in the United Kingdom calculated a Specified Level of Toxicity as 200 parts per million (ppm) for 60 minutes based on animal data. This level is expected to cause severe distress, likely need for medical attention, and possible death in susceptible individuals. The Dangerous Toxic Load, extrapolated to more accurately reflect the brief large exposures that potentially occur in the workplace, is estimated at 12,000 ppm for 1 minute (5).

TOXICOKINETICS AND TOXICODYNAMICS

Hydrofluoric acid is a weak acid with a dissociation constant of 3.53×10^{-4}. It is 1000 times less dissociated than an equimolar amount of hydrochloric acid. Absorption occurs through intact skin, mucous membranes, and gastrointestinal and respiratory tracts. Minor skin damage, including vigorous washing with detergents, may increase dermal absorption (6). Protonation of tissues occurs on dissociation of the hydrogen and fluorine atoms, a process which continues until the acid has been neutralized and the fluorine ion complexes with calcium and magnesium (7).

The liberated fluorine ions concentrate initially at the site of injury. Distribution to bone, blood, and distant soft tissues occurs in the second phase. Autopsy reveals increased fluorine concentration in all tissues. Fluorine is eliminated by both sequestration in bone and renal elimination. The half-life of elimination for fluorine is between 5.1 and 9.0 hours (8,9). Initial elevations in urinary fluoride concentrations after exposure generally approach baseline within 24 hours (10). A direct correlation between air levels of HF and plasma fluorides (11,12), as well as urinary fluorides (13), has been demonstrated. Urinary fluoride has been used to screen workers for excessive exposure (10). A portion of the fluoride ions binds with hydroxyapatite crystals in bone to create a more persistent total body burden of fluoride. This explains the baseline elevation in urinary fluorides of workers chronically exposed to HF in comparison with nonexposed individuals.

PATHOPHYSIOLOGY

The toxicity of HF has two separate mechanisms. The liberation of protons in higher concentration solutions results in extensive liquefactive necrosis of dermal, gastrointestinal, and respiratory tissues. Its relatively low dissociation constant permits deeper tissue penetration and more extensive injury than stronger acids. In addition, the highly electronegative fluorine ion binds avidly to calcium and magnesium, forming insoluble complexes (7). Locally, this manifests as excruciating pain from disruption of transmembrane potentials in nerve fibers. Systemically, it can produce profound hypocalcemia, hypomagnesemia, and hyperkalemia (1,2,14–19). Further pathology may arise from direct cellular toxicity. Fluorine disrupts multiple enzymes, including Na,K–adenosine triphosphatase, adenyl cyclase (20), and 3-hydroxy-3-methylglutaryl coenzyme A reductase (21). Cell death results from disruption of intracellular transport and energy mechanisms. This may cause myocardial injury, as documented in one case. However, concomitant use of adrenergic agents confounds any conclusions from autopsy in that patient (14).

VULNERABLE POPULATIONS

HF is teratogenic and embryotoxic in rats. A study of female superphosphate workers exposed to multiple chemicals, including fluorides, found an increased rate of abnormal pregnancies (22). Large prenatal exposure to fluoride causes mottling of baby teeth in humans (23).

CLINICAL PRESENTATION

Acute Exposure

Dermal and ocular exposures have toxic effects and a rate of onset that is related to the concentration of product, exposure time, and route of exposure. Exposure to concentrations of HF greater than 48% is likely to have significant dermal injury, requiring careful wound assessment. Dermal exposure to high concentrations causes skin burns rapidly and may be fatal. In fatal cases, the product concentration is usually high and involves more than 2.5% total BSA. Industrial accidents involving exposure to large amounts of concentrated HF may cause immediate death (15) or death within hours (10,18,24,25). Immediate pain develops from dermal contact with concentrations of HF greater than 49%, whereas concentrations between 20% and 49% cause fairly rapid onset of symptoms. In contrast, the onset of pain after dilute HF (less than 20%) exposure is delayed up to 24 hours after initial contact, with pain out of proportion to physical findings (26,27).

The skin may be slightly swollen, erythematous, or exhibit whitish-blue discoloration, particularly under the nails. Severe chemical injury leads to blistering and black eschar formation. Occasionally, the skin may show dense, firm white collections from liquefaction of underlying tissues. Even small chemical burns with dilute solutions may be associated with significant morbidity such as severe pain, ocular injury, disfigurement, or disability. Ocular injuries occur from either direct splashes or exposure to HF fumes. Severe corneal abrasions and delayed ulceration are complications from ocular exposure.

Ingestion of a concentrated (typically greater than 20%) solution results in immediate mouth and throat burns, emesis, often profound electrolyte disturbances (15), and death (1). Patients with this degree of exposure often experience syncope, weakness, or altered levels of consciousness. A common misperception is that dilute products (less than 12%) cause acute gastrointestinal injury. In truth, ingestion of a low concentration solution often causes no apparent injury, even on endoscopy (28). Ingestion of a dilute solution may have a 1- to 4-hour period with few symptoms, only to have the patient suddenly deteriorate and die of ventricular dysrhythmia (28). Further, a relatively large ingestion, typically suicidal, is needed to cause death after ingestion of a dilute product (28).

Inhalation exposure produces signs of injury quickly. Pulmonary edema may be delayed for a few hours, but signs of upper respiratory tract injury are present earlier. In one incident, a cloud of HF gas arose from a spill of 53,000 lb anhydrous HF. Local emergency departments subsequently triaged 939 visitors. Most patients complained of ocular, respiratory, and throat irritation (29). Impaired pulmonary function (decreased forced expiratory volume in the first second in 42% of patients), hypoxemia (partial pressure of arterial oxygen less than 80 mm Hg in 17.4% of patients), and hypocalcemia (less than 8.5 mg/dl in 16.3% of patients) were also noted. There were no deaths noted among the 94 patients who were hospitalized.

Ammonium fluoride and ammonium bifluoride are primarily pediatric exposures. Hypocalcemia, hypomagnesemia, recurrent ventricular fibrillation, and death have all occurred after exposure to wheel cleaners containing ammonium bifluoride. Cases involved children spraying each other or ingesting the substance (30,31). External burns were absent in these cases, although endoscopy identified a gastric ulcer in a child who ingested the product. Adult fatalities are described in relation to suicides using similar compounds (32).

Chronic Exposure

Exposure to large amounts of fluoride-containing materials over time may produce a constellation of findings termed *fluorosis*. A classic triad of osteosclerosis, exostoses, and calcifications of ligaments leading to vague, diffuse musculoskeletal pains was described by Roholm in 1937 (33). The teeth exhibit a mottled appearance with chalky patches. Cases of fluorosis have become rare, as water fluoridation and workplace exposures are tightly regulated. U.S. citizens who are not occupationally exposed to fluorides are unlikely to have significant risk of fluorosis. Development of chronic disease requires 20 to 80 mg of fluoride daily for 10 to 20 years (34). The average diet contains 0.25 to 1.50 mg of fluoride daily (35).

DIAGNOSTIC TESTS

Biologic Monitoring

The National Institute for Occupational Safety and Health has recommended limits on preshift and postshift urinary fluoride levels of 4.0 mg/L and 7.0 mg/L, respectively.

Acute Exposure

No laboratory testing is needed for dermal exposure to dilute solutions involving a small surface area. A retrospective review of 237 cases of skin exposure from dilute (6% to 11%) HF found no systemic toxicity (36). Most of these burns involved parts of hands or fingers, the largest involving 8% to 10% total BSA. The only report of severe hypocalcemia from dermal exposure to dilute HF was a 1% to 2% BSA involving intentional intradermal injection of a 7% solution (37).

More intensive monitoring is needed for patients who have ingested HF, have respiratory symptoms, had contact with a product containing more than 20% HF, or in whom more than 1% BSA is involved. These measures provide a safety margin in light of reported deaths associated with burns covering only 2.5% BSA (2). No clear evidence exists to determine the exact risk of systemic toxicity from a given exposure, and other authors may suggest different criteria (14,19).

The goal of testing is to monitor for hypocalcemia and its electrocardiogram (ECG) effects. If available, ionized calcium levels are preferred to total serum calcium because they measure the species of interest and potentially are available more quickly. An ECG allows rapid detection of electrolyte disturbances, as evidenced by peaked T waves, widened QRS, and prolonged QTc. Chvostek's and Trousseau's signs on physical examination provide additional early clues of hypocalcemia.

A chest radiograph is needed in patients with airway irritation or dyspnea. Pulmonary edema may develop rapidly, resulting from either myocardial depression or direct lung injury.

Elevated urine or serum fluoride concentrations are detectable but not readily available for clinical management. Serum concentrations associated with fatality generally exceed 300 μg/dl (2,14,17). However, levels above 600 μg/dl have been reported in survivors (19), with 2100 μg/dl representing the highest serum fluoride concentration reported in a survivor (3). Beyond confirmation of the diagnosis, fluoride concentrations provide little benefit.

TREATMENT

The immediate goals of treatment are to limit skin or gastrointestinal burns and respiratory injury and to treat hypocalcemia. Providers must take care to protect themselves from contamination during examination and treatment. Full personal protective clothing should be used when higher concentrations are involved, but only gloves are likely needed for products of 8% to 12% concentration. The patient's clothes, gowns, and any other items should be handled as hazardous materials.

Decontamination

After *dermal exposure*, the clothing should be removed and skin immediately flushed copiously with water. If potentially involved, the eyes are irrigated with water or saline. Recently, experience with a decontaminant called *hexafluorine* has shown promise as an onsite decontaminant. The solution is amphoteric, polyvalent, and slightly hypertonic. An uncontrolled human trial demonstrated safety and efficacy for skin and eye decontamination (38). However, the lack of a control decontaminant in this study prevents drawing sound conclusions. It is available in France and Germany.

In the case of *ingestion*, initial decontamination can be performed by aspiration with a small nasogastric tube (if very soon after ingestion). A calcium- or magnesium-containing solution (10% calcium gluconate, 30 cc of a magnesium antacid, milk of magnesia, or calcium carbonate) should be given to bind the fluoride ion. Small aliquots are necessary to reduce the risk of vomiting. Emesis is contraindicated due to the caustic nature of HF. Activated charcoal has no role in HF ingestion.

Dermal Injury

The principle of treatment is to provide cationic ions that will bind F^-, the fluoride anion. This reduces tissue injury and relieves pain, but additional therapy for hypocalcemia may be needed. Although a variety of antidotes have been tested [calcium gluconate gel or slurry, calcium carbonate gel, calcium acetate solution, 5% or 10% calcium gluconate injections into affected skin, benzalkonium chloride (Zephiran) soaks, benzethonium chloride (Hyamine) soaks, magnesium gluconate gel, and magnesium hydroxide solution], calcium gluconate preparations are most commonly used. Because penetration of topical compounds to deep tissues is generally poor, penetration enhancers, such as dimethyl sulfoxide, have been tested as well. The addition of dimethyl sulfoxide enhances calcium penetration (39); however, it has a poor safety profile and is unlikely to be approved for this use. Therefore, topical agents are most effective for superficial burns, whereas injections are suggested for deeper injuries refractory to topical therapy. Iontophoretic delivery of calcium chloride in HF-injured mice demonstrated promising results, but human studies are lacking (40).

However, the numerous animal studies performed with fluoride binding agents have yielded conflicting results (27,39–45). Overall, calcium gluconate gel, 2.5%, showed the most consistent improvement with regard to pain relief and wound healing, and 10% calcium gluconate injections often showed harmful effects. *Calcium chloride* should never be injected subcutaneously due to the risk of tissue necrosis. For the same reason, injections of *calcium gluconate* should not exceed a 5% concentration (26). A 2.5% calcium gluconate gel is available commercially, although not all hospitals stock the product. A gel can be formulated in any health facility by adding 3.5 g of calcium gluconate to 5 oz of surgical lubricant. Alternatively, ten calcium carbonate tablets (10 g/tablet) can be crushed and the powder mixed with 20 ml of lubricant, making a slurry (46). Early application yields better results (36). Over time, the fluoride ions in the skin bind irreversibly with dermal calcium, making gel application futile. The mixture may be applied every 4 to 6 hours to the affected area for a 24-hour period. The author uses an occlusive dressing (e.g., place the gel in a latex glove for a hand burn) and mixes the gel with an emollient cream to combat the extreme drying nature of the gel.

If adequate relief is not obtained by topical measures within 60 minutes, consider local injections of 5% calcium gluconate solution, not to exceed 0.5 ml/cm^2. Larger volume injections may compromise blood supply and cause tissue necrosis. Hypercalcemia has been reported with local injections; however, this is rare (47). This technique is limited by pain with injections. In addition, the amount of calcium delivered to the tissues due to the restricted volume may be insufficient to bind the fluoride.

Finger and subungual burns present a difficult challenge. Fascial planes and multiple septations in these areas make injection difficult. Also, the presence of a thick cuticle hinders the topical delivery of calcium to the nail bed. One approach is to remove the fingernail and administer injections into the nail bed, but this technique has produced mixed results (26,46,48). In a low concentration exposure, topical therapy with calcium gluconate gel alone may provide adequate symptom relief. This approach has been effective in case series, both with and without nail removal (36,46,49). Therefore, direct digital injections and nailbed removal are not recommended in most cases.

Intraarterial Infusion and Regional Perfusion

Intraarterial infusion and regional intravenous perfusion of calcium gluconate are techniques used for burns that do not respond to topical therapy. Although prospective, randomized human studies are not available with either technique, persistent severe pain despite the topical application of calcium gluconate gel warrants a more invasive treatment. Both methods provide much higher concentrations of calcium to affected tissues than the topical gel or local injection techniques.

Intraarterial calcium has been used successfully for relief by several authors (50–54). Risks associated with the procedure include arterial spasm, hematoma, nerve injury, and extravasation of calcium, resulting in tissue necrosis. Allen's test should be performed before cannulating the radial artery to confirm adequate collateral flow from the radial and ulnar arteries. Studies using arteriograms have typically advanced the catheter from the radial to the brachial artery to provide an infusion down the ulnar circulation when injuries involved the fourth or fifth digits (51). However, this author has successfully treated ulnar-sided injuries with radial artery infusions. This method is possible in the presence of good collateral flow through the palmar arch.

To make the solution for intraarterial infusion, 10 ml of 10% calcium gluconate is diluted with dextrose 5% in water for a total volume of 50 to 100 ml. The degree of vascular injury from a calcium infusion correlates with the concentration of calcium in the solution (45). Therefore, the solution should not exceed the suggested formulation, and calcium chloride should not be used. The solution is infused over 4 hours. The infusion is repeated up to 3 or 4 times until pain relief is obtained. On average, patients require two or three infusions (51). If symptoms of pain persist beyond 12 hours, additional infusions are unlikely to provide benefit.

Regional perfusion of calcium gluconate is administered using the Bier block technique. It has been used on both upper- and lower-extremity burns with various rates of success (55–59). Intravenous access is obtained in the affected extremity before the procedure. The affected limb is exsanguinated by raising the limb and wrapping it tightly with an Esmarch's bandage. A blood pressure cuff is placed proximally and inflated to a pressure slightly greater than the patient's systolic pressure, thereby preventing blood from reentering the extremity. The infusion is prepared by diluting 10 to 20 ml of 10% calcium gluconate with dextrose 5% in water to a total volume of 40 ml. This is infused intravenously into the exsanguinated limb, resulting in delivery of calcium to all areas of the limb. The cuff pressure is slowly released after 30 to 45 minutes. The patient experiences significant pain from the pressure cuff, exsanguination, and the calcium infusion. Consider procedural sedation for this method. Patients who do not obtain adequate analgesia from any of these techniques should be offered regional nerve blocks with long-acting local anesthetics, if anatomically possible.

Ingestion

Even an ingestion of a dilute HF solution can cause death (28,60,61). Deaths may occur without warning after an initial period of mild gastrointestinal symptoms (28). A retrospective review of 99 cases involving ingestion of dilute products (6% to 8%) revealed gastrointestinal upset in 49 patients and two deaths. Both fatalities occurred within 4 hours (28). All patients with major effects or those who died (N = 3) had intentionally ingested more than 3 oz of a product. An elderly woman attempted suicide by ingestion of dilute HF on two separate occasions. She suffered recurrent ventricular tachycardia on the first attempt and hypocalcemia with a prolonged QTc on both occasions. The patient ultimately survived, exhibiting mild esophageal and gastric burns (15).

Although there is some risk associated with nasogastric tube placement in the context of a caustic injury, decontamination is critical to prevent systemic toxicity from absorbed fluoride ions. The acidic pH of the stomach enhances dissociation of free fluoride ions and heightens the potential for systemic toxicity. Irrigation with small aliquots of calcium-containing solutions may chelate available fluoride ions. Brushite (calcium phosphate) has been shown *in vitro* to bind the highest percentage of fluoride ions in acid pH conditions; however, studies of human safety are lacking (62).

Pediatric ingestions in the home may be initially treated with milk or water dilution, concurrent with seeking medical attention. Emesis is contraindicated due to the caustic nature of HF. Survivors may need consultation with gastroenterology for endoscopy. Higher-concentration solutions are much more likely to cause gastrointestinal injury. The timing of endoscopy is controversial, but as with other caustics, a delay in the procedure beyond 24 hours may be associated with a higher risk of iatrogenic esophageal or gastric perforation.

Ocular Exposure

Few data exist to suggest the optimal treatment for ocular injuries. Exposures may initially appear mild yet result in severe corneal damage. Globe injury may be ongoing and present as delayed corneal ulceration (63). Immediate flushing with normal saline for at least 30 minutes is crucial. Animal models indicate that more prolonged irrigation increases the degree of corneal abrasions (64,65). Case reports in humans suggest using 1% calcium gluconate drops every 2 to 3 hours for 1 to 2 days (63,66). However, a controlled study in rabbits revealed no advantage of 1% calcium gluconate drops or 1% calcium gluconate irrigation over saline irrigation alone (67). Topical steroids, local débridement, and antibiotic drops have all been used in humans with no controlled studies to assess effectiveness. Ophthalmology consultation is warranted with any ocular exposure.

Inhalation Injury

Airway injury may occur from concentrated solutions of HF when splashed on or near the face. Fumes spontaneously emanate from HF solutions greater than 48%. A mass exposure from an HF spill produced nasopharyngeal irritation, cough, and dyspnea (29). Significant exposures may result in rapid pulmonary edema and death (1). Respiratory complaints may prompt the use of calcium gluconate as a 2.5%- or 3.0%-nebulized solution. This is easily made with 1.5 ml of 10% calcium gluconate added to 4.5 ml of water or saline. No guidelines exist regarding the frequency of treatments or endpoints of therapy. Case reports of its use in humans have not revealed any adverse effects (68–70). Literature supporting its efficacy is lacking.

Systemic Toxicity

Hypocalcemia is the primary systemic effect of clinical concern. Systemic toxicity may result from chemical burns of any HF concentration with greater than 1% BSA involvement, burns from high concentrations of HF (greater than 20%) to less than 1% total BSA, ingestion of any HF concentration, or inhalational injuries. Patients may develop life-threatening hypocalcemia, hypomagnesemia, and hyperkalemia. Most deaths due to systemic toxicity have occurred within hours of exposure (2,14,18). Systemic toxicity is often delayed with dilute solutions. Death results from ventricular fibrillation, pulmonary edema, or refractory hypocalcemia or hypomagnesemia. Ventricular fibrillation is frequently recurrent, even in those who ultimately survive their injuries (15).

When systemic toxicity is likely (e.g., large exposure, high HF concentration, or intent for self-harm), intravenous calcium administration should begin before any signs or symptoms of systemic toxicity. The empiric addition, 20 ml of 10% calcium gluconate to the first liter of crystalloid solution, may provide some benefit (71). Much more aggressive therapy is needed if hypocalcemia or its physical signs develop (Chvostek's or Trousseau's signs, ECG-QTc prolongation). Hypocalcemia is treated with 10% calcium chloride, 2 to 4 mg/kg IV in adults or 10 to 30 mg/kg IV in children. Survivors have received up to 266 mEq of calcium in the first 24 hours of exposure (19).

Hypomagnesemia and hyperkalemia also need immediate treatment. The serum magnesium concentration may not accurately reflect the degree of hypomagnesemia. Therefore, the presence of hyporeflexia provides a useful bedside screening tool to determine adequate replacement. Magnesium sulfate can be administered as 2 g in 100 cc of normal saline over 10 minutes. Hyperkalemia may be the proximate cause of death in some HF poisonings. In addition to calcium, insulin, glucose, and sodium bicarbonate may be required to treat hyperkalemia (Chapter 35).

Supportive Care

In addition to chelation of fluoride ions, general wound care measures apply to HF burns. Necrotic tissue requires débridement. Extensive surgical removal of tissue in attempts to remove fluoride ions has been used experimentally (72,73) and in humans for the treatment of systemic toxicity (19,74). No definitive evidence suggests this technique should be routinely used.

Severe pain is common to many HF exposures. Attention to pain control during or shortly after decontamination allows further interventions to take place with maximum patient comfort. Narcotic pain medications are frequently required. Although the effectiveness of antidote therapy is gauged by pain relief, administration of narcotic pain medication is unlikely to mask this endpoint.

Additional care is supportive and may involve treatment of cardiac dysrhythmias, pulmonary edema, and fluid losses from chemical burns covering large surface areas. Patients surviving the initial insult from a significant exposure are at risk for delayed complications, including multisystem organ failure, sepsis, and progressive pulmonary injury.

Management Pitfalls

Hourly or more frequent measurements of serum magnesium and ionized calcium are crucial to guide therapy. Serial ECGs and continuous cardiac monitoring provide an additional window to the metabolic state. Potential airway injury may be overlooked when burns occur to the face or neck. Some effects of hydrofluoric acid may be delayed, especially when less concentrated solutions are involved. Corneal or skin injury can take hours to become apparent.

It is important to perform decontamination in high concentration exposures in addition to using antidotes. Furthermore, the clinician must realize that dermal HF injury can produce systemic effects. Delay in treating the underlying cause of dysrhythmias, such as hypocalcemia, hypomagnesemia, or hyperkalemia, may result in death of the patient.

REFERENCES

1. Blodgett DW, AJ Suruda, Crouch BI. Fatal unintentional occupational poisonings by hydrofluoric acid in the U.S. *Am J Ind Med* 2001;40:215–220.
2. Tepperman PB. Fatality due to acute systemic fluoride poisoning following a hydrofluoric acid skin burn. *J Occup Med* 1980;22:691–692.
3. Bordelon BM, JR Saffle, Morris SE. Systemic fluoride toxicity in a child with hydrofluoric acid burns: case report. *J Trauma* 1993;34:437–439.
4. MacKinnon MA. Hydrofluoric acid burns. *Dermatol Clin* 1988;6:67–74.
5. Meldrum M. Toxicology of hydrogen fluoride in relation to major accident hazards. *Regul Toxicol Pharmacol* 1999;30:110–116.
6. Noonan T, et al. Epidermal lipids and the natural history of hydrofluoric acid (HF) injury. *Burns* 1994;20(3):202–206.
7. Kono K, et al. An experimental study on the biochemical consequences of hydrofluoric acid burns. *Bull Osaka Med Sch* 1982;28:124–133.
8. Pierre F, et al. Effect of different exposure compounds on urinary kinetics of aluminium and fluoride in industrially exposed workers. *Occup Environ Med* 1995;52:396–403.
9. Ekstrand J, Ehrnebo M. The relationship between plasma fluoride, urinary excretion rate and urine fluoride concentration in man. *J Occup Med* 1983;25:745–748.
10. Brown MG. Fluoride exposure from hydrofluoric acid in a motor gasoline alkylation unit. *Am Ind Hyg Assoc J* 1985;46:662–669.
11. Kono K, et al. Serum fluoride as an indicator of occupational hydrofluoric acid exposure. *Int Arch Occup Environ Health* 1992;64:343–346.
12. Lund K, et al. Exposure to hydrogen fluoride: an experimental study in humans of concentrations of fluoride in plasma, symptoms, and lung function. *Occup Environ Med* 1997;54:32–37.
13. Kono K, et al. Urinary fluoride monitoring of industrial hydrofluoric acid exposure. *Environ Res* 1987;42:415–420.
14. Mayer TG, Gross PL. Fatal systemic fluorosis due to hydrofluoric acid burns. *Ann Emerg Med* 1985;14:149–153.
15. Stremski ES, Grande GA, Ling LJ. Survival following hydrofluoric acid ingestion. *Ann Emerg Med* 1992;21(11):1396–1399.
16. Sanz-Gallen P, et al. Hypocalcaemia and hypomagnesaemia due to hydrofluoric acid. *Occup Med (Lond)* 2001;51:294–295.
17. Mullett T, et al. Fatal hydrofluoric acid cutaneous exposure with refractory ventricular fibrillation. *J Burn Care Rehabil* 1987;8:216–219.
18. Chan KM, Svancarek WP, Creer M. Fatality due to acute hydrofluoric acid exposure. *J Toxicol Clin Toxicol* 1987;25(4):333–339.
19. Greco RJ, et al. Hydrofluoric acid-induced hypocalcemia. *J Trauma* 1988;28:1593–1596.
20. Perry HE. Pediatric poisonings from household products: hydrofluoric acid and methacrylic acid. *Curr Opin Pediatr* 2001;13:157–161.
21. Philibert C, et al. Effect of hydrogen fluoride inhalation on lipid metabolism in guinea pigs. *Artery* 1991;18:226–234.
22. Heitland G, Hurlbut KM. Hydrogen fluoride (MEDITEXT Medical Management). In: Heitland G, Hurlbut KM, eds. *TOMES system*. Greenwood Village, CO: Micromedex, Inc., 2003.
23. Dabney BJ. Ammonium bifluoride (REPROTEXT document). In: Dabney BJ, ed. *REPROTEXT system*. Englewood, CO: Micromedex, Inc., 1993.
24. Sheridan RL, et al. Emergency management of major hydrofluoric acid exposures. *Burns* 1995;21:62–64.
25. Braun J, Stoss H, Zober A. Intoxication following the inhalation of hydrogen fluoride. *Arch Toxicol* 1984;56:50–54.
26. Dibbell DG, et al. Hydrofluoric acid burns of the hand. *J Bone Joint Surg Am* 1970;52:931–936.
27. Iverson RE, Laub DR, Madison MS. Hydrofluoric acid burns. *Plast Reconstr Surg* 1971;48:107–112.
28. Kao WF, et al. Ingestion of low-concentration hydrofluoric acid: an insidious and potentially fatal poisoning. *Ann Emerg Med* 1999;34:35–41.
29. Wing JS, et al. Acute health effects in a community after a release of hydrofluoric acid. *Arch Environ Health* 1991;46:155–160.
30. Klasaer AE, et al. Marked hypocalcemia and ventricular fibrillation in two pediatric patients exposed to a fluoride-containing wheel cleaner. *Ann Emerg Med* 1996;28:713–718.
31. Mullins ME, Warden CR, Barnum DW. Pediatric death and fluoride-containing wheel cleaner. *Ann Emerg Med* 1998;31:524–525.
32. Litovitz TL, Smilkstein MJ, Berlin R, et al. 1996 annual report of the American Association of Poison Control Centers Toxic Exposure Surveillance System. *Am J Emerg Med* 1997;15:447–500.
33. Roholm K. *A clinical-hygienic study with a review of the literature and some experimental investigation*. London: H.K. Lewis and Co. Ltd., 1937.
34. Moller PF, Gudjonsson SV. Massive fluorosis of bones and ligaments. *Acta Radiol* 1932;13:269–294.
35. Elliot CG, Smith MD. Dietary fluoride related to fluoride content of teeth. *J Dent Res* 1960;39:93–98.
36. El Saadi MS, et al. Hydrofluoric acid dermal exposure. *Vet Hum Toxicol* 1989;31:243–247.
37. Gallerani M, et al. Systemic and topical effects of intradermal hydrofluoric acid. *Am J Emerg Med* 1998;16:521–522.
38. Mathieu L, et al. Efficacy of hexafluorine for emergent decontamination of hydrofluoric acid eye and skin splashes. *Vet Hum Toxicol* 2001;43:263–265.
39. Seyb ST, et al. A study to determine the efficacy of treatments for hydrofluoric acid burns. *J Burn Care Rehabil* 1995;16:253–257.
40. Yamashita M, et al. Iontophoretic delivery of calcium for experimental hydrofluoric acid burns. *Crit Care Med* 2001;29:1575–1578.
41. Dunn BJ, et al. Hydrofluoric acid dermal burns. An assessment of treatment efficacy using an experimental pig model. *J Occup Med* 1992;34:902–909.
42. Burkhart KK, et al. Comparison of topical magnesium and calcium treatment for dermal hydrofluoric acid burns. *Ann Emerg Med* 1994;24:9–13.
43. Bracken WM, et al. Comparative effectiveness of topical treatments for hydrofluoric acid burns. *J Occup Med* 1985;27:733–739.
44. Harris JC, Rumack BH, Bregman DJ. Comparative efficacy of injectable calcium and magnesium salts in the therapy of hydrofluoric acid burns. *J Toxicol Clin Toxicol* 1981;18:1027–1032.
45. Dowbak G, Rose K, Rohrich RJ. A biochemical and histologic rationale for the treatment of hydrofluoric acid burns with calcium gluconate. *J Burn Care Rehabil* 1994;15:323–327.
46. Chick LR, Borah G. Calcium carbonate gel therapy for hydrofluoric acid burns of the hand. *Plast Reconstr Surg* 1990;86:935–940.
47. Burke WJ, Hoegg UR, Phillips RE. Systemic fluoride poisoning resulting from a fluoride skin burn. *J Occup Med* 1973;15:39–41.
48. Roberts JR, Merigian KS. Acute hydrofluoric acid exposure. *Am J Emerg Med* 1989;7:125–126.
49. Anderson WJ, Anderson JR. Hydrofluoric acid burns of the hand: mechanism of injury and treatment. *J Hand Surg [Am]* 1988;13:52–57.
50. Velvart J. Arterial perfusion for hydrofluoric acid burns. *Hum Toxicol* 1983;2:233–238.
51. Vance MV, et al. Digital hydrofluoric acid burns: treatment with intraarterial calcium infusion. *Ann Emerg Med* 1986;15:890–896.
52. Siegel DC, Heard JM. Intra-arterial calcium infusion for hydrofluoric acid burns. *Aviat Space Environ Med* 1992;63:206–211.
53. Lin TM, et al. Continuous intra-arterial infusion therapy in hydrofluoric acid burns. *J Occup Environ Med* 2000;42:892–897.
54. Pegg SP, Siu S, Gillett G. Intra-arterial infusions in the treatment of hydrofluoric acid burns. *Burns Incl Therm Inj* 1985;11:440–443.
55. Henry JA, Hla KK. Intravenous regional calcium gluconate perfusion for hydrofluoric acid burns. *J Toxicol Clin Toxicol* 1992;30:203–207.
56. Graudins A, Burns MJ, Aaron CK. Regional intravenous infusion of calcium gluconate for hydrofluoric acid burns of the upper extremity. *Ann Emerg Med* 1997;30:604–607.
57. Ryan JM, McCarthy GM, Plunkett PK. Regional intravenous calcium—an effective method of treating hydrofluoric acid burns to limb peripheries. *J Accid Emerg Med* 1997;14:401–404.
58. Isbister GK. Failure of intravenous calcium gluconate for hydrofluoric acid burns. *Ann Emerg Med* 2000;36:398.
59. Gubbay AD, Fitzpatrick RI. Dermal hydrofluoric acid burns resulting in death. *Aust N Z J Surg* 1997;67:304–306.
60. Manoguerra AS, Neuman TS. Fatal poisoning from acute hydrofluoric acid ingestion. *Am J Emerg Med* 1986;4:362–363.
61. Bost RO, Springfield A. Fatal hydrofluoric acid ingestion: a suicide case report. *J Anal Toxicol* 1995;19:535–536.
62. Larsen MJ, Jensen SJ. Inactivation of hydrofluoric acid by solutions intended for gastric lavage. *Pharmacol Toxicol* 1990;67:447–448.
63. Rubinfeld RS, et al. Ocular hydrofluoric acid burns. *Am J Ophthalmol* 1992;114:420–423.
64. McCulley JP. Ocular hydrofluoric acid burns: animal model, mechanism of injury and therapy. *Trans Am Ophthalmol Soc* 1990;88:649–684.
65. McCulley JP, et al. Hydrofluoric acid burns of the eye. *J Occup Med* 1983;25:447–450.
66. Bentur Y, et al. The role of calcium gluconate in the treatment of hydrofluoric acid eye burn. *Ann Emerg Med* 1993;22:1488–1490.
67. Beiran I, Miller B, Bentur Y. The efficacy of calcium gluconate in ocular hydrofluoric acid burns. *Hum Exp Toxicol* 1997;16:223–228.
68. Lee DC, Wiley JF 2nd, Synder JW 2nd. Treatment of inhalational exposure to hydrofluoric acid with nebulized calcium gluconate. *J Occup Med* 1993;35:470.
69. Boyer E, Walker N, Woolf A, Shannon M. Inhalational exposure to hydrogen fluoride treated with nebulized calcium gluconate. *J Toxicol Clin Toxicol* 2000;38:545.
70. Trevino C, Smith G, Ryan M, Arnold T. Nebulized calcium gluconate for the treatment of respiratory exposure to hydrofluoric acid. *J Toxicol Clin Toxicol* 2000;39:509(abst).
71. Trevino MA, Herrmann GH, Sprout WL. Treatment of severe hydrofluoric acid exposures. *J Occup Med* 1983;25:861–863.
72. Scharnweber HC. Treatment of hydrofluoric acid burns of the skin by immediate surgical excision. *IMS Ind Med Surg* 1969;38:179–180.
73. Kohnlein HE, Merkle P, Springorum HW. Hydrogen fluoride burns: experiments and treatment. *Surg Forum* 1973;24:50.
74. Buckingham FM. Surgery: a radical approach to severe hydrofluoric acid burns. A case report. *J Occup Med* 1988;30:873–874.

SECTION

9

Plastics, Plasticizers, and Epoxy Resins

CHAPTER 208

Acrylic Acid and Derivatives

Robert B. Palmer

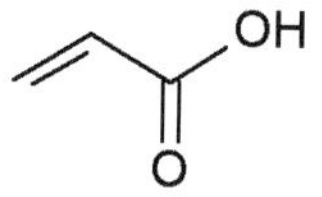

ACRYLIC ACID

Compounds included:	**Acrolein, acrylamide, acrylonitrile, acrylic acid, *n*-butylacrylate, ethylacrylate, ethyl 2-cyanoacrylate, methacrylate, methyl methacrylate**
Molecular weight:	**Acrylic acid, 72.1 g/mol; see Table 1.**
SI conversion:	**Acrylic acid, mg/L × 13.9 = µmol/L**
CAS Registry No.:	**Acrylic acid, CAS 79-10-7; see Table 1.**
Normal levels:	**Not available for clinical use**
Target organs:	**Lung and skin from direct irritant effects. Peripheral neuropathy from some.**
Antidote:	**None**

OVERVIEW

Acrylic acid (2-propenoic acid) is a three-carbon carboxylic acid in which the olefin (double bond) is conjugated with the carbonyl of the carboxyl group (Fig. 1). The nature of the substituent on carbon 2 (the α carbon) determines to a great extent the properties of each ester and the polymer that it forms (1). The chemical structures of acrylic acid derivatives are provided in Table 1. Like most carboxylic acids, acrylic acid is amenable to many chemical derivatizations and conversions resulting in a wide variety of structurally related compounds.

Due to the wide range of applications of acrylic acid derivatives including industrial, medical, hobby, and cosmetic uses, as well as the appearance of many of these compounds as industrial and environmental contaminants, exposure to acrylic acid derivatives is ubiquitous in industrialized countries. Further, the signs and symptoms associated with exposure to these compounds are not pathognomonic.

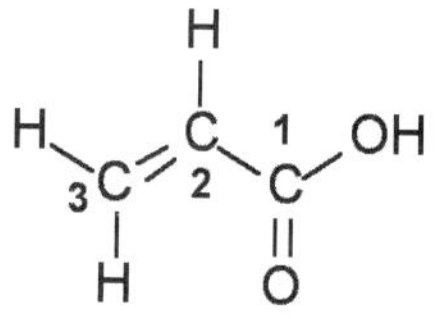

The aldehyde and unsubstituted amide derivatives of acrylic acid (acrolein and acrylamide, respectively) both have toxicologic significance. Esterification of unsubstituted acrylic acid yields the alkyl acrylates such as methacrylate and *n*-butylacrylate commonly used in making polymers. Substitution at the α carbon (the carbon immediately adjacent to the carbonyl) of acrylic acid with a methyl group or nitrile yields the industrially important compounds methacrylate and cyanoacrylate, respectively. Esterification of substituted acrylic acid derivatives is used to create industrially important compounds including methyl methacrylate (MMA), ethyl 2-cyanoacrylate, and many others.

Figure 1. Chemical structure of acrylic acid showing carbon numbering.

Chemical and Physical Properties

Acrylic acid derivatives are of industrial importance primarily as a result of their use in the formation of polymeric plastics, cements, and adhesives. Individual molecules of the unpolymerized acrylic acid derivatives are called *monomers*. When the monomers are covalently linked, a polymer is formed. The monomer is designated by its simple chemical name whereas the polymer is denoted by placing the prefix *poly-* before the compound name (e.g., a polymer of methacrylate is polymethacrylate).

Most of the acrylic acid monomers with lower-molecular-weights are liquids and have a characteristic, often unpleasant,

TABLE 1. Physical characteristics, regulatory guidelines, and toxicity of the acrylic acid derivatives

Compound name, structure, molecular weight (g/mol), CAS Registry No.	Physical description	Exposure guidelines	Common uses	Associated toxicities
Acrolein 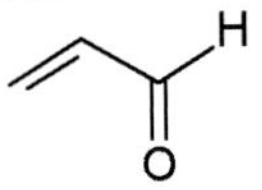 (H; O) 56.1; 107-02-08	Colorless to yellow liquid with a pungent choking odor (odor threshold 0.21 ppm)	PEL (TWA): 0.1 ppm; PEL (STEL): 0.3 ppm; IDLH: 5 ppm	Fuel, pharmaceutical, rubber herbicide, and textile manufacture; common air pollutant	Irritant; burns with high concentrations; CNS depression with high concentrations
Acrylic acid 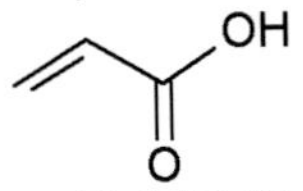 (OH; O) 72.1; 79-10-7	Colorless liquid with a sharp odor	TLV (TWA): 2 ppm	Plastics manufacture; combustion product of some polymers	Corrosive; burns with high concentrations; CNS depression with high concentrations
Methacrylic acid 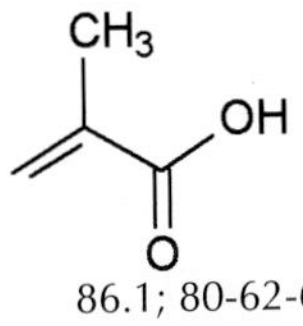 (CH_3; OH; O) 86.1; 80-62-6	Colorless liquid with acrid and repulsive odor	TLV (TWA): 20 ppm	Plastics and resins manufacture; preparation of methyl methacrylate; metabolite of methyl methacrylate	Corrosive; burns with high concentrations; CNS depression with high concentrations
Ethylacrylate 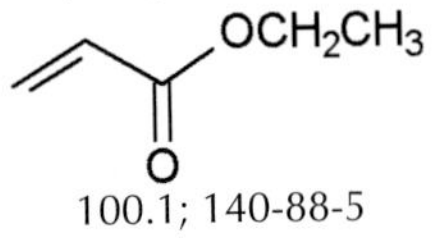 (OCH_2CH_3; O) 100.1; 140-88-5	Colorless liquid with a sharp but fragrant odor (odor threshold 0.00024 ppm)	PEL (TWA): 5 ppm; PEL (STEL): 15 ppm (100 mg/m^3); IDLH: 2000 ppm	Paint manufacture, dirt release agents, thermosetting of acrylic enamels	Irritant; CNS depression with high concentrations
n-Butylacrylate 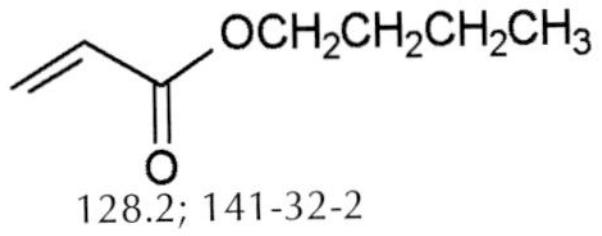 ($OCH_2CH_2CH_2CH_3$; O) 128.2; 141-32-2	Clear colorless liquid with fruity odor	TLV (TWA): 2 ppm (11 mg/m^3)	Plastics manufacture, textile, leather finishes, paints	Irritant; CNS depression with high concentrations
Acrylamide 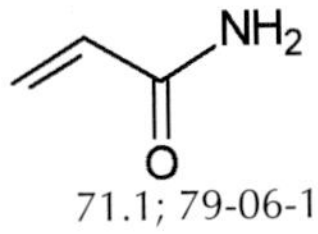 (NH_2; O) 71.1; 79-06-1	Colorless to white flaky crystalline solid; it is odorless	PEL (TWA): 0.03 mg/m^3	Adhesives, dyes, sewage treatment, contact lenses, electrophoresis gels	Irritant; peripheral dying back axonopathy; ocular toxicity; probable carcinogen
Acrylonitrile 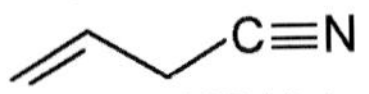 (C≡N) 67.1; 107-13-1	Clear colorless liquid with a garlic-like odor (odor threshold 21.4 ppm)	TLV (TWA): 2 ppm; IDLH: 4,000 ppm; PEL (TWA) 10 ppm	Surface coatings, plastics, adhesives, pesticide fumigants, and as a synthetic intermediate	Irritant; acute: high concentrations may cause seizures, cyanosis and cardiovascular collapse; chronic: headache, confusion, hepatitis, anemia; probable carcinogen
Methyl methacrylate 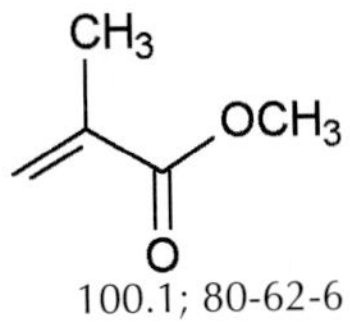 (CH_3; OCH_3; O) 100.1; 80-62-6	Clear colorless liquid with strong fruity odor	PEL (TWA): 100 ppm (410 mg/m^3)	Acrylic production, clear plastics (Lucite, Plexiglas), bone cements, dental sealants, surgical implants, paints, and powdered inks	Irritant; allergic skin sensitization; confusion, irritability, numbness, paresthesia
Ethyl 2-cyanoacrylate 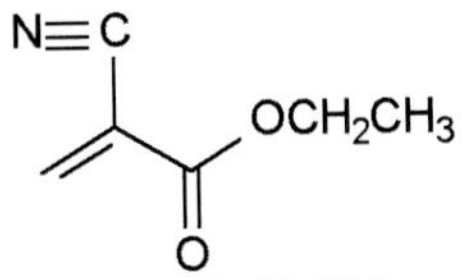 (N≡C; OCH_2CH_3; O) 125.1; 7085-85-0	Clear colorless liquid with strong acrid odor	TLV (TWA): 0.2 ppm (1 mg/m^3)	Fast-drying adhesives (e.g., Krazy Glue), plastics, dentistry, wound closure	Adhesion resulting in physical tears; minor burns as a result of heat release from the polymerization reaction; irritation, histotoxicity, respiratory irritation

CNS, central nervous system; IDLH, immediately dangerous to life and health; PEL, permissible exposure limit; ppm, parts per million; STEL, short-term exposure limit; TLV, threshold limit value; TWA, time-weighted average.

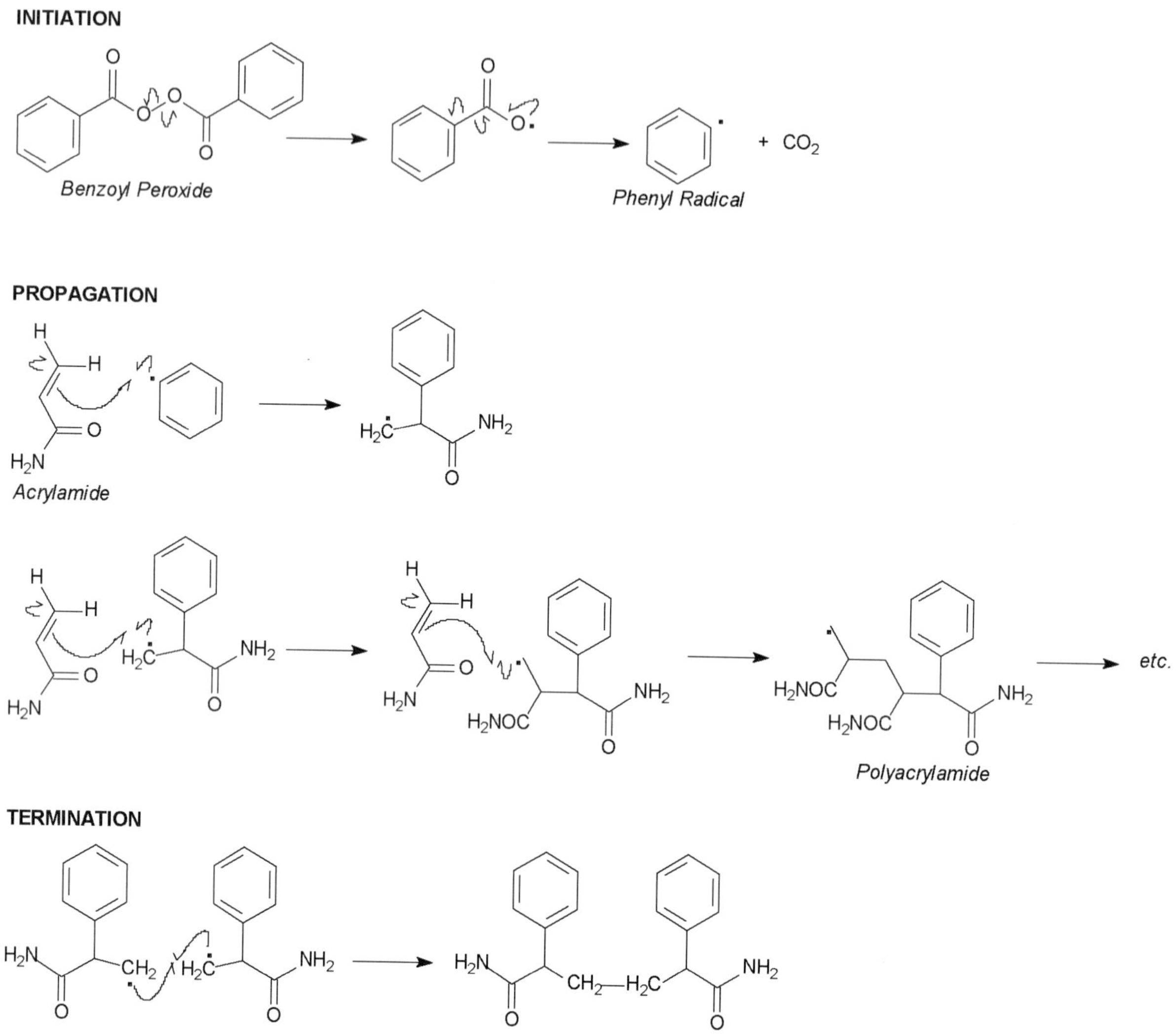

Figure 2. Mechanism of polymerization reactions using acrylamide as an example. Dots represent single unpaired (radical) electrons; single hooked arrows indicate movement of one electron. The initiation step uses benzoyl peroxide, which undergoes hemolytic cleavage of the peroxide linkage, followed by decarboxylation to yield phenyl radical. In the propagation steps, the phenyl radical reacts with the double bond of acrylamide, covalently bonding the two species and creating a radical at the opposite end of the acrylamide double bond. This radical then reacts with another molecule of acrylamide and so on to make the linear polymer. Termination occurs when two radical species react with one another to form a nonradical species. There are many types of termination reactions, but one example is the coupling reaction shown.

odor whereas the esters typically have a fruity smell (Table 1). Acrylamide is a solid at room temperature. The polymers are nonvolatile and therefore have no odor though freshly cured polymer may off-gas monomer for some time giving the mistaken impression that there is odor associated with the polymer.

The reactive site of the acrylic acid derivative monomers in polymerization reactions is the olefin, just as is seen in many other polymerizations such as the formation of polyvinyl chloride and polystyrene. The polymerization reactions involved in acrylic acid derivative polymerization are most often free radical (i.e., one electron) processes (Fig. 2). This series of reactions is started by a peroxide initiator such as benzoyl peroxide, which is converted into a radical most often by a chemical catalyst or ultraviolet light. The benzoyl radical then undergoes decarboxylation yielding a phenyl radical (*initiation*) (Fig. 2). The phenyl radical then creates another radical at the carbon-carbon double bond of the acrylic acid derivative monomer. This radical forms a covalent link with another molecule of monomeric species while simultaneously creating an additional radical electron thereby propagating the process and resulting in covalently bonded monomeric units (*propagation*) (Fig. 2).

The chain of free radical reactions does not proceed at infinitum. The process of polymerization ceases through a number of possible termination reactions that quench radicals. In fact, any collision between two radicals causes formation of a new two-electron covalent bond without the production of another radical species (*termination*) (Fig. 2).

The number of monomer units linked together determines the overall molecular weight of the polymer. Polymeric molecular weight is reported as a range because the precise number of monomeric units involved in the polymer cannot be completely controlled. Cross-linking is the process of covalently bonding separate polymeric chains together through lateral linkages, which makes the polymer become more like a sheet than a chain (Fig. 3).

Commercially available monomeric acrylic acid substances often come as two-component preparations, which are mixed immediately before use. A common such acrylic formula is that

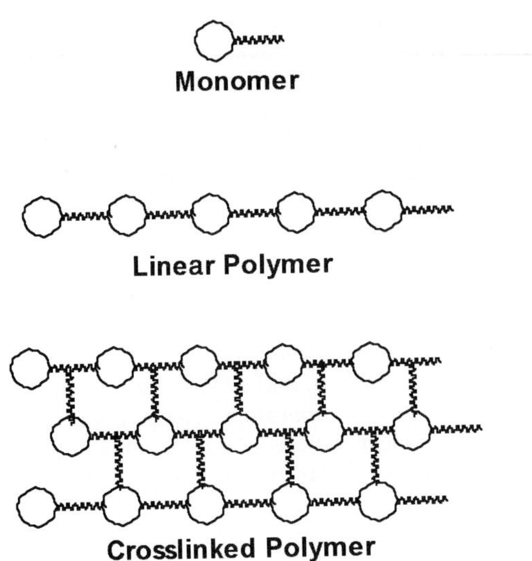

Figure 3. Description of monomer, linear polymerization, and polymer cross-linking.

in which the first component is made up of the liquid acrylic acid monomer stabilized with hydroquinone and a small amount (approximately 2%) of N,N-dimethyl-*p*-toluidine present as a free radical initiator. The second component is generally a powder made of granulated prepolymerized acrylic acid derivative with 2% to 3% benzoyl peroxide present as a radical activator. It is this phase that also contains fillers such as zirconium dioxide, antibiotics such as gentamicin, dyes, and various other additives. When the components are mixed, the free radical chain reactions begin leading to polymerization.

Classification and Uses

MMA is often used as bone cement (e.g., Palacos R Bone Cement). It is supplied as a two-component product (a liquid and a powder), which is mixed shortly before use. The liquid consists of MMA monomer with small amounts of N,N-dimethyl-*p*-toluidine (the cold curing radical initiator) and hydroquinone (prevents premature polymerization). The powder contains ground MMA polymer with benzoyl peroxide (the radical activator) and may contain antibiotics and nonabsorbable fillers such as zirconium dioxide. The orthopedist mixes the components into a dough and applies it to the bone segments to be fixed. This dough then sets to a hard cement-like compound in 5 to 6 minutes. The reaction is markedly exothermic (2). A residual quantity of monomer, usually less than 2%, remains in the final cured polymer (3).

Cyanoacrylates are mostly sold as adhesives. Industrial and consumer grades of adhesives include Superglue, Krazy Glue, Durabond, Eastman 910, and Loctite 494 Superbonder (4). Blais and Campbell described the modifications of cyanoacrylate resulting in improved handling characteristics and mechanical properties (4). Ethyl 2-cyanoacrylate is sold as Krazy Glue and methyl 2-cyanoacrylate is sold as Superglue. Eastman 910 consists of methyl 2-cyanoacrylate monomer modified with a plasticizer (a sebacate), a thickening agent (MMA), and an inhibitor (hydroquinone) as well as $BaSO_4$ to provide radio opacity (4). Aron Alpha consists primarily of monomeric alkyl cyanoacrylate (5).

Commercial preparations are often modified by the addition of substances of high-molecular-weight such as prepolymerized cyanoacrylates, MMA, and polystyrene, as well as fillers including talc, powdered glass, alumina, and fused silica, most of which are not absorbable and can act as embedded foreign bodies in tissue. In addition, some of these preparations incorporate strong desiccants and stabilizers to prevent premature polymerization in multiuse containers. Occasionally, these agents are present in amounts as high as 15% of the total preparation. These compounds are potent irritants; thermal and chemical burns from the additives or incidental to the exothermic reaction that may take place during the curing step are other possible side effects (4).

Methyl, butyl, and other alkyl cyanoacrylates have been used as adhesives (5). Four cyanoacrylates are available for medical use: isobutyl 2-cyanoacrylate (bucrylate), *n*-butyl cyanoacrylate, methyl 2-cyanoacrylate (mecrylate), and 2-octylcyanoacrylate (4). Butyl cyanoacrylate adhesive is sold commercially as Histoacryl and octyl 2-cyanoacrylate is sold as Dermabond. The octyl 2-cyanoacrylate is expected to be less toxic than the methyl or ethyl derivatives as toxicity of the cyanoacrylate esters generally decreases with increasing chain length (6). The primary medical uses for cyanoacrylates include skin closure, particularly during reconstructive surgery of the eyelids and the nose; immobilization of grafts for hair transplants; local hemostasis; closure of gingival flaps in periodontal surgery; and restorative procedures on teeth or on fixed dental prostheses. Cosmetic applications, such as gluing of nail overlays, synthetic eyelashes, eyebrows, small hairpieces, and facial prostheses, also are common (4).

In addition, cyanoacrylate adhesives have been used to treat corneal leaks, to seal aqueous leaks after trauma, and for spontaneous corneal melting (7). Other uses have included temporary tarsorrhaphy for seventh-nerve palsy (7) and facial lacerations (8). Interestingly, cyanoacrylate adhesives are not U.S. Food and Drug Administration approved. Criminalists use vapors of cyanoacrylates to assist with the detection of latent fingerprints on some surfaces (9).

The depolymerization of cyanoacrylic acid ester polymer releasing cyanoacrylate and is likely the major cause of the histotoxicity seen with the cyanoacrylates (10,11). Occupational exposure may lead to an allergic type asthma. Accidental exposure in the eye may lead to corneal damage as a result of mechanical injury. On the skin these compounds lead to a bonding that can often be treated conservatively by simple manipulation. Chronic dermatitis may follow their use on fingernails (12).

Multifunctional acrylates and *methacrylates* are used in photocurable coatings, ultraviolet curing inks, paints, dental sealants, resins, and varnishes. The largest use for polymethacrylate is as a glazing, lighting, or decorative material. Polymethacrylates are also used in the manufacture of dentures, denture bases, and filling materials. In orthodontics, methacrylate polymers are used as pit-and-fissure sealants that are painted over teeth to form physical barriers to tooth decay. Polymethacrylates are also used as bone cement (13,14) in hard and soft contact lenses (1) and the manufacture of artificial nails (9,15,16).

Acrylonitrile has been used as a pesticide fumigant. However, it is currently used principally as a synthetic intermediate for plastics, adhesives, and surface coatings as well as in the synthesis of pharmaceuticals, dyes, and antioxidants.

Acrylamide, which is also known as propanamide, acrylamide monomer, and acrylic amide, has industrial applications including the production of special monomers for grout and dyes, as a sizing agent in the paper and permanent press fabric industries, and in treatment of sewage and wastewater. Polyacrylamides are components of many cosmetics and contact lenses. Acrylamide is also commonly used in biochemistry laboratories for making electrophoresis and chromatography gels. Most toxic exposures to acrylamide occur as a result of fires or during its use as a soil waterproofing agent for mining and tunneling operations (17).

Acrolein is the aldehyde derivative of acrylic acid. It is present as a photooxidation product of 1,3-butadiene and as a component of automobile exhaust and cigarette smoke. Acrolein is also a by-product of solid waste incineration. Monomeric forms of acrolein have been used as a liquid fuel, microbicide, slimicide, herbicide, and as a histologic fixative. Historically, acrolein was used in military poison gas mixtures. Acrolein is present in many foodstuffs and is a combustion by-product frequently encountered by firefighters.

Environmental Exposure

Most of the health and safety aspects of acrylic acid derivatives are due to exposure to the monomeric species. With respect to the polymeric forms, manufacturing processes such as in violent polymerizations can present some risk (1). Acrylics are thermal decomposition products of many synthetic polymers (18,19). Combustion of nitrogen containing monomers or polymers such as those made of cyanoacrylates and acrylamide can release cyanide (18,19).

Accidental environmental exposure is possible outside of a fire or occupational setting. A family of five in Japan drank water contaminated with acrylamide that had leaked into their well from a sewer grouting operation taking place nearby (20). Concentrations of acrylamide in the well were measured to be 400 parts per million (ppm). The three adults had more severe effects than the two children. The adults were reported to experience ataxia, delirium, and hallucinations (visual only in one; visual, auditory and tactile in one). The children, a girl and a boy ages 10 and 13 years, respectively, had milder effects with drowsiness and truncal ataxia in the older child and only peculiar behavior that spontaneously resolved in 3 days in the younger child.

Toxic Dose

Table 1 lists exposure guidelines for several common derivatives of acrylic acid.

MMA has an odor threshold of 0.2 to 0.3 ppm (2). Inhalation of MMA at concentrations of >150 mg/m^3 is expected to produce central nervous system (CNS) effects in humans (21). Workroom air concentrations of MMA and formaldehyde in dental laboratories do not usually exceed the regulatory limits (22). Levels of MMA in the operating room reach 225 ppm during mixing, decreasing to 4 ppm in 6 minutes, and to zero at the time of curing (23). Between 3% to 5% of MMA is unreacted monomer. Paresthesia, numbness, and tingling and coldness in the fingers of the dominantly exposed hand of people manipulating MMA monomer with their bare hands has been reported (24). This is most often in dental technicians making MMA putty molds. Sensory conduction velocities in finger nerves are slowed in conjunction with the numbness (24,25). Furthermore, urine output of MMA in dental technicians suggests percutaneous absorption of the monomer (25) though inhalation may also contribute.

Ethylacrylate exposure at airborne concentrations of 50 to 75 ppm resulted in drowsiness, headache, and nausea (26). Exposure to airborne ethylacrylate concentrations of 4 to 58 mg/m^3 for 5 years showed that 14 of 33 workers complained of autonomic and neurotic symptoms though all had normal electroencephalographic studies (27). Skin sensitization to 4% ethylacrylate in petroleum jelly occurred in 42% of study volunteers (26). Toxic concentrations for other acrylate esters and multifunctional acrylates have not been defined.

Acrylonitrile concentrations as low as 16 ppm for 30 minutes have been reported to cause headache, nausea, and irritability (28). Both inhalation and dermal exposure to acrylonitrile has caused fatalities in humans. The odor threshold for acrylonitrile is 21.4 ppm; however, the onset of olfactory fatigue is rapid, making odor an unreliable warning indicator.

Acrylamide has been studied in more detail than other acrylic acid derivatives. Single or cumulative exposure of 50 to 100 mg of acrylamide can cause neurologic effects and doses more than 300 mg can cause acute CNS and cardiovascular effects. However, because occupational exposure to acrylamide in humans is most often dermal, a defined dose-response relationship is difficult to establish. Multiple studies of workers exposed to acrylamide demonstrate an apparent causal link between exposure and symptoms such as limb pain, numbness and tingling in hands and feet, weakness, and sweaty and peeling skin on the hands (29). Most often, neurologic complaints were seen after exposure to air concentrations of acrylamide in the range of 1 to 5 mg/m^3 (30). These symptoms do not appear to occur at concentrations less than 0.3 mg/m^3, but, as acrylamide concentrations are increased to 0.6 to 0.9 mg/m^3, symptoms become more apparent (30). Exposure to concentrations of 9 mg/m^3 or more is almost certain to result in neurologic effects (30). Acrylamide-induced neuropathy in workers increases over the first year or two of exposure. After approximately 2 years, it appears to reach steady state with axon destruction and lesion repair approximately balancing (30).

Acrolein has a low threshold of irritation (0.25 to 0.5 ppm), which limits the likelihood of chronic exposure. Acute exposure to acrolein results in severe irritation of the skin, eyes, and upper respiratory tract at air concentrations of 1 ppm whereas exposure to 10 ppm of acrolein can be fatal to humans in a short period of time (31). Studies of firefighters have shown that the American Conference of Governmental Industrial Hygienists ceiling value of acrolein (0.1 ppm) may be exceeded during firefighting operations that are typically performed without respiratory protection (32).

PATHOPHYSIOLOGY

Exposure to the acrylic acid derivatives is typically the result of inhalation or direct contact with skin or mucosal surfaces. The most significant toxic manifestations of the acrylic acid derivatives are a result of the monomeric species. Irritation of skin and mucous membranes is the most common manifestation. Skin irritation can be severe and result in chemical burns in high concentration exposures to compounds such as acrolein (31). The irritant effects are a result of local contact and generally not a systemic reaction, though MMA and the multifunctional acrylates are known skin sensitizing agents that can cause an allergic contact dermatitis.

The pulmonary effects of the acrylic acid derivatives become evident after inhalation. Pulmonary edema, which can be delayed in onset, has been reported. Acrylic acid derivatives are well-established causative agents for occupational asthma. Inhalational exposure to high concentrations of most of the acrylic acid derivative monomers can also cause CNS depression.

The primary effects after ingestion of acrylic acid derivatives include direct irritation and possible chemical burning of the gastrointestinal (GI) tract. Nausea, vomiting, and diarrhea are expected consequences. Other effects such as peripheral neuropathy have been reported after ingestion of specific liquid monomeric species.

Typically, the derivatives of acrylic acid are considered nontoxic after polymerization. As a rule of thumb, toxicity decreases with increasing molecular weight of the polymer (1). This being said, there are some effects related to exposure to polymerized species that deserve mention. Ingestion of acrylic acid polymers is unlikely to result in systemic toxicity though mechanical injury from sharp plastic edges or GI obstruction from bulk polymer and irritant or allergic responses to polymer dust are possible. Further, if the polymerization reaction is incomplete or inappropriate ratios of components are used, residual monomers may be trapped in the polymerized matrix. Release of unreacted monomer or monomer derivatives may take place with processing of the polymer. Spontaneous degradation of the polymer may also release monomer or monomer derivatives potentially causing some toxic consequences.

Combustion of monomeric or polymeric forms of derivatives of acrylic acid can release carbon monoxide, cyanide, and oxides of nitrogen if the derivative contains nitrogen and phosgene if the derivative is chlorinated. The agents as toxins are covered in separate chapters and are not discussed further herein.

Parenteral introduction of polymerized acrylates is an embolic risk. Acrylic acid cement embolus of both pulmonary and cerebral arteries has been reported after numerous orthopedic surgical procedures (33–36); however, this is not the only proposed mechanism for intraoperative toxic effects of MMA. Bone implantation syndrome, characterized by bronchoconstriction, hypoxemia, hypotension, pulmonary hypertension, and rarely cardiac arrest, has been tied by some to direct MMA toxicity (34,37). Another postulated mechanism is pulmonary fat embolization (34). Notably, it has been suggested that fat and bone marrow embolism may be related to heat and pressure in the femoral canal during MMA polymer curing (38).

TOXICOKINETICS AND TOXICODYNAMICS

Absorption

The monomeric derivatives of acrylic acid are absorbed through inhalation, ingestion, and dermal contact, though the amount absorbed of each compound varies. Though several attempts have been made to correlate blood concentration, rate of increase, and relative proportions of metabolites of the acrylic acid derivatives with resultant clinical symptoms, none of these studies has demonstrated a clear correlation. Though the route of exposure may play a role in local symptoms, systemic effects such as the neurologic effects in acrylamide exposure, seem to have little or no dependence on exposure route.

MMA, the monomeric component of the polymethyl methacrylate cement used in orthopedic surgery, undergoes hydrolysis to methacrylic acid during hip replacement operations. Kim and Ritter demonstrated methacrylate in the venous blood of patients after cement insertion into the femur and the acetabulum (39). No correlation has been found between MMA or methacrylic acid blood levels and the degree of hypotension (39–41).

Cyanoacrylate monomers are not well absorbed, probably due to their rapid polymerization on exposure to air. This rapid reaction does, however, mean that adhesion to directly exposed tissues is rapid.

Multifunctional acrylates and acrylate esters are absorbed with dermal contact. Reports of ethylacrylate absorption after ingestion and eye contact also exist (42,43). Dermal absorption of multifunctional acrylates has resulted in development of systemic effects and death in laboratory animals with the lower-molecular-weight compounds being better absorbed percutaneously than orally.

Acrylonitrile is well absorbed with inhalation, ingestion, and dermal exposures. An average of 52% of the inhaled dose is retained after exposure to airborne concentrations of 5 to 10 mg/m^3 (44). With exposure to 20 μg/L, an average of 46% of the inhaled dose was retained (43). Acrylonitrile has been absorbed through dermal contact with the forearms of persons working with the compound (43).

Acrylamide is well absorbed after oral, dermal, inhalational, and parenteral exposure, including through intact skin and mucous membranes. Efficient absorption of this compound is demonstrated by the observation that peak blood concentrations occur at approximately 1 hour after exposure (45). It is estimated that human elimination rates of acrylamide are only one-fifth that seen in rats.

Acrolein, the aldehyde derivative of acrylic acid, is absorbed with oral, inhalational, and dermal exposure in humans. One study in dogs demonstrated that 80% of an inhaled dose of acrolein is absorbed in the upper respiratory tract (31).

Distribution

Specific volumes of distribution have not been established in humans for most of the acrylic acid derivatives. Animal studies indicate variable organ distributions with acrylic acid derivative monomers. Orally administered *acrylonitrile* distributes to liver, kidney, brain, spleen, heart, and lung in rats (28). Measurable concentrations are also found in the adrenal cortex and stomach mucosa. *Ethylacrylate* is reportedly widely distributed in rat tissues after a single oral dose (43). Despite acrylonitrile being detected in the brain after oral administration in rats, and the substantial neurologic effects associated with acrylamide ingestion, *acrylamide* does not concentrate in the nervous system (45). The tissue distribution half-life of acrylamide is approximately 5 hours, after which it is detectable in the muscle, skin, liver, and small intestine (45,46).

MMA is sequestered in red blood cells and slowly released into the plasma. Blood cell concentrations are roughly double plasma concentrations, and clearance from plasma is tenfold faster than from blood cells. The partitioning between blood cells and plasma is not unique to MMA. When radiolabeled *acrylonitrile* was given orally and intravenously to rats, the plasma concentrations declined quickly but significant concentrations remained in the red blood cells for approximately 10 days (43). Degradation of ethyl methacrylate appears to occur only in the plasma (47).

Metabolism

As is the case with the overall toxicity profile of the derivatives of acrylic acid, only the monomeric species undergoes significant biotransformation. The polymeric forms are large enough that they are essentially metabolically inert.

In general, the ester derivatives of acrylic acid are hydrolyzed in the GI tract and lungs to form the corresponding acrylic acid and alcohol. Other acrylic acid derivatives undergo biotransformation by P-450 mixed function oxidases to compounds that are then subjected to phase-II conjugation with reduced glutathione and ultimately excreted as the mercapturate derivatives. These transformations occur primarily in the liver and kidneys. Further support of the importance of reduced glutathione conjugation in mitigating toxicity is added by the observation that the neurotoxic effects of acrylamide seem to be enhanced in situations in which reduced glutathione is depleted (45,48,49).

The *multifunctional acrylates* and *MMA* undergo metabolism by coenzyme A to form methacrylic acid, which is a normal intermediate in the Krebs cycle meaning the methacrylic acid metabolites undergo standard lipid metabolism. MMA is ultimately converted to pyruvic acid.

Acrylonitrile is metabolized to cyanide. Interestingly, the overall amount of acrylonitrile metabolism is substantially less in humans than in rodents, and the amount of cyanide produced as a result is greater in rodents than humans (50).

Elimination

MMA has a half-life in whole blood at 20°C of 3 hours. Dental technicians exposed to MMA may develop urine concentrations as high as 373 nmol/mmol creatinine, but this compound is not found in the urine of healthy unexposed controls without a history of specific exposure (51). MMA is also eliminated through exhalation. In a study of rats, 65% of the dose was eliminated in expired air within 2 hours of exposure (52). An additional 18% was exhaled as carbon dioxide over the following 10 days (52).

Ethyl acrylate has an elimination half-life of less than 24 hours (53). Urinary metabolites include thioether conjugates as well as a variety of acid metabolites. The metabolic conversion of ethyl acrylate is fast in blood (half-life 11 to 14 minutes) and follows first-order kinetics (54).

Acrylonitrile is metabolized to mercapturate and related conjugates (44); however, urinary concentration of the metabolites was not deemed useful as an index of exposure. Rats also excrete the majority of acrylonitrile as metabolic conjugates, though after exposures of more than 10 ppm, a small amount of unchanged parent compound is detectable in the urine (50). Elimination of acrylonitrile in humans follows first-order kinetics with a half-life of 8 hours (44). After gavage administration of acrylonitrile in rats, elimination is biphasic with an α elimination half-life of 3.5 to 5.8 hours and a β elimination half-life of 50 to 77 hours (28). This species variability in elimination kinetics may be due in part to the previously mentioned metabolic differences between humans and rodents after acrylonitrile exposure.

Acrylamide is primarily (90% to 95%) excreted in the urine as conjugated metabolite with less than 2% parent compound appearing in the urine (45). Smaller amounts of metabolites are also present in feces, bile, and other biological matrices, still with only small amounts being eliminated as unchanged parent. Acrylamide elimination is biphasic with an α half-life of less than 5 hours and a β half-life of 6 to 8 days (45,46).

Acrolein produces major urinary metabolites of mercapturate and related conjugates in rats (55). However, *in vitro* experiments using liver and lung microsomes have demonstrated formation of other metabolites including glycidylaldehyde and acrylic acid, which may be eliminated through extrarenal mechanisms (43).

VULNERABLE POPULATIONS

Few human data exist regarding acrylic acid derivatives. Though the animal data are conflicting, no evidence exists confirming teratogenicity of MMA in humans. MMA is considered unlikely to be a reproductive hazard in humans with occupational exposure. Multifunctional acrylates do not appear to be potent fetotoxins or teratogens. One human case of menstrual irregularity has been reported after exposure to several acrylates (56). Acrolein is considered a possible reproductive hazard in firefighters (57).

Reports of the teratogenic potential of ethylacrylate in rats are conflicting. Acrylonitrile is well established to be embryotoxic and teratogenic in animals (28,58). Acrylamide causes decreased birth weight in rats, diminished litter size, and increased pre- and postimplantation mortality (58). Both maternal and paternal toxic reproductive effects were also noted. When acrolein was administered by direct intraamniotic injection to rats, birth defects were noted (43). No such defects were found in rabbits receiving acrolein by gavage (59).

CLINICAL PRESENTATION

Systemic Effects

Methylmethacrylate exposure of an operating room nurse produced a sensitivity reaction to the odor of orthopedic cement characterized by hypertension, dyspnea, and generalized erythroderma from which she recovered (2). Complaints of respiratory, cutaneous, and genitourinary problems have been observed in workers exposed to MMA at concentrations of 4 to 49 ppm over an 8-hour time-weighted average (2).

Alkyl cyanoacrylates (ethyl cyanoacrylate, methyl cyanoacrylate) act as allergens, including a type I immunologic response leading to the development of asthma with sneezing, nasal discharge, coughing stridor, and dyspnea beginning several hours after work and not recurring on days off work (5,60).

Ocular Effects

Essentially all of the acrylic acid derivatives cause irritation with ocular contact. Ocular exposure to the hardened polymer may lead to corneal injury due to mechanical damage. Additionally, more concentrated forms of *ethylacrylate* and *acrolein* can potentially cause corrosive injury. Retinal neuronal damage has been suggested as an effect of ocular exposure to *acrylamide* (61). Visual changes (loss of red-green color discrimination) and a hypertensive retinopathy were associated with one severe case of acrylamide poisoning in a patient who developed peripheral neuropathy (16). Persons severely poisoned in an occupational setting may have visual effects as a result of direct ocular damage and/or from cerebellar involvement (29,43,61). Recovery from acrylamide-induced visual damage may or may not be complete (29,43). One patient with long-term postoperative use of a cyanoacrylate adhered eye patch developed endophthalmitis with a fungal infection (62).

Dermal

Nearly all of the acrylic acid derivatives are dermal irritants, though the concentrated methacrylic acid–containing primers used in artificial nail products are corrosive and have caused cutaneous burns. The least significant dermal toxicity is associated with the *cyanoacrylates* whose irritant properties are typically the result of mechanical injury from physically pulling apart adhered skin surfaces. A 2-year-old child bit into a tube of cyanoacrylate glue adhering the lower lip to the lower incisors for more than 12 hours (63,64).

Exposure for prolonged periods or to high concentrations of *acrolein*, *acrylonitrile*, or *acrylic acid* can cause burns that may blister. Chronic exposure has been linked to contact dermatitis and scaly peeling skin for many acrylic acid derivatives including acrylonitrile, acrylamide, multifunctional acrylates, and the cyanoacrylates (43). This has been well established in workers exposed to multifunctional acrylates (43). Chronic dermatitis similar to small plaque parapsoriasis may follow continued use of cyanoacrylate adhesive on fingernails (12).

Polymerization of acrylic bone cement is usually incomplete, leaving small amounts of residual monomer. These monomers penetrate practically all rubber and polyvinyl gloves, except 0.48 mm thick butyl rubber gloves. The use of butyl rubber gloves may prevent the development of contact dermatitis (65). Acquired allergic contact dermatitis from monomeric forms of acrylic acid derivative monomer is well described. This has been shown in strongly positive patch-test reactions to MMA in orthopedic surgeons; however, patients receiving the bone cements rarely become sensitized (9).

In patients sensitive to MMA, potentially irreversible loss of fingernails may be due to an allergic reaction to an acrylic nail preparation (9). There is no apparent cross reactivity of ethyl and *n*-butyl monomers in patients sensitive to MMA (56). However, patients who acquire an allergic contact dermatitis to ethyl methacrylate and butyl methacrylate may also have a positive patch test reaction to MMA monomer (66). A history of skin disease during childhood or allergic conjunctivitis or rhinitis may predispose an individual to the dermatologic effects caused by MMA (24). Paresthesias and tenderness in areas of contact dermatitis frequently outlast the eruption (2).

Cardiovascular

Effects on heart rate, blood pressure, and pulse pressure have been reported after exposure to acrylic acid derivatives. *Acrolein, acrylonitrile, and MMA* are all known to cause tachycardia after inhalation exposure. Hypertension is associated with inhalation of acrolein and has also been reported in a nurse with repeated exposure to 97% MMA bone cement (2). Use of MMA bone cement has resulted in vasodilation with transient hypotension in the patient as well as hypotension and direct cardiotoxicity in the form of atrioventricular blocks (38).

Several cases of intraoperative cardiac arrest have been reported in patients undergoing hip replacements (40,67). One report indicates hypotension occurs intraoperatively in 50% to 80% of total hip replacements (68) though newer techniques in management have likely reduced this rate. The contributing role of fat emboli, micropulmonary emboli, or free MMA in causing these cardiovascular effects is unclear (69). Second-degree atrioventricular block that progressed to a fatal third-degree heart block has been reported during hip arthroplasty using MMA cement (70).

Widened pulse pressure and increased cardiac output has been documented in cases of exposure to *acrylonitrile* (71). Persistently low blood pressure has been reported after long-term exposure to acrylonitrile (71). *Acrylamide* exposure may result in hypotension with cyanosis and cool extremities.

Peripheral Nervous System

Acrylamide is known to cause peripheral neuropathy, which has also been reported with MMA exposure. Toxicity can result from handling the monomer crystalline powder, primarily through cumulative skin absorption (1,56). Once the compound is polymerized, it is nontoxic. A dental technician with extensive and repeated skin and inhalational exposure to MMA monomer developed a generalized sensorimotor peripheral neuropathy of the axonal degeneration type confirmed by nerve biopsy (13).

Acute or chronic exposure may produce neuropathy. Long-term acrylamide exposure produces a motor and sensory polyneuropathy with insidious onset. The peripheral neuropathy is a dying back axonopathy similar to that seen with tri-*o*-cresyl phosphate exposure. It usually begins distally with proximal progression and has a distinct preference toward longer and larger diameter nerve fibers. The usual presentation is as a diffuse but symmetric stocking-glove loss of sensory and motor function. Desquamation of the palms and soles, sweating, and peripheral vasoconstriction are more prominent in acrylamide peripheral neuropathy compared with other occupational toxic neuropathies (13). Early detection typically allows complete recovery (56). However, neurologic effects of weakness, ataxia, and sensory abnormalities may persist with prolonged exposure (56).

Central Nervous System

In severe acute intoxication, confusion and hallucinations may be observed; in moderate subacute intoxication, drowsiness, loss of concentration, and ataxia are seen (1). The presence of ataxia and, occasionally, dysarthria and tremor suggests midbrain and cerebellar involvement (1). Signs and symptoms include weakness, paresthesia, fatigue, lethargy, decreased pinprick sensation, vibratory loss, decreased reflexes, and positive Romberg sign. Severity is worse in distal portions of the extremities. Recovery typically occurs within several months to a year of cessation of exposure, although severe exposures may result in permanent sequelae (1).

MMA may cause irritability, rapid fatigue, and headache in workers engaged in pouring it into forms (72). Concentrations of MMA in this group were 25 to 146 ppm (72). These findings have not been evaluated in controlled studies. Similar symptoms have been described in workers using acrylonitrile.

Panic attacks were reported in one case of a previously healthy 33-year-old man after inadvertent inhalation of cyanoacrylate fumes (73). The authors reported the relationship between exposure and development of the panic disorder as temporal. Over the subsequent 6 months, the attacks reportedly decreased in frequency and severity.

Ethyl acrylate and *n-butyl acrylate* exposures causing drowsiness, headache, and nausea without electroencephalographic changes have been observed (27). Exposure to high concentrations of acrolein, acrylonitrile, acrylamide, and ethyl acrylate is associated with CNS depression. Seizures, autonomic dysfunction, and death have been linked to large exposures.

Gastrointestinal

Nausea, vomiting, and diarrhea are commonly reported after ingestion and prolonged inhalation of derivatives of acrylic acid. Ingestion of acrylic acid derivatives causes GI tract irritation. Stomatitis was reported after contact with MMA (74). Anorexia, alone and in combination with nausea, is known to occur after inhalation of MMA and subchronic exposure to acrylamide. Dental students have developed nausea and anorexia while working with MMA (2).

Respiratory

Most of the acrylic acid derivatives are pulmonary irritants. Because they can also act as sensitizing agents, allergic rhinitis and asthma can result. Occupational asthma has been reported with MMA exposure (60). Acrylamide has resulted in the development of a persistent cough though there were no objective pulmonary findings (20).

MMA causes respiratory irritation at high concentrations. A transient decrease in PaO_2 occurs within seconds after application of MMA and is reversed within minutes (2). The transient hypoxia may be due to fat and bone marrow emboli resulting from the high intramedullary pressure during insertion of the prosthesis (2,69,75). In one study, two cases of intraoperative death occurred during insertion of the hip prosthesis with use of MMA polymer as bone cement. Widespread marrow emboli were found (75).

Heating of *cyanoacrylate* glues as is done in crime laboratories volatilizes the monomer, which can cause respiratory irritation. However, in the absence of actual combustion of the material, cyanide is not released in these vapors (76).

Cyanoacrylates may lead to allergic type asthma. Quirce et al. studied two assembly personnel who worked with cyanoacrylate glue and developed rhinitis and asthma symptoms. Cyanoacrylate exposure induced variable airflow limitation, bronchial hyperresponsiveness, and significant eosinophilia in sputum (77).

Miscellaneous

Hepatotoxicity (inflammation, increased transaminase levels, and elevated bilirubin with clinically apparent jaundice) has been reported with both acute and chronic exposure to many acrylic acid derivatives including acrolein, acrylamide, acrylonitrile, and ethyl acrylate (26). Rats exposed to ethylacrylate at 300 ppm for more than 30 days developed hepatic congestion and cloudy swelling of the liver, which were detected at necropsy (26).

Pancreatitis was reported after ingestion of acrylamide (49). Chronic exposure to acrylonitrile is linked with leukocytosis and decreased red blood cell counts.

Carcinogenesis

In the early 1940s, workers exposed to vapor-phase *ethyl methacrylate and MMA* monomers appeared to experience increased rates of colon cancer 2 decades after their most intense exposures (78). A subsequent cohort study of 2671 men concluded that there was no evidence to conclude that MMA is a human carcinogen (79). Chronic exposure in animals is linked to fibrosarcoma (43).

Chronic intraperitoneal administration of *isobutyl-2-cyanoacrylate* in rats produced an apparent dose-related carcinogenic effect (80). This effect has not been observed in humans. *Multifunctional acrylates* are not strong skin carcinogens but may potentially be absorbed leading to tumors of the viscera (2).

Acrylonitrile is designated as a probable human carcinogen (group 2A) by the International Agency for Research on Cancer (58). Occupational exposure to acrylonitrile has been linked epidemiologically to cancers of the colon, prostate, and respiratory system (58). Further, an increased number of deaths were reported as due to lymphatic, stomach, and lung malignancy (26,58). The presence of confounding factors, methodologies used, and conclusions drawn from these and other studies have been questioned. At present, there is strong evidence to support carcinogenic potential in animals but insufficient data in humans (26).

Acrylamide is a carcinogen in animals; however, occupational assessment has not linked this compound to an increased rate of malignancy in humans. However, one study reported that workers with acrylamide exposures of 0.30 mg/m^3 or more per year had a 2.26-fold increase in the incidence of pancreatic cancer (81,82). At present, acrylamide is classed by the International Agency for Research on Cancer as a group 2A compound (probable human carcinogen) (28).

Acrolein reportedly causes tumors of the respiratory system and urinary bladder in some (83), but not all, animal studies (84). The International Agency for Research on Cancer classification of acrolein is Group 3 (inadequate evidence in both animals and humans) (43,58).

DIAGNOSTIC TESTS

A number of gas and liquid chromatographic methods have been used to quantitate acrylic acid derivatives in biological matrices for kinetic assessment (43,45,58). Levels of these compounds are typically unavailable, however, and are not useful in guiding clinical management of toxic exposure. Determination of mercapturic acid conjugates of acrylic acid derivatives in the urine may be useful as a qualitative index of exposure, but this assessment is quite nonspecific. Whole blood cyanide, blood and urinary thiocyanate, and serum electrolytes lactate are recommended in the assessment of acrylonitrile exposure.

The extent of acrylamide-induced neuropathy can be assessed using nerve conduction studies. Blood and urine concentrations are of little value beyond qualitative proof of exposure (85). Examination of cerebrospinal fluid may have slightly increased protein content in the event of acrylamide exposure (20). Other toxic effects of acrylamide exposure, such as those on the hematopoietic system and the pancreas, should be assessed using standard laboratory analyses. Potential exposure to other acrylic acid derivatives should be assessed using standard laboratory analyses as clinically indicated.

TREATMENT

Management of symptomatic exposure to monomeric forms of acrylic acid derivatives is supportive, as no specific antidote has been proven effective. Treatment of polymeric forms should not be needed unless monomers contaminate or are released from the product. The initial management is to terminate exposure.

Decontamination

Acrylic acid derivative monomers are adsorbed by activated charcoal. Administration of charcoal in the case of ingestion without evidence of corrosive gastric injury or other contraindication is appropriate. There is no role for charcoal after ingestion of polymerized compounds and likely little reason to use multi-dose charcoal even with ingestions of monomeric species. Gastric lavage or gastric aspiration after massive ingestion of acrylonitrile may be beneficial in limiting toxicity from metabolic production of cyanide. Use of gastric lavage to prevent development of peripheral neuropathy in acrylamide ingestion has not been proven helpful and is not recommended.

Enhancement of Elimination

The use of extracorporeal elimination has not been reported.

Antidotes

Intravenous *N*-acetylcysteine therapy may be beneficial in cases of hepatotoxicity from acrylic acid derivatives such as acrylonitrile but has not been proven effective and the appropriate dosing scheme is unknown. The use of the cyanide antidote package may be appropriate in rare cases of acrylonitrile exposure (Chapter 46).

Acrylamide monomer may diminish energy production of distal nerves through progressive blockade of glycolytic enzymes involved in rapid axonal transport (3). Recent studies in rats indicate that *in vivo* activities of glycolytic enzymes remain intact, casting doubt on the hypothesis that acrylamide neuropathy begins with a reduction in metabolic energy (33). Other routes that may result in the secondary loss of metabolic energy involve glutathione conjugation and nicotinamide antagonism (2,14). For these reasons, both N-acetylcysteine and pyridoxine have been suggested for treatment of acrylamide-induced peripheral neuropathy (49,86). However, no clearly discernible benefit has been demonstrated especially after the neuropathy is established.

Additionally, pyruvate was shown to delay the appearance of neurotoxic effects in laboratory animals though there was no difference in outcome and the optimum dose of sodium pyruvate was not established. High doses of methylcobalamin (500 μg/kg) were reported to accelerate recovery from acrylamide-induced peripheral neuropathy in rats (87). After poisoning with acrylamide, recovery was enhanced in animals with partial denervation of muscles with treatment with thioctic acid (88). The significance of these therapies in human poisoning is unknown.

Supportive Care

Respiratory compromise is treated with oxygen with addition of beta-receptor agonists as needed for bronchospasm and standard measures for pulmonary edema. Allergic contact dermatitis from sensitization is managed by ceasing exposure and steroid therapy as needed.

Anaphylaxis may occur, because many of the acrylic acid derivatives can be significantly sensitizing. Anaphylactic reactions to these substances are managed in the standard fashion. To prevent cyanoacrylate-induced dermatitis, the orthopedic cement can be mixed mechanically and applied with a spatula. Also, wearing butyl rubber gloves over two pairs of cotton gloves may help limit exposure. The gloves should be removed as soon as possible and discarded. Skin contamination can be cleaned with alcohol or methylethylketone. Anyone handling the monomeric cement should wash his or her hands with ample soap and water as soon as possible (66).

Bonding of the lips together with sealing of the nostrils may require a tracheotomy (64). Adherence to the corneal conjunctiva and/or eyelid may require copious irrigation of the exposed eye with tepid tap water for at least 15 minutes, application of mineral oil to the external eyelid surface after irrigation, and referral for ophthalmologic evaluation (89). Acetone has been used to remove the adhesive from the fingernails (12) though solvents should not be used in the eyes, mouth, or nose.

Prophylactic administration of isotonic fluids, or even blood, before cement insertion has been suggested to limit the hypotensive response associated with MMA bone cement application. Alternatively, treatment of hypotension with Trendelenburg positioning, isotonic fluid resuscitation, and vasopressors as needed is appropriate (Chapter 37). Cyanide is produced metabolically from acrylonitrile. Combustion of acrylonitrile monomer or polymer produces cyanide as well as carbon monoxide and oxides of nitrogen (90). Data regarding the role of cyanide toxicity in acrylonitrile exposure are conflicting. However, in cases with a consistent clinical picture, and especially those in which cyanide intoxication can be confirmed, administration of the clinically indicated portions of the cyanide antidote kit is reasonable.

REFERENCES

1. Mark HF, McKetta JJ, Othmer DF, et al., eds. *Kirk-Othmer encyclopedia of chemical technology*, 2nd ed. New York: Interscience Publishers/John Wiley and Sons, Inc., 2000.
2. Scolnick B, Collins J. Systemic reaction to methylmethacrylate in an operating room nurse. *J Occup Med* 1986;28:196–198.
3. Autian J. Structure-toxicity relationships of acrylic monomers. *Environ Health Perspect* 1975;11:141–152.
4. Blais P, Campbell RW. Cyanoacrylates in medicine. *Can Med Assoc J* 1982;126:227–228.
5. Nakazawa T. Occupational asthma due to alkyl cyanoacrylate. *J Occup Med* 1990;32:709–710.
6. Mickey BE, Samson D. Neurosurgical applications of the cyanoacrylate adhesives. *Clin Neurosurg* 1981;28:429–444.
7. Diamond JP. Temporary tarsorrhaphy with cyanoacrylate adhesive for seventh-nerve palsy. *Lancet* 1990;335:1039.
8. Watson DP. Use of cyanoacrylate tissue adhesive for closing facial lacerations in children. *BMJ* 1989;299:1014.
9. Cary R. Concise international chemical assessment document 36: methylcyanoacrylate and ethylcyanoacrylate. Geneva: World Health Organization, 2001.
10. Refojo MF, Dohlman CH, Koliopoulos J. Adhesives in ophthalmology: a review. *Surv Ophthalmol* 1971;15:217–236.
11. Thumwanit V, Kedjarune U. Cytotoxicity of polymerized commercial cyanoacrylate adhesive on cultured human oral fibroblasts. *Aust Dent J* 1999;44:248–252.
12. Shelley ED, Shelley WB. Chronic dermatitis simulating small-plaque parapsoriasis due to cyanoacrylate adhesive used on fingernails. *JAMA* 1984;252:2455–2456.
13. Donaghy M, Rushworth G, Jacobs JM. Generalized peripheral neuropathy in a dental technician exposed to methyl methacrylate monomer. *Neurology* 1991;41:1112–1116.
14. Crout DH, Corkill JA, James ML, et al. Methylmethacrylate metabolism in man. The hydrolysis of methylmethacrylate to methacrylic acid during total hip replacement. *Clin Orthop* 1979;90–95.
15. Hecht A. Artificial fingernails: apply with caution. *FDA Consumer Watch* 1988;22:18–21.
16. Kechijian P. Dangers of acrylic fingernails. *JAMA* 1990;236:458.
17. Ellenhorn MJ, Barceloux DG. *Medical toxicology: diagnosis and treatment of human poisoning*. New York: Elsevier, 1988.
18. Yamamoto K. Acute toxicity of the combustion products from various kinds of fibers. *Z Rechtsmed* 1975;76:11–26.
19. Betol E, Mari F, Orzalesi G, et al. Combustion products from various kinds of fibers: toxicological hazards from smoke exposure. *Forensic Sci Int* 1983;22:111–116.
20. Igisu H, Goto I, Kawamura Y, et al. Acrylamide encephaloneuropathy due to well water pollution. *J Neurol Neurosurg Psychiatry* 1975;38:581–584.
21. Gosselin RE , Simth RP, Hodge HCE. *Clinical toxicology of commercial products*, 5th ed. Baltimore: Williams & Wilkins, 1984.
22. Brune D, Beltesbrekke H. Levels of methylmethacrylate, formaldehyde, and asbestos in dental workroom air. *Scand J Dent Res* 1981;89:113–116.
23. McLaughlin RE, Barkalow JA, Allen MS. Pulmonary toxicity of methyl methacrylate vapors: an environmental study. *Arch Environ Health* 1979;34:336–338.
24. Rajaniemi R, Tola S. Subjective symptoms among dental technicians exposed to the monomer methyl methacrylate. *Scand J Work Environ Health* 1985;11:281–286.
25. Rajaniemi R. Clinical evaluation of occupational toxicity of methylmethacrylate monomer to dental technicians. *J Soc Occup Med* 1986;36:56–59.
26. ACGIH. *Documentation of the threshold limit values and biological exposure indices*, 6th ed. Cincinnati, OH: American Conference of Governmental Industrial Hygienists, Inc., 1991.
27. IARC. IARC monographs on the evaluation of carcinogenic risk of chemicals to humans. Lyons, France: International Agency for Research on Cancer, 1986.
28. HSDB. Hazardous Substances Data Bank. *National Library of Medicine*. Englewood, CO: Micromedex, Inc., 1999.
29. Bachmann M, Myers JE, Bezuidenhout BN. Acrylamide monomer and peripheral neuropathy in chemical workers. *Am J Ind Med* 1992;21:217–222.
30. Calleman CJ. The metabolism and pharmacokinetics of acrylamide: implications for mechanisms of toxicity and human risk estimation. *Drug Metab Rev* 1996;28:527–590.
31. Bingham E, Cohrssen B, Powell CHE. *Patty's toxicology*, 5th ed. New York: John Wiley and Sons, Inc., 2001.
32. Lees PS. Combustion products and other firefighter exposures. *Occup Med* 1995;10:691–706.
33. Bernhard J, Heini PF, Villiger PM. Asymptomatic diffuse pulmonary embolism caused by acrylic cement: an unusual complication of percutaneous vertebroplasty. *Ann Rheum Dis* 2003;62:85–86.
34. Fallon KM, Fuller JG, Morley-Forster P. Fat embolization and fatal cardiac arrest during hip arthroplasty with methylmethacrylate. *Can J Anaesth* 2001;48:626–629.
35. Kourani R, Azzi A. Acrylic cement in hip arthroplasty. *Middle East J Anesthesiol* 1986;8:425–435.
36. Schlag G. Mechanisms of cardiopulmonary disturbances during total hip replacement. *Acta Orthop Belg* 1988;54:6–11.
37. Wheelwright EF, Byrick RJ, Wigglesworth DF, et al. Hypotension during cemented arthroplasty. Relationship to cardiac output and fat embolism. *J Bone Joint Surg Br* 1993;75:715–723.
38. Merin RG. Total hip arthroplasty, methyl methacrylate and cardiovascular depression. *JAMA* 1983;249:1354–1355.
39. Kim KC, Ritter MA. Hypotension associated with methyl methacrylate in total hip arthroplasties. *Clin Orthop* 1972;88:154–160.
40. Hyderally H, Miller R. Hypotension and cardiac arrest during prosthetic hip surgery with acrylic bone cement. *Orthop Rev* 1976;5:55–61.
41. Crout DH, Lloyd EJ, Singh J. Metabolism of methyl methacrylate: evidence for metabolism by the valine pathway of catabolism in rat and in man. *Xenobiotica* 1982;12:821–829.
42. Sittig M. *Handbook of toxic and hazardous chemical and carcinogens*, 3rd ed. Park Ridge, NJ: Noyes Publications, 1991.
43. HSDB. Hazardous Substances Data Bank. *National Library of Medicine*. Englewood, CO: Micromedex, Inc., 2000.
44. Jakubowski M, Linhart I, Pielas G, et al. 2-Cyanoethylmercapturic acid (CEMA) in the urine as a possible indicator of exposure to acrylonitrile. *Br J Ind Med* 1987;44:834–840.
45. Miller MJ, Carter DE, Sipes IG. Pharmacokinetics of acrylamide in Fisher-344 rats. *Toxicol Appl Pharmacol* 1982;63:36–44.
46. Tilson HA. The neurotoxicity of acrylamide: an overview. *Neurobehav Toxicol Teratol* 1981;3:445–461.

47. Rijke AM, Johnson RA, Oser ER. On the fate of methyl methacrylate in blood. *J Biomed Mater Res* 1977;11:211–221.
48. Dixit R, Husain R, Mukhtar H, et al. Acrylamide induced inhibition of hepatic glutathione-S-transferase activity in rats. *Toxicol Lett* 1981;7:207–210.
49. Donovan JW, Pearson TO. Ingestion of acrylamide with severe encephalopathy, neurotoxicity and hepatotoxicity. *Vet Human Toxicol* 1987;29:462(abst).
50. Muller G, Verkoyen C, Soton N, et al. Urinary excretion of acrylonitrile and its metabolites in rats. *Arch Toxicol* 1987;60:464–466.
51. Rajaniemi R, Pfaffli P, Savolainen H. Percutaneous absorption of methyl methacrylate by dental technicians. *Br J Ind Med* 1989;46:356–357.
52. Bratt H, Hathaway DE. Fate of methyl methacrylate in rats. *Br J Cancer* 1977;36:114–119.
53. deBethizy JD, et al. The disposition and metabolism of acrylic acid and ethyl acrylate in male Sprague-Dawley rats. *Fundam Appl Toxicol* 1987;8:549–561.
54. NTP. Carcinogenesis studies of ethyl acrylate. National toxicology program technical report #259 (NIH Publication #87-2515). Research Triangle Park, NC: US Department of Health & Human Services, Public Health Service, 1986.
55. Harbison RM. *Hamilton and Hardy's industrial toxicology*, 5th ed. St. Louis, MO: Mosby, 1998.
56. POISINDEX. Acrylates, Multifunctional. Englewood, CO: Micromedex, Inc.
57. McDiarmid MA, Agnew J. Reproductive hazards and firefighters. *Occup Med State of the Art Rev* 1995;10:829–841.
58. RTECS. Registry of Toxic Effects of Chemical Substances. *NIOSH*. Englewood, CO: Micromedex, Inc, 1999.
59. Parent RA, Caravello HECMS, et al. Developmental toxicity of acrolein in New Zealand white rabbits. *Fundam Appl Toxicol* 1993;20:248–256.
60. Lozewicz S, Davison AG, Hopkirk A, et al. Occupational asthma due to methyl methacrylate and cyanoacrylates. *Thorax* 1985;40:836–839.
61. Myers JE, Macun I. Acrylamide neuropathy in a South African factory: an epidemiologic investigation. *Am J Ind Med* 1991;19:487–493.
62. Marcus DM, Hull DS, Rubin RM, et al. Lecythophora mutabilis endophthalmitis after long-term corneal cyanoacrylate. *Retina* 1999;19:351–353.
63. de Fonseka CP. Danger of instant adhesives. *BMJ* 1976;2:1447.
64. de Fonseka CP. Danger of instant adhesives. *BMJ* 1976;2:234.
65. Kassis V, Vedel P, Darre E. Contact dermatitis to methyl methacrylate. *Contact Derm* 1984;11:26–28.
66. Fisher AA. Reactions to acrylic bone cement in orthopedic surgeons and patients. *Cutis* 1986;37:425–426.
67. Durbin FC, Jeffery CC, Jones GB, et al. Cardiac arrest and bone cement. *BMJ* 1970;4:176.
68. Schuh FT, Schuh SM, Viguera MG, et al. Circulatory changes following implantation of methylmethacrylate bone cement. *Anesthesiology* 1973;39:455–457.
69. Gresham GA, Kuczynski A, Rosborough D. Fatal fat embolism following replacement arthroplasty for transcervical fractures of femur. *BMJ* 1971;2:617–619.
70. Learned DW, Hantler CB. Lethal progression of heart block after prosthesis cementing with methylmethacrylate. *Anesthesiology* 1992;77:1044–1046.
71. Buchter A, Peter H. Clinical toxicology of acrylonitrile. *G Ital Med Lav* 1984;6:83–86.
72. Innes DL, Tansy MF. Central nervous system effects of methyl methacrylate vapor. *Neurotoxicology* 1981;2:515–522.
73. Yeragani VK, Pohl R, Balon R. Panic attacks and exposure to chemical agents. *Am J Psych* 1988;145:532.
74. Kanzaki T, Kabasawa Y, Jinno T, et al. Contact stomatitis due to methyl methacrylate monomer. *Contact Derm* 1989;20:146–148.
75. Kepes ER, Undersood PS, Becsey L. Intraoperative death associated with acrylic bone cement: report of two cases. *JAMA* 1972;222:576–577.
76. Gordon ML. Cyanoacrylate warning [Letter]. *J Am Dent Assoc* 1987;115:12.
77. Quirce S, Baeza ML, Tornero P, et al. Occupational asthma caused by exposure to cyanoacrylate. *Allergy* 2001;56:446–449.
78. Walker AM, Cohen AJ, Loughlin JE, et al. Mortality from cancer of the colon or rectum among workers exposed to ethyl acrylate and methyl methacrylate. *Scand J Work Environ Health* 1991;17:7–19.
79. Collins JJ, Page LC, Caporossi JC, et al. Mortality patterns among men exposed to methyl methacrylate. *J Occup Med* 1989;31:41–46.
80. Samson D, Marshall D. Carcinogenic potential of isobutyl 2-cyanoacrylate. *J Neurosurg* 1986;65:571.
81. Collins JJ, Swaen GM, Marsh GM, et al. Mortality patterns among workers exposed to acrylamide. *J Occup Med* 1989;31:614–617.
82. Marsh GM, et al. Mortality patterns in workers exposed to acrylamide: 1994 follow-up. *Occup Environ Med* 1999;56:181–190.
83. Cohen SM, Garland EM, St. John M, et al. Acrolein initiates rat urinary bladder carcinogenesis. *Cancer Res* 1992;52:3577–3581.
84. Parent RA, Caravello HE, Long JE. Two year toxicity and carcinogenicity study of acrolein in rats. *J Appl Toxicol* 1992;12:131–139.
85. Aminoff MJ. Electrophysiologic recognition of certain occupation-related neurotoxic disorders. *Neurol Clin* 1985;3:687–697.
86. Loeb AL, Anderson RJ. Antagonism of acrylamide neurotoxicity by supplementation with vitamin B-6. *Neurotoxicol* 1981;2:625–633.
87. Watanabe T, Kaji R, Oka N, et al. Ultra-high dose methylcobalamin promotes nerve regeneration in experimental acrylamide neuropathy. *J Neurol Sci* 1994;122:140–143.
88. Kemplay S, Martin P, Wilson S. The effects of thioctic acid on motor nerve terminals in acrylamide-poisoned rats. *Neuropathol Appl Neurobiol* 1998;14:275–288.
89. Dean BS, Krenzelok EP. Cyanoacrylates and corneal abrasion. *J Toxicol Clin Toxicol* 1989;27:169–172.
90. Cary R, Evans P, Cocker J, et al. Methylcyanoacrylate and ethyl cyanoacrylate risk assessment document, EH 72/13. Sudbury, Suffolk, UK: HSE Books, 2000.

CHAPTER 209

Epoxides and Epoxy Resins

Robert B. Palmer and Scott D. Phillips

HO–C₆H₄–C(CH₃)₂–C₆H₄–OH

BISPHENOL A

Compounds included:	**Bisphenol A, epichlorohydrin**
Molecular formula and weight:	**Bisphenol A ($C_{15}H_{16}O_2$), 228.29 g/mol; epichlorohydrin (C_3H_5ClO), 92.53 g/mol**
SI conversion:	**µg/L × 0.0044 = µmol/L**
CAS Registry No.:	**106-89-8 (epichlorohydrin); 80-05-7 (bisphenol A)**
Normal levels:	**Not used clinically**
Antidote:	**Cyanide antidote package in rare cases**

OVERVIEW

An epoxide, also called an *oxirane*, is a three-membered ring consisting of one oxygen atom and two carbon atoms. This ring is highly strained and therefore reactive and subject to hydrolysis under acidic and basic conditions. Due to the electron withdrawing characteristics of the oxygen atom, the two carbons in an epoxide have net positive character (though not full positive charges). This unequal distribution of electrons makes the carbon atoms of an epoxide particularly amenable to nucleophilic substitution. When a nucleophile attacks a carbon atom in an epoxide, the bond between the attacked carbon atom and the oxygen of the epoxide ring breaks and the ring oxygen becomes a hydroxyl moiety bonded to the carbon atom of the epoxide

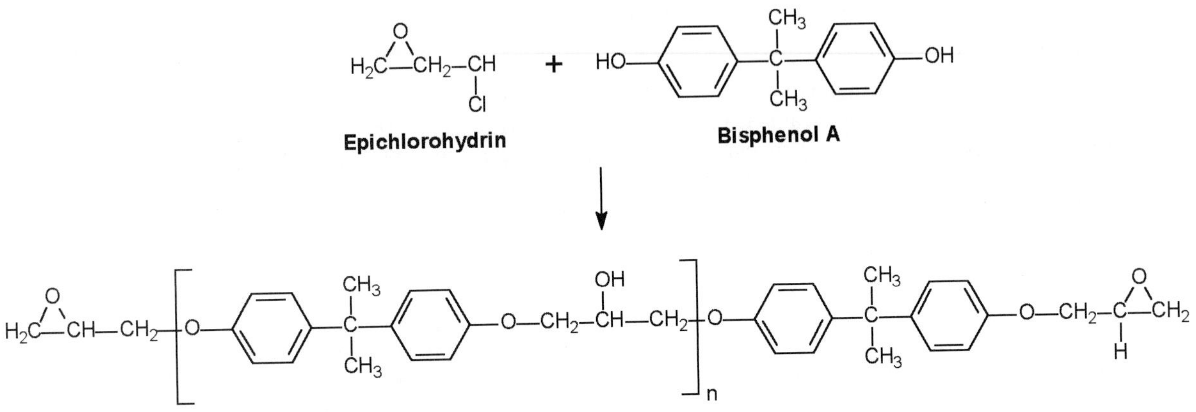

Figure 1. Reaction of epichlorohydrin and bisphenol A to form glycidyl ether adduct epoxy resins of bisphenol A. When n equals one, the adduct is bisphenol A diglycidyl ether.

that was not the subject of nucleophilic attack. The nucleophile remains covalently bonded to the former epoxide carbon it attacked (Fig. 1).

Classification and Uses

Epichlorohydrin (3-chloro-1,2-epoxy propane; chloromethyloxirane) is used not only in the production of epoxy resins but also as a stabilizer in chlorine containing systems and as a solvent in a variety of paints, varnishes, resins, gums, lacquers, and nail enamels (1,2).

Bisphenol A is the most commonly used starting material (along with epichlorohydrin) for epoxy resin production. More than 75% of the resin used in current industrial application is derived from this compound. Bisphenol A is used for many other purposes as well. Approximately 65% of the bisphenol A produced is used to make polycarbonate with 25% going toward epoxy resin manufacture (3). The remaining 10% is used in the production of specialty resins and the manufacture of flame retardants (3). The world production volume of bisphenol A is enormous. The United States alone produces more than 1.1 million tons. Though the major world producers of bisphenol A are Japan, Brazil, Russia, and the United States, other countries including Belgium, Germany, Spain, the Netherlands, and Thailand manufacture significant amounts as well. In 1997 to 1998, it was estimated that the consumption of bisphenol A by the European Union alone was approximately 640,000 tons (3).

Epichlorohydrin and bisphenol A are combined to form the *epoxy resin*. A typical industrial process is to combine bisphenol A, epichlorohydrin, and sodium hydroxide with the appropriate solvents. When the reaction is complete, water is introduced to remove the sodium chloride that forms as a byproduct of the reaction. The residual unreacted epichlorohydrin is recovered at this stage for future use. The reaction products are then steam distilled to further purify the resin. The distillates are filtered and the liquid epoxy resin stored. The epoxy resin is subsequently treated with the curing agent to make the final epoxy product.

Curing agents, which are also called *hardening agents*, are used to covalently link individual molecules of the epoxy resin together to form a large polymeric plastic material. A variety of chemical classes are used for this purpose, with the most common being amines, acid anhydrides, and amides. The conditions under which the curing agent is reacted with the epoxy resin vary and can include either heating or ambient temperature. The specific curing agent selected largely determines the physical characteristics of the final plastic product.

The epoxy resin–derived polymers, which are often simply referred to as *epoxy plastics*, are thermoset plastics (i.e., plastics that are rigid when cool but lose shape when heated). The final product may be a rigid or flexible polymer depending on the specific resin and curing agent used. Typically, these polymers have excellent adhesion properties as they have the polar hydroxyl groups from epoxide opening, low shrinkage, good impact, and moisture resistance and excellent electrical properties.

Uses

Bisphenol A epoxy resin systems (i.e., the resin plus the selected curing agent) have a variety of industrial uses including as adhesives, molding resins, surface coatings, and reinforced plastics (1–3). Systems with resins derived from cycloaliphatic compounds are used in the electrical industry as insulators and encapsulating agents for transformers as well as for coatings for plastics, paper, and metals and in electron microscopy. The triepoxy compound triglycidyl isocyanurate is used for many polyester resins and in solvent-free dry particle paints (4).

Sources of Exposure

Most epoxy resin systems are not naturally occurring. However, the widespread use of the epoxy resins and polycarbonate plastics makes the appearance of these compounds in the environment of industrialized nations no surprise. Most environmental attention has focused on bisphenol A. However, other components of the epoxy resin systems, including diluents, solvents, and curing agents, may also be present in environmental sites. There exist no apparent adverse effects on the environment or on plant or animal life as a result of passive environmental exposure to these compounds.

Small amounts of uncured resins can be found in numerous sources including twist-off bottle caps, film cassettes, metal cosmetic and food containers, brass doorknobs and hooks, plastic tool handles and cleaning gloves, to name a few (1,2). An additional source of exposure to uncured resins is medical equipment (5–7). Uncured epoxy resins are found in vinyl hospital identification bands, insulin pump infusion sets, hemodialysis tubing, ostomy bags, pacemakers, and nasal cannulas.

Bisphenol A is known to leak in minute quantities into food and drink from containers in which these items are stored. This is true for food cans, wine and water bottles, microwave food packaging and polycarbonate baby bottles, and many others (3). Municipal and residential plumbing systems typically use epoxy resin–derived plumbing and adhesives; as a result, bisphenol A is measurable in drinking water (3). Additional sources of bisphenol A include tableware, dental fillings and sealants, coated drugs, and medical adhesives (3,8–10).

Bisphenol A is measurable in packaged foods (3,8,11,12). When the liquid portions in several types of canned vegetables including artichokes, corn, green beans, mixed vegetables, peas, and mushrooms from cans containing epoxy resin linings were analyzed, the highest concentration was estimated to provide a total intake of approximately 80 µg of bisphenol A per kilogram of canned food consumed (3,11). This is well below all established tolerable daily intake amounts. A Japanese study found one brand of canned coffee to contain 127 µg/kg of bisphenol A; the manufacturer reformulated the containers (8). Despite the wide variety of sources, exposure levels are typically far below tolerable daily intake amounts.

In Europe, migration limits (i.e., the amount of a compound that is permitted to migrate into a foodstuff from packaging materials) have been established. The European Commission—Scientific Committee on Food placed a migration limit on bisphenol A at 3 parts per million (ppm) (i.e., 3 mg/kg of food) (3). This agency has also imposed a limit of 1 parts per million (ppm) for bisphenol A diglycidyl ether and its hydrolysis products, which was increased from 0.02 ppm in a controversial decision in 1996. This 1 ppm limit was reconfirmed in 1999, though additional toxicity data were requested (3). The United States has not imposed such limits.

Tolerable daily intakes specify the estimated amount of a compound that can be ingested every day over the course of a lifetime without appreciable health risk. In 1986, the European Commission—Scientific Committee on Food recommended a tolerable daily intake for bisphenol A of 50 µg/kg body weight per day. This value was also adopted by the U.S. Environmental Protection Agency and is based on cancer as the endpoint. A 1998 study published by vom Saal suggested that low levels of bisphenol A (down to 2 µg/kg body weight per day) might have adverse human health effects other than cancer, most notably estrogenic endocrine disrupting effects (13), causing the U.K. Committee on Toxicology to reevaluate the tolerable daily intakes for bisphenol A. Ultimately, the U.K. Committee on Toxicology decided to retain the 50 µg/kg body weight per day limit asserting that the vom Saal study was insufficient to make definitive conclusions. This conclusion has not been confirmed by others (14).

Occupational Safety Precautions

Workers handling epoxy resins and epichlorohydrin should be aware that use of proper protective clothing is essential. Epoxy resins can penetrate rubber, polyethylene, and polyvinyl chloride gloves, though nitrile and nitrile-butatoluene-rubber gloves provided adequate protection for sensitized workers for 48 hours (15). Epichlorohydrin is well-known to rapidly penetrate rubber as well as leather belts, boots, and gloves possibly resulting in chemical burns (1). Extended contact with leather goods soaked with epichlorohydrin has caused severe blistering and tissue necrosis. Rubber or leather items contaminated with epichlorohydrin should be destroyed (1).

Physical and Chemical Properties

The reactivity of the epoxide functional group makes it well suited for the polymerization reactions necessary for making plastics. However, this same reactivity often makes compounds possessing an epoxide moiety strong alkylating agents. Epoxides are known phase I metabolic products of olefins (carbon-carbon double bonds). Metabolically produced epoxides have been established as the carcinogenic species in compounds such as the *Bay region* epoxide metabolites of benzo[a]pyrene. It has been suggested that these compounds alkylate hemoglobin and deoxyribonucleic acid and, as a result, may be genotoxic or carcinogenic (16).

The term *epoxy resin* most often refers to an oligomer that contains more than one epoxide moiety residing at the ends of the oligomeric chains. Though these resins are most often small in molecular weight (e.g., bisphenol A diglicidyl ether; molecular weight = 340 g/mol; Fig. 1), they range to more than 900 g/mol in size. The lower molecular weight resins are liquids whereas those with higher molecular weights are typically either viscous liquids or solids. If it is necessary to reduce the viscosity of an epoxy resin, a reactive diluent or a solvent may be added. A reactive diluent is a low-molecular-weight compound, often a monoglycidyl ether, that may compose up to 15% of the total resin mass. Solvents include methyl ethyl ketone, toluene, xylene, phenyl-, allyl-, and butyl-glycidyl ethers, styrene oxide as well as other compounds. Though the reason for adding a reactive diluent or solvent is largely the same (i.e., decreased viscosity), the distinction is that reactive diluents become covalently incorporated into the final polymer, whereas solvents usually do not.

When treated with an appropriate reagent (called a *curing agent* or *hardener*), the epoxides in the epoxy resins react and covalently bond the curing agent to form a stable three-dimensional polymeric network, which hardens to the final plastic polymer. Curing agents typically have an active (i.e., dissociable) hydrogen atom attached to an oxygen, nitrogen, or sulfur atom. It is the heteroatom (oxygen, nitrogen, or sulfur) that acts as the nucleophile toward the epoxide ring in the curing process. Many types of curing agents are available and include polyamines, anhydrides, and amides. The specific curing agent selected determines the properties of the final plastic product.

Epoxy resins are typically marketed as part of an *epoxy system* (Table 1). The epoxy system consists of two primary parts: (a) the resin, including appropriate solvents or reactive diluents and (b) the curing agent. The two components are usually kept physically separated until use. At the time of use, the resin and the curing agent are combined and the appropriate curing conditions (e.g., heat) are applied. The result is the final epoxy plastic polymer. Some newer epoxy systems used as epoxy coatings have a single component design in which the amine or anhydride curing agent has been modified to reduce sensitization and irritant properties (17).

One of the most widely used classes of curing agents is the amines, which possess a nucleophilic nitrogen atom. Primary or secondary amines can be used and a typical polyamine curing agent will have more than three active amine centers per molecule, which allow for cross linking of multiple epoxy resin molecules in curing. Another common curing agent class is the organic acid anhydrides. A few organic amides are also used as epoxy curing agents.

The reaction between an epoxy resin and the hardening agent can be either a hot cure or a cold cure. Many of the polyamine curing agents react sufficiently well at room temperature (i.e., cold curing conditions). Most often, if a polyamine curing agent is to be used at room temperature, a plasticizer is added to the reaction mixture to help drive the reaction to completion. The most common hot cure hardening agents are anhydrides (1). Cold cure reactions are often used to create flexible plastics and coatings whereas hot cure hardening is used to create high strength epoxy plastics that have improved resistance to heat. In both hot and cold cures, resin, reactive diluent, solvent, and curing agent vapors may be released.

Like many other plastics, the final polymeric substance created from an epoxy resin may also contain additives to improve characteristics of the plastic such as color, moldability, pliability, and resistance to combustion. In many cases (e.g., phthalate plasticizers), these additives are not covalently incorporated

TABLE 1. Example components of epoxy resins systems

Epoxy resins	Curing agent	Reactive diluents	Solvents
Bisphenol A diglycidyl ether	Amines	Phenylglycidyl ether	Methylethyl ketone
Tetrabromobisphenol A diglycidyl ether	Triethylenetetramine	Cresyl glycidyl ether	Toluene
Tetraglycidyl-4,4'-methylene dianiline	Isophorone diamine	Butylglycidyl ether	Xylene
Triglycidyl–para-aminophenol	Xylenediamine	Allylglycidyl ether	Butylglycidyl ether
Ortho-diglycidylphthalate	4,4'-Methylenedianiline	1,4-Butanediol diglycidyl ether	Allylglycidyl ether
4,4-Isopropylidene diphenyl epichlorohydrin	Diaminodiphenylmethane	Neopentyl glycol diglycidyl ether	Phenylglycidyl ether
Vinyl cyclohexene diepoxide	Diethylenetriamine	1,6-Hexanediol diglycidyl ether	Styrene oxide
Triglycidyl isocyanurate	Anhydrides		
	Hexahydrophthalic anhydride		
	Phthalic anhydride		
	Trimellitic anhydride		
	Tetrachlorophthalic anhydride		
	Maleic anhydride		
	Amides		
	Dicyandiamide		

into the polymer of the plastic. Rather, they are physically trapped within the net-like matrix of the polymer. As such, the additives can be leached from the matrix with heat, solvent contact, and simply over time. Because these agents may have inherent toxicity unrelated to the polymer, the complete composition of the plastic product must be considered. The toxicity of plastic additives are considered beyond the scope of this chapter but should not be ignored in the evaluation of a potentially exposed patient. Furthermore, burning of epoxy plastics may produce and liberate a variety of toxins as a result of combustion, including carbon monoxide and cyanide.

Toxic Dose

The threshold limit value–time weighted average for epichlorohydrin set by the American Council of Government Industrial Hygienists is 2 mg/m^3 (0.5 ppm), skin notation (18,19). Though a transitional permissible exposure limit–time weighted average value was set by the U.S. Occupational Safety and Health Administration at 19 mg/m^3 (approximately 5 ppm) averaged over an 8-hour workday, the final rule permissible exposure limit–time weighted average for epichlorohydrin is currently set at 8 mg/m^3 (approximately 2 ppm), skin designation (1,19,20). No short term exposure limit or ceiling limit values have been established. The odor threshold (sweet, pungent) of epichlorohydrin is 10 ppm (4). The immediately dangerous to life and health concentration is 100 ppm.

The no-effect air level for epichlorohydrin is estimated to be 9 ppm, which is close to the odor threshold (1). Humans exposed to epichlorohydrin at 20 ppm for 1 hour reported temporary burning. With air concentrations of 40 ppm, irritant effects lasting up to 48 hours have been reported (1,2,21). At 100 ppm, the immediately dangerous to life and health value for this compound, pulmonary edema and renal lesions have been reported (1,2).

TOXICOKINETICS AND TOXICODYNAMICS

Absorption

Bisphenol A is rapidly absorbed after ingestion. Many of the polyamine curing agents are strongly basic and, as a result, can injure skin and mucosal barriers that may result in systemic absorption. Inhalation and ingestion exposures to epoxy resins have shown effects on the central nervous system within minutes of exposure in laboratory animals (20,22). Epichlorohydrin is absorbed orally, percutaneously, subcutaneously, and through inhalation (18,23). In rodents, the highest tissue concentrations were found in the nose after inhalation and in the stomach after ingestion (19).

Limited kinetic studies of the epoxy resin curing agents have been performed. The kinetics in humans exposed to airborne concentrations of 10, 40, and 80 μg/m^3 of hexahydrophthalic anhydride demonstrated that respiratory uptake of this anhydride is nearly complete and that both plasma and urinary levels of the acid hydrolysis product rapidly increase with onset of exposure and decrease quickly with cessation of exposure (24).

Distribution of the curing agents and resins with corrosive or caustic properties is likely simply a result of entry *via* tissue barrier destruction rather than true organ-specific systemic distribution.

Metabolism and Elimination

In the rat, epichlorohydrin is rapidly metabolized independent of exposure route to water-soluble derivatives that are eliminated primarily in the urine with small amounts through the lungs as carbon dioxide (19). Several of the bisphenol A–derived ethers used as dental sealants can be metabolically converted to release some bisphenol A (25–27). Metabolism of hexahydrophthalic anhydride is hydrolytic and results in the production of hexahydrophthalic acid (24,28,29). This acid is also formed when the anhydride is reacted with water, so the conversion of hexahydrophthalic anhydride to the acid product in exposed humans likely represents a significant amount of chemical degradation.

Animal data indicate rapid elimination of epoxy resins in the urine and feces. Although it does not occur in fish, concern has been expressed regarding the potential for bioaccumulation of bisphenol A in fatty depots such as breast milk fed to human babies (3).

In occupationally exposed humans, hexahydrophthalic anhydride is excreted in the urine primarily as the unconjugated hexahydrophthalic acid (24). As such, it has been suggested that determination of hexahydrophthalic acid might be a useful biological marker for inhalational exposure to hexahydrophthalic anhydride in an occupational setting (24,29,30).

PATHOPHYSIOLOGY

Exposure to epoxy plastics and plastic additives is usually the result of inhalation or direct contact with skin or mucosal surfaces. Though ingestion of pure concentrated epoxy resin components may have significant toxicity, amounts encountered through eating or drinking products stored in cured epoxy containers from which epoxy compounds have leached are unlikely to be of toxicologic significance.

Manufacturing of epoxy resins and plastics and use of the uncured forms of these compounds represent situations in which exposure may occur. In some cases, though the final product is not injurious, synthetic starting materials (e.g., phosgene) may have significant toxicity. Additionally, combustion of monomeric or polymeric forms of derivatives of acrylic acid can release carbon monoxide, cyanide, and oxides of nitrogen if the derivative contains nitrogen and phosgene if the derivative is chlorinated.

After an acute exposure, most of the compounds related to epoxy resins (including reactive diluents, solvents, and curing agents) are irritating or corrosive. Repeated or chronic exposure may also have health consequences ranging from immune reactions due to allergic sensitization as seen with acid anhydride curing agents, to hepatitis, or potentially bladder carcinoma as from heavy exposure to methylenedianiline (31–34).

Though fully cured epoxy plastics are generally considered nontoxic, there are some effects related to exposure to the polymerized species that deserve mention. For example, mechanical injury from sharp plastic edges or gastrointestinal obstruction from bulk polymer and irritant or allergic responses to polymer dust are possible. Furthermore, if the polymerization reaction is incomplete or inappropriate ratios of components are used, the possibility of residual unreacted resin, curing agent, reactive diluent, or solvent being present exists. Release of potentially allergenic compounds may take place with heating, grinding, lathing, and molding of the polymer (31,35).

VULNERABLE POPULATIONS

At high oral doses, epichlorohydrin is linked to fetotoxicity (1,20). Male mice exposed to bisphenol A *in utero* have increased prostate weight and preputial gland size, diminished sperm production, and decreased seminal vesicle size (3,36). However, Cagen found no such effects after prenatal exposure of CF-1 mice to bisphenol A (37). Effects on breast development in female rats and behavioral effects in both genders of rats have been reported after bisphenol A exposure (38,39). These effects have not been observed in cases of human exposure.

CLINICAL PRESENTATION

Systemic Reaction

Epoxy resins and epichlorohydrin may cause allergic contact dermatitis. As a general rule, these compounds may act as allergens causing not only IgE mediated bronchospasm but also induction of IgG formation (1). Many of the organic anhydride curing agents used to harden epoxy resins can also act as sensitizers. It is well-known that the epoxy resin curing agents hexahydrophthalic anhydride and methylhexahydrophthalic anhydride are associated with a high frequency of sensitization symptoms in exposed workers (24,40,41). Anaphylaxis has been reported in sensitized guinea pigs exposed to intravenous hexahydrophthalic anhydride (42,43).

Ocular

Essentially all of the epoxy resins and hardening agents may cause ocular irritation (1). Exposure to high concentrations or for prolonged periods can result in significant caustic injury (1). This is especially true for highly basic compounds such as the polyamine hardening agents as well as for the reactive epoxides and anhydrides. Fumes may cause periorbital edema and conjunctivitis (44). Sensitized workers have reported contact eyelid dermatitis and other allergic symptoms after exposure to epoxy resins and related compounds (45).

An ingestion of methylene dianiline resulted in delayed onset pigmentary retinopathy (46). Within 3 weeks, the patient's vision was limited to the perception of light. Though some gradual recovery occurred, the damage was largely permanent (46).

Dermal

Epichlorohydrin, the epoxy resins and most of the curing agents (e.g., anhydrides, polyamines, and so forth) are dermal irritants and many can cause severe corrosive burns. Irritant dermatitis has been reported with occupational exposure to epoxy resins and is believed to be the result of alkaline curing agents (17,47). Skin sensitization has been reported after occupational exposure (48,49). Development of eczema, photodermatitis, urticaria, persistent itching, vesicles, and erythema multiforme has been reported. Widespread scleroderma with erythema and brown pigmentation was reported in two workers who used an amine curing agent with an epoxy resin (50). A 17-year follow-up of these two persons showed that the sclerotic skin changes disappeared within 5 years and evidence of internal organ involvement was not detected (50–52).

Cardiovascular

Reflex tachycardia associated with pain (e.g., dermal burning), respiratory distress, or hypotension is secondary to hypovolemia. Ingestion of methylene dianiline was associated with hypotension, bradycardia, T-wave inversion, and ST segment abnormalities (46). Experimental animals exposed to epichlorohydrin have developed hypotension (2).

Nervous System

The epoxy resins and curing agents are not known to be primary neurotoxins. Inhalation of large amounts of epoxy resins or curing agents may result in nonspecific central nervous system effects such as diminished level of consciousness or seizures. Three workers were asphyxiated while painting an unventilated underground tank with an epoxy resin–based sealant (53). Experimental animals exposed to high concentrations of epichlorohydrin have displayed somnolence, tremors, ataxia, loss of muscular tone, seizures, respiratory arrest, and death (20,22).

Gastrointestinal

Workers exposed to epichlorohydrin through inhalation and dermal exposure have developed nausea, vomiting, and abdominal pain in the absence of corrosive injury to the gastrointestinal tract (21,54). Ingestion of epichlorohydrin, the epoxy resins, and curing agents may result in effects on the gastrointestinal tract ranging from irritation to severe caustic injury. If polyamine curing agents are ingested, dysphagia, excessive salivation, and chemical burns to the oropharynx and esophagus with subsequent stricture development are possible (55).

Respiratory

Irritation of the upper respiratory tract may result in inflammatory changes of the tongue, epiglottis, and trachea (1). Stridor, dyspnea, dysphagia, and excessive salivation may be observed.

Dry cough, nasal irritation, and burning chest discomfort that resolved without sequelae were reported after inhalation of an epoxy-based dry paint powder (4).

Lower airway effects have also been reported. Fumes and dust particles of epoxy resins and curing agents are associated with cough, bronchospasm, and bronchitis (1,56). These effects, which can be severe, may persist for several days after exposure. Serial pulmonary function tests have shown consistent reversible increases in airway resistance with exposure to amine curing agents (57). This effect was more prominent in smokers.

Inhalation challenge with organic anhydrides can cause severe immediate and delayed-onset occupational asthma. A temporal relationship has been noted in epoxy-related occupational asthma (58). Workers report that earlier in the week, symptoms occur later in the workday, whereas toward the end of the workweek, symptom onset is immediate. In shipyard workers exposed to epoxy paints, presence of lower respiratory symptoms was increased significantly over controls, and a linear relationship was described between duration of exposure to epoxy paints and decrease in forced expiratory volume in 1 second (59). Though similar irritant effects are anticipated with inhalation of epichlorohydrin, this has not been reported in an occupational setting.

The organic acid anhydrides are also irritating to the respiratory tract. This is likely due to hydrolysis of the anhydride to the corresponding carboxylic acid with the concomitant release of heat. The organic acid anhydrides also increase immunoglobulin release (60). Compounds of this class may have some involvement at the IgE-antibody combining site. Trimellitic, methyltetrahydrophthalic, and tetrachlorophthalic anhydrides have been shown to cause IgE mediated responses and bronchial hyperreactivity (58,60). Smokers were at an increased risk of developing a specific IgE mediated bronchial response to tetrachlorophthalic anhydride.

Inhalation exposure to trimellitic anhydride dust and fumes may result in any of four specific clinical syndromes (31): (a) simple irritant respiratory effects, (b) IgE-mediated asthma-rhinitis, (c) *trimellitic anhydride flu* (a late respiratory systemic reaction characterized by cough, dyspnea, myalgia, fever, and chills that typically occurs 4 to 12 hours after exposure), and (d) pulmonary disease–anemia syndrome. This syndrome is the most clinically significant and consists of cough, dyspnea, hemoptysis, hemolytic anemia, and restrictive pulmonary disease. Pulmonary infiltrates may be seen; rarely, the condition can progress to respiratory failure (1,31).

Epoxy sealing paints can also act as simple asphyxiants inside containers. In one case, three workers were killed as a result of asphyxiation while they were painting a nonventilated underground water tank with an epoxy resin sealant (53).

Hepatic

Hepatomegaly has been observed after exposure to epichlorohydrin in both humans and animals (1,54). Abnormalities in liver function have persisted in humans for up to 2 years after a single exposure to an unknown concentration of epichlorohydrin (1).

Some epoxy resin curing agents, especially the aromatic polyamines, have been linked to chemically induced hepatitis. One classic case series describes 84 people who developed hepatitis after eating bread contaminated with methylenedianiline whereas another reports liver injury from a single accidental ingestion (32,46). The former case is known as the *Epping jaundice*. In this case, bread was made with flour contaminated with methylenedialine. Sixteen people died from liver failure.

Dermal exposure to methylenedianiline in an occupational setting has also caused toxic hepatitis (61). Right upper quadrant pain, jaundice, and elevated transaminases may be present with or without hepatomegaly (1,46). The duration of the illness is typically 1 to 7 weeks, but the onset has been delayed as much as 6 weeks. In the case of accidental ingestion of methylenedianiline, transaminases remained elevated for a year (46).

Endocrine Effects

Endocrine modulation by chemicals has become a subject of much debate and research. The growing list of proposed *endocrine-disrupting chemicals* has focused on the modulation of the sex hormones (estrogen and testosterone). However, thyroid, growth hormone, prolactin, and other hormone systems may also be studied. A National Institute for Occupational Safety and Health study in the ovariectomized rat suggests that bisphenol A alters endocrine function (62). Others have suggested that bisphenol A causes prostate gland enlargement, but this finding was not confirmed in a comprehensive three-generation study (14). When compared to estradiol, bisphenol A has only 0.05% to 0.1% of the binding affinity (63). The clinical significance of environmental exposure to bisphenol A and endocrine disruption is questionable.

There are few data on the potential for endocrine modulation from epichlorohydrin. In studies of testicular function in workers with exposure to epichlorohydrin, Milby et al. found no evidence that the cohorts they studied showed any effect on sperm count (64,65).

Glycosuria was reported in one case of methylenedianiline ingestion in a patient with multiple other significant effects (46).

Miscellaneous

Alterations in blood cell counts have been documented in some epoxy resin–related exposures. Hemolytic anemia that resolved over several weeks was observed in workers exposed to fumes containing trimellitic anhydride (55). Pattern and model makers with occupational exposure to epoxy resins may develop lymphocytopenia, though duration of exposure and percentage of time involving exposure were not clearly associated with drop in lymphocyte count (66). Due to their potent sensitizing effects, eosinophilia may occur after exposure to epoxy resins and related compounds (67).

Carcinogenesis

The carcinogenicity of bisphenol A has been studied in rats and mice. The National Toxicology Program concluded that there was no convincing evidence that bisphenol A was carcinogenic in either rats or mice of either gender (68,69).

Several studies have addressed the potential for carcinogenicity of epichlorohydrin in humans. Poor exposure assessments and small sample size compromised the results of all studies. In a study by Tsai et al., there was no excess in cancer deaths, prostate cancer, malignant melanomas, or lung cancer (70). In another study, total cancers (N = 10) were statistically less than expected (71). In a study of lung cancer in workers exposed to epichlorohydrin, Bond et al. performed a nested case-control study among a cohort of 19,608 male chemical workers in the United States (72). Workers who had ever been exposed had a decreased risk of lung cancer, again based on a small sample size. Based on animal data, there are suggestions of tumor formation in the rodent forestomach and nasal cavity (73,74).

DIAGNOSTIC TESTS

A number of gas and liquid chromatographic methods have been used to quantitate epoxy resin–related compounds, including curing agents in workplace air as well as in biological matrices for kinetic assessment (24,29,48,75,76). Though levels of these compounds are typically unavailable and are not useful for clinical management, they can be of some use for biologic monitoring of occupational exposures. Baseline laboratory assessment of kidney, liver, and blood cell counts are recommended due to the potential effects of the epoxy resins on these systems.

Persons removed from situations in which epoxy resins or compounds used in their production were burned may require evaluation of carboxyhemoglobin and cyanide levels. Additional laboratory tests such as electrolytes and arterial blood gases should be performed as clinically indicated. Endoscopic evaluation for corrosive injury may be appropriate after ingestion (Chapter 202).

TREATMENT

Overview of Treatment Strategies

Management of symptomatic exposure to epichlorohydrin, epoxy resins, and curing agents is symptomatic and supportive. The initial step in management is to stop the exposure.

Decontamination

Limiting exposure may include simple removal to fresh air after inhalation. Clothing should be removed. External decontamination with water should be performed as soon as possible.

In the case of a small ingestion of uncured epoxy resins and related compounds, dilution with a small volume (4 to 6 oz) of water or milk is appropriate. Induction of emesis is not recommended due not only to corrosive potential but also to the fact that many of these agents are dissolved in hydrocarbon solvents. Epichlorohydrin is adsorbed by activated charcoal. Activated charcoal should be administered for recent ingestion of an uncured species without evidence of corrosive injury. Potentially severe corrosive injury is expected with ingestion and ocular exposure. There is no role for charcoal after ingestion of polymerized compounds and no reason to use multidose charcoal for ingestion of any epoxy resin–related compound.

Enhancement of Elimination

Extracorporeal techniques for enhanced elimination of epichlorohydrin have not been investigated.

Antidotes

There are no antidotes for epoxy resin poisoning.

Supportive Care

Ocular or skin corrosive injury is managed using standard measures for chemical burns. If pain, lacrimation, photophobia, or other ocular problems persist after adequate decontamination, referral for ophthalmologic evaluation should be considered.

Respiratory compromise is treated with oxygen and inhaled β-adrenergic agonists as needed for bronchospasm. Corticosteroids may be needed for sustained inhibition of inflammation.

Allergic contact dermatitis from sensitization is managed by ceasing exposure and steroid therapy as needed. *Irritant dermatitis* is common with exposure to epoxy resin–related compounds. Affected skin should not be covered after decontamination, except to prevent further contamination in the event of significant burn injury. Many of the epoxy resins and related compounds are potent sensitizing agents and can cause allergic dermatitis. Persons working with these compounds should be aware that epoxy resins are known to penetrate rubber, polyethylene, and polyvinyl chloride gloves (15). Continued exposure from epichlorohydrin-saturated leatherwear has also been documented (2). Workers should use nitrile or nitrile-butatoluene gloves when working with these compounds and wash with ample soap and water as soon as possible after completing work (15).

Dyspnea, hypotension, and *seizures* are treated in the usual manner (Chapters 33, 37, and 40, respectively). Hypotension may result from fluid loss due to corrosive injury. In a case of accidental ingestion of methylene dianline, hypotension may have been caused by a central mechanism or from direct depression of cardiac function (46). If persistent fluid loss and hypotension occurs, surgical intervention may be necessary.

Caustic injuries are treated as other alkaline corrosive agents (Chapter 202).

Cyanide and carbon monoxide poisoning may rarely result from combustion of nitrogen-containing epoxy resins, hardening agents, and fully cured plastics. In cases of persons exposed to such fires in which a consistent clinical picture is present, administration of the clinically indicated portions of the cyanide antidote kit should be considered (Chapter 46).

REFERENCES

1. POISINDEX. Englewood, CO: Micromedex, Inc.
2. Bingham E, Cohrssen B, Powell CHE. *Patty's toxicology*, 5th ed. New York: John Wiley and Sons, Inc. 2001.
3. Lyons G. Bisphenol A: a known endocrine disruptor. Surrey, UK: World Wildlife Federation—European Toxics Programme Report, 2000.
4. Rubinstein B, Shrestha M, Greenberg M. Lack of significant toxicity from acute inhalation of dry paint containing triglycidylisocyanurate (TGIC). *Clin Toxicol* 2002;40:356(abst).
5. Mork MJ. Contact sensitivity from epoxy resin in a hemodialysis set. *Contact Dermatitis* 1979;5:331–32.
6. Fregert S, Persson K, Trulsson L. Hidden sources of unhardened epoxy resin of bisphenol A type. *Contact Dermatitis* 1980;6:446–47.
7. Beck MH, Burrows D, Fregert S, Mendelsohn S. Allergic contact dermatitis to epoxy resin in ostomy bags. *Br J Surg* 1985;72:202–3.
8. Takao Y, Chui LH, Yasuhiro I, et al. Fast screening method for bisphenol A in environmental water and in food by solid-phase microextraction (SPME). *J Health Sci* 1999;45:39–43.
9. Lambert C, Larroque M. Chromatographic analysis of water and wine samples for phenolic compounds released from food contact epoxy resins. *J Chromatogr Sci* 1997;35:57–62.
10. Pulgar R, Olea-Serrano MF, Novillo-Fertrell A, et al. Determination of bisphenol A and related aromatic compounds released from bis-GMA-based composites and sealants by high performance liquid chromatography. *Environ Health Perspect* 2000;108:21–7.
11. Brotons JA, Olea-Serrano MF, Villalobos M, et al. Xenoestrogens released from lacquer coatings in food cans. *Environ Health Perspect* 1995;103:608–12.
12. Kawamura Y, Sano H, Yamada T. Migration of bisphenol A from can coatings to drinks. *J Food Hyg Soc Japan* 1999;40:158–65.
13. Vom Saal FS, Cooke PS, Buchanan DL, et al. A physiologically based approach to the study of bisphenol A and other estrogenic chemicals on the size of reproductive organs, daily sperm production and behaviour. *Toxicol Ind Health* 1998;14:239–60.
14. Tyl RW, Myers CB, Marr MC, et al. Three-generation reproductive toxicity study of dietary bisphenol A in CD Sprague-Dawley rats. *Toxicol Sci* 2002;68:121–46.
15. Blanken R, Nater JP, Veenhoff E. Protection against epoxy resins with glove materials. *Contact Dermatitis* 1987;16:46–7.
16. Kolman A, Chovanec M, Osterman-Golkar S. Genotoxic effects of ethylene oxide, propylene oxide and epichlorohydrin in humans: update review (1990–2001). *Mut Res* 2002;512:173–94.
17. Yokota K, Johyama Y, Yamaguchi K. Occupational dermatoses from one-component epoxy coatings containing a modified polyamine hardener. *Ind Health* 2000;38:269–72.
18. ACGIH. *ACGIH 2002 threshold limit values (TLVs) for chemical substances and physical agents and biological exposure indices (BEIs)*. Cincinnati, OH: American Conference of Governmental Industrial Hygienists, Inc, 2002.
19. IPCS: International Programme on Chemical Safety. *Epichlorohydrin health and safety guide (H&S guide #8)*. Geneva, Switzerland: World Health Organization, 1987.

20. RTECS. Registry of Toxic Effects of Chemical Substances—NIOSH. Englewood, CO: Micromedex, Inc, 1999.
21. Hathaway GJ, Proctor NH, Hughes JP, et al. *Chemical hazards of the workplace*, 4th ed. New York: Van Nostrand Reinhold Company, 1996.
22. Gosselin RE, Smith RP, Hodge HC. *Clinical toxicology of commercial products*, 5th ed. Baltimore, MD: Williams & Wilkins, 1984.
23. Lane JM. Epichlorohydrin. *Vet Hum Toxicol* 1979;21:438–39.
24. Jonsson BAG, Skerfving S. Toxicokinetics and biological monitoring in experimental exposure of humans to gaseous hexahydrophthalic anhydride. *Scand J Work Environ Health* 1993;19:183–90.
25. Hanaoka T, Kawamura N, Hara K, Tsugane S. Urinary bisphenol A and plasma hormone concentrations in male workers exposed to bisphenol A digylcidyl ether and mixed organic solvents. *Occup Environ Med* 2002;59:625–28.
26. Dixit R, Husain R, Mukhtar H, et al. Acrylamide induced inhibition of hepatic glutathione-S-transferase activity in rats. *Toxicol Lett* 1981;7:207–10.
27. Donovan JW, Pearson TO. Ingestion of acrylamide with severe encephalopathy, neurotoxicity and hepatotoxicity. *Vet Human Toxicol* 1987;29:462(abst).
28. Pfaffli P, Savolainen H, Keskinen H. Determination of carboxylic acids in biological samples as their trichloroethyl esters by gas chromatography. *Chromoatographia* 1989;27:483–88.
29. Jonsson B, Skarping G. Method for the biological monitoring of hexahydrophthalic anhydride by the determination of hexahydrophthalic acid in urine using gas chromatography and selected ion monitoring. *J Chromatogr* 1991;572:117–31.
30. Jonsson B, Welinder H, Skarping G. Hexahydrophthalic acid in urine as an index of exposure to hexahydrophthalic anhydride. *Int Arch Occup Environ Health* 1991;63:77–79.
31. Pien LC, Zeiss CR, Leach CL, et al. Antibody response to trimellityl hemoglobin in trimellitic anhydride-induced lung injury. *J Allergy Clin Immunol* 1988;82:1098–103.
32. Kopelman H, Robertson MH, Sanders PG, Ash I. The Epping jaundice. *BMJ* 1966;5486:514–6.
33. Bastian PG. Occupational hepatitis caused by methylenedianiline. *Med J Aust* 1984;141:533–5.
34. Liss GM, Guirguis SS. Follow-up of a group of workers intoxicated with 4,4'- methylenedianiline. *Am J Ind Med* 1994;26:117–24.
35. Ward MJ, Davies D. Asthma due to grinding epoxy resin cured with phthallic anhydride. *Clin Allergy* 1982;12:165–68.
36. Nagel SC, vom Saal FS, Thayer KA, et al. Relative binding affinity-serum modified access (RBA-SMA) assay predicts the relative in vivo bioactivity of the xenoestrogens bisphenol A and octylphenol. *Environ Health Perspect* 1997;105:70–76.
37. Cagen SZ, Waechter JM, Dimond SS, et al. Normal reproductive organ development in CF-1 mice following prenatal exposure to bisphenol A. *Toxicol Sci* 1999;50:36–40.
38. Farobollini F, Porrini S, Dessi FF. Perinatal exposure to the estrogenic pollutant bisphenol A affects behavior in male and female rats. *Pharmacol Biochem Behav* 1999;64:687–94.
39. Colerangle JB, Roy D. Profound effects of the weak environmental estrogen-like chemical bisphenol A on the growth of the mammary gland of noble rats. *J Steroid Biochem Mol Biol* 60:153–60.
40. Grammer LC, Harris KE, Yarnold PR. Effect of respiratory protective devices on development of antibody and occupational asthma to an acid anhydride. *Chest* 2002;121:1317–22.
41. Grammer LC, Shaughnessy MA. Study of employees with anhydride-induced respiratory disease after removal from exposure. *J Occup Environ Med* 1996;38:771–74.
42. Zhao H, Zhang XD, Welinder H, et al. Anaphylactic bronchoconstriction in immunized guinea pigs provoked by inhalation and intravenous administration of hexahydrophthalic anhydride and methyltetrahydrophthalic anhydride. *Allergy* 1997;52:18–26.
43. Lozewicz S, Davison AG, Hopkirk A, et al. Occupational asthma due to methyl methacrylate and cyanoacrylates. *Thorax* 1985;40:836–9.
44. Laurberg G, Christiansen JV. Purpuric allergic contact dermatitis to epoxy resin. *Contact Dermatitis* 1984;11:186–87.
45. Nethercott JR, Nield G, Holness DL. A review of 79 cases of eyelid dermatitis. *J Am Acad Dermatol* 1989;21:223–30.
46. Roy CW, McSorley PD, Syme IG. Methylene dianilene: a new toxic cause of visual failure with hepatitis. *Hum Toxicol* 1985;4:61–6.
47. Jolanki R, Estlander T, Kanerva L. Occupational contact dermatitis and contact urticaria caused by epoxy resins. *Acta Derm Venereol Suppl (Stockh)* 1987;134:90–4.
48. Lindh CH, Jonsson BAG, Welinder H. Biological monitoring of methylhexahydrophthalic anhydride by determination of methylhexahydrophthalic acid in urine and plasma from exposed workers. *Int Arch Occup Environ Health* 1997;70:128–32.
49. Nielsen J, Welinder H, Jonsson B, et al. Exposure to hexahydrophthalic and methylhexahydrophthalic anhydrides—dose response for sensitization and airway effects. *Scand J Work Environ Health* 2001;27:327–34.
50. Yamakage A, Ishikawa H, Saito Y, et al. Occupational scleroderma-like disorder occurring in men engaged in the polymerization of epoxy resins. *Dermatologica* 1980;161:33–44.
51. Ishikawa O, Warita S, Tamura A, et al. Occupational scleroderma. A 17-year follow-up study. *Br J Dermatol* 1995;133:786–9.
52. de Fonseka CP. Danger of instant adhesives. *BMJ* 1976;2:234.
53. Gavino RR, Salva ES, Gregorio SP, et al. Occupational fatalities associated with exposure to epoxy resin paint in an underground tank—Makati, Republic of the Philippines. *MMWR Morb Mortal Wkly Rep* 1990;39:373–80.
54. ACGIH. *Documentation of the threshold limit values and biological exposure indices*, 5th ed. Cincinnati, OH: American Conference of Governmental Industrial Hygienists, Inc, 1986.
55. Rivera M, Nicotra MB, Byron GE, et al. Trimellitic anhydride toxicity. A cause of acute multisystem failure. *Arch Intern Med* 1981;141:1071–4.
56. Nielsen J, Welinder H, Skerfving S. Allergic airway disease caused by methyl tetrahydrophthalic anhydride in epoxy resin. *Scand J Work Environ Health* 1989;15:154–5.
57. Tepper LB. Hazards to health: epoxy resins. *N Engl J Med* 1962;267:821.
58. Venables KM, Taylor AJN. Exposure-response relationships in asthma caused by tetrachlorophthalic anhydride. *J Allergy Clin Immunol* 1990;85:55–58.
59. Rempel D, Jones J, Atterbury M, et al. Respiratory effects of exposure of shipyard workers to epoxy paints. *Br J Ind Med* 1991;48:783–7.
60. Taylor AJ. Acid anhydrides. *Clin Exp Allergy* 1991;21[Suppl 1]:234–40.
61. McGill DB, Motto JD. An industrial outbreak of toxic hepatitis due to methylenedianiline. *N Engl J Med* 1974;291:278–82.
62. Anonymous. *Bisphenol A: reproduction and fertility assessment in CD-1 mice when administered via subcutaneous silastic implants.* ISS NTP-84-015 report, 1984.
63. Makela S, Hyder SM, Stancel GM. Environmental estrogens. In: Oettel M, Schillinger G, eds. *Handbook of experimental pharmacology estrogens and antiestrogens*. Heidelberg: Springer-Verlag, 1998.
64. Milby TH, Whorton D, Stubbs HA, et al. Testicular function among epichlorhydrin workers. *Br J Ind Med* 1981;38:372–73.
65. Milby TH, Whorton D. Epidemiological assessment of occupationally related, chemically induced sperm count suppression. *J Occup Med* 1980;22:77–82.
66. Demers PA, Schade WJ, Demers RY. Lymphocytopenia and occupational exposures among pattern and model makers. *Scand J Work Environ Health* 1994;20:107–12.
67. Aleva RM, Aalbers R, Koeter GH, et al. Occupational asthma caused by a hardener containing an aliphatic and a cycloaliphatic diamine. *Am Rev Respir Dis* 1992;145:1217–18.
68. National Institutes of Health. TR-215 carcinogenesis bioassay of bisphenol A (CAS no. 80-05-7) in F344 rats and $B6C3F_1$ mice (feed study). Available at: http://ntp-server.niehs.nih.gov/htdocs/LT-studies/TR215.html. Accessed August 2003.
69. Haighton LA, Hlywka JJ, Doull J, et al. An evaluation of the possible carcinogenicity of bisphenol A to humans. *Reg Toxicol Pharmacol* 2002;35:238–54.
70. Tsai SP, Gilstrap EL, Ross CE. Mortality study of employees with potential exposure to epichlorhydrin: a 10 year update. *Occup Environ Med* 1996;53:299–304.
71. Olsen GW, Lacy SE, Chamberlin SR, et al. Retrospective cohort mortality study of workers with potential exposure to epichlorohydrin and allyl chloride. *Am J Ind Med* 1994;25:205–18.
72. Bond GG, Flores GH, Shellenberger RJ, et al. Nested case-control study of lung cancer among chemical workers. *Am J Epidemiol* 1986;124:53–66.
73. Wester PW, van der Heijden CA, Bisschop A, et al. Carcinogenicity study with epichlorohydrin (CEP) by gavage in rats. *Toxicology* 1985;36:325–39.
74. Konishi Y, Kawabata A, Denda A, et al. Forestomach tumors induced by orally administered epichlorohydrin in male Wistar rats. *Gann* 1980;71:922–23.
75. Gunderson EC, Anderson CC. A sampling and analytical method for airborne m-phenylenediamine (MPDA) and 4,4'-methylenedianiline (MDA). *Am Ind Hyg Assoc J* 1988;49:531–38.
76. Lindh CH, Jonsson BAG, Welinder HE. Direct measurement if hexahydrophthalic anhydride in workplace air with a transportable Fourier transform infrared spectrometer. *Am Ind Hyg Assoc J* 1996;832–36.

CHAPTER 210

Phthalates and Phthalate Esters

Robert B. Palmer

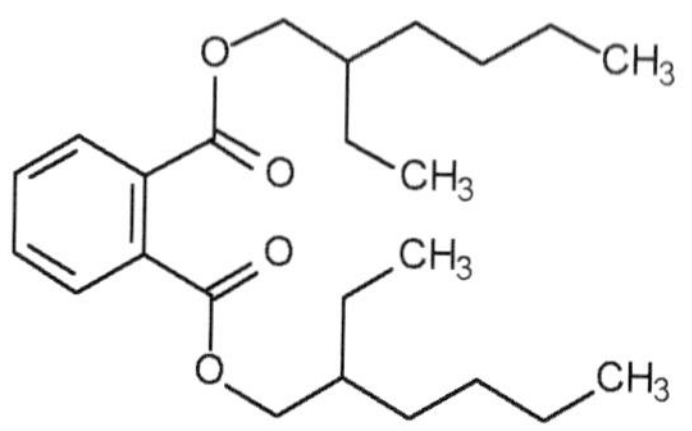

DIETHYLHEXYL PHTHALATE

Compounds included:	Di-*n*-octyl phthalate, diethylhexyl phthalate, phthalic acid anhydride
Molecular formula and weight:	Di-*n*-octyl phthalate ($C_{24}H_{38}O_4$), 390.6 g/mol; diethylhexyl phthalate ($C_{24}H_{38}O_4$), 390.6 g/mol; phthalic acid anhydride ($C_8H_4O_3$), 148.12 g/mol
SI conversion:	Di-*n*-octyl phthalate and diethyhexylphthalate, µg/L × 0.0026 = µmol/L; phthalic acid anhydride, mg/L × 6.8 = µmol/L
CAS Registry No.:	See Figure 1.
Normal levels:	Not used clinically
Target organs:	Liver, kidneys, and reproductive tract in animals
Antidote:	None

OVERVIEW

Plastic is a general term used to describe a wide variety of primarily organic polymers that are capable of being molded, cast, extruded, or drawn into filaments. Due to the formability and wide variety of physical properties, plastics have become ubiquitous in the industrialized world. Exposure to plastics is an everyday occurrence. The annual production volume of one common plasticizer alone, diethylhexyl phthalate, is nearly two million tons (1,2). Although most plastics do not represent a health hazard after polymerization is complete, exposure to other chemical components used in the production of plastics may result in adverse health effects. Other potential sources of toxicity in plastics manufacturing are additives, such as fillers, dyes, and plasticizers. Furthermore, burning of plastics can produce and liberate a variety of toxins as a result of combustion.

Chemical and Physical Characteristics

The two basic classifications of plastics are thermoplastics and thermoset plastics. A thermoplastic can be heated without losing its form. In contrast, a thermoset plastic is rigid when cool but loses its shape when heated. Well over 75% of plastics are thermoplastics, including polyethylene, polystyrene, polyvinyl chloride (PVC), nylon, and many fluorocarbon polymers (e.g., Teflon) (3,4). Included in the thermoset plastics category are polymers such as polyurethane and epoxy resins (3).

Commercially used plastics are typically not simply the polymerized species for which they are named. Multiple additives can be included in the final formulation to tailor the stability, durability, moldability, thermal properties, pliability, color, and so forth. Organic peroxides are common hardening agents in polyester and polyethylene plastics. Hydroquinone, benzophenone, some organolead, organotin, and cadmium compounds are used to stabilize the final plastic product against light and thermal degradation. Organic dyes and inorganic pigments are used to create colored plastics. Flame retardants, including chlorinated and brominated organics and trichloroalkylphosphate esters, may be contained in the plastic. A wide variety of compounds may also be used as fillers in plastic compounds to increase bulk and reduce production costs and to alter physical properties, such as hardness, opacity, electrical properties, and elasticity.

Plasticizers are added to increase pliability of rigid polymers. Organic plasticizers are usually esters, but their carbon skeletons encompass a variety of structural classes, including adipates, sebacates, phthalates, and stearates (3). Of these, one of the most common groups are the di-esters of phthalic acid (1,2-benzene dicarboxylic acid). Typically, these compounds contain two identical alkyl chains on the esters, as in di-*n*-butyl phthalate, dioctyl phthalate, and di(2-ethylhexyl) phthalate (diethylhexyl phthalate). However, mixed esters (e.g., those in which the two chains that make up the ester are not identical), such as benzylbutyl phthalate, are also used (Fig. 1).

Plasticizers, like many of the other plastic additives, are not covalently incorporated into the plastic polymer. Rather, they are physically trapped within the net-like matrix of the polymer. The plasticizer eventually leaches from the polymeric matrix with heat or solvent contact or simply over time. Loss of plasticizer results in the plastic becoming more brittle and cracking. Examples of this phenomenon are automobile vinyl seats and dashboards, which become brittle and crack with age.

Classification

Esters of phthalic acid are commonly used as plasticizers but also are used as solvents and in rubber, cellulose, and polystyrene resins. The two most common di-esters of industrial importance are di-*n*-octyl phthalate and di(2-ethylhexyl) phthalate (also known as *diethylhexyl phthalate*). These isomeric compounds both have two

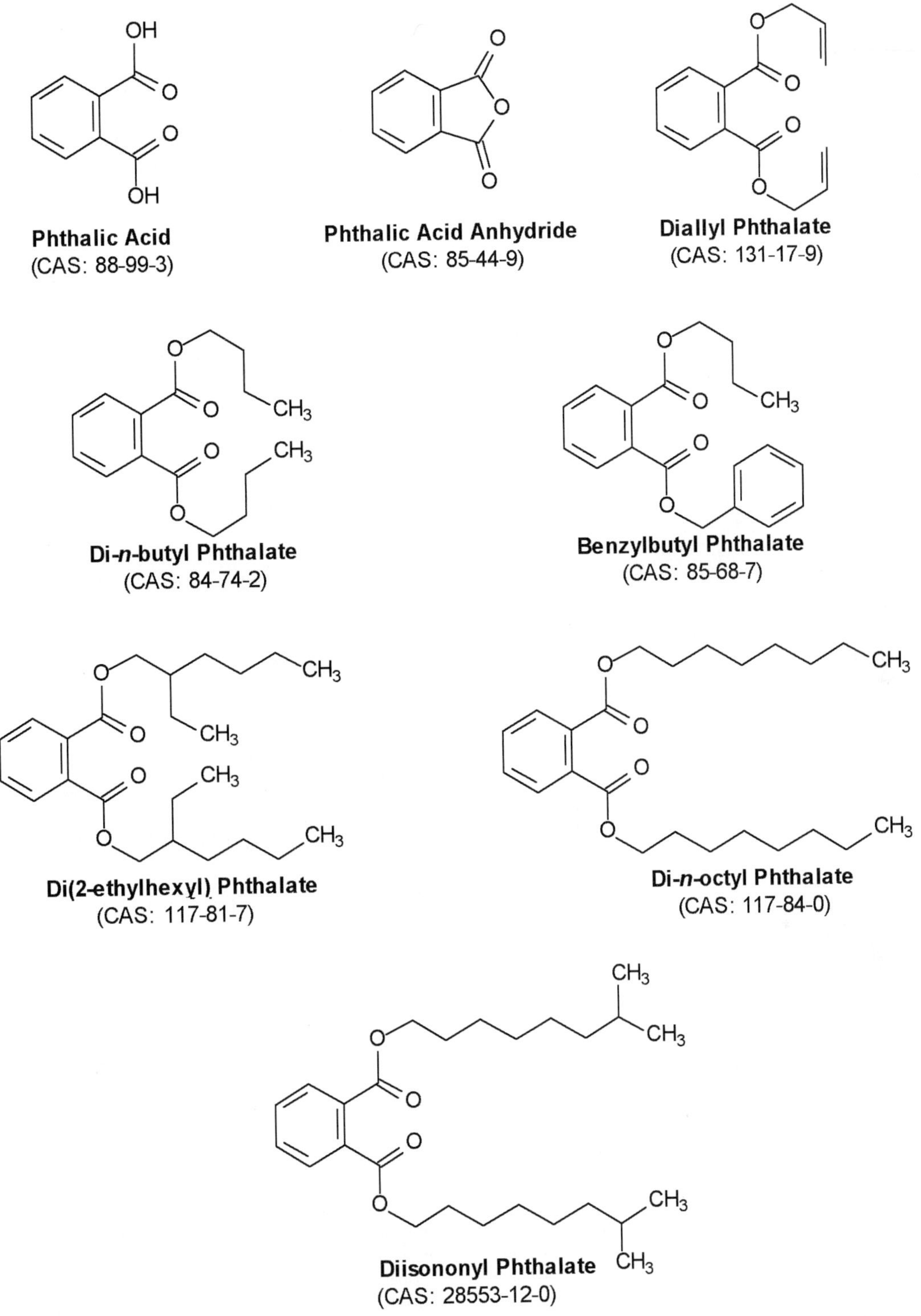

Figure 1. Chemical structures of several important phthalate compounds. The CAS Registry No. for each compound is indicated in parentheses.

eight-carbon chains bonded through ester linkages to phthalic acid. Collectively, these compounds are often referred to simply as *dioctyl phthalates*. The addition of diethylhexyl phthalate to PVC imparts a number of desirable characteristics into the final plastic product, including flexibility, strength, broad-range temperature tolerance, stability to sterilization, resistance to kinking, and optical clarity (1). The phthalic acid esters are prepared by esterification of phthalic acid anhydride and the appropriate eight carbon alcohol (*n*-octanol or 2-ethylhexanol) in the presence of an acid catalyst or elevated temperature (5). Other derivatives are made by reacting phthalic acid anhydride with the appropriate alcohol. Preparation of these compounds can expose workers to phthalic acid anhydride, which is a dermal irritant and a skin sensitizer.

Sources of Exposure

Every person in industrialized society is exposed to phthalate esters daily through ingestion, inhalation, skin contact, and even

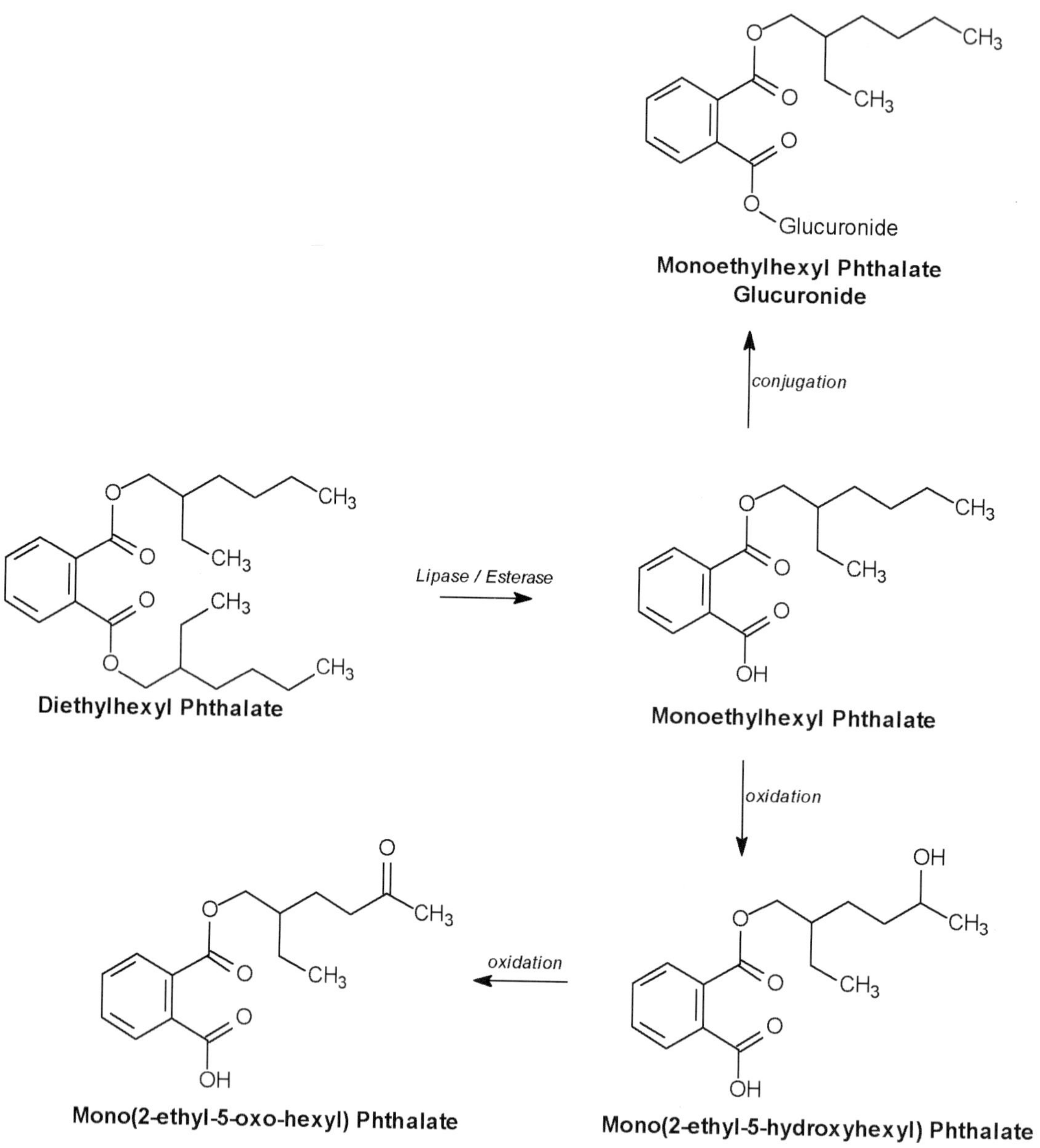

Monoethylhexyl Phthalate Glucuronide

conjugation

Diethylhexyl Phthalate

Lipase / Esterase

Monoethylhexyl Phthalate

oxidation

Mono(2-ethyl-5-hydroxyhexyl) Phthalate

oxidation

Mono(2-ethyl-5-oxo-hexyl) Phthalate

Figure 2. Abbreviated metabolic scheme of diethylhexyl phthalate. The glucuronide conjugation predominates in humans, whereas the oxidatively produced secondary metabolites predominate in rats.

parenteral administration. Ingestion exposure is ubiquitous because phthalate esters enter food during growth, production, processing, or packaging of the foodstuffs, although most seem to come from the packaging materials (1). Many foods are wrapped in PVC plastic, from which the phthalic acid esters leach into the food. This is particularly true of fat-containing foods (dairy products, infant formula, fish, meat, and oils), which have the highest levels because of the lipophilicity of the longer-chain phthalate esters. Other factors, including pH, temperature, and duration of storage also affect leaching rates of plasticizers into foods (1,6–9). Although it is difficult to pinpoint how worldwide amounts of phthalate esters ingested have changed over time due to changes in food production and consumption patterns, it appears that the concentrations of these compounds in infant formula are decreasing (2,10,11). Metabolites derived from other phthalate esters, including the diisononyl, diethyl, dibutyl, and benzylbutyl derivatives, have been detected in human urine, although to a lesser extent than diethylhexyl phthalate (Fig. 2) (12). This is likely a result of the lower production volumes of these other compounds relative to the diethylhexyl ester (1).

Based on the animal studies, although in the absence of firm human data, several countries have taken steps to mitigate potential toxic exposures in human children. Manufacturers in the United States and Canada have removed all phthalates from baby bottle nipples, teethers, and toys intended for mouthing (1,2). Furthermore, many American and Canadian plastics companies have voluntarily substituted diisononyl phthalate for diethylhexyl phthalate in some toys based on the suggested lower toxicity of the diisononyl analog. Of note, many of the data that attempt to quantify exposure in children are inferred rather than experimentally derived. Rates of leaching of plasticizers from nonfood items are estimated based on the amount of time that children mouth nonfood items combined with mouthing studies of diethylhexyl phthalate and diisononyl phthalate in adults (1,13,14). Extrapolation of phthalate content in the object alone is not a reliable indicator of exposure, as phthalate content does not correlate with leaching rate data from mouthing studies (1,15). Public and environmentalist outcry against the use of phthalate esters has also been significant in Europe (7–9,16). A 1990 governmental report from the United Kingdom recommends that phthalate plasticizer containing cling films not be used in conventional ovens, for wrapping food or lining dishes in microwave ovens, or for wrapping food with a high fat content (16).

Inhalation exposure is the second most prevalent source of exposure to phthalate esters because diethylhexyl phthalate adheres well to airborne dust particles. Due to its low vapor pressure and low water solubility, outdoor air and water concentrations are typically much lower than those indoors (1). Estimates for exposure to diethylhexyl phthalate in the U.S. general population are in the range of 3 to 30 mg/kg body weight per day (17–19). Other known exposure routes include occupational, nondietary ingestion and (for diethylhexyl phthalate) medical device exposure.

The diethylhexyl and diisononyl phthalates possess known carcinogenic, developmental, and reproductive toxicity in animals, although diisononyl phthalate is thought to be less toxic than the diethylhexyl derivative (15). Malignancies including leukemia have been reported in experimental animals exposed to diallyl phthalate (20–23). Animal studies have demonstrated that the developing male reproductive tract is sensitive to the phthalate esters. Exposure of female rodents to the phthalate esters causes postimplantation toxicity (1,24). It is believed that the reproductive toxicity and carcinogenicity occur through distinctly different mechanisms. Furthermore, at least for the carcinogenicity, the proposed mechanism of cancer induction in rodents (peroxisome proliferation) is not physiologically relevant to humans. Despite the fact that all assertions of adverse health effect are based on animal studies, Blount et al. (12) concluded that, because the general population in their 2000 study had elevated urinary concentrations of several phthalate metabolites, this represented a potential public health risk.

Parenteral exposure occurs because diethylhexyl phthalate is the most common plasticizer used in PVC medical devices, including medical examination gloves and tubing used in dialysis as well as in blood bags (25,26). This plasticizer not only keeps tubing and bags pliable, but it appears to have membrane-stabilizing effects on the erythrocytes that increase the viable storage time of the blood (25). Although the presence of diethylhexyl phthalate and its monoester metabolite has been confirmed at concentrations exceeding normal population background in adult and infant humans undergoing medical procedures, these levels were severalfold below those required to cause toxic effects in animals (17,27–29). The clinical significance of this observation is unknown. Animal data suggest that exposure to these compounds has adverse effects on the liver, kidneys, heart, lung, and reproductive organs. However, no specific pathology has been noted in humans. Men undergoing hemodialysis have been noted to be sterile and experience testicular atrophy (30). Furthermore, it is common to see polycystic kidney disease in long-term hemodialysis patients, although a true causal link between this pathology and the phthalate plasticizers has not been proven (31,32).

Flexible PVC bags used to store blood products for transfusion may contain dioctyl phthalate as a plasticizer in concentrations as high as 20% to 45% of the final mass of the plastic (1,5,25). Leaching of the plasticizer into the blood products does occur and results in increased lipid peroxidation and decreased vitamin E concentrations in the stored erythrocytes (33,34). Despite these observations, oxidative damage and metabolic acidosis (from either phthalic acid or the monoester derivative metabolically released by cleavage of the esters) do not appear to be clinically limiting factor, even in cases of administration of substantial amounts of blood products.

A toxic response may develop in plastics-manufacturing workers who are exposed to heated or combusted plastic products. In these cases, it is necessary to determine as closely as possible the exact composition of the plastic and other manufacturing agents involved. For example, if a worker is concerned about the health effects of diethylhexyl phthalate exposure, it is prudent to also investigate exposure to PVC, because these compounds are often used together and PVC has known adverse health effects. In instances in which plastic products are burned, a number of potential toxins, including carbon monoxide, cyanide, and phosgene, may be produced, depending on the exact composition of the polymer. Therefore, evaluation of these cases must also include a detailed investigation of all components contacted in the course of the incident in question.

Environmental exposure also occurs. The phthalic acid esters have also been detected as contaminants in industrial organic solvents, including diethyl ether, acetonitrile, and benzene (5,35). Not only are the phthalic acid esters industrial solvent contaminants, they are also environmental contaminants (5,36,37). Dioctyl phthalates are not naturally occurring compounds, and their presence in environmental sources is due to leaching from manmade products, such as dielectric fluids, in which case it has largely replaced polychlorinated biphenyls (35). Although diethylhexyl phthalate can be detected in environmental matrices, concentrations are significantly lower in outdoor air and water compared to indoor air (1).

Concern over environmental exposure is due primarily to the thought that the phthalate ester might bioaccumulate with progression up the food chain (38). However, not all data support this allegation, and it appears more likely that bioaccumulation only occurs in lower animals (39,40). No evidence for bioaccumulation or bioconcentration in humans has been found.

A study of Puerto Rican girls with premature thelarche found serum levels of several phthalates that exceeded corresponding levels in control girls (41). Although a mechanism explaining this observation was not clearly defined and the source of the plasticizers was conjecture, the correlation was statistically significant. The patient history points detailed for occupational exposure assessment also hold true in cases of persons with possible hobby or environmental (e.g., fire-related) complaints. Therefore, a detailed physical examination and a comprehensive occupational, medical, hobby, and environmental exposure history is compulsory in the evaluation of a potentially exposed patient.

Toxic Dose

It is estimated that more than 600,000 workers are exposed to diethylhexyl phthalate and over 100,000 workers are exposed to phthalic anhydride yearly in the United States (42). Workers exposed to phthalic anhydride have shown a variety of effects ranging from cough to bloody nasal discharge and nasal mucosa atrophy (43–45). In most cases, the air contamination consists of phthalic acid and phthalic acid anhydride. Airborne concentrations of phthalic acid were not reported in every case; however, when concentrations in workplace air were in the range of 4 to 5 parts per million (ppm), mucous membrane irritation and conjunctivitis were reliably observed (43–45). Workers have also displayed suspected sensitization responses after repeated or prolonged exposure to phthalic anhydride (43,44). However, it can be difficult to distinguish between chemical irritation and an allergic skin rash.

The regulatory standards and guidelines for phthalic acid esters are provided in Table 1. Threshold limit values and permissible exposure limits for the group are on the order of 1 to 6 ppm. Air concentrations of phthalic acid anhydride in excess of 25 mg/m^3 are known to cause mucous membrane irritation and conjunctivitis (5). The odor threshold for phthalic acid anhy-

TABLE 1. United States regulatory guidelines and standards for major phthalates

Compound	Agency	Description	Concentration, mg/m³ (ppm)
Di-*n*-octyl phthalate	OSHA (air)	PEL-TWA	5 (0.3)
	ACGIH (air)	TLV-TWA	5 (0.3)
		STEL	None
	NIOSH (air)	PEL-TWA ceiling	5 (0.3)
		STEL	10 (0.6)
		IDLH	5000 (313)
Diethylhexyl phthalate	OSHA (air)	PEL-TWA	5 (0.3)
	ACGIH (air)	TLV-TWA	5 (0.3)
	NIOSH (air)	REL-TWA ceiling	5 (0.3)
		STEL	10 (0.6)
		IDLH	5000 (313)
Phthalic acid anhydride	OSHA (air)	PEL-TWA	12 (2)
	ACGIH (air)	TLV-TWA	6 (1)
		STEL	None
	NIOSH (air)	REL-TWA	6 (1)
		IDLH	60 (10)

ACGIH, American Conference of Governmental Industrial Hygienists; IDLH, immediately dangerous to life and health; NIOSH, National Institute for Occupational Safety and Health; OSHA, U.S. Occupational Safety and Health Administration; PEL, permissible exposure limit; ppm, parts per million; REL, recommended exposure limit; STEL, short-term exposure limit; TLV, threshold limit value; TWA, time-weighted average.

dride is below 6 ppm (0.32 to 0.72 mg/m^3) and its strong odor is considered an adequate warning for the prevention of overexposure (5). Because of their low vapor pressures, the odors of the longer-chain phthalate esters tend to be less noticeable. Workplace standards have not been established for phthalic acid or diallyl phthalate.

The amounts of the phthalates generally found in outside water and air are significantly below those found in indoor air (1). The environmental persistence of these esters is expected to be low, as ambient water hydrolyzes the esters fairly quickly. Although the phthalate esters appear to bioaccumulate in lower animals, there is no evidence of bioaccumulation or bioconcentration in humans or other higher life forms (39). A single report associated elevated urinary phthalate concentrations with complications in pregnancy (anemia, toxemia, and preeclampsia) in women who lived near a plastics manufacturing plant (46). These observations have not been independently verified or reported in other investigations.

TOXICOKINETICS AND TOXICODYNAMICS

Absorption

Phthalic acid and the esters of phthalic acid are generally well absorbed orally. Gut absorption of dioctyl phthalates is mostly as the monoester metabolite (1). Many of the lower-molecular-weight phthalates are dermally absorbed. Dermal absorption of the diester phthalates decreases as the alkyl chain length increases beyond four carbons (47). Dioctyl phthalates, which are common in cosmetics, are not appreciably absorbed through the skin (1). In World War II, dibutyl phthalate was used extensively as an insect repellent that was applied as a spray or mist. Although inhalation of the compound regularly occurred during this process, no significant signs of toxicity were reported (48). Inhalation of dioctyl phthalates does not result in significant absorption, likely as a result of its low vapor pressure. However, because dioctylphthalate adheres well to particulate dust in the air, inhalation exposure can occur if the dust is taken into the lungs (1,49). A correlation is found between urinary concentrations of phthalic acid and airborne concentrations of phthalic anhydride in exposed workers (42,50). However, this likely represents a combination of multiple absorption routes (inhalation, dermal contact, and ingestion).

Distribution

Diallyl phthalate and phthalic acid are rapidly distributed after absorption. Although diallyl phthalate concentrates primarily in the liver, kidneys, and bile, phthalic acid distributes more widely (5). In rats, significant concentrations of phthalic acid are detectable in liver, kidney, spleen, adipose tissues, and testes after oral dosing (51). In most cases, the liver is the principal initial repository organ (39). Tissue distribution of other phthalic acid esters likely takes place after ester hydrolysis, making phthalic acid the actual deposited compound (1,39).

Metabolism

The primary mode of metabolism of the phthalic acid esters in humans is ester hydrolysis, which is performed by esterases in the gut, liver, and blood (24). The initial hydrolysis produces the monoester form, which is thought to be the primary toxicant (1,24). For example, in the case of diethylhexyl phthalate, hydrolysis of one of the esters produces the monoester metabolite, monoethylhexyl phthalate. The toxicokinetics of monoethylhexyl phthalate in humans are not well described (1). Secondary metabolites form in some cases, including those from monoethylhexyl phthalate that originate from the diester parent. Secondary monoethylhexyl phthalate metabolites detected in human urine include mono(2-ethyl-5-hydroxyhexyl)phthalate and mono(2-ethyl-5-oxo-hexyl)phthalate (40,52). Because rodents are known to have significantly more intestinal lipase than primates, a larger amount of the potentially toxic monoester metabolite may be produced and absorbed for any given oral dose (1).

As a general rule, the short-chain dialkyl phthalate esters, such as dimethyl phthalate, are excreted either unchanged or as the fully hydrolyzed phthalic acid (39). In contrast, the longer-chain diesters are oxidatively converted to polar monoester derivatives of phthalic acid before excretion (39). A significant interspecies difference is noted with the metabolism of the longer-chain diester compounds. Primates, including humans, as well as some rodents, glucuronidate the exposed phthalic acid carboxylate of the monoesters, whereas rats appear to be unable to perform this conjugation (39). Instead, they oxidatively convert the remaining alkyl side chain to various ketone and carboxylic acid derivatives (39).

Blount et al. (12) reported analysis of the urine of a reference population of 289 adult humans for seven phthalate ester metabolites. It was found that more than 75% of the tested subjects had monoethylhexyl phthalate, monoethyl phthalate, monobenzyl phthalate, and monobutyl phthalate in their urine. In a German study, a set of 85 urine samples from the general population was analyzed for human specific metabolites of phthalate esters as a means of estimating daily intake of the phthalate esters (52). Included in this study were five primary metabolites of phthalate esters and two secondary metabolites of diethylhexyl phthalate. It was extrapolated based on these data that 12% of study subjects had estimated daily intake values that exceeded a tolerable daily intake value of 37 mg/kg body weight per day established by the European Union Scientific Committee for Toxicity, Ecotoxicity and the Environment. The authors concluded, in part, by expressing concern that exposure of the general German populace to phthalate esters appeared much greater than previously suspected.

In a group of seven humans receiving continuous ambulatory peritoneal dialysis, serum concentrations of dioctyl phthalate (0.027 to 0.231 μg/ml) were greater than those of controls (0.016 to 0.025 μg/ml) (29). The source of the plasticizer was reported as leaching from the PVC tubing used in the medical equipment. Another investigator examined infants undergoing exchange transfusion and found undetectable pretransfusion levels of diethylhexyl phthalate at baseline with levels of 6.1 to 21.6 μg/ml after a single transfusion (27). No toxic effects were observed.

Other metabolites are formed to lesser degrees. Small amounts of phthalic acid are converted to carbon dioxide after oral dosing of rats with phthalic acid (51). *Pseudomonas* bacteria perform additional oxidative metabolic transformations on phthalic acid, producing 4,5-dihydroxy phthalic acid (53).

Elimination

Elimination of phthalic acid and the other metabolites of the phthalic acid esters is almost entirely renal and biliary. Approximately 90% of a dose of diethylhexyl phthalate and its monoester-derived metabolites are excreted in the urine and feces within 24 hours (5,38). The elimination half-life of dioctyl phthalate is estimated at 28 minutes after intravenous infusion (54). Elimination of the carbon dioxide metabolite of phthalic acid in expired air accounts for only small amounts of total phthalic acid elimination after oral dosing of rats (5,53). The different metabolic and subsequent excretion profile in rats versus primates for monoethylhexyl phthalate may cause significant differences in elimination half-life in the different species (1).

Despite numerous lipophilic environments in the human body, the esters of phthalic acid generally do not accumulate to an appreciable degree in humans exposed through dietary sources. One investigator states that clearance of the phthalate esters from the body is rapid and there exists only "slight cumulative potential" (39). In a single study in which two human volunteers were dosed with 10 mg/day diethylhexyl phthalate for 4 days, no evidence of accumulation was detected (40). The kinetic profiles of diisononyl phthalate and other dialkyl phthalate esters are expected to be similar, with some variation by route, species, and age at exposure (1).

PATHOPHYSIOLOGY

The acute toxicity of the phthalate esters is believed to be low (1). Most frequently, exposure to these compounds is through dietary sources, although inhalation and direct contact with skin and mucosal surfaces also occur (1,5). In general, phthalic acid and phthalic acid anhydride are moderate irritants and can be corrosive at high concentrations or with prolonged exposure. The irritation associated with phthalic anhydride contact is worse if the contacted areas are moist, presumably as a result of the exothermic aqueous hydrolysis of phthalic anhydride to phthalic acid (43,44). The phthalate esters are mild irritants, and the rough trend of decreasing irritant effect with increasing carbon chain length of the esters seems to hold in going from diallyl to dibutyl to dioctyl esters.

Skin sensitization has been reported with exposure to phthalic anhydride (48,55). However, this does not appear to be a significant issue with the phthalic acid esters. In the case of dioctyl phthalate, which is commonly used in cosmetics, the U.S. Environmental Protection Agency has concluded that skin sensitization does not occur in humans (56).

Although health effects related to chronic phthalate ester exposure in laboratory animals have been reported, human data are lacking. The observed carcinogenic, reproductive, and developmental effects of the phthalate esters seem to be more closely related to the monoester metabolites than the parent compounds (1). The proposed mechanism of carcinogenesis in rodents is peroxisome proliferation (57). The applicability of this mechanism when extrapolated to humans is questionable (18,58).

Combustion of phthalic acid esters alone can release carbon monoxide. Diethylhexyl phthalate is a common plasticizer in PVC (1). Burning this matrix can release not only carbon monoxide but also phosgene. If the phthalate ester is formulated in a plastic matrix containing nitrogen (e.g., a polyamide), cyanide and oxides of nitrogen can form with burning. These agents as toxins are covered in separate chapters and are not discussed further herein.

VULNERABLE POPULATIONS

The phthalate esters enter breast milk, but the clinical significance of this is unknown. The potential reproductive effects of the phthalic acid esters have received a great deal of attention. In animals, phthalic acid esters are known to cause reproductive toxicity, fetal malformation, and fetal death. The potency of these effects depends on the specific phthalate ester involved (12). The potential for these adverse effects to occur in humans is based on extrapolation of animal data. The lack of complete characterization of toxic effects in human exposures has made this an area of significant controversy.

Pregnant rats treated with 15% of an LD_{50} (median lethal dose) of dioctyl phthalate on gestational days 5, 10, and 15 showed significant increases in resorption (27%) and gross fetal abnormalities (22%) (59). Dioctyl phthalate administration in pregnant rats is also known to cause a functional zinc deficiency (60). In pregnant rats that are exposed to dibutyl phthalate and benzylbutyl phthalate, a relationship between dose and frequency of postimplantation loss and fetal malformation was discovered (61,62). Time dependence was also observed for specific malformations in the vertebral column; rib malformation was most often seen with dosing on days 7 to 9, and cleft palate and sternebrae fusion were observed with treatment on days 13 to 15 (61,62). The potency of the reproductive and developmental effects of the phthalates varies. Diethylhexyl phthalate is the most potent, whereas dibutyl phthalate and benzylbutyl phthalate have potencies that are roughly tenfold lower (12). It is noteworthy that fetal toxicity in animals appears at doses of diethylhexyl phthalate at or below amounts that cause mild maternal toxicity (1,2,63). Alternatively stated, after oral exposure, it is possible that fetal toxicity may occur without evidence of maternal toxic effects.

Administration of dibutyl phthalate and diethylhexyl phthalate to pregnant rats causes abnormal fetal development in male pups (64). Some of the monoester metabolites of the phthalate plasticizers, including monobenzyl phthalate, monoethylhexyl phthalate, and monobutyl phthalate, are testicular toxins in animals; specifically, monobenzyl phthalate and monoethylhexyl phthalate are toxic to Sertoli cells (65–68). Teratogenicity of diethylhexyl, dibutyl, and benzylbutyl phthalates and the metabolically produced monobenzyl phthalate and monoethylhexyl phthalates is established in animals (67–71). Genotoxic effects are not limited to developing animals. In adult male mice that are exposed to phthalic acid, abnormal sperm heads and induction of dominant lethal mutations have been observed (72). Another report suggests that the phthalic anhydrides do not induce chromosomal aberrations in culture lines derived from Chinese hamster ovary cells. Effects on spermatogenesis as well as in the testes, epididymis, and sperm of study animals have been reported by other investigators (5). A Russian study suggests that chronic occupational exposure of women working in plastics factories to phthalates in high concentrations is correlated with decreased pregnancy rates and increased probability of spontaneous abortion (24,73).

CLINICAL PRESENTATION

Acute Exposure

With exposure to very high airborne concentrations, mucous membrane irritation and central nervous system (CNS) depression are possible.

Acute oral exposure to dibutyl phthalate (di-*n*-butyl phthalate) has little toxic consequence beyond minor irritation. This is well demonstrated in children who rupture chemiluminescent glow sticks that contain dibutyl phthalate (74,75). Whether the exposure is to the eye, other mucous membranes, gastrointestinal tract, or skin, the resultant irritation is usually minor, resolves with simple irrigation or dilution, and typically does not require referral to a health care facility (74).

Chronic Exposure

Chronic exposure to dibutyl phthalate has been reported (76). It was suggested in one report that workers who are exposed to dibutyl phthalate may display a toxic syndrome consisting of hypertension, pain, reflex disturbances, decreased vestibular function, and hyperbilirubinemia and that this syndrome increases in frequency with length of employment (76). However, because these workers were also exposed to other plasticizers, the case for true causation by the phthalates is difficult to make.

No specific systemic reactions are expected after exposure to the esters of phthalic acid. Workers in whom rhinorrhea, wheezing, and lacrimation had developed over the course of a year while they worked with phthalic acid anhydride had positive patch tests and elevated titers of specific immunoglobulin (Ig) G and IgE antibodies (77,78). In workers who were exposed to tetrachlorophthalic anhydride, specific IgE antibodies were detectable and elevated beyond 5 years after discontinuation of exposure (79).

Ocular contact is associated with irritation with lacrimation, and conjunctivitis is associated with direct ocular contact with essentially all of the phthalic acid ester derivatives. Ocular contact with vapors of diallyl phthalate has a reported association with conjunctivitis (45). These effects are local and not systemically mediated. Interestingly, although human reports of ocular irritation as a result of exposure to dioctyl phthalate exist, this compound did not cause irritation in experimental animals (5,43,44).

Conjunctivitis and eyelid edema developed in rats that were fatally poisoned with oral dosing of dibutylphthalate (80). Only one case of human ingestion resulting in ocular toxicity has been reported (81). In this 1954 report, a worker was alleged to have accidentally ingested 10 g dibutylphthalate. An asymptomatic period of several hours followed by a severe bilateral transient keratitis with eventual loss of the corneal epithelium was described. Due to the strong and bitter odor of the liquid and expected associated difficulty in accidentally ingesting 10 g of the compound, doubt has been expressed regarding the accuracy of the case history (82). Workers who are exposed to mixed vapors containing phthalic anhydride concentrations of 30 mg/m^3 reported conjunctivitis (55,78). Although the conjunctivitis may be persistent, no permanent eye injury or loss of ocular function has been documented (45).

Dermal effects are common. Nearly all of the phthalic acid ester derivatives are minor dermal irritants with acute exposure. The irritant effects generally seem to decrease with increasing alkyl chain length. The common use of the phthalic acid ester compounds in cosmetics and usual lack of significant irritation provide a practical perspective on the lack of significant dermal irritant effects associated with low-concentration exposures to these compounds. The nonester compound, phthalic acid anhydride, is associated with more significant dermal irritation, including severe burns when moist skin is exposed to the compound in a molten state (83). Dermal contact with phthalic acid anhydride results in brown skin pigmentation. Phthalic acid anhydride has also been shown to cause skin sensitization with dermatitis, eczematous lesions, and urticaria (48,55).

The only expected cardiovascular effects after exposure to esters of phthalic acid are the normal physiologic responses to conditions such as hypoxia or hypovolemia from corrosive or hypersensitivity reactions. Neurologic effects do not generally occur after exposure to the esters of phthalic acid. Slight CNS excitation has been reported with exposure to phthalic acid anhydride (84). Ingestion of large amounts of dioctyl phthalate may cause CNS depression (56). Ingestion of dibutyl phthalate may cause dizziness (85). One report of Soviet workers described 32% of the study population as having some neurologic complaint (76). The exact mechanism of this polyneuritis was never fully identified, and the workers studied were exposed to several phthalate ester plasticizers as well as sebacates and adipates.

Gastrointestinal effects include irritation after acute ingestion. However, except in extreme cases, the irritation should be self-limiting and not progress to clinically significant corrosive injury. One paper describing 61 cases of exposure to dibutyl phthalate from glow sticks reported that 63% of the cases were successfully managed at home with soap and water rinses for external contamination and dilution with milk or water for small ingestions (74). None of the patients in this report were treated with activated charcoal, gastric lavage, or whole bowel irrigation. Of slightly greater concern is ingestion of phthalic acid anhydride, which probably has greater potential than the other compounds to cause corrosive injury, especially when in contact with wet skin and mucous membranes (84).

Chronic administration of 890 mg/kg phthalic acid anhydride to rats for 9 weeks produced gastric ulceration (86). Gastric hyperplasia and chronic gastric inflammation were observed in mice with chronic oral administration of 150 to 300 mg/kg diallyl phthalate, and diarrhea developed in rats in subchronic toxicity studies (20). Because of the irritant effects of this class of compounds on mucous membranes, acute ingestions would be expected to cause nausea, vomiting, diarrhea, and possibly gastritis. Severe corrosive injury to the gastrointestinal tract, although remotely possible with large ingestions of phthalic acid anhydride, seems unlikely with the esters of phthalic acid. No human cases of significant corrosive injury or subsequent stricture formation have been reported after ingestion of phthalic acid ester derivatives. Of note, necrotizing enterocolitis has been reported in neonates after exchange transfusion and extracorporeal membrane oxygenation (ECMO) therapy. In these cases, increased serum levels of di(2-ethylhexyl) phthalate were found (27).

Respiratory effects of pulmonary irritation follow exposure to most of the phthalic acid esters and derivatives. Those compounds with higher vapor pressures (e.g., diallyl phthalate) tend to be more irritating to the respiratory tract than those with higher molecular weights (e.g., dioctyl phthalate). The dioctyl phthalate esters adhere well to airborne dust particles. As a result of this "dust transporter" mechanism, inhalation can cause an asthma-like response (49). This response is thought to be the result of the dioctyl phthalate causing inflammation by mimicking prostaglandin release (49). Cyanosis was noted in mice that were given 550 mg/kg phthalic acid intraperitoneally, although this has not been observed in cases of human exposure (87).

The more prominent irritant effects and higher vapor pressure of phthalic acid anhydride make it the most medically significant phthalic acid derivative in terms of inhalation exposure. Upper respiratory tract irritation as well as bronchospasm may occur with each exposure (43,48,78). In the case of workers who are exposed to the chlorinated derivative of phthalic acid anhydride, tetrachlorophthalic anhydride, occupational asthma has recurred as many as 4 years after discontinuation and avoidance of exposure (79).

Renal effects involving increased kidney weight (lacking histologic evidence of tissue damage) developed in chronic feeding studies of dioctyl phthalate to animals (88,89). Rats given up to 890 mg/kg phthalic anhydride for 9 weeks were reported to have nephrosis with severe destruction of the renal tubular epithelium (86). Neither of these renal effects has been noted in human cases. Uremic pruritus in which leaching of dioctyl phthalate from medical supplies was a possible causative agent developed in human hemodialysis patients (28). Polycystic kidney disease has been observed at autopsy of dialysis-dependent patients, and there may be a causal link between this pathology and long-term high exposure to phthalate plasticizers from the medical equipment (90,91). However, this link has not been proven (31).

Hepatic effects include hepatomegaly in rats dosed with dibutyl phthalate for 3 months (92). This effect has also been observed in an inhalational study of diethylhexyl phthalate in rats (93). Mild hepatotoxicity (inflammation, elevation of serum transaminases, hepatomegaly, and proliferation of hepatic peroxisomes with resultant liver cancer) has been reported in rats that were involved in chronic feeding studies of dioctyl phthalate (38,88).

Elevated concentrations of diethylhexyl phthalate and monoethylhexyl phthalate have been recorded in humans undergoing a variety of medical procedures, including cardiac surgery, mechanical ventilation with PVC-containing circuitry, and PVC infusion lines for high lipid-containing parenteral nutrition (94–99). Some investigators have reported that neonatal exposures to diethylhexyl phthalate may exceed exposures in the general population by 1000-fold (1,100). In one study of exposures from exchange transfusions in neonates, diethylhexyl phthalate exposures were measured at 3300 mg/kg per exchange transfusion and monoethylhexyl phthalate exposures were as high as 360 mg/kg per exchange transfusion (100,101). However, with very sick neonates undergoing multiple medical procedures, it is likely that exposures are even higher (2,102).

In human neonates, elevated concentrations of diethylhexyl phthalate have been associated with cholestasis in patients undergoing exchange transfusion or ECMO. However, in at least one study of newborns undergoing exchange transfusion who were exposed to diethylhexyl phthalate as a result of medical procedures no cholestasis was observed (27). This may be a result of the kinetics of metabolism of diethylhexyl phthalate in very young and premature infants being quite different than in adults. Pancreatic lipase systems are not fully matured in human infants until 6 to 12 months of age. Because these enzymes are necessary for the metabolic conversion of the diester parent compound to its monoester metabolite, young age and enzymatic immaturity may provide some degree of protection from toxicity (1).

Although no cases of human ingestion of diallyl phthalate have been reported, hepatic injury, including hepatocellular necrosis, periportal fibrosis, and cirrhosis, did develop in experimental animals (rats and mice) that were exposed to this compound. These effects were demonstrated in rats with acute, subchronic, and chronic oral dosing with diallyl phthalate (20,103).

Carcinogenesis

The carcinogenic potential of the phthalic acid esters has generated substantial debate. In rats and mice, diethylhexyl phthalate is a nongenotoxic hepatocarcinogen (5). The International Agency for Research in Carcinogenesis classifies dioctyl phthalate as carcinogenic in these species (35). The suggested mechanism for this effect is thought to involve peroxisome proliferation. However, it is further suggested that this mechanism is probably not relevant in humans (18,104). With respect to human exposure levels to dioctyl phthalate, the average daily exposure amount (from leaching out of plastic medical supplies) to patients undergoing hemodialysis is 16 times less than the lowest observed effect level for peroxisome proliferation and approximately 100 times less than the lowest observed effect level for development of hepatic tumors in rats (17). Although higher parenteral levels of diethylhexyl phthalate parent compound can be attained with hemodialysis, oral exposure likely results in larger amounts of the monoester metabolite and may therefore be more important toxicologically (1).

Diisononyl phthalate causes kidney and liver cancers in rodents (105). The hepatocarcinogenesis of diisononyl phthalate may also involve peroxisome proliferation (105). The kidney neoplasms may form through a different mechanism that is equally irrelevant in human populations (106).

Diallyl phthalate has been implicated in several malignancies in rodents. Chronic oral administration of this compound caused an increased incidence of hematopoietic tumors in rats and gastric papillomas in mice (5,20). Interestingly, rats did not have an increased incidence of gastric papilloma and mice did not have an increased incidence of hematopoietic tumors. Further, chronic oral administration of 50 to 100 mg/kg diallyl phthalate to female rats increased the incidence of mononuclear cell leukemias, whereas administration of these doses in male rats increased the incidence of lymphomas (20).

Exposure of rats and mice of both genders to 1600 to 25,000 ppm phthalic anhydride for 13 weeks failed to show an increased rate of tumor development (20,22). In general, the carcinogenic risk to humans from at least some of the phthalates appears to be less than that to experimental animals; therefore, many newer studies are evaluating different endpoint assessments of toxicity (1).

LABORATORY

No specific laboratory analyses are recommended for acute exposure to the phthalates. Because there are potential effects on the hematopoietic system, kidneys, and liver with exposure to some of these compounds, baseline cell counts and renal and liver function tests are suggested. As there is no human experience with ingestion of diallyl phthalate and exposure to it is strongly linked to hepatotoxicity in animals, baseline evaluation of liver function seems prudent. Urinalysis as well as serum glucose and electrolytes is also recommended in patients with significant exposure. In patients with notable respiratory involvement, arterial blood gases and chest radiography are appropriate. Other laboratory assessments should be performed as clinically indicated.

The clinician should remember that the phthalates are used as additives in many types of plastics (e.g., PVC) and that these other plastics may have inherent toxicity independent of the phthalate. This is particularly true in cases in which the plastic is burned. Although the primary combustion product of immediate concern from the phthalates is carbon monoxide, other toxins, including phosgene, cyanide, and oxides of nitrogen, may be produced when the rest of the plastic matrix is burned.

PHTHALATE CONCENTRATIONS

Blood levels of the phthalates are typically not readily available and are not useful in guiding clinical management of acute toxic exposure. However, analytic methods for determination of many of these compounds have been reported (52,107,108). Gas chromatographic methods using either flame ionization or mass spectrometric detection have been used to quantitate phthalic acid ester compounds. Most of these methods were designed to detect parent diester compounds. Detection of phthalate metabolites may be a better indicator of exposure, as parent diester may be present in samples as a contaminant from the materials used for the analysis rather than as a result of a true exposure (12,52). An analytic method using high-performance liquid chromatography with tandem mass spectrometric detection has been described (108). This method was validated for eight phthalate metabolites in human urine and was used in the evaluation of phthalate ester compounds and their metabolites in a normal reference population.

Determination of monoester primary metabolites and even oxidative secondary metabolites might be a better marker for exposure monitoring, although this has not been fully validated and is not currently a recommended approach. Although urinary excretion of phthalic acid correlates well with workplace air levels of phthalic anhydride in occupational exposures, this is probably not of significant clinical value in occupational monitoring (50). Of greater utility in monitoring occupational exposure to phthalic anhydride are annual chest radiography and forced expiratory volume examinations with periodic evaluation of liver and renal function (109). In those with a suspected allergic response to phthalic acid anhydride, *in vitro* histamine assessments can be used to confirm the diagnosis (110).

TREATMENT

Management of symptomatic exposure to phthalic acid, phthalic acid anhydride, and the esters of phthalic acid is supportive, as no specific antidote exists. The initial step in management is to terminate the exposure.

Decontamination

Decontamination includes simple removal to fresh air if the exposure was through inhalation and removal of clothing with wet decontamination using soap and water in the case of skin exposure. External decontamination with water should be performed as soon as possible after exposure to limit the severity of the local irritant effects.

Phthalates are adsorbed by activated charcoal. Administration of charcoal in the case of ingestion without evidence of significant corrosive gastric injury or other contraindication is appropriate. Charcoal has no role after ingestion of polymerized compounds (e.g., PVC plastic) even if they do contain phthalate plasticizers. Gastric aspiration after massive ingestion of phthalic anhydride may be beneficial in limiting local corrosive effects if done early but is not a standard therapy. Gastric lavage is likely to be of little benefit.

Removal from the source and administration of oxygen are the only decontamination procedures necessary after inhalation exposure. Inhalation of phthalic anhydride vapors or phthalate esters alone occurs when they are carried on particulate matter. Pulmonary irritation and occupational asthma may develop (43,77,78).

Contact lenses and any jewelry in the exposed areas should be removed. Significant secondary contamination of health care providers by a contaminated patient has not emerged as a concern.

Enhancement of Elimination

Enhanced elimination has not been investigated for these chemicals.

Antidotes

No specific antidote is available for acute phthalate poisoning. If the exposure also involved substances such as cyanide or carbon monoxide (i.e., after combustion), appropriate laboratory assessments and antidotal therapy should be instituted as soon as possible.

Supportive Care

Respiratory effects after inhalation exposure are treated symptomatically. Administration of 100% oxygen should be initiated and bronchospasm treated with inhaled β-adrenergic agonists.

Combustion of pure phthalates produces carbon monoxide. Other potential toxic combustion products depend on the composition of the plastic matrix but can include phosgene, cyanide, and oxides of nitrogen. Specific interventions for management of toxic exposures to these elements should be instituted as clinically indicated.

Allergic contact dermatitis from sensitization to phthalic anhydride is managed by ceasing exposure and by steroid therapy as needed. Endoscopic evaluation for apparent clinically significant corrosive injury is appropriate as detailed in Chapter 202. Should renal or hepatotoxicity become evident, standard supportive measures are indicated. Management of patients with parenteral exposures, such as through dialysis or ECMO, is completely supportive.

No certain correlation between exposure to the phthalate esters and development of cancer or reproductive toxicity in humans has been established. No postexposure therapy exists to prevent carcinogenesis or developmental or reproductive toxicity.

REFERENCES

1. Shea KM, et al. Pediatric exposure and potential toxicity of phthalate plasticizers. *Pediatrics* 2003;111:1467–1474.
2. National Toxicology Program, Center for the Evaluation of Risks to Human Reproduction. NTP-CERHR Expert Panel report on di(2-ethylhexyl)phthalate. Alexandria, VA: U.S. Department of Health and Human Services, 2000.
3. Phillips SD. Plastics. In: Greenberg MI, Hamilton RJ, Phillips SD, eds. *Occupational, industrial, and environmental toxicology*. St. Louis: Mosby–Year Book, 1997.
4. Martinmaa JM. Synthetic polymers: main classes of plastics and their current uses. In: Jarvisalo J, Pfaffi P, Vainio H, eds. *Industrial hazards of plastics and synthetic elastomers*. New York: Alan R. Liss, 1984.
5. POISINDEX. Englewood, CO: Micromedex, Inc.
6. Rubin RJ, Ness PM. What price progress: an update on vinyl blood bags. *Transfusion* 1989;29:358–361.
7. Bradbury J. UK panics over phthalates in babymilk formulae. *Lancet* 1996;347:1541.
8. Petersen JH, Breindahl T. Plasticizers in total diet samples, baby food and infant formulae. *Food Addit Contam* 2000;17:133–141.
9. Scowen P. The facts about the phthalates scare. *Prof Care Mother Child* 1996;6:126–127.
10. United Kingdom Ministry of Agriculture, Fisheries and Food. Phthalates in infant formulae—follow-up survey (Report No. 168). London: Ministry of Agriculture, Fisheries and Food, 1998.
11. McNeal TP, Biles JE, Begley TH, et al. Determination of suspected endocrine disruptors in foods and food packaging. Boston: Annual Meeting of the American Chemical Society, 1998.
12. Blount BC, Silva MJ, Caudill SP, et al. Levels of seven urinary phthalate metabolites in a human reference population. *Environ Health Perspect* 2000;108:979–982.
13. Konemann, WH. Phthalate release from soft PVC bay toys. Report from the Dutch consensus group (RIVM Report No. 613320-002). Bilthoven, The Netherlands: National Institute on Public Health and the Environment, 1998.
14. Juberg DR, Alfano K, Coughlin RJ, et al. An observational study of object mouthing behavior by young children. *Pediatrics* 2001;107:135–142.
15. U.S. Consumer Product Safety Commission. *The risk of chronic toxicity associated with exposure to diisononyl phthalate (DINP) in children's products*. Washington, DC: U.S. Consumer Products Safety Commission, 1998.
16. Plasticizers: continuing surveillance (MAFF Food Surveillance Paper No. 30: ISBNO-11-242905-X). London, HM Stationery Office.
17. Huber WW, Grasl-Kraupp B, Schulte-Hermann R. Hepatocarcinogenic potential of di(2-ethylhexyl)phthalate in rodents and its implications on human risk. *Crit Rev Toxicol* 1996;26:365–481.

18. Doull J, Cattley R, Elcombe C., et al. A cancer risk assessment of di(2-ethylhexyl)phthalate: application of the new US EPA risk assessment guidelines. *Regul Toxicol Pharmacol* 1999;29:327–357.
19. Meek ME, Chan PKL. Bis(2-ethylhexyl)phthalate: evaluation of risks to health from environmental exposure in Canada. *Environ Carcin Ecotoxicol Rev* 1994;C12:179–194.
20. Kluwe WM. Carcinogenic potential of phthalic acid esters and related compounds: structure-activity relationships. *Environ Health Perspect* 1986;65:271–278.
21. Kluwe WM, Haseman JK, Huff JE. The carcinogenicity of di(2-ethylhexyl) phthalate (DEHP) in perspective. *J Toxicol Environ Health* 1983;12:159–169.
22. Kluwe WM, McConnell EE, Huff JE, et al. Carcinogenicity testing of phthalate esters and related compounds by the National Toxicology Program and the National Cancer Institute. *Environ Health Perspect* 1982;45:129–133.
23. Kluwe WM, Haseman JK, Douglas JF, et al. The carcinogenicity of dietary di(2-ethylhexyl) phthalate (DEHP) in Fischer 344 rats and B6C3F1 mice. *J Toxicol Environ Health* 1982;10:797–815.
24. Lovekamp-Swan T, Davis BJ. Mechanisms of phthalate ester toxicity in the female reproductive system. *Environ Health Perspect* 2003;111:139–145.
25. Myhre BA. Toxicological quandary of the use of bis (2-diethylhexyl) phthalate (DEHP) as a plasticizer for blood bags. *Ann Clin Lab Sci* 1988;18:131–140.
26. National Toxicology Program. *NTP report on carcinogens*, 8th ed. Research Triangle Park, NC: National Toxicology Program, 1998.
27. Plonait SL, Nau H, Maier RF, et al. Exposure of newborn infants to di-(2-ethylhexyl)-phthalate and 2-ethylhexanoic acid following exchange transfusion with polyvinylchloride catheters. *Transfusion* 1993;33:598–605.
28. Mettang T, Thomas S, Kiefer T, et al. Uraemic pruritus and exposure to di(2-ethylhexyl) phthalate (DEHP) in haemodialysis patients. *Nephrol Dial Transplant* 1996;11:2439–2443.
29. Mettang T, Thomas S, Kiefer T, et al. The fate of leached di(2-ethylhexyl)phthalate in patients undergoing CAPD treatment. *Perit Dial Int* 1996;16:58–62.
30. Ellenhorn MJ. *Ellenhorn's medical toxicology: diagnosis and treatment of human poisoning*, 2nd ed. Philadelphia: Lippincott Williams & Wilkins, 1996.
31. Woodward KN. Phthalate esters, cystic kidney disease in animals and possible effects on human health: a review. *Hum Exp Toxicol* 1990;9:297–301.
32. Dunnill MS, Millare PR, Oliver D. Acquired cystic disease of the kidney: a hazard of long term intermittent hemodialysis. *J Clin Pathol* 1977;30:868–877.
33. Deepa Devi KV, Manoj Kumar V, Arun P, et al. Increased lipid peroxidation of erythrocytes in blood stored in polyvinyl chloride blood storage bags plasticized with di(2-ethylhexyl) phthalate and the effects of antioxidants. *Vox Sang* 1998;75:198–204.
34. Manojkumar V, Padmakurmaran Nair KG, Santhosh A, et al. Decrease in the concentration of vitamin E in blood and tissues caused by di(2-ethylhexyl) phthalate, a commonly used plasticizer in blood bags and medical tubing. *Vox Sang* 1998;75:139–144.
35. International Agency for Research on Cancer. *IARC: monographs on the evaluation of the carcinogenic risk of chemicals to man*. Geneva: World Health Organization, IARC, 1982.
36. Latini G. Potential hazards of exposure to di(2-ethylhexyl)phthalate in babies: a review. *Biol Neonate* 2000;78:269–276.
37. Fay M, Donohue JM, DeRosa C. ATSDR evaluation of health effects of chemicals. VI. Di(2-ethylhexyl) phthalate. *Toxicol Ind Health* 1999;15:651–746.
38. Gosselin RE, Smith RP, Hodge HC. *Clinical toxicology of commercial products*, 5th ed. Baltimore: Williams & Wilkins, 1984.
39. Kluwe WM. Overview of phthalate ester pharmacokinetics in mammalian species. *Environ Health Perspect* 1982;45:3–9.
40. Schmid P, Schlatter C. Excretion and metabolism of di(2-ethylhexyl)phthalate in man. *Xenobiotica* 1985;15:251–256.
41. Colon I, Caro D, Bourdony CJ, et al. Identification of phthalate esters in the serum of young Puerto Rican girls with premature breast development. *Environ Health Perspect* 2000;108:895–900.
42. Liss GM, Albro PW, Hartle RW, et al. Urine phthalate determinations as an index of occupational exposure to phthalic anhydride and di(2-ethylhexyl)phthalate. *Scand J Work Environ Health* 1985;11:381–387.
43. Hathaway GJ, Proctor NH, Hughes JP, et al. *Chemical hazards of the workplace*, 4th ed. New York: Van Nostrand Reinhold, 1996.
44. Lewis RJ. *Sax's dangerous properties of industrial materials*, 9th ed. New York: Van Nostrand Reinhold, 1996.
45. Grant WM, Schuman JS. *Toxicology of the eye*, 4th ed. Springfield, IL: Charles C Thomas Publisher, 1993.
46. Tabacova S, Little R, Balabaeva L. Maternal exposure to phthalates and complications of pregnancy. *Epidemiology* 1999;10[Suppl]:S127.
47. Elsisi AE, Carter DE, Sipes IG. Dermal absorption of phthalate diesters in rats. *Fundam Appl Toxicol* 1989;70–77.
48. ACGIH. *Documentation of the threshold limit values and biological exposure indices*, 5th ed. Cincinnati: American Conference of Governmental Industrial Hygienists, 1986.
49. Oie L, Hersoung LG, Madsen JO. Residential exposure to plasticizers and its possible role in the pathogenesis of asthma. *Environ Health Perspect* 1997;105:972–978.
50. Pfaffli P. Phthalic acid excretion as an indicator of exposure to phthalic anhydride in the work atmosphere. *Int Arch Occup Environ Health* 1986;58:209–216.
51. Williams DT, Blanchfield BJ. Retention, excretion and metabolism of di-(2-ethylhexyl) phthalate administered orally to the rat. *Bull Environ Contam Toxicol* 1974;11:371–378.
52. Koch HM, Drexler H, Angerer J. An estimation of the daily intake of di(2-ethylhexyl)phthalate (DEHP) and other phthalates in the general population. *Int J Hyg Environ Health* 2003;206:77–83.
53. Goodwin BL. *Handbook of intermediary metabolism of aromatic compounds*. New York: John Wiley and Sons, 1976.
54. Klaassen CD. *Casarett and Doull's toxicology: the basic science of poisons*, 6th ed. New York: McGraw-Hill, 2001.
55. Proctor NH, Hughes JP, Fischman ML. *Chemical hazards of the workplace*, 2nd ed. Philadelphia: JB Lippincott Co, 1988.
56. EPA. *EPA chemical profile on dioctyl phthalate*. Washington, DC: Environmental Protection Agency, 1985.
57. Youseff J, Badr M. Extraperoxisomal targets of peroxisome proliferators: mitochondrial, microsomal and cytosolic effects. Implications for health and disease. *Crit Rev Toxicol* 1998;28:1–33.
58. Melnick RL. Is peroxisome proliferation an obligatory precursor step in the carcinogenicity of di(2-ethylhexyl) phthalate (DEHP)? *Environ Health Perspect* 2001;109:437–442.
59. Singh AR, Lawrence WH, Autian J. Teratogenicity of phthalate esters in rats. *J Pharm Sci* 1972;61:51–55.
60. Peters JM, Taubeneck MW, Keen CL, et al. Di(2-ethylhexyl) phthalate induces a functional zinc deficiency during pregnancy and teratogenesis that is independent of peroxisome proliferator-activated receptor-alpha. *Teratology* 1997;56:311–316.
61. Ema M, Kurosaka R, Amano H, et al. Developmental toxicity evaluation of mono-*n*-butyl phthalate in rats. *Toxicol Lett* 1995;78:101–106.
62. Ema M, Kurosaka R, Amano H, et al. Comparative developmental toxicity of *n*-butyl benzyl phthalate and di-*n*-butyl phthalate in rats. *Arch Environ Contam Toxicol* 1995;28:223–228.
63. Tyl RW, Price CJ, Marr MC, et al. Developmental toxicity evaluation of dietary di(2-ethylhexyl)phthalate in Fischer 344 rats and CD-1 mice. *Fundam Appl Toxicol* 1988;10:395–412.
64. Pirkle JL, Sampson EJ, Needham LL, et al. Using biological monitoring to assess human exposure to priority toxicants. *Environ Health Perspect* 1995;103[Suppl 3]:45–48.
65. Heindel JJ, Powell CJ. Phthalate ester effects on rat Sertoli cell function in vitro: effects of phthalate side chain and age of animal. *Toxicol Appl Pharmacol* 1992;115:116–123.
66. Gray TJ, Beamand JA. Effect of some phthalate esters and other testicular toxins on primary cultures of testicular cells. *Food Chem Toxicol* 1984;22:123–131.
67. Ema M, Harazono A, Miyawaki E, et al. Developmental toxicity of mono-*n*-benzyl phthalate, one of the major metabolites of the plasticizer *n*-butyl benzyl phthalate, in rats. *Toxicol Lett* 1996;86:19–25.
68. Gray LE Jr, Wolf C, Lambright C, et al. Administration of potentially antiandrogenic pesticides (procymidone, linuron, iprodione, chlozolinate, p,p'-DDE, and ketoconazole) and toxic substances (dibutyl- and diethylhexyl phthalate, PCB 169, and ethane dimethane sulphonate) during sexual differentiation produces diverse profiles of reproductive malformations in the male rat. *Toxicol Ind Health* 1999;15:94–118.
69. Ema M, Itami T, Kawasaki H. Teratogenic phase specificity of butyl benzyl phthalate in rats. *Toxicology*. 1993;79:11–19.
70. Shiota K, Chou MJ, Nishimura H. Embryotoxic effects of di-2-ethylhexyl phthalate (DEHP) and di-*n*-buty phthalate (DBP) in mice. *Environ Res* 1980;22:245–253.
71. Foster PM, Thomas LV, Cook MW, et al. Study of the testicular effects and changes in zinc excretion produced by some *n*-alkyl phthalates in the rat. *Toxicol Appl Pharmacol* 1980;54:392–398.
72. Jha AM, Singh AC, Bharti M. Germ cell mutagenicity of phthalic acid in mice. *Mutat Res* 1998;422:207–212.
73. Aldyreva MV, Klimova TS, Iziumova AS, et al. [The effect of phthalate plasticizers on the generative function.] *Gig Tr Prof Zabol* 1975;25–29.
74. Keys N, Erickson T, Lipscomb J. Glow compound exposure. *J Toxicol Clin Toxicol* 1995;33:488(abst 5).
75. Hoffman RJ, Nelson LS, Hoffman RS. Pediatric and young adult exposure to chemiluminescent glow sticks. *Arch Pediatr Adolesc Med* 2002;156:901–904.
76. Milkov LE, Aldyreva MV, Popova TB, et al. Health status of workers exposed to phthalate plasticizers in the manufacture of artificial leather and films based on PVC resins. *Environ Health Perspect* 1973;3:175–178.
77. Maccia CA, Bernstein IL, Emmett EA, et al. In vitro demonstration of specific IgE in phthalic anhydride hypersensitivity. *Am Rev Respir Dis* 1976;113:701–704.
78. Nielsen J, Welinder H, Schutz A, et al. Specific serum antibodies against phthalic anhydride in occupationally exposed subjects. *J Allergy Clin Immunol* 1988;82:126–133.
79. Venables KM, Topping MD, Nunn AJ. Immunologic and functional consequences of chemical (tetrachlorophthalic anhydride)-induced asthma after four years of avoidance of exposure. *J Allergy Clin Immunol* 1987;80:212–218.
80. Krauskopf LG. Studies on the toxicity of phthalates via ingestion. *Environ Health Perspect* 1973;3:61–72.
81. Cagianut B. Corneal erosion and toxic nephritis from ingestion of dibutyl phthalate. *Schweiz Med Wochenschr* 1954;84:1243–1244.
82. Oettel H. Health hazard from synthetic plastics, Naunyn-Schmeideberg. *Arch Exp Pathol Pharmakol* 1957;232:77–132.

83. ITI. *Toxic and hazardous industrial chemicals safety manual*. Tokyo: International Technical Information Institute, 1988.
84. HSDB. *Hazardous substances data bank*. Englewood, CO: Micromedex, 2000.
85. Lefaux R. *CRC: practical toxicology of plastics*. Cleveland: Chemical Rubber Co, 1968.
86. NRC. *National Research Council: drinking water and health*. Washington, DC: National Academy Press, 1977.
87. RTECS. Registry of Toxic Effects of Chemical Substances—NIOSH. Englewood, CO, Micromedex, 1999.
88. Piekacz H. [Effect of dioctyl- and dibutylphthalates on rats during oral administration in prolonged experiments. II. Studies of subacute and chronic toxicity.] *Rocz Panstw Zakl Hig* 1971;22:295–307.
89. Nagasaki A, Tomii S, Tomoiche M. An experimental study on the chronic toxicity of DOP. *Nichieishi* 1975;30:2.
90. Crocker JF, Safe SH, Acott P. Effects of chronic phthalate exposure on the kidney. *J Toxicol Environ Health* 1988;23:433–444.
91. Crocker JF, Belcher SR, Safe SH. Chemically induced polycystic kidney disease. *Prog Clin Biol Res* 140:281–296.
92. Nikonorow M, Mazur H, Piekacz H. Effect of orally administrated plasticizers and polyvinyl chloride stabilizers in the rat. *Toxicol Appl Pharmacol* 1973;26:253–259.
93. Klimisch HJ, Gamer AO, Hellwig J, et al. Di-(2-ethylhexyl) phthalate: a short-term repeated inhalation toxicity study including fertility assessment. *Food Chem Toxicol* 1992;30:915–919.
94. Barry YA, Labow RS, Keon WJ, et al. Perioperative exposure to plasticizers in patients undergoing cardiopulmonary bypass. *J Thorac Cardiovasc Surg* 1989;97:900–905.
95. Roth B, Herkenrath P, Lehmann HJ, et al. Di-(2-ethylhexyl)-phthalate as plasticizer in PVC respiratory tubing systems: indications of hazardous effects on pulmonary function in mechanically ventilated, preterm infants. *Eur J Pediatr* 1988;147:41–46.
96. Latini G, Avery GB. Materials degradation in endotracheal tubes: a potential contributor to bronchopulmonary dysplasia. *Acta Paediatr* 1999;88:1174–1175.
97. Loff S, Kabs F, Witt K, et al. Polyvinylchloride infusion lines expose infants to large amounts of toxic plasticizers. *J Pediatr Surg* 2000;35:1775–1781.
98. Kambia K, Dine T, Gressier B, et al. High-performance liquid chromatographic method for the determination of di(2-ethylhexyl) phthalate in total parenteral nutrition and in plasma. *J Chromatogr B Biomed Sci Appl* 2001;755:297–303.
99. Kambia K, Dine T, Azar R, et al. Comparative study of the leachability of di(2-ethylhexyl) phthalate and tri(2-ethylhexyl) trimellitate from haemodialysis tubing. *Int J Pharm* 2001;229:139–146.
100. Sjoberg P, Bondesson U, Sedin G, et al. Dispositions of di- and mono-(2-ethylhexyl) phthalate in newborn infants subjected to exchange transfusions. *Eur J Clin Invest* 1985;15:430–436.
101. Sjoberg PO, Bondesson UG, Sedin EG, et al. Exposure of newborn infants to plasticizers. Plasma levels of di-(2-ethylhexyl) phthalate and mono-(2-ethylhexyl) phthalate during exchange transfusion. *Transfusion* 1985;25:424–428.
102. Rossi M, Muehlberger M. *Neonatal exposure to DEHP and opportunities for prevention*. Falls Church, VAL Health Care Without Harm, 2000.
103. Eigenberg DA, Carter DE, Schram KH, et al. Examination of the differential hepatotoxicity of diallyl phthalate in rats and mice. *Toxicol Appl Pharmacol* 1986;86:12–21.
104. Ema M, Amano H, Itami T, et al. Teratogenic evaluation of di-*n*-butyl phthalate in rats. *Toxicol Lett* 1993;69:197–203.
105. National Toxicology Program, Center for the Evaluation of Risks to Human Reproduction. NTP-CERHR expert panel report on diisononyl phthalate. Alexandria, VA: U.S. Department of Health and Human Services, 2000.
106. Caldwell DJ. Review of mononuclear cell leukemia in F-344 rat bioassays and its significance to human cancer risk: a case study using alkyl phthalates. *Regul Toxicol Pharmacol* 1999;30:45–53.
107. Koch HM, Gonzalez-Reche LM, Angerer J. On-line clean-up by multidimensional liquid chromatography–electrospray ionization tandem mass spectrometry for high throughput quantification of primary and secondary phthalate metabolites in human urine. *J Chromatogr B Analyt Technol Biomed Life Sci* 2003;784:169–182.
108. Blount BC, Milgram KE, Silva MJ, et al. Quantitative detection of eight phthalate metabolites in human urine using HPLC-APCI-MS/MS. *Anal Chem* 2000;72:4127–4134.
109. Sittig M. *Handbook of toxic and hazardous chemical and carcinogens*, 3rd ed. Park Ridge, NJ: Noyes Publications, 1991.
110. Flaherty DK, Gross CJ, Winzenburger P, et al. In vitro immunologic studies on a population of workers exposed to phthalic and tetrachlorophthalic anhydride. *J Occup Med* 1988;30:785–790.

SECTION

10

Metals

CHAPTER 211

Aluminum

Seth Schonwald

Atomic symbol, atomic number, molecular weight:	**Al, 13, 26.98 g/mol**
Valence state:	**+3**
CAS Registry No.:	**7429-90-5**
Normal levels:	**Less than 10 μg/L (serum)**
SI conversion:	**μg/L × 0.037 = μmol/L**
Target organs:	**Central nervous system after acute exposure in special target groups (e.g., renal failure); bone, pulmonary, and blood with chronic exposure**
Antidote:	**Deferoxamine**

OVERVIEW

Aluminum is an extremely reactive metal element and is always found combined with elements such as oxygen, silicon, or fluorine [e.g., $Al(SO_4)_3$, $AlCl_3$, AlF_3]. Aluminum metal is obtained from bauxite (1) and is commonly found in consumer products as well as industrial applications, such as alums in water treatment and alumina in abrasives and furnace linings. Aluminum phosphide can cause life-threatening toxicity.

Aluminum is contained in numerous consumer products (Table 1) (2–4). Humans are exposed to aluminum in food, water, medicinal products, cooking utensils, and foods prepared or stored in aluminum vessels (5,6). Cooking or storing foods in aluminum pots, foil, or cans increases the aluminum content in some foods because aluminum may dissolve when in contact with salty, acidic, or alkaline food (7). Skin contact with soil, water, metal, antiperspirants, or food additives (e.g., some baking powders) that contain aluminum is another potential source (8).

Uremic patients are at risk for aluminum-related dementia. Prolonged dialysis with aluminum-containing dialysates, possibly combined with oral aluminum hydroxide to control hyperphosphatemia, has produced a characteristic neurotoxicity syndrome termed *dialysis dementia* (9,10). Other populations at risk include infants on parenteral fluids, particularly parenteral nutrition (11,12); burn patients through administration of intravenous albumin, particularly with coexisting renal failure (13); adult parenteral nutrition patients (14); and industrial exposures.

Therapeutic Dose

The normal diet contains 3 to 5 mg/day of aluminum. The total body burden is approximately 30 mg (8). Patients on antacids or phosphate-binding therapy may ingest up to 5 g/dl/day and are in positive balance of 200 to 300 mg/day. Relatively insoluble forms of aluminum include aluminum hydroxide and aluminum phosphate in antacids (e.g., Amphojel 636 mg/30 ml, ALternaGEL 966 mg/30 ml, Maalox 360 mg/30 ml); sucralfate, 207 mg/1000 mg tablet; and Kaopectate, 100 mg/100 ml (13).

TABLE 1. Sources of aluminum exposure

Aluminum hydroxide or phosphate
- Antacids (58)
- Astringents
- Buffered aspirin
- Food additives
- Antiperspirants (59)
- Fumigation (2)

Aluminum sulfate
- Flocculent for water purification and sewage treatment systems
- Paper and pulp industry
- Fireproofing and waterproofing cloth
- Clarifying oils and fats
- Waterproofing concrete
- Antiperspirants
- Tanning leather
- Mordant in dyeing
- Agricultural pesticides
- Intermediate in the manufacture of other chemicals
- Soil conditioner to increase acidity for plants
- Cosmetics and soap (3)

Aluminum metal
- Explosives and fireworks (4)
- Aluminum pots and pans
- Food stored in aluminum foil

Note: Numbers in parentheses correspond to reference numbers.

TABLE 2. U.S. regulatory guidelines and standards for aluminum (Al)

Agency	Description	Concentration (mg/m³)
OSHA	Total dust	
Air	PEL-TWA	15 (as Al)
	Respirable fraction	5 (as Al)
ACGIH	Aluminum metal	
Air	TLV-TWA	10 (as Al dust)
	STEL	None
	Pyro-powders/welding fumes	
	TLV-TWA	5
	STEL	None
	Soluble salts	
	TLV-TWA	2
	STEL	None
	Alkyls	
	TLV-TWA	2
	STEL	None
NIOSH	Total particulate	
Air	REL-TWA	10
	Respirable fraction	
	REL-TWA	5
	STEL	None
	Pyro-powders/welding fumes	
	REL-TWA	5 (as Al)
	STEL	None
	Soluble salts	
	REL-TWA	2 (as Al)
	STEL	None
	IDLH	Not established

ACGIH, American Conference of Governmental Industrial Hygienists; Al, Aluminum; IDLH, immediate danger to life or health; NIOSH, National Institute for Occupational Safety and Health; OSHA, U.S. Occupational Safety and Health Administration; PEL, permissible exposure limit; REL, recommended exposure limit; STEL, short-term exposure limit; TLV, threshold limit value; TWA, time-weighted average.

Toxic Dose

Death has followed occupational exposure to finely powdered metallic aluminum used in paints, explosives, and fireworks. Improved production technology has decreased occupational exposure (6). Regulatory guidelines and standards are shown in Table 2.

TOXICOKINETICS AND TOXICODYNAMICS

Aluminum is poorly absorbed after ingestion or inhalation and is essentially not absorbed through normal skin. Approximately 0.1% of ingested aluminum is absorbed, although absorption of more bioavailable forms can reach 1%. The tenfold range in absorption of aluminum is largely due to the chemical form of aluminum as well as the presence of dietary constituents that can bind and enhance or inhibit its absorption. Gastric acidity and oral citrate favor absorption, and H_2-blockers reduce absorption.

The main mechanism of absorption is probably paracellular passive diffusion. Aluminum binds to ligands in the blood and distributes to every organ, with highest concentrations found in bone (15) and lung tissues. Approximately 89% of serum aluminum is bound to transferrin (16). Aluminum is excreted principally in the urine (17) and, to a lesser extent, in the bile (18).

Aluminum uptake and elimination are maintained in equilibrium in healthy adults. Blood and tissue aluminum levels are increased in people exposed to high levels of aluminum, such as those associated with long-term use of antacids (13). The levels return to normal on cessation of exposure.

PATHOPHYSIOLOGY

The deposition of aluminum in bone may block incorporation of calcium into osteoid, leading to osteomalacia. The prevention of calcium deposition in bone leads to the return of the calcium to the circulation, with a rise in the serum calcium level. The elevated levels in turn inhibit the release of parathyroid hormone by the parathyroid glands (19). Aluminum inhibits osteoclasts and osteoblasts.

Aluminum may contribute to anemia of chronic renal failure (20). Chronic renal failure patients on long-term dialysis may develop high aluminum serum and tissue concentrations, especially in bone. Elevated aluminum levels appear to be an important factor in the pathogenesis of dialysis encephalopathy and renal osteodystrophy (21).

Aluminum-containing, phosphate-binding agents increase gut aluminum absorption and predispose children with renal dysfunction to aluminum toxicity. Children with azotemia (22), infants receiving aluminum-contaminated intravenous solutions (23), and uremic neonates drinking powdered milk with high aluminum content are particularly susceptible to toxicity (24).

VULNERABLE POPULATIONS

Limited animal evidence indicates that aluminum crosses the placenta, accumulates in the fetus, and is distributed to some extent into breast milk (25–27). Developmental toxicity of aluminum includes neurodevelopmental changes and skeletal effects in orally exposed rodents. Neurobehavioral deficits have been observed in mice exposed to aluminum before or after gestation or during weaning (28,29).

CLINICAL PRESENTATION

Aluminum toxicity occurs almost exclusively in patients who are unable to excrete aluminum. The main target organs appear to be the central nervous system and bone. Hypercalcemia, reversible microcytic anemia, vitamin D–refractory osteodystrophy, and progressive encephalopathy may characterize aluminum toxicity.

Respiratory Exposure

Occupational exposure to fine powders of aluminum metal that can deposit in the lung can result in pulmonary fibrosis (aluminosis) (6). Aluminosis and asthma may occur in workers heavily exposed to fine aluminum dust. Severe encephalopathy with incoordination, intention tremor, and cognitive deficits has been reported in aluminum workers with pulmonary fibrosis (30). Symptomatic workers may demonstrate loss of balance and memory loss. A neurologic syndrome observed among workers in the pot room of aluminum smelting plants, previously termed *pot room palsy*, is characterized by incoordination, poor memory, impairment in abstract reasoning, and depression (31). Excesses of lung cancer (32) and bladder cancer (33) have been reported in epidemiologic studies of aluminum workers.

Hemodialysis

Dialysis encephalopathy develops over several months. It initially presents with a mild speech disturbance characterized by stuttering or stammering speech that most frequently occurs immediately after dialysis (34). This is associated with subtle mental changes, such as directional disorientation and personality changes. As the disease progresses, the speech disorder intensifies and is accompanied by twitching, myoclonus, motor apraxia, seizures, visual and auditory hallucinations, and paranoid and suicidal behavior. Ultimately, patients may become immobile, mute, and obtunded. Death may follow 6 to 9 months after onset. If initiated early enough, deferoxamine (DFO) appears to be effective in treating dialysis encephalopathy (35).

Alzheimer's Disease

A possible relationship between aluminum and Alzheimer's disease was proposed more than 30 years ago and remains controversial (36–38). Aluminum levels are increased in the brains of Alzheimer's disease patients. Experimental animals develop neurofibrillary lesions containing aluminum; aluminum also interacts with various components of the pathologic lesions in the brains of Alzheimer's disease patients (39).

Osteomalacia

Osteomalacia has been observed in healthy individuals after long-term use of aluminum-containing antacids and in individuals with kidney disease. There are numerous case reports of osteomalacia and rickets in otherwise healthy infants and adults using aluminum-containing antacids for the treatment of gastrointestinal illnesses (40,41). Aluminum in antacids binds with dietary phosphorus and prevents its absorption, resulting in hypophosphatemia and phosphate depletion. Osteomalacia, increased spontaneous fractures, and pain may be found in dialyzed uremic adults and children exposed to aluminum-contaminated dialysate or oral aluminum-containing, phosphate-binding agents (22,42).

Anemia

Although not observed in patients with normal renal function, microcytic, hypochromatic anemia occurs in individuals with impaired renal function (43). The anemia is unresponsive to iron therapy. The severity of the anemia correlates with plasma and erythrocyte aluminum levels and can be reversed by terminating aluminum exposure and by chelation therapy with DFO.

DIAGNOSTIC TESTS

Aluminum is detected by flameless atomic absorption spectrometry (44). Serum aluminum levels are helpful but do not accurately reflect total body burden because aluminum is highly protein bound. Serum aluminum levels in normal patients are below 10 μg/L and may reach 50 μg/L in chronic dialysis patients without toxicity; levels above 60 μg/L indicate increased absorption. Potential toxicity occurs above 100 μg/L, and clinical symptoms usually are present when serum aluminum levels exceed 200 μg/L (45).

Biologic monitoring involves measurement of the aluminum content in human tissues, especially in blood, urine, and breast milk (46,47). Measurements of aluminum in bone and brain tissue are also available; however, recent (i.e., within 3 years) biologic monitoring data, particularly for aluminum in blood and urine, are limited (1).

Mortality is 18% higher in long-term hemodialysis patients with serum aluminum levels between 1520 and 2220 μmol/L and 60% higher in patients with aluminum levels above 7410 μmol/L. The use of aluminum salts in patients with plasma levels of 1520 μmol/L or higher should be reconsidered (11).

The body burden of aluminum in relation to central nervous system function has been studied among metal inert-gas welders. Objective neurophysiologic and neuropsychological measures and subjective symptomatology indicated mild but unequivocal findings associated in a dose-dependent manner with increased aluminum body burden. The body burden threshold for adverse effect approximates a urinary aluminum value of 4 to 6 μmol/L and a serum value of 0.25 to 0.35 μmol/L (48). There are few data to correlate plasma and bone aluminum levels, suggesting that plasma levels do not necessarily reflect total body aluminum (49). Hair aluminum concentrations are too variable to reliably predict intoxication (50).

Aluminum is radiopaque. Foreign bodies as small as 0.5 mm × 0.5 mm × 1 mm can be clearly visualized when projected away from underlying bone.

Transiliac bone biopsy is the "gold standard" for the diagnosis of aluminum-related bone disease in patients on regular hemodialysis.

TREATMENT

Termination of exposure must be assured in all patients with suspected aluminum toxicity. In people with normal renal function, simply limiting exposure reduces the body burden. Avoidance of aluminum-containing products or coadministration of aluminum compounds and citrate compounds is also recommended for patients with renal failure. Use of non–aluminum-containing, phosphate-binding gels and use of aluminum-free dialysate and parenteral solutions are important (1). The coadministration of an H_2-receptor antagonist, such as ranitidine, can reduce absorption from aluminum-containing phosphate binders, resulting in lower plasma aluminum concentrations.

Decontamination

Gastric lavage is not recommended for acute ingestion of aluminum compounds because of their lack of acute toxicity. The use of activated charcoal would not be expected to improve the outcome of aluminum ingestion.

Enhanced Elimination

Hemodialysis and charcoal hemoperfusion may remove aluminum, including aluminum bound to DFO (51,52). Dialysis facilities should routinely evaluate dialysate delivery systems, including dialysate concentrate transfer and storage devices (53). When elevated serum aluminum levels are found, corrective actions, such as avoiding aluminum-based phosphate binders and initiating chelation therapy, are undertaken.

Antidotal Treatment

The primary antidote is DFO, which has been used to treat dialysis encephalopathy (54) and osteomalacia (Chapter 48) (55). The use of DFO for aluminum-toxic dialysis patients has been suggested for serum aluminum levels between 100 and 200 μg/ml (56). DFO also has been used as a chelation challenge test to diagnose aluminum-related osteodystrophy. After an infusion of DFO, 40 mg/kg over 2 hours, an increase in plasma aluminum concentration of 200 mg/L identified 35 of 37 patients with biopsy-proven, aluminum-related osteodystrophy (57). DFO treatment has been used to facilitate transfer of aluminum from bone into the blood where it can be removed by hemodialysis. Calcium disodium ethylenediaminetetraacetic acid does not appear as effective as DFO.

Hemoglobin levels, mean cell volume, and mean cell hemoglobin concentrations may respond to a 3-month course of DFO. Therapy with DFO significantly improves anemia in patients when sufficient levels of erythropoietin are present to stimulate erythropoiesis. Care must be taken to replete iron stores during therapy to avoid iron deficiency.

REFERENCES

1. ATSDR toxicological profile for aluminum. Atlanta: Agency for Toxic Substances and Disease Registry, Division of Toxicology, 1999:1–393.
2. Budavari S, O'Neil MJ, Smith A, et al. *The Merck index*, 11th ed. Rahway, NJ: Merck & Co., Inc., 1989.
3. HSDB. Hazardous substances data bank. Bethesda, MD: National Library of Medicine, National Toxicology Program (via TOXNET), 1995.
4. Mitchell J, Manning GB, Molyneux M, et al. Pulmonary fibrosis in workers exposed to finely powdered aluminum. *Br J Ind Med* 1961;18:10–20.
5. Lione A. Aluminum toxicology and the aluminum-containing medications. *Pharmacol Ther* 1986;29:255–285.
6. Winship KA. Toxicity of aluminum: a historical review. I. *Adverse Drug React Toxicol Rev* 1992;11:123–141.
7. Abercrombie DE, Fowler RC. Possible aluminum content of canned drinks. *Toxicol Ind Health* 1997;13:649–654.
8. Flarend R, Bin T, Elmore D, et al. A preliminary study of the dermal absorption of aluminium from antiperspirants using aluminium-26. *Food Chem Toxicol* 2001;39:163–168.
9. Chazan JA, Lew NL, Lowrie EG. Increased serum aluminum. An independent risk factor for mortality in patients undergoing long-term hemodialysis. *Arch Intern Med* 1991;151:319–320.
10. Salusky IB, Foley J, Nelson P, et al. Aluminum accumulation during treatment with aluminum hydroxide and dialysis in children and young adults with chronic renal disease. *N Engl J Med* 1991;324:527–531.
11. Sedman A. Aluminum toxicity in childhood. *Pediatr Nephrol* 1992;6:383–393.
12. Klein GL, Alfrey AC, Shike M, et al. Parenteral drug products containing aluminum as an ingredient or a contaminant: response to FDA notice of intent. ASCN/Aspen Working Group on Standards for Aluminum Content of Parenteral Nutrition Solutions. *Am J Clin Nutr* 1991;53:399–402.
13. Progar JJ, May JC, Rains TC, et al. Preparation of an intra-laboratory reference material-determination of the aluminum content of a pooled 5% albumin (human) solution by ETAAS, MFS and ICP-AES. *Biologicals* 1996;24:87–93.
14. Klein GL. Aluminum in parenteral products: medical perspective on large and small volume parenterals. *J Parenter Sci Technol* 1989;43:120–124.
15. Henry PA, Goodman WO, Nudelman RK, et al. Parenteral aluminum administration in the dog. I. Plasma kinetics, tissue levels, calcium metabolism and parathyroid hormones. *Kidney Int* 1984;25:362–369.
16. Ganrot PO. Metabolism and possible health effects of aluminum. *Environ Health Perspect* 1986;65:363–441.
17. Monteagudo FS, Cassidy MJ, Fold PI. Recent developments in aluminum toxicology. *Med Toxicol* 1989;4:1–16.
18. Williams JW, Santiago RV, Peters TG, et al. Biliary excretion of aluminum in aluminum osteodystrophy with liver disease. *Ann Intern Med* 1986;104:782–785.
19. Morissey J, Slatopolsky E. The effect of aluminum on parathyroid hormone secretion. *Kidney Int* 1986;29S:41–48.
20. Wills MR, Savory J. Aluminum and chronic renal failure: sources, absorption, transport, and toxicity. *Crit Rev Clin Lab Sci* 1989;27:59–107.
21. Fournier A, Oprisiu R, Hottelart C, et al. Renal osteodystrophy in dialysis patients: diagnosis and treatment. *Artif Organs* 1998;22(7):530–557.
22. Andreoli SP, Bergstein JM, Sherrard DJ. Aluminum intoxication from aluminum-containing phosphate binders in children with azotemia not undergoing dialysis. *N Engl J Med* 1984;310:1079–1084.
23. Sedman AB, Klein GL, Merritt RJ, et al. Evidence of aluminum loading in infants receiving intravenous therapy. *N Engl J Med* 1985;312:1337–1342.
24. Freundlich M, Zilleruelo G, Faugere MC, et al. Treatment of aluminum toxicity in infantile uremia with deferoxamine. *J Pediatr* 1986;109:140–143.
25. Cranmer JM, Wilkins JD, Cannon DJ. Fetal-placental-maternal uptake of aluminum in mice following gestational exposure: effect of dose and route of administration. *Neurotoxicology* 1986;7:601–608.
26. Golub MS, Domingo JL. What we know and what we need to know about developmental aluminum toxicity. *J Toxicol Environ Health* 1996;48:585–597.
27. Yokel RA. Toxicity of gestational aluminum exposure to the maternal rabbit and offspring. *Toxicol Appl Pharmacol* 1985;79:121–133.
28. Donald JM, Golub MS, Gershwin ME. Neurobehavioral effects in offspring of mice given excess aluminum in diet during gestation and lactation. *Neurotoxicol Teratol* 1989;11:345–351.
29. Golub MS, Germann SL. Aluminum effects on operant performance and food motivation of mice. *Neurotoxicol Teratol* 1998;20:421–427.
30. McLaughlin AIG, Kazantzis G, King E. Pulmonary fibrosis and encephalopathy associated with the inhalation of aluminum dust. *Br J Ind Med* 1962;16:123–125.
31. White DM, Longstretch WT Jr, Rosenstock L, et al. Neurologic syndrome in 25 workers from an aluminum smelting plant. *Arch Intern Med* 1992;152:1443–1448.
32. Gibbs GW, Horowitz I. Lung cancer mortality in aluminum plant workers. *J Occup Med* 1979;21:347–353.
33. Theriault G, Tremblay C, Cordier S, et al. Bladder cancer in the aluminum industry. *Lancet* 1984;1:947–950.
34. Alfrey AC, Mishell MM, Burks J, et al. Syndrome of dyscrasia and multifocal seizures associated with chronic hemodialysis. *Trans Am Soc Artif Intern Organs* 1972;18:257–261.
35. Alfrey AC. Dialysis encephalopathy. *Kidney Int* 1986;29[Suppl 18]:S53–S57.
36. Marcus DL, Wong S, Freedman ML. Dietary aluminum and Alzheimer's disease. *J Nutr Elder* 1992;12:1255–1261.
37. Martyn CN. The epidemiology of Alzheimer's disease in relation to aluminum. In: Chadwick DJ, Whelan J, eds. *Aluminum in biology and medicine*. Chichester, UK: John Wiley & Sons, 1992:69–86.
38. Martyn CN, Osmond C, Edwardson JA, et al. Geographical relation between Alzheimer's disease and aluminum in drinking water. *Lancet* 1989;1:59–62.
39. Armstrong RA, Winsper SJ, Blair JA. Aluminium and Alzheimer's disease: review of possible pathogenic mechanisms. *Dementia* 1996;7:1–9.
40. Carmichael KA, Fallon MD, Dalinka M, et al. Osteomalacia and osteitis fibrosa in a man ingesting aluminum hydroxide antacid. *Am J Med* 1984;76:1137–1143.
41. Woodson GC. An interesting case of osteomalacia due to antacid use associated with stainable bone aluminum in a patient with normal renal function. *Bone* 1998;22:695–698.
42. Mayor GH, Lohr TO, Sanchez TV, et al. Aluminum metabolism and toxicity in renal failure: a review. *J Environ Pathol Toxicol Oncol* 1985;6:43–50.
43. Grutzmacher P, Vlachojannis J, Schoeppe W. Aluminum and renal anemia. *Trace Elem Med* 1991;8:S21–S25.
44. van der Voet GB, de Haas EJ, de Wolff FA. Monitoring of aluminum in whole blood, plasma, serum and water by a single procedure using flameless atomic absorption spectrophotometry. *J Anal Toxicol* 1985;9:97–100.
45. Sedman AB, Wilkening GB, Warady BA, et al. Clinical and laboratory observations. Encephalopathy in childhood secondary to aluminum toxicity. *J Pediatr* 1984;105:836–838.
46. Nieboer E, Gibson BL, Oxman AD, et al. Health effects of aluminum: a critical review with emphasis on aluminum in drinking water. *Environ Rev* 1995;3:29–81.
47. Hawkins NM, Coffey S, Lawson MS, et al. Potential aluminum toxicity in infants fed special infant formula. *J Pediatr Gastroenterol Nutr* 1994;19:377–381.
48. Riihimaki V, Hanninen H, Akila R, et al. Body burden of aluminum in relation to central nervous system function among metal inert-gas welders. *Scand J Work Environ Health* 2000;26(2):118–130.
49. Alfrey AC. Aluminum metabolism. *Kidney Int* 1986;29:[Suppl 18]:S8–S11.
50. Yokel RA. Hair as an indicator of excessive aluminum exposure. *Clin Chem* 1982;28:662–665.
51. Weiss LG, Danielson BG, Fellstrom B, Wikstrom B. Aluminum removal with hemodialysis, hemofiltration and charcoal hemoperfusion in uremic patients after desferrioxamine infusion. A comparison of efficiency. *Nephron* 1989;51:325–329.
52. Ogborn MR, Dorcas VC, Crocker JF. Deferoxamine and aluminum clearance in pediatric hemodialysis patients. *Pediatr Nephrol* 1991;5:62–64.
53. Dialysis patients face dangers from aluminum and other trace elements. *FDA Med Bull* 1992;22(2):8.
54. Arze RS, Parkinson IS, Cartlidge NE, et al. Reversal of aluminum dialysis encephalopathy after desferrioxamine treatment. *Lancet* 1981;2:1116.
55. Brown DJ, Dawborn JK, Ham KN, et al. Treatment of dialysis osteomalacia with desferrioxamine. *Lancet* 1982;2:343–345.
56. Savory J, Berlin A, Courtoux C, et al. Summary report of an international workshop on the role of biological monitoring of aluminum toxicity in man: aluminum analysis in biological fluids. *Ann Clin Lab Sci* 1983;13:444–451.
57. Adhemar JP, Laederich J, Jaudon MC, et al. Removal of aluminum from patients with dialysis encephalopathy. *Lancet* 1980;2:1311.
58. Kaehy WD, Hegg AP, Alfrey AC. Gastrointestinal absorption of aluminum from aluminum-containing antacids. *N Engl J Med* 1977;296:1389–1390.
59. Sax NI, Lewis RJ Sr, eds. *Hawley's condensed chemical dictionary*, 11th ed. New York: Van Nostrand Reinhold Co., 1987:42–51, 1248–1249.

CHAPTER 212

Antimony

Seth Schonwald

ANTIMONY TRISULFIDE

Atomic symbol, atomic number, molecular weight	**Sb; 51; antimony trioxide (Sb_2O_3), 291.50 g/mol; stibine (SbH_3), 124.78**
Valence states:	**Sb^{+3} and Sb^{+5}**
CAS Registry No.:	**7440-36-0 (antimony); 1309-64-4 (antimony trioxide); 7803-52-3 (stibine)**
Normal levels:	**Serum, 0.05 to 0.50 mg/dl; urine, 0.6µl/L**
SI conversion:	**mg/dl × 0.082 = mmol/L**
Target organs:	**Antimony: pneumoconiosis; stibine gas: blood (hemolysis)**
Antidote:	**Dimercapto chelating agents**

OVERVIEW

Antimony is widely used in the production of alloys and is commonly found in ores associated with arsenic (1). It is used in lead storage batteries, solder, sheet or pipe metal, castings, ammunition, cable sheathing, and pewter.

Stibine (SbH_3) is an extremely toxic gas often used as a fumigant. Stibine gas is released when antimony alloys are treated with acids. Patients at risk from the adverse effects of antimony compounds include those treated with antileishmaniasis agents and workers occupationally exposed to dusts and fumes containing antimony (2).

Trivalent antimony compounds were used in the past for the treatment of trypanosomiasis and leishmaniasis but were superseded by the less toxic pentavalent compounds in the 1920s. Pentavalent antimonials remain the main drugs used for the treatment of leishmaniasis (3).

Toxic Dose

U.S. regulatory agency guidelines are shown in Table 1.

For the treatment of leishmaniasis, the Centers for Disease Control and Prevention (CDC) recommends a dose of 20 mg/kg/day with no upper limit on the daily dose of sodium stibogluconate (4). Meglumine antimonate is also used to treat leishmaniasis. The dose is 20 mg/kg/day intramuscularly (IM) for 20 to 28 days. Occasional deaths that may have been due to cardiotoxicity have been reported, but they occurred in association with either doses exceeding CDC recommendations or underlying cardiac disease (5). Occupational inhalation of antimony was associated with an excess of lung cancer in exposed workers with a carcinogenic latency of 20 years (6).

TOXICOKINETICS AND TOXICODYNAMICS

Antimony compounds are poorly absorbed orally. Trivalent antimony compounds rapidly leave the plasma but remain in the circulation bound to erythrocytes. Trivalent antimony readily enters red blood cells, but pentavalent antimony does not (7). They react with the red cell membrane and interfere with hemoglobin function.

The kidney excretes approximately 10% of the trivalent form in 24 hours, and 50% to 60% of the pentavalent form is found in the urine within 24 hours (8). Inorganic trivalent antimony is excreted in the bile after conjugation with glutathione and in the urine. A significant proportion of that excreted in bile undergoes enterohepatic circulation (8).

PATHOPHYSIOLOGY

Antimony is similar to arsenic in its generalized effect and its affinity for sulfhydryl groups on many enzymes. It is primarily an irritant.

VULNERABLE POPULATIONS

Female workers employed in an antimony plant showed an increased incidence of spontaneous late abortions as compared to female workers not exposed to antimony dust (9).

TABLE 1. U.S. regulatory guidelines and standards for antimony

Agency	Description	Antimony metal	Stibine gas
OSHA	PEL-TWA	0.5 mg/m³ (as Sb)	0.1 ppm (0.5 mg/m³)
(air)	STEL	None	None
ACGIH	TLV-TWA	0.5 mg/m³ (as Sb)	0.1 ppm (0.5 mg/m³)
(air)	STEL	None	None
NIOSH	REL-TWA	0.5 mg/m³ (as Sb)	0.1 ppm (0.5 mg/m³)
	STEL	None	None
	IDLH	50 mg/m³ (as Sb)	5 ppm
EPA	Safe Drinking Water Act	6 µg/L	None

ACGIH, American Conference of Government Industrial Hygienists; EPA, Environmental Protection Agency; IDLH, immediate danger to life or health; NIOSH, National Institute of Occupations Safety and Health; OSHA, U.S. Occupational Safety and Health Administration; PEL, permissible exposure limit; ppm, parts per million; REL, recommended exposure limit; STEL, short-term exposure limit; TLV, threshold limit value; TWA, time-weighted average (8 hours).

CLINICAL PRESENTATION

Stibine gas exposure produces a clinical picture similar to that of arsine gas (AsH_3): hemolytic anemia, myoglobinuria, renal failure, weakness, profuse vomiting, nausea, headache, abdominal and low back pain, and hematuria (10). Vomiting is usually prominent.

Meglumine antimonate therapy is associated with pancreatitis, acute renal failure (11), and leukopenia (12). Reversible side effects caused by ingestion of pentavalent antimonial drugs include arthralgia, myalgia, increases in hepatocellular enzymes, and flattening or inversion of T waves on electrocardiogram. A QTc interval greater than 0.50 and development of concave ST segments are ominous signs. A patient has been described with QT prolongation and syncopal episodes related to torsades de pointes after treatment of visceral leishmaniasis with meglumine antimonate (13).

Antimony metal occupational exposure may yield a silicosis-like pneumoconiosis and cardiomyopathy. Workers exposed for 9 to 31 years to dust containing a mixture of antimony trioxide and pentoxide in an antimony smelting plant exhibited chronic cough, bronchitis, emphysema, conjunctivitis, staining of teeth, inactive tuberculosis, and pleural adhesions (14).

Metal fume fever, characterized by chills, fever, cough, sweating, myalgia, headache, weakness, dyspnea, and nausea, may be caused by antimony (Chapter 20). Dermatitis is a well-known complication of occupational antimonial dust exposures (15). One study investigating the immunologic consequences of occupational exposure suggests that antimony disturbs immunohomeostasis in humans observed as aberrant serum cytokine and immunoglobulin levels, which could influence health (16).

DIAGNOSTIC TESTS

Antimony levels may be determined by atomic absorption spectrophotometry. Normal serum values for antimony are 0.05 to 0.50 mg/dl. As leukopenia and pancreatitis may be associated with meglumine antimonate, a baseline complete blood cell count, liver function tests, and amylase should be obtained when initiating therapy. A complete blood cell count and lactate dehydrogenase should be obtained on any potential exposures to stibine gas. A chest radiograph, electrocardiogram, and pulmonary function tests may define pneumoconiosis or cardiomyopathy after prolonged occupational exposures to antimonials.

TREATMENT

Due to its slow rate of absorption, treatment of acute antimony ingestion includes gastric lavage, which may be useful several hours after ingestion. Repeated activated charcoal administration may be useful, although it is unlikely that clinically significant adsorption occurs.

Dialysis may theoretically be useful in removing pentavalent antimony; however, this method of elimination has not been tested in humans.

The role of exchange transfusion is not clear, but may be useful in severe stibine gas exposure with hemolysis. Hydration and monitoring of electrolytes is also vital in treating hemolysis secondary to stibine gas exposure.

ANTIDOTES

Chelation with British antilewisite for serious antimony poisoning is recommended, as in arsenic intoxication. Dimercaptosuccinic acid and dimercaptopropane sulfonic acid have been proposed for the treatment of antimony intoxicants (17). There is no evidence that British antilewisite is useful for stibine gas exposure (18).

REFERENCES

1. Lauwers LF, Roelants A, Rosseel PM, et al. Oral antimony intoxications in man. *Crit Care Med* 1990;18:324–325.
2. de Wolff FA. Antimony and health incriminating stibine in the sudden infant death syndrome is difficult in current evidence. *BMJ* 1995;310:1216–1217.
3. Berman JD. Chemotherapy for leishmaniasis: biochemical mechanisms, clinical efficacy and future strategies. *Rev Infect Dis* 1988;10:560–586.
4. Herwaldt BL, Berman JD. Recommendations for treating leishmaniasis with sodium stibogluconate (Pentostam) and review of pertinent clinical studies. *Am J Trop Med Hyg* 1992;46:296–306.
5. Jones RD. Survey of antimony workers: mortality 1961–1992. *Occup Environ Med* 1994;51:772–776.
6. Schnorr TM, Steenland K, Thun MJ, Rinsky RA. Mortality in a cohort of antimony smelter workers. *Am J Indust Med* 1995;27:759–770.
7. Molokhia MM, Smith H. The behavior of antimony in blood. *J Trop Med Hyg* 1969,72:222–225.
8. Bailly R, Lauwerys R, Buchet JP, et al. Experimental and human studies on antimony metabolism: their relevance for the biological monitoring of workers exposed to inorganic antimony. *Br J Ind Med* 1991;48:93–97.
9. Beljaeva AP. The effect of antimony on reproductive function. *Gig Truda Professional'nye Zabolevanija* 1967;11(1):32–37.
10. Robbins A. Stibine, NIOSH Current Intelligence Bulletin 32. *Vet Hum Toxicol* 1980;22:108–109.
11. Jolliffe DS. Nephrotoxicity of pentavalent antimonials. *Lancet* 1985;1:584.
12. Delgado J, Macias J, Pineda JA, Corzo JE. High frequency of serious side effects from meglumine antimonate given without an upper limit dose for the treatment of visceral leishmaniasis in human immunodeficiency virus type-1-infected patients. *Am J Trop Med Hyg* 1999;61:766–769.
13. Ortega-Carnicer J, Alcazar R, De la Torre M, Benezet J. Pentavalent antimonial-induced torsade de pointes. *J Electrocardiol* 1997;30:143–145.
14. International Agency for Research on Cancer. Some organic solvents, resin monomers and related compounds, pigments and occupational exposures in paint manufacture and painting. *IARC Monogr Eval Carcinog Risks Hum* 1989;47:291–305.
15. White GP, Mathias CG, Davin JS. Dermatitis in workers exposed to antimony in a melting process. *J Occup Med* 1993;35(4):392–395.
16. Kim HA, Heo Y, Oh SY, et al. Altered serum cytokine and immunoglobulin levels in the workers exposed to antimony. *Hum Exper Toxicol* 1999;18(10):607–613.
17. Aaseth J. Recent advances in therapy of metal poisoning with chelating agents. *Hum Toxicol* 1983;2:257–272.
18. Teisinger J. BAL. In: *Occupational health and safety Vol. 1.* New York: McGraw-Hill, 1976:154.

CHAPTER 213

Arsenic and Arsine Gas

E. Martin Caravati

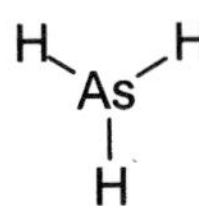

ARSINE

Atomic symbol, atomic number, molecular weight:	**As, 33, 74.92 g/mol**
Valence states:	**0, +3, +5**
CAS Registry No.:	**See Table 1.**
Normal levels:	**Serum less than 5 μg/L; 24-hour urine less than 50 μg/L**
SI conversion:	**μg/L × 13.35 = nmol/L**
Target organs:	**Acute: gastrointestinal tract, heart, peripheral nervous system; chronic: cancer**
Antidotes:	**Dimercaprol, dimercapto-propanesulfonate, succimer**

OVERVIEW

Arsenic is a metalloid that has three oxidation states and forms numerous compounds (Table 1). A wide range of toxicity occurs, depending on the compound, duration of exposure, and dose involved. The trivalent form (arsenite) is considered more toxic. In general, the insoluble salts of arsenic (arsenic trioxide, lead arsenate) and organic alkane arsenates are less toxic than the soluble inorganic arsenic compounds (sodium arsenite, arsenic acid, arsenious acid).

Arsine (AsH_3) is the most potent hemolytic agent encountered in industry and may produce severe anemia and acute renal failure. Exposure is through inhalation. The onset of hemolysis may be delayed up to 24 hours. Delayed peripheral neuropathy from arsine has been reported.

Classification and Uses

Arsenic exposure arises from a remarkable variety of sources (Table 2). Arsenic trioxide [As_2O_3 (Trisenox)] is used as an antineoplastic agent. Organic and inorganic arsenic react with iron and clay in the soil to form insoluble complexes. However, arsenic can leach into the surface water from mine tailings, metal smelters, and soft brown coal combustion. Groundwater has fewer detoxification mechanisms, and the more toxic arsenite can accumulate. Deep wells that tap groundwater contaminated with arsenic provide a source for chronic exposure. Large epidemics of chronic arsenic poisoning from groundwater wells have occurred in Bangladesh, West Bengal (1), Taiwan, Chile, Mexico, Pakistan, and China. Other regions where arsenic well-water contamination is a concern include Argentina, Alaska, and parts of the United States. Arsenic is ingested either by direct consumption of well water or by foods cooked in the water. Bathing is unlikely to be a significant source of exposure in adults.

The average adult consumes less than 1 μg/kg/day of arsenic in the diet. The two most commonly found organic, nontoxic forms of arsenic in food are arsenobetaine and arsenocholine. These organic compounds are found in shellfish, cod, and haddock. Freshwater fish contain up to 2 mg/kg, and lobster contain up to 22 mg/kg. A high-exposure group in Mexico, with average drinking water concentrations of 410 μg/L, was estimated to have a total arsenic daily intake of 12.3 to 16.6 μg/kg. Cooked food accounted for 33% to 44% of the daily intake (1a).

Chromated copper arsenate (CCA)–treated wood for residential purposes contains 2000 to 3000 mg/kg [parts per million (ppm)] arsenic. Soil beneath CCA-treated decks may contain elevated levels of arsenic (2). Hand-to-mouth activity is a potential exposure pathway for children playing in these areas. There are no reports of childhood poisoning from this source, however. The use of sealants can reduce "dislodgeable" arsenic from CCA-treated wood. By 2004, CCA-treated wood should no longer be used to manufacture new residential structures. Burning of CCA-treated wood should be avoided in fireplaces and wood stoves.

Arsenic has been found in association with various folk remedies from India and China. Herbal balls (mixtures of herbs and honey rolled into a ball) imported from China were found to have 0.1 to 36.6 mg of arsenic per ball. The recommended dose is 2 balls/day in warm sine or tea, which may contain up to 73 mg of arsenic (3).

Arsine (hydrogen arsenide, arsenous hydride, arsenic trihydride) is a colorless, flammable, nonirritating gas that evolves from arsenic compounds on addition of an acid (4). The odor threshold is 0.5 ppm and garlic-like and does not provide adequate warning to prevent toxicity from chronic exposure. The vapor density is 2.7 times that of air. Most cases of exposure result from reduction of an inorganic arsenic salt to arsine in the use of acids and metals. Arsine production is facilitated in the presence of zinc. Strong acid and zinc generate nascent hydrogen that reduces arsenic compounds to arsine:

$$As_2O_3 + 6Zn + 12H^+ \rightarrow 2AsH_3 + 3H_2O + 6Zn^{2+}$$

Toxic Dose

Regulatory guidelines and standards for arsenic are provided in Table 3.

ACUTE POISONING

The acute minimum lethal dose in adults is 70 to 200 mg or 1 mg/kg/day. Less than 1 mg/kg of inorganic arsenic can cause serious illness in children. The ingestion of 9 to 14 mg of arsenic trioxide by a 16-month-old child produced significant signs of poisoning, which required chelation therapy (5). A 22-month-old girl ingested 1 oz of 2.27% sodium arsenate ant killer (0.047 mg/kg) and developed vomiting, diarrhea, and lethargy within 30 minutes (6).

Cases of "trivial" exposure to sodium arsenate in an ant killer (As^{5+}) may cause significantly elevated levels of arsenic in a 24-

TABLE 1. Inorganic and organic arsenic compounds relevant to human health

Chemical name	CAS Registry No.	Synonyms and molecular formula	Physical properties (valence state)	Industrial use or biologic occurrence
Arsine	7784-42-1	Arsine,[a] arsenic trihydride, hydrogen arsenide; AsH_3	Colorless, neutral gas; slightly WS (–3)	Organic synthesis; solid-state electronic components; by-product of metal smelting
Arsenic (elemental)	7440-38-2	Gray arsenic, metallic arsenic; As	Gray, shiny, brittle, metallic-looking rhombohedra; WI (0)	Alloys in order to increase hardness and heat resistance
Arsenic trichloride	7784-34-1	Butter of arsenic; $AsCl_3$	Yellowish, oily liquid; WS; decomposes (+3)	Pottery industry; manufacturing of chlorine-containing arsenicals
Arsenic trioxide	1327-53-3	Diarsenic oxide, white arsenic, arsenic sesquioxide, arsenious anhydride; As_2O_3	White, amorphous, or crystalline powder; odorless and tasteless; slowly WS; combines with water to form arsenious acid (+3.	Manufacturing of glass; insecticide; rodenticide; antineoplastic agent
Sodium arsenite	7784-46-5	Arsenious acid, H_3AsO_3; sodium salt, $NaAsO_2$; arsenious acid sodium; metaarsenite	White or grayish hygroscopic powder; very WS (+3)	Veterinary use; insecticide; wood preservative; used in combination with other salts, such as calcium arsenite, lead arsenite, cupric acetoarsenite
Arsenic pentoxide	1303-28-2	Arsenic oxide, arsenic acid, arsenic anhydride; As_2O_5	White, amorphous, deliquescent powder; freely WS; combines with water to form arsenic acid (+5)	Manufacturing of colored glass; insecticide; wood preservative
Lead arsenate	7784-40-9	Arsenic acid, H_3AsO_4; lead (+2) salt; acid lead arsenate; arsenate of lead approximately $PbHAsO_4$	Heavy, white powder; WI; on heating, emits toxic fumes (+5)	Constituent of various insecticides also with other salts; calcium arsenate; sodium arsenate; potassium arsenate
Methylarsonic acid	2163-80-6	Arsenic acid, methylmono-sodium salt, methanearsonic acid, monosodium salt, sodium methylarsonate, sodium methanearsonate; $CH_3AsO(OH)ONa$	White powder; WS	Constituent of various pesticides also as mixture with methylarsonic acid disodium salt; excretion product of mammalian metabolism
Dimethylarsinic acid sodium salt	124-65-2	Arsenic acid, dimethyl-sodium salt, cacodylic acid sodium salt, sodium cacodylate, sodium dimethylarsinate, arsine oxide, hydrosymethylsodium salt; $(CH_3)_2AsO(ONa)$	Colorless crystals; hygroscopic; WS; slightly soluble in ethanol	Constituent of various pesticides; excretion product of mammalian metabolism
Trimethylarsine	593-88-4	Gosio gas; $As(CH_3)_3$	Colorless, neutral gas; slightly WS; decomposes	Produced after metabolic transformation of arsenic compounds by bacteria and fungi, especially in sewage
Arsanilic acid	98-50-0	4-aminobenzenearsonic acid, aminophenylarsine; $NH_2C_6H_4\text{-}AsO(OH)_2$	White, crystalline powder; WS	Stimulator of growth of food-producing animals
Arsenobetaine	—	$(CH_3)_3As^+CH_2COOH$	WS	Organic arsenical compound in marine organisms, "fish arsenic"
Arsenocholine	—	$(CH_3)_3As^+CH_2CH_2OH$	WS	Organic arsenical compound in marine organisms, "fish arsenic"

WI, water insoluble; WS, water soluble.
[a]Chemical abstracts service name.

hour urine collection (range, 3500 to 5300 µg/L). A trivial exposure in an asymptomatic child may have a significant medical risk of arsenic poisoning (7). In 149 calls to a poison center for unintentional exposure, single, low-dose (less than 5 ml) pentavalent arsenate ingestions (less than 3%) of sodium arsenate ant killers were associated with little toxicity. No serum or urine concentrations were obtained, however (8). These products were banned in 1989.

Arsine causes death immediately at 150 to 250 ppm. Exposure to 25 to 50 ppm for 30 minutes or 100 ppm for less than 30 minutes results in extensive hemolysis and death. Symptoms may occur with concentrations as low as 0.15 to 1.50 ppm (0.5 to 5.0 mg/m^3) (9). Exposure to 10 ppm has produced delirium and coma. No pediatric toxicity data are available.

CHRONIC POISONING

The lowest arsenic concentration in drinking water in Bangladesh found to produce dermatologic disease was 103 µg/L (10). There is debate about the toxic threshold for arsenic in drinking water. The frequency of cancerous effects clearly increases at 400 µg/day. Increased mortality from prostate cancer was associated with concentrations of 14 to 166 µg/L in one

TABLE 2. Sources of arsenic

Natural
- Mining release into air, water, and soil
- Fish
- Bivalves
- Seaweed
- Wine
- Some meats and poultry

Industrial
- Clarifier in glass industry
- Wood preservative (copper arsenite)
- Semiconductors (gallium arsenide)
- Desiccants and defoliants
- Cattle and sheep dips
- Smelting of nonferrous metals
- Pigments
- Rodenticides
- Pesticides

Medicinal and herbal
- Arsenic trioxide [As_2O_3 (Trisenox)]
- Fowler's solution (potassium arsenite; discontinued)
- Some Chinese proprietary medicines
- Folk herbal medicines from India and China

Other
- Ironite fertilizer
- Some ceramic glazes
- Python-brand "black snakes" Chinese fireworks
- Museum artifacts preserved with arsenic
- Moonshine
- Opium
- Residential herbicides

TABLE 3. U.S. regulatory guidelines and standards for arsenic (As)

Agency	Description	Concentration
OSHA	Arsenic and inorganic compounds	
(air)	PEL-TWA	10.00 μg/m^3 (as As)
	STEL	None
	Arsenic and organic compounds	
	PEL-TWA	500.00 μg/m^3 (as As)
	STEL	None
	Arsine gas	
	PEL-TWA	0.20 μg/m^3 (0.05 ppm)
	STEL	—
ACGIH	Arsenic and inorganic compounds	
(air)	TLV-TWA	10.00 μg/m^3 (as As)
	STEL	None
	Arsine gas	
	TLV-TWA	0.20 μg/m^3 (0.05 ppm)
	STEL	None
NIOSH	Arsenic	
(air)	REL-Ceiling	2.00 μg/m^3
	STEL	None
	IDLH	5000.00 μg/m^3 (as As)
	Arsine	
	REL-Ceiling	2.00 μg/m^3
	IDLH	9.56 μg/m^3 (3.00 ppm)
EPA	Drinking water standard	10.00 μg/L
FDA	Byproducts of animals treated with veterinary drugs	0.50–2.00 ppm

ACGIH, American Conference of Governmental Industrial Hygienists; EPA, Environmental Protection Agency; FDA, U.S. Food and Drug Administration; IDLH, immediate danger to life or health; NIOSH, National Institute for Occupational Safety and Health; OSHA, U.S. Occupational Safety and Health Administration; PEL, permissible exposure limit; ppm, parts per million; REL, recommended exposure limit; STEL, short-term exposure limit; TLV, threshold limit value; TWA, time-weighted average.

study and appeared to be dose related (11). The National Research Council estimates that a lifetime exposure to drinking water with 10 μg/L of arsenic increases the risk of bladder cancer (12).

TOXICOKINETICS AND TOXICODYNAMICS

Arsenic is readily absorbed via the oral, inhalation, and parenteral routes. Dermal absorption can occur via mucous membranes or abraded skin. The bioavailability for soluble arsenic compounds is 60% to 90% via ingestion or inhalation. Peak serum levels are reached in 60 minutes. Once absorbed, arsenic is distributed to the liver, kidney, muscle, skin, hair, and nails where it binds to sulfhydryl groups. Only small amounts of arsenic cross the blood–brain barrier. Arsenic replaces phosphorus in the bone where it may remain for years. The volume of distribution is 0.2 L/kg.

Pentavalent and trivalent arsenic are interconverted by redox reactions *in vivo*. Most pentavalent arsenic (arsenate) is rapidly reduced by glutathione to the more toxic trivalent species after absorption. "Detoxification" of trivalent arsenic occurs via methylation to monomethylarsenate (MMA) and dimethylarsenate (DMA) primarily in the liver. MMA and DMA are less reactive with tissues than inorganic arsenic and are considered less toxic. Intermediate reduced forms of the methylated metabolites [MMA(III), DMA(III)], which are toxic, have also been detected in the urine.

Large doses of arsenic may overwhelm the methylation process and result in higher levels of the parent compounds and increased tissue deposition. Within 48 hours of acute exposure, 60% to 70% of inorganic arsenic is excreted in the urine as the methylated compounds; 90% is excreted in the urine within 6 days. Urine concentrations remain high for longer periods after chronic exposure. The distribution of urinary arsenic is approximately 10% to 30% inorganic, 10% to 20% MMA, and 60% to 80% DMA (13). With normal renal function, up to 100 mg of arsenic can be excreted daily. Small amounts are excreted in the sweat, feces, and bile. The half-life of inorganic arsenic in blood is approximately 2 hours. The half-life of the methylated metabolites is 5 to 20 hours in urine.

Seafood contains variable amounts of arsenobetaine and arsenocholine, organic arsenic compounds that are nontoxic and rapidly excreted in the urine. No residual toxic metabolites are present. Seaweed and some bivalve mollusks contain arsenosugars that are partly metabolized to dimethylarsinic acid and excreted in the urine. The half-life of organic arsenic is 4 to 6 hours. Total urinary clearance is within 2 days.

Arsine is rapidly absorbed by inhalation, distributed throughout the body, and excreted in the urine. Data on the volume of distribution and elimination half-life of arsine in humans are not available. Elemental arsenic is poorly soluble and considered to have low toxicity.

PATHOPHYSIOLOGY

General Mechanisms

The toxicity of arsenic depends on its form (organic vs. inorganic), valence state, and solubility. Trivalent arsenic is more toxic than pentavalent. Trivalent compounds [arsenite (As^{3+})] bind to sulfhydryl groups and inhibit many enzymatic pathways, including glycolysis, pyruvate dehydrogenase, and the tricarboxylic acid (Krebs) cycle, which results in decreased production of adenosine triphosphate. The arsenates (As^{5+}) replace phosphate molecules ("arsenolysis") and uncouple mitochondrial oxidative phosphorylation. They do not bind thiol groups and are not incorporated into hair or nails.

Arsine causes red blood cell hemolysis by an unknown mechanism. It has been suggested that the oxidation of arsine to arsenic trioxide denatures erythrocyte proteins and causes cell lysis. Other mechanisms of hemolysis may include inhibition of catalase and production of hydrogen peroxide within the cell (14). Arsine is oxidized to trivalent arsenic and arsenous oxide, both human carcinogens.

Gastrointestinal

Arsenic causes dilation of splanchnic vessels and submucosal vesicle formation. Rupture of these vesicles leads to rice-water stools and bleeding. Subsequently, a protein-losing enteropathy may develop. Mucosal inflammation and necrosis of the stomach and small bowel wall can also occur.

Cardiovascular

Fluid loss through capillary leak and diarrhea can lead to hypovolemic shock. Large doses of arsenic can cause QT prolongation, but the mechanism is unclear. Hypokalemia and hypomagnesemia may predispose patients on As_2O_3 chemotherapy to ventricular tachycardia and torsade de pointes (15).

Metabolic and Hepatic

Arsenic is associated with a negative nitrogen balance, hepatic fatty degeneration, central necrosis and cirrhosis, noncirrhotic portal fibrosis, and antagonism of thyroid hormone.

Peripheral Nervous System

Arsenic causes an axonopathy.

Kidney

Renal tubular damage from precipitation of hemoglobin often results in severe renal failure. Arsine may also have a direct toxic effect on the kidney.

VULNERABLE POPULATIONS

Arsenic is U.S. Food and Drug Administration pregnancy category D (arsenic trioxide). Inorganic arsenic crosses the placenta in animals. Teratogenicity has been demonstrated in animals with oral arsenic trioxide and parenteral sodium arsenite. Chronic exposure to high levels of arsenic in drinking water (200 µg/L) is associated with clinically insignificant levels of arsenic in the breast milk (2.3 µg/kg) (16).

A 22-year-old woman at 20 weeks of gestation ingested 340 mg of sodium arsenate. The initial 24-hour urinary arsenic level was 3030 µg/L. Dimercaprol was administered. Fetal heart tones were normal. A healthy infant was delivered at 36 weeks. At birth, 24-hour urinary arsenic levels were less than 50 µg/L in the infant and less than 100 µg/L in the mother. Another case of maternal arsenic ingestion at 30 weeks of gestation resulted in infant death shortly after birth. Arsenic-poisoned pregnant patients have been treated with dimercaprol [British antilewisite (BAL)] and succimer. D-Penicillamine has been associated with teratogenicity (17).

Patients with hematologic malignancies and baseline QT prolongation, hypokalemia, or hypomagnesemia are at increased risk for torsade de pointes or sudden death during treatment with As_2O_3.

ADVERSE EFFECTS

Therapeutic use of As_2O_3 can produce electrocardiographic changes: T wave inversion, T wave alternans, second degree heart block, complete heart block, and QT prolongation. As many as 40% of patients develop a QTc greater than 500 milliseconds (18). Torsade de pointes occurred in 3 of 19 patients receiving As_2O_3 (10 to 20 mg/kg/day) for hematologic malignancies on day 12, 16, and 42 of treatment. Each had normal QTc intervals that became prolonged before the dysrhythmia. Hypokalemia and hypomagnesemia may have contributed to the dysrhythmia (15). Sudden unexplained death occurred in three of ten patients being treated for refractory acute promyelocytic leukemia (19).

Distal polyneuropathy, palmar keratosis, and skin hyperpigmentation occurred in two patients receiving maintenance As_2O_3 chemotherapy at cumulative doses of 280 and 560 mg (20).

CLINICAL PRESENTATION

A detailed clinical history should include occupation, location of residence, source of drinking water, dietary habits (seafood), medications, herbal remedies, hobbies (use of art supplies, pesticides in gardening), and type of wood use in fireplaces or wood stoves. The diagnosis is based on clinical manifestations of poisoning and confirmatory laboratory testing.

Acute and Subacute Exposure

The hallmark of exposure is acute gastrointestinal (GI) illness followed by a sensorimotor peripheral neuropathy. Most patients with an acute ingestion present with acute onset of vomiting, diarrhea, and weakness that may be followed by cardiovascular instability. GI symptoms are less severe in smaller, subacute ingestions (e.g., nutritional or homicidal cases). Peripheral neuropathy is typically delayed days to weeks, begins distally, and ascends in a stocking-glove distribution. It may progress for up to 6 weeks postexposure. Neurologic recovery is prolonged and incomplete. The source of exposure is often not discovered.

General effects of arsenic poisoning include lethargy, weakness, irritability, hypovolemia, and dehydration. Dermal effects include facial edema, delayed-onset desquamation of palms and soles, Mees' lines (uncommon, transverse white lines across nails, representing growth disruption and not arsenic deposition), and keratosis.

GI toxicity includes nausea, vomiting, abdominal pain, and severe watery diarrhea within a few hours of ingestion. Pulmonary effects are acute respiratory distress syndrome and pulmonary edema. Cardiovascular toxicity includes hypovolemic shock, tachycardia, prolonged QT interval, and dysrhythmias.

Renal effects include acute renal tubular necrosis and acidosis, renal insufficiency, proteinuria, hematuria, and oliguria. Hematologic effects are leukocytosis, basophilic stippling, and anemia. Muscle toxicity involves myalgia and rhabdomyolysis. Nervous system toxicity includes confusion, seizures, coma, encephalopathy, and muscle weakness progressing to quadriplegia. Peripheral neuropathy may occur with a latent period of days to weeks and begin with a tingling or "pins and needles" sensation in the hands or feet. The cranial nerves are not affected.

In arsine gas exposure, the onset of symptoms ranges from 2 to 24 hours after exposure. Initial symptoms are nausea, vomiting, and abdominal pain followed hours later by signs of hemolysis. The classic triad is abdominal pain, dark urine, and jaundice. The following signs and symptoms may occur: generalized weakness and malaise, icteric sclera, jaundice, tachycardia, hypotension, nausea, vomiting, abdominal pain, Coombs'-negative hemolytic anemia, dark urine, hemoglobinuria, flank pain, oliguria, anuria, dyspnea, pulmonary edema, and acute oliguric renal failure, which may be reversible over several weeks (21,22).

Neurologic effects of arsine include headache, altered mental status, coma in severe cases, and peripheral sensorimotor neuropathy similar to that observed with inorganic arsenic, which may be delayed 1 to 6 months after exposure (23).

Chronic Exposure

Clinical manifestations vary greatly among patients with similar exposures. Skin lesions, neuropathy, and carcinomas are late findings. Onset of symptoms is dose dependent with a usual latency of weeks to months for neurologic symptoms and years for skin lesions. The majority of patients present with gradual onset of peripheral neuropathy, accompanied by headache, skin changes, and alopecia.

General manifestations include malaise, weakness, anorexia, weight loss, and metallic taste. Skin effects are "raindrops on a dusty road" pigmentation (melanosis) of the trunk and extremities; hyperpigmentation of the tongue, oral mucosa, axilla, groin, and temples; hyperkeratosis of palms and soles (Fig. 1) that are wart-like in texture; alopecia (late); and brittle fingernails and Mees' lines (uncommon). Skin malignancies include intraepidermal (Bowen's disease), basal cell, and squamous cell carcinomas.

Nervous system effects include headache, confusion, dysesthesia, sensory and motor peripheral neuropathy in a stocking-glove distribution, mild dementia, muscular weakness of the extremities, muscle atrophy, and ataxia. Cranial nerves are normal.

Diarrhea and constipation have both been reported. Noncirrhotic portal hypertension, hepatomegaly, and angiosarcoma may develop.

Cough and lung carcinoma secondary to chronic inhalation of high levels of arsenic dust may occur. Cardiovascular manifestations include coronary artery disease, hypertension, and peripheral vascular disease (see Blackfoot Disease).

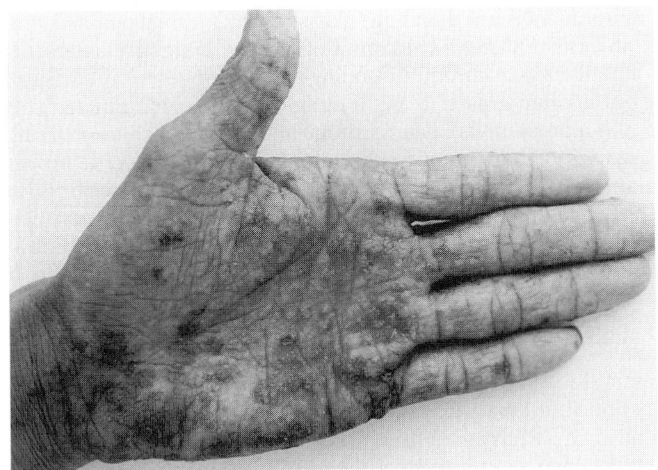

Figure 1. Arsenic keratosis of palms.

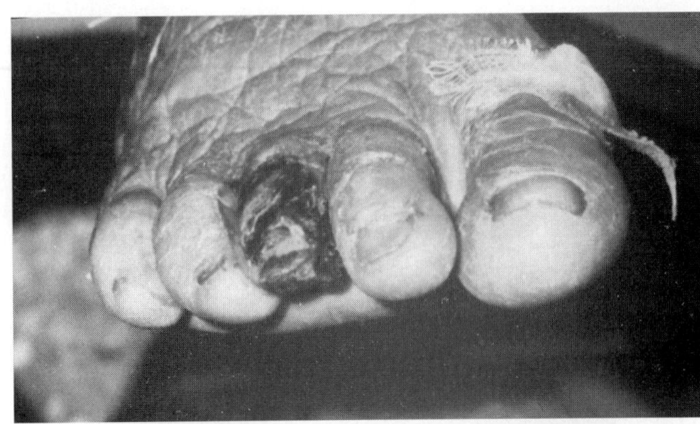

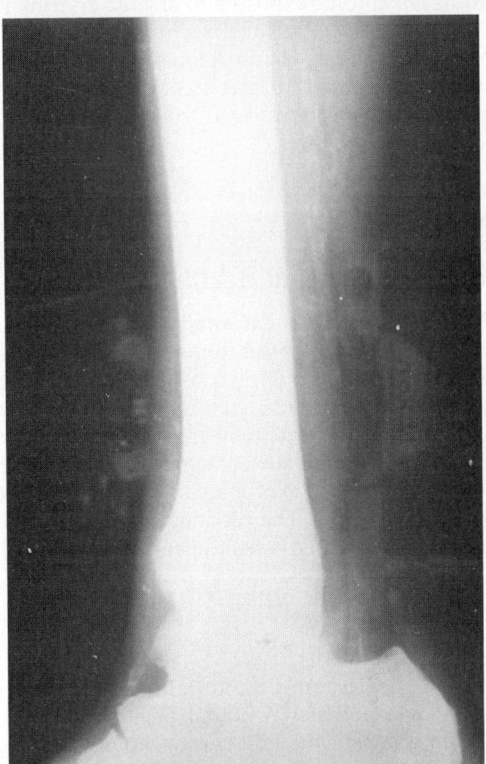

Figure 2. A: Gangrene and autoamputation in patient with blackfoot disease. **B:** Artificial calcifications in leg radiograph of patient with blackfoot disease.

Normocytic or macrocytic anemia, leukopenia, pancytopenia, and basophilic stippling of erythrocytes may develop. Genitourinary effects include carcinoma of the bladder and kidney.

Chronic, low-dose exposure to arsine gas has been associated with anemia, which is proportional to the duration of exposure.

Blackfoot Disease

Blackfoot disease is a unique peripheral vascular disease of the lower extremities that occurs in an area of chronic arsenicosis on the southwest coast of Taiwan. The disease progresses from distal numbness to intermittent claudication, gangrene, and spontaneous amputation (Fig. 2). The incidence of blackfoot disease decreased more than tenfold after bottled water was supplied to the endemic villages (24).

Blackfoot disease appears to be dose dependent and highly associated with the skin manifestations of chronic arsenicosis. The average well-water arsenic concentration ranged from 700 to 930 μg/L in the area. It is estimated that the average daily intake of arsenic by residents of the endemic areas is 1 mg (normal dietary intake is less than 1 μg/kg/day). In addition to arsenic, ergot alkaloids, organic chorines, and humic acid have been identified in the well water of the villages. Nutritional deficiencies, hypertension, and diabetes mellitus may also explain the increased risk of peripheral vascular disease in this population. The induction period is 20 to 30 years. Platelet activation, hypercoagulability, endothelial injury, oxidative stress, and apoptosis may play a role in the pathogenesis. Arteriosclerosis obliterans is present in 70% of patients.

Carcinogenesis

Inorganic arsenic is classified as a human carcinogen. Epidemiologic studies of chronic exposure to arsenic in drinking water suggest that arsenic causes skin, liver, lung, kidney, and bladder cancer. Multiple types of skin cancer may be present at the same time, and the prevalence is dose related. Lung cancer in workers was associated with arsenic trioxide from smelters and pentavalent arsenic from pesticides.

DIAGNOSTIC TESTS

Biologic Monitoring and Health Surveillance

Because hair is subject to external contamination, urinary arsenic is most frequently used to monitor occupational exposure. Dietary sources need to be considered, and care must be taken to avoid contamination from environmental dust, clothing, or skin. The arsenic level most likely to be observed after a 40-hour work-week exposure (Biological Exposure Indexes value) is 50 μg/g creatinine of inorganic arsenic metabolites in end-of-work-week urine. The carcinogen exposure equivalent (EKA) is 50 μg/L inorganic arsenic at end of shift (25).

Acute Exposure

BLOOD ARSENIC LEVEL

A blood arsenic level is rarely useful because of its short half-life in the blood (approximately 2 hours). Serum arsenic levels are detectable only during the first several hours after ingestion. Normal blood levels vary depending on diet and environmental exposure. Serum concentrations range from 3 to 5 μg/L (less than 0.665 μmol/L) in communities with normal arsenic levels in the drinking water. Blood levels averaged 13 μg/L in a community with 393 μg/L arsenic in the drinking water (25).

OTHER LABORATORY TESTS

Anemia, pancytopenia, basophilic stippling, elevated hepatic transaminases, elevated creatine kinase, renal insufficiency, and electrolyte disturbances may be observed.

URINARY ARSENIC LEVEL

The urine contains methylated forms of arsenic that can usually be detected for at least 1 to 3 days after exposure. Large, chronic exposures can be detected in the urine for longer than 96 hours postexposure. "Spot" urine determinations are helpful if elevated but are not a reliable method of determining an elevated body load of arsenic. Twenty-four-hour urine collections are more accurate and may remain elevated for several weeks after exposure. In order to determine whether urinary arsenic is from a toxic (inorganic) or nontoxic (organic, seafood) source, it must be speciated into inorganic and organic fractions.

Urinary As^{3+} and As^{5+} levels are present at approximately 10 hours and return to normal in 20 to 30 hours after exposure. Monomethylarsine and dimethylarsine predominate more than 24 hours after ingestion, peak at 40 to 60 hours, and return to baseline within 6 to 20 days. The half-life of the methylated metabolites is 5 to 20 hours. The presence of dimethylarsinic acid can represent either inorganic or arsenosugar ingestion (26). The latter is present in some seaweed and shellfish and is nontoxic.

ABDOMINAL RADIOGRAPH

Inorganic arsenic is radiopaque, similar to barium, and may be visible on radiograph after acute ingestion.

ELECTROCARDIOGRAM

Prolonged QT interval, abnormal T waves, ventricular bigeminy (27), ventricular tachycardia, ventricular fibrillation, and torsade de pointes may occur.

Chronic Exposure

URINARY ARSENIC LEVEL

Within 4 hours of a seafood meal, urine total arsenic concentrations may be 200 to 1700 μg/L. A common standard for normal is less than 50 μg/L or 25 μg/24 hours of urine in the absence of a seafood diet. Urine levels greater than 200 μg/L are abnormal. Occupational exposure to arsenic trioxide dust resulted in urine concentrations ranging from 20 to 2000 μg/L (25). Residents of Mexico with chronic arsenic poisoning from drinking water averaged urine concentrations of 207 μg/g creatinine inorganic arsenic, 95 μg/g creatinine methylarsonic acid, and 338 μg/g creatinine dimethylarsinic acid (28).

HAIR ARSENIC

Arsenic is deposited in hair after ingestion. It is also deposited by external contamination from water, dust, and cosmetic powders. The source of hair arsenic cannot be determined reliably by examining the hair in cross-section. Both systemically absorbed and externally contaminated arsenic is found throughout the cross-section of hair. External contamination of hair by arsenic is not easily removed by washing. Hair analysis for arsenic is a semireliable method for confirming chronic toxicity. Within 30 hours of ingestion, inorganic arsenic deposits in the hair. Organic arsenic from seafood is not deposited in hair. Arsenic levels in hair are very difficult to interpret because arsenic content varies widely among individual hairs and within the same hair, and there is high interindividual variation in adsorption of arsenic to hair (29).

Normal hair arsenic for people living in a noncontaminated environment is less than 1 μg/g dry weight. Normal people living in an industrial area have a range of 0.02 to 8.17 μg/g. Hair arsenic for patients with chronic poisoning usually ranges from 1 to 5 μg/g but is often greater than 10 μg/g. Arsenic-contaminated soft coal is a problem in Eastern Europe and Asia, and children living downwind from arsenic-contaminated soft coal electric power plants had hair levels up to 10 μg/g. Washing one's hair with arsenic-contaminated water results in significant hair adsorption of arsenic. External contamination has resulted in hair concentrations from 5 μg/g to greater than 1000 μg/g. The degree of poisoning does not correlate well with hair arsenic levels (29).

Arsenic peaks on hair may be indicative of dates of ingestion based on the length from growth site, but this can be unreliable. Variable uptake, in addition to intermittent dosing, may be responsible for distinct peaks along the shaft. Arsenic is also found in sweat, which may contaminate the hair along its length. Hair may not adsorb arsenic from external contamination in an even distribution along the shaft (29).

FINGERNAIL ARSENIC

Arsenic can enter fingernails from the blood or external contamination. There are a paucity of data on the implication of nail arsenic. The average concentration in nails of 50 trauma victims was 0.252 μg/g. Normal is considered less than 1 μg/g (30).

ELECTROMYOGRAPHY

Nerve conduction studies may demonstrate velocity slowing, indicating a distal sensory and motor axonal neuropathy. However, their role in diagnosis is uncertain. Nerve conduction studies were not specific for arsenic neuropathy in a study of 145 patients exposed to arsenic-contaminated well water. Water concentrations ranged from 1 to 4781 μg/L, and urine levels ranged from 6 to 4964 μg/L. Five of six patients with clinical sensory neuropathy had normal nerve conduction velocities. Thirteen patients with elevated arsenic ingestion but no signs of neuropathy had an abnormal nerve conduction velocity (31).

Arsine Gas Exposure

Obtain a urinalysis, complete blood cell count, plasma-free hemoglobin, urine hemoglobin, serum electrolytes, blood urea nitrogen, creatinine, bilirubin, and blood type and screen. Blood and urine arsenic levels can document the occupational exposure but do not influence treatment.

Hematology tests may show Coombs'-negative hemolytic anemia and basophilic stippling (chronic exposure). The urinalysis has proteinuria, urobilinogen, bilirubinuria, red blood cell casts, and hemoglobinuria. Inhalation of arsine gas results in elevated blood and urine arsenic that is not predictive of outcome. Urine concentrations have ranged from 40 to 1900 μg/L in survivors and from 100 to 400 μg/L in three fatalities (25). Arsine air concentrations greater than 15.6 $\mu g/m^3$ (5 ppm) were associated with a urinary arsenic concentration greater than 50 μg/L (32).

Low-dose, chronic gas exposure may result in anemia and basophilic stippling of red blood cells.

Analytic Methods

The standard for arsenic analysis is atomic absorption spectroscopy, which measures total arsenic and does not distinguish among pentavalent, trivalent, or organic arsenic. Arsenic speciation commonly involves separation by liquid chromatography before atomic absorption analysis (30).

Postmortem Considerations

The hair of an individual who dies 6 to 8 hours after an acute ingestion of arsenic generally does not contain arsenic. A range of mean postmortem arsenic concentrations was found in a series of 49 deaths from arsenic overdose: blood, 3.3 mg/L (range, 0.6 to 9.3 mg/L); liver, 29 mg/kg (range, 2 to 120 mg/kg); kidney, 15 mg/kg (range, 0.2 to 70.0 mg/kg); and brain, 1.7 mg/kg (range, 0.2 to 4.0 mg/kg) (30).

Diagnostic Pitfalls

The diagnosis of chronic arsenic poisoning is based on clinical findings. The possibility of external contamination makes the hair arsenic level confirmatory rather than diagnostic. Total urinary arsenic is elevated after consumption of seafood, and patients should avoid seafood consumption for 3 to 4 days before testing. Patients who ingest large amounts of seaweed may have false-positive urine for inorganic arsenic (26).

The differential diagnosis of acute poisoning includes Guillain-Barré syndrome, thallium poisoning, lead poisoning, acute porphyria, marine toxins, and diabetic and alcoholic neuropathies.

TREATMENT

There are several chelating agents that enhance the elimination of arsenic from the body. The decision to chelate and which agent to use is complex and based on multiple factors. Consultation with a physician experienced in the treatment of arsenic poisoning (e.g., a medical toxicologist) or with a poison control center is advised before treatment.

Decontamination

Decontamination has a minor role is arsenic poisoning because acute ingestion often leads to repeated vomiting and chronic exposure has no arsenic available for removal. If arsenic is apparent radiographically in a patient who presents early and is not vomiting, gastric lavage theoretically has value. Activated charcoal does not adsorb inorganic arsenic (33).

Whole bowel irrigation with polyethylene glycol solution may enhance elimination of arsenic from the GI tract after acute ingestion (34). However, this has not been systematically studied. Repeat an abdominal radiograph after the procedure to assess its effectiveness and need for further therapy.

After skin exposure, the patient should be removed from the source of exposure. Contaminated clothing must be removed and double bagged. The skin is washed with soap and water.

In arsine gas areas, self-contained breathing apparatus, a full-face mask, protective clothing, and boots should be worn. Remove the patient from the source of exposure to fresh air. Wash the skin of the victim copiously with soap and water, and transport to a hospital.

Supportive Care

ACUTE OVERDOSE

Symptomatic patients should be hospitalized for stabilization. The acutely symptomatic patient should receive intravenous (IV) isotonic crystalloid fluid replacement for fluid loss. Continuous blood pressure and cardiac monitoring for assessment of potential hypotension, QT prolongation, and dysrhythmias should be instituted immediately. An abdominal radiograph should be obtained to assess the presence of radiopaque arsenic in the GI tract and the need for whole bowel irrigation. Hypokalemia and hypomagnesemia may predispose patients to ventricular tachycardia and torsade de pointes (15), and correction with supplemental potassium and magnesium is important. Quinidine and procainamide should be avoided because they also prolong the QT interval. Isoproterenol shortens the QT interval and may terminate the dysrhythmia. Overdrive pacing may be useful if medical therapy fails.

The reason and source of exposure in arsenic poisoning is often not revealed. A low threshold for psychiatric evaluation is warranted for nonenvironmental exposures. Hemodialysis may be required for renal failure. Disability due to irreversible neurologic dysfunction may require physical therapy, rehabilitation, and long-term care.

ARSINE GAS

Administer IV fluids, provide supplemental oxygen, and initiate cardiac monitoring. Acute hemolysis is treated with IV fluid resuscitation and urinary alkalinization (pH, 7.5 to 8.0) with sodium bicarbonate by adding 50 to 100 mEq to 1 L of 5% dextrose or half-normal saline. Administer IV fluids at a rate to maintain urine output at 2 to 3 cc/kg/hour. Prepare for hemodialysis in the event of renal failure. Severe anemia is treated with transfusion, especially if associated with cardiopulmonary compromise.

Enhancement of Elimination

Arsenic is rapidly cleared from the blood. Multiple-dose activated charcoal is not expected to enhance its elimination from the blood or tissue. Hemodialysis is indicated for enhancing the elimination of arsenic when renal failure is present. The hemodialysis clearance of arsenic is 75 to 87 ml/minute (35). A patient ingested 10 g of sodium arsenate and then developed cardiovascular collapse and anuria. Hemodialysis clearance of arsenic was 85 ml/minute without chelation and 87.5 ml/minute after dimercaprol was administered (36).

In arsine gas exposure, the primary target organ is the red blood cell. Exchange transfusion may eliminate red blood cells and hemoglobin complexed with arsenic. However, no improvement in long-term outcome has been demonstrated compared to regular red cell transfusions for anemia and hemodialysis for renal failure. Exchange transfusion may be considered when plasma free hemoglobin is greater than 1.5 g/dl or a rapid decline in hematocrit occurs. Hemodialysis is often needed for renal failure, hyperkalemia, and volume overload. It does not enhance elimination of arsenic unless renal failure occurs.

Antidotes

Chelation therapy can enhance the elimination of arsenic from the body. Its effectiveness appears to be time dependent. Chelation is expensive and may have serious adverse effects. The decision to institute chelation therapy should be made in conjunction with a medical toxicologist or poison control center. Evidence suggests that the effects of chronic arsenic poisoning do not respond to chelation therapy. Therefore, routine chelation therapy for this presentation without elevated urine arsenic levels is not indicated.

Indications for chelation include (a) severely symptomatic patients after a confirmed acute ingestion (severe diarrhea, hypotension, or abnormal cardiac conduction); therapy should not be delayed by pending blood or urine arsenic levels; (b) symptomatic patients with urinary arsenic greater than 50 μg/L; and (c) asymptomatic patients with a urinary arsenic greater than 200 μg/L.

Patients with significant GI symptoms should be started on a parenteral chelator [BAL or dimercapto-propanesulfonate (DMPS)]. They may be switched to an oral chelator once hemodynamically stable, and the GI tract is properly functioning.

For arsine gas, the major toxicity and cause of mortality is red cell hemolysis and not arsenic poisoning. Therefore, chelation is usually not warranted. It should be considered for extremely high serum or urine levels of arsenic (see the section Treatment).

Dimercaprol (BAL) is administered by deep intramuscular injection only. Details of administration and adverse effects are provided in Chapter 50. Severe poisoning is treated with 3 to 5 mg/kg every 4 to 6 hours for 48 hours, every 6 hours for the next 24 hours, and every 12 hours thereafter. The patient should be switched to an oral chelator (succimer, DMPS) when possible.

In adults, dimercaprol was reported to be of benefit in 10 of 11 cases of arsenic-induced agranulocytosis, with increases in total white blood cell count and greater increases in granulocytes. It was not effective in three cases of arsenic-induced aplastic anemia (37). It was associated with improvement in 70% to 80% of patients with arsenic-induced dermatitis, including the exfoliative type. Disease progression was halted, and healing was accelerated (37). Treatment of established neuropathy with BAL has not been successful (38). It has been suggested that neuropathy may be prevented if therapy is instituted within hours of exposure (39).

In children, dimercaprol was judged effective in a series of 42 children with acute, oral arsenic poisoning, compared with historic controls not treated with dimercaprol. The treatment resulted in a more rapid resolution of symptoms and decreased hospital stay (40).

DMPS (Dimaval, Unithol) is a water-soluble compound with a chemical structure similar to succimer and BAL. It forms a water-soluble complex with arsenic that is less likely to penetrate the central nervous system than the lipophilic BAL-arsenic complex (41). DMPS complexes with monomethlyarsonous acid, increases the urinary excretion of arsenic, and improves the clinical effects of chronic arsenic toxicity. DMPS has also been used as a diagnostic aid (a challenge or provocative test) to approximate the body burden of arsenic in patients suspected of arsenic exposure (42–47).

Details of DMPS administration and adverse effects are provided in Chapter 54. It is available as IV and oral preparations. The adult oral dose is 200 mg three or four times daily in chronic poisoning. For acute poisoning, the dose is 100 to 200 mg IV every 2 to 4 hours. A dose of 1.2 to 2.4 g/day has been suggested in acute poisoning.

In adults in a prospective single-blind, placebo-controlled study, patients ($N = 21$) with chronic arsenicosis were randomized to receive either placebo or DMPS orally (100 mg four times daily) for 1 week, then repeat in weeks 3, 5, and 7 with no medication during the intervening period. The 24-hour urinary excretion of arsenic increased, and significant clinical improvement in weakness, pigmentation, and lung disease was noted. Clinical improvement also occurred in the placebo-treated patients but to a lesser extent. Urinary excretion of arsenic was unchanged in the placebo group. Hematologic parameters, blood chemistry, neuropathy, hepatomegaly, keratosis, and skin histology did not change in either group. This study suggests that DMPS may have clinical benefit for chronic arsenicosis (42).

A patient with severe chronic arsenic poisoning, including a peripheral neuropathy that progressed to facial paresis and quadriparesis, deteriorated despite treatment with oral succimer (30 mg/kg/day) for 2 weeks. Succimer was discontinued, and DMPS was started at 250 mg IV every 4 hours for 12 days. The use of DMPS was associated with increased urinary excretion of arsenic and improvement of the neuropathy in the first 48 hours. The patient's initial blood arsenic level was 5.6 μg/dl. During the first 24 hours of DMPS treatment, urinary arsenic excretion increased from 101 to 300 μg/L. After 1 year, the patient demonstrated mild weakness and paresthesia and was back at work (44).

Succimer [2,3-dimercaptosuccinic acid (Chemet)] chelates extracellular arsenic and is as effective as dimercaprol in eliminating arsenic from tissue in animals. Succimer has been shown to enhance elimination of arsenic in humans after acute exposure (48). It has not been shown to reverse skin lesions or neuropathy.

Details of administration and adverse effects are provided in Chapter 77. The initial dose is 10 mg/kg/dose every 8 hours (30 mg/kg/day) for 5 days, followed by 10 mg/kg every 12 hours for 14 days or until the urinary arsenic level is less than 50 μg/L.

In West Bengal, 21 adults with chronic arsenicosis from drinking contaminated groundwater were randomized to placebo ($N = 10$) or two courses of succimer, 1400 mg/day for 1 week and then 1050 mg/day for 2 weeks. The mean duration of exposure was 15 to 20 years. All had clinical signs of chronic arsenicosis, including neuropathy and hyperkeratosis. Both groups had improved clinical scores at the end of the study, but there was no demonstrable clinical or biochemical difference between the groups (42).

A 46-year-old man ingested approximately 2 g of arsenic in a suicide attempt. After initial improvement, a progressive polyneuropathy developed despite administration of succimer, 300 mg orally every 6 hours for 3 days, beginning 21 hours postingestion. His condition gradually improved over the next 6 months (49).

A critically ill patient secondary to chronic arsenic poisoning did not respond to oral succimer (30 mg/kg/day for 2 weeks) as demonstrated by the lack of increased urinary excretion of arsenic and continued clinical deterioration. It is not known whether this was a result of poor drug absorption or lack of drug efficacy (44).

D-Penicillamine is not typically recommended because of more frequent adverse effects.

Monitoring

The QTc intervals should be monitored in patients with cardiac effects and in patients treated with arsenic trioxide (preferably daily while on therapy). Monitor serum potassium and magnesium, and correct as needed.

Monitor urinary arsenic concentrations while on chelation therapy every few days to assess the effectiveness of enhanced elimination. Chelation may be terminated when the urinary arsenic is less than 50 µg/L.

For arsine gas exposure, monitor the patient's hemoglobin, hematocrit, serum potassium, blood urea nitrogen, and creatinine frequently, depending on the severity of intoxication. Monitor urine output and fluid status closely because renal failure may result in acute volume overload.

REFERENCES

1. Subramanian KS, Kosnett MJ. Human exposures to arsenic from consumption of well water in West Bengal, India. *Int J Occup Environ Health* 1998;4:217–230.

1a. Del Razo LM, Garcia-Vargas GG, Garcis-Salcedo J, et al. Arsenic levels in cooked food and assessment of adult dietary intake of arsenic in the Region Lagunera, Mexico. *Food Chem Toxicol* 2002;40:1423–1431.

2. Stilwell DE, Gorny KD. Contamination of soil with copper, chromium and arsenic under decks built from CCA-treated wood. *Bull Environ Contam Toxicol* 1997;58:22–29.
3. Espinoza EO, Bleasdell B. Arsenic and mercury in traditional Chinese herbal balls. *N Engl J Med* 1995;333:803–804.
4. Parish GG, Glass R, Kimbrough R. Acute arsine poisoning in two workers cleaning a clogged drain. *Arch Environ Health* 1979;34:224–227.
5. Watson WA, Veltri JC, Metcalf TJ. Acute arsenic exposure treated with oral D-penicillamine. *Vet Hum Toxicol* 1981;23:164–166.
6. Cullen NM, Wolf LR, St. Clair D. Pediatric arsenic ingestion. *Am J Emerg Med* 1995;13:432–435.
7. Scalzo AJ, Thompson MW, Peters DW. Asymptomatic presentation of pediatric arsenic ingestion from sodium arsenate ant killer. *Vet Hum Toxicol* 1989;31:340.
8. Kingstrom RL, Hall S, Sioris L. Clinical observations and medical outcome in 149 cases of arsenate ant killer ingestion. *J Toxicol Clin Toxicol* 1993;31:581–591.
9. Fowler BA, Weissberg JB. Arsine poisoning. *N Engl J Med* 1974;291:1171–1174.
10. Anawar HM, Akai J, Mostofa KM, et al. Arsenic poisoning in groundwater: health risk and geochemical sources in Bangladesh. *Environ Int* 2002;27:597–604.
11. Lewis DR, Southwick JW, Oullet-Hellstrom R, et al. Drinking water in Utah: a cohort mortality study. *Environ Health Perspect* 1999;107:359–365.
12. National Research Council (NRC). Arsenic in drinking water: 2001 update. Washington, DC: National Research Council, Subcommittee on Arsenic in Drinking Water, National Academy Press, 2001.
13. Vahter M. Mechanisms of arsenic biotransformation. *Toxicology* 2002;181–182:211–217.
14. Klimecki WT, Carter DE. Arsine toxicity: chemical and mechanistic implications. *J Toxicol Environ Health* 1995;46:399–409.
15. Unnikrishnan D, Dutcher JP, Varshneya N, et al. Torsade de pointes in 3 patients with leukemia treated with arsenic trioxide. *Blood* 2001;97:1514–1516.
16. Concha G, Vogler G, Nermell B, et al. Low-level arsenic excretion in breast milk of native Andean women exposed to high levels of arsenic in the drinking water. *Int Arch Occup Environ Health* 1998;71:42–46.
17. Daya MR, Irwin R, Parshley MC, et al. Arsenic ingestion in pregnancy. *Vet Hum Toxicol* 1989;31:347.
18. Rust DM, Soignet SL. Risk/benefit profile of arsenic trioxide. *Oncologist* 2001;[Suppl 2]:29–32.
19. Westervelt P, Brown RA, Adkins DR, et al. Sudden death among patients with acute promyelocytic leukemia treated with arsenic trioxide. *Blood* 2001;98:266–271.
20. Huang SY, Chang CS, Tang JL, et al. Acute and chronic arsenic poisoning associated with treatment of acute promyelocytic leukemia. *Br J Haematol* 1998;103:1092–1095.
21. Pinto SS. Arsine poisoning: evaluation of the acute phase. *J Occup Med* 1976;18:633–635.
22. Kleinfeld MJ. Arsine poisoning. *J Occup Med* 1980;22:820–821.
23. Frank G. Neurologic and psychiatric disorders following acute arsine poisoning. *J Neurol* 1976;213:59–70.
24. Tseng CH. An overview on peripheral vascular disease in blackfoot disease-hyperendemic villages in Taiwan. *Angiology* 2002;53:529–537.
25. Baselt RC. *Biological monitoring methods for industrial chemicals*, 3rd ed. Foster City, CA: Chemical Toxicology Institute, 1997:30–37.
26. Ma M, Le XC. Effect of arsenosugar ingestion on urinary arsenic speciation. *Clin Chem* 1998;44:539–550.
27. Brayer AF, Callahan CM, Wax PM. Acute arsenic poisoning from ingestion of "snakes." *Pediatr Emerg Care* 1997;6:394–396.
28. Del Rago LM, Garcia-Vargas GG, Vargas H, et al. Altered profile of urinary arsenic metabolites in adults with chronic arsenicism. *Arch Toxicol* 1997;71:211–217.
29. Hindmarsh JT. Caveats in hair analysis in chronic arsenic poisoning. *Clin Biochem* 2002;35:1–11.
30. Baselt RC. *Disposition of toxic drugs and chemicals in man*, 6th ed. Foster City, CA: Chemical Toxicology Institute, 2002:79–82.
31. Kreiss K, Zack MM, Landrigan PJ, et al. Neurologic evaluation of a population exposed to arsenic in Alaskan well water. *Arch Environ Health* 1983;38:116–121.
32. Landrigan PJ, Costello RJ, Stringer WT. Occupational exposure to arsine. An epidemiologic reappraisal of current standards. *Scand J Work Environ Health* 1982;8:169–177.
33. Mitchell RD, Walberg CB, Gupta RC. In vitro adsorption properties of activated charcoal with selected inorganic compounds. *Ann Emerg Med* 1989;18:444–445.
34. Lee DC, Roberts JR, Kelly JJ, et al. Whole-bowel irrigation as an adjunct in the treatment of radiopaque arsenic. *Am J Emerg Med* 1995;13:244–245.
35. Vaziri ND, Upham T, Barton CH. Hemodialysis clearance of arsenic. *J Toxicol Clin Toxicol* 1980;17:451–456.
36. Mathieu D, Mathieu-Nolf M, Germain-Alonso M, et al. Massive arsenic poisoning—effect of hemodialysis and dimercaprol or arsenic kinetics. *Intensive Care Med* 1992;18:47–50.
37. Smith A. "BAL" (British Anti-Lewisite) in the treatment of arsenic and mercury poisoning. *JAMA* 1946;131:824.
38. Heyman A, Pfeiffer JB, Willett RW, et al. Peripheral neuropathy caused by arsenical intoxication. *N Engl J Med* 1956;254:401–409.
39. Jenkins RB. Inorganic arsenic and the nervous system. *Brain* 1966;89:479–498.
40. Woody NC, Kometani JT. BAL in the treatment of arsenic ingestion of children. *Pediatrics* 1948;1:372–378.
41. Moore DF, O'Callaghan CA, Berlyne G, et al. Acute arsenic poisoning: absence of polyneuropathy and after treatment with 2,3-dimercaptopropanesulfonate (DMPS). *J Neurol Neurosurg Psychiatry* 1994;57:1133–1135.
42. Guha Mazumder DN, Ghoshal UC, Saha J, et al. Randomized placebo-controlled trial of 2,3-dimercaptosuccinic acid in therapy of chronic arsenicosis due to drinking arsenic-contaminated subsoil water. *J Toxicol Clin Toxicol* 1998;36:683–690.
43. Reference deleted.
44. Wax PM, Thornton CA. Recovery from severe arsenic-induced peripheral neuropathy with 2,3-dimercapto-1-propanesulphonic acid. *J Toxicol Clin Toxicol* 2000;38:777–780.
45. References deleted.
46. Aposhian HV, Zheng B, Aposhian MM, et al. DMPS-arsenic challenge test. II. Modulation of arsenic species, including monomethylarsonous acid (MMA(III)), excreted in human urine. *Toxicol Appl Pharmacol* 2000;165: 74–83.
47. Aposhian HV. Mobilization of mercury and arsenic in humans by sodium 2,3-dimercapto-1-propane sulfonate (DMPS). *Environ Health Perspect* 1998;106(Suppl 4):1017–1025.
48. Shum S, Whitshead J, Vaughan L, et al. Chelation of organoarsenate with dimercapto succinic acid. *Vet Hum Toxicol* 1995;37:239–242.
49. Lentz K, Hruby K, Druml W, et al. 2,3-Dimercaptosuccinic acid in human arsenic poisoning. *Arch Toxicol* 1981;47:241–243.

CHAPTER 214

Barium

Seth Schonwald

BARIUM NITRATE

Atomic symbol, atomic number, molecular weight:	**Ba, 56, 137.33 g/mol**
Valence state:	**+2**
CAS Registry No.:	**7440-39-3**
Normal levels:	**A serum barium level greater than 20 μg/dl is abnormal (blood).**
SI conversion:	**μg/dl × 0.073 = μmol/L**
Target organs:	**Muscle (paralysis), heart (hypokalemic dysrhythmias)**
Antidote:	**Administration of potassium**

OVERVIEW

Barium was discovered by Sir Humphrey Davy in 1808. It is used in plastics, steels, bricks, tiles, lubricating oils, and jet fuel (Table 1) (1,2). Chemically pure barium sulfate is water insoluble, poorly absorbed orally, and nontoxic to humans. It is used as a benign, radiopaque aid in x-ray diagnosis. Radioactive isotopes of barium may be useful in studying skeletal metabolism as bone-scanning agents (3). The largest natural source of barium is barite ore, which is composed largely of barium sulfate and found in beds or masses in limestone, dolomite, shale, and other sedimentary formations (4).

TOXIC DOSE

Government regulations and standards for barium are shown in Table 2.

Death has resulted from accidental or intentional ingestion of barium salts. Deaths have been attributed to cardiac arrest, severe gastrointestinal (GI) hemorrhage, and to unknown causes (5–7). In one case, a 49-year-old male pharmacist ingested an unknown quantity of barium chloride and died from cardiorespiratory arrest (8). A 61-year-old woman died after undergoing two computed tomography scans of the abdomen with oral administration of barium sulfate. The patient developed nonspecific neurologic and cardiovascular manifestations within hours that led to death a few days later. Elevated levels of barium were found in the blood and cerebrospinal fluid. The most likely mechanism of poisoning was progressive intravasation of barium due to stasis of contrast material related to intestinal obstruction (9). A psychiatric patient survived flaccid paralysis, malignant dysrhythmias, respiratory arrest, and severe hypokalemia after ingesting barium sulfide in ceramic glaze (10).

No studies have described an increased incidence of cancer in humans after exposure to barium.

TABLE 1. Sources of barium

Environmental
- The largest use of mined barite is in oil and gas well drilling.
- The remainder of crude barium sulfate is used in the paint, glass, and rubber industries and in the production of other barium compounds.

Occupational
- Barium metal and its alloys are used as "getters" to remove gases from vacuum tubes.
- Barium carbonate is used as a rodenticide and plays a role in the brick, tile, ceramics, oil drilling, and chemical manufacturing industries.
- Barium chloride is used for chlorine and sodium hydroxide manufacturing, as a flux for aluminum alloys, and in the pigment and textile industries.
- Barium oxide is used to dry gases and solvents, and the hydroxide compound plays a role in glass, synthetic rubber, sugar, and vegetable oil refining.
- Barium sulfate, in the chemically treated, blanc fixe form, is used in high-quality paints, glass, and paper making.

TABLE 2. U.S. regulatory guidelines and standards for barium (Ba)

Agency	Description	Concentration
OSHA		
(air)	PEL-TWA	0.5 μg/m³ (as Ba)
ACGIH	Barium and soluble compounds	
(air)	TLV-TWA	0.5 mg/m³ (as Ba)
	STEL	None
NIOSH	REL	None
(air)	IDLH	50 mg/m³ (as Ba)
EPA		
Water	Maximum allowed concentration	1.0 ppm
FDA		
Water	Quality standard	1.0 ppm

ACGIH, American Conference of Governmental Industrial Hygienists; EPA, Environmental Protection Agency; FDA, U.S. Food and Drug Administration; IDLH, immediate danger to life or health; NIOSH, National Institute for Occupational Safety and Health; U.S. OSHA, Occupational Safety and Health Administration; PEL, permissible exposure limit; ppm, parts per million; REL, recommended exposure limit; STEL, short-term exposure limit; TLV, threshold limit value; TWA, time-weighted average.

TOXICOKINETICS AND TOXICODYNAMICS

Humans are exposed to barium in the air, water, or food. Most barium intake is oral. The GI absorption of barium is less than 5% (11). More than 93% of barium is found in the bones and teeth of humans. It is sometimes found in eyes, lungs, skin, and adipose tissue at less than 1% of total body weight (12).

Approximately 3% of an oral dose in humans is excreted in the urine and most of the remainder in the feces. A man who was injected with barium intravenously (IV) excreted most of the dose in the feces (13). Another case study showed that approximately 9% of an IV dose was excreted in the urine and approximately 84% in the feces (14).

PATHOPHYSIOLOGY

Barium may shift extracellular potassium intracellularly, resulting in extracellular hypokalemia, which is believed to mediate barium-induced paralysis (15). It is unclear whether mechanisms other than hypokalemia contribute to the toxic effects produced by an acute high-level exposure (2).

VULNERABLE POPULATIONS

There does not appear to be an increased incidence of developmental or teratogenic effects when pregnant women are exposed to oral barium sulfate.

CLINICAL PRESENTATION

Case reports and animal studies suggest that acute inhalation, oral, or dermal exposure may be associated with lowered blood potassium levels (16–18). The hypokalemia is due to a shift of potassium intracellularly and is not due to excretion.

Cardiovascular effects of barium after acute ingestion include increased blood pressure, hypokalemic dysrhythmias, direct myocardial damage (19), and changes in heart physiology and metabolism (20).

GI hemorrhage and disturbances, including gastric pain, vomiting, and diarrhea, have been associated with acute ingestion (21). Rare acute intrusion of barium sulfate into the peritoneal space can cause an acute inflammatory tissue response (22). Degeneration of the liver after acute ingestion to barium has been noted (23); however, data are too limited to determine the effect of barium on the liver in humans.

Neuromuscular effects after acute inhalation or ingestion of barium include muscle weakness and hypokalemic paralysis (24,25). Occupational exposure has not been found to result in radiologically apparent barium deposits in skeletal muscle or bone. Areflexic quadriplegia resembling Guillain-Barré syndrome due to barium carbonate poisoning developed in two young patients (26). A 25-year-old man with skeletal muscle weakness, respiratory arrest, rhabdomyolysis, and life-threatening hyperkalemia presented after ingesting a depilatory containing barium sulfide (27). Barium carbonate has also been associated with rhabdomyolysis (28).

Renal failure has been reported in one case study of acute barium inhalation (29). Case studies of humans developing renal failure, renal insufficiency, and renal degeneration after acute oral barium poisoning have been reported (30).

Benign pneumoconiosis (baritosis) occurs in workers exposed to barium by inhalation; however, no respiratory effects were observed in another study of workers exposed to barium carbonate dust (31,32). Respiratory weakness and paralysis due to hypokalemia have followed the acute ingestion of barium (33). Acute intravasation of barium sulfate into the circulatory system of an adult female patient after a barium enema procedure caused the compound to be deposited in blood vessels throughout the body, including the lungs, and resulted in respiratory failure (34). IV administration of barium may also yield respiratory compromise.

DIAGNOSTIC TESTS

After acute intoxication, frequent monitoring of potassium and the potential effects of barium (e.g., electrocardiogram and respiratory function) should occur. Renal function should be determined to assess potential contribution of renal insufficiency.

Barium can be measured in bone, blood, urine, and feces. Levels in blood, urine, and feces vary with daily intake of barium. There are no data correlating bone, blood, urine, or feces levels of barium with specific exposure levels.

Hypokalemia and hypertension are effects usually found in cases of acute and intermediate exposures to relatively high doses of barium. Although it is reasonable to expect the dose level to influence the presence of these effects, there are no data supporting a correlation between dose level and either appearance of or degree of hypokalemia and hypertension.

TREATMENT

Oral Exposure

Contradictions exist in the literature regarding the efficacy or desirability of administering emetics (35). Lavage or emesis has been suggested; however, high concentrations of barium can cause nausea, and emesis should not be induced in cases in which substantial vomiting has already occurred. Administration of oral soluble sulfates may limit barium absorption by forming insoluble barium sulfate (36). The IV administration of sulfate salts should be avoided because barium precipitation in the kidneys can cause renal failure.

Skin Exposure

The patient should be removed from the area, contaminated clothing should be removed, and the patient should wash with mild soap and water. If the eyes or skin are exposed, flush them with water.

Enhancement of Elimination

Infusing saline and inducing saline diuresis may facilitate elimination of barium from the bloodstream. Urine output should be maintained at levels above 3 ml/kg/hour, if possible. Hemodialysis reduces the serum barium concentration and is associated with marked improvement in motor strength during and after hemodialysis (38,39). Hemodialysis should be considered in patients with severe barium toxicity who do not respond to potassium supplementation.

Antidotes

Potassium is an effective antagonist of the cardiotoxic and paralyzing effects of barium in animals and may be a useful antidote in cases of acute human barium poisoning (40). The precise dose is not well established, but large amounts of potassium chloride IV have been required.

Monitoring

Plasma potassium should be monitored, and hypokalemia may be relieved by IV infusion of potassium, as for other causes of hypokalemia (41).

REFERENCES

1. Venugopal B, Luckey TD. *Metal toxicity in mammals*, 2nd ed. New York: Plenum Press, 1978:63–67.
2. Agency for Toxic Substances and Disease Registry, Division of Toxicology. *ATSDR toxicological profile for barium*. Atlanta: ATSDR, 1992:1–163.
3. Spencer RP, Lange RC, Treves S. Use of 135 Ba and 131 Ba as bone scanning agents. *J Nucl Med* 1971;12:216–221.
4. Miner S. Preliminary air pollution survey of barium and its compounds: a literature review, report No. APTD 69-28. Raleigh, NC: U.S. Department of Health, Education and Welfare, Public Health Service; Consumer Protection and Environmental Health Service; Consumer Air Pollution and Control Administration, 1969.
5. Das NC, Singh V. Unusual type of cardiac arrest: case report. *Armed Forces Med J India* 1970;26:344–352.
6. Talwar KK, Sharma BK. Myocardial damage due to barium chloride poisoning. *Indian Heart J* 1979;31:244–245.
7. Downs JC, Milling D, Nichols CA. Suicidal ingestion of barium-sulfide-containing shaving powder. *Am J Forensic Med Pathol* 1995;16:56–61.
8. Jourdan S, Bertoni M, Sergio P, et al. Suicidal poisoning with barium chloride. *Forensic Sci Int* 2001;119:263–265.
9. Pelissier-Alicot AL, Leonetti G, Champsaur P, et al. Fatal poisoning due to intravasation after oral administration of barium sulfate for contrast radiography. *Forensic Sci Int* 1999;106:109–113.
10. Thomas M, Bowie D, Walker R. Acute barium intoxication following ingestion of ceramic glaze. *Postgrad Med J* 1998;74:545–546.
11. Tipton IH, Stewart PL, Martin PG. Trace elements in diets and excreta. *Health Phys* 1966;12:1683–1689.
12. Schroeder HA, Tipton IH, Nason AP. Trace metals in man: strontium and barium. *J Chronic Dis* 1972;25:491–517.
13. Newton D, Rundo J, Harrison GE. The retention of alkaline earth elements in man, with special reference to barium. *Health Phys* 1977;33:45–53.
14. Harrison GE, Carr TEF, Sutton A. Distribution of radioactive calcium, strontium, barium and radium following intravenous injection into a healthy man. *Int J Radiat Biol* 1967;131:235–247.
15. Bradberry SM, Vale JA. Disturbances of potassium homeostasis in poisoning. J *Toxicol Clin Toxicol* 1995;33:295–310.
16. Stewart DW, Hummel RP. Acute poisoning by a barium chloride burn. *J Trauma* 1984;24:768–770.
17. Gupta S. Barium carbonate, hypokalaemic paralysis and trismus. *Postgrad Med J* 1994;70:938–939.
18. Schott GD, McArdle B. Barium-induced skeletal muscle paralysis in the rat, and its relation to human familial periodic paralysis. *J Neurol Neurosurg Psychiatr* 1974;37:32–39.
19. Talwar KK, Sharma BK. Myocardial damage due to barium chloride poisoning. *Indian Heart J.* 1979;31:244–245.
20. Perry HM Jr, Kopp SJ, Perry EF, et al. Hypertension and associated cardiovascular abnormalities induced by chronic barium feeding. *J Toxicol Environ Health* 1989;28:373–388.
21. Lewi Z, Bar-Khayim Y. Food poisoning from barium carbonate. *Lancet* 1964;342–343.
22. Yamamura M, Nishi M, Furubayashi H, et al. Barium peritonitis: report of a case and review of the literature. *Dis Colon Rectum* 1985;28:347–352.
23. McNally WD. Two deaths from the administration of barium salts. *J Am Med Assoc* 1925;84:1805–1807.
24. Gould DB, Sorrell MR, Lupariello AD. Barium sulfide poisoning: some factors contributing to survival. *Arch Intern Med* 1973;132:891–894.
25. Stedwell RE, Allen KM, Binder LS. Hypokalemic paralyses: a review of the etiologies, pathophysiology, presentation, and therapy. *Am J Emerg Med* 1992;10:143–148.
26. Koley TK, Goyal AK, Gupta MD. Barium carbonate poisoning mimicking Guillain-Barré syndrome. *J Assoc Physicians India* 2001;49:656–657.
27. Sigue G, Gamble L, Pelitere M, et al. From profound hypokalemia to life-threatening hyperkalemia: a case of barium sulfide poisoning. *Arch Intern Med* 2000;160:548–551.
28. Johnson CH, Van Tassell VJ. Acute barium poisoning with respiratory failure and rhabdomyolysis. *Ann Emerg Med* 1991;20:1138–1142.
29. Shankle R, Keane JR. Acute paralysis from inhaled barium carbonate. *Arch Neurol* 1988;45:579–580.
30. Wetherill SF, Guarino MJ, Cox RW. Acute renal failure associated with barium chloride poisoning. *Ann Intern Med* 1981;95:187–188.
31. Doig AT. Baritosis: a benign pneumoconiosis. *Thorax* 1976;31:30–39.
32. Essing HG, Buhlmeyer G, Valentin H, et al. [Exclusion of disturbances to health from long years of exposure to barium carbonate in the production of steatite ceramics]. *Arbeitsmedizin Sozialmedizin Praventivmedizin* 1976;11:299–302.
33. Phelan DM, Hagley SR, Guerin MD. Is hypokalemia the cause of paralysis in barium poisoning? *BMJ* 1984;289:882.
34. Cove JK, Snyder RN. Fatal barium intravasation during barium enema. *Radiology* 1974;112:9–10.
35. Bronstein AC, Currance PL, eds. *Emergency care for hazardous materials exposure*. St. Louis: CV Mosby Company, 1988;66:127–128.
36. Haddad LM, Winchester JF, eds. *Clinical management of poisoning and drug overdose*, 2nd ed. Philadelphia: WB Saunders Company, 1990:1129.
37. Reference deleted.
38. Schorn TF, Olbricht C, Schuler A, et al. Barium carbonate intoxication. *Intensive Care Med* 1991;17:60–62.
39. Wells JA, Wood KE. Acute barium poisoning treated with hemodialysis. *Am J Emerg Med* 2001;19:175–177.
40. Foster PR, Elharrar V, Zipes DP. Accelerated ventricular escapes induced in the intact dog by barium, strontium and calcium. *J Pharmacol Exp Ther* 1977;200:373–383.
41. Dreisbach RH, Robertson WO, eds. *Handbook of poisoning: prevention, diagnosis & treatment*, 12th ed. Norwalk, CT: Appleton & Lange, 1987:119–120.

CHAPTER 215

Beryllium

Lee S. Newman and João H. Delgado

Atomic symbol, atomic number, molecular weight:	**Be, 4, 9.01 g/mol**
Valence state:	**+2**
CAS Registry No.:	**7440-41-7**
Normal level:	**Serum, not applicable**
SI conversion:	**μg/L × 110.9 = nmol/L**
Target organs:	**Immune system response (chronic), lungs (chronic)**
Antidote:	**None**

OVERVIEW

Beryllium is the fourth lightest element and possesses a variety of properties that makes it attractive for surprisingly diverse industrial applications. Although it occurs naturally in soil, its threat to human health results from occupational or secondhand exposure. Modern safety regulations have largely eliminated acute beryllium toxicity, at least in the United States. However, ongoing exposure to low-level beryllium continues to pose a significant health threat to workers in the form of *chronic beryllium disease* (CBD), a progressive, systemic hypersensitivity disorder that primarily affects the lungs and lymphatics.

Beryllium is used in many metal and alloy machining industries, including aerospace and aircraft manufacturing, automotive,

TABLE 1. U.S. regulatory guidelines and standards for beryllium

Agency	Description	Concentration (μg/m³)
OSHA[a]	Metal and soluble compounds	
(air)	PEL-TWA	2
	Ceiling	5
	Acceptable maximum peak above ceiling concentration for an 8-h shift	25
ACGIH[b]	TLV-TWA	2
(air)	STEL	10
NIOSH	REL-TWA	0.5
(air)	STEL	None
	IDLH	4 (as beryllium)

ACGIH, American Conference of Governmental Industrial Hygienists; EPA, Environmental Protection Agency; IDLH, immediate danger to life or health; NIOSH, National Institute for Occupational Safety and Health; OSHA, U.S. Occupational Safety and Health Administration; PEL, permissible exposure limit; REL, recommended exposure limit; STEL, short-term exposure limit; TLV, threshold limit value; TWA, time-weighted average.
[a]PEL-TWA is under review. 2002 OSHA Hazard Bulletin indicates that current standard is not protective.
[b]New proposed threshold limit value of 0.2 μg/m³ is under review for 2002 (3).

ceramics, computer, electronics, and defense and nuclear weapons (1). Its use is due to several beneficial properties: high melting point, low density, low coefficient of thermal expansion, high tensile strength, and high stiffness to weight ratio (2). Many of these properties are transferred when small amounts of beryllium are alloyed with copper, aluminum, magnesium, and nickel. Beryllium is present in soils at an average concentration of 6 ppm (2). Coal combustion accounts for more than 90% of ambient air beryllium; however, air concentrations even in urban centers remain quite low (2). Inhalation of beryllium fumes or beryllium-containing dusts in occupational settings accounts for the overwhelming majority of beryllium exposures resulting in toxicity. Exposure can occur during the extraction of beryllium from its ores, during processing into metal alloys or ceramics, from machining of beryllium-containing alloys, and in the recycling of metal alloys.

Toxic Dose

Minimum lethal doses have not been established. However, even brief exposure to more than 10 μg/m³ can cause acute or subacute toxicity and may result in death (2). The minimum dose capable of resulting in chronic pulmonary disease has not been established. U.S. regulatory guidelines and standards are provided in Table 1. It is clear that the current Occupational Safety and Health Administration standard of 2 μg/m³ for an 8-hour time-weighted average is not sufficiently protective. New cases of CBD have occurred in plants that are able to document compliance with this standard (4). CBD has developed in as little as 50 days from first exposure, with exposures as low as 0.02 μg/m³ (8-hour time-weighted average) (5).

TOXICOKINETICS AND TOXICODYNAMICS

Beryllium is not absorbed by the gastrointestinal tract to any significant extent. Inhaled beryllium is primarily cleared by the mucociliary defenses and alveolar macrophages (1). The time course of pulmonary clearance is unknown in humans but probably depends on the dose as well as the solubility of the specific beryllium compound. A study in rats and hamsters using aerosolized BeO demonstrated an average clearance half-life of more than 63 days (6). Systemically absorbed beryllium distributes to bone, liver, and kidneys and is principally excreted in the urine (7). It can also be translocated to local lymph nodes and persist indefinitely in the lung parenchyma.

PATHOPHYSIOLOGY

Beryllium causes chronic pulmonary disease by initiating and perpetuating a cell-mediated immune response. Inhaled beryllium particles that reach the alveoli are phagocytosed by alveolar macrophages capable of presenting beryllium to T lymphocytes. Because of its small size, it is likely that beryllium acts as a hapten, although the exact nature of the beryllium antigen has not been elucidated. Beryllium presentation initiates a cascade of events, which results in the activation of T lymphocytes and the release of Th1 cytokines (tumor necrosis factor-α, interferon gamma, IL-6, IL-2) (8). The persistent cell-mediated response that ensues causes the accumulation of beryllium-sensitized T lymphocytes, macrophages, and other immune effector cells that form the granulomas and mononuclear cell infiltration characteristic of this disease.

Not all workers exposed to beryllium become sensitized. The risk appears to be related to job duties typically associated with higher exposures to airborne beryllium particulates, with certain occupations (i.e., machinists) exhibiting a particularly high risk (4,5). Genetic susceptibility is also a contributing factor. For example, in a case-controlled study involving 77 beryllium-exposed workers, a glutamate substitution at position 69 of the HLA-DPB1 molecule was found to be a risk factor for the development of CBD (9). Of the 33 workers with CBD, 97% had this substitution, compared with only 30% of unaffected workers. More recent studies indicate that this polymorphism is found in approximately 85% of both CBD- and beryllium-sensitized individuals and that homozygosity is more common among those with CBD (10). A polymorphism in the tumor necrosis factor-α promoter region has also been associated with CBD severity (11).

Beryllium may also cause dermal toxicity. Cutaneous exposure can cause a simple irritant dermatitis or atopic dermatitis. Beryllium-containing dermal foreign bodies can cause noncaseating granulomas to form and may need to be excised due to the painful inflammation that they can elicit.

CLINICAL PRESENTATION

Acute Exposure

Inhalational exposure to high concentrations of beryllium results in both upper and lower respiratory tract injury. The spectrum of toxicity includes nasopharyngeal irritation, tracheobronchitis, and chemical pneumonitis. Signs and symptoms include chest pain, cough, dyspnea, and epistaxis and may develop abruptly or over several hours, depending on the dose and solubility characteristics of the beryllium compound.

Chronic Exposure

Chronic inhalational exposure can result in CBD, a systemic granulomatous and mononuclear cell disorder affecting mainly the lungs and thoracic lymph nodes. CBD is characterized by progressive dyspnea on exertion, chest pain, weight loss, fatigue, anorexia, fevers, and night sweats. On physical examination, these patients may exhibit dry crackles on lung auscultation, skin lesions, and lymphadenopathy. With more advanced disease, cyanosis, digital clubbing, and signs of cor pulmonale and right ventricular failure occur. On average, CBD develops 6 to 10 years after exposure, although latencies as long as 30 years and as short as 2 months have been reported (1).

The latency depends, in part, on whether cases are identified at early stages through workplace medical surveillance programs. Some individuals are detected at the time they develop beryllium sensitization but before they have developed CBD. The majority of these individuals progresses to CBD, although it is unknown if all sensitized people ultimately develop CBD. In cross-sectional studies, the frequency of beryllium sensitization and CBD ranges from 2% to 16% of exposed workers. Disease rates in machinists have exceeded 25% in some studies.

Extensive animal data implicate beryllium as a carcinogen, causing lung cancers and osteosarcomas. In humans, several epidemiologic studies have demonstrated a link between beryllium exposure and lung cancer (1,12). It is listed by the International Agency for Research on Cancer as a known human carcinogen.

DIAGNOSTIC TESTS

Biologic Monitoring and Health Surveillance

The current approach to medical surveillance for beryllium sensitization or CBD in the workplace consists of performing blood beryllium lymphocyte proliferation test (BeLPT) on all exposed workers every 2 to 3 years. Baseline chest radiographs with International Labour Organization B-reading and baseline spirometry are also recommended. Although these latter two tests have a much lower positive and negative predictive value than the blood BeLPT, they may detect a few cases missed by initial blood testing. In general, a second confirmatory blood BeLPT is obtained in anyone with an initial positive test. On average, half of such patients already have CBD, even if it is clinically inapparent at the time of diagnosis. Patients who are sensitized but who do not have CBD should be strongly encouraged to remain in medical follow-up because they are at high risk of developing CBD.

Chronic Exposure

The evaluation of patients with suspected CBD involves confirmation of sensitization to beryllium, assessment of physiologic severity, and obtaining specimens for histologic analysis (usually lung tissue obtained by transbronchial biopsy or open lung biopsy). The development of immunologic testing has greatly simplified the work-up of patients suspected of having CBD as well as the workplace monitoring of patients at risk.

The BeLPT is the preferred method of diagnosing sensitization in exposed patients. For this test, lymphocytes are isolated from peripheral blood or from bronchoalveolar lavage specimens and are incubated with $BeSO_4$ and pulsed with tritiated thymidine. Beryllium-sensitized lymphocytes proliferate in response to $BeSO_4$, and this proliferation is measured by the amount of incorporation of radiolabeled thymidine into DNA. Beryllium skin patch testing can also be used to confirm sensitization in equivocal cases only if the individual is not returning to beryllium exposure. The blood BeLPT identifies 80% to 90% of individuals with CBD, making it the preferred method for workplace screening.

Pulmonary function testing may show any number of abnormalities: a predominantly obstructive pattern in one-third of patients; a restrictive pattern in one-fourth of patients; reduced diffusion capacity for carbon monoxide (DL_{CO}), usually with normal airflow and lung volumes in one-third of patients; and mixed disorders of restriction and obstruction (1,13). Measurement of gas exchange, using arterial blood gases at rest and maximum exercise, is more sensitive than DL_{CO} or pulmonary function tests. An abnormally widened alveolar-arterial gradient during exercise may be noted long before abnormalities in either spirometry or DL_{CO} are observed.

Chest radiography is typically normal early in the course of the disease. Diffuse bilateral infiltrates and hilar lymphadenopathy appear as the disease progresses. Conglomerate masses may form in the upper lobes. In later stages, diffuse fibrosis and honeycombing are seen. High-resolution chest computed tomography is more sensitive than plain radiography for detecting these changes, although false-negative studies do occur (14). Findings on computed tomography are similar to those seen with sarcoidosis and include thickened septae, bronchial wall thickening, and small nodules that track along bronchovascular sheaths. A more diffuse nodular pattern is also seen.

Diagnostic Pitfalls

Some CBD patients are mistakenly diagnosed as having other disorders, such as sarcoidosis, asthma, and interstitial lung disease (pulmonary fibrosis). The diagnosis is often missed if a history of beryllium or beryllium-alloy work is not elicited. The blood BeLPT can often correct these misdiagnoses, but in some cases, it necessary to perform a BeLPT with lymphocytes obtained by bronchoalveolar lavage to make the correct diagnosis. Even the bronchoalveolar lavage BeLPT may be falsely negative—this occurs more frequently in smokers. Pathologists often assume erroneously that all lung biopsy specimens from patients with CBD must have noncaseating granulomas. Many patients have only mononuclear cell interstitial infiltrates.

TREATMENT

The goal for treatment of patients with established CBD is to slow disease progression and minimize morbidity. Without treatment, the majority of patients experience gradual worsening of lung function, gas exchange, and symptoms, progressing over the course of months or years. In general, early-stage CBD patients should be monitored over time without treatment to estimate the rate of disease progression. The decision to begin treatment can be a difficult one and is based on the presence of significant symptoms plus objective evidence of abnormal lung function or gas exchange. Evidence to support this approach is based on several case series but no controlled trials.

Corticosteroids are the mainstay of CBD therapy. Although they have numerous potential side effects, they can both reduce morbidity and delay mortality when used correctly. Corticosteroids are usually continued for the rest of the patient's life. Some individuals require use of alternative immunosuppressants, such as methotrexate, for optimal control of symptoms. Supplemental oxygen, bronchodilators, and diuretics are used on an individualized basis. Lung transplantation has also been used in select cases. Other preventive care measures, such as immunization against influenza and pneumococcus, should be optimized.

Beryllium exposure is best managed within the context of prevention rather than treatment of toxic effects. Reducing airborne beryllium to lowest achievable concentrations in the workplace and appropriate screening of at-risk workers are important measures. Although it is considered medically prudent to minimize ongoing exposure for patients who are sensitized or who have CBD, there is little evidence to show that removal at these stages alters outcome.

There are no data on the enhancement of elimination (i.e., chelation) of beryllium in humans.

Pitfalls

A common pitfall is the failure to obtain sufficient baseline clinical data at the time the diagnosis of CBD is made. This information is necessary to accurately assess disease severity and as a point of comparison to determine disease progression. Whenever possible, baseline testing of lung physiology should consist of lung volumes, spirometry, DL_{CO}, and exercise tolerance testing with measurement of arterial blood gases at rest and at peak exertion. Another common management error is the failure to refer the sensitized worker for further clinical evaluation.

REFERENCES

1. Newman LS, Maier LA. Beryllium. In: Sullivan JB, Krieger GR, eds. *Clinical environmental health and toxic exposures*, 2nd ed. Philadelphia: Lippincott Williams & Wilkins, 2001:919–926.
2. Kriebel D, Brain JD, Sprince NL, Kazemi H. The pulmonary toxicity of beryllium. *Am Rev Respir Dis* 1988;137:464–473.
3. American Conference of Governmental Industrial Hygienists. Threshold limit values for chemical substances in the work environment. Cincinnati: American Conference of Governmental Industrial Hygienists, 2002.
4. Kreiss K, Mroz MM, Newman LS, et al. Machining risk of beryllium disease and sensitization with median exposures below 2 μg/m³. *Am J Ind Med* 1996;30:16–25.
5. Kelleher PC, Martyny JW, Mroz MM, et al. Beryllium particulate exposure and disease relations in a beryllium machining plant. *J Occup Environ Med* 2000;43:238–249.
6. Reeves AL, Vorwald AJ. Beryllium carcinogenesis II: Pulmonary deposition and clearance of inhaled beryllium sulfate in the rat. *Cancer Res* 1967;27:446–451.
7. Baselt RC. Beryllium. In: *Disposition of toxic drugs and chemicals in man*, 5th ed. Foster City, CA: Chemical Toxicology Institute, 2000:87–88.
8. Tinkle SS, Schwitters PW, Newman LS. Cytokine production by bronchoalveolar lavage cells in chronic beryllium disease. *Environ Health Perspect* 1996;104S:969–971.
9. Richeldi L, Sorrentino R, Saltini C. HLA-DPb1 glutamate 69: a genetic marker of beryllium disease. *Science* 1993;262:242–244.
10. Wang Z, Farris GM, Newman LS, et al. Beryllium sensitivity is linked to HLA-DP genotype. *Toxicology* 2001;165:27–38.
11. Maier LA, Sawyer RT, Bauer RA, et al. High beryllium-stimulated TNF-α is associated with the –308 TNF–α promoter polymorphism and with clinical severity in chronic beryllium disease. Am J Respir Crit Care Med 2001;164:1192–1199.
12. Freiman DG, Hardy HL. Beryllium disease: the relation of pulmonary pathology to clinical course and prognosis based on a study of 130 cases from the US beryllium case registry. *Hum Pathol* 1970;1:25–44.
13. Andrews JL, Kazemi H, Hardy HL. Pattern of lung dysfunction in chronic beryllium disease. *Am Rev Respir Dis* 1969;100:791–800.
14. Newman LS, Buschman DL, Newell JD Jr, Lynch DA. Beryllium disease: assessment with CT. *Radiology* 1994;190:835–840.

CHAPTER 216
Bismuth

E. Martin Caravati

O⁻ BiO⁺ OH

BISMUTH SUBSALICYLATE

Atomic symbol, atomic number, molecular weight:	**Bi, 83, 208.98 g/mol**
Valence states:	**+3, +5**
CAS Registry No.:	**7440-69-9**
Normal levels:	**Blood, less than 15 μg/L; urine, 5 to 23 μg/L**
SI conversion:	**μg/L × 4.78 = nmol/L**
Therapeutic levels:	**Blood, 5 to 15 μg/L; urine, 20 to 940 μg/L**
Target organs:	**Brain, kidney**
Antidotes:	**Succimer, DMPS**

OVERVIEW

Bismuth salts are used in the treatment of gastric ulcers (bismuth subcitrate), diarrhea, and *Helicobacter pylori* (bismuth subsalicylate). The active ingredient in Pepto-Bismol is bismuth subsalicylate. Between 1973 and 1980, approximately 1000 cases of bismuth-related neurotoxicity and more than 70 deaths were reported in France (1); many cases were also reported in Australia, Belgium, Switzerland, and Spain. In France, the neurotoxicity was associated with the use of a bismuth substrate. Bismuth salts were placed under prescription control, and other restrictions were initiated. In Australia, Canada, France, and Austria, the use of bismuth preparations has been curtailed because of neurotoxicity. In Australia, all preparations of bismuth subgallate for oral administration were withdrawn. In 1980, Austrian authorities withdrew pharmaceutical preparations containing bismuth. In the United States, bismuth subsalicylate was considered safe in doses up to 4.8 g daily. In the United Kingdom, the use of bismuth products was limited to periods of 2 to 4 weeks and dosage to less than 4 g daily (2). The amount of elemental bismuth in most salts ranges from 50% to 75%.

Classification and Uses

Pharmacologically active bismuth compounds are divided into four groups.

Group 1: Simple inorganic compounds, such as bismuth subcarbonate and subnitrate, are insoluble in water in the absence of complexing agents and are minimally absorbed.

Group 2: Lipid-soluble organic compounds and complexes of bismuth, such as bismuth subgallate, are absorbed and may result in elevated bismuth blood concentrations. They are mainly neurotoxic and possibly hepatotoxic.

Group 3: Water-soluble organic compounds and complexes of bismuth, such as bismuth triglycollamate, are absorbed and may result in high bismuth blood concentrations. Renal toxicity is a prominent feature of these compounds.

Group 4: Water-soluble organic complexes of bismuth are decomposed (hydrolyze) in the gastrointestinal (GI) tract and produce simple insoluble bismuth compounds, such as bismuth subchloride and bismuth sulfide. Minimal GI absorption is expected.

Sources of Exposure

The total daily intake via food is approximately 5 to 20 μg for the general population.

OCCUPATIONAL

The principal commercial source of bismuth is lead refining. Bismuth is used in fire detection and safety systems, electrical fuses, and "silvering" mirrors; as a catalyst for making acrylic fibers; in the production of malleable irons; as a carrier for radioactive uranium fuel; as an alloying agent; as an additive (hardener) for lead, tin, and cadmium; and in cosmetics (eye shadow and lipstick). Approximately 77,000 workers are potentially exposed to bismuth in the United States (3). Occupational exposure to bismuth may be through inhalation of airborne dust and dermal contact at metal ore refining facilities and other workplaces. It is one of the least toxic heavy metals, and industrial bismuth poisoning has not been reported.

MEDICINAL

Bismuth subsalicylate/metronidazole/tetracycline hydrochloride (Helidac Therapy) contains bismuth subsalicylate, 262.4 mg, as chewable tablets, in addition to metronidazole and tetracycline hydrochloride.

Pepto-Bismol Original contains bismuth subsalicylate, 262 mg/tablespoon, as a tablet, caplet, or liquid. Pepto-Bismol Maximum Strength Liquid contains bismuth subsalicylate, 525 mg/tablespoon, as a tablet or caplet. The liquid formulas contain salicylate, 130 mg/tablespoon (Original), and salicylate, 236 mg/tablespoon (Maximum Strength). The tablets and caplets each contain approximately 100 mg of salicylate. The product may contain small amounts of lead, which is mined along with bismuth.

Bismuth subsalicylate is an insoluble salt of bismuth and salicylic acid (58% bismuth and 42% salicylate by weight). Bismuth subsalicylate is hydrolyzed in the stomach to form bismuth oxychloride and salicylic acid. Bismuth associates strongly with the gastric mucosa and may be responsible for its cytoprotective properties (4). Dissociation occurs mostly in the stomach. In the small intestine, bismuth reacts with other anions (bicarbonate and phosphate) to form insoluble bismuth subcarbonate and bismuth phosphate salts. In the colon, bismuth salts react with hydrogen sulfide produced by anaerobic bacteria to make bismuth sulfide, a highly insoluble black salt responsible for dark stools.

Bismuth subgallate has been used to treat diarrhea, as an antacid, as a skin protectant, and in dental procedures. It is converted in the GI tract to bismuth sulfide. Less than 1% of the drug is absorbed. DeNol is tripotassium dicitrato bismuthate. Intraoral use of gauze impregnated with bismuth iodide paraffin paste has resulted in systemic absorption and toxicity (5).

HAZARDOUS REACTIVITIES

Bismuth can react with acid to produce toxic fumes. Heating bismuth in air forms bismuth trioxide. Combining bismuth and perchloric acid at temperatures greater than 110°C is explosive. The preparation of a salt from these two chemicals is dangerous.

Toxic Doses

ADULT

The acute ingestion of 1.5 g bismuth sodium triglycollamate (6), 5.4 g colloidal bismuth subcitrate (7), and 7.2 g tripotassium dicitrato bismuthate (8) has resulted in acute renal failure. A study of chronic therapeutic bismuth ingestion in France in the 1970s revealed no difference in dose or duration of treatment between patients who developed encephalopathy and those who did not. Most patients ingested 10 to 15 g/day of bismuth salts for less than 1 year (1).

Doses of 864 mg of bismuth daily as tripotassium dicitrato bismuthate (normal therapeutic dose, 432 mg/day) for 2 months in a patient with renal insufficiency resulted in whole blood concentrations of 880 μg/L and encephalopathy (9). Daily doses of 1 to 4 g of bismuth subsalicylate (Pepto-Bismol) over weeks to months were associated with progressive encephalopathy and gait impairment in a 54-year-old man (10).

PEDIATRIC

Doses of various bismuth salts as low as 100 mg intramuscularly (IM) or 1.5 g orally have been associated with lethargy, abdominal pain, and anuria in children aged 15 months to 19 years (6). A 2-year-old boy ingested 8.4 g of colloidal bismuth subcitrate and developed somnolence and acute renal failure (11). An 8-year-old girl developed acute renal failure during treatment with bismuth sodium triglycollamate (150 mg elemental bismuth twice a day) for approximately 13 weeks over a 5-month period for a total dose of approximately 18 g (6).

TOXICOKINETICS AND TOXICODYNAMICS

Less than 1% of bismuth salts (subsalicylate, subnitrate, subcitrate, subgallate) is absorbed orally. Orally administered bismuth is eliminated in the feces. Bismuth administered parenterally is distributed to brain, lungs, and teeth but is primarily concentrated in the kidney, liver, and bile. It is more than 90% protein bound. Its intermediate half-life is 5 to 11 days, and the terminal half-life is 21 to 72 days. Elimination is primarily urinary and biliary. The renal clearance is 50 ± 18 ml/minute. It is detectable in blood and urine for 5 months after a therapeutic oral dose.

PATHOPHYSIOLOGY

Bismuth binds to α_2-macroglobulin, immunoglobulin M, β-lipoprotein, and haptoglobin in blood. It selectively concentrates in the proximal renal tubule, where it causes necrosis. Characteristic inclusion bodies can be recognized in the nuclei and cytoplasm of the proximal tubule. The abdominal symptoms are believed to be from the precipitation of bismuth sulfide in mesenteric capillaries. Chronic ingestion may result in intracytoplasmic and intranuclear eosinophilic inclusions, especially in the kidney. The acute renal tubular damage may be due to the binding of sulfhydryl groups by bismuth (6). The mechanism of the encephalopathy associated with bismuth is unclear.

VULNERABLE POPULATIONS

Bismuth subsalicylate is U.S. Food and Drug Administration pregnancy category C. Chronic bismuth tartrate has produced animal birth defects. There are no human reports of adverse fetal outcomes after use of inorganic bismuth salts. However, the salicylate component of this drug when used during pregnancy may cause congenital defects. Bismuth subsalicylate should be avoided during breast-feeding because of systemic salicylate absorption (12). Human teratogenesis and carcinogenesis have not been reported.

CLINICAL PRESENTATION

Acute Exposure

GI effects include nausea, vomiting, diarrhea, abdominal pain as well as oral ulcerations (7). Hepatic injury is uncommon but has been reported (6).

Renal function may be impaired with severe nephrosis and acute tubular necrosis with bismuth subcitrate overdose (13). Acute oliguric renal failure developed in a 2-year-old boy 3 days after ingestion of 8.4 g colloidal bismuth subcitrate. His renal function returned to normal by 20 days after exposure (11). Severe proximal tubular injury may cause a Fanconi-like syndrome (6,7).

Neurologic effects include tremors, lethargy, and weakness but are more common after chronic exposures.

CASE STUDY

A 27-year-old man ingested 100 DeNol tablets (colloidal bismuth subcitrate, 120 mg/tablet) and 10 days later developed anorexia, nausea, vomiting, malaise, leg weakness, blurred vision, thirst, and poor urinary output. He was lucid. The bismuth blood level was 260 μg/L at 11 days postexposure. Hemodialysis was performed for 5 days at which time the renal failure and neurologic signs resolved (14).

Chronic Exposure

GI effects include increased salivation, a bluish or brownish discoloration of the gums from bismuth sulfide (bismuth line), black spots in the mucosa and gums, mucous membrane edema, pyorrhea, ulcerative stomatitis, and loss of teeth. Nausea, vomiting, diarrhea, and abdominal pain are common, and hepatitis or hepatocellular necrosis is rare. Therapeutic use is associated with dark discoloration of feces and tongue, headaches, rash, nausea, and vomiting.

Dermatologic effects are a generalized rash (parenteral use) and occasionally permanent discoloration of the skin and mucous membranes. *Renal effects* of acute nephritis, acute tubular necrosis, and renal failure are commonly observed. *Hematologic effects* include granulocytosis and aplastic anemia (rare).

Eight of 59 patients with bismuth-associated encephalopathy of 3 weeks' duration had osteoarticular lesions and fractures of the shoulder and thoracic vertebrae. It was attributed to the trauma of severe, repetitive myoclonus in bedridden, agitated patients (15). Osteoporosis and osteomalacia may follow increased levels of bismuth stored in bone.

Neurologic effects include encephalopathy, which is manifested by confusion, tremor, and motor disturbances after chronic, high-dose therapy (0.7 to 20.0 g for 4 weeks to 30 years) in France and Australia. Myoclonic encephalopathy has been described (16).

Encephalopathy has been reported after large or repetitive ingestions of water- or lipid-soluble salts (2). The encephalopathy is characterized by altered mental status, ataxia, myoclonus, and a specific electroencephalogram (EEG) abnormality (17). Bismuth blood levels range from 150 to 2000 μg/L (18). Clinically, bismuth encephalopathy is separated into two phases (2). The first phase is a prodromal period lasting from 1 week to several months during which cognitive and affective disorders are predominant. The patients are asthenic, somnolent, depressed, and anxious, sometimes with visual hallucinations and even delusions of persecution. Jerky movements are seen in this phase, and disturbances of writing and speech occur more rarely. A second phase of encephalopathy of rapid onset appears over 24 to 48 hours. Four symptoms are constant: confusion progressing to coma or dementia, dysarthria, disturbances of walking and standing, and tremor accompanied by myoclonic jerks. Myoclonic jerks are usually present in this phase. Sometimes they predominate in the upper limbs and distally; at other times, they are diffuse and involve the facial and axial muscles. They are increased by voluntary movements and by stimuli (i.e., change of position, noise).

CASE STUDY

A 54-year-old man took 1 to 4 g/day of bismuth subsalicylate (Pepto-Bismol) for months and developed progressive confusion and memory impairment over a period of 6 weeks. This was followed by onset of coarse postural and intentional hand tremor, myoclonic jerks, involuntary movements, hallucinations, and gait disturbances over 2 to 3 weeks. An extensive encephalopathy evaluation was all normal. The EEG showed bihemispheric slowing. He improved after cessation of bismuth ingestion (10).

DIAGNOSTIC TESTS

During peptic ulcer treatment, urine levels are 20 to 940 μg/L (19). Clinical studies in ulcer patients report a peak blood concentration at 2 to 3 hours postadministration of up to 100 μg/L (20,21). Bismuth salts at an oral dose of 10 to 20 g/day orally for 20 days per month resulted in a median bismuth blood level of 13 μg/L during treatment (22). The mean trough blood bismuth concentration after 2 weeks of 787 mg bismuth subsalicylate (three chewable tablets) four times daily under fasted conditions was 5.1 ± 3.1 μg/L.

Chronic toxicity is associated with a range of blood (50 to 1600 μg/L) and urine (150 to 1250 μg/L) concentrations (23). The median concentration in patients with encephalopathy ranged from 680 to 700 μg/L. A blood bismuth level of 50 to 100 μg/L should be considered an "alarm level." Patients with levels greater than 100 μg/L should cease therapy (22). Symptoms correlate poorly with blood levels; however, decreasing blood levels correlate well with recovery.

The preferred method of quantification of bismuth in urine, blood, or serum is atomic absorption spectrophotometry (detection limit, 1 μg/L) (24,25).

Urinalysis commonly reveals albuminuria, hematuria, and proteinuria.

Bismuth is radiopaque and may be seen on a plain abdominal radiograph of patients with acute ingestion of bismuth tablets (11) or with chronic bismuth encephalopathy (2). Unchewed and undissolved Pepto-Bismol tablets are radiopaque (26). Bismuth may accumulate in the metaphysis of long bones and produce transverse bands on plain radiography similar to lead toxicity or healing rickets (6).

Computed tomography may reveal an increase in density in the cerebral cortex and in the basal ganglia. Hyperdensities in the basal ganglia, cerebellum, and cerebral cortex were most marked when bismuth blood levels exceeded 2000 μg/L. Ventricular dilation may be present. Pathologic findings regressed in a subsequent computed tomography and corresponded to clinical improvement in one case (18,27).

A characteristic EEG in bismuth toxicity displays low voltage and diffuse beta frequencies bilaterally, maximal in the frontal and central areas and accentuated by hyperventilation (28). Epileptic EEG patterns appeared in patients with seizures only when the bismuth blood level was below 1500 μg/L (18).

Diagnostic Pitfalls

Bismuth toxicity should be included in the differential diagnosis of patients with slow-onset encephalopathy. It may mimic Creutzfeldt-Jakob disease, Alzheimer's disease, Ramsay Hunt syndrome, viral encephalopathies, DDT toxicity, alcohol withdrawal, or chronic salicylate intoxication.

Postmortem Considerations

In patients treated with bismuth for syphilis, the highest postmortem tissue levels were found in kidney (33.0 mg/kg), liver (6.8 mg/kg), bile (3.9 mg/L), and urine (1.2 mg/L) (23).

TREATMENT

Treatment of overdose is largely symptomatic and supportive. Dehydration may predispose the patient to renal injury, and adequate hydration should be assured (8). In general, spontaneous recovery from the encephalopathy and renal failure occurs in weeks to months after cessation of exposure. Even after large overdoses, the prognosis is good (10,13,14).

Decontamination and First Aid

A single dose of activated charcoal may be useful in preventing absorption shortly after ingestion but has not been systematically studied.

Enhancement of Elimination

There are no data available indicating that multiple-dose activated charcoal is effective.

Hemodialysis without chelating agents is unlikely to increase bismuth clearance (14). A patient with a blood concentration of 590 μg/L had no detectable elimination of bismuth with hemodialysis alone (8). Peritoneal dialysis has not been demonstrated to enhance bismuth elimination (11).

Antidotes

Acute or chronic toxicity resolves in weeks to months with discontinuation of exposure. Although chelators enhance the elimination of bismuth, treatment has not been shown to improve clinical outcome or limit toxicity.

In animal studies, succimer (Chapter 77) increases urinary excretion and is associated with increased survival and prevention of bismuth uptake by the liver and kidney (25,29). A single dose of 30 mg/kg increased urinary excretion of bismuth 50-fold in human volunteers who had been treated with colloidal bismuth subcitrate. Compared to dimercapto-1-propane sulfonic acid (DMPS), succimer increased blood levels of bismuth during the first 4 hours after succimer dosing (30).

DMPS (Chapter 54) increased urinary excretion of bismuth 50-fold compared to controls in human volunteers who had been treated with colloidal bismuth subcitrate (30). DMPS (300 mg/day orally) led to a tenfold increase in urinary clearance (0.24 to 2.40 ml/minute) of bismuth, with clinical improvement of encephalopathy in a patient with a creatinine clearance of 15 ml/minute (9). It has been associated with a significant increase in bismuth clearance when administered in conjunction with hemodialysis (8). Intravenous (IV) DMPS (250 mg every 4 hours for 48 hours, then 250 mg every 6 hours for 48 hours and 250 mg every 12 hours for another 4 days; total dose, 7 g) in addition to hemodialysis was effective in reducing serum bismuth levels from 640 to 15 μg/L over 6 days in a patient with bismuth subcitrate intoxication and acute renal failure (7). An initial 4-day course of IV DMPS (plus hemodialysis) followed by oral DMPS for 14 days has been recommended for significant acute bismuth intoxication (8).

DMPS administered 250 mg IV every 4 hours for 48 hours and then 250 mg IV every 6 hours for 48 hours increased the elimination of bismuth by hemodialysis with a highly porous polyacrylonitrile membrane (clearance bismuth, 10 to 52 ml/minute). The total bismuth elimination was 600 to 1800 μg/4-hour session (8). It was estimated that 16% of the total amount was eliminated within 16 hours of hemodialysis with DMPS. Early treatment with DMPS and hemodialysis may reduce serum bismuth concentration and prevent renal toxicity (7,8).

Dimercaprol (Chapter 50) enhanced bismuth clearance in two patients with myoclonic encephalopathy (31). It did not increase clearance in a patient treated with dimercaprol, 150 mg IM, for an acute bismuth ingestion. Dimercaprol is not indicated as routine first-line treatment because of its toxicity and its IM route of administration (32).

D-Penicillamine does not appear to facilitate excretion of bismuth (25,33). Although, in a mouse model, D-penicillamine was associated with increased survival (29). Calcium disodium edetate resulted in increased brain bismuth levels in a rat model and is not recommended (25).

Monitoring

Laboratory tests that should be routinely evaluated include a complete blood cell count, serum creatinine, blood urea nitrogen, and urinalysis. Monitoring urine output and creatinine clearance is valuable in determining the extent of renal impairment and the need for hemodialysis. Serum bismuth concentrations should decline after cessation of exposure and reflect improvement in clinical status. Frequent bismuth determinations are not necessary. There are no bismuth concentrations that are absolute indications for instituting chelation or dialysis.

PITFALLS

Because bismuth intoxication is rare, all other reversible causes of renal failure or dementia should also be considered. Inadequate hydration may predispose the patient to more renal injury after acute overdose.

REFERENCES

1. Martin-Bouyer G, Foulon G, Guerbois H, Barin C. Epidemiological study of encephalopathies following bismuth administration per os. Characteristics of intoxicated subjects: comparison with a control group. *J Toxicol Clin Toxicol* 1981;18(11):1277–1283.
2. Winship KA. Toxicity of bismuth salts. *Adverse Drug React Acute Pois Rev* 1982;2:103–121.
3. National Institute for Occupational Safety and Health. National Occupational Exposure Survey 1981–1983. DHHS (NIOSH) Publication No. 89-103, 1989.
4. Bierer DW. Bismuth subsalicylate: history, chemistry and safety. *Rev Infect Dis* 1990;12[Suppl 1]:S3–S8.
5. Bridgeman AM, Smith AC. Iatrogenic bismuth poisoning. Case report. *Aust Dent J* 1994;39:279–281.
6. Urizar R, Vernier RL. Bismuth nephropathy. *JAMA* 1966;198:207–209.
7. Hruz P, Mayr M, Low R, et al. Fanconi's syndrome, acute renal failure, and tonsil ulcerations after colloidal bismuth subcitrate intoxication. *Am J Kidney Dis* 2002;39(3):1–2.
8. Stevens PE, Moore DF, House IM, et al. Significant elimination of bismuth by hemodialysis with a new heavy-metal chelating agent. *Nephrol Dial Transplant* 1995;10:696–698.
9. Playford RJ, Matthews CH, Campbell MJ, et al. Bismuth induced encephalopathy caused by tripotassium dicitrato bismethate in a patient with chronic renal failure. *Gut* 1990;36:359–360.

10. Gordon MF, Abrams RI, Rubin DB, et al. Bismuth subsalicylate toxicity as a cause of prolonged encephalopathy with myoclonus. *Mov Disord* 1995;10:220–222.
11. Islek I, Uysal S, Gok F, et al. Reversible nephrotoxicity after overdose of colloidal bismuth subcitrate. *Pediatr Nephrol* 2001;16:510–514.
12. Briggs GR, Freeman RK, Yaffe SJ. *Drugs in pregnancy and lactation*, 6th ed. Baltimore: Williams & Wilkins, 2002:136–138.
13. Huwez F, Pall A, Lyons D, Stewart MJ. Acute renal failure after one dose of colloidal bismuth subcitrate. *Lancet* 1992;340:1298.
14. Hudson M, Ashley N, Mowat G. Reversible toxicity in poisoning with colloidal bismuth subcitrate. *BMJ* 1989;299:159.
15. Emil J, De Bray JM, Bernat M, et al. Osteoarticular complications in bismuth encephalopathy. *J Toxicol Clin Toxicol* 1981;18:1285–1290.
16. Mendelowitz PC, Hoffman RS, Weber S. Bismuth absorption and myoclonic encephalopathy during bismuth subsalicylate therapy. *Ann Intern Med* 1990;112:140–141.
17. Supino-Veterbo V, Sicard C, Risvegliato M, et al. Toxic encephalopathy due to ingestion of bismuth salts: clinical and EEG studies of 45 patients. *J Neurol Neurosurg Psychiatry* 1977;40:748–752.
18. Buge A, Supino-Viterbo V, Rancirel G, Pontes C. Epileptic phenomena in bismuth toxic encephalopathy. *J Neurol Neurosurg Psychiatry* 1981;44:62–67.
19. Serfontein WJ, Mekel R. Bismuth toxicity in man. II. Review of bismuth blood and urine levels in patients after administration of therapeutic bismuth formulations in relation to the problem of bismuth toxicity in man. *Res Commun Chem Pathol Pharmacol* 1979;26:391–411.
20. Nwokolo CV, Gavy CJ, Smith JT, Pounder RE. The absorption of bismuth from oral dose of tripotassium dicitrate bismuthate. *Aliment Pharmacol Ther* 1989;3:29–39.
21. Lauritsen K, Laursen LS, Rask-Madsen J. Clinical pharmacokinetics of drug used in the treatment of gastrointestinal diseases. I. *Clin Pharmacokinet* 1990;19:11–31.
22. Hillemand P, Palliere M, Laquais B, Bouvet P. Bismuth treatment and blood bismuth levels. *Sem Hop* 1977;53(31–32):1663–1669.
23. Baselt RC. *Disposition of toxic drugs and chemicals in man*, 6th ed. Foster City, CA: Chemical Toxicology Institute, 2002:110–111.
24. Behrendt WA, Groger C, Kuhn D, et al. A study relating to bioavailability and renal elimination of bismuth after oral administration of basic bismuth nitrate. *Int J Clin Pharmacol Ther Toxicol* 1991;29:357–360.
25. Slikkerveer A, Jong HB, Helmich RB, et al. Development of a therapeutic procedure for bismuth intoxication with chelating agents. *J Lab Clin Med* 1992;119:529–537.
26. Woo OF, Jackson GM. Radiopacity of chewable Pepto-Bismol tablets: report of two patients. *Vet Hum Toxicol* 1993;35:317.
27. Gardeur D, Buge A, Rancurel G, et al. Bismuth encephalopathy and cerebral computed tomography. *J Comput Assist Tomogr* 1978;2:436–438.
28. Hasking G, Duggan J. Encephalopathy from bismuth subsalicylate. *Med J Aust* 1982;2:167.
29. Basinger MA, Jones MM, McCroskey SA. Antidotes for acute bismuth intoxication. *J Toxicol Clin Toxicol* 1983;20:159–165.
30. Slikkerveer A, Noach LA, Tytgat GNJ, et al. Comparison of enhanced elimination of bismuth in human after treatment with meso-2,3-dimercaptosuccinic acid and D,L-2,3-dimercaptopropane-1-sulfonic acid. *Analyst* 1998;123:91–92.
31. Molina JA, Calandre L, Bermajo F. Myoclonic encephalopathy due to bismuth salts: treatment with dimercaprol and analysis of CSF transmitters. *Acta Neurol Scand* 1989;79:200–203.
32. Slikkerveer A, Helminth RB, Jong HB, de Wolff TA. Development of a therapeutic procedure for bismuth intoxication using chelating agents. *Hum Exp Toxicol* 1993;12:77–78.
33. Nwokolo CU, Pounder PE. D-Penicillamine does not increase urinary bismuth excretion in patients treated with tripotassium dicitrato bismuthate. *Br J Clin Pharmacol* 1990;30:648–650.

CHAPTER 217

Cadmium

Seth Schonwald

Atomic symbol, atomic number, molecular weight:	**Cd, 48, 112.41 g/mol**
Density:	**8.65 g/cm^3**
Melting point:	**320.9°C**
Valence states:	**0, +1, +2**
CAS Registry No.:	**7440-43-9**
Normal levels:	**Blood: nonexposed, nonsmoking—0.4 to 1.0 μg/L (0.0036 to 0.0089 μmol/L); smoker—1.4 to 4.5 μg/L (0.012 to 0.040 μmol/L); urine: 1 μg/L or lower (0.0089 μmol/L)**
SI conversion:	**μg/L × 0.0089 = μmol/L**
Special concerns:	**Acute respiratory exposure with minimal symptoms initially may develop into pulmonary edema.**
Target organs:	**Kidney (chronic), lung (acute inhalation), gastrointestinal (acute ingestion)**
Antidote:	**An effective chelator for cadmium has not yet been discovered.**

OVERVIEW

Cadmium is a nonessential trace metal that was discovered by Fredrich Stromeyer in 1817. It is present as the metal and in numerous industrial compounds (cadmium acetate, carbonate, chloride, fluoroborate, fluoride, iodide, nitrate, oxide, stearate, sulfate, and sulfide). Environmental contamination in Japan caused a disease called *Itai-Itai* (ouch-ouch), which was characterized by severe arthralgia and osteomalacia in middle-aged, postmenopausal women with low calcium and vitamin D intake. Sources of cadmium arise primarily from human activities (Table 1) (1). Emission control measures have reduced industrial sources in the United States. Cadmium is present in many industrial settings (Table 1) (2,3). Environmental and occupational regulatory limits for cadmium are provided in Table 2 (4).

Toxic Doses

Cadmium has been used as a suicidal agent. The estimated doses ingested in two fatal cases were 25 mg Cd/kg from cad-

TABLE 1. Sources of cadmium

Environmental
- Contaminated foodstuffs (e.g., rice, cigarettes, and soil)
- Fuel combustion
- Disposal of metal-containing products
- Phosphate fertilizer or sewage sludges

Occupational
- The use of cadmium compounds essentially falls into five industrial categories:
  - Active electrode materials in nickel-cadmium batteries (70% of total cadmium use)
  - Pigments used mainly in plastics, ceramics, and glasses (12%)
  - Stabilizers for polyvinyl chloride against heat and light (17%)
  - Engineering coatings on steel and some nonferrous metals (8%)
  - Components of various specialized alloys (2%)
- Smaller sources: zinc and lead smelting, solder, nuclear industry, dental amalgams, electroplated ice trays

mium iodide (5) and 1840 mg Cd/kg from cadmium chloride (6). The cadmium chloride ingestion was 150 g and produced facial edema, vomiting, hypotension, respiratory arrest, metabolic acidosis, pulmonary edema, oliguria, and finally death 30 hours postingestion (6).

Acute occupational inhalation of cadmium has also caused death. Symptoms are initially mild; however, severe pulmonary edema and chemical pneumonitis can culminate in death due to respiratory failure (7). Cadmium has also been implicated in the deaths of workers chronically exposed to dusts (8). Acute, high-level exposures can be fatal, and those who survive may have impaired lung function for years after a single exposure. A 34-year-old worker exposed to cadmium fume from soldering for 1 hour (dose not determined) had persistent impaired lung function when examined 4 years later (9).

No significant increase in cancer rates was found among residents of a cadmium-polluted village in England (10), and no significant increase in prostate, kidney, or urinary tract cancer was found among residents of a cadmium-polluted area of Belgium (11). In a retrospective Japanese study of three areas classified as highly polluted, slightly polluted, or nonpolluted by cadmium, no significant differences were found in cancer mortality (12). A report on 347 copper cadmium alloy workers in the United Kingdom found that cadmium oxide increased mortality from chronic nonmalignant respiratory diseases but did not increase the risks from lung cancer (13). Nonetheless, an International Agency for Research on Cancer working group has designated cadmium as "probably carcinogenic to humans" (14). The Environmental Protection Agency also classifies cadmium as a probable human carcinogen.

TABLE 2. U.S. regulatory guidelines and standards for cadmium (Cd)

Agency	Description	Concentration
OSHA		
(air)	TWA	5.0 μg/m^3
	Action level (8-h TWA)	2.5 μg/m^3
ACGIH		
(air)	TLV-TWA	0.01 mg/m^3 (elemental)
	TLV-TWA	0.002 mg/m^3 (Cd compounds, as Cd)
NIOSH		
(air)	IDLH	9 mg/m^3 (as Cd)

ACGIH, American Conference of Governmental Industrial Hygienists; IDLH, immediate danger to life or health; NIOSH, National Institute for Occupational Safety and Health; OSHA, U.S. Occupational Safety and Health Administration; TLV, threshold limit value; TWA, time-weighted average.

TOXICOKINETICS AND TOXICODYNAMICS

Cadmium metal and cadmium salts have low volatility and exist in air primarily as fine suspended particulate matter. Some soluble cadmium compounds (e.g., cadmium chloride and cadmium sulfate) may undergo limited absorption from particles deposited in the respiratory tree, but the major site of absorption is the alveoli. Approximately 25% of inhaled cadmium is absorbed. Absorption from cigarettes appears to be higher than absorption from cadmium aerosols, probably due to the very small size of particles in cigarette smoke allowing very high alveolar deposition. Only approximately 5% of ingested cadmium is absorbed (15). Cadmium absorption is increased by iron or calcium deficiency and increased dietary fat. Cadmium is not well absorbed dermally.

Cadmium distributes widely throughout the body, with most ending up in the liver and kidney. Plasma cadmium circulates bound primarily to metallothionein and also to albumin and presumably other compounds (16).

Most cadmium that is ingested or inhaled is excreted in the feces and is not absorbed. Absorbed cadmium is excreted very slowly, with urinary and fecal excretion being approximately equal. Cadmium is not known to undergo any direct metabolic conversion, such as oxidation, reduction, or alkylation. Half-times for the human kidney have been estimated between 6 and 38 years and for the human liver at between 4 and 19 years.

PATHOPHYSIOLOGY

The kidney is the main target organ for chronic exposure. Proximal tubular dysfunction characterized by proteinuria, aminoaciduria, and glycosuria occurs. Renal failure is rare. High acute exposure can produce delayed pulmonary edema, progressing to interstitial fibrosis. Chronic effects from cadmium inhalation may include emphysema and chronic bronchitis.

VULNERABLE POPULATIONS

The placenta is a partial barrier to fetal cadmium exposure (17,18). Cadmium concentration in cord blood is about one-half that of maternal blood, including both smoking and nonsmoking women. Cadmium can be excreted in human milk at 5% to 10% of blood levels (19). The health effects of low-level exposure via breast milk are unknown (20). Iron deficiency during pregnancy leads to increased cadmium absorption and body burden (21).

CLINICAL PRESENTATION

Renal Effects

The kidney is the main target organ of cadmium after extended oral or inhalation exposure. Tubular proteinuria has been documented repeatedly in residents of cadmium-polluted areas of Japan (22,23), Belgium (24), and China (25). Workers exposed to cadmium oxide dust and cadmium fumes in factories have a high incidence of proteinuria and decreased glomerular filtration rate (26,27). Significant renal effects may include tubular nephropathy manifested by proteinuria, aminoaciduria, glucosuria, phosphaturia, and calcium wastage. Chronic sequelae may include decreased glomerular filtration rate and increased risk of kidney stones (28). The proteinuria is characterized by low-molecular-weight proteins, indicating proximal tubular damage.

Respiratory Effects

High levels of cadmium oxide fumes or dust are intensely irritating to respiratory tissue, but symptoms can be delayed. Symptoms after acute inhalation may simulate metal fume fever with fever, headache, dyspnea, pleuritic chest pain, conjunctivitis, rhinitis, sore throat, and cough typically developing within 4 to 12 hours of exposure. Noncardiogenic pulmonary edema may appear, which can progress to death. Respiratory failure may ensue in 3 to 10 days. Precise estimates of cadmium dose leading to acute respiratory effects in humans have not been reported.

Long-term pulmonary exposure can cause emphysema; however, early occupational studies did not control for the effects of cigarette smoking. Cadmium may accelerate the development of emphysema in smokers (29). More recent studies that controlled for smoking have reported lung impairment in cadmium-exposed workers (30,31).

Other Health Effects

Ingestion of cadmium in high concentration causes severe irritation to the gastrointestinal epithelium. Acute gastroenteritis is characterized by the sudden onset of vomiting, diarrhea, salivation, cramps, and abdominal pain (32,33). The gastrointestinal symptoms have been caused in children by soft drinks and popsicles. Liver damage occurs after ingestion of high concentrations of cadmium as well.

The cardiovascular system does not appear to be affected after inhalation, although hypertension was associated with increased cadmium levels in one study (34). In some studies, the mortality from cardiovascular disease was actually lower in the cadmium-exposed population (35).

Ingestion of cadmium reduces gastrointestinal uptake of iron, which can result in anemia if dietary iron intake is low. Studies have yielded mixed results on the relationship of dietary cadmium and anemia (3).

Painful bone disorders, including osteomalacia, osteoporosis, and spontaneous and painful bone fractures (Itai-Itai), have been observed in humans chronically exposed to cadmium in food. In the Jinzu river basin in Japan, osteomalacia and Itai-Itai disease were associated with women with poor nutrition and multiparity. Calcium deficiency, osteoporosis, or osteomalacia (36) can also develop in some workers after long-term occupational exposure to high levels of cadmium (37). Effects on bone generally arise only after kidney damage has occurred and are likely to be secondary to changes in calcium, phosphorus, and vitamin D metabolism (3,38). Cadmium exposure has also been associated with "yellow teeth lines" and urinary calculi.

Neurologic effects include dose-dependent slowing of visuomotor functioning on neurobehavioral testing and increased complaints consistent with peripheral neuropathy, impaired equilibrium, and ability to concentrate (39). Cadmium may be a cause of peripheral polyneuropathy in those chronically exposed (40). A 64-year-old man who sustained multiorgan failure after acute exposure to cadmium developed parkinsonian features (41).

DIAGNOSTIC TESTS

The blood concentration of cadmium in exposed workers ranges from 10 to 100 mg/L. Levels above 0.7 μg/dl indicate significant exposure. An outbreak of cadmium intoxication in jewelry factory workers produced a dose–response relationship between blood cadmium levels and symptoms of dyspnea, chest pain, dyscrasia, and dizziness (42). Cadmium in blood may be used to assess recent exposure to cadmium (43).

Cadmium-induced tubular dysfunction is irreversible and is probably best assessed by analyzing α_1-microglobulin in urine (44). When the urinary excretion of cadmium is less than 2 mg/24 hours, the risk of renal injury remains low. The urine level best reflects total body burden. Some authors believe that an increased cadmium level requires the concomitant presence of renal damage.

The most common analytical procedures for cadmium in biologic samples are atomic absorption spectroscopy and atomic emission spectroscopy. The detection limit of urinary cadmium is 0.08 mg/L.

Postmortem concentrations are almost negligible in the liver of neonates and toddlers but increase with age. Postmortem urine levels correlate strongly with levels in the kidney (45).

TREATMENT

The initial care of inhalation exposure to high levels of cadmium includes monitoring for respiratory distress, assisting ventilation as needed, and administering oxygen. If pulmonary edema develops, individuals may need mechanical ventilation, diuretics, intravenous fluids, and possibly steroid medications. Antibiotic therapy is unproven. Monitoring fluid balance (due to kidney function impairment) may also be important.

Ingestion

Oral cadmium exposure is not usually an immediate threat because high doses often induce vomiting. The only known acute fatalities from oral exposure involve acute ingestion of high doses (3). Although vomiting has been recommended after the ingestion (46), concentrated cadmium solutions may be caustic, and esophageal damage could result from induced vomiting. Dilution with water or milk may be helpful but has not been proved. The use of activated charcoal to bind unabsorbed cadmium does not appear to be effective.

Skin Exposure

Dermal or ocular exposure to cadmium compounds may be irritating and is treated by removing contaminated clothing, washing the skin, and thoroughly flushing the eyes.

Respiratory Exposure

Inhalation exposure to high concentrations of cadmium can be particularly dangerous because initial symptoms are often mild. This may allow exposure to continue until a harmful or even fatal dose is received. Severe respiratory symptoms may develop within a few hours of high-dose inhalation. Aside from removing a victim to fresh air and providing supportive care, no effective means have been reported for reducing absorption after inhalation (47).

Antidotes

No means have been proven to reduce the body burden and clinical effects of cadmium in overdose (48), although a variety of chelating agents are being developed. Some sources recommend using ethylenediaminetetraacetic acid; however, ethylenediaminetetraacetic acid may potentiate nephrotoxicity. Succimer may also enhance cadmium excretion after oral intoxication; however, adequate clinical studies in humans are still forthcoming (49,50). British antilewisite (dimercaprol) increases nephrotoxicity and is not indicated (51). In rats, protection from cadmium-induced nephrotoxicity may be possible by continued coadministration of *N*-acetylcysteine, and recovery from advanced nephrotoxicity may be achieved with *N*-acetylcysteine, provided that cadmium exposure is stopped (52).

REFERENCES

1. Elinder CG. Cadmium: uses, occurrence and intake. In: Friberg L, Elinder CG, Kjellstrom T, et al., eds. *Cadmium and health: a toxicological and epidemiological appraisal. Vol. I. Exposure, dose, and metabolism. Effects and response.* Boca Raton, FL: CRC Press, 1985:23–64.
2. Elinder CG. Cadmium as an environmental hazard. *IARC Sci Publ* 1992;118:123–132.
3. Agency for Toxic Substances and Disease Registry, division of toxicology. *ATSDR toxicological profile for cadmium.* Atlanta: ATSDR, 1999:1–440.
4. OSHA. Occupational Safety and Health Administration. 29 CFR 1910.1027(c), 1992.
5. Wisniewska-Knypl JM, Jablonska J, Myslak Z. Binding of cadmium on metallothionein in man: an analysis of a fatal poisoning by cadmium iodide. *Arch Toxicol* 1971;28:46–55.
6. Buckler HM, Smith WD, Rees WD. Self poisoning with oral cadmium chloride. *BMJ* 1986;292:1559–1560.
7. Seidal K, Jorgensen N, Elinder CG. Fatal cadmium induced pneumonitis. *Stand J Work Environ Health* 1993;19:429–431.
8. Friberg L. Health hazards in the manufacture of alkaline accumulators with special reference to chronic cadmium poisoning. *Acta Med Stand* 1950;138[Suppl 240]:1–124.
9. Barnhart S, Rosenstock L. Cadmium chemical pneumonitis. *Chest* 1984;86:789–791.
10. Inskip H, Beral V. Mortality of Shipham residents: 40-year follow-up. *Lancet* 1982;1:896–899.
11. Lauwerys R, De Wals PH. Environmental pollution by cadmium and mortality from renal diseases. *Lancet* 1981;1:383.
12. Shigematsu I. The epidemiological approach to cadmium pollution in Japan. *Ann Acad Med Singapore* 1984;13:231–236.
13. Sorahan T, Lister A, Gilthorpe MS, et al. Mortality of copper cadmium alloy workers with special reference to lung cancer and non-malignant diseases of the respiratory system, 1946–92. *Occup Environ Med* 1995;52:804–812.
14. IARC. Cadmium and certain cadmium compounds. In: *IARC monographs on the evaluation of the carcinogenic risk of chemicals to humans. Beryllium, cadmium, mercury and exposures in the glass manufacturing industry. IARC monographs.* Lyon, France: World Health Organization International Agency for Research on Cancer, 1993;58:119–146, 210–236.
15. Kjellstrom T, Borg K, Lind B. Cadmium in feces as an estimator of daily cadmium intake in Sweden. *Environ Res* 1978;15:242–251.
16. Foulkes EC, Blanck S. Acute cadmium uptake by rabbit kidneys: mechanism and effects. *Toxicol Appl Pharmacol* 1990;102:464–473.
17. Truska P, Rosival L, Balazova G, et al. Blood and placental concentrations of cadmium, lead, and mercury in mothers and their newborns. *J Hyg Epidemiol Microbial Immuno* 1989;133:141–147.
18. Goyer RA. Transplacental transfer of cadmium and fetal effects. *Fundam Appl Toxicol* 1991;16:22–23.
19. Radisch B, Luck W, Nau H. Cadmium concentrations in milk and blood of smoking mothers. *Toxicol Lett* 1987;36:147–152.
20. Abadin HG, Hibbs BF, Pohl HR. Breast-feeding exposure of infants to cadmium, lead, and mercury: a public health viewpoint. *Toxicol Ind Health* 1997;13:495–517.
21. Akesson A, Berglund M, Schutz A, et al. Cadmium exposure in pregnancy and lactation in relation to iron status. *Am J Public Health* 2002;92:284–287.
22. Nogawa K, Kobayashi E, Honda R, et al. Renal dysfunction of inhabitants in a cadmium-polluted area. *Environ Res* 1980;23:13–23.
23. Ishihara T, Kobayashi E, Okubo Y, et al. Association between cadmium concentration in rice and mortality in the Jinzu River basin, Japan. *Toxicology* 2001;163:23–28.
24. Buchet JP, Lauwerys R, Roels H, et al. Renal effects of cadmium body burden of the general population. *Lancet* 1990;336:699–702.
25. Shiwen C, Lin Y, Zhineng H, et al. Cadmium exposure and health effects among residents in an irrigation area with ore dressing wastewater. *Sci Total Environ* 1990;90:67–73.
26. Bustueva KA, Revich BA, Bezpalko LE. Cadmium in the environment of three Russian cities and in human hair and urine. *Arch Environ Health* 1994;49:284–288.
27. Iwata K, Saito H, Moriyama M, et al. Renal tubular function after reduction of environmental cadmium exposure: a ten-year follow-up. *Arch Environ Health* 1993;48:157–163.
28. Savolainen H. Cadmium-associated renal disease. *Ren Fail* 1995;17:483–487.
29. Leduc D, de Francquen P, Jacobovitz D, et al. Association of cadmium exposure with rapidly progressive emphysema in a smoker. *Thorax* 1993;48:570–571.
30. Cortona G, Apostoli P, Toffoletto F, et al. Occupational exposure to cadmium and lung function. In: Nordberg GF, Herber RFM, Alessio L, eds. *Cadmium in the human environment: toxicity and carcinogenicity.* Lyon, France: International Agency for Research on Cancer, 1992.
31. Chan OY, Poh SC, Lee HS, et al. Respiratory function in cadmium battery workers—a follow-up study. *Ann Acad Med Singapore* 1988;17:283–287.
32. Shipman DL. Cadmium food poisoning in a Missouri school. *J Environ Health* 1986;49:89.
33. Nordberg G, Slorach S, Steinstrom T. [Cadmium poisoning caused by a cooled-soft-drink machine.] *Lakartidingen* 1973;70:601–604.
34. Bakshi SK, Chawla KP, Khandekar RN, Raghunath R. Cadmium and hypertension. *J Assoc Physicians India* 1994;42:449–450.
35. Armstrong BG, Kazantzis G. The mortality of cadmium workers. *Lancet* 1983;1:1425–1427.
36. Takebayashi S, Jimi S, Segawa M, Kiyoshi Y. Cadmium induces osteomalacia mediated by proximal tubular atrophy and disturbances of phosphate reabsorption. A study of 11 autopsies. *Pathol Res Pract* 2000;196:653–663.
37. Kazantzis G. Renal tubular dysfunction and abnormalities of calcium metabolism in cadmium workers. *Environ Health Perspect* 1979;28:155–159.
38. Blainey JD, Adams RG, Brewer DB, et al. Cadmium-induced osteomalacia. *Br J Ind Med* 1980;37:278–284.
39. Viaene MK, Masschelein R, Leenders J, et al. Neurobehavioural effects of occupational exposure to cadmium: a cross sectional epidemiological study. *Occup Environ Med* 2000;57:19–27.
40. Viaene MK, Roels HA, Leenders J, et al. Cadmium: a possible etiological factor in peripheral polyneuropathy. *Neurotoxicology* 1999;20:7–16.
41. Okuda B, Iwamoto Y, Tachibana H, Sugita M. Parkinsonism after acute cadmium poisoning. *Clin Neurol Neurosurg* 1997;99:263–265.
42. Baker EL Jr, Coleman C, Peterson WA, et al. Subacute cadmium intoxication in jewelry workers. An evaluation of diagnostic procedure. *Arch Environ Health* 1979;39:173–177.
43. Herber RF, Christensen JM, Sabbioni E. Critical evaluation and review of cadmium concentrations in blood for use in occupational health according to the TRACY protocol. *Int Arch Occup Environ Health* 1997;69:372–378.
44. Jarup L, Persson B, Elinder CG. Blood cadmium as an indicator of dose in a long-term follow-up of workers previously exposed to cadmium. *Scand J Work Environ Health* 1997;23:31–36.
45. Orlowski C, Piotrowski JK, Subdys JK, Gross A. Urinary cadmium as indicator of renal cadmium in humans: an autopsy study. *Hum Exp Toxicol* 1998;17:302–306.
46. Stutz DR, Janusz SJ. *Hazardous materials injuries: a handbook for prehospital care,* 2nd ed. Greenbelt, MD: Bradford Communications Corporation, 1988;21:228–229.
47. EPA. *Recognition and management of pesticide poisonings,* 4th ed. EPA-540/9-88-001. Washington, DC: Environmental Protection Agency, 1989:109–111.
48. Goldfrank LR, Flomenbaum NE, Lewin NA, et al. *Goldfrank's toxicological emergencies,* 5th ed. Norwalk, CT: Appleton & Lange, 1994:1063–1078.
49. Jones MM, Singh PK, Gale GR, et al. Cadmium mobilization in vivo by intraperitoneal or oral administration of monoalkyl esters of meso-2,3-dimercaptosuccinic acid in the mouse. *Pharmacol Toxicol* 1992;70:336–343.
50. Miller AL. Dimercaptosuccinic acid (DMSA), a non-toxic, water-soluble treatment for heavy metal toxicity. *Altern Med Rev* 1998;3:199–207.
51. Goldfrank LR, Flomenbaum NE, Lewin NA, et al. *Goldfrank's toxicological emergencies,* 4th ed. Norwalk, CT: Appleton & Lange, 1990:649–652.
52. Shaikh ZA, Zaman K, Tang W, Vu T. Treatment of chronic cadmium nephrotoxicity by N-acetyl cysteine. *Toxicol Lett* 1999;104:137–142.

CHAPTER 218

Chromium

Seth Schonwald

$$O{=}Cr({=}O)(-OH)-OH$$

CHROMIC ACID

Atomic symbol, atomic number, molecular weight:	**Cr, 24, 51.996 g/mol**
Valence states:	**0, +2, +3, +6**
CAS Registry No.:	**7440-47-3**
Normal levels:	**0 to 10 µg/L**
SI conversion:	**µg/L × 0.0192 = µmol/L**
Special concerns:	**Severe renal injury may arise from relatively small skin exposures.**
Target organs:	**Skin (burns), kidney (renal failure)**
Antidotes:	**British antilewisite (dimercaprol), dimercapto-propane-sulfonic acid (DMPS), *N*-acetylcysteine (NAC), ascorbic acid (none proven)**

OVERVIEW

Chromium was discovered by Louis Vauquelin in 1797. It is used widely in the tanning industry; stainless steel and alloy manufacturing; photography, cement, dye, and lithography industries; and wood preservative production. It is also used for electroplating in automotive and other industries and in the manufacture of safety matches (1,2).

Chromium is an essential trace element required for the maintenance of normal glucose tolerance (3,4). Chromium picolinate, an herbal supplement, has been touted for its weight-losing, cholesterol-lowering, and heart disease–preventing properties (5).

Rare, significant toxicity may occur via dermal exposure from soluble chromic compounds, from aerosolized byproducts of industrial processes, and occasionally as a suicidal agent using oral preparations. Epidemiologic studies have detected an increased incidence of lung cancer in workers exposed to hexavalent chromium compounds (6,7).

Chromium is available commercially in several forms, including chromium polynicotinate, chromium picolinate, chromium-enriched yeast, and chromium chloride. Preparation doses are typically between 15 and 200 µg/day in multivitamins. The recommended dietary intake of chromium (III) is 50 to 200 µg/day.

Toxic Dose

U.S. regulatory guidelines and standards are provided in Table 1. Ingestion of 0.5 to 0.8 g of potassium dichromate may be lethal (2,8). An ingestion of 125 ml of chromic acid by a 33-year-old patient resulted in hypotension, acute renal tubular necrosis, and hepatic failure (9). A 15-year-old patient who ingested a few grains of potassium dichromate died in 12 hours (10). A 35-year-old woman developed severe acidosis, massive gastrointestinal hemorrhage, acute renal failure, and hepatic injury after ingestion of 50 ml of chromic acid and died 12 hours after ingestion (11). A woman who ingested 400 ml of leather tanning solution containing 48 g of basic chromium sulfate died of cardiogenic shock, complicated by pancreatitis and gut mucosal necrosis and hemorrhage (12).

As little as 500 mg of ingested hexavalent chromium (e.g., chromic acid or chromium trioxide) may cause life-threatening toxicity in adults. Trivalent chromium ingestion is generally well tolerated. One exception is chromium sulfate, a particularly corrosive form of trivalent chromium. Up to 1 mg of trivalent chromium per day has not been associated with significant toxicity (13). A 48-year-old man drank 150 ml (22.5 g) of potassium dichromate and was admitted 7 hours after the ingestion. Hemodialysis was promptly undertaken, and the patient survived (14).

TABLE 1. U.S. regulatory guidelines and standards for chromium (Cr)

Agency	Description	Concentration
OSHA (air)	Cr metal and insoluble salts	
	PEL-TWA	1.0 mg/m^3
	Cr (VI) salts	
	PEL-TWA	1.0 mg/m^3
ACGIH (air)	Metal and inorganic compounds	
	TLV-TWA	0.5 mg/m^3 (as Cr)
	STEL	None
	Water-soluble Cr (VI) compounds NOC	—
	TLV-TWA	0.05 mg/m^3
	Insoluble Cr (VI) compounds NOC	
	TLV-TWA	0.01 mg/m^3
NIOSH (air)	Chromium metal and insoluble salts	
	REL-TWA	0.5 mg/m^3
	STEL	None
	IDLH	—
	Chromic acid and chromates	
	REL-TWA	0.001 mg/m^3 (as Cr)
	STEL	None
EPA (water)	Drinking water standard	100 µg/L (water)

ACGIH, American Conference of Governmental Industrial Hygienists; EPA, Environmental Protection Agency; IDLH, immediate danger to life or health; NIOSH, National Institute for Occupational Safety and Health; NOC, not otherwise classified; OSHA, U.S. Occupational Safety and Health Administration; PEL, permissible exposure limit; REL, recommended exposure limit; STEL, short-term exposure limit; TLV, threshold limit value; TWA, time-weighted average.

Long-term exposure to chromium has been associated with lung cancer in workers exposed to ambient air levels of 100 to 1000 times higher than those in nature. Between 1966 and 1986, the childhood leukemia rate in Woburn, Massachusetts, was fourfold higher than the national average. The residents of Woburn may have been exposed to arsenic (70 μg/L) and chromium (240 μg/L) by consuming groundwater contaminated with these metals (15).

Regulatory agencies consider chromium(VI) to be carcinogenic, based on evidence in humans found in chromate production, chromate pigment production, and chromium plating industries (6,16). Chromium(0) and chromium(III) compounds are not classifiable as to their carcinogenicity.

TOXICOKINETICS AND TOXICODYNAMICS

The lungs and gastrointestinal tract absorb chromium compounds. Hexavalent compounds (+6) are more easily absorbed through the lungs compared to trivalent compounds (+3) in part because they traverse biologic membranes more easily (2). Bivalent and trivalent forms (e.g., chromic oxide or sulfate) are relatively insoluble, poorly absorbed, and usually not of clinical importance.

Oral absorption averages 0.5% to 2.0%. In the stomach and after absorption, most hexavalent chromium is reduced to trivalent forms, which accounts for the poor bioavailability of hexavalent chromium(17). Trivalent chromium binds to transferrin and distributes throughout the body (2). Chromium is rapidly excreted mainly by the kidney. The elimination half-life of hexavalent chromium is 15 to 41 hours (18).

PATHOPHYSIOLOGY

Hexavalent chromium is a skin and mucous-membrane irritant as well as a powerful oxidizing agent. Certain hexavalent chromium compounds, such as chromic acid, ammonium dichromate, potassium dichromate, and chromium sulfate, are corrosives (2,19). Chromic acid has a pH of 5, and ammonia dichromate has a pH of 13.

Hexavalent chromium in dichromate compounds binds nonspecifically to proteins and nucleoproteins and is specifically taken up into red cells and platelets. The conversion of hexavalent chromium to trivalent chromium generates free radicals and other species. These reactive intermediates are likely the cause of oxidative DNA damage and genotoxicity of hexavalent chromium compounds (20).

VULNERABLE POPULATIONS

The hexavalent form of chromium crosses the placenta and enters breast milk (21). Limited information suggests that exposure to chromium (VI) may result in complications during pregnancy and childbirth (8).

CLINICAL PRESENTATION

Gastrointestinal Effects

Ingestion of hexavalent chromium compounds, such as chromic acid, usually leads to early abdominal pain, vomiting, diarrhea, and intestinal bleeding. Yellow-green vomitus or hematemesis may be observed. Hepatic necrosis, coagulopathy, and acute tubular necrosis with renal failure may follow, and death may ensue due to circulatory collapse (22,23). An adult who suffered full-thickness burns of the left calf (1% of body surface) from a concentrated chromic acid solution developed nausea and vomiting within 1 hour and anuria within 24 hours (24).

Pulmonary Effects

Inhalation of high levels of hexavalent chromium can cause nasal irritation, sneezing, itching, nosebleeds, ulcers, and "chrome holes" in the nasal septum (25). These effects are associated with occupational use of chromium (VI) for several months to years (26). Dichromate dust can cause conjunctivitis, chronic penetrating lesions of the skin, lacrimation, and ulceration of the nasal septum. Vertigo, thirst, abdominal pain, vomiting, oliguria, anuria, shock, seizures, coagulopathy, intravascular hemolysis, and a hepatorenal syndrome can follow large inhalational doses of dichromate (27). Inhalation of trivalent chromium generally does not cause mucosal irritation.

Dermatologic Effects

Workers handling liquids or solids containing chromium (VI) can develop dermatitis and full-thickness skin ulcers. Certain individuals may be more sensitive to chromium (VI) or chromium (III). Allergic reactions consisting of severe erythema and swelling of the skin have been noted. Systemic contact dermatitis may be associated with oral chromium picolinate (28). A contact dermatitis called *Blackjack disease* may occur in card players and dealers exposed to chromium in green felt (29). Aerosolized hexavalent chromium compounds may cause bronchospasm, hyperemia, and respiratory tract inflammation (30).

Other Effects

Rhabdomyolysis occurred in a 24-year-old body builder who ingested 1200 μg of chromium picolinate over 48 hours (31). Chromium supplements may cause serious renal impairment when ingested in large excess (32).

DIAGNOSTIC TESTS

After ingestion of hexavalent compounds, diagnostic procedures for caustic ingestion may be needed, such as esophagoscopy. Hair chromium concentrations may be helpful in identifying industrial exposure to trivalent chromium (33).

Chromium is measured by flameless atomic absorption spectrometry. Serum concentrations in the general population with no occupational chromium exposure are 1 to 3 nmol/L (0.052 to 0.156 μg/L) (34). Whole blood concentrations of 2 to 3 mg Cr/L are lethal (2).

All patients with significant hexavalent chromium ingestion require intensive monitoring of vital signs, hydration status, complete blood cell count, electrolytes, liver function tests, renal function, and coagulation studies. Chest radiography is recommended after symptomatic exposures to aerosolized hexavalent chromium exposures.

TREATMENT

Chromium toxicity ranges from a small burn to a severe systemic disease with multiple-organ failure. Burns are treated like other burns, with special attention to potential renal injury. Pulmonary effects, such as bronchospasm, are treated as other causes with oxygen and bronchodilator drugs. Circulatory collapse requires vigorous hydration and, in refractory cases, pressor support.

Decontamination and First Aid

Gastrointestinal decontamination is not typically used because hexavalent chromium compounds are caustic. Saline or water dilution may be helpful; however, definitive studies are lacking. Nasogastric lavage with ascorbic acid solution and intravenous doses of ascorbic acid might theoretically reduce hexavalent to trivalent chromium; however, studies to prove clinical efficacy are lacking (35).

Mild dermal exposures to hexavalent compounds require vigorous irrigation with saline solution or water. Chromium dermatitis has occasionally been treated with topical ascorbic acid and 1% aluminum acetate dressings. Early aggressive excision has been suggested as the best method to prevent systemic toxicity after large chromic acid burns (36).

Ocular exposures require extensive saline irrigation, pre- and postirrigation pH testing, slit-lamp evaluation for corneal injury, and ophthalmologic consultation in serious cases.

Extracorporeal Elimination

Survival in at least two cases of chromic acid ingestion and one case of potassium dichromate has reportedly been achieved with vigorous hemodialysis (24). Treatment of chromic acid burns by peritoneal dialysis has not been successful (37).

Other

The clinical efficacy of exchange transfusion has not been established. Severe acute potassium dichromate poisoning has been treated successfully with liver transplantation (38). Intravenous therapy with ascorbic acid after hexavalent chromium ingestion has been recommended in uncontrolled, *in vitro* studies. Theoretically, ascorbic acid may reduce hexavalent chromium to less toxic trivalent chromium.

Antidotes

The efficacy of dimercaprol has not been established. A man who fell into a pool of chromic acid survived with dimercaptopropanesulfonic acid treatment; his urine chromium level rose to 13,614 mg/ml (39). Intravenous *N*-acetylcysteine and hemodialysis were associated with hepatic and renal improvement in an adult who ingested sodium dichromate (40).

REFERENCES

1. Schonwald SN. Chromium. *Clin Toxicol Rev* 1989;11:1–2.
2. Barceloux DG. Chromium. *J Toxicol Clin Toxicol* 1999;37:173–194.
3. Mertz W. Effects and metabolism of glucose tolerance factor. *Nutr Rev* 1975;33:129–135.
4. Anderson RA, Cheng N, Bryden NA. Elevated intakes of supplemental chromium improve glucose and insulin variables in individuals with type 2 diabetes. *Diabetes* 1997;46:1786–1791.
5. Bahadori B, Wallner S, Schneider H, et al. Effect of chromium yeast and chromium picolinate on body composition of obese, non-diabetic patients during and after a formula diet. *Acta Med Austriaca* 1997;24:185–187.
6. Langard S, Vigander T. Occurrence of lung cancer in workers producing chromium pigments. *Br J Ind Med* 1983;40:71–74.
7. Hayes RB, Sheffet A, Spirtas R. Cancer mortality among a cohort of chromium pigment workers. *Am J Ind Med* 1989;16:127–133.
8. Sarayan LA, Reedy M. Chronic determinations in a case of chromic acid ingestion. *J Anal Toxicol* 1988;12:162–164.
9. Varna PP, Jha V, Ghosh AK, et al. Acute renal failure in a case of fatal chromic acid poisoning. *Ren Fail* 1994;16:653–657.
10. Grusz-Harday E. Acute lethal potassium dichromate poisoning. *Bull Int Assoc Forensic Toxicol* 1974;10:7.
11. Loubieres Y, de Lassence A, Bernier M, et al. Acute, fatal, oral chromic acid poisoning. *J Toxicol Clin Toxicol* 1999;37:333–336.
12. van Heerden PV, Jenkins IR, Woods WP, et al. Death by tanning—a case of fatal basic chromium sulphate poisoning. *Intensive Care Med* 1994;20:145–147.
13. Anderson RA. Chromium as an essential nutrient for humans. *Reg Toxicol Pharmacol* 1997;26:S25–S41.
14. Kolacinski Z, Kostrzewski P, Kruszewska S, et al. Acute potassium dichromate poisoning: a toxicokinetic case study. *J Toxicol Clin Toxicol* 1999;37:785–791.
15. Durant JL, Chen J, Hemond HF, Thilly WG. Elevated incidence of childhood leukemia in Woburn, Massachusetts: NIEHS Superfund Basic Research Program searches for causes. *Environ Health Perspect* 1995;103[Suppl 6]:93–98.
16. Hayes RB, Sheffet A, Spirtas R. Cancer mortality among a cohort of chromium pigment workers. *Am J Ind Med* 1989;16:127–133.
17. Donaldson RM, Barreras RF. Intestinal absorption of trace quantities of chromium. *J Lab Clin Med* 1966;68:484–493.
18. Kerger BD, Finley BL, Corbett GE, et al. Ingestion of chromium(VI) in drinking water by human volunteers: absorption, distribution, and excretion of single and repeated doses. *J Toxicol Environ Health* 1997;50:67–95.
19. Michie CA, Hayhurst M, Knobel GJ, et al. Poisoning with a traditional remedy containing potassium dichromate. *Hum Exp Toxicol* 1991;10:129–131.
20. Cohen MD, Kargacin B, Klein CB, Costa M. Mechanisms of chromium carcinogenicity and toxicity. *Crit Rev Toxicol* 1993;23:255–281.
21. Schroeder HA, Balassa JJ, Tipton IH. Abnormal trace metals in man—chromium. J *Chron Dis* 1962;15:941–964.
22. Fristedt B, Lindqvist B, Schutz A, Orrum P. Survival in a case of acute oral chromic acid poisoning with acute renal failure treated by hemodialysis. *Acta Med Scand* 1965;177:153–159.
23. Pedersen RS, Morch PT. Chromic acid poisoning treated with acute hemodialysis. *Nephron* 1978;22:592–595.
24. Stoner RS, Tong TG, Dart R, et al. Acute chromium intoxication with renal failure after 1% body surface area burns from chromic acid. *Vet Hum Toxicol* 1988;30:361.
25. Lin SC, Tai CC, Chan CC, Wang JD. Nasal septum lesions caused by chromium exposure among chromium electroplating workers. *Am J Ind Med* 1994;26:221–228.
26. Kapil V, Krogh J. *Chronic toxicity. Case studies in environmental medicine.* Atlanta: Agency for Toxic Substances and Disease Registry, 1990.
27. Meert KL, Ellis J, Aronow R, Perrin E. Acute ammonium dichromate poisoning. *Ann Emerg Med* 1994;24:748–750.
28. Fowler JF Jr. Systemic contact dermatitis caused by oral chromium picolinate. *Cutis* 2000;65:116.
29. Fisher AA. Blackjack diseases and other chromate puzzles. *Cutis* 1976;18:21–36.
30. Meyers JB. Acute pulmonary complications following inhalation of chromic acid mist. *Ann Ind Hyg Occup Med* 1950;2:742–747.
31. Martin WR, Fuller RE. Suspected chromium picolinate-induced rhabdomyolysis. *Pharmacotherapy* 1998;18:860–862.
32. Cerulli J, Grabe DW, Gauthier I, et al. Chromium picolinate toxicity. *Ann Pharmacother* 1998;32:428–431.
33. Randall JA, Gibson RS. Hair chromium as indices of chromium exposure of tannery workers. *Br J Ind Med* 1989;46:171–175.
34. Brune D, Aitio A, Nordberg G, et al. Normal concentrations of chromium in serum and urine—a TRACY project. *Scand J Work Environ Health* 1993;19[Suppl 1]:39–44.
35. Bradberry SM, Vale JA. Therapeutic review: is ascorbic acid of value in chromium poisoning and chromium dermatitis? *J Toxicol Clin Toxicol* 1999;37:195–200.
36. Matey P, Allison KP, Sheehan TM, Gowar JP. Chromic acid burns: early aggressive excision is the best method to prevent systemic toxicity. *J Burn Care Rehabil* 2000;21:241–245.
37. Lauwerys RR, Hoet P. *Industrial chemical guidelines for biological monitoring*, 2nd ed. Boca Raton, FL: Lewis Publishers, 1993:42–47.
38. Stift A, Friedl J, Langle F, et al. Successful treatment of a patient suffering from severe acute potassium dichromate poisoning with liver transplantation. *Transplantation* 2000;69:2454–2455.
39. Donner A, Meisinger V, Scholtz I, et al. Dimercapto-propane-sulphuric acid (DMPS) in the treatment of an acid copper and an acid chromium poisoning. *Toxicol Lett* 1986;31:154.
40. Vassallo S, Howland MA. Severe dichromate poisoning: survival after therapy with IV N-acetylcysteine and hemodialysis. *Vet Hum Toxicol* 1988;30:347.

CHAPTER 219

Cobalt

Seth Schonwald

COBALT CARBONYL

Atomic symbol, atomic number, molecular weight:	**Co, 27, 58.93 g/mol**
Valence states:	**0, +1, +2, +3, +4, +5**
CAS Registry No.:	**7440-48-4 (cobalt); 10210-68-1 (cobalt carbonyl)**
Normal levels:	**0.1 to 2 μg/L (serum); 0.4 to 1.0 μg/L (urine)**
SI conversion:	**μg/L × 17.0 = nmol/L**
Target organs:	**Lungs (chronic), heart (chronic)**
Antidote:	**None proved**

OVERVIEW

Cobalt was discovered by George Brandt in 1737. Cobalt is used to make alloys (1); as a drier for paint and the porcelain enameling (2) used on steel bathroom fixtures, large appliances, and kitchenware; and in making colored pigments (3). "Hard metal" is a metal alloy with a tungsten carbide and cobalt matrix (4). It is used to make cutting tools because of its hardness and resistance to high temperature. Cobalt alloys are used in orthopedic joints and surgical implants (5–7).

Cobalt carbonyl is a catalyst and an antiknock gasoline additive. In addition to eye, skin, and mucous membrane irritation, it can cause noncardiogenic pulmonary edema. Liver, kidney, and adrenal gland injury may also occur. It may be caustic after ingestion. Cobalt carbonyl can release carbon monoxide on thermal decomposition.

Small amounts of cobalt are added to or naturally occur in foods (3,8). Vitamin B_{12} is a cobalt-containing essential vitamin (9). Important manufactured sources of cobalt are byproducts from the burning of coal (10) and oil; exhaust from cars (11), trucks (12), and aircraft; industrial processes that use the metal or its compounds; and sewage sludge from cities (13).

There is no recommended dietary allowance for cobalt. Food intake is 5.0 to 40.0 μg/day; however, the cobalt content in total diet samples is not known (14). The total body content of cobalt is estimated at 1.1 to 1.5 mg (15).

TABLE 1. U.S. regulatory guidelines and standards for cobalt (Co)

Agency	Description	Concentration (mg/m^3)
OSHA	Metal, dust, and fume	
(air)	PEL-TWA	0.10 (as Co)
ACGIH	Inorganic compounds	
(air)	TLV-TWA	0.02 (as Co)
	STEL	None
NIOSH	Metal, dust, and fume	
(air)	REL-TWA	0.05 (as Co)
	STEL	None
	IDLH	20.00

ACGIH, American Conference of Governmental Industrial Hygienists; IDLH, immediate danger to life or health; NIOSH, National Institute for Occupational Safety and Health; OSHA, U.S. Occupational Safety and Health Administration; PEL, permissible exposure limit; REL, recommended exposure limit; STEL, short term exposure limit; TLV, threshold limit value; TWA, time-weighted average.

Toxic Dose

U.S. regulatory guidelines and standards are shown in Table 1.

Lethal cardiomyopathy was reported in people who consumed large quantities of beer containing cobalt (16,17). The deaths occurred during the early to mid-1960s when breweries in Canada, the United States, and Europe added cobalt to beer as a foam stabilizer; this practice has been discontinued. Death followed ingestion of beer containing 0.04 to 0.14 mg cobalt/kg/day for a period of years (8 to 30 pints of beer each day). Protein-poor diets and cardiac damage from alcohol abuse may have contributed to the illness.

Metallic cobalt and certain cobalt compounds (e.g., cobalt oxide, sulfide, chloride, acetate, and naphthenate) are probable chemical carcinogens related to lung cancer (18). One study found increased lung cancer mortality in workers exposed to cobalt, but the difference was not statistically significant, the characteristic lung diseases commonly found in cobalt workers were not observed, and the workers were exposed to arsenic and nickel as well as cobalt (19).

An 11-year-old boy swallowed two magnets (40% cobalt) and developed vomiting, weight loss, polycythemia, thyromegaly, metabolic acidosis, and cardiomyopathy (20). His serum cobalt level was 4.1 mEq/dl (normal, 0.35 to 1.7 mEq/dl), and his urine cobalt value was 1700 μg/L. An abdominal radiograph showed an opaque mass in the stomach.

TOXICOKINETICS AND TOXICODYNAMICS

Cobalt is absorbed through the lungs (21) and the gastrointestinal tract (22). Gastrointestinal absorption of cobalt in humans varies considerably (18% to 97%) based on the type and dose of cobalt compound given and the nutritional status of the subject

(23). Cobalt has been identified in liver, muscle, lung, lymph nodes, heart, skin, bone, hair, stomach, brain, pancreatic juice, kidneys, plasma, and urinary bladder of nonexposed subjects, with the highest cobalt concentration found in the liver (24). Most elimination of cobalt occurs via the kidney. The half-life of cobalt is several days.

PATHOPHYSIOLOGY

Cobalt is a component of cyanocobalamin (vitamin B_{12}), which is an essential mineral and coenzyme in many enzymatic reactions, including hematopoiesis. Cobalt deficiency can lead to pernicious anemia (25). Cobalamin plays a critical role in the metabolism of one-carbon fragments, including transmethylation to ions of certain metals and metalloids (26).

Both the obstructive and the interstitial syndromes in hard metal disease are responses to the inhalation of cobalt. Histologic abnormalities in subjects chronically exposed to cobalt dust include interstitial pneumonitis (fibrosing alveolitis) with infiltrates of lymphocytes, macrophages, plasma cells, and eosinophils. A more characteristic feature is the presence of multinucleated giant cells of macrophage and monocyte origin within the alveoli and bronchoalveolar lavage fluid (27).

A possible mechanism of myocardial toxicity is the irreversible formation of a cobalt chelate with the sulfhydryl groups of dihydrolipoic acid, inhibiting of two conversions in the tricarboxylic acid cycle (pyruvate to acetyl coenzyme A and alpha-ketoglutarate to succinyl-coenzyme) (8). The resulting inhibition of cellular respiration and oxidative phosphorylation may lead to decreased oxygen uptake by the tissues, resulting in cardiac effects.

VULNERABLE POPULATIONS

Studies in animals suggest that exposure to high amounts of cobalt during pregnancy causes fetal defects. However, birth defects have not been found in children born to mothers who were treated with cobalt for anemia during pregnancy (28).

CLINICAL PRESENTATION

The main target organs for cobalt toxicity appear to be the lungs and heart. Chronic administration may cause goiter and reduced thyroid activity (29). Cobalt is a component of vitamin B_{12} and can induce polycythemia in humans (30).

Pulmonary Effects

Hard metal lung disease is generally found in workers who grind material made from tungsten carbide (31). It can occur as an interstitial lung disease with signs of pulmonary fibrosis and as an obstructive airway syndrome (Chapter 27) (4,32). The acute form of the disease resembles a hypersensitivity reaction with malaise, cough, and wheezing (33,34). The chronic form progresses to cor pulmonale. Hard metal asthma may be an immunoglobulin E antibody–mediated syndrome due to cobalt reactivity. Asthma, interstitial lung disease, and combined asthma and alveolitis are described as occupational health hazards (35).

Cardiac Effects

The abrupt onset of heart failure in high-volume beer drinkers ("beer drinker's cardiomyopathy") in the 1960s was characterized by pericardial effusion, elevated hemoglobin concentrations, and biventricular congestive heart failure (18,19,36). Mortality approached 50%. Industrial cobalt exposure may cause fatal cardiomyopathy in the hard metal industry.

DIAGNOSTIC TESTS

Chronic inhalation exposure levels in humans associated with respiratory effects have been reported, but the minimal chronic exposure levels required to produce these effects have not been identified (35). Respiratory function tests may show evidence of restrictive lung disease and a decrease in diffusion capacity of carbon monoxide. Occupational exposure of humans to cobalt dust has been shown to result in cardiomyopathy, but the exposure levels associated with cardiac effects of inhaled cobalt in humans have not been determined (37).

Cobalt levels are not used in the management of chronic cobalt exposure. Tests to assess respiratory consequences of cobalt exposure include pulmonary function tests, arterial blood gas, chest radiography, and chest computed tomography. Electrocardiogram, chest radiograph, and echocardiography document evidence of cardiomyopathy. A complete blood cell count may be helpful in detecting pernicious anemia. Hair cobalt concentrations do not reliably predict cobalt poisoning (38). A carbon monoxide level should be determined in symptomatic patients with cobalt carbonyl toxicity.

TREATMENT

After ingestion, both ipecac syrup followed by activated charcoal and simply dilution with water (without emesis) have been recommended (39,40). If the eyes are involved, immediate flushing with water should be performed. Skin is washed immediately with soap or mild detergent and water.

Management of patients after acute cobalt exposure includes removal from the contaminated area and removal and isolation of contaminated clothing (41). If the victim is in respiratory distress, ventilation assistance is provided and oxygen administered. Bronchospastic symptoms after acute inhalations of cobalt dust or resulting from chronic hard metal disease may respond to inhaled bronchodilators and steroid therapy (Chapter 27). Lung toxicity after inhalation of cobalt carbonyl involves treatment for bronchospasm or noncardiogenic pulmonary edema as for other agents.

Antidotes

Animal studies have tested various chelating agents in models of cobalt toxicity (42). Animal experiments suggest that *N*-acetylcysteine may be helpful, but there are no human studies to corroborate these findings (41,43). Chelation therapy with calcium disodium ethylenediaminetetraacetic acid or dimercaprol may be useful; however, definitive clinical studies are lacking (42).

REFERENCES

1. Planinsek F, Newkirk JB. Cobalt and cobalt alloys. In: Grayson M, ed. *Kirk-Othmer encyclopedia of chemical technology*, Vol. 6. New York: John Wiley & Sons, Inc., 1979:481–494.
2. Raffn E, Mikkelsen S, Altman DG, et al. Health effects due to occupational exposure to cobalt blue dye among plate painters in a porcelain factory in Denmark. *Stand J Work Environ Health* 1988;14:378–384.
3. ATSDR toxicological profile for cobalt. Atlanta: Agency for Toxic Substances and Disease Registry, Division of Toxicology, 1992:1–165.
4. Davison AG, Haslam IL, Corrin B, et al. Interstitial lung disease and asthma in hard-metal workers: bronchoalveolar lavage, ultrastructural and analytical findings and results of bronchial provocation tests. *Thorax* 1983;38:119–128.
5. Sunderman FW Jr, Hopfer SM, Swift T, et al. Cobalt, chromium, and nickel

concentrations in body fluids of patients with porous-coated knee or hip prostheses. *J Orthop Res* 1989;7:307–315.
6. Stenberg T, Bergman B. Release and uptake of cobalt from cobalt-chromium alloy implants. *Acta Odontol Scand* 1983;41:149–154.
7. Kirk WS. Reprint from the 1987 Bureau of Mines minerals yearbook: cobalt. Washington, DC: United States Department of the Interior, 1987.
8. Taylor A, Marks V. Cobalt: a review. *J Human Nutr* 1978;32:165–177.
9. Elinder CG, Friberg L. Cobalt. In: Friberg L, Nordberg GF, Vouk V, eds. *Handbook on the toxicology of metals*, 2nd ed. New York: Elsevier Science Publishers, 1986:211–232.
10. Mejstrik V, Svacha J. Concentrations of Co, Cd, Cr, Ni, and Zn in crop plants cultivated in the vicinity of coal-fired power plants. *Sci Total Environ* 1988;72:57–67.
11. Abbasi SA, Nipaney PC, Soni R. Environmental status of cobalt and its microdetermination with 7-nitroso-8-hydroxyquinoline-5-sulfonic acid in waters, aquatic weeds and animal tissues. *Anal Lett* 1989;22:225–235.
12. Ondov JM, Zoller WH, Gordon GE. Trace element emissions on aerosols from motor vehicles. *Environ Sci Technol* 1982;16:318–328.
13. Erlandsson B, Ingemansson T, Mattsson S. Comparative studies of radionuclides from global fallout and local sources in ground level air and sewage sludge. *Water Air Soil Pollut* 1983;20:331–346.
14. Jenkins DW. Biological monitoring of toxic trace metals, volume 1. Biological monitoring and surveillance. NTIS PBBl-103475, 1980.
15. Yamagata N, Murata S, Torii T. The cobalt content of human body. *J Radiat Res* 1962;5:4–8.
16. Alexander CS. Cobalt-beer cardiomyopathy: a clinical and pathologic study of twenty-eight cases. *Am J Med* 1972;53:395–417.
17. Morin Y, Tetu A, Mercier G. Cobalt cardiomyopathy: clinical aspects. *Br Heart J* 1971;33:175–178.
18. Jensen AA, Tuchsen F. Cobalt exposure and cancer risk. *Crit Rev Toxicol* 1990;20:427–438.
19. Mur JM, Moulin JJ, Charruyer-Seinerra MP, et al. A cohort mortality study among cobalt and sodium workers in an electrochemical plant. *Am J Ind Med* 1987;11:75–82.
20. Henretig F, Joffe M, Baffa G, et al. Elemental cobalt toxicity and effects of chelation therapy. *Vet Hum Toxicol* 1988;30:372.
21. Foster PP, Pearman I, Ramsden D. An interspecies comparison of the lung clearance of inhaled monodisperse cobalt particles—part II: lung clearance of inhaled cobalt oxide in man. *J Aerosol Sci* 1989;20:189–204.
22. Sorbic J, Olatunbosun D, Corbett WE, et al. Cobalt excretion test for the assessment of body iron stores. *Can Med Assoc J* 1971;104:777–782.
23. Valberg LS, Ludwig J, Olatunkosun D. Alterations in cobalt absorption in patients with disorders of iron metabolism. *Gastroenterology* 1969;56:241–251.
24. Hewitt PJ. Accumulation of metals in the tissues of occupationally exposed workers. *Environ Geochem Health* 1988;10:113–116.
25. Domingo JL. Cobalt in the environment and its toxicological implications. *Rev Environ Contam Toxicol* 1989;108:105–132.
26. Smith IC, Carson BL, ed. *Trace metals in the environment. Volume 6: Cobalt an appraisal of environmental exposure.* Ann Arbor, MI: Ann Arbor Science Publishers, Inc., 1981.
27. Demedts M, Gheysens B, Nagels J, et al. Cobalt lung in diamond polishers. *Am Rev Respir Dis* 1984;130:130–135.
28. Holly RG. Studies on iron and cobalt metabolism. *J Am Med Assoc* 1955;158:1349–1352.
29. Paley KR, Sobel ES, Yalow RS. Effect of oral and intravenous cobaltous chloride on thyroid function. *J Clin Endocrin Metabol* 1958;18:850–859.
30. Duckham JM, Lee HA. The treatment of refractory anemia of chronic renal failure with cobalt chloride. *QJM* 1976;178:277–294.
31. Anttila S, Sutinen S, Paananen M, et al. Hard metal lung disease: a clinical, histological, ultrastructural and X-ray microanalytical study. *Eur J Respir Dis* 1986;69:83–94.
32. Nordberg G. Assessment of risks in occupational cobalt exposures. *Sci Total Environ* 1994;150:201–207.
33. Shirakawa T, Kusaka Y, Fujimura N, et al. The existence of specific antibodies to cobalt in hard metal asthma. *Clin Allergy* 1988;18:451–460.
34. Shirakawa T, Kusaka Y, Fujimura N, et al. Occupational asthma from cobalt sensitivity in workers exposed to hard metal dust. *Chest* 1989;95:29–37.
35. Domingo JL. Cobalt in the environment and its toxicological implications. *Rev Environ Contam Toxicol* 1989;108:105–32.
36. Barceloux DG. Cobalt. *J Toxicol Clin Toxicol* 1999;37:201–206.
37. Horowitz SF, Fischbein A, Matza D. Evaluation of right and left ventricular function in hard metal workers. *Br J Ind Med* 1988;45:742–746.
38. Evans GJ, Jervis RE. Hair as a bio-indicator: limitations and complications in the interpretation of results. *J Radioanal Nucl Chem* 1987;110:613–625.
39. Stutz DR, Janusz SJ. *Hazardous materials injuries—a handbook for pre hospital care*, 2nd ed. Beltsville, MD: Bradford Communications Corp., 1988:254–255.
40. Bronstein AC, Currance PL. *Emergency care for hazardous material exposure.* Washington, DC: The C.V. Mosky Company, 1988:147–148.
41. Llobet JM, Domingo JL, Corbella J. Comparative effects of repeated parenteral administration of several chelators on the distribution and excretion of cobalt. *Res Commun Chem Pathol Pharmacol* 1988;60:225–233.
42. Domingo JL, Llobet JM, Corbella J. The effects of EDTA in acute cobalt intoxication in rats. *Toxicol Eur Res* 1983;5:251–255.
43. Domingo JL, Llobet JM, Tomas JM. N-acetyl-L-cysteine in acute cobalt poisoning. *Arch Farmacol Toxicol* 1985;11:55–62.

CHAPTER 220

Copper

Seth Schonwald

$O{=}S({=}O)(-O^-)-O \cdots Cu^{++}$

COPPER SULFATE

Atomic symbol, atomic number, molecular weight:	**Cu, 29, 63.55 g/mol**
Valence states:	**+1, +2**
CAS Registry No.:	**7440-50-8**
Normal levels:	**70 to 155 mg/dl (serum)**
SI conversion:	**mg/L × 15.7 = μmol/L**
Target organs:	**Gastrointestinal tract (acute), kidney (acute), liver (acute and chronic)**
Antidote:	**None**

OVERVIEW

Copper is most often used as an electrical conductor. It is also used in construction, machinery, and transportation (1). Brass and bronze are alloys of copper. Copper alloys are used in jewelry, bronze sculptures, and coins. In agriculture, copper compounds are used as fungicides.

People may be exposed to copper from beverages in vending machines (2), copper or brass vessels (3), and drinking water (4). Contaminated food and beverages can produce an acute gastrointestinal (GI) illness. Although copper is present as numerous chemical species, the biologic availability and toxicity of copper are probably related to free copper (II) ion activity (1).

Chronic liver disease, diffuse pulmonary fibrosis, and angiosarcoma in workers and children after copper exposure require further confirmation by controlled studies. Wilson's disease is caused by lack of ceruloplasmin, the carrier protein for copper. Biliary excretion is decreased, and copper accumulates in the liver, brain, and other organs.

TABLE 1. U.S. regulatory guidelines and standards for copper (Cu)

Agency	Description	Concentration (mg/m³)
OSHA (air)	Fume	
	PEL-TWA	0.1 (as Cu)
	Dusts and mists	
	PEL-TWA	1.0
ACGIH (air)	Fume	
	TLV-TWA	0.2
	STEL	None
	Dusts and mists	
	TLV-TWA	1.0 (as Cu)
	STEL	
NIOSH (air)	Dusts and mists	
	REL-TWA	1.0 (as Cu)
	STEL	None
	IDLH	100

ACGIH, American Conference of Governmental Industrial Hygienists; IDLH, immediate danger to life or health; NIOSH, National Institute for Occupational Safety and Health; OSHA, U.S. Occupational Safety and Health Administration; PEL, permissible exposure limit; REL, recommended exposure limit; STEL, short-term exposure limit; TLV, threshold limit value; TWA, time-weighted average.

Toxic Dose

The usual intake of copper in the United States population is 1 mg/day. Regulatory guidelines are provided in Table 1.

Copper sulfate has been used to commit suicide. Thirteen of 53 patients died of shock and hepatic or renal complications after ingesting 6 to 637 mg/kg of copper (5). Ingestion of 10 to 20 g of copper sulfate is usually lethal. Renal failure and death may follow ingestion of as little as 1 g of copper sulfate. Hemodialysis has not prevented death in such cases.

A 25-year-old woman was given cupric sulfate, 2.5 g in 1750 ml of water, as an emetic and died 3 days later from acute hemolysis and renal failure due to copper poisoning. The whole blood copper concentration was 5.31 μg/ml (6). A mentally impaired individual died of copper toxicity arising from 275 coins in his stomach. Many coins containing copper were corroded by prolonged contact with gastric fluid, with subsequent absorption and deposition of copper in the liver and kidneys (7).

Copper is not known to cause cancer.

TOXICOKINETICS AND TOXICODYNAMICS

Copper is believed to be absorbed in the stomach and upper intestine. It is poorly absorbed through the skin. Copper binds to plasma albumin and amino acids in the portal blood and is taken to the liver. In the liver, copper is incorporated into the enzyme ceruloplasmin and is released into the plasma. Approximately 7% of copper is bound loosely to albumin, and 93% is bound to the ceruloplasmin. The apparent volume of distribution of copper is 1.95 L/kg. Besides the liver, copper distributes to the kidney, bone, brain, and cornea.

Bile is the major pathway for copper excretion. Approximately 0.1 to 1.3 ng/day is excreted through the bile. The half-life of copper in healthy individuals is approximately 26 days. If a large amount of copper is suddenly released from the liver, it is taken up by erythrocytes, and a hemolytic crisis may occur.

PATHOPHYSIOLOGY

Copper is an essential nutrient that is incorporated into numerous enzymes. These enzymes are involved in hemoglobin formation, carbohydrate metabolism, catecholamine biosynthesis, and cross-linking of collagen, elastin, and hair keratin. There are numerous copper-dependent enzymes, such as cytochrome-*c* oxidase, superoxide dismutase, dopamine β-hydroxylase, and ascorbic acid.

VULNERABLE POPULATIONS

Copper is present in breast milk. Increased fetal mortality occurs in animals exposed to copper; however, similar effects have not been observed in healthy humans or in the offspring of mothers with Wilson's disease. Infants and children younger than 1 year of age may be unusually susceptible to the toxicity of copper. Hepatosplenomegaly has been described in two infant siblings exposed to high levels of copper in tap water (8).

CLINICAL PRESENTATION

Acute ingestion of copper salts causes an acute corrosive injury to the upper GI tract. This is followed in severe cases by renal injury, hemolysis, and liver injury. Death is from multiple-organ failure.

Renal Effects

Copper sulfate ingestion may cause acute renal failure (9) and chronic tubulo-interstitial nephritis (10). Excess copper causes focal necrosis of the proximal tubule. Fanconi syndrome (tubular proteinuria, generalized aminoaciduria, phosphaturia, uricosuria, and hypercalciuria) may result from a direct toxic effect of copper or from associated hemolysis.

Gastrointestinal Effects

Copper sulfate causes a corrosive injury involving rapid onset of nausea, vomiting, diarrhea, and anorexia. Myalgias, abdominal pain, acidosis, and pancreatitis may all occur. It has been suggested that copper poisoning should be considered as a possible cause of chronic GI diseases in countries where copper plumbing is common. Copper may be a factor in the development of childhood cirrhosis (11,12). Centrilobular necrosis of the liver has been seen in severe cases of copper poisoning (13).

Pulmonary Effects

Airborne dusts of inorganic copper have low toxicity. "Vineyard sprayer's lung disease" has been associated with airborne copper sulfate (14). This is a histiocytic granulomatous lung and liver disease occurring after exposure to copper sulfate spray for 2 to 15 years. Metal fume fever probably does not occur after exposure to copper fumes in industry (15).

Hematologic Effects

Hemolysis may occur when large amounts of copper enter the bloodstream, as may occur during dialysis. Individuals with glucose 6 phosphate dehydrogenase deficiency are likely to be susceptible to toxic effects of oxidative stressors, such as copper (16). Methemoglobin formation has also been described after copper exposure (17).

Dermatologic Effects

Copper exposure results in contact allergic dermatitis in some individuals (18). Chronic copper poisoning has occurred after repeated use of a copper-containing topical cream on eczematous skin. The application of copper crystals to granulomatous burn tissue has resulted in chronic poisoning with skin darkening. The use of copper algicidal chemicals in swimming pools can produce green hair by absorption of copper into the hair.

Wilson's Disease

Wilson's disease may cause liver failure, hemolytic anemia, renal tubular dysfunction, and renal stones. Kayser-Fleischer rings are corneal deposits of copper. Wilson's disease can also be associated with central nervous system degenerative changes. Symptoms include poor coordination, psychological impairment, dysarthria, tremor, disturbed gait, and rigidity (19).

Spiritual Water

Overdosage of copper salts is common in developing countries because of its use in traditional preparations. Poisoning is due to the ingestion of "spiritual green water" after distribution to members of spiritual churches. Within a few hours of ingestion, greenish vomiting and abdominal pain are seen. Anuria may supervene within 24 hours. Flapping tremor, toxic psychosis, hemolytic anemia, and jaundice may follow within a few days. Patients have died within a few days (20).

Dialysis and Copper

A syndrome of intravenous copper intoxication due to copper released from tubing during hemodialysis includes nausea, vomiting, abdominal pain, diarrhea, anxiety, and depression (21). Acute hemolytic anemia has been reported in patients exposed to excess copper in the dialysate (22). Although this population is not unusually susceptible to copper toxicity, it is at a high risk of being exposed to high levels of copper.

DIAGNOSTIC TESTS

The corrosive effects after ingestion are assessed and managed as for other caustic ingestions.

Copper is measured by inductively coupled plasma emission spectroscopy. Patients with metal fume fever after exposure to metallic copper have copper levels over 160 mg/dl. The mean value of normal ceruloplasmin is 30 mg/100 ml. The laboratory diagnosis of Wilson's disease is confirmed by decreased serum ceruloplasmin, increased urinary copper content, and elevated hepatic copper concentration.

POSTMORTEM CONSIDERATIONS

Ingestion of 20 to 30 ml of copper sulfate led to a blood copper level of 1.25 mg/ml in a patient who died. Plasma copper concentration in a series of fatal cases involving copper ranged from 9.8 to 46.0 mg/L.

TREATMENT

Treatment of copper poisoning is primarily symptomatic and supportive. Dermatitis may respond to topical steroids. GI decontamination is rarely needed because of vomiting.

Hemodialysis

Although its effect on mortality has not been studied, removal of copper by dialysis may be useful in the early stages of severe poisoning when the metal is still present in the circulation as free copper.

Antidotes

Chelating agents are recommended in severe poisoning, but few human data exist to guide their use. Dimercapto-propanesulfonate prevented the development of renal sequelae of copper intoxication in mice but has not been tested in humans (23). One study suggested that treating copper poisoning with the chelator mercaptodextran could inhibit copper-induced hemolysis and that dimercapto-propanesulfonate might accelerate such hemolysis (24).

Intravenous calcium disodium ethylenediaminetetraacetic acid and intramuscular dimercaprol may be helpful in severe ingestions (25). D-Penicillamine may be administered orally, if tolerated, to patients who are not allergic to penicillin. The copper-chelating drug tetrathiomolybdate, also used in Wilson's disease, has been associated with pancytopenia and has not been recommended for acute copper poisoning (26). Copper chelation with penicillamine (Cuprimine) is an effective therapy in most patients with Wilson's disease, and hepatic transplantation is curative in individuals presenting with irreversible liver failure (27).

REFERENCES

1. ATSDR toxicological profile for copper. Atlanta: Agency for Toxic Substances and Disease Registry, Division of Toxicology, 1990:1–151.
2. Witherell LE, Watson WN, Giguere GC. Outbreak of acute copper poisoning due to soft drink dispenser. *Am J Public Health* 1980;70:1115.
3. Gill JS, Bhagat CI. Acute copper poisoning from drinking lime cordial prepared and left overnight in an old urn. *Med J Aust* 1999;170:510.
4. Eife R, Weiss M, Barros V, et al. Chronic poisoning by copper in tap water: I. Copper intoxications with predominantly gastrointestinal symptoms. *Eur J Med Res* 1999;4:219–223.
5. Chuttani HK, Gupta PS, Gulati S, et al. Acute copper sulphate poisoning. *Am J Med* 1965;39:849–854.
6. Liu J, Kashimura S, Hara K, Zhang G. Death following cupric sulfate emesis. *J Toxicol Clin Toxicol* 2001;39:161–163.
7. Yelin G, Taff ML, Sadowski GE. Copper toxicity following massive ingestion of coins. *Am J Forensic Med Pathol* 1987;8:78–85.
8. Mueller-Hoecker J, Meyer U, Wiebecke B, et al. Copper storage disease of the liver and chronic dietary copper intoxication in two further German infants mimicking Indian childhood cirrhosis. *Pathol Res Pract* 1988;183:39–45.
9. Dash SC. Copper sulphate poisoning and acute renal failure. *Int J Artif Organs* 1989;12:610.
10. Bhowmik D, Mathur R, Bhargava Y, et al. Chronic interstitial nephritis following parenteral copper sulfate poisoning. *Ren Fail* 2001;23:731–735.
11. Muhlendahl K, Lange H. Copper and childhood cirrhosis. *Lancet* 1994;344:1515–1516.
12. Gordon AG. Childhood cirrhosis from copper poisoning in the nineteenth century. *J Pediatr Gastroenterol Nutr* 1988;7:934.
13. Jantsch W, Kulig K, Rumack BH. Massive copper sulfate ingestion resulting in hepatotoxicity. *J Toxicol Clin Toxicol* 1984;22:585–588.
14. Pimental JC, Marques F. "Vineyard sprayer's lung": a new occupational disease. *Thorax* 1969;24:678–688.
15. Borak J, Cohen H, Hethmon TA. Copper exposure and metal fume fever: lack of evidence for a causal relationship. *AIHAJ* 2000;61:832–836.
16. Calabrese EJ, Moore GS. Can elevated levels of copper in drinking water precipitate acute hemolysis in G-6-PD deficient individuals? *Med Hypotheses* 1979;5:493–498.
17. Chugh KS, Singhal PC, Sharma BK. Methemoglobinemia in acute copper sulfate poisoning. *Ann Intern Med* 1975;82:226–227.
18. Barranco VP. Eczematous dermatitis caused by internal exposure to copper. *Arch Dermatol* 1972;106:386–387.
19. Strickland GT, Leu ML. Wilson's disease: clinical and laboratory manifestations in 40 patients. *Medicine* 1975;54:113–137.
20. Akintonwa A, Mabadeje AF, Odutola TA. Fatal poisonings by copper sulfate ingested from "spiritual water." *Vet Hum Toxicol* 1989;31:453–454.
21. Klein WJ Jr, Metz EN, Price AR. Acute copper intoxication. A hazard of hemodialysis. *Arch Intern Med* 1972;129:580–582.
22. Williams DM. Clinical significance of copper deficiency and toxicity in the world population. In: Prasad AS, ed. *Clinical, biochemical and nutritional aspects of trace elements*. New York: Alan R. Liss, Inc., 1982:277–299.
23. Mitchell WM, Basinger MA, Jones MM. Antagonism of acute copper (II)-induced renal lesions by sodium 2,3 dimercaptopropanesulfonate. *Johns Hopkins Med J* 1982;151:283–285.
24. Aaseth J, Benov L, Ribarov S. Mercaptodextran—a new copper chelator and scavenger of oxygen radicals. *Zhongguo Yao Li Xue Bao* 1990;11:363–367.
25. Hantson P, Lievens M, Mahieu P. Accidental ingestion of a zinc and copper sulfate preparation. *J Toxicol Clin Toxicol* 1996;34:725–730.
26. Harpe PL, Walshe JM. Reversible pancytopenia secondary to treatment with tetrathiomolybdate. *Br J Haematol* 1986;6:851–853.
27. Loudianos G, Gitlin JD. Wilson's disease. *Semin Liver Dis* 2000;20:353–364.

CHAPTER 221

Lead

Richard C. Dart, Katherine M. Hurlbut, and Leslie V. Boyer-Hassen

$$H_3CH_2C\text{—}Pb(CH_2CH_3)_2\text{—}CH_2CH_3$$

TETRAETHYL LEAD

Atomic symbol, atomic number, molecular weight:	**Pb, 82, 207.2 g/mol**
Valence states:	**+2, +4**
CAS Registry No.:	**7439-92-1 (elemental)**
Normal levels:	**Less than 10 μg/dl**
SI conversion:	**μg/L × 0.00483 = μmol/L**
Target organs:	**Bone marrow (chronic); peripheral nervous system (chronic); central nervous system (chronic)**
Antidotes:	**British antilewisite (BAL), dimercaprol, succimer, penicillamine, ethylenediaminetetraacetic acid**

OVERVIEW

The element lead is a gray, soft, and malleable metal that exists naturally as a mixture of three isotopes (^{206}Pb, ^{207}Pb, and ^{208}Pb). It forms inorganic (lead acetate, -chloride, and many others) and organic compounds (tetraethyl lead) (Table 1).

Classification and Uses

Lead is a pervasive component of many processes and products (Table 2). Burning, blasting, grinding, or sanding of lead-coated surfaces are the most common causes of adult exposures. Storage batteries and lead-sheltered cable are commonly recycled products. Sheet lead is used to line chemical reaction vessels, for waterproofing and soundproofing, and for radiation shielding. Lead is often used in paints, coatings, and other products because of their bright colors and weather-resistant properties. In the United States, the use of lead in residential paint was banned in 1977.

Red lead (Pb_3O_4) is used as a rustproofer and primer for steel. Lead azide is used in primers and explosives (1). Tetraethyl lead and tetramethyl lead are gasoline additives. The use of leaded gasoline has decreased in many countries but is still used widely in others. The introduction of lead-free gasoline has nearly eliminated lead in the air in the United States, but it is permitted for farm equipment and some marine uses (2).

Environmental and Occupational Exposure

Exposure occurs through the air, water, food, and soil. The concentration of lead in air ranges from 7.6×10^{-5} μg/m^3 in remote areas to more than 10 μg/m^3 near smelters (2). The average maximum level in urban areas in 1984 was 0.36 μg/m^3 (2). Surface water in the United States may contain as much as 5 to 30 μg/L of lead (2). Sources of lead in water include lead pipes or lead solder in pipe joints. Low pH increases the amount of lead in tap water (2). Lead is found in dairy products, meat, fish, poultry, grains, and cereals (2). Naturally occurring soil levels range from approximately 10 μg/g to 30 μg/g (2). The level of lead in soil near urban road areas may reach 2000 to 10,000 μg/g [parts per million (ppm)] and has reached 60,000 μg/g near smelters. The daily intake of lead is 5 to 15 μg/day across all age groups, but may be higher in children due to ingestion of and contact with soil as well as higher minute ventilation rates (2).

Sources of lead in the home include paint, soil, dust, food, water, cosmetics, art materials, toys, and hobbies (3). Household paint and dust remain the major source of childhood lead exposure in the United States and many countries. Peeling and chipping paint may produce dangerous levels of lead in house dust and soil that persist as a hazard even after overpainting or abatement. In the United States, more than 80% of private and public housing units built before 1980 contain at least some lead paint (4).

TABLE 1. Compounds formed by lead

Lead compound	Chemical symbol	Molecular weight (g/mol)
Lead, metal	Pb	207.19
Lead acetate	$Pb(C_2H_3O_2)_2$	325.28
Lead arsenate	$Pb_3(AsO_4)_2$	899.4
Lead azide	$Pb(N_3)_2$	291.23
Lead carbonate (basic white lead)	$2PbCO_3Pb(OH)_2$	775.6
Lead chloride	$PbCl_2$	278.1
Lead chromate (chrome yellow)	$PbCrO_4$	323.18
Lead molybdate	$PbMoO_4$	367.13
Lead monoxide	PbO	223.19
Lead nitrate	$Pb(NO_3)_2$	331.2
Lead oxide (red)	Pb_3O_4	685.57
Lead oxychloride	$PbCl_2{\cdot}2PbO$ (mineral yellow)	519.29
Lead peroxide	PbO_2	239.19
Lead sesquioxide	Pb_2O_3	462.38
Lead silicate	$PbSiO_3$	283.27
Lead stearate	$Pb(C_{18}H_{35}O_2)_2$	774.15
Lead suboxide	Pb_2O	430.38
Lead sulfate	$PbSO_4PbO$	526.44
Lead sulfide	PbS	239.25
Tetraethyl lead	$Pb(C_2H_5)_4$	323.44
Tetramethyl lead	$Pb(CH_3)_4$	267.33

From Keogh JP, Boyer LV. Lead. In: Sullivan JB Jr, Kreiger GR, eds. *Clinical environmental health and toxic exposures*, 2nd ed. Philadelphia: Lippincott Williams & Wilkins, 2001, with permission.

TABLE 2. Sources of lead exposure

Lead smelting	Soldering of lead products
Battery manufacturing	Production of gasoline additives
Welding and cutting operations	Zinc smelting
Construction and demolition	Solid waste combustion
Rubber manufacturing	Organic lead production
Plastics manufacturing	Copper smelting
Printing	Ore crushing and grinding
Firing ranges	Frit manufacturing
Radiator repair	Paint and pigment manufacturing

From Keogh JP, Boyer LV. Lead. In: Sullivan JB Jr, Kreiger GR, eds. *Clinical environmental health and toxic exposures*, 2nd ed. Philadelphia: Lippincott Williams & Wilkins, 2001, with permission.

Parental occupation also contributes to childhood lead exposure (e.g., lead miners, who bring lead dust home on skin and clothes) (5). The prevalence of lead poisoning is increased in black and Hispanic populations (6,7). This greater prevalence may be due to greater dust and soil lead burden as well as lead paint residues in older or dilapidated housing.

Overall, American children are exposed to much lower levels of lead than in the past. The third National Health and Nutrition Examination Survey indicated that among U.S. children from ages 1 through 5, the prevalence of lead levels exceeding 25 µg/dl fell from 9.3% in the 1970s to 0.5% in the 1980s. The prevalence of a blood lead level (BLL) more than 10 µg/dl during the same years dropped from 88.2% to 8.9%, with a further drop in the 1990s to 4.4% (6). In the National Health and Nutrition Examination Survey 1999–2000, 2.2% of children aged 1 to 5 years had BLLs of 10 µg/dl or greater, with a geometric mean BLL of 2.23 µg/dl (8).

In many countries, the challenges of pediatric lead poisoning remain to be addressed. The causes of pediatric lead poisoning are remarkably similar throughout the world (9,9a). This rate is much higher in children adopted from other countries (10).

Toxic Dose

Toxic effects may occur subacutely after a single exposure or more commonly through chronic low-level exposure. A single ingestion of a lead weight can produce high lead levels and severe toxicity or death in children within days. With chronic pediatric lead exposure, toxic effects are noted at a BLL as low as 10 to 15 µg/dl (Table 3). Toxicity at lower levels has been alleged but remains to be proven (11).

In adults, symptoms and signs of lead toxicity usually develop with a BLL above 40 µg/dl. Toxicity has been associated with lower levels (Table 4) (12). An occupational BLL of 40 to 60 µg/dl may produce subtle neurologic effects (13).

Standards and Regulations

Environmental and occupational standards for lead are provided in Table 5. The U.S. Safe Drinking Water Act requires water suppliers to notify customers of lead contamination, to describe the potential hazards of lead and actions being taken, and provide a recommendation as to whether the customer should seek an alternative supply of water (52 *CFR* 41534). Lead is a hazardous waste under the Resource Conservation and Recovery Act (40 *CFR* 260).

Lead-containing paint and certain consumer products bearing lead-containing paint have been banned in the United States. *Lead-containing* is defined by the presence of more than 0.06% lead by weight of the paint or the dried surface (42 *CFR* 44199; 43 *CFR* 8515). Interior surfaces painted before 1975 often contain lead, and the use of exterior lead paint continues. Lead paint removal is regulated by Housing and Urban Development guidelines and by state and local regulations (14,15).

The U.S. Occupational Safety and Health Administration lead standard was extended in 1996 to include the construction and demolition industries. Organic lead compounds are excluded from the lead standard. Currently, organic compounds are covered only by an older standard of 200 µg/m^3 of air. Above the action level for lead of 30 µg/m^3, an employer must provide workers with training, protective clothing, washing facilities, and medical surveillance. The employer must remove from exposure any

TABLE 3. Lowest observed effect levels for lead-induced health effects in children

Lowest observed effect level [blood lead (µg/dl)]	Heme synthesis and hematologic effects	Neurologic effects	Renal effects	Gastrointestinal effects
80–100	—	Encephalopathic signs and symptoms	Chronic nephropathy (aminoaciduria and so forth)	Colic and other overt symptoms
70	Anemia	—	—	—
60	—	Peripheral neuropathies	—	—
50	—	—	—	—
40	Reduced hemoglobin synthesis Elevated coproporphyrin Increased urinary ALA	Peripheral nerve dysfunction (slowed NCVs) CNS cognitive effects —	— — —	— — —
30	Erythrocyte protoporphyrin elevation	Altered CNS electrophysiologic responses, effect on IQ	Vitamin D metabolism interference	—
15	ALA-D inhibition	MDI deficits, reduced gestational age and birth weight (prenatal exposure)	—	—
	Py-5-N activity inhibition	—	—	—
10	—	—	—	—

ALA, aminolevulinic acid; ALA-D, aminolevulinic acid dehydrase; CNS, central nervous system; IQ, intelligence quotient; MDI, mental development index; NCVs, nerve conduction velocities; Py-5-N, pyrimidine-5'-nucleotidase.

Reprinted from Keogh JP, Boyer LV. Lead. In: Sullivan JB Jr, Kreiger GR, eds. *Clinical environmental health and toxic exposures*, 2nd ed. Philadelphia: Lippincott Williams & Wilkins, 2001, with permission.

TABLE 4. Lowest observed effect levels for lead-induced health effects in adults

Lowest observed effect level [blood lead (μg/dl)]	Heme synthesis and hematologic effects	Neurologic effects	Renal effects	Reproductive effects	Cardiovascular effects
100–120	—	Encephalopathic signs and symptoms	—	—	—
80	Anemia	Encephalopathy symptoms	Chronic nephropathy	—	—
60	—	—	—	Reproductive effects in women	—
50	Reduced hemoglobin production	Overt subencephalopathic neurologic symptoms	—	—	—
40	Increased urinary ALA and elevated coproporphyrins	Peripheral nerve dysfunction (slowed nerve conduction)	—	—	—
30	—	—	—	Altered testicular function	Elevated blood pressure (white men, aged 40–59 years)
25–30	Erythrocyte protoporphyrin elevation in men	—	—	—	—
15–20	Erythrocyte protoporphyrin in women	—	—	—	—
<10	ALA-D inhibition	—	—	—	—

ALA, aminolevulinic acid; ALA-D, aminolevulinic acid dehydrase.
From Keogh JP, Boyer LV. Lead. In: Sullivan JB Jr, Kreiger GR, eds. *Clinical environmental health and toxic exposures*, 2nd ed. Philadelphia: Lippincott Williams & Wilkins, 2001, with permission.

worker whose BLL is markedly elevated or who is believed by a physician to need such removal. Workers whose BLL is 50 μg/dl must be removed from exposure immediately; those with a level higher than 40 μg/dl must undergo medical evaluation (16). A Web site (http://www.osha.gov) provides more information.

TOXICOKINETICS AND TOXICODYNAMICS

The kinetics of the uptake, distribution, and equilibration of lead in blood, bone, and soft tissue are complex (17). Three-compartment models that correspond to blood, soft tissue, and bone storage are useful but not always satisfactory in predicting changes in tissue levels. With short-term exposure to a high dose, the BLL may rise and fall relatively quickly (e.g., days), but some of this decline may be due to redistribution rather than excretion. Once a significant burden has been stored in bone, lead has a remarkably long half-life, as long as 10 years in some studies (18). In such a situation, blood and tissue lead levels as well may remain elevated for decades after termination of an exposure. Although chelating agents increase urinary excretion, they also may alter the exchange between body compartments (e.g., across the blood–brain barrier) (19).

TABLE 5. Regulatory guidelines and standards for lead

Agency	Sample or medium	Concentration	Regulation
OSHA	Air	50 μg lead/m^3	Permissible exposure limit for an 8-h workday
ACGIH	Air	150 μg lead/m^3	Time-weighted average for 40-h workweek
EPA	Air	1.5 μg lead/m^3	3-mo average
EPA	Water	50 μg lead/L	Consideration being given to lowering this to 5 μg/L
OSHA	Blood	60 μg/dl	Removal from exposure
OSHA	Blood	40 μg/dl	Medical evaluation required
CDC (EPA)	Blood	10–15 μg/dl	Level of concern in children

ACGIH, American Conference of Governmental Industrial Hygienists; CDC, U.S. Centers for Disease Control and Prevention; EPA, U.S. Environmental Protection Agency; OSHA, U.S. Occupational Safety and Health Administration.
From Keogh JP, Boyer LV. Lead. In: Sullivan JB Jr, Kreiger GR, eds. *Clinical environmental health and toxic exposures*, 2nd ed. Philadelphia: Lippincott Williams & Wilkins, 2001, with permission.

Absorption, Protein Binding, Distribution

Lead is absorbed readily through the lungs. Like other compounds, particulates less than 5 μm in diameter can reach the alveoli for absorption. Larger particles are trapped in airway mucus and produce gastrointestinal (GI) exposure after swallowing. Orally, adults absorb a small amount (20% to 30%), but children absorb up to 50% of ingested lead. Bioavailability may be increased by iron deficiency and other factors. In contrast to inorganic lead, organic lead compounds can be absorbed dermally.

Elimination

In adults, lead is excreted by the kidney at a rate of approximately 30 μg/day (20). With increasing body stores, this amount may reach 200 μg/day (21,22). Excretion may be due both to glomerular filtration and shedding of tubular epithelial cells, in which lead is concentrated (23). The extent of fecal excretion in humans is uncertain. Lead balance studies indicated that fecal lead nearly matched oral intake of lead (20). However, the role of unabsorbed lead in this measurement is unclear. Bile is an important route of excretion in rats, but its importance in humans is unclear (24).

PATHOPHYSIOLOGY

Absorption of ingested lead is influenced by its form and particle size, as well as concurrent iron and calcium absorption (25).

Almost all lead is bound to the red cell after absorption. Lead is distributed extensively throughout tissues, with highest concentrations in bone, teeth, liver, lung, kidney, brain, and spleen (1).

Most absorbed lead is deposited in bone, where it is substituted for calcium in the matrix. It does not seem to damage the bone itself and may act as a "sink," protecting other organs. This, however, also creates a long-term storage depot, allowing the accumulation of lead in the body. Many instances of remobilization of lead and continued toxicity after exposure has ceased have been described.

Lead impairs a variety of enzyme systems. Lead has affinity for sulfhydryl groups and is toxic to zinc- and calcium-dependent enzyme systems. It is estimated that lead must bind to these proteins with K_d of less than 10^{-12} to displace the normal metal ion. For example, the inhibition constant for the enzyme Δ-aminolevulinic acid (ALA-D) is 0.07 pM versus 1.6 pM for the endogenous zinc that is needed for ALA-D activity. Two enzymes in heme synthesis are affected (i.e., inhibited) by lead: the cytoplasmic enzyme ALA-D and ferrochelatase, a mitochondrial enzyme (26). Interference with ALA-D is dose-related, occurs at a BLL between 10 and 20 µg/dl, and is complete at a BLL of 70 and 90 µg/dl (26).

Ferrochelatase catalyzes the transfer of iron from ferritin into protoporphyrin and forms heme (26). Ferrochelatase inhibition by lead results in an increase in coproporphyrin excretion in urine and an increase of protoporphyrin in red blood cells (26). Erythrocyte protoporphyrin concentrations in adults are elevated at a BLL of 25 to 30 µg/dl (26). Heme synthesis is essential not only to hemoglobin but to synthesis of cytochromes needed for all oxidative metabolism.

Lead interferes with deoxyribonucleic acid transcription factors through binding to cysteine sites. It binds and interferes with the ability of calcium to trigger exocytosis of neurotransmitters (27,28). It interferes with calcium-dependent protein kinase C, which regulates many cellular events, such as regulation of cell growth, learning, and memory (28).

Lead also interferes with enzymes important in maintaining the integrity of membranes and affecting steroid metabolism (29). Vitamin D synthesis in renal tubular cells is affected by lead, owing to an interference with a heme-containing hydroxylase enzyme that converts 25-hydroxyvitamin D to 1,25-hydroxyvitamin D (30).

Lead targets motor axons and produces axonal degeneration and segmental demyelination (31). Studies have demonstrated slowed conduction in small motor fibers of the ulnar nerve to be a sensitive marker of subclinical lead neurotoxicity (30,32,33).

PREGNANCY AND LACTATION

Lead crosses the placenta and enters human breast milk (2 to 30 µg/L). Blood levels are generally similar in infants and mothers (33a). Because pregnancy is a period during which maternal calcium stores are mobilized, a significant amount of lead may be transferred simultaneously to the developing fetus (31).

CLINICAL PRESENTATION

Adult

Recognition of adult lead poisoning depends on a high index of suspicion and a thorough patient history. The insidious onset, nonspecific complaints, and lack of diagnostic signs facilitate the missed diagnosis of lead poisoning. A few situations involve brief, intense exposures. Cutting or blasting of lead-coated steel or the use of powered sanding equipment on lead-painted surfaces can produce sudden illness. Severe acute disease has been seen also with ingestion of contaminated food (34) or other lead-containing products and recently was described from intravenous injection of contaminated methamphetamine (35). In this setting, patients may develop an acute encephalopathy that can mimic other neurologic or psychiatric illnesses. Acute colic may be mistaken for appendicitis or other intraabdominal catastrophe.

More commonly, symptoms develop over weeks to months as lead slowly accumulates (Table 4). The patient's history may suggest a variety of GI, rheumatologic, or psychiatric illnesses. Workers in smaller industries or construction tend to have uncontrolled exposures and may be unaware of their exposure. The care with which the physician solicits an occupational and environmental history is critical.

The history can detect processes that disrupt painted or rust-proofed surfaces, including burning or sanding of lead-containing paint, cutting or blasting of structural steel, and welding or burning of rustproofed steel. Small businesses, including radiator repair and the reclaiming of batteries and telephone cables, frequently are conducted with little awareness of the hazards. Indoor firing ranges may expose occupants to high levels of lead when ventilation in the building is imperfect. Hobbies like stained-glass work and ceramics also can pose a risk. The use of lead-glazed pottery (foreign sources) for food or beverages can pose a threat of which affected individuals may be unaware.

Physical findings usually are of little help in diagnosis. Motor weakness may be detectable, and signs of peripheral nerve entrapment may be present. Gingival lead lines are unusual.

CENTRAL NERVOUS SYSTEM

Central nervous system effects can develop after a brief intense exposure or more gradually with lower levels of exposure. Acute encephalopathy usually is associated with a high BLL (more than 150 µg/dl). A subacute or chronic encephalopathy affecting cognitive function and mood is more common than the acute form. Headaches and lassitude are common early symptoms. Sleep disturbances, often with early morning awakening, irritability, and loss of libido, are common. Patients usually respond well to cessation of exposure and chelation therapy.

The central nervous system effects are not confined to symptomatic patients. Lead-exposed workers often have abnormal results on psychometric tests, including cognitive and visuomotor tests. Brass foundry workers with BLLs of 40 to 60 µg/dl had impaired neurobehavioral function, which was correlated to lead exposure over time. A striking reduction in lead exposure and BLLs in the workforce was accompanied by a corresponding functional improvement in the exposed group but not in the control group (36,36a). In Sweden, Mantere et al. (37) showed that psychometric and nerve condition abnormalities developed in workers newly exposed to lead as the BLL rose more than 30 µg/dl.

Early after the introduction of leaded gasoline, numerous cases of severe encephalopathy developed among workers at tetraethyl lead production facilities. Both the rapidity and severity of these intoxications were related to dose absorbed, as organic lead can be absorbed readily through the skin and can pass easily across the blood–brain barrier (30,38).

PERIPHERAL NERVOUS SYSTEM

Lead causes a subtle peripheral axonal neuropathy that affects primarily the motor nerves (27). The neuropathy is more severe in the upper rather than the lower extremity and may cause more severe effects on the dominant side. Although the classic wristdrop of so-called painter's palsy has become rare, subclinical neuropathy has been demonstrated in exposed workers, with effects beginning at BLLs that have been regarded in the past as acceptable for industrial workers. Decreases in ulnar nerve motor conduction velocity are seen at a BLL of 30 to 40 μg/dl. In addition, lead predisposes individuals to nerve entrapment, such as carpal tunnel and tarsal tunnel syndromes (39,40).

CARDIOVASCULAR EFFECTS

Large-scale mortality studies of individuals in the lead-smelting and battery industries have strongly supported the link between lead and hypertension. In an American population between 1946 and 1970, most workers had mean BLLs of 40 to 70 μg/dl. An increase occurred in deaths from renal disease and from hypertensive cardiovascular disease (41). Mortality studies in the United Kingdom and Australia show a similar pattern (42,43). Not all studies of occupational groups have shown an association between blood pressure and lead absorption (44). Little is known about the natural history of the development of hypertension in lead poisoning, its pathophysiology and relation to renal effects, and the effects of intervention.

RENAL EFFECTS

Studies of "moonshine" drinkers in Alabama have shown that gout, hypertension, and renal failure are common outcomes of lead intoxication (45). Lead accumulates in the proximal tubular cells, a process that explains the marked effect on urate excretion. In addition, Fanconi's syndrome (proteinuria, aminoaciduria, and phosphaturia) has been described as the result of lead accumulation. Inclusion bodies have been found in renal tubular cells. These inclusions may represent binding of lead by a renal binding protein that mitigates the effects of lead (46). As toxicity progresses, chronic interstitial nephritis may develop, in some cases progressing to end-stage renal failure. Wedeen has shown increased body burdens of lead in military veterans with hypertension and renal failure, raising the possibility that some cases of unexplained renal failure may be caused by unrecognized lead poisoning (33). However, this finding was not duplicated in a study of members of a health maintenance organization (47,48). Lead interferes with the renin-aldosterone system (29) and may play a role in the development of hypertension.

PULMONARY EFFECTS

Although a recent report identified lead pneumoconiosis in lead miners, no reports have cited pulmonary dysfunction among other intoxicated populations. The changes seen in miners may be due to exposure to silica in the ore (49).

ENDOCRINE EFFECTS

Lead causes decreased serum thyroxine levels, effects on adrenal hormones, and changes in vitamin D levels. However, the mechanisms and clinical significance of such effects have not been elucidated (29).

REPRODUCTIVE EFFECTS

Maternal and paternal occupational exposure to lead has been associated with decreased fertility, spontaneous abortion, stillbirth, and increased infant mortality (50). Only a few modern epidemiologic studies have addressed the effect of lead on reproductive outcome in women. These studies suggest that lower doses of lead may not cause adverse outcomes (51).

Lead readily crosses the placenta and accumulates in the fetus (20). Bellinger et al. correlated cord BLL with the results of developmental assessments in 249 2-year-old children (52). Higher lead levels correlated with poorer developmental scores. This effect was seen at BLL in the 10 to 20 μg/dl range.

Lancranjan et al. (14) demonstrated decreased sperm counts and increased numbers of abnormal sperm in battery-plant workers. Even the plant's office workers were affected, with mean BLL of 23 μg/dl. Workers reported a marked increase in sexual dysfunction. A study among Italian battery-plant workers showed similar findings and supported a direct toxic effect on spermatogenesis rather than an effect mediated by endocrine changes (15).

Pediatric

Young children presenting with possible lead poisoning should be assessed for recognizable sequelae and correlates of exposure. These include a history of such behavioral factors as pica (which increases hand-mouth exposure) and home environmental factors that suggest the availability of lead. Sequelae of poisoning may include lethargy, vomiting, irritability, developmental delay, and failure to thrive, but most children with low-level poisoning have no overtly apparent signs or symptoms (Table 3).

CENTRAL NERVOUS SYSTEM

Acute lead poisoning may produce encephalopathy. Ataxia, altered consciousness, and seizures have been reported in children with a BLL higher than 100 μg/dl, although predicting which children will develop these effects is impossible (53).

The effects of chronic low-level lead poisoning have been addressed through large, complex epidemiologic studies. Although debate remains regarding the threshold of toxicity, the evidence indicates that young children have subtle impairment of neuropsychiatric development when the BLL is elevated. Needleman et al. (54) demonstrated the relationship of a child's lead burden (as evidenced by tooth lead content) with school performance. The lead content of teeth was inversely related to school performance and this effect was maintained at 11-year follow-up (55).

Another major controversy is the lead level at which neurodevelopmental effects may occur. An analysis of the National Health and Nutrition Examination Survey data suggests that a mean BLL of 1.9 μg/dl is associated with cognitive deficits (11). The social implications of this finding, if true, are staggering. More than a million children have a BLL more than 10 μg/dl, and many millions more would have a level more than 1.9 μg/dl (8). Because this study involved a post-hoc analysis of data, there may well be a confounder to explain it.

Few studies have examined the long-term effects of childhood lead poisoning. A study by White et al. (56) among 34 Boston subjects and 20 matched controls 50 years after diagnosis of symptomatic lead poisoning suggested that a permanent pattern of cognitive dysfunction may result from childhood lead poisoning. The study authors suggested that cognitive deficits among previously lead-poisoned adults may explain lower occupational achievement in this group. Ongoing release of skeletal stores of lead may contribute also to central nervous system injury later in life, when mobilization of these stores occurs during pregnancy, lactation, or osteoporosis.

HEMATOLOGIC EFFECTS

Anemia results from impairment of hemoglobin production and from changes in the red cell membrane. Hemoglobin levels may remain normal despite moderately severe intoxication, because enzyme induction may compensate for the effects of lead. The effect of the intoxication may become apparent only when stress is placed on the erythrocyte (e.g., after blood donation) (57). A noticeable rise in hemoglobin concentration is common when lead intoxication resolves. With more severe intoxication, a normochromic, normocytic anemia develops, characterized by the presence of basophilic stippling of erythrocytes on a blood smear. Severe anemia often is a result of the superimposition of a hemolytic process caused, presumably, by membrane changes (29).

RENAL EFFECTS

Few studies have examined the renal effects of lead in children. A study of Romanian children ages 3 to 6 years and an average BLL of 34 µg/dl showed a significant relationship between the BLL and *N*-acetyl-β-D-glucosaminidase (NAG) activity in urine (50).

DIAGNOSTIC TESTS

Environmental Monitoring and Health Surveillance

Lead content can be checked from paint chips, from dust in window wells, or by the use of an x-ray fluorescence detector that analyzes painted surfaces directly. Most states require testing laboratories to report an elevated BLL. Some states monitor clinical lead poisoning through agencies such as poison centers or require the reporting of pediatric or adult lead poisoning to health authorities.

Measurement of BLL is the key to diagnosis. Measurement of blood lead is technically difficult. Local health officials or the poison center may be of help in identifying the appropriate laboratory. The U.S. Occupational Safety and Health Administration maintains a list of laboratories certified to perform measurements for medical surveillance.

Adult

The BLL is the primary test needed for diagnosis and also guides therapy, particularly in the occupational setting. Any worker whose BLL is more than 50 µg/dl must be removed from work immediately; a level more than 40 µg/dl must undergo medical evaluation (16). Routine laboratory work may reveal decreased hemoglobin and hematocrit, but severe anemia is not common. The classic sign of basophilic stippling of erythrocytes rarely is seen. After closure of the epiphyses, "lead lines" of bone growth arrest no longer develop.

Pediatric

Although lead-poisoned children may present for evaluation of failure to thrive, or other health problem, providers in practice today encounter infants and toddlers who appear completely asymptomatic with BLLs in the 1 to 25 µg/dl range. For this reason, the Centers for Disease Control and Prevention (CDC) in 1997 recommended screening of all children at risk for lead poisoning, using the whole-BLL as the diagnostic standard (58). BLLs, rather than erythrocyte protoporphyrin, now are accepted as the primary screening test, because the latter is not sufficiently sensitive to detect BLLs lower than 25 µg/dl, the previously accepted standard (16).

With the national decline in average BLL, the goal of universal blood lead screening among young children is likely to be replaced by targeted screening. High-risk groups that may be targeted include black, low-income, urban, and Hispanic children (59); those with pervasive developmental disorders (60); and those living in geographic regions associated with older housing (61).

The use of standardized screening questionnaires for identification of children at risk for lead poisoning has been proposed but is hindered by the low sensitivity and negative predictive value of most screening questions. Community-specific questionnaires may be of some value, but these must be tested locally before they are used in place of universal blood lead screening (62).

The whole-BLL is the standard for diagnosis of childhood lead poisoning. A classification system based on blood level has been established by the CDC (Table 6) (58). Once an elevated BLL has been recognized, the evaluation depends on the affected child's specific environmental and medical conditions. In most cases, a complete blood count and serum iron determination are indicated. Abdominal radiography may reveal recently ingested paint chips as radiodensities. Long-bone films may show growth arrest lines in children with chronic exposure.

TABLE 6. Classification of childhood lead poisoning and suggested treatment

Class	Blood lead (µg/dl)	Suggested interpretation and action
I	≤9	Normal; rescreen as indicated
IIA	10–14	Educate parents, rescreen in 3 mo, report to health department for community statistics
IIB	15–19	Educate parents, test for and correct iron deficiency, rescreen in 3 mo; if level persists, proceed as for class III
III	20–44	Retest within 1 mo, complete medical evaluation, consider chelation therapy
IV	45–69	Retest within 48 h; complete medical evaluation; begin environmental assessment and medical treatment, including chelation, within 48 h
V	≥70	Medical emergency: retest immediately; hospitalize and begin treatment immediately, identify and remove source of lead

From Turk DS, Schonfeld OJ, Cullen M, et al. Sensitivity of erythrocyte protoporphyrin as a screening test for lead poisoning. *N Engl J Med* 1992;326:137–138, with permission.

TREATMENT

The first step in treatment is to identify the source of exposure, to identify any other individuals (family members or coworkers) who also may have been exposed, and to terminate the exposure. Involvement of local health officials may be essential to confirm the route of exposure and to identify and assess all those at risk. The affected individuals should not return to the work or home activity that caused the poisoning until all risk of further exposure has been eliminated. Treatment of lead poisoning may involve source abatement, behavior modification programs, dietary manipulations, and chelation.

Adult

DECONTAMINATION

Most exposures are chronic and do not need GI decontamination. On occasion, an acute ingestion of a lead-containing foreign body occurs. In this case, GI decontamination is recommended if lead is visualized on abdominal radiograph. Whole bowel irrigation (WBI) often facilitates passage (Chapter 7). Endoscopic removal may be needed if WBI is not effective. The abdominal film is followed to assess clearing of lead.

ANTIDOTES

In cases with minimal symptoms, cessation of exposure may be all that is necessary. Chelation therapy is indicated for the treatment of severe symptoms, such as intractable headache, irritability, and other personality changes; myalgias or arthralgias; and abdominal colic. End-organ damage, as evidenced by neuropathy or nephropathy, also is an indication for intervention.

Even in the absence of symptoms, a markedly elevated BLL may be an indication for therapy. In some severe situations, instituting therapy before test results return may be appropriate as long as other treatable causes have been addressed. The BLL, which is sensitive to recent exposure and to current mobilization of lead from bone stores, should be interpreted in the context of the history of exposure. There are many variations on these basic indications.

There are few prospectively collected data addressing lead toxicity in adults. Anecdotal evidence supports chelation in the treatment of severe symptomatic intoxication. Controversy remains about its value in the setting of asymptomatic or mildly symptomatic intoxication. Although removing lead as rapidly and thoroughly as possible is intuitively attractive, chelating agents may cause unintended harm by redistributing lead into organs or organelles.

Chelation therapy never should be given prophylactically, nor should it be given to a patient in whom lead exposure is ongoing. Once a decision to chelate has been made, therapy should be continued until symptoms have improved and lead levels remain at an acceptable level.

Further detail concerning the use of heavy metal chelators is provided in the antidote section of this book: dimercaprol (BAL; Chapter 50), succimer (Chapter 77), ethylenediaminetetraacetic acid (EDTA; Chapter 45), penicillamine (Chapter 52), and dimercaptopropane sulfonic acid (Chapter 54). $CaNa_2$-EDTA was the mainstay of therapy in the past. Although succimer is not specifically approved for use in adults, it is commonly used to increase lead excretion is both adults and children. Dimercaprol and penicillamine are used much less frequently since succimer became available.

In the presence of severe encephalopathy or when the BLL exceeds 100 µg/dl, treatment should begin with BAL, followed in 4 hours by another dose of BAL and either succimer (if oral administration is tolerated) or $CaNa_2$-EDTA (if intravenous infusion is required). For these severe cases, BAL is typically used every 4 to 6 hours for several doses. It is then phased out and treatment continued with one of the other chelating agents. For less emergent situations or as a continuation of initial therapy, any one of the other agents can be used. Succimer or EDTA is most commonly used. 2,3-Dimercaptopropane sulfonic acid is not widely available is the United States.

Because daily use of any chelator is associated with gradually decreasing amounts of urinary lead excretion, therapy typically is continued for 5 days and then the dose is decreased or interrupted.

MONITORING

Serial lead levels are used to assess the effect of chelation and to watch for rebound of the lead level. Blood levels should be assessed after each round of therapy and weekly thereafter to determine whether rebound is occurring and whether further therapy is warranted.

Pediatric

DECONTAMINATION

Acute lead exposure is more common in children than adults. The ingestion of a lead object can produce life-threatening toxicity within days. GI decontamination may be needed if lead is visualized on abdominal radiograph. WBI often facilitates passage (Chapter 7). Endoscopic removal may be needed if WBI is not effective. The abdominal film is followed to assess clearing of lead.

Environmental decontamination is a crucial element of treatment. Whereas this is also important for adults, for children it is critical that the diagnosis of lead poisoning is followed by prompt placement in a low-risk environment.

ABATEMENT

Separation of poisoned children from the source of exposure is the first priority. Although simple cleanup measures are effective in most cases, in severe cases abatement may involve prolonged hospitalization and the evaluation and removal of siblings to alternative living arrangements. In some cities, health authorities have developed *safe houses* in which families can live until hazards are abated. Because removing lead-containing paint in a poorly controlled fashion can leave an affected home more contaminated with lead dust than before remediation, strict supervision of lead abatement is critical. Guidelines have been developed by the federal department of Housing and Urban Development (63) and should be applied if lead in residential paint exceeds 1.0 µg/cm^2 (5000 ppm) when found on friction-impact surfaces, on protruding surfaces within 3 feet of floor or ground, or in deteriorated condition on any surface (64). Abatement and interim control methods should be instituted also where soil levels exceed 400 ppm and where indoor dust levels exceed 100 µg/ft^2 on floors, 500 µg/ft^2 on interior window sills, 800 µg/ft^2 in window troughs, and 800 µg/ft^2 on exterior surfaces (64).

A retrospective study of St. Louis children with a BLL more than 25 µg/dl showed a greater decline in mean BLL among children whose homes underwent abatement procedures than among those whose homes did not. This effect was more pronounced among children with a higher BLL (greater than 35 µg/dl) (65). A modest decline in BLL occurs after abatement of outdoor soil by greater than 1000 ppm (66), but children who live in homes with elevated floor dust lead levels do not appear to benefit from soil abatement alone (67). Children living in homes that underwent abatement before the 1991 change in CDC blood lead guidelines remain at risk of low-level lead poisoning under the new definition, suggesting that improvement in home lead abatement technology may be necessary (68).

Federal law mandates the disclosure of lead-related information on the sale of all pre-1978 housing in the United States. Under Title X, Section 1018, a home purchaser must receive a lead information pamphlet, the seller must disclose all known lead hazards, purchasers are allowed a 10-day period for lead inspection, and all sales contracts must contain a lead warning statement (69).

ANTIDOTES

Since the release of the CDC's 1991 guidelines for the management of lead poisoning in young children (58), the use of oral and parenteral agents for the chelation of lead has been reconsidered. In 1995, the Committee on Drugs of the American Academy of Pediatrics reviewed the evidence for the use of chelators and recommended that they not be prescribed for children with a BLL less than 25 µg/dl. Those children with levels between 25 and 45 µg/dl should not receive chelation therapy routinely but may benefit from the use of oral chelators in cases in which elevated lead levels persist despite environmental intervention. Children with lead levels between 45 and 70 µg/dl should undergo chelation, usually with oral succimer, and those with encephalopathy or with levels in excess of 70 µg/dl should be admitted to the hospital for parenteral therapy with BAL and EDTA (69a). $CaNa_2$-EDTA does not appear to reduce overall body lead burden for children with moderate lead poisoning when the pretreatment levels are considered (70).

The administration of chelating agents to children is detailed in individual chapters on each agent. In general, succimer (Chemet) is effective in the short-term reduction of moderately elevated BLLs (71,72). It was approved in the United States for lead poisoning in children with a BLL in excess of 45 µg/dl. It was not approved for use in children with a BLL less than 45 µg/dl, but this decision was made principally to prevent the misuse of chelation in children for whom environmental investigation and remediation have not occurred (73). Succimer is typically administered at a higher dose for 5 days, followed by a lower dose for 14 days (Chapter 77), although more intense regimens have been proposed. After this 19-day course, a 2-week rest is used to assess rebound of the BLL.

The efficacy of lead chelation remains controversial. A large well-performed trial involving inner city children with a mean BLL of 26 µg/dl found that succimer chelation produced no improvement in neurodevelopmental indices (TLC study) (74). However, there are still many unanswered questions. Shannon has provided a useful analysis and raised issues for the future (75): (a) the TLC study did not reduce blood lead substantially, with a mean of 4.5 µg/dl in the succimer group compared to controls; (b) only one chelating agent was tested; (c) only neurodevelopmental endpoints were tested; and (d) it is not clear that the group enrolled represents normal practice populations (e.g., mean maternal intelligence quotient was 80). Longer-term studies addressing these issues are necessary to resolve the issue with certainty (76).

Although now rarely necessary, the management of severe pediatric lead poisoning has been described in detail (77–79). With BLLs higher than 70 µg/dl or signs of encephalopathy, therapy involves a combination of agents, beginning with BAL intramuscularly, every 4 hours. Adequate urinary output should be established by hydration, after which $CaNa_2$-EDTA should be added to the treatment by continuous infusion in normal saline or dextrose and water (Chapter 45). $CaNa_2$-EDTA may be administered intramuscularly also in divided doses every 4 hours. This combined therapy is continued for 5 days. Liver and renal function should be monitored during this combined therapy. Rebound can best be assessed 2 days after combined therapy, and a second course of therapy may be required if the BLL rebounds.

MONITORING

Serial lead levels are used to assess the effect of chelation and to watch for rebound of the lead level. Blood levels should be assessed after each round of therapy and weekly thereafter to determine whether rebound is occurring and whether further therapy is warranted.

SUPPORTIVE CARE

For children with a BLL of 10 to 25 µg/dl, specific environmental sources may not be identified readily. To reduce the bioavailability of trace amounts of lead in such cases, several dietary manipulations have been suggested. These include consumption of regular meals, correction of iron deficiency, and increased consumption of calcium and phosphorus. Frequent food consumption over the course of the day (regular meals plus snacks) may inhibit the absorption of lead because of lead chelators and precipitators naturally present in food; in addition, increased caloric intake may help children with failure to thrive. Dietary calcium appears to inhibit the GI absorption of luminal lead by binding to and displacing it from common mucosal carriers, and phosphorus binds lead in the small intestine to form an insoluble complex (80).

Many other substances bind lead. For example, several studies have found that ascorbic acid (vitamin C) reduces the BLL (81). Although animal studies support this intervention, clinical trials have produced mixed results (82), although one clinical trial showed that ascorbic acid was the equal of EDTA in lowering the BLL (83).

The role of iron supplementation in the treatment of lead poisoning is unclear. Evidence from animals suggests that iron deficiency increases the absorption of lead. It is also true that pediatric lead poisoning is associated with iron deficiency. However, it is not clear that iron is appropriate for all lead-poisoned children. The administration of iron to lead-poisoned children may actually decrease the excretion of lead (84). Further, iron therapy improves the scores of lead-poisoned children on the Bayley Development Scale (85). Therefore, iron is likely important therapy for the lead-poisoned child with concurrent iron deficiency. In contrast, it likely has no effect in lead-poisoned children that do not experience concurrent iron deficiency (84).

REFERENCES

1. Stokinger HE. The metals. In: Clayton GD, Clayton FE, eds. *Patty's industrial hygiene and toxicology*. New York: Wiley Interscience, 1981:1687–1728.
2. Agency for Toxic Substances and Disease Registry. *Toxicological profile for lead*. Washington, DC: US Department of Health and Human Services, Public Health Service, Agency for Toxic Substances and Disease Registry, 1999.
3. National Research Council. *Measuring lead exposure in infants, children, and other sensitive populations*. Washington, DC: National Academy Press, 1993.
4. Office of Pollution Prevention and Toxics. *Report on the National Survey of Lead-based Paint in Housing: base report*. Washington, DC: US Environmental Protection Agency, Office of Pollution Prevention and Toxics, 1995. Report no. EPA/747-R95-003.
5. Cook M, Chappell WR, Hoffman RE, et al. Assessment of blood lead levels in children living in a historic mining and smelting community *Am J Epidemiol* 1993;137:447–455.
6. Update: blood lead levels—United States, 1991–1994. *MMWR Morb Mortal Wkly Rep* 1997;46:141–146.
7. Sargent ID, Brown MJ, Freeman JL, et al. Childhood lead poisoning in Massachusetts communities: its association with sociodemographic and housing characteristics. *Am J Public Health* 1995;85:528–534.
8. Anonymous. Second National Report on Human Exposure to Environmental Chemicals. Atlanta: Department of Health and Human Services, National Center for Centers for Disease Control and Prevention. Environmental Health Division of Laboratory Sciences, January 2003. NCEH publication no. 02-0716.
9. Rubin CH, Esteban E, Reissman DB, et al. Lead dust in broken hill homes—a potential hazard for young children? *Aust N Z J Public Health* 2002;26(3):203–7.

9a. Boreland F, Lyle DM, Wlodarczyk J, et al. Lead dust in broken hill homes—a potential hazard for young children? *Aust N Z J Public Health* 2002;26(3):203–207.

10. Anonymous. Elevated blood lead levels among internationally adopted children—United States, 1998. *JAMA* 2000;283:1416–1418.
11. Lanphear BP, Dietrich K, Auinger P, et al. Cognitive deficits associated with blood lead concentrations <10 µg/dl in US children and adolescents. *Pub Health Rep* 2000;115:521–529.
12. Wang Y, Lu P, Chen Z, et al. Effects of occupational lead exposure. *Scand J Work Environ Health* 1985;11:20–25.
13. Hathaway GJ, Proctor NH, Hughes JP, et al. *Chemical hazards of the workplace*, 4th ed. New York: Van Nostrand Reinhold Company, 1996.
14. Lancranjan L, Popescu HI, Gavanescu O, et al. Reproductive ability of workmen occupationally exposed to lead. *Arch Environ Health* 1975;30:396–401.
15. Assennato G, Baser ME, Molinini R, et al. Sperm count suppression without endocrine dysfunction in lead exposed men. *Arch Environ Health* 1986;41:387–390.
16. Turk DS, Schonfeld QJ, Cullen M, et al. Sensitivity of erythrocyte protoporphyrin as a screening test for lead poisoning. *N Engl J Med* 1992;326:137–138.
17. Rabinowitz MB, Wetherill GW, Kopple JD. Kinetic analysis of lead metabolism in healthy humans. *J Clin Invest* 1976;58:260–270.
18. Christoffersson JO, Ahlgren L, Schute A, et al. Decrease of skeletal lead levels in man after end of occupational exposure. *Arch Environ Health* 1986;41:312–318.
19. Cory-Slechta DA, Weiss B, Cox C. Mobilization and redistribution of lead over the course of calcium disodium ethylene diamine tetraacetate chelation therapy. *J Phannacol Exp Ther* 1987;243:804–813.

20. Kehoe RA. Toxicological appraisal of lead in relation to the tolerable concentration in the ambient air. *J Air Pollut Contain Assoc* 1969;19:690–700.
21. Forni A, Cambiaghi G, Secchi GC. Initial occupational exposure to lead. *Arch Environ Health* 1976;31:73–78.
22. Chisolm JJ, Barrett MB, Harrison HV. Indicators of internal dose of lead in relation to derangement in heme synthesis. *Johns Hopkins Med J* 1975;137:612.
23. Bennett WM. Lead nephropathy. *Kidney Int* 1985;28:12–20.
24. Aral F, Yamamura Y, Yamauchi H, et al. Biliary excretion of dimethyl lead after administration of tetraethyl lead in rabbits. *Sangyo Igaku* 1983;25:175–180.
25. Watson WS, Hume R, Moore MR. Oral absorption of lead and iron. *Lancet* 1989;8:236–237.
26. Landrigan P. Current issues in the epidemiology and toxicology of occupational exposure to lead. *Environ Health Perspect* 1990;89:61–66.
27. Krigman MR, Bouldin TW, Mushak P. Lead. In: Spencer PS, Schaumberg HH, eds. *Experimental and clinical neuro toxicology*. Baltimore: Williams & Wilkins, 1980.
28. Godwin HA. The biological chemistry of lead. *Curr Opin Chem Biol* 2001;5:223–227.
29. Cullen MR, Robins JM, Eskenazi B. Adult inorganic lead intoxication: presentation of 31 new cases and a review of recent advances in the literature. *Medicine* 1983;62:221–247.
30. Goyer R. Lead toxicity: from overt to subclinical to subtle health effects. *Health Perspect* 1990;86:177–181.
31. Baltrop D. Transfer of lead to the human foetus. In: Baltrop D, Burland VVL, eds. *Mineral metabolism in paediatrics*. Philadelphia: FA Davis Co, 1968:135–150.
32. Seppalainen A, Hernsberg S, Rock B. Relationship between blood lead levels and nerve conduction-velocities. *Neurotoxicology* 1979;1:313–332.
33. Wedeen RD. In vivo tibial XRF measurement of bone lead. *Arch Environ Health* 1990;45:69–71.

33a. Mattison DR, Nightingale MS, Shiromizu K. Effects of toxic substances on female reproduction. *Environ Health Perspect* 1983;48:43–52.

34. Hershko C, Abrahamov A, Moreb J, et al. Lead poisoning in a West Bank Arab village. *Arch Intern Med* 1984;144:1969–1973.
35. Chandler DB, Norton RL, Kauffman KW, et al. Lead poisoning associated with methamphetamine use, Oregon 1988. *MMWR Morb Mortal Wkly Rep* 1989;38:830–831.
36. Baker EL, Feldman RG, White RA, et al. Occupational lead neurotoxicity: a behavioral and electrophysiological evaluation. *Br J Ind Med* 1984;41:352–361.

36a. Hogstedt C, Hane M, Agrell, et al. Neuropsychological test results and symptoms among workers with well defined long term exposure to lead. *Br J Ind Med* 1983;40:99–105.

37. Mantere P, Hanninen H, Hemberg S, et al. A prospective follow up study on psychological effects in workers exposed to low levels of lead. *Scand J Work Environ Health* 1984;10:43–50.
38. Baker EL, Feldman RG, White RA, et al. Occupational lead in neurotoxicity: improvement in behavioral effects after reduction of exposure. *Br J Ind Med* 1985;42:507–516.
39. Bleecker ML, Lindgren KN, Ford DP. Differential contribution of current and cumulative indices of lead dose to neuropsychological performance by age. *Neurology* 1997;48:639–645.
40. Kajiyama K, Doi R, Sawada J, et al. Significance of subclinical entrapment of nerves in lead neuropathy. *Environ Res* 1993;60:248–253.
41. Cooper WC, Wong O, Kheifets L. Mortality among employees of lead battery plants and lead-producing plants, 1947–1980. *Scand J Work Environ Health* 1985;11:331–345.
42. Fanning D. A mortality study of lead workers, 1926–1985. *Arch Environ Health* 1988,43:247–251.
43. McMichael AJ, Johnson HM. Long-term mortality profile of heavily exposed lead smelter workers. *J Occup Med* 1982;24:375–378.
44. Parkinson DK, Hodgson MJ, Bromet EJ, et al. Occupational lead exposure and blood pressure. *Br J Ind Med* 1987;44:744–748.
45. Morgan JM, Ball GV, Oh SJ, et al. Lead poisoning. *South Med J* 1972;65:278–288.
46. Goering PL, Fowler BA. Mechanisms of renal lead-binding protein protection against lead inhibition of delta-aminolevulinic acid dehydratase. *J Pharmacol Exp Ther* 1985;234:365–371.
47. Baturnen V, Landy E, Maesaka JK, et al. Contribution of lead to hypertension with renal impairment. *N Engl J Med* 1983;309:17–21.
48. Osterloh JD, Selby JV, Bernard BP, et al. Body burdens of lead in hypertensive nephropathy. *Arch Environ Health* 1989;44:304–310.
49. Masjedi MR, Estineh N, Bahadori M, et al. Pulmonary complications in lead miners. *Chest* 1989;96:18–21.
50. Harbison RD. *Hamilton & Hardy's industrial toxicology*, 5th ed. St. Louis, MO: Mosby, 1998.
51. Murphy MJ, Graziano JH, Popovac D, et al. Past pregnancy outcome among women living in the vicinity of a lead smelter in Kosovo, Yugoslavia. *Am J Public Health* 1990;80:33–35.
52. Bellinger D, Leviton A, Waternaux C, et al. Longitudinal analyses of prenatal and postnatal lead exposure and early cognitive development. *N Engl J Med* 1987;316:1037–1043.
53. Davoli CT, Serwint JR, Chisolm JJ. Asymptomatic children with venous lead levels >100 mg/dl. *Pediatrics* 1996;98:965–968.
54. Needleman HL, Gunnoe C, Leviton A, et al. Deficits in psychological and classroom performance of children with elevated dentine lead levels. *N Engl J Med* 1979;300:689–695.
55. Needleman HL, Schell A, Bellinger D, et al. The long term effects of exposure to low doses of lead in childhood. *N Engl J Med* 1990;322:83–88.
56. White RF, Diamond R, Proctor S, et al. Residual cognitive defects 50 years after lead poisoning during childhood. *BMJ* 1993;50:613–622.
57. Grandjean P, Jensen BM, Sand SH, et al. Delayed blood regeneration in lead exposure: an effect on reverse capacity. *Am J Public Health* 1989;79:1385–1388.
58. Centers for Disease Control and Prevention. *Screening young children for lead poisoning: guidance for state and local public health officials*. Atlanta: Centers for Disease Control and Prevention, November 1997.
59. Diermayer M, Hedberg K, Fleming D. Backing off universal childhood lead screening in the USA: opportunity or pitfall? *Lancet* 1994;344:1587–1588.
60. Shannon M, Graef JW. Lead intoxication in children with pervasive developmental disorders. *Clin Toxicol* 1996;34:177–181.
61. Targeted screening for childhood lead exposure in a low prevalence area—Salt Lake County, Utah, 1995–1996. *JAMA* 1997;277:1508–1509.
62. Rooney BL, Hayes EB, Allen BK, et al. Development of a screening tool for prediction of children at risk for lead exposure in a Midwestern clinical setting. *Pediatrics* 1994;93:183–187.
63. US Housing and Urban Development. Lead-based paint: interior guidelines for hazard identification and abatement. *Fed Regist* 1990;55:14556–14789.
64. Guidance on identification of lead-based paint hazards. *Fed Regist* 1995;60(175).
65. Staes C, Matte T, Copley CG, et al. Retrospective study of the impact of lead-based paint hazard remediation of children's blood lead levels in St. Louis, Missouri. *Am J Epidemiol* 1994;39:1016–1026.
66. Weitzman M, Aschengrau A, Bellinger D, et al. Lead-contaminated soil abatement and urban children's blood lead levels. *JAMA* 1993;269:1647–1654.
67. Aschengrau A, Beiser A, Bellinger D, et al. The impact of soil lead abatement on urban children's blood lead levels: phase 11 results from the Boston Lead-in-Soil Demonstration Project. *Environ Res* 1994;67:125–148.
68. Swindell SL, Charney E, Brown MJ, et al. Home abatement and blood lead changes in children with class III lead poisoning. *Clin Pediatr* 1994;33:536–541.
69. Title X, Section 1018 (disclosure rule). *Fed Regist* 1996;61(45).

69a. Treatment guidelines for lead exposure in children. American Academy of Pediatrics Committee on Drugs. *Pediatrics* 1995;96(1 Pt 1):155–160.

70. Markowitz ME, Bijur PE, Ruff H, et al. Effects of calcium disodium. Versenate ($CaNa_2$-EDTA) chelation in moderate childhood lead poisoning. *Pediatrics* 1993;92:265–271.
71. Besunder JB, Anderson RL, Super DM. Short-term efficacy of oral dimercaptosuccinic acid in children with low to moderate lead intoxication. *Pediatrics* 1995;96:683–687.
72. Liebelt EL, Shannon M, Graef JW. Efficacy of oral meso-2,3-dirnercaptosuccinic add therapy for low-level childhood plumbism. *J Pediatr* 1994;124:313–317.
73. Liebelt EL, Shannon MW. Oral chelators for childhood lead poisoning. *Pediatr Ann* 1994;23:616–619.
74. Rogan WJ, Dietrich KN, Ware JH, et al. The effect of chelation therapy with succimer on neuropsychological development in children exposed to lead. *N Engl J Med* 2001;344:1421–1426.
75. Shannon M. Lead poisoning treatment—a continuing need. *J Toxicol Clin Toxicol* 2001;39:661–663.
76. Pocock SJ, Smith M, Baghurse P. Environmental lead and children's intelligence: a systematic review of the epidemiological evidence. *BMJ* 1994;309:1189–1197.
77. Chisolm JJ. Treatment of lead poisoning. *Mod Treat* 1971;8:593–612.
78. Chisolm JJ, Barltrop D. Recognition and management of children with increased lead absorption. *Arch Dis Child* 1979;54:249–262.
79. Piomelli S, Rosen JF, Chisolm JJ, et al. Management of childhood lead poisoning. *J Pediatr* 1984;105:523–532.
80. Sargent ID. Role of nutrition in the prevention of lead poisoning in children. *Pediatr Ann* 1994;23:636–642.
81. Simon JA, Hudes ES. Relationship of ascorbic acid to blood lead levels. *JAMA* 1999;281:2289–2293.
82. Calabrese EJ, Stoddard A, Leonard DA, et al. The effects of vitamin C supplementation on blood and hair levels of cadmium, lead, and mercury. *Ann N Y Acad Sci* 1987;498:347–353.
83. Dawson EB, Harris WA. Effect of ascorbic acid supplementation on blood lead levels. *Abstract. J Am Coll Nutr* 1997;16:480.
84. Wright RO. The role of iron therapy in childhood plumbism. *Curr Opin Pediatr* 1999;11:255–260.
85. Ruff HA, Markowitz ME, Bijur PE, et al. Relationships among blood lead levels, iron deficiency, and cognitive development in two-year-old children. *Environ Health Perspect* 1996;104:180–185.

CHAPTER 222

Lithium

Seth Schonwald

$Li^+ H^-$

LITHIUM HYDRIDE

Atomic symbol, atomic number, molecular weight:	**Li, 3, 6.94 g/mol**
Valence state:	**+1**
CAS Registry No.:	**7580-67-8**
SI conversion:	**mEq/L = mmol/L**
Therapeutic level:	**Serum, 0.6–1.2 mEq/L**
Target organs:	**Neurotoxicity and renal toxicity**
Antidote:	**None**

OVERVIEW

Lithium is the lightest of all metals. It is used in heat transfer applications; however, it is corrosive and requires special handling (1). Lithium hydride is used in dry cells, storage batteries, aircraft alloys, special glasses, and ceramics. Compounds such as $LiAlH_4$ and organolithium reagents (LiMe, LiPh, and so forth) are important reagents in organic chemistry. Lithium hypochlorite (LiOCl) is a pool and spa sanitizer and algicide. Lithium chloride and bromide are used in air conditioning and industrial drying systems. Lithium stearate is used as an all-purpose and high-temperature lubricant (2).

Investigations on aqueous and nonaqueous media have shown that the dust particles of lithium/aluminum alloy are readily soluble in blood serum (3). Lithium carbonate (Li_2CO_3) is used to treat a variety of medical conditions (4). There are three types of pharmacologic lithium poisoning: acute, acute on chronic, and chronic (Chapter 131).

TOXIC DOSE

Regulatory guidelines have not been established for lithium metal but have been for lithium hydride (Table 1). Small doses of lithium metal cause mucous membrane burns. Lithium is not classified as carcinogenic by regulatory agencies (5).

TOXICOKINETICS AND TOXICODYNAMICS

Lithium in industry is available via inhalation and ingestion of materials covered with dust. It is well absorbed orally, and peak levels occur 2 to 4 hours postingestion. Lithium is minimally protein bound and has an apparent volume of distribution of 0.6 L/kg (6). Tissue distribution after ingestion is complex, with preferential uptake in certain compartments (e.g., kidney, thyroid, bone) (7). Lithium is excreted renally (8). The plasma elimination half-life of lithium is 12 to 27 hours and increases to approximately 36 hours in the elderly (secondary to decreased glomerular filtration rate).

TABLE 1. U.S. regulatory guidelines and standards for lithium hydride

Agency	Description	Concentration
OSHA (air)	PEL-TWA	0.025 μg/m³
ACGIH (air)	TLV-TWA	0.025 mg/m³
	STEL	None
NIOSH (air)	REL-TWA	0.025 mg/m³
	IDLH	0.05 mg/m³

ACGIH, American Conference of Governmental Industrial Hygienists; IDLH, immediately dangerous to life and health; NIOSH, National Institute for Occupational Safety and Health; OSHA, U.S. Occupational Safety and Health Administration; PEL, permissible exposure limit; REL, recommended exposure limit; STEL, short-term exposure limit; TLV, threshold limit value; TWA, time-weighted average.

PATHOPHYSIOLOGY

Lithium can substitute for sodium or potassium on several transport proteins, thus allowing lithium entry into cells. Two of the major lithium transporting proteins are the sodium channel and the sodium-proton exchanger (9). The intracellular effects of lithium are multiple. The cyclic adenosine monophosphate signal transduction pathway is a major target for intracellular lithium effects and is important for regulating several kidney functions, including maintenance of normal water balance. Lithium inhibits adenyl cyclase in a number of cell types, including renal epithelia (10).

VULNERABLE POPULATIONS

Lithium crosses the placenta and enters breast milk; however, poisoning appears to have been reported only during use of pharmaceutical preparations.

CLINICAL PRESENTATION

Toxic effects of therapeutic drugs containing lithium are addressed in Chapter 131. Air exposure to lithium hydride can cause mild to severe mucous membrane and corneal injury that may result in permanent scarring. Respiratory irritation and bronchospasm may develop from inhalation.

Severe lithium neurotoxicity occurs almost exclusively in the context of chronic therapeutic administration of lithium and rarely results from acute ingestion of lithium or occupational exposure (11).

Lithium is capable of causing polyuria and secondary polydipsia. Decreased urinary concentrating ability (nephrogenic diabetes insipidus) with a disturbed responsiveness of the distal nephron to the action of antidiuretic hormone (vasopressin) is demonstrable, and the symptoms are largely reversible on cessation of lithium or reduction of the dose. This functional lesion is not always reversible, and the underlying renal histology is a chronic focal interstitial nephropathy (12).

Lithium may inhibit the peripheral conversion of free thyroxine to free triiodothyronine in some susceptible patients (13). Along with its goitrogenic effects, chronic lithium use inhibits thyroid function and may lead to clinical hypothyroidism (14).

DIAGNOSTIC TESTS

Diagnostic testing is directed at evaluation of toxic end-organ effects such as lung, cornea, and burns. Laboratory evaluation of patients with long-term occupational exposures may be appropriate for endocrine and renal effects.

TREATMENT

Management of patients with acute exposure to lithium dusts includes removal from the contaminated area and removal and isolation of contaminated clothing. Bronchospasm is treated in the usual manner with oxygen and bronchodilators.

Burns and mucous membrane exposure are managed with copious irrigation and serial evaluations of potentially caustic injury. After ocular exposure, immediately wipe away any particles, then flush with large amounts of water for at least 15 minutes. If particles are embedded in the skin and cannot be removed, cover the area with U.S. Pharmacopeia grade mineral oil. If particles are not embedded, flush with large amounts of water. No special interventions for lithium burns have been proposed.

Ingestion of lithium metal or lithium hydroxide is caustic. Dilution with water or other water-containing materials may produce a reaction that exacerbates the corrosive activity. Consideration may be given to gastric lavage with a large diameter tube for removal of material and then dilution with large amounts of water. Esophagoscopy may be of assistance in this procedure and to assess extent of damage. Treatment is otherwise symptomatic and supportive. Administration of activated charcoal is not useful because it does not bind to lithium ions and obscures endoscopic findings.

REFERENCES

1. Lithium. The Chemistry Resource Center: British Columbia Institute of Technology Web site. Available at: http://nobel.scas.bcit.ca/resource/ptable/li.htm. Accessed March 2003.
2. Periodic table: lithium. Los Alamos National Library: Chemistry division Web site. Available at: http://pearl1.lanl.gov/periodic/elements/3.html. Accessed March 2003.
3. Bencze K, Pelikan C, Bahemann-Hoffmeister A, et al. Lithium/aluminum alloys. A problem material for biological monitoring. *Sci Total Environ* 1991;101(1–2):83–90.
4. Ilagan MC, Carlson D, Madden JF. Lithium toxicity: two case reports. *Del Med J* 2002;74(6):263–270.
5. Leonard A, Hantson P, Gerber GB. Mutagenicity, carcinogenicity and teratogenicity of lithium compounds. *Mutat Res* 1995;339(3):131–137.
6. Linakis JL, Eisenmesser B. Lithium toxicity. [Emedicine Web site.] Available at: http://www.emedicine.com/emerg/topic301.html. Accessed November 27, 2001.
7. Finley PR, Warner MD, Peabody CA. Clinical relevance of drug interactions with lithium. *Clin Pharmacokinet* 1995;29:172–191.
8. Wang PW, Ketter TA. Pharmacokinetics of mood stabilizers and new anticonvulsants. *Psychopharmacol Bull* 2002;36(1):44–66.
9. Timmer RT, Sands JM. Lithium intoxication. *J Am Soc Nephrol* 1999;10:666–674.
10. Christensen S, Kusano E, Yusufi ANK, et al. Pathogenesis of nephrogenic diabetes insipidus due to chronic administration of lithium in rats. *J Clin Invest* 1985;75:1869–1879.
11. Holroyd S, Smith D. Disabling parkinsonism due to lithium: a case report. *J Geriatr Psychiatry Neurol* 1995;8(2):118–119.
12. Walker RG. Lithium nephrotoxicity. *Kidney Int Suppl* 1993;42:S93–S98.
13. Terao T, Oga T, Nozaki S, et al. Possible inhibitory effect of lithium on peripheral conversion of thyroxine to triiodothyronine: a prospective study. *Int Clin Psychopharmacol* 1995;10(2):103–105.
14. Ozpoyraz N, Tamam L, Kulan E. Thyroid abnormalities in lithium-treated patients. *Adv Ther* 2002;19(4):176–184.

CHAPTER 223

Manganese

Seth Schonwald

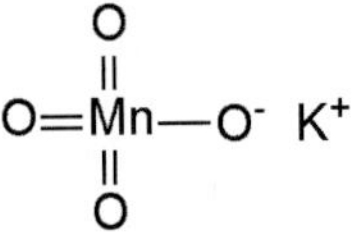

POTASSIUM PERMANGANATE

Atomic symbol, atomic number, molecular weight:	**Manganese, Mn, 25, 54.94 g/mol; potassium permanganate, $KMnO_4$, 158 g/mol**
Valence state:	**7, 4, 2**
CAS Registry No.:	**Manganese, 7439-96-5; potassium permanganate, 7722-64-7**
Normal levels:	**Whole blood, 4 to 14 µg/dl; urine, 0.97–1.07 µg/dl**
SI conversion:	**µg/dl × 0.182 = µmol/L**
Special concerns:	**Potassium permanganate causes rapid onset of caustic injury.**
Target organs:	**Central nervous system**
Antidote:	**None proven to be effective**

OVERVIEW

Manganese is found in rock, soil, water, and food (1). An essential nutrient, it is a cofactor in many enzymatic reactions that involve bone mineralization, protein and energy metabolism, metabolic regulation, protection from free radical species, and the formation of glycosaminoglycans (2). Inhalation or ingestion can lead to adverse health effects. Although *manganism* is a rare condition, it can be the cause of complex nervous system symptoms, such as parkinsonism (3).

Classification and Uses

Metallic manganese (ferromanganese) is used in steel production to improve hardness, stiffness, and strength. It is used in making various steels (carbon, stainless, high-temperature, tool), cast iron, and super alloys (4). Steel making accounts for 85% to 90% of the total demand (5).

Inorganic manganese forms include manganese chloride ($MnCl_2$), manganese sulfate ($MnSO_4$), manganese acetate (MnOAc), manganese phosphate ($MnPO_4$), manganese oxide (MnO_2), and manganese tetroxide (Mn_3O_4). Emphasis has been placed on the health effects of compounds with the Mn(II), Mn(III), or Mn(IV) oxidation states, the forms most often encountered in the environment and workplace (1). Manganese dioxide is used in making dry-cell batteries, matches, fireworks, porcelain, amethyst glass, as well as other manganese compounds (6). Manganese chloride is a precursor for other manganese compounds, a catalyst in the chlorination of organic compounds, in animal feed, and in dry-cell batteries. Manganese sulfate is used as a fertilizer and livestock supplement; it is also used in some glazes, varnishes, ceramics, and fungicides (7).

Potassium permanganate is an oxidizing agent and disinfectant; an antialgal agent; used for metal cleaning, tanning, and bleaching; and used as a fresh flower and fruit preservative. Approximately 80% of its use in the United States is for water purification (7). Another source is *Bazooka*, a cocaine-based street drug contaminated with manganese-carbonate from free-base preparation (8).

Organic manganese compounds include methylcyclopentadienyl manganese tricarbonyl; maneb and mancozeb, both fungicides; and mangafodipir. Methylcyclopentadienyl manganese tricarbonyl is a gasoline additive (9). It is also used as a fuel oil additive and a smoke inhibitor. Maneb and mancozeb are fungicides. In the United States, mancozeb is applied to approximately 80% of onion crops (10). Mangafodipir trisodium is used to improve magnetic resonance imaging (MRI) of the liver and pancreas (11).

Sources of Exposure

Manganese is an essential nutrient found in virtually all diets. Regardless of intake, adults generally maintain stable tissue manganese levels by regulation of absorption and excretion (6). Manganism has been documented in welders and in workers exposed to high levels of manganese dust or fumes in mines or foundries. Extreme examples of psychomotor excitement have been observed in manganese miners and, to a lesser extent, in industrial workers (12).

Exposure to methylcyclopentadienyl manganese tricarbonyl is primarily through inhalation or oral pathways, although dermal exposure is more important for gasoline attendants or mechanics. Exposure to maneb and mancozeb occurs by ingestion, inhalation, or dermal pathways.

Standards

The U.S. Environmental Protection Agency recommends that drinking water not exceed 0.05 parts per million. The U.S. Food and Drug Administration recommends the same level for bottled water. The U.S. Occupational Safety and Health Administration has set limits of 5 mg/m^3 for fumes and 0.2 mg/m^3 for particulate matter as the average amounts of manganese in workplace air over an 8-hour workday (13). The American Conference of Governmental Industrial Hygienists has set a limit of 1 mg/m^3 for manganese fumes and 0.2 mg/m^3 for the average amount of manganese, as either elemental or inorganic compounds, that can be in the air over an 8-hour workday (14).

Toxic Dose

Tissue contact with potassium permanganate produces coagulation necrosis, and oral ingestion may be lethal because of airway edema and obstruction or circulatory collapse (15,16).

Epidemiologic data suggest that manganese concentrations in respirable dust ranging from 0.027 to 0.215 mg/m^3 and 0.14 to 1.59 mg manganese/m^3 in total dust in the workplace can result in measurable neurologic effects (1). Inhalation exposure of 0.215 mg manganese/m^3 (respirable dust) may produce preclinical signs of neurologic change (17).

Information on cancer is scanty, but the results available do not indicate that inorganic manganese is carcinogenic (1), despite causing mutations (18).

Potassium permanganate intoxication occurred in three infant girls (2.5, 2.5, and 5 months of age). The main effects were restlessness, low-grade fever, and inflamed oral mucosa with black-brown discoloration. There was leukocytosis and a left shift. Management included oral and gastric water lavage and milk ingestion. Follow-up revealed no residual abnormalities (19).

A group of 57 children receiving contaminated parenteral nutrition has been reviewed. Eleven had hypermanganesemia and cholestasis. Four of these 11 patients died, and the seven survivors had whole blood manganese concentrations ranging from 34 to 101 μg/L. Four months after terminating exposure, the blood concentration of manganese decreased by a median of 35 μg/L. Two of the seven survivors had movement disorders. An MRI of one survivor revealed bilateral increased signal intensity in the globus pallidus and subthalamic nuclei (20).

TOXICOKINETICS AND TOXICODYNAMICS

Manganese is normally found in human tissue, blood, serum, and urine. Tissue distribution of manganese usually reflects chronic exposure, not acute exposure. The major route of manganese excretion is via the bile although some excretion occurs in urine, milk, and sweat (21). The elimination half-life is about 40 days in normal humans. The half-life is longer in the central nervous system.

PATHOPHYSIOLOGY

The central nervous system is the primary target organ. Although manganese impairs transport systems, enzyme activities, and receptor functions in the central nervous system, the mechanism of neurotoxicity has not been clearly established (22). The mechanism by which manganese leads to selective destruction of dopaminergic neurons is not known. Certain researchers believe that the manganese ion Mn(II) enhances the autoxidation or turnover of various intracellular catecholamines, leading to increased production of free radicals, reactive oxygen species, and other cytotoxic metabolites, along with depletion of cellular antioxidants (23,24).

VULNERABLE POPULATIONS

Manganese is present in the plasma of mothers and the umbilical cord blood of premature and full-term babies. Limited information suggests that higher-than-usual amounts of manganese can cause birth defects (1,25).

CLINICAL PRESENTATION

Neurologic Effects

A 56-year-old welder working with manganese compounds for 30 years developed postural instability and writing clumsiness.

Neurologic findings revealed dystonia of the shoulders and distal limbs as well as signs of parkinsonism (masked face, bradykinesia, rigidity, and retropulsion). Brain MRI showed hyperintensity lesions on T1-weighted images in the bilateral globus pallidus, midbrain, pontine tegmentum, dentate nucleus, and cerebral white matter, which reduced in size and density after 10 months. Manganese poisoning was diagnosed by high levels of both serum and urine, and by marked elevated urinary manganese level after administration of the chelating agent (26). Myoclonic involuntary movement has also been associated with chronic manganese poisoning in a 17-year-old welder (27).

Manganese causes a neurologic disorder that is similar to Parkinson's disease (28). Patients may exhibit an extrapyramidal syndrome characterized by masked facies or facial grimacing; resting tremor in limbs or tremor on extension; bradykinesia; stooped posture; and shuffling gait, often accompanied by propulsion or retropulsion. However, manganism patients have hypokinesia and tremor that is different from Parkinson's patients (29). Other differences from Parkinson's disease have been noted. Patients with manganism may have psychiatric disturbances early in the disease, have a propensity to fall backward when pushed, have less frequent resting tremor than parkinsonian patients, more frequent dystonia, a *cock walk*, and often fail to respond to dopaminergic agonists (30).

Manganese madness includes nervousness, irritability, aggression, and destructiveness, with bizarre compulsive acts such as uncontrollable spasmodic laughter or crying, impulses to sing or dance, or aimless running (31). Patients are aware of their irregular actions but appear incapable of controlling the behavior.

Headaches and dizziness occurred in patients receiving intermittent parenteral nutrition. T1-weighted MRI images have revealed symmetric high-intensity areas in basal ganglia and thalamus in similar cases. After the administration of manganese is stopped, symptoms may disappear and MRI abnormalities may improve (32).

Dermatologic Effects

Potassium permanganate directly damages skin. Maneb and mancozeb can cause skin reactions in people who have allergies to these pesticides. Once the exposure to the pesticide is stopped, the rashes and any other effects resolve.

Gastrointestinal Effects

Corrosive burns to the mouth, esophagus, and trachea can occur after ingestion of potassium permanganate and can be complicated by esophageal or pyloric stenosis (33–35). In severe cases, acute severe injury of the liver, lung, kidneys, and pancreas may develop. Strictures and gastric outlet obstruction may complicate gastrointestinal injury.

Hematologic Effects

Acute acquired methemoglobinemia has followed the ingestion of potassium permanganate (36). Hemolysis has been reported as well.

DIAGNOSTIC TESTS

The normal range of manganese in blood is 4 to 14 μg/dl, 0.97 to 1.07 μg/dl in urine, and 0.15 to 2.65 μg/L in serum. Because manganese is usually excreted promptly, past exposures are difficult to measure. Serial manganese levels rarely assist in the clinical management.

MRI results must be used along with a complete history. MRI is used for patients with signs of severe manganese toxicity, as in manganism, in Parkinson's disease, or in Alzheimer's disease. Manganese accumulates in the globus pallidus of basal ganglia. It can produce hyperintensities that are bilateral, symmetrical, and visible in T1-weighted MRI of different manganese overload conditions. Manganese-exposed workers and patients undergoing total parenteral nutrition had similar MRI studies (37). MRI does not determine the source of exposure and it does not necessarily detect manganese in the brain after exposure has ceased.

TREATMENT

Following acute exposure, *decontamination* includes removal of the patient from the contaminated area, and removal and isolation of contaminated clothing. The eyes are immediately flushed with water for ocular exposure. Skin is washed immediately with soap or mild detergent and water. There are no clinical data consistently documenting benefit from ipecac or dilution after ingestion of metallic, inorganic, or organic manganese.

Ingestion of potassium permanganate is managed as a caustic ingestion with dilution, supportive care, and endoscopy as indicated. If the victim is in respiratory distress, ventilation assistance is provided and oxygen administered. Bronchospastic symptoms following acute inhalation may theoretically respond to inhaled bronchodilators and steroid therapy.

Enhancement of Elimination

Manganese is likely removed by hemodialysis, but its use for poisoning has not been reported. Because this is usually a chronic exposure, enhanced elimination is not expected to be of benefit.

Antidotes

Chelation therapy with agents such as calcium disodium ethylenediaminetetraacetic acid may alleviate some of the neurologic signs of manganism, but the response is often incomplete or transient (38). Calcium disodium ethylenediaminetetraacetic acid reduced the body burden of two elderly patients poisoned by total parenteral nutrition (39). Cyclohexylene-aminotetraacetic acid and dimercaprol-1-propanesulfonic acid sodium salt decreased tissue manganese content in rats following inhalation, but it is unknown whether toxicity was alleviated (40). Treatment with calcium trisodium pentetate decreased serum levels and increased urine excretion of manganese in a 66-year-old man who ingested 10 g (41).

Antiparkinsonian drugs, such as levodopa, have been shown to reverse some of the neuromuscular signs of manganism (42). These drugs produce a variety of side effects, and reports indicate that they are ineffective in improving the symptoms of manganism (43).

Hepatotoxicity arising from potassium permanganate has been treated with *N*-acetylcysteine (15).

REFERENCES

1. Agency for Toxic Substances and Diseases Registry. *Toxicological profile for manganese*. Atlanta: Agency for Toxic Substances and Diseases Registry, Division of Toxicology. 2000:1–504.
2. Wedler FC. Biochemical and nutritional role of manganese: an overview. In: Klimis-Tavantzis DJ, ed. *Manganese in health and disease*. Boca Raton, LA: CRC Press, 1994:1–36.
3. Lee JW. Manganese intoxication. *Arch Neurol* 2000;57(4):597–9.
4. Hazardous Substances Data Bank. Bethesda, MD: National Institutes of Health, National Library of Medicine, 1998.

5. U.S. Geological Survey. *Mineral industry surveys: manganese: 1997 annual review*. Washington, DC: US Geological Survey, US Department of the Interior, 1997.
6. U.S. Environmental Protection Agency. *Health assessment document for manganese. Final draft*. Cincinnati: US Environmental Protection Agency, Office of Research and Development, 1984:EPA-600/8-83-013F.
7. Hazardous Substances Data Bank. Bethesda, MD: National Institutes of Health, National Library of Medicine, 1997.
8. Ensing JG. Bazooka: cocaine-base and manganese carbonate. *J Anal Toxicol* 1985;9:45–46.
9. Davis JM, Jarabek AM, Mage DT, et al. The EPA health risk assessment of methylcyclopentadienyl manganese tricarbonyl (MMT). *Risk Analysis* 1998;18:57–70.
10. Hazardous Substances Data Bank. Bethesda, MD: National Institutes of Health, National Library of Medicine, 1999.
11. Wang C, Gordon PB, Hustvedt SO, et al. MR imaging properties and pharmacokinetics of MnDPDP in healthy volunteers. *Acta Radiologica* 1997;38:665–676.
12. Chu NS, Hochberg FH, Calne DB, et al. Neurotoxicity of manganese. In: Chang L, Dyyer R, eds. *Handbook of neurotoxicology*. New York: Marcel Dekker Inc., 1995:91–103.
13. Occupational Safety and Health Administration. *Limits for air contaminants*. Washington, DC: Occupational Safety and Health Administration, 1998:Table Z-1. Code of federal regulations 29 CFR 1910.1000.
14. American Conference of Governmental Industrial Hygienists. *Threshold limit values and biological exposure indices for 1996–1997*. Cincinnati: American Conference of Governmental Industrial Hygienists, 1998.
15. Young RJ, Critchley JA, Young KK, et al. Fatal acute hepatorenal failure following potassium permanganate ingestion. *Hum Exp Toxicol* 1996;15(3):259–261.
16. Ong KL, Tan TH, Cheung WL. Potassium permanganate poisoning—a rare cause of fatal self poisoning. *J Accid Emerg Med* 1997;14(1):43–45.
17. Roels HA, Ghyselen P, Buchet JP, et al. Assessment of the permissible exposure level to manganese in workers exposed to manganese dioxide dust. *Br J Ind Med* 1992;49:25–34.
18. Gerber GB, Leonard A, Hantson P. Carcinogenicity, mutagenicity and teratogenicity of manganese compounds. *Crit Rev Oncol Hematol* 2002;42(1):25–34.
19. Hershkovitz E, Weizman Z. Potassium permanganate poisoning in infancy. *Harefuah* 1991;120(9):512–513.
20. Fell JM, Reynolds AP, Meadows N, et al. Manganese toxicity in children receiving long-term parenteral nutrition. *Lancet* 1996;347:1218–1221.
21. Environmental Protection Agency. *Drinking water criteria document for manganese*. Cincinnati: Environmental Protection Agency, Office of Health and Environmental Assessment, 1993.
22. Aschner M, Aschner JL. Manganese neurotoxicity: cellular effects and blood-brain barrier transport. *Neurosci Biobehav Rev* 1991;15:333–340.
23. Verity MA. Manganese toxicity: a mechanistic hypothesis. *Neurotoxicology* 1999;20:489–498.
24. Garner CD, Nachtman JP. Manganese catalyzed auto-oxidation of dopamine to 6-hydroxydopamine in vitro. *Chem Biol Interact* 1989;69:345–351.
25. Kilburn CJ. Manganese, malformations and motor disorders: findings in a manganese-exposed population. *Neurotoxicology* 1987;8:421–429.
26. Sato K, Ueyama H, Arakawa R, et al. A case of welder presenting with parkinsonism after chronic manganese exposure [in Japanese]. *Rinsho Shinkeigaku* 2000;40(11):1110–1115.
27. Ono K, Komai K, Yamada M. Myoclonic involuntary movement associated with chronic manganese poisoning. *J Neurol Sci* 2002;199(1–2):93–96.
28. Lander F, Kristiansen J, Lauritsen JM. Manganese exposure in foundry furnacemen and scrap recycling workers. *Int Arch Occup Environ Health* 1999;72(8):546–550.
29. Barbeau A. Manganese and extrapyramidal disorders (a critical review and tribute to Dr. George C. Cotzias). *Neurotoxicology* 1984;5:13–35.
30. Calne DB, Chu NS, Huang CC, et al. Manganism and idiopathic parkinsonism: similarities and differences. *Neurology* 1994;44:1583–1586.
31. Mena I. Manganese poisoning. In: Vinken PJ, Bruyn GW, eds. *Handbook of clinical neurology*. Amsterdam, the Netherlands: North-Holland Publishing Co., 1979:217–237.
32. Masumoto K, Suita S, Taguchi T, et al. Manganese intoxication during intermittent parenteral nutrition: report of two cases. *JPEN J Parenter Enteral Nutr* 2001;25(2):95–99.
33. Southwood T, Lamb CM, Freeman J. Ingestion of potassium permanganate crystals by a three-year-old boy. *Med J Aust* 1987;146(12):639–640.
34. Kochhar R, Das K, Mehta SK. Potassium permanganate induced oesophageal stricture. *Hum Toxicol* 1986;5(6):393–394.
35. Dagli AJ, Golden D, Finkel M, et al. Pyloric stenosis following ingestion of potassium permanganate. *Am J Dig Dis* 1973;18(12):1091–1094.
36. Mahomedy MC, Mahomedy YH, Canham PA, et al. Methaemoglobinaemia following treatment dispensed by witch doctors. Two cases of potassium permanganate poisoning. *Anaesthesia* 1975;30(2):190–193.
37. Lucchini R, Albini E, Placidi D, et al. Brain magnetic resonance imaging and manganese exposure. Review. *Neurotoxicology* 2000;21(5):769–775.
38. Cook DG, Fahn S, Brait KA. Chronic manganese intoxication. *Arch Neurol* 1974;30:59–64.
39. Nagatomo S, Umehara F, Hanada K, et al. Manganese intoxication during total parenteral nutrition: report of two cases and review of the literature. *J Neurol Sci* 1999;162:102–105.
40. Wieczorek H, Oberdorster G. Effects of selected chelating agents on organ distribution and excretion of manganese after inhalation exposure to $^{54}MnCl_2$. I. Injection of chelating agents. *Pol J Occup Med* 1989;2:261–267.
41. Holzgraefe M, Poser W, Kijewski H, et al. Chronic enteral poisoning caused by potassium permanganate: a case report. *J Toxicol Clin Toxicol* 1986;24(3):235–244.
42. Ejima A, Imamura T, Nakamura S, et al. Manganese intoxication during total parenteral nutrition [Letter]. *Lancet* 1992;339:426.
43. Huang CC, Chu NS, Lu CS, et al. Chronic manganese intoxication. *Arch Neurol* 1989;46:1104–1106.

CHAPTER 224

Mercury

Richard C. Dart and John B. Sullivan

$^{+}Hg—CH_3$

METHYL MERCURY

ELEMENTAL MERCURY (quicksilver, hydrargyrum)	
Atomic symbol, atomic number, molecular weight:	**Hg, 80, 200.6 g/mol**
Specific gravity:	**13.59**
Valence state:	**+1, +2**
Density:	**13.59 g/cm^3**
Vapor pressure:	**1.2×10^{-3} mm Hg (20°C)**
SI conversion:	**μg/L × 4.99 = nmol/L**
CAS Registry No.:	**7439-97-6**
INORGANIC MERCURY [mercuric chloride ($HgCl_2$) and others]	
Molecular weight:	**271.5 g/mol**
CAS Registry No.:	**7487-94-7**
ORGANIC MERCURY [methyl mercury ($HgCH_3$)]	
Molecular weight:	**215.62 g/mol**
CAS Registry No.:	**22967-92-6**
THIOMERSAL (thimerosal, $C_9H_9HgNaO_2S$)	
Molecular weight:	**404.8 g/mol**
CAS Registry No.:	**54-64-8**
Normal levels:	**Normal whole blood mercury levels rarely exceed 2.0 μg/dl in unexposed patients.**
Target organs:	**See Table 1.**
Antidotes:	**Dimercaprol, succimer, dimercaptopropane sulfonate (DMPS), penicillamine**

OVERVIEW

Mercury is a metal with unique properties that make it a useful component of industrial processes and consumer products. Once pervasive, its use has been restricted due to its environmental and health effects. The chemical symbol, Hg, is derived from the Greek word hydrargyros, meaning "water silver."

Chemical and Physical Properties

Mercury exists in three chemical forms; each form is addressed individually in this chapter. *Elemental mercury*, also called *quicksilver* or *hydrargyrum*, is the only metal that is liquid at room temperature. This category includes any ionic compound that decomposes into mercury vapor. Unlike other metals or forms of mercury, elemental mercury vaporizes easily at room temperature, saturating the air at 13 to 18 μg/m^3 at 24°C. *Inorganic mercury* has three oxidation states: metallic (0), mercurous (Hg^{+}), and mercuric (Hg^{2+}) [e.g., mercuric chloride ($HgCl_2$) and mercurous chloride (HgCl or Hg_2Cl_2; calomel)]. *Organic mercury* includes both short-chain (e.g., methyl and ethyl mercury) and long-chain (alkyl or aryl) compounds (Table 2).

TABLE 1. Target organs

Elemental	Lungs (inhalation), central and peripheral nervous systems, kidneys
Inorganic	Caustic injury to gastrointestinal tract, kidneys, nervous system effects similar to chronic elemental Hg poisoning
Organic	Central nervous system, congenital abnormalities with prenatal exposure to methyl mercury

TABLE 2. Inorganic and organic mercurial compounds and their uses

Inorganic	Ammoniated mercury ($HgNH_2Cl$)—antiseptic
	Mercuric acetate [$Hg(OOC_2H_3)_2$]—catalyst in organic synthesis, pharmaceuticals
	Mercuric arsenate ($HgNH_3O_4$)—waterproof and antifouling paints
	Mercuric benzoate [$Hg(C_7H_5O_2)_2$]—antisyphilitic
	Mercuric bromide ($HgBr_2$)—medicinal use
	Merbromin (Mercurochrome—25% mercury + 20% bromine)—antiseptic cream mercurous chloride (calomel, mercury monochloride—Hg_2Cl_2)—a laxative
	Mercuric chloride (corrosive sublimate, mercury bichloride)—antiseptic solution
	Mercuric cyanate [fulminate of mercury, $Hg(CNO)_2$]—explosive
	Mercuric cyanide [$Hg(CN)_2$]—antiseptic, photography
	Mercuric oxide, red (red or yellow precipitate Hgo)—pigment, dry batteries
	Mercuric potassium cyanide silvering glass, in mirrors
	Mercuric sulfide—(cinnabar, red vermillion, Chinese red) used in tattoos, combined with cadmium sulfide
	Mercuric salicylate (salicylate mercury)—topical antiseptic
	Mercuric acetate [$Hg(OOC_2H_3)_2$]
	Sublimate ($HgCl_2$)
Organic	Thimerosol (merthiolate—49% mercury)
	Alkyl mercury fungicides: dialkylmercury ethyl mercury (Cresan, Goanosan, Lignasan)
	Phenyl mercury fungicides (Ph Hg +): phenylmercury (Gallotox, Merphenyl, Barbak, Corotrane)
	Alkoxyalkyl mercury fungicides: methoxyethylmercury (MetOEHg + Algalol, Aretan)
	Mercurial diuretics (Mersalyl, Chlormerodrin)

From Mercury. In: Sullivan JB, Krieger GR, eds. *Clinical environmental health and toxic exposures*, 2nd ed. Philadelphia: Lippincott Williams & Wilkins, 2001, with permission.

TABLE 3. Products and industries associated with potential mercury exposure

Elemental mercurials	Fireworks manufacturing
Dental medicine	Fur processing
Batteries	Ink manufacturing
Barometers	Chemical laboratory workers
Boiler makers	Percussion caps and detonators
Calibration instruments	Spermicidal jellies
Caustic soda production	Tannery workers
Carbon brush production	Wood preservatives
Ceramics	Tattooing materials
Chloralkali production	Taxidermists
Ultrasonic amplifiers	Vinyl chloride production
Direct current meters	Embalming preparations
Infrared detectors	Mercury vapor lamps
Electrical apparatus	Antisyphilitic agents
Electroplating	Thermoscopy
Fingerprint detectors	Silvering in mirrors
Silver and gold extraction	Photography
Jewelry	Perfumery and cosmetics
Fluorescent, neon, and mercury arc lamps	Acetaldehyde production
Manometers	**Organic mercurials**
Paints	Bactericides
Paper pulp manufacturing	Embalming preparations
Photography	Paper manufacturing
Pressure gauges	Farmers
Thermometers	Laundry and diaper services
Semiconductor solar cells	External antiseptics
Inorganic mercurials	Fungicides
Disinfectants	Insecticide manufacture
Paints and dyes	Seed handling
Explosives	Wood preservatives
	Germicides

From Mercury. In: Sullivan JB, Krieger GR, eds. *Clinical environmental health and toxic exposures*, 2nd ed. Philadelphia: Lippincott Williams & Wilkins, 2001, with permission.

Classification and Uses

The general population is exposed to mercury primarily by fish consumption and inhalation. Mercury enters the air mainly from mining, ore smelting, and coal burning (1). Levels in the atmosphere range from 3.9 to 50 ng/m^3. Rocks and soils contain 10 to 300 ng/g. Ocean water ranges from 3.0 ng/L to 6 ng/L in coastal waters (1). Surface water usually contains less than 50 ng/L. Microorganisms like *Methanobacterium* create methyl mercury from mercury, promoting accumulation of mercury in fish and humans.

The occupational use of mercury is diverse, but declining in most regions, particularly in developed countries (Table 3). Mercury was previously used in the felt hat industry and in fingerprinting. The use of elemental mercury in mining has become less common. It has been removed from many fungicides, seed dressings, and pharmaceuticals. The predominant use of mercury today is in the manufacture of electrical meters, industrial control instruments, and dry batteries; the production of the chloralkali, antimildew paints; as catalysts; and fungicides. The largest number of exposed workers involves health care providers, dentists, dental technicians, electrical equipment manufacturers, chloralkali producers, and miners (1).

Environmental and occupational standards for mercury are provided in Table 4. The maximum allowable mercury concentration in fish is 1.0 mg/kg in the United States, Finland, and Sweden.

TABLE 4. Regulatory guidelines and standards for mercury and mercury compounds

Agency	Description	Concentration
International:		
WHO		
Guidelines	Drinking water guideline values (applies to all forms of mercury)	0.001 mg/L
Regulations	Permissible to tolerable weekly intake	5 μg/kg total 3.3 μg/kg CH_3Hg
United States regulations:		
Air	Alkyl compounds—PEL, TWA	0.01 mg/m^3
OSHA	Inorganic mercury (skin)	0.05 mg/m^3—TWA
	Alkyl compounds	0.03 mg/m^3 (skin)—STEL
Guidelines		
Air		
ACGIH	Ceiling-alkyl compounds—STEL	0.03 mg/m^3
	Alkyl compound—TWA	0.01 mg/m^3
	Aryl compounds	0.1 mg/m^3
	Metallic mercury and inorganic compounds	0.025 mg/m^3
NIOSH	Aryl or inorganic mercury as mercury—REL for occupational exposure (8-h TWA)	0.1 mg/m^3 ceiling (skin)
	Mercury (organo) alkyl compounds	0.01 mg/m^3—TWA
	Mercury vapor as mercury	0.03 mg/m^3 (skin)—STEL 0.05 mg/m^3 (skin)—TWA
Water		
EPA	Inorganic mercury—lifetime health advisory (adult)	0.002 mg/L
	Inorganic mercury—longer-term health advisory (adult)	0.002 mg/L
	Drinking water equivalent level	0.002 mg/L
	Mercury and phenylmercuric acetate—ambient water quality criteria	
	Human health	
	Water and fish	0.05 μg/L
	Fish only	0.051 μg/L
	Mercury and phenylmercuric acetate as mercury—ambient water Quality criteria for aquatic organisms	
	Acute (1-h average)	Marine, 1.8 μg/L; freshwater, 1.4 μg/L
	Chronic (4-d average)	Marine, 0.94 μg/L; freshwater, 1.77 μg/L
	National primary drinking water regulations	
	MCLGs for inorganic compounds	0.002 mg/L
	MCL for inorganic compounds	0.002 mg/L
Food		
FDA	Action level for poisonous or deleterious substances in human food and animal feed—fish, shellfish, crustaceans, other aquatic animals (fresh, frozen or processed)	1 ppm
	Bottled water	0.002 mg/L

ACGIH, American Conference of Governmental Industrial Hygienists; EPA, U.S. Environmental Protection Agency; FDA, U.S. Food and Drug Administration; MCL, maximum contamination level; MCLG, maximum contamination level goal; NIOSH, National Institute for Occupational Safety and Health; OSHA, U.S. Occupational Safety and Health Administration; PEL, permissible exposure limit; ppm, parts per million; REL, recommended exposure limit; STEL, short-term exposure limit; TWA, time-weighted average; WHO, World Health Organization.
From Mercury. In: Sullivan JB, Krieger GR, eds. *Clinical environmental health and toxic exposures*, 2nd ed. Philadelphia: Lippincott Williams & Wilkins, 2001, with permission.

ELEMENTAL MERCURY

Elemental mercury is diverse and pervasive. It is contained in various meters, switches, pumps, certain surgical tubes, and other medical equipment. Mercury vapor may arise from accidental spills, gold ore processing, heating of metallic mercury, and vacuum cleanup of mercury. Occupations associated with exposure include dental personnel; chloralkali mercury cell operators; electroplaters; manufacturers of explosives; laboratory personnel; pesticide and fungicide production and application workers; manufacturers of batteries and mercury vapor lamps; miners; processors of cinnabar, gold, silver, copper, and zinc; and metallurgists. Dental amalgam is approximately 50% elemental mercury.

Toxic Dose

Because of its poor oral absorption, elemental mercury can be ingested without toxicity. Up to 204 g of elemental mercury have been ingested without systemic toxicity (2). An air concentration of 0.05 mg/m^3 corresponds to urinary and blood levels of approximately 50 μg/L and 30 to 35 μg/L, respectively (3). The U.S. Environmental Protection Agency limit is 1 μg Hg/m^3. Chronic inhalation of mercury vapor concentrations above 1.0 mg/m^3 may produce toxicity (4). Vapor exposure resulting in mercury blood levels of 0.4 to 0.9 mg/L or urine levels of 0.5 to 1.6 mg/L were associated with death (5).

It has been speculated that the small amount of mercury in dental amalgam can cause toxicity. However, the preponderance of evidence continues to support that there are no measurable clinical effects of mercury in patients with dental amalgam (6).

Toxicokinetics and Toxicodynamics

Gastrointestinal (GI) absorption of elemental mercury is less than 0.01% orally, unless GI tract disease has altered the mucosal barrier, allowing increased permeability. In contrast, 75% or more of inhaled elemental mercury is absorbed (7,8). Elimination is primarily urinary and fecal as mercuric ion, with small amounts in breath, sweat, and saliva. Elimination of elemental mercury is dose dependent and biphasic; initially rapid, then slow, with a biological half-life in humans of approximately 60 days.

Pathophysiology

During respiration, elemental mercury crosses the alveolar membrane, enters the circulation, is absorbed into tissues and red blood cells (RBCs), and then is oxidized to the mercuric form (Hg^{+2}). However, this process takes several minutes, and the lipid soluble metal can cross the blood–brain barrier and accumulate in the central nervous system (CNS) before it is oxidized (9,10). Elemental mercury also distributes to other organs and crosses the placenta (11,12). Mercuric ion reacts with protein sulfhydryls to produce nonspecific inhibition of enzyme systems and cellular membrane damage.

Pulmonary injury arises from acute inhalation of high temperature vapor. It also acts as a direct airway irritant and a cellular poison (13–15). The injury is characterized by exudative alveolar and interstitial edema, erosive bronchitis and bronchiolitis with interstitial pneumonitis, and epithelial desquamation. This produces ventilatory dysfunction, such as alveolar distension, interstitial emphysema, pneumatocele formation, pneumothorax, and mediastinal emphysema.

Vulnerable Populations

Mercury inhalation produces similar mercury blood levels in both mother and newborn child (12). Several epidemiologic studies (all with significant methodologic limitations) suggest spontaneous abortion is increased by maternal exposure to mercury (16,17). One study also implicated paternal exposure (18).

Clinical Presentation

The three types of mercury poisoning have different manifestations (Table 5).

ACUTE EXPOSURE

Inhalation. The pulmonary system and CNS are the primary target organs of elemental mercury. The initial effects are nausea, vomiting, fever, chills, headache, tachypnea, dyspnea, metallic taste, cough, chest tightness, abdominal cramps, and diarrhea (13–15). These may subside over a few days or progress to interstitial pneumonitis, bilateral infiltrates, atelectasis, noncardiogenic pulmonary edema, hemoptysis, and interstitial pulmonary fibrosis (15,19,20). Other complications include subcutaneous emphysema, pneumomediastinum, and pneumothorax. Acute intense inhalation, especially in a poorly ventilated area, may result in death.

Children younger than 30 months of age may be particularly susceptible (21). This difference in age-related outcome results

TABLE 5. Comparison of mercury poisoning: elemental, inorganic, organic

	Elemental (Hg^0) (and long-chain or aryl organic mercury)	Inorganic (mercuric chloride)	Organic (methylmercury)
Exposure			
Major	Inhalation	Ingestion	Ingestion
Minor	Injection, ingestion	Dermal, inhalation	Inhalation
Target organ effects			
Primary	Acute—lung (ALI) Chronic—brain (erethism)	Acute—GI (caustic) Chronic—brain (triad)	Acute or chronic—brain (neuropsychiatric)
Other	Kidney, acrodynia	Kidney, acrodynia	Kidney, liver
Diagnostic tests	Blood level (acute) Urine level (acute or chronic)	Blood level (acute) Urine level (acute or chronic)	Blood level (acute or chronic) Urine level
Treatment			
GI decontamination	Rare cases of massive or retained in intestine	None usually due to spontaneous emesis	None, nearly all chronic
Supportive	ALI—oxygen, positive pressure ventilation, and so forth	Volume/hydration for increased losses; hemodialysis for ARF or to increase excretion of Hg:chelator complex	
Chelation	Succimer or DMPS	BAL → succimer or DMPS	Succimer

ALI, acute lung injury (noncardiogenic pulmonary edema); ARF, acute renal failure; BAL, dimercaprol; DMPS, dimercaptopropane sulfonate; GI, gastrointestinal.

from the direct effect of mercury vapor on the lung. Desquamation of bronchial epithelium may cause severe ventilation-perfusion defects and hypoxemia. The obstruction is proportionately greater in infants than older patients because of their smaller airway cross-sectional area (21).

Ingestion. Elemental mercury is poorly absorbed; however, systemic absorption may occur if prolonged contact with compromised GI mucosa occurs (e.g., cantor tube rupture in patient with inflammatory bowel disease) (22). Elemental mercury can also be retained in the appendix, resulting in local inflammation, perforation, and systemic mercury poisoning (23).

Injection. Elemental mercury may be injected subcutaneously or intramuscularly and lead to abscess, embolization, granuloma formation, and systemic absorption with toxic manifestations (24,25). Extravasation at the injection site can produce a severe local inflammatory reaction (26). Granuloma formation with fibrosis and inflammation as a result of systemic mercury absorption has occurred (27). Pulmonary and systemic mercury embolization with an elevated blood mercury level has followed intravenous (IV) injection. Although pulmonary embolization can result in death, most patients develop no sequelae, presumably from the low rate of oxidation of mercury in the blood (24,26,28–30). The kidney may be affected, with white blood cells appearing in the urine. This condition either can resolve spontaneously or progress to renal failure.

CHRONIC EXPOSURE

Inhalation. Chronic inhalation of mercury vapor results in the classic triad of gingivostomatitis, tremor, and neuropsychiatric illness. Tremor has been described as both static/resting and intentional/ataxic. Resting tremor is a fine, trembling motion that is most evident in the upper extremities and occurs when the muscle is at rest. Intentional or ataxic tremor occurs with purposeful movement or as an aggravation of an established static tremor.

Erethism refers to a constellation of neuropsychiatric symptoms. Somatic manifestations include fatigue, insomnia, anorexia, and memory dysfunction. Erethism develops insidiously, beginning with shyness, withdrawal, depression, and loss of confidence, then progresses through nervousness, irritability, timidity, and resentment of being observed. In severe cases, patients may exhibit marked bursts of temper and frequent skin flushing.

Ophthalmic toxicity includes a brown light reflex from the anterior capsule of the lens, opacities of the lens, and vascular changes at the corneoscleral junction (31).

Acrodynia refers to an uncommon idiosyncratic reaction caused by chronic mercury exposure that occurs in infants and children. It involves painful pinkish or red discoloration of the extremities (*pink disease*), swelling, desquamation of the involved areas, as well as anorexia, insomnia, irritability or apathy, lethargy, profuse sweating, photophobia, hypertension, hypotonia, and a generalized rash.

Peripheral nerve and *renal* abnormalities can be identified; however, clinical neuropathy and nephrotoxicity are rare. Peripheral neuropathy (Chapter 26) is uncommon, but workers exposed to mercury vapor may also have subclinical reductions in sensory and peripheral nerve conduction (1). Parkinsonian states, dysarthria, and a syndrome resembling amyotrophic lateral sclerosis have been noted (31).

Diagnostic Tests

Elemental mercury can be effectively monitored in the environment and in workers. If toxicity develops, the diagnosis is made by integrating clinical findings with a history of exposure and mercury levels in the blood or urine. Radiographs may help assess the extent of mercury exposure after ingestion or injection.

ENVIRONMENTAL MONITORING AND HEALTH SURVEILLANCE

Appropriate ventilation of areas in which vapor exposure is possible should prevent toxicity and can be monitored by personal and area air sampling. Mercury vapor concentrations as low as 0.001 mg/m^3 can be detected using electronic devices such as a mercury vapor analyzer. The National Institute for Occupational Safety and Health recommends air sampling using a solid sorbent media, low flow rate, and flameless atomic absorption for detection of elemental mercury concentrations (32).

Appropriate decontamination of a mercury contaminated area includes identification of the extent of contamination; removal of carpets, moldings, and other items capable of retaining mercury; and cleaning of all surfaces with metallic mercury sulfide-converting powder, a chelating compound, and a dispersing agent. A polyurethane coating may be applied, if appropriate. Repeat testing to document decontamination is also important.

Surveillance of occupationally exposed workers should include a medical examination and 24-hour urinary mercury determination every 6 to 12 months. If air monitoring reveals mercury concentrations approaching or exceeding the threshold limit value, the employee should be examined and have a repeat urine mercury level. Hair analysis cannot be recommended for this purpose because of concern with external contamination.

ACUTE EXPOSURE

Whole blood and urine mercury levels are used to confirm exposure. The blood level is useful if measured soon after exposure, but it decreases within days of exposure. It is not a measure of the total body burden. The normal whole blood mercury level is less than 2 µg/dl (without occupational exposure), and urinary mercury concentration is less than 10 µg/L.

Mercury exposure and urinary mercury excretion generally correlate well. The initial urine levels are high and decrease rapidly after exposure is terminated. The most useful test is the 24-hour urinary mercury excretion, which should be less than 50 µg/day. A urinary mercury concentration of 30 to 50 µg/L may be associated with subclinical neuropsychiatric effects; 50 to 100 µg/L can be associated with subclinical tremor; 100 µg/L or greater can be associated with overt neuropsychiatric disturbances; and greater than 200 µg/L is associated with overt tremors (1). A special container is used for urine collection to avoid disinfectants or other contaminants of the collection vessel.

Assessing the total body burden of mercury can be accomplished by a chelation challenge using succimer or D-penicillamine (33). A substantial increase (typically several-fold) in a urinary mercury excretion after administration of a chelator can help identify an increased body burden.

N-Acetyl glucosaminidase (NAG) and β-galactosidase are lysosomal enzymes in renal tubular cells that are being studied as sensitive indicators of renal dysfunction from mercury exposure. Urinary NAG levels correlated with the number of neuropsychologic symptoms among occupational workers exposed to inorganic mercury. Whether NAG is clinically useful as an indicator of clinical effects has not been determined.

Radiography may be able to identify local deposits of mercury after subcutaneous or intramuscular injection. Acute lung injury (noncardiogenic pulmonary edema) is evaluated by chest radiography, arterial blood gases, and ventilation measurements. Chest radiography and computed axial tomography may be useful in determining the location of systemic embolization. Elemental mercury is often evident in the right heart ventricle and pulmonary vasculature for many years (31,34).

CHRONIC EXPOSURE

Diagnostic testing in patients with chronic exposure is similar to acute exposure; however, several tests are not needed. For example, tests of acute lung injury are not usually needed. Urine level testing is used more commonly in this setting than blood testing. There are abundant sulfhydryl groups in hair; thus, mercury hair levels may be 250 to 300 times the RBC concentration. Because ambient elemental mercury can contaminate hair without systemic exposure, these levels are difficult to perform and interpret.

Electromyography and nerve conduction studies may demonstrate peripheral nerve abnormalities (Chapter 26) in patients with chronic mercury exposure. A urine mercury level above 200 μg/L was associated with tremors and impaired hand-eye coordination (35). Tremors have also been described with a blood mercury level of 1 to 2 μg/dl (1).

POSTMORTEM CONSIDERATIONS

A 3-year-old girl died 2 months after playing with elemental mercury. Mercury concentrations at the time of death were 0.16 to 0.86 mg/L in antemortem urine. Postmortem tissue levels were 1.3 mg/kg in brain; 3.7 mg/kg in lung; 3.9 mg/kg in liver; and 14 to 30 mg/kg in kidney (5). Postmortem lung after aspiration 22 years previously showed progressive fibrosis with pleural effusions, pulmonary granulomas, and bronchiectasis (34).

Treatment

Management of the patient with elemental mercury inhalation focuses on immediate removal of the patient from the source of exposure, treatment of pulmonary effects, followed by identification and elimination of the source.

DECONTAMINATION

Inhalation. Treatment is primarily symptomatic and supportive. Airway management with tracheal intubation, mechanical ventilation, and positive end-expiratory pressure may be needed in severe cases. Oxygen and bronchodilators are often needed. Aspiration of mercury is managed with vigorous suctioning, postural drainage, and good pulmonary toilet (34,36). Bronchoscopy may be needed.

Ingestion. Whole-bowel irrigation may be useful in the rare case of massive ingestion and prolonged retention of elemental mercury. Smaller ingestions are not decontaminated due to the low likelihood of toxicity. Abdominal radiographs are used to evaluate whole-bowel irrigation or to follow the passage of ingested mercury. Surgical removal of the affected areas of the intestine should be considered in patients with persistently retained mercury.

Injection. Management of the injection site must be addressed on a case-by-case basis but may include prompt excision, irrigation, and suction to remove mercury droplets (37). Excision of mercury granulomas should be considered (27). Injection of dimercaprol into the wound is not recommended, as it may delay healing (38).

INCREASING MERCURY ELIMINATION

Once absorbed, mercury excretion may be increased by the use of chelation. Although mercury chelation is often recommended, the precise indications and benefits have not been described. For example, no chelating agent has yet been demonstrated to affect outcome. Nevertheless, an increase in elimination is accepted as surrogate endpoint for efficacy and is typically recommended for symptomatic patients and when it is clear that the elimination of the metal can be increased. This is a slippery slope, however, as metal excretion is often highest just after acute exposure. It is difficult to differentiate drug effect from the normal excretion response to high levels of the metal.

Similarly, the role of extracorporeal elimination has not been adequately defined. It appears that chelated mercury is successfully eliminated by hemodialysis and other techniques in the presence of renal insufficiency. Similar to chelation, improvement of outcome has not been demonstrated for multiple-dose activated charcoal, hemoperfusion, or hemodialysis. Nevertheless, extracorporeal techniques can be used when they can increase elimination of the metal without producing serious adverse effects.

Chelation. In the United States, commercially available chelators that have been used for mercury include dimercaprol (British antilewisite; BAL), succimer, and D-penicillamine. DMPS is also effective and used in other countries. Chelators work by binding the metal ionically to a functional group (e.g., the sulfhydryl groups in BAL, succimer, and DMPS).

BAL may be a poor choice because animal studies indicate that it can redistribute mercury from peripheral tissues into the brain (39,40). Succimer is a good choice for elemental mercury poisoning. It causes fewer adverse effects and is more efficient at increasing mercury excretion than penicillamine. Succimer simultaneously enhanced urinary mercury excretion and reduced nephrotoxicity after GI absorption of elemental mercury (41). Because of its side effect profile, penicillamine is reserved for patients that cannot use other agents.

BAL is administered by intramuscular injection and has many adverse effects (Chapter 50). The dose for children and adults is 3 to 5 mg/kg every 4 hours for the first 24 hours, then every 12 hours for the second 24 hours, then once a day for 3 days. A 2-day rest period followed by a treatment course of 5 days is repeated until 24-hour urinary excretion levels are less than 50 μg/L. The BAL-mercury complex is excreted in both the urine and feces and is dialyzable. Serial measurement of urinary mercury helps to assess the effects of chelation therapy. Mercury dissociates from BAL in an acid medium, and maintenance of an alkaline urine may protect the kidneys during chelation therapy (42,43).

Succimer (Chemet) and DMPS (Unithiol) are orally administered analogs of BAL that increase urinary excretion of several metals (Chapters 54 and 77). Succimer and DMPS are predominantly cleared by the kidneys, with peak urinary elimination of the parent drug and its metabolites occurring between 2 and 4 hours after drug administration. Both increase urinary excretion of mercury. Animal and human studies support the increased efficacy, ease of administration, and lower side effect profile of these agents compared to BAL and penicillamine. Succimer capsules can be opened and administered in applesauce to children or via nasogastric tube in severe poisoning cases. Unlike succimer, DMPS is available for IV use. In the United States, DMPS is not U.S. Food and Drug Administration approved but is allowed to be sold for single patients through compounding pharmacists.

Succimer is usually administered using the same dosage regimen as for lead poisoning: 10 mg/kg three times daily for 5 days, then twice daily for another 14 days. The adult dose is 100 to 200 mg orally twice daily. Monitoring of the clinical status and blood and urine mercury excretion is used to guide repeat dosing. Two weeks should be allowed between courses of chelation therapy.

D-Penicillamine (Chapter 52) is less commonly used for mercury poisoning. It is excreted primarily in the urine. Penicillamine may facilitate the absorption of mercury from the GI tract and so should not be given when mercury remains in the GI tract. For less severe elemental and inorganic toxicity in adults, a 5-day course of penicillamine 250 mg orally every 6 hours (children use 100 mg/kg/day divided every 6 hours) has been used.

Endpoint of Chelation. The therapeutic endpoints of chelation are poorly defined. Probably the only objective measurable effect of chelation therapy is enhanced urinary excretion of mercury. A potential endpoint for chelation may be when the patient's urinary mercury concentration approaches baseline or when chelation fails to elicit an increase in mercury excretion.

MONITORING OF TREATMENT

Chest radiographs, arterial blood gases, and pulmonary function should be monitored in patients with pulmonary symptoms. Corticosteroids have been used to prevent or reduce pulmonary fibrosis; however, neither corticosteroids nor prophylactic antibiotics have proved benefits.

INORGANIC MERCURY

Poisoning generally occurs from ingestion; however, mercury salts can be absorbed dermally and through mucous membranes.

Toxic Dose

The reported average lethal dose of mercuric chloride is 1 g (5). In animals, the median lethal dose of mercuric chloride is approximately 1 mg/kg body weight IV. In adults, the lethal dose of mercuric chloride has been estimated to be between 1 and 4 g, although 100 mg causes GI effects. With treatment, individuals have survived much larger doses.

Toxicokinetics and Toxicodynamics

After oral administration, only 7% to 15% of a dose is absorbed, and large amounts remain bound to the GI mucosa. Insoluble compounds may be absorbed after oxidation by intestinal bacteria to more soluble forms. After absorption, the salt ionizes and is initially distributed between RBCs and plasma. Distribution of mercury varies widely. It has been demonstrated by animal autoradiography that mercuric ion accumulates in the renal cortex (44). Mercuric ion does not appear to cross the blood–brain barrier or the placenta initially. However, the brain does take up mercury over time and retains it longer than the kidney (44). Mercuric ion is eliminated from the body mainly in the urine and feces, with small amounts in saliva and sweat. The rate of excretion is biphasic and dose-dependent. Initially, it is rapidly eliminated. Later, it is slowly eliminated, with a half-life in humans of approximately 60 days.

Pathophysiology

The target organs of inorganic mercury are the GI tract and the kidneys. Because it is ionized, little enters the brain (although a few cases of CNS toxicity have been described with chronic mercury ingestion). The causticity of inorganic mercury causes damage throughout the GI tract, including corrosive stomatitis, necrotizing esophagitis, gastritis, and ulcerative colitis. Nephrotoxicity is the result of acute tubular necrosis involving the distal portions of the proximal convoluted tubules (45,46). Oliguria or anuria can develop, usually within 24 hours of acute overdose (47,48).

Vulnerable Populations

Spontaneous abortion may occur in mothers ingesting mercuric chloride. Cataracts, anemia, and renal dysfunction in a newborn followed exposure to mercury prenatally and during nursing (49).

Clinical Presentation

Two main problems arise from acute ingestion of inorganic mercury. First, local and nearly immediate injury to the GI tract causes fluid and electrolyte loss and may result in death. The second is organ damage at the sites of excretion, primarily the kidney. As with elemental mercury exposure, diagnosis depends on integrating characteristic findings with a history of exposure and whole blood mercury concentration and urinary mercury excretion.

HISTORY

GI symptoms are dose related and vary from mild gastritis to severe necrotizing ulceration (50). Ingestion of 100 mg has been associated with a bitter metallic taste, a sensation of throat constriction, substernal burning, gastritis, abdominal pains, nausea, and vomiting (46).

SIGNS

Acute Exposure. Ingestion leads to gastroenteritis, nausea, vomiting, and hematochezia. Renal injury results in a brief initial diuresis followed by renal failure. Oliguria and anuria can develop within 24 hours (12,14,51,52). The patient may die within hours from shock and peripheral vascular collapse due to fluid and electrolyte losses (53). Massive colonic bleeding has occurred 8 to 9 days after ingestion (45). Renal toxicity is always preceded by severe GI symptoms (50). The GI symptoms may be resolving before renal toxicity is detected (45,50). Spontaneous recovery usually occurs 8 to 14 days after ingestion (45,50,54).

Chronic Exposure. Low-level chronic exposure may cause long-term behavioral impairment (55). A metaanalysis of occupational exposure to inorganic mercury (mean urinary mercury level of 32 μg/g creatinine) found a dose-response relationship for several neuropsychiatric abnormalities (56). Workers exposed to inorganic mercury have been shown to have subclinical psychomotor and neuromuscular changes (57,58).

Diagnostic Tests

ACUTE EXPOSURE

In general, blood and urine levels of inorganic mercury are interpreted in the same manner as for elemental mercury. The *whole blood* mercury level is a good measure of acute toxicity because it rises quickly after ingestion and then falls rapidly over several days. A whole blood level above 50 μg/dl is often associated with corrosive gastroenteritis and acute renal insufficiency. Notably, the mercury level may rise slightly above normal after a seafood meal containing mercury.

The relationship of a *urinary mercury* level and clinical findings is based on patients with chronic exposure. Severity of symptoms varies widely among individuals, and the correlation between symptoms and urinary mercury concentration is poor. Occupational exposures that produce neurologic effects are associated with urinary levels of 200 μg/L (1). Often, these effects are reversible after termination of exposure.

Abdominal *radiography* may reveal radiopaque inorganic mercury. A positive radiograph helps confirm the diagnosis, but a negative result does not exclude the presence of mercury.

NAG and *β-galactosidase* are lysosomal enzymes in renal tubular cells. Urinary NAG levels correlated with the number of neuropsychologic symptoms among occupational workers exposed to inorganic mercury. Whether NAG is clinically useful as an indicator of kidney damage has not been determined.

Electromyography and *nerve conduction studies* may demonstrate peripheral nerve abnormalities (Chapter 26) in chronically exposed workers. Urine mercury more than 200 μg/L has been associated with tremors and poor hand-eye coordination (35). Tremors have been associated with a blood mercury level of 1 to 2 μg/dl (1).

Endoscopy is recommended for other corrosive ingestion if signs of injury (drooling, dysphagia, abdominal pain) are present.

POSTMORTEM CONSIDERATIONS

Postmortem examination of patients who died within 48 hours of ingestion of inorganic mercury showed severe hemorrhagic necrosis of the upper GI tract (45).

Treatment

Initial treatment of inorganic mercury ingestion focuses on immediate management of caustic ingestion followed by methods to increase elimination of absorbed mercury.

DECONTAMINATION

Decontamination may not be needed because of repetitive vomiting. If the patient is treated before GI effects develop, cautious gastric lavage should be considered. The clinician must balance the serious potential danger of mercuric chloride with the risk that the procedure may cause injury (perforation) due to early corrosive injury to the esophagus and stomach. A theoretically reasonable approach is to lavage with a protein gastric lavage solution to bind the mercury, along with rinsing the stomach with egg white or concentrated human albumin after the lavage (59). A more practical, albeit unproven, approach is to use activated charcoal, although this may obscure endoscopic findings.

Whole bowel irrigation is a reasonable choice in the unusual case in which mercuric chloride is identified in GI tract, but gastroenteritis has not yet developed. Serial abdominal radiographs are used to follow the course of decontamination.

SUPPORTIVE CARE

The initial corrosive gastroenteritis may result in severe fluid, electrolyte, and blood loss. The patient's intravascular volume status should be monitored closely and losses replaced by crystalloid, colloid, and blood products. Urine output should be maintained at 1 to 2 ml/kg/hour. After the initial few hours, it is critical to distinguish between oliguria due to inadequate volume replacement and oliguria due to developing renal failure. Invasive hemodynamic monitoring may be necessary. As in other caustic ingestions, surgical intervention may be appropriate in patients experiencing severe gastric necrosis or other complications (45,60).

CHELATION TREATMENT

To reduce renal injury, chelation therapy should be initiated immediately. Chelation should not be delayed awaiting laboratory confirmation of poisoning, which may take hours or days. Although succimer, DMPS, penicillamine, and BAL all increase urinary mercury excretion, BAL is often the first choice because oral treatment is prevented by GI effects (Chapter 50). The effectiveness of BAL depends on the promptness of administration and adequacy of dosing (50,61,62). BAL should be administered within 4 hours after ingestion (61). The recommended dose of BAL is 3 to 5 mg/kg every 4 hours for 2 days, followed by 2.5 to 3.0 mg per kg every 6 hours for the next 2 days and then every 12 hours for 7 more days. Another choice for parenteral treatment is DMPS (Chapter 54).

Once oral administration is possible, succimer or penicillamine may be substituted for BAL. The doses are the same as described for elemental mercury. *N*-acetyl-D,L-penicillamine (NAP) has been used in a small number of patients with acute and chronic inorganic and organic mercury toxicity. NAP affects copper balance less than D-penicillamine.

Potential Complications

Renal failure is a common complication of inorganic mercury poisoning. Hemodialysis is used to support the patient. The BAL-mercury complex appears to be dialyzable (63). Some studies indicate that hemodialysis may contribute to the elimination of BAL-Hg in patients with renal failure (47,62,64). There is also evidence from animal studies that BAL-Hg is excreted in the bile.

ORGANIC MERCURY

An organomercurial is a compound in which the mercury atom is covalently bound to a carbon atom. The toxicology of organomercurials is determined by the stability of the covalent bond: short chain alkyl compounds (methyl, ethyl, propyl) are relatively stable, whereas the longer alkyl and aryl (phenyl) mercury compounds are rapidly converted to inorganic mercury. The aryl and long-chain mercury compounds behave like inorganic mercury toxicologically (Table 4) (1). The short-chain alkyl compounds, particularly methyl mercury, are the most toxic organomercurials.

In 1887, diethyl mercury injections were used for the treatment of syphilis but soon were abandoned because of CNS effects. Around 1913, organic mercurial diuretics were introduced and were used for more than 30 years. The antifungal and antibacterial properties of organomercurials prompted their use as seed dressings and ointments. Today, organic mercurials are used chiefly as preservatives and antiseptics. Several mercury compounds (monomethyl mercury chloride, ethyl mercuric chloride, methyl mercuric iodide, and chloromethyl mercury) are used to inhibit fungal growth and delay seed germination. Ingestion of treated seed has been a cause of poisoning from organic mercury. Merbromin (mercurochrome) is still used routinely as a topical antiseptic. Mercury is found in antiseptic solutions (phenylmercuric acetate, phenylmercuric nitrate, phenylmercuric borate, thimerosal, and mercurochrome), ophthalmic products, vaccines, immunoglobulins, nasal sprays, and lyophilized powders.

Mercurochrome (merbromin) was the first organic mercurial antiseptic. Toxicity has included contact dermatitis, epidermal cell damage, and anaphylaxis (65–67). Merbromin is an organic mercury derivative of fluorescein that produces a carmine-red solution. The 2% solution is applied directly to the skin. The lethal IV dose of merbromin in rabbits is 15 to 20 mg/kg. Repeated applications of merbromin to surgical wounds and decubiti have resulted in signs of mercury toxicity and aplastic anemia (68). The ingestion of 20 mL of a 2% solution of merbromin by a 15-year-old child resulted in nausea, vomiting, abdominal pain, dizziness, and elevated blood mercury levels (69). In a retrospective series of 2250 cases of mercurochrome exposure, minor manifestations (nausea, vomiting, abdominal pain, diarrhea) developed in 3.3% of patients, and moderate manifestations developed in 0.4% of patients (doses were not reported) (70).

Thiomersal

Thiomersal (thimerosal, merthiolate) is sodium ethylmercuric thiosalicylate, a bacteriostatic and fungistatic agent that contains 49.6% mercury by weight. Serious adverse effects, including death, have followed parenteral and topical use. Hypersensitivity reactions and allergic conjunctivitis occur occasionally (65).

Thiomersal has been used as a topical antiseptic in concentrations of 0.1% as a preservative in contact lens solutions and as a preservative for vaccines (Chapter 164) and other medical products in concentrations of 0.001% to 0.02% (71). Until 1999, routine pediatric immunization with vaccines containing thiomersal as a preservative could deliver a cumulative dose of 187.5 μg mercury by 6 months of age (71). In addition, the hepatitis B vaccine contained 12.5 μg per dose. As a precautionary measure, several national health organizations have recommended jointly that thiomersal be removed from vaccines (72,73). Currently, no vaccine in the recommended childhood immunization schedule contains thiomersal (71).

Otic irrigation with thiomersal has resulted in elevated serum mercury levels, and, in some cases, signs of mercury poisoning (74). The lethal dose of thiomersal has not been established. Five fatalities resulted from the use of 1000 times the normal concentration of thiomersal in a preparation of chloramphenicol for intramuscular injection (75). An adult who ingested 5 g of thiomersal developed severe GI injury, renal failure, CNS and peripheral nervous system pathology, and elevated blood mercury levels (76). The lethal dose of thiomersal has not been established in children. Ten infants died from treatment of omphaloceles with a tincture of thiomersal (77).

The chronic ingestion of thiomersal by an adult for an unspecified period resulted in agitation, other neurologic effects, and death (78). Respiratory distress and laryngeal obstruction occurred in an adult 30 hours after treating a sore throat with a thiomersal-containing spray (79). Skin patch testing to thiomersal was strongly positive.

A link between thiomersal and autism has been speculated. Relying on methodologically poor retrospective analyses, advocates of this hypothesis note that most patients with autism have been immunized and that many of the individual features of mercury toxicity have correlates in autistic children (80). Confounding is introduced by the fact that nearly all children received immunizations containing thiomersal. Thus, any illness occurring during childhood can be associated with thiomersal. In contrast, information suggests other causes such as strong evidence that complex genetic factors play a major role in etiology (81).

Other Sources

Ingestion of cereals from grain intended for planting and of fish from mercury-polluted streams and rivers is a major source of dietary exposure. Consumption of game birds or their eggs from areas in which methyl mercury fungicides are used can result in exposure. Disinfectant makers, fungicide makers, seed handlers, farmers, lumberjacks, pharmaceutical industry workers, and wood preservers may be exposed to organic mercury compounds in their occupations. In the paper industry, organic mercury compounds are used to control slime. Latex paints may contain phenylmercuric acetate as a preservative. Beginning in 1990, the U.S. Environmental Protection Agency prohibited mercury-containing compounds in interior latex paint.

Another source of organic mercury compound exposure is pharmaceutical product use. Vaginal contraceptive jellies and suppositories may contain phenylmercuric acetate or other organic mercurials that are easily absorbed.

Epidemics of Organomercurial Toxicity

The largest number of cases of human organomercurial poisoning have resulted from contaminated foods. Epidemics have occurred in Minimata Bay and Niigata, Japan; Iraq; Pakistan; Guatemala; Ghana; the United States; and the Soviet Union (82).

JAPAN

In 1956 at Minimata Bay and in 1964 at Niigata, large chronic poisoning of Japanese residents occurred from mercury-containing factory effluent (mercuric chloride) (82). Inorganic mercury was methylated by the fauna in the water and was concentrated as it moved up the food chain. The factories also discharged methyl mercury directly into the water. The elimination half-life of mercury in fish is several hundred days, which concentrates the organic mercury 1000-fold greater than the surrounding water. Mercury levels reached 50 ppm in fish and 85 ppm in shellfish. Because fish were a dietary staple, affected individuals ingested up to 4 mg/day of mercury, which is 40 times the estimated safe daily intake.

IRAQ

In 1956 in northern Iraq and 1960 in central Iraq, wheat grain treated with an ethyl mercury–containing fungicide (Granosan-M) was used to make homemade breads instead of being planted (82). In 1971, an even larger epidemic occurred in Iraq from ingestion of homemade breads made from wheat seed treated with phenylmercuric acetate, methyl mercury dicyanamide, methyl mercury acetate, and ethyl mercury (82). The epidemic resulted in 6500 poisoning cases and 450 deaths.

THE UNITED STATES

In 1969, three children in New Mexico developed organic mercury toxicity after consumption of meat from a hog feed seed grain treated with cyanomethyl mercury guanidine (Panogen).

Toxic Dose

The reported adult toxic dose is 100 mg; however, this is a conservative estimate (5). Unintentional pediatric ingestion of mercurochrome is minimally toxic, producing only GI irritation. Larger ingestion produces more severe toxicity. Acute ingestion of 10 to 60 μg/kg body weight of methyl mercury may be lethal, and chronic daily ingestion of 10 μg/kg may be associated with adverse neurologic and reproductive effects.

Toxicokinetics and Toxicodynamics

ABSORPTION, PROTEIN BINDING, DISTRIBUTION

Oral absorption of organic mercurials is more complete than other forms because of increased lipid solubility. The short-chain alkyl mercury compounds are lipid-soluble, volatile, and well absorbed following inhalation, ingestion, or dermal exposure. Approximately 80% of inhaled short-chain mercury salt vapors are absorbed. Organic mercury antiseptics undergo limited skin penetration; however, poisoning has occurred in rare cases, such as topical application to an infected omphalocele.

More than 90% of methyl mercury is absorbed from the GI tract, as compared with only 15% of inorganic mercury. Methyl mercury distributes widely throughout the body, crosses the placenta, and enters breast milk (83,84). More than 90% of methyl mercury is found in the red cells, with whole blood to plasma ratios of 200 or 300:1 (85). Blood levels equilibrate slowly with tissue levels, making blood the preferred indicator of chronic exposure. Methyl mercury concentrates in the liver, kidney, blood, brain, hair, and epidermis. Newly formed hair avidly incorporates methyl mercury in direct proportion to the blood concentration. The amount of methyl mercury in brain tissue, although less than in the liver and kidney, is greater than the amount of mercury found in the brain after inorganic mercury poisoning.

METABOLISM

After absorption, the carbon-mercury bond is cleaved at differing rates depending on the chemical. The aryl and long-chain mercury bonds degrade readily to yield inorganic mercury; therefore, the toxicity of these compounds is similar to inorganic mercury. In contrast, the strong C-Hg bond of the short-chain mercurials like methyl mercury is cleaved slowly, and inorganic mercury does not play a major role in their toxicity. All tissues except muscle and blood transform organic mercury to an inorganic form. Inorganic mercury is oxidized to the divalent cation in the lungs, RBCs, and liver. This cation, in turn, can be reduced to the elemental form to be exhaled as metallic mercury vapor.

ELIMINATION

The biological half-life of methyl mercury is approximately 70 days (86). In animals, methyl mercury decomposes to carbon and mercury slowly (85), whereas phenyl mercury undergoes rapid breakdown to inorganic mercury within 24 hours (84,87). In humans, the major route of excretion of methyl mercury is biliary/fecal, with less than 10% in the urine (88). A portion undergoes enterohepatic circulation, whereas the remainder is converted to inorganic mercury by the intestinal flora. The enterohepatic recirculation may account for the long biological half-life of methyl mercury (89). This long half-life equates to an excretion rate of 1% per day of the total body burden.

Phenyl mercury is an aryl mercury compound that is metabolized *in vivo* to inorganic mercury and is eliminated primarily fecally for the first few days, with some excretion of the parent compounds in the urine. Later, this shifts to predominantly urinary excretion of inorganic mercury.

Pathophysiology

Mercury binds to sulfhydryl groups, leading to nonspecific inhibition of enzyme systems and alteration of cellular membranes. Likewise, mercury can bind to primary and secondary amine, amide, carboxyl, and phosphoryl groups. Methyl mercury inhibits the enzyme choline acetyltransferase, which catalyzes the final step in acetylcholine synthesis.

The CNS is particularly vulnerable to the toxic effects of methyl mercury. Methyl mercury is highly lipid soluble, which allows rapid penetration of the blood–brain barrier. It may then be transported across the blood–brain barrier as a complex with cysteine by a specific membrane carrier, which may be attributable to its resemblance to an endogenous substrate (90). The resultant neuronal damage is predominantly located within the cerebellar granular layer, the calcarine fissure of the occipital area, and the precentral gyrus. Methyl mercury has been shown to alter brain ornithine decarboxylase levels. Ornithine decarboxylase is an enzyme associated with cellular maturity and neurotransmitter uptake at the presynaptic and postsynaptic adrenergic receptor sites (91).

The congenital form of Minamata disease occurs at lower exposure levels than those associated with adult toxicity and involves diffuse brain involvement that differs from adults. Autopsy data demonstrate cortical and cerebellar atrophy and hypoplasia, corpus callosum hypoplasia, and demyelination of the pyramidal tract (82,92). Microtubule-dependent neuronal migration and cell division may be inhibited. Methyl mercury binds the α- and β-tubulin proteins avidly, inhibiting the polymerization of microtubules. The observed arrest in late mitosis is consistent with microtubule inhibition. This inhibition is specific to small amounts of organic mercury (92).

Vulnerable Populations

Methyl mercury is also a potent teratogen and reproductive toxin. It crosses the placenta, accumulates in the fetus, and is excreted in toxic amounts in breast milk (83,92). The concentration of alkyl mercury in fetal RBCs is 30% higher than in maternal RBCs, and fetal tissue levels are twice the maternal tissue levels (1,93). Maternal milk has 5% of the mercury concentration of maternal blood.

Fetal hemoglobin may increase fetal susceptibility. Congenital damage has been reported in infants born to asymptomatic mothers. In contrast, some mothers have shown signs of mercury intoxication whereas their infants did not, although abnormal neurologic signs in some infants became apparent with time.

Methyl mercury is a teratogen in rats, mice, cats, hamsters, and humans. Some infants born during the Minamata epidemic had a cerebral palsy-like syndrome with severe mental retardation, cerebellar symptoms (ataxia, intention tremor, nystagmus, dysmetria), hypersalivation, hyperkinesia (chorea, athetosis), limb deformities, strabismus, and seizure disorders. Their mothers had few symptoms despite heavy fish consumption.

Clinical Presentation

Most clinical information regarding organic mercury toxicity is derived from methyl mercury poisoning. Methyl mercury toxicity affects the CNS primarily. The classic triad of methyl mercury poisoning is dysarthria, ataxia, and constricted vision fields (94). Its onset is insidious, and it has a poor prognosis. Other signs and symptoms include paresthesia, hearing impairment, and progressive incoordination, loss of voluntary movement, and mental retardation.

Methyl mercury is a cumulative poison. Acute and chronic poisoning present similarly. After acute intoxication, symptoms are usually delayed for several weeks or months. Typically, symptoms worsen for 3 to 10 years, during which time cases may be misdiagnosed. Chronic ingestion becomes apparent after a prolonged period, depending on the dose.

Organic mercurials are mucous membrane irritants. They may cause blistering of the oro- and nasopharynx. Dermatitis of the hands, arms, and face followed by trunk and legs has been described in patients exposed to mercury during all three Iraqi epidemics. It was thought to occur from direct cutaneous contact. Blistering similar to second-degree burns can occur from aryl mercury compounds. Cutaneous application of mercurochrome to burns has been associated with toxicity and death in children.

Methyl mercury toxicity has been defined largely through the knowledge gained from the Japanese and Iraqi epidemics. The effects of methyl mercury poisoning include (1) (a) psychologic—difficulty concentrating, short- and long-term memory loss, emotional lability, depression, decreased intellectual abilities, and ultimately, coma; (b) cerebellar—generalized ataxia with stumbling gait, dysdiadochokinesia, and incoordination; (c) sensory—numbness and stocking-glove paresthesia of distal extremities and mouth, deafness, tunnel vision, visual field constriction, scanning speech with slurring, dysphagia; and (d) motor—spasticity; tremors of hands, face, or legs; and weakness proceeding to paralysis. The initial symptoms are fatigue and perioral/extremity paresthesia, followed by difficulty with hand movements. Sensation and vision disturbances occur next. Electrocardiographic abnormalities (ST segment changes) were noted in approximately one-third of cases from the last Iraqi poisoning.

Ethyl mercury poisoning (1956 and 1960 Iraqi epidemics) produces nausea, vomiting, diarrhea, and abdominal cramps. The clinical syndromes of ethyl mercury and methyl mercury are different. Patients exposed to the ethyl mercury–treated seed experienced polydipsia, polyuria, proteinuria, abdominal pain, nausea, vomiting, and pruritus, especially involving the palms, soles, and genitals often progressing to an exfoliative dermatitis. Involvement of the kidneys, GI tract, and skin are consistent with inorganic mercury toxicity. Methyl mercury rarely produces GI effects. Although patients exhibited slurred speech and ataxia, mentation was not affected in the ethyl mercury patients. Deep musculoskeletal pains and frequent electrocardiographic changes (ST depression, T wave inversion, prolonged QT and PR intervals, and ectopy) also were reported.

Phenyl mercury is much less toxic than methyl mercury because it is less volatile, crosses the placenta and blood–brain barrier more slowly, and is more rapidly excreted. It is metabolized to inorganic mercury and its pattern of toxicity is intermediate between alkyl and inorganic mercury.

SIGNS AND SYMPTOMS

Respiratory Effects. Organic mercurials are mucous membrane irritants. They may cause blistering of the oropharynx and nasopharynx. Significant absorption can occur via inhalation.

Gastrointestinal Effects. Methyl mercury does not usually produce GI effects. Ethyl mercury poisoning can produce nausea, vomiting, diarrhea, and abdominal cramps. Phenyl mercury may produce stomatitis and gum discoloration.

Renal Effects. Clinical nephrotoxicity has not been observed in human methyl mercury poisoning. Mercurial diuretics, methoxyethyl mercury, ethyl mercury, and phenyl mercury compounds have caused renal toxicity, including nephrotic syndrome, albuminuria, and renal failure. An autoimmune response to a mercury-protein complex has been proposed as the cause of nephrotoxicity.

Dermal Effects. Dermatitis consisting of erythroderma and pruritus, initially affecting the hands, arms, and face but followed by involvement of the trunk and legs, has been described in patients exposed to ethyl mercury during the Iraqi epidemics. It was believed to occur from direct cutaneous contact. Blistering similar to second-degree burns can occur from contact with aryl mercury compounds. Cutaneous application of mercurochrome to burns has been associated with toxicity and death in children.

Hematologic Effects. Mercurial diuretics have been associated with thrombocytopenia and agranulocytosis, and phenyl mercury has caused neutropenia.

Diagnostic Tests

ENVIRONMENTAL MONITORING AND HEALTH SURVEILLANCE

Biological monitoring is usually performed using blood. Organic mercurials are more lipid soluble than inorganic forms and tend to concentrate in RBCs. A RBC to plasma ratio of 1:1 is thought to be indicative of inorganic mercury; a RBC to plasma ratio of 10:1 suggests organic mercury toxicity. Despite exposure, blood levels of less than 2 μg/dl may occur in occupationally exposed individuals (1). A history and physical examination help make a diagnosis of organic mercury intoxication. Symptoms may be seen with methyl mercury in the 3 to 5 μg/dl blood concentration range.

ACUTE OR CHRONIC EXPOSURE

Diagnosis of organic mercury toxicity depends on integration of characteristic findings with a history of known or potential exposure and the presence of an elevated whole blood mercury concentration. In addition to an occupational and exposure history and a complete physical examination, neuropsychiatric and nerve conduction studies as well as electromyography should be considered.

Methyl mercury undergoes biliary excretion and enterohepatic recirculation, with 90% eventually being excreted in the feces. Therefore, urinary mercury measurements are not useful. *Blood mercury* levels are normally less than 2 μg/dl. Whole blood mercury concentrations in excess of 20 μg/dl have been associated with symptoms (e.g., paresthesias). The 1999 National Health Survey and Nutrition Examination Survey found that the geometric mean total blood mercury concentration of all women aged 16 to 49 years was 1.2 parts per billion (ppb) (95). For children aged 1 to 5 years the level was 0.3 ppb. The ninetieth percentile level for each group was 6.2 ppb and 1.4 ppb, respectively. A blood mercury level can be elevated for a day or more following a single seafood meal (96).

Hair levels of mercury were used extensively in investigating the Minamata epidemic. Normally, hair mercury levels average 1 to 15 ppm, but those afflicted with the disease had levels of 100 to 700 ppm. The 1999 National Health Survey and Nutrition Examination Survey found that the 90th percentile hair mercury concentration was 1.4 ppm for women and 0.4 ppm for children (95). Hair levels have been used to document temporally remote exposures. However, because of concern about external contamination, hair analysis is not used routinely.

Electromyography and *nerve conduction velocity* may be useful in determining neurologic effects on peripheral nerves (Chapter 26).

N-*Acetyl glucosaminidase* (a lysosomal enzyme) and *retinol-binding protein* (a low-molecular-weight protein) in renal tubular cells are being studied as sensitivity indicators of subclinical renal dysfunction from inorganic mercury exposure. The clinical application of *N*-acetyl glucosaminidase and retinol-binding protein has not yet been determined.

Treatment

Symptomatic and supportive care is the mainstay of treatment for organic mercury intoxication.

DECONTAMINATION

Decontamination is rarely needed because ingestion most often occurs over days or weeks. If a recent acute ingestion has occurred, gastric emptying should be performed. Activated charcoal is expected to bind organic mercury compounds.

Limited data suggest that oral neostigmine may improve motor strength in patients with moderate to severe chronic methyl mercury intoxication (97).

CHELATION

BAL has been ineffective in treating neurologic effects of methyl mercury poisoning (98). The use of BAL in organic mercury poisoning has been discouraged because animal studies showed that BAL redistributed mercury to the brain from other tissue sites (39,40). Animal studies suggest that succimer is effective in reducing the brain concentration of methyl mercury (99) and prevents cerebellar damage in methyl mercury–poisoned animals (100). *N*-acetylcysteine has also been proposed as a chelator for methyl mercury poisoning (101). NAP has been used in a small number of patients with acute and chronic inorganic and organic mercury toxicity. NAP affects copper balance less than D-penicillamine.

ENHANCED ELIMINATION

Repeated oral administration of a nonabsorbable mercury-binding substance (polythiol resin) can interrupt the enterohepatic recirculation of methyl mercury (97,102). Extracorporeal elimination is not expected to be effective because it is rapidly and widely distributed, and a large amount of methyl mercury resides within the RBC.

REFERENCES

1. Agency for Toxic Substances and Disease Registry. Potential for human exposure. In: *Toxicological profile for mercury*. Atlanta: US Department of Health and Human Services, Public Health Service, Agency for Toxic Substances and Disease Registry, April 1993.
2. Wright N, Yeoman WB, Carter GF. Massive oral ingestion of elemental mercury without poisoning. *Lancet* 1980;1(8161):206.
3. Berlin M. Mercury. In: Friberg L, Nordberg G, Vouk V, eds. *Handbook on the toxicology of metals*, vol. 2. New York: Elsevier Science, 1986.
4. Bingham E, Chorssen B, Powell CH, eds. *Patty's toxicology*, vol. 2, 5th ed. New York: John Wiley & Sons, 2001.
5. Baselt RC. *Disposition of toxic drugs and chemicals in man*, 5th ed. Foster City, California: Chemical Toxicology Institute, 2000.
6. Weiner JA, Nylander M, Berglund F. Does mercury from amalgam restorations constitute a health hazard? *Sci Total Environ* 1990;99:1–22.
7. Hursh JB, Clarkson TW, Cherian MG, et al. Clearance of mercury (Hg-197, Hg-203) vapor inhaled by human subjects. *Arch Environ Health* 1976;31:302–309.
8. Cherian MG, Hursh JB, Clarkson TW, et al. Radioactive mercury distribution in biological fluids and excretion in human subjects after inhalation of mercury vapor. *Arch Environ Health* 1978;33:109–114.
9. Magos L. Mercury-blood interaction and mercury uptake by the brain after vapor exposure. *Environ Res* 1967;1:323–337.
10. Magos L. Uptake of mercury by the brain. *Br J Ind Med* 1968;25:315–318.
11. Clarkson TK, Magos L, Greenwood MR. The transport of elemental mercury into fetal tissues. *Biol Neonate* 1972;21:239–244.
12. Lien DC, Todoruk DN, Rajani FIR, et al. Accidental inhalation of mercury vapor: respiratory and toxicologic consequences. *Can Med Assoc J* 1983;129:591–595.
13. Snodgrass W, Sullivan JB, Rumack BH. Mercury poisoning from home gold ore processing. *JAMA* 1981;246:1929–1931.
14. Matthes F, Kirschner R, Yow MD, et al. Acute poisoning associated with inhalation of mercury vapor: report of four cases. *Pediatrics* 1958;22:675–688.
15. Jung PC, Aaronson J. Death following inhalation of mercury vapor at home. *West J Med* 1980;132:539–543.
16. Panova Z, Ivanova S. Changes in ovarian function and some functional liver indices in occupational contact with mercury (I). *Akuch Ginckol Sofica* 1976;15:133–137.
17. Heidam LZ. Spontaneous abortions among dental assistants, factory workers, painters, and gardening workers: a follow-up study. *J Epidemiol Community Health* 1984;38:149–155.
18. Cordier S, Deplan F, Mandereau L, et al. Paternal exposure to mercury and spontaneous abortions. *Obstet Gynecol Survey* 1992;47:152–154.
19. Levin M, Jacobs J, Polos PG. Acute mercury poisoning and mercurial pneumonitis from gold ore purification. *Chest* 1988;94:554–556.
20. Lilis R, Miller A, Lerman Y. Acute mercury poisoning with severe chronic pulmonary manifestations. *Chest* 1985;88:306–309.
21. Jaffe KM, Shurtleff DB, Robertson WO. Survival after acute mercury vapor poisoning. *Am J Dis Child* 1983;137:749–751.
22. Bredfeldt J, Moeller D. Systemic mercury intoxication following rupture of a Miller-Abbott tube. *Am J Gastroenterol* 1978;69:478–480.
23. Birnbaum W. Inflammation of the vermiform appendix by metallic mercury. *Am J Surg* 1947;74:494–496.
24. Conrad ME, Sanford JP, Preston JA. Metallic mercury embolization—clinical and experimental. *Arch Intern Med* 1957;100:59–65.
25. Krohn IT, Solof A, Mobini J, et al. Subcutaneous injection of metallic mercury. *JAMA* 1980;243:548–549.
26. Oliver RM, Thomas MR, Cornaby AJ, et al. Mercury pulmonary emboli following intravenous self-injection. *Br J Dis Chest* 1987;81:76–79.
27. Netscher DT, Friedland JA, Guzewicz RM. Mercury poisoning from intravenous injection: treatment by granuloma excision. *Ann Plast Surg* 1991;26:592–596.
28. Ambre JJ, Welsh MJ, Svare CW. Intravenous elemental mercury injection: blood levels and excretion of mercury. *Ann Intern Med* 1977;7:451–453.
29. Celli B, Kahn MA. Mercury embolism of the lung. *N Engl J Med* 1976;295:883–885.
30. Torres-Alanis O, Garza-Ocanas L, Pineyro-Lopez A. Intravenous self administration of metallic mercury: report of a case with 5-year follow-up. *Clin Toxicol* 1997;35:83–87.
31. Adams CR, Ziegler DK, Lin JT. Mercury intoxication simulating amyotrophic lateral sclerosis. *JAMA* 1983;250:642–643.
32. Casinnelli ME, O'Connor PF, eds. *NIOSH manual of analytic methods*, 4th ed. Cincinnati: DHHS (NIOSH) Publication 94-113, 1994.
33. Aposhian HV. Mobilization of mercury and arsenic in humans by sodium 2,3-dimercapto-1-propane sulfonate (DMPS). *Environ Health Perspect* 1998;106[Suppl 4]:1017–1025.
34. Dzau VJ, Szabos S, Chang YC. Aspiration of metallic mercury: a 22-year follow-up. *JAMA* 1977;238:1531–1532.
35. Shapiro IM, Comblath DR, Sumner AJ, et al. Neurophysiologic and neuropsychologic functions of mercury exposed dentists. *Lancet* 1982;1:1147–1150.
36. Wallach L. Aspiration of elemental mercury: evidence of absorption without toxicity. *N Engl J Med* 1972;287:178–179.
37. Bleach N, McLean LM. The accidental self-injection of mercury: a hazard for glass-blowers. *Arch Emerg Med* 1987;4:53–54.
38. Baruch AD, Hass A. Injury to the hand with metallic mercury. *J Hand Surg* 1984;9A:446–448.
39. Berlin M, Lewander T. Increased brain uptake of mercury caused by 2,3-dimercaptopropanol (BAL) in mice given mercuric chloride. *Acta Pharmacol* 1965;22:1–7.
40. Canty AJ, Kishimoto R. British anti-Lewisite and organo mercury poisoning. *Nature* 1972;253:123–125.
41. Kosnett M, Dutra C, Osterloh J, et al. Nephrotoxicity from elemental mercury: protective effects of dimercaptosuccinic acid. *Vet Hum Toxicol* 1989;31:351.
42. Klaassen CD. Heavy metals and heavy metal antagonists. In: Gilman AG, Goodman LS, Rall TW, et al., eds. *The pharmacological basis of therapeutics*, 7th ed. New York: Macmillan, 1985:1605–1627.
43. Gilman A, Allen RP, Philips FS, et al. The treatment of acute systemic mercury poisoning in experimental animals with BAL, thosorbitol and BAL glucoside. *J Clin Invest* 1946;26:549–556.
44. Berlin M, Ullrebg S. Increased uptake of mercury in mouse brain caused by 2,3-dimercaptopropanol. *Nature* 1963;197:84–85.
45. Sanchez-Sicilia L, Seto DS, Nakamoto S, et al. Acute mercurial intoxication treated by hemodialysis. *Ann Intern Med* 1963;59:692–706.
46. Schreiner GE, Maher JF. Toxic nephropathy. *Am J Med* 1965;38:409–449.
47. Leumann EP, Brandenberger H. Hemodialysis in a patient with acute mercuric intoxication: concentrations of mercury in blood, dialysate, urine, vomitus and feces. *Clin Toxicol* 1977;11:301–308.
48. Tubbs R. Membranous glomerulonephritis associated with mercuric chloride solutions: case report and review of the literature. *BMJ* 1982;77:409–413.
49. Lauwerys R, Bonnier CH, Evrard PH, et al. Prenatal and early postnatal intoxication by inorganic mercury resulting from the maternal use of mercury containing soap. *Human Toxicol* 1987;6:253–256.
50. Troen P, Kaufman SA, Katz KH. Mercuric bichloride poisoning. *N Engl J Med* 1951;244:459–463.
51. Campbell JS. Acute mercurial poisoning by inhalation of metallic vapor in an infant. *Can Med Assoc J* 1948;58:72–75.
52. Teng CT, Breenan JC. Acute mercury vapor poisoning: a report of four cases with radiographic and pathologic correlation. *Radiology* 1959;73:354–361.
53. Winek CL, Fochtman FW, Bricker JD, et al. Fatal mercuric chloride ingestion. *Clin Toxicol* 1981;18:261–266.
54. Fishman AP, Kroop IG, Leiter HE, et al. A management of anuria in acute mercurial intoxication. *N Y State J Med* 1948;48:2363–2396.
55. Williamson AM, Teo RK, Sanderson J. Occupational mercury exposure and its consequences for behaviour. *Int Arch Occup Environ Health* 1982;50:273–286.
56. Meyer-Baron M, Schaeper M, Seeber A. A meta-analysis for neurobehavioral results due to occupational mercury exposure. *Arch Toxicol* 2002;76:127–136.
57. Miller JM, Chaffin DB, Smith RG. Subclinical psychomotor and neuromuscular changes in workers exposed to inorganic mercury. *Am Ind Hyg Assoc* 1975;36:725–733.
58. Rosenman KD, Valciukas JA, Glickman L, et al. Sensitive indicators of inorganic mercury toxicity. *Arch Environ Health* 1986;41:208–215.
59. Berlin M, Ullrebg S. Accumulation and retention of mercury in the mouse. *Arch Environ Health* 1963;6:589–601.
60. Sauder PH, Livardjard F, Jaeger A, et al. Acute mercury chloride intoxication. Effects of hemodialysis and plasma exchange on mercury kinetics. *J Toxicol Clin Toxicol* 988;26:189–197.
61. Longcope WT, Luetscher JA Jr, Calkins E, et al. Clinical uses of 2,3-dimercaptopropanol (BAL). *J Clin Invest* 1946;25:557–567.
62. Doolan PD, Hess WC, Kyle LH. Acute renal insufficiency due to bichloride of mercury. *N Engl J Med* 1953;249:273–276.
63. Giunta F, DiLandro D, Chiaranda M, et al. Severe acute poisoning from the ingestion of a permanent wave solution of mercuric chloride. *Human Toxicol* 1983;2:243–246.
64. Maher JF, Schreiner GE. The dialysis of mercury and mercury-BAL Complex. *Clin Res* 1959;7:298–299.
65. Anonymous. Topical antiseptics and antibiotics. *Med Lett Drug Ther* 1977;19:83–84.
66. Camarasa G. Contact dermatitis from mercurochrome. *Contact Dermatitis* 1976;2:120–121.
67. Galindo PA. Mercurochrome allergy: immediate and delayed hypersensitivity. *Allergy* 1997;52:1138–1141.
68. Slee PH, den Ottolander GJ, de Wolff FA. A case of Merbromin (mercurochrome) intoxication possibly resulting in aplastic anemia. *Acta Med Scand* 1979;205:463–466.
69. Magarey JA. Absorption of mercurochrome. *Lancet* 1993;342:1424.
70. Bryan A, Krenzelok EP. Mercurochrome toxicity? A review of 2,250 exposures. *J Toxicol Clin Toxicol* 1996;34:632.
71. Ball LK, Ball R, Pratt RD. An assessment of thimerosal use in childhood vaccines. *Pediatrics* 2001;5:1–16.
72. American Academy of Pediatrics, Committee on Infectious Diseases and Committee on Environmental Health. Thimerosal in vaccines—an interim report to clinicians. *Pediatrics* 1999;104:570–574.
73. Anonymous. Notice to readers. Thimerosal in vaccines: a joint statement of

the American Academy of Pediatrics and the Public Health Service. *MMWR Morb Mortal Wkly Rep* 1999;48:563–565.

74. U.S. Food and Drug Administration. Mercury toxicity in ear irrigation. *FDA Drug Bull* 1983;13:5–6.
75. Axton JHM. Six cases of poisoning after a parenteral organic mercurial compound (Merthiolate). *Postgrad Med J* 1972;48:417–21.
76. Pfab R, Muckter H, Roider G, et al. Clinical course of severe poisoning with thiomersal. *J Toxicol Clin Toxicol* 1996;34:453–460.
77. Fagan DG. Organ mercury levels in infants with omphaloceles treated with organic mercurial antiseptic. *Arch Dis Child* 1977;52:962–964.
78. Nascimento LOT, Filho GL, Rocha AD. Intoxicacao letal por mercurio atraves da ingestao de "merthiolate." Hurlbut, K, trans. *Rev Hosp Clin Fac Med S Paulo* 1990;45:216–218.
79. Maibach H. Acute laryngeal obstruction presumed secondary to thiomersal (merthiolate) delayed hypersensitivity. *Contact Dermatitis* 1975;1:221–222.
80. Bernard S, Enayati A, Redwood L, et al. Autism: a novel form of mercury poisoning. *Medical Hypotheses* 2001;56:462–471.
81. Wing L, Potter D. The epidemiology of autistic spectrum disorders: is the prevalence rising? *Ment Retard Dev Disabil Res Rev* 2002;8:151–161.
82. Gerstner BH, Huff JE. Selected case histories and epidemiology examples of human poisonings. *Clin Toxicol* 1977;11:131–150.
83. Amin-Zaki L, Elhassani S, Majeed MA, et al. Intra-uterine methylmercury poisoning in Iraq. *Pediatrics* 1974;54:587–595.
84. Gage JC. Distribution and excretion of methyl and phenyl mercury salts. *Br J Ind Med* 1964;21:197–202.
85. Aberg B, Ekman L, Falk R, et al. Metabolism of mey1mercury (^{203}Hg) compounds in man. *Arch Environ Health* 1969;19:478.
86. Suzuki T, Matsumoto N, Miyama T, et al. Placental transfer of mercuric chloride, phenylmercuric acetate and methylmercury acetate in mice. *Ind Health* 1967;5:149–155.
87. Miller VL, Klavano PA, Csonka E. Absorption, distribution and excretion of phenyl mercuric acetate. *Toxicol Appl Pharmacol* 1960;2:344–352.
88. Ekman L, Greitz V, Magi A, et al. Metabolism and retention of methyl-mercury nitrate in man. *Nord Med* 1968;79:450–456.
89. Norseth T, Clarkson TW. Intestinal transport of ^{203}Hg-labeled methylmercury chloride. *Arch Environ Health* 1971;22:568–577.
90. Ballatori N. Transport of toxic metals by molecular mimicry. *Environ Health Perspect* 2002;110[Suppl 5]:689–694.
91. Slotkin TA, Bartolome J. Biochemical mechanisms of developmental neurotoxicity of methylmercury. *Neurotoxicology* 1987;8:65–84.
92. Harda H. Congenital Minamata disease: intrauterine methylmercury poisoning. *Teratology* 1978;18:285–288.
93. Clarkson TW. The pharmacology of mercury compounds. *Annu Rev Pharmacol* 1972;12:375–406.
94. Hunter D, Bonford RR, Russell DS. Poisoning by methylmercury compounds. *Q J Med* 1940;9:193–213.
95. Anonymous. Blood and hair mercury levels in young children and women of childbearing age—United States, 1999. *JAMA* 2001;285:1436–1437.
96. Kershaw TG, Dhahir PH, Clarkson TW. The relationship between blood levels and dose of methylmercury in man. *Arch Environ Health* 1980;35:28–35.
97. Bakir F, Damluji SF, Amin-Zaki L, et al. Methylmercury poisoning in Iraq: an interuniversity report. *Science* 1973;181:230–241.
98. Hay WJ, Rickards AG, McMenemey WH, et al. Organic mercurial encephalopathy. *J Neurol Neurosurg Psychiatry* 1963;26:199–202.
99. Aaseth J. Recent advance in the therapy of metal poisoning with chelating agents. *Hum Toxicol* 1983;2:257–272.
100. Magos L, Peristianis GC, Snowden RT. Postexposure preventive treatment of methylmercury intoxication in rats with dimercaptosuccinic acid. *Toxicol Appl Pharmacol* 1978;45:463–475.
101. Ballatori N, Lieberman MW, Wang W. N-acetylcysteine as an antidote in methylmercury poisoning. *Environ Health Perspect* 1998;106:267–271.
102. Clarkson TW, Small H, Norseth T. The effect of a thiol containing resin on the gastrointestinal absorption and fecal excretion of methylmercury compounds in experimental animals. *Fed Proc* 1971;30:543.

CHAPTER 225

Nickel

Seth Schonwald

$$Ni(C{\equiv}O)_4$$

NICKEL CARBONYL

Atomic symbol, atomic number, molecular weight:	**Ni, 28, 58.71 g/mol**
Valence states:	**–1, 0, +2, +3, +4; +2 is most common**
CAS Registry No.:	**7440-02-0**
Normal levels:	**3 to 7 mg/L (whole blood), 1 to 5 mg/L (serum), 2 to 4 mg/L (urine), 0.1 mg/kg (tissues)**
SI conversion:	**μg/L × 17.0 = nmol/L**
Target organs:	**Skin (allergic), lungs (nickel carbonyl)**
Antidotes:	**Dithiocarb, disulfiram**

OVERVIEW

Nickel was first isolated by Axel F. Cronstedt in 1751. Nickel is widely used in alloys because it imparts properties such as corrosion resistance, heat resistance, hardness, and strength. Most permanent magnets are made of alloys of iron and nickel (1). Alloys of nickel are used in machine parts, electrical wire, armor plating, and coins. Nickel oxide is used in batteries, glassmaking, and pottery glazes. Nickel salts are used in electroplating and to harden oils in soap and margarine. Nickel silvers, nickel alloys with zinc and copper, have a distinctive white color and are used to coat tableware and as electrical contacts. Asthma, urticaria, erythema multiforme, contact dermatitis, and hand eczema may follow use of objects made with nickel.

Nickel carbonyl is a colorless, volatile liquid used in nickel refining. It is the most toxic form of nickel. Immediate symptoms following exposure may include nausea, vertigo, headache, dyspnea, and chest pain (2).

TOXIC DOSE

United States regulatory guidelines and standards are provided in Table 1.

TABLE 1. United States regulatory guidelines and standards for nickel

Agency	Description	Concentration (mg/m^3)
OSHA (air)	Elemental/metal	
	PEL-TWA	1.0
	Nickel carbonyl	
	PEL-TWA	0.007 (as Ni)
ACGIH (air)	Elemental/metal	
	TLV-TWA	1.5 (inhalable fraction)
	STEL	None
	Soluble compound	
	TLV-TWA	0.1 (inhalable fraction)
	STEL	None
	Insoluble compounds	
	TLV-TWA	0.2 (as Ni)
	STEL	None
	Nickel carbonyl	
	TLV-TWA	0.05
	STEL	None
NIOSH (air)	Elemental/metal	
	REL-TWA	0.015
	STEL	None
	IDLH	10
	Nickel carbonyl	
	REL-TWA	0.007 ppm
	STEL	None
	IDLH	2.0
EPA (water)		0.02 mg/kg/d

ACGIH, American Conference of Governmental Industrial Hygienists; EPA, U.S. Environmental Protection Agency; IDLH, immediately dangerous to life or health; NIOSH, National Institute for Occupational Safety and Health; OSHA, U.S. Occupational Safety and Health Administration; PEL, permissible exposure limit; ppm, parts per million; REL, recommended exposure limit; STEL, short-term exposure limit; TLV, threshold limit value; TWA, time-weighted average.

One death from adult respiratory distress syndrome due to inhalation of small particle-size metallic nickel has been reported (3). A fatal case of nickel poisoning by the oral route occurred in a 2-year-old child who ingested 15 g of nickel sulfate crystals (4). Following inhalation of nickel carbonyl above 50 mg/m^3, symptoms referable to the respiratory and nervous system may appear within 30 minutes to 1 hour followed within 24 hours by serious life-threatening events. Fatalities may occur after 4 to 11 days (5).

Ingestion of 0.5 to 2.5 g of nickel sulfate led to transient symptoms and full recovery in 32 workers who drank water contaminated with nickel sulfate, nickel chloride, and boric acid. The intake of 20 to 200 mg of boric acid probably did not contribute to the observed effects (6).

Several studies have found a relationship between increased mortality and nonmalignant respiratory disease and nasal and lung cancers in nickel-exposed workers (7). Nickel refinery dust and nickel subsulfide have been classified by the Environmental Protection Agency as class A human carcinogens (8). Nickel may reasonably be anticipated to be a carcinogen (9). Nickel carbonyl is listed by the International Agency for Research on Cancer as a possible human carcinogen and is classified as a select carcinogen in the Occupational Safety and Health Administration Laboratory Standard.

TOXICOKINETICS AND TOXICODYNAMICS

Nickel is absorbed through the lungs (10), the gastrointestinal tract (11), and the skin (12). Following inhalation, approximately 20% to 35% of nickel deposited in the lungs is absorbed. Pulmonary absorption is dependent on the water solubility of the nickel compound, with higher urinary nickel observed in workers exposed to soluble compounds (nickel chloride, nickel sulfate) than in those exposed to less-soluble compounds (nickel oxide, nickel subsulfide). Nickel carbonyl is the most rapidly and completely absorbed nickel compound in animals and man.

Following ingestion, approximately 27% of the nickel in drinking water was absorbed, whereas only approximately 1% was absorbed when nickel was given with food. Nickel applied directly to the skin can enter the skin without being absorbed into the bloodstream. Increased nickel levels were found in the lungs, nasal septum, liver, and kidneys of workers inhaling nickel (13).

Nickel is primarily excreted in the urine and to a lesser degree in hair, skin, breast milk, and sweat (14). It is associated with low-molecular-weight complexes that have free amino acids as indicated by the ninhydrin reaction.

PATHOPHYSIOLOGY

The physiologic role of nickel has not been unequivocally identified. Nickel may serve as a cofactor in metalloenzymes or metalloproteins, or as a cofactor that facilitates intestinal absorption of iron (Fe^{3+}) (15). Nickel-containing enzymes include urease, hydrogenase, methylcoenzyme M reductase, and carbon monoxide dehydrogenase.

Nickel readily crosses the cell membrane via calcium channels and competes with calcium for specific receptors. Although a deficiency disease for nickel has not been identified in humans, it is an essential element in animals and circumstantial evidence supports its essential status in humans.

PREGNANCY AND LACTATION

The pituitary may accumulate nickel if exposure occurs during pregnancy. Nickel crosses the placenta and accumulates in breast milk. Nickel chloride and nickel carbonyl are teratogenic in animals. However, reproductive effects were not found in a study of women working with nickel carbonyl.

CLINICAL PRESENTATION

Dermal Effects

Contact dermatitis is the most prevalent effect of nickel in the general population. Nickel allergy is the most frequent contact allergen in women. Exposure to nickel in consumer products, especially jewelry, is often the sensitizing exposure. A single oral dose of nickel sulfate can cause dermatitis in nickel-sensitive individuals (16).

An association has been observed between ear piercing and nickel sensitivity (17). In a study in schoolchildren aged 7 to 12 years, the frequency of nickel allergy was 30.8% among girls with pierced ears and 16.3% among girls without pierced ears. Once sensitized, even minimal contact with nickel may cause a reaction. Patch test studies in sensitive individuals using nickel sulfate have shown a dose-response relationship between the amount of nickel and the severity of the test response (18).

Cardiovascular Effects

A 2-year-old child accidentally ingested nickel sulfate crystals (estimated 570 mg nickel/kg). Cardiac arrest occurred 4 hours after ingestion, and the child died 8 hours after exposure (19).

Gastrointestinal Effects

Symptoms of gastrointestinal distress were reported by workers who drank water contaminated with nickel sulfate, nickel chloride, and boric acid. The symptoms included nausea, abdominal cramps, diarrhea, and vomiting. Although the actual contribution of boric acid to these effects is not known, the investigators thought that the boric acid probably did not contribute to the observed effects (20).

Hepatic Effects

A transient increase in serum bilirubin was observed in 3 of 10 workers who were hospitalized after drinking water contaminated with nickel sulfate, nickel chloride, and boric acid (20).

Ocular Effects

Transient homonymous hemianopsia occurred in one man after ingestion of 0.05 mg nickel/kg as nickel sulfate in drinking water.

NICKEL CARBONYL

The acute toxicity of inhaled nickel carbonyl is high. Acute effects occur in two stages, immediate and delayed. Headache, dizziness, shortness of breath, vomiting, and nausea are the initial symptoms of overexposure. The delayed effects (10 to 36 hours) consist of chest pain, coughing, shortness of breath, bluish discoloration of the skin, and, in severe cases, delirium, convulsions, and death. Recovery is protracted and characterized by fatigue on slight exertion. Nickel carbonyl is not regarded as having adequate warning properties (21,22).

DIAGNOSTIC TESTS

With the exception of nickel carbonyl, nickel concentrations in body fluids are not useful indicators of specific health effects (23). For persons exposed to soluble nickel compounds (e.g., nickel chloride, nickel sulfate), an increase in nickel concentration is a signal to reduce exposure, and the absence of increased values indicates nonsignificant exposure. For persons exposed to less-soluble nickel compounds (e.g., nickel subsulfide, nickel oxide), increases in nickel concentrations in body fluids indicate significant absorption, and exposure should be reduced to the lowest level attainable (23).

Electrothermal atomic absorption spectrometry is useful for determination of nickel in urine. The presence of nickel in hair and nails can be determined by the same analytical techniques used for blood and tissue (24).

TREATMENT

Overview

Treatment with fluid and electrolyte replacement is considered necessary only in cases associated with severe vomiting and diarrhea (25). Gastrointestinal decontamination is seldom necessary. Activated charcoal could obscure endoscopic findings. Oral administration of water or milk may help dilute caustic nickel compounds in the stomach (26).

Dermal Exposures

In cases of dermal or ocular exposure, the skin or eyes should be irrigated or washed thoroughly (27). Topical application of chelating agents such as 5-chloro-7-iodoquinolin-8-ol has been used to reduce dermal absorption in nickel-sensitive subjects, but its use may be limited by its toxicity (28). Propylene glycol, petrolatum, and lanolin may reduce the dermal absorption of nickel.

Respiratory Exposure

Nickel carbonyl is the only nickel compound that causes acute poisoning by inhalation. General recommendations include moving the patient to fresh air and monitoring for respiratory distress. Measurement of urinary nickel assists in assessing the severity of poisoning. Inhaled steroids may help in preventing lung damage and edema.

Antidotes

The use of sodium diethyldithiocarbamate (Dithiocarb) as a chelating agent has been suggested (Chapter 53) (29,30). Disulfiram, which is metabolized to two molecules of sodium diethyldithiocarbamate, might also be effective if sodium diethyldithiocarbamate is not available. Data on Dithiocarb and disulfiram have not been subjected to controlled clinical studies (31).

The toxicity of nickel has been mitigated by treatment with other chelating agents. Penicillamine infusion reduced the half time for serum clearance of nickel from 60 to 27 hours in humans who were exposed to nickel sulfate and nickel chloride. Lipophilic chelating agents, such as triethylenetetramine and 1,4,8,11-tetraazacyclotetradecane (Cyclam), were more effective than hydrophilic chelating agents such as ethylenediaminetetraacetic acid, cyclohexanediamine tetraacetic acid, diethylenetriamine pentaacetic acid, and hydroxyethylenediamine triacetic acid (32).

REFERENCES

1. Tien JK, Howson TE. Nickel and nickel alloys. In: Grayson M, Eckroth D, eds. *Kirk-Othmer encyclopedia of chemical technology*, vol. 15, 3rd ed. New York: John Wiley and Sons, Inc. 1981;787–801.
2. Zhicheng S. Acute nickel carbonyl poisoning: a report of 179 cases. *Br J Ind Med* 1986;43:422–424.
3. Rendall REG, Phillips JI, Renton KA. Death following exposure to fine particulate nickel from a metal arc process. *Ann Occup Hyg* 1994;38(6):921–930.
4. Daldrup T, Haarhoff K, Szathmary SC. Toedliche nickel sulfaye-intoxikation. *Berichte zur Serichtlichen Medizin* 1983;41:141–144.
5. Zhicheng S. Acute nickel carbonyl poisoning: a report of 179 cases. *Br J Ind Med* 1986;43:422–424.
6. Sunderman FW, Dingle B, Hopfer SM, et al. Acute nickel toxicity in electroplating workers who accidentally ingested a solution of nickel sulfate and nickel chloride. *Am J Ind Med* 1988;14:257–266.
7. Cornell RG, Landis JR. Mortality patterns among nickel/chromium alloy foundry workers. In: Sunderman FW Jr, Aitio A, Berlin A, eds. *Nickel in the human environment*. Lyon, France: International Agency for Research on Cancer 1984;87–93. International Agency for Research on Cancer scientific publication no. 53.
8. Integrated Risk Information System. Cincinnati: Office of Health and Environmental Assessment, Environmental Criteria and Assessment Office, US Environmental Protection Agency, 1996.
9. US Department of Health and Human Services. *Seventh annual report on carcinogens: summary 1994*. Research Triangle Park, NC: US Department of Health and Human Services, The National Institute of Environmental Health Sciences 1994:262–269.
10. Grandjean P. Human exposure to nickel. In: Sunderman FW Jr, ed. *Nickel in the human environment*. Lyon, France: International Agency for Research on Cancer 1983:469–485. Proceedings of a joint symposium, International Agency for Research on Cancer scientific publication no. 53.
11. Sunderman FW Jr. Mechanisms of nickel carcinogenesis. *Stand J Work Environ Health* 1989;15:1–12.
12. Fullerton A, Andersen JR, Hoelgaard A, et al. Permeation of nickel salts through human skin in vitro. *Contact Dermatitis* 1986;15:173–177.
13. Rezuke WN, Knight JA, Sunderman FW Jr. Reference values for nickel concentrations in human tissues and bile. *Am J Ind Med* 1987;11:419–426.
14. Angerer J, Lehnert G. Occupational chronic exposure to metals. II: Nickel exposure of stainless steel welders—biological monitoring. *Int Arch Occup Environ Health* 1990;62:7–10.
15. Nielsen FH. Possible future implications of nickel, arsenic, silicon, vanadium, and other ultratrace elements in human nutrition. In: Prasad AS, ed. *Clinical, biochemical, and nutritional aspects of trace elements*. New York: Alan R. Liss, 1982;379–404.

16. Veien NK, Hattel T, Justesen O, et al. Oral challenge with nickel and cobalt in patients with positive patch tests to nickel and/or cobalt. *Acta Derm Venereol* 1987;67:321–325.
17. Dotterud LK, Falk ES. Metal allergy in north Norwegian schoolchildren and its relationship with ear piercing and atopy. *Contact Dermatitis* 1994;31:308–313.
18. Eun HC, Marks R. Dose-response relationships for topically applied antigens. *Br J Dermatol* 1990;122:491–499.
19. Daldrup T, Haarhoff K, Szathmary SC. Toedliche nickel sulfaye-intoxikation. *Berichte zur Serichtlichen Medizin* 1983;41:141–144.
20. Sunderman FW, Dingle B, Hopfer SM, et al. Acute nickel toxicity in electroplating workers who accidentally ingested a solution of nickel sulfate and nickel chloride. *Am J Ind Med* 1988;14:257–266.
21. R. J. Safety Co. Web site. Available at: http://www.rjsafety.com/RSMSA.html.
22. US Environmental Protection Agency. *Health assessment document for nickel.* Cincinnati: Environmental Criteria and Assessment Office, Office of Health and Environmental Assessment, Office of Research and Development, 1985. EPA/600/8-83/012F.
23. Sunderman FW Jr. Biological monitoring of nickel in humans. *Stand J Work Environ Health* 1993;19[Suppl 1]:34–38.
24. Takagi Y, Matsuda S, Imai S, et al. Trace elements in human hair: an international comparison. *Bull Environ Contam Toxicol* 1986;36:793–800.
25. Sunderman FW, Dingle B, Hopfer SM, et al. Acute nickel toxicity in electroplating workers who accidentally ingested a solution of nickel sulfate and nickel chloride. *Am J Ind Med* 1988;14:257–266.
26. Bronstein AC, Currance PL. Emergency care for hazardous material exposure. Washington, DC: Mosby, 1988:147–148.
27. Stutz DR, Janusz SJ. *Hazardous materials injuries—a handbook for pre-hospital care,* 2nd ed. Beltsville, MD: Bradford Communications Corporation, 1988;218–219.
28. Gawkrodger DJ, Healy J, Howe AM. The prevention of nickel contact dermatitis. A review of the use of binding agents and barrier creams. *Contact Dermatitis* 1995;32:257–265.
29. Goldfrank LR, Weisman RS, Flomenbaum NE, et al. Goldfrank's toxicologic emergencies, 4th ed. Norwalk, CT: Appleton & Lange, 1990:656–658.
30. Hazardous Substances Data Bank. Bethesda, MD: National Library of Medicine, National Toxicology Information Program, 1996.
31. Bradberry SM, Vale JA. Therapeutic review: do diethyldithiocarbamate and disulfiram have a role in acute nickel carbonyl poisoning? *Clin Tox* 1999;37(2):259–264.
32. Misra M, Athar M, Hasan SK, et al. Alleviation of nickel-induced biochemical alterations by chelating agents. *Fundam Appl Toxicol* 1988;11:285–292.

CHAPTER 226

Phosphorus

Andrew R. Erdman

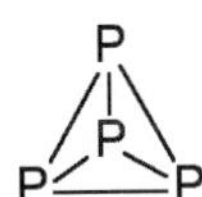

WHITE PHOSPHORUS

Atomic symbol, atomic number, molecular weight:	**White or yellow phosphorus (P_4), 15, 123.92 g/mol**
Valence state:	**3**
CAS Registry No.:	**7723-14-0**
Normal levels:	**Not clinically applicable**
SI conversion:	**1 mg/dL = 0.323 mmol/L**
Special concerns:	**The quiescent stage of toxicity may mislead the clinician into premature discharge or termination of monitoring**
Target organs:	**Multisystem failure arises from ingestion of white phosphorus.**
Antidote:	**None**

OVERVIEW

Elemental phosphorus exists in three forms: black, red, and white (also called *yellow phosphorus* because of impurities). Black phosphorus has a stable structure and has not caused toxicity in humans. Red phosphorus is also fairly stable, poorly absorbed, and hence relatively innocuous, although smoke from burning red phosphorus may cause mucous membrane and respiratory irritation (1). White phosphorus has a single tetrameric structure that is reactive.

White phosphorus can cause devastating burns, severe local gastrointestinal (GI) injury after ingestion, or respiratory damage with inhalation (2–4). Systemic absorption can lead to cardiovascular collapse, hepatic or renal failure, and death (5–7). Chronic, low-level exposure to white phosphorus or its fumes has been associated with oral and mandibular necrosis, a well-described occupational illness referred to as *phossy jaw* (8). Exposure to white phosphorus is uncommon today, primarily because the use of white phosphorus has been severely curtailed through international legislation and trade agreements, and through the development of safer products and manufacturing processes. Exposures still occur in certain industrial settings and in developing countries where regulations are not as strict. Fireworks or munitions, and rodenticide pastes are the more common sources of international exposures (6,9–12).

Properties

White phosphorus is a white or yellowish waxy solid with a garlic-like odor. It must be stored under water because it oxidizes easily and may ignite spontaneously at around 30°C. As it oxidizes, it can give off a faint greenish glow, called *phosphorescence.* It is minimally soluble in water but readily dissolves in bile, fat, and oil. It is easily absorbed orally and through the skin and mucous membranes. Phosphorus combines with various metals (e.g., copper) to form phosphorus salts with considerably less toxicity.

Classification and Uses

Elemental phosphorus exists in combination with other minerals (e.g., as calcium phosphate or fluoroapatite) in phosphate rock, an ore that can be processed to yield elemental white phosphorus (13). Phosphorus has been used in a variety of industries, including the manufacture of matches, munitions, fireworks, and roach or rodent poisons (14). It is also used to make secon-

TABLE 1. United States regulatory guidelines and standards for phosphorus

Agency	Description	Concentration (mg/m^3)
OSHA	PEL-TWA	0.1
(air)	STEL	None
ACGIH	TLV-TWA	0.1
(air)	STEL	None
NIOSH	REL-TWA	0.1
(air)	STEL	None
	IDLH	5.0

ACGIH, American Conference of Governmental Industrial Hygienists; IDLH, immediately dangerous to life or health; NIOSH, National Institute for Occupational Safety and Health; OSHA, U.S. Occupational Safety and Health Administration; PEL, permissible exposure limit; REL, recommended exposure limit; STEL, short-term exposure limit; TLV, threshold limit value; TWA, time-weighted average.

dary compounds such as phosphoric acid or phosphates, which are then used in fertilizers, foods, beverages, cleansers, and a number of other commercial products.

Toxic Dose

Based on retrospective studies, patients ingesting more than approximately 1 mg/kg of white phosphorus are at risk for severe toxicity, and patients ingesting more than 1 g are at risk for death (9,11,15,16). Death has also been reported in children ingesting 1 to 4 phosphorus-containing firecrackers. Mortality rates in patients admitted to the hospital with phosphorus poisoning have ranged from 20% to 50% (6,9,12,17). Mortality appears to be directly related to the amount of phosphorus ingested and ultimately absorbed (9,11,15).

Patients with phosphorus burns covering a large percentage of total body surface area (e.g., 15% to 20%) are at risk for systemic complications, either as a result of absorbed phosphorus or the burns themselves (4). Regulatory workplace guidelines for white phosphorus exposure are listed in Table 1.

TOXICOKINETICS

Because of its lipid solubility, white phosphorus can be absorbed systemically by any route of exposure. It is widely distributed, particularly to the liver and various fatty tissues (16,18–20). The ultimate metabolism or fate of white phosphorus is unclear, but elimination seems to be primarily via renal excretion of various phosphate compounds (21).

PATHOPHYSIOLOGY

Local Effects

Local tissue injury to the cells of the GI tract, skin, or respiratory and mucous membranes is caused by the dual processes of oxidative damage, due to phosphorus's chemical reactivity, and thermal damage, the result of its combustion in the presence of oxygen (3,22,23).

Systemic Effects

White phosphorus is often called a *general protoplasmic poison* (7,9). There are actually several mechanisms underlying its toxic effects, although the relative importance of each is not clear. Phosphorus impairs ribosomal function and protein synthesis, inhibits blood glucose regulation, causes free radical injury and lipid peroxidation, impairs lipoprotein synthesis and triglyceride secretion, and leads to fatty degeneration in a variety of organs (24–30). It is also implicated as an inhibitor of the Krebs cycle (31,32).

CARDIOVASCULAR SYSTEM

Phosphorus directly impairs myocardial contractility and causes vasodilation, leading to hypotension and shock (33,34). This is compounded by concomitant hypovolemia, from vomiting, diarrhea, or fluid loss, and third spacing associated with dermal or GI injury (9,12,17,35). The result is overwhelming cardiovascular collapse. Phosphorus also increases myocardial irritability and the likelihood of dysrhythmias (36). Cardiovascular failure is the most common cause of early deaths from white phosphorus poisoning (7,9,20).

CENTRAL NERVOUS SYSTEM

Central nervous system dysfunction is common with phosphorus toxicity (17). It probably represents a combination of direct neuronal toxicity, cerebral hypoperfusion from shock, and hypoglycemia from hepatic impairment (37). Fatty neuronal infiltration has been noted in the inferior olivary nuclei and may account for much of the neurologic impairment.

HEPATIC INJURY

Hepatic injury may develop in patients who survive the initial cardiovascular and neurologic abnormalities (5–7,9,10,12,15,17,38). It generally develops over the course of several days, but histopathologic changes can be seen within hours (11,16,25,29,39). The damage begins as hydropic or fatty infiltration of hepatocytes, progresses to acute parenchymal inflammation with cellular necrosis, and resolves over the course of days to weeks. In most survivors, there are no permanent hepatic sequelae, although residual fibrosis, scarring, and cirrhosis have been reported (6,12,17,40–42). The damage is generally periportal, but centrilobular or panlobular involvement occurs in some patients (6,16,25,29,40,43). The initial event appears to be impaired lipoprotein synthesis, which results in the intracellular accumulation of lipids and triglycerides, and subsequent fatty degeneration and necrosis (24,26,29,30,44). Hypovolemic shock may exacerbate the injury.

RENAL TOXICITY

Renal toxicity is also common in severely poisoned patients (6,9,15). Whether it is a direct effect of phosphorus or the consequence of shock is unclear.

PHOSSY JAW

Phossy jaw is thought to arise from chronic low-level inhalation of white phosphorus fumes. Some oral or dermal absorption may also contribute (8,14). Such exposures probably result in repeated, direct cytotoxic injury to the tissues of the oral cavity and jaw leading to necrosis of the gums, oral mucosa, and mandible. The disease has been all but eliminated in the U.S. with the implementation of workplace standards.

VULNERABLE POPULATIONS

It is not known whether there are subgroups of patients who are particularly susceptible to phosphorus toxicity. White phosphorus does appear to cross the placenta, and it was once used as an abortifacient (45). No cases, however, of fetotoxicity or teratogenicity have been reported. Fetal mortality is likely to depend on maternal toxicity. Pregnant patients should therefore be managed with aggressive decontamination and supportive measures.

CLINICAL PRESENTATION

The clinical picture of acute white phosphorus toxicity is primarily dictated by the amount and the route of exposure. Dermal contact causes severe chemical burns. Ingestion leads to local GI effects and, if enough phosphorus is absorbed, signs of systemic poisoning. There are scattered reports of systemic human and animal toxicity after large dermal exposures, but it is unclear whether these effects were the result of severe burns or the absorption of phosphorus (4,46).

Burns

White phosphorus can cause severe, deep, and painful chemical burns (2–4,46,47). The wounds may have a distinct garlic odor or emanate smoke as the result of embedded phosphorus particles (2,47). Physical examination findings (presence of white particles, smoke, or a garlic smell) and the historical circumstances or setting of exposure (exploding munitions or chemical spill) generally distinguish these injuries from other types of burns. Wound healing is usually prolonged, and complications, like contractures, are common (3,22,23,48). A few systemic complications peculiar to phosphorus burns include hypocalcemia, hyperphosphatemia, and, rarely, cardiac dysrhythmias (46–49).

Ingestion

Systemic phosphorus poisoning after acute ingestion is often described using three distinct stages. In practice, individual presentations vary—stages may overlap, clinical effects may vary in severity or not occur at all, and interventions may alter the course.

STAGE I

The first signs of poisoning involve the GI tract, although GI effects are not universal (9,17). Nausea, vomiting, diarrhea, and abdominal pain generally develop within minutes to hours of ingestion. The patient's stool or vomitus may have a garlic odor and have occasionally been observed to smoke or phosphoresce (6,7,9,12,17,20). In severe cases, tachycardia, hypotension, and shock may occur (9,20). Neurologic abnormalities such as coma or altered consciousness may develop. Stage I generally lasts several or many hours.

STAGE II

Termed the *quiescent stage*, the patient appears to improve during stage II (5,12,35,50). Despite its name, patients in this stage are rarely asymptomatic—some GI effects or laboratory abnormalities are usually evident (9). Clinical improvement probably represents a waning of direct corrosive effects and precedes the systemic effects of phosphorus. Stage II generally lasts 1 to 3 days.

STAGE III

This stage is marked by clinical deterioration, typically beginning a few days after ingestion and coinciding with the development of end-organ damage from absorbed phosphorus (6,7,9,10,12,15,17,33). Nausea, vomiting, and abdominal pain usually return or worsen. Evidence of liver injury (right upper quadrant abdominal pain, jaundice, elevated bilirubin or serum transaminases, hypoglycemia, and coagulopathy) may develop. Evidence of renal impairment (oliguria or elevated serum creatinine) and central nervous system toxicity (obtundation, delirium, or restlessness) may also occur. Metabolic consequences like acidosis and electrolyte abnormalities are common. Death from multiple organ failure can occur during this stage.

In patients who survive stage III, complete resolution usually requires 1 to 3 weeks. However, laboratory abnormalities persist for months. Long-term sequelae such as hepatic fibrosis and cirrhosis have been reported (6,11,40–42).

DIAGNOSTIC TESTS

There is no single test to confirm the diagnosis. In patients suspected of systemic phosphorus poisoning or the ingestion of a significant amount of white phosphorus, vital signs and cardiac rhythm should be monitored, and serum electrolytes, liver and renal function tests, coagulation parameters, blood glucose, and acid-base status should be measured.

Burns

Phosphorus burns are usually readily apparent and easily diagnosed. Ultraviolet light may help visualize embedded phosphorus particles (3). Patients with burns covering a large area should have serum electrolytes, calcium, and phosphorus measured (46,48,49).

Ingestion

Serum phosphorus levels may be low, elevated, or normal as opposed to patients with large phosphorus burns, in whom phosphorus levels are generally elevated (6,9,17,27,51). Historical elements, including access to fireworks, rodenticide pastes, or other phosphorus-containing products, and physical examination findings, such as smoking or phosphorescent stools/emesis or a garlic odor, may provide diagnostic clues. The clinical course of a patient's illness, particularly the way in which symptoms and stages evolve over time, may also help.

Patients with signs of significant corrosive GI injury or hemorrhage may require endoscopy (12,17,52). A liver biopsy is rarely needed but may reveal steatosis or necrosis involving the periportal areas of the hepatic lobules; other patterns have also been reported (6,16,40,41).

Diagnostic Pitfalls

Diagnostic pitfalls include relying on findings such as smoking or phosphorescent stools or vomitus, or a garlic odor, to make the diagnosis. Although they may be characteristic of phosphorus poisoning, they only occur in a small percentage of patients (9).

TREATMENT

Burns

Treatment depends on rapid decontamination followed by supportive measures. Immediate decontamination in the field improves outcome by removing phosphorus that can continue to oxidize and cause damage (23). Large particles should be brushed off and the wounds irrigated thoroughly with cool water or saline. Any remaining particles should be removed with tissue forceps or surgical debridement. Some authors have proposed using dilute copper sulfate or silver nitrate solutions for irrigation, but the former have been associated with complications such as hemolysis, and the latter may not be readily available (2,47,53–55). Supportive measures are the same as for any burn patient. Patients with dermal injuries exceeding 15% of the total body surface area should be monitored clinically for 24 to 48 hours for the development of systemic phosphorus poisoning. This should include continuous cardiac monitoring and regular determination of fluid status, electrolyte, liver, and renal tests.

Ingestion

There is no specific antidote for phosphorus poisoning, so management depends on rigorous supportive care. Because toxicity and mortality appear to be closely related to the amount of phosphorus absorbed, aggressive decontamination measures are extremely important (6,9,11).

DECONTAMINATION

At least one case series has demonstrated improved survival in patients who received early gastric decontamination (6,56). Gastric lavage is probably the most potentially useful method. Activated charcoal is unlikely to adsorb a significant amount of phosphorus and should not be given unless coingestants are involved. Gastric lavage should be considered in patients with recent, potentially significant phosphorus ingestions (e.g., 1 mg/kg) who have not already vomited repeatedly. Several types of lavage fluid have been proposed, such as potassium permanganate or copper sulfate solutions; however, none of these has been formally studied for safety or efficacy (6,7,9,12,17,35). Ordinary saline or tap water is preferred, followed by an oral dose of mineral oil. Mineral oil, which is not absorbed, helps dissolve the fat-soluble phosphorus and enables it to be passed from the body (7,9,12,17). One animal study reported a benefit with its use (56). Whole bowel irrigation has not been investigated, but should be considered if it appears likely a significant amount of unabsorbed phosphorus remains in the GI tract. Meanwhile, dietary fats and oils should be avoided until the patient has recovered, as they may theoretically enhance absorption (9,12,17,56). Medical personnel should wear protective equipment to avoid secondary contamination and burns from phosphorus particles in the patient's body fluids.

SUPPORTIVE MEASURES AND MONITORING

The patient's airway should be managed and any hypotension treated aggressively. Hypoglycemia and electrolyte abnormalities should be monitored and corrected in the usual manner. A number of specific adjunctive treatments have been proposed, including corticosteroids, *N*-acetylcysteine, exchange transfusions, and others (10,11,57). However, none of these has been proven to provide benefit in humans. Various hepatoprotective agents, such as pentoxyphylline, interferon, and antioxidants (e.g., glutathione and coenzyme Q), are still under investigation in animals (26,28,42,58).

Patients suspected of significant phosphorus toxicity should have cardiac, blood pressure, and oximetry monitoring. Regular measurements of liver and renal function, serum electrolytes, blood glucose, acid-base status, and coagulation status should be performed until patients show evidence of recovery from stage III.

Management Pitfalls

Management pitfalls include failing to perform adequate decontamination measures. Without an effective antidote, and given that the severity of toxicity depends on the amount absorbed, aggressive decontamination should be performed.

Initial improvement may simply represent the quiescent stage of toxicity, and patients may deteriorate precipitously. They should be monitored through stage III or until it becomes clear that no further toxicity may develop.

REFERENCES

1. Marrs TC. Histological changes produced by exposure of rabbits and rats to smokes produced from red phosphorus. *Toxicol Lett* 1984;21(2):141–146.
2. Konjoyan TR. White phosphorus burns: case report and literature review. *Mil Med* 1983;148(11):881–884.
3. Mozingo DW, Smith AA, McManus WF, et al. Chemical burns. *J Trauma* 1988;28(5):642–647.
4. Obermer E. Phosphorus burns. *Lancet* 1943;1:202.
5. Hann RG, Veale RA. A fatal case of poisoning by phosphorus with unusual subcutaneous hemorrhages. *Lancet* 1910;1:163–164.
6. La Due JS, Schenken JR, Kuker LH. Phosphorus poisoning: a report of 16 cases with repeated liver biopsies in a recovered case. *Am J Med Sci* 1944;208:223–234.
7. Simon FA, Pickering LK. Acute yellow phosphorus poisoning. "Smoking stool syndrome." *JAMA* 1976;235(13):1343–1344.
8. Hughs JP, Baron R, Buckland DH, et al. Phosphorus necrosis of the jaw: a present day study. *Br J Ind Med* 1962;19:83–99.
9. Diaz-Rivera RS, Collazo PJ, Pons ER, et al. Acute phosphorus poisoning in man: a study of 56 cases. *Medicine* 1950;29:269–298.
10. Fernandez OU, Canizares LL. Acute hepatotoxicity from ingestion of yellow phosphorus-containing fireworks. *J Clin Gastroenterol* 1995;21(2):139–142.
11. Marin GA, Montoya CA, Sierra JL, et al. Evaluation of corticosteroid and exchange-transfusion treatment of acute yellow-phosphorus intoxication. *N Engl J Med* 1971;284(3):125–128.
12. Rubitsky HJ, Myerson RM. Acute phosphorus poisoning. *Arch Int Med* 1949;83:164–178.
13. Llewellyn TO. *Minerals yearbook*. Washington, DC: U.S. Department of the Interior, Bureau of Mines, 1993.
14. Duerkson-Hughs P, Richter P, Ingerman L, et al. Toxicologic profile for white phosphorus. Washington, DC: Agency for Toxic Substances and Disease Registry, 1997.
15. Fahim FA, el-Sabbagh M, Saleh NA, et al. Biochemical changes associated with acute phosphorus poisoning (in humans). *Gen Pharmacol* 1990;21(6):899–904.
16. Salfelder K, Doehnert HR, Doehnert G, et al. Fatal phosphorus poisoning: a study of forty-five autopsy cases. *Beitr Pathol* 1972;147(4):321–340.
17. McCarron MM, Gaddis GP, Trotter AT. Acute yellow phosphorus poisoning from pesticide pastes. *Clin Toxicol* 1981;18(6):693–711.
18. Cameron JM, Patrick RS. Acute phosphorus poisoning—the distribution of toxic doses of yellow phosphorus in the tissues of experimental animals. *Med Sci Law* 1966;6(4):209–214.
19. Ghoshal AK, Porta EA, Hartroft WS. Isotopic studies on the absorption and tissue distribution of white phosphorus in rats. *Exp Mol Pathol* 1971;14(2):212–219.
20. Winek CL, Collom WD, Fusia EP. Yellow phosphorus ingestion—three fatal poisonings. *Clin Toxicol* 1973;6(4):541–545.
21. Brewer E, Haggerty RJ. Toxic hazards: rat poisons—phosphorus. *N Engl J Med* 1958;258:147–148.
22. Curreri PW, Asch MJ, Pruitt BA. The treatment of chemical burns: specialized diagnostic, therapeutic, and prognostic considerations. *J Trauma* 1970;10(8):634–642.
23. Leonard LG, Scheulen JJ, Munster AM. Chemical burns: effect of prompt first aid. *J Trauma* 1982;22(5):420–423.
24. Barker EA, Smuckler EA, Benditt EP. Effects of thioacetamide and yellow phosphorus poisoning on protein synthesis. *Lab Invest* 1963;12:955–960.
25. Althausen TL, Thoenes E. Influence on carbohydrate metabolism of experimentally induced hepatic changes. *Arch Intern Med* 1932;50:58–75.
26. Pani P, Gravela E, Mazzarino C, et al. On the mechanism of fatty liver in white phosphorus-poisoned rats. *Exp Mol Pathol* 1972;16(2):201–209.
27. McIntosh R. Acute phosphorus poisoning. *Am J Dis Child* 1927;34:595–602.
28. Di Luzio NR. Influence of intravenously administered hexahydrocoenzyme Q4 on liver injury. *Life Sci* 1966;5(16):1467–1478.
29. Ghoshal AK, Porta EA, Hartroft WS. The role of lipoperoxidation in the pathogenesis of fatty livers induced by phosphorus poisoning in rats. *Am J Pathol* 1969;54(2):275–291.
30. Lombardi B, Recknagel RO. Interference with secretion of triglycerides by the liver as a common factor in toxic liver injury. With some observations on choline deficiency fatty liver. *Am J Path* 1962;40:571–586.
31. Kulkybaev GA, Merkusheva NV. [Dynamics of NAD-dependent isocitrate dehydrogenase activity in homogenized rat liver exposed to toxic products of the phosphorus industry]. *Gig Tr Prof Zabol* 1992;(1):21–23.
32. Beloskurskaia GI, Aitbembetov BN, Balmakhaeva RM, et al. The pathogenesis of toxic liver lesions in workers in phosphorus production [in Ukrainian]. *Vrach Delo* 1989;(7):104–106.
33. Pietras RJ, Stavrakos C, Gunnar RM, et al. Phosphorus poisoning simulating acute myocardial infarction. *Arch Intern Med* 1968;122(5):430–434.
34. Talley RC, Linhart JW, Trevino AJ, et al. Acute elemental phosphorus poisoning in man: cardiovascular toxicity. *Am Heart J* 1972;84(1):139–140.
35. Chretien TE. Acute phosphorus poisoning: report of a case with recovery. *N Engl J Med* 1945;232:247–29.

36. Diaz-Rivera RS, Morales FR, Garcia-Palmieri MR, et al. The electrocardiographic changes in acute phosphorus poisoning in man. *Am J Med Sci* 1961;241:758–765.
37. Wertham F. Central nervous system in acute phosphorus poisoning. *Arch Neurol Psych* 1932;28:320–330.
38. Ganote CE, Otis JB. Characteristic lesions of yellow phosphorus-induced liver damage. *Lab Invest* 1969;21(3):207–213.
39. Barone C, Cittadini A, Galeotti T, et al. The effect of intoxication induced in rat liver by carbon tetrachloride, ethionine and white phosphorus on the level of microsomal cytochromes b5 and P-450. *Experientia* 1973;29(1):73–74.
40. Fletcher GF, Galambos JT. Phosphorus poisoning in humans. *Arch Int Med* 1963;112:846–852.
41. Greenberger NJ, Robinson WL, Isselbacher KJ. Toxic hepatitis after the ingestion of phosphorus with subsequent recovery. *Gastroenterology* 1964;47:179–183.
42. Peterson TC, Neumeister M. Effect of pentoxifylline in rat and swine models of hepatic fibrosis: role of fibroproliferation in its mechanism. *Immunopharmacology* 1996;31(2–3):183–193.
43. Burnell JM, Dennis MB Jr, Clayson KJ, et al. Evaluation in dogs of cross-circulation in the treatment of acute hepatic necrosis induced by yellow phosphorus. *Gastroenterology* 1976;71(5):827–831.
44. Seakins A, Robinson DS. Changes associated with the production of fatty livers by white phosphorus and by ethanol in the rat. *Biochem J* 1964;92(2):308–312.
45. Gosselin RE, Smith RP, Hodge HC. *Clinical toxicology of commercial products*, 5th ed. Baltimore: Williams and Wilkins, 1984.
46. Bowen TE, Whelan TJ Jr, Nelson TG. Sudden death after phosphorus burns: experimental observations of hypocalcemia, hyperphosphatemia and electrocardiographic abnormalities following production of a standard white phosphorus burn. *Ann Surg* 1971;174(5):779–784.
47. Chou TD, Lee TW, Chen SL, et al. The management of white phosphorus burns. *Burns* 2001;27(5):492–497.
48. Appelbaum J, Ben-Hur N, Shani J. Subcellular morphological changes in the rat kidney after phosphorus burn. *Pathol Eur* 1975;10(2):145–154.
49. Ben-Hur N, Appelbaum J. Biochemistry, histopathology and treatment of phosphorus burns. An experimental study. *Isr J Med Sci* 1973;9(1):40–48.
50. Jacobinzer H, Raybin HW. Phosphorus poisoning including two fatal case reports. *Arch Ped* 1961;396–402.
51. Blumenthal S, Lesser A. Acute phosphorus poisoning. *Am J Dis Child* 1938;55:1280–1287.
52. Wechsler L, Wechsler RL. Phosphorus poisoning: the latent period and unusual gastrointestinal lesions. *Gastroenterology* 1951;17:279–283.
53. Ben-Hur N, Giladi A, Applebaum J, et al. Phosphorus burns: the antidote: a new approach. *Br J Plast Surg* 1972;25(3):245–249.
54. Mendelson JA. Some principles of protection against burns from flame and incendiary munitions. *J Trauma* 1971;11(4):286–294.
55. Summerlin WT, Walder AI, Moncrief JA. White phosphorus burns and massive hemolysis. *J Trauma* 1967;7(3):476–484.
56. Atkinson HV. The treatment of acute phosphorus poisoning. *J Clin Lab Med* 1921;7:148–150.
57. Bayne JRD, Beck JC, Lowenstein L, et al. Cortisone acetate in the treatment of acute phosphorus poisoning. *Can Med Assoc J* 1952;67:465–467.
58. Gomez N, Andrade R, Roldos F, et al. Use of interferon in hepatic necrosis produced by paraquat and yellow phosphorus: experimental evaluation [in Spanish]. *Acta Gastroenterol Latinoam* 1998;28(2):189–192.

CHAPTER 227

Platinum

Seth Schonwald

CARBOPLATIN

Atomic symbol, atomic number, molecular weight:	**Pt, 78, 195.08 g/mol**
Valence states:	**0, +2, and +4 medically relevant (also +3 through +8)**
CAS Registry No.:	**13454-96-1**
Normal serum level:	**0.003 mg/L (dietary), 30 mg/L (treatment)**
SI conversion:	**1 mg/L = 5.12 μmol/L**
Target organ:	**Kidney**
Antidote:	**None**

OVERVIEW

Platinum was discovered by Julius Scaliger in 1735. Platinum is well known for its use in the chemotherapeutic drugs *cis*-platinum, carboplatin, and oxaliplatin. Their toxicity is addressed separately (Chapter 98). Due to its durability and unreactivity, platinum is used in jewelry and in laboratory equipment. It is used in electrical contacts, to coat missile nose cones, in jet engine fuel nozzles, in dental fillings (1), and in photography. Complex platinum salts are catalysts in the preparation of sulfuric acid in the petroleum and pharmaceutical industries. The platinum in automobile catalytic converters consumes the majority of platinum (2).

The greatest platinum exposure occurs in workers via inhalation and in patients treated with platinum-based antineoplastic agents. Workers exposed to platinum may develop dermatitis and bronchial asthma ascribable to exposure to chloroplatinate (3). Dental technicians working with dental filling alloys may be at higher risk for platinum exposure (4). A health risk assessment of platinum emitted from automotive catalytic converters suggested that no evidence exists that they pose a health risk to the general population (5).

TOXIC DOSE

Regulatory guidelines and standards for the United States are provided in Table 1. A 59-year-old man received a massive cisplatin overdose of 300 mg/m^2. Toxic effects included severe emesis, myelosuppression, renal failure, mental deterioration with hallucinations, dim vision, and hepatotoxicity. Plasmapheresis lowered the platinum concentration from 2979 ng/ml to 185 ng/ml and appeared to be of clinical benefit (6). A 68-year-old woman received a massive overdose of cisplatin without intravenous hydration. Symptoms included severe emesis, myelosuppression, renal failure, and deafness. Plasmapheresis lowered the platinum concentration from more than 2900 ng/ml to 200 ng/ml and appeared to be of clinical benefit. Even after the onset of renal failure, hydration increased urinary excretion of platinum (7).

No data exist to assess the carcinogenic risk of platinum or its compounds in humans (8). The International Agency for Research on Cancer considers *cis*-platinum a group 2A carcinogen.

TABLE 1. United States regulatory guidelines and standards for platinum

Agency	Description	Concentration (mg/m^3)
OSHA		
(air)	PEL-TWA	0.002
ACGIH	Metallic dust	
(air)	TLV-TWA	1
	Soluble platinum salts	
	TLV-TWA	0.002
NIOSH		
(air)	REL-TWA	0.002

ACGIH, American Conference of Governmental Industrial Hygienists; NIOSH, National Institute for Occupational Safety and Health; OSHA, U.S. Occupational Safety and Health Administration; PEL, permissible exposure limit; REL, recommended exposure limit; TLV, threshold limit value; TWA, time-weighted average.

TOXICOKINETICS AND TOXICODYNAMICS

Up to 85% of *cis*-platinum is protein bound, whereas carboplatin is less reactive and only 30% becomes protein bound. Platinum is widely distributed to subcutaneous fat, kidney, bone, pancreas, liver, and hair (9). Erythrocytes represent an important deep compartment for oxaliplatin and a little less for cisplatin. Oxaliplatin is trapped in erythrocytes, and its half-life is identical to that of erythrocytes. In contrast, carboplatin is quickly extruded from erythrocytes.

Carboplatin is largely excreted unchanged in urine. Of the current platinum agents, only carboplatin dosage can be individually adjusted based on creatinine clearance measurement due to its simple renal excretion. Cisplatin renal excretion is more complex, combining reabsorption and secretion processes.

Active cisplatin and oxaliplatin metabolites react with small proteins containing sulfhydryl groups, such as glutathione, cysteine, and methionine, and then with high-molecular-weight proteins, such as albumin. Their terminal half-lives are long, approximately 10 days.

PATHOPHYSIOLOGY

Cis-platinum inhibits DNA synthesis by forming DNA cross-links, denatures the double helix, and covalently binds to DNA bases. Carboplatin is an analog of cisplatin and also covalently links with DNA and interferes with DNA function.

Workplace toxicity results from the potent sensitizing properties of platinum salt complexes but not from platinum itself. These low-molecular-weight compounds (in particular, compounds containing halogen ligands such as chloride) induce immediate hypersensitivity (type I) reactions. Other group VIII metal salts (e.g., palladium and rhodium) are poor skin sensitizers.

PREGNANCY AND LACTATION

Carboplatin and cisplatin are classified as U.S. Food and Drug Administration pregnancy risk category D.

CLINICAL PRESENTATION

Allergic Effects

No convincing evidence exists for sensitization or for other adverse health effects following exposure to metallic platinum. Platinum allergy is induced by a group of charged compounds with reactive ligand systems, the most potent being hexachloroplatinic acid and the chlorinated salts ammonium hexachloroplatinate, potassium tetrachloroplatinate, potassium hexachloroplatinate, and sodium tetrachloroplatinate. Platinum salts act as sensitizers through inhalation or skin contact. Platinum compounds can cause asthma, dermatitis, respiratory symptoms, and anaphylactic shock.

In a study of British refineries, 52 of 91 workers exposed to complex platinum salts reported sneezing, rhinorrhea, chest tightness, wheezing, shortness of breath, and cyanosis; a proportion of these also developed scaly erythematous dermatitis with urticaria (10). Symptoms usually abated soon after stopping exposure. Nasal and conjunctival irritation, sore throat, and rhinitis may also occur.

Potassium Chloroplatinite

Potassium chloroplatinite is a soluble, nonorganic salt of platinum used in photography, in the chemical and electrical industries, in electroplating, and in the manufacture of catalysts. Oliguric renal failure, metabolic acidosis, fever, muscle cramps, gastroenteritis, and rhabdomyolysis have been associated with overdose (11).

DIAGNOSTIC TESTS

Blood and urine platinum levels may be obtained by atomic absorption spectrophotometry. Following blood levels of platinum after exposures has not been shown helpful in management.

TREATMENT

Adequate ventilation is important in preventing significant industrial dust exposures. Bronchospasm following platinum sensitization may respond to β_2-agonist therapy. Decontaminate affected areas by washing thoroughly and treat symptoms supportively. Hemodialysis used to clear platinum after renal insufficiency due to an accidental cisplatin overdosage (205 mg/m^2 instead of 100 mg/m^2) was believed to be of "limited usefulness" (12).

Plasmapheresis has been effective in lowering platinum concentrations in a few cases of severe chemotherapy overdoses.

REFERENCES

1. Schierl R. Urinary platinum levels associated with dental gold alloys. *Arch Environ Health* 2001;56(3):283–286.
2. Ely JC, Neal CR, Kulpa CF, et al. Implications of platinum-group element accumulation along U.S. roads from catalytic-converter attrition. *Environ Sci Technol* 2001;35(19):3816–3822.
3. Shima S, Yoshida T, Tachikawa S, et al. Bronchial asthma due to inhaled chloroplatinate. *Sangyo Igaku* 1984;26(6):500–509.
4. Begerow J, Sensen U, Wiesmuller GA, et al. Internal platinum, palladium, and gold exposure in environmentally and occupationally exposed persons. *Zentralbl Hyg Umweltmed* 1999;202(5):411–424.
5. Merget R, Rosner G. Evaluation of the health risk of platinum group metals emitted from automotive catalytic converters. Review. *Sci Total Environ* 2001;270(1–3):165–173.
6. Jung HK, Lee J, Lee SN. A case of massive cisplatin overdose managed by plasmapheresis. *Korean J Intern Med* 1995;10(2):150–154.
7. Chu G, Mantin R, Shen YM, et al. Massive cisplatin overdose by accidental substitution for carboplatin. Toxicity and management. *Cancer* 1993;72(12):3707–3714.
8. Kazantzis, G. Role of cobalt, iron, lead, manganese, mercury, platinum, selenium, and titanium in carcinogenesis. *Environ Health Perspect* 1981;40:143–161.
9. Vandiver F, Duffield FV, Yoakum A, et al. Determination of human body burden baseline data of platinum through autopsy tissue analysis. *Environ Health Perspect* 1976;15:131–134.
10. Hunter D, Milton R, Perry KM. Asthma caused by the complex salts of platinum. *Br J Ind Med* 1945;2:92–98.
11. Woolf AD, Ebert TH. Toxicity after self-poisoning by ingestion of potassium chloroplatinite. *Review* 1995;13(4):228–244.
12. Lagrange JL, Cassuto-Viguier E, Barbe V, et al. Cytotoxic effects of long-term circulating ultrafiltrable platinum species and limited efficacy of hemodialysis in clearing them. *Eur J Cancer* 1994;30A(14):2057–2060.

CHAPTER 228

Selenium

Seth Schonwald

$HO-Se(=O)-OH$

SELENIOUS ACID

Atomic symbol, atomic number, molecular weight:	**Se, 34, 78.96 g/mol**
Valence states:	**–2, 0, +4, +6**
CAS Registry No.:	**7782-49-2 (selenium); 7783-00-8 (selenious acid).**
Normal levels:	**20 to 200 µg Se/day (urine)**
SI conversion:	**µg/L × 12.66 = nmol/L**
Target organs:	**Gastrointestinal organs, lungs (acute); hair, nails, teeth (chronic)**
Antidote:	**None**

OVERVIEW

Berzelius discovered selenium in 1817. Selenium forms the oxides SeO_2 and SeO_3, the selenious (H_2SeO_3) and selenic (H_2SeO_4) acids, selenite and selenate salts, a nitride, carbide, hydride, two sulfides, and various halides and oxyhalides.

Selenium is extensively used in the vulcanization of rubber, in the manufacture of red glass and some enamels, as a decolorizer of glass, in electronics, and in xerography (1). Selenious acid, a component of gun-bluing solution is the most toxic form of selenium. Medicinal uses of selenium include antidandruff shampoos, dietary supplements, and the treatment of cystic fibrosis.

High blood levels of selenium can result in *selenosis* (2). Symptoms include gastrointestinal upset, hair loss, white blotchy nails, and mild nerve damage. Selenium toxicity is relatively rare; the few reported cases have been associated with industrial accidents and a manufacturing error that led to an excessively high dose of selenium in a supplement (3).

Plant foods are the major dietary sources of selenium in most countries. Most occupational exposures occur in industries that extract, mine, treat, or process selenium-bearing minerals and in industries that use selenium or selenium compounds in manufacturing. In electronics, the semiconductor and photoelectric properties of selenium make it useful in *electric eyes*, photographic exposure meters, and electronic rectifiers. Selenium is used in the preparation of pharmaceuticals. Selenium sulfide is an ingredient in antidandruff shampoos and fungicides (selenium sulfide). Radioactive selenium has been used to visualize difficult malignant tumors (4).

TOXIC DOSE

U.S. regulatory guidelines and standards for selenium may be found in Table 1.

The recommended daily allowance of selenium is 55 µg/day for women and 70 µg/day for men. Accidental selenium human poisonings have caused few fatalities. A 3-year-old boy died 1.5 hours after ingestion of an unknown quantity of selenious acid in a gun-bluing preparation (5). A 15-ml ingestion of gun blue (2% selenious acid) by a 2-year-old (6) and a 30 to 60 ml ingestion by an adult resulted in death (7,8). A 15-year-old girl survived ingestion of sodium selenate (22 mg Se/kg body weight), perhaps because she was forced to vomit soon after exposure (9).

No deaths in the United States have been attributed to chronic oral exposures of selenium or selenium compounds. Most studies in humans and animals have revealed either no association between selenium and cancer or a chemopreventive association. The incidence of nonmelanoma skin cancer is significantly higher in areas of the United States with low soil selenium levels (10).

TOXICOKINETICS AND TOXICODYNAMICS

Selenium compounds are readily absorbed orally. In humans, absorption of sodium selenite or selenomethionine can exceed 80%. Humans also absorb elemental selenium dusts and other selenium compounds, but quantitative inhalation studies have not been done. Selenium accumulates in many organ systems; the highest concentrations are found in the liver and kidney. Selenium concentrations in tissues do not seem to correlate with effects. Blood, hair, and nails may contain selenium. Selenium is primarily eliminated in the urine and feces.

PATHOPHYSIOLOGY

The mechanism of toxicity for selenium has not been demonstrated. One theory is that selenium inactivates sulfhydryl

TABLE 1. United States regulatory guidelines and standards for selenium

Agency	Description	Concentration (mg/m^3)
OSHA (air)	Selenium compounds	
	PEL-TWA	0.2 (as selenium)
	STEL	STEL
ACGIH (air)	Selenium and compounds (sodium selenite, selenious acid)	
	TLV-TWA	0.2 (as selenium)
	STEL	None
NIOSH (air)	Selenium and compounds	
	REL-TWA	0.2
	STEL	None
	IDLH	1.0 (as selenium)
FDA	Bottled water	10 ppb

ACGIH, American Conference of Governmental Industrial Hygienists; FDA, U.S. Food and Drug Administration; IDLH, immediately dangerous to life and health; NIOSH, National Institute for Occupational Safety and Health; OSHA, U.S. Occupational Safety and Health Administration; PEL, permissible exposure limit; ppb, parts per billion; REL, recommended exposure limit; STEL, short-term exposure limit; TLV, threshold limit value; TWA, time-weighted average.

enzymes leading to depression of cellular oxidative processes (11). Selenium is incorporated into four classes of selenoproteins: selenium-specific proteins, proteins incorporating selenocysteine at cysteine codons, proteins incorporating selenomethionine at methionine position in those proteins, and proteins that bind selenide nonspecifically.

VULNERABLE POPULATIONS

No studies have demonstrated that selenium or its compounds are teratogenic in humans. Selenium crosses the placenta and enters breast milk. One study reported that higher plasma selenium levels were associated with less respiratory morbidity in premature infants (12). A Chinese study suggests that selenium supplementation during pregnancy reduced the incidence of pregnancy-induced hypertension (13).

CLINICAL PRESENTATION

In cases of acute toxic exposure to selenium compounds, significant amounts can be eliminated in the breath, causing the characteristic *garlic breath*. Ingestion of selenious acid products causes excessive salivation, garlic odor on the breath, and shallow breathing.

Respiratory Effects

Respiratory distress has occurred after acute inhalation of a high concentration of selenium dioxide (14) and following ingestion of a lethal dose of selenious acid. Signs included bronchial spasm, bronchitis, and pneumonia. Pulmonary congestion and edema, accompanied by focal hemorrhage, have been seen after selenious acid ingestion. The lung may be a target of acute exposure to excess selenium because the metabolite, dimethyl selenide, is exhaled.

Cardiovascular Effects

Following acute inhalation or acute oral exposure to selenium compounds, some cardiovascular signs, such as elevated pulse rate and tachycardia, have been reported in humans.

Gastrointestinal Effects

Gastrointestinal distress, including nausea, vomiting, diarrhea, and abdominal pain, has been reported following ingestion of toxic amounts of aqueous sodium selenate (15). Postmortem examination revealed dilation of, and mucoid fluid in, the stomach and small intestine. High levels of dietary selenium may cause gastrointestinal disturbances in chronically exposed humans. The liver appears to be the primary target organ for the oral toxicity of sodium selenate, sodium selenite, and organic forms of selenium in animals following intermediate and chronic exposure, whereas liver cirrhosis or dysfunction has not been a notable component of the clinical manifestations of chronic selenosis in humans.

Endocrine Effects

One of the most common effects observed following excess selenium intake in animals is a decrease in growth. It is likely that the selenium-induced reduction in growth has an endocrine component.

Dermal Effects

Chronic ingestion of organic selenium compounds can cause hair loss, deformation and loss of nails, and discoloration and excessive decay of teeth. Similar effects occur in livestock after intermediate and chronic exposure to seleniferous plants. Skin rashes, burns, and contact dermatitis have been reported for both acute and chronic exposure to selenium fumes and acute exposures to selenium dioxide (16). Single topical exposures to selenious acid have resulted in purpura, inflammation around hair follicles, and a pustular rash.

Neurologic Effects

Neurologic manifestations in humans, including numbness, paralysis, and hemiplegia, have been observed after chronic oral exposure to high dietary selenium (17).

DIAGNOSTIC TESTS

Selenium can be detected in the blood, feces, urine, hair, and nails. Urinary excretion rates of 20 to 200 µg selenium/day are not associated with either deficiency or toxicity (18). Hair selenium concentrations are often not indicative of dietary exposure. Users of dandruff shampoos containing selenium sulfide may have high levels of selenium in their hair. Toenail samples have also been used as biomarkers of selenium exposure. Clinical symptoms have been associated with excessive blood, urine, and hair levels of selenium in exposed patients.

A fluorometric assay of total selenium in plasma and urine has a detection limit of 10 mg/L. Stable isotope dilution gas chromatography–mass spectrometry can be used for the determination of selenium in urine.

Two endemic diseases, Keshan disease and Kashin-Bek disease, have been reported in selenium-deficient populations in China in which mean hair, blood, and urine selenium levels are low. Keshan disease, manifested as nausea, vomiting of yellowish fluid, and necrosis of the myocardium, has been found in a population with an average whole blood selenium concentration of 0.018 mg/L, an average urinary concentration of 0.007 mg/L, and an average hair selenium concentration of 0.123 µg/g (17).

TREATMENT

Ingestion

In general, only supportive treatment has been recommended for oral exposure to selenious acid, sodium selenate, and selenium dioxide. Because selenious acid (in gun bluing, pH 1) is caustic, lavage and induction of emesis are not recommended. Furthermore, shock, seizures, severe hypotension, and cardiorespiratory arrest may develop rapidly (19). Ingestion of selenious acid is managed similarly to acute acid ingestion (Chapter 201).

Skin

Aggressive dilution with water or saline is indicated after topical exposure to selenious acid. Sodium thiosulfate solution (10%) may decrease pain and necrosis following dermal exposure.

Respiratory Exposure

No specific recommendations have been reported for reducing absorption after acute high-dose exposure to selenium or selenium compounds via inhalation or dermal exposure (20). General procedures to reduce exposure include moving the victim to fresh air, removing contaminated clothing and shoes, and flushing exposed areas with running water.

Antidotes

Chelating agents have not been effective in animal experiments, and both calcium ethylenediaminetetraacetate and dimercaprol may increase the toxic effects of selenium (21). Bromobenzene has been reported to increase the urinary excretion of selenium, but because bromobenzene is also a hepatic toxin, its use is dangerous.

REFERENCES

1. Fishbein L. Environmental selenium and its significance. *Fundam Appl Toxicol* 1983;3:411–419.
2. Koller LD, Exon JH. The two faces of selenium-deficiency and -toxicity are similar in animals and man. *Can J Vet Res* 1986;50:297–306.
3. Raisbeck MF, Dahl ER, Sanchez DA, et al. Naturally occurring selenosis in Wyoming. *J Vet Diagn Invest* 1993;5:84–87.
4. Jereb M, Falk R, Jereb B, et al. Radiation dose to the human body from intravenously administered 75Se-sodium selenite. *J Nucl Med* 1975;16:846–850.
5. Carter RF. Acute selenium poisoning. *Med J Aust* 1966;1:525–528.
6. Nantel AJ, Brown M, Dery P, et al. Acute poisoning by selenious acid. *Vet Hum Toxicol* 1985;27:531–533.
7. Pentel P, Fletcher D, Jentzen J. Fatal acute selenium toxicity. *J Forensic Sci* 1985;30:556–562.
8. Barceloux, DG. Selenium. *Clin Tox* 1999;37(2):145–172.
9. Civil IE, McDonald MJ. Acute selenium poisoning: case report. *New Zealand Med J* 1978;87:354–356.
10. Fleet JC. Dietary selenium repletion may reduce cancer incidence in people at high risk who live in areas with low soil selenium. *Nutr Rev* 1997;55:277–279.
11. Lombeck I, Menzel H, Frosch D. Acute selenium poisoning of a 2-year-old child. *Eur J Pediatr* 1987;146(3):308–312.
12. Darlow BA, Inder TE, Graham PJ, et al. The relationship of selenium status to respiratory outcome in the very low birth weight infant. *Pediatrics* 1995;96:314–319.
13. Han L, Zhou SM. Selenium supplementation in the prevention of pregnancy induced hypertension. *Chi Med J* 1994;107(11):870–871.
14. Wilson HM. Selenium oxide poisoning. *N C Med J* 1962;23:73–75.
15. Koppel C, Baudisch H, Beyer K-H, et al. Fatal poisoning with selenium dioxide. *Clin Toxicol* 1986;24:21–35.
16. Middleton JM. Selenium burn of the eye. Review of a case with review of the literature. *Arch Ophthalmol* 1947;38:806–811.
17. Yang G, Wang-S, Zhou R, et al. Endemic selenium intoxication of humans in China. *Am J Clin Nutr* 1983;37:872–881.
18. Sanz Alaejos M, Diaz Romero C. Urinary selenium concentrations. *Clin Chem* 1993;39(10):2040–2052.
19. Mack RB. The fat lady enters stage left. Acute selenium poisoning. *N C Med J* 1990;51(12):636–638.
20. Gosselin RE, Smith RP, Hodge HC. *Clinical toxicology of commercial products*, 5th ed. Baltimore, MD: Williams & Wilkins, 1984:MDII-64, II-129.
21. Paul M, Mason R, Edwards R. Effect of potential antidotes on the acute toxicity, tissue disposition and elimination of selenium in rats. *Res Commun Chem Pathol Pharmacol* 1989;66(3):441–450.

CHAPTER 229

Silver

Seth Schonwald

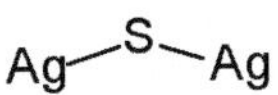

SILVER SULFIDE

Atomic symbol, atomic number, molecular weight:	**Ag, 47, 107.87 g/mol**
Valence state:	**+1**
CAS Registry No.:	**7440-22-4**
Normal serum level:	**Less than 0.05 g/dl**
SI conversion:	**μg/L × 9.27 = nmol/L**
Target organs:	**Lungs (acute), skin (chronic)**
Antidote:	**None**

OVERVIEW

Silver metal and its compounds are used in many commercial and industrial settings. Photographic films and materials account for most consumption. Electrical and electronic products, such as electrical contacts, silver paints, and batteries, are also common sources (1). Silver is a component in brazing alloys and solders, ball bearings, electroplated ware, sterling ware, and jewelry (2,3).

Silver has been used as an antibacterial agent (4). Silver nitrate was used for many years in newborns' eyes to prevent blindness caused by gonorrhea (5), and is used in salves for burn victims (6-8). Some water treatment methods (including water filters) also use a form of silver to kill bacteria. Colloidal silver is popular among alternative medicine enthusiasts and has been marketed as an alternative to antibiotics in health food stores (9). These claims are based on the germicidal properties of silver and anecdotal reports of effectiveness (10).

Argyria is an irreversible blue-grey pigmentation of the skin found in patients who have ingested silver compounds for prolonged periods (11,12). It is commonly caused by impregnation of the skin by small silver particles in workers involved in silver mining, and in the manufacture of silverware, metal alloys, metallic films, electroplating solutions, and photographic processing (13).

The general population is exposed to silver primarily through drinking water and food. Published studies on human inhalation of silver are based predominantly on exposure to elemental silver, silver nitrate, and silver oxide. Inhalation is probably the most important route of occupational exposure. One study estimated that a person developing six rolls of film is exposed to up to 16 g of silver through dermal contact with photographic solutions, if precautions are not taken (14).

Sources of elevated dietary silver include seafood from areas near sewage or industrial sources and crops grown in contaminated soil. Silver has been used in smoking-cessation lozenges and chewing gums (15). Silver acetate in chewing gum is classified as a smoking deterrent (16). High body levels of silver have been reported by this route.

TOXIC DOSES

U.S. regulatory guidelines and standards for silver may be found in Table 1.

There are no reports of death in humans after exposure to silver compounds. Death has been observed in rats after ingestion

TABLE 1. United States regulatory guidelines and standards for silver

Agency	Description	Concentration (mg/m^3)
OSHA	Metal and soluble compounds	
(air)	PEL-TWA	0.01 (as silver)
ACGIH	Silver metal	
(air)	TLV-TWA	0.1
	STEL	None
	Soluble compounds	
	TLV-TWA	0.01 (as silver)
	STEL	None
NIOSH	REL-TWA	0.01
(air)	STEL	None
	IDLH	10 (as silver)
EPA	Drinking water	1.142 mg/L

ACGIH, American Conference of Governmental Industrial Hygienists; EPA, U.S. Environmental Protection Agency; IDLH, immediately dangerous to life or health; NIOSH, National Institute for Occupational Safety and Health; OSHA, U.S. Occupational Safety and Health Administration; PEL, permissible exposure limit; REL, recommended exposure limit; STEL, short-term exposure limit; TLV, threshold limit value; TWA, time-weighted average.

of extremely high amounts of colloidal silver and inorganic silver compounds.

Argyria has reportedly been produced in adults who were given 900 mg of silver orally over a period of 1 year (17). Another study estimated the minimal oral dose for producing agyria to be 25 to 50 g taken over a 6-month period (18).

There are no studies linking cancer to silver or silver compounds in humans or animals.

TOXICOKINETICS AND TOXICODYNAMICS

The predominant routes of occupational exposure to silver are inhalational and dermal, with the dermal route being more important when prolonged contact with silver in solution occurs (as in photographic processing). Several silver compounds are absorbed through intact skin, although the degree of absorption appears low. Silver has been detected in the urine, blood, and body tissues of humans with burns after treatment with topical preparations containing 0.5% silver nitrate to prevent bacterial infection (19). A case of argyria in a woman who applied silver nitrate solution to her gums suggests that absorption across oral mucosa can occur (20).

Following the topical application of silver nitrate for burns, silver was distributed to the muscles, liver, spleen, kidney, heart, and bones in one study (21). An oral dose of silver undergoes a first pass effect through the liver resulting in excretion into the bile, thereby reducing systemic distribution to body tissues (22).

PATHOPHYSIOLOGY

Silver is not an essential mineral supplement and has no known physiologic function. It has a strong affinity for sulfhydryl groups and proteins. The deposition of silver in tissues is the result of the precipitation of insoluble silver salts, such as silver chloride and silver phosphate. These insoluble salts appear to be transformed into soluble silver sulfide albuminates, to form complexes with amino or carboxyl groups in ribonucleic acid, deoxyribonucleic acid, and proteins, or to be reduced to metallic silver by ascorbic acid or catecholamines (23). After oral exposure to silver acetate, silver is eliminated primarily in the feces, with only minor amounts eliminated in the urine (24).

CLINICAL PRESENTATION

Dermal Effects

Irreversible pigmentation of the skin after prolonged exposure to silver is called *argyria*. The pigmentation is described as slate-gray and is most noticeable in areas of skin exposed to light. The pigmentation is not a toxic effect nor is it known to be diagnostic of any other toxic effect; however, the change in skin color can be a cosmetic disfigurement.

Silver can elicit contact dermatitis in humans after dermal exposure to various silver compounds. Acute skin and ocular burns, caused by contact with silver nitrate, have been reported (25).

Respiratory Effects

Inhalation of silver nitrate or oxide can cause upper and lower respiratory tract irritation in humans (26). In one case, inhalation of an unknown form of silver during work with molten silver ingots produced respiratory failure the day after exposure.

Renal Effects

Silver is deposited in the glomerular basement membrane of animals and, therefore, may be expected to affect renal function. Occupational studies in humans, however, are not adequate for establishing a clear relationship between exposure to silver and renal impairment. Silver sulfadiazine has been associated with oliguric renal failure in one report (27).

Neurologic Effects

There are rare reports of neurologic effects in humans. Exposure to silver in a woman who had used nasal drops containing silver nitrate resulted in the deposit of silver in neurons of the central nervous system; however, no toxic effects were observed. Seizures were observed in a schizophrenic patient who had been addicted to silver-containing antismoking pills for years. An extremely high concentration of silver was detected in his serum (28). Neuropathy has been associated with systemic argyria (29).

Gastrointestinal Effects

Workers exposed to silver nitrate and silver oxide in the workplace have reported abdominal pain (30).

DIAGNOSTIC TESTS

No known laboratory tests exist to aid in the identification or management of individuals exposed to silver. Atomic absorption spectroscopy is the most prevalent analytical method to analyze silver in biological tissues and fluids (31). Levels of silver exposure that have led to argyria in humans are poorly documented. Two silver refiners with blood silver levels of 49 μg/L and 74 μg/L were asymptomatic in one report (32). Silver reclamation workers showed no significant symptoms despite the increased presence of silver in the blood, feces, and hair in another study (33) and showed no signs of argyric neuropathy, which has previously been described at blood silver levels as low as 10 μg/L.

In rare cases of intense or prolonged inhalation of silver-containing compounds, chest radiography may be helpful in monitoring respiratory failure.

TREATMENT

As silver compounds have been associated with respiratory irritation and respiratory failure, significant inhalation of silver compounds should be immediately treated with exposure to fresh air and administration of oxygen. There are no known effective treatment regimens regarding argyria. There is no evidence to support the use of charcoal, hemodialysis, hemoperfusion, or antidotal therapy in the management of silver exposures.

REFERENCES

1. Agency for Toxic Substances and Disease Registry. *Toxicological profile for silver*. Atlanta: US Department of Health and Human Services, Public Health Service December 1990:1–157.
2. Sugden P, Azad S, Erdmann M. Argyria caused by an earring. *Br J Plast Surg* 2001;54(3):252–253.
3. Morton CA, Fallowfield M, Kemmett D. Localized argyria caused by silver earrings. *Br J Dermatol* 1996;135(3):484–485.
4. Becker RO, Spadaro JA. Treatment of orthopedic infections with electrically generated silver ions. *J Bone Joint Surg Am* 1978;60-A:871–881.
5. Shaw EB. Questions the need for prophylaxis with silver nitrate. *Pediatrics* 1980;59:792.
6. Humphreys SD, Routledge PA. The toxicology of silver nitrate. *Adverse Drug React Toxicol Rev* 1998;17(2–3):115–143.
7. Iwasaki S, Yoshimura A, Ideura T, et al. Elimination study of silver in a hemodialyzed burn patient treated with silver sulfadiazine cream. *Am J Kidney Dis* 1997;30(2):287–290.
8. Wan AT, Conyers RA, Coombs CJ, et al. Determination of silver in blood, urine, and tissues of volunteers and burn patients. *Clin Chem* 1991;37(10 Pt 1):1683–1687.
9. Fung MC, Bowen DL. Silver products for medical indications: risk-benefit assessment. *J Toxicol Clin Toxicol* 1996;34(1):119–126.
10. Gulbranson SH, Hud JA, Hansen RC. Argyria following the use of dietary supplements containing colloidal silver protein. *Cutis* 2000;66(5):373–374.
11. Newman M, Kolecki P. Argyria in the ED. *Am J Emerg Med* 2001;19(6):525–526.
12. Bouts BA. Images in clinical medicine. Argyria. *N Engl J Med* 1999;340(20):1554.
13. Greene RM, Su WP. Argyria. *Am Fam Physician* 1987;36(6):151–154.
14. Scow K, Goyer M, Nelken L, et al. *Exposure and risk assessment for silver*. Report to US Environmental Protection Agency, Office of Water Regulations and Standards. Cambridge, MA: Arthur D. Little, Inc., 1981:PB85–211993.
15. Shelton D, Goulding R. Silver poisoning associated with an antismoking lozenge [Letter]. *Br Med J* 1979;1(6158):267.
16. Malcolm R, Currey HS, Mitchell MA, et al. Silver acetate gum as a deterrent to smoking. *Chest* 1986;90:107–111.
17. Hill WH, Pillsbury, DM. *Argyria, the pharmacology of silver*. Baltimore: Williams & Wilkins, 1939.
18. Gettler AO, et al. A contribution to the pathology of generalized argyria with a discussion of the fate of silver in the human body. *Am J Pathol* 1927;3:631–652.
19. Bader KF. Organ deposition of silver following silver nitrate therapy of burns. *Plast Reconstr Surg* 1966;37:550–551.
20. Marshall JP II, Schneider RP. Systemic argyria: secondary to topical silver nitrate. *Arch Dermatol* 1977;113:1077–1079.
21. Bader KF. Organ deposition of silver following silver nitrate therapy of burns. *Plast Reconstr Surg* 1966;37:550–551.
22. Furchner JE, Richmond CR, Drake GA. Comparative metabolism of radionuclides in mammals—IV. Retention of silver—110m in the mouse, rat, monkey, and dog. *Health Physics* 1968;15:505–514.
23. Danscher G. Light and electron microscopic localization of silver in biological tissue. *Histochemistry* 1981;71:177–186.
24. East BW, Boddy K, Williams ED, et al. Silver retention, total body silver and tissue silver concentrations in argyria associated with exposure to an antismoking remedy containing silver acetate. *Clin Exp Dermatol* 1980;5:305–311.
25. Moss AP, Sugar A, Hargett NA, et al. The ocular manifestations and functional effects of occupational argyrosis. *Arch Ophthalmol* 1979;97:906–908.
26. Phalen RF, Morrow PE. Experimental inhalation of metallic silver. *Health Phys* 1973;24:509–518.
27. McAlinney PG. Silver sulfadiazine and oliguric renal failure. *Ann Intern Med* 1987;107(2):264.
28. Ohbo Y, Fukuzako H, Takeuchi K, et al. Argyria and convulsive seizures caused by ingestion of silver in a patient with schizophrenia. *Psychiatry Clin Neurosci* 1996;50(2):89–90.
29. Vik H, Andersen KJ, Julshamn K, et al. Neuropathy caused by silver absorption from arthroplasty cement. *Lancet* 1985;1(8433):872.
30. Rosenman KD, Moss A, Kon S. Argyria: clinical implications of exposure to silver nitrate and silver oxide. *J Occup Med* 1979;21:430–435.
31. DiVincenzo GD, Giordano CJ, Schriever LS. Biologic monitoring of workers exposed to silver. *Int Arch Occup Environ Health* 1985;56:207–215.
32. Williams N, Gardner I. Absence of symptoms in silver refiners with raised blood silver levels. *Occup Med (Lond)* 1995;45(4):205–208.
33. Pifer JW, Friedlander BR, Kintz RT, et al. Absence of toxic effects in silver reclamation workers. *Scand J Work Environ Health* 1989;15(3):210–221.

CHAPTER 230

Tellurium

Seth Schonwald

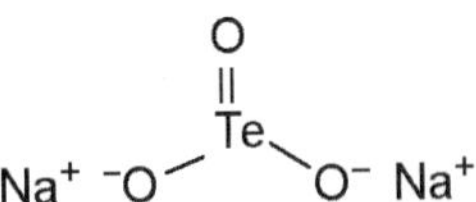

SODIUM TELLURITE

Atomic symbol, atomic number, molecular weight:	**Te, 52, 127.6 g/mol**
Valence states:	**+6, +4, +2**
CAS Registry No.:	**13494-80-9**
Normal levels:	**None**
SI conversion:	**μg/dl × 0.0784 = μmol/L**
Special concerns:	**Toxicity is rare, but there are no available treatments.**
Target organs:	**Central nervous system and skin**
Antidote:	**None**

OVERVIEW

Tellurium is a rare elemental metal similar to selenium. A byproduct of copper refining, it is used as a steel additive and is alloyed with aluminum, copper, lead, or tin. It is a carbide stabilizer and is used in vulcanizing rubber, as a coloring agent in glass and ceramics, and in catalysts for petroleum cracking. It is used with bismuth in thermoelectric devices. Tellurium is a semiconductor material and is slightly photosensitive.

Toxic effects are rare; however, death from ingestion of tellurium compounds occurs. Some have postulated that tellurium plays a role in Alzheimer's disease (1). Tellurium compounds (as may be found in garlic) have been studied regarding their cholesterol-lowering potential (2).

The U.S. Occupational Safety and Health Administration occupational permissible exposure limit is 0.1 mg/m^3 time-weighted average. The recommended exposure limit set by the National Institute for Occupational Safety and Health is 0.1 mg/m^3 for tellurium as a time-weighted average. It is immediately dangerous to life or health at 25 mg/m^3. The American Council of Government Industrial Hygienists has established the threshold limit value at 0.1 mg/m^3 time-weighted average (3).

Humans exposed to as little as 0.01 mg/m^3 may develop *tellurium breath*, which has a garlic-like odor. Acute ingestion of lead telluride or sodium tellurium can cause anhidrosis, nausea, somnolence, inflammation of the gastric mucosa and internal organs, intestinal bleeding, and finally death from respiratory paralysis (rare) (3). A lethal case had a tellurium blood concentration of 801.8 µg/L. The amount ingested was unknown (4).

TOXICOKINETICS AND TOXICODYNAMICS

Tellurium is absorbed by all routes. Animal data indicate that up to 25% of oral tellurium is absorbed (5). After a single exposure, the largest proportion is found in the kidney and bone. With repeated oral dosing, it is found in the heart primarily, followed by kidney, spleen, bone, and lung (6). Tellurium compounds are reduced to the relatively harmless elemental tellurium and methyl telluride. Dimethyl telluride is formed and gives a pungent garlic-like odor to breath, excreta, and the viscera. Tellurium is excreted through the lungs, the urine, the feces, and sweat.

PATHOPHYSIOLOGY

Tellurium caused a highly synchronous primary demyelination of peripheral nerves in developing rats, which was followed by a period of rapid remyelination. The demyelination is related to the inhibition of squalene epoxidase, which blocks cholesterol synthesis and creation of squalene (7).

VULNERABLE POPULATIONS

There are no human data; however, rat studies have shown neurotoxic effects in the developing fetus (8).

CLINICAL PRESENTATION

Acute or chronic exposure to tellurium in humans may cause transient headache, dizziness, somnolence, and anorexia. Peripheral nervous system injury has not been reported in humans (9). Chronic exposure causes neurologic impairment in animals, including hydrocephalus (10), lipofuscinosis, and peripheral demyelinating neuropathy. Tellurium causes demyelination in rats, perhaps by interference of cholesterol synthesis by Schwann's cells (11,12).

Tellurium has been associated with anhidrosis; blue-black discoloration of the face, neck, and hands; hair loss; dry mouth; and metallic taste (13,14).

DIAGNOSTIC TESTS

A lethal case had a tellurium blood concentration of 801.8 µg/L, and 1975.3 µg in the urine (4).

TREATMENT

No effective treatment for poisoning has been reported. Only supportive and symptomatic care is recommended. Dimercaprol has been used in some human cases, but animal data indicate no beneficial effect. *Tellurium breath* has been managed with ascorbic acid (15).

REFERENCES

1. Larner AJ. Alzheimer's disease, Kuf's disease, tellurium and selenium. *Med Hypotheses* 1996;47(2):73–75.
2. Larner AJ. How does garlic exert its hypocholesterolemic action? The tellurium hypothesis. *Med Hypotheses* 1995;44(4):295–297.
3. Material safety data sheet. ESPI Web site. Available at: http://www.espi-metals.com/msds's/leadtelluride.pdf. Accessed March 2003.
4. Shao-hua L. *Poison said to have caused death. Taipei Times* [serial online]. January 18, 2001.
5. Kron T, Hansen C, Werner E. Renal excretion of tellurium after peroral administration of tellurium in different forms to healthy human volunteers. *J Trace Elem Electrolytes Health Dis* 1991;5(4):239–244.
6. Taylor A. Biochemistry of tellurium. *Biol Trace Elem Res* 1996;55(3):231–239.
7. Toews AD, Lee SY, Popko B, et al. Tellurium-induced neuropathy: a model for reversible reductions in myelin protein gene expression. *J Neurosci Res* 1990;26(4):501–507.
8. Duckett S. Teratogenesis caused by tellurium. *Ann N Y Acad Sci* 1972;192:220–221.
9. Olsson Y. Microenvironment of the peripheral nervous system. Uppsala University Web site. Available at: http://www.genpat.uu.se/persons/yo/Microenv/yoindex.html. Accessed: March 2003.
10. Agnew WF, Fauvre FM, Pudenz PH. Tellurium hydrocephalus: distribution of tellurium-127m between maternal, fetal, and neonatal tissues of the rat. *Exp Neurol* 1968;21(1):120–131.
11. Jortner BS. Mechanisms of toxic injury in the peripheral nervous system: neuropathologic considerations. *Toxicol Pathol* 2000;28(1):54–69.
12. Wagner M, Toews AD, Morell P. Tellurite specifically affects squalene epoxidase: investigations examining the mechanism of tellurium-induced neuropathy. *J Neurochem* 1995;64(5):2169–2176.
13. Blackadder ES, Manderson WG. Occupational absorption of tellurium: a report of two cases. *Br J Ind Med* 1975;32(1):59–61.
14. Neuromuscular toxic neuropathies. Neuromuscular disease center Web site. Available at: http://www.neuro.wustl.edu/neuromuscular/nother/toxic.htm. Accessed March 2003.
15. De Meio RH. Tellurium: effect of ascorbic acid on the tellurium breath. *J Ind Hyg Toxicol* 1947;29:393–395.

CHAPTER 231

Thallium

Seth Schonwald

$$Tl^{+}\ {}^{-}O-S(=O)_2-O^{-}\ Tl^{+}$$

THALLIUM SULFATE

Atomic symbol, atomic number, molecular weight:	**Tl, 81, 204.38 g/mol.**
Valence states:	**+1, +3**
CAS Registry No.:	**10031-59-1 (thallium sulfate)**
Normal levels:	**Less than 1 µg/g creatinine in urine**
SI conversion:	**µg/L × 0.0049 = µmol/L]**
Special concerns:	**Small doses cause no symptoms initially but may produce severe effects over several weeks.**
Target organs:	**Gastrointestinal, central and peripheral nervous system, hair loss**
Antidote	**None**

OVERVIEW

Thallium was discovered by Sir William Crookes in 1861. It is a toxic metal that is used in the semiconductor industry, optical systems, and photoelectric cells (1). It is found in smelters and is used in alloys for its anticorrosive properties. Thallium is also used for cardiac imaging, as a depilatory, to treat syphilis, and to manufacture highly refractive optical glass (2). Other products include jewelry pigments, thermometers, and scintillation counters. In 1972, thallium and its compounds were banned for use in pesticides in the United States (3).

Compounds of thallium are generally water-soluble. Humans may be exposed to thallium by ingestion, inhalation, or dermal absorption. Thallium-containing foods, especially homegrown fruits and green vegetables, are the most common sources of exposure. Inhalation of contaminated air near emission sources or in the workplace may contribute to thallium exposure (4).

TOXIC DOSE

Governmental regulations and standards for thallium are shown in Table 1. Ingestion of 54 to 110 mg thallium nitrate/kg resulted in cranial and peripheral neuropathies, and death (5). Examination of nerves obtained on days 7 and 9 demonstrated axonal degeneration with secondary myelin loss. Other studies have noted central-peripheral distal axonopathy (6,7). Two of three subjects who ingested thallous acetate died 1 month later; the dose was not determined (8). The lethal adult dose of thallium has been estimated as 1 g (14 to 15 mg/kg) (9).

A case of severe thallium intoxication was treated with Prussian blue; diuresis enhanced by intravenous fluids; and prolonged, early hemodialysis. In spite of high serum thallium (5240 µg/L), symptoms were minor and recovery complete (10). No studies exist demonstrating that thallium may be a carcinogen in humans or animals.

TOXICOKINETICS AND TOXICODYNAMICS

Animal studies suggest that thallium is well absorbed orally; however, there are few data in humans (11). Thallium is widely distributed after absorption. Thallium tissue levels in a female cancer patient given radioactive thallium nitrate and subsequent thallium sulfate were highest in scalp hair, renal papilla, renal cortex, heart, bone tumor, and spleen. Lower levels were found in the brain (12). Urinary excretion accounted for 15.3% of administered thallium radioactivity, and 0.4% was found in feces. An excretion half-life of 21.7 days has been estimated for thallium (13).

PATHOPHYSIOLOGY

Animal studies suggest that thallium may deplete or inhibit critical enzyme systems. Depletion of succinic dehydrogenase and guanine deaminase is found in rat cerebrum as well as depletion of monoamine oxidase, acid phosphatase, and cathepsin (14). Differential distribution of thallium suggests that some areas of the brain may be affected more severely than others.

TABLE 1. United States regulatory guidelines and standards for thallium

Agency	Description	Concentration (µg/m³)
OSHA (air)	PEL-TWA	0.1 (as thallium)
ACGIH (air)	Thallium and soluble compounds	
	TLV-TWA	0.1 (as thallium)
	STEL	None
NIOSH (air)	REL-TWA	0.1 (as thallium)
	IDLH	15 (as thallium)
EPA (water)	Maximum allow concentration	13 ppb

ACGIH, American Conference of Governmental Industrial Hygienists; EPA, Environmental Protection Agency; FDA, U.S. Food and Drug Administration; IDLH, immediately dangerous to life or health; NIOSH, National Institute for Occupational Safety and Health; OSHA, U.S. Occupational Safety and Health Administration; PEL, permissible exposure limit; ppb, parts per billion; REL, recommended exposure limit; STEL, short-term exposure limit; TLV, threshold limit value; TWA, time-weighted average.

VULNERABLE POPULATIONS

Thallium can cross the human placenta. A retrospective study of 297 children living near a cement plant that discharged thallium into the air demonstrated that congenital malformations and anomalies in the exposed group did not exceed the incidence of expected birth defects (15).

CLINICAL PRESENTATION

Thallium exposure may occur by all routes, but ingestion appears to be the most common. Thallium ingestion can cause acute gastrointestinal symptoms and multiple systemic effects, including respiratory, neurologic, cardiovascular, hepatic and renal damage, and alopecia.

Neurologic Effects

Neurologic effects include peripheral and central nervous system injury after acute oral exposure. Thallium produces distal, predominantly sensory, neuropathy in humans (16). Histological evaluations have shown axonal degeneration and myelin loss. Ataxia, tremor, and multiple cranial palsies have been reported. Numbness of the toes and fingers, a severe "burning feet" sensation, and muscle cramps are common. Convulsions and death can also occur.

Dermal Effects

Hair loss is common; occurs as early as 8 days after exposure; and may involve body hair, full beard, and scalp hair (17). In other instances, body and pubic hair have been spared. Hair loss is temporary, and local skin changes do not occur. Animal studies suggest that thallium affects hair follicles directly or that hair loss is the result of effects of thallium on the sympathetic nervous system (18).

Respiratory Effects

Respiratory effects including alveolar damage, hyaline membrane formation, and pulmonary edema have been reported after oral exposure (19). Thallium may have a direct effect on pulmonary epithelial and endothelial cells.

Cardiovascular Effects

Cardiovascular effects were reported after acute ingestion of 54 to 110 mg thallium nitrate/kg (20). Extensive damage of the myocardium with myofiber thinning, accumulation of lipid droplets, myocardial necrosis, and inflammatory reaction was noted on autopsy. Sinus bradycardia, ventricular dysrhythmias, and T wave anomalies have also been reported. The mechanism of thallium-induced cardiovascular injury is not clear.

Renal Effects

Renal function can be impaired following thallium exposure. Diminished creatinine clearance, a raised blood urea, and proteinuria are common. Tubular necrosis has been reported following ingestion of thallium in humans. However, these effects were reportedly due to infarction rather than a direct affect on kidney tissue.

Gastrointestinal Effects

Ingestion of thallium sulfate causes gastroenteritis, diarrhea or constipation, vomiting, and abdominal pain. Gastrointestinal disturbances were also reported in 189 cases of thallium poisoning from contaminated cabbage in China (21).

The liver may develop centrilobular necrosis and fatty changes (22). Thallium may combine with the sulfhydryl groups in mitochondria, interfering with oxidative phosphorylation. Serum glutamic oxaloacetic transaminase, pyruvic oxaloacetic transaminase, and alkaline phosphatase levels are often elevated.

DIAGNOSTIC TESTS

Thallium levels in urine, blood, and hair have been used to indicate exposure. Typical urine thallium levels in unexposed individuals are below 1 μg/g creatinine (23). Urinary levels in cement workers ranged from less than 0.3 to 6.3 μg/g creatinine in one study. A mean urinary thallium level of 76 μg/L was found in a population living near a cement production plant (24). The blood thallium level reflects recent exposure because it is cleared from the blood rapidly; therefore, it is not a useful means of monitoring human populations for exposure.

The normal concentration range of thallium in human hair is 5 to 10 ng/g. In addition to being incorporated from the blood into hair, thallium may adsorb to the external hair shaft, making it difficult to distinguish the source of elevated hair thallium.

TREATMENT

Treatment for acute, high-level oral exposure is to remove thallium from the gastrointestinal tract quickly, to prevent absorption of any remaining thallium, and to increase its excretion (25). Emptying the stomach by gastric lavage or emesis within the first few hours following exposure has been suggested. After dermal exposure, contaminated clothing should be removed and skin thoroughly washed. After acute inhalation, the victim should be removed from the immediate environment and high-flow, humidified oxygen should be administered (26).

Enhancement of Elimination

Multiple-dose activated charcoal may be administered to adsorb residual thallium; however, its efficacy has not been rigorously proved. Activated charcoal does adsorb thallium *in vitro*.

Hemodialysis or *hemoperfusion* may be beneficial in cases of severe poisoning. Hemodialysis has reduced thallium concentrations in the blood in some cases and only minimally in others (27). Hemoperfusion may give better results than hemodialysis (28).

Antidotes

Prussian blue (potassium ferric ferrocyanide) binds with thallium in the intestine. Details of its administration are provided in Chapter 72. Neither Prussian blue nor its complex with thallium is absorbed systemically. The oral or duodenal administration of this compound effectively prevents absorption and increases fecal excretion. Prussian blue is approved for use in Europe and is in the process of obtaining approval in the United States.

The similarity between thallium and potassium has led some authors to consider the use of sodium polystyrene sulfonate as a potential adsorbent. Although sodium polystyrene sulfonate demonstrates exceptional *in vitro* adsorption of thallium, its greater affinity for potassium probably renders it clinically ineffective (29).

Oral administration of potassium chloride in large doses has been proposed in victims with intact renal function to enhance thallium clearance from tissue stores and to increase renal excretion. Transient worsening of symptoms after this treatment due to the redistribution of thallium into the serum has been noted, however, creating controversy concerning the efficacy of potassium chloride administration.

REFERENCES

1. Hazardous Substances Data Bank. Bethesda, MD: National Library of Medicine, National Toxicology Information Program, 1989.
2. Windholz M, ed. *The Merck index: an encyclopedia of chemicals, drugs, and biologicals*, 10th ed. Rahway, NJ: Merck and Company, Inc., 1983;1324–1325.
3. U.S. Environmental Protection Agency. *Suspended, canceled and restricted pesticides*. Washington, DC: US Environmental Protection Agency, Office of Pesticides and Toxic Substances Compliance, 1985:25.
4. Agency for Toxic Substances and Disease Registry. *Toxicological profile for thallium*. Atlanta: US Department of Health and Human Services, Public Health Service, 1992:1–110.
5. Davis LE, Standefer JC, Kornfeld M, et al. Acute thallium poisoning: toxicological and morphological studies of the nervous system. *Ann Neurol* 1981;10:38–44.
6. Roby DS, Fein AM, Bennett RH, et al. Cardiopulmonary effects of acute thallium poisoning. *Chest* 1984;85:236–240.
7. De Groot G, van Leusen R, van Heijst AN. Thallium concentrations in body fluids and tissues in a fatal case of thallium poisoning. *Vet Hum Toxicol* 1985;27:115–119.
8. Cavanagh JB, Fuller NH, Johnson HR, et al. The effects of thallium salts, with particular reference to the nervous system changes: a report of three cases. *Q J Med* 1974;43:293–319.
9. Gosselin RE, Smith RP, Hodge HC, et al. *Clinical toxicology of commercial products*, 5th ed. Baltimore: Williams & Wilkins, 1984;379–383.
10. Malbrain ML, Lambrecht GL, Zandijk E, et al. Treatment of severe thallium intoxication. *J Toxicol Clin Toxicol* 1997;35(1):97–100.
11. Lie R, Thomas R, Scott J. The distribution and excretion of thallium-204 in the rat, with suggested MPC's and a bioassay procedure. *Health Phys* 1960;2:334–340.
12. Barclay RK, Pencock WC, Karnofsy DA. Distribution and excretion of radioactive thallium in the chick embryo, rat, and man. *J Pharmacol Exp Ther* 1953;107:178–187.
13. U.S. Environmental Protection Agency. *Ambient water quality criteria for thallium*. Washington, DC: US Environmental Protection Agency, Office of Water Regulations and Standards, 1980;EPA-440/5-80-074. NTIS No. PB81-117848.
14. Hasan M, Bajpai VK, Shipstone AC. Electron microscope study of thallium-induced alterations in the oligodendrocytes of the rat area postrema. *Exp Pathol (Jena)* 1977;13:338–345.
15. Dolgner R, Brockhaus A, Ewers U, et al. Repeated surveillance of thallium in a population living in the vicinity of a cement plant emitting dust containing thallium. *Int Arch Occup Environ Health* 1983;52:79–94.
16. Pau PW. Management of thallium poisoning. *Hong Kong Med J* 2000;6(3):316–318.
17. Grunfeld O, Hinostroza G. Thallium poisoning. *Arch Intern Med* 1964;114:132–138.
18. Carson B, Ellis H, McCann J. *Toxicology and biological monitoring of metals in humans*. Chelsea, MI: Lewis Publishers, Inc., 1986:243–254.
19. Roby DS, Fein AM, Bennett RH, et al. Cardiopulmonary effects of acute thallium poisoning. *Chest* 1984;85:236–240.
20. Davis LE, Standefer JC, Kornfeld M, et al. Acute thallium poisoning: toxicological and morphological studies of the nervous system. *Ann Neurol* 1981;10:38–44.
21. Dai-xing Z, Ding-nan L. Chronic thallium poisoning in a rural area of Guizhou Province, China. *J Environ Health* 1985;48:14–18.
22. Cavanagh JB, Fuller NH, Johnson HR, et al. The effects of thallium salts, with particular reference to the nervous system changes: a report of three cases. *Q J Med* 1974;43:293–319.
23. Schaller KH, Manke G, Raithel HJ, et al. Investigations of thallium- exposed workers in cement factories. *Int Arch Occup Environ Health* 1980;47:223–231.
24. Brockhaus A, Dolgner R, Ewers U, et al. Intake and health effects of thallium among a population living in the vicinity of a cement plant emitting thallium containing dust. *Int Arch Occup Environ Health* 1981;48:375–389.
25. Proctor NH, Hughes JP, Fischman ML. *Chemical hazards of the workplace*, 2nd ed. Philadelphia: JB Lippincott Co, 1988.
26. Bronstein AC, Currance PL. *Emergency care for hazardous materials exposure*. St. Louis: Mosby, 1988:211–212.
27. Haddad LM, Winchester JF. *Clinical management of poisoning and drug overdose*, 2nd ed. Philadelphia: WB Saunders, 1990.
28. Proctor NH, Hughes JP, Fischman ML. *Chemical hazards of the workplace*, 2nd ed. Philadelphia: JB Lippincott Co, 1988.
29. Hoffman RS, Stringer JA, Feinberg RS, et al. Comparative efficacy of thallium adsorption by activated charcoal, Prussian blue, and sodium polystyrene sulfonate. *J Toxicol Clin Toxicol* 1999;37(7):833–837.

CHAPTER 232

Tin

Seth Schonwald

TRIPHENYL TIN ACETATE

Atomic symbol, atomic number, molecular weight:	**Sn, 50, 118.71 g/mol**
Valence states:	**+2, +4**
CAS Registry No.:	**7440-31-5**
Normal levels:	**Not applicable**
SI conversion:	**μg/L × 0.0084 = μmol/L**
Special concerns:	**Acute exposure may not produce severe effects for days.**
Target organs:	**Gastrointestinal, brain (acute but delayed onset), lung (chronic)**
Antidote:	**None**

OVERVIEW

Tin has many uses in alloys and is rarely used in its elemental form. Its is used principally in containers, including aerosol cans and food and beverage containers (1). Tin is also used as a reducing agent in chemical processes; in the production of other compounds, such as stannous chloride and stannic oxide; and in the production of organotin compounds.

Inorganic tin compounds have been used to add strength to certain glasses. Inorganic tin compounds serve as the base in certain colors, perfumes, and soaps and as catalysts. Stannic oxide (cassiterite) is used as a polishing compound to produce milky or colored glass and to make fingernail polish (2). Disubstituted organotins are used in the production of plastics, including food wrap in which they act as stabilizers. They are also added to polyurethane foams and silicone to increase their strength and to minimize stickiness (3).

Trisubstituted organotins are used as biocides in agriculture and industry. Tributyltins are used as antifoulants in marine paints (4) and have been restricted by the Organotin Antifouling Paints Control Act, which limits the type of vessel on which these paints can be used. Bis (tributyltin) oxide (TBTO) is used as a preservative for wood products, leather, ropes, fabrics, and paper.

Alloys of tin are used to make dental materials (5), nuclear reactor components, aircraft components, bronze, and brass. Tin is the principal component of pewter (6). Stannous fluoride (SnF_5) is used in toothpaste. Tin is used in superconducting magnets, copper wire, and solder.

TOXIC DOSE

U.S. regulatory guidelines and standards are provided in Table 1. In 1954, the drug diethyltin diiodide (Stalinon) was associated with 100 deaths in French patients who had been treated for osteomyelitis, anthrax, and acne. The primary ingredients were diethyltin diiodide (15 mg/capsule) and linoleic acid. Seventy mg of triethyltin was calculated as the toxic dose ingested over an 8-day period (7). It was proposed that the deaths were caused by triethyltin iodide, which was present as an impurity from the manufacturing process.

No deaths in humans have been reported after either oral or dermal exposure to inorganic tin compounds. Death has occurred after inhalation or oral exposure to organotin compounds. One out of six workers died 12 days after exposure to a mixture of dimethyltin and trimethyltin chloride vapor at a chemical plant (8). Exposure levels were not provided.

No reports have indicated an increased risk of cancer after exposure to inorganic or organotin compounds.

TABLE 1. U.S. regulatory guidelines and standards for tin (Sn)

Agency	Description	Concentration (μg/m³)
OSHA (air)	Inorganic compounds	
	PEL-TWA	2.0 (as Sn)
	Organic compounds	
	PEL–TWA	0.1 (as Sn)
ACGIH (air)	Tin oxide and inorganic compounds	
	TLV-TWA	2.0 (as Sn)
	STEL	None
	Tin organic compounds	
	TLV-TWA	0.1 (as Sn)
	STEL	None
NIOSH (air)	Metal and inorganic compounds	
	REL-TWA	2.0 (as Sn)
	IDLH	100.0
	Organic compounds	
	REL-TWA	0.1 (as Sn)
	IDLH	25.0 (as Sn)

ACGIH, American Conference of Governmental Industrial Hygienists; IDLH, immediate danger to life or health; NIOSH, National Institute for Occupational Safety and Health; OSHA, U.S. Occupational Safety and Health Administration; PEL, permissible exposure limit; REL, recommended exposure limit; STEL, short-term exposure limit; TLV, threshold limit value; TWA, time-weighted average.

TOXICOKINETICS AND TOXICODYNAMICS

There are no studies regarding absorption in humans after oral or dermal exposure to inorganic or organic tin compounds. Limited data from occupational studies suggest organotin may be absorbed to some extent after inhalation. Tin is widely distributed in human tissues; highest concentrations are located in the kidney, liver, lung, and bone (9). In rats, most of an inorganic tin dose is excreted within 48 hours in the feces. Tin has been detected in the urine after inhalation and oral exposure to organotins.

PATHOPHYSIOLOGY

The proposed mechanism for the adverse effects of tin involves inhibition of the hydrolysis of adenosine triphosphate and uncoupling of oxidative phosphorylation in mitochondria (4).

VULNERABLE POPULATIONS

There are not definitive human data indicating that inorganic tin or organotin compounds affect development. Organotin compounds have produced reproductive effects in animals after both inhalation and oral exposures. Oral feeding of TBTO decreases fetal weight, skeletal abnormalities, and cleft palates in mice (10). Toxicokinetic data indicate that the inorganic tin compounds do not transfer to the fetus.

CLINICAL PRESENTATION

Human exposure to tin may occur by inhalation, ingestion, or dermal contact. Gastrointestinal effects have been observed after ingestion of inorganic tin compounds, and ingestion or inhalation of organotin compounds may cause neurologic effects.

Neurologic Effects

Intoxications resulting from Stalinon incidents are characterized by profound neurologic effects. Symptoms appear approximately 4 days after ingestion and include vertigo, headache, photophobia, visual impairment, altered consciousness, and convulsions. Sensory disturbances, hyporeflexia, and incontinence were common. Death occurred in 4 to 10 days as the result of coma or from acute intracranial hypertension. Autopsies revealed diffuse edema in central nervous system white matter (11).

Whereas triethyltin is myelinotoxic, producing edematous and vacuolar changes in the central myelin, trimethyltin is neurotoxic, producing prominent toxic changes in the neurons of the limbic system (e.g., hippocampus, entorhinal cortex) (12,13). Acute trimethyltin has been associated with a limbic cerebellar syndrome (14). Hearing loss, confabulation, hyperphagia, disturbed sexual behavior, nystagmus, partial and tonic-clonic seizures, and a sensory neuropathy characterize this syndrome. Acute short-term memory loss from trimethyltin exposure has also been described. Memory loss gradually improved over the course of several months (15).

Respiratory Effects

A benign form of pneumoconiosis, known as *stannosis*, was observed in workers exposed to stannic oxide dust and fumes for 15 to 20 years (16). No functional impairment or systemic disease was seen. Inorganic tin may cause metal fume fever and has been implicated as a cause of occupational asthma (17).

Five patients developed mucous membrane irritation after inhalation of an interior use latex paint containing the organotin compound TBTO (18,19). After exposure to a mixture of half dimethyltin and half trimethyltin chloride vapor, respiratory depression was noted before the death of an occupationally exposed individual (6).

Gastrointestinal Effects

Gastrointestinal effects of varying severity, consisting of irritation of the mucous membranes of the stomach and intestines, have been observed in humans. This usually occurs after ingestion of inorganic tin by eating food or drinking liquids from tin containers (6,20). Although the corrosive properties of metallic tin salts can produce gastrointestinal disturbances in high dose, poor oral absorption limits systemic toxicity. Liver injury consisting of fatty degeneration has developed in humans and animals exposed by inhalation and in animals after oral exposure to organotin compounds.

Renal Effects

Proximal tubule epithelial degeneration is the major renal change observed in humans after inhalation of organotin compounds. Similar changes are found in animals after inhalation, oral, and dermal exposure to organotins. As with hepatic changes, the possibility that tin compounds may cause renal effects at hazardous waste sites must be considered.

Dermal Effects

Skin and eye irritation have been reported in humans and animals after dermal exposure of acute and intermediate duration to both inorganic tin and organotin compounds. A shipwright developed a delayed bullous irritant dermatitis from contact with paint containing TBTO (21). A patient exposed cutaneously to triphenyltin acetate developed an urticarial eruption (22). Tin compounds may also be contact sensitizers (23).

DIAGNOSTIC TESTS

Tin was measured in an organotin-poisoned patient's urine and blood by a gas chromatography-flame photometric detector and inductively coupled plasma mass spectrometry (24). Determination of tin in blood and urine by neutron activation analysis was reported after two cases of poisoning by triphenyltin acetate (25).

TREATMENT

Because tin toxicity involves a chronic exposure, and animal studies indicate that most of an administered dose of tin is excreted within 48 hours (26), it seems unlikely that efforts to enhance the elimination of tin would be of much benefit. Water may be administered for dilution after ingestion of tin compounds. Emesis is not recommended, as certain organotins may be corrosive.

Dermal and ocular exposure to tin compounds is treated by washing thoroughly with soap and water and flushing the eyes with water.

Antidotes

Neither administration of D-penicillamine to increase urinary tin excretion nor chelation therapy with dimercaprol (British antilewisite) seems to be effective in removing tin from the body.

Supportive Care

Treatment is symptomatic and supportive. Acute lung injury (noncardiogenic pulmonary edema) is treated in the usual manner.

REFERENCES

1. HSDB. Hazardous substances data bank. Bethesda, MD: National Library of Medicine, National Toxicology Information Program, 1989.
2. Windholz M, ed. *The Merck index: an encyclopedia of chemicals, drugs, and biologicals*, 10th ed. Rahway, NJ: Merck and Company, Inc., 1983:1256–1257, 1353–1354.
3. WHO. *Tin and organotin compounds: a preliminary review. Environmental health criteria 15.* Geneva, Switzerland: World Health Organization, 1980.
4. Llewellyn OP. Marine antifouling compositions and their applications. *Ann Occup Hyg* 1972;15:393–397.
5. Barber T, Reisbick MH. Amalgam: past, present, and future. *J Am Dent Assoc* 1973;86:863–869.
6. Agency for Toxic Substances and Disease Registry. *Toxicological profile for tin.* Atlanta: US Department of Health and Human Services, 1992:1–174.
7. Barnes JM, Stoner HB. The toxicology of tin compounds. *Pharmacol Rev* 1959;11:211–231.
8. Rey C, Reinecke HJ, Besser R. Methyltin intoxication in six men: toxicologic and clinical aspects. *Vet Hum Toxicol* 1984;26:121–122.
9. Schroeder HA, Balassa JJ, Tipton IH. Abnormal trace metals in man: tin. *J Chronic Dis* 1964;17:483–502.
10. Davis A, Barale R, Brun G, et al. Evaluation of the genetic and embryotoxic effects of bis(tri-n-butyltin)oxide (TBTO), a broad-spectrum pesticide, in multiple in vivo and in vitro short-term tests. *Mutat Res* 1987;188:65–95.
11. Foncin E, Gruner J. Tin neurotoxicity. In: Vinken P, Bruyn G, ed. *Handbook of clinical neurology. Pt. 1. Intoxications of the nervous system.* New York: North-Holland, 1979:279–290.
12. Chang LW. The neurotoxicology and pathology of organomercury, organolead, and organotin. *J Toxicol Sci* 1990;15[Suppl 4]:125–151.
13. Krigman MR, Silverman AP. General toxicology of tin and its organic compounds. *Neurotoxicology* 1984;5:129–139.
14. Besser R, Kramer G, Thumler R, et al. Acute trimethyl tin limbic cerebellar syndrome. *Neurology* 1987;37:945–950.
15. Yanofsky NN, Nierenberg D, Turco JH. Acute short-term memory loss from trimethyltin exposure. *J Emerg Med* 1991;9:137–139.
16. Dundon CC, Hughes JP. Stannic oxide pneumoconiosis. *Am J Roentgenol Radium Ther* 1950;63:797–812.
17. Shelton D, Urch B, Tarlo SM. Occupational asthma induced by a carpet fungicide-tributyltin oxide. *J Allergy Clin Immunol* 1992;90:274–275.
18. Wax PM, Dockstader L. Tributyltin use in interior paints: a continuing health hazard. *J Toxicol Clin Toxicol* 1995;33:239–241.
19. Acute effect of indoor exposure to paint containing bis(tributyrin) oxide—Wisconsin, 1991. *MMWR Morb Mortal Wkly Rep* 1991;40:280–281.
20. Benoy CJ, Hooper PA, Schneider R. The toxicity of tin in canned fruit juices and solid foods. *Food Cosmet Toxicol* 1971;9:645–656.
21. Lewis PG, Emmett EA. Irritant dermatitis from tri-butyl tin oxide and contact allergy from chlorocresol. *Contact Dermatitis* 1987;17:129–132.
22. Colosio C, Tomasini M, Cairoli S, et al. Occupational triphenyltin acetate poisoning: a case report. *Br J Ind Med* 1991;48:136–139.
23. Menne T, Andersen KE, Kaaber K, et al. Tin: an overlooked contact sensitizer? *Contact Dermatitis* 1987;16:9–10.
24. Gui-Bin J, Qun-Fang Z, Bin H. Tin compounds and major trace metal elements in organotin-poisoned patient's urine and blood measured by gas chromatography-flame photometric detector and inductively coupled plasma-mass spectrometry. *Bull Environ Contam Toxicol* 2000;65:277–284.
25. Manzo L, Richelmi P, Sabbioni E, et al. Poisoning by triphenyltin acetate. Report of two cases and determination of tin in blood and urine by neutron activation analysis. *J Toxicol Clin Toxicol* 1981;18:1343–1353.
26. Hiles RA. Absorption, distribution and excretion of inorganic tin in rats. *Toxicol Appl Pharmacol* 1974;27:366–379.

CHAPTER 233

Uranium

Seth Schonwald

Atomic symbol, atomic number, molecular weight:	**U, 92, 238.03 g/mol**
Valence states:	**+2, +3, +4, +5, +6 (Only the +4 and +6 states are of practical importance.)**
CAS Registry No.:	**7440-61-1**
Normal levels:	**Not applicable**
SI conversion:	**µg/dl × 0.042 = µmol/L**
Target organs:	**Kidney**
Antidotes:	**Sodium bicarbonate, chelating agents**

OVERVIEW

The toxicity of uranium may be divided into its chemical and radiation effects. Uranium compounds are used in photography, as a stain or dye on leather and wood, and as mordants in the silk and wood industries (1). Depleted uranium is used in military equipment (2). Uranium is used in the commercial nuclear power industry and for weapons manufacturing (3). One pound of completely fissioned uranium produces the energy of 1500 tons of coal (4).

Major compounds of uranium include oxides, fluorides, carbides, nitrates, chlorides, acetates, and others. Uranium hexafluoride gas is used to isolate uranium 238 for atomic bombs. Uranium dioxide is used to extend the lives of filaments in large incandescent lamps. Ammonium diuranate is used to produce colored glazes in ceramics. Uranium carbide is a catalyst used for the production of synthetic ammonia (5).

Uranium has 22 isotopes (6). It ultimately decays into the element radium, which then decays to radon, a radioactive gas. Radon gas may seep through house foundations and cause indoor air pollution (7). Radon's isotopes, all of which are radioactive, include mass numbers 200 to 226. "Radon daughters" are fine, solid particles that result from the radioactive decay of radon. They are invisible and odorless and may cause lung cancer after years of respiratory exposure (8).

The National Institute for Occupational Safety and Health and the Occupational Safety and Health Administration have set a recommended exposure limit and a permissible exposure limit of 0.05 mg/m^3 (34 pCi/m^3) for uranium dust, and the Nuclear Regulatory Commission has set an occupational limit of 0.2 mg/m^3 (130 pCi/m^3).

Brief exposure to very high concentrations of uranium hexafluoride resulted in deaths at uranium-processing facilities in 1944 and 1986. The deaths were attributed to the generation of highly toxic hydrofluoric acid and uranyl fluoride (9). Epidemiologic studies of workers at uranium mill and metal-processing plants (where there is little or no increased exposure to radon) showed no increase in deaths attributable to uranium exposure (10). Although gamma radiation is present in all uranium mines, levels rarely exceed the acceptable standard of 5 rad/year.

Renal tubular damage occurs with doses greater than 0.1 mg/kg. A uranium acetate (15 g) ingestion resulted in acute renal failure, refractory anemia, rhabdomyolysis, myocarditis, liver dysfunction with a disproportionate coagulopathy, and paralytic ileus (11).

Uranium itself has not been implicated as a carcinogen; however, uranium miners have higher than expected rates of lung cancer death due to radon and its decay products (12). The International Agency for Research on Cancer has classified radon 222 (^{222}Rn) as a human carcinogen. A subset analysis of the miner data suggests a synergistic effect for combined exposure to ^{222}Rn progeny and cigarette smoke (13). Other factors possibly influencing the relationship between ^{222}Rn progeny exposure and lung cancer include age at exposure, age at risk, exposure rate, sex, other carcinogens, and nonspecific inflammation of the airways (14).

Specific information is not available on the susceptibility of children to the effects of uranium or on whether exposure to uranium affects human reproduction or development. No genetic changes due to radiation have been observed in any human population exposed at any dose of uranium (1).

TOXICOKINETICS AND TOXICODYNAMICS

Absorption of uranium is low by all exposure routes. Systemic absorption from inhaled uranium-containing dusts ranges from 0.76% to 5.00% (16). Gastrointestinal absorption varies from less than 0.1% to 6.0%, depending on the solubility of the uranium compound. Approximately 2% of the uranium in drinking water and dietary sources is absorbed in humans (16).

Uranium is distributed primarily to bone and kidney. Although uranium also distributes to liver, this organ is not a major repository for uranium. The normal adult's body burden is approximately 90 µg—66% in bone, 16% in liver, 8% in kidneys, and 10% in other tissues (17).

Ingested uranium is excreted mostly in the feces; urinary excretion is low. The biologic half-times of soluble uranium compounds (e.g., uranium hexafluoride, uranyl fluoride, uranium tetrachloride, uranyl nitrate hexahydrate) are estimated in days or weeks. Those of the less soluble compounds (e.g., uranium tetrafluoride, uranium dioxide, triuranium octaoxide) are estimated in years (1).

PATHOPHYSIOLOGY

The renal and respiratory effects of uranium are usually attributed to the chemical properties of uranium, whereas the theoretically potential excess cancers are usually attributed to its radiation properties. The pulmonary and renal effects may be due to both chemical and radiation properties, but this relationship has not been demonstrated experimentally (18).

VULNERABLE POPULATIONS

In animals, only 0.01% to 0.03% of an intravenous dose of uranium crossed the placenta (19). No studies were located regarding uranium in breast milk. It is not known if maternal bone stores of uranium (like those of calcium and lead) are mobilized during pregnancy and lactation.

CLINICAL PRESENTATION

Uranium is nephrotoxic. Epidemiologic studies have not found increased mortality in uranium workers due to renal disease (20). Two cases of inhalation and dermal occupational exposures to high concentrations of both soluble and insoluble uranium reported a decreased glomerular filtration rate followed by a return to normal within days (21).

Pulmonary injury, usually noncancerous alveolar epithelium damage of type II cells, can be caused by insoluble reactive chemicals (e.g., uranium tetrafluoride, dioxide, or trioxide and triuranium octaoxide) (22). Studies of uranium workers do not show increased deaths due to uranium-induced diseases of the respiratory system (23). In one case, a man developed myocarditis and rhabdomyolysis after ingestion of uranyl acetate, which resolved over 6 months (12).

After a 5-minute exposure to uranium tetrafluoride fume, a patient developed anorexia, abdominal pain, diarrhea, tenesmus, and pus and blood in the stool (21). A volunteer given a 1-g dose of uranyl nitrate (14.3 mg/kg) experienced acute nausea, vomiting, and diarrhea within hours (24).

DIAGNOSTIC TESTS

There are no specific tests for uranium. The radiation aspects of testing are addressed in Chapter 294. A Geiger counter may help monitor decontamination procedures.

TREATMENT

There are no proven methods for reducing the effects of long-term exposure to uranium. Bicarbonate ion has been administered to increase elimination of uranium (25). Alkalinization of the blood facilitates the renal excretion of uranium and thereby decreases uptake and deposition in critical tissues (kidney, bone). Chelation has limited effectiveness in animals.

In a rat model, ethane-1-hydroxy-1,1-biphosphonate effectively prevented renal damage and mortality after uranium exposure (26). One group found that sodium 4,5-dihydroxybenzene-1,3-disulphonate (Tiron), gallic acid, and diethylamine-tetramine-pentacetic acid were effective agents in dogs (27). Another study found that sodium 4,5-dihydroxybenzene-1,3-disulphonate alone and in conjunction with either diethylamine-tetraamine-pentaacetic acid or ethylenediamine-N,N'-bis(2-hydroxyphenylacetic acid) reduced uranium body burden no more than 35%, indicating that these agents are of limited practical value for the treatment of uranium exposure (28).

REFERENCES

1. Agency for Toxic Substances and Disease Registry, Division of Toxicology. *ATSDR toxicological profile for uranium*. Atlanta: ATSDR, 1999:1–474.
2. EPA. U.S. Environmental Protection Agency Code of Federal Regulation. CFR 421, Subpart AD, 1985.
3. Stokinger HE. Uranium, U. In: Clayton CD, Clayton FE, eds. Industrial *hygiene and toxicology, Vol. 2A*, 3rd ed. New York: John Wiley & Sons, 1981:1995–2013.
4. Lide DR. *Handbook of chemistry and physics*, 74th ed. Boca Raton, FL: CRC Press, 1994:31–32.
5. Hawley GG. *The condensed chemical dictionary*, 10th ed. New York: Van Nostrand Reinhold Co., 1981:1071–1072.
6. Parrington JR, Knox HD, Breneman SL, et al. *Nuclides and isotopes: chart of the nuclides*, 15th ed. San Jose, CA: General Electric Company and KAPL, Inc., 1996.
7. Nazaroff WW, Nero AV, eds. *Radon and its decay products in indoor air*. New York: John Wiley & Sons, 1988.
8. Field RW, Steck DJ, Smith BJ, et al. Residential radon gas exposure and lung cancer: the Iowa radon lung cancer study. *Radiat Res* 1999;151:101–103.
9. Kathren RL, Moore RH. Acute accidental inhalation of uranium: a 38-year follow-up. *Health Phys* 1986;51:609–620.
10. Brown DP, Bloom T. Mortality among uranium enrichment workers. Report to National Institute for Occupational Safety and Health. NTIS PB87-188991. Cincinnati, OH, 1987.
11. Pavlakis N, Pollock CA, McLean G, Bartrop R. Deliberate overdose of uranium: toxicity and treatment. *Nephron* 1996;72:313–317.
12. Samet JM. Radon and lung cancer. *J Natl Cancer Inst* 1989;81:745–757.
13. Band P, Feldstein M, Saccomanno G, et al. Potentiation of cigarette smoking and radiation: evidence from a sputum cytology survey among uranium miners and controls. *Cancer* 1980;45:1273–1277.
14. Field RW. *Radon occurrence and health risk. Occupational medicine secrets*, Philadelphia: Hanley and Belfus, 1999.
15. Reference deleted.
16. Leggett RW, Harrison JD. Fractional absorption of ingested uranium in humans. *Health Phys* 1995;68:484–498.
17. ICRP. International Commission for Radiation Protection. Age-dependent doses to members of the public from intake of radionuclides: part 3, ingestion dose coefficients. *ICRP Publication 69*. Oxford, UK: Pergamon Press, 1995.
18. Dockery DW, Arden P, Xu X. An association between air pollution and mortality in six US cities. *N Engl J Med* 1993;329:1753–1759.
19. Sikov MR, Mahlum DD. Cross-placental transfer of selected actinides in the rat. *Health Phys* 1968;14:205–208.
20. Checkoway H, Pearce N, Crawford-Brown DJ, et al. Radiation doses and cause-specific mortality among workers at a nuclear materials fabrication plant. *Am J Epidemiol* 1988;127:255–266.
21. Zhao S, Zhao FY. Nephrotoxic limit and annual limit of intake for natural U. *Health Phys* 1990;619–623.
22. Wedeen RP. Renal diseases of occupational origin. *Occup Med* 1992;7:449–463.
23. Cragle DL, McLain RW, Qualters JR, et al. Mortality among workers at a nuclear fuels production facility. *Am J Ind Med* 1988;14:379–401.
24. Butterworth A. The significance and value of uranium in urine analysis. *Trans Assoc Ind Med Offrs* 1955;5:30–43.
25. Fisher DR, Kathern RL, Swint MJ. Modified biokinetic model for uranium from analysis of acute exposure of UF6. *Health Phys* 1991;60:335–342.
26. Ubios AM, Braun EM, Cabrini RL. Lethality due to uranium poisoning is prevented by ethane-1-hydroxy-1,1-biphosphonate (EHBP). *Health Phys* 1994;66:540–544.
27. Ortega A, Domingo JL, Gomez M, et al. Treatment of experimental acute uranium poisoning by chelating agents. *Pharmacol Toxicol* 1989;64:247–251.
28. Stradling GN, Gray SA, Moody JC, et al. Efficacy of tiron for enhancing the excretion of uranium from the rat. *Hum Exp Toxicol* 1991;10:195–198.

CHAPTER 234

Vanadium

Seth Schonwald

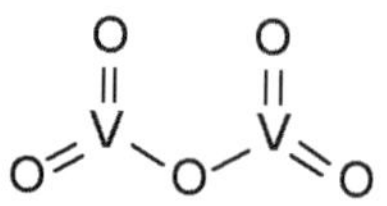

VANADIUM PENTOXIDE

Atomic symbol, atomic number, molecular weight:	**V, 23, 50.94 g/mol**
Valence states:	**−1, 0, +2, +3, +4, +5 (+3, +4, +5 are most common)**
CAS Registry No.:	**7440-62-2**
Normal levels:	**Blood level 1 to 3 μg/L, higher in presence of renal failure**
SI conversion:	**μg/L × 0.0196 = μmol/L**
Target organs:	**Lung and skin from direct irritant effects**
Antidotes:	**None proved; ethylenediaminetetraacetic acid, deferoxamine proposed**

OVERVIEW

Vanadium is named after Vanadis, the Scandinavian goddess of love and beauty. Most vanadium is used to make very strong and durable alloys used widely in the steel industry (1). Vanadium-containing catalysts are used in oxidation reactions to manufacture phthalic anhydride and sulfuric acid and in the production of pesticides and black dyes, inks, and pigments. Vanadium compounds are also used in mercury vapor lamps, paints and varnishes, and corrosion inhibitors in flue gas scrubbers and as components in photographic developers.

Occupational exposure to vanadium and vanadium compounds produces mucous membrane irritation, often accompanied by productive cough, wheezing, rales, chest pain, difficulty in breathing, bronchitis, questionable pneumonia, and rhinitis (2,3).

Vanadium may be an essential dietary requirement, and it may contribute to glucose balance (4). Vanadium is being investigated as a treatment for diabetes (5,6).

Elemental vanadium does not occur in nature, but its compounds exist in many different mineral ores and fossil fuels. The ion is generally bound to oxygen (4). Vanadium pentoxide, for example, is used as a catalyst, dye, and color fixer.

The general population is exposed to vanadium primarily through food. Exposure through inhalation may be important in urban areas where residual fuel oils are burned. Workers are exposed by inhalation in industries processing or using vanadium compounds. People living near vanadium-containing hazardous waste sites may also be exposed to higher levels. People consuming foods grown in soils supplemented with fertilizers or sludge containing vanadium may be exposed to higher concentrations.

Standards

The U.S. Occupational Safety and Health Administration permissible exposure limit is 0.05 mg of vanadium pentoxide/m^3 as a time-weighted average. Direct skin contact with air concentrations of approximately 0.03 mg/m^3 may result in dermal irritation, eczema, generalized rashes (e.g., hives), and contact dermatitis during acute exposures. Direct eye contact with air concentrations as low as 0.018 mg/m^3 may result in irritation, tearing, blurred vision, and a burning sensation of the conjunctiva.

Toxic Dose

There have been no reports of human deaths from vanadium exposure. In one study, workers who had been exposed to vanadium dusts did not show an increased number of cancer deaths, although detailed studies were not performed (7). Federal and international agencies do not list vanadium pentoxide as a carcinogen (8).

TOXICOKINETICS AND TOXICODYNAMICS

Absorption of vanadium occurs after inhalation. Absorption after ingestion is low (9). Vanadium distributes in low levels to human kidney and liver, with less in brain, heart, and breast milk. Higher levels have been detected in hair, bone, and teeth (10). Elimination is primarily in the urine.

PATHOPHYSIOLOGY

Vanadium as vanadate (VO_3^-) inhibits Na^+,K^+–adenosine triphosphatase activity *in vitro* and thus inhibits the sodium-potassium pump (11). This has not been assessed in humans.

VULNERABLE POPULATIONS

Ingestion of vanadium containing soil and dust by children may result in greater exposure than the general population. However, less than 1% of vanadium is absorbed orally. Reproductive studies have not been performed in humans, and data in animals are mixed. Populations in areas with high levels of residual fuel oil use may be exposed to above-background levels of vanadium, both from increased particulate deposition on food crops and soil in the vicinity of power plants and from higher ambient air levels (12).

CLINICAL PRESENTATION

The *respiratory system* is a target organ after acute inhalation exposure of vanadium compounds (13). The mechanism involves interference with alveolar macrophages (14). Clinical effects include mild to moderate respiratory distress and mucosal irritation, resulting in cough, wheezing, chest pain, sore throat, or eye irritation, which can last for several days after exposure. Acute high-concentration inhalation exposure can produce pulmonary edema (15).

Gastrointestinal effects after ingestion of high doses include weight loss, nausea, vomiting, and stomach pain. Green to black discoloration of the tongue, metallic taste, nausea, and diarrhea may occur (16). *Skin contact* may cause dermal irritation, including rash and itching. *Ocular effects* include eye irritation, tearing, and blurred vision after short- and long-term exposures (8). Minor *renal effects* (increased plasma urea and mild histologic changes) have been demonstrated in rat studies after oral exposure to sodium metavanadate ($NaVO_3$) (17). Vanadium has been shown to accumulate transiently in the kidneys after parenteral injection; however, it is difficult to determine the potential for toxicity in humans (18).

DIAGNOSTIC TESTS

The normal blood vanadium concentration is 1 to 3 µg/L. Serum levels are slightly higher. Occupational levels are higher, with serum levels averaging 11 µg/L. Patients with renal failure have higher blood levels.

Pulmonary function testing is appropriate in some cases of symptomatic inhalation exposure. In one case of acute ingestion, magnetic resonance imaging showed lesions in the cortex and subcortex. Focal delta waves were recorded in the parietotemporal region on electroencephalogram.

TREATMENT

After oral exposure, dilution with water or milk has been postulated as one way to decrease absorption (15). Gastric lavage has been suggested as well (19). It has been suggested that activated charcoal be given after significant ingestion of vanadium compounds; however, less than 1% of vanadium is absorbed.

Skin is decontaminated by washing the area with soapy water. For ocular exposure, the eyes are flushed with large amounts of saline or water.

There is no definitive treatment to decrease absorption or increase elimination after inhaling vanadium and its compounds. After acute inhalation exposure to high concentrations of vanadium and its compounds, pulmonary edema may be treated with oxygen and evaluated with serial radiographs (15). Experimental evidence suggests that the administration of steroids may prevent the development of a chemical lung edema.

ANTIDOTES

Enhanced excretion of vanadium was achieved with chelation therapy provided by deferoxamine mesylate in one study (20). Humans or animals with vanadium poisoning have not been helped by the chelating agent dimercaprol (British antilewisite) (21). Intraperitoneal injections of ascorbic acid and of ethylenediaminetetraacetic acid reduced vanadium-induced morbidity in mice and rats (22). In a case of acute ingestion, a patient received deferoxamine mesylate, oral ascorbic acid, plasmapheresis, and dexamethasone (23).

REFERENCES

1. Hilliard HE. Vanadium. The minerals yearbook—minerals and metals. United States Government Printing Office,1987:917–927.
2. Zenz C, Bartlett JP, Theide WH. Acute vanadium pentoxide intoxication. *Arch Environ Health* 1962;5:542–546.
3. Sjoberg SG. Vanadium dust, chronic bronchitis and possible risk of emphysema—a follow-up investigation of workers at a vanadium factory. *Acta Med Scand* 1956;154:381–386.
4. Agency for Toxic Substances and Disease Registry. *Toxicological profile for vanadium*. Atlanta: U.S. Department of Health and Human Services, 1992:1–130.
5. Domingo JL, Sanchez DJ, Gomez M, et al. Oral vanadate and iron in treatment of diabetes mellitus in rats: improvements of glucose homeostasis and negative side-effects. *Vet Hum Toxicol* 1993;35:495–500.
6. Shechter Y, Shisheva A. Vanadium salts and the future treatment of diabetes. *Endeavour* 1993;17:27–31.
7. Orris P, Cone J, McQuilkin S. *Health hazard evaluation report, HETA 80-096-1359, Eureka Company, Bloomington, IL*. Washington, DC: U.S. Department of Health and Human Services, National Institute of Occupational Safety and Health, 1983:NTIS-PB85-163574.
8. Occupational Health Services, Inc. *Material safety data sheet OHS24780—substance: vanadium pentoxide*. New York: Occupational Health Services, 1994.
9. Dimond EG, Caravaca J, Benchimol A. Vanadium: excretion, toxicity, lipid effect in man. *Am J Clin Nutr* 1963;12:49–53.
10. Byrne AR, Kosta L. Vanadium in foods and in human body fluids and tissues. *Sci Total Environ* 1978;10:17–30.
11. Nechay BR, Saunders JP. Inhibition by vanadium of sodium and potassium dependent adenosinetriphosphatase derived from animal and human tissues. *J Environ Pathol Toxicol* 1978;2:247–262.
12. Zoller WH, Gordon GE, Gladney ES, et al. The sources and distribution of vanadium in the atmosphere. In: Kothny EL, ed. *Advances in chemistry series no. 123. Trace elements in the environment*. Washington, DC: American Chemical Society, 1973:31–47.
13. Levy BS, Hoffman L, Gottsegen S. Boilermakers' bronchitis. *J Occup Med* 1984;26:567–570.
14. Castranova V, Bowman L, Wright JR, et al. Toxicity of metallic ions in the lung: effects on alveolar macrophages and alveolar type II cells. *J Toxicol Environ Health* 1984;13:845–856.
15. Stutz DR, Janusz SJ. *Hazardous materials injuries: a handbook for pre-hospital care*, 2nd ed. Beltsville, MD: Bradford Communications Corporation, 1988:406–407.
16. Lewis CE. The biological effects of vanadium. II. The signs and symptoms of occupational vanadium exposure. *AMA Arch Ind Health* 1959;19:497–503.
17. Domingo JL, Llobet JM, Tomas JM, et al. Short-term toxicity studies of vanadium in rats. *J Appl Toxicol* 1985;5:418–421.
18. Bogden JD, Higashino H, Lavenhar MA, et al. Balance and tissue distribution of vanadium after short-term ingestion of vanadate. *J Nutr* 1982;112:2279–2285.
19. HSDB. Hazardous substances databank. Bethesda, MD: National Library of Medicine, National Toxicology Information Program, 1989.
20. Gomez M, Domingo JL, Llobet JM, et al. Effectiveness of chelation therapy with time after acute vanadium intoxication. *J Appl Toxicol* 1988;8:439–444.
21. Lusky LM, Braun HA, Laug EP. The effect of BAL on experimental lead, tungsten, vanadium, uranium, copper and copper-arsenic poisoning. *J Ind Hyg Toxicol* 1949;31:301–305.
22. Jones MM, Basinger MA. Chelate antidotes for sodium vanadate and vanadyl sulfate intoxication in mice. *J Toxicol Environ Health* 1983;12:749–756.
23. Schlake HP, Bertram HP, Husstedt IW, et al. Acute systemic vanadate poisoning presenting as cerebrovascular ischemia with prolonged reversible neurological deficits (PRIND). *Clin Neurol Neurosurg* 1994;96:92–95.

CHAPTER 235
Zinc

Seth Schonwald

Zn=O

ZINC OXIDE

Atomic symbol, atomic number, molecular weight:	**Zn, 30, 65.39 g/mol**
Valence state:	**+2**
CAS Registry No.:	**7646-85-7 (zinc chloride); 1314-13-2 (zinc oxide)**
Normal levels:	**Not applicable**
SI conversion:	**μg/dl × 0.153 = μmol/L**
Target organs:	**Lungs, gastrointestinal**
Antidotes:	**Ethylenediaminetetraacetate, dimercaprol**

OVERVIEW

Zinc is a metallic element discovered by Andreas Marggraf in 1746. It is used widely in alloys for the manufacture of brass and as a protective coating for other metals. Inhalation of zinc oxide is the most common cause of metal fume fever (Chapter 20) (1). Zinc and its alloys are used to make coins in many countries.

Zinc is an essential element. Zinc deficiency is associated with growth retardation, anorexia, delayed sexual maturation, iron deficiency anemia, and alterations of taste (2,3). Zinc compounds are used in sunblock, diaper rash ointment, deodorant, athlete's foot preparation, acne and poison ivy preparation, and antidandruff shampoo. Zinc gluconate has been touted as a cure for the common cold (4). Zinc chloride and zinc sulfate are used as herbicides (5), and zinc phosphide has been used as a rodenticide (Chapter 239) (6). Zinc salts are used as solubilizing agents in many drugs, including insulin (7).

Zinc concentrations in the air are relatively low, except near industrial sources, such as smelters. Occupational exposures to zinc oxide involve pharmaceutical manufacturing, rubber formulation, vulcanizing agents, white pigment, galvanizers, electroplaters, and welders where zinc-containing alloys are heated.

Zinc chloride is used in soldering flux, dry battery cells, oil refining, dentists' cement, and taxidermy. It is a primary ingredient in smoke bombs used for crowd dispersal and is also used in firefighting exercises and by the military. Exposed workers to zinc chloride include military personnel, rubber workers, textile finishers, embalmers, and dental cement makers.

The National Academy of Sciences estimates a recommended daily allowance for zinc of 15 mg/day (men) and 12 mg/day (women). Lower zinc intake has been recommended for infants (5 mg/day) and children (10 mg/day) because of their lower body weights (8). U.S. regulatory guidelines and standards are provided in Table 1.

TOXIC DOSE

Death is rare after acute exposure to zinc compounds. There were 10 deaths among 70 people exposed to a high concentration of zinc chloride smoke in a tunnel during World War II (9). Exposure to zinc oxide, hexachloroethane, calcium silicate, and an igniter were also possible. Two soldiers were exposed to smoke containing zinc chloride and other agents during military training. They died of adult respiratory distress syndrome 25 to 32 days later (10). A firefighter died 18 days after exposure to a smoke bomb (zinc chloride and other substances) in a closed environment; respiratory difficulty from pulmonary fibrosis was the cause of death (11).

The incidence of cancer does not appear to be increased by occupational exposure to zinc (12). An analysis of excess lung cancer associated with a lead and zinc mining and smelting area was elevated in the region but was not associated with environmental levels of lead or zinc (13).

One infant death from bronchopneumonia, resulting from inhalation and possibly ingestion of an unspecified amount of zinc stearate powder, has been reported (14).

TOXICOKINETICS AND TOXICODYNAMICS

Oral absorption after short-term ingestion of zinc supplements ranges from 8% to 81%. Differences in absorption are probably due to the amount of zinc ingested and the amount and kind of food eaten (15,16). Dietary protein appears to facilitate zinc absorption. In plasma, two-thirds of the zinc is bound to albumin; the remainder is bound to other proteins (17). The number

TABLE 1. U.S. regulatory guidelines and standards for zinc

Agency	Description	Concentration
OSHA (air)	Zinc chloride	
	PEL-TWA	1 mg/m^3
	Zinc oxide	
	PEL-TWA	5 mg/m^3 (fume), 15 mg/m^3 (total dust), 5 mg/m^3 (respirable fraction)
ACGIH (air)	Zinc chloride	
	TLV-TWA	1 mg/m^3
	STEL	2 mg/m^3
	Zinc oxide	
	TLV-TWA	5 mg/m^3 (fume)
	STEL	10 mg/m^3 (fume or dust)
NIOSH (air)	Zinc chloride	
	REL-TWA	1 mg/m^3
	STEL	2 mg/m^3
	IDLH	50 mg/m^3
	Zinc oxide	
	REL-TWA	5 mg/m^3 (dust)
	STEL	10 mg/m^3
	Ceiling-TWA	5 mg/m^3 (fume)
	IDLH	500 mg/m^3
EPA	Drinking water	5 mg/L

ACGIH, American Conference of Governmental Industrial Hygienists; EPA, U.S. Environmental Protection Agency; IDLH, immediate danger to life or health; NIOSH, National Institute for Occupational Safety and Health; OSHA, U.S. Occupational Safety and Health Administration; PEL, permissible exposure limit; REL, recommended exposure limit; STEL, short-term exposure limit; TLV, threshold limit value; TWA, time-weighted average.

of binding sites for zinc on albumin and macroglobulin appears to limit the amount of zinc retained by the body. Albumin-bound zinc is correlated with plasma zinc levels.

Zinc is concentrated in the liver after ingestion and is subsequently distributed throughout the body. Muscle and bone contain 90% of total body zinc. Organs containing sizable concentrations of zinc are the liver, gastrointestinal tract, kidney, skin, lung, brain, heart, and pancreas. When plasma zinc levels are high, liver metallothionein synthesis is stimulated, which facilitates the retention of zinc by hepatocytes.

The principal route of excretion of ingested zinc in humans is through the intestine (18). Zinc is mostly secreted via the gut, and the remainder occurs in the urine. Fecal excretion of zinc increases as intake increases (19). Minor routes of elimination include saliva, hair loss, and sweat.

PATHOPHYSIOLOGY

Zinc is an essential nutrient for the function of many metalloenzymes, including alcohol dehydrogenase, alkaline phosphatase, carbonic anhydrase, leucine aminopeptidase, superoxide dismutase, and DNA and RNA polymerase. Zinc is required for normal nucleic acid, protein, and membrane metabolism as well as cell growth and division (1). Zinc phosphide releases phosphine gas, which can enter the blood stream and injure the lungs, liver, kidneys, heart, and central nervous system (20).

VULNERABLE POPULATIONS

An increased incidence of congenital malformations in infants has been associated with maternal zinc deficiency (21). Higher recommended daily allowances are recommended for women during pregnancy and lactation (15 mg/day for pregnant women, 19 mg/day for nursing women during the first 6 months, and 16 mg/day during the second 6 months of nursing).

Zinc enters breast milk but crosses the placenta slowly (22). The *in vitro* transfer of zinc between mother and fetus appears to be bidirectional, with binding in the placenta.

CLINICAL PRESENTATION

Respiratory Effects

Acute exposure to high concentrations of airborne zinc oxide causes metal fume fever, an immune reaction to inhaled metal oxide particles (Chapter 20). Inhaled zinc oxide penetrates alveoli, damages lung tissue, and transiently impairs pulmonary function (23). Inhalation of zinc chloride causes greater damage than zinc oxide. Reported lesions included acute pneumonitis, ulceration of mucous membranes, subpleural hemorrhage, and pulmonary fibrosis. Exposed individuals have died from adult respiratory distress syndrome.

Cardiovascular Effects

In humans, oral exposure of intermediate duration to zinc decreases serum high-density lipoprotein cholesterol levels (24). The decrease in high-density lipoprotein levels may increase the risk of coronary artery disease.

Gastrointestinal Effects

Abdominal pain, vomiting, nausea, esophageal erosions, and gastric hemorrhagic erosion have been observed in humans after acute ingestion of zinc compounds. In most cases, the actual exposure levels are not known. A 15-year-old girl developed epigastric discomfort, gastritis, and hemorrhagic erosion after exposure to 2.6 mg zinc/kg/day as zinc sulfate for 1 week (25). Hepatic effects have not been observed in humans.

Hematologic Effects

Oral chronic exposure to high levels of zinc in humans can cause decreased levels of hemoglobin and hematocrit and microcytic anemia (26,27). The anemia is believed to be the result of zinc-induced copper deficiency. High levels of dietary zinc induce *de novo* synthesis of metallothionein in the intestinal mucosal cells (28). Copper has a higher binding affinity than zinc to metallothionein and replaces zinc.

Dermal and Ocular Effects

Dermal effects depend on the particular zinc salt involved. Zinc oxide creams are used to promote wound healing. Exposure to high concentration zinc oxide dust has resulted rarely in plugging and infection of sebaceous glands. Zinc chloride is irritating to the eyes and skin at high concentration.

DIAGNOSTIC TESTS

Zinc levels vary considerably from one individual to another. Because the zinc level in many biologic and environmental samples is low, it is easy to contaminate the samples. Blood collection tubes have been identified as potential sources of zinc contamination (29).

Atomic absorption spectrometry using a furnace atomizer is a common and simple laboratory technique for zinc analysis of biologic samples, including bone, liver, hair, blood, and urine. It is an economical method for determining trace element composition with good precision, although its sensitivity is not always good at high part per million levels (30).

POSTMORTEM CONSIDERATIONS

Microvascular obliteration, widespread occlusion of the pulmonary arteries, and extensive pulmonary fibrosis were observed at autopsy after death from zinc chloride fume inhalation.

TREATMENT

As zinc salt ingestion typically causes vomiting, ipecac syrup administration is contraindicated after the ingestion of caustic zinc compounds, such as zinc chloride. Although gastric lavage, ingestion of activated charcoal, and cathartics have been recommended to decrease the absorption of zinc, controlled studies have not proved their efficacy. Large amounts of phosphorus and calcium in milk and cheese and phytate in brown bread may reduce absorption of zinc (31). Whole bowel irrigation has been described for zinc sulfate ingestion (32).

The management of patients exposed to large amounts of topical zinc includes removal of the victim from the contaminated area and removal and isolation of contaminated clothing. Excess contaminant is gently brushed away and excess liquids blotted with absorbent material. Exposed skin is washed with water. The eyes should be flushed immediately with water and irrigated with normal saline.

ANTIDOTES

Administration of ethylenediaminetetraacetate to treat humans after exposure to high levels of zinc has been proposed, but experience is lacking. An elevated serum zinc level was reportedly normalized by intravenous (11.5 mg/kg) ethylenediaminetetraacetate in one case (33).

Diethylenetriamine pentaacetic acid and dimercaprol (British antilewisite) have also been reported as antidotes. Dimercaprol was used in a 16-year-old boy who ingested 12 g of metallic zinc (34). The boy reportedly exhibited lethargy and elevated blood zinc concentrations that were reversed after the administration of dimercaprol. Intravenous and nebulized *N*-acetylcysteine increase urinary zinc excretion and decrease plasma levels after inhalation of zinc chloride smoke, but experience is lacking (35).

REFERENCES

1. Agency for Toxic Substances and Disease Registry. *ATSDR toxicological profile for zinc.* Atlanta: U.S. Department of Health and Human Services, Public Health Service, 1994:1–259.
2. Parodi A, Priano L, Rebora A. Chronic zinc deficiency in a patient with psoriasis and alcoholic liver cirrhosis. *Int J Dermatol* 1991;30:45–47.
3. Prasad AS. Clinical spectrum and diagnostic aspects of human zinc deficiency. In: Prasad AS, ed. *Essential and toxic trace elements in human health and disease.* New York: Alan R. Liss, Inc., 1988:3–53.
4. Godfrey JC, Sloane BC, Smith DS, et al. Zinc gluconate and the common cold: a controlled clinical study. *J Int Med Res* 1992;20:234–246.
5. HSDB. *Hazardous substances data bank.* Bethesda, MD: National Library of Medicine, National Toxicology Information Program, 1993.
6. Environmental Protection Agency. Pesticide tolerances for zinc phosphide. *Federal Register* 1991;56:63467–63468.
7. Lloyd TB, Showak W. Zinc and zinc alloys. In: Grayson M, ed. *Kirk-Othmer encyclopedia of chemical technology*, 3rd ed. New York: John Wiley & Sons, 1984;24:835–836.
8. National Academy of Sciences/National Research Council. *Recommended dietary allowances*, 10th ed. Washington, DC: National Academy Press, 1989:195–246.
9. Evans EH. Casualties following exposure to zinc chloride smoke. *Lancet* 1945;2:368–370.
10. Hjortso E, Quist J, Bud M, et al. ARDS after accidental inhalation of zinc chloride smoke. *Intensive Care Med* 1988;14:17–24.
11. Milliken JA, Waugh D, Kadish ME. Acute interstitial pulmonary fibrosis caused by a smoke bomb. *Can Med Assoc J* 1963;8836–8839.
12. Logue JN, Koontz MD, Hattwick MA. A historical prospective mortality study of workers in copper and zinc refineries. *J Occup Med* 1982;24:398–408.
13. Neuberger JS, Hollowell JG. Lung cancer excess in an abandoned lead-zinc mining and smelting area. *Sci Total Environ* 1982;25:287–294.
14. Murray LM. An analysis of sixty cases of drug poisoning. *Arch Pediatr* 1926;43:193–196.
15. Aamodt RL, Rumble WF, Henkin RI. Zinc absorption in humans: effects of age, sex, and food. In: Inglett G, ed. *The nutritional bioavailability of zinc.* Washington, DC: The American Chemical Society, 1983:61–82.
16. Sandstrom B, Cederblad A. Zinc absorption from composite meals: II. Influence of the main protein source. *Am J Clin Nutr* 1980;33:1778–1783.
17. Wastney ME, Aamodt RL, Rumble WF, et al. Kinetic analysis of zinc metabolism and its regulation in normal humans. *Am J Physiol* 1986;251:R398–R408.
18. Reinhold JG, Faradji B, Abadi P, et al. Decreased absorption of calcium, magnesium, and phosphorous by humans due to increased fiber and phosphorous consumption as wheat bread. *Nutr Rev* 1991;49:204–206.
19. Spencer H, Kramer L, Osis D. Zinc metabolism in man. *J Environ Pathol Toxicol Oncol* 1985;5:265–278.
20. HSDB. Hazardous substance database. *Zinc phosphide.* Bethesda, MD: National Library of Medicine, National Toxicology Program (via TOXNET), 1992
21. Sandstead HH. Zinc in human nutrition. In: Bronner F, Coburn JW, ed. *Disorders of mineral metabolism.* New York: Academic Press, 1981:94–159.
22. Beer WH, Johnson RF, Guentzel MN, et al. Human placental transfer of zinc: normal characteristics and role of ethanol. *Alcohol Clin Exp Res* 1992;16:98–105.
23. Blanc P, Wong H, Bernstein MS, et al. An experimental human model of metal fume fever. *Ann Intern Med* 1991;114:930–936.
24. Hooper PL, Visconti L, Garry PJ, et al. Zinc lowers high-density lipoprotein-cholesterol levels. *JAMA* 1980;244:1960–1961.
25. Moore R. Bleeding gastric erosion after oral zinc sulfate. *BMJ* 1978;1:754.
26. Patterson WP, Winkelman M, Perry MC. Zinc-induced copper deficiency: megamineral sideroblastic anemia. *Ann Intern Med* 1985;103:335–386.
27. Gyorffy EJ, Chan H. Copper deficiency and microcytic anemia resulting from prolonged ingestion of over the counter zinc. *Am J Gastroenterol* 1992;87:1054–1055.
28. Cousins RJ. Absorption, transport, and hepatic metabolism of copper and zinc: special reference to metallothionein and ceruloplasmin. *Physiol Rev* 1985;65:238–309.
29. Delves HT. The analysis of biological and clinical materials. *Prog Analyt Atom Spectrosc* 1981;4:1–48.
30. Szpunar CB, Lambert JB, Buikstra JE. Analysis of excavated bone by atomic absorption. *Am J Phys Anthropol* 1978;48:199–202.
31. Pecoud A, Donzel P, Schelling JL. Effects of foodstuffs on the absorption of zinc sulfate. *Clin Pharmacol Ther* 1975;17:469–474.
32. Burkhart KK, Kulig KW, Rumack B. Whole-bowel irrigation as treatment for zinc sulfate overdose. *Ann Emerg Med* 1990;19:1167–1170.
33. Potter JL. Acute zinc chloride ingestion in a young child. *Ann Emerg Med* 1981;10:267–269.
34. Murphy JV. Intoxication following ingestion of elemental zinc. *JAMA* 1970;212:2119–2120.
35. Hjortso E, Quist J, Bud M, et al. ARDS after accidental inhalation of zinc chloride smoke. *Intensive Care Med* 1988;14:17–24.

SECTION

11

Pesticides

CHAPTER 236

Insecticides

Andrew R. Erdman

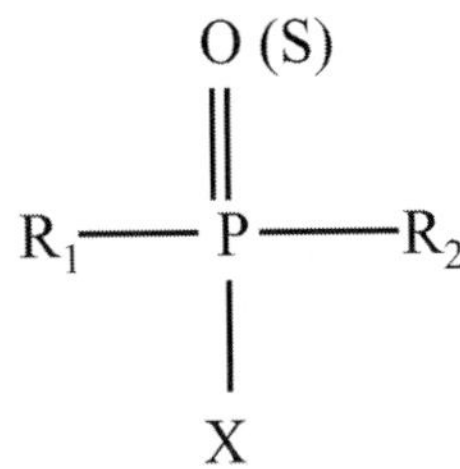

ORGANOPHOSPHATE	
Compounds included:	**Organophosphate insecticides: chlorpyrifos (Dursban), diazinon (Spectracide), dichlorvos (DDVP), fenthion (Baycid), malathion (Cythion), mevinphos (Phosdrin), parathion, diethyl, and many others; carbamate insecticides: aldicarb (Temik), carbaryl (Sevin), propoxur (Baygon), and others; organochlorine insecticides: aldrin (Toxadrin), dieldrin (Quintox), lindane (Kwell), and others**
Molecular formula and weight:	**See Table 1.**
CAS Registry No.:	**See Table 1.**
Special concerns:	**Onset of effects may be delayed after dermal exposure.**
Antidotes:	**Atropine, oximes (pralidoxime, obidoxime)**

OVERVIEW

Insecticides are a diverse group of chemical agents designed to kill and control a broad spectrum of insects. They are used to protect livestock, crops, homes, and communities from the direct damage caused by such insects and from the variety of secondary diseases they may carry. The term *pesticide* is sometimes used interchangeably, but incorrectly, with the term *insecticide*. The former refers to a much broader class of agents used to control not just insects, but any unwanted pest including various animals, plants, or fungi. The term *pesticide* encompasses insecticides, but also rodenticides, herbicides, fumigants, nematocides, algaecides, ascaricides, molluscicides, disinfectants, defoliants, and fungicides.

The development of modern insecticides began in the 1930s with the synthesis of various organochlorines and organophosphorus (OP) compounds. Since that time, tens of thousands of compounds have been developed, including the OP agents, carbamates, organochlorines, pyrethrins and pyrethroids, formamides, avermectins, *N,N*-diethyl-*m*-toluamide, borates, piperonyl butoxide, rotenone, nicotine, arsenicals, thallium compounds, cyanide compounds, and others. The most important and widely used classes of insecticide agents are the OP compounds, carbamates, organochlorines, and pyrethrins/pyrethroids. In general, all four groups work by affecting the well-developed insect nervous system. The mammalian nervous system, however, may also be affected, and because the use of insecticides is so widespread, the potential for human exposures is great.

In 2000, American poison centers reported more than 40,000 exposures to insecticides and approximately six deaths (1). It is likely, however, that this figure significantly underestimates the

TABLE 1. Physical characteristics of selected insecticides

Compound (trade name)	Molecular formula, molecular weight (g/mol), CAS Registry No.
Organophosphate insecticides	
Chlorpyrifos (Dursban)	$C_9H_{11}Cl_3NO_3PS$, 350.58, 2921-88-2
Diazinon (Spectracide)	$C_{12}H_{21}N_2O_3PS$, 304.36, 333-41-5
Dichlorvos (DDVP)	$C_4H_7Cl_2O_4P$, 220.98, 62-73-7
Fenthion (Baycid)	$((CH_3O)_2P(S)OC_6H_3(CH_3)SCH_3)$, 278.33, 55-38-9
Malathion (Cythion)	$C_{10}H_{19}O_6PS_2$, 330.36, 121-75-5
Mevinphos (Phosdrin)	$C_7H_{13}O_6P$, 224.15, 7786-34-7
Parathion, diethyl	$C_{10}H_{14}NO_5PS$, 291.27, 56-38-2
Carbamate insecticides	
Aldicarb (Temik)	$C_7H_{14}N_2O_2S$, 190.27, 116-06-3
Carbaryl (Sevin)	$C_{10}H_7OOCNHCH_3$, 201.22, 63-25-2
Propoxur (Baygon)	$CH_3NHCOOC_6H_4OCH(CH_3)_2$, 209.25, 114-26-1
Organochlorine insecticides	
Aldrin (Toxadrin)	$C_{12}H_8Cl_6$, 364.93, 309-00-2
Dieldrin (Quintox)	$C_{12}H_8Cl_6O$, 380.93, 60-57-1
Lindane (Kwell)	$C_6H_6Cl_6$, 290.85, 58-89-9

actual number of insecticide poisonings because of unrecognized or unreported cases. The U.S. Consumer Product Safety Commission estimated in the early 1990s that there were approximately 20,000 visits to an emergency department annually for pesticide exposures, most of which came from insecticides (2). As many as 3000 to 5000 of these exposures require hospitalization (3). Most of the deaths and severe poisonings from insecticide exposures are the result of OP poisoning, whereas carbamates and organochlorines make up a smaller fraction (4). Most exposures in the United States are accidental, but some are intentional. Exposures in children make up almost one-half of all cases (2).

Exposures to insecticides in countries outside the United States, particularly in developing regions, are a problem of even greater magnitude because of fewer regulations on their manufacture and use; lax or nonexistent workplace training or controls; a greater problem with insect infestations necessitating their use; and poorer access to medical care, decontamination materials, and antidotes. The World Health Organization has estimated an annual incidence of at least 3 million poisonings and more than 200,000 deaths due to insecticides (5). In some countries, such as India, Sri Lanka, Turkey, Taiwan, and parts of Africa, intentional insecticide ingestions are a common form of suicide, due to their relative availability compared to pharmaceuticals (6–9).

CLASSIFICATION AND USES

The categories of insecticides discussed in this chapter include the OP compounds, the carbamates, and the organochlorines. These products are used extensively in a variety of industries, most notably in agriculture, forestry, landscaping, and horticulture. They are used both on livestock and on plants or crops. Many insecticides are used in public areas (e.g., mosquito and fruit fly abatement programs). The people most at risk for exposure are workers involved in their manufacture, packaging, mixing, or application (3). However, a number of compounds can be readily purchased *over the counter* for indoor use, use in household gardens, or on pets. Although generally not as toxic as their commercial counterparts, such products can nonetheless result in serious toxicity.

Accidental poisoning can occur from inhalation and mucous membrane or dermal contact during application periods—most insecticides are applied by spraying, using portable spray devices, automobile mounted sprayers, or airplanes (*crop dusters*). However, significant exposures may also occur from dermal contact with contaminated plants or surfaces even days after application, depending on the product and its environmental persistence. Ingestion of foodstuffs contaminated with insecticide residues may also lead to toxicity. In the United States, pesticides and their application are regulated by the Environmental Protection Agency under the Federal Insecticide, Fungicide, and Rodenticide Act regulations first enacted in 1947.

Intentional exposures are a less common cause of insecticide poisoning, but they often result in greater toxicity. Intentional exposures most often occur by ingestion or injection of the agent.

ORGANOPHOSPHORUS INSECTICIDES

OP agents irreversibly bind to and inhibit the enzyme acetylcholinesterase (AChE). The term *organophosphate* is often used synonymously to describe this broad and diverse class of chemicals, but it is technically incorrect, as many of the constituent have chemical bonds that are not true phosphate bonds.

The first anticholinesterase OP agent (tetraethylpyrophosphate) was synthesized in the 1850s, but its clinical toxicity and potential commercial applications were not recognized initially (3). In the 1930s, diethylfluorophosphate was synthesized, and its toxic effects were noted. This finding impelled the German chemist Schrader to develop parathion and similar agents for use either as pesticides or as chemical warfare agents. More than 50,000 OP chemicals have since been identified, hundreds of which are currently formulated into insecticide products. The commercially available OP products vary in their strength and toxicity (Tables 1 and 2) but in general are far less toxic than the OP compounds developed as chemical weapons. Triorthocresyl phosphate, also an OP agent, has little inherent anticholinesterase activity but has been used as a high-temperature lubricant and plastic softener.

From a toxicologic perspective, the OPs are the most important class of insecticides. OPs account for some 80% of all pesticide-related hospital admissions and are the largest cause of pesticide-related deaths (4,10). In 2000, there were approximately 10,000 exposures to pure OP insecticides reported by U.S. poison centers. Among these, there were five deaths recorded, and approximately 80 cases of major toxicity (1).

Classification and Uses

All OP compounds share a similar chemical structure (Fig. 1). Their central component is a phosphorus atom with a double bond to either oxygen (P=O) or sulfur (P=S), and three side chains. One side chain, the X group or leaving group, differs widely between the OP agents and determines many of its physical and chemical characteristics. The two other side chains, the R_1 and R_2 groups, are typically alkoxy groups but can be almost any aliphatic or aromatic hydrocarbon. These side chains also differ between individual OP agents and account for some variability in their toxicokinetics. Compounds with a sulfur atom (P=S) instead of an oxygen atom (P=O) bound to the phosphorus core are known as *phosphorothioates* or *organothiophosphorus* compounds. Such agents generally have weak inherent toxicity on their own but are metabolized *in vivo* to an OP (oxon) metabolite (P=O) with far greater toxicity. Malathion and parathion

TABLE 2. The relative toxicity of selected organophosphorus and carbamate insecticides, based on a rat lethality model

Organophosphorus agents		
High toxicity (LD_{50} <50 mg/kg)	**Moderate toxicity (LD_{50} = 50–1000 mg/kg)**	**Low toxicity (LD_{50} = >1000 mg/kg)**
Azinphos-methyl (Guthion)	Acephate (Orthene)	Bromophos (Nexagan)
Bomyl (Swat)	Bensulide (Betasan)	Etrimfos (Ekamet)
Carbophenthion (Trithion)	Chlorpyrofos (Dursban, Lorsban)	Iodofenphos (Nuvanol N)
Chlorfenvinphos (Birlane)	Crotoxyphos (Ciodrin)	Malathion (Cythion)
Chlormephos (Dotan)	Cythioate (Proban)	Phoxim (Baythion)
Coumaphos (Co-ral)	DEF (De-Green, E-Z off D)	Propylthiopyrophosphate (Aspon)
Cyanofenphos (Surecide)	Demeton-S-methyl (Metasystox)	Temephos (Abate, Abathion)
Demeton (Systox)	Diazinon (Basudin, Spectracide)	Tetrachlorvinphos (Gardona, Rabon)
Dialifor (Torak)	Dichlorvos (DDVP, Vapona)	
Dicrotophos (Bidrin)	Dimethoate (Cygon)	
Disulfoton (Diasyston)	Edifenphos (EDDP)	
EPN	Ethion (Nialate)	
Famphur (Bo-ana, Warbex)	Ethoprop (Mocap)	
Fenamiphos (Nemacur)	Fenitrothion (Accothion)	
Fenophosphon (Agritox)	Fenthion (Baytex, Entex)	
Isophenfos (Amaze, Oftanol)	Formothion (Anthio)	
Isofluorphate	IPB (Kitazin)	
Mephosfolan (Cytrolane)	Leptophos (Phosvel)	
Methamidophos (Monitor)	Merphos (Folex)	
Methidathion (Supracide)	Naled (Dibrom)	
Mevinphos (Phosdrin)	Phosalone (Zofos)	
Monocrotophos (Azodrin)	Phosmet (Imidan, Prolate)	
Parathion-ethyl	Pirimiphos-ethyl (Dipterex, Dylox, Fernex)	
Parathion-methyl (Penncap-M)	Profenofos (Curacron, Polycron, Selecron)	
Phorate (Thimet)	Propetamphos (Safrotin)	
Phosfolan (Cyolane)	Pyrazophos (Afugan, Curamil)	
Phosphamidon (Dimecron)	Quinalphos (Bayrusil)	
Prothoate (Fac)	Sulprofos (Bolstar)	
Sulfotep (Bladafum)	Thiometon (Ekatin)	
Terbufos (Counter)	Triazophos (Hostathion)	
Tetraethylpyrophosphate (Bladan, TEPP, Tetron)	Tribufos (Butonate)	
	Trichlorfon (Tugon)	

Carbamates		
High toxicity (LD_{50} <50 mg/kg)	**Moderate toxicity (LD_{50} = 50–200 mg/kg)**	**Low toxicity (LD_{50} = >200 mg/kg)**
Aldicarb (Temik)	Bufencarb (Bux)	BPMC (Fenocarb)
Aldoxycarb (Standak)	Carbosulfan	Carbaryl (Sevin)
Aminocarb (Metacil)	Pirimicarb (Pirimor)	Isoprocarb (Etrofolan)
Bendiocarb (Ficam)	Promecarb	MPMC (Meobal)
Carbofuran (Furadan)	Thiodicarb (Larvin)	MTMC (Metacrate, Tsumacide)
Dimetan (Dimetan)	Trimethacarb (Broot)	XMC (Cosban)
Dimetilan (Snip)		
Dioxacarb (Eleocron, Famid)		
Formetanate (Carzol)		
Methiocarb (Mesurol)		
Methomyl (Lannate, Nudrin)		
Oxamyl (Vydate)		
Propoxur (Baygon)		

are two common examples of phosphorothiotes; their respective active metabolites are malaoxon and paraoxon.

OP compounds are either solids or liquids. Solid compounds may be applied as powders when used as an insecticide, but more commonly they are dissolved in a liquid hydrocarbon vehicle for application. The hydrocarbon vehicle enhances the compound's adhesion to and penetration through the insect exoskeleton, and improves its environmental persistence on crops or plants after application. Most commercially available OP products are therefore oily liquids. Whereas some are odorless, many are described as having a garlic-like or kerosene odor of varying strength (11).

Most OP compounds decompose rapidly in the environment by photolysis or hydrolysis. The environmental half-life for

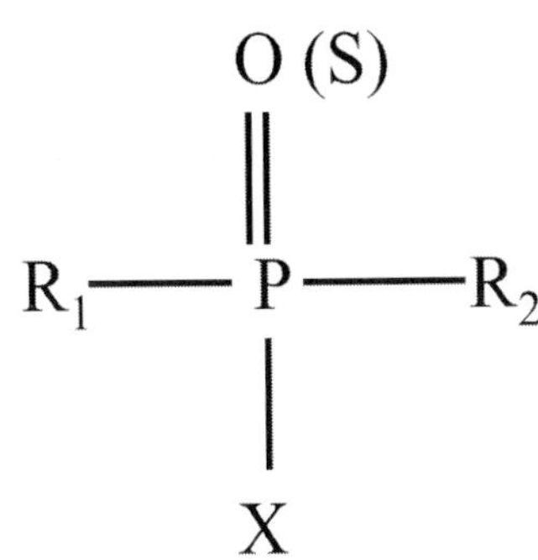

Figure 1. Basic structure of organophosphorus.

most major products is relatively short, typically ranging from hours to days, although some can persist for weeks. Hydrolysis occurs more rapidly at an alkaline pH.

Exposure to OP insecticides can occur by almost any route. Occupational exposures generally occur via direct dermal or mucous membrane contact or by inhalation. Most OP insecticides are not volatile, so exposure by the respiratory route is generally the result of inhalation of aerosolized droplets. Occasionally, accidental exposures may occur with ingestion of contaminated foodstuffs (12,13). Intentional (e.g., suicide) exposures are typically ingestions or parenteral injections of OP compounds.

Toxic Dose

The toxicity of OP compounds varies widely, based on the specific agent, the route and duration of exposure, and patient-specific factors such as genetic differences in OP metabolism and enzyme susceptibility to the agent. The most potent OP compounds are those that have been developed as chemical weapons (e.g., sarin, soman, tabun, VX) (14). Commercial agricultural OP products also have a high toxicity. Animal and household OP products are typically much less potent. An agent's relative toxicity is generally expressed as a measurement of its lethal dose in experimental animals (LD_{50}) (Table 2). There is little human data on toxic dose, but ingestions of as little as a few milliliters of a concentrated solution of some compounds can cause life-threatening toxicity in adults (15).

Toxicokinetics and Toxicodynamics

ABSORPTION

The toxicokinetics of OP agents is complex and varies significantly depending on the agent and its vehicle (16,17). A detailed discussion is beyond the scope of this text, but some general principles are discussed. Many of the differences in the toxicokinetics between various OP compounds are the result of chemical differences in the side chains and core structure.

Most OP compounds are extremely lipophilic, especially the phosphorothioates and compounds containing halogen substitutions (15). They are therefore readily absorbed by passive diffusion, across the lungs and gastrointestinal (GI) tract, with peak blood concentrations occurring within minutes to several hours (16–20). Dermal and mucous membrane absorption tends to be slightly slower, but clinical poisoning can easily develop after prolonged exposures. Powdered compounds are less rapidly absorbed across the skin than liquid agents or agents dissolved in a liquid organic vehicle (21). Abraded, inflamed, or warm, moist skin, or occlusive dressings can dramatically enhance cutaneous absorption. Certain areas of skin are more susceptible than others (e.g., the scrotum and axillae) because of their relatively thin layers and ample blood supply (21,22).

METABOLISM AND ELIMINATION

OP agents are rapidly and widely distributed to various tissues, especially the liver, kidneys, adipose, and tissues rich in lipids, where some agents may accumulate and persist for weeks (18,23,24). The blood elimination half-lives for most of the agents are generally on the order of several hours (18). However, a much longer terminal elimination phase may occur with some of the more fat-soluble agents as the agent slowly leaches back into the blood over time (15,24–30). The overall relationship between an OP agent's reported elimination half-life and the duration of its clinical effects is complex; many of the compounds have active metabolites, tissue-level elimination can vary significantly based on the local content of various detoxification enzyme systems, and once the neuronal AChE has been bound irreversibly, it remains inactive until new enzyme is regenerated.

Most OP agents have direct biological activity, but the phosphorothioates (P=S), such as malathion and parathion, require bioactivation. They undergo oxidative desulfuration, primarily by the cytochrome P-450 system, to form an oxon (P=O) metabolite that possesses much greater toxicity (31–33). The process of bioactivation can slow the onset of effects after exposure (15,23).

Elimination of most agents and their metabolites occurs via a variety of enzyme systems in human plasma, liver, and other organ systems (16,18,31,34). Hydrolysis of the ester bond is one of the more common methods, mediated by various esterases (e.g., carboxylesterase) or paroxonases, which are typically less susceptible to OP inhibition (35,36). Oxidation by the cytochrome P-450 system is another common metabolic pathway. Phosphate-linked hydrolysis and glutathione conjugation may also play a role. The inactive metabolites are excreted in the urine. Various genetic polymorphisms in the detoxification enzyme systems may contribute to individual differences in human susceptibility to the OP agents (37). Chemicals and impurities in the hydrocarbon vehicle of commercial products may alter the elimination of the OP agent.

Pathophysiology

OP agents, or their active metabolites, cause toxicity by inhibiting the function of AChE, the enzyme responsible for hydrolyzing and inactivating the neurotransmitter acetylcholine (ACh) (17,38–45). ACh is vital for the normal transmission of impulses in certain portions of the central nervous system (CNS), in the sympathetic and parasympathetic ganglia, at skeletal neuromuscular junctions, at the parasympathetic nerve terminals innervating certain organ systems and glandular structures, and at the sympathetic nerve terminals innervating sweat glands (Fig. 2). Normally, when cholinergic neurons are depolarized, ACh is released into the synaptic cleft from vesicles stored in the axon terminals (Fig. 3). There it binds to specific postsynaptic receptors, leading to depolarization of the postsynaptic membrane, and further transmission of the impulse or activation of the terminal organ or muscle. Postsynaptic ACh receptors are generally divided into muscarinic and nicotinic subtypes, based on the ability of certain alkaloids (e.g., muscarine or nicotine) to bind and activate them, and based on their mechanism of function (e.g., via G-protein or ligand-gated ion channel).

Normally, ACh is rapidly hydrolyzed to choline and acetic acid in the synaptic cleft by AChE, thus halting further transmission. Accumulation of ACh causes overstimulation of the postsynaptic membranes on neurons, muscles, and glands or organs enervated by the cholinergic neurons. A wide array of systems and functions become overactive. Thus, the resultant clinical findings are based on four main systems affected: the parasympathetic nervous system, sympathetic nervous system, neuromuscular junction, and CNS.

The active site on AChE contains a serine residue with which the OP interacts by phosphorylation (Fig. 4). The serine hydroxyl group gives up its hydrogen to the X group on the OP molecule, which then splits off (hence the name leaving group) as HX. The rest of the OP molecule is then bound covalently to AChE and the enzyme becomes inactive. This initial binding is reversible, but over time one of the R groups may split off, in a process known as aging, and the AChE/OP complex becomes irreversibly bound (46–48). New AChE must be synthesized to replenish its activity. The half-life for the aging process varies among OP agents, ranging from minutes to several days. The rate of aging also influences an agent's toxicity. Spontaneous reactivation of AChE can occur before the aging process, but, by

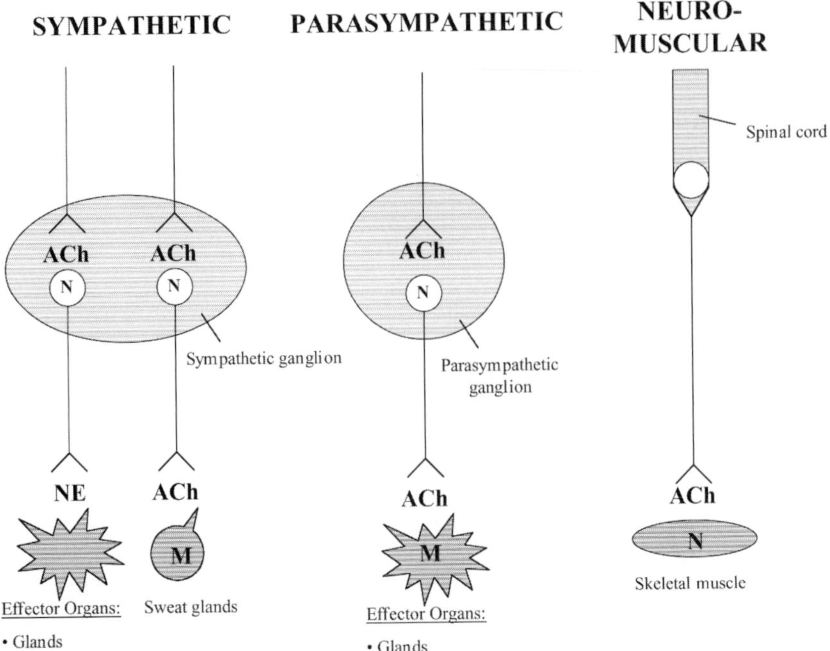

Figure 2. Schematic diagram of peripheral nervous system and sites of acetylcholine (ACh) action. M, muscarinic cholinergic receptors; N, nicotinic cholinergic receptors; NE, norepinephrine.

definition, little occurs after it is complete (49). AChE can also be reactivated before aging by timely treatment with an oxime antidote (e.g., pralidoxime, obidoxime) (50,51).

BUTYRYLCHOLINESTERASE AND ERYTHROCYTE CHOLINESTERASE

The organophosphates bind and inhibit other serine hydrolases, such as butyrylcholinesterase (BChE, also known as plasma cholinesterase or pseudocholinesterase) and erythrocyte cholinesterase (RBC cholinesterase) (11,52). BChE is produced in the liver and can be found in circulating plasma, as well as certain other organs such as the heart or brain. Its endogenous function is not clear, but it is known to play a role in the metabolism of certain xenobiotics (e.g., succinylcholine, cocaine, lidocaine). Erythrocyte cholinesterase is an enzyme similar if not identical to the AChE found at nerve synapses, except that it is bound to the RBC membrane. Both butyrylcholinesterase and erythrocyte cholinesterase can be assayed more readily and easily than synaptic AChE and are used as surrogate markers for the degree of synaptic AChE inhibition.

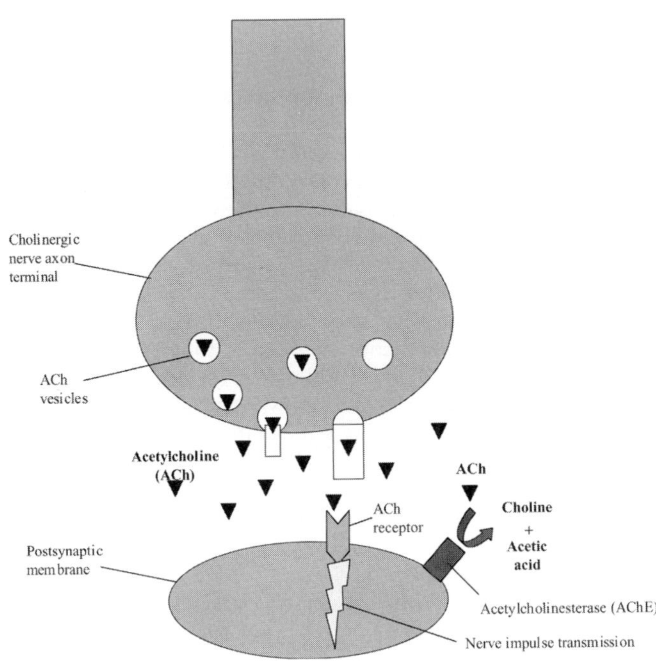

Figure 3. Impulse transmission at cholinergic synapse.

EFFECTS OF EXCESS ACETYLCHOLINE

In the *parasympathetic nervous system*, excessive cholinergic stimulation of nicotinic receptors at the parasympathetic ganglia, and of muscarinic receptors at various exocrine glands and hollow smooth muscle viscera, results in such diverse actions as bladder and bowel stimulation; sphincter relaxation; pupillary constriction; bronchoconstriction; and increased secretion from the lacrimal, salivary (parotid, submaxillary, and sublingual), nasopharyngeal, pancreatic, and bronchial glands. Stimulation of the vagus nerve to the heart can result in bradycardia, although this is sometimes overwhelmed by excessive sympathetic stimulation from a variety of sources.

In the *sympathetic nervous system*, excessive cholinergic stimulation of nicotinic receptors at the sympathetic ganglia may result in catecholamine release and some sympathetic effects, however, these are typically overwhelmed by the effects on the parasympathetic nervous system. Sympathetic signs or symptoms may occasionally predominate. Sweat glands, which are innervated by postganglionic neurons from the sympathetic nervous system, use muscarinic cholinergic receptors and are therefore stimulated by AChE blockade.

At the *neuromuscular junction*, overstimulation of nicotinic receptors on the motor endplate causes myocyte depolarization. As with the paralytic agent succinylcholine, repolarization is thereafter inhibited and the muscle can no longer contract (53).

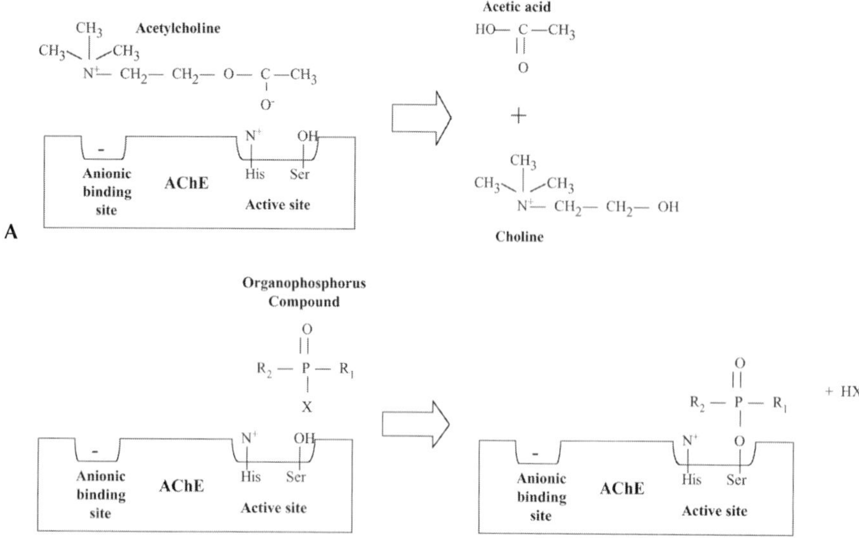

Figure 4. A: Schematic diagram representing the normal action of the enzyme acetylcholinesterase (AChE). **B:** Schematic representing the action of organophosphorus compounds on AChE.

The pathophysiology of OP agents' effects on the CNS is complex and poorly understood. Both muscarinic and nicotinic ACh receptors are present in the mammalian CNS. Earlier reports emphasized the role of muscarinic receptors, but more recent evidence suggests that nicotinic receptors may be important as well. The effects of excessive synaptic ACh may manifest as excitation (seizures, agitation) or suppression (somnolence, coma). The penetration of the blood–brain barrier may also affect the manifestation of CNS symptoms, as can the effects of any coingestants or concomitant hypoxemia or hypotension.

The cardiac effects of OP are unpredictable and reflect the competing effects of multiple influences: vagal stimulation; direct sympathetic stimulation and the effect of circulating catecholamines; and the reflexive or compensatory response to hypoxemia, fluid loss, or CNS agitation.

Significant exposures to OP insecticides can result in four well-described clinical syndromes: (a) acute toxicity from acute high- or intermediate-level exposures or repetitive lower-level exposures of sufficient magnitude, (b) delayed neuromuscular effects days to weeks after acute exposures (also known as *intermediate syndrome*), (c) delayed peripheral neuropathy developing weeks or months after acute exposures (also known as *organophosphate-induced delayed peripheral neuropathy* or OPIDN), and (d) subtle, long-term neuropsychiatric effects (54).

ACUTE TOXICITY

Acute toxicity typically occurs after a single exposure when a significant threshold level of cholinesterase inhibition has been reached. Typically, this occurs when 30% to 50% of AChE has been inhibited, although the percentage varies widely between individuals (52,55). Perhaps more important is the rapidity with which this inhibition occurs (56). This explains why some patients with chronic cumulative exposures do not develop effects as severe as after acute exposures, despite similar enzyme inhibition levels.

CHRONIC OR REPETITIVE EXPOSURES

Occasionally, prolonged or repetitive exposure can produce acute toxic effects; although they are rarely as severe or as rapid in onset as with acute exposures. The pathophysiology of such effects lies partly with the extensive tissue accumulation of some agents and partly with the long period of time required to synthesize new cholinesterase. If the rate of accumulation and hence AChE binding exceeds the body's rate of detoxification and fresh enzyme production, cholinesterase activity levels begin to fall and symptoms develop when each drop below a certain threshold. A degree of tolerance often develops in workers, and thus compared with acute exposures, a greater proportion of cholinesterase must generally be inhibited before effects become evident.

INTERMEDIATE SYNDROME

Intermediate syndrome (IMS) is the delayed development of neuromuscular symptoms in patients recovering from a significant, and often severe, episode of acute OP poisoning (9,57–64). The term *intermediate* is used because the syndrome occurs after the acute cholinergic crisis but before the development of delayed neuropathy. Clinical effects of IMS typically begin 24 to 96 hours after exposure. Almost invariably, patients with IMS have previously experienced significant muscarinic or nicotinic symptoms or a significant fall in cholinesterase activity during the acute episode of poisoning. The incidence of IMS in admitted patients with OP toxicity varies from approximately 10% to 50% (9,63–65).

The etiology and pathophysiology of IMS are poorly understood. It appears to be more commonly associated with some agents than others (e.g., malathion, parathion, fenthion, diazinon, methylparathion, dimethoate, monocrotophos). Some have suggested that it may be due to the redistribution of highly lipophilic agents from adipose tissues as blood levels fall or with fat breakdown (23,57,66,67). Others have speculated that inadequate pralidoxime treatment may be to blame (65,66). Still others have suggested that IMS may not be related to AChE inhibition at all (68). Patients with IMS do not appear to be at any greater risk for developing OPIDN (65).

DELAYED NEUROPATHY

A syndrome termed *OPIDN* may occur 1 to 5 weeks after recovery from the initial toxic exposure to an OP (69–76). The neuropathy may be either motor or sensorimotor and occurs almost exclusively in patients who have had a clinically significant episode of acute poisoning. Only rarely have cases been reported in the absence of acute effects (74). Certain agents have been more frequently implicated, such as triorthocresyl phosphate, parathion, fenthion, chlorpyrifos, malathion, mipafox, merphos, leptophos, cyanophose, and others. Triorthocresyl phosphate was responsible for outbreaks of *Jamaican ginger paralysis*, a type of neuropathy described in the 1930s and associated with the ingestion of a contaminated medicinal agent, Jamaican ginger extract or *Jake* (77).

The pathogenesis of OPIDN does not appear to be due to cholinesterase inhibition (34,78). Rather, the OP-induced phosphorylation and subsequent aging of an enzyme found in nervous tissue, called *neuropathy target esterase*, appear to play a crucial role (79–82). There appears to be a threshold level of neuropathy target esterase inhibition that is required before the effects of OPIDN occur. The phosphorylation of neuronal cytoskeletal proteins may also contribute to the pathophysiology. The role of the hydrocarbon vehicle is unclear.

Axonal degeneration (e.g., Wallerian type) and demyelination are typically found on histopathologic examination, particularly in the larger distal neurons (81). All OP agents in the United States are currently screened for OPIDP before they are considered for registration by the U.S. Environmental Protection Agency.

NEUROBEHAVIORAL AND NEUROPSYCHIATRIC EFFECTS

Numerous reports have suggested that survivors of acute OP poisoning can experience long-term neurobehavioral or psychological sequelae (30,54,83–87). Extrapyramidal manifestations occurring days after poisoning have also been reported (88–90). The pathophysiology of these effects remains unclear. Many of the investigations supporting such sequelae have had significant limitations, and they remain poorly defined. It is important to note that these long-term sequelae generally only develop in patients who experience significant acute exposures.

Chronic low-level exposures to OP agents have also been associated with neuropsychiatric effects, but this issue is controversial. The data are scant and largely based on epidemiologic associations with many confounding variables. A few studies have suggested a correlation between chronic low-level OP exposure in workers and the development of peripheral nervous system toxicity (e.g., hyporeflexia, reduction in vibratory sensitivity) (91,92). Generalized impairments in neuropsychiatric testing have also been reported, as have a variety of mood and anxiety disorders (93–96). An association with chronic fatigue–like symptoms has also been reported (97). Other studies regarding possible neuropsychiatric effects from chronic, low-level exposure are conflicting (98). Well-controlled investigations are needed to characterize the effects further.

Vulnerable Populations

Patients with genetic BChE deficiency may be at increased risk for OP toxicity owing to lower levels of enzyme to compete with OP binding at the neuronal level (99). Genetic variations in carboxylase and some of the other detoxifying enzymes may affect susceptibility, but these have not been well characterized (37). Similarly, the concomitant use of drugs that enhance the metabolic bioactivation (e.g., P-450 inducers) or inhibit the detoxification of various OP agents is expected to enhance their acute toxicity, although the clinical relevance of this is not known.

FETOTOXICITY

Based on animal data, it appears that certain OP agents can cross the placenta and inhibit fetal cholinesterase (100,101). The few reported human cases of pregnant mothers who overdosed on an OP were managed successfully in the usual manner (102,103). Specific reports of fetal toxicity in the absence of maternal toxicity were not found in the literature. Pregnant women with OP poisoning should be managed in the same way as other patients with OP toxicity. The safety and efficacy of administering pralidoxime in the absence of maternal effects has not been studied.

TERATOGENICITY

Animal data on teratogenicity are conflicting and depend on the specific agent. Individual case reports of pregnant women that delivered normal babies after third-term exposure have been published (102,103). Demacarium, echothiophate, and isoglurophate are all U.S. Food and Drug Administration (FDA) pregnancy category C (Appendix I).

Clinical Presentation

ACUTE EXPOSURE

The *onset of clinical effects* depends primarily on the dose, the route of exposure, and the type of compound (i.e., its concentration, lipid solubility, relative toxicity, and direct vs. indirect mechanism of action). Ingestion and inhalation (particularly the latter) result in a more rapid development of symptoms than dermal exposure. After ingestions, symptoms typically occur within 30 to 90 minutes, whereas after dermal exposures they may take 1 to 12 hours (11,104,105). Ingestions generally result in GI symptoms first before the onset of systemic effects; patients with inhalation exposures typically exhibit respiratory effects first, and after ocular exposures, symptoms generally begin in the eyes. Poisoning by agents that require metabolic bioactivation or that are highly lipophilic may result in a greater delay before clinical effects are noted—up to 24 hours in some cases (15). The development of effects can also vary, from progressive (over the course of hours to days) to precipitous deterioration (over the course of minutes). In some cases, deceptively mild initial symptoms may be followed up to 48 hours later by a rapid decline, even despite ongoing antidotal treatment (15).

Clinical poisoning produces a variety of signs and symptoms (Table 3) (9,11,15,25,52,106–110). Their severity varies from mild to life threatening, depending on the exposure dose and potency of the compound (9,106). Large exposures, such as an intentional ingestion, carry the greatest risk for developing severe poisoning (106).

The *classic presentation* of a patient with OP toxicity is often described by the mnemonic SLUDGE (salivation, lacrimation, urination, diaphoresis/defecation, GI motility, emesis) or DUMBELS (defecation, urination, miosis, bronchorrhea/bronchospasm, emesis, lacrimation, and salivation/sweating/seizures). However, these mnemonics neglect the nicotinic and CNS effects of poisoning, understate the clinical significance of the respiratory effects, and fail to account for individual differences in presentation. No single sign or symptom is diagnostic for OP poisoning. Rather, it is the combination of effects and the time course of their evolution that should alert clinicians to the diagnosis.

Clinical effects by receptor type are another method for describing the signs and symptoms of OP toxicity. Poisoning typically represents a dynamic mixture or balance of both muscarinic and nicotinic systems (Table 3). Some patients may present primarily with nicotinic effects before the development of muscarinic effects. However, in severe poisonings, or later in the course of toxicity, muscarinic symptoms typically intervene and a predominantly muscarinic or mixed picture is then observed. Children often display nicotinic and CNS effects (107,108,111).

Although OP poisoning is a disease of cholinergic excess, some patients present, paradoxically, with sympathomimetic rather than cholinergic effects (e.g., tachycardia, hypertension, mydriasis). This is due to excessive stimulation of nicotinic receptors in the sympathetic ganglia or adrenal gland.

TABLE 3. Common effects of acute organophosphorus toxicity

Muscarinic	Nicotinic
Peripheral	
Gastrointestinal	Neuromuscular
Salivation	Muscular fasciculations/twitching
Increased gastrointestinal motility	Cramps
Abdominal cramping/discomfort	Rigidity
Vomiting	Weakness
Diarrhea	Hyporeflexia
Fecal incontinence	Paralysis
Ocular	Hypoventilation
Miosis	Excessive sympathetic output (from stimulation of postganglionic sympathetic neurons and adrenal catecholamine release)
Blurred vision	Mydriasis
Lacrimation	Tachycardia
Respiratory	Hypertension
Rhinorrhea	
Bronchorrhea	
Bronchospasm	
Dyspnea	
Coughing	
Hyperventilation	
Hypoxemia	
Cardiac	
Bradycardia/bradydysrhythmias	
Cardiac conduction delays	
Hypotension	
Genitourinary	
Urination	
Urinary incontinence	
Dermal	
Sweating	
Central nervous system (nicotinic central nervous system receptors may also play a small role)	
Agitation	
Confusion	
Hallucinations	
Somnolence	
Ataxia	
Coma	
Respiratory depression	
Seizures	

Effects by organ system are a third method of assessing OP toxicity. The *cardiac effects* include hypertension or tachycardia from excessive sympathetic outflow, due to direct nicotinic cholinergic stimulation or due to secondary sympathetic outflow caused by a patient's agitation, hypoxemia, or fluid loss (11,15,112). In severe cases, bradycardia and hypotension may predominate (11,15,113,114). Cardiac conduction disturbances and dysrhythmias can also occur (9,112,114–118). Common electrocardiographic findings include QT prolongation, ST segment elevation, varying degrees of atrioventricular block, and PR prolongation. Various ventricular dysrhythmias have been reported but are uncommon.

Respiratory effects include rhinorrhea, excessive nasopharyngeal and bronchial secretions, or pulmonary edema, with evidence of rales, rhonchi, or decreased breath sounds on auscultation (15). Bronchoconstriction can occur, resulting in chest tightness, coughing, wheezing, or decreased air movement on examination. The combination of excessive secretions and narrowed airways can rapidly lead to inadequate gas exchange; this can be exacerbated by any concomitant CNS depression or diaphragmatic weakness. Indeed, respiratory failure is the most common cause of death in patients with severe OP poisoning (8,106). Aspiration pneumonia is also a complication of severe OP poisoning, given the excessive oral and tracheobronchial secretions (106). Noncardiogenic pulmonary edema has also been reported (112).

Neurologic effects include agitation, confusion, dizziness, headache, lethargy, stupor or coma, seizures, muscle fasciculations, weakness, and paralysis. *GI effects* may include salivation, excessive oropharyngeal secretions, nausea, vomiting, abdominal discomfort or cramping, diarrhea or loss of fecal continence, and hyperactive bowel sounds (15). *Ocular effects* include miosis, blurred vision, lacrimation, and occasionally mydriasis.

Nonspecific *laboratory abnormalities* commonly seen in patients with OP poisoning include hyperglycemia and leukocytosis (9,11,106,119–121). Acidosis (due to hypoventilation or hypotension) and hypokalemia are also relatively common (9,106). Mild elevations in liver function tests have been reported, particularly aspartate aminotransferase and lactate dehydrogenase, but it is unclear whether these represent underlying hepatic injury (9,122). Elevated serum amylase and frank pancreatitis have also been reported, as have elevated serum creatine kinase levels in patients with secondary rhabdomyolysis (123,124). In most cases the laboratory abnormalities are not severe.

The *duration of effects* depends on several factors, most important of these are the specific agent, its degree of lipophilicity, and the exposure dose. In most patients, cholinergic symptoms resolve within 2 to 7 days of exposure (106). However, extremely lipophilic agents (e.g., dichlofenthion) may result in prolonged toxicity, up to several weeks in some cases, due to redistribution of the agent from peripheral stores back into the bloodstream (15). Large exposures can also result in significantly prolonged toxicity (106). In some cases, vague, subjective symptoms may persist for months (52).

Other factors affecting duration of illness include the use of oxime therapy and decontamination measures. Oximes in adequate doses can sometimes improve enzyme regeneration and enhance recovery. However, if the OP/AChE complex has had time to age before oxime treatment can be given, symptoms may persist until sufficient AChE can be regenerated via biosynthesis. Inadequate decontamination of patients can result in prolonged absorption, which can also delay the resolution of toxicity.

COMPLICATIONS OF ACUTE TOXICITY

Aspiration pneumonia, various other secondary infections (e.g., urinary tract), and sepsis are common complications of OP poisoning (106). Adult respiratory distress syndrome and multiple organ failure can occur in severely poisoned patients. Rhabdomyolysis and pancreatitis can also occur (123,124).

Reintoxication after a period of initial improvement is also a potentially life-threatening complication, particularly after poisoning by the more lipophilic OP agents (25). Reemergence of both muscarinic and nicotinic symptoms is typical (in contrast to IMS in which neurologic effects predominate) and may occur despite reasonable cholinesterase activity levels.

Mortality in OP poisoning varies. It has been reported to range from approximately 5% to 30% in case series of poisoned patients admitted to the hospital, but it may be higher in certain populations (e.g., suicidal patients) (9,25,106,125,126). Death is most commonly a result of respiratory failure, but occasionally cardiac dysrhythmias and sudden cardiac arrest can occur (8,106).

Hydrocarbon aspiration and subsequent chemical pneumonitis occur as the result of the organic solvent used as a vehicle in some preparations. Patients typically present with coughing; varying degrees of dyspnea or hypoxia; and rales, rhonchi, or wheezing. Radiographic features may take several hours to develop, but typically reveal unilateral or bilateral infiltrates. It may be difficult to distinguish systemic signs of OP poisoning from the effects of aspiration.

CHRONIC OR REPETITIVE EXPOSURES

Symptoms resemble those of acute toxicity, but are usually milder and more insidious in onset. Effects typically include weakness, fatigue, headaches, vague neurologic complaints, miosis, blurred vision, nausea, vomiting, diarrhea, abdominal discomfort, sweating, dyspnea, chest tightness, and occasionally other nicotinic or muscarinic effects. Their onset is variable and depends on the frequency, duration, route, and severity of exposures, as well as the particular OP agent, and various patient-specific factors such as differences in OP susceptibility or metabolism. The diagnosis may be missed due to the nonspecific and protean nature of symptoms, and because a history of exposure may not be as dramatic or readily identifiable.

INTERMEDIATE SYNDROME

IMS is characterized by the development of peripheral neuromuscular symptoms in patients recovering from an episode of OP poisoning (9,58–64). The syndrome typically begins 24 to 96 hours after exposure. Signs include weakness (especially of the proximal musculature), hyporeflexia, and cranial nerve palsies. Interestingly, muscle fasciculations are rare. The neuromuscular effects can progress to frank paralysis with respiratory failure and death (9,64,127). One of the earliest signs of IMS may be the patient's inability to lift his or her head off the bed. Many cases are not diagnosed until significant respiratory insufficiency has developed. Clinical effects usually resolve spontaneously within 1 to 2 weeks of exposure (59,64). Survival is expected with supportive care and mechanical ventilation.

DELAYED NEUROPATHY

Clinical effects of OPIDN typically begin 2 to 3 weeks after an acute OP exposure (69–72,76). Like IMS, OPIDN generally only develops in patients who have exhibited significant acute clinical effects or measurable enzyme inhibition (54). The symptoms typically start in the distal limbs (especially the lower extremities) but can move proximally and into the upper extremities over time. Either motor (e.g., weakness, paralysis) or sensorimotor (e.g., paresthesias, pain, weakness, paralysis) symptoms may occur. Unlike with IMS, neck weakness and cranial palsies are not common. Clinical effects may progress in severity, resulting in ataxia or complete paralysis in some cases. Recovery is variable, with some patients improving spontaneously over months to years and others experiencing permanent or long-term deficits (77).

NEUROBEHAVIORAL AND NEUROPSYCHIATRIC EFFECTS

Long-term neurobehavioral symptoms associated with OP exposures include fatigue, anxiety, depression, restlessness or irritability, confusion, and occasionally frank psychosis. They are generally subtle or mild, begin within days to weeks of an exposure, and resolve spontaneously over the course of several months to a year.

Diagnostic Tests

ACUTE TOXICITY

The diagnosis of OP poisoning may be difficult, particularly in the early stages of poisoning when symptoms may be mild and nonspecific. Confirmation can generally be obtained using measurements of RBC cholinesterase and/or plasma BChE activity—the former is the preferred test in most cases. However, these assays require time, and empiric treatment of the patient should not await the results of confirmatory testing.

As an adjunct to clinical examination, some authors have advocated the use of an *atropine challenge* as a diagnostic aid in patients with suspected OP toxicity (11). A dose of 1 to 2 mg atropine (0.025 mg/kg in children) is administered intravenously (IV) and the patient's clinical response is observed. Patients with muscarinic effects from other causes should improve significantly after atropine. If no clinical improvement occurs, the patient is considered likely to have OP or carbamate poisoning. This therapeutic challenge with atropine has not been studied and is probably neither sensitive nor specific.

Serum, urinary, or tissue levels of most organophosphate insecticides can be performed, provided the offending agent is known or suspected (128). Detectable amounts often persist in the blood for several days and in certain tissues for several weeks. However, the results of specific analysis are generally not readily available, and toxic levels for individual agents have not been established. Hence the clinical use of such measurements is limited. The enzymatic activity level of AChE in neuronal tissues can be assayed, and probably serves as the best representation of the degree of poisoning. However, the procedure requires invasive biopsy sampling and there are no well-recognized standards.

Measurements of *BChE and RBC cholinesterase activity* serve as proxy markers for neuronal AChE activity and are the most useful methods for confirming an OP exposure (11,25,52,129). They can be assayed on routine blood samples and reference values have been established (130–135). In general, BChE levels typically drop more quickly after exposure, whereas RBC cholinesterase takes longer to recover (11). By the time patients present with acute symptoms, both BChE and RBC cholinesterase activity levels are likely to be well below baseline (a 25% decrease is often considered diagnostic). In general, RBC cholinesterase activity levels are more specific, and correlate better with the severity of clinical effects than BChE levels (136). Most laboratories do not have the capabilities to perform rapid in-hospital measurements of cholinesterase activity. Therefore, the use of activity measurements lies primarily in their ability to retrospectively confirm an exposure. Occasionally, activity levels are available quickly enough to assist in ongoing patient management.

Both tests have limitations. One major limitation is that despite their structural and biochemical similarity to neuronal AChE, they are surrogate markers and do not contribute to the clinical toxicity nor do they always correlate with clinical effects (137). In addition, certain OP agents (e.g., diazinon) affect BChE more than they do RBC cholinesterase, whereas others (e.g., parathion) tend to inhibit RBC cholinesterase more (138).

BChE, also referred to as plasma or *pseudo* cholinesterase, is produced by the liver. Exposure to OP insecticides results in a rapid decrease in BChE activity, with a nadir occurring at approximately 24 to 48 hours after exposure (in the absence of treatment) (25,52). There is large inter- and intra-individual variability in baseline activity levels, so the normal reference ranges in most laboratories are broad (up to 300% difference between upper and lower values) (23,133,139–141). As a result, patients who have baseline activity levels in the high-normal range can experience clinical signs of poisoning and still have values that fall above the low-normal level for that same laboratory (52). Results are most helpful when they can be compared to a patient's baseline values. Serial determinations may enhance interpretation.

A number of medical disorders, such as malnutrition, oral contraceptive use, hereditary BChE enzyme deficiency, iron deficiency anemia, hepatic dysfunction, and various chronic disease states can cause a decrease in enzyme activity. Drugs such as succinylcholine, cocaine, and lidocaine, which are metabolized by BChE, may also affect activity levels (142). Patients who work with insecticides chronically may have relatively low baseline levels due to repeated low-level OP exposures. To complicate matters further, BChE may not reflect AChE activity at the neuronal level because of biochemical differences between the two enzymes and differences in the enzyme's location within the body.

After an episode of poisoning, BChE activity levels return to baseline slowly as new enzyme is synthesized in the liver (52). Regeneration of BChE follows an exponential pattern with a recovery half-life of approximately 12 days, and baseline levels of activity are reached approximately 50 days after exposure (143). Oxime administration may enhance the rapidity of enzyme recovery.

Erythrocyte (RBC) cholinesterase, which is bound to the RBC membrane, is biochemically and structurally more similar to the AChE found in neuronal tissues (144). Hence, it is believed to more accurately reflect cholinesterase activity at the neuronal level. Clinical experience indicates that levels do correlate better with the degree of toxicity than BChE activity (25,52,125). There is also less inter- and intra-individual variability (141,145,146). RBC cholinesterase activity levels fall quickly after exposure, although not as quickly as BChE levels, reaching their nadir within 24 to 48 hours (25). Clinical OP effects generally become evident when levels decrease below 50% to 75% of their baseline, and patients with severe poisoning typically have levels below 10% of their baseline (11,25,52,142). However, differences in tissue penetration by the various OP agents and subtle differences in enzyme structure between RBC cholinesterase and neuronal cholinesterase may still result in a disparity between RBC cholinesterase levels and clinical effects (25). As a result, the level of RBC cholinesterase activity does not always predict severity or prognosis in OP poisoning. Indeed, it is likely that the *rate* of inhibition is far more important than absolute amount of inhibition, as evidenced by the observation that patients with chronic, low-level exposures can have decreased cholinesterase activity levels in the absence of significant symptoms. Occasionally, clinical deterioration can occur days after levels have reached their nadir, and even in cases in which activity is beginning to recover; the reason for this is not clear (15).

Although not as severe as BChE, there is still considerable variability in RBC cholinesterase assay values among the population, and temporally within an individual (133,139,140). As a result, patients can experience clinically significant poisoning and still have a RBC cholinesterase level that is within the low normal range (52,56,129,147). RBC cholinesterase activity may also be affected by genetic influences and certain medical conditions, such as anemia or hemolysis, and by ongoing therapy with drugs such as antimalarials or oral contraceptives (148,149). Baseline measurements are an extremely valuable tool when interpreting the results of a single assay. Ideally, serial determinations should be performed.

RBC cholinesterase activity levels take longer to recover after an episode of acute poisoning than do BChE levels. Generally, new RBC production is required to replenish the supply of enzyme once aging has occurred. Hence, it takes up to 120 days for patients to return to their baseline activity level (52,129). The general rule is that levels improve by 0.5% to 1.0% per day (52). Neuronal cholinesterase levels appear to recover more quickly than do RBC levels, because symptoms almost always resolve long before RBC levels reach baseline (11).

Repetitive nerve stimulation testing is a promising modality for assessing the degree of AChE inhibition at the neuromuscular junction both during the acute phase and for IMS (66,150). It provides a relatively accurate, semiquantifiable method of diagnosing and monitoring the nicotinic effects related to OP exposure. Routine *electromyography* may also be a helpful adjunct in the evaluation of OP-induced muscle weakness.

Arterial blood gas and *oximetry* measurements are used to assess the adequacy of the patient's ventilation and oxygenation and may help indicate the need for additional antidotal treatment or endotracheal intubation. Similarly, measurements of *negative inspiratory force* can be valuable in helping the clinician assess the degree of diaphragmatic muscle weakness. *Chest radiography* may help elucidate the extent of any pulmonary secretions or edema, or confirm cases of suspected pulmonary aspiration and hydrocarbon pneumonitis.

An electrocardiogram should be performed in cases of OP poisoning due to the risk of bradydysrhythmias and cardiac conduction abnormalities. *Liver function abnormalities* have been reported after OP exposures and should be monitored after significant exposure. *Serum electrolytes and renal function* should be measured in patients with significant secretions and fluid loss. OP poisoning may occasionally cause either hyper- or hypoglycemia.

CHRONIC OR REPETITIVE EXPOSURE

The diagnosis of OP toxicity due to chronic exposure is often difficult. Measurements of RBC cholinesterase activity are probably the best confirmatory test. A 30% to 50% decrease in activity is generally associated with mild to moderate signs of toxicity. Levels are most helpful if they can be compared to a baseline value, or if they are observed to recover steadily and progressively after removing the patient from exposure. Measurements of BChE activity may also be helpful for evaluating chronic exposures but are less reliable.

Serial measurements of RBC cholinesterase and BChE are often monitored monthly or bimonthly in pesticide workers (138,151–153). In some states, occupational monitoring programs are mandatory. Not only does this enable the clinician to monitor workers for the cumulative effects of repetitive exposure, but also it allows for removal of the patient from work before toxicity develops. A significant drop may also indicate the need for workplace interventions. Workers are generally removed from pesticide work if and when the RBC cholinesterase level falls below 70% of baseline or BChE levels fall below 60% of baseline. They may return to work when the levels rise to above 80%.

DIFFERENTIAL DIAGNOSIS

OP toxicity may be confused with a number of infectious or inflammatory conditions, and particularly with poisonings by other toxic agents. Carbamate insecticides also inhibit AChE and cause an initial clinical syndrome nearly identical to OP poisoning. However, the clinical effects resolve more quickly as described in the following Carbamates section. Drugs such as physostigmine, neostigmine, pyridostigmine, and edrophonium are also carbamates and can cause a similar clinical picture (Chapter 67).

Other agents bind to and stimulate cholinergic receptors directly. Nicotine and its related alkaloids (e.g., coniine, lobeline) activate nicotinic cholinergic receptors. Pilocarpine, carbachol, bethanechol, or methacholine, and muscarine (an alkaloid contained in several species of mushroom) directly activate muscarinic receptors. These syndromes can usually be distinguished from OP poisoning based on exposure history, measurements of RBC or BChE activity, or measurements of the specific agent in urine or blood. Certain medical conditions, such as myasthenia gravis and Eaton-Lambert syndrome, can mimic some of the findings of OP poisoning.

Whenever possible, an effort should be made to identify the exact OP agent responsible in cases of exposure, either from the product label if the package is available, from the material data safety sheet in the case of occupational exposures, or from other databases such as the *Farm Chemical Handbook*.

INTERMEDIATE SYNDROME

The diagnosis of IMS is made based on the clinical history and physical examination (9,58–63). There are no specific diagnostic laboratory tests to confirm the diagnosis, but both plasma and RBC cholinesterase levels are likely to be significantly depressed below baseline. IMS essentially only occurs in patients with a recent clinically significant episode of acute OP poisoning. If performed, an electromyography may reveal tetanic fade and findings consistent with both pre- and postsynaptic involvement (59).

DELAYED NEUROPATHY

The diagnosis of OPIDN is based on a history and physical examination (70–72). The evaluation of peripheral neuropathy is addressed in Chapter 26. There are no specific diagnostic tests to distinguish it from other causes (e.g., alcoholism, diabetes, other toxic agents). The syndrome can be distinguished from IMS by its later onset, the predominance of distal rather than proximal effects, the occasional presence of sensory symptoms, and its duration. Measurements of cholinesterase activity may be normal, as significant enzymatic recovery can occur before the development of neuropathic effects. The electromyography may be suggestive of denervation.

NEUROBEHAVIORAL AND NEUROPSYCHIATRIC EFFECTS

The diagnosis of OP-induced neurobehavioral effects is difficult. There are no diagnostic tests, and the syndrome can easily be confused with other cognitive or psychiatric disorders. Occasionally abnormalities are found on electroencephalography.

DIAGNOSTIC PITFALLS

Making the diagnosis of OP poisoning may be difficult. The classic toxidrome may not be present initially. One potential pitfall is waiting for laboratory confirmation of an exposure (e.g., via measurements of cholinesterase activity) before initiating treatment. Treatment should be administered based on the patient's clinical condition, and response to antidotal treatment may strengthen the diagnosis. Another precaution is that normal cholinesterase activity levels do not rule out OP toxicity. The wide range of *normal* values means that a patient can have a significant decrease in activity but still fall within the normal range.

Treatment

DECONTAMINATION

Patients with ocular exposures should have their eyes irrigated thoroughly with water. All contaminated clothing should be removed and double-bagged. Any exposed areas of skin should then be irrigated thoroughly and washed with soap. Many agents are dissolved in an oily liquid vehicle and may be difficult to remove. Vigorous scrubbing should be avoided to avoid inducing vasodilation and possibly enhancing absorption. Extra attention should be focused on the hair and fingernails. Alcohol-based soaps can help dissolve the insecticide but are generally not readily available. Dilute (0.5%) bleach solutions (10 parts water: 1 part household strength bleach) may inactivate many OP compounds by accelerating their hydrolysis or causing oxidative chlorination but are also not readily available (154).

Gastric decontamination may include aspiration of gastric contents via nasogastric tube if a recent and significant ingestion of a liquid product is suspected. Solid products may require gastric lavage. Ipecac and other emetics should be avoided because of the potential for rapid development of coma or seizures. Activated charcoal appears to bind to some OP agents, and a single dose (1 g/kg) should be administered in most cases. Because atropine treatment can slow intestinal motility, use of a cathartic should be considered in treated patients (if necessary) to enhance intestinal transit and elimination of any remaining OP agent.

Medical personnel should wear appropriate protective gear to prevent self-contamination. Secondary poisoning of rescue workers has been reported after contact with contaminated patients (155,156). A petroleum-based OP can penetrate latex gloves; hence, nitrile or neoprene gloves should be used instead, or alternatively, double-gloving with vinyl gloves. The patient, their clothes, and any bodily fluids may all be contaminated and should be handled appropriately.

ENHANCEMENT OF ELIMINATION

Given the widespread tissue distribution of most OP compounds, it would seem unlikely that extracorporeal measures would be effective. Anecdotal reports of hemoperfusion, hemodialysis, and exchange transfusion to date have been conflicting but with mostly equivocal results (24,157–161).

ANTIDOTES

Atropine is a competitive inhibitor of ACh at the muscarinic cholinergic receptor. It therefore antagonizes the glandular and smooth muscle effects of excessive synaptic ACh. The antimuscarinic effects of atropine can dry excessive secretions; reduce diarrhea, vomiting, and urination; improve sphincteric tone; correct miosis; and improve heart rate, electrical conduction, and blood pressure (11,25,26,28,108,119,162–165). Atropine does not bind to nicotinic receptors, but rare cases of clinical improvement in nicotinic manifestations (e.g., weakness, paralysis) and neuromuscular transmission after its administration have been reported (58,166).

The dose, method of administration, and adverse effects associated with atropine are addressed in detail in Chapter 42. The *primary indication* for atropine administration is excessive bronchial secretions that threaten adequate oxygenation and ventilation. However, patients with significant bradycardia, bradydysrhythmias, or hypotension may also benefit from atropine. The usual starting dose is 2 to 4 mg IV in adults (0.05 mg/kg in children). The dose should be repeated every 2 to 5 minutes as necessary, with increasing incremental doses (e.g., 4 to 8 mg) until effects are sufficiently resolved (e.g., clear lung sounds, adequate oxygenation). Most patients with mild toxicity initially respond to 1 to 10 mg, whereas patients with severe toxicity may require up to 100 mg or more. The major therapeutic endpoint of clinical concern is the control of pulmonary secretions and, perhaps as a secondary goal, the correction of symptomatic bradycardia or bradydysrhythmias.

Atropine has a short half-life relative to most insecticides, so symptoms may recur after its administration. To prevent this, frequent maintenance doses or a continuous infusion should be administered until the patient recovers. Some data suggest that continuous infusions of atropine may be more effective than repeated scheduled boluses (25,26,163,167,168). The usual recommended adult infusion begins at 0.5 to 2.0 mg/hour (0.025 mg/kg/hour for children) and should be titrated to effect. Treatment may be necessary for several days, even weeks in some cases (27,106). Cumulative doses totaling several grams have been required (25,164,169). An adequate hospital supply should be ensured when patients first present for treatment.

Glycopyrrolate has been suggested as an alternative to atropine for control of secretions. It can be administered IV and may have fewer CNS side effects than atropine (170). However, its use has not been extensively evaluated. Scopolamine has also been suggested but remains poorly studied and may have undesirable CNS effects. Nebulized atropine, ipratropium (an inhalable antimuscarinic agent), or β-adrenergic agents may also be administered concurrently to address the pulmonary effects of OP poisoning.

Pralidoxime is a member of a class of drugs known collectively as oximes. When given in adequate doses soon after OP poisoning, oximes may help regenerate active AChE (Chapter 69) (134,162,171–173). However, once aging of the OP:AChE complex has occurred, oximes are no longer effective (46,174).

The oxime group of chemicals also includes obidoxime, asoxime, and trimedoxime. Pralidoxime (2-PAM, Protopam) is currently the only FDA-approved oxime in the United States. Obidoxime is the preferred agent in much of Europe and other parts of the world (23). Oxime-induced reactivation of AChE occurs at both nicotinic and muscarinic sites, so a clinical improvement in nicotinic and muscarinic symptoms can often be achieved (in contrast to atropine, which works almost solely on muscarinic effects). It is not clear to what extent pralidoxime is able to cross the blood–brain barrier and regenerate CNS AChE; theoretically, as a charged quaternary ammonium compound, little should enter the CNS. However, anecdotal cases describe an improvement in CNS effects with its use (175–177).

The data supporting the overall efficacy of pralidoxime for OP insecticide poisoning are limited mostly to case reports or case series and animal data (55,125,164,173,175,176,178–185). Meanwhile, several other case series and trials in humans have suggested that it may not hold any benefit over atropine alone and carries some risk (9,25,126,186–190). However, many of these studies used smaller doses than are generally recommended, and pralixodome may work better for some agents (e.g., parathion, diazinon, dichlorvos, dimethoate) than others (e.g., malathion) (191,192). Continuous infusions may be more efficacious than bolus therapy (164,193). Ultimately, it appears that the efficacy of various oximes is far more complex than commonly perceived, and depends on the individual oxime, the specific OP agent, the relative concentrations of each, and the timing of therapy (173,182). Until more information is available, oxime treatment remains a standard component of care in the United States and is recommended by the World Health Organization and a variety of other sources (194,195).

Because the oximes become ineffective after aging of the OP:AChE complex, pralidoxime should be given as soon as possible after an exposure, preferably within 24 to 48 hours (25,196). However, it may be efficacious later into the course of poisoning, sometimes as many as several days post-exposure (30,65–67,195,197). Some OP agents, such as those used for chemical warfare, have an extremely short aging period, making pralidoxime administration ineffective unless it can be administered immediately after poisoning (Chapter 260).

Oximes are typically administered concomitantly with atropine, and the two drugs may act synergistically. The usual dose of pralidoxime is an IV load of 1 to 2 g over 30 minutes for adults (25 to 50 mg/kg in children), followed by repeated intermittent doses of 1 g (25 mg/kg in children) every 6 to 12 hours as needed, or a continuous maintenance infusion of 500 mg/hour (10 to 20 mg/kg/hour in children). The World Health Organization recommends bolus dosing followed by continuous infusion, (11,28,195,198–201).

The dosage, method of administration, and adverse effects of pralidoxime are addressed in detail in Chapter 69. Treatment should be continued until signs of poisoning have significantly improved. The dose may need to be reduced in patients with renal insufficiency. In patients who do not respond with clinical improvement, there are several possibilities. It may be that an inadequate dose was given, that aging has already occurred, or that a resistant OP agent was responsible for the exposure (e.g., malathion). Or it may be that active OP absorption or tissue redistribution is ongoing. Pralidoxime should be continued in many such situations, as it may be difficult to distinguish the reasons for treatment failure, and because inadequate, delayed, or premature termination of pralidoxime therapy may contribute to development of IMS. Some authors have used serial measurements of RBC cholinesterase to guide pralidoxime therapy.

Diazepam is the anticonvulsant of choice for OP-induced seizures. Even in the absence of seizures, diazepam may act synergistically with other antidotes to improve survival and prevent the development of CNS injury, cardiac effects, or delayed neuropathy (14,162,185,202–206). Prophylactic diazepam should therefore be considered in any patient with significant OP toxicity. The usual dose is 5 to 10 mg IV or intramuscularly in adults (0.1 to 0.2 mg/kg in children). The initial dose may be repeated as clinically indicated for seizures.

Other treatments under investigation for the management of OP poisoning include magnesium, fluoride, and clonidine (207–212). Their use remains experimental.

SUPPORTIVE CARE

The most common cause of death in patients with OP poisoning is respiratory failure. Supplemental oxygen should be given, ideally before atropine administration, as hypoxemia may increase the risk of atropine-induced dysrhythmias (213,214). If ventilation is inadequate, intravenous atropine and inhaled bronchodilators can be tried as previously described, but intubation and mechanical ventilation may be required. Intubation with succinylcholine should be avoided if at all possible because the drug is metabolized predominantly by BChE, and its half-life can be significantly prolonged in OP poisoning (83).

Excessive vagal tone can lead to bradycardia, various bradydysrhythmias, and hypotension. If these are severe, atropine, isotonic fluids, and pressors may be required (Chapter 37). Fluid loss can compound any drop in blood pressure, and the patient's fluid losses should be monitored and replaced as indicated. Caution should be taken to avoid excessive fluid administration as this may exacerbate pulmonary secretions or edema.

Dysrhythmias are treated in the usual fashion. QT prolongation should be managed by correction of any underlying bradycardia, hypoxemia, and electrolyte abnormalities. Supplemental magnesium may be considered. Episodes of torsade de pointes often respond to IV magnesium or electrical overdrive pacing. Seizures should be controlled with diazepam, phenobarbital, and more invasive procedures in refractory patients (Chapter 40). The treatment of hydrocarbon aspiration and any subsequent chemical pneumonitis is discussed elsewhere (Chapter 206).

MONITORING

The patient with a significant OP exposure may deteriorate rapidly (15). Patients with obvious poisoning and those with suspected exposure should receive continuous cardiac monitoring, watching for conduction abnormalities, particularly QT prolongation. Continuous oximetry monitoring is also recommended to look for hypoxemia or hypoventilation. Frequent clinical assessments of pulmonary, cardiac, and neurologic function should be performed and serial cholinesterase levels monitored. Patients should be watched closely until they no longer require atropine or pralidoxime. Symptoms may wax and wane, and, in some cases, patients can deteriorate quickly and unexpectedly. Serious deterioration in clinical condition or cholinesterase activity levels may occur late (hours or even days) in the course of poisoning and despite initial clinical improvement or stabilization with antidotal treatment (25). Patients must be watched carefully until symptoms have completely resolved, and at least 24 to 48 hours have elapsed since the last dose of antidote. Ideally, serial cholinesterase levels should also be improving (15). Symptoms may recur in patients who don contaminated clothing or leather goods (215). Clothes should be washed thoroughly several times and leather goods discarded.

Asymptomatic patients who present after a possible OP exposure should be observed for at least 6 hours. Clinical effects may be delayed in onset after dermatologic exposures to an agent of low fat solubility, and may occur even despite early and adequate decontamination, so consideration should be given to observing such patients for up to 24 hours.

CHRONIC OR REPETITIVE EXPOSURES

Treatment depends on the severity of symptoms. In some cases, removal from the exposure or the institution of improved workplace protective measures may be adequate. Atropine, glycopyrrolate, or other anticholinergic agents can be given if muscarinic symptoms are severe or intolerable. Inhaled β-agonists or anticholinergics may alleviate pulmonary symptoms. There is no evidence to suggest that pralidoxime administration is beneficial, and the AChE/OP enzyme complex is likely to have aged in most cases. Patients should only return to work when RBC cholinesterase levels have returned to near baseline or serial measurements have plateaued.

INTERMEDIATE SYNDROME

Treatment of IMS is supportive. Patients should be monitored closely for the development of respiratory muscle fatigue and progressive hypoxia or hypoventilation (e.g., by measuring neck flexion strength, inspiratory force, and extraocular movements). Mechanical ventilation may be required in some patients. The use of pralidoxime is controversial. Many authors recommend it, but there are little data to support its use (68). The majority of patients recover spontaneously over the course of several days.

DELAYED NEUROPATHY

There is no specific treatment for OPIDN, although animal studies have suggested corticosteroids might be helpful (216). Atropine and pralidoxime do not appear to alter the disease progression or improve symptoms. The prognosis of OPIDN is variable. Patients with mild symptoms may experience significant improvement over time, but those with severe neuropathy are typically left with persistent deficits.

NEUROBEHAVIORAL AND NEUROPSYCHIATRIC EFFECTS

There is no known treatment for OP-induced neurobehavioral effects.

CARBAMATE INSECTICIDES

Carbamates are a diverse group of chemical compounds with a similar structure. Like the OP agents, carbamates inhibit the enzyme AChE. However, the carbamates are generally considered to be less toxic. Carbamates are derivatives of carbamic acid. One of the first recognized agents in this class was physostigmine, an alkaloid isolated from calabar beans in the mid-1800s. In the 1930s, synthetic carbamates began to be developed for use as insecticides. Carbaryl was developed in 1956. A large number of products are currently in use, and, because of their milder toxicity, they are widely available to consumers (Table 2). Certain carbamates, such as physostigmine and pyridostigmine (Chapter 67), neostigmine, and edrophonium, are used medicinally in humans but are not specifically addressed in this chapter. In 2000, American poison centers reported 2700 exposures to pure carbamate insecticides. There were no deaths recorded and only seven cases of major toxicity.

Classification and Uses

Carbamates all share the same basic core structure. Differences in their side chains largely determine their toxicokinetic and toxicodynamic properties (Fig. 5). They are used primarily as broad-spectrum insecticides in the agriculture, landscaping, forestry industries, or home gardening. Thiocarbamates (S-C) and dithiocarbamates (S=C) are generally weak insecticides and are often used as herbicides or fungicides instead. Most carbamates are solids at room temperature and can be applied as dusts or powders. More often they are dissolved in an organic solvent for easier and more effective application.

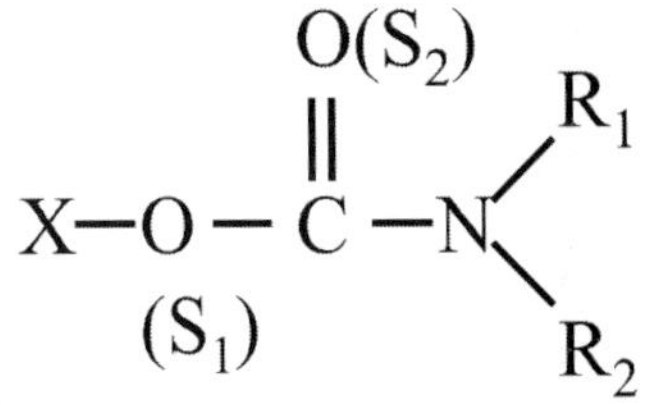

$$X{-}O{-}\overset{\overset{\displaystyle O(S_2)}{\|}}{C}{-}N\begin{matrix} R_1 \\ R_2 \end{matrix} \quad (S_1)$$

Figure 5. Basic chemical structure of a carbamate insecticide.

Exposure to carbamate insecticides can occur by almost any route. Occupational exposures generally occur via direct dermal or mucous membrane contact or by inhalation of aerosolized droplets that form during spray application of the product. Occasionally, accidental exposures may occur with ingestion of contaminated foodstuffs (217,218). This is particularly true with the water-soluble carbamates such as aldicarb, which can accumulate in the water content of certain produce (217). Intentional exposures to carbamates are typically via ingestion or parenteral injection.

Toxic Dose

The toxicity of carbamate insecticides varies widely based on the specific agent and on various patient-specific factors. Human data are inadequate to establish a toxic threshold for individual substances, but ingestions of as little as a few hundred milligrams to a few grams can cause toxicity in an adult (18). The carbamates are divided into three categories of toxicity based on comparisons of their LD_{50} in animal models (Table 2). In general, they are less toxic than most OP insecticides. This is due in part to their relative inability to cross the blood–brain barrier but is also because of their reversible binding and lack of aging. However, cases of severe poisoning and death are not uncommon, particularly after intentional ingestion or exposure (218–221).

Toxicokinetics and Toxicodynamics

Most carbamate insecticides are easily and rapidly absorbed across the skin, lungs, GI tract, and mucous membranes (18,222,223). Some carbamates are more water-soluble (e.g., aldicarb) and therefore absorved more slowly. After ingestion, peak blood levels typically occur within 30 to 60 minutes, but they may peak hours after dermal exposure. Abraded or inflamed skin can enhance cutaneous absorption. Some compounds, known as procarbamates (e.g., thiodicarb), require metabolic conversion *in vivo* to form an active carbamate compound. Exposures to such agents may result in a delay in the onset of clinical effects.

Unlike most OP compounds, the carbamates do not typically penetrate well into the CNS. Most of them are metabolized in the liver by oxidation, hydrolysis, or conjugation (18,224). Both free and conjugated metabolites are then excreted in the urine.

Pathophysiology

ACUTE TOXICITY

Like the OP agents, carbamates bind to and inactivate AChE. However, rather than phosphorylating cholinesterase, they carbamylate it (134,225–227). This carbamate:AChE bond is much less stable and spontaneous decarbamylation occurs readily, resulting in the reactivation of AChE. In addition, the enzyme:inhibitor complex does not undergo the process of aging as it does with

OP agents (228). Nonetheless, the transient inhibition of AChE by a carbamate enables ACh to accumulate at muscarinic and nicotinic receptors in the sympathetic and parasympathetic nervous systems, as well as at neuromuscular junctions and various glandular and smooth muscle organs throughout the body. The resultant clinical picture is similar to OP poisoning, except that the effects are relatively brief and less severe in comparison, and CNS toxicity is less common because of poorer blood–brain barrier penetration.

Rhabdomyolysis, hyperthermia or hypothermia, and acidosis may occur as complications of severe poisoning. Carbamates are commonly dissolved in organic solvents for application, and there is therefore a risk of pulmonary aspiration and hydrocarbon pneumonitis after ingestion. Unlike the OP agents, carbamates do not appear to cause IMS, and instances of delayed or long-term neuropathy and neurobehavioral effects are extremely rare (229,230).

CHRONIC TOXICITY

As with the OP insecticides, frequent chronic or repetitive exposures to carbamates can result in a progressive decline in cholinesterase function and eventually the development of clinical effects. However, this phenomenon is rare because carbamate binding to cholinesterase is reversible and aging does not occur. Chronic or repetitive low-level carbamate exposures have not traditionally been thought to cause significant clinical effects in humans (231,232). However, recent reports reveal a possible association with neurologic complaints (233,234).

Vulnerable Populations

The teratogenic effects of carbamates on the fetus have not been well studied in animals or humans. Fetotoxicity and death have been reported in one case of maternal carbofuran ingestion who was treated with supportive care (235). On postmortem, the fetus appeared normal. Carbamate entry into breast milk has not been described, nor have cases of toxicity in nursing infants.

As with the OP agents, certain patients with a genetic or acquired deficiency or dysfunction in either cholinesterase or the various carbamate-metabolizing enzyme systems may be at risk for acute toxicity.

Clinical Presentation

ACUTE EXPOSURE

The onset of clinical effects after carbamate exposure depends on the dose, the route of exposure, and the type of carbamate (i.e., its concentration, lipid solubility, and relative toxicity). Ingestion, inhalation, and parenteral exposures result in a more rapid onset of effects compared with dermal or ocular exposures. The signs and symptoms of poisoning represent a mixture of muscarinic and nicotinic cholinergic excess, but individual presentations may vary significantly from patient to patient (Table 2) (220,236,237). Most ingestions result in symptoms within 30 to 90 minutes. Dermal exposures typically cause symptoms within several hours, but they may be delayed up to 24 hours in some cases. Patients can deteriorate rapidly with ongoing absorption even after arrival to a medical facility.

Muscarinic receptor stimulation typically produces the same effects as with OP agents. However, significant CNS effects are not common with exposures to carbamate insecticides because of their poor blood–brain barrier penetration. However, agitation and somnolence as the result of hypoxia, hypercarbia, or hypotension can occur in severe poisoning, or as a consequence of coingestants. As with the OP agents, children with carbamate exposures often present with predominantly nicotinic and CNS effects (107).

The duration of symptoms is generally much shorter than with OP poisoning. In most cases symptoms begin to resolve significantly within several hours and often disappear within 24 hours of exposure (238). However, a massive exposure (e.g., suicidal ingestions) or ongoing absorption may produce effects for several days (229,237).

CHRONIC EXPOSURE

Effects due to carbamate accumulation or cumulative inhibition of cholinesterase resemble those of acute toxicity. Chronic exposures have also been reported to cause weakness, anorexia, memory loss, muscle cramps, fasciculations, and symptoms of progressive sensorimotor neuropathy (233,234).

Diagnostic Tests

In most cases, the diagnosis of carbamate poisoning can be made based on a detailed exposure history and the constellation of cholinergic effects, both nicotinic and muscarinic. Measurements of RBC cholinesterase and BChE may be helpful in confirming the diagnosis and guiding therapy (when rapid laboratory turnaround is available). Because carbamate insecticides cause reversible inhibition of AChE without aging, levels of cholinesterase activity return to baseline fairly quickly, coincident with a resolution in clinical effects. As a result, activity measurements should be drawn during the acute phase of illness, the specimen placed immediately on ice, and the assay performed within several hours (to minimize spontaneous decarbamylation and hydrolysis of the agent). The same caveats for OP agents regarding the wide range of *normal* values (and the need for baseline comparison), the influence of other drugs and medical conditions on the results and their imperfect reflection of neuronal cholinesterase activity, also apply with the interpretation of cholinesterase results.

Specific levels of individual carbamate compounds can be measured in blood and other tissues to confirm an exposure, provided the identity of the compound is known or suspected (18). The results are generally not helpful for the acute management of poisoning cases. Such levels may, however, be important for medicolegal or workers compensation purposes.

Treatment

The management of patients with carbamate exposures and toxicity is similar to that for OP compounds. Decontamination and supportive care are identical.

Antidotes do have a role in the management of carbamate toxicity. The indications and doses for *atropine* are the same as with OP toxicity. Given the short duration of effects associated with most carbamate agents, however, maintenance doses or infusions are unlikely to be necessary beyond 24 to 48 hours.

The use of *pralidoxime* for patients with carbamate toxicity is controversial. Some data suggest that pralidoxime may itself inhibit AChE and actually exacerbate the clinical toxicity associated with certain carbamate exposures such as monomethylcarbamate (carbaryl) (219,239–241). In addition, carbamate insecticides do not permanently inhibit AChE. As a result, some authors have argued that oxime treatment is unnecessary. However, in many other cases of carbamate exposure, pralidoxime has been shown to be either beneficial or at least not harmful, and a number of authors still advocate its use (8,236–238,242,242–244).

The monitoring of patients with carbamate toxicity is similar to that for patients with OP toxicity except that recurrent toxicity and IMS do not occur. The patient can therefore be discharged home once symptoms have resolved.

TABLE 4. Classes of common organochlorine insecticides and their constituents

Hexachlorocycloxane isomers	Cyclodienes and related compounds
γ-Hexachlorocyclohexane (lindane, Kwell)	Aldrin (Aldrex, Toxadrin)
DDT and analogues	Chlordane (Octachlor, Toxichlor)
DDT (Ixonex, Neocid)	Dieldrin (Dieldrite, Quintox)
DDD (Rothane)	Dienochlor (Pentac)
DDE	Endrin (Hexadrin)
Chlorbenzilate (Benzilan, Benzochlor)	Endosulfan (Thiodan, Cyclodan)
Dicofol (Kelfane)	Ethylan
Dienochlor	Heptachlor (Drinox)
Methoxychlor (Marlate)	Isobenzan (Telodrin)
	Toxaphene (Alltox)
	Chlordecone and mirex
	Chlordecone (Kepone)
	Mirex (Dechlorane)

DDD, dichlorodiphenyldichloroethane; DDE, dichlorodiphenyldichloroethylene; DDT, dichlorodiphenyltrichloroethane.

TABLE 5. The relative toxicity of selected organochlorine insecticides, based on a rat lethality model

High toxicity (LD_{50} <50 mg/kg)
- Aldrin
- Dieldrin
- Endrin
- Endosulfan

Moderate toxicity (LD_{50} = 50–1000 mg/kg)
- Chlordane
- Dichlorodiphenyltrichloroethane
- Heptachlor
- Kepone
- Lindane
- Mirex
- Toxaphene

Low toxicity (LD_{50} = >1000 mg/kg)
- Ethylan
- Hexachlorobenzene
- Methoxychlor

ORGANOCHLORINE INSECTICIDES

The organochlorine insecticides are a diverse group of complex, cyclic, chlorinated hydrocarbons (Table 4), many of which are still used widely throughout the world, particularly in developing countries, because of their low cost, environmental stability, and efficacy. Dichlorodiphenyltrichloroethane (DDT), the prototypical agent and first organochlorine to be used widely, was synthesized in the late 1800s. Its insecticidal effects went unrecognized until 1939, when Paul Müller discovered its remarkable ability to kill flies (245). DDT was used with great success in worldwide mosquito abatement programs, which led to a significant drop in malaria- and typhus-related mortality. As a result of DDT's public health success and its ease of commercial production, a number of other organochlorine compounds were developed. However, in the 1960s, reports of DDT's environmental persistence began to emerge, along with evidence of its bioconcentration within various animals and its harmful impact on the reproduction of certain bird species (246). So although the organochlorines may be acutely much less toxic to humans than the OP agents or carbamates, many of them have been banned in North America and Europe for ecological reasons; however, their use continues in other parts of the world.

Lindane, the γ-isomer of hexachlorocyclohexane, is another widely used organodichlorine insecticide whose efficacy was first noted in 1942. It has been used extensively as a fumigant for agricultural purposes and is commonly used as a topical medicinal agent for treating humans with scabies or pediculosis (lice). Because of its medicinal use, it is currently the primary organochlorine insecticide of toxicologic concern in the United States.

The organochlorines are less acutely toxic to humans than comparable exposures to an OP or carbamate compound. In 2000, American poison centers reported approximately 2000 exposures to pure organochlorine insecticides (1). There were no deaths recorded and only approximately 40 cases of major toxicity. However, more, large organochlorine exposures can cause significant neurotoxicity, resulting in hyperexcitability, seizures, and even deaths (247–249).

Classification and Uses

The organochlorine insecticides are a group of complex, cyclic chlorinated hydrocarbons, comprising four different categories based on their chemical structure and toxicokinetics (Table 4): (a) hexachlorocyclohexane isomers (e.g., lindane), (b) DDT and its related compounds, (c) cyclodienes (e.g., aldrin, chlordane) and their related compounds, and (d) chlordecone and its precursor mirex. As with the OPs and carbamates, the organochlorine insecticides are frequently classified into categories of relative toxicity, based on their LD_{50} in an animal lethality model (Table 5).

The organochlorine insecticides are solids at room temperature, whereas the chlorinated hydrocarbon solvents and propellants, being of much smaller molecular weight, exist as volatile liquids or gases at room temperature. Most organochlorine insecticides are dissolved in a liquid hydrocarbon vehicle for application. Some, like DDT, can persist for years in soil or water, and accumulate in the animal food chain. Low levels of certain organochlorine compounds are virtually ubiquitous in the enviornment today, and most humans have measurable baseline tissue concentrations.

Lindane is the only organochlorine used medicinally. It is a common, FDA-approved topical agent used to treat patients with pediculosis (lice) or scabies (250) and it is available as a 1% lotion or shampoo. Lindane toxicity can occur as the result of inappropriate dermal use (e.g., large, extended, or repeated applications beyond the normal recommended amount) or after intentional or unintentional ingestion (251–253). Rare cases of seizures have been reported after appropriate therapeutic use (250,254). Inhalational toxicity has been reported in association with its use in home vaporizers.

With the exception of lindane, toxicity from the organochlorine insecticides most often occurs after workplace exposure, usually via inhalation or dermal contact. Accidental ingestion of contaminated foodstuffs is a less common source of poisoning (255). Intentional ingestion of an organochlorine is less common, due to their limited availability.

Toxic Dose

The acute toxic dose of each organochlorine is highly variable. Except for lindane, there is little information in humans. Ingestions of 50 to a few hundred milligrams of lindane can be toxic in children, and a few grams can cause significant toxicity and death in an adult (18,252,256,257). Lindane toxicity can also occur as the result of inappropriate dermal use, but the toxic threshold for transcutaneous toxicity is not known. The usual recommended dose of the 1% shampoo is 1 to 2 oz applied for 4 minutes to hair before thorough rinsing. Occasionally retreatment is necessary 1 week later. The usual recommended dose for the 1% lotion is a complete application over all the skin from the neck down, where it is left on for 8 to 12 hours before thoroughly rinsing off. Rare cases of seizures have been reported after single or therapeutic use (250,253,254,258–261). Dermal absorption may be more efficient when the topical preparations are applied to areas of thinner skin (e.g., scrotum, axillae), warm, moist skin (e.g., under dressings or after a hot shower), or skin that is compromised (e.g., by abrasions, inflammation). Toxicity may also develop with repeated dermal applications, or after products are applied over an extensive surface area or left in place for extended periods of time, as tissue levels accumulate to toxic quantities (260,262).

Toxicokinetics and Toxicodynamics

ABSORPTION AND DISTRIBUTION

All of the organochlorine insecticides are readily absorbed after ingestion or inhalation, with peak levels usually occurring within minutes to hours (18,256). Dermal and mucous membrane absorption is more variable, and depends on the particular agent and its vehicle. Lindane is well absorbed across the skin, and patients with large or repeated dermal applications may develop systemic toxicity (254,260,263–265). Blood lindane levels peak several hours (mean, 6 hours) after dermal application of therapeutic doses; however, peak levels may occur much later with larger exposures (250,254,266). Dermal absorption may be more efficient in areas with thinner skin; in warm, moist environments; or through skin with altered permeability (21,22,260,264). On the other hand, DDT and its analogues [e.g., dichlorodiphenyldichloroethane (DDD), dichlorodiphenyldichloroethylene, chlorbenzylate, dicofol, methoxychlor] are poorly absorbed across the skin but become much more dermally bioavailable when dissolved in an organic solvent (21). Most of the other cyclodienes are well absorbed cutaneously, with the exception of toxaphene (267). Chlordecone and mirex are also dermally well absorbed (18).

Most of the organochlorine insecticides are extremely lipid soluble (18,268). Hence they are widely distributed throughout the body to many tissues where they may accumulate, especially in adipose or lipid-rich neuronal tissue (18,151,269). This property accounts for the numerous reports of acute toxic effects in patients with repeated or prolonged subacute exposures (260,270,271).

METABOLISM AND ELIMINATION

In general, the organochlorines are metabolized in the liver via dechlorination, oxidation, and conjugation (18). Water-soluble metabolites are then renally excreted or eliminated through the biliary tract. Dieldrin undergoes little metabolism and only small amounts are excreted unchanged in the urine. Lindane is rapidly metabolized in the liver, by oxygenation and dehydrohalogenation, to various chlorinated phenols that are then renally excreted in free and conjugated form (18). Chlordecone undergoes reduction, conjugation, and elimination in bile (18,272). A few of the other organochlorine insecticides may exhibit a significant degree of enterohepatic recirculation. In some cases, the metabolites may be more toxic than the parent compound (e.g., the conversion of heptachlor to heptachlor epoxide).

The elimination of the organochlorines also depends on the specific agent. Most agents have prolonged blood elimination half-lives (days to weeks), because they accumulate in fatty tissues and are slowly released or redistributed over time (18). Lindane has a relatively short blood elimination half-life of approximately 18 to 21 hours after therapeutic dosing, due to its rapid metabolism (250,266). However this may be significantly prolonged after overdose or repeated exposure, due to ongoing absorption, tissue accumulation and redistribution, or an overloading of metabolic detoxification pathways (18). For example, blood levels persisted for years in one group of lindane-manufacturing workers (273). Some organochlorines, like DDT, aldrin, dieldrin, chlordane, chlordecone, and mirex, have half-lives of months to years in biological tissues owing to their lipid solubility and slow metabolism. Others, such as methoxychlor, chlorbenzilate, dienchlor, endrin, endosulfan, and toxaphene, are more rapidly eliminated, with half-lives on the order of hours to days.

Vulnerable Populations

Lindane is FDA pregnancy category B (Appendix I) (250). The teratogenic effects of the other organochlorines depend on the agent and are beyond the scope of this chapter. One case of intrauterine fetal demise after the ingestion of lindane has been reported (274). Fetotoxicity from intrauterine exposure to other organochlorines has not been described.

The few human studies available suggest that lindane does enter breast milk in small amounts but is excreted rapidly (250). Many of the other organochlorine compounds have also been reported to be excreted in human breast milk. However, no cases were found of acute neonatal toxicity from breast-feeding infants. The long-term developmental effects are not known.

Little evidence is available, but young children may be at increased risk for organochlorine absorption and toxicity because of their increased surface area to volume ratio, a thinner epidermis, and immature hepatic metabolism. Elderly patients are also at risk due to atrophic skin or hepatic dysfunction. Theoretically, patients with a lower baseline seizure threshold (e.g., concomitant drug therapy, seizure disorder, or structural intracranial lesion) may be at increased risk for organochlorine-related convulsions.

Pathophysiology

The primary target of most organochlorines is the nervous system, particularly the CNS. Despite their chemical and toxicologic differences, most of the organochlorine compounds can be classified into three general pathophysiologic categories based on their mechanism of toxicity in humans and mammals.

LINDANE AND THE CYCLODIENES

Lindane, and the cyclodienes (e.g., aldrin, dieldrin, heptachlor, endrin, chlordane, and endosulfan), act as antagonists to the inhibitory neurotransmitter γ-aminobutyric acid (GABA). Specifically, they bind to and inactivate the $GABA_A$-dependent chloride ion channels (at the same site where picrotoxin binds), preventing the entry of chloride ions into the cell (275–277). This prevents neuronal hyperpolarization, resulting in disinhibition and hence untoward CNS excitation.

DICHLORODIPHENYLTRICHLOROETHANE AND ITS ANALOGS

DDT and its analogs appear to affect axonal sodium channels. By an unknown mechanism, they prevent deactivation or closure of the channels after depolarization in much the same way as the pyrethroids (278,279). This causes a persistent leakage of sodium ions into the neuron after firing, ameliorating the transmembrane potential, and resulting in lower depolarization threshold, spontaneous discharges, and repetitive nerve firing.

CHLORDECONE AND MIREX

The mechanism of chlordecone and mirex toxicity is not clear, but may involve inhibition of various neuronal ion pumps (e.g., sodium-potassium ATPase, or calcium ATPase) (280,281). Unlike the other organochlorine agents, seizures have not been reported with either mirex or chlordecone.

The end result for most significant organochlorine exposures is the development of neuronal dysfunction, typically CNS excitability or seizures, but occasionally CNS depression. Additionally, some organochlorines may sensitize the myocardium to catecholamines, leading to various dysrhythmias and, rarely, cases of sudden death. However, this later phenomenon appears to occur more commonly after inhalation of the volatile chlorinated hydrocarbons used as solvents or propellants, rather than after exposures to the organochlorine insecticides, perhaps because of the more rapid blood levels achieved by the former (Chapter 206).

COMPLICATIONS

Aspiration of the organochlorine insecticides can cause a chemical pneumonitis. Hepatic dysfunction and injury has been reported with exposures to some of the organochlorines, though the mechanism remains unclear. Liver toxicity is more common after chronic exposures.

Clinical Presentation

Clinical toxicity can develop after sufficient acute exposures to any of the organochlorine insecticides. Similar effects can also develop after repeated or prolonged exposures over time, due to their high fat solubility and accumulation in lipid-rich tissues such as the CNS.

ACUTE OR SUBACUTE TOXICITY

Clinical effects generally begin within minutes to several hours after ingestion (typically 1 to 2 hours); after dermal application they typically develop within several hours, but may be delayed much longer (252–254,264). For example, seizures from lindane toxicity may occur several days after application, particularly if absorption is allowed to continue and tissue levels accumulate (261). Clinical effects of toxicity may also lag behind peak blood levels as redistribution to target tissues occurs.

Clinical signs and symptoms of organochlorine toxicity include nausea; vomiting; dizziness; fatigue; headache; agitation; irritability; tremors; fasciculations; paresthesias of the face, mouth, and extremities; and confusion (247,252–255,282–286). Severe toxicity can result in seizures, status epilepticus, coma, and rarely respiratory depression or death (248,255,283,286). With some organochlorines (e.g., lindane), seizures may be the first and only sign of toxicity. This is particularly true after subacute rather than acute overdoses (287). Signs of CNS depression, including somnolence and coma, may occur with certain agents or after severe overdoses (252).

Myocardial sensitization by organochlorines may present as ventricular irritability or dysrhythmias during peak blood drug levels, especially when there is excessive catecholamine stimulation, either endogenous (e.g., fright or pain induced) or exogenous (e.g., pressor administration).

Recovery in patients with acute toxicity typically occurs within 24 to 48 hours of exposure, unless ongoing absorption occurs or complications develop. A few cases of prolonged neurologic effects have been reported after acute overdose (see the following).

COMPLICATIONS

Hyperthermia, acidosis, hypoxemia, and varying degrees of rhabdomyolysis can occur as a complication of excessive muscular hyperactivity (248,288). Hypotension, pulmonary edema, renal and multiple organ failure, disseminated intravascular coagulation, and death have all been reported (257,282,289). Hepatic injury has been associated with a few cases of acute toxicity, but it is unclear to what extent the hydrocarbon vehicle may have contributed. Lindane appears to be hepatotoxic in animals (290).

Aspiration and chemical pneumonitis may present with coughing; varying degrees of dyspnea or hypoxia; and rales, rhonchi, or wheezing. Symptoms may take several hours to develop but can rapidly progress, resulting in severe respiratory distress. Radiographic features may take several hours to develop, but x-rays typically reveal unilateral or bilateral infiltrates. Systemic signs of poisoning can occur in conjunction with aspiration.

A few cases of prolonged peripheral or central neurologic effects have been reported after acute or subacute organochlorine exposure, particularly with lindane (288,291,292). These effects may be due to tissue accumulation and prolonged elimination.

CHRONIC TOXICITY

A few of the organochlorine pesticides have been associated with symptoms of toxicity after chronic exposure, generally in an occupational setting. The agents responsible for chronic toxicity appear to be those with the highest potential for lipid accumulation and lowest metabolism (i.e., compounds that accumulate in tissues with frequent repetitive exposures). It is not clear to what extent the organic solvent vehicle might play a role in the development of chronic toxicity.

Peripheral (e.g., neuropathy) and central (e.g., neurobehavioral or neuropsychiatric) neurologic manifestations have been associated with exposure to certain organochlorines, including lindane, chlordane, heptachlor, aldrin, DDT, and its analogues; however, causality has not been firmly established (293–296). Chlordecone has been associated with a well characterized complex of symptoms including tremors (*Kepone shakes*), weakness, fatigue, anorexia, ataxia, oculomotor findings, neurocognitive or behavioral disturbances, skin rash, slurred speech, and hepatic dysfunction with elevated liver function tests (272,297). Pseudotumor cerebri has been reported with certain agents (272,298). Chronic effects generally begin insidiously after long periods of low-level exposure.

A few of the organochlorines, particularly lindane, have been associated with aplastic anemia and other hematologic abnormalities after long-term exposures (270,294,299,300). The mechanism is not clear. The carcinogenic potential for individual organochlorine agents is beyond the scope of this chapter.

Diagnostic Tests

The diagnosis of organochloride toxicity should be suspected in patients with excitatory CNS symptoms and seizures, particularly if there is a history of working with organochlorine pesticides. Every effort should be made to obtain and confirm the exact ingredients of any pesticide compound to which patients may have been exposed. The differential diagnosis of organochlorine toxicity includes isoniazid, sympathomimetic, anticholinergic, lithium, monoamine oxidase inhibitor, or theophylline toxicity, and various withdrawal syndromes. Medical causes such as meningitis, encephalitis, other infectious diseases, underlying seizure disorders, electrolyte abnormalities, hypoglycemia, and traumatic or neoplastic structural intracranial abnormalities must be ruled out. There are usually no specific clinical findings, although occasionally an unusual odor may be noted, depending on the agent.

There are no readily available diagnostic tests to confirm the diagnosis of organochlorine poisoning. Quantitative levels of the individual agents and their metabolites can be performed by reference laboratories if their identity is known or suspected. Peak blood levels of lindane average approximately 3 ng/ml after a normal application of the shampoo and 24 to 28 ng/ml after total body application of the lotion (250,266). The toxic threshold is not well established and probably differs between individuals. Levels exceeding 20 ng/ml have been associated with symptoms of mild chronic toxicity, such as electroencephalogram changes, twitching, and emotional alterations (294). Levels of 120 to 840 ng/ml have been associated with seizures and severe acute toxicity in case reports (253,256,258,301). Deaths have been reported with blood levels of 1300 ng/ml (289,302). Because of its high fat solubility, CNS levels may be much higher than blood levels (264,303). Measurements of specific levels are generally only useful to confirm an organochlorine exposure retrospectively.

An electrocardiogram may reveal signs of myocardial irritability or dysrhythmias if suspected. Patients with respiratory depression or suspected aspiration should have oxygenation and ventilation checked. Liver function studies and a complete blood count are recommended for patients with large or prolonged exposures. Measurement of serum bicarbonate, creatine kinase, and various electrolytes is important to look for complications of seizures or muscular hyperactivity. Chest radiography should be performed if aspiration is suspected. Because of their degree of chlorination, a few of the organochlorine compounds may be visualized as vague or irregular opacities on radiography. Other studies that may be helpful in assessing patients include a serum chemistry panel to look for electrolyte and glucose abnormalities, kidney function tests to look for renal insufficiency, computed tomography of the brain to rule out structural causes for CNS symptoms, lumbar puncture to look for meningoencephalitis, or electroencephalography to look for underlying seizure foci. Nonspecific electroencephalogram abnormalities are common with significant organochlorine exposures; however, there are no pathognomonic features (294,304).

Treatment

The management of organochlorine exposures and toxicity is symptomatic and supportive.

DECONTAMINATION

Medical personnel should wear appropriate personal protective gear (e.g., gloves, masks, and gowns) to prevent self-contamination. Any contaminated clothing should be removed and double plastic-bagged. Skin should be irrigated and washed with soap and water. Vigorous scrubbing should be avoided to prevent vasodilation and the possibility of increasing absorption.

Ipecac is avoided given the risk for alterations in consciousness and seizures. Nasogastric aspiration may be useful in patients with a recent ingestion of a liquid product. Though its efficacy in organochlorine exposures remains unproven, a dose of activated charcoal may reduce absorption after ingestions.

ENHANCED ELIMINATION

Theoretically the organochlorines, because of their extensive tissue distribution, are not expected to be amenable to extracorporeal removal techniques. However, there is one German report of a patient with lindane toxicity who responded well to hemoperfusion (251).

There is some evidence to suggest that cholestyramine, by binding to bile acids, may enhance the elimination of certain organochlorines (particularly chlordecone) by removing them from the enterohepatic circulation. Its clinical efficacy has been demonstrated in animal models, and human data suggest that it may be beneficial (257,272,305). A dose of 16 g/day is typically recommended.

ANTIDOTES

There are no specific antidotes for any of the organochlorine insecticides.

SUPPORTIVE CARE

Seizures, CNS agitation or depression, and respiratory depression are the primary concerns in most patients. Dysrhythmias due to catecholamine sensitization are extremely rare and may be a theoretical risk. Excessive agitation should be managed aggressively and unnecessary stimulation avoided to limit catecholamine output. Pressors should only be used if absolutely necessary, and agents with the least dysrhythmogenic potential chosen. If dysrhythmias do occur, they should be managed in the usual fashion.

Seizures should be treated initially with benzodiazepines (Chapter 40). Benzodiazepines are preferred because of their specific action as GABA agonists. Phenobarbital or propofol also acts at the GABA receptor and may be considered if benzodiazepines fail to control seizures. Similarly, excessive motor agitation should be managed with the use of benzodiazepines or barbiturates. Antipsychotic agents should be avoided if possible given the potential risk of lowering seizure threshold and because they may exacerbate hyperthermia.

MONITORING

Patients should be watched carefully for the development of toxicity, particularly seizures and other CNS effects. Due to the potential for myocardial sensitization and dysrhythmias, patients should be kept on a continuous cardiac monitor. Seizure precautions should be maintained and the patient's oxygenation monitored.

Organochlorines are well absorbed after ingestion or inhalation, so patients who do not exhibit symptoms within several hours of an acute exposure are unlikely to develop significant effects. After dermal exposure, however, the onset of effects may be delayed. Therefore, consideration should be given to monitoring even asymptomatic patients longer (e.g., up to 24 hours) if a significant dermal exposure has occurred or is suspected.

Patients with toxic effects from organochlorine poisoning can generally be discharged after significant symptomatic improvement has occurred.

REFERENCES

1. Litovitz TL, Klein-Schwartz W, White S, et al. 2000 Annual report of the American Association of Poison Control Centers Toxic Exposure Surveillance System. *Am J Emerg Med* 2001;19:337–95.
2. US Consumer Product Safety Commission. National Electronic Injury Surveillance System (NEISS) estimated injuries associated with pesticide/mothball injuries. Washington: National Injury Information Clearinghouse.
3. Wagner SL. Diagnosis and treatment of organophosphate and carbamate intoxication. *Occ Med* 1997;12:239–49.
4. National Center for Health Statistics. Vital statistics of the United States (for the years 1981–1992), vol. 2, part A ed. Washington: US Public Health Service.
5. Jeyaratnam J. Acute pesticide poisoning: a major global health problem. *World Health Stat Q* 1990;43:139–44.
6. Berger LR. Suicides and pesticides in Sri Lanka. *Am J Public Health* 1988;78:826–8.
7. Agarwal SB. A clinical, biochemical, neurobehavioural, and sociopsychological study of 190 patients admitted to hospital as a result of acute organophosphorus poisoning. *Environ Res* 1993;62:63–70.
8. Tsao TC, Juang YC, Lan RS, et al. Respiratory failure of acute organophosphate and carbamate poisoning. *Chest* 1990;98:631–6.
9. Sungur M, Guven M. Intensive care management of organophosphate insecticide poisoning. *Crit Care* 2001;5:211–5.
10. Environmental Protection Agency. Information statistics. Washington: Environmental Protection Agency, 1980.
11. Namba T, Nolte CT, Jackrel J, et al. Poisoning due to organophosphate insecticides: acute and chronic manifestations. *Am J Med* 1971;50:475–92.
12. Chaudhry R, Lall SB, Mishra B, et al. A foodborne outbreak of organophosphate poisoning. *BMJ* 1998;317:268–9.
13. Wu ML, Deng JF, Tsai WJ, et al. Food poisoning due to methamidophos-contaminated vegetables. *J Toxicol Clin Toxicol* 2001;39:333–6.
14. Sidell FR, Borak J. Chemical warfare agents: II. Nerve agents. *Ann Emerg Med* 1987;16:215–7.
15. Davies JE, Barquet A, Freed VH, et al. Human pesticide poisonings by a fat-soluble organophosphate insecticide. *Arch Environ Health* 1975;30:608–13.

16. Vale JA. Toxicokinetic and toxicodynamic aspects of organophosphorus (OP) insecticide poisoning. *Toxicol Lett* 1998;102–103:649–52.
17. Holmstedt B. Pharmacology of organophosphorus cholinesterase inhibitors. *Pharmacol Rev* 1959;11:567–88.
18. Baselt RC. *Disposition of toxic drugs and chemicals in man*, 6 ed. Foster City, CA: Biomedical Publications, 2002.
19. Griffin P, Mason H, Heywood K, et al. Oral and dermal absorption of chlorpyrifos: a human volunteer study. *Occup Environ Med* 1999;56:10–3.
20. Garfitt SJ, Jones K, Mason HJ, et al. Exposure to the organophosphate diazinon: data from a human volunteer study with oral and dermal doses. *Toxicol Lett* 2002;134:105–13.
21. Idson B. Vehicle effects in percutaneous absorption. *Drug Metab Rev* 1983;14(2):207–22.
22. Franz TJ. Kinetics of cutaneous drug penetration. *Int J Dermatol* 1983;22(9):499–505.
23. Kwong TC. Organophosphate pesticides: biochemistry and clinical toxicology. *Ther Drug Monit* 2002;24:144–9.
24. Martinez-Chuecos J, Jurado MDC, Gimenez MP, et al. Experience with hemoperfusion for organophosphate poisoning. *Crit Care Med* 1992;20:1538–43.
25. Du Toit PW, Muller FO, Van Tonder WM, et al. Experience with the intensive care management of organophosphate insecticide poisoning. *S Afr Med J* 1981;60:227–9.
26. Borowitz SM. Prolonged organophosphate toxicity in a twenty-six month old child. *J Pediatr* 1988;112:302–4.
27. Gerkin R, Curry S. Persistently elevated plasma insecticide levels in severe methylparathion poisoning. *Vet Hum Toxicol* 1987;29:483–4.
28. Karalliedde L, Senanayake N. Organophosphorus insecticide poisoning. *Br J Anaesth* 1989;63:736–50.
29. Sakamoto T, Sawada Y, Nishide K, et al. Delayed neurotoxicity produced by an organophosphorus compound (Sumithion). *Arch Toxicol* 1984;56:136–8.
30. Merrill DG, Mihm FG. Prolonged toxicity of organophosphate poisoning. *Crit Care Med* 1982;10:550–1.
31. Kubistova J. Parathion metabolism in the female rat. *Arch Int Pharmacodyn Ther* 1959;118:308–15.
32. Buratti FM, Volpe MT, Meneguz A, et al. CYP-specific bioactivation of four organophosphorothioate pesticides by human liver microsomes. *Toxicol Appl Pharmacol* 2003;186:143–54.
33. Sams C, Mason HJ, Rawbone R. Evidence for the activation of organophosphate pesticides by cytochromes p450 3A4 and 2D6 in human liver microsomes. *Toxicol Lett* 2000;116:217–21.
34. Costa LG. Basic toxicology of pesticides. *Occ Med* 1997;12:251–68.
35. Costa LG, McDonald BE, Murphy SD, et al. Serum paraoxonase and its influence on paraoxon and chlorpyrifos-oxon toxicity in rats. *Toxicol Appl Pharmacol* 1990;103:66–76.
36. Li WF, Costa LG, Furlong CE. Serum paraoxonase status: a major factor in determining resistance to organophosphates. *J Toxicol Environ Health* 1993;40:337–46.
37. Davies HG, Richter RJ, Keifer M, et al. The effect of human serum paraoxonase polymorphism is reversed with diazinon, soman and sarin. *Nat Genet* 1996;14:334–6.
38. Worek F, Diepold C, Eyer P. Dimethylphosphoryl-inhibited human cholinesterases: inhibition, reactivation and ageing kinetics. *Arch Toxicol* 1999;73:7–14.
39. Adrian ED, Feldberg W, Kilby BA. The cholinesterase inhibiting action of fluorophosphonates. *Br J Pharmacol* 1947;2:56–8.
40. Aldridge WN, Davidson AN. The mechanism of inhibition by organophosphorus compounds. *Biochem J* 1953;55:763–6.
41. Augustinsson KB, Nachmansohn D. Studies on cholinesterase. VI. Kinetics of the inhibition of acetylcholinesterase. *J Biol Chem* 1949;179:543–59.
42. Bagdon RF, DuBois KP. Pharmacologic effects of chlorthion, malathion and tetrapropyl dithionopyrophosphate in mammals. *Arch Int Pharmacodyn* 1955;103:192–9.
43. Barstad JAB. The effect of di-isopropylfluorophosphate on the neuromuscular transmission and the importance of cholinesterase for the transmission of single impulses. *Arch Int Pharmacodyn* 1956;107:21–32.
44. Berry WK. Biochemical mechanism after poisoning with anticholinesterase. *Proc R Soc Med* 1953;46:801–2.
45. Davies DR. Cholinesterases and the mechanism of action of some anticholinesterases. *J Pharm Lond* 1954;6:1–26.
46. Segall Y, Waysbort D, Barak D, et al. Direct observation and elucidation of the structures of aged and nonaged phosphorylated cholinesterase by 31P NMR spectroscopy. *Biochemistry* 1993;32:13441–50.
47. Masson P, Goasdoue JL. Evidence that the conformational stability of "aged" organophosphate-inhibited cholinesterase is altered. *Biochem Biophys Acta* 1986;869:304–13.
48. Berman HA, Decker MM. Kinetic, equilibrium, and spectroscopic studies on dealkylation ("aging") of alkyl organophosphonyl acetylcholinesterase. *J Biol Chem* 1986;261:10646–52.
49. Mason HJ, Waine E, Stevenson A, et al. Aging and spontaneous reactivation of human plasma cholinesterase activity after inhibition by organophosphorus pesticides. *Hum Exp Toxicol* 1993;12:497–503.
50. Davies BR, Green AL. The kinetics of reactivation, by oximes, of cholinesterase inhibited by organophosphorus compounds. *Biochem J* 1956;63:529–35.
51. Wilson IB, Ginsburg S. A powerful reactivator of alkyl phosphate-inhibited acetylcholinesterase. *Biochem Biophys Acta* 1955;18:168–70.
52. Midtling JE, Barnett PG, Coye MJ, et al. Clinical management of field worker organophosphate poisoning. *West J Med* 1985;142:514–8.
53. Karalliedde L, Henry JA. Effects of organophosphates on skeletal muscle. *Hum Exp Toxicol* 1993;289–96.
54. Brown MA, Brix KA. Review of health consequences from high-, intermediate- and low-level exposure to organophosphorus nerve agents. *J Appl Toxicol* 1998;18:393–408.
55. Namba T. Cholinesterase inhibition by organophosphorus compounds and its clinical effects. *Bull WHO* 1971;44:289–307.
56. Summerford WT, Hayes WJ, Johnson JM, et al. Cholinesterase response and symptomatology from exposure to organic phosphorus insecticides. *Arch Ind Hyg Occ Med* 1953;7:383–98.
57. Gadoth N, Fisher A. Late onset of neuromuscular blockade in organophosphorus poisoning. *Ann Intern Med* 1978;88:654–5.
58. Wadia RS, Sadagopan C, Amin RB, et al. Neurological manifestations of organophosphorus insecticide poisoning. *J Neurol Neurosurg Psychiatry* 1974;37:841–7.
59. Senanayake N, Karalliedde L. Neurotoxic effects of organophosphorus insecticides. *N Engl J Med* 1987;316:761–3.
60. Karalliedde L, Senanayake N. Organophosphorus insecticide poisoning. *Br J Anaesth S Afr Med J* 1998:227–9.
61. Samal KK, Sahu CS. Organophosphorus poisoning and intermediate syndrome. *J Assoc Physicians India* 1990;38:181–2.
62. De Bleecker H, Vogelaers D, Ceuterick C, et al. Intermediate syndrome due to prolonged parathion poisoning. *Acta Neurol Scand* 1992;86:421–4.
63. Samuel J, Thomas K, Jesaseelan L, et al. Incidence of intermediate syndrome in organophosphorus poisoning. *J Assoc Physicians India* 1995;43:321–3.
64. He F, Xu H, Qin F, et al. Intermediate myasthenia syndrome following acute organophosphate poisoning—an analysis of 12 cases. *Hum Exp Toxicol* 1998;17:40–5.
65. De Bleecker J, Van Den Neucker K, Colardyn F. Intermediate syndrome in organophosphorus poisoning: a prospective study. *Crit Care Med* 1993;21:1706–11.
66. De Bleecker JL. The intermediate syndrome in organophosphate poisoning: an overview of experimental and clinical observation. *J Toxicol Clin Toxicol* 1995;33:683–6.
67. De Bleecker J, Van den Neucker K, Willems J. The intermediate syndrome in organophosphate poisoning: presentation of a case and review of the literature. *J Toxicol Clin Toxicol* 1992;30:321–9.
68. Sudakin DL, Mullins ME, Horowitz BZ, et al. Intermediate syndrome after malathion ingestion despite continuous infusion of pralidoxime. *J Toxicol Clin Toxicol* 2000;38:47–50.
69. Bidstrup L, Bonnell J, Becket A. Paralysis following poisonings by a new organic phosphorus insecticide (mipafox): report on two cases. *BMJ* 1953;1:1068–72.
70. Moretto A, Lotti M. Poisoning by organophosphorus insecticides and sensory neuropathy. *J Neurol Neurosurg Psychiatry* 1998;64:463–8.
71. Lotti M, Becker CE, Aminoff MJ. Organophosphate polyneuropathy: pathogenesis and prevention. *Neurology* 1984;34:658–62.
72. Senanayake N. Polyneuropathy following insecticide poisoning: a clinical and electrophysiological study. *J Neurol* 1985;203[Suppl]:232.
73. Metcalf DR, Holmes JH. Fenthion and veterinarians: peripheral neuropathy when used in a mixture. *MMWR* 1985;34:26.
74. Kaplan JG, Kessler J, Rosenburg N, et al. Sensory neuropathy associated with Dursban (chlorpyrifos) exposure. *Neurology* 1993;43:2193–6.
75. Argiles AM, Lison D, Lauwerys R, et al. Acute polyneuropathy after malathion poisoning. *Act Neufolo Belg* 1990;90:190–99.
76. De Jager AEJ , van Weerden TW, Houthoff HJ, et al. Polyneuropathy after massive exposure to parathion. *Neurology* 1981;31:603–5.
77. Morgan J, Penovich P. Jamaican ginger paralysis: forty-seven year follow-up. *Arch Neurol* 1978;35:530–2.
78. Lotti M. The pathogenesis of organophosphate neuropathy. *Crit Rev Toxicol* 1992;21:465–87.
79. Abou-Donia MB, Lapadula DM. Mechanism of organophosphorus ester-induced delayed neurotoxicity. *Ann Rev Pharmacol* 1990;30:405–40.
80. Glynn P. Neuropathy target esterase (NTE): molecular characterization and cellular localization. *Arch Toxicol* 1997;19:325–29.
81. Lotti M, Moretto A, Zoppellari R, et al. Inhibition of lymphocyte neuropathy target esterase predicts the development of organophosphate-induced delayed polyneuropathy. *Arch Toxicol* 1986;59:176–9.
82. Johnson MK. Organophosphorus esters causing delayed neurotoxic effects: mechanism of action and structure/activity relationships. *Arch Toxicol* 1975;34:259–88.
83. Selden BS, Curry SC. Prolonged succinylcholine-induced paralysis in organophosphorus insecticide poisoning. *Ann Emerg Med* 1987;16:215–7.
84. Tabershaw IR, Cooper C. Sequelae of acute organic phosphate poisoning. *J Occup Med* 1966;8:5–20.
85. Savage EP, Keefe TJ, Mounce LM, et al. Chronic neurologic sequelae of acute organophosphate pesticide poisoning. *Arch Environ Health* 1988;43:38–45.
86. Rosenstock L, Keifer M, Daniell WE, et al. Chronic central nervous system effects of acute organophosphate pesticide intoxication. *Lancet* 1991;338:223–7.
87. Steenland K, Jenkins B, Ames RG, et al. Chronic neurological sequelae to organophosphate pesticide poisoning. *Am J Public Health* 1994;84:731–6.
88. Bhatt MH, Elias MA, Mankodi AK. Acute reversible parkinsonism due to organophosphate pesticide intoxication. *Neurology* 1999;52:1467.
89. Senanayake N, Sanmuganathan PS. Extrapyramidal manifestations complicating organophosphorus insecticide poisoning. *Hum Exp Toxicol* 1995;14:600–4.
90. Joubert J, Joubert PH. Chorea and psychiatric changes in organophosphate poisoning. *S Afr Med J* 1988;74:32–4.

91. Davignon L, St-Pierre J, Charest G. A study of the chronic effects of pesticides in man. *Can Med Soc J* 1965;92:597–602.
92. Stokes L, Stark A, Marshall E, et al. Neurotoxicity among pesticide applicators exposed to organophosphates. *Occ Environ Med* 1995;52:648–53.
93. Levin HS, Rodnitzky RL, Mick DL. Anxiety associated with exposure to organophosphate compounds. *Arch Gen Psychiatry* 1976;33:225–8.
94. Metcalf RL, Holmes JH. EEG, psychological and neurological alterations in humans with organophosphorus exposures. *Ann N Y Acad Sci* 1969;160:357.
95. Korsak RJ, Kato MM. Effects of organophosphate pesticide exposure on the central nervous system. *Clin Toxicol* 1977;11:83–95.
96. Stephans R, Spurgeon A, Calvert I, et al. Neuropsychological effects of long-term exposure to organophosphates in sheep dip. *Lancet* 1995;345:1135–9.
97. Behan PD. Chronic fatigue syndrome as a delayed reaction to low dose organophosphate exposure. *J Nutrition Environ Med* 1996;6:341–50.
98. Ames RG, Steenland K, Jenkins B, et al. Chronic neurologic sequelae to cholinesterase inhibition among agricultural pesticide applicators. *Arch Environ Health* 1995;50:440–4.
99. Lockridge O, Masson P. Pesticides and susceptible populations: people with butyrylcholinesterase genetic variants may be at risk. *Neurotoxicology* 2000;21:113–26.
100. Abu-qare AW, Abou-donia MB. Inhibition and recovery of maternal and fetal cholinesterase enzyme activity following a single cutaneous dose of methyl parathion and diazinon, alone and in combination, in pregnant rats. *J Appl Toxicol* 2001;21:307–16.
101. Abu-qare AW, Abdel-Rahman A, Brownie C, et al. Inhibition of cholinesterase enzymes following a single dermal dose of chlorpyrifos and methyl parathion, alone and in combination, in pregnant rats. *J Toxicol Environ Health A* 2001;63:173–89.
102. Karalliedde L, Senanayake N, Ariaratnam A. Acute organophosphorus insecticide poisoning during pregnancy. *Human Toxicol* 1988;7:363–4.
103. Carrington da Costa RB, Maul ER, Pimintel J, et al. A case of acute poisoning by methyl demeton in a female 5 months pregnant. *Arch Toxicol Suppl* 1982;5:202–4.
104. Holmes JH, Starr HG, Hanisch RC, et al. Short-term toxicity of mevinphos in man. *Arch Environ Health* 1974;29:84–9.
105. Lokan H, Ross J. Rapid death by mevinphos poisoning while under observation. *Forensic Sci Int* 1981;23:179–82.
106. Emerson GM, Gray NM, Jelinek GA, et al. Organophosphate poisoning in Perth, Western Australia, 1987–1996. *J Emerg Med* 1999;17:273–7.
107. Lifshitz M, Shahak E, Sofer S. Carbamate and organophosphate poisoning in young children. *Pediatr Emerg Care* 1999;15:102–3.
108. Zwiener RJ, Ginsburg CM. Organophosphate and carbamate poisoning in infants and children. *Pediatrics* 1988;81:121–6.
109. Etzel RA, Forthal DN, Hill RH, et al. Fatal parathion poisoning in Sierra Leone. *Bull WHO* 1987;65:645–49.
110. Clay C, Stewart GO. Two unusual presentations of organophosphate poisoning. *Anaesth Intensive Care* 1982;10:279–80.
111. Goldman HTM. Malathion poisoning in a 34-month old child following accidental ingestion. *J Pediatr* 1958;52:76–8.
112. Saadeh AM, Farsakh M, Ali-ali MK. Cardiac manifestations of acute carbamate and organophosphate poisoning. *Heart* 1997;461–4.
113. Namba T, Greenfield M, Grob D. Malathion poisoning: a fatal case with cardiac manifestations. *Arch Environ Health* 1970;21:533–41.
114. Ludomirsky A, Klein H, Sarelli P, et al. Q-T prolongation and polymorphous (torsade de pointes) ventricular arrhythmias associated with organophosphorus insecticide poisoning. *Am J Cardiol* 1982;49:1654–8.
115. Kiss Z, Fazekas T. Arrhythmias in organophosphate poisoning. *Acta Cardiol* 1979;34:323–30.
116. Chuang FR, Jang SW, Lin JL, et al. QTc prolongation indicates a poor prognosis in patients with organophosphate poisoning. *Am J Emerg Med* 1996;14:451–3.
117. Brill DM, Maisel AS, Prabhu R. Polymorphic ventricular tachycardia and other complex arrhythmias in organophosphate insecticide poisoning. *J Electrocardiol* 1984;17:97–102.
118. Wang MH, Tseng CD, Bair SY. Q-T interval prolongation and pleomorphic ventricular tachycardia ("torsade de pointes") in organophosphate poisoning: report of a case. *Hum Exp Toxicol* 1998;17:587–90.
119. Hayes MM, Van der Westhuizen NG, Gelfand M. Organophosphate poisoning in Rhodesia. *S Afr Med J* 1978;54:230–4.
120. Hui K. Metabolic disturbances in organophosphate insecticide poisoning. *Arch Pathol Lab Med* 1983;107:154.
121. Durrant W. Massive glycosuria and ketonuria in organophosphorus poisoning. *Centr Afr J Med* 1978;24:253.
122. Kamal AA, Elgarhy MT, Maklady F, et al. Serum choline esterase and liver function among a group of organophosphorus pesticides sprayers in Egypt. *J Toxicol Clin Exp* 1990;10:427–35.
123. Yeh TS, Wang CR, Wen CL, et al. Organophosphate poisoning complicated by rhabdomyolysis. *J Toxicol Clin Toxicol* 1993;31:497–8.
124. Dressel TD, Goodale RL, Arneson MA, et al. Pancreatitis as a complication of anticholinesterase insecticide intoxication. *Ann Surg* 1979;189:199–204.
125. Durham WF, Hayes WJ. Organic phosphorus poisoning and its therapy. *Arch Environ Health* 1962;5:21–33.
126. DeSilva HJ, Wijewickrema R, Senanayake N. Does pralidoxime affect outcome of management in acute organophosphorus poisoning? *Lancet* 1992;339:1136–8.
127. Routier RJ, Lipman J, Brown K. Difficulty in weaning from respiratory support in a patient with the intermediate syndrome of organophosphate poisoning. *Crit Care Med* 1989;17:1075–6.
128. He F. Biological monitoring of exposures to pesticides: current issues. *Toxicol Lett* 1999;108:277–83.
129. Coye MJ, Barnett PG, Midtling JE. Clinical confirmation of organophosphate poisoning by serial cholinesterase analyses. *Arch Intern Med* 1987;147:438–42.
130. Chai FC, Brown JR, Stopps GI. Human blood cholinesterase activity. *Bull Environ Contam Toxicol* 1978;19:617–23.
131. Worek F, Mast U, Kiderlen D, et al. Improved determination of acetylcholinesterase activity in human whole blood. *Clinica Chimica Acta* 1999;288:73–90.
132. Ellman GL, Courtney D, Andres V, et al. A new and rapid colorimetric determination of acetylcholinesterase activity. *Biochem Pharmacol* 1961;7:88–95.
133. Sanz P, Rodriguez-Vincente MC, Diaz D, et al. Red blood cell and total blood acetylcholinesterase and plasma pseudocholinesterase in humans: observed variances. *Clin Toxicol* 1991;29:81–90.
134. Rotenburg M, Shefi M, Dany S, et al. Differentiation between organophosphate and carbamate poisoning. *Clinica Chimica Acta* 1995;234:11–21.
135. Karlsen RL, Sterri S, Lyngaas S, et al. Reference values for erythrocyte acetylcholinesterase and plasma cholinesterase activities in children, implications for organophosphate intoxication. *Scand J Clin Lab Invest* 1981;41:301–2.
136. Bobba R, Venkataraman BV, Pais P, et al. Correlation between severity of symptoms in organophosphorus poisoning and cholinesterase activity (RBC and plasma) in humans. *Ind J Physiol Pharm* 1996;40:249–52.
137. Craig AB, Woodson GS. Observations on the clinical effects of exposure to nerve gas, I: clinical observations and cholinesterase depression. *Am J Med Sci* 1959;238:13–7.
138. Wilson BW, Sanborn JR, O'Malley MA, et al. Monitoring the pesticide-exposed worker. *Occ Med* 1997;12:347–63.
139. Yager J, McLean H, Hudes M, et al. Components of variability in blood cholinesterase assay results. *J Occ Med* 1976;18:242–4.
140. Mutch E, Blain PG, Williains FM. Interindividual variations in enzymes controlling organophosphate toxicity in man. *Hum Exp Toxicol* 1992;11:109–16.
141. Sidell FR, Kaminskis A. Temporal intrapersonal physiological variability of cholinesterase activity in human plasma and erythrocytes. *Clin Chem* 1975;21:1961–3.
142. Nelson TC, Burritt MF. Pesticide poisoning, succinylcholine, induced apnea and pseudocholinesterase. *Mayo Clin Proc* 1986;61:750–5.
143. Mason HJ. The recovery of plasma cholinesterase and erythrocyte cholinesterase activity in workers after dichlorvos exposures. *Occ Med (London)* 2000;50:343–7.
144. Paleus S. On the localization of the specific cholinesterase in human blood. *Arch Biochem Biophys* 1947;12:153–4.
145. Augustinsson K. The normal variation of human blood cholinesterase activity. *Acta Phys Scand* 1955;35:40–52.
146. Callaway S, Davies DR, Rutland JP. Blood cholinesterase levels and range of personal variation in a healthy adult population. *BMJ* 1951;2:812–6.
147. Hodgson M, Parkinson D. Diagnosis of organophosphate poisoning. *N Engl J Med* 1985;313:329.
148. Johns RJ. Familial reduction in red cell cholinesterase. *N Engl J Med* 1962;267:1344–8.
149. Sidell FR, Kaminskis A. Influence of age, sex, and oral contraceptives on human blood cholinesterase activity. *Clin Chem* 1975;21:1393–5.
150. Besser R, Gutmann L, Dillmann U. End-plate dysfunction in acute organophosphate intoxication. *Neurology* 1989;39:561–7.
151. Coye MJ, Lowe JA, Maddy KJ. Biological monitoring of agricultural workers exposed to pesticides: II. Monitoring of intact pesticides and their metabolites. *J Occup Med* 1986;28(8):628–36.
152. Larsen K, Hanel HK. Effect of organophosphorus compounds on S-cholinesterase in workers removing poisonous depots. *Scand J Work Environ Health* 1982;8:222–6.
153. Dellinger JA. Monitoring the chronic effects of anticholinesterase pesticides in aerial applicators. *Vet Hum Toxicol* 1985;27:427–30.
154. US Army Medical Research Institute of Chemical Defense. *Medical management of chemical casualties handbook*, 3rd ed. Aberdeen Proving Ground, MD: US Army Medical Research Institute of Chemical Defense, 2000.
155. Geller RJ, Singleton KL, Tarantino ML, et al. Nosocomial poisoning associated with emergency department treatment of organophosphate toxicity—Georgia, 2000. *J Toxicol Clin Toxicol* 2001;39:109–11.
156. Koskal N, Buyukbese MA, Guven A, et al. Organophosphate intoxication as a consequence of mouth-to-mouth breathing from an affected case. *Chest* 2002;122:740–1.
157. Windler E, Dreyer M, Runge M. Intoxikation mit dem organophosphat parathion (E-605). *Schweiz Med Wochenschr* 1983;113:861–2.
158. Novikova OV, Druzhinin NV, Kustovskii AV. [Use of hemodialysis in intensive care of organophosphorus insecticide poisoning]. *Anesteziol Reanimatol* 1997;Jan–Feb:74–6.
159. Okonek S, Tonnis HJ, Baldamus CA, et al. Hemoperfusion versus hemodialysis in the management of patients severely poisoned by organophosphorus insecticides and tripyridyl herbicides. *Artif Organs* 1979;3:341–5.
160. Nagler J, Braeckman RA, Willems JL, et al. Combined hemoperfusion-hemodialysis for organophosphate poisoning. *J Appl Toxicol* 1981;1:199–201.
161. de Monchy JGR, Snoek WJ, Sluiter HJ, et al. Treatment of severe parathion intoxication. *Vet Hum Toxicol* 1979;21[Suppl]:115–7.
162. Koplovitz I, Mento R, Matthews C, et al. Dose-response effects of atropine and HI-6 treatment of organophosphorus poisoning in guinea pigs. *Drug Chem Toxicol* 1995;18:119–36.

163. LeBlanc FN, Benson BE, Gilg AD. A severe organophosphate poisoning requiring the use of an atropine drip. *J Toxicol Clin Toxicol* 1986;24:69–76.
164. Singh S, Chaudhry D, Behera D, et al. Aggressive atropinization and continuous pralidoxime (2-PAM) infusion in patients with severe organophosphate poisoning: experience of a northwest Indian hospital. *Hum Exp Toxicol* 2001;20:15–8.
165. Mackey CL. Anticholinesterase insecticide poisoning. *Heart Lung* 1982;11:479–84.
166. Wali FA, Bradshaw EG, Suer AH, et al. Atropine enhances neuromuscular transmission in humans. *Fundam Clin Pharmacol* 1987;1:59–66.
167. Ram JS, Kumar SS, Jayarajan A, et al. Continuous infusion of high doses of atropine in the management of organophosphorus compound poisoning. *J Assoc Physicians India* 1991;39:190–3.
168. Tafuri J, Roberts J. Organophosphate poisoning. *Ann Emerg Med* 1987;16:193–202.
169. Hopmann G, Wanke H. Maximum dose atropine treatment in severe organophosphate poisoning. *Dtsch Med Wochenschr* 1974;99:2106–8.
170. Bardin PG, van Eeden SF. Organophosphate poisoning: grading the severity and comparing treatment between atropine and glycopyrrolate. *Crit Care Med* 1990;18:956–60.
171. Wilson IB. Molecular complementarity and antidotes for alkylphosphate poisoning. *Fed Proc* 1959;18:752–8.
172. Worek F, Kirchner T, Backer M, et al. Reactivation by various oximes of human erythrocyte acetylcholinesterase inhibited by different organophosphorus compounds. *Arch Toxicol* 1996;67:497–503.
173. Willems JL, de Bisschop JP, Verstraete AG, et al. Cholinesterase reactivation in organophosphorus poisoned patients depends on the plasma concentrations of the oxime pralidoxime methylsulphate and of the organophosphate. *Arch Toxicol* 1993;67:79–84.
174. Hobbiger F. Protection against the lethal effects of organophosphates by pyridine-2-aldoxime methiodide. *Br J Pharmacol* 1957;12:438–46.
175. Funckes AJ. Treatment of severe parathion poisoning with pyridine aldoxime methiodide (2-PAM). *Arch Environ Health* 1960;1:404–6.
176. Hiraki K, Namba Y, Taniguchi Y, et al. Effect of 2-pyridine aldoxime methiodide (PAM) against parathion. *Naika Ryoiki* 1958;6:84–97.
177. Lotti M, Becker CE. Treatment of acute organophosphate poisoning: evidence of a direct effect on the central nervous system by 2-PAM (pyridine-2-aldoxime methyl chloride). *J Toxicol Clin Toxicol* 1982;19:121–7.
178. Quinby GE. Further therapeutic experience with pralidoximes in organic phosphorus poisoning. *JAMA* 1964;187:202–6.
179. Jacobinzer H, Raybin HW. Parathion poisoning successfully treated with 2-PAM (pralidoxime chloride). *N Engl J Med* 1961;265:436–7.
180. Kusic R, Jovanovic D, Randjelovic S, et al. HI-6 in man: efficacy of the oxime in poisoning by organophosphorus insecticides. *Hum Exp Toxicol* 1991;10:113–8.
181. Vale JA, Meredith TJ. Organophosphorus poisoning. *BMJ* 1991;302:962–3.
182. Thiermann H, Szinicz L, Eyer F, et al. Modern strategies in therapy of organophosphate poisoning. *Toxicol Lett* 1999;107:233–9.
183. Worek F, Backer M, Thiermann H. Reappraisal of indications and limitations of oxime therapy in organophosphate poisoning. *Hum Exp Toxicol* 1997;16:466–72.
184. Thompson DF, Thompson GD, Greenwood RB, Trammel HL. Therapeutic dosing of pralidoxime chloride. *Drug Intell Clin Pharmacol* 1987;21:590–3.
185. Lotti M. Treatment of organophosphate poisoning. *Med J Aust* 1991;154:51–5.
186. Scott RJ. Repeated asystole following PAM in organophosphate self-poisoning. *Anaesth Intensive Care* 1986;14:458.
187. Delilkan AE, Namazie M, Ong G. Organophosphate poisoning: a Malaysian experience of one hundred cases. *Med J Malaysia* 1984;39:229–33.
188. Samuel J, Peter JV, Thomas K, et al. Evaluation of two treatment regimens of pralidoxime (1 gm single bolus vs. 12 gm infusion) in the management of organophosphorus poisoning. *J Assoc Physicians India* 1996;44:529–31.
189. Cherian AM, Peter JV, Samuel J, et al. Effectiveness of 2PAM (PAM-pralidoxime) in the treatment of organophosphorus poisoning: a randomized, double-blind, placebo-controlled trial. *J Assoc Physicians India* 1997;45:22–4.
190. Sanderson DM. Treatment of poisoning by anticholinesterase insecticides in the rat. *J Pharm Pharmacol* 1961;13:435.
191. Vale JA. Rationale for oxime therapy: pralidoxime as an antidote in insecticide poisoning. *Hum Exp Toxicol* 1996;15:77.
192. Johnson MK, Vale JA, Marrs TC, Meredith TJ. Pralidoxime for organophosphorus poisoning. *Lancet* 1992;340:64.
193. Tush GM, Anstead MI. Pralidoxime continuous infusion in the treatment of organophosphate poisoning. *Ann Pharmacother* 1997;31:441–4.
194. Eddleston M, Szinicz L, Eyer P, et al. Oximes in acute organophosphorus pesticide poisoning: a systematic review of clinical trials. *QJM* 2002;95:275–83.
195. Eddleston M, Roberts D, Buckley N. Management of severe organophosphorus pesticide poisoning. *Crit Care* 2002;6:259.
196. Di Kart WL, Kiestra SH, Sangster B. The use of atropine and oximes in organophosphate intoxication: a modified approach. *J Toxicol Clin Toxicol* 1988;26:199–208.
197. Namba T, Hiraki K. PAM (pyride-2-aldoxime methiodide) therapy for alkylphosphate poisoning. *JAMA* 1958;166:1834–9.
198. Farrar HC, Wells TG, Kearns GL. Use of continuous infusion of pralidoxime for treatment of organophosphate poisoning in children. *J Pediatr* 1990;116:658–61.
199. Schexnayder S, James LP, Kearns GL, et al. The pharmacokinetics of continuous infusion pralidoxime in children with organophosphate poisoning. *J Toxicol Clin Toxicol* 1998;36:549–55.
200. Medicis JJ, Stork CM, Howland MA, et al. Pharmacokinetics following a loading plus a continuous infusion of pralidoxime compared with the traditional short infusion regimen in human volunteers. *J Toxicol Clin Toxicol* 1996;34:289–95.
201. Willems JL, Langenberg JP, Verstaete AG. Plasma concentrations of pralidoxime methylsulphate in organophosphorus poisoned patients. *Arch Toxicol* 1992;66:260–6.
202. Boskovic, Kovacevic V, Jovanovic P. PAM-2 Cl, HI-6, and HGG-12 in soman and tabun poisoning. *Fundam Appl Toxicol* 1984;4(2 Pt 2):S106–S115.
203. Koplovitz I, Gresham VC, Dochtermann LW, et al. Evaluation of the toxicity, pathology, and treatment of cyclohexylmethylphosphonofouridate (CMPF) poisoning in rhesus monkeys. *Arch Toxicol* 1992;66:622–8.
204. Murphy MR, Blick DW, Dunn MA. Diazepam as a treatment for nerve agent poisoning in primates. *Aviat Space Environ Med* 1993;64:110–5.
205. McDonough JH, Jaax NK, Crowley RA, et al. Atropine and/or diazepam therapy protects against soman-induced neural and cardiac pathology. *Fundam Appl Toxicol* 1989;13:256–76.
206. Martin LJ, Doebler JA, Shih T, et al. Protective effect of diazepam pretreatment on soman-induced brain lesion formation. *Brain Res* 1985;325:287–9.
207. Kiss Z, Fazekas T. Organophosphates and torsades de pointes ventricular tachycardia. *J Roy Soc Med* 1983;76:983–4.
208. Petroianu G, Ruefer R. Beta blockade or magnesium in organophosphorus insecticide poisoning. *Anaesth Intensive Care* 1992;20:538–9.
209. Singh G, Avasthi G, Khurana D, et al. Neuropsychological monitoring of pharmacological manipulation in acute organophosphate (OP) poisoning. The effects of pralidoxime, magnesium sulphate and pancuronium. *Electroencephalogr Clin Neurophysiol* 1998;107:140–8.
210. Buccafusco JJ, Aronstam RS. Clonidine protection from the toxicity of soman, an organophosphate acetylcholinesterase inhibitor in the mouse. *J Pharmacol Exp Ther* 1986;239:43–6.
211. Clement JG, Filbert M. Antidote effect of sodium fluoride against organophosphate poisoning in mice. *Life Sci* 1983;32:1803–10.
212. Dehlawi MS, Eldefrawi AT, Eldefrawi ME, et al. Choline derivatives and sodium fluoride protect acetylcholinesterase against irreversible inhibition by DFP and paraoxon. *J Biochem Toxicol* 1994;9(5);261–268.
213. Wills JH, McNamara BP, Fine EA. Ventricular fibrillation in delayed treatment of TEPP poisoning. *Fed Proc* 1950;9:136.
214. Kunkel AM, O'Leary JF, Jones AH. Atropine-induced ventricular fibrillation during cyanosis caused by organophosphorus poisoning. Edgewood Arsenal Technical Report 4711;1973.
215. Clifford NJ, Nies AS. Organophosphate poisoning from wearing a laundered uniform previously contaminated with parathion. *JAMA* 1989;262:3035–6.
216. Baker T, Stanec A. Methylprednisolone treatment of an organophosphorus induced delayed neuropathy. *Toxicol Appl Pharmacol* 1985;79:348–52.
217. Goldman LR, Smith DF, Neutra RR, et al. Pesticide food poisoning from contaminated watermelons in California, 1985. *Arch Environ Health* 1990;45:229–36.
218. Liddle JA, Kimbrough RD, Needham LL. A fatal episode of accidental methomyl poisoning. *Clin Toxicol* 1979;15:159–67.
219. Farago A. Suicidal fatal Sevin poisoning. *Arch Toxicol* 1969;24:309–15.
220. Lima JS, Reis CA. Poisoning due to illegal use of carbamates as a rodenticide in Rio de Janeiro. *J Toxicol Clin Toxicol* 1995;33:687–90.
221. Ameno K, Lee SK, In SW, et al. Blood carbofuran concentrations in suicidal ingestion cases. *Forensic Sci Int* 2001;116:59–61.
222. Casper HH, Pekas JC. Absorption and excretion of radiolabeled l-naphthyl-N-methylcarbamate (carbaryl) by the rat. *N Y Acad Sci* 1971;24:160–66.
223. Peter JV, Cherian AM. Organic insecticides. *Anaesth Intensive Care* 2000;28:11–21.
224. Ryan AJ. The metabolism of pesticidal carbamates. *Crit Rev Toxicol* 1974;1:33–54.
225. Wilson IB, Hatch MA, Ginsburg S. Carbamylation of acetylcholinesterase. *J Biol Chem* 1960;235:2312–5.
226. O'Brien RD. Phosphorylation and carbamylation of cholinesterase. *Ann N Y Acad Sci* 1969;160:204–14.
227. Winteringham FW, Fowler KS. Substrate and dilutional effects on the inhibition of acetylcholinesterase by carbamates. *Biochem J* 1966;101:127–34.
228. Fukuto TR. Mechanism of action of organophosphorus and carbamate insecticides. *Environ Health Perspect* 1990;87:245–54.
229. Yang PY, Tsao TCY, Lin JL, et al. Carbofuran-induced delayed neuropathy. *J Toxicol Clin Toxicol* 2000;38:43–6.
230. Dickoff DJ, Gerber O, Turovsky Z. Delayed neurotoxicity after ingestion of carbamate pesticide. *Neurology* 1987;37:1229–31.
231. Wills JH, Jameson E, Coulston F. Effect of oral doses of carbaryl in man. *Clin Toxicol* 1968;1:265–71.
232. Best EM, Murray BL. Observations on workers exposed to Sevin insecticide: a preliminary report. *J Occ Med* 1962;10:507–17.
233. Umehara F, Izumo S, Arimura K, et al. Polyneuropathy induced by m-tolyl methul carbamate intoxication. *J Neurol* 1991;238:47–8.
234. Branch RA, Jacquez E. Subacute neurotoxicity following long-term exposure to carbaryl. *Am J Med* 1986;80:741–5.
235. Klys MKJ, Pach J, et al. Carbofuran poisoning of pregnant woman and fetus per ingestion. *J Forensic Sci* 1989;34:1413–6.
236. Ekins BR, Geller RJ. Methomyl-induced carbamate poisoning treated with pralidoxime chloride. *West J Med* 1994;161:68–70.

237. Burgess JL, Bernstein JN, Hurlbut K. Aldicarb poisoning. A case report with prolonged cholinesterase inhibition and improvement after pralidoxime therapy. *Arch Int Med* 1994;154:221–4.
238. Lifshitz M, Rotenburg M, Sofer S, et al. Carbamate poisoning and oxime treatment in children. A clinical and laboratory study. *Pediatrics* 1994;93:652–5.
239. Harris LW, Talbot BG, Lennox WJ, Anderson DR. The relationship between oxime-induced reactivation of carbamylated acetylcholinesterase and antidotal efficacy against carbamate intoxication. *Toxicol Appl Pharmacol* 1989;98:128–33.
240. Natoff IL, Reiff B. Effect of oximes on the toxicity of anticholine esterase carbamates. *Toxicol Appl Pharmacol* 1973;25:569–75.
241. Lieske CN, Clark JH, Maxwell DM. Studies on the amplification of carbaryl toxicity by various oximes. *Toxicol Lett* 1992;62:127–37.
242. Kurtz PH. Pralidoxime in the treatment of carbamate intoxication. *Am J Emerg Med* 1990;8:68–70.
243. Mortenson ME. Pharmacological and toxicological considerations in the treatment of carbamate intoxications. *Am J Emerg Med* 1990;8:83–4.
244. Garber M. Carbamate poisoning: the "other" insecticide. *Pediatrics* 1994;79:734–8.
245. Gladwell M. *The mosquito killer*. New York: 2001.
246. Carson R. *Silent spring*. Boston: Houghton Mifflin, 1962.
247. Rowly DL, Rab MA, Hardjotanojo W, et al. Convulsions caused by endrin poisoning in Pakistan. *Pediatrics* 1987;79:928–34.
248. Runhaar EA, Sangster B, Greve PA, et al. A case of fatal endrin poisoning. *Hum Toxicol* 1985;4:241–7.
249. Kintz P, Baron L, Tracqui A, et al. A high endrin concentration in a fatal case. *Forensic Sci Int* 1992;54:177–80.
250. Lindane shampoo [prescribing information]. Alpharma, USP 1%; 2003.
251. Daerr W, Kaukel E, Schmoldt A. [Hemoperfusion—a therapeutic alternative to early treatment of lindane poisoning]. *Deutsch Med Wochenschr* 1985;110:1253–5.
252. Nordt SP, Chew G. Acute lindane poisoning in three children. *J Emerg Med* 2000;18:51–3.
253. Aks S, Krantz A, Hryhrczuk DO, et al. Acute accidental lindane ingestion in toddlers. *Ann Emerg Med* 1995;26:647–51.
254. Fischer TF. Lindane toxicity in a 24-year-old woman. *Ann Emerg Med* 1994;24(5):972–4.
255. Waller K, Prendergast TJ, Slagle A, et al. Seizures after eating a snack food contaminated with the pesticide endrin. The tale of the toxic taquitos. *West J Med* 1992;157:648–51.
256. Starr HG, Clifford NJ. Acute lindane intoxication. *Arch Environ Health* 1972;25:374–5.
257. Jaeger U, Podczeck A, Haubenstock A, et al. Acute oral poisoning with lindane-solvent mixtures. *Vet Hum Toxicol* 1984;26:11–4.
258. Telch J, Jarvis DA. Acute intoxication with lindane (gamma benzene hexachloride). *Can Med Assoc J* 1982;126:662–3.
259. Lee B, Groth P. Scabies transcutaneous poisoning during treatment. *Pediatrics* 1977;59:643.
260. Pramanik AK, Hansen RC. Transcutaneous gamma benzene hexachloride absorption and toxicity in infants and children. *Arch Dermatol* 1979; 115(10):1224–5.
261. Tenenbein M. Seizures after lindane therapy. *J Am Geriatr Soc* 1991;39:394–5.
262. Rasmussen J. The problem of lindane. *J Am Acad Derm* 1981;3:507–16.
263. Solomon LM, Fahrner L, West DP. Gamma benzene hexachloride toxicity: a review. *Arch Dermatol* 1977;113(3):353–7.
264. Solomon BA, Haut SR, Carr EM, et al. Neurotoxic reaction to lindane in an HIV-seropositive patient. An old medication's new problem. *J Fam Pract* 1995;40(3):291–6.
265. Feldmann RJ, Maibach HI. Percutaneous penetration of some pesticides and herbicides in man. *Toxicol Appl Pharmacol* 1974;28(1):126–32.
266. Ginsburg CM, Lowry W, Reisch JS. Absorption of lindane (gamma benzene hexachloride) in infants and children. *J Pediatr* 1977;91:998–1000.
267. Saleh MA. Toxaphene: chemistry, biochemistry, toxicity, and environmental fate. *Rev Environ Contam Toxicol* 1991;118:2–85.
268. Coats JR. Mechanisms of toxic action and structure-activity relationships for organochlorine and synthetic pyrethroid insecticides. *Environ Health Perspect* 1990;87:255–62.
269. Baumann K, Angerer J, Heinrich R, et al. Occupational exposure to hexachlorocyclohexane. *Int Arch Occ Environ Health* 1980;47:119–27.
270. Rugman FP, Cosstick R. Aplastic anemia associated with organochlorine pesticide: case reports and review of the literature. *J Clin Pathol* 1990;43:98–101.
271. Garrettson LK, Guzelien PS, Blanke RV. Subacute chlordane poisoning. *J Toxicol Clin Toxicol* 1984;22:565–71.
272. Cohn WJ, Boylan JJ, Blanke RV, et al. Treatment of chlordecone (kepone) toxicity with cholestyramine. *N Engl J Med* 1978;298:243–8.
273. Jung D, Becher H, Edler L, et al. Elimination of beta-hexachlorocyclohexane in occupationally exposed persons. *J Toxicol Environ Health* 1997;51:23–34.
274. Konje JC, Otolorin EO, Sotunmbi PT, et al. Insecticide poisoning in pregnancy. A case report. *J Reprod Med* 1992;37:992–4.
275. Cole LM, Casida JE. Polychlorocycloalkane insecticide-induced convulsions in mice in relation to disruption of GABA-regulated chloride ionophore. *Life Sci* 1986;39:1855–62.
276. Gant DB, Eldefrawi ME, Eldefrawi AT. Cyclodiene insecticides inhibit GABA-A receptor-regulated chloride transport. *Toxicol Appl Pharmacol* 1987;88:313–21.
277. Sunol C, Vale C, Rodriguez-Farre E. Polychlorocycloalkane insecticide action on GABA- and glycine-dependent chloride flux. *Neurotoxicology* 1998;19:573–80.
278. Holan G. New halocyclopropane insecticides and the mode of action of DDT. *Nature* 1969;221:1025–9.
279. Narahashi T. Nerve membrane as a target for pyrethroids. *Pestic Sci* 1976;7:267–72.
280. Guzelian PS. Comparative toxicology of chlordecone (kepone) in humans and experimental animals. *Ann Rev Pharmacol Toxicol* 1982;22:89–113.
281. Faroon O, Kueberuwa S, Smith L, et al. ATSDR evaluation of health effects of chemicals II. Mirex and chlordecone: health effects, toxicokinetics, human exposure, and environmental fate. *Toxicol Ind Health* 1995;11:1–188.
282. Grimmett WG, Dzendolet I, Whyte I. Intravenous thiodan (30% endosulfan in xylene). *J Toxicol Clin Toxicol* 1996;34:447–52.
283. Carvalho WA, Matos GB, Cruz SLB, et al. Human aldrin poisoning. *Braz J Med Biol Res* 1991;24:883–7.
284. Coble Y, Hildebrandt P, Davis J, et al. Acute endrin poisoning. *JAMA* 1967;202:153–7.
285. Grutsch JF, Khasuwinah A. Signs and mechanisms of chlordane intoxication. *Biomed Environ Sci* 1991;4:317–26.
286. Olanoff LS, Bristow WJ, Colcolough J, et al. Acute chlordane intoxication. *J Toxicol Clin Toxicol* 1983;20:291–306.
287. Ortiz Martinez A, Martinez-Conde E. The neurotoxic effects of lindane at acute and subacute dosages. *Ecotoxicol Environ Saf* 1995;30:101–5.
288. Munk ZM, Nantel A. Acute lindane poisoning with development of muscle necrosis. *Can Med Assoc J* 1977;117:1050–4.
289. Rao CVSR, Shreenivas R, Singh V, et al. Disseminated intravascular coagulation in a case of fatal lindane poisoning. *Vet Hum Toxicol* 1988;30:132–4.
290. Videla LA, Simizu K, Barros SB, et al. Mechanisms of lindane-induced hepatotoxicity: alterations of respiratory activity and sinusoidal glutathione efflux in perfused rat liver. *Xenobiotica* 1991;21:1023–32.
291. Onifer T, Whistnant J. Cerebellar ataxia and neuronitis after exposure to DDT and lindane. *Mayo Clin Proc* 1957;32:67–72.
292. Hall RC. Long-term psychological and neurological complications of lindane poisoning. *Psychosomatics* 1999;40:513–7.
293. Fonseca RG, Resende LA, Silva MD, et al. Chronic motor neuron disease possibly related to intoxication with organochlorine insecticides. *Acta Neurol Scand* 1993;88:56–8.
294. Czegledi-Janko C, Avar P. Occupational exposure to lindane: clinical laboratory findings. *Br J Ind Med* 1970;27:283–6.
295. Kilburn KH, Thornton JC. Protracted neurotoxicity from chlordane sprayed to kill termites. *Environ Health Perspect* 1995;103:691–4.
296. Campbell A. Neurologic complications associated with insecticides and fungicides. *Br Med J* 1952;2:415–7.
297. Martinez AJ, Taylor JR, Dyck PJ, et al. Chlordecone intoxication in man. Part 2: ultrastructure of peripheral nerves and skeletal muscle. *Neurology* 1978;28:631–5.
298. Verderber L, Lavin P, Wesley R. Pseudotumor cerebri and chronic benzene hexachloride (lindane) exposure. *J Neurol Neurosurg Psychiatry* 1991;54:1123.
299. Morgan DP, Roberts RJ, Walter AW, et al. Anemia associated with exposure to lindane. *Arch Environ Health* 1980;35:307–10.
300. Rauch AE, Kowalsky SF, Lesar TS, et al. Lindane (Kwell)-induced aplastic anemia. *Arch Intern Med* 1990;150:2393–5.
301. Dale WE, Curley A, Cueto C. Hexane extractable chlorinated insecticides in human blood. *Life Sci* 1966;5:47–54.
302. Kurt TL, Bost R, Gilliland M, et al. Accidental Kwell (lindane) ingestions. *Vet Hum Toxicol* 1986;28:569–71.
303. Davies JE, Dedhia HV, Morgade C, et al. Lindane poisonings. *Arch Dermatol* 1983;119:142–4.
304. Mayersdorf A, Israeli R. Toxic effects of chlorinated hydrocarbon insecticides on the human electroencephalogram. *Arch Environ Health* 1974;28:159–63.
305. Kassner JT, Maher TJ, Hull KM, Woolf AD. Cholestyramine as an adsorbent in acute lindane poisoning: a murine model. *Ann Emerg Med* 1993;22:1392–7.

CHAPTER 237

Anticoagulant Rodenticides

Luke Yip

See Figure 1.

Compounds included:	**Short-acting rodenticides: warfarin; long-acting rodenticides: brodifacoum, bromadiolone, chlorophacinone, difenacoum, diphacinone.**
Molecular formula and weight:	**See Table 1.**
CAS Registry No.:	**See Table 1.**
Special considerations:	**Most toxic effects involve complications of hemorrhage.**
Antidote:	**Vitamin K**

OVERVIEW

The oral anticoagulants emerged from veterinary research in the 1920s on a hemorrhagic disorder afflicting cattle that consumed spoiled sweet clover hay (1,2). In 1939, Karl Paul Link and his team at the University of Wisconsin identified dicumarol as the hemorrhagic agent. The first therapeutic use of dicumarol in humans began in the 1940s. In the process of developing the ideal rodenticide, Link found warfarin to be more potent and reliable as a rodenticide and it was launched in 1948. Foreign competition with dicumarol in the pharmaceutical market coupled with human studies demonstrating its superiority over dicumarol led to warfarin becoming the oral anticoagulant of choice.

Oral anticoagulants are available in over-the-counter rodenticide products. They may be classified as hydroxycoumarins (e.g., acenocoumarin, bishydroxycoumarin, coumachlor, coumafuryl, dicumarol, ethyl biscoumacetate, fumasol, Panwarfin, phenprocoumon, prolin, warfarin, and warficide) and indanediones (e.g., anisindione diphacinone, diphenadione, phenindione, pindone, and pivalyn).

Warfarin is the prototypic short-acting rodenticide. Due to the emergence of warfarin-resistant rats, *superwarfarins* or long-acting anticoagulants (e.g., brodifacoum, bromadiolone, chlorophacinone, difenacoum, and diphacinone) were developed. The mechanism of action is the same as warfarin. Accidental or intentional exposure to either type of rodenticide anticoagulant has resulted in clinically significant prolonged, sometimes profound, coagulopathy and sometimes death (3–80).

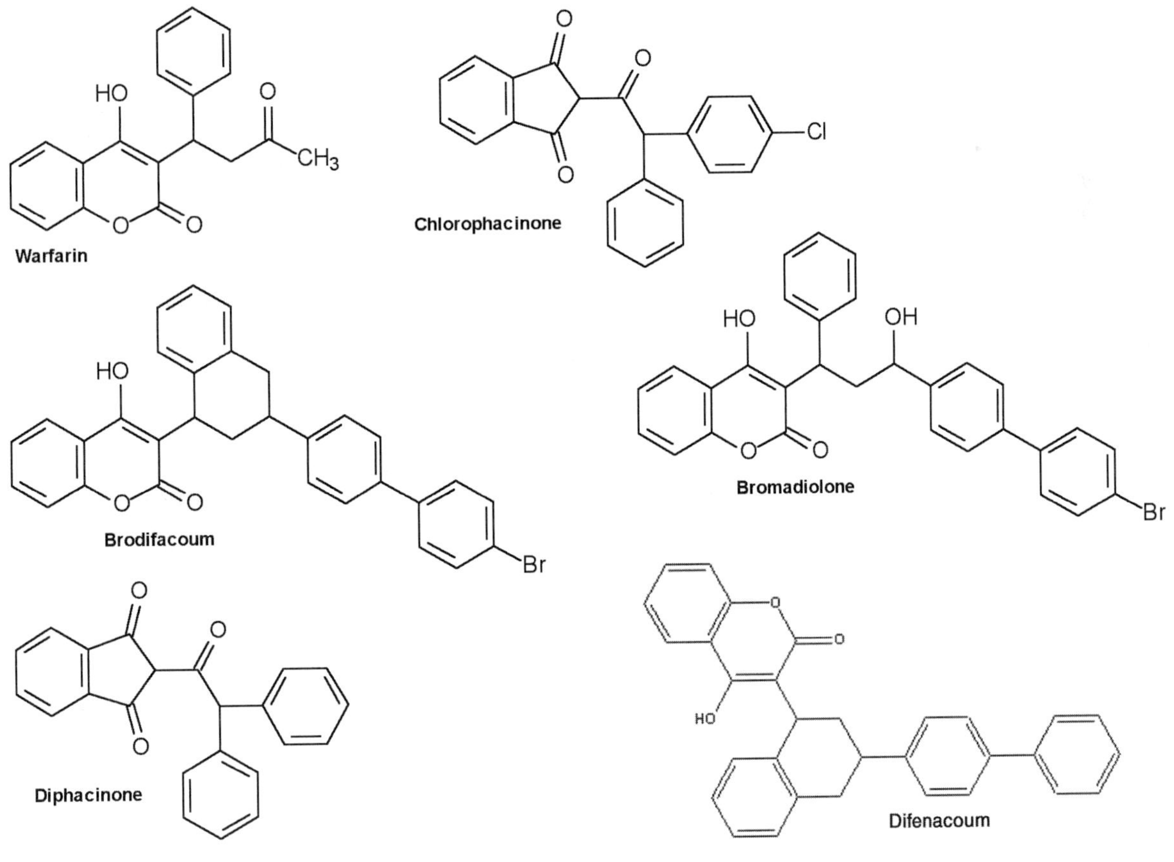

Warfarin

Chlorophacinone

Brodifacoum

Bromadiolone

Diphacinone

Difenacoum

Figure 1. Structures of the anticoagulant rodenticides.

TABLE 1. Physical characteristics and regulatory standards for anticoagulant rodenticides

Compound	Molecular formula, molecular weight (g/mol), CAS Registry No.	Description	Concentration mg/m³ (ppm)
Brodifacoum	$C_{31}H_{23}BrO_3$	OSHA	Not listed
	523.4	ACGIH	
	56073-10-0	NIOSH	
Bromadiolone	$C_{30}H_{23}BrO_4$	OSHA	Not listed
	527.4	ACGIH	
	28772-56-7	NIOSH	
Chlorophacinone	$C_{23}H_{15}ClO_3$	OSHA	Not listed
	374.8	ACGIH	
	3691-35-8	NIOSH	
Difenacoum	$C_{31}H_{24}O_3$	OSHA	Not listed
	444.5	ACGIH	
	56073-07-05	NIOSH	
Diphacinone	$C_{23}H_{16}O_3$	OSHA	Not listed
	340.4	ACGIH	
	82-66-6	NIOSH	
Warfarin	$C_{19}H_{16}O_4$	OSHA PEL-TWA	0.1 (0.008)
	330.3	ACGIH TLV-TWA	0.1 (0.008)
	129-06-6	TLV-STEL	None
		NIOSH REL-TWA	0.1 (0.008)
		REL-STEL	None
		IDLH	100 (8)

ACGIH, American Conference of Governmental Industrial Hygienists; IDLH, immediately dangerous to life or health; NIOSH, National Institute for Occupational Safety and Health; OSHA, U.S. Occupational Safety and Health Administration; PEL, permissible exposure limit; ppm, parts per million; REL, recommended exposure limit; STEL, short-term exposure limit; TLV, threshold limit value; TWA, time-weighted average.

Chemical and Physical Properties

Warfarin is a coumarin derivative and is commercially available as a racemic mixture of R (+) and S (–) warfarin. In the rat, S (–) warfarin is three to seven times more potent than R (+) warfarin in anticoagulant effect (81), whereas in humans, S (–) warfarin is 3.8 times more potent than R (+) warfarin (82).

Superwarfarins are also coumarin derivatives and differ from warfarin by their longer-, higher-molecular-weight polycyclic hydrocarbon side chain (Fig. 1). Their superiority over warfarin rodenticides is high lipid solubility, accumulation in the liver, higher potency on a mole for mole basis, and prolonged duration of action (83–86).

Classification and Uses

Occupational exposure to coumarin anticoagulants (brodifacoum, difenacoum, and warfarin) may result in inhalation or percutaneous coumarin absorption and abnormal vitamin K metabolism in the presence of normal clotting factor activity (25,53). There have also been case reports of brodifacoum toxicity (e.g., epistaxis, mucosal and bleeding wounds, and hematuria) associated with smoking marijuana or crack cocaine mixed with brodifacoum (41,67).

Toxic Doses

Regulatory standards and guidelines are provided in Table 1.

Short-acting (warfarin) compounds have produced lethal toxicity (e.g., bleeding) on an estimated daily dose of 50 mg/day for 8 days (40). Toxicity and death have been reported in infants after percutaneous exposure to talcum powder contaminated with 1.7% to 6.5% warfarin (44). Percutaneous exposure to 0.5% to 6.5% warfarin has resulted in toxicity (25) and death (44).

In adults, an acute single unintentional warfarin ingestion of 1 mg/kg may be considered inconsequential. This dose is expected to result in a therapeutic prothrombin (PT) value within 24 to 48 hours and have an average duration of 5 days (87–89). The minimum pediatric toxic dose may be extrapolated from the therapeutic warfarin loading dose, which is 0.5 to 0.7 mg/kg (90). This dose is expected to result in a therapeutic PT value within 36 to 48 hours.

A typical rodenticide anticoagulant contains 0.025% warfarin or 0.005% brodifacoum (91). A person has to ingest 2.0 to 2.8 g/kg of warfarin or 10 to 14 g/kg of brodifacoum rodenticide to achieve a therapeutic anticoagulant loading dose.

TOXICOKINETICS AND TOXICODYNAMICS

Short-Acting Rodenticides

Warfarin is completely absorbed from the gastrointestinal tract. The maximum plasma level was achieved 2 to 12 hours after a single warfarin dose of 1.5 mg/kg (92,93). Warfarin is extensively bound (97%) to albumin (94). Warfarin is extensively metabolized by the liver and by more than one cytochrome P-450 (CYP) isoenzyme, which stereoselectively hydroxylates warfarin enantiomers. In humans, R (+) and S (–) warfarin metabolism is principally catalyzed by CYP1A2 and CYP2C9, respectively (95). CYP2E1 does not appear to be involved in warfarin metabolism and the R (+) enantiomer may be an inhibitor of S (–) warfarin metabolism.

In human volunteer and overdose studies, warfarin elimination appears to be independent of dose or the route of administration (29,92,93). The mean plasma warfarin half-life is 42 hours and the range is 15 to 58 hours.

Long-Acting Rodenticides

Long-acting compounds are metabolized by hepatic cytochrome P-450 isozymes (e.g., CYP3A4) (83). In adults after intentional brodifacoum ingestion, the mean plasma half-life was 30 days (range, 16 to 62 days) (11,32,70,96,97). In a pediatric case, the plasma brodifacoum half-life was 16 days (3). After intentional chlorophacinone ingestion, the plasma half-life was 6.5 to 22.8 days (12). An intentional difenacoum ingestion resulted in a plasma half-life of 11.5 days (45).

PATHOPHYSIOLOGY

Vitamin K is an essential cofactor in posttranslational modification of prothrombin complex proteins (factors II, VII, IX, and X) and proteins C, S, and Z. In the liver, the inactive coagulation factors are converted to their active forms after carboxylation at the amino terminal end of glutamate residues, forming γ-carboxyglutamates (98,99). They are required for calcium dependent complexing of the clotting proteins to their cofactors on phospholipid surfaces when the coagulation cascade is activated.

Activated protein C and S are anticoagulant proteins that provide control and balance in the coagulation cascade. Protein C, when aided by protein S, inactivates factor Va (platelet coagulation activity) and VIIIa (antihemophilic factor). Depressed protein C activity is associated with hemorrhagic (warfarin) skin necrosis (100–103). Protein Z is a cofactor for the inhibition of factor Xa by protein Z–dependent protease inhibitor.

During γ-carboxylation, the active hydroquinone form of vitamin K is converted to the inactive 2,3-epoxide form. The

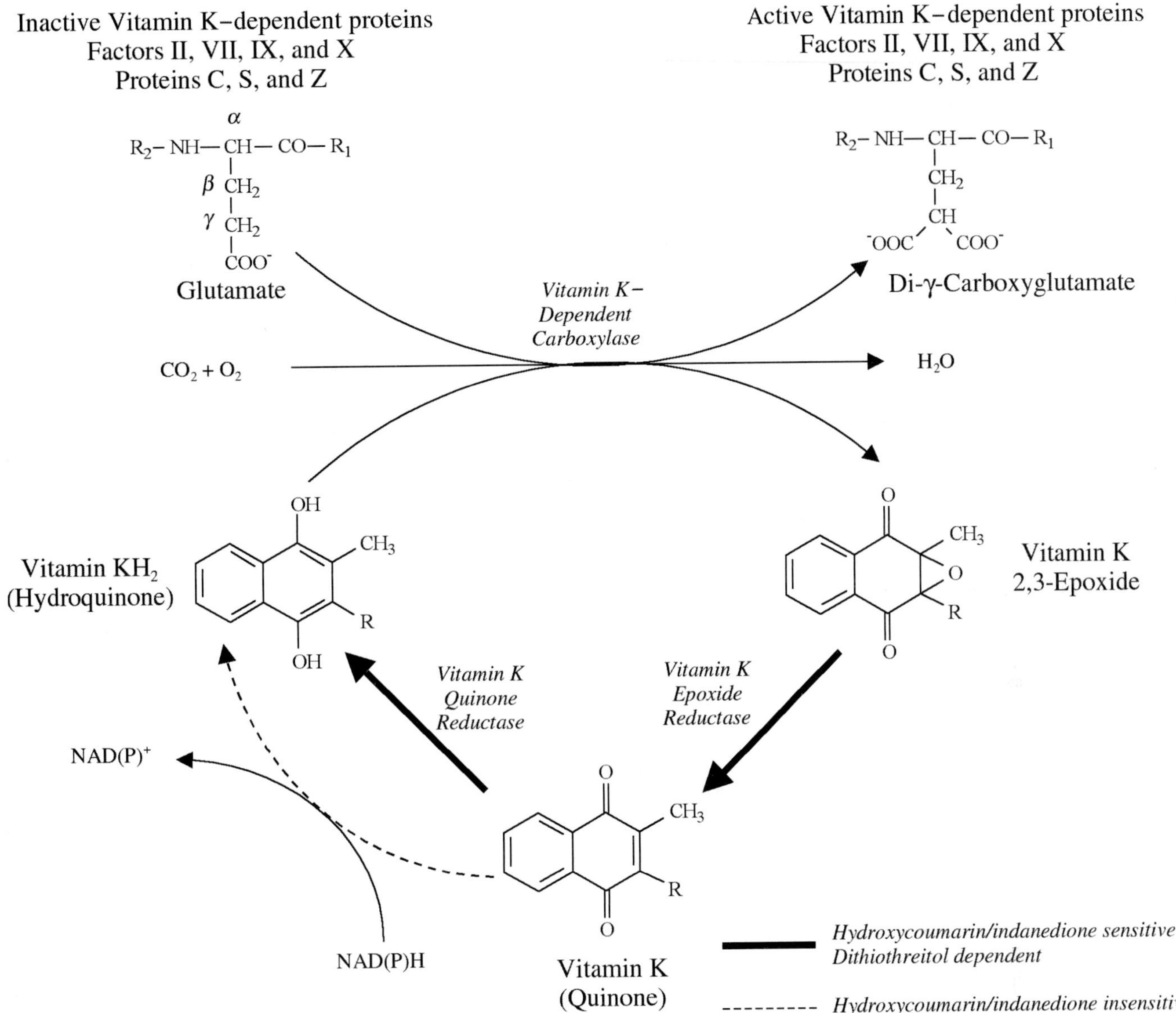

Figure 2. Vitamin K–epoxide cycle.

epoxide, in turn, is reduced back to the active form in two successive reactions (104,105). The first reaction is dithiothreitol dependent and is catalyzed by vitamin K epoxide reductase in which vitamin K 2,3-epoxide is reduced to vitamin K quinone. Vitamin K quinone is then reduced to vitamin K hydroquinone by vitamin K quinone reductase and is dependent on either dithiothreitol or nicotinamide adenine dinucleotide, thus completing the vitamin K–epoxide cycle.

Rodenticide anticoagulants inhibit the dithiothreitol-dependent vitamin K reductase reactions and prevent vitamin K hydroquinone regeneration (104,105), which is evident by the significant increase in serum vitamin K 2,3-epoxide levels and a concurrent increase in the serum vitamin K epoxide-vitamin K ratio (Fig. 2) (106,107). Inhibition of vitamin K reductases indirectly inhibits active prothrombin complex protein formation. Rodenticide anticoagulants inhibit vitamin K regeneration almost immediately, but the anticoagulant effect is delayed until the vitamin K stores are depleted and sufficient active coagulation factors are removed from circulation. The vitamin K turnover rate appears to be 30% to 50% per hour, which means the body stores are replaced every 2 to 3 hours (108) and that the anticoagulant effect is dependent on the coagulation factors' half-lives. Factor VII has the shortest half-life (mean, 5.08 hours; range, 4.83 to 10.08 hours) (109,110). Numerical coagulopathy occurs when factor VII level has decreased by more than 75% of predicted values and in an anticoagulant naïve person, it takes at least 15 hours (three half-lives).

VULNERABLE POPULATIONS

Warfarin is U.S. Food and Drug Administration pregnancy category X (Appendix I). Clinical evidence suggests warfarin is not excreted into breast milk (111). The effects of oral anticoagulants on fertility have not been evaluated.

Warfarin therapy during the first trimester of pregnancy is associated with embryopathy (e.g., nasal cartilage hypoplasia, punctate stippled calcifications of cartilages, and skeletal abnormalities) (112,113). In the late third trimester, exposure to anticoagulants may result in prenatal, perinatal, or postnatal hemorrhages (113–115). Ocular (e.g., optic atrophy, microphthalmia, lens opacities, large prominent eyes, and dilation of the cerebral ventricles associated with blindness) and neurologic (e.g., microcephaly and mental retardation) abnormalities are associated with warfarin therapy at any time during gestation.

Long-acting rodenticides have limited information available. A 21-year-old woman ingested 1.5 kg of a brodifacoum rodenticide over 2 days and developed a marked coagulopathy (42). Vitamin K, fresh frozen plasma (FFP), and phenobarbital therapy were initiated. Pregnancy was diagnosed 33 days after hospital admission and spontaneous abortion occurred 1 week later.

A 19-year-old woman at 22 weeks' gestation ingested brodifacoum rat poison 8 days before presentation (73). Her serum brodifacoum concentration was 220 ng/ml and her hematocrit fell from 31% to 21%. Her subsequent antenatal course was unremarkable on vitamin K therapy. She delivered a 3.12-kg boy at term with Apgar scores of 8 and 9 at 1 and 5 minutes, respectively. Maternal and infant coagulation studies were normal. The infant showed normal development at 1 year.

CLINICAL PRESENTATION

Short-Acting Rodenticides

After an intentional ingestion, a patient typically presents for evaluation after signs and symptoms of excessive anticoagulation are evident and usually involving multiple organ systems. The complications from excessive short-acting anticoagulation (e.g., warfarin) involve bleeding and hemorrhage in nearly any organ system. A list of these effects, in decreasing order of frequency, is provided in Table 2.

Cohort studies of patients on warfarin therapy have shown that risk factors for bleeding are age, sex, duration and intensity of therapy, hypertension, history of gastrointestinal bleeding, previous cerebrovascular accident, alcoholism, and liver disease (116–118). The risk of hemorrhage increases with duration and degree of international normalized ratio (INR) elevation above the therapeutic range and age (117–119).

Apparently trivial injury may result in life-threatening blood loss or bleeding into a closed space (e.g., intracranial). The majority of deaths associated with anticoagulant therapy are due to intracranial hemorrhage. The intracranial hemorrhages in patients on warfarin are twice the size and associated with twice the mortality compared to intracranial hemorrhages in patients not on anticoagulants (120), and intracranial bleeds that occur while on anticoagulants are more likely to enlarge during the initial 24 hours (121).

Long-Acting Rodenticides

The complications from excessive long-acting anticoagulation are similar to the effects of short-acting agents (Table 2). The primarily clinical challenge is that they may produce anticoagulation after a single dose, unlike short-acting agents like coumarin that usually require multiple doses to produce anticoagulation.

Poison information center–based studies suggest normal preschool-aged children with single acute unintentional rodenticide anticoagulant exposure rarely develop any significant laboratory or clinical evidence of excessive anticoagulation, and gastrointestinal decontamination does not appear to alter their clinical outcome (122–126). The incidence of numerical coagulopathy is 0.36% in a healthy child who ingests a long-acting rodenticide anticoagulant (125), which when multiplied by the incidence of major hemorrhage of 1.6% in the first month of anticoagulation (127) gives a 0.0058% risk (5.8 in 100,000 chance) of serious hemorrhage. The risk of a serious bleeding event occurring in the rare child with a transient, minimal increase in PT or INR becomes almost zero.

Adverse Events

Cutaneous and subcutaneous tissue necrosis is a rare complication of coumarin anticoagulant therapy (128,129). The patient is typically an obese woman; lesions are predisposed to generous subcutaneous adipose tissue areas (e.g., breast, thigh, and buttock) and typically appear within 3 to 10 days of initiating anticoagulant therapy. Multiple lesions are unusual, almost every case occurred after the use of loading dose regimes, and necrosis is not associated with hemorrhagic diathesis.

The initial lesion is a painful and tender regional evanescent flush, occasionally edematous and elevated, and often poorly demarcated. Regional petechial hemorrhages soon appear in the involved area, and within hours its center becomes red-blue-black discoloration and edematous with sharp demarcation and irregular contoured borders. Within 24 hours the lesion may be gangrenous and necrotic with hemorrhagic blisters. The skin necrosis may be full thickness and extend into the subcutaneous fat. This is followed by eschar formation and tissue sloughing, leaving deep tissue defects that may heal over several months with extensive scarring. The extent and severity of the lesions are variable; some spontaneously resolve, and others require skin grafts or amputation (130,131). Fatalities have been reported and are due to complications associated with coumarin necrosis (130,132,133). The principal histopathologic feature is thrombosis within the subcutaneous vasculature (133,134).

Purple toes syndrome is characterized by dark blue–tinged bilateral purple discoloration of the feet, especially the plantar surfaces and the sides of the first two toes (135). This may be preceded or accompanied by a red-tinged violaceous nondescript discoloration of the thenar and hypothenar eminences of the hand. The color blanches on direct pressure and fades when the legs are elevated. The toes are painful and tender on examination. The intensity of the discoloration may wax and wane, but the color persists. The pathophysiology remains to be determined. When the clinical syndrome occurs, it is evident within 3 to 8 weeks of initiating anticoagulant therapy. The patient's PT is within the therapeutic range, and there are no associated signs and symptoms of excessive coagulation.

Dermatitis medicamentosa may develop during coumarin therapy and is characterized by maculopapular, vesicular, urticarial, and purpuric eruptions (136). The dermatitis resolves within 1 to 3 weeks after the medication is discontinued and recurs within 2 to 3 weeks if the medication is resumed.

DIAGNOSTIC TESTS

Biologic Monitoring and Health Surveillance

A serum vitamin K 2,3-epoxide level may provide a more sensitive biomarker of industrial coumarin (brodifacoum, difenacoum, and warfarin) exposure or accumulation than the PT, activated partial thromboplastin time (PTT), or INR. The normal serum vitamin K 2,3-epoxide concentration is less than 20 ng/ml after a vitamin K challenge (137). In patients chronically exposed to coumarin anticoagulants, serum vitamin K 2,3-epoxide levels are significantly elevated, whereas the clotting factor activities and antigen levels remain in the normal range (53). This apparent dissociation between the coumarin anticoagulant effects on vitamin K metabolism and clotting factor activity may persist for years after termination of the occupational exposure.

TABLE 2. Manifestations of poisoning by rodenticide anticoagulants[a]

Adult—short acting	Adult—long acting	Child—short acting	Child—long acting
Ecchymoses Hematuria Epistaxis Gingival bleeding Menorrhagia Bleeding wounds Abdominal pain Melena Hematemesis Back pain Hematochezia Purpura or petechiae Anemia Hemoptysis Hematemesis Flank pain Tachycardia Fever Mucosal bleeding Altered mental status Intracranial bleeding (6,7,9,10,20, 21,23–25,27,29, 31,33,37,39, 40,43,49–51,55, 61,63,72,94)	Hematuria Ecchymoses Gingival bleeding Epistaxis Abdominal pain Bleeding wounds Oral mucosa bleeding Melena Flank pain Heme positive stool Hematomas Anemia Decreasing hemoglobin concentrations Intracranial bleeding Vaginal bleeding Back pain Hematochezia Menorrhagia Hemoperitoneum Compartment syndrome Coma Tachycardia Tachypnea Fever Hemoptysis Urethral bleeding Fatigue Headache Seizures (5,8,11–19,22,30,32,34,38,42,45, 47,54,56,58,59,62,64,65,67,68,70,73–80)	Ecchymoses Hematuria Gingival bleeding Anemia Epistaxis Hemarthrosis hematomas Bleeding wounds Abdominal pain Seizures Coma Petechiae Hemorrhagic otitis media Hematemesis Menorrhagia Intracranial bleeding (36,40,44,46,60,71)	Ecchymoses Bleeding wounds Epistaxis Anemia Decreasing hemoglobin concentrations Hematomas Hematuria Intracranial bleeding (3,4,18,26,41,66,69,79)
Uncommon complications	**Uncommon complications**		**Uncommon complications**
Tachypnea Headache Shock Intramural intestinal hematoma Hemobilia Intestinal hemorrhage Groin pain Metrorrhagia Retroperitoneal bleeding Decreasing hemoglobin concentrations (7,9,21,25,28,33,37,40, 49,178)	Mouth ulcer Hypoxia Alveolar hemorrhage Hemothorax Shock Syncope Mesenteric and intramural intestinal hematoma Retroperitoneal hemorrhage Rectal bleeding Metrorrhagia Spontaneous abortion Calyceal hemorrhage Adrenocortical hemorrhage Hepatorenal syndrome Purpura Petechiae Hemarthrosis Rhabdomyolysis Agitation Confusion Lethargy Malaise Anorexia Dizziness Seizures Metabolic acidosis (5,12,19,32,34,35,42,45,47,54,59,67, 74,76–78)		Tachycardia Flank pain Petechial hemorrhage Menorrhagia Hematemesis Hemarthrosis Compartment syndrome Pulmonary hemorrhage (3,4,18,26,41,66,69,79)

[a]Manifestations are present in descending order of frequency.

Acute or Chronic Exposure

The laboratory marker for bleeding diathesis after anticoagulant ingestion is an increase in the PT/PTT or INR, which reflects the reduction of factor VII activity to a critical level. A PT/PTT or INR should be measured in 24 to 48 hours after a significant accidental ingestion. After a deliberate ingestion (i.e., self-harm), the PT/PTT or INR should be obtained immediately and at 24 and 48 hours. Numerical coagulopathy is usually evident between 12 to 24 hours after acute significant warfarin ingestion with the maximal PT occurring 36 to 72 hours postingestion (92). The rate of PT increase is directly related to the warfarin dose, but up to a maximum characteristic for the individual (92,93). Beyond this ceiling, increases in warfarin dosage only increase the duration of PT prolongation. After acute brodifacoum ingestion, numerical coagulopathy is apparent within 24 to 48 hours (126).

An increase in the PT or INR may rarely result from congenital deficiency of a blood-clotting factor or more commonly from an acquired deficiency. The congenital deficiency is usually a single factor, whereas the acquired deficiencies usually affect multiple clotting factors. These deficiencies may be differentiated by specific factor assays. The acquired deficiencies are associated most commonly with liver disease, vitamin K deficiency, oral anticoagulant ingestion, a circulating anticoagulant, and defibrination secondary to intravascular clotting. Patients with severe liver disease often have reduced vitamin K–dependent factors activity as well as factors I, V, XI, and XIII.

Other Tests

Other tests are directed at the potential complications of anticoagulation. Typical tests include a complete blood count, stool guaiac, fibrinogen, and fibrin degradation products. Levels of specific clotting factors may help to distinguish between anticoagulant poisoning, liver dysfunction, and congenital clotting factor deficiency. Testing for specific serum anticoagulant levels may not be available in the acute setting, but help confirm the diagnosis of anticoagulant poisoning. If complications of anticoagulation indicate the need, an electrocardiogram, gastrointestinal endoscopy, and computed tomography of the head may be needed.

Serum vitamin K 2,3-epoxide is a sensitive marker for oral anticoagulant effect and may be diagnostic in surreptitious oral anticoagulant ingestion (53,106). After vitamin K administration, the serum epoxide level peaks within 3 to 4 hours, is dependent on the serum anticoagulant concentration, and accumulates at serum anticoagulant levels that do not produce marked changes in prothrombin time.

Determination of protein induced by vitamin K absence or antagonism for factor II antigen is a useful tool in detecting vitamin K–deficient status among coagulation disorders (41,138). Serum protein induced by vitamin K absence or antagonism for factor II antigen is markedly elevated in the presence of circulating uncarboxylated factor II. Protein induced by vitamin K absence or antagonism for factor II antigen concentration less than 0.15 U/ml is consistent with therapeutic anticoagulation, and concentrations greater than 0.25 U/ml are consistent with profound vitamin K deficiency or warfarin overdose.

The *response to vitamin K_1 and vitamin K_3* may differentiate hypoprothrombinemia of vitamin K deficiency, excessive anticoagulation, congenital clotting factor deficiency, and hepatic dysfunction. Vitamin K deficiency responds promptly to water-soluble vitamin K_3 therapy. Coumarin anticoagulation promptly responds to vitamin K_1 and does not respond to vitamin K_3 therapy. Congenital clotting factor deficiency or hepatic dysfunction does not respond to either vitamin K_1 or K_3 therapy. A circulating anticoagulant is frequently associated with hemophilia and disseminated lupus erythematosus, which does not respond to either vitamin K_1 or K_3 challenge. The patient's PTT remains abnormal when equal amount of normal plasma is mixed with the patient's plasma. Defibrination is associated with reduced fibrinogen and platelets, and elevated fibrin degradation products.

Postmortem Considerations

In a patient who died of complications from phenprocoumon toxicity, phenprocoumon was present in (in descending order) liver, lung, heart blood, venous blood, kidney, and stomach contents (31).

Autopsy findings in patients who died of complications from brodifacoum toxicity include hemarthrosis; pulmonary hemorrhages; renal calyceal hemorrhages; adrenocortical hemorrhage; petechial hemorrhages; subarachnoid, subdural, intraventricular, and intraparenchymal hemorrhages; and diffuse hemorrhagic diatheses (76,79,80). Brodifacoum has been found in blood, lung, liver, bile, spleen, and kidney; the highest concentrations were detected in bile and femoral blood (79,80). However, brodifacoum was not detected in brain or vitreous humor. Postmortem blood and liver specimens may be useful to confirm or diagnose brodifacoum toxicity (34,76,78–80).

A 21-year-old man attempted suicide with brodifacoum 6 months before presenting with seizure and coma, and his head computed tomography showed a lethal intracranial hemorrhage (75). The postmortem serum brodifacoum concentration was 290 ng/ml.

A 39-year-old woman presented with bleeding excoriations and gingivae, multiple hematomas in the oropharynx, bloody stool, hematuria, ecchymoses, INR of 19, PT of 60 seconds, and PTT of 106 seconds (78). Soon after presentation, she developed a severe headache, confusion, and died from subarachnoid hemorrhage despite administration of FFP and vitamin K_1. The postmortem serum brodifacoum concentration was 160 ng/ml.

A 15-year-old woman with a history of menorrhagia, bruising, and prolonged bleeding from sores on her extremities was found dead at home (79). Postmortem examination was remarkable for multicolored ecchymoses; petechial hemorrhages densely concentrated on the shins; subarachnoid, subdural, and intraparenchymal hemorrhages; and acute alveolar hemorrhage. The postmortem brodifacoum concentration in femoral blood was 3919 ng/ml.

TREATMENT

The goal of treatment is to relieve emergent complications such as bleeding, terminate exposure to the agent, and administer vitamin K in selected patients. The suicidal patient should be assessed emergently in a hospital; receive gastrointestinal decontamination; and be admitted for close observation, laboratory monitoring, and expectant treatment. The observation period should be at least 48 hours.

Owing to the extremely low risk of complications, children with a single ingestion of brodifacoum may not require routine hospital referral, gastrointestinal decontamination, and laboratory testing, and parents may be advised simply to seek medical assessment in the unlikely occurrence of unusual bruising or bleeding in their children. However, intentional ingestions, ingestions involving suspected child abuse, and ingestions by children with abnormal neurologic or psychologic development warrant the same management as the suicidal patient.

Decontamination

Although it has not been well studied, a single dose of activated charcoal is recommended after a significant acute ingestion that occurred within the previous few hours. Syrup of ipecac has been reported to cause severe retching and fatal intracranial hemorrhage in a patient with brodifacoum toxicity (77). Gastric lavage, cathartic, and whole bowel irrigation have not been formally studied.

After skin exposure, all areas should be thoroughly washed with soap and water. For respiratory exposure, removal from the source of the exposure is sufficient.

Enhancement of Elimination

Multiple doses of activated charcoal (25 g every 4 hours for six doses) may shorten the terminal elimination half-life of brodifacoum after an intentional ingestion but does not eliminate the need for prolonged vitamin K therapy (139).

Clinical studies have shown that cholestyramine interferes with oral anticoagulant, and presumably rodenticide anticoagulant absorption from the gastrointestinal tract, interrupts its enterohepatic circulation, and decreases the serum half-life of oral anticoagulant (140–142). The typical cholestyramine dose is 50 to 150 mg/kg/dose (adult, 3 to 9 g), and this dose can be repeated every 6 to 8 hours.

Adjunct phenobarbital therapy may induce hepatic cytochrome metabolism of oral anticoagulants and enhance its elimination. The efficacy of this therapy in patients with warfarin poisoning is doubtful because it takes several days for phenobarbital to optimally induce CYP activity, and phenobarbital does not induce the principal isoenzymes in racemic warfarin metabolism (143,144). In addition, the risk of sedation from phenobarbital therapy in a patient prone to hemorrhagic complications should outweigh potential benefits.

There is a case report of phenprocoumon poisoning that was successfully treated with plasmapheresis (145).

Antidotes

The primary antidote for anticoagulant effects is vitamin K. Rodenticide anticoagulant poisoning usually does not become apparent until 24 to 48 hours after ingestion, and its earliest manifestation is numerical coagulopathy (126). Prophylactic vitamin K therapy before laboratory abnormalities develop is not recommended because coagulation factors gradually decline over time and no patient is expected to develop a life-threatening coagulopathy within 24 hours. Vitamin K therapy delays the onset of numerical coagulopathy, which obscures the diagnosis and necessitates prolonged observation. If a significant coagulopathy occurs, it likely lasts for weeks and the prophylactic vitamin K dose does not prevent complications.

Numerical coagulopathy does not necessitate emergency treatment. In selected patients with warfarin poisoning or excessive anticoagulation on warfarin therapy, discontinuation of warfarin and close follow-up with daily or twice daily laboratory coagulation measurements may be acceptable. The majority of excessively anticoagulated patients return to the therapeutic range within 3 days of discontinuing therapy, and patients with therapeutic INRs have complete anticoagulation reversal within 3 to 5 days (146–148). However, the maximal INR decline is delayed for 24 to 36 hours.

Vitamin K may be administered by the oral, subcutaneous, intramuscular, or intravenous route. The preferred route of administration depends on the clinical situation. Intravenous administration results in the most rapid, reliable, and predictable reversal of oral anticoagulant effect and provides 70% of its INR correction within 8 hours (149–152). Intravenous vitamin K_1 results in the fastest INR reduction (153). Oral administration produces a variable response and slower rate of anticoagulation reversal: at least 24 to 48 hours (146,152,154–157). In addition, there appears to be marked differences in the efficacy of anticoagulation reversal between orally administered vitamin K_1 preparations (154,155,157). The volume necessary to deliver a therapeutic vitamin K_1 dose may limit the usefulness of intramuscular and subcutaneous administration; intramuscular injections should be avoided in patients with coagulopathy.

Intravenous vitamin K_1 and prothrombin complex or FFP should be administered to patients with suspected major or life-threatening hemorrhage. Only vitamin K_1 should be administered for treatment of oral anticoagulant toxicity. The physician should anticipate the occurrence of adverse drug events during intravenous vitamin K_1 administration and should be prepared to treat anaphylaxis should it occur. Vitamin K_1 should be diluted with 5% dextrose, 0.9% sodium chloride, or 5% dextrose in 0.9% sodium chloride, and administered at a rate not to exceed 1 mg/minute (158). The recommended initial vitamin K_1 dose is 5 mg for patients with warfarin toxicity and provides complete reversal of anticoagulation in the majority of the situations, irrespective of the INR (159).

One recommended treatment for patients with numerical coagulopathy (INR more than 7.0) or mild hemorrhage who are on warfarin therapy and require partial anticoagulation reversal is intravenous vitamin K_1 0.5 mg (150). A therapeutic INR may be achieved within 24 hours. Patients should be followed with daily INR and repeat vitamin K_1 doses may be necessary. Some clinicians are concerned about administering intravenous vitamin K_1 because of associated anaphylaxis and recommend intravenous administration be reserved for patients with life-threatening hemorrhage (160). A higher vitamin K dose or parenteral administration may be required for partial anticoagulation reversal involving phenprocoumon (161). Oral vitamin K_1 1 to 5 mg failed to decrease the INR to 4.0 at 48 hours in 67% of the patients with an initial INR greater than 6.0, and repeat vitamin K_1 doses may be required. Details regarding the method of administration and complications of vitamin K are provided in Chapter 68.

Gastrointestinal vitamin K_1 absorption is dependent on the presence of bile salts and an energy-dependent saturable process in the proximal portions of the small intestine (162,163). There is marked interindividual variation in absorption (10% to 63%), and intraindividual variation is also evident when the dose is increased from 10 mg to 50 mg (137). The estimated efficiency of vitamin K_1 absorption is 80% (163).

The optimal vitamin K_1 dose for patients with clinically significant coagulopathy after long-acting rodenticide poisoning is not well established. Animal data suggest intravenous vitamin K_1 10 mg/kg every 4 to 8 hours may be necessary in situations of complete vitamin K antagonism (137). One case report suggests a patient with hematuria and gingival bleeding from brodifacoum poisoning (INR 38.2, brodifacoum 170 ng/ml) may be adequately treated with FFP and oral vitamin K_1 7 mg/kg/day divided every 6 hours (11). In maximally brodifacoum anticoagulated rabbits, plasma vitamin K_1 concentration greater than 1.0 µg/ml is necessary to completely reestablish clotting factor synthesis, which is achieved after an intravenous 10 mg/kg dose (137). Prothrombin complex activity increase is evident within 4 hours and peaks 9 hours after vitamin K_1 administration and declines with a half-life of 6 hours. In humans, vitamin K_1 concentration greater than 0.5 μg/ml can be maintained for less than 2 hours after an intravenous, but not an oral, 10 mg dose (137). After oral vitamin K_1 administration, peak plasma level occurs 5 hours after dosing.

Supportive Care

In patients with or suspected major anticoagulant-related hemorrhage, coagulation factors II, VII, IX, and X should be immediately administered. This can be achieved using either prothrombin complex concentrate (PCC) or FFP as adjunct to vitamin K_1 therapy. PCC is a more rapid method of administering clotting factors in doses required to completely reverse coagulopathy regardless of the INR (164). Retrospective studies comparing emergency FFP and PCC therapy in orally anticoagulated patients with life-threatening hemorrhage suggest coagulopathy reversal is more rapid and effective with PCC (165–168).

PCC has been used for the treatment of hemophilia B before the advent of purer factor IX concentrates and recombinant factor IX. PCC is produced by fractionation of pooled plasma and most contain equal quantities of factor II, VII, IX, and X. PCC is available in lyophilized form, and 500 to 1000 U of each factor can be immediately reconstituted in a final volume of 20 ml before administration. The recommended dose for patients with INR 2.0 to 3.9 is 25 U/kg, INR 4.0 to 5.9 is 35 U/kg, and INR greater than 5.9 or life-threatening bleeding is 50 U/kg (159,169). Adverse drug events associated with PCC therapy include thrombosis, disseminated intravascular coagulation, blood-borne pathogens transmission, and allergic reactions. Disseminated intravascular coagulation and uncompensated liver disease are contraindications to PCC therapy.

The recommended FFP dose is 10 to 20 ml/kg for life-threatening bleeding (169). However, there are several disadvantages associated with FFP: the volume of FFP for a 70-kg patient is 700 to 1400 ml and may not be tolerated by patients with marginal cardiovascular reserve. The processing time (e.g., blood specimen for blood grouping, thawing of FFP, transport, and administration) may take at least 1 to 2 hours. FFP quality control is assessed by estimation of factor VIII concentration and the vitamin K–dependent factors are not routinely assayed (167). In one report, the median concentrations of factors II, VII, IX, and X in 20 batches of FFP were 82.5, 92.0, 61.0, and 90.5 U/dl, respectively (167). It can be extrapolated that 15 ml/kg of FFP provides 640 U of factor IX, which raises the factor IX level by 9%. When the INR is greater than 4.0, the factor IX level is often less than 0.20 U/ml and may be less than 0.10 U/ml, which suggests the 15 ml/kg of FFP is inadequate to completely reverse coagulopathy. This was confirmed by one study that showed administration of 800 ml of FFP to patients with INRs between 2.9 and 22.0 failed to raise the median coagulation factors concentrations above 20 U/dl. A small but significant risk of transfusion-related acute lung injury and a finite risk of blood-borne pathogens transmission exist.

Recombinant activated factor VII (rFVIIa) has also been reported to be safe, rapid, and effective in emergency reversal of anticoagulation (170–172). The therapeutic rFVIIa dose ranges from 15 to 90 μg/kg. The advantages of rFVIIa include unlikelihood of blood-borne pathogens transmission, avoidance of the volume constraints of FFP, and substantial reduction in the time for administration and for achieving adequate hemostasis. A limitation of rFVIIa therapy is the inability to monitor or predict hemostatic efficacy because prothrombin times and factor VII activity levels do not correlate. Clinical measures (e.g., cessation of bleeding and stability of hematocrit) are required for monitoring the effectiveness of rFVIIa therapy. Hypercoagulable complications (e.g., myocardial infarction) have been associated with rFVIIa therapy (173).

Acenocoumarol has a short half-life and patients with numerical coagulopathy requiring partial anticoagulation reversal may be managed by withholding one or more of their anticoagulant doses. In one study, patients receiving subcutaneous vitamin K had a greater fall in INR compared to patients who had their anticoagulant withheld (174). However, a similar number of patients in each group reached a *safe* target INR within 24 hours. In contrast, phenprocoumon has a long half-life and patients with numerical coagulopathy may require repeat vitamin K_1 doses to correct their excessive anticoagulation.

Monitoring

Physical examination should focus on signs and symptoms of excessive anticoagulation, which includes epistaxis, gingival bleeding, hematuria, bruising, and ecchymosis; head trauma is of significant concern. Laboratory monitoring of patients that have ingested a long-acting anticoagulant include the PT/PTT or INR. The endpoint of vitamin K therapy for long-acting anticoagulants has been to discontinue therapy at an arbitrary time and obtain serial PT/PTT or INR and observe for its elevation. The disadvantage of this strategy is the patient may be put at risk of bleeding or prolonged hospitalization.

An alternative to the serum coagulation profile is to monitor serum factor VII concentration when vitamin K therapy is withheld (30). A progressive decrease in factor VII levels to 30% of normal indicates the need for further vitamin K therapy. This strategy is limited by the availability of factor VII levels in a timely manner.

The use of serial serum brodifacoum concentrations to determine elimination kinetics and therapeutic endpoints in a patient after an overdose has been suggested (11). The brodifacoum levels can be plotted versus time and are approximated by zero order kinetics (linear decline). Case reports suggest that increased prothrombin times necessitating vitamin K_1 treatments do not occur when the serum brodifacoum concentration is less than 10 ng/ml, which may be a reasonable endpoint for therapy (32,66).

Serum vitamin K 2,3-epoxide is a sensitive marker for oral anticoagulant effect (53,106) and may be a useful guide for vitamin K therapy. It may be reasonable to continue vitamin K therapy until the serum epoxide concentration begins to fall. This strategy is limited to obtaining vitamin K 2,3-epoxide levels within a reasonable time.

Management Pitfalls

Outpatient vitamin K therapy should be considered only in patients who are reliable in taking a large number of pills several times a day for prolonged periods and for periodic follow-up. Serious recurrent coagulopathy and death may occur as a result of poor compliance with outpatient vitamin K therapy (18,30,41,42,45,47,67,76,77).

The INR was developed to assess anticoagulation in patients on coumarin therapy, and FFP therapy makes INR interpretation difficult. The INR is not sensitive to changes in factor IX, which may be an important determinant in anticoagulant-related bleeding outcome, and decreases in INR after FFP therapy actually reflect only partial corrections of anticoagulation (167).

Occult gastrointestinal bleeding in a patient receiving anticoagulant therapy should not be attributed to the anticoagulant; bleeding often indicates the presence of significant intestinal disease (175). Prospective studies have shown a high incidence of underlying major genitourinary tract disease in anticoagulated patients with hematuria, and the degree of coagulation does not appear to correlate with the incidence of hematuria (176,177). In one study, significant genitourinary tract disease (e.g., nephrolithiasis, neoplasms, and papillary necrosis) was identified in 15.6% of patients with more than one episode of microscopic hematuria (176). In another study, significant pathologic condition (e.g., malignancy) was identified in 67% of patients with gross hematuria, and 75% of patients with microscopic hematuria were found to have genitourinary tract disease (e.g., urethritis, calculi, and renal cyst) (177). It is recommended that all episodes of hematuria during anticoagulation therapy should be thoroughly investigated.

The potential widespread tissue distribution and long half-life of brodifacoum raise the theoretical concern that an organ transplanted from a toxic donor is damaged or contains sufficient residual brodifacoum to result in coagulopathy in recipients. However, heart, lungs, liver, pancreas, kidneys, and corneas have been successfully transplanted from donor patients who died of complications from brodifacoum toxicity, and none of the recipients developed a clinically significant coagulopathy in spite of mild postoperative PT/INR elevation in some of the patients (75,77,78).

REFERENCES

1. Link KP. The discovery of dicumarol and its sequels. *Circulation* 1959;19:97–107.
2. Muller RL, Scheidt S. History of drugs for thrombotic disease. Discovery, development, and directions for the future. *Circulation* 1994;89:432–449.
3. Babcock J, Hartman K, Pedersen A, et al. Rodenticide-induced coagulopathy in a young child. A case of Munchausen syndrome by proxy. *Am J Pediatr Hematol Oncol* 1993;15:126–130.
4. Barlow AM, Gay AL, Park BK. Difenacoum (Neosorexa) poisoning. *Br Med J (Clin Res Ed)* 1982;285:541.
5. Barnett VT, Bergmann F, Humphrey H, et al. Diffuse alveolar hemorrhage secondary to superwarfarin ingestion. *Chest* 1992;102:1301–1302.
6. Bates D, Mintz M. Phytonadione therapy in a multiple-drug overdose involving warfarin. *Pharmacotherapy* 2000;20:1208–1215.
7. Bentley WBA. Accidental ingestion of bishydroxycoumarin. Use of vitamin K_1 emulsion in two cases. *JAMA* 1954;156:496–497.
8. Berry RG, Morrison JA, Watts JW, et al. Surreptitious superwarfarin ingestion with brodifacoum. *South Med J* 2000;93:74–75.
9. Bowie EJ, Todd M, Thompson JH Jr, et al. Anticoagulant malingerers (the "Dicumarol-eaters"). *Am J Med* 1965;39:855–864.
10. Breckenridge RT, Kellermeyer RW. A hemorrhagic syndrome due to dicumarol poisoning masquerading as propylthiouracil sensitivity. *Ann Intern Med* 1964;60:1066–1068.
11. Bruno GR, Howland MA, McMeeking A, et al. Long-acting anticoagulant overdose: brodifacoum kinetics and optimal vitamin K dosing. *Ann Emerg Med* 2000;36:262–267.
12. Burucoa C, Mura P, Robert R, et al. Chlorophacinone intoxication. A biological and toxicological study. *J Toxicol Clin Toxicol* 1989;27:79–89.
13. Butcher GP, Shearer MJ, MacNicoll AD, et al. Difenacoum poisoning as a cause of haematuria. *Hum Exp Toxicol* 1992;11:553–554.
14. Casner PR. Superwarfarin toxicity. *Am J Ther* 1998;5:117–120.
15. Chen TW, Deng JF. A brodifacoum intoxication case of mouthful amount. *Vet Hum Toxicol* 1986;28:488.
16. Chong LL, Chau WK, Ho CH. A case of "superwarfarin" poisoning. *Scand J Haematol* 1986;36:314–315.
17. Chow EY, Haley LP, Vickars LM, et al. A case of bromadiolone (superwarfarin) ingestion. *Can Med Assoc J* 1992;147:60–62.
18. Chua JD, Friedenberg WR. Superwarfarin poisoning. *Arch Intern Med* 1998;158:1929–1932.
19. Corke PJ. Superwarfarin (brodifacoum) poisoning. *Anaesth Intensive Care* 1997;25:707–709.
20. Cosgriff SW. Hemorrhage due to self-medication with bishydroxycoumarin. *JAMA* 1953;153:547–548.
21. Eldore A, Zylber-Katz E, Kaplan De-Nour A. Anticoagulant abuse: a psychotic syndrome? *J Nerv Ment Dis* 1979;167:442–446.
22. Exner DV, Brien WF, Murphy MJ. Superwarfarin ingestion. *Can Med Assoc J* 1992;146:34–35.
23. Fantl P, Sawers RJ, Ward HA. Detection of a self-inflicted haemorrhagic disorder. *Med J Aust* 1962;1:246–248.
24. Forbes CD, Prentice CRM, Sclare AB. Surreptitious ingestion of warfarin. *Br J Psychiat* 1974;125:245–247.
25. Fristedt B, Sterner N. Warfarin intoxication from percutaneous absorption. *Arch Environ Health* 1965;11:205–208.
26. Greeff MC, Mashile O, MacDougall LG. "Superwarfarin" (bromodialone) poisoning in two children resulting in prolonged anticoagulation. *Lancet* 1987;2:1269.
27. Green P. Haemorrhagic diathesis attributed to "warfarin" poisoning. *Can Med Assoc J* 1955;72:769–770.
28. Goldsmith JC, Drossman DA, Blatt PM. Hemobilia complicating warfarin therapy. *South Med J* 1979;72:748–750.
29. Hackett LP, Ilett KF, Chester A. Plasma warfarin concentrations after a massive overdose. *Med J Aust* 1985;142:642–643.
30. Hoffman RS, Smilkstein MJ, Goldfrank LR. Evaluation of coagulation factor abnormalities in long-acting anticoagulant overdose. *J Toxicol Clin Toxicol* 1988;26:233–248.
31. Hohler T, Becker J, Meyer zum Buschenfelde KH, et al. Fatal cerebellar haemorrhage due to phenprocoumon poisoning. *Int J Legal Med* 1996;108:268–271.
32. Hollinger BR, Pastoor TP. Case management and plasma half-life in a case of brodifacoum poisoning. *Arch Intern Med* 1993;153:1925–1928.
33. Holmes RW, Love J. Suicide attempt with warfarin, a bishydroxycoumarin-like rodenticide. *JAMA* 1952;148:935–937.
34. Hui CH, Lie A, Lam CK, Bourke C. "Superwarfarin" poisoning leading to prolonged coagulopathy. *Forensic Sci Int* 1996;78:13–18.
35. Huic M, Francetic I, Bakran I, et al. Acquired coagulopathy due to anticoagulant rodenticide poisoning. *Croat Med J* 2002;43:615–617.
36. Hvizdala EV, Gellady AM. Intentional poisoning of two siblings by prescription drugs. *Clin Pediatr* 1978;17:480–482.
37. Ikkala E, Myllyla G, Nevanlinna HR, et al. Haemorrhagic diathesis due to criminal poisoning with warfarin. *Acta Med Scand* 1964;176:201–203.
38. Jones EC, Growe GH, Naiman SC. Prolonged anticoagulation in rat poisoning. *JAMA* 1984;252:3005–3007.
39. Kwaan HC, Simon NM, del Greco F. Hemorrhagic diathesis induced by surreptitious ingestion of coumarin drugs. *Med Clin North Am* 1972;56:263–273.
40. Lange PF, Terveer J. Warfarin poisoning. *U S Armed Forces Med J* 1954;5:872–877.
41. La Rosa FG, Clarke SH, Lefkowitz JB. Brodifacoum intoxication with marijuana smoking. *Arch Pathol Lab Med* 1997;121:67–69.
42. Lipton RA, Klass EM. Human ingestion of a "superwarfarin" rodenticide resulting in a prolonged anticoagulant effect. *JAMA* 1984;252:3004–3005.
43. Maharaj D, Walker ID, Paice B, et al. Surreptitious ingestion of warfarin. *Practitioner* 1986;230:105–108.
44. Martin-Bouyer G, Khanh NB, Linh PD, et al. Epidemic of haemorrhagic disease in Vietnamese infants caused by warfarin-contaminated talcs. *Lancet* 1983;1:230–232.
45. McCarthy PT, Cox AD, Harrington DJ, et al. Covert poisoning with difenacoum: clinical and toxicological observations. *Hum Exp Toxicol* 1997;16:166–170.
46. Mogilner BM, Freeman JS, Blashar Y, et al. Reye's syndrome in three Israeli children. Possible relationship to warfarin toxicity. *Israel J Med Sci* 1974;10:1117–1125.
47. Morgan BW, Tomaszewski C, Rotker I. Spontaneous hemoperitoneum from brodifacoum overdose. *Am J Emerg Med* 1996;14:656–659.
48. Murdoch DA. Prolonged anticoagulation in chlorphacinone poisoning. *Lancet* 1983;1:355–356.
49. Nilsson IM. Recurrent hypoprothrobinaemia due to poisoning with a dicumarol-containing rat-killer. *Acta Haemat* 1957;17:176–182.
50. O'Reilly RA, Aggeler PM. Covert anticoagulant ingestion: study of 25 patients and review of world literature. *Medicine* 1976;55:389–399.
51. O'Reilly RA, Aggeler PM. Surreptitious ingestion of coumarin anticoagulant drugs. *Ann Intern Med* 1966;64:1034–1041.
52. O'Reilly RA, Aggeler PM, Gibbs JO. Hemorrhagic state due to surreptitious ingestion of bishydroxycoumarin. A detailed case study. *N Engl J Med* 1962;267:19–24.
53. Park BK, Choonara IA, Haynes BP, et al. Abnormal vitamin K metabolism in the presence of normal clotting factor activity in factory workers exposed to 4-hydroxycoumarins. *Br J Clin Pharmacol* 1986;21:289–293.
54. Rauch AE, Weininger R, Pasquale D, et al. Superwarfarin poisoning: a significant public health problem. *J Community Health* 1994;19:55–65.
55. Richmond RG, Sawyer WT, Aiello PD, et al. Extreme warfarin intoxication secondary to possible covert drug ingestion. *Drug Intell Clin Pharm* 1988;22:696–699.
56. Ross GS, Zacharski LR, Robert D, et al. An acquired hemorrhagic disorder from long-acting rodenticide ingestion. *Arch Intern Med* 1992;152:410–412.
57. Seidelmann S, Kubic V, Burton E, et al. Combined superwarfarin and ethylene glycol ingestion. A unique case report with misleading clinical history. *Am J Clin Pathol* 1995;104:663–666.
58. Sheen SR, Spiller HA, Grossman D. Symptomatic brodifacoum ingestion requiring high-dose phytonadione therapy. *Vet Hum Toxicol* 1994;36:216–217.
59. Soubiron L, Hantson P, Michaux I, et al. Spontaneous haemoperitoneum from surreptitious ingestion of a rodenticide. *Eur J Emerg Med* 2000;7:305–307.
60. Souid AK, Korins K, Keith D, et al. Unexplained menorrhagia and hematuria: a case report of Munchausen's syndrome by proxy. *Pediatr Hematol Oncol* 1993;10:245–248.
61. Stafne WA, Moe AE. Hypoprothrombinemia due to dicumarol in a malingerer: a case report. *Ann Intern Med* 1951;35:910–911.
62. Stanziale SF, Christopher JC, Fisher RB. Brodifacoum rodenticide ingestion in a patient with shigellosis. *South Med J* 1997;90:833–835.

63. Suwanvecho S, Baker JR. Accidental over-anticoagulation: substitution error by a foreign pharmacy. *Ann Pharmacother* 2000;34:1132–1135.
64. Swigar ME, Clemow LP, Saidi P, et al. "Superwarfarin" ingestion. A new problem in covert anticoagulant overdose. *Gen Hosp Psychiatry* 1990;12:309–312.
65. Tecimer C, Yam LT. Surreptitious superwarfarin poisoning with brodifacoum. *South Med J* 1997;90:1053–1055.
66. Travis SF, Warfield W, Greenbaum BH, et al. Spontaneous hemorrhage associated with accidental brodifacoum poisoning in a child. *J Pediatr* 1993;122:982–984.
67. Waien SA, Hayes D Jr, Leonardo JM. Severe coagulopathy as a consequence of smoking crack cocaine laced with rodenticide. *N Engl J Med* 2001;345:700–701.
68. Wallace S, Worsnop C, Paull P, et al. Covert self poisoning with brodifacoum, a "superwarfarin." *Aust N Z J Med* 1990;20:713–715.
69. Watts RG, Castleberry RP, Sadowski JA. Accidental poisoning with a superwarfarin compound (brodifacoum) in a child. *Pediatrics* 1990;86:883–887.
70. Weitzel JN, Sadowski JA, Furie BC, et al. Surreptitious ingestion of a long-acting vitamin K antagonist/rodenticide, brodifacoum: clinical and metabolic studies of three cases. *Blood* 1990;76:2555–2559.
71. White ST, Voter K, Perry J. Surreptitious warfarin ingestion. *Child Abuse Negl* 1985;9:349–352.
72. Vitellas KM, Vaswani K, Bova JG. Case 3. Spontaneous uroepithelial hemorrhage caused by warfarin overdose. *AJR Am J Roentgenol* 2000;175:881, 884–885.
73. Zurawski JM, Kelly EA. Pregnancy outcome after maternal poisoning with brodifacoum, a long-acting warfarin-like rodenticide. *Obstet Gynecol* 1997;90:672–674.
74. Basehore LM, Mowry JM. Death following ingestion of superwarfarin rodenticide: a case report. *Vet Hum Toxicol* 1987;29:459.
75. Emre S, Kitabayashi K, Miller CM. Successful liver transplantation from a donor with brodifacoum intoxication. *Liver Transpl Surg* 1999;5:509–511.
76. Helmuth RA, McCloskey OW, Doeden DJ, et al. Fatal ingestion of a brodifacoum-containing rodenticide. *Lab Med* 1989;20:25–27.
77. Kruse JA, Carlson RW. Fatal rodenticide poisoning with brodifacoum. *Ann Emerg Med* 1992;21:331–336.
78. Ornstein DL, Lord KE, Yanofsky NN, et al. Successful donation and transplantation of multiple organs after fatal poisoning with brodifacoum, a long-acting anticoagulant rodenticide: case report. *Transplantation* 1999;67:475–478.
79. Palmer RB, Alakija P, de Baca JE, et al. Fatal brodifacoum rodenticide poisoning: autopsy and toxicologic findings. *J Forensic Sci* 1999;44:851–855.
80. Routh CR, Triplett DA, Murphy MJ, et al. Superwarfarin ingestion and detection. *Am J Hematol* 1991;36:50–54.
81. Breckenridge A, Orme ML. The plasma half lives and the pharmacological effect of the enantiomers of warfarin in rats. *Life Sci II* 1972;11:337–345.
82. Breckenridge A, Orme M, Wesseling H, et al. Pharmacokinetics and pharmacodynamics of the enantiomers of warfarin in man. *Clin Pharmacol Ther* 1974;15:424–430.
83. Bachmann KA, Sullivan TJ. Dispositional and pharmacodynamic characteristics of brodifacoum in warfarin-sensitive rats. *Pharmacology* 1983;27:281–288.
84. Leck JB, Park BK. A comparative study of the effect of warfarin and brodifacoum on the relationship between vitamin K_1 metabolism and clotting factor activity in warfarin-susceptible and warfarin-resistant rats. *Biochem Pharmacol* 1981;30:123–128.
85. Lund M. Comparative effect of the three rodenticides warfarin, difenzcoum, and brodifacoum on eight rodent species in short feeding periods. *J Hyg* 1981;87:101–107.
86. Park BK, Leck JB. A comparison of vitamin K antagonism by warfarin, difenacoum, and brodifacoum in the rabbit. *Biochem Pharmacol* 1982;31:3535–3539.
87. Brewer E, Haggerty RJ. Toxic hazards. Rat poisons. I—warfarin. *N Engl J Med* 1957;257:145–146.
88. Shapiro S. Warfarin sodium derivative (Coumadin sodium). An intravenous hypoprothrombinemia-inducing agent. *Angiology* 1953;4:380–390.
89. Udall JA. "No-load" warfarin therapy. *N Engl J Med* 1979;283:1345–1346.
90. Carpentieri U, Nghiem QX, Harris LC. Clinical experience with an oral anticoagulant in children. *Arch Dis Child* 1976;51:445–448.
91. Editorial staff. Long acting anticoagulants. In: Toll LL, Hurlbut KM, eds. POISINDEX system. Greenwood Village, CO: MICROMEDEX (edition expires September 2003).
92. O'Reilly RA, Aggeler PM, Leong LS. The pharmacodynamics of warfarin in man. *J Clin Invest* 1963;42:1542–1551.
93. O'Reilly RA, Aggeler PM, Leong LS. Studies on the coumarin anticoagulant drugs: a comparison of the pharmacodynamics of dicumarol and warfarin in man. *Thromb Diath Haemorrh* 1964;11:1–22.
94. O'Reilly RA, Aggeler PM, Hoag MS. Studies on the coumarin anticoagulant drugs: the assay of warfarin and its biologic application. *Thromb Diath Haemorrh* 1962;8:82–95.
95. Yamazaki H, Shimada T. Human liver cytochrome P450 enzymes involved in the 7-hydroxylation of R- and S-warfarin enantiomers. *Biochem Pharmacol* 1997;54:1195–203.
96. Breckenridge AM, Cholerton S, Hart JAD, et al. A study of the relationship between the pharmacokinetics and the pharmacodynamics of the 4-hydroxycoumarin anticoagulants warfarin, difenacoum and brodifacoum in rabbit. *Br J Pharmacol* 1985;84:81–91.
97. Stanton T, Sowray P, McWaters D, et al. Prolonged anticoagulation with long-acting coumadin derivatives: case report of a brodifacoum poisoning with pharmacokinetic data. *Blood* 1988;72[Suppl 1]:310.
98. Stenflo J, Suttie JW. Vitamin K-dependent formation of the γ-carboxyglutamic acid. *Annu Rev Biochem* 1977;46:157–172.
99. Suttie JW, Jackson CM. Prothrombin structure, activation, and biosynthesis. *Physiol Rev* 1977;57:1–70.
100. Ad-El DD, Meirovitz A, Weinberg A, et al. Warfarin skin necrosis: local and systemic factors. *Br J Plast Surg* 2000;53:624–626.
101. Smirnov MD, Safa O, Esmon NL, et al. Inhibition of activated protein C anticoagulant activity by prothrombin. *Blood* 1999;94:3839–3846.
102. Vigano D'Angelo S, Comp PC, Esmon CT, et al. Relationship between protein C antigen and anticoagulant activity during oral anticoagulation and in selected disease states. *J Clin Invest* 1986;77:416–425.
103. Zimbelman J, Lefkowitz J, Schaeffer C, et al. Unusual complications of warfarin therapy: skin necrosis and priapism. *J Pediatr* 2000;137:266–268.
104. Fasco MJ, Hildebrandt EF, Suttie JW. Evidence that warfarin anticoagulant action involves two distinct reductase activities. *J Biol Chem* 1982;257:11210–11212.
105. Whitlon DS, Sadowski JA, Suttie JW. Mechanism of coumarin action: significance of vitamin K epoxide reductase inhibition. *Biochemistry* 1978;17:1371–1377.
106. Bechtold H, Trenk D, Jahnchen E, et al. Plasma vitamin K_1-2,3-epoxide as diagnostic aid to detect surreptitious ingestion of oral anticoagulant drug. *Lancet* 1983;1:596–597.
107. Shearer MJ, McBurney A, Barkhan P. Effect of warfarin anticoagulation on vitamin-K_1 metabolism in man. *Br J Haematology* 1973;24:471–479.
108. Bjornsson TD, Blaschke TF. Vitamin K_1 disposition and therapy of warfarin overdose. *Lancet* 1978;2:846–847.
109. Frick PG. Studies on the turnover rate of stable prothrombin conversion factor in man. *Acta Haemat* 1958;19:20–29.
110. Loeliger EA, van der Esch B, ter Haar Romeny-Wachter C Ch, et al. Factor VII: its turnover rate and its possible role in thrombogenesis. *Thromb Diath Haemorrh* 1960;4:196–200.
111. Clark SL, Porter TF, West FG. Coumarin derivatives and breast-feeding. *Obstet Gynecol* 2000;95:938–940.
112. Hall JG, Pauli PM, Wilson KM. Maternal and fetal sequelae of anticoagulation during pregnancy. *Am J Med* 1980;68:122–140.
113. Stevenson RE, Burton OM, Ferlauto GJ, et al. Hazards of oral anticoagulants during pregnancy. *JAMA* 1980;243:1549–1551.
114. Ramsay DM. Thromboembolism in pregnancy. *Obstet Gynecol* 1975;45:129–132.
115. Sareli P, England MJ, Berk MR, et al. Maternal and fetal sequelae of anticoagulation during pregnancy in patients with mechanical heart valve prostheses. *Am J Cardiol* 1989;63:1462–1465.
116. Beyth RJ, Quinn LM, Landefeld CS. Prospective evaluation of an index for predicting the risk of major bleeding in outpatients treated with warfarin. *Am J Med* 1998;105:91–99.
117. Fihn SD, Callahan CM, Martin DC, et al. The risk for and severity of bleeding complications in elderly patients treated with warfarin. The National Consortium of Anticoagulation Clinics. *Ann Intern Med* 1996;124:970–979.
118. Palareti G, Leali N, Coccheri S, et al. Bleeding complications of oral anticoagulant treatment: an inception-cohort, prospective collaborative study (ISCOAT). *Lancet* 1996;348:423–428.
119. Meschengieser SS, Fondevila CG, Frontroth J, et al. Low-intensity oral anticoagulation plus low-dose aspirin versus high-intensity oral anticoagulation alone: a randomized trial in patients with mechanical prosthetic heart valves. *J Cardiovasc Surg* 1997;113:910–916.
120. Radberg JA, Olsson JE, Radberg CT. Prognostic parameters in spontaneous intracerebral haematomas with special reference to anticoagulant treatment. *Stroke* 1991;22:571–576.
121. Hart RG, Boop BS, Anderson DC. Oral anticoagulants and intracranial haemorrhage—facts and hypotheses. *Stroke* 1992;26:1471–1477.
122. Ingels M, Lai C, Tai W, et al. A prospective study of acute, unintentional, pediatric superwarfarin ingestions managed without decontamination. *Ann Emerg Med* 2002;40:73–78.
123. Morrissey B, Burgess JL, Robertson WO. Washington's experience and recommendations. Re: anticoagulant rodenticides. *Vet Hum Toxicol* 1995;37:362–363.
124. Mullins ME, Brands CL, Daya MR. Unintentional pediatric superwarfarin exposures: do we really need a prothrombin time? *Pediatrics* 2000;105:402–404.
125. Shepherd G, Klein-Schwartz W, Anderson BD. Acute, unintentional pediatric brodifacoum ingestions. *Pediatr Emerg Care* 2002;18:174–178.
126. Smolinske SC, Scherger DL, Kearns PS, et al. Superwarfarin poisoning in children: a prospective study. *Pediatrics* 1989;84:490–494.
127. Gitter MJ, Jaeger TM, Petterson TM. The bleeding and thromboembolism during anticoagulant therapy: a population-based study in Rochester, Minnesota. *Mayo Clin Proc* 1995;70:806–808.
128. Verhagen H. Local haemorrhage and necrosis of the skin and underlying tissues, during anti-coagulant therapy with dicumarol or dicumacyl. *Acta Med Scand* 1954;148:453–467.
129. Nalbandian RM, Mader IJ, Barrett JL, et al. Petechiae ecchymoses and necrosis of skin induced by coumarin congeners. Rare, occasionally lethal complication of anticoagulant therapy. *JAMA* 1965;192:603–608.
130. Lacy JP, Goodin RR. Warfarin-induced necrosis of skin. *Ann Intern Med* 1975;82:381–382.

131. Robin GC, Levin SM, Freund M. Breast haemorrhage and gangrene during anticoagulant therapy. *Br J Surg* 1963;50:773–774.
132. Kipen CS. Gangrene of the breast—a complication of anticoagulant therapy. Report of two cases. *N Engl J Med* 1961;37:172.
133. Shnider M, D'Souza CR. Cutaneous gangrene: a rare complication of coumarin therapy. *Can J Surg* 1976;19:64–65.
134. Jones RR, Cunningham J. Warfarin skin necrosis. The role of factor VII. *Br J Dermatol* 1979;100:561–565.
135. Feder W, Auerbach R. "Purple toes": an uncommon sequela of oral coumarin drug therapy. *Ann Intern Med* 1961;55:911–917.
136. Schiff BL, Kern AB. Cutaneous reactions to anticoagulants. *Arch Dermatol* 1968;98:136–137.
137. Park BK, Scott AK, Wilson AC, et al. Plasma disposition of vitamin K_1 in relation to anticoagulant poisoning. *Br J Clin Pharmacol* 1984;18:655–662.
138. Umeki S, Umeki Y. Levels of acarboxy prothrombin (PIVKA-II) and coagulation factors in warfarin-treated patients. *Med Lab Sci* 1990;47:103–107.
139. Donovan JW, Ballard JO, Murphy MJ. Brodifacoum therapy with activated charcoal effect on elimination kinetics. *Vet Hum Toxicol* 1990;32:350.
140. Jahnchen E, Meinertz T, Gilfrich HJ, et al. Enhanced elimination of warfarin during treatment with cholestyramine. *Br J Clin Pharmacol* 1978;5:437–440.
141. Meinertz T, Gilfrich HJ, Groth U, et al. Interruption of the enterohepatic circulation of phenprocoumon by cholestyramine. *Clin Pharmacol Ther* 1977;21:731–735.
142. Renowden S, Westmoreland D, White JP, et al. Oral cholestyramine increases elimination of warfarin after overdose. *Br Med J (Clin Res Ed)* 1985;291:513–514.
143. Dayton PG, Tarcan Y, Chenkin T, et al. The influence of barbiturates on coumarin plasma levels and prothrombin response. *J Clin Invest* 1961;40:1797–1802.
144. Parkinson A. Biotransformation of xenobiotics. In: Klaassen CD, ed. *Casarett and Doull's toxicology. The basic science of poisons*, 6th ed. New York: McGraw-Hill, 2001:133–224.
145. Glaser V, Seifert R. Successful therapy of phenprocoumon poisoning with plasmapheresis. *Med Klin* 1998;93:174–176.
146. Cosgriff SW. The effectiveness of an oral vitamin K_1 in controlling excessive hypoprothrombinaemia during anticoagulant therapy. *Ann Intern Med* 1956;45:14–22.
147. Pengo V, Banzato A, Garelli E, et al. Reversal of excessive effect of regular anticoagulation: low oral dose of phytonadione (vitamin K_1) compared with warfarin discontinuation. *Blood Coagul Fibrinolysis* 1993;4:739–741.
148. White RH, McKittrick T, Hutchinson R, et al. Temporary discontinuation of warfarin therapy: changes in the international normalized ratio. *Ann Intern Med* 1995;122:40–42.
149. Andersen P, Godal HC. Predictable reduction in anticoagulant activity of warfarin by small amounts of vitamin K. *Acta Med Scand* 1975;198:269–270.
150. Hung A, Singh S, Tait RC. A prospective randomized study to determine the optimal dose of intravenous vitamin K in reversal of over-warfarinization. *Br J Haematol* 2000;109:537–539.
151. Raj G, Kumar R, McKinney WP. Time course of reversal of anticoagulant effect of warfarin by intravenous and subcutaneous phytomenadione. *Arch Intern Med* 1999;159:2721–2724.
152. Watson HG, Baglin T, Laidlaw SL, et al. A comparison of the efficacy and rate of response to oral and intravenous vitamin K in reversal of over-anticoagulation with warfarin. *Br J Haematol* 2001;115:145–149.
153. Nee R, Doppenschmidt D, Donovan DJ, et al. Intravenous versus subcutaneous vitamin K in reversing excessive oral anticoagulation. *Am J Cardiol* 1999;83:286–288.
154. Crowther MA, Donovan D, Harrison L, et al. Low dose oral vitamin K reliably reverses over-anticoagulation due to warfarin. *Thromb Haemost* 1998;79:1116–1118.
155. Crowther MA, Julian J, McCarty D, et al. Treatment of warfarin-associated coagulopathy with oral vitamin K: a randomized trial. *Lancet* 2000;356:1551–1553.
156. Crowther MA, Douketis JD, Schnurr T, et al. Oral vitamin K lowers the international normalized ratio more rapidly than subcutaneous vitamin K in the treatment of warfarin-associated coagulopathy. *Ann Intern Med* 2002;137:251–254.
157. Pendry K, Bhavnani M, Shwe K. The use of oral vitamin K for reversal of over-warfarinization. *Br J Haematol* 2001;113:839–840.
158. Lefrere JJ, Girot R. Acute cardiovascular collapse during intravenous vitamin K_1 injection. *Thromb Haemost* 1987;58:790.
159. Makris M, Watson HG. The management of coumarin-induced over-anticoagulation. *Br J Haematol* 2001;114:271–280.
160. O'Reilly RA, Kearns P. Intravenous vitamin K_1 injections: dangerous prophylaxis. *Arch Intern Med* 1995;155:2127–2128.
161. Penning-van Beest FJA, Rosendaal FR, Grobbee DE, et al. Course of the international normalized ratio in response to oral vitamin K_1 in patients overanticoagulated with phenprocoumon. *Br J Haematol* 1999;104:241–245.
162. Holland D. Vitamin K_1 absorption by everted intestinal sacs of the rat. *Am J Physiol* 1973;225:360–364.
163. Shearer MJ, McBurney A, Barkhan P. Studies on the absorption and metabolism of phylloquinone (vitamin K_1) in man. *Vitam Horm* 1974;32:513–524.
164. Evans G, Luddington R, Baglin T. Beriplex P/N reverses severe warfarin-induced overanticoagulation immediately and completely in patients presenting with major bleeding. *Br J Haematol* 2001;115:998–1001.
165. Cartmill M, Dolan G, Byrne JL, et al. Prothrombin complex concentrate for oral anticoagulant reversal in neurosurgical emergencies. *Br J Neurosurg* 2000;14:458–461.
166. Fredriksson K, Norrving B, Stromblad LG. Emergency reversal of anticoagulation after intracerebral hemorrhage. *Stroke* 1992;23:972–977.
167. Makris M, Greaves M, Phillips WS, et al. Emergency oral anticoagulant reversal. The relative efficacy of infusions of fresh frozen plasma and clotting factor concentrate on correction of the coagulopathy. *Thromb Haemost* 1997;77:477–480.
168. Nitu IC, Perry DJ, Lee CA. Clinical experience with the use of clotting factor concentrates in oral anticoagulation reversal. *Clin Lab Haematol* 1998;20:363–367.
169. Stainsby D, Cohen H. Use of fresh frozen plasma for over-anticoagulation should not be encouraged. Rapid responses available at: http://www.bmj.com. Accessed March 31, 2003.
170. Deveras RA, Kessler CM. Reversal of warfarin-induced excessive anticoagulation with recombinant human factor VIIa concentrate. *Ann Intern Med* 2002;137:884–888.
171. Lin J, Hanigan WC, Tarantino M, et al. The use of recombinant activated factor VII to reverse warfarin-induced anticoagulation in patients with hemorrhages in the central nervous system: preliminary findings. *J Neurosurg* 2003;98:737–740.
172. Veshchev I, Elran H, Salame K. Recombinant coagulation factor VIIa for rapid preoperative correction of warfarin-related coagulopathy in patients with acute subdural hematoma. *Med Sci Monit* 2002;8:CS98–100.
173. Peerlinck K, Vermylen J. Acute myocardial infarction following administration of recombinant activated factor VII (Novo Seven) in a patient with haemophilia A and inhibitor. *Thromb Haemost* 1999;82:1775–1776.
174. Ortin M, Olalla J, Marco F, et al. Low-dose vitamin K_1 versus short term withholding of acenocoumarol in the treatment of excessive anticoagulation episodes induced by acenocoumarol. A retrospective comparative study. *Haemostasis* 1998;28:57–61.
175. Jaffin BW, Bliss CM, Lamont JT. Significance of occult gastrointestinal bleeding during anticoagulation therapy. *Am J Med* 1987;83:269–272.
176. Culclasure TP, Bray VJ, Hasbargen JA. The significance of hematuria in the anticoagulated patient. *Arch Intern Med* 1994;154:649–652.
177. Schuster GA, Lewis GA. Clinical significance of hematuria in patients on anticoagulation therapy. *J Urol* 1987;137:923–925.
178. Shah P, Kraklow W, Lamb G. Unusual complication of coumadin toxicity. *Wis Med J* 1994;93:212–214.

CHAPTER 238

Fumigants

Jefferey L. Burgess

See Figure 1.

Compounds included:	**Aluminum phosphide, zinc phosphide, methyl bromide, chloropicrin, 1,3-dichloropropene, sulfuryl fluoride, metam-sodium**
Molecular formula and weight:	**See Table 1.**
CAS Registry No.:	**See Table 1.**
Special considerations:	**Toxicity may be delayed after phosphine or methyl bromide exposure.**
Antidote:	**None**

OVERVIEW

Fumigants are gases or volatile liquids used to sterilize products, structures, or soil. They are capable of penetrating soil and structural materials such as wood and generally dissipate readily without leaving toxic residues, although continued off-gassing may pose an exposure risk. Common poisoning scenarios include occupational exposure, excessive application or premature reentry, exposure in structures separate from buildings being fumigated but connected through underground conduits, and, for some of the fumigants, attempted suicide. Fumigants covered in this chapter include aluminum and zinc phosphide, methyl bromide, chloropicrin, 1,3-dichloropropene, sulfuryl fluoride, and metam-sodium. Information on the distribution of use of some of these chemicals in the United States is available from the U.S. Geological Survey at http://water.ca.usgs.gov/pnsp/use92/.

Other chemical agents that are either presently used as fumigants or have at some time been used as fumigants include naphthalene, methylene chloride, chloroform, carbon tetrachloride, ethylene dichloride, ethylene dibromide, dibromochlorpropane, dichloropropane, paradichlorobenzene, ethylene oxide, formaldehyde, acrolein, sulfur dioxide, carbon disulfide, hydrogen cyanide, and acrylonitrile. These chemicals are discussed in other chapters.

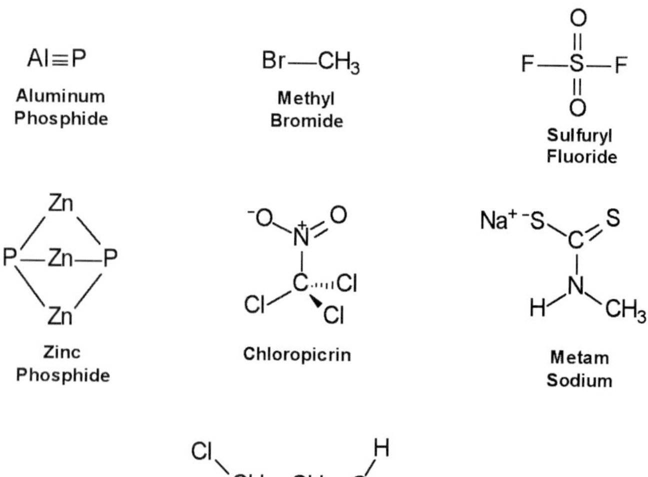

Figure 1. Structures of the fumigants.

PHOSPHINE (ALUMINUM, ZINC PHOSPHIDES)

Phosphine is produced from aluminum, magnesium, and zinc phosphides when they come in contact with water or water vapor. Phosphine (or commonly encountered impurities found with phosphine) has a fishy or garlic smell with an odor threshold of 1.5 to 3.0 parts per million (ppm) (1). Within the fumigant category, phosphine gas is one of the most common causes of poisoning (2).

Classification and Uses

Phosphine may also be produced in illicit methamphetamine laboratories when phosphorous acid is heated in a reducing atmosphere (3,4). Phosphine may be released in the production of acetylene gas and during its use as a doping agent for the manufacture of semiconductors (5).

Aluminum phosphide is frequently used as a grain fumigant. Product formulations have included Al-phos, Celphide, Celphine, Celphos, Detia-Gas-Ex, Fastphos, Fumitoxin, Gastoxin, Max-Kill, Phosfume, Phostoxin, Quickphos, Quick Tox, Synfume, and Weevilcide. It is a commonly used agent for self-poisoning in India (6,7). Commercial formulations of aluminum phosphide often contain ammonium carbamate to reduce the flammability of phosphine gas.

Zinc phosphide is commonly used to kill rodents and moles. Product formulations have included Arrex, Commando, Denkarin Grains, Gopha-Rid, Mouseoff, Phosvin, Pollux, Ridall, Ratol, Rodenticide AG, Zinc-Tox, and ZP Rodent Bait. Zinc phosphide reacts more readily with dilute acid than with water to form phosphine gas (8).

Toxic Dose

Regulatory standards and guidelines are provided in Table 2.

TABLE 1. Physical characteristics of selected chemicals

Compound	Molecular formula	Molecular weight (g/mol)	CAS Registry No.
Aluminum phosphide	AlP	57.96	20859-73-8
Zinc phosphide	P_2Zn_3	258.05	1314-84-7
Chloropicrin	CCl_3NO_2	164.4	76-06-2
1,3-Dichloropropene	$C_3H_4Cl_2$	111	542-75-6
Metam sodium	$C_2H_4NNaS_2$	129.2	137-42-8
Methyl bromide	CH_3Br	94.94	74-83-9
Sulfuryl fluoride	SO2F2	102.06	2699-79-8

TABLE 2. United States regulatory guidelines and standards

		Concentration mg/m³ (ppm)				
Agency	**Description**	**Aluminum phosphide/zinc phosphide (as phosphine)**	**Chloropicrin**	**1,3-Dichloropropene**	**Methyl bromide**	**Sulfuryl fluoride**
OSHA (air)	PEL-TWA	0.4 (0.3)	0.7 (0.1)	None	None	21 (5)
	PEL-ceiling	None	None	None	78 (20)	None
ACGIH (10) (air)	TLV-TWA	0.4 (0.3)	0.7 (0.1)	5 (1)	4 (1)	21 (5)
	STEL	1.4 (1)	None	None	None	42 (10)
NIOSH (air)	REL-TWA	0.4 (0.3)	0.7 (0.1)	5 (1)	None	21 (5)
	REL-STEL	1.4 (1)	None	None	None	42 (10)
	IDLH	70 (50)	13.5 (2)	None	970 (250)	840 (200)
		ppm × 1.39 = mg/m³	ppm × 6.72 = mg/m³	ppm × 4.54 = mg/m³	ppm × 3.88 = mg/m³	ppm × 4.17 = mg/m³

ACGIH, American Conference of Governmental Industrial Hygienists; IDLH, immediate danger to life or health; NIOSH, National Institute for Occupational Safety and Health; OSHA, U.S. Occupational Safety and Health Administration; PEL, permissible exposure limit; ppm, parts per million; REL, recommended exposure limit; STEL, short-term exposure limit; TLV, threshold limit value; TWA, time-weighted average.

Lethality has been reported with aluminum phosphide ingestions as small as 500 mg (7). Ingestion of as little as 4 g of zinc phosphide has been lethal, and survival has occurred after ingestions of up to 50 g (9).

Toxicokinetics and Toxicodynamics

Inhaled phosphine is rapidly absorbed through the lungs. Phosphine gas is also produced after the ingestion of phosphides and their reaction with acidic gastric fluids. Dermal absorption of phosphine gas is insignificant. In the rat, much of the ingested phosphide is eliminated through exhalation as phosphine. Phosphine that is not excreted in the air is excreted in the urine as hypophosphite and phosphite (5).

Pathophysiology

The exact toxic mechanism of action of phosphine is not clearly understood. It noncompetitively inhibits mitochondrial cytochrome oxidase and also inhibits catalase (11,12).

Pregnancy and Lactation

Information on adverse effects in pregnancy or with lactation is limited.

Clinical Presentation

ALUMINUM PHOSPHIDE

After an ingestion of aluminum phosphide, patients may present with profuse vomiting and pain in the upper abdomen, hypotension, tachycardia and other dysrhythmias, altered sensorium, pulmonary edema, jaundice, and renal failure (6,13,14). With severe poisoning, intractable shock is usually present, and death occurs within less than an hour or may require several days (15). Persistent shock that does not respond to fluids and vasopressor support suggests a poor prognosis (16). In severe exposures, almost every organ system of the body may be affected (17).

ZINC PHOSPHIDE

Signs and symptoms of zinc phosphide toxicity include nausea, vomiting, hypotension, dyspnea, and altered mental status. Immediate death results from pulmonary edema. Hepatic, cardiac, and renal injury may occur. Delayed death is often due to cardiotoxicity (9,18). Pancreatitis is an unusual complication (19).

PHOSPHINE

Eye irritation, nausea, vomiting, diarrhea, dizziness, dry cough, shortness of breath, and dizziness may occur immediately after exposure. However, initial symptoms from acute exposure may not occur or may be transient, and findings are often absent on initial physical examination and laboratory testing (2,20). Respiratory toxicity may be the first and only presentation of toxicity. Development of pulmonary edema may be delayed, and respiratory symptoms may persist for weeks to months (4,21).

In severe cases coma, convulsions, hypotension, and pulmonary edema develop. Exposures to phosphine gas can cause gastrointestinal tract symptoms, as well as respiratory, cardiovascular, and central nervous system injury. Prominent clinical manifestations of acute phosphine gas exposure include headache, fatigue, nausea, vomiting, cough, dyspnea, jaundice, paresthesias, ataxia, intention tremor, weakness, and diplopia (22). Exposure may result in dilated pupils (23). On autopsy, fatal cases revealed centrilobular necrosis of the liver, congestive heart failure with pulmonary edema, and focal myocardial necrosis (16,22).

Workers engaged in fumigation of stored grains with phosphine have reported cough, dyspnea, chest tightness, headache, dizziness, numbness, lethargy, anorexia, diarrhea, nausea, epigastric pain, and vomiting (20,24).

Diagnostic Tests

Black stomach contents with garlic-like odor may be seen after large ingestions (25). Metabolic acidosis is common (26). Increased serum transaminases and bilirubin have been observed (6). The electrocardiogram may reveal ST and T wave changes, atrioventricular block, atrial fibrillation, ventricular tachycardia and fibrillation, and a variety of other changes (26,27). An elevated creatine kinase myocardial band isoenzyme (CK-MB) fraction has also been reported in a patient with electrocardiogram changes (22).

Clinical diagnosis can be confirmed by analysis of gastric aspirate or breath, both of which blacken a paper impregnated with 0.1 N silver nitrate (28). Blood phosphine levels are presently difficult to measure and may be absent in postmortem samples (29). Blood aluminum levels may be elevated in patients with severe aluminum phosphide exposure (30).

The blood urea nitrogen and creatinine rise if renal failure ensues. Urinalysis may reveal occult blood, bile, or glucose. Mild elevation of transaminases may also be found, as well as a slight decrease in serum cholinesterase (22). The leukocyte count may be increased (31). Hypokalemia may be observed (32). Intravascular hemolysis and rarely methemoglobinemia may occur (15,33,34). Chromosome rearrangement has been reported in fumigant applicators exposed to phosphine (35).

Treatment

Treatment is primarily symptomatic and supportive.

DECONTAMINATION

The efficacy of gastric decontamination for phosphide ingestion has not been studied. However, if the ingestion occurred immediately before treatment, quantities remaining in the stomach should be removed as effectively as possible by gastric intubation, aspiration, and lavage after all possible precautions have been taken to protect the respiratory tract from aspirated gastric contents. The efficacy of treatment with activated charcoal is unknown.

ENHANCEMENT OF ELIMINATION

Attempts at enhanced elimination have not been reported.

ANTIDOTES

There are no antidotes for phosphine gas exposure.

SUPPORTIVE CARE

Aggressive airway management and circulatory support are critical. However, supportive treatment with fluids, bicarbonate, oxygen, and vasopressors has been unsuccessful in many patients with severe poisoning. Corticosteroids appear to be ineffective (7). Pulmonary edema should be treated symptomatically. Intravenous magnesium sulfate has been attempted with mixed therapeutic results (6,36–38). Renal failure may require dialysis.

For inhalation exposures, the patient may initially be asymptomatic. Development of pulmonary edema may be delayed for up to 18 hours or more (20,31). Patients with clear evidence of exposure should be observed for the development of delayed respiratory symptoms.

METHYL BROMIDE

Methyl bromide is used for both structural and soil fumigation. Synonyms include bromomethane and monobromomethane, and product formulations have included Brom-o-Gas, Bromomethane, Celfume, Dowfume MC-2, Dowfume MC-33, Embafume, Haltox, MB, MeBr, Methogas, Profume, Terr-o-Gas, and Zytox. It has a sweet chloroform-like odor at high concentrations (39). Due to the poor warning properties of methyl bromide, chloropicrin is often added in an attempt to limit exposure. Previously, one of the most common causes of death in California was unauthorized entry into structures under fumigation (40). Due in large part to concern over stratospheric ozone depletion, the U.S. Environmental Protection Agency is phasing out use of methyl bromide by 2005 except for critical agricultural and emergency uses.

Toxic Dose

Regulatory standards and guidelines are provided in Table 2. The lethal concentration for 50% (LC_{50}) for animals ranges from 300 ppm for 5 hours in guinea pigs to 10 ppm for 24 hours in rats (41). Human fatalities have been reported from exposure concentrations as low as 300 to 400 ppm, and harmful effects from exposures at 100 ppm or more. Systemic poisoning has been reported to occur from a 2-week exposure (8 hours per day) at approximately 35 ppm (42).

Toxicokinetics and Toxicodynamics

In rats, major organs of distribution immediately following exposure include fat, lung, liver, adrenals, and kidneys. After ingestion or inhalation, 75% to 85% of the body burden is excreted within 72 hours. Approximately 40% is recovered in the urine as metabolized methyl bromide, and 4% to 20% is exhaled unchanged. Tissue half-lives range from 0.5 to 8.0 hours (39). The half-life of serum bromide ion ranges from 3.5 to 15 days after chronic methyl bromide exposure (41).

Pathophysiology

The toxic mechanism of methyl bromide has not been well defined but may involve formation of reactive intermediates or its alkylating properties (43). Methyl bromide reacts *in vitro* with sulfhydryl groups, and through this mechanism causes progressive and irreversible enzyme inhibition (44).

Vulnerable Populations

Information on adverse effects in pregnancy or with lactation is limited. Mixed, species-specific teratogenicity has been noted in animals.

Clinical Presentation

ACUTE EXPOSURE

Skin exposure to liquid methyl bromide may lead to irritation and blistering, particularly in relatively moist areas. Exposure to methyl bromide at an estimated 10,000 ppm for 40 minutes led to redness and blistering of the skin through penetration of overalls on top of normal daily clothing (45). Eye exposure to liquid has been reported to cause severe corneal burns, although in other cases contact of methyl bromide with the eye either as concentrated vapor or as a splash of liquid resulted in no more than transient irritation and conjunctivitis (46,47).

Inhalation exposure may lead to cough, shortness of breath, nausea, vomiting, dizziness, headaches, fatigue, concentration and memory problems, and visual impairment, including blurry vision, blindness, and loss of green color vision. Other effects of acute exposure may include pulmonary, renal, and mild hepatic injury (41,47,48). Convulsions may occur with severe poisoning and may be refractory in nature (49–51). One case of poisoning in a child resembled Reye's syndrome (52). Although high concentrations of methyl bromide can lead to rapid loss of consciousness, and other symptoms may occur within minutes, symptom onset at lower concentrations is generally delayed several hours and in some cases up to 24 to 48 hours (39).

CHRONIC EXPOSURE

Additional neurologic findings may be reported with chronic exposure or high-level acute exposure including optic atrophy, nystagmus, ataxia, hypo- or hyperreflexia, peripheral neuropathy, paresthesias, dysesthesias, and myoclonus (52–55). The neurologic symptoms in particular can be persistent in nature although they often improve over time (2,50,54,56). One fumigator with predominant dermal exposure to methyl bromide experiencing dermal burns and vesicles on the upper and lower limbs developed progressive weakness of the lower limbs, ataxia, paresthesias, and hyperactive tendon reflexes in the lower limbs 1 week after exposure. Nerve conduction velocity testing was consistent with axonal neuropathy (57).

Diagnostic Tests

Serum, plasma, blood, or urine bromide concentration may be measured after methyl bromide exposure (58–61). In one study, unexposed controls had serum bromide concentrations of 2.5 to 6.6 mg/L, whereas exposed agricultural workers had serum bromide concentrations of 11 to 20 mg/L (58). S-methylcysteine adduct testing may help confirm methyl bromide exposure for up to 10 weeks after exposure (62).

In methyl bromide fumigators, small increases in alkaline phosphate and serum transaminases have been measured in a small number of workers. Serum transaminase levels were correlated with blood bromide levels (63).

Seizures and mental status changes are evaluated in the usual manner (Chapters 30 and 14, respectively).

Treatment

Treatment is supportive. Decontamination is limited to removing the victim from the source of exposure.

ENHANCEMENT OF ELIMINATION

Hemodialysis is effective in removing bromide from the blood but has not been proven to improve clinical condition, although case reports describe neurologic improvement after this treatment (59,64).

ANTIDOTES

There is no antidote for methyl bromide exposure.

SUPPORTIVE CARE

Aggressive airway management and circulatory support are critical. Complications such as pulmonary edema or seizures are treated in the usual manner.

CHLOROPICRIN

Chloropicrin is a colorless, slightly oily liquid with a vapor pressure of 20 mm Hg at 20°C (65). Synonyms include trichloronitromethane, nitrotrichloromethane, and nitrochloroform. Commercial product names include Chlor-O-Pic, Aquinite, Dojyopicrine, Dolochlor, Laracide, Metapicrin, Nemax, Picfume, Pic-Clor, Timberfume, and Tri-Clor. It was used as a tear gas during World War I because of its irritant properties. It has been used as an insecticidal fumigant for cereals and grains and as a soil insecticide. A small amount of chloropicrin is often added to other toxic, odorless fumigants as a deterrent to reentry into fumigated structures, and chloropicrin is also used as a prewarning gas in ship fumigation. The odor detection threshold is considered to be 1.1 ppm (66).

Toxic Dose

Regulatory standards and guidelines are provided in Table 2. A concentration of 4 ppm for a few seconds has been reported to be temporarily disabling because of its irritant effects. Exposure to 15 ppm for the same brief period has been reported to cause respiratory tract injury. Concentrations of 0.3 to 3.7 ppm can lead to painful eye irritation in 3 to 30 seconds. A lethal exposure in humans is approximately 300 ppm for 10 minutes and 120 ppm for 30 minutes, with death usually resulting from pulmonary edema (66).

Toxicokinetics and Toxicodynamics

The water solubility of chloropicrin is low, and its toxicity appears to be similar to chlorine (67).

Pathophysiology

Chloropicrin is an intense irritant. Agents with low water solubility such as chloropicrin tend to damage the lower respiratory tract. In animals, exposure causes moderate to severe degeneration of the respiratory epithelium including the lower respiratory tract (67).

Pregnancy and Lactation

Information on adverse effects in pregnancy or with lactation is not available.

Clinical Presentation

Human exposure may result in eye, nose, and throat irritation; lacrimation; runny nose; chest pain; cough; shortness of breath; nausea; vomiting; abdominal cramping; skin irritation; headache; fatigue; and lethargy (66,68–70). Aspiration causes vomiting and choking (71). An 18-year-old woman was sprayed with chloropicrin and died of pulmonary edema 4 hours later. A friend similarly exposed recovered after 30 days (71). Exposure to chloropicrin as a war gas has resulted in nausea, vomiting, and diarrhea lasting for weeks (72).

Diagnostic Tests

Elevated creatinine phosphokinase levels have been reported after chloropicrin exposure (70). Often, evaluation of pulmonary function with oximetry, arterial blood gases, and chest radiography is needed. Gas chromatography and gas chromatography–mass spectrometry have been used to identify chloropicrin but are not routinely available (71).

Treatment

Treatment is largely symptomatic and supportive.

DECONTAMINATION

For liquid exposure, contaminated clothing should be removed and exposed areas should be flushed with copious amounts of water for at least 15 minutes. After inhalation, the patient should be removed from exposure.

ENHANCEMENT OF ELIMINATION

Attempts at enhanced elimination have not been reported.

ANTIDOTES

No antidotes are available for exposure to chloropicrin.

SUPPORTIVE CARE

For significant exposures, airway management and treatment of bronchospasm and pulmonary edema are critical and performed using the typical indications and interventions (Chapter 33).

1,3-DICHLOROPROPENE

1,3-Dichloropropene is a white to amber colored liquid with a vapor pressure of 28 mm Hg at 20°C and a sweet odor. Synonyms include DCP, 1,3-dichloro-1-propene, and 3-chloroallyl chloride. Product names for 1,3-dichloropropene include Telone II, Telone 2000, DD92, and Dorlone 2000. 1,3-Dichloropropene is used as a soil fumigant for nematodes on numerous food and nonfood crops including bulbs and potatoes.

Toxic Dose

Regulatory standards and guidelines are provided in Table 2. The oral LD_{50} in rats is 110 to 713 mg/kg (73).

Toxicokinetics and Toxicodynamics

After vapor exposure, uptake through the skin is estimated to be approximately 2% to 5% of the absorption through inhalation (74). In rats, the initial elimination half-life for 1,3-dichloropropene in blood ranged from 3 to 27 minutes depending on dose (75). 1,3-Dichloropropene mercapturic acid metabolites have urinary elimination half-lives of approximately 5 hours. Mercapturic acid metabolites are excreted as Z– (45%) and E–1,3-dichloropropene (14%) (76).

Pathophysiology

The toxic mechanism of 1,3-dichloropropene is not well described. Studies of hepatic toxicity in mice suggest that ingested 1,3-dichloropropene is biotransformed via cytochrome P-450, with metabolites inducing liver damage, and that glutathione plays an important role in the detoxification of 1,3-dichloropropene (77).

Pregnancy and Lactation

Information on adverse effects in pregnancy or with lactation is not available.

Clinical Presentation

Exposure to 1,3-dichloropropene may result in acute onset of headache, mucous membrane irritation, dizziness, cough, chest discomfort, nausea, vomiting, and loss of consciousness. Reported persistent symptoms have included headache, abdominal discomfort, chest discomfort, malaise, fatigue, irritability, difficulty concentrating, and decreased libido (73,78). Applicators using 1,3-dichloropropene are potentially exposed orally, dermally, or through inhalation. Dermal exposure may cause edema, erythema, and skin necrosis (46,79).

In one case report of accidental ingestion, 1,3-dichloropropene caused gastrointestinal distress, tachypnea, diaphoresis, hypotension, and tachycardia, followed 11 hours later by bloody diarrhea, metabolic acidosis, hyperglycemia, and worsening hypotension. Within a few hours, acute respiratory distress syndrome, hematologic and hepatorenal functional impairment, and pancreatitis ensued. The patient died of multisystem organ failure 40 hours after ingestion (80).

Diagnostic Tests

Slight elevation of aminotransferases may be observed (78). N-acetyl-S-(cis-3-chloro-2-enyl)-cysteine in urine can be used for biologic monitoring (81,82). Occupational exposure has resulted in increased concentration of urinary N-acetylglucosaminidase and retinol-binding protein.

Treatment

Treatment after inhalation is largely symptomatic and supportive.

DECONTAMINATION

For liquid exposure, exposed areas should be flushed with copious amounts of water for at least 15 minutes. For ingestion, the efficacy of gastric decontamination is not known. Given the potential lethality of ingestion, gastric aspiration may be reasonable if performed soon after ingestion. The role of activated charcoal, but a single dose, is a reasonable intervention.

ENHANCEMENT OF ELIMINATION

Attempts at enhanced elimination have not been reported.

ANTIDOTES

No specific antidote is available for 1,3-dichloropropene poisoning.

SUPPORTIVE CARE

For significant exposures, airway management and treatment of bronchospasm and pulmonary edema are critical and performed using the typical indications and interventions (Chapter 33).

SULFURYL FLUORIDE

Sulfuryl fluoride is a colorless, odorless, nonflammable gas. Synonyms include sulfuric oxyfluoride and sulfuryl difluoride. Sulfuryl fluoride is manufactured under the trade name Vikane. It has been used extensively for structural fumigation against dry wood termites and is currently a popular tent fumigant for insect extermination. It evolves toxic fumes such as hydrofluoric acid when heated (83). Chloropicrin may be added as a warning agent to sulfuryl fluoride before use as a fumigant.

Toxic Dose

Regulatory standards and guidelines are provided in Table 2. One hour LC_{50} concentrations in rats are 3020 to 3730 ppm (84).

Toxicokinetics and Toxicodynamics

The toxicokinetics of human sulfuryl fluoride poisoning have not been well described. Termites exposed to a nonlethal dose of sulfuryl fluoride excrete inorganic sulfate, suggesting release of fluoride (85).

Pathophysiology

Based on insect studies, the toxicity of sulfuryl fluoride may be due to release of fluoride (86).

Vulnerable Populations

Inhalation exposure to sulfuryl fluoride was not teratogenic in either rats or rabbits exposed to levels of up to 225 ppm. Reduced body weights were observed among fetal rabbits exposed at this level, which was believed to be secondary to maternal weight loss (87).

Clinical Presentation

ACUTE EXPOSURE

Exposure to sulfuryl fluoride has caused eye, nose, and throat irritation; pruritus; dyspnea; cough; rhonchi; nausea; vomiting; abdominal pain; weakness; paresthesias; and seizure (83,88,89). In animals, high-dose exposure results in rapid incapacitation, seizures, and death, and focal pulmonary hemorrhages may be found. Low-dose exposure presents with parasympathomimetic findings, including vomiting, diarrhea, abdominal pain, lacrimation, and salivation (83). A similar pattern appears to occur in humans, although not all cases fit these categorizations.

A 19-year-old woman who initially developed cough and chest discomfort worsened 6 hours after the exposure with findings of hyperexcitability, hyperventilation, productive cough, pulmonary edema, carpal/pedal tetany, and cardiac dysrhythmias died 12 hours after exposure. Marked pulmonary edema was found on autopsy (83). A healthy elderly couple entering their home 5 to 8 hours after cessation of fumigation experienced extreme weakness, nausea, and shortness of breath. The following day the husband died after a seizure, and the wife developed a severe interstitial pulmonary edema and experienced a fatal cardiorespiratory arrest 6 days after exposure (89).

CHRONIC EXPOSURE

Chronic occupational exposure may be associated with reduction in odor recognition and reduced performance on cognitive/visual memory testing (90).

Diagnostic Tests

Serum or blood fluoride concentrations are often elevated after sulfuryl fluoride exposure. Fluoride concentrations were 50 mg/L (24 to 36 hours postmortem blood level) and 20 mg/L (antemortem serum level) in two patients who died (83). The serum fluoride level 6 days after exposure in another fatal poisoning was 0.5 ng/L (89). Proteinuria and azotemia may be present (91).

Treatment

DECONTAMINATION

Patients should be immediately removed to fresh air.

ENHANCEMENT OF ELIMINATION

Attempts at enhanced elimination have not been reported.

ANTIDOTES

No proven antidotes are available for sulfuryl fluoride poisoning. In rats exposed to 4000 ppm of sulfuryl fluoride for 45 minutes, pretreatment with calcium gluconate 500 mg/kg intraperitoneal increased survival markedly but did not prevent seizures. Postexposure treatment was not beneficial (92).

SUPPORTIVE CARE

Pulmonary edema, shock, and seizures should be managed symptomatically and supportively. In a study of rats poisoned with sulfuryl fluoride, phenobarbital was more effective than diazepam in reducing the frequency of seizures, and phenytoin made the convulsions more severe and longer in duration (92).

METAM-SODIUM

Metam-sodium is a white crystalline powder applied as an aqueous solution used to fumigate soil, frequently in orchards and field crops. In solution it has a vapor pressure of 21 mm Hg at 25°C (93). Synonyms include sodium methyldithiocarbamate and sodium N-methyldithiocarbamate and it has been sold under the trade names Amvac Metam Sodium, Busan, Metam CLR, Sectagon, Vapam, and VPM. Methylisothiocyanate, the major decomposition product, has a horseradish-like odor.

Toxic Dose

There are no U.S. occupational exposure limits for metam-sodium or methylisothiocyanate. Toxicity may occur after both inhalation and dermal exposure. In animal studies using technical grade (43.7%) metam-sodium, a rabbit dermal LD_{50} of 368 mg/kg and a rat oral LD_{50} of 896 mg/kg have been reported. A rat 4-hour LC_{50} of 4.7 to 5.4 mg/L has been reported for a 32.7% solution (93).

Toxicokinetics and Toxicodynamics

In rats, metam-sodium is rapidly absorbed reaching a peak plasma level in 1 hour, and is excreted in exhaled breath as methylisothiocyanate and carbon disulfide and in the urine as methylisothiocyanate-glutathione conjugates (94).

Pathophysiology

The specific toxic mechanisms of metam-sodium in humans have not been clearly elucidated. The metam-sodium decomposition products (methylisothiocyanate, hydrogen sulfide, carbon disulfide, and monomethylamine) each have inherent toxicity. Metam-sodium may also act through inhibition of cholinesterase (95).

Vulnerable Populations

No information is available on effects of metam-sodium exposure on pregnancy or lactation in humans. In animal studies, metam-sodium is a developmental toxicant (94).

Clinical Presentation

Exposure to metam-sodium vapor may cause respiratory symptoms, skin and eye irritation, headache, nausea, vomiting, abdominal pain, fatigue, and central nervous system depression. One of the best described large-scale releases of metam-sodium followed a 1991 spill into the Sacramento River in California, with resulting exposure of nearby populations to methylisothiocyanate. A number of cases of persistent irritant-induced asthma and asthma exacerbations were reported (96). Skin exposure to metam-sodium or methylisothiocyanate can result in erythema, rash, and blistering including partial thickness burns, as well as allergic contact dermatitis (97,98).

Diagnostic Tests

There are no diagnostic tests specific for metam-sodium exposure.

Treatment

For liquid exposure, exposed areas should be flushed with copious amounts of water for at least 15 minutes. For ingestions, the efficacy of gastrointestinal decontamination has not been determined. Additional care is supportive in nature. There are no specific antidotes available for metam-sodium poisoning.

REFERENCES

1. Beliles RP. Phosphorus, selenium and tellurium. In: Clayton GD, Clayton FE, eds. *Patty's industrial hygiene and toxicology*, 3rd ed. New York: John Wiley and Sons 1981;2A:2121–2140.
2. Burgess JL, Morrissey B, Keifer MC, Robertson WO. Fumigant related illnesses: Washington state's five year experience. *J Toxicol Clin Toxicol* 2000;38:7–14.
3. Willers-Russo LJ. Three fatalities involving phosphine gas, produced as a result of methamphetamine manufacturing. *J Forensic Sci* 1999;44:647–652.
4. Burgess JL. Phosphine exposure from a methamphetamine lab investigation. *J Toxicol Clin Toxicol* 2001;39:165–168.
5. World Health Organization. *Environmental Health Criteria 73: phosphine and selected metal phosphides*. Geneva: International Programme for Chemical Safety, 1988.
6. Chopra JS, Kalra OP, Malik VS, et al. Aluminum phosphide poisoning: a prospective study of 16 cases in one year. *Postgrad Med J* 1986;62:1113–1115.
7. Banjaj R, Wasir HS. Epidemic aluminum phosphide poisoning in Northern India. *Lancet* 1988;1:820–821.
8. von Oettingen EW. The toxicity and potential dangers of zinc phosphide and of hydrogen phosphide (phosphine). *Public Health Rep* 1947;203:1–17.
9. Stephenson JBP. Zinc phosphide poisoning. *Arch Environ Health* 1967;15:83–88.
10. American Conference of Governmental Industrial Hygienists. *Threshold limit values for chemical substances and physical agents and biological exposure indices*. Cincinnati: American Conference of Governmental Industrial Hygienists, 2002.
11. Chefurka W, Kashi KP, Bond EJ. The effect of phosphine on electron transport in mitochondria. *Pestic Biochem Physiol* 1976;6:65–84.
12. Price NR, Mills KA, Humphries LA. Phosphine toxicity and catalase activity in susceptible and resistant strains of the lesser grain borer (*Rhyzopertha dominica*). *Comp Biochem Physiol* 1982;73C:411–413.
13. Misra UK, Tripathi AK, Pandey R, et al. Acute phosphine poisoning following ingestion of aluminum phosphide. *Hum Toxicol* 1988;7:343–345.
14. Goldman JM, Clemens ME, Gibberd FB, et al. Aluminum phosphide ingestion. *Br Med J* 1985;290:1110–1111.
15. Chugh SN, Dushyant, Ram S, et al. Incidence and outcome of aluminum phosphide poisoning in a hospital study. *Indian J Med Res* 1991;94:232–235.
16. Singh S, Dilawandi JB, Vashist R, et al. Aluminum phosphide ingestion. *BMJ* 1985;290:1110–1111.
17. Anger F, Paysant R, Brousse F, et al. Fatal aluminum phosphide poisoning. *J Anal Toxicol* 2000;24:90–92.
18. Rodenberg HD, Chang CC, Watson WA. Zinc phosphide ingestion: a case report and review. *Vet Hum Toxicol* 1989;31:559–562.
19. Sarma PS, Narula J. Acute pancreatitis due to zinc phosphide ingestion. *Postgrad Med J* 1996;72:237–238.
20. Jones AT, Jones RC, Longley EO. Environmental and clinical aspects of bulk wheat fumigation with aluminum phosphide. *Am Ind Hyg Assoc J* 1964;25:376–379.
21. Feldstein A, Heumann M, Barnett M. Fumigant intoxication during transport of grain by railroad. *J Occup Med* 1991;33:64–65.
22. Wilson R, Lovejoy FH, Jaeger RJ, Landrigan PL. Acute phosphine poisoning aboard a grain freighter. *JAMA* 1980;244:148–150.
23. Grant WM. *Toxicology of the eye*, 3rd ed. Springfield, IL: Charles C Thomas Publisher, 1986:733.
24. Misra UK, Bhargava SK, Nag D, et al. Occupational phosphine exposure in Indian workers. *Toxicol Lett* 1988;42:257–263.
25. Hayes WJ, Laws ER, eds. *Handbook of pesticide toxicology, vol. 2. Classes of pesticides*. New York: Academic Press, 1991:657–661.
26. Khosla SN, Handa R, Khosla P. Aluminum phosphide poisoning. *Trop Doct* 1992;22:155–157.
27. Siwach SB, Singh H, Jagdish, et al. Cardiac arrhythmias in aluminum phosphide poisoning studied by on continuous Holter and cardioscopic monitoring. *J Assoc Physicians India* 1998;46:598–601.
28. Mital HS, Mehrotra TN, Dwivedi KK, et al. A study of aluminum phosphide poisoning with special reference to its spot diagnosis by silver nitrate test. *J Assoc Physicians India* 1992;40:473–474.
29. Heyndrickx A, Van Peteghem C, Van den Heede M, et al. A double fatality with children due to fumigated wheat. *Eur J Toxicol* 1976;9:113–118.
30. Garry VF, Good PF, Manivel JC, et al. Investigation of a fatality from nonoccupational aluminum phosphide exposure: measurement of aluminum in tissue and body fluids as a marker of exposure. *J Lab Clin Med* 1993;122:739–747.
31. Schoonbroodt D, Guffens P, Jousten P, et al. Acute phosphine poisoning? A case report and review. *Acta Clin Belg* 1992;47:280–284.
32. Kochar DK, Shubhakaran, Jain N, et al. Successful management of hypokalaemia related conduction disturbances in acute aluminum phosphide poisoning. *J Indian Med Assoc* 2000;98:461–462.
33. Aggarwal P, Handa R, Wig N, et al. Intravascular hemolysis in aluminum phosphide poisoning. *Am J Emerg Med* 1999;17:488–489.
34. Lakshmi B. Methemoglobinemia with aluminum phosphide poisoning [Letter]. *Am J Emerg Med* 2002;20:130–132.
35. Garry VF, Griffith J, Danzl TJ, et al. Human genotoxicity: pesticide applicators and phosphine. *Science* 1989;246:251–255.
36. Siwach SB, Singh P, Ahlawat S, et al. Serum and tissue magnesium content in patients of aluminum phosphide poisoning and critical evaluation of high dose magnesium sulphate in reducing mortality. *J Assoc Physicians India* 1994;42:107–110.
37. Chugh SN, Kumar P, Aggarwal HK, et al. Efficacy of magnesium sulphate in aluminum phosphide poisoning—comparison of two different dosing schedules. *J Assoc Physicians India* 1994;42:373–375.
38. Chugh SN, Kolley T, Kakkar R, et al. A critical evaluation of anti-peroxidant effect of intravenous magnesium in acute aluminum phosphide poisoning. *Magnes Res* 1997;10:225–230.
39. Hayes WJ, Laws ER, eds. *Handbook of pesticide toxicology, vol. 2. Classes of pesticides*. New York: Academic Press, 1991:668–671.
40. Maddy KT, Edmiston S, Richmond D. Illness, injuries, and deaths from pesticide exposures in California 1949–1988. *Rev Environ Contam Toxicol* 1990;114:57–123.
41. Alexeeff GV, Kilgore WW. Methyl bromide. *Residue Rev* 1983;88:101–153.
42. United States Environmental Protection Agency. *Ambient water quality criteria for halomethanes*. EPA 440/5-80-051, 1980:C-34.
43. Garnier R, Rambourg-Schepens MO, Muller A, et al. Glutathione transferase activity and formation of macromolecular adducts in two cases of acute methyl bromide poisoning. *Occup Environ Med* 1996;53:211–215.
44. Lewis SE. Inhibition of SH enzymes by methyl bromide. *Nature* 1948;161:692–693.
45. Zwaveling JH, de Kort WL, Meulenbelt J, et al. Exposure of the skin to methyl bromide: a study of six cases occupationally exposed to high concentrations during fumigation. *Hum Toxicol* 1987;6:491–495.
46. Torkelson TR, Rowe VK. Halogenated aliphatic hydrocarbons containing chlorine bromine and iodine. In: Clayton GD, Clayton FE, eds. *Patty's industrial hygiene and toxicology, vol. 2B. Toxicology*, 3rd ed. New York: John Wiley and Sons 1981:3433–3601.
47. Grant WM. *Toxicology of the eye*, 3rd ed. Springfield, IL: Charles C Thomas Publisher, 1986:607–610.
48. Marraccini JV, Thomas GE, Ongley JP, et al. Death and injury caused by methyl bromide, an insecticide fumigant. *J Forensic Sci* 1983;28:601–607.
49. Hustinx WN, van de Laar RT, van Huffelen AC, et al. Systemic effects of inhalational methyl bromide poisoning: a study of nine cases occupationally exposed due to inadvertent spread during fumigation. *Br J Indust Med* 1993;50:155–159.
50. Deschamps FJ, Turpin JC. Methyl bromide intoxication during grain store fumigation. *Occup Med* 1996;46:89–90.
51. Horowitz BZ, Albertson TE, O'Malley M, et al. An unusual exposure to methyl bromide leading to fatality. *J Toxicol Clin Toxicol* 1998;36:353–357.
52. Shield LK, Coleman TL, Markesbery WR. Methyl bromide intoxication: neurologic features, including simulation of Reye syndrome. *Neurology* 1977;27:959–962.
53. Chavez CT, Hepler RS, Staatsma BR. Methyl bromide optic atrophy. *Am J Ophthalmol* 1985;99:715–719.
54. De Haro L, Gastaut JL, Jouglard J, et al. Central and peripheral neurotoxic effects of chronic methyl bromide intoxication. *J Toxicol Clin Toxicol* 1997;35:29–34.
55. Uncini A, Basciani M, Di Muzio A, et al. Methyl bromide myoclonus: an electrophysiological study. *Acta Neurol Scand* 1990;81:159–164.
56. Herzstein J, Cullen MR. Methyl bromide intoxication in four field-workers during removal of soil fumigation sheets. *Am J Indust Med* 1990;17:321–326.
57. Lifshitz M, Gavrilov V. Central nervous system toxicity and early peripheral neuropathy following dermal exposure to methyl bromide. *J Toxicol Clin Toxicol* 2000;38:799–801.
58. Muller M, Reinhold P, Lange M, et al. Photometric determination of human serum bromide levels—a convenient biomonitoring parameter for methyl bromide exposure. *Toxicol Lett* 1999;107:155–159.
59. Yamano Y, Kagawa J, Ishizu S, et al. Three cases of acute methyl bromide poisoning in a seedling family farm. *Indust Health* 2001;39:353–358.
60. Hurst JA, Tonks CE, Geyer R. An improved X-ray spectrometric method for the determination of bromide in whole blood of workers occupationally exposed to methyl bromide. *J Anal Toxicol* 1994;18:147–149.
61. Tanaka S, Abuku S, Seki Y, et al. Evaluation of methyl bromide exposure on the plant quarantine fumigators by environmental and biological monitoring. *Indust Health* 1991;29:11–21.
62. Buchwald AL, Muller M. Late confirmation of acute methyl bromide poisoning using S-methylcysteine adduct testing. *Vet Hum Toxicol* 2001;43:208–211.
63. Verberk MM, Rooyakkers-Beemster T, de Vlieger M, et al. Bromine in blood, EEG and transaminases in methyl bromide workers. *Br J Indust Med* 1979;36:59–62.
64. Moosa MR, Jansen J, Edelstein CL. Treatment of methyl bromide poisoning with haemodialysis. *Postgrad Med J* 1994;70:733–735.
65. American Conference of Governmental Industrial Hygienists. *Chloropicrin. Documentation of TLVs and BEs*. CD ROM version, 2002.
66. Stokinger HE. Aliphatic nitro compounds, nitrates, nitrites. In: Clayton GD, Clayton FE, eds. *Patty's industrial hygiene and toxicology, 3rd ed. Vol. 2C. Toxicology*. New York: Wiley-Interscience, 1982:4164–4165.
67. Buckley LA, Jiang XZ, James RA, et al. Respiratory tract lesions induced by sensory irritants at the RD50 concentration. *Toxicol Appl Pharmacol* 1984;74:417–429.
68. Goldman LR, Mengle D, Epstein DM, et al. Acute symptoms in persons residing near a field treated with the soil fumigants methyl bromide and chloropicrin. *West J Med* 1987;147:95–98.
69. TeSlaa G, Kaiser M, Biederman L, et al. Chloropicrin toxicity involving animal and human exposure. *Vet Hum Toxicol* 1986;28:323–324.
70. Prudhomme JC, Bhatia R, Nutik JM, et al. Chest wall pain and possible

rhabdomyolysis after chloropicrin exposure: a case series. *J Occup Environ Med* 1999;41:17–22.
71. Gonmori K, Muto H, Yamamoto T, et al. A case of homicidal intoxication by chloropicrin. *Am J Forensic Med Pathol* 1987;8:135–138.
72. Prentiss AM. *Chemicals in war. A treatise on chemical warfare.* New York: McGraw-Hill, 1937:161–163.
73. Hayes WJ, Laws ER, eds. *Handbook of pesticide toxicology. Vol. 2. Classes of pesticides.* New York: Academic Press, 1991:705–708.
74. Kezic S, Monster AC, Verplanke AJ, et al. Dermal absorption of cis-1,3-dichloropropene vapour: human experimental exposure. *Hum Exp Toxicol* 1996;15:396–399.
75. Stott WT, Kastl PL. Inhalation pharmacokinetics of technical grade 1,3-dichloropropene in rats. *Toxicol Appl Pharmacol* 1986;85:332–341.
76. Van Welie RT, van Duyn P, Brouwer DH, et al. Inhalation exposure to 1,3-dichloropropene in the Dutch flower-bulb culture. Part II. Biological monitoring by measurement of urinary excretion of two mercapturic acid metabolites. *Arch Environ Contam Toxicol* 1991;20:6–12.
77. Miyaoka T, Yamashita E, Hasegawa T, et al. Mechanism of 1,3-dichloropropene-induced hepatotoxicity in mice. *J Pesticide Sci* 1990;15:419–425.
78. Flessel P, Goldsmith JR, Kahn E, et al. Acute and possible long-term effects of 1,3-dichloropropene—California. *MMWR Morb Mortal Wkly Rep* 1978;27:50,55.
79. Meulenbelt J, de Vries I. Acute work-related poisoning by pesticides in The Netherlands; a one year follow-up study. *Przeg Lek* 1997;54:665–670.
80. Hernandez AF, Martin-Rubi JC, Ballesteros JL, et al. Clinical and pathological findings in fatal 1,3-dichloropropene intoxication. *Hum Exp Toxicol* 1994;13:303–306.
81. Brouwer EJ, Verplanke AJ, Boogaard PJ, et al. Personal air sampling and biological monitoring of occupational exposure to the soil fumigant cis-1,3-dichloropropene. *Occup Environ Med* 2000;57:738–744.
82. Osterloh JD, Feldman BJ. Urinary protein markers in pesticide applicators during a chlorinated hydrocarbon exposure. *Environ Res* 1993;63:171–181.
83. Scheuerman EH. Suicide by exposure to sulfuryl fluoride. *J Forensic Sci* 1986;31:1154–1158.
84. Vernot EH, MacEwen JD, Haun CC, et al. Acute toxicity and skin corrosion data for some organic and inorganic compounds and aqueous solutions. *Toxicol Appl Pharmacol* 1977;42:417–423.
85. Hayes WJ, Laws ER. *Handbook of pesticide toxicology. Volume 2. Classes of pesticides.* New York: Academic Press, 1991:564.
86. Meikle RW, Stewart D, Globus OA. Fumigant mode of action. Drywood termite metabolism of Vikane fumigant as shown by labeled pool technique. *J Agric Food Chem* 1963;11:226–230.
87. Hanley TR, Calhoun LL, Kociba RJ, et al. The effects of inhalation exposure to sulfuryl fluoride on fetal development in rats and rabbits. *Fundam Appl Toxicol* 1989;13:79–86.
88. Taxay EP. Vikane inhalation. *J Occup Med* 1966;8:425–426.
89. Nuckolls JG, Smith DC, Walls WE, et al. Centers for Disease Control. Fatalities resulting from sulfuryl fluoride exposure after home fumigation—Virginia. *MMWR Morb Mortal Wkly Rep* 1987;36:602–604,609–611.
90. Calvert GM, Mueller CA, Fajen JM, et al. Health effects associated with sulfuryl fluoride and methyl bromide exposure among structural fumigation workers. *Am J Public Health* 1998;88:1774–1780.
91. Rougart JR, Roberts JR. *Recognition and management of pesticide poisonings*, 5th ed. Washington: US Environmental Protection Agency, 1999:161.
92. Nitschke KD, Albee RR, Mattsson JL, et al. Incapacitation and treatment of rats exposed to a lethal dose of sulfuryl fluoride. *Fundamental Applied Toxicol* 1986;7:664–670.
93. Carlock LL, Dotson TA. Metam-sodium. In: *Handbook of pesticide toxicology, 2nd ed. Vol. 2: Agents.* San Diego: Academic Press 2001:1867–1879.
94. Jowa L. Metam: animal toxicology and human risk assessment. In: Fan AM, Chang LW, eds. *Toxicology and risk assessment: principles, methods, and applications.* New York: Marcel Dekker, 1996:619–634.
95. US Environmental Protection Agency. *The determination of whether dithiocarbamate pesticides share a common mechanism of toxicity.* Available at: http://www.epa.gov/oppsrrd1/cumulative/dithiocarb.pdf. Accessed November 19, 2002.
96. Cone JE, Wugofski L, Balmes JR, et al. Persistent respiratory health effects after a metam sodium pesticide spill. *Chest* 1994;106:500–508.
97. Koo D, Goldman L, Baron R. Irritant dermatitis among workers cleaning up a pesticide spill: California 1991. *Am J Indust Med* 1991;27:545–553.
98. Richter G. Allergic contact dermatitis from methylisothiocyanate in soil disinfectants. *Contact Dermatitis* 1980;6:183–186.

CHAPTER 239
Herbicides

Alvin C. Bronstein

See Figure 1.

Compounds included:	**Acrolein, atrazine, carbanilate herbicides (barban, chlorpropham, propham), chlorate salts, chlorophenoxy herbicides [2,4-dichlorophenoxyacetic acid (2,4-D), 2,4,5-trichlorophenoxyacetic acid (2,4,5-T)], dicamba, diquat/paraquat, endothall, glyphosate, metachlor, nitrophenols (dinoseb), substituted ureas, terbutryn**
Molecular formula and weight:	**See Table 1.**
CAS Registry No.:	**See Table 1.**
Normal levels:	**Not applicable**
Antidote:	**None**

OVERVIEW

In the United States, federal regulation of pesticides is under the Federal Insecticide, Fungicide, and Rodenticide Act (FIFRA) and the Federal Food, Drug, and Cosmetic Act (FFDCA) (1,2). The Environmental Protection Agency (EPA) administers FIFRA. Under FIFRA, the EPA regulates the production, registration, periodic reregistration, sale, and use of pesticides for agricultural and nonagricultural purposes. The FFDCA authorizes the EPA to establish pesticide tolerances (maximum residue levels) in food. The U.S. Food and Drug Administration is responsible for the enforcement of these pesticide tolerances (3). In addition, pesticide regulation is coordinated with the U.S. Department of Agriculture and the states (2).

Congress passed the FIFRA in 1947 and amended it several times through 1988 (1). The amendments contained in the Federal Environmental Pesticide Control Act of 1972 moved pesticide control and the FIFRA under the EPA (4). The most recent FIFRA amendments were enacted by the Food Quality Protection Act of 1996. FIFRA, as amended, requires that each manufacturer intending to produce pesticide products for sale, distribution, or use within the United States register each pesticide product and its label with the EPA before its first commercial use. These requirements are predominately federal, with some enforcement delegated to the states. States may impose additional regulations (4).

FIFRA authorizes the EPA to review and register pesticides for specified uses. FIFRA regulations apply to pesticide manu-

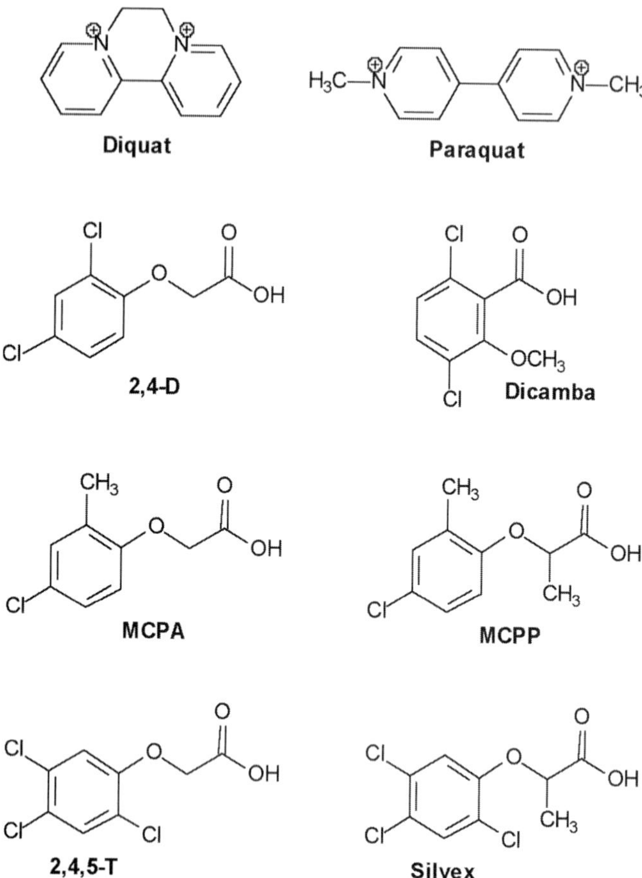

Figure 1. Structures of the selected herbicides.

TABLE 1. Physical characteristics of selected herbicides

Compound (trade name)	Molecular formula	Molecular weight (g/mol)	CAS Registry No.
Acrolein	C_3H_4O	56.1	107-02-8
Atrazine	$C_8H_{14}ClN_5$	215.7	1912-24-9
Carbanilate herbicides			
Barban	$C_{11}H_9Cl_2NO_2$	258.1	101-27-9
Chlorpropham	$C_{10}H_{12}ClNO_2$	213.7	101-21-3
Propham	$C_{10}H_{13}NO_2$	179.2	122-42-9
Chlorate salts			
Sodium chlorate	$ClNaO_3$	106.4	7775-09-9
Calcium chlorate	$CaCl_2O_6$	206.9	10137-74-3
Chlorophenoxy herbicides			
2,4-Dichlorophenoxyacetic acid	$C_8H_6Cl_2O_3$	221	94-75-7
2,4,5-Trichlorophenoxyacetic acid	$Cl_3C_6H_2OCH_2COOH$	255.5	93-76-5
Dicamba	$C_8H_6Cl_2O_3$	221.04	1918-00-9
Diquat	$C_{12}H_{14}N_2$	186.24	2764-72-9
Endothall	$C_8H_{10}O_5$	186.2	145-73-3
Glyphosate	$C_3H_8NO_5P$	169.1	1071-83-6
Metachlor	$C_{14}H_{20}ClNO_2$	269.8	15972-60-8
Nitrophenols (Dinoseb)	$C_{10}H_{12}N_2O_5$	240.22	88-85-7
Paraquat	$C_{12}H_{14}N_2$	186.26	4685-14-7
Substituted ureas			
Diuron	$C_9H_{10}Cl_2N_2O$	233.1	330-54-1
Terbutryn	$C_{10}H_{19}N_5S$	241.4	886-50-0

facturing, formulating, marketing, and distributing. End users (applicators) and pesticide disposal are also covered under the law. According to FIFRA, a *pesticide* is defined as "(1) any substance or mixture of substances intended for preventing, destroying, repelling, or mitigating any pest, (2) any substance or mixture of substances intended for use as a plant regulator, defoliant, or desiccant, and (3) any nitrogen stabilizer" (5). Pesticides include insecticides, herbicides, rodenticides, fungicides, nematicides, and acaricides as well as disinfectants, fumigants, wood preservatives, and plant growth regulators (2).

Pesticide formulations usually contain both "active" and "inert" ingredients. The inert ingredients have their own inherent toxicities. The FIFRA definition for *active ingredient* is essentially the same as for pesticide: an ingredient that prevents, destroys, repels, or mitigates a pest or is a plant regulator, defoliant, desiccant, or nitrogen stabilizer (5). FIFRA requires that the active ingredient together with its percentage by weight must be identified by name on the label. *Inert ingredients* are defined as any product ingredient that does not affect the target pest. FIFRA does not require a manufacturer to list a product's inert ingredients, and this can be problematic. For example, in some products, isopropyl alcohol is an active antimicrobial pesticide. However, in some pesticide formulations, isopropanol is used as a solvent and may be considered an inert ingredient. Inert ingredients are not identified by name and percentage on the label. Many inert ingredients are not inert in a toxicologic sense (6). To help put this issue in better perspective, the EPA issued a notice that encourages manufacturers, formulators, producers, and registrants of pesticide products to voluntarily substitute the term "other ingredients" in place of using the term "inert ingredients" on the label. However, the regulation does not require the manufacturer to list the inert ingredients on the label (7).

To give additional information to the end user, poison center, or medical toxicologist, the EPA classifies pesticides into four categories based on five criteria: oral dose lethal to 50% of experimental animals (LD_{50}), the inhalational [median lethal inhalation concentration (LC_{50})], the dermal LC_{50}, eye effects, and skin effects (8). This signal word scheme is depicted in Table 2.

For category I designations, on the basis of oral, inhalation, or dermal toxicity, the word "poison" must also be on the label. "Poison" must appear in red on a contrasting background with the skull and crossbones in immediate proximity. In addition, a child hazard warning must be on every pesticide label—"keep out of reach of children"—unless the EPA has determined that child access is of low probability. Table 2 shows the criteria for each of the four EPA pesticide toxicity categories. Based on this classification, the following toxicity category appears on the pesticide label.

DEFINITION OF HERBICIDES

Herbicides are a defined subset of pesticides (2). These agents include a broad, varied group of chemical compounds. Herbicides are classified according to their mechanism of action on plants. For many, these mechanisms remain unknown. The structure and activity relationships of the better-known herbicides in regard to plants are summarized in Table 3 (9).

Herbicide exposure most commonly occurs as a result of occupational accidents, intentional ingestions, or low-level chronic exposures that may last for years (10). In 2001, American poison centers reported 9380 herbicide exposures (11). Of these, 2593 (28%) of the herbicide exposures occurred in children younger

TABLE 2. Toxicity categories and pesticide label statements

Toxicity category	I: Danger	II: Warning	III: Caution	IV: Caution
Oral LD_{50}	Up to and including 50 mg/kg	>50–500 mg/kg	>500–5000 mg/kg	>5000 mg/kg
Inhalation LC_{50}	Up to and including 0.2 mg/L	>0.2–2.0 mg/L	>2–20 mg/L	>20 mg/L
Dermal LD_{50}	Up to and including 200 mg/kg	>200–2000 mg/kg	>2000 mg/kg–20,000 mg/kg	>20,000 mg/kg
Eye effects	Corrosive; corneal opacity not reversible within 7 d	Corneal opacity reversible within 7 d; irritation persisting for 7 d	No corneal opacity; irritation reversible within 7 d	No irritation
Skin effects	Corrosive	Severe irritation at 72 h	Moderate irritation at 72 h	Mild or slight irritation at 72 h

LC_{50}, median lethal inhalation concentration; LD_{50}, mean lethal dose.

than 6 years of age. Glyphosate was the identified agent in 47% (4426) of all herbicide exposures, followed by chlorophenoxy herbicides at 22% (2103). Four adult deaths were reported secondary to herbicide exposure—all paraquat. Paraquat accounted for 81 (less than 1%) of all reported herbicide exposures (11).

According to EPA data, there are approximately 890 active ingredients registered as pesticides in the United States (2). In 1999, 2,4-dichlorophenoxyacetic acid (2,4-D) and glyphosate ranked one and two, respectively, in non-farm agricultural use herbicides (12). Table 3 summarizes herbicide mode of action on plants for selected agents (9,10,13,14).

TABLE 3. Selected herbicides and their mode of action on plants

- Photosynthesis inhibitors
  - Anilides
  - Benzimidazoles
  - Biscarbamates
  - Pyridazinones
  - Triazinediones
  - Triazines
  - Triazinones
  - Uracils
  - Substituted ureas
  - Quinones
  - Hydroxybenzonitriles
- Amino acid synthesis inhibitors
  - Glyphosate
  - Sulfonylureas
  - Imidazolinones
  - Bialaphos
  - Glufosinate
- Cell membrane disruptors
  - Bipyridyliums (paraquat and diquat)
  - *p*-Nitrodiphenyl ethers
  - Oxadiazoles
  - *N*-phenylamides
- Lipid synthesis inhibitors
  - Aryloxyphenoxy alkanoic acids
- Cellulose synthesis inhibitors
  - Dichlobenil
- Cell division inhibitors
  - Phosphoric amides
  - Dinitroanilines
- Chlorophyll/carotenoid pigment synthesis inhibitors (interference with photooxidation protection)
  - Pyridazinones
  - Phenoxybenzamines
  - Fluoridone
  - Diflunione
  - 4-Hydroxypyridines
  - Amitrole (3-amino-1,2,4-triazole)
- Inhibition of folate synthesis
  - Methyl [(4-aminophenyl)sulfonyl]carbamate (Asulam)
- Seedling shoot growth inhibitors
  - Metachlor (Lasso)
- Growth regulators (synthetic auxins)
  - Chlorophenoxy compounds (2,4-dichlorophenoxyacetic acid; 2,4,5-trichlorophenoxyacetic acid)
  - Benzoic acid [2,5-dichloro-6-methoxybenzoic acid (Dicamba)]
  - Picolinic acids (Tordon)

CHLOROPHENOXY HERBICIDES

Chlorophenoxy herbicides are chlorinated organic acids. Organic acids, such as acetic, propionic, or butyric acid, serve as the base molecule. The addition of one to three chlorine atoms produces the active herbicide. Some compounds may also have a methyl substitution as part of the chlorophenoxy portion. The chlorophenoxy herbicides usually are manufactured in the form of metal salts, alkylamine salts, or esters to produce materials of low volatility (10). This minimizes their possible spread to nontargeted plants growing nearby. They are known as *selective herbicides* because they kill broadleaf weeds but do not harm grasses.

The best known of this group includes 2,4-D; 2,4,5-trichlorophenoxyacetic acid (2,4,5-T); 2-methyl-4-chlorophenoxyacetic acid; and 2-(2,4,5-trichlorophenoxy) propionic acid. Dicamba, a chlorinated benzoic acid, has a similar structure. It is sometimes grouped with the chlorophenoxy herbicides. All of these chlorinated organic acid compounds have similar biochemical properties.

Chlorophenoxy herbicides are widely used to control broadleaf weeds and woody plants in cereal crops, sugarcane, turf pastures, and non-crop lands (15). These herbicides are absorbed by the roots and leaves within 4 to 6 hours of application (16). They function as plant growth regulators, acting as synthetic auxins (growth-regulating substances) or plant hormones, stimulating rapid but abnormal plant growth reactions similar to 12 naturally occurring indole auxins. Normally, auxins are moved into plant cells by a membrane transporter molecule and removed by facilitated diffusion (17). The chlorophenoxy herbicides are transferred into the cell by the same transporter molecule but are not able to be transported out of the cell, so concentration increases within the cell (13,14,18,19). Rapid growth, stimulated by the herbicide, interferes with nutrient transport and destroys the plant. The plants may develop high levels of nitrates or cyanide before wilting (10).

2,4-Dichlorophenoxyacetic Acid

2,4-D is a widely used chlorophenoxy compound registered as a broadleaf weed herbicide. The herbicidal effects of 2,4-D originally were noted in 1941 (18). More than 60 million lb are used in the United States annually (15). 2,4-D products carry the EPA "DANGER" signal word (8) on the label, primarily because of the herbicide's ability to cause severe eye and dermal irritation.

2,4-D is a white to yellow crystalline, odorless powder with a melting point of 140.5°C. It has a slight phenolic odor. It is a noncombustible solid that is soluble in water and hydrocarbon solvents. 2,4-D may be found in flammable liquids such as hydrocarbon solvents (e.g., xylene) or aqueous vehicles.

There are several methods for the commercial production of 2,4-D. One method involves the chlorination of phenol to form 2,4-dichlorophenol, which is then reacted with monochloroacetic acid to form 2,4-D. Other reactions chlorinate molten phenoxyacetic acid or combine 2,4-dichlorophenol, sodium, and ethyl chloroacetate to produce 2,4-D after ester hydrolysis (20).

TOXIC DOSE

The U.S. Occupational Safety and Health Administration (OSHA) established an inhalational permissible exposure limit (PEL) for 2,4-D of 10 mg/m^3 (21). The National Institute for Occupational Safety and Health (NIOSH) recommended exposure limit (REL) for 2,4-D is 10 mg/m^3 (22). The immediate danger to life or health (IDLH) air concentration value for 2,4-D is 500 mg/m^3 (22).

The American Conference of Governmental Industrial Hygienists (ACGIH) 2003 threshold limit value (TLV)–time-weighted average (TWA) for 2,4-D is 10 mg/m^3. 2,4-D has not been classified as a human carcinogen. Data are inadequate to classify the agent in terms of its carcinogenicity in humans or animals (23).

TOXICOKINETICS AND TOXICODYNAMICS

Chlorophenoxy herbicides appear to demonstrate similar pharmacokinetic profiles (24). Rapid and almost complete absorption occurs after an oral dose (25–29). Differences exist among amine, salt, and ester formulations of 2,4-D. The amine and salt compounds are hydrolyzed and absorbed rapidly (25,27). The ester preparations of 2,4-D demonstrate lower plasma concentrations (26). These compounds are highly bound to plasma proteins (24). Once absorbed, the chlorophenoxy herbicides are distributed to kidneys, liver, gastrointestinal (GI) tract, and the central and peripheral nervous systems.

Oral absorption follows first order kinetics (29,30). This is estimated in humans to be between 1% and more than 27% per hour (27,31). In humans, almost all of a 2,4-D oral dose is absorbed within 24 hours (32). Peak plasma concentrations are reached at between 4 and 24 hours in humans (25,27–29).

Elimination of 2,4-D is rapid. 2,4-D metabolites other than conjugates have not been detected in human urine (27). Approximately 77% of the dose is eliminated unchanged in the urine (27). Five male adult volunteers ingested a single oral dose of 5 mg/kg of 2,4-D. No detectable clinical effects were noted. The average plasma half-life of 2,4-D was 11.6 hours, with a mean urine half-life of 17.7 hours. Eighty-three percent of the ingested oral dose was excreted as the parent compound, and 12.8% of the oral dose was excreted in the urine as an acid-labile conjugate (29,32).

The chlorophenoxy herbicides demonstrate first order elimination kinetics that are dose dependent (30,33). Plasma half-lives range from 10 to 20 hours and may increase to 80 to 120 hours with large, acute poisoning (33). Members of this herbicide group have a relatively small volume of distribution (V_d) (15). The V_d increases with increasing dose. Reflecting this dose-dependent V_d, chlorophenoxy acid herbicide tissue concentrations increase disproportionately with increasing dose, as compared with plasma concentrations. Therefore, increasing the body burden increases the apparent V_d of the chlorophenoxy herbicides. No evidence suggests bioaccumulation (32).

The mean lethal human dose of 2,4-D is approximately 28 g (30,34). Pharmacokinetic studies of a 30.22-kg woman ingesting a mixture of 2,4-D and dicamba in an acute overdose attempt revealed that the V_d was 10.2 L (0.338 L/kg) for 2,4-D and 23.4 L (0.774 L/kg) for dicamba (35). In human volunteers, at a dose of 5 mg/kg, the V_d of 2,4-D is approximately 0.1 L/kg (range, 0.098 to 0.104 L/kg) (27).

Workers exposed to an air concentration of 2,4,-D at 0.1 to 0.2 mg/m^3 had urine concentrations ranging from 3 to 14 mg/L (36). Various studies have found workers to have urinary 2,4-D concentrations ranging from 0.2 to 8.2 mg/L (36). 2,4-D is readily absorbed through the skin. Skin absorption is the major route of exposure for herbicide applicators. Dermal exposure levels are 4 to 50 times greater than those of the inhalational route (33). The most common sources of exposure are found in the manufacture or application of 2,4-D (33).

CLINICAL PRESENTATION

Acute Exposure. Acute chlorophenoxy herbicide toxicity presents a clinical picture of gastroenteritis, including nausea, abdominal pain, GI hypermotility, and diarrhea (sometimes bloody) (10). These compounds have an irritant effect on mucous membranes. Elevations may occur in hepatic enzymes such as lactate dehydrogenase and aspartate aminotransferase (AST). Delayed fever of sudden onset may occur with ingestion (37). At higher doses, muscular and neurologic problems develop (10). Skeletal muscle myotonia (stiff legs, muscle twitching, and spasms) (37); muscle fibrillation; myoglobinuria (36); and rhabdomyolysis may be observed. Central nervous system (CNS) depression, ataxia, miosis, diminished coordination, and paralysis leading to coma are the major CNS findings. Tachycardia is a frequent finding along with the potential for other cardiac dysrhythmias. In one study of chlorophenoxy herbicide overdose patients, 7 of 27 patients developed hypotension (37). Pulmonary edema and hyperventilation have been reported (37,38).

Albuminuria and hemoglobinuria have been seen, which may reflect glomerular or tubular injury (39). Acute renal failure secondary to rhabdomyolysis has occurred after poisoning with 2-(2-methyl-4-chlorophenoxy) propionic acid (38) or 2,4-D (37). Metabolic acidosis has been reported in severe cases (37,40). Ingestion of 2,4-D has been reported to produce hypocalcemia in association with hypophosphatemia and renal failure (41). Hyperkalemia also has been observed (38,39,42). Thrombocytopenia rarely has been seen (38,41). Death usually is due to peripheral vascular collapse (10).

Delayed onset of paresthesias and protracted polyneuropathy have been reported as being due to poisoning with herbicide mixtures containing chlorophenoxy compounds. Onset may be delayed for up to 1 month (43). A polyneuritis-type picture with decreased vibratory and proprioceptive sensation with decreased deep tendon reflexes in the presence of superficial reflexes has been reported (10). Peripheral neuropathies may be seen in acute poisoning survivors or in subacute cases (44,45).

Major target organs are the central nervous and cardiovascular systems (40). Electrocardiogram abnormalities, including flattening or inversion of the T wave, have been reported. Hervonen et al. (46) found reversible damage to the endothelial cells of the blood–brain barrier in rats exposed to 2,4-D. Dudley and Thapar (47) reported autopsy findings in a 76-year-old white man with senile dementia who died 6 days after acute 2,4-D ingestion. Widespread plaques of acute perivascular demyelination and perivascular petechial hemorrhage without cellular infiltration were described. Single intraperitoneal doses of 200 mg/kg in rats produced reversible inhibition of cerebral electrical activity with direct attack on the reticular system. Electroencephalographic changes were seen as early as 24 hours after dosing (48).

Goldstein and Jones (49) were the first to report the development of peripheral neuropathy with electromyelogram abnormalities in three cases after heavy 2,4-D ester dermal exposure. Symptomatology persisted. Recovery was still incomplete several years after exposure. A 39-year-old male farmer who sustained excessive exposure to 2,4-D while spraying crops developed a primary sensory peripheral neuropathy 4 days after exposure (50). Electromyographic and peroneal nerve conduction study results were within normal limits. Symptoms diminished, but the patient continued to experience intermittent numbness of the hands after prolonged use.

Concentrated solutions of 2,4-D (greater than 12%) have been shown to cause severe skin burns in rats and rabbits (51–53). Various authors have reported fatal human poisonings with 2,4-D and its congeners (28,40,52). As stated, the mean adult estimated lethal dose of 2,4-D is 28 g (30,34). Two thousand milligrams of 2,4-D given intravenously produced no symptoms in a patient terminally ill with coccidioidomycosis (53); 3600 mg has caused serious side effects, including fibrillary twitching of the mouth and both upper extremities and generalized hyporeflexia (54). Ingestion of 500 mg over 3 weeks produced no definable symptoms (55), whereas an intentional ingestion of 80 mg/kg caused death in a 23-year-old college student.

Postmortem 2,4-D blood concentrations of 720 mg/L were reported in a 64-year-old white woman who was found comatose and died of pulmonary edema 12 hours after hospital admission (56). In another report, a 26-year-old man ingested 360 ml of Ortho Weed B-Gone M [dimethylamine salts of 2,4-D, 10.8%, 2-(2-methyl-4-chlorophenoxy) propionic acid, 11.6% (77.6% inert ingredients)]; Dexol (chlorpyrifos, 6.7%; in petroleum distillates, 76.8%); and a few granules of warfarin, 0.025%. The patient died approximately 30 hours after admission after four episodes of bradycardia, hypotension, and asystole. Other findings included hyperkalemia, thrombocytopenia, hypocalcemia, and hypophosphatemia. The postmortem concentration of 2,4-D was 389.5 g/ml and of 2-(2-methyl-4-chlorophenoxy) propionic acid was 235.5 g/ml.

Chronic Exposure. Neurotoxicity and hepatic dysfunction are the primary problems reported secondary to chronic exposure to 2,4-D. Chronic neurologic toxicity is due most likely to a direct neurotoxic effect of the chlorophenoxy herbicides (48). 2,3,7,8-Tetrachlorodibenzo-*p*-dioxin (TCDD) contamination may be responsible for other long-term problems as well. Disorders of liver function, such as porphyria, have been reported in chronic occupational exposure cases (57).

Carcinogenicity. The International Agency for Research on Cancer classifies chlorophenoxy herbicides in group 2B: The agent (mixture) is possibly carcinogenic to humans (58).

DIAGNOSTIC TESTING

Patients exposed to chlorophenoxy herbicides require a full biochemical profile, including hepatic enzymes, AST, alanine aminotransferase, γ-glutamyl transpeptidase, and lactate dehydrogenase, electrolytes, glucose, blood urea nitrogen, creatinine, serum aldolase, creatinine phosphokinase, complete blood cell count, and urinalysis. Baseline electrocardiogram and continuous monitoring should be performed because of high probability of cardiac dysrhythmias. Cardiac dysrhythmia should be treated initially with standard advanced cardiac life support protocols.

Chronically exposed patients also require a thyroid profile and vitamin B_{12} and folate determinations to assist in the differentiation of other neurologic diseases. A computerized tomography scan or magnetic resonance imaging of the brain and electroencephalogram may be needed to rule out other possible CNS disease states. Electronystagmography and electromyelogram studies should be undertaken in cases or suspected cases of peripheral neuropathies. Serum or adipose tissue measurements of TCDD may be performed to estimate exposure.

Concentrations of 2,4-D and other chlorophenoxy herbicides in various fluids may be measured with ultraviolet spectrophotometry, high-performance liquid chromatography (34,59), or flame ionization or electron capture gas chromatography (59). The latter two methods appear to be more sensitive and specific (34). Chlorophenoxy concentrations in blood have ranged from 58 to 1220 mg/L in fatal acute overdoses (59). Measuring exposure to dioxin is difficult because of its extremely low concentrations in adipose tissue. It can be measured using gas chromatography-mass spectrometry. Usually, it is measured as picograms per gram of serum lipid.

Adipose tissue sampling or serum measurements for TCDD are the most reliable methods by which to estimate an affected individual's TCDD exposure and body burden. Adipose tissue sampling has been viewed as the most accurate index of TCDD body burden. Recent use of TCDD determinations in the blood lipid component may prove as reliable as the more invasive adipose tissue sampling (60). Preliminary data in Vietnam veterans revealed via adipose tissue sampling that a TCDD blood concentration of 15 pg/g of fat was associated with heavy exposure, with a correlation coefficient (*r*) of +0.89.

Thirty-nine of the aforementioned Missouri residents either exposed to soil TCDD concentrations of 20 to 100 parts per billion (ppb) for 20 or more years or exposed for 6 months or more to soil concentrations of more than 100 ppb underwent adipose tissue sampling for TCDD (61). Their values were compared with those of 57 unexposed controls with adipose tissue sampling obtained during surgical procedures. The mean TCDD concentration in the exposed individuals was 17 parts per trillion (ppt) (range, 2.8 to 750.0 ppt) as compared with a median value of 6.4 (range, 1.4 to 20.2 ppt) in the controls (62). From this study, the half-life of TCDD in humans was estimated to be between 5 and 8 years (62).

TREATMENT

Acutely exposed patients should be removed from the exposure and treated with symptomatic and supportive measures. Special attention should be directed to the respiratory system, with monitoring of airway, breathing, and circulatory status. Supplemental oxygen and intravenous fluids should be given as necessary.

Decontamination. Dermal or ocular contaminated areas should receive prompt irrigation with copious amounts of water (63). Rescue personnel should wear appropriate gloves, boots, and goggles.

Enhancement of Elimination. Various techniques have been advocated to enhance the elimination of the chlorophenoxy herbicides. Because of the relatively low negative logarithm of acid ionization constant (pK_a; 3.3) of the 2,4-D and the chlorophenoxy herbicides, alkaline diuresis has been proposed to enhance the elimination of 2,4-D (64,65). As always, the risk versus benefit of alkaline diuresis must be gauged. Attempts to increase urine volume beyond 100 to 150 ml/hour increase the risk of complications from fluid overload but increase clearance only minimally. Before any alkaline diuresis therapy, hydration status should be documented to ensure that affected patients are well hydrated. Alkaline diuresis should not be attempted in the face of renal failure or impaired renal function.

The usual method for alkaline diuresis is administration of a loading dose of sodium bicarbonate in the range of 1 to 2 mEq/kg body weight. This usually equates to 2 to 3 ampules (88 to 132 mEq). The necessity for coadministration of potassium is controversial. Probably more important is to maintain normal potassium status rather than arbitrarily loading affected patients with potassium. This usually can be accomplished by administration of 20 to 40 mEq of potassium chloride as needed in a crystalloid solution such as 5% dextrose in water. Adequate urine output should be maintained. Optimal urine pH should be kept in the

7.5 to 8.0 range. Overly aggressive alkalinization should be avoided, as should excessive alkalinization of affected patients. Close monitoring of serum and urine pH is required.

Adequate alkalemia should be maintained via administration of additional sodium bicarbonate. A dose of 1 to 2 mEq/kg of sodium bicarbonate periodically, based on pH measurements, usually maintains the alkalemia. Cautious administration of diuretics, such as furosemide or mannitol, may be required to maintain adequate diuresis. Renal function and serum electrolytes need careful, frequent monitoring (66). Alkaline diuresis should not be attempted in patients who have evidence of acute lung injury, cerebral edema, or in those with renal failure.

Supportive Care. Affected patients should be monitored for the development of metabolic acidosis, hyperthermia, seizures, coma, hyperventilation, tachycardia, electrocardiogram abnormalities, vasodilatation, diaphoresis, hypoxia, myotonia, hyperkalemia, myoglobinuria, hepatic dysfunction, or renal failure. Severe hypoxia associated with hyperventilation and normal PCO_2 may result from the uncoupling of oxidative phosphorylation.

Supportive therapy is the mainstay of treatment for acute chlorophenoxy herbicide poisoning. Forced alkaline diuresis for acute poisoning has been advocated, as the chlorophenoxy herbicides are organic acids with a measured pK_a of 3.3 (67). Prescott et al. (67) reported that the renal clearance of 2,4-D increased from 0.14 ml/minute at a urine pH of 5.1 to 5.1 ml/minute at a pH of 8.3. Flanagan et al. (37) reported the positive effect of alkaline diuresis in a series of 41 patients acutely poisoned with chlorophenoxy herbicides and ioxynil (4-hydroxy-3,5-di-iodobenzonitrile). Plasma half-lives were reduced to less than 30 hours with alkaline diuresis. Alkaline diuresis has been recommended in cases of severe poisoning, with coma, acidemia, or total chlorophenoxy herbicide concentrations greater than 0.5 g/L. The 2,4-D pK_a in this study was reported as 2.6 (37).

Rhabdomyolysis is treated with aggressive intravenous fluid therapy to prevent renal insufficiency. Urinary alkalinization is not necessary. Input and output status should be assessed closely.

2,4,5-Trichlorophenoxyacetic Acid

2,4,5-T is a colorless to tan, odorless solid with a melting point of 154° to 155°C. 2,4,5-T is synthesized from the intermediate compound 2,4,5-trichlorophenol. During 2,4,5-trichlorophenol manufacture, 2,4,5-trichlorophenol has the ability to react with itself to produce TCDD. TCDD is one of a family of compounds known collectively as *dioxins*. Dioxins are contaminants of 2,4,5-T and hexachlorophene synthesis (68,69). In addition, dioxins are released in emissions from coal-burning power plants, diesel exhaust, and the incomplete burning of chlorine waste such as polyvinyl chloride plastic and polychlorinated biphenyls. These compounds also are produced naturally in small amounts by volcanoes and forest fires (68,69). TCDD is the best studied of approximately 75 dioxin compounds (68,69). The dioxins, along with related compounds—the furans (polychlorinated dibenzofurans), polychlorinated biphenyls, and polybrominated biphenyls—have been associated in both animal and human epidemiologic studies with an increased risk of cancer and other symptoms such as chloracne (10,25,68,69).

Dioxins bioaccumulate in the food chain, so human exposure usually results from consumption of fish, meat, and dairy products (68,69). Current herbicide-manufacturing processes are designed to remove dioxin contaminants. Because of the dioxin contamination problem during the production of 2,4,5-T, the EPA banned all 2,4,5-T use registrations in March 1985. Before this action, the U.S. Department of Agriculture halted 2,4,5-T use in 1970 on all food crops except rice. The EPA terminated all registrations for the use of this herbicide on rice fields, orchards, sugarcane, rangeland, and other non-crop sites.

The most notorious use of chlorophenoxy herbicide compounds occurred from 1961 to 1971 in the Republic of Vietnam (70). Approximately 19.5 million gallons of phenoxy and other herbicidal agents were applied in 9141 missions. The need for defoliants prompted the use of a variety of herbicide compounds and mixtures. Because of rushed production methods, dioxin contaminants were not uniformly removed during the synthesis process. To avoid clogging problems in the spraying apparatus, the various agents were shipped in color-coded drums (70). The 50:50 mixture of the *N*-butyl esters of 2,4-D and 2,4,5-T was shipped in 55-gallon drums marked with an orange stripe. This herbicide mixture came to be known as *Agent Orange*. It is estimated that the dioxin contamination of Agent Orange ranged from less than 0.05 to 100.0 parts per million (ppm). Other defoliants used in that context included Agent White (triisopropanolamine salts of 2,4-D and picloram) and Agent Blue (cacodylic acid, the arsenical compound $C_2H_7AsO_2$) (70). Because of its dioxin risk, 2,4,5-T was banned in the United States by the EPA in 1979 (69). Millions of pounds of 2,4-D still are used annually in the United States.

TOXIC DOSE

The OSHA PEL for inhalational exposure to 2,4,5-T is 10 mg/m^2 (21). The NIOSH REL is 10 mg/m^3 (22). The IDLH air concentration value for 2,4,5-T is 250 mg/m^3 (22). The ACGIH TLV-TWA is also 10 mg/m^3. 2,4,5-T has the A4 notation by the TLV. 2,4,5-T is not classified as a human carcinogen. Data are inadequate to classify the agent in terms of its carcinogenicity in humans or animals (23).

CLINICAL PRESENTATION

2,4,5-T. In 1971, sludge waste from a hexachlorophene manufacturing plant was mixed with waste oil and sprayed for dust control on dirt roads in residential, recreational, and commercial areas of eastern Missouri near St. Louis (61). By February 1986, 28 separate sites had been found to have TCDD soil concentrations of 1 ppb or more. Using 155 unexposed subjects as controls, Hoffman et al. (61) studied 154 exposed mobile home park residents where the soil TCDD concentration ranged from 1 to 2200 ppb. The exposed residents demonstrated increased frequency of anergy, minor abnormalities in T-cell T4:T8 ratios of less than 1.0, and abnormal T-cell function, suggesting a possible association of long-term TCDD exposure with alterations in cell-mediated immunity. Peak urinary uroporphyrin levels were greater than 13 mg/g of creatinine in 16.3% of the exposed cohort as compared with 7.5% in the controls. Mean urinary uroporphyrins were 9.6 mg/g of creatinine versus 8.4 mg/g of creatinine in those in the unexposed control group. The exposed residents experienced paresthesias of the hands and feet and headaches more than did the controls. Neuropsychological testing failed to find significant differences between the two groups (61).

Seveso, Italy (approximately 20 miles north of Milan, Italy), was the site of a TCDD release over a residential area in 1976. More than 37,000 people may have been exposed to dioxins as a result. No deaths were reported secondary to acute poisoning. Determining etiology of symptoms was confounded by concomitant exposure to release of other compounds. Chloracne appeared almost exclusively in children and young people; most cases resolved spontaneously. Transient lymphopenia and impaired liver function were observed. Subclinical peripheral nerve impairment was observed in 16 of 156 patients with chloracne at 6 years after the dioxin release. No cases of peripheral neuropathy were observed in this group of 156. Long-term epidemiologic studies of the exposed populations are continuing, with special emphasis to define any mutagenic or carcinogenic effects (71).

TCDD. Chloracne is the most common finding in individuals exposed to TCDD (40). In severely contaminated individuals, chloracne can persist for years after exposure (41). Chloracne consists of comedones, cysts, pustules, and abscesses. Hepatic dysfunction, peripheral neuropathy, fat metabolism disorders, elevated serum cholesterol, and porphyria cutanea tarda are the other findings associated most frequently with TCDD exposure in industrial settings (42). Zack and Suskind (40) studied 129 workers exposed to TCDD after a trichlorophenol processing plant explosion in 1949. All employees developed chloracne. The frequency of malignancies was not increased during 30-year follow-up.

Symptoms reported after TCDD exposure included chloracne; severe pain in muscles of upper and lower extremities, shoulders, and thorax; fatigue; nervousness; vertigo; decreased libido; and cold intolerance. Liver impairment, demonstrated by increased prothrombin times, was observed (72). Over time, the symptoms may clear to some degree. Aches and pains in the lower extremities and back, nervousness, fatigue, and dyspnea may continue (72). In a later study of 204 exposed and 163 nonexposed workers, chloracne persisted in 55.7% of those in the exposed group. A positive association was found with GI tract ulcers, but no increased risk of cardiovascular disease, hepatic disease, renal disease, central or peripheral nervous system problems, or malignancies was found (73). In a related study focusing on workers with and without chloracne, the mean duration of chloracne was found to be 26 years. Increased 7-glutamyl transferase concentrations were found in the chloracne group. Abnormal sensory findings also were present in the chloracne group (74).

TCDD has been associated with soft-tissue sarcoma, Hodgkin's disease, non-Hodgkin's lymphoma, gastric cancer, nasal cancer, and liver cancer in various studies (75,76). Rats, mice, and hamsters exposed to TCDD have developed histiocytic lymphomas, fibrosarcomas, and tumors of liver, skin, lung, thyroid, tongue, hard palate, and nasal turbinates (76,77). Initiating or promoting carcinogenesis may be a function of TCDD (78,79).

Fingerhut et al. (15) conducted a retrospective study of a cohort of 5172 workers occupationally exposed to TCDD during production of various chemicals. TCDD serum concentrations were measured in 253 workers. Mortality from all cancers was increased significantly in the cohort. Cancer mortality from stomach, liver, and nasal tumors and from Hodgkin's disease and non-Hodgkin's lymphoma was not significantly different from expected mortality rates in the overall cohort. In a subcohort of 1520 workers with more than 1 year of exposure and more than 20 years' latency since TCDD exposure, mortality was increased significantly from all cancers, specifically from soft-tissue sarcomas and respiratory tract cancers. Confounding variables, such as smoking and exposure to other industrial chemicals, could not be excluded as other potential causes of the cancer mortality rates. Mean TCDD serum concentration adjusted for lipids was 233 pg/g of lipid (range, 2000 to 3000). This compared with 7 pg/g for unexposed individuals. The mean TCDD concentration for 119 workers with 1 year of exposure or more was 418 pg/g, with exposure having occurred 15 to 37 years earlier (15).

Although this study had multiple potential pitfalls, the data indicate probable human risk from TCDD exposure (80). On the basis of this study, the lifetime risk from TCDD-induced soft-tissue sarcoma approximates 2 per 1000. This risk is far greater than the commonly accepted lifetime risk of 1 per 100,000 or 1 per million from exposure for the general public to potential carcinogens (80).

Multiple studies have been conducted of soft-tissue sarcoma incidence among Vietnam veterans (81). A case-control study, including 217 cases of soft-tissue sarcoma and 599 controls, found that Vietnam veterans with higher estimated Agent Orange exposure appeared to be at greater, although not statistically significant, risk for the development of soft-tissue sarcomas (82). An earlier hospital-based case-control study of 234 Vietnam veterans and 13,496 patients in the comparison group failed to find a significant association between soft-tissue sarcomas and previous military service in Vietnam (83). Other studies failed to confirm earlier reports of an association between exposure to chlorophenoxy herbicides and the risk of malignant lymphomas—specifically Hodgkin's and non-Hodgkin's lymphoma from Agent Orange exposure in Vietnam veterans (84–86).

Studies of Vietnam veterans in which the cohort was formed from participants in so-called Operation Ranch Hand failed to show an increased risk of cancer (87,88).These veterans were responsible for spraying chlorophenoxy herbicides (including Agent Orange) during the Vietnam War. The cohort consisted of 995 veterans who flew application aircraft, maintained aircraft and spray equipment, or handled bulk quantities of TCDD-contaminated herbicides for 1 year or more. This cohort was studied and compared with a group of 1200 Vietnam veterans who were not exposed directly. Those in the Ranch Hand group had alkaline phosphatase concentrations averaging 98 U/L, compared with the control group's average concentration of 90 U/L ($p < .01$). No prevalence differences were found in verified skin or systemic malignancies. The median Ranch Hand TCDD concentration was 12.4 ppt as compared with 4.2 ppt in the controls. Of the Ranch Hand group, nonflying enlisted personnel had the highest TCDD concentrations at 23.6 ppt, compared with pilots at 7.3 ppt. No chloracne was found in those in either the Ranch Hand or the control group (87). An earlier study of Vietnam and non-Vietnam veterans found that the mean serum TCDD level was approximately 4 ppt for both groups. This study also suggested that TCDD exposure was higher in Vietnam veterans whose jobs involved handling of herbicides (89).

In a related study, the noncombat mortality in a group of 1261 Ranch Hand veterans was compared with that in a control group of 19,101 Air Force veterans primarily involved in cargo missions. No significant difference in the all-cause standardized mortality ratio was found after adjustment for age, rank, and occupation (88).

Other studies have examined the possible association between phenoxy herbicide exposure and the risk of developing malignant lymphomas in Vietnam veterans. A more recent case-control study of 329 lung cancer cases in Vietnam veterans correlated with Agent Orange exposure failed to find an increased risk of lung cancer associated with Vietnam service (90).

PARAQUAT AND DIQUAT

Paraquat (1,1'-dimethyl-4,4'-dipyridyl) is a bipyridyl compound. It was marketed first in 1962 as a broad-spectrum, nonselective, contact herbicide and desiccant (Fig. 1) after having been described first by Weidel and Rosso in 1882 (91). The redox properties of paraquat were published in 1933. It has been used as a redox indicator under the name of *methyl viologen* since 1933. A yellow solid with a faint ammonia-like odor, its molecular weight is 257.2 D, and its boiling point at 760 mm Hg is 175° to 180°C (347° to 356°F). Paraquat is corrosive to metals and decomposes under ultraviolet light (91). It is a restricted-use herbicide in the United States.

Diquat (1,1'-ethylene-2,2'-dipyridylium dibromide) is a paraquat analog having properties similar to paraquat but different toxic effects. Diquat forms a monohydrate that is a colorless to yellow crystalline substance and has a melting point between 335° and 340°C. Diquat usually is compounded for spraying as diquat dibromide [6,7-dihydrodipyrido (1,2-a: 2',l'-c) pyrazinediium dibromide; $C_{12}H_{12}N_2Br_2$]. Diquat does not produce the pulmonary fibrosis seen in paraquat poisoning.

Uses

Zeneca Agrochemicals manufactures paraquat (Gramoxone) in the United States, China, Mexico, Thailand, Malaysia, and Japan (92). The most common paraquat formulation is a 20% solution (200 mg/dl). Manufacturers' directions usually recommend dilution at approximately 40 times to a 0.5% weight per volume paraquat ion solution (91). Other application procedures suggest a 100 to 200 times dilution for a spray solution. Inhalational poisonings may produce low toxicity because pulmonary absorption is low, as most of the aerosolized particles are larger than 5 mm in diameter and, therefore, are nonrespirable (i.e., do not reach the alveolar barrier) (91,93).

Paraquat may be applied using hand-held knapsack sprayers or vehicles (all terrain vehicles, farm tractors, and high-cycle tractors) with attached spray booms. It may be applied also via aerial spraying (91). Skin exposure is believed to be the most significant route of occupational exposure (91). The most common sources of exposure occur in the manufacture or application of these compounds. The highest risk exists for contamination from spills and splashes during mixing, loading, and maintenance activities. The potential exists for exposure to civilian populations near application sites.

Toxic Dose

The OSHA PEL for *paraquat* (respirable dust) is 0.5 mg/m^3 (83). To prevent skin absorption, skin exposure should be prevented or reduced to the extent necessary in the workplace through the use of gloves, coveralls, goggles, or other appropriate personal protective equipment, engineering controls, and work practices. The ACGIH TLV-TWA is 0.5 mg/m^3 of total dust as the cation and 0.1 mg/m^3 of respirable dust as a fraction of the cation. No short-term exposure limit has been established. The NIOSH REL-TWA is 0.1 mg/m^3 of respirable dust. The IDLH value is 1 mg/m^3. The ACGIH TLV-TWA for paraquat respirable sizes is 0.1 mg/m^3. No ACGIH short-term exposure limit value exists (83). The OSHA and ACGIH TLV-TWA for *diquat* is 0.5 mg/m^3 (83).

For paraquat, mortality from an ingestion of the 20% solution may approach 78% (93). Potential exists for fatality from as little as one mouthful of a 20% solution. Death may be due either to circulatory failure at 3 days after ingestion or progressive irreversible pulmonary fibrosis at 5 to 31 days after ingestion. The minimum lethal human dose is approximately 35 mg/kg (93,94). A mouthful (approximately 20 ml) produces a dose of 55 mg/kg in the average 70-kg adult. A study of 28 paraquat oral poisoning patients reported that one mouthful produced 6 of 12 deaths (50%) from pulmonary fibrosis at 5 to 31 days after ingestion; 11 to 12 (92%) died from circulatory failure within 48 hours after ingesting more than one mouthful (93,94).

Toxicokinetics and Toxicodynamics

The kinetics of paraquat poisoning in humans are similar to those in the canine model, with the peak plasma concentration attained by 2 hours after ingestion (95,96). Plasma concentrations decline quickly as the ion is distributed to the tissues. Absorption of paraquat is believed to take place in the small intestine. Drugs that increase emptying time increase plasma concentrations. Food in the stomach or GI tract may decrease paraquat plasma concentrations. Lung and kidney paraquat concentrations continue to increase even after plasma concentrations seem to stabilize. Lung paraquat accumulation is an energy-dependent process that follows zero order (saturable) kinetics. This system can be blocked by metabolic inhibitors such as cyanide and iodoacetate.

Plasma paraquat concentrations are predictive of survival. Patients whose plasma concentrations do not exceed 2.00, 0.60, 0.30, 0.16, and 0.10 mg/L at 4, 6, 10, 16, and 24 hours, respectively, are likely to survive (97,98). Plasma paraquat concentrations greater than 5 mg/L usually are fatal. In one study of ten cases in Crete, all patients with paraquat concentrations exceeding 5 mg/L died (99). In the same study, two patients with paraquat levels of 2.7 mg/L (approximately 41 hours after ingestion) and 2.8 mg/L (approximately 6 hours after ingestion) did not survive.

Paraquat is excreted unchanged in the urine. Renal elimination is greater than the glomerular filtration rate in individuals with normal creatinine clearance. Paraquat does not appear to bioaccumulate. In animal models, low intravenous or subcutaneous doses are excreted rapidly in the urine (100–103). In the canine model, paraquat is not metabolized (104).

Intravenous paraquat infusions at 30 to 50 mg/kg produced rapid urinary excretion at clearance rates in excess of the glomerular filtration rate, signifying paraquat elimination by active secretion. Doses of 20 mg/kg produced renal failure. The kinetics are described by a three-compartment model, with the lungs as a slow uptake compartment. Paraquat doses high enough to cause renal failure did not produce peak lung concentrations until 15 hours after ingestion. This outcome means that initiation of paraquat removal by hemoperfusion in the first 12 to 15 hours should be helpful. Some have proposed that within the first 24 hours, humans who have ingested paraquat and have urinary paraquat concentrations of more than 10 mg/ml and lower creatinine clearance values should receive hemodialysis or hemoperfusion. Other studies disagree.

Pathophysiology

Paraquat is highly corrosive. It is absorbed poorly after inhalation but is extremely toxic if ingested (105). After paraquat ingestion, edema, burns, or ulceration may be seen in the mucosa of the mouth, pharynx, esophagus, stomach, and intestines (106). Death usually occurs within 48 hours of ingestion of 50 mg/kg; at lower doses, death may be delayed for several weeks (105). Toxicity is due to the bipyridyl compound's pulmonary accumulation, when it accepts an electron and forms a free radical (10). Paraquat ion is transported actively into pulmonary cells. Pulmonary edema or fibrosis is the sequelae of lung uptake (93,106). Lipid peroxidation ensues, and nicotinamide adenine dinucleotide phosphate is depleted (105). Centrizonal hepatic necrosis, proximal renal tubule damage, myocardial damage, and skeletal muscle damage with focal necrosis may be seen. Pancreatic damage and CNS injury may occur. Pulmonary fibrosis usually begins 2 to 14 days after poisoning. With large ingestions (more than 20 mg/kg), pulmonary edema may be seen. Paraquat oxidation produces superoxide (free radical oxygen) ions, which cause mucous membrane lesions and secondary necrosis of the GI tract, liver, pancreas, renal tubules, and adrenal glands by lipid peroxidation.

Two phases of paraquat pulmonary toxicity have been described. In phase 1, type I and type II alveolar epithelial cells are destroyed (107). Alveolitis with extensive pulmonary destruction occurs. Pulmonary edema may develop with the infiltration of polymorphonuclear leukocytes into the lung tissue. Phase II is marked by extensive intraalveolar and interalveolar fibrosis. Normal alveolar architecture is destroyed and replaced by fibrous tissue. Gas exchange is impeded severely, leading to hypoxia and death.

Vulnerable Populations

Paraquat crosses the placenta. Fetal concentration is four to six times that of the mother's. The fetus appears to tolerate maternal paraquat poisoning while it is dependent on the placental circulation and if the gestational age is less than 30 weeks. After that, birth and exposure to atmospheric oxygen result in signs of paraquat poisoning (99,108). Poor late gestation survival may be due to the fact that type II pneumocytes appear between 28 and 32 weeks of gestation (99).

Clinical Presentation

PARAQUAT

The severity of paraquat poisoning symptoms depends on the dose consumed. Most human fatalities are the result of suicide. Individuals consuming large amounts of paraquat usually die within a few days from cardiovascular collapse, whereas those consuming less usually succumb many days to weeks later of irreversible pulmonary fibrosis (93,94,107).

Paraquat ion exposure may cause injuries to the nails, skin, eyes, and nose. These injuries result from exposure to the extremely irritating concentrated solutions before dilution. Paraquat produces a strong irritant action on various types of epithelial tissues. It can cause dryness, erythema, blistering, irritation, and ulceration and fissuring of the skin (109–111). Inhalation may cause epistaxis. Contact dermatitis has been reported after topical exposure. It is believed that paraquat diluted according to manufacturers' recommendations is unlikely to cause skin burns unless spray-soaked clothing is worn for prolonged periods. In one study, 15 consecutive occupational cases of a single skin or eye exposure to paraquat solutions caused only local lesions; no systemic effects were detected in affected patients (112).

Localized discoloration or a transverse white band of discoloration affecting the nail plate may be seen in spray operators (103,104,106). Transverse ridging and furrowing of the nail may progress to an irregular nail deformity and subsequent nail loss. Once exposure stops, normal nail growth usually returns.

Ocular exposure to paraquat concentrate may cause corneal and conjunctival inflammation. Inflammation may develop gradually and progress to maximal damage over a 12- to 24-hour period. Corneal opacification may occur. Frank corneal ulceration and lacrimal duct stenosis has been reported (106). Miosis may be present. Sometimes the severity of these injuries goes relatively unnoticed until symptoms have progressed to corneal scarring and opacification.

Paraquat can be absorbed through the skin. Local and systemic toxicity has been reported after dermal exposure, which may produce local irritation, burns, or systemic effects.

Three stages of paraquat poisoning have been described (87,89,102):

1. Group 1 (mild poisoning): ingestion of less than 20 mg paraquat ion per kg of body weight. Patients may be asymptomatic or experience vomiting and diarrhea. Transient decrement in the carbon monoxide diffusing capacity and vital capacity may be seen. Complete recovery usually occurs.
2. Group 2 (moderate poisoning): ingestion of 20 to 40 mg paraquat ion per kg of body weight. Vomiting and diarrhea are followed by generalized symptomatology of systemic toxicity. All patients develop pulmonary fibrosis. Renal and hepatic failure may be present. Most patients die, but death may be delayed for 2 to 4 weeks.
3. Group 3 (severe poisoning): ingestion of more than 40 mg paraquat ion per kg of body weight. Nausea, vomiting, and diarrhea with marked oropharyngeal and esophageal ulceration are followed by failure of multiple organs (cardiac, respiratory, hepatic, renal, adrenal, pancreatic, and CNS). Cardiotoxicity signs may include ventricular dysrhythmias, hypotension, or cardiorespiratory arrest. Mortality usually is 100%, with death occurring usually in the first 24 hours after ingestion.

Initial symptoms of paraquat ingestion include burning of the mouth, throat, chest, and abdomen. Giddiness, headache, fever, myalgia, bloody diarrhea, and abdominal pain may be present. Urinalysis may show proteinuria, hematuria, or pyuria. Acute tubular necrosis may develop.

DIQUAT

Diquat ingestion, like that of paraquat, damages multiple organ systems. The clinical pattern is different even though diquat and paraquat share common mechanisms of toxicity. Infarction and purpura of the brain stem appear to be specific to diquat poisoning (113,114). Pontine purpura has been reported in three of seven adults who died from diquat ingestion (113,114). Potentially toxic diquat ion doses are in the range of 35 to 105 ml of the 20% solution. Diquat poisoning is characterized by GI tract injury, including burns to the oral mucosa, acute tubular necrosis, and bronchopneumonia. Paralytic ileus is seen more frequently in diquat than in paraquat ion poisoning. Pulmonary fibrosis is not seen in diquat ion poisoning, as diquat is not transported actively by lung tissue. Inhalation may produce nonspecific respiratory distress symptoms. Diquat produces cataracts in rats and dogs but, to date, not in humans. Treatment is similar to that of paraquat ion poisoning. Prompt initiation of charcoal hemoperfusion may be beneficial in minimizing tissue distribution and uptake by target organs.

Diagnostic Tests

Patients exposed to paraquat or diquat should have full evaluation, including hepatic enzymes (AST, alanine aminotransferase, γ-glutamyl transpeptidase, and lactate dehydrogenase), electrolytes, glucose, blood urea nitrogen, creatinine, serum aldolase, complete blood cell count, arterial blood gases, chest radiograph, and urinalysis. Chronically exposed patients also require a thyroid profile, vitamin B_{12}, and folate determination to assist in differentiation of other neurologic diseases.

The dithionite test is a rapid, semiquantitative colorimetric urine test that may be performed to detect paraquat (115). To one volume, add 0.5 volume 1% sodium dithionite (sodium hydrosulfite), add one normal sodium hydroxide. After 1 minute, the color should change: A deep blue reflects paraquat or diquat, with a urinary concentration of less than 0.5 mg/L. Positive or negative controls should be run (115). Urinary diquat is signified by the color green. In either case, the deeper the color, the higher the relative paraquat or diquat concentration is and the worse the prognosis is.

Medical information about paraquat poisoning and urine and plasma sample analysis for paraquat is available 24 hours per day, 7 days per week through the Zeneca Emergency Information Network [1-800-327-8633 (1-800-FASTMED)].

Treatment

Acutely exposed patients should be removed from the source of the exposure and decontaminated as the exposure and condition warrant. Rescue personnel should wear appropriate gloves, boots, and goggles (22).

DECONTAMINATION

Decontamination should be initiated as soon as possible after paraquat ingestion and should be instituted on any suspicion of ingestion. Fuller's earth, bentonite, or activated charcoal should be administered. Desorption of paraquat from the activated charcoal–paraquat complex as it passes through the GI tract is a theoretic (but not confirmed) disadvantage of the use of charcoal (102). Hypercalcemia may occur after the use of fuller's earth (106). The adult dose of bentonite clay (7% suspension) is 100 to 150 g and 2 g/kg for children younger than 12 years of age. The dose for fuller's earth (30% suspension) is 100 to 150 g for adults and 2 g/kg for children younger than 12 years of age.

Gastric lavage should be performed if less than 1 hour has passed since ingestion (102). Because of the high morbidity and mortality associated with paraquat poisoning, the decision to institute gastric lavage more than 1 hour after ingestion must be made on a case-by-case basis. After lavage, one of the aforementioned absorbents should be instilled via lavage tube. Doses may be repeated at 2- to 4-hour intervals.

ENHANCEMENT OF ELIMINATION

Urinary paraquat excretion is 20 to 50 times greater than plasma concentrations (107). Patients with normal renal function after ingestion have a paraquat clearance higher than creatinine clearance. This is due to active tubular secretion and nonionic diffusion additive to the glomerular filtration rate. Paraquat is not reabsorbed from the renal tubules; thus, forced diuresis does not enhance paraquat elimination. Forced diuresis still is advocated because it may reduce the concentration of paraquat in the renal tubules.

Hemodialysis is not effective in treating paraquat or diquat poisoning (116,117). Charcoal hemoperfusion has not been shown to reduce paraquat morbidity or mortality (102). A theoretic benefit is seen in clearing blood paraquat if hemoperfusion can be instituted during the first 2 hours after the poisoning. Neither hemoperfusion nor hemodialysis has been shown to be effective in reducing paraquat or diquat body burden (116,117). Pharmacokinetic data indicate a marked rebound effect from tissue on plasma paraquat levels. Thus, prolonged hemodialysis or hemoperfusion has been advocated by some authors (99).

SUPPORTIVE CARE

Supplemental oxygen should not be given, as this increases paraquat pulmonary toxicity. Late stages of poisoning may require oxygen as pulmonary fibrosis develops. Lung transplantation has not been successful either because the transplanted lung develops paraquat toxicity or other comorbidity factors (107,118,119).

Major prognostic indicators include route of administration (inhalation usually less severe than oral), ingested amount, time of last meal (as food delays absorption and neutralizes paraquat), gastric lesions, renal failure, and plasma paraquat concentrations.

GLYPHOSATE

Glyphosate [(carboxymethylamino)methylphosphonic acid] is an organophosphorus compound that is not a cholinesterase inhibitor. It is used as a broad-spectrum, nonselective, postemergent herbicide to control grasses, broadleaved weeds, and woody plants. Glyphosate products are in EPA toxicity class II (8). Glyphosate is commonly used as the isopropylamine salt. The herbicide is also formulated as a trimethylsulfonium salt. It is supplied as water-soluble concentrates and powders. Glyphosate is marketed under a variety of trade names (Roundup, Touchdown, Bronco, Network, and Kleenup). The commercial product is formulated in water at concentrations between 0.5% and 5.0%. Concentrated Roundup is sold as a 41% concentration before its final dilution as a 1% solution.

Toxic Dose

Occupational health exposure limits have not been established for glyphosate.

Pathophysiology

The toxicity of Roundup has been attributed to both the glyphosate herbicide and to the surfactant (120,121). Uncoupling of oxidative phosphorylation has been proposed as the mechanism of toxicity for glyphosate (122). The toxicity of the surfactant has been reviewed and includes vomiting, diarrhea, hemolysis of red blood cells, hypotension, altered mental status, and pulmonary edema (123). Further study of the mechanism of both glyphosate and the surfactant is required.

Clinical Presentation

Clinical manifestations of ingestion of the product include pharyngitis, vomiting, diarrhea, abdominal pain, hepatic damage, leukocytosis, hypotension, renal damage with oliguria, and erosions of the esophagus, oropharynx, and stomach (120). Ocular exposure can cause conjunctivitis. Inhalation of the mist of the product can cause respiratory irritation. Other dermal contact has caused dermatitis and mild chemical burns. Glyphosate is poorly absorbed from both the GI tract and the skin. In a retrospective study, Tominack et al. (124) described a clinical toxic syndrome after ingestion of a mouthful or more as follows: hypotension, shock, oral esophageal and GI mucosal injury, pulmonary edema, oliguria or anuria, metabolic acidosis, leukocytosis, and fever.

Treatment

As most poisoning from the product occurs by ingestion, clinical management is directed at controlling potential massive GI fluid loss and renal failure. Vomiting is common after ingestion; therefore, inducing emesis is unnecessary. Also, because the product is caustic to the esophagus, inducing emesis is not recommended. Administration of 30 g of activated charcoal may aid in adsorption of glyphosate and the surfactant. Aspiration of the product can produce pulmonary injury with pulmonary edema, so the airway must be protected. Intravenous rehydration is crucial to maintaining blood pressure and urine output.

ACROLEIN

Acrolein (2-propen-1-one, 2-propenal) is a potent herbicide and biocide used to control weeds, algae, and plant growth in irrigation canals and water drainage areas. Acrolein is a clear to yellowish liquid with a pungent odor and is very irritating to the eyes, skin, and mucous membranes.

Exposure occurs mainly by inhalation or dermal-ocular liquid contact by accidental splash. Acrolein is marketed under a variety of trade names, including Magnacide and Magnacide H.

TABLE 4. Health effects from acrolein vapor exposure

Vapor concentration (ppm)	Exposure (min)	Effect
0.25	5	Moderate irritation
1.0	2–3	Ocular and nose irritation
5.5	1	Intolerable
153	10	Potentially fatal

ppm, parts per million.

Human exposure can result in severe dermatitis and burns to the skin, eyes, and mucous membranes.

Toxic Dose

The OSHA PEL is 0.1 ppm or 0.25 mg/m^3 (21). The NIOSH REL is 0.25 mg/m^3, and the NIOSH short-term exposure limit is 0.8 mg/m^3 (22). The IDLH value for acrolein is 2 ppm (22). The ACGIH TLV-Ceiling value is 0.1 ppm (0.23 mg/m^3). Acrolein has not been classified as a human carcinogen. Data are inadequate to classify the agent in terms of its carcinogenicity in humans or animals.

Clinical Presentation

Acrolein vapor and liquid are potent irritants (Table 4). Due to its highly irritating vapor and lacrimator action, humans cannot tolerate vapor concentrations of 0.1 to 1.0 ppm for even short periods. Acute human exposure to high levels (10 ppm) can cause death (125). Pulmonary irritation occurs at levels ranging from 0.17 to 0.43 ppm. The acrolein odor threshold is 0.2 ppm (125).

Splash exposures to the liquid concentrate produce rapid ocular and skin damage. Skin injury from the concentrate can produce edema, erythema, and second-degree burns. Inhalation of the vapor or liquid produces respiratory irritation, mucous membrane irritation, difficulty in breathing, and pulmonary edema. Any splash exposure should be irrigated immediately with water for 15 to 20 minutes.

Chronic acrolein inhalational exposure causes generalized respiratory tract symptoms, including upper and lower respiratory tract irritation. To date, no human reproductive effects have been documented. Acrolein has been reported to cause birth defects in rats when it is injected directly into the embryo (126). No human data are available regarding the possible human carcinogenic effects of acrolein.

ATRAZINE

Atrazine (1-chloro-3-ethylamino-5-isopropylamino-2,4,6-triazine) is a restricted-use triazine herbicide. It is registered as a selective herbicide to control broadleaf and grassy weeds in crops. It is available as dry flowable, flowable liquid, liquid, water dispersible granular, and wettable powder formulations.

OSHA has not established a PEL for atrazine (21). The NIOSH REL for acrolein is 5 mg/m^3 (22). The ACGIH TLV-TWA is 5 mg/m^3. Atrazine has not been classified as a human carcinogen (23). Triazines are considered to be of low toxicity to humans. There are very few reports of human exposure, and most are of multiple agents. The acute oral LD_{50} for atrazine is estimated to be 1780 mg/kg, and that of terbutryn is estimated at 2500 mg/kg (127).

There are no specific tests for atrazine exposure. Atrazine may be detected in urine and biologic tissues by gas chromatography/flame ionization detection (128). Treatment is symptomatic and supportive.

CARBANILATE HERBICIDES

The carbanilate herbicides include barban (3-chlorophenylcarbamic acid chloro-2-butynyl ester), chlorpropham (isopropyl *m*-chlorocarbanilate), and propham (isopropyl-*N*-phenyl carbamate). Chlorpropham is still registered for use by the EPA as a carbanilate–selective preemergence and early postemergence herbicide. Chlorpropham has no occupational health exposure limits established.

These agents are dermal, eye, and respiratory irritants. The carbanilate herbicides are technically carbamates but differ from the insecticide carbamates in that they do not have anti-acetylcholinesterase properties. This is due to the fact that, structurally, they have a large substitution moiety on the nitrogen rather than the oxygen (129). Thus, their toxicity compared with the insecticides is much less different from the dermal sensitizer, although some references state that they do possess weak anticholinesterase properties (130,131).

Treatment is symptomatic and supportive.

CHLORATE SALTS

Sodium chlorate is a inorganic herbicide. Calcium chlorate is also an inorganic herbicide. Sodium and calcium chlorate salts were used as semipermanent soil sterilant herbicides (132). Sodium chlorate herbicide use was canceled by the EPA (133). Only calcium chlorate remains registered. There are no established occupational guidelines or regulations for calcium chlorate.

Pathophysiology

The chlorates oxidize glutathione and hemoglobin. This is followed by glucose 6 phosphate dehydrogenase denaturation and cross-linking of red cell membrane proteins. Time to effect is proportional to dose (134). Alteration in the red cell membrane increases sodium and potassium permeability and results in increased membrane rigidity. Hypoxia secondary to methemoglobinemia is a less important determinant of toxic outcome than hemolysis and disseminated intravascular coagulation, which are followed by renal failure (134). Renal failure is either due to a direct renal toxic effect (135) or secondary to hemolysis. Treatment of chlorate-induced methemoglobinemia with methylene blue is problematic because the chlorate inactivates glucose 6 phosphate dehydrogenase, thus inactivating the pentose phosphate pathway preventing nicotinamide adenine dinucleotide phosphate enzymatic reduction of methemoglobin (134).

Early anoxic death is secondary to methemoglobinemia or disseminated intravascular coagulation, whereas later demise is secondary to renal failure. In a 1979 review of 14 cases of sodium chlorate exposure, only four survived. The cases ranged from 3 to 55 years. The lowest fatal sodium chlorate dose was estimated to be 15 g. One-half of the cases developed cyanosis; cases also developed abdominal pain (36%), diarrhea (21%), dyspnea (21%), coma (12%), and methemoglobin (93%). Renal failure signaled by anuria developed within 48 hours of exposure in one-half of the patients (136). In an elegant rabbit study, the renal toxic effect of chlorate was found to be secondary to a catalytic activation of chlorate by methemoglobin, as rabbits are resistant to hemoglobin oxidation by chlorate and do not develop renal compromise. It is this reaction that is responsible for the renal failure (134).

Chlorates may be inhaled or ingested. Usually a latent period of a few hours is present after significant exposure (137). Heinz bodies have been reported. Findings also include dark urine secondary to methemoglobin production. GI tract irritation has been reported from oral ingestion. Vomiting and diarrhea are possible (138). CNS effects are possible secondary to hypoxia.

Clinical Presentation

Chlorate exposures are marked by the development of methemoglobinemia, hemolysis, and renal failure (134). Hemoglobin oxidation has been demonstrated *in vitro* (134). Chlorate-induced methemoglobinemia may be refractory to methylene blue (134). Cyanosis and methemoglobinemia were noted approximately 5 hours after ingestion of 150 to 200 g of sodium chlorate in a 26-year-old woman. Over the next 14 hours, hemolysis, disseminated intravascular coagulation, and renal shutdown developed. Cyanosis and methemoglobinemia (50%) were present 5 hours postingestion. The patient recovered, but renal function remained impaired (137). In another case, a 48-year-old man inhaled a concentrated sodium chlorate from a sprayer. Inhalation was followed by nausea and vomiting. The next day he developed cyanosis and a 57% methemoglobinemia and renal compromise on the following day. The patient survived (139).

Treatment

Depending on route of exposure, dermal decontamination is recommended. Begin basic and advanced life support. Because of the irritant effects on the GI tract, gastric lavage is problematic. Activated charcoal is of limited value. Treat methemoglobinemia with methylene blue, although the methemoglobinemia may be refractory (134) to methylene blue. In refractory cases, exchange transfusion may be required. Renal failure may require hemodialysis. Monitor renal output and function closely.

ENDOTHALL

Endothall (7-oxabicyclo[2.2.1]heptane-2,3-dicarboxylic acid) is a dicarboxylic acid herbicide available as granules or as a soluble concentrate. The EPA has classified endothall as toxicity class II—moderately toxic. Products containing endothall bear the signal word "WARNING" on the label (8). Endothall is an acid. Occupational guidelines or regulations have not been established for endothall.

Toxicokinetics and Toxicodynamics

Endothall is rapidly absorbed via the GI tract (140,141).

Pathophysiology

Endothall is corrosive to mucous membranes and the GI tract, especially at high concentrations of the free acid. Myocardiopathy and vascular injury leading to shock have been reported in intentional overdose. Seizures and CNS depression and respiratory depression have been reported (140).

Endothall toxicity may be due in part to its structural resemblance to cantharidin. Cantharidin is a toxin produced by blister beetles (142). Mouse studies have shown that cantharidin is toxic by inhibition of protein phosphatases types 1 and 2A. Contraction is increased in mouse myocardial and vascular smooth muscle preparations and increases the phosphorylation state of their regulatory proteins. This may explain the reported myocardial dysfunction in intentional exposures (142).

Clinical Presentation

There are two case reports in the literature of intentional endothall ingestion (140,141). A 23-year-old man ingested 40 ml and developed vomiting with abdominal pain. Gastric decontamination with charcoal and chocolate milk was performed. Symptoms stabilized, but 6 hours later, hematemesis occurred and was followed by acidosis, anuria, disseminated intravascular coagulation, and hypotension and cardiovascular collapse. The patient died 12 hours postingestion (140).

The only other reported case was a 21-year-old, 54-kg man who began vomiting after ingesting two mouthfuls of endothall, 175 g/L, and was found in a semiconscious state. Time of ingestion was unknown. Death ensued 2 hours later. Autopsy findings included focal lung hemorrhages and edema. Hemorrhage of the GI tract was present (141). Blood was assayed for gas chromatography with flame ionization detector. Findings were confirmed by gas chromatography-mass spectrometry. The blood measured 1 mg%; liver, 1.7 mg%. Stomach contents measured 4 mg%.

Treatment

Treatment is decontamination as appropriate and basic and advanced life support. Use of activated charcoal for gastric decontamination is problematic. Monitor renal function and cardiovascular and coagulation status. Be prepared to treat hypovolemic shock.

METACHLOR

Alachlor (Lasso) [2-chloro-2',6'-diethyl-*N*-(methoxymethyl)acetanilide] is a selective pre- and early postemergence herbicide for annual broadleaf control. Alachlor is a mild eye and mucous membrane irritant. Contact dermatitis has been reported. There is no human toxic dose established. The oral LD_{50} in rats is approximately 1800 mg (129). Treatment is symptomatic. Acute allergic reactions are possible.

NITROPHENOLS

Dinoseb (4,6-dinitro-2-sec-butylphenol) use was suspended by the EPA under emergency action to mitigate human exposures in 1986. Dinoseb is extremely toxic to humans. It is absorbed through the skin, GI tract, and lungs (133,143).

Poisoning may present with headache, nausea and vomiting, weakness, chest pain, and fever. Hypotension or hypertension is possible. Tachycardia, tachypnea, acute lung injury, and cyanosis are possible. Cardiovascular collapse, seizures, and coma are possible. Alterations may be found in liver and hepatic function. Ataxia and weakness may be an early finding (144). Methemoglobinemia is also possible.

Treatment includes decontamination and advanced life support as required. Although there are no data to support its use, activated charcoal may be beneficial after acute ingestion. Obtain serum electrolytes, blood urea nitrogen, creatinine, AST, alanine aminotransferase, and arterial blood gases in severely poisoned patients. Close monitoring of acid-base and fluid status is required. Treat methemoglobinemia with methylene blue as needed. If renal failure develops, hemodialysis may be necessary.

SUBSTITUTED UREAS

The substituted ureas (diuron, terbutryn) inhibit photosynthesis by blocking the Hill reaction (145). Diuron is a white, odorless solid. The melting point is 158° to 159°C. The vapor pressure is 3.1×10^{-6} mm Hg at 50°C (132). Hydrocarbon solvent solubility is low.

OSHA has not established a PEL for diuron (21). The NIOSH REL for diuron is 10 mg/m³ (22). The IDLH air concentration value for diuron is not established (22). The ACGIH TLV-TWA for diuron is 10 mg/m³ (23).

Very little information is available on human health effects of these agents. Substituted ureas induce microsomal enzyme function (129). Although this may not be important in most ingestions, one case report of a mixed ingestion of a related substituted urea (monolinuron) and paraquat implicated the substituted urea as the cause of the methemoglobinemia. It is not clear that the methemoglobinemia was related to the substituted urea ingestion (129). These agents are generally considered to be of low toxicity. They may be skin and mucous membrane irritants (129,146). One case was reported of a 31-year-old woman who ingested a mixture of amitrol 30% and diuron 56%. The dose was calculated at 20 mg/kg for the diuron. The patient remained asymptomatic (129).

Treatment is symptomatic and supportive. Monitor for methemoglobinemia.

REFERENCES

1. FIFRA, 40 C.F.R. Sect. 152 (2002).
2. EPA. *1996–1997 pesticide market estimates*. Available at http://www.epa.gov/oppbead1/pestsales/97pestsales/table_of_contents1997.html. Accessed September 2003.
3. FDA. *Compliance policy guidance for FDA staff. Sec. 575.100 pesticide residues in food and feed—enforcement criteria (CPG 7141.01)*. Available at http://www.fda.gov/ora/compliance_ref/cpg/cpgfod/cpg575-100.html. Accessed 9/09/2003.
4. EPA. *Environmental laws that establish EPA's authority*. Available at http://www.epa.gov/history/org/origins/laws.htm. Accessed September 2003.
5. FIFRA, 40 C.F.R. Sect. 152.3, 2002.
6. Yanez L, Ortiz D, Calderon J, et al. Overview of human health and chemical mixtures: problems facing developing countries. *Environ Health Perspect* 2002;110[Suppl 6]:901–909.
7. EPA. *Pesticide registration (PR) notice 97-6*. Available at http://www.epa.gov/opppmsd1/PR_Notices/pr97-6.html. Accessed September 2003.
8. EPA. *Toxicity categories and pesticide label statements*. Available at http://www.epa.gov/pesticides/health/tox_categories.htm. Accessed September 2003.
9. Duke S. Overview of herbicide mechanisms of action. *Environ Health Perspect* 1990;87:263–271.
10. Smith EA, Oehme FW. A review of selected herbicides and their toxicities. *Vet Hum Toxicol* 1991;33:596–608.
11. Litovitz TL, Klein-Schwartz W, Rodgers GC Jr, et al. 2001 annual report the American Association of Poison Control Centers Toxic Exposure Surveillance System. *Am J Emerg Med* 2002;20:391–452.
12. EPA. *1998–1999 pesticide market estimates*. Available at http://www.epa.gov/oppbead1/pestsales/99pestsales/table_of_contents1999.html. Accessed September 2003.
13. Ross MA, Childs D. *Herbicide mode-of-action summary*. Department of Botany and Plant Pathology, Purdue University. Cooperative Extension Service. Available at http://www.farmassist.com/resistance/html/pdf/mode_of_action.pdf. Accessed September 2003.
14. Boerbom C. *Herbicide mode of action reference*. Weed Science, University of Wisconsin. Available at http://ipcm.wisc.edu/uw_weeds/extension/articles/herbmoa.htm. Accessed September 2003.
15. Fingerhut MA, Halperin WE, Marlow BS, et al. Cancer mortality in workers exposed to 2,3,7,8-tetrachlorodibenzo-p-dioxin. *N Engl J Med* 1991;324:212–218.
16. Kennepohl E, Munro IC. Phenoxy herbicides. In: Krieger RI, ed. *Handbook of pesticide toxicology*, 2nd ed. San Diego: Academic Press 2001:1623–1638.
17. Muday GK, DeLong A. Polar auxin transport: controlling where and how much. *Trends Plant Sci* 2001;6:535–542.
18. Stevens JT, Summer DD. Herbicides. In: Hayes WJ Jr, Laws ER Jr, eds. *Handbook of pesticide toxicology*. San Diego: Academic Press, 1991:1317–1408.
19. Kimball, JW. *Auxin*. Available at http://users.rcn.com/jkimball.ma.ultranet/BiologyPages/A/Auxin.html. Accessed September 2003.
20. Hazardous Substances Data Bank. *2,4-D*. Bethesda, MD: National Library of Medicine, Available at http://toxnet.nlm.nih.gov/cgi-bin/sis/search/f?./temp/~egsRLC:1.
21. U.S. Department of Labor. Occupational Safety and Health Administration. Regulations (Standards - 29 CFR) TABLE Z-1 limits for air contaminants. 1910.1000 TABLE Z-1. Available at http://www.osha.gov/pls/oshaweb/owadisp.show_document?p_table=STANDARDS&p_id=9992. Accessed September 2003.
22. National Institute for Occupational Safety and Health (NIOSH). *NIOSH pocket guide to chemical hazards*. Available at http://www.cdc.gov/niosh/npg/npg.html. Accessed September 2003.
23. American Conference of Governmental and Industrial Hygienists. *TLVs and BEIs*. Cincinnati: American Conference of Governmental and Industrial Hygienists, 2003.
24. Arnold EK, Beasley VR. The pharmacokinetics of chlorinated phenoxyacid herbicides: a literature review. *Vet Hum Toxicol* 1989;31:121–125.
25. Erne K. Distribution and elimination of chlorinated phenoxyacetic acids in animals. *Acta Vet Scand* 1966;7:240–256.
26. Bjorklund NE, Erne K. Toxicological studies of phenoxyacetic herbicides in animals. *Acta Vet Scand* 1966;7:364–390.
27. Kohli JD, Khanna RN, Gupta BN, et al. Absorption and excretion of 2,4-dichlorophenoxyacetic acid in man. *Xenobiotica* 1974;4:97–100.
28. Gehring PJ, Betso JE. Phenoxy acids: effects and fate in mammals. *Ecol Bull (Stockh)* 1978;27:122–133.
29. Sauerhoff MW, Braun WH, Blau GE, et al. The fate of 2,4-dichlorophenoxyacetic acid (2,4-D) following oral administration. *Toxicol Appl Pharmacol* 1976;37:136–137.
30. Piper WN, Rose JQ, Leng ML, et al. The fate of 2,4,5-trichlorophenoxyacetic acid (2,4,5-T) following oral administration to rats and dogs. *Toxicol Appl Pharmacol* 1973;26:339–351.
31. Gehring PJ, Kramer CG, Schweta BA, et al. The fate of 2,4,5-trichlorophenoxyacetic acid (2,4,5-T) following oral administration to man. *Toxicol Appl Pharmacol* 1973;26:352–361.
32. Sauerhoff MW, Braun WH, Blau GE, et al. The fate of 2,4-dichlorophenoxyacetic acid (2,4-D) following oral administration to man. *Toxicology* 1977;8:3–11.
33. Libich S, To JC, Frank R, et al. Occupational exposure of herbicide applicators to herbicides used along electric power transmission line of right-of-way. *Am Ind Hyg Assoc J* 1984;45:56–62.
34. Baselt RC. *Disposition of toxic drugs and chemicals in man*, 6th ed. Foster City, CA: Biomedical Publications, 2002:307–309.
35. Young JF, Haley TJ. Pharmacokinetic study of a patient intoxicated with 2,4-dichlorophenoxy acid and 2-methoxy-3,6-dichlorobenzoic acid. *J Toxicol Clin Toxicol* 1977;11:489–500.
36. Kolmodin-Hedman B, Akerblom M. Field application of phenoxy acid herbicides. In: Tordoir WF, van Heemstra EAH, eds. *Field worker exposure during pesticide application*. New York: Elsevier Science, 1980:73–77.
37. Flanagan RJ, Meredith TJ, Ruprah M, et al. Alkaline diuresis for acute poisoning with chlorophenoxy herbicides and ioxynil. *Lancet* 1990;335:454–458.
38. Meulenbelt J, Zwaveling JH, van Zoonen P, et al. Acute MCPP intoxication: report of two cases. *Hum Toxicol* 1988;7:289–292.
39. Friesen EG, Jones GR, Vaughan D. Clinical presentation and management of acute 2,4-D oral ingestion. *Drug Saf* 1990;5:155–159.
40. Osterloh J, Lotti M, Pond SM. Toxicologic studies in a fatal overdose of 2,4 D, MCPP, and chlorpyrifos. *J Anal Toxicol* 1983;7:125–129.
41. Kancir CB, Andersen C, Olesen AS, et al. Marked hypocalcemia in a fatal poisoning with chlorinated phenoxy acid derivatives. *J Toxicol Clin Toxicol* 1988;26:257–264.
42. Keller T, Skopp G, Wu M, et al. Fatal overdose of 2,4-dichlorophenoxyacetic acid (2,4-D). *Forensic Sci Int* 1994;65:13–18.
43. O'Reilly JF. Prolonged coma and delayed peripheral neuropathy after ingestion of phenoxyacetic acid weed-killers. *Postgrad Med* 11984;60:76–77.
44. Berwick P. 2,4-Dichlorophenoxyacetic acid poisoning in man. *JAMA* 1970;214:1114–1117.
45. Wells WDE, Wright N, Yeoman WB. Clinical features and management of poisoning with 2,4-D and mecoprop. *J Toxicol Clin Toxicol* 1981;18:273–276.
46. Hervonen H, Elo HA, Ylitalo P. Blood-brain barrier damage by 2-methyl-4chlorophenoxyacetic acid herbicide in rats. *Toxicol Appl Pharmacol* 1982;65:23–31.
47. Dudley AW, Thapar NT. Fatal human ingestion of 2,4-D, a common herbicide. *Arch Pathol* 1972;94:270–275.
48. Desi I, Sos J, Olasz J, et al. Nervous system effects of a chemical herbicide. *Arch Environ Health* 1962;4:101–108.
49. Goldstein NP, Jones PH. Peripheral neuropathy after exposure to an ester of dichlorophenoxyacetic acid. *JAMA* 1959;171:1306–1309.
50. Berkley MC, Magee KR. Neuropathy following exposure to dimethylamine salt of 2,4-D. *Arch Intern Med* 1963;111:351–352.
51. Mattson JL, Johnson KA, Albee RR. Lack of neuropathologic consequences of repeated dermal exposure to 2,4-dichlorophenoxyacetic acid in rats. *Fundam Appl Toxicol* 1986;6:175–181.
52. Kay JH, Palazzolo BS, Calandra MD. Subacute dermal toxicity of 2,4-D. *Arch Environ Health* 1965;11:648–651.
53. Nielsen K, Kaempe B, Jenson-Holm J. Fatal poisoning in man by 2,4-dichlorophenoxyacetic acid (2,4-D): determination of the agent in forensic materials. *Acta Pharmacol Toxicol* 1965;22:224–234.
54. Seabury JH. Toxicity of 2,4-dichlorophenoxyacetic acid for man and dog. *Arch Environ Health* 1963;7:202–209.
55. Curry AS. Twenty-one uncommon cases of poisoning. *BMJ* 1962;1:687–698.
56. Smith RA, Lewis D. Suicide by ingestion of 2,4-D: a case history demonstrating the prudence of using GC/MS as an investigative rather than a confirmatory tool. *Vet Hum Toxicol* 1987;29:259–261.
57. Bleiberg J, Wallen M, Brodkin R, et al. Industrially acquired porphyria. *Arch Dermatol* 1964;89:793–797.
58. International Agency for Research on Cancer. Chlorophenoxy herbicides. *IARC Monogr Eval Carcinog Risks Chem Man* 1987;41[Suppl 7]:156.
59. Fraser AD, Isner IF, Perry RA. Toxicologic studies in a fatal overdose of 2,4-D, mecoprop, and dicamba. *J Forensic Sci* 1984;29:1237–1241.
60. Kahn PC, Gochfeld M, Nygren M, et al. Dioxins and dibenzofurans in blood and adipose tissue of Agent Orange-exposed Vietnam veterans and matched controls. *JAMA* 1988;259:1661–1667.
61. Hoffman RE, Stehr-Green PA, Webb KB, et al. Health effects of long-term exposure to 2,3,7,8-tetrachlorodibenzo-p-dioxin. *JAMA* 1986;255:2031–2038.
62. Patterson DC, Hoffman RE, Needham LL, et al. 2,3,7,8-Tetrachlorodibenzo-

p-dioxin levels in adipose tissue of exposed persons in Missouri. *JAMA* 1986;256:2683–2686.
63. Bronstein AC, Currance PL. *Emergency care for hazardous material exposures*, 2nd ed. St. Louis: Mosby, 1994:292–295.
64. Prescott LF, Park J, Darrien L. Treatment of severe 2,4-D and mecoprop intoxication with alkaline diuresis. *Br J Clin Pharmacol* 1979;7:111–116.
65. Bradberry SM, Watt BE, Proudfoot AT, et al. Mechanisms of toxicity, clinical features, and management of acute chlorophenoxy herbicide poisoning: a review. *J Toxicol Clin Toxicol* 2000;38:111–122.
66. Reigart JR, Roberts JR. *Recognition and management of pesticide poisonings*, 5th ed. Washington, DC: EPA, Office of Pesticide Programs, 1999:94–98.
67. Prescott LF, Park J, Darrien L. Treatment of severe 2,4-D and mecoprop intoxication with alkaline diuresis. *Br J Clin Pharmacol* 1979;7:111–116.
68. U.S. Department of Health and Human Services. *ASTDR case studies in environmental medicine: dioxin toxicity. Monograph 7.* Washington, DC: U.S. Department of Health and Human Services, Government Printing Office, 1990.
69. Agency for Toxic Substances and Disease Registry (ATSDR). *Toxicological profile for chlorinated dibenzo-p-dioxins (CDDs).* Atlanta: U.S. Department of Health and Human Services, Public Health Service, 1998.
70. Stellman JM, Stellman SD, Weber T, et al. A geographic information system for characterizing exposure to Agent Orange and other herbicides in Vietnam. *Environ Health Perspect* 2003;111:321–328.
71. Reggiani G. Medical problems raised by the TCDD contamination in Seveso, Italy. *Arch Toxicol* 1978;40:161–188.
72. Zack JA, Suskind RS. The mortality experience of workers exposed to tetrachlorobenzodioxin in a trichlorophenol process accident. *J Occup Med* 1980;22:11–14.
73. Suskind RR, Hertzberg VS. Human health effects of 2,4,5-T and its toxic contaminants. *JAMA* 1984;251:2372–2380.
74. Moses M, Lilis R, Crow KD, et al. Health status of workers with past exposure to 2,3,7,8-tetrachlorodibenzo-p-dioxin in the manufacture of 2,4,5-trichlorophenoxyacetic acid: comparison of findings with and without chloracne. *Am J Ind Med* 1984;5:161–182.
75. Hardell L, Sandstrom A. Case-control study: soft tissue sarcomas and exposure to phenoxyacetic acids or chlorophenols. *Br J Cancer* 1979;39:711–717.
76. Kociba R, Keyes D, Beyer J, et al. Results of a two-year chronic toxicity and oncogenicity study of 2,3,7,8-tetrachlorodibenzo-p-dioxin in rats. *Toxicol Appl Pharmacol* 1978;46:279–303.
77. Rao MS, Subbarao V, Prasad JD, et al. Carcinogenicity of 2,3,7,8-tetrachlorodibenzo-p-dioxin in the Syrian golden hamster. *Carcinogenesis* 1988;9:1677–1679.
78. Smith AH, Pearce NE, Fisher DO, et al. Soft tissue sarcoma and exposure to phenoxyherbicides and chlorophenols in New Zealand. *J Natl Cancer Inst* 1984;73:1111–1117.
79. Bailar JC. How dangerous is dioxin? *N Engl J Med* 1991;324:260–262.
80. Hardell L, Bengtsson N, Jonsson V, et al. Aetiological aspects on primary liver cancer with special regard to alcohol, organic solvents and acute intermittent porphyria—an epidemiological investigation. *Br J Cancer* 1984;50:389–397.
81. The Selected Cancers Cooperative Study Group. The association of selected cancers with service in the US military in Vietnam: 11. Soft-tissue and other sarcomas. *Arch Intern Med* 1990;150:2485–2492.
82. Kang H, Enzinger FM, Breslin P, et al. Soft tissue sarcoma and military service in Vietnam: a case-control study. *J Natl Cancer Inst* 1987;79:693–699.
83. Kang HK, Weatherbee L, Breslin PP, et al. Soft tissue sarcomas and military service in Vietnam: a case comparison group analysis of hospital patients. *J Occup Med* 1986;28:1215–1218.
84. Dalager NA, Kang HK, Burt VL, et al. Hodgkin's disease and Vietnam service. *Ann Epidemiol* 1995;5:400–406.
85. Dalager NA, Kang HK, Burt VL, et al. Non-Hodgkin's lymphoma among Vietnam veterans. *J Occup Med* 1991;33:774–779.
86. The Selected Cancers Cooperative Study Group. The association of selected cancers with service in the US military in Vietnam: 1. Non-Hodgkin's lymphoma. *Arch Intern Med* 1990;150:2473–2483.
87. Wolfe WH, Michalek JE, Miner JC, et al. Health status of Air Force veterans occupationally exposed to herbicides in Vietnam: 1. Physical health. *JAMA* 1990;264:1824–1831.
88. Michalek JE, Wolfe WH, Miner JC. Health status of Air Force veterans occupationally exposed to herbicides in Vietnam: 11. Mortality. *JAMA* 1990;264:1832–1836.
89. Centers for Disease Control Veterans Health Studies. Serum 2,3,7,8-tetrachlorodibenzo-p-dioxin levels in US Army Vietnam-era veterans. *JAMA* 1988;260:1249–1254.
90. Mahan CM, Bullman TA, Kang HK, et al. A case-control study of lung cancer among Vietnam veterans. *J Occup Environ Med* 1997;39:740–747.
91. Hart TB. Paraquat-review of safety in agricultural and horticultural use. *Hum Toxicol* 1987;6:13–18.
92. Zeneca Agrochemicals. *Principal products.* Available at http://www.zeneca.com/en/products_services/herbicides.aspx. Accessed September 2003.
93. Smith LL. Mechanism of paraquat toxicity in lung and its relevance to toxicity. *Hum Toxicol* 1987;6:31–36.
94. Bismuth C, Garnier R, Dally S, et al. Prognosis and treatment of paraquat poisoning: a review of 28 cases. *J Toxicol Clin Toxicol* 1982;19:461–474.
95. Rose MS, Lock EA, Smith LL, Wyatt I. Paraquat accumulation tissue and species specificity. *Biochem Pharmacol* 1976;25:419–423.
96. Rose MS, Smith LL. Tissue uptake of paraquat and diquat. *Gen Pharmacol* 1977;8:173–176.
97. Proudfoot AT, Stewart MS, Levitt T, et al. Paraquat poisoning: significance of plasma-paraquat concentrations. *Lancet* 1979;2:330–332.
98. Scherrmann JM, Houze P, Bismuth C, et al. Prognostic value of plasma and urine paraquat concentration. *Hum Toxicol* 1987;6:91–93.
99. Tsatsakis AM, Perakis K, Kournantakis E. Experience with acute paraquat poisoning in Crete. *Vet Hum Toxicol* 1996;38:113–117.
100. Hawksworth GM, Bennett PN, Davies DS. Kinetics of paraquat elimination in the dog. *Toxicol Appl Pharmacol* 1981;57:139–145.
101. Kurisaki E, Sato E. Tissue distribution of paraquat and diquat after oral administration in rats. *Forensic Sci Int* 1979;14:165–170.
102. Daniel JW, Gage JC. Absorption and excretion of diquat and paraquat in rats. *Br J Ind Med* 1966;28:133–136.
103. Murray RE, Gibson JE. Paraquat disposition in rats, guinea pigs and monkeys. *Toxicol Appl Pharmacol* 1974;27:283–291.
104. Bennett PN, Davies DS, Hawkesworth GM. In vitro absorption studies with paraquat and diquat in the dog. *Br J Pharmacol* 1976;58:284.
105. Bismuth C, Garnier R, Baud FJ, et al. Paraquat poisoning—an overview of the current status. *Drug Saf* 1990;5:243–251.
106. Vale JA, Meredith TJ, Buckley BM. Paraquat poisoning: clinical features and immediate general management. *Hum Toxicol* 1987;6:41–47.
107. Pond SM. Manifestations and management of paraquat poisoning. *Med J Aust* 1990;152:256–259.
108. Talbot AR, Fu CC. Paraquat intoxication during pregnancy: a report of 9 cases. *Vet Hum Toxicol* 1988;30:12–17.
109. Hearn CED, Keir W. Nail damage in spray operators exposed to paraquat. *Br J Ind Med* 1971;28:399–403.
110. Joyce M. Ocular damage caused by paraquat. *Br J Ophthalmol* 1969;53:688–690.
111. Karai I, Nakano H, Horiguchi S. A case of lacrimal duct stenosis due to a herbicide paraquat. *Jpn J Ind Health* 1981;23:552–553.
112. Hoffer E, Taitelman U. Exposure to paraquat through skin absorption: clinical and laboratory observations of accidental splashing on healthy skin of agricultural workers. *Hum Toxicol* 1989;8:483–485.
113. Powell D, Pond SM, Allen TB, et al. Hemoperfusion in a child who ingested diquat and died from pontine infarction and hemorrhage. *J Toxicol Clin Toxicol* 1983;20:405–420.
114. Vanholder R, Colardyn F, DeReuck J, et al. Diquat intoxication. Report of two cases and review of the literature. *Am J Med* 1981;70:1267–1271.
115. Braithwaite RA. Emergency analysis of paraquat in biological fluids. *Hum Toxicol* 1987;6:83–86.
116. Proudfoot AT, Prescott LF, Jarvie DR. Haemodialysis for paraquat poisoning. *Hum Toxicol* 1987;6:69-74.
117. Edith CG, Pond SM. Failure of haernoperfusion and haemodialysis to prevent death in paraquat poisoning. *Med Toxicol* 1988;3:64–71.
118. Matthew H, Logan A, Woodruff MFA, et al. Paraquat poisoning. Lung transplantation. *BMJ* 1968;1:759–763.
119. Kalmolz S, Veith FJ, Mollenkopf F, et al. Single lung transplantation in paraquat intoxication. *N Y State J Med* 1984;84:81–85.
120. Menkes D, Temple W, Edwards L. International self-poisoning with glyphosate-containing herbicides. *Hum Exp Toxicol* 1991;10:103–107.
121. Temple WA, Smith NA. Glyphosate herbicide poisoning experience in New Zealand. *N Z Med J* 1992;105:173–174.
122. Talbot AR, Shiaw MH, Huang JS, et al. Acute poisoning with a glyphosate-surfactant herbicide (Round-Up): a review of 93 cases. *Hum Exp Toxicol* 1991;10:1–8.
123. Bartnik F, Kunstler K. Biological effects, toxicology, and human safety. In: Falbe, ed. *Surfactants in consumer products-theory, technology, and application.* New York: Springer-Verlag, 1987:475–499.
124. Tominack RL, Yang GY, Tsai WJ, et al. Taiwan National Poison Center survey of glyphosate—surfactant herbicide ingestions. *J Toxicol Clin Toxicol* 1991;29:91–109.
125. U.S. Environmental Protection Agency. *Integrated risk information system (IRIS):* Acrolein (CASRN 107-02-8). Available at: http://www.epa.gov/iris/subst/0364.htm. Accessed August 2003.
126. Agency for Toxic Substances and Disease Registry. *Toxicological profile for acrolein.* Atlanta: US Public Health Service, Department of Health and Human Services, ATSDR, 1990.
127. Reigart JR, Roberts JR. *Recognition and management of pesticide poisonings*, 5th ed. Washington, DC: EPA, Office of Pesticide Programs, 1999.
128. HSDB. Triazine. Hazardous Substances Data Bank. National Library of Medicine, Bethesda, MD. Available at: http://toxnet.nlm.nih.gov/cgi-bin/sis/search/f?./temp/~j5yunK:1. Accessed July 2003.
129. Stevens JT, Sumner DD. Herbicides. In: Hayes WJ, Laws ER, eds. *Handbook of pesticide toxicology.* San Diego: Academic Press, 1991:1317–1408.
130. HSDB. Cloropropham. Hazardous Substances Data Bank. Bethesda, MD: National Library of Medicine. Available at: http://toxnet.nlm.nih.gov/cgi-bin/sis/search/f?./temp/~gee8DD:1. Accessed July 2003.
131. HSDB. Barban. Hazardous Substances Data Bank. Bethesda, MD: National Library of Medicine. Available at: http://toxnet.nlm.nih.gov/cgi-bin/sis/search/f?./temp/~34MQda:1. Accessed July 2003.
132. HSDB. *Sodium chlorate.* Hazardous Substances Data Bank. Bethesda, MD: National Library of Medicine. Available at: http://toxnet.nlm.nih.gov/cgi-bin/sis/search/f?./temp/~ez3InR:1. Accessed September 2003.
133. EPA. *Status of Pesticides in registration, reregistration, and special review (Rainbow Report).* Special Review and Reregistration Division, Office of Pesticide Programs, 1988. Available at: http://www.epa.gov/docs/Rainbow/98rainbo.pdf. Accessed October 2003.

134. Steffen C, Wetzel E. Chlorate poisoning: mechanism of toxicity. Toxicology. 1993;84:217–231.
135. Oliver J, MacDowell M, Tracey A. The pathogenesis of acute renal failure associated with traumatic and toxic injury. *J Clin Invest* 1955;30:1307–1320.
136. Helliwell M, Nunn J. Mortality in sodium chlorate poisoning. *BMJ* 1979:1119.
137. Steffen C, Seitz R. Severe chlorate poisoning: report of a case. *Arch Toxicol* 1981;48:281–288.
138. HSDB. *Calcium chlorate*. Bethesda, MD: Hazardous Substances Data Bank. National Library of Medicine. Available at: http://toxnet.nlm.nih.gov/cgi-bin/sis/search/f?./temp/~dpW1fI:1. Accessed September 2003.
139. Jackson RC, Elder WJ, McDonnell H. Sodium chlorate poisoning complicated by acute renal failure. *Lancet* 1961;2:1381–1383.
140. Day LC. Delayed death by Endothall, a herbicide. [Abstract]. *Hum Vet Toxicol* 1988;30:366.
141. Allender WJ. Suicidal poisoning by Endothall. *J Analyt Toxicol* 1983;7:79–82.
142. Laidley CW, Cohen E, Casida JE. Protein phosphatase in neuroblastoma cells: [3H]cantharidin binding site in relation to cytotoxicity. *J Pharmacol Exp Ther* 1997;280:1152–1158.
143. HSDB. *Dinoseb*. Hazardous Substances Data Bank. Bethesda, MD: National Library of Medicine. Available at http://toxnet.nlm.nih.gov/cgi-bin/sis/search/f?./temp/~WA2TEd:1. Accessed September 2003.
144. Fikes JD, Lovell RA, Metzler M, et al. Dionseb toxicosis in two dogs. *JAMA* 1989;194:543–544.
145. HSDB. *Diuron*. Hazardous Substances Data Bank. Bethesda, MD: National Library of Medicine. Available at: http://toxnet.nlm.nih.gov/cgi-bin/sis/search/f?./temp/~MqcFxv:7. Accessed September 2003.
146. Liu J. Phenylurea herbicides. In: Krieger RI, ed. *Handbook of pesticide toxicology*, 2nd ed. San Diego: Academic Press, 2001:1521–1528.

CHAPTER 240

Fungicides

Vikhyat S. Bebarta and Scott D. Phillips

H3C, N, H3C, S, S, S, N, CH3, S, CH3

THIRAM

Compounds included:	**Substituted aromatic fungicides: chlorothalonil, hexachlorbenzene, pentachlorophenol; dithiocarbamates: thiram, ferbam, ziram, maneb, zineb, mancozeb; thiobendazoles: benomyl; dicarboximides: captan, folpet, captafol**
Molecular formula and weight:	**See Table 1.**
CAS Registry No.:	**See Table 1.**
Special concerns:	**Thiram may cause a disulfiram-like reaction if alcohol is consumed.**
Antidote:	**None**

OVERVIEW

Fungicides are a diverse group of compounds that interfere with the function or metabolism of fungi. Some fungicides are applied to protect plants from the development of fungi and others destroy the developing mycelium and spores after the plant has been infested. Ongoing research has refined the available agents that are selectively fungicidal. Older agents were nonspecific and significantly toxic to humans. The ideal fungicide is characterized by low toxicity to humans, little toxicity to

TABLE 1. Physiochemical properties of common fungicides

	Molecular formula, molecular weight (g/mol), CAS Registry No.	Vapor pressure at 25°C	Regulatory standards
Chlorothalonil	$C_8Cl_4N_2$; 265.9; 1897-45-6	Less than 0.01 mm Hg	Not listed
Hexachlorobenzene	C_6Cl_6; 284.7; 118-74-1	4.9×10^{-5} mm Hg	
Pentachlorophenol	C_6HCl_5O; 266.3; 87-86-5	0.00011 mm Hg	TLV (TWA) 0.5 mg/m^3; PEL (TWA) 0.5 mg/m^3; REL (TWA) 0.5 mg/m^3
Thiram	$C_6H_{12}N_2S_4$; 240.1; 137-26-8	1.725×10^{-5} mm Hg	TLV (TWA) 1 mg/m^3; PEL (TWA) 5 mg/m^3; REL (TWA) 5 mg/m^3
Maneb	$C_4H_6MnN_2S_4$; 265.2	7.5×10^{-8} mm Hg	NR
Ziram	$C_6H_{12}N_2S_4Zn$; 305.8	0	NR
Benomyl	$C_{14}H_{18}N_4O_3$; 290.3; 17804-35-2	3.7×10^{-9} mm Hg	TLV (TWA) 10 mg/m^3; PEL (TWA) 15 mg/m^3 (total dust), 5 mg/m^3 (respirable fraction)
Captan	$C_9H_8Cl_3NO_2$-S; 300.5; 133-06-2	9×10^{-8} mm Hg	TLV (TWA) 5 mg/m^3; PEL (TWA) 5 mg/m^3
Triphenyltin	$C_{18}H_{16}OSn$; 350; 639-58-7	3.5×10^{-7} mm Hg	Not listed

NR, not reported; PEL, permissible exposure limit; REL, relative exposure limit; TLV, threshold limit value; TWA, time-weighted average.

plants, ability to penetrate spores and mycelium, and limited biodegradation on the plant surface under certain environmental conditions (rain, wind, sunlight, and humidity). Though newer fungicides have less systemic toxicity to humans, no fungicide possesses all of these properties.

The list of fungicides is extensive; therefore the most commonly used fungicides are discussed in this chapter.

SUBSTITUTED AROMATIC FUNGICIDES

Substituted aromatic fungicides, also known as organochlorine fungicides, generally show halogenation of aromatic rings (Fig. 1). Chlorothalonil is a substituted fungicide used to control fungal diseases in vegetables, fruits, turf, and ornamental plants. Hexachlorobenzene, mentioned for historical interest, is used primarily as a seed treatment, especially on wheat. Pentachlorophenol has been used extensively as a preservative of wood, such as telephone poles, and as a fungicide throughout the United States. Because of its toxicity, pentachlorophenol is now a restricted-use agent and is no longer used as a wood preserving agent or as a fungicide available for home use. No cases of intentional poisoning have been reported with chlorothalonil or hexachlorobenzene.

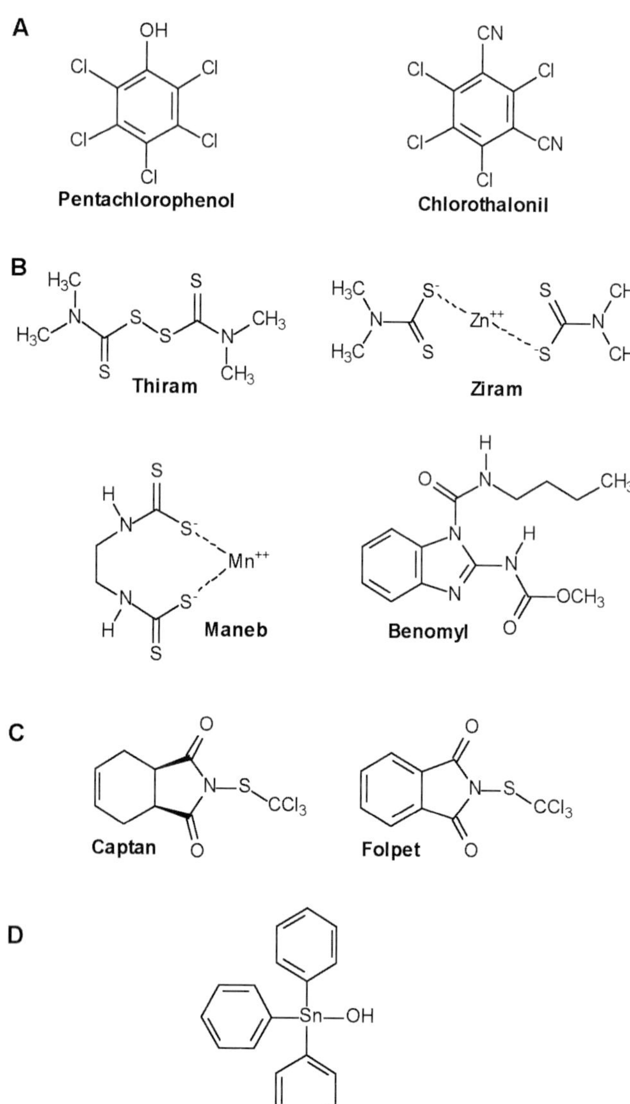

Figure 1. Structures of selected fungicides. **A:** Substituted aromatic compounds. **B:** Dithiocarbamates and carbamates. **C:** Dicarboxamides. **D:** Organotin.

Toxic Dose

Regulatory guidelines and standards are provided in Table 1.

Toxicokinetics and Toxicodynamics

Chlorothalonil and hexachlorobenzene are absorbed well orally and relatively well via inhalation, but they are poorly absorbed dermally. Pentachlorophenol is well absorbed by inhalational, dermal, and oral routes. Once absorbed, it is highly protein bound. In human volunteers, the half-life of elimination from plasma was 30 hours (1). Pentachlorophenol elimination is believed to be first order with some enterohepatic recirculation after ingestion (2).

Vulnerable Populations

There are no human data on chlorothalonil, but it has not been found to be teratogenic in rats and rabbits (3). Hexachlorobenzene crosses the placenta and has been detected in breast milk, and pentachlorophenol is fetotoxic in experimental animals (4,5). Breast-feeding is not recommended.

Clinical Presentation

Chlorothalonil has limited toxicity in humans, though the most common effect is dermatitis, which may be delayed for 48 hours.

Hexachlorobenzene-contaminated flour was associated with porphyria cutanea tarda in Turkey (6). The exposure affected 3000 people and follow-up studies 20 years later demonstrated that some people were still experiencing ill effects including skin changes, hepatomegaly, and hypertrichosis (7).

A common mode of pentachlorophenol exposure is inhalation and may cause irritation of the eyes, nose, and throat and deaths after acute significant inhalation (1). Dermal contact may cause erythema, pain, and exfoliation. Systemic toxicity is related to the ability of pentachlorophenol to uncouple oxidative phosphorylation. This may produce hyperthermia, sweating, hepatotoxicity, altered mental status, and seizures.

Diagnostic Tests

There are no specific diagnostic tests that are helpful. A chest radiograph and pulse oximetry may be needed with patient with pulmonary complaints after an inhalational exposure.

Treatment

Treatment is symptomatic and supportive. In exposed patients, skin and gastrointestinal decontamination should be completed immediately. Dermal exposures should have contaminated clothing removed and exposed skin washed thoroughly with soap and water.

There is no antidote. The contact dermatitis may be treated symptomatically with antihistamines and topical or systemic steroids. Those with inhalational exposure should be removed from the exposure and supplemental oxygen applied.

DITHIOCARBAMATES

Of the groups of fungicides, dithiocarbamates are the most commonly used (Fig. 1). There are three groups of dithiocarbamates:

dithiocarbamates (thiram), metallobisdithiocarbamates (ferbam and ziram), and ethylene bisdithiocarbamates (maneb, zineb, and mancozeb). Unlike the *N*-methyl carbamate insecticides, the carbamate fungicides do not inhibit cholinesterase and therefore do not cause cholinergic symptoms (8).

Toxic Dose

Regulatory guidelines and standards are provided in Table 1.

Toxicokinetics and Toxicodynamics

Detailed data in humans are limited. Thiram is a degradation product of ferbam and ziram and is metabolized to carbon disulfide. Thiram blocks the enzyme aldehyde dehydrogenase for 10 to 14 days. Ethylenethiourea, a byproduct of ethylene bisdithiocarbamates, has an elimination half-life through the kidneys of approximately 100 hours (9).

Vulnerable Populations

Teratogenesis and embryotoxicity have been demonstrated in animal models (10,11). Pregnancy and lactation in humans has not been studied.

Clinical Presentation

Thiram is poorly absorbed dermally, but the small amount absorbed is metabolized to carbon disulfide (12). Significant exposures to thiram may present with headache, delirium, and encephalopathy; these are similar features to carbon disulfide toxicity (13). Thiram also inhibits acetaldehyde dehydrogenase, similar to disulfiram, which is also a dithiocarbamate. Therefore, a disulfiram-like reaction involving vomiting, abdominal pain, hypotension, tremor, and headache may occur after exposure to ethanol (14). Thiram and other dithiocarbamates are mucosal irritants and skin allergens (13). However, ethylene bisdithiocarbamates are even more potent sensitizers than thiram.

Ethylene bisdithiocarbamate fungicides may also cause mucosal irritation. The major concern with these agents is that ethylenethiourea is a breakdown product that has been reported to result in goiters and hyperthyroidism in animals (12). No human thyroid abnormalities have been reported. Maneb contains manganese and may also produce carbon disulfide. Two cases of parkinsonism after significant exposure to maneb have been reported with concern that the manganese may be the causative agent (15,16).

The metallobisdithiocabamates derive their name from the attached metal—ferbam contains iron (Fe), maneb contains manganese (Mn), and ziram contains zinc. They may cause irritation and inhibit alcohol dehydrogenase.

Blood levels are useful to document an occupational exposure; however, they are not useful to guide treatment. No specific laboratory work is needed unless indicated by the clinical presentation (i.e., severe vomiting and diarrhea, and so forth).

Treatment

Treatment is supportive and symptomatic. Whether the exposure is dermal, inhalational, or oral, the main goal is removal from the exposure and decontamination. Irrigation of the skin with soap and water for dermal exposures and supplemental oxygen and beta agonists may be needed for inhalational exposures.

BENOMYL

Benomyl is a thiabendazole that produces its fungicidal effect through inhibition of tubulin formation. It is in the same group as mebendazole and albendazole, the antihelminthic agents (Fig. 1).

Toxic Dose

Regulatory guidelines and standards are provided in Table 1.

Toxicokinetics and Toxicodynamics

Benomyl is poorly absorbed orally and is metabolized to carbendazim, which is also a fungicide. It is primarily excreted in the urine. Carbendazim and benomyl have similar dermal irritant effects.

Vulnerable Populations

Congenital central nervous system malformations, eye anomalies, and fetotoxicity have been reported in animals. Effects on human pregnancy and lactation have not been reported.

Clinical Presentation

The toxicity of benomyl toxicity is dose dependent. Despite being a carbamate derivative, it does not inhibit cholinesterase and cause cholinergic stimulation. Systemic effects have not been reported in humans. Contact dermatitis has been reported and benomyl is known to be particularly irritating to the skin. Benomyl plasma levels are not clinically useful or readily available.

Treatment

Treatment for dermal exposures consists of removing exposed clothing and jewelry and washing the skin and nails vigorously with soap and water.

DICARBOXIMIDES

Dicarboximides form a group of fungicides that are chloralkylthiodicarboximide compounds (Fig. 1). Captan is used in many crops; however, folpet is used only as a preservative in paint. Captafol is no longer available in the United States owing to oncogenicity in laboratory animals.

Toxic Dose

Regulatory guidelines and standards are provided in Table 1.

Toxicokinetics and Toxicodynamics

Captan is rapidly absorbed by the gastrointestinal tract and rapidly metabolized. Its typical half-life in animals ranges from 12 to 18 hours (2). Folpet is also rapidly absorbed from the gastrointestinal tract (17).

Vulnerable Populations

With mixed reports of teratogenicity in rats, rabbits, hamsters, and dogs, captan is not thought to result in birth defects (2). The dicarboximides share the phthalimide nucleus that is the same as in thalidomide, a known teratogen. Thalidomide has not been well studied in humans; however, there are no reported cases of teratogenicity. There are no data on lactation, and breast-feeding is not recommended.

Clinical Presentation

The most common effect is dermatitis (18). Other than diarrhea, dermatitis, eye irritation, and respiratory sensitization, no signs of systemic toxicity directly due to dicarboximides have been reported in humans (19). Plasma levels of these agents are not clinically useful, unless documentation of the exposure is needed. These are not needed unless indicated by signs and symptoms of the patient.

Treatment

Treatment for ingestion of any of the dicarboximides is similar. Remove the patient from exposure and decontaminate with copious amounts of soap and water. Significant ingestions should be treated with activated charcoal.

ORGANOTIN COMPOUNDS

Several alkyl and aromatic derivatives of tin such as triethyltin, dibutyltin, tributyltin, and triphenyltin have been used as fungicides and antifouling agents for ships (Fig. 1). Certain organotins are also used for preservatives for wood, leather, paper, and as stabilizers for plastics. The toxicity of organotins as a group is also addressed in Chapter 232.

Toxicokinetics and Toxicodynamics

Organotin absorption after ingestion depends on the compound and animal species. Monoethyltin is poorly absorbed, short-chained di- and trialkyltins are well absorbed, and triphenyltin absorption is animal species dependent (20). Triphenyltin may be dermally absorbed (21). There is some urinary excretion of organotin in humans (20).

Pathophysiology

Organotins interfere with several mitochondrial enzyme systems and may uncouple oxidative phosphorylation (22) if of sufficient dose.

Vulnerable Populations

Teratogenicity has not been observed in animals and not reported in humans. There are no data on lactation, and breast-feeding is not recommended.

Clinical Presentation

Triphenyltin is responsible for most occupational exposure to organotin compounds (21). It is a potential hepatotoxin if sufficient dose has been absorbed and in some occupational exposures has produced hepatomegaly and elevated liver enzymes. It is also a dermal irritant and may produce headache, nausea, vomiting, and blurred vision. Trialkyltin compounds easily cross the blood–brain barrier producing neurotoxicity, including tremors, headache, weakness, and hyperexcitability. Tetraalkyltins produce similar effects owing to the conversion to trialkyltins *in vivo* (23). All of the organotins, in particular tributyltin, may cause severe chemical burns.

Diagnostic Tests

Qualitative or quantitative levels are helpful for documentation of exposure.

Treatment

The specific treatment for organotin poisoning is primarily symptomatic and supportive. Central nervous system function should be monitored and treated accordingly. Hepatic and renal function should be followed. Dermal, ocular, and mucous membrane irritation and burns are possible. Dermal injuries may respond to topical corticosteroids.

REFERENCES

1. Agency for Toxic Substances and Disease Registry. ATSDR Toxicological profile for pentachlorophenol. Atlanta, GA: Department of Health and Human Services, Public Health Service, Agency for Toxic Substances and Disease Registry, 1994.
2. Phillips SD. Fungicides and biocides. In: Sullivan JB, Krieger GR. *Clinical environmental health and toxic exposures*, 2nd ed. Philadelphia: Lippincott Williams & Wilkins, 2001:1109–1125.
3. Hurlbut KM, Kulig K. Chlorthalonil. POISINDEX system. Greenwood Village, CO: MICROMEDEX. Edition expires 3/2003.
4. Ando M, Hirano S, Itoh Y. Transfer of hexachlorobenzene (HCB) from mother to newborn baby through placenta and milk. *Arch Toxicol* 1985;56(3):195–200.
5. Ekins BR, Hurlbut KM, Esposito-Avella M. Chlorinated hydrocarbon insecticides. POISINDEX system. Greenwood Village, CO: MICROMEDEX. Edition expires 3/2003.
6. Schmid R. Cutaneous porphyria in Turkey. *N Engl J Med* 1960;263:397.
7. Peters HA, Cocmen A, Cripps DJ. Epidemiology of hexachlorobenzene-induced porphyria in Turkey: clinical and laboratory follow-up after 25 years. *Arch Neurol* 1982;39:744.
8. Machemer LH, Pickel M. Carbamate herbicides and fungicides. *Toxicology* 1994;91(1):105–9.
9. Kurttio P, Savolainen K. Ethylenethiourea in air and in urine as an indicator of exposure to ethylenebisdithiocarbamate fungicides. *Scand J Work Environ Health* 1990;16(3):203–207.
10. Khera KS. Ethylenethiourea-induced hindpaw deformities in mice and effects of metabolic modifiers on their occurrence. *J Toxicol Environ Health* 1984;13(4–6):747–756.
11. Robens JF. Teratologic studies of carbaryl, diazinon, norea, disulfiram, and thiram in small laboratory animals. *Toxicol Appl Pharmacol* 1969;15:152–163.
12. Edward IR, Ferry DG, Temple WA. Fungicides and related compounds. In: Hayes WJ, Laws ER. *Handbook of pesticide toxicology*. San Diego: Academic Press, 1991:1409–1470.
13. Dalvi RR. Toxicology of thiram (tetramethylthiuram disulfide): a review. *Vet Hum Toxicol* 1988;30(5):480–482.
14. Garcia de Torres G, Romer KG, Torres Alanis O, Freundt KJ. Blood acetaldehyde levels in alcohol-dosed rats after treatment with ANIT, ANTU, dithiocarbamate derivatives, or cyanamide. *Drug Chem Toxicol* 1983;6(4):317–328.
15. Ferraz HB, Bertolucci PH, Pereira JS, et al. Chronic exposure to the fungicide maneb may produce symptoms and signs of CNS manganese intoxication. *Neurology* 1988;38(4):550–553.
16. Meco G, Bonifati V, Vanacore N, et al. Parkinsonism after chronic exposure to the fungicide maneb (manganese ethylene-bis-dithiocarbamate). *Scand J Work Environ Health* 1994;20(4):301–305.
17. Folpet. National Library of Medicine (U.S.). HSDB hazardous substances data bank: Toxnet (Toxicology Data Network). Bethesda, MD: National Library of Medicine, 2003. Last modified: September 30, 2001.
18. Camarasa G. Difolatan dermatitis. *Contact Dermatitis* 1975;1(2):127.
19. Captan. National Library of Medicine (U.S.). HSDB hazardous substances data bank: Toxnet (Toxicology Data Network). Bethesda, MD: National Library of Medicine, 2003. Last modified: September 15, 2001.
20. Winship KA. Toxicity of tin and its compounds. *Adverse Drug React Acute Poisoning Rev* 1988;7(1):19–38.
21. Colosio C, Tomasini M, Cairoli S, et al. Occupational triphenyltin acetate poisoning: a case report. *Br J Ind Med* 1991;48(2):136–9.
22. Fait A, Ferioli A, Barbieri F. Organotin compounds. *Toxicology* 1994;91(1):77–82.
23. Barnes JM, Stoner HB. Toxic properties of some dialkyl and trialkyl tin salts. *Br J Ind Med* 1959;15:15–22.

CHAPTER 241

Molluscicides

Christopher R. DeWitt and Richard C. Dart

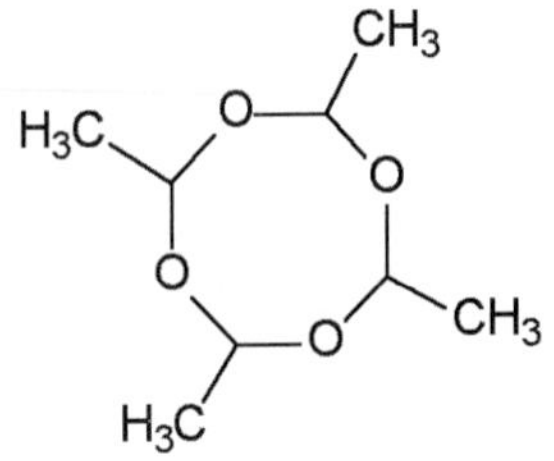

METALDEHYDE

Molecular formula and weight:	$C_8H_{16}O_4$; 176.2 g/mol
CAS Registry No.:	108-62-3
Therapeutic levels:	Unknown
Special concerns:	Seizures
Antidote:	None

OVERVIEW

Molluscicides are a chemically diverse group of compounds, many of which are also used as insecticides, herbicides, and fungicides. Quarternary ammonium compounds and oxidizers such as hydrogen peroxide, chlorine, ozone, and bromine are used. Additionally, several molluscicides are carbamates whereas others contain copper, arsenic, zinc, manganese, or tin compounds. Information regarding toxicity of these substances is covered in their respective chapters.

This chapter focuses on the synthetic molluscicide, metaldehyde. Metaldehyde is a cyclic tetramer of acetaldehyde that was first used as a combustible fuel (still used in Europe) and incidentally found to be molluscicidal. Toxic exposures are usually due to ingestion but may occur via inhalation.

TOXIC DOSE

The toxic dose of metaldehyde is not well studied, but for adults has been suggested to be in the range of 100 mg/kg (1). Occupational standards for metaldehyde have not been established.

TOXICOKINETICS AND TOXICODYNAMICS

There are few data regarding the pharmacokinetics of metaldehyde. It is rapidly absorbed orally.

PATHOPHYSIOLOGY

Acetaldehyde, derived from depolymerization in gastric acid, is thought to produce toxic effects. However, acetaldehyde has not been detected in human poisonings (2,3), but this may be due to the rapid oxidation of acetaldehyde. In mice metaldehyde decreased brain γ-aminobutyric acid levels and increased monoamine oxidase activity (4).

PREGNANCY AND LACTATION

There is no information available for humans.

CLINICAL PRESENTATION

Symptoms generally occur within 3 hours [although they have been delayed up to 48 hours (5)] and include salivation, lethargy, abdominal pain, nausea, vomiting, and diarrhea, progressing to seizures, hyperthermia, coma, and death. Inhalation produces mucous membrane irritation, and inhaling pyrolized metaldehyde has caused noncardiogenic pulmonary edema (6). Memory loss and cognitive dysfunction have been reported after severe poisoning (7).

DIAGNOSTIC TESTS

Blood and urine levels can be performed but are not clinically useful. The typical laboratory studies and other procedures are performed in patients that develop hyperthermia, seizures, or coma.

TREATMENT

Treatment is supportive including airway control, maintenance of vital signs, seizure control with benzodiazepines and barbiturates (Chapter 40), and decontamination.

REFERENCES

1. Booze TF, Oehme FW. Metaldehyde toxicity: a review. *Vet Hum Toxicol* 1985;27(1):11–19.
2. Keller KH, Shimizu G, Walter FG, Olson KR. Acetaldehyde analysis in severe metaldehyde poisoning. *Vet Hum Toxicol* 1991;33:374.
3. Moody JP, Inglis FG. Persistence of metaldehyde during acute molluscicide poisoning. *Hum Exp Toxicol* 1992;11(5):361–362.
4. Homeida AM, Cooke RG. Anti-convulsant activity of diazepam and clonidine on metaldehyde-induced seizures in mice: effects on brain gamma-amino butyric acid concentrations and monoamine oxidase activity. *J Vet Pharmacol Ther* 1982;5(3):187–190.
5. Wilkinson RD. Metaldehyde. *The Practitioner* 1968;200:320.
6. Jay MS, Kearns GL, Stone V, Moss M. Toxic pneumonitis in an adolescent following exposure to Snow Storm tablets. *J Adolesc Health Care* 1988;9(5):431–433.
7. Longstreth WT Jr, Pierson DJ. Metaldehyde poisoning from slug bait ingestion. *West J Med* 1982;137(2):134–137.

CHAPTER 242
Repellents

Christopher R. DeWitt and Richard C. Dart

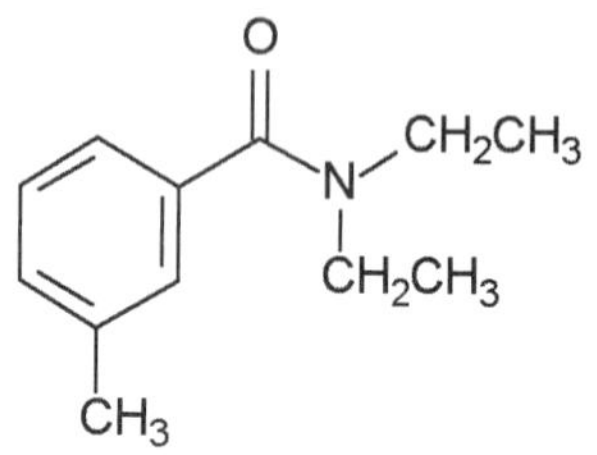

DIETHYLTOLUAMIDE

Compounds included:	**N,N-diethyl-3-methylbenzamide (diethyltoluamide, DEET)**
Molecular formula and weight:	**$C_{12}H_{17}NO$, 191.3 g/mol**
CAS Registry No.:	**134-62-3**
Therapeutic levels:	**None**
Special concerns:	**Rare central nervous system effects**
Antidote:	**None**

OVERVIEW

Repellents are used to keep unwanted animals or insects away from an area. Many substances are used as repellents, including capsaicin, mothballs, citronella, and other essential oils. Pyrethrins and pyrethroids applied to skin and clothing have also been used as deterrents to arthropod bites. Other compounds used as repellants include ethyl hexanediol, indalone, dimethyl phthalate, N-octyl bicycloheptene dicarboximide. However, these are rarely encountered and little information exists regarding toxicities. This chapter focuses on N,N-diethyl-3-methylbenzamide (DEET; formerly N,N-diethyl-m-toluamide), the most widely used insect repellent.

DEET was first marketed in 1957 and is the active ingredient in most insect repellents. It has been used for more than 40 years with a remarkable safety profile (1). The U.S. Environmental Protection Agency estimates that approximately 30% of the U.S. population and more than 200 million people worldwide use DEET-containing products every year (2,3). Despite an incomplete understanding of its mechanism of action, years of comparative testing have failed to find a safer or more effective repellent than DEET (4). It is effective against a broad range of insects including mosquitoes, biting flies, fleas, chiggers, and ticks (1). Marketed products contain 5% to 100% DEET, usually in an alcohol base, and are available in many different preparations. The duration and degree of effectiveness improve with increasing DEET concentrations. However, this effect plateaus, and little additional benefit is gained by using concentrations over 50% (5).

Toxic Dose

Ingestion of 25 to 50 ml of 100% DEET by adults has produced effects ranging from seizures and central nervous system depression to death. Ingestion of up to 100 ml by a 33-year-old woman resulted in coma, hypotension, generalized seizures, and death due to massive bowel infarction (6).

Toxicokinetics and Toxicodynamics

DEET is lipophilic, and based on the presence of symptoms within 30 minutes of ingestion is absorbed rapidly via the gastrointestinal tract (6). Skin absorption is dependent on the concentration, vehicle, skin chemistry and integrity, anatomic site, perspiration, covering (occlusion) of the application area, as well as other factors. The best human study using dermally applied DEET showed approximately 12% (100% DEET) and 20% (15% DEET in ethanol) of the dose was absorbed by 8 hours (7). The average proportion of the applied dose recovered from subjects (after washing the exposed area and removing skin with tape) was 5.6% (100% DEET) and 8.4% (15% DEET in ethanol). Less than 2% was found in the feces and superficial skin. The remainder was recovered in the urine as metabolites. DEET was found in the plasma within 2 hours of application and appeared to have continuous absorption. Plasma levels decreased rapidly within 4 hours of exposure cessation, and levels were not detectable at 16 hours. No studies involving children have been done.

DEET is metabolized by hepatic microsomes via oxidation, hydroxylation, dealkylation, and glucuronidation. Within 12 hours of application, the majority of DEET is excreted in the urine, mainly as metabolites. The amount of the parent compound excreted probably depends on the applied dose (7). Skin and fatty tissues may serve as a reservoir for DEET after repeated excessive dermal applications (8).

Pathophysiology

Although the mechanism of toxicity is unknown, DEET primarily affects the central nervous system. It can also be irritating to the skin, eyes, and mucous membranes.

Pregnancy and Lactation

Animal studies using repeated high doses of DEET during pregnancy show conflicting data regarding infant mortality. However, the only human study showed no differences in gestational age, growth, neurologic performance, death, or congenital abnormalities in infants whose mothers used DEET daily during the second and third trimester compared to controls (9). This study also confirmed that DEET crosses the placenta.

Although there are no studies on DEET in breast-feeding, the Centers for Disease Control and Prevention report no adverse events after use in pregnant or breast-feeding women (10). Additionally, in light of West Nile virus being found in breast milk, the Centers for Disease Control and Prevention recommends DEET use in breast-feeding.

Clinical Presentation

Adverse effects related to DEET are generally related to minor irritation. A study of poison center calls involving more than 9000 DEET exposures showed the majority involved minimal or no symptoms (11). Symptomatic exposures usually involved ocular or inhalation exposure. Unintentional ingestions were least likely to have symptoms. Only 5% required hospitalization with 1 death after a suicidal ingestion. There was no correlation between symptom severity and age or concentration.

However, more serious effects such as bullous skin lesions and scarring have been described (12). Additionally, a recent review demonstrated 20 cases with significant morbidity and six deaths associated with DEET (6,11,13–17). The majority of cases involve children and high-concentration products with excessive prolonged dosing or ingestion. Neurologic findings were predominant including behavioral and mental alterations, ataxia, hypertonicity, seizures, respiratory failure, encephalopathy, and coma.

Cardiovascular effects including bradycardia and hypotension were rarely seen. One report involved anaphylaxis (18), and one of acute psychosis (19). Not all of these cases could definitely be attributed to DEET. In many of these cases information is incomplete and alternative diagnoses were not sought or were discounted. However, there is a similarity in symptomatology whether dermally applied or ingested, suggesting a rare, but real possibility for toxicity.

Drug Interactions

In animals, combined exposure to permethrin and DEET produces more severe toxicity (20). It has been speculatively associated with Gulf War syndrome (21).

Diagnostic Tests

DEET and metabolites can be detected in blood and urine, but toxic levels have not been established and are only useful to confirm exposure. Laboratory testing to exclude alternate causes (central nervous system infection and other intracranial disorders, electrolyte disturbances, and metabolic abnormalities) should be performed (Chapters 9 and 30).

Treatment

Supportive care aimed at airway control and treatment of neurologic symptoms results in full recovery in most cases of serious toxicity. There is no specific treatment, and the majority of symptoms resolve without intervention.

DECONTAMINATION

After ingestion, ipecac should not be administered due to the potentially abrupt onset of seizures. Activated charcoal should be administered within 1 to 2 hours of ingestion. In dermal exposures, the skin should be washed and irrigation used for symptomatic eye exposures.

ENHANCEMENT OF ELIMINATION

Although DEET is likely adsorbed by activated charcoal, the efficacy of multiple dose–activated charcoal has not been investigated. Given its lipophilicity, it is unlikely that DEET is amenable to extracorporeal elimination.

SUPPORTIVE CARE

Seizures are treated with benzodiazepines, followed by phenobarbital and more aggressive interventions as clinically indicated (Chapter 40).

PREVENTION OF TOXICITY

DEET has been used for years with millions of applications. Given the small number of serious adverse reactions, the margin of safety is large. Application should follow recommendations on the package label. Additionally, to minimize the likelihood of side effects, the lowest effective concentration of DEET should be used. The American Academy of Pediatrics recommends DEET concentrations of 10% or less for children (22). Additionally, for children the U.S. Environmental Protection Agency recommends not using DEET in children younger than 2 months old; do not apply to wounds, around mouth or eyes, or on hands; do not saturate skin or use under clothing; wash skin after returning indoors; wash clothing before wearing again; for use on face, apply to adult hands then rub on face (2). Avoiding the outdoors at dusk when mosquitoes are most active, not using combination sunscreen/DEET products when the repellent is not needed, and using barriers to insect bites is also prudent.

REFERENCES

1. Fradin MS. Mosquitoes and mosquito repellents: a clinician's guide. *Ann Intern Med* 1998;128(11):931–940.
2. Office of Pesticide Programs PPaTS. Registration Eligibility Decision (RED): DEET. Washington, DC: Environmental Protection Agency, 1998.
3. Office of Pesticides and Toxic Substances SPRD. N,N-diethyl-m-toluamide (DEET) pesticide registration standard. Washington, DC: Environmental Protection Agency, 1980.
4. Brown M, Hebert AA. Insect repellents: an overview. *J Am Acad Dermatol* 1997;36(2 Pt 1):243–9.
5. Buescher MD, Rutledge LC, Wirtz RA, et al. The dose-persistence relationship of deet against Aedes aegypti. *Mosquito News* 1983;43:364–366.
6. Tenenbein M. Severe toxic reactions and death following the ingestion of diethyltoluamide-containing insect repellents. *JAMA* 1987;258(11):1509–1511.
7. Selim S, Hartnagel RE Jr, Osimitz TG, et al. Absorption, metabolism, and excretion of N,N-diethyl-m-toluamide following dermal application to human volunteers. *Fundam Appl Toxicol* 1995;25(1):95–100.
8. POISINDEX system editorial staff. Insect repellents (management protocol). In: Toll LL, Hurlbut KM, eds. POISINDEX system. Edition expires March 2003.
9. McGready R, Hamilton KA, Simpson JA, et al. Safety of the insect repellent N,N-diethyl-M-toluamide (DEET) in pregnancy. *Am J Trop Med Hyg* 2001;65(4):285–289.
10. Centers for Disease Control and Prevention. West Nile virus and breast-feeding [Web page]. October 7, 2002; Available at http://www.cdc.gov/ncidod/dvbid/westnile/qa/ breastfeeding.htm. Accessed February 2003.
11. Veltri JC, Osimitz TG, Bradford DC, Page BC. Retrospective analysis of calls to poison control centers resulting from exposure to the insect repellent N,N-diethyl-m-toluamide (DEET) from 1985–1989. *J Toxicol Clin Toxicol* 1994;32(1):1–16.
12. Lamberg SI, Mulrennan JA Jr. Bullous reaction to diethyl toluamide (DEET). Resembling a blistering insect eruption. *Arch Dermatol* 1969;100(5):582–586.
13. Osimitz TG, Murphy JV. Neurological effects associated with use of the insect repellent N,N-diethyl-m-toluamide (DEET). *J Toxicol Clin Toxicol* 1997;35(5):435–441.
14. Briassoulis G, Narlioglou M, Hatzis T. Toxic encephalopathy associated with use of DEET insect repellents: a case analysis of its toxicity in children. *Hum Exp Toxicol* 2001;20(1):8–14.
15. Petrucci N, Sardini S. Severe neurotoxic reaction associated with oral ingestion of low-dose diethyltoluamide-containing insect repellent in a child. *Pediatr Emerg Care* 2000;16(5):341–342.
16. Fraser AD, MacNeil A, Theriault M, et al. Analysis of diethyltoluamide (DEET) following intentional oral ingestion of Muscol. *J Anal Toxicol* 1995;19(3):197–199.

17. Hampers LC, Oker E, Leikin JB. Topical use of DEET insect repellent as a cause of severe encephalopathy in a healthy adult male. *Acad Emerg Med* 1999;6(12):1295–1297.
18. Miller JD. Anaphylaxis associated with insect repellent. *N Engl J Med* 1982;307(21):1341–1342.
19. Snyder JW, Poe RO, Stubbins JF, et al. Acute manic psychosis following the dermal application of N,N-diethyl-m-toluamide (DEET) in an adult. *J Toxicol Clin Toxicol* 1986;24(5):429–439.
20. Abu-Qare AW, Abou-Donia MB. Combined exposure to DEET (N,N-diethyl-m-toluamide) and permethrin: pharmacokinetics and toxicological effects. *J Toxicol Environ Health Part B: Critical Reviews* 2003;6:41–53.
21. Riviere JE, Monteiro-Riviere NA, Baynes RE. Gulf War related exposure factors influencing topical absorption of 14C-permethrin. *Toxicol Lett* 2002;135(1–2):61–71.
22. Shelov SP, ed. *Caring for your baby and young child: birth to age 5*. New York: Bantam Books, 1998.

PART

V

Natural Toxins

SECTION

1

Reptiles and Amphibians

CHAPTER 243

Lizards, Newts, and Toads

Christy L. McCowan and E. Martin Caravati

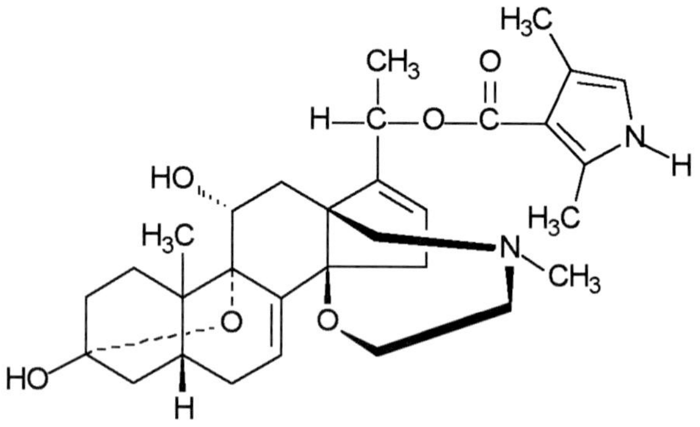

BATRACHOTOXIN

Topics included:	**Gila monsters (*Heloderma* spp.), toads (*Bufo* spp.), poison dart frogs, newts, and salamanders (*Notophthalmus* and *Taricha* spp., others)**
Special concerns:	**Gila monsters: local pain; toads: cardiac dysrhythmias; newts and salamanders: generalized paralysis**
Antidote:	**Toads: digoxin immune Fab**

VENOMOUS LIZARDS

Helodermatids are large, slow-moving lizards that are primarily nocturnal. Adult lizards can reach lengths in excess of 55 cm. The skin has bead-like scales, which can be black or brown in color. The darker colors surround light spots and bars of various other colors ranging from whitish yellow to pink or red (Fig. 1). The lizard has a set of venom glands, which can be found in the lower anterior jaw. The venom empties into the lizard's mouth at the gum line of the teeth of the lower jaw and is drawn up by capillary action to the upper part of the lower teeth and upper jaw.

Heloderma suspectum (reticulate Gila monster) and *H. cinctum* (banded Gila monster) inhabit the southwestern part of the United States. They can be found in southern Utah, Arizona, New Mexico, Nevada, small parts of California, and as far south as the Sonora to the Gulf of California. *H. horridum* (beaded lizard) is native to Mexico and Guatemala and is generally larger than the subspecies found in the United States.

The lizard has a powerful bite, and the teeth may cause several small puncture wounds in the skin of the victim. Envenomation by adult helodermatids produces pain at the bite site and local swelling. Lymphangitis, hypotension, and weakness may occur. No specific antivenom is available. Management consists primarily of wound care, IV fluids, and analgesia.

Chemical and Physical Characteristics

Helodermatidae venom is complex, with constituents similar to those of crotaline snake venom. It contains serotonin, amine oxidase, phospholipase, hyaluronidase, protease, and salivary kallikrein. Unique compounds include arginine ethyl ester hydrolase, gilatoxin, and helothermine. The hemotoxic effects of crotaline snake venom are absent in Helodermatidae venom.

Helothermine has been isolated from *Heloderma horridum horridum* (Mexican beaded lizard) venom. Helothermine has an apparent molecular weight of 25,500 and is composed of approximately 220 amino acid residues. It has an isoelectric point of 6.8 and a unique *N*-terminal amino acid sequence. Helothermine does not appear to affect sodium, potassium, or calcium ion channels. In mice it induces lethargy, partial paralysis of the limbs, and hypothermia (1).

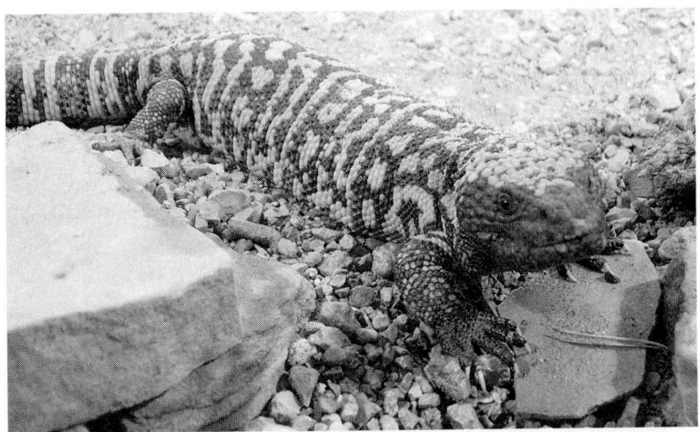

Figure 1. Gila monster (*Heloderma suspectus*). (Courtesy Hogle Zoo, Salt Lake City, UT. http://www.hoglezoo.org.)

Toxic Dose

In general, one adult helodermatid has approximately 15 to 20 mg dried weight venom. The median lethal dose (LD_{50}) of the venom (in mice) is between 0.5 and 1.0 mg/kg (compared to 2.18 mg/kg for the western diamondback rattlesnake). The estimated lethal dose in humans is 5 to 8 mg (2). The lethal activity of the venom is attributed to its proteolytic activity.

Clinical Presentation

The spectrum of toxic effects is described in Table 1. Local effects include marked pain and edema at the bite site. Pain usually reaches its peak between 15 and 45 minutes after venom injection and may persist for 8 to 24 hours. Edema is common, but compartment syndrome has not been described. Necrosis of the affected skin is rare.

Systemic effects, including weakness, anxiety, dizziness, diaphoresis, nausea, vomiting, tinnitus, muscle fasciculations, headache, tachycardia, myocardial infarction, and hypotension, have been reported in severe envenomations (3). Anaphylaxis has also been described (4).

Electrocardiographic (ECG) evidence of an acute anterolateral infarct developed in a previously healthy 23-year-old man after he was bitten by a banded Gila monster. Symptoms developed after admission to the hospital and were not present on initial evaluation in the emergency department. The patient's creatinine kinase rose to 4697 IU, with a positive CPK-MB fraction (5,6). Hypotension and facial and tongue edema developed in a patient who sustained a Gila monster bite to the forearm (7).

Severe anaphylaxis developed in a 44-year-old man after a bite to the right ring finger by a small Gila monster. Facial and tongue edema, inspiratory and expiratory wheezes, and hypotension developed. The patient recovered after treatment with steroids, epinephrine, and diphenhydramine. He had received snake antivenin 20 years earlier. The patient's severe reaction was speculated to be secondary to the development of an acute hypersensitivity reaction from the antigenic similarities between the two venoms (4).

Dyspnea, localized pain at the bite site, and diaphoresis developed in a 29-year-old woman after she was bitten by her pet Gila monster. Frequent profuse vomiting and diarrhea also developed. The patient's medical history was significant for alcohol abuse and a seizure disorder (thought to be secondary to alcoholism). She was treated symptomatically and was discharged home after a 48-hour observation period (8).

TABLE 1. Clinical signs/symptoms associated with 13 Gila monster envenomations

Signs/symptoms	Percent of cases
Pain	82
Tissue edema	77
Erythema	77
Anxiety	73
Nausea/vomiting	69
Weakness	64
Hypotension	62
Leukocytosis	62
Tachycardia	62
Diaphoresis	46
Lymphangitis	23

Adapted from Hooker KR, Caravati EM. Gila monster envenomation. *Ann Emerg Med* 1994;24:731.

Diagnostic Tests

Patients who do not have systemic symptoms do not need laboratory evaluation. Individuals with severe envenomation should have a complete blood count, serum electrolytes, coagulation studies (prothrombin time, activated partial thromboplastin time, International Normalized Ratio, fibrinogen), urinalysis, and an ECG obtained.

Soft-tissue radiographs of the bite area should be considered to evaluate for possible foreign bodies or retained teeth. However, teeth may be difficult to see on plain radiographs (3).

Treatment

No antivenom is commercially available for Gila monster envenomations. Patients should be observed for 6 hours after the bite for signs of systemic toxicity. Intravenous (IV) access should be established for fluid and analgesic administration. Blood pressure and cardiac monitoring are advisable.

FIRST AID

It is important to disengage the lizard as soon as possible while avoiding breaking off any of its teeth into the wound. The lizard's jaw can be pried apart with pliers, a screwdriver, or a crowbar. Other techniques such as cold-water immersion or holding a match under the lizard's lower jaw have also been used to disengage the lizard (9).

ANTIDOTES

No antivenom is available for helodermatid envenomation.

SUPPORTIVE CARE

The local wound should be cleansed, and sterile dressing should be applied. No incision into the wound site should be made; however, the wound should be explored to ensure that no broken teeth remain. Teeth should be removed under local anesthetic. The affected extremity should be elevated for a week. Immobilization of the affected area is not necessary but may help with pain management. Prophylactic antibiotics should be considered when deep puncture wounds are present. Tetanus immunization should be updated as needed. Pain may be severe enough to require narcotic pain medication.

Hypotension generally responds to 10 to 20 ml/kg isotonic fluid boluses. Refractory hypotension can be treated with vasopressors such as dopamine or norepinephrine.

Anaphylaxis should be treated with antihistamines, epinephrine, steroids, and aggressive airway management. The dose of diphenhydramine is 50 mg orally or IV in adults followed by 25 to 50 mg every 4 to 6 hours over the next 48 to 72 hours. The dose in children is 2 mg/kg orally or IV, followed by 5 mg/kg/day in four divided doses over the next 24 to 72 hours. An H_2 antagonist such as famotidine or ranitidine should be considered in addition to diphenhydramine.

In mild cases, 0.3 to 0.5 ml 1:1000 epinephrine can be given subcutaneously and repeated in 20 to 30 minutes. The dose in children is 0.01 ml/kg, with a maximum of 0.5 ml. More severe cases can be treated with IV epinephrine. A continuous infusion may be safer. One milligram of 1:1000 epinephrine is mixed in 250 ml 5% dextrose in water. Infusion is started at 1 mg/minute and titrated to achieve a systolic blood pressure of 100 mm Hg, or a mean arterial pressure of 80 mm Hg. Caution should be used in elderly patients and in individuals with coronary disease. The dosage of methylprednisolone is 1 to 2 mg/kg IV every 6 to 8 hours in adults and children, with a maximum dose of 125 mg.

Thrombocytopenia may develop. Rarely, platelet counts may fall below 100,000, but they usually return to normal levels within 3 days without specific treatment.

TOADS

Toads are found in most places throughout the world; exceptions include Madagascar, New Guinea, New Zealand, and Polynesia (10). Numerous toad species contain toxin (Table 2). Toad venom is secreted into the toad's skin or can be found in the parotid glands behind the toad's eyes. Toxicity can occur if toad skin or secretions are handled or ingested.

The venom of the *Bufo* toad species can cause clinical symptoms that are identical to those of digitalis toxicity. Dried and powdered toad skins have been used as cardiac medications (11,12), hallucinogens (13), expectorants, and diuretics, and also for the treatment of toothaches, sinusitis, and bleeding gums.

Chemical and Physical Characteristics

Toad venom contains many toxins. These include cardioactive substances (bufagins), catecholamines, indolealkylamines, noncardiac sterols, and tetrodotoxin (TTX). Bufagins are cardiotonic sterols that are synthesized from cholesterol (14). They have been found to inhibit sodium, potassium, and adenosine triphosphatase activity (15). This is similar to the action of the cardiac glycosides found in plants (16). Bufotoxins (conjugation products of a specific bufagin with suberylargine) (17) were initially isolated in toads but have also been found in plants and in mushrooms (14,18,19). The catecholamines epinephrine and norepinephrine have also been isolated from toad poison, with epinephrine concentrations as high as 5% documented in some species (17).

The indolealkylamines not only have hallucinogenic effects but have also been shown to cause uterine and intestinal muscle contractions (17). TTXs have been found in the toad *Atelopus oxyrhynchus* (20).

TABLE 2. Toad species that contain toxins

Bufo alvarius	*Bufo bufo gargarizans*	*Bufo peltocephalus*
Bufo americanus	*Bufo formosus*	*Bufo quercicus*
Bufo arenarum	*Bufo fowlerii*	*Bufo regularis*
Bufo asper	*Bufo marinus*	*Bufo valliceps*
Bufo blombergi	*Bufo melanophryniscus*	*Bufo viridis*
Bufo bufo	*Bufo melanostictus*	

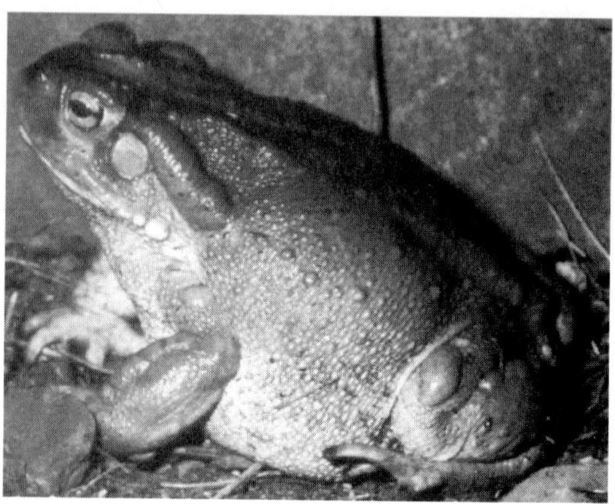

Figure 2. Colorado River toad (*Bufo alvarius*). (Courtesy National Park Service, U.S. Department of the Interior.)

Clinical Presentation

Eye, nose, and throat pain and irritation may follow contact exposure. Some bufagins have local anesthetic effects on mucous membranes. Cardiac effects can resemble those of digitalis toxicity. Cardiac arrest, atrial fibrillation, bradycardia, ventricular fibrillation, right bundle branch block, and hypotension have been described. Respiratory failure has been described, and dyspnea or hyperpnea may develop. Seizures have been reported, as have salivation and vomiting.

Status epilepticus developed in a 5-year-old boy after he put his mouth on a Colorado River toad (*Bufo alvarius*) (Fig. 2). The seizures started within 5 minutes of exposure and lasted for 60 minutes. The boy was successfully treated with diazepam and phenobarbital (21).

Dysrhythmias developed in two children within 4 hours of ingestion of "toad soup." The first child, a 15-month-old boy, initially had a ventricular escape rhythm, which was followed by ventricular fibrillation. Despite treatment with atropine, lidocaine, and cardioversion, he died from persistent bradydysrhythmias. In the second child, a 20-month-old girl, varying degrees of atrioventricular block, ventricular tachycardia, and ventricular fibrillation developed. She was successfully treated with lidocaine, cardioversion, and an internal pacemaker. She was noted to have elevated serum digoxin levels (22).

A 16-year-old male removed and ate approximately 15 toad livers. Bradycardia, hypotension, and a third-degree atrioventricular block developed. Because ingestion of toad livers is not usually associated with toxicity, it was thought that the toxicity was due to the cutaneous exposure of handling the toads (23). Reports have also been published of cardiac dysrhythmias and death after the ingestion of *Bufo marinus* eggs (24).

Bradycardia and hypotension developed in a 25-year-old pregnant woman within 30 minutes of ingestion of approximately 100 ml Chinese herbal tea that contained Ch'an su (dried and powdered toad skins). Sinus tachycardia developed after treatment with atropine, and the patient then went on to develop ventricular tachycardia and intractable ventricular fibrillation. She died approximately 2.5 hours after ingestion (25). Postmortem serum tests showed the presence of a lethal amount of cardiac glycosides.

A topical aphrodisiac (Love Stone, Rock Hard), containing the toxin of the *Bufo gargarizans* toad, has been linked to four human fatalities. Treatment included administration of digoxin Fab. Serum digoxin levels were 0.9 to 2.8 ng/ml (26,27).

Diagnostic Tests

Patients with exposure to toad venom should have continuous cardiac monitoring and serial ECGs obtained. Serum digoxin levels can be used to confirm the presence of toxin but cannot predict the severity of symptoms. Only polyclonal digoxin immunoassays cross-react with the cardiotoxic components found in toad venom. Monoclonal digoxin immunoassays do not cross-react and give false-negative results. All patients should have serum electrolyte levels obtained, especially potassium levels.

Treatment

Mucous membranes should be immediately irrigated after exposure. The irrigating solution should not be swallowed. Exposed skin should be washed thoroughly with soap and water.

DECONTAMINATION

Activated charcoal can be given to patients who are awake and able to protect their airway. It is most effective if given within 1 hour of ingestion.

ENHANCEMENT OF ELIMINATION

The routine use of multiple doses of charcoal is not recommended for toad venom toxicity. A second dose of charcoal can be considered if a patient presents with severe toxicity or when no digitalis Fab fragments are available. Typical doses of charcoal are 25 to 100 g in adults and adolescents, 25 to 50 g in children between the ages of 1 and 12, and 1 g/kg in infants up to the age of 1 (28).

ANTIDOTES

Cardiac dysrhythmias that produce hemodynamic instability can be treated with digitalis Fab fragments. Serum digoxin levels cannot be used to dose digitalis Fab fragments in the setting of bufotoxin toxicity. Empiric treatment with ten vials of digoxin binding fragments has been suggested (27).

Ventricular dysrhythmias should be treated with digoxin Fab. If digoxin Fab is not immediately available, lidocaine or phenytoin may be useful for treatment of ventricular dysrhythmias. The dose of lidocaine is 1.0 to 1.5 mg/kg IV bolus followed by a maintenance drip of 1 to 4 mg/minute in adults. The pediatric dose is 1 mg/kg IV bolus followed by a maintenance drip of 20 to 50 mg/kg/minute. The adult dose of phenytoin is 15 mg/kg (up to 1 g) in adults and children. Infusion should not exceed 0.5 mg/kg/minute. The maintenance dose is 2 mg/kg every 12 hours in adults and 2 mg/kg every 8 hours in children. Phenytoin levels should be measured before administration of the maintenance dose.

Bradydysrhythmias can be treated with standard doses of atropine. The adult dosage is 0.5 to 1.0 mg IV every 5 minutes, with a total dose of 0.04 mg/kg (minimum dose of 0.5 mg). The pediatric dosage is 0.02 mg/kg IV every 5 minutes, with a maximum single dose of 0.05 mg in children and 1.0 mg in adults. The minimum dose of atropine is 0.1 mg in children. The maximum atropine dose is 1 mg in children and 2 mg in adolescents.

Hyperkalemia above 6.5 mEq/L should be treated with digoxin Fab. If digoxin Fab is not available, potassium levels should be lowered using the standard interventions (Chapter 35).

POISON DART FROGS

Poison dart frogs are brightly colored frogs that are found in the tropical rain forests of southern Central America and South America. In general, the frogs are 0.5 to 2.0 in. in length and may have various combinations of red, green, yellow, orange, blue, and black on their skin. Natives in western Colombia have used the toxin secreted by the species *Phyllobates aurotaenia*, *P. bicolor*, and *P. terribilis* to make poison arrows (29).

The toxins produced by *P. terribilis* are thought to be 20 times more toxic than those of the other *Phyllobates* members. No cases of poison dart frog poisoning have been reported. Poison dart frogs secrete several toxins in their skin. These can include pumiliotoxin B, isodihydrohistrionicotoxin, pumiliotoxin C, gephyrotoxin, TTX, and batrachotoxin (30). Batrachotoxin is a depolarizing muscle relaxant that is considered to be 250 times more potent than curare. It has been found in *P. terribilis*, *P. bicolor*, and *P. aurotaenia*.

Pathophysiology

Batrachotoxin causes positive chronotropic and inotropic properties in guinea pig atria. In addition, the toxin has been found to cause dysrhythmias and atrial arrest in isolated guinea pig cardiac muscle preparations. The LD_{50} for batrachotoxin in mice is 2 mg/kg. In comparison, the LD_{50} of TTX in mice is 8 mg/kg, and the LD_{50} of curare is 500 mg/kg (31). One *P. terribilis* is thought to contain up to 1.9 mg batrachotoxin. The lethal dose in humans has been reported to be between 0.02 and 0.2 mg (32).

Batrachotoxin depolarizes electrical membranes through increasing the permeability to sodium ions by stabilizing the sodium channel in an open conformation (33). Morphologically, swelling of the axon is noted at the node of Ranvier, and extracellular fluid accumulation is seen along the axon (34). The plant alkaloids veratridine (*Lilaceae*) and grayanotoxin (*Ericaceae*) produce similar increases in sodium conductance.

NEWTS AND SALAMANDERS

Approximately 340 species of salamanders exist worldwide, with 112 in North America. Newts are a subtype of the salamander family. Unlike salamanders, newts have no costal grooves, and they have a unique arrangement of their palatal teeth on the roof of their mouth. Most salamanders have teeth in their upper and in their lower jaw. In contrast, frogs and toads only have teeth on the upper jaw.

Salamanders can secrete samandarin, which is a potent central nervous system neurotoxin. No fatalities associated with salamander toxin have been reported. Samandarin is thought to open sodium channels irreversibly and can cause seizures and paralysis.

Newts secrete a potent neurotoxin, TTX, in their skin. The newt species found on the U.S. east coast in the Carolinas (*Notophthalmus*) is reported to be less toxic than the west coast varieties (*Taricha*) (35). TTX irreversibly blocks the sodium ion channels that are responsible for nerve and muscle excitability. It is found not only in newts but also in many marine organisms, including puffer fish.

The California newt (*Tarichatorosa*) has been reported to contain a TTX concentration of up to 250 mg per newt (36). Other species that are thought to secrete TTX include *T. pivularis*, *T. granulosa*, *Notophthalmus viridescens*, *Cynops pyrrhogaster*, *C. ensicaudus*, *Triturus vulgaris*, *T. cristatus*, *T. alpestris*, *T. marmoratus*, and *Paramesotriton hongkongensis*. Toxin concentration varies widely between different species (35,37,38). Skin and muscle contain the highest concentration of TTX (37). One report has also been published on the concentration of TTX increasing in *T. granulosa* in association with long-term captivity (39).

Toxic Dose

The minimum lethal dose in 50% of adults has been reported to be approximately 2 mg TTX, which is also the minimum dose needed for toxic symptoms to develop (40).

Toxicokinetics and Toxicodynamics

TTX is adsorbed from the gastrointestinal tract within 5 to 15 minutes (41). Symptoms typically begin approximately 15 to 45 minutes after ingestion; however, onset can occasionally be delayed for several hours (42–44). The peak plasma concentration occurs within 20 minutes after ingestion (41). TTX is widely distributed throughout the body and largely excreted unchanged into the urine (41). The elimination half-life varies from 30 minutes to 3 to 4 hours (45).

Clinical Presentation

Poisoning is caused by ingestion of flesh, viscera, or skin that contains TTX. Ascending paralysis develops, which leads to respiratory paralysis. Onset of symptoms ranges from 10 to 45 minutes but may be delayed for up to 3 hours. Death typically occurs within the first 6 to 24 hours. Most patients who survive beyond 24 hours have full recovery.

Oral paresthesiae often develop with mild poisoning. Severe poisonings are associated with fixed and dilated pupils. Hypotension secondary to vasodilation can occur, and bradycardia and asystole have been reported. Respiratory depression secondary to respiratory muscle paralysis occurs in severe cases.

Vomiting commonly occurs. Diarrhea and salivation have been reported. Paralysis begins in distal extremities and may eventually affect all voluntary muscles. Seizures are rare but have been described. Skin pallor and diaphoresis as well as blistering and desquamation have also been reported.

One case has been reported of a fatal cardiopulmonary arrest that was associated with the ingestion of a 20-cm newt (*T. granulosa*) and alcohol. The patient experienced paresthesiae within 15 minutes and a fatal cardiopulmonary arrest within 2 hours of ingestion (46). A 2-year-old girl bit off approximately 1 cm of the tail of a pet Oregon rough-skinned newt. The tail was not ingested, and the patient's teeth and tongue were brushed with toothpaste after the incident. The child received charcoal and was observed. No adverse events were observed (47).

Diagnostic Tests

Laboratory monitoring is not generally helpful. TTX assays are not widely available.

Treatment

The patient's respiratory function and blood pressure should be supported. Endotracheal intubation and mechanical ventilation may be required until muscle weakness resolves. Activated charcoal can be given to patients who are awake and able to protect their airway. It is most effective if given within 1 hour of ingestion. No antidote is available for TTX poisoning.

REFERENCES

1. Mochca-Morales J, Martin BM, Possani LD. Isolation and characterization of helothermine, a novel toxin from *Heloderma horridum horridum* (Mexican bearded lizard) venom. *Toxicon* 1990;28:299–309.
2. Russell FE, Bogert CM. Gila monster: its biology, venom and bite—a review. *Toxicon* 1981;19:341–359.
3. Hooker KR, Caravati EM. Gila monster envenomation. *Ann Emerg Med* 1994;24:731–735.
4. Caravati EM, Dahl B, Crouch BI. Severe anaphylaxis from Gila monster envenomation. *J Toxicol Clin Toxicol* 1999;37:613(abst).
5. Bou-Abboud CF, Kardassakis DG. Acute myocardial infarction following a Gila monster (*Heloderma suspectum cinctum*) bite. *West J Med* 1988;148:577–579.
6. Preston CA. Hypotension, myocardial infarction, and coagulopathy following Gila monster bite. *J Emerg Med* 1989;7:37–40.
7. Piacentine J, Curry S, Ryan PT. Life-threatening anaphylaxis following Gila monster bite. *Ann Emerg Med* 1986;15:959–961.
8. Heitschel S. Near death from a Gila monster bite. *J Emerg Nurs* 1986;12:259–262.
9. Miller MF. Gila monster envenomation [Letter]. *Ann Emerg Med* 1995;25:720.
10. Lescure J. *Notes du cours "Animaux et toxiques."* Paris: Laboratoire de Zoologie—Reptiles et Amphibians, Museum National d'Histoire Naturelle, 1985.
11. Burton R. *Venomous animals.* London: Colour Library International, 1977.
12. Chern MS, Ray CY, Wu D. Biologic intoxication due to digitalis-like substance after ingestion of cooked toad soup. *Am J Cardiol* 1991;67:443–444.
13. Emboden W. *Narcotic plants.* Macmillan, 1979.
14. Siperstein MD, Murray AW, Titus E. Biosynthesis of cardiotonic sterols from cholesterol in the toad *Bufo marinus*. *Arch Biochem Biophys* 1957;67:154–160.
15. Lichtstein P, Kachalsky S, Deutsch J. Identification of a ouabain-like compound in toad skin and plasma as a bufodienolide derivative. *Life Sci* 1986;38:1261–1270.
16. Palumbo NE, Perri S, Read G. Experimental induction and treatment of toad poisoning in the dog. *J Am Vet Med Assoc* 1975;167:1000–1005.
17. Chen KK, Kovarikova A. Pharmacology and toxicology of toad venom. *J Pharm Sci* 1967;56:1535–1541.
18. Kibmer B, Wichtl M. Bufadienolide aus samen von helleborus odorus. *Planta Med* 1986;2:77–162.
19. Lincoff G, Mitchel DH. *Toxic and hallucinogenic mushroom poisoning.* Dallas: Van Nostrand Reinhold, 1977.
20. Yotsu-Yamishita M, Mebs D, Yasumoto T. Tetrodotoxin and its analogues in extracts from the toad *Atelopus oxyrhynchus* (family: Bufonidae). *Toxicon* 1992;30:1489–1492.
21. Hitt M, Ettinger DD. Toad toxicity. *N Engl J Med* 1986;314:1517.
22. Chi HT, Hung DZ, Hu WH. Prognostic implications of hyperkalemia in toad toxin intoxication. *Hum Exp Toxicol* 1998;17:343–346.
23. Du NT, Due P. Severe toad venom poisoning by dermal absorption. *J Toxicol Clin Toxicol* 2001;39:563(abst).
24. Licht LE. Unpalatability and toxicity of toad eggs. *Herpetologica* 1968;24:93–98.
25. Ko RJ, Greenwald MS, Loscutoff SM. Lethal ingestion of Chinese herbal tea containing Ch'an su. *West J Med* 1996;164:71–75.
26. Brubacher JR, Ravikumar PR, Hoffman RS. Analysis of fatal aphrodisiac known as Love Stone or Rock Hard. *J Toxicol Clin Toxicol* 1995;33:539(abst 139).
27. CDC. Deaths associated with a purported aphrodisiac—New York City, February 1993–May 1995. *MMWR Morb Mortal Wkly Rep* 1995;44:853–861.
28. Chyka PA, Seger D. Position statement: single-dose activated charcoal. American Academy of Clinical Toxicology; European Association of Poisons Centres and Clinical Toxicologists. *Clin Toxicol* 1997;35:721–736.
29. Myers CW, Daly JW, Malkin B. A dangerously toxic new frog (*Phyllobates*) used by Enbera Indians of western Colombia with discussion of blowgun fabrication and dart poisoning. *Bull Am Mus Nat Hist* 1978;101:311–365.
30. Mensah-Dwumah M, Daly JW. Pharmacological activity of alkaloids from poison-dart frogs (Denbrobatidae). *Toxicon* 1978;16:189–194.
31. Daly J, Witkop B. Batrachotoxin, an extremely active cardio and neurotoxin from the Colombian arrow poison frog (*Phyllobates aurotaenia*). *Clin Toxicol* 1971;4:331–342.
32. Daly JW, Myers CW, Warnick JE, et al. Levels of batrachotoxin and lack of sensitivity to its action in poison-dart frogs (*Phyllobates*). *Science* 1980;208:1383–1385.
33. Brown GB. 3H-batrachotoxinin-A benzoate binding to voltage-sensitive sodium channels: inhibition by the channel blockers tetrodotoxin and saxitoxin. *J Neurosci* 1986;6:2064–2070.
34. Moore GR, Boegman RJ, Robertson DM, et al. Acute stages of batrachotoxin-induced neuropathy: a morphologic study of a sodium-channel toxin. *J Neurocytol* 1986;15:573–583.
35. Brodie ED Jr, Hensel JL Jr, Johnson JA. Toxicity of the urodele amphibians *Taricha*, *Notophthalmus*, *Cynops* and *Paramusotriton* (Salamandridae). *Copeia* 1974;2:506–511.
36. Brodie ED Jr. Investigations on the skin toxin of the adult rough-skinned newt, *Taricha granulosa*. *Copeia* 1968;1:307–313.
37. Miyazawa K, Noguchi T. Distribution and origin of tetrodotoxin. *J Toxicol Toxin Rev* 2001;20:11–33.
38. Wakely JF, Fuhrman GJ, Fuhrman FA, et al. The occurrence of tetrodotoxin (Tarichatoxin) in amphibian and the distribution of the toxin in the organs of newts (*Taricha*). *Toxicon* 1966;3:195–203.
39. Hanifin CT, Brodie ED 3rd, Brodie ED Jr. Tetrodotoxin levels of the rough-skin newt, *Taricha granulosa*, increase in long-term captivity. *Toxicon* 2002 Aug;40(8):1149–1153.
40. Noguchi T, Ebesu JSM. Puffer poisoning: epidemiology and treatment. *J Toxicol Toxin Rev* 2001;20:1–10.

41. Kao CY. Tetrodotoxin, saxitoxin and their significance in the study of excitation phenomena. *Pharmacol Rev* 1966;18:997–1049.
42. Chew SK, Goh CH, Wang KW, et al. Puffer fish (tetrodotoxin) poisoning: clinical report and role of anticholinesterase drugs in therapy. *Singapore Med J* 1983;24:168-171.
43. Freeman SE, Turner RJ. Maculotoxin, a potent toxin secreted by Octopus maculosus. *Toxicol Appl Pharmacol* 1970;16:681–690.
44. Laobhripatr S, Limpakarnjanarat K, Sangwonloy O, et al. Food poisoning due to consumption of the freshwater puffer *Tetraodon fangi* in Thailand. *Toxicon* 1990;28:1372–1375.
45. Ogura Y. Some recent problems on fugu-toxin, particularly on crystalline tetrodotoxin. *Seltai No Kagaku* 1958;9:281–287.
46. Bradley SG, Klika LJ. A fatal poisoning from the Oregon rough-skinned newt (*Taricha granulosa*). *JAMA* 1981;246:247.
47. King BR, Hamilton RJ, Kassutto Z. "Tail of newt": an unusual ingestion. *Pediatr Emerg Care* 2000;16:268–269.

CHAPTER 244

Overview of Venomous Snakes of the World

Julian White

Topics included: **Family Colubridae (boomslang, others); family Elapidae (black snake, brown snake, cobra, coral snake, death adder, mamba, taipan, others); family Atracaspidae; family Viperidae, subfamilies Crotalinae (copperhead, cottonmouth snakes, rattlesnakes), Viperinae (gaboon viper, puff adder, Russell viper, saw scaled viper, others)**

Special concerns: **Systemic and local envenoming**

Antidotes: **Antivenoms**

Of the approximately 3000 species of snakes in the world, approximately 600, or 20%, are venomous, nearly all of these possessing specialized teeth (fangs) through which venom can be efficiently delivered to either prey or predators. The vast majority of these venomous snakes fall into just two families, *Elapidae* and *Viperidae*. Venomous snakes are found on all continents except Antarctica, and in tropical waters from East Africa to the Pacific coast of the Americas.

However, in considering the potential danger posed by snakes, it should not be forgotten that some larger nonvenomous snakes, notably some of the pythons and boas, can inflict both unpleasant bites, with a potential for severe local infection, and other, potentially lethal injuries from the crushing effect of coils. The largest boiids have the potential to eat children, and even adults. However, it appears that such feeding attacks on humans are very rare.

A venomous snakebite is the single most important global cause of human injury from venomous and poisonous animals of all types. Precise epidemiologic data are lacking, but most recent estimates published by the World Health Organization point to a global toll of at least 2.5 million bites per year, with 125,000 deaths. The highest toll is in the rural tropics, where snakebites can account for 10% of all hospital beds, can be a major cost for the health system, and are increasingly affecting urban as well as rural populations. There is good evidence that more toxic snake species are invading urban areas, often adapting to the new environment by changing both behavior and diet. This trend suggests the problem of snakebite is likely to expand rather than contract over time.

CLASSIFICATION OF VENOMOUS SNAKES

Venomous snakes are found in four families: Colubridae, Elapidae, Atractaspididae, and Viperidae. The following is a very brief overview of types of venomous snakes. More detail on selected species may be found elsewhere in this book, in other textbooks, notably the *CRC Handbook of Clinical Toxinology of Animal Venoms and Poisons*, and through the clinical toxinology Web site (http://www.toxinology.com).

Family Colubridae

Family Colubridae is the largest family of snakes, with 1864 species in a global distribution (Fig. 1). It is likely to be split into several distinct families in the future. Most colubrid snakes are nonvenomous, lacking either fangs or toxic saliva. A minority of colubrids are venomous, producing either toxic saliva or true venom in venom glands. In the latter, venom is delivered via fangs positioned toward the rear of the mouth (Fig. 2). This position is less effective for biting large predators, such as humans, than the front fangs of most other venomous snakes. It should not be assumed that this renders these snakes universally trivial, because a few species are highly venomous and have caused human deaths. A selection of medically important venomous colubrids is listed in Table 1.

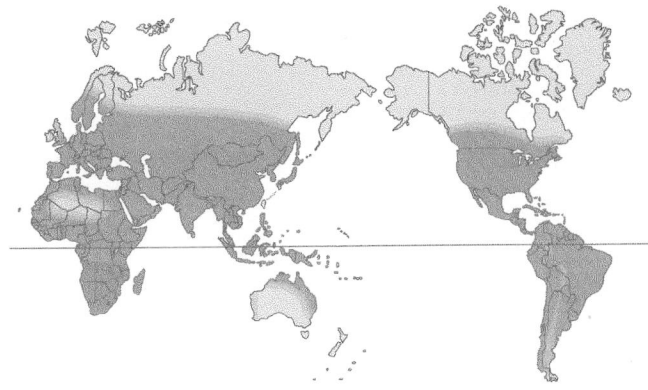

Figure 1. Global distribution of colubrid snakes. (Illustration copyright © by Dr. Julian White.)

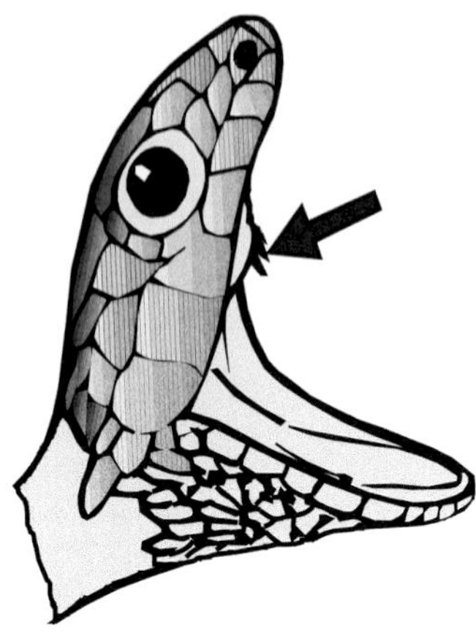

Figure 2. Diagrammatic representation of the typical colubrid snake head, showing fangs placed toward the rear of the mouth. (Illustration copyright © by Dr. Julian White.)

Family Elapidae

Elapid snakes encompass a wide variety of species, with 297 species in a global distribution (Fig. 3), including African and Asian cobras, mambas, kraits, coral snakes, Australian snakes, and sea snakes (60 genera). Their fangs are placed toward the front of the mouth and have limited rotation (Chapter 246). In most species, the fangs have an enclosed groove, acting like a hypodermic needle. The snake has the ability to control venom release, thus it is possible to have a "dry" bite, where minimal venom is released. In general, venom quantities and fang sizes are smaller in elapids compared to vipers of similar length, but elapid venom is often more toxic. There is a common belief, espoused in medical texts in the past, suggesting that elapid bites cause paralysis and viper bites cause bleeding and local tissue injury. This belief is entirely erroneous; many elapids can cause local tissue injury or bleeding, whereas some vipers can cause paralysis. A list of some important elapid snakes is given in Table 2 and their medical effects are addressed in Chapter 246.

TABLE 1. Some major species of medically important colubrid snakes[a]

Scientific name	Common name[b]	Distribution[c]	Clinical effects[d]
Dispholidus typus	Boomslang	CF, SF	C, H, R
Thelatornis spp.	Vine or bird snakes	SF	C, H, R
Rhabdophis spp.	Yamakagashi, red-necked keelback	JA, CK, SE	C, H, R, L
Malpolon monspessulanus	Montpelier snake	NF, ME, EU	?P
Elapomorphus bilineatus	Argentine black-headed snake	SA	H, C
Tachymenis peruviana	Culebra de cola corta	SA	C, H, L

C, coagulopathy; CF, Central and Western Africa; CK, China and Korea; EU, Europe; H, hemorrhagic; JA, Japan; L, significant local tissue reaction (swelling/blisters/hemorrhage/bruising); ME, Middle East; NF, north Africa; P, paralysis; R, renal damage; SA, South America; SE, southeast Asia; SF, southern Africa; V, cardiovascular.
[a]A number of other colubrid snakes may cause envenoming.
[b]Only a single common name is listed, but a variety of common names may exist.
[c]Distribution is approximate only and to continental or subcontinental level; actual distribution may be far more restricted within regions listed.
[d]Only principal or common major clinical effects are listed.

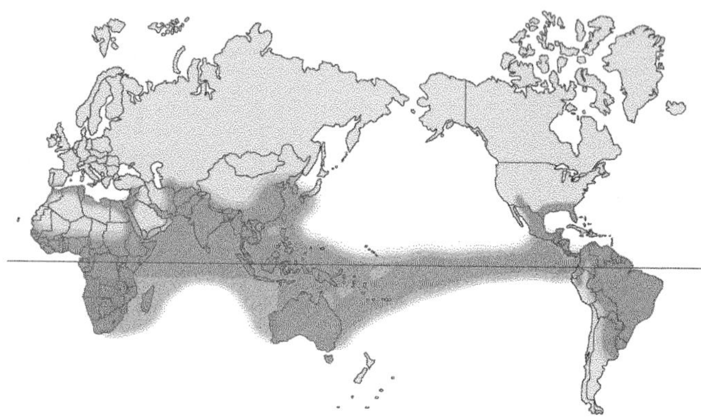

Figure 3. Global distribution of elapid snakes. (Illustration copyright © by Dr. Julian White.)

Family Atracaspididae

Mole or side-fanged vipers in 11 genera have a limited distribution in Africa and the Middle East (Fig. 4). They are fossorial, usually hunting prey beneath the surface, where a standard strike is impossible. They have evolved fangs that come out of the side of the mouth to allow a sideways strike (Fig. 5). This also makes them very difficult to safely pick up behind the head. Most are probably harmless to humans, but a few in the genus *Atractaspis* have toxic venom with unusual components, notably the Sarafotoxins.

Family Viperidae

The vipers are the second venomous snake family of major medical importance globally (Fig. 6). All have mobile fangs in the front of the mouth on hinged maxillae, allowing the fang to fold away against the roof of the mouth when not in use. This has allowed vipers to evolve very long fangs in comparison with elapids. These long fangs are often coupled with large venom glands, allowing large quantities of venom to be injected, but "dry bites" can also occur. There are 33 genera, split into two subfamilies; the typical vipers (Viperinae) and the pit vipers (Crotalinae), so called because they have heat-sensing pit organs towards the front of their head, allowing infrared detection of warm-blooded prey in total darkness. The rattlesnakes are amongst the best known pit vipers. A list of some of the more medically important vipers is given in Table 3.

VENOMS

Venoms are produced in specialized venom glands, usually linked to the base of fangs by a duct. Venom glands have evolved from digestive glands and many venom components bear the hallmark of this ancestry, with components such as phospholipases (PLAs). Venom fulfills three main functions:

- Immobilization of prey
- Digestion of prey
- Deterrence of predators

For the snake, it is the first two functions that are probably most important. Venom components acting to immobilize or

TABLE 2. Some major species of medically important elapid snakes

Scientific name	Common name[a]	Distribution[b]	Clinical effects[c]
Notechis spp., *Tropidechis carinatus*	Tiger snakes, rough scaled snake	AU	P, M, C, R
Hoplocephalus spp.	Broad headed snakes	AU	C
Austrelaps spp.	Copperheads	AU	P, M
Pseudonaja spp.	Brown snakes	AU	C, R, (P)
Pseudechis spp.	Mulga, Papuan black and Collett's snakes	AU	M, R, Ca
Pseudechis spp.	Red bellied black	AU	M
Oxyuranus spp.	Taipans	AU	P, C, M, R
Micropechis ikaheka	New Guinea small eyed snake	AU	P, Ca, M
Acanthophis spp.	Death adders	AU, SE	P
Calliophis spp.	Asian coral snakes	SE	P
Maticora spp.	Asian coral snakes	SE	P
Naja kaouthia	Monocled cobra	SE	L, N, P
Naja siamensis and related spp.	Thai spitting cobra	SE	L, N, (P)
Naja philippinensis	Philippines cobra	SE	P
Ophiophagus hannah	King cobra	SE	P, L
Bungarus spp.	Kraits	SE, IN, CK	P
Naja atra	Chinese cobra	SE, CK	P
Naja naja	Indian cobra	IN	P, L
Walterinnesia aegyptia	Desert black snake	ME, NF	P
Naja haje	Egyptian cobra	NF, ME	P
Boulengeria spp.	Water cobras	CF	P
Naja melanoleuca	Forest cobra	CF, SF	P
Dendroaspis spp.	Mambas	CF, SF	P
Naja mossambica	Mozambique spitting cobra	SF	L, N
Naja nigricolis	Black necked spitting cobra	CF, SF, NF	L, N
Naja nivea	Cape cobra	SF	P
Hemachatus haemachatus	Rinkhals spitting cobra	SF	L, N, P
Aspidelaps spp.	African coral snakes	SF	P
Elapsoidea spp.	African garter snakes	SF	L
Pseudohaje spp.	Tree cobras	SF, CF	L
Paranaja multifasciata	Burrowing cobra	SF, CF	L
Micruroides euryxanthus	American coral snake	NA, CA	P
Micrurus spp.	American coral snakes	SA, CA	P
Enhydrina schistosa	Beaked sea snake	Indo-Pacific oceans	M, P
Aipysurus spp., *Astrotia stokesii, Hydrophis* spp., *Laticauda* spp., *Hydrelaps* spp., *Lapemis* spp., *Pelamis platurus*	Other species of sea snakes	Indo-Pacific oceans; only *Pelamis* is pelagic	M, P

AS, Asia; AU, Australia and New Guinea; C, coagulopathy; CA, Central America; Ca, anticoagulant; CF, Central and Western Africa; CK, China and Korea; EU, Europe; H, hemorrhagic; IN, Indian subcontinent, including Sri Lanka; JA, Japan; L, significant local tissue reaction (swelling/blisters/hemorrhage/bruising); M, myolysis; ME, Middle East; N, necrotoxic or likely to cause significant injury to the bitten area; NA, North America; NF, north Africa; P, paralysis; R, renal damage; SA, South America; SE, southeast Asia; SF, southern Africa.
[a]Only a single common name is listed, but a variety of common names may exist.
[b]Distribution is approximate only and to continental or subcontinental level; actual distribution may be far more restricted within regions listed.
[c]Only principal or common major clinical effects are listed.

digest may have major deleterious effects on bitten humans. Venoms are complex mixtures of toxins. Each toxin may have several distinct actions on diverse body systems, and different toxins may work synergistically to enhance toxicity. The most common measure of venom toxicity, often extrapolated to human envenoming, is the dose of venom that kills 50% of animals (LD_{50}) within a specified time period. Unfortunately, the toxicity of a venom often varies widely with differing test species. Although the LD_{50} is commonly used to define relative dangerousness of different snake species, the rankings so generated are potentially misleading. Nevertheless, in the absence of LD_{50} testing of venoms in humans, such nonhuman LD_{50} is a crude indication of possible relative toxicity. On this basis, the elapid snakes are generally far more toxic than the vipers. It should not

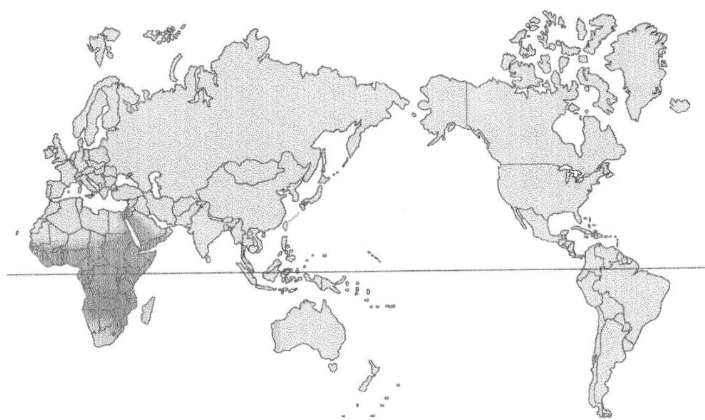

Figure 4. Global distribution of atractaspid snakes. (Illustration copyright © by Dr. Julian White.)

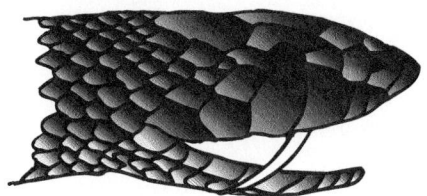

Figure 5. Diagrammatic representation of the head of a typical atractaspid snake, showing the side positioning of the fangs, for sideways strike. (Illustration copyright © by Dr. Julian White.)

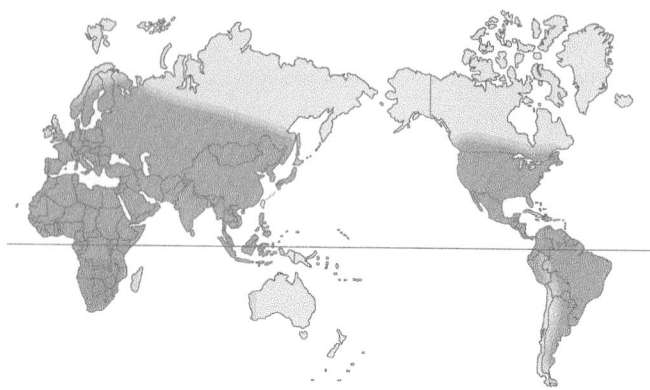

Figure 6. Global distribution of viperid snakes. (Illustration copyright © by Dr. Julian White.)

be forgotten that vipers often produce and inject more venom, which may balance lower venom toxicity. Clinical studies clearly show that in terms of actual numbers of deaths caused by snakebites globally, vipers are more important than elapids.

There are several ways of classifying snake venom components. In this text, a medical classification system is used (Table 4).

Neurotoxins

Neurotoxins are classic venom components causing potentially lethal envenoming in humans. There are many types, widely distributed among venomous animals. Some cause flaccid paralysis, others cause hyperstimulation of portions of the nervous system. The latter are not prominent in snake venoms.

Paralyzing neurotoxins, generally causing flaccid paralysis and respiratory paralysis, are classic snake toxins, responsible for many deaths in rural tropical regions. A broad outline of the mechanism of action is shown in Figure 7. A list of some prominent species with the potential to cause paralysis is shown in Table 5.

TABLE 3. Some major species of medically important viperid snakes

Scientific name	Common name[a]	Distribution[b]	Clinical effects[c]
Viperinae			
Daboia russelli	Russell's viper	SE, IN	C, H, R, M, P, N, L
Echis spp.	Carpet or saw scaled vipers	IN, ME, AS, NF, CF	C, H, R, N, L
Pseudocerastes spp.	Horned vipers	ME, AS	P
Vipera spp. (includes those *Vipera* now assigned to *Macrovipera*)	Vipers	ME, AS, EU, NF	L, H, C, V, R, P
Vipera ammodytes	Long nosed viper	EU, AS	L, P
Cerastes spp.	Horned vipers	NF	L, C
Causus spp.	Night adders	NF, CF, SF	L, P
Atheris spp.	Bush vipers	NF, CF, SF	
Bitis arietans	Puff adder	CF, SF	L, N, C, H, V, R
Bitis gabonica, Bitis nasicornis	Gaboon viper, Rhinoceros viper	CF, SF	L, N, C, H, V, R
Bitis spp.	Other African vipers	NF, CF, SF	L
Crotalinae			
Trimeresurus spp. (includes *Ovophis, Tropidolaemus*)	Green tree pit vipers	SE, CK, JA, IN	L, C, H
Gloydius spp.	Asian pit vipers, including mamushis	SE, CK, JA, AS	L, C, H, N
Calloselasma rhodostoma	Malayan pit viper	SE	L, N, H, C, R
Deinagkistrodon acutus	Hundred pace viper	CK	L, N, H, C
Hypnale spp.	Hump nosed vipers	IN	L
Bothrops asper	Terciopelo	SA	L, N, C, H
Bothrops atrox	Lancehead	SA	L, N, C, H
Bothrops jararaca; B. jararacusu; B. moojeni	Jararaca; Jararacusu; Brazilian lancehead	SA	L, N, C, H, R, M
Bothrops lanceolatus	Fer de Lance	CA	L, N, C, H
Bothrops spp. (includes ex *Bothriopsis* spp.)	Lancehead vipers	SA, CA	L, N, C, H
Atropoides spp.	Jumping pit vipers	CA	L, N
Bothriechis spp.	Palm pit vipers	CA	L, N
Cerriphidion spp.	Montane pit vipers	CA	L, N
Porthidium spp.	Montane pit vipers	CA	L, N
Ophryacus spp.	Horned pit viper	CA	L, N
Lachesis muta	Bushmaster	CA, SA	L, N, C
Crotalus durissus	Neotropical rattlesnake or cascabel	CA, SA	P, M, R, C, H, (L)
Crotalus spp.	Other Central and South American rattlesnakes	CA, SA	P, L, R
Crotalus spp.	North American rattlesnakes	NA	L, N, H, C, (R)
Crotalus scutulatus	Mojave rattlesnake	NA	P, L, (N), (C), (H)
Sistrurus spp.	Pygmy rattlesnakes and massasauga	NA	L, N, (H)
Agkistrodon spp.	Copperhead, cottonmouth, cantil	CA, NA	L, N, C, H, R

AS, Asia; AU, Australia and New Guinea; C, coagulopathy; CA, Central America; CF, Central and Western Africa; CK, China and Korea; EU, Europe; H, hemorrhagic; IN, Indian subcontinent, including Sri Lanka; JA, Japan; L, significant local tissue reaction (swelling/blisters/hemorrhage/bruising); M, myolysis; ME, Middle East; N, necrotoxic or likely to cause significant injury to the bitten area; NA, North America; NF, north Africa; P, paralysis; R, renal damage; SA, South America; SE, southeast Asia; SF, southern Africa; V, cardiovascular.

[a]Only a single common name is listed, but a variety of common names may exist.

[b]Distribution is approximate only and to continental or subcontinental level; actual distribution may be far more restricted within regions listed.

[c]Only principal or common major clinical effects are listed.

TABLE 4. Broad medical classification of snake venom activities

Toxin activity type	Clinical effects
Neurotoxin	Flaccid paralysis
Presynaptic	Resistant to late antivenom therapy
Postsynaptic	Often reversal with antivenom therapy
Anticholinesterase	Fasciculation
Myotoxin	Systemic skeletal muscle damage
Hemostatic system toxins	Interfere with normal hemostasis, causing either bleeding or thrombosis
Hemorrhagins	Damage vascular wall, causing bleeding
Nephrotoxins	Direct renal damage
Cardiotoxins	Direct cardiotoxicity
Necrotoxins	Direct tissue injury at the bite site/bitten limb

Presynaptic neuromuscular junction (NMJ) *neurotoxins* damage the human presynaptic terminal axon. Their action causes a brief period of neurotransmitter release, followed by cessation of all neurotransmitter release, resulting in irreversible paralysis. This manifests clinically as progressive flaccid paralysis. Antivenom therapy cannot reverse such paralysis, which may persist for days, weeks, or occasionally months. However, if administered at the earliest sign of paralysis, antivenom may prevent progression to widespread severe paralysis. As these toxins affect the skeletal NMJ, they affect skeletal muscle only, including respiration, but not cardiac or smooth muscle. They have evolved from PLA_2 toxins, but some are complex multicomponent molecules without residual enzymatic activity. These toxins are particularly found in some snake venoms.

Postsynaptic NMJ neurotoxins also act principally at the skeletal muscle NMJ, causing progressive flaccid paralysis, but act

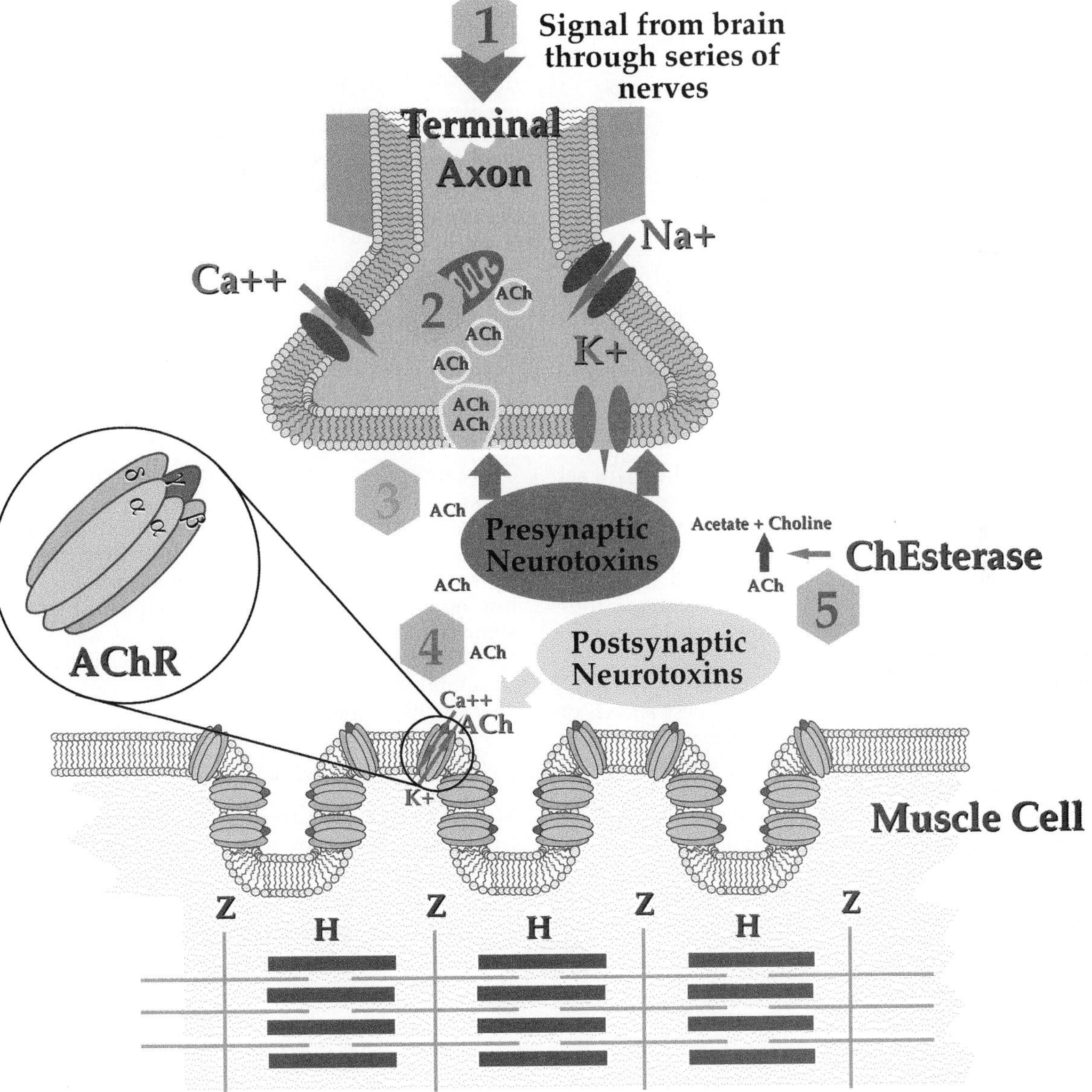

Figure 7. Diagrammatic representation of the site and mode of action of principal paralyzing snake neurotoxins. **1:** Signal arrives at nerve cell ending (terminal axon) from brain. **2:** Neurotransmitter (ACh = Acetyl choline) is released from within nerve cell ending (terminal axon). **3:** ACh leaves terminal axon and crosses the gap (synapse) to the muscle cell well. **4:** The ACh binds to receptors (AChR) on the muscle cell wall, causing changes in the cell, resulting in muscle contraction. **5:** ACh is released from the receptor and broken down by an enzyme (ChEsterase). (Illustration copyright © by Dr. Julian White.)

TABLE 5. Major groups of venomous snakes likely to cause flaccid neurotoxic paralysis

Type of animal	Examples	Type of neurotoxin[a]	Responsiveness to antivenom
Elapid snakes	Kraits	Pre- and post-synaptic	Limited
	Coral snakes	Postsynaptic	Reasonable
	Mambas	Dendrotoxins and fasciculins	Reasonable
	Cobras (some)	Postsynaptic	Reasonable
	King cobra	Postsynaptic	Reasonable
	Death adders	Postsynaptic	Reasonable
	Selected Australian snakes; tiger snakes, taipans, rough scaled snake	Pre- and post-synaptic	Minimal
	Sea snakes	Postsynaptic	Reasonable
Viperid snakes	Mohave rattle-snake (some)	Presynaptic	Limited
	Neotropical rattle-snakes	Presynaptic	Limited
	Sri Lankan Russell's viper	Postsynaptic	Reasonable (only for PulchellaTab)

Limited, only limited or incomplete reversal in most cases; minimal, minimal chance of reversal in most cases; reasonable, reasonable likelihood of reversal.
[a]Definite, predominate, or most likely major site of action in humans.

extracellularly by reversibly binding to the acetylcholine receptor on the muscle end plate. Their effect is therefore reversible with sufficient antivenom therapy and may also be at least partially overcome by the use of anticholinesterases, such as neostigmine, though this often requires repeated dosing.

Presynaptic and postsynaptic synergistic NMJ neurotoxins are found in African mamba snake venoms. The dendrotoxins act presynaptically to increase release of the neurotransmitter, acetylcholine, flooding the NMJ and causing persistent depolarization of the muscle. This action is compounded synergistically by a second set of mamba toxins, the fasciculins, which act as anticholinesterases, preventing removal of the acetylcholine, thus increasing the neurotransmitter concentration and adding to the depolarization neuromuscular blockade and resulting in muscle fasciculation and effective paralysis of skeletal muscle.

A variety of *sodium channel neurotoxins,* the best known of which is tetrodotoxin, is found in such diverse animals as the Australian blue-ringed octopus and the flesh of puffer fish (fugu). A small molecule, tetrodotoxin causes rapid, reversible short-lived flaccid paralysis of skeletal muscle principally by blocking nerve transmission through action on the sodium channels of axons. They are not represented in snake venoms.

Potassium channel neurotoxins are found in a variety of venoms, most notably in some scorpion venoms and cone shell venoms. A variety of potassium channels may be affected, the usual clinical effect being flaccid paralysis, though hypertonic paralysis may also occur. Among snake venoms, only the dendrotoxins are generally considered part of this group.

Excitatory neurotoxins have been found in venoms, especially arthropod venoms such as those from spiders and scorpions, but not snake venoms. These toxins may target diverse parts of the human nervous system, often as an unfortunate byproduct of toxicity designed to immobilize prey species, mostly other arthropods. A good example is the Australian funnel web spider, the principal toxin of which affects arthropod prey, but not most mammals, an unfortunate exception being humans, who are exquisitely susceptible to this venom. Some of these toxins affect neuronal ion channels, though mechanisms of action are still uncertain in many cases.

Autonomic neurotoxins are present in a number of venoms. This includes neurotoxins from the previously mentioned classes, especially the excitatory and ion channel toxins.

Myotoxins

Myotoxins involve two principal types of myotoxic action in venoms: local, at the bite/sting area, and systemic. The latter is of most clinical significance. Systemic myolysins are particularly important in some snake venoms, which in humans may result in potentially lethal myolysis of skeletal muscle. These latter myotoxins are PLA_2 toxins, and in some cases are the same toxins as presynaptic neurotoxins (e.g., notexin from Australian tiger snake venom), mediating myotoxicity through a part of the molecule distinct from the neurotoxic active site. Myotoxins cause extensive membrane and intracellular damage to individual muscle cells, commencing within 60 minutes of reaching their target site, and by 24 hours (in experimental models) cell destruction is complete. However, the basal lamina remains intact, so that after approximately 3 days cellular reconstruction commences, completing around 28 days. There is some evidence that only slow fibers regenerate, not fast fibers. In the process of muscle cell degeneration there is release of cell contents into the circulation, most notably myoglobin, creatine kinase (CK) and potassium. The former may cause secondary renal damage or failure; the latter cardiac dysrhythmia or arrest. Cardiac and smooth muscle appear largely unaffected by venom myolysins. Some principal snakes likely to cause systemic myolysis are listed in Table 6.

Cardiotoxins

There are a number of PLA_2 "cardiotoxins" described from some snake venoms, but these are mostly just general cellular toxins that cause cell damage and tissue necrosis. There are, however, toxins that can directly or indirectly affect the myocardium. These are found in a variety of venoms, notably snake venoms, but indirect cardiac effects are prominent in envenoming by some arthropods (especially scorpions) and marine animals (some jellyfish and cone shells). The mechanisms of action and structural identity of such toxins are diverse and beyond the scope of this chapter.

Coagulopathic Toxins

Many snake venoms have actions on the human hemostatic system. A broad outline of modes of action is given in Table 7 and

TABLE 6. Major groups of venomous animals likely to cause systemic myolysis

Type of animal	Examples
Elapid snakes	Sea snakes
	Selected Australian snakes: tiger snakes, rough scaled snake, taipans, mulga snakes, Collett's snake
	Sea snakes
Viperid snakes	Some South American pit vipers (*Crotalus* spp., selected *Bothrops* spp.)
	Sri Lankan Russell's viper

TABLE 7. Broad classification of types of action of snake coagulopathic and hemorrhagic toxins

Class of toxin	Specific activity
Procoagulants	Factor V activating, factor X activating, factor IX activating, prothrombin activating, fibrinogen clotting
Anticoagulant	Protein C activating, factor IX/X activating protein, thrombin inhibitor, phospholipase 2
Fibrinolytic	Fibrin(ogen) degradation, plasminogen activation
Vessel wall interactive	Hemorrhagins
Platelet activity	Platelet aggregation inducers, platelet aggregation inhibitors
Plasma protein activators	Plasma serine protease inhibitors

Figure 8, whereas Table 8 lists some major species likely to cause coagulopathy.

Although the name *procoagulant* accurately depicts the primary action of these venom toxins, the clinical effects in humans are more complex and subtle. In normal hemostasis, the formation of a blood clot by cross-linking fibrin occurs in a protective platelet plug at the site of hemorrhage. It is therefore protected from dissolution by the fibrinolytic system until vessel wall repair has occurred. Venom procoagulants act outside this structured environment. Fibrinogen is rapidly converted to fibrin, which starts to cross-link, but fibrinolysis is also rapidly activated, so that within minutes of the venom causing microclotting, there is hyperfibrinolysis, causing fibrin to be destroyed as rapidly as it is formed. So powerful is this reaction with some venom procoagulants, notably the prothrombin convertors of some Australian elapid snake venoms, that all circulating fibrinogen can be consumed within 5 to 15 minutes, rendering the patient profoundly anticoagulated and at risk of hemorrhage. If envenoming is severe, there may be a brief period at the outset of procoagulant action, before fibrinolysis is established, when substantial thrombi form and potentially embolize. These may cause diverse and potentially catastrophic effects, notably coronary occlusion leading to cardiac dysrhythmia or arrest. Subsequent fibrinolysis quickly removes such thrombi, so that they are not evident at autopsy in fatal cases. This mechanism is postulated as a cause of the rapid collapse and cardiac problems seen particularly with envenoming by the Australian brown snake. Venom procoagulants are usually multicomponent molecules, sometimes quite large, as seen in some prothrombin convertors, and generally their structure mimics normal components of human hemostasis, particularly part or all of the "prothrombinase" complex (factor Xa, Va, phospholipid, Ca). The specific types of procoagulants are listed in Table 7.

Some venoms contain true *anticoagulants*, components that directly inhibit portions of the clotting cascade, resulting in prolonged clotting times. Although such effects can increase a bleeding tendency, in general the likelihood of major hemorrhage as a result of these direct anticoagulants is less than with the action of the powerful procoagulants mentioned earlier. The precise mechanism of action of the anticoagulants varies between venoms, as does component structure.

Fibrinolytic agents, including proteinases, occur in a number of Viperid snake venoms. Fibrinolytic enzymes split off either the Aα or Bβ, or both, sets of fibrinogen fibrinopeptides. Aα splitting enzymes are principally metalloproteinases, particularly zinc metalloproteinases (metzincin family), which are inactive in the venom gland and activated by cysteine release before a bite. Bβ splitting enzymes are mostly serine proteases, closely related to thrombin-like, protein c–activating and kallikrein-activating snake venom enzymes. The other group of fibrinolytic venom agents are the plasminogen activators, often closely related to the prothrombin activators. Some of the latter also have plasminogen activating activity. The result of all these related agents is rapid thrombus removal and, often, consumption of fibrinogen, thus effectively causing anticoagulation.

Platelet active agents contain a number of components with actions on platelets, either promoting platelet aggregation, or more commonly inhibiting aggregation, through a variety of direct and indirect mechanisms. In clinical terms, both types of action are of importance, in either causing thrombocytopenia, with secondary increased bleeding tendency, or causing inhibition of platelet aggregation, with similar clinical effects. The platelet aggregation inducers are a diverse group of toxins, widely represented in viperid snake venoms; serine proteases, lectins, convulxins, aggregoserpentins, aggretins, von Willebrand's factor agents (botrocetin, bitiscetin, alboaggregins) and the flavocetins. Platelet aggregation inhibitors in snake venoms fall into four classes; α-fibrinogenases, PLA_2, 5'-nucleotidases, and fibrinogen receptor antagonists (disintegrins). The latter group, disintegrins, are the focus of considerable research, because of their many therapeutic possibilities (treating thrombosis, reducing damage from cerebrovascular accidents, platelet protection during heart bypass surgery, potent antineoplastic agents and inhibiting bone resorption). They specifically inhibit integrins of the β_1 and β_2 subfamilies (fibrinogen receptor GIIb/IIIa; vitronectin receptor; fibronectin receptor) and are found principally in viperid snake venoms.

Direct and indirect hemorrhagic activity is a prominent feature of many viper venoms. The viperid zinc metalloproteinases are among the best characterized. They cause capillary leakage by degrading blood vessel basement membranes, resulting in hemorrhagic necrosis. They are related to the disintegrins, containing a disintegrin-like domain, allowing binding to collagen receptors.

SERPIN (plasma SERine Protease INhibitors) inactivators are found in some viperid and colubrid snake venoms. SERPINs are important controlling enzymes for hemostasis, making up 10% of all plasma proteins (e.g., antithrombin III, α_1-proteinase inhibitor) and their inactivation removes checks on thrombosis, clearly synergistic with other hemostatically active venom components.

Nephrotoxins

Renal damage from envenoming is not a rare event, and may follow envenoming by a wide range of venomous animals; as a secondary effect of venom-induced hypotension, causing renal hypoxic damage; or by deposition of byproducts of venom-induced coagulopathy or myolysis. However, at least a few snakes appear to possess primary nephrotoxins in their venom, which can induce severe renal failure. There are also instances, after snakebite, of permanent major renal injury, notably renal cortical necrosis, the etiology of which is uncertain and probably multifactorial.

Necrotoxins

A variety of venomous animals can cause local tissue necrosis at the bite through diverse mechanisms. Some snakes (e.g., many

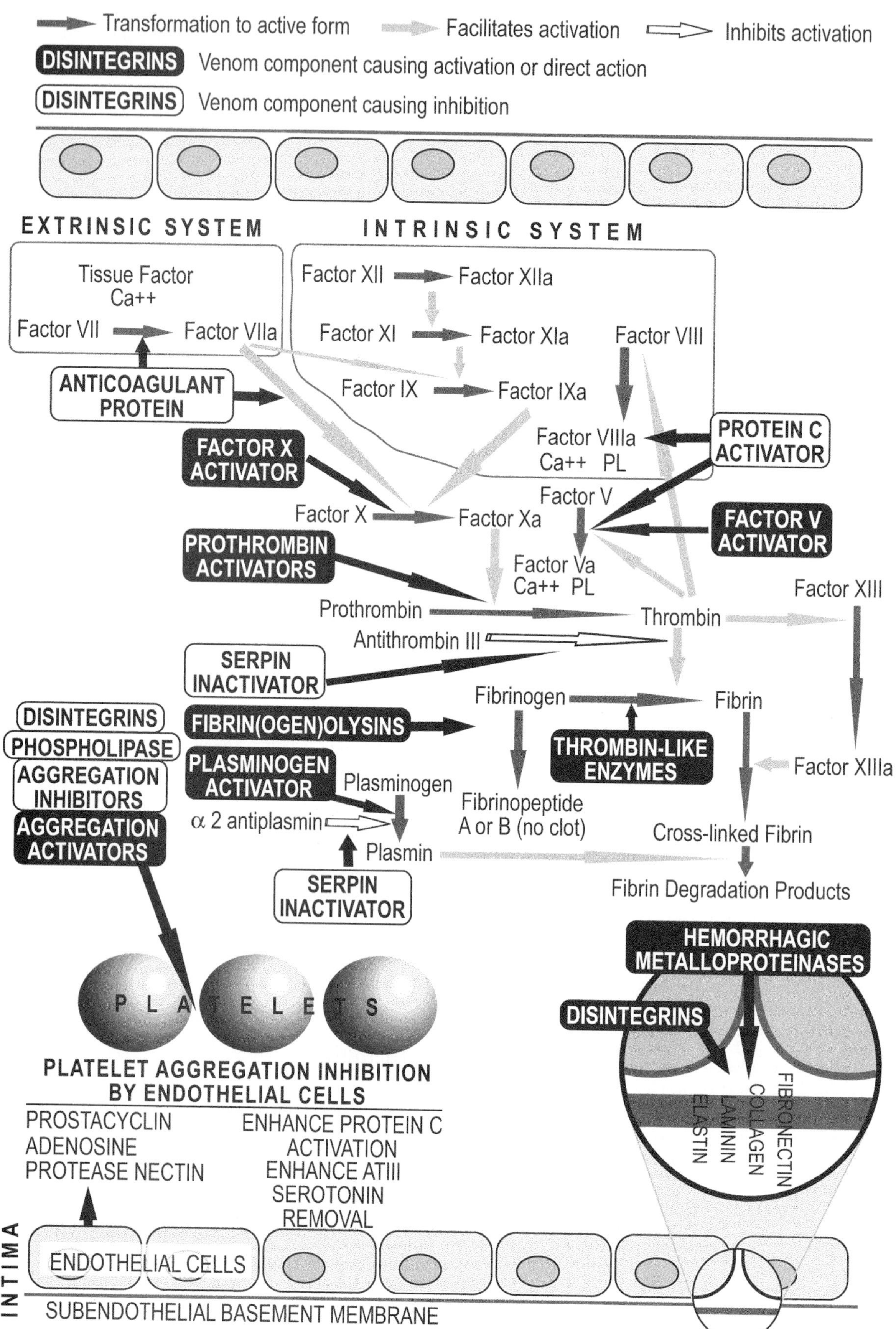

Figure 8. Diagrammatic representation of the sites and mode of action, within blood vessels, of principal snake coagulopathic and hemorrhagic toxins. ATIII, antithrombin III; PL, phospholipase. (Illustration copyright © by Dr. Julian White.)

TABLE 8. Major groups of venomous snakes likely to cause primary coagulopathy

Type of animal	Examples	Type of venom action
Colubrid snakes	Boomslang, vine snake	Procoagulant
	Yamakagashi, red necked keelback	Procoagulant
Elapid snakes	Selected Australian snakes; tiger snakes, rough scaled snake, taipans, brown snakes, broad headed snakes	Procoagulant
	Selected Australian snakes; mulga snakes, Collett's snake, Papuan black snake	Anticoagulant
Viperid snakes	Saw scaled or carpet vipers	Procoagulant, disintegrins, hemorrhagins
	Gaboon vipers and puff adders	Procoagulant, antiplatelet, disintegrins, hemorrhagins
	Russell's vipers	Procoagulant, hemorrhagins
	Malayan pit viper	Procoagulant, antiplatelet, hemorrhagins
	North American rattlesnakes	Procoagulant, fibrinolytic, antiplatelet, disintegrins, hemorrhagins
	North American copperheads	Procoagulant, anticoagulant, fibrinolytic, disintegrins
	South American pit vipers (selected *Bothrops* spp.)	Procoagulant, anticoagulant, fibrinolytic, disintegrins, hemorrhagins
	Asian green pit vipers (selected *Trimeresurus* spp.)	Anticoagulant, fibrinolytic, antiplatelet, disintegrins, hemorrhagins
	Euro-Asian vipers (selected *Vipera* spp.)	Procoagulant, disintegrins, hemorrhagins

vipers, pit vipers, some cobras) commonly cause major local tissue injury, as a result of a variety of different venom effects, including the effects of cytolytic PLA_2 toxins.

Other Venom Components

There are many other components found in venoms, most of which may have little clear clinical effect, but some, such as hyaluronidase, may enhance other venom actions, whereas others, such as histamine, serotonin, and 5-hydroxytryptamine, may have potent, if short-lived, actions. These latter components are particularly prominent in arthropod venoms, notably those of stinging hymenoptera, which also contain specialized small peptides, such as apamin and mellitin (e.g., honey bee venom), which have potent cardiovascular actions. In addition, these peptides may also be highly allergenic, resulting in anaphylaxis on subsequent exposure in sensitive individuals. This is a common problem with honey bee venom, but also with a variety of other bee and wasp venoms and is particularly common with some of the Australian primitive stinging ant venoms (e.g., hopper and inch ants, *Myrmecia* spp.). The importance of these components in relation to human envenoming is unclear, but they may have a role in causation of the nonspecific effects of systemic envenoming, such as headache, nausea, vomiting, abdominal pain, and diarrhea.

It should be remembered that snake venom, like bee venom, can stimulate inappropriate IgE immunity with the potential for fatal anaphylaxis after a subsequent bite. Such anaphylactic deaths after snakebite in sensitized individuals are documented among snake keepers. The components in the venom that cause such sensitization are not defined, and may vary from species to species and person to person.

CLINICAL EFFECTS OF VENOM

Envenoming occurs when the venomous animal, in this case a snake, introduces venom into the prey or predator (classing humans as predators of snakes). In most snakebites, venom is introduced by a fang or fangs making contact with the victim and injecting venom beneath the skin surface, in most cases subcutaneously. Often, some venom is left on the skin surface. Snakes can control venom injection, such that they can bite, even leaving a little venom on the skin surface, yet fail to inject more than a trivial amount of venom—the "dry bite," a phenomenon seen with essentially all snakes. The rate of dry bites varies with species. For North American rattlesnakes, the rate of dry bites is approximately 20%. For Australian taipans, it may be as low as 5%, but the related brown snakes have an 80% dry bite rate. Despite this, this latter group of snakes are the leading cause of death from snakebite in Australia.

The real dangerousness of a snake species is a combination of factors:

- The toxicity of the venom
- The quantity of venom available
- The quantity of venom commonly injected
- The rate of dry bites
- The size of the fangs
- The aggressiveness of the snake
- The likelihood of adverse encounters with humans (this will be determined, in part, by the relative population densities of snakes and humans and the type of lifestyle, accommodation for the humans)

As examples, consider two snake species, the Australian inland taipan and the West African carpet, or saw-scaled, vipers. The inland taipan has the most toxic of all snake venoms and sizable fangs, produces large amounts of venom, and can be swift and aggressive in striking. Technically, it is the most dangerous snake in the world. However, it lives in areas very sparsely populated by humans, is rarely encountered, causes very few bites, and has yet to cause a confirmed fatality. In contrast, the carpet viper has smaller fangs, far less toxic venom, and not much venom. It is found in high numbers in areas with high human populations, where footwear is inadequate to prevent bites, and dwellings readily admit snakes. The result is many deaths because of the inadequate health facilities to treat cases. Precise numbers of deaths are not known, but are considered to exceed 10,000 per year, making this small snake the most prolific killer of humans among all snakes. Therefore, the real dangerousness of a snake is measured more by opportunity than by toxicity. If the inland taipan were to live in similar numbers as carpet vipers in west Africa, there is little doubt it would kill far more people.

Toxicokinetics and Toxicodynamics

The way venoms are introduced by a bite or sting, the depth of injection, quantity involved, the size and action of venom components, size, age, preexisting disease, and postenvenoming activity of the victim will all influence the rate of absorption, clinical effectiveness, and elimination of venom. With a range of

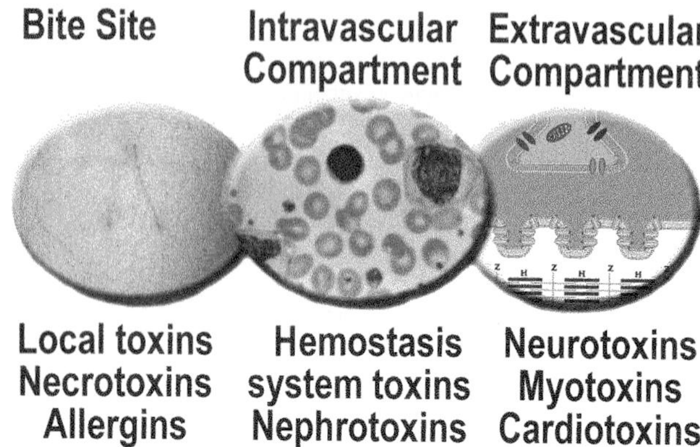

Figure 9. Diagrammatic representation of the three major areas of activity for venoms, illustrating their toxicodynamics. (Illustration copyright © by Dr. Julian White.)

quite different venom components all working at once and in different ways, understanding the pharmacodynamics of envenoming can be difficult. In general terms, however, the speed of onset of action of a particular component is determined by its size and target tissue location. Thus, necrotoxins and other locally active toxins may commence clinical effects almost immediately after the bite or sting, as they are already at their target site, whereas systemically active toxins must first reach the bloodstream (Fig. 9).

Toxins active within the bloodstream rapidly exert their effect, but toxins with extravascular targets, such as neurotoxins and myotoxins, generally have a more delayed onset. The rapidity of effect is also influenced by any latency period between time of binding to the target tissue and onset of detectable action. As an example, presynaptic neurotoxins may have a latency period of 60 minutes, whereas postsynaptic neurotoxins may have almost no latency period; these differences are related in the speed of onset of neurotoxic symptoms and signs. To real clinical circumstances, however, assessment is rarely so simple, for a single venom contains a diverse array of toxins. Again using the neurotoxins as an example, the venom may well contain both pre- and postsynaptic neurotoxins, so there is a continuous onset and development of paralysis, as each type of neurotoxin exerts its effect.

Many venoms are eliminated by the kidneys, explaining why testing urine for venom can be rewarding, and this renal excretion may commence as soon as venom reaches the circulation. Thus, blood levels of venom reflect not just the quantity of venom absorbed, but also the rate of absorption and of excretion. In most cases, when venom is injected by a sting or bite, it is deposited subcutaneously or intradermally. Some snakes, such as large vipers, with long fangs, may occasionally inject deeper, even into muscle. Although direct injection into blood vessels can occur, it seems a rare event, except for some jellyfish, notably species such as the lethal box jellyfish.

Initial Reaction to a Bite

For many snake species, the bite is immediately felt and the victim's attention drawn to the cause of the bite. For most humans, this results in anxiety, which may occasionally be extreme and cause major harm in its own right. Anxiety reactions culminating in fatal myocardial infarction are known after bites by harmless snakes. Anxiety may induce nausea, tachycardia, chest tightness or discomfort, possibly hypotension, and even vomiting, abdominal pain, and collapse. These nonenvenoming effects may be confused with true envenoming.

Many snake species may cause direct injury at the bite site, so local pain, redness, swelling, and even bleeding or blistering may occur. Fang marks may be obvious, as single puncture, dual punctures, or a complex array of multiple tooth marks. Venomous snakes possess many other teeth besides fangs, all of which can leave marks. Multiple bites may produce an even more complex bite pattern. Fangs do not always make clean contact, but may drag through the skin, leaving scratch marks or small lacerations, rather than discrete punctures.

However, some snakes, particularly some elapids, may cause little or no local reaction. The bite may go unnoticed by the victim, who later develops systemic envenoming as the first clue that a snakebite has occurred. If this diagnosis is not considered, great diagnostic confusion may occur. It is common in parts of the rural tropics for humans to be bitten in bed, while asleep, unaware of the bite, only to be discovered dead or paralyzed in the morning by relatives. This is particularly true for krait bites in parts of Asia.

Local Effects of the Bite

Clearly, local effects vary with species of snake. In those species commonly causing significant local reactions, such as most North American rattlesnakes, there is progressive pain, swelling, redness and in more severe cases, blistering, bruising, or active bleeding. The speed of progression of swelling and blistering or bruising is usually indicative of the severity of envenoming in such cases. This has been used to guide antivenom requirements. It is therefore important in these cases to carefully and sequentially document extent of swelling and related effects, including limb circumference. As swelling progresses, there may be significant fluid shifts into the bitten limb, potentially resulting in hypovolemic shock. In some cases, swelling and tissue injury may affect muscle compartments, resulting in true compartment syndrome, with the potential for secondary ischemic damage. Local tissue injury can also cause local necrosis and secondary infection (Chapter 245).

As venom spreads from the bite site, it may cause tenderness or enlargement of draining lymph nodes in the axilla or inguinal region. Persistent local bleeding from the bite area, without sign of normal clotting, is often an indication that systemic envenoming has occurred, with resultant coagulopathy, a complication of some, but not all, types of snakebite.

Systemic Effects of Snakebite

For many snakebites, there may be only local effects, or systemic effects may be largely limited to general effects, such as headache, nausea, vomiting, abdominal pain, or less commonly diarrhea, syncope, or convulsions, the latter most common in children. It may be difficult, initially, to determine if these effects are due to envenoming or an anxiety reaction. However, major collapse or convulsions are more likely due to envenoming. Severe, intractable headache, persistent vomiting, and severe abdominal pain are also more likely to indicate envenoming. Again, the speed of onset and severity of these symptoms may indicate the likely severity of the bite.

Neurotoxic paralysis is usually a result of NMJ pre- and/or postsynaptic neurotoxins, which act systemically rather than locally, affecting voluntary and respiratory muscle. It is a classic effect of many snake venoms, causing delayed-onset paralysis, which may take 1 to 12 or more hours to become evident. There is a progressive flaccid paralysis, often first seen in the cranial nerves, where it is easily missed if not sought by careful examination. Ptosis, partial, then complete ophthalmoplegia,

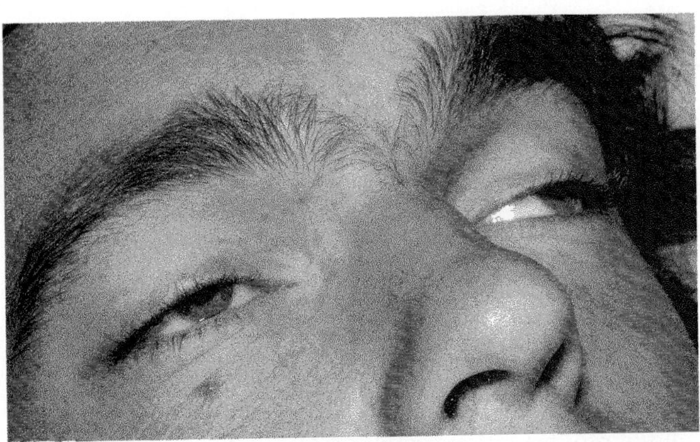

Figure 10. Ptosis and partial ophthalmoplegia, apparent on lateral gaze, as evidence of progressing flaccid neurotoxic paralysis. (Death adder bite; photograph copyright © by Dr. Julian White.)

loss of facial tone, dysarthria, and dysphagia are all common early signs of paralysis (Fig. 10). The pupils may become dilated and unresponsive to light. Progressive weakness of limbs and bulbar function may follow, the latter often requiring intubation and ventilation to protect the airway. Accessory muscles of respiration may become prominent and the patient more agitated or drowsy as hypoxia develops. The diaphragm is often the last muscle to be paralyzed and may not be fully affected for up to 24 hours after a neurotoxic snakebite. If the neurotoxin is extracellular, such as snake postsynaptic neurotoxins, then the paralytic effect may last only a few hours or may be reversible with treatment, such as antivenom or anticholinesterase, but presynaptic paralysis usually involves damage to the terminal axon, so reversal must await regeneration, which may take days, weeks, or months. Table 5 lists snakes commonly causing paralysis.

Cardiovascular effects are secondary to other venom actions, but direct cardiovascular effects, such as hyper- or hypotension, brady- or tachycardia, and cardiac dysrhythmias can occur, particularly in a few snake venoms (e.g., gaboon viper).

Local myotoxins cause local tissue damage, resulting in pain, swelling, and secondary effects, such as compartment syndrome and hypovolemic shock. *Systemic myotoxins*, such as those in some snake venoms, cause progressive myolysis of skeletal muscle resulting in muscle pain, tenderness, weakness that may mimic paralysis, and secondary effects, notably myoglobinemia, myoglobinuria (with potential secondary renal failure), hyperkalemia (with potential secondary cardiac dysrhythmia), and rise in serum enzymes, especially CK, which may reach extraordinary levels. Myoglobinuria gives the classic red to black urine that is dipstick positive for "blood."

Hemostasis effects are distinguishable by detailed coagulation and platelet function studies. However, just three basic syndromes are generally evident: incoagulable blood with bleeding tendency, poorly coagulable or incoagulable blood without clinically apparent bleeding tendency, and thrombotic tendency. The latter is unusual, but is clearly present in envenoming by a viper on the Caribbean island of Martinique, where thrombosis is a common sequelae of envenoming.

Patients with a bleeding tendency may exhibit no clinical signs other than persistent bleeding from the bite site or venipuncture sites, but more commonly there is also bleeding from the gums, and gastrointestinal tract bleeding (manifest as hematemesis or melena) and hematuria may also occur. Bleeding into a major organ or space (e.g., intracranial) produces classic signs, but more localized bleeding, such as into the pituitary (Sheehan's syndrome after Burmese Russell's viper bite), may produce more subtle or delayed signs. Any external breach of vascular integrity, such as insertion of cannulae, may result in prolonged and significant bleeding. It is therefore important to use invasive procedures cautiously in snakebite, and to avoid those with a high risk of causing significant bleeding, such as femoral, jugular, and subclavian punctures or line insertions, surgery of any type, including tracheostomy, and intramuscular injections, until it is clear there is no active coagulopathy present. Table 8 lists snakes commonly causing coagulopathy or bleeding.

The effects of *hemorrhagins* are similar to the more severe effect of hemostatically active toxins, in that they produce clinically apparent bleeding. As the two groups of toxins are usually present together and are synergistic, bleeding can be major. There may be marked bleeding in the bitten area, as other venom components assist tissue breakdown and allow extravasation of blood from vessels damaged by hemorrhagins.

Nephrotoxins, primary or secondary, exert their effect somewhat silently at first, the first indication of problems often being a rapidly falling urine output, accompanied by rising creatinine and urea. In any case of envenoming where renal failure is possible, such as many snakebites, it is therefore advisable to carefully monitor fluid input and output and give an initial intravenous (IV) fluid load.

Other systemic effects may be induced by envenoming by certain species. Of particular note is hemolysis, seen with some snakebites. Liver damage may also occur, after bites or stings by many animals, but is rarely of major significance.

Necrotoxin effects may be rapidly evident, as is seen with some snakebites (e.g., many vipers, pit vipers, some cobras), as progressive swelling, blistering, ecchymosis and darkening of skin, or liquefaction of skin (Fig. 11). Over 24 to 48 hours, this may progress to clear skin necrosis, resulting in deep ulceration, sometimes involving muscle and other deeper tissues. Pain is present in most cases. Local tissue necrosis is historically associated with viper bites in the medical literature, but not elapid bites. However, it is now known that not all vipers cause significant local effects. Neotropical rattlesnakes, in particular, generally cause systemic, not local, effects. Although most elapids cause minimal or comparatively minor local effects, some common species routinely cause moderate to severe local effects, especially necrosis. These latter necrotic elapids are cobras, from both Africa and throughout Asia. In most cases, the local

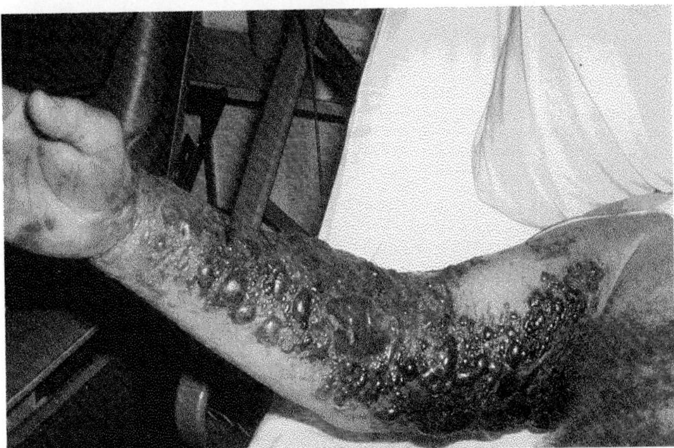

Figure 11. Extensive bleeding, swelling, bullae formation, and developing necrosis. (Rattlesnake bite; illustration copyright © by Dr. David Hardy.)

necrotic effects predominate, not systemic effects such as flaccid paralysis, though both may occur together in individual cases. Most, but not all, cobra species can cause necrosis.

FIRST AID FOR SNAKEBITE

First aid for envenoming is often controversial and frequently based on inadequate experimental or clinical research. The first principle should always be "do no harm." As a general rule, immobilization of the bitten limb is a useful technique to reduce venom transport, as many venom components are of moderate to large molecular weight and lymphatic flow is important in their transport. The use of compression bandaging (Fig. 12) is more controversial, but is apparently beneficial for certain types of snake and spider bites and a few major marine toxins (cone shells, blue ringed octopus). Recent studies with Russell's viper bite in Myanmar have indicated that a modified pressure immobilization technique may be both safe and effective for snakebites causing local tissue injury. Further studies are required to determine if this technique is generally applicable for snakebite.

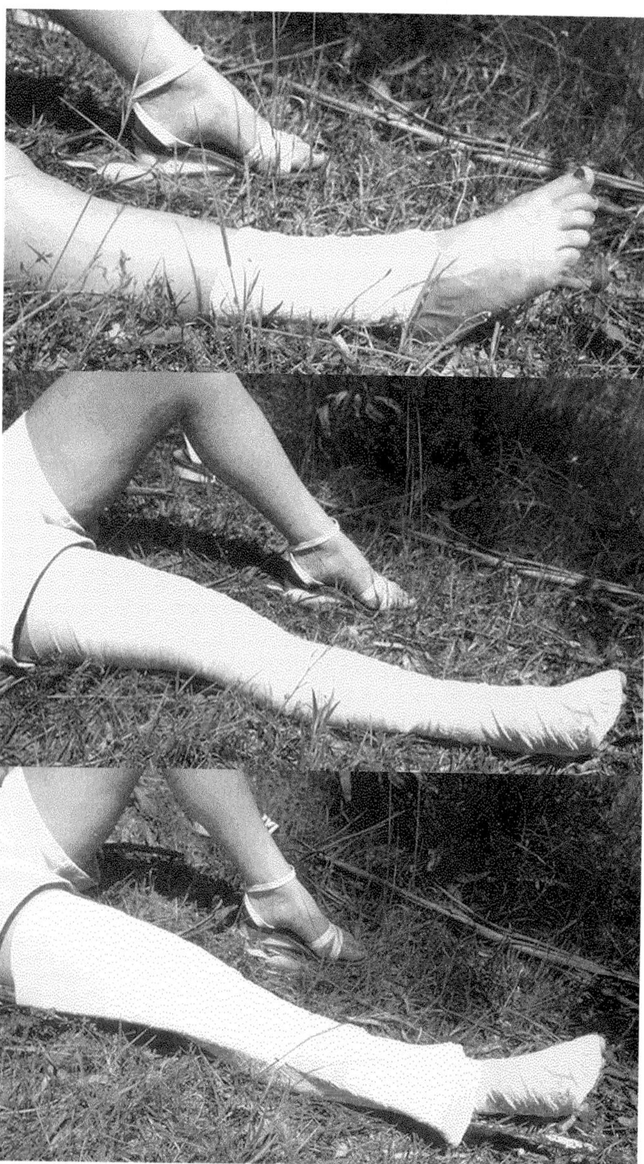

Figure 12. Australian pressure immobilization bandage technique. A broad bandage is first applied over the bite site, at a pressure equivalent to that used for a sprained ankle (i.e., not so tight as to act as a tourniquet). The bandage is then extended over the rest of the limb, over the top of clothing, keeping the limb as still as possible and covering toes/fingers to ensure they are also immobile. Last, the limb is splinted to ensure no movement occurs. Correctly applied, this first aid can safely remain in place for several hours until a suitable medical facility is reached. (Photograph copyright © by Dr. Julian White.)

Until its benefits in bites causing local injury are clarified, the potential risks from pressure immobilization in snakebites likely to cause significant local tissue injury outweigh the possible but unproven benefits of this technique. Unfortunately, this applies to snakebites in most regions, but where the bite is known to have been caused by a non-necrotoxic snake species, then pressure immobilization bandaging is the preferred method. Snakes falling into this latter group include all Australian and New Guinea species, sea snakes, kraits, mambas, coral snakes, selected African cobras, such as forest cobras, and selected Central and South American vipers, notably the neotropical rattlesnakes.

There are some first aid methods known to be either of no value or potentially harmful, and so should not be used. These include tourniquets, cutting and suctioning of the wound, application of chemicals, such as condy's crystals, or the use of cryotherapy or electric shock to the bite site. All these methods are still used in various regions of the world, most commonly for snakebite, despite the evidence that they frequently cause harm without conferring benefit. The use of proprietary suction devices to remove venom is advocated by their manufacturers, but studies of efficacy do not inspire confidence in the technique, as even in optimal circumstances at least 70% of the venom will be left in the victim. Cryotherapy has been clearly shown to be harmful. Electric shock for snakebite, though still promoted by manufacturers of these devices, has been shown to offer no benefit, and its use may delay more appropriate first aid.

MEDICAL TREATMENT OF SNAKEBITE

Most doctors will see few cases of significant envenoming, thus acquiring and maintaining skills in management is problematic. It is therefore advisable, when faced with a case of major envenoming, to seek expert advice at the earliest opportunity, either from a regional expert or from a regional poisons information center, the staff of which may facilitate referral to an appropriate expert.

Diagnosis

Diagnosis is no less crucial in effective management of snakebite than in other areas of medicine, yet is often far from simple. Patients may present with a clear history of a bite or sting and either a good description of their assailant or the assailant itself. The latter may introduce further problems if the snake is still alive. In this situation, although the diagnosis may be clear, some expertise may be required to determine the true identity of the assailant, sometimes crucial in determining which type of antivenom to consider. Equally, the extent of envenoming may not be immediately apparent, and some major types of envenoming, such as paralysis, myolysis, coagulopathy, and renal damage may not be initially evident. Given these obstacles to early accurate diagnosis where the assailant is clearly known, the situation becomes far more complex when the assailant is most uncertain, as is frequently the case.

Children may be unable to give a history of a bite or sting and may present with advanced envenoming, manifest as symptoms and signs that could involve myriad diagnoses. Beware the child with unexplained collapse and convulsions, which might be indicative of major envenoming by a snake. Adults may also be unaware of being bitten, as some snakebites are relatively painless. They later present with symptoms that might indicate a wide range of diagnoses, and the lack of a noted bite may erroneously guide the diagnostic process away from envenoming. Envenoming should be considered in otherwise unexplained collapse, convulsions, flaccid paralysis, autonomic stimulation, myolysis, coagulopathy, thrombosis, hemorrhage, renal failure, chest pain, abdominal pain, nausea and vomiting, headache, local swelling, ecchymosis, and blistering. This list covers only some of the more common effects of snake envenoming.

History

The mix of the following points in history taking will be determined by the circumstances and the nature of the assailant.

- Precise date and time of the incident that might have involved a bite.
- Geographic location at the time of the incident (to narrow down type of snake).
- A description of the snake, if possible.
- A detailed description of how the bite occurred, including how many bites (multiple bites are generally more severe), or the patient's activity at the time an unnoticed bite might have occurred.
- What first aid, if any, was used, its timing after the bite, and patient physical activity both before and after first aid applied (physical activity may decrease first aid effectiveness).
- A list of symptoms observed by the patient and their time of onset and cessation. Specifically ask for symptoms indicative of envenoming by likely snake species.
- A list of any signs noted by those with the patient, including timing of onset and cessation.
- Relevant medical history, including allergy, particularly to animals used to produce antivenom (e.g., horses, sheep, rabbits) and any medications used by the patient. Also inquire about recent use of alcohol or recreational drugs that might affect symptoms or signs.

Physical Examination

It is easy to detect many signs of envenoming if looked for, but even easier to miss them if not considered during examination. Envenoming frequently evolves over time, so repeated examination may be vital in detecting important signs. This is particularly true for systemic effects of envenoming.

- The vital signs should be measured.
- Check the bite or sting site for evidence of bite marks, distance between bite marks (may indicate mouth size for snakebite), multiple bites, local effects such as erythema, edema, blistering, ecchymosis, and necrosis.
- The regional lymph nodes should be palpated for evidence of venom spread (swelling or tenderness).
- Examine for specific venom effects:
  - Flaccid paralysis: ptosis, ophthalmoplegia (partial or complete), pupil dilation, loss of facial tone, limited mouth opening or tongue extrusion, palatal paresis, drooling, limb weakness, gait disturbance, accessory respiratory muscle use, depressed or absent deep tendon reflexes, depressed or absent response to painful stimuli (note the patient still feels the pain, but cannot withdraw due to paralysis, so consideration for patient distress is important), cyanosis, signs of hypoxia, including confusion.
  - Myotoxicity: muscle tenderness, pain on contraction against resistance, weakness (may mimic paralysis), muscle spasm, rarely compartment syndrome signs due to massive muscle swelling. Also check electrocardiogram for evidence of hyperkalemic effects.
  - Cardiotoxicity: cardiac dysrhythmias, arrest, electrocardiogram abnormalities (various).
  - Coagulopathy and hemorrhagins: persistent ooze of blood from bite site, venipuncture sites, bleeding gums, bruising, occasionally signs consistent with a bleed into an internal organ/space (e.g., intracranial, etc.).
  - Nephrotoxicity: usually little to find; check for oliguria or anuria.

Diagnostic Tests

The extent and nature of laboratory tests are determined by the likely type and extent of envenoming and the availability of laboratory resources.

In a basic health facility:

- Urine output: check for hematuria or myoglobinuria (red or black urine; dipstick test positive for blood; simple microscopy for red cells).
- Coagulopathy: 20-minute whole blood clotting test (if poor or absent clot, indicates coagulopathy; requires only needle, syringe, and glass tube or container).
- Venom detection (Australia only at present; in development for Southeast Asia, Brazil): simple commercial enzyme-linked immunosorbent assay–based test for Australian snake venoms (Fig. 13). Best sample is the bite site. If there is systemic envenoming, then urine could be tested, but blood is unreliable as a sample. A positive result indicates both that a snakebite has occurred and the most appropriate antivenom, but is not an indication to give antivenom, as venom can be on the skin, without significant systemic envenoming. A negative result does not exclude snakebite, so is of little diagnostic help.

In a fully resourced hospital:

- Urine output: check for hematuria or myoglobinuria (red or black urine; dipstick test positive for blood; simple microscopy for red cells).
- Blood tests: avoid repeated venipunctures, especially if there may be a coagulopathy; in such cases consider inserting a long line via the cubital fossa, or an arterial line.
- Extended coagulation studies: prothrombin time/international normalized ratio, activated partial thromboplastin time, fibrinogen level, fibrin(ogen) degradation products.

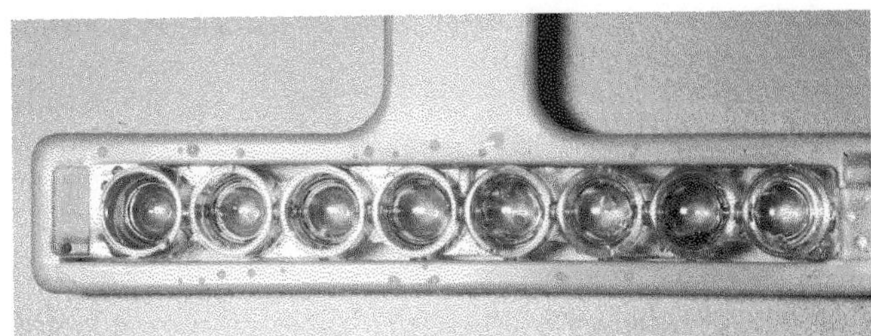

Figure 13. Australian CSL Snake Venom Detection Kit. This commercial kit uses a sandwich enzyme-linked immunosorbent assay to detect snake venom, distinguishing between the five major types of Australian dangerous snakes, allowing use of specific, rather than polyvalent, antivenom. (Photograph copyright © by Dr. Julian White.)

- Complete blood picture: raised white cell count suggestive of envenoming or infection; absolute lymphopenia suggestive of certain types of snake envenoming; hemoglobin level (look for evidence of hemolysis); thrombocytopenia may indicate direct or indirect effect of some snake venoms or secondary disseminated intravascular coagulation.
- Electrolytes and renal function: look for hyperkalemia if there is myolysis or renal failure.
- CK: elevated, sometimes to extreme levels, in presence of myolysis.
- Liver function tests: enzyme levels may be elevated if there is myolysis.
- Arterial blood gas: relevant only if advanced respiratory failure due to neurotoxic paralysis or pulmonary edema. Avoid if there is active coagulopathy present.
- Venom detection: see comments above for a basic health facility.

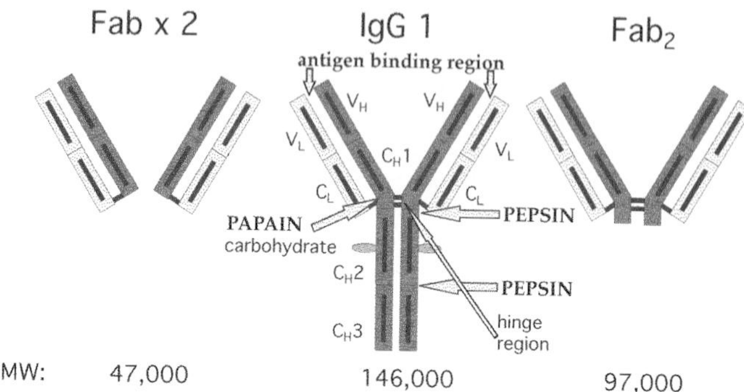

Figure 14. Diagrammatic representation of the three types of antibody or fraction used in antivenoms currently. Ig, immunoglobulin; MW, molecular weight. (Illustration copyright © by Dr. Julian White.)

Requirement for Intensive Care

Major envenoming is often optimally managed in an intensive care setting. The major requirement for intensive care is respiratory support for cases with advanced neurotoxic flaccid paralysis. Respiratory support, including intubation and ventilation, may be needed only for a few hours, but for some snake species, may be required for days, weeks, or months, until the NMJ regenerates. Intubation and ventilation are often required to maintain airway safety, long before there is full respiratory paralysis. Tracheostomy should be avoided until there is complete resolution of any coagulopathy or hemorrhagic tendency; all invasive procedures with the potential to cause bleeding should be avoided for similar reasons.

ANTIVENOMS

Antivenoms are the treatment of choice, where available, for most forms of major envenoming. Old aphorisms suggesting antivenom is more dangerous than envenoming are generally ill-founded and inappropriate. Nevertheless, antivenom therapy carries certain risks and should only be used when clearly indicated. However, for many venomous snakes and in many less developed regions, antivenom is either unavailable or economically impractical.

Antivenoms are specific antidotes to venoms. Virtually all are whole or fractionated animal immunoglobulin (Ig) G raised against a target whole venom, rather than specific venom components. Antivenoms are polyclonal and may contain far more neutralizing activity against some venom components than others. To produce antivenoms, a source of venom for immunizing must be determined. The choice of venoms may strongly influence the clinical efficacy of an antivenom; if only a narrow range of species or species from a small part of a geographic range is used, then the antivenom may lack desired efficacy against bites from a wider range of species.

Antivenoms may be truly monovalent (raised against the venom of a single species of animal), "monovalent" to genus level (cover all or several species within a genus, or occasionally closely related genera), or polyvalent (raised against venoms from a variety of species, usually unrelated apart from a common geographic range). Most commonly, the animal used for immunizing is the horse, but sheep, goats, rabbits, and even chicken egg yolk have been used. Horse-based antivenoms, in particular, have a generally high incidence of adverse reactions, but the rate of reactions is also determined by the degree and quality of refining, particularly removal of non-IgG components, such as albumin, and where IgG has been fractionated, removal of Fc fragment contaminants. Recently, sheep have been used successfully to produce ovine IgG Fab' antivenoms. The three major types of antivenom, based on the degree of fractionation are: whole IgG, $F(ab')_2$, and Fab' (Fig. 14). The recent development of IgY antivenoms and studies of the relative efficiencies of whole IgG versus IgG fractions may yield quite different and more effective antivenoms in the future. Certain venom components appear to be effectively neutralized by IgY antivenom, but other components are best neutralized by whole IgG, raising the possibility of mixed antivenoms, containing IgY and ovine, rather than equine, IgG.

Principles of Antivenom Therapy

The first principle of antivenom therapy is to tailor the dose to the individual situation. From this, it follows that just as the degree of envenoming varies from nil ("dry bite") to severe systemic, so the amount of antivenom required varies from none to potentially large quantities. Most failures of antivenom therapy can be attributed to inadequate dosage or wrong choice of antivenom. The quantity required is determined by the type of snake, not the size of the patient. There are no pediatric doses of antivenom; children require the same amount as adults. Determining how much antivenom to administer requires considerable clinical judgment. For some regions there are guidelines covering common species of snakes. This information is not always available in product literature. It is beyond the scope of this chapter to detail how much of each antivenom to give in any possible clinical case. Consultation with regional, national, or international experts is advised if the appropriate dose is unclear. Lists of available antivenoms and appropriate antivenoms for each snake species are available at http://www.toxinology.com.

The second principle of antivenom therapy is to give it as soon as possible once it is indicated. From this, it follows that in most situations of acute envenoming, the IV route is preferred. This always applies to snakebite, where antivenom should never be given intramuscularly or locally at the bite site.

The third principle is to monitor the effect of antivenom therapy carefully. This includes monitoring both effectiveness in counteracting envenoming and observing for adverse effects of therapy. It is frequently the case that an initial dose of antivenom may be insufficient and that follow-up doses may be required. Some venom may be sequestrated at the bite site, being released over a period of hours or days, necessitating ongoing antivenom therapy. Equally, the type of antivenom influences clearance as well as compartmental distribution. Fab' antivenoms are more rapidly cleared than $F(ab')_2$ or whole IgG antivenoms, so are more likely to require continuous infusion or regular repeated doses. This is particularly so for the new ovine Fab' antivenom for North American rattlesnake bites (Chapters 74 and 245).

Complications of Antivenom Therapy

There are several principal complications of antivenom therapy. *Acute reactions* include anaphylaxis and related early reactions, rash, and febrile reactions (usually related to toxin contamination). *Delayed reactions* include serum sickness. Failure of efficacy is an unrecognized complication that is related to (a) selection of an incorrect antivenom, (b) infusion of an inadequate dose, (c) use of an inappropriate route of administration (intramuscular or local injection when IV was required), (d) commencing therapy too late, (e) use of an expired or poorly stored antivenom (i.e., refrigerated antivenom that has been exposed to prolonged heat), or (f) use of a poor-quality antivenom.

Several methods have been employed to minimize the chance of adverse effects from antivenom therapy. The concept of skin sensitivity testing before administration is flawed in both theory and practice. Such sensitivity testing delays treatment, fails to reliably predict major adverse reactions (e.g., anaphylaxis), potentially sensitizes the patient to antivenom should it be required in the future, and may precipitate an anaphylactic reaction. For these reasons, skin sensitivity testing is not recommended, even though it has been advised by a number of antivenom producers in the past, particularly in North America. The new ovine antivenom available in the United States does not require the use of skin sensitivity testing.

Premedication before antivenom therapy is controversial and is not widely accepted or practiced therapy. Antihistamines and steroids have been shown to have no real benefit in preventing acute antivenom reactions. In addition, antihistamines may induce drowsiness or, occasionally, hyperexcitability, both potentially dangerous in major envenoming. Epinephrine (adrenaline) has been shown to reduce the likelihood of adverse reactions for certain high-risk antivenoms (those that are poorly refined, with a high rate of adverse reactions) in a single trial, but its benefit for other antivenoms is uncertain and it carries clear risks that may outweigh any potential benefits. This is particularly true if the envenoming causes increased bleeding, as seen with many snakebites. Premedication is not currently recommended by antivenom producers. Future studies may better define its role, if any.

Use of Diluted Antivenom Infusions

Most antivenoms should be given IV. Many experts recommend dilution of the antivenom up to 1:10 in a suitable diluent for IV use, such as normal saline or Hartman's solution. The degree of dilution is limited by the volume of antivenom and the size of the patient. Although this technique may be useful, it is not strictly necessary, as studies have shown that IV push neat antivenom does not carry a higher incidence of acute adverse effects. In addition, the latter technique requires the doctor to stay with the patient throughout the antivenom infusion, which increases the chances of rapidly and effectively responding to acute adverse events.

Antivenom should always be given in the expectation that anaphylaxis may occur, even though this complication is rare with well-purified antivenoms. Thus, epinephrine (adrenaline) should always be ready in a syringe or set up as an infusion before commencing antivenom therapy and both staff and equipment for resuscitation should be on hand.

Contraindications to Antivenom Therapy

There are no absolute contraindications to antivenom in the treatment of proven envenoming. However, antivenom therapy is associated with risks, as discussed earlier, so should only be used if the likely benefit outweighs potential adverse effects. Antivenom works best for systemic envenoming. It is generally effective at relieving general systemic symptoms, such as headache and vomiting, and is also effective at reversing coagulopathy and, in most cases, postsynaptic paralysis. It is probably beneficial in treating venom-induced myolysis, even late, but is of uncertain benefit in treating venom-induced renal damage and of little or no use in reversing presynaptic paralysis. Antivenom is less effective in treating local effects of envenoming, but still has a role and certainly should be considered in cases with likely major local effects, as seen with many viper bites.

Certain medications can modify the immune system response, both potentiating the likelihood of an anaphylactic reaction and reducing the effectiveness of treatment for such a reaction, even with epinephrine (adrenaline). Two groups of drugs, the β-adrenergic receptor blockers and angiotensin-converting enzyme inhibitors, have been implicated in this problem. Most published experience relates to anaphylactic reactions to bee stings and radiologic contrast agents, but while not yet verified, it is likely it will also apply to immune reactions to antivenoms. Therefore, patients taking beta-blockers or possibly angiotensin-converting enzyme inhibitors may be at higher risk of major anaphylactic reactions to antivenom. This does not imply they should not be given antivenom, but that indications for antivenom use should be particularly stringent.

Sourcing Antivenoms

For antivenoms required for local species there is usually a common source, often a regional or national antivenom producer. There are significant areas of the world with moderate to high rates of envenoming where antivenom is either in short supply, very expensive, or completely unavailable. There are many venomous snakes for which there is either no specific antivenom or no useable antivenom. For exotic venomous snakes, such as in zoos or private collections, appropriate exotic antivenoms may be unavailable or difficult to source in reasonable time and quantity. A number of major zoos with reptile houses in both North America and Europe stock a range of exotic antivenoms. Poison information centers may also have lists of institutions stocking exotic antivenoms, as well as experts in clinical toxinology who may be consulted on the management of envenoming by exotic animals.

The range of antivenom producers is constantly changing, though the total number of producers is in decline. The names of producers, their contact details and available products are ever changing. Therefore readers are encouraged to seek current information from internet sources, as listed earlier.

NONANTIVENOM TREATMENTS

Although antivenom is often the preferred treatment of significant envenoming, it is not available for all snakes, nor in all areas of the world. Nonantivenom treatments may be effective as adjuncts to antivenom or as alternatives in some situations.

Pharmaceutical

Anticholinesterases may be useful for flaccid neurotoxic paralysis due to postsynaptic snake neurotoxins. They may be used as an adjunct to antivenom or as sole therapy where antivenom is unavailable. First, perform a Tensilon test to determine efficacy.

Fresh frozen plasma may be of value in replacing depleted clotting factors after snakebite coagulopathy, but potentially hazardous if given before neutralization of all circulating venom.

Surgical

Although surgical intervention is rarely appropriate in acute envenoming, some surgical maneuvers are worthy of particular comment. *Fasciotomy*, a technique for releasing local tissue pressure, is generally only warranted to relieve proven (by intracompartmental pressure manometry or by Doppler) intracompartmental syndrome, where failure to do so would be likely to result in significant long-term ischemic injury. Even in this latter, uncommon situation, most likely encountered with some forms of snakebite, any coagulopathy should first be under control. Unwarranted fasciotomy in snakebite, used merely because of extensive tissue swelling, frequently results in long-term cosmetic and functional deformity and is to be avoided.

Bite site wound excision has no substantial evidence to suggest it is effective in immediate envenoming. It is likely to result in short- and long-term complications.

COMPLICATIONS OF VENOMOUS SNAKEBITE

Of the many potential complications of envenoming that may occur, a few particularly common or important varieties are discussed here, most pertaining to snakebite.

Paralysis

Flaccid neurotoxic paralysis is a potentially lethal complication of major envenoming by a variety of venomous snakes (Table 5). It may develop rapidly or be more gradual and insidious in onset. The latter may result in missing early signs, so that diagnosis is not made until paralysis is advanced. There are three principal maneuvers available to manage significant paralysis: intubation and ventilation, administration of antivenom, and administration of anticholinesterases (effective only for postsynaptic-type paralysis).

A fully paralyzed snakebite patient may appear severely cerebrally injured, with fixed dilated pupils, absent reflexes, flaccid tone, and no response to painful stimuli. Nevertheless, the patient may be awake, terrified, and well able to feel painful stimuli. Great care and consideration are required in managing such patients. By manually opening their eyes and moving their head around, they will be able to see their environment and those caring for them. Often, it is possible to find at least some residual muscle movement that can be used to establish communication, even if just indicating "yes" and "no." Aspiration pneumonia and secondary infections are also significant risks in these patients. If the paralysis is presynaptic, then assisted ventilation may be required for weeks or months, necessitating consideration of tracheostomy after 1 to 2 weeks.

Myolysis

Major myolysis is a distinguishing feature of some species (Table 6). Myolysis is most problematic when systemic. Even late administration of antivenom may sometimes speed resolution. Early and maintained good renal throughput, by ensuring adequate hydration, may reduce the chance of secondary renal damage. Hyperkalemia is always a risk in these cases and should be actively sought and vigorously treated if present. At least in the early stages, over the first 1 to 10 days, when muscle breakdown is peaking, it is advisable to avoid procedures that might increase muscle damage, such as active physiotherapy.

Coagulopathy

Although coagulopathy can be a result of envenoming by a wide range of animals, by far the most common cause is snakebite (Table 8). Antivenom is the preferred treatment, giving enough to neutralize expected venom load. In general, replacement therapy (fresh frozen plasma, cryoprecipitate) is unnecessary. Great care is required to avoid iatrogenic bleeding, through injudicious insertion of cannulae. Beware femoral punctures, subclavian and jugular line insertions, and arterial blood gas sampling. For established coagulopathy, where repeat venous sampling is required to titrate antivenom therapy against response, an indwelling line, such as a long line through the cubital vein, may be advantageous.

Necrosis

The single most important aspect of care for necrotic bite wounds is good wound care: keeping the wound clean, elevated, and avoiding early surgical débridement. Infection should be treated with antibiotics targeted to the causative organism, thus culture and sensitivity testing should be routine.

Infection

Although uncommon, tetanus does occasionally develop after snakebite, so tetanus prophylaxis should be routine. Avoid injections in snakebite, however, until any coagulopathy is resolved. In most cases, prophylactic antibiotics are unnecessary. If secondary infection occurs, endeavor to culture the organism and so target antibiotic therapy. If this is impractical, assume a wide possibility of organisms and use an antibiotic combination appropriate to provide wide coverage.

Follow-Up

Although mild envenoming without complications may not warrant follow-up, major envenoming usually does. In particular, patients who have received antivenom should be informed of the symptoms of serum sickness, so that they will report for early assessment should this complication arise. Both major physical and emotional sequelae of envenoming may occur and require extensive follow-up.

SUGGESTED READINGS

Covacevich J, Davie P, Pearn J, eds. *Toxic plants and animals; a guide for Australia.* Brisbane: Queensland Museum, 1987.

Gopalakrishnakone P, Chou LM, eds. *Snakes of medical importance (Asia Pacific region).* Singapore: National University of Singapore, 1990.

Habermehl G. *Venomous animals and their toxins.* Berlin: Springer Verlag, 1981.

Harvey A, ed. *Snake toxins.* London: Pergamon Press, 1991.

Howarth MH, Southee AE, Whyte IM. Lymphatic flow rates and first aid in simulated peripheral snake or spider envenomation. *Med J Aust* 1994:161;695–700.

Junghanss T, Bodio M. *Notfall-handbuch gifttiere.* Stuttgart: Thieme, 1996.

Kamiguti AS, Hay CRM, Theakston RDG, Zuzel M. Insights into the mechanism of haemorrhage caused by snake venom metalloproteinases. *Toxicon* 1996:34(6);627–642.

Kochva E, Bdolah A, Wollberg Z. Sarafotoxins and endothelins; evolution, structure and function. *Toxicon* 1993:31(5);541–568.

Lalloo D, Trevett A, Black J, et al. Neurotoxicity and haemostatic disturbances in patients envenomed by the Papuan black snake (Pseudechis papuanus). *Toxicon* 1994:32(8);927–936.

Markland FS. Snake venoms and the hemostatic system. *Toxicon* 1998:36(12);1749–1800.

Mebs D. *Gifttiere; ein handbuch für biologen, Ttoxikologen, arzte, apotheker.* Stuttgart: Wissenschaftliche Verlagsgesellschaft mbH, 2000.

Meier J, White J, eds. *Handbook of clinical toxicology of animal venoms and poisons.* Boca Raton, FL: CRC Press; 1995.

Minton SA. Bites by non-native venomous snakes in the United States. *Wilderness Envir Med* 1996:4;297–303.

Shier W, Mebs D, eds. *Handbook of toxinology.* New York: Marcel Dekker Inc., 1990.

Sutherland S. *Australian animal toxins.* Melbourne: Oxford University Press, 1983.

Theakston RDG, Warrell DA. Antivenoms: a list of hyperimmune sera currently available for the treatment of envenoming by bites and stings. *Toxicon* 1991:29;1419–1470.

Tun-Pe, Aye-Aye-Mtint, Khin-Ei-Han, et al. Local compression pads as a first aid

measure for victims of bites by Russell's viper (*Daboia russelii siamensis*) in Myanmar. *Trans Roy Soc Trop Med Hyg* 1995:89;293–295.
Warrell DA. The clinical management of snake bites in the south east Asian region. *Southeast Asian J Trop Med Public Health* 1999:30(suppl. 1);1–85.
Warrell DA, Hudson BJ, Lalloo DG, et al. The emerging syndrome of envenoming by the New Guinea small-eyed snake *Microechis ikaheka*. *QJM* 1996:89;523–530.
Weatherall D, Ledingham J, Warrell D, eds. *The Oxford textbook of medicine*, 3rd edition. Oxford: Oxford University Press, 1996.
Weinstein SA, Kardong KV. Properties of Duvernoy's secretions from opisthoglyphous and aglyphous colubrid snakes. *Toxicon* 1994:32(10);1161–1186.
White J. Envenoming and antivenom use in Australia. *Toxicon* 1998:36(11);1483–1492.
White J, Persson H. Snakes. In: Descotes J, ed. *Human toxicology*. Amsterdam: Elsevier, 1996.
Williamson J, Fenner P, Burnett J, et al. *Venomous and poisonous marine animals; a medical and biological handbook*. Sydney: University of NSW Press, 1996.

CHAPTER 245

Crotaline Snakebite

Richard C. Dart and Barry S. Gold

Topics included:	**Family Viperidae; subfamily Crotalinae; genus *Agkistrodon, Crotalus,* or *Sistrurus* (Table 1)**
Normal levels:	**Not clinically available**
Special concerns:	**Local tissue injury and potentially severe coagulopathy, which may develop in a delayed manner.**
Antidote:	**Snake antivenom**

OVERVIEW

The crotaline snakes, also known as the *pit vipers* or *New World vipers*, inhabit North and South America. The crotaline snakes are represented by the rattlesnakes (see Color Plates 1 and 2), pigmy rattlesnakes and massasauga, the copperheads, and water moccasins. The pit vipers inhabit every state in the United States with the exception of Alaska, Hawaii, and Maine. The most common pit viper bite is undoubtedly the copperhead snake. The eastern and western diamondback rattlesnakes cause the most fatalities. The principal crotaline snakes of the United States are provided in Table 1.

A snakebite may occur under a variety of circumstances. Snakes in the wild may bite when stepped on or handled by individuals trying to identify or capture them. Many crotaline snakes are kept in captivity in home zoos or in the illicit snake trade. Still another source of bites is the infamous "rattlesnake rodeos," in which competitive games like "sacking" (a race to stuff the most snakes possible into a burlap bag within 60 seconds) are played for entertainment. Unfortunately, this event can lead to bites and has culminated in death of the human participant. Finally, snakes are still used in a few isolated areas for religious ceremonies.

Classification and Uses

These snakes were previously categorized as the crotalid snakes (family *Crotalidae*). However, the classification nomenclature is now family *Viperidae*, subfamily *Crotalinae*; therefore, the more appropriate term *crotaline* is used to refer to the *Crotalinae* subfamily (1), which includes North American species of *Agkistrodon* (copperhead and cottonmouth snakes), *Crotalus* (rattlesnakes), and *Sistrurus* (massasauga and pigmy rattlesnakes).

Pit vipers have a triangular head and elliptical pupils. Crotalid snakes are also distinguished by two hollow fangs that can be folded against the roof of the mouth, in contrast to the coral snakes, which have shorter, fixed, and erect fangs. The fangs are replaced throughout the life cycle of the snake; consequently, no fangless or defanged snake remains harmless indefinitely (2). The crotaline snakes have bilateral depressions ("pits") located midway between the eye and the nostril, thereby creating the term *pit vipers* (Fig. 1). The pit is a heat-sensitive organ that guides strikes against warm-blooded prey or predators.

Within the pit vipers, the rattle distinguishes the rattlesnake from other crotaline snakes. The rattle is formed by a group of loose, interlocking keratin rings that vibrate against one another when shaken, producing the characteristic buzzing sound. It is speculated that the rattle functions as a warning device to predators (3). One persistent myth states that rattlesnakes always "rattle" before striking. In fact, the successful snake strike often occurs without a warning rattle.

Chemical and Physical Properties

Crotaline venom is a complex enzyme mixture. Its components include molecules ranging from individual metal ions to complex multi-unit proteins with a molecular weight in excess of 150,000 daltons (Table 2). Venom is a highly stable substance, refractory to temperature fluctuations, desiccation, and drugs (4). The venom components can cause local (tissue injury, systemic vascular damage) and systemic effects (hemolysis, fibrinolysis, and neuromuscular dysfunction) depending on the specific snake. Other variables that affect venom composition include season, time since last feeding, age of the snake, and diet.

Epidemiology

The true incidence of snakebites in North America has not been established. Published data would suggest that there are as many as 8000 venomous snakebites annually in the United States (5). However, most experienced clinicians would estimate a smaller number (6). Hospital death reports indicate that there are about 6 deaths per year in the United States (7).

Toxic Doses

The dose of venom that is toxic is unknown. The lethal dose for 50% of a group of experimental animals (LD_{50}) for various venoms has been published and typically varies substantially depending on the laboratory performing the assay. There is also intraspecies variability in the LD_{50}. A single bite can cause injury or even death. Death typically occurs in patients that are bitten

TABLE 1. Crotaline snakes of the United States

Scientific name	Common name
Crotalus	**Rattlesnakes**
C. adamanteus	Eastern diamondback rattlesnake
C. atrox	Western diamondback rattlesnake
C. cerastes	Sidewinder
C.c. cerastes	Mohave desert sidewinder
C. cercobobmus	Sonoran sidewinder
C. laterorepens	Colorado desert sidewinder
C. horridus	Timber rattlesnake
C. lepidus	Rock rattlesnake
C. klauberi	Banded rock rattlesnake
C. lepidus	Mottled rock rattlesnake
C. mithcellii	Speckled rattlesnake
C. pyrrhus	Southwestern speckled rattlesnake
C. stenhensi	Panamint rattlesnake
C. molossus	Blacktail rattlesnake
C. pricei	Twin-spotted rattlesnake
C. ruber	Red diamond rattlesnake
C. scutulatus	Mojave rattlesnake
C. tigris	Tiger rattlesnake
C. viridis	Western rattlesnake
C. abyssus	Great canyon rattlesnake
C. cerberus	Arizona black rattlesnake
C. concolor	Midget faded rattlesnake
C.v. heleri	Southern Pacific rattlesnake
C. lutosus	Great Basin rattlesnake
C. nuntius	Hopi rattlesnake
C.v. viridis	Prairie rattlesnake
C. obscurus	New Mexico ridgenose rattlesnake
C. willardi	Arizona ridgenose rattlesnake
Sistrurus	**Pigmy rattlesnakes and massasauga**
S. catenatus	Massasauga
S.c. catenatus	Eastern massasauga
S.c. ewardsii	Desert massasauga
S.c. tergeminus	Western massasauga
S. miliarius	Pigmy rattlesnake
S.m. barbouri	Dusky pigmy rattlesnake
S.m. miliarius	Caroline pigmy rattlesnake
S.m. steckeri	Western pigmy rattlesnake
Agkistrodon	**Copperhead and cottonmouth**
A. contortrix	Copperhead
A.c. contortrix	Southern copperhead
A.c. laticinctus	Broad-banded copperhead
A.c. mokasen	Northern copperhead
A.c. phaeogaster	Osage copperhead
A.c. pictigaster	Tras-[ecos] copperhead
A. piscivorus	Cottonmouth
A.p. conanti	Florida cottonmouth
A.p. lecuostoma	Western cottonmouth
A.p. piscivorus	Eastern cottonmouth

Modified from Collins JT. *Standard common and current scientific names for Northern American amphibians and reptiles*, 3rd ed. *SSAR Herp Circ* 1990;19:26–33.

by rattlesnakes species and do not receive prompt antivenom treatment. Death after bites by *Agkistrodon* or *Sistrurus* is very unusual.

TOXICOKINETICS AND TOXICODYNAMICS

Snake venom is produced as a complex mixture that varies throughout the life cycle of the snake. Furthermore, most methods to measure venom use immunologic methods. Thus, an antibody must be produced against a group of venom antigens. Some venom components are potent immunologic stimulants and others are not. In short, there is variability within the venom to be measured as well as the technique that measures the venom. Therefore, it is extremely difficult to characterize the toxicokinetics of snake venom and results cannot be extrapolated.

A few general statements about envenomation can be made for clinical purposes. Crotaline snake venom is most commonly injected subcutaneously and occasionally intramuscularly. Absorption usually begins immediately and begins to produce toxic effects within minutes. In rare cases, the onset of effects may be delayed for several hours (8). The metabolism and elimination of snake venom components vary by the individual component and are affected by the injury itself as well as treatment. Some components are excreted rapidly, whereas others can persist for many days. Initial swelling theoretically confines venom locally in the tissues and produces a very prolonged absorption phase.

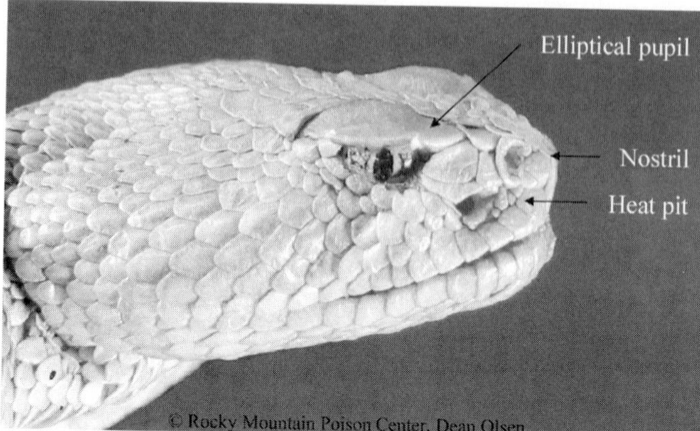

Figure 1. Identifying characteristics of the pit vipers. Features of the crotaline snakes include an elliptical pupil, nostril, and heat pit. (Photograph copyright © 2003 Rocky Mountain Poison and Drug Center.)

PATHOPHYSIOLOGY

The effects of crotaline snakebite can be grouped as local (e.g., pain, swelling, erythema, ecchymosis), coagulopathic (hypofibrinogenemia, thrombocytopenia) and systemic (hypotension,

TABLE 2. Enzymes in North American snake venoms

	Crotalus	*Sistrurus*	*Agkistrodon*
Proteolytic enzymes	+	+	+
Arginine ester hydrolase	+	NK	+
Thrombin-like enzyme	+	NK	+
Collagenase	+	NK	+
Hyaluronidase	+	NK	+
Phospholipase A_2(A)	+	NK	+
Phospholipase B	?	NK	NK
Phosphomonoesterase	+	NK	+
Phosphodiesterase	+	+	+
Acetylcholinesterase	0	0	0
RNAse	+	NK	NK
DNAse	+	NK	NK
5'-Nucleotidase	+	NK	+
NAD-Nucleotidase	0	0	+
L-Amino acid oxidase	+	+	+
Lactate dehydrogenase	NK	NK	NK

+, present; NK, not known.
From Russell FE. *Snake venom poisoning*. Great Neck, NY: Scholium International, 1983:179, with permission; and modified from Gold BS, Dart RC, Barish RA. Bites of venomous snakes. *N Engl J Med* 2002;347:347–356.

altered mental status). The local effects are most common. During a bite, crotaline venom may be deposited intradermally, subcutaneously, intramuscularly, or rarely, into a blood vessel. Crotaline venom first causes local tissue injury, quickly altering blood vessel permeability, and allowing loss of plasma and blood into the surrounding tissue. Electron microscopy shows that venom proteins damage capillary endothelium, resulting in blebs, dilation of the perinuclear space, and plasma membrane destruction (9). Plasma and erythrocytes leak into the tissues, resulting in marked accumulation of fluid in intracellular spaces, which is manifested as edema and ecchymosis. Plasma loss reduces the circulating blood volume and leads to hemoconcentration, hypovolemic shock, and lactic acidosis. Most patients with significant envenomation have hypovolemia.

After absorption into the blood, venom components also consume fibrinogen and platelets, resulting in a coagulopathy, often multicomponent in nature. The most common effects seem to be hypofibrinogenemia and thrombocytopenia. The mechanisms by which a coagulopathy are induced vary by the venom. For example, fibrinogen may be converted by thrombin-like enzymes in the venom, resulting in an unstable fibrin clot. In turn, this "clot" is lysed by the fibrinolytic system, resulting in a consumptive coagulopathy. The mechanisms of coagulopathy are addressed in Chapter 244.

The systemic effects of the crotaline snakes are the most poorly characterized. In some species, specific venom fractions block neuromuscular transmission, leading to ptosis, respiratory failure, and other neurologic effects. Some components also depress cardiovascular function, although their specific role in the clinical effects is unknown. Depression of the central nervous system also occurs in severe cases through undescribed mechanisms.

VULNERABLE POPULATIONS

There are few data available to assess the effect of venom during pregnancy. The few data available suggest that envenomation often causes catastrophic pregnancy outcome, including abruption and spontaneous abortion (10). Most authorities recommend treating the pregnant patient in the same manner as nonpregnant patients, including antivenom administration early in the course of treatment.

Many studies have attempted to address unique aspects of pediatric envenomation by North American crotaline snakes. The most striking aspect of these studies, all retrospective chart reviews, is the similarity of a bitten child to a bitten adult (11–13). Although there can be minor variations in care for the pediatric patient, the dose of antivenom and all major diagnostic and therapeutic decisions are the same for adults and children.

CLINICAL PRESENTATION

Crotaline snakebite results in either in envenomation or a dry bite. Approximately 20% to 25% of crotaline bites are dry: No venom effects develop (14). When venom is injected, the clinical manifestations of poisoning represent a complex interplay between the victim and the many components of the venom. Variables that may affect the severity of clinical effects include the species and size of the snake; the amount of venom injected; the age, size, and co-morbid conditions of the victim; the time elapsed since the bite; and characteristics of the bite (location, depth, and number). The victim's unique susceptibility to the venom also impacts the ultimate severity.

Owing to these factors, the severity of poisoning after a crotalid bite is variable. At least two classification systems for crotaline snakebite have been proposed. However, these are generally insufficient for clinical evaluation. A severity grading system for clinical research has been developed and appears useful; however, it was not designed for clinical care and requires an experienced clinician for its application (15).

The severity of snakebite is best communicated in descriptive terms. The clinically important characteristics to describe are (a) local manifestations, (b) coagulation abnormalities, (c) systemic effects, and (d) the change of venom effects over time. The importance of this final factor cannot be overemphasized. The absence of all three manifestations (local, coagulation, systemic) for a period of 8 to 12 hours after the bite indicates that no venom was injected.

Local Effects

Local effects include the presence of one or more fang marks, localized pain, and progressive edema extending from the bite site (see Color Plates 3 through 6) (14). Although the classic lesion is a pair of fang marks, scratches or small lacerations may be evident instead. In general, swelling becomes apparent within 15 to 30 minutes, but in unusual cases it may not start for several hours (8,16). In severe cases, edema may progress to involve an entire limb within an hour. The edema typically continues to worsen for several hours, although it may continue to expand for a day or more. Edema near an airway or in a muscle compartment may threaten life or limb without the presence of systemic effects.

Progressive ecchymosis may also occur because of leakage of blood into subcutaneous tissue. Ecchymoses may appear within minutes or hours in the area of the snakebite. If untreated, it may become massive (Fig. 2). Hemorrhagic blebs may occur within several hours for similar reasons.

Although uncommon, increased compartment pressure and compartment syndrome may develop. If untreated, this injury can permanently impair the use of the muscles in the compartment. Unfortunately, the classic manifestations of compartment syndrome (pain out of proportion to the apparent injury, pallor, pulselessness, paresthesiae) can be caused by venom in the absence of compartment syndrome (17). The only reliable method to confirm the diagnosis is to perform serial compartment pressure measurements. A fundamental difference between a compartment syndrome in a patient with rattlesnake envenomation compared to trauma is the theoretical combined effect of venom-induced injury and pressure injury (18).

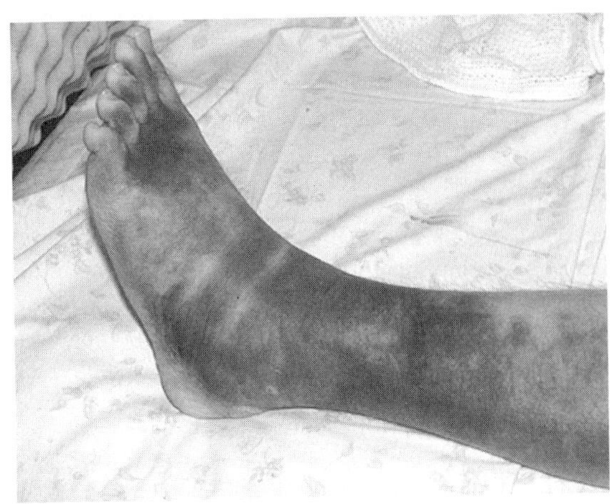

Figure 2. Massive ecchymosis induced by western diamondback snake venom. (Photograph copyright © 2003 by Richard C. Dart, M.D.) (See Color Plate 5.)

TABLE 3. Management of suspected compartment syndrome after crotaline snake envenomation

Determine the intracompartmental pressure.
If not elevated, continue standard management.
If signs of compartment syndrome are present and the compartmental pressure is >30 mm Hg:
 Elevate limb.
 Administer mannitol 1–2 g/kg IV over 30 min.
 Also infuse Polyvalent Crotalidae Antivenin 6 vials IV over 60 min.
 If elevated compartment pressure continues, consider fasciotomy.

Note: Caution: This protocol delivers a high osmotic load.

The typical treatment of compartment syndrome after trauma involves fasciotomy to mechanically relieve the increased intracompartmental pressure. Intense debate surrounds the use of fasciotomy, because it does not prevent the progression of the envenomation syndrome (e.g., coagulopathy) or obviate the need for additional antivenom. Evidence regarding the efficacy of surgical fasciotomy is sparse. Indeed, animal studies indicate that antivenom is the most effective treatment, and that fasciotomy may actually worsen outcome (19).

Therefore, the recommended treatment for venom-induced compartment syndrome is to administer antivenom and mannitol (Table 3) (17,20). If these measures are unsuccessful, fasciotomy is often attempted, but rarely effective. A related effect is increased subcutaneous pressure within a bitten digit. Although not a compartment technically, the skin can act as a compartment and cause very high tissue pressure as swelling progresses. One solution to this problem is to perform a simple procedure termed *digit dermotomy* (17,21).

Coagulation Effects

Although frank bleeding is a rare manifestation of crotaline snakebite, coagulation abnormalities are common. Either platelets or the coagulation cascade may be affected. The coagulation defect may be evident within minutes or be delayed for hours. Thrombocytopenia is more common with rattlesnake bites, especially certain species such as the timber rattlesnake (22). In severe cases, there may be no platelets measurable. The coagulation cascade can be affected through reduction of fibrinogen or other components. The prothrombin time (PT) and international normalized ratio (INR) are often greatly prolonged. Curiously, a normal fibrinogen in conjunction with a prolonged INR may occur (the converse may also occur). The pathophysiology for these presumably incompatible findings is unclear.

Systemic Effects

Early systemic signs of crotaline snake venom poisoning are nausea and vomiting, weakness, oral numbness, or tingling of tongue and mouth. As the envenomation syndrome progresses, tachycardia, dizziness, thrombocytopenia, and myokymia may develop. Hemoconcentration often develops as a result of fluid loss into subcutaneous tissue, followed by a decrease in hemoglobin over several days from blood loss secondary to coagulopathy.

Respiratory compromise is unusual, but does occur. A retrospective chart review of rattlesnake bites from Arizona reported respiratory compromise in 8% of patients and endotracheal intubation in 0.7% of patients. None of the intubations was needed due to an allergic reaction to antivenom (23). It is important to realize that a distal extremity bite can cause airway edema, compromise, and emergent airway management. Airway compromise is often erroneously attributed to local venom injury to the mouth after sucking on the wound. It is well documented to occur as a primary venom effect (24).

Myolysis is another systemic complication of some crotaline snake venoms. In the United States, the canebrake rattlesnake (*C. horridus atricaudatss*) can cause massive increases in creatine kinase (CK). Complications of myolysis (e.g., hyperkalemia) may be fatal (25). The normal course of elevated CK is to peak within a few days and then resolve over a week or more.

Outcome

Although well-established for diseases such as myocardial or cerebral ischemia, the concept that "Time is Tissue" seems underappreciated in the treatment of crotaline snakebite. However, few concepts could be more obvious. It is not unusual for the inexperienced clinician to hesitate in administering antivenom because the initial progression is slow. Indecision allows time for envenomation syndrome to progress.

The few long-term follow-up studies of snakebite that have been performed have all indicated that swelling is the most common long-term morbidity of crotaline snakebite. Spiller evaluated 81 patients with copperhead snake, timber rattlesnake, or other venomous snakebites in adult and pediatric patients. Due to the predominance of copperhead snakes, only nine patients received antivenom. The mean duration of edema (self-reported) was 11.4 days [standard deviation (SD) ± 12 days]. Recurrent edema frequently occurred with limb activity. Of the 37 employed patients, the mean duration of lost work was 14 days (SD ± 18.1 days). Of the 26 patients bitten on the hand or finger, duration of reduced function persisted for a mean of 14.3 days (SD ± 10.4 days) and reduction of hand strength persisted for a mean of 22 days (SD ± 25.5) (26). Similar results have been reported for copperhead snakes (27) as well as other crotaline snakes (28). Unfortunately, no clinical trial has yet tested the effect of antivenom on the local sequelae of crotaline snakebite. However, it is clear that major morbidity occurs and the opportunity for improvement with antivenom exists.

DIAGNOSTIC TESTS

The diagnosis of snakebite is based on the presence of fang marks and a history consistent with exposure to a snake (walking through a field, handling of a snake, etc.). Snake envenomation usually involves the presence of fang marks plus evidence of local or systemic manifestations.

At a minimum, the platelet count and PT or INR should be determined. The presence of an abnormality indicates that systemic absorption of venom has occurred. It is also useful to measure the fibrinogen level, which is occasionally depressed in the presence of a normal PT or INR.

Several other tests should be obtained in patients with signs of progressive envenomation. A complete blood count often reveals a falling hematocrit, although transfusion is very rarely needed. Serum electrolytes and renal function tests are used to monitor for hyperkalemia and renal insufficiency, potential complications of muscle injury. The CK is monitored to evaluate muscle injury. It may become extremely elevated in cases of myolysis (e.g., canebrake rattlesnake) or compartmental syndrome.

DIAGNOSTIC PITFALLS

The most common error is to assume that the initial presentation of the patient represents the ultimate severity of the bite. Many patients progress to much more severe envenomation. Patients discharged with a "dry" bite have subsequently died.

TREATMENT

Treatment of crotaline snakebite may include first aid measures, the administration of antivenom, and the treatment of complications such as compartment syndrome or tissue necrosis. First aid measures are popular, but none has been proven to be effective. Furthermore, the effects of envenomation can be delayed, therefore, all patients with a pit viper bite should go to a health care facility promptly for evaluation.

Decontamination and First Aid Measures

First aid measures are a controversial aspect of snakebite treatment. In general, measures are postulated to work by removing venom (e.g., suction), confining it (e.g., tourniquet), or destroying it (e.g., electric shock). At best, these measures are only partially effective and should never substitute for definitive medical care or delay the administration of antivenom. Table 4 classifies the usefulness of various first aid measures based on numerous animal trials and limited data from humans. The most common first aid measure is suction, with or without an initial incision. A venom suction kit (without incision) has been marketed for many years. Unfortunately, the research evidence suggests that this technique is unlikely to be effective and causes adverse events (29). Some kits contain blades for incision and can injure digital nerves, arteries, and tendons. Incision is not recommended.

Constriction bands may be of some use when medical care is not available or will be delayed. A constriction band is applied circumferentially above the bite to decrease superficial venous and lymphatic flow while maintaining distal pulses and capillary fill. The band should be snug, but loose enough to slide a finger underneath. In theory, a constriction band retards venom absorption, which should increase local tissue injury but reduce the severity of systemic effects. Animal studies and limited human experience suggest that the use of a constriction band delays venom absorption (30).

Other useless and potentially dangerous techniques include electric shock, ice, and tourniquets. Electric shock treatment of the bite site is mentioned only to be condemned. This dangerous procedure is not effective and has resulted in burns and other injuries (31). Other worthless first aid measures include ice-water immersion, which simply adds cold injury to the insult of venom injury. Tourniquets are contraindicated because they obstruct arterial flow and cause ischemia.

TABLE 4. Clinical usefulness of first aid measures for crotaline snakebite

First aid measure	Comments
Likely to be effective	
Immobilization	Multiple animal experiments indicate immobilization reduces systemic absorption of venom.
Possibly effective, but unlikely to be clinically useful	
Incision and suction	In animal experiments, incision and suction are only effective if done immediately.
Suction devices	Suction devices may increase skin necrosis at bite site and have not been demonstrated to improve outcome.
Not effective or clinically useful	
Tourniquets	Decreases absorption, however, adds ischemic injury to venom injury.
Electric shock therapy	All animal studies have showed no effect or harmful effects. Human case reports indicate potential adverse events.
Ice application or ice-water immersion	Adds cold injury to venom injury. Application for short period (i.e., 30 min) unlikely to cause injury. Longer duration increases likelihood of injury.

Emergency Management

In the prehospital phase of care, personnel should immobilize the limb, establish intravenous access in an uninvolved limb, and transport the victim to a medical facility. Most care is consistent with basic life support and advanced life support protocols. The limb should be immobilized at heart level or below until arrival at a facility with antivenom available. Tourniquets and constriction bands should not be applied. If already present, they should not be removed until intravenous access is established and antivenom is available (32).

Initial life-saving care includes management of the airway and hypotension. The airway is managed in the usual manner. Bites to the face are surprisingly common. Furthermore, facial swelling is not an unusual effect of snakebite to other areas of the body. If the patient is hypotensive, initial treatment should include rapid intravenous isotonic fluid infusion. Large volumes may be needed. The limb should be immobilized. The optimal position of immobilization has not been established. In general, the limb is elevated when antivenom is available to encourage absorption and thereby make the venom available for binding by antivenom (Fig. 3). Consultation with a physician or poison center familiar with the management of snake envenomation is recommended for all but the simplest of cases.

Enhancement of Elimination

Extracorporeal measures have not been tested for the acute treatment of snakebite. Given the high molecular weights of many compounds, it seems unlikely that it would substantially alter the clinical course. Hemodialysis may be needed in occasional cases of acute renal failure arising from myoglobinuria.

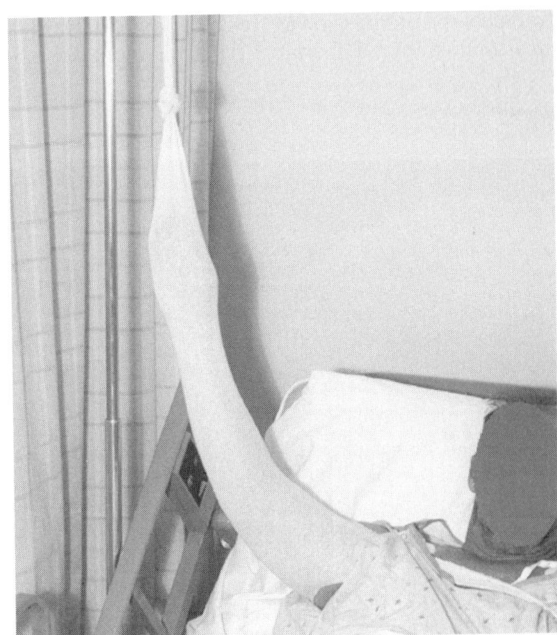

Figure 3. Elevation of the arm after a rattlesnake bite. (Photograph copyright © 2003 by Richard C. Dart, M.D.)

Antidotes

Antivenom is the definitive treatment for North American crotaline snake envenomation. The primary antivenom available in the United States is Crotalidae polyvalent immune Fab (ovine) (FabAV, CroFab). Details regarding its production, method of administration, and adverse effects are provided in Chapter 74. The production of another antivenom, Antivenin (Crotalidae) Polyvalent (Wyeth) for human use was apparently discontinued for human use in 2001 (31). The Wyeth antivenom was a horse-derived and less well-purified product that caused more frequent allergic complications, including anaphylaxis culminating in death (31).

The primary indication for FabAV therapy is the progression of the local, systemic, or coagulopathic effects of snake venom. Progression is defined as worsening of local injury (e.g., pain, ecchymosis, or swelling), laboratory abnormalities (e.g., worsening platelet count, prolonged coagulation times, decreased fibrinogen), or systemic manifestations (e.g., unstable vital signs or abnormal mental status).

Antivenom should be administered only in a critical care facility such as an emergency department or intensive care unit. After reconstitution, the antivenom is initially infused slowly, until it is evident that anaphylaxis will not occur. If a reaction does not develop, the rate should be increased in a stepwise manner until the infusion is complete, typically over 1 hour. Infusion of antivenom should be done under the direct supervision of a physician. If an acute allergic reaction occurs, the infusion should be stopped immediately and antihistamines administered (both H_1- and H_2-receptor blockers). Epinephrine should be added depending on the severity of the reaction (Chapter 34).

The endpoint of antivenom therapy is to establish *initial control*, defined as the arrest of progression of local injury and the improvement of coagulation and systemic signs. A typical dose of FabAV to establish initial control involves two courses of four to six vials, followed by a total of six vials for maintenance therapy (total, 14 to 18 vials). It is important that close patient observation for progression of edema and systemic signs of envenomation be continued after antivenom infusion. Limb circumference should be measured at several sites above and below the bite, and the advancing border of edema should be outlined with a pen every 30 to 60 minutes (Fig. 4). This serves as an index of the progression as well as a guide for further antivenom administration. Laboratory determinations are repeated after each course of antivenom therapy initially and then every 4 to 6 hours after initial control has been established.

The return of venom effect after initial control of the envenomation syndrome has been established is termed *recurrence*. Potentially, there are three forms of recurrence: local, coagulopathy, and systemic, corresponding to the three types of effects that are caused by crotaline snake venom. Systemic recurrence has not been described for FabAV. *Local recurrence* involves the return of swelling after it has apparently been halted by antivenom. Local recurrence is uncommon (33). It usually occurs within 12 to 24 hours of treatment. Local recurrence should be distinguished from other causes of swelling, such as redistribution of edema, infection, and venous thrombosis. All cases reported have involved local recurrence during the patient's hospitalization. Local recurrence after discharge has not been reported. The treatment of local recurrence has not been established. Most physicians have administered an additional dose of FabAV, usually two to six vials.

Coagulopathic recurrence involves the return of prolonged INR, thrombocytopenia, or depressed fibrinogen after they had returned to normal after antivenom administration. Coagulopathic recurrence usually occurs after the patient is discharged. It has been demonstrated for the previous equine Wyeth antivenom as well (34). Thus, the recurrence may go undetected unless coagulation tests are measured after discharge.

Recurrent coagulopathy may partially respond to antivenom administration. If given early, further antivenom may be effective; however, the beneficial effect may be mild or transient (33). For example, routine laboratory testing 2 days after discharge may reveal an asymptomatic thrombocytopenia of 50,000/mm^3 (normal >140,000/mm^3). Additional antivenom may produce a recovery, or only slightly increase the platelet count to 75,000/mm^3. Even if successful, subsequent studies may find that the platelet level falls again. The use of antivenom in such circumstances is controversial. Although coagulation tests are often abnormal, the risk of clinically significant hemorrhage is likely much lower than expected (33,35). Current recommendations suggest that recurrent coagulopathy be treated only if it is extreme and involves more than one coagulation abnormality, or there is evidence of significant bleeding (Fig. 5) (33,35). Most coagulopathy recurrences can be safely managed with observation and serial laboratory monitoring as well as bleeding precautions. Occasionally, patients may need to be hospitalized until it resolves, typically within 2 weeks.

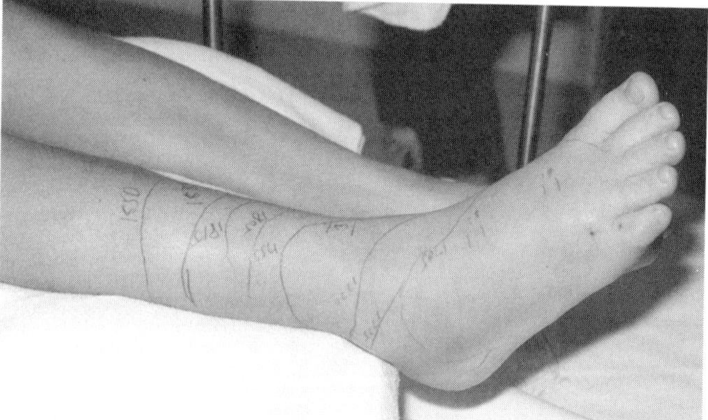

Figure 4. Measurement of swelling after rattlesnake envenomation. This method is performed by simply marking the leading edge of swelling or tenderness with an indelible pen every 15 to 30 minutes. This technique has the advantage of leaving a "map" of the patient's course for subsequent caregivers when the patient is admitted. (Photograph copyright © 2003 by Richard C. Dart, M.D.)

Supportive Care

Attentive supportive care is an important, but often overlooked, aspect of care. Intravascular volume depletion is common in patients with a significant envenomation syndrome. Nearly all patients should receive generous resuscitation with isotonic crystalloid fluids (e.g., 0.9% normal saline). If pressor agents are needed, it is likely that volume resuscitation and antivenom therapy have been insufficient. Vasopressor drugs can be useful, but should be needed for transient periods only. Antivenom is the best treatment for coagulopathy, but blood component replacement is occasionally needed. Blood component replacement should only be given after sufficient quantities of neutralizing antivenom have been administered.

Another complication of snakebite is *compartment syndrome*. Increased compartment pressure may occur when venom is injected into a compartment during a bite. This is usually manifest by severe pain, localized to a compartment that is resistant to narcotic analgesia. The preponderance of animal and human data as well as extensive clinical experience indicates that antivenom without fasciotomy is the optimal treatment (19,20). Recommended management is shown in Table 3.

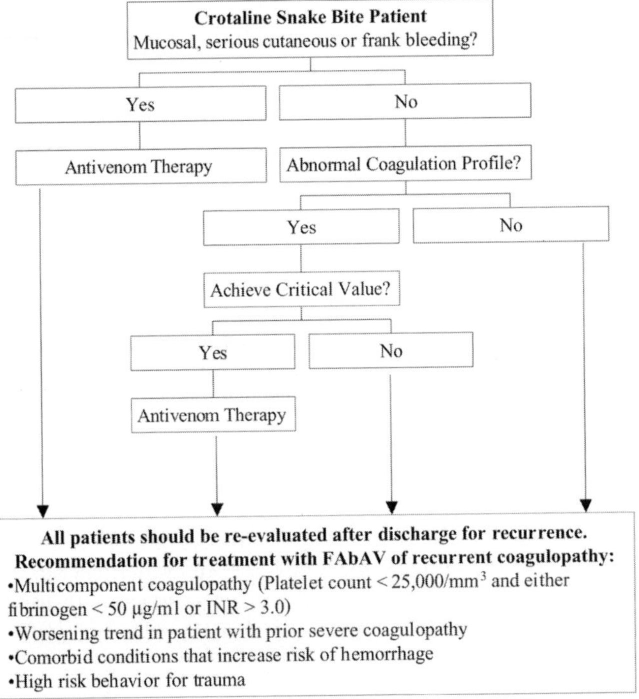

Figure 5. Management of coagulation recurrence after rattlesnake envenomation. INR, international normalized ratio. [Modified from Yip L. Rational use of crotalidae polyvalent immune Fab (ovine) in the management of crotaline bite. *Ann Emerg Med* 2002;39:648–650; and Boyer LV, Seifert SA, Cain JS. Recurrence phenomena after immunoglobulin therapy for snake envenomations: part 2. Guidelines for clinical management with crotaline fab antivenom. *Ann Emerg Med* 2001;37:196–201.]

The wound area should be cleaned and a tetanus booster administered if more than 10 years from the patient's last booster. Blood or wounds should be cultured and antibiotic therapy initiated only if signs of infection are present. The published evidence does not support the use of prophylactic antibiotics (36,37). The use of steroids is also controversial. Several studies suggest lack of efficacy or even deleterious effects. Without evidence of efficacy, steroids should be avoided, except for the treatment of an allergic reaction or serum sickness.

Serum sickness is a type III hypersensitivity reaction that may be seen 7 to 21 days after treatment with a foreign equine or ovine serum (Chapter 74). Serum sickness manifests as fever, rash, arthralgias, and lymphadenopathy. It responds well to a tapering course of prednisone, generally starting at a dose of 60 mg/day, with a rapid taper over a 7- to 10-day period.

Disposition

Patients are ready for discharge when swelling begins to resolve, the coagulopathy has been reversed, and the patient is ambulatory. Once the coagulopathy has resolved, the bitten part (particularly the hand) should be regularly exercised to preserve function and strength. Outpatient follow-up is performed to monitor for serum sickness and infection.

Patients with severe or life-threatening bites and patients receiving antivenom should be admitted to an intensive care unit. The general ward is appropriate for patients with mild or moderate envenomation who have completed or do not require further antivenom therapy.

Patients with dry bites who have been observed for at least 8 hours may be discharged. They should return if pain, swelling, or bleeding develops.

REFERENCES

1. McDiarmid RW, Campbell JA, Toure TA. Snake species of the world: a taxonomic and geographic reference. Washington, DC: The Herpetologists' League, 1999:234–351.
2. Gold BS, Wingert WA. Snake venom poisoning in the United States: a review of therapeutic practice. *South Med J* 1994;579–589.
3. Klauber LM. Rattlesnakes: their habits, life, histories and influence on mankind, vol 2, 2nd ed. San Diego: University of California Press, Zoological Society of San Diego, 1972.
4. Russell FE, Eventor J. Lethality of crude and lyophilized *Crotalus* venom. *Toxicon* 1964;2:81–84.
5. Parrish HM. Incidence of treated snakebites in the United States. *Public Health Rep* 1966;81:269–76.
6. Gold BS, Dart RC, Barish RA. Bites of venomous snakes. *N Engl J Med* 2002;347:347–356.
7. Langley RL, Morrow WE. Deaths resulting from animal attacks in the United States. *Wild Environ Med* 1997;8:8.
8. Hurlbut KM, Dart RC, Spaite D, et al. Reliability of clinical presentation for predicting significant pit viper envenomation. Abstract. *Ann Emerg Med* 1988;17:438–439.
9. Ownby C. Pathology of rattlesnake envenomation. In: Tu AT, ed. *Rattlesnake venoms*. New York: Marcel Dekker, 1982:163–209.
10. Dunnihoo DR, Rush BM, Wise RB, et al. Snakebite poisoning in pregnancy. A review of the literature. *J Reprod Med* 1992;37:653–658.
11. LoVecchio F, DeBus DM. Snakebite envenomation in children: a 10-year retrospective review. *Wilderness Environ Med* 2001;12:184–189.
12. Offerman SR, Bush SP, Moynihan JA, et al. Crotaline Fab antivenom for the treatment of children with rattlesnake envenomation. *Pediatrics* 2002;110:968–971.
13. Shaw BA, Hosalkar HS. Rattlesnake bites in children: antivenin treatment and surgical indications. *J Bone Joint Surg (Am)* 2002;84:1624–1629.
14. Russell FE. *Snake venom poisoning*, 3rd ed. Great Neck, NY: Scholium International, 1983.
15. Dart RC, Garcia RA, Hurlbut KM, et al. Development of a severity score for the assessment of crotalid snakebite. *Ann Emerg Med* 1996;27:321–326.
16. Guisto JA. Severe toxicity from crotalid envenomation after early resolution of symptoms. *Ann Emerg Med* 1995;26:387–389.
17. Hall EL. Role of surgical intervention in the management of crotaline snake envenomation. *Ann Emerg Med* 2001;37:175–180.
18. Garfin SR, Castilionia RR. The effect of antivenin on intramuscular pressure elevations induced by rattlesnake venom. *Toxicon* 1985;23:677–680.
19. Stewart RM, Page CP, Schwesinger WH, et al. Antivenin and fasciotomy/debridement in the treatment of severe rattlesnake bite. *Am J Surg* 1989;158:543–547.
20. Gold BS, Barish RA, Dart RC, et al. Resolution of compartment syndrome after rattlesnake envenomation utilizing non-invasive measures. *J Emerg Med* 2003;24:285–288.
21. Watt CH Jr. Treatment of poisonous snakebite with emphasis on digit dermotomy. *South J Med* 1985;78:694–699.
22. Bond GR, Burkhart KK. Thrombocytopenia following timber rattlesnake envenomation. *Ann Emerg Med* 1997;30:40–44.
23. Brooks DE, Graeme KA, Ruha AM, et al. Respiratory compromise in patients with rattlesnake envenomation. *J Emerg Med* 2002;23:329–332.
24. Hinze JD, Barker JA, Jones TR, et al. Life-threatening upper airway edema caused by a distal rattlesnake bite. *Ann Emerg Med* 2001;38:79–82.
25. Carroll RR, Hall EL, Kitchens CS. Canebrake rattlesnake envenomation. *Ann Emerg Med* 1997;30:45–48.
26. Spiller HA, Bosse GM. Prospective study of morbidity associated with snakebite envenomation. *J Toxicol Clin Toxicol* 2003;41:125–130.
27. Thorson A, Lavonas EJ, Rouse AM, et al. Copperhead envenomations in the Carolinas. *J Toxicol Clin Toxicol* 2003;41:29–35.
28. Dart RC. Sequelae of pit viper envenomation. In: *Biology of pit vipers*. Campbell JA, Brodie ED Jr, eds. Tyler, TX: Selva Publishing, 1992:395–404.
29. Bush SP, Hegewald K, Green SM, et al. Effects of a negative pressure venom extraction device (Extractor) on local tissue injury after artificial rattlesnake envenomation in a porcine model. *Wilderness Environ Med* 2000;11:180–188.
30. Burgess JL, Dart RC, Egen NB, et al. The effects of constriction bands on rattlesnake venom absorption: a pharmacokinetic study. *Ann Emerg Med* 1992;21:1086.
31. Dart RC, McNally J. Efficacy, safety, and use of snake antivenoms in the United States. *Ann Emerg Med* 2001;37:181–188.
32. McKinney PE. Out-of-hospital and interhospital management of crotaline snakebite. *Ann Emerg Med* 2001;37:168–174.
33. Boyer LV, Seifert SA, Cain JS. Recurrence phenomena after immunoglobulin therapy for snake envenomations: part 2. Guidelines for clinical management with crotaline fab antivenom. *Ann Emerg Med* 2001;37:196–201.
34. Bogdan GM, Dart RC, Falbo SC, et al. Recurrent coagulopathy after antivenom treatment of crotalid snakebite. *South Med J* 2000;93:562–566.
35. Yip L. Rational use of crotalidae polyvalent immune Fab (ovine) in the management of crotaline bite. *Ann Emerg Med* 2002;39:648–650.
36. Clark RF, Selden BS, Furbee B. The incidence of wound infection following crotalid envenomation. *J Emerg Med* 1993;11:583.
37. LoVecchio F, Klemens J, Welch S, Rodriguez R. Antibiotics after rattlesnake envenomation. *J Emerg Med* 2002;23:327–328.

CHAPTER 246

Elapid Snakes

Julian White

Topics included:	**Cobras, coral snakes, mambas, kraits, Australian elapid snakes (brown snake, tiger snake, copperhead snakes, mulga, black snake, taipan, others)**
Normal levels:	**Not applicable; Snake Venom Detection Kit detects venom qualitatively**
Special concerns:	**Most common and dangerous effect is paralysis. Local tissue injury or myolysis may occur with some species.**
Antidote:	**Snake antivenom**

OVERVIEW

Elapid or cobra-type snakes are widely distributed and are a major cause of snakebite globally and the only cause of venomous snakebite in Australia, New Guinea, and related areas (distribution maps are provided in Chapter 244). Classically, elapid snakebite is associated with neurotoxic envenoming, not significant local envenoming or coagulopathy. This view is in error. For example, cobras of Africa and Asia more commonly cause local tissue injury than paralysis. In Australia, not all major species cause paralysis, but many cause severe coagulopathy and some cause severe myolysis. Coral snakes cause myolysis more often than paralysis. The same is true for sea snakes. Thus, the classic aphorism, that if there is paralysis, it is an elapid bite, if there is local tissue injury or coagulopathy, it is a viper bite, should be abandoned. This is a crucial understanding because vipers and elapids coexist in most regions of the world.

This chapter provides information on major groups of elapid snakes throughout the world, but apart from a few key species, does not discuss clinical effects and management at a species level. The taxonomy and identification of these snakes are also not discussed in detail. Readers desiring this level of detail should consult the Clinical Toxinology Resources Web site (http://www.toxinology.com).

General Characteristics of Elapid Snakes

Elapid snakes occupy many niches and therefore have evolved into many different forms and sizes, though all have the basic characteristics of snakes. The arrangement of head scales on elapids is generally different from vipers, with fewer but larger scales the rule. There are fewer body scale rows. Body form is generally more slender, and the head less triangular and less distinct from the neck than in vipers. There are clear exceptions to this, such as the death adders of Australasia, which show more viper-like morphology and habits.

Elapid fangs are usually smaller in proportion to body length than in vipers. The fang is anteriorly placed on a minimally mobile maxilla, so that the fang cannot be folded against the roof of the mouth to enable mouth closure. This has probably limited fang length. Again, there are exceptions in fang length, with a few elapids, all large species, having quite long fangs, in some cases exceeding 10-mm length.

Elapid venoms mostly contain at least some toxins with potential for systemic action, the most common being neurotoxins, generally postsynaptic only. A few species, particularly in Australasia, have potent pre- and postsynaptic neurotoxins. Only the cobras have potent toxins causing local tissue injury, but the wide distribution and frequency of human encounters make cobras of great medical significance. A number of elapids have potent myolytic toxins. Only the Australian elapids are known to have potent procoagulant or anticoagulant toxins likely to cause adverse effects in humans.

CLINICAL PRESENTATION

The pattern of clinical effects varies between species. The major possibilities are listed here with characteristic clinical presentation. For each snake group discussed later, each likely clinical effect is only listed by type, without clinical presentation always discussed. The reader is referred back to this section for more detailed clinical presentation.

Neurotoxic Flaccid Paralysis

Neurotoxic flaccid paralysis is first seen as ptosis, then ophthalmoplegia, followed by dysarthria, poor tongue protrusion, dysphagia, drooling, then limb weakness, depressed or absent deep tendon reflexes, and lastly respiratory paralysis. The progression from first signs to full respiratory paralysis may take only a few hours or may take more than 12 hours, depending on the size of the patient, the size of the snake (amount of venom injected), and the species.

There are two major types of neurotoxin: presynaptic and postsynaptic. Presynaptic toxins damage the terminal axon at the neuromuscular junction, so this type of paralysis is not reversed by antivenom therapy. Postsynaptic neurotoxins bind to the acetylcholine receptor at the muscle endplate, and so paralysis may be reversible with antivenom therapy. Mambas cause paralysis by a slightly different mechanism, discussed in the section Mambas.

Myolysis

Myolysis is generally systemic rather than local. It may take several hours, occasionally more than 24 hours, to become clinically apparent. Features include muscle pain and tenderness, muscle weakness, myoglobinuria, elevated plasma creatine kinase (CK) (may be grossly elevated), with the potential for secondary renal failure and hyperkalemia, the latter potentially cardiotoxic.

Coagulopathy

In elapids, essentially restricted to Australian and New Guinea species, even severe coagulopathy may not generate symptoms initially. There are two principal types of elapid coagulopathy; procoagulant and anticoagulant. Procoagulant coagulopathy causes rapid defibrination, with undetectable fibrinogen and grossly elevated fibrin(ogen) degradation products. Defibrination can be complete within 15 to 30 minutes after a bite by some species. Once defibrinated, the patient is at risk of major hemorrhage, but spontaneous hemorrhage is uncommon, though lethal intracranial bleeds have been reported. Platelet counts are usually normal or only slightly reduced, unless there is massive bleeding or development of a secondary disseminated intravascular coagulation. Clinical signs of defibrination are often minor, such as persistent ooze from the bite site, occasionally oozing gums, rare hematemesis or hemoptysis. Prolonged bleeding from venipuncture sites or intravenous line insertion sites is common, and great care should be taken in such procedures.

Anticoagulant coagulopathy is caused by only a very few species. It is characterized by an abnormal international normalized ratio and activated prothrombin time, but normal fibrinogen and degradation products are absent. Platelet count is normal. Pathologic bleeding in these cases is rare. The only clinical sign may be ooze from the bite site.

Renal Damage

Renal damage may be primary, though this has yet to be proven for any elapid snake. More common is secondary renal damage after coagulopathy, myolysis, or a hypotensive episode. Renal injury may manifest as only a slight rise in creatinine in some cases, through to full oliguric or anuric renal failure in others. Renal cortical necrosis, though described, is very rare. Clinical manifestations of early renal failure are few, apart from falling or absent urine output.

Local Tissue Injury

Only cobras are clearly able to cause significant local tissue injury. The bite is usually painful. Over a period of hours to days, an area of skin around the bite site becomes dusky, sometimes bluish-brown, as necrosis develops. There is often a surrounding halo of blistering of the skin, marking the edge of the full necrotic area. This may extend over several days, until the dead skin sloughs. Although more extensive blistering can occur, it is not common. Blood-filled blisters and associated ooze are not characteristic of cobra bite necrosis. The affected area is often painful. There may be swelling, though this is not a universal feature.

Venom Spit Ophthalmia

Only selected cobras spit their venom, often aiming for the eyes of their victim. Venom contacting the eyes causes immediate pain, swelling, and blepharospasm; conjunctival injection and corneal injury can follow. In poorly treated cases, the latter can result in permanent blindness. Systemic envenoming from venom-spit ophthalmia does not appear to occur.

TREATMENT OF ELAPID BITES

There are two accepted types of first aid for elapid snakebite.

Type 1 is for species not likely to cause local tissue injury. The Australian pressure immobilization bandage method is appropriate. It is safer than tourniquets, and when correctly applied, may be left in place for several hours until a hospital or medical center able to treat snakebite is reached. However, it is effective and useable only for bites to limbs. It cannot be used for bites to the body, head, or neck.

The pressure immobilization technique involves a broad bandage applied over the bitten area with a firm, but not occlusive, pressure (approximately the same pressure as used for a sprain). The bandage is then extended to cover as much of the bitten limb as possible, including fingers or toes, over the top of clothing, rather than risking limb movement by removing clothing. The limb is then immobilized using some form of splint. The patient is then carried to transport. The patient should not walk or be otherwise physically active. In Australia, it is important not to wash the bite site, as this may interfere with venom detection tests, but elsewhere, washing the wound gently is acceptable. Be aware of the potential for early syncopal collapse and aspiration of vomitus, so position appropriately on transport to protect the airway. Should respiratory paralysis develop, support ventilation.

Type 2 is for species with the potential to cause local tissue injury. Use of the pressure immobilization bandage has not yet been proven safe for this type of bite. Concern has been expressed that it may increase the pain and probability of serious local tissue injury. Although increased pain has been reported, increased tissue injury has not been reported. For bites where there is a considerable risk of potentially lethal flaccid paralysis and a likely prolonged delay in reaching medical care, then the relative risks of increasing local injury versus delaying onset of systemic envenoming should be considered.

If the pressure immobilization bandage is not going to be used, then gently clean the wound and immobilize the bitten limb with a splint, avoiding direct pressure in the bitten area. Carry the patient to transport. The patient should not walk or be otherwise physically active.

Hospital Management

The degree of urgency required for managing elapid bites is related to the species responsible. Particularly in Australia, there are many small elapid species that are unlikely to cause medically significant effects. However, the size of the snake is not an absolute indicator of harmlessness. Small juveniles of some dangerous species, even at less than 30 cm in length, can inflict potentially lethal bites. In consequence, all elapid bites should be initially managed as potentially severe, requiring urgent full assessment. Only once it is established beyond doubt that the snake was either a minor, nondangerous species or that the bite was minor, with no evidence of systemic or major local envenoming (in the case of cobras), can the patient be reassured and considered for discharge.

DIAGNOSIS

Diagnosis should focus on two aspects: determining if the snake was a species likely to cause medically significant effects, and determining if there is evidence of either local or systemic envenoming. In Australia and New Guinea only, there is a commercial venom detection kit that can identify the broad type of snake from venom left on the skin surface at the bite site. If there is systemic envenoming, it may also detect venom in the urine. Blood is not a reliable sample for this test. Venom can be detected on the skin surface in the absence of systemic envenoming, so a positive test result is not an indication to give antivenom, but does assist in deciding which antivenom to use, if such treatment is otherwise indicated. Similarly, a negative venom detection test does not exclude snakebite. Venom detection kits are being developed for some parts of South East Asia.

In addition to venom detection, in Australia there are published diagnostic algorithms to assist in determining the most likely species of snake involved, based on a constellation of local and systemic effects. Obviously, such a system only works if there is systemic envenoming, but this is reasonable, as only patients with systemic envenoming require antivenom therapy. Similar algorithms have been developed for parts of the Asia-Pacific region and more are being developed for other areas (see www.toxinology.com for updates).

TREATMENT

The principles of snakebite management and antivenom use are provided in Chapter 244. Detailed information on available antivenoms and the species covered is available at http://www.toxinology.com. It is important to remember certain salient points in management.

- Because a patient who is initially well may develop envenoming hours later, frequent repeated assessment (examination and laboratory tests) is important.
- Antivenom is the key instrument of treatment, but should not be used indiscriminately; it should generally only be given to patients with systemic envenoming, the major exception being cobra bites with significant local tissue injury likely.
- Antivenom is the key therapy for coagulopathy, not factor replacement. In patients bitten by species likely to cause coagulopathy, be very careful in establishing vascular access.
- Antivenom may reverse pure postsynaptic paralysis, but will not reverse presynaptic paralysis, so there is no justification for giving large and continuous doses of antivenom in the latter situation. For pure postsynaptic paralysis, anticholinesterases may assist management, but should not replace antivenom therapy if the latter is available. Use the Tensilon test to determine if anticholinesterases will be effective.
- Antivenom may be useful therapy for major myolysis, even more than 24 hours postbite. Any severe snakebite is at potential risk from renal damage; maintain adequate hydration and monitor urine output and renal function.

Snake Venom Spit Ophthalmia

This particular problem caused by spitting cobras (not all cobra species are spitters) requires urgent action to reduce the chance of corneal injury. The eye must be thoroughly and vigorously washed with water or other suitable fluid as soon as possible after the injury. This is the principal first aid for this condition, but should generally be repeated once in a medical facility. Except where slit lamp examination has excluded corneal injury, treat as for corneal abrasions or ulcers, using a suitable topical antibiotic. Topical antivenom is not indicated. Pain may be severe and topical adrenaline eye drops have been suggested as very effective at relieving this pain.

COBRAS

The taxonomy of cobras is still in flux, although it has been somewhat "cleaned up" in recent years. Many distinct species are now recognized, particularly in Asia, where previously most cobras were considered subspecies of the Indian cobra, *Naja naja* (Fig. 1). Cobras of the genus *Naja* are common throughout Africa and Asia, from west Asia through to the Philippines and China, but not Japan, New Guinea, or Australia (Fig. 2). They fall into two major groups medically.

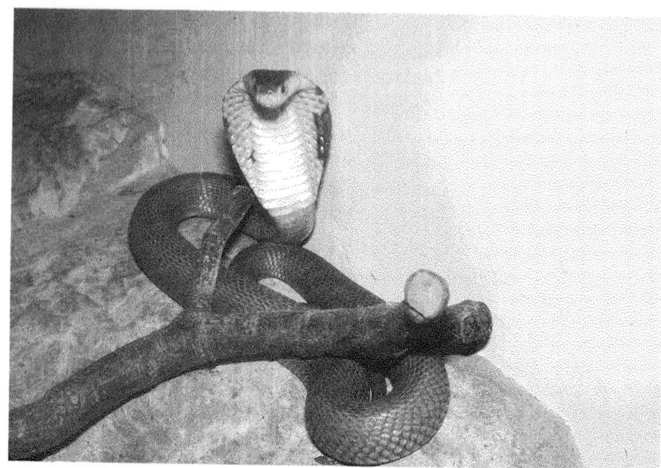

Figure 1. Indian cobra (*Naja naja*). (Original photograph copyright © by Dr. Julian White.) (See Color Plate 7.)

Group 1

Purely neurotoxic cobras (Table 1) are found in Africa and do not generally cause major local reactions, but can cause moderate to severe postsynaptic neurotoxic flaccid paralysis. Bites may cause local pain, though sometimes are almost painless, and local swelling varies from minimal to quite extensive. Some species can also cause blistering (e.g., *N. haje*), but not necrosis. A variable time later, systemic envenoming may develop, characterized by progressive flaccid paralysis, which can progress to full respiratory paralysis. Local necrosis is not a feature of bites. Systemic myolysis and coagulopathy do not occur and secondary renal failure is rare or not reported. Use type 1 first aid (Chapter 244).

Group 2

Cobras causing local tissue injury, with or without neurotoxic paralysis (Table 1), are found in Africa and across Asia. This group encompasses the bulk of cobra species, including many capable of spitting. Some species only rarely cause neurotoxic paralysis, the local tissue injury dominating the clinical presentation. Other species, notably the Philippine cobra, predominantly cause paralysis and cause necrosis uncommonly. Bites are usually painful, with variable swelling, then development of

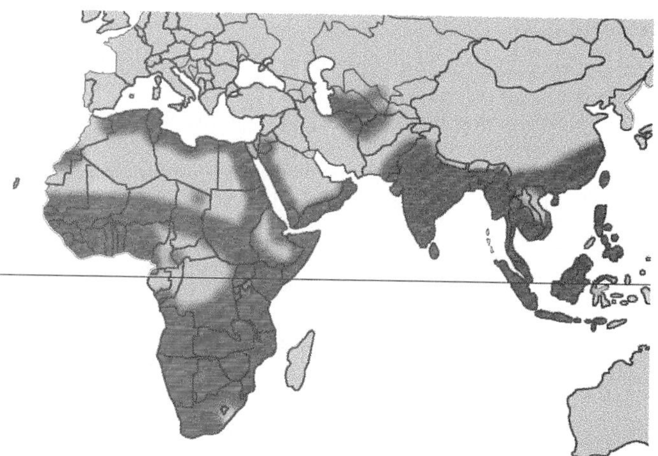

Figure 2. Distribution of cobras globally (genus *Naja*). (Original illustration copyright © by Dr. Julian White.)

TABLE 1. Cobra species classified by clinical effects

Purely neurotoxic cobras			
Egyptian cobra	*N. haje*		Africa
Forest cobra	*N. melanoleuca*		Africa
Cape cobra	*N. nivea*		Africa
Banded cobra	*N. annulifera*		Africa
West Asian cobra	*N. oxiana*		Asia
Cobras causing local necrosis			
Black necked spitting cobra	*N. nigricollis*	Spitter	Africa
Mozambique spitting cobra	*N. mossambica*	Spitter	Africa
Red spitting cobra	*N. pallida*	Spitter	Africa
West African spitting cobra	*N. katiensis*	Spitter	Africa
Chinese cobra	*N. atra*	Spitter (rare)	Asia
Monocellate cobra	*N. kaouthia*		Asia
Indian cobra	*N. naja*		Asia
Philippine cobra	*N. philippinensis*	Spitter	Asia
Samar cobra	*N. samarensis*	Spitter (rare)	Asia
Thai spitting cobra	*N. siamensis*	Spitter	Asia
Javan spitting cobra	*N. sputatrix*	Spitter	Asia
Sumatran spitting cobra	*N. sumatrana*	Spitter	Asia
Mandalay cobra	*N. mandalayensis*	Spitter?	Asia

N., Naja.

blistering, progressing to an area of central skin necrosis, which may be extensive. Use type 2 first aid (Chapter 244).

Antivenom for cobra envenoming is only available for some species. All African species are covered by the South African polyvalent antivenom. Key Asian species, such as *N. kaouthia* and *N. siamensis*, are covered by the Thai Red Cross and Vietnamese antivenoms. Iranian antivenom covers *N. oxiana* bites, and several Indian antivenoms cover *N. naja* bites. Both Chinese and Taiwanese producers have antivenoms covering *N. atra* bites. The Saudis produce an antivenom for *N. haje* bites. For those Asian species not covered by any antivenom officially, consider trying the Thai Red Cross cobra antivenom. The dose of antivenom varies from product to product and is also dictated by the severity of envenoming. All cobra bites with evidence of developing paralysis should be considered for antivenom therapy. In addition, the Tensilon test is appropriate, as paralysis is postsynaptic and may respond to anticholinesterases, as an adjunct to antivenom, not an alternative (except where antivenom is unavailable). Anticholinesterase has been used successfully in the management of respiratory paralysis by Philippine cobra bite.

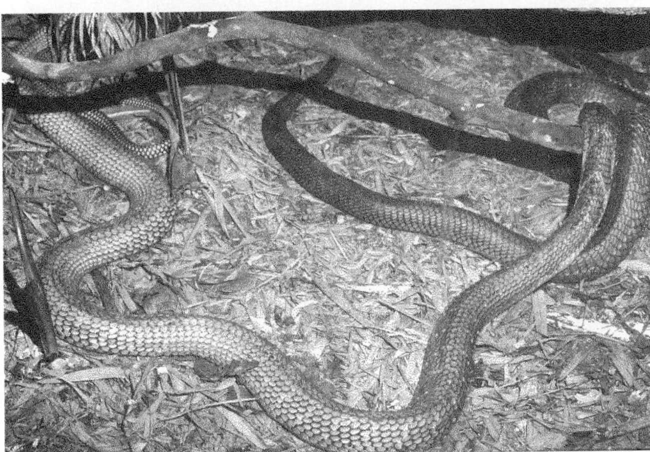

Figure 3. King cobra (*Ophiophagus hannah*). (Original photograph copyright © by Dr. Julian White.)

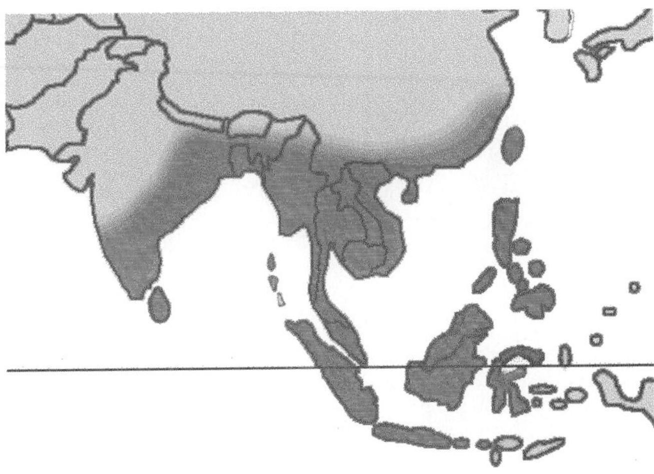

Figure 4. Distribution of the king cobra. (Original illustration copyright © by Dr. Julian White.)

KING COBRA (*OPHIOPHAGUS HANNAH*)

The largest of all venomous snakes, king cobras (Fig. 3) from South East Asia (Fig. 4), can cause rapid severe envenoming, characterized by rapidly progressive flaccid paralysis, local pain and swelling, local necrosis in approximately 15% of cases, and general symptoms such as nausea and vomiting. Use type 1 first aid.

There are several choices in antivenoms, including specific products from the Thai Red Cross and the Vietnamese. Commonwealth Serum Laboratories (CSL) Tiger Snake antivenom has also been used with success. As paralysis is postsynaptic, consider the Tensilon test to determine if anticholinesterases will be of benefit in cases with severe paralysis.

RHINKHALS (*HAEMACHATUS HAEMACHATUS*)

The rhinkhal, an African (Fig. 5) cobra-like elapid, can spit venom and cause both local tissue injury and flaccid paralysis. The South African polyvalent antivenom covers bites by this species. Use type 1 first aid.

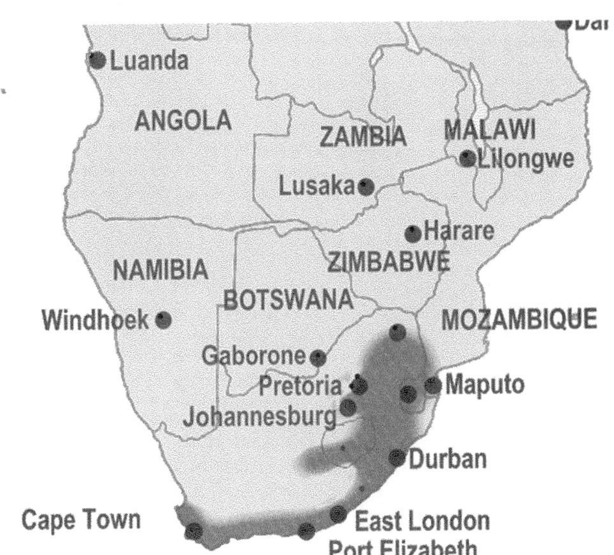

Figure 5. Distribution of rhinkhals (*Haemachatus haemachatus*). (Original illustration copyright © by Dr. Julian White.)

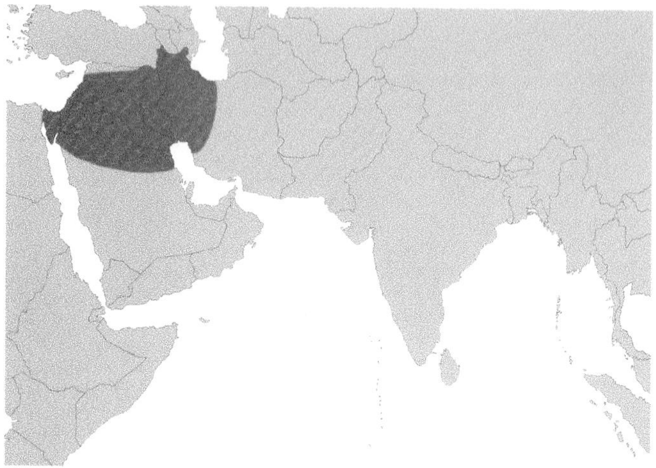

Figure 6. Distribution of black desert cobra (*Walterinnesia aegyptia*). (Original illustration copyright © by Dr. Julian White.)

BLACK DESERT COBRA (*WALTERINNESIA AEGYPTIA*)

The black desert cobra is found in North East Africa through to Iran (Fig. 6), and there is limited reported experience with bites, which may cause local pain, swelling, and systemic features, including headache, nausea, vomiting, and weakness, but there is no clear evidence that either necrosis or major flaccid paralysis is likely. Should major envenoming occur, consider using the South African polyvalent antivenom. Use type 1 first aid.

BURROWING COBRAS (*PARANAJA* SPECIES) AND TREE COBRAS (*PSEUDOHAJE* SPECIES)

There is no case evidence that these African snakes can cause significant envenoming. No specific antivenom is available. Should major envenoming ensue, try the South African polyvalent product. Use type 1 first aid. Tree cobras are treated as for burrowing cobras.

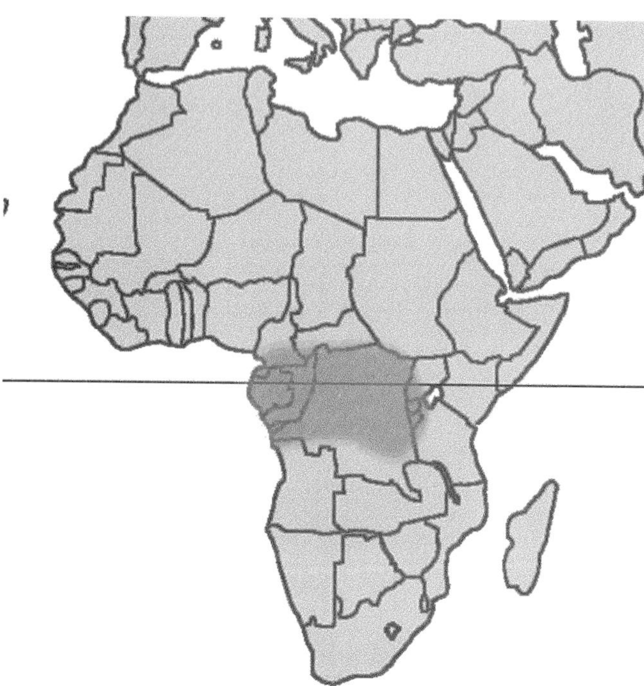

Figure 7. Distribution of water cobras (*Boulengerina*). (Original illustration copyright © by Dr. Julian White.)

WATER COBRAS (*BOULENGERINA* SPECIES)

There is no clear case evidence, but anecdotal reports suggest water snakes (Fig. 7) may cause severe, even fatal envenoming, though the features of such envenoming are unknown. Based on similarities with related species, it is possible that these snakes might cause flaccid paralysis. There is no specific antivenom available, but should major envenoming occur, the South African polyvalent product should be tried. Use type 1 first aid.

MAMBAS

The mambas (genus *Dendroaspis*) of Africa (Fig. 8) can cause lethal envenoming rapidly. In addition to local pain and swelling, neurotoxic features may develop early. The initial manifestations are perioral paresthesiae, progressing swiftly to limb and cranial nerve weakness, followed by respiratory paralysis. Pulmonary edema may occur. General symptoms include headache, nausea, and vomiting. Severe paralysis may develop rapidly, with respiratory failure possible within 15 minutes of a bite. This is more rapid than seen with classic pre- and postsynaptic neurotoxins.

Mamba venoms contain unique synergistic toxins, the dendrotoxins that stimulate axonal release of neurotransmitter, and the fasciculins, that are essentially anticholinesterases, retarding normal destruction and recycling of released neurotransmitter. As a result, there may be not only paralysis, but muscle fasciculation in some cases. The black mamba, *D. polylepis*, is the most potent species; the western green mambas, *D. jamesonii* and *D. viridis* cause less potent paralytic effects, but more severe local swelling. The eastern green mamba, *D. angusticeps*, causes the least severe paralytic effects, but most severe local swelling, occasionally associated with necrosis. Use type 1 first aid.

The South African polyvalent antivenom is considered to cover all mamba species. One Indian antivenom is also claimed

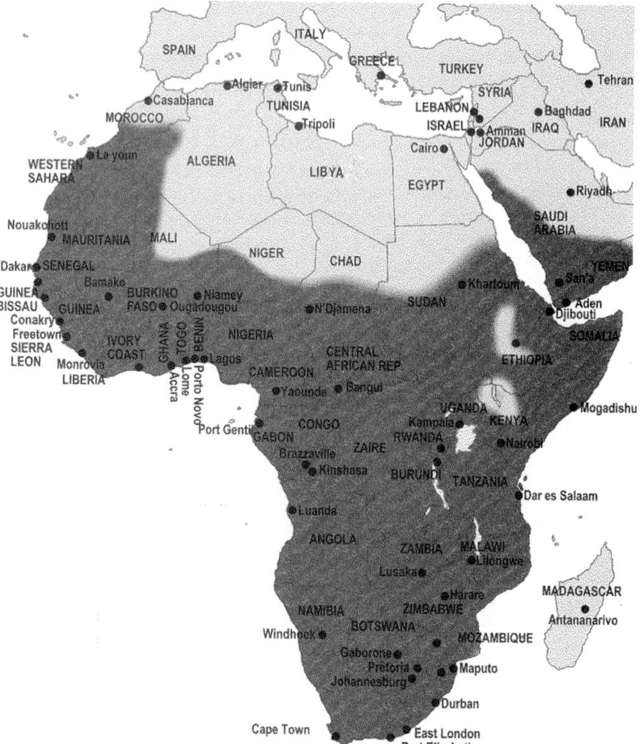

Figure 8. Distribution of mambas (*Dendroaspis*). (Original illustration copyright © by Dr. Julian White.)

TABLE 2. Krait species

Indian krait	*B. caeruleus*	India to Indonesia
Malayan krait	*B. candidus*	South East Asia and Indonesia
Sri Lankan krait	*B. ceylonicus*	Sri Lanka
Banded krait	*B. fasciatus*	North East India to Indonesia
Javan krait	*B. javanicus*	Java
Chinese krait	*B. multicinctus*	Southern China, Taiwan, to Burma
Andaman krait	*B. andamanensis*	Andaman Islands
Himalayan krait	*B. bungaroides*	Northern Indian subcontinent
Red headed krait	*B. flaviceps*	South East Asia to Indonesia
Lesser black krait	*B. lividus*	North East India, Bangladesh, southern China, Bhutan
Burmese krait	*B. magnimaculatus*	Myanmar
Black krait	*B. niger*	North East India, Bangladesh, southern China, Bhutan, Nepal
Sind krait	*B. sindanus*	Northern Indian subcontinent

B., Bungarus.

to cover mamba bites by the producer, but this is unproven and the South African product is preferred.

KRAITS

The kraits (genus *Bungarus*) of Asia (Table 2; Figs. 9 and 10) are a classic cause of progressive flaccid paralysis. Bites vary in severity between species, but all are potentially lethal. The bite may not even be felt and little if any local pain or swelling occurs. Necrosis does not occur. Classic flaccid paralysis develops, generally involving both pre- and postsynaptic neurotoxins (α- and β-bungarotoxins, respectively). At least for the Indian krait, *B. caeruleus*, there are clinical reports suggestive of myolysis, with muscle pain and myoglobinemia, but this has yet to be confirmed with raised CK levels and muscle biopsy. The paralysis may progress to respiratory paralysis and failure over only a few hours, or may take more than 12 hours to reach this stage. In some areas, such as Sri Lanka and India, patients are bitten at night while asleep, so they are unaware of developing paralysis until it is too late to seek help, thus they may be dead or nearly so by the following morning.

There are several antivenoms covering particular krait species. All Indian antivenom producers have products covering the Indian krait, *B. caeruleus*. The Thai Red Cross has an antivenom raised against *B. fasciatus*, said to cover *B. candidus* as well, whereas the Vietnamese have a specific *B. candidus* antivenom. Producers in China and Taiwan make antivenoms covering *B. multicinctus*. However, it should be remembered that antivenom may not be effective at reversing established paralysis caused by kraits because of the presence of presynaptic neurotoxins. Use of the Tensilon test may assist in determining if the paralysis is principally pre- or postsynaptic. If the former, then there is no response and further antivenom to reverse paralysis is probably inappropriate; if the latter, then the Tensilon test shows temporary improvement in paralysis, so further antivenom therapy is worthwhile. For patients with predominantly presynaptic paralysis, with full respiratory paralysis, expect that external ventilation will be required for days to weeks, until the damaged terminal axons regenerate. Use type 1 first aid.

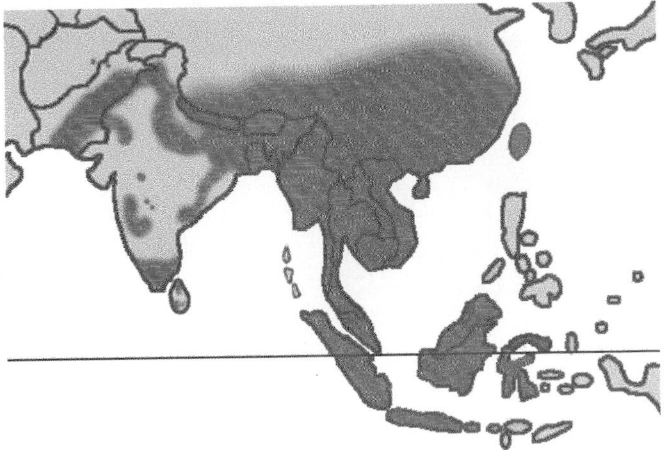

Figure 9. Distribution of kraits (*Bungarus*). (Original illustration copyright © by Dr. Julian White.)

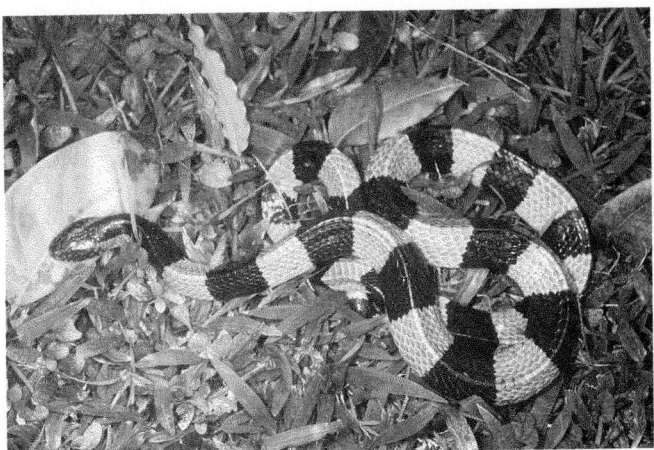

Figure 10. Banded krait (*Bungarus fasciatus*). (Original photograph copyright © by Dr. Julian White.) (See Color Plate 8.)

CORAL SNAKES

Asian Coral Snakes (Genus *Calliophis*) and Long-Glanded Coral Snakes (Genus *Maticora*)

Although most bites by these Asian snakes (Fig. 11) are likely to be minor, they can cause major envenoming, characterized by flaccid paralysis, with lethal respiratory paralysis reported. No antivenom is available, though in a severe case CSL Tiger Snake antivenom might be worth considering. If there is paralysis, a Tensilon test helps determine if anticholinesterases will be of benefit. Use type 1 first aid. The long-glanded coral snakes also inhabit South East Asia. They have caused fatalities, probably from respiratory paralysis in most cases. Treat as for *Calliophis* bites.

American Coral Snakes (Genus *Micrurus, Micruroides*)

Coral snakes of the genus *Micrurus* encompass many species, ranging from the southern part of North America through South America (Fig. 12). Many, but not all species are small, with a low incidence of bites. The Arizona or Sonoran coral snake (*Micruroides euryoxanthus*), a small snake with an average length of 12 to 20 inches, is found in Arizona and New Mexico. The eastern coral snake (*M. fulvius fulvius*; see Color Plate 15) and the Texas coral snake (*M. fulvius tenere*) are larger, with average lengths of 15 to 36 inches. A number of harmless snakes have yellow, black, and red bands that may mimic the coral snake, producing the rhyme "red

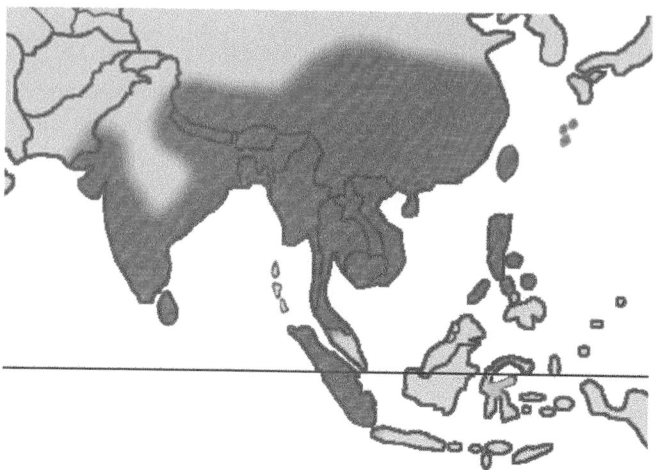

Figure 11. Distribution of Asian coral snakes (*Calliophis*). (Original illustration copyright © by Dr. Julian White.)

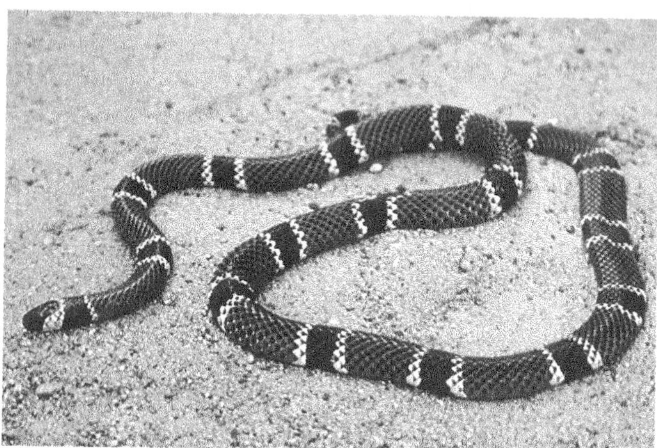

Figure 13. Painted coral snake (*Micrurus corallinus*). (Original photograph copyright © by Dr. Jurg Meier.) (See Color Plate 9.)

on yellow, kill a fellow; red on black, venom lack." This rhyme applies only to coral snakes native to the United States.

Some species cause more frequent bites, with more severe envenoming that is potentially lethal. Most commonly, at least in South America, the major feature is systemic myolysis with the potential for secondary renal damage. Flaccid paralysis can also occur, including full respiratory paralysis. Local tissue injury is not generally a feature of coral snake bites, which are relatively painless and cause little local reaction.

Several antivenoms are available in Central and South America to cover major species, including *M. fulvius*, *M. nigrocinctus*, *M. carincauda*, *M. frontalis*, *M. corallinus* (Fig. 13), *M. spixi*, *M. mipartitus*, *M. alleni*, *M. lemniscatus*, and *M. multifasciatus*. An antivenom is available for treatment of envenomation by *M. f. fulvius* (Eastern coral snake) and *M. f. tenere* (Texas

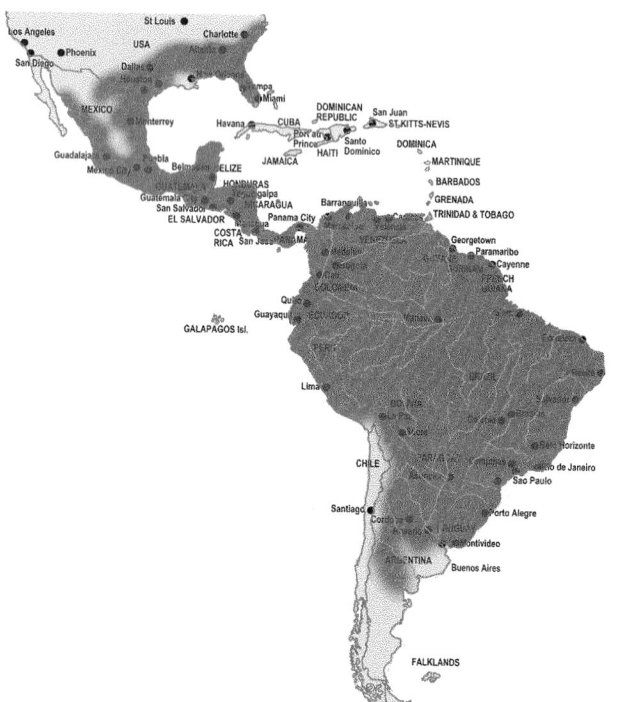

Figure 12. Distribution of American coral snakes (*Micrurus*). (Original illustration copyright © by Dr. Julian White.)

systemic envenoming. As paralysis may be principally postsynaptic, consider the Tensilon test to determine if anticholinesterases will also be of benefit as an adjunct to antivenom. Use type 1 first aid.

South American Coral Snakes (Genus *Leptomicrurus*)

Envenomation and treatment are essentially as for *Micrurus* (Fig. 14).

Shield Nose African Coral Snakes (Genus *Aspidelaps*)

Bites are possibly uncommon by these African snakes (Fig. 15), but may cause severe envenoming, including neurotoxicity, but probably not necrosis. There is no specific antivenom, so treatment is symptomatic and supportive. If paralysis develops, consider the Tensilon test to determine if anticholinesterases will

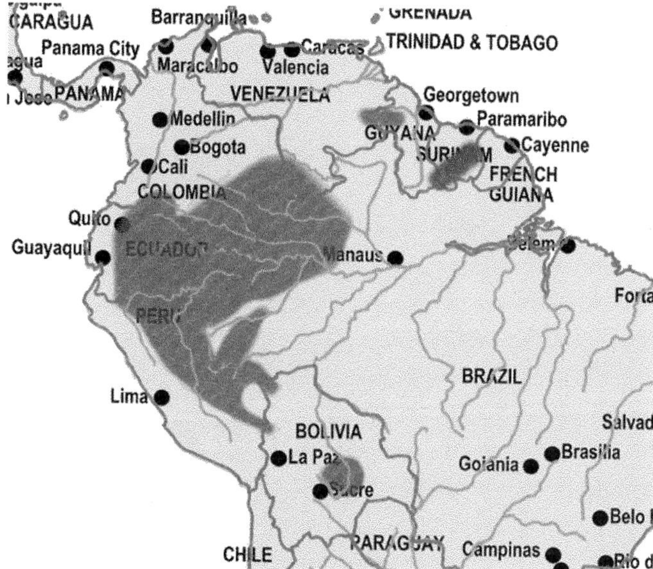

Figure 14. Distribution of coral snakes (*Leptomicrurus*). (Original illustration copyright © by Dr. Julian White.)

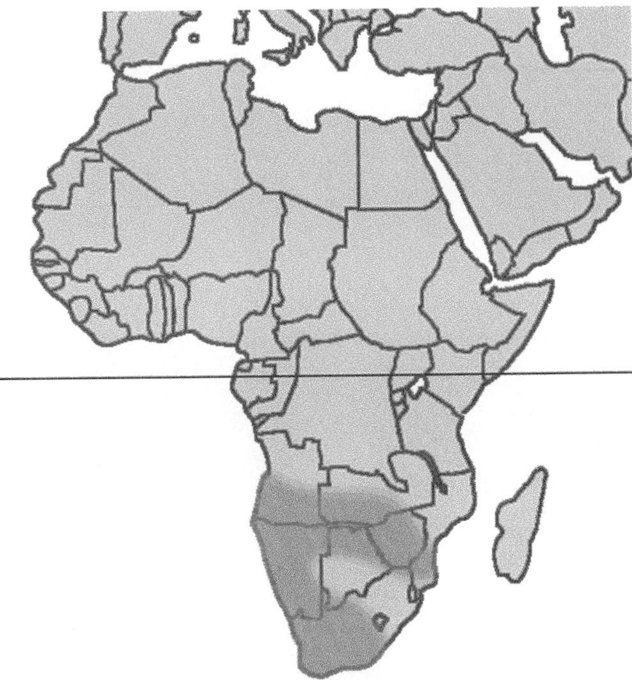

Figure 15. Distribution of shield nose snakes (*Aspidelaps*). (Original illustration copyright © by Dr. Julian White.)

assist in reducing paralytic effects. Use type 1 first aid (see earlier for details).

African Garter Snakes (Genus *Elapsoidea*)

Bites by African garter snakes appear rare and cause local effects, principally pain and swelling, without necrosis. No antivenom is available, so treatment is symptomatic. Use type 1 first aid.

Spotted Harlequin Snake (Genus *Homoroselaps*)

There is little information on bites by spotted Harlequin snakes, but they appear to cause only local effects, including swelling that may be severe as well as lymphangitis and local bleeding. No antivenom is available, so treatment must be symptomatic. Use type 1 first aid.

Bolo (*Ogmodon vitianus*)

This small Fijian elapid is unlikely to cause an effective bite and is considered harmless by the local population. Should envenoming occur, symptomatic treatment only is available, as there is no antivenom. Use Type 1 first aid.

Bougainville Coral Snake (*Parapistocalamas hedigeri*)

This small elapid from Bougainville, New Guinea and the Solomons is not considered dangerous, but lack of case report data precludes definitive assessment. As it is part of the Australian elapid faunal group, it might cause systemic envenoming, such as flaccid paralysis, myolysis, or coagulopathy. Should such effects develop, though there is no specific antivenom, consider using CSL Polyvalent Snake Antivenom. Use Type 1 first aid.

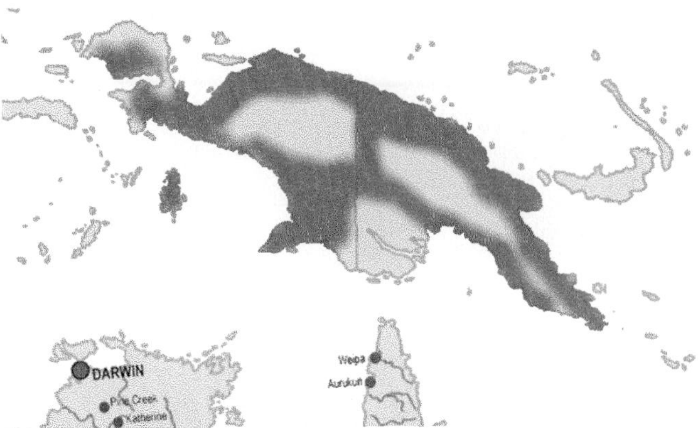

Figure 16. Distribution of New Guinea forest snakes (genus *Toxicocalamus*). (Original illustration copyright © by Dr. Julian White.)

Solomons Coral Snake (*Salomonelaps par*)

Restricted to parts of the Solomon Islands group, this elapid can reach 1 meter in length, so might be capable of causing significant envenoming, but case report data are absent. Although most bites might be minor, they cannot be assumed to be trivial. As it is part of the Australian elapid faunal group, it might cause systemic envenoming, such as flaccid paralysis, myolysis, or coagulopathy. Should such effects develop, though there is no specific antivenom, consider using CSL Polyvalent Snake antivenom. Use Type 1 first aid.

New Guinea Forest Snakes (Genus *Toxicocalamus*)

The clinical effects of these generally small elapids from New Guinea are not well documented. Although most bites are likely to be minor, it cannot be assumed all bites will be trivial, especially if larger specimens are involved. As they are part of the Australian elapid faunal group, they might cause systemic envenoming such as flaccid paralysis, myolysis, or coagulopathy. Should such effects develop, though there is no specific antivenom, consider using CSL Polyvalent Snake antivenom. Use Type 1 first aid.

New Guinea Small-Eyed Snake (*Micropechis ikaheka*)

This large elapid, confined to New Guinea (Fig. 16), is now known to cause severe, sometimes lethal, envenoming. It causes predominantly systemic effects, including flaccid paralysis, myolysis, potentially secondary renal failure, and possibly coagulopathy. Australian polyvalent antivenom appears effective as treatment. Use Type 1 first aid (see earlier for details).

AUSTRALIAN ELAPID SNAKES

This large and diverse group extends into New Guinea and parts of Indonesia. The Australian elapids have a unique status amongst elapids, in the range of systemic effects they may cause, and the rather different approach to management, including use of venom detection. Most of the Australian fauna is not dangerous to humans, but the venomous group includes the most toxic of all snake species. Australia (CSL, Ltd.) produces a range of "specific" antivenoms for each of the five major venom types of Australian snakes, as well as a polyvalent antivenom covering all species. The latter is high volume and expensive and is only

Figure 17. Australian Snake Venom Detection Kit (CSL, Ltd.). (Original illustration copyright © by Dr. Julian White.)

used if the identity of the snake is uncertain or adequate supplies of specific antivenom are unavailable.

The overlap of snake habitats and the use of specific antivenoms make identifying the snake very important. CSL produces a Snake Venom Detection Kit (Fig. 17) that uses a micro–enzyme-linked immunosorbent assay to detect nanogram quantities of venom swabbed from the bite site, or in urine (if there is systemic envenoming). A positive result indicates that venom was present, which type of venom (but not which exact species), and therefore, which type of antivenom is appropriate. However, a positive result does not indicate antivenom should be given. The decision to give antivenom is based on clinical and laboratory evidence of envenoming as described in Table 3.

Laboratory testing, and repeat testing on at least two further occasions, 2 to 3 hours apart, is essential in managing Australian snakebite to avoid missing late-developing envenoming. Antivenom is always given intravenously, without pretesting or premedication, but initial doses vary widely between species. More detail can be found in the *CSL Antivenom Handbook*, available online at http://www.toxinocology.com. All Australian snakes require Type 1 first aid.

Brown Snakes (Genus *Pseudonaja*)

Both in terms of frequency of bites and frequency of deaths, the brown snakes are the most important genus of Australian venomous snakes. They are restricted to mainland Australia, are not found in Tasmania, but have become established in parts of New Guinea (Figs. 18 and 19). Their venom is highly potent, but small fangs and a high rate of dry bites ensure that only approximately 20% of bites develop envenoming. In this group, the characteristic features are minimal or no local pain or swelling and rapid development of systemic effects, in 5 to 30 minutes (sometimes considerably longer), with headache, nausea, vomiting, collapse, convulsions (in small children), and profound defibrination coagulopathy. The latter causes persistent ooze from the bite site. Major hemorrhage into vital organs, especially the brain, occurs rarely. Renal damage or anuric renal failure can develop, even in cases with otherwise mild envenoming. Paralysis occurs rarely, and myolysis never occurs.

All cases with systemic envenoming require antivenom therapy, with a high initial dose (at least 4 to 5 vials), preferably of specific brown snake antivenom (CSL, Australia). Repeat assessment of coagulation is required, and further doses of antivenom

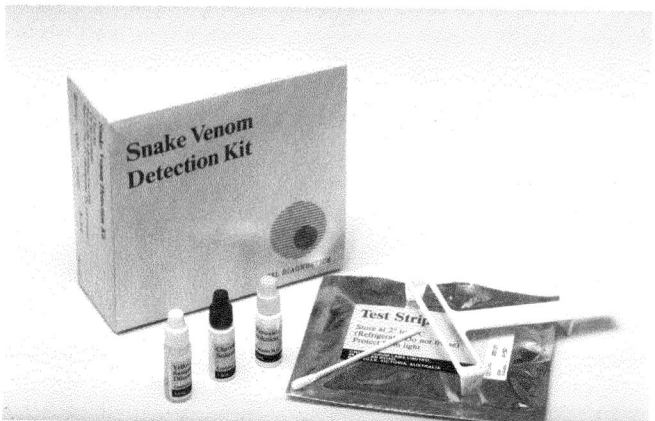

Figure 18. Distribution of brown snakes (genus *Pseudonaja*). (Original illustration copyright © by Dr. Julian White.)

TABLE 3. Indications for use of antivenom in Australia

1. Any degree of flaccid paralysis, including just ptosis, unless this is the only sign and it has been present for at least 6 h.
2. Any degree of significant myolysis, indicated by a creatine kinase (CK) >1500 IU/L (often if an elevated CK is the only feature of envenoming, a rise higher than this will be accepted before starting antivenom therapy).
3. Any degree of significant coagulopathy, indicated by a prolonged blood clotting time, prothrombin time or low fibrinogen, coupled with elevated fibrin(ogen) degradation products. In practice, for snakes causing defibrination, an international normalized ratio >2 is usually accepted as indicating antivenom is required. Beware patients with abnormal results because of preexisting anticoagulant therapy.
4. Any degree of renal failure, unless there is a clear nonenvenoming cause.
5. Any patient with a confirmed snakebite who has had a period of collapse or has had convulsions after the bite.
6. In addition, the presence of headache, nausea/vomiting, or abdominal pain suggests the possibility of systemic envenoming, but if examination and lab results are normal, is not alone sufficient to commence antivenom therapy.

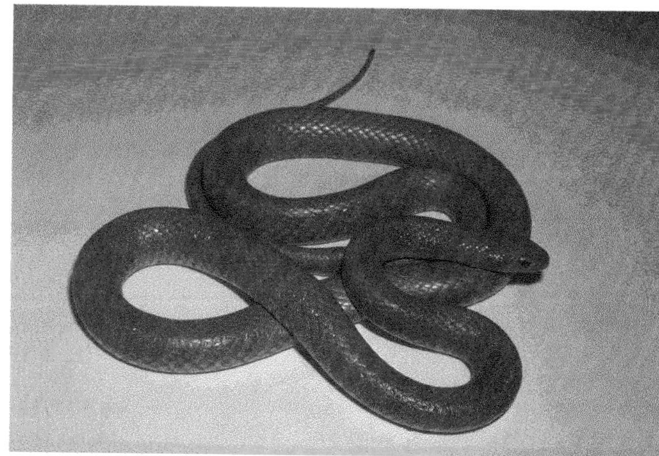

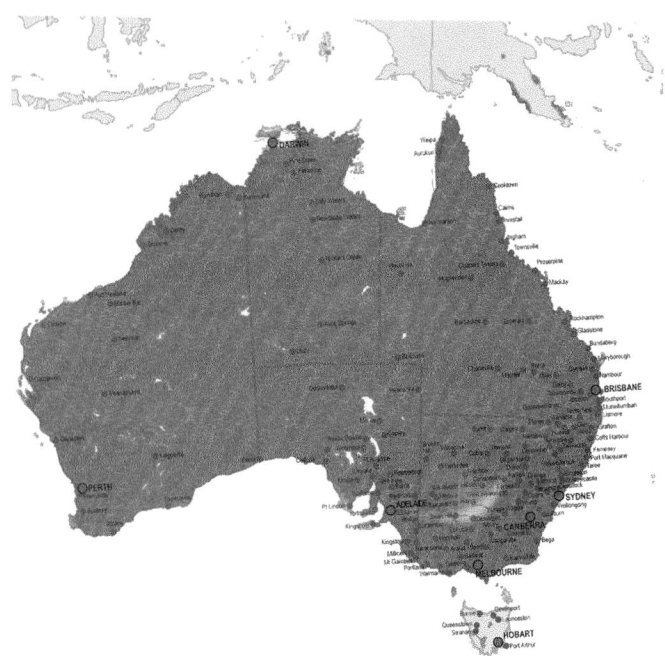

Figure 19. Western brown snake (*Pseudonaja nuchali*). (Original photograph copyright © by Dr. Julian White.)

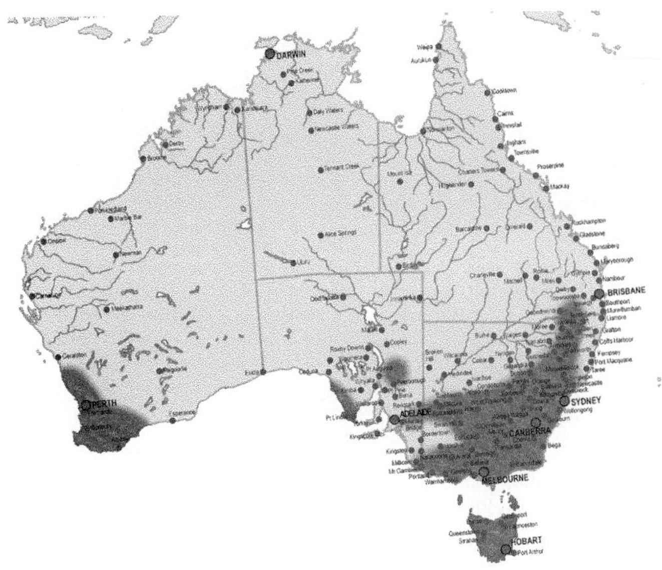

Figure 20. Distribution of tiger snakes (genus *Notechis*). (Original illustration copyright © by Dr. Julian White.)

are often needed if there is no rise in fibrinogen 3 hours after the prior antivenom dose. Coagulation factor replacement is generally inappropriate and is contraindicated if there is evidence of circulating active venom procoagulant.

Tiger Snakes (Genus *Notechis*) and Rough Scaled Snake (Genus *Tropidechis*)

Tiger snakes (Figs. 20 and 21) also have potent venom, but produce more of it than brown snakes. Their venom and larger fangs produce a higher rate of effective envenoming, at least 50%. Bites cause local pain, mild swelling, often with local ecchymosis, but not blistering. Very limited local necrosis occurs, but is rare. Systemic features include the same nonspecific symptoms as brown snakes, as well as defibrination coagulopathy and renal damage. However, tiger snakes also commonly cause pre- and postsynaptic flaccid paralysis and severe myolysis, with CK levels greater than 100,000 in some cases. There is a specific tiger snake antivenom, with an initial dose of 3 to 4 vials for cases with any evidence of systemic envenoming.

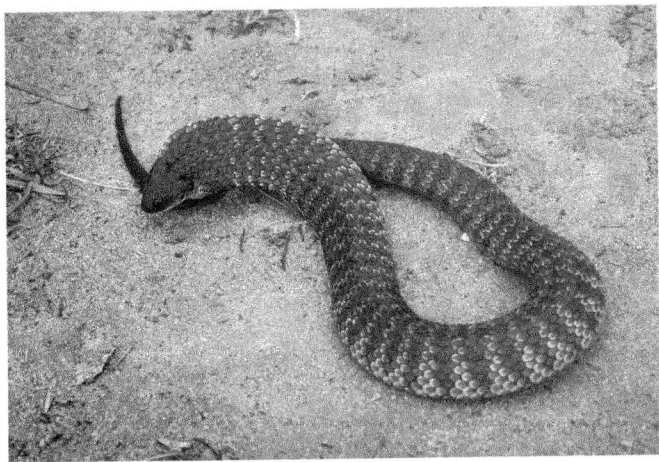

Figure 21. Common tiger snake (*Notechis scutatus*). (Original photograph copyright © by Dr. Julian White.) (See Color Plate 10.)

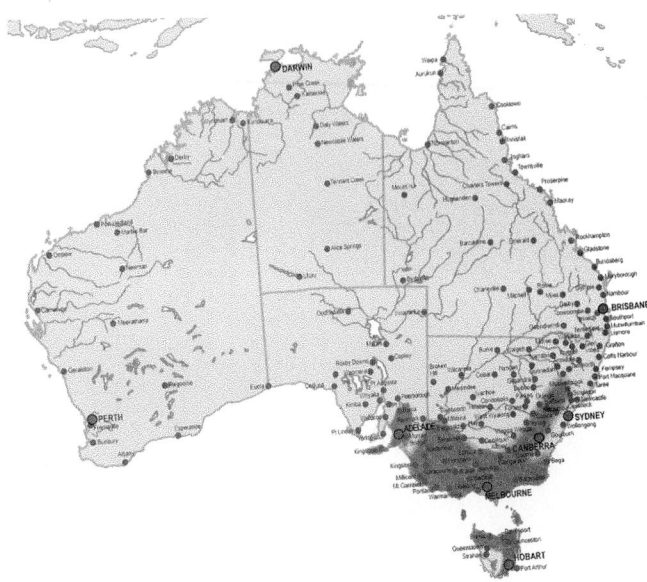

Figure 22. Distribution of copperhead snakes (genus *Austrelaps*). (Original illustration copyright © by Dr. Julian White.)

The rough-scaled snake is treated essentially the same as the tiger snake.

Copperheads (Genus *Austrelaps*)

Australian copperheads (Figs. 22 and 23) are an infrequent and poorly characterized cause of bites. Postsynaptic flaccid paralysis, possibly with myolysis, appears to be the major risk. Defibrination does not occur based on current evidence. Renal damage is a risk in the presence of myolysis. Tiger snake antivenom is considered the best treatment for systemic envenoming, with an initial dose of 2 to 3 vials.

Broad-Headed Snakes (Genus *Hoplocephalus*) (See Color Plate 16)

These medium-sized, largely nocturnal elapids fall within the tiger snake group, but clinically cause only defibrination coagulopathy like the brown snake, with which they are sometimes confused. However, the antivenom of choice is tiger snake antivenom, with an initial dose of 2 to 4 vials, depending on severity of the coagulopathy.

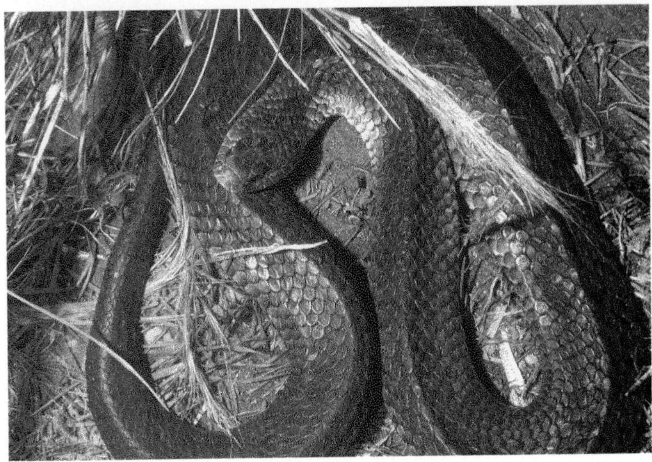

Figure 23. Common copperhead (*Austrelaps superbus*). (Original photograph copyright © by Dr. Julian White.)

Figure 24. Distribution of mulga snakes (*Pseudechis australis* and *butleri*). (Original illustration copyright © by Dr. Julian White.)

Mulga Snakes and Collett's Snake (Genus *Pseudechis*)

These large snakes (Figs. 24, 25, and 26) have moderate-sized fangs, producing large amounts of moderately toxic venom. Clinically, bites cause local pain, often extensive local swelling, without blistering or necrosis and development of systemic envenoming, particularly myolysis, which may be severe. This may result in secondary renal damage or failure. Secondary hyperkalemia can cause cardiac dysrhythmias. Some bites also cause true anticoagulation (without defibrination). Black snake antivenom is the preferred treatment, with 1 vial often sufficient.

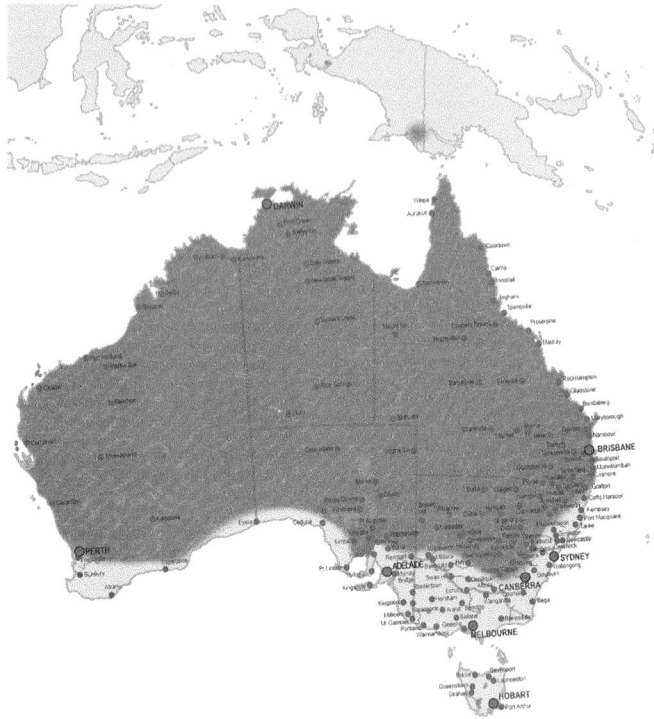

Figure 25. Mulga snake (*Pseudechis australis*). (Original photograph copyright © by Dr. Julian White.) (See Color Plate 11.)

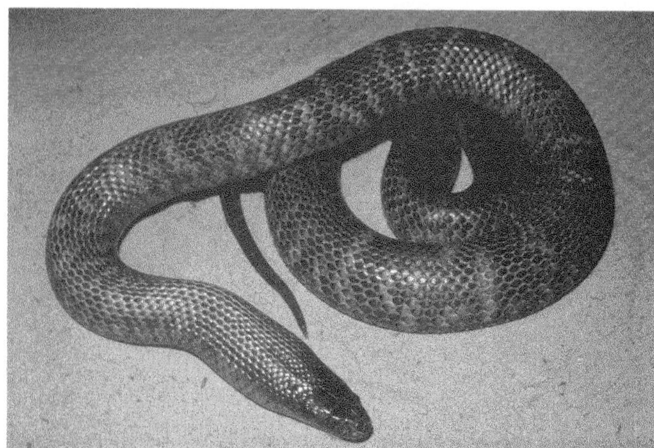

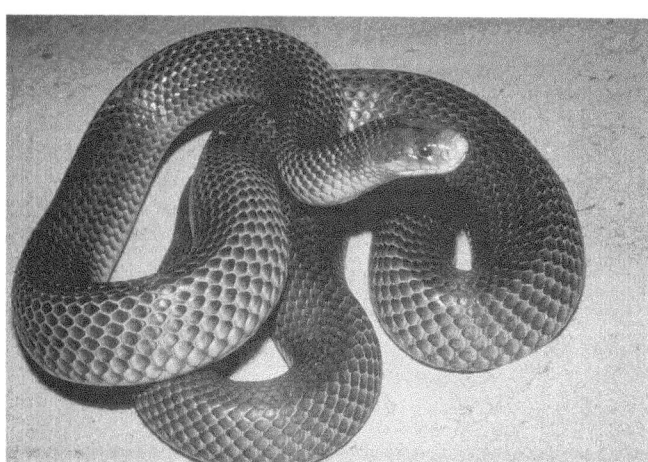

Figure 26. Collett's snake (*Pseudechis colletti*). (Original photograph copyright © by Dr. Julian White.) (See Color Plate 12.)

Black Snakes (Genus *Pseudechis*)

These other members of the *Pseudechis* genus are common in more populated areas (Figs. 27 and 28), with a significant rate of bites, but very low lethality potential compared to other dangerous Australian snakes. Bites often cause local pain, swelling, and general systemic symptoms, but major systemic effects are absent. Myolysis can occur but is rarely severe. Many patients do not require antivenom therapy. If antivenom is needed, tiger snake antivenom is preferred to black snake antivenom. Often, just 1 vial is enough.

Death Adders (Genus *Acanthophis*)

Death adders are the most viper-like of Australian elapids (Figs. 29 and 30), but their bites are classic elapid. They are found in much of mainland Australia, New Guinea, and some western islands of Indonesia. The bite can be painful, but without major swelling or other local effects. The main systemic effect is

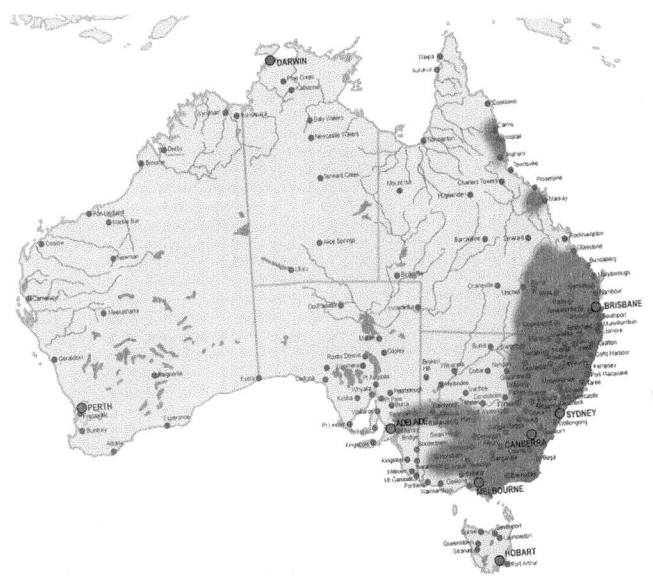

Figure 27. Distribution of black snakes (*Pseudechis porphyriacus* and *gutattus*). (Original illustration copyright © by Dr. Julian White.)

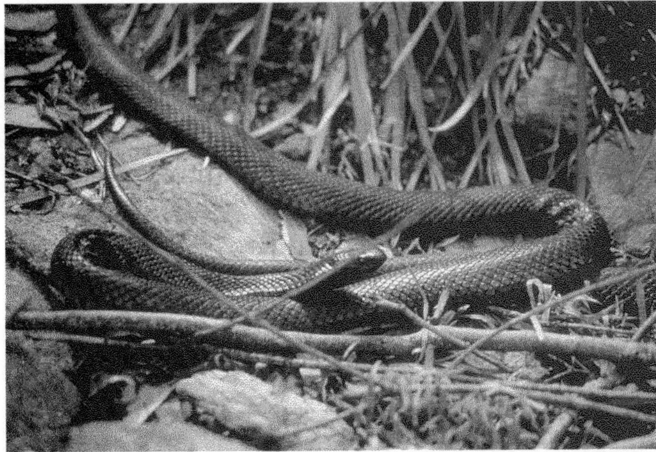

Figure 28. Red-bellied black snake (*Pseudechis porphyriacus*). (Original photograph copyright © by Dr. Julian White.)

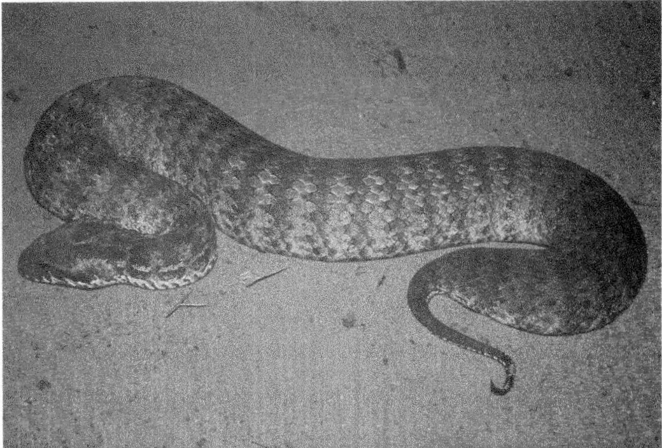

Figure 30. Common death adder (*Acanthophis antarcticus*). (Original photograph copyright © by Dr. Julian White.) (See Color Plate 13.)

postsynaptic flaccid paralysis, which is often reversible with adequate antivenom, either death adder specific or CSL polyvalent. Anticholinesterases can also assist in reducing the effects of paralysis, but should be seen as an adjunct to antivenom, not a replacement.

Taipans (Genus *Oxyuranus*)

The common taipan and the inland taipan (fierce or small-scaled snake) are probably the most deadly snakes in the world (Figs. 31 and 32). They combine agility, size, long fangs, and large amounts of the most potent venoms as a deadly mix. Before development of a specific taipan antivenom, there are only two recorded survivors of taipan bites in Australia. Bites cause rapid development of systemic envenoming in nearly all cases (occasional dry bites do occur). Initially, local pain and mild swelling occur and then onset of profound defibrination coagulopathy, active bleeding, presynaptic flaccid paralysis, renal damage or failure, and myolysis. Renal damage occasionally occurs without other manifestations.

Nearly all cases require antivenom therapy, either using taipan or CSL polyvalent antivenom. Both are high volume and expensive, so for practical reasons most hospitals in Australia and New Guinea choose to stock and use polyvalent antivenom for taipan bites. The initial dose used in Australia is 3 or more vials, with more often given in follow-up if the coagulopathy does not respond after 3 hours. In New Guinea, where antivenom is in short supply, such high doses are not possible and most patients receive only 1 vial in total. Experience there suggests this may result in resolution of the coagulopathy, but over a longer period of time.

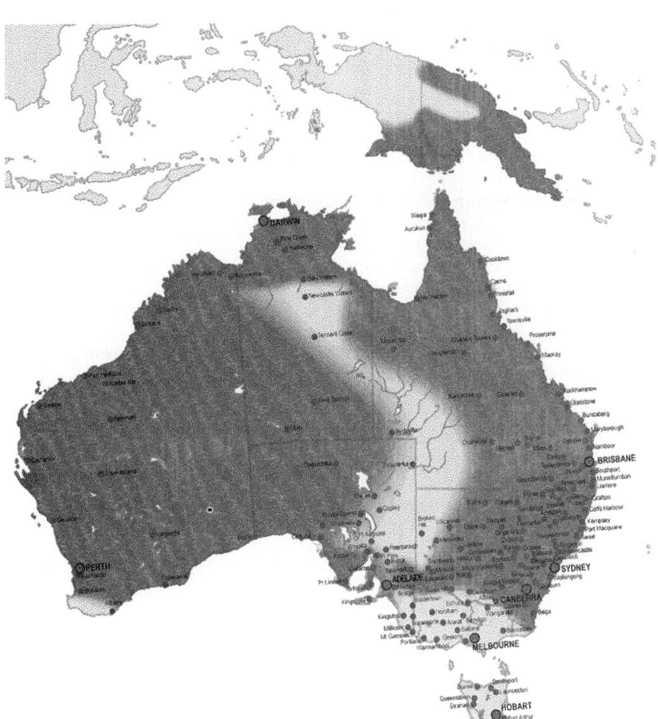

Figure 29. Distribution of death adders (genus *Acanthophis*). (Original illustration copyright © by Dr. Julian White.)

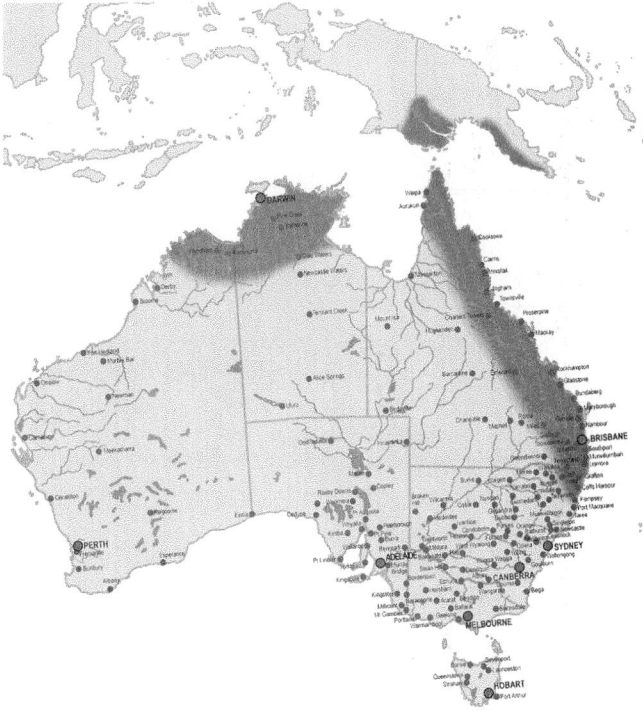

Figure 31. Distribution of common taipans (genus *Oxyuranus scutellatus*). (Original illustration copyright © by Dr. Julian White.)

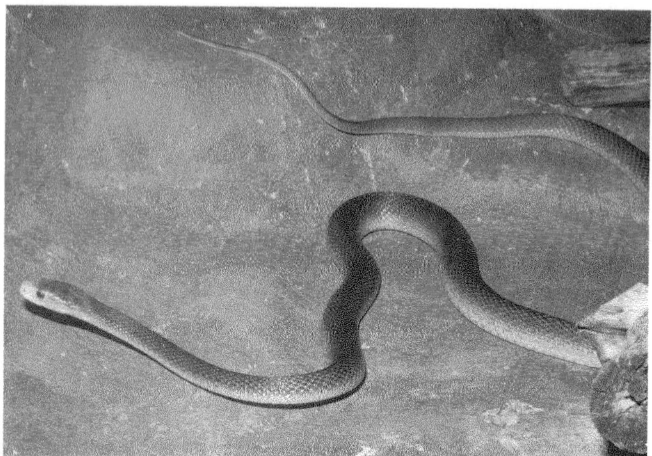

Figure 32. Common taipan (*Oxyuranus scutellatus*). (Original photograph copyright © by Dr. Julian White.) (See Color Plate 14.)

SEA SNAKES

Sea snakes, previously separated in their own family, *Hydrophiidae*, are now considered to be elapids, within the family *Elapidae*, split between the subfamilies *Hydrophiinae* and *Laticaudinae*. Case report data are only available for a few species, but it appears that most sea snakes are capable of inflicting severe, even lethal, bites to humans. Two clear patterns of envenoming are apparent. There are many species of sea snakes found throughout the warmer parts of the Indian and Pacific oceans, from Eastern Africa, to the western shores of the Americas (Fig. 33). Most sea snakes are restricted to areas relatively close to land, including islands, coral cays, and coral reefs, but one species, the pelagic sea snake, can be found in the open ocean, where it may congregate in large groups feeding on schools of fish.

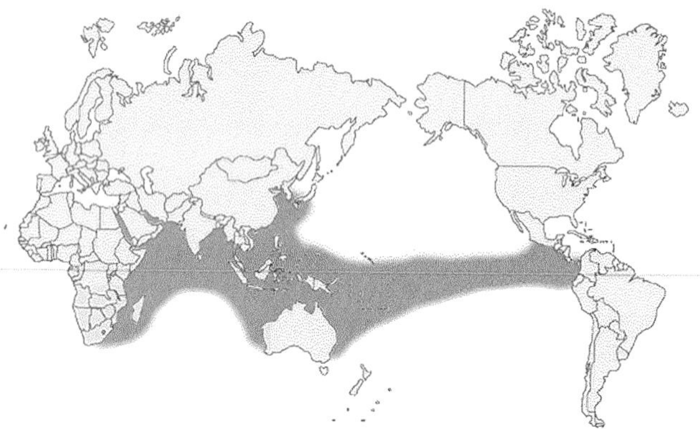

Figure 33. Distribution of sea snakes. (Original illustration copyright © by Dr. Julian White.)

Sea snakes have developed potent venoms, until recently considered the most potent of all snake venoms. Clinically, two distinct actions are apparent; postsynaptic flaccid paralysis and systemic myolysis. Both these problems may occur in a single patient, but more often one feature predominates, usually myloysis. The bite may be painless, with little if any local reaction, though more obvious and symptomatic bites do occur. There may be a quiescent period of up to several hours, until systemic envenoming becomes apparent. Systemic envenoming is manifest as either muscle pain, tenderness, weakness, and myoglobinuria or secondary renal failure, or progressive flaccid paralysis, starting with the cranial nerves, usually as ptosis, potentially progressing to full respiratory paralysis. Both sets of problems can occur simultaneously. Both are potentially lethal.

All cases of systemic envenoming by sea snakes warrant antivenom therapy, using CSL Sea Snake Antivenom. The initial dose varies from 1 to 3 vials depending on severity of envenoming, but failure of response over 3 hours indicates more antivenom may be required, with total doses in severe cases often in the order of 5 to 10 vials. If this antivenom is not available, CSL Tiger Snake or Polyvalent Antivenom has been used, but requires higher doses (3 vials for each vial of specific sea snake antivenom that would have been used). As paralysis is postsynaptic, antivenom in sufficient amount should reverse paralysis. Anticholinesterases can be a useful adjunct to antivenom in such cases. It is unclear how effective antivenom is for systemic myolysis. The cut-off point is not determined, however. Use type 1 first aid.

SUGGESTED READINGS

Bon C, Goyffon M, eds. *Envenomings and their treatments*. Paris: Institute Pasteur, 1995.

Campbell JA, Lamar WW, eds. *The venomous reptiles of Latin America*. Ithaca, NY: Comstock, 1989.

Covacevich J, Davie P, Pearn J, eds. *Toxic plants and animals: a guide for Australia*. Brisbane: Queensland Museum, 1987.

Dart RC, O'Brien PC, Garcia RA, et al. Neutralization of Micrurus distans distans venom by antivenin (Micrurus fulvius). *J Wilderness Med* 1992;3:377–381.

Gopalakrishnakone P, Chou LM, eds. *Snakes of medical importance (Asia-Pacific region)*. Singapore: Singapore University Press, 1990.

Gopalakrishnakone P, ed. *Sea snake toxinology*. Singapore: Singapore University Press, 1994.

Junghanss T, Bodio M. *Notfall-handbuch gifttiere*. Stuttgart: Georg Thieme Verlag, 1996.

Kitchens CS, Van Mierop LHS. Envenomation by the Eastern coral snake (Micrurus fulvius fulvius) a study of 39 victims. *JAMA* 1987;258:1615–1618.

Mebs D. *Venomous and poisonous animals*. Boca Raton, FL: CRC Press, 2002.

Meier J, White J, eds. *Handbook of clinical toxicology of animal venoms and poisons*. Boca Raton, FL: CRC Press, 1995.

Parrish HM, Khan MS. Bites by coral snakes: report of 11 representative cases. *Am J Med Sci* 1967;253:561–568.

Warrell DA, ed. WHO/SEARO Guidelines for the clinical management of snakebites in the Southeast Asian region. *SE Asian J Trop Med Public Health* 1999;30(suppl 1):1–85.

Weis R, McIsaac RJ. Cardiovascular and muscular effects of venom from coral snake, Micrurus fulvius. *Toxicon* 1971;9:219–228.

White J, Persson H. Snakes. In: Descotes J, ed. *Human toxicology*. Amsterdam: Elsevier, 1996:757–802.

White J. *CSL Antivenom Handbook*, 2nd ed. Melbourne: CSL Ltd., 2002.

CHAPTER 247
Viperid Snakes

Julian White

Topics included:	**Eurasian vipers (saw-scaled or carpet, Russell's and others); African vipers and adders (e.g., McMahon's, horned, night, African bush and others); Central and South American pit vipers (Bushmaster, various rattlesnakes, others); Asian pit vipers (hump-nosed vipers, hundred pace snake, Malayan pit viper, mamushi, habu, others)**
Normal levels:	**Not clinically available**
Special concerns:	**Local tissue injury and shock common, as is coagulopathy. Some species cause flaccid paralysis or myolysis.**
Antidote:	**Snake antivenom**

OVERVIEW

Vipers are globally distributed, with the exception of New Guinea, Australia, and associated islands (Chapter 244). They are a major cause of snakebite morbidity and mortality throughout their range. Classically, viper bites are said to cause local tissue injury and hemorrhagic problems. As with related aphorisms about elapid snakes, this simplification is incorrect, as there are important exceptions. Although many vipers do cause both local tissue injury and hemorrhagic effects, some common species cause neither of these effects, but rather cause paralytic and sometimes myolytic effects. Each group of vipers must be considered in its own right when considering clinical effects of bites.

The two types of viper are the basic vipers (subfamily *Viperinae*), which lack heat-sensing organs on the anterior snout, and the "pit vipers" (subfamily *Crotalinae*), which possess such heat-sensing organs. North American pit vipers are addressed in Chapter 245.

General Characteristics of Viperid Snakes

Vipers have evolved into a diverse collection of genera and species occupying many different niches, resulting in a wide variety of sizes and body forms. A typical viper is a robustly built snake, with a broad, generally triangular head, distinct from the narrower neck, with a comparatively short body compared to the stout build. Head scales are generally small and numerous compared to elapids. Although there are a number of exceptions, most vipers have more midbody scale rows than elapid snakes. Unlike some elapids, which have divided anal scales, all vipers (with one exception) have single anal scales.

Because the viper fangs are on a hinged modified maxilla, allowing considerable rotation, the fang can fold away against the roof of the mouth when not in use. This has allowed development of longer fangs than are found in the elapid snakes, which lack this modification. Some vipers have very long fangs, an extreme example being the Gaboon viper (*Bitis gabonica*), whose fangs can exceed 25 mm in length. However, not all vipers have long fangs and some species of great medical importance, such as the saw-scaled or carpet vipers, have only small fangs.

Within the various viper species can be found almost every type of venom component found within snake venoms. These include pre- and postsynaptic neurotoxins, myotoxins, and a bewildering array of toxins affecting blood clotting and blood vessel walls, nephrotoxins, cardiotoxins, toxins causing tissue injury and autonomic toxins. The amount of venom produced varies between species. Some larger vipers, particularly pit vipers such as rattlesnakes, can produce very impressive amounts of venom, far more than virtually all elapids.

CLINICAL EFFECTS OF VIPER BITES

The pattern of clinical effects varies between species and even within species. This fact has major implications in treatment, because an antivenom raised against the venom of a single species may only be effective for bites by members of that species in a restricted part of its range, corresponding to the source of the venom. A classic example is Russell's viper. This important Asian viper is listed as just one species with only two subspecies, yet there are five distinct populations with their own clinical characteristics of envenoming, each requiring its own antivenom. Thus, the clinician faced with a Russell's viper bite from a captive specimen must know from where the snake originated to determine which antivenom is most appropriate. All too often, the snake's keeper is not aware of this distinction, nor the true origin of their snake.

The major possibilities for clinical effects of viper bites are provided in this chapter, with its characteristic clinical presentation. For each snake group discussed later, each likely clinical effect is only listed by type; clinical presentation is not always discussed. The reader is referred back to this section for more detailed clinical presentation.

Neurotoxic Flaccid Paralysis

Though commonly associated with elapid bites, flaccid neurotoxic paralysis can also occur following bites by a few viperid species. Neurotoxic flaccid paralysis is first noted as ptosis, then ophthalmoplegia, followed by dysarthria, poor tongue protrusion, dysphagia, drooling; then limb weakness, depressed or absent deep tendon reflexes; and lastly respiratory paralysis. The progression from first signs to full respiratory paralysis may take only a few hours to more than 12 hours, depending on the size of the patient, the size of the snake (amount of venom injected), and the species.

There are two major types of neurotoxin: presynaptic and postsynaptic. Presynaptic toxins damage the terminal axon at the neuromuscular junction, so this type of paralysis is not reversed by antivenom therapy. Postsynaptic neurotoxins bind to the acetylcholine receptor at the muscle endplate, and so paralysis may be reversible with antivenom therapy.

Myolysis

Clinically important myolysis is generally systemic rather than local, though a number of vipers can cause local myolysis in the bitten area. Systemic myolysis may take several hours, occasionally more than 24, to become clinically apparent. Features include muscle pain, tenderness, and weakness; elevated plasma creatine kinase, which may be grossly elevated; and myoglobinuria, with the potential for secondary renal failure and hyperkalemia, the latter potentially cardiotoxic. Systemic myolysis has not been traditionally associated with viper bites, but is clearly an important feature, even dominant feature, for bites by some vipers, particularly the neotropical (Central and South American) rattlesnakes, and to a lesser extent, Sri Lankan Russell's viper.

Coagulopathy

Although not all vipers cause coagulopathy or hemorrhage, it is a major feature of envenoming by many species, reflecting the wide array of hematologically active toxins spread across viper venoms. The range of possible clinical effects is more limited. The likely clinical effects fit one of the following patterns in most cases:

1. Local ooze or bleeding from the bite area, abnormal coagulation tests with low fibrinogen, elevated degradation products, spontaneous bleeding from gums and other areas.
2. Local bruising of the bite area, sometimes extending up the bitten limb; abnormal coagulation tests, but uncommonly; mild spontaneous bleeding from gums and rarely other areas.
3. Local ooze or bleeding from the bite area, abnormal coagulation tests with low fibrinogen, elevated degradation products, thrombocytopenia, spontaneous bleeding from gums and other areas.
4. Local ooze or bleeding from the bite area or local blood-filled blisters, abnormal coagulation tests, with low fibrinogen, elevated degradation products, spontaneous bleeding from gums and other areas, likelihood of major bleeding into the gut or other organs.
5. Abnormal coagulation tests, with thrombosis formation, including deep venous thrombosis, pulmonary embolus, or infarction of parts of the brain or heart.

Renal Damage

Renal damage may be primary, as seen with Russell's viper bites in Burma. More common is secondary renal damage, following coagulopathy, myolysis, or a hypotensive episode, the latter often associated with hypovolemic shock due to massive fluid shifts into the bitten limb. Renal injury may manifest as only a slight rise in creatinine in some cases, through to full oliguric or anuric renal failure in others. Renal cortical necrosis, though described, is only reported for a few species, such as some major South American pit vipers. Clinical manifestations of early renal failure are few, apart from falling or absent urine output.

Cardiac Toxicity

A few vipers are known to contain cardiotoxins in their venom that can cause cardiac dysrhythmias or arrest in envenomed patients, though this effect is not common. Cardiotoxicity is more commonly a secondary effect of other processes, such as hyperkalemia secondary to severe myolysis.

Local Tissue Injury

Local tissue injury is quite variable in extent and presentation. Most species cause local pain that may be severe, and is often associated with moderate to marked swelling that may ultimately involve the entire bitten limb. Local oozing, bleeding, blistering, and discoloration may all occur, but blister formation does not always imply later development of necrosis. The extent of necrosis varies from none, to superficial skin loss in the bite area, to widespread skin loss. It may involve underlying tissues. In the latter situation, there may be local myolysis or true compartment syndrome. Compartment syndrome is not common and should always be confirmed by intracompartment pressure measurement before considering surgery. In the past, fasciotomy has been performed with alacrity rather than wisdom in many cases, resulting in more extensive tissue injury than might otherwise have occurred.

The development of necrosis often occurs over days rather than hours, but the initiating injury may be more rapid in development. One of the biggest hazards from the tissue injury is hypovolemic shock secondary to massive fluid shifts, particularly apparent in younger children in whom this complication can prove rapidly lethal. Secondary infection of the bitten area is also possible, and for some species, notably some major South American vipers, it appears to be common.

Local Tissue Infection

Although secondary infection of the bitten area is a risk with every snakebite, it is uncommon for most species. Where there is extensive tissue necrosis, opportunistic secondary infection is likely. However, for some vipers, notably some of the South American pit vipers of the genus *Bothrops*, local infection with abscess formation is common in moderate to severe bites.

First Aid for Viper Bites

There are two accepted types of first aid for viper snakebite, described in more detail in Chapter 244. For species not likely to cause local tissue injury, the Australian pressure immobilization bandage method is appropriate. It is safer than tourniquets, and when correctly applied may be left in place for several hours until a hospital or medical center able to treat snakebite is reached. However, it is only effective and useable for bites to a limb. For species with the potential to cause local tissue injury, the pressure immobilization bandage has not yet been proven safe because it may potentially increase the probability of serious local tissue injury. For bites where there is a considerable risk of potentially lethal flaccid paralysis and a likely prolonged delay in reaching medical care, then the relative risks of increasing local injury versus delaying onset of systemic envenoming should be considered, but this is uncommon among vipers, unlike elapids.

Recent research in Myanmar has indicated that a modification of the Australian technique, using a pressure pad locally, may be as effective yet not increase the chance of local tissue injury. If this work is confirmed and extended, it may cause a major rethink about appropriate first aid for snakebite.

TABLE 1. Unsafe and unwise first aid measures

Tourniquets
Cut and suck
Commercial snakebite suction kits
Electric shock
Cryotherapy
Local excision or incision
Amputation
Application of chemicals or patent medicines
Ethanol ingestion
Snake stones
Incantations and spells by witch doctors
Calls to a deity to save the victim

If the pressure immobilization bandage is not going to be used, gently clean the wound and immobilize the bitten limb with a splint, avoiding direct pressure in the bitten area. Carry the patient to transport. The patient should not walk or be otherwise physically active.

Old first aid methods (and some not-so-old methods) abound for snakebite, particularly applied to viper bites. These methods have been shown to be either useless or positively dangerous and should never be used (Table 1).

Hospital Management of Viper Bites

The degree of urgency required for managing viper bites is related to the species responsible. The size of the snake is not an absolute indicator of harmlessness. Small juveniles of some dangerous species, even at less than 30 cm in length, can inflict potentially lethal bites. As a general rule, all viper bites should be initially managed as potentially severe, requiring urgent full assessment. Only once it is established beyond doubt that the snake was either a nondangerous species or that the bite was minor, with no evidence of systemic or major local envenoming, can the patient be reassured and considered for discharge.

TABLE 2. Important aspects of treatment for the viperid snakes

1. A patient who is initially well may develop signs of injury hours later; frequent reassessment, including repeating key laboratory tests (e.g., coagulation tests for species causing coagulopathy, CK for species causing myolysis, creatinine for species causing renal damage) regularly is mandatory.
2. Antivenom is the key instrument of treatment, but should not be used indiscriminately; it should generally only be given to patients with signs of envenoming.
3. In patients bitten by species likely to cause coagulopathy, be very careful in creating vascular access.
4. Antivenom is the key therapy for coagulopathy, not factor replacement.
5. Antivenom may be useful therapy for major myolysis, even more than 24 hours postbite.
6. Antivenom may reverse pure postsynaptic paralysis, but will not reverse presynaptic paralysis, so there is no justification for giving large and continuous doses of antivenom in the latter situation.
7. For pure postsynaptic paralysis, anticholinesterases may assist management, but should not replace antivenom therapy, if the latter is available. Use the Tensilon test to determine if anticholinesterases will be effective.
8. Any severe snakebite is at potential risk from renal damage; maintain adequate hydration and monitor urine output and renal function.
9. Fasciotomy is a last resort treatment for compartment syndrome and should only be used once this condition has been confirmed by pressure measurement.

Diagnosis

Diagnosis should be focused on two aspects: determining if the snake was a species likely to cause medically significant effects and determining if there is evidence of either local or systemic envenoming. Venom detection is not available anywhere as a commercial kit for detecting viper venoms, though work is under way to produce such tests for certain parts of southeast Asia.

Diagnostic algorithms have been developed for a few regions that cover local viperid species (see www.toxinology.com for updates). Experience with the applicability of these diagnostic tools is currently limited. Obviously, such a system only works if there is obvious envenoming, but this is reasonable as only patients with significant envenoming require antivenom therapy.

Treatment

The principles of snakebite treatment are provided in Chapter 244. Detailed information on available antivenoms and the species covered are available on the Internet (www.toxinology.com), which has the most current listings. It is important to remember certain salient points in management (Table 2).

VIPERS (SUBFAMILY VIPERINAE)

Eurasian Vipers (Genera *Vipera, Macrovipera*)

These small- to medium-sized vipers are the classic cause of snakebite in Europe and adjacent parts of western Asia (Figs. 1 and 2). The severity of bites and range of clinical effects are not uniform across the group. They cause mild to severe local swelling and pain, which can be accompanied by blistering, ooze, and even bleeding. Local necrosis can develop but is not common or extensive. Particularly in children, there may be massive fluid shifts into the bitten area, causing shock. Extensive bruising and bleeding beneath the skin can occur. Particularly for *V. berus* in northern Europe and *V. latasti, V. palestinae* (Fig. 3), and *M. lebetina* in western Asia and the Middle East, bites can cause angioneurotic edema and a clinical picture resembling anaphylaxis.

Both *V. berus* and *V. aspis* can cause mild neurotoxic signs, notably ptosis, but more extensive flaccid paralysis does not occur. There may be a mild coagulopathy, less severe than local effects would suggest, but anemia, occasionally profound, may also develop. Renal failure can occur uncommonly. Type 2 first aid should be used.

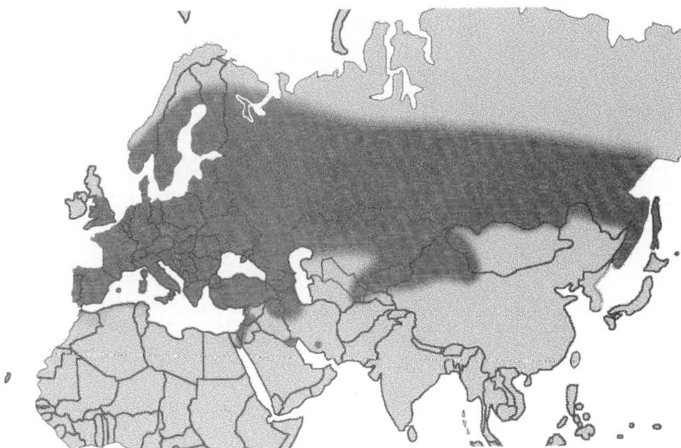

Figure 1. Distribution of Eurasian vipers (genus *Vipera*). (Original illustration copyright © by Dr. Julian White.)

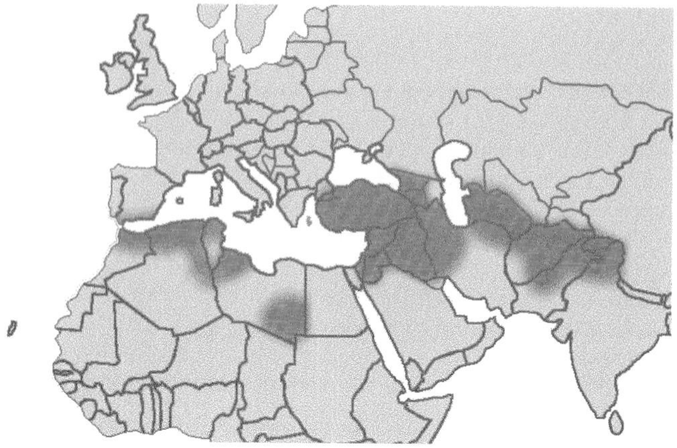

Figure 2. Distribution of Eurasian vipers (genus *Macrovipera*). (Original illustration copyright © by Dr. Julian White.)

V. ammodytes (Fig. 4) from the Balkans contains a potent presynaptic neurotoxin in its venom. Bites by this species may cause less severe local effects, but more significant paralysis. Type 1 first aid should be used.

A variety of antivenoms are available locally for particular species, including the new ovine Fab' antivenom (ViperaTab) for European species, with antivenoms for other species produced in Israel, Iran, Croatia, Serbia, Tunisia, and Morocco.

Saw-Scaled or Carpet Vipers (Genus *Echis*)

Probably the most important genus of snakes in terms of their impact on humankind, these small vipers from Africa through to western Asia (Fig. 5) cause very large numbers of bites within their range, with high morbidity and significant mortality, possibly measured in tens of thousands of cases yearly. Despite their small size, short fangs, and comparatively "nontoxic" venom, their commonness around rural areas ensures frequent bites, accelerated now as these snakes have adapted to urban habitats as well, at least in west Africa.

A typical bite causes local pain, swelling, which may be very extensive, oozing, blistering, and necrosis (10% or more of all cases). Fluid shifts into the bitten limb cause shock. Coagulopathy develops in most cases and can persist, with complete defibrination, for more than a week, associated with bleeding from gums, genitourinary tract, gastrointestinal (GI) tract, and elsewhere. Hemorrhage is the most common cause of death. Renal failure can develop in up to 20% of cases. Thrombocytopenia can occur (most common with *E. coloratus* bites) (Fig. 6). Type 2 first aid should be used.

The most effective treatment is specific antivenom therapy, but this is increasingly unavailable as producers withdraw from the African market. Without antivenom, treatment is supportive: primarily maintaining blood pressure with adequate intravenous fluid infusion, treating anemia, attempting to control coagulopathy with infusions of factor concentrates or similar (of uncertain benefit), managing renal function, and appropriate conservative wound care for the bitten area. Without full control of the coagulopathy, any form of surgical intervention is dangerous. Of the few remaining antivenoms for any *Echis* species, it is now clear that interspecific differences in venom mean that some species are not neutralized by any available antivenom. For African species, only the South African polyvalent antivenom is available, which is thought to have limited value for North African species (*E. pyramidum*). A specific *Echis* antivenom has been made for Nigerian *Echis* (*E. ocellatus*; see Color Plate 24), but availability is uncertain. *Echis* species in west Asia, including India (*E. carinatus*) and the Middle East are more reliably covered by a range of locally produced antivenoms.

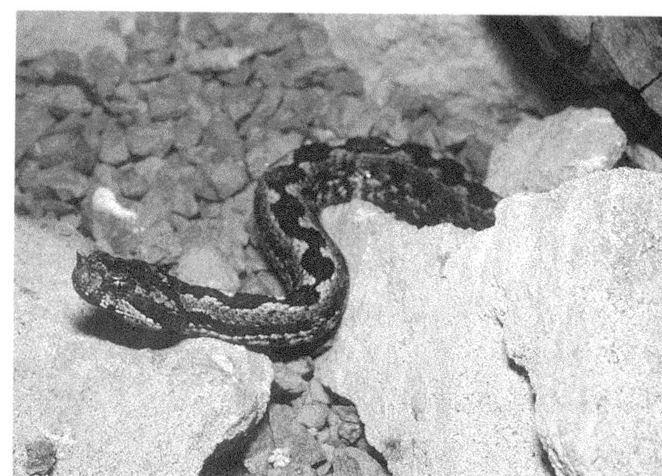

Figure 4. Balkan viper (*Vipera ammodytes*). (Original photograph copyright © by Dr. Julian White.) (See Color Plate 20.)

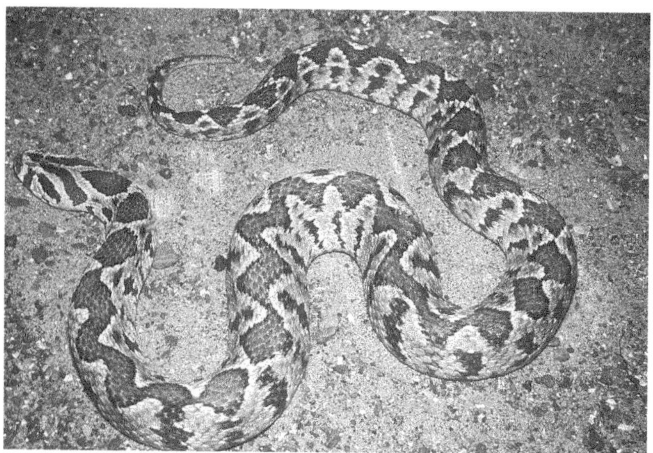

Figure 3. Palestine viper (*Vipera palestinae*). (Original photograph copyright © by Dr. Julian White.) (See Color Plate 19.)

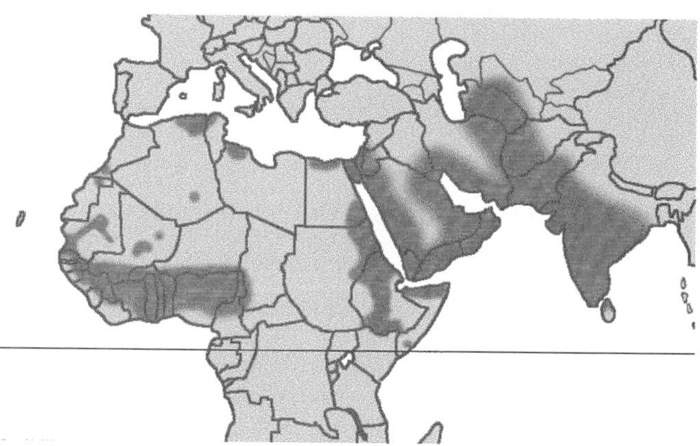

Figure 5. Distribution of saw-scaled vipers (genus *Echis*). (Original illustration copyright © by Dr. Julian White.)

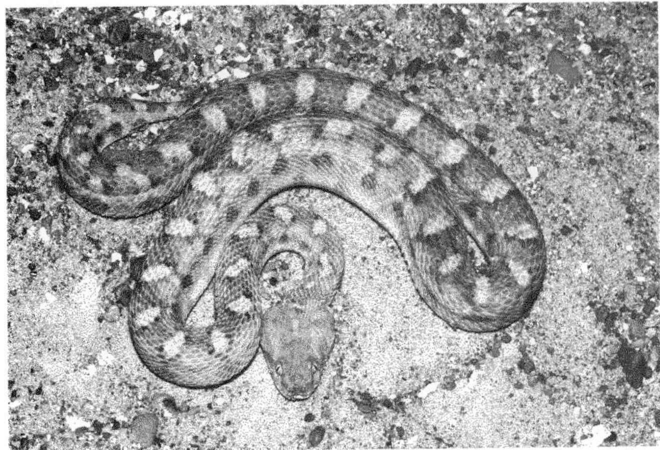

Figure 6. Burton's carpet viper (*Echis coloratus*). (Original photograph copyright © by Dr. Julian White.) (See Color Plate 21.)

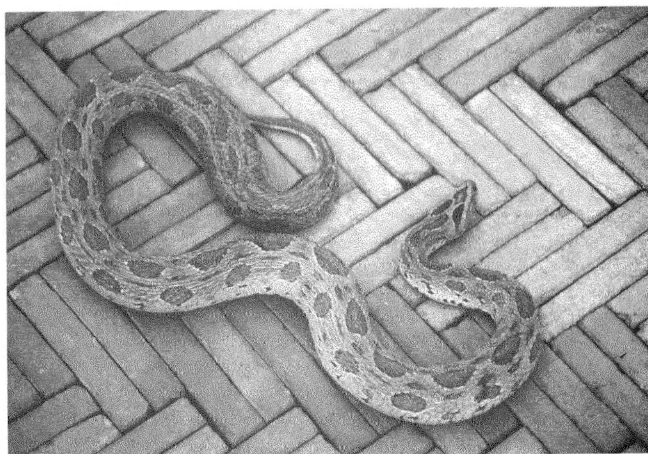

Figure 8. Thai Russell's viper (*Daboia russelii*). (Original photograph copyright © by Dr. Julian White.)

Russell's Viper (*Daboia russelii*)

Sharing almost equal infamy with the saw-scaled vipers, the Russell's viper complex, currently assigned to just one species and two subspecies, is an important cause of snakebite morbidity and mortality across Asia (Fig. 7). Depending on the geographic origin of Russell's viper, the clinical effects can include some or all of the following: local pain, swelling, blistering, oozing, necrosis, coagulopathy, hemorrhagic tendency, intravascular hemolysis, pituitary infarction causing panhypopituitarism (Sheehan's syndrome), renal failure, flaccid paralysis, systemic myolysis, generalized capillary permeability, and shock. Each geographic group of Russell's viper has a distinct venom requiring distinct specific antivenoms. For some races, such distinct antivenoms are either not currently available or are of poor quality. Type 2 first aid should be used.

The Sri Lankan Russell's viper is a major cause of bites in Sri Lanka, especially lethal bites. The most prominent clinical effects are renal damage, neurotoxicity and myotoxicity and intravascular hemolysis; coagulopathy is less marked but spontaneous bleeding can occur. Local necrosis is uncommon. Indian Russell's vipers cause more severe coagulopathy and bleeding, with more severe local effects, including necrosis and fluid shifts resulting in shock. Renal failure, paralysis, and myotoxicity are all reported, but are less common than in Sri Lankan cases. Sheehan's syndrome occasionally occurs, as does intravascular hemolysis.

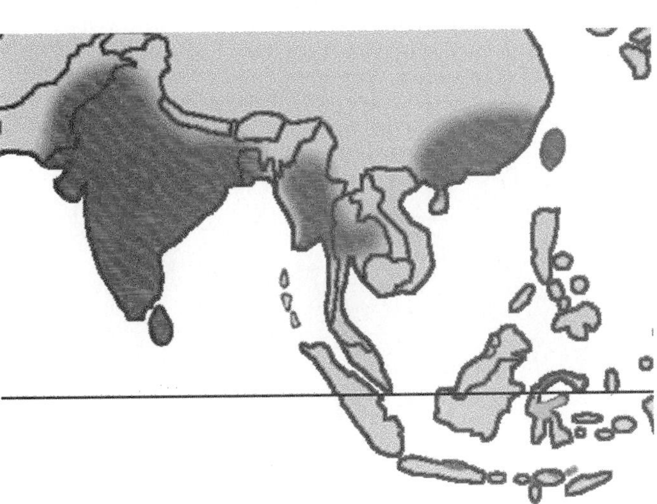

Figure 7. Distribution of Russell's vipers (genus *Daboia*). (Original illustration copyright © by Dr. Julian White.)

Burmese Russell's vipers cause severe coagulopathy, and frequently cause renal failure and generalized capillary permeability associated with shock. Sheehan's syndrome is not uncommon. However, local effects of envenoming are less severe, swelling is often minor, and necrosis rare. Life-threatening systemic envenoming can occur without significant local envenoming. Paralysis and myotoxicity do not occur.

In Indochina (notably Thailand), Russell's viper (Fig. 8) bites cause predominantly severe coagulopathy and bleeding, sometimes with renal failure or intravascular hemolysis, but not Sheehan's syndrome, paralysis, myolysis or capillary changes. Local swelling can occur but necrosis is absent.

Limited experience with Russell's viper bites in southern China indicates they cause severe coagulopathy and bleeding, local swelling and necrosis, occasionally renal failure, but not paralysis or myolysis. Taiwanese Russell's viper bites are associated with coagulopathy, bleeding, renal failure, local swelling, occasionally necrosis, but not paralysis or myolysis. There are insufficient case data to characterize Russell's viper bites in Indonesia.

Antivenom is crucial to the management of Russell's viper bite, but it must be the correct antivenom. In Sri Lanka, a recently produced ovine Fab' antivenom proved very effective in clinical trials, but is not available. Experience with antivenoms to the Indian Russell's viper when used for Sri Lankan envenoming has been disappointing. Their effectiveness for Indian races of this snake is also uncertain, but better than no antivenom. The Burmese make an effective antivenom for their race of snakes, as do the Thai (Thai Red Cross) for Indochinese snakes. This should also be considered for Indonesian Russell's viper bites and probably for Chinese cases. The Taiwanese have a specific antivenom for their race of snakes. In all cases, it should be used promptly in considerable initial doses to maximize the chances of preventing complications of envenoming. In addition to antivenom, it is important to vigorously manage shock with intravenous fluids and pressors if indicated. Fully monitor renal function and output in all cases. A period of dialysis is required if there is renal failure, but even peritoneal dialysis for just a few days has greatly reduced mortality rates in

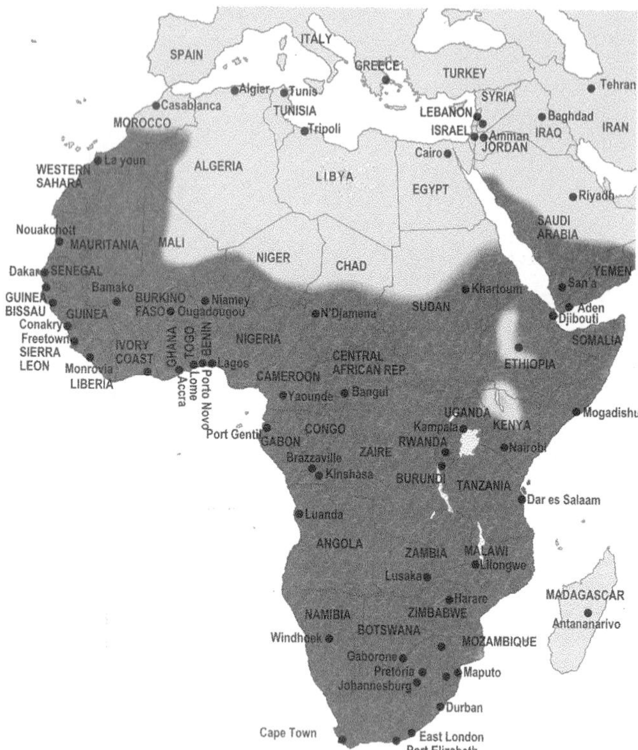

Figure 9. Distribution of African vipers (genus *Bitis*). (Original illustration copyright © by Dr. Julian White.)

southeast Asia. Some doctors have advocated heparin to manage the coagulopathy, but this has not been proven safe or effective by clinical trial and is theoretically dangerous, so cannot be recommended.

African Vipers and Adders (Genus *Bitis*)

African vipers and adders (Fig. 9) vary from small to large, including notorious species such as the puff adder, *Bitis arietans* and the gaboon viper, *B. gabonica*, both popular in private snake collections in North America and Europe. Type 2 first aid should be used. Puff adders (Fig. 10) cause severe local pain, massive swelling, blistering, oozing, extensive necrosis, and sometimes compartment syndrome or underlying muscle necrosis. Fluid shifts can cause shock. Sinus bradycardia, associated with shock, may also be a direct effect of venom components. Spontaneous bleeding occurs, but major coagulopathy with incoagulable blood is not likely. Thrombocytopenia can develop. The South African polyvalent antivenom should be used for envenoming, together with supportive treatment for shock. Beware local infection of the necrotic bite area.

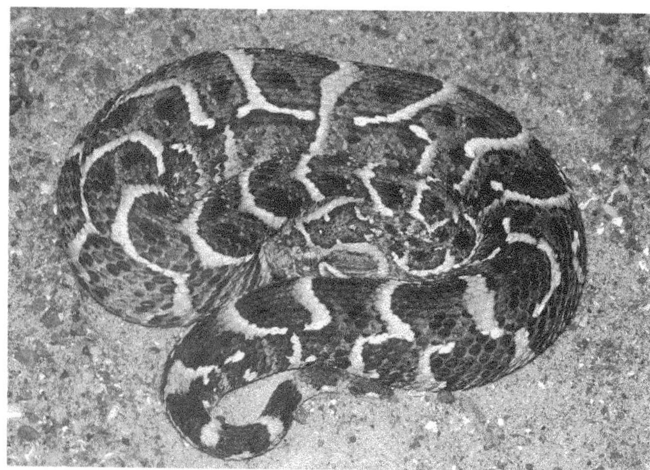

Figure 10. Puff adder (*Bitis arietans*). (Original photograph copyright © by Dr. Julian White.) (See Color Plate 22.)

Gaboon vipers can cause rapid severe local effects, with pain, swelling, blistering, necrosis, and fluid shifts causing shock. The venom is cardiotoxic, causing myocardial damage, bradycardia, atrial tachycardia, ectopic beats, and hypotension. Coagulopathy, with spontaneous bleeding, incoagulable blood, and thrombocytopenia, can occur. Early autopharmacologic effects can cause collapse soon after the bite. Antivenom is essential in treatment (South African polyvalent), sometimes requiring large doses. Supportive treatment is also required. As with puff adders, beware local infection of the bite site.

The rhinoceros viper, *B. nasicornis*, though common in captivity, is poorly characterized clinically. It can cause major envenoming, similar to puff adders or gaboon vipers, and should be treated similarly. Other *Bitis* species include the Berg adder, *B. atropos*, which can cause both local pain and swelling, rarely necrosis, systemic paralytic effects, and GI symptoms, but not coagulopathy. Most other *Bitis* species cause principally local effects, especially pain and swelling, uncommonly necrosis, but not major systemic effects. The South African polyvalent antivenom should be considered for cases with major envenoming, together with supportive and symptomatic treatment, though effectiveness of this antivenom for Berg adder bites is uncertain.

McMahon's Viper (*Eristocophis mcmahoni*)

Bites of this small snake from Western Asia are rarely reported, but fatal cases are recorded. It can cause local swelling with necrosis in severe cases, GI symptoms, possibly shock, and there is at least one case with apparent neurotoxic signs. No specific antivenom exists. Type 2 first aid should be used.

Horned Vipers (Genus *Cerastes*)

Medium-sized North African vipers (Figs. 11 and 12) cause severe, rarely lethal envenoming, with both local pain and swelling. Necrosis is not common. They can also cause mild to severe coagulopathy with bleeding. Several North African and Middle East producers make antivenoms covering bites by these snakes. Type 1 first aid should be used.

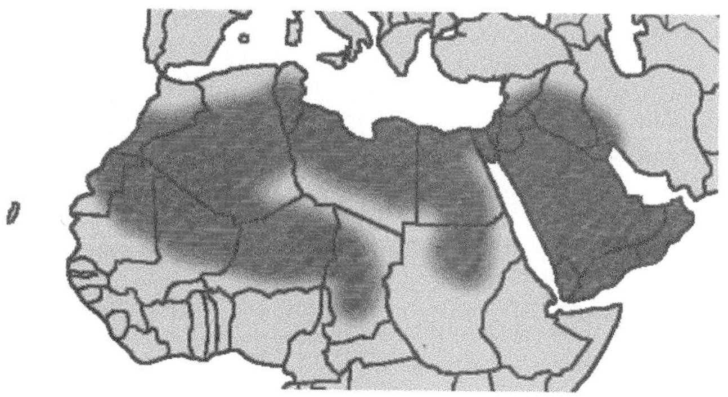

Figure 11. Distribution of horned vipers (genus *Cerastes*). (Original illustration copyright © by Dr. Julian White.)

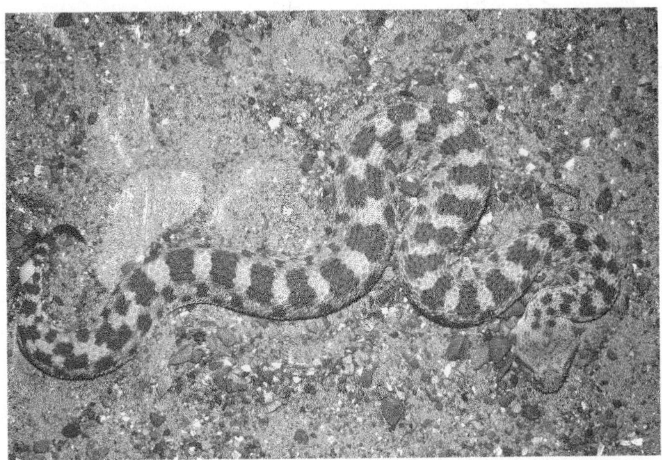

Figure 12. Horned viper (*Cerastes cerastes*). (Original photograph copyright © by Dr. Julian White.) (See Color Plate 23.)

Night Adders (Genus *Causus*)

These small African vipers (Fig. 13) are a major cause of snakebite, but bites are not severe, effects being limited to local pain and swelling without either necrosis or major systemic effects. Antivenom is neither available nor required in most cases. Should more severe envenoming occur, consider the South African polyvalent antivenom. Treat symptomatically. Type 1 first aid should be used.

False Horned Viper (*Pseudocerastes persicus*)

Only very limited case data are available for this species, but these indicate bites are minor, causing local effects only. Treat symptomatically for most cases, although specific antivenom is available from Iran. Type 1 first aid should be used.

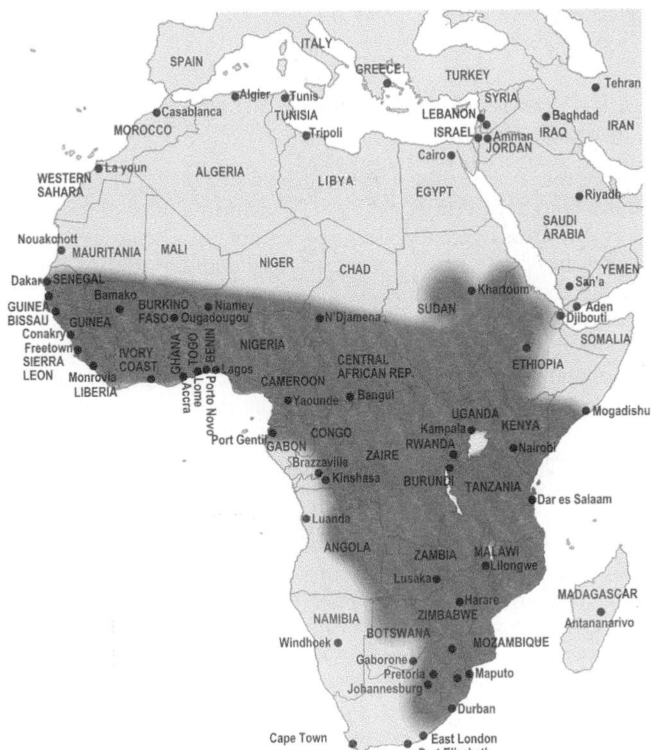

Figure 13. Distribution of night adders (genus *Causus*). (Original illustration copyright © by Dr. Julian White.)

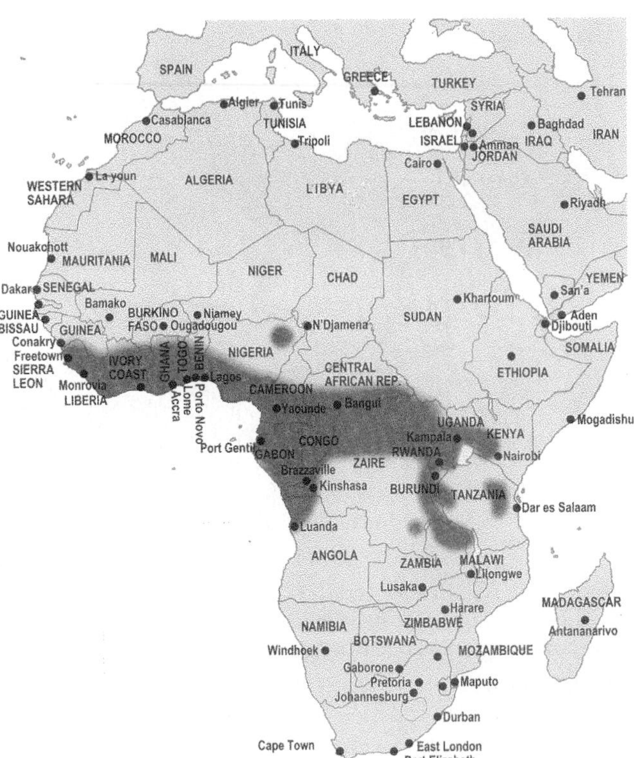

Figure 14. Distribution of bush vipers (genus *Atheris*). (Original illustration copyright © by Dr. Julian White.)

African Bush Vipers (Genera *Atheris, Montatheris,* and *Proatheris*)

Although case data on envenoming by these snakes from Africa (Fig. 14) are sparse, it appears they can cause moderate to severe local pain, swelling, fluid shifts and shock; systemic coagulopathy and fatalities are recorded. Species particularly implicated in major bites are *A. squamiger, A. chlorechis,* and *A. ceratophorus*. No antivenom is available, but the South African anti-*Echis* antivenom is considered to be effective for *Atheris* bites and should be considered in more severe cases. Treatment should be supportive and symptomatic. Type 2 first aid should be used.

Barbour's Bush Viper (*Adenorhinos barbouri*)

Barbour's bush viper is unlikely to cause more than local pain and swelling. No antivenom is available, so treat symptomatically. Type 1 first aid should be used.

Fea's Viper (*Azemiops feae*)

Fea's viper, a small East Asian viper, has rarely been reported to bite, causing only local pain and swelling. It is unclear if it can cause more severe envenoming. No specific antivenom is available. Treat symptomatically. Type 1 first aid should be used.

PIT VIPERS (SUBFAMILY CROTALINAE)

American Pit Vipers (Genus *Agkistrodon*)

Most former members of this genus now reside in *Gloydius*, so that currently there are only three *Agkistrodon* species (Fig. 15):

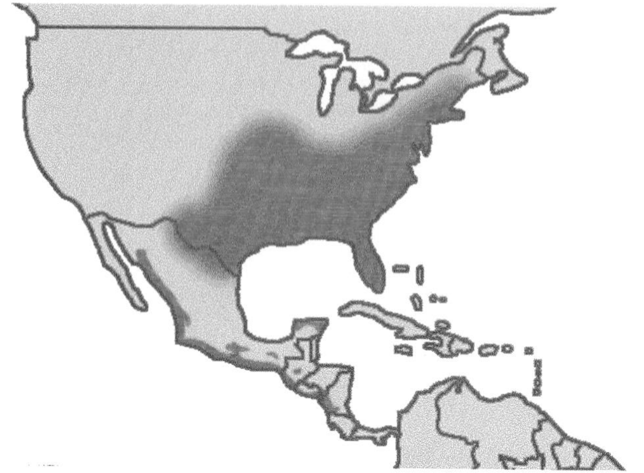

Figure 15. Distribution of American pit vipers (genus *Agkistrodon*). (Original illustration copyright © by Dr. Julian White.)

A. contortrix, *A. piscivorus*, and *A. bilineatus* (Mexican cantil) (Fig. 16). These snakes are considered in detail in the chapter on North American snakebite (Chapter 245). Type 2 first aid should be used.

Jumping Pit Vipers (Genus *Atropoides*)

Jumping pit vipers, small vipers from Central America, are not reported as a significant cause of bites. In the absence of good clinical data, it should be assumed that most bites cause little more than local pain and swelling. In a severe case, swelling may cause fluid shifts and shock. Necrosis cannot be excluded, but is unlikely. Coagulopathy may be minor only. Paralysis and myolysis are not expected, but secondary renal failure might occur in a severe case. Type 2 first aid should be used.

Central and South American Pit Vipers (Genus *Bothriechis*)

There are seven members of this genus of small vipers of Central and northwestern South America, the best known of which is the eyelash viper, *B. schlegelii*. Bites in their native distribution are rarely reported. Most bites are minor, though more severe local or even systemic effects might potentially occur. In the absence of good clinical data, it should be assumed that most bites cause little more than local pain and swelling, though in a severe case, the latter might cause fluid shifts and shock. Necrosis cannot be excluded, but is unlikely. Coagulopathy, if present, may be minor only. Paralysis and myolysis are not expected, but secondary renal failure might occur in a more severe case. Type 2 first aid should be used.

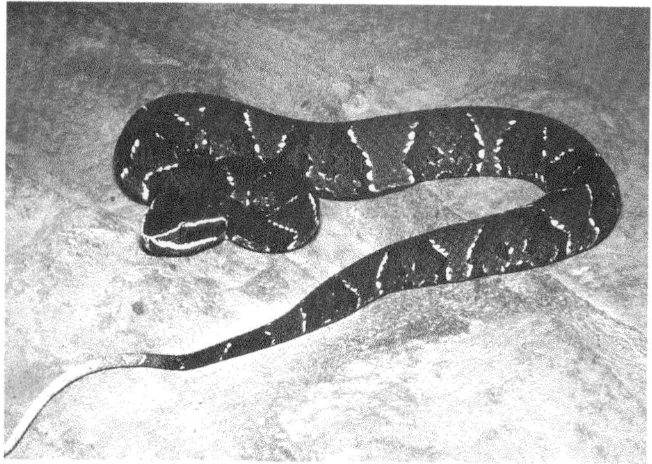

Figure 16. Mexican cantil (*Agkistrodon bilineatus*). (Original photograph copyright © by Dr. Julian White.)

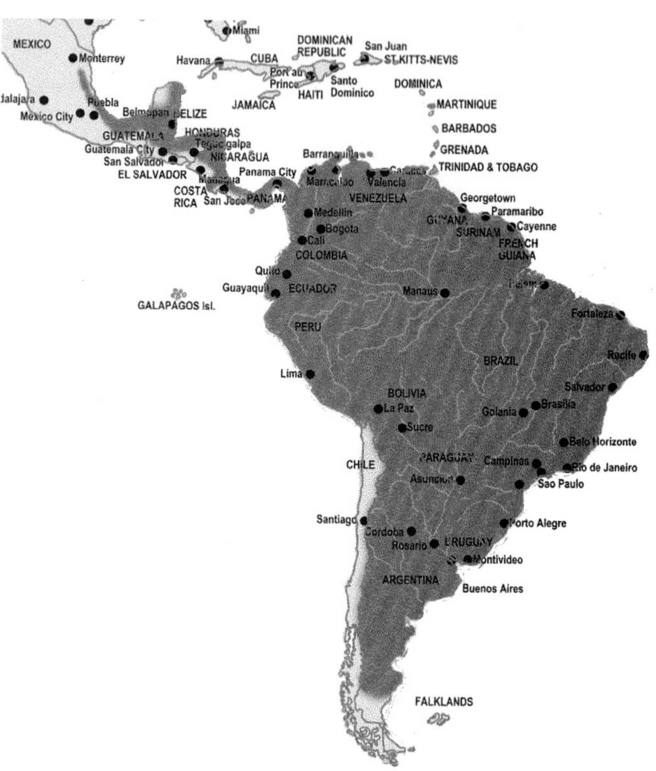

Figure 17. Distribution of lancehead pit vipers (genus *Bothrops*). (Original illustration copyright © by Dr. Julian White.)

South American Lancehead Pit Vipers (Genus *Bothrops*)

This genus contains the greatest number of pit viper species in Central and South America (Fig. 17), including most of the medically important species. Some species are both a frequent cause of bites and cause a high rate of morbidity and mortality. Type 2 first aid should be used.

Bites by *B. alternatus*, the urutu, cause local pain and sometimes severe swelling, with potential for fluid shifts. Ecchymosis and blistering may also develop, the latter often progressing to necrosis. Systemic effects are principally those of coagulopathy and hemorrhage. Renal damage is not commonly reported, but should be considered a risk. A polyvalent antivenom with specific activity against the urutu is available in Brazil.

B. asper, the terciopelo, is also known locally as fer-de-lance, barba amarilla. A major cause of bites within its range, this snake causes local pain and sometimes severe swelling with fluid shifts and shock. Blistering, necrosis, abscess formation, compartment syndrome (10% of cases in one series), as well as systemic envenoming may develop, characterized by coagulopathy, hemorrhagic tendency, bleeding into major organs, shock, and renal failure. In one study, nearly 40% of cases developed renal failure, 10% had cerebral hemorrhages, and more than 80% had severe envenoming. Antivenom therapy is crucial, combined with good supportive care, wound care, and antibiotics to deal with abscesses. The coagulopathy may preclude early surgical attention to any compartment syndrome. Polyvalent antivenoms specifically covering this species are available from Mexico, Costa Rica, and other Central American producers.

B. atrox is known as the fer-de-lance or barba amarilla (as is *B. asper*). Bites by *B. atrox* are in general similar to *B. asper*, as is management. Several producers in Central and South America make polyvalent antivenoms covering this species.

B. jararaca, the jararaca, is probably the most important cause of major snakebite in Brazil. Bites cause rapid development of local and systemic envenoming, including local pain, often severe swelling, blistering, bleeding, necrosis, abscess formation, adenopathy, systemic coagulopathy, hemorrhagic tendency, thrombocytopenia, shock, and renal failure. Antivenom is crucial in management of both local and especially systemic effects. The principal Brazilian polyvalent antivenom is particularly targeted against this species and is considered effective. *B. jararacusu*, the jararacusu, is a larger version of the jararaca in many respects, causing similar local and systemic effects. Treatment is similar. Juvenile specimens less than 50 cm long do not generally cause significant local effects, but still cause the typical major systemic effects, so require antivenom treatment.

B. lanceolatus, the Martinique lancehead, is quite distinctive in clinical effects. Although it causes local pain and sometimes severe swelling, blistering and necrosis are not prominent. The coagulopathy is most unusual, being associated with widespread thrombosis, not hemorrhage. Thrombotic events are well reported, as are pulmonary emboli and thrombotic infarction of vital organs, especially the brain and heart. Antivenom is the obvious treatment and has proven most effective. However, the only product available previously is now in uncertain supply, posing a major management dilemma, especially because use of heparin has not shown significant benefit.

B. moojeni, the Brazilian lancehead, causes clinical effects similar to *B. jararaca* and should be managed in the same way. *B. neuwiedi*, Neuwied's lancehead, is similar to *B. moojeni*, but bites are less commonly severe. There are numerous other *Bothrops* species whose bites are largely undocumented, but should be expected to fall within the clinical spectrum of the species listed above (except the unique Martinique lancehead). Treatment should be similar, except that the smaller species are less likely to cause major local or systemic envenoming, so are less likely to require antivenom therapy.

Malayan Pit Viper (*Calloselasma rhodostoma*)

Widely distributed through Indochina to Burma in the west and Indonesia in the east (Figs. 18 and 19), the Malayan pit viper causes many bites with major morbidity and considerable mortality. Bites cause local pain, often rapid and extensive swelling, commonly with blistering. Fluid shifts can cause shock. Local necrosis can occur, most commonly with bites on digits. Secondary infection occurs, but generally only in cases with necrosis, where it can extend the extent of damage.

Cases with systemic envenoming invariably develop a profound coagulopathy, usually with thrombocytopenia and hemorrhagic tendency. Untreated, this can persist for days to several weeks. Antivenom treatment is crucial in effective management, which should also include supportive care, notably attention to correcting hypovolemic shock, maintaining renal function, and ensuring any wound infection is adequately treated. Fasciotomy is generally contraindicated because of the coagulopathy. Specific antivenom is available from the Thai Red Cross, the Vietnamese, and others. Type 2 first aid should be used.

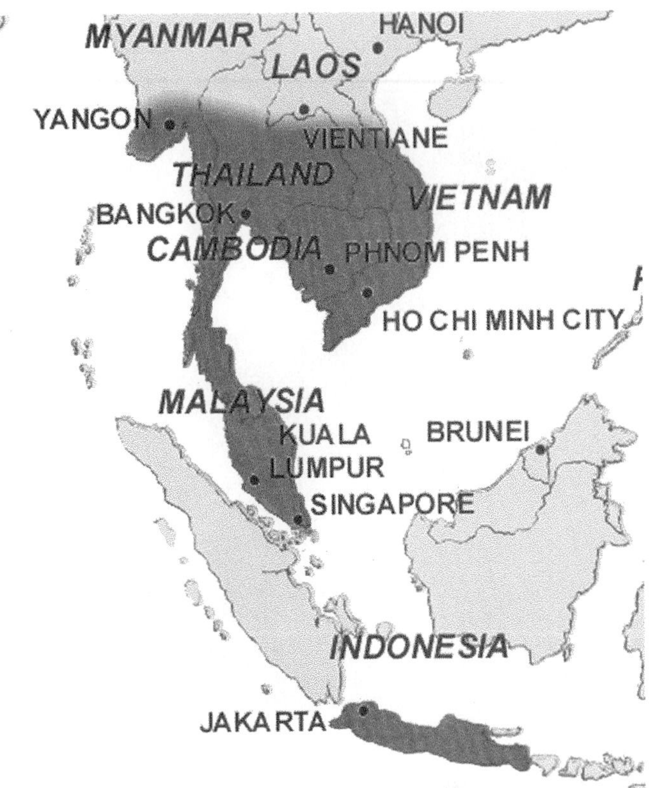

Figure 18. Distribution of Malayan pit viper (genus *Calloselasma*). (Original illustration copyright © by Dr. Julian White.)

Montane Pit Vipers (Genus *Cerrophidion*)

Montane pit vipers, smallish snakes from Central America, are a poorly documented cause of bites. In the absence of good clinical data, it should be assumed that most bites cause little more than local pain and swelling. In a severe case, the latter might cause fluid shifts and shock. Necrosis cannot be excluded, but is unlikely. Coagulopathy, if present, may be minor only. Paralysis and myolysis are not expected, but secondary renal failure might occur in a more severe case. Type 2 first aid should be used.

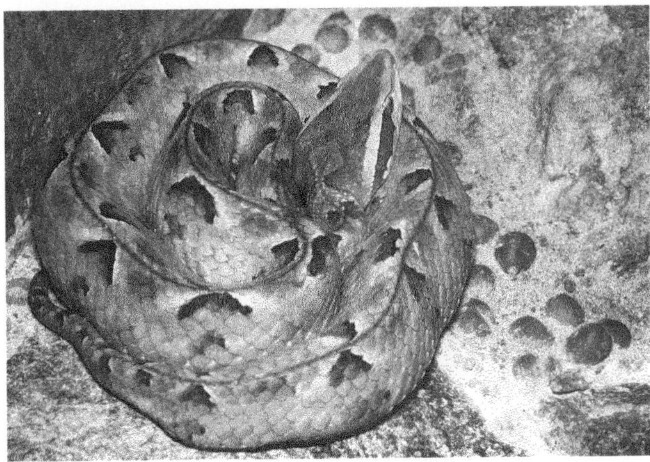

Figure 19. Malayan pit viper (*Calloselasma rhodostoma*). (Original photograph copyright © by Dr. Julian White.) (See Color Plate 24.)

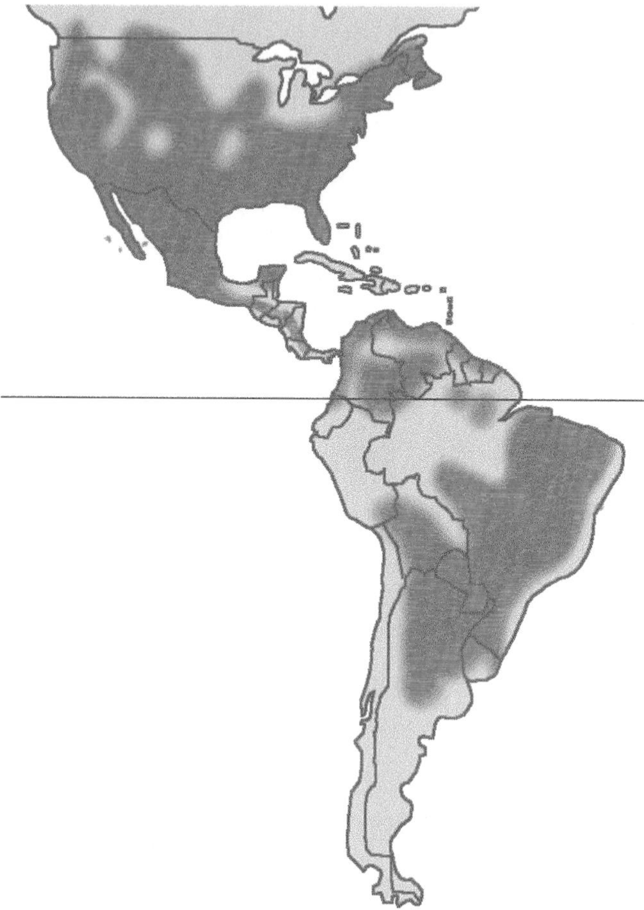

Figure 20. Distribution of rattlesnakes (genus *Crotalus*). (Original illustration copyright © by Dr. Julian White.)

Rattlesnakes (Genus *Crotalus*)

There are two distinct groups of rattlesnakes (Fig. 20): the North American group, causing major local effects and sometimes systemic envenoming, and the Central and South American group (Fig. 21), causing less significant local effects but major systemic effects. The North American crotaline snakes are addressed in Chapter 245.

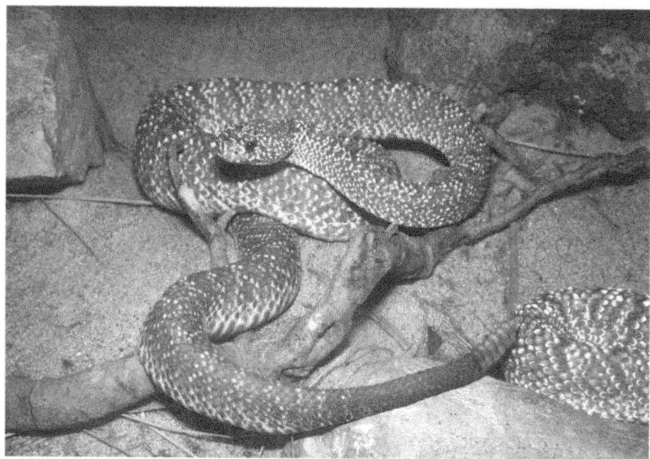

Figure 21. Venezuelan rattlesnake (*Crotalus durissus vegrandis*). (Original photograph copyright © by Dr. Julian White.)

Bites by South American rattlesnakes are typified by the neotropical rattlesnake, *Crotalus durissus terrificus*. Minimal to significant local pain with minimal swelling (occasionally extensive) is present, whereas blistering, bruising, and necrosis do not occur. In more serious bites, major systemic envenoming can be apparent within an hour of the bite, but may be delayed several hours. There may be general symptoms, such as headache, nausea, vomiting, or abdominal pain, but these may all be absent despite major envenoming. Major toxicity is characterized by flaccid paralysis and myolysis. The paralysis usually first presents as ptosis, then ophthalmoplegia, other cranial nerve weakness, sometimes pupil dilation, then progressive skeletal muscle weakness, culminating in respiratory paralysis. First paralytic signs may be evident within 1 hour of the bite. Speed of progression is variable.

Myolysis may also develop early, presenting first as painful or tender muscles, often associated with red to black urine (myoglobinuria). Renal failure, usually anuric, secondary to the myolysis is common and may be associated with potentially lethal hyperkalemia. Death is most often due to intractable cardiac or respiratory arrest. Muscle biopsies show clear evidence of widespread myolysis in such cases. In the past, coagulopathy has not been considered a feature of envenoming by these snakes, but more recent case data from bites by *Crotalus durissus* subspecies from Brazil clearly show that mild to moderate coagulopathy can occur, including defibrination, though major pathologic bleeding is not a feature. Substantial case report data are not available for most species or subspecies in this group, so it is assumed, rather than proven, that all cause similar patterns of envenoming.

Specific and polyvalent antivenoms are available in South and Central America to cover major species, but high initial doses are often required. It is unclear if antivenom can reverse established major paralysis, though it is likely it cannot. Although paralysis is often emphasized in past overviews of bites by these rattlesnakes, setting them apart from their North American cousins, more recent case reports clearly indicate that it is myolysis which is more severe, leading to secondary renal failure and cardiotoxicity. Type 1 first aid should be used.

Hundred Pace Snake (*Deinagkistrodon acutus*)

Restricted to parts of China, Taiwan, and northern Indochina (Fig. 22), this snake is a significant cause of major bites. The bite is painful, with oozing from the bite site. Rapid and severe swelling develops with fluid shifts and shock. Development of blistering and local necrosis is common, especially for bites to digits. There is rapid development of coagulopathy and a hemorrhagic tendency. Antivenom is important in managing envenoming by these snakes, which even so have reported fatality rates as high as 5%. Specific antivenom is produced in Taiwan and China. Correction of hypovolemic shock is also important in management, together with good wound care and avoidance of early surgical intervention. Type 2 first aid should be used.

Mount Mang Pit Viper (*Ermia mangshanensis*)

Restricted to parts of Hunan Province, China, there are no case data on bites by this snake. No specific antivenom is available. Type 2 first aid should be used.

Asian Pit Vipers and Mamushis (Genus *Gloydius*)

Asian pit vipers (formerly in genus *Agkistrodon*) are an important cause of snakebite morbidity and limited mortality within their range in Asia (Fig. 23). Type 2 first aid should be used.

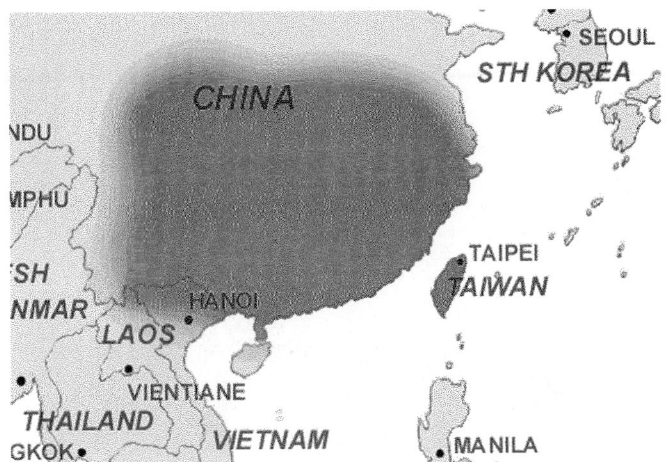

Figure 22. Distribution of hundred pace snake (genus *Deinagkistrodon*). (Original illustration copyright © by Dr. Julian White.)

The mamushis (Japanese mamushi, *G. blomhoffii blomhoffii*; Chinese mamushi, *G. blomhoffii brevicaudus*) are an important cause of major snakebite within their ranges. The Japanese mamushi causes local pain, swelling, the latter sometimes involving the entire bitten limb, with blistering, fluid shifts, and shock. Coagulopathy and bleeding can occur, with ecchymoses and renal failure reported. Mild cranial nerve paresis can develop, though it is rare and full flaccid paralysis does not occur. A specific antivenom is available.

The Chinese mamushi is also a major cause of bites, but local effects are less severe, whereas paralytic effects are sometimes far more prominent, with major, even lethal paralysis reported. Though not confirmed, myolysis seems likely based on case reports of muscle pain and probable myoglobinuria. Renal failure can occur. A specific antivenom is available from Shanghai. In addition to antivenom, supportive treatment, particularly if there is shock, respiratory failure, or renal failure, may be crucial. Because of the likelihood of paralytic effects, Type 1 first aid should be used.

Other members of this genus may cause less severe envenoming. Specific antivenom is available only for *G. intermedius* bites in Iran.

Hump-Nosed Vipers (Genus *Hypnale*)

Limited to Sri Lanka (Fig. 24) and adjacent India (*H. hypnale* only), where *H. hypnale* is a common cause of bites, with local

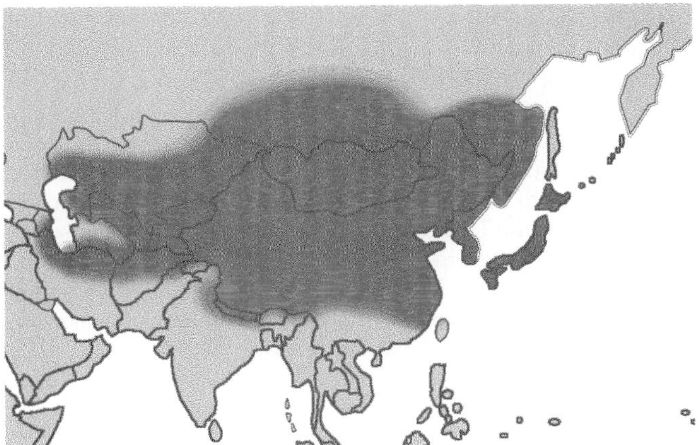

Figure 23. Distribution of Asian pit vipers (genus *Gloydius*). (Original illustration copyright © by Dr. Julian White.)

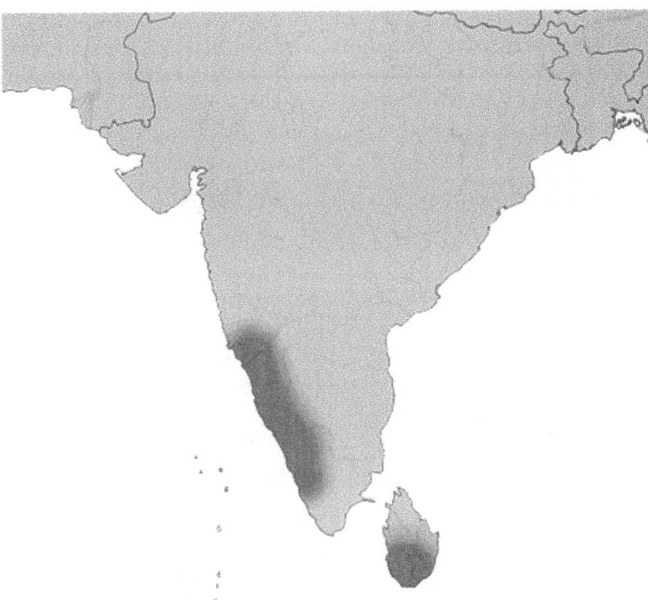

Figure 24. Distribution of hump-nosed vipers (genus *Hypnale*). (Original illustration copyright © by Dr. Julian White.)

pain, swelling, blistering, and systemically, moderate to severe coagulopathy and occasionally renal failure. The coagulopathy can be prolonged over days to more than a week, but major bleeding is not common. No specific antivenom is available, so for most cases treatment is supportive and symptomatic. Type 2 first aid should be used.

Bushmasters (Genus *Lachesis*)

There are three species of bushmasters, ranging from Central America through to Brazil in South America (Fig. 25). *L. muta* is the classic bushmaster. These large snakes are capable of moderate to severe envenoming, but current evidence suggests they are an infrequent cause of bites. Bites are characterized by local pain, swelling, which may be extensive, with potential for fluid shifts and shock. Ecchymoses are common, with local bleeding. Necrosis may occur, but may not be prominent. Apart from hypovolemic shock, the principal systemic feature is coagulop-

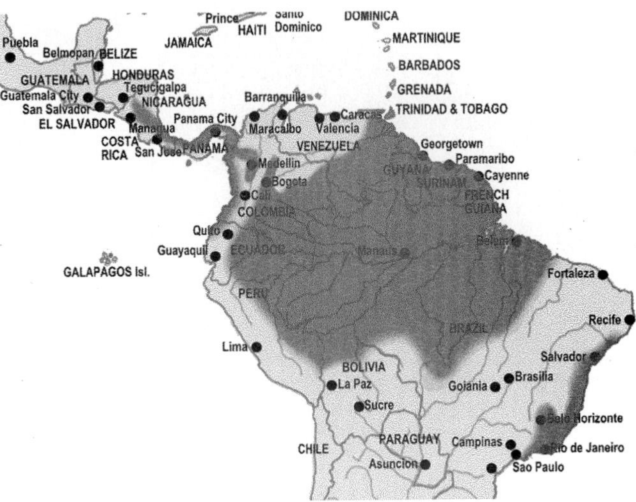

Figure 25. Distribution of bushmasters (genus *Lachesis*). (Original illustration copyright © by Dr. Julian White.)

athy, with fibrinogen consumption and a mild to moderate bleeding tendency. Antivenom is important in management, and several polyvalent products covering bushmasters are available in Central and South America. Correction of hypovolemic shock is also required. Type 2 first aid should be used.

Montane Pit Vipers (Genus *Ophryacus*)

There are little case data available on these two small species from Mexico. It is probable that most bites will cause little more than local pain and swelling, though in a severe case, the latter might cause fluid shifts and shock. Necrosis is unlikely. Coagulopathy is likely to be minor only. Paralysis and myolysis are not expected, but secondary renal failure might occur in a severe case. Type 2 first aid should be used.

Mountain Pit Vipers and Habus (Genus *Ovophis*)

Though case data are scarce for most of these small Asian pit vipers, it appears that they can cause local pain and significant local swelling. Systemic effects of coagulopathy, widespread ecchymoses, and a general hemorrhagic tendency may occur, but not paralysis or myolysis. Fatalities have been reported for some species. No specific antivenom is available. *O. okinavensis* bites have been treated with Japanese habu antivenom. Type 2 first aid should be used.

Hog-Nosed Pit Vipers (Genus *Porthidium*)

Hog-nosed pit vipers are small vipers from Central and South America. There are little case data on the effects of bites. It is probable that most bites cause little more than local pain and swelling. Necrosis is unlikely. Coagulopathy is likely minor only. Paralysis and myolysis are not expected, but secondary renal failure might occur in a severe case. Type 2 first aid should be used.

Habus and Related Pit Vipers (Genus *Protobothrops*)

Despite the generic name, these pit vipers occur in Asia (Fig. 26), the most important members being the Chinese habu, *P. mucrosquamatus*, and Sakishima habu, *P. elegans*. On Okinawa, *P. elegans* is a significant cause of bites, resulting in local pain, swelling, fluid shifts, and shock in severe cases, with necrosis reported (mainly of digits). Coagulopathy, paralysis, and myolysis do not occur. In contrast, in Taiwan and southern China, *P. mucrosquamatus* causes not only moderate to severe local effects, with fluid shifts and shock, but coagulopathy and a hemorrhagic tendency. Coma and convulsions may occur, but necrosis is rare. The Taiwanese make an antivenom specific for this species, but no antivenom is available for *P. elegans* or other members of this genus. Type 2 first aid should be used.

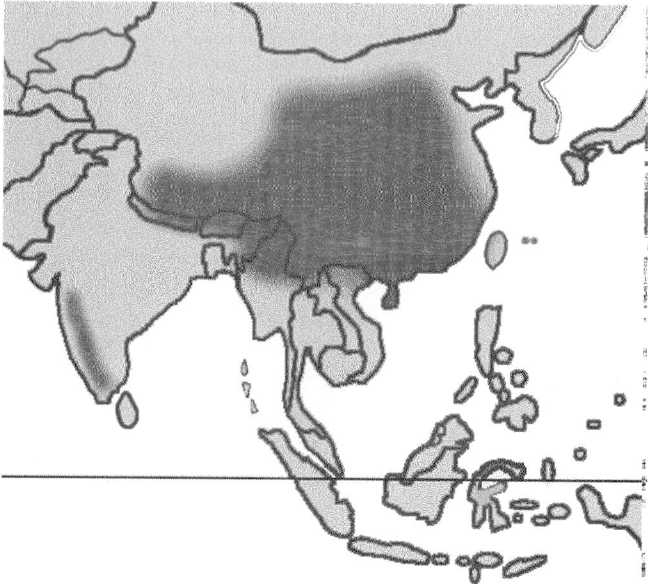

Figure 26. Distribution of habus (genus *Protobothrops*). (Original illustration copyright © by Dr. Julian White.)

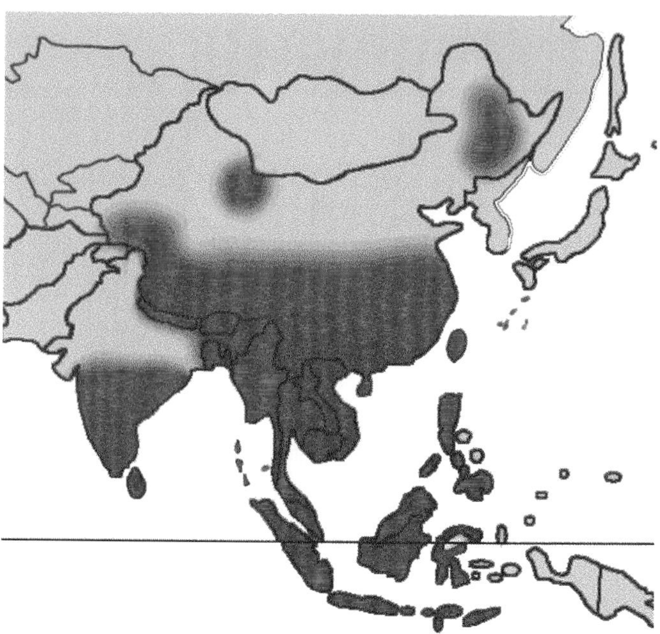

Figure 27. Distribution of green tree pit vipers (genus *Trimeresurus*). (Original illustration copyright © by Dr. Julian White.)

Massasaugas (Genus *Sistrurus*)

Pigmy rattlesnakes and massasaugas are considered in detail in Chapter 245. Type 2 first aid should be used.

Green Pit Vipers (Genus *Trimeresurus*)

This large genus of Asian tree pit vipers (Fig. 27), some but not all of which are green in color, includes some species responsible for many bites, but generally low mortality. Type 2 first aid should be used.

The white-lipped green pit viper, *T. albolabris* (Fig. 28), a common cause of bites across its range, including Bangkok, can cause major local and systemic envenoming, with local pain, swelling, blistering, but only rarely necrosis; systemically, mild to severe coagulopathy can occur, with a hemorrhagic tendency. Shock can occur, but is uncommon. A specific antivenom is available from the Thai Red Cross, but large amounts are sometimes required to reverse coagulopathy.

The habu, *T. flavoviridis* (Fig. 29), from the Okinawa region of Japan where it is a major cause of snakebite, has rather different effects. Local envenoming can be severe, with fluid shifts and shock and necrosis in nearly half of all cases. However, coagulopathy is not seen, nor is there a hemorrhagic tendency, myolysis, or paralysis, most systemic effects relating to secondary effects of hypovolemic shock. The Japanese make a specific antivenom.

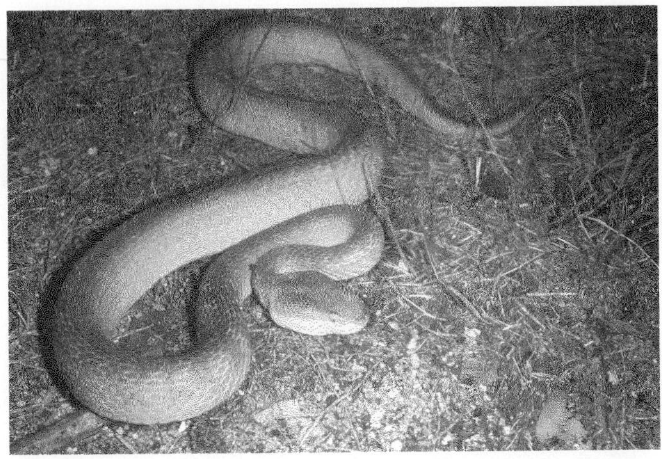

Figure 28. White-lipped green tree viper (*Trimeresurus albolabris*). (Original photograph copyright © by Dr. Julian White.) (See Color Plate 26.)

T. gramineus, the bamboo pit viper of India, is thought to cause considerable numbers of bites, but these are rarely reported so case data are scant. Venom research data suggest bites might cause coagulopathy, but this is not confirmed clinically. Local pain and swelling do occur, and nonspecific GI tract symptoms are reported. No specific antivenom is available, though several Indian antivenoms are claimed to cover this species.

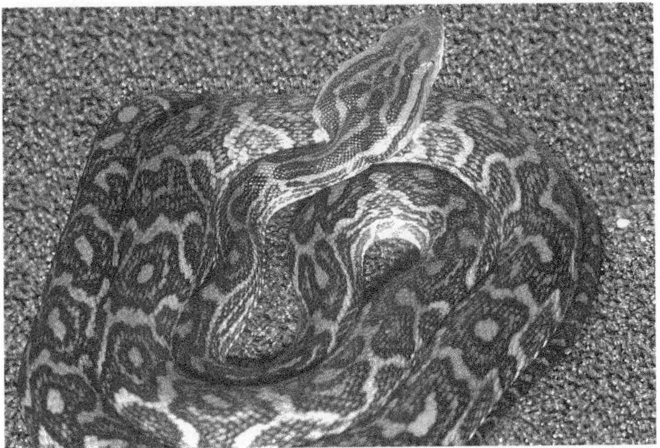

Figure 29. Habu (*Trimeresurus flavoviridis*). (Original photograph copyright © by Dr. Julian White.) (See Color Plate 17.)

Pope's pit viper, *T. popeiorum*, is common but does not appear to cause significant local or systemic effects. *T. purpureomaculatus*, the mangrove pit viper, is common in parts of Malaysia, can cause local pain, swelling, even necrosis and systemically can cause coagulopathy with incoagulable blood and occasionally fatal hemorrhage. There is no specific antivenom, so treatment must be supportive and symptomatic. For coagulopathy, factor concentrates could be considered, but not heparin.

The Chinese bamboo pit viper, *T. stejnegeri*, is a very common cause of bites in Taiwan and adjacent China. However, it is rarely lethal, though it can cause moderate to severe swelling, sometimes with fluid shifts and secondary shock, but only rarely necrosis or coagulopathy. A specific antivenom is available in Taiwan.

Wagler's Pit Vipers (Genus *Tropidolaemus*)

Only two species of this genus are listed, Wagler's pit viper being the best known, also known as the temple pit viper, *Tropidolaemus wagleri* (see Color Plate 18). Bites are often minor, but significant local pain and swelling do occur. Necrosis is rare and coagulopathy is not documented. As no antivenom is available, treatment is supportive and symptomatic. Type 2 first aid should be used.

SUGGESTED READINGS

Bon C, Goyffon M, eds. *Envenomings and their treatments.* Paris: Institute Pasteur, 1995.

Campbell JA, Lamar WW, eds. *The venomous reptiles of Latin America.* Ithaca, NY: Comstock, 1989.

Covacevich J, Davie P, Pearn J, eds. *Toxic plants and animals: a guide for Australia.* Brisbane: Queensland Museum, 1987.

Gopalakrishnakone P, Chou LM, eds. *Snakes of medical importance (Asia-Pacific region).* Singapore: Singapore University Press, 1990.

Gopalakrishnakone P, ed. *Sea snake toxinology.* Singapore: Singapore University Press, 1994.

Junghanss T, Bodio M. *Notfall-handbuch gifttiere.* Stuttgart: Georg Thieme Verlag, 1996.

Mebs D. *Venomous and poisonous animals.* Boca Raton, FL: CRC Press, 2002.

Meier J, White J, eds. *Handbook of clinical toxicology of animal venoms and poisons.* Boca Raton, FL: CRC Press, 1995.

Warrell DA, ed. WHO/SEARO guidelines for the clinical management of snakebites in the Southeast Asian region. *SE Asian J Trop Med Public Health* 1999;30(suppl 1):1–85.

White J, Persson H. Snakes. In: Descotes J, ed. *Human toxicology.* Amsterdam: Elsevier, 1996:757–802.

SECTION

2

Arthropods

CHAPTER 248

Widow Spider Envenomation: Latrodectism

Andis Graudins

OVERVIEW

Widow spiders are members of the genus *Latrodectus* (Araneae: Araneomorphae: Theridiidae). They are perhaps the most clinically significant group of spiders worldwide. In general, Theridiid spiders are referred to as the *comb-footed spiders* and include a number of related genera: *Steatoda*, *Theridion*, and *Argyrodes*. These may be mistaken for widow spiders by untrained observers but present a lesser threat to humans. All Theridiid spiders are typically small to medium sized with a large globular abdomen, relatively small cephalothorax, and long thin legs (1,2). *Latrodectus* spp. are black or dark brown in color with a characteristic hourglass-patterned red mark on the ventral surface of the abdomen. Some species, such as *L. hasselti* (Australian red-back spider), also have a red, pink, or sometimes white stripe (especially in juvenile spiders) on the dorsal surface of the abdomen. The male of these species is considerably smaller than the female and does not pose an envenomation threat to humans (3).

Latrodectus spp. are found on all continents excluding Antarctica. The genus extends up to 50 degrees North latitude in central Europe, 40 degrees North latitude in North America, and as far south as the southern tips of Australia, Africa, and South America (1). Species exist in the Middle East and New Zealand as well as Southeast Asia. Widow spiders are relatively shy and reclusive (3). They exist in natural and in urban environments with a preference for warm, dry, and secluded conditions. This may include the bottom of hay stacks, in farming fields, under wood piles and garden furniture; in corners of garages, barns, and sheds; and in old houses (4).

The true incidence of widow spider bite and envenomation is poorly characterized. In the United States, the poison centers reported 2757 cases of widow spider bite in 1997, with only 0.004% defined as having a "major outcome" (5). In Australia, an estimate of 2000 to 3000 *L. hasselti* (red-back spider) bites per year has been made. Clinically significant *L. hasselti* envenomation requiring antivenom therapy is estimated to occur in approximately 20% of bites (6,7).

Although rarely fatal, envenomation by *Latrodectus* spp. may result in an incapacitating syndrome of severe local, regional, or systemic pain and autonomic features called *latrodectism*. If left untreated, this can last for several days or weeks (1,4).

PATHOPHYSIOLOGY

The venoms of all *Latrodectus* spp. appear to contain similar toxic components. Firstly, envenomation resulting from the bite of any widow spider results in a similar clinical picture regardless of the species of spider. Secondly, widow spider antivenoms produced using the venoms of specific *Latrodectus* spp. reverse the effects of envenomation from other *Latrodectus* spiders in animal models and in the clinical setting (8–11). Finally, all widow spider venoms contain a number of high-molecular-weight insect- and vertebrate-specific toxins, called *latrotoxins*, all of which have a similar mechanism of action (10,12). These latrotoxins have been characterized from the venom of the European widow spider (*L. tredecimguttatus*), but, to date, little is known about the structure of related toxins found in other *Latrodectus* spp. venom (13–18).

Latrotoxins have high binding affinity for neuronal tissues. α-Latrotoxin (α-LTx) is a 120-kd vertebrate-specific toxin that produces envenomation in humans (16,19–21). At least three other insect-specific latroinsectotoxins also exist. These have a similar mechanism of action to that of α-LTx. Two independent, parallel mechanisms of action have been identified for all latrotoxins. These result in massive synaptic vesicle degranulation and neurotransmitter release. First, α-LTx binds to calcium-dependent receptors (neurexin-1α) found on the presynaptic nerve terminal of cell membranes (22,23). In association with this receptor binding, a-LTx combines to form tetramers in the presence of calcium (24). The tetramers insert themselves into the cell membrane and produce ion channels that are permeable to calcium and other divalent cations, resulting in calcium-dependent release of neurotransmitters (24,25). Second, α-LTx binds to latrophilin, a calcium-independent receptor, which can stimulate synaptic vesicle degranulation in the absence of calcium (22,26,27). This probably results from internalization of α-LTx into the cell and subsequent blocking of the mechanism that inhibits vesicle degranulation.

PREGNANCY AND LACTATION

The signs and symptoms of envenomation by a widow spider may mimic those of preeclampsia. Envenomation can cause abdominal contractions and has been associated with premature delivery and spontaneous abortion; however, serious envenomation can occur without adverse effects on the pregnancy (28,29). Maretic et al. treated three women in their second, fourth, and eighth months of pregnancy (28,29). Despite the development of latrodectism, the course of these pregnancies appeared to be unaffected.

At least some concern is warranted, however, because Maretic and Lebez (28) also reported that spontaneous abortion was common in guinea pigs and mice envenomated by the black widow spider, although rats were resistant to venom-induced spontaneous abortion. Because of the potentially severe outcome for the fetus and the relative safety of antivenom, most authors recommend use of antivenom in the pregnant patient with a symptomatic widow spider bite (30).

CLINICAL PRESENTATION

Widow spider envenomation results in an incapacitating syndrome of severe local, regional, or systemic pain and autonomic features called latrodectism (1,4). Fatalities are uncommon, with only one reported in the medical literature since the 1960s. The reported death was very unusual and involved histologically proven myocarditis in a 19-year-old Greek woman with a well-documented bite by *L. mactans tredecimguttatus* (31). The syndrome of latrodectism is clinically similar across continents but may vary in severity depending on the species and size of the spider, the season of the year, and the amount of venom injected (32–38).

The bite of a widow spider is commonly described as initially feeling like a bee sting (4,32,37,39). Local pain, sweating, erythema, and piloerection are noted at the bite site within 1 hour of exposure, but the onset may take longer (4,36,37). Pain is the dominant feature of envenomation and may be out of proportion to clinical signs. Mild tachycardia, hypertension, and pyrexia with regional lymphadenopathy may be apparent. Symptoms may remain isolated to the site of the bite or, less commonly, progress to become regional or systemic (Table 1).

Progression to systemic toxicity with *L. hasselti* bite is estimated to occur in 22% of envenomation cases (1). Similar estimates for other widow spiders have not been made. Systemic envenomation develops over a few hours and peaks at around 24 hours (1,4,6,40,41). The risk of systemic toxicity is greatest at the extremes of age and in those with preexisting chronic medical illnesses (1). Severe abdominal pain mimicking an acute surgical abdomen has been observed and resulted in unnecessary laparotomy (4,42). Priapism may develop (4). Additionally, marked grimacing of the facial muscles, with blepharospasm, and lacrimation (facies latrodectismica) and a feeling of impending doom (pavor mortis) may be observed (4). The natural progression of untreated envenomation is a gradual diminution of symptoms and signs over several days to weeks. Uncommonly, these may persist for months.

A latrodectism-like syndrome has been observed after the bite of the related Theridiid spiders *Steatoda grossa* and *S. nobilis*. This syndrome has been referred to as *Steatodism* and may also present with regional or systemic signs of pain, sweating, and piloerection (43–45). The *in vitro* toxicity of *S. grossa* venom is several-fold less than that of *Latrodectus* spp. (43). This may explain the lack of systemic toxicity after the bite of *Steatoda* spp. Nevertheless, the venom of various *Steatoda* spp. has been shown to have similar in vitro effects on neuronal tissue to those seen with widow spider venom (46–50).

TABLE 1. Symptoms and signs of latrodectism

	Signs and symptoms	
Local and regional effects	Pain	Erythema at bite site
	Piloerection	Localized muscle fasciculation
	Diaphoresis	Regional lymphadenopathy and tenderness
	Regional diaphoresis to bitten or contralateral limb	
Systemic effects	Generalized muscle pain and fasciculation	Vomiting
	Abdominal pain mimicking acute abdomen	Dyspnea
	Diaphoresis	Restlessness
	Tachycardia	Mild pyrexia
	Hypertension	Pavor mortis[a]
	Nausea	Facies latrodectismica[b]
		Priapism

[a]Feeling of impending doom.
[b]Facial muscle grimacing, trismus, blepharoconjunctivitis, and facial erythema.
Data taken from references 1,4,6,32,36,37,41,42,59.

DIAGNOSTIC TESTS

The diagnosis of latrodectism is based on the presence of symptoms and signs consistent with the clinical picture of widow spider envenomation. This may be apparent even in the absence of a definite spider bite. Laboratory tests should only be performed as indicated on general clinical grounds (i.e., to evaluate the differential diagnosis). Nonspecific changes may be seen on biochemical and hematologic testing. These include mild elevations in leukocyte count, lactate dehydrogenase, and creatine phosphokinase (4,40). No specific tests are available to confirm the diagnosis of widow spider envenomation.

TREATMENT

First Aid and General Principles

Latrodectism is rarely life-threatening or fatal. First aid should include reassurance and application of an ice pack to the bite site if pain is present. In asymptomatic patients in whom a widow spider bite is suspected, observation for 3 to 4 hours in the emergency department is indicated. If symptoms do not develop during observation, the patient can be safely discharged and advised to return if symptoms progress slowly over the ensuing hours. If envenomation is present or develops during observation, specific immunotherapy should be considered, as the use of analgesics for pain control alone is usually inadequate.

Antidotes

Antivenom therapy is the most effective treatment available for latrodectism. It should be considered in all individuals with evidence of systemic latrodectism and those with severe regional symptoms. It should be viewed as the primary therapy for patients with distressing features of envenomation (7,36,37,40) and is more effective than opioid analgesia, calcium, or muscle relaxants in terminating symptoms of envenomation. Antivenom therapy significantly reduces the duration of suffering and length of hospital stay when compared to the other therapies mentioned (40,51). Patients complaining of persistent local pain who are unresponsive to opioid analgesia should also receive antivenom in

TABLE 2. Cross-reactivity of *Latrodectus* antivenoms

Venom used for production	Producer	Antivenom composition	Venom cross-neutralization	
			Clinical observations	Mice (*in vivo*)
L. mactans	Merck & Co, Inc, West Point, PA, U.S.A.	Equine IgG	*L. hesperus*[a]	—
	Instituto Nacional de Microbiologia, Buenos Aires, Argentina	Equine IgG	*L. variolus*[a]	—
	Instituto Bioclon, Calzada de Telalpan, Mexico D.F.	Polyvalent equine Fab'2 IgG	*L. bishopi*[a]	—
L. indistinctus	South African Institute for Medical Research, Rietfontein, Edenvale, Transvaal, South Africa	Equine IgG	*L. geometricus*[a]	—
L. hasselti	Commonwealth Serum Laboratories, Melbourne, Australia	Equine Fab'2 IgG fragment	*L. katipo*,[a] *L. tredecimguttatus*,[b] *Steatoda grossa*[c,d]	*L. mactans*,[e,f] *L. hesperus*,[e,f] *L. tredecimguttatus*,[e] *L. lugubris*,[e] *α-LTx*,[e] *Steatoda grossa*[c,d]

IgG, immunoglobulin G; α-LTx, α-latrotoxin.
[a]Normal clinical indication for usage.
[b]Data from Wiener S. Red-back spider bite in Australia: an analysis of 167 cases. *Med J Aust* 1961;2:44–49.
[c]Data from Graudins A, Gunja N, Broady KW, et al. Clinical and in vitro evidence for the efficacy of Australian red-back spider (*Latrodectus hasselti*) antivenom in the treatment of envenomation by a cupboard spider (*Steatoda grossa*). *Toxicon* 2002;40(6):767–775.
[d]Data from South M, Wirth P, Winkel KD. Redback spider antivenom used to treat envenomation by a juvenile *Steatoda* spider [Letter]. *Med J Aust* 1998;169(11–12):642.
[e]Data from Graudins A, Padula M, Broady KW, et al. Evidence for red-back spider antivenom efficacy in the prevention of envenomation by other widow spiders (genus *Latrodectus*). *J Toxicol Clin Toxicol* 2000;38(2):205.
[f]Data from Daly FF, Hill RE, Bogdan GM, Dart RC. Neutralization of *Latrodectus mactans* and *L. hesperus* venom by redback spider (*L. hasseltii*) antivenom. *J Toxicol Clin Toxicol* 2001;39(2):119–123.

view of the fact that their symptoms may otherwise persist for several days. Delayed antivenom administration reverses envenomation in patients who present many hours or days after the onset of symptoms (52–54). Additional information regarding the use of antivenin (*Latrodectus mactans*) from the United States and red-back spider antivenom from Australia is provided in Chapter 76.

Specific *Latrodectus* antivenoms are available in the United States, Mexico, Argentina, South Africa, and Australia (Table 2). These are commonly equine-derived antivenoms that may be either whole immunoglobulin G or Fab'2 fragment formulations. They are often used locally to treat envenomation from a number of *Latrodectus* spp. Clinical observations, as well as in vivo and in vitro experimental studies, have shown that specific antivenoms can be used to treat envenomation from a wide variety of *Latrodectus* spp. around the world (8–11). As a result, these antivenoms should be effective in the treatment of latrodectism in countries that do not possess a local antivenom. Additionally, red-back spider antivenom has been used to treat systemic envenomation after the bite of *S. grossa* (43,44) and effectively prevents and reverses in vitro toxicity of *S. grossa* venom (43).

Most antivenom formulations are administered diluted by slow intravenous infusion. Australian red-back spider antivenom is given intramuscularly for most cases of envenomation but can be administered intravenously in severe cases or in those that are refractory to intramuscular dosing (7,9,37). Symptom relief commonly results after the administration of one ampule of the various antivenom formulations (37,40). Occasionally, two or more ampules must be given. Up to eight ampules of red-back spider antivenom have been safely administered for refractory cases of *L. hasselti* envenomation (6,55). In general, skin testing for horse protein allergy is not indicated. Pretreatment with antihistamines, steroids, or subcutaneous epinephrine is not indicated unless a patient gives a history of preexisting allergy to horse serum. A small number of refractory cases of *L. hasselti* envenomation, primarily with regional pain to an upper limb, have been treated successfully by the administration of red-back spider antivenom directly to the affected limb using a Bier's block technique (56).

The incidence of side effects after antivenom administration is not well documented for most antivenom formulations. The most frequent side effect of antivenom therapy is anaphylaxis (37,40). Nevertheless, it is an uncommon event and more likely to occur with rapid intravenous administration of undiluted or inadequately diluted antivenom. Sutherland and Trinca (37) reported a 0.54% incidence of mild anaphylaxis in 2062 patients who received Australian red-back spider (*L. hasselti*) antivenom and noted that one-half of these cases occurred after the administration of undiluted intravenous antivenom. Similarly, Clark et al. (40) reported the development of urticaria in 5 of 58 patients who received intravenous infusions of North American black widow spider antivenom. Even fewer data exist on the incidence of serum sickness after the administration of widow spider antivenoms. Sutherland and Trinca (37) reported an incidence of 1.7% after the administration of Australian red-back spider antivenom.

Supportive Care

Opioid analgesia should be considered as an adjuvant therapy for pain relief in latrodectism. It is unlikely that this will relieve pain from anything more than the most trivial cases of widow spider envenomation but can be administered before antivenom use.

In the United States, intravenous calcium gluconate has been used as an alternative to antivenom therapy for many years (51). It may provide brief (15 to 30 minutes) symptomatic relief in mild to moderate cases of envenomation. It is rarely effective on its own, and symptoms usually return (40). Calcium gluconate may have a role as an adjunctive therapy to relieve pain before antivenom administration (1). Recommended dosing is 2 to 3 ml 10% calcium gluconate intravenously over a few minutes with continuous cardiac monitoring, repeated in 2-ml increments as necessary (57). No evidence has been found to suggest that this would be more effective than intravenous opioids. Muscle relaxants such as diazepam and methocarbamol have been shown to be ineffective in the relief of muscle spasm resulting from latrodectism and should be avoided (51).

Management Pitfalls

Management pitfalls include failure to consider latrodectism in the differential diagnosis of a patient who presents with an unusual pattern of severe pain or severe abdominal pain in a widow spider endemic region and withholding of widow spider antivenom in cases of moderate to severe envenomation, resulting in unnecessary and prolonged suffering.

REFERENCES

1. White J, Cardoso JL, Fan HW. Clinical toxicology of spider bites. In: Meier J, White J, eds. *Handbook of clinical toxicology of animal venoms and poisons*, 1st ed. Boca Raton, FL: CRC Press, 1995:259–329.
2. York Main B. *Spiders*, 2nd ed. Sydney: Collins, 1984.
3. Sutherland SK. *Latrodectus mactans hasselti*, the Australian red-back spider or jockey spider. In: Sutherland SK, ed. *Australian animal toxins*, 1st ed. Melbourne: Oxford University Press, 1983:242–254.
4. Maretic Z. Latrodectism: variations in clinical manifestations provoked by *Latrodectus* species of spiders. *Toxicon* 1983;21(4):457–466.
5. Litovitz TL, Klein-Schwartz W, Dyer KS, et al. 1997 Annual reports of the American Association of Poison Control Centers Toxic Exposure Surveillance System. *Am J Emerg Med* 1998;16:443–497.
6. Jelinek GA, Banham ND, Dunjey SJ. Red-back spider-bites at Fremantle Hospital, 1982–1987. *Med J Aust* 1989;150(12):693–695.
7. White J. Envenoming and antivenom use in Australia. *Toxicon* 1998;36(11):1483–1492.
8. Keegan HL. Effectiveness of *Latrodectus tredecimguttatus* antivenin in protecting laboratory mice against effects of intraperitoneal injections of *Latrodectus mactans*. *Am J Trop Med Hyg* 1955;4:762–764.
9. Wiener S. Red back spider antivenene. *Med J Aust* 1961;2(2):41–44.
10. Graudins A, Padula M, Broady KW, et al. Evidence for red-back spider antivenom efficacy in the prevention of envenomation by other widow spiders (genus *Latrodectus*). *J Toxicol Clin Toxicol* 2000;38(2):205(abst).
11. Daly FF, Hill RE, Bogdan GM, Dart RC. Neutralization of *Latrodectus mactans* and *L. hesperus* venom by redback spider (*L. hasseltii*) antivenom. *J Toxicol Clin Toxicol* 2001;39(2):119–123.
12. McCrone JD, Netzloff ML. An immunological and electrophoretical comparison of the venoms of the North American *Latrodectus* spiders. *Toxicon* 1965;3:107–110.
13. Grasso A. Preparation and properties of a neurotoxin purified from the venom of black widow spider (*Latrodectus mactans tredecimguttatus*). *Biochimia Biophysica Acta* 1976;439(2):406–412.
14. Grasso A, Alema S, Rufini S, et al. Black widow spider toxin–induced calcium fluxes and transmitter release in a neurosecretory cell line. *Nature* 1980;283:774–776.
15. Grasso A, Pellicia M, Alema S. Characterization of alpha-latrotoxin interaction with rat brain synaptosomes and PC12 cells. *Toxicon* 1982;20:149–156.
16. Grasso A, Senni MI. A toxin purified from the venom of black widow spider affects the uptake and release of radioactive gamma-amino butyrate and N-epinephrine from rat brain synaptosomes. *Eur J Biochem* 1979;102(2):337–344.
17. Frontali N, Ceccarelli B, Gorio A, et al. Purification from black widow spider venom of a protein factor causing the depletion of synaptic vesicles at neuromuscular junctions. *J Cell Biol* 1976;68(3):462–479.
18. Frontali N, Grasso A. Separation of three toxicologically different protein components from the venom of the spider *Latrodectus tredecimguttatus*. *Arch Biochem Biophys* 1964;106:213–218.
19. Rosenthal L, Meldolesi J. Alpha-latrotoxin and related toxins. *Pharmacol Ther* 1989;42(1):115–134.
20. Meldolesi J, Madeddu L, Watanabe O. Studies on alpha-latrotoxin of black widow spider venom and its receptor in presynaptic membranes. *Periodicum Biologorum* 1983;85[Suppl 2]:107–112.
21. Grishin EV. Black widow spider toxins: the present and the future. *Toxicon* 1998;36(11):1693–1701.
22. Geppert M, Khvotchev M, Krasnoperov V, et al. Neurexin I alpha is a major alpha-latrotoxin receptor that cooperates in alpha-latrotoxin action. *J Biol Chem* 1998;273(3):1705–1710.
23. Davletov BA, Shamotienko OG, Lelianova VG, et al. Isolation and biochemical characterization of a Ca2+-independent alpha-latrotoxin–binding protein. *J Biol Chem* 1996;271(38):23239–23245.
24. Orlova E, Rahman MA, Gowen B, et al. Structure of alpha-latrotoxin oligomers reveals that the divalent cation-dependent tetramers form membrane pores. *Nature Struct Biol* 2000;7(1):48–53.
25. Pescatori M, Grasso A. Characterization of the epitope for 4C4.1 mAb on alpha-latrotoxin using phage display-peptide libraries: prevention of toxin-dependent $^{45}Ca^{2+}$ uptake in non-neuronal human embryonic cells transiently expressing latrophilin. *Biochimie* 2000;82(9–10):909–914.
26. Sugita S, Ichtchenko K, Khvotchev M, et al. Alpha-latrotoxin receptor CIRL/latrophilin 1 (CL1) defines an unusual family of ubiquitous G-protein–linked receptors. G-protein coupling not required for triggering exocytosis. *J Biol Chem* 1998;273(49):32715–32724.
27. Krasnoperov V, Bittner MA, Holz RW, et al. Structural requirements for alpha-latrotoxin binding and alpha-latrotoxin–stimulated secretion. *J Biol Chem* 1999;274(6):3590–3596.
28. Maretic Z, Lebez D. *Araneism*. Belgrade, Yugoslavia: Nolit Publishing, 1979.
29. Maretic Z. Epidemiology of envenomation, symptomatology, pathology and treatment. In Bettini S, ed. *Arthropod venoms, handbook of experimental pharmacology*, vol 48. New York: Springer-Verlag, 1978:185–212.
30. Sherman RP, Groll JM, Gonzalez DI, et al. Black widow spider (*Latrodectus mactans*) envenomation in a term pregnancy. *Curr Surg* 2000 Jul 1;57(4):346–348.
31. Pneumatikos IA, Galiatsou E, Goe D, et al. Acute fatal toxic myocarditis after black widow spider envenomation. *Ann Emerg Med* 2003;41:158.
32. Bogen E. Arachnism. *Arch Intern Med* 1926;38:623–632.
33. Keegan HL, Hedeen RA, Whittemore FW. Seasonal variation in venom of black widow spiders. *Am J Trop Med Hyg* 1960;10:477–479.
34. McCrone JD. Comparative lethality of several *Latrodectus* venoms. *Toxicon* 1964;2:201–203.
35. Moss HS, Binder LS. A retrospective review of black widow spider envenomation. *Ann Emerg Med* 1987;16(2):188–192.
36. Muller G. Black and brown widow spider bites in South Africa. A series of 45 cases. *South Afr Med J* 1993;83:399–405.
37. Sutherland SK, Trinca JC. Survey of 2144 cases of red-back spider bites. *Med J Aust* 1978;2:620–623.
38. Wiener S. Red-back spider bite in Australia: an analysis of 167 cases. *Med J Aust* 1961;2:44–49.
39. Ingram WW, Musgrave A. Spider bite (arachnidism): a survey of its occurrence in Australia, with case histories. *Med J Aust* 1933;2:10–15.
40. Clark RF, Wethern-Kestner S, Vance MV, et al. Clinical presentation and treatment of black widow spider envenomation: a review of 163 cases. *Ann Emerg Med* 1992;21(7):782–787.
41. Timms PK, Gibbons RB. Latrodectism—effects of the black widow spider. *West J Med* 1986;144:315–317.
42. White J. Latrodectism as a mimic [Letter]. *Med J Aust* 1985;142:75.
43. Graudins A, Gunja N, Broady KW, et al. Clinical and in vitro evidence for the efficacy of Australian red-back spider (*Latrodectus hasselti*) antivenom in the treatment of envenomation by a cupboard spider (*Steatoda grossa*). *Toxicon* 2002;40(6):767–775.
44. South M, Wirth P, Winkel KD. Redback spider antivenom used to treat envenomation by a juvenile *Steatoda* spider [Letter]. *Med J Aust* 1998;169(11–12):642.
45. Warrell DA, Shaheen J, Hillyard PD, et al. Neurotoxic envenoming by an immigrant spider (*Steatoda nobilis*) in southern England. *Toxicon* 1991;29(10):1263–1265.
46. Cavalieri M, D'Urso D, Lassa A, et al. Characterization and some properties of the venom gland extract of a theridiid spider (*Steatoda paykulliana*) frequently mistaken for black widow spider (*Latrodectus tredecimguttatus*). *Toxicon* 1987;25(9):965–974.
47. Gillingwater TH, Kalikulov D, Ushkaryov Y, et al. Comparison of the effects of alpha-latrotoxin with a partially purified toxin from another theridiid spider, *Steatoda paykulliana*, on exocytosis at mouse neuromuscular junctions. *J Physiol* 1999;520P:40P(abst).
48. Sokolov V, Chanturiia AN, Lishko VK. Channel-forming properties of *Steatoda paykulliana* spider venom. *Biofizika* 1984;29:620–623.
49. Usmanov PB, Kazakov I, Kalikulov D, et al. The channel-forming component of the Theridiidae spider venom neurotoxins. *Gen Physiol Biophys* 1985;4:185–193.
50. Mironov SL, Sokolov Yu V, Chanturiya AN, et al. Channels produced by spider venoms in bilayer lipid membrane: mechanisms of ion transport and toxic action. *Biochim Biophys Acta* 1986;862(1):185–198.
51. Key GF. A comparison of calcium gluconate and methocarbamol (Robaxin) in the treatment of latrodectism (black widow spider envenomation). *Am J Trop Med Hyg* 1981;30(1):273–277.
52. Brown AF. Delayed diagnosis of red-back spider envenomation: a timely reminder. *Med J Aust* 1989;151(11–12):705–706.
53. Allen RC, Norris RL. Delayed use of widow spider antivenin. *Ann Emerg Med* 1995;26(3):393–394.
54. O'Malley GF, Dart RC, Kuffner EF. Successful treatment of latrodectism with antivenin after 90 hours [Letter]. *N Engl J Med* 1999;340(8):657.
55. Graudins A, Vassiliadis J, Dowsett RP. Red-back spider (*Latrodectus mactans hasselti*) envenomation requiring "high dose" antivenom therapy. *J Toxicol Clin Toxicol* 1999;37(5):615(abst).
56. Fatovich DM, Dunjey SJ, Constantine CJ, et al. Successful treatment of red-back spider bite using a Bier's block technique. *Med J Aust* 1999;170:342–343.
57. Binder LS. Acute arthropod envenomation: incidence, clinical features, and management. *Med Toxicol Adverse Drug Exp* 1989;4:163–173.

CHAPTER 249

Recluse Spider and Other Necrotizing Arachnids

Hernán F. Gómez and Gary S. Wasserman

See Figure 1.

Topics included:	**Recluse spiders (*Loxosceles* species); other spiders causing necrotic arachnidism: hobo spider (*Tegenaria agrestis*), yellow sac spider (*Chiracanthium* species), orange argiopa (*Argiope* species), funnel web spider (*Agelenopsis* species) (1), jumping spiders (*Phiddipus* species), wolf spider (*Lycosa* species)**
Molecular weight:	**Sphingomyelinase D, 35,000 g/mol**
Target organs:	**Skin (dermonecrotic arachnidism), red blood cells, coagulation system**
Antidote:	**None proven**

OVERVIEW

Dermonecrotic arachnidism, necrotic arachnidism, and (in South America) *the gangrenous spot of Chile* are terms used to describe necrotic cutaneous lesions induced by arachnids (2–4). A lesion of this type was first described in 1872 (5). It was later proposed by Schamus (Kansas) in 1929 that the bite was associated with *Loxosceles* spp. (2). Linkage of venom from *Loxosceles* spp. and necrotic arachnidism was definitively established in 1947 by Machiavello (4) and later confirmed by Atkins et al. in 1957 (6).

Bites from more than a dozen spider families throughout the world have been reported to result in dermonecrotic lesions in humans (7–12). Six of these families are distributed within the United States (7). This chapter focuses on *Loxosceles* spp., although a brief review of the limited literature of non-*Loxosceles* arachnid species is also included.

Characteristics of *Loxosceles* Spiders

Spiders of the *Loxosceles* spp. are often called *brown, violin,* or *fiddleback* spiders due to the distinctive violin-shaped markings found on the carapace (dorsal surface) of the cephalothorax (Fig. 2). However, the lay term *brown recluse* should be reserved only for *L. reclusa*. Other lay terms given to *Loxosceles* spp. in North America include Apache recluse (*L. apachea*), Arizona recluse (*L. arizonica*), and desert recluse (*L. deserta*) (13). *Loxosceles* spiders vary in length from 1 to 5 cm leg to leg. They range in color from fawn to dark brown. A large spider has a total body length of 1 cm and width of 0.5 cm. The spiders have long, slender legs relative to their body size and are able to move with great speed (2). Other distinctive identifying characteristics are three pairs of eyes, because most other spiders have four pairs (13).

The genus *Loxosceles* is the most venomous and by far the best characterized of dermonecrotic venomous spiders. The most common taxonomy for *Loxosceles* spiders can be described as follows: kingdom: animal, phylum: Arthropoda, class: Archnida, order: Araneae, family: Loxoscelidae, genus: *Loxosceles*. Examples of *Loxosceles* spp. can be found worldwide and include *L. adelaide, L. gaucho, L. intermedia, L. rufescens, L. unicolor, L. laeta,* and numerous other species.

Although a variety of species have been described, the effects of envenomation are indistinguishable from species to species. Amino acid sequence analysis of the dermonecrotic venom component (sphingomyelinase D) has revealed only the most minor

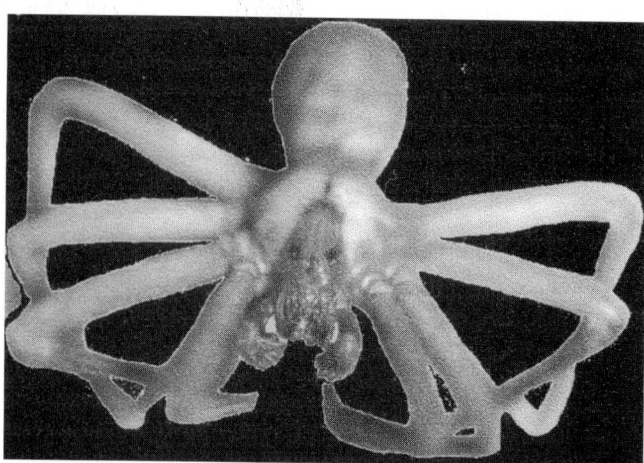

Figure 1. Common appearance of the recluse spider.

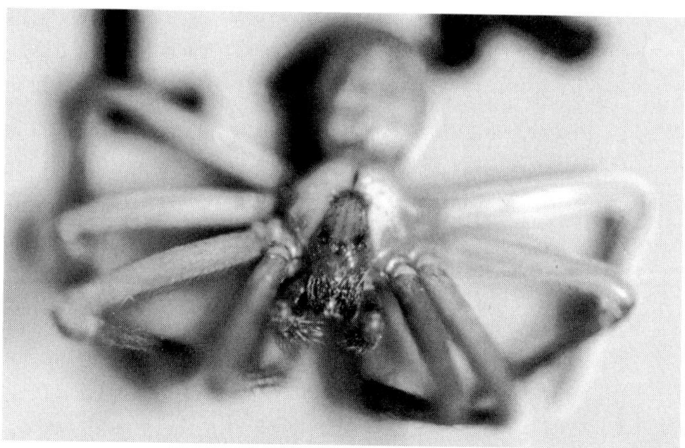

Figure 2. Photograph of *Loxosceles* spider showing characteristic "fiddle" markings on the dorsal surface of the cephalothorax.

sequence differences between species in North and South America (14,15). *L. laeta* is presumed to be among the most potent species because systemic symptoms occur more frequently, with comparatively larger numbers of patient presentations in South America after *L. laeta* envenomation compared to other endogenous species such as *L. intermedia* and *L. gaucho* (16).

Geographic Distribution

The brown spiders of the genus *Loxosceles* can be found in two principal areas: temperate southern Africa northward through the tropics in the Mediterranean region and southern Europe, and the temperate and tropical zones of North and South America (13). *Loxosceles* spp. can also be found on the continent of Australia (13). In continental North America, there are 54 recognized species of *Loxosceles* endemic (13). In addition, United States fauna has been further enriched by two exotic species. The first of these is the South American *L. laeta*, a spider with its original home in western South America. It has been carried by commercial trade, successfully established colonies in Central America, and migrated northward into southern California (13). The second exotic species, *L. rufescens* (originally from North Africa), is now a common spider of the Pacific islands, including the Hawaiian Islands (13).

L. reclusa is the major species responsible for envenomation in the United States (2). Most U.S. *Loxosceles* envenomations occur in the south central regional states, such as Arkansas, Missouri, Kansas, Tennessee, and Oklahoma (2). Other species in North America include *L. apachea*, *L. arizonica*, and *L. deserta* (13). These other domestic species are endemic to southwestern regions of the continental United States.

Habitat

The name *reclusa* is very descriptive of the behavior of *L. reclusa* spiders. Spiders of the genus spin irregular webs, serving as retreats under ground for objects of many kinds, in houses, buildings, and in the human litter around them (13). They are retiring, unaggressive, and nocturnal, inhabiting dark places and not biting unless threatened (2). Bites from these spiders are difficult to induce under experimental conditions (17). Futrell (2) reports multiple incidents of accidentally dropping spiders on her person without suffering a single bite. Similarly, Gertsch (18) mentions collecting hundreds of *Loxosceles* spiders without receiving bites.

In warmer seasonal conditions, *Loxosceles* spiders prefer living in secluded outdoor areas, such as under woodpiles, rocks, and debris (19). During cooler months, these spiders can be found in secluded areas of manmade structures, such as basements, attics, and storage areas. A careful search of homes in certain communities in south-central regions of the United States has revealed the presence of the spider in most domiciles (2). In Chile, a survey of *L. laeta* found homes infested with an average of 163 recluse spiders per home (range, 106 to 222), but no envenomations of the human occupants were reported (20). Thus, the unfortunate interface between human and spider resulting in envenomation likely occurs during accidental physical encounter. Bites usually occur between April and October, when *Loxosceles* spiders are more active indoors, with increased risk of encountering a human (19). The bites can occur anywhere on the body (19). Many bites are thought to occur at night when victims accidentally roll over onto an unsuspecting spider (2,21).

PATHOPHYSIOLOGY

Loxosceles venom is one of the most potent substances found in nature. Like most spiders, *Loxosceles* uses its venom to paralyze its insect prey. Although the precise amount deposited in skin by a spider bite is not known, commercial milking of *Loxosceles* spiders by a single electrical stimulation yields approximately 2 to 3 μg venom (22). This modest amount of venom results in a remarkable spectrum of clinical disease in man. Humans are not its intended victim, and the reason for the evolutionary development of toxic effects noted in humans and other mammalian species is a biologic curiosity. At least 11 major components of the venom have been identified; many are peptides reported to have inherent cytotoxic activity (23,24). Venom components include hyaluronidase (25), which maximizes dermal inflammation by facilitating spread of the venom through tissue from the point of envenomation. In the rabbit model a direct correlation between diffusion of *L. reclusa* venom and extent of dermal inflammation has been definitively established (22). Other components include S-ribonucleotide, phosphohydrolase, alkaline phosphatase, and sphingomyelinase D.

Sphingomyelinase D is responsible for the profound dermal inflammation caused by brown recluse spider bites. Purified sphingomyelinase D alone reproduces the dermal necrotic lesion in the rabbit model. A model summarizing the cellular and molecular basis for tissue events postulated to occur after *Loxosceles* envenomation has been developed (Fig. 3). After envenomation, dermal endothelial and epithelial cells produce and secrete the chemokines interleukin-8 (26–28), growth-related oncogene-α (27,28), and monocyte chemoattractant protein-1 (27). Endothelial cells secrete the cytokine granulocyte/macrophage colony-stimulating factor and express the adhesion molecule E-selectin on the cell surface (26). Neutrophils migrate to the bite site and adhere to intercellular junctions via the E-selectin tethering protein. They are subsequently activated and degranulate, thus resulting in tissue inflammation and necrosis (26). In addition, sphingomyelinase D reacts with cell membrane sphingomyelin, causing release of choline and N-acyl-sphingosine phosphate, resulting in the stimulation of platelet aggregation and serotonin release (24,29–31). Dermal necrosis is exacerbated by the resulting ischemia and marked inflammatory reaction.

The major systemic manifestations are induced by multiple venom effects, including endothelial cell damage, red cell hemolysis, and coagulopathy (29,31). The mediation of systemic loxoscelism involves complex activations of calcium-dependent systems, C-reactive protein, polymorphonuclear leukocytes, serum amyloid P component, antibodies, cytokines, and other reactants (29,30,32–34). Researchers of the Butantan Research Institute (São Paolo) have shown that *Loxosceles* venom–induced erythrocyte lysis is dependent on activation of complement by the alternative pathway. Metalloproteinase activity induced by *Loxosceles* venom causes cleavage of glycophorins from the erythrocyte surface and facilitates complement-mediated lysis (35). Erythrocytes affected by spider venom in turn become activators of complement, resulting in massive hemolysis and ultimately renal failure.

In addition to the local effects, the venom toxins may also provoke a systemic cytokine response resembling that seen in endotoxic shock (36). Epidemiologic studies in Chile and Brazil have shown a mortality of 3.7% and 1.5%, respectively (16,37).

VULNERABLE POPULATIONS

Factors that affect the degree of venom-induced morbidity include the victim's age, location of envenomation, preexisting medical conditions, and immune response of the host. Fortunately, most bite victims have a relatively benign course of illness (38,39). Very young and debilitated patients are at greater

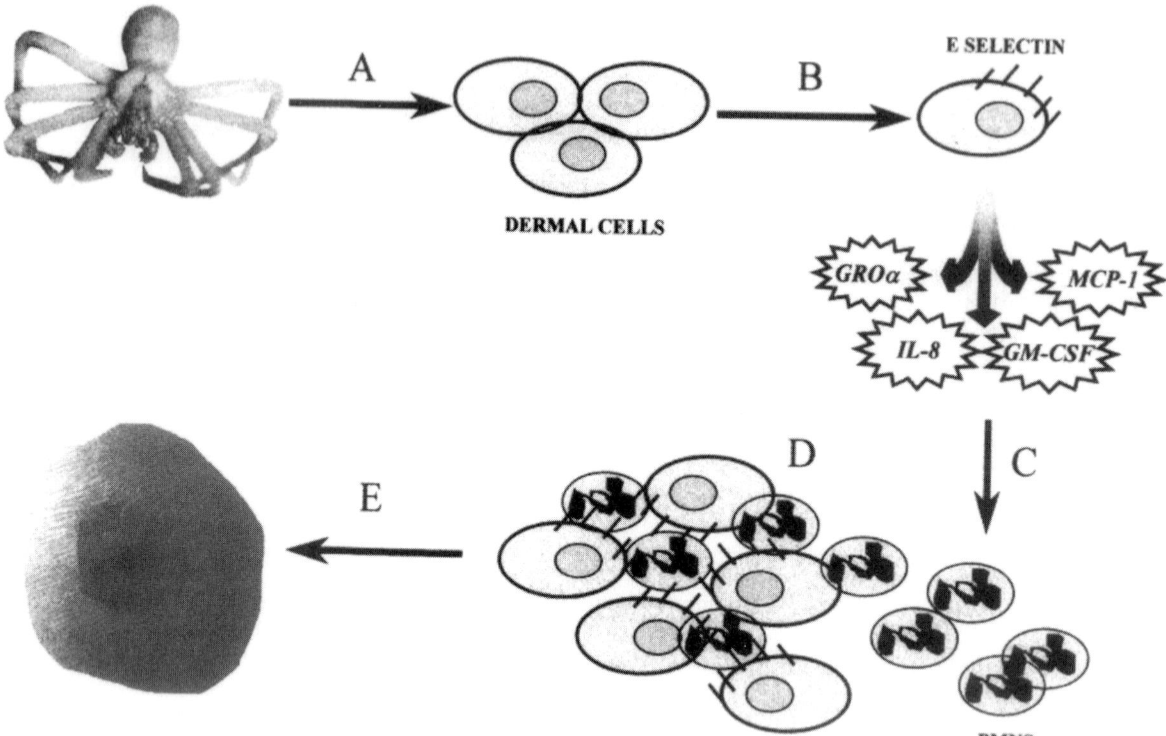

Figure 3. Schematic diagram reviewing the mechanism of *Loxosceles* venom–induced dermal inflammation. **A:** Intradermal deposition of venom. **B:** Induction of the neutrophil-tethering molecule E-selectin on endothelial cell surfaces. **C:** Endothelial and epithelial cell secretion of chemokines interleukin-8 (IL-8), growth-related oncogene-α (GROα), monocyte chemoattractant protein-1 (MCP-1), and granulocyte/macrophage colony-stimulating factor (GM-CSF). PMNS, polymorphonucleocytes. **D:** Neutrophil migration and tethering to endothelial cell surfaces via E-selectin. **E:** Activation band degranulation of neutrophils with resultant tissue injury. (From Gomez HF, Greenfield DM, Miller MM, et al. Direct correlation between diffusion of *Loxosceles reclusa* venom and extent of dermal inflammation. *Acad Emerg Med* 2001;8:309–314, with permission.)

risk for more serious morbidity. The elderly in endemic areas often have relatively limited or no response to envenomation, possibly because of acquired immunity from bites earlier in their lives (40).

Envenomation by the spider *L. reclusa* in five pregnant women proved to have no sustained adverse effects on mother or baby when managed conservatively with low-dose prednisone (41). A striking toxic erythema of the skin, common with the bite of the spider, caused the greatest discomfort and concern for the patients but proved to be entirely tractable. No episodes of hemolysis, disorders of coagulation, or renal damage were discovered. Thus, there is no clinical evidence of any special risk during pregnancy in the event of loxoscelism (41).

CLINICAL PRESENTATION

Local Effects

The clinical presentation of *Loxosceles* envenomation varies from a mild local reaction to systemic symptoms and (on rare occasion) death, depending on the quantity of venom inoculation and a number of host variables. Overall, clinical experience in children and adults points strongly toward individual sensitivity to the toxins of the spider (42).

Most patients do not sense the initial bite or may note a mild pinprick sensation. Within a few hours, the bite site progressively begins to itch and develop mild erythema and edema. A flesh-colored or deep purple/black blister may develop at the site of venom inoculation (19). The area of envenomation may become tender to palpation, and local purpura may be noted. Examination of the area adjacent to the bite site may reveal surrounding erythema and induration, with a morphology that appears gravitational in distribution (Fig. 4).

In more severe lesions, characteristic findings are more readily apparent. The necrotic lesion typically progresses from an appearance of pallor or erythema to a violaceous macule with darkened central areas. The edge of a necrotic lesion is usually uneven as the macule enlarges and the center darkens; the necrotic lesion then generally sinks below skin level (39,43).

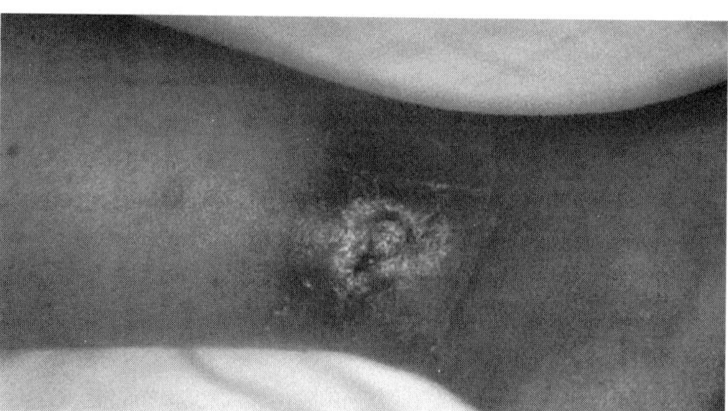

Figure 4. Typical appearance of brown recluse spider bite 12 to 24 hours after envenomation.

Because patients usually do not bring the spider for identification, definitive diagnosis is problematic when clinical findings are restricted to dermal findings alone. This is particularly true in areas that are nonendemic for *Loxosceles* spiders, because the appearance of cutaneous necrosis is not specific for *Loxosceles* envenomation (2–6,10–13,23,44). It is common for clinicians to misinform patients that they have been bitten by a brown recluse bite, even when that patient lives well outside endemic range of *Loxosceles* arachnids (45). It has been suggested (especially in nonendemic areas) that the term *probable arthropod envenomation* (instead of "brown recluse bite") be used when a spider is not captured close to the site of injury at the time of envenomation, assuming that other medical causes of dermonecrotic arachnidism have been excluded (19,46,47).

The central bite may become necrotic in 2 to 4 days and later result in eschar formation (days 4 to 7). The area then becomes indurated, and at 7 to 14 days the central area becomes mummified and the eschar falls off leaving an ulceration (42). The lesion often heals very slowly over 6 to 8 weeks or longer. Lesions seem to be more extensive and have more severe scar formation in areas of fatty tissue, such as the thighs, abdomen, and buttocks (42).

TABLE 1. Differential diagnosis of necrotic arachnidism in the United States

Envenomation from *Loxosceles* species	Herpes simplex
Bites from other U.S. species	Toxic epidermal necrolysis
Tegenaria agrestis (hobo spider)	Ecthyma gangrenosum
Phiddipus species (jumping spider)	Pyoderma gangrenosum
Cheiracanthium species (yellow sac spider)	Pyogenic granuloma
Argiope arantia (orange argiopa)	Sporotrichosis
Lycosa species (wolf spiders)	Focal vasculitis
Peucetia viridans (green lynx spider)	Bedsore
Dolomedes species (fishing spider)	Diabetic ulcer
Bites from other arthropods	Erythema nodosum
Impetigo	Dermatitis of gonococcal arthritis
Soft-tissue trauma	Barbiturate blisters
Contact or chemical dermatitis	Warfarin-induced skin necrosis
Lyme disease	Periarteritis nodosum
Anthrax	Lymphomatoid papulosis
Varicella zoster (shingles)	Tularemia
	Chagas' disease

Modified from Osterhoudt KC, Zaoutis T, Zorc JJ. Lyme disease masquerading as brown recluse spider bite. *Ann Emerg Med* May 2002;39:558–561.

Systemic Effects

Systemic involvement (loxoscelism) is much less common than the local dermal reaction but may be severe and is responsible for all cases that result in death. The systemic response is not necessarily proportional to the severity of the local reaction and vice versa (19). Often, systemic effects are not detected clinically until 24 to 72 hours after the bite. Fever, chills, malaise, weakness, nausea, vomiting, arthralgia, myalgia, rash, seizures, hypotension, disseminated intravascular coagulation (DIC), thrombocytopenia, and hemolysis may develop (42,48–51). Hemolysis may lead to hemoglobinemia; renal failure and ultimately death may be observed in rare cases (48).

DIAGNOSTIC TESTS

The diagnosis of a brown recluse spider bite is a clinical one, based on the morphologic appearance of the cutaneous lesion, consistent patient history, and occurrence in an endemic area. Other arachnids or medical conditions may be the underlying etiology in nonendemic areas (Table 1). The identification of a *Loxosceles*-induced dermonecrotic lesion, as opposed to that induced by other arachnids, or non-necrotic dermal inflammation due to bites or stings from other arthropods, may be very difficult to distinguish in early stages or mild reactions.

In contrast to an isolated skin lesion, the list of natural toxins that cause hemolysis in combination with the discrete characteristic lesion is sharply limited (19). The most common envenomation that induces clinical manifestations similar to those of loxoscelism is coagulopathic (viper) snake envenomation, which can be distinguished clinically by the appearance of at least one fang mark, usually with some blood oozing from the puncture site with rapid progression of swelling and pain.

Presently, there is no routinely available test for the clinician to identify a brown recluse envenomation. Reported histopathologic changes include edema and thickening of the endothelium of blood vessels, collections of inflammatory cells, intravascular coagulation, degeneration of blood vessel walls, and hemorrhage into the dermis and even into the subcutis (2). The accumulation of polymorphonuclear leukocytes is especially marked (2,22).

A passive hemagglutination inhibition test for the diagnosis of North American brown recluse bites was reported in 1993 (52). Although the passive hemagglutination test is sensitive, it is cumbersome to prepare and the results are available only after several (6 to 24) hours (52). Subsequently, a specific North American *Loxosceles* venom enzyme-linked immunosorbent assay (ELISA) was developed for research purposes (14,22). This ELISA was specific for *Loxosceles* spp. venom when relevant amounts of a variety of arthropod venoms were tested (53). The assay has been used to establish the diagnosis in one confirmed case of *L. arizonica* human envenomation (21). An enzyme immunoassay was previously developed and used to detect *L. gaucho* venom in necrotic skin lesions in Brazil (54). Venom has been detected in the hair of a patient with a presumptive case of *Loxosceles* envenomation (55) and in hair shafts and wound aspirates in the animal model (56). A specific ELISA using relatively noninvasive tissue sampling is technically feasible.

Patients with presumed loxoscelism who are monitored in an intensive care unit require serial determinations of complete blood count, platelet count, and urinary hemoglobin. Liver and renal function studies should also be carefully monitored. In addition, victims of systemic loxoscelism should receive a basic work-up for DIC (including prothrombin and partial thromboplastin time, fibrinogen, and D-dimers). Antithrombin III (AT III) is one of the most important physiologic inhibitors of coagulation and is often decreased in coagulopathies. In the setting of coagulopathy, the AT III concentration should be evaluated.

TREATMENT

Overview

A vigilant "support care" approach suffices for the vast majority of bites (57,58). Basic wound care should be provided to prevent secondary bacterial infection from the victim's endogenous dermal colonizing organisms such as *Staphylococcus* or *Streptococcus*. Prophylactic antimicrobials are not generally warranted, although the appearance of the lesion with its marked venom-induced dermal inflammation is often difficult to distinguish clinically from primary or secondary soft-tissue infections. Erythema appearing within the first 12 to 24 hours usually means inflammation rather than infection. No available therapies, applied or injected (locally or parenterally), have ever been proven to alter the clinical course of dermonecrosis once this clinical finding is established. Thus, prudent supportive care and studied avoidance of ineffective or potentially harmful therapies remain the most efficacious therapeutic option.

In a subset of bite victims, serious manifestations of systemic loxoscelism develop. The major life-threatening effects of loxoscelism include hemolysis, DIC, and sepsis. Patients with systemic loxoscelism are admitted to an intensive care unit environment and should receive serial laboratory tests, including a complete blood count, platelet count, and urine hemoglobin or myoglobin. Corticosteroid therapy appears to ameliorate hemolysis. The authors recommend that intravenous methylprednisolone (or equivalent) be administered to adults and children, with a loading dose of 1 to 2 mg/kg ideal body weight followed by 0.5 to 1.0 mg/kg every 6 hours. Alkalinization of the urine and adequate hydration are recommended to prevent renal failure in patients with significant hemoglobinuria.

Bacteremia, septicemia, toxic shock syndrome, and necrotizing fasciitis are serious secondary infection–related complications of loxoscelism. However, infections are not common and usually do not occur during the first 24-hour period after the bite. Equine-derived antivenom products are used in endemic areas of South America for the treatment of severe dermal and systemic forms of loxoscelism. A discussion of experimental antivenom therapies and the role of other therapeutic measures is outlined in Experimental Therapies.

General Wound Care

Basic wound care is directed at preventing the occurrence of secondary complications. By the time the vast majority of patients present to the clinician, the dysregulation of cytokines with resulting inflammation and microvascular injury are well underway. Antibiotics should not be considered a routine part of wound care, although the presence of dermal inflammation as a response to the venom may be extremely difficult to differentiate clinically from a soft-tissue infection. Tetanus prophylaxis is indicated. Any further trauma to the site should be carefully avoided, with palpation limited to that necessary for the clinical examination. Restrictive bindings should be avoided. Needle punctures of areas surrounding the site should be limited to leading edge aspirates if secondary infection is suspected or the occasional need for a dermal biopsy.

It is unlikely that there is an advantage to elevation or immobilization of a bitten extremity, although avoiding a dependent position is helpful because gravity appears to be a variable determining the spread of wound margins (2). Analgesics, such as antiinflammatory medications that affect platelet function, may be avoided because of the potential for bleeding problems in systemic loxoscelism. Acetaminophen is adequate for pain control in most cases. It is the authors' observation that the judicious use of opioids may be required for particularly severe cases of soft-tissue discomfort. Antipruritic or antianxiety medications can be administered as needed.

Treatment of Systemic Manifestations

The major causes of *Loxosceles*-induced morbidity and mortality are hemolysis, DIC, and secondary sepsis. Parenteral corticosteroids appear to attenuate hemolysis as described in Treatment Overview. Corticosteroids may be required for 5 to 10 days; however, tapering can usually begin in 3 to 5 days if hemolysis (and hemoglobinuria) is minimally present. Because the onset of hemolysis may be gradual, a serum "free" hemoglobin and reticulocyte count may be helpful early in the course of evaluation.

Severe hemolytic anemia is an indication for packed red blood cell transfusion. The clinician is advised to determine early in the course of illness if blood component therapy is needed. Cross-matching for blood products during systemic loxoscelism has been problematic due to venom-induced antibody interference (59). In addition, transfusion of whole blood should be avoided because hemolysis appears to be mediated in part via effects of venom on complement (35,59). Caution is also required when treating bleeding or DIC with fresh frozen plasma or cryoprecipitate, because substances in these agents may also interact with venom to worsen hemolysis (59).

AT III is one of the most important physiologic inhibitors of coagulation and is often decreased in coagulopathies. In the setting of coagulopathy, the AT III concentration should be evaluated. AT III is available commercially and should be replaced if the concentration is low. Treatment of coagulopathy is a key component in the management of loxoscelism. Disaster can strike quickly, with third-space blood loss complicating ongoing hemolytic anemia. This unfortunate combination may result in inadequate oxygen delivery to tissue through inadequate circulating red blood cells and hypovolemia.

Unproven or Detrimental Therapies

Throughout the history of *Loxosceles* treatment, various therapies have been proposed and later found to be ineffective and even detrimental in some cases (2). Agents applied or injected locally (corticosteroids, vasodilators, antihistamines, antimicrobials, dextran, and others) have not been shown to reduce or prevent dermonecrosis. Many proposed, but unproven, therapies have been described.

Dapsone is a leukocyte inhibitor that is popular among some clinicians. It has not been found to be an effective therapy in any controlled human or animal investigation. A prospective, randomized, controlled, animal study of *Loxosceles* envenomation did not find a benefit from dapsone, hyperbaric oxygen, or cyproheptadine (60). This lack of efficacy is of concern given that therapeutic doses of dapsone can cause methemoglobinemia and hemolytic anemia, particularly in the pediatric population (Chapter 95) (61). Even if dapsone was shown to be capable of ameliorating the inflammatory cascade induced by envenomation, it is highly unlikely that it could be administered rapidly enough to be of benefit.

Hyperbaric oxygen has no proven benefit in the treatment of *Loxosceles*-induced dermal lesions (60,62). However, it may have theoretic benefit in patients with underlying disease such as diabetes or sickle cell, in which vascular insufficiency may add an unfortunate variable in preventing adequate wound healing.

Nitroglycerin did not reduce dermal necrosis in a randomized, controlled investigation of topical 2% nitroglycerin using a rabbit model. Instead, increased edema, inflammation, and creatine phosphokinase concentrations were found in animals that were treated with nitroglycerin.

Surgical débridement also appears to be ineffective. Early surgical intervention is not helpful because venom diffuses rapidly throughout dermal tissues around the venom inoculation site (22). In general, superficial necrotic lesions of a few centimeters in diameter heal completely with only basic wound care. Scar formation of smaller lesions is usually minimal, although underlying fat necrosis may produce a dimpling effect. Wide surgical excision has been advocated by some, but excision of the bite area may cause delayed wound healing, increase infection, worsen scarring, and ultimately worsen cosmetic outcome (63). The rare large necrotic area may require delayed excision with primary or secondary closure. Cosmetic scar resection is optimally performed after inflammatory effects of the venom have subsided. Skin grafting of a nonhealing necrotic area should be delayed for at least 4 to 12 weeks to allow for neovascularization at the demarcated edges (46).

Management Pitfalls

Bacteremia, septicemia, toxic shock syndrome, and necrotizing fasciitis are all potential secondary complications of loxoscelism. Antimicrobial therapy should be selected to cover anaerobes, *Staphylococcus*, and *Streptococcus* broadly. In the authors' experience secondary infections do not occur until several days after the bite and are almost always secondary to *Staphylococcus* or *Streptococcus* organisms.

Experimental Therapies

Specific treatment for spider bites in South America is routinely provided by polyvalent "antiarachnidic" antiserum produced by Butantan Institute, São Paulo, Brazil (64). The antiserum is raised by immunizing horses with mixtures of venoms from *Tityus serrulatus* and *T. bahiensis* scorpions, as well as *Phoneutria nigriventer* and *L. gaucho* spiders (64). In North America, antivenom therapy is not available, although a few animal studies have shown modest efficacy of intradermally administered anti-*Loxosceles* antibody in the treatment of dermal arachnidism (65–68). Although administration of antibody immediately after dermal inoculation prevents dermonecrotic lesions in animals, the efficacy of this treatment rapidly fades if antibody administration is delayed several hours (65–68). A similar finding was noted with experimental intradermal treatment with Fab (fragment antibody) (69).

The time dependence of intradermal antibody therapy is likely due to the rapid diffusion of venom away from the point of inoculation (thus, physically away from the point of therapeutic intradermal antibody therapy) (22). In addition, the profound release of chemokines and other soluble mediators of inflammation induced by the venom is likely irreversible within minutes to hours after envenomation. Anti-*Loxosceles* antibodies or Fab fragments would likely need to be combined with an agent capable of shutting down the local dysregulated neutrophil activation for the creation of a truly effective dermal antidote. An investigation revealed modest attenuation of dermal inflammation with the intravenous administration of anti–IL-8 monoclonal antibodies (70). The role of parenteral antibody therapy in systemic loxoscelism has not been studied in a prospective controlled fashion due in part to the absence of an adequate animal model to study the systemic effects of *Loxosceles* venom in humans.

OTHER ARACHNIDS REPORTED TO INDUCE DERMAL NECROSIS

At least five other genera of spiders in North America have been reported to cause necrotic lesions in humans, although none as clearly documented and characterized as *Loxosceles* venom (6,8–12,46,57,71) (Table 1). In the United States, this includes *Tegenaria agrestis* (11,72,73), *Chiracanthium* spp. (8,74–77), *Argiope* spp. (8), *Agelenopsis* spp. (50), *Phiddipus* spp. (10), and *Lycosa* spp. (9,78) arachnids. Numerous other arachnids have been identified as a cause of dermonecrotic arachnidism in other parts of the world (79,80). Because there has never been a systematic analysis of venom clinical effects of the vast majority of spiders found in North American fauna, it is quite possible that other arachnid species may induce dermal inflammation.

The differential diagnosis includes bites and stings from a variety of other arthropods. Erythema that evolves into a violaceous macule distinguishes a necrotic envenomation from a non-necrotic bite. In addition, as the macule widens, the edge becomes uneven and the center sinks below skin level; non-necrotic lesions remain edematous, raised, and erythematous (43). It is unusual for the offending spider to be captured and identified by a true expert after a bite. Thus, a generic diagnosis such as "cutaneous necrosis," "necrotic arachnidism," or "necrotic arthropod bite or sting" may be the most accurate diagnosis rather than a definitive one such as "brown recluse bite" or "loxoscelism" (40). This is particularly true in areas where *Loxosceles* spp. are not endemic (45). The clinician should be aware that necrotic wounds have been misdiagnosed as brown recluse spider bites, including those caused by infectious, neoplastic, and other processes (45,47,71,81–88). Some conditions that are misdiagnosed as brown recluse spider envenomation (Table 1), such as the Lyme disease case reported by Osterhoudt et al. (47), require specific treatment. Another example of misdiagnosis involves a 7-month-old child in New York (a nonendemic area) who contracted cutaneous anthrax but was initially diagnosed as having a brown recluse spider bite (88). The sudden appearance of large numbers of "brown recluse spider bites" outside of endemic areas may warrant investigation for cutaneous anthrax by local public health authorities given the current national concerns.

REFERENCES

1. Vetter RS. Envenomation by a spider, *Agelenopsis aperta* (family: Agelenidae) previously considered harmless. *Ann Emerg Med* 1998 Dec;32(6):739–741.
2. Futrell JM. Loxoscelism. *Am J Med Sci* 1992;304:261–267.
3. Macchiavello A. Cutaneous arachnidism or gangrenous spot of Chile. *Pub Health Trop Med* 1947;22:425.
4. Macchiavello A. Cutaneous arachnidism experimentally produced with the glandular poison of *Loxosceles laeta*. *Puerto Rico Trop Med* 1947;23:466.
5. Caveness W. Insect bite complicated by fever. *Nashville J Med* 1872;10: 333.
6. Atkins JA, Wingo CW, Sodeman WA. Probable cause of necrotic spider bite in the Midwest. *Science* 1957;126:73.
7. Geren C, Chan TK, Howell DE, et al. Isolation and characterization of toxins from brown recluse spider venom (*Loxosceles reclusa*). *Arch Biochem Biophys* 1976;174:90–99.
8. Gorham JR, Rheney TB. Envenomation by the spiders *Chiracanthium inclusum* and *Argiope aurantia*. *JAMA* 1968;206:1958–1962.
9. Redman JF. Human envenomation by a lycosid. *Arch Dermatol* 1974;110:111–112.
10. Russell FE. Bite of the spider *Phidippus formossus*: case history. *Toxicon* 1970;8:193–194.
11. Vest DK. Necrotic arachnidism in the Northwest United States and its probable relationship to *Tegenaria agrestis* (Walckenaer) spiders. *Toxicon* 1987;25:175–184.
12. Wong RC, Hughes SE, Voorhees JJ. Spider bites. *Arch Dermatol* 1987;123:98–104.
13. Gertsch WJ, Ennik F. The spider genus *Loxosceles* in North America, Central America, and West Indies (Araneae, Loxscelidae). *Bull Am Mus Nat Hist* 1983;175:265–360.
14. Gomez HF, Miller MJ, Waggener MW, et al. Antigenic cross-reactivity of venoms from medically important North American *Loxosceles* spider species. *Toxicon* 2001;39:817–824.
15. Barbaro KC, Eickstedt, VRD, Mota I. Antigenic cross-reactivity of venoms from medically important *Loxosceles* (*araneae*) species in Brazil. *Toxicon* 1994; 32:113–120.
16. Sezerino UM, Aannin M, Coelho LK, et al. A clinical and epidemiological study of *Loxosceles* spider envenoming in Santa Catarina, Brazil. *Trans Roy Soc Trop Med Hyg* 1998;92:546–548.
17. Russell FE, Waldron WG, Madon MB. Bites by the brown spiders *Loxosceles unicolor* and *Loxosceles arizona* in California and Arizona. *Toxicon* 1969;7:109–117.
18. Gertsch WJ. The spider genus *Loxosceles* in South America (Araneae, Scytodidae). *Bull Am Mus Nat Hist* 1967;136:117–174.
19. Wasserman GS. Brown recluse and other necrotizing spiders. In: Ford MD, Delaney KA, Ling LJ, et al., eds. *Clinical toxicology*. Philadelphia: WB Saunders, 2001:879–884.
20. Schenone H, Rojas A, Reyes H, et al. Prevalence of *Loxosceles laeta* in houses in central Chile. *Am J Trop Med Hyg* 1970;19:564–567.
21. Boyer LV, Theodorou AA, Binsford GJ, et al. Spider on the headboard, child in the unit: severe *Loxosceles arizonica* envenomation confirmed by delayed spider identification and tissue antigen detection. *J Toxicol Clin Toxicol* 2000;38:510(abst).

22. Gomez HF, Greenfield DM, Miller MM, et al. Direct correlation between diffusion of *Loxosceles reclusa* venom and extent of dermal inflammation. *Acad Emerg Med* 2001;8:311–314.
23. Geren CR, Chan TK, Bard BC, et al. Composition and properties of extract of fiddleback spider venom apparatus (*L. reclusa*). *Toxicon* 1973;11:471–479.
24. Rees RS, Nanney LB, Yates RA, et al. Interaction of brown recluse spider venom on cell membranes: the inciting mechanism? *J Invest Dermatol* 1984;83:270–275.
25. Young AR, Pincus SJ. Comparison of enzymatic activity from three species of necrotizing arachnids in Australia: *Loxosceles rufescens, Badumna insignis* and *Lampona cylindrata*. *Toxicon* 2001;39:391–400.
26. Patel KD, Modur V, Zimmerman GA, et al. The necrotic venom of the brown recluse spider induces dysregulated endothelial cell–dependent neutrophil activation. *J Clin Invest* 1994;94:631–642.
27. Gomez HF, Miller MJ, Desai A, et al. *Loxosceles* venom induces production of multiple chemokines by endothelial and epithelial cells. *Inflammation* 1999;23:207–215.
28. Desai A, Gomez HF, Miller MJ, et al. Venom of *Loxosceles deserta* induces activation of NF-KB in endothelial cells. *J Toxicol Clin Toxicol* 1999;37:447–456.
29. Forrester LJ, Barrett JT, Campbell BJ. Red blood cell lysis induced by the venom of the brown recluse spider: the role of sphingomyelinase D. *Arch Biochem Biophys* 1978;187:355–365.
30. Huford DC, Morgan PN. C-reactive protein as a mediator in the lysis of human erythrocytes sensitized by brown recluse spider venom. *Proc Soc Exp Biol Med* 1981;167:493–497.
31. Kurpiewski G, Forrester LJ, Barrett JT, et al. Platelet aggregation and sphingomyelinase D activity of a purified toxin from the venom of *Loxosceles reclusa*. *Biochem Biophys Acta* 1981;678:467–476.
32. Babcock JL, Marmer DJ, Steele RW. Immunotoxicology of brown recluse spider (*Loxosceles reclusa*) venom. *Toxicon* 1986;24:783:790.
33. Gates CA, Rees RS. Serum amyloid P component: its role in platelet activation stimulated by sphingomyelinase D purified from the venom of the brown recluse spider (*Loxosceles reclusa*). *Toxicon* 1990;28:1303–1315.
34. Gertsch WJ. *American spiders*, 2nd ed. New York: Van Nostrand Reinhold, 1979.
35. Tambourgi DV, Morgan BP, De Andrade RMG. et al. *Loxosceles intermedia* spider envenomation induces activation of an endogenous metalloproteinase, resulting in cleavage of glycophorins from the erythrocyte surface and facilitating complement-mediated lysis. *Blood* 2000;95:683–691.
36. Bey TA, Walters FG, Lober W, et al. *Loxosceles arizonica* bite associated with shock. *Ann Emerg Med* 1997;30:701.
37. Schenone H, Saaverdra T, Rojas A, et al. Loxoscelism in Chile. Epidemiologic, clinical, and experimental studies. *Rev Inst Med Trop São Paulo* 1989;31:403–415.
38. Berger R. The unremarkable brown recluse spider bite. *JAMA* 1973;225:1109–1111.
39. Wright SW, Wrenn KD, Murray L, et al. Clinical presentation and outcome of brown recluse spider bite. *Ann Emerg Med* 1997;30:28–32.
40. Wasserman GS. Brown recluse spider envenomations. In Harwood-Nuss AL, Linden CH, Luten RC, et al. (eds). *The clinical practice of emergency medicine*, 2nd ed. Philadelphia: Lippincott–Raven Publishers, 1996:1484–1450.
41. Anderson PC. Loxoscelism threatening pregnancy: five cases. *Am J Obstet Gynecol* 1991;165:1454–1456.
42. Wasserman GS. Loxoscelism (brown recluse spider bites): a review of literature. *Vet Hum Toxicol* 1977;19:256–258.
43. Anderson P. Necrotizing spider bites. *Am Fam Physician* 1982;26:198.
44. Habermehl GG. *Venomous animals and their toxins.* Berlin: Sprinnnder-Verlag, 1981:33–38.
45. Vetter RS, Bush SP. The diagnosis of brown recluse spider bite is overused for dermonecrotic wounds of uncertain etiology [Editorial]. *Ann Emerg Med* 2002;39:544–546.
46. Wasserman G, Anderson P. Loxoscelism and necrotic arachnidism. *J Toxicol Clin Toxicol* 1983;21:451.
47. Osterhoudt KC, Azoutis T, Zorc JJ. Lyme disease masquerading as brown recluse spider bite. *Ann Emerg Med* 2002;39:558–561.
48. Taylor EM, Denny W. Hemolysis, renal failure and death, presumed secondary to the bite of brown recluse spider. *South Med J* 1966;59:1209–1211.
49. Madrigal G, Ercolani R, Wenzl J. Toxicity from a bite of the brown spider. *Clin Pediatr* 1972;11:641–644.
50. Nance W. Hemolytic anemia of necrotic arachnidism. *Am J Med* 1961;31:801–807.
51. Novak R, Kumar M, Thompson E, et al. Severe systemic toxicity from a spider bite in a six-year-old boy. *J Tenn Med Assoc* 1979;72:110–111.
52. Barrett SM, Romine-Jenkins M, Blick KE. Passive hemagglutination inhibition test for diagnosis of brown recluse spider bite envenomation. *Clin Chem* 1993;39:2104–2104.
53. Gomez HF, Krywko DM, Stoecker WV. A new assay for the detection of *Loxosceles* species (brown recluse) spider venom. *Ann Emerg Med* 2002;39:469–474.
54. Cardosa JLC, Wen FH, Franca FOS, et al. Detection by enzyme immunoassay of *Loxosceles gaucho* venom in necrotic skin lesions by spider bites in Brazil. *Trans Roy Soc Trop Med Hyg* 1990;84:608–609.
55. Miller MJ, Gomez HF, Sinder RJ, et al. Detection of *Loxosceles* venom lesional hair shafts and skin application of a specific immunoassay to id tify dermonecrotic arachnidism. *Am J Emerg Med* 2000;18:626–628.
56. Krywko DM, Gomez HF. Detection of *Loxosceles* species venom in derm lesions: a comparison of 4 venom recovery methods. *Ann Emerg M* 2002;39:475–480.
57. Wasserman GS, Anderson PC. Brown recluse spider envenomations. Harwood-Nuss A, Wolfson AB, Linden CH, et al., eds. *The clinical practice emergency medicine*, 3rd ed. Philadelphia: Lippincott Williams & Wilkir 2001:1638–1640.
58. Wright SW, Wrenn KD, Murray L, et al. Clinical presentation and outcom of brown recluse spider bite. *Ann Emerg Med* 1997;30:28–32.
59. Hardman JT, Beck ML, Hardman PK, et al. Incompatibility associated wi the bite of the brown recluse spider (*Loxosceles reclusa*). *Transfusio* 1983;23:233–236.
60. Philips S, Kohn M, Baker D, et al. Therapy of brown spider envenomatior a controlled trial of hyperbaric oxygen, dapsone, and cyproheptadine. *An Emerg Med* 1995;25:363–368.
61. Iserson KV. Methemoglobinemia from dapsone therapy for a suspecte brown spider bite. *J Emerg Med* 1995;3:285–288.
62. Hobbs GD, Anderson AR, Greene JT, et al. Comparison of hyperbaric oxy gen and dapsone therapy for *Loxosceles* envenomation. *Acad Emerg Me* 1996;3:758–761.
63. Rees RS, Altenbern DP, Lynch JB, et al. Brown recluse spider bites: a comparison of surgical excision versus dapsone and delayed surgical excision. *Ann Surg* 1985;202:659–663.
64. Braz A, Minozzo J, Abreu JC, et al. Development and evaluation of the neutralizing capacity of horse antivenom against the Brazilian spider *Loxosceles intermedia*. *Toxicon* 1999;37:1323–1328.
65. Rees R, Shack RB, Withers E, et al. Management of the brown recluse bite. *Plast Recontr Surg* 1981;68:768–773.
66. Bravo M, Oviedo I, Rarias P, et al. Study of anti-*Loxosceles* serum action on hemolytic and ulcero-necrotic cutaneous effects of *Loxosceles laeta* venom. *Rev Med Chil* 1994; 122:625–629.
67. Cole HP, Wesley RE, King LE. Brown recluse envenomation of the eyelid: an animal model. *Ophthal Plast Reconstr Surg* 1995;11:153–164.
68. Rees R, Campbell D, Rieger E, et al. The diagnosis and treatment of brown recluse spider bites. *Ann Emerg Med* 1987;16:945–949.
69. Gomez HF, Mill MJ, Trach JW, et al. Intradermal anti-*Loxosceles* Fab fragments attenuate dermonecrotic arachnidism. *Acad Emerg Med* 1999;6:1195–1202.
70. Whetstone WD, Ernsting K, Warren JS, et al. Inhibition of dermonecrotic arachnidism with interlukin-8 monoclonal antibody. *Acad Emerg Med* 1997;4:337(abst).
71. Russell F. A confusion of spiders. *Emerg Med* 1986;(June 15):8.
72. Vest DK. Envenomation by *Tegenaria agrestis* (Walckenaer) spiders in rabbits. *Toxicon* 1987;25(2):221–224.
73. Anonymous. Necrotic arachnidism—Pacific Northwest, 1988–1996. *MMWR Morb Mortal Wkly Rep* 1996 May 31;45(21):433–436.
74. Krinsky WL. Envenomation by the sac spider *Chiracanthium mildei. Cutis* 1987 Aug;40(2):127–129.
75. Newlands G, Martindale C, Berson SD, et al. Cutaneous necrosis caused by the bite of *Chiracanthium* spiders. *S Afr Med J* 1980 Feb 2;57(5):171–173.
76. Minton SA Jr. Poisonous spiders of Indiana and a report of a bite by *Chiracanthium mildei. J Indiana State Med Assoc* 1972 May;65(5):425–426.
77. Spielman A, Levi HW. Probable envenomation by *Chiracanthium mildei*; a spider found in houses. *Am J Trop Med Hyg* 1970 Jul;19(4):729–732.
78. Atkinson RK, Wright LG. A study of the necrotic actions of the venom of the wolf spider, *Lycosa godeffroyi*, on mouse skin. *Comp Biochem Physiol (C)* 1990;95(2):319–325.
79. Young AR, Pincus SJ. Comparison of enzymatic activity from three species of necrotizing arachnids in Australia: *Loxosceles rufescens, Badumna insignis* and *Lampona cylindrata*. *Toxicon* 2001 Feb–Mar;39(2–3):391–400.
80. St George I, Forster L. Skin necrosis after white-tailed spider bite? *NZ Med J* 1991 May 22;104(912):207–208.
81. Russell FE, Gertsch WJ. For those who treat spider or suspected spider bites [Letter]. *Toxicon* 1983;21:337–339.
82. Kunkel DB. The myth of the brown recluse spider. *Emerg Med* 1985;17:124–128
83. Vetter RS, Visscher PK. Bites and stings of medically important venomous arthropods. *Int J Dermatol* 1998;37:481–496
84. Rosenstein ED, Kramer N. Lyme disease misdiagnosed as a brown recluse bite [Letter]. *Ann Intern Med* 1987;107:782.
85. Nadelman RB, Wormser GP. Erythema migrans and early Lyme disease. *Am J Med* 1995;98[Suppl 4A]:15S–23S
86. Moaven LD, Altman SA, Newnham AR. Sporotrichosis mimicking necrotizing arachnidism. *Med J Aust* 1999;171:865–868
87. Vetter RS, Bush SP. Chemical burn misdiagnosed as brown recluse spider bite. *Am J Emerg Med* 2002;20:68–69.
88. Roche KJ, Chang MW, Lazarus H. Cutaneous anthrax infection. *N Engl J Med* 2001;345:1611.

CHAPTER 250

Scorpion Envenomation

Leslie V. Boyer-Hassen

Topics included:	**Family Buthidae, genus *Centruroides***
Special concerns:	**Most human neurotoxicity is attributable to sodium channel toxins injected intradermally by a stinger at the tip of the scorpion's tail.**
Antidote:	**No commercial product available in United States. Experimental antivenom under development.**

OVERVIEW

Of more than 1000 scorpion species worldwide, the stings of approximately 20 can cause medically important envenomation in humans. All of these species fall within the family Buthidae. The North American buthids of medical importance are members of the genus *Centruroides*. *Centruroides* venom contains a variety of polypeptide ion channel toxins that can, when injected in sufficient quantity, produce a systemic clinical syndrome including profound neurotoxicity. Management may involve intensive supportive care or use of specific antivenom, or both.

In 1998, 12,845 scorpion stings were reported by poison centers in the United States, primarily from Arizona. Of these, 767 were ultimately treated in a health care facility. Outcome data indicate that 6112 cases were mild and 473 cases had moderate to major effects (1). The great majority of severe cases resolve satisfactorily, with only two scorpion-related deaths in Arizona in the past 35 years (2).

Chemical and Physical Properties

Centruroides scorpion venom contains a set of polypeptides directed variously against insect, crustacean, and vertebrate nervous systems. All characterized neurotoxins derived from *Centruroides* venom are active at sites involving ion channels, including those for transport of sodium, potassium, and calcium. Neurotoxicity accordingly varies with the host species, such that envenomation may provoke immediate paralysis in a cricket or neuromotor hyperactivity in a human child.

Centruroides toxins are comprised of 65 to 68 amino acid chains, all of which contain eight highly conserved cysteine residues that are involved in the formation of four disulfide bridges. In Arizona *C. sculpturatus* (also known as *C. exilicauda*) venom, 22 sodium channel toxins fall broadly into three phylogenetically related groups, two of which are specific to insects and one of which is toxic to vertebrates. This last group includes the CsE1 toxin and related peptides, which closely resemble counterparts found in the venom of *C. noxius* and *Tityus serrulatus* and which are believed to be responsible for neurotoxicity in humans (3).

Classification and Uses

Scorpions, like other arachnids, are predators. Venom is stored in a "telson," or bulb, at the tip of the tail, to which is attached a stinger. Venom is injected into prey animals by a tail strike over the scorpion's back at the time of capture to induce paralysis and enable subsequent feeding. Venom is also injected during defensive stings, including those provoked by humans. Because scorpions are predominantly nocturnal, most envenomations occur at night.

In North America, more than 20 *Centruroides* species can be found across the southern United States from California to Florida, as far north as Nebraska and as far south as the southern tip of Mexico. Of these only about eight are of medical importance, however; these are found throughout the western third of Mexico, from the Sierra Madre to the sea, and through Arizona as far north as southern Nevada.

In the United States, occupational exposure to scorpion sting may occur in the exotic pet trade, "scorpion wrangling" for television productions, or the arachnology research setting. Laboratory work may be particularly risky, with stings by more than 40 scorpion species reported during the course of a single taxonomist's studies (4). In Latin American countries where scorpions are used in production of antivenom or tourist items, "alacraneros" (persons who catch scorpions for sale), artisans, and venom scientists and technicians are similarly at risk.

Within their natural geographic range, *Centruroides* scorpions commonly enter homes, putting inhabitants at risk of accidental stings, particularly at night. Scorpions survive travel in tourist baggage or on produce shipments and have been reported to cause envenomations distant from their native geographic regions.

Toxic Dose

A single sting by any scorpion may cause local signs and symptoms. Death, although very rare, has been reported in adults after a single sting by a *Centruroides* scorpion. The only reported death in a U.S. adult in the past 40 years was apparently due to anaphylaxis rather than to neurotoxicity (2).

One sting may be lethal to children. Although neurotoxicity is the most commonly cited cause of death in endemic areas, iatrogenic and allergic deaths have also been reported (2,5,6).

TOXICOKINETICS AND TOXICODYNAMICS

Absorption kinetics and dynamics of scorpion envenomation have not been studied. Stinger length favors intradermal injection in human victims, and prolonged uptake from the site may explain the several-days' duration of pain often noted by adults stung by Centruroides scorpions. On the other hand, children in whom systemic neurotoxicity develops commonly cease complaining of local pain within an hour or two of the sting, suggesting that relatively rapid absorption from pediatric dermis may partially explain the more dramatic systemic presentation in children.

Preliminary observations indicate that, in the absence of antivenom, *Centruroides* venom remains detectable in serum for many hours after envenomation, with a serum half-life of roughly 200 to 500 minutes (7). In the presence of a specific antivenom, the level of unbound scorpion venom in serum drops dramatically. Preliminary human data from Mexican trials of an equine Fab'2 *Centruroides* antivenom indicate an order-of-magnitude decrease in serum levels within 30 to 60 minutes of treatment. This change in level appears to correlate with timing of diminution in systemic toxicity, suggesting that antivenom binding of venom accounts for the more rapid resolution of symptoms in antivenom-treated patients (8).

PATHOPHYSIOLOGY

The principal targets of *Centruroides* venom toxins are voltage-dependent ion channels responsible for nerve conduction. Most clinically important effects in vertebrates appear to arise from two mechanisms. First, slowed inactivation of sodium channels results in potentiation of the neuronal action potential to many times its natural duration. Second, transient shifts in the voltage dependence of activation result in frequent, spontaneous membrane firing. Combined, these two phenomena result in dramatically increased neuronal firing generally (9).

Voltage-dependent ion channel toxicity appears to affect human axonal function generally, resulting in simultaneous sensory (local pain), muscarinic (hypersecretion), nicotinic (tachycardia, hypertension), and neuromotor (cranial and peripheral motor hyperactivity) effects.

VULNERABLE POPULATIONS

Very few reports have been published of severe envenomation in pregnant or lactating women. The author is aware of a single case of systemic envenomation managed with goat-derived antivenom during the third trimester of pregnancy. Serum sickness in this case was managed with corticosteroid treatment 1 week after envenomation, and later pregnancy outcome was normal.

Children are far more susceptible to systemic neurotoxicity than are adults. In case series reported by the Arizona Poison Control System, systemic reactions occur in 26% to 80% of small children, in contrast to 5% to 6% of adults (6,10). Unpublished veterinary experience in southern Arizona suggests that exotic birds and mammals in private and zoo collections may be at heightened risk of mortality from *Centruroides* scorpion envenomation relative to small animals native to the desert southwest.

CLINICAL PRESENTATION

Centruroides scorpion envenomation produces a pattern of neurotoxicity with a spectrum of severity ranging from trivial to life-threatening. Mild envenomation, more common in adults and consisting mainly of local pain, resolves without specific treatment in the course of hours to days. Severe envenomation, more common in small children, may involve neuromotor hyperactivity, pulmonary edema, and ventilatory compromise, occasionally resulting in death.

The pattern of neuromotor hyperactivity in severe envenomation is nearly pathognomonic and includes erratic, yet nearly conjugate, extraocular movements; dysphonic, dysarthric speech or cry; and mixed ballistic and choreiform motor hyperactivity that may mimic seizure but is usually neither symmetric nor accompanied by loss of consciousness. Systemic toxicity peaks roughly 5 hours after scorpion sting (10) and resolves within 24 hours if managed supportively, or within 1 to 4 hours with specific antivenom treatment (10,11).

DIAGNOSTIC TESTS

No diagnostic test is commercially available for the presence of scorpion venom in human tissue. Recent work suggests the utility of venom antigen levels as a research tool and demonstrates a rapid drop in unbound serum toxin after administration of specific antivenom. Consistent with clinical observations, unbound scorpion venom antigen becomes undetectable in serum within 1 hour after treatment with *Centruroides* immune Fab'2 (7,8). Depending on the severity of presentation, chest radiography, pulse oximetry, routine serum electrolytes, and arterial blood gas monitoring may aid in supportive care.

Diagnosis is seldom in doubt when the fully developed manifestations of systemic neurotoxicity are present. Even in the absence of a scorpion, the pattern of cranial and peripheral motor hyperactivity is nearly pathognomonic. Early presentation (less than 4 hours after sting), however, may be misleadingly mild, with predominantly local tenderness indistinguishable from that caused by clinically unimportant scorpions such as *Vejovis* species. Occasionally, the combination of muscarinic and motor findings may mimic organophosphate toxicity, a potential point of confusion in the event of insecticide exposure occasioned by killing of the offending animal. In such a case, cholinesterase levels and prolonged observation may be necessary for final diagnosis.

POSTMORTEM CONSIDERATIONS

Due to the rarity of death in scorpion-envenomated patients, postmortem examination should be directed toward differentiation of death from primary toxicity (e.g., evidence of pulmonary edema or hypoxemia) from that caused by anaphylaxis (e.g., elevated serum tryptase or characteristic airway findings) or by iatrogenic factors (e.g., adverse drug event or airway maintenance misadventure).

TREATMENT

Most scorpion stings result in local pain only and do not require hospital care. Treatment of systemic toxicity, with antivenom or with supportive care alone, has historically involved a risk-benefit analysis dependent on symptom severity, type and availability of antivenom, and proximity to pediatric intensive care, as well as physician and patient perceptions of relative risk. In Mexico, where access to intensive care is low and risk of mortality is high, prompt use of refined equine Fab'2 antivenoms has become the standard of care even in relatively mild cases. In the United States, where intensive care access is greater and risk of mortality is low, the U.S. Food and Drug Administration has never approved any agent for treatment of scorpion envenomation, and whole immunoglobulin G (IgG) scorpion-specific goat antivenom has been associated with risk of acute and delayed serum reactions. Consequently, use of antivenom in the United States, although widely perceived as effective, has not been universally accepted even for severe envenomation (12).

Decontamination and First Aid

Intermittent local application of a single ice cube lessens pain at the sting site.

Enhancement of Elimination

No role is known or postulated in the treatment of scorpion envenomations.

Antidotes

During the course of the last 80 years, at least seven *Centruroides*-specific antivenoms were produced in North America. These included, in Arizona, rabbit and cat serum products between the years 1947 and 1964, followed by a goat serum antivenom produced at Arizona State University (ASU) between the years 1965 and 2000 and still stocked by many Arizona hospitals as of 2002 (13). In Mexico, at least two equine whole immunoglobulin scorpion antivenoms were produced between the 1930s and the early 1990s. These have been replaced by equine "fabotherapeutic" agents produced by IgG cleavage with papain (a mixed Fab/Fab'2 product produced by the Mexican Ministry of Health) or with pepsin ("Alacramyn," a Fab'2 produced by Laboratorios Bioclon, division of Silanes Pharmaceuticals, Mexico City, Mexico). Treatment with ASU goat antivenom, Ministry of Health Fab, and Alacramyn has been reported to result in syndrome resolution within a similar time frame of 1 to 4 hours (10,11).

Dosing of all three agents in current use is most commonly intravenous, one to two vials, with occasional cases requiring an additional vial. Like all serum products, these carry some risk of acute hypersensitivity or anaphylactoid reaction; this has been reported at 4% for the ASU product (14) and at less than 5% for Alacramyn (11). Delayed serum sickness is reported in 61% of ASU antivenom recipients (14). Serum sickness has not been studied after use of "fabotherapeutic" agents, although it is expected to be substantially lower in such cases due to shorter half-life and absence of the immunogenic Fc portion of the IgG molecule. Clinical trials of Alacramyn are scheduled to begin in 2004.

Supportive Care

A patient who is experiencing severe *Centruroides* scorpion envenomation that is treated with sedation and observation may require 6 to 28 hours of intensive care monitoring. Patients managed without specific antivenom may require intensive supportive care, including supplementary oxygen, ventilatory support, and, occasionally, atropine for treatment of excessive airway secretions. Benzodiazepine sedation is commonly used in the intensive care unit setting. Midazolam drip at high doses (ranging from 0.6 to 1.3 mg/kg/hour) may be required to suppress agitation. This approach results, on average, in a 16-hour intensive care stay, during which 12% of patients experience mild hypoxemia (15). Intubation and ventilation for respiratory compromise are occasionally necessary. Patients who present with local pain only (predominantly adults) report improvement with intermittent application of ice to the site. Opiate or acetaminophen/opiate combinations are often used in treatment of local pain, which may last for several days after a sting. It is noteworthy that children with systemic intoxication rarely complain of local pain for more than an hour after the sting. Opiates should, for this reason, be avoided in early pediatric presentation, to minimize ventilatory compromise that may result from combined effects of scorpion venom, sedatives, and narcotics.

Management Pitfalls

Management of scorpion envenomation entails risk of iatrogenic injury from adverse drug events. Patients managed supportively with benzodiazepine sedation incur a 12% risk of hypoxemia (arterial oxygen pressure less than 90%), as well as potential ventilatory failure (15). Those who receive antivenom are at risk of acute (anaphylactic or anaphylactoid) or delayed (serum sickness) immune reactions (14).

REFERENCES

1. Litovitz T, Klein-Schwartz W, Caravati EM, et al. 1998 Annual report of the American Association of Poison Control Centers Toxic Exposure Surveillance System. *Am J Emerg Med* 1999;17:435–487.
2. Boyer L, Heubner K, McNally J, et al. Death from *Centruroides* scorpion sting allergy. *J Toxicol Clin Toxicol* 2001;39:561–562.
3. Corona M, Valdez-Cruz NA, Merino D, et al. Genes and peptides from the scorpion *Centruroides sculpturatus* Ewing, that recognize Na+-channels. *Toxicon* 2001;39:1893–1898.
4. Stockwell SA. Stingers! Scorpions that have stung me. Available at: http://wrbu.si.edu/www/stockwell/stingers/stingers!.html. Accessed September 2002.
5. Stahnke HL. The Arizona scorpion problem. *Arizona Med* 1950;7:23–29.
6. Likes K, Banner W, Chavez M. *Centruroides exilicauda* envenomation in Arizona. *West J Med* 1984;141:634–637.
7. Chase PB, Vazquez HL, Boyer L, et al. Serum levels and urine detection of *Centruroides sculpturatus* venom in significantly envenomated patients. *J Toxicol Clin Toxicol* 2002;40;650.
8. Gonzalez C, Cabral J, Reyes S, et al. Development of an immunoenzymatic assay for the quantification of scorpion venom in plasma. Presentation at 4th reunion of experts in envenomation by poisonous animals, Cuernavaca, 2000.
9. Simard JM. Watt DD. Venoms and toxins. In: Polis GA, ed. *The biology of scorpions*. Stanford, CA: Stanford University Press, 1990:414–444.
10. Curry SC, Vance M, Ryan P, et al. Envenomation by the scorpion *Centruroides sculpturatus*. *J Toxicol Clin Toxicol* 1983–1984;21:417–449.
11. Cabral-Soto J, Escandon-Romero C, Lopez de Silanes J, et al. Comparison of efficacy between two antiscorpion antivenoms. Presentation at 4th reunion of experts in envenomation by poisonous animals, Cuernavaca, 2000.
12. Banner W Jr. A scorpion by any other name is still a scorpion. *Ann Emerg Med* 1999;34:669–670.
13. Stahnke HL. Arizona's lethal scorpion. *Arizona Med* 1972;6:490–493.
14. LoVecchio F, Welch S, Klemens J, et al. Incidence of immediate and delayed hypersensitivity to *Centruroides* antivenom. *Ann Emerg Med* 1999;34:615–619.
15. Gibly R, Williams M, Walter F, et al. Continuous intravenous midazolam infusion for *Centruroides exilicauda* scorpion envenomation. *Ann Emerg Med* 1999;34;620–625.

CHAPTER 251

Other Arthropods

Geoffrey K. Isbister

Topics included:	**Hymenoptera: bees (Apidae), wasps (Vespidae), ants (Formacidae); centipedes (Chilopoda); millipedes (Diplopoda); ticks (Ixodida); beetles (Coleoptera); true bugs (Hemiptera); moths and butterflies (Lepidoptera); walking stick (Phasmatodea); lacewing (Neuroptera)**
Special considerations:	**Arthropods can cause either direct toxicity from venom components or hypersensitivity reactions (e.g., anaphylaxis).**
Antidotes:	**Antivenoms for *Apis mellifera* (honey bee, killer bee), *Lonomia* (caterpillar) stings**

OVERVIEW

Many arthropods in addition to spiders and scorpions cause injuries to humans. This chapter deals mainly with arthropod envenomation by the other major groups that are medically significant. In addition to envenomation, arthropods, mainly Hymenoptera (bees, wasps, and ants), can cause allergic reactions. Hypersensitivity reactions to Hymenoptera account for a large number of venomous animal injuries (1–3). These allergic reactions, which can be triggered by a single sting, differ completely from mass envenomation by Hymenoptera [multiple stings from bees (4) or wasps (5)]. Life-threatening allergic reactions to arthropod stings occur in 0.5% to 4.0% of an exposed population, and the risk is proportional to annual exposure rates (3). Insect venom anaphylaxis almost always begins within half an hour of exposure, with life-threatening allergy usually manifesting within minutes, but may rarely occur as long as 24 hours after the sting. In the latter case the reaction is usually not severe and the rate of progression is relatively slow. Although allergic reactions are considered briefly in this chapter, a detailed discussion of insect allergy and venom immunotherapy is not included.

HYMENOPTERA

The order Hymenoptera contains the bees, wasps, and ants, which are responsible for the majority of cases of insect sting allergy (Fig. 1). Deaths from bee, wasp, and ant stings continue to occur in many countries, including western countries (2,6,7). In most cases, early allergic reactions and anaphylaxis are responsible for death, characterized by hypotension, bronchospasm, and laryngeal edema (8). Bee and wasp sting allergies are not uncommon. These range from localized effects, to generalized urticaria, and finally to systemic effects. Hymenoptera allergic reactions are usually classified into four grades according to the Mueller classification (Table 1).

The majority of species of bees and wasps are solitary creatures and rarely sting humans (9). Only a limited number of groups are responsible for human stings, and an even smaller number live in sufficiently large colonies to be able to cause mass envenomation. These include honey bees (subfamily Apinae), the social bumble bees (subfamily Bombinae) from the family Apidae, and the social wasps—hornets (*Vespa* species), yellow jackets, and paper wasps—from the family Vespidae (9,10).

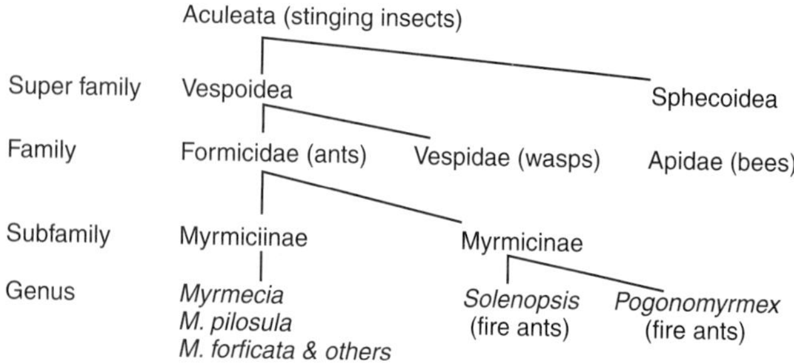

Figure 1. Phylogenetic relationships of common stinging insects, including wasps, ants, and bees. (From Brown SG, Franks, RW, Baldo BA, et al. Prevalence, severity, and natural history of jack jumper ant venom allergy in Tasmania. *J Allergy Clin Immunol* 2003;111:187–192, with permission.)

TABLE 1. Grading of systemic allergic reactions according to the Mueller method

Grade	Clinical effects
I	Generalized urticaria (includes periorbital edema), itching, anxiety, and malaise
II	Angioedema and 2 or more of the following: chest or throat tightness, nausea, vomiting, diarrhea, abdominal pain, dizziness
III	Dyspnea, wheezing, or stridor or 2 or more of the following: dysphagia, dysarthria, hoarseness, weakness, confusion, feeling of impending disaster
IV	Hypotension, collapse, loss of consciousness, incontinence of urine or feces, cyanosis

Adapted from references 3,160,161.

Individuals with a history of systemic allergic reactions to hymenopteran stings should carry an anaphylaxis emergency treatment kit that allows for two doses of epinephrine whenever they are engaged in outdoor activities. Such persons should consult an allergist or clinical immunologist for venom skin testing and venom immunotherapy.

Venom Immunotherapy

More than 20 years of clinical experience, two open-label controlled studies in honeybee and yellow jacket (wasp) sting allergic people (11,12), and one double-blind randomized, placebo-controlled trial in Australia in *Myrmecia pilosula* ("jack jumper") ant sting allergic people (13) have demonstrated the efficacy of venom immunotherapy in preventing sting anaphylaxis in hypersensitive individuals. Conversely, the use of whole body extract (WBE) immunotherapy, probably containing negligible amounts of venom, has been found to be ineffective for the treatment of bee and wasp allergy (11) and of *M. pilosula* ant sting allergy (14). However, WBE continues to be used for the treatment of fire ant sting allergy. Although in one nonrandomized study with poorly matched treatment groups and in one uncontrolled study of immunotherapy with imported fire ants, WBE appeared promising (15,16), there are conflicting assessments as to the therapeutic efficacy of fire ant WBE extracts (17,18). Fire ant stings are usually inflicted by multiple ants, each of which delivers multiple stings. The ability of fire ant sting challenge procedures (which use only one ant at a time) to test treatment efficacy is unknown. Also, no prospective studies of the natural history of untreated fire ant allergy have been published. Therefore, until a rigorously conducted placebo-controlled assessment of fire ant WBE is performed, the efficacy of fire ant WBE immunotherapy remains subject to debate.

Preventive Measures

First-aid kits containing epinephrine should be prescribed to patients who have sustained prior systemic reactions and perhaps to those with large local reactions. EpiPen and EpiPen JR are designed for self-administration of 0.3 and 0.15 mg, respectively, of epinephrine subcutaneously and can be kept in the home, car, or personal belongings.

A warning bracelet or tag should be worn. Sensitized individuals should keep their feet covered outdoors. Bright, flowered clothing and attractive scents, soaps, and shampoos should be avoided. Tight rather than loose clothing should be worn.

Hymenoptera nests in areas around the living space of the sensitized patient should be destroyed. Materials or plants that attract Hymenoptera (e.g., clover, dandelions, uncovered sweet drinks) should be reduced.

Hymenoptera should not be swatted when encountered. Slow retreat or standing still is recommended. If the insect lands on the skin, it should be quickly brushed off.

APIDAE (BEES)

Although many thousands of species of bees exist, only *Apis* spp. (honey bees) form colonies large enough (thousands of worker bees) to be dangerous (9) (Fig. 2). The European honey bee (*A. mellifera*) is subdivided into approximately 24 subspecies, each with different behavioral characteristics such as the quantity of honey that they store or their defensiveness. The majority of mass envenomations are due to the Africanized honey bee (*A. mellifera scutellata*) that was introduced into South America, although other more common and commercially used European honey bee subspecies of *A. mellifera* may also be involved in mass envenomation (4,9,19). In Asia, the giant Asian rock bee (*A. dorsata*) and the Asian honey bee (*A. cerana*) have caused mass envenomations (9). A number of other bees cause stings and allergic reactions, including bumble bees (Bombinae), black bees (Apinae: *Trigona* spp.), and bees of the family Halictidae and Colletidae (20).

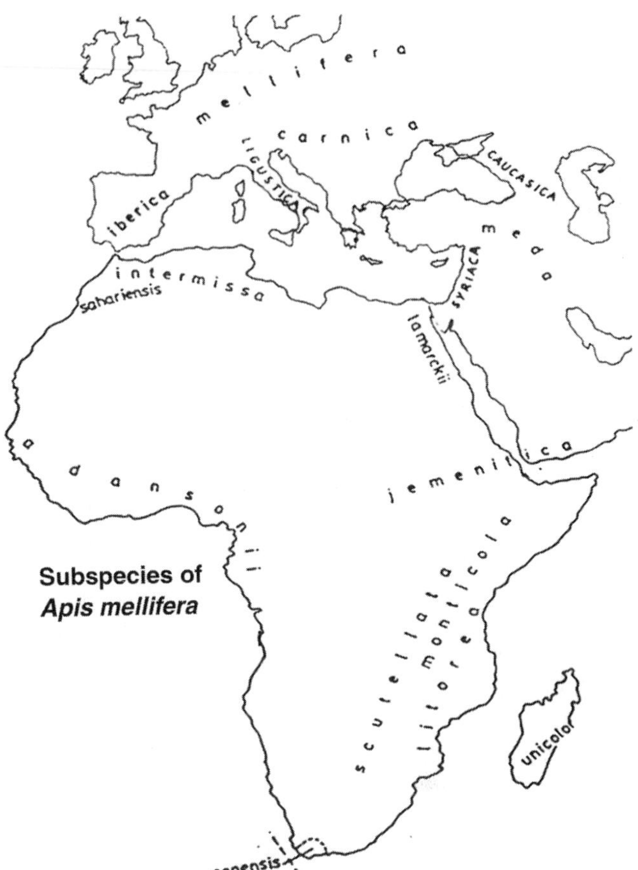

Figure 2. Map of the subspecies of *Apis mellifera* in Europe and Africa. (From Dietz A. Honey bees of the world. In: Graham J, ed. *The hive and the honey bee*. Hamilton, IL: Dadant and Sons, 1992: 23-71, with permission.)

Venoms

The principal components of the venoms of *Apis* spp. are mellitin (35% to 50% by dry weight), which is thought to be the main pain-inducing component, and a phospholipase A_2 (PLA_2; 10% to 20%) (4,9,19). Other components in smaller proportions include hyaluronidases (2% to 3%), apamin, a neurotoxic peptide (3%), mast cell degranulating peptide (2%), and small amounts of histamine and catecholamines (9,19). A study of the lethal activity of venoms from *Apis* spp. demonstrated that the PLA_2 is the most lethal, although mellitin is only slightly less lethal and is likely to be the most important because it makes up over three times the dry weight of venom (21). This investigator also provided evidence that there is no synergistic action between these two major components (21). The anaphylactic effects of venom are mediated by antibodies to PLA_2, hyaluronidase, and, to a lesser extent, mellitin (19).

Clinical Effects

The effects of individual bee stings vary depending on the type of bee and the sensitivity of the victim. Most stings are characterized by initial local pain that may be severe, associated with the development of localized swelling and erythema (9,19,22,23). The pain usually resolves in a number of hours, although redness and swelling may last for 12 to 48 hours. Large local reactions may occur that appear like cellulitis, with erythema and edema peaking at 48 hours and persisting for 7 days (24). Visscher et al. (23) demonstrated that the longer the sting is left in place the greater the wheal area. Importantly, they showed that the method of removal did not change the size of the wheal; thus, the essential treatment is rapid removal of the sting, irrespective of the method of removal.

Numerous local treatments have been suggested, including topical antihistamines, topical aspirin paste, and ice or heat treatment. A randomized controlled trial has demonstrated that topical aspirin paste was no better than ice alone and, in fact, increased the duration of local erythema (22). After a large local reaction, the risk of anaphylaxis is approximately 5% and venom therapy is not effective for preventing large local reactions (25).

Few bees other than honey bees have been studied. One report of stings from Australian native bees, including members of the families Halictidae and Colletidae, showed that they also caused initial moderate to severe pain, followed by variable development of erythema, swelling, and minor blistering (20).

Africanized Honey Bees ("Killer Bees")

Swarms of the Africanized honey bee (*A. mellifera scutellata*) originally escaped in Rio Claro, Brazil, in 1957 and have since spread throughout Latin America and into the southern United States. They reached Mexico in 1985, Texas in 1990, and Phoenix, Arizona, in 1993 (4) (Fig. 3). These bees are a highly successful strain that attack in large numbers and cause mass envenomation. In addition, they can cause anaphylaxis like other honey bees. Multiple stings are necessary to cause death by direct toxicity, usually more than 1000 in the case of bee stings (9). Numerous attacks and possibly almost 1000 deaths have been reported from South and Central America since their introduction (4).

Clinical Effects

In addition to local effects, systemic effects as a result of envenomation usually occur with 20 to 50 simultaneous stings, and more than 500 are usually regarded as necessary to cause death (4). With 20 or more stings, the reaction includes diffuse and widespread edema, a burning sensation in the skin, headache, weakness, dizziness, nausea and vomiting, and lethargy. With increasing numbers of stings and severity, the characteristic features of massive bee envenomation develop that include intravascular hemolysis, acute renal failure, hepatic injury, and rhabdomyolysis (4,9,19).

Less common effects of a severe life-threatening case include acute respiratory distress syndrome, myocardial injury and hypertension (possibly as a result of increased catecholamines), thrombocytopenia, shock, and coma (19). Acute renal failure may develop as a result of acute tubular necrosis secondary to rhabdomyolysis and myoglobinuria, hemoglobinuria, and renal ischemia. Immune mechanisms may also be involved, but the patient is then likely to have had fewer stings and no evidence of intravascular hemolysis or rhabdomyolysis.

Treatment

All stingers should be removed rapidly. Only the time until the stinger is removed is related to increasing severity (23). Studies have shown that the entire contents of domestic bee venom sacs are empty within 2 minutes. In cases of single stings or with only a few stings, symptomatic relief, such as ice and analgesia and brief observation for hypersensitivity, is all that is required.

Hospital admission should be considered for patients with more than 50 bee stings and definitely if hundreds of stings have been sustained. Supportive care is the mainstay of treatment. Initially, a systemic anaphylactic reaction may not be easily distinguished from massive envenomation. In addition to resuscitation, the patient may require the administration of epinephrine, antihistamines, and corticosteroids. The patient should be carefully monitored and observed for generalized urticaria, flushing, angioedema, airway swelling and obstruction, bronchoconstriction, and hypotension.

Early initiation of fluid resuscitation is likely to be beneficial for envenomation and allergic reactions, particularly in the hypotensive patient. Ongoing meticulous fluid therapy is required if acute renal failure develops. Monitoring urine output, hemoglobinuria, serum electrolyte, creatinine, creatine kinase (CK), liver function tests, and urea concentration is essential, as well as repeated urinalysis. Continuous electrocardiographic monitoring may be required initially in severely envenomed patients with dysrhythmias and hyperkalemia. Disseminated intravascular coagulation and the acute respiratory distress syndrome may also occur and should be managed appropriately (9,19).

An ovine antivenom has been developed and tested in mice and in vitro organ systems (26). It appears to neutralize the effects of *A. mellifera* venom, including myotoxic effects in a nerve muscle preparation, PLA_2 activity, and in vivo activity in mice (27). Because venoms from the European and Africanized bees are identical, the antivenom should be effective for all subspecies of *A. mellifera*.

Prevention of Multiple Stings

Because Africanized bees are known to establish their colonies in wall cavities and other protected sites close to homes, it is necessary to ensure that all holes and defects in exterior walls where pipes and conduit enter above ground are properly covered and to maintain garages and sheds similarly. Discarded boxes, junk automobiles, and unused equipment should be removed from yards or sealed. A healthy adult can usually outrun attacking bees because they do not pursue for distances more than 0.25 mile. If possible, the victim should cover the mouth and nose to try to prevent airway stings. Bees can be killed by spraying them with soapy water.

European Honey Bee

European honey bees (*A. mellifera*) and their descendants brought to North America, Australia, and other parts of the world have also caused mass envenomation. Deaths from mass envenomation by *A. mellifera* have been reported in Europe and Hawaii, but in all three cases reported the person either fell on, knocked over, or dropped the bee hive/swarm (4). The clinical effects and treatment are otherwise identical to that with Africanized honey bees.

VESPIDAE (WASPS)

The family Vespidae includes three main types of venomous wasps: hornets (*Vespa* spp.), yellow jackets (*Vespula* spp.), and paper wasps (*Polistes* spp.) (5). Only these three groups exist in

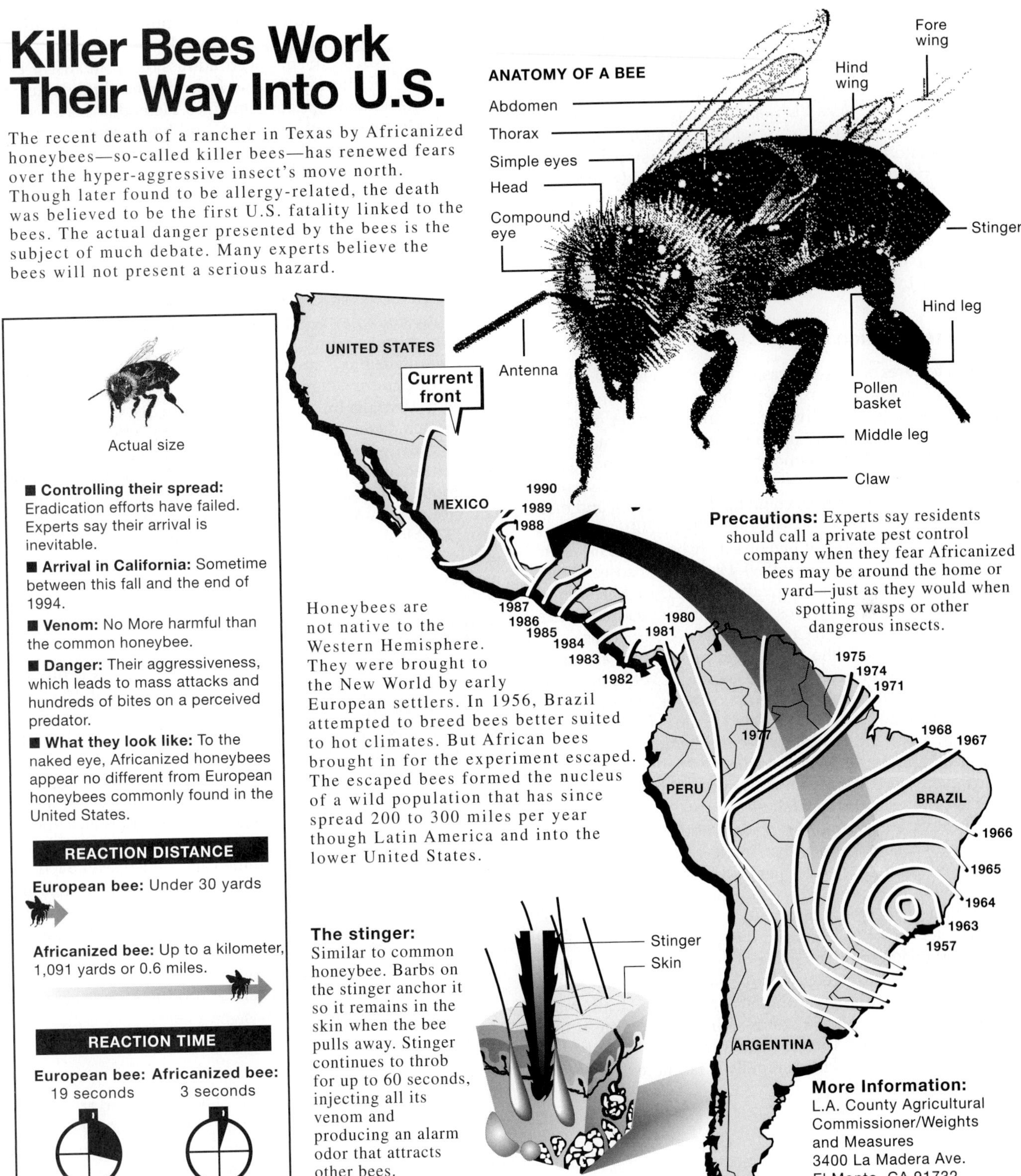
Killer Bees Work Their Way Into U.S.
The recent death of a rancher in Texas by Africanized honeybees—so-called killer bees—has renewed fears over the hyper-aggressive insect's move north. Though later found to be allergy-related, the death was believed to be the first U.S. fatality linked to the bees. The actual danger presented by the bees is the subject of much debate. Many experts believe the bees will not present a serious hazard.
ANATOMY OF A BEE
Abdomen
Thorax
Simple eyes
Head
Compound eye
Antenna
Fore wing
Hind wing
Stinger
Hind leg
Pollen basket
Middle leg
Claw
Actual size
■ Controlling their spread: Eradication efforts have failed. Experts say their arrival is inevitable.
■ Arrival in California: Sometime between this fall and the end of 1994.
■ Venom: No More harmful than the common honeybee.
■ Danger: Their aggressiveness, which leads to mass attacks and hundreds of bites on a perceived predator.
■ What they look like: To the naked eye, Africanized honeybees appear no different from European honeybees commonly found in the United States.
REACTION DISTANCE
European bee: Under 30 yards
Africanized bee: Up to a kilometer, 1,091 yards or 0.6 miles.
REACTION TIME
European bee: 19 seconds
Africanized bee: 3 seconds
UNITED STATES
Current front
MEXICO
1990
1989
1988
1987
1986
1985
1984
1983
1982
1981
1980
1977
1975
1974
1971
1968
1967
1966
1965
1964
1963
1957
PERU
BRAZIL
ARGENTINA
Honeybees are not native to the Western Hemisphere. They were brought to the New World by early European settlers. In 1956, Brazil attempted to breed bees better suited to hot climates. But African bees brought in for the experiment escaped. The escaped bees formed the nucleus of a wild population that has since spread 200 to 300 miles per year though Latin America and into the lower United States.
Precautions: Experts say residents should call a private pest control company when they fear Africanized bees may be around the home or yard—just as they would when spotting wasps or other dangerous insects.
The stinger: Similar to common honeybee. Barbs on the stinger anchor it so it remains in the skin when the bee pulls away. Stinger continues to throb for up to 60 seconds, injecting all its venom and producing an alarm odor that attracts other bees.
Stinger
Skin
More Information:
L.A. County Agricultural Commissioner/Weights and Measures
3400 La Madera Ave.
El Monto, CA 91732

Figure 3. Envenomation. (Adapted from *Los Angeles Times*, August 11, 1993.)

large enough colonies or inject sufficient quantities of venom to cause systemic envenomation (5,9). The *Vespa* wasps include approximately 20 species and are the most dangerous because of their greater venom toxicity and ability to deliver venom. The majority occur in eastern Asia, and only one species, the European hornet (*V. crabro*), occurs in Europe and has been introduced into the United States (5,9). The majority of deaths and reports of severe cases are due to *Vespa* spp., including *V. tropica* and *V. affinis* from Papua New Guinea and southeast Asia and *V. orientalis* from the Middle East and India (5). Three other genera including paper wasps and yellow jackets occur widely throughout the world and have been reported to attack humans (5).

Toxins

Only female wasps can sting. They have unbarbed hollow stings that also serve as an ovipositor in the queen. Vespid venoms contain three types of substances: (a) high-molecular-weight proteins (enzymes such as PLA_2 and hyaluronidases), (b) biologic active amines (histamine, serotonin, tyramine, and catecholamines), and (c) small peptides (kinins, mastoparans, and chemotactic peptides). Immunochemical studies demonstrate that "antigen 5" is the most allergenic, and the phospholipases and hyaluronidases are less active (9). Some wasps have neurotoxins such as mandaratoxin from *V. mandarina*. Mastoparans are reported to cause degranulation of mast cells and stimulation of PLA_2 activity and induce hemolysis.

Clinical Presentation

The clinical features of massive wasp envenomation are similar to those of bee envenomation except that far fewer stings are required. In nonallergic individuals, a small number of stings only cause local effects, including transient pain, erythema, swelling, and pruritus (22). Systemic effects occur with increasing numbers of stings. In moderately severe cases the patient has nonspecific effects, such as nausea, vomiting, fatigue, fever, and malaise. Severe envenomation (usually 20 to 200 stings) is characterized by intravascular hemolysis, rhabdomyolysis, acute renal failure, and hepatic injury (5,9). Hemolysis causes hematuria or hemoglobinuria, anemia, and jaundice (5,9). Rhabdomyolysis presents clinically with muscle aches and cramps, and there is usually a significant rise in CK and lactate dehydrogenase.

Acute renal failure is the most significant feature and may lead to death or chronic renal impairment (5). Vetter et al. (9) demonstrate that it occurs in the majority of cases of mass envenomation. One case demonstrated acute tubular necrosis on biopsy in a patient with intravascular hemolysis with elevated bilirubin, impaired liver function, and acute renal failure (28). However, there is one report from the United States of a patient developing acute renal failure after wasp stings who did not have intravascular hemolysis, rhabdomyolysis, or other features typical of mass envenomation. In this case the renal biopsy demonstrated acute interstitial nephritis that is more likely a result of venom hypersensitivity (29).

Less common effects include acute respiratory distress syndrome, hepatocellular necrosis and dysfunction, hypertension, myocardial damage (perhaps explained by release of endogenous catecholamines by venom PLA_2), shock, coma, and disseminated intravascular coagulation (5,9,28–30). Death may occur with as few as 20 to 50 stings, compared to almost ten times as many bee stings. Time to death varies from 4 hours to 9 days (9). Death that occurs more rapidly is far more likely to be due to acute anaphylaxis.

Diagnostic Tests

Laboratory findings include gross neutrophil leukocytosis and elevated serum enzymes (aspartate aminotransferase, alanine aminotransferase, lactate dehydrogenase, CK, predominantly CK-MM) and creatinine.

Treatment

No specific antivenom is available, and treatment is supportive and symptomatic. All patients with systemic features should be investigated for evidence of envenomation, including renal function, CK, urinalysis, and investigations for hemolysis (full blood count and reticulocyte count). Patients with a history of 20 or more stings, or children with 5 or more stings, should be observed until renal function is assessed.

In severe cases patients need admission to intensive care, with careful monitoring of renal function and fluid status and attention to hematologic abnormalities. Hemodialysis is usually indicated in severe envenomation, and blood component therapy may be required in patients with symptomatic or severe anemia. These individuals may require days to weeks of dialysis, and in some cases they may remain dialysis dependent (5).

ANTS (FORMICIDAE)

More than 10,000 species of ants have been described. Only a few groups of ants are medically significant, although a large number can cause painful stings (1). In Australia, the most medically significant ants are jack jumper and bull ants (*Myrmecia* spp.). They cause a significant number of allergic reactions in southern Australia but are rarely fatal (3,6,31). Other important species include the fire ants (*Solenopsis* spp.), which cause significant problems in North America, and *Rhytidoponera metallica* (green-head ants), which occur in Australia, New Guinea, New Caledonia, and adjacent regions (1). Other less medically important groups include *Odontomachus*, *Cerapachys*, and *Brachyponera* spp. (32). Most species of ants grab onto the skin with their jaws and either sting or spray venom, which causes local pain, itchiness, swelling, and erythema.

Bull Ants and Jumper Ants

Almost 90 described species of bull ants belong to the genus *Myrmecia*, but all except 1 are found only in Australia (33). *M. pilosula*, or the jumper ant (jack jumper), is a common cause of allergic reactions in southern Australia, including Victoria, South Australia, southern New South Wales, and Tasmania (6,34). In Tasmania, it is the single most common reason for patients with allergic reactions (Mueller grades I to IV) to present to an emergency department of one major hospital (3,6). Peptide allergens that are thought to account for most *M. pilosula* immunoglobulin E (IgE)-specific reactions have been identified and cloned (Myr p I, II, and III) (6). A randomized controlled trial has demonstrated that venom immunotherapy is highly effective in preventing severe systemic allergic reactions (13). Local reactions may include intense sharp pain, swelling, and severe itching. Pharmacologic studies suggest that jumper ant venom contains histamine, can stimulate release of cyclooxygenase products, and includes a hemolytic heat-labile factor (35).

Fire Ants

Solenopsis spp. occur in many parts of the world and are a significant medical problem in the United States. A survey of physicians in South Carolina reported 4975 cases of red imported fire ant bites that received medical care in 1990, although only 1% were admitted to the hospital (36) and only one death occurred. The rate of anaphylaxis reported in this study was 2.1% (36). *Solenopsis* spp. have been introduced into other parts of the world and are now established in southern Queensland in Australia (37), with a report of a case of anaphylaxis (32).

S. invicta originated in South America; are native to Brazil, Paraguay, Uruguay, and Argentina; and spread to Alabama in the 1930s, now infesting 12 southern states in the United States (37). Red imported fire ants are inconspicuous, red to brown ants that are difficult to distinguish from other common ant species (32). They are small ants (2 to 6 mm) that occur in grassed areas, gardens, and sites near flowing and still water. Their nests are subterranean but are characterized by an above-ground, dome-shaped mound, which is usually 20 to 30 cm above ground. They are ferocious invading ants and attack in large numbers from a nest (32,37).

Bites by fire ants differ from those of many other ants. Fire ants grab the skin with powerful jaws and then sting in a circle around the bite. Stings from multiple ants are common. Initially, severe local pain and raised wheals occur at the bite site; they resolve within an hour but evolve into sterile pustules over a period of 24 hours. These lesions heal over a week or more and should not be scratched. An enzyme-linked immunosorbent assay has been developed for in vitro measurement of IgE specific for *S. invicta* venom (38). The management of allergic reactions is similar to that of other Hymenoptera, and the role of venom immunotherapy is considered in the section Venom Immunotherapy.

CHILOPODA (CENTIPEDES)

The class Chilopoda or centipedes is widely distributed (39,40). They are nocturnal animals that prefer dark and moist places. A centipede is a multisegmented arthropod, varying in length from 3 to 250 mm with one pair of legs per body segment and one pair of antennae (39–42). The venom apparatus of most centipedes consists of a pair of poison claws, which are the first pair of legs that have been modified into biting appendages (39). The class Chilopoda includes more than 3000 species, which are grouped into four orders: Scolopendromorpha (tropical or giant centipedes), Scutigeromorpha (house or feather centipedes), Geophilomorpha (soil centipedes), and Lithiobiomorpha (rock or garden centipedes) (39,43). The most medically significant centipedes are *Scolopendra* spp. (39,43–47). The venoms of *Scolopendra* spp. are also the most researched (48–50). Only minor effects have been reported from centipedes of the orders Scutigeromorpha and Lithiobiomorpha (39).

Few large series of centipede bites have been reported. Contrary to case reports of severe effects, these series show that most centipede bites cause only minor effects (51–53). Although centipedes were not always identified, it is likely that they were caused by centipedes from the order Scolopendromorpha. Overall, centipede bites resulted in local pain that ranged in severity from mild to severe, associated with erythema and edema. Less common effects were local itchiness, radiating pain, headache, and nausea (51–53). In the majority of cases, the effects resolved within 24 hours. The vast majority of bites occurred on distal limbs (51,52). Although the venom of *S. morsitans* has been reported to be necrotic (54), clinical reports of such are rare (43,47).

Only two deaths can be reasonably attributed to centipede bites. The first was a 7-year-old child who was bitten on the head, although this is a report from early last century (55). The other case was a 21-year-old Thai woman who died from cardiovascular collapse and acute respiratory distress syndrome (56). She had been bitten by centipedes three times in the previous 9 months and had only had local urticarial reactions. On this presentation she had chest discomfort, and hypotension and tachypnea with a generalized urticarial rash. Despite treatment with epinephrine and dexamethasone, she remained hypotensive and pulmonary edema developed. She improved with ventilation and diuretics initially, but 20 hours after admission hypoxia and bilateral pulmonary infiltrates consistent with acute respiratory distress syndrome developed and she died from respiratory failure (56). These effects were probably due to an allergic reaction. Severe effects have been attributed to centipedes, including rhabdomyolysis (47) and Wells' syndrome (57), but in neither case was the centipede collected and expertly identified.

Some evidence has been shown that centipede bites can result in hypersensitivity phenomena. A number of reports have been published of recurrences of effects at the bite site. A man developed acute pain and swelling on two occasions after bites by *S. subspinipes*. Recurrent itching, pain, and swelling developed almost a month later at the bite site (43). Similar effects were reported earlier by Haneveld (58) in which recurrence of pain and swelling developed in 7 of 12 patients from Dutch New Guinea.

Scolopendra Species (Scolopendromorpha)

Scolopendra spp. are the largest centipedes, with some species such as *S. heros* achieving lengths of more than 20 cm (43). They are the most dangerous centipedes worldwide and are credited with at least two deaths (55,56). They are distributed widely, including throughout the Americas, Asia, Australia, and Africa (39). Considerable work has been done on venoms from *Scolopendra* spp. The presence of serotonin and histamine were initially demonstrated (48,59,60). Other toxin components with cardiac and muscarinic effects have been identified (48,50).

The clinical effects of *Scolopendra* are incompletely defined, with only a few case reports and series with definite bites identified by an expert (43–46,51). Bush et al. (43) report a number of bites by *Scolopendra* spp., although four of these occurred in one entomologist. Two bites were by *S. subspinipes,* which causes severe local and radiating pain and significant swelling of the bitten area and the hand. Mild systemic features occurred. The other two bites were by *S. heros* (giant desert centipede) and caused less pain and swelling. After the two bites by *S. subspinipes*, recurrent itchiness and swelling developed at the bite site. The *S. subspinipes* were large centipedes, with the most severe effects occurring with a bite from a 20-cm specimen (43). This suggests that the severity of the effects may be related more to the size of the animal than to the species. The other bite reported by Bush et al. involved a 7-cm *Scolopendra* specimen that caused local pain. The pain resolved within 2 days but required parenteral analgesia in the emergency department. Telephone follow-up revealed that a 3-cm necrotic area developed that sloughed and healed spontaneously (43).

Five definite bites by *Scolopendra* spp. in Brazil caused minor effects (51). A bite by *S. gigantea* in a neonate has been reported from Venezuela. It caused severe pain and extensive erythema and edema at the bite site (45). The child was irritable and inconsolable, but this is likely due to the effects of pain and swelling. The effects diminished within 10 hours and resolved within 72 hours (45). A bite by a *Scolopendra* spp. in Israel caused similar effects, with severe local pain at the bite site (neck) associated with swelling and erythema. Five bites from Japan are consistent with other cases, although in only one case was the centipede identified as *S. subspinipes*. In this case, the patient had severe pain, edema, and redness of the bitten thumb (46). In a prospective Australian study, three of five patients bitten by *Scolopendra* spp. (unpublished data) had severe pain but minimal local swelling and redness. Southcott (40) has also reported two *Scolopendra* bites that caused minor local effects.

Two other cases without definite identifications have caused more severe effects. A 46-year-old woman was bitten on the right foot by a large centipede (14 to 16 cm) that she identified from a photograph as *S. heros* (47). She initially had pain, swelling, numbness, and discoloration of the foot, but over a period of 3 days the whole leg became swollen and tender. She had associated systemic features, with nausea, fever, shortness of breath, and presyncope. She was admitted to the hospital 5 days after the bite with a grossly swollen leg, a small necrotic area at the bite site, acute renal failure, and rhabdomyolysis. Fasciotomies of the leg were required because of increased compartmental pressures. Her renal function improved, but she did not have complete recovery of motor function (47). One report has been published of Wells' syndrome after the bite of an unidentified centipede that resulted in local induration and blistering of the hand (57).

Other Scolopendromorphs

A number of other Scolopendromorphan genera have been reported, including *Otostigmus*, *Cryptops*, *Ethmostigmus*, and *Cormocephalus*. In the Brazilian study of 216 centipede bites, of the 136 with identified centipedes, 79 were by *Cryptops* and 45 by *Otostigmus*. Both of these genera include centipedes under 5 cm, demonstrating that smaller species can cause minor effects. Insufficient details are provided to determine specific effects of these genera.

In an Australian study, there were three bites by the large centipede *Ethmostigmus rubripes*. It caused severe pain and local swelling in all cases, with redness and radiating pain in two cases (unpublished data). This was consistent with the one previous report of a bite by this centipede (61). *E. rubripes* can reach a length of 15 cm, similar to *Scolopendra*. Thus, the size and clinical effects of *E. rubripes* suggest that they are of similar medical significance to *Scolopendra* spp. The venom of *E. rubripes* is toxic to mammals and insects, although the components responsible for toxicity in mammals have not been identified (62). In the same Australian study, there were seven bites by *Cormocephalus* spp., which caused very minor effects, with severe pain in only one case.

Centipedes from Other Orders

Only one detailed report has been published of a bite from the other orders. This is an unusual report of a bite by *Lithobius forficatus*, a common centipede in Britain (63). In this case the centipede appeared to have crawled into the space between the patient's tooth and gum and had bitten the mucosa. This caused mandibular pain, redness, and edema of the gums. The centipede was not found until after the tooth had been extracted (63).

Ingestion and Contact with Centipedes

A 6-month-old Australian child apparently ingested a centipede identified as *Scutigera morpha*. He became pale and lethargic with a marked generalized hypotonia. Reflexes and tests of sensation were normal. He vomited a few times and slowly improved over 48 hours with no specific treatment (64). However, no effects were observed in a more recent report of three cases of ingestion of Scolopendran centipedes (64a). One case has been reported of delayed itchiness, erythema, and the presence of "spines" at the site after contact with a centipede, *C. aurantiipes*. Previous reports have been published of wheal formation after skin contact with the legs of centipedes (65).

Treatment

No antidotes or specific treatment are available for centipede bites. In most cases, the effects are minor and require only symptomatic treatment. The bite site should be cleaned and tetanus prophylaxis provided. The application of ice has been recommended for arthropod bites, but there is some anecdotal evidence that the local application of heat (43) or hot-water immersion may be beneficial (unpublished data) for the pain. Some centipede venoms have been shown to be completely inactivated by heat (62). With more severe pain, either local infiltration with anesthetic or regional anesthesia may be appropriate. Analgesia may also be appropriate.

DIPLOPODA (MILLIPEDES)

The millipedes are a small group that rarely cause injuries to humans. They are slow moving and do not bite aggressively, and their chemical secretions are rarely a hazard to humans (66). They have a long cylindrical body with two pairs of feet attached to each segment (66,67). A few giant species occur in Java and Papua New Guinea that may reach lengths up to 20 cm (66,68). Encounters with millipedes are rare because of the secretive nature of these nocturnal animals.

Although millipedes can produce a broad range of defensive chemical secretions, only a few produce secretions that are more than minor irritants (69). The majority of these are the giant millipedes in tropical regions of the world (66). In addition to producing irritant secretions, giant millipedes are able to spray caustic substances from paired repugnatorial glands found on most body segments (68). They are able to spray up to 80 cm and are able to reach the human eye.

The defensive secretions of giant millipedes contain quinonoids and parabenzoquinones (68,70). The quinonoid secretions appear to cause minor effects when they contact skin, including pain, itching, and local skin eruptions (66). In more severe cases, the skin blisters and peels but usually heals without scarring. Giant millipedes occur in Africa (Nigeria, Tanzania), Papua New Guinea, Irian Jaya, and the Caribbean (including Mexico and Panama). The indigenous cultures of these regions report that spraying of the secretions in the eye causes blindness, although this is not supported by the few reports in the literature (68,69). Despite the relative commonness of some giant millipedes, there are very few reports of skin and eye contact reactions (68,69). Table 2 lists the millipedes that have caused injuries to humans, but many of these are minor skin reactions.

Polyconoceras spp. occur in Papua New Guinea and are nocturnal vegetarian scavengers that can be found in shady areas in daylight (68). In a retrospective series of eight cases, all patients were children (9 months to 7 years), except for one 25-year-old. Clinical effects included a "burn" of the periorbital skin in all eight cases, marked periorbital edema in three cases, conjunctivitis in two cases, and keratitis in one case (68). No cases of blindness were present, and all patients recovered fully with standard topical ophthalmic therapy. Although blindness may occur in situations in which the patient receives no health care, this is unlikely in those who receive appropriate early treatment. Three other injuries have been reported from *Polyconoceras* spp., and in only one case was a small corneal ulcer present (67,69).

TABLE 2. Species of millipedes identified to cause injuries to humans

Species	Country
Rhinocricus lethifer and *R. latespagor*	Haiti
Polyconoceras (Rhinocricidae)	Papua New Guinea
Spirostreptus spp. and *Iulus* spp.	Indonesia
Spirobolus spp.	Tanzania, Nigeria
Orthoporus spp.	Mexico
Tylobolus spp.	United States

Modified from Radford AJ. Millipede burns in man. *Trop Geogr Med* 1975;27:279–287, with additional cases (68,73).

Injuries by other species are less well documented. The millipede *Rhinocridum lethifer* caused severe burning eye pain and persistent periorbital swelling. The pain settled over a few hours, but the swelling took longer to resolve. The surrounding skin had a brown discoloration and blistered, although the skin eventually peeled off and left no scarring (71,72). An 8-year-old child presented with a "black" toe but no other symptoms after removing his foot from his shoe. He had no other problems, and the discoloration gradually faded over weeks. A millipede identified as *Tylobolus* spp. was found in the shoe (73). The red-legged millipede *Metiche tanganyicense* of Kenya has been reported to cause tanning of the skin on contact and can be irritating to mucous membranes (70).

Clinical Effects

The main effect is skin discoloration, which varies depending on the type of millipede. More significant injuries occur when giant millipedes squirt secretions in the eye. This is characterized by initial severe and burning pain. The surrounding skin is usually discolored (tanning) and may blister. This reaction is normally referred to as a *burn* and in more severe cases may cause skin sloughing. A chemical conjunctivitis can occur (68). Periorbital swelling occurs in most cases, peaking after 2 days and lasting for up to 7 days. Conjunctivitis takes up to a week to resolve. All effects resolved, although a slight depigmentation may remain (68).

Treatment

Treatment is similar to that for any chemical burn of the eye and includes irrigation of the eye and periorbital region with water or normal saline, if available. The eye should be carefully inspected for corneal injury with fluorescein eye drops. A topical antibiotic/corticosteroid eye ointment should then be applied (68). Although some authors have recommended eye patching and local anesthetic (69), the periorbital edema usually keeps the eye closed (68).

TICKS (ARACHNIDA: ACARI: MEOSTIGMATA)

Ticks are medically important arthropods. They are vectors for some important infectious diseases, including Lyme disease. A few species are able to cause an envenomation syndrome in humans, which is characterized by paralysis (74). However, tick paralysis is rare and other effects are far more common, including local irritation with or without systemic effects and local or systemic allergic reactions (74–76). Tick paralysis occurs in most parts of the world but is most commonly reported in North America (77) and Australia. The diagnosis of tick paralysis is often mistaken for other neurologic illnesses (77). Fatalities have occurred in Australia and Canada (74).

Ticks belong to the order Acari (class Arachnida). The suborder Ixodida includes three families: Ixoididae (hard ticks), Argasidae (soft ticks), and Nutalliellidae (78). More than 60 of the 820 tick species have been implicated in causing paralysis; the majority of these are hard ticks. The most important species of ticks in veterinary and human medicine are *Dermacentor andersoni* and *D. variabilis* from North America; *Ixodes rubicundus, Rhipicephalus evertsi evertsi*, and *Argas (Pericargas) walkerae* of Africa; and *I. holocyclus* from Australia (78) (Table 3).

Dermacentor andersoni is the most important tick in humans in North America, with cases reported from western Canada, predominantly from southern British Columbia. *D. andersoni* also occurs throughout the western states of the United States, but cases of human paralysis are confined to the northwestern Rocky mountain states (Washington, Montana, Idaho, and Oregon) (77). Between 1900 and 1968, 305 cases of tick paralysis were reported in British Columbia, the majority occurring in the first 27 years. The case-fatality rate was approximately 10%, which is likely to be far greater than in recent years. *D. variabilis*, the dog tick, occurs in the central and eastern United States (i.e., excluding where *D. andersoni* occurs), but the 40 reported cases of tick paralysis due to *D. variabilis* occurred in southern and eastern United States, and not Canada (77). Few other ticks have been reported to cause human paralysis: *Amblyomma maculatum* and *A. americanum* (77).

TABLE 3. Ticks that cause local and generalized paralysis of medical or veterinary importance

Ixodidae	Region
Dermacentor andersoni	Western United States and Canada (British Columbia)
D. variabilis	Central and Eastern United States
Ixodes holocyclus	Eastern Australia
I. cornuatus	Tasmania (Australia) (79)
I. tancitarius	Mexico
I. rubicundus	Africa
Rhipicephalus simus	South Africa, Somalia
R. evertsi evertsi	Africa

Ixodes holocyclus occurs along the eastern coast of Australia and is responsible for significant medical effects in humans. More than 20 species are present in Australia, but envenomation has only been reported with *I. holocyclus*, except for a single case by *I. cornuatus* in Tasmania (79). Twenty deaths from tick paralysis were reported in Australia before 1945, the majority in children under 3 years of age (75), which is more than for either the red back spider or the Australia funnel web spider (80). No further deaths have occurred since the introduction of advanced life support techniques and intensive care units (74). Approximately one to five severe envenomations occur in Eastern Australia each year in children.

Toxins

It has been demonstrated that tick saliva contains the neurotoxins that are responsible for paralysis (78). The salivary secretions from *D. andersoni* cause neuromuscular paralysis due to a presynaptic effect of the toxins (77). Studies with *I. holocyclus* venom demonstrate that paralysis from this species results from the inhibition of acetylcholine release at the neuromuscular junction (81,82), possibly similar to *D. andersoni*. This study also demonstrated that low temperatures prevent the effects of the venom/paralysis (81). It has been suggested that there are centrally acting neurotoxins in tick saliva because of the early ataxia that develops in Australian tick paralysis and that reflexes have been abolished in animal studies, with only minor effects on neuromuscular transmission.

Numerous attempts have been made to isolate the neurotoxins from *D. andersoni* and *I. holocyclus* (77,78). Studies of *I. holocyclus* venom have concluded that the neurotoxin is proteinaceous in nature with a molecular weight of 40 to 80 kd (78). Similar toxins have been reported from *R. evertsi evertsi* and *A. walkerae*, which also cause an ascending flaccid paralysis, although it is suggested that this results from abnormalities in nerve conduction rather than presynaptic involvement (78). Studies have isolated neurotoxins that have been termed *holocyclotoxins* (HT-1, HT-2, and HT-3). These neurotoxins of approximately 5 kd are similar to peptide neurotoxins from spiders and scorpions (78).

Clinical Presentation

The first signs of tick paralysis usually occur 4 to 5 days after attachment of the tick. They may continue to worsen for up to 48 hours after the tick is removed. In the majority of cases in children, there is a generalized lower motor neuron paralysis. The first effects are usually in the lower limbs, with initial ataxia and then weakness of the legs. This may be preceded by paresthesiae of the legs. Some children may initially present with ataxia, and tick paralysis is an important differential diagnosis in children who present with ataxia. Weakness ascends to involve the upper limbs, neck, and trunk muscles. The facial and bulbar muscles may also be affected and cause ptosis, squint, extraocular muscular paralysis, dysarthria, cough, and stridor. In severe cases respiratory muscle paralysis and death occur unless there is intervention (74,75,83).

In some cases, there may be local paralysis, which is most commonly of the facial nerve (80,83,84), but paralysis of the frontalis and orbicularis oculi muscles alone has been reported (84). A delayed facial nerve palsy occurred a day after 44 engorged ticks were removed from an adult male (80).

Allergic reactions to Australian ticks are well reported (75,83–85) and have been classified based on skin prick testing and radioimmunoassay testing (76). Allergic reactions to other tick species are less well reported. Gauci et al. (76) divided their series of 42 patients into various tick bite reactions, including local effects (small and large), allergic/anaphylactic effects, and atypical effects. A modified classification with clinical descriptions is included in Table 4. They demonstrated that all of the allergic/anaphylactic and atypical reactions were IgE mediated and 73% of the large reactions were associated with IgE specific for tick allergens. However, only 12.5% of the small reactions were associated with tick allergens. In addition, a heavy tick exposure (more than 10 ticks) or atopic status was significantly associated with tick allergy. This study suggests that ticks can cause a range of allergic reactions, from large local reactions to severe systemic allergy, that appear to be type I hypersensitivity reactions, as well as atypical hypersensitivity reactions (76).

TABLE 4. Summary of tick bite reactions based on effects of *Ixodes holocyclus*, the Australian paralysis tick; not including paralytic effects

Tick bite reaction	Clinical syndrome/features
Small local	Painful, pruritic, erythematous, and papular lesion at the bite site lasting minutes to hours that may persist for up to 3 days. An itchy spot at the site may last for several weeks.
Large local	Painful, erythematous lesion (minutes to hours) generally >50 mm diameter and persisting for 1 wk or more. Swelling and erythema contiguous with bite site, and the pain and inflammation may be severe.
Allergic/anaphylactic	Mild: urticaria, erythema, and pruritus distant from the bite site. Severe: generalized urticaria, angioedema, laryngeal edema, bronchospasm (wheeze, cough, dyspnea), hypotension, collapse, and loss of consciousness within 1 hr of tick bite (usually soon after tick removal).
Atypical	Large local reaction in combination with headache, nausea, lethargy, and arthralgia 12–24 h after removal of tick, persisting for 1 wk or more.

Modified from Gauci M, Loh RK, Stone BF, et al. Australian reactions to the Australian paralysis tick, *Ixodes holocyclus*: diagnostic evaluation by skin test and radioimmuoassay. *Clin Exp Allergy* 1989;19:279–283.

COLEOPTERA

The beetles (Coleoptera) represent the greatest number of species, with approximately 300,000 species worldwide (86). Occasionally, beetles cause injury to humans, resulting from (a) a bite or the beetle lodging in a body cavity (e.g., external auditory canal), (b) the effects of toxic secretions, or (c) irritation from the effects of hairs of larvae (86). Arguably, the most serious effects result from contact with vesicating beetles. A number of beetle families are well known for causing blistering to human skin after contact, including the Meloidae, Oedemeridae, and Staphylinidae. When threatened, bombardier beetles (family Carabidae) are able to emit a defensive spray of heated benzoquinones from the tip of the abdomen (87). This may cause initial burning pain and a throbbing ache for several hours associated with a yellow-brown discoloration (88).

Meloidae

The Meloidid beetles have been known from ancient times to cause blistering reactions and produce a defensive agent called *cantharidin* (89). This is commonly known as *Spanish fly* and is obtained from the beetle *Lytta vesicatoria* that occurs in the Mediterranean region (86). Other species in the family occur throughout Asia, North America, and Australia. Cantharidin was used widely in medicine in the past but has largely been abandoned (86). Recent interest has been shown in cantharidin as a chemotherapeutic agent because it is an inhibitor of protein phosphatases 1 and 2A, which have key roles in cell cycle progression (90). Ingestion of *Mylabris dicincta* beetles in Zimbabwe by a 4-year-old girl caused hematuria and abdominal pain (91).

Oedemeridae

Beetles of the family Oedemeridae, or false blister beetles, are the smallest and least known of the vesicating beetles, although they may be more common than realized (86,92). Most cases have come from the Pacific and Caribbean regions. *Ananca* spp. has been reported to cause blistering and rashes in New Guinea and the Solomon Islands (86,93). *Thelyphassa lineata* was reported to cause a blistering dermatosis (tense unilocular lesions with clear fluid and minimal surrounding erythema) in 74 members of the New Zealand Army (94). A blistering reaction from Hawaii was caused by *T. apicata* (95). *Oxacis* and *Oxycopis* spp. from the Caribbean and Central America have caused dermatitis and vesicular lesions (96).

Genus *Paederus* (Staphylinidae)

Beetles of the genus *Paederus* (whiplash rove beetles) occur on many continents, including South America, Asia, Africa, Europe, and Australia (97–101). Paederus beetles are small, elongated beetles (5 to 10 mm) that favor swamps and stream banks. They are attracted to light, and large numbers often appear after heavy rainfall (86,101). Contact with these beetles causes pain, erythema, and vesicle formation; however, this only occurs if the beetle is crushed or damaged because the injury is caused by a toxic alkaloid pederin that is in the hemolymph of the beetle (86,98).

Pederin is one of the most complex insect toxins (89). The major difference to other families of vesicating beetles is that the lesions take 12 to 96 hours to develop, rather than 2 to 3 hours after cantharidin contact (98). Blistering and pain resolve over 7 days, and the area slowly heals over a period of weeks (98). An epidemic of 40 cases due to *P. australis* has been reported from northern Australia (101). Four patients required inpatient admission (101). Similar cases have been reported in most parts of the world. Millard suggested that immediate washing of the area with soapy water or a fat solvent after exposure may reduce the effects; however, most patients are not aware of the contact at the time because it is relatively painless (98). Preventative measures are needed in regions where there are large numbers of beetles and beetles should not be squashed against the skin (101).

Tenebrionidae

The family Tenebrionidae includes a large number of beetles that have defensive secretions. More than 100 species have been investigated, and the majority contain quinonoid compounds (89). Some species, such as *Blaps* spp., whose defensive secretions contain quinines, are known to cause blistering reactions (86).

HEMIPTERA (TRUE BUGS)

The Hemiptera are a large group of insects with more than 55,000 species. Although few cause human injuries, they are well-known as serious plant pests, vectors of plant viruses, and vectors of disease in humans and animals (102). Many bugs are able to cause painful bites, including plant-feeding bugs (Miridae and Lygaeidae) and many water bugs: backswimmers (Notonectidae), water scorpions (Nepidae), and fishkillers (Belostomatidae) (1).

Reduviidae (Assassin Bugs)

The family Reduviidae are predatory arthropods that do not feed on vertebrate blood (non–blood sucking). One important subfamily, Triatominae, feeds on vertebrate blood and includes the vectors of South American trypanosomiasis (103). A number of reduviids have been reported to cause effects in humans. In most cases there is moderate to severe pain at the bite site, which is followed by local swelling and wheal formation (1,103). In some cases there is persistent dull pain or urticaria, or both. No major effects have been reported.

Cimicidae (Bed Bugs)

Bed bugs such as *Cimex* spp. are pests and can cause urticaria. The insects deposit a drop of liquid on the skin when they bite, which causes local and distant urticaria (1,89).

LEPIDOPTERA

The Lepidoptera are the order of insects that include moths and butterflies, of which caterpillars are the larvae. *Lepidopterism* refers to injuries from insects belonging to the order Lepidoptera. The larvae of butterflies (Rhopalocera) very rarely have stinging hairs, except for a few species of Nymphalidae—species of *Vanessa* and *Euvanessa* of North America and Europe, which only cause mild urticaria (93). Thus, the majority of important cases of lepidopterism are due to the larvae of members of the suborder Heterocera (moths) (93,104,105).

Clinical Presentation

Lepidopterism includes contact, penetration, inhalation, and ingestion of any part or structure of a lepidopteran, from any stage in its life cycle (104). By far the most common injury or reaction is skin or eye contact with the hairs or spines of caterpillars, the larval stage of the Lepidoptera (104). The hairs can also be woven into the cocoons by some species, and in these cases the cocoon may be responsible for skin irritation or urticaria (106). Occasionally, the effects of the various stages of larvae on humans are referred to as *erucism* rather than *lepidopterism*, which is then reserved for the effects of adult moths and butterflies.

Lepidopterism is historically classified into two major types of reactions/injuries: stinging and urticarial reactions (104,107–109). Stinging caterpillars tend to have hollow spines that contain and inject venom when skin contact occurs. The effects include burning, severe pain and, less commonly, systemic effects (108,110–113). The second type of reaction results from exposure to "itchy" caterpillars, which have nonvenomous hairs that produce mechanical irritation (105), dermatitis (109,114,115), or foreign body reactions on contact (105). Numerous caterpillars cause intermediate or mixed effects in which such a simple classification is unhelpful (93,104,107). In most cases, it is best simply to describe the effects of different caterpillars. One study of skin irritations from caterpillars in the United States, including a number of families of irritant caterpillars, demonstrated that early and delayed reactions occur and that the severity is dependent on the sensitivity of the individual and is usually worse in atopic individuals (116). A more recent study with *Euproctis* spp. supports this and suggests that the early reactions are likely to be due to mechanical, toxic, and allergic reactions and the delayed reactions are allergic in origin (117).

Because caterpillar species cause wide-ranging clinical effects, local knowledge of the lepidopteran fauna is important in treating lepidopterism. Only a few appear to cause major problems (105), including *Euproctis*, *Thaumatopoea*, *Hylesia*, *Automeris*, *Lonomia*, *Megalopyge*, *Lonomia*, and *Latoia*. Some groups are confined to a small region and therefore cause considerable problems locally or occasionally epidemics despite the rarity of reports (109,118). In some cases it is apparent that the effects are mainly toxic, such as stinging caterpillars—*Megalopyge*, *Lonomia*, *Doratifera*, and *Hylesia*—and in other cases the mechanism is likely to be allergic, such as with the classic urticating caterpillars—*Euproctis*, *Lymantria*, and *Thaumatopoea*.

Euproctis Species (Lymantriidae)

Euproctis spp. are well known for causing epidemics of itchy reactions or dermatitis (104,109,114,119–124). The genus includes species throughout Europe, Asia, and Australia. The clinical effects are similar for different species, although some components of the spicule venoms differ slightly (125). In many cases the person does not recall contact and the diagnosis is based on the presence of caterpillar in the proximity of the person or circumstantial evidence. Because the hairs or spicules of *Euproctis* spp. are able to detach from the caterpillar, not only can the dermatitis result from contact with the caterpillar, but also from contact with airborne hairs (109).

The mechanism of dermatitis is not fully characterized. In the past it has been suggested that there is a mechanical reaction to the spicules (similar to fiberglass) and chemical irritation resulting from the venom contained in the spicules (114,126). de Jong et al. (126) investigated the effects of cutaneous application of spicules from *E. chrysorrhoea* in humans. Untreated hairs caused early skin reactions characterized by erythematous and wheal-like papules. Heat treatment (to denature proteinaceous toxins) and saline extraction only reduced the skin-irritating properties, suggesting that mechanical trauma and a toxic injury caused the clinical effects. A study in human volunteers demonstrated that immediate and delayed-type reactions occur with cutaneous application of *E. pseudoconspersa*, with some people having no response, some having delayed responses only, and some having immediate and delayed reactions (117). In addition they identified a venom fraction that caused similar reactions to the crude venom. This fraction did not contain histamine but did contain a large-molecular-weight (20 to 40 kd) substance. The authors suggest that in addition to mechanical injury from the spicule and chemical injury from venom components, an immediate and delayed-type allergic reaction contributed to the dermatitis (117).

The clinical effects of *Euproctis* spp. are similar, but there is large variability in individual human responses. This may be due to varying sensitivity to the allergens in the venom. *Euproctis* spp. contact results in a dermatitis that is characterized by a papulourticarial rash, usually on the exposed skin, or may be more extensive if clothing is contaminated with hairs. The lesions are usually 3 to 5 mm in size and may be papules or, less commonly, vesicles or pustules (119). The rash can develop immediately or, more commonly, hours to days after contact, making the diagnosis difficult. The rash usually lasts approximately 3 days, but in severe cases excoriation and secondary infection may be present (120). Contact with the eyes can result in conjunctivitis and in severe cases can produce ophthalmia nodosa. Rarely, some patients experience rhinitis, which is likely a result of inhalation of the caterpillar hairs. Many patients present with dermatitis of unknown cause, and a thorough history is required to determine the source. Diagnosis can be confirmed by sticky tape testing. This involves applying sticky tape to the rash and then putting the sticky tape on a microscope slide and looking for caterpillar hairs under low-power microscopy (109,127).

Treatment is usually symptomatic but must include removal of the source of exposure. In addition removal of the hairs by sticky tape application (which may also be diagnostic) is important. Topical aspirin paste appeared to be beneficial in one patient in a study, and topical lidocaine and oral antihistamines may provide some relief (109).

Thaumatopoea Species (Thaumatopoeidae)

Thaumatopoea spp. include a number of processionary caterpillars that occur across Europe and Africa. The term *processionary* refers to their habit of proceeding head to tail. A number of *Thaumatopoea* spp., including the oak processionary caterpillars (*T. processionea*), pine processionary caterpillars (*T. pityocampa* and *T. wilkinsoni*), and *T. jordana*, have been reported to cause painful and itchy rashes (128,129). The larva of *Thaumatopoea* spp. are densely covered in urticating hairs or spicules that are continuously shed and become airborne (128). Reactions to these caterpillars are usually due to airborne hairs, making the diagnosis difficult. A 28-kd protein thaumatopoein isolated from *T. wilkinsoni* causes the identical cutaneous reaction as the hair extract (130). Further research also demonstrated that the urticating hairs of *Thaumatopoea* caterpillars may be an important cause of airborne insect allergy, because 4 of 21 pine forest workers had a positive enzyme-linked immunosorbent assay directed against pine processionary extract (131). In addition, there was a reaction to a larger-molecular-weight substance in addition to thaumatopoein (131).

The clinical effects of *Thaumatopoea* larval hair contact are similar to those of other urticating caterpillars, with itchy erythema and papular rashes in exposed areas of skin. The effects are often severe enough to prevent sleep but usually resolve over 24 to 48 hours. Epidemics are common, and a number of outbreaks in military personnel have been reported (128,129). The onset of effects is approximately 2 hours after exposure, although this is difficult to determine because of the airborne nature of the caterpillar hairs (128). Treatment is symptomatic, and prevention of further cases is more important. Once a source is identified and destroyed, the number of cases decreases rapidly (128).

Lymantria dispar (Lymantriidae)

Lymantria dispar, or the gypsy moth caterpillar, occurs worldwide but has been mainly reported in epidemics in the United States (127,132,133). A massive infestation of this moth occurred in the northeastern part of the United States in 1981, and coincidentally thousands of cases of pruritic rashes were reported. Although the majority were not confirmed, it is likely that many of these rashes were due to contact with the gypsy moth caterpillar or its airborne hairs (127). The reactions involved an itchy papular rash that sometimes took hours to days to develop. The symptoms ranged from mild pruritic rashes to severe intense itch that prevented people from sleeping (127).

In volunteer closed-patch testing studies, the effects were similar to those reported in the epidemic: pruritic, erythematous, papular, and occasionally vesicular inflammation (133). In addition, these studies demonstrated that only sensitive individuals reacted to the caterpillar hairs (133,134). Another study showed that there was a much higher risk of developing a rash in high infestation areas (risk ratio 6.5) (132). Other associated risk factors for developing a rash included a previous rash or history of caterpillar exposure, hay fever, and hanging out the washing (airborne caterpillar hairs can get trapped in clothing and cause reactions when the clothing is worn) (132).

The effects of *Lymantria dispar* are similar to those of *Euproctis* spp., with mainly delayed hypersensitivity reactions that develop more commonly and are more severe in sensitive individuals (history of hay fever or atopy). Sticky tape testing may help confirm the diagnosis (127). Treatment is also problematic because topical treatments and oral antihistamines may not be effective. Systemic corticosteroids have been tried in more severe cases (133).

Lophocampa caryae

The hickory tussock caterpillar *L. caryae* occurs across most of the eastern United States and causes itchy reactions or dermatitis similar to *Euproctis* and *Lymantria*. In one large series of *L. caryae* exposures, erythema and itchiness occurred associated with caterpillar hairs in the skin that resolved within 24 hours (135). The clinical course and treatment are similar to those of urticating caterpillars, and the spines can be removed with sticky tape.

Hemileuca maia (Saturniidae)

The buck moth (*H. maia*) occurs in the United States and has been responsible for epidemics of caterpillar stings (118). A number of *Hemileuca* spp. from the family of giant silkworm moths (Saturniidae) occur in the United States (105), but most reports are from stings by *H. maia*, which occurs from Maine to Wisconsin and south to Florida, Louisiana, and Texas (111,118). Preliminary work on the venom extract of *H. maia* suggested that it did not contain histamine or serotonin and that the irritative properties may be due to a proteolytic enzyme (116). The clinical effects of stings by *H. maia* are characterized by an acute, painful papulovesicular dermatitis, associated with local bruising and edema (116,118). In a report of 19 cases, typical caterpillar reactions occurred in young males who trod on the caterpillar (118). They presented with a painful dermatitis on the plantar surface of the foot. Linear clusters of vesicles with surrounding bruising and edema usually occurred. The rash and swelling generally took 2 to 3 days to resolve. Some patients had tender lymphadenopathy, extensive swelling, and fever (118).

Lonomia Species (Saturniidae)

Lonomia caterpillars are the most medically important caterpillars in the world and occur throughout South America (110,136–140). *L. achelous* is found in the Amazon region in Venezuela and Northern Brazil, whereas *L. obliqua* occurs in southern Brazil and has reached epidemic proportions (139). In addition to severe local pain, envenomation by this caterpillar results in systemic effects, including renal failure, coagulopathy, and bleeding (110,138,139). Procoagulant activity has been identified in the hemolymph of both major *Lonomia* caterpillars. The crude hemolymph of *L. achelous* had two different prothrombin activator activities. It was able to activate prothrombin directly, independent of the prothrombinase complex, whereas the other activity was stimulated by factor V, calcium ions, and phospholipase (141). A crude extract from the bristles of *L. oblique* had procoagulant activity due to prothrombin and factor X activators (142). A serine protease prothrombin activator (Lopap) has been isolated from *L. obliqua* (142). Lopap generated thrombin from prothrombin and was able to clot purified human fibrinogen and plasma (143). In rats it also caused thrombocytopenia, inhibited platelet aggregation, and caused congestion and hemorrhage in renal glomeruli and necrosis in renal distal tubules (143).

A series of 105 cases of *L. obliqua* envenomation described the frequency of various clinical effects (139) (Table 5). Envenomation causes consumption of fibrinogen and coagulopathy, similar to some snake envenomation syndromes. Anuric renal failure has also been reported, requiring dialysis in many cases, and has a high mortality (136). In early series it was reported in up to 18% of cases (136). However, renal failure was not found in a more recent series, although this may be a result of antivenom treatment in most of the patients. The mechanism of renal damage remains unclear, although it is postulated that it may be a result of early fibrin deposition in the renal microcirculation. Evidence of fibrin deposition is likely to resolve within 48 hours and may not be identified on a renal biopsy. This could explain the relatively mild changes in renal histology out of proportion to the severe clinical picture (136). Intracerebral hemorrhage can also occur after *Lonomia* stings and has a high mortality (110,137). Coagulopathy, bleeding, acute renal failure, and premature labor developed in a 37-week pregnant woman. She delivered a slightly hypoxic baby, and then postpartum bleeding and hypotension developed. She had ongoing renal failure and slowly improved over weeks (138).

TABLE 5. Clinical and laboratory effects of *Lonomia obliqua* envenomation

Clinical or laboratory finding	Frequency (%)
Local pain	95
Headache	64
Nausea and vomiting	35
Local hyperemia	33
Dizziness	25
Hemorrhagic manifestations	23
Gingival mucosal hemorrhage	11
Ecchymosis	9
Bleeding from recent wounds	6
Epistaxis	4
Hematemesis	4
Hematuria	2
Fibrinogen	
Normal (>1.5 g/L)	16
0.51–1.50 g/L	14
<0.5 g/L	70
Renal failure	0

From Zannin M, Lourenco DM, Motta G, et al. Blood coagulation and fibrinolytic factors in 105 patients with hemorrhagic syndrome caused by accidental contact with *Lonomia obliqua* caterpillar in Santa Catarina, Southern Brazil. *Thromb Haemost* 2003;89:355–364, with permission.

An antivenom has been developed for *L. obliqua* and is now available in Brazil (144). The antivenom appears to be effective in reducing the coagulopathy and bleeding (145). The mainstay of therapy in *Lonomia* stings is now antivenom and supportive care. Delayed presentation may still result in acute renal failure or significant hemorrhage, which may require prolonged hospital care.

Megalopyge opercularis (Megalopygidae)

M. opercularis is arguably the most important stinging caterpillar in the United States. Most reports of stinging caterpillar envenomations involve this American puss caterpillar (111–113,146), the larva of the flannel moth (*M. opercularis*). *M. opercularis* is also known as the *woolly slug*, and in various regions of the United States and Mexico it is also known as the *tree asp*, *Italian asp*, *nasty worm*, *opossum bug*, *el perrito* (little dog), and *bicho peludo negro* (black hairy bug) (147). The species is confined to the southern United States and Mexico (147). Stings were first reported in 1913 in Texas, but a number of epidemics have been reported since that time (111–113,147).

Stings by *M. opercularis* cause severe local pain, erythema, and swelling. A characteristic "grid-like" mark is usually present at the sting site (112). Radiating pain occurs in about one-fourth of patients (112). Other local and regional features include paresthesiae, muscle spasms, numbness, arthralgia, myalgia, chest pain, and abdominal pain (111,112,148). Less commonly, systemic symptoms occur, including lymphadenopathy, headache, nausea, "shock-like" symptoms, and convulsions (112,113). Treatment is mainly supportive and symptomatic, and patients may require parenteral analgesia for severe and regional pain. Numerous topical treatments have been used, but there is no evidence that any of these is effective.

Doratifera Species and *Thosea penthima* (Limacodiae)

A number of stinging caterpillars in Australia belong to the family Limacodidae (cup moths). The most widespread and important group is from the genus *Doratifera*; it has four raised tubercles at each end of the body, and when the caterpillar is disturbed they erect a cluster of spines on the tubercles (93,149). Exposures to these caterpillars cause a reaction consisting of severe stinging, erythema, and wheal formation that resolves within 24 hours and is consistent with an acute toxic reaction rather than an allergic response (1,93,104,107,149). *T. penthima*, known as the *billygoat plum stinging caterpillar*, is another Australian limacodid that causes severe acute pain reactions and in one case caused radiating pain that required parenteral analgesia but resolved within 24 hours (108).

Chelepteryx collesi (Anthelidae)

The white-stemmed gum moth or *C. collesi* occurs in central eastern Australia, including Canberra and Sydney. These caterpillars are large and cylindrical, reaching lengths of 10 cm, with black, white, and reddish-brown markings (104). They are covered with tufts of short, dark stiff hairs (106,150). With pupation of the larva, these hairs are woven into the cocoon with the hairs protruding outward, making the cocoons just as important a cause of contact reactions. The hairs are easily able to penetrate human skin (104).

Exposure to the caterpillar or cocoon results in local, transient pain and the presence of multiple hairs at the site (104,151). Removal of the hairs is universally unsuccessful, with the majority breaking off and remaining embedded in the removal process. No adverse effects were associated with the presence of these spines, and in some cases, they may be present for up to 2 months (151). The spines have not been formally investigated, but they appear to cause very minor mechanical trauma that in most cases has been confirmed by repeated handling by numerous entomologists in Australia (93,104,149,150). In rare cases they are responsible for early acute allergic reactions (106), but in the only reported series there were no delayed hypersensitivity reactions in 13 definite and 13 probable cases (151).

Hylesia Species

Caripito itch is a pruritic dermatitis that is more common in Central and South America (152,153). It is caused by contact with the urticating abdominal hairs of the adult female moths of the genus *Hylesia* and persists for 7 to 14 days.

Ophthalmia Nodosa from Lepidopteran Hairs

Ophthalmia nodosa is defined as an ocular inflammatory reaction resulting from contact with arthropod hairs or vegetable material (105,154,155). The name is derived from the fact that the reaction is often characterized by a nodular conjunctivitis. Species of moths that cause ophthalmia nodosa include *Thaumatopoea* spp., *Euproctis* spp., and *Dendrolimus punctatus* (154,155). Caterpillar hairs may enter the eye from direct contact or may be blown into the eye. Initially, there is intense inflammation with periorbital edema and irritant/allergic dermatitis, and subsequent significant conjunctivitis may occur (154). Penetration of the cornea results in a localized or nummular keratitis, depending on the number of hairs involved. A latent asymptomatic period may occur. The hairs are able to migrate into the eye, and the free hairs cause intense inflammation in the anterior uvea. The reaction may be severe enough to produce a hypopyon and nodules on the iris or in the conjunctiva (154). The severity of the reaction is mainly determined by the number of hairs, and as many hairs as possible should be removed initially (154). Referral to an ophthalmologist is essential for ongoing management.

Caterpillar Ingestion

Only two case reports of caterpillar ingestion have been published, from Pittsburgh (156,157). In some cases, the description of the caterpillar was consistent with the hickory tussock moth or *L. caryae*. Cases ranged from swallowing caterpillars or parts thereof, oropharyngeal contact with the caterpillar, and contact with the cocoon. In the larger reported series of 26 children, all were symptomatic. The most common symptoms were dysphagia (88%), then local erythema (85%), pain (69%), edema (65%), drooling (58%), pruritus (58%), and shortness of breath (4%) (156). All patients recovered after 48 hours, and none had major sequelae. In all cases of caterpillar ingestion and some cases of oropharyngeal contact, the child underwent laryngoscopy and esophagoscopy (156). Hair removal was difficult and required magnification. Treatment should be symptomatic. The role of endoscopy is unclear because some children require no treatment and the hairs slowly extrude themselves.

OTHER ARTHROPODS

The order Phasmatodea includes the leaf-eating insects that resemble leaves or sticks. The majority are not harmful to humans. An important exception is the southern walking stick, or *Anisomorpha buprestoides*, which occurs in the United States (Texas). This insect has two venom-secreting glands and when agitated can discharge the venom at a desired target. In one report an 8-year-old boy was sprayed in the eye by a southern walking stick, and immediate pain and blurred vision developed (158). He had corneal and conjunctival epithelial defects that resolved over 6 days with no sequelae.

Neuroptera

The only reports of injuries from the order Neuroptera (lacewings) are from the larvae of Chrysopidae. Bites by these larvae cause minor effects, including a small puncture and stinging, with associated erythema, and in some cases induration and papule formation (159).

REFERENCES

1. Southcott RV. Some harmful Australian insects. *Med J Aust* 1988;149:656–662.
2. McGain F, Harrison J, Winkel KD. Wasp sting mortality in Australia. *Med J Aust* 2000;173:198–200.
3. Brown SG, Franks RW, Baldo BA, et al. Prevalence, severity, and natural history of jack jumper ant venom allergy in Tasmania. *J Allergy Clin Immunol* 2003;111:187–192.
4. Franca FO, Benvenuti LA, Fan HW, et al. Severe and fatal mass attacks by 'killer' bees (Africanized honey bees—*Apis mellifera scutellata*) in Brazil: clinicopathological studies with measurement of serum venom concentrations. *QJM* 1994;87:269–282.
5. Barss P. Renal failure and death after multiple stings in Papua New Guinea. Ecology, prevention and management of attacks by vespid wasps. *Med J Aust* 1989;151:659–663.
6. Brown SGA, Wu Q, Kelsall GR, et al. Fatal anaphylaxis following jack jumper ant sting in southern Tasmania. *Med J Aust* 2001;175:644–647.
7. Rhoades RB, Stafford CT, James FK Jr. Survey of fatal anaphylactic reactions to imported fire ant stings. Report of the Fire Ant Subcommittee of the American Academy of Allergy and Immunology. *J Allergy Clin Immunol* 1989;84:159–162.
8. Incorvaia C, Pucci S, Pastorello EA. Clinical aspects of Hymenoptera venom allergy. *Allergy* 1999;54[Suppl 58]:50–52.
9. Vetter RS, Visscher PK, Camazine S. Mass envenomations by honey bees and wasps. *West J Med* 1999;170:223–227.
10. Meier J. Biology and distribution of Hymenopterans of medical importance, their venom apparatus and venom composition. In: *Clinical toxicology of animal venoms and poisons*, 1st ed. Boca Raton, FL: CRC Press, 1995:331–348.
11. Hunt KJ, Valentine MD, Sobotka AK, et al. A controlled trial of immunotherapy in insect hypersensitivity. *N Engl J Med* 1978;299:157–161.
12. Muller U, Thurnheer U, Patrizzi R, et al. Immunotherapy in bee sting hypersensitivity. Bee venom versus wholebody extract. *Allergy* 1979;34:369–378.
13. Brown SG, Wiese MD, Blackman KE, et al. Ant venom immunotherapy: a double-blind, placebo-controlled, crossover trial. *Lancet* 2003;361:1001–1006.
14. Weiner JM, Baldo BA, Donovan GR, et al. Allergy to jumper ant (*Myrmecia pilosula*) stings in south-eastern Australia. *Ann Allergy Asthma Immunol* 1995;74:60.
15. Freeman TM, Hylander R, Ortiz A, et al. Imported fire ant immunotherapy: effectiveness of whole body extracts. *J Allergy Clin Immunol* 1992;90:210–215.
16. Tankersley MS, Walker RL, Butler WK, et al. Safety and efficacy of an imported fire ant rush immunotherapy protocol with and without prophylactic treatment. *J Allergy Clin Immunol* 2002;109:556–562.
17. Hoffman DR, Jacobson RS, Schmidt M, et al. Allergens in Hymenoptera venoms. XXIII. Venom content of imported fire ant whole body extracts. *Ann Allergy* 1991;66:29–31.
18. Stafford CT, Wise SL, Robinson DA, et al. Safety and efficacy of fire ant venom in the diagnosis of fire ant allergy. *J Allergy Clin Immunol* 1992;90:653–661.
19. Robertson ML. Multiple bee stings. *Emerg Med* 1998;10:151–155.
20. Morris B, Southcott RV, Gale AE. Effects of stings of Australian native bees. *Med J Aust* 1988;149:707–709.
21. Schmidt JO. Toxinology of venoms from the honeybee genus *Apis*. *Toxicon* 1995;33:917–927.
22. Balit CR, Isbister GK, Buckley NA. Randomised controlled trial of topical aspirin in the treatment of bee and wasp stings. *J Toxicol Clin Toxicol* 2003;(in press).

23. Visscher PK, Vetter RS, Camazine S. Removing bee stings. *Lancet* 1996;348:301–302.
24. Mauriello PM, Barde SH, Georgitis JW, et al. Natural history of large local reactions from stinging insects. *J Allergy Clin Immunol* 1984;74:494–498.
25. Reisman RE. Insect stings. *N Engl J Med* 1994;331:523–527.
26. Jones RGA, Corteling RL, To HP, et al. A novel Fab-based antivenom for the treatment of mass bee attacks. *Am J Trop Med Hyg* 1999;61:361–366.
27. Jones RGA, Lee L, Landon J. The effects of specific antibody fragments on the "irreversible" neurotoxicity induced by Brown snake (*Pseudonaja*) venom. *Br J Pharmacol* 1999;126:581–584.
28. Thiruventhiran T, Goh BL, Leong CL, et al. Acute renal failure following multiple wasp stings. *Nephrol Dial Transplant* 1999;14:214–217.
29. Zhang R, Meleg-Smith S, Batuman V. Acute tubulointerstitial nephritis after wasp stings. *Am J Kidney Dis* 2001;38:E33.
30. Watemberg N, Weizman Z, Shahak E, et al. Fatal multiple organ failure following massive hornet stings. *J Toxicol Clin Toxicol* 1995;33:471–474.
31. McGain F, Winkel KD. Ant sting mortality in Australia. *Toxicon* 2002;40:1095–1100.
32. Solley GO, Vanderwoude C, Knight GK. Anaphylaxis due to red imported fire ant sting. *Med J Aust* 2002;176:521–523.
33. Ogata K, Taylor RW. Ants of the genus *Myrmecia fabricus*: a preliminary review and key to the named species (Hymenoptera: Formicidae: Myrmeciinae). *J Nat History* 1991;25:1623–1673.
34. Douglas RG, Weiner JM, Abramson MJ, et al. Prevalence of severe ant-venom allergy in southeastern Australia. *J Allergy Clin Immunol* 1998;101:129–131.
35. Matuszek MA, Hodgson WC, Sutherland SK, et al. Pharmacological studies of jumper ant (*Myrmecia pilosula*) venom: evidence for the presence of histamine, and haemolytic and eicosanoid-releasing factors. *Toxicon* 1992;30:1081–1091.
36. Schuman SH, Caldwell ST. 1990 South Carolina Physician Survey of tick, spider and fire ant morbidity. *J S C Med Assoc* 1991;87:429–432.
37. McCubbin KI, Weiner JM. Fire ants in Australia: a new medical and ecological hazard. *Med J Aust* 2002;176:518–519.
38. Ponder RD, Stafford CT, Kiefer CR, et al. Development of an enzyme-linked immunosorbent assay for measurement of fire ant venom-specific IgE. *Ann Allergy* 1994;72:329–332.
39. Minelli A. Secretions of centipedes. In: *Arthropod venoms*, 1st ed. Berlin: Springer-Verlag, 1978:73–85.
40. Southcott RV. Arachnidism and allied syndromes in the Australian region. *Records of the Adelaide Children's Hospital* 1976;1:97–186.
41. McKeown KC. Centipedes and centipede bites. *Australian Museum Magazine* 1930;4:59–60.
42. Harvey MS, Yen AL. *Worms to wasps: an illustrated guide to Australia's terrestrial invertebrates.* Melbourne: Oxford University Press, 1989.
43. Bush SP, King BO, Norris RL, et al. Centipede envenomation. *Wilderness Environ Med* 2001;12:93–99.
44. Mumcuoglu KY, Leibovici V. Centipede (Scolopendra) bite: a case report. *Isr J Med Sci* 1989;25:47–49.
45. Rodriguez-Acosta A, Gassette J, Gonzalez A, et al. Centipede (*Scolopendra gigantea* Linneaus 1758) envenomation in a newborn. *Rev Inst Med Trop Sao Paulo* 2000;42:341–342.
46. Mohri S, Sugiyama A, Saito K, et al. Centipede bites in Japan. *Cutis* 1991;47:189–190.
47. Logan JL, Ogden DA. Rhabdomyolysis and acute renal failure following the bite of the giant desert centipede *Scolopendra heros. West J Med* 1985;142:549–550.
48. Gomes A, Datta A, Sarangi B, et al. Pharmacodynamics of venom of the centipede *Scolopendra subspinipes dehaani* Brandt. *Indian J Exp Biol* 1982;20:615–618.
49. Mohamed AH, Abu-Sinna G, El Shabaka HA, et al. Proteins, lipids, lipoproteins and some enzyme characterizations of the venom extract from the centipede *Scolopendra morsitans. Toxicon* 1983;21:371–377.
50. Mohamed AH, Zaid E, El Beih NM, et al. Effects of an extract from the centipede *Scolopendra moristans* on intestine, uterus and heart contractions and on blood glucose and liver and muscle glycogen levels. *Toxicon* 1980;18:581–589.
51. Knysak I, Martins R, Bertim CR. Epidemiological aspects of centipede (Scolopendromorphae: Chilopoda) bites registered in greater S. Paulo, SP, Brazil. *Rev Saude Publica* 1998;32:514–518.
52. Lin TJ, Yang CC, Yang GY, et al. Features of centipede bites in Taiwan. *Trop Geogr Med* 1995;47:300–302.
53. Uppal SS, Agnihotri V, Ganguly S, et al. Clinical aspects of centipede bite in the Andamans. *J Assoc Physicians India* 1990;38:163–164.
54. Cohen E, Quistad GB. Cytotoxic effects of arthropod venoms on various cultured cells. *Toxicon* 1998;36:353–358.
55. Pineda EV. A fatal case of centipede bite. *J Med Assoc* 1923;3:59–61.
56. Lersloompleephunt N, Eakthunyasakul S, Sittipunt C, et al. Severe hypotension and adult respiratory distress syndrome (ARDS) following centipede bite. In: *Proceedings of the 5th Asia-Pacific Congress on Animal, Plant and Microbial Toxins.* Thailand: International Society on Toxinology, 2003.
57. Friedman IS, Phelps RG, Baral J, et al. Wells' syndrome triggered by centipede bite. *Int J Dermatol* 1998;37:602–605.
58. Haneveld GT. Centipede bites. *BMJ* 1957;592.
59. Welsh JH, Batty CS. 5-Hydroxytryptamine content of some arthropod venoms and venom containing parts. *Toxicon* 1963;1:165.
60. Gomes A, Datta A, Sarangi B, et al. Occurrence of histamine and histamine release by centipede venom. *Indian J Med Res* 1982;76:888–891.
61. Sutherland SK, Tibballs J. Venomous arthropods of medical importance, other than spider and ticks. In: *Australian animal toxins*, 2nd ed. Melbourne: Oxford University Press, 2001:489–533.
62. Menez A, Zimmerman K, Zimmerman S, et al. Venom apparatus and toxicity of the centipede *Ethmostigmus rubripes* (Chilopoda, Scolopendridae). *J Morphol* 1990;206:303–312.
63. Gelbier S, Kopkin B. Pericoronitis due to a centipede. A case report. *Br Dent J* 1972;133:307–308.
64. Barnett PL. Centipede ingestion by a six-month-old infant: toxic side effects. *Pediatr Emerg Care* 1991;7:229–230.
64a. Balit CR, Hervey MS, Isbister GK. Prospective study of centipede stings in Australia. *J Toxicol Clin Toxicol* 2003;41:699.
65. Lawrence RF. *The centipedes and millipedes of southern Africa. A guide.* Cape Town, Rotterdam, 1984.
66. Eisner T, Alsop D, Hicks K, et al. Defensive secretions of millipedes. In: *Arthropod venoms*, 1st ed. Berlin: Springer-Verlag, 1978:41–72.
67. Haneveld GT. Eye lesions caused by the exudate of tropical millepedes I. Report of a case. *Trop Geogr Med* 1958;10:165–167.
68. Hudson BJ, Parsons GA. Giant millipede 'burns' and the eye. *Trans R Soc Trop Med Hyg* 1997;91:183–185.
69. Radford AJ. Millipede burns in man. *Trop Geogr Med* 1975;27:279–287.
70. Wood WF, Shepherd J, Chong B, et al. Ubiquinone-O in defensive spray of African millipede. *Nature* 1975;253:625–626.
71. Loomis HT. The millipedes of Hispaniola with descriptions of a new family, new genera and new species. *Bull Museum Comparative Zool Harvard* 1936;80:1–191.
72. Loomis HT. New millipedes from Haiti. *J Washington Acad Sci* 1941;31:190–193.
73. Shpall S, Frieden I. Mahogany discoloration of the skin due to the defensive secretion of a millipede. *Pediatr Dermatol* 1991;8:25–27.
74. White J. Clinical toxicology of tick bites. In: *Clinical toxicology of animal venoms and toxins*, 1st ed. Boca Raton, FL: CRC Press, 1995:191–203.
75. Banfield JF. Tick bites in man. *Med J Aust* 1966;2:600–601.
76. Gauci M, Loh RK, Stone BF, et al. Allergic reactions to the Australian paralysis tick, *Ixodes holocyclus*: diagnostic evaluation by skin test and radioimmunoassay. *Clin Exp Allergy* 1989;19:279–283.
77. Murnaghan MF, O'Rourke FJ. Tick paralysis. In: *Arthropod venoms*, 1st ed. Berlin: Springer-Verlag, 1978:419–464.
78. Masina S, Broady KW. Tick paralysis: development of a vaccine. *Int J Parasitol* 1999;29:535–541.
79. Tibballs J, Cooper SJ. Paralysis with *Ixodes cornuatus* envenomation. *Med J Aust* 1986;145:37–38.
80. Miller MK. Massive tick (*Ixodes holocyclus*) infestation with delayed facial-nerve palsy. *Med J Aust* 2002;176:264–265.
81. Cooper BJ, Spence I. Temperature-dependent inhibition of evoked acetylcholine release in tick paralysis. *Nature* 1976;263:693–695.
82. Thurn MJ, Gooley A, Broady KW. Identification of the neurotoxin from the Australian paralysis tick, *Ixodes holocyclus*. In: *Recent advances in toxinology research*, vol 2. Singapore: Venom and Toxin Research Group, National University of Singapore, 1992:243–256.
83. Pearn J. The clinical features of tick bite. *Med J Aust* 1977;2:313–318.
84. Hamilton DG. Tick paralysis: a dangerous disease in children. *Med J Aust* 1940;1:759–765.
85. Trinca JC. Insect allergy: results of a five year survey. *Med J Aust* 1964;2:659–663.
86. Southcott RV. Injuries from Coleoptera. *Med J Aust* 1989;151:654–659.
87. Dean J, Aneshansley DJ, Edgerton HE, et al. Defensive spray of the bombardier beetle: a biological pulse jet. *Science* 1990;248:1219–1221.
88. Chee PG, Dunkley SM. Boiling beetles. *Med J Aust* 2002;177:685.
89. Weatherston J, Percy JE. Venoms of Coleoptera. In: *Arthropod venoms*. Berlin: Springer-Verlag, 1978:511–554.
90. Sakoff JA, Ackland SP, Baldwin ML, et al. Anticancer activity and protein phosphatase 1 and 2A inhibition of a new generation of cantharidin analogues. *Invest New Drugs* 2002;20:1–11.
91. Tagwireyi D, Ball DE, Loga PJ, et al. Cantharidin poisoning due to "blister beetle" ingestion. *Toxicon* 2000;38:1865–1869.
92. Nicholls DS, Christmas TI, Greig DE. Oedemerid blister beetle dermatosis: a review. *J Am Acad Dermatol* 1990;22:815–819.
93. Lee D. *Arthropod bites and stings and other injurious effects.* Sydney: School of Public Health and Tropical Medicine, University of Sydney, 1975.
94. Christmas TI, Nicholls D, Holloway BA, et al. Blister beetle dermatosis in New Zealand. *NZ Med J* 1987;100:515–517.
95. Samlaska CP, Samuelson GA, Faran ME, et al. Blister beetle dermatosis in Hawaii caused by *Thelyphassa apicata* (Fairmaire). *Pediatr Dermatol* 1992;9:246–250.
96. Fleisher TL, Fox I. Oedemerid beetle dermatitis. *Arch Dermatol* 1970;101:601–605.
97. Armstrong RK, Winfield JL. *Paederus fuscipes* dermatitis; an epidemic on Okinawa. *Am J Trop Med Hyg* 1969;18:147–150.
98. Millard PT. Whiplash dermatitis produced by the common rove beetle. *Med J Aust* 1954;1:741–744.
99. George AO, Falope ZF. An epidemic of *Paederus* dermatitis in southern Nigeria. *Contact Dermatitis* 1989;20:314–315.
100. Sendur N, Savk E, Karaman G. *Paederus* dermatitis: a report of 46 cases in Aydin, Turkey. *Dermatology* 1999;199:353–355.
101. Todd RE, Guthridge SL, Montgomery BL. Evacuation of an aboriginal com-

munity in response to an outbreak of blistering dermatitis induced by a beetle (*Paederus australis*). *Med J Aust* 1996;164:238–240.

102. Weatherston J, Percy JE. Venoms of Rhyncota (Hemiptera). In: *Arthropod venoms*. Berlin: Springer-Verlag, 1978:489–509.
103. Cook ML, Lee DJ. Effects on humans of bites of Australian non-bloodsucking reduviid bugs. *Med J Aust* 1977;2:833–835.
104. Southcott RV. Lepidopterism in the Australian region. *Records of the Adelaide Children's Hospital* 1978;2:87–173.
105. Kawamoto F, Kumada N. Biology and venoms of Lepitdoptera. In: *Insect poisons, allergens and other invertebrate venoms*. New York: Marcel Dekker, 1984.
106. Mulvaney JK, Gatenby PA, Brookes JG. Lepidopterism: two cases of systemic reactions to the cocoon of a common moth, *Chelepteryx collesi*. *Med J Aust* 1998;168:610–611.
107. Southcott RV. Moths and butterflies. In: *Toxic plants and animals: a guide for Australia*, 1st ed. Brisbane: Queensland Museum, 1987:243–256.
108. Isbister GK, Whelan PI. Envenomation by the billygoat plum stinging caterpillar (*Thosea penthima*). *Med J Aust* 2000;173:654–655.
109. Balit CR, Ptolemy HC, Geary MJ, et al. Outbreak of caterpillar dermatitis caused by airborne hairs of the mistletoe browntail moth (*Euproctis edwardsi*). *Med J Aust* 2001;175:641–643.
110. Arocha-Pinango CL, de Bosch NB, Torres A, et al. Six new cases of a caterpillar-induced bleeding syndrome. *Thromb Haemost* 1992;67:402–407.
111. Everson GW, Chapin JB, Normann SA. Caterpillar envenomations: a prospective study of 112 cases. *Vet Hum Toxicol* 1990;32:114–119.
112. Stipetic ME, Rosen PB, Borys DJ. A retrospective analysis of 96 "asp" (*Megalopyge opercularis*) envenomations in Central Texas during 1996. *J Toxicol Clin Toxicol* 1999;37:457–462.
113. McGovern JP, Barkin GD, McElhenney TR, et al. *Megalopyge opercularis*: observations of its life history, natural history of its sting in man, and report of an epidemic. *JAMA* 1961;175:1155–1158.
114. Dunlop K, Freeman S. Caterpillar dermatitis. *Australas J Dermatol* 1997;38:193–195.
115. Scholz A, Russell R, Geary M. Investigation of caterpillar dermatitis in school children. *New South Wales Public Health Bull* 1993;4:65–66.
116. Goldman L, Sawyer F, Levine A, et al. Investigative studies of skin irritations from caterpillars. *J Invest Dermatol* 1960;34:67–79.
117. Natsuaki M. Immediate and delayed-type reactions in caterpillar dermatitis. *J Dermatol* 2002;29:471–476.
118. Walker RB, Thomas T, Cupit D, et al. An epidemic of caterpillar sting dermatitis in a rural West Virginia community. *West Virginia Med J* 1993;89:58–60.
119. Blair CP. The browntail moth, its caterpillar and their rash. *Clin Exp Dermatol* 1979;4:215–222.
120. Hellier FF, Warin RP. Caterpillar dermatitis. *BMJ* 1967;2:346–348.
121. Cleland JB. Papulo-urticarial rashes caused by the hairlets of caterpillars of the moth (*Euproctis edwardsi newm*). *Med J Aust* 1920;169–170.
122. Natsuaki M. Study on patients with caterpillar dermatitis in Itami city hospital. *Jpn J Entomol Zool* 1995;7:87–90.
123. Ogata K. Studies on the Far Eastern urticating moth, *Euproctis flava* Bremer, as a pest of medical importance. III. Epidemiological notes [text in Japanese with English summary]. *Jpn J Sanit Zool* 1958;9:228–234.
124. Frankel S. Severe urticaria caused by a moth *Euproctis* sp. (Lepidoptera: Lymantriidae). *Papua New Guinea Med J* 1976;18:149–151.
125. de Jong MC, Kawamoto F, Bleumink E, et al. A comparative study of the spicule venom of *Euproctis* caterpillars. *Toxicon* 1982;20:477–485.
126. de Jong MC, Bleumink E, Nater JP. Investigative studies of the dermatitis caused by the larva of the brown-tail moth (*Euproctis chrysorrhoea* Linn). I. Clinical and experimental findings. *Arch Dermatol Res* 1975;253:287–300.
127. Shama SK, Etkind PH, Odell TM, et al. Gypsy-moth-caterpillar dermatitis. *N Engl J Med* 1982;306:1300–1301.
128. Hesler LS, Logan TM, Benenson MW, et al. Acute dermatitis from oak processionary caterpillars in a U.S. military community in Germany. *Milit Med* 1999;164:767–770.
129. Kozer E, Lahat E, Berkovitch M. Hypertension and abdominal pain: uncommon presentation after exposure to a pine caterpillar. *Toxicon* 1999;37:1797–1801.
130. Lamy M, Pastureaud MH, Novak F, et al. Thaumetopoein: an urticating protein from the hairs and integument of the pine processionary caterpillar (*Thaumetopoea pityocampa* Schiff., Lepidoptera, Thaumetopoeidae). *Toxicon* 1986;24:347–356.
131. Werno J, Lamy M, Vincendeau P. Caterpillar hairs as allergens. *Lancet* 1993;342:936–937.
132. Tuthill RW, Canada AT, Wilcock K, et al. An epidemiologic study of gypsy moth rash. *Am J Public Health* 1984;74:799–803.
133. Beaucher WN, Farnham JE. Gypsy-moth-caterpillar dermatitis. *N Engl J Med* 1982;306:1301–1302.
134. Etkind PH, Odell TM, Canada AT, et al. The gypsy moth caterpillar: a significant new occupational and public health problem. *J Occup Med* 1982;24:659–662.
135. Kuspis DA, Rawlins JE, Krenzelok EP. Human exposures to stinging caterpillar: *Lophocampa caryae* exposures. *Am J Emerg Med* 2001;19:396–398.
136. Burdmann EA, Antunes I, Saldanha LB, et al. Severe acute renal failure induced by the venom of *Lonomia* caterpillars. *Clin Nephrol* 1996;46:337–339.
137. Duarte AC, Crusius PS, Pires CA, et al. Intracerebral haemorrhage after contact with *Lonomia* caterpillars. *Lancet* 1996;348:1033.
138. Fan HW, Cardoso JL, Olmos RD, et al. Hemorrhagic syndrome and acute renal failure in a pregnant woman after contact with *Lonomia* caterpillars: a case report. *Revista do Instituto de Medicina Tropical de Sao Paulo* 1998;40:119–120.
139. Zannin M, Lourenco DM, Motta G, et al. Blood coagulation and fibrinolytic factors in 105 patients with hemorrhagic syndrome caused by accidental contact with *Lonomia obliqua* caterpillar in Santa Catarina, Southern Brazil. *Thromb Haemost* 2003;89:355–364.
140. Arocha-Pinango CL, Layrisse M. Fibrinolysis produced by contact with a caterpillar. *Lancet* 1969;1:810–812.
141. Guerrero B, Arocha-Pinango CL. Activation of human prothrombin by the venom of *Lonomia achelous* (Cramer) caterpillars. *Thromb Res* 1992;66:169–177.
142. Reis CV, Portaro FC, Andrade SA, et al. A prothrombin activator serine protease from the *Lonomia obliqua* caterpillar venom (Lopap) biochemical characterization. *Thromb Res* 2001;102:427–436.
143. Reis CV, Farsky SH, Fernandes BL, et al. In vivo characterization of Lopap, a prothrombin activator serine protease from the *Lonomia obliqua* caterpillar venom. *Thromb Res* 2001;102:437–443.
144. Isbister GK, Graudins A, White J, et al. Antivenom treatment in arachnidism. *J Toxicol Clin Toxicol* 2003;41:291–300.
145. Rocha-Campos AC, Goncalves LR, Higashi HG, et al. Specific heterologous F(ab')2 antibodies revert blood incoagulability resulting from envenoming by *Lonomia obliqua* caterpillars. *Am J Trop Med Hyg* 2001;64:283–289.
146. Pinson RT, Morgan JA. Envenomation by the puss caterpillar (*Megalopyge opercularis*). *Ann Emerg Med* 1991;20:562–564.
147. McMillan CW, Purcell WR. The puss caterpillar, alias woolly slug. *N Engl J Med* 1964;271:147–149.
148. Neustater BR, Stollman NH, Manten HD. Sting of the puss caterpillar: an unusual cause of acute abdominal pain. *South Med J* 1996;89:826–827.
149. McKeown KC. *Australian insects. An introductory handbook.* 1942:262.
150. Common IFB. *Moths of Australia.* Melbourne University Press, 1990.
151. Balit CR, Geary MJ, Russell RC, et al. Prospective study of the clinical effects of exposure to the white-stemmed gum moth (*Chelepteryx collesi*). *J Toxicol Clin Toxicol* 2002;40:378–379(abst).
152. Dinehart SM, Archer ME, Wolf JE Jr, et al. Caripito itch: dermatitis from contact with *Hylesia* moths. *J Am Acad Dermatol* 1985;13:743–747.
153. Fernandez G, Morales E, Beutelspacher C, et al. Epidemic dermatitis due to contact with a moth in Cozumel, Mexico. *Am J Trop Med Hyg* 1992;46:560–563.
154. Watson PG, Sevel D. Ophthalmia nodosa. *Br J Ophthalmol* 1966;50:209–217.
155. Horng CT, Chou PI, Liang JB. Caterpillar setae in the deep cornea and anterior chamber. *Am J Ophthalmol* 2000;129:384–385.
156. Lee D, Pitetti RD, Casselbrant ML. Oropharyngeal manifestations of lepidopterism. *Arch Otolaryngol Head Neck Surg* 1999;125:50–52.
157. Pitetti RD, Kuspis D, Krenzelok EP. Caterpillars: an unusual source of ingestion. *Pediatr Emerg Care* 1999;15:33–36.
158. Paysse EA, Holder S, Coats DK. Ocular injury from the venom of the Southern walkingstick. *Ophthalmology* 2001;108:190–191.
159. Southcott RV. Injuries from larval Neuroptera. *Med J Aust* 1991;154:329–332.
160. Mueller UR. *Insect sting allergy. Clinical picture, diagnosis and treatment.* New York: Gustav Fischer, 1990.
161. Mosbech H. Clinical toxicology of hymenopteran stings. In: *Clinical toxicology of animal venoms and poisons*, 1st ed. Boca Raton, FL: CRC Press, 1995:349–359.

SECTION

3

Marine Animals

CHAPTER 252

Marine Envenomation and Poisoning

Geoffrey K. Isbister

Invertebrates, venomous:	**Portuguese man-of-war, fire coral, box jellyfish, true jellyfish, sea nettle, sea anemones, sea urchins, starfish, sea cucumbers, sponges, bristleworms, cone snails, and blue-ringed octopus**
Vertebrates, venomous:	**Stingrays**
Vertebrates, poisonous:	**Fish poisonings, sea snakes addressed in Chapter 246**

OVERVIEW

A remarkable array of marine organisms are either venomous or poisonous to humans. This chapter addresses the invertebrate and vertebrate organisms in the following order:

Invertebrates, venomous
- Phylum Cnidaria (formerly Coelenterates)
  - Hydrozoa: Portuguese man-of-war, hydroids, fire corals
  - Cubozoa: Box jellyfish
  - Scyphozoa: True jellyfish (sea nettle; mauve stinger; hair, blubber, moon jellyfish; sea lice)
  - Anthozoa: Sea anemones
- Phylum Echinodermata
  - Echinoidea: Sea urchins
  - Asteroidea: Starfish
  - Holothuroidea: Sea cucumber
- Phylum Porifera: Sponges
- Phylum Annelida: Bristleworms
- Phyllum Mollusca: Cone snails and the blue-ringed octopus

Vertebrates, venomous
- Silurformes: Catfish
- Scorpaenidae: Stonefish, scorpionfish, rockfish, lionfish, soldierfish, bullrout
- Trachinidae: Weeverfish
- Rajiformes: Stingrays
- Other venomous fish: Scats, zebrafish, rabbitfish, Port Jackson shark

Vertebrates, poisonous
- Puffer fish
- Ciguatera
- Shellfish poisoning: Paralytic, neurotoxic, diarrhetic, amnesic, scombroid, azasperacid
- Other marine poisoning: Clupeotoxin, palytoxin, ichthyocrinotoxication, ichthyohepatotoxication, sea hare, Pfiesteria dinoflagellates

Marine animals are divided into venomous and poisonous marine creatures. Venomous animals produce venom in a specialized gland, which the animal can then apply or inject parenterally into another organism using a specialized apparatus. Venom is a mixture of mainly protein and peptide toxins and is not a pure substance (1). In contrast, poisonous animals may have special glands that produce toxins but more often accumulate toxic compounds from the environment in their bodies. These substances are referred to as *poisons* and have to be ingested to be effective because the animal lacks an apparatus to deliver them (1).

Toxins are pure compounds that are the constituents of venoms or poisons. The clinical effects of toxins depend on their site of action and may be neurotoxic, hematoxic, cytotoxic, or myotoxic, to list some common effects (1–4). Marine venoms contain toxins that are usually heat labile and large-molecular-weight proteins. Marine poisons generally consist of heat- and gastric acid–stable metabolic byproducts of lower molecular weight (1).

Epidemiology

One study in the United States reviewed more than 6 years of aquatic animal exposures reported to poison information centers. The study demonstrated that the most common exposures were jellyfish stings (31%); stingrays (16%); venomous fish stings (28%), including lionfish, catfish, and others; and gastropods (6%) (5). These figures are most likely biased to more severe injuries, not including common minor injuries such as sea bather's eruption, Physalia envenomation, and sea urchin injuries, in which many people would not seek medical assistance.

In the United States, there are thousands of cases of minor jellyfish stings each year from *Physalia physalis* (Portuguese man-of-war) and *Chrysaora* species (spp.) (1), and similarly in Australia, there are thousands of injuries by bluebottles (*Physalia utriculus*). A retrospective study from Victoria, a southern state of Australia with a population of approximately five million people, described 205 cases from 1995 to 2000 presenting to emergency departments (Victorian Emergency Minimum Dataset). The most common injuries were from fish species (40.5%), stingrays (22.4%), and jellyfish stings (20.5%) (6). This study demonstrates the rarity of these injuries in colder climates. The large proportion of venomous fish stings is likely a bias, because the majority of jellyfish stings are minor and patients would not seek medical attention. In tropical northern Australia, the numbers of cases are far higher, with a predominance of jellyfish stings. In two prospective studies over a period of 1 year presenting to an emergency department, there were 40 jellyfish stings (7) and 23 venomous fish and stingray injuries (8). Similarly, in far north Queensland over a period of 1 year, 128 patients coded as marine stings were seen in the emergency department of one hospital; the vast majority were jellyfish stings (9). These studies are also biased to severe cases.

Deaths have been reported from envenomation by many types of marine animals, including sea snakes, many types of jellyfish, cone snails, stonefish, other venomous fish, and the blue-ringed octopi (*Hapalochlaena* spp.) (1,2,10). Deaths have been documented after stingray injuries but are almost always a result of thoracic or abdominal trauma (11,12).

Classification: Invertebrates

The invertebrates that are responsible for human envenomation are found in only five phyla: Cnidaria (jellyfish), Porifera (sponges), Echinodermata, Mollusca (including octopi and cone snails), and Annelida (1,2). The large phylum Cnidaria contains approximately 10,000 named species (1,2). The phylum was previously known as the *Coelenterates*. It contains the jellyfish, sea anemones, corals, hydroids, and related groups (13). Cnidaria have a radial structure with attached tentacles. They can be either single organisms or exist in a colony of organisms, such as occurs with *Physalia* spp. They can range in size from microscopic forms to massive jellyfish such as *Cyanea*, in which a specimen with a bell size of 2 m has been recorded (13). The biology and ecology of these creatures are still poorly understood and continue to be problematic in attempting to predict jellyfish swarms and their impact on humans.

The four classes in the Cnidaria phylum are as follows: Hydrozoa, Scyphozoa (true jellyfish), Cubozoa (box jellyfish), and Anthozoa (1,2), and all four contain venomous species (Table 1). Approximately 100 species are medically significant. First aid and treatment are discussed, following information on the known medically important jellyfish.

The phylum Echinodermata contains organisms with pentamerous (five-part) radial symmetry and includes sea urchins (class: Echinoidea), starfish (Asteroidea), and sea cucumbers (Holothuroidea). Echinoderms contain a variety of toxins, including steroid glycosides and terpenes, but only a few of these animals are able to cause injuries or envenomation in humans. The important members of the group are the crown-of-thorns starfish (*Acanthaster planci*) and a number of sea urchin species (1). Most injuries from these animals are a result of careless handling of the animals or treading on them in shallow waters. In subtropical and tropical regions, injuries are common, but in most cases simple removal of spines is all that is required, and serious envenomation is rare (1).

The phyllum Mollusca contains unsegmented soft-bodied invertebrates that include the snails and slugs, chitons, bivalves, octopi, squids, and related species (1,13). Two classes of mol-

TABLE 1. Classification of common jellyfish and clinical effects

Organism	Distribution	Clinical syndromes
Hydrozoa		
Physalia spp.	*P. physalis* Portuguese man-of-war (Atlantic), Pacific man-of-war and *P. utriculus* (Australia)	Variable severity from minor to life threatening; local intense pain lasting 1 h and linear erythematous or urticarial cutaneous eruptions
Hydroids	Tropical and temperate waters worldwide	Immediate local pain followed by itching over 30 min and painful wheals or urticaria developing, lasting for up to 1 wk
Millepora (fire coral)	Worldwide	Similar effects to the feather hydroids but less likely to cause delayed effects
Gonionemus spp.	Japan and Eastern Russia	Three clinical syndromes: painful effects similar to those of Irukandji syndrome, a respiratory form with acute upper respiratory effects and a mixed form
Olindias spp.	South America	Immediate local pain lasting hours and wheals/urticaria for days that may be round rather than linear
Cubozoa (box jellyfish)		
Chirodropidae	Indo-Pacific region, east coast of America	Immediate severe local pain and linear eruptions; cardiac effects and death with severe stings, typified by the *Chironex fleckeri* in Australia
Carybdidae	Indo-Pacific region	Majority cause local effects; some cause the Irukandji syndrome (*Carukia barnesi*) characterized by delayed generalized pain associated with tachycardia, hypertension, sweating, piloerection, agitation, and, rarely, pulmonary edema
Scyphozoa (true jellyfish)		
Cyanea spp. (hair jellyfish)	Worldwide, colder oceans	Majority cause short-lived moderate pain, less commonly local blistering and systemic effects
Catostylus spp. (blubber jellyfish)	Mainly Indo-Pacific region	Minor sting, not medically significant
Chrysaora quinquecirrha (sea nettle)	Worldwide, well known from North America	The majority cause immediate cutaneous pain that subsides over a few hours, similar to *Physalia* spp.
Pelagia noctiluca (mauve stinger)	Worldwide, important in Mediterranean	Immediate, transient localized pain, associated with wheals, itching, and edema, which usually blister and can continue to cause problems for weeks
Aurelia spp. (moon jellyfish)	Mediterranean, Australia, and America	Local pain, mild to severe, lasting less than 1 h
Thimble jellyfish (*Linuche unguiculata*)	Mainly east coast of America	Intensely pruritic, vesicular or maculopapular eruption affecting skin surfaces covered by swim wear occurring 1–24 h after exposure
Anthozoa		
Sea anemone	Worldwide	Immediate local pain of variable severity

lusks have a venom apparatus, the gastropods (cone snails and nudibranchs) and the cephalopods (octopi).

Classification: Vertebrates

The most important marine vertebrates causing envenomation are the sea snakes, venomous fish, and stingrays. Sea snakes are addressed in Chapter 246. Venomous fish and stingrays have venomous spines that cause mechanical trauma in addition to introducing venom into the wound. The spines are associated with the cells that produce the toxins that are released when the spine sheath is ruptured on entering the skin.

Venomous fish are found in tropical and, less commonly, temperate oceans. Many venomous fish are now kept in private aquariums (14–17). Important groups of venomous fish include catfish (Siluriformes), stonefish (Synanceiidae), weeverfish (Trachinidae), and scorpion and lionfish (Scorpaenidae). The clinical effects of stings range in severity from minimal or minor effects with some types of catfish and other fish with nonvenomous spines to severe with stonefish envenomation (2,8). In many cases, the associated trauma is more significant than the envenomation itself, and, in all cases, secondary infection with marine organisms is an important complication. The venoms of many of these fish have been investigated, including the isolation of a number of pharmacologically active toxins (18). Surprisingly few incidents of fish stings have been reported and almost no large series, despite the commonness of these injuries in commercial fishermen. It has been observed that the pain is not reduced in those who experience repeated stings, indicating that individuals do not become immunologically desensitized to the venom (8,19).

Marine Poisoning

Worldwide, marine poisoning causes more problems than marine envenomation, with rates of marine poisoning exceeding 1200 per 100,000 people annually in parts of the Pacific (20,21). These rates are most likely due to the fact that marine animals are an important part of human diets in many parts of the world, particularly the Pacific, and therefore large numbers of people are potentially exposed to marine poisons.

The three most important conditions that may occur after consumption of seafood are tetrodotoxin (TTX) poisoning, ciguatera, and paralytic shellfish poisoning (PSP). These conditions are caused by a group of toxins that mainly affect voltage-gated sodium channels in myelinated and unmyelinated nerves. Ciguatera is the most common marine poisoning but is rarely fatal, and puffer fish (TTX) poisoning, although far less common, is more likely to be lethal. Numerous marine toxins exist, and there is ongoing research into the structure, isolation, and function of these toxins.

CNIDARIA

Pathophysiology

Cnidariae have a unique stinging apparatus referred to as the *nematocyst*. Each creature has thousands of nematocysts, mainly on the tentacles, but also in smaller numbers on the bell or body of the creature. The number of nematocysts ranges up to millions on long tentacles for species such as *Chironex* and *Cyanea*, or they may be grouped in "batteries" of nematocysts, as is observed with *Physalia* spp. (13). A species of jellyfish may have several types of nematocysts, containing different types of venom and used for different processes, such as prey capture (26). The complete set of nematocysts for a species is referred to as the *cnidome*, and preliminary research suggests that the cnidome is species specific and can thus be used to help identify the creature (27).

Each nematocyst contains a very small amount of venom, sometimes highly potent, and a coiled-up harpoon-like mechanism (Fig. 1). A physical or chemical stimulus triggers the release of the hollow, sharply pointed thread-like tube from the contained nematocyst (1,2,26). This process is extremely rapid (thousandths of a second) and results in the thread-like tube penetrating the skin and delivering venom subcutaneously (1,2,28).

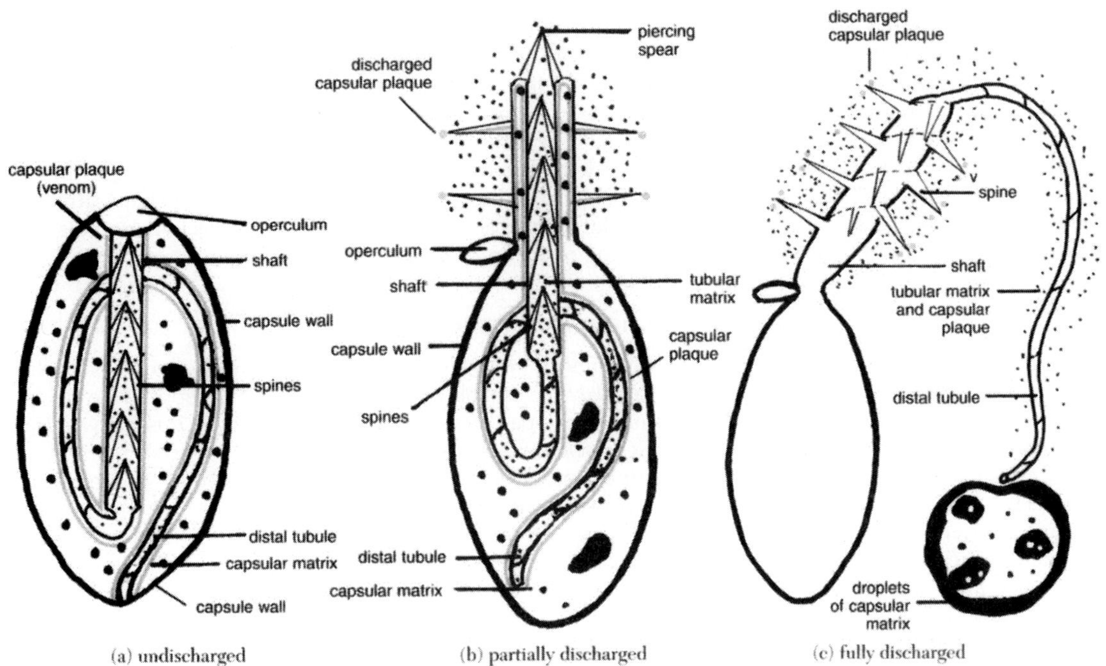

Figure 1. Image of a nematocyst before and after firing. (From Williamson JA, Fenner PJ, Burnett JW, et al. *Venomous and poisonous marine animals.* Sydney: New South Wales Press, 1996, with permission.)

Clinical Presentation

A wide variety of clinical syndromes result from jellyfish envenomation (Table 1).

HYDROZOA

The class Hydrozoa has worldwide distribution and includes *Physalia* spp. (Portuguese and Pacific man-of-war and bluebottle), the hydroids, *Millepora* (stinging corals), limnomedusae, and Gonionemus (1,2,13). *Physalia* spp. cause many thousands of human envenomations in Florida (22), South America (23), parts of Asia and Africa, Australia (24), and Portugal (1). This widely distributed group of jellyfish has several important species. The taxonomy of this group is still not entirely resolved, making it difficult to determine the effects of species in different regions. The best known member is *P. physalis*, or the Portuguese man-of-war, that occurs in the Atlantic. It is a multitentacled hydrozoan colony rather then a single jellyfish. The smaller, Pacific man-of-war is similar but may possibly be a separate species. The third member is the Australian bluebottle, or *P. utriculus*, which is a single-tentacled jellyfish that should not be confused with the Pacific man-of-war. *P. utriculus* is attributed with numerous stings in Australia, although recent examination of specimens suggests that at least some stings in eastern Australia may be from *P. physalis*.

Physalia occur in swarms in shallow water and usually cause stings in the surf or when they are washed up on shore. *P. physalis* have large gas-filled floats, which suspend multiple tentacles, up to 30 m in Atlantic specimens. The nematocysts occur on the tentacles but not on the float. The Atlantic variety occurs in the Atlantic Ocean and Caribbean Sea, whereas the smaller Pacific variety is distributed across the Pacific and Indian Oceans.

The feather or stinging hydroids (also fireweeds) are plume-like, sessile animals that constitute the major group of hydrozoans (order Leptomedusae). They occur in tropical and in temperate waters worldwide, commonly attached to wrecks and wharves (2). Coastal storms can break off hydroid branches and infest a local swimming area. Like other jellyfish, hydroids have nematocysts that are responsible for the sting on contact with the creature (1).

Several hydroid species from the family Aglaopheniidae cause discomfort in humans, including *Lytocarpus philippinus* (Indo-Pacific region, Atlantic Ocean, and the Mediterranean) and *Aglaophenia cupressina* (Indo-Pacific region including the Philippines and northern Australia). *Lytocarpus* and *Aglaophenia* are often referred to as *fireweeds* (2) and have feather-like branches lined with nematocyst-bearing polyps (2). Other stinging hydroids include two from the family Haleciidae: *Halecium beani* from Australia and *Nemalecium lighti* from Brazil (2,25).

Physalia Species

Physalia stings range in severity from minor to occasionally severe and life-threatening envenomation. They cause immediate, intense pain that often fades over an hour. The pain may persist for many hours, particularly with *P. physalis*. The sting causes a characteristic linear erythematous or "beaded" urticarial cutaneous eruption (1,2,23,24,29); the spacing of the "ladder"-like appearance can vary depending on the contraction of the tentacle at the time of the sting (13). Respiratory distress and death have occurred after *P. physalis* envenomation (22,30). The severity of the local injuries can vary significantly from simple erythematous and urticarial lesions, to vesicular, hemorrhagic, and necrotic lesions, and, in severe cases, this can result in permanent scarring (13). Acute regional vascular insufficiency has been reported after jellyfish stings in two suspected *Physalia* envenomations, with severe sequelae in one case (31). First aid and treatment are discussed in Treatment.

Hydroids

Hydroid stings are generally minor but can occur after even superficial contact, such as brushing past the creature, and are known to reef workers. In the majority of cases, contact causes immediate local pain, but there is a report of only a mild burning sensation initially (2,25). This is followed by the rapid development of an itchy, painful wheal and urticaria over 30 to 60 minutes. More extensive contact may lead to blistering, erythematous, and edematous papular reaction or the development of a "haemorrhagic and zosteriform" reaction (1,2,32). The wheals may last days to a week but do not leave a permanent mark. Similar effects have been reported in the Indo-Pacific region (2) and more recently in Brazil (25). First aid treatment consists of blotting the area carefully with a dry tissue. Vinegar inhibits nematocyst discharge in *L. philippinus*, but studies on other species are required (2). Analgesia with ice packs or medication is appropriate.

Millepora (Fire Corals)

These animals appear similar to hard corals, but they are relatively smooth. These creatures are widely distributed in shallow tropical waters and, due to their innocuous appearance, may be mistaken for seaweed (2). They have tiny nematocyst-bearing tentacles that protrude from numerous minute surface gastropores. Research on *Millepora* venoms have demonstrated that they have hemolytic and dermonecrotic effects and can induce death in mice injected with extract from the fire coral. A study on nematocyst extracts from *M. complanata* shows that it causes calcium-dependent smooth muscle contraction (33).

The effects of contact with the tentacles are similar to those with hydroid stings, but in the majority of cases persistent reactions do not occur (2). Immediate localized burning or stinging pain occurs, and over the course of an hour an initially small red mark progresses to urticarial wheals. The pain generally resolves within 2 hours with no specific treatment, and in most cases there is no further reaction. Although blistering is rare, the urticarial lesions may become infected, leading to pustular lesions that occasionally become necrotic (2,13). More severe effects from the Red Sea have been reported that resulted in well-demarcated painless necrosis at the sting site after the initial itchy, painful, and erythematous reaction (34). Treatment is similar to that for hydroids and other minor jellyfish stings, with drying of the area and ice packs.

Other Hydrozoans

A number of other medically important hydrozoans exist, including *Gonionemus* and *Olindias* (2). *Gonionemus* spp. cause envenomation in Japan (*G. oshoro*) and the east coast of Russia (*G. vertens*). *Gonionemus* causes a clinical syndrome similar to the Irukandji syndrome seen in Australia (see Irukandji Syndrome) but includes some respiratory features. It has been reported in large case series from Russia and also in Japan (2). In the most recent series of 648 cases, three clinical forms were distinguished. The painful form was most similar to Irukandji syndrome with an initial sting and local erythema, which was followed 15 to 20 minutes later by severe pain in the muscles, joints, abdomen, chest, and back. Associated nonspecific features occurred, such as weakness, fatigue, motor anxiety, and fever (2). The effects resolved over 2 to 3 days (2). A respiratory form was also reported in which allergic catarrhal symptoms developed, including rhinitis, lacrimation, hoarseness, cough, and dyspnea, which lasted for a few hours to days (2). The third form was a mixed syndrome of the painful and the respiratory forms. Similar effects have been reported from Japan by Otsuru (2).

Olindias spp. are also reported to cause stings. The most important is *O. sambaquiensis* in the coastal waters of eastern South America, including Brazil, Uruguay, and Argentina (2,23,35). It is likely to be responsible for many hundreds of stings annually in Argentina in the Monte Hermoso region, and swarming usually occurs in January and February (2). Few confirmed stings by these jellyfish have been reported (23,35). *Olindias* cause immediate burning pain that may last for several hours associated with short linear welts (zigzag lines) or irregular white welts with surrounding erythema (2). A more recent report of five cases, four with confirmed stings with identification of the organism, described stings causing round erythematous and edematous reactions associated with only mild pain (23).

CUBOZOA (BOX JELLYFISH)

The box jellyfish, or class Cubozoa, are characterized by having a bell or body that is shaped similarly to a cube, with tentacles attached to each of the four corners. The class includes two important orders: Chirodropidae and Carybdidae. Members of these orders not only differ morphologically but appear to cause very different patterns of envenomation.

Chirodropidae

Chirodropid box jellyfish are multitentacled jellyfish. They have many tentacles (up to 15) arising from complex pedalia (2). The Indo-Pacific chirodropids have some of the most toxic venoms known, but the characterization of the toxins and exact mechanism of action remain unclear because of the difficulties in extracting the venom from nematocysts and the lability of the venom components (36,37). *Chironex fleckeri* is the most important chirodropid and has been responsible for more than 60 deaths in Australia (2,7). *Chiropsalmus* spp. are more widely distributed and less well understood but have also been reported to cause deaths in the Indo-Pacific region (2,38).

C. fleckeri is often described as the world's most venomous animal (2,7). It is found along the northern coast of Australia, although it is unclear if it occurs outside of this region. It has caused at least 60 fatalities in the past century and continues to cause deaths in healthy children in northern Australia (7). Systemic envenomation and death can rapidly occur (often within 20 minutes) after skin contact with tentacles in excess of 6 to 7 m (2,7). A primary cardiotoxic mechanism is postulated. The venom causes an overload of intracellular calcium in cardiac myocytes, possibly as a result of increased Na^+ influx into the cell (39). *In vivo* experiments in rats using purified nematocyst extract have confirmed this, with intravenous venom causing rapid death due to hypotension, even in artificially ventilated animals (unpublished observations). Earlier work in animals demonstrated that *C. fleckeri* venom causes dermatonecrotic, hemolytic, and lethal effects (40,41). However, hemolysis has not been documented in humans, with death and skin damage being the two important effects (42). After this, two myotoxins were isolated from the venom, and myotoxicity has been confirmed in isolated muscle preparations (36).

The clinical effects of *Chironex* stings are well characterized in studies correlating positive nematocyst stings with effects. The majority of cases are mild to moderate, causing immediate, sometimes severe, pain and skin welts (7). The skin reactions may be quite severe with formation of wheals, vesicles, and darkened reddish-brown or purple whip-like flare patterns with stripes of 8 to 10 mm in width (pathognomonic cross-hatched pattern) (7). In severe cases, blistering followed by superficial necrosis occurs that can ultimately result in significant permanent scarring. Localized delayed hypersensitivity reactions have been reported in approximately 60% of cases, characterized by a papular urticarial reaction along the linear stings (7).

Chiropsalmus quadrigatus has been responsible for deaths in the Philippines and Japan, and possibly other parts of the Indo-Pacific region (2,10). Deaths have been reported in Malaysia and Brunei, but it is unclear whether these are *Chironex*-like jellyfish or *Chiropsalmus* spp. The clinical effects of *Chiropsalmus* spp. include moderate to severe localized pain associated with linear wheals and inflammation, similar to *Chironex* stings.

C. quadrumanus is a small, transparent jellyfish 2 to 6 cm in diameter that occurs along the southeastern coastline of the United States (10) down into South America (23). The rapid death of a 5-year-old child after a sting has been attributed to *C. quadrumanus* based on nematocysts scraped from the skin and the geographic distribution of the jellyfish (38). In this case, the child had an acute cardiac dysrhythmia and evidence of pulmonary edema and died within 40 minutes of the sting (38). A series of 20 stings by *C. quadrumanus* (8 confirmed stings) in Brazil demonstrated that stings are characterized by intense local pain, long linear marks (similar to *Chironex*), and systemic effects (nausea, vomiting, malaise, and respiratory distress) (23).

Carybdidae

Carybdidae jellyfish are also box shaped but only have one tentacle attached to each pedalium (corner of the box). The group is typified by *Carukia barnesi* from Australia, which causes Irukandji syndrome (2,7,43), but other carybdids include *Carybdea* spp. and Morbakka types (*Tamoya virulenta*) (2). The clinical effects of jellyfish in this group vary, with some causing Irukandji-like effects and others producing more localized linear stings.

C. barnesi is the best characterized of the carybdids and causes the Irukandji syndrome. It is a small carybdeid jellyfish (1.5 to 2.5 cm) with a transparent bell (44). The effects of this jellyfish have been well described by correlation of stings from both identified specimens (45) and in patients in whom nematocysts have been collected from the sting site (9). *C. barnesi* occurs in far north Queensland and is responsible for many stings and closure of beaches in the wet season (9,43). Stings occur sporadically and depend on local weather patterns. Irukandji syndrome is described in detail below.

A number of *Carybdea* spp. have been identified, and the clinical effects have been characterized in some cases. *C. alata* is responsible for hundreds to thousands of stings each year in Hawaii, but no deaths have been reported (46,47). In the majority of cases, stings result in severe localized pain and linear erythematous skin eruptions that resolve within an hour to a day (46,47). Occasionally, patients experience persistent pain and rash (46). Although there is one report of a patient developing an Irukandji-like syndrome, the jellyfish causing the sting was not seen or identified (2), and the absence of any other reports suggests that this is unlikely with *C. alata* (46,47).

C. rastoni ("Jimble") occurs in many parts of the Indo-Pacific region and has been reported to cause stings in southern and western Australia (1), Hawaii (46), Japan, and Malaysia, at least. Stings from these jellyfish cause immediate local pain with a papular wheal and red flare (1). *Tamoya* spp. ("Morbakka") are large carybdids that occur in tropical Australia (48), the Indo-Pacific, the Gulf of Oman, and West Africa. They cause severe pain and leave a cross-hatched pattern similar to stings by *Chironex* jellyfish (48). No deaths have been reported.

Irukandji Syndrome

The Irukandji syndrome was first described in the 1940s and is characterized by generalized pain, hypertension, nausea, vomiting, and anxiety (43,44). Initially, the sting causes mild local pain and a patch of erythema and may not even be noticed by the patient (43). Approximately 20 to 30 minutes later, severe generalized pain in the abdomen, back, chest, and muscles occurs. The pain is associated with systemic features, including tachycardia, hypertension, tachydysrhythmias, sweating, piloerection, agitation, and, in severe cases, pulmonary edema (43,44).

Heroic experiments by Jack Barnes, in which he stung himself and two others with jellyfish and developed severe Irukandji syndrome, established that *C. barnesi* at least caused the syndrome (45). A more recent study confirmed that the majority of cases of Irukandji syndrome in far north Queensland were due to *C. barnesi* (9), but other cubozoan jellyfish are likely to cause the same or similar clinical effects. In 2002, two deaths were attributed to the Irukandji syndrome (9,48). Considerable controversy has arisen regarding attribution in the first case (48), and, although nematocysts were obtained from the patient in the second case, they were from an unknown jellyfish, highlighting the lack of information on these organisms (9). At least in Australia, other carybdid jellyfish are undoubtedly responsible for Irukandji-like effects (9).

Cardiac Effects of Cubozoan Stings

The difficulty in correctly attributing the effects of jellyfish stings and the delayed effects of some stings has meant that the effects of many cubozoan jellyfish remain unknown. Cardiac toxicity appears to be the mechanism of rapid death in *Chironex* stings, but the effects appear to be all or none. Cardiac effects are rare in patients who present to the hospital with only severe local pain (7), but in patients with a rapid fatal outcome it is apparent that severe myocardial dysfunction is present (49), consistent with the cardiac effects of the venom (50). In addition, it is well recognized that *C. barnesi* can cause myocardial depression with elevated troponin I concentrations and abnormal electrocardiograms (T-wave inversion and ST-segment depression), and, in severe cases, pulmonary edema develops with systolic dysfunction on echocardiogram (9,43). It is unclear whether the cardiac dysfunction is a result of the hypercatecholaminergic state or a primary cardiotoxic effect (9,51).

Cardiac effects are not confined to *Chironex* and *Carukia* jellyfish stings. Reports have been published of elevated troponin levels, pulmonary edema, and cardiac failure in cases in which nematocysts from unknown jellyfish have been retrieved (9,52), including a death in Australia (9).

SCYPHOZOA (TRUE JELLYFISH)

The class Scyphozoa includes some of the most well-known jellyfish and represents the true jellyfish. The important and common members are *Cyanea* spp. (hair jellyfish), *Catostylus* spp. (blubber jellyfish), *Chrysaora quinquecirrha* (sea nettle), the *Rhizostoma*, *Pelagia noctiluca* (mauve stinger), the thimble jellyfish (*Linuche unguiculata*), and *Aurelia* spp. (1,2).

Chrysaora Species (Sea Nettle)

Chrysaora spp. have a worldwide distribution but are most familiar in North America, in the Chesapeake Bay, where *C. quinquecirrha*, the North American sea nettle, is abundant and a cause of stings (1,2,13). *Chrysaora* spp., or sea nettles, are found in tropical and temperate waters, including the Atlantic coast of the United States, the coast of Brazil and Argentina, and the western Pacific Ocean in Japan and the Philippines (2,13). An estimated 500,000 annual jellyfish envenomations occur in the Chesapeake Bay and 60 to 200,000 in Florida, but there are no large series of envenomations despite extensive research into the venom (53–55).

In the majority of cases, the effects are minor, with immediate cutaneous pain that subsides over a few hours, similar to *Physalia* spp. It has been reported that touching the fishing tentacle is more painful than touching the mesenteric tentacles closer to the bell (55). Earlier reports from the Philippines described more severe effects. One report appeared of vascular insufficiency after a *Chrysaora* sting (31) and a case of mononeuritis with hyperimmune serum to *Chrysaora* after a *C. quinquecirrha* sting (2). Corneal stings are uncommon but can cause lacrimation; photophobia and delayed increased intraocular pressure may occur 1 to 2 days later as a result of acute iridocyclitis (56).

Cyanea Species (Hair Jellyfish)

Cyanea spp., or hair jellyfish, have a flat saucer-like bell and many hair-like tentacles that trail from the medusa (57). The tentacles break off easily, and free tentacles can still sting. Some species of *Cyanea* can grow to massive proportions; they occur in open and colder oceans (1) and have a worldwide distribution (2). Reports of the severity of effects vary, with only mild effects reported from Chesapeake Bay in the United States and in Australia (2). In these cases, localized pain develops over minutes and only lasts for 10 to 20 minutes (1,55). The pain is associated with a spreading erythema that fades and may leave zigzag lines. More severe local effects have been reported, with blistering and hemorrhagic lesions (2,13). Systemic effects have been reported in children, with mainly nausea, backache, and abdominal pain (58), and another case in which the patient lost consciousness (32). Corneal injuries after *Cyanea* stings are well documented (32,56,59).

Catostylus Species (Blubber Jellyfish)

Catostylus spp. are the common blubber jellyfish, which occur mainly in the Indo-Pacific region. These jellyfish are unlikely to cause more than slight pain on contact and are not medically significant (1,2).

Pelagia Species (Mauve Stingers)

Pelagia spp., or the mauve stingers, occur worldwide; they are a common cause of stings in the Mediterranean (60) and are also known from Australia (1). The jellyfish is named because it phosphoresces at night. It is usually a deep-water jellyfish but approaches the shoreline in larger colonies. Stings by *Pelagia* spp. cause immediate but transient localized pain associated with a wheal, itching, and localized swelling or edema (1). The lesions usually blister and can continue to cause problems for weeks. One severe anaphylactic reaction to a jellyfish that was likely to be the mauve stinger has been reported (61). One case of Guillain-Barré syndrome is associated with a probable *P. noctiluca* sting (62). In this patient, paresthesia, proximal muscle weakness, and gait ataxia developed in the week after the sting.

Nerve conduction studies performed 2 months after the sting revealed a prominent demyelinating neuropathy with conduction block. The clinical effects resolved after 6 months, and the nerve conduction studies improved. The authors proposed that the syndrome was due to an aberrant immune response to the jellyfish venom (62).

Aurelia Species (Moon Jellyfish)

Aurelia spp. (moon jellyfish) are found in many regions of the world, including the Mediterranean shores and Atlantic Ocean. Although reports from the Australian region suggest that local pain and wheal formation are minor after contact with *Aurelia* spp. (32), more recent reports from America and Israel suggest that significant local effects can occur (63,64). In one case, a definite sting by *A. aurita* caused immediate local pain for 30 minutes and piloerection, followed by urticaria at the site after a few minutes (64). Other effects included ulceration at the sting site, which then crusted over but remained hyperpigmented for a few weeks (64). *A. aura* occurs commonly along the shores of the Mediterranean and causes mild to moderate local envenomation, with immediate pain, localized swelling, wheal formation, and urticaria (63).

Sea Bather's Eruption and *Linuche unguiculata*

Sea bather's eruption is often described using the misnomer *sea lice*. It has been reported predominantly in the Florida Keys. It is an intensely pruritic, vesicular, or maculopapular eruption primarily affecting skin surfaces covered by swim wear (65) that occurs 1 to 24 hours after exposure. The condition is best characterized around Florida and in the Mexican Caribbean (65–67), where there is good evidence that the responsible jellyfish is *L. unguiculata* (thimble jellyfish). However, it has also been reported from other regions. A number of outbreaks on Long Island have been attributed to the sea anemone *Edwardsiella lineata* (68). The condition is not reported to any degree in the Indo-Pacific region.

One study demonstrated that all three stages of the scyphozoan *L. unguiculata* can cause sea bather's eruptions, although its effects can differ slightly between contact with the larvae, the ephyrae, and the medusa (66). The majority of cases occur between March and May and correspond with the life cycle of the jellyfish. Divers may be afflicted on the neck when floating in water churned by boat propellers that have ground floating jellyfish into fragments. The effects begin after a few minutes to 24 hours of ocean exposure, and usually no stinging sensation occurs. The condition is characterized by itchy, erythematous papules that are distributed on the areas of skin covered by the bathing suit, swimming cap, or wet suit or between large folds of skin such as the axillae (2). The major clinical effect is pruritus, which may continue for days to weeks (66) but resolves spontaneously. Systemic effects may occur uncommonly and appear to be more common in children (65).

Treatment has included antihistamines and antipruritic agents, but they usually give temporary relief. Topical steroids can be used. All treatment may be disappointing in severe cases. Changing swim wear and showering are probably effective in preventing stings.

ANTHOZOA

The class Anthozoa of the phylum Cnidaria is the largest class of jellyfish. They are less medically important than other groups. They include the sea anemones, stony (true) corals, and soft corals. The hard and soft coral are a large and important group of organisms that all have stinging nematocysts but rarely cause more than minor effects (2). However, coral cuts are a common underwater injury. The initial reactions to coral abrasions are a stinging pain (may be more severe if envenomation is present), erythema, and pruritus. The skin abrasion is usually rapidly surrounded by an erythematous wheal, which fades over 1 to 2 hours. Most important, there is a risk of marine infection, including cellulitis with lymphangitis, reactive bursitis, local ulceration, and wound necrosis. In general, the wound heals slowly over weeks. *Coral poisoning* usually refers to systemic malaise, fever, diarrhea, and general inanition associated with a coral wound. Coral cuts should be cleaned as soon as possible (within 3 hours) with a soft bristle brush, fresh water, and a mild antiseptic (2). Foreign bodies should be removed promptly because of the risk of foreign body granulomata. The wound should be closed only with adhesive strips.

Sea Anemones

The sea anemones belong to the taxonomic order Actiniaria. They are common and attractive seashore creatures, often found in tidal pools, where the unwary may brush up against them or inquisitively touch them. They have numerous nematocysts on their tentacles or wavy fronds. However, despite the toxicity of their venoms, little morbidity results from sea anemone stings. Stings are characterized by immediate local pain like any other jellyfish sting, but the severity can vary enormously. The pain may last for hours, and local tenderness may remain for days. Local effects include wheals and, in more severe cases, vesicular eruptions. Systemic effects are uncommon, and treatment is symptomatic. Sea anemone stings from many parts of the world have been reported, including *Actinodendron pulmosum* from the Barrier Reef in Australia, which can cause significant stings (1,2). One report has appeared of fulminant hepatic failure associated with a sea anemone sting (69). The patient experienced local pain initially, and hepatic failure developed within 48 hours. The patient's serum was positive for immunoglobulin G against *Condylactis* spp. (69).

Diagnosis

The majority of jellyfish stings are minor. Simple first-aid measures and symptomatic relief are all that are required. However, in severe and potentially life-threatening cases treatment should be directed at initial resuscitation and then reversal of the effects of venom if possible. All cases of envenomation with severe effects should be observed for at least 8 hours.

DIAGNOSIS AND CONFIRMATION OF JELLYFISH STINGS

Research into the effects and treatment of different jellyfish stings has been slowed by the difficulty in correctly attributing clinical effects to specific jellyfish because they are rarely caught at the time of the sting. Scraping the skin over the area of the sting allows the collection of any remaining nematocysts, which can then be identified under the microscope. The skin scraping should be put in 1% to 4% formalin, which is the best means of retrieving nematocysts but can be slightly painful. It is the only method of collecting nematocysts from bell stings (e.g., *C. barnesi*) because of the small numbers (9). Sticky-taping the sting site is less painful and is appropriate for predominantly tentacular stings. This method simply requires placing adhesive tape over the sting site and then carefully pulling the tape. The adhesive tape should next be applied to a microscope slide for later identification. This technique has been validated for diagnosis and research into *Chironex* stings (7,70). It is also an appropriate technique for *Physalia* stings and has been used less frequently in jellyfish that cause less severe effects (7,9,70).

Each species of cubozoan has several types of nematocysts, with the complete complement present being termed the *cnidome* (27). The cnidomes are equivalent to "fingerprints" for jellyfish, which allow other clinical envenoming syndromes to be correctly correlated with jellyfish species. For common jellyfish, the nematocysts can be identified easily, but for more uncommon jellyfish or in areas where stings are uncommon these should be examined by an expert who has access to the cnidomes of medically significant jellyfish.

Treatment

FIRST AID AND DECONTAMINATION

Various methods have been suggested for the first aid of jellyfish stings. However, there is increasing evidence to support a safe and effective approach to the majority of jellyfish stings, including the use of hot water (either hot showers or hot-water immersion), topical decontaminants, and removal of remaining jellyfish tentacles. Some previously recommended therapies such as cold packs (71) and pressure immobilization bandages (72) need review.

Although the deactivation of the remaining nematocysts is important, the use and type of topical decontaminants for jellyfish stings remain controversial in some regions. The sting site or tentacles should not be washed with fresh water because it is believed that its hypotonicity may stimulate nematocyst discharge. After the deactivation of nematocysts, the remaining tentacular material should be removed with either forceps or double gloves. Reports have certainly been published of secondary stings in rescuers removing tentacles.

Acetic acid 5% (vinegar) is the decontaminant treatment of choice for *C. fleckeri* stings and should be poured liberally over the sting site for at least 30 seconds (7). The value of acetic acid is less clear in other jellyfish stings. In minor stings in which heat may be simpler and more effective, topical decontaminants are less likely to be used. Alternative decontaminants include isopropyl alcohol (40% to 70%) and a baking soda slurry or sodium bicarbonate for *Chrysaora* and *Cyanea* (73).

A number of studies have suggested that hot-water showers or hot-water immersion are more effective (24,46,47,74) than the previous advice of cold packs (71). Cubozoan venoms are heat labile, and *C. fleckeri* venom is inactivated by heat to above 43°C (37). This has now been supported in a number of small clinical studies investigating the value of warm-water therapy (24,46,47,74). One controlled trial demonstrated that hot-water showers were more effective in reducing pain than cold packs in jellyfish stings in Florida (74). More recently, a randomized trial in Australia showed that hot showers reduced pain and treatment duration better than cold packs for *Physalia* (bluebottle) stings (24). A randomized trial of volunteers stung by *C. alata* in Hawaii also demonstrated that hot-water immersion was more effective than either papain meat tenderizer or vinegar (47). These clinical studies support the effectiveness of hot-water treatment in cubozoan jellyfish and *Physalia* stings. Pressure immobilization bandages are not recommended for any jellyfish envenomation, and studies have demonstrated that they may in fact increase nematocyst discharge (72,75).

SUPPORTIVE CARE

Minor stings require only symptomatic treatment. In many cases, the effects begin to resolve before transport to the hospital. First-aid treatments such as hot water (45°C) should be instigated if they are not already being used. Other symptomatic treatment such as oral or parenteral analgesia may be required. Prophylactic antibiotics are not indicated, but the wound should be carefully cleaned. For more severe local stings, such as in *C. fleckeri* or more severe *Physalia* stings, significant local injury may develop. These wounds should be managed similarly to partial-thickness burns. Corneal envenomations can be irrigated with an isotonic solution and treated judiciously with topical steroids. Delayed hypersensitivity reactions are best treated with topical corticosteroids (7). Anaphylaxis from jellyfish envenomations should be treated by maintaining the airway and cardiovascular system, and epinephrine as required.

Chironex Jellyfish

The majority of cases cause pain and linear eruptions. Initial treatment should be symptomatic, including oral and parenteral analgesia for pain. The requirement for opioid analgesia is far less than that for Irukandji syndrome and was only required in 1 of 23 nematocyst-positive cases in one series (7). Treatment for severe *Chironex* envenomation consists of standard resuscitative measures and sheep-derived antivenom specific for *C. fleckeri* (Commonwealth Serum Laboratories, Melbourne, Australia). The antivenom has never been tested in controlled trials, and its efficacy is unclear in human envenomation (76). In addition, animal studies have produced conflicting evidence regarding its effectiveness (76). The rapid onset of cardiotoxicity in clinical envenomation suggests that antivenom should be given very early (within minutes) and possibly in large doses (6 ampules or more) to prevent death (76).

Verapamil has been suggested as an adjunct therapy for *Chironex* envenomation. However, despite initial evidence in animal models, it has more recently been shown to increase morbidity and mortality in a piglet model (44,50). Because there are also concerns about using a negative inotrope and potentially prodysrhythmic agent in patients with severe myocardial dysfunction, it cannot be recommended.

Irukandji Syndrome

Treatment of Irukandji syndrome is mainly symptomatic and based on primarily anecdotal evidence. Opioid analgesia is almost universally required, and large doses are often used. Although many agents have been given, pethidine should be avoided to prevent norpethidine toxicity and myocardial depression with the large doses used (43,44). Pulmonary edema is treated as for other causes of noncardiogenic pulmonary edema. Cardiac dysfunction returns to normal within 3 to 4 days (44).

Magnesium sulfate infusion has been used in Australia to treat severe Irukandji syndrome (77). A 26-year-old man had significant envenomation with elevated cardiac troponin I (6.4 mg/L), hypertension, and generalized pain. Intravenous magnesium was given (10 mmol loading dose and 5 mmol per hour infusion), and he had resolution of sympathetic features and almost complete relief of pain. The infusion was continued until 20 hours after the sting. A recurrence of hypertension occurred when the rate was reduced early in the course. The mechanism for the therapeutic benefit of magnesium may be either its benefit in hypercatecholaminergic states (77) or that magnesium interferes with calcium influx into cells. However, controlled studies are required before magnesium can become a standard treatment for Irukandji syndrome.

ECHINOIDEA (SEA URCHINS)

The globular body of sea urchins is covered with calcareous spines of many sizes and shapes, some of which contain venom glands. Between the spines are small pincer-like organs called *pedicellariae*, which also serve as a venom apparatus. Sea urchins are found in all oceans, but most commonly in the tropics.

Clinical Presentation

Traumatic injury by penetration of the spines occurs in all cases. In the majority of cases, sea urchins have solid spines that cause localized pain but no envenomation. The spines often break off in the wound and are difficult to remove, sometimes requiring surgical removal. In some cases the spine may remain embedded and cause persistent local symptoms (78) or secondary infection and granuloma formation (2). All patients should have a radiograph to determine if there is any retained spine or whether spines have penetrated joints or bone. It appears that the spines are simply resorbed in some cases. Like any spinous injury, the spine may enter a joint, which rapidly induces severe synovitis. Wounds from black sea urchin spines may leave a black discoloration of the skin.

In the small group of sea urchins that can cause envenomation, the venom apparatus varies from short sharp spines with venom glands on their tips (*Asthenosoma* spp.) to longer and hollow spines that can inject venom (*Diadema* spp.) to the triple-jawed pedicellariae (mobile grasping organs) of some species (2). Contact with venomous species usually causes pain that exceeds that expected for a similar mechanical injury, supporting envenomation as a component of the injury. Immediate and intense burning pain usually occurs, associated with a bleeding puncture wound and local erythema. The pain generally resolves over a period of hours. Systemic features have been reported, including nausea, vomiting, paresthesiae, muscular paralysis, hypotension, and respiratory distress (2,79). Sea urchins with pedicellariae have been reported to cause more severe effects (2).

ASTEROIDEA (SEA STARS)

Most sea stars only cause a minor traumatic injury and are not medically significant, but the crown-of-thorns sea star (*A. planci*) causes more severe effects. *A. planci* is found on most reefs in the Indo-Pacific region, and there have been large outbreaks in Japan and Australia (2). The animals are covered with sharp, rigid spines that can passively deliver a variety of substances when they penetrate skin. The toxic substances are a mixture of venom produced in special glandular tissue, mucus, bacteria, and dermal tissue. The local effects are similar to those of sea urchin stings with initial severe burning pain that lasts approximately 1 to 2 hours, associated with bleeding, erythema, and mild edema. The region may become dusky or discolored, particularly with multiple spine injuries. Systemic effects are uncommon but have been reported (1,2).

HOLOTHURIOIDEA (SEA CUCUMBERS)

Sea cucumbers are able to produce a toxin that is concentrated in the tentacular organs. The creatures do not have a venom apparatus, but direct contact may induce a contact dermatitis, which is usually mild due to dilution with sea water. In some regions of the world, sea cucumbers are eaten, but they have not been reported to cause major problems because they are either dried or nontoxic species. Injuries to the corneas and conjunctivae are of more consequence and may cause intense inflammation.

TREATMENT OF ECHINODERM INJURIES

Treatment of echinoderm stings is mainly symptomatic and, in line with other marine spine injuries, immersion in hot water is recommended for up to 30 to 90 minutes if there is evidence of envenomation (78). The extremity should be examined radiologically and broken spines or pedicellariae removed surgically as soon as possible before they migrate into deeper tissues. It has been suggested for sea urchin spines that bolus ejection of lidocaine into the lateral surfaces of an involved phalanx, then incising over the apex with a scalpel, can propel the spine out of an injured digit (80). Treatment of systemic symptoms is supportive, and analgesia may be needed. Granuloma formation may require excision.

PORIFERA (SPONGES)

The phylum of Porifera, or sponges, includes thousands of species of sedentary marine organisms that are the simplest of the multicellular organisms with a primitive tissue organization (13,81). They are composed of horny, elastic skeletons with spicules of silicon dioxide or calcium carbonate embedded in the connective tissue matrices. The term *Porifera* means pore bearers, which describes the external surface of the animal, which is perforated by small holes. The external shape of a Porifera may be well defined in more complex animals, but, in more primitive species, the animal has a far less defined morphology (2,13).

Pathophysiology

Although some sponges are horny and cause abrasions when handled, contact with chemical substances in the sponge also appears to cause the reactions (81). Sponges do not have a specialized venom gland, but many species produce crinotoxins (slimes or surface liquids), and a few species can cause skin irritation and dermatitis (2,13). Little evidence is available to suggest that hypersensitivity or allergy plays a role in this dermatitis, although patch testing has produced anaphylactoid reactions (82). Although there are a number of studies on the toxins produced by the sponges, the majority involved intravenous injection of the toxic substances into laboratory animals (13). The clinical relevance of these studies to contact effects in humans is unclear. Extracts of different marine sponges have also been shown to have antimicrobial, paralytic, antispasmodic, hypotensive, and neuroexcitatory effects (81,83). A study in South Australia of the toxicity of crinotoxin to skin demonstrated that two factors were involved but was unable to define this any further (13,57).

A more recent study investigated the properties of the extract and spicules of *Neofibularia mordens* (83). This study demonstrated that two different effects are likely to cause the response to skin contact with the sponge. The initial burning or stinging sensation is likely to be the result of contact with various neuroexcitatory substances that are present in the sponge extract (83). The second effect, which is much slower in onset, is probably the result of the intrusion of the silicon spicules into the skin. This would explain the slower onset and longer duration of the urticaria that occurs with sponge injuries, because the silicon is unlikely to be dissolved by metabolic processes (83). The effects of sponges in other regions of the world are similar, and it is likely that the mechanism of clinical effects is similar. Contact with some sponges causes no initial sensation and gradual onset of dermatitis, and it is possible that in these cases the injury is due entirely to the tiny spicules of silicon from the sponge breaking off in the skin.

Clinical Presentation

The clinical effects of sponge injuries vary considerably and are referred to as *stinging sponge dermatitis*. Usually no initial sensation occurs after contact with a sponge, but after a few minutes to hours, there is localized stinging and itching (2,82). The stinging or itching sensation generally increases in intensity over 2 to 3 days and may become almost unbearable. In some cases, there may be an initial prickly or burning sensation, which is characteristic of stings by *N. mordens* from southern Australia (83). Initially, erythema occurs at the contact site, which may then form papules, vesicles, or bullae. In some cases, there may be local swelling and edema and occasionally regional joint stiffness. In more severe cases, desquamation occurs approximately 3 weeks after the contact and has been reported with *N. mordens* (57,83). The effects may be persistent for days to weeks.

Few cases of sponge stings have been reported (13,57,83), and the majority occur in divers or persons collecting sponges (83). In Australia and New Zealand, significant reactions can occur after contact with *N. mordens* and *Lissodendoryx*. *N. mordens* causes the most severe stings in the Australasian region. Other *Neofibularia* spp. occur in northern Australia, as do *Haliclona* spp. Stings from several sponges have been reported in the United States, Hawaii, and the Caribbean Islands, including *Tedania ignis* (fire sponge), *Fibula nolitangere*, and *Microciona prolifera* (red sponge) (2,82,84). Stings from *T. ignis* are similar in severity to those of *N. mordens*. One case of erythema multiforme has been reported 10 days after contact with a sponge (85). Application of sponge extract to the rabbit cornea results in opacity and blindness, demonstrating the potential hazard to eyes (57,83). Direct contact of sponge material with the eye or contamination of the eye with the fingers may cause significant corneal injury or iritis. Skin plaques and postinflammatory pigmentation have been reported to persist for months (82).

Treatment

Numerous treatments have been suggested for the treatment of sponge injuries. However, it appears that these injuries generally run their natural course over weeks irrespective of various interventions (2). Decontamination of the contact region is likely to be the most important treatment. Attempts can be made to remove the spicules once the skin has been washed, but this may be difficult and in many cases impossible due to the size of these spicules. Some authors have suggested adhesive tape (73).

Other treatments are the same as those for other irritant contact dermatitides. Local treatment with cold packs may help relieve the symptoms, and oral or parenteral analgesia may be required. No evidence has supported the use of antihistamines, topical anesthetics, or corticosteroids (82). Topical steroid creams may be useful for severe cases but should not be applied if there is any evidence of infection.

Another condition consisting of an irritant skin rash is often referred to as *Mediterranean sponge diver's disease*. However, this condition is due to contact with co-inhabiting sea anemone on the sponge and is not a direct result of injury by the sponge (2).

ANNELIDA (BRISTLEWORMS)

Phylum Annelida includes the bristleworms, which are segmented marine worms covered with bristle-like setae that become erect on contact (13). These setae or spines easily detach from the worm and are able to penetrate human skin (86). Stings have been reported in many parts of the world, including Florida and the Caribbean waters (86). Initially, there is a burning sensation, followed by intense skin inflammation with a reddened urticarial rash. More severe effects such as necrosis are rare, but localized soft-tissue edema and itchiness may occur. In some cases, the effects may last for many weeks, although pain is unlikely to be problematic after 2 to 3 days.

MOLLUSCA (CONE SNAIL SHELLS)

Cone snail shells (*Conus* spp.) are beautiful, univalve creatures that are found mainly in the warmer regions of the Indo-Pacific, with the majority occurring in the Pacific Ocean (91%) (1). A few species occur in more temperate regions. *Conus* are venomous predators that have developed an effective mechanism for immobilizing fast-moving prey. The venom that they produce consists of a potent mixture of neurotoxic components, which has allowed these animals to overcome their lack of physical agility. Cone snails are often classified according to their feeding behavior: (a) piscivorous, (b) molluskivorous, or (c) vermivorous (87). The venoms are a complex mixture of small peptides and proteins, the conotoxins, which each have a high affinity and specificity for particular receptor targets (88,89). They have a broad range of pharmacologic effects, including blockade of Na^+, Ca^+, and K^+ channels and antagonism at nicotinic and serotonin receptor sites (89).

Clinical Presentation

Stings by cone snails are rare, with few published cases in the literature (1,90). Most cases are due to *Conus geographus*, although other *Conus* spp. have been implicated, including *C. omaria*, *C. textile*, and *C. marmoreus* (1). Although the fatality rate has been estimated to be almost 40% (90), the paucity of published reports suggests that this may be biased due to the mild cases not being published (1). Envenomations usually occur when there is prolonged contact with the shell or if the shell is significantly interfered with and occurs on the hand or finger.

Most reports are of *C. geographus*, which are characterized by local pain, numbness, and flaccid paralysis. The sting causes sharp pain, often described as equivalent to a bee sting in reported cases. The local pain is soon followed by numbness at the sting site. With significant envenomation the onset of effects is rapid. Localized numbness spreads proximally up the limb, usually to the shoulder, throat, and lips. Partial paralysis can develop in as rapid a time as 30 minutes, which then progresses to complete paralysis of voluntary muscles and to respiratory failure (1). The latter is believed to cause death, although coma is also reported. Less severe cases cause muscle pain, partial paralysis, or ataxia, or, in mild cases, only local effects. The numbness and weakness usually persist for a few days in survivors. Very few reports of other *Conus* spp. have been published, and, although some may be similar to *C. geographus*, the diversity in venom composition, feeding habits, and prey suggests that the effects may vary with species (88).

Treatment

No effective first-aid measures or antidotes are available. Treatment is symptomatic and supportive. The critical intervention is maintenance of the airway and oxygenation.

MOLLUSCA (BLUE-RINGED OCTOPUS)

The only cephalopods (octopi) that have been reported to cause significant envenomation belong to the genus *Hapalochlaena*, the

Australian blue-ringed octopus (2). Uncommon reports have appeared of poisoning from the ingestion of the flesh of some cephalopods in Japan (91). Fewer than 20 bites of the Australian blue-ringed octopus (*Hapalochlaena* spp.) have been reported in the literature over the last 50 years, with two known fatalities (32,92). The octopus can inject its neurotoxin, which it stores in modified venom glands. The neurotoxin was initially called *maculotoxin* until it was demonstrated that it was identical to TTX (93).

Clinical Presentation

The bite is usually painless but causes local bleeding with small puncture marks. They typically occur on the upper extremities because, in most cases, the patient is bitten while handling the animal. The first symptoms of envenomation may be generalized paresthesiae or nausea, dizziness, and malaise, and the onset is usually rapid (92,94). Neurologic features then develop, including flaccid paralysis, jerky muscular movements in some cases, and finally respiratory failure typical of TTX poisoning (2,92).

Treatment

The pressure immobilization technique (pressure bandage with immobilization) is recommended for cone snail shell and paralytic octopus envenomations. This technique is accomplished by wrapping the limb with a lymphatic occlusive bandage and then applying a splint (95). The wrap is maintained until the victim is brought to a medical facility where advanced life support can be provided. Other treatment is the same as for puffer fish poisoning, including supportive care, admission to intensive care, and mechanical ventilation. Full recovery is usual.

SILURIFORMES (CATFISH)

Approximately 1000 species of catfish inhabit fresh and salt water, although many do not contain venomous spines (2). People at risk from catfish stings include fishermen and, less commonly, water-sports participants. Worldwide, saltwater fishermen have sustained many serious envenomations from the Arabian Gulf catfish (*Aurius thalasinus*) and the Oriental or striped catfish (*Plotosus lineatus*), which possess potent marine toxins.

Table 2 lists catfish that have been implicated in envenomation (4). Eel-tailed catfish (Plotosidae) occur in the Indo-Pacific region and live in marine, estuarine, and freshwater enviroments. The striped catfish, *P. lineatus*, is an important member of this family and can cause severe pain requiring hospitalization (2), including stings in northern Australia (8). Forktailed catfish (Ariidae) also occur worldwide and cause only minor effects (8). Other families have a more restricted distribution, such as the family Ictaluridae (genus *Ictalurus* and *Noturus*), which includes the common freshwater catfish from North America, the Carolina madtom (*Noturus furiosus*) (96), the brown bullhead (*I. nebulosus*), the channel catfish (*I. punctatus*), the blue catfish (*I. furcatus*), and the catfish (*N. catus*) (2,96). The family Siluridae occurs throughout Europe and Asia and are large catfish, some species reaching up to 4 m in length (4).

TABLE 2. Catfish families implicated in envenomation

Family	Examples	Distribution
Ariidae	*Arius* spp.	Worldwide
Bagridae	*Liobagrus reini, Pseudobagrus*	Asia, Africa, Japan
Clariidae	*Clarias batrachus*	Indo-Pacific and India
Doradidae	*Pterodoras granulosus, Centrochir crocodili*	Fresh waters of South America
Heteropneustidae	*Heteropneustes fossilis*	India
Ictaluridae	*Ictalurus* and *Noturus*	America, from Canada to Guatemala
Pimelodidae	*Pimelodus clarias*	South America to Mexico
Plotosidae	*Plotosus lineatus, Cnidoglanis megastoma, Tandanus bostocki*	Indo-Pacific region and Australia
Siluridae	—	Africa and Asia

From Halstead BW. *Poisonous and venomous marine animals of the world,* 2nd ed. Princeton, NJ: Darwin Press, 1988, with permission.

Pathophysiology

Catfish have a single spine in the dorsal fin and spines in each of the pectoral fins that can inflict painful wounds. The venom glands are attached in the leading edges of the spines and are contained within integumentary sheaths. Penetration of the spine into the skin and subdermal tissues simultaneously causes the rupture of the spine integument, and venom is then injected into the wound (2). Many spines also have a series of razor-sharp teeth that act as barbs, making extraction of these structures difficult. The spines normally lie flat against the side of the fish but extend when the fish is frightened or agitated (2,96).

Some studies on catfish venoms have appeared, mainly from the more dangerous species such as *P. lineatus*, but the relevance of these to human envenomation is unclear. Components of *P. lineatus* produced muscular spasm, respiratory distress, neurotoxicity, hemolysis, and death in laboratory animals, but these effects are rarely reported in humans (1). Crinotoxins are proteinaceous toxins found in catfish epidermal secretions that coat the entire body, including the fins, and are now thought to play a part in spinous envenomation (1). Crinotoxins have been reported in at least two types of catfish (*A. thalasinus* and *P. lineatus*) (97,98). They can be introduced into the wound during envenomation and may be responsible for severe pain in fish handlers by merely coming in contact with the fish (2).

Clinical Presentation

The clinical effects of catfish stings vary enormously. Although fatalities have been attributed to catfish, this seems unlikely, and in one case it was secondary to septicemia (99). The effects of catfish stings range from a simple traumatic puncture injury to severe pain associated with envenomation (8,96,100–102). In most cases, localized pain is the major symptom, but it may radiate in more severe cases. The pain usually subsides within an hour, but with more severe envenomation, such as with some marine catfish (e.g., *P. lineatus*), the pain may persist for up to 48 hours.

Local effects may be confined to a puncture mark but in more severe cases may cause bleeding, edema, and erythema (8,96,100–102). Occasionally, the spine may break off and have to be removed. The most significant complication of catfish injuries is secondary infection, including large wound infections, tendon sheath infections, and septic arthritis (101,103). Although many catfish have nonvenomous spines, injuries still have a significant risk of infection (104).

STONEFISH (*SYNANCEIA* SPECIES)

Stonefish (*Synanceia* spp.) belong to the family Synanceiidae and include the Australian estuarine stonefish (*S. trachynis*), the

Indian stonefish (*S. horrida*), and the reef stonefish (*S. verrucosa*). They occur throughout tropical and warm temperate oceans, including the central Pacific, west through the Indo-Pacific and east to the African coast. Stonefish are stationary bottom dwellers that camouflage themselves well. The majority of human encounters occur when they are trodden on. They are often found in shallow water, which is where most injuries occur.

Pathophysiology

The venom apparatus of stonefish is highly developed and consists of paired venom glands that are associated with the 13 dorsal spines of the fish (1). Each spine of *S. trachynis* produces approximately 6 mg venom, with a total of up to 88 mg per fish (105). Many toxins have been isolated from the three major species. Early work demonstrated that the venom was heat labile and contained components that caused cardiotoxicity, myotoxicity, and neurotoxicity (105,106). Ongoing research has demonstrated that the venoms of *Synanceia* spp. are highly complex, with multiple components and enzymatic effects (76). It has been demonstrated that the venom of the Australian stonefish causes calcium influx into murine cortical neurons (107). *In vivo* work with the same venom shows that there is an initial hypertensive response to intravenous injection of venom followed by a depressor response (78). These effects are reversed *in vitro* and *in vivo* by stonefish antivenom (78,107).

Like most of the work on toxins isolated from venomous fish, the clinical relevance of these studies is unclear (1,2). Although the venom of *S. trachynis* has been reported to cause myotoxicity, cardiotoxicity, and neurotoxicity (78), these effects are rarely seen with human envenomation. Marine venom research has also been complicated by differences in methodology and in the effects caused by lyophilized compared to milked venom, making comparison between the species difficult (108).

Clinical Presentation

Few confirmed reports of stonefish envenomations have appeared. It is thought that they can cause fatal effects, but this conclusion is not based on well-documented definite stings (109,110). The clinical effects are characterized by immediate severe and increasing local pain that may radiate proximally. Significant local swelling and erythema are usually present (2,8,109–111).

Systemic effects occur in more severe cases, including sweating, nausea, and hypotension, and even syncope may occur. However, systemic effects are more likely due to severe pain, although transient pulmonary edema has been reported in one patient (110). Extensive tissue necrosis is unlikely and usually secondary to infection if it occurs (2) (often associated with retained spine material). Whether there are regional variations in severity of stonefish envenoming remains to be ascertained.

Treatment

Stonefish antivenom is the only currently available antivenom for venomous fish stings. It is a horse-derived Fab'2 antivenom produced by Commonwealth Serum Laboratories in Australia against *S. trachynis* (76). The antivenom was first developed in 1959 and has been shown to reverse the lethal, vascular permeability, cardiovascular, and hemolytic effects in animal studies (76,78,106). Each ampule of antivenom contains 2000 units, which should neutralize 20 mg venom. The antivenom is recommended for intramuscular administration, but there is increasing evidence from other antivenoms that the intravenous route is more appropriate.

It has been suggested that stonefish antivenom may be effective for other venomous fish stings, based on its reversal of *in vitro* and *in vivo* venom effects in animals, such as the soldierfish (*Gymnapistes marmoratus*) and lionfish (*Pterois volitans*) (78,112,113), but there is currently no clinical evidence to support this conclusion. A study of bullrout (*Notesthes robusta*) venom in Australia demonstrated no reaction with stonefish antivenom (19).

SCORPAENIDAE (SCORPIONFISH, ROCKFISH, AND LIONFISH)

Scorpionfish (Scorpaenidae) occur worldwide but most commonly in tropical and temperate oceans and seas. At least 80 members of the family have been implicated in envenomation. The scorpionids are a diverse group of fish, with differing habitats and ability to camouflage; they may be stationary fish or slow-moving swimmers (2). Their venom apparatus varies between species, with most having 10 to 15 dorsal spines, 2 pelvic, and 3 anal spines associated with venom glands.

Pterois volitans (Lionfish)

Lionfish are probably the most commonly reported fish to cause stings in the United States because they are kept in aquariums (14,16,17). They occur in all oceans, but outside of aquarium-related injuries, the majority of stings occur in the tropics, both Indo-Pacific and Mediterranean. They are one of the most colorful venomous fish, with large fan-like fins, and go by many common names, including "lionfish" and "butterfly cod."

Venom extracted from the stinging spines has similar effects *in vitro* and *in vivo* to other marine toxins. It produces contraction in chick biventer cervicis muscle and causes an increased intracellular Ca^{2+} in murine cortical neurons (107). Earlier work on *P. volitans* venom demonstrated that it causes a biphasic response in the anesthetized rat that appears to be the result of protein toxins acting on muscarinic cholinergic receptors and adrenoceptors (113). In addition, it was demonstrated that stonefish antivenom reversed the majority of effects of the venom *in vivo* and *in vitro* (113).

In three poison center studies from the United States reporting a total of 101 lionfish stings, almost all occurred on the hand or fingers as a result of a lionfish kept in an aquarium (14,16,17). Severe local pain was universal (14,16,17) and radiated to the affected extremity in about one-fifth of patients in the study by Kizer et al. (14). Swelling up to two to three times normal size occurred in 30% to 60% of patients (14,17). Less commonly, vesicles at the sting site occurred.

In one series, 6 of 45 patients were reported to have systemic effects, including nausea, diaphoresis, dyspnea, chest and abdominal pain, generalized weakness, hypotension, and syncope (14). However, the retrospective nature of a study including calls to a poison center makes it difficult to determine the significance of systemic effects and whether they were a result of venom-mediated effects or secondary to pain (14).

Gymnapistes marmoratus (Soldierfish or Cobbler)

Soldierfish occur in southern Australia and are characterized by a lack of scales on the head and body (114). The venom apparatus consists of 13 dorsal, 3 anal, 2 pectoral, and 4 opercular spines. The venom has been shown to cause similar effects to stonefish venom (107), with significant cardiovascular effects mediated by muscarinic receptors and adrenoceptors (115). Stonefish antivenom has been shown to reverse venom effects *in vitro* and in anesthetized rats (112). No confirmed reports have been published of envenomation by *G. marmoratus*, but unpublished cases suggest that the effects are similar to those of other fish stings, although less severe.

Scorpaena Species

Scorpaena spp. are responsible for stings in many parts of the world (2,14). *S. guttata*, or sculpin, is a common edible fish found on the Pacific coast. Stings are common on the hands of fishermen who encounter sculpin that are caught in nets with other fish, and the effects are similar to those of other scorpaenidae. *S. ergastulorum* (red rock cod) occurs in eastern Australia and is commonly handled by fishermen. It has spines on the dorsum and head and is reported to cause mild pain with scratches. However, severe pain after puncture injuries has been reported associated with pallor, writhing, vomiting, and collapse, although the systemic effects are likely to be secondary to pain (116).

Notesthes robusta (Bullrout)

The bullrout occurs in slow-moving streams and tidal estuaries in coastal waters of eastern Australia and belongs to the Scorpaenidae family. It is responsible for seasonal stings (November to January). They occur in rocks and weeds and usually cause injuries to the feet. They have 15 spines that erect when the fish is disturbed (117). A report of 16 cases described the main effect to be severe pain that radiated up the affected limb (117). Almost all stings are on the feet because the fish is a bottom dweller in muddy river shallows. Despite the severe pain only minor swelling occurs (117), but radiating pain appears to be common. An algesic substance has been identified in *N. robusta* venom, which is a 170-kd protein that consistently caused pain in human subjects and has been called *nocitoxin* (19).

Other scorpionids include *Centropogon australis* (Fortescue), *Neosebastes* spp., and *Hypodytes carinatus* (ocellated waspfish), which appear to cause similar effects (2,114).

TRACHINIDAE (WEEVERFISH)

Weeverfish are all marine fish found in the Mediterranean, European coastal areas, Black Sea, and Pacific Ocean off the coast of Chile (2). Four species are found in Europe, including the greater weeverfish (*Trachinus draco*) and the lesser weeverfish (*Echiichtis vipera*) (2). Weeverfish are bottom dwellers that sting when stepped on. The greater weeverfish is a large deep sea fish that usually only stings fishermen who handle the fish in nets (4,118). The lesser weeverfish is responsible for stings on beaches in the United Kingdom (119). Weeverfish have five obviously visible dorsal spines and a few less visible ones that are responsible for stings (2). These spines are able to pierce a leather boot.

A number of studies on the venoms of weeverfish have shown them to be proteinaceous and highly labile venoms (2,120). Studies of venom from *T. draco* demonstrated that the venom had hemolytic properties and was lethal in a mouse model. The hemolytic properties and lethal effects were abolished by heat or proteolytic enzyme treatment (120). Dracotoxin, a hemolytic toxin, has been isolated from *T. draco* (121). The venom of the lesser weeverfish, *E. vipera*, has also been shown to contain a lethal fraction (122).

The literature remains confusing in regard to the severity of stings by weeverfish. Three deaths from weeverfish stings were reported from the late eighteenth century and nineteenth century, but they were likely to be a result of secondary infection (123). The majority of case series and reports suggest that severe pain is the main feature, although persistent local inflammation may occur for up to a week with greater weeverfish. One study of stings included 39 cases on beaches in Wales that were followed up. This demonstrated that the majority of stings cause only moderate effects (119). In 18 patients, pain lasted for less than 1 hour, and in only 8 did pain last longer than 6 hours. Half of the patients reported that their feet felt abnormal after 24 hours, one patient had an embedded spine removed, and one patient developed a painful lump that discharged after 4 weeks.

Hot-water immersion for 5 to 20 minutes was used in 24 of 39 patients, and 23 reported improvement (119). A number of stings by the greater weeverfish from the Mediterranean have been reported (2,118). In a report of three cases, the sting caused severe pain that was helped by hot-water immersion but ultimately required opioid analgesia (118). One patient was followed up, which demonstrated that local inflammatory effects can take a week or more to resolve (118). In France, 31 cases of weeverfish stings were reported in which pain was universal, swelling occurred in a majority, and other symptoms were less common (124).

STINGRAYS (ORDER: RAJIFORMES)

Stingrays have a characteristic dorsoventrally flattened appearance with pectoral flaps (fins) that they use for propulsion. The gills are confined to the ventral surface (4). Stingrays can cause significant trauma and envenomation (8,11,125–131).

The suborder Myliobatoidea includes a number of ray families that include the venomous rays (Table 3), five marine families, and one fresh-water group. In temperate regions, including Australia (130) and the West Coast of the United States (131,132), Urolophidae (round stingrays or stingarees) are commonly implicated. The family Dasyatidae (stingrays or whiprays) are another important family in tropical regions, including northern Australia, the Indo-Pacific region, and the southeast coast of the United States (8,126,132,133).

The venom apparatus of stingrays is a whip-like striking organ (spine) attached to the dorsal surface of the creature. These creatures rest on the bottom, often buried in the sand. The sting victim can then tread on the stingray, causing the tail to whip upward reflexively and thrust the spines into the victim. The sting can produce a significant laceration and, less commonly, a puncture wound. The traumatic wound itself is dangerous and increases the risk of infection. Venom is

TABLE 3. Families of venomous stingrays

Family	Common name	Examples	Distribution
Dasyatidae	Stingrays or whiprays	*Dasyatis, Taeniura, Urogymnus*	Worldwide
Potamotrygonidae	River rays	*Potamotrygon*	South America
Gymnuridae	Butterfly rays	*Gymnura*	America
Urolophidae	Round stingrays or stingarees	*Urolophus*	Worldwide
Myliobatidae	Devil rays or bat rays	*Aetobatus narinari, Myliobati*	Worldwide
Rhinopteridae	Cow-nosed rays	Rhinoptera	America and Europe

From Williamson JA, Fenner PJ, Burnett JW, et al. *Venomous and poisonous marine animals.* Sydney: New South Wales Press, 1996; and Halstead BW. *Poisonous and venomous marine animals of the world,* 2nd ed. Princeton, NJ: Darwin Press, 1988, with permission.

simultaneously injected. Little work has been done on the venoms of stingrays because the venom is difficult to obtain and extract from the animals. Russell et al. (132) demonstrated that the venom caused cardiovascular collapse as well as neurologic effects when injected intravenously and intraperitoneally to rats.

Clinical Presentation

The majority of injuries occur to the lower limb when the stingray is trodden on in shallow water. Injuries to the hands occur when stingrays are caught. Divers have sustained injuries to the chest or abdomen that are far more significant (8,11,125,128). Similar to other venomous fish, the spine can occasionally break off in the wound.

Envenomation causes intense local pain resulting from the trauma and the antalgic effects of the venom. The pain can radiate proximally and may last for a number of hours. Significant hemorrhage is common, and the wound often becomes swollen and red. Systemic effects have been reported, but in the majority of cases these can be accounted for by severe pain.

The most significant problem with stingray injuries is that the length and size of the spine mean that there can be significant trauma to limbs or, more important, penetrating trauma to other body cavities (8,11,125,128). Abdominal or thoracic trauma is made worse by the presence of toxins that prevent healing and can cause infection if not treated early. Secondary infection is the other major concern after stingray injuries, particularly wounds penetrating joint or tendon spaces and wounds that are not cleaned or managed appropriately initially.

OTHER VENOMOUS FISH

Scats (Family Scatophagidae)

Scats are less well-known but can cause significant pain. They occur in the Indo-Pacific Ocean, where they usually inhabit inshore, coastal areas, often near cities in the Australasian region (1,4). In northern Australia, stings from the most common species, the silver scat, striped butterfish, or spadefish (*Selenotoca multifasciata*) have been reported (8,134). Stings cause immediate severe pain that peaks after approximately 5 to 15 minutes and lasts up to an hour but has minimal other local effects. Spadefish have become popular aquarium fish, particularly in the United States (1), although there are no reports of stings.

Enoplus armatus ("Old Wife" or Zebrafish)

Zebrafish have been implicated in spine injuries, but no studies of the spines have confirmed that the fish has a venom apparatus. Most injuries cause minor pain, but more severe effects have been reported (135).

Rabbitfish or Happy Moments (Family Siganidae)

Rabbitfish occur in the tropical regions of the Indo-Pacific Ocean. *Siganus* spp. are reported to cause severe pain that may last for hours (2), which is similar to scorpaenids.

Heterodontus portusjacksoni (Port Jackson Shark)

H. portusjacksoni is an Australian shark that has venomous spines at the front of each of its dorsal fins. Fisherman may be injured by these spines when the fish moves about on a line. The spines cause significant jagged wounds, and there are three reports of muscle weakness of the affected limb being associated with the injuries (135).

MANAGEMENT OF VENOMOUS FISH INJURIES

The treatment of venomous fish stings includes managing the envenomation and the traumatic injury. In many cases the venom-mediated effects are more significant and medical treatment is most appropriate, but with large traumatic wounds the latter takes priority. Treatment consists of reversing the effects of venom, relieving pain, and preventing infection.

First Aid

All wounds should be immediately irrigated and visible pieces of the spine or integumentary sheath removed. First-aid measures should include control of any hemorrhage and hot-water immersion therapy. Hot-water immersion should be done as soon as possible. The affected limb should be immersed in hot water [113°F (45°C)] for 30 to 90 minutes or until pain is relieved. The temperature should first be tested with the unaffected limb. Many of the toxins appear to be heat labile, although it is unclear if this is the reason that hot water appears to be effective treatment. Hot-water immersion has been shown to be at least partially effective in almost all venomous fish stings in a number of studies (8,14,118,119). During hot-water immersion, the wound can be explored and foreign material removed.

Supportive Care

If the pain does not respond to hot-water immersion, adequate analgesia is required. Local infiltration of the wound with local anesthetic (without epinephrine) or a regional nerve block is often more effective with severe pain and has been reported for lionfish, catfish, and bullrout envenomation (117,136,137). Great care must be taken with hot water once the sting site or limb has been anesthetized to prevent burns. Antivenom is available for stonefish envenomation and is discussed in Stonefish (Synanceia Species).

Optimal wound outcome depends not only on removal of foreign material but also on consideration of secondary bacterial infection. Deep wounds or obviously infected injuries should be cultured. Soft-tissue radiography should be used to visualize calcified matter. Lacerations caused by stingray envenomations should be left open for delayed primary closure or, rarely, sutured loosely, ensuring adequate drainage. Inpatient therapy may also be required in patients with deep wounds, long delays in wound care, wounds with retained foreign material, or spine penetration of sterile body cavities.

The use of prophylactic antibiotics remains controversial. Although some authors routinely recommend prophylactic antibiotics (73), increasing evidence shows that this is unnecessary. The few large series of venomous fish stings, and the experience of aquarium workers, is that most injuries are minor and do not require antibiotics (8,11,96). A retrospective review of stingray envenomations in the United States also demonstrated no benefit of prophylactic antibiotics (15). Antibiotics should be considered if the wound is large, considerable foreign material is present, or there is a delay in presentation. It is essential that patients who are discharged from the hospital are followed up for at least 24 to 48 hours and that any sign of infection is treated early.

In patients with obvious infection after a venomous fish sting, appropriate culture should be taken and correct antimicrobial therapy initiated. Because marine microorganisms usually require special selective media, the clinician should inform the microbiology laboratory that a marine-acquired organism might be present. In one study, a delay between admission and initiation of antibiotic treatment of 24 hours for established marine infection resulted in a mortality of 33%, whereas a delay of 72 hours resulted in almost 100% mortality (138).

Many marine wound infections are polymicrobial, and skin flora still remain the commonest organisms involved. Initially, empiric therapy should be started based on the clinical condition and the need for early antibiotic therapy, which is well established in definite marine infections in patients who are at risk (diabetes, liver disease, iron overload, or immunosuppressed) (138). A penicillinase-resistant penicillin or a first-generation cephalosporin is appropriate to cover skin flora. This agent should be used in conjunction with a tetracycline, a quinolone (e.g., ciprofloxacin), or a third-generation cephalosporin (e.g., ceftazidime) for marine-acquired injuries, where *Vibrio* infection is the most important consideration. Alternatively, in fresh-water infections, in which *Aeromonas* is more important, the recommended antibiotics are sulfamethoxazole-trimethoprim, a quinolone, a third-generation cephalosporin, or imipenem.

TABLE 4. Clinical grading system for tetrodotoxin poisoning

Grade of poisoning	Clinical features	Onset
Grade 1	Perioral numbness and paresthesiae, with or without gastrointestinal symptoms (mainly nausea)	5–45 min
Grade 2	Lingual numbness, numbness of face, and other areas (distal); early motor paralysis and incoordination; slurred speech; normal reflexes	10–60 min
Grade 3	Generalized flaccid paralysis, respiratory failure, aphonia and fixed/dilated pupils; patient remains conscious	15 min to several hours
Grade 4	Severe respiratory failure and hypoxia; hypotension, bradycardia, and cardiac dysrhythmias; unconsciousness may occur	15 min to 24 h

Modified from Fukuda A, Tani I. Records of puffer poisonings. *Nippon Igaku oyobi Kenko Hoken* 1941;(3528):7–13; and Isbister GK, Son J, Wang F, et al. Puffer fish poisoning: a potentially life-threatening condition. *Med J Aust* 2002;177:650–653.

PUFFER FISH POISONING

TTX poisoning is the commonest lethal marine poisoning and is most often the result of ingesting puffer fish or "fugu" in Japan. Puffer fish poisoning is confined mainly to southeast Asia and is more common in Japan, where fugu is a delicacy and commonly consumed (139–141). Before 1950, 100 deaths per year were reported in Japan (142). Although improved legislation of marketing and preparation of the fish has reduced the incidence of puffer fish poisoning in Japan, it remains the commonest cause of fatal food poisoning there because of unlicensed cooks and untrained preparation of the fish (139,142). A 4-year-old child died from puffer fish poisoning in Australia, and the frequency of poisoning is increasing there (143).

Pathophysiology

TTX poisoning occurs from ingestion of a broad range of bony fish from families in the order Tetraodontiformes, most importantly from the family Tetraodontidae (puffer fish) (142). TTX is present in increasingly higher concentrations in the skin, intestines, ovary, and liver of the fish (139). TTX has also been isolated from xanthid crabs, and there have been a number of cases of TTX poisoning after the ingestion of the eggs or flesh of crabs (144,145). TTX is a guanidinium toxin and a selective blocker of voltage-sensitive sodium channels that prevents conduction in motor and sensory nerves by blocking sodium channels at the nodes of Ranvier (142,146). It blocks Na^+ channels at concentrations over the single nanomolar range and thereby exhibits effects on action potential generation and impulse conduction.

Nerve conduction studies in single cases of TTX poisoning have indicated that TTX equally and reversibly affected myelinated nerve fibers throughout the entire length of the axon (147). In a series of four patients with TTX poisoning, neurophysiologic investigation was undertaken within 24 hours of ingestion and the results compared to previously established normative data (143). Each patient had profound abnormalities in parameters dependent on Na^+ channel function. Nerves in these four patients were of high threshold, had slow conduction, and exhibited reduced amplitude compound potentials, indicating that some axons were unable to conduct at all. The effect on amplitude was greater in sensory neurons compared to motor axons, which was consistent with the prominence of sensory symptoms (dysesthesiae and numbness) over motor involvement (weakness) in the patients (143).

Clinical Presentation

TTX poisoning causes perioral numbness and paresthesiae, distal limb numbness and paresthesiae, ataxia, dizziness, and muscle weakness. It is usually associated with nausea and less commonly vomiting. In more severe cases, respiratory muscle paralysis, coma, and cardiovascular toxicity (hypotension and dysrhythmias) occur. A clinical grading system has been developed for TTX poisoning and is shown in Table 4 (1,143).

TTX poisoning has a rapid onset of effects that is correlated with the ultimate severity. In moderately severe cases symptoms occur within 90 minutes. In reported fatal cases and severe poisoning, symptoms have almost always developed within 1 to 2 hours (148).

Treatment

Puffer fish poisoning has caused many deaths, particularly in Japan, and no antidote or antivenom is available. The mainstay of treatment is careful observation and serial neurologic examination to determine progression of more severe effects such as respiratory failure. Supportive care and admission to an intensive care unit are required in more severe cases to prevent complications from coma, muscle paralysis, and cardiovascular effects. Atropine is indicated for bradycardia.

Neostigmine has been suggested to be an effective treatment in a number of case reports and series of TTX poisoning (149,150). Although individual case reports support its efficacy, this has not been confirmed in controlled trials. The postulated mechanism of anticholinesterase treatment suggested by proponents is that TTX causes a competitive reversible blockade of the motor endplate, in addition to its effects on nerve conduction (141). Other case reports demonstrated that neostigmine had no effect (151), and animal studies show that TTX appears to have no effect at the neuromuscular junction (152).

Awareness of TTX poisoning is important for health professionals because of its potential severity and the importance of instituting early supportive care. It has been suggested that patients with all but the mildest cases (grade I) (Table 4) should be admitted for observation until the peak of effects has passed. After 24 hours it is extremely unlikely that life-threatening effects will develop in patients who are not already severely poisoned. With good supportive care, there should be no untoward outcomes if the diagnosis is made early.

CIGUATERA POISONING

Ciguatera is the most common foodborne illness associated with the ingestion of fish and, although rarely fatal, affects far more people than puffer fish poisoning (153–161). It is endemic throughout the subtropical and tropical parts of the Indo-Pacific region and the Caribbean (153–161) but is occurring more commonly in nonendemic areas because reef fish can be shipped or flown to distant locations (1).

Ciguatera results from the ingestion of certain tropical and subtropical finfish that have accumulated ciguatoxins (CTX), either by ingesting other toxic fish or by eating benthic (bottom-dwelling) algae (153,162). CTX arise from the biotransformation of less polar compounds (gambiertoxins) that are produced by the marine dinoflagellate *Gambierdiscus toxicus* (162) that lives on macroalgae, usually attached to dead coral. CTX and their metabolites are then concentrated in the food chain, as carnivorous fish eat the smaller herbivorous fish that ingest the dinoflagellates. Humans sit at the top of this marine food chain (154,162).

A large number of fish have been implicated in ciguatera, but only a few are regularly involved (162). Although a number of herbivorous fish, such as the Acanthurids (surgeonfish) and corallivorous Scarids (parrotfish), are primary vectors for the toxins, they are rarely caught for human consumption (154). More commonly, carnivorous fish cause human poisoning. The common reef fish involved in the Pacific and Caribbean are listed in Table 5. Fish that contain CTX do not smell, taste, or appear any different to other fish, and detection of CTX in reef fish remains a problem (162).

Pathophysiology

CTX are heat-stable, lipid-soluble, polyether toxins, and more than 20 precursor gambiertoxins and CTX have been identified in *G. toxicus*, herbivorous, and carnivorous fish (162). The two major classes of CTX are Pacific ciguatoxins (P-CTX) and Caribbean CTX, which appear to underlie the regional differences in the clinical effects of ciguatera (154). P-CTX-1 is the dominant CTX found in carnivorous fish in the Pacific and is tenfold more toxic (causes ciguatera at concentrations of 0.1 mg/kg fish flesh) than the gambiertoxins found in *G. toxicus* and of the main Caribbean CTX, Caribbean CTX-1 (162). A third class has now been identified that appears to be responsible for the different pattern of effects seen in the Indian Ocean (154).

CTX are the most potent known Na^+ channel toxins in mammals and activate voltage-sensitive sodium channels at nanomolar and picomolar concentrations (154). CTX cause a hyperpolarizing shift of the voltage dependence of channel activation that causes sodium channels to open at resting membrane potentials. This then leads to the spontaneous firing of various nerve types as TTX-sensitive Na^+ channels are activated. The increased spontaneous activity, membrane excitability, and instability of various nerves cause the neurologic manifestations of the condition. Brevetoxin [neurotoxic shellfish poisoning (NSP)] and CTX share the same binding site on voltage-sensitive sodium channels. Although maitotoxins and scaritoxin (re-identified as P-CTX-4A) have previously been implicated in the pathogenesis of ciguatera, this is unlikely to be the case.

Clinical Presentation

Ciguatera is rarely fatal but causes significant acute and occasionally persistent effects. It is characterized by moderate to severe gastrointestinal effects (vomiting, diarrhea, and abdominal cramps), neurologic effects (myalgia, paresthesiae, burning of skin on contact with cold water, back pain, ataxia, and headache), and, to a lesser extent, cardiovascular effects (155–161). Studies from many parts of the Indo-Pacific and Atlantic regions demonstrate that the proportion of clinical effects varies in different regions, but the characteristic combination of effects is similar (157,158,163).

The commonest clinical features and the frequency of these effects based on several large studies in different regions are listed in Table 6 (155–160). In the Pacific, the neurologic features

TABLE 5. Fish species implicated in cases of ciguatera from Pacific regions and the Caribbean

Fish family	Included fish and common names
Muraenids	Moray eels
Lutjanids	Red bass, snappers
Serranids	Sea bass and groupers, includes coral trout from the Great Barrier Reef
Epinephelids	Cod, including flowery cod and spotted cod
Lethrinids	Emperors and scavengers
Scombrids	Mackerel, including tunas, Spanish mackerel
Carangids[a]	Jacks and scads
Sphyraenids[a]	Barracuda

[a]Specific problems in the Caribbean.
From Meier J, White J. *Handbook of clinical toxicology of animal venoms and poisons.* Boca Raton, FL: CRC Press, 1995; and Lewis RJ. The changing face of ciguatera. *Toxicon* 2001;39:97–106, with permission.

TABLE 6. Frequency of clinical effects in cases of ciguatera from Pacific regions and the Atlantic

Clinical features	Frequency range (%)
Gastrointestinal features	
Diarrhea	50–78
Abdominal pain	47–70
Vomiting	30–38
Nausea	26–55
Neurologic effects	
Myalgia	56–83
Paresthesiae (mouth, hands, and/or feet)	52–91
Arthralgia	62–86
Cold allodynia (burning on contact with cold)	55–94
Headache	50–74
Ataxia	38–54
Dizziness or vertigo	38–62
Other effects	
Loss of energy/asthenia/weakness	60–90
Pruritus	42–78
Perspiration	34–43
Mood disorders	23–50
Bradycardia	9–16
Eye pain	22–41
Dental pain	25–43
Dysuria	10–26
Skin rash	0–26

Data from references 1,153,155–160,168,221.

predominate, whereas the gastrointestinal features predominate in the Caribbean Sea (154). In the Indian Ocean is a third cluster of symptoms characterized by hallucinations, incoordination, loss of equilibrium, depression, and nightmares (154). The differences are most likely due to different CTX, but differing dose and individual susceptibility may also play a role.

The *gastrointestinal effects* usually develop first but are occasionally delayed up to 12 hours and resolve within 24 hours. Neurologic features develop over a 24-hour period, with paresthesiae and numbness of the lips occurring early. In one study of 219 cases in Queensland, Australia, there was an "incubation" period of about 2 to 8 hours, and effects had developed in 90% of patients within 12 hours, although in a few cases it took longer than 24 hours (157). The onset time varied significantly, even between individuals who consumed the same fish (157).

Neurologic effects are very common, with paresthesiae, cold allodynia, or numbness occurring in more than 90% of all patients. Paresthesiae develop in the extremities and perioral1y. Cold allodynia or dysesthesia associated with contact with cold water or objects is almost pathognomonic of ciguatera and is not a true temperature reversal. A study of 50 patients demonstrated that these neurologic symptoms were associated with objective signs of polyneuropathy, with 80% having abnormal temperature sensation, more than half having abnormal pinprick and vibration sensation (stocking-glove distribution), and a third having diminished light touch sensation (153). Tendon areflexia only occurred in 10%, and cerebellar signs were rare. Although this was a small study and probably biased by including more severe cases, it suggests that the polyneuropathy of ciguatera is a predominantly sensory, length-dependent neuropathy of mixed large- and small-fiber involvement with prominent small-fiber dysfunction (153). Neurologic symptoms may persist for as long as 6 months and with repeated exposure can persist longer.

The *clinical course* is one of acute illness that resolves without lasting effect. It is estimated that approximately 3% to 20% have chronic effects of ciguatera poisoning (164). These effects are characterized by fatigue and loss of energy, arthralgia (especially knees, ankles, shoulders, and elbows), myalgia, headache, and pruritus (157). The symptoms often fluctuate and are difficult to treat. In addition, mood disorders, including depression and anxiety, can be associated with the acute and chronic forms. In contrast to some venom-induced illnesses, immunity is not conferred by repeated exposure; rather, sensitization to the toxins appears to occur (157). It appears that persons with a previous history of exposure have a more rapid onset of effects. In addition, eating other fish species not usually associated with ciguatera and even chicken sometimes appears to provoke a recurrence. Most unusual is that alcohol consumption may cause a recurrence, as occurred in 28% of cases in Queensland (157). Alcohol also appears to increase the severity of the acute illness.

Diagnostic Tests

Currently, no laboratory method is available to confirm ciguatera ingestion. A pilot study demonstrated that a neuroblastoma cell bioassay for seafood toxins detected elevated concentrations in 40% of symptomatic patients with a history of seafood ingestion (165). However, until a more sensitive and specific test is available, the diagnosis should be made on the history and symptoms. A number of methods have been used for the identification of CTX in the flesh of the fish, but this has usually been completely eaten or lost.

Treatment

No specific evidence-based treatment is available for acute ciguatera poisoning, and good supportive care, including appropriate rehydration (intravenous if required), observation, and symptomatic relief, is the mainstay of therapy. Uncommon cardiovascular complications, such as symptomatic bradycardia or severe hypotension, require treatment with atropine or intravenous fluids (153). For delayed and chronic effects, a number of agents have been used with variable success.

Mannitol therapy had been accepted as the treatment of choice for ciguatera because it was initially suggested in an uncontrolled study of 24 patients (166). The initial study was supported by case reports, several nonrandomized studies, and a randomized but not double-blinded study (153). The lack of benefit for mannitol was shown in a double-blinded randomized controlled trial, which compared mannitol treatment to normal saline in 50 patients with ciguatera (153). At 24 hours, some improvement of symptoms was reported in 96% of mannitol-treated patients and 92% of normal saline-treated patients. The prevalence of polyneuropathic symptoms and signs had reduced by about half in both groups. The groups did not differ in requirement for additional treatment, and treatment satisfaction in the two groups was equal. Discomfort or pain at the infusion site occurred in 84% of patients treated with mannitol compared to 36% treated with normal saline (p = .015). The study demonstrates that mannitol was no more useful than normal saline but caused more side effects (153). A study on CTX-intoxicated rats using mannitol found that mannitol did not reverse the effects of CTX on nerve conduction (167).

Supportive care is used for neuropathic pain, dysesthesiae, and pruritus associated with ciguatera. Amitriptyline has been used in a small series of patients and a number of case reports with symptomatic improvement. It is postulated that the beneficial effect is a result of sodium channel modulation (168–170). Tocainide was reported effective in three patients, and mexiletine has been suggested, also based on its sodium channel action (171). Gabapentin improved symptoms of dysesthesiae, pruritus, and shooting pain when administered 1 month after the event (172). Cessation of the medication resulted in a recurrence of symptoms initially, and then after 3 weeks of further treatment only minor symptoms remained off treatment. Nifedipine has also been used with some success (170). These agents have not been tested in controlled trials. It is important that controlled trials are undertaken before any of these agents are routinely recommended, especially in the light of the initial mistaken effectiveness of mannitol in acute treatment.

SHELLFISH POISONING

Contamination of shellfish is a medical and an economic problem that affects many fisheries, especially in temperate regions, including Japan, Southeast Asia (173), Central (174) and North America (175,176), North Africa (177), and Europe (32,178). Shellfish are the vectors for a number of illnesses, including infections (viral and bacterial), allergies, and toxin poisoning. Viral and bacterial infections are the most common cause of shellfish-related illness, including *Salmonella*, *Vibrio* spp., Norwalk, and Hepatitis A (1). In addition, heavy metal poisoning can result in contaminated areas because the filters that feed shellfish concentrate heavy metals in a similar way that they concentrate toxins. The epidemiology of shellfish poisoning is not well known, and different types of shellfish poisoning occur in different regions of the world. In the United States, toxic shellfish poisoning accounts for approximately 1.1% of foodborne illness or 7.4% of marine intoxications (1).

Four major toxic syndromes result from the ingestion of shellfish. They are produced by different microorganisms (1,21).

1. *PSP* is caused by saxitoxin and gonyautoxins (GTXs) and their derivatives and results in a clinical syndrome with paralysis similar to that of TTX poisoning. It is the commonest form of shellfish poisoning.
2. *Neurotoxic shellfish poisoning* is caused by brevetoxins and results in neuroexcitatory effects.
3. *Diarrhetic shellfish poisoning* (DSP) is caused by okadaic acid (OA) and its derivatives and results in severe gastroenteritis and fluid loss.
4. *Amnesic or encephalopathic shellfish poisoning* is caused by domoic acid and results in severe gastroenteritis associated with confusion, memory loss, headaches, and coma.

PARALYTIC SHELLFISH POISONING

PSP is the most common form of toxin-related disease associated with shellfish ingestion and occurs in many parts of the world. Deaths continue to occur from PSP in many countries (1), particularly in children, in whom the case-fatality rate has been greater than 50% (179,180). The incidence appears to have increased over the last 30 years, with its appearance in parts of the world where it has not previously been reported (181). However, ciguatera is still a far more common condition (21,181). The clinical syndrome is almost indistinguishable from TTX poisoning, consistent with the similarities between TTX and PSP toxins (1,181).

PSP is most commonly associated with the ingestion of bivalve shellfish (mussels, oysters, and clams) that have ingested, by filter feeding, large amounts of toxic microalgae or dinoflagellates (181). The process of filter feeding that these organisms use means that the toxins are concentrated in the shellfish. Predators of shellfish, such as crabs and fish, can also contain the toxins. A number of crab species, mainly from the family Xanthidae, also contain paralytic shellfish toxins and have been responsible for human deaths after ingestion (182–185). Xanthid crab poisoning is discussed here as well due to the same toxins being involved.

Pathophysiology

Since the recognition of PSP, a number of toxins have been identified that are responsible for the effects of poisoning, the paralytic shellfish toxins. The principal member of the group is saxitoxin, which is similar to TTX but is far more potent (146). Saxitoxin and its derivatives are water-soluble, heat-stable, tetrahydropurine compounds that are some of the most potent neurotoxins known (1,181). These toxins block TTX-sensitive Na^+ channels, preventing entry of Na^+ into cells, which disrupts nerve conduction and results in paralysis and sensory nerve abnormalities (146,186). Many of the derivatives have been called *GTXs* after the dinoflagellates *Gonyaulax* spp. (now *Alexandrium* spp.) that produce these toxins. Saxitoxin is the most potent blocker of sodium channels except for GTX III on a molar and weight basis (1). One mouse unit (MU) is the amount of toxin that kills a mouse weighing 20 g in 15 minutes by intraperitoneal injection; it is equivalent to 0.18 μg saxitoxin (187) and forms the basis of a mouse bioassay. The specific toxicity of saxitoxin is usually expressed as 5500 ± 500 MU (MU/mg; i.e., 1 mg pure saxitoxin hydrochloride kills approximately 5500 mice) (182). The effects of these toxins in humans have been demonstrated in a patient with PSP who had nerve conduction studies with prolonged distal latencies, reduced conduction velocities, and a moderate reduction in sensory and motor amplitudes in peripheral nerves (188).

The paralytic shellfish toxins are initially produced by toxic microalgae. A number of species of marine microalgae have been associated with PSP, including *Alexandrium* spp., *Pyrodinium bahamense* var *compressum*, and *Gymnodinium catenatum* (1,181). These toxic dinoflagellates are often associated with sea discoloration known as *red tides*, an association that has been recognized since biblical times (1). However, there is often a lead time between the toxic algal blooms and the onset of clinical illness, and not all outbreaks of PSP are associated with toxic blooms.

Clinical Presentation

The mortality of PSP from the most recent series is 5.9% worldwide (137 deaths in 2334 cases) but ranges from 0 to 44%, with a far higher rate in children, particularly those under the age of 6 (1). The clinical effects develop over 30 minutes to 3 hours (median 1 hour) (1,181). The rapidity of progression is correlated with the severity of poisoning, with paralysis and respiratory failure rapidly developing in severe cases (1,179,181), similar to TTX poisoning (189).

A clinical grading system is provided in Table 7. Paresthesia is usually the first effect that is noted, with tingling and numbness of the tongue and lips that then spreads to the face, neck, fingers, and toes. Sensation and proprioception are distorted, and the patient describes a feeling of dizziness, "floating," or disequilibrium (1). With progression, generalized paresthesiae and weakness of the upper and lower limbs occur, and the patient becomes uncoordinated and ataxic. These symptoms are usually associated with headache, nausea, and vomiting. Hypersalivation and diaphoresis may also occur. Most patients remain conscious and alert. In severe cases dysphagia, dysarthria, diplopia, and respiratory failure develop. Death usually occurs within 12 hours and has been reported within 2 to 3 hours in fulminant untreated cases. In less severe cases, the clinical effects have taken 2 to 3 days to resolve, although weakness may persist for up to a week (1,181). Poisoning with xanthid crabs causes similar clinical effects (182,185).

Diagnostic Tests

Shellfish are most commonly tested for toxins using a mouse bioassay or immunoassay, which can be supplemented by more

TABLE 7. Clinical features of paralytic shellfish poisoning based on severity

Mild
Paresthesiae and numbness: mouth, lips and throat, facial, distal upper and lower limbs
Headache
Nausea and vomiting
Dizziness, feeling of lightheadedness or floating feeling
Moderate-severe
Weakness progressing to paralysis of limbs
Ataxia
Dysarthria, dysphagia
Diplopia
Life threatening
Muscle paralysis
Respiratory failure

Modified from Meier J, White J. *Handbook of clinical toxicology of animal venoms and poisons.* Boca Raton, FL: CRC Press, 1995; and Lehane L. Paralytic shellfish poisoning: a potential public health problem. *Med J Aust* 2001;175:29–31.

analytic techniques. A capillary electrophoresis method with ultraviolet (CE-UV) detection was initially described for the separation and determination of un-derivatized toxins associated with PSP (190). GTX, often found in toxic shellfish and dinoflagellates, can also be identified in a single ultraviolet (CE-UV) study together with neosaxitoxin and saxitoxin (190). Since that time, various other methods have been developed and continue to improve the detection of these toxins.

Treatment

The treatment of PSP is supportive and similar to TTX poisoning. Decontamination may be useful if administered early, but this is unlikely, and there is no evidence that it is effective in shellfish poisoning. Antibodies to saxitoxin have been investigated but are currently not available for treatment (1). Close observation of patients with early or moderate poisoning is important so that progressing paralysis and respiratory failure can be treated early and effectively.

Prevention of PSP is important, and various monitoring programs are used in different parts of the world. The California shellfish monitoring program has detected early toxic dinoflagellate blooms and enabled health agencies to issue special guidelines, close commercial harvesting areas, alert the shellfishing public, and take other public health measures (191). Similar programs exist in other parts of the world, including Australia (1), the Adriatic Sea, and Morocco (177).

DIARRHETIC SHELLFISH POISONING

DSP is characterized by a severe gastroenteritis and is not associated with neurologic effects (1). Three classes of DSP toxins, derived from the dinoflagellate *Dinophysis* spp., have been identified in shellfish: (a) OA and dinophysistoxins, (b) pectenotoxins, and (c) yessotoxins (192), although the third group has been reclassified as nondiarrheal. After the initial discovery of DSP toxins in Japan, they were found to be widely distributed, occurring in all coastal regions of western Europe (178,193), in South America (194), and in New Zealand (195).

The onset of symptoms is usually 30 minutes to 2 hours (rarely up to 12 hours). The major symptoms are nausea, vomiting, diarrhea, and abdominal cramps. In severe cases, the diarrhea causes dehydration, and in the elderly it can lead to hypovolemic shock. No deaths have been reported, but OA has been implicated in gastric cancer (196). It is a tumor promoter and an inhibitor of protein phosphatases and protein synthesis. OA induces deoxyribonucleic acid adducts, suggesting that it may be carcinogenic, and evidence suggests that it may induce tumors via an epigenetic mechanism (197). Management is the same as for other causes of severe diarrheal food poisoning (Chapter 253).

AZASPIRACID POISONING

Azaspiracid poisoning is the most recently discovered toxic syndrome resulting from shellfish ingestion. It was first reported in 1995 in the Netherlands after ingestion of shellfish that had been cultured on the west coast of Ireland (192,198). Its effects in animals are distinctly different from those caused by OA, the representative DSP toxin, confirming that it is a different form of shellfish poisoning (198). Azaspiracid poisoning is caused by a different class of polyether toxins, the azaspiracids that are produced by marine dinoflagellates and accumulate in the shellfish. The symptoms in humans are similar to those of DSP, with nausea, vomiting, severe diarrhea, and stomach cramps (192). One study suggests that, like OA, they are tumorigenic (198).

NEUROTOXIC SHELLFISH POISONING

NSP is less common and has a more restricted distribution than PSP and clinically is milder and more like ciguatera. Human poisoning has been reported from the west coast of Florida (1), North Carolina (175), and New Zealand (199). NSP is caused by eating filter-feeding shellfish (oysters, clams, coquinas, and other bivalve mollusks) that contain brevetoxins produced by the marine dinoflagellate *Gymnodinium brevis*. The distribution of shellfish containing brevetoxin includes other regions, such as the Gulf of Mexico, where it is responsible for fish kills (174).

Pathophysiology

Brevetoxins are lipid-soluble polyether toxins that have a unique structure and pharmacologic effect (200). Brevetoxins cause toxicity in the nanomolar to picomolar concentration range *in vivo* and *in vitro*. They enhance sodium entry into cells via voltage-sensitive sodium channels in a similar way to CTX and bind at site 5 similar to CTX. They have an excitatory effect produced by sodium entry causing nerve cell depolarization and resting membrane potentials (200).

Clinical Presentation

NSP is characterized by paresthesiae, temperature reversal, myalgia, vertigo, and ataxia in association with gastrointestinal effects, including abdominal pain, nausea, and diarrhea. Other effects, including burning pain in the rectum, headache, bradycardia, and dilated pupils, have been reported. The health problems caused by *G. brevis* are associated with a red tide bloom seen along the Florida, Texas, Gulf of Mexico, New Zealand, and North Carolina coasts. Proliferation of the dinoflagellate occurs mostly in October and November and results in massive fish kills (174,175). Treatment is symptomatic and supportive, and the clinical effects are usually mild.

AMNESIC SHELLFISH POISONING

Amnesic shellfish poisoning (encephalopathic shellfish poisoning) is a toxic encephalopathy associated with severe memory loss and confusion that is caused by the ingestion of mussels contaminated with domoic acid. Only one outbreak has occurred in humans (176), but mass deaths of sea birds and marine mammals have since been attributed to domoic acid–containing fish (201).

Pathophysiology

Domoic acid is a natural, heat-stable, water-soluble neuroexcitatory amino acid produced by microscopic algae (*Nitzschia* spp.). It impersonates the normal neurotransmitter glutamic acid, resulting in neuronal damage. Domoic acid is considered to be a natural "excitotoxin," an agent that overstimulates but does not destroy cells. The source of domoic acid in the Canadian outbreak appears to have been *Nitzschia pungens*, a pennate phytoplanktonic diatom that was present in extensive blooms in the Cardigan River estuary in November and December 1987.

N. pungens produces domoic acid in cell culture. Domoic acid has also been found in razor clams (*Siliqua patula*) and in the viscera of the Dungeness crab (*Cancer magister*) along the coasts of

Washington and Oregon (202) and also on the Pacific coast of Mexico, where it has caused massive poisoning of sea birds and mammals (174). Studies have demonstrated that domoic acid permeates benthic and pelagic marine animals during algal blooms in the western United States (203). Extracts of seaweed containing domoic acid have been used as an ascaricidal agent in Japan for many years, but no adverse effects have been reported. The dose (20 mg) of domoic acid ingested in Japanese seaweed extract was much lower than the doses ingested in the Canadian mussel poisoning outbreak (60 to 290 mg).

Clinical Presentation

In 1987, an outbreak (107 cases reported) of an acute illness after ingestion of mussels contaminated with domoic acid was reported (176,204). Gastrointestinal symptoms (vomiting, abdominal cramps, diarrhea) within the first 24 hours were followed in 48 hours by unusual neurologic abnormalities (headache, loss of short-term memory, confusion, disorientation, disordered eye movements, mutism, purposeless chewing and grimacing, seizures, myoclonus, coma) (176). Additional signs included profuse respiratory secretions, hemodynamic instability, cardiac dysrhythmias, and hiccups.

Persistent neurologic abnormalities, including anterograde amnesia with relative preservation of other cognitive functions, were demonstrated in 14 of the most severely affected patients (204). Four patients died (all elderly), all of whom had focal neural necrosis and loss of the amygdala and hippocampus (204). No cases of human poisoning have been reported since that time (201), but significant concern has been shown because of the severity of the illness and the number of persons affected (1). Diagnosis should be based on the only clinical case series in which the combination of gastrointestinal and neurologic features characterized by memory loss and confusion had to be present. The median onset was 5.5 hours, and the gastrointestinal symptoms tended to precede the neurologic effects. Younger patients were more likely to have diarrhea, and older and male patients were more apt to have memory loss.

Diagnostic Tests

Cranial computed tomographic scans may be normal. Electroencephalography may demonstrate generalized slow-wave activity. Mussels can be tested for the presence of domoic acid by a mouse bioassay and high-performance liquid chromatography (176). The relative preservation of intellect and higher cortical functions distinguishes the mussel-induced intoxication syndrome from Alzheimer's disease. The absence of confabulation, together with the relatively well-preserved frontal lobe function, is atypical of the amnesic syndrome associated with alcohol-induced Korsakoff's syndrome (204).

Treatment

Treatment is supportive and symptomatic, and patients should be hospitalized in an intensive care unit where neurologic dysfunction can be monitored closely. Intubation and mechanical ventilation may be required. Kynurenic acid administered before domoic acid in animals has provided protection against convulsions and lethality, but further studies are required (205).

SCOMBROID POISONING

Scombroid poisoning is due to the ingestion of fish that contain high concentrations of histamine, previously referred to as *scombrotoxin*. The histamine accumulates during spoilage of the fish and thus differs from other marine poisonings, such as ciguatera, in which toxin accumulation occurs in the live fish. Clinical scombroid poisoning is very similar to an acute allergic reaction; the diagnosis is often missed by clinicians, and in some cases the syndrome is erroneously labeled as an allergic reaction to the fish (206).

A number of fish in the Scombridae family can result in scombroid poisoning, including tuna, bonito, skipjack, mackerel, saury, needlefish, kingfish, wahoo, and albacore. Other dark-meat fish not belonging to the Scombridae that are also implicated include the amberjack (yellowtail or Kahala, mahi mahi, dolphin fish), bluefish (*Pomatomus saltatrix*) (207), kahawai, anchovy, herring, and Western Australian salmon (*Arripis truttaceus*) (206). In Hawaii, the fish most frequently implicated is mahi mahi (*Coryphaena hippurus*).

Pathophysiology

If scombroid are inadequately preserved, bacteria break down endogenous histidine in the fish tissue to form high levels of histamine and the toxic substance, saurine. The fish usually need to be left at room temperature for some time for this to occur, but scombroid has been reported to occur when fish stored on ice for 2 days were left at room temperature for only 3 to 4 hours (208).

Clinical Presentation

Within minutes to hours of ingesting the fish, the patient develops signs and symptoms of a severe histamine-mediated reaction, including diffuse erythema of the face that resembles sunburn, giant urticaria, pruritus or a hot burning sensation, dizziness, throbbing headache, nausea, vomiting, abdominal cramps, and diarrhea. In severe cases, bronchospasm, respiratory distress, and hypotension occur. The symptoms generally are self-limited, subsiding in 8 to 10 hours.

Diagnostic Tests

The diagnosis is based on the clinical presentation and is confirmed by analysis of the fish for histamine content (206). Histamine levels in normal fresh fish should be less than 1 mg/dl or 1 mg/100 g. Levels of 20 mg/100 g in some species have been reported to produce symptoms (209). The Food and Drug Administration has established 50 mg/dl as the hazard action level for histamine in tuna. Demonstration of levels greater than 100 mg/dl is diagnostic for histamine fish poisoning. Concentrations of histamine and its metabolite, *N*-methylhistamine, in the urine were 9 to 20 times and 15 to 20 times normal, respectively, in one series of poisoned patients, confirming that histamine was the causative agent (210).

Treatment

The mainstay of treatment is antihistamines, which are best administered parenterally and rapidly alleviate the effects (210). Major toxicity may require the same aggressive management as for acute anaphylaxis (206). A recommended treatment has been suggested and is presented in Table 8 (206). Chronic persistent symptoms, such as headache, abdominal cramps, and diarrhea, may respond to oral cimetidine, 300 mg every 6 hours, and there is one report of symptoms that resolved within 48 hours with cimetidine (211). Fluids and bronchodilators should be administered as required.

Because histamine and the scombrotoxins are heat stable, cooking (drying, heating, smoking) does not alter the poisoned fish, nor does freezing, salting, or marinating fish that are already contaminated. Effective prevention of scombroid poi-

TABLE 8. Recommended treatment of scombroid poisoning

Degree of poisoning	Clinical features	Treatment
Mild	Rash only or brief flushing tachycardia	Observe for 2 h; consider parenteral antihistamines if condition fails to improve or worsens.
Moderate	Rash and persistent flushing, tachycardia, headache and/or gastrointestinal symptoms	Basic life support ABC, O_2 intravenous access, parenteral antihistamines (H_1 and H_2 antagonists). Repeat if necessary; consider oral activated charcoal if present within 1 h; overnight admission if symptoms slow to resolve.
Severe	Any of the above and/or bronchospasm and/or hypotension and/or airway compromise and/or angioedema	Basic life support ABC, O_2, and/or advanced life support; intravenous fluids; adrenaline; parenteral antihistamine (H_1 and H_2 antagonists). Repeat as necessary; consider oral activated charcoal within 1 h; nebulized bronchodilators; hospital admission.

Adapted from Smart DR. Scombroid poisoning. A report of seven cases involving the Western Australian salmon, *Arripis truttaceus. Med J Aust* 1992;157:748–751.

soning requires proper handling and storage of fish (rapid refrigeration). Histamine formation usually appears negligible in fish stored at 0°C.

OTHER MARINE POISONINGS

Clupeotoxism

Clupeotoxin fish poisoning is caused by ingestion of plankton-eating fish (herrings, sardines) and is distinguished from ciguatera and other fish poisoning by its severity and high fatality rate (212). An unusual or sharp metallic taste is usually present, associated with nausea, vomiting, diarrhea, and abdominal cramps. A number of neurologic features occur, including dilated pupils, paresthesiae, muscle cramps, paralysis, and coma. Death often occurs with severe cases. Outbreaks have been reported from the Caribbean and the Indo-Pacific region (1). The toxin involved is not known because samples are difficult to obtain. One study following the death of a woman in Madagascar suggests that palytoxin may be the cause, but this remains to be confirmed (212). Treatment is supportive.

Palytoxin poisoning

Palytoxin is one of the most potent toxins known and was originally found in zoanthid anemones (*Palythoa* spp.) (1,213). Because it can form pores in cells, it acts as a hemolysin and alters the functioning of excitable cells (213). In excitable cells, it induces the activity of a small conductance nonselective cationic channel, which then triggers the activation of voltage-dependent Ca^{2+} channels and the Na^+/Ca^{2+} exchange. This causes neurotransmitter release by nerve terminals and contraction of smooth and skeletal muscle (213). Palytoxin has other actions, including causing influx of H^+ into cells and increasing intracellular Ca^{2+} in cardiac myocytes independent of its other actions.

Ingestion of animals that incorporate palytoxin into their flesh, including crabs (214) and some fish (215), has resulted in palytoxin poisoning. Palytoxin poisoning followed the ingestion of serranid fish (*Epinephelus* spp.) in Japan, which resulted in severe muscle and lower back pain and black urine. Serum creatine phosphokinase concentrations in the patients were high (700 to 23,800 IU/L), and recovery took more than a month (215).

Ichthyocrinotoxication

Ichthyocrinotoxication occurs after ingestion of secretions from the skin of lampreys, hagfish, moray eels, toadfish, puffer fish, porcupine fish, and trunkfish. Abdominal pain, nausea, vomiting, diarrhea, and weakness may follow.

Ichthyohepatotoxication

Ichthyohepatotoxication occurs after ingestion of fish liver, usually from tropical sharks, and is probably due to an excessive dose of vitamin A. Severe headaches, neurologic symptoms, nausea, vomiting, and diarrhea may occur (216).

Sea Hares

Sea hares are a group of marine gastropod mollusks of the order Aplysiomorpha, including *Dolabella auricularia* from Fiji ("veata") and *Aplysia kurodai* from Japan. Very few poisonings by these animals have been reported. Poisoning by *D. auricularia* can cause vomiting, tachypnea, tremor, diarrhea, limb pain, tingling, restlessness, muscle fasciculations, disturbed coordination, fever, and hallucinations, but normal sensation. Recovery occurred in one patient after 6 days with some residual perioral muscle twitching (217). Sea hare poisoning in humans may be a form of subacute organic bromine intoxication.

Treatment is symptomatic and supportive. Sodium or ammonium chloride therapy may have a theoretic basis for use but has not been tried (217). Poisoning by ingestion of *A. kurodai* has also been reported to cause acute liver damage and sustained elevations of transaminases. Liver biopsy demonstrated apoptotic hepatocytes (218). Ingestion of sea hare eggs has also been reported to cause liver injury (219).

Pfiesteria

Pfiesteria spp. are estuarine dinoflagellates that appear to be responsible for massive fish deaths and associated human illnesses in the southeastern United States (220). It is thought that these dinoflagellates can produce a water-soluble toxin that is responsible for the effects in fish (ulcers, disorientation, and eventually death) and in humans (paresthesiae, arthralgia, myalgia, headache, nausea, abdominal pain, memory problems, and emotional changes), but no toxin has been isolated despite significant investigation. The effects appear to be due to direct contact with the dinoflagellate. Despite the considerable hysteria that peaked in 1997, the condition does not appear to be as significant as first thought (221).

REFERENCES

1. Meier J, White J. *Handbook of clinical toxicology of animal venoms and poisons*, 1st ed. Boca Raton, FL: CRC Press, 1995.
2. Williamson JA, Fenner PJ, Burnett JW, et al. *Venomous and poisonous marine animals*, 1st ed. Sydney: University of New South Wales Press, 1996.
3. Auerbach PS. Marine envenomations. *N Engl J Med* 1991;325:486–493.
4. Halstead BW. *Poisonous and venomous marine animals of the world*, 2nd (revised) ed. Princeton, NJ: Darwin Press, 1988.
5. Hanley M, Tomaszewski C, Kerns W. The epidemiology of aquatic envenomations in the US: most common symptoms and animals. *J Toxicol Clin Toxicol* 2000;38:512(abst).
6. Taylor DM, Ashby K, Winkel KD. An analysis of marine animal injuries presenting to emergency departments in Victoria, Australia. *Wilderness Environ Med* 2002;13:106–112.

7. O'Reilly GM, Isbister GK, Lawrie PM, et al. Prospective study of jellyfish stings from tropical Australia, including the major box jellyfish *Chironex fleckeri*. *Med J Aust* 2001;175:652–655.
8. Isbister GK. Venomous fish stings in tropical northern Australia. *Am J Emerg Med* 2001;19:561–565.
9. Huynh TT, Seymour J, Pereira P, et al. Severity of Irukandji syndrome and nematocyst identification from skin scrapings. *Med J Aust* 2003;178:38–41.
10. Fenner PJ, Williamson JA. Worldwide deaths and severe envenomation from jellyfish stings. *Med J Aust* 1996;165:658–661.
11. Fenner PJ, Williamson JA, Skinner RA. Fatal and non-fatal stingray envenomation. *Med J Aust* 1989;151:621–625.
12. Wright-Smith RJ. A case of fatal stabbing by a stingray. *Med J Aust* 1945;2:466–467.
13. Southcott RV. The neurologic effects of noxious marine creatures. In: *Topics on tropical neurology*. Philadelphia: FA Davis Co, 1975:165–258.
14. Kizer KW, McKinney HE, Auerbach PS. Scorpaenidae envenomation. A five-year poison center experience. *JAMA* 1985;253:807–810.
15. Dougherty T, Greene T, Lee DC. Stingray envenomations and antibiotic use: a pilot study. *J Toxicol Clin Toxicol* 2001;39:564(abst).
16. Aldred B, Erickson T, Lipscomb J. Lionfish envenomations in an urban wilderness. *Wilderness Environ Med* 1996;7:291–296.
17. Trestrail JH III, al Mahasneh QM. Lionfish string experiences of an inland poison center: a retrospective study of 23 cases. *Vet Hum Toxicol* 1989;31:173–175.
18. Church JE, Hodgson WC. The pharmacological activity of fish venoms. *Toxicon* 2002;40:1083–1093.
19. Hahn ST, O'Connor JM. An investigation of the biological activity of bullrout (*Notesthes robusta*) venom. *Toxicon* 2000;38:79–89.
20. Brusle J. Ciguatera fish poisoning—a review; sanitary and economic aspects. *INSERM:Paris* 1992.
21. White J, Warrell D, Eddleston M, et al. Clinical toxicology—where are we now? *J Toxicol Clin Toxicol* 2003;41.
22. Stein MR, Marraccini JV, Rothschild NE, et al. Fatal Portuguese man-o'-war (*Physalia physalis*) envenomation. *Ann Emerg Med* 1989;18:312–315.
23. Haddad V Jr, da Silveira FL, Cardoso JL, et al. A report of 49 cases of cnidarian envenoming from southeastern Brazilian coastal waters. *Toxicon* 2002;40:1445–1450.
24. Bowra J, Gillett M, Morgan J, et al. Randomised crossover trial comparing hot showers and icepacks in the treatment of *Physalia* envenomation. *Emerg Med* 2002;14:A22(abst).
25. Marques AC, Haddad V Jr, Esteves MA. Envenomation by a benthic Hydrozoa (Cnidaria): the case of *Nemalecium lighti* (Haleciidae). *Toxicon* 2002;40:213–215.
26. Hessinger DA. Nematocyst venoms and toxins. In: *Biology of nematocysts*. San Diego: Academic Press, 1988.
27. Carrette T, Alderslade P, Seymour J. Nematocyst ratio and prey in two Australian cubomedusans, *Chironex fleckeri* and *Chiropsalmus* sp. *Toxicon* 2002;40:1547–1551.
28. Lotan A, Fishman L, Zlotkin E. Toxin compartmentation and delivery in the Cnidaria: the nematocyst's tubule as a multiheaded poisonous arrow. *J Exp Zool* 1996;275:444–451.
29. Burnett JW, Calton GJ. Jellyfish envenomation syndromes updated. *Ann Emerg Med* 1987;16:1000–1005.
30. Burnett JW, Gable WD. A fatal jellyfish envenomation by the Portuguese man-o'-war. *Toxicon* 1989;27:823–824.
31. Williamson JA, Burnett JW, Fenner PJ, et al. Acute regional vascular insufficiency after jellyfish envenomation. *Med J Aust* 1988;149:698–701.
32. Cleland JB, Southcott RV. Injuries to man from marine invertebrates in the Australian region. National Health and Medical Reseach Council. Special Report Series 12. Canberra, 1965.
33. Rojas A, Torres M, Rojas JI, et al. Calcium-dependent smooth muscle excitatory effect elicited by the venom of the hydrocoral *Millepora complanata*. *Toxicon* 2002;40:777–785.
34. Sagi A, Rosenberg L, Ben Meir P, et al. "The fire coral" (*Millepora dichotoma*) as a cause of burns: a case report. *Burns Incl Therm Inj* 1987;13:325–326.
35. Kokelj F, Mianzan H, Avian M, et al. Dermatitis due to *Olindias sambaquiensis*: a case report. *Cutis* 1993;51:339–342.
36. Ramasamy S, Isbister GK, Seymour JE, et al. The in vitro effects of two chirodropid (*Chironex fleckeri* and *Chiropsalmus* sp.) venoms: efficacy of box jellyfish antivenom. *Toxicon* 2003;41:711.
37. Carrette TJ, Cullen P, Little M, et al. Temperature effects on box jellyfish venom: a possible treatment for envenomed patients? *Med J Aust* 2002;177:654–655.
38. Bengtson K, Nichols MM, Schnadig V, et al. Sudden death in a child following jellyfish envenomation by *Chiropsalmus quadrumanus*. Case report and autopsy findings. *JAMA* 1991;266:1404–1406.
39. Mustafa MR, White E, Hongo K, et al. The mechanism underlying the cardiotoxic effect of the toxin from the jellyfish *Chironex fleckeri*. *Toxicol Appl Pharmacol* 1995;133:196–206.
40. Baxter EH, Marr AG. Sea wasp (*Chironex fleckeri*) venom: lethal, haemolytic and dermonecrotic properties. *Toxicon* 1969;7:195–210.
41. Freeman SE, Turner RJ. A pharmacological study of the toxin in a Cnidarian, *Chironex fleckeri* Southcott. *Br J Pharmacol* 1969;35:510–520.
42. Currie B. Clinical implications of research on the box-jellyfish *Chironex fleckeri*. *Toxicon* 1994;32:1305–1313.
43. Little M, Mulcahy RF. A year's experience of Irukandji envenomation in far north Queensland. *Med J Aust* 1998;169:638–641.
44. Bailey PM, Little M, Jelinek GA, et al. Jellyfish envenoming syndromes: unknown toxic mechanisms and unproven therapies. *Med J Aust* 2003;178:34–37.
45. Barnes JH. Cause and effect in Irukandji stingings. *Med J Aust* 1964;1:897–904.
46. Thomas CS, Scott SA, Galanis DJ, et al. Box jellyfish (*Carybdea alata*) in Waikiki: their influx cycle plus the analgesic effect of hot and cold packs on their stings to swimmers at the beach: a randomized, placebo-controlled, clinical trial. *Hawaii Med J* 2001;60:100–107.
47. Nomura JT, Sato RL, Ahern RM, et al. A randomized paired comparison trial of cutaneous treatments for acute jellyfish (*Carybdea alata*) stings. *Am J Emerg Med* 2002;20:624–626.
48. Fenner PJ, Hadok JC. Fatal envenomation by jellyfish causing Irukandji syndrome. *Med J Aust* 2002;177:362–363.
49. Lumley J, Williamson JA, Fenner PJ, et al. Fatal envenomation by *Chironex fleckeri*, the north Australian box jellyfish: the continuing search for lethal mechanisms. *Med J Aust* 1988;148:527–534.
50. Tibballs J, Williams D, Sutherland SK. The effects of antivenom and verapamil on the haemodynamic actions of *Chironex fleckeri* (box jellyfish) venom [see Comments]. *Anaesth Intensive Care* 1998;26:40–45.
51. Little M, Mulcahy RF, Wenck DJ. Life-threatening cardiac failure in a healthy young female with Irukandji syndrome. *Anaesth Intensive Care* 2001;29:178–180.
52. McD TD, Pereira P, Seymour J, et al. A sting from an unknown jellyfish species associated with persistent symptoms and raised troponin I levels. *Emerg Med (Fremantle)* 2002;14:175–180.
53. Houck HE, Lipsky MM, Marzella L, et al. Toxicity of sea nettle (*Chrysaora quinquecirrha*) fishing tentacle nematocyst venom in cultured rat hepatocytes. *Toxicon* 1996;34:771–778.
54. Lin WW, Lee CY, Burnett JW. Effect of sea nettle (*Chrysaora quinquecirrha*) venom on isolated rat aorta. *Toxicon* 1988;26:1209–1212.
55. Burnett JW, Calton GJ. Venomous pelagic coelenterates: chemistry, toxicology, immunology and treatment of their stings. *Toxicon* 1987;25:581–602.
56. Glasser DB, Noell MJ, Burnett JW, et al. Ocular jellyfish stings. *Ophthalmology* 1992;99:1414–1418.
57. Southcott RV, Coulter JR. The effects of the southern Australian marine stinging sponges, *Neofibularia mordens* and *Lissodendoryx* sp. *Med J Aust* 1971;2:895–901.
58. Barnes JH. Observations on jellyfish stingings in Northern Queensland. *Med J Aust* 1960;2:993–999.
59. Mitchell JH. Eye injuries due to jellyfish (*Cyanea annaskala*). *Med J Aust* 1962;2:303–305.
60. Maretic Z, Russell FE, Ladavac J. Epidemic of stings by the jellyfish *Pelagia noctiluca* in the Adriatic. *Toxicon* 1979;17:115.
61. Togias AG, Burnett JW, Kagey-Sobotka A, et al. Anaphylaxis after contact with a jellyfish. *J Allergy Clin Immunol* 1985;75:672–675.
62. Pang KA, Schwartz MS. Guillain-Barré syndrome following jellyfish stings (*Pelagia noctiluca*). *J Neurol Neurosurg Psychiatry* 1993;56:1133.
63. Benmeir P, Rosenberg L, Sagi A, et al. Jellyfish envenomation: a summer epidemic. *Burns* 1990;16:471–472.
64. Burnett JW, Calton GJ, Larsen JB. Significant envenomation by *Aurelia aurita*, the moon jellyfish. *Toxicon* 1988;26:215–217.
65. Wong DE, Meinking TL, Rosen LB, et al. Sea bather's eruption. Clinical, histologic, and immunologic features. *J Am Acad Dermatol* 1994;30:399–406.
66. Segura-Puertas L, Ramos ME, Aramburo C, et al. One Linuche mystery solved: all 3 stages of the coronate scyphomedusa *Linuche unguiculata* cause sea bather's eruption. *J Am Acad Dermatol* 2001;44:624–628.
67. Segura PL, Burnett JW, Heimer DLC. The medusa stage of the coronate scyphomedusa Linuche unguiculata ("thimble jellyfish") can cause sea bather's eruption. *Dermatology* 1999;198:171–172.
68. Freudenthal AR, Joseph PR. Sea bather's eruption. *N Engl J Med* 1993;329:542–544.
69. Garcia PJ, Schein RM, Burnett JW. Fulminant hepatic failure from a sea anemone sting. *Ann Intern Med* 1994;120:665–666.
70. Currie BJ, Wood YK. Identification of *Chironex fleckeri* envenomation by nematocyst recovery from skin. *Med J Aust* 1995;162:478–480.
71. Exton DR, Fenner PJ, Williamson JA. Cold packs: effective topical analgesia in the treatment of painful stings by *Physalia* and other jellyfish. *Med J Aust* 1989;151:625–626.
72. Little M. Is there a role for the use of pressure immobilisation bandages in the treatment of jellyfish envenomation in Australia? *Emerg Med (Fremantle)* 2002;14:171–174.
73. Auerbach PS. Marine envenomation. In: *Wilderness medicine: management of wilderness and environmental emergencies*, 3rd ed. St. Louis: Mosby, 1995:1327–1374.
74. Lopez EA, Weisman RS, Bernstein J. A prospective study of the acute therapy of jellyfish envenomations. *J Toxicol Clin Toxicol* 2000;38:512(abst).
75. Seymour J, Carrette T, Cullen P, et al. The use of pressure immobilization bandages in the first aid management of cubozoan envenomings. *Toxicon* 2002;40:1503.
76. Currie BJ. Marine antivenoms. *J Toxicol Clin Toxicol* 2003;41:301–308.
77. Corkeron MA. Magnesium infusion to treat Irukandji syndrome. *Med J Aust* 2003;178:411.
78. Burnett JW, Burnett MG. Sea urchins. *Cutis* 1999;64:21–22.
79. Linaweaver PG. Toxic marine life. *Milit Med* 1967;132:437–442.
80. Burnett JW. Bolus ejection: a method for removing sea urchin spines. *Ann Emerg Med* 2002;39:94–95.

81. Southcott RV. Sponges. In: *Toxic plants and animals: a guide for Australia*, 1st ed. Brisbane: Queensland Museum, 1987:73–78.
82. Burnett JW, Calton GJ, Morgan RJ. Dermatitis due to stinging sponges. *Cutis* 1987;39:476.
83. Flachsenberger W, Holmes NJ, Leigh C, et al. Properties of the extract and spicules of the dermatitis inducing sponge *Neofibularia mordens* Hartman. *J Toxicol Clin Toxicol* 1987;25:255–272.
84. Yaffee HS. Irritation from red sponge. *N Engl J Med* 1970;282:51.
85. Yaffee HS, Stargardter S. Erythema multiforme from *Tedania ignis*. *Arch Dermatol* 1963;87:601.
86. Auerbach PS. Marine envenomations. *N Engl J Med* 1991;325:486–493.
87. Kohn AJ. Feeding biology of gastropods. *Mollusca* 1983;5:1–63.
88. Olivera BM, Rivier J, Scott JK, et al. Conotoxins. *J Biol Chem* 1991;266:22067–22070.
89. McIntosh JM, Jones RM. Cone venom—from accidental stings to deliberate injection. *Toxicon* 2001;39:1447–1451.
90. Yoshiba S. An estimation of the most dangerous species of cone shell *Conus geographus* venoms lethal dose in humans. *Jpn J Hyg* 1984;39:565.
91. Kawabata T, Halstead BW, Judefind TF. A report of a series of recent outbreaks of unusual cephalopod and fish intoxications in Japan. *Am J Trop Med Hyg* 1957;6:935–939.
92. Walker DG. Survival after severe envenomation by the blue-ringed octopus (*Hapalochlaena maculosa*). *Med J Aust* 1983;2:663–665.
93. Sheumack DD, Howden ME, Spence I, et al. Maculotoxin: a neurotoxin from the venom glands of the octopus *Hapalochlaena maculosa* identified as tetrodotoxin. *Science* 1978;199:188–189.
94. Edmonds C. A non-fatal case of blue-ringed octopus bite. *Med J Aust* 1969;2:601.
95. Sutherland SK, Coulter AR, Harris RD. Rationalisation of first-aid measures for elapid snake bite. *Lancet* 1979;1:183–186.
96. Das SK, Johnson MB, Cohly HH. Catfish stings in Mississippi. *South Med J* 1995;88:809–812.
97. Shiomi K, Takamiya M, Yamanaka H, et al. Toxins in the skin secretion of the oriental catfish (*Plotosus lineatus*): immunological properties and immunocytochemical identification of producing cells. *Toxicon* 1988;26:353–361.
98. Al Hassan JM, Thomson M, Ali M, et al. Vasoconstrictor components in the Arabian Gulf catfish (*Arius thalassinus*, Ruppell) proteinaceous skin secretion. *Toxicon* 1986;24:1009–1014.
99. McKinstry DM. Catfish stings in the United States: case report and review. *J Wilderness Med* 1993;4:293–303.
100. Blomkalns AL, Otten EJ. Catfish spine envenomation: a case report and literature review. *Wilderness Environ Med* 1999;10:242–246.
101. Murphey DK, Septimus EJ, Waagner DC. Catfish-related injury and infection: report of two cases and review of the literature. *Clin Infect Dis* 1992;14:689–693.
102. Scoggin CH. Catfish stings. *JAMA* 1975;231:176–177.
103. Mann JW, Werntz JR. Catfish stings to the hand. *J Hand Surg* 1991;16:318–321.
104. Andrews CJ, Morris A, Pearn JH. Catfish trauma [Letter]. *Med J Aust* 1991;155:130.
105. Wiener S. Observations on the venom of the stonefish (*Synanceia trachynis*). *Med J Aust* 1959;1:620–627.
106. Kreger AS. Detection of a cytolytic toxin in the venom of the stonefish (*Synanceia trachynis*). *Toxicon* 1991;29:733–743.
107. Church JE, Moldrich RX, Beart PM, et al. Modulation of intracellular Ca2+ levels by Scorpaenidae venoms. *Toxicon* 2003;41:679–689.
108. Church JE, Hodgson WC. Dose-dependent cardiovascular and neuromuscular effects of stonefish (*Synanceia trachynis*) venom. *Toxicon* 2000;38:391–407.
109. Wiener S. Stone-fish sting and its treatment. *Med J Aust* 1958;2:218–222.
110. Lehmann DF, Hardy JC. Stonefish envenomation. *N Engl J Med* 1993;329:510–511.
111. Phleps DR. Stone-fish poisoning. *Med J Aust* 1960;1:293–294.
112. Church JE, Hodgson WC. Stonefish (*Synanceia* spp.) antivenom neutralises the in vitro and in vivo cardiovascular activity of soldierfish (*Gymnapistes marmoratus*) venom. *Toxicon* 2001;39:319–324.
113. Church JE, Hodgson WC. Adrenergic and cholinergic activity contributes to the cardiovascular effects of lionfish (*Pterois volitans*) venom. *Toxicon* 2002;40:787–796.
114. Southcott RV. Australian venomous and poisonous fishes. *Clin Toxicol* 1977;10:291–325.
115. Hopkins BJ, Hodgson WC. Cardiovascular studies on venom from the soldierfish (*Gymnapistes marmoratus*). *Toxicon* 1998;36:973–983.
116. Watkins ABK. Bullrout stings. *Med J Aust* 1969;2:212.
117. Patkin M, Freeman D. Bullrout stings. *Med J Aust* 1969;2:14–16.
118. Halpern P, Sorkine P, Raskin Y. Envenomation by *Trachinus draco* in the eastern Mediterranean. *Eur J Emerg Med* 2002;9:274–277.
119. Briars GL, Gordon GS. Envenomation by the lesser weever fish. *Br J Gen Pract* 1992;42:213.
120. Chhatwal I, Dreyer F. Biological properties of a crude venom extract from the greater weever fish *Trachinus draco*. *Toxicon* 1992;30:77–85.
121. Chhatwal I, Dreyer F. Isolation and characterization of dracotoxin from the venom of the greater weever fish *Trachinus draco*. *Toxicon* 1992;30:87–93.
122. Perriere C, Goudey-Perriere F, Petek F. Purification of a lethal fraction from the venom of the weever fish, *Trachinus vipera* C.V. *Toxicon* 1988;26:1222–1227.
123. Russell FE. Marine toxins and venomous and poisonous marine animals. In: *Advances in marine biology*, vol III. London: Academic Press, 1965:255–384.
124. de Haro L, Prost N, Arditti J, et al. Efficacy of local temperature variation in the treatment of Mediterranean fish envenomations: experience of the Marseilles Poison Center during summer 1999. EAPCCT XX International Congress abstract. *J Toxicol Clin Toxicol* 2000;38:225.
125. Cadzow WH. Puncture wound of the liver by stingray spines. *Med J Aust* 1960;1:936–937.
126. Barss P. Wound necrosis caused by the venom of stingrays. Pathological findings and surgical management. *Med J Aust* 1984;141:854–855.
127. Cross TB. An unusual stingray injury—the skindiver at risk. *Med J Aust* 1976;2:947–948.
128. Weiss BF, Wolfenden HD. Survivor of a stingray injury to the heart. *Med J Aust* 2001;175:33–34.
129. Ho PL, Tang WM, Lo KS, et al. Necrotizing fasciitis due to *Vibrio alginolyticus* following an injury inflicted by a stingray. *Scand J Infect Dis* 1998;30:192–193.
130. Pacy H. Stingray and catfish injuries in New South Wales. *Med J Aust* 1962;1:119–120.
131. Russell FE. Stingray injuries: a review and discussion of their treatment. *Am J Med Sci* 1953;N.S. 226:611–622.
132. Russell FE, Panos TC, Kang LW, et al. Studies of the mechanism of death from stingray venom : a report of two fatal cases. *Am J Med Sci* 1958;235:566–584.
133. Ikeda T. Supraventricular bigeminy following a stingray envenomation: a case report. *Hawaii Med J* 1989;48:162, 164.
134. Cameron AM, Endean R. Venom glands in scatophagid fish. *Toxicon* 1970;8:171–178.
135. Southcott RV. Notes on stings of some venomous Australian fishes. *Med J Aust* 1970;2:722–725.
136. Garyfallou GT, Madden JF. Lionfish envenomation. *Ann Emerg Med* 1996;28:456–457.
137. Pacy H. Australian catfish injuries with report of a typical case. *Med J Aust* 1966;2:63–65.
138. Klontz KC, Lieb S, Schreiber M, et al. Syndromes of *Vibrio vulnificus* infections. Clinical and epidemiologic features in Florida cases, 1981–1987. *Ann Intern Med* 1988;109:318–323.
139. Tsunenari S, Uchimura Y, Kanda M. Puffer poisoning in Japan—a case report. *J Forensic Sci* 1980;25:240–245.
140. Kanchanapongkul J. Puffer fish poisoning: clinical features and management experience in 25 cases. *J Med Assoc Thai* 2001;84:385–389.
141. Ellis RM, Jelinek GA. Never eat an ugly fish: three cases of tetrodotoxin poisoning from Western Australia. *Emerg Med* 1997;9:136–142.
142. Kaku N, Meier J. Clinical toxicology of fugu poisoning. In: *Handbook of clinical toxicology of animal venoms and poisons*, 1st ed. Boca Raton, FL: CRC Press, 1995:75–83.
143. Isbister GK, Son J, Wang F, et al. Puffer fish poisoning: a potentially life-threatening condition. *Med J Aust* 2002;177:650–653.
144. Tsai YH, Hwang DF, Chai TJ, et al. Occurrence of tetrodotoxin and paralytic shellfish poison in the Taiwanese crab *Lophozozymus pictor*. *Toxicon* 1995;33:1669–1673.
145. Kanchanapongkul J, Krittayapoositpot P. An epidemic of tetrodotoxin poisoning following ingestion of the horseshoe crab *Carcinoscorpius rotundicauda*. *Southeast Asian J Trop Med Public Health* 1995;26:364–367.
146. Kao CY. Tetrodotoxin, saxitoxin and their significance in the study of excitation phenomena. *Pharmacol Rev* 1966;18:997–1049.
147. Kan SK, Chan MK, David P. Nine fatal cases of puffer fish poisoning in Sabah, Malaysia. *Med J Malaysia* 1987;42:199–200.
148. Oda K, Araki K, Totoki T, et al. Nerve conduction study of human tetrodotoxication. *Neurology* 1989;39:743–745.
149. Torda TA, Sinclair E, Ulyatt DB. Puffer fish (tetrodotoxin) poisoning: clinical record and suggested management. *Med J Aust* 1973;1:599–602.
150. Sorokin M. Puffer fish poisoning. *Med J Aust* 1973;1:957.
151. Tibballs J. Severe tetrodotoxic fish poisoning. *Anaesth Intensive Care* 1988;16:215–217.
152. Southcott RV. Australian venomous and poisonous fishes. *Clin Toxicol* 1977;10:291–325.
153. Schnorf H, Taurarii M, Cundy T. Ciguatera fish poisoning: a double-blind randomized trial of mannitol therapy. *Neurology* 2002;58:873–880.
154. Lewis RJ. The changing face of ciguatera. *Toxicon* 2001;39:97–106.
155. Bagnis R, Kuberski T, Laugier S. Clinical observations on 3009 cases of ciguatera (fish poisoning) in the South Pacific. *Am J Trop Med Hyg* 1979;28:1067–1073.
156. Bagnis R, Legrand AM. Clinical features on 12,890 cases of ciguatera (fish poisoning) in French Polynesia. In: *Progress in venom and toxin research*, 1st ed. Singapore: National University of Singapore and International Society of Toxinology, Asia Pacific Section, 1987:372–377.
157. Gillespie NC, Lewis RJ, Pearn JH, et al. Ciguatera in Australia: occurrence, clinical features, pathophysiology and management. *Med J Aust* 1986;145:584–590.
158. Johnson R, Jong EC. Ciguatera: Caribbean and Indo-Pacific fish poisoning. *West J Med* 1983;138:872–874.
159. Narayan Y. Fish poisoning in Fiji. *Fiji Med* 1980;8:567–574.
160. Lawrence DN, Enriquez MB, Lumish RM. Ciguatera fish poisoning in Miami. *JAMA* 1980;244:254–258.
161. Morris JG, Lewin P, Smith WC, et al. Ciguatera fish poisoning: epidemiology of the disease on St. Thomas U.S. Virgin Islands. *Am J Trop Med Hyg* 1982;31:574–578.

162. Lehane L, Lewis RJ. Ciguatera: recent advances but the risk remains. *Int J Food Microbiol* 2000;61:91–125.
163. Lewis RJ, Chaloupka MY, Gillespie NC, et al. An analysis of the human response to ciguatera in Australia. Proceedings of the Sixth International Coral Reef Symposium. 3, 67-71, Australia, 1988.
164. Goonetilleke A, Harris JB. Envenomation and consumption of poisonous seafood. *J Neurol Neurosurg Psychiatry* 2002;73:103–109.
165. Matta J, Navas J, Milad M, et al. A pilot study for the detection of acute ciguatera intoxication in human blood. *J Toxicol Clin Toxicol* 2002;40:49–57.
166. Palafox NA, Jain LG, Pinano AZ, et al. Successful treatment of ciguatera fish poisoning with intravenous mannitol. *JAMA* 1988;259:2740–2742.
167. Purcell CE, Capra MF, Cameron J. Action of mannitol in ciguatoxin-intoxicated rats. *Toxicon* 1999;37:67–76.
168. Lange WR, Snyder FR, Fudala PJ. Travel and ciguatera fish poisoning. *Arch Intern Med* 1992;152:2049–2053.
169. Calvert GM, Hryhorczuk DO, Leikin JB. Treatment of ciguatera fish poisoning with amitriptyline and nifedipine. *J Toxicol Clin Toxicol* 1987;25:423–428.
170. Davis RT, Villar LA. Symptomatic improvement with amitriptyline in ciguatera fish poisoning. *N Engl J Med* 1986;315:65.
171. Lange WR, Kreider SD, Hattwick M, et al. Potential benefit of tocainide in the treatment of ciguatera: report of three cases. *Am J Med* 1988;84:1087–1088.
172. Perez CM, Vasquez PA, Perret CF. Treatment of ciguatera poisoning with gabapentin. *N Engl J Med* 2001;344:692–693.
173. Holmes MJ, Teo SL. Toxic marine dinoflagellates in Singapore waters that cause seafood poisonings. *Clin Exp Pharmacol Physiol* 2002;29:829–836.
174. Sierra-Beltran AP, Cruz A, Nunez E, et al. An overview of the marine food poisoning in Mexico. *Toxicon* 1998;36:1493–1502.
175. Morris PD, Campbell DS, Taylor TJ, et al. Clinical and epidemiological features of neurotoxic shellfish poisoning in North Carolina. *Am J Public Health* 1991;81:471–474.
176. Perl TM, Bedard L, Kosatsky T, et al. An outbreak of toxic encephalopathy caused by eating mussels contaminated with domoic acid. *N Engl J Med* 1990;322:1775–1780.
177. Taleb H, Vale P, Blaghen M. Spatial and temporal evolution of PSP toxins along the Atlantic shore of Morocco. *Toxicon* 2003;41:199–205.
178. Kumagai M, Yanagi T, Murata M, et al. Okadaic acid as the causative toxin of diarrhetic shellfish poisoning in Europe. *Agric Biol Chem* 1986;50:2853–2857.
179. Rodrigue DC, Etzel RA, Hall S, et al. Lethal paralytic shellfish poisoning in Guatemala. *Am J Trop Med Hyg* 1990;42:267–271.
180. Roy RN. Red tide and outbreak of paralytic shellfish poisoning in Sabah. *Med J Malaysia* 1977;31:247–251.
181. Lehane L. Paralytic shellfish poisoning: a potential public health problem. *Med J Aust* 2001;175:29–31.
182. Llewellyn LE, Endean R. Paralytic shellfish toxins in the xanthid crab (*Atergatis floridus*) collected from Australian coral reefs. *J Wilderness Med* 1991;2:118–126.
183. Hashimoto Y, Konosu S, Yasumoto T, et al. Occurrence of toxic crabs in Ryukyu and Amami Islands. *Toxicon* 1967;5:85–90.
184. Llewellyn LE, Dodd MJ, Robertson A, et al. Post-mortem analysis of samples from a human victim of a fatal poisoning caused by the xanthid crab, *Zosimus aeneus*. *Toxicon* 2002;40:1463–1469.
185. Llewellyn LE. Human fatalities in Vanuatu after eating a crab (*Daira perlata*). *Med J Aust* 2001;175:343–344.
186. Ritchie JM, Rogart RB. The binding of saxitoxin and tetrodotoxin to excitable tissue. *Rev Physiol Biochem Pharmacol* 1977;79:1–50.
187. Schantz EJ. Historical perspective on paralytic shellfish poisoning. In: *Seafood toxins*. Washington, DC: American Chemical Society, 1984:99–111.
188. Long RR, Sargent JC, Hammer K. Paralytic shellfish poisoning: a case report and serial electrophysiologic observations. *Neurology* 1990;40:1310–1312.
189. Isbister GK, Son J, Lin CS, et al. Puffer fish poisoning : a poorly recognised and potentially life-threatening condition in Australia. 6th Asia-Pacific Congress on Animal, Plant and Microbial Toxins. Cairns, 2002.
190. Thibault P, Pleasance S, Laycock MV. Analysis of paralytic shellfish poisons by capillary electrophoresis. *J Chromatogr* 1991;542:483–501.
191. Price DW, Kizer KW. California's paralytic shellfish poisoning prevention program 1927–1989. 1-36. California Department of Health Services, 1990.
192. James KJ, Furey A, Lehane M, et al. First evidence of an extensive northern European distribution of azaspiracid poisoning (AZP) toxins in shellfish. *Toxicon* 2002;40:909–915.
193. Vale P, et al. First confirmation of human diarrhoeic poisonings by okadaic acid esters after ingestion of razor clams (*Solen marginatus*) and green crabs (*Carcinus maenas*) in Aveiro Lagoon, Portugal and detection of okadaic acid esters in phytoplankton. *Toxicon* 2002;40:989–996.
194. James KJ, Lehane M, Moroney C, et al. Azaspiracid shellfish poisoning: unusual toxin dynamics in shellfish and the increased risk of acute human intoxications. *Food Addit Contam* 2002;19:555–561.
195. Yasumoto T, Takizawa A. Fluorometric measurement of yessotoxins in shellfish by high-pressure liquid chromatography. *Biosci Biotechnol Biochem* 1997;61:1775–1777.
196. Suganuma M, Fujiki H, Suguri H, et al. Okadaic acid: an additional non-phorbol-12-tetradecanoate-13-acetate-type tumor promoter. *Proc Natl Acad Sci U S A* 1988;85:1768–1771.
197. Creppy EE, Traore A, Baudrimont I, et al. Recent advances in the study of epigenetic effects induced by the phycotoxin okadaic acid. *Toxicology* 2002;181–182:433–439.
198. Ito E, Satake M, Ofuji K, et al. Multiple organ damage caused by a new toxin azaspiracid, isolated from mussels produced in Ireland. *Toxicon* 2000;38:917–930.
199. Ishida H, Muramatsu N, Nukaya H, et al. Study on neurotoxic shellfish poisoning involving the oyster, *Crassostrea gigas*, in New Zealand. *Toxicon* 1996;34:1050–1053.
200. Baden DG. Brevetoxins: unique polyether dinoflagellate toxins. *FASEB J* 1989;3:1807–1817.
201. Vale P, Sampayo MAM. Domoic acid in Portuguese shellfish and fish. *Toxicon* 2001;39:893–904.
202. Wekell JC, Gauglitz EJ Jr, Barnett HJ, et al. Occurrence of domoic acid in Washington state razor clams (*Siliqua patula*) during 1991–1993. *Nat Toxins* 1994;2:197–205.
203. Lefebvre KA, Bargu S, Kieckhefer T, et al. From sanddabs to blue whales: the pervasiveness of domoic acid. *Toxicon* 2002;40:971–977.
204. Teitelbaum JS, Zatorre RJ, Carpenter S, et al. Neurologic sequelae of domoic acid intoxication due to the ingestion of contaminated mussels. *N Engl J Med* 1990;322:1781–1787.
205. Glavin GB, Pinsky C, Bose R. Mussel poisoning and excitatory amino acid receptors. *Trends Pharmacol Sci* 1989;10:15–16.
206. Smart DR. Scombroid poisoning. A report of seven cases involving the Western Australian salmon, *Arripis truttaceus*. *Med J Aust* 1992;157:748–751.
207. Etkind P, Wilson ME, Gallagher K, et al. Bluefish-associated scombroid poisoning. An example of the expanding spectrum of food poisoning from seafood. *JAMA* 1987;258:3409–3410.
208. Chen KT, Malison MD. Outbreak of scombroid fish poisoning, Taiwan. *Am J Public Health* 1987;77:1335–1336.
209. CDC. Scombroid: fish poisoning—Illinois, South Carolina. *MMWR Morb Mortal Wkly Rep* 1989;39:140–147.
210. Morrow JD, Margolies GR, Rowland J, et al. Evidence that histamine is the causative toxin of scombroid-fish poisoning. *N Engl J Med* 1991;324:716–720.
211. Auerbach PS. Persistent headache associated with scombroid poisoning: resolution with oral cimetidine. *J Wilderness Med* 1990;1:279–283.
212. Onuma Y, Satake M, Ukena T, et al. Identification of putative palytoxin as the cause of clupeotoxism. *Toxicon* 1999;37:55–65.
213. Frelin C, Van Renterghem C. Palytoxin. Recent electrophysiological and pharmacological evidence for several mechanisms of action. *Gen Pharmacol* 1995;26:33–37.
214. Yasumoto T, Yasumura D, Ohizumi Y, et al. Palytoxin in two species of xanthid crab from Philippines. *Agric Biol Chem* 1986;50:163–167.
215. Taniyama S, Mahmud Y, Terada M, et al. Occurrence of a food poisoning incident by palytoxin from a serranid *Epinephelus* sp. in Japan. *J Nat Toxins* 2002;11:277–282.
216. Holliman CJ. Something fishy. Prehospital management of toxic seafood ingestions. *Emerg Med Serv* 1994;32–37.
217. Sorokin M. Human poisoning by ingestion of a sea hare (*Dolabella auricularia*). *Toxicon* 1988;26:1095–1097.
218. Sakamoto Y, Nakajima T, Misawa S, et al. Acute liver damage with characteristic apoptotic hepatocytes by ingestion of *Aplysia kurodai*, a sea hare. *Intern Med* 1998;37:927–929.
219. Hino K, Mitsui Y, Hirano Y. Four cases of acute liver damage following the ingestion of a sea hare egg. *J Gastroenterol* 1994;29:679.
220. Miller TR, Belas R. *Pfiesteria piscicida*, *P. shumwayae*, and other *Pfiesteria*-like dinoflagellates. *Res Microbiol* 2003;154:85–90.
221. Karalis T, Gupta L, Chu M, et al. Three clusters of ciguatera poisoning: clinical manifestations and public health implications. *Med J Aust* 2000;172:160–162.

SECTION

4

Bacterial Foodborne Illness

CHAPTER 253

Bacterial Foodborne Illness

Steven A. Seifert

Compounds included (Table 1):	***Bacillus cereus, Campylobacter* species, *Clostridium botulinum, Clostridium perfringens, Escherichia coli, Listeria monocytogenes, Salmonella* species, *Shigella* species, *Staphylococcus aureus, Yersinia enterocolitica***
SI conversion:	**Not applicable**
Normal levels:	**Not applicable**
Special concerns:	**Dehydration, sepsis**
Antidote:	**None; selected infections are treated with antibiotics (Table 16).**

OVERVIEW

Foodborne illness may follow ingestion of foods contaminated with bacteria, algae, protozoa, viruses, parasites, and other organisms, as the result of food sensitivities or chemical or drug contamination. Foodborne illness is an important cause of acute morbidity and increased short-term mortality. The Centers for Disease Control and Prevention (CDC) estimates that in 1998 foodborne bacteria alone produced 76 million illnesses, 325,000 hospitalizations, and 5000 deaths in the United States (1). Approximately 600 outbreaks of foodborne illness are reported to the CDC every year (2). In addition, infections with *Salmonella, Campylobacter,* and *Yersinia enterocolitica* are associated with increased long-term mortality (3).

When faced with the symptoms of acute gastrointestinal (GI) illness, structural, functional, and metabolic causes must also be considered. Because incubation periods of foodborne illness may be quite long, with many meals and other activities occurring in the interim, the association between contaminated food intake may not be made or may be erroneous. Evaluating the differential diagnosis and initiating treatment before a definitive diagnosis is available are significant clinical challenges.

Bacterial organisms are the most common cause of foodborne illness and may be the result of either direct action of the organism or the action of endo- or exotoxins. The incubation period depends on whether there is a preformed exotoxin, which generally produces symptoms sooner than illness that results from organisms that must first reproduce and elaborate a toxin in the GI tract. *Salmonella* was the most commonly reported foodborne poisoning reported to the CDC between 1993 and 1997 (4). Other common bacterial causes included *Escherichia coli, Clostridium perfringens, Shigella, Staphylococcus aureus, Bacillus cereus, Campylobacter* species (spp.), *Streptococcus* (group A), *Listeria monocytogenes, Clostridium botulinum, Vibrio parahaemolyticus,* and *Y. enterocolitica. Salmonella* and *E. coli* were responsible for the greatest number of deaths (4). Because of their similarities, the diagnostic tests and management of bacterial foodborne illness are addressed as a group in the sections at the end of this chapter.

Marine agents and toxins may produce similar symptoms (Chapter 252). Common parasitic causes of diarrhea include *Giardia, Cryptosporidium,* and *Entamoeba histolytica.* Rotavirus is the most common cause of acute diarrhea among children, accounting for one-fourth of all cases, but many other viruses can cause diarrhea as well, including Norwalk-like viruses, enteric adenoviruses, astroviruses, and calciviruses.

Prevention

Prevention of foodborne illness is preferred to treatment. It is especially important for human immunodeficiency virus (HIV)–positive patients. A review of school-related illness concluded, "Strengthening food safety measures in schools would better protect students and school staff from outbreaks of foodborne illness. Infection control policies, such as training and certification of food handlers in the proper storage and cooking of foods, meticulous hand washing, and paid sick leave for food handlers with gastroenteritis, could make meals safer for American students" (5).

Food Irradiation

Food irradiation reduces biologic food contamination and related foodborne illness. Approximately 170 irradiation facilities exist worldwide. Food irradiation has been approved for use in the United States in selected foods since 1963 (6). One advantage of irradiation is that it can be used after packaging, thus minimizing handling after treatment (6). In the United States, the source of ionizing energy is ^{66}Co contained in stain-

TABLE 1. Approach to the diagnosis and management of infectious diarrhea

Causative agent	Patient age groupings	Selected symptoms			Incubation period	Duration of illness	Mode of transmission
		Vomiting	Fever	Diarrhea			
Bacillus cereus and *Staphylococcus aureus*	All	Common	Rare	Usually not prominent	1–6 h	<24 h	Food
Campylobacter jejuni	All groups, especially <1 yr old and young adults	Variable	Variable	May be dysenteric	3–5 d (1–7 d)	1–4 d, occasionally 10 d	Food, water, pets, fecal-oral
Enterotoxigenic *Escherichia coli*	Adults, infants, children	Occasional	Variable	Watery to profuse watery	12–72 h	3–5 d	Food, water, PTP, fecal-oral
Enteropathogenic *E. coli*	Infants	Variable	Variable	Watery to profuse watery	2–6 d	1–3 wk	Food, water, PTP, fecal-oral
Enteroinvasive *E. coli*	Adults	Occasional	Common	May be dysenteric	2–3 d	1–2 wk	Food, water, PTP, fecal-oral
Enterohemorrhagic *E. coli*	<10 yr (50%), 15 mo–73 yr	Common	Rare or mild	First watery, then grossly bloody	3–5 d	7–10 d (1–12 d)	Food, PTP, fecal-oral
Salmonella	All groups, especially infants and young children	Occasional	Common	Loose, watery, occasionally bloody	8–48 h	3–5 d	Food, water, fecal-oral
Shigella	All groups, especially 6 mo–10 yr	Occasional	Common	May be dysenteric	1–7 d	4–7 d	Food, water, PTP, fecal-oral
Yersinia enterocolitica	All groups, especially older children and young adults	Occasional	Common	Mucoid, occasionally bloody	2–7 d	1 d–3 wk (average 9 d)	Food, water, PTP, pets, fecal-oral
Vibrio cholerae	All groups	Common	Variable	May be profuse and watery	9–72 h	3–4 d	Fecal-oral, food, water

PTP, person-to-person.
From CDC. Lew JF, et al. *MMWR Morb Mortal Wkly Rev* 1990;39:1–13, with permission.

less steel rods in racks that emit gamma rays (7). Technically, food irradiation is a "food additive" under the 1958 Food Additives Amendment to the Federal Food, Drug and Cosmetic Act of 1938 (8). The American Dietetic Association (ADA) has declared that "food irradiation enhances the safety and quality of the food supply and helps protect consumers" (9).

Ionizing radiation passes through the food and destroys harmful bacteria and other organisms. Viruses, spores, prions, and preformed toxins are resistant to the effects of irradiation (6). Food irradiation, therefore, does not replace proper storage and handling of food, and irradiated foods may still become contaminated by preformed toxins or spores before irradiation and by organisms after irradiation. Negligible loss of nutrients and sensory qualities occurs, there is no residue, and the small amount of energy absorbed by the food is retained as a minimal increase in temperature. A small number of radiolytic products are generated by this process, but less than that generated by traditional heating (10). A U.S. Food and Drug Administration review found no evidence that unique radiolytic products are produced during irradiation (11). Treated food or its packaging does not become a source of ionizing radiation, as the ionizing energy is too low to induce the release of neutrons. In the United States, irradiated foods sold to consumers must be identified with an international symbol (Radura) and terminology that describes the process on product labels.

The increase in cost of irradiating foods is estimated at $0.02 to $0.03 per pound for fruits and vegetables and $0.03 to $0.08 per pound for meats (7). Some concern exists with regard to safety issues related to irradiating facilities. Radioactive material must be transported, stored, used, and protected. Low-level radioactive waste is generated when ^{66}Co has lost approximately 90% of its activity (15 to 20 years). Because fusion or fission is not occurring, a "meltdown" is not possible, and removal of the radiation source renders the facilities useable for any purpose. When consumers are informed regarding the irradiation process and safety issues, most prefer irradiated to nonirradiated foods (12).

DIFFERENTIAL DIAGNOSIS OF BACTERIAL FOODBORNE ILLNESS

Foodborne illness presents with certain characteristic clinical manifestations. These manifestations may help identify the causative agent. Marine organism causes are not included.

Acute Gastroenteritis

Acute gastroenteritis includes primary presenting symptoms of abdominal pain, vomiting, diarrhea, and dysentery (bloody diarrhea), with or without fever. Vomiting may prevent oral intake, leading rapidly to dehydration, especially when diarrhea contributes to fluid losses. Diarrhea may be debilitating or fatal even in the absence of vomiting. Diarrhea kills about four million people in developing countries each year and remains a problem in developed countries as well. In the United States, children less than 5 years of age experience more than 20 million episodes of diarrhea each year, leading to several million doctor visits, 200,000 hospitalizations, and approximately 400 deaths. More than 10,000 children worldwide die each day from associated diarrhea. Much of this morbidity is the result of the dehydration associated with acute watery diarrhea. Most hospitalizations and deaths due to diarrhea occur in the first year of life.

If sought, a causative agent for gastroenteritis with diarrhea can be found in 60% to 80% of cases, although rates of less than 10% are commonly reported in clinical practice. An approach to the diagnosis and management of infective diarrhea can be found in Figure 1. Comparisons of outbreaks of bacterial, par-

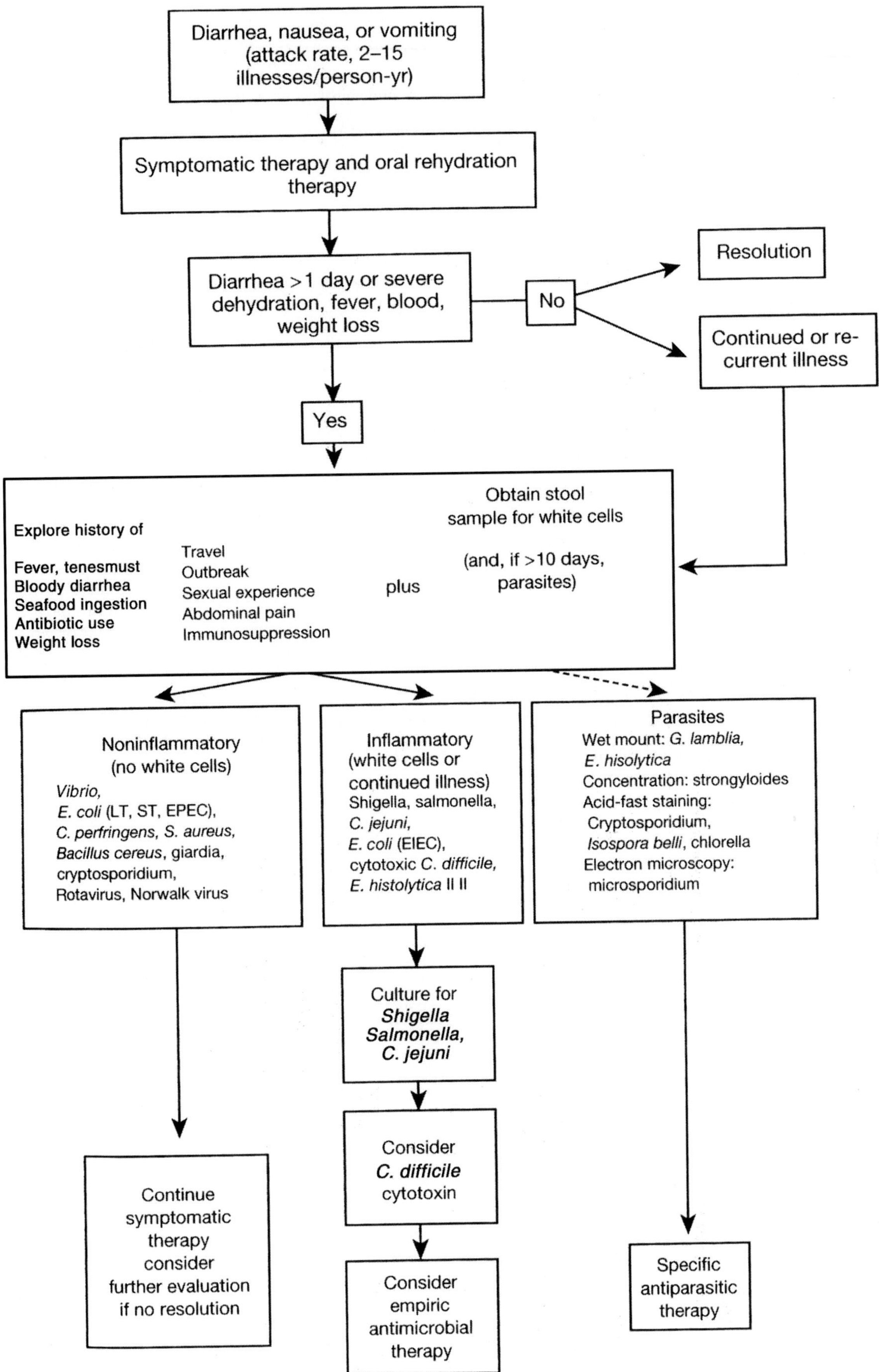

Figure 1. Approach to the diagnosis and management of infectious diarrhea.

TABLE 2. Information relevant to outbreaks of parasitic gastroenteritis

Causative agent	Patient age groupings	Selected symptoms: Fever	Diarrhea	Abdominal	Incubation period	Duration of illness	Mode of transmission
Balantidium coli	Unknown	Rare	Occasional mucus or blood	Mild to severe pain	Unknown	Unknown	Good, water, fecal-oral
Cryptosporidium	Children, adults with AIDS	Occasional	Profuse, watery	Occasional cramping	1–2 wk	4 d–3 wk	Food, water, PTP, pets, fecal-oral
Entamoeba histolytica	All groups, adults	Variable	Occasional mucus or blood	Colicky pain	2–4 wk	Weeks–months	Food, water, fecal-oral
Giardia lamblia	All groups, children	Rare	Loose, pale, greasy stools	Cramps, bloating, flatulence	5–25 d	1–2 wk to months and years	Food, water, fecal-oral
Isospora belli	Adults with AIDS	Unknown	Loose stools	Unknown	9–15 d	2–3 wk	Fecal-oral

AIDS, acquired immunodeficiency syndrome; PTP, person-to-person.
Modified from CDC. Lew JF, et al. *MMWR Morb Mortal Wkly Rev* 1990;39:1–13.

asitic, and viral gastroenteritis are summarized in Tables 1, 2, and 3.

Diarrhea without fever is characteristic of agents that produce preformed toxins, including *B. cereus*, *C. perfringens*, enterotoxigenic *E. coli*, *S. aureus*, and some viruses (13). Diarrhea with fever is characteristic of foodborne illness caused by invasive organisms, including *Campylobacter* spp., invasive *E. coli*, *Salmonella* spp., *Shigella* spp., *V. parahaemolyticus*, *Yersinia* spp., and some viruses (13).

Examination of the stool can assist in distinguishing the etiology of diarrhea. Blood is characteristic of invasive organisms, including invasive *E. coli*, *Salmonella* spp., and *Shigella* spp. Gross blood is often visible, but testing for occult blood may be required. The finding of blood is not pathognomonic for invasive bacterial illness. Persistent diarrhea of any cause may irritate the rectal mucosa and cause bleeding. Fecal leukocytes are typical of bacterial illness, including *C. jejuni*, invasive *E. coli*, *Shigella* spp., *Salmonella* spp., typhoid fever, *V. parahaemolyticus*, and *Y. enterocolitica*. Leukocytes may also be seen with inflammatory conditions such as ulcerative colitis. In typhoid fever, mononuclear cells predominate, whereas polymorphonuclear cells are seen with the others. Very few leukocytes are seen with cholera, noninvasive *E. coli*, and viral illness (14).

The timing and epidemiology of symptoms in relation to ingestion of a suspected food source may also assist in the differential diagnosis. Short incubation periods (less than 6 hours) are typical of preformed toxins and infections with *S. aureus*, *B. cereus* (type I), and enterotoxigenic *E. coli* (15). Roundworm and larval infections also produce rapid symptoms. A knowledge of which foods are likely sources of particular organisms may also assist in the diagnosis (Table 4). An incubation period of 6 to 24 hours is more typically seen with *B. cereus* (type II), *C. perfringens*, invasive *E. coli*, and *Salmonella* spp. Noninvasive *E. coli*, *Shigella* spp., *Vibrio cholerae*, and botulinum toxin usually have an incubation period of 1 to 3 days, and *C. jejuni* and *Yersinia* spp., may have incubation periods of up to a week.

An obvious epidemic of similar cases with a common exposure helps to rule out structural, functional, and metabolic etiologies. When an illness occurs as part of a multipatient exposure, rapid determination of the incubation period, the source food, and the likely agent is often possible. In addition, when the incubation period can be demonstrated to be short, most viruses,

TABLE 3. Information relevant to outbreaks of viral gastroenteritis

Causative agent	Patient age groupings	Selected symptoms: Vomiting	Fever	Incubation period	Duration of illness	Mode of transmission[a]
Astrovirus	Young children and elderly people	Occasional	Occasional	1–4 d	2–3 d; occasionally 1–14 d	Food, water, fecal-oral
Calicivirus	Infants, young children, and adults	Common for infants; variable for adults	Occasional	1–3 d	1–3 d	Food, water, nosocomial, fecal-oral
Enteric adenovirus	Young children	Common	Common	7–8 d	8–12 d	Nosocomial, fecal-oral
Norwalk virus	Older children and adults	Common	Rare or mild	18–48 h	12–48 h	Food, water, PTP, ?air, fecal-oral
Rotavirus, group A	Infants and toddlers	Common	Common	1–3 d	5–7 d	Water, PTP, ?food, ?air, nosocomial, fecal-oral
Rotavirus, group B	Children and adults	Variable	Rare	56 h (average)	3–7 d	Water, PTP, fecal-oral
Rotavirus, group C	Infants, children, and adults	Unknown	Unknown	24–48 h	3–7 d	Fecal-oral

PTP, person-to-person, ?, not confirmed.
[a]Diarrhea is common and is usually loose, watery, and nonbloody when associated with gastroenteritis.
From CDC. Lew JF, et al. *MMWR Morb Mortal Wkly Rep* 1990;39:1–13, with permission.

TABLE 4. Relation between food source and chemical or bacterial organism

Organism/toxin	Food source
Bacillus cereus	Type I: fried rice, cooked rice, noodles, pasta, pastries; type II: meats, vegetables, sauces, puddings, milk/milk products
Campylobacter	Contaminated water, unpasteurized milk, poultry
Capsaicin	Peppers
Clostridium botulinum	Home-canned vegetables, fish, meats, honey, corn syrup
Clostridium perfringens	Poultry, heat-processed meats, gravy
Escherichia coli	Contaminated water, cattle/cattle-related food products (milk, beef, yogurt, cheese), apple cider
Listeria monocytogenes	Cabbage, cheese, pasteurized milk, raw vegetables
Metabisulfites	Wines, salad bars, fruit, juices, shrimp
Monosodium glutamate (MSG)	Flavor enhancers, Chinese food, meats, canned foods, other fast foods
Salmonella spp.	Poultry, un-/under-cooked eggs, sprouts, pets (chicks, ducklings, all reptiles)
Shigella spp.	Poor hygiene practices, mechanical vectors (e.g., housefly)
Staphylococcus spp.	Proteinaceous foods (cream-filled baked goods), prepared foods, meats, pastries, salads, skin-infected individuals
Tartrazine	Yellow food coloring
Tyramine	Wines, aged cheese
Vibrio cholerae	Water, enteric contact
Yersinia spp.	Pork, pasteurized and unpasteurized milk, buttermilk, pets

fungal, algal, and parasitic infections (other than roundworms and larvae) can also be eliminated from the differential diagnosis, because their incubation periods are longer.

Required for diagnosis of epidemic food poisoning are two or more cases with a common exposure and a well-defined and similar symptomatology within the exposed group. Additional factors to consider are whether some individuals may have altered susceptibility, whether the exposure was similar in timing and route for all contacts, and complicating factors of multiple foods ingested in-common. Contacting local and state health departments permits early, thorough investigation of potential additional cases of suspected foodborne illness. Health departments are also often capable of arranging for food analysis for toxins or organisms by a variety of methods that are not typically available in acute-care hospitals (16,17). Determination of organism and strain through deoxyribonucleic acid analysis also aids in tracing the origin of foodborne illness. Although epidemic foodborne illness is usually the result of improper storage and handling of food or inadvertent contamination (18), intentional poisoning has been reported (19,20). One incident involved 12 laboratory workers intentionally poisoned by *Shigella dysenteriae* (19). In other incidents, more than 16,000 cases of illness were traced to contamination of a dairy tank by unpasteurized milk (18), and a political sect produced 751 cases of illness by contaminating common food sources with *Salmonella typhimurium* in an act of political sabotage (20). The ease of culturing pathogenic strains of common bacterial agents and of contaminating common food sources mandates improved surveillance of epidemics of GI illness.

Neurologic Effects

Neurologic symptoms of blurred vision, diplopia, dysarthria, dysphagia, and descending paralysis are typical of botulinum toxin. A history of ingestion of home-canned fruits and vegetables or commercial fish products, a predisposing wound, or ingestion of honey by a child less than 1 year of age, combined with such neurologic symptoms, is highly suspicious, and the diagnosis of botulism should be made presumptively, as aggressive early treatment is required.

Seizures are typical of *Shigella*. Marine toxins also commonly produce neurologic symptoms and signs (Chapter 252). Conditions presenting with neurologic toxicity that may be confused with possible food poisoning include plant toxins, such as poison hemlock and buckthorn, as well as myasthenia gravis, tick paralysis, Eaton-Lambert syndrome, heavy metals, diphtheria, atypical Guillain-Barré syndrome, and carbon monoxide poisoning. Headache is commonly reported after the ingestion of foodborne contaminants, such as monosodium glutamate (MSG), metabisulfites, tyramine, and tartrazine, and in scombroid poisoning.

Nephrotoxicity

Nephrotoxicity from ingested foods is uncommon. *E. coli* O157:H7 may produce acute gastroenteritis, hemolysis and anemia, thrombocytopenia, and azotemia: the hemolytic-uremic syndrome (HUS). Other exposures and conditions may produce this syndrome, including estrogen-containing contraceptives, cyclosporine-A and mitomycin-C (21). Occasionally, acute renal insufficiency is seen in patients with aberrant ingestion-related behavior. In the case of Vichy water, Worcestershire sauce, milk, licorice, and rhubarb, such high quantities of food are ingested that one component reaches nephrotoxic levels (Table 5).

Traveler's Diarrhea

Although a heat-labile enterotoxin derived from *E. coli* is the most common cause of traveler's diarrhea, site and season may predispose the traveler to diarrhea associated with other causative bacteria (22) (Table 6). These infections are most commonly acquired through ingestion of contaminated food and water but may be transmitted by person-to-person contact. Many beaches around the world are contaminated with sewage and fecal microorganisms. Most episodes of traveler's diarrhea can be allowed to run their course with symptomatic treatment alone

TABLE 5. Nephrotoxic foods

Probable renal lesion	Food	Toxic component
Chronic interstitial nephritis	Vichy water, Worcestershire sauce	Fluoride unknown
Hypercalcemia (milk-alkali syndrome)	Milk	Calcium
Hemoglobinuric tubular necrosis	Fava or broad beans (*Vicia faba* L)	Divicine and isouramil
Myoglobinuric tubular necrosis	Licorice	Glycyrrhizic acid (hypokalemia)
	Wild birds (chaffinch, quail, or European robin	?Cicutoxin
Nephrotoxic tubular necrosis	Djenkol beans (*Pithecolabium lobatum*)	?Djenkolic acid
	Bile of the grass carp (*Clenopharyngodon idellus*)	?Cyprinol
Oxalosis	Rhubarb (*Rheum rhaponticum*)	Oxalic acid

Adapted from Abuelo JG. *Arch Intern Med* 1990;150:505–510.

TABLE 6. Causative organisms, epidemiologic aspects, and current methods of detection in traveler's diarrhea

Causative organism	Epidemiologic features (geographic and seasonal distribution)	Detection methods
Enterotoxigenic *Escherichia coli*	Worldwide, summer	Research laboratory
Invasive *E. coli*	Unusual cause of food-borne illness	Research laboratory
Shigella spp.	Worldwide, summer	Stool culture
Salmonella spp.	Worldwide, summer	Stool culture
Aeromonas spp.	Worldwide, summer	Stool culture
Plesiomonas shigelloides	Worldwide, summer, fish source	Stool culture
Campylobacter jejuni	Worldwide, all year, especially winter	Stool culture
Vibrio cholerae	Indian subcontinent and South America	Stool culture using TCBS media
Vibrio parahaemolyticus	Coastal areas, summer	Stool culture using TCBS media
Viral agents (e.g., rotavirus)	Worldwide, all year, especially winter	Rotavirus antigen test
Cryptosporidium spp.	Waterborne disease, particularly in Russia	Stool parasite examination
Giardia lamblia	Mountainous areas, Russia	Stool parasite examination
Entamoeba histolytica	Areas with markedly reduced hygienic standards	Stool parasite examination

TCBS, triosulfate-citrate-bile salts-sucrose (agar).
Adapted from DuPont HL. *Drugs* 1993;45:917–927.

and no need to isolate the pathogen. Exceptions are bloody diarrhea (dysentery) and diarrhea that lasts more than 7 days. Therapy of traveler's diarrhea based on clinical features is listed in Tables 7 and 8 (22).

TABLE 7. Agents for treatment of traveler's diarrhea in adults

Agent	Dosage	Comments
Attapulgite	3 g initially, then 3 g after each loose stool or every 2 h (whichever comes first) for a total of 9 g/d	Nonabsorbed; use should be safe during pregnancy
Bismuth subsalicylate	1 oz every 30 min for a total of 8 oz/d	Salicylate is absorbed
Loperamide	4 mg initially, then 2 mg after each loose stool (not to exceed 16 mg/d)	Avoid use in cases of dysentery
Trimethoprim-sulfamethoxazole	320/1600 mg once or 160/800 mg twice a day for 3 d	Use of loading dose followed by standard doses for 3 d is most effective
Fluoroquinolone		
Norfloxacin	800 mg once or 400 mg twice a day for 3 d	Efficacy of administration of fluoroquinolones as a loading dose followed by 3 d therapy has not been studied
Ciprofloxacin	1000 mg once or 500 mg twice a day for 3 d	
Ofloxacin	600 mg once or 300 mg twice a day for 3 d	

Adapted from Ericsson CD, DuPont HL. *Clin Infect Dis* 1993;16:616–626.

TABLE 8. Approach to treatment of traveler's diarrhea in adults

Severity of diarrhea	Preferred treatment[a]	Comments
Mild (1–2 loose stools/24 h tolerable symptoms)	None	Attapulgite, bismuth subsalicylate, or loperamide could be used
Moderate (>3 loose stools/24 h tolerable symptoms)	Loperamide	Attapulgite or bismuth subsalicylate could be used: 3-day antimicrobial therapy is necessary if symptoms persist for >2 d
Moderate to severe (>3 loose stools/24 h distressing symptoms)	Loperamide plus single-dose antimicrobial therapy	Continue standard dosing of antimicrobial agent for 3 d if symptoms clearly are no better after 12 h
Severe [>3 loose stools/24 h (incapacitating symptoms) *or* fever *or* bloody stools]	Loading dose of antimicrobial agent plus standard doses for 3 d	Avoid use of loperamide

[a]Rehydration is assumed.
Adapted from Ericsson CD, DuPont HL. *Clin Infect Dis* 1993;16:616–626.

Other Food-Related Illness

Mushrooms are capable of producing acute GI illness, with or without additional toxicity (Chapter 257). Spicy foods, such as capsaicin-containing peppers or horseradish, may induce severe oropharyngeal or abdominal pain and syncope (23,24).

MSG may produce a syndrome characterized by burning, facial pressure, headache, flushing, chest pain, and, to a lesser extent, nausea and vomiting. Angioedema and life-threatening reactive airway disease may occur rarely (25,26). In susceptible individuals there is a dose-response relationship to the severity of symptoms (27). Symptoms usually last about an hour. Although typically described as a component of Chinese cooking, MSG is also found in "flavor enhancers" (28), in processed meats, and in some canned foods.

Tyramine is found in wines, aged cheese, and other foods. It is normally inactivated by monoamine oxidase in the GI tract. In patients who are taking monoamine oxidase inhibitors, a tyramine reaction may develop, characterized by headache and severe hypertension.

Canthaxanthine is a naturally occurring orange carotenoid that does not have vitamin A properties. It has been used therapeutically to impart an orange-brown tone to the skin. It has not been shown to be acutely toxic, carcinogenic, or mutagenic in animals. In humans, there is a 12% to 14% incidence of retinopathy—manifested by yellow retinal deposits in the retina with minimal effects on vision—in individuals who consume canthaxanthine. This effect is dose related and has an incidence of 100% after a cumulative dose of 60 g (29). Some glare effect is reported, and prolonged dark adaptation may be seen on examination, but most patients remain asymptomatic (30). Canthaxanthine may impart an orange color to the serum and interferes with carotene and vitamin A laboratory determinations. Reversibility of deposits after discontinuation of canthaxanthine is slow and variable (31).

Type I hypersensitivity reactions, immunoglobulin E and non–immunoglobulin E mediated, may occur to otherwise uncontaminated foods. Eggs, fish, milk, nuts, peanuts, soy, and shellfish are common allergens. Reactions to metabisulfites can produce flushing, hypotension, and bronchospasm. These agents are used as preservatives in wines and fruits.

INTESTINAL INFECTIONS IN IMMUNOCOMPROMISED HOSTS

In patients infected by HIV, diarrhea can be a presenting manifestation of acquired immunodeficiency syndrome (AIDS) or a life-threatening complication. The diarrhea may be accompanied by fever, malaise, and marked weight loss and may be severely disabling and fatal (32). Such diarrhea may be present in HIV-infected patients who have no other clinical evidence of the AIDS (33,34). Etiologies include (a) cytomegalovirus, *E. histolytica*, and *Cryptosporidium* in one series (32); (b) *Campylobacter* spp., herpes simplex virus, and *Neisseria gonorrhoeae* in another study (33); (c) *C. jejuni* (34); and (d) *C. jejuni*, *Salmonella*, and *L. monocytogenes*; in descending order of frequency, they were especially noted to be associated with the AIDS patients' diarrhea group.

Patients with AIDS and diarrhea have lower numbers of OKT4 cells and a higher incidence of enteric pathogens and extraintestinal opportunistic infections (32). Direct HIV infection of mucosa epithelial cells may be a possible cause of diarrhea. HIV-positive patients often harbor more than one pathogen (33).

Acquired Immunodeficiency Syndrome or Human Immunodeficiency Virus Enteropathy

AIDS enteropathy is a chronic, well-established diarrhea (over 1 month's duration) for which no infectious cause can be determined after complete evaluation, including duodenal biopsy with electron microscopy of the small bowel, and is found in patients with advanced HIV infection. Occult enteric pathogens (*Mycobacterium avium-intracellulare* and *Microsporidia*) may be found. Villous atrophy and crypt hyperplasia may be related to T-cell dysfunction (35,36).

Cyanobacteria-Like Bodies

Cyanobacteria-like bodies are found in immunocompromised patients and travelers to tropical regions after ingestion of contaminated water. Symptoms include fatigue, malaise, and low-grade fever followed by explosive, watery diarrhea. Treatment is supportive. Diarrhea usually resolves even in patients with AIDS (37).

Anaerobiospirillum Species

Anaerobiospirillum, a genus of spiral bacteria with bipolar tufts of flagella, may produce a chronic diarrhea in humans (38–40). Transfer from pets may occur. The organism can be cultured under anaerobic conditions. It has a potential for invasiveness and pathogenicity, especially in compromised hosts (41,42).

Treatment of Human Immunodeficiency Virus–Positive Patients

Patients infected with HIV may require prolonged antimicrobial therapy. Even then, specific therapy may be no more effective in reducing the diarrhea than symptomatic treatment with diphenoxylate hydrochloride (43). Weight loss and malabsorption may persist and even progress despite the elimination of potential pathogenic organisms. Control of the diarrhea with symptomatic therapy may add the least to the suffering of the patient (43). In patients with AIDS or HIV enteropathy, anecdotal case reports suggest that immune serum globulin, somatostatin, spiramycin, and hyperimmune bovine colostrum may be useful in long-standing chronic cryptosporidiosis.

SPECIFIC PATHOGENS CAUSING BACTERIAL FOOD POISONING

Bacillus cereus

B. cereus is an aerobic to facultative gram-positive motile rod that is found in a variety of sites. It can form endospores that are resistant to heat and cold. The incidence of *B. cereus*–related diseases is increasing. Although *B. cereus* can be cultured from many foods, it is only the enterotoxin-producing strains that cause human disease. Two distinct illness patterns occur. Type I toxin is associated primarily with contaminated fried and cooked rice, noodles, pasta, and pastries (44). Type II illness is associated with contaminated meats, vegetables, sauces, puddings, milk, and milk products (44).

PATHOPHYSIOLOGY

The type I enterotoxin (emetic toxin) is called *cereulide* (44). The toxin is resistant to heat, pH, and proteolysis. Type II enterotoxin (diarrheal toxin) is heat labile and is produced in the small intestine during the growth of vegetative cells (45). Diarrheal illness is produced by a number of enterotoxins, including the protein complexes hemolysin BL and nonhemolytic enterotoxin and enterotoxic proteins (enterotoxin T and cytotoxin K) (46). In addition to the primary enterotoxins, phospholipase C, β-lactimases, proteases, and collagenases act as co-virulence factors (47).

CLINICAL PRESENTATION

Type I toxin has an incubation period of 1 to 6 hours (48). It typically causes abdominal pain and vomiting, but diarrhea may occur as well. Liver injury has also been reported (49). Illness from type I enterotoxin is more likely to cause serious illness, although symptoms are usually mild and last less than 24 hours with either form of illness. Fatalities occur rarely (49).

Type II disease has an incubation period of 6 to 24 hours (48). Abdominal pain and diarrhea are common, as is nausea, but vomiting usually does not occur. Fever is uncommon with either type (48).

DIAGNOSTIC TESTS

Differentiating *B. cereus* from other causes of foodborne illness may be difficult. Several commercial immunoassay-based kits are available to detect enterotoxin. The BCET-RPLA kit (Oxoid, Hampshire, England, United Kingdom) uses reverse passive latex agglutination to detect a component of type II toxin. An enzyme-linked immunosorbent assay (ELISA) is available from Tecra Diagnostics (New South Wales, Australia) (49,50) that also detects a component of type II toxin. Type I toxin is less immunogenic and difficult to detect immunochemically. Bioassays have been developed for detecting type I toxin (51). Culturing more than 10^5 organisms from the suspected food source confirms the diagnosis (48).

TREATMENT

The principles of treatment are described in Treatment of Acute Foodborne Gastroenteritis. Antibiotics are generally not indicated for *B. cereus*, as the symptoms are caused by already formed enterotoxins that are present in the food. Further, the clinical illness produced is usually mild and the course generally short; however, immunocompromised patients may require antibiotic therapy.

Campylobacter Species

Campylobacter is a genus of microaerophilic, spirally curved, gram-negative rods (52,53). It is a major cause of bacterial enteritis and has been implicated in ulcer formation and fetal loss. In

1996, it was the leading cause of bacterial foodborne disease, with an incidence of 25 per 100,000 population (54). Overall, it is responsible for 3% to 6% of all diarrheal illness in the United States and is a major cause of traveler's diarrhea. Important constituents of the genus include *C. pylori (Helicobacter)* and *C. jejuni. C. coli, C. fetus*, and *C. upsaliensis* are rare causes of illness. Children less than 5 years of age are particularly susceptible (53,55,56). Primary sources of *Campylobacter* are contaminated water (57), unpasteurized milk (58), and poultry (59). Contact of other foods with raw poultry can result in cross-contamination and infection (60). *Campylobacter*-like organisms are also found in homosexual men with diarrhea.

PREGNANCY AND LACTATION

A toxin produced by the bacterium is believed responsible for increased rates of abortion in sheep and goats (61–63), guinea pigs (64), and mice (65). Many case reports have been published of miscarriage and perinatal deaths in infected women (66–71). However, colonization does not occur more frequently in women who have a spontaneous abortion than in those with uncomplicated pregnancies (72), and it is uncertain how much the risk of abortion is increased as a result of *Campylobacter* infection.

Human milk may contain immunoglobins against *Campylobacter*. Breast-feeding may reduce the incidence of *Campylobacter*-associated gastroenteritis (73,74).

CLINICAL PRESENTATION

The incubation period is 3 to 5 days, with a 1-day prodrome of headache, myalgia, and malaise, followed by nausea, severe abdominal cramping, profuse watery diarrhea that contains blood in 50% of infected individuals by day two, and usually high fever. Vomiting is minimal. Because of the often intense abdominal pain, *Campylobacter* infection may mimic appendicitis (53). If untreated, symptoms last 1 to 2 weeks. Relapses in untreated patients occur in approximately 25%. Antibiotic treatment shortens the average duration of symptoms, reduces the incidence of relapse, and is therefore indicated in suspected or confirmed infections.

Immunocompromised patients are particularly predisposed to recurrent or chronic *C. jejuni* infection (53 other species may also infect HIV patients) (75). Extraintestinal illness may follow *C. jejuni* enteritis, including reactive arthritis, Reiter's syndrome, Guillain-Barré syndrome, and pancreatitis (53). In women with suspected *Campylobacter* infection, antibiotic treatment has been proposed to minimize fetal risk (76). The risk to the neonate born to a chronic *Campylobacter*-infected mother is unclear. In a study of 85 *C. pylori*–positive women, their newborn infants did not have an increased risk of *C. pylori* infection or associated gastritis during the first year of life (77).

DIAGNOSTIC TESTS

Definitive diagnosis is made by culturing the organism. The organism can be detected by polymerase chain reaction techniques (78). Blood is present in the stool in 50% of cases by the second day, and large numbers of fecal leukocytes are usually seen on microscopic examination of the stool, as with most bacterial enteritis.

TREATMENT

In addition to the standard symptomatic and supportive care of bacterial diarrhea, antibiotics for *C. jejuni* infection include erythromycin or azithromycin. Alternatively, a fluoroquinolone, tetracycline, or gentamicin can be used. Drug resistance is an increasing problem. A combination of ampicillin plus a fluoroquinolone can be used (79). For *C. pylori*, the usual treatment includes triple therapy with amoxicillin or tetracycline, a metronidazole, and a bismuth compound (80).

Clostridium botulinum

C. botulinum is a spore-forming, anaerobic, gram-positive bacillus that produces botulinum toxin. Variants *C. barati* and *C. butyricum* also produce human disease. The toxin has eight serotypes, with seven (A, B, C_α, C_β, E, F, and G) known to produce illness in humans. The toxin is a single polypeptide chain that undergoes proteolysis, generating heavy (molecular weight 100,000) and light (molecular weight, 50,000) chains linked by disulfide bonds. Spores germinate in an anaerobic environment in a pH greater than 4.6, and are heat resistant. The toxin is heat labile and can be destroyed by heating at a temperature of 100°C (212°F) for 10 minutes. Because of the lower boiling point of water at higher altitudes, increased boiling times or pressure cooking must be used to ensure destruction of the toxin. Commercial food processing accounts for only 2% of cases, with the majority being the result of home-canning errors, typically involving vegetables, fish, and meats. Serotype A is generally found west of the Mississippi (81) and type B east of it (82). Serotype E is found primarily in the Pacific Northwest and is particularly associated with consumption of fish (83).

Three general types of clinical disease occur. Foodborne botulism occurs as a result of the ingestion of preformed toxin. Infant botulism results from the organism elaborating toxin in the infant's immature GI tract, which lacks bile, gastric acids, and organisms (84,85) that would inhibit clostridial reproduction in an older person. This form has rarely been reported in adults. Wound botulism occurs as the result of *C. botulinum*–contaminated wounds, with absorption of toxin. It is a relatively uncommon cause of illness, with a median of four cases of foodborne botulism, three cases of wound botulism, and 71 cases of infant botulism reported to the CDC yearly (86). Concern has been shown that botulinum toxin may be used as a biological weapon (87).

PATHOPHYSIOLOGY

The dichain botulinum toxin binds to the cell membrane and is taken into the cell by endocytosis. Inside the cell, the toxin prevents release of acetylcholine from the presynaptic junction, impairing cholinergic nerve transmission at all acetylcholine-dependent synapses in the peripheral nervous system (88–90). This blockade is dose dependent, and results in acute symmetric voluntary muscle dysfunction and paralysis that can progress to respiratory muscle paralysis and death (91).

CLINICAL PRESENTATION

Clinical Diagnosis. The diagnosis of botulism is often missed on initial presentation because of nonspecific initial GI symptoms and the rarity of the disease. Approximately 70% of cases involve only one victim, and only 10% of cases involve more than two victims (92). Botulism should be suspected in any patient presenting with descending weakness and paralysis. The differential diagnosis includes other poisonings (carbon monoxide, aminoglycosides, anticholinergics, heavy metals, magnesium toxicity, organophosphate insecticides, plants, mushrooms, paralytic shellfish poisoning, elapid envenomation) and medical conditions (cerebrovascular accidents, Guillain-Barré syndrome, diphtheria, Eaton-Lambert syndrome, myelopathies, multiple sclerosis, myasthenia gravis, poliomyelitis). Patients with botulism may have a mildly positive response to cholinergic agents such as edrophonium, but it is usually less than that seen with myasthenia gravis, and the test is not diagnostic (Table 9).

TABLE 9. Differential diagnosis of botulism

Disease	Fever	Eye signs	Ascend descend	Symmetric asymmetric	Motor sensory autonomic	Comment
Botulism	–	Yes	Descend bulbar	Symmetric	Motor > autonomic	DTR absent late, ptosis late
Guillain-Barré	+	No	Ascend bulbar	Symmetric	Motor > sensory	Abnormal CSF, DTR absent
Fisher type		Yes			Autonomic	Early, previous URI
Poliomyelitis	+	No	Ascend bulbar	Asymmetric focal	Motor	Abnormal CSF, DTR absent early
Paralytic shellfish	–	No	Ascend	Symmetric	Motor = sensory	History, onset within 30–60 min
Tick paralysis	–	No	Ascend	Symmetric	Motor > sensory	Presence of tick
Diphtheria	+	No	Ascend	Symmetric	Motor	Membrane in pharynx
Myasthenia gravis	–	Yes	Descend bulbar	Symmetric	Motor autonomic	Ptosis early, fatigue
Lead	–	No	Ascend	Symmetric	Motor	History
Arsenic	–	No	Ascend	Symmetric distal	Sensory > motor	History
Periodic familial paralysis	–	No	Ascend	Symmetric	Motor	Family history
	Does not affect muscles of respiration					

+, present; –, absent; CSF, cerebrospinal fluid; DTR, deep tendon reflexes; URI, upper respiratory infection.
Adapted from Mofenson HC, et al., eds. *PP/T News*. MMWC Poison Control Center 1989;8:139.

The diagnosis of botulism is made by finding at least one of the following: (a) culture of the organism (e.g., from stool or a wound); (b) the detection of botulinum toxin in serum, stool, or food source; (c) typical electromyographic findings (repetitive nerve stimulation producing an incremental increase of small, compound muscle action potentials); or (d) compatible symptoms in someone exposed to a known source (87). The toxin (in adult foodborne disease) may not be detectable after the first several days. Examination of the wound in wound botulism is not diagnostic.

Foodborne Botulism. Botulinum toxin is the most potent toxin known, with as little as 0.05 µg (a lick) being potentially fatal (Table 10). Botulinum toxin is capable of producing disease regardless of the route of exposure (i.e., foodborne, wound, intestinal, inhalation) (91). Clinical features of foodborne botulism, such as incubation period, severity, and case-fatality rates, vary by serotype. Type A generally has an incubation period of 0 to 7 days; type B, 0 to 5 days; and type E, 0 to 2 days (92), although the incubation period is directly related to the amount of the exposure. As such, the index case in an outbreak usually occurs in the most heavily exposed individual. Initial GI symptoms may be particularly prominent with type E toxin. Approximately 67% of patients with type A require intubation, compared with 52% with type B and 39% with type E (92). The case fatality rate is 12% for type A and 10% for B and E (93–95).

Botulism presents with nonspecific GI symptoms of nausea and vomiting, progressing to involvement of the bulbar muscles, with diplopia, dysarthria, dysphonia, and dysphagia. Dizziness, fatigue, and sore throat are commonly reported, and cranial nerve deficits, facial paresis, ptosis, and ophthalmoplegia are common signs. Pupils are commonly dilated and fixed, helping differentiate botulism from Guillain-Barré and its descending Miller-Fisher variant. Also, sensory findings are notably absent in botulism and commonly present in other neurologic disorders. Muscle weakness progresses distally, eventually reaching the respiratory muscles and producing respiratory paralysis and death. Respiratory failure, when it occurs, usually develops within 12 hours of the onset of oculomotor (cranial nerve III) paralysis. The central nervous system and axonal nerve conduction are unaffected (90), and fever is usually absent.

TABLE 10. Relative lethality of selected toxins

Toxin	Source	MLD(µg/kg mouse)	No. of molecules causing death
Botulinum toxin	Bacteria	0.0003	2×10^7
Tetanus toxin	Bacteria	0.001	8×10^7
Diphtheria toxin	Bacteria	0.03	6×10^9
Batrachotoxin	Frog	2.0	5×10^{13}
Taipoxin	Snake	2.0	6×10^{11}
Ricin	Plant	3.0	6×10^{11}
Conotoxin	Snail	5.0	4×10^{13}
Tetrodotoxin	Fish	8.0	3×10^{14}
Saxitoxin	Dinoflagellate	9.0	3×10^{14}
α-Latrotoxin	Spider	10.0	9×10^{11}
β-Bungarotoxin	Snake	14.0	8×10^{12}
Cobrotoxin	Snake	75.0	1×10^{14}
Curare	Plant	500	2×10^{16}
DFP	Synthetic nerve gas	1000	7×10^{16}
Sodium cyanide	Chemical	10,000	2×10^{18}

DFP, diisopropyl fluorophosphate; MLD, minimum lethal dose.
Adapted from Middlebrook JL. *J Toxicol Toxin Rev* 1980;5:177–190.

Infant Botulism. Infant botulism is the most common form and usually involves children under 1 year of age. Ingestion of honey was associated with 34.7% of hospitalized cases (96). The onset of symptoms may be insidious. The presentation is of a "floppy" child with a diffuse decrease in muscle tone, decreased deep tendon reflexes, diminished gag reflex, and cranial nerve findings on examination. Constipation is common. Fever usually does not occur, and, in contrast to adult foodborne botulism, GI symptoms are usually absent. Although thought to be a possible explanation for some cases of sudden infant death syndrome, not one of 248 infants with sudden infant death syndrome was found to be culture positive for *C. botulinum* in a prospective study (97).

Wound Botulism. Wound botulism most commonly occurs in intravenous (IV) drug abusers, particularly among black tar heroin users (98,99) and in patients with contaminated crush wounds. The incubation period is 4 to 18 days (100), followed by the typical neurologic findings and often fever, but without GI symptoms.

TREATMENT

Foodborne Botulism. Admission to a hospital is indicated whenever botulism is suspected. Treatment consists of GI decontamination, administration of the specific antitoxin, possibly the use of hyperimmune globulin, and meticulous symptomatic and supportive care. Aggressive respiratory support is essential. Controlled, anticipatory intubation is indicated when the decline in vital capacity approaches 30% of predicted. The period of recovery from paralysis may be prolonged.

Removal of the spores and toxin from the GI tract should be attempted, even days after exposure. Activated charcoal has been shown to adsorb *C. botulinum* type A toxin *in vitro* (101). Gastric lavage or whole bowel irrigation should be considered for recent ingestion of a known or suspected contaminated food.

Antitoxin is available as a monovalent (A, B, E, or F), bivalent (AB), or trivalent (ABE) formulation from the CDC and experimental pentavalent or heptavalent antitoxins from the military. Trivalent antitoxin is preferred if the serotype is unknown, should be administered as soon as possible after the clinical diagnosis has been made, and should not be delayed for the results of microbiologic testing. A review of 132 cases found lower case-fatality rates and shorter duration of illness in patients who received trivalent antitoxin (95). The antitoxin is an equine-based immunoglobulin G. Anaphylaxis is reported in 1.9% (94,102), and skin testing and appropriate measures for managing potential hypersensitivity reactions should be available. Serum sickness occurs in 9% to 17% of cases (103). The antitoxin generally prevents progression of muscle weakness, but does not reverse existing paralysis. Because antitoxin is only available from the CDC, early notification is essential in timely acquisition and administration. The CDC prefers to be notified through its designated contact in the appropriate state health department, although there are direct lines if necessary (404-639-2206; after hours, 404-639-2888).

Infant Botulism. In infant botulism, circulating levels of the toxin are very low. Antitoxin has not been shown to be clinically useful and is not recommended. Human botulism immunoglobulin may be useful (104,105). The role of antibiotics has not been clearly demonstrated. Children have recovered without antitoxin or antibiotics, and spores and toxin have been detected in the stool for months after clinical recovery in infants treated with antibiotics and antitoxin. Aggressive respiratory and nutritional support may be required. Recovery is usually slow.

Wound Botulism. In wound botulism, the wound should be débrided. The efficacy of antitoxin is not well established but probably should be used. The role of antibiotics has not been clearly demonstrated with regard to botulism, but they are usually prescribed for local infection.

Clostridium perfringens

C. perfringens is found in poultry and heat-processed meats and gravy. It produces heat-labile enterotoxins. The toxins bind to a protein receptor in cell membranes, producing a conformational change that affects permeability for molecules less than 200,000 daltons (106). *C. perfringens* enterotoxin is the virulence factor responsible. It is a single polypeptide chain with a molecular weight of 3500 daltons that binds to receptors on the target epithelial cells (107). Illness can be prevented by heating food to greater than 100°C (212°F) (108).

CLINICAL PRESENTATION

Illness with *C. perfringens* is usually mild and self-limiting. After an incubation period of 8 to 24 hours, abdominal cramping, nausea, and diarrhea generally develop. Headache was reported in 42%, and fever occurred in 19% of patients in one case series (109). Vomiting occurred in 13% (109) to 30% (110) of patients. Headache was reported in 42% of 230 patients in one series (109). Blood is usually present in the stool. Symptoms generally resolve within 24 hours.

DIAGNOSTIC TESTS

The organism can be cultured from vomitus, stool, or food source, but this is usually not required or helpful. A *C. perfringens* isolate can be classified by plasmid profiling, ribotyping, and macrorestriction analysis by pulsed-field gel electrophoresis (111–113). The enterotoxin gene can be identified by polymerase chain reaction (111,114,115), and Western blotting (116), the enterotoxin itself by latex agglutination (111), and antibodies to the enterotoxin can be detected in human serum by an ELISA (117).

TREATMENT

Antibiotic treatment is usually not required. Type C *C. perfringens* has been associated with necrotic enteritis and a high mortality and is the result of a β-toxin (118). This toxin is degraded by proteolytic enzymes such as trypsin. In individuals with normal production of pancreatic trypsin who avoid trypsin inhibitors such as sweet potatoes, necrotic disease generally does not develop.

Escherichia coli O157:H7

The most common source of *E. coli* O157:H7 is cattle and includes all cattle-related food products, such as beef, milk, yogurt, and cheese. One outbreak was traced to unpasteurized apple cider. Water contaminated with fecal material from cattle or humans is another common source (119–121). Frequent *E. coli* O157:H7 epidemics occur in the United States, most commonly in the summer months, corresponding to the peak incidence of positive cattle stool cultures (122). The infectious dose of *E. coli* O157:H7 is less than 1000 organisms (123). Proper cooking of beef, pasteurization of milk and apple cider, and proper preparation, storage, and handling of other dairy products are essential in preventing illness.

PATHOPHYSIOLOGY

E. coli O157:H7 is a gram-negative rod that produces a toxin similar to that produced by *S. dysenteriae* type I, referred to as a *Shiga-like toxin* (SLT). At least two types of SLT with variants (124) and more than 50 *E. coli* O serotype strains exist. Other organisms may also produce SLTs. In addition to intestinal injury, the toxin is believed to gain access to the renal glomerular endothelium after intestinal absorption and then produce ribosomal inactivation and cell death. Numerous other effects, including activation of the coagulation cascade, platelet binding, and the production of cytokines, can occur (125,126).

CLINICAL PRESENTATION

The incubation period is 24 to 72 hours. Typically, acute diarrhea develops that lasts for 3 to 4 days and often becomes bloody. In patients in whom more serious illness will develop, vomiting and low-grade fever progress to altered mental status. Patients who progress to severe renal and central nervous system effects tend to develop antibodies to a larger number of *E. coli* serogroups than those with moderate or mild impairment (127). In its most severe form, an HUS develops, characterized by a microangiopathic hemolytic anemia, thrombocytopenia, and acute, oliguric renal failure. Liver and pancreatic injury may also occur, and approximately 10% of children present with a generalized seizure at the onset of HUS (128). Attack rates are lower in those with long-term exposure to *E. coli* sources, suggesting that partial immunity may occur (129) and help explain why HUS is most commonly seen in children less than 6 years of age and frequently in children less than 2 years of age.

DIAGNOSIS

Early diagnosis and aggressive supportive care improve outcome. A high index of suspicion and active surveillance for *E. coli* O157:H7 should be maintained. Fecal leukocytes are seen in one-third to two-thirds of patients. *E. coli* O157:H7 can be identified through stool culture. Recovery of the organism declines after the first week (130). An enzyme-based immunoassay and polymerase chain reaction test may detect SLT in the stool (131).

TREATMENT

Treatment of HUS requires meticulous attention to fluid and electrolyte balance and early peritoneal or hemodialysis for renal failure, acidosis, or fluid overload. Approximately 50% of patients with HUS require peritoneal or hemodialysis (132). Transfusion may be required if the hemoglobin concentration declines below 6 g/dl and is required in 75% of cases (132). Thrombocytopenia and coagulation abnormalities may also need to be corrected.

Seizures are managed in the usual manner, starting with benzodiazepines (Chapter 40), and renal hypertension can be controlled with short-acting antihypertensives such as nifedipine. Various therapies have been tried in HUS, including IV immunoglobulin, fresh frozen plasma, antiplatelet agents, fibrinolytics, and heparin. None has been proven effective (133). Plasmapheresis has been used in HUS after renal transplant. Plasma exchange therapy in three patients with HUS was followed by mild illness and early resolution of symptoms. Various inflammatory cytokines were lower in patients treated with plasma exchange (134).

Antibiotics do not change the course or outcomes in children with postdiarrheal HUS (135) and may increase the incidence of HUS in elderly patients (136), either by allowing faster growth of resistant organisms in the absence of competing organisms or by liberating bacterial cytotoxins (137). Antimotility drugs may also increase the incidence of HUS (132). HUS is more likely to develop in those with bloody diarrhea (132), and oliguria lasting more than 2 weeks, anuria lasting longer than 1 week, or severe extrarenal disease is a marker of higher morbidity and mortality. The acute mortality from HUS is approximately 5%, with another 5% progressing to end-stage renal failure or chronic, residual central nervous system effects (21). Currently, a number of experimental therapies are in development, including synthetic SLT receptors attached to a chromosorb and oriented carbohydrates that bind to SLT and prevent uptake into target cells (138,139).

Listeria monocytogenes

L. monocytogenes is a facultative intracellular bacterium that causes disease primarily in pregnant women, neonates, and immunocompromised patients. The bacterium is ubiquitous, appearing in streams, sewage, soil, domestic and wild animals, fowl, and humans. Carrier rates are approximately 5% in healthy adults and higher in special risk groups. *Listeria* can penetrate the placenta and produce intrauterine infections. *L. monocytogenes* organisms can remain in pasteurized milk even after proper processing. Recent epidemics of listeriosis resulted from the consumption of cabbage, cheese, pasteurized milk (140), and raw vegetables.

DIAGNOSIS

An initial study of human listeriosis suggests that detection of antibodies against listeriolysin O, an extracellular hemolysin, may aid in the diagnosis of listeriosis, especially when bacteria have not been isolated (141). Listeriolysin O appears to be produced by all pathogenic strains of *L. monocytogenes*. Prior agglutination tests and complement fraction tests have been nonspecific. Immunosuppression increases the risk of listeriosis. Total rise is 33% (142).

TABLE 11. Intravenous antibiotics suggested for treating *Listeria*: dosages and dosage intervals

Antibiotic	Dosage per day	Interval (h)
Ampicillin	200–300 mg/kg	Every 4
Penicillin G	24,000–48,000 U/kg	Every 4
Gentamicin	5–6 mg/kg	Every 6–8
Tobramycin	5–6 mg/kg	Every 6–8
Erythromycin	40–60 mg/kg	Every 6
Tetracycline	15 mg/kg	Every 6
Doxycycline	3 mg/kg intravenous load, then 1.5 mg/kg	Every 12
Sulfamethoxazole and trimethoprim	15 and 75 mg/kg	Every 8
Vancomycin	2 g	Every 12

Adapted from Gellin BG, Broome CV. *JAMA* 1989;261:1313–1318.

CLINICAL COURSE

In healthy adults and children, *L. monocytogenes* produces a mild flu-like syndrome, with GI symptoms and myalgias resolving in several days. Meningitis and sepsis characterized by nausea, vomiting, headache, and fever may develop in immunocompromised patients. Perinatal infections can cause either perinatal meningitis or intrauterine fetal demise.

TREATMENT

IV antibiotics suggested for listeriosis treatment are found in Table 11.

Salmonella Species

Salmonella is a gram-negative bacillus. The most common species in the United States include *S. enteritidis* and *S. typhimurium*. Species found in reptiles include *S. arizonae*, *S. chameleon*, *S. java*, and *S. marinum* (143). Infections are associated with cattle, domestic animals, and poultry (in particular, uncooked or undercooked eggs) and in sprouts (144,145). Raw eggs are found as an ingredient in numerous foods, including chocolate mousse, eggnog, egg creams, Caesar salad dressing, and hollandaise sauce. The potential for undercooking exists when eggs are prepared "sunny side up" or are poached. Household pets may harbor *Salmonella*. Aside from poultry, such as chicks and ducklings, all reptiles (e.g., turtles, lizards, snakes, iguanas) are capable of harboring the organism and producing disease as well. In the United States, nearly 100,000 cases of *Salmonella* infections are caused by contact with reptiles. The widespread use of antibiotics in animal feed is believed to have contributed to the development of multiple drug-resistant strains.

Chronic diarrheal syndromes frequently involve multidrug-resistant *Salmonella* (146). Infection with multidrug-resistant *S. typhimurium* results in hospitalization rates that are twice those of other foodborne *Salmonella* infections and have a tenfold higher case-fatality rate (147). Nontyphoidal *Salmonella* infection has also been associated with increased fetal loss in pregnancy (148). Typhoid and paratyphoid fevers are caused by *S. typhi* and *S. paratyphi*, respectively. They are endemic in developing countries with poor sanitation (149,150). The majority of cases occur in South and Southeast Asia (151), and most cases in the industrialized world are related to international travel to endemic regions. Vaccines are being tested in humans (152) and animals (153) for protection of animal flocks, but they are not completely protective.

CLINICAL PRESENTATION

Young children are particularly susceptible. The highest incidence of salmonellosis occurs in children less than 5 years of age. Nearly 25% are less than 1 year of age (154,155). Specifically, most patients who contract reptile-associated salmonellosis are infants and young children, and infants are particularly prone to invasive illness, including osteomyelitis, sepsis, and meningitis (156). Immunocompromised individuals, especially HIV-infected persons, are at increased risk for infection with *S. typhi* and *S. paratyphi* (157).

The incubation period of *S. enteritidis* is 12 to 36 hours, followed by fever, vomiting, and diarrhea, and is inversely related to dose (158). Symptoms gradually diminish over 3 to 5 days (158). With *S. typhi* or *S. paratyphi*, the incubation is 10 to 14 days and may be as long as 3 days to 2 months. With typhoid or paratyphoid fevers, the diarrhea is classically described as appearing like "pea soup." Fever, malaise, headache, and myalgias follow. The fever predictably ascends in a stepwise fashion over 3 to 4 days, plateaus, and then slowly returns to normal. Bradycardia relative to the fever may be present, and hepatosplenomegaly is a common finding. Blanching, maculopapular erythematous lesions ("rose spots") approximately 2 mm in size occur on the upper abdomen in 30% of cases.

DIAGNOSIS

Definitive diagnosis is made by culturing the organism from the stool.

TREATMENT

Antimotility drugs should be avoided because they increase the risk of invasive disease (159). Antibiotics are not required unless there are signs of systemic illness or prolonged or severe symptoms or in immunocompromised individuals and in young children. Infants less than 3 months have an increased risk of complications and require aggressive antibiotic treatment (160). Although *Salmonella* spp. have historically been sensitive to fluoroquinolones and second- and third-generation cephalosporins, multidrug-resistant strains are becoming more frequent (161) and drug sensitivities may be required for proper antibiotic selection.

Shigella Species

Shigellosis is caused by a gram-negative rod. The species includes *S. boydii*, *S. dysenteriae*, *S. flexneri*, and *S. sonnei* (162). *Shigella* most frequently occurs in children below 5 years of age. Day-care centers are associated with epidemic spread (163), and it is a cause of 4% to 7% of traveler's diarrhea (164). The most common organism infecting children is *S. sonnei*, whereas *S. flexneri* is more common in elderly patients and homosexual men (165,166). HIV infection is an important risk factor for shigellosis (167). The organism is found in contaminated food and water (168). A very small inoculum (10 to 200 organisms) is capable of causing infection (169). It is spread by poor hygiene, such as inadequate hand-washing (170,171). Person-to-person contact and mechanical vectors, such as the housefly, spread infection (172,173). *Shigella* has also been used as a means of intentional food poisoning (19,20).

CLINICAL PRESENTATION

The incubation period is usually 24 to 48 hours. Illness begins with the rapid onset of fever, crampy abdominal pain, and diarrhea. Profuse and watery stools often contain blood and mucus. Fluid loss may result in significant dehydration (171,174), especially in neonates (163). Febrile seizures may occur early in the course in children. They are usually generalized and self-limited (174,175). Seizures and other neurologic symptoms, such as delirium, hallucinations, and meningismus, may precede GI symptoms, making diagnosis difficult (171,176–178).

Encephalopathy and cerebral edema may occur (178,179–181). Other complications include intestinal obstruction (182), appendicitis (183), colonic perforation, and intra-abdominal abscesses (184). Symptoms generally resolve in 5 to 7 days. *S. flexneri* is characterized by a more prolonged course than *S. sonnei* (165,166). Shigellosis may produce fatalities. Risk factors for fatality include age less than 1 year, altered mental status, bacteremia, hyponatremia, hypoproteinemia, ileus, and thrombocytopenia (163,185).

DIAGNOSIS

The white blood cell count is frequently below 10,000 cells per cubic millimeter with a high band count (186). Fecal leukocytes are routinely observed, and the stool often contains blood. Definitive diagnosis is made by culturing the organism.

TREATMENT

Antibiotic therapy shortens the course, lessens the severity, decreases the incidence of complications, and shortens the period of fecal shedding, which may reduce epidemic spread. Azithromycin, ceftriaxone, trimethoprim-sulfamethoxazole, and fluoroquinolones are generally effective (187,188), although the incidence of drug-resistant strains is increasing. Trimethoprim-sulfamethoxazole is generally the drug of choice. Ampicillin (not amoxicillin) or tetracycline (in adults) is an alternative. In drug-resistant strains, a fluoroquinolone or azithromycin (in children) may be the preferred agent (189).

Antidiarrheal agents are not recommended and may worsen the illness (169). Vaccines are in clinical trials. Preliminary data suggest adequate immunogenic response and efficacy in young adults (190,191), but adverse reactions may occur at a relatively high rate (22%) (192).

Staphylococcus aureus

Although the organism is heat sensitive, food poisoning from *S. aureus* is the result of preformed, heat-stable enterotoxins, classified as types A, B, C, D, and E. Type A toxin is the most common in the United States. *Staphylococcus* toxins have a molecular weight of approximately 28,000 and are water soluble. The enterotoxins are formed when food remains at temperatures of 10 to 45°C for more than 4 hours (193). Most pathogenic strains are coagulase positive, but coagulase-negative strains have been reported (194). The toxins produce an inflammatory response in GI mucosa, leading to cell injury and death. Sources of exposure include proteinaceous food, especially unrefrigerated cream-filled baked goods, and individuals with staphylococcal infections. Skin contamination may not be clinically obvious, and contamination of food may come from poor hygiene practices of food handlers who are unaware of their carrier status (193).

CLINICAL COURSE

Because illness is caused by a preformed toxin, the incubation period is usually short, between 2 and 6 hours. The type of enterotoxin affects the severity of the disease. Type B enterotoxin is associated with more severe illness, resulting in 46% of patients seeking hospital care, compared with 5% with type A toxin (193). Abdominal pain, nausea, vomiting (sometimes violent), and diarrhea are common. Subjective fever was reported in 16% of 2992 cases during 131 outbreaks (193), but significant temperature elevation is rare (195). Headache was reported in 11% of cases in a large series (193). Duration of symptoms is usually less than 24 hours.

Exposure to enterotoxin may also occur in an aerosolized form and has potential as a war or terrorism agent. The incubation period is between 3 and 12 hours, and symptoms frequently include cough and dyspnea. The aerosol-incapacitating dose is smaller than the ingested dose (approximately 30 ng inhaled vs. 200 ng ingested), with a lethal inhalation dose of approximately 1.7 mg. Most patients recover within 1 to 2 weeks, with less than 1% mortality (196,197).

DIAGNOSIS

Detection of specific *S. aureus* isolates can be accomplished by restriction fragment length polymorphisms analysis by pulsed-field gel electrophoresis (198,199). Latex agglutination, deoxyribonucleic acid probe (200), and ELISA immunoassays can also detect staphylococcal enterotoxins in food and biologic fluids (201).

TREATMENT

Treatment is comprised primarily of supportive care of vomiting and diarrhea. Antibiotic treatment is not effective in altering the course of the illness unless systemic staphylococcal infection occurs. Immunocompromised patients may be at greater risk.

Yersinia enterocolitica

Y. enterocolitica is an invasive gram-negative coccobacillus. *Y. enterocolitica* 0:3 is emerging as an important pathogen in the United States, particularly among black infants and children who consume chitterlings, an ethnic food that is often prepared by blacks for holiday meals. Raw chitterlings are an important vehicle for transmitting infection (202). It has also been reported in the consumption of buttermilk (203). Wild and domestic animals both harbor this organism. It contaminates the food chain because of its frequency in farm animals. Outbreaks follow ingestion of tofu and unpasteurized as well as pasteurized milk. The organism can replicate at refrigerator temperatures.

CLINICAL COURSE

Infections by *Y. enterocolitica* result in three clinical types of illness, depending on the patient's age. In patients under 5 years of age, a self-limited gastroenteritis generally develops with variable amounts of diarrhea and fever. In a recent outbreak, the dysentery-like picture was characterized by fever (93%), abdominal pain (86%), diarrhea (83%), vomiting (41%), sore throat (22%), rash (22%), bloody stools (20%), and joint pain (15%). In older children mesenteric adenitis and ileitis, which mimics appendicitis, often develop. In 10% of confirmed cases in the above outbreak, patients underwent laparotomy for suspected appendicitis (204). In adults, bacteremia, hepatic abscess, Reiter's syndrome, glomerulonephritis, polyarthritis, arthralgias, or erythema nodosum may develop. Intestinal perforation, peritonitis, and gangrene of the small bowel have been reported after *Y. enterocolitica* infections.

Y. enterocolitica, using deferoxamine as a siderophore, can transfer iron across its membranes for its metabolic needs. Iron loading increases the virulence of *Y. enterocolitica*. Iron overload and deferoxamine therapy are independent predisposing factors for systemic infections with *Y. enterocolitica* (205). Iron enrichment may similarly have been a factor in *Y. enterocolitica* bacteremia cases and endotoxic shock associated with red blood cell transfusions in the United States and Australia (206,207).

DIAGNOSIS

Diagnosis by stool culture requires the special culture technique of cold enrichment. Serologic examination of paired sera also helps establish the diagnosis.

TREATMENT

This disease is usually self-limiting. Tetracycline is reserved for severe, protracted cases. Trimethoprim-sulfamethoxazole is also effective. Little medical literature is available to guide antibiotic therapy.

DIAGNOSTIC TESTS FOR ACUTE FOODBORNE GASTROENTERITIS

Supplementary laboratory studies in the assessment of the patient with acute diarrhea are rarely needed. However, serum electrolytes should be measured when there are signs of significant dehydration or abnormal electrolyte concentrations, or with prolonged symptoms. Stool examination and cultures are indicated for dysentery but are not needed to initiate treatment in the usual case of acute watery diarrhea in the immunocompetent patient. White blood cells in the stool are suggestive of a bacterial enteritis. They may be seen on a standard Gram stain, but methylene blue is simpler and demonstrates them as well. Preformed toxins can be detected by immunoassays and other methods. The culturing of greater than 10^5 organisms per gram of material is presumptive evidence of infection (48).

Instructions for collection of stool specimens are listed in Table 12. Stool osmolality may be useful in selected cases. Diarrhea caused by defective electrolyte absorption or by excessive electrolyte secretion by intestinal epithelial cells is called *secretory diarrhea*. In secretory diarrhea the fecal fluid should be rich in electrolytes because secretion of electrolytes or failure to absorb electrolytes is the primary cause of the diarrhea. By contrast, osmotic diarrhea is caused by the osmotic effect of poorly absorbed solutes that are ingested in the diet or as medications. Secretory and osmotic diarrhea can be differentiated by measurement of fecal electrolytes. The monovalent electrolyte composition of fecal fluid can be estimated by the sum of the sodium and potassium concentrations, multiplied by a factor of 2 to account for associated anions. When this value is subtracted from fecal osmolality, the "osmotic gap" is derived; the osmotic gap should be large in osmotic diarrhea and small in secretory diarrhea. The osmotic gap is calculated using the theoretic osmolality of fecal fluid as it exits the rectum, which is the same as plasma osmolality of 290 mOsm/kg (208).

In phenolphthalein-induced secretory diarrhea an osmotic gap is less than 50 mOsm/kg. In osmotic diarrhea caused by polyethylene glycol, magnesium hydroxide, lactulose, or sorbitol, the osmotic gap is usually greater than 50 mOsm/kg. The osmotic gaps are more often over 140 mOsm/kg and frequently over 200 mOsm/kg (208).

TREATMENT OF ACUTE FOODBORNE GASTROENTERITIS

The primary symptoms of food poisoning are vomiting and diarrhea. Control of vomiting may or may not be necessary. With ill-

TABLE 12. General instructions for collection of stool specimens

Instructions for collecting specimens	Type of agent to be tested		
	Virus	Bacterium	Parasite
When to collect	Within 48–72 h after onset of illness	During period of active diarrhea (preferably as soon after onset of illness as possible)	Any time after onset of illness (preferably as soon after onset of illness as possible)
How much to collect	As much stool sample from each of 10 ill persons as possible (at least 10 ml each person); samples from 10 controls can also be submitted	Two rectal swabs or swabs of fresh stool from each of 10 ill persons; samples from 10 controls can also be submitted	A fresh stool sample from each of 10 ill persons; samples from 10 controls can also be submitted
Method of collection	Place fresh stool specimens (liquid preferable), unmixed with urine, in clean, dry containers (e.g., urine specimen cups)	For rectal swabs, moisten each of 2 swabs in Cary-Blair medium first, then insert sequentially 1.0–1.5 in. in rectum and gently rotate; place both swabs into the same Cary-Blair medium tube; break off top portions of swab sticks and discard	Collect a bulk stool specimen, unmixed with urine, in a clean container; place a portion of each stool sample into 10% formalin and polyvinyl alcohol preservatives at a ratio of 1 part stool to 3 parts preservative; mix well
Storage of specimen after collection	Immediately refrigerate at 4°C; *do not freeze* if electron microscopy is anticipated	Immediately refrigerate at 4°C if testing is to be done within 48 h after collection; otherwise freeze samples at 70°C	Store at room temperature or refrigerate at 4°C; *do not freeze*
Transportation	Keep refrigerated; place bagged and sealed specimens on ice or with frozen refrigerant packs in an insulated box; send by overnight mail; *do not freeze*	Refrigerate as directed for viral specimens; for frozen samples: place bagged and sealed samples on dry ice; mail in insulated box by overnight mail	Refrigerate as directed for viral specimens; for room-temperature samples: mail in waterproof containers; *do not freeze*

From CDC. Lew JF, et al. *MMWR Morb Mortal Wkly Rep* 1990;39:1–13, with permission.

ness of short duration, most patients can tolerate a brief period of decreased oral intake. When diarrhea is profound, when symptoms persist beyond 24 to 48 hours, in the very young or old, or in patients with concomitant illnesses, control of vomiting ameliorates dehydration and allows oral rehydration.

A controversial issue is whether control of diarrhea is beneficial or may delay clearance of the toxin or infectious agent. Diphenoxylate with atropine may prolong symptoms and the duration of some bacterial infections. Antibiotic therapy of bacterial food poisoning generally is not effective in treating a preformed toxin but may be useful in decreasing the severity and duration of bacterial agents that must first reproduce in the GI tract to cause illness. Although the use of ampicillin in *Salmonella* infection has been shown to prolong organism recovery in the stool, clinical symptoms resolve more quickly. No good evidence has shown that such treatment results in a chronic carrier state. Other antibiotics, such as the floxacillins, have been shown to shorten the clinical course and the period of bacterial recovery in the stool (209).

Vomiting

In the child with vomiting, oral rehydration should proceed with small, frequent volumes at first (e.g., 5 ml every minute). Careful administration with a spoon or syringe helps guarantee gradual progression in the amount taken. Often, simultaneous correction of dehydration lessens the frequency of vomiting. Because dehydration may occur more rapidly and be more difficult to appreciate clinically in children, the need for pharmacologic suppression of vomiting in children under 2 should prompt an evaluation of the need for hospitalization and IV hydration. In the older child and adult, antiemetics can be used more freely.

Acute Diarrhea in Children

Infants with acute diarrhea are more apt to dehydrate than are older children. Young children have a higher metabolic rate, have a higher rate of insensible loss because they have a higher body surface–weight ratio, and are dependent on others for fluid. The most accurate assessment of fluid status is acute weight change, but the patient's premorbid weight is often unknown. The clinical signs and symptoms of mild dehydration (3% to 5% fluid deficit) include increased thirst and slightly dry mucous membranes. Moderate dehydration (6% to 9% fluid deficit) is associated with loss of skin turgor, tenting of skin when pinched, and dry mucous membranes. Signs and symptoms of severe dehydration (10% fluid deficit) are severe lethargy or altered state of consciousness, prolonged skin tenting and skin retraction time (greater than 2 seconds), cool and poorly perfused extremities, and decreased capillary refill. Rapid, deep breathing (respiratory compensation for metabolic acidosis), prolonged skin retraction time, and decreased perfusion are more reliably predictive of dehydration than is a sunken fontanel or absence of tears. A good correlation has been reported between time of capillary refill and fluid deficit. However, fever, ambient temperature, and age can affect capillary refill time as well.

Oral Rehydration Therapy

The treatment of acute diarrhea (in contrast to diarrhea lasting 2 weeks or longer) is aimed primarily at watery diarrhea rather than bloody diarrhea (dysentery). Oral rehydration therapy (ORT) encompasses two phases of treatment: (a) the rehydration phase in which water and electrolytes are given as oral rehydration solution (ORS) to replace existing losses and (b) the maintenance phase, which includes replacement of ongoing fluid and electrolyte losses and adequate dietary intake. Although ORT implies rehydration alone, the definition has been broadened to include maintenance fluid therapy and nutrition.

Rehydration therapy is based on the degree of dehydration. For the mildly dehydrated patient (3% to 5% fluid deficit), oral rehydration should commence with a fluid containing 50 to 90 mEq/L sodium. The amount of fluid administered should be 50 ml/kg over a period of 2 to 4 hours. Using a teaspoon, syringe, or medicine dropper, the caregiver should initially provide small volumes of fluid (e.g., 1 tsp) and then gradually increase the amount as tolerated. After 2 to 4 hours, hydration status should be reassessed. If the patient is rehydrated, treatment should progress to the maintenance phase of therapy. If the patient is still dehydrated, the fluid deficit should be re-estimated and rehydration therapy should begin again.

For the moderately dehydrated patient (6% to 9% fluid deficit), oral rehydrating solution should be administered by the same procedures as used for the mildly dehydrated patient. The initial amount of fluid administered for rehydration should be increased to 100 ml/kg, administered over 2 to 4 hours.

Severe dehydration (10% fluid deficit, shock, or near shock) is a medical emergency. IV rehydration should begin immediately. Repeated infusions of Ringer's lactate solution, normal saline, or a similar solution, 20 ml/kg IV, should be administered until pulse, perfusion, and mental status return to normal. This treatment may require two IV lines or alternate access sites (e.g., venous cutdown, femoral vein, intraosseous infusion). When the patient's level of consciousness returns to normal, he or she can take the remaining estimated deficit by mouth.

For patients with acute diarrhea, but without signs of dehydration, the rehydration phase of therapy should be omitted and maintenance therapy started immediately. The dose of ORS should be 1 ml for each gram of diarrheal stool. Alternatively, stool losses can be approximated by administering 10 ml/kg for each watery or loose stool passed, and 2 ml/kg fluid should be administered for each episode of emesis. Excess fluid losses during maintenance therapy can be replaced either with low-sodium ORS (containing 40 to 60 mEq/L sodium) or with ORS containing 75 to 90 mEq/L sodium. When the latter type of fluid is used, an additional source of low-sodium fluid is recommended (e.g., breast milk, formula, or water).

Oral therapy has now become the mainstay of World Health Organization efforts to decrease diarrhea morbidity and mortality. Diarrheal disease control programs have been established in more than 100 countries worldwide (Tables 13, 14, and 15).

Oral Rehydrating Solutions

ORS can be used to treat diarrhea regardless of the patient's age, causative pathogen, or initial sodium values. Many physicians continue to prescribe a variety of "clear liquids" to treat patients with diarrhea instead of an appropriately composed ORS. "Clear fluids" can cause osmotic diarrhea and electrolyte imbalance, and they often contain inadequate sodium bicarbonate and excess sugar for appropriate replacement of stool losses.

Studies in Dhaka and Calcutta have confirmed that the addition of glucose to sodium-containing solutions results in net movement of salt and water from the intestinal lumen to the bloodstream of patients with severe cholera. These studies suggest that the use of a glucose-electrolyte solution provides safe, effective, and practical maintenance therapy for severely dehydrated patients who typically required IV rehydration to correct shock. Glucose-based ORS does not reduce the duration of illness or the volume of stool output. Early feeding, however, can reduce the severity, duration, and nutritional consequences of diarrhea. Providing additional drinking water at the bedside of rehydrated patients allows for excretion of any excess salt intake. More importantly, oral therapy allows fluid losses to be replaced in a timely manner and on a volume-for-volume basis with rehydration solution.

TABLE 13. Comparison of electrolyte-glucose concentrations of solutions commonly administered at home

Clear liquids	Na (mEq/L)	K (mEq/L)	HCO_3 (mEq/L)	Glucose (g/L)	Osmolarity (mmol/L)
Cola	2	0.1	13	50–150 glucose and fructose	550
Ginger ale	3	1	4	50–150 glucose and fructose	540
Apple juice	3	20	0	100–150 glucose and fructose	700
Chicken broth	250	5	0	0	450
Tea	0	0	0	0	5
Gatorade	20	3	3	45 glucose and other sugars	330

Adapted from CDC. *MMWR Morb Mortal Wkly Rep* 1992;41:6.

TABLE 14. Comparison of electrolyte and carbohydrate concentrations of commercial oral rehydration solution (ORS) and solutions commonly administered at home

	Commercial ORS (manufacturer)			
Component of solution[a]	WHO[b]	Pedialyte[c] (Ross)	Rehydralyte[c] (Ross)	Ricelyte[c] (Mead Johnson)
Sodium (mEq/L)	90	45	75	50
Potassium (mEq/L)	20	20	20	25
Chloride (mEq/L)	80	35	65	45
Citrate (mEq/L)	30	30	30	34
Glucose (g/L)	20	25	25	—
Rice-syrup solids (g/L)	—	—	—	30

WHO, World Health Organization.
[a]Composition of solutions taken from package inserts.
[b]WHO-ORS is dispensed in packets. This product is considered optimal. Manufactured and distributed in the United States by Jianas Brothers, Kansas City, MO.
[c]Pedialyte, Rehydralyte, and Ricelyte are dispensed in premixed liquid form.
Adapted from CDC. *MMWR Morb Mortal Wkly Rep* 1992;41:7.

Oral Rehydration Solution Guidelines

A key factor in the excellent therapeutic and safety record of ORT has been the development of simple rules that can be successfully taught by hospital and community clinical medical staff. Several approaches are effective, but all guidelines include communicating to the parent or guardian rules enabling him or her to mix the solution appropriately. These guidelines also permit the amount of oral solution administered to be related to the condition of the child and the frequency of stools. In addition, all rules encourage the parent or guardian to begin appropriate dietary liquids and foods early in the maintenance phase.

Availability of Oral Rehydration Solution in the United States

When caretakers are asked to mix ORS from packets at home, detailed written and oral instructions should be given. With premixed solutions, the concentration can be ensured, but cost can limit access. The bicarbonate component of the World Health Organization-ORS has been replaced with the bicarbonate precursor, citrate, because it has a longer shelf life. In the past 5

TABLE 15. Diarrhea treatment chart

Degree of dehydration	Signs[a]	Rehydration therapy (within 4 h)	Replacement of stool fluid losses	Dietary therapy[b]
Mild (3–5%)	Slightly dry buccal mucous membranes, increased thirst	ORS 50 ml/kg	10 ml/kg or 0.5–1.0 cup of ORS for each diarrheal stool	Human milk feeding, or half- or full-strength lactose-containing milk or undiluted lactose-free formula
Moderate (6–9%)	Sunken eyes, sunken fontanel, loss of skin turgor, dry buccal mucous membranes	ORS 100 ml/kg	Same as above	Same as above
Severe (>10%)	Signs of moderate dehydration with one of the following: rapid thready pulse, cyanosis, cold extremities, rapid breathing, lethargy, coma	IV fluids (Ringer's lactate), 20 ml/kg/h until pulse, perfusion, and mental status return to normal; then 50–100 ml/kg of ORS	Same as above	Same as above

ORS, oral rehydration solution.
[a]If no signs of dehydration are present, rehydration therapy is not required. Proceed with maintenance therapy and replacement of stool losses.
[b]Infants and children who receive solid food can continue their usual diet, but foods high in simple sugars and fats should be avoided.
Adapted from CDC. *MMWR Morb Mortal Wkly Rep* 1992;41:14.

years, American manufacturers of ORS have altered their formulations to contain lower, more appropriate concentrations of carbohydrate. The sodium concentrations of the fluids have also increased compared with previously available ORS.

When fluids with more than 60 mEq/L sodium are used for maintenance, other low-sodium fluids, such as breast milk, diluted or undiluted infant formula, or water, need to be administered as well to prevent sodium overload. The most widely used solutions in the United States, Pedialyte and Ricelyte, contain 45- and 50-mEq/L sodium, respectively. These fluids are intended for maintenance of hydration and prevention of dehydration in clinical practice. Pedialyte, Ricelyte, and other similar low-sodium solutions can be used for rehydration when the alternative is physiologically inappropriate liquids or IV fluids. When the rate of fluid loss is very high (e.g., above 10 ml/kg/hour), solutions with 75 to 90 mEq/L are recommended for rehydration.

One advantage of cereal-based ORS, at least in developing countries, is that these solutions can be easily prepared at home. The solutions require time and effort to prepare, and they can become contaminated if left unrefrigerated. Standardization of cereal-based solutions may prove difficult. The practice of early feeding reduces the severity, duration, and nutritional consequences of diarrhea.

Home Use of Oral Rehydration and Maintenance Solutions

Management of acute diarrhea should begin at home (Tables 13 and 14). Families with infants and small children should be encouraged to keep a supply of ORS at home at all times and to use the solution when diarrhea first occurs in the child. Regardless of the type of fluid used, an appropriate diet should be administered as well.

The most crucial aspect underlying home management of diarrhea is the need to administer increased volumes of appropriate fluids, as well as to maintain adequate caloric intake. Medications, other treatments, or inappropriate home remedies should be avoided. Infants should be offered more frequent feedings at the breast or bottle, and children should also be given more fluids.

Limitations of Oral Rehydration Therapy

ORT is not sufficient therapy for some cases of bloody diarrhea (dysentery), because patients with bloody diarrhea may have a bacterial or parasitic infection that requires treatment with an antimicrobial agent. Patients in shock or near shock should be treated initially with IV fluid (Table 15). Also, patients with intestinal ileus should not be given oral fluids until bowel sounds are audible.

Many patients with clinically significant acute diarrhea have concomitant vomiting. Nevertheless, greater than 90% can be successfully rehydrated or maintained with oral fluids when small volumes of ORS (4 to 10 ml) are administered every 1 to 2 minutes, with a gradual increase in the amount consumed. A frequent mistake is to allow a thirsty child to drink large volumes of ORS fluids (*ad libitum*) from a cup or a bottle; the caretaker should be instructed to administer ORS in small amounts via a spoon, syringe, cup, or feeding bottle. Continuous, slow nasogastric infusion of ORS via a feeding tube can be helpful for the child who is vomiting.

Stool output greater than 10 ml/kg/hour is associated with a lower rate of success of oral rehydration, although these data are derived from a study performed among patients who had cholera. In general, no patient should be denied ORT simply because of a high diarrheal fluid loss rate, because most patients respond well when administered adequate replacement fluid. In these individuals, subtle differences in substrate and electrolyte composition of oral solutions play a critical role in the success of therapy.

The presence of glucose or reducing substances in the stools, accompanied by a dramatic increase in stool output with the administration of ORS, is an indication of glucose malabsorption. The presence of stool-reducing substances alone is not sufficient to make the diagnosis, because this is a common finding among patients with diarrhea and does not indicate failure of oral therapy. Patients with true glucose malabsorption show an immediate reduction in stool output when IV therapy is begun instead of oral therapy. Malabsorption of lactose, maltose, and sucrose can also occur because of deficiencies of their respective enzymes or starvation associated with the lack of enzyme induction.

Breast-fed infants should continue nursing on demand. For bottle-fed infants, full-strength, lactose-free, or lactose-reduced formulas should be administered immediately on rehydration in amounts sufficient to satisfy energy and nutrient requirements. Patients with true lactose intolerance have exacerbation of diarrhea when a lactose-containing formula is introduced. The presence of low pH (below 6.0) or reducing substances (greater than 5%) in the stool in the absence of clinical symptoms is not diagnostic of lactose intolerance; this diagnosis is indicated by more severe diarrhea on introduction of lactose-containing foods. If lactose intolerance occurs, appropriate therapy includes temporary reduction or removal of lactose from the diet.

Dietary Therapy of Acute Diarrhea

Although dehydration is the most serious direct effect of diarrhea, adverse nutritional consequences also can occur when nutritional management is not appropriate. Acute diarrhea can endanger the nutritional status of affected children because (a) anorexia and food withdrawal interfere with adequate intake; (b) carbohydrates, fats, proteins, and micronutrients are often malabsorbed; (c) excess urinary and stool nitrogen losses are likely, even with subclinical infections; and (d) metabolic demands are generally higher with fever and systemic illness.

Older children who are accustomed to eating a variety of table foods should continue receiving a regular diet; cereal-milk and cereal-legume diets have been used successfully for the dietary management of these children. Other recommended foods include starches (e.g., rice, potatoes, noodles, crackers, and bananas), cereals (e.g., rice, wheat, and oat cereals), soup, yogurt, vegetables, and fresh fruits. Foods to be avoided are those that are high in simple sugars, which can exacerbate diarrhea by osmotic effects. These foods include soft drinks, undiluted apple juice, Jell-O, and presweetened cereals. In addition, foods high in fat may not be tolerated because of their tendency to delay gastric emptying. Although there have been no controlled trials concerning its efficacy, the "BRAT" diet (*b*ananas, *r*ice, *a*pplesauce, and *t*oast) has long been used as a dietary management tool among pediatric practices in the United States. To the extent that it included starches and fruits, it is a reasonable dietary recommendation. Prolonged use of the BRAT diet or a protracted course of diluted formulas can result in inadequate energy and protein content in the recovering child's diet.

Drug Therapy of Acute Diarrhea

Antimicrobial agents (Table 16) and other drugs have limited usefulness in the management of acute diarrhea. Viral agents are the predominant cause of acute diarrhea. Watery diarrhea and vomiting in a child under 2 years of age most likely represent viral gastroenteritis and therefore do not require antimicrobial therapy.

Bloody diarrhea or the presence of white blood cells on methylene blue stain of the stool specimen suggests a bacterial agent causing invasive mucosal damage and indicates that stool cultures should be performed to identify the organism. Other clinical clues suggesting infectious diarrhea amenable to antimicrobial therapy include a history of recent antibiotic use (in which case *Clostridium difficile* should be suspected), exposure to children in day-care centers where *Giardia* or *Shigella* is prevalent, recent foreign travel, and an immunodeficiency, and the infectious cause of the diarrhea should be diligently evaluated. Antibiotics should be considered when dysentery or a high fever is present, when watery diarrhea lasts for more than 5 days, or when stool cultures, microscopy, or epidemic setting indicate an agent for which specific treatment is required. The use of ciprofloxacin has been shown to reduce clinical severity and shorten the course of infections with *Shigella* and *Salmonella* without prolonging organism shedding or creation of a carrier state (209,210).

Use of adsorbents (e.g., Kaolin-Pectin), antimotility agents (e.g., loperamide), antisecretory drugs, or toxin binders (e.g., cholestyramine) is a common practice in many developed and developing countries. Available data do not demonstrate their effectiveness in reducing diarrhea volume or duration. Stool water losses are unchanged, and electrolyte losses may increase. Side effects of these drugs are well known, including opiate-induced ileus, drowsiness and nausea due to atropine effects, and binding of nutrients and other drugs. Reliance on antidiarrheal agents shifts the therapeutic focus away from appropriate fluid, electrolyte, and nutritional therapy; can interfere with oral therapy; and can unnecessarily add to the economic cost of the illness. Little evidence exists to support the use of nonspecific drug therapy in children, and much information exists to the contrary.

A typical 30-ml dose of bismuth subsalicylate (Pepto-Bismol) yields 303 mg bismuth, 258 mg salicylate, and 10.2 mg sodium. Two Pepto-Bismol tablets contain 303 mg bismuth, 204 mg salicylate, 0.6 mg sodium, and 280 mg calcium (211). Reye's syndrome has been reported in patients whose only exposure to salicylates was to bismuth subsalicylate (212). The CDC states that it is prudent to avoid all compounds containing salicylate for presumed viral illnesses (including most cases of gastroenteritis) in children (213). The routine use of bismuth subsalicylate as adjunctive therapy for gastroenteritis with three or more watery stools in a 24-hour period may be unsafe (214). Hypercalcemia can also develop after large doses of Pepto-Bismol tablets (215,216).

Doses of 30 to 90 ml Pepto-Bismol providing a total ingestion of 5.2 to 9.4 g/day bismuth every 2 hours were ingested by a 45-year-old man with watery diarrhea. After 7 days of therapy, lethargy, dysarthria, and myoclonic jerking of the facial and axial muscles developed. The clinical course progressed from stupor to coma and death. Blood and urinary bismuth concentrations were 95 nmol/L (normal less than 48 nmol/L) and 14,164 nmol/L (normal less than 479 nmol/L), respectively (217). Daily doses of 2.1 g and 4.2 g bismuth subsalicylate for 3 weeks resulted in dark tongues, dark stools, and mild tinnitus (218). After bismuth subsalicylate ingestion encephalopathy developed in a patient with a blood bismuth concentration of 344.5 nmol/L (219).

TABLE 16. Role of antibiotics in specific causes of bacterial gastroenteritis

Role of antibiotics	Enteropathogen
Always indicated	*Shigella*, enteroinvasive *Escherichia coli*,[a] cholera
Indicated in certain clinical settings or hosts	*Salmonella, Campylobacter*, enteropathogenic *E. coli*, enterotoxigenic *E. coli, Clostridium difficile*
Unclear	Enterohemorrhagic *E. coli*, enteroadherent *E. coli, Aeromonas* spp., *Plesiomonas shigelloides*, noncholera *Vibrio* spp.

[a]Based on the microbiologic and clinical similarity to *Shigella*; controlled studies are not available.
Adapted from Ashkenazi S, Cleary TG. *Pediatr Infect Dis J* 1991;10:140–148.

REFERENCES

1. Mead PS, Slutsker L, Dietz V, et al. Food-related illness and death in the United States. Emerging infectious diseases (serial online). 1999;5(5):607–625. Available at: http://www.cdc.gov/ncidod/eid/vol5no5/mead.htm. Accessed May 2003.
2. Tan BJ. Food poisoning: a pediatric detective story. *Contemp Pediatr* 1990;8:211–228.
3. Helms M, Vastrup P, Gerner-Smidt P, et al. Short and long term mortality associated with foodborne bacterial gastrointestinal infections: registry based study. *BMJ* 2003;326:357–359.
4. Olsen SJ, Mackinnon LC, Goulding JS, et al. Surveillance for foodborne disease outbreaks—United States, 1993–1997. *MMWR Morb Mortal Wkly Rep* 2000;49:SS1–SS51.
5. Daniels NA, MacKinnon L, Rowe SM, et al. Foodborne disease outbreaks in United States schools. *Pediatr Infect Dis J* 2002;21(7):623–628.

6. Shea KM. Technical report: irradiation of food. *Pediatrics* 2000;106:1505-1510.
7. Wood OB, Bruhn CM. Position of the American Dietetic Association: food irradiation. *J Am Diet Assoc* 2000;100(2):246–253.
8. Pauli GH, Tarantino LM. FDA regulatory aspects of food irradiation. *J Food Prot* 1995;58:209–212.
9. ADA. Position of the American Dietetic Association: food irradiation. *ADA Rep* 2000;100(2):246–253.
10. Lagunas-Solar MC. Radiation processing of foods: an overview of scientific principles and current status. *J Food Prot* 1995;58:186–192.
11. US Department of Health and Human Services, Food and Drug Administration. Irradiation in the production, processing, and handling of food. *Fed Regist* 1986;51:13376–13399.
12. Fox JB, Lakritz L, Hampson J, et al. Gamma irradiation effects on thiamin and riboflavin in beef, lamb, pork, and turkey. *J Food Sci* 1995;60:596–598.
13. Grady GF, Keush GT. Pathogenesis of bacterial diarrheas. *N Engl J Med* 1971;285:831–841, 891–900.
14. Harris JC, Dupont JL, Hornic RB. Fecal leukocytes in diarrheal illness. *Ann Intern Med* 1972;76:697–703.
15. Taylor WR, Schell WL, Wells JG, et al. A foodborne outbreak of enterotoxigenic *Escherichia coli* diarrhea. *N Engl J Med* 1982;306:1093–1095.
16. Goossens H, Giesendorf BA, Vandamme P, et al. Investigation of an outbreak of *Campylobacter upsaliensis* in day care centers in Brussels: analysis of relationships among isolates by phenotypic and genotypic typing methods. *J Infect Dis* 1995;172:1298–1305.
17. MMWR. Surveillance for epidemics. *MMWR Morb Mortal Wkly Rep* 1990;38:694–696.
18. Ryan CA, Nickels MK, Hargrett-Bean NT, et al. Massive outbreak of antimicrobial-resistant salmonellosis traced to pasteurized milk. *JAMA* 1987;258(22):3269–3274.
19. Kolavic SA, Kimura A, Simons SL, et al. An outbreak of *Shigella dysenteriae* type 2 among laboratory workers due to intentional food contamination. *JAMA* 1997;278:396–398.
20. Torok TJ, Tauxe RV, Wise RP, et al. A large community outbreak of salmonellosis caused by intentional contamination of restaurant salad bars. *JAMA* 1997;278:389–395.
21. Pickering LK, Obrig TG, Stapleton FB. Hemolytic-uremic syndrome and enterohemorrhagic *Escherichia coli*. *Pediatr Infect Dis J* 1994;13:459–475.
22. DuPont HL, Ericsson CD. Prevention and treatment of traveler's diarrhea. *N Engl J Med* 1993;328:1821–1827.
23. Graham DY, Smith JL, Opekun AT. Spicy food and the stomach: evaluation by endoscopy. *JAMA* 1988;260:3473–3475.
24. Spitzer DR. Horseradish horrors—Sushi syncope. *JAMA* 1988;259:218–219.
25. Allen DH, Baker GJ. Chinese restaurant asthma. *N Engl J Med* 1981;305:1154–1155.
26. Squire EN. Angioedema and monosodium glutamate. *Lancet* 1987;1:988.
27. Yang WH, Drouin MA, Herbert M, et al: The monosodium glutamate symptom complex: assessment in a double-blind, placebo-controlled, randomized study. *J Allergy Clin Immunol* 1997;99:757–762.
28. Bellisls F. Effects of monosodium glutamate on human food palatability. *Ann N Y Acad Sci* 1998;855:438–441.
29. Metge P, Mandirac-Bonnefoy C, Bellaube P. The saurismose retinienne à la canthaxanthine. *Bull Mem Soc Fr Ophthalmol* 1984;95:547–549.
30. Barker FM. Canthaxanthin retinopathy. *J Toxicol Cut Ocular Toxicol* 1988;7:223–236.
31. Harnois C, Samson J, Malenfant M, et al. Canthaxanthin retinopathy. *Arch Ophthalmol* 1989;107:538–540.
32. Smith PD, Lane HC, Gill VJ, et al. Intestinal infections in patients with acquired immunodeficiency syndrome (AIDS). Etiology and response to therapy. *Ann Intern Med* 1988;108:328–333.
33. Laughon E, Druckman DA, Vernon A, et al. Prevalence of enteric pathogens in homosexual men with and without acquired immunodeficiency syndrome. *Gastroenterology* 1988;94:984–993.
34. Perlman DM, Ampell NM, Schifman RB, et al. Persistent *Campylobacter jejuni* infections in patients infected with human immunodeficiency virus (HIV). *Ann Intern Med* 1988;109:540–546.
35. Archer DL. Food counseling should be given to all persons infected with the human deficiency virus. *J Infect Dis* 1990;161:358–359.
36. Greenson JK, Belitsos PC, Yardley JH, et al. AIDS enteropathy: occult enteric infections and duodenal mucosal alteration in chronic diarrhea. *Ann Intern Med* 1991;114:366–372.
37. Hale D, Aldeen W, Carroll K. Diarrhea associated with cyanobacteria-like bodies in an immunocompetent host. An unusual epidemiological source. *JAMA* 1994;271:144–145.
38. Harland WA, Lee FD. Intestinal spirochaetosis. *BMJ* 1967;3:718–719.
39. Kaplan LR, Taceuchi A. Purulent rectal discharge associated with a non-treponemal discharge. *JAMA* 1979;241:52–53.
40. Shera AG. Specific granular lesions associated with intestinal spirochaetosis. *Br J Surg* 1962;50:68–77.
41. Rifkin GD, Opdyke JE. *Anaerobiospirillum succiniproducens* septicemia. *J Clin Microbiol* 1981;13:811–813.
42. Schlaes DM, Dul MJ, Lerner PI. *Anaerobiospirillum* bacteremia. *Ann Intern Med* 1982;97:63–64.
43. Johanson JF, Sonnenberg A. Efficient management of diarrhea in the acquired immunodeficiency syndrome (AIDS). *Ann Intern Med* 1990;112:942–948.
44. Granum PE, Lund T. *Bacillus cereus* and its food poisoning toxins. *FEMS Microbiol Lett* 1997;157:223–228.
45. Granum PE. *Bacillus cereus* and its toxins. *J Appl Bacteriol* 1994;23[Suppl]:61S–66S.
46. Guinebretiere MH, Broussolle V, Nguyen-The C. Enterotoxigenic profiles of food-poisoning and food-borne *Bacillus cereus* strains. *J Clin Microbiol* 2002;40(8):2053–2056.
47. Kotiranta A, Lounatmaa K, Haapasalo M. Epidemiology and pathogenesis of *Bacillus cereus* infections. *Microbes Infect* 2000;2:189–198.
48. CDC. *Bacillus cereus* food poisoning associated with fried rice at two child day care centers—Virginia, 1993. *Morb Mortal Wkly Rep* 1994;43(10):177–178.
49. Mahler H, Pasi A, Kramer JM. Fulminant liver failure in association with the emetic toxin of *Bacillus cereus*. *N Engl J Med* 1997;336:1142–1148.
50. Fermanian C, Lapeyre C, Fremy J-M. Production of diarrheal toxin by selected strains of *Bacillus cereus*. *Int J Food Microbiol* 1996;30:345–358.
51. Andersson MA, Mikkola R, Helin J. A novel sensitive bioassay for detection of *Bacillus cereus* emetic toxin and related depsipeptide ionophores. *Appl Environ Microbiol* 1998;64:1338–1343.
52. Gorbach SL. Bacterial diarrhea and its treatment. *Lancet* 1987;2:1378–1382.
53. Peterson MC. Clinical aspects of *Campylobacter jejuni* infections in adults. *West J Med* 1994;161:148–152.
54. MMWR. Foodborne diseases active surveillance network, 1996. *JAMA* 1997;227(17):1344–1345.
55. Chowdhury MNH, Bact D, Al-Eissa YA. *Campylobacter* gastroenteritis in children in Riyadh, Saudi Arabia. *J Trop Pediatr* 1992;38:158–161.
56. Murga H, Huicho L, Guevara G. Acute diarrhea and *Campylobacter* in Peruvian children: a clinical and epidemiologic approach. *J Trop Pediatr* 1993;39:338–341.
57. CDC. *Campylobacter* enteritis–New Zealand, 1990. *MMWR Morb Mortal Wkly Rep* 1991;40:116–117, 123.
58. Wood RC, MacDonald KL, Osterholm MT. Campylobacter enteritis outbreaks associated with drinking raw milk during youth activities. A 10-year review of outbreaks in the United States. *JAMA* 1992;268(22):3228–3230.
59. Deming MS, Tauxe RV, Blake PA, et al. *Campylobacter* enteritis at a university: transmission from eating chicken and from cats. *Am J Epidemiol* 1987;126:526–534.
60. CDC. Outbreak of *Campylobacter* enteritis associated with cross-contamination of food—Oklahoma, 1996. *MMWR Morb Mortal Wkly Rep* 1998;47:129–131.
61. Anderson KL, Hamoud MM, Urbance JW, et al. Isolation of *Campylobacter jejuni* from an aborted caprine fetus. *J Am Vet Med Assoc* 1983;183:90–92.
62. Diker KS, Istanbulluoglu E. Ovine abortion associated with *Campylobacter jejuni*. *Vet Rec* 1986;118:307.
63. Diker KS, Sahal M, Aydin N. Ovine abortion associated with *Campylobacter coli*. *Vet Rec* 1988:122:87.
64. Coid CR, O'Sullivan AM, Dore CJ. Variations in the virulence, for pregnant guinea pigs, of campylobacters isolated from man. *L Med Microbiol* 1987;23:187–189.
65. O'Sullivan AM, Dore CJ, Boyle S, et al. The effect of *Campylobacter* lipopolysaccharide on fetal development in the mouse. *J Med Microbiol* 1988;26:101–105.
66. Denton KJ, Clarke T. Role of *Campylobacter jejuni* as a placental pathogen. *J Clin Pathol* 1992;45:171–172.
67. Gilbert GL, Davoren RA, Cole ME, et al: Midtrimester abortion associated with septicaemia caused by *Campylobacter jejuni*. *Med J Aust* 1981;1:585–586.
68. Gribble MJ, Salit IE, Isaac-Renton J, et al. *Campylobacter* infections in pregnancy. Case report and literature review. *Am J Obstet Gynecol* 1981;140:423–426.
69. Pines A, Goldhammer E, Bregman J, et al. *Campylobacter* enteritis associated with recurrent abortions in agammaglobulinemia. *Acta Obstet Gynecol Scand* 1983;62:279–280.
70. Sauerwein RW, Bisseling J, Horrevorts AM. Septic abortion associated with *Campylobacter fetus* subspecies fetus infection: case report and review of the literature. *Infection* 1993;21:331–333.
71. Simor AE, Karmali MA, Jadavji T, et al. Abortion and perinatal sepsis associated with *Campylobacter* infection. *Rev Infect Dis* 1986;8:397–402.
72. Munday PE, Porter R, Falder PF, et al. Spontaneous abortion an infectious aetiology? *Br J Obstet Gynecol* 1984;91:1177–1180.
73. Ruiz Palacios GM, Calva JJ, Pickering LK, et al. Protection of breast-fed infants against *Campylobacter* diarrhea by antibodies in human milk. *J Pediatr* 1990;116:707–713.
74. Thomas JE, Austin S, Dale A, et al. Protection by human milk IgA against *Helicobacter pylori* infection in infancy. *Lancet* 1993;342:121.
75. Snijders F, Kuijper EJ, de Wever B, et al. Prevalence of *Campylobacter*-associated diarrhea among patients infected with human immunodeficiency virus. *Clin Infect Dis* 1997;24(6):1107–1113
76. Goh J, Flynn M. *Campylobacter jejuni* in pregnancy. *Aust N Z J Obstet Gynaecol* 1992;32:246–248.
77. Blecker U, Lanciers S, Keppens E, et al. Evolution of *Helicobacter pylori* positivity in infants born from positive mothers. *J Pediatr Gastroenterol Nutr* 1994;19:87–90.
78. Giesendorf BA, Quint WG. Detection and identification of *Campylobacter* spp. using the polymerase chain reaction. *Cell Mol Biol* 1995;41:625–638.
79. Anon. The choice of antibacterial drugs. *Med Lett Drugs Ther* 2002;43(1111–1112):69–78.

80. Rautelin H, Vaara M, Renkonen OV, et al. In vitro activity of antifungal azoles against *Helicobacter pylori*. *Eur J Clin Microbiol Infect Dis* 1992;11:273–274.
81. MacDonald KL, Spengler RF, Hatheway CL, et al. Type A botulism from sautéed onions: clinical and epidemiologic observations. *JAMA* 1985;253:1275–1278.
82. Barker WH, Weissman MD, Dowell VR, et al. Type B botulism outbreak caused by a commercial food product. *JAMA* 1977;237:456–459.
83. MacDonald KL, Cohen ML, Blake PA. The changing epidemiology of adult botulism in the United States. *Am J Epidemiol* 1986;124(5):794–799.
84. Hentges D. The intestinal flora and infant botulism. *Rev Infect Dis* 1979;1:668–673.
85. Thompson JA, Glascow LA, Warpinski JR, et al. Infant botulism. Clinical spectrum and epidemiology. *Pediatrics* 1980;6:9336–9942.
86. Shapiro RL, Hatheway C, Swerdlow DL. Botulism in the United States: a clinical and epidemiologic review. *Ann Intern Med* 1998;129:221–228.
87. Arnon SS, Schechter R, Inglesby TV, et al. Botulinum toxin as a biological weapon: medical and public health management. *JAMA* 2001;285:1059–1070.
88. Sheridan RE. Gating and permeability of ION channels produced by *Botulinum* toxin types A and E in PC12 cell membranes. *Toxicon* 1998;36:703–717.
89. Simpson LL. *Botulinum* toxin: a deadly poison sheds its negative image. *Ann Intern Med* 1996;125:616–617.
90. Simpson LL. The origin, structure, and pharmacological activity of *Botulinum* toxin. *Pharm Rev* 1981;33:155–188.
91. Robinson RF, Nahata MC. Management of botulism. *Ann Pharmacother* 2003;37(1):127–131.
92. Woodruff BA, Griffin PM, McCroskey LM, et al. Clinical and laboratory comparison of botulism from toxin types A, B, and E in the United States, 1975–1988. *J Infect Dis* 1992;166:1281–1286.
93. LeCour H, Ramos H, Almeida B, et al. Food borne botulism: a review of 13 outbreaks. *Arch Intern Med* 1988;148:578–580.
94. Morris JG Jr, Hatheway CL. Botulism in the United States, 1979. *J Infect Dis* 1980;142:302–305.
95. Tacket CO, Shandera WX, Mann JM, et al. Equine antitoxin use and other factors that predict outcome in type A foodborne botulism. *Am J Med* 1984:794–798.
96. Arnon SS, Midura TF, Damus K, et al. Honey and other environmental risk factors for infant botulism. *J Pediatr* 1979;94:331–336.
97. Byard RW, Moore L, Bourne AJ, et al. *Clostridium botulinum* and sudden infant death syndrome: a 10-year prospective study. *J Paediatr Child Health* 1992;28:156–157.
98. Passaro DJ, Werner B, McGee J, et al. Wound botulism associated with black tar heroin among injecting drug users. *JAMA* 1998;279:859–863.
99. Swedberg J, Wendel TH, Deiss F. Wound botulism. *West J Med* 1987;147:335–338.
100. Merson MH, Dowel VR. Epidemiologic, clinical and laboratory aspects of wound botulism. *N Engl J Med* 1973;289:1005–1010.
101. Gomez HF, Johnson R, Guven H, et al. Adsorption of botulinum toxin to activated charcoal with a mouse bioassay. *Ann Emerg Med* 1995;25:818–822.
102. Badhey H, Cleri DJ, D'Amato RF, et al. Two fatal cases of type E adult foodborne botulism with early symptoms and terminal neurologic signs. *J Clin Microbiol* 1986;23:616–618.
103. Black RE, Gunn RA. Hypersensitivity reactions associated with botulinal antitoxin. *Am J Med* 1980;69:567–570.
104. Frankovich TL, Arnon SS. Clinical trial of botulism immune globulin for infant botulism. *West J Med* 1991;154:103.
105. Metzger JF, Lewis GE Jr. Human derived immune globulin for the treatment of botulism. *Rev Infect Dis* 1979;1:689–692.
106. McClane BA. An overview of *Clostridium perfringens* enterotoxin. *Toxicon* 1996;34:1335–1343.
107. Brynestad S, Granum PE. *Clostridium perfringens* and foodborne infections. *Int J Food Microbiol* 2002;74(3):195–202.
108. Shandera WX, Tackett CO, Blake PA. Food poisoning due to *Clostridium perfringens* in the United States. *J Infect Dis* 1983;147:167–170.
109. Hook D, Jalaludin B, Fitzsimmons G. *Clostridium perfringens* food-borne outbreak: an epidemiological investigation. *Aust NZ J Public Health* 1996;20:119–122.
110. Parikh AI, Jay MT, Kassam D, et al. Clostridium perfringens outbreak at a juvenile detention facility linked to a Thanksgiving holiday meal. *West J Med* 1997;166(6):417–419.
111. Lukinmaa S, Takkunen E, Siitonen A. Molecular epidemiology of *Clostridium perfringens* related to food-borne outbreaks of disease in Finland from 1984 to 1999. *Appl Environ Microbiol* 2002;68(8):3744–3749.
112. Schalch B, Bjorkroth J, Eisgruber H, et al. Ribotyping for strain characterization of *Clostridium perfringens* isolates from food poisoning cases and outbreaks. *Appl Environ Microbiol* 1997;63:3992–3994.
113. Schalch B, Sperner B, Eisgruber H, et al. Molecular methods for the analysis of *Clostridium perfringens* relevant to food hygiene. *FEMS Immunol Med Microbiol* 1999;24:281–286.
114. Arcieri R, Dionisi AM, Caprioli A, et al. Direct detection of *Clostridium perfringens* enterotoxin in patients' stools during an outbreak of food poisoning. *FEMS Immunol Med Microbiol* 1999;23:45–48.
115. Miwa N, Masuda T, Terai K, et al. Bacteriological investigation of an outbreak of *Clostridium perfringens* food poisoning caused by Japanese food without animal protein. *Int J Food Microbiol* 1999;49:103–106.
116. Sparks SG, Carman RJ, Sarker MR, et al. Genotyping of enterotoxigenic *Clostridium perfringens* fecal isolates associated with antibiotic-associated diarrhea and food poisoning in North America. *J Clin Microbiol* 2001;29(3):883–888.
117. Kim Y, Lee K, Ryu S. A survey of human serum samples for antibody against *Clostridium perfringens* type A enterotoxin in humans in Korea. *Int J Food Microbiol* 1998;41:239–241.
118. Granum PE. *Clostridium perfringens* toxins involved in food poisoning. *Int J Food Microbiol* 1990;10:101–111.
119. Deschenes G, Casenave C, Grimont F, et al. Clusters of haemolytic uremic syndrome due to unpasteurized cheese. *Pedatr Nephrol* 1996;10:203–205.
120. Griffin PM, Tauxe RV. The epidemiology of infections caused by *Escherichia coli* 0157:H7, other enterhemorrhagic *E. coli* and the associated hemolytic uremic syndrome. *Epidemiol Rev* 1991;13:60–98.
121. Swerdlow DL, Woodruff BA, Brady RC, et al. A waterborne outbreak in Missouri of *Escherichia coli* O157:H7 associated with bloody diarrhea and death. *Ann Intern Med* 1992;117:812–819.
122. Hancock DD, Besser TE, Kinsel ML, et al. The prevalence of *Escherichia coli* O157:H7 in dairy and beef cattle in Washington State. *Epidemiol Infect* 1994;113:199–207.
123. Consensus Conference. Consensus conference statement: *Escherichia coli* O157:H7 infections—an emerging national health crisis, July 11–13, 1994. *Gastroenterology* 1995;108:1923–1934.
124. Bitzan M, Ludwig K, Klemt M, et al. The role of *Escherichia coli* O157 infections in the classical (enteropathic) haemolytic uraemic syndrome: results of a Central European, multicentre study. *Epidemiol Infect* 1993;110:183–196.
125. Karpman D, Andreasson A, Thysell J, et al. Cytokines in childhood hemolytic uremic syndrome and thrombotic thrombocytopenic purpura. *Pediatr Nephrol* 1995;9:694–699.
126. Van de Kar NC, van Hinsbergh VW, Brommer EJ, et al. The fibrinolytic system in the hemolytic uremic syndrome: in vivo and in vitro studies. *Pediatr Res* 1994;36:257–264.
127. Kulkarni H, Goldwater PN, Martin A, et al.. Escherichia coli 'O' group serological responses and clinical correlations in epidemic HUS patients. *Comp Immunol Microbiol Infect Dis* 2002;25(4):249–268.
128. Siegler RL, Pravia AT, Christofferson RD, et al: A 20-year population-based study of postdiarrheal hemolytic uremic syndrome in Utah. *Pediatrics* 1994;94:35–40.
129. Olsen SJ, Miller G, Kennedy M, et al. A waterborne outbreak of *Escherichia coli* O157:H7 infections and hemolytic uremic syndrome: implications for rural water systems. *Emerg Infect Dis* 2002;8(4):370–375.
130. Tarr PI, Neill MA, Clausen CR, et al. *Escherichia coli* O157:H7 and the hemolytic uremic syndrome: importance of early cultures in establishing the etiology. *J Infect Dis* 1990;162:553–556.
131. Brian MJ, Frosolono M, Murray BE, et al. Polymerase chain reaction for diagnosis of enterohemorrhagic *Escherichia coli* infection and hemolytic-uremic syndrome. *J Clin Microbiol* 1992;30:1801–1806.
132. Boyce TG, Swerdlow DL, Griffin PM. *Escherichia coli* O157:H7 and the hemolytic-uremic syndrome. *N Engl J Med* 1995;333:364–368.
133. Siegler RL. Management of hemolytic-uremic syndrome. *J Pediatr* 1988;112:1014–1020.
134. Nakatani T, Tsuchida K, Yoshimura R, et al. Plasma exchange therapy for the treatment of *Escherichia coli* O-157 associated hemolytic uremic syndrome. *Int J Mol Med* 2002;10(5):585–588.
135. Proulx F, Turgeon JP, Delage G, et al. Randomized, controlled trial of antibiotic therapy for *Escherichia coli* O157:H7 enteritis. *J Pediatr* 1992;121:299–303.
136. Carter AO, Borczyk AA, Carlson JAK, et al. A severe outbreak of *Escherichia coli* O157:H7-associated hemorrhagic colitis in a nursing home. *N Engl J Med* 1987;317:1496–1500.
137. Tarr PI, Neill MA, Christie DL, et al. *Escherichia coli* O157:H7 hemorrhagic colitis [Letter]. *N Engl J Med* 1988;318:1697.
138. Nishikawa K, Matsuoka K, Kita E, et al. A therapeutic agent with oriented carbohydrates for treatment of infections by Shiga toxin-producing *Escherichia coli* O157:H7. *Proc Natl Acad Sci U S A* 2002;99(11):7669–7674.
139. Trachtman H, Christen E. Pathogenesis, treatment, and therapeutic trials in hemolytic uremic syndrome. *Curr Opin Pediatr* 1999;11(2):162–168.
140. Dalton C, Austin C, Sobel J, et al. An outbreak of gastroenteritis and fever due to *Listeria monocytogenes* in milk. *N Engl J Med* 1997;336:100–105.
141. Berche P, Reich KA, Bonnichon M, et al. Detection of anti-listeriolysin 0 for serodiagnosis of human listeriosis. *Lancet* 1990;335:624–627.
142. Pigrau C, Almiran B, Pahissa A, et al. Clinical presentation and outcome in cases of listeriosis. *Clin Infect Dis* 1993;17:143–146.
143. Sanyal D, Douglas T, Roberts R. *Salmonella* infection acquired from reptilian pets. *Arch Dis Child* 1997;77:345–346.
144. Mishu B, Griffen PM, Tauxe RV, et al. *Salmonella enteritidis* gastroenteritis transmitted by intact chicken eggs. *Ann Intern Med* 1991;115:190–194.
145. Mohle-Boetani JC, Farrar JA, Werner SB, et al. *Escherichia coli* 0147 and *Salmonella* infections associated with sprouts in California, 1996–1998. *Ann Intern Med* 2001;135:239–247.
146. Cody SH, Abbott SL, Marfin AA, et al. Two outbreaks of multidrug-resistant *Salmonella* serotype *typhimurium* DT 104 infections linked to raw-milk cheese in northern California. *JAMA* 1999;281:1805–1810.
147. WHO. Emergence of multidrug-resistant salmonella. *WHO Drug Inf* 1997;11:21.
148. Scialli AR, Rarick TL. Salmonella sepsis and second-trimester pregnancy loss. *Obstet Gynecol* 1992;79:820–821.

149. Butler T, Islam A, Kabir I, et al. Patterns of morbidity and mortality in typhoid fever dependent on age and gender: review of 552 hospitalized patients with diarrhea. *Rev Infect Dis* 1991;13:85–90.
150. Ellis ME, Moosa A, Hillier V. A review of typhoid fever in South African black children. *Postgrad Med J* 1990;66:1032–1036.
151. Zenilman JM. Typhoid fever. *JAMA* 1997;278:847–850.
152. Levine MM, Ferreccio C, Abrego P, et al. Duration of efficacy of Ty21a, attenuated *Salmonella typhi* live oral vaccine. *Vaccine* 1999;17[Suppl 2]:S22–S27.
153. Feberwee A, de Vries TS, Hartman EG, et al. Vaccination against *Salmonella enteritidis* in Dutch commercial layer flocks with a vaccine based on a live *Salmonella gallinarum* 9R strain: evaluation of efficacy, safety, and performance of serologic *Salmonella* tests. *Avian Dis* 2001;45(1):83–91.
154. Barkin RM. Acute infectious diarrheal disease in children. *J Emerg Med* 1985;3:1–9.
155. Schutze GE, Kirby RS, Flick EL, et al. Epidemiology and molecular identification of *Salmonella* infections in children. *Arch Pediatr Adolesc Med* 1998;152:659–664.
156. CDC. Reptile-associated salmonellosis—selected states, 1996–1998. *MMWR Morb Mortal Wkly Rep* 1999;48:1010–1013.
157. Gotuzzo E, Frisancho O, Sanchez J, et al. Association between the acquired immunodeficiency syndrome and infection with *Salmonella typhi* or *Salmonella paratyphi* in an endemic typhoid area. *Arch Intern Med* 1991;151:381–382.
158. Glynn JR, Palmer SR. Incubation period, severity of disease, and infecting dose: evidence from a *Salmonella* outbreak. *Am J Epidemiol* 1992;136:1369–1377.
159. Smith DF, Smith CC, Douglas JG, et al. Severe salmonellosis related to oral administration of anti-diarrheal drugs. *Scot Med J* 1990;35:176–177.
160. Wittler RR, Bass JW. Nontyphoidal *Salmonella* enteric infections and bacteremia. *Pediatr Infect Dis J* 1989;8:364–367.
161. Carnevale R, Molbak K, Bager F, et al. Fluoroquinolone resistance in *Salmonella*: a web discussion. *Clin Infect Dis* 2000;31:128–130.
162. Pelletier AR, Finger RF, Sosin DM. Shigellosis in Kentucky, 1986 through 1989. *South Med J* 1991;84:818–821.
163. Huskins WC, Griffiths JK, Faruque ASG, et al. Shigellosis in neonates and young infants. *J Pediatr* 1994;125:14–22.
164. Taylor DN, Echeverria P. Etiology and epidemiology of travelers' diarrhea in Asia. *Rev Infect Dis* 1986;8[Suppl 2]:S136–S141.
165. Halpern Z, Dan M, Giladi M, et al. Shigellosis in adults: epidemiologic, clinical, and laboratory features. *Medicine* 1989;68:210–217.
166. Tauxe RV, McDonald RC, Hargrett-Bean NH, et al. The persistence of *Shigella flexneri* in the United States: increasing role of adult males. *Am J Public Health* 1988;78:1432–1435.
167. Baer JT, Vugia DJ, Reingold AL, et al. HIV infection as a risk factor for shigellosis. *Emerg Infect Dis* 1999;5(6):820–823.
168. CDC. *Shigella sonnei* outbreak associated with contaminated drinking water—Island Park, Idaho, August 1995. *MMWR Morb Mortal Wkly Rep* 1996;45:229–231.
169. CDC. Shigellosis—technical information. Available at: http://www.cdc.gov/ncidod/dbmd/diseaseinfo/shigellosis_g.htm. Accessed 2000.
170. Hedberg CW, Levine WC, White KE, et al. An international foodborne outbreak of shigellosis associated with a commercial airline. *JAMA* 1992;268:3208–3212.
171. Zajdowicz T. Epidemiologic and clinical aspects of shigellosis in American forces deployed to Saudi Arabia. *South Med J* 1993;86:647–650.
172. Cohen D, Green M, Block C, et al. Reduction of transmission of shigellosis by control of houseflies *(Musca domestica)*. *Lancet* 1991;337:993–997.
173. Levine OS, Levin MM. Houseflies *(Musca domestica)* as mechanical vectors of shigellosis. *Rev Infect Dis* 1991;13:688–696.
174. Daoud AS, Zaki M, Al-Mutairi G, et al. Childhood shigellosis: clinical and bacteriological study. *J Trop Med Hygiene* 1990;93:275–279.
175. Lahat E, Katz Y, Bistritzer T, et al. Recurrent seizures in children with *Shigella*-associated convulsions. *Ann Neurol* 1990;28:393–395.
176. Diercks DB, Friedland LR, Ernst AA. Hallucinations as the initial presentation of shigellosis. *Pediatr Emerg Care* 2000;16:99–101.
177. Khan WA, Dhar U, Salam MA, et al. Central nervous system manifestations of childhood shigellosis: prevalence, risk factors, and outcome. *Pediatrics* 1999;103(2)(abst). Avaiable at: http://www.pediatrics.org/cgi/content/full/103/2/e18. Accessed June 2003.
178. Mulligan K, Nelson S, Friedman HS, et al. Shigellosis-associated encephalopathy [Letter]. *Pediatr Infect Dis J* 1992;11:889–890.
179. Ferrera PC, Jeanjaquet MS, Mayer DM. *Shigella*-induced encephalopathy in an adult. *Am J Emerg Med* 1996;14:173–175.
180. Goren A, Freier S, Passwell JH. Lethal toxic encephalopathy due to childhood shigellosis in a developed country. *Pediatrics* 1992;89:1189–1193.
181. Perles Z, Bar-Ziv J, Granot E. Brain edema: an underdiagnosed complication of *Shigella* infection. *Pediatr Infect Dis J* 1995;14:1114–1115.
182. Bennish ML, Azad AK, Yousefzadeh D. Intestinal obstruction during shigellosis: incidence, clinical features, risk factors, and outcome. *Gastroenterology* 1991;101:626–634.
183. Nussinovitch M, Shapiro RP, Cohen AH, et al. Shigellosis complicated by perforated appendix [Letter]. *Pediatr Infect Dis J* 1993;12:352–353.
184. Miron D, Sochotnick I, Yardeni D, et al. Surgical complications of shigellosis in children. *Pediatr Infect Dis J* 2000;19:898–900.
185. Bennish ML, Harris JR, Wojtyniak BJ, et al. Death in shigellosis: incidence and risk factors in hospitalized patients. *J Infect Dis* 1990;161:500–506.
186. Ashkenazi S, Amir Y, Dinari G, et al. Differential leukocyte count in acute gastroenteritis: an aid to early diagnosis. *Clin Pediatr* 1983;22:356–358.
187. DuPont HL. Guidelines on acute infectious diarrhea in adults. *Am J Gastroenterol* 1997;92:1962–1975.
188. Guerrant RL, Van Gilder T, Steiner TS, et al. Practice guidelines for the management of infectious diarrhea: IDSA guidelines. *Clin Infect Dis* 2001;32:331–351.
189. Khan WA, Seas C, Dhar U, et al. Treatment of shigellosis: V. Comparison of azithromycin and ciprofloxacin: a double-blind, randomized, controlled trial. *Ann Intern Med* 1997;126:697–703.
190. Cohen D, Ashkenazi S, Green MS, et al. Double-blind vaccine-controlled randomized efficacy trial of an investigational *Shigella sonnei* conjugate vaccine in young adults. *Lancet* 1997;349:155–159.
191. Fries LF, Montemarano AD, Mallett CP, et al.. Safety and immunogenicity of a proteosome–*Shigella flexneri* 2a lipopolysaccharide vaccine administered intranasally to healthy adults. *Infect Immun* 2001;69(7):4545–4553.
192. Kotloff KL, Taylor DN, Sztein MB, et al. Phase I evaluation of delta virG *Shigella sonnei* live, attenuated, oral vaccine strain WRSS1 in healthy adults. *Infect Immun* 2002;70(4)2016–2021.
193. Holmberg SD, Blake PA. Staphylococcal food poisoning in the United States: new facts and old misconceptions. *JAMA* 1984;251:487–489.
194. Udo EE, Al-Bustan MA, Jacob LE, et al. Enterotoxin production by coagulase-negative staphylococci in restaurant workers from Kuwait City may be a potential cause of food poisoning. *J Med Microbiol* 1999;48:819–823.
195. Cunha BA. Staphylococcal food poisoning. *Emerg Med* 1988;20:117–126.
196. Eitzen EM Jr. Education is the key to defense against bioterrorism [Editorial]. *Ann Emerg Med* 1999;34:221–223.
197. Franz DR, Zajtchuk R. Biological terrorism: understanding the threat, preparation, and medical response. *Disease-a-Month* 2000;46:125–190.
198. Shimizu A, Fujita M, Igarashi J, et al. Characterization of *Staphylococcus aureus* cogaulase type VII isolates from staphylococcal food poisoning outbreaks (1980–1995) in Tokyo, Japan, by pulsed-field gel electrophoresis. *J Clin Microbiol* 2000;38(10):3746–3749.
199. Suzuki Y, Saito M, Ishikawa N. Restriction fragment length polymorphisms analysis by pulsed-field gel electrophoresis for discrimination of *Staphylococcus aureus* isolates from foodborne outbreaks. *Int J Food Microbiol* 1999;46:271–274.
200. Jackson GJ. Public health and research perspectives on the microbial contamination of foods. *J Anim Sci* 1990;68(3):884–891.
201. Mukhin DN, Chatterjee S. A receptor-based immunoassay to detect *Staphylococcus* enterotoxin B in biological fluids. *Anal Biochem* 1997;245:213–217.
202. Lee LA, Taylor J, Carter GP, et al. *Yersinia enterocolitica* 0:3: an emerging cause of pediatric gastroenteritis in the United States. *J Infect Dis* 1991;163:660–663.
203. Abraham M, Pai Madhukar, Kang Gagandeep, et al. An outbreak of food poisoning in Tamil Nadu associated with *Yersinia enterocolitica*. *And J Med Res* 1997;106:465–468.
204. Lee LA, Taylor J, Carter GP, et al. Yersinia enterocolitica 0:3: an emerging cause of pediatric gastroenteritis in the United States. *J Infect Dis* 1991;163:660–663.
205. Cover TL, Aber RC. *Yersinia enterocolitica*. *N Engl J Med* 1989;321:16–24.
206. CDC. *Yersinia enterocolitica* bacteremia and endotoxic shock associated with red blood cell transfusions—United States, 1991. *MMWR Morb Mortal Wkly Rev* 1991;40:176–178.
207. Munro R, Lye A. *Yersinia enterocolitica* bacteraemia after blood transfusion. *Med J Aust* 1990;152:280.
208. Eherer AF, Fordtran JS. Fecal osmotic gap and pH in experimental diarrhea of various causes. *Gastroenterology* 1992;103:545–551.
209. Mathai D, Kudva GC, Keystone JS, et al. Short course ciprofloxacin therapy for enteric fever. *J Assoc Physicians India* 1993;41(7):428–430.
210. Pithie AD, Wood MJ. Treatment of typhoid fever and infectious diarrhea with ciprofloxacin. *J Antimicrob Chemother* 1990;26[Suppl F]:47–53.
211. DuPont HL. Bismuth subsalicylate in the treatment and prevention of diarrheal disease. *Drug Intell Clin Pharm* 1987;221:687–693.
212. Horwitz ES, Barrett MJ, Bregman D, et al. Public Health Service study of Reye's syndrome and medications: report of the main study. *JAMA* 1987;257:1905–1911.
213. Barrett MJ. Association of Reye's syndrome with use of Pepto-Bismol (bismuth subsalicylate). *Pediatr Infect Dis* 1986;5:611.
214. Abramson JS, Givner LB, Woods CR Jr. Bismuth in infants with watery diarrhea. *N Engl J Med* 193;329:1762.
215. Levine RA. Risk of hypercalcemia from prophylaxis of traveler's diarrhea. *JAMA* 1983;249:1151–1152.
216. Pickering LK, Feldman S, Ericsson CD, et al. Absorption of salicylate and bismuth from a bismuth subsalicylate–containing compound (Pepto-Bismol). *J Pediatr* 1981;99:654–656.
217. Mendelowitz PC, Hoffman RS, Wacher S. Bismuth absorption and myoclonic encephalopathy during bismuth subsalicylate therapy. *Ann Intern Med* 1990;112:140–141.
218. DuPont HL, Ericsson CD, Johnson PC, et al. Use of bismuth subsalicylate for the prevention of traveler's diarrhea. *Rev Infect Dis* 1990;12[Suppl 1]:564–567.
219. Hasking GJ, Duggan JM. Encephalopathy from bismuth salicylate. *Med J Aust* 1982;2:167.

SECTION

5

Plants

CHAPTER 254

Introduction to Plants

Richard C. Dart

OVERVIEW

Poisoning from plants is a common fear but an extremely rare event. It is true that a few plant species in certain localities can produce serious toxicity, including oleander (*Nerium oleander*), foxglove (*Digitalis purpurea*), jequirity pea (*Abrus precatorius*), castor bean (*Ricinus communis*), water hemlock (*Cicuta maculata*), Jerusalem cherry (*Solanum pseudocapsicum*), tree tobacco (*Nicotiana glauca*), jimsonweed (*Datura stramonium*), false hellebore [*Veratrum* species (spp.)], plants containing pyrrolizidine alkaloids (e.g., *Senecio longilobus* teas), autumn crocus (*Colchicum autumnale*), and hepatotoxic mushrooms (*Amanita phalloides*, *Amanita virosa*). In most cases, exceptional circumstances are required to produce severe poisoning. Each year, a few deaths from plant poisonings occur in the United States. For example, brewing a tea from a misidentified plant can concentrate and increase the bioavailability of the poisons it contains, leading to more rapid and severe toxicity.

Poisoning from individual plant species is addressed in Chapter 255. Mycotoxins are addressed in Chapter 256, mushrooms in Chapter 257, and herbs and indigenous remedies in Chapter 258.

Plant Identification

A working relationship with a botanist or the local poison control center represents a valuable resource to optimize therapy. As soon as a toxic ingestion is recognized, a portion of the plant, including reproductive parts, should be taken to the appropriate place (e.g., nursery, botanist, emergency department) for identification. Visual recognition of oleander, foxglove, jimsonweed seed pod, castor bean, and jequirity bean is important. Willis has tabulated common poisonous plants in North America according to their site of toxic action (Table 1) (1).

Toxic Dose

Nonpoisonous plants that do not generally cause symptoms are listed in Table 2. Henry has compiled a review of the possibly fatal amount of some plants (Table 3) (2).

PHYSICAL EXAMINATION

In many cases, the identity of the plant involved is unknown. A few plants produce effects that may assist in the diagnosis of the cause. However, the most common effects produced by plants are gastrointestinal (GI) irritation, manifested by abdominal discomfort, nausea, and vomiting. Table 4 provides a partial list of plants known to cause GI irritation. Pokeweed (*Phytolacca americana*) and holly bush (*Ilex* spp.) are common causes of gastroenteritis. The toxalbumin-containing plants castor bean (*R. communis*) and jequirity bean (*A. precatorius*) produce a severe gastroenteritis and, rarely, multiorgan failure.

Cardiovascular Toxicity

Cardiovascular abnormalities can be caused by the common oleander (*N. oleander*), lily-of-the-valley (*Convallaria majalis*), foxglove (*D. purpurea*), and yellow oleander (*Thevetia peruviana*), which contain cardiac glycosides resembling digitalis (Chapter 255).

Neurologic Toxicity

Convulsions suggest toxicity from water hemlock (*Cicuta* spp.) ingestions produce convulsions within 30 to 60 minutes of exposure. Chinaberry (*Melia azedarach*), moonseed (*Menispermum canadense*), and *Coriaria myrtifolia* contain potential convulsants. Occasionally, convulsions have resulted from serious ingestions of *Aconitum* (monkshood), *Taxus* (yew), and *Veratrum* plant species.

Nicotine and nicotine-like toxicity is produced by plant species that contain nicotine-like toxins, including the golden chain tree (*Laburnum anagyroides*), tree tobacco (*N. glauca*), Indian tobacco (*Lobelia inflata*), and poison hemlock (*Conium maculatum*). Nausea, vomiting, salivation, and abdominal cramps begin soon after exposure and are followed by headache, confusion, tachycardia, mydriasis, fever, and ataxia.

Anticholinergic effects are produced by plants that contain atropine-like chemicals (Table 5). Atropine, scopolamine, and hyoscyamine appear in a variety of plants, the most common of

TABLE 1. Common poisonous plants native to and cultivated in North America

Name	Toxic parts	Toxic compounds
Anticholinergics		
Deadly nightshade (*Atropa belladonna*)	All	Atropine and related compounds
Henbane (*Hyoscyamus niger*)	All	Hyoscyamine, hyoscine, atropine
Jimsonweed (angel's trumpet, thorn apple; *Datura stramonium*)	All	Hyoscyamine, hyoscine, atropine
Lantana (bunchberry; *Lantana* spp.)	Berries, leaves	Lantadene
Cardiac toxins		
Azalea (*Rhododendron* spp.)	All	Grayanotoxins
Death camus (black snakeroot; *Zigadenus* spp.)	All	Zygadenine, veratrine
False hellebore (corn lily; *Veratrum californicum*)	All	Veratrum alkaloids
Foxglove (*Digitalis purpurea*)	Leaves, seeds	Digitalis glycosides
Green hellebore (American white hellebore; *Veratrum viride*)	All	Veratrum alkaloids
Japanese pieris (*Pieris japonica*)	All	Grayanotoxins
Larkspur (*Delphinium ambiguum*)	All	Delphinin and other alkaloids
Lily-of-the-valley (*Convallaria majalis*)	All	Convallarin, convallamarin
Monkshood (aconite; *Aconitum* spp.)	Leaves, roots, seeds	Aconitine, aconine
Mountain laurel (*Kalmia latifolia*)	All	Grayanotoxins
Oleander (*Nerium oleander*)	All	Oleandrin, oleandrosine
Yew (*Taxus* spp.)	All parts except flesh of berry	Taxine
Central nervous system stimulants		
Chinaberry (*Melia azedarach*)	All	A resinoid
Water hemlock (*Cicuta maculata*)	All parts, especially roots	Cicutoxin
Western water hemlock (*Cicuta douglasii*)	All parts, especially roots	Cicutoxin
Cyanogenic glycosides		
Cherry laurel (*Prunus laurocerasus*)	Foliage, pits	Amygdalin
Choke cherry (*Prunus virginiana*)	Foliage, pits	Amygdalin
Elderberry (*Sambucus nigra*)	Foliage, pits	Amygdalin
Hydrangea spp.	All	Hydrangin
Dermatitis producing		
Poinsettia (*Euphorbia pulcherrima*)	All	Vesicant sap
Poison ivy (*Rhus toxicodendron*)	All	Oleoresin
Poison oak (*Toxicodendron* spp.)	All	Oleoresin
Gastrointestinal irritants		
Amaryllis (*Hippeastrum puniceum*)	Bulb	Lycorine
Autumn crocus (*Colchicum autumnale*)	All	Colchicine
Daffodil, narcissus, jonquil (*Narcissus* spp.)	All parts	Lycorine, narcissine
Daphne (*Daphne* spp.)	All	Daphnin, narcissine
Holly (*Ilex* spp.)	Berries	Ilicin
Horsechestnut (buckeye; *Aesculus hippocastanum*)	Nut	Esculin
Hyacinth (*Hyacinthus orientalis*)	Bulb	Narcissine
Iris (blue flag; *Iris* spp.)	Bulb, leaves	Irritant resins
Mistletoe (*Phoradendron flavescens*)	All parts, especially berries	Sympathomimetic amines
Oak (*Quercus* spp.)	Acorns	Tannins
Poinsettia (*E. pulcherrima*)	Sap	Irritant
Pokeweed (inkberry; *Phytolacca americana*)	All	Resins, saponins, alkaloids
Privet (*Ligustrum* spp.)	All	Not known
Snowberry (waxberry; *Symphoricarpos albus*)	Berries	Loturidine
Snowdrop (*Galanthus nivalis*)	Bulb	Narcissine, lycorine
Wisteria (*Wisteria* spp.)	Seeds, pods	Wisterin, resin
Nicotinics		
Laburnum (golden chain; *Laburnum anagyroides*)	All	Cystine
Lobelia (cardinal flower; *Lobelia* spp.)	All	Lobeline
Poison hemlock (*Conium maculatum*)	All	Coniine
Tobacco (*Nicotiana* spp.)	All	Nicotine
Oxalates		
Caladium (*Caladium* spp.)	All	Calcium oxalate
Dumbcane (*Dieffenbachia* spp.)	All	Calcium oxalate
Elephant's ear (*Colocasia* spp.)	All	Calcium oxalate
Jack-in-the-pulpit (*Arisaema triphyllum*)	All parts except rhizome	Calcium oxalate
Philodendron	All	Calcium oxalate
Pothos (*Scindapsus aureus*)	All	Calcium oxalate
Rhubarb (*Rheum rhaponticum*)	Leaves	Oxalic acid and soluble oxalates
Skunk cabbage (*Symplocarpus foetidus*)	All	Calcium oxalate
Solanine		
Black nightshade (*Solanum nigrum*)	Leaves, fruit	Solanine, alkaloids
Jerusalem cherry (*Solanum pseudocapsicum*)	Leaves, fruit	Solanine, alkaloids
Potato (*Solanum tuberosum*)	Sprouts, sun-greened tuber	Solanine, alkaloids
Toxalbumins		
Black locust (black acacia; *Robinia pseudoacacia*)	All parts except flowers	Robin, robitin
Castor bean (*Ricinus communis*)	All parts (mainly)	Ricin
Jequirity bean (rosary pea; *Abrus precatorius*)	Seeds	Abrin

spp., species.
Adapted from Willis GA. *Medicine North America.* 1990:1753–1759.

TABLE 2. Nonpoisonous houseplants that generally do not cause symptoms

Common name	Botanical name
African violet	*Episcia reptans*
Aluminum plant	*Pilea cadierei*
Aralia	*Fatsia japonica*
Baby tears	*Helxine soleirolii*
Bird's nest fern	*Asplenium nidus*
Bridal veil	*Tradescantia*
Coleus X hydrus	*Coleus*
Corn plant	*Dracaena fragrans*
Creeping Charlie[a]	*Lysimachia nummularia*
Creeping Charlie[a]	*Pilea nummularifolia*
Creeping Jenny	*Lysimachia*
Dracaena indivisa	*Cordyline indivisa*
Dwarf schefflera	*Schefflera arboricola*
Emerald ripple	*Peperomia caperata*
Fiddleleaf fig	*Ficus lyrata*
Gardenia	*Gardenia jasminoides*
Grape ivy	*Cissus rhombifolia*
Jade plant	*Crassula argentea*
Parlor palm	*Chamaedorea elegans*
Peacock plant	*Calathea*
Piggyback begonia	*Begonia hispida*, variant *Cucullifera*
Piggyback plant	*Tolmiea menziesii*
Prayer plant	*Maranta leuconeura*
Rubber tree	*Ficus elastica "Decora"*
Schefflera, umbrella plant	*Brassaia actinophylla*
Snake plant	*Sansevieria trifasciata*
Spider plant	*Chlorophytum comosum*
String of hearts	*Ceropegia woodii*
Swedish ivy	*Plectranthus verticillatus*
Velvet plant	*Gynura aurantiaca*
Wandering Jew	*Tradescantia albiflora*
Wandering Jew (red and green)	*Zebrina pendula*
Wax plant	*Hoya carnosa*
Zebra plant	*Aphelandra squarrosa*

[a]There are species in this group that are poisonous.

TABLE 3. Common fatal plants

Plant	Toxic principle	Possibly fatal amount (in an adult)
Ackee (*Blighia sapida*)	Hypoglycin	1 fruit
Apple or pear seeds (*Pyrus* spp.)	Amygdalin (cyanogenic glycoside)	50 seeds
Castor oil plant (*Ricinus communis*)	Ricin	1 bean
Death cap (*Amanita phalloides*)	Amanitin, phalloidin (cyclopeptides)	1 mushroom
Galerina spp. mushrooms	Amanitin-type cyclopeptide	1 mushroom
Gyromitra spp. mushrooms	Monomethylhydrazine	1 mushroom
Hemlock water dropwort (*Oenanthe crocata*)	Oenanthetoxin	1 root
Holly (*Ilex aquifolium*)	Ilicin	30 berries
Jequirity (*Abrus precatorius*)	Abrin	1 bean
Oleander (*Nerium oleander*)	Oleandrin (cardiac glycoside)	1 leaf
Stone fruit kernels (*Prunus* spp.)	Amygdalin (cyanogenic glycoside)	30 kernels
Yew (*Taxus baccata*)	Taxine A and B (cardiac glycosides)	50 needles

spp., species.
Adapted from Henry JA. *Eur Assoc Pois Cont Center Newsletter*, 1985 May.

TABLE 4. Some primary gastrointestinal irritants

Plant	Toxic parts
Aloe spp.	All parts
Amaryllis (*Hippeastrum equestre*)	Bulb
Baneberry (*Actaea* spp.)	All parts, especially berries
Barberry (*Berberis vulgaris*)	Root, root bark
Bellyache bush (*Jatropha gossypifolia*)	Fruit
Bittersweet, American (*Celastrus scandens*)	All parts
Boxwood (*Buxus* spp.)	Leaves, stems
Buttercup (*Ranunculus* spp.)	All parts
Chinaberry (*Melia azedarach*)[a]	Fruits, leaves
Christmas rose (*Helleborus niger*)	All parts, especially rootstocks, leaves
Coral plant (*Jatropha multifida*)	Fruit
Crown of thorns (*Euphorbia milii*)	All parts
Daffodil (*Narcissus pseudonarcissus*)	All parts, especially bulb
Daphne (*Daphne mezereum*)[a]	All parts, especially bark, fruit
Desert potato (*Jatropha macrorhiza*)	Root
English ivy (*Hedera helix*)	All parts
Euonymus (*Euonymus* spp.)	All parts
Four o'clocks (*Mirabilis jalapa*)	Roots, seeds
Holly (*Ilex* spp.)	Berries; leaves less toxic
Hyacinth (*Hyacinthus orientalis*)	Bulb
Iris (*Iris*)	Bulb leaves
Marsh marigold (*Caltha palustris*)	All parts
Mayapple (*Podophyllum peltatum*)[a]	Green fruit, roots, foliage
Mistletoe (*Phoradendron flavescens*)[a]	All parts, especially berries
Pokeweed (*Phytolacca americana*)[a]	All parts
Privet (*Ligustrum* spp.)	Berries, leaves
Purging nut (*Jatropha curcas*)	Seeds, perhaps leaves
Purple rattlebox (*Daubentonia longifolia*)	Seeds
Pyracantha (*Pyracantha* spp.)	Berries (mild)
Tung nut (*Aleurites fordii*)	Nut
Wisteria (*Wisteria sinensis*)	Pods
Yew (*Taxus* spp.)[a]	All parts except fleshy red aril

spp., species.
[a]Anecdotally, fatalities have been associated with large ingestions.

which are jimsonweed (*D. stramonium*), deadly nightshade (*Atropa belladonna*), henbane (*Hyoscyamus niger*), angel's trumpet (*Brugmansia* spp., formerly *Datura suaveolens*), and matrimony vine (*Lycium halimifolium*). Clinical manifestations of toxicity are similar to those of classic atropine poisoning, with headache, nausea, dry skin and mouth, tachycardia, mydriasis, and urinary retention.

Hallucinations (Table 6) may be caused by nutmeg (*Myristica fragrans*), the ergot fungus (*Claviceps purpurea*), morning glory seeds (*Ipomoea violacea*), peyote (*Lophophora williamsii*), *Mimosa* spp., psilocybin-containing mushrooms (e.g., *Psilocybe* or *Panaeolus* spp.), ibotenic acid–containing mushrooms (e.g., *Amanita muscaria*), marijuana (*Cannabis* spp.), and any anticholinergic drug.

Nephrotoxicity

Renal injury may indicate chronic ingestion of the rhubarb plant, which contains soluble oxalate crystals. Decreased renal function also occurs secondary to the hepatorenal syndrome seen after *A. phalloides* poisoning. Autumn crocus (*C. autumnale*), podophyllum resin, and *Cortinarius* mushrooms can produce primary renal dysfunction. Nephrotoxic plants are listed in Table 7 (3).

TABLE 5. Hyoscyamine- and hyoscine-containing plants (alkaloids with a tropane nucleus)

Scientific name	Common names	Description	Distribution	Poisonous component
Datura stramonium	Tolguacha, apple of Peru, jimsonweed, Jamestown weed, devil's apple, thorn apple, devil's trumpet, stinkweed, loco seeds, locoweed	Large, erect plant; funnel-shaped white or purple flowers; spreading branches; hard, prickly, ovate; many-seeded fruit	Cultivated or noncultivated fields; widespread in the United States	Hyoscyamine (leaves, roots, seeds), hyoscine (roots).
Hyoscyamus niger	Henbane, black henbane	Tall, erect, multibranched stem having fetid odor; yellowish flowers; encapsulated seeds	Common in the United States	Hyoscyamine, hyoscine.
Atropa belladonna	Belladonna, deadly nightshade	Fleshy, erect stem; hairy leaves; purple flowers; purple-black, many-seeded berry when ripe	Cultivated in the eastern United States; rarely survives in wild form	Hyoscyamine (throughout plants).
Lycium halimifolium	Matrimony vine	Vine or shrub; bell-shaped flowers; ovoid, orange-red berry	Northern United States	Hyoscyamine.
Cestrum nocturnum, Cestrum diurnum	Night-blooming jessamine	Large, attractive shrubs; fragrant trumpet flowers; small berry	Coastal plains in south and southwest United States	Atropine (?), gastroenterotoxin.
Mandragora officinarum	Mandrake	Native Mediterranean plant whose leaves resemble lettuce	Greece and Mediterranean countries	Roots, fruit, and leaves contain hyoscyamine, scopolamine, pseudohyoscyamine, and mandragorine.

Adapted from Goldfrank L, Melinek M. *Hosp Physician* 1979;15:40.

Hepatic Toxicity

Hepatotoxic mushrooms are well described. Less well known are the pyrrolizidine alkaloids, which produce hepatic failure both sporadically (e.g., when ingested as teas from *S. longilobus*) and epidemically (e.g., consumption of cereals contaminated by *Crotalaria* or *Heliotropium* seeds). Akee fruit, a South African tuber (*Callilepis laureola*), and sassafras root also cause hepatic dysfunction in severe cases.

Other Effects

Plants of abuse are listed in Table 8 (4).

TABLE 6. Major hallucinogenic plants and their active principles

Plant	Family	Active principle
Cannabis sativa	Cannabinaceae	Tetrahydrocannabinol
Lophophora williamsii	Cactaceae	Mescaline
Piptadenia species	Leguminosae	Substituted tryptamines
Mimosa species	Leguminosae	Substituted tryptamines
Virola species	Myristicaceae	Substituted tryptamines
Banisteriopsis species	Malpighiaceae	Harmaline, harmine
Peganum harmala	Zygophyllaceae	Harmaline, harmine
Tabernanthe iboga	Apocynaceae	Ibogaine
Ipomoea violacea	Convolvulaceae	*d*-Lysergic acid amide, *d*-isolysergic acid amide
Turbina corymbosa	Convolvulaceae	*d*-Lysergic acid amide, *d*-isolysergic acid amide
Datura species	Solanaceae	Scopolamine
Methysticodendron amesianum	Solanaceae	Scopolamine
Amanita muscaria	Agaricaceae	Pantherine, ibotenic acid
Psilocybe mexicana	Agaricaceae	Psilocybin

Adapted from Farnsworth NR. *Science* 1986;162:1090.

TOXIC PLANT SUBSTANCES

Toxic plant substances belong to a relatively few broad categories of compounds. Major groupings of these compounds include alkaloids, glycosides, proteinaceous compounds, organic acids, alcohols, resins and resinoids (including phenolics), mineral toxins, and nonorganic compounds (Tables 9 and 10).

Alkaloids

1. The belladonna type (tropane or atropine alkaloids) such as belladonna (*Atropa*), jimsonweed (*Datura*), henbane (*Hyoscyamus*), mandrake (*Mandragora*), and coca tree (*Erythroxylum*)

TABLE 7. Nephrotoxic plants

Plant	Scientific name	Toxic compounds
Autumn crocus	*Colchicum autumnale*	Colchicine
Castor bean	*Ricinus communis*	Ricin and recinine
Daphne	*Daphne mezereum*	Daphnin, vesicant resin, and mezerenic acid anhydride
Herbal remedies	Exact plants unknown	Unknown
Impila	*Callilepis laureola*	Atractyloside
Marking nut tree	*Semecarpus anacardium*	Phenolic constituents
Poison mushrooms	*Amanita phalloides* and *Cortinarius* species	Amatoxin cyclopeptides
Rosary pea	*Abrus precatorius*	Abrin and abric acid
?	*Securidaca longipedunculata*	Methyl salicylate, saponins, tannins, and gaultheria
Water hemlock	*Cicuta maculata*	Cicutoxin

Adapted from Abuelo JG. *Arch Intern Med* 1990;150:505–510.

TABLE 8. Plants of abuse

Plant	Part used	Toxic agent
Argyreia nervosa	Seed	Ergoline hallucinogens
Atropa belladonna	Seed	Tropane alkaloids
Banisteriopsis species	Various	Harmaline (hallucinogen)
Cola nitida	Seed	Caffeine
Datura species	Seed	Tropane alkaloids
Hyoscyamus niger	Whole plant	Tropane alkaloids
Ilex paraguariensis	Leaf	Caffeine
Lophophora	—	—
Mandragora officinarum	Whole plant	Tropane alkaloids
Methysticodendron amesianum	Stems/leaf	Tropane alkaloids
Mimosa hostilis	Root	Phenylamine hallucinogens
Olmedioperebea sclerophylla	Fruit	Unknown hallucinogen
Passiflora incarnata	Stem/leaf	Harmaline (hallucinogen)
Peganum harmala	Seed	Harmaline (hallucinogen)
Piper methysticum	Root	Methysticin/kawain
Piptadenia colubrina	Seed	Phenylamine hallucinogens
Piptadenia excelsa	Seed	Phenylamine hallucinogens
Piptadenia macrocarpa	Seed	Phenylamine hallucinogens
Piptadenia peregrina	Seed/bark	Phenylamine hallucinogens
Salvia divinorum	Leaf	Unknown hallucinogen
Sophora secundiflora	Seed	Cytosine (stimulant)
Tabernanthe iboga	Root	Ibogaine (hallucinogen)
Trichocereus pachanoi	Cactus	Mescaline
Virola calophylla	Bark	Phenylamine hallucinogens

Adapted from Spoerke DG, Hall AH. *Emerg Clin North Am* 1990;8:579–593.

2. The groundsel type (pyrrolizidine alkaloids) such as groundsel (*Senecio*), blue devil (*Echium*), and heliotrope (*Heliotropium*)
3. Hemlock type (pyridine or piperidine alkaloids) such as poison hemlock (*Conium*) and Indian tobacco (*Lobelia*)
4. Nicotine or tobacco type (pyridine alkaloids) such as tobacco (*Nicotiana*) and horsetail (*Equisetum*)
5. Caffeine or caffeine type (purine alkaloids) such as coffee (*Coffea*); chocolate, "cola," and cocoa (*Theobroma*); and tea (*Camellia*)
6. Quinine type (quinoline alkaloids) such as the quinone tree (*Cinchona*) and globe thistle (*Echinops*)
7. Opium or morphine type (isoquinoline alkaloids) such as opium poppy (*Papaver*), blood root (*Sanguinaria*), squirrel corn (*Dicentra*), goldenseal (*Hydrastis*), and fumitory (*Corydalis*)
8. Ergot type (indole or indolizidine alkaloids) such as ergot (*Claviceps*), magic mushroom (*Psilocybe*), locoweed (*Astragalus*), Carolina jessamine (*Gelsemium*), and strychnine (*Strychnos*)
9. Lupine type (quinolizidine alkaloids—cytosine type) such as lupines (*Lupinus*), golden chain (*Laburnum*), false indigo (*Baptisia*), Scotch broom (*Cytisus*), and Kentucky coffee tree (*Gymnocladus*)
10. Tomato or solanine type (steroidal, glycoalkaloids) such as tomato (*Lycopersicon*), Irish potato (*Solanum*), and nightshades (*Solanum*)
11. Veratrum type (steroid alkaloids) such as false hellebore (*Veratrum*) and death camus (*Zigadenus*)
12. Larkspur type (diterpenoid alkaloids) such as larkspur (*Delphinium*) and monkshood (*Aconitum*)
13. Mescaline type (phenylalanine alkaloids) such as peyote (*Lophophora*) and ephedra (*Ephedra*)

Glycosides

1. Cyanogenic (cyanogenic glycoside) aglycone is hydrocyanic acid (e.g., amygdalin in seeds or pits of wild cherry, peach, apricot, apple, and almond), which on hydrolysis yields sugar, cyanide, and benzaldehyde. Amygdalin from ground-up apricot pits is laetrile.
2. Steroid glycosides: Sugar is joined to a steroid molecule such as (a) cardiac glycosides [Chapter 120; e.g., foxglove (digoxin, *D. purpurea*), lily-of-the-valley (*Convallaria*), ouabain (*Strophanthus*), dogbane (*Apocynum*), milkweed (*Ascle-*

TABLE 9. Plant toxins

Toxin	Source	Chemistry	Mode of action
Sodium channels			
Lipophilic toxins			
Veratridine	Plant rhizome *Veratrum album* (Liliaceae) or seeds of *Schoenocaulon officinale*	Alkaloid	Hyperexcitability resulting from reversible membrane depolarization
Aconitine	Monk's hood: *Aconitum napellus* (Ranunculaceae)	Alkaloid	Cardiac dysrhythmia, repetitive firing of nerve
Grayanotoxins	Leaves of *Rhododendron, Kalmia, Leucothoe* (Ericaceae)	Diterpenoid	Membrane depolarization
Pyrethrins	Chrysanthemum flower: *Chrysanthemum cinerarifolium*	Organic ester	Insecticidal; lethal convulsive paralysis in insects; also used historically in humans as stimulant, aphrodisiac
Calcium channels			
Ryanodine	Plant: *Ryania speciosa* (Flacourtiaceae)	Alkaloid	Insecticidal; causes muscle contracture
Glutamate-gated channels			
Ibotenic acid	Fly agaric mushroom: *Amanita muscaria*	Amino acid	Depolarization of cells possessing glutamate receptors
Kainic acid	Red alga: *Digenea simplex*	Cyclic amino acid	Depolarization of crayfish and insect muscle
Domoic acid	Alga: *Nitzschia pungens* found in blue mussel, *Mytilus edulis*; seaweed: *Chondria armata*	Cyclic amino acid	Excitotoxic; causes amnesia
Acromelic acid	Mushroom: *Clitocybe* species	Cyclic amino acid	After systemic administration in rats, causes forced hind limb extension, seizures, wet-dog shakes, degeneration of spinal interneurons

Adapted from Adams ME, Swanson G. *Trends Neurosci Suppl* 1994.

TABLE 10. Plant toxins

Toxin	Source	Chemistry	Mode of action
Acetylcholine receptors			
Nicotine	Tobacco: *Nicotiana tabacum*	Alkaloid	CNS stimulant: decreases skeletal muscle tone; nausea and vomiting at high doses
Anatoxin-A	Freshwater cyanobacterium: *Anabaena flosaquae*	Bicyclic alkaloid	Flaccid paralysis
Muscarinic (agonist)			
Muscarine	Fly agaric mushroom: *Amanita muscaria*	Quaternary ammonium-substituted alkaloid	Stimulates parasympathetic system, smooth muscle; slows heart rate; CNS arousal
Arecoline	Betel nut: *Areca catechu*	Tertiary amine-substituted alkaloid	Stimulates parasympathetic system, smooth muscle; slows heart rate; CNS arousal
Pilocarpine	Leaves of plant: *Pilocarpus* species	Tertiary amine-substituted alkaloid	Stimulates parasympathetic system, smooth muscle; slows heart rate; CNS arousal
Muscarinic (antagonist)			
Scopolamine (hyoscine)	Henbane: *Hyoscyamus niger* or *Scopolia carniolica*	Alkaloid	Depression of salivary and bronchial secretion and sweating; pupil dilation; increases heart rate at higher doses
Atropine	Deadly nightshade: *Atropa belladonna*; jimsonweed: *Datura stramonium*	Alkaloid	Depression of salivary and bronchial secretion and sweating; pupil dilation; increases heart rate at higher doses
GABA receptor agonists			
Muscimol	Fly agaric mushroom: *Amanita muscaria*	Alkaloid; cyclic GABA analog	Hallucinogenic; potentiates morphine-induced analgesia
Glycine receptor			
Strychnine	Seed: *Strychnos nux vomica*	Heterocyclic alkaloid	CNS convulsant; acts primarily on spinal cord and brain stem
Transmitter reuptake (GABA)			
Guvacine	Seeds of betel nut: *Areca catechu* (Palmae)	Nicotinic acid analogs	Anticonvulsant
Catecholamines			
Cocaine	Leaves of coca plant: *Erythroxylon coca*	Benzoylmethylecgonine	Stimulates CNS; vasoconstrictor
Adenosine triphosphatase			
Digitoxin	Foxglove: *Digitalis purpurea*	Glycoside	Cardiac acceleration

CNS, central nervous system; GABA, γ-aminobutyric acid.

pias), and oleander (*Nerium*)]; and (b) saponin (saprogenic) glycosides [e.g., pokeweed (*Phytolacca*), English ivy (*Hedera*)]. Steroid glycosides cause GI irritation; aglycones are hemolytic.

3. Coumarin glycosides: sugar attached to a coumarin aglycone such as Ohio buckeye (*Aesculus glabra*) and yellow and white sweet clover (*Melilotus* spp.) produces anticoagulation.
4. Anthraquinone and mustard oil glycosides are cathartics and GI irritants.

Proteinaceous Compounds

1. Proteins: phytotoxins (toxalbumins) such as abrin [seeds of rosary bean (*Abrus precatorius*)] and ricin [castor bean (*R. communis*) seeds].
2. Polypeptides: amatoxins, phallotoxins, and phalloidin in *A. phalloides*.
3. Amines such as *Lathyrus* contain aminopropionitrile that causes the degeneration of motor tracts of spinal cord. Mistletoe berries contain tyramine and phenylethylamine, which cause acute gastroenteritis, cardiovascular collapse.

Oxalates

The leaves, stems, and roots of many plants contain oxalates. Rhubarb leaves contain up to 1% soluble sodium and potassium oxalates. Other plants containing high amounts of insoluble calcium oxalates in their leaves include dieffenbachia, philodendron, and sorrel. Insoluble calcium oxalate crystal needles are contained in raphides, then bundled into elongated idioblasts that fire the needles as projectiles when force, such as chewing, is applied (Fig. 1). Highest levels are found in the families Polygonaceae (*Rheum, Rumex*), Chenopodiaceae (*Halogeton glomeratus*), Spinacia, Oxalidaceae (*Oxalis coirnua*), Portulacaceae (*Portulaca*), and Ficoidaceae (*Tetragonia*). Ingestion of a small amount of plant parts with high oxalate concentrations usually causes only mild irritation of the mouth and esophageal mucosa. More pronounced GI effects may follow ingestion of

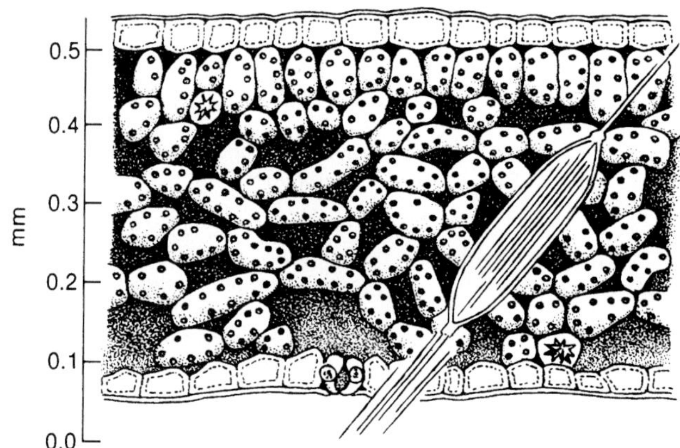

Figure 1. Diagrammatic section of leaf of dieffenbachia showing needle-like crystals of calcium oxalate inside the specialized bivented idioblast situated in the spongy mesophyll. Two druses are also shown. (Adapted from Dore WC. *JAMA* 1963;185:1045.)

large amounts of soluble oxalate such as spinach, rhubarb, and dieffenbachia (5).

Alcohols

Cicutoxin from *C. maculata*, water hemlock, is a convulsant, and tremetol from white snakeroot (*Eupatorium rugosum*) produces trembling in cattle.

Resins and Resinoids

Phenolic resins: tetrahydrocannabinol from *Cannabis sativa*.
Resinoids: urushiol (from poison ivy, poison oak, and poison sumac) and hypericin (from *Hypericum perforatum*, St. John's wort).
Phenolics: gossypol (seed oil of *Gossypium*). Is a male contraceptive.

Mineral Toxins

Weed species [goosefoot, *Chenopodium album*, and pigweed, (*Amaranthus* spp.)] accumulate potassium nitrate.

DIAGNOSTIC TESTS

If the patient is symptomatic, obtain blood for electrolytes and complete blood cell count and perform renal and hepatic function tests and urinalysis. Toxic analyses should be done on samples of emesis or lavage fluid, blood, and urine. Electrocardiographic monitoring is indicated in cardiac glycoside poisonings (*D. purpurea, N. oleander*) and anticholinergic or cholinergic ingestions.

TREATMENT

Decontamination

The majority of casual ingestions require no specific therapy. Emesis is preferred to lavage because plant particles are difficult to remove by gastric tube from children. Activated charcoal absorbs most alkaloids well and should be administered in almost all symptomatic cases.

Elimination Enhancement

Most plant poisonings respond to supportive care. Hemoperfusion has been used after *A. phalloides* and *Podophyllum* poisonings, but its precise role remains controversial.

Antidotes

Few antidotes to plant poisonings are available. Laetrile toxicity has been successfully treated with use of the cyanide kit (Chapter 46). Digoxin-specific Fab fragments have been administered to symptomatic patients who ingested digitalis-containing plants (Chapter 49).

REFERENCES

1. Willis GA. *Common poisoning by plants. Medicine North America.* 1990:1753–1759.
2. Henry JA. *Eur Assoc Pois Cont Centers Newsletter* 1985.
3. Abuelo JG. Renal failure. *Arch Intern Med* 1990;150:505–510.
4. Spoerke DG, Hall AH. Plants and mushrooms of abuse. *Emerg Med Clin North Am* 1990;8:579–593.
5. Fassett DW, Chap IC. *Oxalates in toxicants occurring naturally in foods*, 2nd ed. Washington, DC: National Academy of Sciences, 1973.

CHAPTER 255

Plants

E. Martin Caravati, Christy L. McCowan, and Scott W. Marshall

Topics included:	**See Table 1.**
Molecular formula and weight:	**See Table 2.**
CAS Registry No.:	**See Table 2.**
Special concerns:	**Many plants have delayed onset of toxic effects due to slower release of toxin from plant material.**
Antidotes:	**There are no antidotes for most plant toxins. Toxins with anticholinergic effects can be treated with physostigmine. Toxicity from cardiac glycosides can be treated with digoxin immune Fab in some cases.**

GENERAL PLANT TOXICOLOGY

The toxicity of plants can be examined from the perspective of the toxicity they cause (e.g., cardiovascular), the toxins they contain (e.g., *Veratrum* alkaloids), or their common groupings (e.g., houseplants). Chapter 254 addresses plants from the perspective of clinical presentation. This chapter addresses the perspectives of toxin and known plant ingestions.

There are thousands of poisonous plant species. *Philodendron* species are the most common exposures reported to U.S. poison centers, followed by *Dieffenbachia, Euphorbia, Capsicum*, and *Ilex* species (1). In 2001, more than 100,000 plant exposures were reported to U.S. poison control centers. Approximately 70% were in children younger than 6 years of age, and 7% of exposures were treated in a health care facility (2). Each year, a few deaths from plant poisonings occur in the United States. The most important potentially serious exposures follow ingestion of cardiac glycosides (e.g., oleander), anticholinergics (e.g., jimsonweed), solanine (e.g., green potato, nightshade), jequirity pea (*Abrus precatorius*), water hemlock, Jerusalem cherry (*Solanum pseudocapsicum*), tree tobacco (*Nicotiana glauca*), false hellebore (*Veratrum* species), and plants containing pyrrolizidine alkaloids (e.g., *Senecio longilobus* teas).

TABLE 1. Topics included

Houseplants (mistletoe, holly, dumbcane, poinsettia)
Beans and seeds (castor beans, guar gum, jequirity bean, *Jatropha* seeds, *Mucuna pruriens*, golden banner, lupine bean, mescal bean, sunflower seeds)
Food plants and bulbs (pepper; garlic; ackee fruit; betel nut; white chameleon; mate; thujone and absinthe; rhubarb; potatoes, tomato, and solanine; autumn crocus; cassava; amygdalin; fava beans; cycads; cotton seed)
Moist woodland plants and trees (goldenseal, hellebore, death camus, water hemlock)
Herbs (chaparral, pyrrolizidine alkaloids, ginseng, oil of melaleuca, eucalyptus oil, sassafras, cinnamon oil, oil of citronella, oil of cloves, pennyroyal oil, feverfew, licorice)
Wildflowers, weeds, and natural herbs (mayapple and podophyllum, nicotine, pokeweed, jimsonweed, poison hemlock, buckthorn, snowberry, buckeye, dog's mercury, baneberry, white snakeroot)
Ornamental shrubs and trees (rhododendron, common oleander, yellow oleander, lantana, yew)
Plants cultivated for flowers (*Aconitum* species, foxglove, lily-of-the-valley, sweet pea, Carolina yellow jessamine)
Psychoactive and hallucinogenic plants (nutmeg, peyote cactus, morning glory family, khat, yohimbine)

The amount of toxins present in plants is variable not only among species, but also among the various parts of an individual plant. For example, the entire plant is toxic in the case of jimsonweed (*Datura*) or monkshood (*Aconitum*), but for water hemlock (*Cicuta*), the roots and lower stems are toxic. In rhubarb (*Rheum*), the blade of the leaf is toxic but not the leaf stalk. In some cases, the toxicity of a plant can change depending on the age of the plant. Deadly nightshade (*Solanum*) increases in toxicity as the plant ages by accumulating the toxin in the fruit. Larkspur (*Delphinium*) is more toxic early and becomes less toxic as the season progresses. Because toxicity may vary among different plants within members of a particular plant family, identification of the individual plant genus and species is important. For example, in the nightshade family, three distinct types of alkaloids are found depending on the plant: tropane type in *Atropa*, nicotine type in *Nicotiana*, and steroid type in *Solanum*. A portion of the plant, including stem, leaf, flower, and fruit, should be taken to an appropriate location (e.g., nursery, botanist, emergency department) for identification. A working relationship with a botanist or the local poison control center is a valuable resource for poisonous plant identification.

TABLE 2. Physical characteristics of selected plant toxins

Toxin	CAS Registry No.	Common name	Molecular formula	Molecular weight (g/mol)
Abrin	1393-62-0	Jequirity bean	NR	65,000 (A chain, 30,000; B chain, 35,000)
Aconitine	302-27-2	*Aconitum* species	$C_{34}H_{47}NO_{11}$	645.7
Amygdalin	29883-15-6	Cyanogenic plants	$C_{20}H_{27}NO_{11}$	457.4
Anabasine	—	Tobacco	$C_{10}H_{14}N_2$	162.234
Arecoline	63-75-2	Betel nut	$C_8H_{13}NO_2$	155.2
Atropine	51-55-8	Jimsonweed	$C_{17}H_{23}NO_3$	289.3736
Capsaicin	404-86-4	Pepper	$C_{18}H_{27}NO_3$	305.4
Cathinone	71031-15-7	Khat	$C_9H_{11}NO$	149.1
Chelidonine	476-32-4	Snowberry	$C_{20}H_{19}NO_5$	353.4
Colchicine	64-86-8	Autumn crocus, mayapple	$C_{22}H_{25}NO_6$	399.4
Coniine	458-88-8	Poison hemlock	$C_8H_{17}N$	127.23
Digitoxin	71-63-6	Foxglove	$C_{41}H_{64}O_{13}$	764.9
Eugenol	97-53-0	Oil of clove	$C_{10}H_{12}O_2$	164.2
Glycyrrhizic acid	—	Licorice root	$C_{42}H_{62}O_{16}$	822.9
Gossypol	303-45-7	Cotton seed	$C_{30}H_{30}O_8$	518.6
Hydrastine	118-08-1	Goldenseal	$C_{21}H_{21}NO_6$	383.4
Hyoscyamine	101-31-5	Jimsonweed	$C_{17}H_{23}NO_3$	289.37
Hypoglycin	NR	Ackee fruit	NR	NR
Isoergine	50-37-3	Morning glory	$C_{20}H_{25}N_3O$	323.4
Linamarin	554-35-8	Cassava	$C_{10}H_{17}NO_6$	247.25
Lobeline	—	Tobacco	$C_{22}H_{27}NO_2$	337.46
Mercurialine	74-89-5	Dog's mercury	CH_5N	31.06
Mescaline	54-04-6	Peyote	$C_{11}H_{17}NO_3$	211.3
Myristicin	607-91-0	Nutmeg	$C_{11}H_{12}O_3$	192.2
Nicotine, anabasine, lobeline	—	Tobacco	$C_{10}H_{14}N_2$	162.23
Oleandrin	465-16-7	Common oleander	$C_{32}H_{48}O_9$	576.7
Oxalate	144-62-7	Dumbcane, rhubarb, others	$C_2H_2O_4$	90.03
Parthenolide	1405-86-3	Feverfew	$C_{15}H_{20}O_3$	248.3
Peruvoside	1182-87-2	Yellow oleander	$C_{30}H_{44}O_9$	548.67
Podophyllotoxin	518-28-5	Mayapple	$C_{22}H_{22}O_8$	414.4
Protoanemonin	108-28-1	Baneberry	$C_5H_4O_2$	96.08
Pulegone	89-82-7, 8007-44-1	Pennyroyal	$C_{10}H_{16}O$	152.24
Ricin	9009-86-3	Castor bean	NR	66,000
Scopolamine	138-12-5	Jimsonweed	$C_{17}H_{21}NO_4$	303.36
Solanine	121-54-0	Potato, tomato	$C_{27}H_{42}ClNO_2$	448.1
Sparteine	90-39-1	Lupine bean	$C_{15}H_{26}N_2$	234.4
Thujone	546-80-5	Absinthe	$C_{10}H_{16}O$	152.2
Veratridine	60-70-8	Hellebore	$C_{27}H_{39}NO_2$	409.6
Yohimbine	146-48-5	NR	$C_{21}H_{26}N_2O_3$	354.4

NR, not reported.

TABLE 3. Plant toxins by site of action

Toxin	Source	Chemistry	Mode of action
Sodium channels: lipophilic toxins			
Veratridine	Plant rhizome of *Veratrum album* (Liliaceae) or seeds of *Schoenocaulon officinale*	Alkaloid	Hyperexcitability resulting from reversible membrane depolarization
Aconitine	Monkshood [*Aconitum napellus* (Ranunculaceae)]	Alkaloid	Cardiac dysrhythmia, repetitive firing of nerve
Grayanotoxins	Leaves of *Rhododendron, Kalmia, Leucothoe* (Ericaceae)	Diterpenoid	Membrane depolarization
Pyrethrins	Chrysanthemum flower (*Chrysanthemum cinerarifolium*)	Organic ester	Insecticidal; lethal convulsive paralysis in insects; also used historically in humans as stimulant, aphrodisiac
Calcium channels			
Ryanodine	*Ryania speciosa* (Flacourtiaceae)	Alkaloid	Insecticidal; causes muscle contracture
Glutamate-gated channels			
Ibotenic acid	Fly agaric mushroom (*Amanita muscaria*)	Amino acid	Depolarization of cells possessing glutamate receptors
Kainic acid	Red alga (*Digenea simplex*)	Cyclic amino acid	Depolarization of crayfish and insect muscle
Domoic acid	Alga: *Nitzschia pungens* found in blue mussel, *Mytilus edulis*; seaweed: *Chondria armata*	Cyclic amino	Excitotoxic; causes amnesia
Acromelic acid	Mushroom (*Clitocybe* spp.)	Cyclic amino acid	After systemic administration in rats, causes forced hind limb extension, seizures, wet-dog shakes, degeneration of spinal interneurons
Acetylcholine receptors			
Nicotine	Tobacco (*Nicotiana tabacum*)	Alkaloid	CNS stimulant: decreases skeletal muscle tone; nausea and vomiting at high doses
Anatoxin-A	Freshwater cyanobacterium (*Anabaena flos-aquae*)	Bicyclic alkaloid	Flaccid paralysis
Muscarinic (agonist)			
Muscarine	Fly agaric mushroom (*A. muscaria*)	Quaternary ammonium-substituted alkaloid	Stimulates parasympathetic system, smooth muscle; slows heart rate; CNS arousal
Arecoline	Betel nut (*Areca catechu*)	Tertiary amine-substituted alkaloid	Stimulates parasympathetic system, smooth muscle; slows heart rate; CNS arousal
Pilocarpine	Leaves of *Pilocarpus* spp.	Tertiary amine-substituted alkaloid	Stimulates parasympathetic system, smooth muscle; slows heart rate; CNS arousal
Muscarinic (antagonist)			
Scopolamine (hyoscine)	Henbane (*Hyoscyamus niger*) or *Scopolia carniolica*	Alkaloid	Depression of salivary and bronchial secretion and sweating; pupil dilation; increases heart rate at higher doses
Atropine	Deadly nightshade (*Atropa belladonna*), jimsonweed (*Datura stramonium*)	Alkaloid	Depression of salivary and bronchial secretion and sweating; pupil dilation; increases heart rate at higher doses
GABA receptor agonist			
Muscimol	Fly agaric mushroom (*A. muscaria*)	Alkaloid, cyclic GABA analog	Hallucinogenic; potentiates morphine-induced analgesia
Glycine receptor			
Strychnine	Seeds of *Strychnos nux-vomica*	Heterocyclic alkaloid	CNS convulsant; acts primarily on spinal cord and brain stem
Transmitter reuptake: GABA			
Guvacine	Seeds of betel nut [*A. catechu* (Palmae)]	Nicotinic acid analogs	Anticonvulsant
Catecholamines			
Cocaine	Leaves of coca plant (*Erythroxylon coca*)	Benzoylmethylecgonine	Stimulates CNS, vasoconstriction
Adenosine triphosphatase			
Digitoxin	Foxglove (*Digitalis purpurea*)	Glycoside	Cardiac acceleration
Ouabain (Strophanthin G)	Seeds of *Strophanthus gratus*	Glycoside	Ataxia, rapid breathing, cardioacceleration, tremor, convulsions
Toxins with unknown targets			
Cycasin	Seeds of cycad (*Cycas revoluta*)	b-D-Glucopyranoside	Neurotoxic; might be causal agent in slow neurodegenerative disease; western Pacific amyotrophic lateral sclerosis and parkinsonism; dementia complex

CNS, central nervous system; GABA, γ-aminobutyric acid; spp., species.
Adapted from Adams ME, Swanson G. *Trends Neurosci Suppl* 1994.

PLANT TOXINS BY CLASS

Toxic plant substances belong to a relatively few broad categories of compounds. Major groupings of these compounds include alkaloids, glycosides, proteinaceous compounds, organic acids, alcohols, and resins and resinoids (including phenolics) (3). Many plant toxins have ion channel or neuromuscular receptor activity that is responsible for toxic effects (Table 3).

Alkaloids

The alkaloids are a heterogeneous group of plant compounds. The name derives from the bitter taste and mild alkaline nature

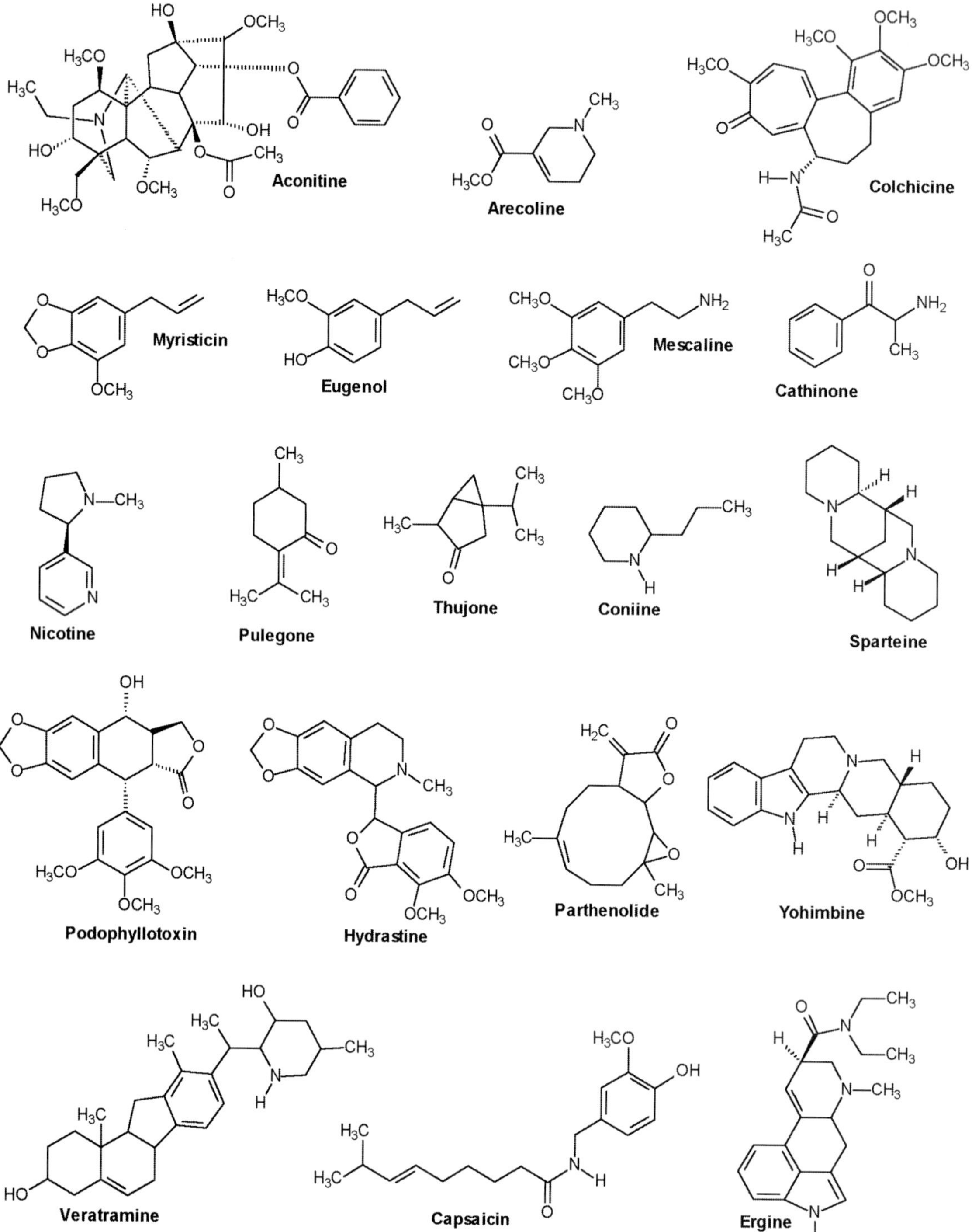

Figure 1. Chemical structures of plant toxins. (*continued*)

of the chemicals (3). The molecular structure usually contains a ring-like structure and nitrogen (Fig. 1). Most of the alkaloids affect the central nervous system (CNS), and some have psychoactive properties (e.g., mescaline). The major types of alkaloids in plant toxicity are listed below:

1. Belladonna type (tropane or atropine alkaloids): belladonna (*Atropa*), jimsonweed (*Datura*), henbane (*Hyoscyamus*), mandrake (*Mandragora*), and coca tree (*Erythroxylum*)
2. Groundsel type (pyrrolizidine alkaloids): groundsel (*Senecio*), blue devil (*Echium*), and heliotrope (*Heliotropium*)
3. Hemlock type (pyridine or piperidine alkaloids): poison hemlock (*Conium*) and Indian tobacco (*Lobelia*)
4. Nicotine or tobacco type (pyridine alkaloids): tobacco (*Nicotiana*) and horsetail (*Equisetum*)
5. Caffeine or caffeine type (purine alkaloids): coffee (*Coffea*); chocolate, cocoa (*Theobroma*); and tea (*Camellia*)
6. Quinine type (quinoline alkaloids): quinine tree (*Cinchona*) and globe thistle (*Echinops*)
7. Opium or morphine type (isoquinoline alkaloids): opium poppy (*Papaver*), blood root (*Sanguinaria*), squirrel corn (*Dicentra*), goldenseal (*Hydrastis*), and fumitory (*Corydalis*)

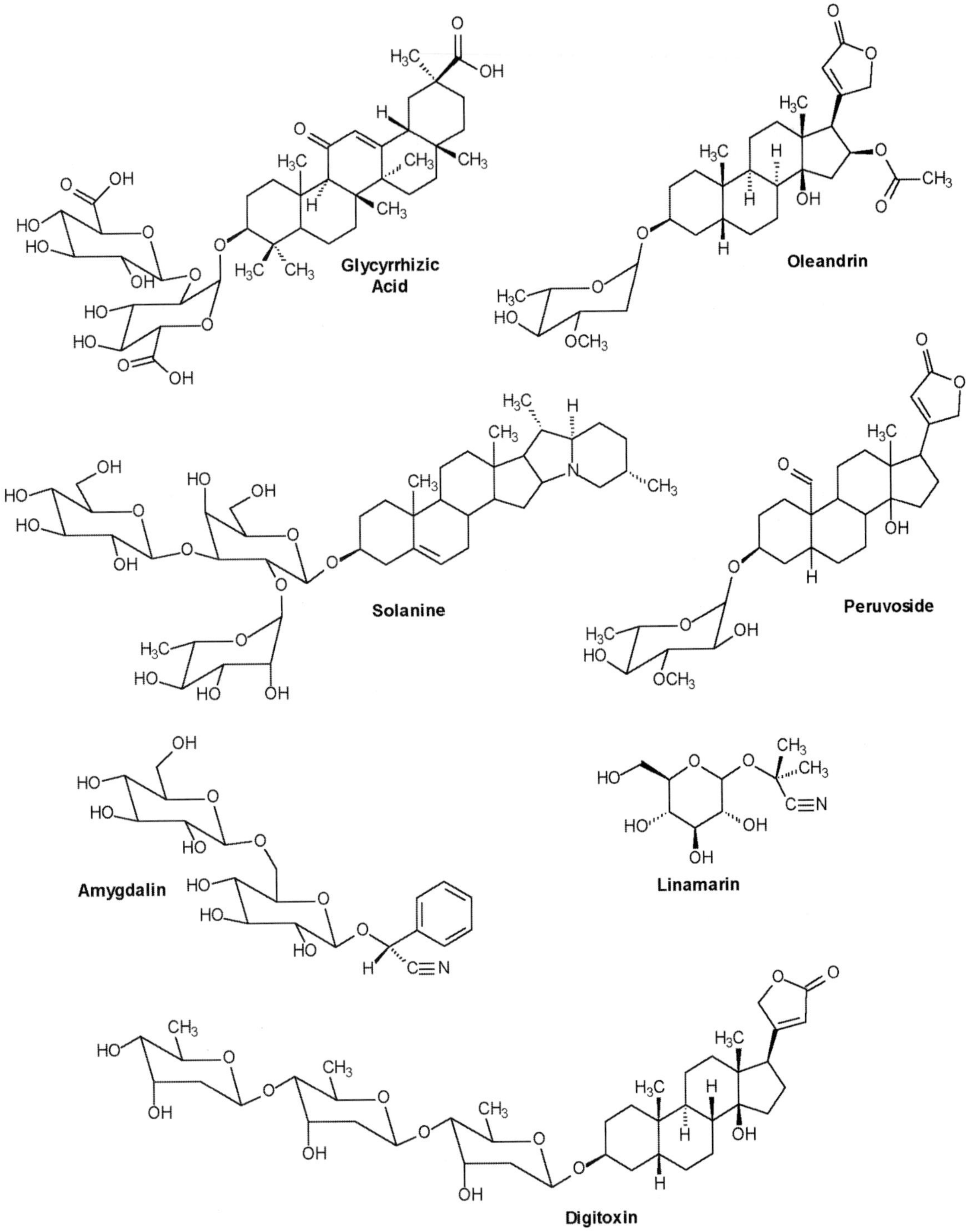

Glycyrrhizic Acid

Oleandrin

Solanine

Peruvoside

Amygdalin

Linamarin

Digitoxin

Figure 1. (*continued*)

8. Ergot type (indole or indolizidine alkaloids): ergot (*Claviceps*), magic mushroom (*Psilocybe*), locoweed (*Astragalus*), Carolina jessamine (*Gelsemium*), and strychnine (*Strychnos*)
9. Lupine type (quinolizidine alkaloids—cytisine type): lupines (*Lupinus*), golden chain (*Laburnum*), false indigo (*Baptisia*), Scotch broom (*Cytisus*), and Kentucky coffee tree (*Gymnocladus*)
10. Tomato or solanine type (steroidal, glycoalkaloids): tomato (*Lycopersicon*), Irish potato (*Solanum*), and nightshades (*Solanum*)
11. Veratrum type (steroid alkaloids): false hellebore (*Veratrum*) and death camus (*Zigadenus*)
12. Larkspur type (diterpenoid alkaloids): larkspur (*Delphinium*) and monkshood (*Aconitum*)
13. Mescaline type (phenylalanine alkaloids): peyote (*Lophophora*) and ephedra (*Ephedra*)

Glycosides

1. Cyanogenic glycosides: Amygdalin is found in the seeds or pits of wild cherry, peach, apricot, apple, and almond and on hydrolysis yields sugar, cyanide, and benzaldehyde. Laetrile is the amygdalin obtained from ground-up apricot

pits and was promoted as an anticancer therapy. Plants that contain cyanide-releasing compounds include hydrangea (*Hydrangea*), flax (*Linum*), elderberry (*Sambucus),* and wild cherry (*Prunus*).

2. Steroid glycosides: The sugar is joined to a steroid molecule. Plants that contain cardiac glycosides (Chapter 122) include foxglove (digoxin, *Digitalis purpurea*), lily-of-the-valley (*Convallaria*), ouabain (*Strophanthus*), dogbane (*Apocynum*), milkweed (*Asclepias*), and oleander (*Nerium*). Plants that contain saponin (sapogenic) glycosides include pokeweed (*Phytolacca*) and English ivy (*Hedera*). They primarily cause gastric irritation.
3. *Coumarin glycosides*: The sugar is attached to a coumarin aglycone. Some plants include Ohio buckeye (*Aesculus glabra*) and yellow and white sweet clover (*Melilotus* species). These plants are usually harmless but may form dicoumarin compounds (anticoagulants) under moldy conditions, which has resulted in cattle fatalities from hemorrhage.
4. Anthraquinone and mustard oil glycosides: Senna (*Cassia* fistulose) and *Aloe* species contain anthraquinones and are cathartics. Mustard oils are gastrointestinal (GI) tract irritants.

Proteinaceous Compounds

1. Proteins: phytotoxins (toxalbumins), such as abrin, found in seeds of rosary bean *(A. precatorius)* and ricin found in the castor bean (*Ricinus communis* seeds).
2. Amines: Aminopropionitrile (*Lathyrus*) may cause degeneration of motor tracts of the spinal cord ("lathyrism"); mistletoe berries (tyramine, phenylethylamine) are associated with acute gastroenteritis and cardiovascular collapse (European mistletoe).

Oxalates

The leaves, stems, and roots of many plants contain oxalates (Table 4). Rhubarb leaves contain up to 1% soluble sodium and potassium oxalates. Other plants containing high amounts of insoluble calcium oxalates in their leaves include dieffenbachia, philodendron, and sorrel. Insoluble calcium oxalate crystal needles are contained in raphides, which are bundled into elongated idioblasts that fire the needles as projectiles when force is applied (chewing). Ingestion of a small amount of plant parts with high oxalate concentrations usually causes only mild irritation of the mouth and esophageal mucosa. More pronounced GI effects may follow ingestion of large amounts of soluble oxalate: spinach, rhubarb, and dieffenbachia (4). An 11-month-old chewed on the leaves of a philodendron plant and developed oropharyngeal erosions and dysphagia. Esophageal erosions and stricture were observed 16 days postingestion. The patient died 17 days after exposure (5).

TABLE 4. Selected plants that contain oxalates

Name	Toxic parts	Toxic compounds
Caladium (*Caladium* spp.)	All	Calcium oxalate
Dumbcane (*Dieffenbachia* spp.)	All	Calcium oxalate
Elephant's ear (*Colocasia* spp.)	All	Calcium oxalate
Jack-in-the-pulpit (*Arisaema triphyllum*)	All parts except rhizome	Calcium oxalate
Philodendron	All	Calcium oxalate
Pothos (*Scindapsus aureus*)	All	Calcium oxalate
Rhubarb (*Rheum rhaponticum*)	Leaves	Oxalic acid and soluble oxalates
Skunk cabbage (*Symplocarpus aureus*)	All	Calcium oxalate

Alcohols

Cicutoxin from *Cicuta maculata* (water hemlock) is a proconvulsant, and tremetol from white snakeroot (*Eupatorium rugosum*) produces trembling in cattle.

Resins and Resinoids

Tetrahydrocannabinol from *Cannabis sativa* is a phenolic resin. Urushiol (from poison ivy, poison oak, and poison sumac) and hypericin (from *Hypericum perforatum,* St. John's wort) are resinoids. Gossypol is a phenol compound from the cotton seed (seed oil of *Gossypium*) and has been found to decrease sperm count.

DIAGNOSTIC TESTS

Serum or urine concentrations are not routinely available for plant toxins and are not expected to contribute to patient management. Cardiac glycoside–containing plants (e.g., foxglove, oleander) may cross-react with digoxin assays and can confirm the exposure. However, serum digoxin levels may not correlate with clinical toxicity, as many of the plant cardiac glycosides cannot be measured.

If the patient is symptomatic, obtain blood for electrolytes and complete blood cell count. Renal and hepatic function tests and urinalysis should be obtained with exposures to potentially nephrotoxic and hepatotoxic plants. Electrocardiographic monitoring is indicated in cardiac glycoside poisonings (*D. purpurea, Nerium oleander*) and anticholinergic or cholinergic ingestions.

TREATMENT

Gastrointestinal Decontamination

The efficacy of gastric emptying techniques for plant ingestions has not been studied. Although not specifically studied for plant toxins, activated charcoal has been demonstrated to adsorb cardiac glycosides (6) and may be beneficial in adsorbing plant alkaloids. Administration of activated charcoal is generally recommended for potentially toxic plant ingestions.

Elimination Enhancement

Most plant poisonings respond to supportive care, and the toxins are not dialyzable. Hemoperfusion has been used for *Podophyllum* (mandrake) poisonings, but its precise role remains controversial (7).

Antidotes

Few antidotes to plant poisonings are available. Digoxin-specific Fab fragments have been administered to symptomatic patients who ingested digitalis-containing plants. Physostigmine may be useful for anticholinergic syndrome. Refer to the individual plant section for specific antidote recommendations.

HOUSEPLANTS

Mistletoe (*Phoradendron flavescens, Viscum album*)

Mistletoe is a semiparasitic perennial houseplant that grows chiefly on oak trees. It grows as a 1- and 4-ft bush in the oak branches and is distinguished from the oak by light green leaves and hairy stems. Small white berries grow in grape-like clusters. Several species are present in the United States, including the familiar Christmas mistletoe (*Phoradendron flavescens*). All parts of the plants are poisonous. The dominant European mistletoe species is *Viscum album*. It contains viscotoxins that cause vasoconstriction, bradycardia, and negative inotropic effects when administered parenterally to cats (7a).

TOXIC DOSE

Based on limited case study data, ingestion of fewer than six leaves or berries of American mistletoe appears to cause only occasional mild GI upset (8).

CLINICAL PRESENTATION

Ingestion of large quantities of berries causes gastroenteritis. Anecdotal reports suggest that European mistletoe (*V. album*) is cardiotoxic. Symptoms begin less than 6 hours after ingestion. Most unintentional exposures to American mistletoe involve children who rarely develop symptoms (9). In a retrospective review of 14 symptomatic exposures to American mistletoe reported to three U.S. poison centers, six patients developed GI symptoms, two developed mild drowsiness, one 21-month-old child developed ataxia, and one 13-month-old child developed a seizure. The dose associated with the pediatric seizure was unknown (8). All patients became symptomatic within 6 hours of ingestion.

TREATMENT

There are no specific antidotes to mistletoe toxicity. Patients who manifest dysrhythmias or electrolyte imbalance should be hospitalized for observation overnight. Asymptomatic patients may be discharged after several hours of observation.

Holly (*Ilex* Species)

The genus *Ilex* contains 300 to 350 species found throughout regions with temperate and tropical climates where they grow as deciduous and evergreen shrubs and trees. They have bright green leaves, often with hard teeth on the leaf margins, which discourage leaf consumption. The red or black berries (Christmas holly) are attractive ornaments, especially to curious children. *Ilex* species produce GI distress in some, but not all, ingestions. Treatment is supportive.

Dumbcane (*Dieffenbachia*)

A popular ornamental houseplant that has broad, shiny leaves and grows to 6 ft, this tropical American native has leaves that may be spotted or variegated; it grows well indoors. It contains calcium oxalate and compact bundles of needle-shaped crystals (raphides) that extrude in response to mechanical forces such as chewing (10).

CLINICAL PRESENTATION

Dieffenbachia species cause salivation and severe swelling of the lips, mouth, and tongue, which may lead to interference with swallowing and breathing. Bullae of the tongue and mouth may develop (11).

TREATMENT

Usually demulcents (milk, water) and cold packs are all that is required for symptomatic relief. The most severe sequelae appears to be the potential for respiratory obstruction, which progresses over the first 6 hours. Only those patients with significant edema require direct medical observation. Otherwise, only symptomatic care with topical agents (e.g., Cepacol) is necessary. Severe cases require more potent analgesics. Admission criteria should be based on the presence of respiratory obstruction and the ability to maintain fluid balance. Diphenhydramine may be used as a topical anesthetic.

Poinsettia (*Euphorbia pulcherrima*)

Poinsettia is a popular indoor Christmas ornamental houseplant with large (3 to 7 in.) alternating leaves and prominent red, pink, yellow, or cream bracts clustered at the tops of the stems. Poinsettia toxicity is limited to local irritation, contact dermatitis, mucosal burns, and keratoconjunctivitis from the sap. Treatment is supportive, as in dumbcane (*Dieffenbachia*) exposure.

BEANS AND SEEDS

Castor Bean (*Ricinus communis*)

The castor plant is a member of the Euphorbiaceae (spurge) family. It is a large shrub (4 to 12 ft high) with wide palmate green-red leaves (Fig. 2). Soft-spined brown capsules are found clustered together on the central stalk and contain three mottled seeds. It is grown commercially for its oil. Castor "beans" are decorative, hard-shelled seeds that contain the potent toxalbumin ricin. It is also known as *palma Christi* and *mole bean*. The beans need to be chewed or crushed for the ricin to be available for local or system effects. Attempts to extract the ricin for malicious use have been noted in the media. In general, toxicity from chewing and ingesting a few beans consists of acute gastroenteritis and dehydration. Treatment is supportive (12,13).

TOXIC DOSE

The lethal dose of ricin in humans has been estimated to be 1 mg/kg body weight (14). This corresponds to eight seeds. Ingestion of two seeds caused protracted nausea and vomiting in a 12-year-old boy (15). Ingestion of 30 partially chewed seeds by a 21-year-old patient resulted in severe hemorrhagic gastritis and dehydration (14). Because of the potential of anaphylaxis, one seed may be fatal.

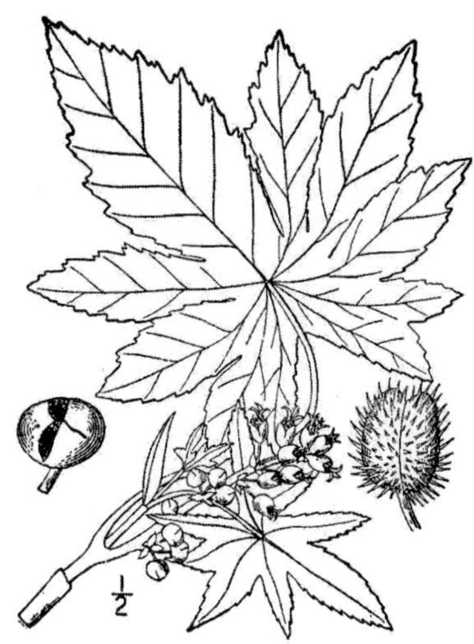

Figure 2. Castor plant. (From USDA-NRCS PLANTS database/Britton NL, Brown A. *Illustrated flora of the northern states and Canada. Vol. 2.* 1913:461, with permission.)

PHARMACOKINETICS

The urinary elimination half-life was calculated to be 8 days in one case report (14).

PATHOPHYSIOLOGY

The toxicity of this plant results from the effects of ricin, which is one of the most toxic parenteral substances in the plant kingdom. Ricin is a glycoprotein that contains two polypeptide chains held together by a single disulfide bond. Chain B is a lectin that binds to the surface of the cell to facilitate toxin entry into the cell. Chain A disrupts protein synthesis by activating the 60S ribosomal subunit (16). Hence, its toxic effects are delayed and widespread. The pulp of the seed contains allergenic glycoproteins, which cause allergic dermatitis, rhinitis, and asthma in sensitized industrial workers. In addition, the leaves, stem, and seeds contain potassium nitrate and hydrocyanic acid. Castor oil increases peristalsis of the small intestine by the action of ricinoleic acid on the small intestine. The oil extract of the castor bean contains the ricinoleic acid; the fibrous portion contains the toxic protein ricin.

CLINICAL PRESENTATION

Toxic effects from ricin usually require several hours to develop. Allergic reactions in sensitized individuals may occur immediately after exposure. The most common initial symptoms result from GI irritation and include burning in the alimentary tract, nausea, vomiting, diarrhea, and colicky abdominal pain. In severe poisoning, these symptoms progress to hemorrhagic gastritis and dehydration. Hepatotoxicity has occurred 3 days after ingestion (15,17).

A review of 424 cases of castor bean intoxication revealed symptoms including acute gastroenteritis, fluid and electrolyte depletion, GI bleeding, hemolysis, and hypoglycemia. Fourteen patients died due to hypovolemic shock (12). The clinical severity of the intoxication cannot be predicted on the basis of the number of beans ingested.

DIAGNOSTIC TESTS

Obtain a complete blood cell count, serum electrolytes, liver function tests, and urinalysis. Hematuria and elevated free serum hemoglobin have been reported in a 4-year-old girl who ingested four seeds (18). Delayed hepatotoxicity has been reported. Serum ricin concentrations are not routinely available and do not help in management. It may be detected by radioimmunoassays for forensic or medical-legal reasons.

TREATMENT

GI decontamination techniques have not been studied for bean ingestions. Intact seeds are too large to pass through a nasogastric or gastric lavage tube. They should pass through the GI tract intact. Gastric emptying via induction of emesis with ipecac should be considered for ingestions younger than 30 minutes old, particularly if the beans are chewed. Whole bowel irrigation should be considered for all ingestions unless the patient is hemodynamically unstable. The ability of activated charcoal to bind ricin is unknown.

Supportive care includes maintenance of fluid, and electrolyte balance is the most important aspect of supportive care. Most patients respond well to intravenous (IV) fluid and electrolyte replacement and recover without complications or permanent sequelae.

Elimination enhancement is unlikely to be effective. Ricin is not dialyzable, and little is excreted in the urine. Therefore, hemodialysis or forced diuresis is not indicated.

There are no antidotes to ricin.

Symptomatic patients should be hospitalized. Asymptomatic patients may be discharged with instructions to return immediately if symptoms develop. Asymptomatic pediatric patients who have ingested more than several beans should be observed for at least 4 to 6 hours postingestion. Daily outpatient follow-up for several days after ingestion is important for patients who actually chewed castor beans to identify hepatotoxicity (17).

Guar Gum (*Cyamopsis tetragonolobus* Taub)

Guar gum, also known as *Indian cluster bean* and *guar plant*, belongs to the legume family. Synonyms include burtonite v-7-e, cyamopsis gum, decorpa, Guarem, guar flour, gum cyamopsis, gum guar, jaguar gum a-20-d, jaguar no. 124, and jaguar plus. It is a nitrogen-fixing annual that bears pods, each containing a number of seeds. Native to tropical Asia, the plants grow throughout India and Pakistan and have been growing in the United States since the early 1900s. It has been used in the management of hypercholesterolemia and as an over-the-counter diet pill. It contains approximately 80% guaran. The viscosity of guar gum varies in proportion to the degree of galacto cross-linking. In Australia, the galacto diet pills were banned in 1985. The U.S. Food and Drug Administration (FDA) has taken similar measures (19).

CLINICAL PRESENTATION

Esophageal and small bowel obstruction have been reported after use of Cal-Ban 3000, guar gum "diet pills" in tablet and capsule formulations. Nine of 18 individuals reported to the FDA had preexisting disorders (esophageal obstruction, esophageal or gastric disorders) (19).

TREATMENT

Management has included endoscopic removal from the esophagus or stomach. This is difficult because of its tenacious sticky consistency. Surgery has been required for small bowel obstruction.

Jequirity Bean (*Abrus precatorius*)

A. precatorius is a tropical vine-like plant of the legume family. Common names include jequirity bean, rosary pea, precatory bean, prayer vine, Buddhist rosary bead, Indian bead, Seminole bead, prayer head, crab's eye, weather plant, lucky bean, and ojo de pajaro. The seeds, roots, and leaves are poisonous. It can be found in parts of southern Florida. The practice of using the beans to make decorative jewelry or rosary necklaces is illegal in the United States. The plant is widely distributed in Sri Lanka, and the seeds are used in traditional games played during the Sri Lankan New Year (20). Extracts of the plant have been used as an herbal remedy in Zimbabwe in the treatment of urinary schistosomiasis (20).

The seeds are potentially extremely toxic. They are 3 to 8 mm long, ovoid, hard, and colorful. One-third is a scarlet red and the rest a shiny black with a seed stalk scar. The seed of another tropical vine, the coral berry (*Rhynchosia phaseoloides*), produces a seed that is similar in appearance but appears to be nontoxic. It can be distinguished from the jequirity bean by the seed stalk scar location on the red portion of the seed (3).

TOXIC DOSE

The amount of toxin available in one seed may cause severe toxicity in children. The toxin is released by chewing or otherwise breaking the hard covering of the seed. An adult homogenized 20 seeds in a blender, drank a portion of the mixture, and died (21).

PATHOPHYSIOLOGY

The jequirity bean contains *N*-methyltryptophan, abric acid, glycyrrhizin (the active principle of licorice), a lipolytic enzyme, and abrin. Structurally, abrin has the same two-subunit configuration as ricin. It is a lectin glycoprotein. These compounds are known to agglutinate erythrocytes *in vitro*. Abrin is a severe mucous membrane irritant, resulting in ulcerations and bleeding of the GI tract. It also may produce hemoagglutination and focal necrosis of the liver and kidney after systemic absorption.

CLINICAL PRESENTATION

Serious abrin ingestion produces a severe gastroenteritis with an onset of several hours to 5 days after consumption. It is characterized by vomiting, abdominal cramps, hematemesis, and bloody diarrhea. Hemolysis, hemagglutination, and hypovolemic shock may occur and cause subsequent renal failure. Drowsiness, seizures, hypertension, and pulmonary edema have been reported. Symptoms may last as long as 10 days. Mortality rate is 5% and may occur up to 14 days after exposure (20).

A 13-year-old boy ate two or more beans and 5 days later developed vomiting, diarrhea, and crampy abdominal pain. He developed hypertension (180/120 mm Hg), tachycardia [pulse, 164 beats/minute (bpm)], and pulmonary edema. He was treated with mechanical ventilation, diuretics, and vasodilators and was discharged home on the fourth hospital day (20).

DIAGNOSTIC TESTS

Elevated hepatic transaminases and serum bilirubin may occur. A chest radiograph may reveal pulmonary edema.

TREATMENT

GI decontamination techniques have not been studied for bean ingestion. Because one or two chewed seeds may be life-threatening, aggressive decontamination appears warranted. Gastric emptying techniques, such as induction of emesis with ipecac or gastric lavage, should be considered for ingestions less than 1 hour old. Whole bowel irrigation should be considered for all ingestions unless the patient is hemodynamically unstable. The ability of activated charcoal to bind abrin is unknown.

Supportive care includes IV administration of fluids to correct hypovolemia. There is no effective method to increase elimination. There is no antidote for abrin toxicity. Monitoring includes hematocrit, electrolytes, serum creatinine, and vital signs in symptomatic patients for at least 24 hours.

Jatropha Seeds

The black seeds of unripe *Jatropha* fruit are known in the Philippines as *tuba-tuba*. Children commonly ingest them. A prospective study described vomiting, abdominal pain, nausea, muscle twitching, weakness, salivation, and sweating after ingestion. Most patients were discharged in 24 to 48 hours with only supportive therapy. The toxicity may be due to the ricin (a toxalbumin) and tannic acid content (22).

Mucuna Pruriens

An outbreak of acute toxic psychosis in Mozambique followed ingestion of the seeds of *Mucuna pruriens*, also known as *feijao nacaca* in Mozambique and as *cowitch*, *cowhage*, *kaunch*, and *pica-pica* in other countries. The seeds contain levodopa, *N,N*-dimethyltryptamine, bufotenine, 5-methoxy-*N,N*-dimethyltryptamine, and other alkaloids. Assay of *Mucuna* has detected levodopa yields of 3.1% to 6.1% of the mature seed (22a). Casual contact with the pod produces an erythematous, pruritic macular lesion believed to be an immediate hypersensitivity reaction (23).

Golden Banner/Buffalo Pea (*Thermopsis* Species)

Golden banner, also known as *false lupine*, *buck bean*, *buffalo pea*, *buffalo bean*, *yellow bean*, and *mountain thermopsis*, belongs to the legume family. Various *Thermopsis* species are found in the foothills and plains of the Rocky Mountains. These plants are herbaceous with leaves containing three leaflets; bright yellow, pea-like flowers; and a flat, pea-like pod (Fig. 3). They bloom from May to July and after 2 to 3 weeks develop long pods. The seeds contain the highest plant concentration of quinolizidine alkaloids. Symptoms may follow ingestion of the flowers or blossoms. *Thermopsis rhombifolia* contains anagyrine, thermopsine, rhombfoline, cytisine, *N*-methylcytisine, 5-6-dehydrolupanine, and lupanine. The two principal alkaloids of the group are anagyrine and thermopsine. Cytisine, the primary toxin of *Laburnum anagyroides* (golden chain), has nicotine-like activity and produces CNS excitation, ataxia, and respiratory paralysis (3). No specific toxic dose is known for humans, but a "handful" of seeds produces symptoms.

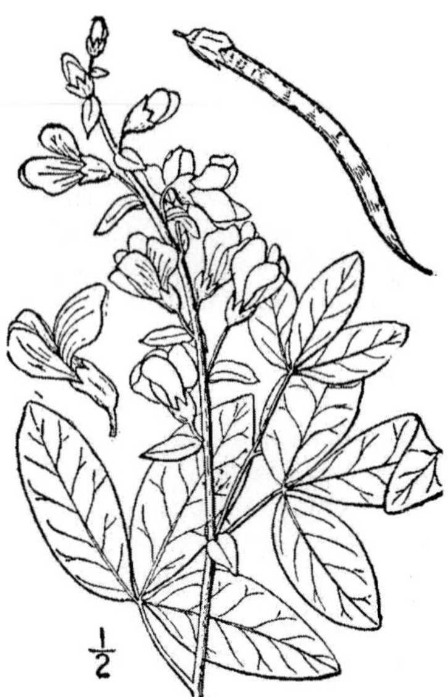

Figure 3. Allegheny mountain golden banner (*Thermopsis mollis*). (From USDA-NRCS PLANTS database/Britton NL, Brown A. *Illustrated flora of the northern states and Canada. Vol. 2.* 1913:343, with permission.)

CLINICAL PRESENTATION

Symptoms seen in quinolizidine alkaloid poisoning include abdominal pain, cramping, vomiting, convulsions, and death through respiratory paralysis. A review of 23 suspected *Thermopsis* exposures found that vomiting was the most common effect, followed by dizziness, abdominal pain, drowsiness, headache, oral irritation, tachycardia, and tremor (24). A serious cytisine case could exhibit nausea, abdominal pain, vomiting, stupor, giddiness, muscular weakness, incoordination, and ataxia followed by respiratory paralysis. Headaches occur within 4 to 6 hours postingestion and usually clear within 12 to 24 hours.

TREATMENT

Children should be observed for at least 4 hours for vomiting, lethargy, and tachycardia. There is no specific antidote, and treatment is supportive, with IV fluids and antiemetics.

Lupine Beans

Lupines are legumes cultivated extensively in Australia, South America, Eastern Europe, and the Mediterranean as supplemental feed for livestock. Humans ingest lupines as bean dishes, appetizers, or in high-fiber breads, pastas, and biscuits containing lupine flour (25). Approximately 100 different species of lupine are found in the United States and are commonly known as the *blue bonnet*. Only some species are poisonous. The beans are very bitter, and human toxicity is rare.

CLINICAL PRESENTATION

There are two forms of lupine toxicity: an alkaloid-induced syndrome and a mycotoxin (phomopsin)–induced hepatoxicosis (lupinosis). Quinolizidine alkaloids are present in lupine plants, and the beans are responsible for acute lupine toxicity. Fatalities among children and four moderately severe acute anticholinergic reactions have been reported. A motor neuron disease–like presentation associated with chronic and excessive consumption of lupine beans containing high levels of alkaloids has been observed (25).

A 72-year-old woman drank a glass of extract made from lupine beans and developed vomiting, diaphoresis, mydriasis, generalized weakness, and mild tachycardia. Symptoms resolved in 12 hours. Oxo-sparteine and sparteine were identified in the extract by gas chromatography-mass spectrometry (Fig. 1) (26).

TREATMENT

There is no specific antidote. Treatment is supportive.

Mescal Bean (*Sophora secundiflora*)

The mescal bean is a member of the legume family and is a woody evergreen shrub native to the southwestern United States and adjacent Mexico. The seeds are approximately 1 cm long and yellow to scarlet in color. The seeds are used as a good luck charm. The major toxic compound is cotinine, a quinolizidine alkaloid that pharmacologically resembles nicotine. There are no human reports of toxicity from the seed.

Sunflower Seed Syndrome

Ingestion of large amounts of unhusked sunflower seeds may result in obstipation, rectal pain with defecation, and a "crunchy" sensation on rectal examination. Attempts to defecate enhance the symptoms (27). Rectal impaction has occurred in children that required removal by endoscopic biopsy forceps and rectal irrigation (28). Disimpaction may require general anesthesia.

FOOD PLANTS AND BULBS

Pepper (*Capsicum* Species)

The pungency of peppers is the sum of the concentration and potencies of five compounds (29). Topical capsaicin has been used for the treatment of neuralgia associated with herpes zoster infection (30) and psoriasis (31). Substance P is released from cutaneous sensory nerve endings and is increased in the regional skin in psoriasis. Capsaicin (Fig. 1) depletes substance P through inducing degeneration of primary sensory neurons (thus relieving itching) (31), diabetic neuropathy (32), pruritus related to hemodialysis (33), and posttraumatic amputation stump pain (34). In diabetics receiving angiotensin converting enzyme inhibitors, topical capsaicin may enhance the angiotensin converting enzyme inhibitor cough (35). Workers exposed to hot chili cayenne peppers (*Capsicum annum*) may experience an increase in cough ("chili workers' cough") (36). Capsaicin, the active principle of the hot peppers (genus *Capsicum*), has been a subject of child abuse when a split jalapeno pepper was placed in the child's mouth, resulting in burning of the mouth, throat, and stomach and burning at the anus (37).

Black pepper [*Piper nigrum* (Piperaceae)] contains terpinoids (*d*-limonene, *l*-pinene, linalool, and philadendrone), which are reported to be potential carcinogens in animals (38). Intragastric administration of red or black pepper is associated with a significant increase in gastric acid and pepsin secretion, mucosal exfoliation, and potassium loss (39).

PATHOPHYSIOLOGY

Capsaicin affects cutaneous sensory neurons through substance P, which depolarizes unmyelinated type C and thinly myelinated A neurons. The symptoms are due to nerve receptor stimulation and not local skin injury (40).

CLINICAL PRESENTATION

Peeling of chili peppers in New Mexico is performed manually, causing burning pain, irritation, and erythema. Such "chili burns" are improved after immersion into cool tap water and vegetable oils (41). "Hunan hand" is a contact dermatitis resulting from the direct handling of chili peppers containing capsaicin (40).

Eight patients died due to aspiration of pepper. Seven deaths involved homicides. These deaths occurred in different states (42). A 4-year-old boy with a history of pica aspirated table pepper with subsequent respiratory arrest, severe anoxia, and death (43).

TREATMENT

Several home remedies have been suggested. Immersion in cool tap water seems to provide some immediate but transient relief, whereas immersion in vegetable oil provides less immediate but better long-lasting relief (41). Other remedies include immersion in vinegar (acetic acid 5%) and application of lidocaine gel (2%) to the affected area.

Garlic (*Allium sativum*)

Garlic, also known as *stinking rose, rustic treacle, nectar of the gods,* and *camphor of the poor* belongs to the Liliaceae family. It is a perennial bulb with a tall, erect flowering stem. The plant produces pink to purple flowers that bloom from July to September. The bulb is odoriferous. Garlic has been used as a medicine in many cultures, as reported in folk medicine literature. It has been used as an antipyretic, antibiotic, antifungal, and antiviral agent. It may affect antifibrinolytic activity in humans, decrease atherosclerotic plaque formation, and decrease lipid and cholesterol levels in humans (44–47). Most of these claims have not been subjected to controlled clinical studies.

Garlic contains approximately 0.5% of a volatile oil comprised of sulfur-containing compounds (diallyl disulfide, diallyl trisulfide, and methylallyl trisulfide). The enzyme allinase converts alliin (5-allyl-L-cysteine sulfoxide) to 2-propenesulfenic acid, which dimerizes to form allicin. Allicin gives the pungent characteristic odor to crushed garlic and probably is the cause of skin reactions.

CLINICAL PRESENTATION

Adverse effects include asthma (48), contact dermatitis, tearing, and second-degree skin burns (49). Ingestion of several cloves can cause GI upset.

TREATMENT

Management is supportive and symptomatic. Topical burns respond to cleansing with water and sterile dressings.

Ackee Fruit (*Blighia sapida*)

The ackee tree grows in Africa, the West Indies, and Jamaica. It is a tropical evergreen tree with a straw-colored fruit approximately 10 cm wide and 100 g in weight. The fruit is edible when ripe, but unripe fruit contains the amino acid hypoglycin A (L-2-aminomethylenecyclopropylpropionic acid). It inhibits gluconeogenesis and causes hypoglycemia (50). It also produces vomiting (Jamaican vomiting sickness), CNS depression, and seizures (51). It is metabolized to the active metabolite methylenecyclopropane acetic acid. Methylenecyclopropane acetic acid inhibits acyl coenzyme A dehydrogenases, which results in accumulation of serum carboxylic acids. Accumulation of carboxylic acids is a possible explanation for the clinical course of Jamaican vomiting sickness (52).

Potential risk behaviors for ackee poisoning include selection and cooking of unripe ackee; purchase of tampered, forcibly opened ackee; and reuse of the water in which unripe ackee has been cooked (53). Undernutrition is also believed to be associated with both susceptibility to and severity of toxic hypoglycemic syndrome, particularly among children in Jamaica.

CLINICAL PRESENTATION

Nausea, intractable vomiting, and abdominal pain usually occur several hours after ingestion of the unripe fruit. This is followed by lethargy, seizures, coma, metabolic acidosis (lactate), and hypoglycemia. Death may occur 2 to 12 hours after exposure.

PREGNANCY AND LACTATION

Hypoglycin A has been associated with a high incidence of fetal resorption and malformations (encephalocele syndactyly and stunted growth) in rats. These teratogenic effects may be due to the metabolite of hypoglycin, methylene cyclopropane acetic acid (54). This may have been a factor in the cause of 33 neonatal human stillborn and neonatal deaths, with anencephaly, spina bifida, and hydrocephalus observed out of an estimated 54,400 total births in Jamaica between September 1986 and August 1987 (55).

TREATMENT

Gastric emptying and activated charcoal have not been studied, but vomiting is usually a presenting symptom. Altered mental status or seizures should be empirically treated with supplemental glucose. Treatment is supportive, with correction of electrolyte disturbances, acidosis, and hypoglycemia.

Betel Nut (*Areca catechu* L.)

The areca nut, commonly known as *betel nut*, grows on the areca palm tree (*Areca catechu*). It is the oldest known masticatory used by Asians. Many older Cambodian refugee women in the United States chew betel nut quid, a combination of areca nut, betel leaf (from Piper beetle), lime paste, and leaf tobacco. The women are easily identified because the quid causes the teeth to turn black-brown and stains the tongue and oral mucosa. The lime that is part of the betel quid hydrolyzes arecoline into arecaidine, a CNS stimulant that, in combination with the essential oil of the betel pepper (a mixture of phenols and terpene-like constituents), accounts for the euphoric properties of the betel quid when absorbed from the buccal mucosa (56). Betel nut is also known as *supari* in India. The Indian Ministry of Information has issued a health warning and has banned all advertisements for supari because of its association with oral cancer (57).

TOXIC DOSE

One to two "quids" produce tachycardia. Hypertension may be seen in new chewers (58). Five to six quids may cause salivation, sweating, tremor, tachycardia, bronchospasm, and hypotension (59).

PATHOPHYSIOLOGY

Arecoline, the main constituent of betel nut (Fig. 1), produces widespread cortical arousal similar to the action of acetylcholine. This arousal from arecoline administration is associated with an elevation of acetylcholine concentrations in the CNS (60). It is a potent diaphoretic; it stimulates the salivary, lacrimal, gastric, pancreatic, and intestinal glands and the mucosal cells of the respiratory tract; increases muscle tone; slows the heart rate; constricts the pupils of the eyes; and mimics the action of acetylcholine in the body. Approximately six reduced pyridine alkaloids are present in these nuts. Arecaidine may have carcinogenic effects and may be a factor in the associated increased incidence of oral cancer (61).

CLINICAL PRESENTATION

Most betel nut–related effects are transient and mild in nature. However, betel nut can produce significant cholinergic, neurologic, cardiovascular, and GI manifestations. It produces various autonomic and neuropsychiatric effects, including tachycardia, flushing, warmth, cholinergic activation, alertness, and euphoria. The Taiwan Poison Control Center reviewed 17 cases of acute betel nut exposure and found the most common manifestations were tachycardia/palpitations (seven patients); tachypnea/dyspnea (six patients); hypotension and sweating (five patients); vomiting, dizziness, and chest discomfort (four patients); abdominal colic, nausea, numbness, and coma (three patients); and acute myocardial infarction (two patients). Symptom onset was within 1 hour of exposure in all patients. Recovery occurred within 24 hours (59). Bronchospasm, pulmonary edema, and death have also been reported. Chronic use may result in tolerance, psychosis, and withdrawal symptoms (62).

TREATMENT

There are no specific antidotes. Symptomatic patients should have cardiac monitoring. Management is supportive. The use of atropine for cholinergic manifestations of betel nut toxicity has not been studied.

White Chameleon (*Atractylis gummifera*)

White chameleon is a tuber with long serrated leaves (thistle). It is located around the Mediterranean Sea (Greece, Italy, Spain, Portugal, North Africa). It is also used to prepare an extract from the root as a traditional medicine for oxyuriasis. The leaves secrete a gum that is used by children as chewing gum. Poisoning due to *Atractylis gummifera* has been due to ingestion of the root.

PATHOPHYSIOLOGY

A. gummifera contains two toxic glucosides, atractyloside and 4-carboxy-atractyloside. These norditerpenes have structural similarities to the aconitine-delphinidine alkaloids. Both are inhibitors of mitochondrial adenosine nucleotide translocation, resulting in inhibition of oxidative phosphorylation and disturbance of the Krebs cycle oxidative reactions (63).

CLINICAL PRESENTATION

Patients may appear 1 to 2 days after ingestion in coma, with epigastric pain and vomiting. The liver is enlarged. The patient then proceeds into respiratory failure, renal insufficiency, hypoglycemia, and liver failure. Postmortem examination of the liver reveals a diffuse necrosis of the hepatic parenchyma with collapse of the interstitial connective tissue (63,64). The prognosis is usually poor, and death often results.

TREATMENT

Treatment is symptomatic and supportive. There are no antidotes.

Maté (*Ilex paraguariensis*)

Maté, also known as *yerba maté, Paraguay tea, St. Bartholomew's tea,* and *Jesuit's tea,* is a beverage, not a plant. It is prepared from the leathery leaves of *Ilex paraguariensis,* a species of holly that is found in South America. In areas where maté is drunk, it largely replaces coffee and tea. The leaves are plunged into hot water.

Yerba maté contains phenylpropanoids, including caffetannin, yielding caffeic acid when hydrolyzed, chlorogenic acid, neochlorogenic acid, and isochlorogenic acid. The beverage contains caffeine (approximately 2%), theobromine, and theophylline. Heavy use of yerba maté has been associated with a high risk of esophageal cancer. This may be due to the hot drinks rather than the alkaloids (65).

Thujone and Absinthe (*Artemisia absinthium*)

Wormwood (*Artemisia absinthium*) is a perennial shrub native to Europe but also grown in the northeast and north-central United States. The leaves and stems are covered with fine silky hairs, and the plant grows to a height of approximately 3 ft. The small flowers are green-yellow, and the indented leaves have a silver-gray color. In the first century, a wine fortified with extract of wormwood was described as "absinthites" by Pliny the Elder. A stronger drink, with 70% to 80% alcohol by volume, was developed by a Frenchman who sold the recipe to M. Pernod in 1797 (66).

The compound in absinthe that appeared to produce hallucinations and psychosis was thujone (Fig. 1). Thujone is a terpene. It occurs in a variety of plants, including tansy (*Tanacetum vulgare*) and sage (*Salvia officinalis*) as well as in all trees of the arborvitae group (e.g., white cedar, *Thuja occidentalis*). Wormwood is a bitter plant. The bitterness is due to a compound called *absinthin* ($C_{30}H_{40}O_6$).

CLINICAL PRESENTATION

Ingestion of absinthe may lead to a group of neurologic symptoms described as "absinthism" and characterized by digestive disorders, thirst, restlessness, vertigo, tremor, numbness of extremities, diminished intellect, delirium, paralysis, and death. Fifteen grams of the volatile oil can cause convulsions and coma in humans.

TREATMENT

Treatment is symptomatic and supportive. Some countries have banned absinthe (66,67).

Rhubarb (*Rheum rhaponticum*)

Rhubarb is a garden vegetable plant with large, leathery, heart-shaped leaves and a reddish color. The leaf blade is the toxic part of the plant, containing somewhat less than 1% soluble oxalates. The stalks have much lower oxalate levels and therefore are edible. Cooking does not make rhubarb leaves edible. The soluble oxalates are readily absorbed from the GI tract. Systemic formation of calcium oxalate may produce hypocalcemia; precipitation of insoluble salts in the renal system may lead to kidney dysfunction and electrolyte imbalance.

CLINICAL PRESENTATION

Early symptoms result from the mucosal irritant effect of oxalate on the GI tract and include sore throat, nausea, vomiting, anorexia, diarrhea, and abdominal pain. GI symptoms are not always present in rhubarb poisoning. Kidney dysfunction and electrolyte imbalance are the major causes of death and appear after signs of GI distress develop. Anuria, oliguria, proteinuria, hematuria, and oxaluria are present in severe cases. Paresthesias, tetany, hyperreflexia, muscle twitches, and muscle cramps reflect hypocalcemia.

TREATMENT

Mucous membrane irritation can be treated with demulcents (milk, water) and cold packs. The symptomatic patients should receive a complete blood cell count and serum electrolytes, including calcium and kidney function tests (creatinine, urinalysis). Kidney function may deteriorate over the first week. IV calcium may be necessary to reverse the oxalate-induced hypocalcemia. In an adult, the dose is 10 ml of 10% calcium gluconate intravenously with cardiac monitoring over a 10-minute period and repeated if symptoms, signs, and electrocardiographic evidence (e.g., shortened QT interval) persist.

Potatoes, Tomatoes, and Solanine Toxicity

Species of *Solanum* contain the toxic glycoalkaloid solanine (Fig. 1, Table 5). Ripe fruit contains the least amount of solanine. The highest concentrations occur in areas of high metabolic rate such as the sprouts, green skin, and stems.

CLINICAL PRESENTATION

GI and neurologic symptoms predominate depending on the amount ingested. Vomiting, headache, and flushing are the most common symptoms reported in children ingesting plant parts. Deaths have been associated with consumption of toxic potatoes, but those reports involved malnourished patients who may not have received adequate care. Headache, abdominal pain, vomiting, thirst, restlessness, and apathy preceded death.

TREATMENT

There is not a specific antidote. Those patients with neurologic signs or orthostatic changes should be admitted for at least 24 hours of observation. Treatment is supportive.

Autumn Crocus (*Colchicum autumnale*)

The autumn crocus, also known as *meadow saffron*, belongs to the lily family and contains colchicine in all parts of the flower (0.1% to 0.6%). It flowers in the fall, as opposed to the true crocus, which flowers in the spring. Colchicine (Fig. 1) has well-known dose-related toxicity, which includes abdominal pain, hemorrhagic gastroenteritis, metabolic acidosis, and aplastic anemia (68).

CLINICAL PRESENTATION

A 44-year-old man ingested 40 flowers of *Colchicum autumnale* and developed severe abdominal pain and vomiting 2 hours after exposure. He received gastric lavage and activated charcoal. He developed diarrhea 14 hours after exposure. His GI symptoms continued for 3 days. His serum colchicine concentration was 3.8 ng/ml at 6 hours postingestion (normal range, 0.3 to 2.4 ng/ml). The patient had an elevated creatine kinase (534 U/L) and mild elevation of serum aspartate aminotransferase and alanine aminotransferase. He responded to IV fluids and antiemetics (69).

Two patients ate autumn crocus after confusing it with a wild garlic popular in Central Europe. One patient had nausea, vomiting, and diarrhea for 3 days. The other patient developed multisystem organ failure and died 48 hours after ingestion of the leaves. Postmortem examination revealed hemorrhagic pulmonary edema, hypocellular bone marrow, centrilobular fatty necrosis of the liver, and proximal convoluted tubule necrosis of

TABLE 5. Solanine- and solanidine-containing plants

Scientific name	Common name	Description	Distribution	Poisonous component
Solanum dulcamara	European bittersweet, blue nightshade, woody nightshade, climbing nightshade	Shrub or slender vine, purple flowers, bright red berry, various seeds	Along fences, streams, ditches; most common in the east and north-central United States	Solanine
Solanum nigrum or *Solanum americanum*	Black nightshade, poison berry, common nightshade	Multibranched vines or bushes, white flowers, purple-black berries	In fields, woods, waste places; widespread in the United States	Solanine, other glycoalkaloids
Solanum tuberosum	Irish potato, common potato	Vines, "eyes" and sprouts, peelings or tubers exposed to light turning green	Mainly in northeast, northwest United States	Solanine, solanidine
Solanum pseudocapsicum	Jerusalem cherry, natal cherry	Ornamental plant; orange, cherry-like berries	Various species throughout the United States	Solanine, solanidine
Solanum villosum	Hairy nightshade	—	—	Solanocapsine
Solanum aculeatissimum	Devil's apple, bull nettle	—	—	—
Solanum triflorum	Three-flowered nightshade, cut-leafed nightshade	—	—	—
Solanum melongena	Eggplant	—	—	—
Solanum carolinense	Horse nettle	—	—	—
Solanum gracile	Bull nettle, wild tomato	—	—	—
Solanum eleagnifolium	White horse nettle, silver leaf nightshade, tropillo	—	—	—
Solanum sodomeum	Apple of Sodom, popalo	—	—	—
Solanum rostratum	Buffalo burr, sand burr, Colorado burr, Texas thistle	—	—	—
Solanum intrusum Soria	Garden huckleberry, wonderberry	—	—	—
Lycopersicon esculentum	Tomato	Vines and suckers of tomato plant	Worldwide	Glycoalkaloids of solanine type
Solandra spp.	Trumpet flower, chalice vine	Large, showy yellow or white flowers	Greenhouse or warmest parts of the United States	Solanine type
Physalis heterophylla	Ground cherry	Perennial, solitary flowers; many-seeded	Eastern North America	—
Physalis longifolia	Husk tomato	Yellow berry	Weed meadows, pastures	—

spp., species.
Adapted from Foldfrank L, Melinic M. *Hosp Physician* 1979;15:25.

the kidney. The concentration of colchicine in the bile was 7.5 mg/L, and it was undetectable in the blood (70).

TREATMENT

There are no specific antidotes available. Management is the same as colchicine toxicity (Chapter 169). Activated charcoal may be administered, but its efficacy is unknown. Respiratory support should be provided and electrolyte and fluid imbalances corrected. Granulocyte colony-stimulating factor [filgrastim (Neupogen)] is useful in treating pancytopenia after a colchicine overdose. A 19-year-old patient received a single dose (300 μg) of granulocyte colony-stimulating factor. The pancytopenia resolved, and the patient recovered (71). Ingestion of plant material or seeds may have delayed absorption, and the toxic effects can be delayed, so observation for 12 hours after exposure is recommended.

Cyanogenic Plants

Cyanogenic glucosides are present in significant concentrations in a variety of plants and plant parts (Table 6). Naturally occurring enzymes present in plant parts, such as fruit pits, hydrolyze the glycosides, and release hydrogen cyanide. Hydrolysis of amygdalin [active ingredient of *l*-mandelonitrile-β-glucoronic acid (Laetrile)] by the enzyme emulsin results in gentiobiose (a sugar), benzaldehyde (an aldehyde), and hydrogen cyanide. β-Glucosidase, which is present in the human GI tract, nuts, seeds, fruit pits, and vegetables, converts amygdalin to hydrogen cyanide in the human gut.

In general, pits, seeds, or kernels must be chewed or crushed for cyanide to be released in the gut. Sources of common cyanogenic glycosides include three compounds.

Bitter almonds (*Prunus dulcis*) and apricot seeds (*Prunus armeniaca*) have high concentrations of *amygdalin*, whereas peach, plum, pear, and apple pits have smaller amounts. The

TABLE 6. Cyanogenic plants

- Christmas berry
- Velvet grass
- *Linum* species
- *Prunus* species (leaves, bark, seeds)
  - Cherry laurel
  - Western chokeberry
  - Mountain mahogany
  - Pin cherry
  - Wild black cherry
  - Chokecherry
  - Plum
  - Bitter almond
  - Peach
  - Apricot
- *Sorghum* species
  - Johnson grass
  - Sorghum
  - Sudan grass
  - Arrow grass
- Pear (seeds)
- Apple (seeds)
- Crab apple (seeds)
- Jetberry bush (jet bead)
- Elderberry (leaves and shoots)
- Hydrangea (leaves and buds)
- Bamboo (sprouts)
- Cassava (beans and roots)
- Cycad nut
- Lima beans (black beans from Puerto Rico and tropical countries; not those grown in the United States)

Adapted from Kingsbury JM. *Poisonous plants of the United States and Canada.* Englewood Cliffs, NJ: Prentice-Hall Inc., 1964:26.

average amount of cyanide in bitter almonds and apricot seeds is 4.7 mg/g and 2.9 mg/g, respectively (72,73).

Prunasin is present in the cherry laurel and the primary metabolite of orally administered amygdalin. It is produced at the mucosal absorption site by a true "first pass" effect. *Linamarin* is a cyanogenic glycoside found in cassava and certain lima beans (cyanide content varies among species, with black Puerto Rican beans being the most lethal). Linase or acid hydrolysis yields hydrocyanic acid from linamarin (Fig. 1).

CASSAVA (*MANIHOT ESCULENTA*)

Cassava (*Manihot esculenta*) has been estimated as the second largest carbohydrate crop in the world. It forms a majority of the diet for millions of people. The main toxin is the cyanogenic glycoside, which occurs in varying amounts in all parts of the cassava plant. Cassava is often eaten without processing during the dry season when the diet is completely dominated by cassava due to a lack of other food items. Dietary cyanide exposure from cassava results from consumption of insufficiently processed roots (to remove cyanide), probably from liberation of cyanide from ingested linamarin. The detoxification mechanism for cyanide in the body converts cyanide to the far less toxic thiocyanate. The substrate for this reaction is sulfur originating from proteins in the diet.

Clinical Presentation. Cyanide intake from a cassava-dominated diet has been proposed as a contributing factor to two forms of nutritional neuropathies: tropical ataxic neuropathy and epidemic spastic paraparesis described from Mozambique, Tanzania, and Zaire. Tropical ataxic neuropathy has occurred in Nigeria, was found among adult males, and resulted in ataxia. A low dietary protein intake resulting in sulfur deficiency was proposed as a contributing factor (74).

Epidemic spastic paraparesis mainly affected women and children in Mozambique (1102 cases in 1981) and Zaire during droughts and resulted in a spastic paralysis of both legs. The spastic paraparesis epidemic, also known as *konzo*, constitutes a distinct upper motor neuron disease entity, probably caused by a toxic effect from insufficiently processed cassava under adverse dietary circumstances. The uniform clinical findings in 39 cases, ages 4 to 46 years, consisted of abrupt, symmetric, isolated, and permanent, but not progressive, damage to the upper motor neurons (75).

Treatment. Treatment for the neuropathies is supportive and symptomatic.

AMYGDALIN

Pharmacokinetics. Amygdalin (Fig. 1) is minimally protein bound and distributed in the extracellular department. It is rapidly filtered by the kidney, with small hepatic clearance (76). Amygdalin is eliminated with a half-life of approximately one-half hour. Of an orally administered "therapeutic" amygdalin dose, 62% to 96% is excreted within the first 24 hours (77).

Toxic Dose. Ingestion of 45 ml (10.5 g) Laetrile caused severe headache, dizziness, coma, and convulsions within 8 minutes (78). An estimated ingestion of 500 to 2500 mg of amygdalin by an 11-month-old child caused vomiting and listlessness within one-half hour, followed quickly by obtundation, depressed respirations, and shock (79). Consumption of 48 apricot kernels as a milkshake caused vomiting, headache, flushing, diaphoresis, and lightheadedness after 1 hour, which rapidly subsided after ipecac-induced emesis at an emergency department (80). Ingestion of 20 to 40 apricot kernels resulted in similar symptoms plus disorientation, reversal of which required sodium nitrite and thiosulfate (81). Ingestion of 12 bitter almonds produced vomiting, abdominal pain, coma, lactic acidosis, and transient pulmonary edema starting within 15 minutes (73).

Clinical Presentation. The clinical picture of amygdalin poisoning mimics cyanide poisoning. The rapid onset of dyspnea, cyanosis, vomiting, diaphoresis, weakness, lightheadedness, and excitement followed by convulsions, stupor, disorientation, paralysis, weakness, coma, and cardiovascular collapse characterizes cyanide toxicity. Symptoms typically start within one-half hour of consumption and progress quickly.

Wild apricot seed ingestion causes the sudden onset of vomiting and crying, followed by fainting, lethargy, or coma in children in Turkey (82). Skin eruptions, hepatosplenomegaly, and progressive neuromuscular weakness have been associated with Laetrile treatment (83).

A 41-year-old woman ingested approximately 30 apricot kernels (15 g) and within 20 minutes developed generalized weakness and numbness. Initial vital signs were blood pressure, 90/78 mm Hg; pulse, 100; and respirations, 36. She was pale and diaphoretic. A mild metabolic acidosis developed, and she was treated with sodium nitrite and sodium thiosulfate with immediate improvement in mental status. The whole blood cyanide was 43.1 μmol/L (normal, less than 15.8 μmol/L). The plasma thiocyanate was 448 μmol/L (normal, 172 to 344 μmol/L). She was treated with a continuous infusion of sodium thiosulfate at 2 g/hour for 24 hours and survived (84).

Treatment. Treatment is the same as cyanide poisoning (Chapter 185). Mild to moderate ingestions may require only decontamination and supportive care. Activated charcoal has a relatively low binding capacity for cyanide.

FAVA BEANS (*VICIA FABA*) AND FAVISM

Fava bean, also known as *broadbean*, comes from a coarse, erect annual vine without tendrils. The fruit is up to 14 in. long and consists of a thick many-seeded legume. The large seeds are compressed or globular and variously colored from green to purple or blue. *Vicia faba* is widely cultivated in Canada and often grown as an ornamental vine in the United States. It is of European origin and often cultivated there.

The hemolytic syndrome associated with favism has been recognized since antiquity. Approximately 10% to 20% of glucose 6 phosphate dehydrogenase (G6PD)–deficient individuals who consume fava beans experience fava crises. A high incidence of low activity G6PD variants is typical of the Mediterranean area and the Middle East as well as Taiwan and south China. Approximately 12% of black men are G6PD deficient. The sensitivity to favism by individuals with G6PD deficiency is poorly understood.

Clinical Presentation. The first symptoms of favism are malaise, generalized weakness to severe lethargy, nausea and vomiting, headache, and lumbar or abdominal pain. Chills, tremors, and fever are often present. After a delay of up to 48 hours, jaundice appears, accompanied by enlargement of the spleen and liver. A few hours after fava bean intake hemoglobinuria begins and may continue for several days. Anemia and reticulocytosis follow. In most cases, the hemolysis is self-limited. During an acute episode, the measured G6PD levels may be normal (85).

Treatment. Favism usually consists of a self-limited to low-grade hemolytic anemia, mild or no hemoglobinuria, and slight jaundice. It may require no treatment or only supportive therapy with hydration to maintain urine output and diuresis to prevent precipitation of hemoglobin in the kidneys. If anemia is life-threatening, transfusion is required.

CYCADS (*CYCAS CIRCINALIS*)

The false sago palm is a tropical plant with palm-like leaves that grow outward encircling a central trunk. The seeds have been used as a dietary staple for the Chamorro indigenous population of the Mariana Islands in the western Pacific (86). The leaves and seeds of the false sago palm contain a glycoside, cycasin, and an unusual nonprotein amino acid, α-amino-β-methylamino propionic acid (BMAA). BMAA is chemically similar to β-*N*-oxalyl-amino-alanine, a toxin found in the pea *Lathyrus sativus* associated with a motor or neuron disease in India.

Evidence links the motor neuron disease parkinsonism in Guam to BMAA. Cycad was the main source of edible starch among the Chamorros before and during World War II. Motor neuron disease accompanied by parkinsonism and dementia was common among Chamorros in this area. Modern processing methods remove more than 80% of the total BMAA content from the seeds. Therefore, even when cycad flour is eaten regularly, it is unlikely that it causes the amyotrophic lateral sclerosis and parkinsonism dementia complex of Guam (87,88). Cycad ingestion by sheep and cattle in Australia produces ataxia and liver necrosis (89).

Treatment of the amyotrophic lateral sclerosis and parkinsonism dementia syndrome is symptomatic and supportive. If children ingest the seeds, syrup of ipecac or gastric emptying may reduce the exposure.

COTTON SEED (*GOSSYPIUM* SPECIES)

Gossypol is a pigment present in various parts of the cotton plant. In the 1960s, attention began to be paid to the antifertility activity of gossypol when farmers in some rural areas of China developed fatigue and a burning sensation on the face, hands, and other exposed parts of the body. This was given the name "Hanchuan fever" because it was first recognized in Hanchuan county. The farmers called it "burning fever." Epidemiologists showed that patients with this burning fever had consumed homemade unheated cottonseed oil containing gossypol. Many couples from these areas were found to be infertile. The women had amenorrhea, and the men had oligospermia or azoospermia. Gossypol has since been considered as a possible male contraceptive or a therapeutic agent for some gynecologic diseases. The use of gossypol, 50 mg/week, resulted in abrupt decreases in sperm counts after 3 months. Hypokalemia due to renal potassium loss has been observed. Sperm morphology and count often return to normal values approximately 3 months after gossypol use is discontinued (90).

MOIST WOODLAND PLANTS AND TREES

Goldenseal (*Hydrastis canadensis* L.)

Goldenseal is a stout perennial found deep in rich woods from Vermont to Arkansas in the United States. The five- to nine-lobed plant palmate leaves can grow to 10 in. (Fig. 4). It produces dark red berries in April and May from green-white flowers. The rhizomes are golden yellow and knotted in appearance. It is also known as *eye balm, eye root, ground raspberry, Indian dye, jaundice root, orange root, turmeric root, yellow Indian paint, yellow puccoon,* and *yellow root.*

Goldenseal contains the alkaloids hydrastine (approximately 4%; Fig. 1) and berberine (up to 6%), with smaller amounts of hydrastinine, canadine, and related alkaloids. It has been used as a uterine hemostatic. Berberine has weak antibiotic activity and some antineoplastic activity. It had the reputation of being able to prevent the detection of morphine, marijuana, or cocaine in urine samples. Studies have found no basis for this belief.

Hydrastine can cause hypertension, seizures, and death from respiratory failure. Large doses of the plant irritate the mouth and throat and cause nausea, vomiting, diarrhea, and paresthesias. Treatment is supportive.

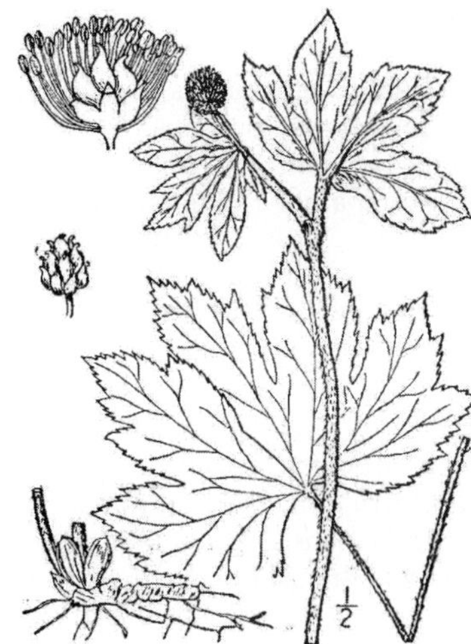

Figure 4. Goldenseal. (From USDA-NRCS PLANTS database/Britton NL, Brown A. *Illustrated flora of the northern states and Canada. Vol. 2.* 1913:85, with permission.)

Hellebore (*Veratrum viride*)

Hellebore (*Veratrum viride*) is a tall perennial herb 4 to 6 ft in height with alternate pleated leaves (Fig. 5). It is a native of moist woodlands in the southeast United States but is also found in Canada and the northern United States. *Veratrum californicum* is a similar perennial herb found in the coniferous forests of the Pacific coast and northern Rockies. Common names include *skunk cabbage* and *corn lily. V. album* is found in Europe, and the pulverized root has been marketed as a sneezing powder (91). All parts of the plant are poisonous.

PATHOPHYSIOLOGY

Veratrum alkaloid production varies among species. *V. viride* contains substantial amounts of the hypotensive alkaloids,

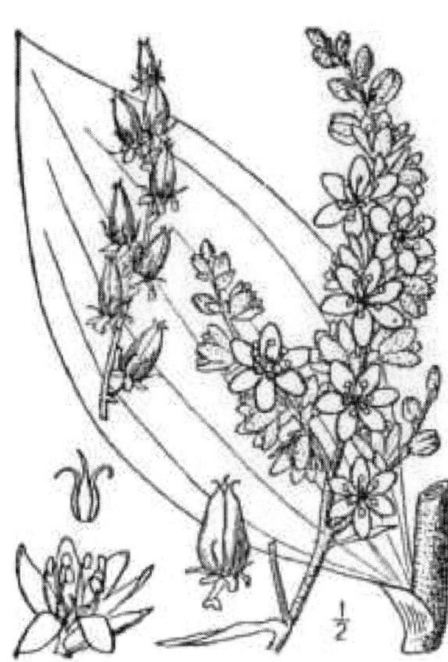

Figure 5. Green false hellebore (*Veratrum viride* Ait.) (From USDA-NRCS PLANTS database/Britton NL, Brown A. *Illustrated flora of the northern states and Canada. Vol. 1.* 1913:494, with permission.)

whereas *V. californicum* contains little. Veratramine (Fig. 1) causes release of γ-aminobutyric acid, perhaps by increasing the permeability of the nerve terminals to sodium. The afferent vagal fibers of the coronary sinus and left ventricle appear to be most sensitive to the depolarizing effects of *Veratrum* alkaloids. Reflex cardiac parasympathetic stimulation results in bradycardia and hypotension.

CLINICAL PRESENTATION

GI distress usually develops within 60 minutes of ingestion. Abdominal pain, vomiting, diaphoresis, blurred vision, and confusion may occur. Mydriasis, bradycardia, hypotension, and syncope have been reported. Massive ingestions may result in heart block and ventricular dysrhythmias. Eye contact may cause lacrimation, conjunctival irritation, and erythema. Symptoms usually resolve within 24 hours.

TREATMENT

Cardiac monitoring should be done for symptomatic patients due to the possibility of dysrhythmias. Atropine may reverse bradycardia. IV fluids and vasopressors may be required for blood pressure support.

Death Camus (*Zigadenus* Species)

Death camus, also known as *black snakeroot*, is a perennial herb with narrow, grass-like leaves and thick horizontal rootstock. Yellow or whitish-green flowers form along the top of a central stalk (Fig. 6). Most poisonings involve ingestion of the bulbs, which are mistaken for onion but lack the characteristic onion odor. Most reported poisonings have been from the western United States. The bulbs and blossoms are toxic.

Zigadenus species contain *Veratrum*-like ester alkaloids that produce bradycardia, hypotension, GI distress, and CNS depression similar to hellebore. Consumption of one-half to two bulbs produced nausea, vomiting, abdominal pain, and bradycardia within 1 hour (92). Treatment is similar to that for hellebore. Atropine is administered for symptomatic bradycardia. Hypotension should be treated with IV fluids and vasopressors. Symptomatic patients should be observed for 24 hours on a cardiac monitor.

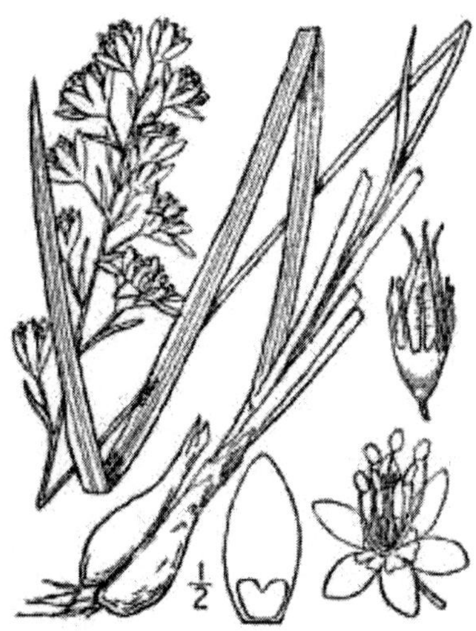

Figure 6. Mountain death camus. (From USDA-NRCS PLANTS database/Britton NL, Brown A. *Illustrated flora of the northern states and Canada. Vol. 1.* 1913:491, with permission.)

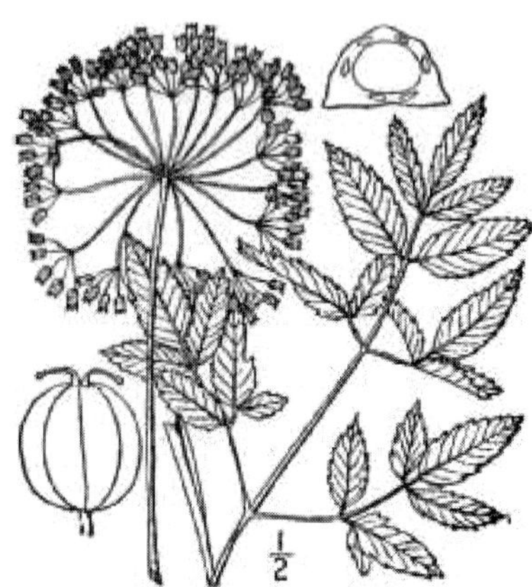

Figure 7. Spotted water hemlock (*Cicuta maculate*). (From USDA-NRCS PLANTS database/Britton NL, Brown A. *Illustrated flora of the northern states and Canada. Vol. 2.* 1913:658, with permission.)

Water Hemlock (*Cicuta* Species)

Water hemlock is a perennial weed that has multiple, thick tuberous roots and a hollow stalk reaching 8 ft high and grows along moist areas, such as marshes and streams, throughout the United States. The leaves are several inches long with saw-toothed borders (Fig. 7). Small, white clustered flowers appear in an umbrella shape in June and July. It is very similar in appearance to poison hemlock except that the leaves are not as finely divided, and there is little or no purple blotching on the lower stem. The odor is similar to wild carrot, and the root is similar to wild parsnip. Slicing of the root reveals chambers and an oily yellowish fluid that contains the long-chain toxic alcohol, cicutoxin. Other common names include *cowbane, false parsley*, and *snakeroot*. The hemlock water dropwort (*Oenanthe crocata*) is indigenous in the United Kingdom and has caused death after ingestion (93). Because of its resemblance to other edible plants, human poisoning is more common than with other poisonous plants. All parts of the plant are poisonous, but the root is the most toxic.

PATHOPHYSIOLOGY

Cicutoxin is a long-chain unsaturated alcohol and an isomer of oenanthetoxin. It is absorbed through the skin and GI tract. It is a CNS stimulant. It is believed to cause stimulation of cholinergic receptors in the basal ganglia and brain stem, resulting in seizures. Hypotension usually results from hypovolemia. Mortality has been reported as high as 30% (94).

CLINICAL PRESENTATION

Severe nausea, vomiting, and abdominal pain usually begin 15 to 90 minutes after ingestion. This is often followed within 1 hour by mydriasis, seizures, and coma (95,96). Salivation, diaphoresis, flushing, dizziness, opisthotonus, and hemiballismus have also been reported (94).The patient may progress to status epilepticus, respiratory arrest, and death. Rhabdomyolysis and renal failure may develop, probably secondary to prolonged seizure activity (97).

DIAGNOSTIC TESTS

Thin-layer chromatography, high-performance liquid chromatography (HPLC), and mass spectrometry techniques have been described for identifying oenanthetoxin (*Oenanthe* species) (98). Obtain a complete blood cell count, serum electrolytes, creatine kinase, creatinine, and urinalysis on symptomatic patients.

TREATMENT

There are no specific antidotes. IV access should be established and seizure precautions instituted. Patients presenting within 1 hour of ingestion should be administered oral activated charcoal and observed for at least 4 to 6 hours. Symptomatic patients should be admitted and observed. Patients often present after seizure activity, which should be treated with benzodiazepines (e.g., diazepam, 5 to 10 mg intravenously, in an adult, titrated to response). Patients refractory to high doses of benzodiazepines should receive phenobarbital as a second-line anticonvulsant. IV crystalloid fluids should be administered to correct volume depletion and to ensure adequate urine output. Alkalinization of the urine (urine pH, 7.5 to 8.0) with sodium bicarbonate should be instituted for evidence of rhabdomyolysis. There are no data on elimination enhancement of either cicutoxin or oenanthotoxin.

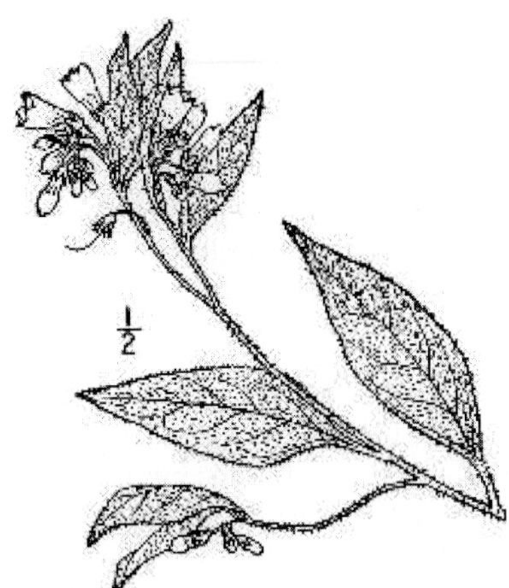

Figure 8. Prickly comfrey (*Symphytum asperum* Lepechin). (From USDA-NRCS PLANTS database/Britton NL, Brown A. *Illustrated flora of the northern states and Canada. Vol. 3.* 1913:92, with permission.)

HERBS

Chaparral (*Larrea tredentata, Larrea divaricata*)

The chaparrals (chaparral, creosote bush, greasewood, hediondilla) are a group of closely related wild shrubs found in the deserts of the American Southwest and Mexico. Chaparral is derived from the ground leaves of the creosote bush. It is found in health food stores as leaflets and twigs. Chaparral has been used by Native Americans in teas, capsules, and tablet form for a variety of disorders. Nordihydroguaiaretic acid and related lignans appear to be antioxidants at the cellular levels. Nordihydroguaiaretic acid also inhibits collagen- and adenosine-5'-diphosphate–induced platelet aggregation and platelet adhesiveness in aspirin-treated patients. Chronic ingestion of chaparral may be associated with acute or chronic hepatotoxicity. In December 1992, the United States issued a public warning after four cases of hepatitis (99,100). Cessation of use may lead to improvement in liver function.

Pyrrolizidine Alkaloids

The pyrrolizidine alkaloid herbs comprise 180 compounds that occur in at least eight plant families. Four genera—*Heliotropium, Crotalaria, Senecio,* and *Symphytum*—have accounted for most toxic ingestions. The last genus includes common comfrey (*Symphytum officinale*), prickly comfrey (*Symphytum asperum*) (Fig. 8), and Russian comfrey (*Symphytum uplanicum*) (101). Comfrey has been used by herbalists as a demulcent, an antihemorrhagic, an antirheumatic, and an antiinflammatory agent. The dried roots and the dried or fresh leaves are used, taken orally, or applied topically. Comfrey may be the most widely recognized source of dietary pyrrolizidine alkaloids in developed countries (101).

TOXIC DOSE

Consumption of herbal teas for up to several years may produce liver toxicity. A high level of comfrey consumption as salad is approximately five to six leaves daily. Intake from comfrey tea is at the same level. The average alkaloidal content of the leaves is 1 mg per leaf. Alkaloid intake may vary from 1 to 6 mg/day. In fatal cases, the total intake ranged from 6 to 167 mg/kg body weight; in nonfatal cases of veno-occlusive disease, it was 2 to 27 mg/kg body weight. Comfrey root tea can yield as much as 26 mg of the alkaloids per day. Comfrey papain capsules can contain as much as 2.9 ng/day total pyrrolizidine alkaloids (102).

PATHOPHYSIOLOGY

An essential structural requirement for toxicity is the presence of the unsaturated pyrrolizidine ring structure (103). The hepatotoxic alkaloids have a 1,2-double bond in the pyrrolizidine ring. The pyrrolizidine alkaloids occur as free bases and *N*-oxides. The latter are reduced to the free bases in the GI tract and have similar toxicity when ingested. Saturated pyrrolizidine alkaloids do not exhibit toxicity. The pyrrolizidine nucleus is dehydrogenated in the liver to the corresponding pyrrole, which is chemically reactive and serves as a biologic alkylating agent. Pyrroles cause a similar toxic picture in animals to that seen with the parent pyrrolizidines. The alkaloids in themselves are not toxic and are largely cleared from the body in 24 hours. They are activated in the liver where they are metabolized by mixed-function oxidase to pyrrolic dehydroalkaloids, which are the reactive alkylating agents. These metabolites induce the liver cell necrosis and vascular lesions characterized by primary pulmonary hypertension (103).

The characteristic hepatic veno-occlusive lesion and the endothelial proliferation, arterial medial hypertrophy pulmonary arterial hypertension, right ventricular hypertrophy, and cor pulmonale are probably due to the release of pyrrole metabolites by the liver (104).

PREGNANCY AND LACTATION

Use of herbal comfrey tea throughout pregnancy (one cup of tea per day; total exposure of 0.125 mg of senecionine per kg) led to the birth of an infant with fatal hepatic veno-occlusive disease (102). No studies are available on the presence of pyrrolizidine alkaloids in the milk of lactating women.

CLINICAL PRESENTATION

Large doses over several days produce occlusion of hepatic venules and a clinical picture similar to Reye's syndrome. It is characterized by vomiting and progressive encephalopathy. Jaundice, ascites, hepatomegaly, hypoglycemia, and massive elevations of serum aminotransferase levels are prominent features. A more insidious form of the disease has been found in epidemic settings and is characterized by anorexia, malaise, weight loss, hepatomegaly, and splenomegaly. Jaundice and bleeding are uncommon in this form (105).

DIAGNOSTIC TESTS

Liver biopsy demonstrates centrilobular hemorrhagic necrosis with occlusion of the hepatic venules. Hepatic sinusoids and central veins are congested, but the hepatic architecture remains intact. Extensive portal and sinusoidal fibrosis may be present.

Laboratory findings include massive elevation of serum aminotransferases, hyperbilirubinemia, hypoglycemia, leukocytosis, and coagulopathy.

TREATMENT

There are no specific antidotes, and management is supportive. It consists of correcting the coagulopathy, hypoglycemia, and encephalopathy often seen with hepatic failure.

Ginseng (*Panax quinquefolium*)

Ginseng is one of the most popular and best known herbal remedies in Oriental medicine. The recommended daily dose for dried ginseng root is 0.5 to 2.0 g. In general, commercial ginseng preparations are not well defined, and they are known to contain a large number of substances. The most characteristic compounds in the ginseng roots are the ginsenosides, and most biologic effects have been ascribed to these compounds. Ginsenosides, being glycosylated steroids, are very difficult to analyze and quantify in small amounts (106).

PREGNANCY AND LACTATION

No reproductive studies are available that address the safety of ginseng use during pregnancy. A 30-year-old woman ingested ginseng throughout pregnancy and early lactation. She experienced repeated premature uterine contractions during late pregnancy and noted increased and thicker hair growth on her head, face, and pubic area. Her full-term baby had thick, black pubic hair, hair over the entire forehead, and swollen red nipples (107).

CLINICAL PRESENTATION

Hypertension has been associated with chronic use (108). A patient developed cerebral arteritis after ingestion of a large quantity of ginseng extract (approximately 25 g drug weight) (109). Siegel described ginseng abuse syndrome consisting of hypertension, nervousness, sleeplessness, skin eruptions, and morning diarrhea. The subjects took an average of 3 g of ginseng root per day. The symptoms usually occurred after 1 to 3 weeks of daily ingestion (110).

TREATMENT

Treatment is supportive.

Oil of Melaleuca (Tea Tree Oil)

Oil of melaleuca is promoted as a remedy for certain skin conditions. Melaleuca oil is extracted from the leaves of the Australian native tree *Melaleuca alternifolia* (the tea tree) and contains 50% to 60% terpenes and related alcohols. It has been used as an antiseptic and antifungal agent. Terpin-4-ol is a hydrocarbon of the terpene class with possible antimicrobial properties. Ingestion of 100% melaleuca oil by a 23-month-old child led to confusion, inability to walk, disorientation, ataxia, and a eucalyptus-like odor on the breath. Recovery followed 5 hours after ingestion (111).

Eucalyptus Oil

Adults and children may develop vomiting, CNS depression, premature ventricular contractions, and apnea with as little as a swallow of eucalyptus oil (112). Ingestion of "taste" amounts seems to be relatively harmless. This observation should be confirmed. Survival has been reported with ingestion of 21 to 30 ml in an 8-year-old child, 23 ml in an adult, and 120 to 240 ml in a treated adult (113). A boy ingested 10 ml and survived with supportive care. He was seen within 30 minutes of ingestion and was deeply comatose, with miosis, absent deep tendon reflexes, and shallow, irregular respiration. His breath had a strong odor of eucalyptus (114).

Sassafras (*Sassafras albidum*)

Teas from the root bark of the sassafras tree contain safrole (4-alkyl-1,2-methylene dioxybenzene). The aromatic oil contains 80% safrole. An adult ingested 5 ml of sassafras oil. Within 1 hour, vomiting, "shakiness," flushing, and tachycardia were observed. The patient recovered (115). A 72-year-old woman drank ten cups of sassafras teas daily. She developed diaphoresis and hot flashes that resolved on cessation of drinking the tea (116).

Cinnamon Oil

Cinnamon oil contains local mucous membrane irritants such as cinnamaldehyde. It is easily obtained from pharmacies in 5- to 10-ml amounts for use as a flavoring agent and in craft items.

Prolonged skin contact over 48 hours produced superficial partial-thickness burns (117). A 7-year-old boy ingested 2 oz (approximately 6 ml) of oil of cinnamon and immediately felt a burning sensation in his mouth, chest, and stomach, lasting for approximately 15 minutes. He then developed double vision, dizziness, and vomiting and collapsed. After ipecac and activated charcoal, he developed diarrhea, more vomiting, dizziness, abdominal cramps, and burning in the rectal area. The white blood cell count was 29,800/mm^3. GI symptoms and sleepiness persisted for 5 hours (118).

Cinnamon oil abuse in young adolescents follows sucking on toothpicks or fingers dipped in cinnamon oil. A rush or sensation of warmth, facial flushing, and oral burning may be experienced. No residual symptoms have been observed (119).

Oil of Citronella

Oil of citronella is a fragrant, volatile oil obtained by distillation from fresh grass of *Cymbopogon nardus* Rendle or *Cymbopogon winterianus* Jowitt (family Gramineae). The main constituents are geraniol and citronellol. Countries producing this oil include Sri Lanka, Indonesia, and Taiwan. Ceylon oil has 10% citronellol and 18% geraniol, and Java oil has 35% citronellol and 21% geraniol. Citronella oil is used in perfumery, insect repellents, and other veterinary products.

A child of 21 months drank 3 teaspoons of a preparation containing oil of citronella. The child developed cyanosis, seizures, vomiting, and died in 5 hours. The child had been given an emetic of salt and water that may have contributed to the clinical course (120). Treatment is symptomatic.

Oil of Cloves

Clove oil is obtained from the dried flower buds or leaves of the *Syzygium aromaticum* (*Eugenia caryophyllus*) tree of the myrtle family (Myrtaceae) and contains approximately 70% to 90% of eugenol (Fig. 1) with a number of impurities. Clove oil is obtained without prescription for the treatment of toothaches, as a flavoring agent in foods and pharmaceuticals, in the manufacture of textiles, and in herbal medicines. Eugenol is a phenol that inhibits prostaglandin synthesis and uncouples oxidative phosphorylation. Like acetaminophen, it is metabolized by glucuronide and sulfate conjugates in the liver.

Consumption of 5 to 15 ml of oil of cloves may induce a high anion gap acidosis, seizures, coagulopathy, acute liver damage, behavioral changes, and coma. A clove oil spill may lead to a stinging erythematous reaction, with diminished sweating and reduced sensation in the affected areas. Animal studies suggest

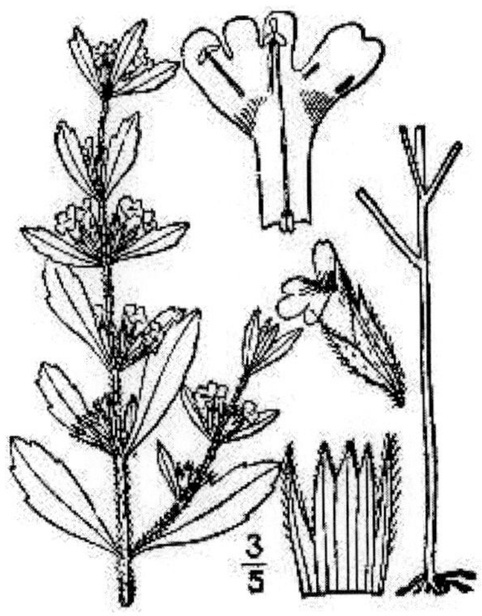

Figure 9. American false pennyroyal [*Hedeoma pulegioides* (L.)]. (From USDA-NRCS PLANTS database/Britton NL, Brown A. *Illustrated flora of the northern states and Canada. Vol. 3.* 1913:136, with permission.)

that the hepatic damage is reversed by *N*-acetylcysteine. Evidence for this in humans is not available. Treatment is symptomatic and supportive (121,122).

Pennyroyal Oil (*Mentha pulegium, Hedeoma pulegioides*)

Pennyroyal oil is a volatile oil derived from *Mentha pulegium* and *Hedeoma pulegioides* (Fig. 9), which are indigenous plants present from Canada to Florida and west to Nebraska (pennyroyal, squaw mint, mosquito plant). Herbalists use pennyroyal oil as an abortifacient and to induce menses. The usual doses are 0.12 to 0.60 ml. Toxic effects usually result from the misuse of the herb in folk medicine. Pulegone is the ketone cyclohexanone, which constitutes 85% of pennyroyal oil and produces direct hepatic damage (Fig. 1). A toxic metabolite, menthofuran, is produced by hepatic metabolism. Glutathione is depleted, leading to hepatic necrosis.

TOXIC DOSE

A dose of pennyroyal oil, 10 ml, produced GI distress; 15 to 30 ml caused fatal hepatic necrosis (123). Ingestion of greater than 5 ml by an adult is considered potentially toxic.

CLINICAL PRESENTATION

Pennyroyal oil consumption produces direct toxic effects on the GI tract and the liver. Depending on the dose, the clinical presentation includes nausea, vomiting, abdominal pain, burning of the throat, and dizziness usually within 2 hours of ingestion, followed by liver dysfunction. In fatal cases, hepatomegaly, coagulation abnormalities, and renal failure, as well as hypotension, consumptive coagulopathy, and massive hepatic necrosis, have developed (123,124). Multiple grand mal seizures occurred within a 24-hour period after the ingestion of 40 pennyroyal tablets over 4 days (125).

Two infants were fed home-brewed mint tea. One developed fulminant hepatic failure and cerebral edema and died. The serum menthofuran concentration was 10 ng/ml. The other infant developed hepatic dysfunction and severe epileptic encephalopathy and survived. The serum pulegone was 25 ng/ml, and menthofuran was 41 ng/ml. The home-brewed tea was used to treat colic and was made from "mint plants" that contained pennyroyal oil (126).

TREATMENT

Although clinical experience is limited, patients who ingest more than 5 to 10 ml of pennyroyal oil should receive acetylcysteine therapy (Chapter 64) because evidence exists that it depletes glutathione. Patients should have a complete blood cell count, electrolytes, creatinine, liver function tests, urinalysis, and coagulation profiles. Hepatic necrosis usually occurs within 24 hours. Such patients should be observed for development of bleeding secondary to coagulation abnormalities and treated with platelet packs, fresh frozen plasma, and blood transfusions as necessary. Seizures are self-limited and should respond to diazepam.

Feverfew

Feverfew [*Tanacetum parthenium* (synonyms, *Chrysanthemum parthenium, Leucanthemum parthenium, Pyrethrum parthenium*), featherfew, midsummer daisy, nosebleed, Santa Maria] is a short, bushy perennial that grows 15 to 60 cm tall along fields and roadsides. Its yellow-green leaves and yellow flowers resemble those of chamomile (Fig. 10). The flowers bloom from July to October. It has been used for the treatment of disorders often controlled by aspirin such as fever, rheumatic inflammations, and migraine headache (127). Feverfew is taken orally either as fresh leaves or in tablets.

The plant is rich in sesquiterpene lactones, principally parthenolide (Fig. 1). It appears to inhibit platelet aggregation, histamine release from mast cells, and the production of prostaglandins, thromboxanes, and leukotrienes. Symptoms such as mouth ulcers, swollen lips, and abdominal pain have been experienced. Management is supportive. There are no controlled studies on its use during pregnancy or lactation (128).

Licorice Root (*Glycyrrhiza glabra*)

Licorice root has been claimed to have many medicinal properties. The principal toxic component is 10% to 20% glycyrrhizic acid (Fig. 1). Consumption of 100 g of commercial licorice (0.3% glycyrrhizic acid) is equivalent to a dose of 300 mg glycyrrhetic acid. Glycyrrhizic acid inhibits both the hepatic and renal 11-β hydroxysteroid dehydrogenase enzyme, which converts active cortisol to the inactive 11-dehydro product, cortisone, and is present in the kidneys, gonads, placenta, lungs, and intestinal mucosa. A daily dose of 10 mg glycyrrhizic acid is probably safe in healthy adults. Approximately two to four licorice twist can-

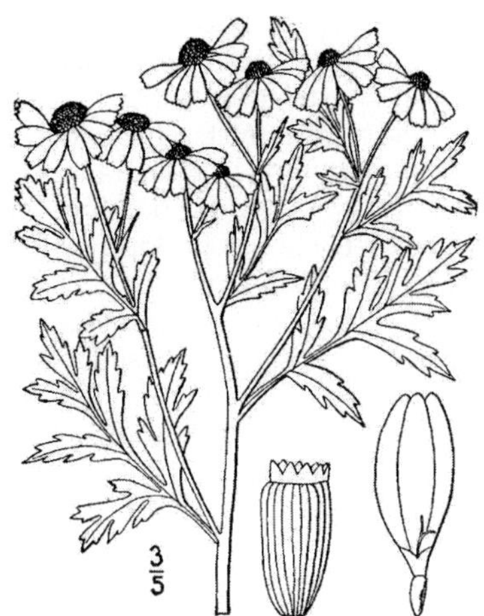

Figure 10. Feverfew (*Tanacetum parthenium*). (From USDA-NRCS PLANTS database/Britton NL, Brown A. *Illustrated flora of the northern states and Canada. Vol. 3.* 1913:159, with permission.)

dies can contain approximately 100 g of licorice (700 mg glycyrrhizinic acid) and, when ingested daily for weeks to months, may be toxic. Licorice candy, licorice flavored soft drinks, medicinals, chewing tobacco, and chewing gum may be toxic when excessive amounts are consumed chronically.

CLINICAL PRESENTATION

Chronic excess consumption of licorice leads to weakness, edema, weight loss, hypertension, hypokalemia, and confusion. A syndrome of pseudoprimary hyperaldosteronism has occurred after chronic ingestion (129,130).

DIAGNOSTIC TESTS

Glycyrrhetic acid may be detected in the blood by enzyme-linked immunosorbent assay techniques. After two to four licorice twists daily for 2 to 4 weeks, plasma glycyrrhetic acid concentrations may reach 480 ng/ml. Hyponatremia, severe life-threatening hypokalemia, hypomagnesemia, and elevated creatine kinase may occur.

TREATMENT

Obtain a careful history of dietary sources of licorice in patients with hypertension and hypokalemia, with or without muscle weakness. Stop all licorice intake. Monitor serum electrolytes, fluid balance, and acid-base status. Obtain an electrocardiogram (ECG) and cardiac monitoring, if necessary, in patients with electrolyte imbalances. Advise patients with hypertension or circulatory disorders to avoid licorice intake. Many confections are made with artificial flavorings that taste like licorice but contain no licorice root extract.

WILDFLOWERS, WEEDS, AND NATURAL SHRUBS

Mayapple and Podophyllum Resin

Mayapple (mandrake, *Podophyllum peltatum*) is a perennial plant belonging to the Berberidaceae (bayberry) family. Identifying features include a horizontal fleshy rootstock; thick, fibrous roots; and large, circular, multilobed leaves (Fig. 11). Single flowers produce a yellow fruit on ripening. Mayapple is found in wet meadows, open woodlands, and disturbed areas along roadsides, often in groups, from Quebec to Florida and west to southern Ontario, Minnesota, and Texas. The roots have been used medicinally as a cathartic by American Indians. Since 1942, podophyllum resin, which is an extract of the dried rhizomes and roots, has been used to topically cure warts, especially condyloma acuminatum. Etoposide is a semisynthetic derivative of podophyllotoxin that is used in the treatment of many cancers (131).

The podophyllum resin extract, which often but incorrectly has been named podophyllin (132), contains at least 16 active physiologic compounds, including podophyllotoxin (Fig. 1), picro-podophyllin (*cis*-isomer of podophyllotoxin), α- and β-pellatins, and quercetin (133). Podophyllum resin is a potent spindle poison that blocks mitosis in metaphase, similar to colchicine. Most human poisonings result from either topical application or ingestion of the commercial extract. Overexposure causes neurologic, GI, and hematologic toxicity that occasionally results in fatalities. Rarely, poisoning results from consumption of unripe fruit or plant parts and causes primarily diarrhea. The ripe fruit does not produce toxicity.

TOXIC DOSE

The lethal dose to 50% of experimental animals of podophyllotoxin is 33 mg/kg in mice and 15 mg/kg in rats (134). Death has resulted from the ingestion of as little as 350 mg, whereas survival

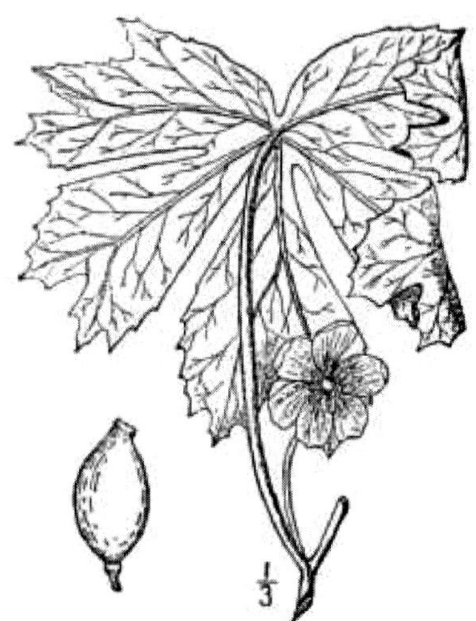

Figure 11. Mayapple (*Podophyllum peltatum*). (From USDA-NRCS PLANTS database/Britton NL, Brown A. *Illustrated flora of the northern states and Canada. Vol. 2.* 1913:130, with permission.)

occurred with reported quantities as large as 2.8 g (135) and 10 g (136). The podophyllum content of commercial resin extracts ranges from 5% to 25%. The level of toxicity has been calculated from animal and human studies to occur when the podophyllum dose exceeds 300 mg/m^2 body surface area (137). A recommendation subsequently was made to limit 20% podophyllum resin application to 2 ml; however, toxic effects may be produced at concentrations as low as 100 mg/m^2. Bone marrow suppression and a severe motor sensory neuropathy developed in a 20-year-old woman when 3 ml of a 20% podophyllum resin solution was applied to condyloma acuminatum and was not washed off after use (138). The calculated dose was 150 mg (100 mg/m^2).

PREGNANCY AND LACTATION

Podofilox is FDA pregnancy risk category C (Appendix I). Fetal death and premature labor have been associated with the use of podophyllum resin extract (139).

CLINICAL PRESENTATION

Features of systemic toxicity include nausea, vomiting, fever, obtundation, coma, hypotension, oliguria, hyperpnea, adynamic ileus, peripheral neuropathy, and death. Symptoms may be delayed up to 13 hours (136). A child received syrup of ipecac for ingestion of 10 ml of an 8% podophyllum resin solution. She was comatose, hypotensive, and hyperpyrexic on returning to the emergency department 9 hours postingestion (140). Poisoning has been described secondary to adulteration of herbal products (141).

CNS effects include changes in sensorium and peripheral neuropathies. In serious cases, lethargy and obtundation develop after 12 hours and may progress to convulsions, confusion, delirium, and prolonged coma (137). Over the course of the first several days, a symmetric motor sensory peripheral neuropathy develops distally and is characterized by profound bilateral weakness in upper and lower extremities. In addition, loss of deep tendon reflexes, vibration, position sense, and distal light touch occurs (140). Changes in sensorium may require up to 10 to 15 days to clear (142). Peripheral neuropathies resolve much more slowly than CNS symptoms and sequelae may be present months to years after the incident.

Cardiac effects include sinus tachycardia and hypertension in an adult who swallowed podophyllin liquid, mistaking it for cough syrup (143). Postural hypotension has also been noted and may complicate recovery (138,144).

Pulmonary effects are not major. Direct pulmonary toxicity has not been reported, although tachypnea may occur, most likely as a result of respiratory compensation for a metabolic acidosis. The generalized weakness seen in severe poisonings may contribute to respiratory depression and necessitate intubation in comatose patients. Previously, hyperventilation was believed to result from direct central neurogenic stimulation (145).

Renal failure has developed despite normal renal perfusion, which may represent a direct toxic effect to the kidney (136). Glycosuria and pyuria have been reported, but renal failure is uncommon. GI effects have included paralytic ileus within several days of exposure, which can persist for 2 weeks (146). Nausea, vomiting, and abdominal pain are common features of podophyllum toxicity. Dermal effects include irritation of skin and mucosal membranes. Severe ulcerations or persistent neuropathies may develop (147).

DIAGNOSTIC TESTS

Electroencephalograms show bilateral slowing primarily in the delta range. Bone marrow aspiration in several poisoning cases revealed sudden maturational arrest of both erythroid and myeloid precursors. Initially, a profound leukocytosis may be present (55,450/mm^3 in one case) along with metamyelocytes and immature band forms, which show hyperchromatism and cytoplasmic vacuolization (137,146). The leukocyte and platelet counts reached nadir by the fourth or fifth day. Severe poisoning has resulted in mild to moderately elevated levels of creatine kinase and hepatic aminotransferases as well as hypocalcemia; however, liver dysfunction has not been significant.

TREATMENT

Symptomatic patients should be hospitalized. Children who ingest potentially toxic quantities (e.g., one swallow or 5 ml of the 20% podophyllum resin solution) should be directly observed for at least 8 hours (140).

The usual measures of decontamination (activated charcoal) should be used for patients seen within a few hours of exposure. All patients who ingest podophyllum resin should be decontaminated. Any topical podophyllum resin solution should be removed from the skin with soap and water.

For elimination enhancement, hemodialysis probably is not effective because of the high lipid solubility of podophyllum resin. Hemoperfusion rapidly decreases plasma podophyllotoxin concentrations, with an extraction ratio of 0.75 (7); however, the pharmacokinetics and plasma podophyllotoxin levels are not well enough understood to indicate whether hemoperfusion alters clinical outcome.

Supportive care includes monitoring of serum electrolytes, fluid status, and serum calcium levels, which should be followed closely. Check for metabolic acidosis in all patients who are hyperventilating. Symptomatic patients should be observed for at least 24 hours. Although fever occurs with overdose, its presence also may indicate infection in patients whose susceptibility to infection peaks around 4 to 5 days postexposure. All patients who deteriorate during this period should have blood drawn for culture. Clinical judgment dictates the necessity of broad-spectrum antibiotics. In severe poisonings, complete blood cell counts, platelet counts, and coagulation profiles should be determined daily because hematologic suppression reaches a peak within 4 to 5 days. Replacement therapy (platelet packs, red blood cell transfusion) may be necessary.

Nicotine (*Nicotiana* and *Lobelia* Species)

Nicotine and similar alkaloids are found in a variety of species. Sources of commercial tobacco are *Nicotiana tabacum* and *Nicotiana rustica*. These varieties, as well as tree tobacco (*N. glauca*) and wild tobacco (*Nicotiana trigonophylla*), are members of the Solanaceae family.

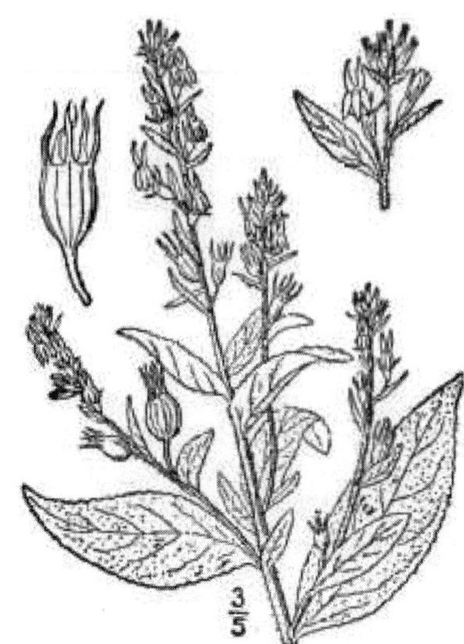

Figure 12. Indian tobacco (*Lobelia inflata* L.). (From USDA-NRCS PLANTS database/Britton NL, Brown A. *Illustrated flora of the northern states and Canada. Vol. 3.* 1913:303, with permission.)

Wild tobacco is a branching annual plant of dry southwestern American stream beds and flats. Identifying features include long, tubular white flowers that open at night. Tree tobacco is an ornamental shrub or small evergreen tree that grows wild in California and Florida. The loosely branching tree, which can grow 6 to 18 ft high, has pithy stems, ovate leaves, and yellow flowers. Indian tobacco (*Lobelia inflata*, family Lobeliaceae), grows in the eastern United States. This annual plant has simple alternate leaves with inconspicuous blue flowers arranged in a terminal raceme (Fig. 12). Several other Lobelia species (*Lobelia cardinalis, Lobelia siphilitica, Lobelia berlandieri*) are native species of moist woodlands.

TOXIN

N. tabacum contains nicotine as its major toxic alkaloid. The concentration in tobacco leaves ranges from 1.5% to 4.0% by dry weight. Cigarettes and cigars have an average nicotine content of 1% to 2% (10 to 20 mg of nicotine). *N. glauca* contains the alkaloid anabasine [1-(3-pyridyl) piperidine], which is pharmacologically similar to nicotine (Fig. 1). Anabasine is a minor alkaloid in the common tobacco plant but is present in the *N. glauca* leaf at a concentration of 1.3% by weight.

L. inflata contains at least 14 different piperidine alkaloids of which lobeline is the principal one with a concentration of approximately 0.3%. The emetic alkaloids, lobelanine and lobelanidine, also are present. Lobeline is similar to nicotine. The dried herb was used by eastern North American Indians as a purgative and emetic. The North American Indians also incorporated the herb into tobacco leaves for smoking. Lobeline sulfate has been advocated in tablets as a tobacco substitute to aid in breaking the smoking habit, but its efficacy is questionable.

CLASSIFICATION AND USES

Nicotine is a water-soluble alkaloid [(*S*)-3-(1-methyl-2-pyrrolidinyl)pyridine] and has an alkaline negative logarithm of acid ionization constant of 8.5 (Fig. 1). Structurally, nicotine belongs to the pyridine/piperidine alkaloid class. Nicotine has been used as a pesticide, but safer chemicals have largely replaced the more toxic nicotine products (e.g., Black Flag 40), although such products have been identified in malicious poisonings (148).

Nicotine has been used as an animal neuromuscular blocking agent, but most zoos have replaced it with safer agents.

TOXIC DOSE

The estimated lethal adult dose of nicotine is 60 mg (three to six cigarettes). The extraction of the nicotine from five to ten cigarettes in hot water and the administration of the fluid as an enema resulted in a moderately severe poisoning (149). Although most cases of cigarette consumption by children result in no to mild symptoms, severe poisoning have been reported after the ingestion of two cigarettes by 9- and 10-month-old infants (150). Flaccidity, bradycardia, and sinoatrial block developed in an infant who reportedly ingested one-half of a cigarette (151). Exposure to transdermal nicotine patches has produced clinical symptoms in children, with an estimated nicotine dose less than or equal to 0.10 mg (0.01 mg/kg body weight) (152).

PHARMACOKINETICS

Nicotine is well absorbed from the skin, lungs, and GI tract, and poisonings have been documented from all three routes of exposure. Peak nicotine levels in smokers appear approximately 10 minutes after inhalation (153). Nicotine appears to be poorly absorbed in the acid pH of the stomach, and in fact, some nicotine excretion occurs into the stomach (154). However, clinical ingestion of liquid nicotine pesticides (40% nicotine) has resulted in death within 5 to 10 minutes (155,156), and nicotine toxicity is characterized by a rapid onset of action (30 to 60 minutes). Dermal absorption of a 95% nicotine solution resulted in coma and respiratory failure. The bioavailability of nicotine in ingested cigarettes has not been studied.

Intravenously administered nicotine in doses commonly found in cigarettes has a volume of distribution of 1.7 times body weight (157). The terminal elimination half-life is 86 to 110 minutes. Approximately 80% to 90% of administered nicotine is metabolized by the liver into inactive compounds, such as cotinine and nicotine-1'-*N*-oxide, which are then excreted by the kidney. At least in administered doses corresponding to cigarette smoking, the amount excreted unchanged by the kidney varies with urinary pH (23% in acid urine, 2% in alkaline urine) (157).

PATHOPHYSIOLOGY

Initially, nicotine stimulates the sympathetic and parasympathetic ganglia via a direct acetylcholinergic-like action on the ganglion. This stimulatory phase may be brief and is followed by prolonged ganglionic blockade resulting from persistent depolarization. Similar excitatory-inhibitory phases occur in the cardiovascular system and CNS and at the neuromuscular junction.

PREGNANCY AND LACTATION

In experimental piglets, consumption of *N. glauca* produces congenital defects, including cleft palate and limb defects. The principal alkaloid of the common tobacco plant, nicotine, apparently is not the teratogenic agent. Anabasine is a more likely candidate because of its structural similarity to other known piperidine teratogens (e.g., coniine and γ-coniceine) (158).

CLINICAL PRESENTATION

The onset of symptoms usually is rapid (15 to 30 minutes) after acute liquid ingestion, beginning with GI distress (vomiting, nausea, salivation, abdominal pain, diarrhea). Symptoms in mild poisonings resolve in several hours; in severe poisoning, 24 hours may be required. Nicotine gum and transdermal patches may have a delayed onset and prolonged effects.

Neurologic effects include headache, diaphoresis, ataxia, lightheadedness, weakness, confusion, and, in severe poisoning, convulsions and coma. Miosis, lacrimation, bronchorrhea, loss of deep tendon reflexes, fasciculations, and paralysis may be seen. Paralysis of respiratory muscles may occur and necessitate intubation (159). Transient hypertension and tachycardia may be followed by hypotension, bradycardia, and cardiovascular collapse.

Tree tobacco leaves (*N. glauca*) can produce nicotine-like poisoning, with initial hypertension and coma followed by neuromuscular blockade and respiratory failure requiring intubation for 24 hours (160). Symptoms, however, were delayed (1.5 hours to onset of symptoms), perhaps because of slower absorption of anabasine. Postmortem examination in a case associated with *N. glauca* ingestion revealed only pulmonary edema and aspiration pneumonia. Anabasine was found in similar concentrations within the liver, lung, brain, kidney, and myocardium (10 to 15 µg/ml). Urine and gastric contents contained the greatest anabasine concentrations (161).

Green tobacco sickness is an occupational disease associated with picking green tobacco in a moist environment. Characteristic symptoms include headache, pallor, nausea, vomiting, weakness, lightheadedness, and abdominal pain. The disease is self-limited and resolves by the following day. Cigarette smokers rarely display symptoms of green tobacco sickness, suggesting that a tolerance to nicotine may be developed through chronic smoking (162).

DIAGNOSTIC TESTS

Comprehensive urine toxicology screens are able to detect nicotine and its metabolite cotinine but are not commonly reported unless specifically requested. Serum levels are also available but have little use in acute management. Leukocytosis and glycosuria may be seen, but most laboratory values are normal. Analytic HPLC methods for detecting anabasine have been developed (163).

TREATMENT

Charcoal and lavage are preferable to syrup of ipecac because of rapid onset of nicotine effects. When to administer decontamination measures to children who sample cigarettes remains an unresolved question. Most children only taste the tobacco and develop no symptoms. Ingestion of more than one-half to one cigarette may lead to symptoms, and consumption of more than two cigarettes may cause serious effects (150). Hence, decontamination measures are reasonable for those children who eat more than one cigarette and who are not spontaneously vomiting. Multiple-dose charcoal and whole bowel irrigation can be considered for ingestions of gum or transdermal patches. All skin contaminated with nicotine solutions or patches should be thoroughly washed with a nonalkaline soap and cool water. Acidification of the urine is not recommended.

Respiratory failure represents the greatest risk to life, so an initial evaluation must be done to ensure adequate ventilation. Patients with altered sensorium should receive cardiac monitoring, oxygen, and arterial blood gases in addition to the usual doses of glucose and naloxone. The initial hypertension and tachycardia should not be aggressively treated unless they represent a definite risk because bradycardia and hypotension often follow. Patients should be observed for at least 4 to 6 hours to rule out delayed toxicity or up to 12 to 24 hours for ingestion of gum tablets or transdermal patches. Atropine may improve bradycardia and hypotension but does not reverse neuromuscular weakness. Mecamylamine, a specific antagonist of nicotinic effects, has limited usefulness, as it is only available in an oral dosage form.

Pokeweed (*Phytolacca americana*)

Pokeweed (*Phytolacca americana*) is a large, shrub-like perennial herb that regrows from a long, fleshy taproot each spring. Common names include pokeberry, poke, inkberry, pigeonberry, American cancer, scoke, and garget. Characteristic features include purple-

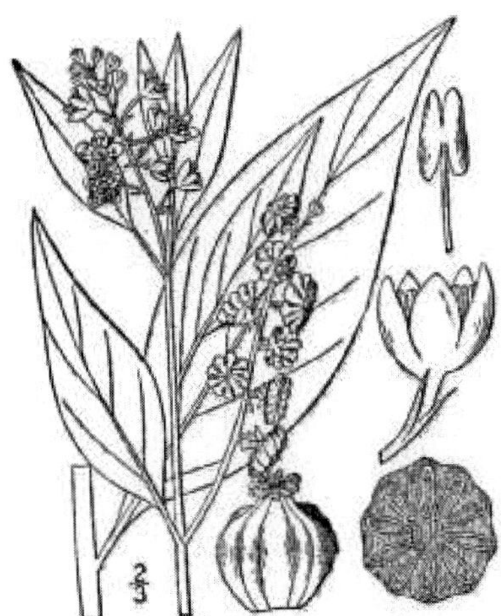

Figure 13. Pokeweed. (From USDA-NRCS PLANTS database/Britton NL, Brown A. *Illustrated flora of the northern states and Canada. Vol. 2.* 1913:26, with permission.)

green leaves with smooth margins and sharp tips; round clusters of black berries appear in late summer (Fig. 13). Pokeweed is a native weed of the eastern United States and grows abundantly in rich, moist areas in open fields and roadsides. Occasionally, it grows on the West Coast. The Indians used it for a purgative and for relief from rheumatism. Folk remedies include use as a salve and bronchodilator. Poke salad is a regional delicacy of the rural southern United States. Young, tender leaves are collected in the spring; these leaves are boiled twice, the washing water is discarded, and the leaves are rinsed carefully before ingestion.

Controversy continues over whether any part of the plant is edible. There is no question that toxicity varies among susceptible individuals, parts of the plant, and time of year. The root is the most toxic plant part. Hemorrhagic gastritis and hypotension in a 43-year-old woman who ingested a pokeroot herbal tea have been observed (164). In order of decreasing toxicity are the leaves, the stems, and the berries. Green berries are more toxic than mature ones, whereas young leaves may be less toxic than older ones. Double washing of pokeweed leaves apparently does not guarantee edibility. Of 46 campers who ate "properly prepared" pokeweed on a New Jersey nature expedition, 20 developed gastroenteritis (165).

PATHOPHYSIOLOGY

The plant contains a powerful GI irritant, phytolaccine, which causes symptoms ranging from a burning sensation of the alimentary tract to severe hemorrhagic gastritis. As the plant matures, this toxin increases in concentration. Five nonspecific mitogens have been isolated by salt extraction (166). These mitogens have hemagglutinating, as well as mitotic, activity, and they vary in concentration throughout the growing season. In four of five children exposed to pokeweed, a significant *in vivo* increase in the number of both immature and mature plasma cells has been noted (167). Noncardioactive steroids and triterpenoid glycosides (termed *saponins*) also are present in significant quantities. Their exact role in pokeweed toxicity is not known. Although not readily absorbed through the uninjured GI tract, the presence of the phytolaccine enhances their absorption. Saponins may potentiate GI toxicity and, when administered parenterally, produce vasodilation (168).

CLINICAL PRESENTATION

Early GI symptoms predominate in pokeweed poisoning, and severity depends on the type of ingestion. Symptoms in an outbreak of poke salad poisoning included nausea (86%), stomach cramps (86%), vomiting (81%), headache (52%), dizziness (48%), burning of mouth or stomach (38%), and diarrhea (29%). The mean onset of illness was 3 hours (range, 30 minutes to 5.5 hours) and the duration was 1 to 48 hours (165). Poisoning from poke salad tea and poke root tea is more severe and immediate (15 to 30 minutes). Symptoms include lethargy, weakness, respiratory depression, convulsions, paresthesias, syncope, blurred vision, vertigo, sweating, salivation, and urgency. Peripheral and central cholinergic symptoms have been suggested as a prominent part of severe intoxication (169).

Death has been reported in the literature from a large ingestion of poke berries. Death of a 5-year-old girl who crushed a large number of berries and drank the resulting juice has been reported (170); however, a pokeberry pancake breakfast for a group of boy scouts resulted only in a few cases of mild diarrhea (171). Ingestion of raw pokeweed leaves produced a Mobitz type I heart block associated with vomiting that resolved with administration of promethazine (172).

TREATMENT

The efficacy of gastric emptying or activated charcoal in pokeweed ingestion has not been studied. Therapy should be directed toward maintaining fluid and electrolyte balance. Serious intoxications involve ingestion of pokeweed teas and usually result in significant GI symptoms within 1 hour. These patients should be hospitalized and monitored for secondary hypotension and electrolyte imbalance. Symptoms rarely last more than 36 hours, and there have been no reports of long-term sequelae. There are no antidotes to pokeweed toxins. Because of the prominence of cholinergic symptoms, atropine has been considered beneficial by some, but there has been no documentation of its usefulness.

Jimsonweed (*Datura stramonium*)

Datura species (*Datura stramonium*, *Datura sanguinea*, *Datura aurea*), commonly referred to as *jimsonweed*, grow as a weed throughout the United States, particularly in rich, disturbed soils such as barnyards. Otherwise known as *thorn apple*, *stinkweed*, *Jamestown weed*, *datura*, *devil's apple*, *devil's trumpet*, *loco seed*, *apple of Peru*, *melpitte*, or *green dragon*, this common annual weed grows 3 to 6 ft high and emits a rank odor. It has a simple, large, white taproot and a strong, dichotomous stem. The leaves are large, waxy, and dark green with pointed margins and scalloped borders. Attractive, white tubular flowers bloom in late spring and grow 3 to 4 in. long. Later, a 2-in.-long green burr-like fruit appears, which ripens in early fall (Fig. 14). The dried pod may contain up to five hundred 2- to 3-mm kidney-shaped seeds.

There are more than a dozen species of this naturalized Asian plant (168), with *D. stramonium* being most common in the eastern United States. Its toxic, mind-altering properties have been known since ancient times; references have been noted in Homer's *Odyssey* and Shakespeare's *Romeo and Juliet* and *Anthony and Cleopatra* (173). The "cursed hebenon" of Shakespeare's *Hamlet* probably was the anticholinergic poison henbane. Historical accounts in the United States date back to 1676 when British soldiers sent to Jamestown to put down the Bacon rebellion mistakenly ate *Datura*, "the effect of which was a very pleasant comedy, for they turned natural fools upon it for several days" (174). The effects reportedly lasted 11 days, much longer than expected for a single mistaken ingestion. It has been proposed that aboriginal rock paintings of the California Chumash Indians were produced by shamans under the influence of hallucinogens because the polychrome paintings show designs similar to those induced by *Datura* species (jimsonweed) (175).

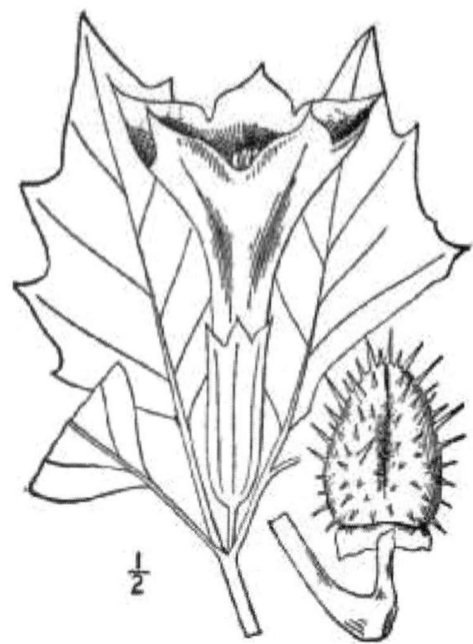

Figure 14. Jimsonweed (*Datura stramonium*). (From USDA-NRCS PLANTS database/Britton NL, Brown A. *Illustrated flora of the northern states and Canada. Vol. 3.* 1913:169, with permission.)

A case of *Datura* poisoning in a 3-year-old child occurred more than 200 years ago (176). Over-the-counter asthma preparations (e.g., Asthmador, Barter's Powder, Kinsman's Asthmatic Powder, Green Mountain Asthmatic Compound, Haywood's Powder) have been marketed for years and abused by the teenage population. The most common intoxication now involves teenagers seeking the mind-altering properties of the seeds, which appear in the autumn (hence the name "autumnal high") (177). Based on calls to a regional poison control center, the typical patient is 17 years of age (range, 11 to 28 years) and ingests seeds and perhaps other substances to experience their hallucinogenic effects (178). European species include *D. sanguinea*, *Brugmansia arborea*, and *D. aurea* and cause anticholinergic symptoms similar to those produced by *D. stramonium* (179).

DESCRIPTION AND TOXICITY

The toxins in *Datura* species are tropane belladonna alkaloids (atropine, hyoscyamine, scopolamine), which possess strong anticholinergic properties (180). Mass spectrometric analysis in a fatal case of *Datura* tea intoxication revealed that hyoscyamine and scopolamine were the chief biochemical constituents (181). The exact concentration of specific alkaloids varies among species as well as with cultivation, environmental, and storage factors. Such alkaloids are easily absorbed from mucous membranes, skin, and intestinal tract. Hyoscyamine and scopolamine are metabolized in the liver by hydrolysis and excreted unchanged in the kidney (177).

Deadly nightshade (*Atropa belladonna*) contains the alkaloid L-hyoscyamine, which represents approximately 75% of total alkaloid content, with most of the remainder being scopolamine. The roots and leaves have the highest total alkaloid content (0.6% and 0.4%, respectively), followed by seeds and berries. Stems have an approximate total alkaloid concentration of 0.05% by weight.

Henbane (*Hyoscyamus niger*) contains tropane alkaloids in all parts, with the leaves containing from 0.05% to 0.15% of the total alkaloid content. Like *A. belladonna*, most of the alkaloids are L-hyoscyamine, with the rest primarily scopolamine (L-hyoscine).

Mandrake (*Mandragora officinarum*) contains L-hyoscyamine and scopolamine in all plant parts as well as small amounts of the unidentified alkaloid mandragorine.

TOXIC DOSE

All parts of the *Datura* plant are poisonous. Toxic effects have been reported after ingestion of teas brewed from plant parts (181), ingestion of leaves and flowers (173,179,182), and smoking of stramonium cigarettes (183). Seed ingestion is the most common route of toxicity. In case studies, the history of ingestion has not been reliably predicted. Based on calculations of hyoscyamine content, 50 to 100 *Datura* seeds contain the equivalent of 3 to 6 mg of atropine, which causes severe intoxication on ingestion (174). Atropine is a racemic mixture of hyoscyamine (the L-isomer is physiologically active). Hall analyzed *Brugmansia suaveolens* (formerly *Datura suaveolens*; angel's trumpet) flowers and concluded that paralysis and convulsions were likely after ingestion of six flowers or the tea from nine flowers (182). Consumption of one-half to two seed pods and alcohol produced symptoms of atropine poisoning that lasted 18 hours to 9 days. Blurred vision was the most persistent symptom (165).

CLINICAL PRESENTATION

Datura ingestion produces the classic presentation of anticholinergic poisoning syndrome described by the phrase "blind as a bat, hot as a hare, dry as a bone, red as a beet, and mad as a hatter (wet hen)." Symptoms typically begin within 2 to 6 hours after ingestion (184), but consumption of *Datura* tea has resulted in symptoms within 5 to 10 minutes (182). Progressive effects from cigarettes prepared from *D. stramonium* were reviewed and indicated that dryness of the mouth is the earliest sign of intoxication followed by pupillary dilation (183).

The classic presentation of a severe intoxication is fever, erythema, dilated pupils, blurred vision, delirium, and hallucination. Based on a review of case studies, Gowdy listed the following frequencies: hallucinations (83%), disorientation (54%), dilated pupils (54%), dry mucous membranes (46%), fever (31%), ataxia (26%), rapid pulse (20%), and amnesia and flush (19%) (183). Hallucinations usually involve simple images in natural colors, in contrast with the brilliant displays seen with lysergic acid diethylamide (LSD). The presence of bowel sounds and diaphoresis suggests an adrenergic (cocaine, amphetamine) poisoning rather than an anticholinergic (jimsonweed) one. Tactile hallucinations are uncommon but may involve crawling insects. Seizures occur but are uncommon (182,185,186). Fatalities usually result from trauma or drowning rather than direct toxic effects (176,183,184).

Symptoms usually resolve in 24 to 48 hours, although pupillary dilation may continue up to 1 week. Patients often are amnesic for any events between ingestion and recovery, and this can last up to 24 hours (187). Fatalities as a result of medical complications of overdose are rare but have been reported in children (188).

Corn picker's pupil is an occupational disease in which jimsonweed in a corn field is pulverized by the harvesting process and causes mydriasis for several days after mechanical harvesting (189,190).

Deadly nightshade (*Solanum dulcamara*) poisoning is uncommon. Ingestion of berries produced typical atropine-like delirium, hallucinations, tachycardia, fever, and amnesia as well as diffuse hypertonia (191). Consumption of ten mandrake fruits (*M. officinarum*) caused confusion, tachycardia, mydriasis, blurred vision, and facial flushing that resolved in 20 hours (192).

DIAGNOSTIC TESTS

Concentrations of tropane alkaloids in body fluids are generally unavailable, although gas chromatography-mass spectrometry methods have been described (193). Elevations of aspartate aminotransferase, lactate dehydrogenase, bilirubin levels, and prothrombin time have been reported (185); however, no liver biopsy has been reported, and an autopsy case showed only subcapsular petechiae on the liver (181). Electroencephalographic changes include prominent lambda activity, increased slow wave activity, and a bizarre high voltage pattern.

TREATMENT

Most patients respond well to supportive and protective measures. The patient should be placed in a calm, reassuring environment with a familiar person. Pharmacologic intervention should be limited to those patients who do not respond to a calm environment and present a danger to themselves or others.

Gastric emptying and activated charcoal may be useful in patients seen within several hours postingestion, although this has not been studied. Generally, the tropane alkaloids are well absorbed in solution. Their anticholinergic properties may delay absorption of vegetable matter and seeds (171,194).

The antidote for anticholinergic poisoning is physostigmine (Chapter 67). The initial adult dose is 1 to 2 mg (0.01 to 0.03 mg/kg) intramuscularly or intravenously over 2 to 5 minutes. Improvement usually occurs within 15 to 20 minutes. A second dose may be repeated in 20 to 30 minutes. Repeated doses should be given only if symptoms reappear. Watch for signs of cholinergic excess (bradycardia, heart block, excessive secretions). Because symptoms usually abate in 24 hours, often only three to four doses are needed (185).

Diazepam has been used for agitation, but care must be exercised not to heavily sedate these patients. Because of their anticholinergic properties, phenobarbital, phenothiazines, and haloperidol should not be used. Vital signs should be monitored every 15 to 20 minutes until improvement is noted. Hypertension usually is transient and requires no therapy. Hyperthermia may be treated with a cooling blanket or a sponge bath. Catheterization may be necessary for urinary retention. Baseline liver function tests, creatine kinase, prothrombin time, and urinalysis for myoglobin should be performed on those patients with increased muscle tone, seizures, or hyperthermia. Patients requiring physostigmine should be admitted for at least 24 hours of observation. Patients who exhibit CNS symptoms (e.g., disorientation, hallucinations, or delusions) should be observed until those symptoms resolve. Patients with mild symptoms may be discharged from the emergency department after 4 to 6 hours of observation if symptoms are improving.

Poison Hemlock (*Conium maculatum*)

Poison hemlock (*Conium maculatum*) grows as a luxuriant weed along roadsides, ditches, and open areas throughout the United States, especially in the north. Also known as *poison fool's parsley, California fern*, and *Nebraska fern*, poison hemlock is a biennial weed that has a large taproot and lacy, fern-like leaves that reach 8 to 10 ft in height (Fig. 15). The stems are hollow and hairless. The leaves are multiply pinnate and deeply divided into minute leaflets. The flowers are white and clustered into multiple umbrella-shaped groups.

Alkaloid content varies significantly among species, plant parts, and geographic locations. As the plant matures, alkaloid concentration increases in the stems, leaves, and fruit, but the roots consistently contain the largest alkaloid concentrations.

Poisonings usually result from mistaken identification as a natural food. The plant may be mistaken for wild carrots, the leaves for parsley, and the seeds for anise; however, the bitter taste of the plant usually discourages consumption. This plant was used by the early Greeks as a means of suicide (168).

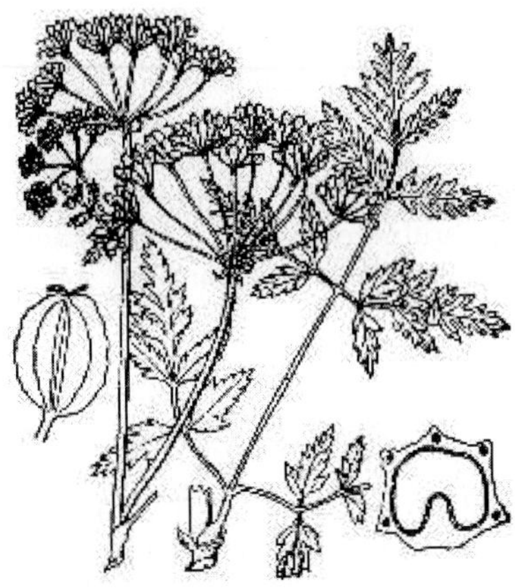

Figure 15. *Conium maculatum.* (From USDA-NRCS PLANTS database/Britton NL, Brown A. *Illustrated flora of the northern states and Canada. Vol. 2.* 1913:653, with permission.)

Socrates probably died from *Conium* poisoning, as was the custom in Greek executions, although the characteristic ascending paralysis and terminal asphyxia of *Conium* poisoning are not well described in historical accounts (195).

PATHOPHYSIOLOGY

Conium toxicity results from piperidine alkaloids, which are structurally related to the pyridine nicotine (Fig. 1). These propylpiperidine alkaloids are among the simplest alkaloids and appear in other plant families (Crassulaceae, Punicaceae). Five alkaloids have been isolated from *Conium* (196). Symptoms appear similar to those of nicotine poisoning.

The mechanism of action of these alkaloids is twofold. The most serious effect occurs at the neuromuscular junction where they act as nondepolarizing blockers similar to curare. Death, when it occurs, is usually caused by respiratory failure. As a result of their action at the autonomic ganglia, the toxins produce biphasic nicotinic effects, including salivation, mydriasis, and tachycardia followed by bradycardia.

PREGNANCY AND LACTATION

In experiments, feeding livestock fresh green *Conium* plants results in congenital joint and spinal abnormalities similar to those of crooked calf disease seen after lupine ingestion (196,197).

CLINICAL PRESENTATION

Toxicity to animals has been widely reported in the veterinary literature and includes ataxia, salivation, convulsions, and coma. Based on their structural similarity to nicotine and on data in animals, these alkaloids produce initial stimulation, tremor, ataxia, mydriasis, nausea, vomiting, and sore throat followed by cardiorespiratory depression, bradycardia, paralysis, coma, and ascending paralysis. Death results from respiratory failure. The usual absence of convulsions distinguishes coniine toxicity from the more deadly *Cicuta* (water hemlock) poisoning. Recent case studies describe nonneurologic features in hemlock poisoning, including rhabdomyolysis and acute tubular necrosis (198).

TREATMENT

Because no antidote exists for coniine poisoning, treatment is supportive. Respiratory support and gastric decontamination should be instituted immediately. Anticonvulsants should be administered as needed. Alkaline diuresis may be useful in preventing renal failure from rhabdomyolysis and myoglobinuria.

Buckthorn (*Karwinskia humboldtiana*)

Buckthorn (*Karwinskia humboldtiana*), also known as *coyotillo, wild cherry*, or *tullidora*, is a woody shrub or small tree with opposite stalked leaves 1 to 3 in. long. A brownish-black berry matures from clusters of greenish flowers and contains a pit. This poisonous shrub grows along canyons and gullies of the southwestern United States and northern and central Mexico. The common buckthorn (*Rhamnus* species) is an ornamental plant used as a hedge and is now naturalized in the eastern United States. A small deciduous tree (also known as *Rhamnus purshiana*) is a native species of the Pacific Northwest.

PATHOPHYSIOLOGY

The seeds of *K. humboldtiana* contain an unidentified neurotoxin that produces an ascending paralysis similar to Guillain-Barré syndrome (Chapter 8). Injection of the toxin into experimental animals produces a segmental demyelination of peripheral nerves, probably as a result of disruption of Schwann's cell metabolism (199). Common buckthorn (*Rhamnus*) contains glycosides that are strong cathartics.

CLINICAL PRESENTATION

Chronic consumption of *K. humboldtiana* caused a progressive, symmetric polyneuropathy that resulted in flaccid quadriplegia and respiratory insufficiency complicated by pneumonia (200). Sural nerve biopsy revealed segmental demyelination. A slow but progressive recovery resulted in restoration of function with persistent reflex deficits. Exposure to *Rhamnus* causes primarily diarrhea but no serious symptoms.

DIAGNOSTIC TESTS

Although assays for buckthorn toxicity are not commonly available, the presence of *K. humboldtiana* toxins in blood has been determined with thin-layer chromatography in children presenting with acute ascending paralysis (201).

TREATMENT

Supportive care is the mainstay of treatment. Decontamination is not necessary.

Snowberry (*Symphoricarpos albus* or *Symphoricarpos racemosus*)

Snowberry (*Symphoricarpos albus* or *Symphoricarpos racemosus*) is a low-growing deciduous shrub that grows in woodlands and open areas of the northern United States and Canada. In Europe, the species is cultivated as an ornamental hedge. Flowers are pink and bell shaped, growing in small clusters along the main stem (Fig. 16). The white, waxy berries mature in late summer and fall and often remain on the shrub after the leaves drop.

The alkaloid chelidonine has been isolated from *S. albus* but does not account for its toxicity (202). Additional compounds reported to be present include aesculin, sitosterol saponins, tannins, terpenes, triglycerides, sugars, coumarins, flavonoids, and secologanin, but which, if any, cause adverse effects remains unknown.

CLINICAL PRESENTATION

Most children who ingest snowberries remain asymptomatic. Vomiting, difficulty in urination, and induction of a semicomatose state have been the only reported complications (203,204). Heavy consumption of snowberries before 1900 was reported to cause GI distress, delirium, and obtundation but no fatalities (205).

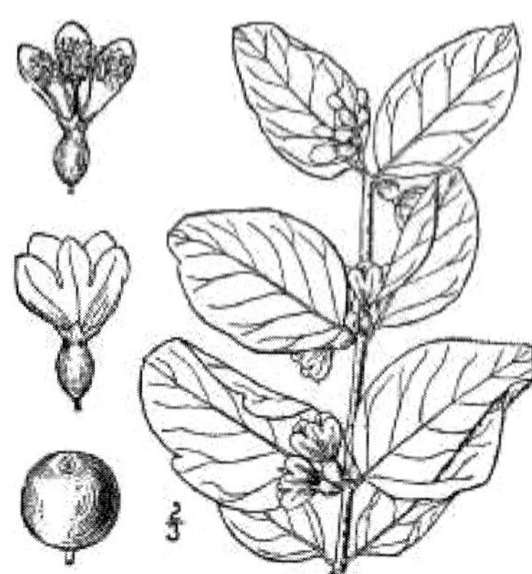

Figure 16. Common snowberry (*Symphoricarpos albus*). (From USDA-NRCS PLANTS database/Britton NL, Brown A. *Illustrated flora of the northern states and Canada. Vol. 3.* 1913:276, with permission.)

DIAGNOSTIC TESTS

Specific diagnostic tests for snowberry toxicity are not available, as the compounds responsible for toxicity have yet to be elucidated.

TREATMENT

Treatment is supportive. Decontamination probably is not necessary unless more than several berries have been ingested.

Buckeye (*Aesculus* Species)

Buckeye (*Aesculus* species) refers to a genus of deciduous trees and shrubs that contain palmately divided leaflets (toothed margins) on long stalks. Yellow, red, and white flowers produce a characteristic three-compartment fruit surrounded by a leathery husk, which encloses brown, glossy seeds. Commonly known as *horse chestnut*, *Aesculus hippocastanum* is widely planted as an ornamental shade tree (Fig. 17). Other species include *Aesculus californica* (California buckeye), *Aesculus sylvatica* (painted buckeye), *Aesculus parviflora* (bottlebrush buckeye), *Aesculus pavia* (red buckeye), *A. glabra* (Ohio buckeye), and *Aesculus octandra* (yellow buckeye). These plants range from the central and eastern temperate zone of North America westward to the Gulf Coast and California and northward to southern Ontario, southwestern Quebec, and Newfoundland.

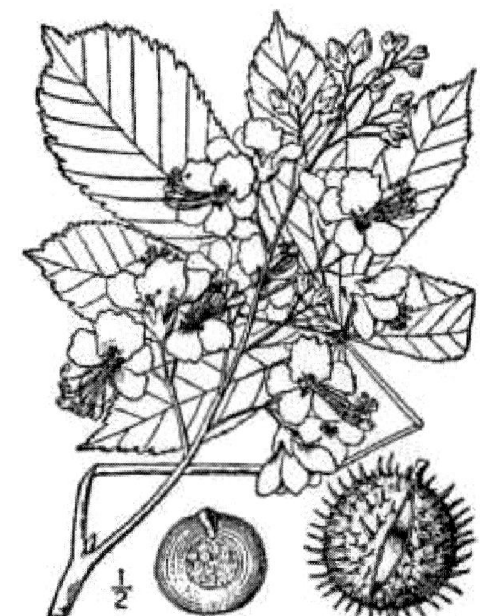

Figure 17. Horse chestnut (*Aesculus hippocastanum*). (From USDA-NRCS PLANTS database/Britton NL, Brown A. *Illustrated flora of the northern states and Canada. Vol. 2.* 1913:498, with permission.)

CLINICAL PRESENTATION

This genus contains a mixture of saponins known collectively as *aesculin*, which is capable of causing weakness, ataxia, dilated pupils, nausea, vomiting, and obtundation. The seeds and twigs contain the toxic principle. Most ingestions of horse chestnut by children result in no symptoms. GI distress is the most common symptom complex.

TREATMENT

Treatment is supportive and is focused mainly on fluid and electrolyte replacement and general therapy for gastroenteritis.

Dog's Mercury (*Mercurialis perennis*)

Dog's mercury (*Mercurialis perennis*) is a common woodland plant found in Britain with serrate, opposite leaves and clusters of flowers on a central stalk. The American species is *Mercurialis annual*, which is a common weed found in uncultivated areas. The active principle is mercurialine, a volatile basic oil.

CLINICAL PRESENTATION

Ingestion of a tea made from *M. perennis* produced severe gastroenteritis and trace hemoglobinuria without liver or renal dysfunction (206). Pronounced anisocytosis was present in blood smears, but no changes in hemoglobin concentration occurred. Hemolysis, hepatic centrilobular necrosis, and GI distress do occur in animal poisoning but have not been reported in human poisoning to date.

TREATMENT

Treatment is supportive.

Baneberry (*Actaea rubra*)

Baneberry (*Actaea rubra*) is a tall perennial herb with thick roots and large, compound leaves comprised of toothed edges that is found from Alaska to California, east through Canada and the United States to the Atlantic, and south through the Rockies to New Mexico. Common names include red baneberry, snakeberry, white cohosh, doll's eyes, and coral berry.

The rootstock, sap, and berries contain glycosides or essential oils that produce a direct irritant and vesicant effect on skin and mucous membranes. Hallucinogenic effects have also been reported (207). The toxic constituent of baneberry has yet to be isolated but is reputedly protoanemonin.

CLINICAL PRESENTATION

Ingestion of the berries produces gastroenteritis within one-half hour of a six-berry ingestion. Confusion, headache, and distorted visual perception occurred, followed in 1 hour by tachycardia, abdominal pain, lethargy, dry mouth, and eructations. Symptoms resolved by 3 hours postingestion (207).

TREATMENT

Treatment is generally supportive. GI decontamination measures are reasonable if undertaken within the first several hours after ingestion.

White Snakeroot (*Eupatorium rugosum*)

White snakeroot (*E. rugosum*) is a perennial plant found growing in wooded and shaded areas of the southern, midwestern, and eastern United States. It matures in late summer and early autumn and has large ovate toothed leaves on long stalks with clusters of white composite flowers (Fig. 18). Common names include fall poison, richweed, Indian sanicle, white sanicle, deerwort, boneset, poolwort, squaw weed, white top, stevia, and snow thoroughwort.

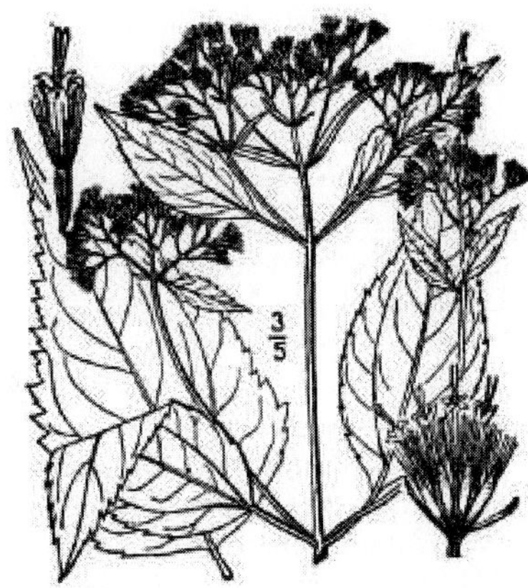

Figure 18. White snakeroot (*Ageratine altissima* L). (From USDA-NRCS PLANTS database/Britton NL, Brown A. *Illustrated flora of the northern states and Canada. Vol. 3.* 1913:361, with permission.)

The entire plant contains the higher alcohol tremetol and certain glycosides, which accumulate in the milk of cows grazing on this plant (208). The afebrile epidemic illness known as *milk sickness* results from ingestion of contaminated milk. In colonial times and particularly during the first half of the nineteenth century, milk sickness caused numerous deaths. The rayless goldenrod (*Haplopappus heterophyllus*) in the Southwest also contains tremetol and causes milk sickness (209).

TOXICOKINETICS AND TOXICODYNAMICS

Three distinct higher alcohols, tremetone, dehydrotremetone, and hydroxytremetone, are found in white snakeroot (210). Evidence exists that microsomal enzyme activation is necessary for these compounds to become toxic (211).

PREGNANCY AND LACTATION

Evidence of toxin excretion by lactating livestock exists, but no human cases have been reported.

CLINICAL PRESENTATION

Milk sickness is an insidious disease causing weakness, nausea, vomiting, tremors, headache, constipation, dizziness, delirium, and in serious cases, coma, convulsions, and death. Recovery is often prolonged, and relapse may occur. Autopsy has revealed fatty degeneration of the liver and kidney. Modern milk-processing procedures have eliminated milk sickness, but consumption of unprocessed milk represents a potential danger.

Anorexia, abdominal pain, and repeated vomiting have been described. Muscular tremors are common. In terminal cases, delirium and coma preceded death (168). A characteristic acetone odor on the breath may appear as the disease progresses.

TREATMENT

Management of toxicity is generally supportive. Levels for tremetol are not routinely available. Acute toxic effects are unlikely; hence, decontamination measures are not necessary. There is no antidote for snakeroot toxicity.

ORNAMENTAL SHRUBS AND TREES

Rhododendron (*Rhododendron ponticum*)

Grayanotoxins are known to occur in the honey produced from the nectar of *Rhododendron ponticum* growing on the mountains of the eastern Black Sea region of Turkey and in Japan, Nepal, Brazil, and some parts of North America and Europe. Turkish honey from the Black Sea coast occasionally contains concentrations of acetylandromedol (andromedotoxin) high enough to cause poisoning. The substance is obtained by bees from some species of *Rhododendron* that they then incorporate into their honey. Typical of the poisoning are GI symptoms and marked, life-threatening bradycardia and hypotension (212).

CLINICAL PRESENTATION

A 33-year-old woman ingested tea made from fresh rhododendron leaves and complained of weakness, dizziness, blurred vision, nausea, and vomiting. She was hypotensive and bradycardic and experienced a transient episode of complete atrioventricular (AV) dissociation. Her hypotension improved with IV fluids alone. She was asymptomatic the following day when she was discharged (213).

Symptoms after honey ingestion (2 to 5 teaspoonfuls) by 23 people in Turkey began within 30 minutes and up to 2 hours after ingestion and included nausea, vomiting, sweating, dizziness, hypotension, bradycardia, and impairment of consciousness. Changes in the ECG include bradycardia, junctional rhythm, complete AV blocks, and Wolff-Parkinson-White syndrome with sinus bradycardia. ECGs were normal in 24 hours. Patients regained consciousness or felt better in 30 minutes to 6 hours and recovered completely in 1 or 2 days. Bradycardia responded to atropine (214).

Common Oleander (*Nerium oleander*)

Common oleander, or *N. oleander,* belongs to the Apocynaceae (dogbane) family. *N. oleander* is an evergreen shrub that grows to be 20 to 25 ft high. The leaves are long and narrow, with a pointed tip. The flowers are funnel shaped and may be yellow, rose-pink, red-purple, or white in color. The plant is native to Japan and the Mediterranean. It can be found in Hawaii and in the southern part of the United States.

N. oleander contains numerous cardiac glycosides. The Greeks recorded that oleander was poisonous to "all four-footed beasts" (215). Oleander has been used as rodenticides, insecticides, and also as a remedy for indigestion, malaria, and venereal diseases. There are also reports of its use as an abortifacient and for treatment of mental disorders. Aqueous extracts of the plant are used to treat cancer in Turkey.

More than 400 naturally occurring cardiac glycosides have been detected in the plant kingdom. Table 7 lists the natural sources of concentrated cardiac glycosides (168). *N. oleander* contains oleandrin (Fig. 1), oleandroside, and neriin. All parts of the plant (whether green or dry) contain cardiac glycosides (168). The total cardiac glycoside content is believed to be the highest during April and May when the plant is flowering (216). The toxicity from ingestion varies depending on the amount and part of plant that is ingested. Toxicity is also dependent on the season, humidity, and age of plant. Serious toxicity from children tasting whole plant material is rare. Elevated digitoxin serum levels confirm toxicity but cannot guide management because of cross-reactivity.

TOXIC DOSE

Pharmacokinetic calculations in a 40-kg adult who ingested oleander tea showed that 5 to 15 leaves of oleander were required to achieve lethal levels (217).

PATHOPHYSIOLOGY

Cardiac glycosides inhibit the Na^+,K^+–adenosine triphosphate (Na^+,K^+-ATP) pump. This causes a decrease in intracellular potassium and interferes with electrical conduction by reducing the normal resting membrane potential, decreases the myocardial cell's ability to function as a pacemaker, and may result in a complete loss of normal myocardial electrical function. In severe poisoning, asystole may ensue, and the myocardium may lose its responsiveness to electrical pacing. The toxicity of cardiac glycosides resembles digitalis poisoning.

TABLE 7. Major sources of naturally occurring cardiac glycosides

Family	Scientific name	Common name
Dogbane family (Apocynaceae)	*Carissa spectabilis*	Wintersweet
	Carissa acokanthera	Bushman's poison
	Cerbera manghas	Sea mango
	Plumeria rubra	Frangipani
	Nerium oleander	Common oleander
	Thevetia peruviana	Yellow oleander
Lily family (Liliaceae)	*Convallaria majalis*	Lily-of-the-valley
	Urginea maritima	Sea onion
Figwort family (Scrophulariaceae)	*Digitalis purpurea*	Foxglove
Milkweed family (Asclepiadaceae)	*Asclepias fruticosa*	Balloon cotton
	Asclepias curassavica	Redheaded cotton bush
	Calotropis procera	King's crown
	Cryptostegia grandiflora	Rubber vine
Bufonidae[a]	*Bufo marinus*	Cane toad

[a]Radford DF, Giles AD, Hinds JA, et al. Naturally occurring cardiac glycosides. *Med J Aust* 1986;144:540–544.

From Kingsbury JM. *Poisonous plants of the United States and Canada.* Englewood, NJ: Prentice-Hall Inc., 1964, with permission.

CLINICAL PRESENTATION

The most common symptoms that are observed with cardiac glycoside plant toxicity are nausea, vomiting, bradycardia with AV block, hypotension, lethargy, and dizziness. Seizures, hypertension, coma, and electrolyte imbalances have been reported with ingestions but are rare.

Serious cardiotoxicity usually results in ventricular ectopy, conduction delays, and cardiovascular collapse. Conduction delays can persist 3 to 6 days (218,219). A 45-year-old woman developed sinus bradycardia after ingesting oleander leaves, prazepam, and flunitrazepam in a suicide attempt. The patient recovered after decontamination (220).

A 42-year-old woman developed sinus bradycardia and an AV block after an oleander smoke inhalation. Her serum digoxin level was 0.3 ng/ml 48 hours after the exposure (221). A 66-year-old woman ingested unprocessed *N. oleander.* Initially, the patient developed a heart rate of 20 bpm with periods of asystole that lasted up to 4 seconds. The patient then developed paroxysmal atrial tachycardia with a heart rate of 140 bpm (222).

A 30-year-old woman died after ingesting a tea made from oleander leaves. The patient initially developed nausea and vomiting and complained of numbness to her tongue. The patient developed bradycardia (30 bpm), tachypnea, and hypotension approximately 10 hours after ingestion. The patient died despite aggressive resuscitation. The postmortem digoxin level was 6.4 ng/ml (223).

A woman ingested seven *N. oleander* seeds and had a serum digoxin level of 5.69 nmol/L 8 hours later. The patient had nausea, vomiting, and stomach cramps. Her ECG showed a rate of 40 bpm, depressed ST segments, and preterminal inverted T waves. The patient was treated with atropine. The patient was discharged after 5 days, and her ECG still showed ST-segment depression (224).

A 13-month-old child presented with first degree AV block and bradycardia after ingesting oleander. The serum digoxin level was 6.1 nmol/L approximately 21 hours after the initial symptoms. The patient gradually recovered from the ingestion (225).

DIAGNOSTIC TESTS

Antidigoxin antiserum cross reacts with glycosides of digoxigenin that share the aglycone portion of digoxin. Cross-reactivity with the digoxin radioimmunoassay is believed to occur with both foxglove and oleander (226). However, serum digoxin levels may not correlate to clinical toxicity, as many of the plant cardiac glycosides cannot be measured. Patients with a significant ingestion should have cardiac monitoring and serum potassium levels followed closely.

TREATMENT

Serious toxicity from children tasting whole plant material is rare. A child who ingests less than one leaf or flower can be treated with close observation at home. Induction of emesis can be considered. Any child or adult who ingests more than one leaf or flower should be referred for medical treatment. Patients who ingest a significant amount of *N. oleander* should receive charcoal and have an ECG and serum electrolytes obtained. Markers of severe toxicity include hyperkalemia, elevated digoxin levels, conduction blocks, and ventricular ectopy. Patients who exhibit toxicity should be admitted for at least 24 hours. Patients with a significant ingestion should be observed with continuous cardiac monitoring for at least 12 hours. Cardiac monitoring can be discontinued when the patient's rhythm returns to a normal sinus rhythm.

Decontamination is commonly performed using activated charcoal for patients who are awake and able to protect their airway. It is most effective if given within 1 hour of ingestion. A second dose of charcoal can be considered if a patient presents with severe toxicity, a large ingestion, or when digitalis Fab fragments are not available.

The antidote for cardiac glycoside poisoning is digoxin immune Fab (Chapter 49). Digoxin Fab should be used in patients who develop hemodynamically significant dysrhythmias or hyperkalemia. Serum digoxin levels cannot be used to calculate a dose of digoxin Fab for cardiac glycoside toxicity from plants. Empiric treatment with digitalis Fab fragments is suggested for symptomatic patients. Potassium levels greater than 6.5 mEq/L should be treated with digitalis Fab fragments. If Fab is not available, potassium levels should be lowered using the standard measures (Chapter 35).

Cardiac dysrhythmias can be treated with standard doses of atropine for bradycardia (Chapter 42). Lidocaine or phenytoin may be useful for treatment of ventricular dysrhythmias unresponsive to digitalis Fab fragments. The dose of lidocaine is 1.0 to 1.5 mg/kg IV bolus followed by a maintenance drip of 1 to 4 mg/minute in adults. The pediatric dose is 1 mg/kg IV bolus followed by a maintenance drip of 20 to 50 μg/kg/minute. The loading dose of phenytoin is 15 mg/kg (up to 1 g) in both adults and children. Infusion should not exceed 0.5 mg/kg/minute. The maintenance dosage is 2 mg/kg every 12 hours in adults, and 2 mg/kg every 8 hours in children. Phenytoin levels should be measured before administration of the maintenance dose.

Yellow Oleander (*Thevetia peruviana*)

Yellow oleander (*Thevetia peruviana*) belongs to the family Apocynaceae. It is an evergreen tree that can grow to more than 30 ft in height. It has dense branches, and its leaves are long and narrow. Leaves can grow to 6 in. in length and are dark green and glossy. Yellow oleander has bright orange or yellow flowers that are 2 to 3 in. long and form clusters at the ends of the branches. The fruit resembles a small irregular-shaped apple and is approximately 1 in. across (227,228). The plant is native to tropical America and is widespread in the southern United States and Hawaii. Like common oleander, the plant contains cardiac glycosides.

Yellow oleander is used mostly as an ornamental plant. However, various parts of the plant have been used as insecticides, rodenticides, and fish poisons (229–232). The glycosides were used to treat heart failure and atrial fibrillation in the 1930s. Their use was discontinued because of the high GI and cardiac toxicity of the plant (233,234). Toxicity has been documented with accidental exposures, suicide and homicide attempts, and inhalation of smoke from burning oleander.

TOXIC DOSE

One to two fruits are potentially lethal in children (227), and eight to ten seeds are considered to be lethal in adults. A retrospective study of 13 patients who had intentionally ingested yellow oleander seeds revealed that patients who ingested less than two seeds developed few symptoms. Ingestion of more than two seeds caused GI and cardiovascular symptoms. Patients who took less than four seeds or who presented within 4 hours of ingestion could be treated symptomatically and did well with supportive treatment. Markers of poor outcome included the ingestion of more than four seeds or a delay in presentation (235).

TOXICOKINETICS AND TOXICODYNAMICS

Cardiac glycosides include thevetin A and B (cerebroside); α-L-thevetosides; glucosyl- and gentiobiosyl-x-L-thevetosides of digitoxigenin, cannogenin, cannogenol, uzarigenin; x-L-acofrioside, c-nor-D-homo-cardenolide; and peruvoside (Fig. 1) (236–238). The most toxic glycosides in yellow oleander are (in order of decreasing toxicity): peruvoside, ruvoside, thevetin A, nerifolin, cerebrin, and thevetin B (239). Peruvoside and thevetin A and B produce effects similar to digitalis but have a more rapid onset of action (232,240). Digoxin radioimmunoassays may confirm the presence of cardiac glycosides due to cross-reactivity with digoxin (241).

Yellow oleander does not lose its toxicity, even when dried (242). It is well absorbed orally in animals (243). The cardiac glycosides in yellow oleander have a more rapid onset of action than does digitalis (244). The glycosides from oleander undergo extensive enterohepatic cycling (240). The amount of glycoside per plant part is 0.07% in the leaves, 0.045% in the fruit, 4.8% in the seed kernel, and 0.036% in the sap (245).

PATHOPHYSIOLOGY

Cardiac glycosides inhibit the Na^+,K^+-ATP pump. This causes a decrease in intracellular potassium and interferes with electrical conduction by reducing the normal resting membrane potential. This decreases the myocardial cell's ability to function as a pacemaker. Acute poisoning may result in a complete loss of normal myocardial electrical function.

PREGNANCY AND LACTATION

Thevetin, the active glycoside of yellow oleander, may cross the placenta.

CLINICAL PRESENTATION

The most common symptoms that are observed with cardiac glycoside plant toxicity are bradycardia with AV block, hypotension, lethargy, dizziness, and GI upset. Nausea and vomiting usually occur within several hours of the ingestion. The cardiac glycosides in yellow oleander have a quicker onset of action than digoxin. Paresthesias, weakness, hypertonia, and excessive salivation have also been associated with yellow oleander toxicity (246,247). Seizures, hypertension, coma, and electrolyte imbalances have been reported with ingestions but are rare. A study of 300 intentional yellow oleander ingestions showed that 46% of patients developed some type of dysrhythmia, 49% had bradycardia, 39% had ischemic changes on their ECG, and 12% noted palpitations (248).

An 18-month-old child ingested a yellow oleander fruit. The child developed heart block and bradycardia. The child was treated symptomatically and released 4 days later (249). A 3-year-old girl was brought to a physician because of persistent vomiting after playing under a yellow oleander tree earlier that day. The child was diaphoretic, weak, and had a heart block. The child suffered a cardiac arrest and died en route to a hospital (241).

DIAGNOSTIC TESTS

Serum digoxin levels may not correlate with clinical toxicity, as many of the plant cardiac glycosides cannot be measured. Patients with a significant ingestion should have cardiac rhythm and serum potassium levels followed closely. A study of 351 patients showed that most symptomatic patients had conduction defects at the sinus node or the AV node. Patients with an AV block had a mean cardiac glycoside level of 2.88 nmol/L (range, 1.25 to 4.46). The mean for patients with sinus node dysfunction was 2.68 nmol/L (range, 1.82 to 3.84). Patients with both an AV block and sinus node dysfunction had a mean level of 3.10 nmol/L (range, 2.24 to 4.16) (250). Patients with moderate toxicity had PR prolongation, which proceeded to AV dissociation. Patients with severe toxicity died from persistent ventricular fibrillation.

TREATMENT

The treatment of yellow oleander toxicity is similar to that of digoxin toxicity (Chapter 122). The optimal dose of digoxin immune Fab is unknown in symptomatic *Thevetia* ingestions. One study of oleander ingestions examined the effect of digoxin immune Fab on cardiac toxicity. The treatment group consisted of 33 patients with conduction defects or dysrhythmias who received digoxin immune Fab. Fifteen of the 33 patients reverted to a normal sinus rhythm within 2 hours. In comparison, only 2 out of 32 patients in the control group reverted to a normal sinus rhythm (233). Further indications, dose, method of administration, and adverse effects of digoxin Fab are provided in Chapter 49.

Lantana (*Lantana camara*)

Also known as *red or yellow sage, Lantana camara* belongs to the Verbenaceae family. It is a woody shrub plant that is common in topical areas (251). It is considered one of the ten most noxious weeds in the world (252). There are more than 150 different species, varieties, and cultivars (253). The plant produces multicolored flowers, which start in April and May and persist until November. Most varieties of *Lantana* are native to subtropical and tropical America (253).

There have been multiple reports of poisoning in grazing animals that have caused widespread livestock losses in South Africa, Australia, India, Mexico, and the United States. *L. camara* appears to be the most widespread and toxic to animals (254).

TOXIC DOSE

There is no toxic dose established in humans. The amount of lantadenes found in a toxic dose of lantana leaves was estimated to be 3 mg/kg (253). In 17 reported cases of human ingestion, four patients developed symptoms. The ingested amounts were not known (255). The total lantadene concentration of the plant varies from 0.2% in the spring to 1.4% to 1.7% in the late summer and early fall. The flowers, fruits, and shoots have no detectable lantadene in July and August, whereas the plant leaves were found to contain 0.6% by dry weight of lantadene A (256). However, there have been reports of serious toxicity and death when unripe berries are ingested in the spring or fall (255).

There have been reports of poisonings in children who have ingested unripe berries. Ripe berries appear to be nontoxic in children.

PATHOPHYSIOLOGY

The components believed to cause toxicity are lantadenes. Both lantadene A and B have been isolated. There have been conflicting reports of toxicity of these compounds. Studies suggest that purified lantadene A and B are not toxic, whereas reduced lantadene A may be toxic. However, other impurities may be responsible for the hepatotoxicity, as some studies have shown that even reduced lantadene A did not cause hepatotoxicity (252,257). Lantadene B appears to be pharmacologically inactive.

CLINICAL PRESENTATION

Vomiting, respiratory distress, dilated pupils, ataxia, lethargy, coma, diarrhea, depressed deep tendon reflexes, weakness, cyanosis, and death have been described after the ingestion of unripe berries. Onset of symptoms varies between 2.5 to 6.0 hours. No toxicity has been described from ingestion of the leaves of lantana.

A 2.5-year-old girl ate an unknown amount of unripe berries and became lethargic approximately 6 hours later. She developed vomiting, ataxia, unconsciousness and coma with depressed respirations, pinpoint pupils, and cyanosis. No decontamination occurred. The patient was treated with adrenal steroids, epinephrine, oxygen, and general supportive care but died approximately 90 minutes after arriving at the hospital (255).

TREATMENT

Ingestions of unripe berries require oral decontamination. Patients should also be treated if it is unknown if the berry is ripe or not. Patients should be observed for 4 to 6 hours after the ingestion. Ingestion or chewing of leaves does not require any treatment other than observation.

Yew (*Taxus* Species)

The yew (*Taxus brevifolia*) is a native tree from northern California to Alaska and Montana. It has drooping branches and alternate branchlets with needle-like leaves approximately 2 cm long. Hard seeds are surrounded by a fleshy red cup (aril). *Taxus canadensis* is native to the eastern United States (Fig. 19).

PATHOPHYSIOLOGY

The main toxins are the alkaloids taxine A and taxine B. They are found in all parts of the tree except the fleshy red part of the berry. Several taxine alkaloids have been isolated and characterized by HPLC, mass spectroscopy, and nuclear magnetic resonance. Current evidence suggests that their chief action is on cardiac myocytes, resulting in heart failure (258).

CLINICAL PRESENTATION

Ingestion may result in hypotension, bradycardia, depressed myocardial contractility, and conduction delay similar to digitalis poisoning (259). A 5-year-old girl ate an unknown amount of yew leaves and berries and presented 3 hours later with lethargy, hypotension, and complete heart block. A transcutaneous external cardiac pacemaker was successful in increasing her heart rate with subsequent improvement in blood pressure (260).

Fatalities from ingestion of yew leaves have been reported (261). Most unintentional ingestions result in either no symp-

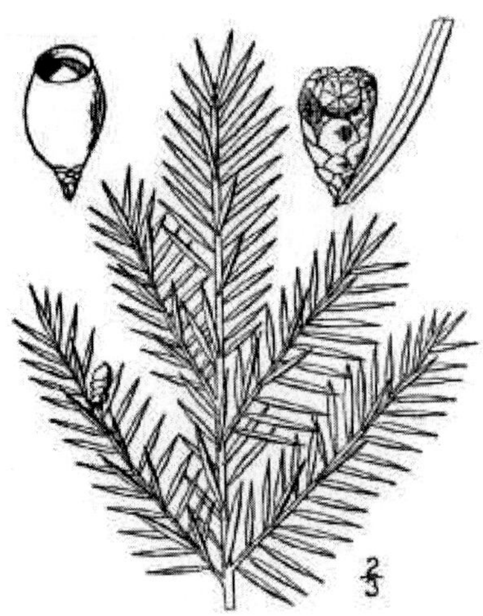

Figure 19. Canada yew (*Taxus canadensis*). (From USDA-NRCS PLANTS database/Britton NL, Brown A. *Illustrated flora of the northern states and Canada. Vol. 1.* 1913:67, with permission.)

toms or mild GI distress (262). Patients usually display symptoms within 3 to 4 hours of exposure.

TREATMENT

Ingestion of a few berries does not require decontamination. Large or intentional ingestions should receive activated charcoal and cardiac monitoring for 4 to 6 hours.

PLANTS CULTIVATED FOR FLOWERS

Aconitum Species and Aconite

Aconitum belongs to the Ranunculaceae (buttercup) family. It is a perennial herb that can reach 1 to 5 ft in height. It has palmate leaves and a tuberous root. The flowers are blue or white and are symmetric with a prominent upper hood. There are more than 170 different species of *Aconitum* in China alone. *Aconitum napellus* can be found in the wild in both North America and Europe. *Aconitum columbianum* is found in the western United States and Canada. The leaves of both of these species resemble delphiniums. *Aconitum lycoctonum* can grow to 6 ft and is native to Europe. *Aconitum* contains diterpene and norditerpene alkaloids, which are potent poisons.

Most poisonings occur when these plants are used in herbal remedies or are mistaken for parsley or the roots of horseradish or celery. *Aconitum ferox* extract has been used in India to make poison arrows (263). *A. napellus* was used until the eighteenth century as a medicinal remedy (263). This species is still used in India as an herbal remedy and also to increase the intoxicating effects of alcohol (264). Its use has also been implicated in murder (265). *Aconitum sungpanase, Aconitum carmichaeli, and Aconitum kusnezoffii* are all used in Chinese herbal remedies (264,266). There have been more than 600 aconite poisonings in 30 years reported in China from the use of herbal preparations (267–269).

A. napellus contains between 0.4% to 0.8% diterpene alkaloids (270). The aconitine (Fig. 1) concentration in a fresh *A. napellus* plant is between 0.3% and 2.0% in the tuber and 0.2% and 1.2% in the leaves (271). The highest concentration of aconitine in the plants tubers is found in the winter months (263).

TOXIC DOSE

The minimum lethal dose of aconitine is 3 to 6 mg (263). It is estimated that 1 g of fresh *A. napellus* contains 2 to 20 mg of aconitine. After ingestion of 5 to 10 mg of pure aconitine, a patient noted a bitter taste in the oropharynx, became symptomatic, and recovered (272).

TOXICOKINETICS AND TOXICODYNAMICS

Aconitum species contain both diterpene (C-20) and norditerpene (C-19) alkaloids (273,274). The C-20 diterpenes are low in toxicity, whereas the C-19 norditerpenes are much more toxic. If the ester functions of norditerpenes are hydrolyzed, the toxicity is decreased to that of the diterpenes. Therefore, the toxicity of a particular plant depends on the ratio of diterpenes to norditerpenes (263).

Aconitine can be absorbed orally (275), through mucous membranes, and through undamaged skin. Handling of plants, leaves (276), or tubers can produce toxicity (263). Aconitine has a rapid onset of action when ingested and has a sharp, bitter taste (272).

PATHOPHYSIOLOGY

Aconite alkaloids have been shown to have antiinflammatory effects in animal studies (277). Aconite slows the heart through a vagal action, which may be treated with atropine (278). Aconite also has been shown to produce a spontaneous auricular rate increase and spontaneous ventricular beats. The roots of *A. carmichaeli* contain four glycans. Together, these glycans have prominent hypoglycemic effects in normal and alloxan-produced hypoglycemic mice (279).

CLINICAL PRESENTATION

Symptoms of aconite poisoning develop quickly, usually within 10 to 20 minutes. Initially, patients complain of a tingling or burning sensation in the fingers and toes. The patient then develops sweats and chills, generalized paresthesias, dry mouth, numbness, and a feeling of intense cold. Late symptoms of poisoning include vomiting, diarrhea, skeletal muscle paralysis, cardiac dysrhythmias, and intense pain. Death typically results from ventricular dysrhythmias or respiratory paralysis within 1 to 6 hours after ingestion (range, minutes to 4 days) (280). A characteristic feature of aconite poisoning is skin paresthesias followed by numbness.

Miosis, diplopia, yellow-green vision, airway constriction, and difficulty swallowing and speaking have been reported. Cardiovascular effects include hypotension, vagal slowing, cardiac dysrhythmias, and ventricular fibrillation. Cardiac dysrhythmias can include multifocal premature ventricular contractions, ventricular tachycardia, and torsade de pointes (281–283).

Respiratory effects include pulmonary edema and respiratory paralysis. Neurologic toxicity includes burning and tingling sensation of the lips, tongue, fingers, and toes, most prominent in the face. Patients may develop muscle fasciculations, tonic-clonic seizures, and ataxia. Nausea, vomiting, and diarrhea and increased salivation may be present in the early stages of toxicity. Generalized weakness may progress to skeletal muscle paralysis. Dermatitis has been reported in pharmaceutical workers who are exposed to the plant.

A 36-year-old patient consumed an alcoholic drink, which contained aconitine. The patient developed lethargy and swollen, numb skin within 30 minutes. The patient then developed diarrhea, vomiting, spasms, was unable to speak and died within 8 hours (284).

A 35-year-old man ingested a tuber of *Aconitum brachypodium.* He developed nausea, abdominal pain, sweating, and an unsteady gait within 10 minutes and 90 minutes postingestion (284). A 35-year-old man developed cardiac dysrhythmias and hypotension after ingesting 3 or 4 rootstocks of *A. napellus.* The patient developed polymorphic ventricular tachycardia, which resolved after treatment with a bolus and continuous infusion of magnesium (285). Two out of three adults who were exposed to *Aconitum* root developed severe dysrhythmias (286). One patient, a 60-year-old man, developed fatal ventricular fibrillation 3 hours after ingestion; the other patient survived after treatment with high-dose phenytoin.

DIAGNOSTIC TESTING

Profuse vomiting and diarrhea may necessitate monitoring and replacement of fluids and electrolytes. An ECG and cardiorespiratory monitoring should be performed.

TREATMENT

In general, the treatment of aconite poisoning is symptomatic after decontamination. There is no antidote available. Because of the rapid onset, the prognosis after ingestion is usually poor (263). Respiratory support is often necessary due to the paralysis of respiratory muscles. In addition, copious vomiting and diarrhea may dictate fluid and electrolyte replacement.

Activated charcoal may be given to patients who are awake and able to protect their airway. It is most effective if given within 1 hour of ingestion. In general, cardiac dysrhythmias have been found to be refractory to drug management. Many different agents have been used, including atropine, quinidine (287), dichloroisoproterenol, digitalis, parasympathomimetics, inorganic ions (288,289), and mexiletine (290). Lidocaine and direct current cardioversion were unsuccessful in a number of Hong Kong cases (269,282,291). Atropine has been used to treat bradycardia due to vagal stimulation (292,293).

Foxglove (*Digitalis purpurea*)

Foxglove (*D. purpurea*) belongs to the snapdragon family, Scrophulariaceae. Foxglove is a biennial herb that can grow to be 4 ft tall. It has gray-green toothed leaves. It usually flowers between June and September. Foxglove has tubular and bell-shaped flowers that range in color from white to yellow, to a pink or purple color (Fig. 20). Foxglove is native to Europe and can be found in the United States, including Hawaii.

There are more than 400 different cardiac glycosides present in plants (294). Cardiac glycosides are combinations of an aglycone or genin (e.g., digoxigen, digitoxigenin), with one to four molecules of sugar (e.g., digitoxose or 2,6-dideoxyhexose). The leaves of foxglove are ground and milled to make *Digitalis* leaf. This is used for medicinal purposes. The cardiac glycosides in *D. purpurea* are hydrolyzed to digitoxin (Fig. 1), gitoxin, and gitalin. Small amounts of digoxin are formed by liver metabolism. The toxicity from foxglove can last up to 4 or 5 days due to the long serum half-life of digitoxin.

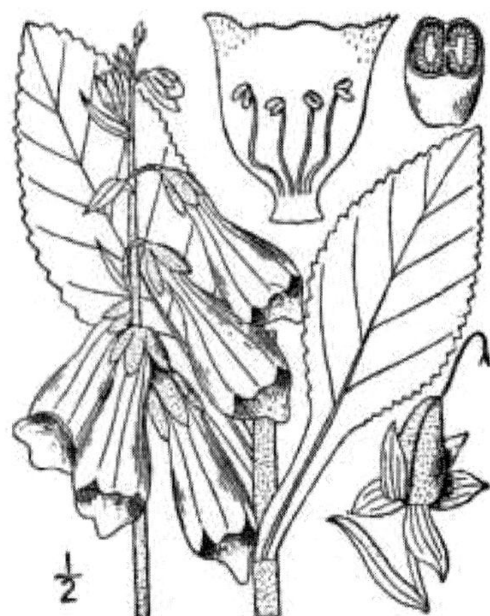

Figure 20. Purple foxglove (*Digitalis purpurea* L). (From USDA-NRCS PLANTS database/Britton NL, Brown A. *Illustrated flora of the northern states and Canada. Vol. 3.* 1913:204, with permission.)

Toxicity varies depending on the amount and part of plant that is ingested as well as the season, humidity, and age of plant. Serious toxicity from children tasting whole plant material is rare. Elevated digitoxin serum levels confirm toxicity but cannot guide management because of cross-reactivity.

TOXICOKINETICS AND TOXICODYNAMICS

Cardiac glycosides inhibit the Na^+,K^+-ATP pump. This causes a decrease in intracellular potassium and interferes with electrical conduction by reducing the normal resting membrane potential. This decreases the myocardial cell's ability to function as a pacemaker and may result in a complete loss of normal myocardial electrical function. In severe poisoning, asystole may ensue, and the myocardium may lose its ability to respond to electrical pacing.

CLINICAL PRESENTATION

The most common symptoms that are observed with cardiac glycoside plant toxicity are bradycardia with AV block, hypotension, lethargy, dizziness, and GI upset. Seizures, hypertension, coma, and electrolyte imbalances occur rarely.

A 36-year-old woman ingested foxglove and developed nausea, vomiting, abdominal pain, and cardiovascular shock. The patient's heart rate dropped to 38 bpm. The serum concentrations of the cardiac glycosides peaked the first day and then gradually decreased. The patient was treated with atropine, dimethicone, alginic acid, and metoclopramide (295). A 31-year-old woman and her husband ingested an herbal laxative, which mistakenly contained *Digitalis lantana* (instead of plantain). The woman's serum digoxin level was 4.2 ng/ml, and her husband's was 5.2 ng/ml (296).

A 46-year-old Asian woman ingested four large foxglove leaves and developed nausea, vomiting, lethargy, dizziness, and weakness approximately 4 hours later. She also developed a junctional bradycardia and an intermittent second degree AV block. The patient's serum digoxin level was 0.8 ng/ml, with a normal serum potassium level. Administration of two vials of digoxin immune Fab at 24 and 48 hours postingestion produced no improvement (297).

An 85-year-old man ingested 1 cup of tea that contained foxglove. The patient reported weakness, nausea, vomiting, and yellow halos around objects within a few hours. Initially, the ECG showed a normal sinus rhythm with prolonged PR intervals and ST depression. The patient developed ventricular tachycardia, and on day 2, he developed a junctional rhythm with a heart rate of 40 bpm and frequent premature ventricular contractions. Serum digitoxin levels peaked at 59 ng/ml on day 3. By day 4, the patient denied any further nausea or visual symptoms, and by day 6, the ECG had reverted to a normal sinus rhythm (298).

DIAGNOSTIC TESTS

Foxglove does not contain digoxin. There may be some cross-reactivity between the digoxin assay and other cardiac glycosides contained in foxglove (298). Serum levels do not correlate with clinical toxicity, as many of the plant glycosides cannot be measured. All foxglove ingestions should have the ECG and serum potassium levels followed closely.

TREATMENT

Any patient who has ingested foxglove should have GI decontamination, an ECG, and serum electrolytes obtained. Patients with signs of toxicity should be admitted for at least 24 hours.

Patients with a significant ingestion should be observed with continuous cardiac monitoring for at least 12 hours. The management of foxglove ingestion is similar to oleander poisoning, as described above (Chapters 49 and 122).

Lily-of-the-Valley (*Convallaria majalis*)

Convallaria majalis, or lily-of-the-valley, belongs to the Liliaceae (lily) family. It is an herbaceous perennial. It has two or three basal, broad leaves, which can be up to 8 in. in length. The flowers are bell-shaped and originate from the central stalk (Fig. 21). The flowers can be white or pale pink and are fragrant. The plant has been cultivated in Europe for its fragrance and can also be found throughout the United States. All parts of the plant contain convallarin and convallamarin, which are cardiac glycosides (299).

Convallatoxins are believed to be less potent than digoxin or digitalis. The toxicity from ingestion varies depending on the amount and part of the plant as well as the season, humidity, and age of plant. All parts of *C. majalis* contain cardiac glycosides, which range in concentration from 0.2% to 0.4% in the dried leaves to 0.5% in the flowers and seeds. Significant concentrations of the cardiac glycosides have not been found in the fruit pulp of the plant (300).

A review of 2639 exposures to *C. majalis* found that only 6.1% of patients experienced any symptoms, with three patients (0.1%) developing severe symptoms. Children younger than 6 years of age accounted for 93% of exposures (301). Although most ingestions in children are asymptomatic, significant conduction disturbances (grade I/II AV block) have been described in children ingesting small amounts of *C. majalis* (302). Serious toxicity from children tasting whole plant material is rare.

TOXICOKINETICS AND TOXICODYNAMICS

Cardiac glycosides inhibit the Na^+,K^+-ATP. This decreases intracellular potassium, interferes with electrical conduction, decreases the myocardial cell's ability to function as a pacemaker, and may result in a complete loss of normal myocardial electrical function. In severe poisonings, asystole may ensue, and the myocardium may lose its ability to respond to electrical pacing. The toxicity of cardiac glycosides resembles digitalis poisoning.

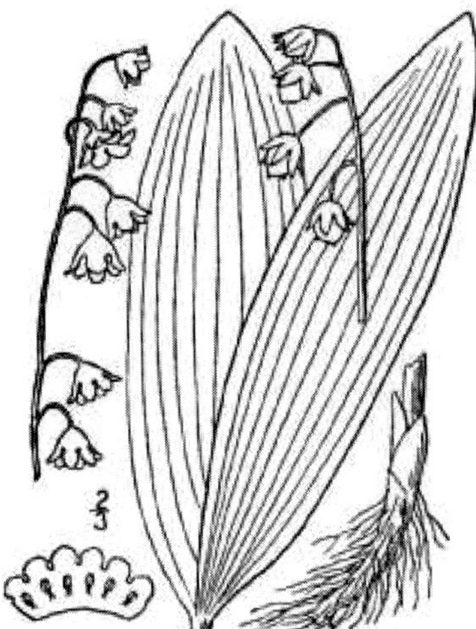

Figure 21. European lily-of-the-valley (*Convallaria majalis* L). (From USDA-NRCS PLANTS database/Britton NL, Brown A. *Illustrated flora of the northern states and Canada. Vol. 1.* 1913:522, with permission.)

CLINICAL PRESENTATION

The most common symptoms that are observed with cardiac glycoside plant toxicity are bradycardia with AV block, hypotension, lethargy, dizziness, and GI upset. Seizures, hypertension, coma, and electrolyte imbalances occur rarely. A 6-year-old boy ingested eight to ten *C. majalis* flowers. The initial ECG showed an incomplete right bundle-branch block and a PQ time of 0.17 seconds. After gastric lavage and activated charcoal, the PQ time increased to 0.2 seconds. There were no dysrhythmias (302). Another 6-year-old boy ingested one to two flowers of lily-of-the-valley. His ECG revealed sinus rhythm at a rate of 110 bpm and a PQ time of 0.18 seconds. The patient's PQ time increased to 0.4 seconds after gastric lavage. No dysrhythmias were detected (302).

A 4-year-old boy developed four episodes of grade II AV block after chewing on a *C. majalis* leaf (302). Tachycardia developed in three children after they ingested *C. majalis* (300). A 5-year-old child ingested 15 berries of *C. majalis* and developed vomiting (300).

DIAGNOSTIC TESTING

Serum digoxin levels may not correlate to clinical toxicity, as many of the plant cardiac glycosides cannot be measured. Patients with significant ingestions should have cardiac monitoring and serum potassium levels followed closely.

TREATMENT

Any patient with a significant ingestion of *C. majalis* should have an ECG and serum potassium obtained. Patients with signs of toxicity should be admitted for at least 24 hours. Patients with a significant ingestion should be observed with continuous cardiac monitoring for at least 12 hours. The management of *C. majalis* ingestion is similar to digoxin poisoning (Chapters 49 and 122).

Sweet Pea (*Lathyrus odoratus*) and Lathyrism

Sweet pea (*Lathyrus odoratus*) belongs to the family Fabaceae. The sweet pea is an annual climbing plant, which can reach heights greater than 6 ft. Its leaves are approximately 2 in. long. The leaves are elliptic and are comprised of a pair of leaflets. The flower comes in many different colors. The flowers are approximately 2 in. wide, with one to four flowers on each stem. The plant produces a 2-in. long legume, which is flat. The peas are eaten raw or cooked in the form of flour. The ingestion of a moderate amount of peas in this species does not usually produce poisoning.

There are more than 100 different species of *Lathyrus* in Europe and the United States. Many members of this species have been associated with toxicity in animals. These include *Lathyrus hirsutus, Lathyrus latifolius, L. odoratus, Lathyrus pusillus, Lathyrus sphaericus, Lathyrus splendens, Lathyrus laetiflorus, Lathyrus alefeldii, Lathyrus sylvestris,* and *Lathyrus tingitanus*. Excessive ingestion of the peas has been associated with lathyrism. Animals usually develop a collagen tissue disorder that has been termed *osteolathyrism*, whereas humans develop a neurologic disorder called *neurolathyrism* (303).

PATHOPHYSIOLOGY

All parts of the plants, especially the peas, are believed to contain β-aminopropionitrile and α-γ-aminobutyric acid. β-Aminopropionitrile is not present in the *Lathyrus* species that cause toxic effects in humans; however, it is believed to be the main toxin responsible for osteolathyrism in animals. The nitriles of β-aminopropionitrile replace amino acids during collagen synthesis. The abnormal collagen has a poor tensile strength and has been associated with skeletal deformities and aortic aneurysms in animals (304,305).

Human toxicity is believed to be secondary to the neurotoxin β-*N*-oxalylamino-L-alanine. It is structurally similar to the neurotransmitter glutamate (306). β-*N*-oxalylamino-L-alanine is a potent excitatory neurotransmitter, and it has been hypothesized that it may disrupt the CNS neurotransmitter activity of glutamate.

CLINICAL PRESENTATION

Human lathyrism has been described since the time of Hippocrates. It has also been described in World War II prisoner-of-war and concentration camps. It has been recognized as a public health problem in India. A slow weak pulse, respiratory depression, seizures, and paralysis have been described. The characteristic posture for lathyrism shows the patient's feet turned in and the toes turned down. Symptoms usually appear after 4 to 8 weeks.

In concentration camps, lathyrism occurred in prisoners who consumed approximately 300 g of *L. sativus* every day for 3 months and occurred preferentially in young males. Symptoms included spasticity, ataxia, and paraplegia. Of the patients who developed neurolathyrism, 80% had upper motor neuron lesions, 15% had both upper and lower lesions, and 5% had peripheral neuropathies (307). Skeletal bone abnormalities were also described; however, it is unclear whether these resulted from the secondary stresses produced by the neurologic lesions (308). Patients were noted to have motor and sensory complaints in the lower extremities, GI distress, bladder and sexual dysfunction, insomnia, and short-term memory loss (309). There are no reports of acute toxicity from a single ingestion of *Lathyrus*.

TREATMENT

Treatment consists of supportive care. Decontamination is not necessary for childhood ingestions.

Carolina Yellow Jessamine (*Gelsemium sempervirens*)

Yellow jessamine (*Gelsemium sempervirens*) belongs to the family Loganiaceae. It is an evergreen vine with a woody stem, which can grow to be more than 20 ft. The leaves are dark green and shiny and are 1 to 3 in. long (Fig. 22). The flowers come in yellow clusters and are funnel shaped. The vine is found in the southeastern United States and is also cultivated in California, where it is used as a fence plant (294). The roots and rhizome have been made into an extract, which has been used for pain relief for such conditions as trigeminal neuralgia and migraines. It has also been used as an emetic, a CNS depressant, and a treatment for fever (310–313).

TOXIC DOSE

The minimum lethal human exposure is unknown. A patient ingested approximately five blossoms and became obtunded (314). There is one report of three people dying after ingesting *Gelsemium*-containing honey. There were an abundance of yellow jessamine flowers in the area used by the bees. The honey was never analyzed (316).

PATHOPHYSIOLOGY

Yellow jessamine contains indole alkaloids. The main components are gelsemine, gelsemicine, and sempervirine (317,318). These compounds primarily affect the CNS. The toxins interfere with the motor nerve endings by binding to the acetylcholine receptor (315). This can lead to respiratory arrest. In addition, yellow jessamine also belongs to the same plant family that contains strychnine. Some alkaloids in yellow jessamine may resemble strychnine, which blocks the glycine receptors in the spinal cord (294).

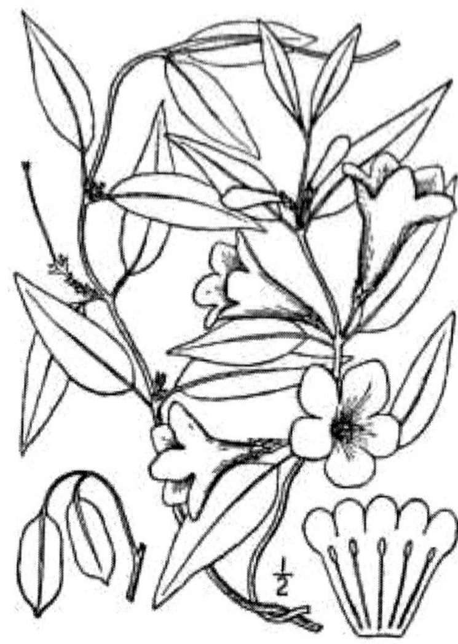

Figure 22. Carolina yellow jessamine (*Gelsemium sempervirens* L.) (From USDA-NRCS PLANTS database/Britton NL, Brown A. *Illustrated flora of the northern states and Canada. Vol. 2.* 1913:730, with permission.)

CLINICAL PRESENTATION

Poisoning may cause headache, vomiting, dizziness, muscular weakness or rigidity, dyspnea, bradycardia, or seizures. Most reports of toxicity were published before 1900 when herbalists used the plant to induce abortions. A 3.5-year-old girl was noted to develop a wide-based gait, bilateral ptosis, and generalized weakness after ingesting approximately five blossoms of yellow jessamine. The child became obtunded within 1 hour, and all symptoms had resolved by 9.5 hours. The child also complained of headache, dry mouth, dysphagia, blurry vision, and light-headedness (315).

TREATMENT

The onset of toxicity is usually 15 to 30 minutes after ingestion. Gastric lavage should be considered for ingestion times of less than 1 hour. Oral decontamination with charcoal is the preferred treatment. Activated charcoal may be given to patients who are awake and able to protect their airway. Charcoal is most effective if given within 1 hour of ingestion.

PSYCHOACTIVE AND HALLUCINOGENIC PLANTS

Nutmeg

Nutmeg is a common spice that is obtained from the tree *Myristica fragrans* (family Myristicaceae). *Myristica* is grown in Grenada and is also found in the South Pacific and East Indies (319). The tree produces a nutmeg apple, which is similar to an apricot. Two spices, nutmeg and mace, can be obtained from the fruit. Both of these spices are used as narcotic hallucinogens.

Nutmeg comes from the dried seed of *M. fragrans,* and mace comes from the dried, fleshy, scarlet covering of the seed (aril). Mace has a flavor that is similar to nutmeg (320). Nutmeg is comprised of 20% to 40% nutmeg butter (fixed oil), and 8% to

15% essential oils (320,321). The volatile oils present in both nutmeg and mace are believed to be the main source of toxicity. Once the volatile oils have been removed, the psychological effects of the nut are no longer present. The volatile oils are comprised of mixtures of allylbenzene derivatives (myristicin, elemicin, safrole) and terpenes (321).

Multiple psychogenic effects have been associated with nutmeg toxicity. Hallucinations (similar to those seen with phencyclidine) usually cause distortions in time, color, and space (319). Nutmeg intoxication also can give a sense of euphoria, detachment from reality, and a feeling of loss of limbs (320,322). In addition, nutmeg can cause anxiety and a sense of dread (323).

Nutmeg has been used as an herbal remedy for GI disorders, rheumatism, madness, and flatulence. It has also been used as an emetic, abortifacient, and as an aphrodisiac (320). Reports of nutmeg toxicity are much more common than mace toxicity.

TOXIC DOSE

Nine teaspoons per day of nutmeg has been used to control diarrhea associated with medullary carcinoma. However, this dose did cause toxic symptoms (324). Toxicity can be seen with small doses of the volatile oil (0.4 to 4.0 ml) or with 5 to 30 g of ground nut (one nutmeg weighs approximately 6 g).

In adults, a dose of 400 mg of myristicin was associated with mild cerebral stimulation (325). A dose of 18.5 g was noted to cause excitement and a feeling of impending doom (324). A dose of 28 g was noted to cause severe anxiety, palpitations, a sense of dread, and hallucinations (323). There is one case report of an 8-year-old boy ingesting two nutmegs. The boy subsequently became comatose and died approximately 24 hours after ingestion (326).

TOXICOKINETICS AND TOXICODYNAMICS

The components of the volatile oils of nutmeg are believed to produce psychogenic effects. These effects may be due to the combination of myristicin (Fig. 1) with other compounds that are present in its volatile oils such as elemicin, eugenol, safrole, and borneol (325). It is postulated that the metabolism of myristicin and elemicin may change these compounds to their amino derivatives. One probable derivative of myristicin is 3-methoxy-4,5,-methylenedioxyamphetamine, whereas elemicin may be metabolized to 3,4,5-trimethoxyamphetamine. Both of these compounds are psychoactive compounds that are related to amphetamine and have clinical effects that are similar to LSD (319). It is unknown what percentage of myristicin and elemicin are metabolized into these compounds (320).

PREGNANCY AND LACTATION

Nutmeg is FDA pregnancy risk category C (Appendix I). A 29-year-old woman at 30 weeks' gestation mixed 1 tablespoon (7 g) of grated nutmeg in a cookie recipe and ate several cookies. She developed signs of anticholinergic toxicity. The fetal heart rate was increased for approximately 12 hours. A healthy infant was born 10 weeks later (322).

CLINICAL PRESENTATION

Symptoms begin approximately 3 to 8 hours after ingestion and consist of periods of delirium alternating with stupor over the next 6 to 24 hours. Most people recover within 24 hours; however, in some cases, complete recovery may take several days (320,324,327). Hypothermia has been described (320,328). Initial excitation is followed by extreme drowsiness, which can persist for 24 hours or more (325,329,330). One report describes muscle weakness and ataxia in a 13-year-old girl who ingested 15 to 24 g of nutmeg over 3 hours and smoked marijuana. Her symptoms resolved after treatment with 50 g of activated charcoal (329).

Dry mouth, blurred vision, headache, thirst, flushing, and miosis have been reported. Miosis is more common than mydriasis (330) but is not a reliable sign of toxicity (331). Tachycardia is common. Blood pressure may be slightly elevated; however, severe hypotension with cyanosis and shock has also been reported (332). Tachypnea may occur.

Nausea, vomiting, and burning epigastric pain may occur. Urinary retention has been reported (322). Dermatologic effects have included flushing (333), hives (320), dry skin (322), and increased sweating (334).

Initial CNS excitation is followed by drowsiness. Hallucinations, euphoria, distortions of time and space, detachment from reality, sensation of loss of limbs, anxiety, and a sense of doom have all been reported.

DIAGNOSTIC TESTS

Laboratory parameters are usually normal, and levels for myristicin or elemicin are not routinely available. One case report recorded a myristicin level of 2 μg/ml 8 hours after ingestion of 14 to 21 g of nutmeg powder by an adult. Another case report measured a postmortem level of myristicin of 4 μg/ml after an estimated ingestion of 560 to 840 mg/kg of nutmeg (335). Abnormal liver function tests have been noted in cats and dogs (325) but not in humans (330).

TREATMENT

Management of toxicity is generally supportive. Activated charcoal may be useful shortly after ingestion, although it has not been studied. There is no specific antidote for nutmeg toxicity. Treatment includes controlling nausea and vomiting, maintaining blood pressure, and keeping the patient calm. Benzodiazepines may be used for patients who are hallucinating. Antiemetics are useful in the treatment of nausea and vomiting. Hypotension is rare, and the use of vasopressors has not been necessary. Seizures have not been described with nutmeg toxicity.

MANAGEMENT PITFALLS

The initial presentation may resemble anticholinergic toxicity with tachycardia, dry mouth, and altered mental status. However, physostigmine is not of benefit and may be potentially harmful.

Peyote Cactus (Mescaline)

The peyote cactus, *Lophophora williamsii*, family Cactaceae, can be found in dry areas, cliffs, and rocky slopes in the southwestern United States and on the Mexican plateau. The peyote cactus is a small, spineless cactus that has pink (sometimes white or yellow) flowers. Its length does not usually exceed 15 to 20 cm. It has a cylindric stalk that has horizontal wrinkles and is gray-brown in color. The stalk is less visible because it grows beneath the surface of the ground. The peyote "button," located on top, consists of the dried, brownish-gray part of the cactus.

Mescaline is the major hallucinogen among at least 16 active β-phenylethylamine and isoquinoline alkaloids (Fig. 1). Peyote is comprised of approximately 1% to 6% mescaline, with each button containing approximately 45 mg of mescaline (336). It takes between 6 and 12 buttons to produce a hallucinogenic response. Ingestion of peyote initially causes nausea and vomiting, which is followed by CNS and sympathetic stimulation and hallucinations. Deaths from peyote are rare and are usually the result of psychotic, suicidal, or homicidal behavior.

CLASSIFICATION AND USES

The primary hallucinogenic alkaloid is mescaline (3,4,5-trimethoxyphenethylamine). It is a phenylethylamine similar to methylenedioxymethamphetamine. Peyote cactus is used primarily for its hallucinogenic effects. It is also used for religious purposes by American Indian tribes, usually as a tea brewed from the cactus button (337). Dried slices of the cactus are called *mescal buttons*. Common street names include Big Chief, mesc, and peyote. Capsules of ground cactus buttons contain approximately 6% mescaline and may be purchased in the illicit drug market. LSD may be substituted for mescaline by illicit drug manufacturers or dealers.

TOXIC DOSE

Approximately 5 mg/kg of mescaline is needed to produce hallucinogenic effects. Higher doses produce more sympathomimetic effects. A typical adult dose is 250 to 500 mg. No deaths have been reported from the direct physiologic effects of mescaline.

TOXICOKINETICS AND TOXICODYNAMICS

Peyote is rapidly absorbed after ingestion (338). The onset of action is between 30 minutes and 2 hours, and peak blood levels occur 2 hours after ingestion. The duration of effect usually ranges from 6 to 12 hours but may last up to 14 hours.

Mescaline binds to liver proteins but not to plasma proteins (338). It is rapidly and widely distributed into the peripheral tissues. The volume of distribution is not specifically known but is believed to be on the order of several liters per kilogram. It is metabolized in the liver by mescaline oxidase into numerous inactive metabolites. These include 3,4,5-trimethoxyphenylacetic acid; 3,4,5-trimethoxybenzoic acid; 3,4-dihydroxy-5-methoxy-phenylacetyl glutamine; 3-hydroxy-4,5-dimethoxyphenethylamine; *N*-acetylmescaline; and *N*-acetyl-3,4-dimethoxy-5-hydroxyphenethylamine (338–340). Sixty percent of mescaline is excreted unchanged in a 24-hour urine, and the rest is excreted as metabolites (339,340).

PATHOPHYSIOLOGY

The mechanism of action of mescaline is unknown. Hallucinogenic effects are believed to be due to stimulation of serotonin and dopamine receptors in the CNS.

PREGNANCY AND LACTATION

Mescaline is considered to be a potential human teratogen (341). There are no data on excretion into breast milk.

CLINICAL PRESENTATION

Mescaline produces hallucinations and symptoms of CNS and sympathetic stimulation. Mild elevations in pulse, blood pressure, respiratory rate, and temperature may be noted. Nausea and vomiting commonly precede the hallucinogenic effects. The clinical presentation may mimic an anticholinergic syndrome.

Mydriasis, salivation, and blurred vision are common. Palpitations may occur.

Nausea and vomiting, abdominal cramps, and diarrhea are common. GI effects may persist for several days. Antidiuretic effects and polyuria have been noted.

Headaches, dizziness, ataxia, tremors, weakness, hallucinations, and paresthesias have been noted. Anxiety, auditory and visual hallucinations, emotional instability, paranoia, and flashbacks may occur.

Piloerection, flushing, and diaphoresis can occur. Shivering, tremors, increased muscle tone, hyperreflexia, and weakness may occur.

DIAGNOSTIC TESTS

Qualitative analysis for mescaline or its metabolites is sufficient for diagnosis of toxicity. Tolerance to mescaline does occur, and blood levels may not correlate with clinical effect. A 500-mg dose of mescaline hydrochloride produced an average blood concentration of 3.8 mg/L at 2 hours after ingestion in 12 volunteers (342). A postmortem mescaline blood concentration of 9.7 mg/L was found in an adult who jumped from a height of 600 ft while under the influence of mescaline (342).

TREATMENT

Ingestion of peyote (mescaline) is rarely life-threatening. Emesis with human ingestion is common and may limit toxicity. Patients exhibiting toxicity should have blood pressure monitoring and should be observed in a monitored setting until symptoms resolve. A patient can be discharged home if they remain asymptomatic for 4 hours. Symptomatic patients should be monitored for suicidal, homicidal, or psychotic behavior.

Activated charcoal may be given to patients who are awake and able to protect their airway. Due to the rapid absorption of mescaline, it is most effective if given within 1 hour of ingestion.

Mild increases in blood pressure, pulse, and temperature may be noted; however, this usually resolves with treatment of anxiety, agitation, and hallucinations. Severe agitation can be treated with 5 to 10 mg of diazepam (orally or intravenously) in adults and 0.1 to 0.3 mg/kg in children (up to a maximum dosage of 10 mg). The dose can be repeated every 10 to 60 minutes up to a total dosage of 30 mg in adults. Psychosis in adults can be treated with neuroleptics, such as haloperidol, given orally or intravenously at a dose of 5 to 10 mg. The dose of haloperidol can be repeated as needed in 10 to 60 minutes.

Morning Glory Family (Convolvulaceae)

Certain varieties of the morning glory family have seeds that possess hallucinogenic properties similar to LSD (Table 8). Certain species, *Ipomoea violacea* and *Turbina corymbosa,* were used by the Aztecs for religious ceremonies. Consumption of morning glory seeds was popularized in the 1960s by teenagers and young adults who ingested the seeds for their hallucinogenic properties. Common street names include heavenly blue, blue star, and flying saucers. Other members of the Convolvulaceae family also have hallucinogenic properties when ingested. *Argyreia nervosa*, or wood rose, has been used by Hawaiians as a hallucinogen. In addition, the ergot alkaloids found in the fungus *Claviceps purpurea* are identical to those found in the morning glory family.

CLASSIFICATION AND USES

The psychotomimetic indole compounds found in the morning glory family include isoergine, chanoclavine, elymoclavine, lysergol, ergonovine, and penniclavine (343). Ergine is the major alkaloid present in this family (Fig. 1). Its potency is approximately 10% of that of LSD. Chanoclavine and elymoclavine are not believed to have any psychotomimetic effects. The seeds are dark brown to black, wedge shaped, and 3 to 4 mm long.

TOXIC DOSE

Varieties of *I. violacea* have similar indole alkaloid contents. The seeds must be pulverized or chewed for absorption of the alkaloids to occur (344). A dose of 20 to 40 seeds produces restlessness, increased awareness, and increased socialization, followed by relaxation for several hours rarely associated with hallucinations. A dose of 100 to 150 seeds produces effects similar to ingestion of 75 to 150 μg/kg of LSD—spatial distortions, hallu-

TABLE 8. Hallucinogenic/nonhallucinogenic species of the morning glory family

Botanical name	Horticultural name (varieties)
Hallucinogenic properties	
Ipomoea violacea	Heavenly blue, pearly gates, wedding bells, flying saucers, summer skies, blue star
No hallucinogenic properties	
Ipomoea purpurea	Crimson rambler, convolvulus major, sunrise serenade, Rose Marie, Tinkerbell's petticoat
Ipomoea nil	Scarlett O'Hara, candy pink, cornell, royal crown, darling
Ipomoea alba	Moon vines
Ipomoea x sloteri	Cardinal climber
Ipomoea quamoclit	Cypress vine
Ipomoea coccinea; variant, *Ipomoea hederifolia*	Mina sanguinea
Convolvulus tricolor	Royal marine

Adapted from Der Marderosian A. Psychotomimetic indoles in the Convolvulaceae. *Am J Pharm* 1967;139:21.

cinations, enhanced imagery, and mood elevations for 1 to 4 days; relaxation and sleep follow. A dose of 200 to 250 seeds produces effects similar to ingestion of 200 to 500 μg/kg of LSD. Patients experience euphoria and great philosophic insight; they may have nausea, vomiting, abdominal pain, lethargy, and paresthesias.

T. corymbosa seeds are less potent than *I. violacea* seeds. This species contains approximately 40% of isoergine and less than 20% of the concentration of the more potent ergine when compared with *I. violacea*. One *A. nervosa* seed contains approximately the same amount of ergine that is present in 75 to 100 *I. violacea* seeds (345).

Ingestion of 250 *I. violacea* seeds produced dilated pupils, hyperreflexia, facial erythema, emotional lability, and a dissociative state within 3 hours of ingestion. Approximately 2 hours later, the patient developed tension and anxiety. Symptoms resolved approximately 6 hours postingestion. No hallucinations were reported (346).

CLINICAL PRESENTATION

The effects of the morning glory family are similar to those of LSD. Symptoms are dose dependent and may include hallucinations, euphoria, special distortions, panic reactions, marked paranoia, persistent changes in perception and sensation, and violent behavior. Adverse effects include nausea, vomiting, numbness, cool extremities, lethargy, and uterine stimulation. There is a report of hypotension with IV injection (347). In addition, suicidal behavior has resulted from panic reactions, prolonged dissociative reactions, and schizophrenic breakdowns (348).

TREATMENT

Treatment is similar to that of LSD ingestion. The patient should be placed in a safe environment to prevent self-harm. Most symptoms resolve within 8 hours. Diazepam may be used if sedation is required.

Khat (Cathinone)

Khat (quat, qat, mirra) is the common name for the plant *Catha edulis,* an evergreen bush in the family of Celastraceae. It grows in southwestern Arabia and in east Africa between Sudan and Madagascar. Wild khat may grow to 20 m, but most cultivated trees are approximately 5 m tall. The young branches and shoots of the tree are harvested and sold in bunches. Bunches are wrapped up tightly in plastic to preserve the leaves. Unless frozen, much of the potency of the plant is lost within 24 to 48 hours after harvesting (349). The plant and leaves contain sympathomimetic alkaloids, and its potency is determined by the phenylalkylamine content. Most of the toxic effects of khat are due to large single doses in conjunction with chronic use.

CLASSIFICATION AND USES

The main active ingredient is cathinone (benzylketoamphetamine), which constitutes up to 0.3% of the plant (Fig. 1). Khat is used primarily as a stimulant. It plays a prominent role in socialization in the countries where it is grown. Users may consume 100 to 200 g of leaves over a 3- to 4-hour period. Historically, khat has been used to treat fatigue, depression, obesity, and gastric ulcers (350). It also has anorectic properties.

TOXIC DOSE

The usual dose is 100 to 200 g of fresh leaves chewed all at once. The juice of the leaves is swallowed, and the leaves are retained in the cheek and later expelled (351). The toxicity of khat is limited because of the limited plant content, slow release of alkaloid during chewing, and the rapid breakdown of cathinone. However, cardiovascular complications during routine use may occur in the elderly or people who take khat while exercising. Most toxic effects are seen after large single doses during chronic use.

TOXICOKINETICS AND TOXICODYNAMICS

The active components of khat are absorbed orally by chewing the leaves. The peak plasma concentrations of cathinone, cathine, and norephedrine are reached in 127 minutes, 183 minutes, and 200 minutes, respectively (352). The pharmacologic effects of khat start as soon as the leaves are chewed, and the effects last approximately 2 hours after chewing has stopped. The volume of distribution is unknown but believed to be similar to amphetamine, which has a volume of distribution of 3 to 6 L/kg.

Cathinone is metabolized by keto-reduction to norephedrine and norpseudoephedrine at an approximate ratio of 9:1 (353). A small amount of cathinone is excreted by the kidney unchanged (0.6% to 3.3%). Up to 52% of oral doses of cathinone isomers are recovered in 24-hour urine samples as aminoalcohol metabolites (353). Cathine is also primarily excreted in the urine: 40% of an oral dose within 6 hours and 84.6% within 24 hours (354). The elimination half-life of cathinone (given as khat) is approximately 4 hours (352).

PATHOPHYSIOLOGY

Sympathomimetic alkaloids are the main active components in khat. The most common alkaloids consist of the phenylpropylamines cathinone, cathine, and (–)-norephedrine. In general, 100 g of fresh khat contains approximately 36 mg of cathinone, 120 mg of cathine, and 8 mg of (–)-norephedrine. In addition, khat also contains low concentrations of phenylpentenylamines such as merucathinone, pseudomerucathine, and merucathine (349).

Cathinone is the main active ingredient in khat. In general, the phenylalkylamines in khat are similar to sympathomimetic amines, such as ephedrine and amphetamines, that release neurotransmitters from presynaptic nerve endings. These neurotransmitters lead to the indirect activation of both peripheral and central catecholaminergic pathways (355).

PREGNANCY AND LACTATION

Khat use during pregnancy has been associated with low-birth-weight infants. It has been shown to decrease uteroplacental flow (356) and may contribute to hypertensive disease of pregnancy (357). No teratogenic effects have been associated with khat in humans. Its dopaminergic effects might inhibit prolactin secretion and decrease breast milk production; however, plasma prolactin levels appear unchanged (358).

CLINICAL PRESENTATION

Khat may increase heart rate, blood pressure, temperature, and respirations. Chemosis, dry mouth, stomatitis, dilated pupils, and pseudoexophthalmus have all been observed. Hypertension and tachycardia with palpitations have been described. Dysrhythmias and acute myocardial infarction are rare. Respiratory effects include tachypnea (359), dyspnea (360), and pulmonary edema (361). Diaphoresis and flushing (361) have been described. Nausea, gastritis, and ulcers can occur. Urinary retention can occur.

Common neurologic effects include anorexia, headache, hyperactivity, insomnia, and tremors as well as depression, panic attacks, and anxiety. Chronic use may result in paranoid psychosis. Cathinone may be addictive.

DIAGNOSTIC TESTS

Cathinone, norephedrine, and norpseudoephedrine can all be detected by HPLC analysis of urine (353). These substances may be misidentified as amphetamines or phenylpropanolamine on common screening tests because of cross-reactivity. Other laboratory tests are used as described for amphetamines (Chapter 174).

TREATMENT

Treatment for khat ingestion is largely symptomatic. Symptomatic patients should be placed on a monitor, have an ECG obtained, and have vital signs monitored frequently. Most symptoms resolve in 4 to 6 hours. Patients with persistent vital sign abnormalities, evidence of end-organ ischemia, or psychiatric symptoms should be admitted for observation.

Activated charcoal may be given to patients who are awake and able to protect their airway. It is most effective if given within 1 hour of ingestion. Urinary acidification is not recommended for treatment of sympathomimetic overdose.

The complications of agitation, cardiovascular overstimulation, and seizures are treated as for amphetamines (Chapter 174). Agitation is treated with benzodiazepines, which are also generally effective in reducing many cardiovascular effects and terminating seizures. Hyperthermia can be treated with cooling blankets, IV fluids, sponging, and bladder and gastric lavage with cool fluids (Chapter 38).

Yohimbine (*Pausinystalia yohimbe*)

Yohimbine is an indole derivative that is extracted from the bark of the West African tropical plant (*Corynanthe yohimbe*). It can be found in Congo, Cameroon, and Gabon. Treatment of overdoses is largely symptomatic. The most common side effects include hypothermia, tachycardia, hypertension, hallucinations, anxiety, and vasodilation. There is not a specific antidote for yohimbine toxicity. Clonidine has been used to counteract the effect of yohimbine in experimental studies. However, more testing needs to be done before the routine use of clonidine can be recommended (362).

CLASSIFICATION AND USES

Yohimbine is an indole alkaloid and an α_2-adrenoreceptor antagonist (Fig. 1). It is used as an aphrodisiac and mild hallucinogen. It has been used to treat male erectile dysfunction. In veterinary medicine, it is a reversal agent for xylazine. It has been on the U.S. Department of Agriculture unsafe herb list since 1977 (363). The action of yohimbine is similar to that of reserpine and opposite of the action of clonidine. It has been used as an antidote for clonidine overdoses, although it is not FDA approved for this use (364). It is available in tablet form (5 mg) as Aphrodyne (United States), Yocon (Germany, Canada), and Prowess Plain (United Kingdom). It is also available as a dietary supplement.

TOXIC DOSE

The adult therapeutic dosage for impotence is 5 mg three times a day. A dose of 0.1 mg/kg can produce stimulant effects. A dose of 15 to 20 mg may produce mild elevations in systolic blood pressure (365). A 38-year-old man ingested 350 mg of yohimbine (no other coingestions) and developed atrial fibrillation with a ventricular rate of 150 bpm (366). A 16-year-old girl ingested 250 mg of yohimbine and developed weakness, generalized paresthesias, decreased coordination, and a dissociative state within 20 minutes (367). A 42-year-old man ingested 16.2 mg of yohimbine and developed acute renal failure (creatinine, 8.9 mg/dl) and a lupus-like syndrome with a generalized cutaneous skin rash (368).

TOXICOKINETICS AND TOXICODYNAMICS

Yohimbine is absorbed rapidly after oral ingestion and has a half-life of 7 to 11 minutes (369,370). Oral bioavailability is 7% to 87% (mean, 33%) depending on the patient (369). Yohimbine has a volume of distribution of 0.3 to 3.0 L/kg. Most of yohimbine (82%) is bound to plasma proteins. Yohimbine undergoes extensive first-pass metabolism in the liver. The major metabolites of yohimbine are 11-hydroxy-yohimbine (active metabolite) and 10-hydroxy-yohimbine (minor metabolite) (371). Less than 1% of yohimbine is excreted unchanged into the urine over a 24-hour period (370,371). The half-life is 0.6 hours.

PATHOPHYSIOLOGY

Yohimbine is a selective competitive antagonist of α_2-adrenergic receptors and at high concentrations may interact with α_1-adrenoreceptors and serotonin and dopamine receptors. Yohimbine potentiates the release of norepinephrine and increases sympathetic outflow, which increases peripheral sympathetic activity (372).

CLINICAL PRESENTATION

The effects of yohimbine include nausea, vomiting, diarrhea, hypothermia, mydriasis, flushing, vasodilation, hypertension, tachycardia, orthostatic hypotension, and palpitations. A possible case of renal failure from yohimbine ingestion has been reported (368).

Neurologic effects include nervousness and reversible paresthesias in legs and feet. Retrograde amnesia and confusion has been reported in a yohimbine overdose (366). Anxiety and mild hallucinations may occur if smoked or used in a tea.

A 38-year-old man ingested 350 mg of yohimbine (no other coingestions) and developed atrial fibrillation with a ventricular rate of 150 bpm. The atrial fibrillation resolved by the next day. The patient was also noted to have confusion, lethargy, and retrograde amnesia. The retrograde amnesia lasted for 4 days (366).

A 16-year-old girl ingested 250 mg of yohimbine and developed weakness, generalized paresthesias, decreased coordination, and a dissociative state within 20 minutes. She had a blood pressure of 150/80 mm Hg and a heart rate of 116 bpm 30 hours after ingestion. She also had a fine tremor in the extremities and a blotchy erythematous rash on her back. The patient had an elevated serum norepinephrine level. Symptoms resolved within 36 hours with bed rest (367).

A 42-year-old man ingested 16.2 mg of yohimbine and developed acute renal failure (creatinine, 8.9 mg/dl) and a lupus-like syndrome with a generalized cutaneous skin rash. The patient's condition improved with hydration over a 2-week period (368).

DIAGNOSTIC TESTS

There is no toxic serum blood level established. A 10-mg oral dose produces a peak blood concentration of 289 μg/L at 1 hour and 115 μg/L at 4 hours (373).

TREATMENT

Activated charcoal may be given to patients after overdose who are awake and able to protect their airway. It is probably most effective if given within 1 hour of ingestion, although this has not been studied.

The complications of agitation, cardiovascular overstimulation, and seizures are treated as for stimulants (Chapter 174). Agitation is treated with benzodiazepines, which are also generally effective in reducing many cardiovascular effects. Hyperthermia can be treated with cooling blankets, IV fluids, sponging, and bladder and gastric lavage with cool fluids (Chapter 38).

Although there is not a specific antidote for yohimbine toxicity, clonidine has been used to counteract the effect of yohimbine in experimental studies. However, more testing needs to be done before the routine use of clonidine can be recommended (362). Clonidine, 0.1 mg orally in an adult, may be useful for anxiety and mild to moderate hypertension. The preferred treatment for hypertensive emergencies is nitroprusside (Chapter 36).

REFERENCES

1. Krenzelok EP, Jacobsen TD. Plant exposures . . . a national profile of the most common plant genera. *Vet Hum Toxicol* 1997;39:248–249.
2. Litovitz TL, Klein-Schwartz W, Rodgers GC, et al. 2001 annual report of the American Association of Poison Control Centers Toxic Exposure Surveillance System. *Am J Emerg Med* 2002;20:391–452.
3. Toxic plant substances. The chemistry of poisonous and medicinal plants. In: Blackwell WH. *Poisonous and medicinal plants*. Englewood Cliffs, NJ: Prentice-Hall, 1990:34–52.
4. Fassett DW, Chap IC. *Oxalates in toxicants occurring naturally in foods*, 2nd ed. Washington, DC: National Academy of Sciences, 1973.
5. McIntire MS, Guest JR, Porterfield JF. Philodendron—an infant death. *J Toxicol Clin Toxicol* 1990;28:177–183.
6. Neuvonen PJ, Elfving SM, Elonen E. Reduction of adsorption of digoxin, phenytoin, and aspirin by activated charcoal in man. *Eur J Clin Pharmacol* 1978;13:213–222.
7. Heath A, Mellstrand T, Ahlmin J. Treatment of podophyllin poisoning with resin hemoperfusion. *Hum Toxicol* 1982;1:373–378.
7a. Smythies JR, Robinson CR, Al-Zahid SA. On the tertiary structure and mechanism of action of the viscotoxins. *Ala J Med Sci* 1976;13:240–246.
8. Spiller HA, Willias DB, Gorman SE, et al. Retrospective study of mistletoe ingestion. *J Toxicol Clin Toxicol* 1996;34:405–408.
9. Krenzelok EP, Jacobsen TD, Aronic JM. American mistletoe exposures. *Am J Emerg Med* 1997;15:516–520.
10. Dore WC. Crystalline raphides in the toxic houseplant *Dieffenbachia*. *JAMA* 1963;185:1045.
11. Drach G, Maloney WA. Toxicity of the common houseplant *Dieffenbachia:* report of a case. *JAMA* 1963;184:1047–1048.
12. Challoner KR, McCarron MM. Castor bean intoxication. *Ann Emerg Med* 1990;19:1177–1183.
13. Rauber A, Heard J. Castor bean toxicity re-examined: a new perspective. *Vet Hum Toxicol* 1985;27:498–502.
14. Kopferschmitt J, Flesch F, Lugnier A, et al. Acute voluntary intoxication by ricin. *Hum Toxicol* 1983;2:239–242.
15. Malizia E, Sarcinelli L, Andreucci G. Ricinus poisoning, a familiar epidemy. *Acta Pharmacol Toxicol* 1977;41[Suppl 2]:351–361.
16. Olsnes S, Kozlov JV. Ricin. *Toxicon* 2001;39:1723–1728.
17. Palatnick W, Tenenbein M. Hepatotoxicity from castor bean ingestion in a child. *J Toxicol Clin Toxicol* 2000;38:67–69.
18. Henry GW, Schwenk GR, Bohnert PG. Umbrellas and moe beans: a warning about acute ricin poisoning. *J Indiana Med Assoc* 1981;43:572–573.
19. Lewis JH. Esophageal and small bowel obstruction from guar gum-containing "diet pills." Analysis of 26 cases reported to the Food and Drug Administration. *Am J Gastroenterol* 1992;87:1424–1428.
20. Fernando C. Poisoning due to *Abrus precatorius* (jequirity bean). *Anaesthesia* 2001;56:1178–1180.
21. Davis JH. *Abrus precatourius* (rosary pea): the most common lethal plant poison. *J Fla Med Assoc* 1978;65:189–191.
22. Makalinao IP. A descriptive study on the clinical profile of *Jatropha* seed poisoning. *Vet Hum Toxicol* 1993;35:330.
22a. Infante ME, Perez AM, Simoo MR, et al. Outbreak of acute toxic psychosis attributed to *Mucuna pruriens*. *Lancet* 1992;336:1129.
23. Anonymous. *Mucuna pruriens*-associated pruritius-New Jersey. *MMWR Morb Mortal Wkly Rep* 1985;48:732.
24. McGrath-Hill CA, Vicas IM. Case series of *Thermopsis* exposures. *J Toxicol Clin Toxicol* 1997;35:659–665.
25. Lowen RJ, Alam FKA, Edgar JA. Lupin bean toxicity. *Med J Aust* 1995;162:256–257.
26. Tsiodras S, Shin RK, Christian M, et al. Anticholinergic toxicity associated with lupine seeds as a home remedy for diabetes mellitus. *Ann Emerg Med* 1999;33:715–717.
27. Phillips RW, Moses FR. Sunflower seed syndrome: a prickly proctological problem. *Ann Emerg Med* 1991;20:1049–1050.
28. Purcell L, Gremse DA. Sunflower seed bezoar leading to fecal impaction. *South Med J* 1995;88:87–88.
29. Cordell GA, Araujo DE. Capsaicin: identification, nomenclature and pharmacotherapy. *Ann Pharmacother* 1993;27:330–331.
30. Don PC. Topical capsaicin for treatment of neuralgia associated with herpes zoster infection. *J Am Acad Dermatol* 1988;18:1135–1136.
31. Kurkcuoglu N, Alaybeyi F. Topical capsaicin for psoriasis. *Br J Dermatol* 1990;123:549–550.
32. Ross DR, Varepapa RJ. Treatment of painful diabetic neuropathy with topical capsaicin. *N Engl J Med* 1989;321:474–475.
33. Breneman DL, Cardose JS, Kaufmann PS, et al. Topical capsaicin for treatment of pruritus related to hemodialysis. *Clin Pharmacol Ther* 1989;45:188.
34. Weintraub M, Golik A, Rubio A. Capsicum for treatment of post-traumatic amputation stump pain. *Lancet* 1990;336:1003–1004.
35. Kakas JF Jr. Topical capsaicin induces cough in patients receiving ACE inhibitors. *Ann Allergy* 1990;65:322.
36. Blanc P, Liu D, Juarez C, et al. Cough in hot pepper workers. *Chest* 1991;99:27–32.
37. Tominack RL, Spyker DA. Capsicum and capsaicin—review: case report of the use of hot peppers in child abuse. *J Toxicol Clin Toxicol* 1987;25:591–601.
38. El-Mofty MM, Soliman AA, Abdel-Gawad AF, et al. Carcinogenicity testing of black pepper *(Piper nigrum)* using the Egyptian toad *(Bufo regularis)* as a quick biological test animal. *Oncology* 1988;45:247–252.
39. Myers BM, Smith JL, Graham DY. Effect of red pepper and black pepper on the stomach. *Am J Gastroenterol* 1987;82:211–214.
40. Williams SR, Clark RF, Dunford JW. Contact dermatitis associated with capsaicin. Hunan hand syndrome. *Ann Emerg Med* 1995;25:713–715.
41. Jones LA, Tandberg D, Troutman WG. Household treatment for "chili burns" of the hand. *J Toxicol Clin Toxicol* 1987;25:483–491.
42. Cohle SD, Trestrail JD III, Graham MA, et al. Fatal pepper aspiration. *Am J Dis Child* 1988;1242:633–636.
43. Sheahan K, Page DV, Kemper T, et al. Childhood sudden death secondary to accidental aspiration of black pepper. *Am J Forensic Med Pathol* 1988;9:51–57.
44. Roser D. Garlic. *Lancet* 1990;335:114–115.
45. Kleijnen J, Knipschild P, Ter Piet G. Garlic, onions and cardiovascular risk factors. A review of the evidence for human experiments with emphasis on commercially available preparations. *Br J Clin Pharmacol* 1989;28:535–544.
46. Bordia A. Effect of garlic on blood lipids in patients with coronary heart disease. *Am J Clin Nutr* 1991;34:2100–2103.
47. Ariga T, Oshiba S, Tamad T. Platelet aggregation inhibition in garlic. *Lancet* 1981;1:150–151.
48. Lybarger JA, Gallagher JS, Pulver DW, et al. Occupational asthma induced by inhalation and ingestion of garlic. *J Allergy Clin Immunol* 1982;69:948–957.
49. Lachter J, Babich JP, Brookman JC, et al. Garlic: a way out of work. *Medicine* 2003;168:499–500.
50. Feng PC, Patrick SJ. Studies of the action of Hypoglycin-A, an hypoglycaemic substance. *Br J Pharmacol* 1958;13:125–130.
51. Bressler R. The unripe ackee: forbidden fruit. *N Engl J Med* 1976;295:500–501.
52. Tanaka K. Jamaican vomiting sickness. *N Engl J Med* 1976;295:461–467.
53. CDC. Toxic hypoglycemic syndrome—Jamaica 1989–1991. *MMWR Morb Mortal Wkly Rep* 1992;41:53–55.
54. Persaud TVN. Foetal abnormalities caused by the active principle of the fruit of *Blighia sapida* (ackee). *West Indian Med J* 1967;16:193–197.
55. Golding J, Foster-Williams K, Coard K, et al. A cluster of central nervous system defects in Jamaica. *Hum Exp Toxicol* 1990;9:13–16.
56. Pickwell SM, Schimelpfening S, Palinkas LA. "Betelmania." Betel quid chewing by Cambodian women in the United States and its potential health effects. *West J Med* 1994;160:326–330.
57. Anonymous. Mangla betel nut warning. *Lancet* 1993;341:810–819.
58. Chu NS. Cardiovascular responses to betel chewing. *J Formosa Med Assoc* 1993;92:835–837.
59. Deng JF, Ger J, Tsai WJ, et al. Acute toxicities of betel nut: rare but probably overlooked events. *J Toxicol Clin Toxicol* 2001;39:355–360.
60. Chu NS. Effects of betel chewing on electroencephalographic activity: spectral analysis and topographic mapping. *J Formosa Med Assoc* 1994;93:167–169.
61. Ashby J, Styles JA, Boyland E. Betel nuts, arecaidine, and oral cancer. *Lancet* 1979;1:112.

62. Wiesner DM. Betel-nut withdrawal. *Med J Aust* 1987;146:453.
63. Georgiou M, Siandidou L, Hatzis T, et al. Hepatotoxicity due to *Atractylis gummifera* L. *J Toxicol Clin Toxicol* 1988;26:487–493.
64. Nogue S, Sanz P, Botey A, et al. Insuffisance renale aigue due a une intoxication par le chardona glu *(Atractylis gummifera). Presse Medicale* 1992;21:130.
65. de Stefani E, Munoz N, Esteve J, et al. Maté drinking, alcohol, tobacco, diet and esophageal cancer in Uruguay. *Cancer Res* 1990;5:426–431.
66. Arnold WN. Vincent van Gogh and the thujone connection. *JAMA* 1988;260:3042–3044.
67. Arnold WN. Absinthe. *Sci Am* 1989;260:112–117.
68. Milne ST, Meek PD. Fatal colchicine overdose: report of a case and review of the literature. *Am J Emerg Med* 1998;16:603–608.
69. Danel VC, Wiart JD, Hardy GA, et al. Self-poisoning with *Colchicum autumnale* L. flowers. *J Toxicol Clin Toxicol* 2001;39:409–411.
70. Klintschar M, Beham-Schmidt C, Radner H, et al. Colchicine poisoning by accidental ingestion of meadow saffron (*Colchicum autumnale*): pathological and medicolegal aspects. *Forensic Sci Int* 1999;106:191–200.
71. Katz R, Chuang LC, Sutton JD. Use of granulocyte colony-stimulating factor in the treatment of pancytopenia secondary to colchicine overdose. *Ann Pharmacother* 1992;26:1087–1088.
72. Holzbecher MD, Moss MA, Ellenberger HA. The cyanide content of laetrile preparations, apricot, peach and apple seeds. *J Toxicol Clin Toxicol* 1984;22:345.
73. Shragg TA, Albertson TE, Fisher CJ. Cyanide poisoning after bitter almond ingestion. *West J Med* 1982;136:65–69.
74. Osuntokun RO, Durooju JE, McFarlane WJ. Plasma aminoacids in the Nigeria nutritional ataxic neuropathy. *BMJ* 1968;3:647–649.
75. Howlett WP, Brubaker GR, Mlingi N, et al. Konzo, an epidemic upper motor neuron disease studied in Tanzania. *Brain* 1990;113:223–235.
76. Rauws AG, Olling M, Timmerman A. The pharmacokinetics of amygdalin. *Arch Toxicol* 1982;49:311–319.
77. Moertel CG, Ames MM, Kovach JS, et al. A pharmacologic and toxicological study of amygdalin. *JAMA* 1981;245:591–594.
78. Sadoff L, Fuchs K, Hollander J. Rapid death associated with laetrile ingestion. *JAMA* 1978;239:1582.
79. Humbert JR, Tress JH, Braico KT. Fatal cyanide poisoning. Accidental ingestion of amygdalin. *JAMA* 1977;238:482.
80. Townsend WA, Boni B. Cyanide poisoning from ingestion of apricot kernels. *MMWR Morb Mortal Wkly Rep* 1975;24:427.
81. Rubino MJ, Davidoff F. Cyanide poisoning from apricot seeds. *JAMA* 1979;241:359.
82. Sayre JW, Kaymakcalan S. Cyanide poisoning of apricot seeds among children in central Turkey. *N Engl J Med* 1964;270:1113–1115.
83. Smith FP, Butler TP, Cohan S, et al. Laetrile toxicity: a report of two cases. *JAMA* 1977;238:1361.
84. Suchard JR, Wallace KL, Gerkin RD. Acute cyanide toxicity caused by apricot kernel ingestion. *Ann Emerg Med* 1998;32:742–744.
85. Hasler J, Lee S. Acute hemolytic anemia after ingestion of fava beans. *Am J Emerg Med* 1992;11:560–561.
86. Spencer PS. Guam ALS/parkinsonism—dementia. A long-lasting neurotoxic disorder caused by "slow toxin(s)" in food? *Can J Neurol Sci* 1987;14:347–357.
87. Duncan MW, Kopin IJ, Garruto MM, et al. 2-Amino-3-(methylamino) propionic acid in cycad-derived form is an unlikely cause of amyotrophic lateral sclerosis/parkinsonism. *Lancet* 1988;2:631–632.
88. Duncan MW, Steele JC, Kapin IJ, et al. 2-Amino-3-(methylamino) propionic acid (BMAA) in cycad flour: an unlikely cause of amyotrophic lateral sclerosis and parkinsonism—dementia (ALS-PD) of Guam. *Neurology* 1990;40:767–772.
89. Hall WTK. Cycad (*Zamia*) poisoning in Australia. *Aust Vet J* 1987;64:149–150.
90. Wu D. An overview of the clinical pharmacology and therapeutic potential of gossypol as a male contraceptive agent and in gynaecological disease. *Drugs* 1989;38:333–341.
91. Fogh A, Kulling P, Wichstrom E. Veratrum alkaloids in sneezing powder. A potential danger. *J Toxicol Clin Toxicol* 1983;20:175–179.
92. Spoerke DG, Spoerke SE. Three cases of *Zigadenus* (death camus) poisoning. *Vet Hum Toxicol* 1979;21:346–347.
93. Mitchell MI, Rutledge PA. Hemlock water dropwort poisoning. A review. *J Toxicol Clin Toxicol* 1978;12:417–426.
94. Starreveld E, Hope CE. Cicutoxin poisoning (water hemlock). *Neurology* 1975;25:730–734.
95. Miller MM. Water hemlock poisoning. *JAMA* 1933;101:852–853.
96. Landers D, Seppi K, Blauer W. Seizures and death on a White River float trip. Report of water hemlock poisoning. *West J Med* 1985;142:637–640.
97. Carlton BE, Tufts D, Girard DE. Water hemlock poisoning complicated by rhabdomyolysis and renal failure. *J Toxicol Clin Toxicol* 1979;14:87–93.
98. King LA, Lewis MJ, Parry D. Identification of ownanthotoxin and related compounds in hemlock water dropwort poisoning. *Hum Toxicol* 1985;4:355–364.
99. Nightingale SL. Public warning about herbal product "chaparral." *JAMA* 1993;269:328.
100. CDC. Chapparal-induced toxic hepatitis in California and Texas 1992. *MMWR Morb Mortal Wkly Rep* 1992;41:812–814.
101. Ridker PM, McDermott WW. Comfrey herb tea and hepatic occlusive disease. *Lancet* 1989;1:657–658.
102. Roulet M, Laurini R, Rivier L, et al. Hepatic veno-occlusive disease in newborn infant of a woman drinking herbal tea. *J Pediatr* 1988;112:433–436.
103. Abbott PJ. Comfrey: assessing the low-dose health risk. *Med J Aust* 1988;149:678–682.
104. Huxtable RJ. Activation and pulmonary toxicity of pyrrolizidine alkaloids. *Pharmacol Ther* 1990;47:371–389.
105. Mohabbat O, Younos MS, Merzad AA, et al. An outbreak of hepatic veno-occlusive disease in northwestern Afghanistan. *Lancet* 1976;2271–2272.
106. Cui J, Garle M, Eneroth P, et al. What do commercial ginseng preparations contain? *Lancet* 1994;344:134.
107. Koren G, Randor S, Martin S, et al. Maternal ginseng use associated with neonatal androgenization. *JAMA* 1990;264:2866.
108. Siegel RK. Ginseng and high blood pressure. *JAMA* 1980;243:32.
109. Ryu SJ, Shien YY. Ginseng-associated cerebral arteritis. *Neurology* 1995;45:829–830.
110. Siegel RK. Ginseng abuse syndrome: problems with the panacea. *JAMA* 1979;241:1614–1615.
111. Jacobs MR, Hornfeldt CS. Melalueca oil poisoning. *J Toxicol Clin Toxicol* 1994;32:461–464.
112. Spoerke DG, Vandenberg S, Smolinske S, et al. Eucalyptus oil. 14 cases of exposure. *Vet Hum Toxicol* 1989;31:166–168.
113. Mack RD. Fair dinkum roala kruisine—eucalyptus oil poisoning. *N C Med J* 1988;49:599–600.
114. Patel S, Wiggins J. Eucalyptus oil poisoning. *Arch Dis Child* 1980;55:405.
115. Grande GA, Dannewitz SR. Symptomatic sassafras oil ingestion. *Vet Hum Toxicol* 1987;29:463.
116. Haines JD Jr. Sassafras tea and diaphoresis. *Postgrad Med* 1991;9:75–76.
117. Sparks T. Cinnamon oil burn. *West J Med* 1985;142:835.
118. Pilapil VR. Toxic manifestations of cinnamon oil ingestion in a child. *Clin Pediatr* 1989;28:276.
119. Perry PA, Dean BS, Krenzelok EP. Cinnamon oil abuse by adolescents. *Vet Hum Toxicol* 1990;32:162–163.
120. Mant AK. Association proceedings. VI. A case of poisoning by oil of citronella. *Med Sci Law* 1961;112:170–171.
121. Hartnoll G, Moore D, Douek D. Near fatal ingestion of oil of cloves. *Arch Dis Child* 1993;69:392–393.
122. Lane BW, Ellenhorn MJ, Vulbert TV, et al. Clove oil ingestion in an infant. *Hum Exp Toxicol* 1991;10:291–294.
123. Sullivan JB Jr, Rumack BH, Thomas H Jr, et al. Pennyroyal oil poisoning and hepatotoxicity. *JAMA* 1979;242:2873–2874.
124. Vallance WB. Pennyroyal poisoning: a fatal case. *Lancet* 1955;2:850–851.
125. Early DF. Pennyroyal: a rare cause of epilepsy. *Lancet* 1961;2:580–581.
126. Bakerink JA, Gospe SM Jr, Dimand RJ, et al. Multiple organ failure after ingestion of pennyroyal oil from herbal tea in two infants. *Pediatrics* 1996;98:944–947.
127. Murphy JJ, Heptinstall S, Mitchell JRA. Randomized double-blind placebo-controlled trial of feverfew in migraine prevention. *Lancet* 1988;2:189–192.
128. Baldwin CA, Anderson LP, Phillipson JD. What pharmacists should know about feverfew. *Pharm J* 1987;239:237–238.
129. Brayley J, Jones J. Life-threatening hypokalemia associated with excessive licorice ingestion. *Am J Psychiatry* 1994;151:617–618.
130. Woolf A. Licorice root poisoning. *Clin Toxicol Rev* 1994;16:1–2.
131. Damayanthi Y, Lown JW. Podophyllotoxins: current status and recent developments. *Curr Med Chem* 1998;5:205–252.
132. Gruber M. *Podophyllum* versus podophyllin. *J Am Acad Dermatol* 1984;10:302–303.
133. Tosenstein G, Tosenstein H, Freeman M, et al. *Podophyllum*, a dangerous laxative. *Pediatrics* 1976;57:419–421.
134. Sullivan M, Follis RH, Hilgartner M. Toxicology of podophyllin. *Proc Soc Exp Biol Med* 1951;77:269–272.
135. Clark ANG, Parosonabe MJ. A case of *Podophyllum* poisoning with involvement of the nervous system. *BMJ* 1957;2:1155–1157.
136. Cassidy DE, Drewry J, Fanning JP. *Podophyllum* toxicity: a report of a fatal case and a review of the literature. *J Toxicol Clin Toxicol* 1982;19:35–44.
137. Moher LM, Mauer SA. *Podophyllum* toxicity. Case report and literature review. *J Fam Pract* 1979;9:237–240.
138. Rate RG, Leche J, Chervenak C. Podophyllin toxicity. *Ann Intern Med* 1979;90:723.
139. Powell LC. *Condyloma acuminatum*. *Clin Obstet Gynecol* 1972;15:948.
140. Campbell AN. Accidental poisoning with podophyllin. *Lancet* 1985;11:206–207.
141. But PP, Tomlinson B, Cheung KO, et al. Adulterants of herbal products can cause poisoning. *BMJ* 1996;313:117.
142. Dobb GJ, Edis RH. Coma and neuropathy after ingestion of herbal laxative containing podophyllin. *Med J Aust* 1984;140:495–496.
143. Holdright DR, Jahangiri M. Accidental poisoning with podophyllin. *Hum Exp Toxicol* 1990;9:55–56.
144. McFarland MF, MacFarland J. Accidental ingestion of *Podophyllum*. *J Toxicol Clin Toxicol* 1981;18:973–977.
145. Balucani M, Zellers PD. *Podophyllum* resin poisoning with complete recovery. *JAMA* 1964;189:639.
146. Stoehr GP, Peterson AL, Taylor WJ. Systemic complications of local podophyllin therapy. *Ann Intern Med* 1978;89:362–363.
147. Mack RB. Living mortals run mad. Mandrake (*Podophyllum*) poisoning. *N C Med J* 1992;53:98–99.

148. Nicotine poisoning after ingestion of contaminated ground beef—Michigan, 2003. *MMWR Morb Mortal Wkly Rep* 2003;52:413–416.
149. Garcia-Estrada H, Fischman CM. An unusual case of nicotine poisoning. *J Toxicol Clin Toxicol* 1977;10:391–393.
150. Malizia E, Andreucci G, Alfani F, et al. Acute intoxication with nicotine alkaloids and cannabinoids in children from ingestion of cigarettes. *Hum Toxicol* 1983;2:315–316.
151. Gyllensward A, Nordbring F. Tobacco poisoning with sino-auricular block. *Acta Paediatr* 1953;42:356–359.
152. Woolf A, Burkhart K, Caraccio T, et al. Childhood poisoning involving transdermal nicotine patches. *Pediatrics* 1997;99:E4.
153. Armitage AK, Dollery CT, George CF, et al. Absorption and metabolism of nicotine from cigarettes. *BMJ* 1975;4:313–316.
154. McGuigan MA. Nicotine. *Clin Toxicol Rev* 1982;4:1–2.
155. Moore HW. Poison case report of the month. Acute nicotine poisoning. *SC Med Assoc J* 1962;58:445.
156. McNally WD. A report of seven cases of nicotine poisoning. *J Lab Clin Med* 1922;8:83–85.
157. Rosenburg J, Benowitz NL, Jacob P, et al. Disposition kinetics and effects of intravenous nicotine. *Clin Pharmacol Ther* 1980;28:517–520.
158. Keller RF, Crowe MW. Congenital deformities in swine induced by wild tree tobacco, *Nicotiana glauca*. *J Toxicol Clin Toxicol* 1983;20:47–58.
159. Oberst BB, McIntyre RA. Acute nicotine poisoning. *Pediatrics* 1953;11:338–340.
160. Manoguerra AS, Freeman D. Acute poisoning from the ingestion of *Nicotiana glauca*. *J Toxicol Clin Toxicol* 1982–1983;19:861–864.
161. Shaw RF. *A fatality involving anabasine.* (Abstract) California Association of Toxicologists Annual Meeting, Feb 2, 1985. Reported in CAT Newsletter, Spring 1985.
162. Ghelback SH, Wiliams WA, Perry LD, et al. Green tobacco sickness. An illness of tobacco harvesters. *JAMA* 1974;229:1880–1883.
163. Steenkamp PA, van Heerden FR, van Wyk BE. Accidental fatal poisoning by *Nicotiana glauca*: identification of anabasine by high performance liquid chromatography/photodiode array/mass spectrometry. *Forensic Sci Int* 2002;127:208–217.
164. Lewis WH, Smith PR. Pokeroot herbal tea poisoning. *JAMA* 1979;242:2759–2760.
165. Callahan R. Plant poisonings—New Jersey. *MMWR Morb Mortal Wkly Rep* 1981;30:65.
166. Waxdal MJ. Isolation, characterization and biological activities of five mitogens from pokeweed. *Biochemistry* 1974;18:3671–3676.
167. Barker BE, Parnes P, La Marche. Peripheral blood plasmacytosis following systemic exposure to *Phytolacca americana* (pokeweed). *Pediatrics* 1966;38:490–493.
168. Kingsbury JM. *Poisonous plants of the United States and Canada*. Englewood, NJ: Prentice-Hall, 1964:33.
169. Jaeckle KA, Freeman FR. Pokeweed poisoning. *South Med J* 1981;5:639–640.
170. Hardin JW, Arena JM. Human *Poisoning from native and cultivated plants*, 2nd ed. Durham, NC: Duke University Press, 1974:74.
171. Edwards N, Rogers G. Pokeberry pancake breakfast or it's gonna be a great day. *Vet Hum Toxicol* 1982;24[Suppl]:135–137.
172. Hamilton RJ, Shih RD, Hoffman RS. Mobitz type I heart block after pokeweed ingestion. *Vet Hum Toxicol* 1995;37:66–67.
173. Weintraub S. Stramonium poisoning. *Postgrad Med* 1960;28:364–367.
174. Brown JK, Malone MH. "Legal highs"—constituents, activity, toxicology, and herbal folk lore. *J Toxicol Clin Toxicol* 1978;12:1–31.
175. Wellman KE. North American Indian rock art and hallucinogenic drugs. *JAMA* 1978;239:1524–1527.
176. Rush B. An account of the effects of the stramonium or thorn apple. *Clin Pediatr* 1973;12:50–53.
177. Moore DW. The autumnal high: jimson weed in North Carolina. *N C Med J* 1976;37:492–494.
178. Klein-Schwartz W, Oderda GM. Jimsonweed intoxication in adolescents and young adults. *Am J Dis Child* 1984;138:737–739.
179. Belton PA, Gibbons DO. *Datura* intoxication in West Cornwall. *BMJ* 1979;1:585–586.
180. Hudson MJ. Acute atropine poisoning from ingestion of *Datura rosei*. *N Z Med J* 1973;77:245–248.
181. Urich RW, Bowerman DL, Levisky JA. *Datura stramonium*: a fatal poisoning. *J Forensic Sci* 1982;27:948–954.
182. Hall RW, Popkin MK, McHenry LE. Angel's trumpet psychosis: a central nervous system anticholinergic syndrome. *Am J Psychiatry* 1977;134:312–314.
183. Gowdy JM. Stramonium intoxication: a review of symptomatology in 212 cases. *JAMA* 1972;221:585–587.
184. Hayman HJ. *Datura* poisoning. The angel's trumpet. *Pathology* 1985;17:465–466.
185. Mikolich JR, Paulson GW, Cross CJ. Acute anticholinergic syndrome due to jimson weed ingestion. Clinical and laboratory observation in six cases. *Ann Intern Med* 1975;83:321–325.
186. Rosen CS, Lechner M. Jimson weed intoxication. *N Engl J Med* 1967;267:448–450.
187. Johnson RT. Jimson weed toxicity. *Clin Med* 1977;84:14–15.
188. Blattner RJ. Jimson weed poisoning. Stramonium intoxication. *J Pediatr* 1962;61:941–943.
189. Thompson HS. Cornpicker's pupil: jimson weed mydriasis. *J Iowa Med Soc* 1971;61:475–478.
190. Savitt DL, Robets JR, Siegel EG. Anisocoria from jimson weed. *JAMA* 1986;255:1439–1440.
191. Trabattoni G, Visintini D, Terzano GM, et al. Accidental poisoning with deadly nightshade berries. A case report. *Hum Toxicol* 1984;3:513–516.
192. Vlachos P, Poulos L. A case of mandrake poisoning. *J Toxicol Clin Toxicol* 1982;19:521–522.
193. Namera A, Yashiki M, Hirose Y, et al. Quantitative analysis of tropane alkaloids in biological materials by gas chromatography-mass spectrometry. *Forensic Sci Int* 2002;130:34–43.
194. Levy R. Jimson weed poisoning. *Ann Intern Med* 1976;84:223.
195. Ober WB. Did Socrates die of hemlock poisoning? *N Y State J Med* 1977;77:254–258.
196. Keeler RF, Balls LD. Teratogenic effects in cattle of *Conium maculatum* and *Conium* alkaloids and analogs. *J Toxicol Clin Toxicol* 1978;12:49–64.
197. Panter KE, James LF, Gardner DR. Lupines, poison-hemlock and *Nicotiana* spp: toxicity and teratogenicity in livestock. *J Nat Toxins* 199;8:117–134.
198. Rizzi D, Basile C, Di Maggio A, et al. Clinical spectrum of accidental hemlock poisoning: neurotoxic manifestations, rhabdomyolysis and acute tubular necrosis. *Nephrol Dial Transplant* 1991;6;939–943.
199. Mitchell J, Weller RO, Evans H, et al. Buckthorn neuropathy. Effects of intraneural injection of *Karwinskia humboldtiana* toxins. *Neuropathol Appl Neurobiol* 1978;4:85–97.
200. Calderon-Gonzalez R, Rizzi-Hernandez H. Buckthorn polyneuropathy. *N Engl J Med* 1967;277:69–71.
201. Martinez HR, Bermudez MV, Rangel-Guerra RA, et al. Clinical diagnosis in *Karwinskia humboldtiana* polyneuropathy. *J Neurol Sci* 1998;154:49–54.
202. Szaufer M, Kowalewski Z. Chelidonine from *Symphoricarpos albus*. *Phytochemistry* 1978;17:1446–1447.
203. Lewis WH. Snowberry (*Symphoricarpos*) poisoning in children. *JAMA* 1979;242:2663.
204. Lamminpaa A, Kinos M. Plant poisonings in children. *Hum Exp Toxicol* 1996;15:245–249.
205. Amyot TE. Poisoning by snowberries. *BMJ* 1885;1:986.
206. Rugman F, Melchan J, Edmondson J. *Mercurialis perennis* (dog's mercury) poisoning. A case of mistaken identity. *BMJ* 1983;287:1924.
207. Bacon AE. An experiment with the fruit of red baneberry. *Rhodora* 1903;5:77–79.
208. Couch JF. Tremetol, the compound that produced "trembles" (milk sickness). *J Am Chem Soc* 1929;51:3617.
209. Zalkow LH, Burke H, Cabot G, et al. Toxic constituents of rayless goldenrod. *J Med Pharm Chem* 1962;5:1342.
210. Bonner WA, DeGraw JI. Ketones from "white snakeroot" *Eupatorium urticaefolium*. *Tetrahedron* 1962;18:1295.
211. Beier RC, Norman JO, Irvin TR, et al. Microsomal activation of constituents of white snakeroot (*Eupatorium rugosum* Houtt) to form toxic products. *Am J Vet Res* 1987;48:583–585.
212. von Malottki K, Wiechmann HW. Acute life-threatening bradycardia: food poisoning by Turkish wild honey. *Dtsch Med Wochenschr* 1996;121:936–938.
213. Meier KH, Hemmich RS. Bradycardia and complete heart block after ingestion of rhododendron tea. *Vet Hum Toxicol* 1992;34:351.
214. Yavuz H, Ozel A, Akkus I, et al. Honey poisoning in Turkey. *Lancet* 1991;337:789–790.
215. Kirtikar, KR. The poisonous plants of Bombay. *J Bombay Natural Hist Soc* 1897;11:251–261.
216. Karawya MS, Balbaa SI, Khayyal SE. Estimation of cardenolides in *Nerium oleander*. *Planta Med* 1973; 23:70–73.
217. Osterloh J, Harold S, Pond S. Oleander interference in the digoxin radioimmunoassay in a fatal ingestion. *JAMA* 1982;247:1596–1597.
218. Chin D, Wei-liang C. Auricular tachycardia with auriculo-ventricular block in oleander leaf poisoning. *Chin Med J* 1957;75:74–77.
219. Spevak L. Dva slucaja trovanja cajem od oleanderrovog lisca. *Arh Hig Rada* 1975;26:147–150.
220. Tracqui A, Kintz P, Branche F, et al. Confirmation of oleander poisoning by HPLC/MS. *Int J Legal Med* 1998;111:32–34.
221. Khasigian P, Everson G, Bellinghausen R, et al. Poisoning following oleander smoke inhalation. *J Toxicol Clin Toxicol* 1998;36:456–457(abst).
222. Graeme KA, LoVecchio FA, Selden BS, et al. Cardiotoxicity from ingestion of unprocessed *Nerium oleander* leaves treated with FAB fragments. *J Toxicol Clin Toxicol* 1998;36:457(abst).
223. Haynes BE, Bessen HA, Wightman WD, et al. Oleander tea: herbal draught of death. *Ann Emerg Med* 1985;14:350–353.
224. Romano GA, Mombelli G. Intoxikation mit oleanderblattern. *Schweiz Med Wschr* 1990;120:596–597.
225. Gupta A, Joshi P, Jortani SA, et al. A case of nondigitalis cardiac glycoside toxicity. *Ther Drug Monitor* 1997;19:711–714.
226. Nickel SL, Staba EJ. Suitability of antidigoxin antiserum for digoxin in plant extracts. *Lloydia* 1977;40:230–235.
227. Tampion J. *Dangerous plants*. New York: Universe Books, 1977.
228. Chopra RN, Mukerjee B. The pharmacological action of "thevetin"—a glucoside occurring in *Thevetia neriifolia* (yellow oleander). *Ind J Med Res* 1933;20:903–912.
229. Oji O, Okafor QE. Toxicological studies on stem bark, leaf and seed kernel of yellow oleander (*Thevetia peruviana*). *Phytother Res* 2000;14:133–135.
230. Oji O, Madubuike FN, Ojimelukwe PC, et al. Rodenticide potential of *Thevetia peruviana*. *J Herbs Spices Medicinal Plants* 1994;2:3.

231. Pahwa R, Chatterjee VC. The toxicity of yellow oleander (*Thevetia neriifolia juss*) see kernels to rats. *Vet Hum Toxicol* 1990;32:561–564.
232. Morton J. *Plants poisonous to people in Florida and other warm areas*. Miami: Hurricane House, 1971.
233. Eddleston M, Warrell DA. Management of acute yellow oleander poisoning. *Q J Med* 1999;92:483–485.
234. Eddleston M, Ariaratnam CA, Meyer WP, et al. Epidemic of self-poisoning with seeds of the yellow oleander tree (*Thevetia peruviana*) in northern Sri Lanka. *Trop Med Int Health* 1999;4:266–273.
235. Saraswat DK, Garg PK, Saraswat M. Rare poisoning with cerebra *Thevetia* (yellow oleander). Review of 13 cases of suicidal attempt. *J Assoc Physicians India* 1992;40:628–629.
236. Abe F, Yamauchi T, Nohara T. C-nor-d-homo-cardenolide glycosides from *Thevetia neriifolia*. *Phytochemistry* 1992;31:251–254.
237. Thilagar S, Thirumalaikolundusubramanian P, Gopalakrishnan S, et al. Possible yellow oleander toxicity in a neonate. *Indian Pediatr* 1986;23:393.
238. Kyerematen G, Hagos M, Weeratunga G, et al. The cardiac glycosides of *Thevetia ovata* A.DC. and *Thevetia nereifolia* juss. ex Stend. *Acta Pharm Suec* 1985;22:37–44.
239. Ahlawat SK, Agarwal AK, Wadhwa S. Rare poisoning with cerebra *Thevetia* (yellow oleander): a report of three cases. *Trop Doc* 1994;24:37–38.
240. Langford SD, Boor PJ. Oleander toxicity: an examination of human and animal toxic exposures. *Toxicol* 1996;109:1–13.
241. Ansford AJ, Morris H. Fatal oleander poisoning. *Med J Aust* 1981;1:360–361.
242. Seawright AA. Cardiac glycosides. In: *Animal health in Australia. Vol. 2. Chemical and plant poisons*. Canberra, Australia: Australian Govt Publ Service, 1982:19–21.
243. Arnold HL, Middleton WS, Chen KK. The action of thevetin, a cardiac glucoside, and its clinical application. *Am J Med Sci* 1935;189:193–206.
244. Middleton WS, Chen KK. Clinical results from oral administration of thevetin, a cardiac glucoside. *Am Heart J* 1936;11:75–88.
245. Saravanapavananthan N, Ganeshamoorthy J. Yellow oleander poisoning—a study of 170 cases. *Forensic Sci Int* 1988;26:247–250.
246. Bhattacharya SK, Somani PN, Srivastava PK. Cardiac changes in *Thevetia nerifolia* poisoning. *Acta Cardiol* 1976;31:169–174.
247. Kakrani AL, Rajput CS, Khandare SK, et al. Yellow oleander seed poisoning with cardiotoxicity. A case report. *Indian Heart J* 1981;33:31–33.
248. Bose TK, Basu RK, Biswas B, et al. Cardiovascular effects of yellow oleander ingestion. *J Ind Med Assoc* 1999;97:407–410.
249. Vince JD, Salamon B, Tan G, et al. Digoxin type toxicity from ingestion of *Thevetia peruviana* or the case of the betel nut that wasn't. *Papua New Guinea Med J* 1984;27:167–169.
250. Eddleston M, Ariaratnam CA, Sjostrom L, et al. Acute yellow oleander (*Thevetia peruviana*) poisoning: cardiac arrhythmias, electrolyte disturbances, and serum cardiac glycoside concentrations on presentation to hospital. *Heart* 2000;83:301–306.
251. Gopinath C, Ford EJH. The effect of *Lantana camara* on the liver of sheep. *J Path* 1969;9:75–85.
252. Sharma OP, Makkar HPS, Dawra R. A review of the noxious plant *Lantana camara*. *Toxicon* 1988;26:975–987.
253. Ghisalberti EL. *Lantana camara* l. (Verbenaceae). *Filoterapia* 2000;71:467–486.
254. Seawright AA. Cobalt ineffective against experimental *Lantana* poisoning. *Aust Vet J* 1963;39:249.
255. Wolfson SL, Solomons TWG. Poisoning by fruit of *Lantana camara*: an acute syndrome observed in children following ingestion of the green fruit. *Am J Dis Child* 1964;107:173.
256. Sharma OP, Makkar HPS, Pal RN, et al. Lantadene A content and toxicity of the lantana plant (*Lantanacamara* Linn.) to guinea pigs. *Toxicon* 1980;18:485–488.
257. Sharma OP. *Isolation and purification of* Lantana camara *toxins and their toxicity to guinea pigs*. 55th Annual Meeting of Society of Biological Chemists (India) held at Trivandrum, Dec 15–18, 1986.
258. Wilson CR, Sauer J, Hooser SB. Taxines: a review of the mechanism and toxicity of yew (*Taxus* spp.) alkaloids. *Toxicon* 2001;39:175–185.
259. Schulte T. Lethal intoxication with leaves of the yew tree (*Taxus baccata*). *Arch Toxicol* 1975;34:153–158.
260. Cummins RO, Haulman J, Quan L, et al. Near-fatal yew berry intoxication treated with external cardiac pacing and digoxin-specific FAB antibody fragments. *Ann Emerg Med* 1990;19:38–43.
261. Sinn LE, Porterfield JF. Fatal taxine poisoning from yew leaf ingestion. *J Forensic Sci* 1991;36:599–601.
262. Krenzelok EP, Jacobsen TD, Aronis J. Is the yew really poisonous to you? *J Toxicol Clin Toxicol* 1998;36:219–223.
263. Frohne D, Pfander HJ. *A colour atlas of poisonous plants. A handbook for pharmacists, doctors, toxicologists, and biologists*. London: Wolfe Publishing Ltd., 1983.
264. Chan TYK. Aconitine poisoning: a global perspective. *Vet Hum Toxicol* 1994b;36:326–328.
265. Lewin L. *Die gifte in der weltgeschichte*. Berlin: J Springer, 1920:536.
266. Chan TYK, Tse LKK, Chan JCN, et al. Aconitine poisoning due to Chinese herbal medicines: a review. *Vet Hum Toxicol* 1994;36:452–455.
267. Chan TYK, Tomlinson B, Critchley JA. Aconitine poisoning following the ingestion of Chinese herbal medicines: a report of eight cases. *Aust N Z J Med* 1993;23:268–271.
268. Tai YT, But PP, Young K, et al. Adverse effects from traditional Chinese medicine [Letter]. *Lancet* 1993;341:892.
269. But PPH, Tai YT, Young K. Three fatal cases of herbal aconite poisoning. *Vet Hum Toxicol* 1994;36:212–215.
270. Budavari, ed. *The Merck index*, 11th ed. Rahway, New Jersey: Merck & Company, Inc., 1989.
271. Bentz H. *Nutztiervergiftungen*. Jena, Germany: Erkennung und Verhutung, G Fisch, 1969:361.
272. Fiddes FS. Poisoning by aconitine. A report of two cases. *BMJ* 1958;2:779–780.
273. Wang R, Chen YZ. Diterpenoid alkaloids of *Aconitum sungpanase*. *Planta Medica* 1987;53:544–546.
274. Arlandini E, Ballabio M, Gioia B, et al. N-deethylaconitine from *Aconitum napellus* ssp vulgare. *J Natl Prod* 1987;50:937–939.
275. Druckrey H. Todliche medizinale aconitin-vergiftung. *Samml Vergiftungsfallen* 1943;44;13:21–26.
276. Brugsch H. Vergiftungen im Kindesalter. Stuttgart, Germany: Ferdinand Enke, 1956:144–146.
277. Luo B, Kobayashi S, Kimura I, et al. Inhibitory effects on angiogenesis and pouch fluid exudation by aconite alkaloids in adjuvant-induced inflammation of the mouse. *Phytotherapy Res* 1991;5:231–233.
278. Wedd AM, Tenney SM. Effects of aconite on cold blooded heart. *Proc Soc Exp Biol Med* 1953;84:199–203.
279. Konno C, Murayama M, Sugiyama K, et al. Isolation and hypoglycemic activity of aconitans A, B, C, and D, glycans of *Aconitum carmichaeli* roots. *Planta Medica* 1985;51:160–163.
280. Mack R. Play it again, Voltaire—aconite (monkshood) poisoning. *N C Med J* 1985;46:518–519.
281. Tai YT, But PP, Young K, et al. Cardiotoxicity after accidental herb-induced aconite poisoning. *Lancet* 1992;340:1254–1256.
282. Tomlinson B, Chan TYK, Chan JCN, et al. Herb-induced aconitine poisoning. *Lancet* 1993;341:370–371.
283. Yi-gu Z, Guang-zhao H. Poisoning by toxic plants in China. Report of 19 autopsy cases. *Am J Forensic Med Pathol* 1988;9:313–319.
284. Felgenhauer N, Zilker T, Dorfmann N. Severe intoxication with aconitum. *J Toxicol Clin Toxicol* 1999;37:416(abst).
285. Deraemaeker C, DeSchuiteneer E, Goossens E, et al. Severe accidental aconitum poisoning: case report. *Przeglad Lekarski* 1995;52:213(abst).
286. Heistracher P, Pillat B. Electrophysiologische Untersuchungern uber die Wirkung von Chinidin auf die Aconitinvergiftung von Herzmuskelfasern. *Arch Exp Path Pharm* 1962;244:48.
287. Fitzpatrick AJ, Crawford M, Allan RM, et al. Aconite poisoning managed with a ventricular assist device. *Anaesth Intensive Care* 1994;22:714–717.
288. Lucchesi BR. The action of dichloroisoproterenol (DCI) and several other pharmacological agents upon the aconitine-induced ventricular arrhythmia in the isolated rabbit heart. *J Pharm Exp Ther* 1962;137:291.
289. Mladoveanu C, Vasilco O, Gheorghu P. Le sulfate de magnesium et le chlorure de calcium dans les intoxications experimentales ave de l'aconitine. *Arch Int Pharmcodyn* 1939;53:494.
290. Poy JY, Racle JP, Benkhadra A, et al. Intoxication par l'aconitine. Troubles du rythme cardiaque traites avec succes par la mexiletine. *Cah Anesthesiol* 1986;34:429–433.
291. Tai YT, Lau CP, But PP, et al. Bidirectional tachycardia induced by herbal aconite poisoning. *Pacing Clin Electrophysiol* 1992;15:831–839.
292. French G. Aconitine-induced cardiac arrhythmias. *Br Heart J* 1958;20:140.
293. Scherf D, Blumenfeld S, Taner D, et al. The effect of diphenylhydantoin (Dilantin) sodium on atrial flutter and fibrillation provoked by focal application of aconitine or delphinine. *Am Heart J* 1960:60:936–947.
294. Fuller TC, McClintock E. *Poisonous plants of California*. Berkeley, CA: University of California Press, 1986.
295. Lacassie E, Marquet P, Martin-Dupont S, et al. A non-fatal case of intoxication with foxglove, documented by means of liquid chromatography-electrospray-mass spectrometry. *J Forensic Sci* 2000;45:1154–1158.
296. LoVecchio F, Seby MV, Johnson D. Digitalis poisoning following the ingestion of an herbal dietary supplement. *J Toxicol Clin Toxicol* 1998;36:457.
297. Porter R, Schultz D, Robertson WO. Alternative medicine toxicity: digitalis poisoning! *J Toxicol Clin Toxicol* 1999;37:617.
298. Dickstein ES, Kunkel FW. Foxglove tea poisonings. *Am J Med* 1980;69:167–169.
299. Moxley RA, Schneider NR, Steinegger DH, et al. Apparent toxicosis associated with lily-of-the-valley (*Convallaria majalis*) ingestion in a dog. *J Am Vet Med Assoc* 1989;195:485–487.
300. Bruneton J. *Toxic plants. Dangerous to humans and animals*. Paris: Lavoisier Publishing, 1999.
301. Krenzelok EP, Jacobsen TD, Aronis JM. Lily-of-the-valley (*Convallaria majalis*) exposures: are the outcomes consistent with the reputation? *J Toxicol Clin Toxicol* 1996;34:601.
302. Haugen S, Bryne E, Falke M, et al. Grade I-II atrioventricular block following lily-of-the-valley (*Convallaria majalis*) intake: a report of three cases. *J Toxicol Clin Toxicol* 2001;39:303.
303. Weaver AL, Spittell JA. Lathyrism. *Mayo Clin Proc* 1964;39:485–489.
304. Lalich JJ, et al. Production of aortic rupture in turkey poults fed beta-aminopropionitrile. *Arch Path* 1957;64:643–648.
305. Cheeke PR, Shull LR. *Natural toxicants in feeds and poisonous plants*. Westport, CT: AVI Publishing Company, Inc., 1985.
306. Mehta T, Zarghami NS, Cusick PK, et al. Tissue distribution and metabolism of the *Lathyrus sativus* neurotoxin, L-3-oxalylamino-2-aminopropionic acid in the squirrel monkey. *J Neurochem* 1976;27:1327–1331.
307. Streifler M, Cohn PF. Chronic central nervous system toxicity of the chickling pea (*Lathyrus sativus*). *J Toxicol Clin Toxicol* 1985;18:1513–1517.

308. Paissios CS, Demopoulos T. Human lathyrism: a clinical and skeletal study. *Clin Orthop* 1982;23:236–249.
309. Spencer PS, Roy DN, Ludolph A, et al. Lathyrism: evidence for role of the neuroexcitatory aminoacid BOAA. *Lancet* 1986;2:1066–1067.
310. Krochmal A, Krochmal C. A guide to the medicinal plants of the United States. New York: Quadrange, New York Times Book Co., 1973.
311. Lewis W, Elvin-Lewis M. *Medical botany. Plants affecting man's health*. New York: Wiley & Sons, 1977.
312. Leung A. *Encyclopedia of common natural ingredients used in food, drugs, and cosmetics*. New York: Wiley & Sons, 1980.
313. Reynolds JEF, ed. *Martindale: The extra pharmacopoeia* (electronic version). Englewood, CO: Micromedex, Inc., 2000.
314. Blaw M, Adkisson M, Garriott J, et al. Poisoning with Carolina jessamine, *Gelsemium sempervirens* (L) Ait. *J Pediatr* 1979;94:998–1001.
315. Reference deleted.
316. Chestnut V. *Principal poisonous plants of the United States*. USDA, Division of Botany, Bulletin 20, 1898.
317. Perkins K, Payne W. *Guide to the poisonous and irritant plants of Florida*. Gainesville, FL: University of Florida, Circular 441, Cooperative Extension Service, Inst Food and Agric Sci, 1978.
318. Swan G. *An introduction to the alkaloids*. New York: Wiley & Sons, 1967.
319. Mack RB. Toxic encounters of the dangerous kind. *N C Med J* 1982;43:439.
320. Anon. The pharmacology of nutmeg. *Lawrence Rev Natl Prod* 1984;5:13–14.
321. Kalbhen DA. Nutmeg as a narcotic. *Angew Chem Internat Edit* 1971;10:370–374.
322. Lavy G. Nutmeg intoxication in pregnancy. A case report. *J Reprod Med* 1987;32:63–64.
323. Abernethy MK, Becker LB. Acute nutmeg intoxication. *Am J Emerg Med* 1992;10:429–430.
324. Venables GS, Evered D, Hall R. Nutmeg poisoning. *BMJ* 1976;1:96.
325. Truitt EB, Callaway E, Braude MC, et al. The pharmacology of myristicin: a contribution to the psychopharmacology of nutmeg. *J Neuropsych* 1961;2:205–210.
326. Cushny AR. Nutmeg poisoning. *Proc Royal Soc Med* 1908;1:39–44.
327. Painter JC, Shanor SP, Winek CL. Nutmeg poisoning—a case report. *J Toxicol Clin Toxicol* 1971;4:1–4.
328. Panayotopoulos DJ, Chisholm DD. Hallucinogenic effect of nutmeg. *BMJ* 1970;1:754.
329. Sangalli BC, Chiang W. Toxicology of nutmeg abuse. *J Toxicol Clin Toxicol* 2000;38:671–678.
330. Payne RB. Nutmeg intoxication. *N Engl J Med* 1963;269:36–38.
331. Brenner N, Frank OS, Knight E. Chronic nutmeg psychosis. *J Royal Soc Med* 1993;86:179–180.
332. Green RC. Nutmeg poisoning. *JAMA* 1959;171:1342–1344.
333. Shafran I. Nutmeg toxicology. *N Engl J Med* 1976;294:849.
334. Faguet RA, Rowland KF. Spice cabinet intoxication. *Am J Psychiatry* 1978;135:860–861.
335. Hentschel H, Greyer H, Stein U. Ingestion of nutmeg (*Myristica fragrans*). *J Toxicol Clin Toxicol* 2000;38:234(abst).
336. Kulberg A. Substance abuse: clinical identification and management. *Pediatr Clin North Am* 1986;33:325–361.
337. Duke JA. *CRC handbook of medicinal herbs*. Boca Raton, FL: CRC Press, 1985.
338. Aboul-Enein HY. Mescaline: a pharmacological profile. *Am J Pharm* 1973;145:125–128.
339. Demish L, Kaczmarczyk P, Seiler N. 3,4,5-Trimethoxybenzoic acid, a new mescaline metabolite in humans. *Drug Metab Dispos* 1978;6:507–509.
340. Charalampous KD, Walker KE, Kinross-Wright J. Metabolic fate of mescaline in man. *Psychopharmacology* 1966;9:48–63.
341. Gilmore HT. Peyote use during pregnancy. *South Dakota J Med* 2001;54:27–29.
342. Baselt RC. *Disposition of toxic drugs and chemicals in man*, 6th ed. Foster City, CA: Chemical Toxicology Institute, 2002:637–638.
343. Hofman A, Tscherter H. Isolierung von Lysergsaure-Alkaloiden aus der mexickanischen Zauberdroge Ololiuqui (Rivea Corymbosa L. Hallier F). *Experientia* 1960;46:414.
344. Der Marderosian A. Psychotomimetic indoles in the Convolvulaceae. *Am J Pharm* 1967;139:19–26.
345. Brown JK, Malone MH. "Legal highs"—constituents, activity, toxicology, and herbal folklore. *J Toxicol Clin Toxicol* 1978;12:1–31.
346. Ingram AL. Morning glory seed reaction. *JAMA* 1964;190:107–108.
347. Fink PJ, Goldman MJ, Lyons I. Morning glory seed psychosis. *Arch Gen Psychiatry* 1966;15:209–213.
348. Cohen S. Suicide following morning glory seed ingestion. *Am J Psychiatry* 1964;120:1024–1025.
349. Geisshusler S, Brenneisen R. The content of psychoactive phenylpropyl and phenylpentenylkhatamines in *Catha edulis* forsk of different origin. *J Ethnopharmacol* 1987;19:269–277.
350. Al-Meshal IA. Effect of (-)-cathinone, an active principle of *Catha edulis* forssk (khat) on plasma amino acid levels and other biochemical parameters in male Wistar rats. *Phytotherapy Res* 1988;2:63–66.
351. Kalix P. *Catha edulis*, a plant that has amphetamine effects. *Pharm World Sci* 1996;18:69–73.
352. Widler P, Mathys K, Brenneisen R, et al. Pharmacodynamics and pharmacokinetics of khat: a controlled study. *Clin Pharmacol Ther* 1994;55:556–562.
353. Brenneisen R, Geisshusler S, Schorno X. Metabolism of cathinone to (–)-norephedrine and (–)-norpseudoephrine. *J Pharm Pharmacol* 1986;38:298–300.
354. Maitai CK, Mugera GM. Excretion of the active principle of *Catha edulis* (Miraa) in human urine. *J Pharm Sci* 1975;64:702–703.
355. Kalix P. The pharmacology of khat. *Gen Pharmacol* 1984;15:179–187.
356. Jansson T, Kristiansson G, Qirbi A. Effect of khat on uteroplacental blood flow in awake, chronically catheterized late-pregnant guinea pigs. *J Ethnopharmacol* 1988;23:19–26.
357. Drake PH. Khat-chewing in the Near East. *Lancet* 1988;1:532–533.
358. Nencini P, Ahmed AM. Khat consumption: a pharmacological review. *Drug Alcohol Depend* 1989;23:19–29.
359. Nencini P, Ahmed A, Amiconi G, et al. Tolerance develops to sympathetic effects of khat in humans. *Pharmacology* 1984;28:150–154.
360. Giannini AJ, Miller NS, Turner CE. Treatment of khat addiction. *J Sub Abuse Treat* 1992;9:379–382.
361. Halbach H. Medical aspects of chewing khat leaves. *Bull World Health Org* 1972;47:21–29.
362. Charney DS, Heninger GR, Redmond DE. Yohimbine induced anxiety and increased noradrenergic function in humans: effects of diazepam and clonidine. *Life Sci* 1983;33:19–29.
363. Tyler VE. *The new honest herbal*. Philadelphia: Stickley Company, 1987.
364. Roberge RJ, McGuire SP, Krenzelok EP. Yohimbine as an antidote for clonidine overdose. *Am J Emerg Med* 1996;14:678–680.
365. Ingram CG. Some pharmacologic actions of yohimbine and chlorpromaeine in man. *Clin Pharm Ther* 1962;3:345–352.
366. Varkey S. Overdose of yohimbine [Letter]. *BMJ* 1992;304:548.
367. Linden CH, Vellman WP, Rumack B. Yohimbine: a new street drug. *Am Emerg Med* 1985;14:1002–1004.
368. Sandler B, Aronson P. Yohimbine-induced cutaneous drug eruption, progressive renal failure, and lupus-like syndrome. *Urology* 1993;41:343–345.
369. Guthrie SK, Hariharan M, Grunhaus LJ. Yohimbine bioavailability in humans. *Eur J Clin Pharmacol* 1990;39:409–411.
370. Owen JA, Nakatsu SL, Fenemore J, et al. The pharmacokinetics of yohimbine in man. *Eur J Pharmacol* 1987;32:577–582.
371. Sturgill MG, Grasing KW, Rosen RC, et al. Yohimbine elimination in normal volunteers is characterized by both one- and two-compartment behavior. *J Cardiovasc Pharmacol* 1997;29:697–703.
372. Shannon M, Neuman MI. Yohimbine. *Pediatr Emerg Care* 2000;16:49–50.
373. Bagheri H, Picault P, Schmitt L, et al. Pharmacokinetic study of yohimbine and its pharmacodynamic effects on salivary secretion in patients treated with tricyclic antidepressants. *Br J Clin Pharm* 1994;37:93–96.

CHAPTER 256

Mycotoxins and Toxigenic Fungi

Daniel L. Sudakin

AFLATOXIN B_1

Molecular weight:	**312.29 g/mol**
Normal or therapeutic levels:	**Not available**
Special concerns:	**Carcinogenesis, food safety, acute hepatic injury**
Target organs:	**Gastrointestinal tract and liver after acute exposure, hepatocellular carcinoma with chronic exposure**
Antidote:	**None**

T-2 TOXIN

Molecular weight:	**466.53 g/mol**
Normal or therapeutic levels:	**Not available**
Special concerns:	**Food safety, chemical warfare**
Target organs:	**Gastrointestinal tract and hematopoietic system after acute exposure**
Antidote:	**None**

Fungi are ubiquitous. In addition to their allergenic and infectious properties, certain fungi can produce mycotoxins. *Mycotoxins* are secondary products of fungal metabolism that can produce biologic effects in other organisms. Most historical accounts of human mycotoxicoses have followed ingestion. This chapter focuses on two clinically important mycotoxins: aflatoxins and trichothecenes.

AFLATOXINS

Overview

Aflatoxins are frequently detected as natural contaminants of food and other agricultural commodities. Food-borne exposure to aflatoxin B_1 (AFB_1) has been implicated in association with acute hepatic injury in humans as well as carcinogenesis. At least 18 structurally related variants have been identified, the most potent of which is AFB_1.

The major *Aspergillus* species of fungi that can produce aflatoxins are *Aspergillus flavus* and *Aspergillus parasiticus*, both of which are found worldwide. Some strains of *A. flavus* and *A. parasiticus* do not produce aflatoxin, and the presence of these species in food or feed does not necessarily imply aflatoxin contamination (1). *Aspergillus versicolor* is another toxigenic species that is commonly found indoors (2). It can produce sterigmatocystin (Fig. 1), a structural precursor to aflatoxin, which is less potent than AFB_1 (3). Sterigmatocystin has been detected on water-damaged building materials (4) but has not been detected in bioaerosols (5).

STANDARDS

The action level for AFB_1 in food in the United States is 20 parts per billion (ppb), and in milk it is 0.5 ppb as the less potent metabolite aflatoxin M_1 (AFM_1). The European Union is in the process of harmonizing limits and regulations for aflatoxins in human foods, with maximum admissible levels ranging from 2 to 15 ppb for cereals, nuts, and dried fruits (6). There are no regulatory standards for occupational exposure to aflatoxins.

TOXIC DOSE

Acute aflatoxicosis in children and adults has been associated with an estimated daily consumption of 2 to 6 mg of aflatoxin (7). Carcinogenic doses of AFB_1 and AFM_1 have not been established. AFB_1 can cross the placenta (8), but reproductive or teratogenic effects have not been reported in human studies.

Toxicokinetics and Toxicodynamics

The liver is the predominant site of metabolic transformation of AFB_1 (Fig. 2). Cytochrome P-450 3A4 and 1A2 catalyze the epoxidation of AFB_1 to a highly reactive intermediate AFB_1 exo-8,9-epoxide (9). This intermediate binds with high affinity to

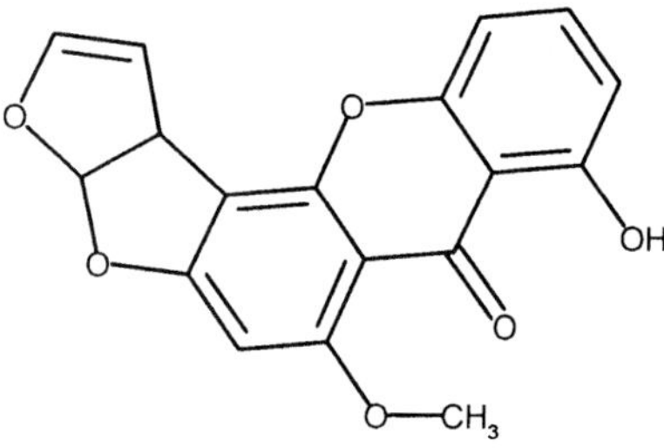

Figure 1. Sterigmatocystin.

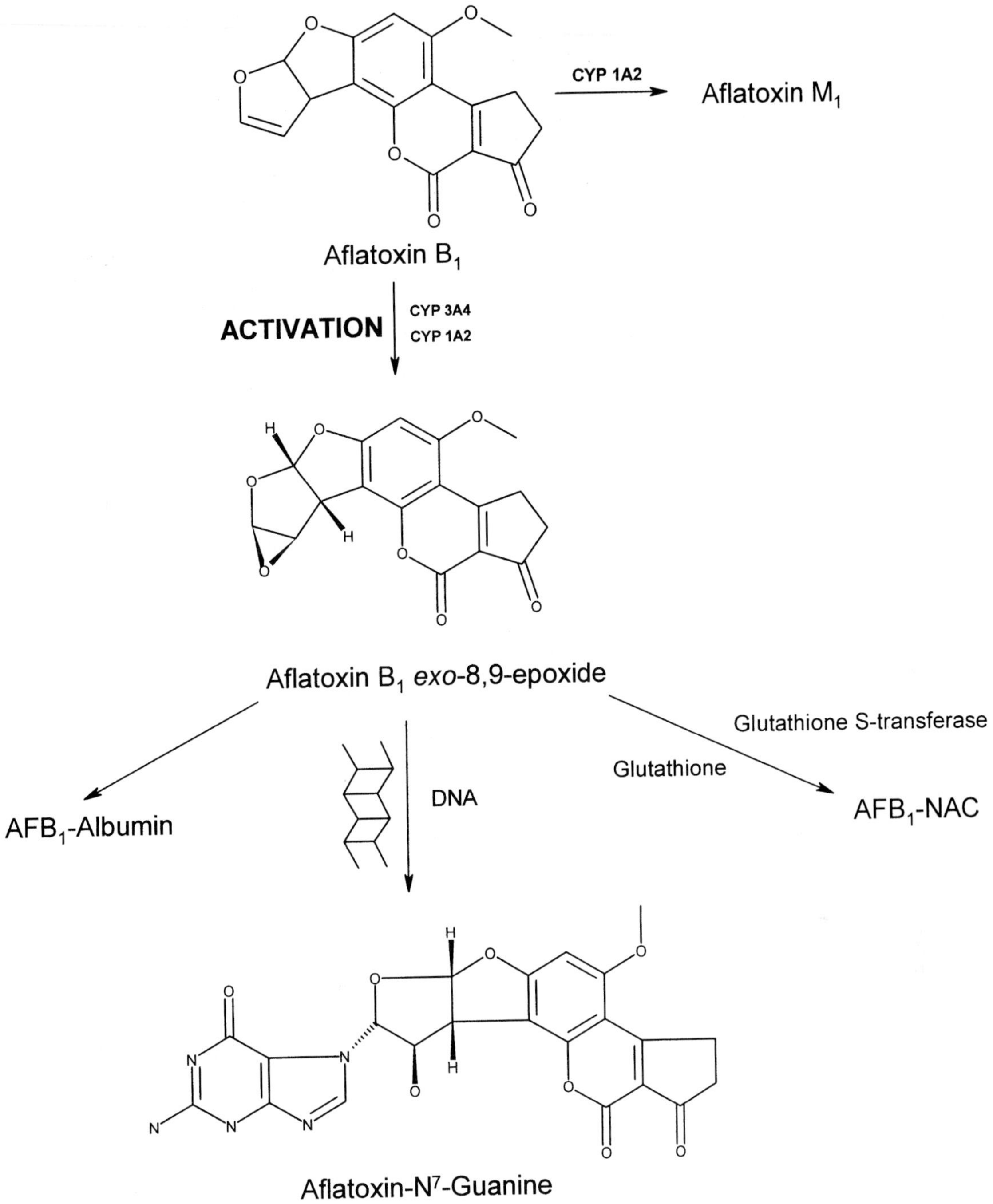

Figure 2. Metabolism and covalent binding of Aflatoxin B_1. AFB_1-NAC, aflatoxin B_1–mercapturic acid.

guanine bases in DNA to form guanyl-N^7 adducts (10). The epoxide may also form adducts to lysine residues in albumin (11) and other cellular proteins (12). Less than 5% of an ingested dose of AFB_1 binds to serum albumin (11,13). Detoxification pathways involve conjugation reactions of the reactive epoxide with glutathione (GSH) to form AFB_1–mercapturic acid, catalyzed by GSH-*S*-transferase (12). Cytochrome 1A2 can carry out other oxidation reactions to AFB_1, resulting in the conversion to AFM_1, which does not interact with DNA (9).

Toxicokinetic parameters of AFB_1 have not been well studied in humans. Approximately 5% of ingested AFB_1 appears in urine as the AFM_1 metabolite (14,15). The biologic half-life of aflatoxin-N^7-guanine adducts is relatively short, approximately 8 hours (16). Short half-lives have also been reported for AFM_1– and AFB_1–mercapturic acid conjugates (17). Biliary and fecal excretion of aflatoxin is significant in some animal species and may be important pathways in humans (18).

The formation of DNA adducts explains the toxicodynamic effects of AFB_1. These adducts can give rise to guanine to thymine transversion mutations (19). Studies on the *p53* tumor suppressor gene, the most common mutated gene detected in many human cancers, have identified a high frequency of guanine to thymine transversions with an apparent clustering at codon 249 (20). Although controversy exists as to whether this mutation is a specific marker for aflatoxin-associated hepatocellular carcinoma (HCC) (21), there is sufficient evidence for the carcinogenicity of AFB_1 (22).

Acute cytotoxic effects from high-level AFB_1 exposure may be mediated by binding to functional cellular proteins. Animal studies have shown effects on enzymes involved in glycolysis and gluconeogenesis as well as inhibition of cellular transport proteins (12).

Pathophysiology

The liver is the primary target of toxicity. Extensive centrilobular necrosis has been described, commencing in the perivenular zone (zone 3) and extending to periportal zones (zone 1) (23). Bile duct proliferation and metaplasia are also prominent findings (7,23). Giant cell infiltration of the liver has been consistently reported as well as cholestasis in severe cases (24). The liver injury from acute AFB_1 exposure can lead to acute liver failure.

Vulnerable Populations

AFM_1 may be secreted in human breast milk and was detected in up to 37% of samples obtained in one developing country (25). The risks to infants and neonates from this route of exposure have not been studied. Several studies have identified hepatitis B virus infection as a risk factor for HCC. The interaction between aflatoxin and hepatitis B virus is likely an explanatory factor in the high rates of HCC that are found in regions where both risk factors are prevalent (26).

Clinical Presentation

Early symptoms of hepatic injury from acute aflatoxicosis include abdominal pain, anorexia, malaise, and low-grade fever (27). Icterus and jaundice develop within several days, followed by abdominal distention, vomiting, ascites, and edema (7,24). Massive gastrointestinal (GI) bleeding frequently occurs in fatal cases (7,27). Mortality rates from acute aflatoxicosis range from 10% to 76% (23,24,27). The chronic effect of aflatoxin is primarily carcinogenesis, which presents as the underlying tumor type.

Diagnostic Tests

Laboratory tests of liver function confirm the extent of hepatic injury in acute aflatoxicosis. Aspartate and alanine aminotransferase are frequently elevated to levels exceeding 5000 IU/L (23). Bilirubin levels are also increased (24). In cases of liver failure, elevation of prothrombin time, metabolic acidosis, and hypoglycemia are characteristic signs (23,28).

Biomarkers of recent exposure to aflatoxin include urinary aflatoxin-N^7-guanine and AFM_1, both of which show a dose-dependent relationship between dietary intake and excretion (17). A single 24-hour urinalysis may not be adequate to measure recent exposure to aflatoxin because of variations in dietary intake and urinary excretion over time (29). Due to the longer half-life of circulating albumin (2 to 3 months), serum AFB_1-albumin adducts have also been used as a biomarker of chronic exposure to aflatoxin in human studies (30).

Treatment

Treatment of acute aflatoxicosis requires identification of and removal from the source of exposure. AFB_1 strongly adsorbs to activated charcoal *in vitro* (31). A single dose of activated charcoal is indicated in cases of recent ingestion. Aggressive supportive management is indicated in all suspected cases. Patients with acute hepatic injury should be managed in typical fashion (Chapter 17). Hemodialysis and hemoperfusion have not been studied but are not expected to enhance elimination. There are no published reports of liver transplantation.

No antidotes have been identified. Given the role of GSH in the detoxification of AFB_1 exo-8,9-epoxide, *N*-acetylcysteine may have a protective effect against mutagenesis by increasing intracellular GSH levels (32). A recent animal investigation found reduced hepatic injury when *N*-acetylcysteine was coadministered with high daily doses of AFB_1 (33).

Several studies have investigated modulators of aflatoxin metabolism and bioavailability and their role in reducing the risk of HCC. The dithiolethione antischistosomal drug oltipraz induces phase II enzymes, such as GSH-*S*-transferase, which detoxifies the AFB_1 exo-8,9-epoxide (34). Oltipraz may also prevent the epoxidation of AFB_1 through competitive inhibition of CYP 1A2 (35). Other chemoprevention trials have explored the potential efficacy of chlorophylls and their water-soluble salts (chlorophyllins) at preventing the genotoxicity of aflatoxin by reducing its oral bioavailability (16,36).

TRICHOTHECENES

Overview

The trichothecenes are mycotoxins produced by certain fungi in the indoor and outdoor environment (Table 1). Trichothecenes of importance with respect to food contamination include deoxynivalenol (vomitoxin) and T-2 toxin. Trichothecenes are nonvolatile compounds, and their environmental fate may be influenced by competing fungi and bacteria that may metabolize them or inhibit their production (37,38).

There are few studies of trichothecenes in humans. The largest epidemic of food-borne disease in humans that has been associated with trichothecene ingestion occurred in the former Soviet Union and was termed *alimentary toxic aleukia* (39). Famine conditions forced the population to consume grain contaminated with toxigenic fungi (*Fusarium poae, Fusarium sporotrichioides*) that produced high levels of T-2 toxin (39). The outbreak was characterized by progressive leukopenia, thrombocytopenia, and necrotic lesions of the GI tract (39).

Clinical trials have evaluated the trichothecene anguidine (diacetoxyscirpenol) as a chemotherapeutic agent (40), although dose-dependent adverse effects and a lack of efficacy led to its abandonment. Due to their potent blistering properties, purified trichothecenes have also been investigated because of their potential misuse as agents of chemical warfare (41). T-2 toxin was implicated in the "Yellow Rain" attacks in Southeast Asia; however, a United Nations investigation concluded that the evidence was inconclusive (42).

Trichothecenes are detected throughout the world in agricultural commodities as well as commercial foods (43). Recent studies have focused on exposure to toxigenic fungi (particularly *Stachybotrys chartarum*) in the indoor environment. The prevalence of fungi capable of producing trichothecenes indoors is not known. In one study of toxigenic fungi in bulk, surface, and air samples from residences in a North American city, *S. chartarum* was detected in the majority of homes of unaffected individuals (44).

TABLE 1. Examples of fungi capable of trichothecene production

Fusarium graminearum	*Memnoniella echinata*
Fusarium moniliforme	*Myrothecium roridum*
Fusarium poae	*Stachybotrys chartarum*
Fusarium sporotrichioides	

The assessment of exposure to trichothecenes is complex because the production of mycotoxins by a toxigenic species is strain dependent and affected by environmental conditions. Some toxigenic fungi (including *S. chartarum*) do not produce trichothecenes (45). Of those toxigenic fungi that can produce trichothecenes, the quantity is influenced by factors including temperature (39), humidity, and growth substrate (46).

STANDARDS

The U.S. Food and Drug Administration has issued an advisory level of 1 parts per million (mg/kg) for deoxynivalenol in finished wheat products intended for human consumption. A joint expert committee of the Food and Agriculture Organization and World Health Organization has recommended a provisional maximum tolerable daily intake of 60 ng/kg body weight per day for T-2 toxin and HT-2 toxin, alone or in combination (43).

TOXIC DOSE

In phase I clinical trials, intravenous doses of diacetoxyscirpenol exceeding 2.4 mg/m^2/day were associated with adverse effects (40). On review by the International Agency for Research on Cancer, toxins derived from *Fusarium* species (including T-2 toxin, deoxynivalenol, nivalenol) were not classifiable as to their carcinogenicity to humans (group 3) (22). There are no human studies on reproductive or teratogenic effects.

Toxicokinetics and Toxicodynamics

Most studies have been conducted in animals, and it is unknown whether these data are predictive of toxicokinetics in humans. Bioavailability of ingested T-2 toxin is poor in several animal species as a result of physiologic instability, first-pass metabolism (47), and detoxification by gut microorganisms (48). T-2 toxin penetrates intact skin slowly (49,50), and the risk of systemic toxicity from dermal exposure is low (50). There are no studies that have measured the systemic bioavailability of trichothecenes from inhaled fungal spores.

Animal studies indicate that orally or parenterally administered T-2 toxin does not bioaccumulate (47). Short elimination half-lives have been reported for T-2 toxin (less than 30 minutes) (47) and deoxynivalenol (3 to 5 hours) (51). *In vitro* studies of human blood suggest that carboxylesterases may be important in the hydrolysis of T-2 toxin to more polar and less toxic metabolites (52).

Trichothecenes are potent inhibitors of eukaryotic protein synthesis (53). The 12,13-epoxide group common to trichothecenes is necessary for protein synthesis inhibition, although certain substitutions of the ring structure lead to enhanced effects on the elongation and termination phase (53). The more potent trichothecenes (including T-2 toxin) inhibit the initiation of protein synthesis (54).

Pathophysiology

Immunomodulatory effects of trichothecenes have been described in animal studies and human *in vitro* studies (55,56). Local cytotoxic effects on the GI mucosa have been demonstrated after oral or intravenous administration of trichothecenes in animal studies, resulting in a loss of vascular functional integrity and fluid losses into the gut (57).

Vulnerable Populations

Acute pulmonary hemorrhage in infants was purportedly associated with residential exposure to *S. chartarum* and other toxigenic fungi (58). A detailed analysis of this report was conducted by the Centers for Disease Control and Prevention (CDC), which found methodologic shortcomings and concluded that the association was not confirmed (59). The role of *S. chartarum* or trichothecenes in infant pulmonary hemosiderosis and hemorrhage cannot be determined based on the available data (60). The CDC has developed a clinical case definition that is specific for acute idiopathic pulmonary hemorrhage in infants (61).

Clinical Presentation

Acute effects of trichothecene extracts or materials heavily contaminated with toxigenic fungi include irritant contact dermatitis after skin exposure (62,63). After ingestion of foods contaminated with significant levels of trichothecenes, symptoms of mild to moderate abdominal pain develop within 15 minutes to 1 hour (64,65). Throat irritation and diarrhea have also been frequently described after ingestion. GI symptoms usually resolve within 12 hours (64).

After chronic ingestion, four clinical stages have been described (39). The first stage includes irritation and inflammation of the GI mucosa, leading to abdominal pain, vomiting, and diarrhea, which may last 3 to 9 days. The second stage extends over 2 to 8 weeks and is latent; symptoms are not prominent, but progressive anemia, thrombocytopenia, and leukopenia with relative lymphocytosis develop. With persistent exposure, the third stage involves infectious complications and petechial hemorrhages on the skin and mucous membranes. Necrotic lesions develop along the GI tract, and regional lymph node enlargement becomes prominent. Blood abnormalities become more severe, and the erythrocyte sedimentation rate is significantly elevated. Very few cases reaching the third stage survive. The fourth stage is convalescence and resolution of necrotic lesions and hematologic abnormalities.

Some studies have reported pulmonary disease (66) and nonspecific building-related symptoms (67–69) in association with exposure to toxigenic fungi (particularly *S. chartarum*) in nonindustrial building environments with a history of moisture problems. Assessing the role of trichothecenes or other mycotoxins in these studies is complicated by ill-defined case definitions, a lack of objective exposure or response indicators, and inadequate assessment of confounders. The weight of the scientific evidence does not currently support a causal relationship between inhalation exposure to trichothecenes in the indoor environment and specific health effects (70–73).

Diagnostic Tests

Analytic techniques using gas chromatography with mass spectrometry have been developed for certain trichothecenes in human blood and urine (74,75); however, these methods have not been used in epidemiologic studies. Serologic testing for antibodies specific to toxigenic fungi does not provide accurate information on exposure to trichothecenes, as the immunoglobulin is directed toward fungal antigens, not mycotoxins. Furthermore, cross-reactivity in laboratory assays exists between *S. chartarum* antigens and fungi that are commonly found in the outdoor environment (76). Abnormalities in lymphocyte subset analysis have been reported in some studies (67), but consistent and specific findings have not been identified (77). Based on the available data, the most appropriate diagnostic test to evaluate hematologic and immune parameters associated with trichothecene exposure is a complete blood cell count with differential.

Treatment

No specific therapies for trichothecene mycotoxicosis have been identified. Dexamethasone has been associated with improved animal survival after low- and high-dose exposure to T-2 toxin (78) but has not been investigated in humans. Standard supportive measures are indicated for symptomatic cases, after removal from the source of exposure, and after decontamination has taken place.

The skin may be effectively decontaminated after T-2 exposure by washing with an aqueous soap solution (49,79). Polyethylene glycol 300 is also effective at removing large doses of T-2 toxin from the skin (49). Decontamination is most effective when treatment is carried out within minutes of dermal exposure.

T-2 toxin is tightly adsorbed onto activated charcoal and has been associated with improved animal survival when administered with oral or parenteral doses of T-2 toxin (80). These findings suggest that activated charcoal may decrease absorption and enhance elimination of toxin. A single dose of activated charcoal is probably warranted after acute trichothecene ingestion. The role of repeated doses of activated charcoal is not known but may be of theoretic benefit. Other methods to enhance elimination have not been studied.

Laboratory monitoring should include serial evaluations of the complete blood cell count for leukopenia, thrombocytopenia, and anemia. The development of significant immune suppression warrants neutropenic precautions. After ingestion, careful examination of the oral mucous membranes and GI tract is warranted to evaluate for the presence of necrotic lesions. Lesions involving the oropharynx or esophagus may lead to airway compromise, which should be monitored in an intensive care unit.

REFERENCES

1. Denning DW. Aflatoxin and human disease. *Adverse Drug React Acute Poisoning Rev* 1987;6:175–209.
2. Hunter CA, Grant C, Flannigan B, et al. Mould in buildings: the air spora of domestic dwellings. *Int Biodeterioration* 1988;24:81–101.
3. Wang JS, Groopman JD. DNA damage by mycotoxins. *Mutat Res* 1999;424:167–181.
4. Tuomi T, Reijula K, Johnsson T, et al. Mycotoxins in crude building materials from water-damaged buildings. *Appl Environ Microbiol* 2000;66:1899–1904.
5. Fischer G, Muller T, Schwalbe R, et al. Species-specific profiles of mycotoxins produced in cultures and associated with conidia of airborne fungi derived from biowaste. *Int J Hyg Environ Health* 2000;203:105–116.
6. European Commission. Commission regulation number 1525/98 of 16 July 1998 amending regulation (EC) No 194/97 of 31 January 1997 setting maximum levels for certain contaminants in foodstuffs. *Off J Eur Community* 1998;201:43–46.
7. Krishnamachari KA, Bhat RV, Nagarajan V, et al. Hepatitis due to aflatoxicosis. An outbreak in Western India. *Lancet* 1975;1:1061–1063.
8. Denning DW, Allen R, Wilkinson AP, et al. Transplacental transfer of aflatoxin in humans. *Carcinogenesis* 1990;11:1033–1035.
9. Guengerich FP, Johnson WW, Shimada T, et al. Activation and detoxication of aflatoxin B1. *Mutat Res* 1998;402:121–128.
10. Guengerich FP. Forging the links between metabolism and carcinogenesis. *Mutat Res* 2001;488:195–209.
11. Sabbioni G, Ambs S, Wogan GN, et al. The aflatoxin-lysine adduct quantified by high-performance liquid chromatography from human serum albumin samples. *Carcinogenesis* 1990;11:2063–2066.
12. McLean M, Dutton MF. Cellular interactions and metabolism of aflatoxin: an update. *Pharmacol Ther* 1995;65:163–192.
13. Gan LS, Skipper PL, Peng XC, et al. Serum albumin adducts in the molecular epidemiology of aflatoxin carcinogenesis: correlation with aflatoxin B1 intake and urinary excretion of aflatoxin M1. *Carcinogenesis* 1988;9:1323–1325.
14. Cheng Z, Root M, Pan W, et al. Use of an improved method for analysis of urinary aflatoxin M1 in a survey of mainland China and Taiwan. *Cancer Epidemiol Biomarkers Prev* 1997;6:523–529.
15. Zhu JQ, Zhang LS, Hu X, et al. Correlation of dietary aflatoxin B1 levels with excretion of aflatoxin M1 in human urine. *Cancer Res* 1987;47:1848–1852.
16. Egner PA, Wang JB, Zhu YR, et al. Chlorophyllin intervention reduces aflatoxin-DNA adducts in individuals at high risk for liver cancer. *Proc Natl Acad Sci U S A* 2001;98:14601–14606.
17. Groopman JD, Kensler TW. The light at the end of the tunnel for chemical-specific biomarkers: daylight or headlight? *Carcinogenesis* 1999;20:1–11.
18. de Vries HR, Maxwell SM, Hendrickse RG. Aflatoxin excretion in children with kwashiorkor or marasmic kwashiorkor—a clinical investigation. *Mycopathologia* 1990;110:1–9.
19. Bailey EA, Iyer RS, Stone MP, et al. Mutational properties of the primary aflatoxin B1-DNA adduct. *Proc Natl Acad Sci U S A* 1996;93:1535–1539.
20. Hsu IC, Metcalf RA, Sun T, et al. Mutational hotspot in the p53 gene in human hepatocellular carcinomas. *Nature* 1991;350:427–428.
21. Lasky T, Magder L. Hepatocellular carcinoma p53 G > T transversions at codon 249: the fingerprint of aflatoxin exposure? *Environ Health Perspect* 1997;105:392–397.
22. IARC. *Mycotoxins. Some naturally occurring substances: food items and constituents, heterocyclic aromatic amines and mycotoxins, vol. 56.* Lyon, France: International Agency for Research on Cancer, 1993:397–488.
23. Chao TC, Maxwell SM, Wong SY. An outbreak of aflatoxicosis and boric acid poisoning in Malaysia: a clinicopathological study. *J Pathol* 1991;164:225–233.
24. Tandon BN, Krishnamurthy L, Koshy A, et al. Study of an epidemic of jaundice, presumably due to toxic hepatitis, in Northwest India. *Gastroenterology* 1977;72:488–494.
25. Coulter JB, Lamplugh SM, Suliman GI, et al. Aflatoxins in human breast milk. *Ann Trop Paediatr* 1984;4:61–66.
26. Ross RK, Yuan JM, Yu MC, et al. Urinary aflatoxin biomarkers and risk of hepatocellular carcinoma. *Lancet* 1992;339:943–946.
27. Ngindu A, Johnson BK, Kenya PR, et al. Outbreak of acute hepatitis caused by aflatoxin poisoning in Kenya. *Lancet* 1982;1:1346–1348.
28. Olson LC, Bourgeois CH Jr, Cotton RB, et al. Encephalopathy and fatty degeneration on the viscera in northeastern Thailand. Clinical syndrome and epidemiology. *Pediatrics* 1971;47:707–716.
29. Groopman JD, Hall AJ, Whittle H, et al. Molecular dosimetry of aflatoxin-N7-guanine in human urine obtained in Gambia, West Africa. *Cancer Epidemiol Biomarkers Prev* 1992;1:221–227.
30. Wild CP, Turner PC. Exposure biomarkers in chemoprevention studies of liver cancer. *IARC Sci Publ* 2001;154:215–222.
31. Decker WJ, Corby DG. Activated charcoal adsorbs aflatoxin B1. *Vet Hum Toxicol* 1980;22:388–389.
32. De Flora S, Bennicelli C, Camoirano A, et al. In vivo effects of N-acetylcysteine on glutathione metabolism and on the biotransformation of carcinogenic and/or mutagenic compounds. *Carcinogenesis* 1985; 6:1735–1745.
33. Valdivia AG, Martinez A, Damian FJ, et al. Efficacy of N-acetylcysteine to reduce the effects of aflatoxin B1 intoxication in broiler chickens. *Poult Sci* 2001;80:727–734.
34. Kwak MK, Egner PA, Dolan PM, et al. Role of phase 2 enzyme induction in chemoprotection by dithiolethiones. *Mutat Res* 2001;480–481:305–315.
35. Wang JS, Shen X, He X, et al. Protective alterations in phase 1 and 2 metabolism of aflatoxin B1 by oltipraz in residents of Qidong, People's Republic of China. *J Natl Cancer Inst* 1999;91:347–354.
36. Breinholt V, Arbogast D, Loveland P, et al. Chlorophyllin chemoprevention in trout initiated by aflatoxin B(1) bath treatment: an evaluation of reduced bioavailability vs. target organ protective mechanisms. *Toxicol Appl Pharmacol* 1999;158:141–151.
37. Jesenska Z, Sajbidorova I. T-2 toxin degradation by micromycetes. *J Hyg Epidemiol Microbiol Immunol* 1991;35:41–49.
38. Cooney JM, Lauren DR, di Menna ME. Impact of competitive fungi on Trichothecene production by *Fusarium graminearum*. *J Agric Food Chem* 2001;49:522–526.
39. Joffe AZ. Effects of fusariotoxins in humans. In: Joffe AZ, ed. Fusarium *species: their biology and toxicology.* New York: John Wiley and Sons, 1986:225–292.
40. Murphy WK, Burgess MA, Valdivieso M, et al. Phase I clinical evaluation of anguidine. *Cancer Treat Rep* 1978;62:1497–1502.
41. Wannemacher RW, Weiner SL. Trichothecene mycotoxins. In: Sidell FR, Takafuji ET, Franz DR, eds. Medical aspects of chemical and biological warfare. Washington, DC: Borden Institute, Walter Reed Army Medical Center, 1997:655–676.
42. United Nations. Chemical and bacteriological (biological) weapons: report of the secretary general. A/36/613. New York: United Nations, 1981.
43. Food and Agriculture Organization. Joint FAO/WHO Expert Committee on Food Additives. Lyon, France: World Health Organization, Food and Agriculture Organization, 2001:1–33.
44. Dearborn DG, Yike I, Sorenson WG, et al. Overview of investigations into pulmonary hemorrhage among infants in Cleveland, Ohio. *Environ Health Perspect* 1999;107[Suppl 3]:495–499.
45. Jarvis BB, Hinkley SF. Analysis for *Stachybotrys* toxins. In: Johanning E, Yang CS, eds. *Bioaerosols, fungi, and mycotoxins: health effects, assessment, prevention and control.* Latham, NY: Eastern New York Occupational Health Program, 1999:232–239.
46. Nikulin M, Pasanen AL, Berg S, et al. *Stachybotrys* atra growth and toxin production in some building materials and fodder under different relative humidities. *Appl Environ Microbiol* 1994;60:3421–3424.
47. Yagen B, Bialer M. Metabolism and pharmacokinetics of T-2 toxin and related trichothecenes. *Drug Metab Rev* 1993;25:281–323.
48. Swanson SP, Helaszek C, Buck WB, et al. The role of intestinal microflora in the metabolism of trichothecene mycotoxins. *Food Chem Toxicol* 1988;26:823–829.
49. Fairhurst S, Maxwell SA, Scawin JW, et al. Skin effects of trichothecenes and their amelioration by decontamination. *Toxicology* 1987;46:307–319.
50. Maxwell SA, Brown RF, Upshall DG. The in vitro penetration and distribution of T-2 toxin through human skin. *Toxicology* 1986;40:59–74.
51. Prelusky DB, Veira DM, Trenholm HL, et al. Excretion profiles of the mycotoxin deoxynivalenol, following oral and intravenous administration to sheep. *Fundam Appl Toxicol* 1986;6:356–363.

52. Johnsen H, Odden E, Johnsen BA, et al. Metabolism of T-2 toxin by blood cell carboxylesterases. *Biochem Pharmacol* 1988;37:3193–3197.
53. Feinberg B, McLaughlin CS. Biochemical mechanism of action of trichothecene mycotoxins. In: Beasley VR, ed. *Trichothecene mycotoxicosis: pathophysiological effects.* Boca Raton, FL: CRC Press Inc., 1989:27–35.
54. Murthy MR, Radouco-Thomas S, Bharucha AD, et al. Effects of trichothecenes (T-2 toxin) on protein synthesis in vitro by brain polysomes and messenger RNA. *Prog Neuropsychopharmacol Biol Psychiatry* 1985;9:251–258.
55. Bondy GS, Pestka JJ. Immunomodulation by fungal toxins. *J Toxicol Environ Health B Crit Rev* 2000;3:109–143.
56. Thuvander A, Wikman C, Gadhasson I. In vitro exposure of human lymphocytes to trichothecenes: individual variation in sensitivity and effects of combined exposure on lymphocyte function. *Food Chem Toxicol* 1999;37:639–648.
57. Schiefer HB, Beasley VR. Effects on the digestive system and energy metabolism. In: Beasley VR, ed. *Trichothecene mycotoxicosis: pathophysiologic effects.* Boca Raton, FL: CRC Press Inc., 1989:61–89.
58. Etzel RA, Montana E, Sorenson WG, et al. Acute pulmonary hemorrhage in infants associated with exposure to *Stachybotrys* atra and other fungi. *Arch Pediatr Adolesc Med* 1998;152:757–762.
59. From the Centers for Disease Control and Prevention. Update: pulmonary hemorrhage/hemosiderosis among infants—Cleveland, Ohio, 1993–1996. *JAMA* 2000;283:1951–1953.
60. Epidemiology Program Office, Centers for Disease Control. Report of the CDC working group on pulmonary hemosiderosis/hemorrhage. Atlanta: Centers for Disease Control and Prevention, 1999.
61. From the Centers for Disease Control and Prevention. Pulmonary hemorrhage in infants. *JAMA* 2001;286:786.
62. Andrassy K, Horvath I, Lakos T, Toke Z. [Mass incidence of mycotoxicoses in Hajdu-Bihar county]. *Mykosen* 1980;23:130–133.
63. Mortimer PH, Campbell J, di Menna ME, et al. Experimental myrotheciotoxicosis and poisoning in ruminants by verrucarin A and roridin A. *Res Vet Sci* 1971;12:508–515.
64. Wang ZG, Feng JN, Tong Z. Human toxicosis caused by moldy rice contaminated with *Fusarium* and T-2 toxin. *Biomed Environ Sci* 1993;6:65–70.
65. Bhat RV, Beedu SR, Ramakrishna Y, et al. Outbreak of trichothecene mycotoxicosis associated with consumption of mould-damaged wheat production in Kashmir Valley, India. *Lancet* 1989;1:35–37.
66. Hodgson MJ, Morey P, Leung WY, et al. Building-associated pulmonary disease from exposure to *Stachybotrys chartarum* and *Aspergillus versicolor. J Occup Environ Med* 1998;40:241–249.
67. Johanning E, Biagini R, Hull D, et al. Health and immunology study following exposure to toxigenic fungi (*Stachybotrys chartarum*) in a water-damaged office environment. *Int Arch Occup Environ Health* 1996;68:207–218.
68. Croft WA, Jarvis BB, Yatawara CS. Airborne outbreak of trichothecene toxicosis. *Atmospheric Environ* 1986;20:549–552.
69. Cooley JD, Wong WC, Jumper CA, et al. Correlation between the prevalence of certain fungi and sick building syndrome. *Occup Environ Med* 1998;55:579–584.
70. Fung F, Clark R, Williams S. *Stachybotrys*, a mycotoxin-producing fungus of increasing toxicologic importance. *J Toxicol Clin Toxicol* 1998;36:79–86.
71. Robbins CA, Swenson LJ, Nealley ML, et al. Health effects of mycotoxins in indoor air: a critical review. *Appl Occup Environ Hyg* 2000;15:773–784.
72. Page EH, Trout DB. The role of *Stachybotrys* mycotoxins in buildings related illness. *AIHAJ* 2001;62:644–648.
73. Terr AI. *Stachybotrys*: relevance to human disease. *Ann Allergy Asthma Immunol* 2001;87:57–63.
74. Begley P, Foulger BE, Jeffery PD, et al. Detection of trace levels of trichothecenes in human blood using capillary gas chromatography-electron-capture negative-ion chemical-ionization mass spectrometry. *J Chromatogr* 1986;367:87–101.
75. Black RM, Clarke RJ, Read RW. Detection of trace levels of trichothecene mycotoxins in human urine by gas chromatography-mass spectrometry. *J Chromatogr* 1986;367:103–115.
76. Halsey JF. Performance of a *Stachybotrys chartarum* serology panel. Western Society of Allergy, Asthma, and Immunology annual meeting, 2000.
77. Johanning E, Landsbergis P. Clinical findings related to indoor fungal exposure—review of clinic data of a specialty clinic. In: Johanning E. ed. *Bioaerosols, fungi and mycotoxins: health effects, assessment, prevention and control.* Latham, NY: Eastern New York Occupational Health Program, 1999:70–78.
78. Shohami E, Wisotsky B, Kempski O, et al. Therapeutic effect of dexamethasone in T-2 toxicosis. *Pharm Res* 1987;4:527–530.
79. Bunner BL, Wannemacher RW Jr, Dinterman RE, et al. Cutaneous absorption and decontamination of [3H]T-2 toxin in the rat model. *J Toxicol Environ Health* 1989;26:413–423.
80. Fricke RF, Jorge J. Assessment of efficacy of activated charcoal for treatment of acute T-2 toxin poisoning. *J Toxicol Clin Toxicol* 1990;28:421–431.

CHAPTER 257

Mushrooms

Seth Schonwald

See Figure 1.

Compounds included: **See Table 1.**

Special considerations: **Ingestion of a mixture of mushroom types may produce a mixed picture of toxicity.**

Antidotes: **Group I: thioctic acid, silibinin, penicillin, *N*-acetylcysteine; group II: pyridoxine; group IV: atropine**

OVERVIEW

Although only approximately 2% of the 5000 mushroom species in the United States are poisonous, serious poisonings continue to result from the inability of patients to distinguish toxic from nontoxic mushrooms. The often-repeated dictum "there are old mushroom hunters and bold mushroom hunters, but there are no old, bold mushroom hunters" is an appropriate admonition. The actual incidence of mushroom toxicity is difficult to estimate because poisoning often occurs in clusters and state laws do not require the reporting of adverse reactions from mushroom ingestion.

Poisonous mushrooms contain toxins that are as diverse as the mushrooms themselves. The clinical syndromes caused by poisoning involve multiple organ systems, and progression of clinical signs is often directly related to the quantity eaten. Diagnostic detection of the toxins is rarely an option; rather, diagnosis is based on a history of possible exposure and identification of mushroom species in the stomach contents and environment.

TABLE 1. Compounds included

Group I (cyclopeptide group): *Amanita phalloides* ("death cap"), *Amanita verna* ("deadly agaric," fool's mushroom), *Amanita virosa* ("destroying angel"), *Amanita bisporigera* ("white destroying angel"), *Galerina autumnalis, Galerina marginata,* and *Galerina venenata*
Group II (monomethylhydrazine group): *Amanita muscaria* ("fly agaric") and *Amanita pantherina* ("panther cap," "false blusher")
Group III (coprine group): *Gyromitra* species
Group IV (muscarine group): *Clitocybe* and *Inocybe* species, *A. muscaria,* and *A. pantherina*
Group V (ibotenic acid and muscimol group): *Coprinus atramentarius* ("ink cap")
Group VI (hallucinogen group): *Psilocybe, Panaeolus, Gymnopilus, Stropharia,* and *Conocybe*
Group VII (gastrointestinal irritant group): *Chlorophyllum molybdites* and many others
Group VIII (renal failure group): *Cortinarius* species

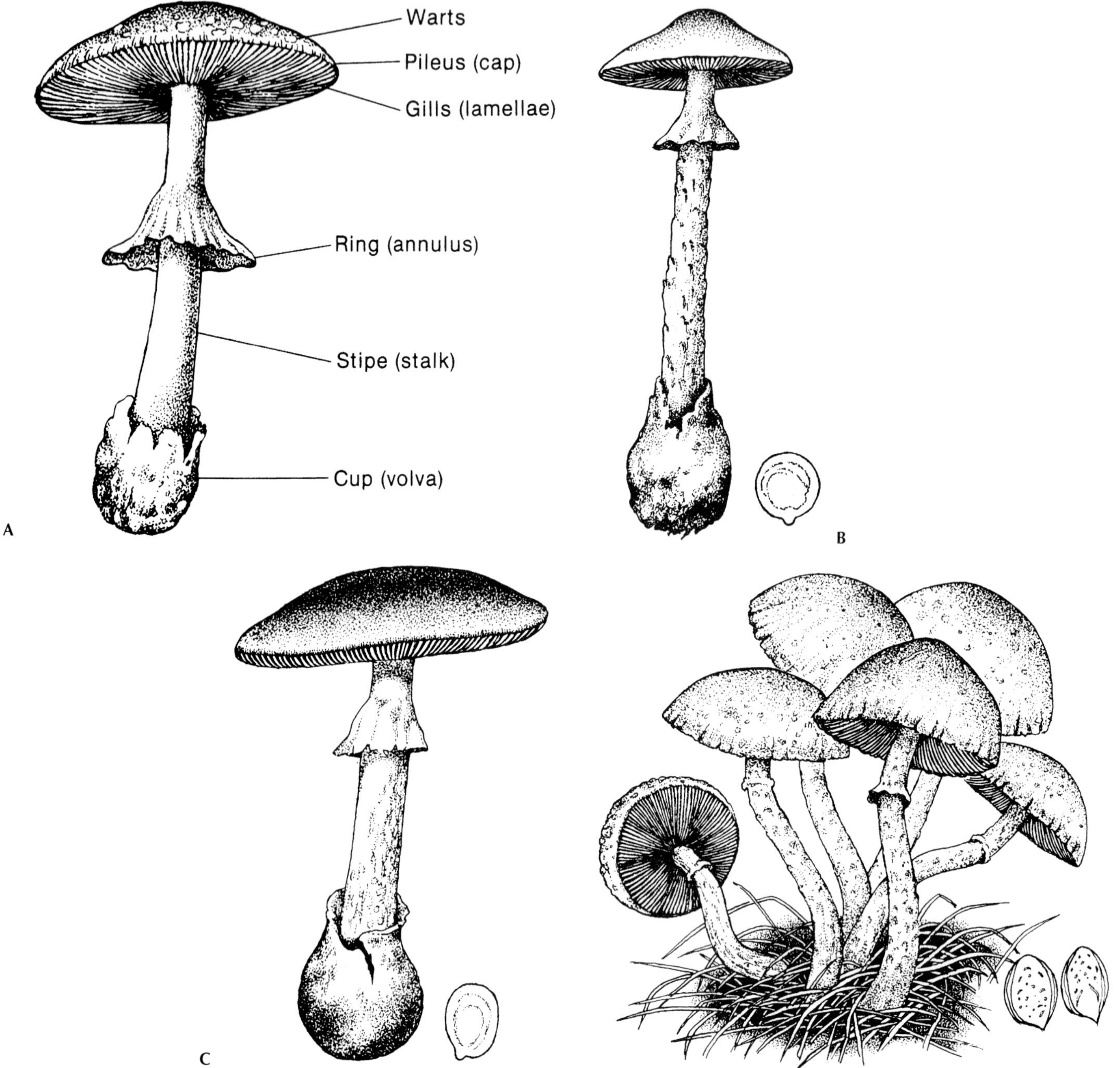

Figure 1. The mushrooms. **A:** Composite of the mushroom. Basic structure of an *Amanita* mushroom. **B:** Destroying angel (*Amanita virosa*). **C:** Death cap (*Amanita phalloides*). **D:** *Galerina marginata*. (*continued*)

Treatment is usually based on clinical signs, as most mushroom toxins are without an antidote (1).

Chemical and Physical Characteristics

The distribution and structural characteristics of a mushroom may aid in its identification (Table 2); however, the distribution of mushrooms changes over time, and local information should augment national information. The mushroom portion of the fungus is the reproductive structure that grows from an underground mycelium as a densely packed cap and stipe (stalk) of interwoven hyphal strands. This structure contains the spores that germinate and form new mycelia. Variation in size, shape, color, and spore and other microscopic structures aids in the identification of mushroom species (Fig. 1).

Mycelia are an extensive network of minute underground tubules (i.e., hyphae) that extend several hundred feet and live for years in the pursuit of nutrients. At times, a specific mycelium develops a mutually beneficial relationship with higher plant roots, and together they are known as a *mycorrhiza*.

Two higher fungus divisions, Basidiomycetes and Ascomycetes, contain the poisonous mushroom species. Because fungi contain no chlorophyll, they must obtain their nutrients from decaying organic matter (as a saprophyte) or from living organisms (as a parasite).

Classification and Identification

Mushrooms are generally divided into seven groups based on target organ and the onset of symptoms (Fig.1). Because ade-

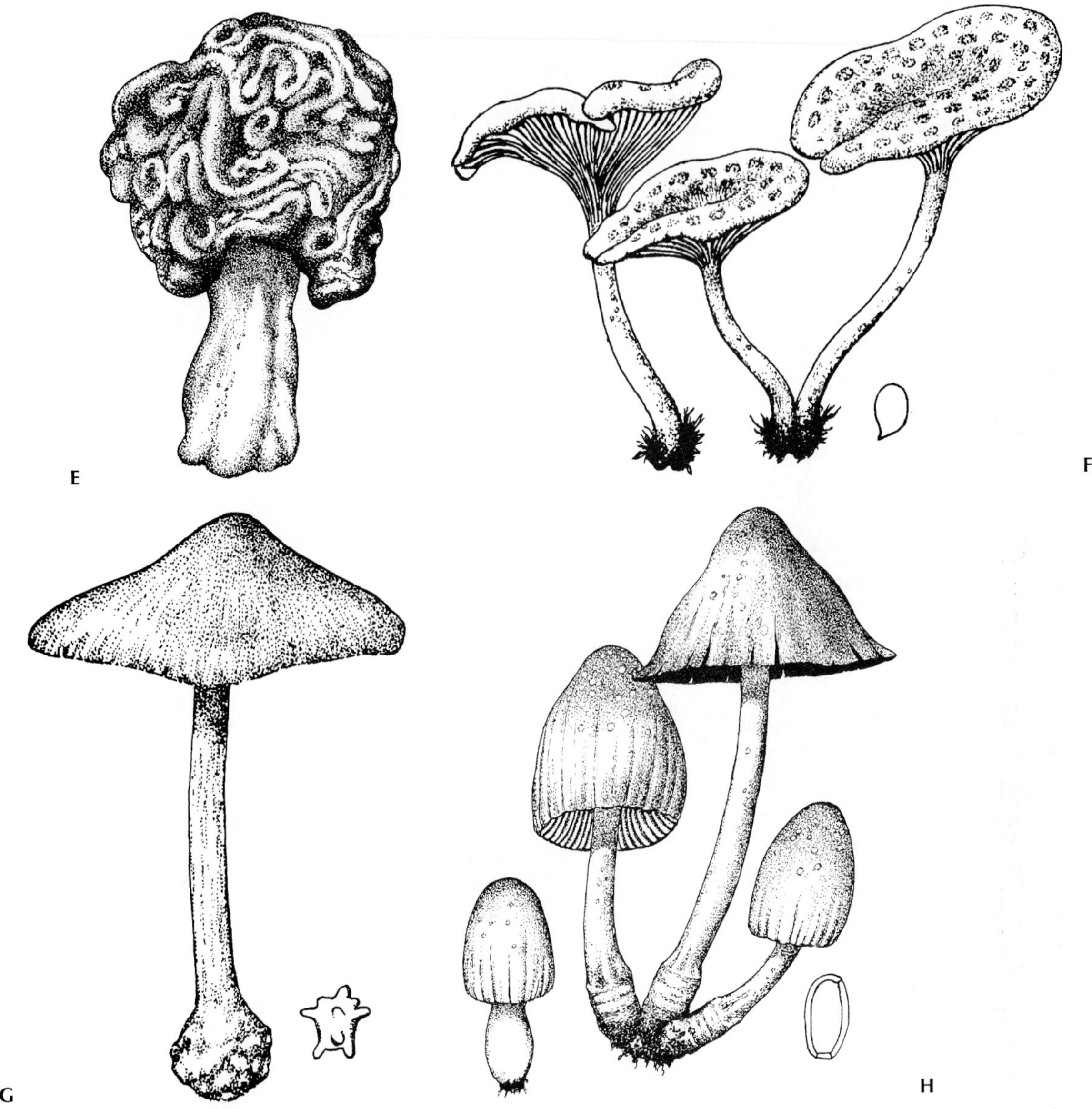

Figure 1. (*continued*) E: False morel (*Gyromitra esculenta*). **F:** *Clitocybe dealbata.* **G:** Turnip-bulb inocybe (*Inocybe napipes*). **H:** Inky cap (*Coprinus atramentarius*). (*continued*)

quate mushroom specimens are often unavailable for identification, a clinical classification provides an excellent mechanism to guide medical treatment (Fig. 2). Individual variations in susceptibility and the coingestion of other mushroom species may limit the usefulness of this classification. The best aid to treatment remains the accurate identification of the species involved. This often requires an experienced mycologist and a microscope.

There are no visible signs present on all mushrooms to indicate toxicity. The distinguishing characteristics of each mushroom must be learned species by species. The *annulus* is a ring of tissue (skirt) left on the stalk when the veil covering the gill breaks. The *pileus* is the mushroom cap. *Spores* are minute, uniquely shaped reproductive units that are analogous to seeds in higher plants. The application of Meltzer's reagent aids in the differentiation of spore species. Spores that turn blue after contact with Meltzer's reagent are referred to as *amyloid* and those that do not turn blue are called *nonamyloid.*

A *partial veil* is a membrane that covers the gills of some immature mushrooms. The remnant is the annulus that remains on the stipe. Occasionally the partial veil adheres to the cap margin (i.e., appendiculate margin). A *universal veil* is a membrane that covers the entire immature mushroom. After maturation, the mushroom expands, breaking through the universal veil. Some species leave a remnant at the base of the stipe known as the *volva. Gills* or *lamellae* are vertical plates on the undersurface of the cap on which spores form and are released.

Assessing Toxicity

Because of limited knowledge, species variation, and individual susceptibility, a priori determination of clinical effects is difficult. The seriousness of toxicity depends on a number of variables. Some mushrooms require cooking (e.g., *Clitocybe nuda*) to remove toxins; however, deadly amatoxins are not altered by

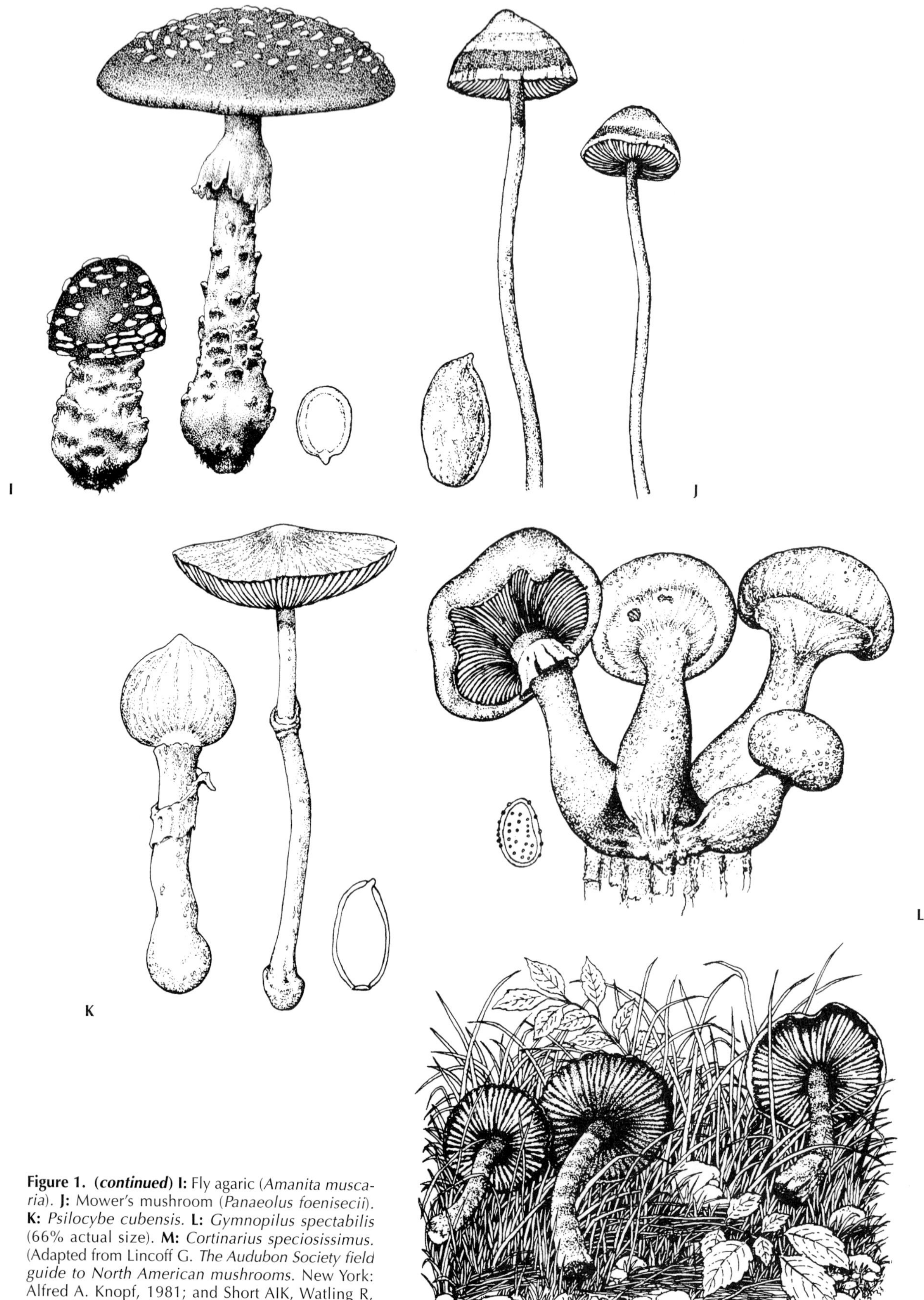

Figure 1. ***(continued)*** **I:** Fly agaric (*Amanita muscaria*). **J:** Mower's mushroom (*Panaeolus foenisecii*). **K:** *Psilocybe cubensis.* **L:** *Gymnopilus spectabilis* (66% actual size). **M:** *Cortinarius speciosissimus.* (Adapted from Lincoff G. *The Audubon Society field guide to North American mushrooms.* New York: Alfred A. Knopf, 1981; and Short AIK, Watling R, MacDonald MK, et al. *Lancet* 1980;2:942.)

TABLE 2. Distribution and structural characteristics of toxic North American mushroom species

Genus and species	Distribution	Season	Pileus	Spore Print	Amyloid reaction
Group I: cyclopeptide poisoning					
Amanita					
Amanita bisporigera	E NA, Pac coast (rare)	Sp, S, F	White	White	Positive
Amanita virosa (destroying angel)	E NA, Pac coast (rare)	Sp, S, F	White	White	Positive
Amanita verna (death angel)	E NA, Pac coast (rare)	Sp, S, F	White	White	Positive
Amanita phalloides (death cap)	Rare—E NA, PNW, Pac coast	S, F	Pale yellow-green to green	White	Positive
Amanita brunnescens	E NA	S, F	Brown with white margin	White	Positive
Amanita pantherina (see also group V)	Common; widely, especially RM, PNW	Sp, S, F	Light brown to brown with buff or yellowish margin	White	Negative
Galerina					
Galerina autumnalis	Common, widely	Late F, early Sp	Dark brown to leathery light tan	Rust brown	Negative
Galerina venenata	Rare—PNW	Late F, W	Cinnamon brown	Rust brown	Negative
Group II: monomethylhydrazine poisoning					
Gyromitra					
Gyromitra californica	Common, RM, PNW, PSW	Early Sp	Tan to red-brown	Brown	Negative
Gyromitra brunnea	Common, E NA	Early Sp	Chocolate brown, white beneath	Brown	Negative
Gyromitra esculenta	Common, widely, especially RM, PNW	Late Sp	Brown to red-brown	Brown	Negative
Group III: disulfiram-like poisoning					
Coprinus					
Coprinus atramentarius	Common, widely	S, F	Light gray-brown (exhibits deliquescence)	Black	Negative
Group IV: muscarine poisoning					
Inocybe	Common, widely, woodlands	S, F	Brown to dark brown	Brown	Negative
Inocybe napipes					
Inocybe fastigiata					
Inocybe patouillardii					
Inocybe lanuginose					
Inocybe geophylla			White to lilac	Clay brown	Negative
Clitocybe					
Clitocybe dealbata	Common, widely	S, F	Dull white	White	Negative
Clitocybe rivulosa					
Clitocybe trunicola					
Panaeolus					
Panaeolus separatus	Common, widely	Sp, S, F	Light gray to dull gray-white	Black	Negative
Gymnopilus					
Gymnopilus spectabilis	Common, widely	Sp, S, F, early W	Buff yellow to yellow-orange	Rusty orange	Negative
Gymnopilus luteus					
Gymnopilus decurrens					
Gymnopilus validipes					
Gymnopilus aeruginosus					
Gymnopilus viridans					
Also reported					
Gymnopilus stropharia	—	—	—	—	—
Gymnopilus copelandia	—	—	—	—	—
Group V: isoxazole derivatives: ibotenic acid and muscimol poisoning					
Amanita					
Amanita muscaria	Common, widely, especially in N Eng, Pac coast, RM	Sp, S, F	Orange or straw yellow (N Eng) to bright red (Pac coast; often with pileal warts)	White	Negative
Amanita pantherina	Common, widely, especially in RM, PNW	Sp, S, F	Light brown to brown with buff or yellowish-white margin	White	Negative
Group VI: hallucinogens					
Psilocybe[a]					
Psilocybe cubensis	Rare, Florida	Late W to F	Whitish to pale yellow	Purple-brown	Negative
Psilocybe baeocystis	Oregon, Washington	W to F	—	Purple-brown	Negative
Psilocybe semilanceata	PNW, Britain	F, W	Buff-gray to gray-green	Purple-brown	Negative
Psilocybe stuntzii	PNW	F, W	Brown to ochre	Dark purple	Negative
Psilocybe mexicana	—	—	—	—	—
Psilocybe quebecensis	—	—	—	—	—
Panaeolus venenosus					
Panaeolus campanulatus	Common, widely	Sp, S, F	Gray, speckled dark purple-brown	Black	Negative
Panaeolus foenisecii	Common, widely	Sp, S, F	Dark brown or reddish brown to tan or light gray-brown	Purple-brown	Negative

(continued)

TABLE 2. (*continued*)

Genus and species	Distribution	Season	Pileus	Spore Print	Amyloid reaction
Group VII: gastrointestinal irritants					
Agaricus					
Agaricus hondensis	Common, widely	S, F	White-brown, gray-brown	Chocolate brown	Negative
Boletus					
Boletus luridus	Rare, NE, SE, mid W	S, F	Mixed, many colors	Olive-brown	Negative
Boletus eastwoodiae	Rare, Pac coast	F	Dark to red-brown	Olive-brown	Negative
Boletus satanas	Rare, Pac coast	F	Dark to red-brown	Olive-brown	Negative
Boletus sensibilis	—	—	—	Olive-brown	Negative
Chlorophyllum					
Chlorophyllum molybdites	Common, widely	Sp, S, F	White with buff scales	Green	Negative
Entoloma					
Entoloma lividum	Common, widely	S, F	Tan	Salmon pink	Negative
Gomphus					
Gomphus floccosus	Common, widely	—	—	Smoky gray to black	Negative
Hebeloma					
Hebeloma crustuliniforme	Rare, widely	F	Brown to cream at margin	Yellow to olive-brown	Negative
Hebeloma mesophaeum	Common, widely	Sp, S, F	Brown	Yellow to olive-brown	Negative
Lactarius species[b]	Common, widely	Sp, S, F	Variable	White to yellow	Positive
Naematoloma					
Naematoloma fasciculare	Common, especially PNW, SE	Sp, F, W	Yellow to orange-yellow	Purple-brown	Negative
Omphalatus					
Omphalatus olearius	E NA, S, Pac coast	S, F	Yellow-orange to bright orange	White	Negative
Paxillus					
Paxillus involutus	Common, widely	S, F	Red-brown	Clay-brown, yellow-brown	Negative
Ramaria (coral fungus)					
Ramaria formosa	Common, widely	F, W	Pink to light orange (coral branches)	Red-brown	Negative
Rhodophyllus (*Rhodophyllus sinuatus*; see *E. lividum*—same species)					
Russula					
Russula emetica	Common, widely	S, F	Bright red	White	Negative
Russula densifolia	Common, widely, especially E NA	S, F	White to gray	White	Positive
Scleroderma (puffball fungi) species	Common, especially E NA	S, F	Gleba (spore mass): purple to purple-brown; surface: tan to white	Brown	Negative
Tricholoma species	Common, widely, especially NE, RM, PNW, mid W	F	Gray-brown	White	Negative

E NA, eastern North America; F, fall; mid W, middle western states; N Eng, New England; NE, northeastern states; negative, spores do not turn blue in Melzer's reagent; Pac coast, Pacific coast; PNW, Pacific Northwest; positive, spores turn blue in Melzer's reagent; PSW, Pacific Southwest; RM, Rocky Mountain states; S, summer; SE, southeastern states; Sp, spring; W, winter.

[a]The stalks of hallucinogenic *Psilocybe* species stain blue with bruising.

[b]Beware of all *Lactarius* species that stain lilac when bruised and emit latex from the gills.

Adapted from Geehr EC. Toxic plant ingestions. In: Auerbach PS, Geehr EC, eds. *Management of wilderness and environmental emergencies.* New York: Macmillan, 1983.

any method of preparation. The toxicity of the *Coprinus atramentarius* species requires the ingestion of alcohol within several days of consumption. Concurrent ingestion does not cause adverse symptoms.

For other species, only a large ingestion or consumption on consecutive days (e.g., early morel or *Verpa bohemica*) produces toxic effects. Some species (e.g., *Paxillus involutus*) are poisonous in one geographic area but edible in another. Some mushrooms are edible when they are young or fresh but toxic when old, decayed, or traumatized, similar to some fruits and vegetables (e.g., potatoes). Some mushroom toxins (e.g., phallotoxin) are severely toxic when injected but nontoxic when given orally because of poor absorption. Amatoxin concentrations vary both between species (some edible species have minute amounts) and within the same species.

GENERAL APPROACH

Points of history to obtain should include a history of ingestion, how many types of mushrooms were ingested, the time

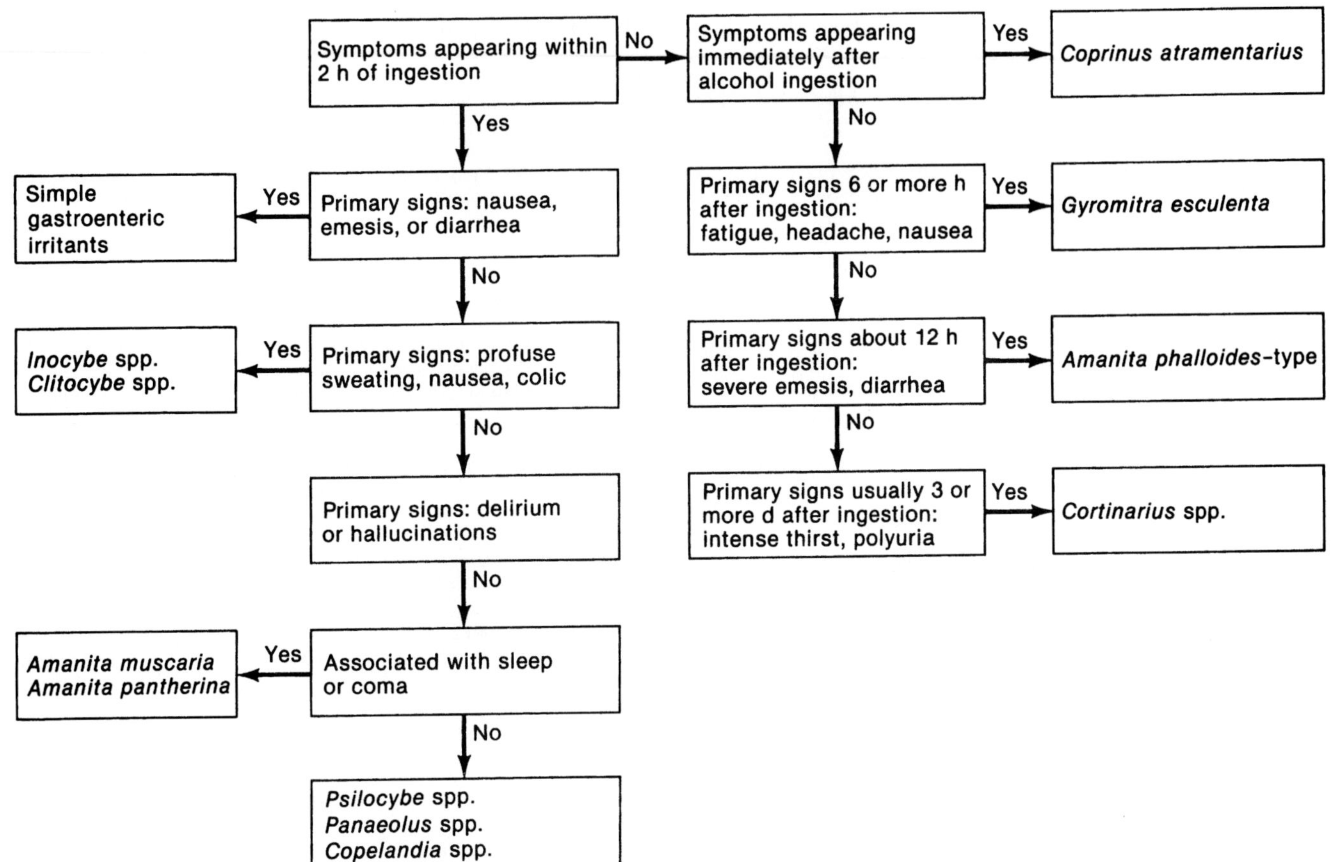

Figure 2. Differential diagnosis of mushroom intoxications by symptoms. (Adapted from Lampe KF. *Paediatrician* 1977;6:290.)

of ingestion, other people that may have eaten them, and details of the patient's current symptoms. Obtain a history of symptom presentation with emphasis on chronology. Potentially lethal mushrooms usually produce symptoms 6 hours or longer after ingestion, whereas nonlethal mushrooms produce symptoms within 6 hours (Fig. 2). However, keep in mind that a variety of mushrooms could have been eaten, and early symptoms do not rule out a potentially serious poisoning.

Try to perform a preliminary identification of mushroom and spores. Mycologists can assist with mushroom identification by telephone. Prepare a spore print if possible. If the ingested mushroom is suspected to be in the cyclopeptide group (i.e., *Amanita phalloides* and *Galerina autumnalis*), admit the patient, and follow hepatic and renal functions until recovery. Consider the use of specific antidotes when indicated (see specific mushroom groups below).

PITFALLS

"Mushroom poisoning" may actually represent an allergic reaction or food poisoning. Symptoms actually may be secondary to pesticides sprayed on the mushroom, secondary to edible mushrooms being laced with drugs (i.e., phencyclidine), or from a concomitant medical or surgical disease.

Never assume that all people ingesting the same mushroom must become ill. Never assume that a deadly *Amanita* has not been eaten if symptoms occur within 6 hours of ingestion. Patients should not be discharged without follow-up after recovering from gastrointestinal (GI) symptoms when those symptoms developed more than 6 hours postingestion.

In most cases of mushroom poisoning, supportive care and close follow-up can lead to a favorable outcome. It is always recommended to contact your regional poison center for assistance with any mushroom ingestion (Appendix V).

CYCLOPEPTIDE POISONING (GROUP I)

The cyclopeptide amatoxins contained within certain species of *Amanita* and *Galerina* can cause severe hepatorenal dysfunction and gastritis. *A. phalloides* causes more than 50% of all mushroom poisonings. The *Amanita* genus accounts for 95% of mushroom-related fatalities. Appropriately, *A. phalloides* has been named the *death cap*, whereas several other species (e.g., *Amanita virosa*, *Amanita verna*, *Amanita bisporigera*, and *Amanita ocreata*) are known as the *destroying angel*.

A. phalloides is the predominant European poisonous mushroom. Frequently, this mushroom is ingested when it is mistakenly identified as *Tricholoma equestre*. Several other *Amanita* species (e.g., *A. virosa*, *A. verna*, *Amanita brunnescens*, *A. ocreata*, and *A. bisporigera*) are more prevalent than *A. phalloides* in the United States. Many patients consider themselves experts and have consumed wild mushrooms on previous occasions without adverse effects. Rarely, fatalities have resulted from other

TABLE 3. Distinguishing characteristics of toxic *Amanita* species

Characteristic	*Amanita verna*	*Amanita virosa*	*Amanita bisporigera*	*Amanita tenuifolia*	*Amanita ocreata*	*Amanita phalloides*
Cap						
Size	2–5 in. across	2–5 in. across	1.5–3.5 in. across	2.50–3.25 in. across	2–5 in.? across	2.5–6.0 in. across
Shape and color	Convex, viscid, smooth, no warts, white, at times discoloring in age to cream on disk; no color change when touched with 3–10% KOH (or NaOH) solution	Convex to broadly umbonate, viscid, smooth, no warts, white, discoloring in age to pinkish cream or pale gray-brown (in some cases); staining yellow in KOH (or NaOH)	Convex, viscid, smooth, no warts, white; discoloring in age to pinkish cream; staining yellow in KOH (or NaOH)	Convex, viscid, smooth, shining when dry, no warts, white; becoming yellowish on disk with age or on drying; no data with KOH	Convex, viscid, smooth, no warts, white; discoloring in age to buff, pinkish, or pale brownish; staining yellow in KOH (or NaOH)	Convex, viscid, smooth, no warts, yellowish green to greenish brown; paler toward margin, with flattened radiating hairs
Gills	Free or attached to stalk by a line; white	Free or attached to stalk by a line; white	Free or attached to stalk by a line; white	Adnate; white	Free or attached to stalk by a line; white	Free or attached to stalk by a line; white
Stalk	3–8 × 0.25–0.75 in. enlarging downward to basal bulb; smooth to floccose; white	3–8 × 0.25–0.75 in. enlarging downward to basal bulb; floccose; white	3–5 × 0.25–0.75 in. enlarging downward to basal bulb; smooth to finely floccose; white	3 × 0.25–0.50 in. enlarging downward to basal bulb; smooth and shining white	3–8 × 0.25–0.75 in.? enlarging downward to basal bulb; floccose?; white	3–5 × 0.5–0.8 in. enlarging downward to basal bulb; smooth; off-white to gray or greenish yellow
Annulus	Superior, pendant, membranous, persistent, white	Superior, pendant, membranous, lacerated to partly free, white	Superior, pendant, membranous, persistent, white	Superior, pendant, membranous, persistent, white	Superior, pendant, membranous, persistent, white	Superior, pendant, membranous, persistent, white
Volva	1+ in. high, membranous, persistent, sac-like, white	1+ in. high, membranous, persistent, sac-like, white	1+ in. high, membranous, persistent, sac-like, white	1+ in. high, membranous, persistent, sac-like, white	1+ in. high, membranous, persistent, sac-like, white	1+ in. high, membranous, persistent, sac-like, white
Spores	White spore print 8–11 × 7–9 μm (L/W ratio >1.35), elliptical with distinct apiculus, thin-walled, amyloid (turns blue in Melzer's reagent)	White spore print 8–10 μm (L/W ratio <1.25), typically subglobose with distinct apiculus, thin-walled, amyloid	White spore print 7–10 μm, globose, with distinct apiculus, thin-walled, amyloid; two per basidium (all others in chart have four-spored basidia)	White spore print 12 × 5 μm, cylindrical with distinct apiculus, thin-walled, amyloid	White spore print 9–14 μm, ovoid to subellipsoid with distinct apiculus, thin-walled, amyloid	White spore print 8–11 × 7–9 μm with distinct apiculus, subglobose, thin-walled, amyloid

Adapted from Lincoff G, Mitchel DH. *Toxic and hallucinogenic mushroom poisoning. A handbook for physicians and mushroom hunters.* New York: Van Nostrand Reinhold, 1977.

North American mushroom species belonging to the *Galerina* genus (e.g., *G. autumnalis*, *Galerina marginata*).

Amanita Species

A. phalloides appears to be spreading rapidly along the east and west coasts of the United States. Although the mature *A. phalloides* mushroom often has a distinctive olive-green cap, white gills, and veil at the base of the stem, even experts, especially in its immature stages, can misidentify it. Other toxic species have white gills and caps and are difficult to distinguish from one another with the unaided eye.

Although trauma may alter distinguishing characteristics, certain physical mushroom structures of the toxic *Amanita* species are reviewed here as an aid to emergency department management and not as a guide for mushroom hunters (Table 3). These include a ring around the stalk ("ring of death"), a cup or volva at the bottom of the stalk ("cup of death"), white spores and usually white gills, gills that physically do not attach to the stalk (twisting off the stalk should leave the gills intact), and thin-walled spores that have a positive (blue) amyloid reaction to Meltzer's reagent.

Galerina Species

Galerina compounds include at least seven cyclic heptapeptides (phalloidins), eight cyclic octapeptides (amatoxins), and five virotoxins (e.g., alaviroidin, viroisin, desoxoviroidin, viroidin, and deoxoviroisin). Although phalloidin is a potent parenteral animal hepatotoxin, it has poor oral bioavailability and probably is not involved in human poisoning. *Phallotoxins* are bicyclic peptides containing cysteine, whereas *virotoxins* are monocyclic peptides containing D-serine. Characteristics of toxic species are provided in Table 4.

Toxic Dose

One to three fresh mushrooms (50 g) probably contain sufficient quantities of amatoxin to be lethal.

TABLE 4. Characteristics of toxic *Galerina* species

Characteristic	*Galerina autumnalis*	*Galerina marginata*	*Galerina venenata*
Cap			
Size	1.0–2.5 in. across	2/3–1.5(3) in. across	0.5–1.5 in. across
Shape and color	Convex, becoming plane or with slightly obtuse umbo; smooth; viscid, with separable pellicle; margin striate when moist; dark brown (when moist) to ochre tawny, fading to buff or pale yellow on drying and in age, disk at times remaining darker	Obtuse to convex, becoming broadly convex, plane, or slightly umbonate; smooth; moist but not viscid; margin striate when moist; margin extending somewhat beyond gills; dark brown when moist, fading to yellowish or dull tan, disk at times remaining darker	Convex to broadly convex; smooth; moist but not viscid; margin wavy and split in age; pale bay-brown to reddish cinnamon-brown
Gills	Adnate or with slight decurrent tooth; close; light brown at first, becoming rusty brown at maturity	Adnate to subdecurrent; close; yellowish to pallid brown when young, becoming tawny or darker at maturity	Attached; subdistant; golden brown to dull cinnamon
Stalk			
Size	(1.25)2.0–3.5 × 1/8–1/3 in.	(4/5)1.25–2.50 × 1/8–1/3 in.	1.25–1.50 × 1/8–1/4 in.
Shape and color	Equal to subclavate; hollow; dry; brown streaked with white fibrils; white mycelial covering about base	Equal to slightly enlarged downward; hollow; dry; brown to reddish brown or darker; white mycelial covering about base	Equal; dry; hairless; brownish; white mycelium just at base
Annulus (ring; partial veil)	Almost fibrillose, superior, evanescent, thin, white, hairy ring	Submembranous to fibrillose, median to superior, often evanescent, becoming brown from spores	Hairy band-like ring above middle of stalk
Spores	Brown to rusty brown spore print 8.5–10.5 × 5.0–6.5 μm ovate—elliptical, with apiculus, wrinkled to rough depression near base (by apiculus) and wrinkled exosporium	Brown to rusty brown spore print 8–10 × 5–6 μm ovate—elliptical, with apiculus, warty-wrinkled with base and wrinkled exosporium	Rusty brown spore print 8–11 × 6.0–6.5 μm ovate—elliptical, with apiculus, roughened, near base of spore

Adapted from Lincoff G, Mitchel DH. *Toxic and hallucinogenic mushroom poisoning. A handbook for physicians and mushroom hunters.* New York: Van Nostrand Reinhold, 1977.

Toxicokinetics and Toxicodynamics

Amatoxins are rapidly absorbed from the GI tract and can subsequently be detected by radioimmunoassay in the serum and urine of poisoned patients. Amatoxins may remain in the gastric aspirate more than 48 hours, probably because of their biliary excretion, but they disappear from serum within 24 hours. Both enterohepatic circulation and resorption of glomerular filtrate potentially augment toxicity.

Amatoxins are excreted rapidly in the urine. Urine concentrations reflect serum concentrations several hours previously. In dogs, 85% of α-amanitine is excreted within 6 hours, with a calculated elimination half-life of 22 hours. Blood and amniotic fluid samples taken from a woman in the eighth month of pregnancy suggested that amatoxins do not cross the placental barrier.

Pathophysiology

Amatoxins and phallotoxins are responsible for major toxicity in this class. Amatoxins inhibit RNA polymerase II within the nucleoplasm at very low concentrations and interfere with both RNA and DNA transcription. Those cells with the highest replication rates and most direct contact with the amatoxins (e.g., liver, kidney, and intestinal cells) develop necrosis. Amatoxins are not altered by any method of food preparation.

Phallotoxin, the other toxin isolated from death cap, binds with high affinity to microfilamentous structures (in particular, to F-actin), which stimulates the polymerization of G-actin, stabilizes the F-actin filaments, irreversibly polymerizes actin filaments, and causes cholestasis.

The liver is the target organ for *A. phalloides* toxins; it is presented by fatty degeneration, acute toxic dystrophy, and centrilobular necrosis. Of the amatoxins, α-amanitine is the chief component and, together with β-amanitine, probably produces the hepatorenal syndrome seen with mushroom ingestions. Amatoxin concentrations vary significantly among species, with some American samples of *A. virosa* containing small amounts of amatoxin.

A. bisporigera appears to be the most toxic American species, and *A. verna* contains variable amounts of amatoxins. Generally, other toxic *Amanita* species contain less amatoxin. Interestingly, the *Galerina* species, similar to the toxic *Amanita* species, can produce a fatal hepatorenal dysfunction, and yet they contain no phallotoxins. This observation further supports the concept that amatoxins are the primary toxic constituents.

Vulnerable Populations

Maternal poisonings are rare, and medical decisions of abortion or liver transplantation in this critical situation frequently are based on laboratory data. In one case, a 22-year-old woman in the eleventh week of pregnancy ingested *A. phalloides* mushrooms. Management consisted of intravenous (IV) hydration and administration of silymarin and *N*-acetylcysteine. No fetal damage was observed, and birth and development of the infant proceeded without incident (2).

Clinical Presentation

Typically, 6 to 24 hours (average, 10 to 12 hours) pass between the ingestion of amatoxin and the onset of symptoms. This delayed onset is an important, but not sensitive, sign of cyclopeptide ingestion. Most nonlethal mushrooms produce toxic effects soon after ingestion. Presumably, the latent period represents the time required for the amatoxins to bind to intranuclear RNA polymerase II and disrupt protein synthesis. Characteristically, cyclopeptide poisoning has three stages.

GASTROENTERITIS PHASE

A profuse, cholera-like diarrhea characterized by the abrupt onset of severe abdominal pain, nausea, vomiting, and bloody diarrhea marks the onset of toxicity. Usually, this phase lasts approximately 24 hours. Fever, tachycardia, hyperglycemia, dehydration, and electrolyte imbalance may complicate this phase.

LATENT PHASE

With adequate fluid and electrolyte replacement, a remission of symptoms occurs with a subclinical elevation of serum hepatic aminotransferase enzymes. If mushroom-related toxicity is not suspected during this 12- to 24-hour latent phase, the patient may be misdiagnosed as having gastroenteritis and discharged.

HEPATORENAL PHASE

Within 3 to 4 days of ingestion, hepatic dysfunction becomes clinically obvious, and jaundice, delirium, confusion, hypoglycemia, and coma develop despite appropriate supportive care. Coagulopathy, metabolic acidosis, conduction abnormalities, hemorrhage, and sepsis frequently complicate severe cases. Renal failure is present in most fatal cases and occasionally may be the dominant feature. Renal toxicity results from direct nephrotoxicity, hypovolemia, or both.

SYSTEMIC EFFECTS

Cardiovascular and central nervous system (CNS) effects are believed to be secondary to hepatorenal failure. Autopsies have demonstrated cerebral edema and cerebellar tonsillar herniation with fatty infiltration and mild hemorrhage of the subendocardial region. Neuropathologic changes, as well as cardiovascular changes, are variable and nonspecific, especially in view of the hyperpyrexia, sepsis, and cardiovascular collapse seen in terminal cases. Severe ileus may complicate the hepatorenal phase in *A. phalloides* or *Galerina* poisoning (3).

Mortality rates vary from 10% to 40% because of the wide variation in the amount of toxin ingested, individual susceptibility, and the patient's condition on admission. Previous estimates of a 90% mortality rate vastly overrated *Amanita* toxicity. Death usually results from hepatorenal failure 3 to 7 days postingestion. In most fatalities, encephalopathy, coma, and renal insufficiency have developed.

In a European studies of *Amanita* toxicity, the mortality rate of children younger than 10 years of age approached 50%. A 4-year-old child in a coma after ingesting *A. phalloides* received an orthotopic liver transplant (OLT) 70 hours after ingestion and regained consciousness in 24 hours (4). *A. virosa* ingestions have been associated with toxic hepatitis (5) and occasional deaths due to fulminant liver failure (6).

Diagnostic Tests

ANALYTIC METHODS

The Meixner test is a field test for the presence of amatoxins that is highly sensitive, but negative results do not guarantee edibility. The test is based on the acid-catalyzed reaction of amatoxin with lignin. A drop of freshly squeezed "juice" from the mushroom in question is placed on a sheet of newsprint paper. After the location of the spot has been marked and the area dried using a blow dryer, a drop of concentrated hydrochloric acid is placed on the spot. The paper should turn blue in the presence of amatoxin.

Specific detection of amanitines in body fluids is necessary for an early diagnosis of poisoning with *Amanita* mushrooms. A liquid chromatography-mass spectrometry assay after immunoaffinity extraction has been described (7). Thin-layer chromatography assays have been developed with documented standards to detect α-amanitine levels at approximately 50 μg/ml (8). Radioimmunoassay techniques have been developed to detect amatoxin levels as low as 0.5 ng/ml in gastric, serum, and urine samples.

BLOOD LEVELS

Blood levels may identify *Amanita*; however, concentrations may not correlate with toxicity. Amatoxins are found in the serum as late as 30 hours after ingestion in concentrations of 0.5 to 24.0 ng/ml.

Treatment

DECONTAMINATION

Induction of emesis is not beneficial more than 4 hours after ingestion. The delay in time for presentation beyond 4 hours after ingestion is a common occurrence because of the delayed toxicity of amatoxin. Activated charcoal and cathartics have been recommended, but their exact role has not been defined. Potentially, such therapy is efficacious because of enterohepatic circulation of the amatoxin within the first 36 hours. Serial activated charcoal need not be continued more than 48 hours postingestion.

ENHANCEMENT OF ELIMINATION

Ongoing controversy concerns the value of extracorporeal elimination. Plasmapheresis (9), peritoneal dialysis, hemodialysis (10), and hemoperfusion (11) have yielded occasional successes but inconsistent results (12). A new detoxication method, the molecular adsorbent recirculating system, for protein-bound substances in patients with liver failure and grade III and IV hepatic encephalopathy has been introduced.

Molecular adsorbent recirculating system is performed with an albumin-containing dialysate, which is recycled in a closed loop that contains a charcoal cartridge, an anion exchanger resin adsorber, and a conventional hemodialyzer. With dialysis using an albumin-containing dialysate, protein-bound substances, which are usually not sufficiently dialyzable, can be eliminated. The treatment increases the rate of toxin elimination to the extent that the toxic exposure of hepatocytes is minimized (13).

SUPPORTIVE MEASURES

Initial treatment requires the restoration of fluid and electrolyte balance. Obtunded patients should receive IV glucose immediately because of the common complication of hypoglycemia. Patients have presented to an emergency department in cardiac arrest resulting from fluid loss and massive GI hemorrhage. Fresh frozen plasma and vitamin K may be needed in addition to packed red blood cell transfusions and balanced electrolyte infusions. The differential diagnosis and management of acute liver failure is described in Chapter 17.

OLT can be performed in cases of severe hepatic failure (14). Once hepatic coma develops, the chances of survival with medical therapy alone are remote (15). Candidates for OLT include patients who experience progression to stage II encephalopathy or beyond; prolongation of prothrombin time greater than two times the normal despite vigorous replacement with fresh frozen plasma; and serum bilirubin levels greater than 25 mg/dl (16). Other patients with findings, such as acidosis, hypoglycemia, GI hemorrhage, and hypofibrinogenemia after marked serum aminotransferase elevation, should be considered for urgent liver transplantation without waiting for progression to advanced hepatic encephalopathy, azotemia, or jaundice.

Additional suggested criteria for transplantation after *Amanita* poisoning include peak prothrombin time less than 10% (100 seconds), factor V concentration less than 10%, lactic acidosis, GI bleeding, and age younger than 12 years. When OLT may be indicated, there does not appear to be a risk of intoxication to the transplanted liver because no further circulating amatoxins are detected after day 4 (17). Guidelines for surveillance of patients who may need OLT should include repeated clinical examinations, prothrombin times, factor V, pH, blood lactose, electroencephalography, and liver echography (18).

In one report, three experiences with liver transplantation after *A. phalloides* poisoning were analyzed. Cardiac problems were found in all patients during the postoperative period. It was hypothesized that amatoxins have cardiotoxic effects. Pancreatitis, disseminated intravascular coagulation, GI bleeding, and acute renal failure (ARF) were found in all patients (19).

ANTIDOTES

A variety of substances have been suggested for the treatment of *Amanita* poisoning: silibinin, penicillin G, rifampicin, thioctic acid, insulin, human growth hormone, cytochrome-*c*, acetylcysteine, aucubin, hyperbaric oxygen, and vitamin C. None of these drugs has been tested in controlled clinical trials.

Thioctic acid is a coenzyme of the Krebs cycle and has few adverse effects except for hypoglycemia. It has been used extensively in Eastern Europe since 1968 and has been credited with lowering mortality (20). The dose is 50 to 150 mg every 6 hours titrated to clinical response. Studies in animals have not documented the beneficial effect of thioctic acid, and its efficacy remains unproven.

Silibinin is a constituent of the extract silymarin derived from the milk thistle *Silybum marianum*. Studies in animals suggest that this derivative reduces hepatic damage even when given 24 hours after *A. phalloides* administration, perhaps through inhibition of amatoxin uptake by hepatocytes. Silybin, 20 to 48 mg/kg/day, in humans has shown promise as a clinical antidote to acute poisoning; however, further studies paying attention to the amount of ingested mushroom and time elapsed before administration of treatment are needed to clarify its role in this indication (21).

One study supported silybin, administered either as monochemotherapy or in drug combination, and acetylcysteine as monochemotherapy as the most effective therapeutic modes (22). In a retrospective, uncontrolled Austrian study, the administration of IV silibinin (20 to 50 mg/kg/day in four doses) and penicillin was associated with a favorable outcome in all but one of 18 *A. phalloides* cases (23).

Penicillin appears to displace amatoxin from plasma protein-binding sites, allowing for increased renal excretion. It also may inhibit the penetration of amatoxin into hepatocytes. In one retrospective clinical study of 205 patients, dosages of 300,000 to 1 million U of benzyl penicillin daily tended to be more often associated with survival than less than 300,000 U/day (24). Despite experimental data, the overall survival of patients treated with penicillin is not impressively higher than that of the total population.

Acetylcysteine in high doses has reportedly been used to successfully treat *A. phalloides* poisoning in humans (25); however, this intervention was unsuccessful in at least one rat study (26).

MONITORING

Routine laboratory tests for symptomatic cases include a complete blood cell count, electrolytes, blood urea nitrogen, creatinine, prothrombin time, bilirubin urinalysis, and blood glucose. Determinations should be repeated daily until clinical improvement occurs. Serum hepatic aminotransferases generally are lower in survivors than nonsurvivors, but they are not accurate predictors of survival. Elevated serum amylase levels have been reported in up to 50% of *A. phalloides* poisonings. Blood ammonia levels are not elevated until the advanced stages of hepatic failure.

MONOMETHYLHYDRAZINE POISONING (GROUP II)

The genus *Gyromitra* contains some of the most prized edible mushrooms of all, the morels. Gyromitrin is one of nine different hydrazones found in variable amounts in *Gyromitra* species. Its hydrolysis to monomethylhydrazine (MMH; a compound used for rocket fuel) causes gastritis. Less often, hemolysis, hepatorenal dysfunction, coma, convulsions, and death occur after ingestion. Not all species of *Gyromitra* contain the relatively unstable gyromitrin, and concentration varies dramatically even within the same species.

Gyromitra esculenta is a serious health hazard in Poland, where improper consumption accounts for nearly one-fourth of mushroom-related fatalities. There are at least eight species of *Gyromitra* (including *G. esculenta*) in the United States that contain variable amounts of gyromitrin. All are nongilled fungi. Caps are yellow-brown to dark-red and have irregularly wrinkled, deep, convoluted tops. The cap size varies between 1 and 5 inches.

Lycoperdon (puffballs) are mushroom species belonging to the Basidiomycetes family (27,28). Puffballs are usually safe, but may produce nausea and vomiting 6 to 12 hours after exposure and respiratory symptoms (e.g., shortness of breath), fever, myalgia, and fatigue within 3 to 7 days after inhalation and ingestion (29). The respiratory symptoms (lycoperdonosis) may include symptoms of pneumonia and widespread nodular densities on lung radiography. One puffball species (*Lycoperdon marginatum*) can produce psychoactive effects (30).

Toxic Dose

The lethal dose of gyromitrin in adults is estimated to be from 20 to 50 μg/kg. Two patients who ate approximately ten *G. esculenta* mushrooms developed moderate liver damage with signs of hemolysis. One patient was treated with combined hemodialysis and hemoperfusion together with pyridoxine, 25 mg/kg, and symptomatic therapy (31).

Pathophysiology

Gyromitrin is the most toxicologically important of the nine hydrazones isolated from *G. esculenta*. Structurally, gyromitrin is an aldehyde that hydrolyzes in the body to MMH. Gyromitrin is heat labile, although simple parboiling does not guarantee edibility. Toxic concentrations vary with climatic conditions, as well as other undetermined variables, so that people who previously have consumed them without difficulty may develop adverse reactions.

Clinical Presentation

Humans who ingest gyromitrin develop gastroenteritis 6 to 8 hours later, similar to those who eat amatoxin-containing mushroom species. Symptoms may include dizziness, fatigue, nausea, vomiting, severe headache, and abdominal pain. In mild cases, vomiting may persist for several hours, but nonspecific symptoms may persist for several days. Jaundice, convulsions, coma, and death may follow severe cases of *G. esculenta* poisoning (32). In severe cases, hepatic failure may develop over the next several days, complicated by hypoglycemia and hypovolemia. Most gyromitrin ingestions result in mild symptoms. Progression of symptoms is a poor prognostic sign and suggests hepatic involvement.

Diagnostic Tests

ANALYTIC METHODS

Ultraviolet spectrophotometric methods have been developed to detect gyromitrin after extraction by thin-layer chromatography. MMH can be detected using gas-liquid chromatography.

BLOOD LEVELS

Blood levels do not always correlate well with clinical presentation. Methemoglobin may be detected early in the course of the poisoning and is an indicator of MMH exposure. Free hemoglobin may be detected early in the poisoning. Few clinical studies have evaluated methemoglobinemia in *G. esculenta* poisoning (33).

OTHER TESTS

In severe cases, baseline laboratory analysis should include a complete blood cell count, electrolytes, creatinine, liver function tests (including prothrombin time), glucose, and urinalysis (including a screen for hemoglobinuria).

Treatment

DECONTAMINATION

Most patients present long after methods of decontamination are expected to be beneficial. The use of activated charcoal is a reasonable treatment modality, although no human or animal data are available to guide the therapy. Ipecac or lavage may be used if the patient presents within 4 hours of ingestion when the usual precautions are observed.

ENHANCEMENT OF ELIMINATION

No extracorporeal methods have been studied in human gyromitrin toxicity.

SUPPORTIVE MEASURES

Depletion of fluids, electrolytes, and glucose is the most common complication of severe gyromitrin poisoning. Rarely, coma and convulsions may compromise the airway, requiring ventilatory support. Seizures are initially treated in the typical manner with benzodiazepines and more aggressive measures as clinically indicated (Chapter 40). However, pyridoxine should also be administered as described in antidotes.

Gyromitrin-induced hepatic encephalopathy requires the same supportive treatment used in *A. phalloides* poisoning and other causes of acute liver failure (Chapter 17). Drugs that require cytochrome P-450 metabolism (e.g., phenobarbital) may have exaggerated effects because of gyromitrin-induced disruption of the cytochrome P-450 pathway and should be used with caution.

ANTIDOTES

Pyridoxine (25 mg/kg up to a daily adult dose of 15 to 20 g) has been recommended for the neurologic symptoms of gyromitrin poisoning based on the similarity between gyromitrin and hydrazine toxicity. Pyridoxine increases the formation of γ-aminobutyric acid (GABA) in the presence of toxic levels of isoniazid and its hydrazine, but the activation of GABA transamination by pyridoxine may actually lead to decreased brain GABA. Which effect predominates in humans remains to be documented.

Although sensory neuropathies have been reported in chronic megavitamin overdose, large pyridoxine doses have few reported side effects (34). Doses administered for CNS effects of gyromitrin toxicity are similar to those used for isoniazid toxicity. More details regarding the indications, adverse events, and method of administration for pyridoxine are provided in Chapter 71.

COPRINE POISONING (GROUP III)

The North American species *C. atramentarius* ("inky cap") produces coprine, a toxin that interacts with ethanol to cause a disulfiram-like reaction. Although hyperacetaldehydemia is present in coprine toxicity, similar to the disulfiram-ethanol reaction, disulfiram has not been consistently isolated from *C. atramentarius*. The exact toxic mechanism remains unclear because elevated aldehyde levels alone do not reproduce either coprine or disulfiram-ethanol toxicity in experimental animals. Instead, the toxic component probably is a derivative of glutamine.

Coprinus species are gilled fungi with convex to parabolic caps that often fold over the stalk like an umbrella. The common name "inky cap" derives from the propensity of the gills to dissolve into an inky, black fluid on maturity.

Pathophysiology

The fungal toxin coprine blocks the enzyme acetaldehyde dehydrogenase, which stops the metabolism of ethanol at the acetaldehyde stage. It acts very similarly to the drug disulfiram used in the treatment of alcoholism. If ethanol is not consumed with the meal, these fungi may be edible. The *Coprinus* species do not contain disulfiram.

Clinical Presentation

Sensitivity to ethanol occurs as soon as 2 hours (average, 3 to 6 hours) after the consumption of *Coprinus* mushrooms and may last up to 72 hours. Typically, symptoms begin soon after ethanol ingestion (15 to 20 minutes) and spontaneously resolve in 3 to 6 hours. The intensity of symptoms is related to the quantity of mushrooms and ethanol ingested as well as the time elapsed between mushroom and ethanol consumption.

Common symptoms include severe headache, facial flushing, paresthesias, lightheadedness, orthostatic hypotension, vomiting, palpitations, tachycardia, diaphoresis, and chest pain. Shock, metabolic acidosis, cardiac dysrhythmias, and myocardial infarction have complicated disulfiram-ethanol reactions. Such adverse symptoms represent a theoretic danger in coprine-ethanol interactions, especially in patients with underlying cardiovascular disease.

Treatment

DECONTAMINATION

These measures are usually unnecessary, especially because spontaneous vomiting frequently occurs, and the reaction rarely lasts more than several hours.

ENHANCEMENT OF ELIMINATION

No methods to enhance elimination have been used clinically. The use of hemodialysis to remove alcohol has theoretic benefit only in the critically ill patient.

SUPPORTIVE MEASURES

Adequate fluid and electrolyte management are the most important aspects of supportive care. Reactions usually are mild and self-limited. Patients should be warned to avoid all alcohol-containing products (including cold remedies and medical elixirs) for 72 hours. Phenothiazine antiemetics should be avoided because their α-adrenergic–blocking properties may exacerbate hypotension.

Coprine toxicity should be treated similarly to the disulfiram-ethanol reaction. Hypotension and cardiac dysrhythmias present the most immediate threat to life. Patients with vital sign abnormalities or those with cardiovascular disease should receive cardiac monitoring, oxygen, and an IV line. Hypotension should be treated with isotonic fluid infusion followed by a vasopressor for refractory patients (Chapter 37).

ANTIDOTES

Propranolol has been recommended for the treatment of supraventricular tachycardia and anxiety (10 to 15 mg orally) but is not well tested. Antihistamines, ascorbic acid, and iron salts have not been effective in human trials, at least in the disulfiram-ethanol reaction.

MUSCARINE POISONING (GROUP IV)

Only three genera of mushrooms (*Amanita*, *Inocybe*, and *Clitocybe*) are reported to contain muscarine, whereas several other genera (*Boletus*, *Hebeloma*, *Mycena*, and *Omphalotus*) are suspected of containing muscarine. Elevated levels of liver function tests and hypokalemia have been observed after jack o'lantern mushroom poisoning (*Omphalotus illudens*). Muscarine was first isolated from *Amanita muscaria* in 1868; however, this mushroom contains such toxicologically insignificant amounts that other physiologically dissimilar compounds are responsible for *A. muscaria* toxicity.

Clitocybe are widely distributed species that occasionally inhabit lawns and parks. They often are found in close association with other genera of fungi, making identification difficult. They have white-tan to gray caps, fleshy central stalks, and adnate to decurrent gills. *Inocybe* mushrooms are usually found in oak and pine woods. They are small, brown mushrooms with conical, fibrillose caps and adnate whitish to tobacco-brown gills.

Ingestion of *Clitocybe* or *Inocybe* mushrooms usually produces a mild cholinergic excess syndrome within 30 minutes. Serious toxicity is relatively unusual, perhaps because of the inaccessible habitat of some toxic species, poor oral bioavailability of muscarine, and general unattractiveness as a forage food. This type of mushroom poisoning is the only one for which atropine is a specific antidote.

Toxic Dose

A series of muscarine mushroom poisonings from southern France between 1973 and 1998 yielded 248 incidents involving 483 patients (41 children between 1 and 14 years of age). The average onset of symptoms was 2 hours. The most frequent signs were perspiration (96% of patients), vomiting (70%), diarrhea (62%), hypotension (36%), abdominal pain (32%), miosis (25%), blurred vision (22%), bradycardia (20%), rhinorrhea (6%), and lacrimation (6%) (35).

Ingestions of nine jack o'lantern mushrooms (*O. illudens*) by 14 people led to vomiting in eight, diarrhea in five, and weakness in two; tiredness and the feeling of being cold occurred in eight. Recovery was complete within 18 hours (36). Seven adults who ingested jack o'lantern mushrooms experienced nausea, vomiting, abdominal cramping, diarrhea, weakness, dizziness, and diaphoresis. All symptoms began within 15 to 90 minutes after ingestion. Three had mildly elevated liver function tests; one had hypokalemia requiring potassium supplementation. All were given IV fluids and oral activated charcoal. They were discharged the following day (37).

After ingestion of the mushroom *Inocybe tristis*, a 2-year-old girl had sudden onset of diarrhea, vomiting, stupor, and miosis. Subsequently, she developed excessive hypertension, a purpuric rash, and transient hepatic, muscular, renal, and cutaneous damage. The patient completely recovered after supportive therapy (38).

Pathophysiology

Muscarine is responsible for the parasympathomimetic effects of *Inocybe* and *Clitocybe*. Physiologically, muscarine stimulates postganglionic cholinergic fibers, producing increased muscle tone and gastrourinary activity, bradycardia, miosis, diaphoresis, and salivation. Muscarine is heat stable, so that cooking does not produce edible species.

Clinical Presentation

Typically, symptoms from this group of mushrooms begin within 15 minutes to 1 hour, with headache, nausea, vomiting, and abdominal pain followed by salivation, lacrimation, diarrhea, diaphoresis, miosis, and blurred vision. Bronchoconstriction may lead to dyspnea and wheezing. The presence of diaphoresis is an important diagnostic sign and strongly suggests muscarinic poisoning unless hypovolemic shock is present.

Elevated liver function tests have been reported in *Clitocybe* ingestions. Cardiovascular effects include bradycardia, hypotension, and shock. Symptoms are usually mild and generally abate within 2 to 6 hours. Death is uncommon.

Ingestion of jack o'lantern mushrooms (*O. illudens*) has led to vomiting, diarrhea, weakness, tiredness, and the feeling of being cold. Recovery is complete within 18 hours. Abdominal cramping, dizziness, and diaphoresis may also occur. Pantherina poisoning syndrome is characterized by CNS dysfunction (39).

Treatment

DECONTAMINATION

Syrup of ipecac may be given to alert patients if they present within several hours of ingestion, although spontaneous vomiting may preclude its use. Activated charcoal may be useful. Patients who remain asymptomatic need not be decontaminated unless a toxic coingestion is suspected.

ENHANCEMENT OF ELIMINATION

No extracorporeal methods have been shown to enhance the elimination of muscarine mushrooms.

SUPPORTIVE MEASURES

Although rare, death may result from the inability to control respiratory secretions, bronchospasm, and cardiovascular collapse. Such patients require oxygen, suctioning IV lines, cardiac monitoring, and, if indicated, intubation. Symptoms resolve within 24 hours, so that observation beyond that time is rarely necessary. Be sure to watch for fluid depletion and treat accordingly. Elevated levels of liver function tests and hypokalemia have been observed after jack o'lantern mushroom poisoning (*O. illudens*).

ANTIDOTES

Atropine may be used to dry secretions by antagonizing the effect of muscarine (Chapter 42). A useful starting IV dose is 0.2 mg for children younger than 2 years of age, 0.3 mg for children 2 to 4 years of age, 0.4 mg for children 4 to 10 years of age, 0.6 mg for children 10 to 14 years of age, and 0.8 to 1.0 mg for adults. Additional smaller doses may be given, adjusted to the clinical response. Drying of secretions should be used as an endpoint, along with rhythm monitoring, to prevent excessive atropinization.

IBOTENIC ACID AND MUSCIMOL POISONING (GROUP V)

A. muscaria and *Amanita pantherina* are the two major North American species that contain psychoactive isoxazole derivatives. As with hallucinogenic psilocybin mushrooms (group VI), the onset of CNS symptoms occurs in 30 to 60 minutes. Isoxazole compounds produce alterations in visual perception rather than formed hallucinations seen with the indole derivatives (psilocybin and psilocin).

A. muscaria contains only minute amounts of muscarine, and the syndrome caused by its ingestion cannot be characterized as cholinergic or anticholinergic. Occasionally, both these species are intentionally ingested for their psychoactive properties.

A. muscaria (fly agaric) is white, has gills free from the stalk, and a 3- to 4-inch orange-red cap with distinctive white to pale yellow warts on top. An annulus and a distinguishing volva of concentric rings are present, slightly differing from those of other *Amanita* species. *A. pantherina* is most abundant during the rainy seasons of spring, summer, and fall. It has the distinctive pileal warts, white gills, annulus, and bulbous volva as at the stalk's base of *A. muscaria* but possesses more sheathing. The pileus (cap) is tan to yellow-brown to dark brown.

Toxic Dose

The threshold for development of CNS disturbance in humans is approximately 6 mg of muscimol or 30 to 600 mg of ibotenic acid (40).

Pathophysiology

The isoxazole compounds, ibotenic acid, and its decarboxylated derivative muscimol account for most (e.g., muscle spasm, confusion, intoxication, drowsiness, and sleep), but not all, of the symptoms of poisoning. Ibotenic acid is structurally similar to glutaminic acid and mimics its effects in animals. Ibotenic acid is rapidly converted to muscimol, which structurally resembles GABA. Both isoxazole derivatives can be detected in the urine within 1 hour of ingestion.

Muscimol has high affinity for GABA receptor sites and imitates the action of GABA-B in animals and humans, inhibiting and controlling the recruitment and multiplication of nerve impulses mediated by many positive neurotransmitters (41). Determination of clinical toxicity by ingestion history is complicated by the fact that considerable variation occurs both in individual isoxazole compounds and in total isoxazole content within the same species.

A. pantherina often contains compounds, in addition to ibotenic acid and muscimol (found also in *A. muscaria*), such as stizolobic and stizolobinic acid, in concentrations that may be clinically significant. These compounds are related to L-dopa oxidation products and can produce anticholinergic effects (42–44). *A. muscaria* appears to contain a greater concentration of isoxazole compounds (0.17% to 1.00% dry weight) than *A. pantherina* (0.02% to 0.53%).

Clinical Presentation

Depending on the amounts of isoxazole compounds consumed, symptoms may appear within 30 minutes to several hours and include dizziness, ataxia, euphoria, muscle twitches, and initial psychic stimulation followed by a dream-filled sleep. More severe ingestions produce visual disturbances, fever, confusion, myoclonus, mydriasis, seizures, and coma. Death from these mushrooms is extremely rare (45).

The primary effects are CNS depression and stimulation, which may alternate. Symptoms usually begin with drowsiness followed by a state of confusion, with ataxia, dizziness, and euphoria resembling alcohol intoxication, and may proceed to increase activity, illusions, or even manic excitement. These periods of excitement may alternate with periods of somnolence, deep sleep, or stupor (44). Symptoms are transient, last approximately 6 hours, and rarely simulate either a cholinergic or anticholinergic syndrome. Vomiting is not a prominent part of the clinical picture. Some patients may have residual headaches for days.

Treatment

DECONTAMINATION

Measures of gastric decontamination (e.g., syrup of ipecac/lavage, charcoal) may be useful within the first several hours of ingestion, although agitation may make these procedures technically difficult. For this reason, activated charcoal alone or ipecac is preferred to lavage in the alert patient.

ENHANCEMENT OF ELIMINATION

No extracorporeal methods to enhance elimination have been used clinically.

SUPPORTIVE MEASURES

General supportive care is the mainstay of treatment because most ingestions require observation and no medications. Short-acting hypnotic agents should be used with caution because studies suggest that isoxazole compounds potentiate their effect by inhibiting the formation of microsomal enzymes. Nonpharmacologic intervention is preferred unless seizures or airway compromise necessitates treatment. *A. pantherina* often contains compounds in addition to ibotenic acid and muscimol that can produce anticholinergic effects.

ANTIDOTES

Atropine most likely exacerbates symptoms and should not be given. Experimentally, muscimol symptoms are not ameliorated by physostigmine.

HALLUCINOGENIC MUSHROOMS (GROUP VI)

The use of hallucinogenic mushrooms predates the arrival of the Spaniards to the New World. The Aztecs consumed a substance called teonanacatl (God's flesh) in religious ceremonies. Later, *Psilocybe mexicana* was discovered to be the active component of teonanacatl. The use of mushrooms by people native to the Americas to produce mystical revelations during religious ceremonies continued into the twentieth century.

The psilocybin-containing species known to cause the majority of toxic exposures are *Psilocybe*, *Panaeolus*, *Copelandia*, *Gymnopilus*, *Pluteus*, and *Conocybe*. The main toxin is psilocybin. Psilocybin and the less stable psilocin were isolated in 1958 from mushrooms used in Mazatec Indian ceremonies in the state of Oaxaca, Mexico. These compounds have lysergic acid diethylamide–like properties and produce alterations of autonomic function, motor reflexes, behavior, and perception. During the 1960s, Aldous Huxley and Carlos Castaneda popularized recreational ingestion of psilocybin-containing mushrooms in the western United States.

Patients typically present with dysphoric and sympathomimetic symptoms that are transient, lasting less than 12 hours. The adolescent substance abuser when seen in a state of panic may have ingested hallucinogenic mushrooms possibly with simultaneous lysergic acid diethylamide (also known as *LSD*), alcohol, phencyclidine (also known as *PCP*), and marijuana (46). The potential for self-inflicted or accidental trauma during periods of altered behavior represents the greatest health hazard, although persistent psychiatric symptoms have been rarely reported.

Classification and Uses

The principal hallucinogenic mushrooms in North America are found primarily in the Pacific Northwest, Hawaii, Texas, and Florida and are grouped into three genera. *Panaeolus* mushrooms have a thin stalk, dark purple to black spores, and a convex to parabolic pileus. The North American *Psilocybe* species has long thin stalks with a conical or bell-shaped pileus and dark brown to purple-brown spores. Characteristically, the stalk turns blue on handling, and common names include liberty cap, blue legs, and magic mushrooms. *Gymnopilus* mushrooms have a broad yellow to orange cap, a thick stalk, and rusty orange spores and usually grow in the woods on buried logs.

A number of other plants can be considered agents of abuse and are often taken in combination with other pharmacologically active substances (Chapters 177 and 255). This group includes jimsonweed (*Datura stramonium*); nutmeg (*Myristica fragrans*); morning glory (*Ipomoea tricolor*—active ingredients include various amides of lysergic acid; ololiuqui (*Rivea corymbosa*)—active ingredients include indole alkaloids in the seeds; khat (*Catha edulis*); and peyote (*Lophophora williamsii*) (47).

Toxic Dose

Agitation and hallucination were reported after ingestion of ten mushrooms in one case; however, another patient complained of only abdominal pain after consuming 200 mushrooms (48). The concentration of active ingredients in these species is so low that consumption of one or two mushroom caps does not result in symptoms. Most patients have eaten large quantities to experience the psychotomimetic effects.

Pathophysiology

The active constituents of hallucinogenic mushrooms probably are indole compounds derived from tryptamine. Psilocybin and its less stable metabolite psilocin are the best known active compounds, but their effects may not entirely explain the range of symptoms caused by hallucinogenic mushrooms. Wide variation occurs in clinical response.

Clinical Presentation

Patients usually present within 4 hours of ingestion with symptoms of lightheadedness, weakness, and anxiety that began 30 to 60 minutes after ingestion. Most symptoms resolve within 4 hours, and persistence of dysphoric symptoms past 12 hours is rare. Persistent neurologic symptoms comprised primarily of flashback phenomena are well recognized but are uncommon complications of psilocybin ingestion.

Mydriasis and blurred vision are common, but other sympathomimetic signs, such as tachycardia, hypertension, and hyperreflexia, are seen in less than one-half of emergency department patients. Dysphoria, disorientation, ataxia, agitation, and aggressive behavior may appear after ingestions. Antisocial behavior represents the greatest danger to life. Hallucinations occur in less than one-half of patients who ingest these mushrooms. Visual hallucinations are more common than auditory hallucinations; however, alterations in perception occur in almost all patients and involve primarily distortion of shapes and colors.

Coma, convulsions, hyperthermia, and death have been reported after large ingestions in small children. Adult seizures also have been reported in psilocybin intoxication. Several cases of IV administration of psilocybin extract have been associated with vomiting, myalgias, hyperpyrexia, hypoxemia, and mild methemoglobinemia.

Diagnostic Tests

Mild elevations of lactate dehydrogenase, serum aspartate aminotransferase, and alkaline phosphatase have been reported but probably are not clinically important.

Treatment

DECONTAMINATION

Although recommended by some authorities, decontamination measures may be technically difficult, and most patients can be managed by supportive care alone. Within 2 hours of ingestion, gastric emptying may be used in the alert patient, but in series in which decontamination measures have not been used, no complications have been reported. The one exception is the rare case of a large ingestion in a small child.

ENHANCEMENT OF ELIMINATION

No methods to enhance elimination have been used clinically.

SUPPORTIVE MEASURES

Most patients who ingest psilocybin-containing mushrooms do not present to a hospital and usually suffer no ill effects. For those who do go to a hospital, dysphoria is the major complaint, and a quiet, supportive environment (darkened room with familiar faces) and calm reassurance are all that are usually necessary. There are no specific antidotes for hallucinogenic mushrooms. Diazepam (oral or IV) may be needed for sedation, and chlorpromazine should be reserved for frank hallucinations.

GASTROINTESTINAL IRRITANTS (GROUP VII)

The rapid onset of GI distress is the most common adverse reaction to mushroom ingestion. A large group of mushrooms, including *Agaricus* species, *Amanita brunnescens*, *Boletus sensibilis*, *Chlorophyllum molybdites*, *Entoloma* species, *Hebeloma crustuliniforme* ("poison pie"), *Naematoloma fasciculare*, *Paxillus involutus*, *Ramaria formosa*, *Ramaria gelatinosa*, *Scleroderma* species, and *Tricholoma* species, are capable of producing such unpleasant, but seldom dangerous, reactions.

In general, symptoms appear within 2 hours of ingestion and include malaise, weakness, nausea, vomiting, and diarrhea that may turn bloody. Fluid and electrolyte imbalance and the coingestion of hepatotoxic mushrooms (e.g., group I or II) represent the greatest danger. The clinical course of isolated ingestion of group VII mushrooms is usually mild, with resolution occurring within 24 hours.

Toxic Dose

A 6-year-old girl who ingested an unknown quantity of *C. molybdites* (*Lepiota morgani*) presented with hypotension, lethargy, and shallow respirations. This followed an episode of abdominal pain and diarrhea that began 1.5 hours after ingestion. She was treated symptomatically with IV fluids, pressor amines, activated charcoal, ranitidine, and penicillin G. She recovered in 3 days (49).

Pathophysiology

Because most GI irritants remain unidentified, most mechanisms of action are also unknown. Many reactions are idiosyncratic, and allergic reactions have been proposed as a possible mechanism. No cases of anaphylactic reactions to mushroom ingestions have been reported despite the fact that the diversity of higher fungi suggests that haptens may be present.

The structures of the toxins within this group have not been elucidated except for those of *C. molybdites*, *Gomphus floccosus*, and *Lactarius* species. Cooking appears to inactivate many gastritis-inducing mushroom toxins but does not guarantee the absence of side effects.

Clinical Presentation

This group represents a large variety of unrelated toxins that cause similar symptoms. Symptoms generally begin 30 to 90 minutes after consumption. All cause varying degrees of digestive upset, characterized by diarrhea, vomiting, and abdominal cramps. Symptoms typically clear in 3 to 4 hours and complete recovery several days later. Some cases of fatality have been recorded, but these are usually cases in which large quantities of mushrooms have been consumed or if the patients were young children (50).

Mature *C. molybdites* specimens ("green parasol") are easily recognized by their gills, which are green because of mature spore deposits. Ingestion of these mushrooms generally produces a self-limited gastroenteritis (51) characterized by nausea, vomiting, abdominal pain, and diarrhea within 1 to 3 hours of consumption. Initially, the stool is watery, but subsequently, bloody diarrhea develops along with fecal leukocytes. Shaking chills, diffuse abdominal pain, and myalgias occasionally are present, and symptoms resolve within 24 to 48 hours.

GI hemorrhage with disseminated intravascular coagulation has followed ingestion of *C. molybdites* (52). A 6-year-old girl developed hypovolemic shock after ingesting *C. molybdites* mushrooms (49). GI-irritant mushrooms can produce severe toxicity in pediatric patients who have a limited capacity for fluid loss before becoming hypovolemic.

Clitocybe nebularis ("clouded agaric" or "clouded funnel cap") and *Tricholomopsis platyphylla* (53) are usually considered edible but may cause gastroenteritis in a limited number of susceptible people. Typically, the symptoms of nausea, vomiting, lightheadedness, headache, and diarrhea begin 2 to 6 hours after ingestion and resolve in 24 to 48 hours. *Entoloma lividum* has been associated with the rapid onset of gastroenteritis (chills, nausea, vomiting, crampy abdominal pain) and mild elevation of hepatic aminotransferase levels. Acute symptoms resolve within 12 hours, and loose stools improve within 48 hours.

Treatment

Gut decontamination is generally unnecessary, as vomiting occurs spontaneously. No methods to enhance elimination have been used clinically.

SUPPORTIVE MEASURES

Treatment is supportive. Fluid and electrolyte imbalance is the most common serious adverse effect. Most symptoms resolve within 24 to 48 hours with supportive care. Antiemetics may be helpful.

MANAGEMENT PITFALLS

The most important diagnostic point is to exclude group I (cyclopeptide) and group II (gyromitrin) poisonings through history and either specimen identification or spore analysis. GI irritants and hepatotoxic mushrooms may be coingested.

CORTINARIUS (GROUP VIII)

Cortinarius species poisoning is characterized by a delayed ARF. The main features of this severe poisoning are still poorly known and often overlooked (54). Several species of the genus *Cortinarius* (e.g., *Cortinarius speciosissimus*, *Cortinarius orellanus*, *Cortinarius splendens*, and *Cortinarius venenosus*) have produced irreversible renal failure in European and Japanese patients. Some patients later required renal transplantation to restore normal kidney function. Poisoning by this mushroom group first was reported in Poland and subsequently has been reported from Scotland, France, Switzerland, Finland, and Sweden.

Although *Cortinarius* toxicity has not been reported in the United States, many representatives of this genus do appear in North America. They have robust, colored (purple, orange, greenish yellow) fruit bodies with characteristic rusty orange gills, a partial veil hanging over the gills, a thick stalk with striae, and a bulbous base.

Toxic Dose

Twenty-six young men ingested mushroom soup made only with *C. orellanus*. They were hospitalized 10 to 12 days after the incident. Twelve presented with acute tubulointerstitial nephritis with ARF; eight required hemodialysis; nine were given corticosteroids. Of these 12, eight patients recovered rapidly, and four suffered from chronic renal failure for several months (55).

Pathophysiology

Two bipyridyl toxins, orelline and orellanine, have been isolated from *C. orellanus*, but the mechanism of action and its pharmacokinetics are not well understood. These 2,2-bipyridine compounds are structurally related to paraquat and diquat. Cooking or drying does not reduce toxicity.

Clinical Presentation

Typically, gastritis appears approximately 36 hours postingestion and is followed by anorexia, headache, chills, thirst, myalgias, lumbar pain, burning thirst, and oliguria over the next week. In one series of 12 patients poisoned with *C. orellanus*, after a latent period of between 2 to 5 days, the patients complained of asthenia, intense thirst, and digestive and neurologic disorders. Leukocyturia was detected in all patients but without proteinuria.

The incidence of ARF in this series varied from 30% to 46%. Renal failure depends on individual sensitivity, preexisting nephropathy, and the cumulated dose of toxin ingested. Early and severe interstitial fibrosis, marked interstitial edema, and tubular epithelial necrosis are the most characteristic renal lesions (56).

In one series, ingestion of *Cortinarius rubellus* and *C. orellanus* resulted in permanent renal failure in four out of five patients after a latent period of approximately 10 days (57.) A few cases of poisoning involving hepatocellular damage have been reported after *C. orellanus* ingestion, but no liver damage has been demonstrated in *C. speciosissimus* poisoning cases.

Diagnostic Tests

The presence of normal liver function together with delayed ARF (up to 20 days after ingestion), abdominal pain, and burning thirst characterize the toxic syndrome. Orellanine, the toxin believed to cause tubulointerstitial nephritis, and orelline may be isolated from urine, serum, and feces (58). Orellanine can be detected by fluorometry after thin-layer chromatography (59).

Treatment

Measures of gastric decontamination (e.g., syrup of ipecac/lavage, charcoal, cathartics) may be useful within the first several hours of ingestion. The use of hemodialysis for supportive care may reduce fatalities (60). Clinical evidence supporting hemoperfusion remains anecdotal.

Supportive Care

The mainstay of treatment is supportive care with careful management of fluid and electrolyte balance. Hospitalization may be prolonged because of slow return of kidney function. In the more severe cases, irreversible renal disease occurs, requiring kidney transplantation.

REFERENCES

1. Tegzes JH, Puschner B. Toxic mushrooms. *Vet Clin North Am Small Anim Pract* 2002;32:397–407.
2. Boyer JC, Hernandez F, Estorc J, et al. Management of maternal *Amanita phalloides* poisoning during the first trimester of pregnancy: a case report and review of the literature. *Clin Chem* 2001;47:971–974.
3. Feldman R. Probable *Amanita phalloides* poisoning with pseudo-obstructive, paralytic ileus (Ogilvie's syndrome). *Pol Arch Med Wewn* 2001;106:1169–1173.
4. Kern C, Zilker T, Clarmann M. *Successful liver transplantation in a child after* Amanita *poisoning*. Proc Eur Assoc Pois Cont Centers Toxicol XV Congress, Istanbul, Turkey, May 24–27 1992:126.
5. Lim JG, Kim JH, Lee CY, et al. *Amanita virosa* induced toxic hepatitis: report of three cases. *Yonsei Med J* 2000;41:416–421.
6. Chaiear K, Limpaiboon R, Meechai C, et al. Fatal mushroom poisoning caused by *Amanita virosa* in Thailand. *Southeast Asian J Trop Med Public Health* 1999;30:157–160.
7. Maurer HH, Schmitt CJ, Weber AA, et al. Validated electrospray liquid chromatographic-mass spectrometric assay for the determination of the mushroom toxins alpha- and beta-amanitin in urine after immunoaffinity extraction. *J Chromatogr B Biomed Sci Appl* 2000;748:125–135.
8. Stijve T, Seeger T. Determination of alpha-, beta-, and gamma-amanitin by high performance thin-layer chromatography in *Amanita phalloides* (Vaill. ex Fr.) secr. from various origin. *Z Naturforsch (C)* 1979;34:1133–1138.
9. Jander S, Bischoff J, Woodcock BG. Plasmapheresis in the treatment of *Amanita phalloides* poisoning: II. A review and recommendations. *Ther Apher* 2000;4:308–312.
10. Sabeel AI, Kurkus J, Lindholm T. Intensive hemodialysis and hemoperfusion treatment of *Amanita* mushroom poisoning. *Mycopathologia* 1995;131:107–114.
11. Parish RC, Doering PL. Treatment of *Amanita* mushroom poisoning: a review. *Vet Hum Toxicol* 1986;28:318–322.
12. Mullins ME, Horowitz BZ. The futility of hemoperfusion and hemodialysis in *Amanita phalloides* poisoning. *Vet Hum Toxicol* 2000;42:90–91.
13. Shi Y, He J, Chen S, et al. MARS: optimistic therapy method in fulminant hepatic failure secondary to cytotoxic mushroom poisoning—a case report. *Liver* 2002;22[Suppl 2]:78–80.
14. Burton JR Jr, Ryan C, Shaw-Stiffel TA. Liver transplantation in mushroom poisoning. *J Clin Gastroenterol* 2002;35:276–280.
15. Klein AS, Hart J, Brens JJ, et al. *Amanita* poisoning: treatment and the role of liver transplantation. *Am J Med* 1989;66:187–193.
16. Pinson CW, Daya MR, Benner KG, et al. Liver transplantation for severe *Amanita phalloides* mushroom poisoning. *Am J Surg* 1990;159:493–499.
17. Jaeger A, Jehl F, Flesch F, et al. Amatoxin kinetics in *Amanita phalloides* poisoning. *Vet Hum Toxicol* 1989;31:360.
18. Jaeger A, Kopferschmitt J, Flesch F, et al. *Liver transplantation for* Amanita *poisoning*. Proc Eur Assoc Pois Cont Cent Toxicol XV Congress, Istanbul, Turkey, May 24–27, 1992:103.
19. Forro M, Mandli T. Liver transplantation after *Amanita phalloides* poisoning from the viewpoint of anesthesia and intensive care based on three cases. *Orv Hetil* 2003;144:269–273.
20. Roldan EJ, Perez Lloret A. Thioctic acid in *Amanita* poisoning. *Crit Care Med* 1986;14:753–754.
21. Wellington K, Jarvis B. Silymarin: a review of its clinical properties in the management of hepatic disorders. *BioDrugs* 2001;15:465–489.
22. Enjalbert F, Rapior S, Nouguier-Soule J, et al. Treatment of amatoxin poisoning: 20-year retrospective analysis. *J Toxicol Clin Toxicol* 2002;40:715–757.
23. Hruby K, Csomos G, Fuhrmann M, et al. Chemotherapy of *Amanita phalloides* poisoning with intravenous silibinin. *Hum Toxicol* 1983;2:183–195.
24. Floersheim GL, Weber O, Tschumi P, et al. Clinical death-cap (*Amanita phalloides*) poisoning: prognostic factors and therapeutic measures. Analysis of 205 cases. *Schweiz Med Wochenschr* 1982;112:1164–1177.
25. Montanini S, Sinardi D, Pratico C, et al. Use of acetylcysteine as the life-saving antidote in *Amanita phalloides* (death cap) poisoning. Case report on 11 patients. *Arzneimittelforschung* 1999;49:1044–1047.
26. Schneider SM, Michelson EA, Vanscoy G. Failure of N-acetylcysteine to reduce alpha amanitin toxicity. *J Appl Toxicol* 1992;12:141–142.
27. Lincoff G, Mitchel DH. *Toxic and hallucinogenic mushroom poisoning. A handbook for physicians and mushroom hunters*. New York: Van Nostrand Reinhold, 1977:156–157.
28. Lewis WH, Elvin-Lewis MPF. *Medical botany. Plants affecting man's health*. New York: John Wiley, 1977:398.
29. Vachuska C, Vachuska P. "Puff ball madness" or "How low can you go to get high." The spore print. *J Los Angeles Mycolog Soc #201*, 1994.
30. Henriksen NT. Lycoperdonosis. *Acta Paediatr Scand* 1976;65:643–645.
31. Zilker T, Clarmann M, Felgenhaser N, et al. *A rarity in Western Europe: a mushroom poisoning with* Gyromitra esculenta. Proc XIV Internet Congress Eur Assoc Pois Control Centers, Milan, Italy, Sept 25–29, 1990:98.
32. Michelot D, Toth B. Poisoning by *Gyromitra esculenta*—a review. *J Appl Toxicol* 1991;11:235–243.
33. Lincoff G, Mitchell DH. Toxic and hallucinogenic mushroom poisoning. A handbook for physicians and mushroom hunters. New York: Van Nostrand Reinhold, 1977:19,49–61, 190–191.
34. Albin RL, Albers MD, Greenberg HS, et al. Acute sensory neuropathy from pyridoxine overdose. *Neurology* 1987;37:1729–1732.
35. de Haro L, Prost N, David JM, et al. Syndrome sudorien ou muscarinien: expérience du Centre Antipoison de Marseille. *Presse Méd* 1999;28:1069–1070.
36. Cochran KW. Mushroom poisoning case registry. *JAMA* 1984;252:1685.
37. Vanden Hoek LL, Erickson T, Hryhorczuk D, et al. Jack o'lantern mushroom poisoning. *Ann Emerg Med* 1991;20:559–561.
38. Amitai I, Peleg O, Ariel I, et al. Severe poisoning in a child by the mushroom *Inocybe tristis*, Malencon and Bertault. *Isr J Med Sci* 1982;18:798–801.
39. Michelot D, Melendez-Howell LM. *Amanita muscaria*: chemistry, biology, toxicology, and ethnomycology. *Mycol Res* 2003;107:131–146.
40. Waser FG. The pharmacology of *Amanita muscaria*. In: Efron, DH Holmstedt, B, Kline NS, eds. *Ethnopharmacoplogical search for psychoactive drugs*. U.S. Public Health Service Publication, No. 1645, 1979:419–439.
41. Page LB. Mushroom toxins and the nervous system: some facts and speculations. *McIlvainea* 1984;6:39–43.
42. Chilton WS, Ott J. Toxic metabolites of *Amanita pantherina*, *A. cothurnata*, *A. muscarina* and other *Amanita* species. *Lloydia* 1976;39:150–157.
43. Clitton WS, Hsu CP, Zdybak WT. Stizolobic and stizolobinic acid: L-dopa oxidation products of *A. pantherina*. *Phytochemistry* 1974;13:1179–1181.
44. Benjamin DR. Mushroom poisoning in infants and children. The *Amanita pantherina/muscarina* group. *J Toxicol Clin Toxicol* 1992;30:13–22.
45. Chilton WS. Chemistry and mode of action of mushroom toxins. In: Rumack BH, Salzman E, eds. *Mushroom poisoning: diagnosis and treatment*. West Palm Beach, FL, CRC Press Inc., 1978:87, 124.
46. Schwartz PH, Smith DE. Hallucinogenic mushrooms. *Clin Pediatr* 1888;27:70–73.
47. Spoerke DG, Hall AH. Plants and mushrooms of abuse. *Emerg Clin North Am* 1990;8:579–593.
48. Francis J, Murray VG. Review of enquiries made to the NPIS concerning *Psilocybe* mushroom ingestion 1973–1981. *Hum Toxicol* 1983;2:349–352.
49. Stenklyft PH, Augenstein WL. *Chlorophyllum molybdites*-severe mushroom poisoning in a child. *J Toxicol Clin Toxicol* 1990;28:159–168.
50. Poisonous mushrooms. Available at http://www.botany.hawaii.edu/faculty/wong/BOT135/Lect19.htm. Accessed September 2003.
51. Lehmann PF, Khazan U. Mushroom poisoning by *Chlorophyllum molybdites* in the Midwest United States. Cases and a review of the syndrome. *Mycopathologia* 1992;118:3–13.
52. Levitan D, Macy JI, Weissman J. Mechanism of gastrointestinal hemorrhage in a case of mushroom poisoning by *Chlorophyllum molybdites*. *Toxicon* 1981;19:179–180.
53. Goos RD, Shoop CR. A case of mushroom poisoning caused by *Tricholomopsis platyphylla*. *Mycologia* 1980;72:433–435.
54. Saviuc P, Garon D, Danel V, et al. Cortinarius poisoning. Analysis of cases in the literature. *Nephrologie* 2001;22:167–173.
55. Bouget J, Bousser J, Pats B, et al. Acute renal failure following collective intoxication by *Cortinarius orellanus*. *Intensive Care Med* 1990;16:506–510.
56. Duvic C, Hertig A, Herody M, et al. Acute renal failure following ingestion of *Cortinarius orellanus* in 12 patients. Initial presentation and progress over a period of 13 years. *Presse Med* 2003;32:249–253.
57. Svendsen BS, Gjellestad A, Eivindson G, et al. Serious mushroom poisoning by *Cortinarius* and *Amanita virosa*. *Tidsskr Nor Laegeforen* 2002;122:777–780.
58. Moore B, Burton BT, Lindgren J, et al. *Cortinarius* mushroom poisoning resulting in anuric renal failure. *Vet Hum Toxicol* 1991;33:360.
59. Andar C, Rapior S, Delpech N, et al. Laboratory confirmation of *Cortinarius* poisoning. *Lancet* 1989;1:213.
60. Danel VC, Saviuc PF, Garon D. Main features of *Cortinarius* spp. poisoning: a literature review. *Toxicon* 2001;39:1053–1060.

CHAPTER 258

Herbal and Indigenous Remedies

Christopher R. DeWitt and Richard C. Dart

Compounds included:	**Aconite, anticholinergic plants, aristolochia, Ayurvedic medicines, betel nut, blister beetle (Spanish fly), cardiac glycosides, Chinese patent medicines, Chinese cucumber root, colloidal silver, ephedra, ginkgo biloba, ginseng, heavy metals, hepatic toxins, kava, khat, Kombucha "mushroom," nutmeg and mace, podophyllin, pyrrolizidine alkaloids, pennyroyal, rattlesnake capsules, shark cartilage, St. John's wort, wormwood (absinthe), and others (Table 1)**
Special concerns:	**Herbs may produce myriad toxicities and contain unpredictable dosages.**
Antidotes:	**Digoxin Fab, heavy metal chelating drugs, amiodarone and flecainide, *N*-acetylcysteine**

OVERVIEW

A tremendous variety of plants, animals, and minerals are used as medications throughout the world (Table 1). It is not unusual for patients who use traditional medicines to seek advice and treatment with traditional ethnic practitioners before resorting to more conventional medical advice. Physicians must be alert to the possibility of unusual poisonings in such patients. In most developed nations, immigrant neighborhoods have local ethnic stores that carry familiar products imported from the respective home country, including traditional foods, utensils, medicines, and cosmetics. Importation of these items appears to be unregulated in part because many of these items have never been tested for possible health hazards. Indigenous remedies that are plant derived are addressed in more detail in Chapter 255.

HISTORY OF INDIGENOUS REMEDIES

Indigenous remedies have been used for millennia, dating back to 1500–2000 B.C. It is not surprising that many medicines used today, such as morphine, cocaine, colchicine, reserpine, vincristine, and paclitaxel (Taxol), were initially derived from plants. Although safety studies on most natural products are lacking, most are relatively safe and have only mild side effects if used correctly. The beneficial effects of many products are anecdotal and based on years of use in traditional medicine. They are often used as "adaptogens" to combat stress and return the body to a normal state and indicated for a variety of conditions involving multiple organ systems. Individual ingredients may be complex mixtures of chemicals, and the exact active constituents and mechanisms of action are often not known.

Only recently has the efficacy of herbal products been studied. Of the thousands of herbs used, only a handful, such as *Ginkgo biloba*, saw palmetto, garlic, and kava, have been studied in a randomized, controlled fashion. Effectiveness of traditional remedies lies beyond the scope of this chapter, which focuses mainly on remedies of known or potential toxicity (Table 1).

The World Health Organization estimates that 80% of the world population relies primarily on traditional medicine, with a major part involving the use of plant extracts or active constituents (1). Herbal medicines are likely the most common type of indigenous remedy. The botanic definition of an *herb* is a leafy plant without woody stems. However, the term *herbal product* includes nonherb plant materials, animal products, minerals, and other substances. Hence, the term *herbal* is ill defined and may be used to refer to a variety of "traditional" or "natural" remedies.

The use of herbal medicines is becoming increasingly more common in the United States. A 1997 survey estimated that 12% of American adults had used an herbal medicine in the past 12 months, an increase of 380%, compared with 1990 (2). Although only one-third the size of the European market, the estimated size of the U.S. herb industry was $1.5 billion in 1995 and was growing at 15% per year (3). Americans currently spend approximately $4 billion on botanicals and herbs (4). A study of patients presenting to the emergency department at an urban teaching hospital found that 22% of respondents reported using herbal products (5). Most herbal medicines in the United States are considered dietary supplements and are not subjected to the same standards used for drugs under the Federal Food, Drug, and Cosmetic Act. Currently, there is mounting concern over product safety and the poor regulation of the herbal industry. Critics of the industry have proposed new legislation regarding the regulation of dietary supplements (6–8).

Although considered safe by many people, herbs contain pharmacologically active substances, and many herbal products have been shown to cause adverse effects and death. As usage increases, so do reports of poisoning and adverse reactions (9). Poisoning from herbal medications is often due to one of the following (10):

1. Persistent use of highly toxic herbs
2. Misidentification of herbs such that a toxic herb is mistaken for a harmless variety
3. Substitution of herbs with more toxic and often cheaper ingredients
4. Use of larger than recommended doses—because patients often perceive herbs as safe, they may consume excessive quantities under the misconception that "more is better"

TABLE 1. Selected herbals, usage, and potential toxicities

Herb name/botanical source (scientific name)	Common names	Usage	Active/toxic ingredients	Potential toxicity
Aconite (*Aconitum carmichael, Aconitum kusnezoffii, Aconitum napellus*)	Chuanwu, caowu, monkshood, wolfbane, bushi, fuzi, bachnag	Rheumatism, bruises, fractures, hemiplegia, diarrhea, abdominal pain	Aconite alkaloids	Ventricular dysrhythmias, paresthesias, weakness, nausea, vomiting
Alfalfa (*Medicago sativa*)	Lucerne, phytoestrogen	Diuretic, asthma, arthritis	Saponins	Photosensitivity
Allspice (*Pimenta dioica*)	Clove pepper, Jamaica pepper, pimento	Topically for tooth pain or antiseptic	Eugenol	Large doses: GI distress, seizures
Aloe (*Aloe vera, Aloe spp.*)	Burn plant, elephant's gall, lily of the desert, miracle plant	Dried juice of leaf: laxative; gel within leaf: topically for inflammation, burns, wound healing	Dried juice of leaf: anthracene; gel: carboxypeptidase, salicylate, magnesium lactate	Dried juice of leaf: diarrhea, abdominal pain; gel: none
Aristolochia (*Aristolochia spp.*)	Birthwort, snakeroot, guangfangi, pelican flower	Aphrodisiac, immune stimulant, GI colic	Aristolochic acid	GI distress, fibrosing interstitial nephritis, nephropathy, urothelial cancer
Arnica (*Arnica spp.*)	Leopard's bane, mountain tobacco, wolf's bane	Inflammation, immune stimulant	Sesquiterpenoid lactones	GI distress, inhibits platelet function, tachycardia, drowsiness, coma, death
Astragalus (*Astragalus membranaceus, Astragalus mongholicus*)	Astragali, membranous milk vetch, Mongolian milk	Respiratory infections, immune stimulant, antioxidant	Multiple constituents	None
Autumn crocus (*Colchicum autumnale, Colchicum speciosum, Colchicum vernum*)	Crocus, meadow saffron, mysteria, naked ladies, wonder bulb	Arthritis, gout	Colchicine	GI distress, bone marrow suppression, multiorgan failure, death
Basil (*Ocimum basilicum*)	Common basil, holy basil, St. Joseph wort	Antispasmodic, snake and insect bites, colds, warts	Multiple constituents	Hypoglycemia
Bee pollen/pollen collected from legs and body of bee	Buckwheat pollen, maize pollen, pine pollen	Appetite stimulant, premature aging, hay fever, diuretic, alcohol intoxication	Depends on plant source	Allergic reactions
Bee venom [*Apis mellifera* (honeybee), *Bombus terrestris* (bumblebee), *Vespula maculata* (hornet, wasp)]	*Apis venenum purum*, bee sting, wasp venom	Arthritis, neuralgias, desensitization to stings, tendonitis	Multiple constituents	Injection site irritation, allergic reactions
Beeswax (*Apis cerana, A. mellifera*)	White wax, yellow wax	Diarrhea, pain relief, hiccups	D-002 (high-molecular-weight alcohols)	Allergic reactions
Belladonna (*Atropa belladonna, Atropa belladonna acuminata*)	Deadly nightshade, devil's cherries, dwayberry, great morel naughty man's cherries, poison black cherries	Asthma, antispasmodic, sedative, Parkinson's disease, motion sickness	Hyoscyamine, scopolamine	Anticholinergic effects
Betacarotene	Provitamin A	Vitamin A source	Carotenoids	Skin discoloration with prolonged use
Betel nut (*Areca catechu*)	Areca nut, betel quid, pinag	CNS stimulant, schizophrenia	Arecoline	Cholinergic effects, red staining of mouth, oral cancer
Bitter melon (*Momordica charantia*)	African cucumber, balsam pear, bitter apple, karela, wild cucumber	Diabetes	*p*-Insulin	Possibly hypoglycemia
Black cohosh (*Cimicifuga racemosa, Actaea racemosa, Actaea macrotys*)	Baneberry, black snakeroot, bugwort, phytoestrogen, squawroot	Premenstrual syndrome, labor induction, abortifacient, snake bites	Multiple constituents	GI distress, dizziness, headache
Black tea (*Camellia sinensis*)	Chinese tea	Stimulant, headache, GI disorders	Caffeine	GI distress, headache, anxiety, palpitations, tachycardia
Blue cohosh (*Caulophyllum thalictroides*)	Blue ginseng, papoose root, squawroot, yellow ginseng	Premenstrual syndrome, labor induction, abortifacient	Multiple constituents, *N*-methylcytosine (similar to nicotine)	GI distress, chest pain, hypertension
Brewer's yeast (*Saccharomyces cerevisiae*)	Medicinal yeast	Diarrhea, diabetes, B vitamin and protein source	—	Migraine headache, abdominal discomfort
Buckthorn (*Rhamnus frangula, Rhamnus catharticus*)	Alder buckthorn, black dogwood, European buckthorn, hartshorn, highwaythorn	Laxative	Anthraquinones	Diarrhea; chronic use: hypokalemia, albuminuria, hematuria
Calabar bean (*Physostigma venenosum*)	Chop nut, ordeal bean, physostigma	Constipation, cholera, tetanus	Physostigmine	Cholinergic effects
Camphor (*Cinnamomum camphora*)	Camphora, cemphire, laurel camphor	Topically as an analgesic, warts, cold sores, respiratory disorders, "coining"	Camphor	Orally: GI distress, confusion, delirium, hallucinations, seizures, coma, death

(*continued*)

TABLE 1. (*continued*)

Herb name/botanical source (scientific name)	Common names	Usage	Active/toxic ingredients	Potential toxicity
Cantharidin/blister beetles	Spanish fly, blister beetle	Aphrodisiac	Cantharidin	Orally: irritation, GI distress, renal toxicity
Capsicum (*Capsicum spp.*)	African chilies, cayenne, chili pepper, Louisiana sport pepper, paprika, Tabasco pepper	Stimulate digestion; improve circulation; topically: neuropathies, muscle aches	Capsaicinoid constituents; capsaicin causes substance P release	Orally: GI irritation, diaphoresis, lacrimation, rhinorrhea; topically: burning, irritation, dermatitis
Cascara (*Rhamnus purshiana*)	Bitter bark, buckthorn, dogwood bark, yellow bark	Laxative	Cascarosides A and B	Diarrhea; chronic use: hypokalemia, albuminuria, hematuria
Castor bean (*Ricinus communis, Ricinus sanguines*)	African coffee tree, castor seed, Mexico weed, wonder tree	Birth control, laxative, syphilis	Ricin	Ingestion of chewed whole beans: GI distress, hypovolemia, hepatic and renal damage, cardiovascular collapse, death
Cat's claw (*Uncaria guianensis, Uncaria tomentosa*)	Samento, uña de gato	GI disorders, viral infections, HIV, wound healing, arthritis	Rhynchophylline	Headache, dizziness, vomiting
Catnip (*Nepeta cataria*)	Catmint, catswort, field balm	Insomnia, migraines, colds, GI disorders, smoked for euphoria	Nepetalactone	Headache, vomiting, sedation
Chamomile (*Matricaria recutita*)	German chamomile, manzanilla	Sleep aid, GI disorders	Allergens, coumarin	Allergic reactions, vomiting, possible anticoagulant effect
Chan Su (*Bufo bufo gargarizans, Bufo melanos*)	Chan Su, kyushin, lushenwan	Antiinflammatory, analgesic, skin infections	Cardiac glycoside (bufandienolides)	GI distress, hyperkalemia, cardiac dysrhythmias
Chaparral (*Larrea divaricata, Larrea tridentate*)	Creosote bush, greasewood, hediondilla	Arthritis, cancer, venereal disease, colds, weight loss	Nordihydroguaiaretic acid	Hepatotoxicity
Chinese cucumber root (*Trichosanthes kirilowii*)	Chinese snake gourd, compound Q, tian hua fen, trichosanthes	HIV infection, abortion induction, cough, fever	Trichosanthin, "TAP 29," trichosanthin, momorcharin	Seizures, pulmonary and cerebral edema, cerebral hemorrhage, allergic reactions, death
Choline/trimethylethanolamine	Choline bitartrate, choline chloride, intrachol, lipotropic factor	Liver disease, hypercholesterolemia, depression, dementia, TPN-associated hepatic steatosis	Choline	GI distress, diaphoresis, fishy body odor
Chondroitin/chondroitin 4-sulfate	Chondroitin sulfate	Osteoarthritis	Glycosaminoglycan	GI distress, edema, allergic reactions
Chromium	Chromium chloride, chromium picolinate, chromium 3	Diabetes, hypercholesterolemia, weight loss	Chromium	Cognitive dysfunction; chronic high doses: anemia, thrombocytopenia, hemolysis, hepatic dysfunction, renal failure
Cinchona (*Cinchona calisaya, Cinchona ledgeriana, Cinchona pubescens*)	Chinarinde, Jesuit's bark, quinine, red cinchona bark	Appetite stimulation, varicose veins, colds, leg cramps	Quinine	Quinine poisoning
Clove oil and dried plant (*Syzygium aromaticum*)	Caryophylli, carophyllum	GI disorders; expectorant; topically: toothache	Eugenol	Smoking: respiratory tract injury, pulmonary edema; oil: CNS depression, seizure
Coca (*Erythroxylum coca*)	Bolivian coca, java coca, spadic	Anesthetic, stimulant	Cocaine	Cocaine poisoning
Cod liver oil	Omega-3 fatty acids	Hyperlipidemia, hypertension, coronary artery disease, arthritis	Omega-3 fatty acids, vitamin A and D	Nausea; loose stools; chronic use: malignant melanoma in women, vitamin A and D toxicity
Coenzyme Q-10/ Ubiquinone, ubidecarenone, mitoquinone	Coenzyme Q, CO Q10, Q10	CHF, angina, diabetes, hypertension, prevention of doxorubicin cardiotoxicity, immune stimulation, mitochondrial dysfunction, antioxidant	Coenzyme Q-10	GI distress
Cola nut (*Cola acuminata*)	Bisy nut, guru nut, kola nut	Stimulant	Caffeine	GI distress, headache, anxiety, palpitations, tachycardia
Colloidal minerals/anhydrous aluminum silicates	Bioelectrical minerals, clay suspension, plant-derived liquid minerals	Trace mineral supplement, diabetes, arthritis	Anhydrous aluminum silicates, may contain heavy metals	None reported

(*continued*)

TABLE 1. (*continued*)

Herb name/botanical source (scientific name)	Common names	Usage	Active/toxic ingredients	Potential toxicity
Colloidal silver/silver in suspending agent	Silver protein	Infections, HIV, respiratory disorders	Silver	Argyria, neurologic deficits, renal damage
Comfrey (*Symphytum officinale*)	Ass ear, black root, blackwort, gum plant, slippery root	Orally: ulcers, diarrhea, respiratory disorders; topically: analgesic	Pyrrolizidine alkaloids	Hepatic veno-occlusive disease
Cranberry (*Vaccinium macrocarpon, Vaccinium oxycoccos*)	American cranberry, European cranberry, mossberry	Urinary tract infections	Proanthocyanidin	None
Creatine/N-amidinosarcosine	Creatine monohydrate	Athletic performance, neuromuscular disorders, CHF	Creatine converted *in vivo* to creatinine	GI distress, possible dehydration, elevation of serum creatinine despite normal renal function
Dandelion (*Taraxacum officinale*)	Blowball, cankerwort, lion's tooth, wild endive	Gallstones, indigestion, laxative	Taraxacin	None
Danshen (*Salvia bowelyana, Salvia miltiorrhiza, Salvia przewalskii, S. yunnanensis*)	Ch'ih shen, red root sage, red sage, saliva root, tan-shen	Circulation, cardiovascular, and menstrual disorders; bruising	Protocatechualdehyde, 3,4-dihydroxyphenyllactic acid, salvianolic acid, tanshinone	Pruritus, upset stomach, decreased platelet aggregation
Devil's claw (*Harpagophytum procumbens*)	Grapple plant, wood spider	Arteriosclerosis, arthritis, dyspepsia, menstrual disorders	Iridoid glycosides, harpagoside	Diarrhea
Dehydroepiandrosterone	Prasterone	Reversing aging, weight loss, improve strength, erectile dysfunction	Dehydroepiandrosterone converted to precursor of androgens and estrogens	Acne, hair loss, hirsutism, hypertension, hepatic dysfunction, mania
Digitalis (*Digitalis purpurea, Digitalis lanata*)	Foxglove, dead man's bells, fairy cap, lady's thimble	Congestive heart failure, atrial fibrillation, diuretic, asthma	Cardiac glycosides	GI distress, yellow-green vision, hyperkalemia, weakness, cardiac dysrhythmias
Dong quai (*Angelica sinensis*)	Chinese angelica, dang gui, dong qua, phytoestrogen	Menstrual disorders, menopause, hypertension	Coumarin constituents	Photosensitivity, photodermatitis, anticoagulant effect
Echinacea (*Echinacea angustifolia, Echinacea pallida, Echinacea purpurea*)	American cone flower, comb flower, snakeroot	Immunostimulant for infection treatment and prevention	Allergens	Allergic reactions, nausea, vomiting
Elderberry (*Sambucus nigra*)	Baccaae, black elder, elkhorn, sambuci sambucus	Influenza treatment	Multiple constituents	GI distress
Ephedra (*Ephedra spp.*)	Ephedrae herba, herbal ecstasy, ma huang, Mormon tea, yellow horse	Weight loss, stimulant, respiratory conditions	Ephedrine, pseudoephedrine, phenylpropanolamine	Anxiety, headache, GI distress, tachycardia, hypertension, palpitations, myocardial infarction, ischemic and hemorrhagic stroke, death
Ergot (*Claviceps purpurea*) (Chapter 102)	Cockspur rye, hornseed, smut rye	Obstetric and gynecologic bleeding	Ergot alkaloids	Nausea; vomiting; long-term use: thrombosis, stroke, seizures, ergotism
Evening primrose oil (*Oenothera spp.*)	Fever plant, king's cureall, sun drop	Premenstrual syndrome, arthritis, hypercholesterolemia	γ-Linolenic acid	Nausea, headache, decreased platelet aggregation
Feverfew (*Tanacetum parthenium*)	Altamisa, bachelor's button, featherfew, Santa Maria	Headaches, migraines, menstrual irregularities, arthritis, asthma	Multiple constituents	GI distress; oral ulcers; decreased platelet activity; "post-feverfew syndrome": anxiety, headaches, insomnia after discontinuation
Flaxseed (*Linum usitatissimum*)	Linseed, winterlien	Constipation, hypercholesterolemia	Soluble fiber; linolenic, linoleic, and oleic acid	Diarrhea, possibly decreased platelet aggregation
Garlic (*Allium sativum*)	Ail, ajo, camphor of the poor, rust treacle, stinking rose	Hypertension, hyperlipidemia, infections	Alliin, allicin, ajoene	GI distress, body odor, contact dermatitis, decreased platelet aggregation
Germander (*Teucrium chamaedrys*)	Wild germander, wall germander	GI disorders, fever, mouthwash, weight loss	Furan-containing neoclerodane diterpenoids, teucrin A	Hepatitis, hepatic necrosis, death
Ginger (*Zingiber officinale*)	African ginger, gingembre, ginger root, zingiberis rhizoma	Nausea, motion sickness, hyperemesis gravidarum	Gingerols	GI distress, prolongation of bleeding time
Ginkgo (*Ginkgo biloba*)	Adiantifolia, bai guo ye, fossil tree, kew tree, maidenhair tree, salisburia	Dementia, cerebral vascular insufficiency, sexual dysfunction, acute mountain sickness, asthma	Flavonoids, terpenoids, organic acids	Leaf: GI distress, headache, dizziness, allergic reactions, decreased platelet aggregation; seeds: GI distress, seizures, death

(*continued*)

TABLE 1. (*continued*)

Herb name/botanical source (scientific name)	Common names	Usage	Active/toxic ingredients	Potential toxicity
Ginseng (*Panax ginseng, Panax quinquefolius*) (see also Siberian ginseng)	Siberian ginseng, American ginseng, ren shen	Adaptogen, improving stamina, immune function, cognitive function	Ginsenosides	Insomnia; GI distress; possibly "ginseng abuse syndrome": anxiety, hypertension, insomnia after discontinuation
Glucosamine	Glucosamine hydrochloride, glucosamine sulfate	Arthritis	Some products may be derived from shellfish	Mild GI upset, possibly insulin resistance
Goat's rue (*Galega officinalis*)	French honeysuckle, French lilac, Italian fitch	Diabetes, diuretic	Galegine	Possibly hypoglycemia
Goldenseal (*Hydrastis canadensis*)	Eye root, goldenroot, ground raspberry, Indian plant, yellow root	Upper respiratory infections, GI disorders	Hydrastine, berberine	GI distress; kernicterus; in large overdose: bradycardia, hypotension, seizures, paralysis, death
Goldenthread (*Coptis chinensis, Coptis japonica*)	Chuenlin, cankerroot, coptis	GI disorders	Berberine displaces bilirubin	Neonatal hyperbilirubinemia
Gotu kola (*Centella asiatica, Centella coriacea*)	Brahma-buti, hydrocotyle, Indian pennywort, marsh penny, white rot	Improving memory, reducing fatigue, wound healing	Triterpene acids	GI distress, pruritus, photosensitivity
Grape seed (*Vitis vinifera, Vitis coignetiae*)	Activin, muskat	Circulatory disorders, wound healing	Procyanidins	None
Grapefruit (*Citrus paradisi*)	Paradisapfel, pomelo	Cholesterol reduction, weight loss, cancer prevention	—	Possibly decreases hematocrit
Green tea (*Camellia sinensis*)	Chinese tea	Improves cognition, GI disorders	Polyphenols, caffeine	GI distress, headache, anxiety, palpitations, tachycardia
Guarana (*Paullinia cupana*)	Brazilian cocoa, paullinia, zoom	Weight loss, stimulant, aphrodisiac	Caffeine	GI distress, painful urination, headache, anxiety, palpitations, tachycardia
Hawthorn (*Crataegus laevigata*)	Aubepine, crategi folium, hagedorn, maybush, whitehorn	Cardiovascular and GI disorders, sedative	Flavonoids, procyanidins	GI distress, headache, palpitations, agitation
Hemlock (*Conium maculatum*)	California fern, carrot weed, poison-hemlock, wild carrot	Sedative, antispasmodic	Coniceine, coniine	Salivation, mydriasis, drowsiness, rigidity, paralysis, cardiovascular collapse, death
Henbane (*Hyoscyamus niger*)	Devil's eye, fetid nightshade, hen bell, poison tobacco	GI disorders	Hyoscyamine, scopolamine	Anticholinergic effects
Holly (*Ilex aquifolium, Ilex opaca, Ilex vomitoria*)	Christ's thorn, holy tree, hulver bush	Diuretic, digestive disorders, expectorant, purgative	Saponins	GI distress
Iboga (*Tabernanthe iboga*)	None	Aphrodisiac, hallucinogen, stimulant, treatment of alcohol and drug addiction	Indole alkaloids	Cholinergic effects, hallucinations
Indian snakeroot (*Rauwolfia serpentina*) (Chapter 124)	Chandrika, covanamilpori, rauwolfia, sarpagandha, snake root	Hypertension, psychosis, insomnia, peripheral vascular disorders	Rauwolfia alkaloids, reserpine	GI distress, lethargy, bradycardia, hypotension
Indian tobacco (*Lobelia inflata*)	Asthma weed, lobelia, pukeweed, wild tobacco	Asthma, sedative, smoking cessation	α-Lobeline (similar to nicotine)	Similar to nicotine poisoning
Jimsonweed (*Datura stramonium*)	Angel trumpet, devil's apple, Jamestown weed, locoweed, nightshade, thorn-apple	Asthma, bronchitis, hallucinogen	Atropine, hyoscyamine, scopolamine	Anticholinergic effects (Chapter 10)
Juniper (*Juniperus communis*)	Common juniper berry, zimbro	GI and urinary disorders, abortifacient	Terpinen-4-ol	Renal irritation, albuminuria, hematuria
Kava (*Piper methysticum*)	Ava, awa, kava kava, kawa, kew, yagona	Anxiety, insomnia, epilepsy, psychosis, depression, headaches, respiratory infections	Kava lactones	GI distress, headache, drowsiness, hepatotoxicity, skin discoloration
Kelp (*Ascophyllum nodosum, Fucus spp.*, brown seaweed spp.)	Black tang, bladder fucus, bladderwrack, fucus, rockweed	Iodine deficiency, thyroid disorders, arthritis	Iodine	Exacerbation of hyperthyroidism
Khat (*Catha edulis*)	Abyssinian tea, gat, kat, tohai, tschut	Stimulant	Cathine	Euphoria, manic behavior, insomnia, hypertension, tachycardia
Levant berry (*Anamirta cocculus*)	Fish berries, Indian berry, louseberry, poisonberry	Vertigo, epilepsy, malaria, topically for scabies	Picrotoxin	GI distress, agitation, seizures, muscle spasms, death
Licorice (*Glycyrrhzia glabra*)	Gancao, Chinese licorice, glycyrrhiza	Upper airway and gastric irritation, liver disease	Glycyrrhizic and glycyrrhetinic acids	Mineralocorticoid excess, hypertension, sodium retention, hypokalemia

(*continued*)

TABLE 1. (*continued*)

Herb name/botanical source (scientific name)	Common names	Usage	Active/toxic ingredients	Potential toxicity
Lily-of-the-valley (*Convallaria majalis*)	Lily-of-the-valley, constancy, convallaria	Cardiac insufficiency, dysrhythmias, urinary tract infections	Cardiac glycosides	GI distress, visual color disturbances, cardiac dysrhythmias
Mandrake (*Mandragora officinarum*)	European mandrake, mandragora, Satan's apple	Hallucinogen	Hyoscyamine, scopolamine	Anticholinergic effects
Melatonin	MEL, MLT, pineal hormone	Sleep aid, circadian rhythm disturbances, dementia, depression	Melatonin	Headache, drowsiness, abdominal cramps
Milk thistle (*Silybum marianum*)	Holy thistle, lady's thistle, silybin, silymarin	Liver disease, *Amanita phalloides* poisoning	Silymarin	Mild GI discomfort
Myrrh (*Commiphora molmol, Commiphora myrrha, Commiphora erythraea*)	Bol, commiphora, didin, heerabol	Indigestion, ulcers, colds, asthma, topically for wounds	Volatile oil, mucilage	Dermatitis; large doses: diarrhea
Nutmeg (*Myristica fragrans*)	Mace, muscadier, nuez moscada	GI disorders, insomnia, abortifacient, hallucinogen	Multiple volatile oils, myristicin	GI distress, hallucinations, anticholinergic effects
Nux vomica (*Strychnos nux-vomica*)	Poison nut, Quaker buttons, strychnos seed	Impotence, GI disorders, appetite stimulant	Strychnine and brucine	Muscular spasms resulting in respiratory muscle failure, rhabdomyolysis, acidosis
Oleander (*Nerium oleander, Thevetia peruviana*)	Common oleander, rose bay, rose laurel, yellow oleander	Cardiac conditions, asthma, epilepsy	Cardiac glycosides: oleandroside, nerioside, digitoxigenin	GI distress, weakness, hyperkalemia, cardiac dysrhythmias
Oregano (*Origanum vulgare*)	Carvacrol, mountain mint, wild marjoram, wintersweet	Respiratory and GI disorders, dysmenorrhea, urinary infections	Carvacrol, thymol	Large doses: GI distress
Papaya or papain (*Carica papaya*)	Melon tree, papaw, plant protease concentrate, vegetable pepsin	Antiinflammatory, digestive aid, topically for wounds	Proteolytic enzymes	Large oral doses: gastritis, esophageal perforation
Para-aminobenzoic acid	Aminobenzoate potassium, vitamin B_{10}, vitamin H	Skin disorders, sunscreen, infertility, hair-loss prevention	Para-aminobenzoic acid	GI distress; large doses: hepatic toxicity
Parsley (*Petroselinum crispum*)	Common parsley, garden parsley	GI and urinary disorders, abortifacient	Myristicin, apiole	Large doses: myristicin (hallucinations, bradycardia, hypotension, paralysis), apiole (hemolytic anemia, thrombocytopenia)
Passion flower (*Passiflora incarnata*)	Apricot vine, maypop, passion vine, water lemon	Insomnia, anxiety, antispasmodic, analgesic	Multiple constituents	Sedation, vasculitis
Pennyroyal leaf or oil (*Hedeoma pulegioides, Mentha pulegium*)	American pennyroyal, European pennyroyal, lurk-in-the-ditch, squaw balm	GI disorders, diuretic, abortifacient	Pulegone, menthofuran, isopulegone	GI distress, agitation, lethargy, seizures, hallucinations, pulmonary edema, hepatotoxicity, death
Peppermint oil (*Mentha piperita*)	Menthae piperitae, aetheroleum	Colds, GI disorders, headache	Menthol	Oral irritation, laryngeal spasm, allergic reactions
Periwinkle (*Vinca minor*)	Earlyflowering, evergreen, myrtle, vincae minoras herba, wintergreen	Improving memory and concentration, diarrhea, vaginal discharge, throat ailments	Vincristine	Vincristine toxicity
Peyote (*Lophophora williamsii*)	Devil's root, mescal buttons, mescaline, sacred mushroom	Fever, rheumatism, hallucinogen	Mescaline	Nausea, vomiting, hallucinations, anxiety, paranoia, mydriasis, hypertension, tachycardia
Podophyllum (*Podophyllum hexandrum, Podophyllum pelatum*)	American mandrake, devil's apple, mayapple, baijiaolian	Wart removal, cathartic, snake bite	Podophyllotoxin	Inhibition of protein synthesis and mitosis, GI distress, confusion, incoordination, neuropathy, bone marrow suppression, embryotoxic
Pokeweed (*Phytolacca americana*)	American nightshade, American spinach, cancer jalap, coakum, pigeonberry, poke, red weed	Emetic, rheumatism, inflammation, skin infection, dysmenorrhea	Saponin glycosides, mitogens	GI distress, GI bleeding, salivation, seizures, respiratory failure, leukocytosis, death
Pomegranate (*Punica granatum*)	Granada, grenadier, shi liu gen pi	Intestinal worms, abortifacient	Polyphenols, fatty acids, piperidine alkaloids, tannins	GI distress, temporary blindness, strychnine-like effects

(*continued*)

TABLE 1. (*continued*)

Herb name/botanical source (scientific name)	Common names	Usage	Active/toxic ingredients	Potential toxicity
Precatory bean (*Abrus precatorius*)	Black-eyed Susan, Buddhist rosary bead, jequirity bean, rosary pea	Abortifacient, oral contraceptive, analgesic	Abrin (similar to ricin)	Ingestion of chewed whole beans: GI distress, hypovolemia, hepatic and renal damage, cardiovascular collapse, death
Rhubarb (*Rheum spp.*)	Da huang, garden rhubarb, rhei	GI disorders	Anthraquinones	Diarrhea, uterine contractions
Rose hip (*Rosa spp.*)	Dog rose, hip berry, hop fruit, wild boar fruit	Vitamin C supplement, colds, GI disorders	Pectin, citric acid, malic acid	GI upset
Rosemary (*Rosmarinus officinalis*)	Compass plant, old man, polar plant	Dyspepsia, abortifacient, cough, headache	Essential oils: cineole, borneol, camphor	Large doses: GI distress, seizure, coma
Royal jelly/from *Apis mellifera* (honeybee)	Bee saliva, bee spit, honey bee milk	General health tonic	Secretions from bee glands	Allergic reactions
Rue (*Ruta graveolens*)	Garden rue, herbygrass, rutae folium	Menstrual disorders, abortifacient, dyspepsia	Furocoumarins, alkaloids	GI irritation, sleep disorders, abortion, renal and hepatic injury
Saffron (*Crocus sativus*)	Autumn crocus, Indian saffron, safran	Asthma, insomnia, cough, sedative	Crocin, picrocrocin, crocetin	Large doses: GI distress, abortion, bleeding
Sage (*Salvia officinalis, Salvia lavandulaefolia*)	Common sage, garden sage, sauge, Spanish sage	Digestive problems, dysmenorrhea, appetite stimulant	Thujone	Large doses: hallucinations, psychosis, delirium, seizures, GI distress
Saint John's wort (*Hypericum perforatum*)	Amber, demon chaser, goatweed, hypericum, klamath weed, tipton weed	Depression, anxiety, sleep disorders	Hypericin, hyperforin	Insomnia, anxiety, GI distress, photosensitivity, possibly serotonin syndrome, P-450 induction
Sassafras (*Sassafras albidum*)	Ague tree, cinnamon wood	Urinary tract disorders, tonic	Volatile oils: safrole	Diaphoresis; large doses: hallucinations, hypertension, tachycardia, stupor, abortion, possibly carcinogenic
Saw palmetto (*Serenoa repens*)	American dwarf palm tree, cabbage palm, sabal	Benign prostatic hypertrophy, diuretic, sedative, antiinflammatory	Volatile and fatty oils	GI distress
Scotch broom (*Cytisus scoparius*)	Bannal, broom, hogweed, scoparium	Cardiovascular disorders	Sparteine: negative inotropic and chronotropic effects	Large doses: headache, dizziness, weakness, sedation
Skullcap (*Scutellaria lateriflora*)	Blue pimpernel, helmet flower, mad weed, Quaker bonnet	Stroke, fever, general tonic, seizures	Flavonoids, volatile oil	Large doses: confusion, stupor, seizure, possibly hepatotoxicity
Senna (*Senna alexandrina*)	Alexandrian senna, Indian senna, true senna	Laxative	Anthraquinones	Diarrhea
Shark cartilage (*Squalus acanthias*)	—	Cancer prevention and treatment, arthritis, wounds	—	Nausea, vomiting, constipation
Siberian ginseng (*Eleutherococcus senticosus*) (see also Ginseng)	Ci wu jia, devil's bush, eleuthera, ginseng, wild pepper	Adaptogen, improving stamina, immune function, cognitive function, blood pressure control	Eleutherosides A – M	Occasionally slight drowsiness, anxiety, irritability, palpitations, hypertension, tachycardia, false elevation of serum digoxin levels
Squill (*Urginea indica, Urginea maritima, Urginea scilla*)	Red squill, white squill, sea onion	Heart failure, arrhythmias, diuretic, asthma, bronchitis	Cardiac glycosides: bufadienolides, scillaren A, proscillaridin A	GI distress, cardiac dysrhythmias
Superoxide dismutase	SOD	Increase lifespan, antiinflammatory	—	None
Sweet clover (*Melilotus altissimus, Melilotus officinalis*)	Common melilot, king's clover, yellow sweet clover	Venous insufficiency, thrombophlebitis	Coumarinic acids converted to coumarins when dried and dicumarol when allowed to spoil	Anticoagulant effect
Tea tree oil (*Melaleuca alternifolia*)	Australian tea tree oil, melaleuca oil	Topically: antiseptic, skin infections, insect bites	Multiple terpenoid constituents	Ingestion: confusion, sedation, coma
Tonka beans (*Dipteryx odorata*)	Coumarouna odorata, cumaru, torquin bean	General tonic, aphrodisiac	Coumarin	Anticoagulant effect
Valerian (*Valeriana spp.*)	Amantilla, baldrian, garden heliotrope, *Valeriana officinalis*	Insomnia, anxiety, sedative	Valepotriates and volatile oils	Sedation, headache, insomnia, benzodiazepine-like withdrawal
Water hemlock (*Cicuta spp.*)	Beaver poison, false parsley, wild parsnip	Migraine headache, menstrual pain, worm infestation	Cicutoxin	Cholinergic effects
White cohosh (*Actaea alba*)	Baneberry, doll's eye, snakeberry	Stimulate menstruation	Toxic glycosides and essential oil	GI distress, tachycardia, delirium, hallucinations, circulatory failure

(*continued*)

TABLE 1. (*continued*)

Herb name/botanical source (scientific name)	Common names	Usage	Active/toxic ingredients	Potential toxicity
White hellebore (*Veratrum album*)	European hellebore, langwort	Cholera, gout, hypertension	Toxic ester-alkaloids; protoveratrine A and B inactivate sodium channels	Nausea, vomiting, salivation, bradycardia, hypotension, paralysis, death
Willow bark (*Salix spp.*)	Basket willow, purple osier, violet willow, white willow	Fever, headache, antiinflammatory, analgesic	Salicylates	None reported
Wintergreen leaf (*Gaultheria procumbens*)	Boxberry, deerberry, mountain tea, wax cluster	Analgesic, antiinflammatory, asthma	Galutherin converts to methyl salicylate with drying	Large doses: salicylate toxicity
Witch hazel (*Hamamelis virginiana*)	Hazel, snapping tobacco, spotted elder	Diarrhea, respiratory disorders, topically for skin inflammation	Tannins	Nausea, vomiting, contact dermatitis
Wormwood (*Artemisia absinthe*)	Absinthe, green ginger	Aphrodisiac, flavoring alcoholic beverages, wound healing, GI complaints	Thujone	Hallucinations, psychosis, delirium, seizures, GI distress
Yarrow (*Achillea millefolium*)	Achilee, bloodwort, green arrow, nosebleed, wound wort	Colds, diarrhea, fever, antispasmodic, toothache, wounds	Multiple constituents, salicylic acid	Contact dermatitis
Yew (*Taxus baccata*)	Chinwood, Pacific yew, western yew	Promote menstruation, abortifacient, cancer treatment	Alkaloids; taxine B inhibits sodium and calcium currents	Large doses: nausea, vomiting, weakness, bradycardia, hypotension, death
Yohimbine (*Pausinystalia yohimbe*)	Johimbi, yohimbehe	Aphrodisiac, sexual dysfunction, hallucinogen, muscle growth	Yohimbine	Low doses: anxiety, tremor, hypertension, tachycardia; high doses: hypotension, cardiac failure, paralysis, death

CHF, congestive heart failure; CNS, central nervous system; GI, gastrointestinal; HIV, human immunodeficiency virus; spp., species; TPN, total parenteral nutrition.
Adapted from Jellin JM, Gregory PJ, Batz F, et al. *Pharmacist's letter/prescriber's letter natural medicines comprehensive database*, 4th ed. Stockton, CA: Therapeutic Research Faculty, 2002.

5. Variability in the amount of active ingredients caused by poor processing and the inherent biologic variability in the amount of active ingredient in the plant
6. Faulty processing such as inadequate boiling time for products containing aconitine

Additional reasons for toxicity include the lack of childproof containers, potential for malicious tampering, unexpected interactions of multiple components (Chinese herbal medications can contain more than 20 different herbs), underlying illness predisposing the patient to toxicity (e.g., hemolysis from *Acalypha indica* or *Salix caprea* in patients with glucose 6 phosphate dehydrogenase deficiency) (9), and metabolic differences among ethnicities (e.g., Asian vs. whites). Besides the direct risks of toxicity and drug interactions, patients may forego or delay effective conventional treatments in favor of herbs that have no demonstrated efficacy (11). Because uncommon reactions and embryotoxic, fetotoxic, and carcinogenic effects may go unnoticed by individual practitioners (11,12), health care providers are encouraged to report adverse reactions to the U.S. Food and Drug Administration (FDA) MedWatch program (1-800-FDA-1088 or https://www.accessdata.fda.gov/scripts/medwatch/).

Raw herbs can be taken whole, ground into powder, or made into a decoction (concentrated extract prepared by boiling the herb in water until reduced to a small volume) or a tea (prepared by steeping the raw herbs in hot water) (9). Ko suggests that the type of preparation can aid in determining the expected toxicity (9). Raw, unprocessed herbs are likely to cause toxicity from the naturally occurring medicinal compounds. Toxicity from decoctions can be due to chemical reactions between different herbs, heat-stable medicinal compounds, and organic or inorganic contaminates. Herb teas generally have a lower concentration of active ingredients, and adverse reactions are often due to chronic consumption. Additionally, toxicity can differ if the product is imported or manufactured domestically. Foreign products can have large batch-to-batch inconsistencies and may contain toxic adulterants such as other botanicals, microorganisms, microbial toxins, pesticides, heavy metals, and drugs (12). Domestic products may contain vitamins and minerals that are not commonly used in traditional Chinese medicines, or producers may "standardize" an active ingredient by adding synthetic chemicals that mimic the natural compound. Additionally, products with the same name may contain different ingredients. Chinese herbalists may use the same name for products that contain different ingredients to tailor remedies to each individual patient (13).

CLINICAL PRESENTATION

Acute Exposure

Joubert and Mathibe have summarized acute poisoning from traditional medicines as presenting with one of three major clinical syndromes (14):

1. Gastrointestinal (GI) irritation is the most common presentation. It may affect either the upper or lower, or the entire, GI tract. Upper GI symptoms may vary from mild epigastric discomfort and nausea to severe vomiting with dehydration. Diarrhea of varying severity and even frank bleeding from the GI tract may occur. Many traditional

TABLE 2. Psychoactive substances used in herbal preparations

Ingredient	Scientific name	Active ingredients	Usage	Effects
Bufo toad secretions	*Bufo* spp.	Bufotenin	Secretions smoked or ingested as hallucinogen	Hallucinogen
California poppy	*Eschscholtzia californica*	Isoquinoline alkaloids	Smoke as marijuana substitute	Probably none
Catnip	*Nepeta cataria*	Nepetalactone	Smoke or tea as marijuana substitute	Euphoriant
Cinnamon	*Cinnamomum camphora*	Unknown	Smoke with marijuana	Mild stimulant
Coca leaves	*Erythroxylum coca*	Cocaine	Chewed as stimulant	Stimulant
Cola nut	*Cola* spp.	Caffeine	Smoke, tea, or capsules as stimulant	Stimulant
Damiana	*Turnera diffusa*	Unknown	Smoke as marijuana substitute	Mild stimulant
Guarana	*Paullinia cupana*	Caffeine	Capsules or tea as stimulant	Stimulant
Hemlock	*Conium maculatum*	Coniceine, coniine	Tea or ingested as sedative	Sedative, cholinergic effects
Hops	*Humulus lupulus*	Humulene, myrcene, β-caryophylline, farnesene	Smoke or tea as sedative and marijuana substitute	Mild sedative
Iboga	*Tabernanthe iboga*	Indole alkaloids	Tea or chewed as hallucinogen	Hallucinogen
Juniper	*Juniper macropoda*	Unknown	Smoke as hallucinogen	Hallucinogen
Kava	*Piper methysticum*	Kava lactones	Smoke or tea as marijuana substitute	Hallucinogen
Khat	*Catha edulis*	Cathine, cathinone	Tea, chew	Stimulant
Lobelia	*Lobelia inflata*	Lobeline	Smoke or tea as marijuana substitute	Mild euphoriant
Mandrake	*Mandragora officinarum*	Scopolamine, hyoscyamine	Tea as hallucinogen	Anticholinergic effects
Maté tea	*Ilex paraguayensis*	Caffeine	Tea as stimulant	Stimulant
Mormon tea	*Ephedra nevadensis*	Ephedra	Tea as stimulant	Stimulant
Morning glory	*Ipomoea violacea, Ipomoea purpurea, Ipomoea corymbosa*	Lysergic acid hydroxyethylamide	Seeds crushed and ingested as hallucinogen	Hallucinogen
Nutmeg	*Myristica fragrans*	Myristicin, volatile oils	Tea as hallucinogen	Hallucinogen
Passion flower	*Passiflora incarnata*	Harmine alkaloids	Smoke, tea, or capsules as marijuana substitute	Mild stimulant
Peyote	*Lophophora williamsii*	Mescaline	Chewed or tea as hallucinogen	Hallucinogen
Periwinkle	*Catharanthus roseus*	Indole alkaloids	Smoke or tea as euphoriant	Hallucinogen
Prickly poppy	*Argemone mexicana*	Protopine, bergerine, isoquinilines	Smoke as euphoriant	Analgesic
Scotch broom	*Cytisus* spp.	Sparteine	Smoke as marijuana substitute	Mild euphoriant
Snakeroot	*Rauwolfia serpentina*	Reserpine	Smoke or tea as tobacco substitute	Sedative
Thorn apple	*Datura stramonium*	Atropine, scopolamine	Smoke or tea as tobacco substitute or hallucinogen	Anticholinergic effects
Tobacco	*Nicotiana* spp.	Nicotine	Smoke as tobacco	Strong stimulant
Valerian	*Valeriana officinalis*	Valepotriates, volatile oils	Tea or capsules as sedative	Sedative
Wild lettuce	*Lactuca sativa*	Unknown	Smoked as opioid substitute	Possibly analgesic, sedative
Wormwood	*Artemisia absinthium*	Thujone	Smoke or tea as relaxant	Sedative
Yohimbine	*Corynanthe yohimbe*	Yohimbine	Smoke or tea as stimulant	Mild hallucinogen

Adapted from Siegel RK. Herbal intoxication. *JAMA* 1976;236:474.

medicines are purgatives used to "clean out" the body, and many herbal remedies are administered as enemas.

2. Hepatic or renal toxicity is the second syndrome and is often associated with metabolic disturbances.
3. Central nervous system (CNS) involvement usually reflects cerebral irritation, and patients can be confused or may even hallucinate. Examples of psychoactive substances found in herbal preparations are shown in Table 2.

Adverse Events

Adverse reactions to herbal remedies can be further classified to include both acute and chronic effects (11). *Type A reactions* are pharmacologically predictable and usually dose dependent such as the induction of hypertension and anxiety by yohimbine, the major alkaloid in yohimbe bark preparations. *Type B reactions* are idiosyncratic reactions that occur in only a minority of patients but can be serious and potentially fatal; for example, normal doses of yohimbine were associated with bronchospasm and increased mucus production in a patient with severe allergic dermatitis and with progressive renal failure and a lupus-like syndrome in another patient. *Type C reactions* develop during long-term therapy such as muscular weakness due to hypokalemia in long-term users of herbal anthranoid laxatives. *Type D reactions* consist of delayed effects such as carcinogenicity and teratogenicity. Some herbs are known to have carcinogenic and teratogenic potential.

TOXICITY OF SELECTED HERBS AND REMEDIES

Aconite

Aconites are the dried root stocks or tubers of *Aconitum* plants (15). In Hong Kong, they are known as *chuanwu* (*Aconitum carmichaeli*) or *caowu* (*Aconitum kusnezoffii*) and as *monkshood* or *wolfsbane* (*Aconitum napellus*) in Europe and the United States. They have been used to treat rheumatism, bruises, fractures, hemiplegia, diarrhea, and abdominal pain. The root stock is the most toxic part of the plant and is processed to decrease toxicity, usually by soaking or boiling. The principal toxic ingredients are C19-diterpenoid alkaloids (aconitine, mesaconitine, and hypaconitine) (16). Toxicity has occurred after 0.2 mg of aconitine or 6 g of processed prescription root stocks (15).

The pathophysiology of aconitine alkaloids includes binding to sodium channels in excitable tissues, thereby causing persistent activation and sodium influx during the plateau phase of depolarization (17). Muscarinic activation can also lead to bradydysrhythmias and hypotension (17). The effects on the heart are predictably similar to cardiac glycosides (15). However, unlike cardiac glycosides, aconites also affect the muscular and nervous systems. Patients generally present with abdominal pain, nausea and vomiting, paresthesias that begin in the mouth and tongue and spread to the extremities, generalized muscle weakness that can progress to tetraparesis, cardiovascular abnormalities (hypotension, bradycardia, heart blocks, ventricular ectopy and dysrhythmias), acidosis, and hypokalemia (10,15). Seizures have also been reported (18). Death is usually from refractory ventricular dysrhythmias. Symptoms can occur within 3 minutes to several hours after ingestion, and ventricular dysrhythmias are most likely to occur within the first 24 hours.

Treatment is supportive, and patients should have cardiac monitoring for at least 24 hours (18). Bradycardia can be treated with atropine. Hypotension is treated with isotonic crystalloidal fluid boluses and inotropic support. Ventricular dysrhythmias can be refractive to defibrillation, and no antidysrhythmic drug has been uniformly effective. However, in a series of 17 patients with aconite-induced ventricular dysrhythmias, amiodarone followed by flecainide was most effective at suppressing ventricular tachycardia, whereas lidocaine was ineffective in all patients (15). One case was managed successfully with a ventricular assist device (19).

Anticholinergic Plants

Plants, such as belladonna, henbane, jimsonweed, and mandrake, contain alkaloids such as scopolamine, hyoscyamine, or atropine. These are often used to treat GI and respiratory disorders or as hallucinogens. Additionally, these plants may be adulterants in other herbal preparations (20). The anticholinergic effects are also addressed in Chapters 10 and 255. Patients present with signs and symptoms of anticholinergic toxicity, including confusion, agitation, tachycardia, dry flushed skin, fever, mydriasis, dry mouth, urinary retention, and decreased bowel sounds. Treatment is generally supportive, including benzodiazepines for sedation. Severe poisoning may require airway support and ventilation. Physostigmine reversed anticholinergic effects. However, because of the possibility of potentiating seizures and dysrhythmias, it should be used only in severely poisoned patients in whom the diagnosis is in question and benefits of administration outweigh risks (Chapter 67).

Aristolochia

Aristolochia (e.g., *Aristolochia fangchi*) is also known as *birthwort*, *snakeroot*, *guangfangi*, and *pelican flower*. It is used as an aphrodisiac, an immune stimulant, and for GI colic. An outbreak of rapidly progressive interstitial renal fibrosis was seen in Belgium when *Aristolochia fangchi* was substituted for another herb in a weight-loss preparation (21,22). More than 100 patients have developed nephropathy, with 40% progressing to end-stage renal failure (23). A high prevalence of urothelial cancer was also observed in patients with end-stage nephropathy (23). Aristolochic acid, the toxic ingredient, appears to produce dose-dependent toxicity and is classified as a genotoxic carcinogen (23).

Ayurvedic Medicines (Bhasmas)

In India, Ayurdeva is a widely practiced type of traditional medicine. This discipline uses preparations such as vegetable products, animal products, minerals, precious stones (e.g., pearls, diamonds), and metals (most often lead, mercury, arsenic, copper, gold, silver, iron, and zinc) (24–26). Modern pharmaceuticals are prescribed even by traditional healers. Ayurvedic healers frequently administer penicillin, analgesics, antipyretics, and corticosteroids (27).

Ayurvedic traditional medicinal preparations, known as *bhasmas* and commonly used in Asia, are applied locally or administered orally for systemic use. In Ayurvedic medicine, lead is regarded as an aphrodisiac, and its reputed role may have been to counter the impotence associated with autonomic neuropathy in the diabetic male (28). Bhasmas are fine ashes of metals and a variety of natural products (oyster shells, conches, and herbs) (24). The ingredients are subjected to several cycles of heating, cooling, and grinding until the preparation turns to a fine ash. All contain polycyclic aromatic hydrocarbons. They may be significantly contaminated with benzo[*a*]pyrene, a chemical carcinogen (29). Like many indigenous remedies, Ayurvedic products in India also suffer from lack of quality control, allowing contamination, adulteration, and herb misidentification (24). Putative therapeutic uses of some Ayurvedic bhasmas are summarized in Table 3.

Gymnema (e.g., *Gymnema sylvestre*) has been used by Ayurvedic practitioners in India for centuries either alone or as a compound of "Tribang shia," a mixture of tin, lead, zinc, *G. sylvestre* leaves, neom (*Melia azadirachta*) leaves, *Enicostemma littorale*, and jambul (*Eugenia jambolana*) seeds (30). It has also been used in traditional African medicines. *Gymnema* appears to have hypoglycemic activity through a mechanism similar to sulfonylurea medications, but the exact mechanism has not been established (30).

Betel Nut

The areca nut, commonly known as *betel nut*, grows on the Areca palm tree (*Areca catechu*) and may be the most widely used stimulant in the world. Believed to have originated on the Malay Peninsula, it is the oldest known masticatory used by Asians. More than 200 million people worldwide, including people in Western countries, chew betel (31). It is used as a mild stimulant, similar to

TABLE 3. Therapeutic uses of Ayurvedic bhasmas

Common name	Ingredient	Major use
Made from iron		
Lauha	Iron	Anemia, weakness, cough
Kashees	Iron sulfate	Anemia, weakness, cough, leprosy
Mandoor	Filth of iron	Anemia, jaundice, infection
Made from copper		
Tamra	Copper	Asthma, cough, piles
Swarnmakshik	Copper pyrite	Angina pectoris, antiseptic
Mayurchandrika	Copper sulfate	Spleen enlargement, cough, indigestion, paralysis, leprosy
Made from lead		
Nag	Lead	Paralysis and leprosy
Made from natural products		
Abarakh	Mica	Tuberculosis, cough, anemia
Panna	Beryl	Anemia, cough, weakness
Muktashukti	Oyster shell	Diabetes, respiratory disease
Shankh	Conches	Vomiting, asthma, liver and spleen disorders
Varatika	Kawrie	Tuberculosis, leprosy
Mrigashringa	Horn	Asthma, joint pain, chest pain, cough

Adapted from Jani JP, et al. *Hum Exp Toxicol* 1991;10:347–350.

caffeine or tobacco, and as a digestive aid. The nut may be chewed by itself but more commonly is made into a quid known as *pan*. A *quid* is a combination of areca nut and lime paste (calcium hydroxide) that is wrapped in a leaf from the betel pepper (from *Piper betle*), hence the name betel nut (32). The betel pepper is similar to kava pepper (*Piper methysticum*) (33). Leaf tobacco and aromatic spices may also be added to the quid.

Betel juice is red, and chronic use creates dark stains on the teeth, gingiva, and oral mucosa. Many societies regard the color change as cosmetically appealing (33). Chewing is associated with oral leukoplakia, submucous fibrosis, and squamous cell carcinoma (33). Betel use also appears to be addictive (32).

Arecoline, a cholinomimetic alkaloid similar to acetylcholine, is a major constituent of the betel nut. It is a potent diaphoretic. It stimulates the salivary, lacrimal, gastric, pancreatic, and intestinal glands and the mucosal cells of the respiratory tract; increases muscle tone and muscle movement throughout the body; slows the heart rate; and produces pupillary constriction. Arecoline can also trigger asthma attacks (34) and has been linked to cardiovascular disease and diabetes (31). In high doses, it causes seizures and death (35). The lime that is part of the betel quid hydrolyzes the arecoline into arecaidine, a CNS stimulant that, in combination with the essential oil of the betel pepper, accounts for the euphoric properties (36). A milk-alkali syndrome has also been attributed to the calcium hydroxide component (37). Treatment for betel toxicity is supportive and similar to other stimulants. Theoretically, anticholinergic medicines may be of benefit.

Blister Beetle (Spanish Fly)

One of the best known traditional medicines responsible for poisoning is the blister beetle. There are more than 2000 species of beetle, including Spanish fly (*Cantharis vesicatoria*), that contain the toxic ingredient cantharidin. The beetles are found in southern Europe, the United States, and South Africa and are usually black and yellow in color, although they can be black and red or all black (38). The ovaries, soft tissues, and blood of blister beetles have the highest concentrations of cantharidin (39). Crystals of cantharides are colorless, odorless, glistening, and water insoluble (39). They are soluble in oils, which help dissolve the toxin and increase intestinal absorption (39).

The beetles are ground into a powder that has been used as an abortifacient, wart remover (topically), and diuretic agent in veterinary medicine. Spanish fly has classically been used as an aphrodisiac. This was based on the observation that the irritant effects of near-toxic doses could cause priapism in men and pelvic congestion and uterine bleeding in women (39).

Cantharidin is extremely toxic and causes damage to nearly every organ system. It acts as a vesicant on epithelial linings (GI tract, urinary tract, skin) and leads to a separation of cells in the skin and liver similar to acantholysis (40,41). Elevated hepatic transaminases has been reported (42).

Symptoms after application of a toxic quantity of cantharidin to the skin can result in a full spectrum of toxicity, ranging from inflammation followed by blistering within 4 to 5 hours to death within 12 hours (39). Handling the beetles, crushing them on the skin, or applying their vesiculating fluid to the genitals can result in blisters on the skin of the penis, scrotum, and labia (43).

Burning of the lips, mouth, and pharynx may begin minutes after ingestion (42). Ulceration and excoriation of the lips and buccal mucosa develop with perilabial encrustations of blood. The tongue becomes swollen. Nausea, vomiting, and diarrhea may begin within 5 minutes to 1 hour, accompanied by midline abdominal pain and tenderness and by hematemesis. Vesiculation of the esophagus, stomach, and intestinal tract can occur (42). Acidosis and hypotension due to severe fluid loss can result. Genitourinary involvement is prominent with patients demonstrating hematuria (gross and microscopic) and proteinuria. Renal failure and acute tubular necrosis may ensue (42). Poisoning can cause pulmonary edema and subpleural hemorrhages (39). Myocardial and subendocardial hemorrhages are documented at autopsy (44). Cardiac dysrhythmias, including sinus tachycardia and bradycardia, ventricular tachycardia, and ventricular fibrillation, may be seen (39,45). The electrocardiogram may show elevations of the ST segments in lead II, III, AVF, and V_1 to V_3, with T-wave inversion in V_2 and V_3 (42). Altered mental status, coma, and seizure can also occur in severe poisonings (42).

The toxic dose is unknown. Death has occurred after ingesting 10 mg (39), but patients have survived after ingestions of 175 mg (42). Toxicity and death have also occurred after ingesting whole beetles (38) and within 12 hours of topical application (39).

Treatment is symptomatic and supportive, with particular attention to airway control, fluid replacement, and maintenance of vital signs. Decontamination after ingestion is unlikely to be helpful due to vomiting. Charcoal administration may interfere with esophagoscopy attempts needed to delineate damage to the upper GI tract. Intravenous hydrocortisone and antibiotics have been administered, but further work remains to confirm their usefulness (45). Skin lesions should be cleansed with acetone, ether, fatty soap, or alcohol because these substances dissolve or dilute the cantharidin (43). Lesions then should be thoroughly washed with soap and water. Calamine lotion containing a steroid may be useful. Hemodialysis may be needed for renal failure but does not increase excretion of toxin.

Cardiac Glycosides

Various plants contain cardiac glycosides that can poison the user. Examples include foxglove (*Digitalis purpurea* or *Digitalis lanata*), oleander (*Nerium oleander* or *Thevetia peruviana*), lily-of-the-valley (*Convallaria majalis*), and squill (*Urginea* species). These agents are used to treat heart conditions and asthma and as diuretics; they are addressed in more detail in Chapter 255. Chan Su, venom derived from the skin and venom gland of the toad *Bufo bufo gargarizans* or *Bufo melanos*, is a traditional herbal remedy that is also found in the Chinese patent medicine (CPM) *lushenwan* (46). It contains cardioactive steroids of the bufandienolide class (47) and is used as an antiinflammatory or analgesic agent, an aphrodisiac, and topically for skin infections. Additionally, the venom contains the hallucinogen bufotenin (47), lending to the practice of "toad-licking" to get "high" (48). Toad venoms are also included in Chapter 243.

Cardiac glycosides have a narrow therapeutic window. Ingestion of herbs or preparations containing these substances can result in "digoxin-like" toxicity, including nausea, vomiting, hyperkalemia, digoxin-like changes on the electrocardiogram, ventricular dysrhythmias, and death. Laboratory assays for digoxin display varying, weak cross-reactivity with nondigoxin cardiac glycosides (49). Digoxin-specific Fab fragments have been used to treat poisoning from nondigoxin cardiac glycosides, including oleander (50), foxglove extract (51), and bufandienolide (47). Treatment is similar to that for digoxin toxicity, including digoxin-specific Fab fragments (Chapter 49).

Chinese or Asian Patent Medicines

CPMs are mixtures of multiple products used to treat a variety of conditions. They may contain herbal extracts, minerals, animal parts, and medications such as acetaminophen or salicylates. Toxic herbal ingredients, such as aconite, borneol (similar to camphor), *Bufo* toad secretions (bufotoxin), and strychnine, are common (9). Additionally, they may contain cinnabar (mercuric sulfide), realgar (arsenic sulfide), and litharge (lead oxide) as part of the traditional formula (9). The mixtures are formulated into tablets, capsules, powders, and liquids that are available in herbal stores, often with non-English labeling.

Many of these medicines are manufactured in foreign countries with poor regulation. These medications may have completely unrelated ingredients yet be marketed under the same name. Subsequently, they are susceptible to adulteration and contamination with undeclared pharmaceuticals and heavy metals. Testing of 260 Asian patent medications from California herbal stores found 17 containing undeclared pharmaceuticals (ephedrine, chlorpheniramine, methyltestosterone, and phenacetin were the most common) and 85 containing lead [up to 319 parts per million (ppm)], arsenic (up to 114,000 ppm), and mercury (up to 5070 ppm) (52). Almost one-third of tested products contained undeclared pharmaceuticals or heavy metals that could be potentially harmful. Thus, the exact ingredients are often not known, and multiple cases of toxicity related to adulterants, mislabeling, and misuse have been reported.

Nan Lien Chui Fong Toukuwan, now withdrawn from the market in most countries, is responsible for the majority of reported poisonings from CPMs in western countries (10). Several cases of agranulocytosis have resulted from use of preparations containing undeclared pharmaceuticals (53,54). Aminopyrine, phenacetin, phenylbutazone, indomethacin, mefenamic acid, diazepam, hydrochlorothiazide, dexamethasone, cinnabar, and other heavy metals were identified as adulterants in products from various manufacturers and countries (10).

Jin Bu Huan (JBH) is used to treat insomnia and as an analgesic. Several herbs may be marketed under the name JBH. Cases of toxicity in the United States related to a JBH product that was mislabeled by the Chinese manufacturer were likely the result of excessively high concentrations of the active ingredient levo-tetrahydropalmatine (55). Acute poisoning in three pediatric patients resulted in sedation, respiratory depression, flaccid tone, and bradycardia requiring intubation and atropine administration (55). Additionally, chronic use in ten adults resulted in hepatitis with mixed cholestatic and cytotoxic features (55,56). The FDA subsequently banned importation of JBH.

Cases of heavy metal poisoning from CPMs are also reported (10). Calomel (mercuric chloride) toxicity and death from Tse Koo Choy, Qing Fen, and Chen Fen have occurred (57). Arsenic and mercury have been found in traditional Chinese herbal balls (58), and arsenic poisoning followed the use of various medications for asthma (59). Lead and thallium poisoning have also been observed (60,61).

Various topical treatments contain essential oils, including oil of wintergreen or methyl salicylate. Pak Fa Oil (40% oil of wintergreen, 30% menthol, 6% camphor), Hung Fa Oil (67% oil of wintergreen, 22% turpentine oil), and Kwan Loong Medicated Oil (15% oil of wintergreen, 25% menthol, 10% camphor) are a few examples (10). Ingestion of these oils has resulted in salicylate poisoning (62). Toxicity is also possible after topical application of methyl salicylate in infants and young children or application over damaged skin.

Chinese Cucumber Root

Extracts of Chinese cucumber root, *Trichosanthes kirilowii*, have been used as an abortifacient and more recently as an infection treatment in human immunodeficiency virus. The constituents trichosanthin and protein "TAP 29" may selectively kill human immunodeficiency virus–infected cells (63), and human clinical trials have been initiated (64). Trichosanthin and other components show antitumor, cytotoxic, abortifacient, and ribosome-inhibitory activity (63,64). Trichosanthin and root extracts are taken orally or administered via intramuscular or intravenous routes. However, trichosanthin and root extracts are extremely toxic, especially when administered parenterally. The intravenous median lethal dose in mice for root extract is 2.26 mg and 0.236 mg for trichosanthin (64). Injections can cause anaphylaxis, fever, pulmonary and cerebral edema, seizures, cardiac damage, cerebral hemorrhage, and death (63).

Colloidal Silver

Colloidal silver is a mixture of silver nitrate, sodium hydroxide, gelatin, and water. It is used both orally and topically for a variety of conditions. Because inorganic silver is germicidal, it is often used to treat infections. Silver compounds inactivate enzymes via formation of hemisilver sulfides and denature proteins causing precipitation (65). Oral or topical use of colloidal silver can produce an irreversible bluish discoloration of the skin known as *argyria* (66). Excessive use of silver can produce diffuse silver deposition in visceral organs, renal damage, and neurologic deficits (vertigo, gait disturbances, hypesthesia, and weakness) (65). The FDA does not consider colloidal silver safe or effective (67). There is no specific antidote, and treatment is supportive.

Ephedra

Ephedra species, known as *Ma Huang*, *herbal ecstasy*, or *Mormon tea*, contain ephedra alkaloids consisting primarily of ephedrine, pseudoephedrine, and small amounts of phenylpropanolamine (68). Dried plant parts or extracts are used as a stimulant and for respiratory conditions. More recently, ephedra has been used in weight loss and "energy" products. Although uncommon, adverse events are similar to those of other adrenergic stimulants, including stroke, myocardial infarction, seizure, cardiac arrest, and death. These have occurred in patients without underlying disease after using "recommended doses" of products containing ephedra (69). Patients with underlying cardiovascular disease are more likely to experience adverse effects (70) and should avoid ephedra use. However, it remains to be proved that ephedra-containing products taken by healthy patients at recommended doses cause significant toxicity (7,70,71). Signs and symptoms of poisoning are similar to other sympathomimetics and are treated in similar fashion (Chapter 99).

Ginkgo Biloba Leaf

The *Ginkgo* is the world's oldest living tree species, and preparations have been used in traditional Chinese medicine for more than a thousand years (72). The leaves were used to treat asthma and chilblains, and the seeds were used as a digestive aid. Ginkgo has been used in the Western world since the 1960s, and leaf extracts are one of the most widely prescribed medications in Europe, where both oral and intravenous forms are available (72). Ginkgo is one of the best-selling herbal supplements in the United States.

Flavonoids and terpenoids found in the leaf are associated with various pharmacologic actions. It is believed that constituents work synergistically to scavenge free radicals, prevent oxidative damage, reduce lipid peroxidation, decrease inflammation, decrease platelet aggregation, and improve circulation (73). Leaf extracts are taken mainly for memory impairment, dementia, tinnitus, and vascular insufficiency. Studies on the effectiveness of ginkgo for these conditions have shown superiority to placebo (12,74). However, methodologic flaws, differences in dosing, conflicting evidence, and clinical insignificance of benefits make conclusions difficult (12,74).

Ginkgo is generally considered safe (75). Adverse effects are generally mild, including GI upset, nausea, vomiting, and headache (74). Large doses are associated with restlessness, diarrhea, lack of muscle tone, and weakness (73). Ginkgo use has been associated with spontaneous subdural hematomas and increased bleeding time (76). A 70-year-old man taking aspirin suffered a spontaneous hyphema after taking ginkgo (77). Its effects on platelet aggregation in combination with aspirin, nonsteroidal antiinflammatory drugs, or anticoagulants may increase bleeding risks (72,73,75,78).

Ginseng (*Panax*)

Ginseng (*Panax ginseng* native to Asia, and *Panax quinquefolius* native to North America) is one of the world's most popular herbal remedies. It has a wide variety of uses such as stimulating immune function, improving concentration and cognitive function, treating diabetes, and as a general health tonic and adaptogen (improves well being and increases resistance to stress). In fact, the genus name *Panax* is derived from the Greek words for "all healing," and the shape of the root resembles that of a person and is believed to befit any part of the body (79). Ginseng should not be confused with Siberian ginseng (*Eleutherococcus senticosus*), which belongs to the same family as *Panax* and is used to treat similar complaints but has a different chemical composition and is not as widely used (80).

Ginseng root, the applicable part of *Panax*, contains many pharmacologically active constituents, with the ginsenosides (triterpenoid saponins) considered the most important (81). Saponin content varies between *P. ginseng* and *P. quinquefolius* and varies depending on the age of the plant, location, season, and method of curing (82). Ginseng appears to have immunomodulatory, anticancer, hypoglycemic, antihypertensive, smooth muscle relaxation, androgenic, estrogen-like, platelet aggregation, and CNS stimulation and inhibition effects (81,82). Dose-finding studies have not been done, but 0.5 to 2.0 g of dry root or 200 to 600 mg of extract per day is used for short-term therapy (74). If used long-term, doses should not exceed the equivalent of 1 g of dry root per day (74).

Coon and Ernst recently reviewed the safety of ginseng (79). Use appears relatively safe with few adverse effects reported. GI and sleep-related effects are reported most commonly but do not appear to be more common than with placebo. More serious effects [e.g., mastalgia; Stevens-Johnson syndrome; mania; cerebral arteritis; pneumonitis; and interactions with loop diuretics (decreased effectiveness), phenelzine (headache, tremulousness, and mania), and warfarin (decreased international normalized ratio)] have been associated with ginseng. However, the authors suggest that because of difficulty in determining causal relationship and the potential for contamination, adulteration, and mislabeling, the bulk of the data should be evaluated with caution. Because neonatal death has been reported, use during pregnancy and lactation is not recommended (82). Finally, chronic excessive use has been reported to cause "ginseng abuse syndrome" (diarrhea, insomnia, agitation, hypertension, and tachycardia) (83). However, there is debate as to whether this actually occurs (79,81).

Heavy Metals

As evidenced by the CPMs, heavy metal poisoning has resulted from use of indigenous remedies. Preparations may contain heavy metals as part of the traditional recipe, or they may be present as adulterants. Numerous reports of heavy metal poisoning from myriad products exist, especially from lead. Hai Ge Fen (clamshell powder) and other Chinese medicines have been sources of lead poisoning (60,84,85). Azarcon (lead tetroxide; a bright orange-colored powder) and greta (lead oxide; a mustard-colored powder) are Mexican folk remedies used to treat a variety of GI ailments collectively referred to as *empacho.* A 1982 survey estimated that 7% to 12% of Hispanic families from Mexico use these remedies (86). Cases of lead toxicity and death have been reported with use (86–89).

Paylooah, an orange-red powder, may contain lead and arsenic and has resulted in elevated lead levels (87,90). It is used in China and Southeast Asia for childhood fever and rash (90). Ayurvedic remedies have also resulted in lead poisoning (87,91). They may also contain various other metals such as gold, silver, copper, zinc, iron, tin, and mercury (91). The Asian-Indian folk remedies Ghasard, Bola Goli, and Kandu may also contain lead and cause poisoning and death (26,92).

Kohl and Surma, traditional eye makeup in India, Africa, and the Middle East, contain more than 50% lead (93–95). Poisoning may occur when children get the substance on their hands and subsequently put them in his or her mouth.

Hepatic Toxins

The liver is the major site for biotransformation and appears to be the most common target of serious herbal toxicity (96). Because of this, just as with traditional medications, there are risks of herb-induced hepatotoxicity. There are two major types of herb-induced hepatotoxicity (9): (a) hepatitis due to direct toxic effects on hepatocytes, with dose dependency or idiosyncratic reactions that are most often immune modulated (97); and (b) veno-occlusive disease.

Diagnosis of herb-induced hepatotoxicity can be difficult, and physicians must question patients carefully regarding herbal use. However, even when a history of herbal use is elicited, cause and effect may still be elusive because of mislabeling, adulterants, and multiple constituents. Perharic et al. reported nine patients with liver injury associated with Chinese herbal medicines (98). Forty-three different ingredients were identified in the medications, but they were unable to isolate the toxins responsible. Often, there are no specific diagnostic tests, but uncommon patterns of liver injury (zonal necrosis; necrotic lesions with steatosis or bile duct injury; and vascular injury, especially veno-occlusive disease) should raise suspicion of an herbal etiology (99). Occasionally, diagnosis may be established by urine or serum screening tests, as with pyrrolizidine urine metabolites (100), or serum measurements of pennyroyal constituents (101). Table 4 demonstrates herbal remedies associated with liver injury. The diagnostic approach to acute liver failure injury is addressed in Chapter 17.

Kava

Kava refers to both the rhizome and extracts of or tea made from the rhizome of the pepper plant *P. methysticum*. Kava is a shrub native to islands in the South Pacific that is used recreationally in traditional ceremonies and social gatherings (102). It has also been used as a treatment for gonorrhea, syphilis, and cystitis, and as a sleep aid (102). Today it is used mainly as an anxiolytic. Kava produces a calm tranquil state but does not affect thoughts or memory (103). A recent metaanalysis of randomized, controlled trials showed that kava extract was efficacious in treating anxiety, compared with placebo (104). It has also been shown to be as effective as prescription anxiety agents but nonaddictive (105).

TABLE 4. Herbal products associated with liver injury

Herb (scientific name)	Toxic ingredient	Effects
Camphor (*Cinnamomum camphora*)	Cyclic terpenes	Abnormal liver tests, encephalopathy
Carp bile (*Ctenopharyngodon idellus, Cyprinus carpio*)	Cyprinol	Abnormal liver tests and renal failure, hepatic necrosis (rats)
Cascara (*Rhamnus purshiana*)	? Anthracene glycoside	Cholestatic hepatitis
Chaparral (*Larrea divaricata, Larrea tridentate*)	Nordihydroguaiaretic acid	Cholestasis, cholangitis, chronic hepatitis, cirrhosis
Chinese herbal medicines	Many (? *Paeonia, Dictamnus dasycarpus, Scutellaria, Glycyrrhizin*)	Liver injury, veno-occlusive disease, chronic cholestasis
Clove oil (*Syzygium aromaticum*)	Eugenol	Dose-dependent hepatotoxin
Comfrey (*Symphytum officinale*)	Pyrrolizidine alkaloids	Veno-occlusive disease
Greater celandine (*Chelidonium majus*)	? Isoquinoline alkaloids	Cholestatic hepatitis, fibrosis
Germander (*Teucrium chamaedrys*)	Furan-containing neoclerodane diterpenoids, teucrin A	Acute and chronic hepatitis, necrosis, fibrosis, cirrhosis
Impila (*Callilepis laureola*)	Potassium atractylate–like compound	Hepatic necrosis
Isabgol	Not identified	Giant cell hepatitis (one report)
Jin Bu Huan	Levo-tetrahydropalmatine	Acute and chronic hepatitis, cholestatic hepatitis, fibrosis
Kava (*Piper methysticum*)	Kava lactones	Diffuse hepatocellular necrosis, intrahepatic cholestasis, fulminant hepatic failure
Kombucha mushroom tea	Yeast-bacteria aggregate	Liver injury
Ma huang (*Ephedra* spp.)	Ephedrine	Acute hepatitis, autoimmune hepatitis
Margosa oil (*Azadirachta indica*)	Not identified	Reye's syndrome
Mediterranean glue thistle (*Atractylis gummifera*)	Atractyloside	Diffuse hepatic necrosis
Pennyroyal oil (*Hedeoma pulegioides, Mentha pulegium*)	Pulegone, menthofuran, isopulegone	Hepatocellular necrosis
Sassafras (*Sassafras albidum*)	Safrole	Hepatocellular carcinogen (animals)
Shark cartilage	Not identified	Abnormal liver tests
Teas: gordolobo yerba tea (*Senecio longiloba, Senecio auresus, Senecio vulgaris, Senecio spartoides*), Maté tea (*Ilex paraguariensis*), T'u-san-chi (*Gynura segetum*)	Pyrrolizidine alkaloids	Veno-occlusive disease
Valerian (*Valeriana* spp.)	Not identified	Abnormal liver tests
Venencapsan (*Aesculus hippocastanum*)	Aesculin or coumarin	Portal inflammation and mild steatosis

Note: See also Chapter 17.
Adapted from Stedman C. Herbal hepatotoxicity. *Semin Liver Dis* 2002;22:195–206.

The active components are kava lactones, which are believed to affect γ-aminobutyric acid A receptors (105). Although the exact mechanism of action is not known, kava has been found to have sedative, anxiolytic, anticonvulsant, local anesthetic, spasmolytic, and analgesic effects (106). With use, there appears to be a low incidence of side effects (mainly GI symptoms and dermopathy) that are reversible on discontinuation (107). Stevinson et al. summarized studies suggesting kava does not impede cognitive or motor performance nor interact with alcohol or benzodiazepines (102). However, most studies are small, and some evidence is conflicting. They suggested that until further information is available kava should not be used with alcohol or anxiolytics, and use cannot be considered safe while driving or operating machinery. There is one case report of disorientation and lethargy in a patient using both kava and alprazolam (108). Extrapyramidal symptoms have also been described with kava use (109).

Liver injury is the most feared complication of kava use. Although hepatotoxicity appears to be rare, the FDA recently released a consumer advisory regarding kava use and liver injury (110). Because of hepatitis, cirrhosis, and hepatic failure progressing to liver transplant, kava has been removed from the market in several countries (110). Toxicity has occurred at doses of kava extract ranging from 60 to 400 mg/day (recommended dose range, 60 to 120 mg/day) and after several days to 2 years of use (111). Other than supportive care and discontinuation of use, there is no specific treatment.

Khat

In East Africa and Arabian countries, khat, *Catha edulis*, is used and abused for depression, fatigue, obesity, and as a euphoriant. Fresh stems and leaves are chewed and the juice swallowed. Leaves lose their potency 1 day after picking (112). The active ingredients are cathine (norpseudonephrine) and cathionine (α-aminopropiophenone), which have stimulant effects that fall between those of caffeine and amphetamine (113). Red khat contains more cathinone than the white and fresh leaves more than dried (113). Adverse effects of khat include those typical of adrenergic stimulants: euphoria, mania, anxiety, hypertension, tachycardia, cerebral hemorrhage, myocardial infarction, and pulmonary edema (114). Treatment is similar to that for amphetamine toxicity (Chapter 174). Insomnia, malaise, and lack of concentration may occur after use as a rebound phenomenon (113). Chronic use is associated with hypertension (114) and oral cancer (115). The United States, Switzerland, and several other countries have prohibited the use of khat.

Kombucha "Mushroom"

Kombucha tea is a popular health beverage made by incubating the Kombucha "mushroom" in sweet black tea. Although advocates of Kombucha tea have attributed many therapeutic effects to the drink, its beneficial and adverse effects have not been determined scientifically (116). Beneficial effects attributed to consumption of Kombucha tea include prevention of cancer, relief of arthritis, treatment of insomnia, stimulation of hair growth, and immune system stimulant (it is popular among people with human immunodeficiency virus) (117).

The Kombucha mushroom is actually not a mushroom but a symbiotic colony of several species of yeast and bacteria that are bound together by a surrounding thin membrane (118). Kombucha tea is a mixture of yeast and bacteria (i.e., *Bacterium xylinum, Bacterium gluconicum, Pichia fermentans,* and *Acetobacter ketogenum*) and products of bacterial fermentation (116). The tea can contain up to 1.5% alcohol and a variety of other metabolites (e.g., ethyl acetate, acetic acid, and lactate) (117). Additionally, pathogenic organisms, such as *Aspergillus* and anthrax, can incubate during the preparation process (119). There are at least two commercial producers of Kombucha mushrooms in the United States. Sharing of the mushrooms is believed to have helped to promote its popularity in the United States (117).

Drinking this tea in quantities typically consumed (approximately 4 oz daily) may not cause adverse effects in healthy people, but the potential health risks are unknown for those with preexisting health problems or those who drink excessive quantities of the tea (120). Two cases of unexplained severe lactic acidosis, including one death, and one case of hepatitis have been associated with use of the tea (117,118). Topical application for pain relief has resulted in cutaneous anthrax (121).

The FDA has evaluated the practices of the commercial producers of the Kombucha mushroom and has found no pathogenic organisms or hygiene violations (122). However, because the tea is produced under varying conditions in individual homes, contamination with pathogenic organisms is possible.

Because of the acidity of Kombucha tea, it should not be prepared or stored in containers made from materials such as ceramic or lead crystal, which both contain toxic elements that can leach into the tea (117). Health care professionals should consider consumption of Kombucha tea in the differential diagnosis of people with unexplained lactic acidosis. Treatment is supportive.

Nutmeg and Mace

Nutmeg and mace are derived from *Myristica fragrans*, an evergreen tree native to the Spice Islands and cultivated in the Caribbean. The tree produces a fruit similar in appearance to a peach and contains a nut covered in a red net-like aril. The dried nut is used to make nutmeg, and the dried aril yields mace. Nutmeg is most commonly used as a spice but has been used to treat GI disorders, as an abortifacient, and topically as an analgesic. Nutmeg has psychoactive properties and has been intentionally used as a hallucinogen (123–125).

Both nutmeg and mace contain an essential oil that is believed to be the active component. The nut is comprised of 8% to 15% essential oil (126), which is a complex mixture of aromatic and terpene components (124). Myristicin, a component of the oil, was believed to be responsible for the psychoactive effects, but debate surrounds this issue (126). The mechanism of nutmeg effects is not clear. Effects may be due to the metabolism of myristicin and other constituents to amphetamine-like compounds and to monoamine oxidase inhibition, but this is also debated (124).

Five to 20 g (one to three nuts or 2 tablespoons of powder) of nutmeg appears to be required for pharmacologic activity (126). Doses used to treat diarrhea may be in this range (127). Symptoms generally appear 3 to 8 hours after ingestion. Signs and symptoms of intoxication include euphoria, anxiety, fear, hallucinations (usually visual but also auditory and tactile), headache, drowsiness, dry mouth, nausea, vomiting, paresthesias, numbness, blurred vision, tachycardia, hypotension, and nystagmus (124). Symptoms may be mistaken for anticholinergic effects; however, nutmeg typically causes miosis (125). Symptomatic and supportive care is generally all that is required. Symptoms generally resolve within 24 hours but may persist for days with large ingestions. Two deaths have been associated with nutmeg (128,129).

Podophyllin

The dried roots, rhizomes, and resin of *Podophyllum hexandrum* and *Podophyllum peltatum* (American mandrake, devil's apple, mayapple, baijiaolian) have been used orally as cathartics and topically for wart removal. Major active components are the lignan derivatives, including podophyllotoxin (130). Podophyllin is a spindle poison blocking cell division and inhibiting mitochondrial activity (131). Toxicity may occur with oral or topical administration and generally occurs within 12 hours (131). Acute poisoning produces effects similar to colchicine, antineoplastic agents, arsenic, and ricin. Signs and symptoms of toxicity include abdominal pain, nausea, vomiting, hematemesis, hematochezia, renal failure, bone marrow depression, peripheral neuropathy, seizures, altered mental status, coma, paralysis, acidosis, and death (130). *Podophyllum* is also a suspected teratogen (132). Treatment is symptomatic and supportive, including decontamination. Improvement after hemoperfusion has been reported (133), but failure of improvement is also reported (134).

Pyrrolizidine Alkaloids

Pyrrolizidine alkaloids are found in more than 200 species of plants known to be ingested by humans (135). Species most often related to human poisoning are *Heliotropium, Senecio, Crotalaria,* and *Symphytum.* Pyrrolizidine alkaloids are dose-dependent hepatotoxins typically causing veno-occlusive disease and fibrosis or cirrhosis (99). Pyrrolizidine alkaloids are metabolized by the liver cytochrome P-450 system to reactive intermediates that alkylate hepatic macromolecules (136). Certain metabolites are capable of producing pulmonary toxicity leading to pulmonary artery hypertension and right ventricular hypertrophy (137). Trichodesmine, a metabolite of pyrrolizidine alkaloids, also demonstrates neurotoxicity (138). Liver injury can occur after chronic use or a single exposure, and symptoms may have an acute or insidious onset (100). The most common presentation is chronic ingestion and progressive fibrosis. Patients often present with ascites, hepatomegaly, elevated liver enzymes, and occasionally portal hypertension (100). Complete recovery is possible, but the mortality rates may be as high as 30% to 40%. Infants may be more prone to toxicity (100). Treatment is primarily supportive. *N*-acetylcysteine may be beneficial (139).

Pennyroyal

Pennyroyal oil, derived from the leaves of *Hedeoma pulegioides* or *Mentha pulegium,* is used mainly for menstrual regulation and as an abortifacient. Although uncommon, toxicity from pennyroyal oil is well recognized with multiple reports of adverse effects and death (140). Anderson et al. reported two cases of toxicity related to pennyroyal and reviewed the literature (101). Patients invariably presented with GI effects, with some reports of seizures, coma, cardiac arrest, disseminated intravascular coagulation, and multiorgan failure. Toxicity has occurred after ingestion of 10 ml, and death from hepatic failure ensued after ingestion of 15 ml (101). Pennyroyal contains pulegone, which in combination with its metabolites is theorized to cause glutathione depletion and subsequent toxicity (140). *N*-acetylcysteine therapy has been recommended and used to treat poisoning from pennyroyal (101,141), but definitive evidence of benefit is lacking. Treatment of ingestion should focus on decontamination, supportive care, and early initiation of *N*-acetylcysteine therapy as used in acetaminophen toxicity.

Rattlesnake Capsules

Rattlesnake-capsule ingestion is a common practice among Mexican-Americans in the Los Angeles area. It is a Mexican folk remedy used to treat cancer, diabetes, arthritis, and skin disorders. The reptile is decapitated, skinned, dried in the sun, pulverized, placed in capsules, and sold under various names—*vibora de cascabel, polvo de vibora,* and *carne de vibora*—without prescription in *farmacias. Salmonella arizonae* infections may follow its use (142–147).

Shark Cartilage

Because it was believed that sharks do not get cancer, ingestion and rectal administration of shark cartilage has been used to prevent cancer (148). However, malignant tumors have been found to occur in sharks (149). Preliminary evidence suggests that shark cartilage may actually have anticancer effects (150). Shark cartilage is made up of 40% proteins, 5% to 20% glycosaminoglycans, and calcium salts (149). Side effects of use have included nausea, vomiting, constipation, hypotension, dizziness, hypercalcemia, hyperglycemia, altered mental status, decreased sensation, generalized weakness (150), and possibly hepatitis (151).

St. John's Wort

St. John's wort (*Hypericum perforatum*) has been used both orally and topically to treat a wide variety of conditions. Its most popular use is as an antidepressant. Hypericin and hyperforin are believed to be the active constituents. Hypericin inhibits catechol *O*-methyltransferase and monoamine oxidase *in vitro* (152). However, in a nonhuman primate model, hypericin was not found to cross the blood–brain barrier (153). Hyperforin inhibits serotonin, dopamine, and norepinephrine reuptake (154), but St. John's wort appears to have a different mode of action from conventional antidepressant medications (155). Side effects are minimal, but hypomania and mania have been reported, and serotonin syndrome has been described in patients using other serotonergic medications (152). It is recommended that physicians wait at least 1 week after discontinuing St. John's wort before initiating therapy with selective serotonin reuptake inhibitors (156). St. John's wort also induces the cytochrome P-450 system, which could interfere with metabolism of other medications (78). The evaluation and treatment of serotonin syndrome is the same as that of other causes (Chapter 24).

Wormwood

Wormwood or *Artemisia absinthium* has been used as an aphrodisiac, for wound healing, and an aid to various GI complaints. During the 1800s, particularly in France, extract of wormwood with its licorice-like flavor and emerald-green color was used to make an alcoholic drink known as *absinthe*. Absinthe became popular with artists such as Vincent van Gogh and Henri de Toulouse-Lautrec (157). It is believed that absinthe contributed to van Gogh's death (158). Chronic consumption produces absinthism, a syndrome of stomach irritation, vertigo, psychosis, hallucinations, insomnia, and seizures. In addition to seizures, rhabdomyolysis and renal failure have been described after ingestion of 10 ml of oil of wormwood (159). Wormwood is also porphyrogenic (160). Because of toxicity, absinthe has been banned in the United States since 1912 but is still available in other countries and via the World Wide Web.

Wormwood contains a volatile oil comprised mainly of thujone (α-thujone and β-thujone), which is responsible for toxicity. Because of structural similarity to tetrahydrocannabinol, thujone was believed to bind to the same CNS receptors (161). However, a recent experiment suggests that α-thujone acts on the γ-aminobutyric acid A receptor similar to picrotoxin, and toxicity could be alleviated by diazepam, phenobarbital, and ethanol (160).

Herb-Drug Interactions

Based on a 1997 U.S. survey, nearly 1 in 5 adult patients taking prescription medications were also taking herbs or high-dose vitamins, leading to an estimated 15 million patients that were at risk for adverse interactions (2). Thirty-eight percent of these patients did not discuss their use of alternative therapies with their physician. Often, patients do not consider herbal preparations as medicines. Therefore, physicians must ask specifically about their use. However, physicians are often unaware of concomitant use as well as the potential for drug interactions. Well-documented herbal-drug interactions are lacking (78), and there is even less understanding of herb-herb interactions or the effects of underlying disease on herbal metabolism and pharmacology. Additionally, induction of cytochrome P-450 enzymes by prescription medications or alcohol may increase toxic herbal metabolites, resulting in liver injury (99). Table 5 lists some known and potential herb-drug interactions.

SUMMARY

Poisoning and adverse reactions from herbal products are expected to increase as their use and availability continue to rise. Although most products pose no danger to users when prepared and used correctly, there are insufficient data regarding safety and efficacy for nearly all indigenous and herbal remedies. Considered "natural" and safe by many patients, herbs and folk remedies can cause significant toxicity. Patients, health care providers, and even herbalists may be unaware that these products have pharmacologic activity with the potential for adverse effects, interactions with other medications and herbal preparations, and death. Additionally, certain disease states put patients at greater risk for adverse effects. Many patients do not consider herbs or folk remedies as medications and, therefore, take excessive doses or use for durations longer than recommended. Huxtable has recommended that patients not take large quantities of any one herb and to avoid use in infants, if pregnant or attempting to become pregnant, or if nursing (162).

Product manufacturing is poorly regulated, and industry standards are lacking. Labeling may be inaccurate and claims of efficacy unfounded. Products may not contain reported ingredients and may be contaminated with other botanicals, microorganisms, microbial toxins, pesticides, heavy metals, and drugs (11). It is not uncommon for Chinese medications to have completely different ingredients yet share the same name. Unqualified and misleading sources of information (Web sites, books, and herbal-store employees) may provide medical advice that is incorrect and potentially harmful. Finally, patients may forego or delay known effective treatments in favor of alternative therapies without demonstrated benefit.

Because world travel has become common and relatively easy, many traditional remedies are no longer "indigenous." Health care providers may see patients that use products from a variety of countries. Because many patients do not consider herbs or folk remedies as "medicines," they may not volunteer their use during routine history taking. Health care providers should ask specifically about herbal and alternative therapy use

TABLE 5. Herb-drug interactions

Herb	Drug	Effect
Betel nut (*Areca catechu*)	Antipsychotics	Extrapyramidal symptoms
	Cholinergic medications	Potentiation of effects
Bitter melon (*Momordica charantia*)	Sulfonylureas	Possibly hypoglycemia
Cardiac glycosides: foxglove (*Digitalis purpurea* or *Digitalis lanata*), oleander (*Nerium oleander* or *Thevetia peruviana*), lily-of-the-valley (*Convallaria majalis*), squill (*Urginea* spp.), Chan Su (*Bufo bufo gargarizans* or *Bufo melanos*)	Digoxin, beta-blockers, calcium-channel blockers	Potentiation of digoxin effects, atrioventricular nodal blocks
Chamomile (*Matricaria recutita*)	Aspirin, antiplatelet agents, anticoagulants	Possibly increased bleeding risk
Coenzyme Q-10	Warfarin	Decreased effectiveness
Danshen (*Salvia miltiorrhiza*)	Warfarin, aspirin, antiplatelet agents	Increased INR, increased bleeding risk
	Digoxin	False elevation of serum digoxin level
Devil's claw (*Harpagophytum procumbens*)	Warfarin	Purpura
Dong quai (*Angelica sinensis*)	Warfarin, aspirin, antiplatelet agents	Increased INR, increased bleeding risk
Echinacea (*Echinacea* spp.)	Cyclosporin, corticosteroids	May offset immunosuppressant effects
Ephedra (*Ephedra* spp.)	Caffeine, decongestants	Tachycardia, hypertension
Feverfew (*Tanacetum parthenium*)	Aspirin, antiplatelet agents, anticoagulants	Possibly increased bleeding risk
Garlic (*Allium sativum*)	Aspirin, antiplatelet agents, anticoagulants	Increased bleeding risk, increased INR
Germander (*Teucrium chamaedrys*)	Cytochrome 3A4 inducers (e.g., Phenobarbital)	Increased toxic herbal metabolites
Ginger (*Zingiber officinale*)	Aspirin, antiplatelet agents, anticoagulants	Increased bleeding risk
Ginkgo (*Ginkgo biloba*)	Aspirin, antiplatelet agents, anticoagulants	Increased bleeding risk
Ginseng (*Panax* spp.)	Warfarin	Decreased INR
Ginseng (*Eleutherococcus senticosus*)	Digoxin	False elevation of serum digoxin level
Grapefruit (*Citrus paradisi*)	Medications with cytochrome 3A4 metabolism (i.e., calcium-channel blockers, carbamazepine, cyclosporin, diazepam, diltiazem, indinavir, saquinavir, tacrolimus, warfarin)	Increased plasma concentrations of medications
Kava (*Piper methysticum*)	Ethanol, sedatives	Potentiates sedation
Kelp (*Ascophyllum nodosum, Fucus* spp., brown seaweed spp.)	Thyroxine	Hyperthyroidism
Licorice (*Glycyrrhzia glabra*)	Antihypertensives	Decreased effectiveness
	Corticosteroids	Potentiation of drug effects
	Digoxin	Potentiation of drug effects
	Diuretics	Hypokalemia, offset effects of potassium-sparing diuretics
Papaya (*Carica papaya*)	Warfarin	Increased INR
Psyllium (*Plantago ovata*)	Digoxin	Decreased serum digoxin levels
	Lithium	Decreased serum lithium level
Pyrrolizidine alkaloid containing herbs	Cytochrome 3A4 inducers (e.g., Phenobarbital)	Increased toxic herbal metabolites
St. John's wort (*Hypericum perforatum*)	Digoxin	Decreased area under the curve
	Medications with serotonergic effects	Serotonin syndrome
	MAO inhibitors	Possibly potentiation of drug effects
	Medications with P-450 metabolism (oral contraceptives, cyclosporin, theophylline, protease inhibitors)	Decreased effectiveness
Shankhapushpi (Ayurvedic mixed-herb syrup)	Phenytoin	Decreased serum phenytoin levels
Thujone-containing herbs: wormwood (*Artemisia absinthe*), sage (*Salvia officinalis, Salvia lavandulaefolia*)	Anticonvulsants	Lower seizure threshold
Tonka beans (*Dipteryx odorata*)	Warfarin	Increased INR
Valerian (*Valeriana officinalis*)	Ethanol, sedatives	Potentiates sedation
Yohimbine (*Pausinystalia yohimbe*)	Antihypertensives	Decreased effectiveness
	MAO inhibitors	Insomnia, headache, tremor
	Caffeine, decongestants, tricyclic antidepressants	Hypertension

INR, international normalized ratio; MAO, monoamine oxidase.
Adapted from Fugh-Berman A. Herb-drug interactions. *Lancet* 2000;355:134–138; Miller LG. Selected clinical considerations focusing on known or potential drug-herb interactions. *Arch Intern Med* 1998;158:2200–2211; Stedman C. Herbal hepatotoxicity. *Semin Liver Dis* 2002;22:195–206; and Jellin JM, Gregory PJ, Batz F, et al. *Pharmacist's letter/prescriber's letter natural medicines comprehensive database*, 4th ed. Stockton, CA: Therapeutic Research Faculty, 2002.

and recognize the possibility for adverse effects. Adverse effects should be reported to FDA MedWatch at 1-800-FDA-1088 or https://www.accessdata.fda.gov/scripts/medwatch/.

REFERENCES

1. Akerele O. Summary of WHO guidelines for the assessment of herbal medicines. *Herbal Gram* 1993;28:13–20.
2. Eisenberg DM, Davis RB, Ettner SL, et al. Trends in alternative medicine use in the United States, 1990–1997: results of a follow-up national survey. *JAMA* 1998;280:1569–1575.
3. Marwick C. Growing use of medicinal botanicals forces assessment by drug regulators. *JAMA* 1995;273:607–609.
4. Mitka M. Web site showcases science-based information on herbs, other supplements. *JAMA* 2003;289:829–830.
5. Hung OL, Shih RD, Chiang WK, et al. Herbal preparation use among urban emergency department patients. *Acad Emerg Med* 1997;4:209–213.
6. Fontanarosa PB, Rennie D, DeAngelis CD. The need for regulation of dietary supplements—lessons from ephedra. *JAMA* 2003;289:1568–1570.
7. Fleming GA. The FDA, regulation, and the risk of stroke. *N Engl J Med* 2000;343:1886–1887.
8. Marcus DM, Grollman AP. Botanical medicines—the need for new regulations. *N Engl J Med* 2002;347:2073–2076.
9. Ko RJ. Causes, epidemiology, and clinical evaluation of suspected herbal poisoning. *J Toxicol Clin Toxicol* 1999;37:697–708.

10. Chan TY, Critchley JA. Usage and adverse effects of Chinese herbal medicines. *Hum Exp Toxicol* 1996;15:5–12.
11. De Smet PA. Health risks of herbal remedies. *Drug Saf* 1995;13:81–93.
12. De Smet PA. Herbal remedies. *N Engl J Med* 2002;347:2046–2056.
13. Sanders D, Kennedy N, McKendrick MW. Monitoring the safety of herbal remedies. Herbal remedies have a heterogeneous nature. *BMJ* 1995;311:1569.
14. Joubert PH, Mathibe L. Acute poisoning in developing countries. *Adverse Drug React Acute Poisoning Rev* 1989;8:165–178.
15. Tai YT, But PP, Young K, et al. Cardiotoxicity after accidental herb-induced aconite poisoning. *Lancet* 1992;340:1254–1256.
16. Chan TY, Tomlinson B, Tse LK, et al. Aconitine poisoning due to Chinese herbal medicines: a review. *Vet Hum Toxicol* 1994;36:452–455.
17. Yeih DF, Chiang FT, Huang SK. Successful treatment of aconitine induced life threatening ventricular tachyarrhythmia with amiodarone. *Heart* 2000;84:E8.
18. Chan TY, Tomlinson B, Critchley JA. Aconitine poisoning following the ingestion of Chinese herbal medicines: a report of eight cases. *Aust N Z J Med* 1993;23:268–271.
19. Fitzpatrick AJ, Crawford M, Allan RM, et al. Aconite poisoning managed with a ventricular assist device. *Anaesth Intensive Care* 1994;22:714–717.
20. Chan TY. Anticholinergic poisoning due to Chinese herbal medicines. *Vet Hum Toxicol* 1995;37:156–157.
21. Vanherweghem JL, Depierreux M, Tielemans C, et al. Rapidly progressive interstitial renal fibrosis in young women: association with slimming regimen including Chinese herbs. *Lancet* 1993;341:387–391.
22. Vanhaelen M, Vanhaelen-Fastre R, But P, et al. Identification of aristolochic acid in Chinese herbs. *Lancet* 1994;343:174.
23. Nortier JL, Martinez MC, Schmeiser HH, et al. Urothelial carcinoma associated with the use of a Chinese herb (*Aristolochia fangchi*). *N Engl J Med* 2000;342:1686–1692.
24. Gogtay NJ, Bhatt HA, Dalvi SS, et al. The use and safety of non-allopathic Indian medicines. *Drug Saf* 2002;25:1005–1019.
25. McElvaine MD, Harder EM, Johnson L, et al. Lead poisoning from the use of Indian folk medicines. *JAMA* 1990;264:2212–2213.
26. Saryan LA. Surreptitious lead exposure from an Asian Indian medication. *J Anal Toxicol* 1991;15:336–338.
27. Dolan G, Jones AP, Blumsohn A, et al. Lead poisoning due to Asian ethnic treatment for impotence. *J R Soc Med* 1991;84:630–631.
28. Keen RW, Deacon AC, Delves HT, et al. Indian herbal remedies for diabetes as a cause of lead poisoning. *Postgrad Med J* 1994;70:113–114.
29. Jani JP, Raiyani CV, Mistry JS, et al. Polycyclic aromatic hydrocarbons in traditional medicinal preparations. *Hum Exp Toxicol* 1991;10:347–350.
30. Gymnema. In: DerMarderosian A, Beutler J, eds. *The Review of natural products*, 2nd ed. St. Louis: Facts and Comparisons, 2002:320–321.
31. Trivedy C, Warnakulasuriya S, Peters TJ. Areca nuts can have deleterious effects. *BMJ* 1999;318:1287.
32. Warnakulasuriya S, Trivedy C, Peters TJ. Areca nut use: an independent risk factor for oral cancer. *BMJ* 2002;324:799–800.
33. Norton SA. Betel: consumption and consequences. *J Am Acad Dermatol* 1998;38:81–88.
34. Taylor RF, al-Jarad N, John LM, et al. Betel-nut chewing and asthma. *Lancet* 1992;339:1134–1136.
35. Betel nut. In: DerMarderosian A, Beutler J, eds. *The review of natural products*, 2nd ed. St. Louis: Facts and Comparisons, 2002:77–78.
36. Burton-Bradley BG. Arecaidinism: betel chewing in transcultural perspective. *Can J Psychiatry* 1979;24:481–488.
37. Wu KD, Chuang RB, Wu FL, et al. The milk-alkali syndrome caused by betel nuts in oyster shell paste. *J Toxicol Clin Toxicol* 1996;34:741–745.
38. Tagwireyi D, Ball DE, Loga PJ, et al. Cantharidin poisoning due to "Blister beetle" ingestion. *Toxicon* 2000;38:1865–1869.
39. Till JS, Majmudar BN. Cantharidin poisoning. *South Med J* 1981;74:444–447.
40. Weakley D, Eikenbinder J. The mechanics of cantharidin acantholysis. *J Invest Dermatol* 1962;39:39–45.
41. Graziano MJ, Waterhouse AL, Casida JE. Cantharidin poisoning associated with specific binding site in liver. *Biochem Biophys Res Commun* 1987;149:79–85.
42. Oaks W, DiTunno J, Magnani T, et al. Cantharidin poisoning. *Arch Intern Med* 1960;105:574–582.
43. Burnett JW, Calton GJ, Morgan RJ. Blister beetles: "Spanish fly." *Cutis* 1987;40:22.
44. Nickolls L, Teare D. Poisoning by cantharidin. *BMJ* 1954:1384–1386.
45. Ewart WB, Rabkin SW, Mitenko PA. Poisoning by cantharides. *Can Med Assoc J* 1978;118:1199.
46. Tomlinson B, Chan TY, Chan JC, et al. Toxicity of complementary therapies: an eastern perspective. *J Clin Pharmacol* 2000;40:451–456.
47. Brubacher JR, Ravikumar PR, Bania T, et al. Treatment of toad venom poisoning with digoxin-specific Fab fragments. *Chest* 1996;110:1282–1288.
48. Lyttle T, Goldstein D, Gartz J. *Bufo* toads and bufotenin: fact and fiction surrounding an alleged psychedelic. *J Psychoactive Drugs* 1996;28:267–290.
49. Nelson L, Perrone J. Herbal and alternative medicine. *Emerg Med Clin North Am* 2000;18:709–722.
50. Safadi R, Levy I, Amitai Y, et al. Beneficial effect of digoxin-specific Fab antibody fragments in oleander intoxication. *Arch Intern Med* 1995;155:2121–2125.
51. Rich SA, Libera JM, Locke RJ. Treatment of foxglove extract poisoning with digoxin-specific Fab fragments. *Ann Emerg Med* 1993;22:1904–1907.
52. Ko RJ. Adulterants in Asian patent medicines. *N Engl J Med* 1998;339:847.
53. Brooks PM, Lowenthal RM. Chinese herbal arthritis cure and agranulocytosis. *Med J Aust* 1977;2:860–861.
54. Ries CA, Sahud MA. Agranulocytosis caused by Chinese herbal medicines. Dangers of medications containing aminopyrine and phenylbutazone. *JAMA* 1975;231:352–355.
55. Horowitz RS, Feldhaus K, Dart RC, et al. The clinical spectrum of Jin Bu Huan toxicity. *Arch Intern Med* 1996;156:899–903.
56. Woolf GM, Petrovic LM, Rojter SE, et al. Acute hepatitis associated with the Chinese herbal product jin bu huan. *Ann Intern Med* 1994;121:729–735.
57. Kang-Yum E, Oransky SH. Chinese patent medicine as a potential source of mercury poisoning. *Vet Hum Toxicol* 1992;34:235–238.
58. Espinoza EO, Mann MJ, Bleasdell B. Arsenic and mercury in traditional Chinese herbal balls. *N Engl J Med* 1995;333:803–804.
59. Tay CH, Seah CS. Arsenic poisoning from anti-asthmatic herbal preparations. *Med J Aust* 1975;2:424–428.
60. Chan H, Billmeier GJ Jr, Evans WE, et al. Lead poisoning from ingestion of Chinese herbal medicine. *J Toxicol Clin Toxicol* 1977;10:273–281.
61. Schaumburg HH, Berger A. Alopecia and sensory polyneuropathy from thallium in a Chinese herbal medication. *JAMA* 1992;268:3430–3431.
62. Chan TY, Lee KK, Chan AY, et al. Poisoning due to Chinese proprietary medicines. *Hum Exp Toxicol* 1995;14:434–436.
63. Chinese cucumber root. In: Jellin J, Gregory P, Batz F, et al., eds. *Pharmacist's letter/prescriber's letter natural medicines comprehensive database*, 4th ed. Stockton, CA: Therapeutic Research Faculty, 2002:328–329.
64. Chinese cucumber. In: DerMarderosian A, Beutler J, eds. *The review of natural products*, 2nd ed. St. Louis: Facts and Comparisons, 2002:165–166.
65. Fung MC, Bowen DL. Silver products for medical indications: risk-benefit assessment. *J Toxicol Clin Toxicol* 1996;34:119–126.
66. Colloidal silver. In: Jellin J, Gregory P, Batz F, et al., eds. *Pharmacist's letter/prescriber's letter natural medicines comprehensive database*, 4th ed. Stockton, CA: Therapeutic Research Faculty, 2002:382–383.
67. Over-the-counter drug products containing colloidal silver ingredients or silver salts. Department of Health and Human Services (HHS), Public Health Service (PHS), Food and Drug Administration (FDA). Final rule. *Federal Register* 1999;64:44653–44658.
68. Ephedra. In: Jellin J, Gregory P, Batz F, et al., eds. *Pharmacist's letter/ prescriber's letter natural medicines comprehensive database*, 4th ed. Stockton, CA: Therapeutic Research Faculty, 2002:497–500.
69. Haller CA, Benowitz NL. Adverse cardiovascular and central nervous system events associated with dietary supplements containing ephedra alkaloids. *N Engl J Med* 2000;343:1833–1838.
70. Haller C, Benowitz N. Dietary supplements containing ephedra alkaloids. *N Engl J Med* 2001;344.
71. Traub SJ, Hoyek W, Hoffman RS. Dietary supplements containing ephedra alkaloids. *N Engl J Med* 2001;344.
72. Ginkgo. In: DerMarderosian A, Beutler J, eds. *The review of natural products*, 2nd ed. St. Louis: Facts and Comparisons, 2002:281–284.
73. Ginkgo leaf. In: Jellin J, Gregory P, Batz F, et al., eds. *Pharmacist's letter/prescriber's letter natural medicines comprehensive database*, 4th ed. Stockton, CA: Therapeutic Research Faculty, 2002:586–590.
74. Ernst E. The risk-benefit profile of commonly used herbal therapies: ginkgo, St. John's wort, ginseng, echinacea, saw palmetto, and kava. *Ann Intern Med* 2002;136:42–53.
75. Miller LG. Herbal medicinals: selected clinical considerations focusing on known or potential drug-herb interactions. *Arch Intern Med* 1998;158:2200–2211.
76. Rowin J, Lewis SL. Spontaneous bilateral subdural hematomas associated with chronic *Ginkgo biloba* ingestion. *Neurology* 1996;46:1775–1776.
77. Rosenblatt M, Mindel J. Spontaneous hyphema associated with ingestion of *Ginkgo biloba* extract. *N Engl J Med* 1997;336:1108.
78. Fugh-Berman A, Ernst E. Herb-drug interactions: review and assessment of report reliability. *Br J Clin Pharmacol* 2001;52:587–595.
79. Coon JT, Ernst E. *Panax ginseng*: a systematic review of adverse effects and drug interactions. *Drug Saf* 2002;25:323–344.
80. *Eleutherococcus*. In: DerMarderosian A, Beutler J, eds. *The review of natural products*, 2nd ed. St. Louis: Facts and Comparisons, 2002:236–238.
81. Ginseng, *Panax*. In: Jellin J, Gregory P, Batz F, et al., eds. *Pharmacist's letter/prescriber's letter natural medicines comprehensive database*, 4th ed. Stockton, CA: Therapeutic Research Faculty, 2002:593–597.
82. Ginseng, *Panax*. In: DerMarderosian A, Beutler J, eds. *The review of natural products*, 2nd ed. St. Louis: Facts and Comparisons, 2002:285–289.
83. Siegel RK. Ginseng abuse syndrome. Problems with the panacea. *JAMA* 1979;241:1614–1615.
84. Hill GJ, Hill S. Lead poisoning due to hai ge fen. *JAMA* 1995;273:24–25.
85. Markowitz SB, Nunez CM, Klitzman S, et al. Lead poisoning due to hai ge fen. The porphyrin content of individual erythrocytes. *JAMA* 1994;271:932–934.
86. CDC. Lead poisoning from Mexican folk remedies—California. *MMWR Morb Mortal Wkly Rep* 1983;32:554–555.
87. CDC. Lead poisoning associated with use of traditional ethnic remedies—California, 1991–1992. *MMWR Morb Mortal Wkly Rep* 1993;42:521–524.
88. Bose A, Vashistha K, O'Loughlin BJ. Azarcon por empacho—another cause of lead toxicity. *Pediatrics* 1983;72:106–108.
89. CDC. Childhood lead poisoning associated with Tamarind candy and folk remedies—California, 1999–2000. *MMWR Morb Mortal Wkly Rep* 2002;51:684–686.
90. CDC. Folk remedy-associated lead poisoning in Hmong children—Minnesota. *MMWR Morb Mortal Wkly Rep* 1983;32:555–556.

91. Prpic-Majic D, Pizent A, Jurasovic J, et al. Lead poisoning associated with the use of Ayurvedic metal-mineral tonics. *J Toxicol Clin Toxicol* 1996;34(4):417–423.
92. CDC. Lead poisoning-associated death from Asian Indian folk remedies—Florida. *MMWR Morb Mortal Wkly Rep* 1984;33:643–645.
93. Parry C, Kohl EJ. A lead-hazardous eye makeup from the third world to the first world. *Environ Health Perspect* 1991;94:121–123.
94. Ali AR, Smales OR, Aslam M. Surma and lead poisoning. *BMJ* 1978;2:915–916.
95. Aslam M, Healy MA, Davis SS, Ali AR. Surma and blood lead in children. *Lancet* 1980;1:658–659.
96. Pillans PI. Toxicity of herbal products. *N Z Med J* 1995;108:469–471.
97. Brent J. Three new herbal hepatotoxic syndromes. *J Toxicol Clin Toxicol* 1999;37:715–719.
98. Perharic L, Shaw D, Leon C, et al. Possible association of liver damage with the use of Chinese herbal medicine for skin disease. *Vet Hum Toxicol* 1995;37:562–566.
99. Stedman C. Herbal hepatotoxicity. *Semin Liver Dis* 2002;22:195–206.
100. Steenkamp V, Stewart MJ, Zuckerman M. Clinical and analytical aspects of pyrrolizidine poisoning caused by South African traditional medicines. *Ther Drug Monit* 2000;22:302–306.
101. Anderson IB, Mullen WH, Meeker JE, et al. Pennyroyal toxicity: measurement of toxic metabolite levels in two cases and review of the literature. *Ann Intern Med* 1996;124:726–734.
102. Stevinson C, Huntley A, Ernst E. A systematic review of the safety of kava extract in the treatment of anxiety. *Drug Saf* 2002;25:251–261.
103. Norton SA. Herbal medicines in Hawaii from tradition to convention. *Hawaii Med J* 1998;57:382–386.
104. Pittler MH, Ernst E. Efficacy of kava extract for treating anxiety: systematic review and meta-analysis. *J Clin Psychopharmacol* 2000;20:84–89.
105. Bilia AR, Gallon S, Vincieri FF. Kava-kava and anxiety: growing knowledge about the efficacy and safety. *Life Sci* 2002;70:2581–2597.
106. Kava. In: Jellin J, Gregory P, Batz F, et al., eds. *Pharmacist's letter/prescriber's letter natural medicines comprehensive database*, 4th ed. Stockton, CA: Therapeutic Research Faculty, 2002:759–761.
107. Ernst E. Safety concerns about kava. *Lancet* 2002;359:1865.
108. Almeida JC, Grimsley EW. Coma from the health food store: interaction between kava and alprazolam. *Ann Intern Med* 1996;125:940–941.
109. Schelosky L, Raffauf C, Jendroska K, et al. Kava and dopamine antagonism. *J Neurol Neurosurg Psychiatry* 1995;58:639–640.
110. Center for Food Safety and Applied Nutrition, USFDA. Kava-containing dietary supplements may be associated with severe liver injury. Available at http://www.cfsan.fda.gov/~dms/addskava.html. Accessed August 2003.
111. Ernst E. Second thoughts about kava. *Am J Med* 2002;113:347–348.
112. Randall T. Khat abuse fuels Somali conflict, drains economy. *JAMA* 1993;269:12, 15.
113. Khat. In: DerMarderosian A, Beutler J, eds. *The review of natural products*, 2nd ed. St. Louis: Facts and Comparisons, 2002:364–366.
114. Khat. In: Jellin J, Gregory P, Batz F, et al., eds. *Pharmacist's letter/prescriber's letter natural medicines comprehensive database*, 4th ed. Stockton, CA: Therapeutic Research Faculty, 2002:761–762.
115. Soufi HE, Kameswaran M, Malatani T. Khat and oral cancer. *J Laryngol Otol* 1991;105:643–645.
116. Kombucha. In: DerMarderosian A, Beutler J, eds. *The review of natural products*, 2nd ed. St. Louis: Facts and Comparisons, 2002:371–372.
117. CDC. Unexplained severe illness possibly associated with consumption of Kombucha tea—Iowa, 1995. *MMWR Morb Mortal Wkly Rep* 1995;44:892–893, 899–900.
118. Perron AD, Patterson JA, Yanofsky NN. Kombucha "mushroom" hepatotoxicity. *Ann Emerg Med* 1995;26:660–661.
119. Kombucha tea. In: Jellin J, Gregory P, Batz F, et al., eds. *Pharmacist's letter/prescriber's letter natural medicines comprehensive database*, 4th ed. Stockton, CA: Therapeutic Research Faculty, 2002:767–768.
120. CDC. Unexplained severe illness possibly associated with consumption of Kombucha tea—Iowa, 1995. From the Centers for Disease Control and Prevention. *JAMA* 1996;275:96–98.
121. Sadjadi J. Cutaneous anthrax associated with the Kombucha "mushroom" in Iran. *JAMA* 1998;280:1567–1568.
122. Food and Drug Administration. FDA cautions consumers on "Kombucha mushroom tea." Washington, D.C.: U.S. Department of Health and Human Services, Public Health Service, Food and Drug Administration, 1995.
123. Abernethy MK, Becker LB. Acute nutmeg intoxication. *Am J Emerg Med* 1992;10:429–430.
124. Sangalli BC, Chiang W. Toxicology of nutmeg abuse. *J Toxicol Clin Toxicol* 2000;38:671–678.
125. Sjoholm A, Lindberg A, Personne M. Acute nutmeg intoxication. *J Intern Med* 1998;243:329–331.
126. Nutmeg. In: DerMarderosian A, Beutler J, eds. *The review of natural products*, 2nd ed. St. Louis, MO: Facts and Comparisons, 2002:468–469.
127. Nutmeg and mace. In: Jellin J, Gregory P, Batz F, et al., eds. *Pharmacist's letter/prescriber's letter natural medicines comprehensive database*, 4th ed. Stockton, CA: Therapeutic Research Faculty, 2002:925–927.
128. Cushny A. Therapeutical and pharmacological section: nutmeg poisoning. *Proc R Soc Med* 1908;1:39–44.
129. Stein U, Greyer H, Hentschel H. Nutmeg (myristicin) poisoning—report on a fatal case and a series of cases recorded by a poison information centre. *Forensic Sci Int* 2001;118:87–90.
130. Podophyllum. In: Jellin J, Gregory P, Batz F, et al., eds. *Pharmacist's letter/prescriber's letter natural medicines comprehensive database*, 4th ed. Stockton, CA: Therapeutic Research Faculty, 2002:1014–1016.
131. Podophyllum. In: DerMarderosian A, Beutler J, eds. *The review of natural products*, 2nd ed. St. Louis: Facts and Comparisons, 2002:512–513.
132. Karol MD, Conner CS, Watanabe AS, et al. Podophyllum: suspected teratogenicity from topical application. *J Toxicol Clin Toxicol* 1980;16:283–286.
133. Slater GE, Rumack BH, Peterson RG. Podophyllin poisoning. Systemic toxicity following cutaneous application. *Obstet Gynecol* 1978;52:94–96.
134. Cassidy DE, Drewry J, Fanning JP. Podophyllum toxicity: a report of a fatal case and a review of the literature. *J Toxicol Clin Toxicol* 1982;19:35–44.
135. Batchelor WB, Heathcote J, Wanless IR. Chaparral-induced hepatic injury. *Am J Gastroenterol* 1995;90:831–833.
136. Cooper RA, Huxtable RJ. The relationship between reactivity of metabolites of pyrrolizidine alkaloids and extrahepatic toxicity. *Proc West Pharmacol Soc* 1999;42:13–16.
137. Huxtable RJ. Activation and pulmonary toxicity of pyrrolizidine alkaloids. *Pharmacol Ther* 1990;47:371–389.
138. Huxtable RJ, Yan CC, Wild S, et al. Physicochemical and metabolic basis for the differing neurotoxicity of the pyrrolizidine alkaloids, trichodesmine and monocrotaline. *Neurochem Res* 1996;21:141–146.
139. Stewart MJ, Steenkamp V. Pyrrolizidine poisoning: a neglected area in human toxicology. *Ther Drug Monit* 2001;23:698–708.
140. Pennyroyal. In: DerMarderosian A, Beutler J, eds. *The review of natural products*, 2nd ed. St. Louis: Facts and Comparisons, 2002:498–499.
141. Buechel DW, Haverlah VC, Gardner ME. Pennyroyal oil ingestion: report of a case. *J Am Osteopath Assoc* 1983;82:793–794.
142. Cone LA, Boughton WH, Cone LA, et al. Rattlesnake capsule-induced *Salmonella arizonae* bacteremia. *West J Med* 1990;153:315–316.
143. Waterman SH, Juarez G, Carr SJ, et al. *Salmonella arizonae* infections in Latinos associated with rattlesnake folk medicine. *Am J Public Health* 1990;80:286–289.
144. Babu K, Sonnenberg M, Kathpalia S, et al. Isolation of salmonellae from dried rattlesnake preparations. *J Clin Microbiol* 1990;28:361–362.
145. Riley KB, Antoniskis D, Maris R, et al. Rattlesnake capsule-associated *Salmonella arizonae* infections. *Arch Intern Med* 1988;148:1207–1210.
146. Bhatt BD, Zuckerman MJ, Foland JA, et al. Disseminated *Salmonella arizonae* infection associated with rattlesnake meat ingestion. *Am J Gastroenterol* 1989;84:433–435.
147. Noskin GA, Clarke JT. *Salmonella arizonae* bacteremia as the presenting manifestation of human immunodeficiency virus infection following rattlesnake meat ingestion. *Rev Infect Dis* 1990;12:514–517.
148. Lane I, Comac L. *Sharks don't get cancer.* Garden City, NY: Avery Publishing Group, 1992.
149. National Cancer Institute. Cartilage (bovine and shark). Available at: http://www.cancer.gov/cancerinfo/pdq/cam/cartilage. Accessed August 2003.
150. Shark cartilage. In: Jellin J, Gregory P, Batz F, et al., eds. *Pharmacist's letter/prescriber's letter natural medicines comprehensive database*, 4th ed. Stockton, CA: Therapeutic Research Faculty, 2002:1142–1144.
151. Ashar B, Vargo E. Shark cartilage-induced hepatitis. *Ann Intern Med* 1996;125:780–781.
152. St. John's wort. In: Jellin J, Gregory P, Batz F, et al., eds. *Pharmacist's letter/prescriber's letter natural medicines comprehensive database*, 4th ed. Stockton, CA: Therapeutic Research Faculty, 2002:1180–1184.
153. Fox E, Murphy RF, McCully CL, et al. Plasma pharmacokinetics and cerebrospinal fluid penetration of hypericin in nonhuman primates. *Cancer Chemother Pharmacol* 2001;47:41–44.
154. Chatterjee SS, Bhattacharya SK, Wonnemann M, et al. Hyperforin as a possible antidepressant component of hypericum extracts. *Life Sci* 1998;63:499–510.
155. Fornal CA, Metzler CW, Mirescu C, et al. Effects of standardized extracts of St. John's wort on the single-unit activity of serotonergic dorsal raphe neurons in awake cats: comparisons with fluoxetine and sertraline. *Neuropsychopharmacology* 2001;25:858–870.
156. Waksman J, Heard K, Joliff H, et al. Serotonin syndrome associated with the use of St. John's wort and paroxetine. 2000;35:521.
157. Arnold WN. Absinthe. *Sci Am* 1989;260:112–117.
158. Arnold WN. Vincent van Gogh and the thujone connection. *JAMA* 1988;260:3042–3044.
159. Weisbord SD, Soule JB, Kimmel PL. Poison on line—acute renal failure caused by oil of wormwood purchased through the Internet. *N Engl J Med* 1997;337:825–827.
160. Hold KM, Sirisoma NS, Ikeda T, et al. Alpha-thujone (the active component of absinthe): gamma-aminobutyric acid type A receptor modulation and metabolic detoxification. *Proc Natl Acad Sci U S A* 2000;97:3826–3831.
161. del Castillo J, Anderson M, Rubottom GM. Marijuana, absinthe and the central nervous system. *Nature* 1975;253:365–366.
162. Huxtable RJ. The myth of beneficent nature: the risks of herbal preparations. *Ann Intern Med* 1992;117:165–166.

PART VI

Mass Incidents

CHAPTER 259

Hazardous Materials Incidents

Jefferey L. Burgess

Definitions of hazardous materials include the following: a substance (solid, liquid, or gas) capable of creating harm to people, property, and the environment (1); and any material or substance that in normal use can be damaging to the health and well-being of humans (2). The U.S. Department of Transportation and U.S. Environmental Protection Agency (EPA) have published lists of chemicals designated as hazardous materials (3,4). Hazardous materials incidents include airborne releases of gas and vapor, spills of solid and liquid material, and explosions and fires resulting in chemical release to the environment. These incidents result in an on-site response commonly including firefighters in specially trained hazardous materials teams. Only a fraction of hazardous materials incidents involve clinically significant human exposure, and they generally result in only limited morbidity or mortality (5). In a limited number of incidents, however, large numbers of individuals may be exposed, and the potential for severe and persistent medical sequelae of exposure is an important concern (6,7). The term *chemical disaster* refers to an incident in which the capability to respond is overwhelmed. Disasters may require local, regional, national, or international assistance depending on their size and complexity. Table 1 provides a partial list of worldwide major chemical disasters.

Hazardous materials incidents can be challenging to handle. Unlike most other poisonings, rescuers and caregivers face a risk of exposure to chemicals remaining on a contaminated patient. In addition, a vast number of potential chemicals are involved, so it is unlikely that the treating medical professional will have previous experience with a specific chemical. It also may be difficult to find information on the toxicity of many chemicals, particularly information addressing the inhalation and dermal exposure routes that most frequently occur in hazardous materials incidents. Most medical professionals have limited experience in estimating the extent of exposure to individuals present at the incident site. Incidents are unexpected, and appropriate planning is therefore difficult. Communication from the incident scene to the medical treatment facility may be limited; as a result, only scant information about the nature and extent of exposure may be available to the medical team. In many incidents, the exposure may be unknown initially (8). However, the majority of hazardous materials incidents involve a relatively small number of victims. In a multistate study, the mean number of victims per incident in 1998 was four (9). Therefore, the victims of most hazardous materials incidents can be treated by a single health care facility.

This chapter provides a general overview of evaluation and treatment of patients exposed during hazardous materials incidents. Many excellent publications provide additional information, including an extensive set of materials produced by the U.S. Agency for Toxic Substances and Disease Registry (ATSDR) (10–12). An Advanced HAZMAT Life Support course is offered internationally (http://www.ahls.org/). Nonproprietary hazardous materials databases are available on the Web, including those compiled by the National Library of Medicine (http://toxnet.nlm.nih.gov/). Biological agents and radioactive substances are not included in this chapter. Chemical warfare agents represent a special hazard that is addressed in Chapter 260.

INCIDENCE

Although a number of country-specific hazardous materials incident registries exist, there are no reliable data on worldwide occurrence. However, there are organizations tracking or providing information on such incidents internationally. The University of Wales Institute in Cardiff, United Kingdom is designated by the World Health Organization (WHO) as an International Clearing House for Major Chemical Incidents (http://www.healthchem.uwic.ac.uk/). It investigates pollution incidents throughout the world. The International Programme on Chemical Safety is a cooperative program of the United Nations Environment Programme, the International Labour Organisation, and the WHO. The main roles of the International Programme on Chemical Safety are to establish the scientific health and environmental risk assessment basis for safe use of chemicals and to strengthen national capabilities for chemical safety (13).

In the United States, the EPA reported in its Toxic Release Inventory that more than 7 billion pounds of chemicals were released into the environment in the year 2000 alone (14). The National Response Center, the point of contact for reporting all oil, chemical, radiologic, biological, and etiologic discharges into the environment in the United States and its territories, reported 32,185 incidents in 2002, an increase of 18% since 1992 (15). Hazardous materials incidents are more likely to occur in certain industries, although there is regional variation. In Washington State, 33% of incidents occurred in the trucking service, pulp paper and paperboard mills, sanitary services, and electric light and power and petroleum refining industries. However, the 30% of incidents with reported human exposure were most likely to occur in elementary and secondary schools, private households, sanitary services, trucking services, and eating and drinking places. When ranked on the basis of total incidents per number of employees, the industries with the highest incident rates were agricultural chemical manufacturing, petroleum refining, industrial and miscellaneous chemical manufacturing, electric light and power, and pulp paper and paperboard mills (16).

The ATSDR collects information on nonpetroleum product hazardous materials incidents. For 1998, 13 state health departments (Alabama, Colorado, Iowa, Minnesota, Mississippi, Missouri, New York, North Carolina, Oregon, Rhode Island, Texas, Washington, and Wisconsin) collected data for the Hazardous Substance Emergency Event Surveillance (HSEES) system. Of the 5987 reported incidents, 79% occurred at fixed facilities and accounted for 86% of reported injuries, and 21% occurred during transportation. Of fixed-facility incidents, 42% were reported as involving a reaction chamber in which chemicals are processed, 11% involved ancillary process equipment, 11% involved storage above ground, 9% involved piping, 9% involved material handling, and 18% involved more than one area or the area was unknown. Of transportation-related incidents, 14% involved transport by rail, 82% occurred during other forms of ground transport, and 4% involved water, air, or pipeline transport. Only one substance was released in 96.5% of incidents, two substances in 2.1% of incidents, and more than two in 1.4% of all incidents. Of these incidents, 405 (6.8%) involved injurious human exposure, resulting in a total of 1533 victims, including 36 deaths, and 537 incidents required evacuations (9).

TABLE 1. Hazardous materials incidents resulting in more than 50 fatalities

Year	Location	Origin of accident	Products involved	Deaths	Injuries
1984	India, Bhopal	Leakage	Methyl isocyanate	2800	50,000
1989	USSR, Acha Ufa	Explosion (pipeline)	Gas	575	623
1984	Mexico, St. J. Ixhuatepec	Explosion (storage tank)	LPG	>500	2500
1975	India, Chasnala	Industry	—	431	
1993	Columbia, Remeios	Release	Crude oil	430	
1983	Egypt, Nile River	Explosion (transport)	LPG	317	44
1979	USSR, Novosibirsk	Plant	Chemicals	300	
1993	Thailand, Bangkok	Fire (toy factory)	Plastics	240	547
1998	Cameroon, Yaoundi	Transport accident	Petroleum products	220	130
1978	Spain, San Carlos	Road transport	Propylene	216	200
1992	Mexico, Guadalajara	Explosion (sewers)	Hydrocarbon oil, gas	>206	>1500
1994	Egypt, Drowka, Durunka	Flash flood	Burning oil	>200	
1991	Thailand, Bangkok	Transport accident	Dynamite, detonators	171	100
1988	UK, North Sea	Explosion, fire (platform)	Oil, gas	167	
1982	Venezuela, Tacoa	Explosion (tank)	Fuel oil	>153	500
1990	India, Basti	Food poisoning	Sulplios	150	>150
1991	Italy, Livorno	Transport accident	Naphtha	141	
1996	China, Shaoyang	Explosion (storage)	Explosives	125	400
1991	Korea, Pyongyang	Explosion	Dynamite	>120	
1980	Turkey, Danaciobasi	Use/application	Butane	107	
1995	Korea, Taegu	Explosion (subway)	LPG	101	140
1988	Pakistan, Islamabad	Explosion (storage)	Explosives	>100	3000
1995	Brazil, Boqueiro	Explosion (store)	Ammunition	100	
1995	India, Madras	Transport accident	Fuel	~100	23
1991	Ethiopia, Addis Ababa	Explosion	Ammunition	100	200
1990	India, near Patna	Leakage, transport accident	Gas	100	100
1984	Romania	Factory	Chemicals	100	100
1978	Mexico, Xilatopec	Explosion (road transport)	Gas	100	200
1991	India, Medran	Transport accident	Inflammable liquid	93	25
1984	Brazil, Cubatao	Pipeline explosion	Gasoline	89	
1993	China, Kuiyong	Fire (doll factory)		81	19
1980	Iran, Deh-Bros Org	Fire, explosion	Dynamite	80	45
1970	Japan, Osaka	Explosion (subway)	Gas	79	425
1994	China, Zhuhai	Fire (textile factory)		76	150
1983	India, Dhurabari	Fire	Oil	76	>60
1994	China, Guangix	Explosion (storage)	Dynamite, explosives	73	99
1988	USSR, Arzamas	Explosion (rail transport)	Explosives	73	230
1991	China, Dongguang	Fire (textile industry)		71	
1993	China, Baohe	Explosion	Natural gas	70	
1991	Thailand, Bangkok	Explosion	Gas	>63	
1988	Mexico, Mexico City	Explosion	Fireworks	62	87
1993	China, Shuangpai	Explosion		61	
1996	Haiti	Poisoned medicine	Diethylene glycol	>60	
1996	Afghanistan, Kabuhl	Explosion (store)	Ammunition	60	>125
1994	Nigeria, Onitsha	Fire (road transport)	Fuel oil	60	
1985	India, Tamil Nadu	Transport	Gasoline	60	
1984	Pakistan, Gahri Dhoda	Explosion (pipeline)	Gas	60	
1977	South Korea, Iri	Explosion (rail transport)	Dynamite	57	1300
1987	China, Guangxi Province		Methyl alcohol	55	3600
1980	Thailand, Bangkok	Explosion	Explosives	54	353
1993	Venezuela, Tejerias	Explosion (sewers)	Gas	53	35
1979	Turkey, Istanbul	Explosion (marine transport)	Crude oil	52	>2
1973	Indonesia, Djakarta	Fire, explosion	Fireworks	52	24
1990	Thailand, Bangkok	Transport accident	LPG	>51	>54
1980	USA, Alaska	Platform fire	Oil	51	
1980	Spain, Ortuella	Explosion	Propane	51	

LPG, liquified petroleum gas.
Adapted from United Nations Environment Programme. Awareness and Preparedness for Emergencies on a Local Level Disasters Database. Available at: http://www.uneptie.org/pc/apell/disasters/lists/disasterdate.html. Accessed February 2003.

The most frequently reported substances released include flammable gases and liquids, sewage, unknown materials, ammonia, butadiene, carbon monoxide, chlorine, ethylene glycol, hydrochloric acid, mercury, oxides of nitrogen, polychlorinated biphenyls, sodium hydroxide, sulfur dioxide, sulfuric acid, and vinyl chloride (15). The substances most frequently reported to HSEES for 1998, including sulfur dioxide, ammonia, sulfuric acid, and butadiene, are listed in Table 2. However, chlorine, ammonia, and acids were the most common substances or categories associated with human injuries (9). These data differ somewhat from hazardous materials incidents reported to an American poison center, where carbon monoxide, pepper spray, ammonia, natural gas, chlorine, sulfuric acid, hydrochloric acid, and mercury were the most common exposure agents (5). When chemicals are com-

TABLE 2. The 50 most commonly released chemicals reported by Hazardous Substance Emergency Event Surveillance (HSEES) System—1998

Chemical	Incidents
Sulfur dioxide	494
Ammonia	374
Sulfuric acid	143
Butadiene	142
Paint or coating NOS	137
Hydrochloric acid	132
Mercury	127
Sodium hydroxide	127
Indeterminate[a]	114
Benzene	112
Chlorine	100
Freon 22	83
Mixture: H_2S/SO_2	78
Mixture: NO/NO_2	75
Ethylene	71
Ethylene glycol	70
Hydrogen sulfide	70
Carbon monoxide	62
Nitric oxide	62
Polychlorinated biphenyls	59
Sodium hypochlorite	53
Mixture: benzene/butadiene	46
Solvent NOS	43
Nitrogen fertilizer	40
Phosphoric acid	38
Methylene chloride	37
Corrosive NOS	35
Mixture: α-pinene/β-pinene/methyl mercaptan/terpene	35
Nitric acid	34
Adhesive NOS	32
Toluene	32
Hydrogen peroxide	31
Pesticide NOS	31
Nitrogen dioxide	30
Resin solution	27
Ethanol	26
Hydrofluoric acid	26
Xylene	26
Acid NOS	25
Methanol	25
Perchloroethylene	25
Diesel fuel	24
Ink NOS	24
Mixture: $H_2S/NO/NO_2/SO_2$	24
Urea-ammonium nitrate fertilizer	24
Potassium hydroxide	23
Propylene	23
Nitrogen, phosphorus, potassium fertilizer	22
Isopropanol	21
Ethylene oxide	20

NOS, not otherwise specified.
[a]Unable to assign a standardized name for the substance.
Data from Hazardous Substances Emergency Event Surveillance System 1998 database, Agency for Toxic Substances and Disease Registry Available at: http://www.atsdr.cdc.gov/HS/HSEES/annual98.html. Accessed January 2003.

bined into categories by mechanism of action and exposure type, irritant chemicals, unknown chemicals, and solvents are frequently encountered, as listed in Table 3. As demonstrated in one study, the route of human exposure in these incidents is overwhelmingly by inhalation (73% of incidents), and mixed dermal/inhalation exposure (13% of incidents), with dermal exposure alone less common (7% of incidents), and ingestion uncommon (8). The high prevalence of respiratory exposure in hazardous materials incidents also has been reported elsewhere (17).

TABLE 3. Hazardous materials incidents by chemical exposure type

Chemical	Incidents	Exposures[a]	Transports[b]	% Transported
Unknown	16	171	101	59
Irritant, high water solubility	14	189	156	83
Irritant, low water solubility	8	216	175	81
Solvents (volatile organics)	6	44	6	14
Pesticides	5	38	14	37
Chemical asphyxiants	5	25	24	96
Metals	3	26	3	12
Simple asphyxiants	2	354	1	<1
Radioactive	1	9	0	0
Other/mixed	10	48	21	44
Total	**70**	**1120**	**501**	**45**

[a]Individuals with reported chemical exposures.
[b]Exposure victims transported to a health care facility.
From Burgess JL, Pappas GP, Robertson WO. Hazardous materials incidents: the Washington Poison Center experience and approach to exposure assessment. *J Occup Environ Med* 1997;39:760–766, with permission.

In a limited number of cases, chemical contamination may not be apparent initially. Certain circumstances are suggestive of chemical release and subsequent human exposure. Accidents at industrial or agricultural sites and involving chemical transport should be considered high risks for chemical contamination, as should suspected terrorism and mass-casualty incidents. Strong or caustic odors suggest chemical exposure, although their presence does not prove the existence of a toxic concentration of chemicals, and their absence does not rule out contamination. Patients should also be considered at risk for contamination if they exhibit cholinergic syndromes (Chapter 13), irritant mucous membrane symptoms, chemical burns, soiling of skin or clothing with unidentified liquids or powders, or intentional overdoses with industrial products.

CLINICAL PRESENTATION

Given the broad spectrum of hazardous materials, the clinical presentation after specific exposure varies tremendously. In the ATSDR-HSEES data, individual symptoms are collected along with limited outcome data. Consistent with the predominant inhalation route of exposure, the most common symptoms involve the respiratory system and eye irritation, followed by skin irritation, gastrointestinal symptoms, and headache (Table 4). In 1998, 2% of exposure victims died, 15% were treated and released at the incident site, 66% were treated at a hospital and either directly discharged or observed but not admitted, 9% were admitted, and 8% were treated by a private physician (9). However, determining whether many of the exposure victims required or benefited from medical evaluation is difficult.

The HSEES study results are comparable to data from the State of Washington evaluating 202 subjects in 87 incidents, with predominantly minor injuries and no deaths reported. The most common acute symptoms included headache (40%), cough (33%), itchy or irritated eyes (32%), sore or dry throat (32%), chest or lung irritation (26%), dizziness or lightheadedness (25%), and nausea

TABLE 4. Type of injury reported by Hazardous Substance Emergency Event Surveillance (HSEES) System—1998

Type of injury	Injuries[a]	(%)
Chemical burns	95	(3.4)
Heart problems	42	(1.5)
Dizziness /central nervous system[b]	200	(7.2)
Eye irritation	354	(12.7)
Headache	239	(8.6)
Heat stress	11	(0.4)
Gastrointestinal problems	267	(9.6)
Respiratory system	901	(32.4)
Shortness of breath	153	(5.5)
Skin irritation	298	(10.7)
Thermal burns	44	(1.6)
Trauma	123	(4.4)
Other	56	(2.0)
Total	**2783**	**(100.0)**

[a]A victim can have had more than one injury.
[b]Central nervous system symptoms.
Data from Hazardous Substances Emergency Event Surveillance System 1998 database, Agency for Toxic Substances and Disease Registry. Available at: http://www.atsdr.cdc.gov/HS/HSEES/annual98.html. Accessed January 2003.

or vomiting (20%). The most common persistent symptoms (for a minimum of 8 days) included fatigue (10%), sputum or phlegm production (8%), sore or dry throat (8%), stuffy or runny nose (8%), and cough (8%) (Fig. 1). Persistent medical symptoms were reported in 25% of subjects, and 9% left work or school for more than 2 days owing to the exposure. Medical intervention was reported in 58% of subjects for whom medical records were available, and objective abnormalities, including transient elevations in blood pressure, were found in 72%. Subjects with dermal exposures, greater chronic ingestion of alcohol, and previous treatment with psychiatric medications were more likely to report persistent symptoms. Divorced, widowed, or separated subjects, asthmatic subjects, and those having initial dermal symptoms were more likely to miss work or school for more than 2 days. Of patients evaluated at a health care facility, subjects with an inhalation exposure and those decontaminated at the scene were less likely to be treated or have objective abnormalities (5).

Chemical incidents provoke extreme fear among the public and may result in large numbers of victims who suffer only from mass sociogenic illness or collective hysteria (18–20). Information on the toxicity of the involved chemicals may help rule out

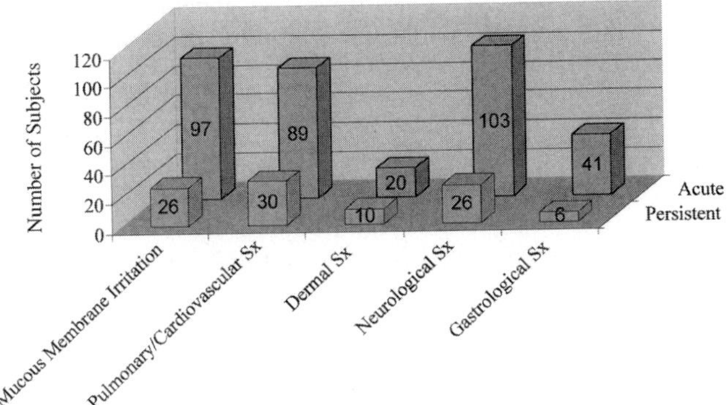

Figure 1. Acute (within 60 minutes) and persistent (8 days or longer) physiologic symptoms (Sx) in 202 subjects after hazardous materials incidents. (Adapted from Burgess JL, Kovalchick DF, Lymp JF, et al. Risk factors for adverse health effects after hazardous materials incidents. *J Occup Environ Med* 2001;43:558–566.)

contamination in these patients. Even in incidents without direct toxicity from chemical exposure, persistent psychological morbidity may occur. In published studies on psychological effects of acute chemical exposures, victims had increased stress and psychological complaints (21–24). Subjects involved in disasters had significantly higher test scores in depression and anxiety (23), as well as higher distress and lower perceived control (21). Some physical effects of exposures can also be explained by elevated psychological distress (22,24).

INCIDENT PLANNING AND RESPONSE

Planning for hazardous materials incidents is essential to providing appropriate treatment. It is advisable to include scenarios requiring treatment of contaminated patients during preparedness drills. The extent of equipment, training, and preparedness required for decontamination of each chemically contaminated patient will differ. In 1986, the U.S. Congress enacted the Superfund Amendments and Reauthorization Act (SARA). Under SARA, Title III established the Emergency Planning and Community Right-to-Know Act, in which each state was required to establish a State Emergency Response Commission (SERC) to oversee and review plans and preparations made by Local Emergency Planning Committees (LEPCs). The EPA subsequently published the Hazardous Materials Planning Guide (NRT-1), updated in 2001 (http://yosemite.epa.gov/oswer/cepoweb.nsf/content/serc-lepc-publications.htm), to assist LEPCs in meeting their legal obligations (25). Major trauma centers and hospitals should be actively engaged and participate in these plans with clearly delineated roles and responsibilities to provide the appropriate level of care for chemically exposed and contaminated patients. Those health care facilities identified by the LEPC for care of chemically contaminated patients should have a higher level of preparedness, as should hospitals near major industrial sites, agricultural activities, and transportation routes. Any plan must include contingencies for contamination sources within the hospital and for emergency department evacuation.

For hospitals participating in the emergency response to a hazardous substance release, the U.S. Occupational Safety and Health Administration (OSHA) Hazardous Waste Operations Emergency Response standards require staff training, as well as a plan that includes procedures for decontaminating patients and appropriate personal protective equipment for hospital staff (26). The Joint Commission on Accreditation of Healthcare Organizations requires institutions to have procedures describing the specific precautions, procedures, and protective equipment used during emergency response to hazardous materials and waste spills or exposures (27). Specifically, any institution with an emergency department should have plans for treatment of a contaminated patient. However, a study of Washington State hospital-based emergency care facilities found that only 52 (55%) had protocols for handling medical facility contamination and potential evacuation arising during the management of contaminated patients (28). In a study of U.S. Level I trauma centers, 6% acknowledged having all equipment required for safe decontamination; 83% of the facilities had hazardous materials response plans, but less than one-third of these were considered complete; and only 58% of the trauma centers had performed a single drill (29). A similar lack of preparation is expected in other states and countries.

Although it is impossible to predict the exact type of incident that may occur, an emergency department should be prepared for commonly released chemicals and more unusual chemicals stored or used in industrial sites located in its vicinity. Material safety data sheets (MSDSs) contain basic chemical, reactivity, and toxicology data and are kept on file by an employer for each hazardous substance used in the facility (30). On review of the MSDS, the health

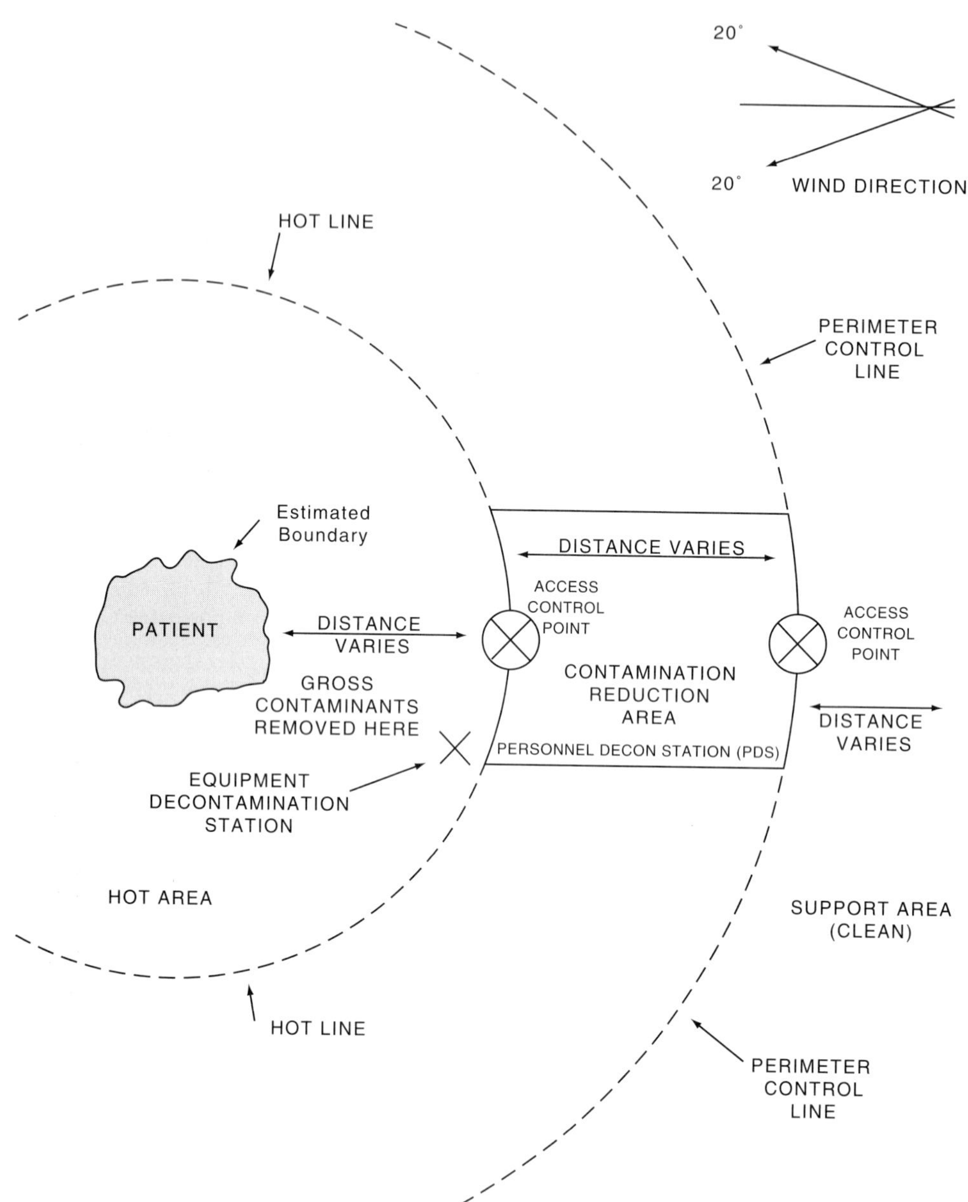

Figure 2. Organization of hazardous materials incident area. (Adapted from Paparek PJ Jr, Karbus J, and subcommittee members, Subcommittee on Medical and Emergency Response in Managing Victims of Hazardous Materials Release. Los Angeles County Department of Health Services, 1988.)

care provider may encounter the words "trade secret" as a category of chemical constituents for a particular product. Current regulation allows the manufacturers to protect their formulations under certain circumstances. In the event that such information is needed by the health care professional, contact can be made with the manufacturer using the 24-hour emergency number listed on the MSDS. This chemical constituent information must be released to health care providers on request while treating an exposed patient. Emergency departments can obtain copies of these MSDS and keep them on file. The EPA requires companies of all sizes that use sufficient quantities of certain flammable and toxic substances to develop a risk-management program, which includes among other things a hazard assessment that details the potential effects of an accidental release, an accident history of the last 5 years, an evaluation of worst-case and alternative accidental releases, and an emergency response program that spells out emergency health care, employee training measures, and procedures for informing the public and response agencies (e.g., the local fire department) should an accident occur. The plans must be revised and resubmitted every 5 years (31). However, chemical releases may occur with chemicals not covered by the Risk Management Program.

Chemical releases of significant size generally result in a resource-intensive site response, including hazardous materials teams that are trained and equipped to work safely in a hazardous environment. These teams are usually formed within fire departments, public agencies, and industry. The response to the incident includes the designation of a "hot" or exclusion zone, a "warm" or contamination-reduction zone, and a "cold" or support area (Fig. 2). Depending on the substance released and the nature of the exposure, on-site decontamination procedures may be necessary for both victims and emergency medical services (EMS) personnel (Fig. 3). Protective clothing may be essential for those involved in rescue and triage procedures. Decontamination should be performed before transport, except in patients with life-threatening injuries who require immediate transport. Shelter-in-place or evacuation of adjacent populations may be required. Patients may self-report to nearby medical care facilities, which can result in the need for decontamination and triage at the hospital before evaluation and

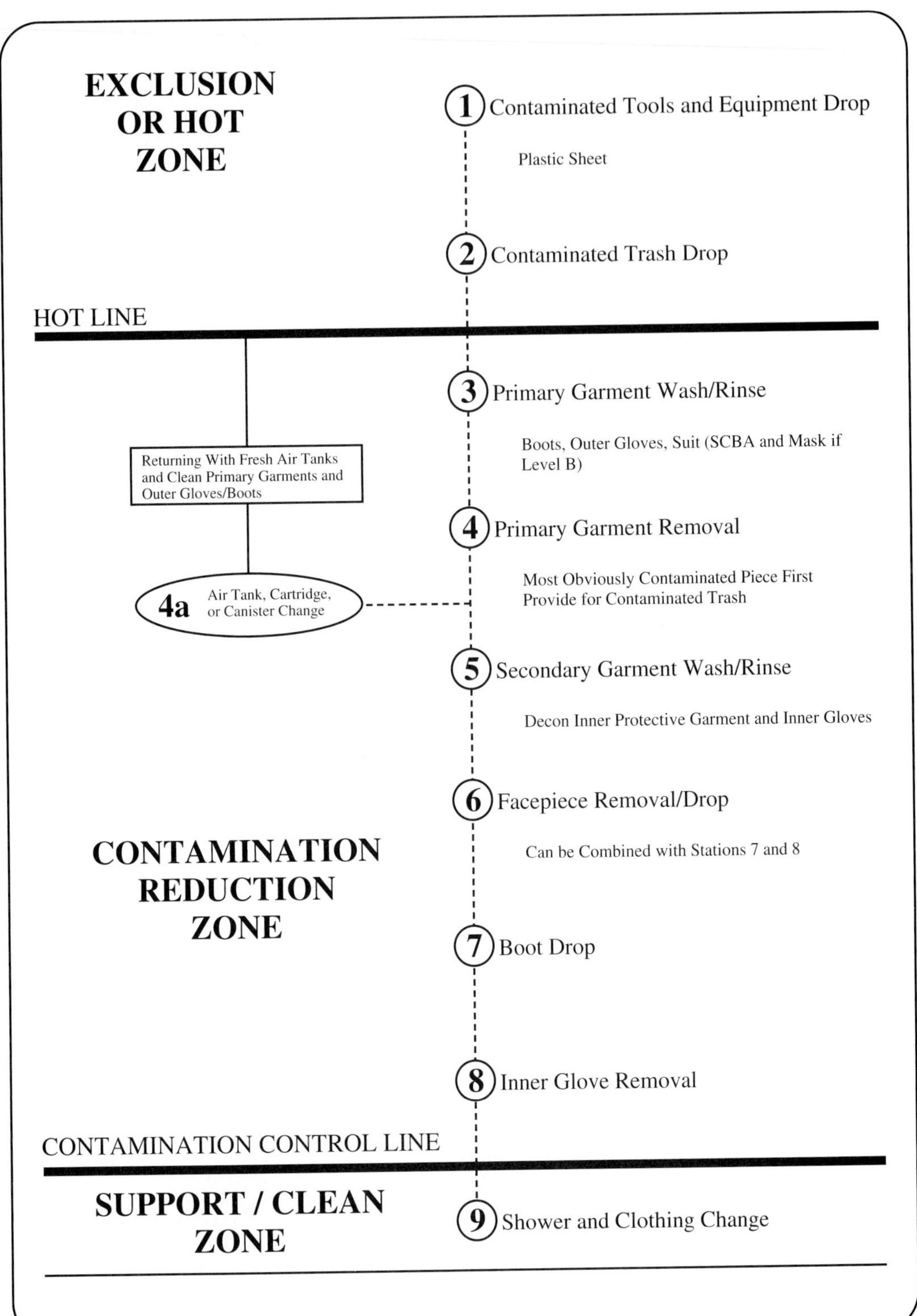

Figure 3. Nine-step personnel decontamination. SCBA, self-contained breathing apparatus.

treatment. Emergency care facilities have been shut down owing to concern over chemical contamination of the facilities after care of patients without prior decontamination (32).

For health care providers, part of the preparation for hazardous materials incidents involves compilation of a list of local and national resources with emergency contact phone numbers. Local resources include, but are not limited to, fire departments (specifically, hazardous materials teams); local police and state patrol; city, county, and state health departments; local and state environmental agencies; port authorities (including airports); local and state departments of transportation; water departments; LEPCs; the SERC; and local and state government. Each state has an emergency management division or equivalent that can serve as a central coordinating agency for incidents requiring multiagency response. Some states have dedicated response teams for radioactive substances release. National resources for hazardous materials incident planning and response are listed in Table 5.

TABLE 5. U.S. resources for hazardous materials incident planning and response

Resource	Contact	Services provided
Agency for Toxic Substances and Disease Registry (ATSDR)	(404) 498-0120; http://www.atsdr.cdc.gov/	24-h emergency number for health-related support in hazardous materials emergencies, including onsite assistance.
American Society for the Prevention of Cruelty to Animals (ASPCA) Animal Poison Control Center (an allied agency of the University of Illinois)	(888) 426-4435	24-h consultation with veterinary toxicologists concerning animal poisonings or chemical contamination. Provides diagnostic recommendations and treatment protocols. Can provide an emergency response team to investigate incidents and perform laboratory analysis (a fee may be required).
Centralized Scheduling and Information Desk (operated under the Department of Homeland Security)	(800) 368-6498	24-h consultation service for threats and releases pertaining to chemical and biological agents.
Chemical Transportation Emergency Center (CHEMTREC)	(800) 424-9300	24-h emergency number connecting with manufacturers and/or shippers. Advice provided on handling, rescue gear, decontamination considerations, etc. Also provides access to the Chlorine Emergency Response Plan (CHLOREP).
Federal Emergency Management Agency	(202) 566-1600; http://www.fema.gov/	A federal agency responsible for building and supporting a national emergency management system. Provides 24-h response for disasters. Consult Web site for education and training opportunities on emergency preparedness for emergency personnel and general public.
Regional Offices:		
Region I (CT, MA, ME, NH, RI, VT)	(617) 223-9540	
Region II (NJ, NY, PR, VI)	(212) 680-3600	
Region III (DC, DE, MD, PA, VA, WV)	(215) 931-5608	
Region IV (AL, FL, GA, KY, MS, NC, SC, TN)	(770) 220-5200	
Region V (IL, IN, MI, MN, OH, WI)	(312) 408-5500	
Region VI (AR, LA, NM, OK, TX)	(940) 898-5399	
Region VII (IA, KS, MO, NE)	(816) 283-7061	
Region VIII (CO, MT, ND, SD, UT, WY)	(303) 235-4800	
Region IX (AZ, CA, Guam, HI, NV)	(510) 627-7100	
Region X (AK, ID, OR, WA)	(425) 487-4600	
National Pesticide Information Center (NPIC) (US, PR, VI) (cooperative effort of Oregon State University and the EPA)	(800) 858-7378; http://npic.orst.edu	Provides information on pesticide products, recognition and management of pesticide poisoning, toxicology, and environmental chemistry. Directs callers for pesticide incident investigation, emergency human and animal treatment, safety practices, cleanup and disposal, and laboratory analyses. Supplies general information on regulation of pesticides in the United States.
National Pesticides Information Retrieval System (NPIRS) and the State Pesticide Information Retrieval System (NSPIRS) (CERIS, Center for Environmental and Regulatory Information at Purdue University)	(765) 494-6616; http://ceris.purdue.edu/npirs/	Contact information for help in searching NPIRS database to get fact sheets on pesticides, insecticides, fungicides, and state and federally registered chemicals (fee for service).
National Response Center and Terrorist Hotline (U.S. Coast Guard)	(800) 424-8802 or (202) 267-2675; http://www.nrc.uscg.mil/	A federal 24-h hotline for reporting oil and chemical spills where hazardous materials are responsible for death, serious injury, property damage in excess of $50,000, continuing danger to life and property, or known or suspected terrorist threats (bombings, bomb threat, suspicious letters or packages, and incidents related to the intentional release of chemical/biological/radioactive agents).
Nuclear Regulatory Commission	(800) 368-5642; http://www.nrc.gov/	Contact number to report a safety concern involving a nuclear facility or radioactive materials.
Oak Ridge National Laboratories (ORNL)	(865) 574-3000; http://www.ornl.gov/	Offers in-depth training courses on radiation safety and management of radiation victims.
Poison Center (regional)	(800) 222-1222	24-h response number providing information on health effects of poisonings and consultation with medical toxicologists.
Radiation Emergency Assistance Center/Training Site (REAC/TS)	(865) 576-3131; http://www.orau.gov/reacts/	Provides emergency consultation for accidents involving radioactive materials.
Transportation Technology Center, Inc. (TTCI) (a wholly owned subsidiary of the Association of American Railroads)	(800) 933-4882	Contact number during business hours for Hazmat services. Will refer to the appropriate regional Bureau of Explosives (BOE) Inspector for technical questions about railway transportation of hazardous materials. For emergencies, call CHEMTREC (800-424-9300).
U.S. Environmental Protection Agency (EPA)	(202) 564-4700; http://www.epa.gov/	Environmental response teams available for technical assistance.
Regional Offices:		
Region I (CT, MA, ME, NH, RI, VT)	(617) 918-1111 or intraregional only; (800) 372-7431	
Region II (NJ, NY, PR, VI)	(212) 637-3000	
Region III (DC, DE, MD, PA, VA, WV)	(215) 814-5000 or intraregional only; (800) 438-2474	
Region IV (AL, FL, GA, KY, MS, NC, SC, TN)	(404) 562-9900 or intraregional only; (800) 241-1754	
Region V (IL, IN, MI, MN, OH, WI)	(312) 353-2000 or intraregional only; (800) 621-8431	
Region VI (AR, LA, NM, OK, TX)	(214) 665-2200 or intraregional only; (800) 887-6063	
Region VII (IA, KS, MO, NE)	(913) 551-7000 or intraregional only; (800) 223-0425	

(continued)

TABLE 5. (*continued*)

Resource	Contact	Services provided
Region VIII (CO, MT, ND, SD, WY, UT)	(303) 312-6312 or intraregional only; (800) 227-8917	
Region IX (AS, AZ, CA, GU, HI, MH, MP, NV)	(415) 947-8021	
Region X (AK, ID, OR, WA)	(206) 553-1200 or intraregional only; (800) 424-9346	
U.S. EPA RCRA, Superfund, and EPCRA Call Center	(800) 424-9346; http://www.epa.gov/epaoswer/hotline	Available 9:00 a.m. to 5:00 p.m. (EST). Provides information on several Environmental Protection Agencies (EPA) including questions regarding the Resource Conservation and Recovery Act (RCRA), which includes the Underground Storage Tank (UST) program; the Comprehensive Environmental Response, Compensation and Liability Act (CERCLA or Superfund); the Oil Program; the Emergency Planning and Community Right-to-Know Act (EPCRA); and the accidental release prevention provisions of the Clean Air Act (CAA).

Adapted from Agency for Toxic Substances and Diseases Registry. Managing Hazardous Materials Incidents: A Planning Guide for the Management of Contaminated Patients, Vol. 1. Atlanta: US Department of Health and Human Services, Agency for Toxic Substances and Diseases Registry 2000. Available at: http://www.atsdr.cdc.gov/mhmi.html. Accessed February 2003.

PERSONAL PROTECTIVE EQUIPMENT

Individuals responding to a hazardous materials incident must wear personal protective equipment to prevent their exposure to hazardous materials. The type and extent of protective equipment required vary from incident to incident, and such equipment may be required on a more limited basis in health care facilities treating contaminated patients. The EPA describes four levels of personal protective equipment, and they include respiratory and dermal protection components (33).

Level A ensemble provides the highest level of skin, respiratory, and eye protection. The ensemble is comprised of positive-pressure, full-face (covers eyes, nose, and mouth) self-contained breathing apparatus (SCBA) or positive-pressure supplied-air respirator with escape SCBA, totally encapsulated chemical suits that are liquid and vapor tight, and inner and outer chemical-resistant gloves and boots. Early suits were made of single materials, such as butyl rubber or neoprene, that exhibit different types of chemical compatibility. More recent suits have a composite design (multilayer) of several different types of material, providing a greater degree of chemical resistance to a wider range of chemicals.

Level B protection should be used for circumstances requiring the highest level of respiratory protection and a lesser degree of dermal protection. In general, level B suits provide splash protection only. Level B ensemble includes positive-pressure, full-facepiece SCBA or positive pressure supplied-air respirator with escape SCBA, inner and outer chemical-resistant gloves, and outer chemical-resistant boots.

Level C protection is required when the concentration and type of airborne substances are known, and the criteria for using air-purifying respirators are met. Typically, this level of protection includes full-face air-purifying respirators, inner and outer chemical-resistant gloves, hard hat, and chemical-resistant boots. The difference between level C and level B protection is the type of equipment used to protect the respiratory system, assuming the same type of chemical-resistant clothing is used. Level C protection cannot be used in oxygen-deficient (below 19.5%) atmospheres, because no additional oxygen is provided to the wearer.

Level D equipment provides the lowest level of protection. Level D protection may be sufficient when no contaminants are present or work operations preclude splashes, immersion, or the potential for unexpected inhalation or contact with hazardous levels of chemicals. Appropriate level D protective equipment ensemble may include gloves, coveralls, safety glasses, face shield, and chemical-resistant, steel-toe boots or shoes.

In general, a completely unknown or highly toxic potential exposure would require level A protection. An incident involving a chemical that does not have significant dermal absorption could be handled using level B protection. Firefighter turn-out gear is not designed to provide full chemical protection. Level C protection should only be used in very controlled settings, and level D only in incidents without risk of air or skin contamination. Several free and proprietary databases contain decontamination information, including the Hazardous Substances Data Bank (HSDB; http://toxnet.nlm.nih.gov/) under Chemical Safety and Handling (34).

CHEMICAL IDENTIFICATION

The first step in responding to a hazardous materials incident call is to identify the chemical(s) involved. In some cases, this information is immediately apparent, but in many incidents, the identity of the offending agent is never determined (8). Chemical identification can often be accomplished using a number of different techniques. Some help to identify groups of chemicals, and others provide very specific information. If time permits, it is useful to cross-check different means of identification to ensure that they agree. In some incidents, it will be necessary to begin the decontamination and supportive care before full identification of the offending agent.

Known Chemical

In case the chemical released is known, the information obtained should include (a) the exact spelling of the chemical(s), (b) the form (solid/liquid/gas) and concentration of the chemical(s), (c) the composition of the mixture (e.g., many organophosphates are in a hydrocarbon base, and the specific components should be identified), and (d) the manufacturer of the chemical(s). Because a chemical may have many names, or synonyms, it also may be useful to record Chemical Abstracts Registry or Registry of Toxic Effects of Chemical Substances numbers for each chemical.

Placards and Labels

Placards and labels are required for all chemical containers over a specific volume or weight. A placard is a diamond-shaped sign displayed on trucks, trailers, shipping containers, and railroad cars. They are 10 in. square and coded by symbol and color (Fig. 4). In North America, the Emergency Response Guidebook [http://hazmat.dot.gov/gydebook.htm (35)] can be used for

Transport Canada Transports Canada

The Marks of Safety

Canada

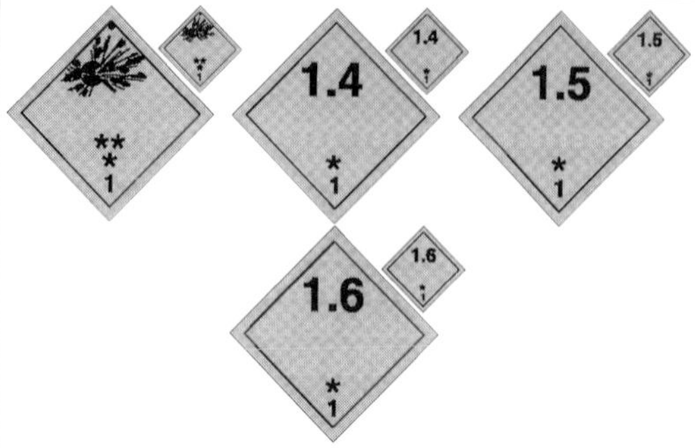

CLASS 1 - Explosives

1.1 - A substance or article with a mass explosion hazard.

1.2 - A substance or article with a fragment projection hazard, but not a mass explosion hazard.

1.3 - A substance or article which has a fire hazard along with either a minor blast hazard or a minor projection hazard or both, but not a mass explosion hazard.

1.4 - A substance or article which presents no significant hazard; explosion effects are largely confined to the package and no projection or fragments of appreciable size or range are to be expected.

1.5 - A very insensitive substance which nevertheless has a mass explosion hazard like those substances in 1.1.

1.6 - An extremely insensitive substance which does not have a mass explosion hazard.

Commonly used in mining and construction operations (example: blasting agents).

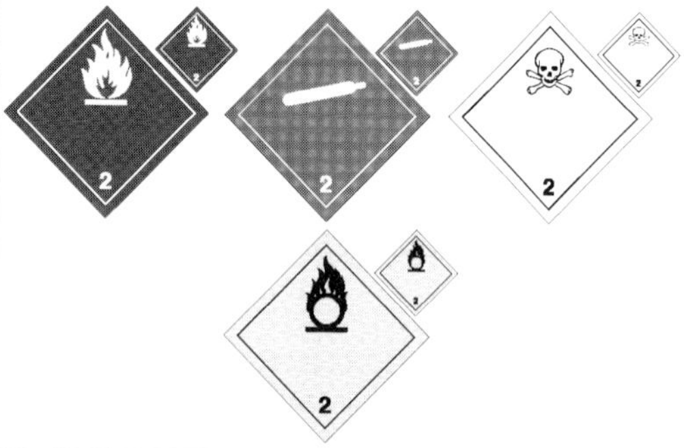

CLASS 2 - Gases

2.1 - Flammable Gas.

Commonly used as fuel (example: propane).

2.2 - Non-Flammable, Non-Toxic Gas.

Commonly used in food refrigeration (example: nitrogen).

2.3 - Toxic Gas.

Commonly used in pulp bleaching (example: sulphur dioxide).

2.2 (5.1) - Oxygen and oxidizing gases.

CLASS 3 - Flammable Liquids

A liquid which has a closed-cup flash point not greater than 60.5° C.

Commonly used as fuel (example: gasoline, ethanol, fuel oil (diesel)).

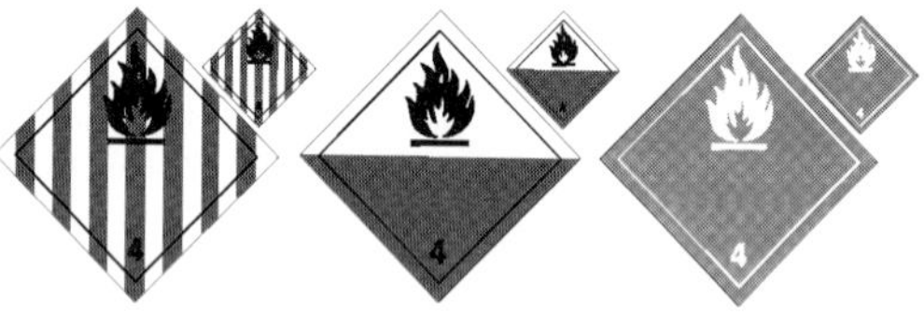

CLASS 4 - Flammable Solids, Substances liable to spontaneous combustion; Substances that on contact with water emit flammable gases (water-reactive substances)

4.1 - A solid that under normal conditions of transport is readily combustible, or would cause or contribute to fire through friction or from heat retained from manufacturing or processing, or is a self-reactive substance that is liable to undergo a strongly exothermic reaction, or is a desensitized explosive that is liable to explode if they are not diluted sufficiently to suppress their explosive properties.

Commonly used in lacquers (example: nitrocellulose).

4.2 - A substance liable to spontaneous combustion, under normal conditions of transport, or when in contact with air, liable to spontaneous heating to the point where it ignites. Commonly used in rocket fuel (example: diethylzinc).

4.3 - A substance that, on contact with water, emits dangerous quantities of flammable gases or becomes spontaneously combustible on contact with water or water vapour.

Commonly used in heat exchangers (valves) (example: sodium).

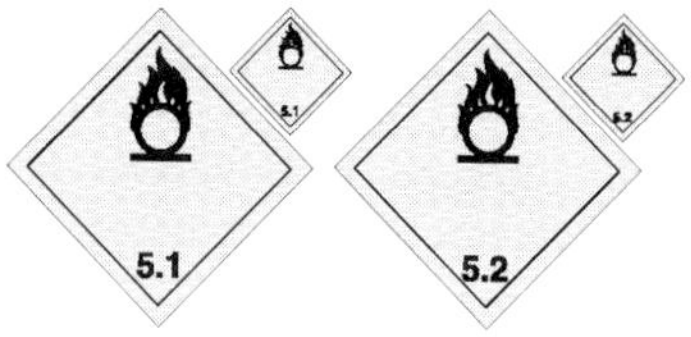

CLASS 5 - Oxidizing Substances and Organic Peroxides

5.1 - A substance which causes or contributes to the combustion of other material by yielding oxygen or other oxidizing substances whether or not the substance itself is combustible.

Commonly used in fertilizers (example: ammonium nitrate).

5.2 - An organic compound that contains the bivalent "-O-O-" structure which is a strong oxidizing agent and may be liable to explosive decomposition, be sensitive to heat, shock or friction, react dangerously with other dangerous goods or may cause damage to the eyes.

Commonly used in automobile body shops as body filler (example: dibenzoyl peroxide).

A

Figure 4. Hazardous materials placards and labels. **A:** Classes 1–5. *(continued)*

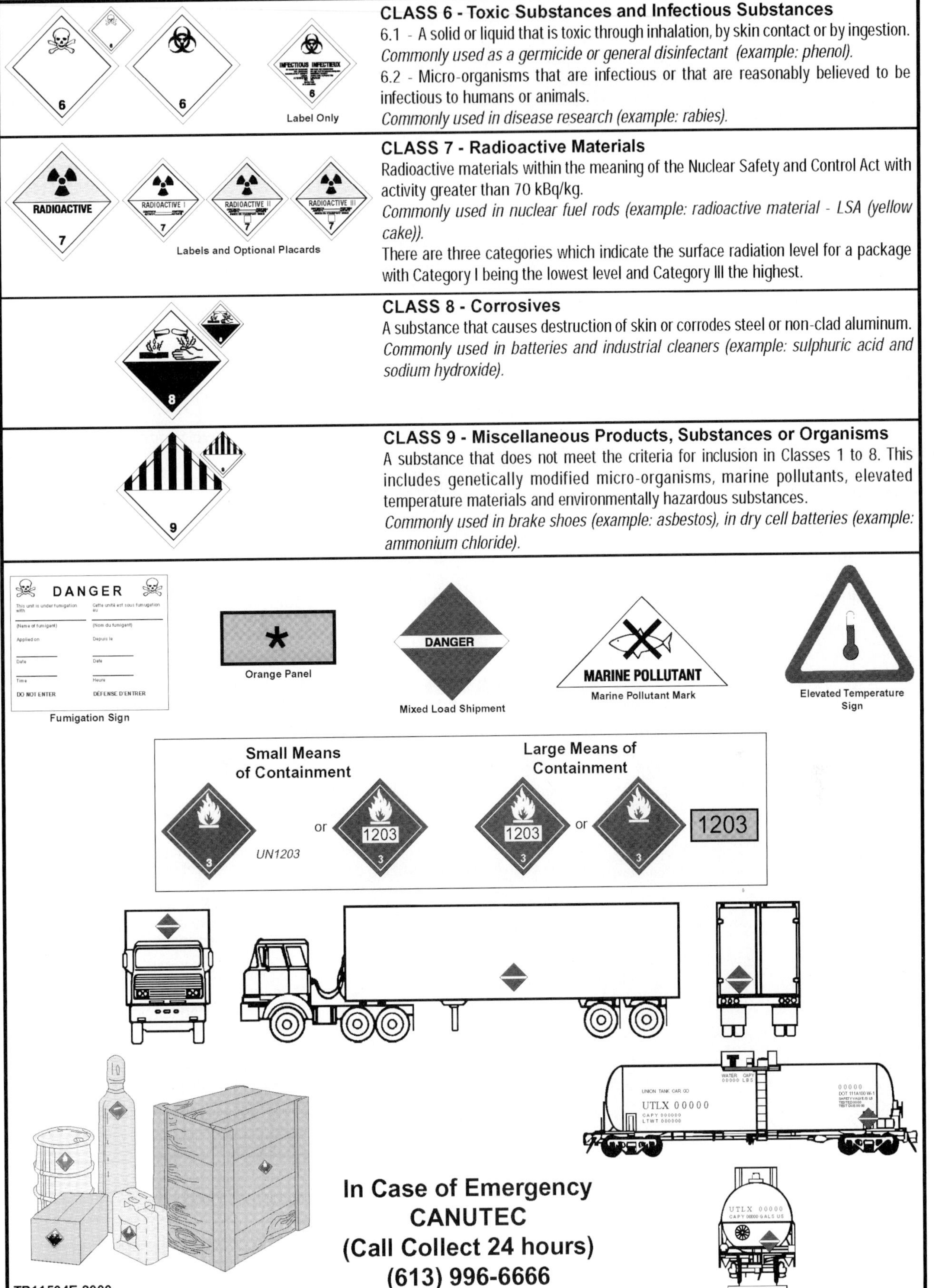

CLASS 6 - Toxic Substances and Infectious Substances
6.1 - A solid or liquid that is toxic through inhalation, by skin contact or by ingestion.
Commonly used as a germicide or general disinfectant (example: phenol).
6.2 - Micro-organisms that are infectious or that are reasonably believed to be infectious to humans or animals.
Commonly used in disease research (example: rabies).
Label Only
CLASS 7 - Radioactive Materials
Radioactive materials within the meaning of the Nuclear Safety and Control Act with activity greater than 70 kBq/kg.
Commonly used in nuclear fuel rods (example: radioactive material - LSA (yellow cake)).
There are three categories which indicate the surface radiation level for a package with Category I being the lowest level and Category III the highest.
RADIOACTIVE
Labels and Optional Placards
CLASS 8 - Corrosives
A substance that causes destruction of skin or corrodes steel or non-clad aluminum.
Commonly used in batteries and industrial cleaners (example: sulphuric acid and sodium hydroxide).
CLASS 9 - Miscellaneous Products, Substances or Organisms
A substance that does not meet the criteria for inclusion in Classes 1 to 8. This includes genetically modified micro-organisms, marine pollutants, elevated temperature materials and environmentally hazardous substances.
Commonly used in brake shoes (example: asbestos), in dry cell batteries (example: ammonium chloride).
DANGER
DO NOT ENTER
DÉFENSE D'ENTRER
Fumigation Sign
Orange Panel
DANGER
Mixed Load Shipment
MARINE POLLUTANT
Marine Pollutant Mark
Elevated Temperature Sign
Small Means of Containment
Large Means of Containment
UN1203
or
1203
UTLX 00000
In Case of Emergency
CANUTEC
(Call Collect 24 hours)
(613) 996-6666
TP11504E 2000
B

Figure 4. (*continued*) **B:** Classes 6–9. (See Color Plate 34.)

immediate reference and is carried by almost every first responder vehicle. The chemicals are identified by their NA (North American) or UN (United Nations) four-digit identification number. However, not all chemical transportation vehicles are placarded. Placards are required for any quantity of the following classes of materials: Explosives, Poisons, Radioactive III, and Flammable Solids-Use No Water. In all other cases, placards are required only for greater than 1000-lb quantities loaded at a single location. Placards designated DANGEROUS indicate a mix of hazard classes. Labels are much smaller (4 in. square) than placards and are placed on individual packages. The National Fire Protection Association placards rank the health, fire, and reactivity hazards of a chemical through the assignment of a numeric value between 0 and 4 (Fig. 5). They may contain a special hazard symbol in the lower quadrant. Container shape may be suggestive of certain classes of hazardous materials but not individual chemicals.

Material Safety Data Sheets

In the United States, MSDSs are required by law to be available in every business where the products are used. MSDSs are also extremely useful when a product has a commercial name and cannot otherwise be identified. Shipping papers are required to accompany the transport of hazardous materials. The American Chemistry Council provides a service (CHEMTREC 1-800-424-9300) for identification and response to chemicals produced by member companies. The ATSDR has a 24-hour emergency response number (1-404-498-0120) and may be able to provide additional information. The Internet continues to provide rapid identification of chemicals as well through the provision of MSDSs.

CAMEO

Computer-Aided Management of Emergency Operations (CAMEO) is a system of software applications produced by the EPA and National Oceanic and Atmospheric Administration (NOAA) to plan for and respond to chemical emergencies (36). One component of CAMEO is the Response Information Data Sheets, prepared by NOAA after consultation with several recognized technical resources. Although the Response Information Data Sheet information is complete, it is not available for all chemicals. Within the United States, primary users include firefighters, SERCs, Tribal Emergency Response Commissions, LEPCs, industry, schools, environmental organizations, and police departments. CAMEO has been translated into French and Spanish, was selected by the United Nations Environment Programme (http://www.unep.org) as a tool for helping developing nations prepare for and respond to chemical accidents, and is part of the United Nations Environment Programme's Awareness and Preparedness for Emergencies at the Local Level program.

Odor and Color

Certain chemicals have easily identified odors, such as the "rotten egg" or sulfur smell of hydrogen sulfide. The American Industrial Hygiene Association publication *Odor Thresholds for Chemicals with Established Occupational Health Standards* provides information on odors and odor thresholds for a number of

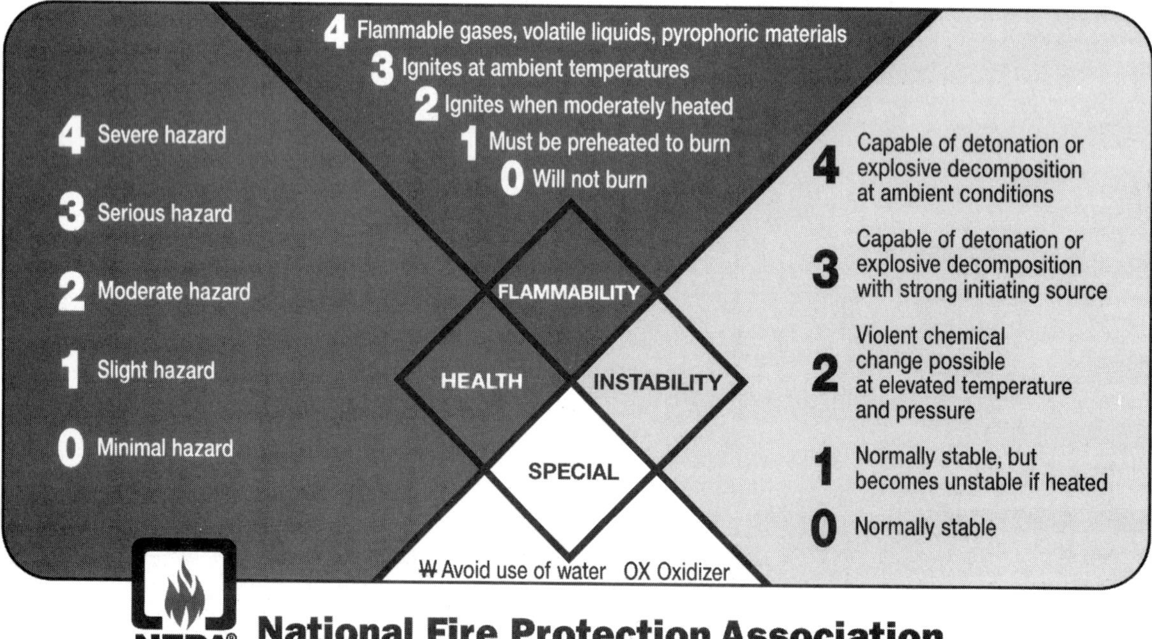

Figure 5. National Fire Protection Association (Quincy, MA) placard (reproduced with permission). (See Color Plate 35.)

chemicals (37). However, there is a tremendous range of ability to detect odors within any population; certain individuals may be unable to perceive the odor of certain chemicals, as is the case with cyanide (38), and olfactory fatigue may occur (39). Many online databases have odor information, including HSDB and the U.S. Coast Guard Chemical Hazards Response Information System (CHRIS; http://www.chrismanual.com/) (34,40). Certain gases and vapors have characteristic colors, such as the yellow-green of chlorine, red-brown for mixed oxides of nitrogen and red fuming nitric acid, and purple for iodine.

Combustion

Where there is fire, there is a possibility for hazardous materials exposure. Carbon monoxide is present in nearly every fire where there is even a minimal component of incomplete combustion. Often, the products of combustion are more toxic than the chemicals supporting the fire. For example, phosgene is produced from the combustion of certain chlorinated hydrocarbons and can cause delayed pulmonary injury. HSDB provides product of combustion data under the Chemical Safety and Handling, Toxic Combustion Products section.

Chemical Reactions

In certain instances, the exposure that an individual receives is based on chemical interactions and the subsequent liberation of gases and vapors. It is often difficult, without extensive chemistry background, to predict the reaction products released as a result of fire, explosion, or transportation accident. It must be kept in mind that the chemicals released in a hazardous materials incident may in fact be different than those that were initially present. To assist responders with this difficult issue, NOAA has created the Chemical Reactivity Worksheet (http://response.restoration.noaa.gov/chemaids/react.html), which predicts the outcome product of chemicals that are allowed to mix (41).

EXPOSURE ASSESSMENT

One of the greatest challenges in handling a hazardous materials incident is estimating the extent of chemical exposure through inhalation and skin absorption. Using the information collected from the on-site teams, it is often possible to estimate the extent of individual chemical exposures. The extent of exposure provides essential information in predicting the medical outcome of the exposure and therefore helps guide decisions on the need for hospital transport and subsequent diagnostic testing and treatment. Exposure assessment makes use of information on the extent of chemical release, chemical characteristics, patient signs and symptoms, and additional information whenever possible. Where a range of possible chemical exposure concentrations can be established, comparison with established exposure limits can help to determine whether exposure to this range of chemical concentrations could result in significant injury. These exposure assessment techniques are most useful for inhalation exposures, with less application for dermal exposures. For a number of systemically absorbed chemicals, dermal exposure may result in a significant delay in absorption, thereby complicating the use of symptoms as a means of estimating initial exposure and requiring an extended observation period (42).

Comparative Values

It is necessary to compare estimated or measured exposures to acceptable exposure limits to understand the significance of the exposure and to make on-scene medical evaluation and treatment decisions. OSHA publishes permissible exposure limits (PELs) that are legally enforceable workplace limits (http://www.osha-slc.gov/SLTC/pel/). They represent the maximum concentration averaged over an 8-hour workday period that workers can be exposed to on a continuous basis. Exposures below these concentrations for 8 hours or less per day (up to 40 hours per week) are considered not to be dangerous for the great majority of workers.

Threshold limit values (TLVs) are exposure limits published by the American Conference of Governmental Industrial Hygienists. The TLV includes an 8-hour time-weighted average (TLV-TWA), "to which nearly all workers may be repeatedly exposed, day after day, without adverse effect" (43). The short-term exposure limit (TLV-STEL) commonly referred to as *STEL*, is a 15-minute average concentration that should not be exceeded at any time and should not occur more than four times during an 8-hour shift, separated by at least an hour between excursions above the TLV-TWA. The STEL represents "the concentration to which workers can be exposed continuously for a short period of time without suffering from 1) irritation, 2) chronic or irreversible tissue damage, or 3) narcosis of sufficient degree to increase the likelihood of accidental injury, impair self-rescue or materially reduce work efficiency" (43). The ceiling limit (TLV-C) is "the concentration that should not be exceeded during any part of the working exposure" (43). These values are guidelines and are not enforceable under current regulation. OSHA also publishes STEL and ceiling limits for some chemicals. Exposures significantly exceeding the STEL or ceiling limit may warrant medical evaluation.

Immediately dangerous to life and health (IDLH) concentrations are published by National Institute for Occupational Safety and Health (NIOSH) and "represent the maximum concentration from which, in the event of a respirator failure, one could escape within thirty minutes without a respirator and without experiencing any escape impairing (e.g., severe eye irritation) or irreversible health effects" (44). These concentrations are higher than the STEL. Exposures at or above the IDLH concentrations generally warrant medical examination. The suitability of using IDLH concentrations for estimating the hazard of chemical releases is controversial (45).

Other exposure limits include Emergency Response Planning Guidelines levels (ERPGs) and Acute Exposure Guideline Levels (AEGLs). The American Industrial Hygiene Association publishes ERPGs, which are divided into three categories. The ERPG-2 values are defined as "The maximum airborne concentration below which it is believed that nearly all individuals could be exposed for up to one hour without experiencing or developing irreversible or other serious health effects or symptoms which could impair an individual's ability to take protective action" (46). The ERPG-3 values are set to prevent life-threatening health effects, and the ERPG-1 values are set to prevent discomfort (46). The EPA develops the AEGLs, which provide exposure limits for time periods ranging from 30 minutes to 8 hours. Exposure at or above the AEGL-1 level could cause noticeable discomfort; exposure at or above the AEGL-2 level irreversible or other serious, long-lasting effects or impaired ability to escape; and exposure at or above the AEGL-3 level life-threatening effects or death. Final AEGLs will be published by the National Research Council, National Academy of Sciences after peer review.

When a chemical exposure concentration can be estimated or measured, then that concentration should be compared with the selected exposure limits. For the limited duration of most hazardous materials incidents (less than 8 hours), exposure below the PEL or TLV-TWA is considered safe, significantly exceeding the STEL is potentially dangerous, and at or above the IDLH is potentially lethal. These comparisons are only part of the exposure assessment process, and all sources of information, including patient symptoms, should be considered.

All forms of exposure assessment have practical limitations, and each incident and individual exposure should be evaluated on a case-by-case basis. Certain individuals, such as asthmatics, may have a greater sensitivity to low-level chemical exposures and may develop symptoms at exposure concentrations below PEL and TLV-TWA levels. These exposure limits were developed for healthy adult workers, and other exposure levels, such as the EPA National Ambient Air Quality Standards (47), ERPGs, and AEGLs, should be considered for the general population. However, these values have only been developed for a limited number of chemicals.

Extent of Release

The extent of chemical exposure will depend on the quantity of chemical available. If the quantity of a chemical released is known, then it is possible to calculate whether this quantity released into a known or estimated confined area would pose a problem after volatilization or diffusion had occurred. A calculation of chemical mass divided by room volume will yield an estimated maximum exposure concentration, which can be compared to occupational exposure limits. However, chemical concentrations may not be evenly distributed across the space, and any degree of ventilation will reduce overall exposure. Concentrations resulting from chemical release into open air can be modeled, as described under Air Modeling.

Observations

When firefighters approach a hazardous materials incident, they do so from uphill and upwind. This gives them time to assess the situation and determine the type of personal protective equipment needed for the response. Certain clues, such as dead animals, unresponsive individuals, or a visible vapor cloud at the scene, suggest a highly toxic chemical concentration.

Chemical Characteristics

Chemical characteristics that are especially useful in the evaluation of exposure include vapor pressure and odor threshold. *Vapor pressure* is defined as "the pressure (often expressed in millimeters of mercury, mm Hg) characteristic at any given temperature of a vapor in equilibrium with its liquid or solid form" (2). Chemicals with higher vapor pressures evaporate more easily; an example of such a chemical is acetone, with a vapor pressure of 180 mm Hg at 20°C (44). Vapor pressure calculations are useful to establish "ballpark" limits on the extent of exposure. For practical purposes in hazardous materials incidents, vapor pressure calculations will be useful primarily for estimating inhalation exposure to liquid spills. In the absence of generation of aerosols, the vapor pressure gives a theoretical maximum concentration to which a nearby individual could be exposed. In most circumstances, it is unlikely that vapor pressure would ever be reached, unless the exposure occurred in a confined space or other location with extremely poor ventilation. Vapor pressures are usually provided at room temperature, and although formulas are available for calculating vapor pressure at various other temperatures, it is difficult to use vapor pressure to estimate possible exposure at environmental temperature extremes.

An easily obtained reference with vapor pressures for a variety of chemicals is the NIOSH Pocket Guide (http://www.cdc.gov/niosh/npg/npg.html) (44). The vapor pressure measurement (in mm Hg) can be approximated in parts per million (ppm) by multiplying by 1300. Conversion from ppm to milligrams/cubic meter of air (mg/m^3) can then be made as needed, using the formula mg/m^3 = (ppm)(mw)/24.45, where *mw* is the molecular weight of the chemical. The ppm or mg/m^3 values are then compared with standard occupational exposure limits. In general, after conversion to similar units, chemicals with a vapor pressure near or below the PEL would not be considered toxic for the short exposure intervals typically seen during hazardous materials incidents. Exposure to chemicals with vapor pressures significantly exceeding IDLH concentrations is much more likely to result in injury. The vapor density will determine whether in general the gas or vapor will be heavier (vapor density greater than 1) or lighter (vapor density less than 1) than air and therefore whether it will collect in below-grade areas, such as tunnels or depressions.

Odor Thresholds

Odor thresholds can also provide useful information to "ballpark" exposures, by suggesting that exposures are occurring at concentrations below the odor threshold if no odor is detected and concentrations above the odor threshold if the odor is detected. Odor threshold values may be obtained from publications and databases (34,37,40). The use of odor threshold to estimate exposure is problematic owing to several factors. Many individuals lack the ability to detect certain odors, such as cyanide (38,48). A number of chemicals, such as hydrogen sulfide, can cause olfactory fatigue (39). Given these limitations, detection of odor can still provide information that can be compared with published exposure limits. Lack of detection of chemicals with odor thresholds near or below their PEL, particularly in a group of individuals, would suggest that their exposure would not be considered toxic for the short exposure intervals typically seen during hazardous materials incidents. Detection of odors with exposure to chemicals with odor thresholds significantly exceeding IDLH concentrations is much more likely to result in injury.

Patient Symptoms

Despite the variability in individual responses to hazardous materials, symptoms such as mucous membrane irritation, headache, lightheadedness, and other complaints can be very useful in determining exposure. For example, exposure to arsine with gastrointestinal complaints suggests a serious poisoning mandating aggressive medical care (49). Irritant water-soluble chemicals will interact with moist mucous membranes, producing such symptoms as burning eyes and irritation of the nose, throat, and upper respiratory tract, and therefore have good warning properties. Examples of moderate to highly water-soluble irritant or corrosive chemicals include ammonia, sulfur dioxide, and acid gases, such as hydrochloric acid. Lack of symptoms in this type of exposure essentially rules out significant exposure. Chemicals with lower water solubility, or with significant systemic toxicity at concentrations below those causing irritation, cannot be evaluated in the same fashion. Patients exposed to low water-solubility agents, such as oxides of nitrogen, phosphine, phosgene, and mercury, may present with limited or no initial symptoms, followed hours later with significant pulmonary toxicity (50–54). Concern over the exposure alone can result in symptoms, such as has been described in episodes of mass sociogenic illness (18,55–57). Therefore, presence of symptoms does not always indicate that significant exposure has occurred.

The use of symptoms to provide additional information on the extent of exposure is most useful for inhalation exposures. In dermal exposures, initial symptoms may not occur owing to delayed absorption, with significant toxicity occurring at a later time. Identification of the specific chemical exposure is important in these instances to determine whether skin absorption of the chemical occurs and what eventual toxicity could be expected.

Site Sampling

Site sampling involves the measurement of chemical concentrations at the hazardous materials incident site. Monitoring instruments include colorimetric tubes, which can provide immediate information on specific chemicals, oxygen and combustible gas indicators that detect the presence of a contaminant gas but do not identify the specific one(s), and more advanced direct-read instruments. Even if this information is available, it is important to remember that the chemical concentration in the area sampled may be different than the concentration in another area where victims have been exposed. Using analytical instrumentation specific to the contaminant of interest can be extremely useful in incidents where chemical concentrations are found to be significantly below toxic concentrations or below detectable limits, or conversely where high concentrations are found. Results of direct monitoring may change rapidly over time and space, and cannot be used to forecast conditions before or after monitoring has been initiated, or potentially in locations even a short distance away from the monitoring location.

Air Modeling

A number of free and proprietary air-modeling programs are available to estimate chemical concentrations after a release. One of the CAMEO modules is the Area Locations of Hazardous Atmospheres (ALOHA) air dispersion model, used to estimate airborne pollutant concentrations downwind from the source of a spill. Once a description of an accidental chemical release is entered into the model, ALOHA displays a "footprint" diagram representing the area at risk, as well as graphs of indoor and outdoor pollutant concentrations for specified locations. ALOHA footprints can be plotted on electronic maps. Air release modeling provides general exposure estimates, but again, care should be taken in using these estimates to determine individual exposure, owing to the complexity of an actual release and lack of uniform concentrations throughout the chemical plume. Modeling is most useful in making decisions at a population level, including the need for evacuation or shelter-in-place. It is not pertinent to indoor hazardous materials releases.

Unknown Exposures

Unknown exposures constitute a significant percentage of incidents evaluated by hazardous materials teams (8). Unknown exposures are less amenable to exposure assessment. Protocols have been established to help prehospital personnel handle unidentified chemical exposures, and it is important to prepare for such incidents during planning and drills (12).

POISON CENTERS

Poison centers can play a major role in helping to facilitate evaluation and treatment of hazardous materials exposure victims. Poison center staff are familiar with drug, occupational, and environmental exposures and generally have extensive reference materials. They are available 24 hours a day and are already familiar to and trusted by medical professionals. Poison centers can also maintain databases on hazardous materials incidents for a region to facilitate information gathering on the types of exposures likely to happen in the future and gather enough experience to learn from what is otherwise a widely scattered and relatively infrequent occurrence for a specific locality. A list of poison center roles in hazardous materials incident response is provided in Table 6.

TABLE 6. The poison center role in hazardous materials emergencies

1. Participate in a coordinated, community-specific response plan with clearly designated responsibilities and defined procedures when a hazardous materials emergency occurs.
2. Assist incident responders in identifying and assessing the threat to health and environment.
3. Facilitate the linkage between toxicologic expertise and information resources with incident responders and the emergency management system; the goal for such ties is to arrive at appropriate decisions dealing with health and environmental risks.
4. Assist in the mobilization of medical resources to provide rescue and emergency care of the injured or ill from exposure to toxic release.
5. Provide appropriate medical management information to medical personnel treating victims.
6. Be a mechanism by which health effects from exposures can be accurately followed up and documented.
7. Be the designated toxicologic focal point for dissemination of accurate, clear, consistent, and appropriate information to the public during toxic incidents.
8. Offer educational programs and opportunities to medical and public safety personnel on control, management, and response to hazardous chemical incidents.
9. Evaluate toxicologic information and data on hazardous materials and become an accessible repository of this information and data.
10. Become involved in a surveillance role to help identify and remove undetected environmental toxic hazards from the community.

Poison centers should be prepared to provide first responders, authorities, and mass media (e.g., local and national radio, television) with information on the substance released, including toxic effects, treatment measures, and how to avoid or minimize exposure. Ideally, poison centers should have access to a wide range of expertise, including medical toxicologists, chemists, industrial (or occupational) hygienists, environmental and industrial toxicologists, occupational health specialists, and hazardous wastes and materials specialists. Problems with communication are common in hazardous materials incidents, and planning should emphasize means of preserving accurate communication between all the parties involved in a site response. Specifically, paramedics and treating physicians often do not receive all the necessary information from the scene to estimate exposures and make appropriate treatment decisions. This is one particularly important area where using a poison center as an intermediary between on-site teams and medical professionals can help ensure the transmission of correct information. First-responder use of a hazardous materials information service at a regional poison center was associated with a reduction from 81% to 15% of exposure victims transported to a health care facility (58).

Medical toxicologists experienced in chemical exposures may be available with local poison centers, or through other local, state, or federal agencies. They may be called on to rapidly provide chemical toxicity information and medical management information to first responders, paramedics, and hospitals. This information should include guidelines for decontamination and how to obtain and administer antidotes.

A number of regional poison centers and other health agencies have developed specialized response systems for hazardous materials incidents (58–61). Poison centers participating in the International Program for Chemical Safety, some of which will have specialized expertise, are listed on the program's Web site (http://www.who.int/pcs/chem_incid_main.html). As mentioned, the University of Wales Institute in Cardiff, United Kingdom has been designated by the WHO as an International Clearing House for Major Chemical Incidents (http://www.healthchem.uwic.ac.uk/).

MEDICAL TREATMENT

Treatment decisions will fall into three major categories: decontamination, supportive care, and definitive treatment of victims. In general, medical treatment will follow this order, although it is best to be flexible when warranted medically. In certain cases, such as with cyanide exposure, definitive treatment may need to be provided immediately. Because treatment capabilities will commonly differ from the prehospital to the hospital setting, these two arenas are discussed separately.

Prehospital Treatment

The EMS providers responding to a hazardous materials incident have five goals:

1. To protect themselves and other responders from any significant toxic exposure.
2. To obtain accurate information on the identity and health effects of the hazardous materials and the appropriate prehospital evaluation and medical care for victims.
3. To minimize continued exposure of the victim and secondary contamination of health care personnel by ensuring that proper decontamination (if necessary) has been completed before transport to a hospital.
4. To provide appropriate prehospital emergency medical care consistent with their certification.
5. To prevent unnecessary ambulance or other transport vehicle contamination.

Patient decontamination may be carried out on an individual basis in small-scale incidents, or in a more organized fashion for large hazardous materials incidents involving multiple exposures, as outlined in Figure 3. In general, any gas or vapor exposure without liquid or solid chemical exposure will not require decontamination. However, chemicals may be adsorbed onto the patient's clothing, and for malodorous chemicals it may be useful to remove and store the clothing in plastic bags placed one within the other (double bagging). For instance, exposure to carbon monoxide or methane requires removal from exposure, and if indicated, further medical treatment, but it does not require decontamination. If there is any doubt about the potential for secondary contamination (exposure to others through chemical off-gassing or direct dermal contact with chemicals remaining on the patient), the patient should be decontaminated. Most solid and liquid exposures will require removing the patient's clothing and washing the skin with either water or soap and water. With exposure to a water-reactive chemical, excess solid material should be rapidly removed before irrigation.

Victims who are able and cooperative may assist with their own decontamination. Exposed or irritated skin and hair should be flushed with water for at least 15 minutes. Oily or lipophilic substances, such as many organophosphate pesticide products, should be washed with soap and flushed with water. Exposed eyes should be rinsed for a minimum of 15 minutes with clean water or sterile isotonic solutions, after removal of contact lenses if present. If a corrosive material is suspected, or if pain or injury is evident, irrigation should be continued while transferring the victim. A contaminated appendage can be washed without wetting the whole body if that is the only part contaminated. Patients with chemical burns receiving prompt decontamination at the scene have been shown to have less full-thickness skin injury and shorter hospital stays than do patients whose decontamination was delayed until arrival at the hospital (62).

If the patient requires rapid medical treatment, transport and treatment should not be delayed by providing definitive decontamination. Removal of clothing, followed by a rapid rinse, will remove most of the chemical contaminant in a minimal amount of time. If decontamination cannot be achieved before transport to a medical facility, placing the patient in a chemical-resistant bag with his or her head and IV site access exposed will prevent contamination of the ambulance. Helicopter transport of incompletely decontaminated patients from a hazardous materials incident may be problematic. With the release of volatile chemicals from a contaminated patient, the flight crew could experience difficulty in breathing or seeing. Also, the area of the incident needs to be clearly communicated to the flight crew to avoid traveling through an unsafe area. Furthermore, the downdraft from the helicopter could increase exposure to chemical vapors or fumes at the incident scene.

After decontamination, supportive care is the mainstay for most chemical exposures, starting with the ABCs (airway, breathing, circulation). The extent of supportive and definitive care will depend on the nature of the chemical. Chemical toxicity can be grouped into four major categories.

1. Simple asphyxiants cause toxicity by displacing oxygen from the atmosphere. No special treatment is needed, other than removing the patient from the exposure, supplying supplemental oxygen, and giving supportive care. Examples of simple asphyxiants include nitrogen, helium, methane, and acetylene.
2. Systemic asphyxiants interfere with oxygen transfer and cellular uptake within the body. In addition to the treatment listed above, specific antidotal therapy may be required. Examples of systemic asphyxiants include carbon monoxide, cyanide, hydrogen sulfide, and sodium azide.
3. The third group consists of irritants and corrosives, and examples include acids and bases. After decontamination, no additional treatment may be required, although specific chemical exposures may require more in-depth care. Patients with bronchospasm should be treated with aerosolized bronchodilators.
4. The fourth category, other chemicals, may or may not require antidotal therapy, and treatment should be based on the toxicity of each specific chemical.

Emergency Department Treatment

Emergency departments need to be prepared to treat contaminated victims from hazardous materials incidents. A survey of hospital safety officers revealed that 47% of responding hospitals had received chemically contaminated patients during 1994, ranging from one to 20 patients with an average of 4.9 patients for those hospitals specifying the number treated (63). Secondary contamination of emergency care providers from treatment of patients exposed to hazardous materials has also been described (64–67). Exposure may occur from dermal contact with chemicals remaining on the patient or through inhalation of volatile contaminants or particulates. A number of "worried well" concerned patients without symptoms and not requiring decontamination may also seek emergency care after a hazardous materials incident (68).

The degree of decontamination performed in the prehospital environment will vary with the team providing hazardous materials response and the patient's medical condition. Ideally, decontamination should be performed before hospital transport, but in some cases, particularly when the patient appears unstable, prehospital decontamination may be deferred to hospital personnel. In addition, exposed patients may transport themselves to the hospital without prior prehospital evaluation or decontamination, a situation that without adequate preparation may lead to hospital evacuation. Strong or unpleasant odors from chemically contaminated patients can also result in hospital staff illness, even if the chemical concentrations in air are below levels normally considered to be injurious. In general, toxic liquids and solids pose a dermal contact hazard to emergency department staff, and only volatile liquid or solid contamination poses a risk of significant exposure through inhalation.

Guidance materials have been published to help hospitals manage hazardous materials incidents (11,12). Protocols are also available for treatment of exposure to radioactive materials (69). Emergency departments should devise contaminated patient protocols appropriate to their setting, provide employees with appropriate training, practice these protocols during chemical incident drills, and carefully review both training sessions and actual incidents to improve future performance (11,64,66,70–73).

Contaminated Patient Protocol

The emergency department staff has three primary goals in managing a hazardous materials exposure victim who may be contaminated or has not been adequately decontaminated before arrival at the hospital:

1. To isolate the chemical contamination.
2. To appropriately decontaminate and treat the patient(s) while protecting hospital staff, other patients, and visitors.
3. To reestablish normal service as quickly as possible.

These goals should be accomplished concurrently. Medical care may be required before complete isolation of the chemical contamination, although rapid institution of personal protection of health care providers should precede intervention. Medically necessary care, such as stabilization of a traumatized victim of a motor vehicle accident, should not be delayed owing to contamination with relatively low toxicity substances. However, a critically ill patient with chemical contamination posing a significant secondary exposure hazard requires that caregivers be protected while they are providing treatment. In such an instance, basic life support may be provided during initial protected decontamination, and advanced life support may follow immediately thereafter.

A hazardous materials template protocol for dealing with contaminated patients, which may be modified according to local needs, is described in Table 7 (74). If adequate prior decontamination has taken place, then patients with inhalation and dermal chemical exposure can be treated without special precautions. The first steps in handling contaminated patients in the emergency department are to recognize the presence of chemical contamination, identify the hazardous substance if possible, and determine its level of toxicity and risk for secondary contamination. Triage personnel should be trained to recognize high-risk situations for chemical contamination of patients.

Ideally, either a portable outside decontamination unit or an internal decontamination facility with separate ventilation and water containment is available. Particularly in cold weather conditions, decontamination units should be supplied with warm running water. Portable curtains can provide protection from wind and personal privacy during decontamination. The protocol assumes there is either a separate waste water containment system or that the waste water treatment company for the hospital has the capacity to treat the low concentrations of chemical contaminants produced from decontamination of exposed patients, as contrasted with larger-volume primary spills. Alternatively, plastic pools or commercially available specialized decontamination stretchers can be used for decontamination, and the waste water kept in sealed containers for later disposal.

The amount of contamination on a patient is generally much less than is present at the actual site of chemical release. Unless significant solid and liquid chemical contamination of the emergency department has occurred, it is unlikely that volatilization of chemicals from a contaminated patient would result in injury to hospital staff. Most hazardous material exposure victims are exposed by inhalation only (8) and are unlikely to have enough residual chemical present to present a risk to hospital personnel, although strong odors may be present. In one study of 72 emergency department patients exposed to hazardous materials, positive predecontamination swabs analyzed by a certified analytical chemistry laboratory using gas chromatography/mass spectrometry were seen for pesticides and polychlorinated biphenyls only (72). In a study of hospital staff decontaminating mannequins soaked with volatile solvents, personal breathing zone exposure monitoring demonstrated chemical concentrations well within acceptable occupational exposure limits (75). Removing clothing should substantially decrease the amount of chemical contamination and risk of secondary contamination. However, it is not unusual for chemicals with strong odors to elicit a symptomatic response in hospital staff, even at concentrations generally considered nontoxic.

The minimum level of personal protection required for hospital decontamination will vary depending on the chemical contaminant and its concentration. Respiratory protection is only necessary when toxic vapors are at concentrations high enough to cause potentially harmful effects to staff, a situation that is extremely uncommon. After clothing removal, a contaminated patient poses minimal inhalation risk when decontamination is performed outside of the emergency department. However, if a patient is placed in a poorly ventilated treatment room, personnel without respiratory protection could develop symptoms from inhalation of off-gassing vapors from clothing, skin, or vomitus.

All emergency departments included in emergency response plans for hazardous materials incidents, through agreements with industries or hazardous waste sites, LEPCs, or other organizations, must meet OSHA requirements [29 CFR 1910.120(q)] for both training and response to hazardous materials (26), as it is likely that at some time they will be faced with a chemically exposed patient without prior decontamination. Under these regulations, emergency medical personnel expected to decontaminate victims exposed to a hazardous substance must be trained at a minimum to the first responder operations level. Additional guidance on regulations concerning hospitals and emergency response to hazardous substances is available in an OSHA informational booklet (76).

OSHA regulations require level B protection (positive-pressure SCBA and splash-protective chemical resistant clothing) for response to an unknown hazard. However, these regulations should not be interpreted to require the use of such protection for treatment of contaminated patients in all hospitals. Hazards associated with use of level B protection include increased weight, improper use of the equipment,

TABLE 7. Emergency department (ED) guidelines for the care of chemically contaminated patients

Objective	Plan of action	Comments
Isolation		
Protect the ED staff and patients from exposure	ISOLATE THE CONTAMINATED PATIENT AND KEEP OR MOVE HIM/HER OUTSIDE IF POSSIBLE. Personnel should wear protective equipment if in the isolation area (see Treatment section of this table).	Keep victim outside patient care and waiting areas until decontamination is completed if possible. It is best to at least initiate decontamination outside before entering the hospital, including removal of clothing and initial brief rinse.
	If decontamination must be performed indoors and a fully equipped decontamination room is not available, use a single large patient room (preferably one that is not used often) to limit ED contamination. Maintain ventilation to the decontamination area. Avoid "sealing the room," which may create an enclosed space environment, augmenting inhalation exposures to hospital personnel. However, consider risk to other hospital occupants if air from the room is recycled to other areas of the hospital. If escaping vapors pose a risk to other staff or patients, they should be isolated or evacuated and patients discharged or transferred.	It may be necessary to initiate treatment before decontamination is accomplished, although personnel should be protected in advance. Limit number of personnel involved.
	Remove nonessential and nondisposable equipment from the decontamination area. Establish and secure zones with yellow tape on the floor, including decontamination zone (warm) and clean zone (cold) to prevent unauthorized entry until cleanup has been completed.	Use hospital security to help prevent nonauthorized personnel from entering or leaving contaminated areas. If liquid or solid contamination was tracked into the ED, then affected areas should be outlined with yellow tape and secured.
Notification	Notify appropriate hospital personnel. Examples include maintenance, security, hospital supervisor, ED director. Contact external agencies (e.g., the poison center) as required.	Establish contact list before actual incident. If the incident occurs within the hospital, fire department and Hazmat teams may be needed.
Minimize risk to staff	Consider staff to be potentially contaminated if they provided care and had direct dermal contact before decontamination with a patient with liquid or solid on skin or clothes.	Contact the poison center or other consultant to determine need for staff decontamination.
	Move staff noticing irritant or other symptoms without direct patient contact to fresh air.	
Communication	Communicate frequently with supervisor, security, staff, and departmental administration.	Brief ED staff regarding the chemicals involved, expected toxicity, and protection needed.
	Notify hospital administrator and public information officer for hospital.	The evacuation may well be a media event.
Determine need for evacuation	Assess extent and toxicity of chemical contamination.	EVACUATION IS RARELY INDICATED. In most instances, isolation of the contamination will be required, but a complete evacuation will not be necessary. Odor is not a reliable predictor of toxicity.
	If low risk for toxicity, continue operation of department, institute cleanup, and restore to normal operations. If highly toxic, more extensive isolation or evacuation may be required.	Reasons to consider evacuation: 1. Primary spill of toxic chemical in ED 2. Nearby Hazmat incident threatening hospital 3. Patient contaminated with **highly** toxic volatile chemical and not decontaminated before entry
	If symptoms are noted outside of the isolation area or the situation warrants urgent decision making without time to identify the hazardous substance, then consider evacuation.	
	Determine who is responsible for making the evacuation decision. Contact local fire department for assistance as needed.	
Implement evacuation	Establish alternate triage and treatment sites in appropriate locations and a transfer route to assure patients with emergent needs have access to emergency services.	Alternate site should be identified in disaster plan. Consider the possibility of the hospital itself as a Hazmat incident site.
	If time permits, assign a staff member to take responsibility for organization and movement of essentials, including equipment, crash carts, staff roster, patient log, personal belongings, and telephone triage references, as well as log book, suture cart, splint cart, and mobile lighting.	
	Determine alternate source if unable to relocate essential equipment and carts owing to contaminated environment.	
	Notify Central Supply, hospital supervisor, and Critical Care of needs and status.	
	Consult pharmacy regarding antidotes and other medications, including controlled substances, in alternate site.	
Preserve essential communications	Contact emergency medical services system re: divert status and switchboard to divert calls to new location.	Moving ED to a new location may limit ability to accept patients by ambulance.
	If necessary, contact alternate hospital to assume base station functions, and inform other hospitals of situation.	Alternate hospital should be identified in disaster plan.
Treatment		
Life-saving intervention	Evaluate patient, determine urgency for care, and initiate lifesaving procedures in decontamination area or triage.	May occur at same time as, or before, decontamination.
Determine toxicity and appropriate treatment, including need for decontamination.	Assess chemical toxicity and determine appropriate treatment through identification of specific chemical (if known), form of material, and routes and duration of exposure.	Contact the poison center or consultants, such as CHEMTREC, ATSDR, or local industry for additional information.
	Decontamination is required for toxic solid and liquid exposures, but usually is not necessary for noncorrosive gas and vapor exposures.	Material Safety Data sheets help identify the chemical, but may not have correct treatment information.

(*continued*)

TABLE 7. (*continued*)

Objective	Plan of action	Comments
Protect staff	IF POSSIBLE, ALLOW THE PATIENT TO DECONTAMINATE SELF, OR USE A SPECIALLY TRAINED AND EQUIPPED DECONTAMINATION TEAM. Otherwise, wear PPE when assisting the contaminated victim. Gloves, goggles, mask, and disposable gowns provide some degree of protection. Select additional PPE, including chemical-resistant gloves and clothing, based on the chemical hazard.	Local fire departments may be recruited to assist in decontamination. Sources of additional information on appropriate PPE include Hazmat teams, industrial hygienists, medical toxicologists, chemical manufacturers, and retail PPE outlets.
Patient decontamination	REMOVE PATIENT'S CLOTHING AND PLACE IN PLASTIC BAGS. If stable, have patient remove clothes and shower with soap and water in decontamination shower. If victim must sit or lie down, place chair (washable surface) or stretcher in shower area. Wash from victim's head to feet. Decontaminate open wounds first, and avoid contamination of unexposed skin. Surgical drapes may help protect unexposed skin. Decontaminate exposed area: Flush exposed areas with soap and water for 10–15 min, with gentle sponging (surgical sponge) to avoid skin breakdown. Irrigate exposed eyes with saline 10–15 min. Clean under nails with scrub brush or plastic nail cleaner. Gently irrigate contaminated open wounds with water or saline an additional 5–10 min.	Double bag contaminated clothing, linens, and gloves in red biohazard bags, then seal and label. Take special precaution with exposures to concentrated acids, caustics, or oily or lipid-soluble liquids (pesticides). For special circumstances, staff should consider additional or different PPE (for preplanning, consider possible sources of contamination from nearby industry). Patient ingestion of toxic materials warrants special care in gastric decontamination (if indicated) and staff protection.
Supportive care	Assess ABCs, establish airway and breathing, and provide supplemental oxygen as indicated.	
Antidotal treatment	Determine if antidotal treatment would be effective and available. Administer as indicated.	Anticipate need for antidotes based on chemicals used in local industry.
Staff decontamination	Decontaminate personnel with direct skin contact with the chemical contaminant. Move other symptomatic staff to fresh air.	Staff without direct dermal contact with the contaminated patient or clothing do not require decontamination.
Large exposures	For significant and very large exposures, or if staff are untrained in use of protective equipment or protective equipment is unavailable, contact local fire department for assistance.	Emergency departments should use chemical exposure scenarios for drills with local fire departments.
Reestablish normal operations		
Decontaminate facility	Ventilate the contaminated area with large fans if available, moving air outside and away from occupied areas. Clean spills with soap and water after removing gross particulates. Use existing hazardous materials spill protocols.	Fire departments may assist in facility decontamination. For significant contamination, use an environmental cleanup service (available 24 h, preestablished contract) if hospital resources are limited or fire department assistance is not practical.
Chemical monitoring	Consider chemical-specific monitoring if indicated and appropriate equipment available.	Usually not necessary, but fire department may provide.
Authorize reentry	Obtain appropriate agency clearance prior to reentry, if required or if adequacy of hospital decontamination is uncertain.	Determine agency and 24-h contact number before incident.
Communication	Contact all individuals and sites contacted previously at initiation of incident to provide notification of reopening.	Involve hospital administration and public information officer.
Debriefing	Debrief staff regarding signs and symptoms from the specific chemical exposure and risks posed to them, if any. Discuss incident. Revise protocol as needed.	Consider how to better identify chemical contamination.

ATSDR, U.S. Agency for Toxic Substances and Disease Registry.
From Burgess JL, Kirk M, Borron SW, et al. Emergency department hazardous materials protocol for contaminated patients. *Ann Emerg Med* 1999;34:205–212, with permission from Elsevier.

problems with donning and doffing, and decreased dexterity. Other options include having patients perform self-decontamination if they are capable of doing so, designating a local fire department hazardous materials team to assist in or perform the decontamination, and proceeding with decontamination with less than level B protection if such assistance is not available within a suitable time interval based on the patient's condition. It should be kept in mind that hazardous materials teams may be involved in the on-scene response and therefore not available to assist in hospital-based decontamination. Hospitals frequently receiving contaminated casualties or in high-risk areas may need to consider additional training and equipment, such as specialized chemical-resistant clothing and respirators.

Emergency department evacuation is rarely necessary and can generally be avoided by recognizing chemical contamination and adequately decontaminating the patient outside the emergency department, or using an appropriately designed room within the emergency department. Moving a contaminated patient outside or to a dedicated decontamination room with separate ventilation and establishing proper ventilation, such as with large fans, are usually sufficient to prevent exposure to other patients. Ventilation fans should be positioned to exhaust air to an appropriate outside location, and doors to "clean" areas should be closed as necessary. If evacuation has already occurred, the emergency department can be rapidly reoccupied after adequate ventilation. Primary spills of hazardous volatile liquids or solids that cannot be quickly controlled may require facility evacuation. If a fire department has been involved in the emergency department incident, the final decision to reopen the facility may be that of the fire chief. A close working relationship between the fire chief, emergency department personnel, and toxicology consultants is therefore essential.

Supportive Care

Many patients exposed to hazardous materials may not need any therapy other than decontamination, if required. Standard supportive care should be provided as needed.

ABCS

The patient's airway, breathing, and circulation should be evaluated and supported as indicated. Tracheal intubation should be performed as needed. Patients with bronchospasm should be treated with aerosolized bronchodilators. The possibility of enhanced risk of cardiac dysrhythmias in hypoxic patients treated with catecholamines should be kept in mind. Coma, seizures, hypotension, or ventricular dysrhythmias should be treated in a standard fashion. Cardiac monitoring and an intravenous line should be placed as soon as possible in all patients who are unconscious, obtunded, or hypotensive, or who may become so. Patients exposed to substances that may cause cardiac sensitization or intravascular hemolysis will also require monitoring and establishing of intravenous access.

EYE EXPOSURE

Care should be taken that any contact lenses have been removed and adequate eye irrigation has been completed. For acidic and basic exposures, the pH of the conjunctival fluid should be normalized if possible. After testing of visual acuity, the eyes should be examined for corneal damage using a magnifying device or a slit lamp and fluorescein stain. Small corneal defects may be treated with ophthalmic ointment or drops, analgesic medication, and an eye patch. An ophthalmologist should be immediately consulted for patients who have significant corneal injury.

INGESTION EXPOSURE

Treatment of hazardous materials ingestions should be chemical specific. Potential therapies include gastric lavage and administration of activated charcoal. Not all chemicals will bind efficiently to charcoal. If a corrosive material is suspected, then activated charcoal should be avoided and endoscopy considered to evaluate the extent of gastrointestinal tract injury.

Laboratory Tests

Depending on the chemical exposure and the patient's symptoms and signs of toxicity, useful routine tests may include a complete blood count, glucose, electrolytes, renal function tests, liver enzymes, urinalysis, and electrocardiogram. Chest radiographs are recommended for symptomatic inhalation exposure, and measurements of arterial blood gases for ventilated patients or suspected hypoxemia.

Disposition and Follow-Up

Hospitalization should be considered for all patients with a suspected serious exposure and those with persistent or progressive symptoms. If there is a possibility of delayed onset of symptoms, the patient should be observed for an extended period or admitted to the hospital. Follow-up instructions should be provided to return to the emergency department or a private physician for additional testing as needed, to reevaluate initial findings, or for persistence or development of new symptoms.

Post-incident debriefing should be provided to hospital staff, patients, and their families. Failure to address the concerns of the individuals exposed to hazardous materials may result in more persistent morbidity. When specific identification of involved compounds is not possible, appropriate patient follow-up should be recommended, and exposed staff should be invited to seek follow-up with occupational medicine or toxicology consultation for persistent or new-onset symptoms.

Reporting

If a work-related incident has occurred, a workers' compensation claim should be filed. If the incident occurred in the workplace, discussing it with company leaders may prevent future incidents. If a public health risk exists, then the appropriate public agencies should be notified. When appropriate, patients should be informed that they may request an evaluation of their workplace from OSHA or a corresponding state agency.

Antidotes

There are no specific antidotes for most chemical exposures. For the limited number of chemicals with an available antidote, adequate supplies must be readily available. A partial list of antidotes is provided in Table 8. Additional information on the use of these antidotes is provided in the antidote section of this book (Chapters 42 through 77).

Common Problems

A number of problems have been commonly observed in the treatment of chemical exposure victims. Failure may occur in communication between police, firefighters, and ambulance and hospital services, particularly concerning the identification of the chemical substance and its toxicity. Protective clothing is rarely provided for emergency department staff and is generally not provided for the police. Emergency departments may not have effective decontamination facili-

TABLE 8. Recommended hazardous materials antidotes

Antidote	Indication
Atropine	Organophosphate pesticides
Calcium gluconate (gel and IV)	Hydrofluoric acid and fluoride toxicity
Cyanide antidote kit[a] (or hydroxocobalamin)	Cyanide
Methylene blue	Methemoglobin forming agents
Oxygen	Carbon monoxide
Pralidoxime or other oximes	Organophosphate pesticides
Pyridoxine	Hydrazine

[a]Includes amyl nitrite, sodium nitrite, and sodium thiosulfate.
Adapted from Walter FG, Klein R, Thomas RG. Advanced HAZMAT Life Support: Provider Manual, 2nd ed. Tucson, AZ: University of Arizona Emergency Medicine Research Center, 2000.

ties available, and those that are available may not comply with those recommended by hospital accreditation regulations. In addition, although a poison center may be able to provide help, it will not be able to prepare information in advance of the patient's arrival at a hospital if it is not notified by first responders (66).

TRIAGE

In a disaster, triage generally occurs on site and at the hospital. On-site triage is involved with rapid evaluation, stabilization, and evacuation of victims. During hospital triage, victims are reevaluated to determine the most appropriate treatment for them.

On-Site Triage

On-site EMS workers triage victims to appropriate treatment and transportation areas. They are triaged and tagged where they lie and then transported to "immediate" or "delayed" transportation areas, where they are given whatever medical care is available. In a mass-casualty disaster, field resuscitation is limited to airway maintenance, hemorrhage control, and correcting mechanical problems, such as stabilizing suspected spinal injuries. Immediate goals are to rescue and remove the injured and to separate potentially salvageable victims from the moribund or dead. Rapid classification of injury and tagging establish priorities for stabilization and evacuation of the most critically injured. Color-coded tags (attached to the great toe or wrist) indicate the severity of injury. This color-code system must remain uniform throughout all stages of triages. Special requisitions for laboratory tests and x-rays should be part of the tag. An internationally adopted system is as follows (77):

Red (immediate care, critically injured) requires immediate life support and is first priority for hospital transport.

Yellow (intermediate care, significant injury that is not immediately life threatening) requires definitive care and is second priority for evacuation.

Green (walking wounded, minor or no injuries) requires little or no treatment and should be directed to the area for delayed hospital transportation.

Black [expectant (unsalvageable) or dead] denotes survival is unlikely, even with the best of care. Analgesics should be administered but not life support, and these victims have the lowest priority for transport.

Paramedics identify and label the dead and cover the remains and personal effects. The medical examiner directs removal and preservation of bodies and parts for identification. Prior plans should include disposition and handling of dead victims found on site. A temporary morgue can be set up. Arrangement can be made for non-EMS personnel to transport such victims at a later time.

Casualty collection points are the second stage in the triage process and the final station for all victims at the disaster site. Such points should be established in a safe place, with easy access to both the flow of victims and traffic lanes. Before patients are evacuated, the on-scene medical officer or staff proceeds with a more definitive triage, stabilization, and treatment of injured patients. Treatment varying from first aid to lifesaving measures may need to be performed before evacuation (78).

The on-scene medical officer in charge should ensure that patient dispatch proceeds smoothly. Appropriate matching of individual hospital resources with the patient load to be received is critical, because an overload of critically injured patients may occur at one hospital while another hospital receives minimally injured individuals. All this requires constant communication between the various hospitals and the on-scene command post.

Hospital Triage

The final stage of the triage process for casualties occurs at hospitals. The first wave of victims may arrive within 30 minutes after an incident. These individuals generally have minor injuries and come of their own volition. They may easily overload the hospital facilities, interfering with the care of more severely affected patients arriving later (78).

The hospital receiving and triage area should not be established in the emergency department. A large, open area (a lobby or predesignated outer space) frees up the emergency department for use as a resuscitation area. The entry point provides rapid access to all treatment areas. Traffic is one way only: Emergency vehicles unload victims and depart rapidly. The hospital triage officer is stationed at the entry point and reviews the triage tags of the victims. Misdiagnosis and deterioration may occur owing to inaccurate field tagging. The triage officer will designate the priority in which victims will receive treatment and to which treatment area the victim is to go (77).

A disaster may force rearrangement of the entire hospital for maximum efficiency. Suggested treatment areas defined in a disaster plan include a resuscitation area, critical care treatment areas, immediate care area, ambulatory treatment area, and expectant category area set up to care for the dying. A temporary supplemental morgue may be required if there is a large number of deceased patients. After proper decontamination of the surviving victims, laboratory work, radiographs, and surgery may be indicated. Plans should include allocation of such resources in an emergency (77).

ACKNOWLEDGMENT

I would like to thank Gary D. Gordon of the Boeing Fire Department for his thoughtful suggestions and review of the chapter.

REFERENCES

1. NFPA 473: Standard for Professional Competencies for EMS Personnel Responding to Hazardous Materials Incidents. National Fire Protection Association, Quincy, MA; 1992.
2. Lewis RJ. *Hawley's condensed chemical dictionary*, 12th ed. New York: Van Nostrand Reinhold Co., 1993.
3. Code of Federal Regulations, Title 49, Part 172. Washington: US Government Printing Office, 1994.
4. U.S. Environmental Protection Agency Superfund. Available at: http://www.epa.gov/superfund/programs/er/hazsubs/lauths.htm. Accessed January 2003.
5. Burgess JL, Kovalchick DF, Lymp JF, et al. Risk factors for adverse health effects following hazardous materials incidents. *J Occup Environ Med* 2001;43:558–566.
6. Mehta PS, Mehta AS, Mehta SJ, et al. Bhopal tragedy's health effects: a review of methyl isocyanate toxicity. *JAMA* 1990;264:2781–2787.
7. Wagner GN, Clark MA, Koenigsberg EJ, Decata SJ. Medical evaluation of the victims of the 1986 Lake Nyos disaster. *J Forensic Sci* 1988;33:899–909.

8. Burgess JL, Pappas GP, Robertson WO. Hazardous materials incidents: the Washington Poison Center experience and approach to exposure assessment. *J Occup Environ Med* 1997;39:760–766.
9. Hazardous Substances Emergency Event Surveillance System 1998 database, Agency for Toxic Substances and Disease Registry. Available at: http://www.atsdr.cdc.gov/HS/HSEES/annual98.html. Accessed January 2003.
10. Agency for Toxic Substances and Diseases Registry. Managing Hazardous Materials Incidents: A Planning Guide for the Management of Contaminated Patients, Vol. 1. Atlanta: US Department of Health and Human Services, Agency for Toxic Substances and Diseases Registry 2000. Available at: http://www.atsdr.cdc.gov/mhmi.html. Accessed February 2003.
11. Agency for Toxic Substances and Disease Registry. Managing Hazardous Materials Incidents, Vol. II, Hospital Emergency Departments: A Planning Guide for the Management of Contaminated Patients. Atlanta: US Department of Health and Human Services, Agency for Toxic Substances and Disease Registry, 2000. Available at: http://www.atsdr.cdc.gov/mhmi.html. Accessed February 2003.
12. Agency for Toxic Substances and Disease Registry. Managing Hazardous Materials Incidents, Vol. III, Medical Management Guidelines for Acute Chemical Exposures. Atlanta: US Department of Health and Human Services, Agency for Toxic Substances and Disease Registry, 2000. Available at: http://www.atsdr.cdc.gov/mhmi.html. Accessed February 2003.
13. International Programme on Chemical Safety Web site. Available at: http://www.who.int/pcs/chem_incid_main.html. Accessed January 2003.
14. US Environmental Protection Agency Toxics Release Inventory, 2000. Available at: http://www.epa.gov/triexplorer/chemical.htm. Accessed January 2003.
15. US Coast Guard National Response Center, 2002 data. Available at: http://www.nrc.uscg.mil/incident97-02.html. Accessed February 2003.
16. Burgess JL, Kovalchick DF, Harter L, et al. Hazardous materials events: an industrial comparison. *J Occup Environ Med* 2000;42:546–553.
17. Kales SN, Polyhronopoulos GN, Castro MJ, et al. Injuries caused by hazardous materials accidents. *Ann Emerg Med* 1997;30:598–603.
18. Baker P, Selvey D. Malathion-induced epidemic hysteria in an elementary school. *Vet Hum Toxicol* 1992;34:156–160.
19. Gamino LA, Elkins GR, Hackney KU. Emergency management of mass psychogenic illness. *Psychosomatics* 1989;30:446–449.
20. Selden BS. Adolescent epidemic hysteria presenting as a mass casualty, toxic exposure incident. *Ann Emerg Med* 1989;18:892–895.
21. Baum A, Fleming I. Implications of the psychological research on stress and technological accidents. *Am Psychol* 1993;48:665–672.
22. Dayal HH, Baranowski T, Li Y, et al. Hazardous chemicals: psychological dimensions of the health sequelae of a community exposure in Texas. *J Epidemiol Community Health* 1994;48:560–568.
23. Bowler RM, Mergler D, Huel G, et al. Psychological, psychosocial, and psychophysiological sequelae in a community affected by a railroad chemical disaster. *J Trauma Stress* 1994;7:601–624.
24. Kovalchick D, Burgess JL, Kyes KB, et al. Psychological effects of hazardous materials exposures. *Psychosom Med* 2002;64:841–846.
25. US Environmental Protection Agency. NRT-1: Hazardous Materials Planning Guide, 2001 Update. Available at: http://yosemite.epa.gov/oswer/ceppoweb.nsf/content/serc-lepc-publications.htm. Accessed February 2003.
26. Code of Federal Regulations Title 29, Part 1910.120. Washington: US Government Printing Office, 1995.
27. *Comprehensive Accreditation Manual for Hospitals: The Official Handbook.* Oakbrook Terrace, IL: Joint Commission on Accreditation of Healthcare Organizations, updated November 2002.
28. Burgess JL, Blackmon GM, Brodkin CA, et al. Hospital preparedness for hazardous materials incidents and treatment of contaminated patients. *West J Med* 1997;167:387–391.
29. Ghilarducci DP, Pirrallo RG, Hegmann KT. Hazardous materials readiness of United States level 1 trauma centers. *J Occup Environ Med* 2000;42:683–692.
30. Code of Federal Regulations Title 59:6126-6184 Hazard Communication 29 CFR Parts 1910, 1915, 1917, 1918, 1926, and 1928. Washington: US Government Printing Office, 1994.
31. US Environmental Protection Agency Risk Management Program. Available at: http://yosemite.epa.gov/oswer/ceppoweb.nsf/content/RMPoverview.htm. Accessed January 2003.
32. Burgess JL. Hospital evacuations due to hazardous materials incidents. *Am J Emerg Med* 1999;17:50–52.
33. US Environmental Protection Agency Emergency Response. Available at: http://www.epa.gov/superfund/programs/er/hazsubs/equip.htm. Accessed January 2003.
34. Hazardous Substances Data Bank. Available at: http://toxnet.nlm.nih.gov/. Accessed January 2003.
35. US Department of Transportation Emergency Response Guidelines 2000. Available at: http://hazmat.dot.gov/gydebook.htm. Accessed January 2003.
36. US Environmental Protection Agency, National Oceanic and Atmospheric Administration. Computer-Aided Management of Emergency Operations (CAMEO). Available at: http://www.epa.gov/ceppo/cameo/. Accessed January 2003.
37. Odor Thresholds for Chemicals with Established Occupational Health Standards. Fairfax, VA: American Industrial Hygiene Association, 1993.
38. Gonzalez ER. Cyanide evades some noses, overpowers others. *JAMA* 1982;248:2211.
39. Ahlborg G. Hydrogen sulfide poisoning in shale oil industry. *AMA Arch Indust Hyg Occup Med* 1951;3:247–266.
40. US Coast Guard Chemical Hazards Response Information System (CHRIS). Available at: http://www.chrismanual.com/. Accessed January 2003.
41. US National Oceanic and Atmospheric Administration. The Chemical Reactivity Worksheet. Available at: http://response.restoration.noaa.gov/chemaids/react.html. Accessed February 2003.
42. Garfitt SJ, Jones K, Mason HJ, et al. Oral and dermal exposure to propetamphos: a human volunteer study. *Toxicol Lett* 2002;134:115–118.
43. American Conference of Governmental Industrial Hygienists. Threshold Limit Values for Chemical Substances and Physical Agents and Biological Exposure Indices. Cincinnati: 2002.
44. NIOSH Pocket Guide to Chemical Hazards. National Institute for Occupational Safety and Health, DHHS (NIOSH) Publication No. 97-140. Washington: US Government Printing Office, July 2001. Available at: http://www.cdc.gov/niosh/npg/npg.html. Accessed January 2003.
45. Alexeeff GV, Lipsett MJ, Kizer KW. Problems associated with the use of immediately dangerous to life and health (IDLH) values for estimating the hazard of accidental chemical releases. *Am Ind Hyg Assoc* 1989;50:598–605.
46. The AIHA 2002 Emergency Response Planning Guidelines and Workplace Environmental Exposure Level Guides Handbook. Fairfax, VA: American Industrial Hygiene Association, 2002.
47. Code of Federal Regulations, Title 40, Part 50. Washington: US Government Printing Office, 1992.
48. Peden NR, Taha A, McSorley PD, et al. Industrial exposure to hydrogen cyanide: implications for treatment. *Br Med J (Clin Res Ed)* 1986;293:538.
49. Wilkinson SP, McHugh P, Horsley S, et al. Arsine toxicity aboard the Asiafreighter. *BMJ* 1975;3:559–563.
50. Jones AT, Jones RC, Longley EO. Environmental and clinical aspects of bulk wheat fumigation with aluminum phosphide. *Am Ind Hyg Assoc J* 1964;25:376–379.
51. Schoonbroodt D, Guffens P, Jousten P, et al. Acute phosphine poisoning? A case report and review. *Acta Clin Belg* 1992;47:280–284.
52. Morgan WK. "Zamboni disease." Pulmonary edema in an ice hockey player. *Arch Intern Med* 1995;155:2479–2480.
53. Kanluen S, Gottlieb CA. A clinical pathologic study of four adult cases of acute mercury inhalation toxicity. *Arch Pathol Lab Med* 1991;115:56–60.
54. Lim SC, Yang JY, Jang AS, et al. Acute lung injury after phosgene inhalation. *Korean J Intern Med* 1996;11:87–92.
55. McLeod WR. Merphos poisoning or mass panic? *Aust N Z J Psychiatry* 1975;9:225–229.
56. Krug SE. Mass illness at an intermediate school: toxic fumes or epidemic hysteria? *Pediatr Emerg Care* 1992;8:280–282.
57. Cole TB, Chorba TL, Horan JM. Patterns of transmission of epidemic hysteria in a school. *Epidemiology* 1990;1:212–218.
58. Burgess JL, Keifer MC, Barnhart S, et al. The Hazardous Materials Exposure Information Service: development, analysis, and medical implications. *Ann Emerg Med* 1997;29:248–254.
59. Mrvos R, Dean BS, Krenzelok EP. A poison center's emergency response plan. *Vet Hum Toxicol* 1988;30:138–140.
60. Murray V, Goodfellow F. Mass casualty chemical incidents—towards guidance for public health management. *Public Health* 2002;116:2–14.
61. Geller RJ, Lopez GP. Poison center planning for mass gatherings: the Georgia Poison Center experience with the 1996 Centennial Olympic Games. *J Toxicol Clin Toxicol* 1999;37:315–319.
62. Leonard LG, Scheulen JJ, Munster AM. Chemical burns: effect of prompt first aid. *J Trauma* 1982;22:420–423.
63. Cone DC, Davidson SJ. Hazardous materials preparedness in the emergency department. *Prehosp Emerg Care* 1997;1:85–90.
64. Huff JS. Lessons learned from hazardous materials incidents. *Emerg Care Q* 1991;7:17–22.
65. Merritt NL, Anderson MJ. Malathion overdose: when one patient creates a departmental hazard. *J Emerg Nurs* 1989;15:463–465.
66. Thanabalasingham T, Beckett MW, Murray V. Hospital response to a chemical incident: report on casualties of an ethyldichlorosilane spill. *BMJ* 1991;302:101–102.
67. Nozaki H, Hori S, Shinozawa Y, et al. Secondary exposure of medical staff to sarin vapor in the emergency room. *Intensive Care Med* 1995;21:1032–1035.
68. Wing JS, Brender JD, Sanderson LM, et al. Acute health effects in a community after a release of hydrofluoric acid. *Arch Environ Health* 1991;46:155–160.
69. Leonard RB, Ricks RC. Emergency department radiation accident protocol. *Ann Emerg Med* 1980;9:462–470.
70. Cox RD. Decontamination and management of hazardous materials exposure victims in the emergency department. *Ann Emerg Med* 1994;23:761–770.
71. Kirk MA, Cisek J, Rose SR. Emergency department response to hazardous materials incidents. *Emerg Med Clin North Am* 1994;12:461–481.
72. Lavoire FW, Coomes T, Cisek JE, et al. Emergency department external decontamination for hazardous chemical exposure. *Vet Hum Toxicol* 1992;34:61–64.

73. Levitin HW, Siegelson HJ. Hazardous materials. Disaster medical planning and response. *Emerg Med Clin North Am* 1996;14:327–348.
74. Burgess JL, Kirk M, Borron SW, et al. Emergency department hazardous materials protocol for contaminated patients. *Ann Emerg Med* 1999;34:205–212.
75. Schultz M, Cisek J, Wabeke R. Simulated exposure of hospital emergency personnel to solvent vapors and respirable dust during decontamination of chemically exposed patients. *Ann Emerg Med* 1995;26:324–329.
76. Hospitals and Community Emergency Response—What You Need to Know. Emergency Response Safety Series, US Department of Labor, Occupational Safety and Health Administration. OSHA 3152. 1997. Available at: http://www.osha.gov/Publications/OSHA3152/osha3152.html. Accessed February 2003.
77. Dwyer BJ, Cheu D. Emergency medical response to civilian disasters. *Emerg Med Rep* 1990;11:169–176.
78. Waeckerle JF. Disaster planning and response. *N Engl J Med* 1991;324:815–821.

CHAPTER 260

Chemical Warfare Agents

Daniel C. Keyes

Compounds included:	**Nerve agents [sarin (GB), soman, tabun (GA), VX]; vesicant agents (mustards, arsenicals, phosgene oxime); incapacitating agents (psychotomimetic agents); lung-damaging agents (choking agents)**
Molecular formula and weight:	**See Table 1.**
CAS Registry No.:	**See Table 1.**
Special concerns:	**Nerve gases cause rapid onset of toxicity after aerosol exposure, but skin exposure may produce delayed onset of toxicity.**
Antidotes:	**Atropine, oximes (pralidoxime, obidoxime), diazepam**

OVERVIEW

Terrorism has become a reality of life in many countries. News reports frequently remind us of those individuals and groups who are intent on injuring and killing noncombatants in the name of a cause, for personal satisfaction, or for power. The March 1995 sarin nerve agent attack on the Tokyo subway system resulted in a heightened level of concern in the United States for such an attack on domestic soil. Since the attacks on the World Trade Center in 1993 and September 2001, the United States has entered into a new era of awareness of terrorism threat.

Although there are a variety of potential weapons for terrorism, only a few are likely for use in a nonmilitary setting. Dr. Alexei Yablokov, an expert on nuclear security and former science advisor to President Boris Yeltsin, testified before the National Security House Subcommittee in 1997 about the existence of "nuclear suitcase bombs" in the former Soviet Union and the lack of knowledge of their current location (1). Each suitcase is attributed to a 1-kiloton nuclear weapon. It is assumed that nuclear weapons might be difficult for a terrorist group to bring into the United States and detonate. Radioactive materials could, however, be incorporated into an explosive device and thus constitute a greater threat, but this is also considered unlikely.

Chemical and biological agents are much more likely to be used and thus are considered to be highly significant threats by the U.S. Federal Bureau of Investigation. Of these, only chemical agents have been used in a nonmilitary setting with significant consequences. It is now considered a question of *when*, not *if*, a terrorist using chemical weapons will strike in many countries.

HISTORY OF BIOLOGICAL AND CHEMICAL WARFARE

Nonconventional weapons have been used throughout history. The Greeks used animal corpses to pollute the water wells used by the enemy. In the Middle Ages, invading armies catapulted bodies laden with plague and other diseases against besieged populations (2). The United States, Britain, and France have all used blankets laden with smallpox to infect Native Americans. In World War I, biological and chemical weapons became important tools of the continental armies. At Ypres, Belgium, the Germans instituted the first use of chemical agents in warfare. In April 1915, they released 168 tons of chlorine gas along enemy lines. Five miles of allied lines were opened, but the Germans did not expect such a result, and they did not take advantage of the success. They later implemented mustard gas also. There were approximately 1 million chemical casualties in World War I, with approximately 5% of those being fatalities.

Since the early 1970s, the number of terrorist acts has increased. Many of these have involved the use of explosive devices; however, the use of chemical and biological materials is increasing (Fig. 1). In 1972, a group called the Order of the Rising Sun were found to have 30 to 40 kg of typhoid bacteria cultures with which they intended to attack the water supplies of Chicago, St. Louis, and other cities in the Midwest. The 1984 attack by the Bhagwan cult was an attempt to influence local elections by spraying salmonella onto salad bars at community restaurants in Oregon. In that event, 45 victims were admitted to area hospitals and 751 people became ill. No fatalities were reported. These two events were more isolated in nature.

TABLE 1. Physical and chemical properties of the nerve agents

Agent	Molecular formula, molecular weight (g/mol), CAS Registry No.	LCt_{50} (mg/min/m^3)	Volatility (mg/m^3 at 25°C)	Vapor density (air = 1)	Topical LD_{50} (mg)
Tabun (GA)	$C_5H_{11}N_2O_2P$; 162.12; 77-81-6	400	610	5.63	1000
Sarin (GB)	$(CH_3)_2CHOP(CH_3)OF$; 140.11; 107-44-8	100	22,000	4.86	1700
Soman (GD)	$C_7H_{16}FO_2P$; 182.17; 96-64-0	50	3900	6.33	100
VX	$C_{11}H_{26}NO_2PS$; 267.37; 50782-69-9	10	10.5	9.20	10

LCt_{50}, the dose that kills 50% of unprotected humans expressed as a concentration per cubic meter and with a 1-minute exposure.
Modified from Holstege CP, Kirk M, Sidell FR. Chemical warfare. Nerve agent poisoning. *Crit Care Clin* 1997;13:923–942.

In the early 1980s, a man named Chizuo Matsumoto changed his name to Asahara and established the Aum Association of Mountain Wizards. After a trip to meet the Dalai Lama, he decided to establish a world religion and changed the name of his organization to Aum Supreme Truth or Aum Shinrikyo. This organization grew to a membership of 20,000 members and an estimated wealth of $1 billion. The group became increasingly authoritative, requiring absolute submission to its leader, Asahara. The group carried out assassinations of opponents and developed facilities to manufacture nerve agents and biological terrorist weapons.

In June 1994, the group attempted to assassinate three judges in Matsumoto, Japan. The assassination team released sarin nerve agent in the residential community where the judges lived. The attack involved a truck with a device to release sarin. Although the judges were not killed, seven people died and 280 were injured.

On March 20, 1995, Aum Shinrikyo launched a chemical attack on the Tokyo subway (3). They put dilute sarin nerve agent into lunch boxes and other containers disguised as lunch bags. The terrorists used umbrellas with sharpened points to puncture the containers during the morning rush hour on three subway lines. This tragic event caused 11 deaths and approximately 5500 injuries among the commuters and emergency responders (4). The nearest hospital, St. Luke's International Hospital, saw 641 of the victims. Approximately 85% of the victims bypassed the emergency medical system and presented directly to hospitals without decontamination. Fortunately, the weekly grand rounds were taking place at St. Luke's hospital and a large part of the medical staff was present when patients began arriving (5).

There were important delays in determining the identity of the poison involved and in reporting this information to the hospitals. Medical personnel contacted the poison center, but this agency had not been informed of the nature of the toxin. Initially, it was assumed that the victims had been exposed to carbon monoxide or possibly cyanide vapor. A physician from Matsumoto correctly noted from news coverage that this was similar to the incident that had occurred in his city several months previously. He contacted colleagues in Tokyo with the identity of the agent within 2 hours of the subway attack (6).

The Tokyo sarin incident demonstrated a concept commonly discussed by disaster response planners. Approximately 80% of victims present directly to hospitals without the intervention of hazmat or other prehospital personnel. A typical time for response and set-up for a hazmat incident is 1 hour. This time is a minimum realistic time because of the sequence of activities that must occur: notification, response, hot-zone and perimeter setup, assembly of decontamination stations, and initiation of victim triage. In most cases, ambulatory victims do not wait for this period for treatment or transportation to a medical facility. The most realistic option for an individual on the scene would be to obtain private transportation to the nearest emergency room. As a result of the public self-referral to area hospitals, health facilities require decontamination facilities, personal protective equipment (PPE), antidotes, and disaster plans to respond to such an incident, and must not rely on emergency medical system for these actions.

Physicians are key participants in the response to a chemical agent attack. After a terrorist incident, the great majority of patients present to hospitals without the benefit of decontamination or treatment at the scene by emergency medical system

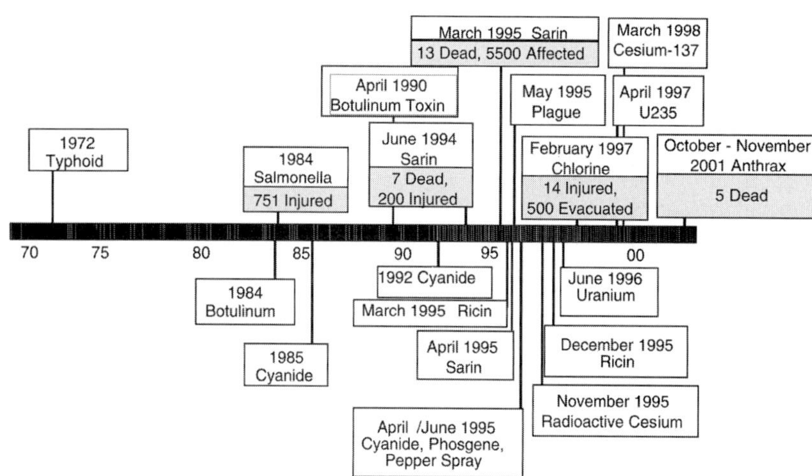

Figure 1. Chemical, biological, and nuclear terrorist incidents in the United States and abroad since 1970. [Soldier Biological and Chemical Command (SBC-COM), 2003 Domestic Preparedness Training Program materials.]

Abbreviation	*Common Name*	*Proper Name*
GA	Tabun	Ethyl N-dimethylphosphoramidocyanidate 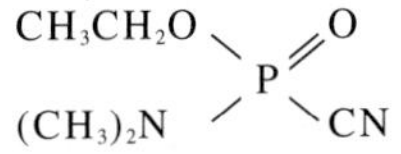 $CH_3CH_2O \backslash \quad //O$ P $(CH_3)_2N \; / \quad \backslash CN$
GB	Sarin	Isopropyl methylphosphonofluoridate 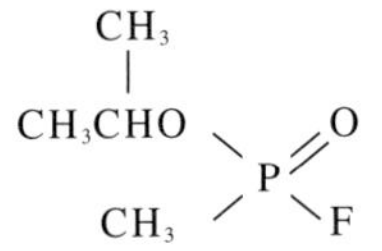 CH_3 $\vert$ $CH_3CHO \; \backslash \quad //O$ P $CH_3 \; / \quad \backslash F$
GD	Soman	1,2,2-trimethylpropyl methylphosphonofluoridate (Pinacolyl methylphosphonofluoridate) 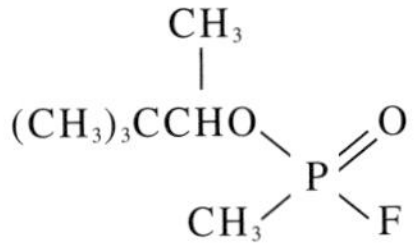 CH_3 $\vert$ $(CH_3)_3CCHO \backslash \quad //O$ P $CH_3 / \quad \backslash F$
GE	—	Isopropyl ethylphosphonofluoridate 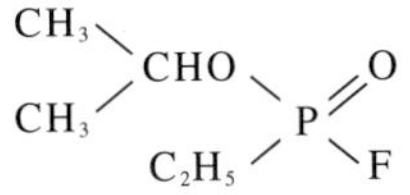 $CH_3 \backslash$ $CHO \; \backslash \quad //O$ $CH_3 /$ P $C_2H_5 \; / \quad \backslash F$
GF	—	Cyclohexyl methylphosphonofluoridate 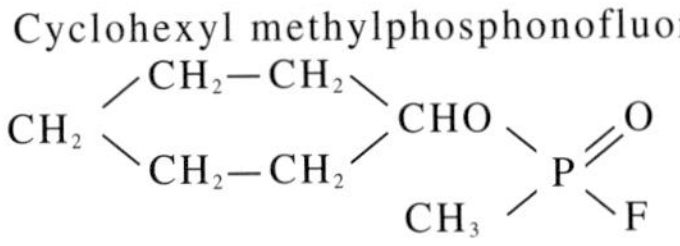 $/CH_2-CH_2\backslash$ $CH_2 \qquad CHO \; \backslash \quad //O$ $\backslash CH_2-CH_2/ \qquad P$ $CH_3 \; / \quad \backslash F$
VX	—	O-Ethyl S-[2-(diisopropylamino)ethyl] methylphosphonothioate 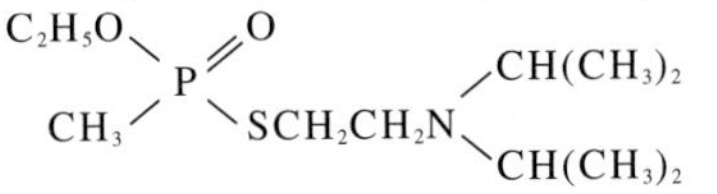 $C_2H_5O \backslash \quad //O$ $P \qquad /CH(CH_3)_2$ $CH_3 / \quad \backslash SCH_2CH_2N$ $\backslash CH(CH_3)_2$
VE	—	O-Ethyl S-[2-(diethylamino)ethyl] ethylphosphonothioate 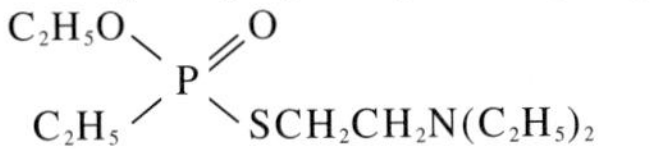 $C_2H_5O \backslash \quad //O$ P $C_2H_5 / \quad \backslash SCH_2CH_2N(C_2H_5)_2$
VG	—	O O-Diethyl S-[2-(diethylamino)ethyl] phosphorothioate 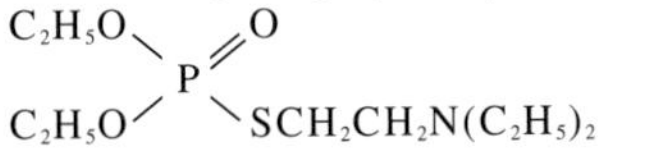 $C_2H_5O \backslash \quad //O$ P $C_2H_5O / \quad \backslash SCH_2CH_2N(C_2H_5)_2$
VM	—	O-Ethyl S-[2-(diethylamino)ethyl] methylphosphonothioate 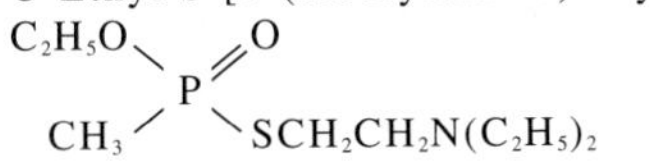 $C_2H_5O \backslash \quad //O$ P $CH_3 / \quad \backslash SCH_2CH_2N(C_2H_5)_2$

Figure 2. Formulas of nerve agents. (Adapted from Ballantyne B, Marust C, eds. *Clinical and experimental toxicology of organophosphates and carbamates.* Oxford: Butterworth-Heinemann, 1992.)

personnel. This means that medical personnel and hospitals must plan to be able to respond to such an incident. The agents that are discussed here include tabun, sarin, soman, and VX.

NERVE AGENTS

The nerve agents include tabun (GA), sarin (GB), VX, and soman. Their biologic and physical properties are provided in Table 1 and Figure 2.

The modern use of nerve agents began in World War II (7). A chemist named Gerhard Schrader was working on the development of organophosphate (OP) insecticides in 1936 when he developed the first nerve agent, tabun (GA). This was followed by sarin, named for the initials of the scientists involved in its creation (GB) (8). The German Ministry of Defense established a large production facility at Dyhernfurth. This facility produced tabun and sarin beginning in 1942 (8). Toward the end of the war, the Soviets captured the Dyhernfurth facility, dismantled it, and moved it to the former Soviet Union where production continued.

The nerve agents differ in their potential toxicities (Table 1). The LCt_{50} refers to the dose that kills 50% of unprotected humans expressed as a concentration per cubic meter and with a 1-minute exposure. The first three agents, tabun, sarin, and soman, are considered volatile agents, with characteristics that allow their suspension in air from a properly designed dissemination device. The larger vapor density of VX is manifested by its highly viscous nature, with a consistency similar to motor oil.

Difference between Organophosphorus Nerve Agents and Insecticides

Although many similarities exist between the OP insecticides and the nerve agents in terms of their pathophysiology and treatment, there are some differences. In cases of volatile nerve agent exposure, patients who do not present to the hospital with symptoms are not likely to become ill later. Several of the OP insecticides differ in this respect. Some agents such as fenthion and chlorfenthion may cause late onset of symptoms 12 or more hours after exposure due to their strong lipophilicity. The nerve agent VX can also cause severe symptomatology late after the exposure; however, the G agents (tabun, sarin, soman) typically have an onset of symptoms within minutes.

Another difference with the OP insecticides is in the development of sequelae. The chronic neuropathy associated with the OP insecticides does not appear to occur with the nerve agents. This is possibly due to the lack of effect on the neurotoxic esterase by nerve agents. A difference with respect to the dosing of atropine exists between the nerve agents and the insecticides. As noted in the following, OP insecticides may require extremely large doses of atropine, whereas nerve agents rarely require more than 20 to 30 mg of atropine.

Toxic Dose

A *sarin* dose of 2 μg/kg intravenously (IV) produced no symptoms in human subjects. The red cell cholinesterase was depressed to 28% of control values. No spontaneous recovery was seen. 2PAMCl 2.5 to 25 mg/kg was administered at 1 to 5 hours after sarin, resulting in reactivation of approximately 40% of the erythrocyte cholinesterase (RBC-ChE) (11,12).

Oral *VX* administration of 4.0 μg/kg resulted in a few symptoms (diarrhea, transient nausea) within 3 to 4 hours. The RBC cholinesterase was depressed to 70% below normal values. Spontaneous recovery occurred in some subjects within 24 to 48 hours. Pralidoxime chloride IV, 5 to 30 mg/kg, was administered at 5 to 48 hours after VX. All subjects exhibited reactivation of 70% of the inhibited enzyme. With an IV *VX* infusion of 1.5 μg/kg, most subjects experienced some lightheadedness and dizziness; some had nausea and vomiting within 1 hour. An increase in heart rate and blood pressure was observed at 3 hours. RBC cholinesterase was depressed to approximately 20% of normal in subjects with symptoms and to 28% of normal in asymptomatic subjects. Spontaneous recovery of RBC cholinesterase was observed at 1% per hour over 70 hours. Pralidoxime chloride 2.5 to 25 mg/kg IV at 0.5 to 24 hours after VX resulted in reactivation of 70% of the inhibited enzyme.

Pathophysiology

The general pathophysiology of acetylcholine, acetylcholinesterase, and acetylcholinesterase inhibition is addressed in detail in Chapter 236. Briefly, the neurotransmitter acetylcholine becomes attached to acetylcholinesterase (AChE) by weak ionic bonds. At the esteratic site, acetylcholine is cleaved into two simple molecules: acetate and choline. This enzyme has a high turnover number (number of substrate molecules that it catalyzes per unit time). Acetate goes into intermediate metabolism, and choline is taken up presynaptically and recycled by combination with acetyl CoA. It is catalyzed by the enzyme choline acetyltransferase, to form more acetylcholine.

Organophosphorus and carbamate compounds are attracted to this esteratic site of acetylcholinesterase, and, as a result of this attraction, acetylcholine cannot enter. This blocks the cleaving of the neurotransmitter and causes acetylcholine accumulation in the synapse. Carbamates attach to both the anionic and esteratic sites. A portion of the carbamate is immediately cleaved off. The enzyme remains inactive during the time in which the carbamate remains carbamoylated to this esteratic site. This hydrolysis step may take 1 hour in the case of the pharmaceutical agent physostigmine, or several hours in the case of pyridostigmine. Carbamate inactivation of acetylcholinesterase is always reversible.

In contrast to the carbamates, most organophosphates attach only to the esteratic site of acetylcholinesterase. Nerve agents and organophosphorus insecticides combine with the hydroxyl group of a serine residue, leaving an inactive phosphorylated form of the enzyme. Depending on the size of the alkyl group on the organophosphate molecule, hydrolytic cleavage may take a long time to occur, or may not occur at all. If this bond becomes permanent, the enzyme remains inactivated definitively. New enzyme must be synthesized for the synapse to function normally once again. In the case of red blood cells, this period of regeneration corresponds to the life of the cell, or 120 days.

Wherever acetylcholine excess is found, there are symptoms of cholinergic excess (Chapter 236). Acetylcholine is the neurotransmitter at the neuromuscular endplate and for the parasympathetic nervous system. It is also the neurotransmitter at the ganglionic level for the sympathetic and parasympathetic nervous systems. As a result of this, neurotransmitter excess is manifested in the sympathetic and parasympathetic nervous system. Ganglionic, nicotinic cholinergic excess can result in tachycardia, hypertension, and mydriasis, which may be misleading for the clinician who expects to see the classic cholinergic (muscarinic) findings.

Clinical Presentation

The primary diagnosis of exposure to nerve agents is based on the signs and symptoms of victims. The majority of exposed patients presents with miosis in the case of the volatile agents. Victims of VX exposure usually do not manifest miosis. The more severely intoxicated patients present with vomiting and seizures. Observation of these effects should provoke the inclusion of nerve agent exposure in the mind of the treating physician. The combination of miosis and muscle fasciculation is considered pathognomonic of organophosphate exposure. If several patients present with the same symptoms, this should cause the physician and hospital staff to consider the possibility of a terrorist attack with these agents. If a chemical attack occurs, one would expect that the majority of victims would arrive within a short period of time (hours) during the same day as the exposure.

The cholinergic symptoms are listed in Table 2. It is of special importance to include the important findings of bronchorrhea and bronchoconstriction in one's effort to remember this toxic syndrome. These are the principal causes of death in organophosphate poisoning. The resolution of pulmonary and bronchial complications constitutes the primary endpoint of treatment. The common mnemonic SLUDGE (*s*alivation, *l*acrimation, *u*rination, *d*iaphoresis/defecation, *G*I motility, *e*mesis) leaves out this important endpoint and should not be used for teaching health care providers the characteristics of the cholinergic (muscarinic) toxic syndrome.

Vapor exposures tend to primarily affect the areas they have contact with, eyes (miosis) or lungs (bronchoconstriction) (Table 3). In contrast, dermal application of the same agent often produces local effects of fasciculation and sweating. Systemic effects may follow and may be delayed (Table 4).

SARIN

A 52-year-old man was exposed to sarin nerve agent and developed the following signs: cyanosis, seizures, labored respirations, miosis, muscle fasciculations, marked salivation, and rhinorrhea. He was treated with atropine (14 mg in 1 day), pralidoxime chloride (2 g in 150 ml normal saline IV) given three times over the first 2 hours, oxygen, assisted ventilation, and nasogastric suction. The patient recovered within several days after a period of emotional lability but died of an acute myocardial infarction 18 months later.

TABLE 2. Signs and symptoms of nerve agent poisoning

Site of action	Signs and symptoms
After local exposure	
Muscarinic	
Pupils	Miosis, marked, usually maximal (pinpoint), sometimes unequal
Ciliary body	Frontal headache, eye pain on focusing, blurring of vision
Nasal mucous membranes	Rhinorrhea, hyperemia
Bronchial tree	Tightness in chest, bronchoconstriction, increased secretion, cough
Gastrointestinal	Occasional nausea and vomiting
After systemic absorption (depending on dose)	
Bronchial tree	Tightness in chest, with prolonged wheezing expiration suggestive of bronchoconstriction or increased secretion, dyspnea, pain in chest, increased bronchial secretion, cough, cyanosis, pulmonary edema
Gastrointestinal	Anorexia, nausea, vomiting, abdominal cramps, epigastric and substernal tightness (cardiospasm) with "heartburn" and eructation, diarrhea, tenesmus, involuntary defecation
Sweat glands	Increased sweating
Salivary glands	Increased salivation
Lacrimal glands	Increased lacrimation
Heart	Bradycardia
Pupils	Miosis, occasionally unequal, later maximal miosis (pinpoint)
Ciliary body	Blurring of vision, headache
Bladder	Frequency, involuntary micturition
Nicotinic	
Striated muscle	Easy fatigue, mild weakness, muscular twitching, fasciculations, cramps, generalized weakness/flaccid paralysis (including muscles of respiration) with dyspnea and cyanosis
Sympathetic ganglia	Pallor, transitory elevation of blood pressure followed by hypotension
Central nervous system	Immediate (acute) effects: generalized weakness, depression of respiratory and circulatory centers with dyspnea, cyanosis, and hypotension; convulsions, loss of consciousness, and coma
	Delayed (chronic) effects: giddiness, tension, anxiety, jitteriness, restlessness, emotional lability, excessive dreaming, insomnia, nightmares, headaches, tremor, withdrawal and depression, bursts of slow waves of elevated voltage in electroencephalogram (especially on hyperventilation), drowsiness, difficulty concentrating, slowness of recall, confusion, slurred speech, ataxia

Adapted from Army FM8-285, Navy NAVMED P-5041, Air Force AFM 160-11 Field Manual. The treatment of chemical agent casualties and conventional military chemical injuries. Washington: Departments of the Army, the Navy, and the Air Force; February 28, 1990.

Three adults experienced a sudden onset of rhinorrhea and slight respiratory discomfort, miosis, eye pain, increase in salivation, scattered wheezes, and rhonchi. Symptoms were mild, no treatment was given, and the RBC cholinesterase (lowest values 20% to 40% of normal) spontaneously recovered in 20 (plasma cholinesterase) to 90 days (RBC cholinesterase) (13,14).

Two adults accidentally exposed to sarin vapor (0.09 mg/m^3) exhibited RBC cholinesterase levels of 19% and 84%, respectively, and developed fixed extremely miotic pupils (15). No other signs or symptoms developed, and neither man required treatment. Recovery to normal cholinesterase activity was gradual over a 90-day period. Pupillary reflexes were not detectable 11 days after exposure. The miotic pupils dilated slowly over a 30- to 45-day period (16). Inhibition of red cell cholinesterase activity appears to be directly related to the dose of sarin. After exposure to sarin at a concentration of 2.73 mg/m^3 for 2 minutes, one of two subjects manifested a 23% RBC cholinesterase inhibition. Pupillary contraction remained constant for 24 hours (17). Workers exposed to sarin three or more times within the previous 6 years developed long-term brain abnormalities reflected in the electroencephalogram (18–20).

TABLE 3. Effects of vapor exposure to nerve agents[a]

Exposure to small amount (local effects)
- Miosis
- Rhinorrhea
- Slight bronchoconstriction/secretions (slight dyspnea)

Exposure to moderate amount (local effects)
- Miosis
- Rhinorrhea
- Bronchoconstriction/secretions (moderate to marked dyspnea)

Exposure to large amount
- As above plus the following:
- Loss of consciousness
- Convulsions (seizures)
- Generalized fasciculations
- Flaccid paralysis
- Apnea
- Involuntary micturition/defecation

[a]Onset within seconds to several minutes after onset of exposure.
Adapted from Sidell FR. In: Somani SM, ed. *Chemical warfare agents.* San Diego: Academic Press, 1992:155–194.

SOMAN

There are few cases of soman poisoning. A 33-year-old male laboratory technician was working with 1 ml of 25% (V/V) soman solution and broke the pipette, splashing a small amount into and around his mouth. "He immediately washed his face and rinsed his mouth with water and was brought to the emergency room . . . about 5 to 10 minutes after the accident. He complained of impending doom and immediately collapsed. His physical examination revealed him to be comatose with labored respirations and he was slightly cyanotic. He had miosis . . . markedly injected conjunctiva, marked oral and nasal secretions, moder-

TABLE 4. Effects of dermal exposure to nerve agents

Minimal exposure
- Increased sweating at site of exposure
- Muscular fasciculations at site of exposure

Moderate exposure
- Increased sweating at site
- Muscular fasciculations at site
- Nausea, vomiting, and diarrhea
- Feeling of generalized weakness
- May be precipitant in onset after long (4–18 h) asymptomatic interval

Severe exposure
- The previous may be present
- Loss of consciousness (may be precipitous in onset after asymptomatic interval)
- Convulsions (seizures)
- Generalized fasciculations
- Flaccid paralysis
- Apnea
- Involuntary micturition/defecation

Adapted from Sidell FR. In: Somani SM, ed. *Chemical warfare agents.* San Diego: Academic Press, 1992:155–194.

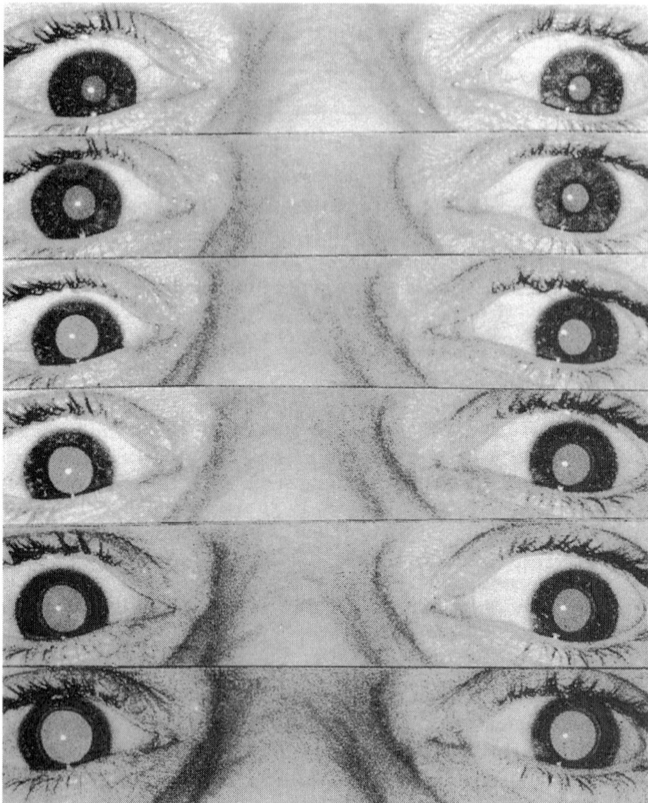

Figure 3. Prolonged miosis after accidental exposure to soman. As with other volatile agents, miosis tends to be predominant and is prolonged. This fascinating series of photographs was taken by Dr. Frederick Sidell to demonstrate the long duration of miosis after soman exposure. These photographs were taken over a 62-day period in which the patient was maximally dark-adapted, then a flash photograph was taken of the pupil faster than its ability to constrict. (From Sidell FR, M.D., 1974, with permission.)

ate trismus and nuchal rigidity, prominent muscular fasciculations, and hyperactive deep-tendon reflexes. Except for tachycardia, his heart, lungs, and abdomen were normal" (14).

After a total of 12 mg of atropine as well as pralidoxime, bronchoconstriction became less severe; however, he could not be intubated because of trismus. He received a tracheostomy and awoke after approximately 30 minutes. His hospital course was described as difficult with persistent fasciculations, nausea, weakness, and restlessness. Although previous publications referred to worsening cholinergic symptomatology with the use of phenothiazines, he was given a dose of Phenergan. He later developed torticollis that responded to diphenhydramine (21,22). A remarkable feature of this case was the requirement of anticholinergic therapy for 5 more weeks (Fig. 3). Scopolamine was administered with varying effects during the hospital course. The drug seemed more beneficial at the beginning, and detrimental toward the end of his medical care (23).

Diagnostic Tests

CHOLINESTERASE MEASUREMENT

There are two types of cholinesterases in the blood, which are not identical to the tissue enzyme but provide an accessible source for measuring body cholinesterase activity. The two types are serum or butyrylcholinesterase (BChE) and erythrocyte (RBC) cholinesterase. BChE is also described as serum or *pseudocholinesterase*. The RBC cholinesterase is thought to be a more representative marker for tissue AChE activity. Cholinesterase levels may vary depending on ethnicity and other genetic factors, nutritional status, and underlying disease states. Considerable variation occurs between individuals.

Studies that have attempted to relate symptoms of toxicity to AChE levels have found a greater correlation to RBC cholinesterase than to BChE (23,24). Many OP insecticides preferentially inhibit BChE, whereas nerve agents such as VX tend to inhibit RBC cholinesterase to a greater degree (13,25). Once inhibited, BChE is resynthesized more rapidly than RBC cholinesterase, which takes approximately 120 days to return to normal, or 1% per day (26). BChE requires approximately 50 days to return to normal levels. BChE less than 20% of predicted was a useful prognostic indicator for poor outcome in the Tokyo sarin terrorist attack (27).

Symptoms vary in the degree that they relate to serum cholinesterase levels. Eye and airway signs are caused principally by direct exposure and have little correlation to RBC-AChE levels (28–30).

AGENT IDENTIFICATION

A capillary column gas chromatography–mass spectrometry method is available for tabun determinations. Gas chromatography retention indices have been determined for 22 chemical warfare agents (32).

Treatment

Treatment of nerve agents should always follow proper decontamination of the victims (discussed in the following section). If contaminated patients are brought into the hospital, many of the staff members may become secondarily contaminated and develop injury from exposure to the nerve agent involved (33).

DECONTAMINATION

PPE refers to special garments designed to protect the members of the decontamination team against exposure to the toxic materials. The components of PPE include suits, eye protection, boots, gloves, and respiratory devices. There are various types of PPE available depending on the agent involved and the risk of exposure. Not all hospital staff members require sophisticated PPE provided that victims are adequately decontaminated before entering the hospital. All personnel who work with decontaminated patients should work in a well-ventilated environment and use basic universal precautions including the use of a face mask. Universal precautions do not prevent the inhalation of a nerve agent; however, they do minimize the risk of secondary contamination from splash and small amounts of contaminants that might not be removed from the victim.

The use of more sophisticated PPE is required by any personnel who is involved in decontamination and also for those involved with the initial triage of victims. Those who use this type of equipment are required to receive appropriate training as mandated by the U.S. Occupational Safety and Health Administration (29 CFR 1910.120 and 19410.134), and also in some cases by the National Institute for Occupational Safety and Health, the U.S. Environmental Protection Agency, and Joint Commission on Accreditation of Healthcare Organizations.

Decontamination is the process of physically removing toxic substances from a victim, equipment, or supplies. In the hospital setting, it is imperative to avoid the introduction of contaminated elements into the clinical setting. In most cases, victims arrive at the hospital nearest to the incident with no prior decontamination. Institutions should have a plan for decontaminating victims of hazardous material incidents, including those involving terrorist nerve agents. In the terrorist sarin incident in Tokyo, many hos-

TABLE 5. Recommended nerve agent treatment (Soldier Biological and Chemical Command, 2003)

Type of exposure	Presentation	Antidotal therapy	Observation
Mild vapor (GA, GB, BD) exposure	Nasal congestion with mild shortness of breath; miosis	One Mark I kit or 2 mg atropine, 1 g 2PAMCl[a]	Miosis may not reverse with treatment
Mild liquid (VX) exposure	Localized sweating and fasciculations	One Mark I kit or 2 mg atropine, 1 g 2PAMCl	—
Moderate vapor or liquid exposure	More severe respiratory distress, muscular weakness	One or two Mark I kits or 2–4 mg atropine, 1 g 2PAMCl intravenous drip over 30 min[a]	—
Severe vapor or liquid exposure	Unconscious, possibly seizing or flaccid, possibly apneic or severe symptoms	Three Mark I kits or 6 mg atropine and 1 g 2PAMCl initially[a]	May repeat atropine as needed and 2PAMCl in 1 h

[a]See text for the unique features of soman intoxication.

pital personnel were secondarily contaminated due to their involvement in removing clothing or working in poorly ventilated environments. At one research institution, the Keio University School of Medicine, 13 people developed symptoms of secondary contamination from off-gassing of the nerve agent (33).

For the volatile agents such as sarin, the decontamination is nearly complete with the simple removal of clothing and jewelry by the decontamination team. Use of large amounts of low-pressure water adequately completes the decontamination along with the use of soap and a gentle brush to assist in the removal of fat-soluble substances. Decontamination is most ideally undertaken outdoors near the hospital emergency department. This outdoor setting is especially suitable for areas of the United States with milder weather. Indoor facilities are necessary in conditions of severe winter weather. Security personnel should have a plan to direct traffic to this area, and to prevent entry of persons into other parts of the hospital. Signs, the presence of security personnel, and locking access points help to assure the proper flow of traffic.

Bleach solutions have been advocated for use in decontaminating victims of chemical agents. Although there may be some benefit to the use in certain circumstances, for example, immediately after a mustard exposure, it is not necessary for this to be done to living victims in the setting of a nerve agent exposure. Cadavers exposed to nerve agents may require special hypochlorite treatment, however. Simple soap and water are adequate for other circumstances. In a large-scale exposure such as the sarin attack in Tokyo—in which more than 600 patients arrived within the first hours after the incident—concern over use of hypochlorite is inappropriate. The simple removal of clothing and jewelry outside of the facility by properly protected decontamination personnel essentially eliminates the secondary contamination problems experienced in the Tokyo incident.

SUPPORTIVE CARE

The acute management of the patient with nerve agent exposure involves rapid establishment of a patent airway. The major cause of death is hypoxia resulting from pulmonary and bronchial involvement with the toxin. In cases of severe bronchoconstriction and bronchorrhea, it may be necessary to provide atropine before other interventions are attempted. Endotracheal intubation may be difficult without the application of atropine due to the extremely high airway resistance resulting from bronchoconstriction, on the order of 50 to 70 cm H_2O. This is higher than the pressure allowed by the *pop-off* valve of most bag-valve mask devices.

Patients who respond to treatment initially begin to show small skeletal muscle movements. They progress to spontaneous, random movements of the limbs and then a struggle against the ventilation. These may be alternating periods of spontaneous breathing and apnea. Weakness and obtundation may persist for 1 or more days. Miosis and subtle mental change may persist for weeks (34–36).

ANTIDOTES

Three pharmaceutical agents are considered essential in the management of nerve agent exposure and OP insecticide intoxication: atropine, pralidoxime, and diazepam (or other benzodiazepines).

Atropine. *Atropine* is an agent with both systemic and central effects to combat the effects of acetylcholine excess at muscarinic sites. Atropine dosing should begin with typical advanced cardiac life support doses of 1 to 2 mg but may require much more than the usual amounts after this initial test-dose (Table 5). Lack of response to normal doses of atropine supports the diagnosis of OP toxicity. Patients with severe muscarinic effects require larger amounts of atropine. The endpoint of atropine administration is the clearing of bronchial secretions and decreasing ventilatory resistance. This is an essential point to remember, because heart rate and pupil diameter are not useful parameters for monitoring the response to treatment with this antidote. Nebulized bronchodilators such as albuterol are not as effective as atropine at treating nerve agent exposure, due to the need for an anticholinergic effect (7).

Typical doses for atropine in severely intoxicated nerve agent casualties are in the range of 5 to 15 mg (14,37). This is in sharp contrast to the much larger doses required in organophosphate insecticide intoxication, in which several grams of atropine may be required in the first days of treatment (38,39). In cases of severe organophosphate poisoning, an IV drip is implemented to meet the continuing requirement for atropinization (40). The OP insecticides may be sequestered in lipid compartments or may require a greater time for metabolism. Hence the need for prolonged treatment in many cases of poisoning by these agents. The method of administration, contraindications, and adverse effects associated with atropine are addressed in Chapter 42.

The U.S. military supplies kits containing the two most important antidotes for nerve agent exposure, atropine and pralidoxime. The military kit, known as the *Mark I*, consists of two autoinjector pens. The smaller autoinjector contains 2 mg of atropine for intramuscular administration. The autoinjector mechanism provides remarkable rapid absorption (Fig. 4). After the atropine is administered, the pralidoxime is administered in the same fashion either to the same thigh or to the opposite side. The atropine autoinjectors each contain 2 mg of atropine citrate. Such kits are also available commercially for civilian use (Meridian Medical Technologies, St. Louis, MO). These autoinjectors permit rapid intramuscular injection of antidote through protective clothing and underlying garments. Military medical personnel carry additional atropine autoinjectors and are trained to add

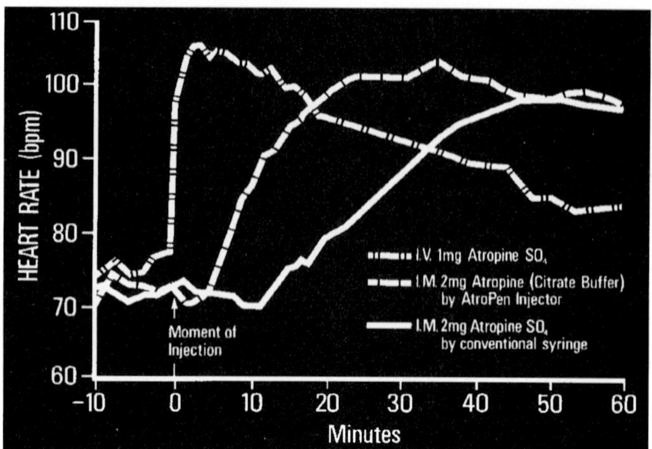

Figure 4. Absorption of atropine administered by autoinjector device. The authors used heart rate to demonstrate the effect of atropine administration given either intravenously, intramuscularly, or by autoinjector. The graph illustrates the effectiveness of the device. Intravenous administration causes an effect more rapidly but has a shorter duration of action.

more atropine as required based on the endpoints of good control of respiratory secretions and adequate respiratory effort (41).

Oximes. The oximes (pralidoxime, obidoxime) are nucleophilic substances that reactivate the acetylcholinesterase inhibited by OP toxins. An oxime should be administered before aging occurs. Aging occurs at different time intervals from exposure for different nerve agents. For example, sarin requires several hours to age, whereas soman ages in only 2 to 6 minutes and VX takes more than 2 days (Table 6). The time for complete aging is approximately 10 times the half-life, and treatment with an oxime may be useful up to this point.

Once the oxime has regenerated acetylcholinesterase, the enzyme resumes its critical role in the breakdown of acetylcholine, normalizing neurotransmission. This brings about the improvement of nicotinic symptoms such as fasciculations, muscle twitching, and the return to normal muscle strength. Pralidoxime as the chloride (2PAMCl) or mesylate (P2S) probably is best administered in a dose of 30 mg/kg body weight over a 30-minute period every 4 to 6 hours, preferably by IV injection, but it can also be given by intramuscular injection (Table 5). Oxime concentrations more than 4 μg/ml can be maintained for 3 to 6 hours after intramuscular injections of 30 mg/kg body weight of either oxime (chloride or mesylate). Alternatively, 2-PAM (chloride or mesylate) can be given as a continuous infusion at a rate of 550 mg/hour (8 mg/kg/hour) after the injection of 30 mg/kg/body weight on two occasions 4 hours apart (38). PAM should be continued as long as the OP compound or its active metabolite is present in the body. The method of administration, precautions, and adverse effects of the oximes are provided in Chapter 69.

TABLE 6. Aging

Agents	Aging half-life
Tabun	46 h
Sarin	5.2–12 h
VX	>12 d
Soman	40 sec to 10 min
Paraxon	2.1–5.4 d

Adapted from Dunn MA, Sidell RF. *JAMA* 1989;262:649–652.

Benzodiazepines. Benzodiazepines (diazepam, lorazepam, others) should be used to treat the seizures induced by the nerve agents. This can be administered IV or through the use of an autoinjector. Military sources suggest that in patients manifesting symptoms of severe toxicity, benzodiazepines should be administered even before seizures are evident. If three of the MARK I kits are administered (due to more severe symptomatology), diazepam should be administered immediately after completing the administration with the autoinjector kits. With the exception of benzodiazepines, conventional treatment modalities for seizures are considered ineffective in this setting, including phenytoin (42).

Treatment of nerve agent casualties should be based on the initial signs and symptoms, and modified appropriately when the actual agent is defined. If the exposure was a volatile agent, such as sarin or soman, the patients are symptomatic within the first hour of exposure to the toxin. This usually means that patients who are not symptomatic when they are evaluated at the hospital are not likely to become serious exposure victims. For the case of the liquid exposure of VX, patients may not become symptomatic for up to 18 hours and therefore should be observed for a much longer period of time. If the exposure history is not certain, it is prudent to institute the longer observation period for these patients. The degree of symptomatology determines the dose of the antidotal therapy (Table 5).

PYRIDOSTIGMINE PRETREATMENT

The use of atropine and the oximes may be insufficient for protection against the toxic effects of GD (soman), even if they are administered immediately after the agent. Soman exhibits rapid *aging* (within minutes). As Dunn and Sidell have emphasized (43), even with training and the ability to don a mask rapidly, soldiers on a chemical battlefield may be at risk for absorbing up to five times the lethal dose of GD during a chemical attack. The *protective ratio* (43,44) is the factor by which a treatment raises the lethal dose of a toxic agent. Antidotes have not yet been devised that can raise the protective ratio sufficiently high in humans to counteract the lethal effects of GD. Therefore, a preexposure treatment has been sought. Pretreatment is not effective against sarin and VX challenge. When used for soman challenge, it should be followed by atropine and an oxime.

Pyridostigmine by itself does not provide protection without the use of the antidotes (atropine/oximes). It is an antidote *enhancer* rather than a *true* treatment. It appears to enhance the efficacy of the antidotes within 1 to 3 hours after taking the first tablet. Maximal benefit appears to develop with time and may be reached when a tablet is taken every 8 hours (41).

The U.S. Army provides a pyridostigmine bromide (30 mg) pretreatment set of tablets (21 total) packaged in a blister pack, to be taken one every 8 hours, enough for 7 days. One tablet is taken orally with water (41).

PITFALLS

It is essential for institutions to prepare for large numbers of casualties. Atropine may be obtained as a powdered form, which may be compounded in the hospital pharmacy. The powdered drug has a much longer shelf life than does the atropine-containing solution. One alternative is to have enough atropine solution on hand for 30 to 40 casualties, and use the powdered form after the initial stock is completed. Compounding of atropine solution from the powdered form can be initiated in the pharmacy after the first cases arrive at the hospital.

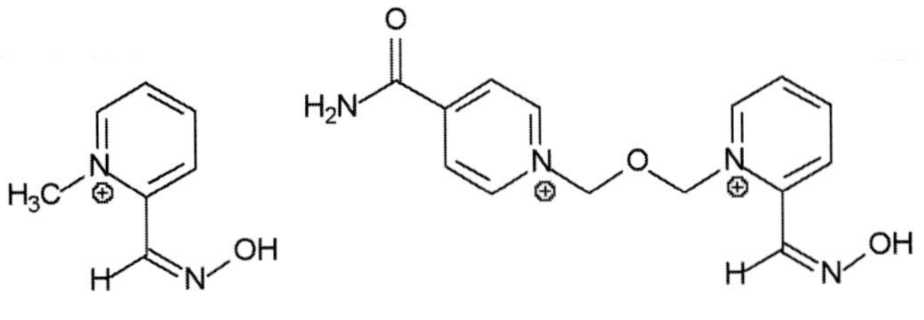

Figure 5. Oxime acetylcholinesterase reactivators. 2-PAM, pralidoxime.

In the United States, the only oxime widely available is pralidoxime. The data for pralidoxime with soman are rather unique. In an experiment using rat, monkey, and human muscle tissue, Clement demonstrated that pralidoxime is ineffective in the treatment of soman poisoning. Hence, the agent most commonly used in the United States would not be useful for treatment of this particular poison. The lethal dose for soman is approximately 50 mg. One problem with soman is the extremely rapid aging time. Aging occurs in approximately 2 minutes, making the application of an agent such as pralidoxime essentially useless.

The bispyridinium oximes offer some promise as a treatment for soman. The structure includes an additional oxime ring: a nitrogen-substituted benzene ring with a side group. By combining oximes into larger molecules, antidotes have been developed that are effective against nerve agents. One such agent is HI-6 (Fig. 5). Hamilton investigated the efficacy of the bispyridinium agent HI-6 after giving monkeys five times an LD_{50} of soman. Three out of four monkeys survived using the newer oxime (45). One of the interesting aspects of this case was the fact that acetylcholinesterase inhibition was the same for the monkeys that survived and those that died. Thus, some factor is involved in the efficacy of the bispyridinium agent other than acetylcholinesterase reactivation. Some have suggested that it is the brain cholinesterase that makes the difference in survival. However, in a study involving rat brain homogenate cholinesterase activity, essentially no improvement enzyme reactivation could be found from pralidoxime (46). The mechanisms involved in oxime antidotal efficacy are still to be fully elucidated (47). There is not a perfect oxime reactivator that is effective for all agents. However, a combination of oxime agents would offer a more complete spectrum of protection (48).

VESICANT AGENTS

The vesicant agents include the sulfur mustards, nitrogen mustards, arsenicals, and phosgene oxime (Table 7). They act on the eyes, mucous membranes, lungs, skin, and blood-forming organs. They incapacitate many more people than they kill. In World War I, approximately 5% of victims died from exposure to chemical agents (41,49–67,69–72,74,76,79,80). Some vesicants have a faint odor; others are odorless. Odor is not a useful way to detect these agents because one may be intoxicated if within olfactory distance of the source. Smells reported by patients, however, can provide useful information on which to base a diagnosis. Lewisite (L) and phosgene oxime cause immediate pain on contact. Sulfur mustard and nitrogen mustards are insidious in action, with little or no pain at the time of exposure. Signs of injury may not appear for several hours (41,49,50). Metabolites may be found in the urine (81–83). Physical properties of the vesicants are delineated in the U.S. Army Field Manual (50,52–56).

TABLE 7. Vesicants or blister agents

Sulfur mustards	
HD	2,2'-Di(chloroethyl) sulfide
Nitrogen mustards	
HN-1	2,2-Dichlorotriethylamine
HN-2	2,2-Dichloro-*N*-methyldiethylamine
HN-3	2,2,2-Trichlorotriethylamine
Arsenicals	
MD	Methyldichloroarsine
PD	Phenyldichloroarsine
ED	Ethyldichloroarsine
L	Lewisite (dichloro [2-chlorovinyl] arsine)
Oximes	
CX	Phosgene oxime (dichloroformoxime)
Mixtures of mustards and arsenicals	
HL	Mustard-lewisite mix: 63% L and 37% HD, by weight
HT	Mustard-T(*bis*-[2-chloroethyl sulfide] monoxide) mix 60% HD and 40% T by weight—not in production

Mustards were named for their pungent mustard-garlic odor (84–86). Mustard gas was first used offensively by the German army at Ypres, Belgium, in July 1917 (84–86). This led to the use of nicknames: Yperite (French after Ypres), Lost (German after the name of two chemists Lommel and Steinkopf who were able to mass produce the substance), Yellow-Cross (after the markings on the mustard-containing shell cases), and HS (Hun Stuff) (84). From July 1917 to the end of World War I, British casualties from mustard gas amounted to at least 125,000 with approximately 1859 deaths (84). In World War II, no chemical agents were used, but from 1945 to 1948 large stockpiles of chemical weapons, including mustard gas, were dumped into the Baltic Sea. Corrosion weakened the containers, and the shells broke when they were brought on board fishing trawlers, leading to mustard gas poisoning of 23 fishermen in 1984 (56). Finally, mustard gas appeared to have been used by Iraqi forces during the Iran-Iraq conflict (57,58,64,65,69,74). Exposure to mustard agents continues to be a risk for workers at chemical weapon storage facilities (87). The long-term sequelae of mustard exposure for veterans exposed during World War I have been the subject of ongoing debate (88). These agents were verified as having been used in the Iran-Iraq conflict as well (89).

Pathophysiology

Sulfur mustard consists of two ethyl groups bound together around an atom of sulfur. The terminal H bonds have been replaced by chlorine atoms. Mustards are powerful alkylating agents and react with amino, thiol, carboxyl, hydroxyl, and primary phosphate groups (Fig. 6) (49,90). As a result of its alkylating and electrophilic properties, mustard gas is able to change the structure of nucleic acids, cellular membranes, and proteins (56). Mustard gas causes a cross-linking of the two complementary strands in the deoxyribonucleic acid molecule by a monofunctional alkylation of the nitrogenous bases. This cross-linking prevents the separation of the strands required for normal replications of the deoxyribonucleic acid molecule and so interferes with deoxyribonucleic acid syntheses and cellular division (56). Indigenous antioxidants may play a limited role in natural protection against this type of mustard injury (91). Mustard gas may induce long-term mutagenic and carcinogenic changes (56,61,63).

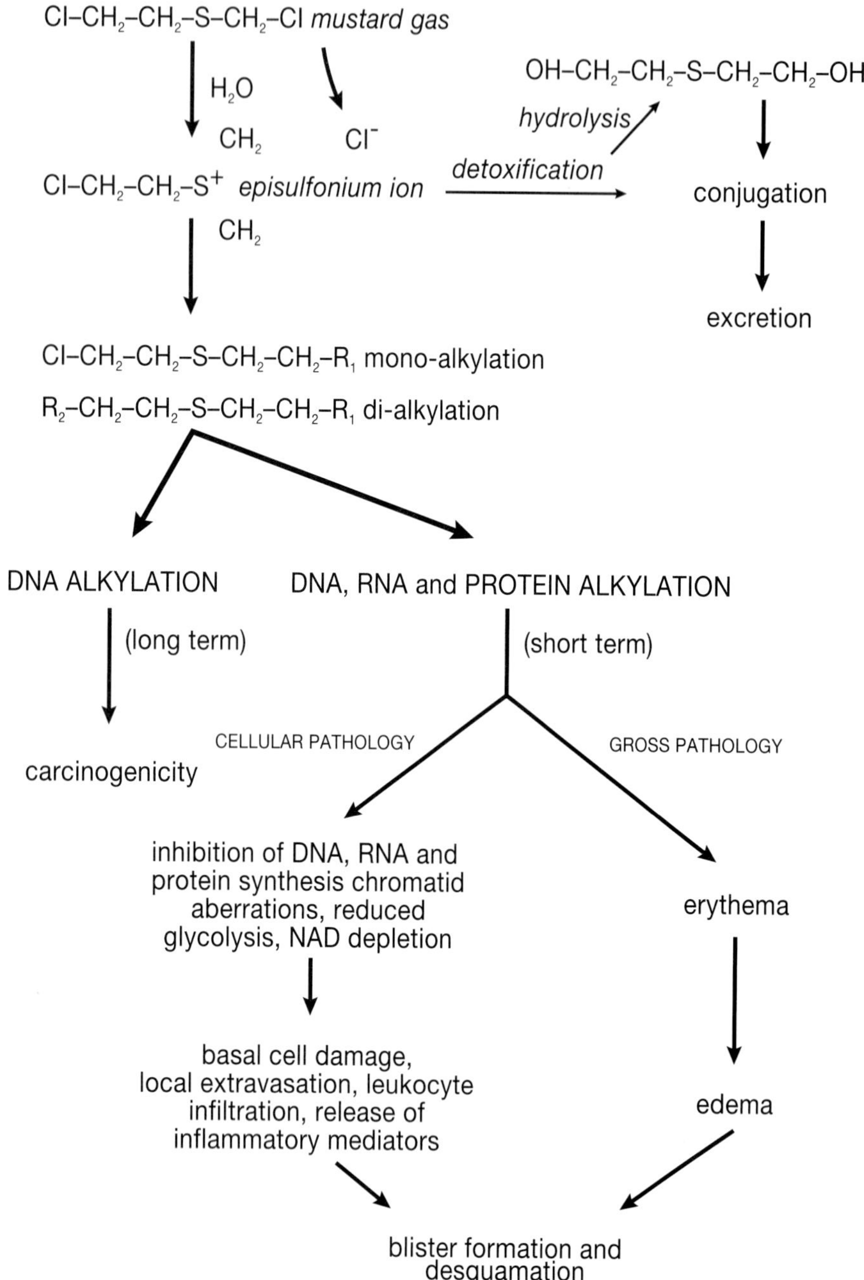

Figure 6. Proposed mechanism of action of mustard gas–induced lesions. (Adapted from Wormser U. *Trends Pharmacol Sci* 1991;12:164-167.)

Vulnerable Populations

There are not useful data available for the mustard as a war agent; however, related therapeutic agents (e.g., nitrogen mustards) cause birth defects when administered to pregnant patients (92).

Clinical Presentation

SULFUR MUSTARD

Mustard gas (either vapor or liquid) causes damage to the skin, eyes, respiratory system, and gastrointestinal tract, as well as having a general effect on the body similar to that of radioactive radiation. Ingestion of food or water contaminated by liquid mustard produces nausea and vomiting, pain, bloody diarrhea, and prostration resulting from dehydration (54,56).

Skin effects appear after a delay after exposure and are described in Table 8. Ocular effects including conjunctival irritation, lacrimation, photophobia, dryness, pain, blepharospasm, and corneal ulceration may develop after a delay of 4 to 6 hours. The injury from mustard is limited to the anterior segment of the eye (93). The periocular area is red and edematous. In severe cases, blindness may occur. Recovery from a mild conjunctivitis may take 1 to 2 weeks; from a severe conjunctivitis, 2 to 5 weeks; and from mild corneal involvement, 2 to 3 months. A delayed keratopathy may develop decades later (94).

Pulmonary effects are also delayed. After a delay of 24 hours, inhalation of the gas produces hoarseness initially, which may progress to loss of voice (41). A cough (worse at night) appears early, and later becomes productive. Fever, dyspnea, and moist rhonchi and rales may develop. Bronchopneumonia frequently intervenes. Symp-

TABLE 8. Typical development of mustard skin lesion

Effect	Time after vapor exposure[a]
Earliest appearance of erythema	1 h
Definite erythema	2–3 h
Raised erythema (edema)	8–12 h
Pinhead vesication	13–22 h
Vesicles coalescing into blisters	16–48 h
Maximum blisters or necrosis	42–72 h
Complete skin surface denudation	6–9 d
Removal of scab	20–28 d
Complete healing	22–29 d

[a]Vapor cup exposure of forearm in healthy adult male volunteers at air temperature of 26°C with relative humidity of 51%. Exposure was 10 minutes with vapor cup containing 5- to 10-mg liquid mustard. Precise vapor concentration is not known. Adapted from Smith WJ, Dunn MA. *Arch Dermatol* 1991;127:1207–1213.

toms may persist for 1 or more years. The distinct features of bronchospasm on the one hand and chronic chemical injury and bronchitis on the other represent two independent syndromes resulting from inhalation exposure to this agent, although they can both be present in the same individual (95). Bronchoalveolar lavage reveals typical features of these two disease processes (96).

Systemic effects, including dizziness, anorexia, lethargy, and general malaise, may follow exposure. Although hemoglobin values, leukocyte, differential and platelet counts, lactate dehydrogenase and aspartate aminotransferase, and serum creatinine levels are usually normal, fatalities may follow severe exposure and are largely due to respiratory complications (55,65).

Long-term effects include eye problems, and recurrent bronchopneumonia may persist for many months. Exposure of human research subjects to the mustard gases during World War II has led to a number of long-term health effects: asthma, chronic bronchitis, emphysema, chronic laryngitis, corneal opacities, chronic conjunctivitis, and ocular keratitis. The Institute of Medicine has cited other health problems for which substantial causal relationship with exposure to sulfur or nitrogen mustard exists, including respiratory cancer (especially nasopharyngeal, laryngeal, and lung), skin cancer, pigmentation abnormalities of the skin, chronic skin ulceration and scar formation, recurrent ulcerative disease of the eye (including opacities), bone marrow depression, psychologic disorders, and scarring of the scrotum or penis which may result in sexual dysfunction (97).

Sister chromatid exchanges, a measure of mutagenicity and carcinogenicity, were present in increased rates in the lymphocytes of fishermen exposed to leaky mustard gas shells (66). Follow-up studies of workers in British mustard gas manufacture suggest an increase in the death rate from respiratory tract malignancies (63); similarly, an increased death rate from respiratory tract malignancies has been observed in Japanese and German mustard gas factories (55,61). Only a marginal increase in lung cancer was found in exposed servicemen from the United States 46 years later (98).

NITROGEN MUSTARD

In single exposures, nitrogen mustard irritates the eyes in doses that do not significantly damage the skin or respiratory tract. Respiratory tract symptoms and signs may be similar to those after exposure to mustard gas. Residual effects may include a persistent cough and low-grade fever for a few weeks. Severe exposure may terminate in a fatal pneumonia (41).

In humans, ingestion of 2 to 6 mg of a nitrogen mustard may result in nausea and vomiting. Animals develop severe hemorrhagic diarrhea (41).

Systemic effects of nitrogen mustard exposure after absorption from the skin or respiratory or gastrointestinal tracts may exert profound effects on the hematopoietic and lymphoid tissue. Degenerative bone marrow changes may be detected within 12 hours and may progress to severe aplasia. There may be a transient leukocytosis for a few hours, followed by severe lymphopenia, granulocytopenia, thrombocytopenia, and a moderate anemia.

ARSENICAL VESICANTS

Arsenical vesicants are more dangerous as liquids than as vapors. The liquids cause severe burns of the eyes and skin. Skin effects include stinging pain that is usually felt in 10 to 20 seconds after contact with liquid arsenical vesicants. In a few minutes, it becomes a deep, aching pain. In approximately 5 minutes, a gray area of dead epithelium appears, resembling that seen in corrosive burns. The pain lessens in 48 to 72 hours. Erythema and blisters are similar to the other vesicants. If the arsenical vesicant burn is large and deep, there may be considerable necrosis of tissue, gangrene, and slough.

Liquid arsenical vesicants cause severe damage to the eye, including the cornea, iris, and conjunctivae; this may terminate in permanent residual damage or blindness.

Respiratory lesions are similar to those after mustard gas. Pulmonary edema and pleural effusion may be observed. There have been no human cases of poisoning by vapors of arsenical vesicants. Systemic effects, including pulmonary edema, diarrhea, restlessness, weakness, hypothermia, and hypotension, have been observed in animals.

PHOSGENE OXIME

Phosgene oxime or dichloroformoxime has a disagreeable penetrating odor. It may be a liquid or a colorless, low-melting-point solid, soluble in water (41,49).

Phosgene oxime is irritating to the mucous membranes of the eyes and nose. Within 30 seconds, exposure to liquid or vapor can produce pain and skin necrosis at the site of contact. The original blanched area becomes brown in 24 hours, followed by eschar formation in 1 week; the eschar sloughs in approximately 3 weeks. Healing may be delayed for several months.

Diagnostic Tests

SULFUR MUSTARD

A method for quantitation of exposure to mustard gas was used to test urine samples of Iranian patients, victims of an alleged mustard gas attack in March 1984. The method analyzes thiodiglycol (2,2'-thiodiethanol) in the urine (83). The method is sensitive to 1 ng/ml. Thiodiglycol values may also be obtained from analyses of the skin, a possible retrospective method for verifying exposure to mustard gas (83). Unmetabolized mustard gas has been analyzed by a gas chromatography–mass spectrometry method (81,82).

Soil, metal fragments, and wool collected from and in the vicinity of a chemical warfare spill in Northern Iraq analyzed by gas chromatography–mass spectrometry techniques (full scanning, selective ion monitoring, thermal desorption) have yielded *bis*-(2-chloroethyl) sulfide (mustard); thiodiglycol; and other sulfides and other volatile breakdown products, including 1,4-oxathiane, 1,4-dithiane, and ethene 1,1-thio-bis. Sulfur mustard may persist in the soil for weeks if the ambient temperature and rainfall are both low. 1,4,6-Trinitrotoluene and tetryl suggest explosive components (99).

Urine thiodiglycol levels found in Iranians ranged from 5 to 336 ng/ml in one study (83) and from 1 to 30 ng/ml in another (80).

Treatment

SULFUR MUSTARD

Decontamination

1. If erythema has not appeared, known or likely skin areas of contamination may be decontaminated with immediate use of prewetted pad wipes (hydroxyethane 72%, phenol 10%, sodium hydroxide 5%, ammonia 0.2%, and water) and a pad impregnated with chloramine B. Cut away and discard hair contaminated with liquid mustard. If the above substances are not available, use 0.5% aqueous sodium hypochlorite solution for decontamination of the skin and hair. Wash off the decontaminating solutions within 3 to 4 minutes.
2. If erythema of the skin has appeared, soap and water are the best decontaminant.
3. Contaminated clothing should be promptly removed outside the treatment facility to prevent more severe burns and to lessen the vapor hazard to patients and attendants. Dermabrasion has been described as a treatment modality but requires further evaluation before use as definitive treatment (100).

Skin Erythema. If skin erythema is mild, no treatment is required. If pruritus exists, use topical steroid creams or compound calamine lotion (containing 1% each of phenol and menthol).

Skin Blisters. If the blisters have been broken, remove the ragged roof; if not broken, drain under aseptic conditions. Clean the area with tap water or saline with application of petrolatum gauze when the areas are small. For large blisters, apply thick layer of 10% mafenide acetate or silver sulfadiazine burn cream. Appropriate antibiotic drugs may be given locally or systemically as indicated.

Skin Pain. Intense burning pain during skin healing may not be controlled by antihistamines or opioids. Considerable relief has been observed with the use of carbamazepine 200 mg three times daily (50).

Eye Exposure. Self-aid should be performed within 2 minutes after exposure. Sterile petroleum jelly is used to prevent the lid margins from sticking together.

Mustard Conjunctivitis. Mild lesions may require little treatment. A steroid antibiotic eye ointment can be applied. Ophthalmic ointment such as 5% boric acid ointment provides lubrication and minimal antibacterial effects. If injuries are more severe, edema of the lids, photophobia, and blepharospasm may obstruct and alarm the patient. The lids may be gently forced open to provide assurance that the patient is not blinded. Pain is controlled by systemic narcotic analgesics. Severe photophobia and blepharospasm are treated with one drop of atropine sulfate solution (1%) instilled in the eye three times daily. To prevent infection, a few drops of 15% solution of sodium sulfacetamide should be instilled every 4 hours. Other antibacterial ointments may be substituted. Do not bandage the eye; the lids should not be allowed to stick together. Keep the patient in a darkened room. Dark glasses or an eyeshade may be worn for photophobia.

Infected Mustard Burns of the Eye. If infection develops, start with several drops of 15% solution of sodium sulfacetamide every 2 hours. Take cultures. Apply specific antibacterial preparations. Irrigate to remove accumulated exudate. Do not use local anesthetics. Refer to an ophthalmologist.

Respiratory Tract. Mild respiratory tract injury with hoarseness and sore throat only usually requires no treatment. Cough may be relieved by codeine-containing cough syrups. Laryngitis and tracheitis may be treated symptomatically with steam or sterile cool mist inhalations. For more severe respiratory tract injury, hospitalize. Treat chemical pneumonitis initially with broad-spectrum antibiotics. Perform culture and sensitivity studies on sputum. Use appropriate specific antibiotics. Severely affected patients may need assisted ventilation and oxygen-enriched air. Simple mouthwashes can be used for the oropharynx (54).

Systemic Mustard Poisoning. Atropine subcutaneously (0.4 to 0.8 mg) may be useful in reducing gastrointestinal activity. Discomfort and restlessness may be treated with sedatives but may also be a manifestation of hypovolemic shock from severe systemic injury. If severe systemic poisoning is present (vomiting, diarrhea, leukopenia, hemoconcentration, shock), maintain adequate nutritional status and replace loss of fluid and electrolytes. Monitor leukocytes and hemoglobin. For significant drops in the leukocyte count, isolation and appropriate antibiotics may be necessary. Sodium thiosulfate in a dose of 35 g IV (500 mg/kg) if given within 20 to 30 minutes of exposure may prevent or reduce damage from mustard. However, mustard gas is an alkylating agent that binds strongly to protein x, and it is unlikely that sodium thiosulfate is effective after a severe exposure. A monoclonal antibody that binds sulfur mustard is under development (101).

Most patients exposed to mustard gas recover completely. Only a small proportion have long-term eye or lung damage (50).

NITROGEN MUSTARD

Skin. Liquid nitrogen mustards are absorbed through the skin slower than mustards. Decontamination should be performed within 2 to 3 hours of exposure even if erythema is already present and no liquid nitrogen mustard is visible on the skin.

Eyes. Treat as with mustard gas. Lesions and symptoms may be more severe than with mustard; frequent instillations of atropine may be required for pain due to spasms of ciliary and orbicular muscles.

Respiratory. Treat as for mustard gas exposure.

Systemic. Frequent hematologic evaluations (hematocrit, peripheral blood counts, and platelets) are required. Vomiting and diarrhea require IV fluids with electrolyte or volume expanders. Isolate against infection. Use antibiotics vigorously as indicated. Use sedatives, opiates, and atropine with care.

ARSENICAL VESICANTS

Skin. If seen before actual vesication has occurred, dimercaprol (BAL) ointment should be tried, rubbed in with the fingers, allowed to remain at least 5 minutes, and then washed off with water. BAL may cause temporary stinging, itching, or urticarial wheals. Treatment of erythema, blisters, and denuded areas is similar to that for mustard lesions. For larger skin area exposure (more than 20% of body surface area or less than 20% if deep lesion), hospitalization is required. Débride wound, and treat with 10% mafenide acetate burn cream or silver sulfadiazine burn cream.

Eyes. Treatment is largely symptomatic. Occlusive dressings or pressure on the globe should be avoided. Atropine sulfate ointment, sodium sulfacetamide solution, and sterile petrolatum may be applied as indicated.

TABLE 9. Treatment protocol for British antilewisite (2,3-dimercapto-1-propanol) (dimercaprol)

Antidote/action	Dose	Overdose symptoms, management
Lifesaving in acute poisoning of arsenicals (except arsine) and solutions of organic Hg compounds. Also for chronic As or Au poisoning. Action by displacing the metal from its combination with sulfhydryl groups of enzyme proteins. Toxicity rating 4; very toxic. [Probable oral lethal dose is 50–500 mg/kg or 1 teaspoon to 1 ounce for 150-lb (70-kg) person.]	Intramuscularly into buttocks in dosage of 0.5 ml/25 lb body weight (commercial preparation of 10% British antilewisite in peanut oil) up to maximum of 4.0 ml. Repeat in 4, 8, 12 h. For severe cases, interval shortened to 2 h.	Consistent objective response in rise in systolic and diastolic blood pressure plus tachycardia (rapid heartbeat). Nausea and sometimes vomiting; headache; burning sensation of lips, mouth; feeling of constriction in throat, chest, hands; conjunctivitis, tearing, salivation; hand tingling; burning sensation in penis; sweating forehead and hands; abdominal pain; tremors; lower back pain; anxiety, weakness, and restlessness; tachycardia (rapid heartbeat) and elevated arterial blood pressure; persistent fever in children; occasional painful sterile abscesses at injection sites; coma and convulsions at high dose (in children, this occurs at 10, 25, and 40.5 mg/kg) (recovery prompt). Management symptoms usually subside in 30–90 min; intramuscular use of 1:100 solution epinephrine HCl (0.1–0.5 ml) or oral ephedrine sulfate (25–50 mg).

Adapted from Munro NB, et al. *Environ Health Perspect* 1990;89:205–215.

Respiratory. Treatment is similar to that after exposure to mustards.

Systemic Effects. Systemic treatment is indicated for the following: cough with dyspnea and frothy sputum, and signs of pulmonary edema or skin covering, skin burn the size of the palm of the hand not decontaminated within 15 minutes; skin contamination by a liquid arsenical vesicant covering 5% or more of body surface with signs of gray or dead-white blanching of skin or erythema developing within 30 minutes. Treatment includes local BAL ointment and intramuscular injection of BAL in oil (10%) (Tables 9 and 10). Further information on BAL is provided in Chapter 50. Treat shock supportively.

PHOSGENE OXIME

Treatment is symptomatic and supportive. If possible, flood the contaminated area as soon as possible with copious amounts of water. Recommended control limits are listed in Table 11. (See Vesicant Agents.)

TABLE 10. Chemical weapons, their effects, and treatment for exposure to them[a]

Agent	Toxicity	Signs and symptoms	Antidote	Care
Riot control agents (tear gas), CN (Mace), CS	Rarely life-threatening	Nose and eye irritation, coughing, mild dyspnea. Large dose: retching, burns.	None	Symptomatic treatment
Blister agents, nitrogen mustard, and sulfur mustard	Delayed effects; large dose life-threatening if untreated	Erythema; vesication; burns; eye, lung, and skin damage; respiratory effects; leukopenia; thrombocytopenia; decrease in RBCs; sepsis.	None; decontamination within 2 min to prevent tissue damage	Burn care, eye therapy, pulmonary support
Nerve agents: GA (tabun), GB (sarin), GD (soman), VX	Immediately life-threatening	Eye, nose, lung, and GI effects. Large dose: almost immediate loss of consciousness, convulsions, cessation of respiration, flaccid paralysis, copious nasal and oral secretions, intense bronchoconstriction.	Atropine sulfate, pralidoxime (Protopam) chloride	Administration of antidotes, ventilation, administration of diazepam (Valium)
Phosgene	Delayed effects possibly life-threatening if untreated	Eye and respiratory system irritation, dyspnea, massive pulmonary edema, hypotension, hypovolemia, bronchospasm, bronchosecretions, right ventricular failure, infection.	None	Close observation for at least 4 h, symptomatic treatment
Cyanide, hydrocyanic acid, cyanogen chloride	Immediately life-threatening	Inhalation: convulsions, death. Ingestion: dizziness, nausea, vomiting, weakness, respiratory distress, loss of consciousness, convulsions, apnea, death.	Amyl nitrite, sodium nitrite, sodium thiosulfate	Administration of antidotes, supplemental oxygen
Incapacitating agents				
Narcotic congeners[b] (e.g., fentanyl), tranquilizers[b]	Possibly life-threatening	Hypotension, paralysis, loss of consciousness.	None	Observation, symptomatic treatment
BZ (QNB)	Rarely life-threatening	Sedation, confusion, hallucinations, disorientation, impaired memory, incoherent speech, manifestations of cholinolytic activity.	Physostigmine salicylate (Antilirium)	Administration of antidote, observation, and reassurance in quiet place

GI, gastrointestinal; RBCs, red blood cells.
[a]Adapted from Sidell FR. *Postgrad Med* 1990;88:70–84.
[b]Nonmilitary use only.

TABLE 11. Recommended control limits for selected chemical agents[a]

Chemical agent[b]	General population (mg/m³)		Workers (mg/m³)	
Nerve agents[c]				
GA, GB	0.000003	(3×10^6)	0.0001	(1×10^4)
VX	0.000003	(3×10^6)	0.00001	(1×10^5)
Vesicants[d]				
H, HD, HT[e]	0.0001	(1×10^4)	0.003	(3×10^3)
L	0.003	(3×10^3)	0.003	(3×10^3)
Averaging time	72 h		8 h	

[a]Adapted from *MMWR Morb Mortal Wkly Rep* 1988;37:72–79.
[b]Protection against exposure to agents in aerosol and liquid form must be sufficient to prevent direct contact with the skin and eyes.
[c]GA, tabun or ethyl *N,N*-dimethylphosphoramidocyanidate; GB, sarin or isopropyl methylphosphonofluoridate; VX, *S*-(2-diisopropylaminoethyl) O-ethyl methyl phosphonothiolate.
[d]H or HD, sulfur mustard or di-2-chloroethyl sulfide; HT, *Bis*(2-chloroethylthioethyl) ether (T) in a mixture with sulfur mustard; L, lewisite or dichloro (2-chlorovinyl) arsine.
[e]Data supporting the ability to monitor for H at 0.0001 mg/m³ at all sites should be developed. HT is measured as HD.

BLOOD AGENTS (CYANOGENS)

The cyanogens include hydrogen cyanide (AC), cyanogen chloride (CNCl), and arsine (SA). The use of cyanide agents was initiated by the French in 1916 with the use of shells filled with AC (49,84). Cyanide had extreme volatility; its vapor was lighter than air. Therefore, it was almost impossible to establish a lethal concentration in the field by this means of delivery. To overcome this problem, cyanogen chloride and cyanogen bromide were produced; these vapors were heavier than air (41,49,84,86).

Pathophysiology

Blood agents produce their effects by interfering with oxygen use at the cellular level. Inhalation is the usual route of entry. CK also has a choking effect (41).

Clinical Presentation

The cyanogen agents release AC and produce the effects of cyanide. These are described in detail in Chapter 185. Typically, either death occurs rapidly or recovery takes place within a few minutes after removal from the toxic atmosphere. With high concentrations, there is increased depth of respiration within a few seconds, violent seizures after 20 to 30 seconds, cessation of regular respiration within 1 minute, occasional shallow gasps, and asystole within a few minutes. With moderate exposure, vertigo, nausea, and headache appear early and are followed by seizures and coma. Long exposure to low concentrations may result in tissue anoxia and central nervous system damage. Coma and seizures may follow and persist for hours or days. There is residual damage as evidenced by irrationality, altered reflexes, and ataxia that may last for a few weeks or longer. Mild exposure may produce headache, vertigo, and nausea, but recovery is complete.

CK produces a combination of signs from AC and lung irritation. Exposure may be followed by immediate intense irritation of the nose, throat, and eyes, with coughing, tightness in the chest, and lacrimation. There may be dizziness and dyspnea. Unconsciousness, failing respiration, and death may supervene in a few minutes. Seizures, retching, involuntary urination, and defecation may occur. Pulmonary edema may develop.

Diagnostic Tests

TREATMENT

Decontamination. The patient must be removed from the exposure. A standard protective mask with a fresh filter gives adequate protection against field concentrations of a blood agent vapor. A protective overgarment and mask are needed when exposed to or handling AC. CK has systemic effects similar to AC, but it also has local irritant effects on the eyes, upper respiratory tract, and lungs (41). It may induce severe inflammatory changes in the bronchioles and congestion and edema in the lungs.

Antidotes. The antidotes for cyanide toxicity are sodium nitrite and sodium thiosulfate. The dose and method of administration are the same as other sources of cyanide toxicity (Chapter 46). Do not use amyl nitrite under an oxygen mask because of the risk of an explosion (102).

Although not used in the United States, other agents such as dicobalt edetate (United Kingdom) and dimethylaminophenol (Germany) have been used (see Antidotes section): (a) Dicobalt edetate (toxic to liver and kidneys) directly fixes the cyanide ion: 300 mg in 20 mg of solution (kelocyanor) given IV. Repeat according as circumstances may require. Follow with IV sodium thiosulfate 25 g in 50% solution slowly. (b) Dimethylaminophenol, a methemoglobin former: 250 mg in 5 ml IV. Repeat according as circumstances may require. Follow by sodium thiosulfate 25 g in a 50% solution (Chapter 51). (May induce a high methemoglobin value.)

Studies in cyanide-poisoned beagle dogs suggest that dimethylaminophenol 5 mg/kg and hydroxylamine hydrochloride 50 mg/kg were the only drugs able to reverse the lethal effects of cyanide poisoning when administered by the intramuscular route. Sodium nitrite, amyl nitrite, and sodium thiosulfate do not appear to be effective by the intramuscular route. Further studies are indicated to pursue this finding for military or civilian use (102).

Supportive Care. The lung irritant effects of CK are treated as with the choking agents [e.g., phosgene (CG)].

PSYCHOTOMIMETIC AGENTS

Many drugs act on the central nervous system to produce incapacitation. Few are potent or safe, or possess the necessary physical and chemical properties to make them useful as potential chemical agents. Of these few, 3-quinuclidinyl benzilate (an atropine-like drug; BZ) and lysergic acid diethylamide (Chapter 177) are of interest (86).

Pathophysiology

BZ appears to block the action of acetylcholine peripherally and centrally, but unlike atropine, it produces predominantly central rather than peripheral effects (49). High doses produce a toxic delirium that renders the individual unable to perform any task. BZ is a crystalline solid at normal temperatures, and there is no device available to detect it. Prevention is best accomplished with a protective mask.

Clinical Presentation

One to 2 hours after exposure, BZ produces dilation of the pupils, dry mouth, and increased heart rate, which are later followed by ataxia and drowsiness. In approximately 6 or 7 hours, these symptoms diminish to be replaced by a confused mental state with delusions, hallucinations, and aimless behavior that may last for several days. The mydriasis may last for 3 days.

Treatment

Usually symptomatic treatment is all that is necessary. Remove dangerous objects or anything that may be swallowed. Heat stroke may occur in tropical climates. Maintain fluid intake.

LUNG-DAMAGING AGENTS (CHOKING AGENTS)

Chemicals that primarily attack lung tissue causing pulmonary edema are known as *lung-damaging* or *choking agents* (103). They include the following: CG, diphosgene, chlorine, and chloropicrin. The best known of these agents is CG. Agents of this group irritate the bronchi, trachea, larynx, pharynx, and nose, and this, together with acute pulmonary edema, contributes to the sensation of choking (41,49,84,86,104–107).

Chloropicrin (108) (CCl_3NO_2) is a colorless, slightly oily liquid used as a fumigant for cereals and grains, a soil insecticide, and a chemical warfare agent. It produces a severe irritation to the eyes, mucous membranes, and lungs. A lethal exposure in humans is approximately 119 ppm for 30 minutes with death resulting from pulmonary edema. Residual spray may induce a dry cough.

Chlorine was the first chemical agent used as an offensive military weapon, and it initiated the age of chemical warfare in April 1915, when the German army released a greenish yellow cloud and caused the death of 5000 Allied soldiers and the wounding of 10,000 more (84). On December 22, 1915, at Ypres, the German army initiated the second major chemical, CG, and this caused the gassing of 1069 men with 116 deaths from acute pulmonary edema. More than 80% of all chemical agent fatalities in World War I were from CG (86). Diphosgene, basically CG with chloroform grafted onto it, was created after World War I as an attempt to improve on CG, but by the 1930s was superseded by the nerve agents (86). Chloropicrin was used in World War I because of its irritant action on skin and mucous membranes (49).

Phosgene and Diphosgene

CG (carbonyl chloride) is a colorless gas at room temperature and atmospheric pressure. It has an odor of newly cut hay. The vapor is heavier than air and may remain in trenches, valleys, and woods for some time, depending on atmospheric conditions. A standard field protective mask or a gas-particulate filter gives adequate protection against lung-damaging agents.

TOXIC DOSE

Exposure doses less than 25 ppm/minute can be regarded as harmless. Exposure of patients to mild doses of 50 to 150 ppm/minute should receive steroids by inhalation and systemically. They should be observed for at least 8 hours and if chest radiographs are normal, they can be discharged. If no radiographs are available, continue observation for 24 hours. Doses more than 150 ppm/minute of CG induce clinical pulmonary edema. Doses more than 300 ppm/minute are life endangering (105,106,109).

PATHOPHYSIOLOGY

Damage to the bronchiolar epithelium, development of patchy areas of emphysema, partial atelectasis, and edema of the perivascular connective tissue precede massive pulmonary edema (41,49). The trachea and bronchi are usually normal in appearance after CG exposure. This contrasts with the findings in chlorine and chloropicrin poisoning in which both structures may show serious damage to the epithelial lining with desquamation.

CLINICAL PRESENTATION

Initially, there may be mild irritation of the eyes and throat with some coughing, choking, feeling of tightness in the chest, nausea and occasional vomiting, headache, and lacrimation. A latent period follows during which the patient may be relatively symptom free without chest signs, lasting from 30 minutes to 48 hours.

Thereafter, in those developing severe pulmonary damage, progressive pulmonary edema develops rapidly with shallow rapid respiration, cyanosis, and a painful paroxysmal cough producing copious amounts of frothy white or yellowish liquid. Examination of the chest reveals increasing diminution of breath sounds with rales and rhonchi throughout the lung fields. Distress, apprehension, dyspnea, and cyanosis increase. Hypovolemia, hypoxia, and circulatory failure may then lead to death.

DIAGNOSIS

Irritation of the nose and throat by CG may be mistaken for upper respiratory tract infection. Difficulty in breathing and complaints of tightness of the chest may suggest nerve-agent poisoning or an acute asthmatic attack. The noncardiac pulmonary edema may be confused with the edema associated with heart failure. Diagnosis depends on a definite history of exposure to CG. Arterial blood gases confirm clinical status.

A radiograph of the chest during approximately one-half of the clinical latent period may indicate incipient toxic pulmonary edema much earlier than clinical signs and symptoms (105). CG indicator badges are used at Bayer/Germany (106).

TREATMENT

Rest during the latent stage is important because any activity between exposure and the onset of pulmonary symptoms and/or signs greatly increases the likelihood of death. Cough is treated with codeine phosphate (30 to 60 mg).

Humidified oxygen should be administered. Early use of positive airway pressure [intermittent positive pressure breathing, positive end–expiratory pressure, mask (*positive end–expiratory pressure mask*)], or, if necessary, intubation with or without a ventilator may delay or minimize the pulmonary edema and reduce hypoxemia.

Withhold sedatives until adequate oxygenation is assured and facilities for possible respiratory assistance are available. Do *not* use atropine, barbiturates, analeptics, or antihistamines.

Antibiotics are reserved for acquired bacterial bronchitis or pneumonitis. Do not use prophylactically. Diuretics are largely ineffective against toxic pulmonary edema (106,109), but they may be helpful in combination with positive end–expiratory pressure by reducing interstitial edema.

Steroids used soon (within 15 minutes preferably) after exposure may lessen the severity of the edema. Once preliminary edema has evolved, steroids are much less effective. The initial dose is five times that conventionally used in asthma, followed by approximately one-half the dose for 12 hours, and then standard asthma dosages for the subsequent 72 hours until the risk of pulmonary edema has passed. Use betamethasone valerate, beclomethasone dipropionate, or dexamethasone sodium phosphate.

ANTIDOTE

There is no antidote against CG. N-acetylcysteine and other free radical scavengers have been suggested for use in treating lung and other injuries in mustard gas exposure (110–112). Treatment is otherwise largely supportive.

LACRIMATING AGENTS

Riot control agents are aerosol-dispersed chemicals that produce eye, nose, mouth, skin, and respiratory tract irritation. Most of these symptoms resolve by 30 minutes postexposure. Both ocular and mucous membrane symptoms may persist for 24 hours. The three currently used agents are 1-chloroacetophenone, 2-chlorobenzylidenemalononitrile, and dibenz([b,fl]-1,4-oxazepine. Serious systemic toxicity is rare.

These lacrimators are relatively nontoxic except when dispersed in a confined, nonventilated space. *1-Chloroacetophenone* is the most toxic lacrimator and has accounted for at least five deaths resulting from pulmonary injury and/or asphyxia (113,114). *2-Chlorobenzylidenemalononitrile* is a lacrimator 10 times more potent than 1-chloroacetophenone and is less toxic. *Dibenz[b,fl]-1,4-oxazepine* is the most potent lacrimator with the least systemic toxicity.

Clinical Presentation

Respiratory tract toxicity usually affects the upper airway; rhinorrhea, nasal irritation and congestion, bronchorrhea, sore throat, cough, sneezing, unpleasant taste, and burning of the mouth occur immediately after exposure and rapidly resolve within minutes. Prolonged concentrated or closed space exposure can produce the low airway effects of acute laryngotracheobronchitis (115).

Skin burning and sometimes erythema occur after exposure to lacrimators.

Diagnostic Tests

A significant leukocytosis (i.e., more than 20,000 white blood cells/cm^3) may occur after exposure to 1-chloroacetophenone and can last for several days (115,116).

Treatment

The immediate priority is removal from exposure and establishment of an airway. Patients with respiratory distress should receive oxygen, an evaluation of airway patency and ventilation, an IV line, and cardiac monitoring. Obtain arterial blood gases and a chest radiograph.

DECONTAMINATION

Remove all contaminated clothing, and seal it in a plastic bag. Medical personnel should use disposable rubber gloves when handling contaminated clothes. The eyes should be irrigated copiously with saline for 15 to 20 minutes. Contaminated skin should be washed thoroughly with mild liquid soap and water. Only a saline irrigation should be used over vesiculated skin.

SUPPORTIVE CARE

The eyes should be examined for corneal abrasions and treated with oral analgesics, topical antibiotics (sulfacetamide), and mydriatics as needed. Vesiculated skin is treated like a second-degree chemical burn. Patients with respiratory distress should be admitted if symptoms persist several hours. These patients should be observed for the development of bronchospasm and pneumonia (e.g., serial chest radiographs, arterial blood gases). Prophylactic antibiotics and steroids probably are not effective. Humidified oxygen may provide symptomatic relief.

REFERENCES

1. Public Broadcasting System (PBS). An interview with Alexei 1999. PBS online and WGBH/FRONTLINE. Complete interview available at http://www.PBS.org.
2. Newardk T. *Medieval warfare*. London, England: Bloomsbury Books: 1988.
3. Kaplan DE, Marshall A. *The cult at the end of the world: the terrifying story of the Aum Doomsday Cult, from the subways of Tokyo to the nuclear arsenals of Russia*. Crown Publishing, 1996.
4. Morita H, Yanagisawa N, Nakajima T, et al. Sarin poisoning in Matsumoto, Japan. *Lancet* 1995;346:290–293.
5. Okumura T, Suzuki K, Fukuda A, et al. The Tokyo subway sarin attack: disaster management, part 2: hospital response. *Acad Emerg Med* 1998;5(6):618–24.
6. Okumura T, Suzuki K, Fukuda A, et al. The Tokyo subway sarin attack: disaster management, part 1: community emergency response. *Acad Emerg Med* 1998;5(6):613–7.
7. Sidell FR. Nerve agents. In: Zajtchukk R, Bellamy RF, eds. *Textbook of military medicine*. Washington: Office of the Surgeon General, 1997.
8. Paxman HR. *A higher form of killing*. New York: Hill and Wang; 1982:53.
9. Reference deleted.
10. Reference deleted.
11. Grob D. The manifestations and treatment of poisoning due to nerve gas and other organic phosphate anticholinesterase compounds. *Arch Intern Med* 1956;98:221–238.
12. Grob D, Harvey JC. Effects in man of the anticholinesterase compound sarin (isopropyl methyl phosphorofluoridate). *J Clin Invest* 1958;37:350–68.
13. Sidell FR, Groff WA. The reactivatibility of cholinesterase inhibited by VX and sarin in man. *Toxicol Appl Pharmacol* 1974;27:241–52.
14. Sidell FR. Soman and sarin: clinical manifestations and treatment of accidental poisoning by organophosphates. *Clin Toxicol* 1974;7:1–17.
15. Rengstorff RH. Accidental exposure to sarin: vision effects. *Arch Toxicol* 1985;56:201–3.
16. Oberst FW, Koon WS, Christensen MK, et al. Retention of inhaled sarin vapor and its effect on red blood cell cholinesterase activity in man. *Clin Pharmacol Ther* 1968;9:421–7.
17. Rubin LS, Goldberg MN. Effect of sarin on dark adaptation in man. Threshold change. *J Appl Physiol* 1957;11:439–444.
18. Duffy FH, Burchfiel JL, Bartels PH, et al. Long-term effects of an organophosphate upon the human electroencephalogram. *Toxicol Appl Pharmacol* 1979;47:161–76.
19. Burchfield JL, Duffy FH. Organophosphate neurotoxicity: chronic effects of sarin on the electroencephalogram of monkey and man. *Neurobehav Toxicol Teratol* 1982;4:767–778.
20. Burchfield JL, Duffy FH, Sim VM. Persistent effects of sarin and dieldrin upon the primate electroencephalogram. *Toxicol Appl Pharmacol* 1976;35:365–379.
21. Arterberry JD, Bonifaci RW, Nash EW, et al. Potentiation of phosphorus insecticides by phenothiazine derivative. *JAMA* 1962;182:848.
22. Weiss LR, Orzel RA. Enhancement of toxicity of anticholinesterases by central depressant drugs in rats. *Toxicol Appl Pharm* 1967;10:334.
23. Kechum JS, Sidell FR, Crowell EB, et al. Atropine, scopolamine and Ditran: comparative pharmacology and antagonists in man. *Psychopharmacology (Berlin)* 1973;28:121.
24. Grob D, Lilienthal JL Jr, Harvey AM, et al. The administration of di-isopropyl fluorophosphate (DFP) to man, I: effect on plasma and erythrocyte cholinesterase; general systemic effects; use in study of hepatic function and erythropoieses; and some properties of plasma cholinesterase. *Bull Johns Hopkins Hosp* 1947;81:217–244.
25. Sim VM. Variability of different intact human skin sites to the penetration of VX. Edgewood Arsenal, MD: Medical Research Laboratory; 1962. Chemical Research and Development Laboratory Report 3122.
26. Grob D, Harvey AM. The effects and treatment of nerve gas poisoning. *Am J Med* 1953;14:52–63.
27. Okumura T, Takasu N, Ishimatsu S, et al. Report on 640 victims of the Tokyo subway sarin attack. *Ann Emerg Med* 1996;28:129–35.
28. Harvey JC. Clinical observations on volunteers exposed to concentrations of GB. Edgewood Arsenal, MD: Medical Research Laboratory; 1952. Medical Laboratory Research Report 144.
29. Craig AB, Woodson GS. Observations on the effects of exposure to nerve gas, I: clinical observations and cholinesterase depression. *Am J Med Sci* 1959;238:13–7.
30. Sidell RF. Clinical considerations in nerve agent intoxication. In: Somani SM, ed. *Chemical warfare agents*. New York: Academic Press; 1992:163.
31. Reference deleted.
32. D'Agostino PA, Provost LR. Gas chromatographic retention indices of chemical warfare agents and stimulants. *J Chromatogr* 1985;331:47–54.
33. Nozaki H, Hori S, Shinozawa Y, et al. Secondary exposure of medical staff to sarin vapor in the emergency room. *Intens Care Med* 1995;21:1032–5.
34. Fischetti M. Gas vaccine. Bioengineering immunization could shield against nerve gas. *Sci Am* 1991;153:154.
35. Orma PS, Middleton RK. Aerosolized atropine as an antidote to nerve gas. *Ann Pharmacother* 1992;26:937–938.
36. Doctor BP, Blick DW, Recht KM, et al. Protection of rhesus monkey against soma toxicity by pretreatment with cholinesterase. Proceedings of the 4th International Symposium: Protection against Chemical Warfare Agents. Stockholm, Sweden: June 8–12, 1992; 335–340.
37. Ward JR. Case report: exposure to a nerve gas. In: Whittenberger JL, ed. *Artificial respiration: theory and applications*. New York: Harper & Row; 1962:258–265.
38. Vale JA, Meredith TJ, Health A. High dose atropine in organophosphorus poisoning. *Postgrad Med J* 1990;66:881.

39. Chew LS, Chee KT, Yeo JM, et al. Continuous atropine infusion in the management of organophosphorus insecticide poisoning. *Singapore Med J* 1971;12:80–85.
40. LeBlanc FN, Benson BE, Gilg AD. A severe organophosphate poisoning requiring the use of an atropine drip. *Clin Toxicol* 1986;24:69–76.
41. Departments of the Navy, Army, and Air Force. Potential military chemical/biological agents and compounds. December 12, 1990; FM 3-9, NAV/FAC:467.
42. Soldier Biological and Chemical Command (SBCCOM). Domestic Preparedness Training Program materials; 2003.
43. Dunn MA, Sidell FR. Progress in medical defense against nerve agents. *JAMA* 1989;262:649–652.
44. Munro NB, Watson AP, Ambrose KR, Griffin GD. Treating exposure to chemical warfare agents: implications for health care providers and community emergency planning. *Environ Health Perspect* 1990;89:205–215.
45. Hamilton MG, Lundy PM. HI-6 therapy of soman and tabun poisoning in primates and rodents. *Arch Toxicol* 1989;63(2):144–149.
46. Kassa J, Cabal J. A comparison of the efficacy of a new asymmetric bispyridinium oxime BI-6 with currently available oximes and H oximes against soman by in vitro and in vivo methods. *Toxicol* 1999;132(2–3):111–8.
47. Van Helden HP, Busker RW, Melchers BP, et al. Pharmacological effects of oximes: how relevant are they? *Arch Toxicol* 1996;70(12):779–86.
48. Kassa J. Review of oximes in the antidotal treatment of poisoning by organophosphorus nerve agents. *J Toxicol Clin Toxicol* 2002;40(6):803–16.
49. JSP 312: Medical manual of defense against chemical agents. Ministry of Defense. London: Her Majesty's Stationery Office; 1987:4-2-4-3.
50. Murray VSG, Volans GN. Management of injuries due to chemical weapons. Most patients exposed to mustard gas recover completely. *BMJ* 1991;302:129–130.
51. Reference deleted.
52. Sidell FR. What to do in case of an unthinkable chemical warfare attack or accident. *Postgrad Med* 1990;88(7):70–84.
53. Shalit I. Chemical warfare and disasters: medical organization and treatment. In: Reis ND, Dolve E, eds. *Manual of disaster medicine, civilian and military*. Berlin: Springer Verlag, 1989:113–123.
54. Newman-Taylor AJ, Marris AJR. Experience with mustard gas casualties. *Lancet* 1991;337:242.
55. Wormser U. Toxicology of mustard gas. *Trends Pharmaceut Sci* 1991;12:164–167.
56. Aasted A, Darre E, Wolf HC. Mustard gas: clinical, toxicological and mutagenic aspects based on modern experience. *Ann Plastic Surg* 1987;19:330–333.
57. Balali-Mood M. Sulfur mustard poisoning in the Iran-Iraq war. *Clin Pharmacol Ther* 1990;47:183–184.
58. Willems JL. Clinical management of mustard gas casualties. *Ann Med Mitt Belg* 1989;3[Suppl 1]:1–61.
59. Papirmeister B, Feister AJ, Robinson SI, et al. Medical defense against mustard gas: toxic mechanisms and pharmacological implications. Boca Raton, FL: CRC Press, 1991:1–42.
60. Watson AP, Jones TD, Griffin GD. Sulfur mustard as a carcinogen: application of relative potency analyses to the chemical warfare agents H, HD and HT. *Regul Toxicol Pharmacol* 1989;10:1–25.
61. Yanagida J, Hozawa S, Ishioka S, et al. Somatic mutation in peripheral lymphocytes of former workers at the Okunojima poison gas factory. *Jpn J Cancer Res* 1988;79:1276–1286.
62. Requena L, Requena C, Sanchez M, et al. Chemical warfare. Cutaneous lesions from mustard gas. *J Am Acad Dermatol* 1988;19:529–536.
63. Easton DF, Peto J, Doll R. Cancers of the respiratory tract in mustard gas workers. *Br J Indust Med* 1988;45:652–659.
64. Somani SM, Babu SR. Toxicodynamics of sulfur mustard. *Int J Clin Pharmacol Ther Toxicol* 1989;27:419–435.
65. Sohrabpour H. Observation and clinical manifestations of patients injured with mustard gas. *Med J Islamic Rep of Iran* 1987;1:32–37.
66. Goldman M, Jacre JC. Lewisite. Its chemistry, toxicology and biological effects. *Rev Environ Contam Toxicol* 1989;110:76–114.
67. Papirmeister B, Gross CL, Meier HL, et al. Molecular basis for mustard induced vesication. *Fund Appl Toxicol* 1985;5:S134–S149.
68. Reference deleted.
69. Heyndrickx B. Report and conclusion of the biological samples of men intoxicated by war gases sent to the Department of Toxicology of the State University of Ghent for toxicological investigation; 1986:553–582.
70. Balali-Mood M, Farhoodi M, Panjvani FK. Report of three fatal cases of war gas poisoning. Proceedings of the 2nd World Congress on new compounds in biological and chemical warfare. Ghent, Belgium: International Association of Forensic Toxicologists, 1993:475–482.
71. Jones GB. From mustard gas to medicines: the history of modern cancer chemotherapy. *Chem Heritage/CHF* 1998;15(2):8–9, 40–42.
72. Balali-Mood M, Navaeian A. Clinical and paraclinical findings in 233 patients with sulfur mustard poisoning. Proceedings of the 2nd World Congress on new compounds in biological and chemical warfare. Ghent, Belgium: International Association of Forensic Toxicologists, 1986:464–473.
73. Reference deleted.
74. Balali M. First report of delayed toxic effects of yperite poisoning in Iranian fighters. In: Heyndricks B, ed. Terrorism: Analysis and detection of explosives. Proceedings of the 2nd World Congress on new compounds in biological and chemical warfare. Ghent, Belgium: International Association of Forensic Toxicologists, 1986.
75. Reference deleted.
76. Vde Keyser H, Geerts ML, Colardyn F, et al. [Skin damage caused by the effect of nitrogen mustard gas]. *Hautarzt* 1986;37(8):467–471.
77. Reference deleted.
78. Reference deleted.
79. Heyndrickx B, ed. Proceedings of the Second World Congress. New compounds in biological and chemical warfare: toxicological evaluation. Industrial chemical disasters. Civil protection and treatment. Ghent: The International Association for Toxicology. 23rd European International Meeting on Terrorism: Analysis and Detection of Explosives; August 24–27, 1986.
80. Heyndrickx A, Heyndrickx B. [Toxicologic research on neurotoxic gas in samples from intoxicated soldiers]. *Arch Belges* 1984;Suppl:147–154.
81. Drasch G, Kretschmer E, Kauert G, et al. Concentrations of mustard gas [bis(2-chloroethyl)sulfide] in the tissues of a victim of a vesicant exposure. *J Forens Sci* 1987;32(6):1788–1793.
82. Vycudilik W. Detection of bis(2-chlorethyl) sulfide lyperite in urine by high resolution gas chromatography/mass spectrometry. *Forensic Sci Int* 1987;35:67–71.
83. Wils ERJ, Hulst AG, Van Laar J. Analysis of thiodiglycol in urine of victims of an alleged attack with mustard gas. II. *J Anal Toxicol* 1988;12:15–19.
84. Harris C, Paxman J. *A higher form of killing. The secret story of chemical and biological warfare*. New York: Hill & Want, 1982:1–3,17–20,187–188,206–210,274.
85. Douglass JD Jr, Livingston NC. *America the vulnerable. The threat of chemical/biological warfare. The new shape of terrorism and conflict*. Lexington, MA: Lexington Books, 1987:4–5,204.
86. Compton JAF. *Military chemical and biological agents. Chemical and toxicological properties*. Caldwell, NJ: Telford Press, 1987:87–134,253–335,458.
87. Davis KG, Aspera G. Exposure to liquid sulfur mustard. *Annals Emerg Med* 2001;37(6):653–656.
88. Bullman T, Kang H. A fifty year mortality follow-up study of veterans exposed to low level chemical warfare agent, mustard gas. *Annals of Epidemiology* 2000;10(5):333–8.
89. Benschop HP, van der Schans GP, Noort D, et al. Verification of exposure to sulfur mustard in two casualties of the Iran-Iraq conflict. *J Anal Toxicol* 1997;21(4):249–251.
90. Dacre JC, Goldman M. Toxicology and pharmacology of the chemical warfare agent sulfur mustard. *Pharmacological Reviews* 1996;48(2):289–326.
91. Naghii MR. Sulfur mustard intoxication, oxidative stress and antioxidants. *Military Medicine* 2002;167(7):573–575.
92. Editorial staff. *Mustard gas*. In: Toll LL, Hurlbut KM, eds. POISINDEX system. Greenwood Village, CO: MICROMEDEX (edition expires 09/2003).
93. Solberg Y, Alcalay M, Michael B. Ocular injury by mustard gas. *Surv Ophthalmol* 1997;41(6):P461–466.
94. Blodi FC. Mustard gas keratopathy. *Internat Ophthal Clin* 1971;11:1–13.
95. Blanc PD. The legacy of war gas. *Am J Med* 1999;106:689–670.
96. Emad A, Gholam RR. Characteristics of bronchoalveolar lavage fluid in patients with sulfur mustard gas–induced asthma or chronic bronchitis. *Am J Medicine* 1999;(106):625–628.
97. Pechura CM, Rall DP, ed. Veterans at risk. The health effects of mustard gas and lewisite. Committee to Survey the Health Effects of Mustard Gas and Lewisite. Institute of Medicine. Washington: National Academy Press, 1993.
98. Norman JE Jr. Lung cancer mortality in World War I veterans with mustard-gas injury: 1919–1965. *JNCI* 1975;54:311–317.
99. Hay A, Roberts G. The use of poison gas against the Iraqi Kurds: analysis of bomb fragments, soil and wool samples. *JAMA* 1990;263:1065–1066.
100. Rice P, Brown RF, Lam DG, et al. Dermabrasion—a novel concept in the surgical management of sulphur mustard injuries. *Burns* 2000;26(1):34–40.
101. Lieske CN, Klopcic RS, Gross CL, et al. Development of an antibody that binds sulfur mustard. *Immunol Lett* 1992;31:117–122.
102. Vick JA, Froehlich H. Treatment of cyanide poisoning. *Milit Med* 1991;156:330–339.
103. Army Field Manual No. 3-9. Potential military chemical/biological agents and compounds. Washington: December 12, 1990:14–17,46–47,71.
104. Wang Y-T, Lee LKH, Poh S-C. Phosgene poisoning from a smoke grenade. *Eur J Respir Dis* 1987;70:126–128.
105. Diller WF. Early diagnosis of phosgene overexposure. *Toxicol Ind Health* 1985;1:73–80.
106. Diller WF. Therapeutic strategy in phosgene poisoning. *Toxicol Ind Health* 1985;1:93–99.
107. Sjogren B, Plato N, Alexandersson R, et al. Pulmonary reactions caused by welding-induced decomposed trichloroethylene. *Chest* 1991;99:237–238.
108. Proctor NH, Hughes JP, Fischman ML. *Chemical hazards of the workplace*, 2nd ed. New York: Van Nostrand Rheinhold, 1989:149.
109. Diller WF, Zantz R. A literature review: therapy for phosgene poisoning. *Toxicol Ind Health* 1985;1:117–128.
110. Anderson DR, Byers SL, Vesely KR. Treatment of sulfur mustard (HD)-induced lung injury. *J Appl Toxicol* 2000;20[Suppl 1]:S129–32.
111. Atkins KB, Lodhi IJ, Hurley LL, et al. N-acetylcysteine and endothelial cell injury by sulfur mustard. *J Appl Toxicol* 2000;20[Suppl 1]:S125–8.
112. Cowan FM, Broomfield CA, Smith WJ. Inhibition of sulfur mustard-increased protease activity by niacinamide, N-acetyl-L-cysteine or dexamethasone. *Cell Biol Toxicol* 1992;8(2):129–38.
113. Stein AA, Kirwan WE. Chloroacetophenone (tear gas) poisoning. A clinico-pathologic report. *J Forensic Sci* 1964;9:374–382.

114. Chapman AJ, White C. Death resulting from lacrimatory agents. *J Forensic Sci* 1978;23:527–530.
115. Thorburn KM. Injuries after use of the lacrimatory agent chloroacetophenone in a confined space. *Arch Environ Health* 1982;37:182–186.
116. Park S, Giammonia ST. Toxic effects of tear gas on an infant following prolonged exposure. *Am J Dis Child* 1972;123:245–246.

SUGGESTED READING

Compton JAF. *Military chemical and biological agents. Chemical and toxicological properties.* Caldwell, NJ: Telford Press, 1987:458.

Departments of the Army, the Navy, and the Air Force. Field manual. Treatment of chemical agent casualties and conventional military chemical injuries. Army FM 8-285, Navy Navmed P-4051, Air Force AFM 160-11; February 1990.

Douglass JD Jr, Livingstone NC. *America the vulnerable. The threat of chemical/biological warfare.* Lexington, MA: Lexington Books, 1987:204.

Harris R, Paxman J. *A higher form of killing. The secret story of chemical and biological warfare.* New York: Hill & Wand, 1982:274.

Maynard RL, Beswich FW. Organophosphorus compounds as chemical warfare agents. In: Ballantyne B, Marris TC, eds. *Clinical and experimental toxicology of organophosphates and carbamates.* Oxford: Butterworth-Heinemann, 1992:373–385.

Medical Management of Chemical Casualties course. Office of the Surgeon General and US Army Medical Research Institute of Chemical Defense; January 1992.

JSP 312: Medical manual of defense against chemical agents, 6th ed. Ministry of Defense (United Kingdom). London: Her Majesty's Stationery Office; 1987. Second Impression 1990. D/Med (Fond S) (2)/10/11.

JSP 312: Medical manual of defense against chemical agents, 5th ed. Ministry of Defense. London: Her Majesty's Stationery Office; 1972. First published 1939. A/24/Gen/4392.

NATO handbook on the concept of medical support in NBC environments. A MED P-7(A). Unclassified. August 1982.

Potential military chemical/biological agents and compounds. Headquarters, Departments of the Army, Navy, and Air Force; December 12, 1990. FM 3-9, NAVFAC P-467, AFR 355-7.

Proceedings of the 4th International Symposium on Protection Against Chemical Warfare Agents. Stockholm, Sweden: National Defense Research Establishment; June 8–12, 1992. 82 Umea, Sweden. Department of NBC Defense S-901.

Sidell FR. What to do in case of an unthinkable chemical warfare attack or incident. *Postgrad Med* 1990;88:70–84.

Somani SM, ed. *Chemical warfare agents.* San Diego: Academic Press, 1992:443.

Appendices

APPENDIX I
Pregnancy Categories of United States Food and Drug Administration

Since 1975, the U.S. Food and Drug Administration (FDA) has required manufacturers to label their drugs with pregnancy classifications. These products must be classified under one of five letter categories: A, B, C, D, or X. These categories are meant to inform the prescriber about the information available on that drug and its general implications. There are several caveats to remember when using this information:

1. Although the category designation is likely accurate at the time that a drug is introduced, package labeling is not frequently updated, and the FDA pregnancy category in the product literature may be out of date.
2. It is often assumed that drugs labeled as category X pose the greatest pregnancy risk; however, this is not always the case. Category X involves a risk/benefit assessment, which could vary according to the individual patient.
3. It is often assumed that a higher label (e.g., category A vs. category C) indicates a "better" safety record in pregnancy. However, category C actually indicates a lack of information. A drug could be category A or X in reality but initially be classified as category C.

Category	Description
A	Adequate, well-controlled studies in pregnant women have not shown an increased risk of fetal abnormalities.
B	Animal studies have revealed no evidence of harm to the fetus; however, there are no adequate and well-controlled studies in pregnant women. *Or* Animal studies have shown an adverse effect, but adequate and well-controlled studies in pregnant women have failed to demonstrate a risk to the fetus.
C	Animal studies have shown an adverse effect, and there are no adequate and well-controlled studies in pregnant women. *Or* No animal studies have been conducted, and there are no adequate and well-controlled studies in pregnant women.
D	Studies—adequate, well-controlled or observational—in pregnant women have demonstrated a risk to the fetus. However, the benefits of therapy may outweigh the potential risk.
X	Studies—adequate, well-controlled or observational—in animals or pregnant women have demonstrated positive evidence of fetal abnormalities. The use of the product is contraindicated in women who are or may become pregnant.

APPENDIX II

Some Drug/Poison Concentrations and Mass/Amount Concentration Conversion Factors*,†

Robert J. Flanagan

Analyte	"Therapeutic" or "normal" plasma concentration (less than)	Plasma concentration associated with acute serious toxicity[a]	Relative atomic or formula mass	Mass/amount conversion	Amount/mass conversion
Abacavir	5 mg/L	—	286.3	mg/L × 3.49 = μmol/L	μmol/L × 0.286 = mg/L
Acamprosate	1 mg/L	[Not known]	180.2	mg/L × 5.54 = μmol/L	μmol/L × 0.180 = mg/L
Acebutolol	2 mg/L	15 mg/L	336.4	mg/L × 2.97 = μmol/L	μmol/L × 0.336 = mg/L
Diacetolol[b]	5 mg/L	90 mg/L	308.4	mg/L × 3.24 = μmol/L	μmol/L × 0.308 = mg/L
Acecainide (*N*-acetyl-procainamide)	12 mg/L	25 mg/L	277.4	mg/L × 3.60 = μmol/L	μmol/L × 0.277 = mg/L
Acecarbromal	20 mg/L	[Not known]	279.1	mg/L × 3.58 = μmol/L	μmol/L × 0.279 = mg/L
Aceclofenac: see also Diclofenac[b]	5 mg/L	[Not known]	354.2	mg/L × 2.82 = μmol/L	μmol/L × 0.354 = mg/L
Acemetacin: see also Indometacin[b]	2.5 mg/L	[Not known]	415.8	mg/L × 2.41 = μmol/L	μmol/L × 0.416 = mg/L
Acenocoumarol	0.2 mg/L	—	353.3	mg/L × 2.83 = μmol/L	μmol/L × 0.353 = mg/L
Acetaldehyde	0.2 mg/L	[Not known]	44.1	mg/L × 22.7 = μmol/L	μmol/L × 0.044 = mg/L
Acetaminophen: see Paracetamol					
Acetazolamide	15 mg/L	30 mg/L	222.2	mg/L × 4.50 = μmol/L	μmol/L × 0.222 = mg/L
Acetohexamide	100 mg/L (diabetics)	—	324.4	mg/L × 3.08 = μmol/L	μmol/L × 0.324 = mg/L
Hydroxyhexamide[b]	50 mg/L (diabetics)	—	326.4	mg/L × 3.06 = μmol/L	μmol/L × 0.326 = mg/L
Acetone (urine): see also 2-Propanol[b]	10 mg/L (1 g/L in ketosis) urine 10 mg/L (2 g/L in ketosis) 80 mg/L[c]	[Not known]	58.1	g/L × 17.21 = mmol/L	mmol/L × 0.058 = g/L
Acetonitrile: see also Cyanide[b]	—	50 mg/L	41.1	mg/L × 24.3 = μmol/L	μmol/L × 0.041 = mg/L
N-acetyl-L-cysteine (NAC)	0.9 g/L (peak during infusion) 0.1 g/L (postinfusion)	—	163.2	g/L × 6.13 = mmol/L	mmol/L × 0.163 = g/L
l-α-Acetylmethadol	0.1 mg/L	[Not known]	353.5	mg/L × 2.83 = μmol/L	μmol/L × 0.354 = mg/L
Noracetylmethadol[b]	0.2 mg/L	[Not known]	339.5	mg/L × 2.95 = μmol/L	μmol/L × 0.340 = mg/L
Dinoracetylmethadol[b]	0.3 mg/L	[Not known]	325.5	mg/L × 3.07 = μmol/L	μmol/L × 0.326 = mg/L
N-Acetylprocainamide: see Acecainide					
o-Acetylsalicylic acid: see Aspirin					
Aciclovir	5 mg/L	—	225.2	mg/L × 4.44 = μmol/L	μmol/L × 0.225 = mg/L
Acrivastine	0.5 mg/L	[Not known]	348.4	mg/L × 2.87 = μmol/L	μmol/L × 0.348 = mg/L
Acrylonitrile: see Cyanide[b]					
Acyclovir: see Aciclovir					
Adrenaline	0.2 μg/L		183.2	μg/L × 5.46 = nmol/L	nmol/L × 0.183 = μg/L
Adriamycin: see Doxorubicin					
Ajmaline	1 mg/L	[Not known]	326.4	mg/L × 3.06 = μmol/L	μmol/L × 0.326 = mg/L
Albuterol: see Salbutamol					
Alcuronium	5 mg/L	[Not known]	667.9	mg/L × 1.50 = μmol/L	μmol/L × 0.668 = mg/L
Aldrin: see also Dieldrin[b]	0.1 mg/L	—	364.9	mg/L × 2.74 = μmol/L	μmol/L × 0.365 = mg/L
Alfentanil	2 mg/L (IV infusion)	—	416.5	mg/L × 2.40 = μmol/L	μmol/L × 0.417 = mg/L
Allobarbitone (allobarbital)	5 mg/L	30 mg/L	208.2	mg/L × 4.80 = μmol/L	μmol/L × 0.208 = mg/L
Allopurinol	20 mg/L	[Not known]	136.1	mg/L × 7.35 = μmol/L	μmol/L × 0.136 = mg/L
Oxypurinol[b]	20 mg/L	[Not known]	152.1	mg/L × 6.57 = μmol/L	μmol/L × 0.152 = mg/L
Alphaprodine	1 mg/L	—	261.4	mg/L × 3.83 = μmol/L	μmol/L × 0.261 = mg/L
Alphachloralose: see Chloralose					
Alprazolam	0.1 mg/L	0.2 mg/L	308.8	mg/L × 3.24 = μmol/L	μmol/L × 0.309 = mg/L
Alprenolol	0.2 mg/L	2 mg/L	249.4	mg/L × 4.01 = μmol/L	μmol/L × 0.249 = mg/L
4-Hydroxyalprenolol[b]	0.2 mg/L	[Not known]	265.4	mg/L × 3.77 = μmol/L	μmol/L × 0.265 = mg/L
Aluminium (urine)	15 μg/L urine 200 μg/L[c]	60 μg/L	27.0	μg/L × 0.037 = μmol/L	μmol/L × 27.0 = μg/L
Amantadine	1 mg/L	4 mg/L	151.3	mg/L × 6.61 = μmol/L	μmol/L × 0.151 = mg/L
Amethocaine: see Tetracaine					

*Data also available at http://www.leeds.ac.uk/acb/annals/.
†Achiral methods used unless otherwise indicated.

Analyte	"Therapeutic" or "normal" plasma concentration (less than)	Plasma concentration associated with acute serious toxicity[a]	Relative atomic or formula mass	Mass/amount conversion	Amount/mass conversion
Amikacin	25 mg/L	30 mg/L	585.6	mg/L × 1.71 = μmol/L	μmol/L × 0.586 = mg/L
Amiloride	50 μg/L	[Not known]	229.6	μg/L × 4.36 = nmol/L	nmol/L × 0.230 = μg/L
Amineptine	2 mg/L	[Not known]	337.5	mg/L × 2.96 = μmol/L	μmol/L × 0.338 = mg/L
7-Pentanoate metabolite[b]	1 mg/L		309.5	mg/L × 3.23 = μmol/L	μmol/L × 0.310 = mg/L
Aminoglutethimide	25 mg/L	—	232.3	mg/L × 4.30 = μmol/L	μmol/L × 0.232 = mg/L
5-Aminolevulinate (urine)	5 mg/L 6 mg/L (females)[c] 15 mg/L (males)[c]		131.1	mg/L × 7.63 = μmol/L	μmol/L × 0.131 = mg/L
4-Aminopyridine: see Fampridine					
Aminopyrine	20 mg/L	[Not known]	231.3	mg/L × 4.32 = μmol/L	μmol/L × 0.231 = mg/L
4-Aminosalicylate	250 mg/L	[Not known]	153.1	mg/L × 6.53 = μmol/L	μmol/L × 0.153 = mg/L
N-Acetyl-4-aminosalicylate[b]	150 mg/L	[Not known]	195.1	mg/L × 5.13 = μmol/L	μmol/L × 0.195 = mg/L
Amiodarone	2 mg/L	[Not known]	645.3	mg/L × 1.55 = μmol/L	μmol/L × 0.645 = mg/L
Noramiodarone[b]	2 mg/L	[Not known]	617.3	mg/L × 1.62 = μmol/L	μmol/L × 0.617 = mg/L
Amisulpride	1 mg/L	5 mg/L	369.5	mg/L × 2.71 = μmol/L	μmol/L × 0.370 = mg/L
Amitriptyline: see also Nortriptyline[b]	0.3 mg/L	1 mg/L	277.4	mg/L × 3.60 = μmol/L	μmol/L × 0.277 = mg/L
Amlodipine	50 μg/L	[Not known]	408.9	μg/L × 2.45 = nmol/L	nmol/L × 0.409 = μg/L
Amobarbital: see Amylobarbitone					
Amodiaquine	50 μg/L	[Not known]	355.9	μg/L × 2.81 = nmol/L	nmol/L × 0.356 = μg/L
Amoxapine	0.1 mg/L	0.5 mg/L	313.8	mg/L × 3.19 = μmol/L	μmol/L × 0.314 = mg/L
8-Hydroxyamoxapine[b]	0.5 mg/L	[Not known]	329.8	mg/L × 3.03 = μmol/L	μmol/L × 0.330 = mg/L
Amoxicillin	15 mg/L	[Not known]	365.4	mg/L × 2.74 = μmol/L	μmol/L × 0.365 = mg/L
d-Amphetamine	0.2 mg/L	1 mg/L	135.2	mg/L × 7.40 = μmol/L	μmol/L × 0.135 = mg/L
Ampicillin	20 mg/L	[Not known]	349.4	mg/L × 2.53 = μmol/L	μmol/L × 0.349 = mg/L
Amrinone	4 mg/L	[Not known]	187.2	mg/L × 5.34 = μmol/L	μmol/L × 0.187 = mg/L
4-Aminophenol (urine)	10 mg/L (occupational aniline exposure)		109.1	mg/L × 9.17 = μmol/L	μmol/L × 0.109 = mg/L
Amphotericin B	100 mg/L	[Not known]	924.1	mg/L × 1.08 = μmol/L	μmol/L × 0.924 = mg/L
Amsacrine	5 mg/L	—	393.5	mg/L × 2.54 = μmol/L	μmol/L × 0.394 = mg/L
Amygdalin: see also Cyanide[b]	1 mg/L (oral dose) 1200 mg/L (IV dose)	—	457.4	mg/L × 2.19 = μmol/L	μmol/L × 0.457 = mg/L
Amylobarbitone	5 mg/L	20 mg/L	226.3	mg/L × 4.42 = μmol/L	μmol/L × 0.226 = mg/L
Anileridine	0.5 mg/L	[Not known]	352.5	mg/L × 2.84 = μmol/L	μmol/L × 0.353 = mg/L
Aniline (urine): see also 4-Aminophenol[d]	1 mg/L[c]		93.1	mg/L × 10.7 = μmol/L	μmol/L × 0.093 = mg/L
Antimony (whole blood)	10 μg/L	200 μg/L	121.8	μg/L × 8.20 = nmol/L	nmol/L × 0.122 = μg/L
(urine)	1.2 μg/L	20 μg/L			
Antipyrine: see Phenazone					
Aprindine	2.5 mg/L	3 mg/L	322.5	mg/L × 3.10 = μmol/L	μmol/L × 0.323 = mg/L
Aprobarbitone (aprobarbital)	15 mg/L	60 mg/L	210.2	mg/L × 4.76 = μmol/L	μmol/L × 0.210 = mg/L
Arsenic (total)[e]	10 μg/L	50 μg/L	74.9	μg/L × 13.35 = nmol/L	nmol/L × 0.075 = μg/L
(total, whole blood)	10 μg/L	50 μg/L			
(total, urine)	10 μg/L	200 μg/L			
Aspirin (as salicylate[b])	300 mg/L	500 mg/L	138.1 (salicylate)	mg/L × 0.0072 = mmol/L	mmol/L × 138 = mg/L
Astemizole	0.1 mg/L	[Not known]	458.6	mg/L × 2.18 = μmol/L	μmol/L × 0.459 = mg/L
Atenolol	1 mg/L	10 mg/L	266.3	mg/L × 3.76 = μmol/L	μmol/L × 0.266 = mg/L
Atorvastatin	0.1 mg/L	[Not known]	558.6	mg/L × 1.79 = μmol/L	μmol/L × 0.559 = mg/L
Atracurium	5 mg/L	[Not known]	929.1	mg/L × 1.07 = μmol/L	μmol/L × 0.929 = mg/L
Atrazine	—	1 mg/L	215.7	mg/L × 4.63 = μmol/L	μmol/L × 0.216 = mg/L
Atropine (*d,l*-hyoscyamine)	20 μg/L	200 μg/L	289.4	μg/L × 3.46 = nmol/L	nmol/L × 0.289 = μg/L
Azapropazone	80 mg/L	[Not known]	336.4	mg/L × 2.97 = μmol/L	μmol/L × 0.336 = mg/L
Azathioprine: see 6-Mercaptopurine[b]					
Azithromycin	2 mg/L	[Not known]	749.0	mg/L × 1.34 = μmol/L	μmol/L × 0.749 = mg/L
AZT: see Zidovudine					
Baclofen	1 mg/L	2 mg/L	213.7	mg/L × 4.68 = μmol/L	μmol/L × 0.214 = mg/L
Barbitone (barbital)	30 mg/L	300 mg/L	184.2	mg/L × 5.43 = μmol/L	μmol/L × 0.184 = mg/L
"Barbiturates": see individual compounds					
Barium	1 μg/L	[Not known]	137.3	μg/L × 7.28 = nmol/L	nmol/L × 0.137 = μg/L
(urine)	5 μg/L				
Bendiocarb: see 2,2-Dimethyl-1,3-benzodioxol-4-ol (DMBD)[d]					
Bendrofluazide (bendroflumethiazide)	20 μg/L	[Not known]	421.4	μg/L × 2.37 = nmol/L	nmol/L × 0.421 = μg/L
Benoxaprofen	50 mg/L	[Not known]	301.7	mg/L × 3.31 = μmol/L	μmol/L × 0.302 = mg/L
Benzene (whole blood)	0.2 μg/L (nonsmokers) 0.6 μg/L (smokers)	1000 μg/L	78.1	μg/L × 12.8 = nmol/L	nmol/L × 0.078 = μg/L
γ-Benzene hexachloride: see Lindane					

Analyte	"Therapeutic" or "normal" plasma concentration (less than)	Plasma concentration associated with acute serious toxicity[a]	Relative atomic or formula mass	Mass/amount conversion	Amount/mass conversion
Benzhexol	50 µg/L	200 µg/L	301.5	µg/L × 3.32 = nmol/L	nmol/L × 0.302 = µg/L
Benzoate	0.01 g/L (dietary)	0.5 g/L (neonates)	122.1	g/L × 8.19 = mmol/L	mmol/L × 0.122 = g/L
Benzonatate	0.5 mg/L	[Not known]	603.7	mg/L × 1.66 = µmol/L	µmol/L × 0.604 = mg/L
Benztropine	0.2 mg/L	0.4 mg/L	307.4	mg/L × 3.25 = µmol/L	µmol/L × 0.307 = mg/L
Benzyl alcohol: see also Benzoate[b]	—	50 mg/L (neonates)	108.1	mg/L × 9.25 = µmol/L	µmol/L × 0.108 = mg/L
Benzylpenicillin	10 mg/L				
Bepridil	2.5 mg/L	[Not known]	334.4	mg/L × 2.99 = µmol/L	µmol/L × 0.334 = mg/L
Beryllium	0.3 µg/L	[Not known]	366.6	mg/L × 2.73 = µmol/L	µmol/L × 0.367 = mg/L
(urine)	1 µg/L	[Not known]	9.01	µg/L × 110.9 = nmol/L	nmol/L × 0.009 = µg/L
Betaxolol	50 µg/L				
Bethanidine	0.5 mg/L	[Not known]	307.4	µg/L × 3.25 = nmol/L	nmol/L × 0.307 = µg/L
Bezafibrate	3 mg/L	[Not known]	177.3	mg/L × 5.64 = µmol/L	µmol/L × 0.177 = mg/L
γ-BHC: see Lindane		[Not known]	361.8	mg/L × 2.76 = µmol/L	µmol/L × 0.362 = mg/L
Biperiden	0.1 mg/L	[Not known]	311.5	mg/L × 3.21 = µmol/L	µmol/L × 0.312 = mg/L
Bismuth (whole blood)	10 µg/L (dietary)	100 µg/L	209.0	µg/L × 4.78 = nmol/L	nmol/L × 0.209 = µg/L
Bisoprolol	0.1 mg/L	[Not known]	325.5	mg/L × 3.07 = µmol/L	µmol/L × 0.326 = mg/L
Bopindolol	15 µg/L	[Not known]	380.5	µg/L × 2.63 = nmol/L	nmol/L × 0.381 = µg/L
Borate	7 mg/L (dietary)	20 mg/L	58.8	mg/L × 17.0 = µmol/L	µmol/L × 0.059 = mg/L
Boron	0.2 µg/L	[Not known]	10.8	µg/L × 92.6 = nmol/L	nmol/L × 0.011 = µg/L
Brallobarbitone (brallo-barbital)	8 mg/L	40 mg/L	287.1	mg/L × 3.48 = µmol/L	µmol/L × 0.287 = mg/L
Bretylium	5 mg/L	[Not known]	243.4	mg/L × 4.11 = µmol/L	µmol/L × 0.243 = mg/L
Brodifacoum	—	100 µg/L	523.4	µg/L × 1.91 = nmol/L	nmol/L × 0.523 = µg/L
Bromazepam	0.2 mg/L	1 mg/L	316.2	mg/L × 3.16 = µmol/L	µmol/L × 0.316 = mg/L
Bromide	10 mg/L (dietary)	500 mg/L (inorganic bromide exposure) 40 mg/L (organobromine alkylating agents)	79.9	mg/L × 12.52 = µmol/L	µmol/L × 0.080 = mg/L
Bromisoval	20 mg/L	40 mg/L	223.1	mg/L × 4.48 = µmol/L	µmol/L × 0.223 = mg/L
Bromocriptine	1 µg/L	—	645.6	µg/L × 1.55 = nmol/L	nmol/L × 0.646 = µg/L
Bromomethane: see Bromide[b]					
Bromoxynil	—	20 mg/L	276.9	mg/L × 3.61 = µmol/L	µmol/L × 0.277 = mg/L
Bromperidol	20 µg/L	[Not known]	420.3	µg/L × 2.38 = nmol/L	nmol/L × 0.420 = µg/L
Brompheniramine	50 µg/L	[Not known]	319.2	µg/L × 3.13 = nmol/L	nmol/L × 0.319 = µg/L
Brotizolam	50 µg/L	[Not known]	393.7	µg/L × 2.54 = nmol/L	nmol/L × 0.394 = µg/L
Buflomedil	20 µg/L	40 mg/L	307.4	mg/L × 3.25 = µmol/L	µmol/L × 0.307 = mg/L
Buformin	0.6 mg/L (diabetics)	1 mg/L	157.2	mg/L × 6.36 = µmol/L	µmol/L × 0.157 = mg/L
Bupivacaine	0.8 mg/L (epidural)	1.5 mg/L	288.4	mg/L × 3.47 = µmol/L	µmol/L × 0.288 = mg/L
Buprenorphine	5 µg/L (oral)	200 µg/L	467.6	µg/L × 2.14 = nmol/L	nmol/L × 0.468 = µg/L
Bupropion	0.4 mg/L	4 mg/L	239.7	mg/L × 4.17 = µmol/L	µmol/L × 0.240 = mg/L
Buspirone	5 µg/L	[Not known]	385.5	µg/L × 2.59 = nmol/L	nmol/L × 0.386 = µg/L
Busulfan	2 mg/L	—	246.3	mg/L × 4.06 = µmol/L	µmol/L × 0.246 = mg/L
Butanone (whole blood)	10 mg/L (occupational exposure)	500 mg/L	72.1	mg/L × 13.9 = µmol/L	µmol/L × 0.072 = mg/L
(urine)	5 mg/L[c]				
Butaperazine	3 mg/L	[Not known]	409.6	mg/L × 2.44 = µmol/L	µmol/L × 0.410 = mg/L
Butethal: see Butobarbitone					
Butobarbitone (butobar-bital)	15 mg/L	60 mg/L	212.2	mg/L × 4.71 = µmol/L	µmol/L × 0.212 = mg/L
Butorphanol	2 µg/L	[Not known]	327.5	µg/L × 3.05 = nmol/L	nmol/L × 0.328 = µg/L
Butoxyacetate (urine)	100 mg/L[c]		132.2	mg/L × 6.75 = µmol/L	µmol/L × 0.148 = mg/L
2-Butoxyethanol: see Butoxyacetate[d]					
Butriptyline	0.2 mg/L	1 mg/L	293.5	mg/L × 3.41 = µmol/L	µmol/L × 0.294 = mg/L
Norbutriptyline[b]	0.2 mg/L	1 mg/L	279.5	mg/L × 3.58 = µmol/L	µmol/L × 0.280 = mg/L
Butyl nitrite: see Nitrite[b]					
4-*tert*.-Butylphenol: see 4-(1,1-Dimethylethyl)phenol					
Cadmium (whole blood)	5 µg/L	20 µg/L	112.4	µg/L × 8.90 = nmol/L	nmol/L × 0.112 = µg/L
(urine)	5 µg/L	20 µg/L			
Caffeine	15 mg/L (dietary)	60 mg/L	194.2	mg/L × 5.14 = µmol/L	µmol/L × 0.194 = mg/L
Camazepam	0.6 mg/L	2 mg/L	371.8	mg/L × 2.69 = µmol/L	µmol/L × 0.372 = mg/L
Camphor	—	1 mg/L	152.2	mg/L × 6.57 = µmol/L	µmol/L × 0.152 = mg/L
Canrenone	0.25 mg/L	[Not known]	340.5	mg/L × 2.94 = µmol/L	µmol/L × 0.341 = mg/L
Captopril	1 mg/L	5 mg/L	217.3	mg/L × 4.60 = µmol/L	µmol/L × 0.217 = mg/L
Captopril disulfide[b]	0.5 mg/L	[Not known]	432.6	mg/L × 2.31 = µmol/L	µmol/L × 0.433 = mg/L
Carazolol	20 µg/L	[Not known]	298.4	µg/L × 3.35 = nmol/L	nmol/L × 0.298 = µg/L
Carbamazepine	12 mg/L	30 mg/L	236.3	mg/L × 4.23 = µmol/L	µmol/L × 0.236 = mg/L
Carbamazepine-10,11-epoxide[b]	6 mg/L	15 mg/L	252.3	mg/L × 3.96 = µmol/L	µmol/L × 0.252 = mg/L
Carbaryl	—	5 mg/L	201.2	mg/L × 4.97 = µmol/L	µmol/L × 0.201 = mg/L
Carbenoxolone	30 mg/L	[Not known]	570.8	mg/L × 1.75 = µmol/L	µmol/L × 0.571 = mg/L

Analyte	"Therapeutic" or "normal" plasma concentration (less than)	Plasma concentration associated with acute serious toxicity[a]	Relative atomic or formula mass	Mass/amount conversion	Amount/mass conversion
Carbidopa	0.4 mg/L	[Not known]	226.3	mg/L × 4.42 = μmol/L	μmol/L × 0.226 = mg/L
Carbimazole: see Methimazole[b]					
Carbon disulfide: see 2-Thiothiazolidine-4-carboxylate[d]					
Carbon monoxide (carboxyhemoglobin saturation: see Chapter 80, Table 8)					
Carbon tetrachloride (whole blood)	0.07 mg/L[c]	0.5 mg/L (2 h postexposure)	153.8	mg/L × 6.50 = μmol/L	μmol/L × 0.154 = mg/L
Carboplatin: see also Platinum[d]	30 mg/L	—	371.3	mg/L × 2.69 = μmol/L	μmol/L × 0.371 = mg/L
Carbromal: see also Bromide[b]	10 mg/L	40 mg/L	237.1	mg/L × 4.22 = μmol/L	μmol/L × 0.237 = mg/L
Carisoprodol: see also Meprobamate[b]	5 mg/L	30 mg/L	260.3	mg/L × 3.84 = μmol/L	μmol/L × 0.260 = mg/L
Carteolol	0.1 mg/L	[Not known]	292.4	mg/L × 3.42 = μmol/L	μmol/L × 0.292 = mg/L
Carvedilol	0.3 mg/L	[Not known]	406.5	mg/L × 2.46 = μmol/L	μmol/L × 0.407 = mg/L
Cathine	1 mg/L	[Not known]	151.2	mg/L × 6.61 = μmol/L	μmol/L × 0.151 = mg/L
Cathinone: see also Norephedrine[b]	—	1 mg/L	149.2	mg/L × 6.70 = μmol/L	μmol/L × 0.149 = mg/L
Cefuroxime	200 mg/L	[Not known]	424.4	mg/L × 2.36 = μmol/L	μmol/L × 0.424 = mg/L
Celiprolol	1 mg/L	[Not known]	379.5	mg/L × 2.64 = μmol/L	μmol/L × 0.380 = mg/L
Celecoxib	1 mg/L	[Not known]	381.4	mg/L × 2.62 = μmol/L	μmol/L × 0.381 = mg/L
Cephaloridine	50 mg/L	—	415.5	mg/L × 2.41 = μmol/L	μmol/L × 0.416 = mg/L
Cetirizine	1 mg/L	[Not known]	388.9	mg/L × 2.57 = μmol/L	μmol/L × 0.389 = mg/L
Chloral (hydrate): see 2,2,2-Trichloroethanol[b]					
Chloralose	—	50 mg/L	309.5	mg/L × 3.23 = μmol/L	μmol/L × 0.310 = mg/L
Chlorambucil	0.3 mg/L	[Not known]	304.2	mg/L × 3.29 = μmol/L	μmol/L × 0.304 = mg/L
Chloramphenicol	25 mg/L	40 mg/L	323.1	mg/L × 3.10 = μmol/L	μmol/L × 0.323 = mg/L
Chlordane (total)	0.001 mg/L (dietary)	1 mg/L	409.8	μg/L × 2.44 = nmol/L	nmol/L × 0.410 = μg/L
Chlordecone	—	0.5 mg/L	490.6	mg/L × 2.04 = μmol/L	μmol/L × 0.491 = mg/L
Chlordiazepoxide: see also Nordazepam,[b] Demoxepam[b]	2 mg/L	10 mg/L	299.8	mg/L × 3.33 = μmol/L	μmol/L × 0.300 = mg/L
Chlorguanide: see Proguanil					
Chlorhexidine	0.2 mg/L (topical)	2 mg/L	505.5	mg/L × 1.98 = μmol/L	μmol/L × 0.506 = mg/L
Chlormethiazole (clomethiazole)	2 mg/L (oral)	10 mg/L	161.6	mg/L × 6.19 = μmol/L	μmol/L × 0.162 = mg/L
Chlormezanone	10 mg/L	40 mg/L	273.7	mg/L × 3.65 = μmol/L	μmol/L × 0.274 = mg/L
Chlorobenzene	0.5 mg/L (industrial exposure)	[Not known]	112.6	mg/L × 8.88 = μmol/L	μmol/L × 0.113 = mg/L
Chloroethane (whole blood)	—	20 mg/L	64.5	mg/L × 15.5 = μmol/L	μmol/L × 0.065 = mg/L
Chloroform (whole blood)	200 mg/L (anesthesia) 0.01 mg/L (dietary)	—	119.4	mg/L × 8.38 = μmol/L	μmol/L × 0.119 = mg/L
4-Chloro-2-methylphenoxyacetate	—	0.5 g/L	200.6	g/L × 4.99 = mmol/L	mmol/L × 0.201 = g/L
2-(4-Chloro-2-methylphenoxy)propionate	—	0.5 g/L	214.6	g/L × 4.66 = mmol/L	mmol/L × 0.215 = g/L
Chlorophacinone	—	0.1 mg/L	374.8	mg/L × 2.67 = μmol/L	μmol/L × 0.375 = mg/L
Chloroprocaine	5 mg/L	[Not known]	270.7	mg/L × 3.69 = μmol/L	μmol/L × 0.271 = mg/L
Chloroquine: see also Norchloroquine[b]	0.3 mg/L	1 mg/L	319.9	mg/L × 3.13 = μmol/L	μmol/L × 0.320 = mg/L
Chlorothiazide	10 mg/L (oral)	[Not known]	295.7	mg/L × 3.38 = μmol/L	μmol/L × 0.296 = mg/L
Chlorphenesin carbamate	20 mg/L	[Not known]	245.7	mg/L × 4.07 = μmol/L	μmol/L × 0.246 = mg/L
Chlorpheniramine	0.05 mg/L	0.5 mg/L	274.8	mg/L × 3.64 = μmol/L	μmol/L × 0.275 = mg/L
Chlorphentermine	0.5 mg/L	[Not known]	183.7	mg/L × 5.44 = μmol/L	μmol/L × 0.184 = mg/L
Chlorpromazine: see also Promazine[b]	0.5 mg/L	2 mg/L	318.9	mg/L × 3.14 = μmol/L	μmol/L × 0.319 = mg/L
Chlorpropamide	400 mg/L (diabetics)	—	276.7	mg/L × 3.61 = μmol/L	μmol/L × 0.277 = mg/L
Chlorprothixene	0.05 mg/L	0.1 mg/L	315.9	mg/L × 3.17 = μmol/L	μmol/L × 0.316 = mg/L
Chlorpyriphos	—	0.2 mg/L	350.6	mg/L × 2.85 = μmol/L	μmol/L × 0.351 = mg/L
Chlorthalidone	2 mg/L	[Not known]	338.8	mg/L × 2.95 = μmol/L	μmol/L × 0.339 = mg/L
Chlorzoxazone	40 mg/L	[Not known]	169.6	mg/L × 5.90 = μmol/L	μmol/L × 0.170 = mg/L
Chromium	0.35 μg/L	[Not known][f]	52.0	μg/L × 19.2 = nmol/L	nmol/L × 0.052 = μg/L
(urine)	0.25 μg/L				
Cimetidine	4 mg/L	20 mg/L	252.3	mg/L × 3.96 = μmol/L	μmol/L × 0.252 = mg/L
Cineole	—	[Not known]	154.3	mg/L × 6.48 = μmol/L	μmol/L × 0.154 = mg/L
Cinnarizine	0.2 mg/L	[Not known]	368.5	mg/L × 2.71 = μmol/L	μmol/L × 0.369 = mg/L
Ciprofloxacin	5 mg/L	[Not known]	331.4	mg/L × 3.02 = μmol/L	μmol/L × 0.331 = mg/L
Cisapride	0.1 mg/L	[Not known]	466.0	mg/L × 2.15 = μmol/L	μmol/L × 0.466 = mg/L
Cisplatin: see also Platinum[d]	5 mg/L	—	300.1	mg/L × 3.33 = μmol/L	μmol/L × 0.300 = mg/L
Citalopram	0.3 mg/L	1 mg/L	324.4	mg/L × 3.08 = μmol/L	μmol/L × 0.324 = mg/L
Norcitalopram[b]	0.2 mg/L		310.4	mg/L × 3.22 = μmol/L	μmol/L × 0.310 = mg/L

Analyte	"Therapeutic" or "normal" plasma concentration (less than)	Plasma concentration associated with acute serious toxicity[a]	Relative atomic or formula mass	Mass/amount conversion	Amount/mass conversion
Clemastine	5 μg/L	[Not known]	343.9	μg/L × 2.91 = nmol/L	nmol/L × 0.344 = μg/L
Clenbuterol	0.1 μg/L	[Not known]	277.2	μg/L × 3.61 = nmol/L	nmol/L × 0.277 = μg/L
Clobazam	1 mg/L	5 mg/L	300.7	mg/L × 3.33 = μmol/L	μmol/L × 0.301 = mg/L
Norclobazam[b]	4 mg/L	20 mg/L	286.7	mg/L × 3.49 = μmol/L	μmol/L × 0.287 = mg/L
Clofibrate	250 mg/L	—	242.7	mg/L × 4.12 = μmol/L	μmol/L × 0.243 = mg/L
Clomethiazole: see Chlormethiazole					
Clomipramine	0.4 mg/L	1 mg/L	314.9	mg/L × 3.18 = μmol/L	μmol/L × 0.315 = mg/L
Norclomipramine[b]	0.8 mg/L	2 mg/L	300.8	mg/L × 3.32 = μmol/L	μmol/L × 0.301 = mg/L
Clonazepam	0.08 mg/L	1 mg/L	315.7	mg/L × 3.17 = μmol/L	μmol/L × 0.316 = mg/L
Clonidine	2 μg/L	10 μg/L	230.1	μg/L × 4.35 = nmol/L	nmol/L × 0.230 = μg/L
α-Clopenthixol: see Zuclopenthixol					
Clorazepate: see also Nordazepam[b]	20 μg/L	[Not known]	314.7	μg/L × 3.18 = nmol/L	nmol/L × 0.315 = μg/L
Clotiazepam	0.5 mg/L	[Not known]	318.8	mg/L × 3.14 = μmol/L	μmol/L × 0.319 = mg/L
Clozapine	1 mg/L	2 mg/L	326.8	mg/L × 3.06 = μmol/L	μmol/L × 0.327 = mg/L
Norclozapine[b]	1 mg/L	2 mg/L	312.8	mg/L × 3.20 = μmol/L	μmol/L × 0.313 = mg/L
Cobalt	0.4 μg/L	[Not known]	58.9	μg/L × 17.0 = nmol/L	nmol/L × 0.060 = μg/L
(urine)	1 μg/L				
Cocaine	0.3 mg/L	1 mg/L	303.4	mg/L × 3.30 = μmol/L	μmol/L × 0.303 = mg/L
Benzoylecgonine[d]	1 mg/L		289.4	mg/L × 3.46 = μmol/L	μmol/L × 0.289 = mg/L
Codeine: see also Morphine[b]	0.3 mg/L	1 mg/L	299.4	mg/L × 3.34 = μmol/L	μmol/L × 0.299 = mg/L
Colchicine	4 μg/L (oral dose)	20 μg/L	399.4	μg/L × 2.50 = nmol/L	nmol/L × 0.399 = μg/L
Copper (total)[g]	0.6–1.6 mg/L	5 mg/L (not Wilson's disease)	63.6	mg/L × 15.7 = μmol/L	μmol/L × 0.064 = mg/L
(urine)	60 mg/L	100 mg/L (Wilson's disease)			
Cotinine (from nicotine)	0.01 mg/L (nonsmokers)		176.2	mg/L × 5.67 = μmol/L	μmol/L × 0.176 = mg/L
Coumafuryl	—	0.25 mg/L	298.3	mg/L × 3.35 = μmol/L	μmol/L × 0.298 = mg/L
Creatine	10 mg/L (endogenous) 20–130 mg/L (dietary supplement)	[Not known]	131.1	mg/L × 7.63 = μmol/L	μmol/L × 0.131= mg/L
Cresols: see Methylphenols					
Cromoglycate (cromolyn)	10 μg/L	[Not known]	468.4	μg/L × 2.13 = nmol/L	nmol/L × 0.468 = μg/L
Cumene	1 μg/L (environmental)	[Not known]	120.2	μg/L × 8.32 = nmol/L	nmol/L × 0.120 = μg/L
Cyamemazine	0.5 mg/L	[Not known]	323.5	mg/L × 3.09 = μmol/L	μmol/L × 0.324 = mg/L
Cyanide (whole blood): see also Thiocyanate[b]	0.2 mg/L (nonsmokers) 0.5 mg/L (heavy smokers)	5 mg/L (1 mg/L inhalation)	26.0	mg/L × 38.5 = μmol/L	μmol/L × 0.026 = mg/L
Cyclizine	0.25 mg/L	1 mg/L	266.4	mg/L × 3.75 = μmol/L	μmol/L × 0.266 = mg/L
Norcyclizine[b]	0.025 mg/L	[Not known]	252.4	mg/L × 3.96 = μmol/L	μmol/L × 0.252 = mg/L
Cyclobarbitone (cyclobarbital)	5 mg/L	30 mg/L	236.3	mg/L × 4.23 = μmol/L	μmol/L × 0.236 = mg/L
Cyclobenzaprine	0.04 mg/L	0.4 mg/L	275.4	mg/L × 3.63 = μmol/L	μmol/L × 0.275 = mg/L
Cyclohexane	0.4 mg/L (occupational exposure)	[Not known]	84.2	mg/L × 11.9 = μmol/L	μmol/L × 0.084 = mg/L
Cyclopropane	100 mg/L (anesthesia)	—	42.1	mg/L × 23.8 = μmol/L	μmol/L × 0.042 = mg/L
Cyclosporin (ciclosporin; whole blood)	0.4 mg/L	—	1203	mg/L × 0.83 = μmol/L	μmol/L × 1.203 = mg/L
Cyproheptadine	50 μg/L	[Not known]	287.4	μg/L × 3.48 = nmol/L	nmol/L × 0.287 = μg/L
Cytarabine	0.5 mg/L	—	243.2	mg/L × 4.11 = μmol/L	μmol/L × 0.243 = mg/L
2,4-D: see 2,4-Dichlorophenoxyacetate					
Danazol	0.2 mg/L	—	337.5	mg/L × 2.96 = μmol/L	μmol/L × 0.338 = mg/L
Dantrolene	3 mg/L	[Not known]	314.3	mg/L × 3.18 = μmol/L	μmol/L × 0.314 = mg/L
Dapsone	5 mg/L	20 mg/L	248.3	mg/L × 4.03 = μmol/L	μmol/L × 0.248 = mg/L
DCPP: see 2-(2,4-Dichlorophenoxy)propionate					
DDT: see 1,1,1-Trichloro-di-(4-chlorophenyl)ethane					
Debrisoquin(e)	0.2 mg/L	[Not known]	175.2	mg/L × 5.70 = μmol/L	μmol/L × 0.175 = mg/L
DEET: see *N,N*-diethyl-3-methylbenzamide					
Deferoxamine: see Desferrioxamine					
Demoxepam	3 mg/L	10 mg/L	286.7	mg/L × 3.49 = μmol/L	μmol/L × 0.287 = mg/L
N_1-Desalkylflurazepam: see Flurazepam					
Desferrioxamine	15 mg/L	[Not known]	560.7	mg/L × 1.78 = μmol/L	μmol/L × 0.561 = mg/L
Desflurane	20 mg/L (whole blood)	—	168.0	mg/L × 5.95 = μmol/L	μmol/L × 0.168 = mg/L
Desipramine	0.3 mg/L	1 mg/L	266.4	mg/L × 3.75 = μmol/L	μmol/L × 0.266 = mg/L
Desloratadine: see Loratadine					
Dexamethasone	0.2 mg/L	[Not known]	392.5	mg/L × 2.55 = μmol/L	μmol/L × 0.393 = mg/L
Dexfenfluramine	50 μg/L	200 μg/L	231.3	mg/L × 4.32 = μmol/L	μmol/L × 0.231 = mg/L
Nordexfenfluramine[b]	25 μg/L	100 μg/L	203.3	mg/L × 4.92 = μmol/L	μmol/L × 0.203 = mg/L
Dextromethorphan	0.2 mg/L	1 mg/L	271.4	mg/L × 3.70 = μmol/L	μmol/L × 0.271 = mg/L
Dextromoramide	0.1 mg/L	0.2 mg/L	392.5	mg/L × 2.55 = μmol/L	μmol/L × 0.393 = mg/L

Analyte	"Therapeutic" or "normal" plasma concentration (less than)	Plasma concentration associated with acute serious toxicity[a]	Relative atomic or formula mass	Mass/amount conversion	Amount/mass conversion
Dextropropoxyphene	0.4 mg/L	1 mg/L	339.5	mg/L × 2.95 = μmol/L	μmol/L × 0.340 = mg/L
Norpropoxyphene[b]	1.5 mg/L	3 mg/L	325.5	mg/L × 3.07 = μmol/L	μmol/L × 0.326 = mg/L
Diacetolol: see Acebutolol					
4,4'-Diaminodiphenylmethane: see 4,4'-Methylenedianiline					
Diamorphine: see Heroin, Morphine[b]					
Diazepam: see also Nordazepam,[b] Temazepam[b]	2 mg/L	5 mg/L	284.7	mg/L × 3.51 = μmol/L	μmol/L × 0.285 = mg/L
Diazinon	—	0.5 mg/L	304.4	mg/L × 3.29 = μmol/L	μmol/L × 0.304 = mg/L
Diazoxide	50 mg/L	100 mg/L	230.7	mg/L × 4.33 = μmol/L	μmol/L × 0.231 = mg/L
Dibenzepin	0.5 mg/L	5 mg/L	295.4	mg/L × 3.39 = μmol/L	μmol/L × 0.295 = mg/L
Dichloroacetate	300 mg/L (postinfusion)	[Not known]	128.9	mg/L × 7.76 = μmol/L	μmol/L × 0.129 = mg/L
1,4-Dichlorobenzene	20 μg/L (environmental exposure)	[Not known]	147.0	μg/L × 6.80 = nmol/L	nmol/L × 0.147 = μg/L
2,5-Dichlorophenol (urine)[d]	100 mg/L (occupational exposure)		163.0	mg/L × 6.13 = μmol/L	μmol/L × 0.163 = mg/L
Dichloromethane (whole blood): see also Carbon monoxide[b]	1 mg/L[c]	200 mg/L	84.9	mg/L × 11.8 = μmol/L	μmol/L × 0.085 = mg/L
2,4-Dichlorophenoxyacetate	—	0.5 g/L	221.0	g/L × 4.52 = mmol/L	mmol/L × 0.221 = g/L
2-(2,4-Dichlorophenoxy)propionate	—	0.5 g/L	235.1	g/L × 4.25 = mmol/L	mmol/L × 0.235 = g/L
Dichlorprop: see 2-(2,4-Dichlorophenoxy)propionate					
Diclofenac	2.5 mg/L	50 mg/L	296.2	mg/L × 3.38 = μmol/L	μmol/L × 0.296 = mg/L
Dicoumarol	30 mg/L	70 mg/L	336.3	mg/L × 2.97 = μmol/L	μmol/L × 0.336 = mg/L
Dicyclomine (dicycloverin)	0.1 mg/L	0.5 mg/L	309.5	mg/L × 3.23 = μmol/L	μmol/L × 0.310 = mg/L
Dieldrin	5 μg/L (dietary)	300 μg/L	380.9	μg/L × 2.63 = nmol/L	nmol/L × 0.381 = μg/L
Diethylcarbamazine	0.2 mg/L	[Not known]	199.3	mg/L × 5.02 = μmol/L	μmol/L × 0.199 = mg/L
Diethyldithiocarbamate: see Dithiocarb					
Diethyl ether (whole blood)	500 mg/L (anesthesia)	—	74.1	g/L × 13.50 = mmol/L	mmol/L × 0.074 = g/L
N,N-Diethyl-3-methylbenzamide (DEET)	3 mg/L (topical)	200 mg/L	191.3	mg/L × 5.23 = μmol/L	μmol/L × 0.191 = mg/L
Diethylpropion	0.01 mg/L	2 mg/L	205.3	mg/L × 4.87 = μmol/L	μmol/L × 0.205 = mg/L
Diethyltoluamide: see *N,N*-Diethyl-3-methylbenzamide					
Difenacoum	—	0.5 mg/L	444.5	mg/L × 2.25 = μmol/L	μmol/L × 0.445 = mg/L
Diflunisal	150 mg/L	300 mg/L	250.2	mg/L × 4.00 = μmol/L	μmol/L × 0.250 = mg/L
Digitoxin	30 μg/L	60 μg/L	765.0	μg/L × 1.31 = nmol/L	nmol/L × 0.765 = μg/L
Digoxin	2 μg/L	4 μg/L	780.9	μg/L × 1.28 = nmol/L	nmol/L × 0.781 = μg/L
Dihydrocodeine	0.25 mg/L	1 mg/L	301.4	mg/L × 3.32 = μmol/L	μmol/L × 0.301 = mg/L
Dihydroergotamine	10 μg/L	[Not known]	583.7	μg/L × 1.71 = nmol/L	nmol/L × 0.584 = μg/L
Diltiazem	0.4 mg/L	2 mg/L	414.5	mg/L × 2.41 = μmol/L	μmol/L × 0.415 = mg/L
Dimethadione	1 g/L	[Not known]	129.1	g/L × 7.75 = mmol/L	mmol/L × 0.129 = g/L
N,N-Dimethylacetamide: see *N*-Methylacetamide (NMA)[d]					
2,2-Dimethyl-1,3-benzodioxol-4-ol (urine)	0.8 mg/L (occupational bendiocarb exposure)	[Not known]	166.2	mg/L × 6.02 = μmol/L	μmol/L × 0.166 = mg/L
4-(1,1-Dimethylethyl)phenol (urine)	2 mg/L[c]		150.2	mg/L × 6.66 = μmol/L	μmol/L × 0.150 = mg/L
N,N-Dimethylformamide: see *N*-Methylformamide (NMF)[d]					
Dimethylsulfoxide (DMSO)	2 g/L (topical)	[Not known]	78.1	g/L × 12.8 = mmol/L	mmol/L × 0.078 = g/L
Dimethylsulfone[b]	1 g/L (topical DMSO)	[Not known]	94.1	g/L × 10.6 = mmol/L	mmol/L × 0.094 = g/L
N,N-Dimethyltryptamine	1 μg/L	[Not known]	188.3	μg/L × 5.31 = nmol/L	nmol/L × 0.188 = μg/L
4,6-Dinitro-2-methylphenol (DNOC)	—	40 mg/L	198.1	mg/L × 5.05 = μmol/L	μmol/L × 0.198 = mg/L
1,4-Dioxane	12 mg/L (occupational exposure)	[Not known]	88.1	mg/L × 11.4 = μmol/L	μmol/L × 0.088 = mg/L
β-Hydroxyethoxyacetate (urine)[d]	0.5 g/L (occupational exposure)		120.1	g/L × 8.33 = mmol/L	mmol/L × 0.120 = g/L
Dioxin: see 2,3,6,7-Tetrachlorodibenzodioxin					
Diphenhydramine	0.5 mg/L	5 mg/L	255.4	mg/L × 3.92 = μmol/L	μmol/L × 0.255 = mg/L
Diphenoxylate	10 μg/L	[Not known]	452.6	μg/L × 2.21 = nmol/L	nmol/L × 0.453 = μg/L
Diphenylhydantoin: see Phenytoin					
Dipipanone	0.05 mg/L	0.2 mg/L	349.5	mg/L × 2.86 = μmol/L	μmol/L × 0.350 = mg/L
Diprophylline	20 mg/L	40 mg/L	254.3	mg/L × 3.93 = μmol/L	μmol/L × 0.254 = mg/L
Dipyridamole	2 mg/L	4 mg/L	504.6	mg/L × 1.98 = μmol/L	μmol/L × 0.505 = mg/L
Dipyrone: see 4-Methyaminophenazone[b]					
Diquat	—	0.4 mg/L	184.2	mg/L × 5.42 = μmol/L	μmol/L × 0.184 = mg/L
Disopyramide	5 mg/L	[Not known]	297.5	mg/L × 3.36 = μmol/L	μmol/L × 0.298 = mg/L
Nordisopyramide[b]	5 mg/L		255.5	mg/L × 3.91 = μmol/L	μmol/L × 0.256 = mg/L

Analyte	"Therapeutic" or "normal" plasma concentration (less than)	Plasma concentration associated with acute serious toxicity[a]	Relative atomic or formula mass	Mass/amount conversion	Amount/mass conversion
Disulfiram: see also Dithiocarb[b]	0.5 mg/L	5 mg/L	296.5	mg/L × 3.37 = μmol/L	μmol/L × 0.297 = mg/L
Dithiocarb	1.5 mg/L	[Not known]	148.3	mg/L × 6.74 = μmol/L	μmol/L × 0.148 = mg/L
DMAC: see *N,N*-Dimethylacetamide					
DNOC: see 4,6-Dinitro-2-methylphenol					
Dobutamine	20 μg/L	[Not known]	301.4	μg/L × 3.32 = nmol/L	nmol/L × 0.301 = μg/L
Domperidone	20 μg/L	[Not known]	425.9	μg/L × 2.35 = nmol/L	nmol/L × 0.426 = μg/L
Dosulepin: see Dothiepin					
Dothiepin	0.3 mg/L	1 mg/L	295.5	mg/L × 3.38 = μmol/L	μmol/L × 0.297 = mg/L
Nordothiepin[b]	0.3 mg/L	1 mg/L	281.5	mg/L × 3.55 = μmol/L	μmol/L × 0.282 = mg/L
Doxapram	5 mg/L	[Not known]	378.5	mg/L × 2.64 = μmol/L	μmol/L × 0.379 = mg/L
Doxazosin	0.2 mg/L	[Not known]	451.5	mg/L × 2.21 = μmol/L	μmol/L × 0.452 = mg/L
Doxepin	0.3 mg/L	1 mg/L	279.4	mg/L × 3.58 = μmol/L	μmol/L × 0.279 = mg/L
Nordoxepin[b]	0.3 mg/L	1 mg/L	265.4	mg/L × 3.77 = μmol/L	μmol/L × 0.265 = mg/L
Doxorubicin	20 μg/L	—	543.5	μg/L × 1.84 = nmol/L	nmol/L × 0.544 = μg/L
Doxycycline	10 mg/L	30 mg/L	444.5	mg/L × 2.25 = μmol/L	μmol/L × 0.445 = mg/L
Doxylamine	0.2 mg/L	0.5 mg/L	270.4	mg/L × 3.70 = μmol/L	μmol/L × 0.270 = mg/L
Droperidol	50 μg/L	[Not known]	379.4	μg/L × 2.64 = nmol/L	nmol/L × 0.379 = μg/L
Dyphylline: see Diprophylline					
Efavirenz	5 mg/L	[Not known]	315.7	mg/L × 3.17 = μmol/L	μmol/L × 0.316 = mg/L
Emetine	0.1 mg/L	0.5 mg/L	480.7	mg/L × 2.08 = μmol/L	μmol/L × 0.481 = mg/L
Enalapril: see Enalaprilat[b]					
Enalaprilat	0.1 mg/L	[Not known]	348.5	mg/L × 2.87 = μmol/L	μmol/L × 0.349 = mg/L
Encainide	0.1 mg/L (1 mg/L slow metabolizers)	[Not known]	352.5	mg/L × 2.84 = μmol/L	μmol/L × 0.353 = mg/L
O-Desmethylencainide[d]	0.2 mg/L	[Not known]	338.5	mg/L × 2.95 = μmol/L	μmol/L × 0.339 = mg/L
3-Methoxy-*O*-desmethylencainide[d]	0.2 mg/L	[Not known]	368.5	mg/L × 2.71 = μmol/L	μmol/L × 0.369 = mg/L
Endosulfan	—	1 mg/L	406.9	mg/L × 2.46 = μmol/L	μmol/L × 0.407 = mg/L
Endrin	3 μg/L (dietary)	10 μg/L	380.9	μg/L × 2.63 = nmol/L	nmol/L × 0.381 = μg/L
Enflurane (whole blood)	100 mg/L (anesthesia)	—	184.5	mg/L × 5.42 = μmol/L	μmol/L × 0.185 = mg/L
Enoximone	0.5 mg/L	[Not known]	248.3	mg/L × 4.03 = μmol/L	μmol/L × 0.248 = mg/L
Enoximone sulfoxide[d]	1 mg/L	[Not known]	264.3	mg/L × 3.78 = μmol/L	μmol/L × 0.264 = mg/L
Ephedrine	0.2 mg/L	[Not known]	165.2	mg/L × 6.05 = μmol/L	μmol/L × 0.165 = mg/L
Epinephrine: see Adrenaline					
Ergometrine	1 μg/L	[Not known]	325.4	μg/L × 3.07 = nmol/L	nmol/L × 0.325 = μg/L
Erythromycin	8 mg/L	12 mg/L	733.9	mg/L × 1.36 = μmol/L	μmol/L × 0.734 = mg/L
Esmolol	2 mg/L	[Not known]	295.4	mg/L × 3.39 = μmol/L	μmol/L × 0.295 = mg/L
Estazolam	0.2 mg/L	[Not known]	294.7	mg/L × 3.39 = μmol/L	μmol/L × 0.295 = mg/L
Eterobarb: see Monomethoxymethylphenobarbitone,[b] Phenobarbitone[b]					
Ethambutol	6 mg/L	10 mg/L	204.3	mg/L × 4.89 = μmol/L	μmol/L × 0.204 = mg/L
Ethanol	—	0.5 g/L (children) 2 g/L (adolescents/adults)	46.1	g/L × 21.7 = mmol/L	mmol/L × 0.046 = g/L
Ethchlorvynol	20 mg/L	100 mg/L	144.6	mg/L × 6.92 = μmol/L	μmol/L × 0.145 = mg/L
Ether: see Diethyl ether					
Ethinamate	10 mg/L	50 mg/L	167.2	mg/L × 5.98 = μmol/L	μmol/L × 0.167 = mg/L
Ethmozin: see Moricizine					
Ethosuximide	100 mg/L	250 mg/L	141.2	mg/L × 7.08 = μmol/L	μmol/L × 0.141 = mg/L
Ethotoin	50 mg/L	[Not known]	204.2	mg/L × 4.90 = μmol/L	μmol/L × 0.204 = mg/L
Ethoxyacetate (urine)	50 mg/L[c]		104.1	mg/L × 9.61 = μmol/L	μmol/L × 0.104 = mg/L
Ethoxyethanol: see Ethoxyacetate[d]					
2-Ethoxyethyl acetate: see Ethoxyacetate[d]					
Ethyl acetate: see Ethanol[b]					
Ethylbenzene: see Mandelate[d]					
Ethyl chloride: see Chloroethane					
Ethylene glycol: see also Oxalate[d]	—	0.5 g/L (4 h postingestion) 0.2 g/L (24 h postingestion)	62.1	g/L × 16.1 = mmol/L	mmol/L × 0.062 = g/L
Ethylmorphine	1 mg/L	[Not known]	313.4	mg/L × 3.19 = μmol/L	μmol/L × 0.313 = mg/L
Etidocaine	1.5 mg/L (epidural)	—	276.4	mg/L × 3.62 = μmol/L	μmol/L × 0.276 = mg/L
Etomidate	0.5 mg/L	[Not known]	244.3	mg/L × 4.09 = μmol/L	μmol/L × 0.244 = mg/L
Etodolac	25 mg/L	[Not known]	287.4	mg/L × 3.48 = μmol/L	μmol/L × 0.287 = mg/L
Etoposide	6 mg/L	—	588.6	mg/L × 1.70 = μmol/L	μmol/L × 0.589 = mg/L
Eugenol (total hydrolyzed)	7 mg/L (dietary)	[Not known]	164.2	mg/L × 6.09 = μmol/L	μmol/L × 0.164 = mg/L
Famotidine	0.3 mg/L (oral dose) 1 mg/L (IV injection)	[Not known]	337.4	mg/L × 2.96 = μmol/L	μmol/L × 0.337 = mg/L
Fampridine (4-aminopyridine)	0.1 mg/L	0.2 mg/L	94.1	mg/L × 10.6 = μmol/L	μmol/L × 0.094 = mg/L
Famprofazone: see Methylamphetamine[b]					
Felbamate	200 mg/L	[Not known]	238.2	mg/L × 4.20 = μmol/L	μmol/L × 0.238 = mg/L

Analyte	"Therapeutic" or "normal" plasma concentration (less than)	Plasma concentration associated with acute serious toxicity[a]	Relative atomic or formula mass	Mass/amount conversion	Amount/mass conversion
Felodipine	10 µg/L	[Not known]	384.3	µg/L × 2.60 = nmol/L	nmol/L × 0.384 = µg/L
Fenbufen	60 mg/L	[Not known]	254.3	mg/L × 3.93 = µmol/L	µmol/L × 0.254 = mg/L
Fenethylline: see also Amphetamine[b]	50 µg/L	[Not known]	341.4	µg/L × 2.93 = nmol/L	nmol/L × 0.341 = µg/L
Fenfluramine	0.2 mg/L	0.5 mg/L	231.3	mg/L × 4.32 = µmol/L	µmol/L × 0.231 = mg/L
Norfenfluramine[b]	0.1 mg/L	0.2 mg/L	203.3	mg/L × 4.92 = µmol/L	µmol/L × 0.203 = mg/L
Fenitrothion	—	1 mg/L	277.2	mg/L × 3.61 = µmol/L	µmol/L × 0.277 = mg/L
2-Methyl-4-nitrophenol (urine)[d]	—	1 mg/L	153.1	mg/L × 6.53 = µmol/L	µmol/L × 0.153 = mg/L
Fenofibrate	15 mg/L	[Not known]	360.8	mg/L × 2.77 = µmol/L	µmol/L × 0.361 = mg/L
Fenoprofen	60 mg/L	[Not known]	242.3	mg/L × 4.13 = µmol/L	µmol/L × 0.242 = mg/L
Fenoprop: see 2-(2,4,5-Trichlorophenoxy)propionate					
Fenoterol	5 µg/L	[Not known]	303.4	µg/L × 3.30 = nmol/L	nmol/L × 0.303 = µg/L
Fentanyl	30 µg/L (anesthesia)	—	336.5	µg/L × 2.97 = nmol/L	nmol/L × 0.337 = µg/L
Fexofenadine (terfenadine acid metabolite)	400 µg/L	1000 µg/L	503.7	µg/L × 1.99 = nmol/L	nmol/L × 0.504 = µg/L
Flecainide	0.7 mg/L	1 mg/L	414.4	mg/L × 2.41 = µmol/L	µmol/L × 0.414 = mg/L
Fenthion	—	1 mg/L	278.3	mg/L × 3.59 = µmol/L	µmol/L × 0.278 = mg/L
Fluconazole	10 mg/L	—	306.3	mg/L × 3.26 = µmol/L	µmol/L × 0.306 = mg/L
Flumazenil	0.3 mg/L	[Not known]	303.3	mg/L × 3.30 = µmol/L	µmol/L × 0.303 = mg/L
Flunarizine	0.1 mg/L	[Not known]	404.5	mg/L × 2.47 = µmol/L	µmol/L × 0.405 = mg/L
Flunitrazepam	20 µg/L	200 µg/L	313.3	µg/L × 3.19 = nmol/L	nmol/L × 0.313 = µg/L
Fluoride (serum)	0.2 mg/L	2 mg/L	19.0	mg/L × 52.6 = µmol/L	µmol/L × 0.019 = mg/L
(urine)	2 mg/L 4 mg/L[c]				
5-Fluorouracil	0.3 mg/L	0.4 mg/L	130.1	mg/L × 7.69 = µmol/L	µmol/L × 0.130 = mg/L
Fluoxetine	0.5 mg/L	1 mg/L	309.3	mg/L × 3.23 = µmol/L	µmol/L × 0.309 = mg/L
Norfluoxetine[b]	0.5 mg/L	1 mg/L	295.3	mg/L × 3.39 = µmol/L	µmol/L × 0.295 = mg/L
Flupenthixol	15 µg/L	[Not known]	434.5	µg/L × 2.30 = nmol/L	nmol/L × 0.435 = µg/L
Fluphenazine	20 µg/L	100 µg/L	437.5	µg/L × 2.29 = nmol/L	nmol/L × 0.438 = µg/L
Flurazepam	0.02 mg/L	0.5 mg/L	387.9	mg/L × 2.58 = µmol/L	µmol/L × 0.388 = mg/L
N_1-Desalkylflurazepam[b]	0.2 mg/L	1 mg/L	288.9	mg/L × 3.46 = µmol/L	µmol/L × 0.289 = mg/L
Flurbiprofen	15 mg/L	[Not known]	244.3	mg/L × 4.09 = µmol/L	µmol/L × 0.244 = mg/L
Fluvastatin	0.5 mg/L	[Not known]	411.5	mg/L × 2.43 = µmol/L	µmol/L × 0.412 = mg/L
Fluvoxamine	0.3 mg/L	5 mg/L	318.3	mg/L × 3.14 = µmol/L	µmol/L × 0.318 = mg/L
Fomepizole	50 mg/L	[Not known]	82.1	mg/L × 12.2 = µmol/L	µmol/L × 0.082 = mg/L
Formaldehyde: see also Formate[b]	4 mg/L (occupational exposure)		30.0	mg/L × 33.3 = µmol/L	µmol/L × 0.030 = mg/L
Formate	10 mg/L		46.0	mg/L × 21.7 = µmol/L	µmol/L × 0.046 = mg/L
Fosphenytoin: see Phenytoin[b]					
Frusemide (furosemide)	10 mg/L	30 mg/L	330.8	mg/L × 3.02 = µmol/L	µmol/L × 0.331 = mg/L
Gabapentin	6 mg/L	50 mg/L	171.2	mg/L × 5.84 = µmol/L	µmol/L × 0.171 = mg/L
Galantamine	0.1 mg/L	[Not known]	287.4	mg/L × 3.50 = µmol/L	µmol/L × 0.287 = mg/L
Gallopamil	0.1 mg/L	[Not known]	484.6	mg/L × 2.06 = µmol/L	µmol/L × 0.485 = mg/L
Gemfibrozil	25 mg/L	[Not known]	250.3	mg/L × 4.00 = µmol/L	µmol/L × 0.250 = mg/L
Gentamicin	10 mg/L	15 mg/L	449–477		
Germanium	1 µg/L (dietary)	[Not known]	72.6	µg/L × 13.8 = nmol/L	nmol/L × 0.073 = µg/L
GHB: see 4-Hydroxybutyrate					
Glibenclamide	0.05 mg/L (diabetics)	0.1 mg/L	494.0	mg/L × 2.02 = µmol/L	µmol/L × 0.494 = mg/L
Gliclazide	4 mg/L (diabetics)	—	323.4	mg/L × 3.09 = µmol/L	µmol/L × 0.323 = mg/L
Glipizide	1 mg/L (diabetics)	2 mg/L	445.5	mg/L × 2.24 = µmol/L	µmol/L × 0.446 = mg/L
Glutethimide	5 mg/L	30 mg/L	217.3	mg/L × 4.60 = µmol/L	µmol/L × 0.217 = mg/L
Glyburide: see Glibenclamide					
Glyceryl trinitrate	20 µg/L	[Not known]	227.1	µg/L × 4.40 = nmol/L	nmol/L × 0.227 = µg/L
Glycol ethers: see 2-Butoxyethanol, 2-Ethoxyethanol					
Glycopyrrolate	1 µg/L (oral dose) 10 µg/L (IM dose)	[Not known]	318.4	µg/L × 3.14 = nmol/L	nmol/L × 0.318 = µg/L
Glyphosate	—	0.5 g/L	169.1	g/L × 5.91 = mmol/L	mmol/L × 0.169 = g/L
Gold	0.0001 mg/L (dietary)		197.0	mg/L × 5.08 = µmol/L	µmol/L × 0.197 = mg/L
(total, serum)	3 mg/L (therapy)	10 mg/L			
(total, urine)	2 mg/L (therapy)				
Granisetron	50 µg/L	[Not known]	312.4	µg/L × 3.20 = nmol/L	nmol/L × 0.312 = µg/L
Griseofulvin	2.5 mg/L	[Not known]	352.8	mg/L × 2.83 = µmol/L	µmol/L × 0.353 = mg/L
Guanethidine	10 µg/L	[Not known]	198.3	µg/L × 5.04 = nmol/L	nmol/L × 0.198 = µg/L
Guaifenesin	2 mg/L	50 mg/L	198.2	mg/L × 5.05 = µmol/L	µmol/L × 0.198 = mg/L
Guanfacine	5 µg/L	[Not known]	246.1	µg/L × 4.06 = nmol/L	nmol/L × 0.246 = µg/L
Halazepam: see also Nordazepam[b]	0.2 mg/L	[Not known]	352.7	mg/L × 2.84 = µmol/L	µmol/L × 0.353 = mg/L
Halofantrine	50 µg/L	[Not known]	500.4	µg/L × 2.00 = nmol/L	nmol/L × 0.500 = µg/L
Haloperidol	0.2 mg/L	1 mg/L	375.9	mg/L × 2.66 = µmol/L	µmol/L × 0.376 = mg/L

Analyte	"Therapeutic" or "normal" plasma concentration (less than)	Plasma concentration associated with acute serious toxicity[a]	Relative atomic or formula mass	Mass/amount conversion	Amount/mass conversion
Halothane (whole blood)	50 mg/L (anesthesia)	—	197.4	mg/L × 5.06 = μmol/L	μmol/L × 0.197 = mg/L
Trifluoroacetate (urine)[d]	2.5 mg/L[c]		114.0	mg/L × 8.77 = μmol/L	μmol/L × 0.114 = mg/L
γ-HCH: see Lindane					
Heparin	1 USP unit/ml	—	[h]		
Heptabarbitone (heptabarbital)	5 mg/L	30 mg/L	250.3	mg/L × 4.00 = μmol/L	μmol/L × 0.250 = mg/L
Heptachlor	1 μg/L (dietary)	[Not known]	373.3	mg/L × 2.68 = μmol/L	μmol/L × 0.373 = mg/L
Heroin: see also Morphine[b]	0.1 mg/L	—	369.4	mg/L × 2.71 = μmol/L	μmol/L × 0.369 = mg/L
6-Acetylmorphine[b]	0.15 mg/L	—	327.4	mg/L × 3.05 = μmol/L	μmol/L × 0.327 = mg/L
Hexachlorobenzene	100 μg/L (dietary) 150 μg/L[c]	200 μg/L	284.8	μg/L × 3.51 = nmol/L	nmol/L × 0.285 = μg/L
γ-Hexachlorocyclohexane: see Lindane					
Hexachlorophene	1 mg/L	[Not known]	406.9	mg/L × 2.46 = μmol/L	μmol/L × 0.407 = mg/L
Hexane (*n*-Hexane): see also 2,5-Hexanedione[b]	10 μg/L (environmental)	[Not known]	86.2	μg/L × 11.6 = nmol/L	nmol/L × 0.086 = μg/L
2,5-Hexanedione (+ 4,5-dihydroxy-2-hexanone; urine)	5 mg/L[c]		[h]		
2-Hexanone: see 2,5-Hexanedione[b]					
Hexobarbitone (hexobarbital)	5 mg/L	20 mg/L	236.3	mg/L × 4.23 = μmol/L	μmol/L × 0.236 = mg/L
Hippurate (urine)	0.2 g/L (dietary) 2 g/L[i]		179.2	g/L × 5.59 = mmol/L	mmol/L × 0.179 = g/L
Hydralazine	1 mg/L	[Not known]	160.2	mg/L × 6.24 = μmol/L	μmol/L × 0.160 = mg/L
Hydrochlorothiazide	0.5 mg/L	[Not known]	297.7	mg/L × 3.36 = μmol/L	μmol/L × 0.298 = mg/L
Hydrocodone	0.05 mg/L	0.2 mg/L	299.4	mg/L × 3.34 = μmol/L	μmol/L × 0.299 = mg/L
Hydrogen sulfide: see Sulfide					
Hydromorphone	0.05 mg/L	0.2 mg/L	285.3	mg/L × 3.51 = μmol/L	μmol/L × 0.285 = mg/L
4-Hydroxybutyrate	1 mg/L	250 mg/L	104.1	mg/L × 9.61 = μmol/L	μmol/L × 0.104 = mg/L
Hydroxychloroquine: see also Norchloroquine[b]	0.5 mg/L	2 mg/L	335.9	mg/L × 2.98 = μmol/L	μmol/L × 0.336 = mg/L
1-Hydroxypyrene (urine)	4 μg/L[j]	[Not known]	218.3	μg/L × 4.58 = nmol/L	nmol/L × 0.218 = μg/L
Hydroxyzine	0.1 mg/L	1 mg/L	374.9	mg/L × 2.67 = μmol/L	μmol/L × 0.375 = mg/L
d,l-Hyoscyamine: see Atropine					
Hyoscine (scopolamine)	2 μg/L	200 μg/L	303.4	μg/L × 3.30 = nmol/L	nmol/L × 0.303 = μg/L
Ibogaine	2 mg/L	[Not known]	310.4	mg/L × 3.22 = μmol/L	μmol/L × 0.310 = mg/L
O-Desmethylibogaine[b]	2 mg/L	[Not known]	296.4	mg/L × 3.37 = μmol/L	μmol/L × 0.296 = mg/L
Ibuprofen	50 mg/L	250 mg/L	206.3	mg/L × 4.85 = μmol/L	μmol/L × 0.206 = mg/L
Imipramine: see also Desipramine[b]	0.3 mg/L	1 mg/L	280.4	mg/L × 3.57 = μmol/L	μmol/L × 0.280 = mg/L
Indometacin (indomethacin)	5 mg/L	[Not known]	357.8	mg/L × 2.79 = μmol/L	μmol/L × 0.358 = mg/L
Indoramin	0.1 mg/L	[Not known]	347.5	mg/L × 2.88 = μmol/L	μmol/L × 0.348 = mg/L
Insulin (human, free)[k]	1 μg/L (25 mU/L; fasting nondiabetic) 1.5 μg/L (40 mU/L; nonfasting nondiabetic) 17 μg/L (450 mU/L; insulin-treated diabetic)	40 μg/L (1000 mU/L; insulin-treated diabetic)	5807	μg/L × 0.172 = nmol/L	nmol/L × 5.807 = μg/L
"C-peptide" (from proinsulin)	4 μg/L		ca. 3200		
Iodide (urine)	0.5 mg/L	[Not known]	126.9	mg/L × 7.88 = μmol/L	μmol/L × 0.127 = mg/L
Ioxynil	—	20 mg/L	370.9	mg/L × 2.70 = μmol/L	μmol/L × 0.371 = mg/L
Iproniazid	5 mg/L	[Not known]	179.2	mg/L × 5.58 = μmol/L	μmol/L × 0.179 = mg/L
Iridium	20 ng/L	[Not known]	192.2	ng/L × 5.20 = pmol/L	pmol/L × 0.192 = ng/L
Iron (serum)	0.5–1.8 mg/L	5 mg/L (children) 8 mg/L (adults)	55.8	mg/L × 17.9 = μmol/L	μmol/L × 0.056 = mg/L
Irbesartan	50 mg/L	[Not known]	428.5	mg/L × 2.33 = μmol/L	μmol/L × 0.429 = mg/L
Isoamyl nitrite: see Nitrite[b]					
Isobutyl nitrite: see Nitrite[b]					
Isoflurane (whole blood)	20 mg/L (anesthesia)	—	184.5	mg/L × 5.42 = μmol/L	μmol/L × 0.185 = mg/L
Isoniazid	20 mg/L	40 mg/L	137.1	mg/L × 7.29 = μmol/L	μmol/L × 0.137 = mg/L
Isoprenaline	10 μg/L	[Not known]	211.3	μg/L × 4.73 = nmol/L	nmol/L × 0.211 = μg/L
Isopropanol: see 2-Propanol					
Isoproterenol: see Isoprenaline					
Isosorbide 2,5-dinitrate	50 μg/L	[Not known]	236.1	μg/L × 4.24 = nmol/L	nmol/L × 0.236 = μg/L
Isosorbide 2-mononitrate[b]	25 μg/L	[Not known]	190.1	μg/L × 5.26 = nmol/L	nmol/L × 0.190 = μg/L
Isosorbide 5-mononitrate[b]	100 μg/L	[Not known]	190.1	μg/L × 5.26 = nmol/L	nmol/L × 0.190 = μg/L

Analyte	"Therapeutic" or "normal" plasma concentration (less than)	Plasma concentration associated with acute serious toxicity[a]	Relative atomic or formula mass	Mass/amount conversion	Amount/mass conversion
Isotretinoin	4 μg/L (dietary) 1 mg/L (oral dose)	[Not known]	300.4	mg/L × 3.33 = μmol/L	μmol/L × 0.300 = mg/L
4-Oxoisotretinoin[b]	2 mg/L (oral dose)	[Not known]	315.4	mg/L × 3.17 = μmol/L	μmol/L × 0.315 = mg/L
Isoxsuprine	20 μg/L	[Not known]	301.4	μg/L × 3.32 = nmol/L	nmol/L × 0.301 = μg/L
Isradipine	0.1 mg/L	[Not known]	371.4	mg/L × 2.69 = μmol/L	μmol/L × 0.371 = mg/L
Itraconazole	5 mg/L	[Not known]	705.7	mg/L × 1.42 = μmol/L	μmol/L × 0.706 = mg/L
Hydroxyitraconazole[b]	10 mg/L	[Not known]	721.7	mg/L × 1.39 = μmol/L	μmol/L × 0.722 = mg/L
Kanamycin	30 mg/L	—	484.5	mg/L × 2.06 = μmol/L	μmol/L × 0.485 = mg/L
Kavain (Kava, Kawain)	0.1 mg/L	[Not known]	230.3	mg/L × 4.34 = μmol/L	μmol/L × 0.230 = mg/L
4'-Hydroxykavain[b]	0.5 mg/L	[Not known]	246.3	mg/L × 4.06 = μmol/L	μmol/L × 0.246 = mg/L
Ketamine	5 mg/L	10 mg/L	237.7	mg/L × 4.21 = μmol/L	μmol/L × 0.238 = mg/L
Ketanserin	1 mg/L	[Not known]	395.4	mg/L × 2.53 = μmol/L	μmol/L × 0.395 = mg/L
Ketazolam: see also Nordazepam[b]	20 μg/L	[Not known]	368.8	μg/L × 2.71 = nmol/L	nmol/L × 0.369 = μg/L
Ketobemidone	0.05 mg/L (oral dose) 1 mg/L (IV dose)	0.5 mg/L —	247.3	mg/L × 4.04 = μmol/L	μmol/L × 0.247 = mg/L
Ketoconazole	10 mg/L	[Not known]	531.4	mg/L × 1.88 = μmol/L	μmol/L × 0.531 = mg/L
Ketoprofen	20 mg/L	[Not known]	254.3	mg/L × 3.93 = μmol/L	μmol/L × 0.254 = mg/L
Ketorolac	5 mg/L	[Not known]	255.3	mg/L × 3.92 = μmol/L	μmol/L × 0.255 = mg/L
Ketotifen	2 mg/L	[Not known]	309.4	mg/L × 3.23 = μmol/L	μmol/L × 0.309 = mg/L
LAAM: see *l*-α-Acetylmethadol					
Labetalol	0.3 mg/L	2 mg/L	328.4	mg/L × 3.05 = μmol/L	μmol/L × 0.328 = mg/L
Lamivudine	10 mg/L	[Not known]	229.3	mg/L × 4.36 = μmol/L	μmol/L × 0.229 = mg/L
Lamotrigine	10 mg/L	30 mg/L	256.1	mg/L × 3.90 = μmol/L	μmol/L × 0.256 = mg/L
Lansoprazole	1 mg/L	[Not known]	369.4	mg/L × 2.71 = μmol/L	μmol/L × 0.369 = mg/L
Lead (whole blood)	100 μg/L	600 μg/L	207.2	μg/L × 0.00483 = μmol/L	μmol/L × 207.2 = μg/L
Levetiracetam	100 mg/L	[Not known]	170.2	mg/L × 5.88 = μmol/L	μmol/L × 0.170 = mg/L
Levodopa	5 mg/L	[Not known]	197.2	mg/L × 5.01 = μmol/L	μmol/L × 0.197 = mg/L
Levomepromazine: see Methotrimeprazine					
Levorphanol	20 μg/L	[Not known]	257.4	μg/L × 3.89 = nmol/L	nmol/L × 0.257 = μg/L
Lignocaine (lidocaine)	5 mg/L	8 mg/L	234.3	mg/L × 4.27 = μmol/L	μmol/L × 0.234 = mg/L
Monoethylglycinexylidide[b]	2 mg/L	[Not known]	206.3	mg/L × 1.85 = μmol/L	μmol/L × 0.206 = mg/L
Lindane (γ-HCH)	1 μg/L (dietary) 25 μg/L[c]	1 mg/L	290.8	μg/L × 3.44 = nmol/L	nmol/L × 0.291 = μg/L
(whole blood)	10 μg/L[l]				
Lisinopril	0.1 mg/L	[Not known]	405.5	mg/L × 2.47 = μmol/L	μmol/L × 0.406 = mg/L
Lithium	8 mg/L	10 mg/L	6.94	mg/L × 0.144 = mmol/L	mmol/L × 6.94 = mg/L
Lofepramine: see also Desipramine[b]	10 μg/L		419.0	mg/L × 2.39 = μmol/L	μmol/L × 0.419 = mg/L
Loperamide	5 μg/L	[Not known]	477.1	μg/L × 2.10 = nmol/L	nmol/L × 0.477 = μg/L
Loprazolam	20 μg/L	[Not known]	464.9	μg/L × 2.15 = nmol/L	nmol/L × 0.465 = μg/L
Loratadine	0.1 mg/L	[Not known]	382.9	mg/L × 2.61 = μmol/L	μmol/L × 0.383 = mg/L
Desloratadine (descarboxyethylloratadine)[b]	0.1 mg/L	[Not known]	310.8	mg/L × 3.22 = μmol/L	μmol/L × 0.311 = mg/L
Lorazepam	0.3 mg/L	1 mg/L	321.2	mg/L × 3.11 = μmol/L	μmol/L × 0.321 = mg/L
Lorcainide	0.2 mg/L	[Not known]	370.9	mg/L × 2.70 = μmol/L	μmol/L × 0.371 = mg/L
Norlorcainide[b]	1.5 mg/L	[Not known]	328.9	mg/L × 3.04 = μmol/L	μmol/L × 0.329 = mg/L
Lormetazepam	20 μg/L	[Not known]	335.2	μg/L × 2.98 = nmol/L	nmol/L × 0.335 = μg/L
Losartan	2 mg/L	[Not known]	422.9	mg/L × 2.36 = μmol/L	μmol/L × 0.423 = mg/L
Losigamone	4 mg/L	[Not known]	254.7	mg/L × 3.93 = μmol/L	μmol/L × 0.255 = mg/L
Loxapine: see also Amoxapine[b]	0.1 mg/L	1 mg/L	327.8	mg/L × 3.05 = μmol/L	μmol/L × 0.328 = mg/L
8-Hydroxyloxapine[b]	0.2 mg/L	[Not known]	343.8	mg/L × 2.91 = μmol/L	μmol/L × 0.344 = mg/L
Lysergic acid diethylamide (LSD)	—	2 μg/L	323.4	μg/L × 3.09 = nmol/L	nmol/L × 0.323 = μg/L
Magnesium[g]	12–32 mg/L	85 mg/L	24.3	mg/L × 0.041 = mmol/L	mmol/L × 24.3 = mg/L
Malathion	—	0.5 mg/L	330.4	mg/L × 3.03 = μmol/L	μmol/L × 0.330 = mg/L
Mandelate (urine)	0.005 g/L (dietary) 2 g/L[c]		152.1	g/L × 6.57 = mmol/L	mmol/L × 0.152 = g/L
Manganese	0.5–1.5 μg/L	[Not known]	54.9	μg/L × 18.2 = nmol/L	nmol/L × 0.055 = μg/L
(whole blood)	4–12 μg/L				
Maprotiline	0.5 mg/L	1 mg/L	277.4	mg/L × 3.60 = μmol/L	μmol/L × 0.277 = mg/L
Normaprotiline[b]	0.5 mg/L	[Not known]	263.4	mg/L × 3.80 = μmol/L	μmol/L × 0.263 = mg/L
Mazindol	20 μg/L	[Not known]	284.8	μg/L × 3.51 = nmol/L	nmol/L × 0.285 = μg/L
MBK: see 2-Hexanone					

Analyte	"Therapeutic" or "normal" plasma concentration (less than)	Plasma concentration associated with acute serious toxicity[a]	Relative atomic or formula mass	Mass/amount conversion	Amount/mass conversion
MbOCA: see 4,4'-Methylenebis(2-chloroaniline)					
MCPA: see 4-Chloro-2-methylphenoxyacetate					
MCPP: see 2-(4-Chloro-2-methylphenoxy)propionate					
MDA: see Methylenedioxyamphetamine (Methylenedianiline in occupational context)					
MDEA: see Methylenedioxyethylamphetamine					
MDMA: see Methylenedioxymethylamphetamine					
Mebutamate	10 mg/L	[Not known]	232.3	mg/L × 4.30 = μmol/L	μmol/L × 0.232 = mg/L
Meclizine	0.1 mg/L	[Not known]	391.0	mg/L × 2.56 = μmol/L	μmol/L × 0.391 = mg/L
Mecoprop: see 2-(4-Chloro-2-methylphenoxy)propionate					
Medazepam: see also Diazepam,[b] etc.	1 mg/L	[Not known]	270.8	mg/L × 3.69 = μmol/L	μmol/L × 0.271 = mg/L
Mefenamic acid	20 mg/L	25 mg/L	241.3	mg/L × 4.14 = μmol/L	μmol/L × 0.241 = mg/L
Mefloquine	2.5 mg/L	—	379.3	mg/L × 2.64 = μmol/L	μmol/L × 0.379 = mg/L
MEK: see Butanone					
Melatonin	0.2 μg/L (endogenous) 200 μg/L (therapy)	[Not known]	232.3	μg/L × 4.30 = nmol/L	nmol/L × 0.232 = μg/L
Melperone	0.2 mg/L	[Not known]	263.4	mg/L × 3.80 = μmol/L	μmol/L × 0.263 = mg/L
Meperidine: see Pethidine					
Mephenesin	20 mg/L	[Not known]	182.2	mg/L × 5.49 = μmol/L	μmol/L × 0.182 = mg/L
Mephenytoin	2 mg/L	4 mg/L	218.3	mg/L × 4.58 = μmol/L	μmol/L × 0.218 = mg/L
5-Ethyl-5-phenylhydantoin[b]	20 mg/L	40 mg/L	204.3	mg/L × 4.89 = μmol/L	μmol/L × 0.204 = mg/L
Mephobarbital: see Methylphenobarbitone					
Mepindolol	0.1 mg/L	[Not known]	262.4	mg/L × 3.81 = μmol/L	μmol/L × 0.262 = mg/L
Mepivacaine	10 mg/L (epidural)	—	246.4	mg/L × 4.06 = μmol/L	μmol/L × 0.246 = mg/L
Meprobamate	25 mg/L	50 mg/L	218.3	mg/L × 4.58 = μmol/L	μmol/L × 0.218 = mg/L
Meptazinol	0.2 mg/L (oral)	20 mg/L	233.4	mg/L × 4.28 = μmol/L	μmol/L × 0.233 = mg/L
Mequitazine	50 μg/L	[Not known]	322.5	mg/L × 3.10 = μmol/L	μmol/L × 0.323 = mg/L
6-Mercaptopurine	0.2 mg/L	1 mg/L	152.2	mg/L × 6.57 = μmol/L	μmol/L × 0.152 = mg/L
Mercury (whole blood)	10 μg/L	50 μg/L	200.6	μg/L × 4.99 = nmol/L	nmol/L × 0.201 = μg/L
(urine)	10 μg/L	100 μg/L			
Mescaline	—	2 mg/L	211.3	mg/L × 4.73 = μmol/L	μmol/L × 0.211 = mg/L
Mesoridazine	1 mg/L	5 mg/L	386.6	mg/L × 2.59 = μmol/L	μmol/L × 0.387 = mg/L
Sulforidazine[b]	0.5 mg/L	[Not known]	402.6	mg/L × 2.48 = μmol/L	μmol/L × 0.403 = mg/L
Metaclazepam	0.4 mg/L	[Not known]	393.7	mg/L × 2.54 = μmol/L	μmol/L × 0.394 = mg/L
Metformin	4 mg/L (diabetics)	40 mg/L	129.2	mg/L × 7.74 = μmol/L	μmol/L × 0.129 = mg/L
Methadone	0.1 mg/L (single dose) 1 mg/L (maintenance therapy)	1 mg/L	309.5	mg/L × 3.23 = μmol/L	μmol/L × 0.310 = mg/L
Methadyl acetate: see *l*-α-Acetylmethadol					
d-Methamphetamine: see *d*-Methylamphetamine					
Methanol: see also Formate[b]	0.002 g/L (dietary)	0.5 g/L (2 h postingestion) 0.2 g/L (6 h postingestion)	32.0	g/L × 31.25 = mmol/L	mmol/L × 0.032 = g/L
(urine)	0.03 g/L[c]				
Methapyrilene	0.1 mg/L	4 mg/L	261.4	mg/L × 3.83 = μmol/L	μmol/L × 0.261 = mg/L
Methaqualone	5 mg/L	10 mg/L	250.3	mg/L × 4.00 = μmol/L	μmol/L × 0.250 = mg/L
Metharbitone (metharbital): see Barbitone[b]					
Methimazole (from carbimazole)	3 mg/L	[Not known]	114.2	mg/L × 8.76 = μmol/L	μmol/L × 0.114 = mg/L
Methocarbamol	50 mg/L	250 mg/L	241.2	mg/L × 4.15 = μmol/L	μmol/L × 0.241 = mg/L
Methohexitone (methohexital)	10 mg/L (anesthesia)	—	262.3	mg/L × 3.81 = μmol/L	μmol/L × 0.262 = mg/L
Methomyl	—	1 mg/L	162.2	mg/L × 6.17 = μmol/L	μmol/L × 0.162 = mg/L
Methotrexate	1 mg/L (24 h postdose) 0.45 mg/L (48 h postdose)	—	454.5	mg/L × 2.20 = μmol/L	μmol/L × 0.455 = mg/L
Methotrimeprazine	0.2 mg/L	[Not known]	328.5	mg/L × 3.04 = μmol/L	μmol/L × 0.329 = mg/L
4-Methoxyamphetamine (PMA)	—	0.4 mg/L	165.2	mg/L × 6.05 = μmol/L	μmol/L × 0.165 = mg/L
Methoxyflurane (whole blood)	200 mg/L (anesthesia)	—	165.0	mg/L × 6.06 = μmol/L	μmol/L × 0.165 = mg/L
2-(6-Methoxynaphthyl)acetic acid	100 mg/L	[Not known]	216.3	mg/L × 4.62 = μmol/L	μmol/L × 0.216 = mg/L
4-Methsuximide	0.1 mg/L		203.2	mg/L × 4.92 = μmol/L	μmol/L × 0.203 = mg/L
Normethsuximide[b]	40 mg/L	[Not known]	189.2	mg/L × 5.28 = μmol/L	μmol/L × 0.189 = mg/L
N-Methylacetamide (NMA; urine)	65 mg/L[l]	—	73.1	mg/L × 13.7 = μmol/L	μmol/L × 0.073 = mg/L
4-Methylaminophenazone (from dipyrone)	20 mg/L	[Not known]	217.3	mg/L × 4.60 = μmol/L	μmol/L × 0.217 = mg/L

Analyte	"Therapeutic" or "normal" plasma concentration (less than)	Plasma concentration associated with acute serious toxicity[a]	Relative atomic or formula mass	Mass/amount conversion	Amount/mass conversion
d-Methylamphetamine: see also *d*-Amphetamine[b]	0.1 mg/L	1 mg/L	149.2	mg/L × 6.70 = μmol/L	μmol/L × 0.149 = mg/L
Methyl bromide: see Bromide[b]					
Methyl *tert.*-butyl ether (MTBE)	2 mg/L (inhalation)	[Not known]	88.2	mg/L × 11.3 = μmol/L	μmol/L × 0.088 = mg/L
tert.-Butanol[b]	2 mg/L (MTBE inhalation)		74.2	mg/L × 13.5 = μmol/L	μmol/L × 0.074 = mg/L
Methyl *n*-butyl ketone: see 2-Hexanone					
α-Methyldopa	5 mg/L	10 mg/L	211.2	mg/L × 4.73 = μmol/L	μmol/L × 0.211 = mg/L
4,4'-Methylenebis(2-chloroaniline; total hydrolyzed, urine)	35 μg/L[l]		267.2	mg/L × 3.74 = μmol/L	μmol/L × 0.267 = mg/L
4,4'-Methylenedianiline (total, urine)	88 μg/L[l]		198.3	mg/L × 5.04 = μmol/L	μmol/L × 0.198 = mg/L
Methylenedioxyamphetamine	—	1 mg/L	179.2	mg/L × 5.58 = μmol/L	μmol/L × 0.179 = mg/L
Methylenedioxyethylamphetamine	—	1 mg/L	207.3	mg/L × 4.82 = μmol/L	μmol/L × 0.207 = mg/L
Methylenedioxymethylamphetamine	—	1 mg/L	193.3	mg/L × 5.17 = μmol/L	μmol/L × 0.193 = mg/L
Methyl ethyl ketone: see Butanone					
α-Methylfentanyl	—	2 μg/L	350.5	μg/L × 2.85 = nmol/L	nmol/L × 0.351 = μg/L
N-Methylformamide (NMF; urine)	15 mg/L[c]		59.1	mg/L × 16.9 = μmol/L	μmol/L × 0.059 = mg/L
Methylhippurates (total, urine)	2 g/L[c]		193.2	g/L × 5.18 = mmol/L	mmol/L × 0.193 = g/L
Methyl isobutyl ketone: see 4-Methyl-2-pentanone					
4-Methyl-2-pentanone (urine)	3.5 mg/L[c]		100.2	mg/L × 9.98 = μmol/L	μmol/L × 0.100 = mg/L
Methylphenidate	0.1 mg/L	[Not known]	233.3	mg/L × 4.29 = μmol/L	μmol/L × 0.233 = mg/L
Methylphenobarbitone (methylphenobarbital): see also Phenobarbitone[b]	4 mg/L	8 mg/L	246.3	mg/L × 4.06 = μmol/L	μmol/L × 0.246 = mg/L
Methylphenols (total)	—	50 mg/L	108.1	mg/L × 9.25 = μmol/L	μmol/L × 0.108 = mg/L
4-Methylphenol (urine)	200 mg/L (dietary)				
4-Methylpyrazole: see Fomepizole					
Methylsalicylate (as salicylates)	—	500 mg/L	138.1 (salicylate)	mg/L × 0.0072 = mmol/L	mmol/L × 138.1 = mg/L
4-Methylthioamphetamine	—	0.2 mg/L	181.3	mg/L × 5.52 = μmol/L	μmol/L × 0.181 = mg/L
Methyprylon(e)	10 mg/L	50 mg/L	183.2	mg/L × 5.46 = μmol/L	μmol/L × 0.183 = mg/L
Metoclopramide	0.15 mg/L	[Not known]	299.8	mg/L × 3.34 = μmol/L	μmol/L × 0.300 = mg/L
Metocurine	0.4 mg/L	[Not known]	652.8	mg/L × 1.53 = μmol/L	μmol/L × 0.653 = mg/L
Metoprolol	0.5 mg/L	5 mg/L	267.4	mg/L × 3.74 = μmol/L	μmol/L × 0.267 = mg/L
Metronidazole	20 mg/L	[Not known]	171.2	mg/L × 5.84 = μmol/L	μmol/L × 0.171 = mg/L
Mexiletine	2 mg/L	4 mg/L	179.3	mg/L × 5.58 = μmol/L	μmol/L × 0.179 = mg/L
Mianserin	0.1 mg/L	0.5 mg/L	264.4	mg/L × 3.78 = μmol/L	μmol/L × 0.264 = mg/L
MIBK: see 4-Methyl-2-pentanone					
Midazolam	0.25 mg/L	1 mg/L	325.8	mg/L × 3.07 = μmol/L	μmol/L × 0.326 = mg/L
Milnacipran	0.5 mg/L	[Not known]	246.4	mg/L × 4.10 = μmol/L	μmol/L × 0.246 = mg/L
Milrinone	0.4 mg/L	[Not known]	211.2	mg/L × 4.73 = μmol/L	μmol/L × 0.211 = mg/L
Minaprine	0.1 mg/L	[Not known]	298.4	mg/L × 3.35 = μmol/L	μmol/L × 0.298 = mg/L
Minoxidil	30 μg/L (topical) 200 μg/L (oral dose)	[Not known]	209.3	μg/L × 4.78 = nmol/L	nmol/L × 0.209 = μg/L
Mirtazapine	0.05 mg/L	[Not known]	265.4	mg/L × 3.77 = μmol/L	μmol/L × 0.265 = mg/L
Normirtazapine[b]	0.04 mg/L	[Not known]	251.4	mg/L × 3.98 = μmol/L	μmol/L × 0.251 = mg/L
Mizolastine	1 mg/L	[Not known]	432.5	mg/L × 2.31 = μmol/L	μmol/L × 0.433 = mg/L
MMMP: see Monomethoxymethylphenobarbitone					
MOCA: see 4,4'-Methylenebis(2-chloroaniline)					
Moclobemide	2 mg/L	20 mg/L	268.7	mg/L × 3.72 = μmol/L	μmol/L × 0.269 = mg/L
Modafinil	10 mg/L	[Not known]	273.4	mg/L × 3.66 = μmol/L	μmol/L × 0.273 = mg/L
Molindone	0.5 mg/L	[Not known]	276.4	mg/L × 3.62 = μmol/L	μmol/L × 0.276 = mg/L
Molsidomine	0.2 mg/L	[Not known]	242.2	mg/L × 4.13 = μmol/L	μmol/L × 0.242 = mg/L
Molybdenum	5 μg/L	[Not known]	95.9	μg/L × 10.4 = nmol/L	nmol/L × 0.096 = μg/L
Monomethoxymethylphenobarbitone (MMMP)	[Not known]	[Not known]	276.3	mg/L × 3.62 = μmol/L	μmol/L × 0.276 = mg/L
Moricizine	1 mg/L	[Not known]	427.5	mg/L × 2.34 = μmol/L	μmol/L × 0.428 = mg/L
Morphine (free)	0.05 mg/L (single dose) 0.5 mg/L (chronic therapy)	0.3 mg/L	285.3	mg/L × 3.51 = μmol/L	μmol/L × 0.285 = mg/L
Morphine-6-glucuronide[b]	0.1 mg/L	[Not known]	461.5	mg/L × 2.17 = μmol/L	μmol/L × 0.462 = mg/L

Analyte	"Therapeutic" or "normal" plasma concentration (less than)	Plasma concentration associated with acute serious toxicity[a]	Relative atomic or formula mass	Mass/amount conversion	Amount/mass conversion
4-MP: see Fomepizole					
6-MP: see 6-Mercaptopurine					
4-MTA: see 4-Methylthioamphetamine					
Nabumetone: see 2-(6-Methoxynaphthyl)acetic acid[b]					
NAC: see *N*-Acetyl-L-cysteine					
Nadolol	0.4 mg/L	[Not known]	309.4	mg/L × 3.23 = μmol/L	μmol/L × 0.309 = mg/L
Naftidrofuryl (nafronyl)	0.5 mg/L	[Not known]	383.5	mg/L × 2.61 = μmol/L	μmol/L × 0.384 = mg/L
Nalbuphine	0.2 mg/L	[Not known]	357.5	mg/L × 2.80 = μmol/L	μmol/L × 0.358 = mg/L
Nalidixic acid	30 mg/L	40 mg/L	232.2	mg/L × 4.31 = μmol/L	μmol/L × 0.232 = mg/L
(urine)	200 mg/L				
Nalmefene	100 μg/L	[Not known]	339.4	μg/L × 2.95 = nmol/L	nmol/L × 0.339 = μg/L
Naloxone	100 μg/L	[Not known]	327.4	μg/L × 3.05 = nmol/L	nmol/L × 0.327 = μg/L
Naltrexone	50 μg/L	[Not known]	341.4	μg/L × 2.93 = nmol/L	nmol/L × 0.341 = μg/L
Nandrolone	10 μg/L (IM dose)	[Not known]	274.4	μg/L × 3.64 = nmol/L	nmol/L × 0.274 = μg/L
(urine)	1 μg/L (endogenous)				
Naproxen	100 mg/L	500 mg/L	230.3	mg/L × 4.34 = μmol/L	μmol/L × 0.230 = mg/L
Nedocromil	25 μg/L	[Not known]	371.4	μg/L × 2.69 = nmol/L	nmol/L × 0.371 = μg/L
Nefazodone	1 mg/L	[Not known]	470.0	mg/L × 2.13 = μmol/L	μmol/L × 0.470 = mg/L
Nefopam	0.2 mg/L	5 mg/L	253.3	mg/L × 3.95 = μmol/L	μmol/L × 0.253 = mg/L
Neostigmine	10 μg/L (oral)	[Not known]	223.3	μg/L × 4.48 = nmol/L	nmol/L × 0.223 = μg/L
Netilmicin	10 mg/L	15 mg/L	475.6	mg/L × 2.10 = μmol/L	μmol/L × 0.476 = mg/L
Nicardipine	0.5 mg/L	[Not known]	479.5	mg/L × 2.09 = μmol/L	μmol/L × 0.480 = mg/L
Nicardipine "pyridine metabolite"[b]	0.1 mg/L		477.5	mg/L × 2.09 = μmol/L	μmol/L × 0.478 = mg/L
Nickel	1.3 μg/L	[Not known]	58.7	μg/L × 17.0 = nmol/L	nmol/L × 0.059 = μg/L
(urine)	6 μg/L				
Nicotine: see also Cotinine[d]	0.01 mg/L (nonsmokers) 0.05 mg/L (smokers)	1 mg/L	162.2	mg/L × 6.17 = μmol/L	μmol/L × 0.162 = mg/L
Nicoumalone: see Acenocoumarol					
Nifedipine	0.2 mg/L	[Not known]	346.3	mg/L × 2.89 = μmol/L	μmol/L × 0.346 = mg/L
Niflumic acid	40 mg/L	[Not known]	282.2	mg/L × 3.54 = μmol/L	μmol/L × 0.282 = mg/L
Nilvadipine	10 μg/L	[Not known]	385.4	μg/L × 2.59 = nmol/L	nmol/L × 0.385 = μg/L
Nimesulide	10 mg/L	[Not known]	308.3	mg/L × 3.24 = μmol/L	μmol/L × 0.308 = mg/L
4-Hydroxynimesulide[b]	5 mg/L	[Not known]	324.3	mg/L × 3.08 = μmol/L	μmol/L × 0.324 = mg/L
Nimodipine	30 μg/L	[Not known]	418.5	μg/L × 2.39 = nmol/L	nmol/L × 0.419 = μg/L
Nisoldipine	10 μg/L	[Not known]	388.4	μg/L × 2.57 = nmol/L	nmol/L × 0.388 = μg/L
Nitrazepam	0.2 mg/L	1 mg/L	281.3	mg/L × 3.55 = μmol/L	μmol/L × 0.281 = mg/L
Nitrate	2 mg/L	[Not known]	62.0	mg/L × 1.61 = μmol/L	μmol/L × 0.062 = mg/L
Nitrendipine	0.1 mg/L	[Not known]	360.4	mg/L × 2.77 = μmol/L	μmol/L × 0.360 = mg/L
Nitrite	2.5 mg/L	[Not known]	46.0	mg/L × 21.7 = μmol/L	μmol/L × 0.046 = mg/L
(urine)	—	10 mg/L			
Nitrofurantoin	2 mg/L	3 mg/L	238.2	mg/L × 4.20 = μmol/L	μmol/L × 0.238 = mg/L
Nitroprusside: see Cyanide,[b] Thiocyanate[b]					
Nitrous oxide	100 mg/L (anesthesia)	—	44.0	mg/L × 22.7 = μmol/L	μmol/L × 0.044 = mg/L
Nizatidine	1 mg/L	[Not known]	331.5	mg/L × 3.02 = μmol/L	μmol/L × 0.332 = mg/L
NMA: see *N*-Methylacetamide					
NMF: see *N*-Methylformamide					
Nomifensine (total hydrolyzed)	4 mg/L	[Not known]	238.3	mg/L × 4.20 = μmol/L	μmol/L × 0.238 = mg/L
Noradrenaline (norepinephrine)	2 pg/L	[Not known]	169.2	pg/L × 5.91 = fmol/L	fmol/L × 0.169 = pg/L
Norchloroquine	0.3 mg/L	[Not known]	291.9	mg/L × 3.43 = μmol/L	μmol/L × 0.292 = mg/L
Nordazepam (nordiazepam): see also Oxazepam[b]	2 mg/L	5 mg/L	270.7	mg/L × 3.69 = μmol/L	μmol/L × 0.271 = mg/L
Norephedrine: see Phenylpropanolamine					
Norepinephrine: see Noradrenaline					
Nororphenadrine: see Tofenacin					
Norpseudoephedrine: see Cathine					
Northiaden = nordothiepin: see Dothiepin					
Nortriptyline	0.3 mg/L	1 mg/L	263.4	mg/L × 3.80 = μmol/L	μmol/L × 0.263 = mg/L
Obidoxime	10 mg/L	[Not known]	288.2	mg/L × 3.47 = μmol/L	μmol/L × 0.288 = mg/L
Olanzapine	0.2 mg/L	[Not known]	312.4	mg/L × 3.20 = μmol/L	μmol/L × 0.312 = mg/L
Omeprazole	5 mg/L	[Not known]	345.4	mg/L × 2.90 = μmol/L	μmol/L × 0.345 = mg/L
Ondansetron	0.3 mg/L	[Not known]	293.4	mg/L × 3.41 = μmol/L	μmol/L × 0.293 = mg/L
Opipramol	0.5 mg/L	2 mg/L	363.5	mg/L × 2.75 = μmol/L	μmol/L × 0.364 = mg/L
Orphenadrine: see also Tofenacin[b]	1 mg/L	5 mg/L	269.4	mg/L × 3.71 = μmol/L	μmol/L × 0.269 = mg/L
Ouabain	0.2 μg/L	[Not known]	584.7	μg/L × 1.71 = nmol/L	nmol/L × 0.585 = μg/L
Oxalate	2.5 mg/L (dietary, etc.)	4 mg/L	90.0	mg/L × 11.1 = μmol/L	μmol/L × 0.090 = mg/L

Analyte	"Therapeutic" or "normal" plasma concentration (less than)	Plasma concentration associated with acute serious toxicity[a]	Relative atomic or formula mass	Mass/amount conversion	Amount/mass conversion
Oxandrolone	1 mg/L	[Not known]	306.4	mg/L × 3.26 = μmol/L	μmol/L × 0.306 = mg/L
Oxatomide	0.1 mg/L	[Not known]	426.6	mg/L × 2.34 = μmol/L	μmol/L × 0.427 = mg/L
Oxazepam	1 mg/L	5 mg/L	286.7	mg/L × 3.49 = μmol/L	μmol/L × 0.287 = mg/L
Oxazolam: see also Nordazepam[b]	0.4 mg/L	[Not known]	328.8	mg/L × 3.04 = μmol/L	μmol/L × 0.329 = mg/L
Oxcarbazepine	1 mg/L		252.3	mg/L × 3.96 = μmol/L	μmol/L × 0.252 = mg/L
10-Hydroxycarbazepine[b]	30 mg/L	[Not known]	254.3	mg/L × 3.93 = μmol/L	μmol/L × 0.254 = mg/L
Oxpentifylline (pentoxifylline)	5 mg/L	[Not known]	278.3	mg/L × 3.59 = μmol/L	μmol/L × 0.278 = mg/L
1-(5-Hydroxyhexyl)-3,7-dimethylxanthine[d]	10 mg/L		280.3	mg/L × 3.57 = μmol/L	μmol/L × 0.280 = mg/L
1-(3-Carboxypropyl)-3,7-dimethylxanthine[d]	10 mg/L		266.3	mg/L × 3.76 = μmol/L	μmol/L × 0.266 = mg/L
Oxprenolol	0.5 mg/L	5 mg/L	265.4	mg/L × 3.77 = μmol/L	μmol/L × 0.265 = mg/L
Oxybutynin	20 μg/L	[Not known]	358.5	μg/L × 2.79 = nmol/L	nmol/L × 0.359 = μg/L
Oxycodone	0.05 mg/L	0.5 mg/L	315.4	mg/L × 3.17 = μmol/L	μmol/L × 0.315 = mg/L
Oxymetholone	20 μg/L	[Not known]	332.5	μg/L × 3.01 = nmol/L	nmol/L × 0.333 = μg/L
Oxyphenbutazone	100 mg/L	200 mg/L	324.4	mg/L × 3.08 = μmol/L	μmol/L × 0.324 = mg/L
Oxytetracycline	10 mg/L	30 mg/L	460.4	mg/L × 2.17 = μmol/L	μmol/L × 0.460 = mg/L
Oxytocin	0.2 μg/L	—	1007	μg/L × 0.99 = nmol/L	nmol/L × 1.007 = μg/L
Paclitaxel	10 mg/L	—	853.9	mg/L × 1.17 = μmol/L	μmol/L × 0.854 = mg/L
Pancuronium	1 mg/L	—	572.9	mg/L × 1.75 = μmol/L	μmol/L × 0.573 = mg/L
Pantoprazole	5 mg/L	[Not known]	383.4	mg/L × 2.60 = μmol/L	μmol/L × 0.383 = mg/L
Papaverine	2 mg/L	[Not known]	339.4	mg/L × 2.95 = μmol/L	μmol/L × 0.339 = mg/L
Paracetamol	30 mg/L	200 mg/L (4 h postingestion) 30 mg/L (16 h postingestion)	151.2	mg/L × 0.00662 = mmol/L	mmol/L × 151 = mg/L
Paraldehyde: see also Acetaldehyde[b]	0.3 g/L	0.5 g/L	132.2	g/L × 7.56 = mmol/L	mmol/L × 0.132 = g/L
Paraquat	—	0.6 mg/L (6 h postingestion) 0.1 mg/L (24 h postingestion)	186.3	mg/L × 5.38 = μmol/L	μmol/L × 0.186 = mg/L
Parathion	0.2 mg/L (occupational exposure)	[Not known]	291.3	mg/L × 3.43 = μmol/L	μmol/L × 0.291 = mg/L
4-Nitrophenol (urine)[d]	0.5 mg/L[c]		139.1	mg/L × 7.19 = μmol/L	μmol/L × 0.139 = mg/L
Paroxetine	0.1 mg/L	1 mg/L	329.4	mg/L × 3.04 = μmol/L	μmol/L × 0.329 = mg/L
PCP: see Phencyclidine (Pentachlorophenol in occupational/environmental context)					
Pefloxacin	10 mg/L	25 mg/L	333.4	mg/L × 3.00 = μmol/L	μmol/L × 0.333 = mg/L
Pemoline	5 mg/L	[Not known]	176.2	mg/L × 5.68 = μmol/L	μmol/L × 0.176 = mg/L
Penbutolol	1 mg/L	[Not known]	291.4	mg/L × 3.43 = μmol/L	μmol/L × 0.291 = mg/L
Penfluridol	25 μg/L	[Not known]	524.0	μg/L × 1.91 = nmol/L	nmol/L × 0.524 = μg/L
D-Penicillamine	10 mg/L	[Not known]	149.2	mg/L × 6.70 = μmol/L	μmol/L × 0.149 = mg/L
Pentachlorophenol	0.2 mg/L (dietary)	30 mg/L	266.3	mg/L × 3.75 = μmol/L	μmol/L × 0.266 = mg/L
(total)	1 mg/L[c]				
(total, urine)	0.3 mg/L[c]				
Pentazocine	0.2 mg/L (oral) 1 mg/L (subcutaneous)	1 mg/L	285.4	mg/L × 3.50 = μmol/L	μmol/L × 0.285 = mg/L
Pentobarbitone (pentobarbital)	5 mg/L	20 mg/L	226.3	mg/L × 4.42 = μmol/L	μmol/L × 0.226 = mg/L
Pentoxifylline: see Oxpentifylline					
Perazine	0.2 mg/L	0.5 mg/L	339.5	mg/L × 2.95 = μmol/L	μmol/L × 0.340 = mg/L
Perhexiline	1 mg/L	2 mg/L	277.5	mg/L × 3.60 = μmol/L	μmol/L × 0.278 = mg/L
4-Hydroxyperhexiline[b]	2 mg/L		293.5	mg/L × 3.41 = μmol/L	μmol/L × 0.294 = mg/L
Pericyazine	50 μg/L	100 μg/L	365.5	μg/L × 2.74 = nmol/L	nmol/L × 0.366 = μg/L
Perphenazine	30 μg/L	[Not known]	404.0	μg/L × 2.48 = nmol/L	nmol/L × 0.404 = μg/L
Pethidine	0.6 mg/L	2 mg/L	247.3	mg/L × 4.04 = μmol/L	μmol/L × 0.247 = mg/L
Norpethidine[b]	0.3 mg/L	0.5 mg/L	233.3	mg/L × 4.29 = μmol/L	μmol/L × 0.233 = mg/L
Phenacetin	20 mg/L	[Not known]	179.2	mg/L × 5.58 = μmol/L	μmol/L × 0.179 = mg/L
Phenazocine	10 μg/L	[Not known]	321.5	μg/L × 3.11 = nmol/L	nmol/L × 0.322 = μg/L
Phenazone	50 mg/L	[Not known]	188.2	mg/L × 5.31 = μmol/L	μmol/L × 0.188 = mg/L
Phencyclidine	—	0.3 mg/L	243.4	mg/L × 4.11 = μmol/L	μmol/L × 0.243 = mg/L
Phendimetrazine	0.3 mg/L	[Not known]	191.3	mg/L × 5.23 = μmol/L	μmol/L × 0.191 = mg/L
Phenelzine	0.02 mg/L	0.5 mg/L	136.2	mg/L × 7.34 = μmol/L	μmol/L × 0.136 = mg/L

Analyte	"Therapeutic" or "normal" plasma concentration (less than)	Plasma concentration associated with acute serious toxicity[a]	Relative atomic or formula mass	Mass/amount conversion	Amount/mass conversion
Phenformin	0.3 mg/L (diabetics)	—	205.3	mg/L × 4.87 = μmol/L	μmol/L × 0.205 = mg/L
Pheniramine	1 mg/L	4 mg/L	240.4	mg/L × 4.16 = μmol/L	μmol/L × 0.240 = mg/L
Phenmetrazine	0.3 mg/L	1 mg/L	177.3	mg/L × 5.64 = μmol/L	μmol/L × 0.177 = mg/L
Phenobarbitone (phenobarbital)	40 mg/L	100 mg/L	232.2	mg/L × 4.31 = μmol/L	μmol/L × 0.232 = mg/L
Phenol (total hydrolyzed) (urine; total hydrolyzed)	0.1 mg/L (dietary, etc.) 1 mg/L (dietary, etc.) 300 mg/L[c]	50 mg/L	94.1	mg/L × 0.011 = mmol/L	mmol/L × 94.1 = mg/L
Phenprocoumon	3 mg/L	5 mg/L	280.3	mg/L × 3.57 = μmol/L	μmol/L × 0.280 = mg/L
Phensuximide	20 mg/L	80 mg/L	189.2	mg/L × 5.29 = μmol/L	μmol/L × 0.189 = mg/L
Phentermine	0.5 mg/L	2 mg/L	149.2	mg/L × 6.70 = μmol/L	μmol/L × 0.149 = mg/L
Phentolamine	10 μg/L	[Not known]	281.4	μg/L × 3.55 = nmol/L	nmol/L × 0.281 = μg/L
Phenylbutazone: see also Oxyphenbutazone[b]	150 mg/L	300 mg/L	308.4	mg/L × 3.24 = μmol/L	μmol/L × 0.308 = mg/L
Phenylephrine	0.1 mg/L	1 mg/L	167.2	mg/L × 5.98 = μmol/L	μmol/L × 0.167 = mg/L
Phenylethylamine (phenethylamine)	0.2 mg/L (endogenous)	[Not known]	121.2	mg/L × 8.25 = μmol/L	μmol/L × 0.121 = mg/L
Phenylpropanolamine (norephedrine)	0.5 mg/L	2 mg/L	151.2	mg/L × 6.61 = μmol/L	μmol/L × 0.151 = mg/L
Phenytoin	20 mg/L	40 mg/L	252.3	mg/L × 3.96 = μmol/L	μmol/L × 0.252 = mg/L
Pholcodine	0.2 mg/L	[Not known]	398.5	mg/L × 2.51 = μmol/L	μmol/L × 0.399 = mg/L
Phytomenadione (vitamin K_1)	0.5 mg/L	[Not known]	450.7	mg/L × 2.22 = μmol/L	μmol/L × 0.451 = mg/L
Physostigmine	5 μg/L	[Not known]	275.4	μg/L × 3.63 = nmol/L	nmol/L × 0.275 = μg/L
Pimozide	20 μg/L	[Not known]	461.6	mg/L × 2.17 = μmol/L	μmol/L × 0.462 = mg/L
Pinazepam: see also Nordazepam[b]	0.1 mg/L	[Not known]	308.8	mg/L × 3.24 = μmol/L	μmol/L × 0.309 = mg/L
Pindolol	0.1 mg/L	1 mg/L	248.3	mg/L × 4.03 = μmol/L	μmol/L × 0.248 = mg/L
Pirenzepine	0.3 mg/L	[Not known]	351.4	mg/L × 2.85 = μmol/L	μmol/L × 0.351 = mg/L
Piritramide	0.1 mg/L	[Not known]	430.6	mg/L × 2.32 = μmol/L	μmol/L × 0.431 = mg/L
Piracetam	60 mg/L	[Not known]	142.2	mg/L × 7.03 = μmol/L	μmol/L × 0.142 = mg/L
Piroxicam	20 mg/L	[Not known]	331.3	mg/L × 3.02 = μmol/L	μmol/L × 0.331 = mg/L
Pizotifen (pizotyline)	10 μg/L	[Not known]	295.5	μg/L × 3.38 = nmol/L	nmol/L × 0.296 = μg/L
Platinum	0.003 mg/L (dietary) 30 mg/L (therapy)	—	195.1	mg/L × 5.12 = μmol/L	μmol/L × 0.195 = mg/L
PMA: see 4-Methoxyamphetamine					
Polybrominated biphenyls	2 mg/L	[Not known]	h		
Polychlorinated biphenyls	0.01 mg/L (dietary, etc.)	0.4 mg/L	h		
Polycyclic aromatic hydrocarbons (PAHs): see 1-Hydroxypyrene					
Potassium (no hemolysis)	0.13–0.18 g/L		39.1	g/L × 25.6 = mmol/L	mmol/L × 0.039 = g/L
Practolol	5 mg/L	[Not known]	266.3	mg/L × 3.76 = μmol/L	μmol/L × 0.266 = mg/L
Prajmalium (prajmaline)	0.5 mg/L	[Not known]	369.6	mg/L × 2.71 = μmol/L	μmol/L × 0.370 = mg/L
Pralidoxime	4 mg/L	[Not known]	137.1	mg/L × 7.29 = μmol/L	μmol/L × 0.137 = mg/L
Prazepam: see also Nordazepam[b]	10 μg/L		324.8	μg/L × 3.08 = nmol/L	nmol/L × 0.325 = μg/L
Prazosin	0.1 mg/L	[Not known]	383.4	mg/L × 2.61 = μmol/L	μmol/L × 0.383 = mg/L
Prednisolone	1 mg/L	[Not known]	360.5	mg/L × 2.77 = μmol/L	μmol/L × 0.361 = mg/L
Prilocaine	5 mg/L	—	220.3	mg/L × 4.54 = μmol/L	μmol/L × 0.220 = mg/L
Primaquine	0.2 mg/L	[Not known]	259.4	mg/L × 3.86 = μmol/L	μmol/L × 0.259 = mg/L
Carboxyprimaquine[b]	2 mg/L	[Not known]	274.4	mg/L × 3.64 = μmol/L	μmol/L × 0.274 = mg/L
Primidone: see also Phenobarbitone[b]	12 mg/L	40 mg/L	218.3	mg/L × 4.58 = μmol/L	μmol/L × 0.218 = mg/L
Probenecid	200 mg/L	[Not known]	285.4	mg/L × 3.50 = μmol/L	μmol/L × 0.285 = mg/L
Procainamide: see also Acecainide[b]	8 mg/L	12 mg/L	235.3	mg/L × 4.25 = μmol/L	μmol/L × 0.235 = mg/L
Procaine	20 mg/L	—	236.3	mg/L × 4.23 = μmol/L	μmol/L × 0.236 = mg/L
Prochlorperazine	0.05 mg/L	0.3 mg/L	373.9	mg/L × 2.67 = μmol/L	μmol/L × 0.374 = mg/L
Procyclidine	0.5 mg/L	2 mg/L	287.4	mg/L × 3.48 = μmol/L	μmol/L × 0.287 = mg/L
Progabide	1.2 mg/L	[Not known]	334.8	mg/L × 2.99 = μmol/L	μmol/L × 0.335 = mg/L
Progabide "acid metabolite"[b]	2.5 mg/L	[Not known]	335.8	mg/L × 2.98 = μmol/L	μmol/L × 0.336 = mg/L
Proguanil	0.4 mg/L	[Not known]	253.7	mg/L × 3.95 = μmol/L	μmol/L × 0.254 = mg/L
Cycloguanil[b]	0.2 mg/L	[Not known]	251.7	mg/L × 3.97 = μmol/L	μmol/L × 0.252 = mg/L
Promazine	0.4 mg/L	2 mg/L	284.4	mg/L × 3.52 = μmol/L	μmol/L × 0.284 = mg/L
Promethazine	0.1 mg/L	1 mg/L	284.4	mg/L × 3.52 = μmol/L	μmol/L × 0.284 = mg/L
Propafenone	1 mg/L	3 mg/L	341.5	mg/L × 2.93 = μmol/L	μmol/L × 0.342 = mg/L
5-Hydroxypropafenone[b]	1 mg/L	[Not known]	357.5	mg/L × 2.80 = μmol/L	μmol/L × 0.358 = mg/L
Norpropafenone[b]	0.5 mg/L	[Not known]	327.5	mg/L × 3.05 = μmol/L	μmol/L × 0.328 = mg/L
1,2-Propanediol	1 g/L (as vehicle)	4 g/L	76.1	g/L × 13.1 = mmol/L	mmol/L × 0.076 = g/L

Analyte	"Therapeutic" or "normal" plasma concentration (less than)	Plasma concentration associated with acute serious toxicity[a]	Relative atomic or formula mass	Mass/amount conversion	Amount/mass conversion
2-Propanol: see also Acetone[b]	—	2.5 g/L	60.1	g/L × 16.63 = mmol/L	mmol/L × 0.060 = g/L
Propantheline	20 μg/L	[Not known]	368.5	μg/L × 2.71 = nmol/L	nmol/L × 0.369 = μg/L
Propofol	10 mg/L	[Not known]	178.3	mg/L × 5.61 = μmol/L	μmol/L × 0.178 = mg/L
Propoxyphene: see Dextropropoxyphene					
Propranolol	0.2 mg/L	2 mg/L	259.3	mg/L × 3.86 = μmol/L	μmol/L × 0.259 = mg/L
Propylene glycol: see 1,2-Propanediol					
Propylhexedrine	0.01 mg/L	0.5 mg/L	155.3	mg/L × 6.44 = μmol/L	μmol/L × 0.155 = mg/L
Propylthiouracil	5 mg/L	—	170.2	mg/L × 5.88 = μmol/L	μmol/L × 0.170 = mg/L
Protriptyline	0.2 mg/L	1 mg/L	263.4	mg/L × 3.80 = μmol/L	μmol/L × 0.263 = mg/L
Pseudoephedrine	1 mg/L	10 mg/L	165.2	mg/L × 6.05 = μmol/L	μmol/L × 0.165 = mg/L
Pyrilamine	[Not known]	5 mg/L	285.4	mg/L × 3.50 = μmol/L	μmol/L × 0.285 = mg/L
Pyridostigmine	0.2 mg/L	[Not known]	181.3	mg/L × 5.52 = μmol/L	μmol/L × 0.181 = mg/L
Pyrimethamine	1 mg/L	[Not known]	248.7	mg/L × 4.02 = μmol/L	μmol/L × 0.249 = mg/L
Quazepam	0.2 mg/L	[Not known]	386.8	mg/L × 2.59 = μmol/L	μmol/L × 0.387 = mg/L
Quetiapine	0.6 mg/L	[Not known]	383.5	mg/L × 2.61 = μmol/L	μmol/L × 0.384 = mg/L
Quinalbarbitone	5 mg/L	20 mg/L	238.3	mg/L × 4.20 = μmol/L	μmol/L × 0.238 = mg/L
Quinapril	1 mg/L	[Not known]	438.5	mg/L × 2.28 = μmol/L	μmol/L × 0.439 = mg/L
Quinaprilat[b]	3 mg/L	[Not known]	410.5	mg/L × 2.44 = μmol/L	μmol/L × 0.411 = mg/L
Quinidine	5 mg/L	8 mg/L	324.4	mg/L × 3.08 = μmol/L	μmol/L × 0.324 = mg/L
Quinine	0.3 mg/L (dietary) 16 mg/L (malaria patients)	8 mg/L (naïve subjects)	324.4	mg/L × 3.08 = μmol/L	μmol/L × 0.324 = mg/L
Ranitidine	2 mg/L	[Not known]	314.4	mg/L × 3.18 = μmol/L	μmol/L × 0.314 = mg/L
Rapacuronium	10 mg/L	[Not known]	597.9	mg/L × 1.72 = μmol/L	μmol/L × 0.598 = mg/L
Desacetylrapacuronium[b]	1 mg/L		555.9	mg/L × 1.80 = μmol/L	μmol/L × 0.556 = mg/L
Reboxetine	2 mg/L	[Not known]	313.4	mg/L × 3.19 = μmol/L	μmol/L × 0.313 = mg/L
Remacemide	2 mg/L	[Not known]	268.3	mg/L × 3.73 = μmol/L	μmol/L × 0.268 = mg/L
Desglycinylremacemide[b]	0.3 mg/L		211.3	mg/L × 4.73 = μmol/L	μmol/L × 0.211 = mg/L
Remifentanil	50 μg/L	[Not known]	367.5	μg/L × 2.72 = nmol/L	nmol/L × 0.368 = μg/L
Remoxipride	5 mg/L	[Not known]	371.3	mg/L × 2.69 = μmol/L	μmol/L × 0.371 = mg/L
Reserpine	10 μg/L	[Not known]	608.7	μg/L × 1.64 = nmol/L	nmol/L × 0.609 = μg/L
Ricin	10 μg/L (IV dose)	—	[h]		
Rifampicin (rifampin)	5 mg/L	—	823.0	mg/L × 1.22 = μmol/L	μmol/L × 0.823 = mg/L
Desacetylrifampicin[b]	10 mg/L	[Not known]	781.0	mg/L × 1.28 = μmol/L	μmol/L × 0.781 = mg/L
Rimiterol	10 μg/L	[Not known]	223.3	μg/L × 4.48 = nmol/L	nmol/L × 0.223 = μg/L
Risperidone	50 μg/L	[Not known]	410.5	μg/L × 2.44 = nmol/L	nmol/L × 0.411 = μg/L
9-Hydroxyrisperidone[b]	100 μg/L	[Not known]	426.5	μg/L × 2.34 = nmol/L	nmol/L × 0.427 = μg/L
Ritodrine	40 μg/L	[Not known]	287.4	μg/L × 3.48 = nmol/L	nmol/L × 0.287 = μg/L
Ritonavir	20 mg/L	—	721.0	mg/L × 1.39 = μmol/L	μmol/L × 0.721 = mg/L
Rivastigmine	200 μg/L	[Not known]	250.3	μg/L × 4.00 = nmol/L	nmol/L × 0.250 = μg/L
Rizatriptan	0.1 mg/L	[Not known]	269.3	mg/L × 3.71 = μmol/L	μmol/L × 0.269 = mg/L
Rocuronium	10 mg/L (IV infusion)	[Not known]	529.8	mg/L × 1.89 = μmol/L	μmol/L × 0.530 = mg/L
Rofecoxib	5 mg/L	[Not known]	314.4	mg/L × 3.18 = μmol/L	μmol/L × 0.314 = mg/L
Ropivacaine	5 mg/L	[Not known]	274.4	mg/L × 3.64 = μmol/L	μmol/L × 0.274 = mg/L
Rosiglitazone	1 mg/L	[Not known]	357.4	mg/L × 2.80 = μmol/L	μmol/L × 0.357 = mg/L
Salbutamol	20 μg/L (inhaled dose) 200 μg/L (oral dose)	[Not known]	239.3	μg/L × 4.18 = nmol/L	nmol/L × 0.239 = μg/L
Salicylamide (as salicylates)	50 mg/L	[Not known]	138.1 (salicylate)	mg/L × 0.0072 = mmol/L	mmol/L × 138 = mg/L
Salmeterol	5 μg/L (inhaled dose)	[Not known]	415.6	μg/L × 2.41 = nmol/L	nmol/L × 0.416 = μg/L
Scopolamine: see Hyoscine					
Secobarbital: see Quinalbarbitone					
Selenium[g]	45–120 μg/L	400 μg/L	79.0	μg/L × 12.66 = nmol/L	nmol/L × 0.079 = μg/L
(urine)	30 μg/L 100 μg/L (occupational exposure)				
Sertindole	100 μg/L	[Not known]	441.0	μg/L × 2.27 = nmol/L	nmol/L × 0.441 = μg/L
Dehydrosertindole[b]	70 μg/L		439.0	μg/L × 2.28 = nmol/L	nmol/L × 0.439 = μg/L
Sertraline	0.3 mg/L	[Not known]	306.2	mg/L × 3.27 = μmol/L	μmol/L × 0.306 = mg/L
Norsertraline[b]	0.5 mg/L	[Not known]	292.2	mg/L × 3.42 = μmol/L	μmol/L × 0.292 = mg/L
Sevoflurane (blood)	200 mg/L (anesthesia)	—	200.1	mg/L × 5.00 = μmol/L	μmol/L × 0.200 = mg/L
Sildenafil	0.5 mg/L	[Not known]	474.6	mg/L × 2.11 = μmol/L	μmol/L × 0.475 = mg/L
Norsildenafil[b]	0.3 mg/L		460.6	mg/L × 2.17 = μmol/L	μmol/L × 0.461 = mg/L
Silicon	300 mg/L	[Not known]	28.1	mg/L × 35.6 = μmol/L	μmol/L × 0.028 = mg/L
Silver (whole blood)	0.3 μg/L	[Not known]	107.9	μg/L × 9.27 = nmol/L	nmol/L × 0.108 = μg/L
(urine)	0.8 μg/L				
Sodium	3.11–3.29 g/L	—	23.0	g/L × 43.5 = mmol/L	mmol/L × 0.023 = g/L
Sotalol	2 mg/L	20 mg/L	272.4	mg/L × 3.67 = μmol/L	μmol/L × 0.272 = mg/L

Analyte	"Therapeutic" or "normal" plasma concentration (less than)	Plasma concentration associated with acute serious toxicity[a]	Relative atomic or formula mass	Mass/amount conversion	Amount/mass conversion
Spironolactone: see also Canrenone[b]	0.2 mg/L	[Not known]	416.6	mg/L × 2.40 = μmol/L	μmol/L × 0.417 = mg/L
Stavudine	1 mg/L	[Not known]	224.2	mg/L × 4.46 = μmol/L	μmol/L × 0.224 = mg/L
Stiripentol	5 mg/L	[Not known]	234.3	mg/L × 4.27 = μmol/L	μmol/L × 0.234 = mg/L
Streptomycin	20 mg/L	40 mg/L	581.6	mg/L × 1.72 = μmol/L	μmol/L × 0.582 = mg/L
Strontium (serum)	30 μg/L	[Not known]	87.6	μg/L × 11.4 = nmol/L	nmol/L × 0.088 = μg/L
(urine)	300 μg/L				
Strychnine	—	0.5 mg/L	334.4	mg/L × 2.99 = μmol/L	μmol/L × 0.334 = mg/L
Styrene (whole blood; see also Mandelate[d])	0.6 mg/L (occupational exposure)	[Not known]	104.1	mg/L × 9.61 = μmol/L	μmol/L × 0.104 = mg/L
Succinylcholine: see Suxamethonium					
Sufentanil	20 μg/L	—	386.6	μg/L × 2.59 = nmol/L	nmol/L × 0.387 = μg/L
Sulfamethoxazole	60 mg/L	200 mg/L	253.3	mg/L × 3.95 = μmol/L	μmol/L × 0.253 = mg/L
N-Acetylsulfamethoxazole[b]	—	100 mg/L	295.3	mg/L × 3.39 = μmol/L	μmol/L × 0.295 = mg/L
Sulfinpyrazone	10 mg/L	[Not known]	404.5	mg/L × 2.47 = μmol/L	μmol/L × 0.405 = mg/L
Sulindac	5 mg/L	[Not known]	356.4	mg/L × 2.81 = μmol/L	μmol/L × 0.356 = mg/L
Sulindac sulfide[b]	10 mg/L	[Not known]	340.4	mg/L × 2.94 = μmol/L	μmol/L × 0.340 = mg/L
Sulfide (whole blood)	0.05 mg/L (dietary)	0.1 mg/L	32.1	mg/L × 31.2 = μmol/L	μmol/L × 0.032 = mg/L
Sulfite (urine)	6 mg/L		80.0	mg/L × 12.5 = μmol/L	μmol/L × 0.080 = mg/L
Sulpiride	0.5 mg/L	[Not known]	341.4	mg/L × 2.93 = μmol/L	μmol/L × 0.341 = mg/L
Sulthiame	12 mg/L	20 mg/L	290.4	mg/L × 3.44 = μmol/L	μmol/L × 0.290 = mg/L
Sultopride	5 mg/L	[Not known]	354.5	mg/L × 2.82 = μmol/L	μmol/L × 0.355 = mg/L
Sumatriptan	30 μg/L	[Not known]	295.4	μg/L × 3.39 = nmol/L	nmol/L × 0.295 = μg/L
Suramin	150 mg/L	[Not known]	1291	mg/L × 0.77 = μmol/L	μmol/L × 1.29 = mg/L
Suxamethonium	5 mg/L (infusion)	—	291.3	mg/L × 3.43 = μmol/L	μmol/L × 0.291 = mg/L
2,4,5-T: see 2,4,5-Trichlorophenoxyacetate					
Taxol A: see Paclitaxel					
Tacrolimus	20 μg/L	—	804.0	mg/L × 1.24 = μmol/L	μmol/L × 0.804 = mg/L
Talinolol	1 mg/L	[Not known]	363.5	mg/L × 2.75 = μmol/L	μmol/L × 0.364 = mg/L
Tamoxifen	0.5 mg/L	[Not known]	371.5	mg/L × 2.69 = μmol/L	μmol/L × 0.372 = mg/L
TCDD: see 2,3,6,7-Tetrachlorodibenzodioxin					
Temazepam	1 mg/L	5 mg/L	300.7	mg/L × 3.33 = μmol/L	μmol/L × 0.301 = mg/L
Tenoxicam	15 mg/L	[Not known]	337.4	mg/L × 2.96 = μmol/L	μmol/L × 0.337 = mg/L
Terazosin	0.1 mg/L	[Not known]	387.4	mg/L × 2.58 = μmol/L	μmol/L × 0.387 = mg/L
Terbinafine	2 mg/L	[Not known]	291.4	mg/L × 3.43 = μmol/L	μmol/L × 0.291 = mg/L
Norterbinafine[b]	2 mg/L	[Not known]	277.4	mg/L × 3.60 = μmol/L	μmol/L × 0.277 = mg/L
Terbutaline	30 μg/L	[Not known]	225.3	μg/L × 4.44 = nmol/L	nmol/L × 0.225 = μg/L
Terfenadine: see also Fexofenadine[b]	10 μg/L	40 μg/L	471.7	μg/L × 2.12 = nmol/L	nmol/L × 0.472 = μg/L
Terodiline	0.6 mg/L	[Not known]	281.4	mg/L × 3.55 = μmol/L	μmol/L × 0.281 = mg/L
Tetracaine	0.2 mg/L (topical)	[Not known]	264.3	mg/L × 3.78 = μmol/L	μmol/L × 0.264 = mg/L
4-Butylaminobenzoate[d]	1 mg/L (topical tetracaine)		193.2	mg/L × 5.18 = μmol/L	μmol/L × 0.193 = mg/L
2,3,6,7-Tetrachlorodibenzodioxin (TCDD)	5 ng/L (dietary)	[Not known]	322.0	ng/L × 3.11 = pmol/L	pmol/L × 0.322 = ng/L
Tetrachloroethylene (whole blood)	1 mg/L[c]	10 mg/L	165.8	mg/L × 6.03 = μmol/L	μmol/L × 0.166 = mg/L
Tetracycline	10 mg/L (IV dose)	30 mg/L	444.4	mg/L × 2.25 = μmol/L	μmol/L × 0.444 = mg/L
Tetraethyllead: see Lead					
Δ^9-Tetrahydrocannabinol (THC)	0.01 mg/L (passive inhalation) 0.2 mg/L (single "joint")	[Not known]	314.5	mg/L × 3.18 = μmol/L	μmol/L × 0.315 = mg/L
Tetrahydrofuran (urine)	8 mg/L[c]		72.1	mg/L × 13.9 = μmol/L	μmol/L × 0.072 = mg/L
Tetrazepam	1 mg/L	[Not known]	288.8	mg/L × 3.46 = μmol/L	μmol/L × 0.289 = mg/L
Thalidomide	7 mg/L	[Not known]	258.2	mg/L × 3.87 = μmol/L	μmol/L × 0.258 = mg/L
Thallium (whole blood)	2 μg/L	50 μg/L	204.4	μg/L × 4.89 = nmol/L	nmol/L × 0.204 = μg/L
(urine)	2 μg/L	200 μg/L			
Theobromine	15 mg/L	30 mg/L	180.2	mg/L × 5.55 = μmol/L	μmol/L × 0.180 = mg/L
Theophylline: see also Caffeine in neonates[b]	20 mg/L	40 mg/L	180.2	mg/L × 5.55 = μmol/L	μmol/L × 0.180 = mg/L
Thiabendazole	10 mg/L	[Not known]	201.3	mg/L × 4.97 = μmol/L	μmol/L × 0.201 = mg/L
Thiocyanate	4 mg/L (nonsmokers) 20 mg/L (heavy smokers) 100 mg/L (nitroprusside therapy)	120 mg/L	58.1	mg/L × 17.2 = μmol/L	μmol/L × 0.058 = mg/L
Thiopentone (thiopental): see also Pentobarbitone[b]	5 mg/L	20 mg/L	242.3	mg/L × 4.13 = μmol/L	μmol/L × 0.242 = mg/L
Thioridazine: see also Mesoridazine[b]	1.5 mg/L	2 mg/L	370.6	mg/L × 2.70 = μmol/L	μmol/L × 0.371 = mg/L

Analyte	"Therapeutic" or "normal" plasma concentration (less than)	Plasma concentration associated with acute serious toxicity[a]	Relative atomic or formula mass	Mass/amount conversion	Amount/mass conversion
2-Thiothiazolidine-4-carboxylate (TTCA; urine)	8 mg/L[c]		163.2	mg/L × 6.13 = μmol/L	μmol/L × 0.163 = mg/L
Thiothixine	0.1 mg/L	[Not known]	443.6	mg/L × 2.25 = μmol/L	μmol/L × 0.444 = mg/L
Tiagabine	1 mg/L	[Not known]	375.6	mg/L × 2.66 = μmol/L	μmol/L × 0.376 = mg/L
Tiapride	5 mg/L	[Not known]	328.4	mg/L × 3.05 = μmol/L	μmol/L × 0.328 = mg/L
Tiaprofenic acid	100 mg/L	[Not known]	260.3	mg/L × 3.84 = μmol/L	μmol/L × 0.260 = mg/L
Ticlopidine	1 mg/L	—	263.8	mg/L × 3.79 = μmol/L	μmol/L × 0.264 = mg/L
Tilidate	0.1 mg/L	[Not known]	273.4	mg/L × 3.66 = μmol/L	μmol/L × 0.273 = mg/L
Nortilidate[b]	0.2 mg/L	[Not known]	259.4	mg/L × 3.86 = μmol/L	μmol/L × 0.259 = mg/L
Tilidine: see Tilidate					
Timolol	0.2 mg/L	[Not known]	316.4	mg/L × 3.16 = μmol/L	μmol/L × 0.316 = mg/L
Tin	30 μg/L	[Not known]	118.7	μg/L × 0.0084 = μmol/L	μmol/L × 118.7 = μg/L
Tinidazole	60 mg/L	[Not known]	247.3	mg/L × 4.04 = μmol/L	μmol/L × 0.247 = mg/L
Tizanidine	15 μg/L	[Not known]	253.7	μg/L × 3.94 = nmol/L	nmol/L × 0.254 = μg/L
Tobramycin	8 mg/L	12 mg/L	467.5	mg/L × 2.14 = μmol/L	μmol/L × 0.468 = mg/L
Tocainide	10 mg/L	25 mg/L	192.3	mg/L × 5.20 = μmol/L	μmol/L × 0.192 = mg/L
Tofenacin (nororphenadrine)	0.1 mg/L	0.5 mg/L	255.4	mg/L × 3.92 = μmol/L	μmol/L × 0.255 = mg/L
Tolazoline	0.5 mg/L	[Not known]	160.2	mg/L × 6.24 = μmol/L	μmol/L × 0.160 = mg/L
Tolbutamide	200 mg/L (diabetics)	400 mg/L	270.3	mg/L × 3.70 = μmol/L	μmol/L × 0.270 = mg/L
Tolmetin	80 mg/L	[Not known]	257.3	mg/L × 3.89 = μmol/L	μmol/L × 0.257 = mg/L
Toluene (whole blood): see also Hippurate[d]	1 mg/L[c]	10 mg/L	92.1	mg/L × 10.86 = μmol/L	μmol/L × 0.092 = mg/L
2-Methylphenol[d] (urine)	3 mg/L[c]		108.1	mg/L × 9.25 = μmol/L	μmol/L × 0.108 = mg/L
Topiramate	30 mg/L	[Not known]	339.4	mg/L × 2.95 = μmol/L	μmol/L × 0.339 = mg/L
Tramadol	1 mg/L	[Not known]	263.4	mg/L × 3.80 = μmol/L	μmol/L × 0.263 = mg/L
Tranexamate	50 mg/L	[Not known]	157.2	mg/L × 6.36 = μmol/L	μmol/L × 0.157 = mg/L
Tranylcypromine	0.1 mg/L	0.3 mg/L	133.2	mg/L × 7.51 = μmol/L	μmol/L × 0.133 = mg/L
Trazodone	2 mg/L	[Not known]	371.9	mg/L × 2.69 = μmol/L	μmol/L × 0.372 = mg/L
Triamcinolone acetonide	50 μg/L (IM dose) 2 μg/L (intranasal dose)	[Not known]	434.5	μg/L × 2.30 = nmol/L	nmol/L × 0.435 = μg/L
Triamterene	3 mg/L	[Not known]	253.3	mg/L × 3.95 = μmol/L	μmol/L × 0.253 = mg/L
Triazolam	20 μg/L	40 μg/L	343.2	μg/L × 2.91 = nmol/L	nmol/L × 0.343 = μg/L
2,2,2-Tribromoethanol	—	50 mg/L	282.8	mg/L × 3.54 = μmol/L	μmol/L × 0.283 = mg/L
Trichloroacetate (urine)	100 mg/L[c]		163.4	mg/L × 6.12 = μmol/L	μmol/L × 0.163 = mg/L
1,1,1-Trichloro-di-(4-chlorophenyl)ethane (DDT; total)	0.04 mg/L (dietary)	1 mg/L	354.5	mg/L × 2.82 = μmol/L	μmol/L × 0.355 = mg/L
1,1-Dichloro-di-(4-chlorophenyl)ethene (DDE)[d]	0.2 mg/L (dietary)		318.0	mg/L × 3.14 = μmol/L	μmol/L × 0.318 = mg/L
1,1,1-Trichloroethane (whole blood)	0.5 mg/L[c]	10 mg/L	133.4	mg/L × 7.50 = μmol/L	μmol/L × 0.133 = mg/L
2,2,2-Trichloroethanol (whole blood)	10 mg/L 5 mg/L[c]	50 mg/L	149.4	mg/L × 6.69 = μmol/L	μmol/L × 0.149 = mg/L
Trichloroethylene (whole blood): see also Trichloroacetate,[d] 2,2,2-Trichloroethanol[b]	—	10 mg/L	131.4	mg/L × 7.61 = μmol/L	μmol/L × 0.131 = mg/L
2,4,5-Trichlorophenoxyacetate	—	0.5 g/L	255.5	g/L × 3.91 = mmol/L	mmol/L × 0.256 = g/L
2-(2,4,5-Trichlorophenoxy)propionate	—	0.5 g/L	269.5	g/L × 3.71 = mmol/L	mmol/L × 0.270 = g/L
Trifluoperazine	50 μg/L	100 μg/L	407.5	μg/L × 2.45 = nmol/L	nmol/L × 0.408 = μg/L
Triflupromazine	0.1 mg/L	0.5 mg/L	352.4	mg/L × 2.84 = μmol/L	μmol/L × 0.352 = mg/L
Trihexyphenidyl: see Benzhexol					
Trimebutine	3 mg/L	[Not known]	387.5	mg/L × 2.58 = μmol/L	μmol/L × 0.388 = mg/L
Nortrimebutine[b]	3 mg/L		373.5	mg/L × 2.68 = μmol/L	μmol/L × 0.374 = mg/L
Trimeprazine	0.4 mg/L	[Not known]	298.5	mg/L × 3.35 = μmol/L	μmol/L × 0.299 = mg/L
Trimethadione: see also Dimethadione[b]	40 mg/L	—	143.1	mg/L × 6.99 = μmol/L	μmol/L × 0.143 = mg/L
Trimethobenzamide	2 mg/L	[Not known]	388.5	mg/L × 2.57 = μmol/L	μmol/L × 0.389 = mg/L
Trimethoprim	5 mg/L	20 mg/L	290.3	mg/L × 3.44 = μmol/L	μmol/L × 0.290 = mg/L
3,4,5-Trimethoxyphenethylamine: see Mescaline					
Trimipramine	0.5 mg/L	1 mg/L	294.4	mg/L × 3.40 = μmol/L	μmol/L × 0.294 = mg/L
Nortrimipramine[b]	0.5 mg/L	1 mg/L	280.4	mg/L × 3.57 = μmol/L	μmol/L × 0.280 = mg/L
Tripelennamine	0.2 mg/L	[Not known]	255.4	mg/L × 3.92 = μmol/L	μmol/L × 0.255 = mg/L
Triprolidine	50 μg/L	[Not known]	278.4	μg/L × 3.59 = nmol/L	nmol/L × 0.278 = μg/L

Analyte	"Therapeutic" or "normal" plasma concentration (less than)	Plasma concentration associated with acute serious toxicity[a]	Relative atomic or formula mass	Mass/amount conversion	Amount/mass conversion
2-Thiothiazolidine-4-carboxylate (TTCA; urine)	8 mg/L[c]		163.2	mg/L × 6.13 = μmol/L	μmol/L × 0.163 = mg/L
Tropisetron	50 μg/L	[Not known]	284.4	μg/L × 3.52 = nmol/L	nmol/L × 0.284 = μg/L
TTCA: see 2-Thiothiazolidine-4-carboxylate					
Tubocurarine	3 mg/L	[Not known]	611.7	mg/L × 1.63 = μmol/L	μmol/L × 0.612 = mg/L
Tungsten	35 μg/L	[Not known]	183.8	μg/L × 5.44 = nmol/L	nmol/L × 0.184 = μg/L
Uranium	50 ng/L (urine)	—	238.0	ng/L × 4.20 = pmol/L	pmol/L × 0.238 = μg/L
Valacyclovir: see Aciclovir					
Valproate	100 mg/L	500 mg/L	144.2	mg/L × 6.93 = μmol/L	μmol/L × 0.144 = mg/L
Valpromide: see Valproate					
Vanadium	50 μg/L	[Not known]	50.9	μg/L × 19.6 = nmol/L	nmol/L × 0.051 = μg/L
(urine)	1 μg/L				
Vancomycin	30 mg/L	—	1449	mg/L × 0.69 = μmol/L	μmol/L × 1.449 = mg/L
Vecuronium	0.5 mg/L	[Not known]	557.8	mg/L × 1.79 = μmol/L	μmol/L × 0.558 = mg/L
Venlafaxine	0.1 mg/L	[Not known]	277.4	mg/L × 3.60 = μmol/L	μmol/L × 0.277 = mg/L
O-Desmethylvenlafaxine[b]	0.3 mg/L	[Not known]	263.4	mg/L × 3.80 = μmol/L	μmol/L × 0.263 = mg/L
Verapamil	0.2 mg/L	2 mg/L	454.6	mg/L × 2.20 = μmol/L	nmol/L × 0.455 = μg/L
Norverapamil[b]	0.2 mg/L	2 mg/L	440.6	mg/L × 2.27 = μmol/L	μmol/L × 0.441 = mg/L
Vidarabine	10 mg/L	[Not known]	267.3	mg/L × 3.74 = μmol/L	μmol/L × 0.267 = mg/L
Vigabatrin	45 mg/L	[Not known]	129.2	mg/L × 7.74 = μmol/L	μmol/L × 0.129 = mg/L
Viloxazine	4 mg/L	[Not known]	237.3	mg/L × 4.21 = μmol/L	μmol/L × 0.237 = mg/L
Vinblastine	0.4 mg/L	—	811.0	mg/L × 1.23 = μmol/L	μmol/L × 0.811 = mg/L
Vincristine	0.4 mg/L	—	825.0	mg/L × 1.21 = μmol/L	μmol/L × 0.825 = mg/L
Vitamin K_1: see Phytomenadione					
Warfarin	7 mg/L	10 mg/L	308.3	mg/L × 3.25 = μmol/L	μmol/L × 0.308 = mg/L
Xamoterol	0.2 mg/L	[Not known]	339.4	mg/L × 2.95 = μmol/L	μmol/L × 0.339 = mg/L
Xipamide	20 mg/L	[Not known]	354.8	mg/L × 2.82 = μmol/L	μmol/L × 0.355 = mg/L
Xylenes (total, whole blood): see also Methylhippurates[d]	0.01 mg/L (environmental) 1.5 mg/L[c]	[Not known]	106.2	mg/L × 9.42 = μmol/L	μmol/L × 0.106 = mg/L
Yohimbine	0.3 mg/L	[Not known]	354.5	mg/L × 2.82 = μmol/L	μmol/L × 0.355 = mg/L
Zaleplon	0.1 mg/L	[Not known]	305.3	mg/L × 3.28 = μmol/L	μmol/L × 0.305 = mg/L
Zidovudine (AZT)	1 mg/L	—	267.2	mg/L × 3.74 = μmol/L	μmol/L × 0.267 = mg/L
Zipeprol	0.1 mg/L	[Not known]	384.5	mg/L × 2.60 = μmol/L	μmol/L × 0.385 = mg/L
Zileuton	5 mg/L	[Not known]	236.3	mg/L × 4.23 = μmol/L	μmol/L × 0.236 = mg/L
Zimelidine	0.3 mg/L	[Not known]	317.2	mg/L × 3.15 = μmol/L	μmol/L × 0.317 = mg/L
Norzimelidine[b]	0.5 mg/L	[Not known]	303.2	mg/L × 3.30 = μmol/L	μmol/L × 0.303 = mg/L
Zinc[g]	0.7–1.6 mg/L	5 mg/L	65.4	mg/L × 15.3 = μmol/L	μmol/L × 0.065 = mg/L
(urine)	0.3–0.6 mg/L				
Ziprasidone	0.2 mg/L	[Not known]	412.9	mg/L × 2.42 = μmol/L	μmol/L × 0.413 = mg/L
Zolmitriptan	20 μg/L	[Not known]	287.4	mg/L × 3.48 = μmol/L	μmol/L × 0.287 = mg/L
Norzolmitriptan[b]	10 μg/L		273.4	mg/L × 3.66 = μmol/L	μmol/L × 0.273 = mg/L
Zolpidem	0.3 mg/L	3 mg/L	307.4	mg/L × 3.25 = μmol/L	μmol/L × 0.307 = mg/L
Zomepirac	5 mg/L	[Not known]	291.7	mg/L × 3.43 = μmol/L	μmol/L × 0.292 = mg/L
Zonisamide	20 mg/L	30 mg/L	212.2	mg/L × 4.71 = μmol/L	μmol/L × 0.212 = mg/L
Zopiclone	0.1 mg/L	[Not known]	388.8	mg/L × 2.57 = μmol/L	μmol/L × 0.389 = mg/L
Zotepine	50 μg/L	[Not known]	331.9	μg/L × 3.01 = nmol/L	nmol/L × 0.332 = μg/L
Zoxazolamine	15 mg/L	[Not known]	168.6	mg/L × 5.93 = μmol/L	μmol/L × 0.167 = mg/L
Zuclopenthixol	0.1 mg/L	0.3 mg/L	401.0	mg/L × 2.49 = μmol/L	μmol/L × 0.401 = mg/L

[a]Dash indicates that concentration that could be associated with serious toxicity may be no greater than "therapeutic" concentration in other patients.
[b]Active metabolite/decomposition product.
[c]Deutsche Forschungsgemeinschaft suggested "action level" (1996).
[d]Metabolite/decomposition product.
[e]Recent ingestion of fish or shellfish renders total arsenic measurements uninterpretable.
[f]Toxicity of chromium dependent on oxidation state.
[g]True normal range—deficiency more common problem than poisoning, except in Wilson's disease, with which serious copper poisoning can occur at relatively low plasma copper concentrations because of ceruloplasmin deficiency.
[h]No accurate relative molecular mass.
[i]Suggestive of recent toluene exposure, but dietary benzoate may give elevated hippurate excretion.
[j]Occupational exposure (greatly increased after topical use of coal tar products).
[k]Human insulin, 1 mU, is contained in 0.03846 μg of the first International Standard (1986).
[l]Suggested United Kingdom Health and Safety Executive "health guidance value" (1996).

APPENDIX III

Système International Conversion Factors for Frequently Used Laboratory Components

Table III-1
Système International Conversion Factors for Frequently Used Laboratory Components[a]

System*	Component	Traditional Reference Interval†	Traditional Unit‡	Conversion Factor	SI Reference Interval†	SI Unit	Significant Digits§	Suggested Minimum Increment
S	Copper	70–140	μg/dL	0.1574	11.0–22.0	μmol/L	XX.X	0.2 μmol/L
U	Copper	<40	μg/24 hr	0.0574	<0.6	μmol/d	X.X	0.2 μmol/d
P	Corticotropin (ACTH)	20–100	pg/mL	0.2202	4–22	pmol/L	XX	1 pmol/L
S	Creatine							
	Male	0.17–0.50	mg/dL	76.25	10–40	μmol/L	X0	10 μmol/L
	Female	0.35–0.93	mg/dL	76.25	30–70	μmol/L	X0	10 μmol/L
U	Creatine							
	Male	0–40	mg/24 hr	7.625	0–300	μmol/d	XX0	10 μmol/L
	Female	0–80	mg/24 hr	7.625	0–600	μmol/d	XX0	10 μmol/d
S	Creatine kinase (CK)	0–130 (37°C)	Units/L	1.00	0–130	U/L	XXX	1 U/L
S	Creatine kinase isoenzymes, MB fraction	>5 in myocardial infarction	%	0.01	>0.05	1	X.XX	0.01
S	Creatinine	0.6–1.2	mg/dl **(Dual report)**	88.40	50–110	μmol/L	XX0	10 μmol/L
U	Creatinine	Variable	g/24 hr **(Dual report)**	8.840	Variable	mmol/d	XX.X	0.1 mmol/d
S, U	Creatinine clearance	75–125	mL/min **(Dual report)**	0.01667	1.24–2.08	mL/s	X.XX	0.02 mL/s
U	Cystine	10–100	mg/24 hr	4.161	40–420	μmol/d	XX0	10 μmol/d
P	Digoxin, therapeutic	0.5–2.2	ng/mL **(Dual report)**	1.281	0.6–2.8	nmol/L	X.X	0.1 nmol/L
		0.5–2.2	μg/L **(Dual report)**	1.281	0.6–2.8	nmol/L	X.X	0.1 nmol/L
S	Estradiol, male >18 y	15–40	pg/mL **(Dual report)**	3.671	55–150	pmol/L	XXX	1 pmol/L
P	Ethyl alcohol	>100	mg/dL	0.2171	>22	mmol/L	XX	1 mmol/L
P	Fibrinogen	200–400	mg/dL	0.01	2.0–4.0	g/L	X.X	0.1 g/L
P	Follicle-stimulating hormone (FSH)							
	Female	2.0–15.0	mIU/mL	1.00	2–15	IU/L	XX	1 IU/L
	Peak production	20–50	mIU/mL	1.00	20–50	IU/L	XX	1 IU/L
	Male	1.0–10.0	mIU/mL	1.00	1–10	IU/L	XX	1 IU/L
U	Follicle-stimulating hormone (FSH)							
	Follicular phase	2–15	IU/24 hr	1.00	2–15	IU/d	XXX	1 IU/d

[a]Adapted from JAMA 1995;274:97–98.

*P represents plasma; B, blood; S, serum; U, urine; CSF, cerebrospinal fluid; RBCs, red blood cells; and WBCs, white blood cells.

†These reference values are not intended to be definitive since each laboratory determines its own values. They are provided for illustration only.

‡Traditional units should be reported parenthetically after the SI units *only* for those units marked "Dual report."

§"Significant digits" refers to the number of digits used to describe the reported results. XX implies that results expressed to the nearest whole number are meaningful; XX0, that results are only meaningful when rounded to the nearest 10, and that results reported to lower numbers or decimal points are beyond the sensitivity of the procedure.

(continued)

Table III-1 (Continued)

System*	Component	Traditional Reference Interval†	Traditional Unit‡	Conversion Factor	SI Reference Interval†	SI Unit	Significant Digits§	Suggested Minimum Increment
	Midcycle	8–40	IU/24 hr	1.00	8–40	IU/d	XXX	1 IU/d
	Luteal phase	2–10	IU/24 hr	1.00	2–10	IU/d	XXX	1 IU/d
	Menopausal women	35–100	IU/24 hr	1.00	35–100	IU/d	XXX	1 IU/d
	Male	2–15	IU/24 hr	1.00	2–15	IU/d	XXX	1 IU/d
S	γ-Glutamyltransferase (GGT)	0–30 (30°C)	Units/L	1.00	0–30	U/L	XX	1 U/L
P	Glucose	70–110	mg/dL **(Dual report)**	0.05551	3.9–6.1	mmol/L	XX.X	0.1 mmol/L
B	Hemoglobin Male	14.0–18.0	g/dL	10.0	140–180	g/L	XXX	1 g/L
	Female	11.5–15.5	g/dL	10.0	115–155	g/L	XXX	1 g/L
S	Immunoglobulins IgG	500–1200	mg/dL	0.01	5.00–12.00	g/L	XX.XX	0.01 g/L
	IgA	50–350	mg/dL	0.01	0.50–3.50	g/L	XX.XX	0.01 g/L
	IgM	30–230	mg/dL	0.01	0.30–2.30	g/L	XX.XX	0.01 g/L
	IgD	<6	mg/dL	10	<60	mg/L	XX0	10 mg/L
	IgE 0–3 y	0.5–1.0	U/mL	2.4	1–24	μg/L	XX	1 μg/L
	3–80 y	5–100	U/mL	2.4	12–240	μg/L	XX	1 μg/L
S	Iron Male	80–180	μg/dL **(Dual report)**	0.1791	14–32	μmol/L	XX	1 μmol/L
	Female	60–160	μg/dL **(Dual report)**	0.1791	11–29	μmol/L	XX	1 μmol/L
S	Iron-binding capacity	250–460	μg/dL **(Dual report)**	0.1791	45–82	μmol/L	XX	1 μmol/L
S	Lactate dehydrogenase (L → P)	50–150 (37°C)	Units/L	1.00	50–150	U/L	XXX	1 U/L
			Wroblewski units/mL	0.482	. . .	U/L	XXX	1 U/L
S	Lactate dehydrogenase isoenzymes LD_1	15–40	%	0.01	0.15–0.40	1	X.XX	0.01
	LD_2	20–45	%	0.01	0.20–0.45	1	X.XX	0.01
	LD_3	15–30	%	0.01	0.15–0.30	1	X.XX	0.01
	LD_4 and LD_5	5–20	%	0.01	0.05–0.20	1	X.XX	0.01
	LD_1	10–60	Units/L	1	10–60	U/L	XX	1 U/L
	LD_2	20–70	Units/L	1	20–70	U/L	XX	1 U/L

(continued)

Table III-1 (Continued)

System*	Component	Traditional Reference Interval†	Traditional Unit‡	Conversion Factor	SI Reference Interval†	SI Unit	Significant Digits§	Suggested Minimum Increment
	LD_3	10–45	Units/L	1	10–45	U/L	XX	1 U/L
	LD_4 and LD_5	5–30	Units/L	1	5–30	U/L	XX	1 U/L
B	Lead, toxic	>60	µg/dL **(Dual report)**	0.04826	>2.90	µmol/L	X.XX	0.05 µmol/L
			mg/dL **(Dual report)**	48.26	. . .	µmol/L	X.XX	0.05 µmol/L
U	Lead, toxic	>80	µg/24 hr **(Dual report)**	0.004826	>0.40	µmol/d	X.XX	0.05 µmol/d
P	Lipids, total	400–850	mg/dL **(Dual report)**	0.01	4.0–8.5	g/L	X.X	0.1 g/L
P	Lipoproteins Low-density (LDL), as cholesterol	50–190	mg/dL **(Dual report)**	0.02586	1.30–4.90	mmol/L	X.XX	0.05 mmol/L
	High-density (HDL), as cholesterol Male	30–70	mg/dL **(Dual report)**	0.02586	0.80–1.80	mmol/L	X.XX	0.05 mmol/L
	Female	30–90	mg/dL **(Dual report)**	0.02586	0.80–2.35	mmol/L	X.XX	0.05 mmol/L
S	Magnesium	1.8–3.0	mg/dL **(Dual report)**	0.4114	0.80–1.20	mmol/L	X.XX	0.02 mmol/L
P	Phenytoin, therapeutic	10–20	mg/L	3.964	40–80	µmol/L	XX	5 µmol/L
P	Phosphatase, acid (prostatic)	0–3	King-Armstrong units/dL	1.77	0–5.5	U/L	X.X	0.05 U/L
			Bodansky units/dL	5.37	0–16.1	U/L	X.X	0.5 U/L
S	Phosphatase, alkaline	30–120	Units/L	1.00	30–120	U/L	XXX	1 U/L
			Bodansky units/dL	5.37	161–644	U/L	XXX	1 U/L
			King-Armstrong units/dL	7.1	213–852	U/L	XXX	1 U/L
S	Phosphate (as phosphorus)	2.5–5.0	mg/dL **(Dual report)**	0.3229	0.80–1.60	mmol/L	X.XX	0.05 mmol/L
S	Potassium	3.5–5.0	mEq/L	1.00	3.5–5.0	mmol/L	X.X	0.1 mmol/L
P	Progesterone Follicular phase	<2	ng/mL	3.180	<6	nmol/L	XX	2 nmol/L
	Luteal phase	2–20	ng/mL	3.180	6–64	nmol/L	XX	2 nmol/L
S	Protein, total	6–8	g/dL	10.0	60–80	g/L	XX	1 g/L
CSF	Protein, total	<40	mg/dL	0.01	<0.40	g/L	X.XX	0.01 g/L
U	Protein, total	<150	mg/24 hr	0.001	<0.15	g/d	X.XX	0.01 g/d
S	Sodium	135–147	mEq/L	1.00	135–147	mmol/L	XXX	1 mmol/L
S	Sodium ion	135–147	mEq/L	1.00	135–147	mmol/L	XXX	1 mmol/L
U	Sodium ion	Diet dependent	mEq/24 hr	1.00	Diet dependent	mmol/d	XXX	1 mmol/d

(continued)

Table III-1 (Continued)

System*	Component	Traditional Reference Interval†	Traditional Unit‡	Conversion Factor	SI Reference Interval†	SI Unit	Significant Digits§	Suggested Minimum Increment
U	Steroids Hydroxycorticosteroids (as cortisol) Female	2–8	mg/24 hr	2.759	5–25	μmol/d	XX	1 μmol/d
	Male	3–10	mg/24 hr	2.759	10–30	μmol/d	XX	1 μmol/d
U	17-Ketogenic steroids (as dehydro-epiandrosterone) Female	7–12	mg/24 hr	3.467	25–40	μmol/d	XX	1 μmol/d
	Male	9–17	mg/24 hr	3.467	30–60	μmol/d	XX	1 μmol/d
U	17-Ketosteroids (as dehydroepian-drosterone) Female	6–17	mg/24 hr	3.467	20–60	μmol/d	XX	1 μmol/d
	Male	6–20	mg/24 hr	3.467	20–70	μmol/d	XX	1 μmol/d
U	Ketosteroid fractions Androsterone Female	0.5–3.0	mg/24 hr	3.443	1–10	μmol/d	XX	1 μmol/d
	Male	2.0–5.0	mg/24 hr	3.443	7–17	μmol/d	XX	1 μmol/d
	Dehydroepiandrosterone Female	0.2–1.8	mg/24 hr	3.467	1–6	μmol/d	XX	1 μmol/d
	Male	0.2–2.0	mg/24 hr	3.467	1–7	μmol/d	XX	1 μmol/d
	Etiocholanolone Female	0.8–4.0	mg/24 hr	3.443	2–14	μmol/d	XX	1 μmol/d
	Male	1.4–5.0	mg/24 hr	3.443	4–17	μmol/d	XX	1 μmol/d
				58.07	580–870	μmol/L	XX0	10 μmol/L
P	Testosterone Female	<0.6	ng/mL **(Dual report)**	3.467	<2 0	nmol/L	XX.X	0.5 nmol/L
	Male	4.0–8.0	ng/mL **(Dual report)**	3.467	14.0–28.0	nmol/L	XX.X	0.5 nmol/L
S	Thyroxine (T_4)	4–11	μg/dL **(Dual report)**	12.87	51–142	nmol/L	XXX	1 nmol/L
S	Thyroxine-binding globulin (TBG), as thyroxine	12–28	μg/dL **(Dual report)**	12.87	150–360	nmol/L	XX0	10 nmol/L
S	Thyroxine, free	0.8–2.8	ng/dL **(Dual report)**	12.87	10–36	pmol/L	XX	1 pmol/L

(continued)

Table III-1 (Continued)

System*	Component	Traditional Reference Interval†	Traditional Unit‡	Conversion Factor	SI Reference Interval†	SI Unit	Significant Digits§	Suggested Minimum Increment
S	Triiodothyronine (T_3)	75–220	ng/dL	0.01536	1.2–3.4	nmol/L	X.X	0.1 nmol/L
S	Urate (as uric acid)	2.0–7.0	mg/dL	59.48	120–420	µmol/L	XX0	10 µmol/L
U	Urate (as uric acid)	Diet dependent	g/24 hr	5.948	Diet dependent	mmol/d	XX	1 mmol/d
S	Urea nitrogen	8–18	mg/dL **(Dual report)**	0.3570	3.0–6.5	mmol/L of urea	X.X	0.5 mmol/L
U	Urea nitrogen	12–20 (diet dependent)	g/24 hr **(Dual report)**	35.70	430–700	mmol/L of urea	XX0	10 mmol/d
U	Urobilinogen	0–4.0	mg/24 hr	1.693	0.0–6.8	µmol/d	X.X	0.1 µmol/d
S	Zinc	75–120	µg/dL	0.1530	11.5–18.5	µmol/L	XX.X	0.1 µmol/L
U	Zinc	150–1200	µg/24 hr	0.0153	2.3–18.3	µmol/d	XX.X	0.1 µmol/d

APPENDIX IV

Pediatric Emergency Drugs

Generic drug name (trade name)	Preparation	Dose and route of administration	Toxicity of adverse effects	Contraindications
Acetaminophen (Tylenol, Panadol, Tempra, APAP)	Drops: 80 mg/0.8 ml; elixir: 80, 120, 160, 325 mg/5 ml; liquid: 160 mg/5 ml; suppository: 120, 125, 325, 600, 650 mg; tablets: 325, 500, 650 mg	10–15 mg/kg/dose PO q4h; maximum, 5 doses in 24 h	Hepatic toxicity in overdose; nausea, vomiting, diaphoresis, malaise	Recent (4 h) acetaminophen dose
Acetylsalicylic acid (ASA, aspirin)	Tablets: 65, 75, 200, 300, 325, 500, 600, 650 mg; suppository: 60, 65, 130, 150, 195, 200, 300, 325, 600 mg	10–15 mg/kg PO q4h; maximum, 60–80 mg/kg in 24 h or 3.6 g in 24 h	Anaphylactic shock, rash, bleeding, Reye's syndrome, salicylism-nausea, vomiting, tinnitus, hearing impairment, headache, dizziness, drowsiness, hyperpnea, hyperventilation, tachycardia, sweating, thirst	Contact with varicella or influenza illness, known hypersensitivity, severe bleeding disorder, coagulopathy, severe liver damage, concomitant anticoagulation therapy, peptic ulcer disease
Adenosine (Adenocard)	Injection: 6 mg/2 ml	0.1 mg/kg rapid IV bolus; may increase by 0.05 mg/kg increments to maximum of 0.25 mg/kg or 12 mg/dose; repeat with careful monitoring	Hypotension, chest pain or pressure, dyspnea, tingling, heart block, dysrhythmias	Second or third degree AV block, sick sinus syndrome, hypersensitivity, theophylline
Albuterol (Proventil, Ventolin)	MDI: 90 µg/puff; inhalation solution: 5 mg/ml (0.5%) or unit dose, 2.5 mg/3 ml, normal saline	MDI: 1–2 puffs q5min to maximum of 12 puffs; nebulization: 0.15–0.30 mg/kg/dose q15–20min	Tremor, dizziness, headache, nausea, tachycardia, hypertension, paradoxic bronchospasm	Hypersensitivity, tachycardia >180–200 beats/min
Amiodarone (Cordarone)	Injection: 50 mg/ml	5 mg/kg IV push for cardiac arrest; infuse over 20–60 min for wide complex tachycardia	Bradycardia, hypotension, vomiting, dysrhythmias, photosensitivity	Cardiogenic shock, second or third degree block, severe sinus bradycardia
Atropine	Injection: 0.05, 0.1, 0.3, 0.4, 0.5, 0.8, 1.0 mg/ml	0.01–0.03 mg/kg IV q2–5min to a maximum of 1–2 mg; minimum dose, 0.1 mg	Paradoxic bradycardia, tachydysrhythmias	Tachydysrhythmias
Calcium chloride	Injection: 100 mg/ml	10–30 mg/kg slowly IV, preferably central line	Tissue necrosis if extravasates	Hypercalcemia, cardiac glycoside poisoning
Charcoal	Powder: 15, 30, 40, 120, 240 g; suspension: 12.5 g/60 ml, 15 g/75 ml, 24 g/120 ml	1–2 g/kg PO; maximum dose, 50 g in 24 h	Constipation, aspiration	None
Chloral hydrate	Syrup: 250, 500 mg/5 cc; suppository: 324, 500, 648 mg	15–50 mg/kg PO, PR depending on desired effect; maximum dose, 2 g in 24 h	Prolonged sedation	Hepatic failure
Cimetidine	Injection: 150 mg/ml	20–40 mg/kg IV divided q6h	Diarrhea, dizziness, somnolence, headache, confusion, cardiac dysrhythmias with rapid IV bolus	Known hypersensitivity
Dexamethasone (Decadron)	Injection: 4, 10, 20, 24 mg/ml	0.25–0.50 mg/kg IV q6h for airway edema; 0.6 mg/kg IM once for croup	Multiple effects with long-term use (see prednisone)	Systemic fungal infections, known hypersensitivity, caution in immunosuppressed individuals
Diazepam (Valium)	Injection: 5 mg/ml	Neonates: 0.1–0.3 mg/kg IV q15–30min; children: 0.2–0.5 mg/kg IV q15–30min; maximum dose, 10 mg; administer slowly over 5–10 min; 0.3–0.5 mg/kg PR	Drowsiness, fatigue, ataxia, apnea, bradycardia, hypotension, venous thrombosis or phlebitis, pain at injection site	Known hypersensitivity to diazepam, acute narrow-angle glaucoma; use in a monitored setting only

(*continued*)

Generic drug name (trade name)	Preparation	Dose and route of administration	Toxicity of adverse effects	Contraindications
Digoxin	Injection: 100, 250 μg/ml	10–40 μg/kg IV (complex dosing schedule—consult cardiology text)	Conduction disturbances, dysrhythmias, anorexia, nausea, vomiting, diarrhea, blurred or yellow vision, sweating	V fib, bradycardia, high grade AV block, bypass tract present
Diphenhydramine (Benadryl, Genahist)	Injection: 10, 50 mg/ml; capsules: 25, 50 mg; elixir/syrup: 12.5 mg/5 ml; tablets: 25, 50 mg	5 mg/kg per 24 h PO, IM divided q6h; for anaphylaxis: 1–2 mg/kg slow IV push; maximum, 300 mg in 24 h	CNS depression, incoordination, hallucinations, coma, urticaria, hypotension, tachycardia, headache, epigastric distress, thickening of bronchial secretions	Altered mental status, newborn or preterm infants, known hypersensitivity
Dobutamine	Injection: 12.5 mg/ml; do not add to alkaline solutions	2.5–15.0 μg/kg/min; maximum, 40 μg/kg/min	Increased heart rate, increased blood pressure, ventricular ectopic activity, hypotension, phlebitis, nausea, angina, palpitations, headache, dyspnea	Idiopathic hypertrophic subaortic stenosis, known hypersensitivity, use in monitored setting only
Dopamine	Injection: 40, 80, 160 mg/ml; inactivated if added to alkaline solution	5–20 μg/kg/min, depending on desired effect	Ectopic beats, nausea, vomiting, tachycardia, angina, palpitations, dyspnea, headache, hypotension, vasoconstriction, aberrant conduction, bradycardia, widened QRS	Pheochromocytoma, uncorrected tachydysrhythmias or V fib, uncorrected hypovolemia; use in monitored setting only
Epinephrine	Injection: 1:1000 (1 mg/ml)	Infusion: 0.1–0.4 μg/kg/min, 0.01 mg/kg SQ; maximum, 0.3 ml = 0.3 mg	Palpitations, tachycardia, sweating, nausea, vomiting, cardiac dysrhythmias	No contraindication in life-threatening situations; tachydysrhythmias
	Injection: 1:10,000, 1:1000	0.01 mg/kg/dose IV q5min; second dose or via endotracheal tube increase to 0.1 mg/kg	Palpitations, tachycardia, sweating, nausea, vomiting, cardiac dysrhythmias	None in life-threatening situations; tachydysrhythmias; use in a monitored setting only
Fentanyl (Sublimaze)	Injection: 50 μg/ml	1–3 μg/kg/dose IV q30–60min	Respiratory depression, apnea, muscle rigidity, circulatory depression, bradycardia, nausea, vomiting, cardiopulmonary arrest	Known intolerance; use in monitored setting only
Fluids	Normal saline	20 ml/kg boluses IV as needed	Pulmonary edema, IV infiltration, fluid overload	Use judiciously in congestive heart failure and renal failure
Furosemide (Lasix)	Injection: 10 mg/ml; oral: 10 mg/ml, 40 mg/5 ml; tablets: 20, 40, 80 mg	1–2 mg/kg IM, IV q6–12h PRN; maximum dose, 600 mg in 24 h; 2 mg/kg PO	Electrolyte depletion, alkalosis, hyperuricemia, hypotension, dehydration, tinnitus, hearing loss	Anuria, known hypersensitivity, caution in hepatic disease
Glucagon	Injection: 1-, 10-mg vials (1 U/mg)	Neonates: 0.3 mg/kg IM, IV q4h PRN; children: 0.03–0.10 mg/kg IM, IV, SQ q20min; maximum, 1 mg	Nausea and vomiting	Known hypersensitivity, pheochromocytoma, suspected insulinoma
Glucose	10%, 25% dextrose in water	Infants: 2–4 ml/kg 10% dextrose in water IV push; older than 1 mo of age: 2 ml/kg of 25% dextrose in water IV push	Hyperglycemic	Bedside determination of normoglycemia
Hydralazine (Apresoline)	Injection: 20 mg/ml; tablets: 10, 25, 50, 100 mg	0.1–0.2 mg/kg IM, IV q4–6h (hypertensive crisis)	Lupus-like illness (rare), headache, anorexia, nausea, vomiting, diarrhea, palpitations, tachycardia, angina, hypotension, skin flushing, rash, abdominal pain	Known hypersensitivity, coronary artery disease, mitral valve disease, caution in renal disease
Ibuprofen (Advil, Motrin, Nuprin)	Liquid: 100 mg/5 ml; tablets: 200, 300, 400, 600, 800 mg	10–15 mg/kg/dose PO q4–6h	GI hemorrhage, ulcer formation with chronic use, dizziness, nervousness, rash, tinnitus, decreased appetite, edema, bleeding	Known hypersensitivity, syndrome of nasal polyps, angioedema, bronchospasm with ASA or other NSAID, GI hemorrhage or ulcer disease
Insulin	Regular: 100 U/ml	0.1 U/kg IV bolus then 0.1 U/kg/h IV infusion	Sweating, syncope, altered mental status, hypoglycemia	Hypoglycemia
Ipecac	1.5%, 2% syrup	6–12 mo; 10 ml PO; 1–12 yr of age: 15–30 ml PO; >12 yr of age: 30–60 ml PO; repeat once in 20 min if no emesis	Aspiration, failure to prevent drug absorption	Children <6 mo of age, caustic ingestions, hydrocarbon ingestion, gypsum weed ingestion, coma or seizures
Ipratropium bromide (Atrovent)	Inhalation solution: 250, 500 μg/dose; MDI: 18 μg/dose	250–500 μg q4h nebulized or 2 puffs via MDI q4–6h; maximum, 12 doses in 24 h	Palpitations, nervousness, dizziness, headache, nausea, vomiting, tremor, blurred vision, dry mouth	Hypersensitivity, narrow-angle glaucoma, bladder neck obstruction

(continued)

Generic drug name (trade name)	Preparation	Dose and route of administration	Toxicity of adverse effects	Contraindications
Ketamine	Injection: 10, 50, 100 mg/ml	1–2 mg/kg IV, 2–4 mg/kg IM	Emergence reactions, vivid imagery, hallucinations, delirium, confusion, hypertension, tachycardia, hypotension dysrhythmias, apnea with rapid IV bolus, laryngospasm, diplopia, nystagmus, muscle twitching	Any patient in whom blood pressure elevation or increased intracranial pressure is hazardous, known hypersensitivity; use in monitored setting only
Ketorolac (Toradol)	Injection: 30, 60 mg	0.5–1.0 mg/kg/dose IV or IM 9–6 h; maximum, 60 mg	GI hemorrhage, ulcer formation with chronic use, edema, nausea, dyspepsia, diarrhea, nervousness, dizziness, headache, sweating	Known hypersensitivity, syndrome of nasal polyps, angioedema, bronchospasm with ASA or other NSAID use; not officially approved for use in children
Lidocaine	Injection (in D_5W): 2, 4, 8, 10, 20 mg/ml; drip: 40, 100, 200 mg/ml	Loading dose: 1 mg/kg IV q5–10min until dysrhythmia controlled or maximum dose, 5 mg; maintenance: 20–50 μg/kg/min IV	CNS excitation, seizures, vomiting, bradycardia, hypotension	Hypersensitivity to amide-based local anesthetics, Wolff-Parkinson-White syndrome or severe AV block, seizures; use in a monitored setting only
Lorazepam (Ativan)	Injection: 2, 4 mg/ml; refrigeration suggested	0.05–0.10 mg/kg IM or IV; may repeat q15–20min; maximum, 1 mg/dose to total of 4 mg	CNS depression, pain at injection site, hypotension, hypertension, partial airway obstruction, arterial spasm if injected intraarterially	Known hypersensitivity to lorazepam or propylene glycol, acute narrow-angle glaucoma; use in a monitored setting only
Long-acting epinephrine (Sus-Phrine)	Injection: 1 : 2000 (5 mg/ml)	0.005 ml/kg SQ; maximum, 0.15 ml q8–12h	Palpitations, tachycardia, sweating, nausea, vomiting, cardiac dysrhythmias	Tachycardia, rhythm disturbances, vomiting
Meperidine (Demerol)	Injection: 10, 25, 50, 75, 100 mg/ml; syrup: 50 mg/5 ml; tablets: 50, 100 mg	1–2 mg/kg IM or IV q2–4h	Vomiting, dystonic reactions, paradoxic crying, constipation, hypotension, seizures from toxic intermediary metabolites, respiratory depression	Known hypersensitivity, concomitant use of monoamine oxidase inhibitors
Methohexital (Brevital)	Injection: 0.5-, 2.5-, 5.0-g vials	1 mg/kg/dose IV	Circulatory depression, respiratory depression, cardiopulmonary arrest, thrombophlebitis, laryngospasm, bronchospasm, nausea, emesis, abdominal pain, skeletal muscle hyperactivity	Porphyria, known hypersensitivity to barbiturates, if general anesthesia is contraindicated; use in a monitored setting only
Methylprednisolone (Solu-Medrol), hydrocortisone (Solu-Cortef)	Injection: 20, 40, 62.5, 80, 125 mg/ml; single-dose vials of 100, 250, 500, 1000 mg	2 mg/kg IV q6–8h; 4–8 mg/kg IV q6h; maximum dose, 250 mg	Sodium and fluid retention, peptic ulcer formation, myopathy, adrenocortical insufficiency, impaired mineralocorticoid secretion, mood lability, suppression of growth and development (full range of effects beyond the scope of this text)	Do not use in preterm infants when preparation contains benzyl alcohol; systemic fungal or other infections; known hypersensitivity; caution in immunosuppressed patients
Midazolam (Versed)	Injection: 1, 5 mg/ml	0.1 mg/kg IM, IV; 0.3 mg/kg PR; 0.5 mg/kg PO; 0.4–0.6 mg/kg intranasal	Respiratory depression, hypotension, bradycardia	Caution when used with benzodiazepines; use in a monitored setting only
Morphine	Injection: 2, 4, 5, 8, 10, 15 mg/ml	0.1–0.2 mg/kg IM, SQ, IV q2–4h; maximum, 15 mg/dose	CNS and respiratory depression, nausea, vomiting, hypotension, bradycardia, increased intracranial pressure, miosis, biliary or urinary spasm, stiff chest syndrome, histamine release	Altered mental status, hypotension, bradycardia, apnea, or respiratory depression; use in monitored setting only
Naloxone (Narcan)	Injection: 0.4, 1 mg/ml	0.05–0.10 mg/kg SQ, IM, IV	Nausea, vomiting, sweating, tachycardia, hypertension, tremulousness, seizure, cardiopulmonary arrest	Known hypersensitivity
Nifedipine (Adalat, Procardia)	Capsules: 10, 20 mg; sustained release: 30, 60, 90 mg	0.25–0.50 mg/kg PO q6–8h; maximum, 30 mg/dose or 180 mg/d	Hypotension, dizziness, flushing, headache, nausea, peripheral edema, tachycardia, syncope	Known hypersensitivity; not officially approved for use in children
Nitroglycerin (Nitrostat, Nitro-Bid)	Injection: 0.5, 0.8, 5, 10 mg/ml; must be diluted in D_5W or normal saline for infusion	0.025–20.0 μg/kg/min continuous IV infusion; maximum, 5 μg/kg/min for children; no fixed optimum dose, titrate to response	Headache, hypotension, tachycardia, nausea, vomiting, palpitations	Known hypersensitivity, hypotension, uncorrected hypovolemia, increased intracranial pressure, constrictive pericarditis, cardiac tamponade, inadequate cerebral circulation

(*continued*)

Generic drug name (trade name)	Preparation	Dose and route of administration	Toxicity of adverse effects	Contraindications
Nitroprusside (Nipride)	50-mg vials; mix only with D_5W	0.3–10.0 μg/kg/min; not to exceed 6 μg/kg/min in neonates; mix in D_5W and cover with aluminum foil	Cyanide toxicity with prolonged use, methemoglobinemia, tachyphylaxis, profound hypotension, nausea, vomiting, headache, anxiety, dysrhythmias, metabolic acidosis, altered mental status	Compensatory hypertension secondary to AV shunt or coarctation of the aorta; use in monitored setting only
Norepinephrine (Levarterenol, Levophed)	Injection: 1 mg/ml	0.1 μg/kg/min initially; titrate to desired effect	Severe peripheral and visceral vasoconstriction, decreased renal perfusion and urine output, tissue hypoxia, lactic acidosis, skin necrosis with extravasation, cardiac dysrhythmias	Hypotension secondary to blood volume deficits, mesenteric or peripheral thromboses; use in monitored setting only
Octreotide (Sandostatin)	Injection: 0.5, 0.1, 0.5 μg/ml	1–10 μg/kg SQ, IM, or IV q12h	Dysrhythmias, conduction abnormalities, sinus bradycardia	Hypersensitivity
Phenobarbital	Injection: 30-, 60-, 65-, 75-, 120-, 130-mg/ml; 120-mg vials	10–20 mg/kg IV initially, no faster than 1 mg/kg/min, then 5–10 mg/kg IV q20min until seizure controlled or maximum dose, 40 mg/kg; 10 mg/kg IM	CNS depression, particularly somnolence; hypoventilation; apnea	Known hypersensitivity, marked impairment of liver function, porphyria, respiratory disease with dyspnea or obstructions
Phenytoin	Injection: 50 mg/ml	15–20 mg/kg IV initially, not faster than 1 mg/kg/min, maximum, 50 mg/min; successive doses, 5–10 mg/kg IV q30min until seizure controlled or maximum dose, 25 mg/kg or 1000 mg in 24 h	Local tissue irritation, hypotension with rapid administration, cardiovascular collapse, CNS depression, crystallization of drug in IV tubing	Known hypersensitivity, sinus bradycardias, AV block, signs of toxicity/ataxia, nystagmus
Prednisone (Pediapred, Prelone)	Oral solution: 1, 3, 5 mg/ml; tablets: 1, 2.5, 5, 10, 20, 25, 50 mg	1–2 mg/kg PO BID or QD	See methylprednisolone	See methylprednisolone
Pyridoxine	Injection: 100 mg/ml	70 mg/kg IV for seizure	Chronic administration associated with neurologic abnormalities	No documented pyridoxine deficiency
Racemic epinephrine (Vaponefrin)	2.25% solution	0.05 ml/kg diluted to 3 cc with normal saline nebulized q1–4h; maximum, 0.5 ml/dose	Palpitations, tachycardia, sweating, nausea, vomiting, cardiac dysrhythmias, rebound stridor	Tachydysrhythmias; no contraindications in life-threatening situations; use in a monitored setting only
Verapamil (Calan, Isoptin)	Injection: 2.5 mg/ml	0.1–0.3 mg/kg IV q15min × 2 doses; maximum, 5 mg	Constipation, dizziness, hypotension, bradycardia, AV block	Children <1 yr of age, severe left ventricular dysfunction, hypotension, sick sinus syndrome, second or third degree AV block, atrial fibrillation or flutter with a bypass tract; use in a monitored setting only

ASA, aspirin; AV, atrioventricular; CNS, central nervous system; D_5W, 5% dextrose in water; GI, gastrointestinal; MDI, metered-dose inhaler; NSAID, nonsteroidal antiinflammatory drug; V fib, ventricular fibrillation.

APPENDIX V

American, Australian, Canadian, and European Poison Centers

ALABAMA

Alabama Poison Center, Tuscaloosa

2503 Phoenix Drive
Tuscaloosa, AL 35405
Emergency telephone: (800) 462-0800 (AL only) or (205) 345-0600
E-mail address: jfisher@alapoisoncenter.org

Regional Poison Control Center

THE CHILDREN'S HOSPITAL
1600 7th Avenue South
Birmingham, AL 35233
Emergency telephone: (800) 292-6678 (AL only), (205) 933-4050 or (205) 939-9201
E-mail address: bill.king@chsys.org

ALASKA

Oregon Poison Center

Oregon Health Sciences University
3181 SW Sam Jackson Park Road, CB550
Portland, OR 97201
Emergency telephone: (800) 222-1222 or (503) 494-8968
E-mail: N/A

ARIZONA

Arizona Poison and Drug Information Center

Arizona Health Sciences Center, Room 1156
1501 North Campbell Avenue
Tucson, AZ 85724
Emergency telephone: (800) 362-0101 (AZ only) or (520) 626-6016
E-mail address: mcnally@pharmacy.arizona.edu

Banner Poison Control Center

Good Samaritan Regional Medical Center
1111 E. McDowell—Ancillary 1
Phoenix, AZ 85006
Emergency telephone: (800) 362-0101 (AZ only) or (602) 253-3334
E-mail address: poisoncenter@bannerhealth.com

ARKANSAS

Arkansas Poison and Drug Information Center

College of Pharmacy
University of Arkansas for Medical Sciences
4301 W. Markham, Mail Slot 522-2
Little Rock, AR 72205
Emergency telephone: (800) 376-4766
E-mail address: N/A

CALIFORNIA

California Poison Control System—Fresno/Madera Division

Children's Hospital Central California
9300 Valley Children's Place, MB 15
Madera, CA 93638-8762
Emergency telephone: (800) 876-4766 (CA only)
E-mail: dstrong@calpoison.org

California Poison Control System—Sacramento Division

UC Davis Medical Center
2315 Stockton Boulevard
Sacramento, CA 95817
Emergency telephone: (800) 876-4766 (CA only)
E-mail: jalsop@calpoison.org

California Poison Control System—San Diego Division

University of California, San Diego, Medical Center
200 West Arbor Drive
San Diego, CA 92103-8925
Emergency telephone: (800) 876-4766 (CA only)
E-mail: amanoguerra@ucsd.edu

California Poison Control System—San Francisco Division

UCSF Box 1369
San Francisco, CA 94143-1369
Emergency telephone: (800) 876-4766 (CA only)
E-mail: pcctk@itsa.ucsf.edu

COLORADO

Rocky Mountain Poison and Drug Center

777 Bannock, MC 0180
Denver, CO 80204-4507
Emergency telephone: (800) 332-3073 (CO only/outside metro area) or (303) 739-1123 (Denver metro)
E-mail: rdart@rmpdc.org

CONNECTICUT

Connecticut Poison Control Center

University of Connecticut Health Center
263 Farmington Avenue
Farmington, CT 06030-5365
Emergency telephone: (800) 343-2722 (CT only) or (860) 679-4540
E-mail: mccormick@nso.uchc.edu

DELAWARE

The Poison Control Center

Children's Hospital of Philadelphia
34th and Civic Center Blvd.
Philadelphia, PA 19104-3309
Emergency telephone: (800) 722-7112 or (215) 590-2100
E-mail: land@email.chop.edu

DISTRICT OF COLUMBIA

National Capital Poison Center

3201 New Mexico Avenue, Suite 310
Washington, DC 20016
Emergency telephone: (800) 222-1222 or (202) 625-3333
E-mail: pc@poison.org

FLORIDA

Florida Poison Information Center—Jacksonville

655 West Eighth Street
Jacksonville, FL 32209
Emergency telephone: (800) 282-3171 (FL only) or (904) 244-4480
E-mail: schauben@ufl.edu

Florida Poison Information Center—Miami

University of Miami, Department of Pediatrics
Jackson Memorial Medical Center
P.O. Box 016960 (R-131)
Miami, FL 33101
Emergency telephone: (800) 282-3171 (FL only) or (305) 585-5253 or (305) 585-8417
E-mail: rweisman@med.miami.edu

Florida Poison Information Center—Tampa

Tampa General Hospital
P.O. Box 1289
Tampa, FL 33601
Emergency telephone: (800) 282-3171 (FL only) or (813) 844-4444
E-mail: vsperanza@mindspring.com

GEORGIA

Georgia Poison Center

Hughes Spalding Children's Hospital
Grady Health System
80 Jesse Hill Jr. Drive SE
P.O. Box 26066
Atlanta, GA 30335-3801
Emergency telephone: (800) 222-1222 or (404) 616-9000 (Metro Atlanta)
E-mail: lope8573@dhr.state.ga.us

HAWAII

Rocky Mountain Poison and Drug Center

777 Bannock, MC 0180
Denver, CO 80204-4507
Emergency telephone: (800) 941-4411 (Oahu) or (800) 362-3585 (outer islands, Kauai, Maui, Molokai, and Hawaii)
E-mail: rdart@rmpdc.org

IDAHO

Rocky Mountain Poison and Drug Center

777 Bannock, MC 0180
Denver, CO 80204-4507
Emergency telephone: (800) 860-0620
E-mail: rdart@rmpdc.org

ILLINOIS

Illinois Poison Center

222 S. Riverside Plaza, Suite 1900
Chicago, IL 60606
Emergency telephone: (800) 222-1222 or (312) 906-6186
E-mail: Khughes@mchc.com

INDIANA

Indiana Poison Center

Methodist Hospital
Clarian Health Partners
I-65 at 21st Street
Indianapolis, IN 46206-1367
Emergency telephone: (800) 382-9097 (IN only) or (317) 962-2323
E-mail: mshowalt@clarian.com

IOWA

Iowa Statewide Poison Control Center

St. Luke's Regional Medical Center
2910 Hamelton Blvd. Lower A
Sioux City, IA 51104
Emergency telephone: (800) 222-1222 or (712) 277-2222
E-mail: KalinLB@stlukes.org

KANSAS

Mid-America Poison Control Center

University of Kansas Medical Center
3901 Rainbow Blvd., Room B-400
Kansas City, KS 66160-7231

Emergency telephone: (800) 332-6633 (KS only) or (913) 588-6633
E-mail: N/A

KENTUCKY

Kentucky Regional Poison Center

Medical Towers South, Suite 847
234 Gray Street
Louisville, KY 40202
Emergency telephone: (800) 722-5725 or (502) 589-8222
E-mail: henry.spiller@nortonhealthcare.org

LOUISIANA

Louisiana Drug and Poison Information Center

University of Louisiana at Monroe
College of Pharmacy, Sugar Hall
Monroe, LA 71209-6430
Emergency telephone: (800) 256-9822 (LA only) or (318) 362-5393
E-mail: mryan@ulm.edu

MAINE

Northern New England Poison Center

Maine Medical Center
22 Bramhall Street
Portland, ME 04102
Emergency telephone: (800) 442-6305 (ME only) or (207) 871-4720
E-mail: simonk@mmc.org

MARYLAND

Maryland Poison Center

University of Maryland at Baltimore
School of Pharmacy
20 North Pine Street, PH 772
Baltimore, MD 21201
Emergency telephone: (800) 492-2414 (MD only) or (410) 706-7701
E-mail: Banderso@rx.umaryland.edu

National Capital Poison Center

3201 New Mexico Avenue, NW, Suite 310
Washington, DC 20016
Emergency telephone: (800) 222-1222 or (202) 625-3333
E-mail: pc@poison.org

MASSACHUSETTS

Regional Center for Poison Control and Prevention

300 Longwood Avenue
Boston, MA 02115
Emergency telephone: (800) 682-9211 (MA and RI only) or (617) 232-2120
E-mail: woolf@hub.tch.harvard.edu

MICHIGAN

Children's Hospital of Michigan

REGIONAL POISON CONTROL CENTER
4160 John R Harper Professional Office Building, Suite 616
Detroit, MI 48201
Emergency telephone: (800) 764-7661 (MI only) or (313) 745-5711
E-mail: dmcpcc@dmc.org

DeVos Children's Hospital

REGIONAL POISON CENTER
100 Michigan, NE, Suite 203
Grand Rapids, MI 49503
Emergency telephone: (800) 222-1222
E-mail: john.trestrail@spectrum-health.org

MINNESOTA

Hennepin Regional Poison Center

Hennepin County Medical Center
701 Park Avenue
Minneapolis, MN 55415
Emergency telephone: (800) 222-1222 or (612) 347-3141
E-mail: mnpoison@yahoo.com

MISSISSIPPI

Mississippi Regional Poison Control Center

University of Mississippi Medical Center
2500 N. State Street
Jackson, MS 39216
Emergency telephone: (800) 222-1222 or (601) 354-7660
E-mail: mhughes@pharmacology.umsmed.edu

MISSOURI

Missouri Regional Poison Center

7980 Clayton Road, Suite 200
St. Louis, MO 63117
Emergency telephone: (800) 366-8888 or (314) 772-5200
E-mail: michael_thompson@ssmhc.com

MONTANA

Rocky Mountain Poison and Drug Center

777 Bannock, MC 0180
Denver, CO 80204-4507
Emergency telephone: (800) 525-5042 (MT only)
E-mail: rdart@rmpdc.org

NEBRASKA

The Poison Center

Children's Hospital
8200 Dodge Street
Omaha, NE 68114

Emergency telephone: (800) 955-9119 or (402) 955-5555
E-mail: jmcvoy@chsomaha.org

NEVADA

Oregon Poison Center

Oregon Health Sciences University
3181 SW Sam Jackson Park Road, CB550
Portland, OR 97201
Emergency telephone: (800) 452-7165 or (503) 494-8968
E-mail: N/A

Rocky Mountain Poison and Drug Center

777 Bannock, MC 0180
Denver, CO 80204-4507
Emergency telephone: (800) 446-6179 (NV only)
E-mail: rdart@rmpdc.org

NEW HAMPSHIRE

New Hampshire Poison Information Center

Dartmouth-Hitchcock Medical Center
One Medical Center Drive
Lebanon, NH 03756
Emergency telephone: (800) 222-1222 or (603) 650-8000
E-mail: Linda.A.Courtemanche@hitchcock.org

NEW JERSEY

New Jersey Poison Information and Education System

65 Bergen Street
Newark, NJ 07107
Emergency telephone: (800) 222-1222 or (973) 643-2993
E-mail: info@njpies.org

NEW MEXICO

New Mexico Poison and Drug Information Center

MSC09 5080
1 University of New Mexico
Albuquerque, NM 87131-0001
Emergency telephone: (800) 432-6866 or (505) 272-2222
E-mail: jebenson@salud.unm.edu

NEW YORK

Central New York Poison Center

750 East Adams Street
Syracuse, NY 13210
Emergency telephone: (800) 252-5655 (NY only) or (315) 476-4766
E-mail: storkc@upstate.edu

Finger Lakes Regional Poison and Drug Information Center

University of Rochester Medical Center
601 Elmwood Avenue, Box 321
Rochester, NY 14642
Emergency telephone: (800) 222-1222 or (585) 275-3232
E-mail: poison_center@urmc.rochester.edu

Long Island Regional Poison and Drug Information Center

Winthrop University Hospital
259 First Street
Mineola, NY 11501
Emergency telephone: (800) 222-1222, (516) 542-2323, or (516) 663-2650
E-mail: pcontrol@winthrop.org

New York City Poison Control Center

NYC Bureau of Labs
455 First Avenue
Room 123, Box 81
New York, NY 10016
Emergency telephone: (800) 210-3985, (212) 340-4494, (212) POI-SONS or (212) VEN-ENOS
E-mail: bobhoff@pol.net

Western New York Regional Poison Control Center

Children's Hospital of Buffalo
219 Bryant Street
Buffalo, NY 14222
Emergency telephone: (800) 888-7655 or (716) 878-7654
E-mail: wnypoison@hotmail.com

NORTH CAROLINA

Carolinas Poison Center

Carolinas Medical Center
5000 Airport Center Parkway, Suite B
Charlotte, NC 28208
Emergency telephone: (800) 848-6946 or (704) 355-4000
E-mail: marsha.ford@carolinashealthcare.org

NORTH DAKOTA

Hennepin Regional Poison Center

Hennepin County Medical Center
701 Park Avenue
Minneapolis, MN 55415
Emergency telephone: (800) 222-1222
E-mail: mnpoison@yahoo.com

OHIO

Central Ohio Poison Center

700 Children's Drive, Room L032
Columbus, OH 43205
Emergency telephone: (800) 682-7625 or (614) 228-1323
E-mail: centralohiopoisoncenter@chi.osu.edu

Cincinnati Drug and Poison Information Center

Regional Poison Control System
3333 Burnet Avenue
Vernon Place—3rd Floor
Cincinnati, OH 45229
Emergency telephone: (800) 872-5111 (OH only) or (513) 636-5111
E-mail: siegeleg@email.uc.edu

Greater Cleveland Poison Control Center

11100 Euclid Avenue
Cleveland, OH 44106-6010
Emergency telephone: (888) 231-4455 (OH only) or (216) 231-4455
E-mail: mdr2@po.cwru.edu

OKLAHOMA

Oklahoma Poison Control Center

Children's Hospital at Oklahoma Medical Center
940 N.E. 13th Street, Room 3510
Oklahoma City, OK 73104
Emergency telephone: (800) 764-7661 (OK only) or (405) 271-5454
E-mail: lee-mcgoodwin@ouhsc.edu

OREGON

Oregon Poison Center

Oregon Health Sciences University
3181 SW Sam Jackson Park Road, CB550
Portland, OR 97201
Emergency telephone: (800) 452-7165 (OR only) or (503) 494-8968
E-mail: N/A

PENNSYLVANIA

Pittsburgh Poison Center

Children's Hospital of Pittsburgh
3705 Fifth Avenue
Pittsburgh, PA 15213
Emergency telephone: (800) 222-1222 or (412) 681-6669
E-mail: krenzee@chplink.chp.edu

The Poison Control Center

Children's Hospital of Philadelphia
34th & Civic Center Blvd.
Philadelphia, PA 19104-3309
Emergency telephone: (800) 722-7112 or (215) 590-2100
E-mail: land@email.chop.edu

PUERTO RICO

San Jorge Children's Hospital Poison Center

Calle San Jorge #252
Santurce, Puerto Rico 00912
Emergency telephone: (800) 222-1222 or (787) 726-5674
E-mail: info@poisoncenter.net

RHODE ISLAND

Regional Center for Poison Control and Prevention

300 Longwood Avenue
Boston, MA 02115
Emergency telephone: (800) 682-9211 (MA and RI only) or (617) 232-2120
E-mail: woolf@hub.tch.harvard.edu

SOUTH CAROLINA

Palmetto Poison Center

College of Pharmacy
University of South Carolina
Columbia, SC 29208
Emergency telephone: (800) 922-1117 (SC only) or (803) 777-1117
E-mail: palmettopc@cop.sc.edu

SOUTH DAKOTA

Hennepin Regional Poison Center

Hennepin County Medical Center
701 Park Avenue
Minneapolis, MN 55415
Emergency telephone: (800) 222-1222 (MN and SD)
E-mail: mnpoison@yahoo.com

TENNESSEE

Middle Tennessee Poison Center

501 Oxford House
1161 21st Avenue South
Nashville, TN 37232-4632
Emergency telephone: (800) 288-9999 (TN only) or (615) 936-2034 (Greater Nashville)
E-mail: kim.barker@mcmail.vanderbilt.edu

Southern Poison Center

University of Tennessee
875 Monroe Avenue, Suite 104
Memphis, TN 38163
Emergency telephone: (800) 288-9999 (TN only) or (901) 528-6048
E-mail: pchyka@utmem.edu

TEXAS

Central Texas Poison Center

Scott and White Memorial Hospital
2401 South 31st Street
Temple, TX 76508
Emergency telephone: (800) POISON-1 (TX only) or (254) 724-7401
E-mail: dborys@swmail.sw.org

North Texas Poison Center

Texas Poison Center Network

Parkland Health and Hospital System
5201 Harry Hines Blvd.
Dallas, TX 75235
Emergency telephone: (800) 222-1222
E-mail: gsheph@parknet.pmh.org

South Texas Poison Center

The University of Texas Health Science Center—San Antonio
Department of Surgery, Mail Code 7849
7703 Floyd Curl Drive
San Antonio, TX 78229-3900
Emergency telephone: (800) 222-1222
E-mail: stpc@uthscsa.edu

Southeast Texas Poison Center

The University of Texas Medical Branch
3.112 Trauma Building
Galveston, TX 77555-1175
Emergency telephone: (800) 222-1222 or (409) 765-1420
E-mail: mellis@utmb.edu

Texas Panhandle Poison Center

1501 S. Coulter
Amarillo, TX 79106
Emergency telephone: (800) 222-1222 or (806) 354-1466
E-mail: ppc@nwths.com

West Texas Regional Poison Center

Thomason Hospital
4815 Alameda Avenue
El Paso, TX 79905
Emergency telephone: (800) 764-7661 (TX only) or (915) 534-3804
E-mail: edinfo@poisoncenter.org

UTAH

Utah Poison Control Center

410 Chipeta Way, Suite 230
Salt Lake City, UT 84108
Emergency telephone: (800) 222-1222 or (801) 581-2151
E-mail: barbara.crouch@hsc.utah.edu

VERMONT

Northern New England Poison Center

Maine Medical Center
22 Bramhall Street
Portland, ME 04102
Emergency telephone: (800) 442-6305 (ME only) or (207) 842-7222
E-mail: simonk@mmc.org

VIRGINIA

Blue Ridge Poison Center

University of Virginia Health System
PO Box 800774
Charlottesville, VA 22908-0774
Emergency telephone: (800) 451-1428 (VA only) or (434) 924-5543
E-mail: N/A

National Capital Poison Center

3201 New Mexico Avenue, NW, Suite 310
Washington, DC 20016
Emergency telephone: (800) 222-1222 or (202) 625-3333
E-mail: pc@poison.org
E-mail: N/A

Virginia Poison Center

Medical College of Virginia Hospitals
Virginia Commonwealth University
P.O. Box 980522
Richmond, VA 23298-0522
Emergency telephone: (800) 552-6337 (VA only) or (804) 828-9123

WASHINGTON

Washington Poison Center

155 NE 100th Street, Suite 400
Seattle, WA 98125-8012
Emergency telephone: (800) 732-6985 (WA only) or (206) 526-2121
E-mail: bobbink@wapc.org

WEST VIRGINIA

West Virginia Poison Center

3110 MacCorkle Ave, S.E.
Charleston, WV 25304
Emergency telephone: (800) 222-1222 or (304) 388-4211
E-mail: escharman@hsc.wvu.edu

WISCONSIN

Children's Hospital of Wisconsin Poison Center

P.O. Box 1997, Mail Station 677A
Milwaukee, WI 53201-1997
Emergency telephone: (800) 815-8855 (WI only) or (414) 266-2222
E-mail: ernest@mcw.edu

WYOMING

The Poison Center

Children's Hospital
8200 Dodge Street
Omaha, NE 68114
Emergency telephone: (800) 222-1222
E-mail: jmcvoy@chsomaha.org

AUSTRALIA

New South Wales Poisons Information Centre

The Children's Hospital at Westmead
Locked Bag 4001

Westmead, NSW 2145
Emergency telephone: 61-2-9845-3111
E-mail: poison@chw.edu.au

BELGIUM

Brussels + 32 70 245245

BRAZIL

Centro de Informação Toxicologica do

RIO GRANDE DO SUL
Rua Domingos Crescêncio 132 - 8° Andar
Porto Alegre, RS 90650-090
Emergency telephone: 800-780-200
E-mail: cit@pro.via-rs.com.br

CANADA

Poison and Drug Information Service

Foothills Medical Centre
1403 29th Street, NW
Calgary, Alberta T2N 2T9
Emergency telephone: (800) 332-1414 (Alberta only) or (403) 670-1414
E-mail: ingrid.vicas@calgaryhealthregion.ca

Poison Information Centre

IWK Health Centre
5850 University Avenue
P.O. Box 3070
Halifax, Nova Scotia B3J 3G9
Emergency telephone: (800) 565-8161 or (902) 428-8161
E-mail: wenda.macdonald@iwk.nshealth.ca

Ontario Regional Poison Centre

Children's Hospital of Eastern Ontario
401 Smythe Road
Ottawa, Ontario KIH 8LI
Emergency telephone: (800) 267-1373 or (613) 737-1100
E-mail: poison@cheo.on.ca

Quebec Poison Control Center

Aile "L" 1er etage
1050 chemin Sainte-Foy Quebec
Quebec G1S 4L8
Emergency telephone: (800) 463-5060 or (418) 565-8090
E-mail: capq@inspq.qc.ca

Ontario Regional Poison Control Center

The Hospital for Sick Children
555 University Avenue
Toronto, Ontario M5G 1X8
Emergency telephone: (800) 268-9017 (Ontario only) or (416) 813-5900
E-mail: ontregpc@sickkids.on.ca

B.C. Drug and Poison Information Centre

1081 Burrard Street
Vancouver, BC V6Z1Y6
Emergency telephone: (800) 657-8911 or (604) 682-5050
E-mail: daws@dpic.bc.ca

EIRE

Dublin +353 1 8379 964

FRANCE

Lille +33 0320 44 44 44
Paris +33 140 37 0404
Strasbourg +33 388 37 3737

GERMANY

Berlin +49 30 19240
Munich +49 89 19420

GREECE

Athens +30 1 779 3772

ITALY

Milan +39 266 1010 29
Rome +39 630 54343

NETHERLANDS

Utrecht +31 302 74 8888

NEW ZEALAND

National Poisons Centre

Dunedin School of Medicine
P.O. Box 913
Dunedin, New Zealand
Emergency telephone: 0800 764 766
E-mail: poisons@otago.ac.nz

POLAND

Krakow +48 1221 3710

PORTUGAL

Lisbon +351 1795 0143

RUSSIA

Moscow +7 095 928 7541

SPAIN

Madrid +34 1 562 0420

SWEDEN

Stockholm +46 8 610 0522

SWITZERLAND

Zurich +41 1 251 5151

TURKEY

Ankara +90 44 33 7001

UNITED KINGDOM

UK National Poisons Information Service 0870 600 6266

Calling this number will direct you to the centre responsible for your area. Individual centres can also be contacted on the following numbers. The UK National Teratology Service is on 0191 232 1525. If dialing internationally, all UK telephone numbers are prefixed by a +44:

BELFAST
01232 240 503 (UK—Northern Ireland)

BIRMINGHAM
0121 507 5588 (UK—England)

CARDIFF
01222 709901 (UK—Wales)

EDINBURGH
0131 536 2300 (UK—Scotland)

LONDON
0207 635 9191 (UK—England)

NEWCASTLE
0191 282 0300 (UK—England)

Index

Note: Page numbers followed by *f* indicate figures; page numbers followed by *t* indicate tables.